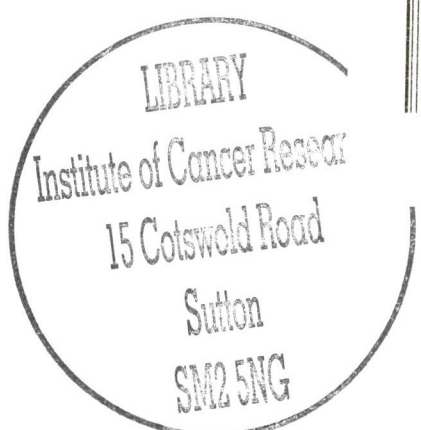

Institute of Cancer Research Library

Sutton

Please return this book by the last date stamped below

10. JUL 2007		
18. JUN. 2008		
12. FEB. 2009		

Dedication

This book is dedicated to our patients and their families whose courage and trust enabled them to choose a difficult, dangerous, and sometimes unproven therapy which offered the only chance in their fight against a fatal disease. Today, many thousands of patients are alive after a successful hematopoietic cell transplantation which would have been impossible without the fortitude of our patients, who took risks and thereby paved the way for the increasing application of this therapy. The progress in the area of clinical transplantation of hematopoietic cells would not have been possible without the dedicated, tireless work of the nurses and the supporting staff in the many transplant units around the world.

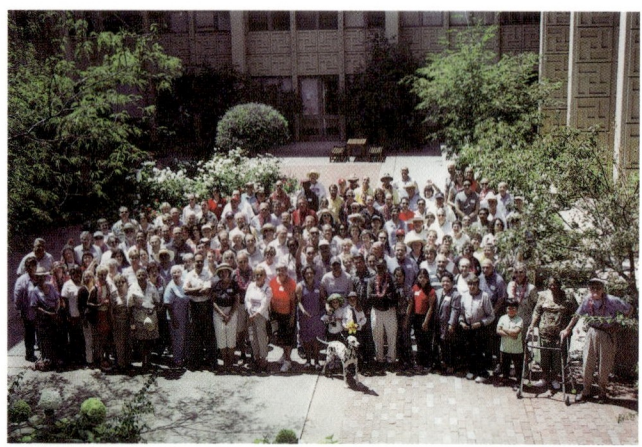

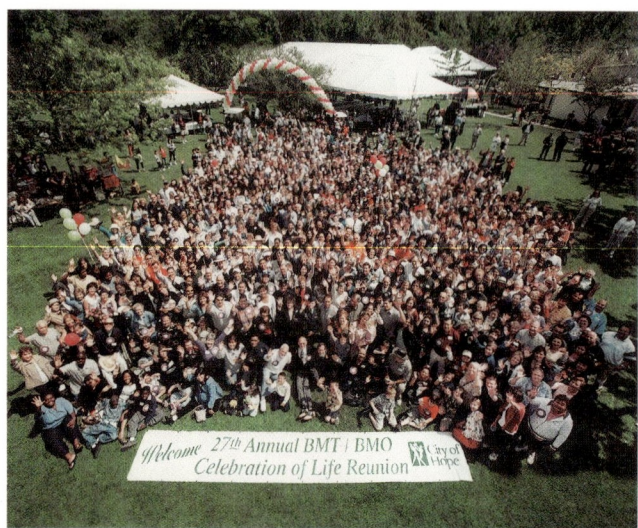

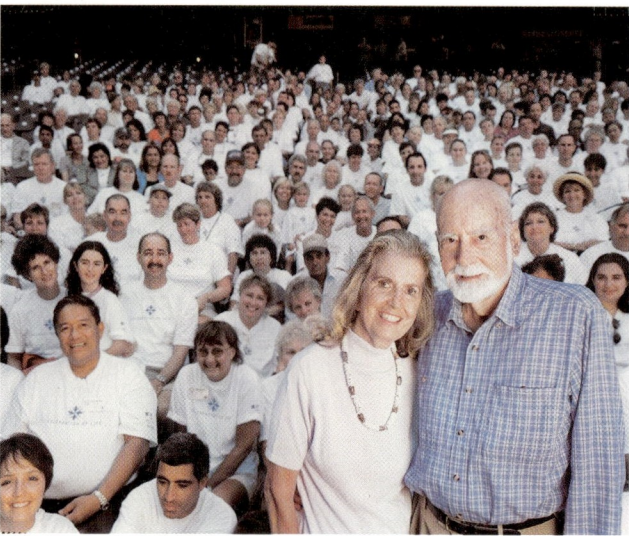

Thomas' Hematopoietic Cell Transplantation

Edited by

Karl G. Blume, MD
Professor of Medicine
Division of Bone Marrow Transplantation
Department of Medicine
Stanford University
Stanford, California

Stephen J. Forman, MD
Director, Department of Hematology and Bone Marrow Transplantation;
Staff Physician, Division of Medical Oncology and Therapeutics Research
City of Hope Comprehensive Cancer Center
Duarte, California

Frederick R. Appelbaum, MD
Member and Director, Clinical Research Division
Fred Hutchinson Cancer Research Center;
Professor and Head, Division of Medical Oncology
University of Washington School of Medicine
Seattle, Washington

THIRD EDITION

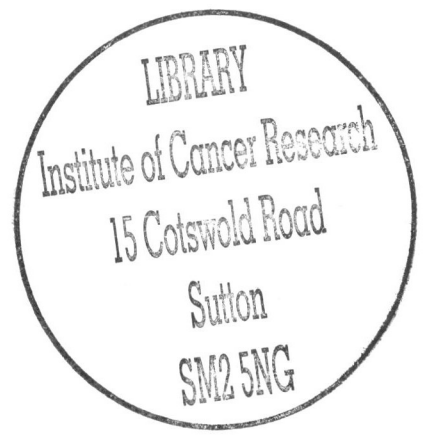

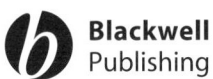
Blackwell Publishing

© 1994, 1999 by Blackwell Science Ltd
© 2004 by Blackwell Publishing Ltd
Blackwell Publishing, Inc., 350 Main Street, Malden, Massachusetts 02148-5020, USA
Blackwell Publishing Ltd, 9600 Garsington Road, Oxford OX4 2DQ, UK
Blackwell Publishing Asia Pty Ltd, 550 Swanston Street, Carlton, Victoria 3053, Australia

The right of the Authors to be identified as the Authors of this Work has been asserted in accordance with the Copyright, Designs and Patents Act 1988.

All rights reserved. No part of this publication may be reproduced, stored in a retrieval system, or transmitted, in any form or by any means, electronic, mechanical, photocopying, recording or otherwise, except as permitted by the UK Copyright, Designs and Patents Act 1988, without the prior permission of the publisher.

First published 1994
Second edition 1999
Third edition 2004
Reprinted 2004

Library of Congress Cataloging-in-Publication Data

Thomas' hematopoietic cell transplantation/edited by Karl G. Blume, Stephen J. Forman, Frederick R. Appelbaum.—3rd ed.
   p. ; cm.
Rev. ed. of: Hematopoietic cell transplantation/edited by E. Donnall Thomas, Karl G. Blume, Stephen J. Forman. 2nd ed. c1999.
Includes bibliographical references and index.
ISBN 1-4051-1256-5
1 Hematopoietic stem cells—Transplantation.
[DNLM: 1 Hematopoietic Stem Cell Transplantation.   2 Transplantation Immunology.
WH 380 T457 2004]
   I. Title: Hematopoietic cell transplantation.   II. Thomas, E. Donnall.   III. Blume, Karl G.   IV. Forman, Stephen J.
   V. Appelbaum, Frederick R.   VI. Hematopoietic cell transplantation.
RD123.5.B652 2004
617.4'4—dc21   2003012534

ISBN 1-4051-1256-5

A catalogue record for this title is available from the British Library

Set in 8.75/11pt Times Roman by Graphicraft Limited, Hong Kong
Printed and bound in Denmark by Narayana Press, Odder

Commissioning Editor: Maria Khan
Managing Editor: Rupal Malde
Editorial Assistant: Katrina Chandler
Production Editor: Fiona Pattison
Production Controller: Kate Charman

For further information on Blackwell Publishing, visit our website:
http://www.blackwellpublishing.com

Contents

Contributors, ix
Preface to the First Edition, xvi
Preface to the Second Edition, xvii
Preface to the Third Edition, xviii
Tribute, xix
List of Abbreviations, xxi

SECTION 1

Scientific Basis for Hematopoietic Cell Transplantation

1. A History of Bone Marrow Transplantation, 3
   E. Donnall Thomas
2. Uses and Growth of Hematopoietic Cell Transplantation, 9
   Mary M. Horowitz
3. Overview of Hematopoietic Cell Transplantation Immunology, 16
   Paul J. Martin
4. Histocompatibility, 31
   Eric Mickelson & Effie W. Petersdorf
5. Functional Evolution of the Major Histocompatibility Complex, 43
   Lakshmi K. Gaur
6. The Hematopoietic Microenvironment, 53
   Claudio Brunstein & Catherine M. Verfaillie
7. Molecular Aspects of Stem Cell Renewal, 62
   Peter M. Lansdorp
8. Biology of Hematopoietic Stem and Progenitor Cells, 69
   Markus G. Manz, Koichi Akashi & Irving L. Weissman
9. Expansion of Hematopoietic Stem Cells, 96
   Colleen Delaney, Robert Andrews & Irwin Bernstein
10. Methods for Gene Transfer: Genetic Manipulation of Hematopoietic Stem Cells, 107
    Thomas Moritz & David A. Williams
11. Clinical Trials of Gene Marking and Gene Therapy Using Hematopoietic Stem Cells, 118
    Donald B. Kohn & Gay M. Crooks
12. Pharmacological Basis for High-Dose Chemotherapy, 130
    James H. Doroshow & Timothy Synold
13. Preparative Regimens and Modification of Regimen-Related Toxicities, 158
    William I. Bensinger & Ricardo Spielberger
14. Radiotherapeutic Principles of Hematopoietic Cell Transplantation, 178
    Brenda Shank & Richard T. Hoppe
15. Radioimmunotherapy and Hematopoietic Cell Transplantation, 198
    Dana C. Matthews & Frederick R. Appelbaum
16. Pharmacology and the Use of Immunosuppressive Agents after Hematopoietic Cell Transplantation, 209
    Nelson J. Chao
17. T-Cell Depletion to Prevent Graft-vs.-Host Disease, 221
    Robert J. Soiffer
18. Documentation of Engraftment and Characterization of Chimerism Following Hematopoietic Cell Transplantation, 234
    Eileen Bryant & Paul J. Martin
19. Antibody Mediated Purging, 244
    John G. Gribben
20. Pharmacologic Purging of Bone Marrow, 254
    O. Michael Colvin
21. Molecular Inhibition of Gene Expression in Hematopoietic Cells, 258
    Joanna B. Opalinska & Alan M. Gewirtz
22. The Detection and Significance of Minimal Residual Disease, 272
    Jerald P. Radich & Marilyn L. Slovak
23. Pathology of Hematopoietic Cell Transplantation, 286
    George E. Sale, Howard M. Shulman & Robert C. Hackman
24. Mechanisms of Tolerance, 300
    Megan Sykes
25. The Experimental Basis for Hematopoietic Cell Transplantation for Autoimmune Diseases, 324
    Judith A. Shizuru
26. Murine Models for Graft-vs.-Host Disease, 344
    Robert Korngold & Thea M. Friedman
27. The Pathophysiology of Graft-vs.-Host Disease, 353
    James L.M. Ferrara & Joseph Antin
28. Graft-versus-Tumor Responses, 369
    Alexander Fefer
29. Adoptive Immunotherapy with Antigen-Specific T Cells, 380
    Stanley R. Riddell & Philip D. Greenberg

30 Autologous Graft-vs.-Host Disease, 405
Allan D. Hess & Richard J. Jones

31 Biostatistical Methods in Hematopoietic Cell Transplantation, 414
Joyce C. Niland

32 Outcomes Research in Hematopoietic Cell Transplantation, 434
Stephanie J. Lee

SECTION 2

Patient-Related Issues in Hematopoietic Cell Transplantation

33 The Evaluation and Counseling of Candidates for Hematopoietic Cell Transplantation, 449
Karl G. Blume & Michael D. Amylon

34 Clinical and Administrative Support for Hematopoietic Cell Transplant Programs, 463
Laura L. Adams & Angela A. Johns

35 Nursing Issues in Hematopoietic Cell Transplantation, 469
Rosemary C. Ford, Judy Campbell & Juanita Madison

36 The Patient's Perspective, 483
Susan K. Stewart

37 Ethical Issues in Hematopoietic Cell Transplantation, 488
David S. Snyder

38 Psychosocial Issues in Hematopoietic Cell Transplantation, 497
Michael A. Andrykowski & Richard P. McQuellon

39 Assessment of Quality of Life in Hematopoietic Cell Transplantation Recipients, 507
Karen Syrjala

40 Sexuality after Hematopoietic Cell Transplantation, 519
D. Kathryn Tierney

SECTION 3

Sources of Hematopoietic Cells for Human Transplant

41 Hematopoietic Cell Procurement, Processing and Transplantation: Regulation and Accreditation, 531
Phyllis I. Warkentin, Lewis Nick & Elizabeth J. Shpall

42 Hematopoietic Cell Donors, 538
Dennis L. Confer

43 Cord Blood Hematopoietic Cell Transplantation, 550
Hal E. Broxmeyer & Franklin O. Smith

44 *In Utero* Transplantation, 565
Alan W. Flake & Esmail D. Zanjani

45 Mobilization of Autologous Peripheral Blood Hematopoietic Cells for Support of High-Dose Cancer Therapy, 576
Judith Ng-Cashin & Thomas Shea

46 Peripheral Blood Hematopoietic Cells for Allogeneic Transplantation, 588
Norbert Schmitz

47 Cryopreservation of Hematopoietic Cells, 599
Scott D. Rowley

48 Recombinant Growth Factors after Hematopoietic Cell Transplantation, 613
Jürgen Finke & Roland Mertelsmann

49 Hematopoietic Cell Donor Registries, 624
Jeffrey W. Chell

SECTION 4

Complications and Their Management

50 Graft-vs.-Host Disease, 635
Keith M. Sullivan

51 Bacterial Infections, 665
John R. Wingard & Helen L. Leather

52 Fungal Infections after Hematopoietic Cell Transplantation, 683
Janice (Wes) M. Y. Brown

53 Cytomegalovirus Infection, 701
John A. Zaia

54 Herpes Simplex Virus Infections, 727
James I. Ito

55 Varicella-Zoster Virus Infections, 732
Ann M. Arvin

56 Epstein–Barr Virus Infection, 749
Richard F. Ambinder

57 Other Viral Infections after Hematopoietic Cell Transplantation, 757
Michael Boeckh

58 Gastrointestinal and Hepatic Complications, 769
Simone I. Strasser & George B. McDonald

59 Neurological Complications of Hematopoietic Cell Transplantation, 811
Harry Openshaw

60 Blood Group Incompatibilities and Hemolytic Complications of Hematopoietic Cell Transplantation, 824
Margaret R. O'Donnell

61 Principles of Transfusion Support before and after Hematopoietic Cell Transplantation, 833
Jeffrey McCullough

62 Immunological Reconstitution following Hematopoietic Cell Transplantation, 853
Robertson Parkman & Kenneth I. Weinberg

63 Vaccination of Hematopoietic Cell Transplant Recipients, 862
Clare A. Dykewicz

64 Pulmonary Complications after Hematopoietic Cell Transplantation, 873
David A. Horak

65 Nutritional Support of Hematopoietic Cell Recipients, 883
Sally Weisdorf-Schindele & Sarah Jane Schwarzenberg

66 Pain Management, 894
Jonathan R. Gavrin & F. Peter Buckley

67 Oral Complications, 911
Mark M. Schubert, Douglas E. Peterson & Michele E. Lloid

68 Growth and Development after Hematopoietic Cell Transplantation, 929
Jean E. Sanders

69 Delayed Complications after Hematopoietic Cell Transplantation, 944
Mary E.D. Flowers & H. Joachim Deeg

70 Secondary Malignancies after Hematopoietic Cell Transplantation, 962
Smita Bhatia & Ravi Bhatia

SECTION 5

Allogeneic Transplantation for Acquired Diseases

71 Allogeneic Hematopoietic Cell Transplantation for Aplastic Anemia, 981
George E. Georges & Rainer Storb

72 Allogeneic Transplantation for Paroxysmal Nocturnal Hemoglobinuria, 1002
Robert P. Witherspoon

73 Allogeneic Transplantation for Chronic Myeloid Leukemia, 1007
Frederick R. Appelbaum

74 Hematopoietic Cell Transplantation for Juvenile Myelomonocytic Leukemia, 1018
Robert A. Krance

75 Allogeneic Hematopoietic Cell Transplantation for Adult Patients with Acute Myeloid Leukemia, 1025
Keith E. Stockerl-Goldstein & Karl G. Blume

76 Allogeneic Transplantation for Acute Myeloid Leukemia in Children, 1040
David A. Margolis & James T. Casper

77 Allogeneic Hematopoietic Cell Transplantation for Acute Lymphoblastic Leukemia in Adults, 1055
Stephen J. Forman

78 Allogeneic Transplantation for Acute Lymphoblastic Leukemia in Children, 1067
Stella M. Davies, Norma K.C. Ramsay & John H. Kersey

79 Allogeneic Transplantation for Myelodysplastic and Myeloproliferative Disorders, 1084
Jeanne E. Anderson

80 Allogeneic Hematopoietic Cell Transplantation for Multiple Myeloma, 1096
David G. Maloney & Gösta Gahrton

81 Allogeneic Transplantation for Lymphoma and Chronic Lymphocytic Leukemia, 1105
Issa Khouri & Richard Champlin

82 Hematopoietic Cell Transplantation from HLA Partially Matched Related Donors, 1116
Claudio Anasetti & Andrea Velardi

83 Hematopoietic Cell Transplantation from Unrelated Donors, 1132
Effie W. Petersdorf

84 Management of Relapse after Allogeneic Transplantation, 1150
Robert H. Collins, Jr

85 Nonmyeloablative Therapy and Hematopoietic Cell Transplantation for Hematologic Disorders, 1164
Brenda M. Sandmaier & Rainer Storb

86 Allogeneic Hematopoietic Cell Transplantation for Solid Tumors, 1177
Richard W. Childs & Ramaprasad Srinivasan

SECTION 6

Autologous Transplantation for Acquired Diseases

87 Autologous and Allogeneic Hematopoietic Cell Transplantation for Hodgkin's Disease, 1191
Philip J. Bierman & Auayporn Nademanee

88 Autologous Hematopoietic Cell Transplantation for Non-Hodgkin's Lymphoma, 1207
Sandra J. Horning & James O. Armitage

89 Autologous Hematopoietic Cell Transplantation for Acute Myeloid Leukemia, 1221
Anthony S. Stein & Stephen J. Forman

90 Autologous Hematopoietic Cell Transplantation for Acute Lymphoblastic Leukemia, 1238
   Charles A. Linker
91 Autologous Hematopoietic Cell Transplantation for Chronic Myeloid Leukemia, 1250
   Ravi Bhatia & Philip B. McGlave
92 Autologous Hematopoietic Cell Transplantation for Multiple Myeloma, 1262
   Laurence Catley & Kenneth Anderson
93 Autologous Hematopoietic Cell Transplantation for AL Amyloidosis, 1283
   Raymond L. Comenzo & Morie A. Gertz
94 Hematopoietic Cell Transplantation for Breast Cancer, 1298
   Karen H. Antman
95 Hematopoietic Cell Transplantation in Germ Cell Tumors, 1308
   Brandon Hayes-Lattin & Craig R. Nichols
96 Hematopoietic Cell Transplantation in Ovarian Carcinoma, 1320
   Patrick J. Stiff
97 Hematopoietic Cell Transplantation for Neuroblastoma, 1333
   Katherine K. Matthay
98 Hematopoietic Cell Transplantation for Brain Tumors, 1345
   Ira J. Dunkel & Jonathan L. Finlay
99 Hematopoietic Cell Transplantation for Pediatric Patients with Solid Tumors, 1354
   Allen R. Chen & Curt I. Civin
100 AIDS and Hematopoietic Transplantation: HIV Infection, AIDS, Lymphoma and Gene Therapy, 1369
   John A. Zaia, J. Scott Cairns & John J. Rossi
101 Hematopoietic Stem Cell Transplantation for Autoimmune Diseases, 1385
   Alan Tyndall & Alois Gratwohl
102 Prevention and Therapy of Relapse following Autologous Hematopoietic Cell Transplantation, 1394
   Robert S. Negrin

SECTION 7

Allogeneic Transplantation for Inherited Disease

103 Marrow Transplantation in Thalassemia, 1409
   Guido Lucarelli & Reginald A. Clift
104 Hematopoietic Cell Transplantation for Sickle Cell Disease, 1417
   Mark C. Walters
105 Hematopoietic Cell Transplantation for Immunodeficiency Diseases, 1430
   Trudy N. Small, Wilhelm Friedrich & Richard J. O'Reilly
106 Hematopoietic Cell Transplantation for Osteopetrosis, 1443
   Peter F. Coccia
107 Hematopoietic Cell Transplantation for Storage Diseases, 1455
   Charles Peters
108 Hematopoietic Cell Transplantation for Macrophage and Granulocyte Disorders, 1471
   Rajni Agarwal
109 Hematopoietic Cell Transplantation for Fanconi Anemia, 1483
   John E. Wagner, Margaret L. MacMillan & Arleen D. Auerbach

SECTION 8

The Future

110 Hematopoietic Cell Transplantation in the 21st Century, 1507
   Ernest Beutler

SECTION 9

Colorplates, *facing page 296*
Robert C. Hackman

Index, 1511

Contributors

Laura L. Adams, BS
Administrative Director, Blood and Marrow Transplant Program, Stanford Hospital and Clinics, Stanford, California

Rajni Agarwal, MD
Assistant Professor, Staff Physician, Division of Pediatric Hematology–Oncology–Bone Marrow Transplantation, Department of Pediatrics, Stanford University School of Medicine, Stanford, California

Koichi Akashi, MD, PhD
Assistant Professor, Department of Cancer Immunology and AIDS, Dana-Farber Cancer Institute, Boston, Massachusetts

Richard F. Ambinder, MD, PhD
James B. Murphy Professor of Oncology, Director, Hematologic Malignancies Division, Kimmel Comprehensive Cancer Center, Johns Hopkins School of Medicine, Baltimore, Maryland

Michael D. Amylon, MD, FACP
Professor of Pediatrics, Division of Pediatric Hematology–Oncology, Department of Pediatrics, Stanford University School of Medicine, Stanford, California

Claudio Anasetti, MD
Member, Clinical Research Division, Fred Hutchinson Cancer Research Center; and Professor, University of Washington School of Medicine, Seattle, Washington

Jeanne E. Anderson, MD
Katmai Oncology Group, Anchorage, Alaska

Kenneth Anderson, MD
Dana-Farber Cancer Institute, Boston, Massachusetts

Robert Andrews, MD
Associate Member, Fred Hutchinson Cancer Research Center; and Associate Professor, University of Washington School of Medicine, Seattle, Washington

Michael A. Andrykowski, PhD
Department of Behavioral Science, University of Kentucky College of Medicine, Lexington, Kentucky

Joseph Antin, MD
Dana-Farber Cancer Institute, Boston, Massachusetts

Karen H. Antman, MD
Professor of Medicine, Columbia University, Herbert Irving Comprehensive Cancer Center, New York, New York

Frederick R. Appelbaum, MD
Member and Director, Clinical Research Division, Fred Hutchinson Cancer Research Center; and Professor and Head, Division of Medical Oncology, University of Washington School of Medicine, Seattle, Washington

James O. Armitage, MD
Dean, College of Medicine, Joe Shapiro Professor of Medicine, University of Nebraska Medical Center, Omaha, Nebraska

Ann M. Arvin, MD
Professor of Pediatrics, Microbiology and Immunology, Department of Pediatrics, Infectious Disease Division, Stanford, University School of Medicine, Stanford, California

Arleen D. Auerbach, PhD
Director of the Laboratory of Human Genetics and Hematology, The Rockefeller University, New York, New York

William I. Bensinger, MD
Member, Fred Hutchinson Cancer Research Center; and Professor of Medicine, University of Washington, Seattle, Washington

Irwin Bernstein, MD
Member and Program Head, Pediatric Oncology, Fred Hutchinson Cancer Research Center; and Professor and Division Head, Pediatric Hematology/Oncology, University of Washington School of Medicine, Seattle, Washington

Ernest Beutler, MD
Department of Molecular and Experimental Medicine, The Scripps Research Institute, La Jolla, California

Ravi Bhatia, MD
Staff Physician; Director, Stem Cell Biology Program, Division of Hematology and Bone Marrow Transplantation, City of Hope National Medical Center, Duarte, California

Smita Bhatia, MD, MPH
Staff Physician; Director, Epidemiology and Outcomes Research, Division of Pediatric Hematology/Oncology and Bone Marrow Transplantation, City of Hope National Medical Center, Duarte, California

Philip J. Bierman, MD
Associate Professor of Medicine, Department of Internal Medicine, Section of Oncology and Department Hematology, University of Nebraska Medical Center, Omaha, Nebraska

Contributors

Karl G. Blume, MD, FACP
Professor of Medicine, Division of Bone Marrow Transplantation, Department of Medicine, Stanford University School of Medicine, Stanford, California

Michael Boeckh, MD
Assistant Member, Program in Infectious Diseases, Fred Hutchinson Cancer Research Center; and Assistant Professor, University of Washington School of Medicine, Seattle, Washington

Janice (Wes) M.Y. Brown, MD
Assistant Professor, Divisions of Bone Marrow Transplantation and Infectious Diseases, Department of Medicine, Bone Marrow Transplantation Program, Stanford University School of Medicine, Stanford, California

Hal E. Broxmeyer, PhD
Chairman and Mary Margaret Walther Professor of Microbiology and Immunology, Professor of Medicine, Scientific Director, the Walther Oncology Center, Indiana University School of Medicine, Cancer Research Institute, Indianapolis, Indiana

Claudio Brunstein, MD
Medical Fellow, Division of Hematology, Oncology and Transplantation, Department of Medicine, University of Minnesota, Minneapolis, Minnesota

Eileen Bryant, PhD
Associate Member, Fred Hutchinson Cancer Research Center, Seattle, Washington

F. Peter Buckley, MB, FRCA
Interim Director, Multidisciplinary Pain Center; and Associate Professor, Department of Anesthesiology, University of Washington School of Medicine; and Associate Member, Fred Hutchinson Cancer Research Center, Seattle Washington

J. Scott Cairns, PhD
Targeted Interventions Branch, Division of AIDS, National Institute of Allergy and Infectious Diseases, Bethesda, Maryland

Judy Campbell, RN, OCN
Nurse Specialist, Long Term Follow-up Department, Seattle Cancer Care Alliance, Seattle, Washington

James T. Casper, MD
Professor of Pediatrics, Section of Pediatric Hematology–Oncology–Transplantation, Department of Pediatrics, Medical College of Wisconsin, Children's Hospital of Wisconsin, Milwaukee, Wisconsin

Laurence Catley, MBBS, FRACP, FRCPA
Dana-Farber Cancer Institute, Boston, Massachusetts

Richard Champlin, MD
Anderson Cancer Center, Houston, Texas

Nelson J. Chao, MD
Professor of Medicine and Immunology, Duke University Medical Center, Durham, North Carolina

Jeffrey W. Chell, MD
Chief Executive Officer, National Marrow Donor Program, Minneapolis, Minnesota

Allen R. Chen, MD, PhD, MHS
The Sidney Kimmel Comprehensive Cancer Center at Johns Hopkins and the Department of Pediatrics, Assistant Professor of Pediatrics and Oncology, Johns Hopkins University School of Medicine, Baltimore, Maryland

Richard W. Childs, MD
Hematology Branch, National Heart, Lung and Blood Institute, National Institutes of Health, Bethesda, Maryland

Curt I. Civin, MD
The Sidney Kimmel Comprehensive Cancer Center at Johns Hopkins and the Department of Pediatrics, Professor of Pediatrics and Oncology, Johns Hopkins University School of Medicine, Baltimore, Maryland

Reginald A. Clift, FIMLS
Senior Staff Scientist (Emeritus), Clinical Research Division, Fred Hutchinson Cancer Research Center, Seattle, Washington

Peter F. Coccia, MD
Ittner Professor of Pediatrics; and Chief, Section of Pediatric Hematology/Oncology; and Director, Pediatric Bone Marrow Transplantation Program; and Vice-Chairperson, Department of Pediatrics, University of Nebraska Medical Center, Omaha, Nebraska

Robert H. Collins Jr., MD
Professor of Internal Medicine, Director, Hematopoietic Cell Transplantation, University of Texas Southwestern, Medical Center at Dallas, Dallas, Texas

O. Michael Colvin
Duke University Comprehensive Cancer Center, Durham, North Carolina

Raymond L. Comenzo, MD
Associate Attending, Hematology Service, Department of Medicine, Memorial Sloan-Kettering Cancer Center, New York, New York

Dennis L. Confer, MD
Clinical Professor of Medicine, University of Minnesota; and Chief Medical Officer, National Marrow Donor Program, Minneapolis, Minnesota

Gay M. Crooks, MD
Associate Professor, Departments of Pediatrics, Keck USC School of Medicine, Childrens Hospital, Los Angeles, California

Stella M. Davies, MB, BS, PhD, MRCP
Jacob G. Schmirdlapp Endowed Chair and Professor of Pediatrics; and Director, Blood and Marrow Transplantation Program, Division of Hematology/Oncology, Cincinnati Children's Hospital Medical Center, Cincinnati, Ohio

H. Joachim Deeg, MD
Member, Clinical Research Division, Fred Hutchinson Cancer Research Center; and *Professor of Medicine, University of Washington School of Medicine, Seattle, Washington*

Colleen Delaney, MD, MSc
Research Associate, Fred Hutchinson Cancer Research Center, Seattle, Washington

James H. Doroshow, MD, FACP
Chairman, Department of Medical Oncology and Therapeutics Research, Associate Director for Clinical Investigation, City of Hope Comprehensive Cancer Center, Duarte, California

Ira J. Dunkel, MD
Memorial Sloan-Kettering Cancer Center, Department of Pediatrics, New York, New York

Clare A. Dykewicz, MD, MPH
Medical Epidemiologist, Centers for Disease Control and Prevention, Atlanta, Georgia

Alexander Fefer, MD
Professor of Medicine, University of Washington; and *Member, Fred Hutchinson Cancer Research Center, Seattle, Washington*

James L.M. Ferrara, MD
Professor of Medicine and Pediatrics; and *Director, Blood and Marrow Transplantation Program, University of Michigan Comprehensive Cancer Center, Ann Arbor, Michigan*

Jürgen Finke, MD
Department of Internal Medicine I, Hematology and Oncology, Freiburg University Medical Center, Freiburg, Germany

Jonathan L. Finlay, MB, ChB
The New York University Cancer Institute, New York University Medical Center, New York, New York

Alan W. Flake, MD
Professor of Surgery and Obstetrics and Gynecology, University of Pennsylvania; and *Ruth and Tristram Colket Professor of Pediatric Surgery, Director, Institute for Surgical Science, Children's Hospital of Philadelphia, Abramson Research Center, Philadelphia, Pennsylvania*

Mary E.D. Flowers, MD
Assistant Member, Fred Hutchinson Cancer Research Center; and *Assistant Professor, University of Washington School of Medicine, Seattle, Washington*

Rosemary C. Ford, RN, BSN, OCN
Nurse Manager, Transplant Clinic, Seattle Cancer Care Alliance, Seattle, Washington

Stephen J. Forman, MD
Director, Department of Hematology and Bone Marrow Transplantation; and *Staff Physician, Division of Medical Oncology and Therapeutics Research, City of Hope Comprehensive Cancer Center, Duarte, California*

Thea M. Friedman, PhD
Instructor, Department of Microbiology and Immunology, Kimmel Cancer Center, Jefferson Medical College, Philadelphia, Pennsylvania

Wilhelm Friedrich, MD
Professor of Pediatrics, Department of Pediatrics, University Children's Hospital Ulm, University of Ulm, Ulm, Germany

Gösta Gahrton, MD, PhD
The Karolinska Institutet, Huddinge Sjukhus/Huddinge University Hospital, Stockholm, Sweden

Lakshmi K. Gaur, PhD
Principal Investigator, University of Washington National Primate Research Center, University of Washington, Seattle, Washington

Jonathan R. Gavrin, MD
Associate Director for Clinical Anesthesia, Harborview Medical Center; and *Associate in Clinical Research, Fred Hutchinson Cancer Research Center;* and *Associate Professor, Department of Anesthesiology;* and *Adjunct Associate Professor, Department of Internal Medicine, University of Washington School of Medicine, Seattle, Washington*

George E. Georges, MD
Assistant Member, Program in Transplantation Biology, Clinical Research Division, Fred Hutchinson Cancer Research Center; and *Assistant Professor, University of Washington School of Medicine, Seattle, Washington*

Morie A. Gertz, MD
Professor of Medicine, Mayo Medical School; and *Chair, Division of Hematology, Mayo Clinic, Rochester, Minnesota*

Alan M. Gewirtz, MD
Doris Duke Distinguished Clinical Professor in Medicine and Pathology, University of Pennsylvania School of Medicine, Philadelphia, Pennsylvania

Alois Gratwohl, MD
Professor and Head, Division of Haematology, Department of Internal Medicine, University of Basle, Kantonsspital, Basle, Switzerland

Philip D. Greenberg, MD
Member, Fred Hutchinson Cancer Research Center; and *Professor of Medicine and Immunology, University of Washington School of Medicine, Seattle, Washington*

John G. Gribben, MD, DSc
Associate Professor of Medicine, Harvard Medical School, Division of Medical Oncology, Dana-Farber Cancer Institute, Boston, Massachusetts

Robert C. Hackman, MD
Member, Fred Hutchinson Cancer Research Center; and Associate Professor, Departments of Pathology and Laboratory Medicine, University of Washington, Seattle, Washington

Brandon Hayes-Lattin, MD
Oregon Health and Science University, Division of Hematology and Medical Oncology, Portland, Oregon

Allan D. Hess, PhD
Professor of Oncology, Immunology and Pathology, Sidney Kimmel Comprehensive Cancer Center, The Johns Hopkins University School of Medicine, Baltimore, Maryland

Richard T. Hoppe, MD, FACR
Henry S. Kaplan and Harry Lebeson Professor in Cancer Biology and Chairman, Department of Radiation Oncology, Stanford University School of Medicine, Stanford, California

David A. Horak, MD
Director, Department of Pulmonary and Critical Care Medicine, City of Hope National Medical Center, Duarte, California

Sandra J. Horning, MD
Professor of Medicine, Stanford University Medical Center, Division of Oncology, Palo Alto, California

Mary M. Horowitz, MD, MS
Scientific Director, International Bone Marrow Transplant Registry, Autologous Blood and Marrow Transplant Registry; Robert A. Uihlein Jr. Professor of Hematologic Research, Medical College of Wisconsin, Milwaukee, Wisconsin

James I. Ito, MD
Director, Department of Infectious Diseases, City of Hope National Medical Center, Duarte, California

Angela A. Johns, RN, BSN, MPA
Clinical Director, Adult Stem Cell Transplant Program, Duke University Health System, Durham, North Carolina

Richard J. Jones, MD
Professor of Oncology, Sidney Kimmel Comprehensive Cancer Center, The Johns Hopkins University School of Medicine, Baltimore, Maryland

John H. Kersey, MD
University of Minnesota Cancer Center, Minneapolis, Minnesota

Issa Khouri, MD
Associate Professor of Medicine, Department of Blood and Marrow Transplantation, University of Texas, Old Anderson Cancer Center, Houston, Texas

Donald B. Kohn, MD
Departments of Pediatrics and Molecular Microbiology & Immunology, Keck USC School of Medicine, Childrens Hospital, Los Angeles, California

Robert Korngold, PhD
Department of Microbiology and Immunology, Kimmel Cancer Center, Jefferson Medical College, Philadelphia, Pennsylvania

Robert A. Krance, MD
Professor Pediatrics and Medicine, Baylor College of Medicine; and Director Pediatric Stem Cell Transplantation Program, Texas Children's Hospital, Houston, Texas

Peter M. Lansdorp, MD, PhD
Scientist, Terry Fox Laboratory, British Columbia Cancer Agency; and Professor, Department of Medicine, University of British Columbia, Vancouver, BC, Canada

Helen L. Leather, B. Pharm, BCPS
Clinical Pharmacy Specialist BMT/Leukemia, Shands at the University of Florida; and Clinical Associate Professor, College of Pharmacy, University of Florida, Gainesville, Florida

Stephanie J. Lee, MD MPH
Assistant Professor of Medicine, Dana-Farber Cancer Institute, 44 Binney Street, Boston, Massachusetts

Charles A. Linker, MD
Clinical Professor of Medicine, Director, Hematologic Malignancies and Bone Marrow Transplant Program, University of California, San Francisco, A 502, 400 Parnassus Ave., San Francisco, California

Michele E. Lloid, RDH, MS
Oral Medicine, Seattle Cancer Care Alliance, Seattle, Washington

Guido Lucarelli, MD
Director, International Project on Transplantation in Thalassemia, Bone Marrow Transplant Center, Hospital of Pesaro, Pesaro, Italy

Margaret L. MacMillan, MD
Assistant Professor of Pediatrics, Division of Blood and Marrow Transplantation, Director of Unrelated Donor Program, University of Minnesota, Minneapolis, Minnesota

Juanita Madison, RN, MSN, AOCN
Oncology Nurse Specialist, Amgen Inc., Maple Valley, Washington

David G. Maloney, MD, PhD
Associate Member, Fred Hutchinson Cancer Research Center; and Associate Professor, University of Washington School of Medicine, Seattle, Washington

Markus G. Manz, MD
Institute for Research in Biomedicine (IRB), Bellinzona, Switzerland

David A. Margolis, MD
Associate Professor of Pediatrics, Section of Pediatric Hematology–Oncology–Transplantation, Department of Pediatrics, Medical College of Wisconsin, Children's Hospital of Wisconsin, Milwaukee, Wisconsin

Paul J. Martin, MD
Member, Fred Hutchinson Cancer Research Center; and Professor, University of Washington School of Medicine, Seattle, Washington

Katherine K. Matthay, MD
Department of Pediatrics, University of California School of Medicine, San Francisco, California

Dana C. Matthews, MD
Associate Member, Fred Hutchinson Cancer Research Center; and Associate Professor of Pediatrics, University of Washington School of Medicine, Seattle, Washington

Jeffrey McCullough, MD
Department of Laboratory Medicine and Pathology, University of Minnesota, Minneapolis, Minnesota

George B. McDonald, MD
Member, Fred Hutchinson Cancer Research Center; and Professor of Medicine, Division of Gastroenterology, University of Washington School of Medicine, Seattle, Washington

Philip B. McGlave, MD
Professor of Medicine, Director, Division of Hematology, Oncology and Transplantation, Department of Medicine; and Associate Director of Experimental Therapeutics, University of Minnesota Cancer Center; and Cecil J. Watson Land Grant Chair in Medicine, University of Minnesota, Minneapolis, Minnesota

Richard P. McQuellon, PhD
Comprehensive Cancer Center of Wake Forrest University, Bowman Gray School of Medicine, Medical Center Boulevard, Winston-Salem, North Carolina

Roland Mertelsmann, MD, PhD
Professor, Department of Internal Medicine I, Head of Department of Hematology and Oncology, Freiburg University Medical Center, Freiburg, Germany

Eric Mickelson, BSc
Associate Staff Scientist, Fred Hutchinson Cancer Research Center, Seattle, Washington

Thomas Moritz, MD
Department of Internal Medicine (Cancer Research), West German Cancer Center, University of Essen Medical School, Essen, Germany

Auayporn Nademanee, MD
Associate Clinical Director, Division of Hematology and Bone Marrow Transplantation, City of Hope National Medical Center, Duarte, California

Robert S. Negrin, MD
Associate Professor of Medicine, Division of Bone Marrow Transplantation, Department of Medicine, Stanford University School of Medicine, Stanford, California

Judith Ng-Cashin, MD
The University of North Carolina at Chapel Hill, Old Clinic Building, Chapel Hill, North Carolina

Craig R. Nichols, MD
Oregon Health and Science University, Division of Hematology and Medical Oncology, Portland, Oregon

Lewis Nick, RN, BSN, MT(ASCP)
Technical Director, Accreditation Program, Foundation for the Accreditation of Cellular Therapy, University of Nebraska Medical Center, Omaha, Nebraska

Joyce C. Niland, PhD
Professor and Chair, Information Sciences, City of Hope National Medical Center, Duarte, California

Margaret R. O'Donnell, MD
City of Hope National Medical Center, Division of Hematology and Bone Marrow Transplantation, Duarte, California

Joanna B. Opalinska, MD
Adiunkt, Department of Hematology, Pommeranian Medical Academy, ul. Unii Lubelskiej 1, Szczecin, Poland

Harry Openshaw, MD
City of Hope National Medical Center, Duarte, California

Richard J. O'Reilly, MD
Chairman, Department of Pediatrics, Chief, Marrow Transplantation Service, Memorial Sloan-Kettering Center, New York, New York

Robertson Parkman, MD
Head, Division of Research Immunology/Bone Marrow Transplantation, Childrens Hospital Los Angeles; and Professor of Pediatrics, Molecular, Microbiology and Immunology, University of Southern California School of Medicine, Los Angeles, California

Charles Peters, MD
Associate Professor of Pediatrics, Division of Hematology, Oncology, Blood and Marrow Transplantation, University of Minnesota School of Medicine, Minneapolis, Minnesota

Effie W. Petersdorf, MD
Member, Fred Hutchinson Cancer Research Center, Division of Clinical Research; and Professor of Medicine, University of Washington, Seattle, Washington

Douglas E. Peterson, DMD, PhD
Professor and Chair, Department of Oral Diagnosis, School of Dental Medicine, University of Connecticut Health Center, Farmington, Connecticut

Jerald P. Radich, MD
Member, Program in Genetics and Genomics, Fred Hutchinson Cancer Research Center; and Associate Professor, Division of Medical Oncology, University of Washington School of Medicine, Seattle, Washington

Norma K.C. Ramsay, MD
MMC 366, 420 Delaware St SE, Minneapolis, Minnesota

Stanley R. Riddell, MD
Member, Fred Hutchinson Cancer Research Center; and Professor of Medicine, University of Washington School of Medicine, Seattle, Washington

John J. Rossi, PhD
Professor of Molecular Biology, Department of Molecular Biology, Beckman Research Institute of City of Hope, Duarte, California

Scott D. Rowley, MD, FACP
Chief, Adult Blood and Marrow Transplant Program, Hackensack University Medical Center, Hackensack, New Jersey; and Clinical Associate Professor of Medicine, University of New Jersey School of Medicine, Newark, New Jersey

George E. Sale, MD
Member, Fred Hutchinson Cancer Research Center; and Professor, Department of Pathology, University of Washington, Seattle, Washington

Jean E. Sanders, MD
Member, Clinical Research Division; and Director, Pediatric Hematopoietic Stem Cell Transplantation, Fred Hutchinson Cancer Research Center; and Professor of Pediatrics, University of Washington, Seattle, Washington

Brenda M. Sandmaier, MD
Associate Member, Program in Transplantation Biology, Clinical Research Division, Fred Hutchinson Cancer Research Center; and Associate Professor, University of Washington School of Medicine, Seattle, Washington

Norbert Schmitz, MD
Professor of Medicine, Department of Hematology, AK St. Georg, Hamburg, Germany

Mark M. Schubert, DDS, MSD
Professor, Oral Medicine, School of Dentistry, University of Washington; and Director, Oral Medicine, Fred Hutchinson Cancer Research Center, Seattle, Washington

Sarah Jane Schwarzenberg, MD
Associate Professor, Pediatric Gastroenterology, Hepatology and Nutrition, University of Minnesota School of Medicine, Minneapolis, Minnesota

Brenda Shank, MD, PhD, FACR
Medical Director, J.C. Robinson, MD Regional Cancer Center, Doctors Medical Center, San Pablo; and Clinical Professor, Radiation Oncology Department, University of California, San Francisco Medical School, San Francisco, California

Thomas Shea, MD
Division of Hematology/Oncology, Department of Medicine, University of North Carolina, Chapel Hill, North Carolina

Judith A. Shizuru, PhD, MD
Assistant Professor of Medicine, Division of Bone Marrow Transplantation, Department of Medicine, Stanford University School of Medicine, Stanford, California

Elizabeth J. Shpall, MD
Professor of Medicine, University of Texas, Medical Director, Cell Therapy Laboratory, MD Anderson Cancer Center, Houston, Texas

Howard M. Shulman, MD
Member, Fred Hutchinson Cancer Research Center; and Professor, Department of Pathology, University of Washington, Seattle, Washington

Marilyn L. Slovak, PhD
Director, Cytogenetics, City of Hope National Medical Center, Duarte, California

Trudy N. Small, MD
Associate Attending, Department of Pediatrics, Bone Marrow Transplantation Service, Memorial Sloan-Kettering Cancer Center, New York, New York

Franklin O. Smith, MD
Children's Hospital Medical Center, Cincinnati, Ohio

David S. Snyder, MD
Division of Hematology/Bone Marrow Transplantation, City of Hope National Medical Center, Duarte, California

Robert J. Soiffer, MD
Associate Professor of Medicine, Harvard Medical School; and Chief, Division of Hematologic Malignancies, Dana-Farber Cancer Institute, Boston, Massachusetts

Ricardo Spielberger, MD
City of Hope National Medical Center, Kaiser BMT Program, Duarte, California

Ramaprasad Srinivasan, MD, PhD
Urologic Oncology Branch, National Cancer Institute, National Institutes of Health

Anthony S. Stein, MD
Staff Physician, Chair, Acute Myeloid Leukemia Program, City of Hope Comprehensive Cancer Center, Division of Hematology and Bone Marrow Transplantation, Duarte, California

Susan K. Stewart
Executive Director, Blood & Marrow Transplant Information Network, Highland Park, Illinois

Patrick J. Stiff, MD
Professor of Medicine and Pathology, Director, BMT Program, Loyola University Medical Center, Maywood, Illinois

Keith E. Stockerl-Goldstein, MD
Assistant Professor of Medicine, Division of Bone Marrow Transplantation, Stanford University Medical Center, Stanford, California

Rainer Storb, MD
Member and Head, Program in Transplantation Biology, Clinical Research Division, Fred Hutchinson Cancer Research Center; and Professor of Medicine, University of Washington School of Medicine, Seattle, Washington

Simone I. Strasser, MBBS, MD, FRACP
The A.W. Morrow Gastroenterology and Liver Centre, Royal Prince Alfred Hospital, Camperdown, New South Wales, Australia

Keith M. Sullivan, MD
James B. Wyngaarden Professor of Medicine, Chief, Division of Medical Oncology and Transplantation, Department of Medicine; Director, Center for Cancer Survivor and Outcomes Research, Duke University Medical Center, Durham, North Carolina

Megan Sykes, MD
Professor of Surgery and Medicine—Harvard Medical School, Bone Marrow Transplantation Section, Transplantation Biology Reseach, Surgical Service, Massachusetts General Hospital/Harvard Medical School, Boston, Massachusetts

Timothy Synold, DPharm
Department of Medical Oncology and Therapeutics Research, Co-Director, Pharmacoanalytic Core Facility, City of Hope Comprehensive Cancer Center, Duarte, California

Karen Syrjala, PhD
Associate Member, Clinical Research Division, Fred Hutchinson Cancer Research Center; and Associate Professor, Department of Psychiatry and Behavioral Sciences, University of Washington School of Medicine, Seattle, Washington

E. Donnall Thomas, MD
Member, Fred Hutchinson Cancer Research Center; and Professor Emeritus, University of Washington School of Medicine; and Nobel Laureate, Medicine/Physiology 1990, Seattle, Washington

D. Kathryn Tierney, RN, PhD(c)
Oncology Clinical Nurse Specialist, Division of Blood and Marrow Transplantation, Stanford University Medical Center, Stanford, California

Alan Tyndall, MD
Professor and Head, Department of Rheumatology, University of Basle, Felix Platter Spital, Basle, Switzerland

Andrea Velardi, MD
Professor, Department of Clinical and Experimental Medicine, Section of Hematology and Clinical Immunology, Perugia University School of Medicine, Perugia, Italy

Catherine M. Verfaillie, MD
Professor of Medicine, Division of Hematology, Oncology and Transplantation, Department of Medicine, Director, Stem Cell Institute, University of Minnesota, Minneapolis, Minnesota

John E. Wagner, MD
Professor of Pediatrics, Division of Blood and Marrow Transplantation, Department of Pediatrics; and Clinical Director, Stem Cell Institute, University of Minnesota, Minneapolis, Minnesota

Mark C. Walters, MD
Blood and Marrow Transplantation Program, Children's Hospital and Research Center, Oakland; and the Department of Pediatrics, University of California, San Francisco School of Medicine, San Francisco, California

Phyllis I. Warkentin, MD
Professor of Pathology and Pediatrics, University of Nebraska Medical Center, Omaha, Nebraska

Kenneth I. Weinberg, MD
Division of Research Immunology/Bone Marrow Transplantation, Children's Hospital Los Angeles; and Associate Professor of Pediatrics, Molecular, Microbiology and Immunology, University of Southern California School of Medicine, Los Angeles, California

Sally Weisdorf-Schindele, MD
Idaho Pediatric Gastroenterology, P.A., Boise, Idaho

Irving L. Weissman, MD
Beekhuis Professor of Cancer Biology, Director, Stanford Institute of Cancer/Stem Cell Biology and Medicine; and Professor, Departments of Pathology, Developmental Biology and by courtesy, Biology, Stanford University Medical Center, Stanford, California

David A. Williams, MD
Beatrice C. Lampkin Chair and Professor of Pediatrics; and Director, Division of Experimental Hematology, Cincinnati Children's Hospital Research Foundation; and Associate Chair for Translational Research Cincinnati Children's Hospital Medical Center; and University of Cincinnati College of Medicine, Cincinnati, Ohio

John R. Wingard, MD
Professor of Medicine, Director, Blood and Marrow Transplant Program, Associate Director of Clinical and Translational Research of the University of Florida Shands Cancer Center, Division of Hematology/Oncology, Gainesville, Florida

Robert P. Witherspoon, MD
Member, Fred Hutchinson Cancer Research Center; and Associate Professor of Medicine, University of Washington School of Medicine; and Medical Director, Transplant Clinic, Seattle Cancer Care Alliance, Seattle, Washington

John A. Zaia, MD
Professor of Virology, Department of Virology, Beckman Research Institute of City of Hope, Duarte, California

Esmail D. Zanjani, PhD
Professor, Department of Medicine, University of Nevada-Reno, Reno, Nevada

Preface to the First Edition

The widespread application of bone marrow transplantation (BMT) to the treatment of a steadily increasing number of life-threatening hematological, oncological, hereditary, and immunological disorders is the culmination of more than four decades of research by many investigators. Early attempts in the 1950s to transplant living cells from one individual to another were carried out in the face of considerable skepticism. It was generally accepted as axiomatic that the immunological barrier to "foreign tissue" could never be overcome.

The horrors of Nagasaki and Hiroshima spurred interest in studies of the lethal effects of irradiation. It was discovered that mice given total body irradiation in doses lethal to the marrow could be protected from death by shielding the spleen or by an infusion of marrow, and that the marrow of such animals contained living cells of donor origin. These observations suggested that patients with leukemia might be given a lethal exposure of total body irradiation, which would destroy the malignant cells along with remaining normal marrow. The exposure would also destroy the immune system, making it possible to protect against lethality by a transplant of normal marrow cells.

The theory was correct, but results were disappointing. Because the procedure was both unproved and dangerous, only those patients who had no other options were considered. Except for a few patients with an identical twin donor, there were no survivors beyond a few months. Understanding of the human leukocyte antigen (HLA) system was not yet available, and little was known about the complication we now call graft-versus-host disease (GVHD). Thus, after a brief period of enthusiasm, most investigators abandoned this seemingly hopeless pursuit. Fortunately, work in animal models continued. Studies in inbred rodents defined the genetics of the major histocompatibility system and the fundamental rules of transplantation biology. Immunosuppressive drugs were developed to limit the severity of the immune reactions between donor and host. Demonstration of successful marrow transplants in the canine model using littermates matched for the major histocompatibility complex set the stage for successful transplantation of marrow between human siblings. Thus, it is clear that a long series of experimental studies in animals ultimately made human marrow transplantation possible.

By the late 1960s, much was known about the HLA system, more effective antibiotics were available, and platelet transfusions were becoming routine. Thus began the modern era of human BMT. THe past 25 years have witnessed an almost exponential growth in the number of transplants being performed and the number of diseases being considered for BMT. Initially, most grafts employed marrow from an HLA-identical sibling. Autologous marrow, long known to be effective in animal systems, is now being used with increasing frequency following intensive cancer chemotherapy. Hematopoietic progenitor cells from the peripheral blood are now being used for BMT, either alone or to supplement marrow. As a result of increasing national and international cooperation, large panels of volunteer marrow donors of known HLA type are becoming available to patients whose own marrow cannot be used or who do not have a family donor.

Currently, thousands of transplants are being performed each year world-wide. With the demonstration that marrow could be transplanted and that the cure rate would be substantial, the logical step was taken to treat patients early during the course of their respective disease (i.e. in leukemia when the burden of malignant cells was relatively low and when the patient was in excellent clinical condition). With improved patient selection, development of improved tissue typing methods, availability of potent antimicrobial agents, advances in supportive care, and improved prevention of GVHD, the results of BMT have continued to improve.

Marrow transplantation is now being applied to a long list of diseases with a wide range of results depending on the disease, the type of transplant, and the stage of the disease. For some of the diseases, BMT has already proven to be the most effective therapy (e.g., some leukemias and severe aplastic anemia), whereas for others it is the only available curative treatment (e.g., thalassemia). In very rare genetic disorders, one successful BMT may establish the success of the treatment. For other more common disorders, controlled trials are necessary to define the proper role of allogeneic or autologous BMT, or therapy not involving BMT.

Only through rigorous study and long-term follow-up can novel approaches be confirmed as effective (or ineffective). For those working in the field of marrow transplantation, a source of intellectual satisfaction has been the interdisciplinary nature of the studies. A view of the wide-ranging disciplines involved can be gleaned by reading the chapter titles for this book. A successful BMT program is always a team effort. There must be cooperation between blood banks, referring physicians, radiation oncologists, immunologists, and physicians from many subspecialties. A dedicated support staff of technicians, data managers, and, above all, nurses, is crucial. The nursing team in particular is responsible for the day-to-day care of patients. Nurses not only provide the bedside management of complex protocol studies, but also bear the burden of emotional support through the difficult hospital period. They are the most readily available source of information for the patients and families day and night. Without a strong nursing team, the entire BMT program is jeopardized.

Most important are the patients who come to the transplant center with the courage to accept days, weeks, and sometimes months of discomfort in the hope of surviving a fatal disease. We must ensure that we acknowledge and respect the dignity and individuality of each patient, that we provide adequate information for informed decision making and then include patients and families in the decision process. The greatest reward for clinical investigators is to see patients reintegrated into their personal, social, and professional lives, free of their disease and its complications.

Stephen J. Forman
Karl G. Blume
E. Donnall Thomas
Summer, 1993

Preface to the Second Edition

During the five-year period since the first edition of this book was published, an enormous amount of new scientific information has been generated through experimental research and through clinical trials. This growth in knowledge is reflected by the doubling in the volume of this book and a 50 percent increase in the number of new chapters. The selection of a new title *Hematopoietic Cell Transplantation* became necessary because bone marrow is no longer the major source of allogeneic and autologous hematopoietic cells. Hematopoietic stem cells from peripheral blood collections and from umbilical cord blood are rapidly gaining clinical importance for hematologic and immunologic reconstitution following myeloablative, high-dose therapies for malignant and non-malignant, hereditary or acquired life-threatening disease.

It would be impossible to identify a single scientific observation as the leading contribution to the progress made during the past five years. Exciting new data have been reported in all areas of preclinical and clinical research: New histocompatibility antigens for optimal donor selection have been described, novel concepts have been developed to eradicate the underlying malignancies, engineering of allogeneic and autologous grfts has been further developed, previously unavailable drugs for post-transplant immunosuppression and for the prevention or therapy of infectious complications have been tested. The indication list for high-dose therapy and hematopoietic cell transplantation has been extended and the long-term evaluation and management of transplant recipients has been further defined.

Still, the editors would caution the young investigator that "breakthroughs" do not occur. Each step towards a cure has to be earned through thoughtfully designed and carefully conducted pre-clinical experiments and clinical trials. Single institution studies require confirmation through prospective randomized trials, each needing several years before a new concept can be fully accepted as a proven advance.

The editors hope that the new edition will serve as a resource for physicians and many other members of health care teams at transplant centers and for new and established investigators in the area of hematopoietic cell transplantation and related fields of research; in brief, for everyone who wishes to learn about this exciting field which is now at the beginning of its fifth decade of development as a curative treatment modality for disorders with an otherwise poor prognosis.

E. Donnall Thomas
Karl G. Blume
Stephen J. Forman
Summer, 1998

Preface to the Third Edition

Ten years after the first and five years following the publication of the second edition of this textbook, the editors and the publisher, Blackwell Publishing, present now the third edition. Because of the continued impressive growth of knowledge in the field of hematopoietic cell transplantation, a new and completely revised book was needed to document and critically review the scientific progress made during the past five years.

The editors wish to emphasize several changes in the third edition compared to the second edition. *First*, the title of the book has been changed to honor the pioneering work of E. Donnall Thomas, the 1990 Nobel Laureate in Physiology or Medicine (see Tribute, p. xix). *Second*, the reader will find ten new chapters which deal with new experimental or clinical research observations while four prior chapters have been deleted. Topics for the new chapters include stem cell expansion, the theory and application of non-myeloablative regimens followed by allogeneic hematopoietic cell transplantation, the experimental basis for transplantation for autoimmune diseases, long-term complications and others. *Third*, we have again tried to avoid overlap and contradiction between chapters, however, following academic principles, we have allowed the expression of opposing views and opinions in certain areas, for example, on the topic of plasticity of embryonic and adult stem cells.

The editors are indebted to the publishing house which again has produced a high quality product in a timely fashion for the international community of investigators at all professional levels and disciplines in the field of hematopoietic cell transplantation. Finally, this book would not have been possible without the dedicated work of our assistants Sara E. Clark, Stephen J. Loy and Kristine A. Logan.

Karl G. Blume
Stephen J. Forman
Frederick R. Appelbaum
Spring 2003

Tribute

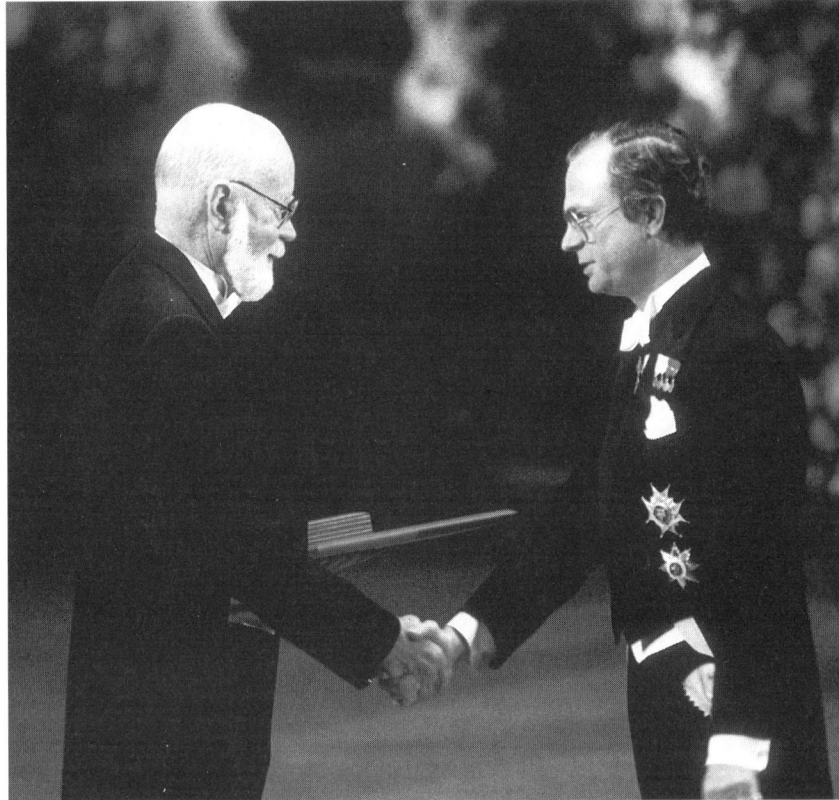

Dr. E. Donnall Thomas and King Carl Gustaf of Sweden. Dr. Thomas and Dr. Joseph Murray (not shown in the picture) shared the Nobel Prize for Physiology or Medicine, 1990, recognizing the field of organ transplantation. Dr. Thomas was honored for endeavors in experimental and clinical bone marrow transplantation. Their prizes emphasize the importance of patient-related research.

As noted in the Preface to this third edition, our textbook's title has been changed to honor Dr. E. Donnall Thomas. This change is altogether fitting given that he is the single individual most responsible for creating the subject of this book.

Don was born on March 15, 1920, the son of a solo general practitioner in a small Texas village. He recalls as a child accompanying his father to his small office and to patients' homes. As Don has mentioned, between he and his father, they span the period from horse and buggy house calls to our modern high-tech medicine. He received his BA and MD from the University of Texas and that is where he met his wife, Dottie. Besides raising three children and eight grandchildren together, Dottie has been Don's partner in every aspect of his professional life, from working in the laboratory, to editing manuscripts and administering grants. Anyone who has been lucky enough to work with Don knows that if he is the father of marrow transplantation, then Dottie is, without question, the mother.

Don graduated from Harvard Medical School in 1947 and completed his internship and residency at Peter Brent Brigham Hospital in Boston. It was while in medical school that Don first became interested in normal and malignant hematopoiesis. During those years, Sydney Farber was initiating his first studies of the use of antifolates to treat children with acute leukemia and Don witnessed the very first patient to achieve a remission with this approach. He was exposed to the pioneering work of Allan Erslev and his search for erythropoietin. Most importantly, he learned of Leon Jacobsen and his studies showing that shielding the spleen protected mice from the otherwise lethal effects of total body irradiation. As data emerged that a similar irradiation protection effect could be achieved by transferring bone marrow from a non-irradiated to an irradiated mouse, Don became convinced of the clinical potential of marrow transplantation.

In 1955, Don moved to Cooperstown, New York, and the Imogene Basset Hospital, a Columbia University affiliate, where he began working on marrow transplantation, both in the canine model and in humans, with Dr. Joseph Farrebee. In 1957, Don published the first report in human patients showing that complete remissions of leukemia could be achieved using total body irradiation followed by infusion of marrow from an identical twin. At that time, there was little understanding of the principles of human histocompatibility and so attempts to expand these studies to patients without identical twins were uniformly unsuccessful. These failures were the stimulus for a long series of experiments conducted by Don in the canine model showing it was possible to expose dogs to supralethal doses of irradiation and rescue them by reinfusing their own marrow, that the marrow could be cryopreserved, and that large doses of peripheral blood could substitute for marrow. But attempts at allogeneic transplantation in this outbred species continued to fail because of graft-versus-host disease or graft rejection.

In 1963, Don moved to Seattle and the University of Washington to become the first head of the Division of Oncology. There he developed techniques for rudimentary histocompatibility typing in the dog and by the mid-1960s showed that by selecting matched donors and using methotrexate post-transplant, it was possible to successfully transplant marrow between matched littermates in almost every case. At the same time, based on the work of Dausset, Payne, Amos and others, the understanding of human histocompatibility also dramatically increased and so, in the late 1960s, Don made the decision to return to the subject of allogeneic transplantation in humans. He began to assemble a team of physicians, nurses and support personnel (many of whom are still part of the current Seattle Transplant Program) and obtained a program project grant from the National Cancer Institute. In November 1968, Dr. Robert Good and his colleagues carried out the first marrow transplant from a matched sibling for an infant with immunodeficiency and in March 1969, Don performed the first matched sibling donor transplant for a patient with leukemia.

The Seattle Transplant Program was originally housed at the Seattle Public Health Hospital but in 1972, when the hospital was faced with closure by the federal government, the Program moved to Providence Hospital. In 1975, Don and his team moved to the newly created Fred Hutchinson Cancer Research Center, a move that provided Don with increased space, resources and scientific collaborations. That same year, he and his colleagues published their classic *New England Journal of Medicine* paper summarizing the field of allogeneic transplantation and particularly the early Seattle experience. These results demonstrated not only the feasibility of the procedure, but also that there was a plateau on the survival curves following transplantation, suggesting that some of these patients were cured with this novel technique. Don continued to lead the Clinical Research Division of the Center and its transplant program until his partial retirement in 1989. Yet he continues to work writing manuscripts, delivering lectures and participating in research discussions at the Center.

Appropriately, Don has received almost every possible award for his work, including the American Society of Hematology's Henry M. Stratton Award, the General Motor's Kettering Prize, the American Society of Oncology's Karnofsky Award, the Presidential Medal of Science, and of course, the 1990 Nobel Prize in Medicine which he shared with Joseph Murray. With each award, Don has always emphasized how much his work was a team effort. He invariably mentions the contributions of Rainer Storb, Dean Buckner, Reg Clift, Paul Neiman, Alex Fefer, and Bob Epstein, who helped form the original Seattle Transplant Team, and of Ted Graham, who moved with Don from Cooperstown to help in the animal research. Don never fails to credit the nursing and support staff who played such a critical role in these efforts, and he always acknowledges the patients and their families who have been true partners in his work.

Although Don is most noted for his pioneering scientific achievements, for those of us who have been fortunate enough to work with him, Don is equally admired for the way in which he achieved his success. He has always been focused, hardworking and uncompromising in his laboratory and clinical research. He can be a demanding critic and holds others accountable for their actions, yet at the same time he has always been generous with his ideas, loyal to his employees and quick to deflect praise to his coworkers. Although he has dedicated an enormous amount of himself to a life in medical science, he has managed to maintain a great deal of balance. He has traveled widely as a visiting lecturer, donated time to professional organizations and supported local and international charities. He and Dottie are avid and expert hunters and fishers and have a close and loving extended family.

It is difficult to think of many other fields of modern medicine that are so much the result of a single man's work. Don's vision and dedication have changed the lives of literally hundreds of thousands of patients. By naming this textbook for him, we are joining those patients, and the many nurses, physicians and staff privileged to work in the field he created, in thanking Don both for what he has accomplished and for the way he has done it.

List of Abbreviations

AA	aplastic anemia	BC	blood culture
AABB	American Association of Blood Banks	BCNU	1,3-*bis*(2-chloroethyl)-1-nitrosourea
AAV	adeno-associated virus	BDP	beclomethasone 17, 21-dipropionate
ABMT	autologous bone marrow transplant	BEAC	BCNU, etoposide, cytarabine and cyclophosphamide
ABMTR	Autologous Blood and Marrow Transplant Registry	BEAM	BCNU, etoposide, cytosine arabinoside, melphalan
ABW	actual body weight	BFU-E	burst-forming units-erythroid
ACD	acid-citrate-dextrose	BLS	bare lymphocyte syndrome
ACIF	anticomplement immunofluorescence	BM	bone marrow
ACIP	Advisory Committee on Immunization Practices	BMC	bone marrow cell
AD	autoimmune disease	BMDW	Bone Marrow Donors Worldwide
ADA	adenosine deaminase	BMEC	bone marrow microvascular endothelial cell
ADCC	antibody-dependent cell-mediated cytotoxicity	BMHC	bone marrow hematopoietic cell
ADL	activities of daily living	BMP	bone morphogenic protein
ADP	adenosine diphosphate	BMT	bone marrow transplantation
ADV	adenovirus	BOOP	bronchiolitis obliterans organizing pneumonia
AFM	doxorubicin, fluorouracil and methotrexate	bpRNA	basepair RNA
AG	antigenemia assay	BrdU	bromo-deoxyuridine
AGM	aorta-gonad-mesonephros	BSA	body surface area/bovine serum albumin
aHCT	autologous hematopoietic cell transplantation	BSE	bovine spongiform encephalopathy
AHRQ	Agency for Health Care Research and Quality	BU	busulfan
AIBW	adjusted ideal body weight	BUN	blood urea nitrogen
AICD	activation-induced cell death	CA	cyclophosphamide and doxorubicin
AIDS	acquired immune deficiency syndrome	CAF	cyclophosphamide, doxorubicin and fluorouracil
ALDH	aldehyde dehydrogenase	CALGB	Cancer and Leukaemia Group B
ALG	antilymphocyte globulin	CAP	College of American Pathologists
ALL	acute lymphoblastic leukemia	CB	cord blood
ALS	antilymphocyte serum	CBC	complete blood count *or* cord blood cell
ALT	alanine aminotransferase	CBER	Center for Biologic Evaluation and Research
AMBTR	Autologous Blood and Marrow Transplant Registry	CBHC	cord blood hematopoietic cell
AML	acute myeloid leukemia	CBP	cyclophosphamide, BCNU and cisplatin
ANA	antinuclear antibody	CBSC	cord blood stem cell
ANC	absolute neutrophil count	CBV	cyclophosphamide, BCNU and etoposide
AP	alkaline phosphatase	CC	complete chimerism
APACHE	Acute Physiology, Age, Chronic Health Evaluation	CCG	Children's Cancer Group
APC	antigen-presenting cell	CCR	continuous complete remission
APL	acute promyelocytic leukemia	CD	cluster designation
AR	aldehyde reductase	CDAD	*Clostridium difficile* associated diarrhea
ARA-C	cytosine arabinoside	CDC	Centers for Disease Control
ARA-G	guanine arabinoside	cdd	cytotoxic double deficient (mouse)
ARC	American Red Cross	CDK	cyclin dependent kinase
ARDS	acute respiratory distress syndrome	CDR3	complementarity determining region 3
ARS	antigen recognition site	CDRH	Center for Devices and Radiological Health
ASBMT	American Society for Blood and Marrow Transplantation	CEA	carcinoembryonic antigen
		CFC	colony-forming cell
ASHI	American Society for Histocompatibility and Immunogenetics	CFU	colony-forming unit
		CFU-GEMM	colony-forming unit–granulocyte/erythrocyte/macrophage/megakaryocyte
ATG	antithymocyte globulin		
ATP	adenosine triphosphate	CFU-GM	colony-forming unit–granulocyte/macrophage
ATRA	all *trans* retinoic acid	CFU-S	colony-forming unit–spleen
AUC	area-under-the-curve	CGD	chronic granulomatous disease
BACT	BCNU, cytosine arabinoside, cyclophosphamide, thioguanine	cGMP	cyclic guanosine monophosphate
		cGTP	current Good Tissue Practices
BAL	bronchoalveolar lavage	CHOEP	cyclophosphamide, doxorubicin, vincristine, etoposide and prednisone
BAVC	BCNU, amsacrine, etoposide		

CHOP	cyclophosphamide, doxorubicin, vincristine and prednisone	DTPA	diethylenetriaminepentaacetic acid
CHVmP/BP	cyclophosphamide, doxorubicin, teniposide, prednisone, bleomycin and vincristine	E	early
		EAE	experimental autoimmune encephalomyelitis
CIK	cytokine induced killer	EBMT	European Group for Blood and Marrow Transplantation
c-kitL	c-kit ligand	EBNA	Epstein–Barr (virus) nuclear antigen
CLIP	class II invariant chain peptide	EBV	Epstein–Barr virus
CLL	chronic lymphocytic leukemia	EBV-BLCL	Epstein–Barr virus immortalized B lymphoblastoid cell line
CLP	common lymphocyte progenitor		
CMA	cyclophosphamide, mitoxantrone and melphalan	EBV-LPD	Epstein–Barr virus-associated lymphoproliferative disorder
CMF	cyclosphosphamide, methotrexate and fluorouracil		
CML	chronic myeloid leukemia or cell-medicated lympholysis	EC	epirubicin and cyclophosphamide
CML-CP	CML in chronic phase	ECG	electrocardiogram
CMML	chronic myelomonocytic leukemia	ECM	extracellular matrix
CMP	common myeloid progenitor	ECP	extracorporeal photopheresis
CMV	cytomegalovirus	EFS	event-free survival
CMVIg	cytomegalovirus immunoglobulin	EIAV	equine infectious anaemia virus
CMV-IP	cytomegalovirus-associated interstitial pneumonia	ELISA	enzyme-linked immunosorbent assay
CNNU	1-(2-chloroethyl)-3-cyclohexyl-1-nitrosurea	ENSG	European Neuroblastoma Study Group
CNS	central nervous system or clinical nurse specialist	ENU	N-ethyl-N-nitrosourea
CONSORT	Consolidated Standards of Reporting Trials	EORTC	European Organization for Research and Treatment of Cancer
COX	cyclo-oxygenase	EPO	erythropoietin
CR	complete remission or complete response	ER	endoplasmic reticulum
CREG	crossreactive group	ES	embryonic stem
CS	chondroitin-sulfate	ET	essential thrombocythemia
CSF	colony-stimulating factor	ETP	early thymic progenitor
CSP	cyclosporine	EWOG	European Working Group
CT	computerized tomography	F	female
CTCb	cyclophosphamide, thiotepa and carboplatin	FAC	fluorouracil, doxorubicin and cyclophosphamide
CTL	cytotoxic T lymphocyte	FACS	fluorescence activated cell sorter
CTLA-4	cytotoxic T-lymphocyte antigen 4	FACT	Functional Assessment of Chronic Illness Therapies or Foundation for the Accreditation of Cellular Therapy
CTLp	cytotoxic T-lymphocyte precursor		
CVAD	cyclophosphamide, vincristine, doxorubicin, decadron	FAH	final adult height
CVC	central venous catheter	FAHCT	Foundation for the Accreditation of Hematopoietic Cell Therapy (2001 renamed FACT)
CVS	chorionic villous sampling		
CY	cyclophosphamide	FAI	free androgen index
DAG	diacylglycerol	FAMA	fluorescent-antibody staining of membrane antigen
DC	dendritic cell	FasL	Fas ligand
DCC	data coordinating center	FC	facilitator cell
DFA	direct fluorescence antigen/direct fluorescent antibody	FCS	fetal calf serum
DFCI	Dana-Farber Cancer Institute	FDA	Food and Drug Administration
DFS	disease-free survival	FDCA	Food, Drug and Cosmetic Act
DHAP	cisplatin, cytarabine and decadron	FEC	fluorouracil, epirubicin and cyclophosphamide
DHFR	dihydrofolate reductase	FEV	forced expiratory volume
DIC	disseminated intravascular coagulopathy	FGF	fibroblast growth factor
DLA	dog leukocyte antigen	FGF-7	fibroblast growth factor 7 (a.k.a. KGF)
DLCL	diffuse large B cell lymphoma	FHCRC	Fred Hutchinson Cancer Research Center
DLCO	diffusion capacity	FIRST	Fully Integrated Research Standards and Technology
DLI	donor lymphocyte infusion	FISH	fluorescence in situ hybridization
DMB	dimethylbusulfan	FIV	feline immunodeficiency virus
DMS	dimethylsulfide	FKBP	FK506-binding protein
DMSO	dimethylsulfoxide	FL	fetal liver
$DMSO_2$	dimethylsulfone	Flt3L	Flt3 ligand
DNA	deoxyribonucleic acid	FN	fibronectin
DNAse	deoxyribonuclease	FRET	fluorescence resonance energy transfer
DNR	do not resuscitate	FSH	follicle-stimulating hormone
DOTA	1,4,7,10-tetra-azacyclododecane-N, N^1, N^{11} N^{111}-tetracetic acid	FTE	full-time equivalent
		FTOC	fetal thymic organ culture
DR	death receptor	5-FU	5-fluorouracil
DS	dermatan sulfate	FVC	forced vital capacity
DSMB	Data and Safety Monitoring Board	GAD	glutamic acid decarboxylase
dsRNA	double stranded RNA	GAG	glycosaminoglycans
DST	donor-specific transfusion	GALV	gibbon ape leukemia virus

GCRC	General Clinical Research Center	HSV	herpes simplex virus
G-CSF	granulocyte colony-stimulating factor	HSV-1	herpes simplex virus, type 1
GCT	giant cell tumor	HSV-tk	herpes simplex virus thymidine kinase
GDP	guanosine diphosphate	HTLV-1	human T-cell lymphotropic virus 1
GEGMO	Group d'Etudes de la Greffe de Moelle Osseuse	HUS	hemolytic uremic syndrome
GELA	Groupe d'Etude des Lymphomes de Adulte	HUVEC	human umbilical cord endothelial cell
GeMCRIS	Genetic Modification Clinical Research Information System	HVEM	herpesvirus entry mediator
		HVG	host-vs.-graft
GFP	green fluorescent protein	IAP	inhibitor of apoptosis
GFR	glomerular filtration rate	IBC	Institutional Biosafety Committees
GH	growth hormone	IBMTR	International Bone Marrow Transplant Registry
GI	gastrointestinal	IBW	ideal body weight
GIMEMA	Gruppo Italiano Malattie Ematologiche Maligne dell' Adulto	IC	initiating cell
		ICAM	intracellular adhesion molecule
GITMO	Gruppo Italiano Trapianti di Midolio Osseo	ICBTR	International Cord Blood Transplant Registry
GlyCAM-1	glyosylation-dependent cell adhesion molecule	ICE	ifosfamide, carboplatin and etoposide regimen
GM-CSF	granulocyte macrophage colony-stimulating factor	ICH	International Conference on Harmonization
GMP	guanosine monophosphate *or* granulocyte macrophage progenitor *or* Good Manufacturing Practices	ICOS	inducible costimulator
		ICU	intensive care unit
		Id	idiotype
GnRH	gonadotropin-releasing hormone	IDE	investigational device exemption
GRE	glucocorticoid response elements	IDM	infectious disease marker
GSH	glutathione	IDSA	Infectious Disease Society of America
GST	glutathione-*S*-transferase	IE	immediate early
GTP	guanosine triphosphate	IF	involved-field
GVH	graft-vs.-host	IFN	interferon
GVHD	graft-vs.-host disease	Ig	immunoglobulin
GVHR	graft-vs.-host reaction	IGF-I	insulin-like growth factor I
GVL(E)	graft-vs.-leukemia *or* lymphoma (effect)	IgH	immunoglobulin heavy chain
GVT	graft-vs.-tumor	IL	interleukin
GVT(E)	graft-vs.-tumor (effect)	IL-1RA	IL-1 receptor antagonist
H	histocompatibility	IL-2R	IL-2 receptor
H&E	hematoxylin and eosin	Im	imidazole
HA	hyaluronic acid	IM	intramuscular/intramuscularly
HAMA	human antimouse antibody	IMPDH	inosine monophosphate dehydrogenase
Hb	hemoglobin	IND	investigational new drug
HBsAg	hepatitis B surface antigen	INSS	International Neuroblastoma Staging System
HBV	hepatitis B virus	IP	interstitial pneumonia
4-HC	4-hydroperoxycyclophosphamide	IP_3	inositol-1,4,5-triphosphate
HC	hematopoietic cell *or* hydroxycyclophosphamide	IPI	International Prognostic Factors Index
HCFA	Health Care Financing Administration	IPS	interstitial pneumonia syndrome
HCT	hematopoietic cell transplantation	IPSS	International Prognostic Scoring System
HCT/Ps	human cells, tissues and cellular and tissue-based products	IRB	Institutional Review Board
		IRES	internal ribosome entry site
HCV	hepatitis C virus	IRF	interferon regulatory factor
HCW	health care worker	ISCT	International Society for Cellular Therapy
HD	Hodgkin's disease	ISHAGE	International Society for Hematotherapy and Graft Engineering (2001 renamed ISCT)
HEPA	high-efficiency particulate air		
HES	hydroxyethyl starch	IST	immunosuppressive therapy
HHV-6	human herpesvirus 6	ITAM	immunoreceptor tyrosine-based activation motifs
Hib	*Haemophilus influenzae* type b	ITIM	immunoreceptor tyrosine-based inhibitory motifs
HIPAA	Health Insurance Portability and Accountability Act	IU-HCT	*in utero* hematopoietic cell transplantation
HIV	human immunodeficiency virus	IV	intravenous/intravenously
HLA	human leukocyte antigen	IVIg	intravenous immunoglobulin
Hp	hydroxypyrrole	JACIE	Joint Accreditation Committee of ISHAGE-Europe and EBMT
HPC	hematopoietic progenitor cell		
HPLC	high-pressure liquid chromatography	JAK-3	Janus kinase 3
HPV	human papillomavirus	JCAHO	Joint Commission on Accreditation of Health Care Organizations
HRQOL	health-related quality of life		
HRSA	Health Resources and Services Administration	JCML	juvenile chronic myelogenous leukemia
HRT	hormone replacement therapy	KGF	keratinocyte growth factor (a.k.a. FGF-7)
HS	heparin sulfate	KIR	killer immunoglobulin-like receptor
HSC	hematopoietic stem cell		
HSCT	hematopoietic stem cell transplantation		

KLH	keyhole limpet hemocyanin	MPD	myelin-basic protein
KTLS	cKit⁺Thy1.1^lo Lin^−/lo Sca-1⁺cKit⁺	MPO	myeloperoxidase
L	late	MPP	multipotent progenitor
LAK	lymphokine-activated killer	MPS	mucopolysaccharidosis
LB	lumbar puncture	MPSV	myeloproliferative sarcoma virus
LBP	LPS binding protein	MRC	Medical Research Council
LD	linkage disequilibrium	MRD	minimal residual disease *or* matched-related donor
LDH	lactate dehydrogenase	MRI	magnetic resonance imaging
LFA-1	leukocyte function-associated antigen-1	mRNA	messenger ribonucleic acid
LFR	limited field irradiation	MRP	multidrug resistance-associated protein
LFS	leukemia-free survival	MRSA	methicillin-resistant *Staphylococcus aureus*
LGL	large granular lymphocyte	MSC	mesenchymal stem cell
LH	lutenizing hormone	MSCH	mouse spinal cord homogenate
LIF	leukemia inhibitory factor	MSKCC	Memorial Sloan Kettering Cancer Center
LMP	latent membrane protein	MTD	maximum tolerated dose
LNA	locked nucleic acid	mTOR	mammalian target of rapamycin
LPS	lipopolysaccharide	MTX	methotrexate
LT	long-term	MUD	matched-unrelated donor
LTC-IC	long-term culture initiating cells	MUGA	multigated acquisition
LTMC	long-term marrow cultures	MuMLV	Moloney murine leukemia virus
LTR	long-terminal repeats	NAB	natural antibody
LY	life year	NASBA	nucleic acid sequence-based amplification
M	male	NCCN	National Comprehensive Cancer Network
MAB	monoclonal antibody	NCIC	National Cancer Institute of Canada
Mac-1	macrophage antigen-1	NCM	nurse case manager
MAdCAM-1	mucosal addressin cell adhesion molecule	NCR	natural cytotoxicity receptor
MALT	mucosa associated lymphoid tissue	N-D-N	nucleotide-diversity-nucleotide
MAPC	mesenchymal associated progenitor cell	NF-1	neurofibromatosis type 1
MAPK	mitogen activated protein kinase	NF-AT	nuclear factor of activated T cells
MBN	myeloblastin	NGFR	nerve growth factor receptor
MC	mixed chimerism	NGVL	National Gene Vector Laboratory
MCL	mantle cell lymphoma	NHL	non-Hodgkin's lymphoma
MCMV	murine cytomegalovirus	NHLBI	National Heart, Lung and Blood Institute
MCP-1	monocyte chemoattractant protein-1	NIH	National Institutes of Health
M-CSF	macrophage colony-stimulating factor	NK	natural killer
MDR	multidrug resistant	NM	nonmyeloablative
MDS	myelodysplastic syndrome	NMDP	National Marrow Donor Program
MEAC	minimum effective analgesic concentration	NO	nitric oxide
MEL	melphalan	NOD	nonobese diabetic
MEP	megakaryocyte erythrocyte progenitor	NOD-SCID	nonobese diabetic mice with severe combined immunodeficiency syndrome
MGDF	megakaryocyte growth and development factor	NP	nucleoside phosphorylase
MGMT	O⁶-methylguanine DNA methyltransferase	NPM	nurse program manager
mHA	minor histocompatibility antigen	NS	natural suppressor (cells)
MHC	major histocompatibility complex	NSAID	nonsteroidal anti-inflammatory drug
MIBG	metaiodobenzylguanidine	NZB	New Zealand black (mouse)
MIRD	medical internal radiation dose	NZW	New Zealand white (mouse)
MKP	megakaryocyte progenitor	O⁶-BG	O⁶-benzyl-guanine
MLC	mixed lymphocyte culture	OBA	Office of Biotechnology Activities
MLR	mixed lymphocyte reaction	ODN	oligodeoxynucleotide
MLV	murine leukemia virus	OMB	Office of Management and Budget
MM	multiple myeloma	OMIM	Online Mendelian Inheritance in Man database
MMF	mycophenolate mofetil	OPM	oropharyngeal mucositis
MMP	matrix metalloproteinase	O-PRISM	oncologic pediatric risk of mortality
MMR	measles–mumps–rubella	OR	odds ratio
MMRD	mismatched related donor	OS	overall survival
MMUD	mismatched unrelated donor	PACT	Psychosocial Assessment of Candidates for Transplantation Scale
MNC	mononuclear cell	PAS	periodic-acid Schiff
MOG	myelin oligodendrocyte glycoprotein	PB	peripheral blood
MP	methylprednisolone	PBC	peripheral blood cell
MPA	mycophenolic acid	PBHC	peripheral blood hematopoietic cell
MPB	mobilized peripheral blood		
mPBPC	mobilized peripheral blood progenitor cells		

PBHCT	peripheral blood hematopoietic cell transplantation	Rh	rhesus
PBL	peripheral blood lymphocyte	RHC	residual host cell
PBMC	peripheral blood mononuclear cell	RHu	recombinant human
PBP	penicillin-binding protein	RHuEPO	recombinant human erythropoietin
PBPC	peripheral blood progenitor cell	RHuG-CSF	recombinant human granulocyte colony-stimulating factor
PBPCT	peripheral blood progenitor cell transplantation	RHuGM-CSF	recombinant human granulocyte macrophage colony-stimulating factor
PBS	primer binding site	RIA	radioimmunoassay
PBSC	peripheral blood stem cell	rIL	recombinant interleukin
PBSCT	peripheral blood stem cell transplantation	RISC	RNAi induced silencing complex
PCP	*Pneumocystis carinii* pneumonia	RNA	ribonucleic acid
PCR	polymerase chain reaction	RNAi	RNA interference
PDQ	Physician Data Query	RNase H	ribonuclease H
PEG	pegylated bovine	RR	relative rate *or* relative risk
PFS	progression-free survival	RRT	regimen-related toxicity
PG	proteoglycans	RSCA	reference strand mediated conformation analysis
PGD	preimplantation genetic diagnosis	RSCH	rat spinal cord homogenate
pgk	phosphoglycerokinase	RSV	respiratory syncytial virus
PGS	primitive germline cell	RT_3U	resin triiodothyronine uptake
Ph	Philadelphia (chromosome)	RT-PCR	reverse transcription-polymerase chain reaction
PHA	phytohemagglutan A	SAA	severe aplastic anemia
PHN	post-herpetic neuralgia	SAE	severe adverse event
PHS	Public Health Services	SBA-E-	soy bean agglutinin and E-rosette depletion
PI	phosphoinositol *or* principal investigator	SBA	soy bean agglutinin
$PI4,5-P_2$	phosphoinositide-4,5-diphosphate	SBT	sequencing-based typing
PKC	protein kinase C	SC	subcutaneous *or* subcutaneously
PLP	proteolipid protein	SCF	stem cell factor
PLPHA	post-lumbar puncture headache	SCID	severe combined immunodeficiency syndrome
PLS	Psychosocial Levels System	SCN	severe chronic neutropenia
PMC	persistent mixed chimerism	SDF-1	stromal derived factor-1
PMRD	partially matched-related donor	SEB	*Staphylococcal enterotoxin* B
PNA	peptide nucleic acid	SEER	Surveillance, Epidemiology and End Results
PNH	paroxysmal nocturnal hemoglobinuria	SF-36	Short Form 36
POG	Pediatric Oncology Group	SFFV	spleen focus-forming virus
PORT	Patient Outcomes Assessment Research Team	Shh	sonic hedgehog
PR	partial remission *or* partial response	SI	stimulation index
PR3	proteinase 3	siRNA	short interfering RNA
PSC	pluripotent stem cell	SIV	simian immunodeficiency virus
PSE	prednisone	SLE	systemic lupus erythematosus
PSGL-1	P-selectin glycoprotein ligand-1	SLF	steel factor
PTLD	post-transplant lymphoproliferative disease	SNP	single nucleotide polymorphism
PUVA	psoralen and ultraviolet light A	SOP	standard operating procedure
PV	polycythemia vera	SOS	sinusoidal obstruction syndrome
PVP	polyvinylpyrrolidone	SRC	SCID-repopulating cell
PWM	pokeweed mitogen	SSOP	sequence-specific oligonucleotide probe
Py	pyrrole	SSP	sequence-specific primer
QALY	quality-adjusted life year	SSRI	selective serotonergic reuptake inhibitor
Q-FISH	quantitative fluorescence *in situ* hybridization	ST	short-term
QOL	quality of life	STAT	signal transduction and activator of transcription
Q-PCR	quantitative PCR	sTNFR	soluble form of the TNF-α receptor
Q-TWiST	quality time without symptoms of toxicity	STR	short tandem repeat
RA	refractory anemia	SWOG	South-West Oncology Group
RAC	Recombinant DNA Advisory Committee	T1DM	type 1 diabetes mellitus
RAEB	refractory anemia with excess blasts	T_3	triiodothyronine
RAEB-T	refractory anemia with excess blasts in transformation	T_4	thyroxine
RAIT	radioimmunotherapy	TAA	tumor associated antigens
RARS	refractory anemia with ringed sideroblasts	TAC	taxotere, doxorubicin and cyclophosphamide
RBC	red blood cell	TAI	thoracoabdominal irradiation
RCC	renal cell carcinoma *or* ratios of costs to charge	TAM	total body irradiation, Ara-C and melphalan
RCT	randomized controlled trial	TAP	transporter associated with antigen processing
rFBN	recombinant fibronectin fragment	TBI	total body irradiation
RFLP	restriction fragment length polymorphism	Tc	cytotoxic T
RFS	relapse-free survival		

Tc1	cytotoxic T type 1 subset	TSH	thyroid-stimulating hormone
Tc2	cytotoxic T type 2 subset	TT	thiotepa
TCD	T-cell depletion	TTP	thrombotic thrombocytopenic purpura
TCD-BM	T-cell-depleted bone marrow	UCB	umbilical cord blood
TCR	T-cell receptor	UCBT	umbilical cord blood transplantation
TDM	therapeutic drug monitoring	UCLA	University of California at Los Angeles
TdT	terminal deoxynucleotidyl transferase	URD	unrelated donor
TED	Transplant Essential Data	URI	upper respiratory infection
TERS	Transplant Evaluation Rating Scale	v/v	volume in volume
TERT	telomere-reverse transcriptase	VCAM	vascular cell adhesion molecule
TFO	triple helix forming oligodeoxynucleotide	VEGF	vascular endothelial growth factor
TGF	transforming growth factor	VLA	very-late antigen
T$_H$	T-helper	VNTR	variable number of tandem repeat
T$_H$1	T-helper type 1 subset	VOD	veno-occlusive disease
T$_H$2	T-helper type 2 subset	VP16	etoposide
TIL	tumor infiltrating lymphocytes	VRE	vancomycin resistant enterococci
TK	thymidine kinase	VSV	vesicular stomatitis virus
TLI	total lymphoid irradiation	VSV-G	vesicular stomatitis virus G protein
TLR	toll-like receptor	VZIG	varicella-zoster immunoglobulin
Tm	melting temperature	VZV	varicella-zoster virus
TMC	transient mixed chimerism	w/v	weight in volume
TNC	total nucleated cells	WAS	Wiskott–Aldrich syndrome
TNF	tumor necrosis factor	WASp	Wiskott–Aldrich syndrome protein
TNFR	TNF-α receptor	WBC	white blood cell/white blood cell count
TNM	Tumor, Node, Metastasis classification	WGA	wheat germ agglutinin
TPO	thrombopoietin	WHO	World Health Organization
TREC	T-cell receptor excision circle	WMDA	World Marrow Donor Association
TRF	telomere restriction fragment	XSCID	X-linked severe combined immunodeficiency syndrome
TRM	treatment-related mortality *or* transplant-related mortality	ZIG	zoster immunoglobulin
TSC	totipotent stem cell	ZIP	zoster immunoplasma

Section 1

Scientific Basis for Hematopoietic Cell Transplantation

1

E. Donnall Thomas

A History of Bone Marrow Transplantation

History means different things to different people. The use of fire began about 500,000 years ago, and recorded history began only about 3 millennia ago. On this time scale any history of bone marrow transplantation (BMT) occupies only a moment in time. It seems strange that our knowledge of the functions of the bone marrow is less than 2 centuries old, and the knowledge of transplantation of bone marrow is confined to the last half century. History as defined in this chapter will be restricted to those findings that led to clinical BMT. It will not deal with solid organ transplantation, extensive studies in mice or with the advances in immunology and immunosuppressive drugs except as related to clinical marrow transplantation.

Attempts to employ marrow for therapeutic purposes began in 1939 and 1940 [1,2]. However, infusions of a few milliliters of marrow were not attempts at transplantation, and no useful results were seen. During World War II, some very interesting experiments were carried out by Rekers and colleagues [3] in the then classified laboratories of the atomic energy commission at Rochester, NY. When these studies were published in 1950, they were found to be carefully conducted trials of infusion of bone marrow from normal dogs into dogs exposed to 350 R. The investigators found no significant effect on pancytopenia nor on survival. They were not aware that at least twice this exposure is necessary to provide sufficient immunosuppression to achieve engraftment. Thus, they failed in their attempts to achieve marrow recovery by intravenous marrow infusion.

The beginning

The seminal studies, first published in 1949, were those of Jacobson and colleagues [4] who found that a mouse would survive otherwise lethal irradiation if the spleen were exteriorized and protected from the irradiation. They found that an intraperitoneal injection of spleen cells (an hematopoietic organ in the mouse) would achieve the same result. Lorenz et al. [5] extended these observations by demonstrating a similar protective effect by an infusion of bone marrow cells.

At first it was hypothesized that this "irradiation protection" effect was due to some kind of hormone or growth factor contained in the infusion. Most of these early studies involved measuring death at 30 days after lethal irradiation. Infusions of preparations from a donor of different H2 type were effective when survival was measured at 30 days. Such a result favored a humoral mechanism since it would not be expected if incompatible cells were involved. However, in 1954 Barnes and Loutit [6] reported that mice protected with syngeneic marrow survived beyond 100 days. However, mice given allogeneic marrow (A into CBA) survived at 30 days ("academic survivors") but died thereafter of a "secondary disease".

Another argument in favor of a hormonal effect was that "cell free" extracts contained the protective effect. The investigators did not yet appreciate the very small number of cells required for transplantation in the syngeneic situation. Barnes and Loutit [7] sounded a warning against the hormonal hypothesis when they noted that the "cellular hypothesis" had not been excluded as an explanation of the irradiation protective effect.

The demise of the humoral hypothesis became inevitable in 1955 with a publication by Main and Prehn in the *Journal of the National Cancer Institute* [8]. It was a well-known fact that a skin graft between H2 incompatible strains of mice would be rejected in 10–12 days. Main and Prehn, however, were able to overcome this rejection problem by giving mice lethal irradiation and marrow from an H2 incompatible (BALB/cAnN into DBA/2JN) strain. Subsequently, a skin graft from the donor strain placed on a surviving marrow recipient was accepted indefinitely. Trentin was able to show that the tolerance of the graft was specific for the marrow donor strain [9]. Survival of the graft could be explained only by the persistence of cells of the donor strain leading to "tolerance".

Proof that these animals protected against lethal irradiation by marrow infusion were true radiation chimeras came from several sources. In 1956 Nowell et al. [10] described growth and continued function of rat marrow cells in X-irradiated mice. Most convincingly Ford et al. [11] showed that the marrow of lethally irradiated mice given infusions of syngeneic marrow marked by the T6 chromosome was made up of cells of the cytogenetic type of the donor.

Early clinical studies

At this point it became evident that marrow transplantation might be of use not only in irradiation protection but also in therapeutic application to marrow aplasia, leukemia and other diseases of the marrow and lymphoid system. In 1956 Barnes et al. [12] described the treatment of mice with leukemia by lethal irradiation and marrow transplantation.

In Cooperstown, NY, Thomas and Ferrebee and their colleagues [13] had already begun comparable studies in terminal patients with hematological malignancies. In 1957 they reported six patients treated with irradiation and intravenous infusion of marrow from a normal individual. Only one patient showed a transient marrow graft. These failures were duplicated by many investigators and in 1970 Bortin [14] was able to compile a list of approximately 200 attempts at allogeneic marrow grafting, all of which had failed.

The first attempts at autologous marrow transplantation appeared at about this time. In 1958 Kurnick and colleagues [15] described two patients with metastatic malignancy whose marrow was collected and stored by freezing. Following intensive regional radiation therapy the

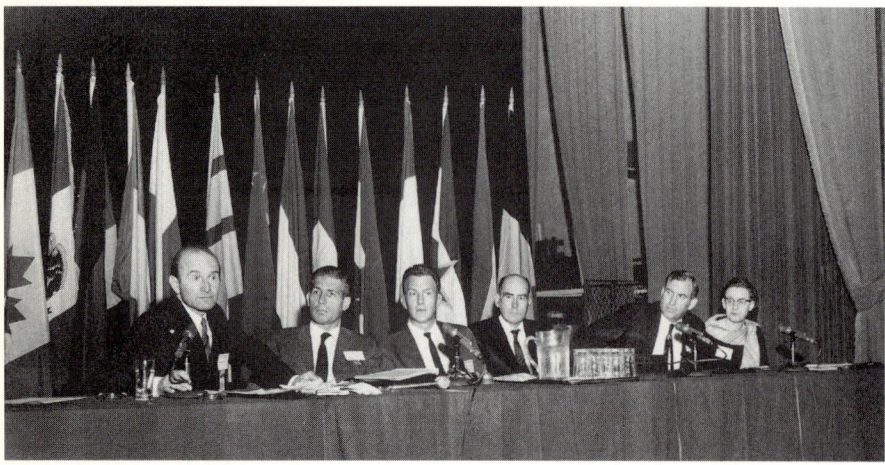

Fig. 1.1 A symposium on bone marrow transplantation (BMT) in Paris in 1971. From left to right: George Mathé, Dirk van Bekkum, George Santos, Don Thomas, Charles Congdon, Delta Uphoff.

marrows were thawed and infused intravenously. One patient died but the other showed recovery after moderate pancytopenia. In 1959 McGovern et al. [16] reported three patients with leukemia whose marrow was stored at the time of remission. They were treated with 500 R total body irradiation (TBI) followed by infusion of thawed marrow. Two died and one achieved a remission. In Philadelphia an autologous marrow graft was carried out after high-dose chemotherapy in a patient with lymphoma. In 1997 this patient was reported to be alive without disease 31 years later [17].

The authors of these early attempts at autologous marrow grafting pointed out the difficulty of defining the role of the infused marrow in hematological recovery in view of the uncertainty about whether marrow recovery was due to the infused marrow or to regeneration of the patient's own *in situ* marrow. Whether or not contamination of the infused marrow with malignant cells contributed to recurrence of malignancy also could not be evaluated. These parameters are as difficult to evaluate now as they were then.

In 1959, Thomas et al. [18] reported an identical twin with terminal leukemia who was given 850 R (748 cGy) TBI from opposing cobalt-60 sources and an intravenous infusion of marrow from the normal twin. This dose of irradiation would be expected to produce prolonged pancytopenia and death [19]. However, she showed prompt recovery and disappearance of leukemia for 4 months. This study demonstrated that lethal irradiation followed by compatible marrow could have an antileukemic effect even in advanced leukemia. Most importantly, it showed that compatible marrow infused intravenously could restore marrow function in human beings after lethal irradiation.

Also in 1959 Mathé et al. [20] reported the infusion of marrow into patients exposed to potentially lethal irradiation in a reactor accident. Subsequent analysis raised doubt about whether there had been a therapeutic effect [21]. Nevertheless, this experience gave a great boost to interest in marrow transplantation and attracted many investigators to the field.

One of the driving spirits of the early studies was Charles Congdon of the Oak Ridge National Laboratory, TN. In 1957 he organized an informal series of conferences at Oak Ridge, TN. The early results of these conferences were published in abstract form in small leaflets called *Fundamental and Clinical Aspects of Radiation Protection and Recovery*. From 1964 to 1970 the abstracts appeared under the title *Experimental Hematology*. These small booklets may be difficult to find but are well worth the effort. They list the authors and the investigations of that early time. There was life before Medline. In 1971 these meetings were organized into The International Society for Experimental Hematology that publishes the modern journal *Experimental Hematology* (Fig. 1.1).

Advances from animal studies

Thus, it was soon recognized that marrow grafting in humans would be very difficult. Many investigators therefore turned to animal studies for definition and resolution of the problems. Much early information came from the work of Billingham, Brent, Medawar and their colleagues [22]. They studied induction of tolerance in newborn mice. In the course of these studies they described the syndrome of "runt disease" in newborn mice given allogeneic cells. The principles they established were to prove the same as for "secondary disease" in irradiated mice and, eventually, for graft-vs.-host disease (GVHD) in humans.

In 1959, Billingham and Brent [23] published a landmark study of runt disease in newborn mice and Billingham [24] described in detail the biology of the graft-vs.-host reactions. They noted the following:

- Syngeneic cells did not result in runt disease.
- Persistence of allogeneic cells in the recipient was necessary for the development of runt disease.
- The severity and incidence of runt disease were determined by antigenic differences between donor and host.
- Tolerance could occur in the absence of runt disease.
- The severity of runt disease was enhanced by cells already sensitized by exposure to host strain cells.

The principles they elaborated were applicable to all studies of hematopoietic cell transplantation (HCT).

The mouse has been used widely in studies of transplantation biology. Numerous studies in the murine system are cited in a book by van Bekkum and de Vries [25]. The availability of inbred strains has permitted extensive studies of genetic factors in transplantation. Uphoff [26] showed that the severity of the secondary disease after irradiation and marrow grafting was controlled by genetic factors. Uphoff [27] and Lochte and colleagues [28] showed that methotrexate (MTX) could prevent or ameliorate the secondary disease now known as GVHD.

The dog has been used frequently for transplantation and surgical studies. Dogs are outbred animals comparable to humans. They come in large families permitting study of inherited factors. Studies in dogs first demonstrated the utility of autologous marrow grafts [29,30]. Marrow from dogs was collected and set aside. The marrow donor group and the control group were then given lethal or supralethal irradiation. The control animals invariably died while those treated with their own marrow promptly recovered. Obviously, this type of study could not be done with human beings.

Successful cryopreservation of marrow had been accomplished by freezing in glycerol [31] using the Polge–Smith–Parkes technique. Careful step-wise removal of the glycerol was essential before infusion of the cells. Cavins *et al.* [32] showed that canine marrow could be cryopreserved by freezing in dimethylsulfoxide (DMSO), thawed and injected intravenously without removal of the DMSO. This technique was to become standard for autologous marrow transplantation. Goodman and Hodgson [33] had shown that mice could be protected against lethal irradiation by infusion of blood cells. Cavins *et al.* [34] showed that autologous canine buffy coat cells from the peripheral blood could be collected, cryopreserved in DMSO and infused after lethal irradiation with subsequent recovery of marrow function. Practical application of peripheral blood cells for transplantation had to await better methods of centrifugation for separation of buffy coat cells and techniques for mobilizing stem cells into the blood.

The dog was a most informative model for the extensive studies of allogeneic marrow grafting in an outbred species. Ferrebee *et al.* [35] reported the first allogeneic marrow graft in an irradiated dog. Four dogs were given 400 R on each of 3 days. One control and two dogs given marrow from unrelated dogs died of the acute irradiation syndrome. The male dog given marrow from a female littermate engrafted, and the leukocyte nuclei showed female "drumsticks" characteristic of the donor.

Thomas *et al.* [36,37] carried out a series of studies of irradiation and allogeneic marrow grafting in the dog. Allogeneic graft recipients showed all of the problems that were soon to be recognized in human patients. The problems were graft failure, graft rejection, GVHD and/or death from opportunistic infections. A few animals did not develop these problems and became long-term survivors with marrow cells of donor type. Presumably these survivors had donors fortuitously of sufficient histocompatibility to permit long-term survival. In 1960, methods for selecting compatible donors were unknown.

Early studies of marrow grafting after irradiation were carried out with non-human primates. Autologous marrow grafts were effective in protecting monkeys against lethal irradiation [38]. After allogeneic marrow grafting they developed early severe secondary disease [38] which was somewhat reduced by treatment with antilymphocyte serum [39]. In Rhesus monkeys it was shown that blood transfusions given before irradiation interfered with acceptance of an allogeneic graft [40]. In the dog prior transfusions from histocompatible donors also prevented successful engraftment [41].

Despite being studies in primates, marrow grafting in non-human primates was not very helpful for application to human patients. The non-human primates were expensive and difficult to work with. Therefore, the number of subjects studied was small. Also, they were not available in families. Survival studies were difficult because of infection and parasitism in wild-caught animals [42].

In 1960 Medawar and Burnett received the Nobel Prize for the discovery "of acquired immunological tolerance." When the prize was announced, my wife, Dottie, and I were attending a transplantation meeting in Switzerland. The joy and celebration knew no bounds. Not only were we honoring the winners but also recognizing that transplantation biology had become a recognized field of scientific endeavor.

Advances in knowledge of histocompatibility

Techniques for defining tissue antigens in humans were crucial to the development of BMT. In 1954, Miescher and Fauconnet [43] recognized antibodies induced by transfusion or pregnancy that reacted with antigens on white blood cells. In 1958 Dausset and van Rood and their colleagues [44,45] recognized that human leukocyte antigens (HLAs) followed genetic principles of inheritance. Numerous studies followed designed to elucidate the role of these antigens in transplantation. HLA proved to be of minimal value in the prediction of the outcome of skin grafts [46,47].

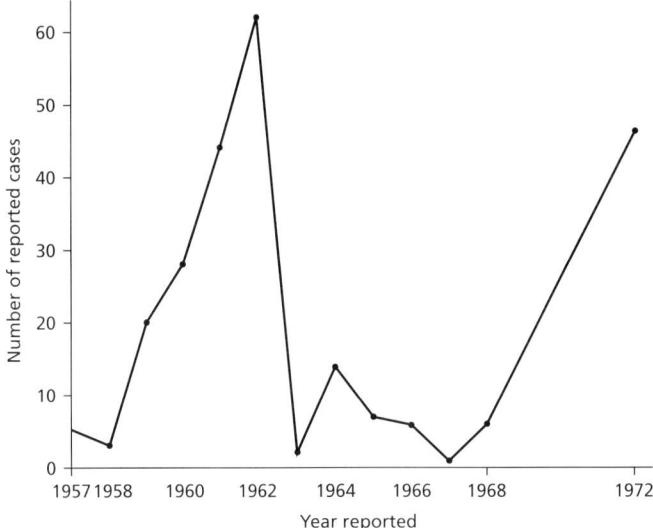

Fig. 1.2 Number of reported cases of bone marrow transplantation (BMT) by year. Adapted from Bortin [14].

Epstein *et al.* [48] developed typing sera for dog leukocyte antigens (DLAs). Storb and colleagues [49,50] studied dogs given lethal irradiation and a marrow graft from a littermate. They showed that marrow grafts between mismatched littermates always failed. Grafts between DLA-matched donors and recipients showed much improved survival. The administration of a short course of MTX for immunosuppression after grafting improved long-term survival of matched recipients to 90% or better [51]. Thus, studies in dogs illustrated the importance of DLA-matching. At about the same time, Singal, Mickey and Terasaki [52] reported that the outcome of kidney grafts between siblings was highly dependent on HLA-matching. Taken together these studies showed that matching for leukocyte antigens would be essential in human marrow grafting.

Renewed clinical studies

After all the disappointments of clinical marrow transplants in the late 1950s and 1960s there was general pessimism about the field, and many of the early investigators had moved on to other studies (Fig. 1.2 [14]). Nevertheless, improvements in transfusion medicine, treatment of infections and, especially, improved understanding of the importance of HLA-typing encouraged a renewed attack on clinical application of marrow grafts.

The first good news came from studies of children with an immunological deficiency. Because of their disease, these children could not reject a foreign graft. Therefore immunosuppression before grafting should not be necessary. In November 1968 Gatti *et al.* [53] performed the first successful allogeneic graft in a patient with severe combined immunodeficiency. Two similar successes were reported immediately thereafter [54,55]. All three patients were alive and well 25 years later [56].

In late 1967 the Seattle marrow transplantation team received a grant to support clinical marrow transplantation. The following year was spent assembling and training a team of nurses, technicians, dieticians, etc., who were to be dedicated to patients undergoing intensive therapy and marrow transplantation with a special emphasis on post-transplant clinical care. The first transplant by this team was carried out in March of 1969 [57]. The patient was a 46-year-old man with the blastic crisis of chronic myeloid leukemia. Initial tissue typing showed the patient's sister to be an HLA match. After an irradiation exposure of a calculated midline dose of 954 cGy, marrow was infused intravenously. Engraftment by donor cells was evident in 13 days. The patient developed mild GVHD controlled by MTX. Subsequently, he developed fever and died after 56 days. Autopsy showed cytomegalovirus pneumonia. There was no evidence of leukemia or GVHD. This patient showed successful engraftment and control of GVHD but illustrated the problem of opportunistic infection. Thus began the Seattle marrow transplant team's long series of patients given marrow grafts from HLA-matched siblings.

In 1972, Thomas et al. [58] reported the first experience with allografting of marrow for severe aplastic anemia. The first four patients were referred for BMT after failure of conventional therapy with steroids and multiple transfusions. Since these patients did not involve the problem of eradication of a malignant disease, they were prepared with immunosuppression using four large doses of cyclophosphamide (CY) following the regimen of Santos et al. [59]. All four grafts were initially successful. One patient died of GVHD and one died of graft rejection. Two patients became long-term survivors.

In 1975, the Seattle team published a Medical Progress review in the *New England Journal of Medicine*, which was to become a highly cited article [60]. That article reviewed the rationale and experimental background for marrow transplantation. It emphasized the importance of histocompatibility and the possibility of using unrelated donors. It described the preparation of the patient, the technique of marrow transplantation and the importance of supportive care. It described the use of HLA-matched siblings in 37 patients with aplastic anemia and 73 with leukemia who had reached an advanced stage of their disease before transplantation. Death from recurrent disease, opportunistic infection and GVHD was analyzed. Most importantly, the report described a number of survivors.

In 1977, the Seattle team reported 100 patients with end-stage acute leukemia treated by chemotherapy, TBI and allogeneic marrow transplantation [61]. Thirteen of these patients became long-term survivors. Also, by 1977 the time of follow-up of transplanted patients was long enough to show a change in the shape of the survival curve, indicating a plateau suggesting that some patients were cured of their disease [62].

The survival of some patients transplanted in a terminal stage of their disease raised the possibility of transplantation earlier in the course of the disease. Transplantation before the development of drug resistance and before the complications of advanced disease might be expected to improve survival. In 1979, two reports described marrow grafts for patients with acute myeloid leukemia transplanted in first remission [63,64]. As expected, survival was greatly improved and approximately 50% of the patients became long-term survivors.

In the 1970s there was a renewed interest in autologous marrow transplantation since it represented a way to avoid the problems of GVHD and in theory could be used for every patient. Numerous high-dose combination chemotherapy regimens were tried as preparation for the autologous graft. There was uncertainty about whether or not the autologous marrow was necessary for marrow reconstitution after the preparative regimen. Further, when malignancy recurred after grafting, it was impossible to tell whether it came from remaining malignant cells in the patient or from contamination of the infused autologous marrow. Investigators were therefore forced to depend on empiric observation to determine the effectiveness of the autologous transplant [65–67]. A randomized trial of high-dose CY with or without autologous marrow showed a profound pancytopenia in both groups [68]. However, the marrow infusion was not necessary since hematological recovery occurred in both groups at an equal rate. In a randomized study after a more myelotoxic high-dose combination chemotherapy (BACT) Appelbaum et al. [69] were able to show a more rapid hematological recovery in patients given cryopreserved autologous marrow than in controls not given marrow. Randomized trials still are the only effective way to evaluate autologous marrow transplantation.

Mathé [70] had coined the term "adoptive immunotherapy" to indicate the possibility that lymphoid elements in the engrafted marrow might react against malignant cells in the patient to aid in eradication of the remaining malignant cells. Initial attempts to evaluate the possibility that GVHD might include a graft-vs.-leukemia effect were unrewarding [60]. However, when enough cases had been accumulated, Weiden et al. [71] were able to demonstrate that the more severe the GVHD the less likely was recurrence of leukemia.

In the 1970s a major concern was the limitation of allogeneic grafting to HLA-matched sibling pairs. Obviously only about one-fourth of the patients would have a suitable marrow donor. Because of the complexity of the HLA system finding a matched unrelated donor was a formidable task. In 1979, Hansen et al. [72] performed the first successful marrow graft from an unrelated donor for a patient with leukemia. A young patient with refractory acute leukemia did not have a matched sibling. Quite by chance it was found that one of our hematology technicians had an HLA type that matched the patient. The graft was successful without GVHD until the leukemia recurred 2 years later. This patient's experience stimulated the formation of the National Marrow Donor Program.

History is now

It seems prudent to conclude this "history" at the end of the 1970s. By that time marrow grafting was recognized as a legitimate subject for research and as a form of therapy for patients with a variety of hematological diseases. Many investigators were attracted to the field, and many institutions established marrow transplant programs. The tremendous progress since 1980 is the subject of the remaining chapters of this book and is described by investigators who carried out much of the work.

The use of donor leukocytes or cord blood cells has become a routine part of transplantation. Clinical transplants, whether of marrow, peripheral blood or cord blood, have always employed mixtures of many cell types. Therefore, these are not stem cell transplants but are hematopoietic cell transplants.

The use of donor lymphocytes to cure recurrent leukemia and the use of non-myeloablative preparative regimens are but a few of the advances that are also current subjects of research. We are just beginning to appreciate the importance of the microenvironment, the cytokines and the multitude of genes regulating cell division and senescence. The plasticity of stem cells opens entirely new areas of investigation.

The large number of patients being treated should permit reliable statistical analyses so that proper comparisons can be made of marrow transplantation vs. other forms of therapy, or of different regimens for marrow transplantation. However, large group studies analyzed by intent to treat are plagued by the fact that many patients do not get the assigned treatment. Each advance with new agents, such as imatinib mesylate (STI571, Gleevec®), forces us to redefine the role of HCT. Each advance will require carefully conducted randomized trials. Perhaps in another two decades these topics will become subjects for another "historical review".

References

1 Osgood EE, Riddle MC, Mathews TJ. Aplastic anaemia treated with daily transfusions and intravenous marrow. *Ann Intern Med* 1939; **13**: 357–67.

2 Morrison M, Samwick AA. Intramedullary (sternal) transfusion of human bone marrow. *JAMA* 1940; **115**: 1708–11.

3 Rekers PE, Coulter MP, Warren S. Effect of transplantation of bone marrow into irradiated animals. *Arch Surg* 1950; **60**: 635–67.

4 Jacobson LO, Marks EK, Robson MJ, Gaston EO, Zirkle RE. Effect of spleen protection on mortality following X-irradiation. *J Laboratory Clin Med* 1949; **34**: 1538–43.

5 Lorenz E, Uphoff D, Reid TR, Shelton E. Modification of irradiation injury in mice and guinea pigs by bone marrow injections. *J Natl Cancer Inst* 1951; **12**: 197–201.

6 Barnes DWH, Loutit JF. What is the recovery factor in spleen [Letter] *Nucleonics* 1954; **12**: 68–71.

7 Barnes DWH, Loutit JF. Spleen protection: the cellular hypothesis. In: Bacq ZM, ed. *Radiobiology Symposium*. London: Butterworth, 1955.

8 Main JM, Prehn RT. Successful skin homografts after the administration of high dosage X-radiation and homologous bone marrow. *J Natl Cancer Inst* 1955; **15**: 1023–9.

9 Trentin JJ. Mortality and skin transplantability in X-irradiated mice receiving isologous or heterologous bone marrow. *Proc Soc Exp Biol Medical* 1956; **92**: 688–93.

10 Nowell PC, Cole LJ, Habermeyer JG, Roan PL. Growth and continued function of rat marrow cells in X-radiated mice. *Cancer Res* 1956; **16**: 258–61.

11 Ford CE, Hamerton JL, Barnes DWH, Loutit JF. Cytological identification of radiation chimaeras. *Nature* 1956; **177**: 452–4.

12 Barnes DWH, Corp MJ, Loutit JF, Neal FE. Treatment of murine leukaemia with X-rays and homologous bone marrow. Preliminary communication. *Br Med J* 1956; **2**: 626–7.

13 Thomas ED, Lochte HL Jr, Lu WC, Ferrebee JW. Intravenous infusion of bone marrow in patients receiving radiation and chemotherapy. *N Engl J Med* 1957; **257**: 491–6.

14 Bortin MM. A compendium of reported human bone marrow transplants. *Transplantation* 1970; **9**: 571–87.

15 Kurnick NB, Montano A, Gerdes JC, Feder BH. Preliminary observations on the treatment of post-irradiation hematopoietic depression in man by the infusion of stored autogenous bone marrow. *Ann Intern Med* 1958; **49**: 973–86.

16 McGovern JJ Jr, Russel PS, Atkins L, Webster EW. Treatment of terminal leukemic relapse by total-body irradiation and intravenous infusion of stored autologous bone marrow obtained during remission. *N Engl J Med* 1959; **260**: 675–83.

17 Haurani FI. Thirty-one-year survival following chemotherapy and autologous bone marrow in malignant lymphoma. *Am J Hematol* 1997; **55**: 35–8.

18 Thomas ED, Lochte HL Jr, Cannon JH, Sahler OD, Ferrebee JW. Supralethal whole body irradiation and isologous marrow transplantation in man. *J Clin Invest* 1959; **38**: 1709–16.

19 Cronkite EP, Bond VP. *Radiation Injury in Man*. Oxford: CC Thomas & Blackwell Scientific Publications, 1960.

20 Mathé G, Jammet H, Pendic B et al. Transfusions et greffes de moelle osseuse homologue chez des humains irradiés a haute dose accidentellement. *Rev Franc Etudes Clin et Biol* 1959; **iv**: 226–38.

21 Andrews GA. Criticality accidents in Vinca, Yugoslavia, and Oak Ridge, Tennessee. *Am J Roentgenol Radium Ther Nucl Medical* 1965; **93**: 56–74.

22 Billingham RE, Brent L, Medawar PB. 'Actively acquired tolerance' of foreign cells. *Nature* 1953; **172**: 603–6.

23 Billingham RE, Brent L. Quantitative studies on tissue transplantation immunity. IV. Induction of tolerance in newborn mice and studies on the phenomenon of runt disease. *Philos Trans R Soc Lond B Biol Sci* 1959; **242**: 477.

24 Billingham RE. The biology of graft-versus-host reactions. *The Harvey Lectures*. New York: Academic Press, 1966: 21–78.

25 van Bekkum DW, de Vries MJ. *Radiation Chimaeras*. London: Logos Press Limited, 1967.

26 Uphoff DE. Genetic factors influencing irradiation protection by bone marrow. I. The F1 hybrid effect. *J Natl Cancer Inst* 1957; **19**: 123–5.

27 Uphoff DE. Alteration of homograft reaction by A-methopterin in lethally irradiated mice treated with homologous marrow. *Proc Soc Exp Biol Medical* 1958; **99**: 651–3.

28 Lochte HL Jr, Levy AS, Guenther DM, Thomas ED, Ferrebee JW. Prevention of delayed foreign marrow reaction in lethally irradiated mice by early administration of methotrexate. *Nature* 1962; **196**: 1110–1.

29 Alpen EL, Baum SJ. Modification of X-radiation lethality by autologous marrow infusion in dogs. *Blood* 1958; **13**: 1168–75.

30 Mannick JA, Lochte HL Jr, Ashley CA, Thomas ED, Ferrebee JW. Autografts of bone marrow in dogs after lethal total-body radiation. *Blood* 1960; **15**: 255–66.

31 Barnes DWH, Loutit JF. The radiation recovery factor: preservation by the Polge–Smith–Parkes technique. *J Natl Cancer Inst* 1955; **15**: 901–5.

32 Cavins JA, Kasakura S, Thomas ED, Ferrebee JW. Recovery of lethally irradiated dogs following infusion of autologous marrow stored at low temperature in dimethyl-sulphoxide. *Blood* 1962; **20**: 730–4.

33 Goodman JW, Hodgson GS. Evidence for stem cells in the peripheral blood of mice. *Blood* 1962; **19**: 702–14.

34 Cavins JA, Scheer SC, Thomas ED, Ferrebee JW. The recovery of lethally irradiated dogs given infusions of autologous leukocytes preserved at –80°C. *Blood* 1964; **23**: 38–43.

35 Ferrebee JW, Lochte HL Jr, Jaretzki A III, Sahler OD, Thomas ED. Successful marrow homograft in the dog after radiation. *Surgery* 1958; **43**: 516–20.

36 Thomas ED, Ashley CA, Lochte HL Jr et al. Homografts of bone marrow in dogs after lethal total-body radiation. *Blood* 1959; **14**: 720–36.

37 Thomas ED, Collins JA, Herman EC Jr, Ferrebee JW. Marrow transplants in lethally irradiated dogs given methotrexate. *Blood* 1962; **19**: 217–28.

38 Crouch BG, van Putten LM, van Bekkum DW, de Vries MJ. Treatment of total-body X-irradiated monkeys with autologous and homologous bone marrow. *J Natl Cancer Inst* 1961; **27**: 53–65.

39 Merritt CB, Darrow CC II, Vaal L, Rogentine GN Jr. Bone marrow transplantation in rhesus monkeys following irradiation. Modification of acute graft-versus-host disease with antilymphocyte serum. *Transplantation* 1972; **14**: 9–20.

40 van Putten LM, van Bekkum DW, de Vries MJ, Balner H. The effect of preceding blood transfusions on the fate of homologous bone marrow grafts in lethally irradiated monkeys. *Blood* 1967; **30**: 749–57.

41 Storb R, Epstein RB, Rudolph RH, Thomas ED. The effect of prior transfusion on marrow grafts between histocompatible canine siblings. *J Immunol* 1970; **105**: 627–33.

42 van der Waay D, Zimmerman WMTh. Problems in the Sanitation of Monkeys for Whole-Body Irradiation Experiments. *Proceedings of the International Symposium on Bone Marrow Therapy and Chemical Protection in Irradiated Primates 1962*. 1962: 231–40.

43 Miescher PP, Fauconnet M. Mise en évidence de différents groupes leucocytaires chez l'homme. *Schweiz Med Wochenschr* 1954; **84**: 597–9.

44 Dausset J. Iso-ieuco-anticorps. *Acta Haematol* 1958; **20**: 156–66.

45 van Rood JJ, Eernisse JG, van Leeuwen A. Leukocyte antibodies in sera from pregnant women. *Nature* 1958; **181**: 1735–6.

46 Rapaport FT, Lawrence HS, Thomas L et al. Cross-reactions to skin homografts in man. *J Clin Invest* 1962; **41**: 2166–72.

47 Dausset J, Rapaport FT, Legrand L et al. Studies on transplantation antigens (HL-A) by means of skin grafts from 90 children onto their fathers [French]. *Nouv Rev Fr Hematol* 1969; **9**: 215–29.

48 Epstein RB, Storb R, Ragde H, Thomas ED. Cytotoxic typing antisera for marrow grafting in littermate dogs. *Transplantation* 1968; **6**: 45–58.

49 Storb R, Epstein RB, Bryant J, Ragde H, Thomas ED. Marrow grafts by combined marrow and leukocyte infusions in unrelated dogs selected by histocompatibility typing. *Transplantation* 1968; **6**: 587–93.

50 Storb R, Rudolph RH, Thomas ED. Marrow grafts between canine siblings matched by serotyping and mixed leukocyte culture. *J Clin Invest* 1971; **50**: 1272–5.

51 Storb R, Epstein RB, Graham TC, Thomas ED. Methotrexate regimens for control of graft-versus-host disease in dogs with allogeneic marrow grafts. *Transplantation* 1970; **9**: 240–6.

52 Singal DP, Mickey MR, Terasaki PI. Serotyping for homotransplantation. XXIII Analysis of kidney transplants from parental versus sibling donors. *Transplantation* 1969; **7**: 246–58.

53 Gatti RA, Meuwissen HJ, Allen HD, Hong R, Good RA. Immunological reconstitution of sex-linked lymphopenic immunological deficiency. *Lancet* 1968; **ii**: 1366–9.

54 Bach FH, Albertini RJ, Joo P, Anderson JL, Bortin MM. Bone-marrow transplantation in a patient with the Wiskott–Aldrich syndrome. *Lancet* 1968; **2**: 1364–6.

55 deKoning J, van Bekkum DW, Dicke KA et al. Transplantation of bone-marrow cells and fetal thymus in an infant with lymphopenic immunological deficiency. *Lancet* 1969; **i**: 1223–7.

56 Bortin MM, Bach FH, van Bekkum DW, Good RA, van Rood JJ. Twenty-fifth anniversary of the first successful allogeneic bone marrow transplants. *Bone Marrow Transplant* 1994; **14**: 211–2.

57 Buckner CD, Epstein RB, Rudolph RH et al. Allogeneic marrow engraftment following whole body irradiation in a patient with leukemia. *Blood* 1970; **35**: 741–50.

58 Thomas ED, Buckner CD, Storb R et al. Aplastic anaemia treated by marrow transplantation. *Lancet* 1972; **i**: 284–9.

59 Santos GW, Sensenbrenner LL, Burke PJ et al. Marrow transplantation in man following cyclophosphamide. *Transplant Proc* 1971; **3**: 400–4.

60 Thomas ED, Storb R, Clift RA et al. Bone-marrow transplantation. *N Engl J Med* 1975; **292**: 832–43, 895–902.

61 Thomas ED, Buckner CD, Banaji M et al. One hundred patients with acute leukemia treated by chemotherapy, total body irradiation, and allogeneic marrow transplantation. *Blood* 1977; **49**: 511–33.

62 Thomas ED, Flournoy N, Buckner CD et al. Cure of leukemia by marrow transplantation. *Leuk Res* 1977; **1**: 67–70.

63 Thomas ED, Buckner CD, Clift RA *et al.* Marrow transplantation for acute nonlymphoblastic leukemia in first remission. *N Engl J Med* 1979; **301**: 597–9.
64 Blume KG, Beutler E. Allogeneic bone marrow transplantation for acute leukemia [Letter]. *JAMA* 1979; **241**: 1686.
65 Gorin NC, Najman A, David R *et al.* Autogreffe de moelle osseuse après chimiothérapie lourde. Etude de la cinétique de réparation médullaire et sanguine sur 12 malades. *Mèmoire* 1978; **7**: 4105–10.
66 Spitzer G, Dicke KA, Verma DS, Zander A, McCredie KB. High-dose BCNU therapy with autologous bone marrow infusion: preliminary observations. *Cancer Treat Rep* 1979; **63**: 1257–64.
67 Dicke KA, Spitzer G, Peters L *et al.* Autologous bone-marrow transplantation in relapsed adult acute leukaemia. *Lancet* 1979; **1**: 514–7.
68 Buckner CD, Rudolph RH, Fefer A *et al.* High-dose cyclophosphamide therapy for malignant disease. Toxicity, tumor response, and the effects of stored autologous marrow. *Cancer* 1972; **29**: 357–65.
69 Appelbaum FR, Herzig GP, Ziegler JL *et al.* Successful engraftment of cryopreserved autologous bone marrow in patients with malignant lymphoma. *Blood* 1978; **52**: 85–95.
70 Mathé G, Amiel JL, Schwarzenberg L, Catton A, Schneider M. Adoptive immunotherapy of acute leukemia: experimental and clinical results. *Cancer Res* 1965; **25**: 1525–31.
71 Weiden PL, Flournoy N, Thomas ED *et al.* Antileukemic effect of graft-versus-host disease in human recipients of allogeneic-marrow grafts. *N Engl J Med* 1979; **300**: 1068–73.
72 Hansen JA, Clift RA, Thomas ED *et al.* Transplantation of marrow from an unrelated donor to a patient with acute leukemia. *N Engl J Med* 1980; **303**: 565–7.

2

Mary M. Horowitz

Uses and Growth of Hematopoietic Cell Transplantation

Introduction

The first successful transplantations of allogeneic hematopoietic cells were performed in 1968 in three children with congenital immune deficiency diseases [1–4]. In each instance, hematopoietic cells were collected from the marrow of sibling donors who were genotypically identical or closely matched to the recipient for human leukocyte antigens (HLAs). Since then, thousands of patients have received hematopoietic cell transplantations (HCTs) to treat life-threatening malignant and nonmalignant diseases. Current estimates of annual numbers of HCTs are 45,000–50,000, worldwide (Fig. 2.1). Reasons for widespread use include proven and potential efficacy in many diseases, better understanding of the appropriate timing of transplantation and patient selection, greater availability of donors, greater ease of hematopoietic cell collection, and improved transplantation strategies and supportive care leading to less transplantation-related morbidity and mortality.

Changing indications for HCT

HCT has efficacy in many diseases (Table 2.1). In some, transplantation corrects congenital or acquired defects in blood cell production and/or immune function. In others, it restores hematopoiesis after high-dose (myeloablative) cytotoxic therapy for malignancy and/or provides potent anticancer adoptive immunotherapy. In the 1970s, more than half of the diseases for which HCT was performed were nonmalignant disorders: 40% were for aplastic anaemia and 15% for immune deficiencies. Fewer than half were for cancers and these were mostly for advanced acute leukemia. In the 1970s, Thomas and colleagues showed convincingly that some patients with refractory acute leukemia could achieve long-term leukemia-free survival with high-dose therapy and HLA-identical sibling transplantation [5,6]. Better outcome was subsequently demonstrated in patients transplanted in first or second remission [7–9]. Syngeneic and allogeneic HCTs were shown to produce cytogenetic remissions and long-term leukemia-free survival in chronic myeloid leukemia (CML) in the late 1970s and early 1980s [10–12].

Use of allogeneic HCT for leukemia treatment increased dramatically in the 1980s. By 1985, about 75% of allogeneic transplantations were for leukemia, with approximately equal numbers for CML, acute myeloid leukemia (AML) and acute lymphoblastic leukemia (ALL); over 90% were from HLA-identical sibling donors. Introduction of alternative therapies for CML has led to recent decreases in use of HCT for this disease [13–15] with the appropriate relative roles of transplantation and nontransplantation therapies for this disease still to be determined. However, leukemia treatment still accounts for about 70% of allogeneic HCT procedures (Fig. 2.2) (Statistical Center of the International Bone Marrow Transplant Registry [IBMTR] and Autologous Blood and Marrow Transplant Registry [ABMTR], unpublished data).

Experimental and clinical evidence of a dose–response effect of lymphoma therapy led to trials of autologous HCT for non-Hodgkin's lymphoma in the middle 1980s [16–18]. Results were promising and there was rapid acceptance of autotransplants as salvage therapy in persons failing conventional chemotherapy for lymphoma followed by increasing use as consolidation of primary therapy in patients with high-risk disease. The rationale of dose-intensification led to application of autotransplants to many hematologic and nonhematologic cancers over the past 10 years. One striking development was a dramatic increase in their use for breast cancer in the early 1990s. Breast cancer accounted for 16% of autotransplants done in 1989–90 and 40% in 1994–95 [19]. However, results of randomized clinical trials in early and advanced breast cancer were disappointing [reviewed in 20–22]. In 1999, the use of HCT for breast cancer declined dramatically and in 2001 breast cancer accounted for <5% of autotransplants in North America. Treatment of solid tumors still accounts for about 15% of autotransplants (Fig. 2.2) (Statistical Center of the IBMTR and ABMTR, unpublished data).

In 1996, a randomized trial comparing high-dose therapy and autologous HCT with conventional therapy for multiple myeloma indicated a significant survival benefit with autotransplantation [23]. Autologous HCT for myeloma increased dramatically after this report; multiple myeloma now accounts for 30–40% of autotransplants (Fig. 2.2) (Statistical Center of the IBMTR and ABMTR, unpublished data).

The most common indications for allogeneic and autologous HCT in North America in 2001 are shown in Fig. 2.2. Sixty-nine percent of allogeneic HCTs are for leukemia or preleukemia: 28% for AML, 17% for ALL, 11% CML, 9% for myelodysplastic or myeloproliferative

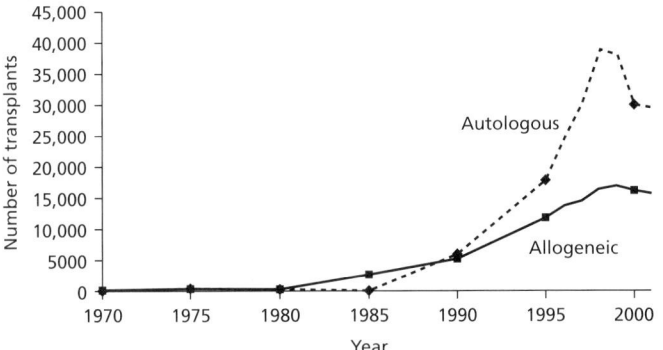

Fig. 2.1 Numbers of allogeneic and autologous hematopoietic cell transplantations (HCTs) performed yearly, worldwide. Courtesy of the Statistical Center of the IBMTR and ABMTR.

Table 2.1 Diseases in which autologous and/or allogeneic hematopoietic cell transplants (HCTs) may be used.

Malignant	Nonmalignant
Leukemia/preleukemia	Severe aplastic anemia
Chronic myeloid leukemia	Paroxysmal nocturnal hemoglobinuria
Myeloproliferative syndromes (other than CML)	Hemoglobinopathies
Acute myeloid leukemia	Thalassemia major
Acute lymphoblastic leukemia	Sickle cell disease
Juvenile chronic myeloid leukemia	Congenital disorders of hematopoiesis
Myelodysplastic syndromes	Fanconi anemia
Therapy-related myelodysplasia/leukemia	Diamond–Blackfan syndrome
Kostmann agranulocytosis	Familial erythrophagocytic histiocytosis
Chronic lymphocytic leukemia	Dyskeratosis congenita
Non-Hodgkin's and Hodgkin's lymphoma	Shwachman–Diamond syndrome
Multiple myeloma	SCID and related disorders
Solid tumors	Wiskott–Aldrich syndrome
Breast cancer	Inborn errors of metabolism
Neuroblastoma	
Ovarian cancer	
Small cell lung cancer	
Testicular cancer	

CML, chronic myeloid leukemia; SCID, severe combined immunodeficiency syndrome.

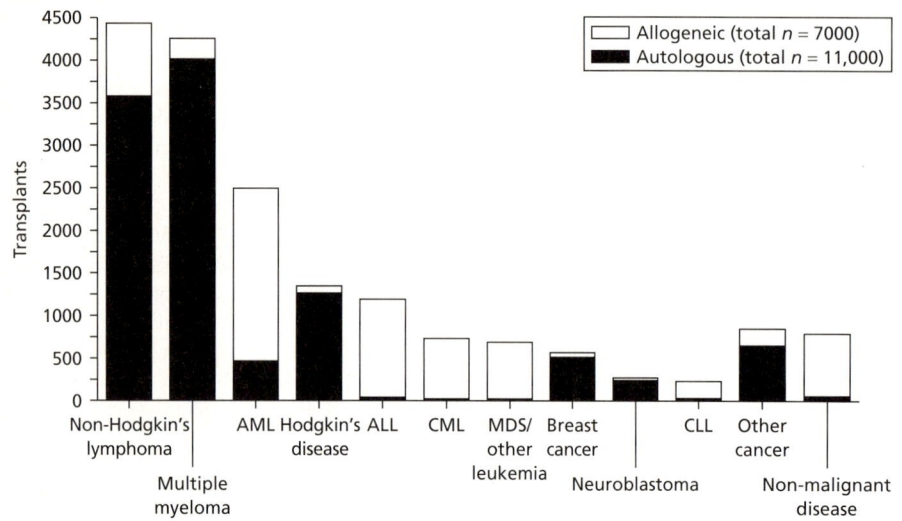

Fig. 2.2 Indications for hematopoietic cell transplantation (HCT) in North America, 2001. Courtesy of the Statistical Center of the IBMTR and ABMTR.

syndromes and 4% for other leukemias. Twenty percent are for other cancers including non-Hodgkin's lymphoma (12%), multiple myeloma (3%), Hodgkin's disease (<1%) and other cancers (4%). The remainders are for aplastic anemia (3%), immune deficiencies (2%) and other diverse nonmalignant disorders (6%). The most common indications for autotransplants are multiple myeloma (34%), non-Hodgkin's lymphoma (33%), Hodgkin's disease (12%), leukemia (5%), neuroblastoma (3%) and other cancers (Statistical Center of the IBMTR and ABMTR, unpublished data).

There is increasing interest in using HCT in several diseases where transplantation was not or rarely used in the past, some with promising results in either anecdotal reports or Phase II studies. These include sickle cell disease [24], inborn errors of metabolism [25,26], chronic lymphocytic leukemia [27,28], solid tumors such as ovarian cancer [29] and small cell lung cancer [30], and autoimmune diseases such as multiple sclerosis, systemic lupus erythematosus and severe rheumatoid arthritis [31]. These diseases currently account for <4% of HCT, allogeneic or autologous. However, their prevalence is high and, if subsequent trials confirm efficacy, the numbers of persons treated with HCT could increase dramatically. Several large trials of HCT for autoimmune disease are being conducted in Europe and in the USA. Additionally, hematopoietic cells are ideal candidates as vehicles for gene therapy, and their use in this capacity is being explored in several settings [32].

Changes in patient selection

In the 1970s marrow transplants were often applied as desperate measures for desperate situations. Not infrequently, patients came to transplantation with longstanding, refractory cancers, active infection, after receiving multiple transfusions, and with poor performance status.

The available graft-vs.-host disease (GVHD) prophylaxis was not optimal, nor were supportive care measures, especially antiviral and antifungal therapy. Not surprisingly, these procedures were associated with high risks of graft failure, GVHD, infectious and noninfectious pneumonitis, nonpulmonary infections and other complications, all leading to high transplant-related mortality. Much of the acceptance and growth of transplantation is attributable to better understanding of factors leading to improved transplantation outcomes, especially selection of appropriate patients for transplantation at a point in their disease course when transplantation is most likely to be of benefit. Many studies in diverse diseases demonstrate that HCTs done earlier are associated with lower risks of both transplant-related mortality and disease recurrence. Transplantation is increasingly applied as first or second line rather than as "last chance" therapy. In the 1970s, only 18% of HCTs for leukemia were done in first remission or first chronic phase while 34% were done for advanced disease (beyond second remission for acute leukemia, in accelerated or blast phase for CML). In contrast, in 2000–01, about 60% of transplants for AML, ALL and CML were done in patients in first remission or first chronic phase and only 15% were for advanced disease (Statistical Center of the IBMTR and ABMTR, unpublished data). Although delay beyond first remission may be appropriate for patients with standard-risk ALL or good risk AML (who may have good outcomes with conventional therapy), or for older patients with CML and a good response to imatinib mesylate (STI571, Gleevec®), young patients with CML and AML are probably best served by allogeneic transplantation done soon after diagnosis if a suitably matched donor is available. Such a strategy is not only associated with better outcome but decreases the chance that patients will develop an intervening complication (refractory relapse, life-threatening infection or organ toxicity) that will preclude transplantation. A trend toward earlier transplantation over the past decade was seen particularly in CML, where in 1984–85 the median interval between diagnosis and HLA-identical sibling transplantation was 17 months but in 2000–01 was 7 months (Statistical Center of the IBMTR and ABMTR, unpublished data). This may change as more physicians and patient opt for initial treatment with imatinib mesylate.

There has also been a trend for earlier use of autotransplants. In 1989, the median interval between diagnosis and autotransplantation for non-Hodgkin's lymphoma was 23 months; in 2000–01, it was 18 months (Statistical Center of the IBMTR and ABMTR, unpublished data). Similarly, in 1990, the median interval between diagnosis and autologous transplantation for multiple myeloma was 18 months; in 2000–01, it was 8 months.

Earlier treatment accounts, in part, for the fact that patients in 2000–01 were less likely to have poor performance status at the time of transplantation than in the 1970s. About 40% of patients transplanted in 1974–79 had pretransplant Karnofsky scores <80% compared to 10% in 2000–01 (Statistical Center of the IBMTR and ABMTR, unpublished data).

HCT is now used in much older patients than in the 1970s, when the median age of transplant recipients was 17 years and <5% were older than 40 years. In 2000–01, the median age of allograft recipients was 34 years and of autograft recipients, 49 years (Statistical Center of the IBMTR and ABMTR, unpublished data). This is important since the onset of the diseases for which HCT is most frequently used is usually in older adulthood, often in the 6th decade. Ability to apply HCT in older patients makes it a useful treatment for many more patients. Autotransplants have been successfully used in patients older than 70 years. Seventy percent of autotransplant recipients in 2000–01 were over the age of 40 years and 20% were older than 60 years. Allogeneic HCT is also being used in older patients, with the introduction of better GVHD prophylaxis and supportive care. Forty percent of allograft recipients in 2000–01 were older than 40 years in contrast to only 27% in 1994–95. Fifteen percent of the allogeneic HCTs done in 2000–01 were in patients older than 50 years. Several studies suggest that, among adults over the age of 30, increasing age has only modest effects on transplantation outcome, at least up to the age of 50 [33–35]. One approach being investigated that has the potential to increase use of allografts in older adults is reduced intensity or nonmyeloablative pretransplant conditioning. This strategy uses conditioning as immune suppressive therapy to allow donor cell engraftment rather than as high-dose anticancer therapy. The approach relies on immune-mediated graft-vs.-tumor effects for long-term disease control (see Chapters 85 & 86). First reported in the late 1990s, these nonmyeloablative transplants now account for about 30% of allografts registered with the IBMTR, though data on long-term outcome or efficacy relative to conventional HCT are lacking.

Hematopoietic cell sources

In the 1970s and early 1980s essentially all HCTs used cells collected from the marrow of closely HLA-matched related donors. The few transplantations done with HLA-mismatched related donors were associated with high risks of graft failure, GVHD and poor outcome, except, in some series, when the disparity was limited to a single HLA antigen [36,37]. This limited application of HCT to the 25–30% of patients with an HLA-matched relative. Several developments dramatically increased the applicability of HCT to patients without HLA-identical relatives, including the use of autologous cells, collected either from marrow or blood, and the use of unrelated donors.

Autologous transplantation

Although a few autologous transplantations were done before the 1970s, the approach of collecting cells from a patient before high-dose therapy with reinfusion afterwards did not generate much enthusiasm until the middle to late 1980s [38]. The appeal of the approach rested in its applicability, since it did not require a donor, allowing dose-intensification with hematopoietic cell support in many patients with chemotherapy-sensitive cancers. Autotransplants also had lower transplant-related mortality since GVHD did not occur and immune recovery was more rapid than after allografting. Although immune-mediated antitumor effects were also absent, and there was some concern about reinfusing cancer cells with the graft, early trials showed good results in persons with lymphoma failing other therapies. The technology diffused rapidly in the late 1980s, becoming the treatment of choice for persons with relapsed lymphoma and increasingly used for other chemotherapy-sensitive but infrequently cured cancers including acute leukemia, multiple myeloma, and selected solid tumors.

An important development allowing diffusion of the technology was the demonstration that hematopoietic cell grafts could be collected from peripheral blood in a limited number of leukaphereses after mobilization with chemotherapy or growth factors such as granulocyte (G)- or granulocyte macrophage (GM) colony-stimulating factor (CSF) [39–41]. The resulting hematopoietic cell products contained large numbers of progenitor cells and led to faster hematopoietic recovery after transplantation. It also eliminated the need for a marrow harvest in an operating room. While in 1989–90, 85% of autotransplants used cells collected from marrow, in 2000–01, <5% used marrow cells alone (Statistical Center of the IBMTR and ABMTR, unpublished data). In contrast to allogeneic transplantation, which is still done largely in academic, tertiary care medical centers, autotransplants were soon used in the community setting partly because of the ease with which the hematopoietic cell product could be obtained, and partly because of the more rapid hematopoietic and immune recovery and lower frequency of transplant-related complications compared to allografting. Despite the recent large decrease in numbers of autotransplants for breast cancer (see above), numbers of autotransplants still exceed numbers of allotransplants (Fig. 2.1).

Allogeneic transplantation

There were anecdotal reports of successful HCTs using HLA-matched unrelated donors as early as 1973 [42–44] but the polymorphism of human HLA made the feasibility of finding such a donor for an individual patient low. In the middle 1980s several national and international groups organized marrow donor registries with panels of HLA-typed volunteers agreeing to serve as donors for unrelated patients. There are now about eight million HLA-typed volunteer donors, worldwide (see Chapter 49). Accessing these donors is facilitated by their listing in a compendium by Bone Marrow Donors Worldwide (BMDW), a collaborative effort of many national registries coordinated by the Europdonor group [45]. After determining the existence of potential donors of suitable HLA type in BMDW, donors are accessed, according to the policies of the registry in which they are listed, for further typing and evaluation. The largest national registry is the US National Marrow Donor Program (NMDP), which has more than 3 million donors on its file [46]. Currently, Caucasian patients have an 80% or greater chance of finding an HLA-matched (as defined by serologic typing for HLA-A and -B and DNA typing for HLA-DR) donor through existing donor panels. Because of greater HLA-polymorphism and fewer ethnically similar donors, patients in other groups have lower probabilities of finding an HLA-matched unrelated donor. Establishment of large donor panels dramatically increased use of unrelated donor transplantation. While in 1985 <10% of allogeneic HCTs were from unrelated donors, in 2000–01, >30% were from unrelated donors. There are about 1400 unrelated donor transplantations yearly in the USA. In some settings, survival after unrelated donor transplantation is similar to that after HLA-identical sibling transplantation, although risks of graft failure and GVHD are higher [47–53]. Unrelated donor HCT is associated with longer delays between diagnosis and transplantation, partly because of time needed for the donor search and evaluation process and partly because of reluctance to use this more difficult transplantation approach early in disease.

Recent experimental and clinical studies suggest that umbilical cord blood, which is rich in hematopoietic progenitors, may be a good source of allogeneic hematopoietic cells for persons without a suitable marrow donor [54–57] (see Chapter 43). To be useful, there must be a large supply of cord blood units readily available. Several cord blood banks are now established with about 100,000 units cryopreserved worldwide. The advantage of cord blood cell (CBC) transplantation is rapid availability of a graft without need for screening, typing and collecting cells from live donors and the potential to target under-represented ethnic groups for collection and storage. There are some data suggesting that CBC transplantation has less potential for severe GVHD, even with some degree of donor-recipient HLA mismatch, than marrow transplants, although this advantage remains to be proven. About 3500 CBC transplants have been done, mostly from unrelated donors and mostly in children. CBC transplants now account for about 15% of the allografts done in patients younger than 20 years old. Hematopoietic recovery after CBC transplantation may be slow and predictable engraftment in adults remains to be demonstrated in large numbers of patients; however, enthusiasm for this approach is great and use of CBC transplants is expected to grow rapidly over the next few years, particularly for treatment of children.

Use of relatives partially matched for HLAs is another way of offering HCTs to more people (see Chapter 82). About 10% of allografts are from relatives sharing one HLA-haplotype and mismatched for one or more antigens on the unshared haplotype. Results with more than one antigen disparity on the unshared haplotype have been disappointing and there has been little increase in the numbers of these transplants over the past 10 years. Recent studies, however, suggest that the approach may be successful if T-cell-depleted grafts containing high doses of CD34 cells are administered [58,59].

If alternative donor HCTs, whether from unrelated volunteers, unrelated cord blood or HLA-mismatched relatives, were to be applied in all or most indications currently considered appropriate for HLA-identical sibling transplantation, there would be about 12,000–15,000 such transplants yearly in the USA. This is far more than the estimated 6000 now being done. It remains to be seen whether increasing awareness of the availability of unrelated donor marrow transplantation or the use of CBC transplants will increase these numbers.

Most allogeneic HCTs still use cells collected from marrow. For many years there was reluctance to use cells collected from peripheral blood because of the large numbers of mature T lymphocytes in blood-derived grafts, the cells that mediate GVHD. However, in 1995, three centers reported rapid hematopoietic recovery and acceptable acute GVHD after HLA-identical related peripheral blood allografts in a small number of patients [60–62]. Rapid increase in allogeneic peripheral blood HCTs followed. About 50% of allogeneic HCTs now use cells obtained by leukapheresis. Several randomized trials have compared results of peripheral blood and marrow HCTs in the related donor setting [63–66]. Some, but not all, suggest an early survival advantage with peripheral blood HCT in patients with advanced disease and some, but not all, suggest an increased risk of chronic GVHD with peripheral blood HCT. Blood-derived grafts might be expected to replace marrow for most transplants in the near future as has happened with autotransplants, although some concerns still exist regarding chronic GVHD and donor safety.

Transplantation regimens and supportive care

Historically, with the exception of some transplantations for immune deficiencies, infusion of hematopoietic cell was preceded by intensive immune suppressive and/or cytotoxic therapy. This treatment is aimed at eliminating malignant cells and, in the case of allografts, host immune cells that mediate rejection. In the 1970s and the 1980s most HCTs for malignant disease used a combination of high-dose cyclophosphamide (CY) and total body irradiation (TBI), with or without other drugs, for pretransplant conditioning. According to data reported to the IBMTR and the ABMTR, there has been a trend away from the high-dose radiation regimens used in the 1980s and the early 1990s. As noted above, about 30% of allotransplants are done using reduced intensity regimens, about 30% using high-dose TBI with CY or other high-dose chemotherapy, about 30% using busulfan and CY with or without other drugs and the remainder with a variety of high-dose chemotherapy regimens. High-dose therapy regimens in autotransplants vary according to the underlying disease but only a minority include TBI. Another important change in allogeneic HCT strategy has occurred in the approach to post-transplant immune suppression. In the 1970s and the early 1980s, methotrexate (MTX) was used. In the middle 1980s, cyclosporine (CSP) was substituted for MTX in many centers. In the middle 1980s, a regimen combining MTX and CSP was introduced, which proved to be superior to either MTX or CSP alone for preventing GVHD [67,68]. IBMTR/ABMTR data indicate that this is now the most common GVHD prophylaxis regimen. The risk of grade II–IV acute GVHD after HLA-identical sibling HCT decreased from 45% to 30% between the 1970s and the 1990s, with most of the decrease being in the most severe manifestations (Fig. 2.3) (Statistical Center of the IBMTR and ABMTR, unpublished data). Better prevention of cytomegalovirus (CMV) disease through use of CMV-negative or filtered blood products for CMV-negative patients and prophylaxis, or early treatment with ganciclovir in CMV-positive patients, reduced the incidence of CMV interstitial pneumonitis, a lethal complication of allogeneic transplantation, from about 10% to 3% (Fig. 2.3) (Statistical Center of the IBMTR and ABMTR, unpublished data). Noninfectious interstitial pneumonitis also decreased, possibly from decreased use of MTX and unfractionated radiation. Use of peripheral blood hematopoietic cell and post-transplant growth factors has hastened hematopoietic recovery and decreased hospital stays after autografts. Some of the latter are now done, at least partly, in the outpatient setting. The net effect of these and other changes has been a decrease in transplant-related mortality after HLA-identical sibling HCT, according to

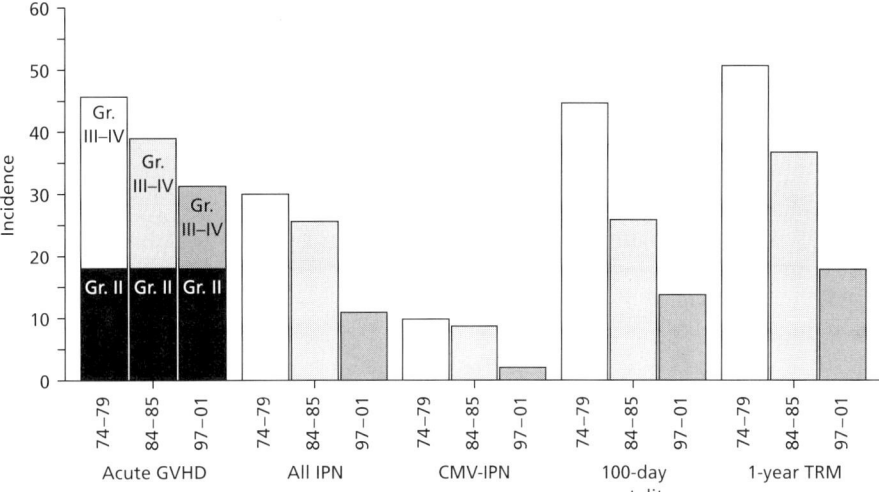

Fig. 2.3 Incidence of acute graft-vs.-host disease (GVHD), interstitial pneumonitis (IPN) due to all causes, IPN due to cytomegalovirus (CMV), and 100-day overall mortality and 1-year transplant-related mortality (TRM) after human leukocyte antigen (HLA)-identical sibling hematopoietic cell transplantation (HCT) among patients reported to the International Bone Marrow Transplant Registry (IBMTR) by year of HCT. Courtesy of the Statistical Center of the IBMTR and ABMTR.

IBMTR/ABMTR data, from about 50% in 1974–79 to about 20% in 1997–2001 (Fig. 2.3) (Statistical Center of the IBMTR and ABMTR, unpublished data). Transplant-related mortality after autotransplants is even lower, about 10% after autotransplants for leukemia and 5–10% after autotransplants for lymphoma and solid tumors (Statistical Center of the IBMTR and ABMTR, unpublished data).

Long-term survivors

The increasing use of HCT and better outcome of recipients means increasing numbers of long-term transplant survivors. There are now about 100,000 persons surviving 5 years or more after transplantation, and that number will grow rapidly. Most 5-year survivors are well, off all immune suppression and leading normal lives. Some data suggest that, at least in patients receiving transplants for AML and aplastic anemia, mortality rates return to that of an age- and sex-matched general population by 5–8 years post-transplant [69]. However, transplant recipients remain at risk for late complications long after HCT [69,70]. These include late infections, cataracts, abnormalities of growth and development, thyroid disorders, chronic lung disease and avascular necrosis. All of these are more frequent in patients with chronic GVHD. There is also an increased incidence of leukemias, myelodysplasias and solid tumors in transplant recipients compared to the general population [71–77]. Second cancers and other complications may not all be due to HCT *per se* but also due to the chemotherapy and/or radiation preceding the HCT. Regardless, lifelong surveillance is necessary, as is increased awareness of late complications among the many nontransplant physicians who will care for these patients.

References

1 Bach FH, Albertini RJ, Joo P, Anderson JL, Bortin MM. Bone-marrow transplantation in a patient with the Wiskott–Aldrich syndrome. *Lancet* 1968; **2**: 1364–6.

2 Gatti RA, Meuwissen HJ, Allen HD, Hong R, Good RA. Immunological reconstitution of sex-linked immunological deficiency. *Lancet* 1968; **2**: 1366–9.

3 Good RA, Meuwissen HJ, Hong R, Gatti RA. Successful marrow transplantation for correction of immunological deficit in lymphopenic agammaglobulinemia and treatment of immunologically induced pancytopenia. *Exp Hematol* 1969; **19**: 4–10.

4 De Konig J, Dooren LJ, Van Bekkum DW, van Rood JJ, Dicke KA, Radl J. Transplantation of bone-marrow cells and fetal thymus in an infant with lymphopenic immunological deficiency. *Lancet* 1969; **1**: 1223–7.

5 Thomas ED, Storb R, Clift RA *et al*. Bone marrow transplantation. *N Engl J Med* 1975; **292**: 832–43 and 895–902.

6 Thomas ED, Buckner CD, Banaji M *et al*. One hundred patients with acute leukemia treated by chemotherapy, total body irradiation, and allogeneic marrow transplantation. *Blood* 1977; **49**: 511–33.

7 Thomas ED, Buckner CD, Clift RA *et al*. Marrow transplantation for acute nonlymphoblastic leukemia in first remission. *N Engl J Med* 1979; **301**: 597–9.

8 Blume KG, Beutler E, Bross KJ *et al*. Bone marrow ablation and allogeneic marrow transplantation in acute leukemia. *New Engl J Med* 1980; **302**: 1041–6.

9 Bortin MM, Gale RP, Kay HEM, Rimm AA. Bone marrow transplantation for acute myelogenous leukemia: factors associated with early mortality. *J Am Med Assoc* 1983; **249**: 1166–75.

10 Fefer A, Cheever MA, Greenberg PD *et al*. Treatment of chronic granulocytic leukemia with chemoradiotherapy and transplantation of marrow from identical twins. *N Engl J Med* 1982; **306**: 63–8.

11 Speck B, Bortin MM, Champlin R *et al*. Allogeneic bone marrow transplantation for chronic myelogenous leukemia. *Lancet* 1984; **1**: 665–8.

12 Thomas ED, Clift RA, Fefer A *et al*. Marrow transplantation for the treatment of chronic myelogenous leukemia. *Ann Intern Med* 1986; **104**: 155–63.

13 Kantarjian H, Sawyers C, Hochhaus A *et al*. Hematologic and cytogenetic responses to imatinib mesylate in chronic myelogenous leukemia. *N Engl J Med* 2002; **346**: 645–52.

14 Talpaz M, Silver RT, Druker BJ *et al*. Imatinib induces durable hematologic and cytogenetic responses in patients with accelerated phase chronic myeloid leukemia: results of a phase 2 study. *Blood* 2002; **99**: 1928–37.

15 Sawyers CL, Hochhaus A, Feldman E *et al*. Imatinib induces hematologic and cytogenetic responses in patients with chronic myelogenous leukemia in myeloid blast crisis: results of a phase II study. *Blood* 2002; **99**: 3530–9.

16 Philip T, Biron P, Maraninchi D *et al*. Massive chemotherapy with autologous bone marrow transplantation in 50 cases of bad prognosis non-Hodgkin's lymphoma. *Br J Haematol* 1985; **60**: 599–609.

17 Armitage JO, Gingrich RD, Klassen LW *et al*. Trial of high-dose cytarabine, cyclophosphamide, total-body irradiation and autologous marrow transplantation for refractory lymphoma. *Cancer Treat Rep* 1986; **70**: 871–5.

18 Philip T, Armitage JO, Spitzer G *et al*. High-dose therapy and autologous bone marrow transplantation after failure of conventional chemotherapy in adults with intermediate-grade or high-grade non Hodgkin's lymphoma. *N Engl J Med* 1985; **316**: 1493–8.

19 Antman KH, Rowlings PA, Vaughan WP *et al*. High-dose chemotherapy with autologous HSC support for breast cancer in North America. *J Clin Oncol* 1997; **15**: 1870–9.

20 Nieto Y, Champlin RE, Wingard JR *et al*. Status of high-dose chemotherapy for breast cancer: a review. *Biol Blood Marrow Transplant* 2000; **6**: 476–95.

21 Antman KH. High-dose chemotherapy in breast cancer. The end of the beginning? *Biol Blood Marrow Transplant* 2000; **6**: 469–75.

22 Armstrong DK, Davidson NE. Dose intensity for breast cancer. *Oncology* 2001; **15**: 701–12.

23 Attal M, Harousseau JL, Stoppa AM *et al*. A prospective, randomized trial of autologous bone marrow transplantation and chemotherapy in multiple myeloma. Intergroupe Francais du Myelome. *N Engl J Med* 1996; **335**: 91–7.

24 Walters MC, Patience M, Leisenring W *et al*. Bone marrow transplantation for sickle cell disease. *N Engl J Med* 1996; **335**: 369–76.

25 Krivit W, Lockman LA, Watkins PA, Hirsch J, Shapiro EG. The future for treatment by bone marrow transplantation for adrenoleukodystrophy, metachromatic leukodystrophy, globoid cell leukodystrophy and Hurler syndrome. *J Inherited Metabol Dis* 1995; **18**: 398–412.

26 Krivit W, Shapiro EG, Peters C *et al*. Hematopoietic stem-cell transplantation in globoid-cell leukodystrophy. *N Engl J Med* 1998; **338**: 1119–26.

27 Michallet M, Archimbaud E, Bandini G *et al*. for the European Group for Blood and Marrow Transplantation and the International Bone Marrow Transplant Registry. HLA-identical sibling bone marrow transplantation in younger patients with chronic lymphocytic leukemia. *Ann Intern Med* 1996; **124**: 311–5.

28 Khouri IF, Keating MJ, Vriesendrop HM *et al*. Autologous and allogeneic bone marrow transplantation for chronic lymphocytic leukemia: preliminary results. *J Clin Oncol* 1994; **12**: 748–58.

29 Stiff PJ, Veum-Stone J, Lazarus HM *et al*. High dose chemotherapy and autologous hematopoietic stem cell transplantation for ovarian carcinoma in North America: a report from the Autologous Blood and Marrow Transplant Registry. *Ann Int Med* 2000; **133**: 504–15.

30 Rizzo JD, Elias AD, Stiff PJ *et al*. Autologous stem cell transplantation for small cell lung cancer. *Bone Marrow Transplant* 2002; **8**: 273–80.

31 Burt RK, Slavin S, Burns WH, Marmont AM. Induction of tolerance in autoimmune diseases by hematopoietic stem cell transplantation: getting closer to a cure? *Blood* 2002; **99**: 768–84.

32 Kohn DB. Gene therapy for genetic haematological disorders and immunodeficiencies. *J Intern Med* 2001; **249**: 379–90.

33 Ringdén O, Horowitz MM, Gale RP *et al*. Outcome after allogeneic bone marrow transplant for leukemia in older adults. *J Am Med Assoc* 1993; **270**: 57–60.

34 Miller CB, Piantadosi S, Vogelsang GB *et al*. Impact of age on outcome of patients with cancer undergoing autologous bone marrow transplant. *Blood* 1996; **14**: 1327–32.

35 Kusnierz-Glaz CR, Schlegel PG, Wong RM *et al*. Influence of age on the outcome of 500 autologous bone marrow transplant procedures for hematologic malignancies. *J Clin Oncol* 1997; **15**: 18–25.

36 Beatty PG, Clift RA, Mickelson EM *et al*. Marrow transplantation from related donors other than HLA-identical siblings. *N Engl J Med* 1985; **313**: 765–71.

37 Ash RC, Horowitz MM, Gale RP *et al*. Bone marrow transplantation from related donors other than HLA-identical siblings: effect of T-cell depletion. *Bone Marrow Transplant* 1991; **7**: 443–52.

38 Appelbaum FR, Herzig GP, Ziegler JL, Graw RG, Levine AS, Deisseroth AB. Successful engraftment of cryopreserved autologous bone marrow in patients with malignant lymphoma. *Blood* 1978; **52**: 85–95.

39 Reiffers J, Bernard P, David B *et al*. Successful autologous transplantation with peripheral blood haemopoietic cells in a patient with acute leukaemia. *Exp Hematol* 1986; **14**: 312–5.

40 Korbling M, Dorken B, Ho AD, Pezzuto A, Hunstein W, Fliedner TM. Autologous transplantation of blood-derived hemopoietic stem cells after myeloablative therapy in a patient with Burkitt's lymphoma. *Blood* 1986; **67**: 529–32.

41 Kessinger A, Armitage JO, Landmark JD, Weisenberger DD. Reconstitution of human hematopoietic function with autologous cryopreserved circulating stem cells. *Exp Hematol* 1986; **14**: 192–6.

42 Speck B, Zwaan FE, van Rood JJ, Eernisse JG. Allogeneic bone marrow transplantation in a patient with aplastic anemia using a phenotypically HLA-identical unrelated donor. *Transplantation* 1973; **16**: 24–8.

43 O'Reilly RJ, Dupont B, Pahwa S *et al*. Reconstitution in severe combined immunodeficiency by transplantation of marrow from an unrelated donor. *N Engl J Med* 1977; **297**: 1311–8.

44 Hansen JA, Clift RA, Thomas ED, Buckner CD, Storb R, Giblett ER. Transplantation of marrow from an unrelated donor to a patient with acute leukemia. *N Engl J Med* 1980; **303**: 565–7.

45 Oudshoorn M, Leeuwen A, van Zanden HGM, van Rood JJ. Bone marrow donors worldwide: a successful exercise in international cooperation. *Bone Marrow Transplant* 1994; **14**: 3–8.

46 Dodson KL, Coppo PA, Confer DL. The National Marrow Donor Program: improving access to hematopoietic stem cell transplantation. *Clinical Transplants* 1999: 121–7.

47 Ash RC, Casper JT, Chitambar CR *et al*. Successful allogeneic transplantation of T-cell depleted bone marrow from closely HLA-matched unrelated donors. *N Engl J Med* 1990; **32**: 485–94.

48 Kernan NA, Bartsch G, Ash RC *et al*. Analysis of 462 transplantations from unrelated donors facilitated by the National Marrow Donor Program. *N Engl J Med* 1993; **328**: 593–602.

49 Casper J, Camitta B, Truitt R *et al*. Unrelated bone marrow donor transplants for children with leukemia or myelodysplasia. *Blood* 1995; **85**: 2354–63.

50 Petersdorf EW, Longton GM, Anasetti C *et al*. The significance of HLA-DRB1 matching on clinical outcome after HLA-A, B, DR identical unrelated donor marrow transplantation. *Blood* 1995; **86**: 1606–13.

51 Szydlo R, Goldman JM, Klein JP *et al*. Results of allogeneic bone marrow transplants for leukemia using donors other than HLA-identical siblings. *J Clin Oncol* 1997; **15**: 1767–77.

52 Hansen JA, Gooley TA, Martin PJ *et al*. Bone marrow transplants from unrelated donors for patients with chronic myeloid leukemia. *N Engl J Med* 1998; **338**: 962–8.

53 Davies SM, DeFor TE, McGlave P *et al*. Equivalent outcomes in patients with chronic myelogenous leukemia after early transplantation of phenotypically matched bone marrow from related or unrelated donors. *Am J Med* 2001; **110**: 339–46.

54 Kurtzberg J, Laughlin M, Graham ML *et al*. Placental blood as a source of hematopoietic stem cells for transplantation into unrelated recipients. *N Engl J Med* 1996; **335**: 157–66.

55 Gluckman E. The therapeutic potential of fetal and neonatal hematopoietic stem cells. *N Engl J Med* 1996; **335**: 1839–40.

56 Wagner JE, Kernan NA, Steinbuch M, Broxmeyer HE, Gluckman E. Allogeneic sibling umbilical-cord-blood transplantation in children with malignant and non-malignant disease. *Lancet* 1995; **346**: 214–9.

57 Rubinstein P, Carrier C, Scaradavou A *et al*. Outcomes among 562 recipients of placental-blood transplants from unrelated donors. *N Engl J Med* 1998; **339**: 1565–77.

58 Aversa F, Tabilio A, Velardi A *et al*. Treatment of high-risk acute leukemia with T-cell-depleted stem cells from related donors with one fully mismatched HLA haplotype. *N Engl J Med* 1998; **339**: 1186–93.

59 Ruggeri L, Capanni M, Urbani E *et al*. Effectiveness of donor natural killer cell alloreactivity in mismatched hematopoietic transplants. *Science* 2002; **295**: 2097–100.

60 Bensinger WI, Weaver CH, Appelbaum FR *et al*. Transplantation of allogeneic peripheral blood stem cells mobilized by recombinant human granulocyte colony-stimulating factor. *Blood* 1995; **85**: 1655–8.

61 Körbling M, Przepiorka D, Huh YO *et al*. Allogeneic blood stem cell transplantation for refractory leukemia and lymphoma: potential advantage of blood over marrow allografts. *Blood* 1995; **85**: 1659–65.

62 Schmitz N, Drege P, Suttorp M *et al*. Primary transplantation of allogeneic peripheral blood progenitor cells mobilized by filgrastim (granulocyte colony-stimulating factor). *Blood* 1995; **85**: 1666–72.

63 Blaise D, Kuentz M, Fortanier C *et al*. Randomized trial of bone marrow versus lenograstim-primed blood cell allogeneic transplantation in patients with early-stage leukemia: a report from the Société Française de Greffe de Moelle. *J Clin Oncol* 2000; **18**: 537–71.

64 Bensinger WI, Martin PJ, Storer B *et al*. Transplantation of bone marrow as compared with peripheral-blood cells from HLA-identical relatives in patients with hematologic cancers. *N Engl J Med* 2001; **344**: 175–81.

65 Schmitz N, Beksac M, Hasenclever D *et al*. Transplantation of mobilized peripheral blood cells to HLA-identical siblings with standard-risk leukemia. *Blood* 2002; **100**: 761–7.

66 Couban S, Simpson DR, Barnett MJ *et al*. A randomized multicenter comparison of bone marrow and peripheral blood in recipients of matched sibling allogeneic transplants for myeloid malignancies. *Blood* 2002; **100**: 1525–31.

67 Storb R, Deeg HJ, Whitehead J *et al*. Methotrexate and cyclosporine compared with cyclosporine alone for prophylaxis of acute graft-versus-host disease after marrow transplantation for leukemia. *N Engl J Med* 1986; **314**: 729–35.

68 Storb R, Deeg HJ, Pepe M *et al*. Methotrexate and cyclosporine versus cyclosporine alone for prophylaxis of graft-versus-host disease in patients given HLA-identical marrow grafts for leukemia: long-term follow-up of a controlled trial. *Blood* 1989; **73**: 1729–34.

69 Socié G, Veum-Stone J, Wingard JR *et al*. Long-term survival and late deaths after allogeneic bone marrow transplantation. *New Engl J Med* 1999; **341**: 14–21.

70 Duell T, van Lint MT, Ljungman P *et al*. Health and functional status of long-term survivors of bone marrow transplantation. EBMT Working Party on Late Effects and EULEP Study Group on Late Effects, European Group for Blood and Marrow Transplantation. *Ann Intern Med* 1997; **126**: 184–92.

71 Witherspoon RP, Fisher LD, Schoch G *et al*. Secondary cancers after bone marrow transplantation for leukemia and aplastic anemia. *N Engl J Med* 1989; **321**: 784–9.

72 Miller JS, Arthur DC, Litz CE, Neglia JP, Miller WJ, Weisdorf DJ. Myelodysplastic syndrome after autologous bone marrow transplantation. An additional late complication of curative cancer therapy. *Blood* 1994; **83**: 3780–6.

73 Darrington DL, Vose JM, Anderson JR *et al.* Incidence and characterization of secondary myelodysplastic syndrome and acute myelogenous leukemia following high-dose chemoradiotherapy and autologous stem-cell transplantation for lymphoid malignancies. *J Clin Oncol* 1994; **12**: 2527–34.

74 Traweek ST, Slovak ML, Nademanee P, Brynes RK, Niland JC, Forman SJ. Clonal karyotypic hematopoietic cell abnormalities occurring after autologous bone marrow transplantation for Hodgkin disease and non-Hodgkin lymphoma. *Blood* 1994; **84**: 957–63.

75 Deeg HJ, Socié G, Schoch G *et al.* Malignancies after marrow transplantation for aplastic anemia and Fanconi anemia: a joint Seattle and Paris analysis of results in 700 patients. *Blood* 1996; **87**: 386–92.

76 Curtis RE, Rowlings PA, Deeg HJ *et al.* Solid cancers after bone marrow transplantation. *N Engl J Med* 1997; **336**: 897–904.

77 Socié G, Curtis RE, Deeg HJ *et al.* New malignant diseases after allogeneic marrow transplantation for childhood acute leukemia. *J Clin Oncol* 2000; **18**: 348–57.

3

Paul J. Martin

Overview of Hematopoietic Cell Transplantation Immunology

Introduction

Immunology plays a central role in allogeneic hematopoietic cell transplantation (HCT). Any appreciation of the immunological mechanisms involved in engraftment, graft-vs.-host disease (GVHD), control of malignancy, the development of tolerance and immune reconstitution requires some understanding of the immunogenetic basis for immune reactions provoked by grafting tissue from one individual to another. Insight into the cellular basis of alloreactivity requires an understanding of immune recognition, the development of the immune system and the nature of immune responses. This chapter will serve to introduce the reader to the immunology of HCT. Citations are made to selected references and reviews from recent literature and to other chapters that provide detailed information.

Fundamental differences between marrow transplantation and solid organ transplantation

HCT differs fundamentally from grafting of most other organs. In solid organ transplantation, the graft generally contains only limited numbers of cells with immunologic function. The primary clinical concern rests with preventing rejection by the recipient immune system. Life-long administration of immunosuppressive medication is generally required to prevent rejection not only by cellular and humoral mechanisms in the recipient at the time of transplantation, but also by elements generated from recipient-derived immunologic precursors after transplantation.

The preparative regimen administered before HCT (see Chapters 12–15) eliminates most, though not all, precursors and mature elements of the recipient immune system. The graft contains large numbers of precursors and mature cellular elements that replace those of the recipient. Thus, the immune system in the recipient is generated by the graft and originates from the donor. The primary clinical concerns rest not only with preventing graft rejection by recipient cells that survive the conditioning regimen, but also with preventing donor cells from causing immune-mediated injury (GVHD) in the recipient, while allowing immunologic reconstitution for recognition and control of pathogens. Immunosuppressive medications (see Chapter 16) are administered after transplantation primarily to prevent GVHD. Eventually it becomes possible to discontinue such treatment. The subsequent persistence of engraftment and the absence of GVHD, together with recovery of host immune defenses, indicate that a state of immunological "tolerance" has been achieved between the donor and recipient.

Transplantation antigens

Genes that encode major histocompatibility antigens

Immune reactions provoked by grafting tissue from one individual to another are caused by transplantation or histocompatibility antigens (see Chapters 4 & 5). Genes encoding transplantation antigens are located both within and outside the major histocompatibility complex (MHC). The human MHC is located on the short arm of chromosome six and contains a series of genes encoding two distinct types of highly polymorphic cell surface glycoproteins termed human leukocyte antigen (HLA). HLA class I antigens contain a single polymorphic α chain noncovalently associated with β_2-microglobulin. HLA class I antigens encoded by three loci termed HLA-A, HLA-B and HLA-C are known to provoke immune reactions in HCT. The role of antigens encoded by other class I loci has not yet been defined. As of 2002, 219 HLA-A alleles, 436 HLA-B alleles and 97 HLA-C alleles with protein-changing exon polymorphisms have been described [1].

HLA class II antigens are encoded by three clusters of loci (HLA-DR, -DQ and -DP) and contain a single polymorphic (DQ and DP) or non-polymorphic (DR) α chain noncovalently associated with a polymorphic β chain. The α chains of HLA-DR, DQ and DP antigens are encoded by the respective *DRA*, *DQA1* and *DPA1* genes, while the β chains are encoded by the respective *DRB*, *DQB1* and *DPB1* genes. Four distinct *DRB* genes, termed *DRB1*, *DRB3*, *DRB4* and *DRB5*, encode polymorphic HLA-DR β chains. Antigens encoded by *DRB1*, *DQ* and *DP* genes are known to provoke reactions in HCT. The role of antigens encoded by *DRB3*, *DRB4* and *DRB5* genes has not yet been defined. As of 2002, 312 HLA-DRB1 alleles, 17 DQA1 alleles, 42 DQB1 alleles, 12 DPA1 alleles and 90 DPB1 alleles with protein-changing exon polymorphisms have been described [1].

HLA matching

The genes encoding HLA class I and class II antigens are tightly linked, such that they are inherited in families as "haplotypes" with low recombination frequencies. An HLA-matched sibling can be readily identified by an informative family study, especially if family members are HLA-heterozygous and if the parental haplotypes can be identified by reliable markers and clearly assigned by segregation analysis. For a given patient there is a 0.25 probability that any one sibling inherited the same paternal haplotype and the same maternal haplotype, thereby being "HLA-genotypically identical." Siblings identified this way are identical not only for the polymorphisms detected by HLA typing, but also for all other polymorphisms in the MHC.

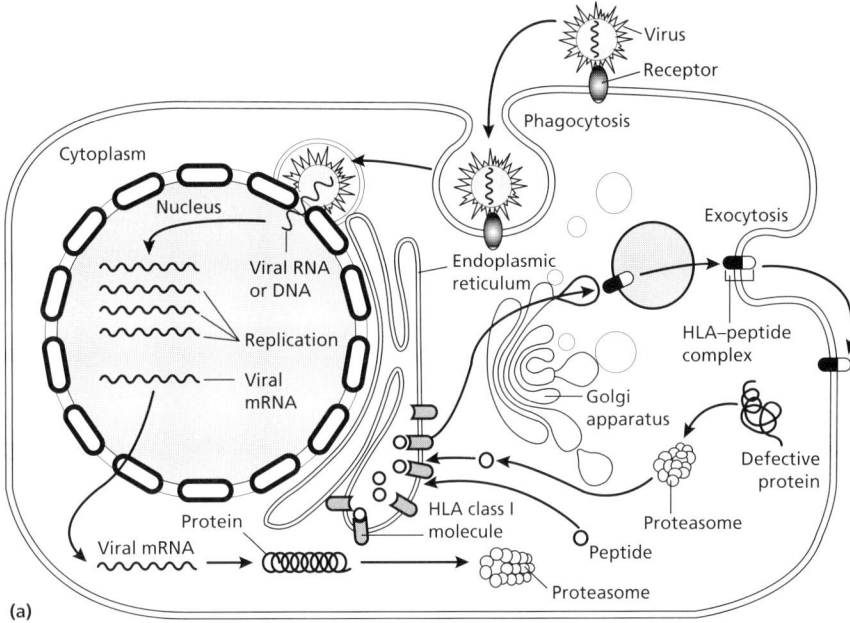

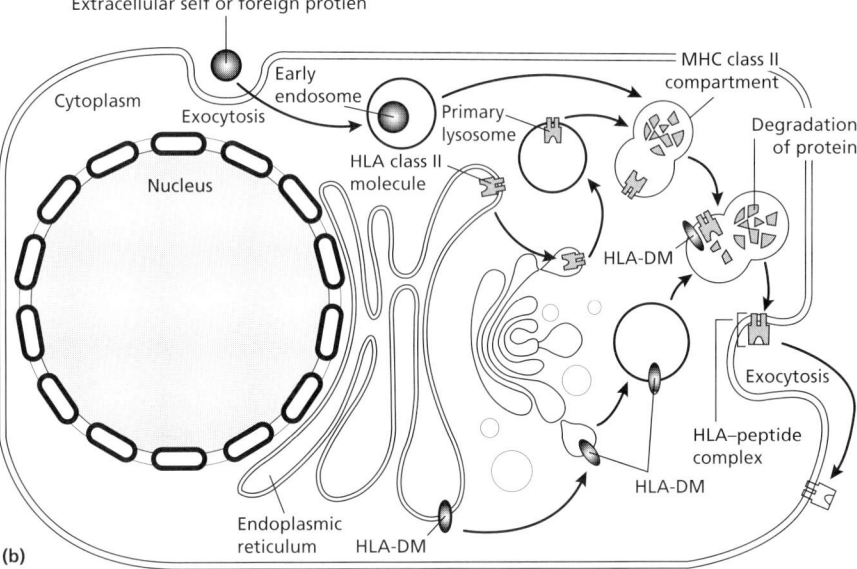

Fig. 3.1 Mechanisms of peptide presentation by major histocompatibility complex (MHC) class I and class II molecules. (a) Peptide presentation by MHC class I molecules occurs through degradation of endogenous and exogenous (e.g. viral) proteins in the cytosol. Peptides degraded by proteasomes are transported from the cytosol into the endoplasmic reticulum and inserted into the binding groove of MHC class I molecules, which are then transported through the Golgi apparatus to the cell surface.
(b) Peptide presentation by MHC class II molecules occurs through degradation of extracellular proteins in primary lysosomes. MHC class II molecules are synthesized in the endoplasmic reticulum and delivered through the Golgi apparatus to the lysosomal compartment. HLA-DM molecules are delivered through transport vesicles to the same compartment where they facilitate loading of peptide into the binding groove of MHC class II molecules, which are then transported to the cell surface. Adapted from Klein and Sato [2] with permission. Copyright (2000), Massachusetts Medical Society. All rights reserved.

The term "HLA-matched" has a different significance when applied to unrelated individuals. In this context, matching can be defined only with respect to the polymorphisms encompassed by the testing. Unrelated individuals who are HLA-phenotypically identical can have disparity that is not detected by the methods used for HLA typing. Serologically indistinguishable antigens are encoded by multiple alleles whose gene products can elicit alloimmune T-cell responses, and disparity within HLA-A, -B, -C, -DR, -DQ or -DP loci can occur in regions not encompassed by routine laboratory testing. In addition, unrelated individuals nearly always have disparity at other loci within the MHC, unlike HLA-genotypically identical siblings. Because of the highly polymorphic nature of HLA antigens, the probability that two unrelated individuals will have the same HLA-A, -B, -C, -DR, -DQ and -DP alleles is extremely low.

Structure of HLA

MHC class I and class II antigens have similar structures [2,3]. The general structure consists of a floor formed by eight antiparallel β strands overlaid by two α-helices in parallel orientation to each other, leaving a groove or cleft between them for binding of small peptides. The polymorphic residues of HLA molecules are located primarily in the β-strand floor and in positions on the α-helices that point into the groove between the two helices.

MHC class I [4] and class II [5] molecules bind short peptides for display at the cell surface where they can be recognized by T cells [6,7] (Fig. 3.1 [2]). Peptides that bind MHC class I molecules are generated in the cytosol. Ubiquitin-modified proteins in the cytosol are degraded by proteasomes, and the resulting peptides are transferred into the lumen of the endoplasmic reticulum by an adenosine triphosphate (ATP)-dependent transport mechanism. Proteasome-mediated cleavage mechanisms have not yet been fully defined, but there appears to be a preference for generation of short peptides that contain a hydrophobic or basic residue at the carboxy terminus. The transport mechanism functions most efficiently with peptides containing 8–12 amino acids with a hydrophobic residue at the carboxy terminus. Binding of peptides to MHC class I molecules in the lumen of the endoplasmic reticulum is dictated by the way that the side chains of specific "anchor" residues of the peptide fit into "pockets" formed by polymorphic residues lining the groove between the α-helices of the class I molecule. Thus each specific MHC molecule displays a characteristic preference for peptides with distinctive anchor residues. For example, HLA-A2 molecules preferentially bind nine-mer peptides with leucine or methionine at position two and valine or leucine at the carboxy terminal position nine, while HLA-B35 molecules preferentially bind peptides with proline at position two and a hydrophobic residue at position nine.

Peptides that bind MHC class II molecules generally originate from extracellular proteins that are taken into cells by endocytosis. Acidification of endosomes activates proteases that degrade internalized proteins into peptides. Peptides bind MHC class II molecules when endosomes fuse with vesicles containing newly synthesized membrane proteins being transported to the cell surface. Binding of peptides to MHC class II molecules is dictated by the way that the side chains of specific residues of the peptide fit into pockets formed by polymorphic residues lining the groove between the α-helices of the class II molecules.

Minor histocompatibility antigens

Minor histocompatibility antigens (mHAs) originate from polymorphic proteins encoded by genes outside the MHC [8,9]. These proteins are processed either through the cytosolic pathway to generate peptides that are presented at the cell surface by MHC class I molecules or through the endosomal pathway to generate peptides that are presented by MHC class II molecules. Recognition of a minor antigen by T cells is specified both by the polymorphic peptide and the MHC molecule to which it is bound. Polymorphisms producing a single amino acid substitution in a peptide presented by MHC molecules can be sufficient to generate a T-cell alloimmune response in the absence of any MHC disparity. Only a few mHAs have been defined biochemically. Genetic studies in mice have identified more than 40 loci that encode mHAs, each typically having two known alleles.

Human genomes contain an enormous number of polymorphisms. mHAs originate from loci that contain polymorphisms encoding peptides that can provoke alloimmune responses. Because these loci are distributed throughout the entire genome, siblings other than identical twins always have some disparity for mHAs, even when they are HLA-matched. The general population has a greater diversity of minor histocompatibility alleles than any given family. For this reason, the probability of minor antigen disparity is higher between unrelated individuals than between siblings.

Innate and adaptive immune responses

Transplantation evokes both innate [10] and adaptive or acquired immune responses. In general, the innate immune system is poised for immediate responses against pathogens, whereas acquired immune responses are activated more slowly over a period of days. The receptors involved in innate immunity are encoded directly in the germ line and typically recognize invariant molecules involved in the pathogenic effects or survival of invading organisms. The receptors involved in adaptive immunity are encoded by rearrangement and selection of germ-line genes and typically recognize foreign "nonself" epitopes, regardless of whether they originate from a pathogenic organism or not. Innate immune responses are activated without proliferation of the effector cells, whereas adaptive immune responses are activated through clonal expansion of precursors followed by differentiation into effectors. Innate immune responses regulate adaptive immune responses through activation of dendritic cells that are primarily responsible for presentation of antigens. In this way, innate immunity serves as an alarm that signals the "danger" [11] posed by an invading organism, thereby evoking an adaptive immune response against the organism.

Regulation of natural killer cell responses

Natural killer (NK) cells are a component of the innate immune system [12]. These cells are characterized by expression of CD (cluster of differentiation) 56 and CD16 and by absence of CD3. NK cells mediate their effects through cytotoxic activity and production of cytokines such as interferon-gamma (IFN-γ), tumor necrosis factor-alpha (TNF-α) and granulocyte macrophage colony-stimulating factor (GM-CSF). The importance of NK cells for transplantation comes from their ability to recognize MHC class I alloantigens. Human NK cells collectively express at least four different types of activating receptors and at least two types of inhibitory receptors. Killer immunoglobulin-like receptors (KIRs) with cytoplasmic tails containing immunoreceptor tyrosine-based activation motifs (ITAM) and certain C-type lectins in the CD94 family activate NK cells after binding to MHC molecules. NKG2D is an NK activating receptor that recognizes MHC class I-like molecules that are expressed in response to cellular stress. Other activating receptors recognize ligands that have not yet been defined. KIRs with cytoplasmic tails containing immunoreceptor tyrosine-based inhibitory motifs (ITIM) and other C-type lectins in the CD94 family inhibit activation of NK cells. Genes that encode both activating and inhibitory KIRs are located in a cluster on the short arm of chromosome 19, while genes that encode members of the CD94 family are located in a cluster on the short arm of chromosome 12.

The balance of activation and inhibitory signals mediated through cell surface receptors regulates NK function, and inhibitory signals dominate the effect of activation signals (Fig. 3.2 [13]). Individual NK cells must each have at least one inhibitory receptor that recognizes a ligand expressed by the host. The expression of this receptor prevents the NK cell from killing targets that have the inhibitory ligand, which is often a MHC class I molecule. In this way, self-MHC molecules shield potential targets from attack by NK cells [14]. When the self-MHC molecule that binds the inhibitory receptor is absent, for example, on a tumor cell or

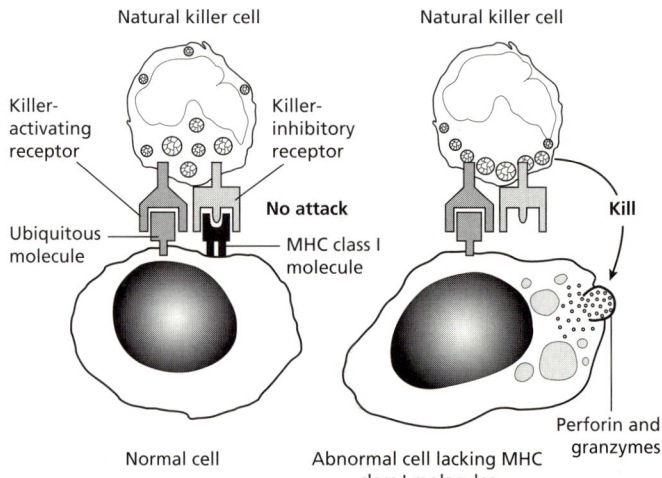

Fig. 3.2 Activation and inhibition of natural killer (NK) cells. A variety of cell surface ligands can bind killer-activating receptors on NK cells. Normal cells express major histocompatibility complex (MHC) class I molecules that bind to killer inhibitory receptors on NK cells, thereby overriding the activation signal and preventing a cytotoxic attack. Abnormal cells that lack MHC class I molecules are susceptible to attack by NK cells because the activation signal is not blocked by inhibitory signals delivered through killer inhibitory receptors. Adapted from Delves PJ and Roitt [13] with permission. Copyright (2000), Massachusetts Medical Society. All rights reserved.

virally infected target, the NK cell is activated, and the target cell is killed.

Self-tolerance and alloantigen recognition by T cells

Molecules used for recognition of antigens

Adaptive immune responses are orchestrated and mediated by T and B lymphocytes [13]. In T cells, immune recognition is mediated by the T-cell receptor (TCR); in B cells, immune recognition is mediated by immunoglobulin molecules. In general, each T cell and B cell expresses only one type of receptor for recognizing antigen epitopes. Both types of cells utilize similar mechanisms for generating an enormous diversity of clonally distributed receptors. This diversity is generated initially by somatic rearrangements that link V (variable), D (diversity), and J (joining) segments in various combinations to encode distinct receptors.

Selection of T cells in the thymus

Precursors destined to become T cells originate from stem cells in the bone marrow and migrate to the thymus (Fig. 3.3 [13]). Within the thymus, developing T cells that express receptors capable of recognizing foreign peptide antigens in association with the organism's own "self"-MHC molecules survive and are selected for export to the peripheral blood, lymph nodes, spleen and other organs [15,16]. This process of "positive selection" is mediated primarily by thymic cortical epithelial cells. Before export to the periphery, developing T cells that express receptors with high affinity for peptide-MHC complexes or "self"-antigens on adjacent cells are deleted by a process termed "negative selection" [17]. Negative selection is mediated most efficiently by marrow-derived dendritic cells and also by thymic medullary epithelium. Interactions with thymic epithelial cells can also cause developing T cells to become nonresponsive or "anergic" to self-MHC molecules [18], and cortical epithelium can induce the development of regulatory T cells that can suppress responses against self-MHC molecules [19,20]. Negative selection, induction of nonresponsiveness and generation of regulatory T cells in the thymus represent the principal "central" mechanisms for establishing self-tolerance (see Chapter 24). Mechanisms of central tolerance cannot explain the absence of responses against antigens expressed exclusively in tissues outside the thymus.

Presentation of self-antigens by immature dendritic cells outside the thymus in the absence of alarm signals from an innate immune response has been proposed as a major mechanism of "peripheral" tolerance to explain why T cells that recognize extrathymic tissue-specific antigens do not cause immunological injury under normal conditions [21–25]. After activation by immature dendritic cells, T cells proliferate vigorously, but they are then deleted, become anergic, or differentiate as regulatory T cells [26]. Alarm signals from an innate immune response induce maturation of antigen-presenting cells (APCs) and convert otherwise tolerogenic signals into a productive adaptive immune response.

Differences in responses against major and minor antigens

Immune responses against major histocompatibility antigens differ greatly from responses against mHAs. Generation of an *in vitro* response against major histocompatibility antigens does not require *in vivo* priming, and the precursor frequency of T cells that respond to any given major histocompatibility antigen has been estimated to be as high as 1–10%. Major histocompatibility antigens also induce alloimmune antibody responses detectable by serologic testing. Generation of an *in vitro* response against mHAs requires *in vivo* priming. The precursor frequency of T cells that respond to MHC-identical stimulators with disparity for multiple mHAs after priming has been estimated at 0.01–0.10%. mHAs generally do not induce alloimmune antibody responses detectable by serologic testing.

At least two mechanisms might account for differences in the strength of immune responses against major histocompatibility antigens as compared to mHAs. First, MHC molecules encoded by any given allele contain a variety of different peptides, whereas any given mHA involves a single specific peptide. For this reason, the variety of epitopes and numbers of responding T cells are far greater for major histocompatibility

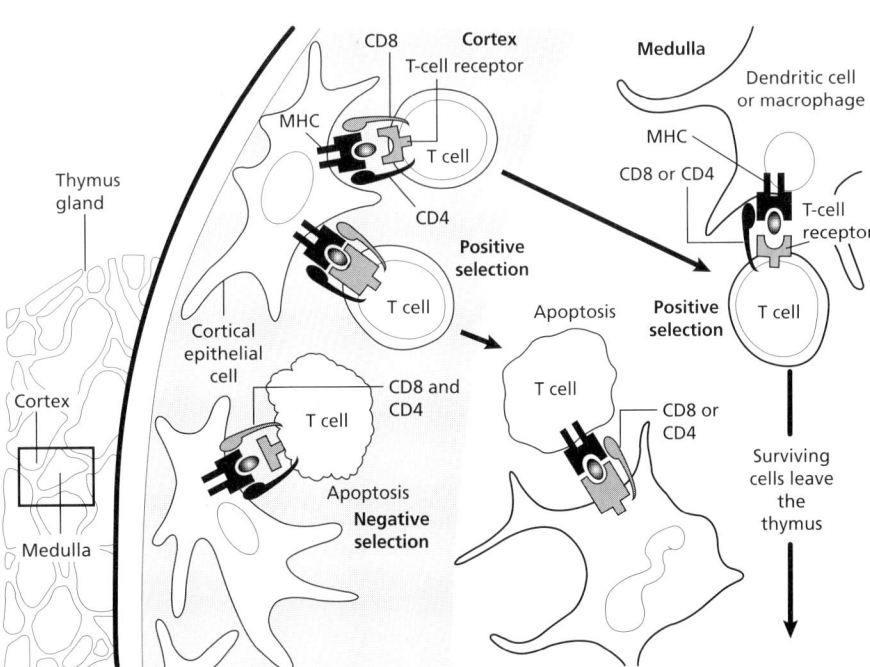

Fig. 3.3 Positive and negative selection of T cells in the thymus. T cells must pass two tests as they develop the ability to express a receptor that recognizes major histocompatibility complex (MHC)/peptide complexes. First, immature T cells that express both CD4 and CD8 must have a receptor that recognizes an MHC/peptide complex on thymic cortical epithelial cells in order to survive. Those that fail this test die through apoptosis, as shown for the cell at the lower left. Those that pass this test are positively selected to travel to thymic medulla where expression of CD4 or CD8 is lost, as shown for the cells at the upper left. Maturing T cells that express CD4 or CD8 and have a receptor that binds too well with an MHC/peptide complex on medullary dendritic cells are negatively selected and die through apoptosis, as shown for the cell at the lower right. Maturing T cells that express CD4 or CD8 and have a receptor that bind weakly with an MHC/peptide complex on medullary dendritic cells escape negative selection and are exported to the periphery, as shown for the cell at the upper right. Adapted from Delves PJ and Roitt [13] with permission. Copyright (2000), Massachusetts Medical Society. All rights reserved.

antigens than for mHAs. Second, certain major histocompatibility determinants are present on all MHC molecules encoded by a given allele, independent of the peptides that are bound between the α-helices [27], whereas any given minor histocompatibility epitope is present only on the small fraction of MHC molecules that contain a specific polymorphic peptide. For this reason, the cell surface density of epitopes can be much greater for major histocompatibility antigens than for mHAs.

Activation of T-cell responses by alloantigens

Interactions between APCs and T cells

Dendritic cells, B cells and macrophages function as APCs. Among these, dendritic cells have by far the most potent activity as APCs. Activation of an alloimmune response begins with binding between MHC/peptide complexes on APCs and the TCR on T cells [28]. Interaction between TCR and MHC/peptide complexes requires close apposition between T cells and APCs. Adhesive interactions [29] exemplified by the respective binding of CD11a/CD18 (leukocyte function-associated antigen-1 [LFA-1]) and CD2 on T cells with CD54 (intracellular adhesion molecule-1 [ICAM-1]) and CD58 (LFA-3) on APCs help to overcome the repulsive forces created by the net negative surface charge of these cells.

Optimal activation of a T-cell immune response typically involves three-way interactions between APCs, CD4 cells and CD8 cells. CD4 cells are activated by mature dendritic cells that present MHC class II alloantigens and mHAs bound to self-MHC class II molecules. Direct binding between MHC class II molecules on APCs and CD4 molecules on T cells facilitates this interaction. Activation of CD4 cells by antigen increases expression of CD154, also known as CD40 ligand or gp39 [30,31]. CD154 on activated CD4 cells binds to CD40 on APCs, which causes APCs to increase expression of CD86, also known as B7-2. CD86 molecules on APCs bind to CD28 on T cells [32], providing "costimulation" signals that augment TCR signaling. CD8 cells are activated by mature dendritic cells that present MHC class I alloantigens and mHAs bound to self-MHC class I molecules. Direct binding between MHC class I molecules on APCs and CD8 molecules on T cells facilitates this interaction. CD4 cells help CD8 responses by increasing costimulation through APCs and by secretion of cytokines such as interleukin 2 (IL-2).

Signal transduction leading to activation of T cells

Signal transduction in T cells leads to transcriptional activation of numerous genes by AP-1, NFκB, and the nuclear factor of activated T cells (NF-AT). In broad outline, the process begins by the formation of "immunological synapses" that concentrate TCR/CD3 complexes, CD2 and CD4 or CD8 within small regions of the membrane [33,34]. Molecules associated with the cytoplasmic domains of TCR/CD3 complexes and CD4 or CD8 assemble as a scaffold that initiates a cascade of protein tyrosine phosphorylation events leading to activation of p21 *ras* and phospholipase Cγ. The p21 *ras* pathway activates expression of Fos, which functions as a component in the AP-1-promoter complex for transcription of *IL-2* and other genes involved in activation. Phospholipase Cγ cleaves phosphoinositide-4,5-diphosphate (PI4,5-P$_2$) in the plasma membrane to form diacylglycerol (DAG) and inositol-1,4,5-triphosphate (IP$_3$). DAG activates protein kinase C (PKC) isoforms that regulate p21 *ras* and NFκB. In the nucleus, NFκB family members function as transcriptional regulators for numerous cytokine genes, including *IL-2*. IP$_3$ releases Ca^{2+} from intracellular stores and allows influx of extracellular Ca^{2+}, thereby activating calcineurin, an enzyme with serine/threonine phosphatase activity. Activated calcineurin dephosphorylates NF-AT, which is then translocated from the cytosol to the nucleus where it activates transcription in conjunction with AP-1. Cyclosporine (CSP) and tacrolimus bind to intracellular proteins, forming drug/protein complexes that inhibit the enzymatic activity of calcineurin, thereby interfering with signal transduction in T cells after stimulation with antigen.

Signal transduction through costimulation has not been fully characterized, but appears to involve several pathways leading to increased production of cytokines through activation of Jun, which functions as a component in the AP-1 promoter complex [35]. In addition, CD28 signaling increases production of IL-2 by stabilizing IL-2 messenger RNA (mRNA).

Outcomes after activation of T cells

Activation of peripheral T cells can produce at least three qualitatively distinct results. TCR signaling together with appropriate costimulation signals results in production of IL-2, followed by differentiation into effectors [29,36]. TCR signaling during the S phase of the cell cycle, and interactions between Fas ligand (FasL) and Fas can cause apoptosis or activation-induced cell death, resulting in deletion [37]. With suboptimal TCR signaling or suboptimal costimulation, T-cell activation can induce a state of anergy characterized by lack of IL-2 production [38].

Complex mechanisms regulate costimulation during an immune response [39]. Costimulation of resting T cells occurs through CD28, while costimulation of activated T cells occurs through the inducible costimulator (ICOS) protein. Certain molecules that have homology with TNF can also provide costimulation through binding to T cells. Activation of T cells induces the expression of CD152, also known as CTLA-4, a second ligand for binding CD80. The high avidity of binding between CD152 and CD80 competitively limits the degree of signaling through CD28 in activated T cells. In addition, signaling through CD152 inhibits activation of T cells through induction of phosphatase activity that counteracts the kinase cascade induced by signaling through the TCR. T-cell responses may also be inhibited by ligation of other molecules that have homology with CD28.

T-cell effector functions

Activated T cells differentiate into effector cells that produce cytokines and mediate cytotoxic activity. Under *in vitro* conditions, both CD4 cells and CD8 cells can be induced to differentiate according to characteristic response patterns of cytokine production [40]. In the presence of IL-12 produced by monocytes or activated dendritic cells, T cells are stimulated to differentiate into effectors that produce "type 1" cytokines, including IFN-γ and lymphotoxin, which activate proinflammatory macrophages. In the presence of IL-4, activated T cells are stimulated to differentiate into effectors that produce "type 2" cytokines, including IL-4 and IL-5, which activate B-cell proliferation and differentiation.

Both CD4 cells and CD8 cells can differentiate into cytotoxic effectors. The cytotoxic effector function of T lymphocytes can be mediated by two mechanisms [41]. One of these involves cell surface interactions between FasL expressed on activated cytotoxic T lymphocytes (CTLs) and Fas expressed on cells targeted for lysis. The other involves exocytosis of granules containing perforin and granzymes from CTL effectors. Perforin facilitates transport of granzymes into the cytosol of cells recognized by CTLs. Both mechanisms induce apoptosis in target cells.

T cells exhibit two general types of immune responses *in vivo* (Fig. 3.4 [29]) [42]. "Primary" responses occur when immunologically "naive" cells first encounter a specific antigen. The immune response after an initial encounter with antigen develops during a period of approximately 1 week and results in the expansion of specific clones of effectors having receptors capable of recognizing the antigen. This initial expansion is

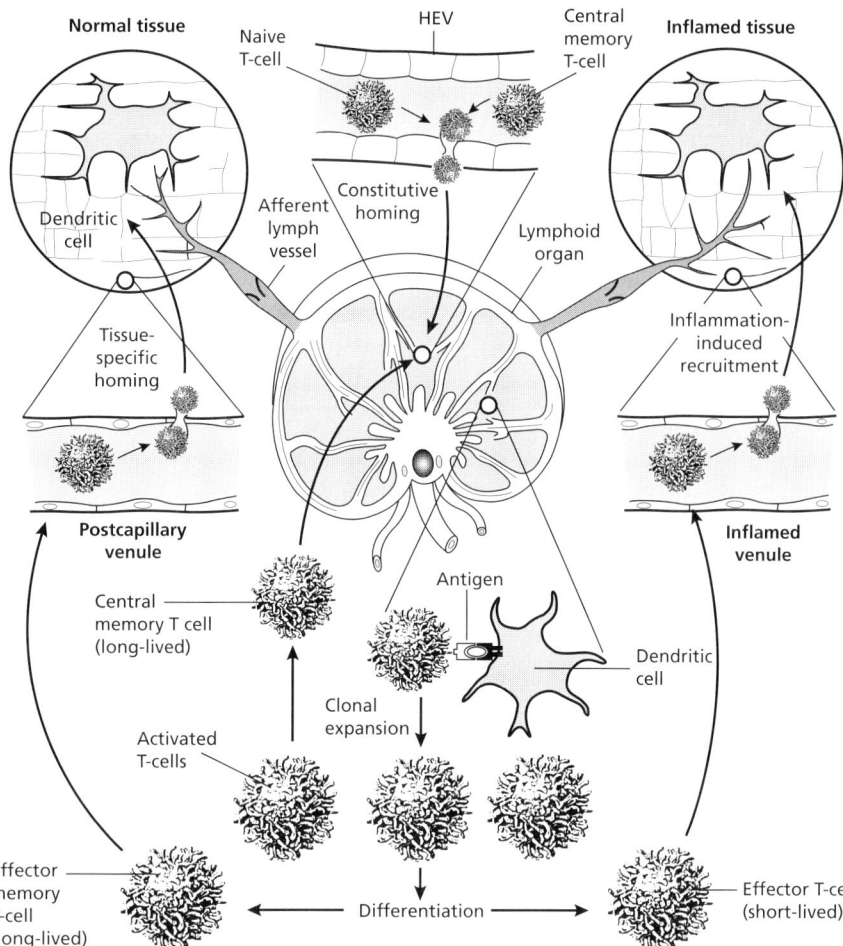

Fig. 3.4 Migration of naive and memory T cells. Naive T cells (top center) adhere to high-endothelial venules in lymph nodes and then percolate through the lymph node to efferent lymphatics leading to the thoracic duct where they return to the blood for recirculation. Activated dendritic cells (upper right) migrate to lymph nodes through afferent lymph vessels, where they present antigen to naive T cells (bottom center). During activation and clonal expansion, naive T cells differentiate into short-lived effector T cells that migrate directly to inflamed tissues (upper right). The response to antigen also gives rise to long-lived effector memory T cells that patrol tissues through specific homing mechanisms (upper left). Activated T cells also give rise to long-lived central memory T cells with migratory behavior resembling that of naive T cells. Adapted from von Andrian and Mackay [29] with permission. Copyright (2000), Massachusetts Medical Society. All rights reserved.

followed by regression as the antigen is cleared. "Memory" T cells emerge from precursors that are distinct from effectors and can be divided into two distinct subsets. The "central" memory population resembles the antigen-inexperienced naive T-cell population, whereas the "effector" memory population resembles the antigen-experienced effector T-cell population. Memory cells are generally characterized by selection for high TCR affinity, increased expression of adhesion molecules and altered migratory patterns with distinctive cytokine production and response profiles, and more rapid turnover when compared to naive cells. Memory cells remain poised to respond quickly after a repeated encounter with antigen. "Secondary" responses by memory cells develop during a period of several days and show greater intensity than the original primary response.

A variety of regulatory T-cell populations have been defined in different experimental systems [43]. In general, these cells originate in the thymus and have distinct cell surface phenotypes. They are activated by specific antigens, but they do not proliferate rapidly after stimulation. They inhibit the response of other cells through nonspecific contact-dependent mechanisms or through the secretion of cytokines such as transforming growth factor beta (TGF-β) and IL-10.

Selection of donors for allogeneic HCT

The immunogenetic relationship between the donor and recipient profoundly influences the outcome of HCT, much more so than with solid organ transplants. Within the constraints of current practice, however, these differences are most apparent when analyzing immunologic outcomes, such as graft rejection and the incidence and severity of GVHD, and are less apparent when analyzing disease-free survival (DFS). Best results are seen after transplantation from HLA-genotypically identical sibling donors, but only 30% of patients have such a donor. Some patients without an HLA-identical sibling have an HLA-haploidentical family member with limited disparity between the nonshared haplotypes (see Chapter 82). Previous studies have shown that patients receiving an HLA-haploidentical transplant incompatible for a single HLA-A, -B or -DR antigen can have DFS similar to that of patients with marrow from HLA-genotypically identical siblings donors (see Chapter 82). Patients receiving transplants incompatible at two or three of these loci have a significantly lower probability of survival (see Chapter 82).

HCT from HLA-phenotypically matched unrelated donors is an alternative for patients who lack a donor in the family (see Chapter 83). Unrelated HCT has been made feasible by the development of large registries of HLA-typed individuals willing to serve as hematopoietic cell donors. With registries currently available in the USA and in other countries, it is now possible to identify an HLA-A, B-phenotypically matched DRB1 allele-matched unrelated donor for at least 70% of patients [44]. If a single HLA-A, -B or -DRB1 disparity were allowed, then it would be possible to identify a donor for many more patients. Under certain circumstances, DFS for patients with HLA-A, -B, -C, -DRB1 and -DQB1 allele-matched unrelated donors may be comparable to that for similar patients with HLA-genotypically identical sibling donors (see Chapter 83).

Outcomes influenced by genetic disparity between the donor and recipient

Engraftment

Graft rejection after HCT may be manifested as either the lack of initial engraftment or the development of pancytopenia and marrow aplasia after initial engraftment. In humans, rejection, drug toxicity, sepsis and certain viral infections can all cause graft failure. The key findings that support a diagnosis of rejection in a patient with graft failure are the absence of donor cells and the presence of recipient T cells. The durable persistence of donor cells makes rejection unlikely, even when recipient T cells can be detected.

Experiments in animal models have demonstrated that both NK cells and T cells can mediate allogeneic marrow graft rejection [45]. Briefly summarized, NK-mediated rejection does not involve immunologic priming and occurs within 1–2 days after transplantation. The effectors have a life span of less than 1 week but are highly resistant to irradiation. In rodents, NK-mediated rejection can be overcome by treatment of the recipient with cyclophosphamide (CY) before the transplant [46]. Because NK precursors are sensitive to irradiation, NK-mediated rejection can also be overcome by split dose irradiation of the recipient, with an interval of 1 week between two irradiation exposures. Rejection mediated by unprimed T cells does not occur until 7–8 days after transplantation. Rejection by T cells can be enhanced by priming or transfusion-induced sensitization before the transplant. T-cell effectors have a longer life span than NK cells and are generally more sensitive to radiation than NK cells. Experiments in animal models can be established in ways that allow recipient NK cells, T cells or both to be involved in causing marrow graft rejection.

Mechanisms by which recipient NK cells or T cells might cause marrow graft rejection have not been fully elucidated. Although it seems intuitively obvious that cell-mediated cytotoxicity might be involved, recipients deficient in perforin, granzyme-B or FasL function can reject an allogeneic marrow graft [47–50]. These results indicate redundancy in the mechanisms by which recipient effectors can kill donor hematopoietic cells. This hypothesis was supported by observations that NK cells from certain strains of mice could not mediate marrow graft rejection when perforin and FasL-mediated mechanisms of cytotoxicity were both absent [51]. Because hematopoietic stem cells do not express Fas under steady-state conditions, any potential involvement of a FasL-mediated mechanism in marrow graft rejection would require the induction of Fas expression, possibly through exposure to IFN-γ or TNF-α. Alternatively, TNF-α released by CTLs or NK cells could have a direct suppressive or cytotoxic effect on hematopoietic stem cells.

The increased risk of rejection associated with transfusion-induced sensitization and the decreased risk of rejection associated with the use of higher levels of total body irradiation (TBI) before the transplant clearly implicate recipient T cells as effectors that can mediate HCT rejection in humans. In support of this hypothesis, recipient-derived T cells with anti-donor HLA-specific cytotoxic activity have been isolated from the blood of patients with graft failure after HLA-mismatched HCT. A delayed onset of rejection and an occurrence of rejection after grafting from an HLA-identical donor would argue against a role for NK cells in causing rejection. NK-mediated rejection also seems unlikely among patients who have received high-dose CY before the transplant, if it is assumed that this agent has similar effects on human and murine NK cells. Studies have not yet determined whether NK cells can reject NK-incompatible grafts in humans when the conditioning regimen does not include CY.

The risk of graft failure depends on the degree of genetic disparity between the donor and recipient. In particular, graft failure has been associated with HLA class I disparity after unrelated marrow transplantation [52]. The association between HLA class I disparity and graft failure has been observed primarily among patients with chronic myeloid leukemia (CML) and other diseases that are not treated with intensive chemotherapy before referral for transplant. The risk of graft rejection is also greatly increased by transfusion or pregnancy-induced alloimmunization of the recipient against the donor before the transplant. Alloimmunization presumably occurs when a fetus or transfusion donor happens to have transplantation antigens in common with the donor. Sensitization of the recipient against some alloantigens can be detected by the presence of antibodies that recognize donor T cells or B cells. After sensitization, rejection may be caused either by memory T cells that survive the conditioning regimen or by antibody-mediated destruction of donor cells.

The use of more intensive conditioning regimens can reduce the risk of rejection by eliminating a greater proportion of recipient T cells before the transplant. Post-transplant administration of immunosuppressive agents such as methotrexate (MTX) [53] and possibly CSP decreases the risk of rejection by interfering with the function of recipient cells that survive the conditioning regimen. Donor T cells can also play a critical role in preventing rejection primarily by recognizing any surviving recipient T cells and eliminating them through a perforin-mediated cytotoxic mechanism [54]. Under certain experimental conditions, donor NK cells and T cells that do not cause GVHD can prevent rejection.

A variety of methods can be used to produce mixed reconstitution with both donor and recipient marrow cells after nonmyeloablative conditioning in animals and humans (see Chapters 85 & 86). These methods generally include pretransplant conditioning with an amount of TBI or busulfan (BU) that is sufficient to ablate a significant fraction of hematopoietic stem cells in the recipient, together with the administration of immunosuppressive agents to prevent rejection. In animals, rejection can be prevented by administration of agents that block costimulation of T cells after the transplant, resulting in durable mixed chimerism [32,55–58]. In humans, a pretransplant regimen of low-dose BU or TBI and the immunosuppressive nucleoside analog fludarabine is sufficient to prevent rejection of an MHC-match graft if the graft contains T cells and if immunosuppressive medications are administered after the transplant. After engraftment has been established, the immunosuppressive medications can be withdrawn, permitting donor T cells to eliminate residual hematopoietic cells and T cells of the recipient, thereby converting mixed chimerism to full donor chimerism. In some ways, this type of transplant resembles a controlled form of transfusion-induced GVHD, where the primary targets of the disease are recipient hematopoietic cells and T cells. In this case, hematopoietic cells in the graft prevent marrow failure and death.

Acute GVHD

The development of GVHD represents a major determinant of outcome after allogeneic HCT (see Chapter 50). This complication is initiated by donor T cells that recognize recipient alloantigens (see Chapters 26 & 27). Donor CD8 cells are activated when there is recipient disparity for MHC class I antigens and also when disparate peptides or mHAs of the recipient are presented by MHC class I molecules that are identical between the donor and recipient. Donor CD4 cells are activated when there is recipient disparity for MHC class II antigens and also when disparate peptides or mHAs are presented by MHC class II molecules that are identical between the donor and recipient.

Donor T cells are strongly activated by alloantigens directly expressed by recipient APCs that remain after the pretransplant conditioning regimen [59–63]. MHC class I molecules on donor dendritic cells can "cross-present" exogenous peptides acquired though phagocytosis of necrotic cells [24,64], but results with one well-studied donor-recipient strain combination suggest that this indirect pathway for presentation of mHAs to CD8 cells does not play a prominent role in the pathogenesis of GVHD [65,66]. Activation of donor CD4 cells also occurs through recognition of MHC class II alloantigens on recipient APCs [67], since tissues outside the hematopoietic system ordinarily do not express MHC class II molecules at high levels. Donor CD4 cells might also be activated by recipient minor antigens indirectly expressed by donor APCs.

The pretransplant conditioning regimen greatly increases susceptibility of the recipient to GVHD. Within as little as 6 h after irradiation, dendritic cells increase their expression of CD86, initiating the maturation process that resembles activation by alarm signals from an innate immune response [66]. The initial activation of donor cells induced by alloantigens on mature recipient dendritic cells occurs as early as 24 h after the transplant and is followed by rapid, IL-2-dependent clonal proliferation and differentiation into effectors. Proliferation and differentiation of activated donor T cells can be maintained in the absence of recipient dendritic cells.

During the effector phase of GVHD, activated T cells from both the CD4 and CD8 subsets produce proinflammatory cytokines, and both subsets also generate CTLs. No single effector mechanism can account for the entire clinical spectrum of acute GVHD (see Chapters 26, 27 & 50). In some patients, the disease presents as a syndrome of high-grade fever, confluent erythematous rash, and vascular leak with pulmonary infiltrates and edema during the first 10 days after the transplant. In this situation, the disease can be viewed appropriately as a "cytokine storm" [68] that generally shows striking improvement after treatment with high-dose glucocorticoids. In most patients, however, the disease presents in much less dramatic fashion with a slowly progressive morbilliform rash or with anorexia, nausea and vomiting. Whether cytokine storm plays a role in these more typical cases of acute GVHD without overt systemic toxicity remains to be determined.

Events leading to cytokine storm include epithelial damage to the gastrointestinal tract, which facilitates translocation of endotoxin into the blood stream [69,70]. Macrophages that have been primed by alloactivated T cells show exquisite sensitivity to endotoxin, producing inflammatory cytokines such as TNF-α and IL-1, which contribute to tissue injury [69,71–74]. Primed macrophages also produce nitric oxide, which depletes iron from epithelial cells, causing a cytostatic effect that exacerbates tissue injury [75]. Nitric oxide also contributes to immunosuppression associated with GVHD. Administration of antibodies that neutralize TNF-α and IL-1 can prevent early death related to severe GVHD following very high TBI exposure in mice [67]. In humans, however, attempts to neutralize these cytokines individually have not produced any major clinical benefit [76].

Cytokines play complex roles in the pathogenesis of GVHD. For example, activated T cells produce IFN-γ, which makes macrophages highly sensitive to stimulation by endotoxin [69]. On the other hand, GVHD is exacerbated by the neutralization of IFN-γ and by the use of donor T cells that cannot produce IFN-γ [77–79]. These results suggest that IFN-γ actually has a protective role in mice with acute GVHD (see below). Some studies have suggested that GVHD is more severe when caused by T cells polarized to produce type 1 cytokines as compared to type 2 cytokines. It is now clear that both cell types contribute to the pathogenesis of GVHD, although with different patterns of organ involvement in mice [80,81]. Type 1 cells cause intestinal pathology, whereas type 2 cells cause pathologic changes in the skin, gut and liver. The presence of eosinophils in duodenal biopsies from patients with GVHD supports the involvement of type 2 cells in the pathogenesis of the disease [82].

Cell-mediated cytotoxic mechanisms clearly contribute to the pathogenesis of GVHD, particularly in recipients prepared with lower amounts of TBI [83]. In mice, GVHD is less severe when induced by perforin-deficient donor T cells as compared to wild type donor T cells [84,85]. In a model of GVHD caused by disparity for mHAs, recipients transplanted with FasL-deficient donor T cells developed cachexia, but inflammatory lesions in the skin and liver were absent, and the profound B-lymphoid hypoplasia associated with GVHD did not occur. The severity of hepatic GVHD was reduced in Fas-deficient recipients, but the severity of GVHD in other organs was increased [86]. Neutralization of FasL prevented hepatic lesions in wild-type recipients but had no effect on intestinal GVHD, while neutralization of TNF-α improved intestinal GVHD but had no effect on hepatic GVHD [87]. Neutralization of both FasL and TNF-α prevented GVHD in all organs. These results suggest that the mechanisms leading to tissue damage vary among different organs.

Cytokines and cell-mediated mechanisms of cytotoxicity interact to regulate the severity of GVHD. Triggering of Fas on recipient cells by FasL on donor cells causes production of IL-18 through a caspase-1-dependent mechanism [88]. IL-18, in turn, increases expression of Fas on donor T cells, making these cells susceptible to FasL-mediated apoptosis in the presence of IFN-γ [89]. The absence of IL-18 production might explain the paradoxically increased severity of GVHD in the skin and intestinal tract of Fas-deficient recipients [86]. A reduced susceptibility of donor T cells to FasL-mediated apoptosis might explain the increased severity of GVHD caused by IFN-γ-deficient T cells [77,79]. Likewise, administration of IL-12 or IFN-γ to recipients after the transplant might decrease the severity of GVHD by increasing the susceptibility of donor T cells to FasL-mediated apoptosis [90].

Under certain conditions, activated donor NK cells have been shown to reduce the severity of GVHD. Mechanisms proposed to explain this effect include production of TGF-β or IL-4 by donor NK cells or rapid elimination of recipient dendritic cells by donor NK cells after the transplant [91–93]. Donor $CD25^+CD4^+$ regulatory T cells can also reduce the severity of GVHD in mice [94–96]. GVHD can be ameliorated by adding large numbers of regulatory T cells to the graft and exacerbated by removal of these cells from the graft. The ability of regulatory T cells to prevent GVHD was partly mediated by their ability to produce IL-10.

Clinical studies have shown that the risk of acute GVHD depends primarily on the degree of genetic disparity between the recipient and donor. The risk of GVHD is greater with unrelated donors than with related donors, both because of unavoidable MHC disparity and an increased probability of minor antigen disparity with unrelated donors. In North American populations, the risk of GVHD is increased more by a single HLA class II disparity than by a single HLA class I disparity [97]. In Japanese populations, HLA-A, -B, -C and -DRB1 disparities are associated with similarly increased risks of GVHD [98]. In both populations, the risk of GVHD is higher with multiple disparities than with a single disparity. Alloimmunization of the donor by prior pregnancy or possibly by transfusion has also been associated with an increased risk of GVHD, probably caused by "memory" T cells with specificity for antigens shared by the fetus or transfusion donor and the transplant recipient. GVHD might also be exacerbated when T cells recognize alloantigens having epitopes that resemble those produced by certain pathogens [99].

The type of post-transplant immunosuppression and compliance with the prophylactic regimen influence the risk of GVHD. The most effective regimens currently in widespread use include a calcineurin inhibitor (CSP or tacrolimus) combined with MTX (see Chapter 16). Multidrug regimens are more effective than single-drug regimens. Acute GVHD can be prevented by removing mature T cells from the donor marrow (see Chapter 17). In HLA-identical recipients given no post-transplant immunosuppression, the incidence of grades II–IV acute GVHD can be decreased from ≥80% with unmodified marrow to ≤20% when >98% of T cells are removed. The benefit brought about by a reduced risk of GVHD, however, is offset by increased risks of graft failure and recurrent leukemia and by delayed immune reconstitution (see below). For this reason, removal of T cells from the donor marrow to prevent GVHD has not appreciably improved DFS after the transplant.

Research studies are attempting to determine whether the donor cells that cause GVHD can be distinguished from those needed to prevent rejection, eliminate malignant progenitors or initiate immune reconstitution. In the past, most clinical trials have employed methods aimed at global T-cell depletion, even though GVHD is initiated by the relatively small subset of donor cells that recognize recipient histocompatibility antigens. In the future, it may be possible to prevent GVHD by specific depletion of donor T cells that recognize recipient alloantigens [100–105], by interference with costimulatory signals needed for optimal activation [106–113] or by infusion of regulatory T cells. In addition, the severity of GVHD might also be decreased with the use of agents that protect gastrointestinal integrity after the conditioning regimen [114] or by neutralizing endotoxin and other agents that activate innate immunity [115].

Chronic GVHD

The biological mechanisms leading to chronic GVHD are not as well understood as those leading to acute GVHD, and the relationship between acute and chronic GVHD is not entirely clear. Although acute GVHD has been recognized as a risk factor for chronic GVHD, not all cases of acute GVHD evolve into chronic GVHD, and chronic GVHD can develop in the absence of any prior overt acute GVHD. In the skin, the initial phase of chronic GVHD is characterized by an intense mononuclear inflammatory infiltrate with destructive changes at the dermal–epidermal junction, accompanied by irregular acanthosis, hyperkeratosis or atrophy. Evolution of the disease is characterized by increasing dermal fibrosis, ultimately resulting in dermal sclerosis (see Chapter 23). Other pathognomonic hallmarks of chronic GVHD include destruction of tubuloalveolar glands and ducts in the skin, salivary and lacrimal glands and respiratory epithelium, and destruction of bile ducts in the liver.

A "chronic GVHD" syndrome resembling systemic lupus erythematosis in mice has been extensively studied, but the manifestations of this disease differ from chronic GVHD in humans [116]. Chronic GVHD characterized by cutaneous scleroderma has been described with a limited number of donor–recipient strain combinations. In one carefully studied model, skin thickening and deposition of type-1 collagen was preceded by infiltration with donor T cells and activated macrophages that had increased expression of TGF-β_1 [117]. In this model, the development of fibrosis could be prevented by administration of a neutralizing antibody against TGF-β.

Graft-vs.-leukemia effects

Myelosuppression represents the dose-limiting toxicity of many agents used for the treatment of malignancy. By circumventing this limitation, HCT allows the administration of chemotherapy and irradiation at doses two-to-threefold higher than would otherwise be possible. It has been recognized, however, that the therapeutic advantage of allogeneic HCT results not only from the ability to deliver more intensive treatment but also from antineoplastic effects mediated by the graft (see Chapters 28 & 29). Clinical evidence for a graft-vs.-leukemia effect (GVLE) came initially from retrospective observations that leukemic relapse occurred less frequently in patients who developed GVHD compared to those who did not [118].

Other clinical observations have supported the concept that certain cells in an allogeneic marrow graft can help to eliminate malignant cells that survive the conditioning regimen. Removal of T cells in the donor marrow has been associated with an increased risk of relapse. The risk of relapse after T-cell-depleted marrow transplantation for acute leukemia is comparable to the risk in patients who do not develop GVHD after transplantation with unmodified marrow [119]. Thus, the increased risk of relapse associated with T-cell depletion in patients with acute leukemia could simply reflect a decreased incidence of GVHD. These data suggest that the occurrence of GVHD *per se* can have an antileukemic effect. Removal of T cells from the graft causes a strikingly increased risk of recurrent malignancy among patients with a pretransplant diagnosis of CML. Multivariate analyses have shown that the increased relapse risk cannot be explained entirely by a decreased incidence of GVHD [120]. In patients with CML, donor T cells may therefore exert an antileukemic effect that is independent of overt GVHD.

Efforts to gain a therapeutic advantage from interventions designed to increase GVLEs have had mixed success. Among patients with high-risk malignancies, the administration of nonirradiated peripheral blood buffy coat cells from the marrow donor during the first 4 days after transplantation caused an unacceptably high risk of GVHD and transplant-related mortality [121]. Among patients who have recurrent malignancy after transplantation, remissions can occasionally be induced simply by stopping the administration of immunosuppressive medications. In patients who do not have GVHD, remissions can be more reliably induced by infusion of donor lymphocytes (see Chapter 84) [122,123]. Remissions are most often induced in patients with CML in chronic phase, myeloma or myelodysplasia. Remissions occur much less frequently in patients with acute leukemia. GVHD and transient marrow aplasia are frequent complications of donor lymphocyte infusions.

Multiple mechanisms are likely to account for the antileukemic effects associated with GVHD. Thus alloantigens expressed by malignant cells can serve as direct targets for GVHD effector cells, or GVHD may activate other effectors such as NK cells and lymphokine-activated killer cells that have cytotoxic activity against leukemic cells [124]. Finally, certain cytokines elaborated during GVHD may have effects on the proliferation and differentiation of malignant cells. From a clinical standpoint, the central question is whether GVLEs can be separated from GVHD. Studies with mice have suggested that perforin and TNF-α-mediated cytotoxic mechanisms might have particular importance for GVLEs [125,126]. FasL-mediated cytotoxic mechanisms were neither necessary nor sufficient for activity against the tumors used for testing in mice. On the other hand, it is of interest that donor CD4 cells appear to have a prominent role in control of CML in humans [127]. Since perforin does not play a dominant role in the cytotoxic activity of CD4 cells, these results suggest that perforin-independent mechanisms might be important for GVLEs in patients with CML.

With new insights gained from ongoing laboratory research, future clinical trials might demonstrate the feasibility of manipulating the immune system to prevent leukemic relapse without increasing the morbidity and mortality caused by GVHD [102,128]. Donor NK cells or NK-T cells might be especially well suited for this purpose [124,129]. Alternatively, it might be possible to produce GVLEs through the use of donor-derived T cells that recognize mHAs of the recipient [130] or other antigens selectively expressed by malignant cells of the recipient [131,132]. At late time points after the transplant, when large numbers of recipient dendritic cells are no longer present, infusion of donor effector cells that recognize minor antigens with expression limited to lymphoid or hematopoietic cells of the recipient might also produce potent antitumor effects without causing GVHD (see Chapter 29).

Development of tolerance

GVHD is caused entirely by the progeny of mature donor T cells in the graft at the time of transplant, and rejection is caused entirely by the progeny of recipient T cells that survive the conditioning regimen. T cells that develop in the recipient thymus after HCT do not cause acute GVHD or rejection. Those that express receptors for recipient alloantigens are eliminated or induced into anergy through interactions with thymic epithelial cells. Any marrow-derived dendritic cells of the recipient that survive in the thymus after the transplant can also help to eliminate developing T cells that recognize recipient alloantigens. The presence of donor marrow-derived dendritic cells in the thymus prevents the development of T cells that could recognize and destroy the graft. The failure of negative selection mechanisms in the thymus might allow development of cells that recognize MHC class II antigens, thereby causing chronic GVHD [133]. In the absence of chronic GVHD, prophylactic immunosuppressive treatment can be discontinued without complications.

Donor-derived T helper and T cytotoxic cells that recognize recipient alloantigens can be detected by *in vitro* assays in all patients after allogeneic HCT regardless of whether clinically evident GVHD has occurred or not [134,135]. Characteristics that determine the extent of immunologic injury caused by these cells have not been defined. To some extent, donor T cells that recognize recipient alloantigens must be subject to the same mechanisms that induce peripheral tolerance in autoreactive T cells that emerge from the thymus. Induction of anergy, development of regulatory cells or suppressor cells, and activation-induced cell death or clonal exhaustion are possible mechanisms that prevent or limit the immunologic injury that would otherwise be caused by donor T cells that recognize recipient alloantigens [136,137]. Inflammatory mediators present at the time of the transplant can interfere with induction of tolerance in donor T cells that recognize recipient alloantigens [138].

In the future, HCT may be developed as a method for facilitating transplantation of other tissues from the same donor (see Chapter 24). In one experimental approach, mature T cells in the recipient are depleted through the administration of antibodies before the transplant. Donor T cells administered as part of the graft help to inactivate or eliminate any remaining recipient T cells that can recognize donor alloantigens [139,140]. Negative selection by marrow-derived cells and epithelial cells in the thymus ensures that T cells developing after the transplant are tolerant of histocompatibility antigens of both the donor and the recipient. The presence of donor marrow-derived cells in the recipient thymus is sufficient to prevent the development of T cells that could recognize a solid organ graft from the same donor, and complete elimination of recipient marrow cells is not necessary. In fact, complete elimination of recipient marrow cells could have deleterious effects on immune reconstitution unless the donor and recipient had some degree of MHC-compatibility so that T cells positively selected by interactions with MHC molecules on the thymic epithelium can recognize antigens presented by the same MHC molecules on peripheral dendritic cells. Preservation of recipient marrow cells together with the donor marrow allows complete MHC incompatibility between the donor and recipient without jeopardizing immune function after the transplant, thereby considerably broadening the availability of donors.

Immune reconstitution

Pathways of T-cell reconstitution

After HCT, all patients develop profound immunodeficiency as a consequence of the preparative regimen, the effects of donor T cells and the administration of immunosuppressive medications. Reconstitution with donor cells corrects this immunodeficiency (see Chapter 62). Reconstitution of T cells can occur both through thymus-independent expansion of the mature T-cell population in the graft and through maturation of marrow-derived cells in the recipient thymus [141,142]. Clinical and experimental studies have indicated that initial reconstitution of T cells after transplantation occurs primarily through proliferation of mature donor T cells in the graft [143–145], and the contribution of new T cells from the thymus becomes apparent later. Production of new T cells in the thymus persists throughout life but declines gradually with age [146].

Irradiation and GVHD impair recovery of thymic function after the transplant, with more profound effects in adults than in children [147–149]. The thymic pathway of T-cell reconstitution is more important for recovery of CD4 cells than for CD8 cells [145,150]. For these reasons, the balance between contributions from the thymus-independent and thymus-dependent pathways of T-cell reconstitution depends on the age of the patient, the number of T cells in the graft, the time interval from transplant, and the expression of CD4 or CD8.

The time for restoration varies for different components and functions of the immune system. In recipients transplanted with unmodified marrow from an HLA-identical sibling, proliferative responses to phytohemagglutinin begin to reach the normal range after approximately 4–6 months; the number of peripheral blood CD4 cells begins to reach the normal range after 7–9 months; and production of immunoglobulin G as measured by *in vitro* assays recovers after 7–9 months. Recovery of immune responses is delayed by several months in recipients transplanted with T-cell-depleted marrow [151,152], and recovery of CD4 cells is accelerated when hematopoietic growth factor-mobilized stem cells are used for transplantation [153,154]. Long-term reconstitution of immunity against certain pathogens probably represents the acquisition of new memory cells generated by exposure to antigens after the transplant.

During the first 3 months after HCT, selective proliferation among different T cells in the thymus-independent pathway of reconstitution causes severe skewing in the distribution of TCRs among repopulating T cells [155,156]. During this time, the spectrum of *TCR* gene rearrangements remains abnormally limited and unstable. Changes in the T-cell repertoire during this period of time most likely result from antigen-driven proliferation, especially in patients with GVHD [157].

Naive T cells produced through the thymus-dependent pathway of reconstitution have a normal spectrum of TCR gene rearrangements. Throughout the first 3 years after the transplant, progeny of mature T cells in the graft are gradually replaced by T cells that originated through maturation of marrow cells in the thymus [157]. With this replacement, the spectrum of *TCR* gene rearrangements gradually becomes normal. The rate at which the spectrum of *TCR* gene rearrangements returns to normal depends on the number of mature T cells in the graft and the level of thymic function. Thymus-dependent dilutional replacement of cells that originated from the thymus-independent pathway would be expected to occur more slowly with grafts that contain a large number of mature T cells and more rapidly with grafts that contain small numbers of mature T cells [158,159]. Abnormalities in the spectrum of *TCR* gene rearrangements can persist for more than 3 years in patients with severely impaired thymic function. For reasons that are not yet clear, the spectrum of *TCR* gene rearrangements also remains abnormal in patients with persistent mixed chimerism, even in the absence of GVHD [155]. The diversity of immunoglobulin gene rearrangements in B cells is also reduced after HCT. One mechanism for this effect is related to an abnormally low rate of somatic mutation in rearranged immunoglobulin genes during B-cell development after HCT [160].

Effects of GVHD on immune reconstitution

GVHD impairs T cell immune reconstitution through at least four distinct mechanisms. First, GVHD causes injury to thymic epithelium [148], thereby reducing T-cell reconstitution and diversification of the TCR repertoire through the thymus-dependent pathway. Second, GVHD decreases the total number of T cells that can be accommodated within the periphery, perhaps by causing microenvironmental abnormalities that reduce the number of functional peripheral T-cell niches [161]. Third, stimulation by recipient alloantigen induces expression of FasL and Fas, resulting in activation-induced apoptosis in a large fraction of donor T cells that recognize recipient alloantigens [162]. Fourth, during GVHD, donor T cells that do not recognize recipient alloantigens are induced to express Fas and become susceptible to fratricidal or bystander apoptosis caused by donor T cells that express FasL [162]. Both acute and chronic GVHD block B lymphopoiesis. Patients with chronic GVHD do not develop immunocompetence until chronic GVHD resolves [163].

Opportunistic infections as an indicator of impaired immune reconstitution

Opportunistic infections are a key clinical indicator of immunodeficiency after HCT. Pathogens involved in opportunistic infections prominently include the Epstein–Barr virus (EBV) (see Chapter 56), cytomegalovirus (CMV) (see Chapter 53), adenovirus (see Chapter 57) and fungal organisms (see Chapter 52). The development of lymphoproliferative disorders caused by EBV infection is a particularly striking example of opportunistic infection associated with immunodeficiency after HCT. The risk of this often-fatal complication is increased among adults who receive a T-cell-depleted graft from an unrelated donor followed by immunosuppression with antithymocyte globulin and steroids after the transplant [164,165]. Risk factors for CMV infection, fungal infection [166] and adenovirus infection [167] are very similar. Prolonged lymphopenia represents a common thread among these risk factors. In particular, CD4 lymphopenia has been strongly correlated with the risk of opportunistic infections after HCT [152,168]. In addition, more subtle abnormalities of T-cell function are likely to increase the risk of opportunistic infections. Examples include qualitative defects in T-cell signal transduction [169] and reduced production of TNF-α by activated CMV-specific CD8 cells [170].

Approaches for enhancement of immune reconstitution

Under certain conditions, EBV-specific immunity can be reconstituted and regression of EBV-associated lymphoproliferative disorders can be induced by infusion of a relatively small number of donor lymphocytes [171]. Alternatively, immune responses against specific pathogens can be reconstituted by infusion of antigen-specific T-cell lines [172] or T-cell clones (see Chapter 29). Immune reconstitution might also be accelerated through a variety of other strategies. Administration of keratinocyte growth factor has been shown to protect thymic epithelium from the effects of irradiation and GVHD, thereby improving immune reconstitution through the thymus-dependent pathway after the transplant [173,174]. Thymic epithelium is a source of IL-7, a growth factor involved in production of T cells and maintenance of T-cell homeostasis in the periphery [175]. Exogenous administration of this cytokine does not reverse the effects of GVHD on thymic stromal function but can enhance T-cell production through direct effects on T cells as they develop in the thymus [176]. IL-7 can also increase the number of T cells and enhance T-cell function through direct effects on peripheral T cells [176,177]. The potential effects of IL-7 on GVHD are still under study [178,179]. Finally, administration of synthetic oligodeoxynucleotides containing unmethylated cytosine-guanine motifs can expand naive and memory populations by preventing T-cell death [180].

In most recipients without chronic GVHD, immunologic function has recovered sufficiently to allow responses after administration of diphtheria, pertussis and tetanus vaccine and pneumococcal vaccine at 1 year after HCT (see Chapter 63) [181]. To some extent, antigen-experienced donor T cells contribute to this immune reconstitution, and responses in the recipient after the transplant can be enhanced by vaccination of the donor before the transplant [182]. Administration of live viral vaccines, such as measles, mumps, rubella and oral polio, is deferred until at least 2 years after transplantation, even in healthy recipients, as a precaution to avoid inadvertent infection with these attenuated strains. These vaccines should not be given to patients with chronic GVHD or to anyone taking immunosuppressive medications.

Summary and conclusions

Although this overview of the immunology of HCT has focused on the individual outcomes of engraftment, GVHD, control of malignancy, tolerance and immune reconstitution, these remain highly interconnected as different aspects of a single overall process. For this reason, the evaluation of interventions designed to influence one particular immunologic outcome of HCT will require equivalent scrutiny of other immunologic outcomes. Historically, clinical HCT has evolved from the biomedical knowledge and understanding gained from animal studies. Murine models have the advantages of well-defined immunogenetics and a wealth of reagents for dissecting the cellular and humoral mechanisms involved in HCT immunobiology, while canine and nonhuman-primate models more closely mimic the immunological and medical challenges of HCT in a large outbred species. The wide range of experimental manipulations afforded by animal models has enabled rapid progress in the biomedical understanding of HCT immunology in all of its interconnected complexity. These insights provide a rational foundation for the ongoing development of HCT as a therapeutic modality in humans.

References

1 http://www.anthonynolan.org.uk/HIG
2 Klein JK, Sato A. The HLA system. First of two parts. *N Engl J Med* 2000; **343**: 702–9.
3 Madden DR. The three-dimensional structure of peptide-MHC complexes. *Annu Rev Immunol* 1995; **13**: 587–622.
4 Shastri N, Schwab S, Serwold T. Producing nature's gene-chips: the generation of peptides for display by MHC class I molecules. *Annu Rev Immunol* 2002; **20**: 463–93.
5 Robinson JH, Delvig AA. Diversity in MHC class II antigen presentation. *Immunol* 2002; **105**: 252–62.
6 Germain RN. MHC-dependent antigen processing and peptide presentation: providing ligands for T lymphocyte activation. *Cell* 1994; **76**: 287–99.
7 Joyce S, Nathenson SG. Alloreactivity, antigen recognition and T-cell selection: three diverse T-cell recognition problems with a common solution. *Immunol Rev* 1996; **154**: 59–103.
8 Perreault C, Decary F, Brochu S, Gyger M, Belanger R, Roy D. Minor histocompatibility antigens. *Blood* 1990; **76**: 1269–80.
9 Simpson E, Scott D, James E et al. Minor H antigens: genes and peptides. *Eur J Immunogenet* 2001; **28**: 505–13.
10 Medzhitov R, Janeway C. Innate Immunity. *N Engl J Med* 2000; **343**: 338–44.
11 Matzinger P. Tolerance, danger, and the extended family. *Annu Rev Immunol* 1994; **12**: 991–1045.
12 Farag SS, Fehinger TA, Ruggeri L, Velardi A, Caligiuri MA. Natural killer cell receptors. New biology and insights into the graft versus leukemia effect. *Blood* 2002; **100**: 1935–47.
13 Delves PJ, Roitt IM. The immune system. First of two parts. *N Engl J Med* 2000; **343**: 37–49.
14 Renard V, Cambiaggi A, Vely F et al. Transduction of cytotoxic signals in natural killer cells: a general model of fine tuning between activatory and inhibitory pathways in lymphocytes. *Immunol Rev* 1997; **155**: 205–21.
15 Vukmanovic S. The molecular jury: deciding whether immature thymocytes should live or die. *J Exp Med* 1996; **84**: 305–9.
16 Goldrath AW, Bevan MJ. Selecting and maintaining a diverse T-cell repertoire. *Nature* 1999; **402**: 255–62.
17 van Meerwijk JPM, Marguerat S, Lees RK, Germain RN, Fowlkes BJ, MacDonald HR. Quantitative impact of thymic clonal deletion on the T-cell repertoire. *J Exp Med* 1997; **185**: 377–83.
18 Vandekerckhove BA, Namikawa R, Bacchetta R, Roncarolo MG. Human hematopoietic cells and thymic epithelial cells induce tolerance via different mechanisms in the SCID-hu thymus. *J Exp Med* 1992; **175**: 1033–43.
19 Jordan MS, Boesteanu A, Reed AJ et al. Thymic selection of CD4$^+$CD25$^+$ regulatory T cells induced

by an agonist self-peptide. *Nat Immunol* 2001; **2**: 283–4.

20 Bensinger SJ, Bandeira A, Jordan MS, Caton AJ, Laufer TM. Major histocompatibility complex class II-positive cortical epithelium mediates the election of CD4+25+ immunoregulatory T cells. *J Exp Med* 2001; **194**: 427–38.

21 Kamradt T, Mitchison NA. Tolerance and autoimmunity. *N Engl J Med* 2001; **344**: 655–64.

22 Lechler R, Ng WF, Steinman RM. Dendritic cells in transplantation: friend or foe? *Immunity* 2001; **14**: 357–68.

23 Steinman RM, Nussenzweig MC. Avoiding horror autotoxicus. The importance of dendritic cells in peripheral T cell tolerance. *Proc Nat Acad Sci U S A* 2002; **99**: 351–8.

24 Sauter B, Albert ML, Francisco L, Larsson M, Somersan S, Bhardwaj N. Consequences of cell death: exposure to necrotic tumor cells, but not primary tissue cells or apoptotic cells, induces the maturation of immunostimulatory dendritic cells. *J Exp Med* 2000; **191**: 423–34.

25 Huang F-P, Platt N, Wykes M *et al*. A discrete subpopulation of dendritic cells transports apoptotic intestinal epithelial cells to T cell areas of mesenteric lymph nodes. *J Exp Med* 2000; **191**: 435–44.

26 Hawiger D, Inaba K, Dorsett Y *et al*. Dendritic cells induce peripheral T cell unresponsiveness under steady state conditions *in vivo*. *J Exp Med* 2001; **194**: 769–79.

27 Smith PA, Brunmark A, Jackson MR, Potter TA. Peptide-independent recognition by alloreactive cytotoxic T lymphocytes (CTL). *J Exp Med* 1997; **185**: 1023–33.

28 Garcia KC, Teyton L, Wilson IA. Structural basis of T cell recognition. *Annu Rev Immunol* 1999; **17**: 369–97.

29 von Andrian UH, Mackay R. T-cell function and migration. Two sides of the same coin. *N Engl J Med* 2000; **343**: 1020–34.

30 Sayegh MH, Turka LA. The role of T-cell costimulatory activation pathways in transplant rejection. *N Engl J Med* 1998; **338**: 1813–21.

31 Grewal IS, Flavell RA. CD40 and CD154 in cell-mediated immunity. *Annu Rev Immunol* 1998; **16**: 111–35.

32 Lang TJ, Nguyen P, Peach R, Gause WC, Via CS. *In vivo* CD86 blockade inhibits CD4+ T cell activation, whereas CD80 blockade potentiates CD8+ T cell activation and CTL effector function. *J Immunol* 2002; **168**: 3786–92.

33 Lanzavecchia A, Sallusto F. Antigen decoding by T lymphocytes: from synapses to fate determination. *Nat Immunol* 2001; **2**: 487–92.

34 Bromley SK, Burack WR, Johnson KG *et al*. The immunological synapse. *Annu Rev Immunol* 2001; **19**: 375–96.

35 Frauwirth KA, Thompson CB. Activation and inhibition of lymphocytes by costimulation. *J Clin Invest* 2002; **109**: 295–9.

36 Jenkins MK, Khoruts A, Ingulli E *et al*. *In vivo* activation of antigen-specific CD4 T cells. *Annu Rev Immunol* 2001; **19**: 23–45.

37 Li XC, Strom TB, Turka LA, Wells AD. T cell death and transplantation tolerance. *Immunity* 2001; **14**: 407–16.

38 Lechler R, Chai JG, Marelli-Berg F, Lombardi G. The contributions of T-cell anergy to peripheral T-cell tolerance. *Immunology* 2001; **103**: 262–9.

39 Carreno BM, Collins M. The B7 family of ligands and its receptors: new pathways for costimulation and inhibition of immune responses. *Annu Rev Immunol* 2002; **20**: 29–53.

40 Carter LL, Dutton RW. Type 1 and type 2: a fundamental dichotomy for all T-cell subsets. *Curr Opin Immunol* 1996; **8**: 336–42.

41 Russell JH, Ley TJ. Lymphocyte-mediated cytotoxicity. *Annu Rev Immunol* 2002; **20**: 323–70.

42 Sprent J, Surh CD. T cell memory. *Annu Rev Immunol* 2002; **20**: 551–79.

43 Battaglia M, Blazar BR, Roncarolo M-G. The puzzling world of murine regulatory T cells. *Microbes and infection*. 2002; **4**: 559–66.

44 Tiercy JM, Bujan-Lose M, Chapuis B *et al*. Bone marrow transplantation with unrelated donors: what is the probability of identifying an HLA-A/B/Cw/DRB1/B3/B5/DQB1-matched donor? *Bone Marrow Transplant* 2000; **26**: 437–41.

45 Murphy WJ, Kumar V, Bennett M. Acute rejection of murine bone marrow allografts by natural killer cells and T-cells. Differences in kinetics and target antigens recognized. *J Exp Med* 1987; **166**: 1499–509.

46 Cudkowicz G, Bennett M. Peculiar immunobiology of bone marrow allografts. I. Graft rejection by irradiated responder mice. *J Exp Med* 1971; **134**: 83–102.

47 Baker MB, Podack ER, Levy RB. Perforin- and Fas-mediated cytotoxic pathways are not required for allogeneic resistance to bone marrow grafts in mice. *Biol Blood Marrow Transplant* 1995; **1**: 69–73.

48 Aguila HL, Weissman IL. Hematopoietic stem cells are not direct cytotoxic targets of natural killer cells. *Blood* 1996; **87**: 1225–31.

49 Graubert TA, Russel JH, Ley TJ. The role of granzyme B in murine models of acute graft-versus-host disease and graft rejection. *Blood* 1996; **87**: 1232–7.

50 Jones M, Komatsu M, Levy RB. Cytotoxically impaired transplant recipients can efficiently resist major histocompatibility complex–matched bone marrow allografts. *Biol Blood Marrow Transplant* 2000; **6**: 456–64.

51 Taylor MA, Ward B, Schatzle JD, Bennett M. Perforin- and Fas-dependent mechanisms of natural killer cell-mediated rejection of incompatible bone marrow cell grafts. *Eur J Immunol* 2002; **32**: 793–9.

52 Petersdorf EW, Hansen JA, Martin PJ *et al*. Major-histocompatibility-complex class I alleles and antigens in hematopoietic-cell transplantation. *N Engl J Med* 2001; **345**: 1842–4.

53 Deeg HJ, Storb R, Weiden PL *et al*. Cyclosporin A and methotrexate in canine marrow transplantation: engraftment, graft-versus-host disease, and induction of intolerance. *Transplantation* 1982; **34**: 30–5.

54 Martin PJ, Akatsuka Y, Hahne M, Sale G. Involvement of donor T-cell cytotoxic effector mechanisms in preventing allogeneic marrow graft rejection. *Blood* 1988; **92**: 2177–81.

55 Ito H, Kurtz J, Shaffer J, Sykes M. CD4 T cell-mediated alloresistance to fully MHC-mismatched allogeneic bone marrow engraftment is dependent on CD40–CD40 ligand interactions, and lasting T cell tolerance is induced by bone marrow transplantation with initial blockade of this pathway. *J Immunol* 2001; **166**: 2970–81.

56 Adams AB, Durham MM, Kean L *et al*. Costimulation blockade, busulfan, and bone marrow promote titratable macrochimerism, induce transplantation tolerance, and correct genetic hemoglobinopathies with minimal myelosuppression. *J Immunol* 2001; **167**: 1103–11.

57 Kean LS, Durham MM, Adams AB *et al*. A cure for murine sickle cell disease through stable mixed chimerism and tolerance induction after non-myeloablative conditioning and major histocompatibility complex-mismatched bone marrow transplantation. *Blood* 2002; **99**: 1840–9.

58 Taylor PA, Lees CJ, Wilson JM *et al*. The combined effects of calcineurin inhibitors or sirlimus with anti-CD40L mAb on alloengraftment under non-myeloablative conditions. *Blood* 2002; **100**: 3400–7.

59 Hilgard HR, Martinez C, Good RA. Production of runt disease in tolerant mice by the injection of syngeneic lymphoid cells. *J Exp Med* 1965; **122**: 1017–27.

60 Sprent J, Miller JF. Interaction of thymus lymphocytes with histoincompatible cells. I. Quantitation of the proliferative response of thymus cells. *Cellular Immunol* 1972; **3**: 361–84.

61 Steinmuller D, Shelby J. Lymphoid target cell replacement and refractoriness to graft-versus-host disease. *Transplantation* 1980; **30**: 313–4.

62 Mowat AM. Evidence that Ia+ bone-marrow-derived cells are the stimulus for the intestinal phase of the murine graft-versus-host reaction. *Transplantation* 1986; **42**: 141–4.

63 Kosaka H, Surh CD, Sprent J. Stimulation of mature unprimed CD8+ T cells by semiprofessional antigen-presenting cells *in vivo*. *J Exp Med* 1992; **176**: 1291–302.

64 Heath WR, Carbone FR. Cross-presentation, dendritic cells, tolerance and immunity. *Annu Rev Immunol* 2001; **19**: 47–64.

65 Shlomchik WD, Couzens MS, Tang CB *et al*. Prevention of graft versus host disease by inactivation of host antigen-presenting cells. *Science* 1999; **285**: 412–5.

66 Zhang Yi, Louboutin J-P, Zhu J, Rivera AJ, Emerson SG. Preterminal host dendritic cells in irradiated mice prime CD8+ T cell-mediated acute graft-versus-host disease. *J Clin Invest* 2002; **109**: 1335–43.

67 Teshima T, Ordemann R, Reddy P. Acute graft-versus-host disease does not require alloantigen expression on host epithelium. *Nat Med* 2002; **8**: 553–5.

68 Hill GR, Ferrara JL. The primacy of the gastrointestinal tract as a target organ of acute graft-versus-host disease: rationale for the use of cytokine shields in allogeneic bone marrow transplantation. *Blood* 2000; **95**: 2754–9.

69 Nestel FP, Price KS, Seemayer TA, Lapp WS. Macrophage priming and lipopolysaccharide-triggered release of tumor necrosis factor alpha during graft-versus-host disease. *J Exp Med* 1992; **175**: 405–13.

70 Hill GR, Crawford JM, Cooke DR, Brinson YS, Pan L, Ferrara JL. Total body irradiation and acute graft-versus-host disease: the role of gastrointestinal damage and inflammatory cytokines. *Blood* 1997; **90**: 3204–13.

71 Piguet PF, Grau GE, Allet B, Vassali P. Tumor necrosis factor/cachectin is an effector of skin and gut lesions of the acute phase of graft-vs.-host disease. *J Exp Med* 1987; **166**: 1280–9.

72 Speiser DE, Bachmann MF, Frick TW *et al*. TNF receptor p55 controls early acute graft-versus-host disease. *J Immunol* 1997; **158**: 5185–90.

73 Hill GR, Teshima T, Gerbitz A *et al.* Differential roles of IL-1 and TNF-α on graft-versus-host disease and graft versus leukemia. *J Clin Invest* 1999; **104**: 459–67.

74 Cooke KR, Hill GR, Crawford JM *et al.* Tumor necrosis factor-alpha production to lipopolysaccharide stimulation by donor cells predicts the severity of experimental acute graft-versus-host disease. *J Clin Invest* 1998; **102**: 1882–91.

75 Nestel FP, Greene RN, Kichian K, Ponka P, Lapp WS. Activation of macrophage cytostatic effector mechanisms during acute graft-versus-host disease: release of intracellular iron and nitric oxide-mediated cytostasis. *Blood* 2000; **96**: 1836–43.

76 Antin JH, Weisdorf D, Neuberg D *et al.* Interleukin-1 blockade does not prevent acute graft versus host disease. Results of a randomized, double blind, placebo-controlled trial of interleukin 1 receptor antagonist in allogeneic bone marrow transplantation. *Blood* 2002; **100**: 3479–82.

77 Murphy WJ, Welniak LA, Taub DD, Wiltrout RH, Taylor PA, Vallera DA. Differential effects of the absence of interferon-γ and IL-4 in acute graft-versus-host disease after allogeneic bone marrow transplantation in mice. *J Clin Invest* 1998; **102**: 1742–8.

78 Ellison CA, Fischer JM, HayGlass KT, Gartner JG. Murine graft-versus-host disease in an F1-hybrid model using IFN-γ gene knockout donors. *J Immunol* 1998; **161**: 631–40.

79 Yang YG, Qi J, Wang MG, Sykes M. Donor-derived interferon-γ separates graft-versus-leukemia effects and graft-versus-host disease induced by donor CD8 T cells. *Blood* 2002; **99**: 4207–15.

80 Liu J, Anderson BE, Robert ME *et al.* Selective T-cell subset ablation demonstrates a role for T1 and T2 cells in ongoing acute graft-versus-host disease: a model system for the reversal of disease. *Blood* 2001; **98**: 3367–75.

81 Nikolic B, Lee S, Bronson RT, Grusby MJ, Sykes M. Th1 and Th2 mediate acute graft-versus-host disease, each with distinct end-organ targets. *J Clin Invest* 2000; **105**: 1289–98.

82 Daneshpouy M, Socie G, Lemann M, Rivet J, Gluckman E, Janin A. Activated eosinophils in upper gastrointestinal tract of patients with graft-versus-host disease. *Blood* 2002; **99**: 3033–40.

83 Jiang Z, Podack E, Levy RB. Major histocompatibility complex-mismatched allogeneic bone marrow transplantation using perforin and/or Fas ligand double-defective CD4+ donor T cells: involvement of cytotoxic function by donor lymphocytes prior to graft-versus-host disease pathogenesis. *Blood* 2001; **98**: 390–7.

84 Baker MB, Altman NH, Podack ER, Levy RB. The role of cell-mediated cytotoxicity in acute GVHD after MHC-matched allogeneic bone marrow transplantation in mice. *J Exp Med* 1996; **183**: 2645–56.

85 Baker MB, Riley RL, Podack ER, Levy RB. Graft-versus-host disease-associated lymphoid hypoplasia and B cell dysfunction is dependent upon donor T-cell-mediated Fas-ligand function, but not perforin function. *Pro Natl Acad Sci U S A* 1997; **94**: 1366–71.

86 van Den Brink MR, Moore E, Horndasch KJ *et al.* Fas-deficient lpr mice are more susceptible to graft-versus-host disease. *J Immunol* 2000; **164**: 469–80.

87 Hattori K, Hirano T, Miyajima H *et al.* Differential effects of anti-Fas ligand and anti-tumor necrosis factor alpha antibodies on acute graft-versus-host disease pathologies. *Blood* 1998; **91**: 4051–5.

88 Itoi H, Fujimori Y, Tsutsui H *et al.* Fas ligand-induced caspase-1-dependent accumulation of interleukin-18 in mice with acute graft-versus-host disease. *Blood* 2001; **98**: 235–7.

89 Reedy P, Teshima T, Kukuruga M *et al.* Interleukin-18 regulates acute graft-versus-host disease by enhancing Fas-mediated donor T cell apoptosis. *J Exp Med* 2001; **194**: 1433–40.

90 Yang YG, Dey BR, Sergio JJ, Pearson DA, Sykes M. Donor-derived interferon-γ is required for inhibition of acute graft-versus-host disease by interleukin 12. *J Clin Invest* 1998; **102**: 2126–35.

91 Asai O, Longo DL, Tian ZG *et al.* Suppression of graft-versus-host disease and amplification of graft-versus-tumor effects by activated natural killer cells after allogeneic bone marrow transplantation. *J Clin Invest* 1998; **101**: 1835–42.

92 Zeng D, Lewis D, Dejbakhsh-Jones S *et al.* Bone marrow NK1.1− and NK1.1+ T cells reciprocally regulate acute graft versus host disease. *J Exp Med* 1999; **189**: 1073–81.

93 Ruggeri L, Capanni M, Urbani E, Perruccio K, Shlomchik WD, Tosti A. Effectiveness of donor natural killer cell alloreactivity in mismatched hematopoietic transplants. *Science* 2002; **295**: 2097–100.

94 Taylor PA, Lees CJ, Blazar BR. The infusion of *ex vivo* activated and expanded CD4+ CD25+ immune regulatory cells inhibits graft-versus-host disease lethality. *Blood* 2002; **99**: 3493–9.

95 Hoffmann P, Ermann J, Edinger M, Fathman G, Strober S. Donor-type CD4+CD25+ regulatory T cells suppress lethal acute graft-versus-host disease after allogeneic bone marrow transplantation. *J Exp Med* 2002; **196**: 389–99.

96 Cohen JL, Trenado A, Vasey D, Klatzmann D, Salomon BL. CD4+CD25+ immunoregulatory T cells. *J Exp Med* 2002; **196**: 401–6.

97 Petersdorf EW, Gooley TA, Anasetti C *et al.* Optimizing outcome after unrelated marrow transplantation by comprehensive matching of HLA class I and II alleles in the donor and recipient. *Blood* 1998; **92**: 3515–20.

98 Morishima Y, Sasazuki T, Inoko H *et al.* The clinical significance of human leukocyte antigen (HLA) allele compatibility in patients receiving a marrow transplant from serologically HLA-A, HLA-B, and HLA-DR matched unrelated donors. *Blood* 2002; **99**: 4200–6.

99 Burrows SR, Khanna R, Burrows JM, Moss DJ. An alloresponse in humans is dominated by cytotoxic T lymphocytes (CTL) cross-reactive with a single Epstein–Barr virus CTL epitope: implications for graft-versus-host disease. *J Exp Med* 1994; **179**: 1155–61.

100 Cohen JL, Boyer O, Salomon B *et al.* Prevention of graft-versus-host disease in mice using a suicide gene expressed in T lymphocytes. *Blood* 1997; **89**: 4636–45.

101 Lake-Bullock MHV, Bryson JS, Jennings CD, Kaplan AM. Inhibition of graft-versus-host disease. Use of a T-cell-controlled suicide gene. *J Immunol* 1997; **158**: 5079–82.

102 Bonini C, Ferrari G, Verzeletti S *et al. HSV-TK* gene transfer into donor lymphocytes for control of allogeneic graft-versus-leukemia. *Science* 1997; **276**: 1719–24.

103 Tiberghien P, Ferrand C, Lioure B *et al.* Administration of herpes simplex-thymidine kinase-expressing donor T cells with a T-cell-depleted allogeneic marrow graft. *Blood* 2001; **97**: 63–72.

104 Drobyski WR, Morse HC III, Burns WH, Casper JT, Sanford G. Protection from lethal murine graft-versus-host disease without compromise of alloengraftment using transgenic donor T cells expressing a thymidine kinase suicide gene. *Blood* 2001; **97**: 2506–13.

105 Maury S, Salomon B, Klatzmann D, Cohen JL. Division rate and phenotypic differences discriminate alloreactive and nonalloreactive T cells transferred in lethally irradiated mice. *Blood* 2001; **98**: 3156–8.

106 Gribben JG, Guinan EC, Boussiotis VA *et al.* Complete blockade of B7 family-mediated costimulation is necessary to induce human alloantigen-specific anergy: a method to ameliorate graft-versus-host disease and extend the donor pool. *Blood* 1996; **87**: 4887–93.

107 Van Gool SW, Vandenberghe P, de Boer M, Ceuppens JL. CD80, CD86 and CD40 provide accessory signals in a multiple-step T-cell activation model. *Immunol Rev* 1996; **153**: 47–83.

108 Blazar BR, Sharpe AH, Taylor PA *et al.* Infusion of anti-B7.1 (CD80) and anti-B7.2 (CD86) monoclonal antibodies inhibits murine graft-versus-host disease lethality in part via direct effects on CD4+ and CD8+ T-cells. *J Immunol* 1996; **157**: 3250–9.

109 Blazar BR, Taylor PA, Panoskaltsis-Mortari A *et al.* Blockade of CD40 ligand–CD40 interaction impairs CD4+ T-cell-mediated alloreactivity by inhibiting mature donor T-cell expansion and function after bone marrow transplantation. *J Immunol* 1997; **158**: 29–39.

110 Saito K, Sakurai J, Ohata J. *et al.* Involvement of CD40 ligand-CD40 and CTLA4-B7 pathways in murine acute graft-versus-host disease induced by allogeneic T cells lacking CD28. *J Immunol* 1998; **169**: 4225–31.

111 Buhlmann JE, Gonzalez M, Ginther B *et al.* Cutting edge: sustained expansion of CD8+ T cells requires CD154 expression by Th cells in acute graft versus host disease. *J Immunol* 1999; **162**: 4373–6.

112 Blazar BR, Taylor PA, Panoskaltsis-Mortari A, Sharpe AH, Vallera DA. Opposing roles of CD28: B7 and CTLA-4: B7 pathways in regulating *in vivo* alloresponses in murine recipients of MHC disparate T cells. *J Immunol* 1999; **162**: 6368–77.

113 Tamada K, Tamura H, Flies D *et al.* Blockade of LIGHT/Ltβ and CD40 signaling induces allospecific T cell anergy, preventing graft-versus-host disease. *J Clin Invest* 2002; **109**: 549–57.

114 Krijanovski OI, Hill GR, Cooke KR *et al.* Keratinocyte growth factor separates graft-versus-leukemia effects from graft-versus-host disease. *Blood* 1999; **94**: 825–31.

115 Cooke KR, Gerbitz A, Crawford JM *et al.* LPS antagonism reduces graft-versus-host disease and preserves graft-versus-leukemia activity after experimental bone marrow transplantation. *J Clin Invest* 2001; **107**: 1581–9.

116 Via CS, Shearer GM. T-cell interactions in autoimmunity. Insights from a murine model of graft-versus-host disease. *Immunol Today* 1988; **9**: 207–13.

117 Zhang Y, McCormick LL, Desai SR, Wu C, Gilliam AC. Murine sclerodermatous graft-versus-host disease, a model for human scleroderma. Cutaneous cytokines, chemokines, and immune cell activation. *J Immunol* 2002; **168**: 3088–98.

118 Weiden PL, Flournoy N, Thomas ED *et al.* Antileukemic effect of graft-versus-host disease in human recipients of allogeneic-marrow grafts. *N Engl J Med* 1979; **300**: 1068–73.

119 Horowitz MM, Gale RP, Sondel PM et al. Graft-versus-leukemia reactions after bone marrow transplantation. *Blood* 1990; **75**: 555–62.

120 Goldman JM, Gale RP, Horowitz MM et al. Bone marrow transplantation for chronic myelogenous leukemia in chronic phase. Increased risk for relapse associated with T-cell depletion. *Ann Int Med* 1988; **108**: 806–14.

121 Sullivan KM, Storb R, Buckner CD et al. Graft-versus-host disease as adoptive immunotherapy in patients with advanced hematologic neoplasms. *N Engl J Med* 1989; **320**: 828–34.

122 Guglielmi C, Arcese W, Dazzi F et al. Donor lymphocyte infusion for relapsed chronic myelogenous leukemia: prognostic relevance of the initial cell dose. *Blood* 2002; **100**: 397–405.

123 Marks DI, Lush R, Cavenagh J et al. The toxicity and efficacy of donor lymphocyte infusions given after reduced intensity conditioning allogeneic stem cell transplantation. *Blood* 2002; **100**: 3108–14.

124 Zeng D, Hoffmann P, Lan F, Huie P, Higgins J, Strober S. Unique patterns of surface receptors, cytokine secretion, and immune functions distinguish T cells in the bone marrow from those in the periphery: impact on allogeneic bone marrow transplantation. *Blood* 2002; **99**: 1449–57.

125 Tsukada N, Kobata T, Aizawa Y, Yagita H, Okumura K. Graft-versus-leukemia effect and graft-versus-host disease can be differentiated by cytotoxic mechanisms in a murine model of allogeneic bone marrow transplantation. *Blood* 1999; **93**: 2738–47.

126 Schmaltz C, Alpdogan O, Horndasch KJ et al. Differential use of Fas ligand and perforin cytotoxic pathways by donor T cells in graft-versus-host disease and graft-versus-leukemia effect. *Blood* 2001; **97**: 2886–95.

127 Alyea EP, Soiffer RJ, Canning C et al. Toxicity and efficacy of defined doses of CD4$^+$ donor lymphocytes for treatment of relapse after allogeneic bone marrow transplant. *Blood* 1998; **91**: 3671–80.

128 Litvinova E, Maury S, Boyer O, Bruel S, Benard L, Boisserie G. Graft-versus-leukemia effect after suicide-gene-mediated control of graft-versus-host disease. *Blood* 2002; **100**: 2020–5.

129 Baker J, Verneris MR, Ito M, Shizuru JA, Negrin RS. Expansion of cytolytic CD8$^+$ natural killer T cells with limited capacity for graft-versus-host disease induction due to interferon-γ production. *Blood* 2001; **97**: 2923–31.

130 Fontaine P, Roy-Proulx G, Knafo L, Baron C, Roy DC, Perreault C. Adoptive transfer of minor histocompatibility antigen-specific T lymphocytes eradicates leukemia cells without causing graft-versus-host disease. *Nat Med* 2001; **7**: 789–94.

131 Dolstra H, Fredrix H, Maas F et al. A human minor histocompatibility antigen specific for B cell acute lymphoblastic leukemia. *J Exp Med* 1999; **189**: 301–8.

132 Scheibenbogen C, Letsch A, Thiel E et al. CD8 T cell responses to Wilms' tumor gene encoded protein WT1 and proteinase 3 in patients with acute myeloid leukemia. *Blood* 2002; **100**: 2132–7.

133 Parkman R. Clonal analysis of murine graft-vs-host disease. I. Phenotypic and functional analysis of T lymphocyte clones. *J Immunol* 1986; **136**: 3543–8.

134 van Els CA, Bakker A, Zwinderman AH, Zwaan FE, van Rood JJ, Goulmy E. Effector mechanisms in graft-versus-host disease in response to minor histocompatibility antigens. I. Absence of correlation with cytotoxic effector cells. *Transplantation* 1990; **50**: 62–6.

135 van Els CA, Bakker A, Zwinderman AH, Zwaan FE, van Rood JJ, Goulmy E. Effector mechanisms in graft-versus-host disease in response to minor histocompatibility antigens. II. Evidence of a possible involvement of proliferative T-cells. *Transplantation* 1990; **50**: 67–71.

136 Rocha B, Grandien A, Freitas AA. Anergy and exhaustion are independent mechanisms of peripheral T-cell tolerance. *J Exp Med* 1995; **181**: 993–1003.

137 Lanoue A, Bona C, von Boehmer H, Sarukhan A. Conditions that induce tolerance in mature CD4$^+$ T-cells. *J Exp Med* 1997; **185**: 405–14.

138 Ehl S, Hombach J, Aichele P et al. Viral and bacterial infections interfere with peripheral tolerance induction and activate CD8$^+$ T cells to cause immunopathology. *J Exp Med* 1998; **187**: 763–74.

139 George JF, Sweeney SD, Kirklin JK, Simpson EM, Goldstein DR, Thomas JM. An essential role for Fas ligand in transplantation tolerance induced by donor bone marrow. *Nat Med* 1998; **4**: 333–5.

140 Umemura A, Morita H, Li XC, Tahan S, Monaco AP, Maki T. Dissociation of hemopoietic chimerism and allograft tolerance after allogeneic bone marrow transplantation. *J Immunol* 2001; **167**: 3043–8.

141 Mackall CL, Hakim FT, Gress RE. T-cell regeneration: all repertoires are not created equal. *Immunol Today* 1997; **18**: 245–51.

142 Haynes BF, Markert ML, Sempowski GD, Dhavalkumar DP, Hale LP. The role of the thymus in immune reconstitution in aging, bone marrow transplantation, and HIV-1 infection. *Annu Rev Immunol* 2000; **18**: 529–60.

143 Storek J, Witherspoon RP, Storb R. T-cell reconstitution after bone marrow transplantation into adult patients does not resemble T-cell development in early life. *Bone Marrow Transplant* 1995; **16**: 413–25.

144 Vavassori M, Maccario R, Moretta A et al. Restricted TCR repertoire and long-term persistence of donor-derived antigen-experienced CD4$^+$ T-cells in allogeneic bone marrow transplantation recipients. *J Immunol* 1996; **157**: 5739–47.

145 Heitger A, Nikolaus N, Hannelore K et al. Essential role of the thymus to reconstitute naive (CD45RA$^+$) T-helper cells after human allogeneic bone marrow transplantation. *Blood* 1997; **90**: 850–7.

146 Mackall CL, Punt JA, Morgan P, Farr AG, Gress RE. Thymic function in young/old chimeras: substantial thymic T cell regenerative capacity despite irreversible age-associated thymic involution. *Eur J Immunol* 1998; **28**: 1886–93.

147 Storek J, Joseph A, Espino G, Dawson MA, Douek DC, Sullivan KM. Immunity of patients surviving 20–30 years after allogeneic or syngeneic bone marrow transplantation. *Blood* 2001; **98**: 3505–12.

148 Weinberg K, Blazar BR, Wagner JE et al. Factors affecting thymic function after allogeneic hematopoietic stem cell transplantation. *Blood* 2001; **97**: 1458–66.

149 Lewin SR, Heller G, Zhang L, Rodriques E, Skulsky E, van den Brink MRM. Direct evidence for new T-cell generation by patients after either T-cell-depleted or unmodified allogeneic hematopoietic stem cell transplantations. *Blood* 2002; **100**: 2235–42.

150 Mackall CL, Stein D, Fleisher TA et al. Prolonged CD4 depletion after sequential autologous peripheral blood progenitor cell infusions in children and young adults. *Blood* 2000; **96**: 754–62.

151 Lucas KG, Small TN, Heller G, Dupont B, O'Reilly RJ. The development of cellular immunity to Epstein–Barr virus after allogeneic bone marrow transplantation. *Blood* 1996; **87**: 2594–603.

152 Small TN, Avigan D, Dupont B et al. Immune reconstitution following T-cell depleted bone marrow transplantation: effect of age and posttransplant graft rejection prophylaxis. *Biol Blood Marrow Transplant* 1997; **3**: 65–75.

153 Storek J, Witherspoon RP, Maloney DG, Chauncey TR, Storb R. Improved reconstitution of CD4 T-cells and B cells but worsened reconstitution of serum IgG levels after allogeneic transplantation of blood stem cells instead of marrow. *Blood* 1997; **89**: 3891–3.

154 Storek J, Dawson MA, Storer B et al. Immune reconstitution after allogeneic marrow transplantation compared with blood stem cell transplantation. *Blood* 2001; **97**: 3380–9.

155 Wu CJ, Chillemi A, Alyea EP et al. Reconstitution of T-cell receptor repertoire diversity following T-cell depleted allogeneic bone marrow transplantation is related to hematopoietic chimerism. *Blood* 2000; **95**: 352–9.

156 Verfuerth S, Peggs K, Vyas P, Barnett L, O'Reilly RJ, Mackinnon S. Longitudinal monitoring of immune reconstitution by CDR3 size spectratyping after T-cell-depleted allogeneic bone marrow transplant and the effect of donor lymphocyte infusions on T-cell repertoire. *Blood* 2000; **95**: 3990–5.

157 Hazenberg MD, Otto SA, de Pauw ES et al. T-cell receptor excision circle and T-cell dynamics after allogeneic stem cell transplantation are related to clinical events. *Blood* 2002; **99**: 3449–53.

158 Talvensaari K, Clave E, Douay C et al. A broad T-cell repertoire diversity and an efficient thymic function indicate a favorable long-term immune reconstitution after cord blood stem cell transplantation. *Blood* 2002; **99**: 1458–64.

159 Eyrich M, Croner T, Leiler C et al. Distinct contributions of CD4$^+$ and CD8$^+$ naive and memory T-cell subsets to overall TCR-repertoire complexity following transplantation of T-cell depleted CD34 selected hematopoietic progenitor cells from unrelated donors. *Blood* 2002; **100**: 1915–8.

160 Glas AM, van Montfort EH, Storek J et al. B-cell-autonomous somatic mutation deficit following bone marrow transplant. *Blood* 2000; **96**: 1064–9.

161 Dulude G, Roy DC, Perreault C. The effect of graft-versus-host disease on T cell production and homeostasis. *J Exp Med* 1999; **189**: 1329–42.

162 Brochu S, Rioux-Masse B, Roy J, Roy DC, Perreault C. Massive activation-induced cell death of alloreactive T cells with apoptosis of bystander postthymic T cells prevents immune reconstitution in mice with graft-versus-host disease. *Blood* 1999; **94**: 390–400.

163 Storek J, Wells D, Dawson MA, Storer B, Maloney DG. Factors influencing B lymphopoiesis after allogeneic hematopoietic cell transplantation. *Blood* 2001; **98**: 489–91.

164 Small TN, Papadopoulos EB, Boulad F, Black P, Castro-Malaspina H, Childs BH. Comparison of immune reconstitution after unrelated and related T-cell-depleted bone marrow transplantation: effect of patient age and donor leukocyte infusions. *Blood* 1999; **93**: 467–80.

165 Curtis RE, Travis LB, Rowlings PA, Socie G, Kingma DW, Banks PM. Risk of lymphoproliferat-

165 ive disorders after bone marrow transplantation: a multi-institutional study. *Blood* 1999; **94**: 2208–16.
166 Marr KA, Carter RA, Boeckh M, Martin P, Corey L. Invasive aspergillosis in allogeneic stem cell transplant recipients. Changes in epidemiology and risk factors. *Blood* 2002; **100**: 4358–66.
167 Chakrabarti S, Mautner V, Osman H, Collingham KE, Fegan CD, Klapper PE. Adenovirus infections following allogeneic stem cell transplantation. The incidence and outcome in relation to graft manipulation, immunosuppression and immune recovery. *Blood* 2002; **100**: 1619–27.
168 Storek J, Gooley T, Witherspoon RP, Sullivan KM, Storb R. Infectious morbidity in long-term survivors of allogeneic marrow transplantation is associated with low CD4 T cell counts. *Am J Hematol* 1997; **54**: 131–8.
169 Pignata C, Sanghera JS, Soiffer RJ *et al*. Defective activation of mitogen-activated protein kinase after allogeneic bone marrow transplantation. *Blood* 1996; **88**: 2334–41.
170 Ozdemir E, St. John LS, Gillespie M *et al*. Cytomegalovirus reactivation following allogeneic stem cell transplantation is associated with the presence of dysfunctional antigen-specific CD8+ T cells. *Blood* 2002; **100**: 3690–7.
171 O'Reilly RJ, Small TN, Papadopoulos E, Lucas K, Lacerda J, Koulova L. Adoptive immunotherapy for Epstein–Barr virus-associated lymphoproliferative disorders complicating marrow allografts. *Semin Immunopathol* 1998; **20**: 455–91.
172 Einsele H, Roosnek E, Rufer N *et al*. Infusion of cytomegalovirus (CMV)-specific T cells for the treatment of CMV infection not responding to antiviral chemotherapy. *Blood* 2002; **99**: 3916–22.
173 Chung B, Barbara-Burnham L, Barsky L, Weinberg K. Radiosensitivity of thymic interleukin-7 production and thymopoiesis after bone marrow transplantation. *Blood* 2001; **98**: 1601–6.
174 Min D, Taylor PA, Panoskaltsis-Mortari A *et al*. Protection from thymic epithelial cell injury by keratinocyte growth factor: a new approach to improve thymic and peripheral T-cell reconstitution after bone marrow transplantation. *Blood* 2002; **99**: 4592–600.
175 Fry TJ, Mackall CL. Interleukin-7: from bench to clinic. *Blood* 2002; **99**: 3892–904.
176 Mackall CL, Fry TJ, Bare C, Morgan P, Galbraith A, Gress RE. IL-7 increases both thymic-dependent and thymic-independent T-cell regeneration after bone marrow transplantation. *Blood* 2001; **97**: 1491–7.
177 Fry TJ, Christensen BL, Komschlies KL, Gress RE, Mackall CL. Interleukin-7 restores immunity in athymic T-cell-depleted hosts. *Blood* 2002; **97**: 1525–33.
178 Alpdogan O, Schmaltz C, Muriglan SJ *et al*. Administration of interleukin-7 after allogeneic bone marrow transplantation improves immune reconstitution without aggravating graft-versus-host disease. *Blood* 2001; **98**: 2256–65.
179 Sinha ML, Fry TJ, Fowler DH, Miller G, Mackall CL. Interleukin-7 worsens graft-vs-host disease. *Blood* 2002; **100**: 2642–9.
180 Davila E, Velez MG, Heppelmann CJ, Celis E. Creating space: an antigen-independent, CpG-induced peripheral expansion of naive and memory T lymphocytes in a full T cell compartment. *Blood* 2002; **100**: 2537–45.
181 Avigan D, Pirofski LA, Lazarus HM. Vaccination against infectious disease following hematopoietic stem cell transplantation. *Biol Blood Marrow Transplant* 2001; **7**: 171–83.
182 Vavassori M, Maccario R, Moretta A, Comoli P, Wack A, Locatelli F. Restricted TCR repertoire and long-term persistence of donor-derived antigen-experienced CD4+ T cells in allogeneic bone marrow transplantation recipients. *J Immunol* 1996; **157**: 5739–47.

4

Eric Mickelson & Effie W. Petersdorf

Histocompatibility

Introduction

The transplantation of tissues between two genetically dissimilar individuals almost universally results in an immune reaction leading to graft rejection unless immunosuppressive medications are given. The immunologic reactivity, involving activation of T lymphocytes and B lymphocytes, results from differences between the transplant host and donor for cell surface determinants known as histocompatibility antigens. Histocompatibility antigens that provoke the strongest transplant reactions are encoded by a series of genes that reside in a discrete chromosomal region termed the major histocompatibility complex (MHC). Antigens encoded by MHC genes are expressed on virtually all nucleated cells. The MHC controls immune responsiveness in all vertebrate species and MHC genes have been highly conserved throughout vertebrate evolution (see Chapter 5). The human MHC was first recognized in the early 1950s following observations that sera from patients with febrile transfusion reactions could cause the agglutination of leukocytes from their transfusion donors, as well as other individuals [1]. Subsequent studies showed that leukocyte antibodies could also be found in the sera of multiparous women. The term *HLA* was derived by combining the human-1 (*HU*-1) and leukocyte antigen (*LA*) designations used by Dausset and Payne, respectively, to describe the newly discovered leukocyte antigen system [1–5]. Since 1964 a series of 13 collaborative international histocompatibility workshops has greatly extended our knowledge of the HLA system and contributed to the standardization of HLA-typing methods as well as HLA nomenclature.

During an immune response cells of the immune system interact through recognition of cell surface molecules encoded by genes of the human MHC. T cells recognize foreign antigens presented as peptide fragments in association with MHC molecules. Before T cells can recognize an antigen, that antigen must be processed by an antigen-presenting cell, bound to a "self" MHC molecule, and transported to the cell surface. Many different peptide antigens can be processed and presented to T cells, including those derived from bacteria, viruses, toxins and foreign cells and tissues, as well as from autologous tissue and cellular products. Definition of the peptide-binding motifs that characterize HLA molecules provides important information on the role of the HLA system in peptide presentation, immune responsiveness and disease susceptibility [6–8]. The role of the MHC in antigen presentation helps explain the extensive polymorphism of the MHC at the population level: the greater the polymorphism of the MHC, the greater the array of foreign peptides that can be presented to the immune system. Thus, MHC genes can influence T-cell immune responsiveness by the selection of antigens that can be bound and presented for T-cell recognition. MHC molecules have a major effect in transplantation due to the fundamental role they play in T-cell activation and initiation of an alloresponse.

With the advent of DNA typing methods, it is now possible to define each class of HLA molecule by its unique sequence [9]. The remarkable diversity among genes of the HLA system has greatly exceeded expectations. An appreciation of HLA polymorphism is clearly important to an understanding of how histocompatibility antigens function as transplantation determinants.

HLA genes: structure and function

HLA antigens are encoded by a series of closely linked genes located at position p21.3 on the short arm of chromosome 6. Genes of the HLA region span approximately 4000 kb of DNA, equivalent to 0.1% of the human genome, and are clustered in three distinct regions designated class I, class II and class III (Fig. 4.1). With the recent mapping of the class I-like gene associated with hemachromatosis (Hfe), the outer boundary of the MHC may extend an additional 4000 kb telomeric of HLA-F [10]. Genes within the class I and class II regions share structural and functional properties and are considered to be part of the immunoglobulin gene superfamily. Although distinct in sequence and structure, both class I and class II genes encode polypeptides that are critical in controlling T-cell recognition and determining histocompatibility in transplantation.

A characteristic feature of HLA genes is their extreme polymorphism (Tables 4.1 & 4.2). HLA diversity is a reflection of the primary immunological function of MHC molecules, i.e., to bind and present antigenic peptides for recognition by antigen-specific T-cell receptors (TCRs). The differential structural properties of HLA class I and class II molecules account for their respective roles in activating different populations of T lymphocytes. Cytotoxic (Tc) T lymphocytes recognize antigenic peptides presented by HLA class I molecules, while helper (TH) T lymphocytes recognize antigenic peptides presented by HLA class II molecules. HLA class I and class II molecules are characterized by distinctive α and β polypeptide subunits that combine to form αβ heterodimers characteristic of the mature molecule. Class I molecules were originally defined by typing with alloantisera and class II molecules defined by testing in functional assays, such as the mixed lymphocyte culture (MLC) reaction [11,12].

Class I genes: HLA-A, -B, -C, -E, -F, -G

At least 17 loci including several pseudogenes exist in the HLA class I region (Fig. 4.1). Three of these loci, termed class *Ia*, encode HLA-A, -B and -C alloantigens that constitute the major class I determinants important for matching in tissue transplantation. Genes of the *HLA-A, -B*

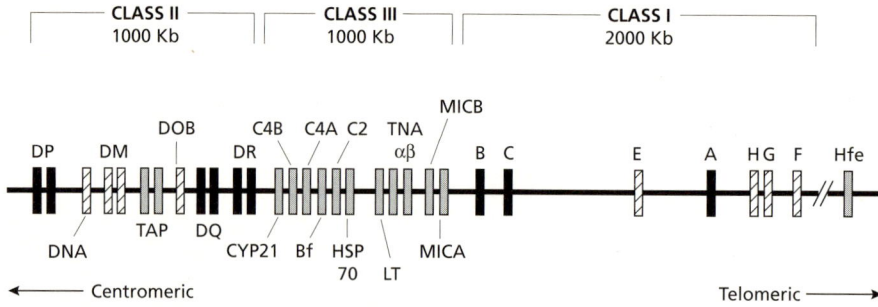

Fig. 4.1 The human major histocompatibility complex (MHC) on the short arm of chromosome 6. The class II *HLA-DP*, *DNA*, *DM*, *DOB*, *DQ*, *DR* genes and the class I *HLA-B*, *-C*, *-E*, *-A*, *-H*, *-G* and *-F* genes are shown in black; those encoding classical transplantation antigens are shown as solid bars, others are cross-hatched. Other HLA region-associated genes are shown in blue: transporter of antigenic peptides (*TAP*); 21-hydroxylase (*CYP21*; also termed *21-OH* or P450-*C21B*); complement component C4; properidin factor B of the alternate complement pathway (*Bf*); complement component C2; heat-shock protein (*HSP70*); tumor necrosis factor (*TNF*) complex with TNF-α, TNF-β and lymphotoxin-A (*LTA*); *MICB*; *MICA*; and the hemachromatosis gene (*Hfe*). The distance from the *HLA-F* gene telomeric to the *Hfe* gene is approximately 4000 kb.

Table 4.1 Class I HLA antigens and alleles.

A locus		B locus				C locus	
Antigens[†]	Allele(s)	Antigens	Allele(s)	Antigens	Allele(s)	Antigens	Allele(s)
A1	A*0101-08	B7	B*0702;0704-26	B52(5)	B*5201-03	Cw1	Cw*0102-04
A2	A*0201-49	B703	B*0703	B53	B*5301-02	Cw2	Cw*0202-04
A3	A*0301-08	B8	B*0801-13	B54(22)	B*5401-02	Cw10(w3)	Cw*0302; 0304
A23(9)[‡]	A*2301-06	B13	B*1301-07	B55(22)	B*5501-10	Cw9(w3)	Cw*0303
A24(9)	A*2402-31	B14	B*1401-06	B56(22)	B*5601-07	Cw3	Cw*0305-12
A9	A*2410	B15	B*1501-64	B57(17)	B*5701-07	Cw4	Cw*0401-08
A25(10)	A*2501;03	B18	B*1801-05	B58(17)	B*5801-06	Cw5	Cw*0501-04
A26(10)	A*2601-17	B27	B*2701-07; 2709-23	B59	B*5901	Cw6	Cw*0602-07
A10	A*2502	B2708	B*2708	B67	B*6701-02	Cw7	Cw*0701-14
A11	A*1101-09	B35	B*3501-37	B73	B*7301	Cw8	Cw*0801-09
A29(19)	A*2901-04	B37	B*3701-05	B78	B*7801-05	—[§]	Cw*1202-07
A30(19)	A*3001-09	B38(16)	B*3801-07	B81	B*8101	—	Cw*1301
A31(19)	A*3101-05	B39(16)	B*3901-24	—[§]	B*8201	—	Cw*1402-04
A32(19)	A*3201-06	B40	B*4001-35	—	B*8301	—	Cw*1502-10
A33(19)	A*3301-06	B41	B*4101-05			—	Cw*1601-02; 1604
A34(10)	A*3401-04	B42	B*4201-02			—	Cw*1701-03
A36	A*3601-02	B44(12)	B*4402-24			—	Cw*1801-02
A43	A*4301	B45(12)	B*4501-04				
A66(10)	A*6601-04	B46	B*4601-02				
A68(28)	A*6801-02; 6804-11; 6813-19	B47	B*4701-03				
A69(28)	A*6901	B48	B*4801-07				
A28	A*6803;12	B49(21)	B*4901-03				
A74(19)	A*7401-05	B50(21)	B*5001-02;5004				
A80	A*8001	B51(5)	B*5101-24				

[†]Antigens are defined by alloantisera. Antigens listed in parentheses are broadly defined public specificities subsequently split into two or more subtypic antigens.
[‡]Allele(s) encoding the corresponding antigen expressed at the cell surface.
[§]For some HLA antigens defined by DNA typing methods, no corresponding alloantigen has been defined by alloantisera or cellular typing.

and -C loci show a striking degree of sequence and structural homology with one another and all are highly polymorphic. More than 400 alleles, for example, have been defined at the *HLA-B* locus [9] (summarized in Table 4.1). More recently, three additional class I genes, *HLA-E*, *-F* and *-G*, have been defined [13–15]. These genes, termed class *Ib* genes, encode cell-surface molecules that have different patterns of expression. HLA-G molecules are found only on the placental trophoblast, HLA-F molecules are found in the trophoblast and possibly other tissues, while

Table 4.2 Class II HLA antigens and alleles.

DRB1 locus		DQB1 locus		DPB1 locus	
Antigens[†]	Allele(s)	Antigens	Allele(s)	Antigens	Allele(s)
DR1	DRB1*0101-07	DQ5(1)	DQB1*0501-04	DPw1	DPB1*0101
DR15(2)[‡]	DRB1*1501-11	DQ6(1)	DQB1*0601-17	DPw2	DPB1*0201-02
DR16(2)	DRB1*1601-08	DQ2	DQB1*0201-03	DPw3	DPB1*0301
DR17(3)	DRB1*0301; 0304-05	DQ7(3)	DQB1*0301;0304	DPw4	DPB1*0401-02
DR18(3)	DRB1*0302-03	DQ8(3)	DQB1*0302;0305; 0310	DPw5	DPB1*0501
DR3	DRB1*0306-18	DQ9(3)	DQB1*0303	DPw6	DPB1*0601
DR4	DRB1*0401-38	DQ3	DQB1*0306-09	—[§]	DPB1*0801-8901[¶]
DR11(5)	DRB1*1101-41	DQ4	DQB1*0401-02		
DR12(5)	DRB1*1201-07				
DR13(6)	DRB1*1301-47				
DR14(6)	DRB1*1401-40				
DR7	DRB1*0701-04				
DR8	DRB1*0801-23	DQA1 locus		DPA1 locus	
DR9	DRB1*0901				
DR10	DRB1*1001	—[§]	DQA1*0101-06	—[§]	DPA1*0103-07
		—	DQA1*0201	—	DPA1*0201-03
		—	DQA1*0301-03	—	DPA1*0301-02
		—	DQA1*0401	—	DPA1*0401
		—	DQA1*0501-05		
		—	DQA1*0601		

†Antigens are defined by alloantisera. Antigens listed in parentheses are broadly defined public specificities subsequently split into two or more subtypic antigens.
‡Allele(s) encoding the corresponding antigen expressed at the cell surface.
§For some HLA antigens defined by DNA typing methods, no corresponding alloantigen has been defined by alloantisera or cellular typing.
¶Eighty-one additional DPB1 alleles have been defined (DPB1*0801-8901) for which no corresponding alloantigens have been defined.

HLA-E molecules are ubiquitously expressed. The function of HLA-E, F and G molecules is not fully known, but they appear at least in part to serve as ligands for natural killer (NK) cell receptors and thus may regulate NK function [16,17]. Their potential role in transplantation is the subject of current investigation (see Chapters 82 & 83).

Class I *HLA-A*, *-B* and *-C* genes are each comprised of eight exons and seven intervening introns. Exon 1 is a leader sequence; exons 2, 3 and 4 encode the α1, 2 and 3 domains of the class I molecule, respectively; exon 5 encodes the *trans*-membrane portion of the molecule; and exons 6, 7 and 8 encode the cytoplasmic tail. HLA class I molecules consist of a single polymorphic α (heavy) chain of approximately 338–341 residues in length, which is noncovalently bound at the cell surface to a $β_2$-microglobulin light chain (Fig. 4.2; see also Plate 4.1, *facing p. 296*). The gene for $β_2$-microglobulin is located outside of the HLA complex on chromosome 15. Structurally, class I molecules are comprised of two α-helical regions overlaying an eight strand antiparallel β-pleated sheet that forms the groove for peptide binding [6] (Fig. 4.3a; see also Plate 4.2, *facing p. 296*).

Nucleotide substitutions within exons two and three of class I genes are not distributed randomly, but are concentrated in discrete hypervariable regions (Fig. 4.4). Polymorphic sites within the α1 and α2 domains facilitate the binding of peptide fragments for presentation to the TCR [18]. These polymorphic sites also determine the allospecificity of the molecule and form the basis for their classification as HLA alloantigens (see Table 4.1).

Class II genes: HLA-DR, -DQ, -DP

The HLA class II region is comprised of nine distinct genes: *DRA*, *DRB1*, *DRB3*, *DRB4*, *DRB5*, *DQA*, *DQB*, *DPA* and *DPB*. The class II region also contains functionally related genes (*TAP* and *LMP*) that play a role in the loading of class I molecules with peptides. Six additional class II genes or gene fragments have been described but these are either nonfunctional pseudogenes or do not encode proteins known to participate in transplant-related immune interactions. Class II genes have been collectively referred to as *HLA-D* region genes since they were initially described in the mid-1970s after the description of the *HLA-A* and *-B* (1965) and *-C* (1971) loci. Class II genes are divided into five families, designated *DR*, *DQ*, *DO*, *DN* and *DP*, based on their degree of sequence homology and their location within the *HLA-D* region. As with class I genes, class II *HLA-DR*, *-DQ* and *-DP* genes show a striking degree of polymorphism, with more than 270 alleles thus far defined at the *DRB1* locus [9].

Class II molecules consist of a single polymorphic (DQ and DP) or nonpolymorphic (DR) α chain noncovalently bound to a polymorphic β chain (Fig. 4.3b; see also Plate 4.2, *facing p. 296*) [7]. The β chains of HLA-DR, -DQ and -DP antigens are encoded by the *DRB*, *DQB* and *DPB* genes, respectively. Polymorphic HLA-DR β chains are encoded by four distinct *DRB* genes termed *DRB1*, *DRB3*, *DRB4* and *DRB5*. *HLA-DRB* genes are inherited as a genetic unit, or *haplotype*. Within the *HLA-DRB* region variable numbers of genes are expressed from one haplotype to another (Fig. 4.5). For example, DRB haplotypes that type as DR1

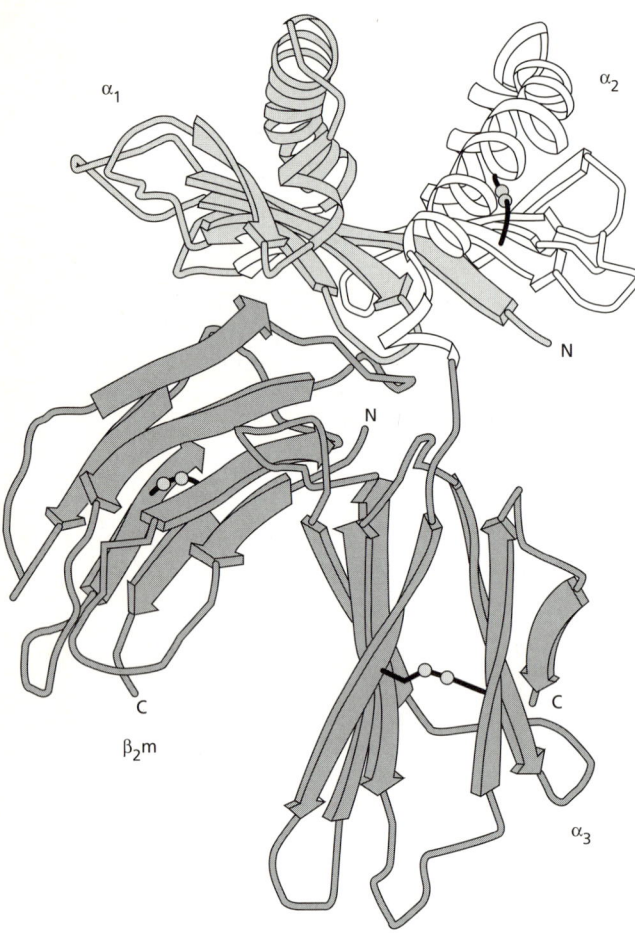

Fig. 4.2 Schematic representation of an HLA class I molecule. Ribbon diagram of a class I molecule showing the four domains. The α_3 and β_2 microglobulin domains proximal to the cell membrane are shown at the bottom and the polymorphic α_1 and α_2 domains are shown at the top. The β-strands are indicated as wide arrows while α-helical portions are shown as coiled ribbons. (*See also Plate 4.1, facing p. 296.*)

include four genes: a polymorphic *DRB1* gene, a nonpolymorphic *DRA* gene and two pseudogenes. In contrast, DRB haplotypes that type as *DR3* include five genes: a polymorphic *DRB1* gene, a nonpolymorphic *DRA* gene, a polymorphic *DRB3* gene and two pseudogenes. Further polymorphism within the *HLA-D* region can result from *trans* pairing of a polymorphic DQ α chain encoded by one parental chromosome with a polymorphic DQ β chain encoded by the other parental chromosome.

Polymorphic sites within class II molecules are localized in specific regions of the α1 and β1 domains of the α and β chains, respectively, to enable binding of a large array of peptides [18,19]. The polymorphic α1 and β1 domains also determine the allospecificity of the class II molecule (summarized in Table 4.2). Antigens encoded by *DRB1* and *DQB* genes are known to be potent stimulators of immune reactions in hematopoietic cell transplantation (HCT) [20,21].

Class III genes

The HLA class III region is comprised of at least 62 genes that span approximately 1 Mb of DNA, located between the HLA class II and class I regions. Although class III genes are located within the MHC complex, they are notably different from class I and class II genes. Class III genes encode a diverse group of proteins that include complement components, tumor necrosis factor, transport proteins and heat shock proteins. The role of class III cytokine genes in transplantation is under active investigation [22].

HLA nomenclature

The naming of HLA genes and the alleles encoded by different HLA loci has been delegated to the World Health Organization Nomenclature Committee for Factors of the HLA System [9]. HLA nomenclature has evolved in concert with the application of molecular typing technology to the study of HLA genes. Names were originally assigned based on the analysis of phenotype by serology. Thus, the *HLA-B* locus allele B*4402 encodes a molecule recognized serologically as B44. In this designation, *HLA-B* defines the genetic locus, the *asterisk* separates the locus name from the allele name, the digits *44* indicate the broadly defined serological specificity, and the digits *02* uniquely identify the allele that encodes the B44 alloantigen. A silent substitution in an HLA gene that does not translate into a molecular variant is designated by a fifth digit. For example, HLA-A*68011 and A*68012 indicate two forms of the A*6801 allele that differ for a single nucleotide that does not alter the encoded protein.

Characteristics of the HLA genetic system

Haplotypes

HLA genes are closely linked to one another within the MHC and are generally inherited *en bloc* as a genetic unit. The series of HLA alleles occurring on a single chromosome 6 is termed a *haplotype* and the combination of two parental haplotypes inherited by an individual com-

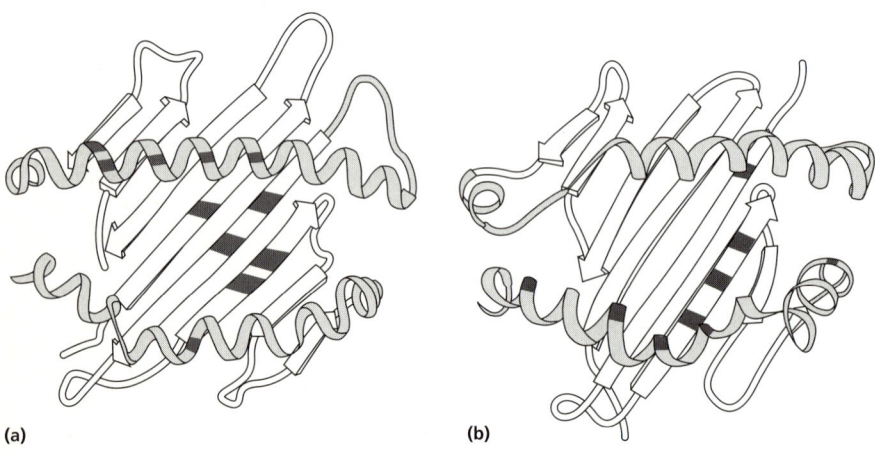

Fig. 4.3 The location of polymorphic sites in the antigen-binding cleft of HLA class I and class II molecules. Schematic representation of an HLA class I molecule (a) and an HLA class II molecule (b) as seen from the top surface. The α1 and α2 domains (class I) and α1 and β1 domains (class II) form the sides of the antigen-binding cleft. Polymorphic sites with maximum amino acid variation from allele to allele are shown as colored bars. (*See also Plate 4.2, facing p. 296.*)

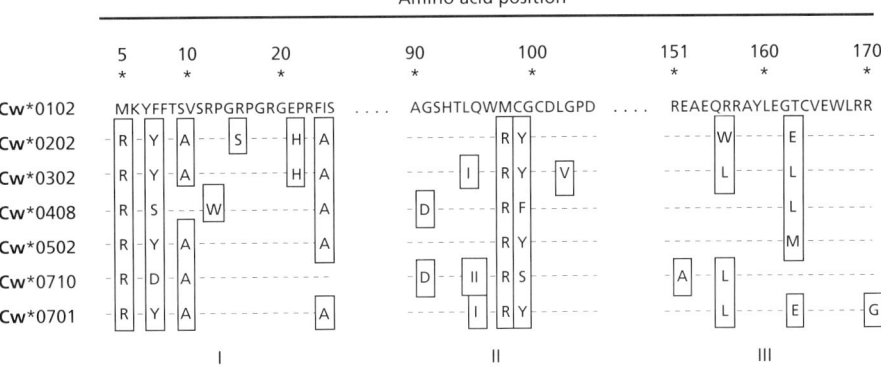

Fig. 4.4 Variable sites within a class I molecule. Sequence alignment of seven *HLA-C* alleles illustrating the clustering of amino acid substitutions in hypervariable regions (indicated by roman numerals, *bottom*). The polymorphisms map to sites on the floor (I) and within the antigen-binding groove (II, III) of the class I molecule (see Fig. 4.3a and Plate 4.2, *facing p. 296*). The consensus sequence (the most common amino acids found at a given position) is shown for the Cw*0102 allele.

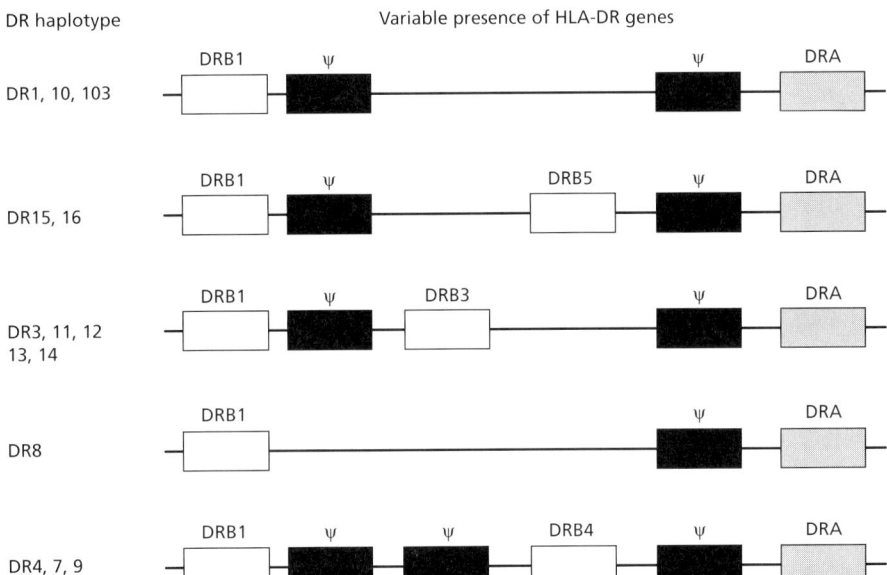

Fig. 4.5 Variable expression of DRB genes according to HLA haplotype. Open boxes, DRB genes; hatched boxes, nonpolymorphic *DRA* gene; shaded boxes, pseudogenes (Ψ).

prises that individual's HLA *genotype*. Because the HLA system is highly polymorphic, most individuals are heterozygous for two different parental alleles at each HLA locus. For a given HLA locus, the antigens encoded by the two HLA alleles are codominantly expressed, and a heterozygous individual will therefore possess two different antigens at that locus. The polymorphism displayed by HLA genes, coupled with their tendency to be strongly linked to one another, have important implications in donor–recipient histocompatibility matching for HCT.

HLA antigens show characteristic variation from one racial group to another. The frequencies of individual HLA alleles vary greatly within a population and between populations. For example, the allele encoding *HLA-B8* is very common in Caucasian populations (gene frequency, 7.7–16.3%) but very infrequent in Asian populations (gene frequency, 0.0–0.2%). Conversely, the allele encoding *HLA-B46* is common in Asian populations (gene frequency, 4.7–12.5%) but virtually absent in Caucasians. The diversity that characterizes HLA molecules presents a formidable problem from a donor–recipient histocompatibility perspective.

Linkage disequilibrium

Certain HLA alleles are found associated with one another more frequently than would be predicted by chance alone; conversely, other alleles are rarely if ever found associated with one another. This nonrandom association of HLA alleles is termed positive or negative *linkage disequilibrium* (LD). The exact basis for LD is unknown. Possible explanations include mutations, racial admixture and positive selection. The latter hypothesis argues that an evolutionary advantage derives from the association of certain HLA alleles and that this advantage is sufficient to offset the randomizing effects of genetic recombination, mutation and genetic drift [23]. Table 4.3 shows representative HLA haplotypes that characterize five different racial groups [24]. For the purposes of finding an HCT donor, strong LD between two or more HLA loci (e.g. *HLA-A1*, *-B8*, *-DR3* in Caucasian-Americans) can be of major benefit to a patient, since matching for two of the loci (e.g. *-A1*, *-B8*) will very often determine matching for the third (e.g. *-DR3*). Patients possessing HLA haplotypes with less strongly linked alleles will have more difficulty finding donors.

HLA typing: a historical perspective

There has been a dramatic advance in the laboratory methods used to define HLA genes and alloantigens during the past 20 years. The following section presents a brief historical overview of the evolution in technology, which has culminated in the current and widespread use of DNA-based typing methods for the definition of HLA alleles.

Serology

Historically, HLA class I antigens were defined by serologic methods utilizing a complement-dependent microcytotoxicity assay and panels of alloantisera containing HLA antibodies [25]. These antisera were highly

Table 4.3 HLA haplotype frequencies in selected populations. Data summarized from Mori et al. [24].

Population	HLA-A, B, DR haplotype	Haplotype frequency (%)
Caucasian-American	A1, B8, DR3	5.2
	A3, B7, DR2	2.6
	A2, B44, DR4	2.2
Asian-American	A33, B58, DR3	1.6
	A33, B44, DR6	1.5
	A24, B52, DR2	1.4
African-American	A30, B42, DR3	1.7
	A1, B8, DR3	1.2
	A3, B7, DR2	0.8
Latin-American	A2, B35, DR8	1.8
	A29, B44, DR7	1.7
	A1, B8, DR3	1.7
Native-American	A1, B8, DR3	4.7
	A3, B7, DR2	2.7
	A2, B44, DR2	2.0

Table 4.5 Definition of HLA-DRB1 antigens.

Public	Private
DR1	
DR2	DR15
	DR16
DR3	DR17
	DR18
DR4	
DR5	DR11
	DR12
DR6	DR13
	DR14
DR7	
DR8	
DR9	
DR10	

selected for HLA specificity and were usually obtained from multiparous women immunized to HLA alloantigens through pregnancy. Serologic typing showed that HLA alloantigens characteristically express multiple specificities or epitopes. Epitopes shared by more than one distinct antigen are referred to as *public specificities*, whereas epitopes unique to a single antigen are referred to as *private specificities*. These private specificities are also termed *splits* of the public antigen. The public specificity A19, for example, is shared by several distinct antigens: A29, A30, A31, A32, A33 and A74 (Table 4.4). Clusters of serologically crossreactive HLA-A and -B antigens can be classified as belonging to *crossreactive groups* (CREGs) (Table 4.4). Antigens within a CREG are presumed to share one or more public epitopes in addition to their individual and unique private epitope(s). The classification of public and private antigens into CREGs constitutes a basis for donor–recipient matching in HCT. Although CREGs were not originally defined for class II specificities, a similar classification scheme can be constructed for HLA-DRB1 antigens (Table 4.5). The serologically defined DR2 antigen, for example, corresponds to a public specificity that can be split into the DR15 and DR16 private specificities. An increasing number of class I and class II alleles are definable by DNA-based typing methods but not by serologic methods. To bridge the transition in nomenclature from serological to DNA-based typing methods, "serologically equivalent" designations have been defined [26].

Table 4.4 HLA-A and B crossreactive antigen groups (CREGs).*

HLA-A locus	HLA-B locus
A1, A3, A11, A36	B5, B18, B35, B51, B52, B53, B70, B71, B72, B78
A23, A24, A9	B12, B21, B44, B45, B49, B50, B4005
A25, A26, A34, A66, A43, A10	B14, B64, B65
	B8, B59
A19, A29, A30, A31, A32, A33, A74	B15, B46, B57, B58, B62, B63, B70, B71, B72, B75, B76, B77
A2, A28, A68, A69	B16, B38, B39, B67
	B7, B27, B42, B73
	B7, B22, B54, B55, B56, B67
	B7, B40, B41, B48, B60, B61, B81
	B13, B47

*CREGs defined by the National Marrow Donor Program (NMDP). Antigens within a given box are members of the same HLA-A or -B locus CREG and share a common public specificity (epitope); antigens from different boxes belong to different CREGs. A donor–recipient incompatibility for antigens within the same box (e.g. B13 vs. B47) represents a *minor* mismatch. A donor–recipient incompatibility for antigens from different boxes (e.g. B18 vs. B21) represents a *major* mismatch. Certain antigens (e.g. HLA-A80) are not part of any defined CREG. HLA-B7 is a member of three different CREGs.

Cellular typing

A second method of HLA typing has involved testing T cells *in vitro* for their ability to recognize certain HLA antigens. The most commonly used cellular assay is the MLC reaction, a test in which disparity for class II HLA-D region antigens leads to lymphocyte activation and proliferation [11,12]. Cells that proliferate in an MLC reaction belong to the T$_H$ subset. The strength of the proliferation measured in an MLC test correlates roughly with the degree of HLA-D region incompatibility [27].

Whereas the MLC reaction primarily measures proliferation of CD4$^+$ T cells responding to class II antigens, the predominant alloimmune response to class I antigens occurs among CD8$^+$ cytotoxic T lymphocytes (CTLs). CTL responses can be measured in bulk culture in a test system known as the cell-mediated lympholysis (CML) assay. The CML assay is a two-step procedure beginning with an activation phase in which responder cells are cultured with irradiated stimulator cells. After incubation for 6–10 days, the responder cells are tested against chromium-51 labeled target cells. Cytotoxicity is measured by chromium release and used to assess the degree of functional class I disparity between two individuals.

DNA typing methods

The development of DNA-based typing methods for the analysis of HLA genes has greatly advanced our knowledge of MHC diversity, the role of class I and II molecules in the immune response, and the factors important in the selection of volunteer unrelated donors for transplantation. Most typing methods currently in use in clinical and research laboratories are based on the amplification of specific HLA genes from genomic DNA using the polymerase chain reaction (PCR). PCR-based typing methods provide either direct determination of the entire coding region sequence of an allele (e.g. sequencing-based typing [SBT]) or partial sequence information, which allows inference of the HLA allele (e.g. sequence-specific oligonucleotide probe [SSOP] hybridization or sequence-specific primer [SSP] typing). These methods have clarified the relationship between HLA genes and their encoded antigens. For a given HLA locus (e.g. *HLA-A*), the gene variant at that locus is termed the allele (e.g. A*0201), and the alleles expressed by the two parental haplotypes constitute the genotype (e.g. A*0201, *0301). Each HLA allele, consisting of a unique nucleotide sequence, encodes the corresponding unique HLA molecule expressed at the cell surface. HLA molecules are characterized and classified by their reaction with HLA antibodies, and are hence referred to as HLA antigens. The combination of two antigens at a given locus, encoded by the alleles of the two parental chromosomes, is termed the phenotype (e.g. *HLA-A2, -A3*). Because of the broadly reactive nature of HLA antibodies, two or more unique sequences (e.g. HLA-A*0201, *0205 and *0213) may have the same serologically defined phenotype (e.g. *HLA-A2*).

DNA-based typing methods vary according to the level of discrimination they provide in defining the nucleotide sequence of an HLA gene. When the DNA typing method allows identification of a serologically defined antigen-equivalent (e.g. HLA-A2), the method is termed *"low-resolution"*. For example, SSOP hybridization methods employing a restricted number of probes may provide only limited sequence information about a particular HLA gene, equivalent to that achievable by serology. Typing methods that provide information beyond the serologic level but short of the allele level are termed *"intermediate-resolution"*. For example, an SSOP method that employs a wider array of probes might identify the presence of either HLA-A*0201 *or* *0209 in an amplified DNA sample, but is unable to discriminate one allele from the other. This intermediate-resolution result would be characterized as "HLA-A*02" or "HLA-A*0201/09". Typing methods that generate nucleotide sequence information allowing precise identification of an HLA allele (e.g. HLA-A*0201) are termed *"high-resolution"*. High-resolution typing results may be achieved by direct automated sequencing of an HLA gene (SBT) or by the use of large panels of oligonucleotide probes that test all known regions of variability within a gene. In order to interpret HLA typing results and select donors for transplantation, it is necessary to know whether the typing was carried out at low-, intermediate- or high-resolution. A patient and donor who are "matched" for HLA-A and -B *antigens* by low-resolution typing methods may be mismatched for *HLA-A* and/or *-B alleles* (see Chapter 83).

DNA amplification strategies for HLA typing

Amplification of an HLA gene by PCR involves the use of *locus-specific*, *group-specific* or *allele-specific* primers. *Locus-specific* primers amplify all alleles encoded at a given locus but not others outside of that locus. In heterozygous samples, both alleles are coamplified (e.g. in an *HLA-DR2, 4*-positive sample both the *DR2* and the *DR4* alleles are coamplified). *Group-specific* primers are designed to amplify a group of alleles sharing a common polymorphism (e.g. a primer specific for the *HLA-DR4* group of alleles will only amplify the *HLA-DR4* allele in a heterozygous *HLA-DR4,8*-positive sample). *Allele-specific* primers may be used to amplify a single allele. For example, in a sample that is *HLA-DR4*-homozygous but heterozygous for two different *HLA-DR4* alleles (e.g. HLA-DRB1*0401, *0405), the HLA-DRB1*0401 allele can be amplified and analyzed independent of the HLA-DRB1*0405 allele. Strategies for HLA typing can thus be built on a step-wise process that first uses locus-specific primers to amplify and analyze both alleles in a sample, followed by group-specific or allele-specific amplification to isolate one of the two alleles for further characterization.

Sequence-specific primers

In the SSP method, a panel of amplification primers is designed to detect all known polymorphisms encoded by an HLA locus or group of alleles [28–33]. PCR reactions are first performed for each of the primer pairs. The PCR products are then electrophoresed on a gel and the presence or absence of a PCR product of the appropriate size is scored (Fig. 4.6). Assignment of an HLA type is made by examining the pattern of positive and negative PCR reactions. Advantages of the SSP method include its relatively low cost, its technical simplicity and the speed with which low-resolution typing can be achieved. High-resolution level typing requires as many primers as there are polymorphisms and large numbers of PCR reactions are therefore necessary, increasing both assay time and cost.

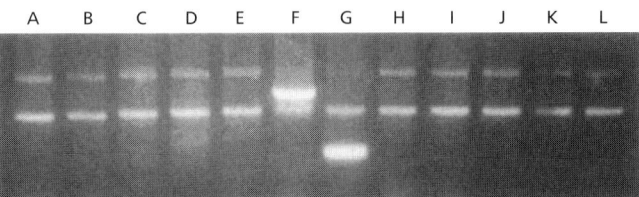

Fig. 4.6 Sequence-specific primer (SSP) typing. Genomic DNA from a single sample was amplified with a panel of HLA-C primer pairs, electrophoresed on an agarose gel, stained with ethidium bromide and visualized with UV translumination. All primer pair amplicons (lanes A through L) showed amplification of the 796 base pair (bp) fragment from the internal control primers, demonstrating successful PCR conditions in each sample. The sample was typed as Cw*06 and Cw*07 by the identification of specific amplification products in lane F (1062 bp fragment specific for Cw*0701/0702/0703) and lane G (304 bp fragment for Cw*06).

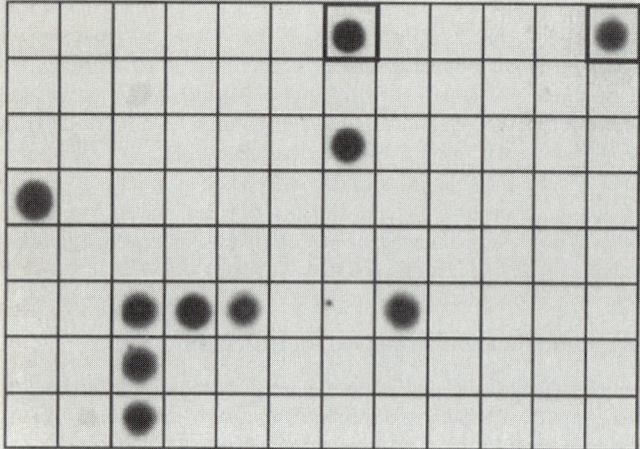

Fig. 4.7 Sequence-specific oligonucleotide probe (SSOP) typing. Genomic DNAs of 12 known control samples and 82 unknown samples were amplified with HLA-A locus specific primers, blotted on a series of nylon membranes and probed with a panel of HLA-A locus probes. Positive hybridization of probes labeled with alkaline phosphatase was detected by chemiluminescence and exposure to X-ray film. In this example, a probe specific to a sequence found only in A*29 and A*43 at codons 62 and 63 of exon 2 showed positive hybridization with two control samples (outlined in bold) and eight of the unknown test samples.

Sequence-specific oligonucleotide probe (SSOP) hybridization

SSOP hybridization methods can be applied to both low- and high-resolution HLA typing [34–44]. With this method, the HLA gene of interest is amplified by PCR and immobilized on nylon membranes. Oligonucleotide probes labeled with a reporter molecule (either radioactive or nonradioactive) are then allowed to hybridize to the membranes. Probes with sequences complementary to the membrane-bound DNA will hybridize, while those with as little as a single nucleotide mismatch will not (Fig. 4.7). The pattern of positive and negative hybridization is used to deduce the HLA type of the target DNA. In this method, only the known polymorphic sites in an HLA gene are probed and, therefore, no information is obtained for regions of the gene not defined by the sequence-specific probes. Although novel patterns of probe hybridization may indicate the possible presence of a new allele, alleles with polymorphisms outside of the probed regions may escape detection. Since many samples being examined for a given HLA gene can be tested on the same set of membranes, the SSOP method is particularly well suited to high volume HLA typing.

The above procedure describes the *forward blot* SSOP method. In a second format, the *reverse blot* method, the sequence-specific probes are immobilized on a solid phase support [45–47]. Sample DNA is labeled during PCR amplification and allowed to hybridize to the immobilized panel of probes. As with forward SSOP, HLA alleles are deduced from the pattern of positive and negative probe reactions (Fig. 4.8).

Sequencing

Sequencing methods provide the highest resolution typing of HLA alleles [48–53]. HLA genes and alleles can be sequenced from cloned templates (cDNA) or directly from PCR-amplified genomic DNA. These methods use either radioactive or fluorescent labels to detect nucleotide substitutions among HLA genes. Automated fluorescent sequencing has emerged as a powerful approach to typing HLA genes. The HLA gene is first amplified in a PCR reaction. Cycle sequencing of the PCR product is then

Fig. 4.8 SSOP reverse probe format typing. Genomic DNA was amplified with DRB locus specific biotinylated primers and hybridized to a panel of probes for DRB1, DRB3, DRB4 and DRB5 sequences immobilized on a nylon membrane strip. The pattern of positive hybridization reactions, detected by color formation, was interpreted with a computerized analysis program. The sample was typed as DRB1*15 or *16 by the presence of band A, DRB1*04 by bands B and C, DRB4*01 by band D, and DRB5*0101 or *0104 by bands E and F.

performed using primers which are labeled with a fluorescent label (*dye primer*, usually 5′ primer). Alternatively, the dideoxynucleotides ddATP, ddTTP, ddGTP, ddCTP can be individually labeled with fluorescent label (*dye terminator*). In dye primer sequencing, the label is incorporated into the 5′ end of the HLA sequence, whereas in dye terminator sequencing the addition of a labeled dideoxynucleotide at the 3′ end terminates the sequencing reaction. In both approaches the sequencing reaction is electrophoresed on a polyacrylamide gel using an automated sequencer. The fluorescent signals are captured and interpreted as a sequence of DNA bases by a computer program (Fig. 4.9). Assignment of the HLA allele(s) is performed by comparing the derived sequence to all known sequences for a given gene.

Sequencing methods can be applied to large-scale typing of populations and are particularly well-suited for the definitive characterization of newly defined alleles. Future developments in instrumentation, chemistry and automated allele analysis should enable this method to be more widely available for routine clinical use.

Reference strand mediated conformation analysis

Reference strand mediated conformation analysis (RSCA) is a novel

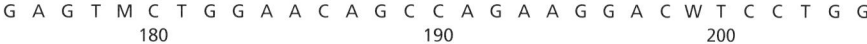
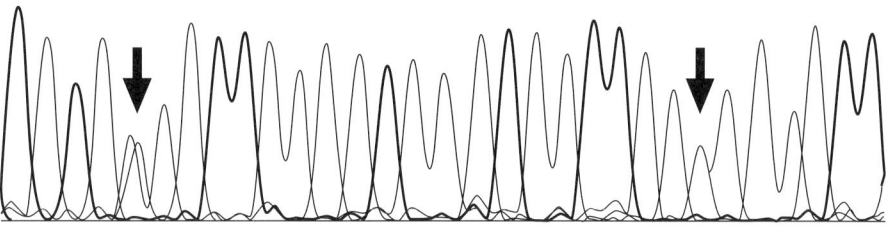

Fig. 4.9 DNA sequencing-based typing (SBT). The partial sequence chromatogram shows polymorphic positions 179 and 199 (arrows) of DRB1 exon 2 (residues 60 and 67) from an HLA-DRB1*0801,1201-positive sample. The genomic DNA was sequenced using direct automated dye primer fluorescent chemistry on an Applied Biosystems Model 377 sequencer (ABI, Inc., Foster City, CA). The laser induced fluorescent signal emitted from each sequenced fragment is captured and interpreted by software and identified on the chromatogram above the peak as an A, C, G, or T nucleotide base, except at heterozygous positions. Using the IUB codes, heterozygous position 179 has M, indicating signals from A (DRB1*0801) and C (DRB1*1201) while the W at position 199 indicates T (DRB1*0801) and A (DRB1*1201) were incorporated.

approach for high-resolution DNA typing and donor matching [54,55]. This technique uses a fluorescein-labeled reference DNA that has been PCR-amplified from the HLA gene of interest. The reference DNA is allowed to hybridize to locus-specific PCR products from the test samples. Duplex formation occurs when there is complementarity between the reference and test nucleotide sequences. Each antisense nucleotide strand is uniquely different and thus the mobility of the duplex on gel electrophoresis can be used for discrimination. This method allows the detection of single nucleotide substitutions within a given sequence and the rapid assessment of donor–recipient identity.

Oligonucleotide arrays

Oligonucleotide array technology combines standard nucleic acid hybridization approaches with innovative high-density DNA array technology. Initially developed to improve sequencing efforts in the Human Genome Project, the oligonucleotide array technology has been successfully applied to many fields of molecular biology, including large-scale gene discovery, monitoring the expression of thousands of genes, mutation and polymorphism detection, as well as the mapping of genomic clones.

Oligonucleotide array technology for HLA typing is particularly well-suited for the detection of complex polymorphisms in heterozygous individuals [56]. Multiple regions of polymorphisms in many HLA genes can be simultaneously assessed. Oligonucleotide probes can be designed to all known substitutions or to all four potential nucleotides and, thereby, enable detection of new sequence polymorphisms. Redundancy of probe sequences allows combinations of alleles to be distinguished in heterozygous individuals. Arrays are well-suited to the analysis of very large populations for multiple polymorphic genes.

Selection of typing methods to support allogeneic HCT

In addition to the methods described above, restriction fragment length polymorphism (RFLP) analysis [57], heteroduplex analysis [58,59] and single strand conformation polymorphism [60,61] have been developed and applied to clinical HLA testing and the study of the MHC. The selection of one or more DNA-based typing methods is largely determined by typing volume and the resolution required for clinical matching. The importance of HLA-matching and its impact on the clinical outcome for patients undergoing unrelated HCT (see Chapter 83) emphasizes the need for high-resolution typing capability for the final selection of a donor. At the same time, however, time constraints and the requirements for high-throughput typing technology must be considered, particularly in cases of high-risk unrelated transplant candidates who require the rapid identification of a suitable donor. Histocompatibility guidelines for unrelated HCT have recently been revised to accommodate DNA-based typing methods [62]. Informatic systems to facilitate automated data analysis and reporting are being actively developed. These systems will not only enable the accurate interpretation of complex sets of HLA data but will also promote the donor search process within large volunteer registries [63].

Clinical applications

With the establishment of DNA-based methods for clinical HLA typing, the importance of correlating previous serologic designations with new allele designations has emerged as a major issue. This is especially true in the field of unrelated donor HCT. Currently the National Marrow Donor Program, the world's largest volunteer registry, contains at least four million donors (see Chapter 49). Algorithms for equating serologically defined specificities with DNA-defined alleles have been developed, allowing access to donors in the registry who have been previously typed by outdated serologic methods. Each HLA allele is given a name or a *search determinant*, which encompasses a broader family of alleles [62]. This nomenclature facilitates donor identification as long as serologically typed donors are present in the registry. The search process will be made more efficient and accurate with the use of DNA method for upfront typing of newly recruited donors.

Identification of unrelated donors for HCT

A suitable donor can be identified for approximately 50–80% of patients for whom an unrelated donor search is initiated. The likelihood of identifying a donor is increased if the donor and patient share the same ethnic or racial background. The chances of finding a matched donor are also increased when the patient has two common extended HLA haplotypes and genotypes. Strong positive LD between HLA-B and -C and between HLA-DR and -DQ increases the probability that an HLA-A, -B, -DR-matched donor will also be matched for HLA-C and -DQ [20,21,64–67]. Conversely, mismatching at HLA-B or HLA-DR increases the chance of HLA-C or HLA-DQ mismatching, respectively. When an HLA-A, -B, -DR-matched donor is not available and selection must be made among mismatched donors, then avoidance of HLA-B or HLA-DR mismatching may help to decrease the total number of mismatches.

HLA-DP is now known to function as a transplantation determinant [68,69]. HLA-DP maps 400 kb centromeric to HLA-DQ (Fig. 4.1 and [10]). The weak LD between HLA-DP and HLA-A, -C, -B, -DR, -DQ leads to a high frequency of HLA-DP disparity among donor–recipient pairs who are matched for other HLA genes. If HLA-DP typing is performed prospectively for the purposes of donor identification, an average of six HLA-A, -C, -B, -DR, -DQ matched donors must be HLA-DP typed to yield one matched donor. In general, prospective typing and matching for HLA-DP is most useful when there is no clinical urgency to perform the transplant and when there are several five-locus HLA-A, -C, -B, -DR, -DQ matched donors who are equally suitable with respect to non-HLA variables, including CMV sero-status.

Definition of a mismatch

As described above, the availability of DNA-based typing methods provides two major "levels" of definitions of HLA genes. The "low" resolution level defines the serological-equivalent of the antigen (e.g. HLA-A2 vs. -A11), whereas the "high" resolution level defines nucleotide sequence disparity between individuals who are otherwise serologically matched (e.g. A*0201 vs. A*0205).

Traditionally, mismatching between serologically detectable HLA-A and -B antigens has been termed "minor" (CREG) if the antigens share serological crossreactive epitopes (Table 4.4). Examples of CREG mismatches include HLA-A2 and -A28, and HLA-B60 and -B61. An equivalent nomenclature is not available for HLA-C because of the lack of informative sera for many HLA-C gene products [64]. A "major" HLA-A or -B antigen mismatch occurs when the antigens do not show serological crossreactivity. Examples of major mismatches are HLA-A1 and -A2, and HLA-B8 and -B44.

Serologically detectable mismatches at HLA-DR can be defined in two ways. The term "minor" mismatch has been used to describe mismatching between the antigen subtypes, or splits, of a given parent antigen. Examples of HLA-DR minor mismatches include DR15 and DR16 (splits of DR2); DR11 and DR12 (splits of DR5); DR13 and DR14 (splits of DR6); and DR17 and DR18 (splits of DR3). The term "major" HLA-DR mismatch has been used to describe mismatches between two parent antigens (or between their respective subtypes). Examples of major mismatches include DR1 and DR2; DR3 and DR4; DR15 and DR17.

Vector of incompatibility

In 1994, Anasetti and Hansen [70] demonstrated the relevance of the vector of HLA compatibility in risk of graft failure and acute graft-vs.-host disease (GVHD) in related haploidentical transplants. The vector (sometimes referred to as the "direction" of the mismatch) can be defined for host-vs.-graft (HVG) and graft-vs.-host (GVH) alloreactivity. The presence of donor antigens or alleles not shared by the recipient determines HVG allorecognition. The presence of recipient antigen or alleles not shared by the donor provides the immunological basis for GVH allorecognition. Examples of HVG and GVH vector mismatches are provided in Table 4.6.

Mismatching between a donor and recipient can be described as "bidirectional" if both HVG and GVH vectors are present at a given HLA locus. Mismatching is called "unidirectional" if one but not the other vector is present. Unidirectional mismatching in the GVH vector occurs when the donor is homozygous and the recipient is heterozygous and shares one allele or antigen with the donor (e.g. patient A*0201, *0205 vs. donor A*0201, *0201). Unidirectional mismatching in the HVG vector occurs when the patient is homozygous and the donor is heterozygous and shares one allele with the patient (e.g. patient A*0201, *0201 vs. donor A*0201, *0205).

Table 4.6 Vector of mismatch.

		Examples	
Vector	Definition	Donor	Recipient
HVG	Presence of donor alleles or antigens not present in the recipient	B*0801,4402[†] B*0801,4402[‡]	B*0801,4405 B*0801,0801
GVH	Presence of recipient alleles or antigens not present in the donor	B*0801,4402[†] B*0801,0801[‡]	B*0801,4405 B*0801,4405

[†]These combinations contain bi-directional (both HVG and GVHD) mismatch vectors.
[‡]Unidirectional mismatches.
GVH, graft-vs.-host; GVHD, graft-vs.-host disease; HVG, host-vs.-graft.

Minor histocompatibility antigens

While MHC genes and their encoded proteins represent the major barrier to tissue transplantation, disparity for antigens encoded by genes outside the MHC, termed minor histocompatibility antigens (mHA), can also provoke significant alloimmune responses. mHA are small endogenous polymorphic peptides that are recognized by T cells in an MHC-restricted manner. In comparison to MHC-region genes, the genes that encode mHA are much less polymorphic; however, the total number of mHA-encoding loci throughout the genome is predicted to be very large. To date, 11 different human mHA have been defined biochemically, seven of which are encoded by genes located on the Y chromosome and four by genes located on at least three different autosomes. The latter mHA have been termed HA-1, HA-2, HA-3 and HA-8 [71].

The extent to which donor–recipient incompatibility for mHA results in graft rejection and/or GVHD in human HCT is an area of ongoing research. Among patients receiving HCT from an HLA-identical sibling, mismatching for HA-1 has been shown to be associated with an increased risk of acute GVHD in one study [72] but not in another [73]. Disparity for CD31, a platelet-endothelial-cell adhesion molecule encoded by a gene residing on chromosome 17, has been reported to be associated with an increased risk of GVHD among patients receiving HCT from HLA-identical sibling donors [74,75]. The results of a separate study, however, did not identify CD31 as a significant risk factor for GVHD [76]. The typing and matching of patients and prospective donors for mHA prior to HCT might be advantageous for transplant outcome, but practical considerations will likely limit its implementation in the selection of potential donors. Only a few of the mHA that are predicted to exist can be defined by current laboratory methods. Moreover, the identification of suitable related and unrelated donors is already limited by the requirement for HLA-matching, and the further requirement for mHA matching would significantly reduce the number of available donors [77]. See Chapter 3 for further discussion of mHA and their role in HCT.

Impact of donor compatibility on clinical outcome after unrelated HCT

Substantial new information is now available on the role of donor HLA matching in unrelated HCT (see Chapter 83 for a comprehensive review) [64–69,78]. The clinical utility of DNA-based typing methods for donor selection is twofold: (i) the identification and prioritization of well-matched donors (more complete and accurate matching is associated with lower risks of graft failure and GVHD and with improved survival); and (ii) identification and avoidance of donors mismatched for multiple alleles (multilocus disparity is associated with increased risks of graft failure,

GVHD and mortality). The minimal requirements for HLA matching can vary depending on the clinical situation. Recent data demonstrate that in the absence of allele-matched donors the use of donors with a single allele mismatch may not necessarily lower survival [65–67]. The factors that govern whether a gene mismatch is likely to be tolerable are highly complex and depend on the specific donor–recipient allele or antigen mismatch, the transplant procedure (conditioning and immunosuppressive regimen) and other non-HLA variables. Comprehensive examination of class I and class II disparities in ethnically diverse transplant populations is needed in order to understand how qualitative and quantitative differences between mismatches can aid in the identification of permissible mismatches.

Conclusion

Genes of the HLA system encode a complex array of histocompatibility molecules that play a central role in immune responsiveness and in determining the outcome of tissue transplantation. The primary goal of histocompatibility testing for patients undergoing HCT is the identification of a suitable HLA-matched donor to reduce the risk of post-transplant complications resulting from HLA incompatibility. The recent advent of DNA-based methods that allow discrimination of HLA genes at the allele level has enhanced our ability to perform typing and matching with precision and speed. The extensive polymorphism of the HLA system, however, makes the selection of an optimally matched donor a challenging endeavor. New data demonstrate that the permissibility of an HLA mismatch is shaped by a complex interaction of qualitative and quantitative differences in the HLA sequences between the donor and recipient. Current experience indicates that it is possible to achieve excellent clinical results with a less than perfectly matched donor. Identification of the elements that define tolerable mismatches will permit increased availability of unrelated donor and mismatched family member donor HCT to patients who lack a genotypically identical sibling.

References

1. Dausset J. Leuco-agglutinins. IV. Leuco-agglutinins and blood transfusion. *Vox Sang* 1954; **4**: 190–8.
2. van Rood JJ, van Leeuwen A. Leucocyte grouping. A method and its application. *J Clin Invest* 1963; **42**: 1382–90.
3. Payne R, Tripp M, Weigle J, Bodmer W, Bodmer J. A new leukocyte isoantigenic system in man. *Cold Spring Harbor Sym Quant Biol* 1964; **29**: 285–95.
4. Amos DB. Nomenclature for factors of the HL-A system. *Science* 1968; **160**: 659–60.
5. Bodmer WF. HLA. What's in a name? A commentary on HLA nomenclature development over the years. *Tissue Antigens* 1997; **46**: 293–6.
6. Bjorkman PJ, Saper MA, Samrowi B et al. Structure of the human class I histocompatibility antigen, HLA-A2. *Nature* 1987; **329**: 506–12.
7. Brown JH, Jardetzky TS, Gorga JC et al. Three-dimensional structure of the human class II histcompatibility antigen HLA-DR1. *Nature* 1993; **364**: 33–9.
8. Horn GT, Bugawan TL, Long CM, Erlich HA. Allelic sequence variation of the HLA-DQ loci: relationship to serology and to insulin-dependent diabetes susceptibility. *Proc Natl Acad Sci U S A* 1988; **85**: 6012–6.
9. Bodmer JG, Marsh SGE, Albert ED et al. Nomenclature for factors of the HLA system, 2000. *Tissue Antigens* 2001; **57**: 236–83.
10. Rhodes DA, Trowsdale J. Genetics and molecular genetics of the MHC. *Rev Immunogenetics* 1999; **1**: 21–31.
11. Bain B, Vas MR, Lowenstein L. The development of large immature cells in mixed leukocyte cultures. *Blood* 1964; **23**: 108–16.
12. Bach FH, Hirschhorn K. Lymphocyte interaction: a potential histocompatibility test *in vitro*. *Science* 1964; **143**: 813–4.
13. Geraghty DE, Wei X, Orr HT et al. HLA-F: an expressed HLA gene composed of a class I coding sequence linked to a novel transcribed repetitive element. *J Exp Med* 1990; **171**: 1–19.
14. Geraghty DE, Koller BH, Orr HT. A human major histocompatibility complex class I gene that encodes a protein with a shortened cytoplasmic segment. *Proc Natl Acad Sci U S A* 1987; **84**: 9145–9.
15. Koller BH, Geraghty DE, Shimizu Y et al. A novel HLA class I gene expressed in resting T lymphocytes. *J Immunol* 1988; **141**: 897–904.
16. Mandelboim O, Pazmany L, Davis DM et al. Multiple receptors for HLA-G on human natural killer cells. *Proc Natl Acad Sci U S A*, 1997; **94**: 14666–70.
17. Lee N, Llano M, Carretero M et al. HLA-E is a major ligand for the natural killer inhibitory receptor CD94/NKG2A. *Proc Natl Acad Sci U S A*, 1998; **95**: 5199–204.
18. Rammensee H-G. Chemistry of peptides associated with MHC class I and class II molecules. *Current Opinion Immunol* 1995; **7**: 85–96.
19. Marshall KW, Liu AF, Canales J et al. Role of the polymorphic residues in HLA-DR molecules in allele-specific binding of peptide ligands. *J Immunol* 1994; **152**: 4946–57.
20. Petersdorf EW, Longton GM, Anasetti C et al. The significance of HLA-DRB1 matching on clinical outcome after HLA-A, B, DR identical unrelated donor marrow transplantation. *Blood* 1995; **86**: 1606–13.
21. Petersdorf EW, Longton GM, Anasetti C et al. Definition of HLA-DQ as a transplantation antigen. *Proc Natl Acad Sci U S A* 1996; **93**: 15,358–63.
22. Socie G, Loiseau P, Tamouza R et al. Both genetic and clinical factors predict the development of graft-versus-host disease after allogeneic hematopoietic stem cell transplantation. *Transplantation* 2001; **72**: 699–706.
23. Begovich AB, McClure GR, Suraj VC et al. Polymorphism, recombination, and linkage disequilibrium within the HLA class II region. *J Immunol* 1992; **148**: 249–58.
24. Mori M, Beatty PG, Graves M et al. HLA gene and haplotype frequencies in the North American population. *Transplantation* 1997; **64**: 1017–27.
25. National Institutes of Health. NIH lymphocyte microcytotoxicity technique. In: *NIAID Manual of Tissue Typing Techniques*. Publication no. NIH 80–545. Atlanta: Department of Health, Education, and Welfare, 1979.
26. Schreuder GM, Hurley CK, Marsh SG et al. The HLA dictionary 1999. A summary of HLA-A-B-C-DRB1/3/4/5-DQB1 alleles and their association with serologically-defined HLA-A-B-C-DR, and -DQ antigens. *Hum Immunol* 1999; **60**: 1157–81.
27. Termijtelen A, Erlich HA, Braun LA et al. Oligonucleotide typing is a perfect tool to identify antigens stimulatory in the mixed lymphocyte culture. *Hum Immunol* 1991; **31**: 241–5.
28. Browning MJ, Krausa P, Rowan A et al. Tissue typing the HLA-A locus from genomic DNA by sequence-specific PCR. Comparison of HLA genotype and surface expression on colorectal tumor cell lines. *Proc Natl Acad Sci U S A* 1993; **90**: 2842–5.
29. Krausa P, Bodmer JG, Browning M. Defining the common subtypes of HLA-A9, A10, A28 and A19 by use of ARMS/PCR. *Tissue Antigens* 1993; **42**: 91–9.
30. Bunce M, Welsh KI. Rapid DNA typing for HLA-C using sequence-specific primers (PCR-SSP). Identification of serological and nonserologically defined HLA-C alleles including several new alleles. *Tissue Antigens* 1994; **43**: 7–17.
31. Sadler AM, Petronzelli F, Krausa P et al. Low-resolution DNA typing for HLA-B using sequence-specific primers in allele or group specific ARMS/PCR. *Tissue Antigens* 1994; **44**: 148–54.
32. Guttridge MG, Burr C, Klouda PT. Identification of HLA-B35, B53, B18, B5, B78 and B17 alleles by the polymerase chain reaction using sequence-specific primers (PCR-SSP). *Tissue Antigens* 1994; **44**: 43–6.
33. Hein J, Bottcher K, Grundmann R, Kirchner H, Bein G. Low resolution DNA typing of the HLA-B5 cross-reactive group by nested PCR-SSP. *Tissue Antigens* 1995; **45**: 27–35.
34. Bugawan TL, Begovich AB, Erlich HA. Rapid HLA DPB typing using enzymatically amplified DNA and nonradioactive sequence-specific ologonucleotide probes. *Immunogenetics* 1990; **32**: 231–41.
35. Petersdorf EW, Smith AG, Mickelson EM, Martin PJ, Hansen JA. Ten HLA-DR4 alleles defined by sequence polymorphisms within the DRB1 first domain. *Immunogenetics* 1991; **33**: 267–75.
36. Dominguez O, Coto E, Martinez-Naves E, Choo SY, Lopez-Larrea C. Molecular typing of HLA-B27 alleles. *Immunogenetics* 1992; **36**: 277–82.
37. Yoshida M, Kimura A, Numano F, Sasazuki T. Polymerase chain reaction-based analysis of polymorphism in the HLA-B gene. *Hum Immunol* 1992; **34**: 257–66.
38. Rufer N, Breur-Vriesendorp BS, Tiercy J-M et al. High-resolution histocompatibility testing of a group of sixteen B44-positive, ABDR serologically matched unrelated donor–recipient pairs: analysis of serologically undisclosed incompatibilities by cellular techniques, isoelectric focusing, and HLA oligotyping. *Hum Immunol* 1993; **38**: 235–9.

39 Molkentin J, Gorski J, Baxter-Lowe LA. Detection of 14 HLA-DQB1 alleles by oligotyping. *Hum Immunol* 1991; **31**: 114–22.
40 Allen M, Liu L, Gyllensten U. A comprehensive polymerase chain reaction-oligonucleotide typing system for the HLA-class I A locus. *Hum Immunol* 1994; **40**: 25–32.
41 Gao XJ, Jakobsen IB, Serjeanson SW. Characterization of HLA-A polymorphism by locus-specific polymerase chain reaction amplification and oligonucleotide hybridization. *Hum Immunol* 1994; **41**: 267–79.
42 Levine JE, Yang SY. SSOP typing of the Tenth International Histocompatibility Workshop: reference cell lines for HLA-C alleles. *Tissue Antigens* 1994; **44**: 174–83.
43 Fernandez-Vina MA, Lazaro AM, Sun Y et al. Population diversity of B-locus alleles observed by high resolution DNA typing. *Tissue Antigens* 1995; **45**: 153–68.
44 Hurley CK, Baxter-Lowe LA, Begovich AB et al. The extent of HLA class II allele level disparity in unrelated bone marrow transplantation: analysis of 1259 National Marrow Donor Program donor–recipient pairs. *Bone Marrow Transplant* 2000; **25**: 385–93.
45 Erlich HA, Bugawan T, Begovich A et al. HLA-DR, DQ & DP typing using PCR amplification and immobilized probes. *Eur J Immunogen* 1991; **18**: 33–5.
46 Scharf SJ, Griffith RL, Erlich HA. Rapid typing of DNA sequence polymorphism at the HLA-DRB1 locus using the polymerase chain reaction and non-radioactive oligonucleotide probes. *Hum Immunol* 1991; **30**: 190–201.
47 Bugawan TL, Apple R, Erlich HA. A method for typing polymorphism at the HLA-A locus using PCR amplification and immobilized oligonucleotide probes. *Tissue Antigens* 1994; **44**: 137–47.
48 Santamaria P, Lindstrom AL, Boyce-Jacino MT et al. HLA class I sequence-based typing. *Hum Immunol* 1993; **37**: 39–50.
49 Versluis LF, Rozemuller E, Tonks S et al. High-resolution HLA-DPB typing based upon computerized analysis of data obtained by fluorescent sequencing of the amplified polymorphic exon 2. *Hum Immunol* 1993; **38**: 277–83.
50 Domena JD, Little A-M, Arnett KL et al. A small test of a sequence-based typing method: definition of the B*1520 allele. *Tissue Antigens* 1994; **44**: 217–24.
51 Petersdorf EW, Hansen JA. A comprehensive approach for typing the alleles of the HLA-B locus by automated sequencing. *Tissue Antigens* 1995; **46**: 73–85.
52 Yao Z, Keller E, Scholz S et al. Identification of two major HLA-B44 subtypes and a novel B44 sequence: oligotyping and solid phase sequencing of PCR products. *Hum Immunol* 1995; **42**: 54–60.
53 Kotsch K, Wehling J, Blasczyk R. Sequencing of HLA class II genes based on the conserved diversity of the non-coding regions: sequencing based typing of HLA-DRB genes. *Tissue Antigens* 1999; **53**: 486–97.
54 Arguello R, Avakian H, Goldman JM, Madrigal JA. A novel method for simultaneous high resolution identification of HLA-A, HLA-B and HLA-Cw alleles. *Proc Natl Acad Sci U S A* 1996; **93**: 10,961–5.
55 Madrigal JA, Arguello R, Gallardo D et al. High resolution HLA class I and II typing for unrelated bone marrow donors. *Eur J Immunogenet* 1997; **24**: 70 [Abstract].
56 Guo Z, Gatterman MS, Hood L, Hansen JA, Petersdorf EW. Oligonucleotide arrays for high-throughput SNPs detection in the MHC class I genes: HLA-B as a model system. *Genome Res* 2002; **12**: 447–57.
57 Marcadet A, O'Connell P, Cohen D. Standardized Southern blot workshop technique. In: Dupont B, ed. *Immunobiology of HLA*, Vol. 1. New York: Springer-Verlag, 1989: 553–60.
58 Clay TM, Bidwell JL, Howard MR, Bradley BA. PCR-fingerprinting for selection of HLA matched unrelated marrow donors. Collaborating centres in the IMUST Study. *Lancet* 1991; **337**: 1049–52.
59 Tong JR, Hammad A, Rudert WA, Trucco M, Hsia S. Heteroduplexes for HLA-DQB1 identity of family members and kidney donor–recipient pairs. *Transplantation* 1994; **57**: 741–5.
60 Orita M, Suzuki Y, Sekiya T, Hayashi K. Rapid and sensitive detection of point mutations and DNA polymorphisms using polymerase chain reaction. *Genomics* 1989; **5**: 874–9.
61 Blasczyk R, Hahn U, Wehling J, Huhn D, Salama A. Complete amplification followed by direct sequencing or single-strand conformation polymorphism analysis. *Tissue Antigens* 1995; **46**: 86–95.
62 Hurley CK, Wade JA, Oudshoorn M et al. A special report: histocompatibility testing guidelines for hematopoietic stem cell transplantation using volunteer donors. *Tissue Antigens* 1999; **53**: 394–406.
63 Helmberg W, Zhan R, Keller E et al. Virtual DNA analysis as a platform for interlaboratory exchange of HLA DNA typing results. *Tissue Antigens* 1999; **54**: 379–85.
64 Petersdorf EW, Longton GM, Anasetti C et al. Association of HLA-C disparity with graft failure after marrow transplantation from unrelated donors. *Blood* 1997; **89**: 1818–23.
65 Sasazuki T, Juj G, Morishima Y et al. Effect of matching of class I HLA alleles on clinical outcome after transplantation of hematopoietic stem cells from an unrelated donor. *N Engl J Med* 1998; **339**: 1177–85.
66 Petersdorf EW, Gooley TA, Anasetti C et al. Optimizing outcome after unrelated marrow transplantation by comprehensive matching of HLA class I and II alleles in the donor and recipient. *Blood* 1998; **82**: 3515–20.
67 Petersdorf EW, Hansen JA, Martin PJ et al. Major-histocompatibility-complex class I alleles and antigens in hematopoietic cell transplantation. *N Engl J Med* 2001; **345**: 1794–800.
68 Petersdorf EW, Gooley T, Malkki M et al. The biological significance of HLA-DP gene variation in hematopoietic cell transplantation. *Br J Haematol* 2001; **112**: 988–94.
69 Varney MD, Lester S, McCluskey J, Gao X, Tait BD. Matching for HLA DPA1 and DPB1 alleles in unrelated bone marrow transplantation. *Human Immunol* 1999; **60**: 532–8.
70 Anasetti C, Hansen JA. Effect of HLA incompatibility in marrow transplantation from unrelated and HLA-mismatched related donors. *Transfus Sci* 1994; **15**: 221–30.
71 Simpson E, Roopenian D. Report of the Second International Symposium on Minor Histocompatibility Antigens: Seattle, 2002. In: Hansen JA, Dupont B, eds. *HLA 2002: Immunobiology of the Human MHC (Proceedings of the 13th International Histocompatibility Workshop and Conference)*. Seattle, WA: IHWG Press, 2002: in press.
72 Goulmy E, Schipper R, Pool J et al. Mismatches of minor histocompatibility antigens between HLA-identical donors and recipients and the development of graft-versus-host disease after bone marrow transplantation. *N Engl J Med* 1996; **334**: 281–5.
73 Lin M-T, Gooley T, Hansen JA et al. Absence of statistically significant correlation between disparity for the minor histocompatibility antigen HA-1 and outcome after allogeneic hematopoietic cell transplantation (Letter to the editor). *Blood* 2001; **98**: 3172–3.
74 Behar E, Chao NJ, Hiraki DD et al. Polymorphism of adhesion molecule CD31 and its role in acute graft-versus-host disease. *N Engl J Med* 1996; **334**: 286–91.
75 Grumet FC, Hiraki DD, Brown BW et al. CD31 mismatching affects marrow transplantation outcome. *Biol Blood Marrow Transplant* 2001; **7**: 503–12.
76 Nichols WC, Antin JH, Lunetta KL et al. Polymorphism of adhesion molecule CD31 is not a significant risk factor for graft-versus-host disease. *Blood* 1996; **88**: 4429–34.
77 Martin PJ. Applicability of matching for minor histocompatibility antigens in human bone marrow transplantation. In: Roopenian DC, Simpson E, eds. *Minor Histocompatibility Antigens: from the Laboratory to the Clinic*. Georgetown, Washington, DC: Landis Bioscience, 2000: 97–103.
78 Ferrara GB, Bacigalupo A, Lamparelli T et al. Bone marrow transplantation from unrelated donors: the impact of mismatches with substitutions at position 116 of the human leukocyte antigen class I heavy chain. *Blood* 2001; **98**: 3150–5.

5

*Lakshmi K. Gaur**

Functional Evolution of the Major Histocompatibility Complex

Introduction

The major histocompatibility complex (MHC) is a multigene family that includes several highly polymorphic loci and plays a cardinal role in the defense of vertebrates against parasites and other pathogens [2]. It is by far the most polymorphic gene cluster known and is divided into three regions, classes I, II and III, each region containing multiple genes. Class I and class II gene products are directly associated with immune reactions whereas class III gene products play an indirect role. The extraordinary polymorphism at class I and class II has become a target of intensive scrutiny for the last three decades. What are the functions of these class I and class II gene clusters that require such an extensive diversity? The primary function of class I and class II molecules is to "present" antigenic peptides to the T cells of the immune system. However, there are subtle differences in what and how they present the antigenic peptides that are facilitated by the structural differences within these two classes of molecules. MHC class I molecules are expressed on all nucleated cells and bind to intracellularly processed antigenic peptides, for example viral peptides, and thus provide the context for recognition of foreign proteins by cytotoxic T lymphocytes (CTLs). Whereas the MHC class II molecules are expressed constitutively on a few specialized cells, termed antigen-presenting cells (APCs), and primarily present peptides that have been digested from external sources and internalized by APCs, such as macrophages, B cells and dendritic cells, to CD4$^+$ T helper cells. After elegantly deciphering that the function of MHC is to bind foreign antigens and present them to the T lymphocytes [3], Doherty and Zinkernagel speculated that MHC polymorphism could be maintained by heterozygote advantage [4,5].

Over 1500 allelic variants have been identified to date at these multiple MHC loci in humans (referred to as human leukocyte antigens [HLAs]) and include 957 class I and over 630 class II alleles (see http://www.ebi.ac.uk/imgt/hla/) [6]. This genetic polymorphism is the basis for structural variation in MHC molecules both within individuals and between individuals within a species, which accounts for the complex and diverse functional interactions by which different MHC proteins bind a wide array of antigenic peptides. Further, this structural diversity has shown evolutionary conservation in several mammalian species studied to date. One of the unique features in the evolution of the MHC is the presence of distinct allelic lineages within a species that are recapitulated in another related species [7]. In other words, certain polymorphisms persisted as the MHC has evolved across species. This striking finding implies functional selection and evolutionary mechanisms that are quite ancient. Detailed analysis of MHC nucleotide and amino acid sequences has led to several hypotheses to account for the generation and maintenance of this polymorphism, including the speculation by Doherty and Zinkernagel [5]. Understanding the evolutionary history of MHC allelic lineages has the potential to clarify fundamental functional properties intrinsic to these loci.

Allelic diversity

The MHC class I and class II molecules are cell surface heterodimers with four extra cellular domains and gene encoding for them is located on the short arm of chromosome 6 (Fig. 5.1; see also Plate 5.1, *facing p. 296*). There are at least 10 class I members (*HLA-A, -B, -C, -E, -F, -G, -H, -J, -K, -L* in humans) and numerous class II loci in a long stretch of contiguous genes across the short arm of chromosome 6 (6p21.31). The generation of this genetic diversity perhaps required numerous gene duplications, including tandem duplications. In the later situation more than one locus duplicates. Based on their structural similarities it was speculated that all MHC genes are perhaps derived from a common ancestral gene. In this scheme, the class I lineage evolved as a single three-domain polypeptide while the class II lineage evolved as a series of codependent α and β polypeptides [8]. In humans, the class II α-β linkage clusters have evolved into four main clusters termed *DR, DQ, DP, DM* and *DO* and within each cluster multiple loci represent additional gene duplications, some of which are currently functional and some of which are pseudogenes.

Figure 5.2 (see also Plate 5.3, *facing p. 296*) illustrates the two-layer polymorphism of the MHC loci where the classical class I (*HLA-A, -B* and -*C*) and class II genes (for the three regions *HLA-DR, -DQ* and -*DP*) are shown. Extraordinary polymorphism is evident for class I loci 274, 519 and 133 alleles at *A, B* and *C* loci, respectively. Among class II genes, except for *DRA*, all other loci are highly polymorphic. As a consequence of multiple gene duplication events, the number of MHC genes is variable between individuals. Although there are nine *DRB* loci identified, not all of them are present in every individual. A variable number of *HLA-DRB* genes appear in different combinations. The pattern of *DR* haplotypes is shown in Table 5.1 (see also Plate 5.2, *facing p. 296*) where every individual carries in addition to a *DRB1* locus a second expressed *DRB* locus (*DRB3, DRB4* and/or *DRB5*) with the exception of *DR8* and *10*. For instance, the *HLA-DR2* haplotype (*DR15* and *DR16* group of alleles) expresses *DRB1* and *B5* genes, *HLA-DR3, 11, 12, 13* and *14* haplotypes express *DRB1* and *B3* genes, while *HLA-DR4, HLA-DR7* and *HLA-DR9* haplotypes express *DRB1* and *B4* genes. Most *HLA-DR1* and *HLA-DR8* haplotypes express only the *DRB1* gene. Certain *DR1* group alleles show association with *DRB5* in certain populations. All haplotypes possess the DRB9 pseudogene. The nonpolymorphic *DRA* gene is linked to a varying number of *DRB* genes in different *DR* haplotypes [9].

*Adapted from the previous version by Gaur & Nepom [1]

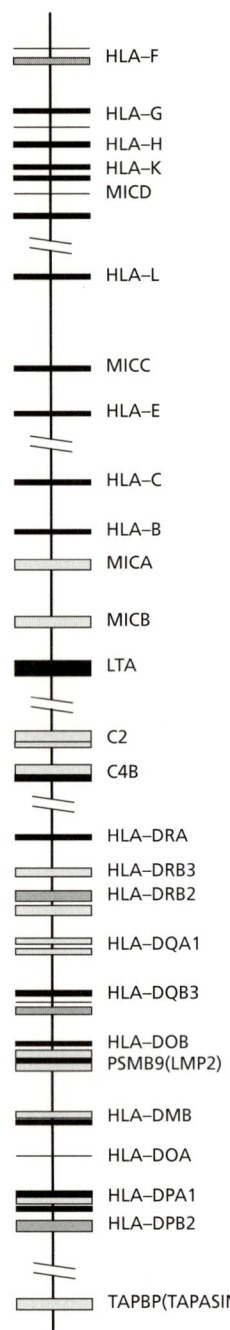

Fig. 5.1 Localization and organization of HLA class I and class II genes on the short arm of chromosome 6 (6p21.31). Selected class I and class II genes are shown not to scale from (HLA-F) telomere towards centromere (tapasin). (Adapted in part from http://www.path.cam.ac.uk/~mch/map/MainMapPage.html) (See also Plate 5.1, *facing p. 296*.)

Patterns of diversification

This diversity in gene number is but a small part of MHC polymorphism. For example, hundreds of alleles occur at some of the individual functional class I and class II alleles (500 alleles at *HLA-B* and >320 at *HLA-DRB1* alone). While certain clusters of alleles are highly homologous, others differ by multiple substitutions. For example, *HLA-DR2*, *3* and *4* differ from each other at 18–20 amino acids, as do HLA class I alleles such as *HLA-A2* and *-A3*. There are subtle differences in the allelic diversity between class I and class II loci. In class I the polymorphic α_1–α_2 domains encoded by the second and third exons, respectively, form the peptide-binding groove, where most of the sequence polymorphisms are located. Within class II the pattern of diversification is twofold; one in *DP* and *DQ* regions, a combinatorial-dimer formation is a possibility since polymorphisms occur both in α and β chain encoding genes. However, it is the *DRB* loci with at least four functional and five pseudogenes that contribute to the bulk of class II polymorphism as evidenced by the 400 *DRB* allelic variants in humans (Fig. 5.2; see also Plate 5.3, *facing p. 296*). Interestingly, in the *DR* region, the *DRA* gene remained monomorphic while *DRB* genes have evolved in a manner reminiscent of the way class I genes diverged [10].

Within each *MHC-DRB* locus, variation occurs prominently within the second exon, while other exons are largely invariant. This is also true for other class II genes. The second exon of the *MHC-DRB* genes encode discrete sequence motifs, which can be used as a basis for lineage assignments to determine genetic and evolutionary relationships. For instance all DRB1*04 group of alleles are expected to share sequence motifs at the first hypervariable region (HVR_I), in addition to the linkage with the DRB4 locus. HVR_I falls within the part of the exon encoding β-pleated sheet platform structure underlying the MHC-antigen binding groove: Codons 6–53 encode β-pleated sheet. However, motif conservation between allelic variants was also apparent at HVR_{III} and codons contributing to this region are known to form part of the α-helical cleft of the peptide-binding groove [11,12]. Allelic alignments within the *HLA-DRB* display a pattern of shared sequence identities that could be grouped based on homologies at either β-pleated sheet encoding sequences or sequences encoding the α-helical region (codons 54–78) and revealed different evolutionary histories when subjected to phylogenetic analyzes [13–15]. A similar analysis using selected *HLA-DRB* and old world monkey *DRB* sequences for codons 6–53, encoding the β-pleated sheet (Fig. 5.3a; see also Plate 5.4, *facing p. 296* [16]) and codons 54–78, encoding the α-helix (Fig. 5.3b; Plate 5.4) corroborate these earlier observations [14]. In the phylogenetic trees for the β-pleated sheet the sequences cluster according to homologies in HVR_I. This pattern corresponds to the serological *HLA-DR52* grouping (*DR3, 5, 6* and *8*) which supports a common ancestry for the *DR8* and *52* haplotype and the *DR53* associated group (*DR4* and *9*). In contrast, in the tree based on codons 54–78 (encoding the α-helix) the *DR* specificities are intermixed. However, there are exceptions in assuming group specific allelic designations. For example, owing to their HVR_I, which are identical to *DR4* alleles, DRB1*1122 and DRB1*1410 show branch relation to the *DR4* group of alleles (Fig. 5.3a; Plate 5.4). This pattern is not evident when sequences from α-helical regions are aligned (Fig. 5.3b; Plate 5.4). These alleles do not share the linkage with the *DRB4* locus but are linked to the *DRB3* locus, which is characteristic of *DR11* and *14* alleles. HLA-DRB1*0103, 0402, 0414,1301 and 1302 also form a close cluster, all having a very similar nucleotide sequence pattern from codons 54–78. Earlier it was shown that when nucleotide sequences from the relatively nonpolymorphic third exon were used in the alignment, the sequences clustered in accordance with the β-pleated sheet sequences [14].

Interestingly, these findings are not limited to HLA alone. The loci that are polymorphic in humans are also polymorphic in other primates, and the allelic divergence is just as extensive. This pattern of polymorphism, with the presence of multiple DRB loci and a limited locus diversification for DQ and DP molecules, is also seen in other mammalian species [14–22]. Further, certain human lineages seem to bear ancient roots. Numerous examples are available where certain alleles in different species bear close resemblance to contemporary human alleles. For instance, the macaque and baboon DRB1*4 group of alleles cluster with the HLA DRB1*04 alleles; similarly, macaque and baboon DRB1*13 alleles cluster with the *HLA-DRB3*-associated *DRB1* alleles (Fig. 5.3a; Plate 5.4).

Functional Evolution of the MHC

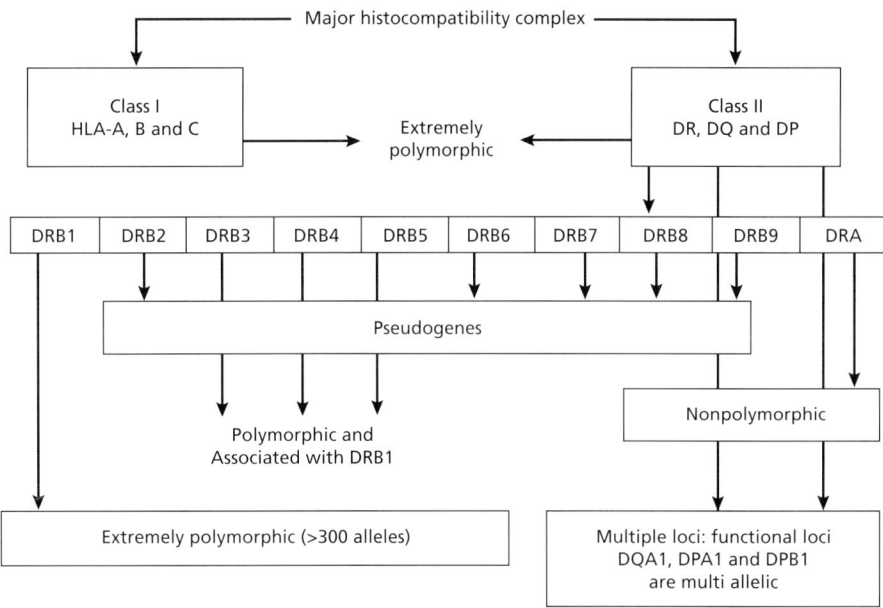

Fig. 5.2 Two layer polymorphism of the major histocompatibility loci: multiple loci and multiple alleles. DR region with a variation in the number of DRB genes compared to the conserved number of DQ and DP genes is intriguing. The duplication and recombination events have affected other class II genes differently. DP and DQ clusters present a possibility of combinatorial dimers since polymorphism occurs both in α and β chain encoding genes. (See also Plate 5.3, facing p. 296.)

Table 5.1 Organization of *DRB* haplotypes. (See also Plate 5.2, facing p. 296)

DRB1 allelic groups	DRB2	DRB3	DRB4	DRB5	DRB6	DRB7	DRB8	DRB9
DR3, 11, 12, 13 & 14		X						X
DR4, 7 & 9			X			X	X	X
DR1*, 15 & 16				X	X			X
DR1, 10					X			X
DR8								X

Some examples are provided in the *MHC-DRB* second exon sequence alignment (Fig. 5.4; see also Plate 5.5, *facing p. 296*, [14,15,20,23]).

Evolutionary conservation of polymorphisms

One of the most intriguing aspects of this extensive polymorphism is its evolutionary history. The existence of vast numbers of alleles in populations, marked by a considerable amount of nucleotide sequence diversity between the alleles, has been a focus of evolutionary analysis for years [7,8,24,25]. Although the accumulation of nucleotide substitutions by mutation following species inception seems *a priori*, a plausible explanation for the presence of such extensive polymorphism, interspecies comparative studies have yielded alternative explanations [8,24–29]. Allelic specificities present in one species are often present in others (Fig. 5.4, *Plate 5.5*); indeed, the evolution of MHC alleles does not correlate with inception of a species. Instead, a group of major alleles is represented in the phylogeny from one species to another, with the subsequent accumulation of additional mutations. This is evidenced by the presence of contemporary human alleles in evolutionarily distant species [8,21,27–32]. A few examples of this can be seen where macaque and baboon *DR4*, *DR13* alleles cluster with their human homologues (Figs 5.3 & 5.4, *Plates 5.4 & 5.5*). Such a *trans*-species mode of evolution enables individual MHC alleles to accumulate mutations and diverge significantly from each other without needing a high mutation rate that could accelerate the diversification of alleles [27]. It was estimated that the mutation rate of MHC loci is not higher than that of most other genetic loci [33] and alternative mechanisms, such as gene conversion and interlocus genetic exchange, have been suggested [34–36]. If new species were formed from small numbers of individuals expressing a set of particular genetic variants, these variants would serve as wild type in the new species. The further diversification of the species by additional mutational mechanisms would generate subsequent polymorphisms not shared by different populations.

Phylogenetic studies based on molecular comparisons in various species, from rodents [24,37] to chimpanzees [15,22,23,26,27], have been used to analyze patterns of MHC diversification. Nonhuman primate species with known divergence rates from humans are excellent models for these studies and have led to the remarkable finding that individual patterns of alleles in humans are more related by sequence to similar alleles in nonhuman primates than they are to other human alleles at the same locus. Both Fig. 5.3a (*Plate 5.4*) and Plate 5.6 (*facing p. 296*) illustrate this, for the selected old world monkey alleles. For instance, macaque-*DR4* alleles (Mane-DRB1*04a and Mane-DRB1-*04b) clearly cluster with *HLA-DR4* alleles. These observations corroborate the *trans*-species hypothesis espoused by Jan Klein, according to which the evolution of MHC alleles does not begin at the inception of a species; rather, a group of major alleles is passed on in phylogeny from one species to another [7,24]. How is this polymorphism generated and why is it maintained across species barriers? This Chapter will illustrate the generation and maintenance of this diversity by analysis of the *DRB* loci, in which there are multiple *DRB* functional and pseudogenes.

Patterns of diversification

Within each *MHC-DRB* locus, variation occurs prominently within the second exon, while other exons are largely invariant. As summarized in Fig. 5.4 (*Plate 5.5*) and Plate 5.6 (*facing p. 296*), a detailed sequence comparison of the three hypervariable region sequence alignments from humans and nonhuman primates illustrates the second exon polymorphism [21,38], and highlights its segmental nature. The alignments show

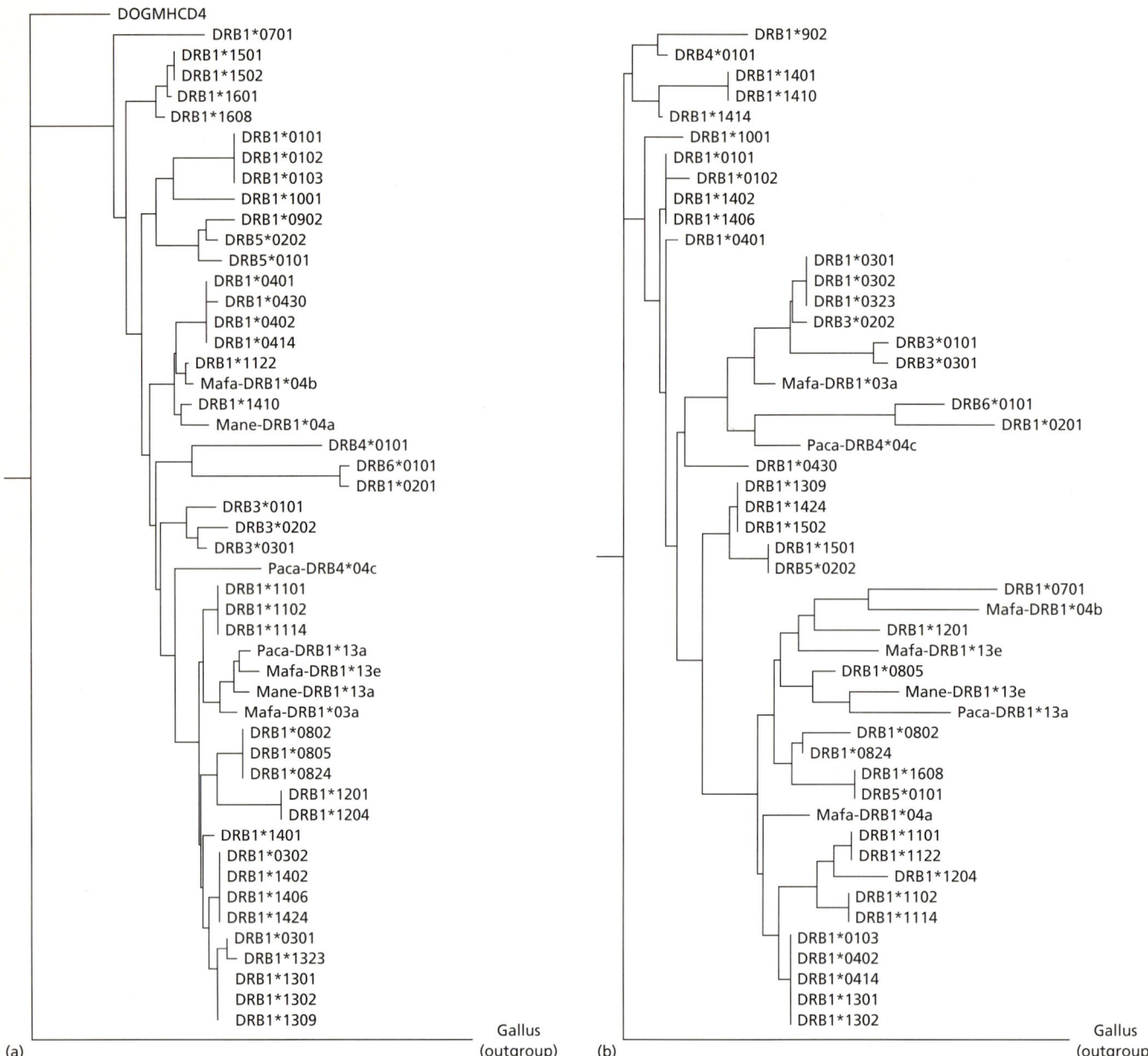

Fig. 5.3 Parsimony trees showing relationships between nucleotide sequences of the second exons of human DRB (denoted simply as DRB followed by the corresponding locus number) and for nonhuman DRB alleles (species designations in the prefix) from a set of closely related primates. Sequences for residues 6–53, encoding the β-pleated sheet (left, a) and residues 54–78, encoding the α-helix (right, b) were analyzed separately. One or more allelic variants from each major allelic group were selected and phylogenetic trees were created using PHYLIP (the PHYLogeny Inference Package) program neighboring joining/UPGMA method to construct the trees on the website http://hiv-web.lanl.gov/content/hiv-db/CONTAM/TreeMaker/TreeMaker.html [16]. Sequence motifs in the β-pleated sheet appear to reflect a common ancestry while shared sequences encoding α-helix segments may have recombined into the framework of different alleles by segmental transfer after the divergence of ancestral allelic lineages. These results indicate that two segments of the second exon have different evolutionary histories. Included are sequences from nonhuman primate species (Mane, *Macaca nemestrina*; Mafa, *M. fascicularis*; Paca, *Papio cynocephalus anubis*. Bird, *Gallus* MHC sequence was used as outgroup). Interestingly, the old world monkey (OWM) sequences cluster with several HLA alleles, suggesting both sequence and motif conservation. (*See also Plate 5.4, facing p. 296.*)

conservation of short stretches of sequences among the four species. Comparisons between various *DRB* loci, between alleles of each locus, and of various alleles between species, lead to the following observations: (i) nonhuman primate *MHC-DRB* regions are highly polymorphic and, like the human MHC, contain multiple loci, both functional and silenced; (ii) extensive allelic diversity exists in both functional and pseudogenes [15,21,39,40]; (iii) certain contemporary human alleles are present among the non-human primates (examples: Fig. 5.3 (Plate 5.4) and Plate 5.6, *facing p. 296*); and (iv) there is a striking conservation of sequence motifs between alleles, loci and species. Thus, in addition to identifying the presence of numerous contemporary alleles in evolutionarily distant species, which suggested that allelic polymorphisms predate speciation, a striking conservation of sequence motifs, particularly within HVR_{III} was noted. That is, the accumulation of certain allelic variants that are very similar or identical between species is congruent with Klein's *trans*-species hypothesis [7,24]. However, the unit displaying the *trans*-species properties is predominantly each hypervariable region cluster rather than an allele *per se*.

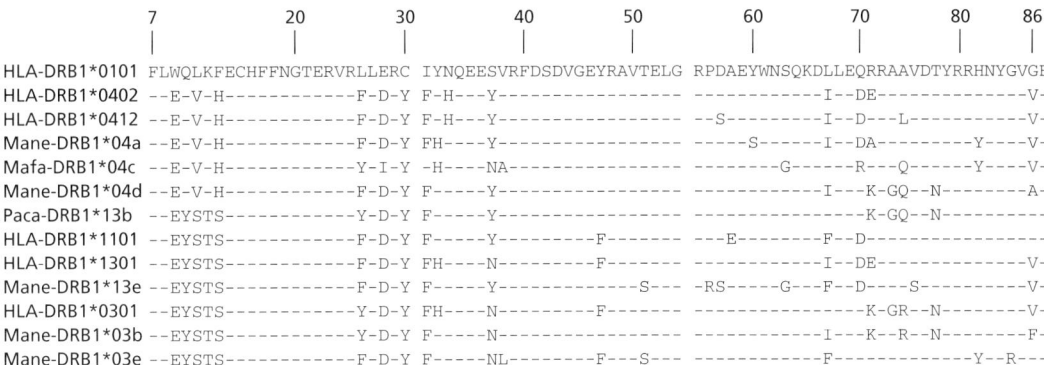

Fig. 5.4 DRB second exon sequence alignment to demonstrate allelic lineages predate speciation. DRB1*04 and DRB1*13 alleles from macaques (Mane, *Macaca nemestrina*; Mafa, *M. fascicularis*) and a baboon (Paca, *Papio cynocephalus anubis*) were aligned with human contemporary human alleles. More examples from published literature see [14,15,20,23]. (*See also Plate 5.5, facing p. 296.*)

Plate 5.6 (*facing p. 296*) and Fig. 5.3 (*Plate 5.4*) clearly demonstrate the phenomenon of shared residues within a species, between loci and between distantly related species, which was observed and reported in numerous species by several investigators. How were these shared polymorphisms generated? Several possibilities exist, such as hypermutation, which was repudiated [41], genetic exchange, overdominant selection and/or frequency dependent selection (that is, these sequence "motifs" could have simply emerged by common descent or independently). Let's first examine sequence convergence.

Sequence convergence

Convergence in DNA sequences is defined as an event where a particular nucleotide at a site is restored through successive substitutions. There are many examples of short stretches of sequences occurring between alleles, loci and species that illustrate the complexity of this phenomenon which can partly be resolved by statistical applications [10,42,43]. Convergence mechanisms are illustrated by the shared motif EYSTS (residuals 9–13), which is shared between the *DR3, 11, 13* and *14* lineages. Synonymous (silent) substitutions are often observed in this sequence, and in cattle Ser11 is specified by codon TCT and in the horse by codon AGT [44]. Changing the former codon into the latter would require passing through intermediates, either codons ACT or TGT, which specify different amino acids. A similar relationship is also true of position 13. By definition this is convergent evolution, as two species arrived at the same phenotype from different starting points [45]. In addition to EYSTS, there are several other first, second and third hypervariable sequence motifs that were conserved across the species barrier (some are shown in Plate 5.6 (*facing p. 296*) and Fig. 5.4; *Plate 5.5*). Similar examples are found elsewhere; for example, in *DQA*, where there is strong selection for leucine found at position 63 in all the species studied (L. Gaur, unpublished observations), despite first place substitutions. This type of convergent evolution may account for up to a dozen shared polymorphisms in the second exon sequences of *DRB* or other class II loci.

The theory of convergence is easiest to explain for functional sites in the antigen-binding region of MHC molecules, as sequence convergence among different species suggests that these species have common selection pressures, such as exposure to common pathogens. Convergence mechanisms require that a particular nucleotide at a site be restored through successive substitutions. If a site undergoes only one substitution there is no possibility of convergence and sequences remain diverse. A good example for this is codon 86 polymorphism [23,46] and the balancing selection of residue 57 among class II alleles [10,47,48]. However, unlike these, a shared motif often requires five or more convergent substitutions. That is, for convergence to prevail, both the conditions, number of substitutions per site and the number of sites involved, must be met. Takahata [49] argues that this seemingly unlikely convergence in motifs may be possible because change from one motif to another necessarily includes several intermediates, and the fact that such intermediates do exist [44] suggests that they can play their functional roles equally well. It will be interesting to find if several intermediates exist for those alleles where all three hypervariable regions are conserved, or whether these alleles were generated as a result of multiple evolutionary mechanisms that include sequence convergence. Indeed, there are instances where all three hypervariable regions were conserved across species barrier [15]; for example, HLA-DRB1*1122 and Mafa-DRB1*04b (Plate 5.6, *facing p. 296*) share all three motifs with one codon exception. Alternatively, gene conversion events might foster the motif conservation [10,33,37,50,51] in addition to convergent mechanisms.

Segmental exchange/recombination

Clusters of sequences have persisted for long evolutionary periods, not only conserved between allelic variants within a species but also between loci across species barriers [38]. Plate 5.6 (*facing p. 296*) illustrates this finding. Thus, two distinct patterns of sequence maintenance are evident in evolution: (i) an underlying strong segmental motif conservation represented in multiple allelic lineages, suggestive of some kind of segmental exchange as one of the favorable mechanisms of maintaining successful sequence motifs; (ii) variation within alleles by certain point mutations consistent with convergent mechanisms of evolution based on functional selection, presumably subsequent to speciation.

The observation that a limited set of hypervariable region sequences are used in nature at the β chain loci to generate a large number of alleles was originally deduced from alignments of human and/or rodent MHC class II β chain genes [14,22,23,52,53]. Examples bearing such features between *HLA-DRB1* allelic variants include HLA-DRB1*0103, 0402, 1102 and 1301, which have identical hypervariable regions (Fig. 5.3b (*Plate 5.4*) & Plate 5.6, *facing p. 296*). Motif sharing could be seen between the same locus alleles, between loci, and between species. Despite numerous examples (a few can be seen in Figs 5.3b & 5.4 (*Plates 5.4 & 5.5*) and Plate 5.6, *facing p. 296*) pointing out the shared sequences across species barriers, the segmental exchange is hard to prove since it is difficult to show the origin of donor sequence. As per the use of tree topologies, it was argued that the use of short stretches of sequences in these analyses might render biased interpretation due to stochastic error [10]. Gaur and coworkers have presented partial evidence in favor of segmental exchange as a mechanism for generating such *trans*-species segments by demonstrating alleles with deleted segments from the second exon HVR$_{III}$ α-helical regions from *DRB6* locus alleles in various primates [15,21]. These sequences lacked HVR$_{III}$ (Plate 5.6, *facing p. 296*). We obtained such sequences from three species of old world monkeys.

Such conservation of sequence stretches between alleles (segmental polymorphism) was also found in rodents by other investigators. It was suggested that genetic mechanisms, such as gene conversion, which lead to segmental exchanges of DNA stretches from one gene to another, also play a major role in generating mouse class I MHC polymorphism [54,55]. Although segmental exchange was not featured in the original formulation of the *trans*-species hypothesis, the phenomenon of shared sequences suggests that recombinatorial events between sequences could be one of the ways either to generate the polymorphism by intergenic shuffling or for maintaining successful motifs in evolution.

Mechanisms to maintain polymorphism

In summary, there are four major observations with respect to the generation of *DRB* polymorphism. First, significant variation is largely limited to the second exon encoding a single functional domain; second, within this single domain different segmental motifs have distinct evolutionary histories; third, there is a remarkable *trans*-species conservation of short sequence elements that appear to arise from intergenic exchange mechanisms, particularly at the HVR$_{III}$ region; fourth, additional convergent changes, including within the HVR$_I$ segments often used to describe allelic lineages, contribute to a complex pattern of hypervariable region relationships. The overall percentage of similarities between the *DRB* allelic variants suggest a strong conservation of certain polymorphic residues, while other polymorphic residues remain mostly species specific. The latter are the group specific polymorphic clusters in the second exon of *DRB*. There are several types of evolutionary and statistical models that have been discussed in the context of MHC evolution to help explain both the strong motif conservation and the diverse patterns of motif interchange which persist in a highly polymorphic array. These types and patterns are discussed below.

Such long-term polymorphisms can be maintained only by some form of balancing selection [49], and there is evidence of such selection on the antigen-binding regions [11,12,56] of both class I and class II MHC molecules [41,57]. The known primary function of MHC molecules is presentation of peptides to T lymphocytes, which provide immune surveillance and protection. Selection occurs at regions of the MHC involved in the binding of these peptides, hence, the primary force for selection must be imposed by the nature of the antigenic peptides that are bound [58]. Two important aspects of the polymorphism may help us understand the functional importance of preservation of this polymorphism. First, regions of variation are the regions conserved. The nucleotide substitutions for both class I and class II sites are predominantly of the amino acid altering variety. These nonsynonymous substitutions are almost three times greater than that of synonymous (silent) substitutions [30,41,57]. Second, it is important to know that the majority of the polymorphic residues are crucial for peptide binding [41,57].

Frequency-dependent selection

One of most the popular early hypotheses for maintenance of MHC diversification was frequency-dependent selection [59,60]. This hypothesis was derived from data suggesting association of certain HLA alleles with particular chronic diseases, even in heterozygous conditions. One of the frequency-dependent selection models, the pathogen adaptation model [59,60], is based on the assumption that host individuals carrying new antigens which have arisen recently by mutation will be at an advantage because viruses will not yet have had the time to adapt to infecting the cells carrying a new antigen. In such a model, a new mutant allele at an MHC locus initially has a selection advantage over old alleles, so that the rate of incorporation of mutant alleles into the population increases. However, while this model generates a higher rate of nonsynonymous (amino acid replacing) substitutions than synonymous (silent) substitutions, it does not explain either the high degree of polymorphism nor long persistence of polymorphic alleles [41], both of which could be explicitly explained in terms of overdominant selection as proposed by Hughes and Nei [41,57].

Heterozygote advantage

Hughes and Nei [41,57] argue that overdominant selection or heterozygote advantage may account for the persistence of polymorphism. That heterozygotes at MHC loci can have an advantage is readily understood in terms of the antigen presentation function of MHC molecules, as noted above. The amino acid sequence variability in both class I and class II molecules shows evidence for positive selection [41,57,61,62] as one or more sites at these variable regions interact with either peptide and/or T-cell receptors [11,56]. In their original description of the MHC role for presentation of foreign antigens to T cells, Zinkernagel and Doherty [63] suggested that MHC polymorphism could be maintained by heterozygote advantage. Elucidation of a class I structure by X-ray crystallography by Bjorkman *et al.* [11] identified the peptide-binding site or antigen recognition site (ARS) of the class I molecule, providing a molecular solution to this model. If the MHC molecules are subjected to overdominant selection and the ARS is responsible for this selection, the rate of amino acid altering substitutions are expected to be greater than that of silent substitutions [41,57]. This appears to be the case. Figure 5.5 (*see also Plate 5.7, facing p. 296*) presents a computer derived molecular model for three MHC class I amino acid sequences for two macaques and a baboon compared with human class I. Structures were modeled using the Insight II software package from MSI (Molecular Simulation Inc., now Accelrys). Models were based on published crystalline structure [64]. The human HLAA2 crystalline structure has all amino acid backbones with known variation marked on its ribbon structure with the white color balls. Variations within the same positions were displayed by different primate sequences.

Substitutions that favor amino acid altering changes at sites which interact with peptides or T-cell receptors are consistent with the hypothesis that a strong selection operates to maintain a balanced polymorphism over long evolutionary periods.

Despite eliciting great insights into the maintenance of MHC polymorphisms, the overdominant selection method (or the *trans*-species hypothesis) falls short of offering plausible mechanisms for generation of MHC diversity, nor can it explain the high rate of nonsynonymous substitutions among various class II pseudogenes (for example, DRB6).

Intraexonic recombination

While it is reasonable to assume that some of the polymorphisms may have arisen by point mutations followed by subsequent selection [65], numerous examples are available in support of genetic exchange of coding sequences in the β1 domain for class II alleles in rodents [52,66] to primates [13,21,50,51,67,68]. Direct evidence in the form of localized deletion of α-helical regions was obtained from baboon and macaque *DRB6*-like loci second exon sequences (Plate 5.6, *facing p. 296*) [21], implicating segmental exchange of MHC-encoded *DRB* gene fragments as one of the evolutionary mechanisms both for generating and maintaining MHC diversity. Segmental recombination was at this site in *DRB* second exons and is presumably not limited to the *DRB6* pseudogene. For example, the HLA-DRB1*1415 gene sequence is consistent with recombination between DRB1*1404 and DRB1*0802, or DRB1*0804 alleles

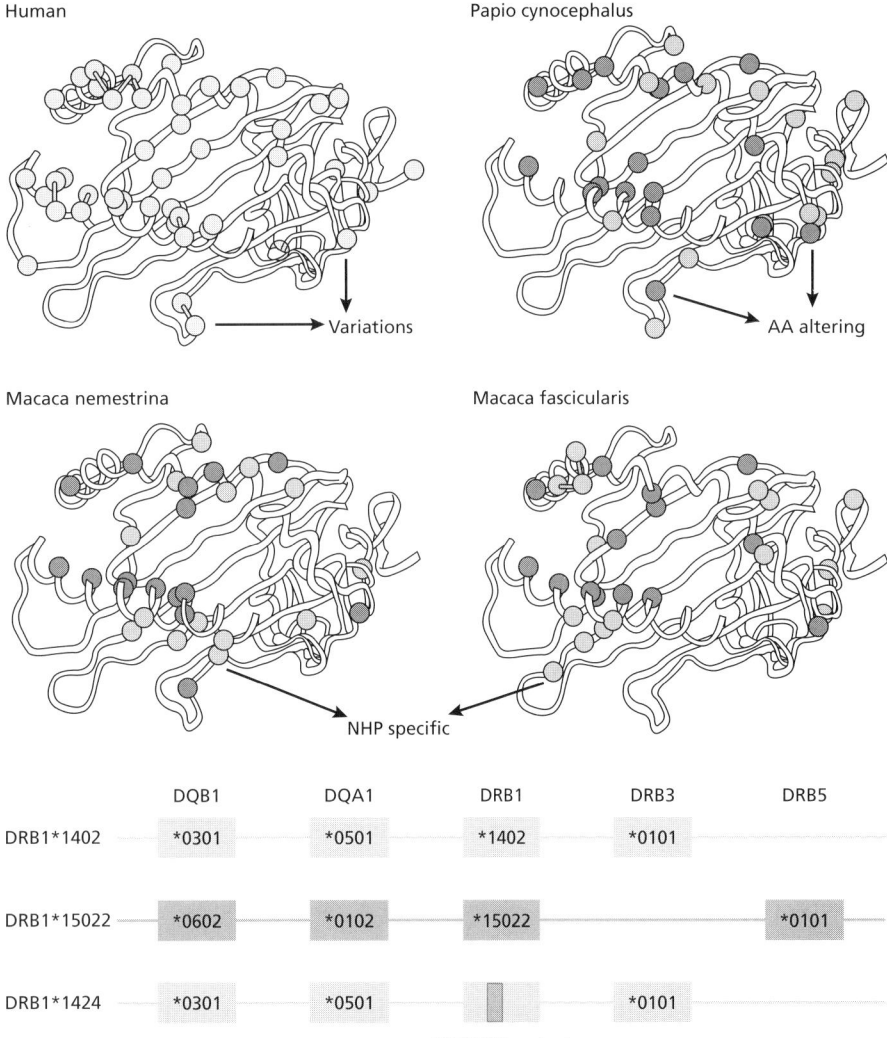

Fig. 5.5 Comparison of class I molecular modeling representation from the old world monkey (OWM) species and humans highlighting the pattern of substitution in three species of OWM. The human HLA class I A2 crystalline structure (63) has all amino acid backbones with known variation (HLA-A locus alleles) marked on its ribbon structure with the light shaded balls. The other three molecules are models of a baboon (*Papio cynocephalus*), pigtailed (*M. nemestrina*) and cynomolgus (*M. fascicularis*) macaques. Variations within the same positions are seen in these three species. The darker points on the models indicate amino acid identities within the nonhuman primate species that are different from the most known human sequence at points where polymorphism is known to occur. The dark gray points in the ribbon structures indicate novel amino acids at points that are conserved in humans. (*See also Plate 5.7, facing p. 296.*)

Fig. 5.6 An example of segmental exchange: a DR14-DR15 recombinant on DR14 background. Donor sequence most likely is from DR15022. Other alternative donor sequence would be DRB5*0202. (*See also Plate 5.8, facing p. 296.*)

at this second exon site [69], and similarly the DRB1*0415 sequence may derive from DRB1*0401/DRB1*11 recombination [70]. A typical major histocompatibility typing laboratory quandary is presented in Fig. 5.6 (*see also Plate 5.8, facing p. 296*). One of the HLA typings, upon molecular typing, presented ambiguous results that resembled both *DR14* and *15*, but *DRB5* allelic variant was lacking from this individual. The presence of *DRB3*, DQA1*0501 and DQB1*0301 indicated a *DRB3*-associated *DRB1* allele. Nucleotide sequence of the second exon of this variant revealed a sequence identity at the α-helical region of DRB1*1502 possibly due to a gene conversion/segmental exchange between DRB1*1402 and DRB1*15022 (Fig. 5.6; *Plate 5.8*). Allelic variant DRB1*1309 arose from a similar segmental exchange. The sequences DRB1*1309, 1424 formed clusters with group specificity with other *DR13, 14* and *15* groups of alleles when sequences containing residues 6–54 were aligned but clustered with DRB1*1502 when α-helical sequences were aligned.

Thus, it is likely that mutation was probably responsible for HVR_I diversification, while intraexon recombination may have largely contributed to the conservation of HVR_{III} [71]. This supports the concept that two distinct phenomena, namely segmental exchange and mutation events, generate and maintain the genetic diversity. While successful motifs persist over long evolutionary periods by shuffling sequence segments, it is possible that the point mutations are required to introduce requisite diversity from time to time as required for proper adaptation to evade pathogens [57,72].

Functional evolution

Each of these evolutionary mechanisms that generate and maintain specific polymorphisms are based on functional selection, in which MHC–peptide interactions are crucial. From a structural perspective, therefore, the selective pressures that are reflected in the MHC protein are likely to cluster in regions of MHC–peptide contact. As noted above, this appears to be the case, as peptide contact residues within the MHC binding groove are highly polymorphic, whereas MHC residues outside the groove are highly conserved. Many of these key polymorphic residues implicated in peptide interactions are encompassed in the sequences discussed above, which are made up of segmental motifs that show evolutionary conservation. One would be tempted to speculate a functional conservation across the species barrier should the peptide contact sites be conserved between species; Plate 5.9 (*facing p. 296*) illustrates conservation of peptide contact sites across the species barrier. In other words, the sites that are the basis for functional allelic specificity are identical to sites of segmental evolutionary conservation. This strongly implies that the evolutionary pressure for segmental allelic conservation and exchange is based on specific peptide-binding properties selected for MHC function.

In this paradigm, conserved peptide-binding properties of the MHC molecule correspond to conserved allelic sequences. The MHC sites that define specific peptide-binding interactions can be grouped according to functional interactions based on spatial alignments in the MHC molecule.

Key polymorphic MHC residues cluster into discrete pockets within the peptide-binding groove, where they determine the preferential binding of peptide–amino acid "anchor" residues, essential for high-avidity peptide–MHC complex formation. In the three dimensional structure of MHC molecules these key pocket residues are not necessarily colinear, so that amino acids from both α and β chains, as well as nonadjacent β chain residues, together provide the necessary specificity for each pocket.

Plate 5.9 (*facing p. 296*) presents a cross-sectional representation of three peptide-binding pockets highlighting the key polymorphic residues, which within *HLA-DRB1* alleles, account for specificity. These residues are aligned with the corresponding sequence from selected nonhuman primates, which illustrates the high degree of homology preserved for these pockets.

Not shown in the Fig. 5.4 is pocket 1, a glycine to valine polymorphism at residue 86, which is conserved across species barrier [46,48,73,74]. For example, in pocket 1, a glycine to valine polymorphism at residue 86 among different human alleles influences the peptide–amino acids bound. Large, bulky, hydrophobic residues are accommodated when residue 86 is glycine; smaller peptide–amino acids are accommodated when residue 86 is valine. In different macaques–*DRB* sequences residue 86 [15] is either glycine, phenylalanine or alanine, and the other pocket 1 residues 82, 85, 89 and 90 are, like in humans, nonpolymorphic, recapitulating a parallel set of binding preferences [73,74]. A more extensive illustration of such functional conservation is seen with pocket 9. The key β-chain polymorphisms at noncontiguous residues 9, 37, 57, 60 and 61 form a functional unit. The corresponding amino acid sequence at these five residues varies considerably. For example, EYDYW, which occurs in DRB1*0401 in humans, also occurs in macaque DRB sequences as well in a red wolf; ENDYW occurs both in HLA-DRB1*0301 and *1301, and also in certain macaque alleles (in fact, one of nonhuman primate sequences, MafaDRB1*03, is identical to the HLA-DRB1*0301 at all three pockets selected); the human *DR8* variant with "nonaspartic acid" at codon 57, EYSYW, also occurs identically in macaques. The charge polymorphism at codon 57, which distinguishes between these motifs in humans, has a major functional role in selection of peptide binding and disease susceptibility [47,48,75]. Precise conservation of identical pocket residues amongst different macaque alleles illustrates the importance of maintenance of this functional dimorphism.

The strong sequence conservation at each of these peptide-binding pockets implies a clear functional bias for their restricted set of suitable amino acid residues. It is likely that this selection is based either on an evolutionary need to recognize some fundamental conserved peptide or, alternatively, that the pockets have evolved a highly successful motif capable of binding a variety of peptide patterns. In the latter model, several structural options may have evolved for solving a recurring problem—such as binding amino acids that might have positive, negative or hydrophobic characteristics. In order to maintain the capability for each option, the structural solutions are fixed within a population as discrete polymorphisms. During evolution, the conservation of these multiple individual solutions (alleles) may represent a selective pressure to maintain multiple binding options. There is also likely a structural constraint due to the coevolution of linked structural features, in that separate amino acid polymorphisms within a binding pocket are interdependent on other amino acids within the same pocket.

This concept of interdependent functional elements composing specific binding pockets underlies the selective pressure for segmental conservation of allelic motifs in HLA molecules. It implies a strong requirement for fundamental structural solutions to the need for a wide range of peptide recognition specificities, and implies that the highly conserved motifs presently found in multiple species are the successful solution to this need. *Trans*-species evolution in the MHC is segmental, reflecting the relationship between residues that determine these successful binding motifs.

Perhaps the best example of this type of sequence conservation is in the amino acid residues that encompass pocket 4 of the DR molecule. As shown in Plate 5.9 (*facing p. 296*) this pocket is bounded by key polymorphic residues at 13 and 26, on the floor of the β-chain, and by residues 70, 71, and 74 on the α-helical loop along the side and the top of the pocket. The size of the residues at positions 13, 26, and 74 largely determines the change in size of pocket 4 and, therefore, the availability for binding to amino acids of reciprocal size. At the same time, the charge of residues 70 and 71 strongly influences the ability of charged peptide–amino acids to be accommodated in this same pocket. Thus, the polymorphisms at each of these noncontiguous locations together form discrete binding properties.

The key charged residues in these motifs are encoded at residues 70–71 of the *DR* β chain, and are localized within the HVR_{III} segment. As discussed previously, the $DRB1$-HVR_{III} segment is notable for its strong *trans*-specific conservation of polymorphisms and genetic evidence suggests that intergenic exchange mechanisms have provided for the distribution of this fixed sequence element among multiple genes.

Conclusions

Polymorphism is the hallmark of the MHC. Generation of this polymorphism through segmental intergenic exchange mechanisms which are *trans*-specific, as well as both convergent and divergent intraspecific sequence changes, have generated a complex tapestry of interwoven sequence elements which encode a set of structural motifs used in MHC–peptide binding and T-cell interaction. The structural dilemma faced by an MHC molecule is immense: too avid a peptide interaction risks hyperresponsiveness, crossreactivity and autoimmunity; too weak an interaction risks nonresponsiveness, infection and immunodeficiency. Levels of expression must both be tissue-specific and inducible, able to adjust in response to extra cellular stimuli. Most importantly, the spectrum of recognition specificities must encompass a universe of pathogens, so solutions to these challenges must be robust and generalizable. Analysis of the evolutionary history of MHC gene sequences and interpretation in the context of MHC structure and function illustrate a remarkable solution in which the strict conservation of segmental polymorphisms across species is a key adaptation unique to the HLA complex.

However, evolution is beyond this segmental polymorphism. Clearly several duplication, recombination and contraction events must have occurred during evolution of the *DR* region. Compared to this complexity of distinct *DR* haplotypes and the nonpolymorphic status of the *DRA* locus the conserved number of *DQ* and *DP* genes is intriguing. It is tempting to speculate that the reason for this difference may be related to different evolutionary constraints acting on the antigen-presenting function of different class II molecules.

References

1 Gaur L, Nepom G. Functional evolution of the major histocompatibility complex. In: Forman SJ, Blume KG, Thomas ED, eds. *Hematopoietic Cell Transplantation*, 2nd edn. Boston, MA: Blackwell Science, 1998: 38–47.

2 Ayala FJ, Escalante A, O'Huigin C, Klein J. Molecular genetics of speciation and human origins. *Proc Natl Acad Sci U S A* 1994; **91**(15): 6787–94.

3 Zinkernagel RM, Doherty PC. Immunological surveillance against altered self components by sensitised T lymphocytes in lymphocytic choriomeningitis. *Nature* 1974; **251**(5475): 547–8.

4 Doherty PC, Zinkernagel RM. Enhanced immunological surveillance in mice heterozygous at the H-2 gene complex. *Nature* 1975; **256**(5512): 50–2.

5. Doherty PC, Zinkernagel RM. A biological role for the major histocompatibility antigens. *Lancet* 1975; **1**(7922): 1406–9.
6. Robinson J, Waller M, Parham P, Bodmer J, Marsh S. IMGT/HLA database: a sequence database for the human major histocompatibility complex. *Nucl Acids Res* 2001; **29**: 210–3.
7. Klein J. Origin of major histocompatibility complex polymorphism: the *trans*-species hypothesis. *Hum Immunol* 1987; **19**(3): 155–62.
8. Lawlor DA, Ward FE, Ennis PD, Jackson AP, Parham P. HLA-A and B polymorphisms predate the divergence of humans and chimpanzees. *Nature* 1988; **335**(6187): 268–71.
9. Böhme J, Andersson M, Andersson G, Möller E, Peterson PA, Rask L. HLA-DR β genes vary in number between different DR specificities, whereas the number of DQ β genes is constant. *J Immunol* 1985; **135**: 2149–55.
10. Yeager M, Hughes AL. Evolution of the mammalian MHC. Natural selection, recombination, and convergent evolution. *Immunol Rev* 1999; **167**: 45–58.
11. Bjorkman PJ, Saper MA, Samraoui B, Bennett WS, Strominger JL, Wiley DC. The foreign antigen binding site and T cell recognition regions of class I histocompatibility antigens. *Nature* 1987; **329**: 512–8.
12. Brown JH, Jardetsky TS, Gorga JC et al. Three-dimensional structure of the human class II histocompatibility antigen HLA-DR1. *Nature* 1993; **364**: 33–9.
13. Gyllensten U, Sundvall M, Ezcurra I, Erlich HA. Genetic diversity at class II DRB loci of the primate MHC. *J Immunol* 1991; **146**(12): 4368–76.
14. Gyllensten UB, Sundvall M, Erlich HA. Allelic diversity is generated by intraexon sequence exchange at the DRB1 locus of primates. *Proc Natl Acad Sci U S A* 1991; **88**: 3686–90.
15. Gaur LK, Nepom GT, Snyder KE et al. MHC-DRB allelic sequences incorporate distinct intragenic trans-specific segments. *Tissue Antigens* 1997; **49**(4): 342–55.
16. Felsenstein J. PHYLIP: PHYLogeny Inference Package version 3.2. *Cladistics* 1989; **5**: 164–6.
17. Brandle U, Ono H, Vincek V et al. *Trans*-species evolution of MHC-DRB haplotype polymorphism in primates: organization of DRB genes in the chimpanzee. *Immunogenetics* 1992; **36**(1): 39–48.
18. Bontrop RE, Otting N, de Groot NG, Doxiadis GG. Major histocompatibility complex class II polymorphisms in primates. *Immunol Rev* 1999; **167**: 339–50.
19. Bontrop RE, Otting N, Niphuis H, Noort R, Teeuwsen V, Heeney JL. The role of major histocompatibility complex polymorphisms on SIV infection in rhesus macaques. *Immunol Lett* 1996; **51**(1–2): 35–8.
20. Bontrop RE, Otting N, Slierendregt BL, Lanchbury JS. Evolution of major histocompatibility complex polymorphisms and T-cell receptor diversity in primates. *Immunol Rev* 1995; **143**: 33–62.
21. Gaur LK, Nepom GT. Ancestral major histocompatibility complex DRB genes beget conserved patterns of localized polymorphisms. *Proc Natl Acad Sci U S A* 1996; **93**(11): 5380–3.
22. Gustafsson K, Germana S, Hirsh F, Pratt K, LeGuern C, Sachs SH. Structure of miniature swine class II DRB genes: conservation of hypervariable amino acid residues between distantly related mammalian species. *Proc. Natl Acad Sci U S A* 1990; **87**: 9898–02.
23. Andersson L, Sigurdardottir S, Borsch C, Gustafsson K. Evolution of MHC polymorphism: extensive sharing of polymorphic sequence motifs between human and bovine DRB alleles. *Immunogenetics* 1991; **33**(3): 188–93.
24. Figueroa F, Gunther E, Klein J. MHC polymorphism pre-dating speciation. *Nature* 1988; **335**(6187): 265–7.
25. Mayer WE, Jonker M, Klein D, Ivanyi P, van Seventer G, Klein J. Nucleotide sequences of chimpanzee MHC class I alleles: evidence for *trans*-species mode of evolution. *Embo J* 1988; **7**(9): 2765–74.
26. Kenter M, Otting N, Anholts J, Jonker M, Schipper R, Bontrop RE. MHC-DRB diversity of the chimpanzee (Pan troglodytes). *Immunogenetics* 1992; **37**(1): 1–11.
27. Kasahara M, Klein D, Fan WM, Gutknecht J. Evolution of the class II major histocompatibility complex alleles in higher primates. *Immunol Rev* 1990; **113**: 65–82.
28. Gaur LK, Heise ER, Hansen JA, Clark EA. Conservation of HLA class I private epitopes in macaques. *Immunogenetics* 1988; **27**(5): 356–62.
29. Gaur LK, Hughes AL, Heise ER, Gutknecht J. Maintenance of DQB1 polymorphisms in primates. *Mol Biol Evol* 1992; **9**(4): 599–609.
30. Gaur LK, Heise ER, Thurtle PS, Nepom GT. Is DQB2 functional among nonhuman primates? In: Klein J, Klein D, eds. *Molecular Evolution of the Major Histocompatibility Complex*. NATO ASI Series H, 1991: 221–9. Springer-Verlag, Berlin, Heidelberg.
31. Gaur LK, Heise ER, Ting JP. Conservation of the promoter region of DRA-like genes from nonhuman primates. *Immunogenetics* 1992; **35**(2): 136–9.
32. Gaur LK, Pandarpurkar M, Anderson J. DQA-DQB linkage in old world monkeys. *Tissue Antigens* 1998; **51**(4) (Part 1): 367–73.
33. Hayashida H, Miyata T. Unusual evolutionary conservation and frequent DNA segment exchange in class I genes of the major histocompatibility complex. *Proc Natl Acad Sci U S A* 1983; **80**(9): 2671–5.
34. Ohta T. Allelic and nonallelic homology of a supergene family. *Proc Natl Acad Sci U S A* 1982; **79**(10): 3251–4.
35. Mellor AL, Weiss EH, Ramachandran K, Flavell RA. A potential donor gene for the *bm1* gene conversion event in the C57BL mouse. *Nature* 1985; **306**: 792–5.
36. Lopez de Castro JA, Strominger JL, Strong DM, Orr HT. Structure of crossreactive human histocompatibility antigens HLA-A28 and HLA-A2: possible implications for the generation of HLA polymorphism. *Proc Natl Acad Sci U S A* 1982; **79**(12): 3813–7.
37. McConnell TJ, Talbot WS, McIndoe RA, Wakeland EK. The origin of MHC class II gene polymorphism within the genus Mus. *Nature* 1988; **332**(6165): 651–4.
38. Gaur LK, Nepom GT, Snyder KE, Anderson JM, Heise R. Conserved sequence motifs create a pattern of MHC genetic diversification within primate DRB lineages. In: Charron DEDK, ed. *Genetic Diversity of HLA. Functional and Medical Implications*. Paris, 1997: 267–9. EDK, Medical + Scientific International Publishers.
39. Bontrop RE, Broos LA, Pham K, Bakas RM, Otting N, Jonker M. The chimpanzee major histocompatibility complex class II DR subregion contains an unexpectedly high number of β-chain genes. *Immunogenetics* 1990; **32**(4): 272–80.
40. Corell A, Morales P, Varela P et al. Allelic diversity at the primate major histocompatibility complex DRB6 locus. *Immunogenetics* 1992; **36**(1): 33–8.
41. Hughes AL, Nei M. Pattern of nucleotide substitution at major histocompatibility complex class I loci reveals overdominant selection. *Nature* 1988; **335**(6186): 167–70.
42. Takahata N, Nei M. Allelic genealogy under overdominant and frequency-dependent selection and polymorphism of major histocompatibility complex loci. *Genetics* 1990; **124**(4): 967–78.
43. Kriener K, O'Huigin C, Tichy H, Klein J. Convergent evolution of major histocompatibility complex molecules in humans and new world monkeys. *Immunogenetics* 2000; **51**(3): 169–78.
44. Klein J, O'Huigin C. Class II B MHC motifs in an evolutionary perspective. *Immunol Rev* 1995; **143**: 89–111.
45. Gustafsson K, Andersson L. Structure and polymorphism of horse MHC class II DRB genes: convergent evolution in the antigen binding site. *Immunogenetics* 1994; **39**(5): 355–8.
46. Titus-Trachtenberg EA, Rickards O, De Stefano GF, Erlich HA. Analysis of HLA class II haplotypes in the Cayapa Indians of Ecuador: a novel DRB1 allele reveals evidence for convergent evolution and balancing selection at position 86. *Am J Hum Genet* 1994; **55**(1): 160–7.
47. Kwok WW, Domeier ME, Johnson ML, Nepom GT, Koelle DM. HLA-DQB1 codon 57 is critical for peptide binding and recognition. *J Exp Med* 1996; **183**: 1253–8.
48. Nepom BS, Nepom GT, Coleman M, Kwok WW. Critical contribution of β chain residue 57 in peptide binding ability of both HLA-DR and -DQ molecules. *Proc Natl Acad Sci U S A* 1996; **93**(14): 7202–6.
49. Takahata N. MHC diversity and selection (Review). *Immunol Rev* 1995; **143**: 225–47.
50. Gorski J, Mach B. Polymorphism of human Ia antigens: gene conversion between DR β loci results in a new HLA-D/DR specificity. *Nature* 1986; **322**: 67–70.
51. Sigurdardottir S, Borsch C, Gustafsson K, Andersson L. Exon encoding the antigen-binding site of MHC class II β-chains is divided into two subregions with different evolutionary histories. *J Immunol* 1992; **148**(3): 968–73.
52. She JX, Boehme SA, Wang TW, Bonhomme F, Wakeland EK. Amplification of major histocompatibility complex class II gene diversity by intraexonic recombination. *Proc Natl Acad Sci U S A* 1991; **88**(2): 453–7.
53. Lundberg AS, McDevitt HO. Evolution of major histocompatibility complex class II allelic diversity: direct descent in mice and humans. *Proc Natl Acad Sci U S A* 1992; **89**(14): 6545–9.
54. Bregegere F. A directional process of gene conversion is expected to yield dynamic polymorphism associated with stability of alternative alleles in class I histocompatibility antigens gene family. *Biochemie* 1983; **65**: 229–37.
55. Pease LR. Diversity in H2 genes encoding antigen-presenting molecules is generated by interactions between members of the major histocompatibility complex gene family (Review). *Transplantation* 1985; **39**: 227–31.
56. Brown JH, Jardetzky T, Saper MA, Samraoui B, Bjorkman PJ, Wiley DC. A hypothetical model of

foreign antigen binding site of class II histocompatibility molecules. *Nature* 1988; **332**: 845–50.

57 Hughes AL, Nei M. Nucleotide substitution at major histocompatibility complex class II loci: evidence for overdominant selection. *Proc Natl Acad Sci U S A* 1989; **86**(3): 958–62.

58 Klein J, Takahata N. The major histocompatibility complex and the quest for origins. *Immunol Rev* 1990; **113**: 5–25.

59 Bodmer WF. Evolutionary significance of the HLA system (Review). *Nature* 1972; **237**: 139–45.

60 Snell GD. The H-2 locus of the mouse: observations and speculations concerning its comparative genetics and its polymorphism. *Folia Biol* 1968; **14**: 335–58.

61 Holmes N, Ennis P, Wan AM, Denney DW, Parham P. Multiple genetic mechanisms have contributed to the generation of the HLA-A2/A28 family of class I MHC molecules. *J Immunol* 1985; **139**: 936–41.

62 N'Guyen CR, Sodoyer J, Trucy T, Strachan T, Jordan BR. The HLA-Aw24 gene: sequence surroundings, and comparison with the HLA-A2 and HLA-A3 genes. *Immunogenet* 1985; **21**: 479–89.

63 Zinkernagel RM, Doherty PC. Restriction of *in vitro* T cell-mediated cytotoxicity in lymphocytic choriomeningitis within a syngeneic or semi allogeneic system. *Nature* 1974; **248**(450): 701–2.

64 Gao GF, Tormo J, Gerth UC *et al*. Crystal structure of the complex between human CD8alpha (α) and HLA-A2. *Nature* 1997; **387**(6633): 630–4.

65 Gustafsson K, Wiman K, Emmoth E *et al*. Mutations and selection in the generation of class II histocompatibility antigen polymorphism. *EMBO J* 1984; **3**: 1655–61.

66 Mengle-Gaw L, McDevitt HO. Genetics and expression of mouse Ia antigens. *Annu Rev Immunol* 1985; **3**: 367–96.

67 Bell JI, Denney J, Foster L, Belt T, Todd JA, McDevitt HO. Allelic variation in the DR subregion of the human major histocompatibility complex. *Proc Natl Acad Sci U S A* 1987; **84**: 6234–8.

68 Coppin HL, Avoustin P, Fabron J *et al*. Evolution of the HLA-DR1 gene family. Structural and functional analysis of the new allele 'DR-BON'. *J Immunol* 1990; **144**(3): 984–9.

69 Fogdell A, Olerup O. A novel DRB1 allele (DRB1*1415) formed by interallelic crossing over between the DRB1*1404 and the DRB1*0802 or 0804 alleles. *Tissue Antigens* 1994; **43**: 327–9.

70 Tiercy J-M, Gebuhrer L, Betuel H, Mach B, Jeannet M. A new HLA-DR4 allele with a DR11 α-helix sequence. *Tissue Antigens* 1993; **41**: 97–101.

71 Ohta T. Role of diversifying selection and gene conversion in evolution of major histocompatibility complex loci. *Proc Natl Acad Sci U S A* 1991; **88**(15): 6716–20.

72 Sigurdardottir S, Borsch C, Gustafsson K, Andersson L. Exon encoding the antigen-binding site of MHC class II β-chains is divided into two subregions with different evolutionary histories. *J Immunol* 1992; **148**: 968–73.

73 Ong B, Willcox N, Wordsworth P *et al*. Critical role for the Val/Gly86 HLA-DR β dimorphism in autoantigen presentation to human T cells. *Proc Natl Acad Sci U S A* 1991; **88**: 7734–7.

74 Busch R, Hill CM, Hayball JD, Lamb JR, Rothbard JB. Effect of natural polymorphism at residue 86 of the HLA-DR β chain on peptide binding. *J Immunol* 1991; **147**: 1292–8.

75 Todd JA, Bell JI, McDevitt HO. HLA DQ β gene contributes to susceptibility and resistance to insulin-dependent diabetes mellitus. *Nature* 1987; **329**: 599–604.

6

Claudio Brunstein & Catherine M. Verfaillie

The Hematopoietic Microenvironment

Introduction

Hematopoiesis takes place in adult life in the bone marrow (BM) microenvironment. The BM microenvironment is composed of a multitude of cells, both of mesenchymal and hematopoietic origin, that produce cell surface, extracellular matrix (ECM) and soluble factors that in concert are responsible for the regulation of proliferation and quiescence, differentiation, and retention in and recruitment to the BM of hematopoietic stem cells (HSCs) and hematopoietic progenitor cells (HPCs). Although a number of these factors have been molecularly characterized, the exact mechanisms that govern HSC self-renewal are still unknown. This chapter will address the different components of the hematopoietic microenvironment, and what is known about their role in the hematopoietic process.

Hematopoietic microenvironments throughout development

During embryogenesis hematopoiesis takes place sequentially in the yolk-sac and/or aorta-gonad-mesonephros (AGM) region, followed by the fetal liver until it finally localizes exclusively to the BM. Hematopoietic cells are detected in the in the yolk sac at embryonic day 8 (e8) in the mouse, and between 3 and 4 weeks in the human as pools of nucleated erythrocytes in close proximity with endothelial cells [1]. At approximately the same gestational age, hematopoietic cells can be detected adjacent to the aortic endothelium in the AGM region [2,3]. Whether cells from the yolk sac seed the AGM region, or *vice versa*, or whether these represent independent populations of HSCs is still a topic of debate. However, cells from both tissues can repopulate the hematopoietic system in the mouse [3,4].

Cells from either the yolk sac or the AGM, or both, seed the fetal liver at approximately 4–5 weeks of gestation in humans and β_9 in the mouse. Between 10 and 15 weeks in humans and β_{11}–β_{12} in the mouse, hematopoietic cells can be detected in the BM, the spleen and the thymus. During fetal life, liver and BM contribute differently to hematopoiesis. The fetal liver produces predominantly erythroid cells, vital to the fetus, while the BM produces predominantly granulocytes [1].

Little is known about the mechanism(s) that determine changes in localization of hematopoiesis during embryonic and fetal life. Microenvironmental differences play a role in the regulation of this process. For instance, fetal liver epithelium is crucial for the support of hematopoiesis during the initial stages of development. However, factors, such as oncostatin-M, produced by hematopoietic cells induce terminal differentiation of the hepatocytes rendering them nonsupportive for hematopoiesis [5]. The onset of hematopoiesis in the BM coincides with sequential changes in the BM microenvironment. Initially, the bones are devoid of hematopoietic cells, and consist of chondrocytes and endothelial cells in the perichondral limb mesenchyme. Subsequently, there is chondrolysis followed by the development of a vascular bed still in the absence of detectable hematopoiesis. The first hematopoietic progenitors can be observed in the BM between 10.5 and 15 weeks of human gestational age. Over the next few weeks there is progressive bone calcification and proliferation of hematopoietic progenitors with the development of dense areas of hematopoiesis [6]. Seeding of the BM during embryologic life is subject to similar signals as is seen during adult life. Animals that are null for the chemokine receptor CXCR4 or its ligand, stroma-derived factor 1 (SDF1α), develop fetal liver hematopoiesis but not BM hematopoiesis [7,8]. Likewise, β_1-integrin$^{-/-}$ HSCs can not migrate into the BM, even though they proliferate and differentiate appropriately in the fetal liver [9]. Additional qualitative and quantitative differences in other adhesion receptors on HSCs and HPCs may also be responsible for differences in their homing and proliferation capabilities during specific periods of gestational life [10,11].

The adult BM microenvironment

Normal steady-state hematopoiesis takes place in the BM. A complex interplay between soluble cytokines, chemokines and growth factors, as well as adhesive interactions between HSCs/HPCs and hematopoietic supportive cells and ECM components in the BM microenvironment are thought to orchestrate the behavior of HSCs/HPCs (Fig. 6.1).

Cellular components of the hematopoietic microenvironment

BM, fetal liver, AGM and yolk sac contain a variety of cells that serve to support hematopoiesis. These consist of mesenchymal cells, including fibroblasts and myofibroblasts, adipocytes, osteoblasts, as well as endothelial cells and HSC-derived macrophages. Most if not all of these cell-types regulate HSCs/HPCs via production of cytokines and growth factors, production of ECM components, and direct interaction with HSCs/HPCs.

The function of the different cell types has been evaluated through creation of cell lines, and testing their ability to allow self-renewal and/or differentiation of HSCs/HPCs *in vitro*. More than 20 years ago, Dexter and colleagues showed that "stromal" cells generated from mouse BM could support hematopoiesis *in vitro* [12]. Stromal cells are generated by plating BM mononuclear cells in culture vessels. Within 2–4 weeks a confluent layer of mixture of adherent cells is generated with development of areas of hematopoietic cell proliferation and differentiation

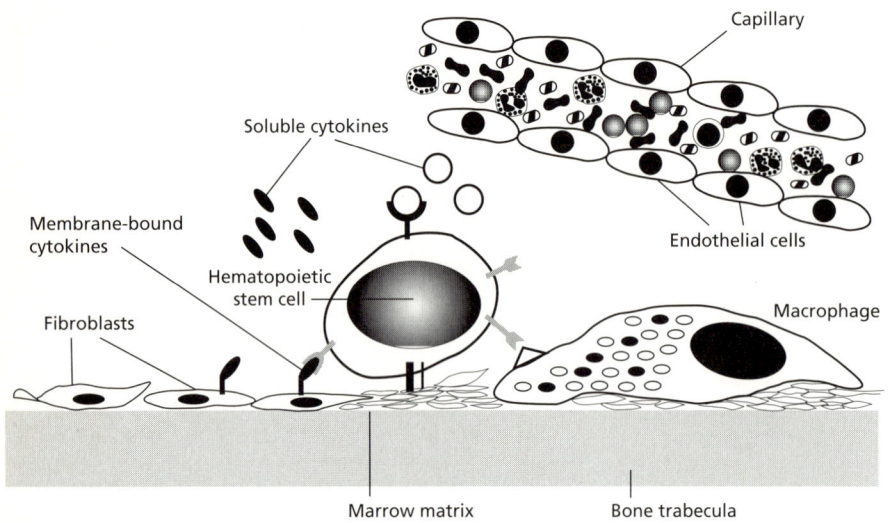

Fig. 6.1 The behavior of HSC/HPC is regulated by a complex interplay between soluble cytokines, chemokines and growth factors as well as adhesive interactions between HSC/HPC and hematopoietic supportive cells and extracellular matrix (ECM) components in the bone marrow microenvironment.

between the stromal elements. These hematopoietic areas have the appearance under phase contrast microscope of cobble stone areas. Since then, cell lines representing different components of these mixed stromal feeders have been generated, and their ability to support hematopoiesis examined.

Fibroblasts/myofibroblasts

A large number of cell lines with fibroblast/myofibroblast characteristics has been generated from ontogenically different tissues, including the yolk sac [13], AGM region [14,15], fetal liver [16] and adult BM [17] that support one or more functions of hematopoiesis. Interestingly, although several cell lines have been generated from the AGM region in the mouse, only some support HSCs/HPCs, while others do not [14,15]. Likewise, among a series of cell lines generated from murine fetal liver, only some support primitive HSCs/HPCs [16]. Some studies have shown that the ability of murine HSCs/HPCs to form cobble stone areas when cultured on fibroblast feeders correlates with the hematopoietic supportive ability of the feeder [18,19], suggesting that cell–cell or cell–ECM interactions play an important role in HSC/HPC survival and proliferation. However, there is also evidence that these same feeders may support HSCs/HPCs plated in transwells above the feeder, supporting the notion that at least some of the factors important for HSC/HPC survival and proliferation can be secreted [20,21]. Why some but not all myofibroblast feeders support hematopoiesis is currently unknown. Evaluation of the cytokine profile elaborated by the different feeders has not identified significant differences between supportive and nonsupportive feeders [16]. Therefore, differences in expression of other yet to be defined soluble factors, ECM components or cell surface ligands must be responsible for the ability of some but not other feeders to support hematopoiesis [22].

Osteoblasts

A second cell population thought to play a role in regulating hematopoiesis are osteoblasts. The most primitive hematopoietic cells are located adjacent to cortical bone, while more differentiated cells are located at a distance of the cortex. Clusters of neutrophil progenitors can often be seen adjacent to bone trabeculas [23]. When isolated from BM and cultured *in vitro*, osteoblasts, like many other cell types in the BM microenvironment, produce a number of cytokines important for hematopoiesis, including transforming growth factor beta (TGF-β), tumor necrosis factor (TNF), colony stimulating factors (CSFs), c-kit ligand (c-kitL), leukemia inhibitory factor (LIF), and several interleukins (ILs). As is true for myofibroblasts and endothelial cells, these secreted factors can influence hematopoietic cells *in vitro* [24,25]. The interesting finding that the more primitive HPCs can be found lining the bone cortex may also suggest that direct HPC/osteoblast interactions *via* the adhesive ligands ALCAM and NCAM, expressed on osteoblasts, may play a role in the regulation of hematopoiesis [26].

Adipocytes

Adipocytes are normal constituents of the BM microenvironment. Early studies showed that maturing granulocytes cluster in and around areas of fat cell aggregations suggesting that they might be important for HSC/HPC differentiation. The mechanisms underlying adipocytes-mediated regulation of hematopoiesis was unclear until recently. It is now believed that preadipocytes support hematopoiesis in culture, while mature adipocytes produce less macrophage CSF, c-kitL, IL-6 and LIF, with an associated decline in hematopoietic supportive ability [27]. This suggests that terminal differentiation to mature adipocytes inhibits hematopoiesis. Recent studies have shown that adipocytes secrete a number of factors, including leptin [28] and adiponectin, which inhibit adipocyte differentiation, but support myelopoiesis in stroma-based cultures [29,30]. Interestingly, delta-like (dLk), a transmembrane protein containing epidermal growth factor-like repeat motifs homologous to the delta/serrate family, which is also a negative regulator of adipocyte differentiation, promotes the cobblestone area colony formation and influences B-cell differentiation in stromal cultures [31–33].

Endothelial cells

Already during the earliest steps of the development of the hematopoietic system [1], hematopoietic cells and endothelial cells colocalize [2], attesting to their common ancestor, the hemangioblast [34]. This interaction is maintained in postnatal life. The BM is highly vascularized, and islands of active hematopoiesis can often be seen adjacent to endothelial cells. Whether a hemangioblast persists in postnatal human BM is not known, although a recent study has indicated that such a cell may persist in murine postnatal BM [35]. Endothelial cells selected from the BM can be cultured *in vitro*, and display characteristics of microvascular endothelial cells (BM microvascular endothelial cells or BMECs) [36]. Such endothelial cell feeders support proliferation and differentiation of HSCs/HPCs *in vitro* [36]. Likewise, endothelial cells generated from other hematopoietic supportive environments, such as the AGM region [37] and the yolk sac [38], support hematopoiesis *in vitro*. In contrast, human umbilical cord endothelial cells (HUVECs) do not support hematopoiesis. Interestingly, there is also evidence that other types of microvascular endothelial cells support hematopoiesis *in vitro* [39], suggesting that the ability of this type of endothelial cells to support hematopoiesis is not solely related to the tissue of origin. Again, the nature of factors that support HSC/HPC proliferation are unknown and comparative studies on different microvascular endothelial cell lines and, for instance, HUVECs should be informative.

In addition, endothelial cells constitute a barrier between the circulation and the BM microenvironment. BM endothelial cells express a number of adhesive ligands, including vascular cell adhesion molecule 1 (VCAM-1), the ligand for very-late antigen 4 (VLA-4, CD49d/CD29, $\alpha_4\beta_1$-integrin) [40], intracellular adhesion molecule 1 (ICAM-1), the ligand for LFA1 (CD11b/CD18) [41], and selectins [42]. Expression of these ligands are up-regulated by ionizing irradiation and inflammatory cytokines [43]. These molecules play an important role in regulating entry and exit of HSCs/HPCs in the BM, which will be discussed below.

ECM components

A variety of ECM molecules are found in the BM microenvironment, among which fibronectin (FN) and proteoglycans (PGs) appear to be more important for hematopoiesis.

Fibronectin

FN is a glycoprotein, containing multiple domains to which cells can bind via integrins, as well as heparin-binding domains to which cells adhere via glycosaminoglycans (GAGs) [44]. Adhesion of HSCs, HPCs and more mature hematopoietic cells to FN serves not only to anchor them in the BM microenvironment [45] but also to regulate their proliferative behavior [46]. β_1-integrins on HSCs/HPCs allow adhesion to purified FN. The VLA-5 and VLA-4 receptors present on committed HPCs support adhesion to both the RGD site and CS1 site on FN, whereas more primitive CD34$^+$ cells bind more exclusively via their VLA-4 receptor to the CS1 domain [47]. It is believed that these interactions are important for retaining HSCs/HPCs in the BM and aid in the homing of HSCs/HPCs to the BM. Chronic myeloid leukemia (CML) is a disease characterized by premature egress of primitive and committed CD34$^+$ cells in the blood. Consistent with the notion that VLA-4/VLA-5/FN interactions may be important for retaining HSCs/HPCs in the BM, integrins present on CD34$^+$ cells from the BM of patients with CML do not support interaction with stroma, FN and either RGD or CS1 [48,49]. Aside from playing a role in retaining HSCs/HPCs in the BM, studies over the last decade have also shown that integrin interactions with FN may play a role in HSC/HPC survival, proliferation and differentiation [46,50,51], which will be discussed later in this chapter.

Proteoglycans and glycosaminoglycans

PGs are complex molecules consisting of a core protein to which one or more GAGs are attached [52]. GAGs are long, negatively charged, unbranched polysaccharide chains composed of repeating sulfated disaccharide units. PGs are made by a variety of cells and can either be secreted in the ECM, or be present on the cell surface. Chondroitin-sulfate (CS) GAGs, heparin sulfate (HS) GAGs, dermatan sulfate (DS) GAGs, as well as hyaluronic acid (HA), can be found in the BM microenvironment [53,54].

In 1988, two groups showed that HS-GAGs in BM stromal feeders bind hematopoietic supportive cytokines, including IL-3 and granulocyte macrophage colony-stimulating factor (GM-CSF) [55,56]. Since then several other cytokines that bind to HS-GAGs have been described, among them several ILs, chemokines, fibroblast growth factors (FGFs), and members of the TGF-β/bone morphogenic protein (BMP) family, all known to be important in regulating diverse functions of HSCs/HPCs. That HS-GAGs are important in the regulation of HSCs was shown in studies in which GAGs were removed from stromal cultures, leading to decreased generation of colony forming cells (CFCs) [57]. Subsequent studies in which HS-GAGs were purified from fibroblast feeders and added to *in vitro* HPC/HSC cultures showed that compared with cytokine-only cultures, the combination of cytokines and HS-GAGs improved significantly the maintenance of primitive long-term culture initiating cells (LTC-IC) as well as SCID-repopulating cells (SRC) [58,59]. For adequate support of hematopoiesis, HS-GAGs need to be 6-*O*-sulfated on the glucosamine residues [60]. Such 6-*O*-sulfated HS-GAGs support not only the binding of hematopoiesis supportive cytokines and other ECM components such as thrombospondin, but also CD34$^+$ cells themselves, leading the authors of these studies to speculate that HS-GAGs may be an important orchestrator of the "stem cell niche" [22,60,61]. The receptor responsible for CD34$^+$ cell binding to HS-GAGs is currently unknown.

Other ECM components

The BM microenvironment also contains thrombospondin, a glycoprotein produced by platelets, endothelial cells and fibroblasts [62], to which cells bind via the CD36 receptor. CD34$^+$ cells that express CD36 interact with thrombospondin. However, the functional consequences have not been studied [63]. Several types of collagen are present in the hematopoietic microenvironment of fetal liver, fetal BM, and adult BM. Fibroblasts produce collagen-I and collagen-III. Type IV collagen is produced by endothelial cells and organized in a sheet-like mesh, which constitutes the major part of basement membranes where it colocalizes with laminin. HSCs/HPCs obtained from postnatal BM cannot readily interact with collagens or laminin, due to lack of appropriate integrin expression or affinity [10,49]. However, CD34$^+$ cells from CML BM express functional $\alpha_2\beta_1$- and $\alpha_6\beta_1$-integrins allowing them to interact with collagen-IV and laminin, and it has been speculated that this may allow them to migrate out of the BM microenvironment into the peripheral blood (PB) [49]. Likewise, HSCs/HPCs in fetal liver also express $\alpha_2\beta_1$- and $\alpha_6\beta_1$-integrins, which may allow them to exit the liver and gain access to the BM [64]. Several matrix metalloproteinases (MMPs) have been detected in different cells within the BM [65]. MMP-2 and MMP-9, important for degradation of basement membranes, are expressed by circulating CD34$^+$ cells and leukemic hematopoietic cells, but not resting BM derived CD34$^+$ cells [66]. This expression pattern is consistent with the notion that aside from the appropriate complement of adhesion receptors that allow CD34$^+$ cells to interact with components of basement membranes, MMPs needed for degradation of the basement membrane are required for hematopoietic cell egress from the BM to the PB.

Cell surface adhesive ligands

Aside from ECM molecules, cell surface expressed ligands are also involved in recruiting HSCs/HPCs from the PB in the BM, and retaining them in the BM. VCAM-1 is expressed on BM endothelial cells [67] and fibroblasts found in subosteal regions. VCAM-1 serves as the ligand for VLA-4. Blocking anti-VCAM-1 antibodies inhibit homing of HSCs/HPCs to the BM, and the VLA-4/VCAM-1 interaction appears to be the predominant cell–cell interaction required for HSCs/HPCs to gain access to the BM [68]. In contrast to microvascular endothelial cells in most organs, BM endothelial cells constitutively express VCAM-1 [40]. Following radiation or chemotherapy, treatment with IL-1α or TNF-α, levels of VCAM-1 on both endothelial cells and fibroblasts are increased [67]. Expression of VCAM-1 is down regulated significantly when HSCs/HPCs are mobilized using granulocyte colony-stimulating factor (G-CSF), apparently as a result of proteolysis by neutrophil derived elastase and cathepsin-G [69]. It has been postulated that this allows egress of HSCs/HPCs from the BM to the blood. Therefore, it appears

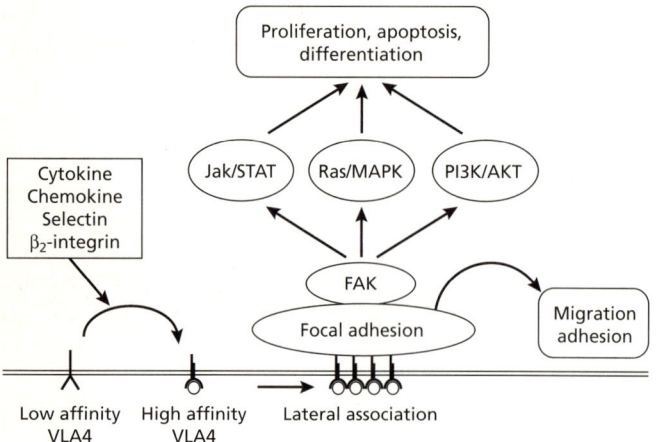

Fig. 6.2 HSC/HPC express several types of adhesion receptors, including members of the integrin family, selectins and sialomucins, which are responsible for regulating migration, adhesion, proliferation and survival of HSC/HPC.

that VCAM-1 serves as the gatekeeper for HSCs/HPCs to gain access to the BM and leave the BM. ICAM-1 is also expressed on BM endothelial cells. Like VCAM-1, ICAM-1 expression is regulated by inflammatory cytokines such as IL-1α and TNF-α [70]. CD34+ cells interact with ICAM-1 via the LFA-1 receptor [41].

Adhesion receptors

Adhesion receptors on HSCs/HPCs regulate their trafficking in and out of the BM and, like cytokine receptors, play a role in regulating their proliferation, differentiation and survival. The three major classes of adhesion receptors that are important for HSC/HPC trafficking and HSC/HPC proliferation and survival are the integrin family, selectins and sialomucins (Fig. 6.2).

Integrins are transmembrane receptors consisting of noncovalently associated heterodimeric α and β subunits, of which there are more than 24 known combinations. Integrins have a long extracellular domain formed by the α/β interface that interacts with ECM or cell surface adhesive ligands, a short transmembrane domain and a short C-terminal cytoplasmic tail that does not have intrinsic kinase activity [71]. Integrins mediate adhesion between cells and ECM or cell surface expressed ligands, are required for cell migration, and can act as signaling receptors. They relay information from the extracellular milieu to the cell, influencing cell proliferation, differentiation and survival [72], as well as from the cell to the extracellular milieu, affecting ECM composition and integrin affinity [73]. Such signaling includes cytoskeletal changes without impact on transcriptional events as well as signals that affect gene transcription, which is mediated by initial activation of focal adhesion kinase or the related PYK2 [74], and which leads to activation of the Janus kinase (JAK)-signal transduction and activator of transcription (STAT), mitogen activated protein kinase (MAPK) and phosphoinositol (PI)-3-kinase pathway [75–77]. HSCs/HPCs express β_1- and β_2-integrins [78].

Selectins (L-, E- and P-selectin) are a family of membrane proteins that mediate adhesive interactions under shear with their respective ligands [79,80]. E-selectin is expressed on endothelial cells and platelets, P-selectin on platelets and L-selectin on neutrophils as well as HSCs/HPCs [81,82]. The ligands for these receptors are not all characterized, although they generally fall within the family of sialylated, fucosylated lactosamines displayed on O-linked carbohydrates [83]. Multiple ligands for L-selectin have been described, such as several glycoproteins reactive with the monoclonal antibody MECA 79 including glyosylation-dependent cell adhesion molecule (GlyCAM-1), the endothelial cell expressed CD34, mucosal addressin cell adhesion molecule (MAdCAM-1), and P-selectin glycoprotein ligand-1 (PSGL-1) [84–86]. Ligands for E-selectin and P-selectin include PSGL-1 and CD44 [86,87]. In contrast to integrins, little is known regarding signaling via selectins, even though some reports have shown that the intracellular domain of selectins may interact with α-actinin [88], may activate the nonreceptor tyrosine kinase c-Src [89], as well as the MAP kinase cascade [90], leading among other things to activation of integrin receptors.

Finally, HSCs/HPCs express several sialomucins, including CD34, CD43, CD45RA, PSGL-1 and CD164 [91]. Sialomucins are highly glycosylated polypeptides, densely substituted with sialylated mainly O-linked carbohydrate side chains linked to serine and threonine residues, some of which serve as ligands for selectins (PSGL-1, GlyCAM-1, CD34, and MAdCAM-1) [92]. Like integrins sialomucins serve to allow homing and retention of HSCs/HPCs in the BM, and engagement of sialomucins affects HSC/HPC differentiation, proliferation and survival [91]. The signal pathways activated by mucin receptors are not as well understood as for integrins. The cytoplasmic tails of mucin receptors do not have intrinsic kinase or other enzymatic function. Mucins may interact via ezrin and moesin to the cell cytoskeleton, and may activate the protein tyrosine kinase, the phospholipase C/phosphoinositides signaling pathways and the MAPK pathways [93–96].

Role of adhesion receptors in homing and retention of HSCs/HPCs in the BM

The process of extravasation has been most extensively studied in neutrophil egress from the vasculature into tissues in response to inflammation. It is generally believed that the initial event involves "rolling" of leukocytes over endothelial cells via selectins and β_2-integrins, which results in activation of β_1-integrins responsible for subsequent firm adhesion to endothelium and migration between endothelial cells into tissues [97]. Similar events may also be responsible for the "homing" of HSCs/HPCs to BM. As has been shown for neutrophils, interactions under flow between CD34+ cells and endothelial cells or stromal feeders are mediated by selectins [11], β_2- and β_1-integrins [41] whereas firm adhesion to endothelium, stromal feeders, VCAM-1 or FN is mediated by the VLA-4 and VLA-5 integrins [41,45,98]. As for leukocytes, the affinity of β_1-integrins is increased by inside out signaling in response to activation of other adhesion receptors, including selectins and sialomucins [99], cytokines and growth factors [100–102], and chemokines [103] (Fig. 6.3).

The homing process *in vivo* has been evaluated in syngeneic murine transplantation models and in models in which human CD34+ cells are transplanted into nonobese diabetic with severe combined immunodeficiency syndrome (NOD-SCID) mice. Several studies have suggested a dominant role for the VLA-4/VCAM-1 pathway in the homing of both murine and human HSCs/HPCs [40,103,104]. That β_1-integrins are important for localizing and retaining HSCs/HPCs in the BM is obvious from studies in β_1-integrin$^{-/-}$ mice, where hematopoiesis occurs normally in the fetal liver, but does not relocate to the BM [9]. β_1-integrin$^{-/-}$ HSCs also do not engraft in the BM [68]. Treatment of mice or nonhuman primates with anti-α4 antibodies or anti-VCAM-1 antibodies results in the mobilization of HSCs/HPCs in the blood [40,105] and, conversely, preincubation of HSCs/HPCs with blocking anti-α$_4$- or anti-β$_1$-integrin antibodies results in failure of HSCs/HPCs to engraft in the BM [45]. CD34+ cells obtained from the blood following mobilization with G-CSF express lower levels of VLA-4 with lower affinity [106,107], which along with the decreased levels of VCAM-1 [69] may be responsible for egress of CD34+ cells from the BM. The VLA-4/VCAM-1 interaction is augmented following activation of the CXCR4 receptor as a result of stimulation by SDF-1α. The role of VLA-5, a chemokine present at high concentrations in the BM and known to play a role in homing, is less

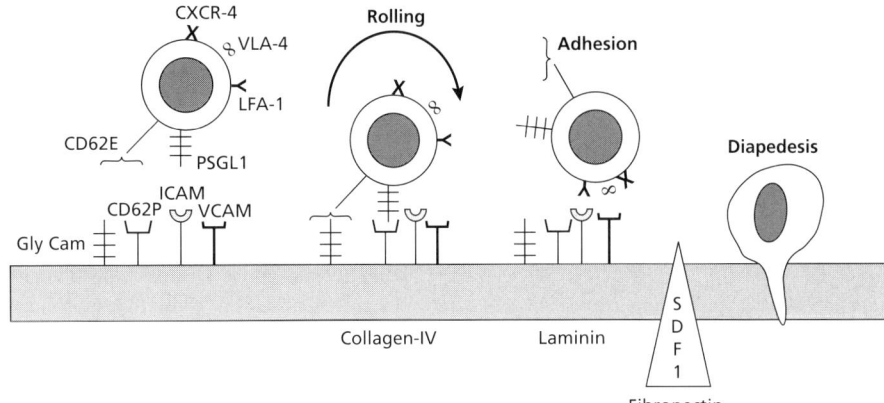

Fig. 6.3 β_1-integrins are expressed on HSC/HPC. However, presence of integrins does not translate into function, as this is dependent on the affinity of the receptor. The affinity of β_1-integrins on HSC/HPC is modulated by inside out signaling cascades initiated by activation of other adhesion receptors including selectins and sialomucins, cytokines and growth factors such as SCF and IL3, and chemokines, such as SDF-1α.

clear. In some but not all studies evaluating murine HSC homing and engraftment, VLA-5 appears only minimally involved in homing [68,108], whereas homing and engraftment of human CD34+ cells in NOD-SCID BM depends at least in part on the VLA-5 receptor [109].

LFA-1 is known to aid in "rolling" of cells over endothelium, a step necessary to allow firm interactions between cells and endothelium via VLA-4/VCAM-1 prior to migration of cells between endothelial cells [97]. Although CD34+ cells express LFA-1, and LFA-1 can mediate rolling of CD34+ cells under flow *in vitro*, CD18$^{-/-}$ murine BM cells home normally into wild-type animals [68]. Likewise, hematopoiesis is not impaired in patients with leukocyte adhesion deficiency due to a defect in CD18 expression [110]. Hence, compared to β_1-integrins, LFA-1 plays a less prominent role in hematopoietic progenitor–BM interactions, and rolling of HSCs/HPCs *in vivo* can be mediated by VLA-4/VCAM-1 interactions.

In murine transplantation models, loss of E- and P-selectin results in only a 50% reduction in rolling and homing in the BM, and complete inhibition of HSC/HPC homing requires blocking of the VLA-4/VCAM-1 interaction [68]. However, several studies have suggested that homing of human CD34+ cells to murine BM is almost completely blocked by inhibiting the ability of cells to interact with E- and P-selectin [11].

Role of adhesion receptors in progenitor proliferation and differentiation

Aside from playing a role in homing and retention of HSCs/HPCs in the BM, β_1-integrin engagement initiates signals that influence proliferation, differentiation and survival of HSCs/HPCs. Several studies have shown that interaction between HSCs/HPCs and FN inhibits their proliferation [46,111,112], whereas other studies have shown that engagement of β_1-integrins results in enhanced proliferation [100–102,113]. Although these studies at first appear contradictory, closer examination of the methods used to assess the effect of integrin engagement on HSC/HPC proliferation shows that the concentrations of cytokines used differ significantly. In fact, addition of high concentrations of a number of cytokines, including c-kitL and IL-3 was shown to override the inhibition of proliferation seen following integrin engagement in the presence of low concentrations of cytokines, representing perhaps more physiological levels of cytokines [111,112,114]. Other studies found that engagement of integrins also serves as an antiapoptotic signal [50,114,115]. This characteristic is clinically being exploited in murine oncoretroviral vector-mediated gene therapy protocols for HSCs/HPCs. As integration of murine leukemia virus (MLV)-based retroviruses requires that HSCs/HPCs undergo cell mitosis, culture for 2–4 days is required, which is commonly associated with HSC loss, in part due to apoptosis. This can be counteracted by plating cells on FN or the synthetic FN fragment, CH296 [50,115].

The molecular mechanisms underlying integrin-mediated effects on HSC/HPC proliferation and cell survival are less well understood than in adherent cell types. Nevertheless, effects of integrin engagement on protein levels of cell cycle regulatory molecules, including p27^{kip-1}, even though the signal pathways leading to altered levels in p27^{kip1} are not yet known [111,112].

The other family of adhesion receptors that affects cell survival and proliferation is the sialomucin family. Engagement of CD43, CD164 and PSGL-1 on committed HPCs can lead to cell apoptosis, while engagement on more primitive HSCs/HPCs may result in cell quiescence [116–119], while engagement of CD34 on hematopoietic cells leads to prevention of terminal differentiation of myeloid cells seen after enforced expression of CD34 [120]. Which signal pathways are involved in these effects is not known.

Cytokines

A large number of cytokines, growth factors and chemokines have been identified that influence hematopoiesis. Few cytokines are made exclusively by cells in the BM microenvironment; most are produced both by cells in and outside of the BM, whereas yet others, such as IL-3 and erythropoietin (EPO), are made exclusively by cells outside of the BM. The role of cytokines in hematopoiesis is discussed at length in Chapters 45 & 48. Cytokines are also mentioned in this chapter on the BM microenvironment because of the complex interplay between cytokines and other components of the BM microenvironment, which is crucial for the normal hematopoietic process. For instance, as discussed in the section above, the effect of a given cytokine in isolation on HSC/HPC proliferation and differentiation may differ from what is observed when, in addition to cytokine stimulation, adhesion receptors are engaged [101,111,113,114]. Conversely, as discussed earlier, the functional status of adhesion receptors is influenced by cytokine-mediated signals [100,102,103,111]. Therefore, a number of *in vitro* studies in which each of the components is evaluated individually cannot recapitulate the complexity of hematopoiesis *in vivo*. Because the effect of an individual cytokine is modulated by the presence or absence of other cytokines, chemokines or growth factors, combinatorial presentation of cytokines affect HSC/HPC behavior in a manner distinct from that of single cytokines [60]. Therefore, the concept that GAGs and other ECM molecules in the BM serve to orchestrate specific niches where certain cytokines are presented in tightly controlled concentrations and combinations to HSCs, HPCs and more mature cells is important when considering the *in vivo* effects of cytokines [55,56,60]. Discussed elsewhere too is the notion that cytokine-mediated signals may be affected by coengagement of members of the Notch-family of receptors [121], again demonstrating that the complexity of the BM microenvironment affects the final action resulting from cytokine receptor stimulation. Finally, some cytokines, such as kit-L [122] and macrophage-CSF [123], exist in a membrane bound form and secreted form, and the influence exerted on HSCs/HPCs by the membrane bound form differs from that of the soluble molecule.

Despite the cloning of more than 50 cytokines and growth factors known to be present in the BM microenvironment, and the knowledge gained regarding their effects in combination with adhesion events and other signaling events that occur in the BM, we still do not know how HSC self-renewal vs. differentiation is governed. This will likely require that global gene and protein expression patterns in cells present in stem cell niches and committed progenitor niches are characterized. Initial studies in this area have identified a large number of known genes, not previously associated with hematopoiesis, as well as novel genes to be expressed in long-term repopulating stem cell supportive cell lines [22]. These novel insights will likely greatly enhance our understanding of the tightly regulated hematopoietic process in the next 5–10 years.

BM stromal cells as therapeutics

The majority of stromal cells in BM are of the mesenchymal lineage. Mesenchymal stem cells (MSC) were initially described by Fridenshtein [124]. He showed that when BM aspirates were plated with fetal calf serum (FCS) at limiting cell numbers, colonies consisting of adherent fibroblast cells developed that could differentiate into bone and adipocytes. Since then several investigators have shown that these cells can form osteoblasts, chondrocytes, adipocytes, hematopoietic supportive fibroblasts and skeletal myocytes [125–130]. Most investigators have purified MSC based on their ability to adhere to culture vessels when cultured in the presence of fetal calf serum. Caplan isolated monoclonal Abs SH2 and SH4 that when used in combination can isolate MSC [125,126], whereas Gronthos, Simmons and colleagues purified these cells based on the expression of Stro-1 [127,131].

As MSC differentiate into multiple mesodermal cell types, they might be used to treat disorders of bone, cartilage and hematopoietic supportive fibroblasts. When transplanted into preimmune fetal sheep, human MSC derived osteoblasts and chondroblasts, as well as fibroblasts, have been detected for several months [129]. It is less clear what the degree of engraftment is when MSC are transplanted postnatally. Because of their size, the majority of cells are retained in the lung vasculature, and only small numbers of cells can be detected in other organs, such as BM or spleen [132]. However, there is evidence that MSC may enhance engraftment of small numbers of umbilical cord blood progenitors in NOD-SCID mice, a finding that has led to the development of human clinical trials. Whether MSC could be used to restore the function of hematopoietic stroma following radiation and/or chemotherapy is not known. Although some studies have suggested that hematopoietic stroma is donor-derived following BM transplantation [133], several well-controlled studies have suggested that that may not be the case [134,135]. However, the number of MSC present in a BM graft is low [126], and studies aimed at testing whether infusion of large numbers of MSC will lead to engraftment in hematopoietic stroma compartment are ongoing.

MSC contribution, albeit at low levels, to bone and cartilage formation in the preimmune fetal sheep model, has also led to clinical trials in which MSC are used to treat osteogenesis imperfecta, with clinical improvement in the symptoms of the disease [135,136]. Finally, there is an ever-expanding body of studies indicating that MSC may also be capable of differentiating in cells outside of the classical limb bud mesodermal cell lineages, including cardiac muscle [137], neuroectoderm [138–141] and endoderm [141]. The mechanism(s) underlying this perceived greater potency of MSC is currently not understood. Also not known at this time is whether BM-derived MSC will ultimately be suitable for therapy of tissues other than bone, cartilage or fibroblasts. Extensive additional *in vitro* and *in vivo* studies will be needed to evaluate this hypothesis.

Conclusion

This chapter demonstrates that significant new insights have been gained over the last 5–10 years in the role different constituents of the BM microenvironment play in the regulating of HSC/HPC entry into and exit from the BM, HSC/HPC proliferation and differentiation. It should also be obvious from the discussion above that many processes are still not fully understood. With the advent of novel molecular techniques, which will allow evaluation of the complement genes that are expressed in HSCs as well as in the BM microenvironment and the gaging of their activation status, it is likely that rapid progress will be made in further deciphering the factors that govern HSC self-renewal, homing and mobilization. Finally, the mesenchymal stromal cells have gained prominence because of their putative therapeutic potential. Intensive studies ongoing in many laboratories around the world will likely demonstrate within the next 5–10 years whether this promise can be translated into clinically relevant therapies.

References

1 Tavassoli M. Embryonic and fetal hemopoiesis: an overview. *Blood Cells Mol Dis* 1991; **17**: 282–6.

2 Tavian M, Coulombel L, Luton D, Clemente H, Dieterlen-Lievre F, Peault B. Aorta-associated CD34[+] hematopoietic cells in the early human embryo. *Blood* 1996; **87**: 67–76.

3 Medvinsky A, Dzierzak E. Definitive hematopoiesis is autonomously initiated by the AGM region. *Cell* 1996; **86**: 899–908.

4 Yoder M, Hiatt K. Engraftment of embryonic hematopoietic cells in conditioned newborn recipients. *Blood* 1997; **89**: 2176–84.

5 Miyajima A, Kinoshita T, Tanaka M, Kamiya A, Mukouyama Y, Hara T. Role of oncostatin M in hematopoiesis and liver development. *Cytokine Growth Factor Rev* 2000; **11**: 177–83.

6 Charbord P, Tavian M, Humeau L, Peault B. Early ontogeny of the human marrow from long bones: an immunohistochemical study of hematopoiesis and its microenvironment. *Blood* 1996; **87**: 4109–17.

7 Ma Q, Jones D, Borghesani P *et al.* Impaired B-lymphopoiesis myelopoiesis and derailed cerebellar neuron migration in CXCR4- and SDF-1- deficient mice. *Proc Natl Acad Sci U S A* 1998; **95**: 9448–53.

8 Nagasawa T, Hirota S, Tachibana K *et al.* Defects of B-cell lymphopoiesis and bone-marrow myelopoiesis in mice lacking the CXC chemokine PBSF/SDF-1. *Nature* 1996; **382**: 635–8.

9 Hirsch E, Iglesias A, Potocnik AJ, Hartmann U, Fassler R. Impaired migration but not differentiation of haematopoietic stem cells in the absence of beta-1 integrins. *Nature* 1996; **380** (6570): 171–5.

10 Roy V, Verfaillie CM. Expression and function of cell adhesion molecules on fetal liver, cord blood and bone marrow hematopoietic progenitors: implications for anatomical localization and developmental stage specific regulation of hematopoiesis. *Exp Hematol* 1999; **27**: 302–12.

11 Hidalgo A, Weiss LA, Frenette PS. Functional selectin ligands mediating human CD34[+] cell interactions with bone marrow endothelium are enhanced postnatally. *J Clin Invest* 2002; **110**: 559–69.

12 Dexter TM. Haemopoiesis in long-term bone marrow cultures. *A Rev Acta Haematol* 1979; **62**: 299–305.

13 Yoder M, Papaioannou V, Breitfeld P, Williams D. Murine yolk sac endoderm- and mesoderm-derived cell lines support *in vitro* growth and differentiation of hematopoietic cells. *Blood* 1994; **83**: 2436–44.

14 de Bruijn MF, Ma X, Robin C, Ottersbach K, Sanchez MJ, Dzierzak E. Hematopoietic stem cells localize to the endothelial cell layer in the midgestation mouse aorta. *Immunity* 2002; **16**: 673–83.

15 Kusadasi N, Oostendorp RA, Koevoet WJ, Dzierzak EA, Ploemacher RE. Stromal cells from murine embryonic aorta-gonad-mesonephros

region, liver and gut mesentery expand human umbilical cord blood-derived CAFC (week 6) in extended long-term cultures. *S Leukemia* 2002; **16**: 1782–90.
16. Wineman J, Moore K, Lemischka I, Muller-Sieburg C. Functional heterogeneity of the hematopoietic microenvironment: rare stromal elements maintain long-term repopulating stem cells. *Blood* 1996; **87**: 4082–90.
17. Sutherland HJ, Eaves CJ, Lansdorp PM, Thacker JD, Hogge DE. Differential regulation of primitive human hematopoietic cells in long-term cultures maintained on genetically engineered murine stromal cells. *Blood* 1991; **78**: 666–78.
18. Coloumbel L, Eaves A, Eaves C. Enzymatic treatment of long-term marrow cultures reveals the preferential location of primitive hematopoietic progenitors in the adherent layer. *Blood* 1983; **62**: 291–300.
19. Moore KA, Hideo E, Lemischka IR. In vitro maintenance of highly purified transplantable hematopoietic stem cells. *Blood* 1997; **89**: 4337–437.
20. Verfaillie C. Direct contact between progenitors and stroma is not required for human *in vitro* hematopoiesis. *Blood* 1992; **79**: 2821–6.
21. Punzel M, Gupta P, Roodell A, Mortari F, Verfaillie C. Factor S secreted by AFT024 fetal liver cells following stimulation with human cytokines are important for human LTC-IC growth. *Leukemia* 1999; **13**: 1079–84.
22. Hackney JA, Charbord P, Brunk BP, Stoeckert CJ, Lemischka IR, Moore KA. A molecular profile of a hematopoietic stem cell niche. *Proc Natl Acad Sci U S A* 2002; **99**: 13,061–6.
23. Deldar A, Lewis H, Weiss L. Bone lining cells and hematopoiesis: an electron microscopic study of canine BM. *Anat Rec* 1985; **213**: 187–201.
24. Cheng S, Lecanda F, Davidson M et al. Human osteoblasts express a repertoire of cadherins which are critical for BMP-2 induced osteogenic differentiation. *J Bone Miner Res* 1998; **13**: 633–41.
25. Taichman R, Emerson S. Human osteoblasts support hematopoiesis through the production of granulocyte colony-stimulating factor. *J Exp Med* 1994; **179**: 1677–86.
26. Nelissen JM, Torensma R, Pluyter M et al. Molecular analysis of the hematopoiesis supporting osteoblastic cell line U2-OS. *Exp Hematol* 2000; **28**: 422–32.
27. Gimble JM, Robinson CE, Wu X, Kelly KA. The function of adipocytes in the bone marrow stroma: an update. *Bone* 1996; **19**: 421–8.
28. Fantuzzi G, Faggioni R. Leptin in the regulation of immunity, inflammation, and hematopoiesis. *J Leukoc Biol* 2000; **68**: 437–46.
29. Yokota T, Oritani K, Takahashi I et al. Adiponectin, a new member of the family of soluble defense collagens, negatively regulates the growth of myelomonocytic progenitors and the functions of macrophages. *Blood* 2000; **96**: 1723–32.
30. Yokota T, Meka C, Medina K et al. Paracrine regulation of fat cell formation in bone marrow cultures via adiponectin and prostaglandins. *J Clin Invest* 2002; **109**: 1303–10.
31. Moore K, Pytowski B, Witte L, Hickling D, Lemischka I. Hematopoietic activity of a stromal cell transmembrane protein containing epidermal growth factor-like repeat motifs. *Proc Natl Acad Sci U S A* 1997; **94**: 4011–6.
32. Ohnoa N, Izawaa A, Hattorib M, Kageyamac R, Sudoa T. DLK inhibits stem cell factor-induced colony formation of murine hematopoietic progenitors Hes-1: independent effect. *Stem Cells* 2001; **19**: 7109–16.
33. Bauer SR, Ruiz-Hidalgo MJ, Rudikoff EK, Goldstein J, Laborda J. Modulated expression of the epidermal growth factor-like homeotic protein DLK influences stromal-cell pre-B-cell interactions, stromal cell adipogenesis, and pre-B-cell interleukin-7 requirements. *J Clin Invest* 2002; **109**: 1303–10.
34. Choi K. Hemangioblast development and regulation. *Biochem Cell Biol* 1998; **76**: 947–56.
35. Grant MB, May WS, Caballero S et al. Adult hematopoietic stem cells provide functional hemangioblast activity during retinal neovascularization. *Nat Med* 2002; **8**: 607–12.
36. Candal F, Rafii S, Parker J et al. BMEC-1: a human bone marrow microvascular endothelial cell line with primary cell characteristics. *Microvasc Res* 1996; **52**: 221–9.
37. Ohneda O, Fennie C, Zheng Z et al. Hematopoietic stem cell maintenance and differentiation are supported by embryonic aorta-gonad-mesonephros region-derived endothelium. *Blood* 1998; **92**: 908–16.
38. Fennie C, Cheng J, Dowbenko D, Young P, Lasky L. CD34$^+$ endothelial cell lines derived from murine yolk sac induce the proliferation and differentiation of yolk sac CD34$^+$ hematopoietic progenitors. *Blood* 1995; **86**: 4454–65.
39. Brandt J, Galy A, Luens K et al. Bone marrow repopulation by human marrow stem cells after long-term expansion culture on a porcine endothelial cell line. *Exp Hematol* 1998; **26**: 950–9.
40. Papayannopoulou T, Craddock CBN, Priestley G, Wolf S. The VLA4/VCAM adhesion pathway defines contrasting mechanisms of lodging of transplanted murine hematopoietic progenitors between bone marrow and spleen. *Proc Natl Acad Sci U S A* 1995; **92**: 9647–53.
41. Teixido J, Hemler ME, Greenberger JS, Anklesaria P. Role of β_1- and β_2-integrins in the adhesion of human CD34^{hi} stem cells to bone marrow stroma. *J Clin Invest* 1992; **90**(2): 358–67.
42. Kansas G. Selectins and their ligands: current concepts and controversies. *Blood* 1996; **88**: 3259–68.
43. Shirota T, Tavassoli M. Alterations of bone marrow sinus endothelium induced by ionizing irradiation: implications in the homing of intravenously transplanted marrow cells. *Blood Cells* 1992; **18**: 197–204.
44. Potts J, Campbell I. Fibronectin structure and assembly. *Curr Opin Cell Biol* 1994; **6**: 648–55.
45. Williams D, Rios M, Stephens C, Patel V. Fibronectin and VLA-4 in haematopoietic stem cell-microenvironment interactions. *Nature* 1991; **352**: 438–41.
46. Hurley RW, McCarthy JB, Verfaillie CM. Direct adhesion to bone marrow stroma via fibronectin receptors inhibits hematopoietic progenitor proliferation. *J Clin Invest* 1995; **96**: 511–21.
47. Verfaillie CM, Benis A, Iida J, McGlave PB, McCarthy JB. Adhesion of committed human hematopoietic progenitors to synthetic peptides from the C-terminal heparin-binding domain of fibronectin: cooperation between the integrin $\alpha_4\beta_1$ and the CD44 adhesion receptor. *Blood* 1994; **84**: 1802–11.
48. Gordon M, Dowding C, Riley G, Goldman J, Greaves M. Altered adhesive interactions with marrow stroma of haematopoietic progenitor cells in chronic myeloid leukaemia. *Nature* 1987; **328**: 342–6.
49. Verfaillie CM, McCarthy JB, McGlave PB. Mechanisms underlying abnormal trafficking of malignant progenitors in chronic myelogenous leukemia: decreased adhesion to stroma and fibronectin but increased adhesion to the basement membrane components laminin and collagen type IV. *J Clin Invest* 1992; **90**: 1232–41.
50. Nolta J, Smogorzewska E, Kohn D. Analysis of optimal conditions for retroviral mediated transduction of primitive human hematopoietic cells. *Blood* 1995; **86**: 101–9.
51. Patel V, Lodish H. A fibronectin matrix is required for differentiation of murine erythroleukemia cells into reticulocytes. *J Cell Biol* 1987; **105**: 3105–14.
52. Fedarko N. Isolation and purification of proteoglycans. *EXS* 1994; **70**: 9–15.
53. Wright T, Kinsella M, Keating A, Singer J. Proteoglycans in human long-term bone marrow cultures. Biochemical and ultrastructural analyzes. *Blood* 1986; **67**: 133–41.
54. Gupta P, McCarthy J, Verfaillie C. Marrow stroma derived proteoglycans combined with physiological concentrations of cytokines are required for LTC-IC maintenance. *Blood* 1996; **87**: 322–39.
55. Gordon M, Riley G, Watt S, Greaves M. Compartmentalization of a haematopoietic growth factor (GM-CSF) by glycosaminoglycans in the bone marrow microenvironment. *Nature* 1987; **326**: 133–41.
56. Roberts R, Gallagher J, Spooncer E, Allen T, Bloomfield F, Dexter T. Heparan sulphate bound growth factors: a mechanism for stromal cell mediated haemopoiesis. *Nature* 1988; **332**: 376–9.
57. Spooncer E, Gallagher JT, Krizsa F, Dexter TM. Regulation of haemopoiesis in long-term bone marrow cultures. IV. Glycosaminoglycan synthesis and the stimulation of haemopoiesis by β-D-xylosides. *J Cell Biol* 1983; **96**: 510–4.
58. Gupta P, Oegema TR, Brazil JJ, Dudek AZ, Slungaard A, Verfaillie CM. Human LTC-IC can be maintained for at least 5 weeks *in vitro* when interleukin-3 and a single chemokine are combined with O-sulfated heparan sulfates. Requirement for optimal binding interactions of heparan sulfate with early-acting cytokines and matrix proteins. *Blood* 2000; **95**: 147–55.
59. Lewis ID, Almeida-Porada GJ, Lemischka IR, Moore KA, Zanjani ED, Verfaillie CM. Long-term repopulating cord blood stem cells are preserved after *ex-vivo* culture in a noncontact system. *Blood* 2001; **97**: 3441–9.
60. Gupta P, Oegema TR, Brazil JJ, Dudek AZ, Slungaard A, Verfaillie CM. Structurally specific heparan sulfates support primitive human hematopoiesis by formation of a multimolecular stem cell niche. *Blood* 1998; **92**: 4641–51.
61. Quesenberry PJ, Crittenden RB, Lowry P et al. In vitro and *in vivo* studies of stromal niches. *Blood Cell* 1994; **2**: 97–104.
62. Bornstein P. Thrombospondins. Structure and regulation of expression. *FASEB J* 1992; **6**: 3290–6.
63. Long M, Dixit V. Thrombospondin functions as a cytoadhesion molecule for human hematopoietic progenitor cells. *Blood* 1990; **75**: 2311–21.
64. Roy V, Miller JS, Verfaillie CM. Phenotypic and functional characterization of committed and primitive myeloid and lymphoid hematopoietic precursors in human fetal liver. *Exp Hematol* 1997; **25**: 387–94.

65 Marquez-Curtis LA, Dobrowsky A, Montano J et al. Matrix metalloproteinase and tissue inhibitors of metalloproteinase secretion by haematopoietic and stromal precursors and their production in normal and leukaemic long-term marrow cultures. Br J Haematol 2001; 115: 595–604.

66 Janowska-Wieczorek A, Marquez LA, Dobrowsky A, Ratajczak MZ, Cabuhat ML. Differential MMP and TIMP production by human marrow and peripheral blood CD34+ cells in response to chemokines. Exp Hematol 2000; 28: 1274–85.

67 Mazo IB, von Andrian UH. Adhesion and homing of blood-borne cells in bone marrow microvessels. J Leukoc Biol 1999; 66: 225–32.

68 Papayannopoulou T, Priestley GV, Nakamoto B, Zafiropoulos V, Scott LM. Molecular pathways in bone marrow homing. Dominant role of $\alpha_4\beta_1$ over β_2-integrins and selectins. Blood 2001; 98: 2403–11.

69 Levesque JP, Takamatsu Y, Nilsson SK, Haylock DN, Simmons JP. Vascular cell adhesion molecule-1 (CD106) is cleaved by neutrophil proteases in the bone marrow following hematopoietic progenitor cell mobilization by granulocyte colony-stimulating factor. Blood 2001; 98: 1289–97.

70 Gaugler MH, Squiban C, Mouthon MA, Gourmelon P, van der Meeren A. Irradiation enhances the support of haemopoietic cell transmigration, proliferation and differentiation by endothelial cells. Br J Haematol 2001; 113: 940–50.

71 Larson R, Springer T. Structure and function of leukocyte integrins. Immunol Rev 1990; 114: 181–9.

72 Howe A, Aplin A, Alahari S, Juliano R. Integrin signaling and cell growth control. Curr Opin Cell Biol 1998; 10: 220–31.

73 Hughes P, Pfaff M. Integrin affinity modulation. Trends Cell Biol 1998; 8: 359–67.

74 Guan J. Focal adhesion kinase in integrin signaling. Matrix Biol 1997; 16: 195–200.

75 Morino N, Mimura T, Hamasaki K et al. Matrix/integrin interaction activates the mitogen-activated protein kinase p44erk-1 and p42erk-2. J Biol Chem 1995; 270: 269–78.

76 Meng F, Lowell CA. A β_1-integrin signaling pathway involving Src-family kinases, Cbl and PI-3 is required for macrophage spreading and migration. EMBO 1998; 17: 4391–403.

77 Xie B, Zhao J, Kitagawa M et al. Focal adhesion kinase activates Stat1 in integrin-mediated cell migration and adhesion. J Biol Chem 2001; 276: 19,512–23.

78 Coulombel L, Auffray I, Gaugler M, Rosemblatt M. Expression and function of integrins on hematopoietic progenitor cells. Acta Haematol 1997; 97: 13–21.

79 McEver R. Selectin–carbohydrate interactions during inflammation and metastasis. Glycoconj J 1997; 14: 585–93.

80 Tedder T, Steeber D, Chen A, Engel P. The selectins: vascular adhesion molecules. FASEB J 1995; 9: 866–70.

81 Dercksen M, Gerritsen W, Rodenhuis S et al. Expression of adhesion molecules on CD34+ cells: CD34+ L-selectin+ cells predict a rapid platelet recovery after peripheral blood stem cell transplantation. Blood 1995; 85: 3313–21.

82 Frenette P, Wagner D. Insights into selectin function from knock-out mice. Thromb Haemost 1997; 78: 60–9.

83 Varki A. Selectin ligands: will the real ones please stand up? J Clin Invest 1997; 100: S31–3.

84 Dowbenko D, Andalibi A, Young P, Lusis A, Lasky L. Structure and chromosomal localization of the murine gene encoding GLYCAM 1. A mucin-like endothelial ligand for L-selectin. J Biol Chem 1993; 268: 4525–34.

85 Baumhueter S, Dybdal N, Kyle C, Lasky L. Global vascular expression of murine CD34: a sialomucin-like endothelial ligand for L-selectin. Blood 1994; 84: 2554–64.

86 McEver R, Cummings R. Role of PSGL-1 binding to selectins in leukocyte recruitment. J Clin Invest 1997; 100: S97–101.

87 Dimitroff CJ, Lee JY, Fuhlbrigge RC, Sackstein R. A distinct glycoform of CD44 is an L-selectin ligand on human hematopoietic cells. Proc Natl Acad Sci U S A 2000; 97: 13,841–6.

88 Dwir O, Kansas GS, Alon R. Cytoplasmic anchorage of L-selectin controls leukocyte capture and rolling by increasing the mechanical stability of the selectin tether. J Cell Biol 2001; 1155: 145–56.

89 Piccardoni P, Sideri R, Manarini S et al. Platelet/polymorphonuclear leukocyte adhesion: a new role for SRC kinases in Mac-1 adhesive function triggered by P-selectin. Blood 2001; 98: 108–16.

90 Hu Y, Szente B, Kiely JM, Gimbrone MAJ. Molecular events in transmembrane signaling via E-selectin. SHP2 association, adaptor protein complex formation and ERK1/2 activation. J Biol Chem 2001; 276 (4859): 4–53.

91 Simmons PJ, Levesque JP, Haylock DN. Mucin-like molecules as modulators of the survival and proliferation of primitive hematopoietic cells. Ann N Y Acad Sci 2001; 938: 196–206.

92 Lasky L. Sialomucin ligands for selectins. A new family of cell adhesion molecules. Princess Takamatsu Symp 1994; 24: 81–104.

93 Orlando RA, Takeda T, Zak B et al. The glomerular epithelial cell anti-adhesin podocalyxin associates with the actin cytoskeleton through interactions with ezrin. J Am Soc Nephrol 2001; 12: 1589–98.

94 Tada J, Omine M, Suda T, Yamaguchi N. A common signaling pathway via Syk and Lyn tyrosine kinases generated from capping of the sialomucins CD34 and CD43 in immature hematopoietic cells. Blood 1999; 93: 3723–35.

95 Gordon MY, Marley SB, Davidson RJ et al. Contact-mediated inhibition of human haematopoietic progenitor cell proliferation may be conferred by stem cell antigen, CD34. Hematol J 2000; 1: 77–86.

96 Zhu X, Price-Schiavi SA, Carraway KL. Extracellular regulated kinase (ERK)-dependent regulation of sialomucin complex/rat Muc4 in mammary epithelial cells. Oncogene 2000; 19: 4254–61.

97 Steeber DA, Tedder TF. Adhesion molecule cascades direct lymphocyte recirculation and leukocyte migration during inflammation. Immunol Res 2001; 22: 299–317.

98 Verfaillie C, Blakolmer K, McGlave P. Purified primitive human hematopoietic progenitor cells with long-term in vitro repopulating capacity adhere selectively to irradiated BM stroma. J Exp Med 1990; 172: 509–20.

99 Janowska-Wieczorek A, Majka MK, Baj-Krzyworzeka M et al. Platelet-derived microparticles bind to hematopoietic stem/progenitor cells and enhance their engraftment. Blood 2001; 98: 3143–9.

100 Levesque JP, Leavesley DI, Niutta S, Vadas M, Simmons PJ. Cytokines increase human hemopoietic cell adhesiveness by activation of very late antigen (VLA)-4 and VLA-5 integrins. J Exp Med 1995; 181: 1805–14.

101 Levesque J, Haylock D, Simmons P. Cytokine regulation of proliferation and cell adhesion are correlated events in human CD34+ hemopoietic progenitors. Blood 1996; 88: 1168–76.

102 Schofield K, Rushton G, Humphries M, Dexter T, Gallagher J. Influence of interleukin-3 and other growth factors on $\alpha_4\beta_1$-integrin-mediated adhesion and migration of human hematopoietic progenitor cells. Blood 1997; 90: 1858–66.

103 Peled A, Kollet O, Ponomaryov T et al. The chemokine SDF-1 activates the integrins LFA-1, VLA-4, and VLA-5 on immature human CD34+ cells: role in transendothelial/stromal migration and engraftment of NOD/SCID mice. Blood 2000; 95: 3289–96.

104 Gothot A, van der Loo JC, Clapp DW, Srour EF. Cell cycle-related changes in repopulating capacity of human mobilized peripheral blood CD34+ cells in nonobese diabetic/severe combined immune-deficient mice. Blood 1998; 92: 2641–9.

105 Papayannopoulou T, Nakamato B. Systemic treatment of primates with anti-VLA4 leads to an immediate egress of hemopoietic progenitors to periphery. Proc Natl Acad Sci U S A 1993; 90: 9374–9.

106 Prosper F, Stroncek D, McCarthy JB, Verfaillie CM. Mobilization and homing of peripheral blood progenitors is related to reversible downregulation of $\alpha_4\beta_1$-integrin expression and function. J Clin Invest 1998; 101(11): 2456–67.

107 Mohle R, Murea S, Kirsch M, Haas R. Differential expression of L-selectin VLA-4 and LFA-1 on CD34+ progenitor cells from bone marrow and peripheral blood during G-CSF-enhanced recovery. Exp Hematol 1995; 23: 1535–44.

108 van der Loo J, Xiao X, McMillin D, Hashino K, Kato I, Williams D. VLA-5 is expressed by mouse and human long-term repopulating hematopoietic cells and mediates adhesion to extracellular matrix protein fibronectin. J Clin Invest 1998; 102: 1051–61.

109 Giet O, Huygen S, Beguin Y, Gothot A. Cell cycle activation of hematopoietic progenitor cells increases very late antigen-5-mediated adhesion to fibronectin. Exp Hematol 2001; 29: 515–24.

110 Anderson D, Springer T. Leukocyte adhesion deficiency: an inherited defect in the Mac-1 LFA-1 and p15095 glycoproteins. Ann Rev Med 1987; 38: 175–84.

111 Jiang Y, Prosper F, Verfaillie CM. Opposing effects of engagement of integrins and stimulation of cytokine receptors on cell cycle progression of normal human hematopoietic progenitors. Blood 2000; 95: 846–54.

112 Jiang Y, Zhao RCH, Verfaillie CM. Inactivation of the cyclin-dependent kinase inhibitor, p27, is responsible for overriding the integrin-mediated inhibition of CML CD34+ cells. Proc Natl Acad Sci U S A 2000; 97: 10,538–43.

113 Schofield K, Humphries M, de Wynter E, Testa N, Gallagher J. The effect of $\alpha_4\beta_1$-integrin binding sequences of FN on growth of cells from human hematopoietic progenitors. Blood 1998; 91: 3230–8.

114 Kapur R, Cooper R, Zhang L, Williams DA. Crosstalk between $\alpha_4\beta_1/\alpha_5\beta_1$ and c-kit results in opposing effect on growth and survival of hematopoietic cells via the activation of focal adhesion kinase, mitogen-activated protein kinase, and Akt signaling pathways. Blood 2001; 97: 1975–81.

115 Moritz T, Dutt P, Xiao X et al. Fibronectin improves transduction of reconstituting hemato-

115 poietic stem cells by retroviral vectors: evidence of direct viral binding to chymotryptic carboxy-terminal fragments. *Blood* 1996; **88**: 855–62.
116 Zannettino A, Buhring H, Niutta S, Watt S, Benton M, Simmons P. The sialomucin CD164 (MGC-24v) is an adhesive glycoprotein expressed by human hematopoietic progenitors and bone marrow stromal cells that serves as a potent negative regulator of hematopoiesis. *Blood* 1998; **92**: 2613–21.
117 Bazil V, Brandt J, Tsukamoto A, Hoffman R. Apoptosis of human hematopoietic progenitor cells induced by crosslinking of surface CD43 the major sialoglycoprotein of leukocytes. *Blood* 1995; **86**: 502–11.
118 Bazil V, Brandt J, Chen S *et al*. A monoclonal antibody recognizing CD43 (leukosialin) initiates apoptosis of human hematopoietic progenitor cells but not stem cells. *Blood* 1996; **87**: 1272–81.
119 Levesque JP, Zannettino AC, Pudney M. PSGL-1-mediated adhesion of human hematopoietic progenitors to P-selectin results in suppression of hematopoiesis. *Immunity* 1999; **11**: 369–78.
120 Fackler MJ, Krause DM, Smith OM, Civin CI, May WS. Full-length but not truncated CD34 inhibits hematopoietic cell differentiation of M1 cells. *Blood* 1995; **85**: 3040–7.
121 Ohishi K, Varnum-Finney B, Bernstein ID. Delta-1 enhances marrow and thymus repopulating ability of human CD34[+] CD38[−] cord blood cells. *J Clin Invest* 2002; **110**: 1165–74.
122 Bernstein A, Forrester L, Reith AD, Dubreuil P, Rottapel R. The murine W/c-kit and Steel loci and the control of hematopoiesis. *Semin Hematol* 1991; **28**: 138–66.
123 Tsuboi I, Revol V, Blanchet JP, Mouchiroud G. Role of the membrane form of human colony-stimulating factor-1 (CSF-1) in proliferation of multipotent hematopoietic FDCP-mix cells expressing human CSF-1 receptor. *Leukemia* 2000; **14**: 1460–6.
124 Fridenshtein A. Stromal bone marrow cells and the hematopoietic microenvironment. *Arkh Patol* 1982; **44**: 3–11.
125 Haynesworth SE, Barber MA, Caplan IA. Cell surface antigens on human marrow-derived mesenchymal cells are detected by monoclonal antibodies. *Bone* 1992; **13**: 69–80.
126 Pittenger MF, Mackay AM, Beck SC *et al*. Multilineage potential of adult human mesenchymal stem cells. *Science* 1999; **284**: 143–7.
127 Gronthos S, Graves S, Ohta S, Simmons P. The STRO-1[+] fraction of adult human bone marrow contains the osteogenic precursors. *Blood* 1994; **84**: 4164–73.
128 Prockop D. Marrow stromal cells as stem cells for nonhematopoietic tissues. *Science* 1997; **276**: 71–4.
129 Liechty KW, MacKenzie TC, Shaaban AF *et al*. Human mesenchymal stem cells engraft and demonstrate site-specific differentiation after *in utero* transplantation in sheep. *Nat Med* 2000; **6**: 1282–6.
130 Wakitani S, Saito T, Caplan A. Myogenic cells derived from rat bone marrow mesenchymal stem cells exposed to 5-azacytidine. *Muscle Nerve* 1995; **18**: 1417–26.
131 Gronthos S, Simmons P. The biology and application of human bone marrow stromal cell precursors. *J Hematoth* 1996; **5**: 15–26.
132 Gao J, Dennis JE, Muzic RF, Lundberg M, Caplan AI. The dynamic *in vivo* distribution of bone marrow-derived mesenchymal stem cells after infusion. *Cells Tissues Organs* 2001; **169**: 12–20.
133 Keating A, Singer JW, Killen PD *et al*. Donor origin of the *in vitro* haematopoietic microenvironment after marrow transplantation in man. *Nature* 1982; **298**: 280–3.
134 Simmons PJ, Przepiorka D, Thomas ED, Torok-Storb B. Host origin of marrow stromal cells following allogeneic bone marrow transplantation. *Nature* 1987; **328**: 429–33.
135 Awaya N, Rupert K, Bryant E, Torok-Storb B. Failure of adult marrow-derived stem cells to generate marrow stroma after successful hematopoietic stem cell transplantation. *Exp Hematol* 2002; **30**: 937–42.
136 Horwitz EM, Prockop DJ, Fitzpatrick LA *et al*. Transplantability and therapeutic effects of bone marrow-derived mesenchymal cells in children with osteogenesis imperfecta. *Nat Med* 1999; **5**: 309–15.
137 Horwitz EM, Gordon P, Koo W *et al*. Isolated allogeneic bone marrow-derived mesenchymal cells engraft and stimulate growth in children with osteogenesis imperfecta: implications for cell therapy of bone. *Proc Natl Acad Sci U S A* 2002; **25**: 8932–7.
138 Tomita S, Li R, Weisel R *et al*. Autologous transplantation of bone marrow cells improves damaged heart function. *Circulation* 1999; **100** (Suppl. II): 247–56.
139 Kopen G, Prockop D, Phinney D. Marrow stromal cells migrate throughout forebrain and cerebellum, and they differentiate into astrocytes after injection into neonatal mouse brains. *Proc Natl Acad Sci U S A* 1999; **96**: 10,711–6.
140 Woodbury D, Schwarz EJ, Prockop DJ, Black IB. Adult rat and human bone marrow stromal cells differentiate into neurons. *J Neurosci Res* 2000; **15**: 364–70.
141 Jiang Y, Jahagirdar B, Reyes M *et al*. Pluripotent nature of adult marrow derived mesenchymal stem cells. *Nature* 2002; **418**: 41–9.

7

Peter M. Lansdorp

Molecular Aspects of Stem Cell Renewal

Introduction

Several factors have led to intensive investigations of the hematopoietic system over the last several decades. The hematopoietic system represents the prototype of a self-renewing biological system in that large numbers of blood cells have to be produced daily in order to compensate for the loss of relatively short-lived mature blood cells. The relative ease at which blood and marrow samples can be obtained and single cell suspensions prepared have greatly facilitated *in vitro* and *in vivo* experimentation with hematopoietic cells. Techniques to purify increasingly rare cells on the basis of cell surface antigens or functional properties have been refined and are available to most researchers. A large number of purified recombinant proteins and other molecules with activity on various hematopoietic cells have been discovered and become available as are various *in vitro* and *in vivo* assays to measure functional properties of hematopoietic cells. Together, these advances have allowed various studies with purified cells and molecules, some of which have revealed unexpected characteristics of stem cell "candidates". From such studies, it has become clear that hematopoietic stem cells (HSCs) can no longer be considered a homogeneous population of cells but represent a heterogeneous population of cells with diverse functional properties. This is most strikingly illustrated by the pronounced developmental changes in functional properties of purified "candidate" stem cell populations and the age-related changes in the length of telomeric DNA in hematopoietic cells. While debates and reports on stem cell properties and purification techniques may have appeared academic from a clinical point of view, it has become clear that limited engraftment and failure of stem cell transplants may result from properties of HSCs that are predictable and, increasingly, measurable. In this chapter, molecular aspects related to the self-renewal of HSCs are reviewed. No attempt is made to cover the extensive literature in this general area. Instead, selected studies and the author's personal view on the topics are presented in the hope that this approach will benefit the design of future studies of stem cell biology and hematopoietic cell transplantation (HCT).

The stem cell hierarchy

A recurrent theme in laboratory experimental hematology over the last 40 years has been the redefinition of what HSCs are based on changes and improvements in assays. The trend has invariably been towards the identification of cells with a lower frequency than was previously reported or proposed [1]. The inevitable conclusion of this trend will no doubt be the identification of the fertilized egg as the "mother of all stem cells". A recent paper indicating that mesenchymal stem cells with properties of embryonic stem cells can be obtained by culture of adult bone marrow [2] (see also Chapter 6) indicates that we are approaching this conclusion. What could be the explanation for the seemingly endless debates and the apparent inability of an extensive field to agree on basic principles? Perhaps the success of bone marrow transplantation is part of the explanation. Transplantation of a limited number of blood or bone marrow derived HSCs reproducibly results in complete regeneration of hematopoiesis in suitably conditioned recipients. While the minimum number of HSCs required for sustained human engraftment is not known, it has been shown that a single purified HSC in the mouse can reconstitute hematopoiesis [3]. This remarkable fact has supported the definition of HSCs as "pluripotent cells with self-renewal potential". Implicit in this definition is that the two daughter cells derived from the cell division of a single parental HSC are essentially indistinguishable from that parental cell. Despite experimental evidence to the contrary, the central dogma and current paradigm in experimental hematology has remained that perhaps the frequency, but not HSCs themselves, are subject to significant molecular changes. In a way, it is understandable that experimental hematologists hate to part with the "self-renewal" concept. After all, "self-renewal" allows for, at least in theory, external control of HSC properties and net "expansion" of HSCs in the laboratory and this has been the goal of more than a few grant proposals. Furthermore, inclusion of "relative" in the definition of "self-renewal" certainly complicates models of stem cell biology and hematopoiesis. Could hematopoietic tissues indeed contain a spectrum of "stem" cells, each endowed with a different replicative potential and related functional properties? Intriguingly, this idea does provide an explanation for the remarkable observation that "very primitive" mesenchymal stem cells can be isolated from adult bone marrow, muscle and brain [4]. Perhaps such rare primitive stem cells were sequestered during early development in a microenvironment that does not support further cell division and differentiation. Only when released from environmental constraints (e.g. by an innovative experimental hematologist) and subjected to appropriate conditions would such cells show their extensive developmental potential. Strikingly, the isolation of such cells and the exploitation of their potential in clinical meaningful ways is currently one of the most exciting areas in experimental medicine.

Hematopoiesis: how many stem cell divisions?

The realization that stem cells are subject to pronounced developmental changes has focused attention on the question "how many times can stem cells divide"? Unfortunately, no techniques to address this important question are currently available, and possible answers range from <100 times [1] to >5000 times [5,6]. The total number of blood cells required for life-long maintenance of normal levels of blood cells can be calculated to be in the order of 4.10^{16} cells ($\sim 10^{12}$ cells/day $\times$ 365 days $\times$ 100 years). In principle, only 55 divisions of a single cell would satisfy this need (2^{55} = 4.10^{16}) and presumably many hundreds of different HSCs are contributing to hematopoiesis at any given time. It seems that an absolute replicative potential of <100 cell divisions per HSC can easily accommodate both the known apoptosis of cytokine-deprived committed progenitor cells and the remarkable regenerative capacity of HSCs displayed in response to marrow injury and in (serial) transplantation experiments. An important related question is how many HSC clones are actually present in normal adults. Because genetic markers such as point mutations can occur at any given cell division, the presence of such a clonal marker does not allow conclusive identification of a single HSC clone. For example, in patients with paroxysmal nocturnal hemoglobinuria (PNH), the presence of a mutation in the *PIG-A* gene is often used to identify the abnormal HSC "clone" [7]. However, such a mutation could have occurred relatively early in development, e.g. before the major expansion of HSC numbers in early childhood [8]. As a result, many hundreds of adult HSC clones would be expected to show the mutation and "clonal" marker. Conversely, when a mutation takes place very late in the stem cell hierarchy, only committed progenitors could be affected resulting in the transient appearance of a clonal marker in the peripheral blood. The transient presence of *BCR-ABL* fusion genes in the circulation of normal individuals could be an example of such a late occurrence [9]. Presumably the likelihood of *PIG-A*, *BCR-ABL* or other mutations will be directly related to the number of cells at risk: relatively few in early development and many in adult tissues.

The notion that HSC's have a limited replicative potential is supported by several observations. Both the *in vivo* regenerative capacity [10,11] and the *in vitro* expansion potential [12,13] of HSCs appear to be under developmental control (see also below). Most HSCs in adult tissue are quiescent cells in line with expectations if HSCs have only a limited replicative potential and are lacking self-renewal properties in an absolute sense. The loss of telomere repeats in adult hematopoietic cells (including purified "candidate" HSCs), relative to fetal hematopoietic cells [14], also fits a model that postulates a finite and limited replicative potential of HSCs [1,15].

Development and organization of hematopoietic tissue

The hematopoietic system has been subdivided into a hierarchy of three distinct populations [16,17]. In this model the most mature cells are morphologically identifiable as belonging to a particular lineage and have very limited proliferative potential. The cells in this most mature compartment are derived from committed progenitor cells with a higher but finite proliferative potential. Committed progenitor cells in turn are produced by a population of multipotential HSCs with variable "self-renewal" potential.

Hematopoiesis in embryos is first observed in "blood islands" in the yolk sac. Blood island precursor cells are mesenchymal cells derived from the primitive streak region of the early blastoderm. In the mouse, the yolk sac does not contain precursors of adult hematopoiesis, which can first be found in the aorta-gonad-mesonephros (AGM) region at day 10 in gestation [18]. From the AGM region, hematopoiesis appears to move to the fetal liver before reaching its final destination in the marrow. The concept of subsequent waves of progenitor cells seeding different tissues is compatible with various observations. However, the origin and number of cells seeding a particular hematopoietic niche still needs to be defined. Interestingly, some cells from yolk sac, fetal liver and marrow are all capable of producing spleen colonies in irradiated adult recipients [10]. This observation, together with the questionable use of spleen colony assays to measure HSCs [19], is probably responsible for what appears to be an incomplete appreciation of the development changes in the biological properties of primitive hematopoietic cells. Results showing that cells from early stages of development can function, to a large extent, in adult hosts and vice versa [20], illustrate a remarkable functional adaptive capacity or "plasticity" of hematopoietic cells at various stages of development. However, in the mouse, cells giving rise to spleen colonies upon transplantation into lethally irradiate recipients (colony forming unit-spleen or CFU-S) from different tissues were found to be qualitatively different in that the number of CFU-S per individual spleen colony decreased during ontogeny [10]. In these experiments, yolk sac CFU-S could be "passaged *in vivo*" seven times, fetal liver CFU-S four to six times and marrow CFU-S from young and adult mice up to three times [10]. These findings support developmental changes in stem cell self-renewal properties and/or a decreasing and limited replicative potential of HSCs (see below).

Several more recent observations provide further evidence of ontogeny-related differences between populations of primitive hematopoietic cells at various stages of development (reviewed in [13,21]). In general, fetal cells have a higher turnover rate and a higher replating potential than their functional counterparts from adult marrow. This observation is illustrated in Fig. 7.1 [12,22] which shows the production of CD34+ cells in culture from "candidate" HSCs with a CD34+CD45RA^lo CD71^lo phenotype purified from, respectively, human bone marrow, cord blood and fetal liver. Using identical growth factors and culture conditions, no

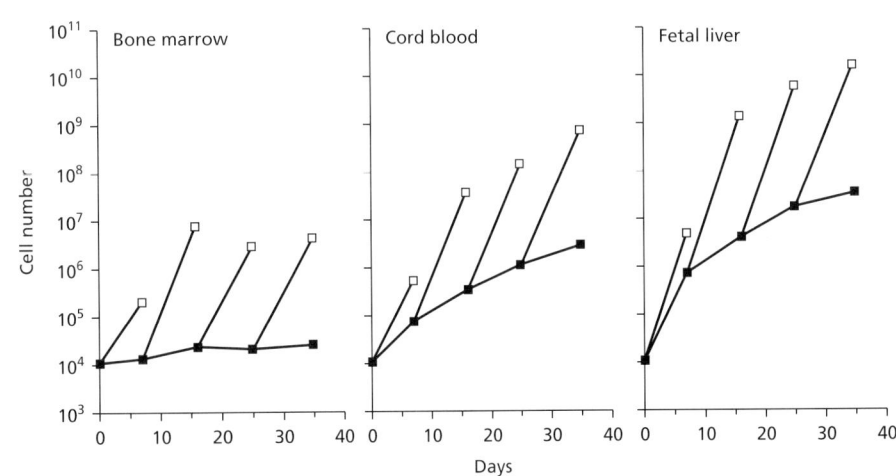

Fig. 7.1 Ontogeny-related differences in production of CD34+ cells in culture. Human candidate hematopoietic stem cells (HSCs) with a CD34+CD45RA^lo CD71^lo phenotype were purified from bone marrow, umbilical cord blood and fetal liver, and cultured in serum-free culture medium supplemented with interleukin 6 (IL-6), IL-3, stem cell factor and erythropoietin (Epo) as described [22]. Cultures (1 mL each) were initiated with 10^4 sorted cells. At the indicated time interval the total number of nucleated (□) and CD34+ cells (■) present in the cultures was calculated from the cell counts and the percentage of viable CD34+ cells measured by flow cytometry. All CD34+ cells from bone marrow cultures and fractions of the CD34+ cells from cord blood and fetal liver cultures were sorted and used for continuation of the cultures. Reproduced with permission from Lansdorp *et al.* [12].

significant production of CD34⁺ cells was observed in cultures initiated with adult bone marrow HSCs, whereas the number of CD34⁺ cells in cultures of fetal liver HSCs increased several 1000-fold. As the same number of cells was cultured under identical conditions, these observations point to intrinsic differences between the candidate HSCs themselves. Developmental switches have also been described in the immune system (reviewed in [23]). The switches from embryonic to fetal to adult hemoglobin in red cells reflect overall changes in the chromatin of HSCs that could also affect their biological properties upon transplantation. Because such developmental switches are likely, many assumptions about HSCs in adults need experimental verification. For example, it is currently not clear that adult HSCs have a similar potential to produce lymphoid progenitors as their fetal counterparts. Indeed, the lymphoid potential of HSCs in adults could be entirely derived from a small residual population of cells in adult tissue with "fetal" characteristics.

Molecular control of stem cell fate

Of fundamental interest to experimental hematologists and developmental biologists are the mechanisms that control the fate of HSCs. At any point in time, a "stem" cell has a choice to contribute either to the immediate future (by differentiating and producing committed progenitor cells) or to the more distant requirements for mature cells (by undergoing a functional self-renewal division). It has been proposed that such decisions at the level of pluripotent HSCs can be depicted as stochastic processes that are intrinsic to the cells [16,24]. If this concept is correct, the distinction between HSC's with limited and extensive *in vivo* repopulation potential will likely remain elusive as the critical distinction between the cells, the number of actual self-renewal divisions executed *in vivo*, would be governed by chance. This possibility is certainly in agreement with the difficulties encountered by many investigators in purifying repopulating HSC's to homogeneity. However, as was outlined above, the situation is more complex as self-renewal properties of HSCs are also subject to developmental control. Furthermore, it seems likely that the two daughter cells resulting from cell division of a single HSC may each differ in functional properties. Such asymmetric cell divisions are key in animal development [25] and need to be taken into account in models of HSC biology and hematopoiesis [26].

What factors are involved in stem cell fate decisions? The dramatic clinical effect of cytokines such as erythropoietin, granulocyte colony-stimulating factor (G-CSF), stem cell factor, thrombopoietin and others have underscored the important and critical role that cytokines play in the proliferation and differentiation of committed hematopoietic progenitor cells. However, attempts to modulate cell fate decisions in early hematopoietic cells using cytokines have invariably been unsuccessful [24,26–28]. Perhaps the primary role of cytokines and the microenvironment in HSC biology is to provide an essential but primarily permissive environment required for survival, proliferation and differentiation. If growth factors or factors in the microenvironment do not dictate stem cell fate decisions, what factors do? Important clues to this crucial question have been obtained by studies of the expression of homeobox genes in human hematopoietic cells [29]. It was found that expression of *Hox* genes is restricted to the most primitive hematopoietic progenitors and that overexpression of *Hox*B4 in murine HSC's results in a remarkable expansion of cells with long-term lympho-myeloid repopulating potential [30,31]. Involvement of *Hox* genes in stem cell biology is particularly striking because *Hox* genes are better known as key regulators of patterning along the body axis of developing embryos [32]. Does the involvement of *Hox* genes indicate developmental regulation of stem cell function? Are homeobox genes, the genes regulated by *Hox* genes or the regulators of *Hox* genes, the ultimate regulators of stem cell fate? What other transcription factors are involved [33,34]? To what extent are such genes subject to extracellular regulation? Can models be derived that incorporate the essential components involved in transcriptional control of stem cell fate and can this information be used to manipulate HSCs *ex vivo* in a way that is clinically meaningful? The answers to these questions are eagerly awaited. However, given the known complexity of transcriptional regulation and the well-known difficulties to assay stem cell function, a detailed understanding of the molecular control of stem cells may not be achieved in the near future.

Telomere structure and function

Without extremely reliable mechanisms to duplicate and segregate complete copies of genomes into daughter cells, life in any form could not exist. It seems certain that given this fundamental importance, many factors and pathways involved in securing the fidelity of DNA replication and chromosome segregation remain to be uncovered [35]. Increasingly, the important role of telomeres in maintaining chromosome integrity in mammalian cells is being recognized. Telomeres are the physical ends of eukaryotic chromosomes and contain both DNA and protein [36]. The DNA component of telomeres in all vertebrates consist of $(TTAGGG)_n$. Telomeres distinguish intact from broken chromosomes, stabilize chromosome ends and provide protection against nuclear degradation and end-to-end fusion events [37]. Telomeres are furthermore involved in the positioning of chromosomes within the nucleus and are also important for chromosome segregation [38].

Forty years ago, Hayflick suggested that most normal human cells are unable to divide indefinitely but are programmed for a given number of cell divisions [39]. In 1990, several papers described loss of telomeres with replication and with age and suggested that progressive telomere shortening could explain Hayflick's original observation [40–42]. This model was confirmed by subsequent studies showing that transfer of the telomerase reverse transcriptase gene could prevent telomere erosion and resulted in immortalizing of the cells that Hayflick studied in most detail: normal diploid human fibroblasts [43,44]. Since then, many papers have appeared that are compatible with the notion that telomere shortening limits the number of times most normal diploid cells can divide (for review see [45]).

Telomeric DNA is lost in human cells via several mechanisms that are related to DNA replication, remodeling and repair. Causes of telomere loss include the "end replication problem" [46,47], the nucleolytic processing of 5′ template strands following DNA replication to create a 3′ single strand overhang [48,49] and failed repair of oxidative DNA damage to telomeric DNA [50–52]. The relative contribution of these different causes of telomere shortening to the overall decline in telomere length with age is not known and most likely varies between cell types, between individuals and with age.

To compensate for the inevitable loss of telomere repeats with each cell division, certain cells express telomerase. Telomerase is a ribonucleoprotein containing the reverse transcriptase telomerase protein (hTERT) and the telomerase RNA template component (hTERC) as essential elements. In addition, a number of proteins have been described that are important for telomerase assembly (sub) nuclear localization [53] and stability (reviewed in [54]). Telomerase is capable of extending the 3′ ends of telomeres. Telomerase levels are typically high in immortal cells that maintain a constant telomere length such as the stem cells of the germline in the testis and embryonic stem cells. For reasons that remain to be precisely defined, the telomerase activity that is readily detected in human candidate HSCs [55] (reviewed in [56]) appears to be insufficient to maintain the telomere length in these cells. Nevertheless, existing telomerase levels in HSC are functionally important as is highlighted in patients with the disorder *Dyskeratosis congenita*. Patients with the autosomal dominant form of this disease have one normal and one mutated copy of the telomerase RNA template gene [57]. As expected, such patients show a modest reduction in telomerase levels, yet they eventually typically suffer from marrow failure, immune deficiencies or cancer and rarely live past the age of 50 [54,57–59]. These findings are in stark contrast to those in the mouse where complete lack of telomerase activity is tolerated for up to six generations [60]. An emerging consensus is that telomere shortening evolved as a checkpoint mechanism in long-lived mammals that controls unlimited and life-threatening proliferation of organ-specific stem cells and lymphocytes [61]. Current data are compatible with a model in which telomerase levels in human HSC are tightly regulated and sufficient to elongate only a limiting number of short telomeres. As a result, the telomere length in human HSCs declines with cell proliferation and with age, eventually triggering replicative senescence or, more likely, apoptosis.

Telomeres in the hematopoietic system

Since the important original observation that telomeres in adult blood leukocytes are significantly shorter as compared to germ-line material (sperm) from the same donor [62], the decline of somatic telomeres has been documented in three ways. The original observation was confirmed [42,63], it was shown that telomeres in various tissues were shorter in older donors [40,41] and telomere shortening was documented during *in vitro* culture of human cells [41,64]. In 1994, it was reported that cells produced in culture by highly purified human "candidate" HSCs from fetal liver, cord blood and adult bone marrow could be distinguished by reproducible differences in telomere length and that these cells showed a measurable decline in telomere length upon culture *in vitro* (Fig. 7.2 [14]). In the years that followed these initial reports, a large number of papers have appeared that have greatly refined our understanding of telomere shortening in human nucleated blood cells (reviewed in [56]). Studies in this general area have been facilitated by the development of quantitative fluorescence *in situ* hybridization (FISH) techniques to measure the telomere length in suspension cells using flow cytometry ("flow FISH" [65,66]). With this technique, it was shown that the age-related decline in telomere length in lymphocytes is much more pronounced than in granulocytes and that rapid telomere shortening early in life is followed by a much more gradual decline thereafter (Fig. 7.3 [8]).

If one assumes that the number of cell divisions between HSCs and granulocytes is relatively constant throughout life and that telomere shortening in HSCs is (i) primarily resulting from replication and (ii) relatively constant with each cell division, the telomere length in granulocytes can be used as a surrogate marker for the average telomere length in the "average" HSC clone. While the telomere length in leukocytes shows an overall decline with age [8,67], the telomere length at any given age in humans is very heterogeneous as is illustrated in Fig. 7.3. This variation appears to be primarily genetically determined [8,68]. For example, monozygous twins of over 70 years of age were shown to have very similar telomere length in both granulocytes and lymphocytes whereas such values in dizygotic twins differed more but not as much as between unrelated individuals [8].

Using further refinements in the flow FISH method (Baerlocher and Lansdorp, unpublished), it was recently shown that the rapid decline early in life is followed by a slow decline until the age of 50–60 years after which the decline again accelerates. The decline in both granulocytes and lymphocytes is nonlinear and fits a cubic curve. The pronounced decline in telomere length in specific T and NK cells could trigger apoptosis in these cells during a normal lifetime and compromise immune responses in the elderly. In contrast, granulocytes show a much more modest decline in telomere length with age and critical telomere shortening in HSCs during normal hematopoiesis does not seem very plausible. More likely, the total production of blood cells from a single HSC is primarily determined by differentiation into committed progenitor cells and not by replicative senescence. Furthermore, the occasional loss of individual stem cells via telomere shortening is not expected to impact on overall hematopoiesis (or on the overall telomere length in granulocytes) as long as an excess of HSCs exists in the marrow. Nevertheless, the age-related loss of telomeres in granulocytes, the (modest) loss of telomeres following allogeneic transplantation [56,69] and the aplastic anaemia that follows partial telomerase deficiency [54] all indicate that telomerase levels in normal HSCs are limiting and that the proliferation of HSCs is ultimately also limited by progressive telomere shortening.

The number of mature "end" cells, such as granulocytes, produced by an individual HSC could be highly variable as it appears primarily determined by the stochastic processes that regulate self-renewal and differentiation. Even a limited number of additional self-renewal divisions in a HSC will greatly increase cell output. Especially if provided with a proliferative advantage, individual HSCs can produce a staggering number of cells. This phenomenon is illustrated in clonal proliferative disorders such PNH and chronic myeloid leukemia (CML). However, even in CML, clonally expanded Philadelphia-positive stem cells eventually appear to encounter a telomere crisis [70]. Unfortunately, with a large number of cells to select from, the genetic instability triggered by the loss of functional telomeres appears to facilitate the emergence of subclones with additional genetic abnormalities, more malignant properties and higher levels of telomerase.

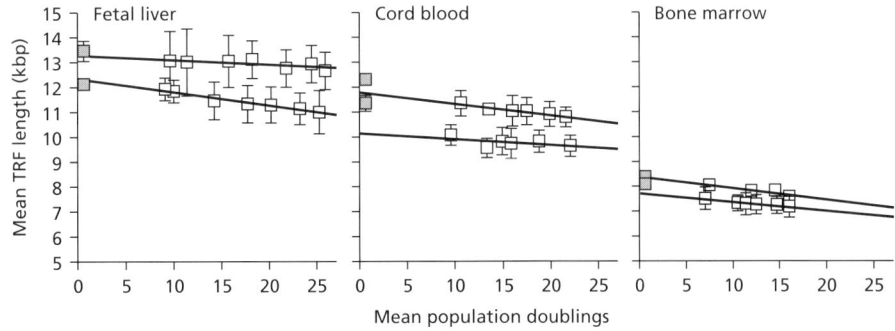

Fig. 7.2 Loss of telomeric DNA in cells from cultures of purified human candidate hematopoietic stem cell (HSCs) with a CD34$^+$CD45RA^{10}CD7^{10} phenotype from fetal liver, cord blood and bone marrow. The purified cells were cultured in serum-free medium supplemented with a mixture of cytokines to stimulate their proliferation and obtain sufficient numbers of cells for telomere restriction fragment (TRF) length measurements by Southern analysis. The mean ±SE of TRF measurements for two different donors of each tissue is shown for the cells produced in culture (□) as well as for the total nucleated cells from each donor before culture and cell purification (■). Reproduced with permission from Vaziri *et al*. [14]. Copyright (1994), National Academy of Sciences, USA.

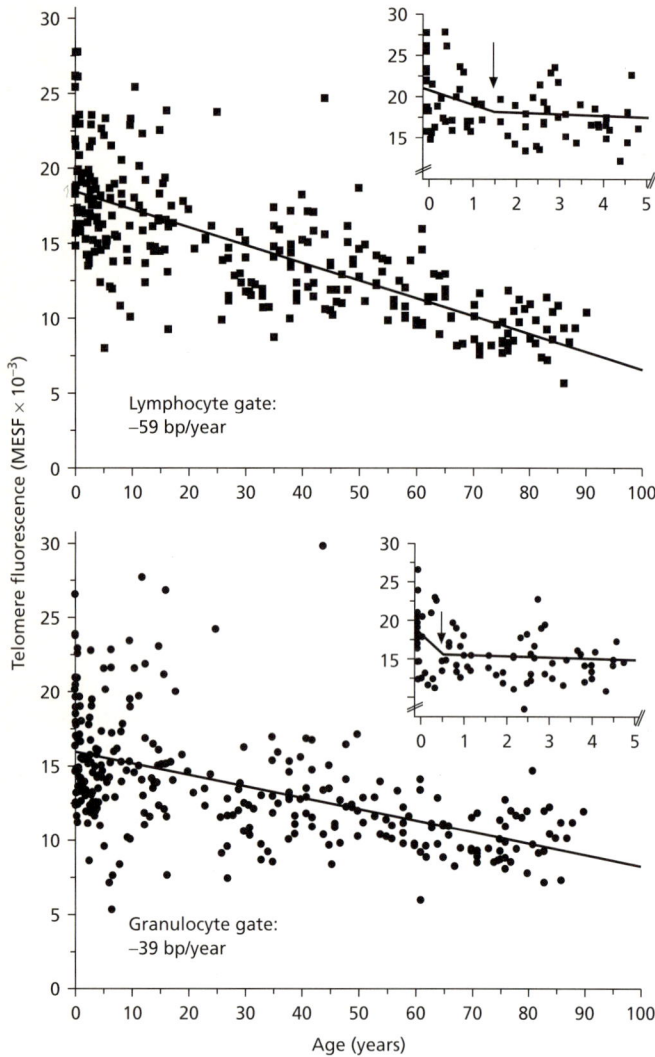

Fig. 7.3 Age-related loss of telomere length in lymphocytes and granulocytes from peripheral blood of normal individuals measured by flow fluorescence *in situ* hybridization (FISH). The specific telomere fluorescence of lymphocytes and granulocytes was analyzed after gating on these cells based on light scatter properties and DNA fluorescence. Note the heterogeneity in telomere fluorescence values, the overall decline in telomere fluorescence with age in both cell types and the higher rate of telomere attrition in lymphocytes. In this study it was found that a bi-segmented line resulted in a significantly better fit with the data than the linear fit shown on the left. Inserts show the results of bi-segmented fit analysis for lymphocytes (top) and granulocytes (bottom). Arrows indicate the optimal intersection of calculated regression lines which for both cell types was before 2 years of age. Reproduced with permission from Rufer *et al.* [8]. Copyright, the Rockefeller University Press.

The telomere checkpoint

Most human somatic cells, including HSCs, express limiting levels of telomerase and, as a result, telomere shortening effectively limits their proliferative potential. Most likely, telomere shortening evolved as a checkpoint function to suppress tumor growth specifically in long-lived species. The function of this "telomere checkpoint" may help explain poorly understood aspects of stem cell biology including stem cell "exhaustion" in aplastic anaemia and other proliferative disorders. Cells may bypass the telomere checkpoint by expressing high levels of telomerase or by inactivating downstream signaling events, e.g. by loss of p53 function. Some cells, including subsets of B cells, may avoid the telomere checkpoints altogether and this process could make these cells more vulnerable to tumor development. Loss of p53 function also inactivates the telomere checkpoint. This is expected to be a rare event as both copies of the normal p53 allele in a cell must typically be lost or mutated in order to continue proliferation in the presence of many short and dysfunctional telomeres [71]. Loss of p53 function allows survival of cells with dysfunctional telomeres. The resulting chromosome fusions result in chromosome breakage and, as a result, in the loss and amplification of genes [72]. This leaves us with a paradox: telomere shortening can act both as a tumor suppressor mechanism (by imposing limits to the replication of somatic cells) and as a tumor promoter mechanism (by favoring genetic instability once cells have reached their telomere imposed limit in replicative potential). Whether tumor growth is suppressed or promoted by progressive telomere shortening may depend on the number of cells that encounter such a telomere crisis and the genetic changes acquired by such cells prior to this encounter.

Conclusions

In this chapter, molecular aspects related to stem cell renewal were discussed. The emphasis has been on developmental changes in the functional properties of HSCs and on the loss of telomeric DNA in HSCs. It is clear that, despite much progress over the last several decades, we are left with many questions. Some of the most urgent are: How many times *can* HSCs divide and what *is* the actual replicative potential of HSCs at various stages of development? To what extent are factors in the microenvironment (i.e., cytokines) capable of modulating self-renewal properties of HSCs? What are the mechanisms controlling the turnover time of HSCs in steady state hematopoiesis and during hematopoietic regeneration? Are differences in the replicative history of HSCs reflected in their anatomical location, cytokine response and mobilization properties? Do microenvironmental niches exist that stimulate telomerase expression in HSC to levels that prevent telomere shortening altogether? Are such niches rare or limiting? Hopefully, the answers to some of these important questions will become available soon.

Studies with cultured hematopoietic cells have shown that the formation of hematopoietic colonies, as well as the proliferation and survival of various hematopoietic cells, typically requires the presence of "hematopoietic growth factors", many of which have been cloned over the last decade and produced for clinical trials (reviewed in Chapters 43 & 48). The availability of recombinant growth factors has led to frantic research efforts over the past decade to achieve clinically useful manipulation of blood-cell production *in vitro*. Two sets of observations that were discussed in this chapter cast doubt about the feasibility of some of the perceived applications of *ex vivo* "expansion" and should probably be taken into account when laboratory or clinical experiments involving limited numbers of HSCs are contemplated. First, there are the observations indicating that currently ill-defined, intrinsic (genetic) mechanisms with a developmental component control the fate of HSCs. Second, hematopoietic cells, including purified HSCs, appear to loose telomeric DNA with each cell division [14]. The studies of telomeres have focused attention on possible genetic limitations in the replicative potential of somatic cells including HSCs and such restrictions are compatible with most experimental evidence produced in clinical and laboratory studies. In view of these considerations, it seems prudent to use reasonably large numbers of HSCs for transplantation, especially from adult donors [73]. Although the number of HSCs in fetal liver or cord blood is small, such cells are likely to be superior in terms of replicative potential. This genetic superiority must be balanced against practical disadvantages including the small number of cells available for transplantation. The small size of fetal or neonatal stem cell grafts is expected to compromise clinical results especially in the presence of histocompatibility differences between donor and recipient [74]. Possibly, this limitation could be addressed by more effective immunosuppression and conditioning regimens. In addition, the outcome of fetal liver and cord blood transplants could possibly be improved by increasing the number of cells in the transplant, for example by culture *ex vivo*.

References

1 Lansdorp PM. Self-renewal of stem cells. *Biol Blood Marrow Transplant* 1997; **3**: 171–8.

2 Jiang Y, Jahagirdar BN, Reinhardt RL et al. Pluripotency of mesenchymal stem cells derived from adult marrow. *Nature* 2002; **418**(6893): 41–9.

3 Osawa M, Hanada KI, Hamada H et al. Long-term lymphohematopoietic reconstitution by a single CD34-low/negative hematopoietic stem cell. *Science* 1996; **273**: 242–5.

4 Jiang Y, Vaessen B, Lenvik T et al. Multipotent progenitor cells can be isolated from postnatal murine bone marrow, muscle, and brain. *Exp Hematol* 2002; **30**(8): 896–904.

5 Potten CS, Loeffler M. Stem cells. attributes, cycles, spirals, pitfalls and uncertainties. Lessons for and from the crypt. *Development* 1990; **10**: 1001–20.

6 Rubin H. The disparity between human cell senescence *in vitro* and lifelong replication *in vivo*. *Nat Biotechnol* 2002; **20**(7): 675–81.

7 Karadimitris A, Luzzatto L. The cellular pathogenesis of paroxysmal nocturnal haemoglobinuria. *Leukemia* 2001; **15**: 1148–52.

8 Rufer N, Brummendorf TH, Kolvraa S et al. Telomere fluorescence measurements in granulocytes and T lymphocyte subsets point to a high turnover of hematopoietic stem cells and memory T cells in early childhood. *J Exp Med* 1999; **190**: 157–67.

9 Bose S, Deininger M, Gora-Tybor J et al. The presence of typical and atypical *BCR-ABL* fusion genes in leukocytes of normal individuals: biologic significance and implications for the assessment of minimal residual disease. *Blood* 1998; **92**: 3362–7.

10 Moore MAS, Metcalf D. Ontogeny of the haemopoietic system; yolk sac origin of *in vivo* and *in vitro* colony forming cell in the developing mouse embryo. *Br J Haematol* 1970; **18**: 279–86.

11 Pawliuk R, Eaves C, Humphries RK. Evidence of both ontogeny and transplant dose-regulated expansion of hematopoietic stem cells *in vivo*. *Blood* 1996; **88**: 2852–8.

12 Lansdorp PM, Dragowska W, Mayani H. Ontogeny-related changes in proliferative potential of human hematopoietic cells. *J Exp Med* 1993; **178**: 787–91.

13 Lansdorp PM. Developmental changes in the function of hematopoietic stem cells. *Exp Hematol* 1995; **23**: 187–91.

14 Vaziri H, Dragowska W, Allsopp RC et al. Evidence for a mitotic clock in human hematopoietic stem cells: loss of telomeric DNA with age. *Proc Natl Acad Sci U S A* 1994; **91**: 9857–60.

15 Lansdorp PM. Telomere length and proliferation potential of hematopoietic stem cells. *J Cell Sci* 1995; **108**: 1–6.

16 Till JE, McCulloch EA, Siminovitch L. A stochastic model of stem cell proliferation, based on the growth of spleen colony-forming cells. *Proc Natl Acad Sci U S A* 1964; **51**: 29–36.

17 Metcalf D. *The Hemopoietic Colony Stimulating Factors*. Amsterdam: Elsevier, 1984.

18 de Bruijn MF, Ma X, Robin C et al. Hematopoietic stem cells localize to the endothelial cell layer in the midgestation mouse aorta. *Immunity* 2002; **16**(5): 673–83.

19 Ploemacher RE, Brons RHC. Separation of CFU-S from primitive cells responsible for reconstitution of the bone marrow hemopoietic stem cell compartment following irradiation: evidence for a pre-CFU-S cell. *Exp Hematol* 1989; **17**: 263–6.

20 Fleischman RA, Mintz B. Development of adult bone marrow stem cells in H-2-compatible and-incompatible mouse fetuses. *J Exp Med* 1984; **159**: 731–45.

21 Zon LI. Developmental biology of hematopoiesis. *Blood* 1995; **86**: 2876–91.

22 Lansdorp PM, Dragowska W. Long-term erythropoiesis from constant numbers of $CD34^+$ cells in serum-free cultures initiated with highly purified progenitor cells from human bone marrow. *J Exp Med* 1992; **175**: 1501–9.

23 Jane SM, Cunningham JM. Molecular mechanisms of hemoglobin switching. *Int J Biochem Cell Biol* 1996; **28**: 1197–209.

24 Ogawa M. Differentiation and proliferation of hematopoietic stem cells. *Blood* 1993; **81**: 2844–53.

25 Knoblich JA. Asymmetric cell division during animal development. *Nat Rev Mol Cell Biol* 2001; **2**: 11–20.

26 Brummendorf TH, Dragowska W, Zijlmans JMJM et al. Asymmetric cell divisions sustain long-term hematopoiesis from single-sorted human fetal liver cells. *J Exp Med* 1998; **188**: 1117–24.

27 Mayani H, Dragowska W, Lansdorp PM. Lineage commitment in human hemopoiesis involves asymmetric cell division of multipotent progenitors and does not appear to be influenced by cytokines. *J Cell Physiol* 1993; **157**: 579–86.

28 Fairbairn LJ, Cowling GJ, Reipert BM et al. Suppression of apoptosis allows differentiation and development of a multipotent hemopoietic cell line in the absence of added growth factors. *Cell* 1993; **74**: 823–32.

29 Sauvageau G, Lansdorp PM, Eaves CJ et al. Differential expression of homeobox genes in functionally distinct $CD34^+$ subpopulations of human bone marrow cells. *Proc Natl Acad Sci U S A* 1994; **91**: 12 223–7.

30 Sauvageau G, Thorsteinsdottir U, Eaves CJ et al. Overexpression of *Hox*B4 in hematopoietic cells causes the selective expansion of more primitive populations *in vitro* and *in vivo*. *Genes Dev* 1995; **9**: 1753–65.

31 Antonchuk J, Sauvageau G, Humphries RK. *Hox*B4-induced expansion of adult hematopoietic stem cells *ex vivo*. *Cell* 2002; **109**: 39–45.

32 Krumlauf R. *Hox* genes in vertebrate development. *Cell* 1994; **68**: 191–201.

33 Orkin SH, Zon LI. Hematopoiesis and stem cells: plasticity versus developmental heterogeneity. *Nat Immunol* 2002; **3**: 323–8.

34 Georgopoulos K. Haematopoietic cell-fate decisions, chromatin regulation and ikaros. *Nat Rev Immunol* 2002; **2**: 162–74.

35 Hoeijmakers JHJ. Genome maintenance mechanisms for preventing cancer. *Nature* 2001; **411**: 366–74.

36 Blackburn EH. Switching and signaling at the telomere. *Cell* 2001; **106**: 661–73.

37 Sandell LL, Zakian VA. Loss of a yeast telomere: arrest, recovery and chromosome loss. *Cell* 1993; **75**: 729–39.

38 Dernberg AF, Sedat JW, Cande WZ et al. Cytology of telomeres. In: Blackburn EH, Greider CW, eds. *Telomeres*. Cold Spring: Harbor Laboratory Press, 1995: 295–338.

39 Hayflick L, Moorhead PS. The serial cultivation of human diploid strains. *Exp Cell Res* 1961; **25**: 585–621.

40 Hastie ND, Dempster M, Dunlop MG et al. Telomere reduction in human colorectal carcinoma and with ageing. *Nature* 1990; **346**: 866–8.

41 Harley CB, Futcher AB, Greider CW. Telomeres shorten during ageing of human fibroblasts. *Nature* 1990; **345**: 458–60.

42 de Lange T, Shiue L, Myers R et al. Structure and variability of human chromosome ends. *Mol Cell Biol* 1990; **10**: 518–27.

43 Bodnar AG, Ouellette M, Frolkis M et al. Extension of life span by introduction of telomerase into normal human cells. *Science* 1998; **279**: 349–53.

44 Vaziri H, Benchimol S. Reconstitution of telomerase activity in normal human cells leads to elongation of telomeres and extended replicative life span. *Curr Biol* 1998; **8**: 279–82.

45 Mathon NF, Lloyd AC. Cell senescence and cancer. *Nature Rev Cancer* 2001; **1**: 203–13.

46 Watson JD. Origin of concatameric T4 DNA. *Nat New Biol* 1972; **239**: 197–201.

47 Olovnikov AM. A theory of marginotomy. The incomplete copying of template margin in enzymic synthesis of polynucleotides and biological significance of the phenomenon. *J Theor Biol* 1973; **41**: 181–90.

48 Wellinger RJ, Ethier K, Labrecque P et al. Evidence for a new step in telomere maintenance. *Cell* 1996; **85**: 423–33.

49 Makarov VL, Hirose Y, Langmore JP. Long G tails at both ends of human chromosomes suggest a C strand degradation mechanism for telomere shortening. *Cell* 1997; **88**: 657–66.

50 Kruk PA, Rampino NJ, Bohr VA. DNA damage and repair in telomeres: relation to aging. *Proc Natl Acad Sci U S A* 1995; **92**: 258–62.

51 Petersen S, Saretzki G, von Zglinicki T. Preferential accumulation of single-stranded regions in telomeres of human fibroblasts. *Exp Cell Res* 1998; **239**: 152–60.

52 Lansdorp PM. Repair of telomeric DNA prior to replicative senescence. *Mech Ageing Dev* 2000; **118**: 23–34.

53 Wong JMY, Kusdra L, Collins K. Subnuclear shuttling of human telomerase induced by transformation and DNA damage. *Nat Cell Biol* 2002; **4**: 1–6.

54 Collins K, Mitchell JR. Telomerase in the human organism. *Oncogene* 2002; **21**: 564–79.

55 Chiu C-P, Dragowska W, Kim NW et al. Differential expression of telomerase activity in hematopoietic progenitors from adult human bone marrow. *Stem Cells* 1996; **14**: 239–48.

56 Ohyashiki JH, Sashida G, Tauchi T et al. Telomeres and telomerase in hematologic neoplasia. *Oncogene* 2002; **21**: 680–7.

57 Vulliamy T, Marrone A, Goldman F et al. The RNA component of telomerase is mutated in autosomal dominant dyskeratosis congenita. *Nature* 2001; **413**: 432–5.

58 Dokal I. Dyskeratosis congenita. A disease of premature ageing. *Lancet* 2001; **358** (Suppl.): S27.

59 Mitchell JR, Wood E, Collins K. A telomerase component is defective in the human disease dyskeratosis congenita. *Nature* 1999; **402**: 551–5.

60 Blasco MA, Lee H-W, Hande MP et al. Telomere shortening and tumor formation by mouse cells lacking telomerase RNA. *Cell* 1997; **91**: 25–34.

61 Maser RS, DePinho RA. Connecting chromosomes, crisis, and cancer. *Science* 2002; **297**: 565–9.

62 Cooke HJ, Smith BA. Variability at the telomeres of the human X/Y pseudoautosomal region. *Cold Spring Harb Symp Quant Biol* 1986; **51**: 213–9.

63 Allshire RC, Gosden JR, Cross SH et al. Telomeric repeat from T. thermophila cross-hybridizes with human telomeres. *Nature* 1988; **332**: 656–9.

64 Counter CM, Avilion AA, LeFeuvre CE et al. Telomere shortening associated with chromosome instability is arrested in immortal cells which express telomerase activity. *EMBO J* 1992; **11**: 1921–9.

65 Rufer N, Dragowska W, Thornbury G et al. Telomere length dynamics in human lymphocyte subpopulations measured by flow cytometry. *Nat Biotechnol* 1998; **16**: 743–7.

66 Baerlocher GM, Mak J, Tien T et al. Telomere length measurements by fluorescence in situ hybridization and flow cytometry: tips and pitfalls. *Cytometry* 2002; **47**: 89–99.

67 Frenck RW Jr, Blackburn EH, Shannon KM. The rate of telomere sequence loss in human leukocytes varies with age. *Proc Natl Acad Sci U S A* 1998; **95**: 5607–10.

68 Slagboom PE, Droog S, Boomsma DI. Genetic determination of telomere size in humans: a twin study of three age groups. *Am J Hum Genet* 1994; **55**: 876–82.

69 Rufer N, Brummendorf TH, Chapuis B et al. Accelerated telomere shortening in hematological lineages is limited to the first year following stem cell transplantation. *Blood* 2001; **97**: 575–7.

70 Brummendorf TH, Holyoake TL, Rufer N et al. Prognostic implications of differences in telomere length between normal and malignant cells from patients with chronic myeloid leukemia measured by flow cytometry. *Blood* 2000; **95**: 1883–90.

71 Martens UM, Zijlmans JMJM, Poon SSS et al. Short telomeres on human chromosome 17p. *Nat Genet* 1998; **18**: 76–80.

72 de Lange T. Telomere dynamics and genome instability in human cancer. In: Blackburn EH, Greider CW, eds. *Telomeres*. Cold Spring: Harbor Laboratory Press, 1995: 265–93.

73 Awaya N, Baerlocher GM, Manley TJ et al. Telomere shortening in hematopoietic stem cell transplantation: a potential mechanism for late graft failure? *Biol Blood Marrow Transplant* 2002; **8**: 597–600.

74 Sierra J, Storer B, Hansen JA et al. Transplantation of marrow cells from unrelated donors for treatment of high-risk acute leukemia: the effect of leukemic burden, donor HLA-matching, and marrow cell dose. *Blood* 1997; **89**: 4226–35.

Markus G. Manz, Koichi Akashi & Irving L. Weissman

8 Biology of Hematopoietic Stem and Progenitor Cells

Stem cells can be defined as single cells that carry the capacity of both self-renewal and differentiation [1–3]. Hematopoietic stem cells (HSCs) are therefore blood-forming cells that, at the single cell level, can duplicate by self-renewal as well as produce all types of differentiated blood cells [2,4,5]. There are three theoretical and two practical ways to define HSCs.
1 Prospectively isolate single cells that can self-renew and differentiate in a clonal fashion [4–7].
2 Introduce chromosomal markers into cells, and demonstrate that a common and unique chromosomal marker is present in all blood cell lineages as well as the cells that can generate them long-term [2,8].
3 Establish a culture system wherein single cells can self-renew and give rise to all blood cell types.

Unfortunately, these definitions are rarely followed by practitioners of clinical transplantation or scientists studying the biology and plasticity of stem cells. There are many claims that HSCs can turn into stem cells and daughter cells of other tissues, again simply on the basis of bone marrow transplants (some enriched for HSC) [9–18]. It is therefore important from the beginning to use the terminology accurately, as one cannot expect every reader of the scientific and clinical literature to discern that unpurified rather than rigorously purified stem cells were used in the clinical and/or scientific investigations, which results in misconceptions and mistakes.

The principal property that distinguishes stem cells from progenitor cells is their ability to undergo limitless or limited self-renewal [1,5,19–22]. In essence, self-renewal means that the cells can divide without undergoing discernible differentiation, and that they possess properties that allow large numbers of self-renewing cell divisions to occur over the lifespan of a host in a regulated fashion. Poorly regulated or unregulated self-renewal is a property that all cancers have, and we call those cells within a cancer that have self-renewal capacity cancer stem cells [23]. Therefore it is important for the reader to keep in mind that the major distinguishing property of normal and neoplastic stem cells is their capability of self-renewal, and therefore it becomes important to understand whether the genetic expression pathways that lead to self-renewal are novel in normal HSCs, or might be shared between different classes of tissue-specific multipotent stem cells, and might be acquired by cancer cell progenitors as they emerge as cancer stem cells [23].

A word on nomenclature. Although the founders of this field—Till, McCulloch and their colleagues—called their first candidate stem cell a pluripotent stem cell [24–27], recent revisions in the nomenclature now distinguish stem cell hierarchies. *Totipotent stem cells* are single cells that can give rise to every tissue of the embryo, the extraembryonic tissues and the developing adult; so far, only the zygote has that property [28,29]. *Pluripotent stem cells* are cells that can give rise to stem and progenitor cells of all tissues, but lack the capacity to give rise to extraembryonic tissues; cells of the inner cell mass of the blastocyst stage of embryogenesis (the latest preimplantation step) appear to be pluripotent, and successful culture of these cells results in pluripotent embryonic stem (ES) cell lines [28–30]. At the time of writing, there are two published reports of identification of pluripotent stem cells in the adult [13,31; see below]. *Multipotent stem cells* are single cells, like the HSC, that can self-renew and differentiate into more than one cell type in a particular tissue lineage: HSC, central nervous system (CNS) stem cells, peripheral nervous system stem cells and perhaps liver stem cells, epidermal/hair follicle stem cells and muscle stem cells are leading examples of purified and enriched populations of these multipotent stem cell types [1,19,32–38]. *Unipotent stem cells* exist in each germline, where self-renewal and differentiation leads only to one or another type of gamete; but there exists in every chordate embryo/fetus a class of germline stem cells that are bipotent prior to colonization of the genital ridges, taking their unipotent specificity from the sex of the genital ridge in which they make their unipotent commitment. In this terminology there can also be multipotent, oligopotent and unipotent progenitor cells, which are differentiated from stem cells by their failure to undergo extended self-renewal.

History of HSC isolation

Following the demonstration that just lethal doses of whole body irradiation caused death by hematopoietic failure, and that hematopoietic failure could be averted either by shielding hematopoietic organs or by transplantation of unirradiated bone marrow [39–41], the critical study that set the stage for the concept of HSC was the demonstration that the injected bone marrow reconstituted the hematopoietic system rather than provided radiation repair factors [42–44]. In our view, the seminal study in the HSC field began with the observation by Till and McCulloch that transplantation of limiting numbers of bone marrow cells into just lethally irradiated mice gave rise to colonies of the spleen that contained all elements of the myeloerythroid (but not lymphoid) lineages and that the number of colonies was proportional to the number of bone marrow cells injected [24].

Two experiments followed these observations that opened the field to stem cell biology and changed the thinking of the hematology community: first, preirradiation of the marrow donor at doses that would allow the survival of some cells that had random chromosome translocations or inversions resulted in the finding that each spleen colony was the product of a clonogenic precursor [2]; and, second, at least some of these colonies contained cells that also contained spleen colony-forming cells, as well as cells that could be radioprotective [2,26,45]. Later, it was shown that the daughter cells of some of these spleen colony-forming cells included

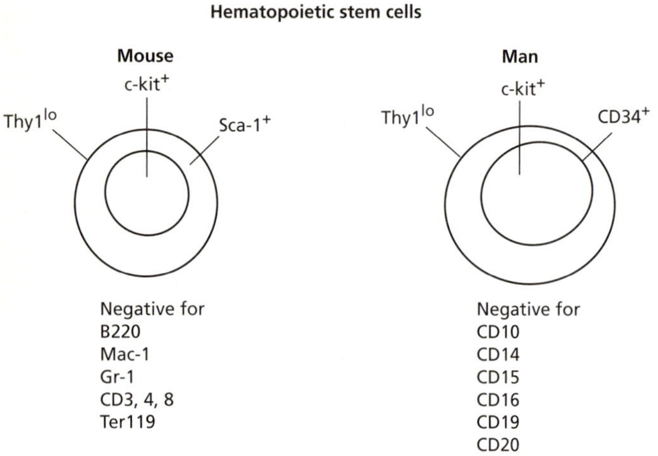

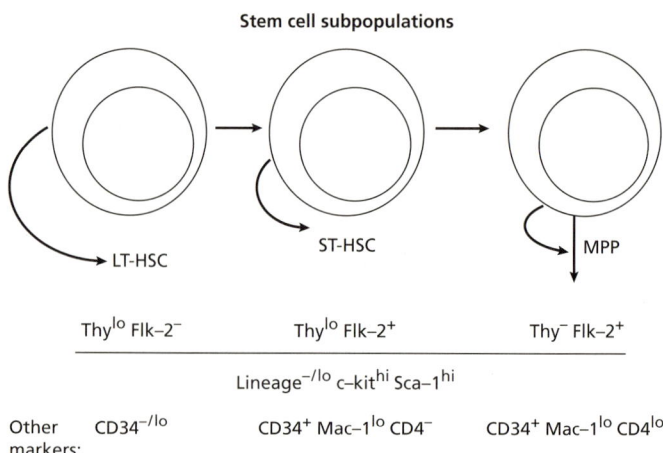

Fig. 8.1 Clonogenic multipotent progenitors have a distinctive marker profile. Shown are surface phenotypes of hematopoietic stem cells (HSCs) in human and mouse.

Fig. 8.2 Flk-2 and Thy-1.1 delineate a pathway of hematopoietic stem cell (HSC) differentiation. Surface expression of Flk-2 is upregulated and Thy-1.1 is downregulated as HSC self-renewal capacity diminishes. LT-HSC, long-term hematopoietic stem cells; MPP, multipotent progenitors; ST, short-term. (Courtesy of Julie Christensen PhD, Department of Pathology, Stanford University School of Medicine, Stanford CA94305.)

lymphocytes [27]. From these experiments it was clear that there had to exist in the bone marrow single cells capable of self-renewal and full differentiation to hematopoietic fates. It was subsequently demonstrated that at least two classes of spleen colony-forming cells existed: those that peaked at days 8–10 and were the progeny, mainly, of nonstem cell oligopotent progenitors; and those that peaked in size at days 12–14, which were believed to include much more primitive progenitors and stem cells [46,47]. Recently, following the isolation of both stem and progenitor cells it is clear that most of the day 8–10 spleen colonies are derived from committed myeloid progenitors [48; see below], whereas the day 12–14 colonies are derived from hematopoietic stem cells, multipotent but self-renewing progenitors, and some left-over committed myeloid progenitors [48–52; see below]. Nevertheless, the impact of these elegant studies by the Till, McCulloch, Becker, Wu and Siminovitch group established the field of hematopoietic stem and progenitor cell biology by *in vivo* assessment and first introduced genetic marking to show the unequivocal existence of HSCs [2]. These important experiments were carried out mainly in the 1960s, before the discovery of monoclonal antibodies [53] or the development of high-speed multiparameter fluorescence activated cell sorters [54]. The eventual isolation of HSCs required not only these innovations, but also the development of *in vitro* and *in vivo* assays for the identification and quantification of clonogenic precursors of T-cell lineage [55], B-cell lineage [56] and myeloerythroid lineages [57–60]. While many important enrichments of these precursors were accomplished using cell sorting with monoclonal antibodies [61], it was not until a simultaneous analysis of all lineages was coupled with quantitative reconstitution of irradiated mice by limiting numbers of candidate HSCs that one could show that HSCs could be prospectively isolated rather than retrospectively inferred by chromosome marking [50,52,56].

As shown in Fig. 8.1, we have isolated both mouse and human HSCs, and they share the properties of being Thy-1$^+$ and lineage marker negative (Lin$^-$); both express c-*kit*, albeit mouse at higher levels than human, and mice in addition express the Sca-1 (stem cells antigen 1) marker [50,52,62,63]. We have isolated human HSCs that are of the phenotype CD34$^+$Thy-1$^+$Lin$^-$ [64,65]. The human HSC were enriched for all clonogenic assays (T, B and myeloid), and were efficient at restoration of the human hematolymphoid organs in SCID-hu mice [64]. Mouse long-term (LT) HSC are totally lineage negative and, in addition, do not express surface Flk2/Flt3, the receptor for the Flt3 ligand [66,67], whereas just downstream of the mouse LT-HSC are successive stages of multipotent progenitors that increasingly lose self-renewal capacity; their surface phenotypes are shown in Fig. 8.2 [50,66,67]. Human LT-HSC are, in addition, CD38 negative to low, but the full surface marker arrays of human short-term (ST) HSC and multipotent progenitors (MPP) are not yet fully worked out [64,68–72]. In both species, a search for other HSCs in the hematopoietic tissues was carried out: in mice the Sca-1$^-$, Lin$^+$, c-*kit*$^-$,Thy-1$^-$ or Thy-1^{hi} subsets did not, in the context of bone marrow transplantation, contain any long-term multilineage hematopoietic potential [63]. In the human, CD34$^-$, Lin$^+$ or Thy-1$^-$ cells also do not contain any *in vitro* or *in vivo* long-term multilineage hematopoietic precursor potential [64,65,71,73] although some groups believe CD34$^-$CD38$^-$ human HSC exist [74–76]. In mice transplantation of limit dilution or single LT-HSC results reproducibly in a high frequency of hosts (5–40%) showing long-term multilineage reconstitution, with self-renewal of HSC, including its expansion to full normal levels, for the life of the host [4–7,77]. The bone marrow of allogeneic human HSC transplants contains self-renewed HSC that also work in serial transplantation in SCID-hu mice [64]. Thus, in both mouse and human, HSC that self-renew as well as differentiate to all blood cell lineages can be prospectively isolated as single clonogenic precursors.

Properties of mouse hematopoietic stem cells and other multipotent progenitors

Using the markers shown in Fig. 8.2, we have shown that transplantation of single or limit dilution or small numbers of LT-HSC results in both HSC expansion and lifelong self-renewal, through at least four or five serial transplant generations [77]. Transplantation of either ST-HSC or MPP results in transient expansion (or self-renewal) of those cell populations, with robust transient multilineage reconstitution after which residual host HSC recover [6,50,67]. These cells have ended their productive lifespan rather than enter quiescence [50]. It is important to point out that no matter how many ST-HSCs or MPPs are transplanted, at no time is there any measurable differentiation from the short-term cells into the long-term pool [51].

In the normal steady state about 8% of LT-HSCs randomly enter cell cycle each day, whereas higher percentages of ST-HSC and MPP are in cell cycle at any time [78]. Interestingly, when steady-state bone marrow LT-HSCs are isolated according to their position in the cell cycle, 2N vs.

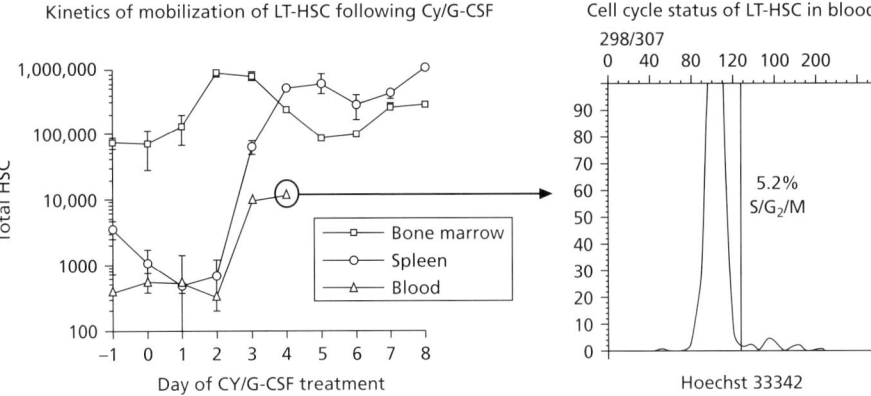

Fig. 8.3 The total number of long-term hematopoietic stem cells (LT-HSCs) in the bone marrow, spleen and blood of mice on successive days of CY/G-CSF treatment. Total bone marrow hematopoietic stem cells (HSCs) were calculated by assuming that the femurs and tibias (less the epiphyses) contained 15% of all bone marrow in the mouse. Total HSC in the blood was calculated by assuming that the total blood volume was 1.8 mL. Cell cycle status of LT-HSC in blood was determined by Hoechst DNA stain. (From [81] with permission.)

greater than 2N cellular DNA content, the 2N class of cells is highly efficient, at both limit dilution and at higher numbers of cells, at providing radioprotection and long-term multilineage reconstitution, whereas the dividing subsets (>2N DNA content) are less efficient at reconstitution, and are similarly less efficient at homing directly to the bone marrow rather than the spleen or liver [79,80]. Following transplantation, a much higher fraction of LT-HSCs remain in cell cycle in the radioprotected host, and this period can extend at least 4–5 months after transplantation [51,77–79]. Given the poor transplantability of cycling HSCs, it is conceivable that protocols that test the "stemness", of stem cell transplants by serial transplantation could be affected by this artefact, and that a much higher proportion of reconstituted HSCs remain in cycle because of the lingering effects of radiation and reconstitution [77–79]. Therefore, experiments that are designed to measure the lifespan of expanding and self-renewing HSCs by transplantation should be carried out in ways that remove the induced cell cycle phenomenon from consideration.

Although in the steady state only a small fraction of LT-HSCs are in cell cycle, this ratio can be dramatically altered by a number of circumstances. For example, upon transplantation into irradiated hosts probably every HSC that lands in a hematopoietic microenvironment undergoes, at least initially, symmetrical self-renewing cell divisions to expand the HSC pool. In addition, the techniques used to mobilize HSCs into the bloodstream usually operate by first causing all HSCs to enter the cell cycle nonrandomly [80–82]. As shown in Fig. 8.3, treatment of a mouse with cyclophosphamide (CY) (which should kill no more than 4–8% of LT-HSC, but should have a dramatic effect on both multipotent progenitors and oligolineage progenitors [see below] because they are largely in cell cycle), followed by granulocyte-colony stimulating factor (G-CSF) treatment, results in every HSC entering cell cycle leading to an increase in the steady state number of LT-HSC about 12- to 15-fold [81]. Even bleeding of mice, up to 25% or 50% of their blood volume two or three times in a week, results in a measurable increase in the fraction of HSC in the cell cycle (S. Cheshier & I.L. Weissman, unpublished data). It is of interest that only rare HSCs express the message for either the G-CSF receptor or the erythropoietin receptor [21,83], and therefore the effects of G-CSF or erythropoietin on the entry of HSCs into the cell cycle are likely to be indirect rather than direct. As shown in Fig. 8.3, expanding HSC numbers reach a steady state at a 12- to 15-fold increase, indicating that positive and negative feedbacks on the regulation of HSC cell division must exist, but at the time of writing their nature and mechanisms are unknown.

HSCs must go through many self-renewing cell divisions over the life of an animal, and it is reasonable to wonder if they are susceptible to a natural limit on the number of cell divisions they can undergo, often called the "Hayflick limit" [84] and whether HSC have a special mechanism for maintaining the ends of their chromosomes, called telomeres,

to avoid programmed cell senescence resulting from critical telomere shortening events [85,86; see also Chapter 7]. This issue is complex. Mouse LT-HSCs exhibit very high levels of telomerase activity, rivaling that of the immortalized human cell line 293 [87], but in both mouse and human, telomere length declines in the progeny of HSCs that have undergone a large number of cell divisions, usually in response to radiation and transplant recovery [77,88]. Therefore, the high telomerase activity in HSCs [87] is not sufficient to prevent at least some telomere shortening through several cell division cycles. In the absence of a functional telomerase-reverse transcriptase (TERT) component, the progeny of dividing HSCs lose telomeres much more rapidly, confirming that the telomerase in normal HSCs is functioning to maintain telomere length [22,77].

However, transgenic mouse strains that overexpress the TERT component of the telomerase complex at high levels in HSC do not reduce the length of their telomeres, even following successive induced cell cycles by transplantation. Nevertheless, these HSCs still lose transplantation activity after the fourth or fifth serial HSC transplant generation [22]. This *loss* of transplantability with HSCs that retain telomeres points to other phenomena limiting the transplantation of these cells, including perhaps the persistent entry into cell cycle, programmed cell lifespans independent of telomere length, or random factors associated with transplantation and/or cell division [51,77,89].

Programmed cell death or senescence of HSCs need not occur only as a result of extensive numbers of HSC cell divisions. There are several genetic loci that regulate, in mice, both the frequency of HSC and the frequency of HSC that are in cell cycle [90,91]. These loci can be mapped to several distinct chromosomes, but to date none of the genes on those chromosomes involved in regulating HSC frequencies have been isolated or characterized. One genetic program that likely regulates HSC numbers is that leading to programmed cell death inhibitable by the antiapoptotic protein BCL2 (and by extension, its antiaptoptotic gene relatives such as BCL-x). In mice that have enforced high level expression of hBCL2 in HSC, the steady-state levels of HSCs are increased four- to fivefold, and the competitive repopulation activity of these HSCs, cotransplanted with CD45 congenic HSCs into the same irradiated host, is high [92,93]. Therefore, it is likely that programmed cell death is one regulator of HSC numbers, and it is yet to be determined what stimuli to HSCs enact the programmed death pathway inhibitable by BCL2.

There are several genes whose expression is required to initiate hematopoiesis, hematopoiesis and angiogenesis, or angiogenesis resulting in failed hematopoiesis; these include *AML-1* (also known as *RUNX-1* [94], *SCL1-TAL* [95], *FLK1* [96,97]. It is unclear whether these genes act directly within HSCs, within their immediate precursors to generate HSCs, or if they act on other cell populations that have a role in the survival or stimulation of HSCs, or, as in the case of a developing vasculature, if they regulate the movement of HSCs or their precursors from one part of the body to another [98]. Reverse transcriptive unilateral polymerase chain reaction (RT-PCR) analysis of highly purified HSCs, or the use of highly purified HSC mRNA probes to interrogate extensive mouse cDNA libraries has revealed that at least some of these genes are expressed intrinsically in HSCs [99–101]. It is important to point out that many factors could be playing a part in the movement of pre-HSCs or HSCs during the embryonic and fetal stages of development, and factors affecting the release of cells from a particular microenvironment, their movement through tissues or the bloodstream, the recognition of endothelium in tissues, and their homing to stem cell niches could easily be read out as genes affecting HSCs without directly affecting either their development or their self-renewal capacity (see below).

Genetic pathways for the self-renewal of HSCs

Self-renewal is the single distinguishing characteristic between LT-HSCs and the rest of the multipotent and oligopotent progenitors in the hematopoietic system (see Chapter 7). While LT-HSCs can be expanded in a variety of situations *in vivo*, the attempt to expand rigorously purified mouse or human HSCs *in vitro* with conventional cytokines such as steel factor (SLF), thrombopoietin (TPO), interleukin 11 (IL-11), IL-6, IL-3 and Flt3L, alone or in combination in serum-containing medium has never resulted in more than a minor expansion in HSCs by phenotype, and little or no expansion by function [102–108]. Many investigators were led astray by the expansion of cells expressing CD34 markers, but a broad variety of non-HSCs are also CD34 positive, and these cells were the result of proliferation of HSCs and progenitors coupled with cell differentiation. The introduction of the antiapoptosis protein BCL2 into HSCs in mice allowed HSCs to survive serum-free culture conditions, and so the response of LT-HSCs to factors in the absence of serum —which clearly contains differentiating factors, such as monocyte/macrophage-colony stimulating factor (M-CSF), G-CSF, granulocyte monocyte-colony stimulating factor (GM-CSF) and others could be studied [92,93]. Any combination of these cytokines and others when added to these BCL2 containing HSC led to a massive burst of proliferation and progenitor expansion by most HSCs, but no detectable HSC self-renewal [92,93]. These HSCs could respond to three factors as single factors *in vitro*: SLF, IL-3 and TPO [93]. HSCs responding to IL-3 give large bursts of proliferation with concomitant maturation along the myeloid and mast cell lineages, without self-renewal of HSCs. Stimulation with TPO led to mild proliferation, and dedicated differentiation along the megakaryocytic lineage; interestingly, RT-PCR analysis of mRNA from HSCs and highly purified myeloid progenitors revealed that HSCs might have the highest expression of the TPO receptor c-mpl, of any of these cell populations [21,83,109]. One might have hoped that the HSC response to SLF alone might have been self-renewing divisions, as mutations in the *SLF* gene lead to the mouse Sl phenotype [110–113], and mutation in its receptor, *c-kit*, lead to the W phenotype [114,115]. Both of these mutations cause fetal or early neonatal lethality, usually because of profound anemia. However, the response of single highly purified LT-HSC to SLF in serum-free medium was proliferation without detectable self-renewal, but with maturation through both common lymphoid and common myeloid progenitor pathways [93; see below]. Some early experiments indicated that other factors might be involved in HSC expansion; e.g. activation of the Notch-1 receptor mimicked by retroviral transduction with the intracellular activated form of Notch-1, occasionally led to the generation of mouse cell lines with many of the characteristics of HSCs, although this response was neither general nor robust [116,117]. Provision of *Hox*B4 as a retroviral insert to semipurified mouse hematopoietic progenitors led to vigorous proliferation and at least some retention of hematopoietic multilineage and long-term reconstituting activity *in vitro* and *in vivo* [118,119], although rigorous demonstration that this

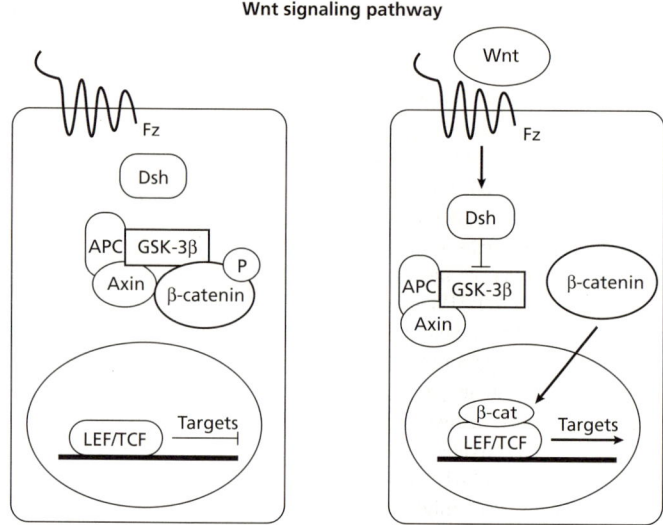

Fig. 8.4 The Wnt signaling pathway. On the left is a cell that has not received a Wnt signal. The axin-APC-GSK3β complex holds β-catenin in the complex, phosphorylates its N-terminal serines, and prepares it for proteolysis. The lef/tcf proteins bind their DNA motifs and repress transcription. On the right, Wnt binds the Fzd ectodomain, activating the cytoplasmic Dsh protein. The activated Dsh inhibits GSK3β phosphorylation of β-catenin, which builds up in the cytoplasm as bound and free forms. The free form can translocate to the nucleus where it complexes to lef/tcf elements, activating transcription. (Courtesy of Tannishtha Reya, Department of Pharmacology and Cancer Biology, Duke University Medical Center, Durham, NC.)

outcome was caused by expansion of HSCs alone, rather than provision of other signals that in addition enable their engraftment has not yet been established [119–121]. The addition of semipurified members of the Wnt family to enriched CD34+ cells led to vigorous proliferation and expansion of CD34+ cells, but again this was not carried out in a way that allows the conclusion that HSC expansion had occurred [122].

Highly purified LT-HSCs, however, contain transcripts of the LEF/TCF family of transcription factors (K. Li, I.L. Weissman & S. Cheshier, unpublished data). Lef and TCF are DNA binding and bending proteins that, alone, are gene repressors, but when they are associated with nuclear β-catenin proteins, form a transcriptionally active complex for those genes that have Lef/TCF DNA binding sites [reviewed in 23]. Lef is a nonredundant critical factor for early B-lineage cells, and at least part of its action is through provision of antiapoptotic stimuli to cells in the pro- and pre-B lineage [23]. The activation of LEF/TCF proteins by β-catenin results from signaling through the Wnt/Fzd/Dsh/GSK-3β/β-catenin pathway (Fig. 8.4). As shown in Fig. 8.4, Wnt, a highly hydrophobic protein binds to surface frizzled (Fzd), a 7TM protein, in combination with a low-density lipoprotein associated receptor, usually LRP 5 [23]. Binding of Wnt to Fzd leads to activation of disheveled (Dsh), which acts on a multimolecular cytoplasmic complex of adenomatous polyposis colon (APC), axin, GSK-3β and associated β-catenin (Fig. 8.4). The action of Dsh on this complex is to prevent GSK-3β phosphorylation of N-terminal residues on β-catenin, and also allows β-catenin to dissociate from the complex [23]. GSK-3β phosphorylated β-catenin is targeted for ubiquitination and proteosomal digestion [23]. Unphosphorylated free β-catenin appears to build up, and some may translocate to the nucleus where it becomes available for binding to Lef/TCF factors and activation of transcription.

The addition of partially or fully purified Wnt3A to highly purified LT-HSCs in serum-free medium, with or without SLF, results in clonal and massive proliferation of HSCs. *In vitro*, these HSCs go through at least a 300-fold expansion and up to 50% of the expanded progeny are cells of the LT-HSC phenotype [123,124]. The expanded cells of the LT-HSC phenotype, on a cell per cell basis, are functional HSCs as assayed by transplantation *in vivo* [123,124]. Transfection of β-catenin forms lacking the N-terminal phosphorylation sites similarly drives LT-HSC into massive and prolonged expanding cell divisions, and 300- to 3000-fold expansions of LT-HSCs both by phenotype and by function upon transplantation have been recorded [124]. Inhibitors of Wnt signaling even blocked SLF and other cytokine-mediated proliferation of LT-HSCs [124]. When LT-HSCs are transfected with a reporter of LEF/TCF + β-catenin activity in the nucleus and then transplanted into lethally irradiated hosts, LT-HSCs reading out the reporter are retained *in vivo* long term, whereas myeloid progenitors derived from these LT-HSCs do not express the reporter [124]. Taken together, these results indicate that the Wnt/Fzd/β-catenin pathway is likely to be an important pathway, and perhaps the only pathway utilized by LT-HSCs in self-renewing cell division. When activated by Wnt 3A, LT-HSCs upregulate expression of both Notch-1 and *Hox*B4 and so these and other genes implicated in the self-renewal of HSCs might make up a complex pathway.

The *bmi-1* gene is a member of the polycomb family, which have a role in silencing gene expression by site-specific deacetylation of histones associated with those genes [125]. *Bmi-1* is expressed in high levels in mouse and human LT-HSC, and mice made mutant for the *BMI-1* gene have a profound defect in the transplantation and self-renewal of LT-HSCs [99,125]. The two transcripts of the p16 locus, P16INK4A and P19ARF, are overexpressed selectively in the hematopoietic tissues in the *Bmi*-mutant mice, thus implicating a role of *Bmi-1* in downregulation of genes whose expression is contrary to self-renewal of hematopoietic stem cells [126]. These could include decreased viability, enforced differentiation or direct regulation or inhibition of genes involved in the self-renewing pathways such as those of the Wnt/Fzd/β-catenin and Notch pathways [23,116,117,124]. *Bmi-1* mutants do not show differences in expression in either *Hox*A9 or *Hox*B4, genes that also have some role in HSC functions (M. Clarke, *et al*. unpublished data).

Migration of hematopoietic stem cells

Hematopoietic capacity is known to be present in the adult mouse at highest levels in bone marrow, at about one-tenth that level in spleen, and at 1/100 the level of bone marrow or less in blood [127]. In those early experiments, the ability of marrow transplants or of tissue transplants to retain erythropoiesis could not be assigned directly to actions of HSCs. There was no clear explanation as to why hematopoietic activity might be present in organs other than the bone marrow, and certainly not in the blood. It was only when clinical hematopoietic cell transplantation groups described the phenomenon of hematopoietic activity increasing in the blood of cytotoxic drug-treated individuals that the possibility of HSC mobilization into the blood was considered [128]. Empirical protocols using CY plus cytokines such as G-CSF, GM-CSF, SLF alone or in combination with G-CSF, IL-1, IL-3, and various combinations of the above led to efficient mechanisms to mobilize hematopoietic cells into the bloodstream [129–133]. While at the early stages, this activity was measured in terms of *in vitro* tests for hematopoietic colony-forming cells (CFCs), CFC assays alone are not specific for HSC vs. oligolineage progenitor activities [48,64]. However, there could be no doubt that HSCs were involved when mobilized peripheral blood (MPB) transplants were used in myeloablated hosts, resulting in both early and sustained hematopoiesis. When CY and G-CSF are used in the mouse model, wherein one can analyze directly the daily changes in marrow, spleen and blood, it is clear that nearly every HSC and MPP enters cell cycle rapidly [81]. These reach a steady state in the marrow, at which time the cells appear rapidly in blood and spleen [81]. At all times the HSCs appearing in the blood have 2N amount of DNA, indicating that they are not pro-

liferating in the blood; in fact the fold increase in their numbers would have ruled out a blood-only expansion of the HSC pool [81,82]. Bromodeoxyuridine (BrdU) labeling of mice during the expansion phase of HSC in the "mobilized" bone marrow results in virtually every HSC incorporating this nucleoside into their chromosomal DNA and, interestingly, just 1 or 2 days later the 2N HSCs found in the blood are all labeled with BrdU (Fig. 8.3) [81,82]. Thus, mobilization appears to result as a consequence of marrow HSC proliferation, and accumulation of emigrant HSCs in extramedullary sites such as spleen, liver and blood [81,82]. The proliferation that precedes mobilization has been described above, and it is notable that the cytokines (e.g. G-CSF) that show high efficiency in the mobilization process do not have receptors on native HSCs [21,83,101]. In the early phases of mobilization there is a rise in cells of the myelomonocytic series, and it has been shown that the elaboration locally by myeloid cells of matrix metalloproteinases such as MMP9 can serve to cleave cell–cell interaction molecules known to be active between HSCs and marrow stroma [134]. Similarly, elaboration of the chemokine IL-8 occurs, and infusion of IL-8 alone can cause a significant and rapid mobilization of HSCs [135,136]. The actual nature of molecules involved in HSC release is not clear, although it is known that HSCs express integrin $\alpha_4\beta_1$ that allows them to attach to hematopoietic stromal cell VCAM-1 [137–141]. Also, HSCs express the c-*kit* receptor that allow HSCs to bind to, at least, cell surface SLF on stroma. Although HSCs have a number of other members of the adhesion and integrin family members, the role of each of these in cell proliferation, detachment from stroma, local emigration into sinusoids, movement through the bloodstream, margination on distant blood vessels, transendothelial migration at these vessel sites, and localization to microniches that support LT-HSC are still unclear. In the adult mouse, homing of infused HSCs appears to involve both cell surface integrin $\alpha_4\beta_1$ and cell surface CXCR4, a receptor for the chemokine SDF-1 [142–144]. Of all known chemokines, adult mouse HSCs migrate *in vitro* only in response to SDF-1, and this is chemotactic movement [144]. It is of historical interest that fibroblasts or epithelial cells adhering to culture dishes could be synchronized by their stage of the cell cycle by shaking the dishes; only cells in the M phase of mitosis had released their attachment sites to the dish and could be detached easily. It is conceivable that the intracellular fluid dynamics might be sufficient to sweep away unbound HSCs at the M phase of cell division, as it is clear from the previous findings that mobilized HSCs found in the bloodstream must have been nonrandomly released into the blood just after M phase [82]. However released, coinfusion of labeled HSCs and labeled red blood cells (RBCs) from mobilized blood into the blood of same stage mobilized animals results in the rapid emigration of HSCs out of the blood, with retention of RBCs in the vessels [82]. In fact, most HSCs are gone by 1 min, and do not reappear in the bloodstream within the next several hours. These HSCs nonrandomly home to hematopoietic sites in immobilized animals: bone marrow, spleen and liver (Fig. 8.5). This observation fits with previous studies on the rapid egress of infused lymphocytes out of the bloodstream into tissues via recognition of particular vascular addressins for which they have cognate homing receptors [145,146]; and the rapid egress from the bloodstream of other nucleated cells such as monocytes [147]. There are similar HSC, MPP and myeloid progenitor fluxes in normal mice. To maintain the approximate 100 HSCs found in the blood of mice, given a residence time in the blood of 5 min or less would require fluxes of well over tens of thousands of HSCs and MPPs per day. It is not yet clear whether these cells are passing through the blood in one pass or if they form a specialized pool of HSCs and MPPs that marginate for more than a few hours, yet have a higher probability of reentering the blood than cells resident in deep marrow niches. If HSCs found in the blood are also derived from dividing HSCs, nearly one out of every two daughter cells from a self-renewing HSC division would have to enter the bloodstream.

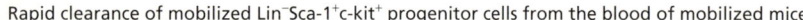

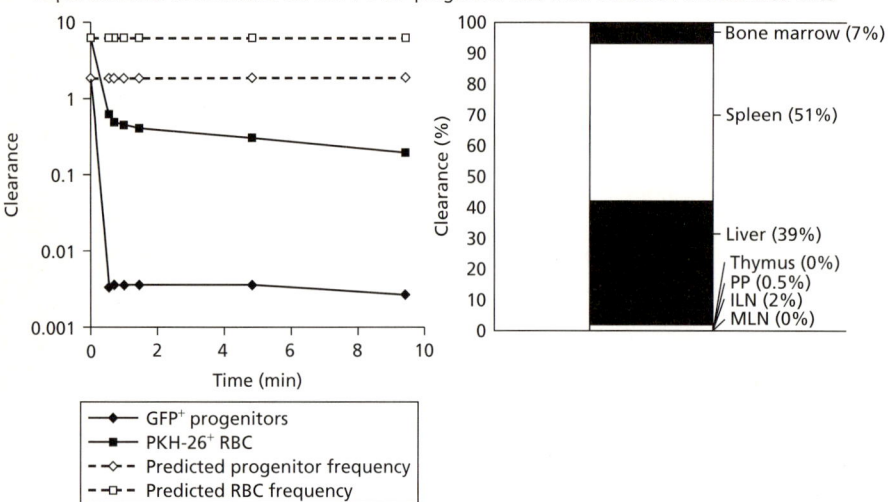

Fig. 8.5 Rapid clearance of mobilized hematopoietic progenitor cells from the bloodstream. Clearance from the blood of eGFP+ progenitors and PKH-26+ red blood cells (RBC), and predicted progenitor and RBC frequencies, respectively. *In vivo* homing to different organs of mobilized and consecutively transplanted hematopoietic progenitor and stem cells 3 h after injection. (From [80] with permission.)

This interpretation of the fate of recently self-renewed HSCs calls for a deeper examination of hematopoietic niches in the marrow; niches that commit recently entering HSCs into the myeloid or lymphoid pathways need not be adjacent to the HSC niche if the daughter cells of HSCs are constantly migrating. This finding also has potential significance when one considers claims of plasticity of stem cells in one or more tissues [5]. While this topic will be covered in greater depth in a later section of this chapter, if tens of thousands of HSCs are fluxing through tissues every day, finding HSC activity in those tissues might only result from these itinerant HSCs, rather than transdifferentiation of local tissue-specific stem cells into hematopoietic fates [5].

Ontogeny and aging of hematopoietic stem cells

It is tacitly assumed that HSCs derive from the embryonic mesoderm. In mammals, the first site of definable blood cells appears to be the yolk sac blood islands, in mice at about E7.5 [148,149]. (Although the terminology used for development from the time of conception is E 1–21 [for mouse], in fact the transition from the embryo to fetus, at organogenesis, is about 8–9 days postconception [dpc], and so hereafter we use the dpc abbreviation.) At that time mouse yolk sacs contain cells capable of responding *in vitro* to produce hematopoietic CFC [148,149]. The yolk sac connects to the developing embryo/fetus [150,151] about a day later via the development of the umbilical vein, which feeds into the developing fetal liver. At very nearly that dpc8–E8.5 time interval, hematopoietic cells appear in and around the dorsal aorta of the developing fetus [reviewed in 152]. Transplantation of dpc8–9 yolk sac blood island cells into the yolk sac cavity of dpc8 allogeneic hosts results in mice that have lifelong presence of donor-derived day 10 CFU-S in marrow as well as thymocytes [98]. At about dpc10–11 hematopoiesis begins in the fetal liver in the mouse, and continues there throughout fetal life (Fig. 8.6a).

Where do the first HSC develop? At dpc3.5 the blastocyst implants into the uterus, and its inner cell mass appears to be a population of pluripotent cells without defined commitments [150,151]. Between dpc3.5 and dpc5.5, gastrulation occurs with the formation of the three germ layers [150,151]. It is still a mystery whether the developing postgastrulation mesoderm cells emigrate separately to yolk sac and embryo to give rise to independent origins of hematopoiesis; or if only one of these sites is the initial site of commitment to hematopoiesis, the later appearance of hematopoiesis at the other site resulting from migration [98,152–154]. One reason that seemed to indicate separate origins for extraembryonic (yolk sac) hematopoiesis and intraembryonic hematopoiesis was the fact that yolk sac erythropoiesis resulted in the production of embryonic and fetal hemoglobins, while lifelong hematopoiesis resulted in the production of mainly adult hemoglobin [153,155]. These were called, respectively, primitive and definitive hematopoiesis [155]. However, there has been no direct experiment that assessed the origin of these two kinds of hematopoiesis at the clonal cellular level, and so there is still much to be done to clarify these cell lineages. There is obviously a close association of hematopoiesis and angiogenesis in both the developing blood islands and the developing dorsal aorta, and there is good evidence that mutant mice lacking the cell surface receptors for angiogenic peptides fail to develop either hematopoietic or angiogenic cells [96,156].

While these experiments are largely taken to indicate that a bipotent stem cell for both lineages called the hemangioblasts exists that can give rise to both angiogenic stem cells and HSCs, prospective isolation of *in vivo* hemangioblasts has not yet been shown rigorously. It is possible that mutant mice that cannot make blood vessels properly, cannot make blood because primitive stem cells travel via the blood, or that blood vessels make factors important for hematopoiesis. There is an interesting point coming out of embryonic stem cell biology that might be relevant to these issues. ES cells are derived from the inner cell mass of blastocysts, and likely represent pluripotent stem cells at approximately dpc3.5 age. They are maintained as pluripotent cells by the addition of LIF (leukemia inhibitory factor) to their cultures, at least in mouse ES lines [157]. Removal of LIF from these pluripotent ES lines results in the onset of hematopoiesis and during this development, at about 4 days, cells capable of *in vitro* hematopoiesis emerge, which express some markers shared with HSCs (J. Domen & I. Weissman, unpublished data). This interval, 3.5 + 4.0 days, correlates in developmental time to about dpc7.5, when HSC first appear in yolk sac blood islands [98,158]. Thus, these two systems appear in parallel to produce embryonic HSCs.

The next stage of hematopoiesis beyond the embryonic stage is the fetal stage and the first site of fetal hematopoiesis appears to be the fetal liver [149]. The numbers of HSCs increase logarithmically from dpc11 to E15 within the fetal liver, but even though hematopoiesis keeps expanding in the liver, fetal liver HSC numbers level off after dpc15 [62,159,160]. At dpc16 hematopoiesis appears in the fetal spleen in mice, and at dpc18 in the fetal bone marrow.

The initiation of fetal liver hematopoiesis is blocked in mice with mutations in integrin $\alpha_4\beta_1$ (VLA-4) or integrin $\alpha_5\beta_1$ (VLA-5) [161,162].

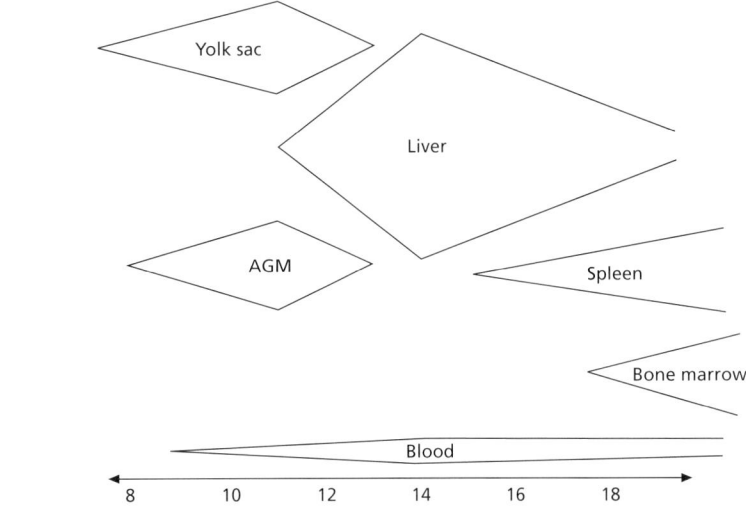

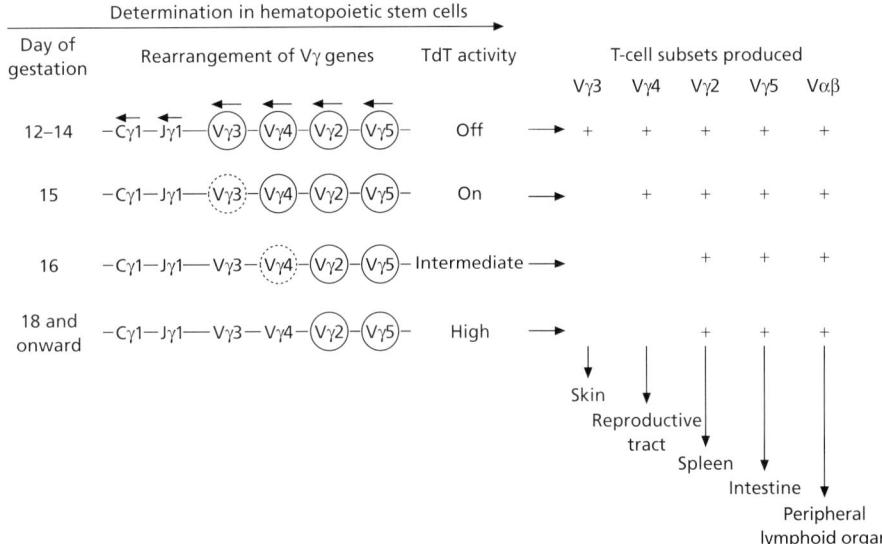

Fig. 8.6 (a) The ontogeny of hematopoietic progenitors. The sites of hematopoiesis in the fetus and neonate are shown. (Courtesy of Julie Christensen PhD, Department of Pathology, Stamford University School of Medicine, Stanford CA94305, and Sean Morrison, PhD, Department of Internal Medicine and Department of Cell and Developmental Biology, University of Michigan.) (b) A model of chromosomal determinative events at the level of hematopoietic stem cells that concern T-cell development. Determination of T-cell receptor gene rearrangement and N-nucleotide insertion at the level of hematopoietic stem cells is shown. Circles indicate Vγ genes open to V-J rearrangement. Broken circles indicate Vγ genes undergoing chromosomal closure to the recombination machinery. Vγ genes without circles represent closed loci which are not accessible for the recombination machinery. The outcome of T-cell development and distribution is shown on the right. (From [380] with permission.)

Because integrins are involved in cell migration, it is reasonable to propose that immigration of these cells into the fetal liver might require steps that include expression of $\alpha_4\beta_1$, or induce the expression of integrin $\alpha_5\beta_1$ at this stage of the liver. Integrin $\alpha_4\beta_1$ is used by trafficking HSCs throughout life to enter sites of hematopoiesis [141], and so the endowment of expression of integrin $\alpha_4\beta_1$ permits fetal liver HSCs to be assayed by transplantation in fetuses or adults. It is important to note that neither yolk sac blood island HSCs nor ES-derived HSCs in their native state can be transplanted into adult irradiated mice. It has been reported that the transition of yolk sac HSCs and ES-derived HSCs from that embryonic stage to the fetal stage can be facilitated by enforced expression by HoxB4 in these cells [118]. Therefore, there are important clues how embryonic HSCs, presumably capable of primitive hematopoiesis, can develop into fetal HSCs capable of definitive hematopoiesis.

During the various stages of fetal HSC functions, it seemed possible that waves of HSCs emerged from tissues such as the fetal liver at specific time points to be accepted by and to engraft in secondary sites such as fetal spleen, fetal bone marrow and lymphoid sites such as the thymus [98]. However, HSCs are found constitutively in the blood throughout fetal life, and it must be the preparedness of the developing organs such as the spleen, marrow and thymus that results in the movement of hematopoiesis to those sites (J.C. Christensen & I.L. Weissman, unpublished data).

A detailed examination of HSCs in the developing fetal liver with respect to T-cell developmental potentials has revealed that even at the level of HSCs changes are occurring that show that HSCs develop in a quantal but dynamic process [163]. Developing T cells gain their specificity and their function in a coordinated series of molecular events, including selection of which class of T-cell receptor genes are rearranged and selected, and to which distant sites the T cells will migrate (Fig. 8.6b). Within the thymus during fetal development the first T cells to emerge use products of the T-cell receptor Vγ3 and T-cell receptor (δ) gene families, to be followed by use of the T-cell receptor γ Vγ2 and Vγ5 and T-cell receptor αβ gene families (Fig. 8.6b). In mice the T-cell receptor V genes at the γ locus that must rearrange to be expressed are, extending from the most proximal site of potential rearrangements, Vγ3, Vγ4, Vγ2 and then Vγ5 (Table 8.1). The first T cells to emerge in the thymus are Vγ3 cells, which colonize the skin only during fetal life [164]. While Vγ3 T-cell development is shutting down in the thymus, Vγ4 T-cell development arises, and these T cells will migrate during their fetal life to the presumptive female genital tract epithelia and the tongue epithelium of both sexes (Fig. 8.6b) [163,164]. The development of Vγ4 T cells ceases at about day 16 or 17 of fetal life, to be replaced by the almost simultaneous onset of Vγ2 T cells which will inhabit lymph nodes and secondary lymphoid sites such as the spleen, and Vγ5 T cells which

Table 8.1 Analysis of hematopoietic stem cell (HSC)-derived cells in single HSC-transplanted mice. Frozen sections of the indicated tissues from single GFP⁺ HSC-transplanted mice were analyzed for the presence of GFP⁺CD45⁻ cells. (From [5] with permission.)

Tissue	Sections examined	Cells examined (approx.)	GFP⁺ non-hematopoietic cells
Brain	60	13,200,000	1
Liver	18	470,000	7
Kidney	24	990,000	0
Gut	24	360,000	0
Skeletal muscle	23	2355	0
Cardiac muscle	14	4346	0
Lung	12	23,000	0

will inhabit the entire gastrointestinal tract, and αβ T cells which are largely restricted to lymphoid tissues.

The kinetics of T-cell development from T-cell precursors can be studied with the use of fetal thymic organ cultures (FTOCs), although it should be noted that these cannot be physiological cultures. When single clonogenic E12 fetal liver HSCs are added to FTOCs, those thymuses produce Vγ3, then Vγ4, then Vγ2, then Vγ5, and TCRαβ T cells (Fig. 8.6b) [163]. When E14 fetal liver HSCs are placed at clonal levels into the same stage FTOC, Vγ3 T cells do not emerge, but the rest of the repertoire is developed. When E16 or older HSC are added to FTOC, including adult bone marrow HSC, neither Vγ3 nor Vγ4 T cells are produced, but the Vγ2, Vγ5 and T-cell αβ repertoire is developed [163]. Finally, E12 fetal liver HSC added directly into the adult thymus cannot produce the fetal program of Vγ3 and Vγ4 T cells, but can produce the mature program of Vγ2, Vγ5 and TCRαβ cells [163].

Taken together, these studies indicate that at probably each HSC cell division within the fetal liver, HSCs are changing (usually reducing) their developmental fates that would only be read out when their progeny entered the fetal thymus, and the change in these fates and the read-out of these fates is dependent upon factors within HSCs and within the thymus microenvironment [163]. After birth, and at least into young adulthood in mice, the numbers of LT-HSCs, ST-HSCs and MPPs are regulated at a relatively constant level. Thereafter there is a gradual loss of cells of the MPP phenotype, and an increase in both the number of LT-HSCs and the fraction of LT-HSCs that are in the cell cycle [89], most dramatically seen in the marrow of geriatric mice.

Does hematopoiesis only derive from HSC and do HSC only give rise to blood?

Once the phenotype of HSCs had been established in mice, it became possible to test whether hematopoietic tissues such as bone marrow harboured any cell population more primitive than HSCs that could continually contribute to hematopoiesis. Only Thy-1^{lo}, but not Thy-1^{hi} or Thy-1⁻ marrow cells contain transplantable hematopoietic progenitors [63]. Likewise, hematopoietic capacity rested in Sca-1⁺ but not Sca-1⁻ cells, and Lin⁻ to Lin^{lo} but not Lin⁺ cells, and c-kit⁺ but not c-kit⁻ cells, providing strong evidence that in the context of hematopoietic cell transplantation, these were the only sources of hematopoiesis in the young adult mouse [63]. This did not rule out the possibility that a rare, more primitive population existed that could not give rise to hematopoietic cells in the timespan of a competitive repopulation experiment, although it would be hard to understand how that population was missed. Nevertheless, several experiments provide evidence for a bone marrow population capable of widespread differentiation to daughter cells of all germ layers, including hematopoietic cells [13,31]. It should be noted that these experiments have not yet been independently replicated, and the possibility of cell fusion rather than cell differentiation to explain how bone marrow cells can give rise to various outcomes such as epithelial tissues and neural tissues has not at the time of writing been ruled out [165].

In one experiment, a population of cells freshly isolated from bone marrow as small cells that are Lin⁻ and which upon transplantation do not divide over a 2-day period, and that home with remarkable efficiency to bone marrow have been reported to give rise to a variety of tissues from all three germ layers [13]. It has been reported that as few as one cell transplanted from this population into secondary hosts along with radio-protective doses of marrow cells allows the appearance of daughter cells in the hematopoietic series, in widespread epithelia and other tissues [13]. Taking a completely different approach, Verfaillie et al. have found that stromal cultures from adult mouse bone marrow can at late intervals give rise to pauciclonal or clonal populations after the usual primary culture crisis period, and these multipotent adult progenitor cells (MAPCs) upon transplantation into adults give rise to donor-derived hematopoiesis and representatives of virtually every tissue [31]. The transplantation of these cells at the level of 1–12 cells into mouse blastocysts showed robust contribution of donor-derived cells to virtually all cell types in the mice developing from such chimeric blastocysts [31]. Both of these experiments can be interpreted that there exists in adults a population of pluripotent cells similar to inner cell mass pluripotent cells in their capability to differentiate to daughter cells of the mesodermal, endodermal and ectodermal lineages. It is also possible at the time of writing that the cells in both experiments are not pluripotent but fusigenic, and that it is fusion rather than differentiation that accounts for the presence of donor markers in all lineages [165,166].

These and other experiments should be taken in a larger context. As shown in Fig. 8.7, the usual characterization of cell lineage outcomes goes from *totipotency* in the fertilized egg to *pluripotency* of inner cell mass cells to the derivation of germline stem cells on the one hand and, alternatively, somatic stem cells on the other. It is unknown if there exist pluripotent stem cells that survive beyond the blastocyst period. Until recently, several experiments seemed to indicate that by day 4.5 or 5.5 of mouse gestation, cells have lost the capability of responding to the blastocyst microenvironment by contributing to multiple cell lineages (pluripotency) [150,151]. Whether there exists between pluripotent blastocyst cells and multipotent, largely lineage-specified stem cells a pluripotent precursor that survives into adulthood is unknown. It is conceivable that germline stem cells that do not land in genital ridges (where they commit to a protogametic fate) can survive into adulthood and remain pluripotent [1]. More direct experiments are required to test for the tissue localization of pluripotent populations such as MAPC, if they exist *in vivo* rather than as an *in vitro* generated but unique population. Other experiments that seem to show ready transdifferentiation of adult stem cells or multipotent stem cells of one tissue type into the tissues of the others are at this point still in question. There have been reports that bone marrow hematopoietic cells give rise to brain cells, that brain stem cell populations can give rise to blood, that fat cells can give rise to neurons and mesenchymal fates, that muscle stem cells can give rise to hematopoietic and myogenic outcomes, and a host of others [9–18,167,168]. What has been lacking in most of these experiments is the demonstration that the transplanted population was in fact a stem cell purified to homogeneity that could give rise at the clonal level to two different tissue types, and that the tissue types that had been generated were robustly characterized as functional mature cells of that tissue without cell fusion.

Attempts to repeat the experiments showing transdifferentiation of CNS stem cells to hematopoietic tissues have thus far failed. A reexam-

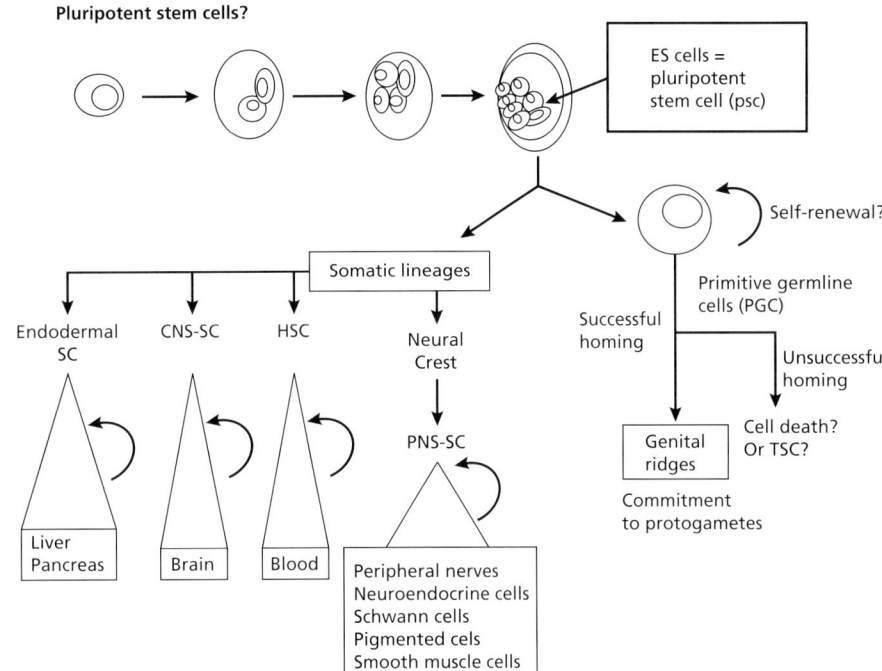

Fig. 8.7 Model of pluripotent stem cell (PSC) generation of germline and somatic progenitor cells. PSC can diverge into primitive germline cells (PGCs) and to tissue-specific stem cells. A possible source of residual totipotent stem cells (TSCs) is depicted. The organ and tissue-specific stem cells are developed as CNS-SL, HSC, PNS-SC, etc. (Adapted from [19] with permission).

Table 8.2 Analysis of partner-derived GFP+ cross-engrafting cells in parabiotic mice. Frozen sections of the indicated tissues from nontransgenic partners parabiotic pairs were analyzed for the presence of GFP+CD45− cells. (From [5] with permission.)

Tissue	Sections examined	Cells examined (approx.)	Partner-derived nonhematopoietic cells
Brain	30	3,189,000	0
Liver	9	174,100	0
Kidney	8	101,000	0
Gut	8	399,000	0
Skeletal muscle	32	3037	0
Cardiac muscle	10	2014	0
Lung	6	226,000	0

ination of the cells in muscle that give rise to blood show them to be CD45 positive committed HSCs, separable from muscle progenitors that, on their own, give rise to muscle [169,170]. In some circumstances, regenerating muscle following an injury can incorporate cells whose markers are expressed in the regenerated muscle tissue, and the most common transplantable source of these cells is bone marrow [10,11]. While some claims have been made that these are derived from HSCs, in fact single purified HSCs, even over long intervals, cannot contribute to muscle or any other tissue, except a rare set of liver cells in irradiated hosts (Plate 8.1, *facing p. 296*; Tables 8.1 and 8.2) [5]. In another example, liver regeneration of hepatocytes bearing markers from injected purified HSCs, following multiple rounds of selection through liver toxicity can occur [168], but recent evidence (M. Grompe, unpublished data) indicates that these are mainly a result of cell fusion events between some progeny of the hematopoietic stem cells, and some precursor of liver cells [165,166]. We had previously proposed that cases of transdifferentiation of one tissue specific stem cell to another tissue specific stem cell might not really be transdifferentiation, but differentiation from a more pluripotent precursor [1]. That possibility is still viable. In some circumstances neural cultures derive from single adult mouse brain ependymal cells can, upon implantation into blastocysts, contribute to many lineages, although hematopoiesis is not one of them [171].

The many claims that transdifferentiation could occur represents a problem in stem cell biology—a young field. Most new investigators to the field have not felt compelled to purify the populations to homogeneity, transplant single cells, populations of cells of apparent phenotypic and functional homogeneity, and have not marked cells retrovirally or with other genetic markers to follow the fate of clonogenic precursors. In fact, bone marrow is not the same as HSCs, but is a population of mature or maturing cells, and certainly includes at least two or three stem and progenitor populations: HSCs, mesenchymal stem cells (MSCs) and endothelial precursors, which might really be MSCs [31]. The term "plasticity" has been used many times to describe formerly unexpected outcomes from cell transplantations, this may not be the most accurate term, if transdifferentiation cannot occur. Perhaps the unexpected outcomes are always derived from a class of previously unappreciated adult pluripotent cells, or perhaps the normal developmental fates of MSCs are not yet appreciated.

A few other tissue-specific stem cells have been isolated or enriched: these include human CNS stem cells [38], peripheral nervous system stem cells [32], MSCs [31] and pluripotent ES cells [172–174]. Other multipotent precursors have been enriched dramatically, but it is not yet sure whether they are stem cells—the most prominent among these being epidermal or skin stem cells [175].

Lineage committed hematopoietic progenitor cells

Considerations for the definition/isolation of hematopoietic progenitors

The developmental process from HSCs to mature cells must involve developmental intermediates that have lost stem cell potentials but are not yet terminally differentiated. An important question is in which sequence lineage commitment occurs. The immediate progeny of HSCs and/or MPPs might be oligopotent progenitors that have some but not all developmental options or monopotent progenitors that are committed to one single mature cell type. Several findings are suggestive for the existence of oligopotent progenitors. First, the lack of lymphocyte in patients with severe combined immunodeficiency syndromes (SCID) was taken as evidence for the existence of oligopotent, lymphoid committed progenitor cells or lymphoid stem cells. However, the loss of lymphocytes caused by adenosine deaminase (ADA) deficiency [176,177] or by mutations of the common cytokine receptor γ-chain (γc) [178,179] does not necessarily imply a common progenitor. Rather, several lymphoid cell types or their progenitors might be most susceptible to the induced alterations [180] or might be dependent on the same signal transduction mechanisms. This same caution needs to be applied to the interpretation of hematopoietic phenotypes of genetically altered mice, as mutants of Ikaros [181] or Notch-1 [182] that could either be essential factors for a common or multiple different progenitors [183].

Second, leukemia cells can be viewed as cells that are arrested at early developmental stages but have gained self-renewal capacity. The occurrence of leukemias that either coexpress antigens normally associated with myeloid or lymphoid cell types (mixed lineage leukemias) or that harbour two leukemia populations of clonal origin (bilineal leukemias) could be taken as evidence for the existence of bipotent B-myeloid or T-myeloid progenitors [184–192]. However, leukemia clones could be derived from HSCs, from MPPs, or from restricted progenitors that, because of their altered gene expression profile, display cell surface gene products which are normally not present at these developmental stages.

Third, the fact that single cells in bone marrow give rise to colonies that contain all myeloid but no lymphoid progeny *in vitro* (colony-forming unit–granulocyte/erythrocyte/macrophage/megakaryocyte, CFU-GEMM) or *in vivo* (mixed CFU-S) is suggestive for the existence of oligopotent myeloid progenitors. However, cells that give multimyeloid read out could also be multipotent but did not find the conditions to read out progeny [59,193–195].

In light of these problems, several prerequisites need to be met to define restricted progenitors in a developmental hierarchy. First, in order to prospectively identify candidate populations, they need to be isolated to highest possible homogeneity/purity. Second, if a population shows oligopotent differentiation activity, it must be demonstrated that at least some single cells within this population give oligopotent read-out, i.e. that this population is not a mixture of different monopotent progenitors. Third, it further needs to be shown that single oligopotent progenitors are not HSCs or MPPs. These prerequisites are difficult to achieve. At any given time point, progenitor cells might underlie intrinsic "stochastic" random commitment events, might not find suitable microenvironments to read-out in all their possibilities or might even not read out at all [196–198]. However, by applying the above criteria, we and others were able to identify oligopotent developmental intermediates in mice and humans. These data strongly support the hypothesis that multipotent hematopoietic progenitors first lose their self-renewal ability and consecutively commit to either the lymphoid or myeloid developmental pathway. Although not formally proven, based on frequency, cycling status and *in vitro* and *in vivo* expansion potential of bone marrow lymphoid and myeloid committed progenitors, it seems possible that all hematopoiesis develops through either a common lymphoid or common myeloid developmental stage.

Common lymphoid progenitor cells and lymphoid development

Lymphoid cell development from HSCs is dependent on externally provided differentiation, growth and survival factors. Of those, IL-7 might be most important. Its cognate high-affinity receptor is a complex composed of the IL-7Rα chain [199] and the γc chain [179,200]. Neutralizing antibodies to IL-7 or genetic ablation of either IL-7 or IL-7Rα inhibit both T- and B-cell development *in vivo* [201,202]. Targeted deletion of the γc gene leads to the loss of T and B cells and the additional loss of natural killer (NK) cells [203–205], presumably because of the impaired formation not only of the IL-7R, but also the IL-2R and IL-15R that might be nonredundant cytokines for NK cell development [206–208]. Furthermore, mice that lack Jak3, a signal transduction molecule associated with γc [209,210], display a similar phenotype as the γc-deficient mice [211–213]. Also, patients with genetic defects in Jak3 show similar defects in lymphoid development as patients with γc gene disruptions (X-SCID) [214,215]. Based on these data, IL-7 is recognized as a nonredundant cytokine for both T- and B-cell development that could act as a proliferation factor, a survival factor and/or could initiate lineage specific developmental programs. IL-7R is expressed in both developing T and B cells, and in mature T cells [216,217]. In genetically modified mice that are either IL-7Rα$^{-/-}$, γc$^{-/-}$ or IL-7$^{-/-}$, T-cell progenitors express low levels of Bcl-2, an antiapoptotic protein [218]. However, incubation of T cells from IL-7$^{-/-}$ mice with recombinant IL-7 results in the upregulation of Bcl-2 [219] and enforced expression of Bcl-2 in either IL-7Rα$^{-/-}$ or γc$^{-/-}$ mice lead to significant rescue of αβT-cell development [20,219,220]. Therefore, a critical role of IL-7 in developing and mature αβT cells is the promotion of survival via expression of Bcl-2 or other antiapoptotic proteins as possibly Bcl-Xγ [221]. However, enforced expression of Bcl-2 was not sufficient to rescue B-cell development and γδ T-cell development [20,92,219]. Here, IL-7R mediated signals are necessary for the rearrangement of immunoglobulin heavy chain V segments via *Pax*-5 gene activation [222,223] and for V-J recombination of γδ TCR genes via Stat5 [224,225]. Therefore IL-7R signaling can either lead to the transmission of "trophic" survival signals in the T-cell lineage or "mechanistic" differentiation and proliferation signals in the B and γδ T-cell lineage, respectively. Thus, it was reasonable to search for oligopotent common lymphoid progenitors (CLPs) within the Lin$^-$IL-7Rα$^+$ fraction in adult mouse bone marrow. We identified a population of Lin$^-$IL-7Rα$^+$Thy-1$^-$Sca-1^{lo}c-*kit*^{lo} cells that also express γc, indicating that this population possesses functional IL-7R (Fig. 8.8) [20]. In contrast, both LT-HSC and ST-HSC populations are IL-7Rα$^-$. In both *in vitro* and *in vivo* assays, Lin$^-$IL-7Rα$^+$Thy-1$^-$Sca-1^{lo}c-*kit*^{lo} cells completely lack myeloid differentiation activity [20]. Also no day 8 and day 12 CFU-S activity could be detected [20,48]. These CLPs possess rapid and potent T, B and NK cell-restricted differentiation activity in reconstitution assays. Injection of 1000 CLP could generate 0.6–1.1 × 10^7 CD3$^+$ spleen T cells by 4–6 weeks, and 1.4 × 10^7 B220$^+$ spleen B cells by 2 weeks *in vivo*. CLP-derived T- and B-cell generation peaks 7–10 days earlier than similar numbers of T and B cells derived from the same number of HSCs [20]. However, in contrast to HSC-derived cells, numbers of CLP-derived T and B cells begin to decline after 4–6 weeks, suggesting that this population has no or limited self-renewal activity. Using a two-step assay we demonstrated that CLPs contain clonogenic progenitors for both T and B cells. Single cells were cultured in methylcellulose in the presence of SLF, IL-7 and Flt-3 ligand to expand cell numbers, and a portion of the day 3 colonies were picked up and injected directly into the thymus. Those injected into the thymus differentiated into all stages of T-cell development and, in some cases, differentiated into both T and B lineage cells. The further cultured cells formed B-lineage colonies composed of pro-B and pre-B cells [20]. Therefore, the defined CLPs matches the criteria for the definition of oligopotent progenitor cells. Accordingly, CLPs exist downstream of ST-HSCs in normal hematopoiesis.

Based on their frequency in bone marrow, their cycling status and their *in vivo* T, NK and B-cell generation potential, CLPs theoretically could be a developmental intermediate for most if not all mature lymphoid cells. The commitment of CLP to either the T or B lineage may be determined simply by the microenvironment which CLPs encounter. However, it is still unclear whether CLPs are an indispensable stage of T- and

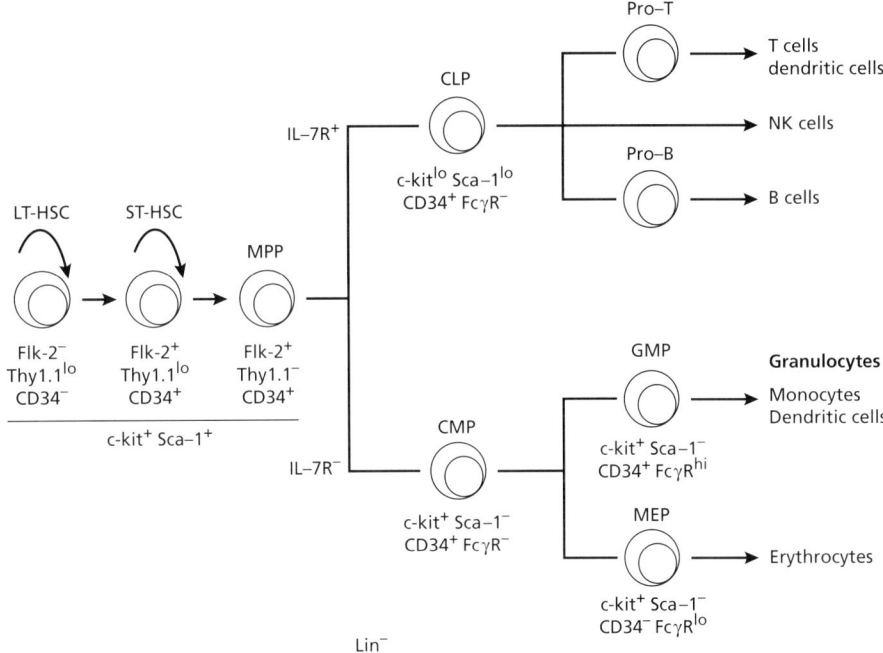

Fig. 8.8 A current map of the mouse hematopoietic lineage. Long-term hematopoietic stem cell (LT-HSC) self-renew for life, while their downstream short-term (ST)-HSC self-renew for 6–8 weeks. Further downstream progenitors have been prospectively isolated to phenotypic, functional and for the more mature cells, gene expression profile homogeneity. CLP, common lymphocyte progenitor; CMP, common myeloid progenitor; GMP, granulocyte/macrophage progenitor; MEP, megakaryocyte/erythrocyte progenitor.

B-cell development. The earliest thymic progenitors (DN1, double negative 1 cells) are $CD4^{lo}CD8^-CD44^+CD25^-$ c-kit^+ cells [226–229] and therefore closely resemble the phenotype of HSCs. Most of these early thymic progenitors are T-cell committed (pro-T cells); however, some cells within this population are capable of differentiating into B, NK and dendritic cells (DCs) and, at a low frequency, into myeloid cells [229] but their clonal origin has not been established [228–230]. Whether the earliest thymic progenitor population contains a small number of recently homed CLPs that, within this microenvironment, preferentially differentiate into T cells, or whether CLPs commit to the T-cell lineage while still in bone marrow and successively home to the thymus [231] is unknown.

In a recent report, Allman et al. [232] suggest that thymopoiesis is maintained through early thymic progenitors (ETPs) that might develop from bone marrow progenitors more closely related to HSCs and not via a CLP-dependent pathway. This is based on findings that some cells (ETPs) within the DN1 fraction do not express IL-7Rα at high levels, have some myeloid potential, give rise to T and B cells with kinetics that resemble those of ST-HSCs [67] more closely than that of CLPs, and that were present at near-normal frequencies in Ikaros$^{-/-}$ mice while CLPs were not detectable by phenotype. While these data add important information on possible alternative T-cell developmental pathways, they do not assess directly how many of ETPs or mature T cells are CLP-derived or whether most thymopoiesis is independent of CLPs. Both HSCs and CLPs might home to the thymus where T-cell commitment might immediately be initiated and thymus homing receptors might be lost. Therefore, until formally proven, it is reasonable to believe that ETPs are progeny of recently homed HSCs rather than CLPs. Whether most mature T cells are produced directly through HSCs or via CLPs will then depend on their trafficking through blood and homing to thymus. Of note, CLPs cotransplanted in addition to HSCs in autologous or allogeneic transplantation models, can rescue mice from otherwise lethal cytomegalovirus (mCMV) infections [381], providing evidence for the robust *and* functional T and/or NK cell reconstitution capacity of CLPs *in vivo*. The issue of progenitor commitment to the T-cell lineage in bone marrow vs. thymus is further complicated by the observation that, at least in experimental settings, extrathymic T-cell development can occur.

Recently, a $Thy-1.2^{hi}CD2^-CD16^+CD44^{hi}Lin^-$ committed T-cell progenitor population (CTPs) in bone marrow was described that, *in vitro* and upon transplantation generated TCRαβ$^+$ CD4$^+$ and CD8$^+$ T cells, but no other hematopoietic lineages [233,234]. In these studies extrathymic, i.e. peripheral lymphoid tissue and bone marrow T-cell reconstitution was earlier and more robust than thymic reconstitution, and progeny T cells showed an atypical $CD44^{hi}CD45RB^{hi}$ phenotype [234]. The lineal relations of CTPs to CLPs and to thymic T-cell progenitors as well as the relevance of extrathymic T-cell development in healthy hematopoiesis still needs to be established.

Similar to T-cell development, the exact lineage relationship between CLPs and the earliest defined B-cell progenitors remain unclear. B-cell progenitors were divided into prepro-B cells (fraction A0, $AA4.1^+CD4^{lo}B220^-HSA^-$; A1, $AA4.1^+CD4^+B220^+HSA^-$; A2, $AA4.1^+CD4^-B220^+HSA^-$); and pro-B cells (fraction B, $B220^+CD43^+HSA^+6C3/BP-1^-$; C, $B220^+CD43^+HSA^+6C3/BP-1^+$) [235–237]. Some fraction A0 cells express c-*kit* and Sca-1 and can give rise not only to B cell but also to myeloid and T-cell progeny. Therefore they might contain MPPs. The majority of fraction A1 cells are c-*kit*$^-$, lack myeloid potential but minor T-cell potential can be detected after intrathymic injection. Pro-B cells are B-lineage committed, rearrange D_H-J_H genes (fraction B) and undergo V-DJ recombination (fraction C). In view of their T- and B-cell read-out capacity, the A0 or A1 fraction could contain CLPs. Because different markers were used for their isolation, a direct comparison of the populations is not possible. However, a majority of A0 and A1 fraction cells do not express IL-7Rα, while IL-7Rα is expressed on fraction A2 cells. These issues need to be addressed by further studies, and these cells need to be tested at the clonal level.

In humans, evidence for a T/NK bipotential precursor population in fetal thymus [238] and a terminal deoxynucleotidyl transferase (TdT) positive candidate lymphoid precursor population in CD34$^+$ bone marrow cells has been reported [239]. However, clonal analysis was not carried out. A subpopulation of the CD34$^+$TdT$^+$ cells express the neutral endopeptidase CD10 [240]. Later it was shown that fetal and adult bone marrow Lin$^-$CD34$^+$Thy-1$^-$CD38$^+$CD10$^+$ cells contain clonal progenitors of B, NK and dendritic cells [241]. As a population these cells gives rise to T cells in the SCID-hu thymus assay but could not generate myeloid progeny [241]. In another report it was shown that cord blood CD34+CD38−CD7+ cells contain clonal B, NK and dendritic cell precursors; however, T-cell read out was not evaluated [242]. Therefore, both studies suggest but do not formally demonstrate the existence of CLPs in humans. IL-7 signaling might not be essential for normal B-cell development in humans because B cells can be generated without IL-7 *in vitro* [243], and disruption of the IL-7R *in vivo* causes T-cell but not consistently B-cell deficiencies [244,245; reviewed in 240]. Therefore, it is of interest to know whether human early lymphoid progenitors in analogy to mouse CLPs express IL-7Rα and depend on IL-7 signaling. Indeed, Lin−CD34+CD38+CD10+ cells can be subdivided into a CD10+IL-7Rα− and a CD10loIL-7Rα+ fraction, with the latter being highly enriched in clonal B-cell progenitors (K. Akashi *et al.*, unpublished data; M. Manz *et al.*, unpublished data). It is important to determine whether CD10loIL-7Rα+ cells or CD10+IL-7Rα− cells contain both T and B-cell progenitors and whether thymus seeding cells share some of these phenotypes [for review of human early thymocyte development see 246].

Common myeloid progenitor cells and myeloid development

The fact that IL-7Rα expressing cells in mouse bone marrow contain CLP and hold no myeloid differentiation activity [20], suggests that complementary progenitors common to all myeloid cells may exist in the IL-7Rα negative cell fraction. In addition, we had noted that the Sca-1− subset of Thy-1loLin− cells contained myeloerythroid progenitors [52]. Therefore, to exclude HSCs and CLPs we searched for myeloid progenitors within the Lin−IL-7Rα−Sca-1−c-*kit*+ bone marrow fraction. We identified three myeloid progenitor populations:

1 FcγRloCD34+ common myeloid progenitor cells (CMPs) and their lineal descendants;
2 FcγRloCD34− megakaryocyte/erythrocyte progenitor cells (MEPs); and
3 FcγRhiCD34+ granulocyte/macrophage progenitor cells (GMPs) [21].

These three myeloid progenitor subsets likely represent the major pathways for myeloid cell differentiation because they contain the vast majority of myeloid progenitor activity in steady state bone marrow. CMPs give rise to all myeloid colonies *in vitro* including CFU-Mix; GMP give rise to CFU-G and CFU-M as well as CFU-GM; and the MEPs give rise to BFU-E (burst-forming unit, erythroid), CFU-Meg as well as CFU-MegE, each with high cloning efficiency. We demonstrated that CMPs as a population differentiate *in vitro* into cells with MEP and GMP phenotype and function [21]. Furthermore, the majority of single CMPs generate both GM- and MegE-related progeny. Upon *in vivo* transfer, the three cell populations give short-term but not long-term read-out corresponding to their *in vitro* activities, indicating that they have only limited if any self-renewal activity [48].

MEP contain radioprotective cells for lethally irradiated mice housed under infection control conditions [48]. Lethally irradiated mice injected with MEPs, CMPs, ST-HSCs or MPPs show transient donor-derived hematopoiesis sufficient to allow reconstitution with residual host HSC to sustain survival [48,50,92]. In addition, the majority of day 8 CFU-S activity resides within the MEP population, but is absent from GMP [48], supporting previous findings that day 8–9 CFU-S are largely erythroid [46,52,247]. Our data also confirm previous findings that the majority of day 12 CFU-S activity resides not within lineage-committed progenitors but within the more primitive HSC populations with some activity in CMPs and MEPs [46,50,52]. Neither B nor T-cell differentiation activity was detectable in either MEPs or GMPs. CMPs could not generate T cells; however, a small number of B-cell progeny were detectable *in vitro* and *in vivo* [21]. Accordingly, it is important to determine whether the CMP fraction contains a minority of bipotent B-cell/myeloid progenitors, or whether some minor B-cell progenitor population share surface phenotype with CMPs (see below). We have recently isolated a pure population of megakaryocyte progenitors (MKP) in mice. These Lin−c-*kit*+Sca-1−CD34+CD9+CD41+ cells are highly efficient at producing megakaryocyte CFC *in vitro*, micromegakaryocyte loci *in vivo*, and donor-derived platelet production *in vivo*, while they are devoid of erythrogenic activity [248].

As in the case of CLPs, multiple studies suggested the existence of human oligopotent myeloid progenitors [249–255]. Recently, we were able to identify human bone marrow and cord blood cell populations that are counterparts of the mouse CMPs, GMPs and MEPs [256]. They are negative for multiple mature lineage markers (including early lymphoid markers that might define human CLPs as CD7, CD10 or IL-7Rα) and all are CD34+CD38+. They are distinguished by the expression of CD45RA, an isoform of the CD45 cell-surface tyrosine phosphatase that can negatively regulate at least some classes of cytokine receptor signaling [257], and IL-3Rα, a receptor that upon activation supports proliferation and differentiation of primitive progenitors [93,196,258]. CD45RA−IL-3Rαlo (CMPs), CD45RA+IL-3Rαlo (GMPs) and CD45RA−IL-3Rα− (MEPs) show high myeloid cloning efficacy but low long-term (stromal hematopoietic) culture-initiating cell (LTC-IC) capacity, indicating that they do not self-renew. Although FcγR II–III (CD16/CD32) expression distinguishes mouse CMPs and GMPs, it was not detectable on any of the human myeloid progenitor populations; and all human clonal myeloid progenitors are positive for CD34 while mouse MEP are CD34− [21]. Interestingly, in mouse myeloid progenitors IL-3Rα as well as CD45RA expression were both negative to low in MEPs, intermediate in CMPs and positive in GMPs, without providing sufficient discrimination to clearly set a cut-off level between the different cellular fractions. As with the mouse myeloid progenitors, CMPs give rise to MEPs and GMPs *in vitro* and a significant proportion of CMPs have clonal granulocyte/macrophage and megakaryocyte/erythrocyte read-out potential. We did not test T-cell differentiation ability; however, no *in vitro* B or NK cell read-out could be detected. However, some B cells might develop from large numbers of transplanted CMPs. As in the case of mouse CMPs, it is important to clarify whether the CMP population contains oligopotent B/myeloid progenitors, or monopotent B-cell progenitors that share CMP phenotypes but do not read out in our *in vitro* assay, or whether *in vivo* B-cell read-out was because of small numbers of contaminating B-cell progenitors in the large number of transplanted cells (see below).

Lineage commitment in fetal hematopoiesis

While fetal liver (FL) HSCs show major similarities to adult HSCs, some phenotypic and functional differences exist [159,259–261]. Remarkably, FL-HSCs possess some cell fate potentials such as the generation of Vγ3+ and Vγ4+ T cells [163] and B-1a lymphocytes [262] that are not detectable in adult HSCs. Therefore it was important to determine the phenotype and developmental capacities of fetal liver CLP and CMP. We recently identified FL-CLPs (Lin−IL-7Rα+B220−/loSca-1loc-*kit*lo) [263], and the myeloid progenitors FL-CMPs (Lin−IL-7Rα−Sca-1−c-*kit*+AA4.1−FcγRloCD34+), FL-GMPs (Lin−IL-7Rα−Sca-1−c-*kit*+AA4.1−FcγRhiCD34+) and FL-MEPs (Lin−IL-7Rα−Sca-1−c-*kit*+AA4.1−FcγRloCD34−) [264] that show high similarities to their adult counterparts. However, some significant differences in proliferative potential colony-forming activity and lineage differentiation capacities exist. Of special note, FL-CLPs generate CD45+CD4+3−LTβ+ cells that are candidate initiators of lymph node and Peyer's patch formation [265–267]. About 5% of these IL-7R+ FL-CLPs differentiated into macrophages as well as into B cells, at least *in vitro*. Interestingly, the FL-CLPs fail to express Pax5, a suppressor of macrophage development [268] while adult marrow CLPs that lack myeloid potential are Pax5+ [263]. Conversely, although FL-CMP and downstream FL-MEPs or FL-GMPs do not give rise to T cells, FL-CMPs possess some *in vitro* and *in vivo* B-cell potential. A close relation between B-cell and macrophage development for adult and fetal hematopoiesis was suggested before (see below). It can therefore be speculated that during commitment to the lymphoid or myeloid lineage in FL hematopoiesis, the developmental capacity for macrophages and B cells might be the last to be lost in commitment to either the lymphoid or myeloid lineage.

Alternative developmental pathways

If HSCs commit to lymphoid or myeloid lineages in an intrinsic "stochastic" manner, as proposed for myeloerythroid differentiation *in vitro* [196,197], it is possible that besides CLPs and CMPs either bipotent B-cell/myeloid, or T-cell/myeloid progenitors, or both might exist.

In support of a B/macrophage progenitor, it was demonstrated that several B-cell lines can be modified to produce cells with features of macrophages by *in vitro* manipulations [269–271]. Importantly, transfection of v-raf into B-cell lines established from Eµ-*myc* transgenic mice could convert them into macrophages that maintained the identical rearrangement of an IgH gene [270]. This observation suggests that latent developmental potentials that are not accessible under normal conditions might be regained through genetic alteration. Indeed, we have shown that CLPs, which under normal conditions never generate myeloid read-out, produced granulocytes and macrophages after they were genetically engineered to express the human IL-2 receptor β chain (hIL-2Rβ) or the granulocyte/macrophage colony-stimulating factor receptor (GM-CSFR) and were stimulated with the cognate ligands [272]. This was blocked by enforced expression of Pax5 (M. Kondo, A. King and I.L. Weissman, unpublished observation).

Also *in vitro*, single FL cells could be demonstrated to give rise to both B/myeloid and T/myeloid progeny [195,273,274]. In these experiments using a FTOC system in the presence of 60% O_2 for single cell read-out, Kawamoto *et al*. [274] detected B/T/myeloid, B/myeloid, T/myeloid, but never T/B bipotent progenitors from FL cells populations [274]. These findings led them to the proposal that T/B cell development might not be as closely linked as T/myeloid or B/myeloid development [275]. However, in these high O_2 concentration cultures, only ~5% of single Lin$^-$Sca-1$^+$c-*kit*$^+$ HSCs gave rise to multilineage (T/B/myeloid) outcomes, suggesting that this system is not reproducible enough to demonstrate all differentiation capacities of HSCs. Also, differentiation into T/myeloid or B/myeloid lineages might simply be because of the "random" commitment of HSCs in these culture conditions. Alternatively, T/B committed bipotent progenitors might not be contained in the Lin$^-$Sca-1$^+$c-*kit*$^+$ population but only in the Lin$^-$Sca-1^{lo}c-*kit*^{lo} CLP fraction [20,263]. Recently, bipotent B/macrophage progenitors were also described at a very low frequency (~0.02%) in adult hematopoiesis *in vitro* [276], supporting the hypothesis that a B/macrophage developmental line might be conserved beyond fetal hematopoiesis.

From the above data, it might have seemed possible that alternative bipotent lymphoid/myeloid developmental pathways in genetically unaltered hematopoietic development exist. However, studies suggesting this developmental pathway in postnatal hematopoiesis are derived from *in vitro* data only. To evaluate the *in vivo* relevance in hematopoiesis, such progenitors need to be prospectively isolated, and it is important to test how robust these progenitors will reconstitute the respective hematopoietic branches *in vivo* as already shown for fetal and adult CLP and myeloid progenitors [21,48,248,256,263,264,277,278].

Dendritic cell development

Dendritic cells (DCs) are bone marrow-derived leukocytes that were initially defined as nonmacrophage cell populations with high antigen presentation capacities and their ability to prime naive T cells [279–281]. To date, with their numbers still growing, multiple DC subpopulations that differ in tissue distribution, surface marker expression and functional capacities have been described in humans and laboratory mice [reviewed in 282,283]. From an evolutionary point of view, DCs might belong to the myeloid as well as to the lymphoid lineage because they link the innate and adaptive immune response. Based on current data, two opposing models of DC ontogeny can be suggested: either the mature DC subpopulation is determined at the level of an early hematopoietic progenitor or, alternatively, immature DCs retain the capacity to mature to distinct DC subpopulations in response to different environmental instructions.

In mice, two major DC subpopulations are distinguishable by their expression of the CD8α chain [284]. It was reported that early intrathymic progenitors (TP) (CD4^{lo}CD44$^+$CD25$^-$c-*kit*$^+$) and thymic pro-T cells (CD44$^+$CD25$^+$c-*kit*$^+$) contain precursors capable to differentiate into CD8α$^+$ DCs *in vivo* [230,285]. Therefore, and because the majority of thymic DCs and only a minority of secondary lymphoid organ DCs express CD8α$^+$, the CD8α$^+$ DCs had been considered to be related to the T-lymphoid lineage and were therefore termed "lymphoid DCs" in contrast to the CD8α$^-$ "myeloid DCs". This model seemed to be supported, but not directly demonstrated, in mice deficient for the transcription factors RelB [286], PU.1 [287] and Ikaros [288] that lack only CD8α$^-$ DC. However, other mutants as in c-*kit*$^{-/-}$, γc$^{-/-}$ [289] and Notch1$^{-/-}$ [290] mice, showed a developmental dissociation of CD8α$^+$ DC and T cells. We and others therefore tested DC developmental potentials in adult and fetal lymphoid and myeloid committed progenitors. Surprisingly, CD8α$^+$ and CD8α$^-$ DCs were produced both by highly purified CLPs and CMPs with similar efficacy on a per cell basis, therefore disproving the concept of CD8α$^+$ "lymphoid" and CD8α$^-$ "myeloid" derived DCs in mice [263,278,290,291]. Furthermore, beyond CLPs and CMPs, DC developmental potential is conserved in the lymphoid lineage in pro T cells and in the myeloid lineage in GMPs, but it is lost once B-cell or megakaryocyte/erythrocyte commitment occurs [278,290].

In contrast to mice wherein DCs or their precursors are usually isolated from the lymphoid organs or bone marrow, human DCs and their precursors have usually been isolated from peripheral blood and only in rare cases from blood-forming organs, making direct comparisons difficult [for review see 283]. However, DCs could be generated from total CD34$^+$ progenitor populations, lymphoid restricted progenitor populations and from peripheral blood monocytes, suggesting that in analogy to mice, DC developmental potential is conserved in myeloid and lymphoid restricted lineages [241,242,292–296]. Recently, an immediate DC precursor population that upon stimulation can produce high amounts of interferon α, displays a set of distinct pattern recognition receptors and can mature into DCs *in vitro*, was identified in humans [297–301] and later in mice [302–304]. This DC subpopulation was termed plasmacytoid DCs or DC2 [305]. It was postulated that plasmacytoid DCs are derived from lymphoid committed progenitors because some of these cells isolated from different tissues express mRNA usually found in the lymphoid lineage as pre-Tα, Igλ-like 14.1 and Spi-B [306,307]. Furthermore, CD34$^+$ progenitor cells transduced with Id2 and Id3 (inhibitors of basic helix-loop-helix transcription factor binding) cannot differentiate into T cells, B cells [308,309] and into plasmacytoid DCs, but do differentiate into other DC populations [307]. However, Olweus *et al*. [254] had previously described DCs that display a surface phenotype similar to plasmacytoid DCs, although other features as IFN-α production were not evaluated. *In vitro*, these cells could be generated from an M-CSF receptor positive progenitor cell fraction that is largely restricted to granulomonocytic read out [253], arguing for their development from the myeloid lineage.

Taken together, DCs are developing along a lymphoid and myeloid pathway *in vitro* and *in vivo*. By using simple assays as immunophenotyping or functional read out as MLR and cytokine production, we did not detect differences in lymphoid precursor and myeloid precursor derived CD8α⁺ DC fraction DCs [278]. This is an unexpected finding, because it suggests developmental redundancy for DCs. Of note, DC developmental capacities in CLPs and pro T cells correlate with their latent myeloid developmental potential that can be "rescued" by artificial introduction and activation of the IL-2β or GM-CSF receptor [272,310]. It would therefore be important to characterize the signals that are involved to retain DC developmental capacities in the otherwise exclusively lymphoid or myeloid committed progenitor cells. Activation of the Flt3 tyrosine kinase could be one of them [382]. Furthermore, it still needs to be conclusively determined whether other DC subpopulations such as plasmacytoid DCs segregate with the lymphoid and/or myeloid lineage.

Gene expression profiles of HSC

Several powerful technologies have allowed the characterization of transcripts in defined cells, populations of cells, tissues and organs. These technical advances allow for reductionist approaches to understand the complexity of RNA transcripts found in these cells or tissues, and how the transcriptional profile changes upon differentiation, self-renewal or other functional events. One of the most powerful technologies is gene microarray analysis, wherein a high fraction of all known genes (or oligonucleotides) in the species are placed in clonal microarrays, and the transcripts (e.g. from purified HSCs) are labeled with one fluorochrome are compared quantitatively with a control set of transcripts, perhaps that same population under another physiological condition, or whole bone marrow or other interesting populations. Using these techniques, several genes expressed by either mouse fetal liver HSCs, adult mouse bone marrow HSCs or even human HSCs have been described [99,100]. Gene subtractions or other differential expression techniques have revealed a subset of genes that appear to be expressed in HSCs, but not broadly elsewhere. In fact, some genes have been found that are expressed in HSCs and neurosphere cultures (highly enriched for CNS stem cells) [101], or HSCs and ES cells, or all three [109].

These gene expression arrays cannot detect important events that are essentially post-translational, e.g. the phosphorylation and dephosphorylation of proteins in signal transduction pathways, or the changes in subcellular location of proteins such as β-catenin under conditions when they are held within the degradation complex, or attached to the cytoplasmic face of cadherins [23], or allowed to be free in the cytoplasm and appear in the nucleus [23]. Most of the oligolineage progenitors downstream of mouse HSCs [20,21] and human HSCs [241,242,256] have been isolated to homogeneity, and in some instances a comparison of their gene expression profiles reveals important clues as to genes responsible for particular commitments to differentiated fates [101; see below]. It is reasonable to expect that the reductionist approach to cataloging genes in this way will reveal many new clues about stem cell behaviors, but it will require a similar cataloging of cellular proteins (proteomics) to begin to reveal cell protein modifications that lead one to identify important pathways in stem cell behaviors.

Gene expression profile of stem and progenitor cells

An important question is how the progeny of multipotent cells adopt one fate from a choice of several. Lineage commitment and subsequent differentiation of multipotent cells should involve the selective activation and silencing of particular gene expression programs. There are single or pairs of transcription factors that have "master" roles in hematopoiesis in altering the phenotype of hematopoietic cells under defined circumstances. Combinatorial control is operated at the level of two or more lineage-specific regulators. This transcriptional control might be more complicated, considering protein–protein interactions mounted by the formation of multiprotein hematopoietic-specific protein complexes [311], and changes in the expression levels of transcription factors [312]. Furthermore, as in the case of cytokine signals, roles in transcription factors are also sometimes redundant. Finally, single multipotential progenitors appear to coexpress transcription factors and cytokine receptors related to multiple lineages [313].

Changes in chromatin structure, allowing access for RNA polymerase to initiate transcription, is essential for genetic programs to be transcribed [314,315]. The activation of chromatin structure can occur prior to significant expression of genes [316]. It has been hypothesized that a wide-open chromatin structure is maintained in early hematopoietic progenitors, enabling multilineage-affiliated programs to be accessible [317]. This phenomenon of open chromatin in early hematopoietic progenitors could lead to "promiscuous" expression of genes affiliated with multiple lineages in stem or progenitor cells prior to their lineage determination [109,318–320].

Promiscuous expression of multiple myeloid or lymphoid genes in hematopoietic branchpoints [83]

In a multipotential myeloid cell line, FDCP-mix, activation of the β-globin locus control region occurs prior to erythroid commitment [321]. Transcriptional enhancers for the immunoglobulin heavy chain, the CD3beta component of the T-cell receptor [322], and the myeloperoxidase (MPO) genes [323] are also DNase I hypersensitive in this cell line. Single cells of this cell line coexpress a variety of genes related to granulocyte/monocyte (GM) and megakaryocyte/erythrocyte (MegE) lineages, including MPO and β-globin by single cell RT-PCR studies [313]. Coexpression of MPO and β-globin was also found in a fraction of human Lin⁻CD34⁺ cells [313] and mouse intraembryonic hematopoietic progenitors in the aorta-gonad-mesonephros region [324].

Prospectively purified LT-HSC, oligopotent progenitors and lineage-committed progenitors have been used for a definitive sampling of the transcriptional profiles of cells at these particular stages of physiological hematopoiesis. The expression patterns of lineage-affiliated genes in each stage of hematopoiesis are largely consistent with their known functions. Using semiquantitative RT-PCR assay targeted for each purified population, SCL (Stem cell leukemia) [325,326] is expressed in HSCs and all myeloid progenitors. GATA-2 [327] and c-mpl are expressed in HSCs, CMPs and MEPs, but not in GMPs [21,83,109]. Other megakaryocyte/erythroid (MegE)-related genes such as NF-E2 [326], GATA-1 [328,329] and the Epo receptor are expressed in CMPs and MEPs but not in GMPs, and their expression levels are highest in MEPs [83]. Granulocyte-affiliated transcription factor, C/EBPα [330] is expressed in HSCs, CMPs and GMPs but not in MEPs, and its expression level is highest in GMPs [83]. All of these genes are expressed in CMPs, but not in CLPs or other late lymphoid progenitors, suggesting potential roles for each in myeloid-specific cell fate decisions. In contrast, the lymphoid-related transcription factor, Aiolos [331] is not expressed in any myeloid progenitors, nor in HSCs. Ikaros, an Aiolos partner nuclear factor, thought initially to be a lymphoid-specific transcription factor [181,332], is expressed in HSCs and all stages of hematopoiesis [333]. Interestingly, expression of Aiolos first appears at the CLP stage, and is highest in T- and B-cell progenitors [21,83]. Lymphoid-related GATA-3 [334] and Pax-5 [268] are expressed at a low level in adult marrow CLPs but not in myeloid progenitors and fetal liver CLPs [21,263].

These data provide a clearer view of gene expression regulation in hematopoietic development. First, the expression of many myeloid and lymphoid genes is mutually exclusive in each pathway. Second, CMPs express both MegE and GM-affiliated genes, and CLPs express both T and B lymphoid genes, although CMPs and CLPs have not committed to myeloid and lymphoid sublineages, respectively [21,83]. These data are consistent both with the priming hypothesis [335] and a model wherein chromatin is open prior to commitment, but the transcripts from that open chromatin are not critical for maturation [83].

The view of myeloid or lymphoid promiscuity has been significantly extended by using an oligonucleotide microarray analysis targeted for purified CMPs and CLPs. Genome-wide profiling by using microarray methods revealed that CMPs and CLPs coexpress a vast majority of GM and MegE-affiliated genes, and T, B and NK lymphoid genes, respectively [109]. Furthermore, coexpression of both GM and MegE-related genes in CMPs and of both T and B lymphoid genes in CLPs have been formally demonstrated at the level of single cells [83]. By using RT-PCR analysis targeted for single cells, CMPs coexpress MegE-related β-globin, EpoR, NF-E2 and GM-related MPO, G-CSFR and PU.1, while CLPs coexpress B-cell-related λ5 and/or Pax-5 and T-cell-related CD3δ and/or GATA-3 [83]. These results indicate that the expression of lineage-related genes can precede commitment, and suggest that the "promiscuous" expression of multiple lineage-related genes may allow a flexibility of commitment at these oligopotent stages: for differentiation towards T- and B-cell lineages in CLPs, and towards GM and MegE lineages in CMPs.

It is still unclear whether the primary mechanism of hematopoietic commitment could be operated first by opening chromatin at programmed sites, or whether the "priming" seen in promiscuous transcription patterns results from the presence of open chromatin and transcription factors that can form "sterile" transcripts. None the less, in priming stages, multiple differentiation programs might collaborate or compete with each other until one becomes dominant. These programs should include cross-talk among transcription factors or transcriptional complexes, because transcription factor activity can be potentiated [330] or suppressed [336,337] by interaction with other transcription factors. Changes in levels of key transcription factors [312,338] may also be critical for the lineage decision. Cross-talk between different cytokine signals may also be important, as single progenitors coexpress multiple cytokine receptors. Furthermore, fluctuations of gene expression of multiple differentiation programs in progenitors may lead to different differentiation outcomes in the microenvironment. In this context, both intrinsic and extrinsic factors could play a part in lineage determination.

Downregulation of genes irrelevant to committed lineages as a critical mechanism of lineage restriction

According to the "priming" model, commitment could be dependent on two independent molecular events: upregulation of differentiation programs related to selected lineages and the transcriptional abrogation of master control genes in the unselected lineages.

A striking example is Pax-5, a key molecule for restriction to B-cell lineage [268]. In normal hematopoiesis, Pax-5 expression initiates at the CLP stage, and is upregulated in proB cells, but undetectable in pro-T cells or myeloid cells. Expression of Pax-5 in pro-B cells is important not to differentiate into other lineage cells, because pro-B cells from Pax-5-deficient mice (Pax-5$^{-/-}$ pro-B cells) can differentiate into T cells, NK cells, granulocytes, macrophages and osteoclasts as well as B cells [268]. Pax-5$^{-/-}$ pro-B cells rearrange the D-J locus of IgH genes and express other pro-B related genes. Thus, even after a set of B lineage-associated genes begin to be transcribed, differentiation programs for other lineages are still accessible. Conversely, if Pax-5 is ectopically expressed in myeloid progenitors, enforced Pax-5 suppresses myeloid development presumably blocking signals from myelomonocytic cytokine receptors such as G-CSFR and GM-CSFR [339].

Similarly, enforced expression of PU.1 in pro-T cells can block T-cell differentiation [340]. Ectopic GATA-1 expression in GMPs also inhibits differentiation into granulocyte/monocyte lineages, but induces trans-differentiation into megakaryocytes and erythrocytes (H. Iwasaki, S. Mizuno, R.A. Wells *et al.*, unpublished data). A similar phenomenon is observed in ectopic cytokine receptors. Ectopic IL-2Rβ or GM-CSFR signals into CLPs can reprogram cells to myelomonocytic transdifferentiation [272].

These data indicate that termination of lineage-related gene expression is equally important for completion of lineage commitment. First, in committed progenitors, abrogated differentiation programs for unselected lineages are not totally erased after commitment, but could be reactivated by "instructive" signals including ectopic cytokine receptors and transcription factors. For example, GMPs might be restricted to GM lineages simply because GATA-1 is downregulated, and CLPs are likely lymphoid-restricted because they downregulate myeloid cytokine receptors. Second, differentiation programs into committed lineages can be operated on condition that transcription factors for unselected lineages are downregulated, as Pax-5 and PU.1 inhibit myeloid and T-cell differentiation programs, respectively.

Thus, hierarchically organized epigenetic programs that regulate transcription factors and cytokine receptors are critical to maintain hematopoietic homeostasis.

Transplantation of HSC in mouse and humans

It is fair to say that the field of bone marrow transplantation, later called hematopoietic cell transplantation (HCT), has provided one of the most striking medical advances in our lifetime and, similarly, the desire to understand cells involved in such transplants has opened the field of stem cell biology, first to hematopoietic stem cells, but then to other tissue-specific stem cells. It is important at the outset, however, to make sure that the scientific and clinical community uses the appropriate nomenclature for the type of transplant used, as misconceptions as to the cell type transplanted leads to misconceptions about the scientific or clinical results obtained [28,29]. Thus, the transplantation of complex mixtures of hematopoietic cells in bone marrow or mobilized peripheral blood is not the same as transplanting purified HSCs.

Clinical HCTs have been used for a variety of purposes, but the primary use is the ability to regenerate the hematopoietic tissues of a cancer patient who had received otherwise lethal doses of a myeloablative regimen of chemoradiotherapy [341,342]. Other uses have been the correction of inherited or acquired hematopoietic cell defects and dysplasias, and in animals the induction of transplantation tolerance to other cells tissues or organs cotransplanted from the HSC donor, the hematopoietic cell donor, and also the reversal of autoimmune disease [19; see Chapter 25].

It was not clear whether HSCs could replace HCT, as it was not clear whether a rapid and sustained regeneration of a particular hematopoietic outcome could be accomplished with the primitive HSCs alone, without having oligolineage progenitors in the transplant. Several experiments demonstrated in mice and in humans that HSCs are the principal cells that are functional in the transplant setting, and that by varying cell dose one could achieve both rapid and sustained regeneration of hematopoietic tissues (Fig. 8.8) [343]. Prospective isolation of HSCs with multiple markers allows the possibility that grafts would consist solely of HSCs, and of no other contaminating cells. There are two important advantages, at least theoretically, to the transplantation of HSCs rather than HCT-removal of cancer cells and removal of T cells. Autologous HCT from cancer patients can be accompanied by transplantation of the patient's cancer cells; in some diseases such as stage 4 breast cancer and many lymphomas the HCT populations to be transplanted that are contaminated with cancer cells varies from 20 to 40% of all transplants [344–346]. In patients with multiple myeloma, contamination of the graft is the rule and not the exception [347]. Therefore it was important to test whether positive selection of HSCs will eliminate or purge cancer cells. One such test is shown in Fig. 8.9.

Deliberate spiking of MPB with cell lines representing human breast cancer, human non-Hodgkin's lymphoma (NHL) and human myeloma

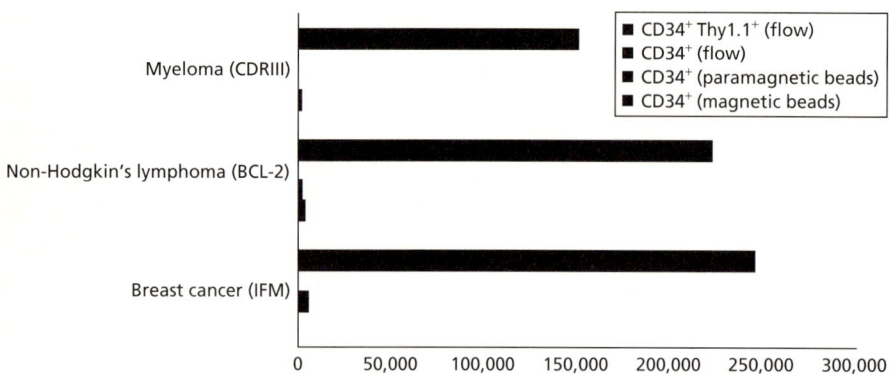

Fig. 8.9 Comparison between CD34 only and CD34⁺ Thy-1 isolation of human stem and progenitor cells in terms of fold depletion of human cancer cells. Mobilized peripheral blood (1.6×10^{10}) was spiked with 1.2×10^8 cancer cells (T47D breast cancer, SU DHL 6 non-Hodgkin's lymphoma (NHL) cells, or RPMI-LAV myeloma cells) prior to cell sorting. The CD34⁺ Thy-1 cells were flow sorted with a modified high-flow cytometer, as were the first CD34 flow sort test. The other devices were a commercial paramagnetic bead coupled Mab passed through magnetized steel mesh, and the last on a large magnetic bead device. Breast cancer cells were analyzed by immunofluorescence microscopy for cytokeratin, the NHL by Igh-BCL2 real time polymerase chain reaction (PCR), and the myeloma by CDR III real time PCR. The data are represented as fold reductin of cancer cells from the sorted CD34 or CD34⁺ Thy-1 cells. (E. Hanania, unpublished data.)

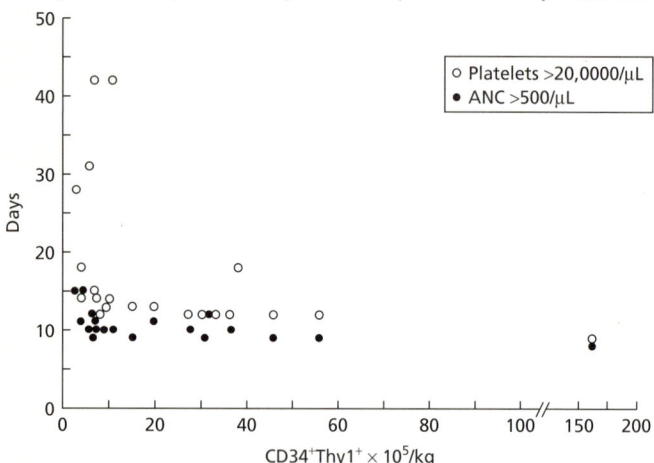

Fig. 8.10 Transplantation of highly purified human hematopoietic stem cells (HSCs) in patients with metastatic breast cancer. Shown are the times to engraftment of neutrophils (absolute neutrophil count [ANC >500/μL]) following transplantation with purified CD34⁺ Thy1-1⁺ hematopoietic stem cells. (E. Hanania, unpublished data.)

was performed, and four methods of HCT/HSC isolates were carried out to determine the full reduction of contaminating cancer cells. Two independent methods to identify breast cancer cells were used: a visual test for cells carrying breast cell cytokeratins, and a flow-based method. Myeloma and B-cell lymphoma representative cells were detected by a DNA PCR technique specific for the immunoglobin heavy chain rearrangements in these B lineage cells. All three techniques have a sensitivity of 10^{-5}–10^{-6}.

Three techniques were used to isolate cells based on CD34 markers only, one of which is flow-based and two of which use pure magnetic labeled anti-CD34 antibodies followed by a magnetic devised based separation. Over 10^5-fold reductions of contaminating cancer cells were accomplished with the multiparameter cell sorting of CD34⁺Thy⁺ cells from MPB, whereas the other techniques were at least two to three orders of magnitude less efficient (Fig. 8.9).

The data in Fig. 8.10 show the result of one of three clinical trials in terms of time to engraftment of absolute neutrophil count (ANC) >500 and platelets >20,000/μL of blood [344,345,348]. These are very similar to the times to achieve this level of engraftment using unmanipulated MPB as the HCT transplant. A dose–response for mouse HSC in syngeneic transplants is similar (Fig. 8.11) [343]. Even in acute myeloid leukemia (AML), HSC can be separated from leukemic stem cells by surface markers [349]. Therefore, the stage is set to test whether transplantation of cancer-depleted HSCs will lead to clinical benefits when compared to transplantation of cancer-containing unmanipulated HCT grafts.

Allogeneic HCT transplants have been plagued from the beginning by the appearance of graft-vs.-host disease (GVHD) as a result of contaminating T cells [350]. Mice receiving allogeneic HSCs have little or no contaminating T cells, and never develop GVHD [343,351]. Dose–response comparisons of purified HSC transplants in syngeneic, in the matched unrelated donor (MUD) allogeneic, and in the fully allogeneic circumstances have been carried out and, for the most part, doses of HSCs sufficient to allow rapid and sustained engraftment can be achieved without contaminating T cells (Fig. 8.12) [351; see Chapter 25]. However, at lower HSC doses, the number of HSCs required for engraftment can be 10 times higher than that required for syngeneic HSC engraftment (Fig. 8.12) [343]. In these cases one can achieve nearly equal levels of engraftment at the same HSC dose between the syngeneic and allogeneic models if the allogeneic hosts had received either monoclonal antibodies that eliminate NK and T-cell populations [351,352], or facilitator cells (FCs) [353–355]. Inclusion of donor FC populations with HSCs eliminates host residual T and NK cells, whereas in the absence of such FC or antibodies that eliminate T and NK populations, the hosts have persistent T-cell chimerism that represent both donor and host, while the B-cell lineage and the myeloid lineages are entirely from the donor in the myeloablative setting [351–353]. There are two kinds of FCs found in mouse bone marrow and lymphoid tissues: classic CD8α⁺TCR⁺CD3⁺ T cells and CD8α⁺TCR⁻CD3⁻ FCs [353–355]. The immunocompetent CD8α⁺TCR⁺ T cells have some capacity for GVHD disease, and so there is great interest in understanding the nature and function of CD8α⁺TCR⁻CD3⁻ FCs [353]. There are two other kinds of cells that share this phenotype: CD8α positive immature dendritic cells and Veto cells [353,356,357]. We have proposed that all three cell types are in fact a single cell class, and that it is only the assays that makes one believe that they are different lymphoid cell subsets [353]. This view is strengthened by the recent findings of Steinman et al. [358] that CD8α⁺ dendritic cells that do not have active or appropriate costimulation can in fact lead to the inactivation or disappearance of T cells (and, we propose, NK cells) that have receptors which recognize them. Thus, a cell that facilitates

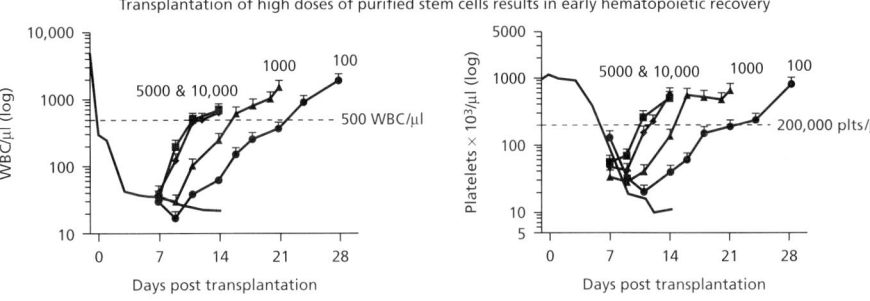

Fig. 8.11 Hematopoietic recovery in lethally irradiated C57BL/Ka mice syngeneically transplanted with different doses of purified HSCs. Irradiated mice were injected with 100 (solid circles), 1000 (triangles), 5000 (solid triangles) or 10,000 (squares) HSCs. Shown are the recovery kinetics for white blood cell (WBC), and platelet counts. (From [343] with permission.)

KTLS cell dose	Days to reach 500 WBC/μl (10% of normal)	200,000 plts/μl (20% of normal)
10,000	11	11
5000	11	12
1000	15	14
100	22	23

KTLS ... c-kit$^+$ Thy-1.1^{lo} Lin$^{-/lo}$ Sca-1$^+$ cells

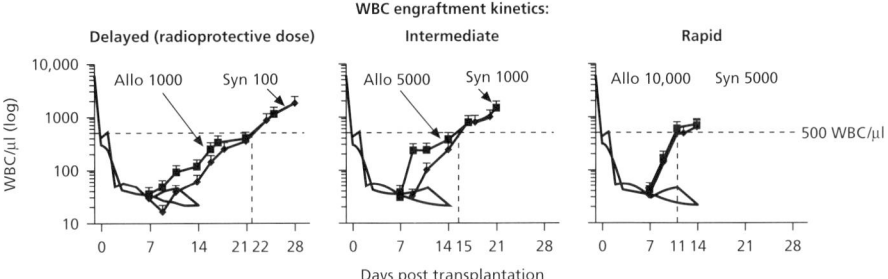

Fig. 8.12 Engraftment kinetics of allogeneic vs. congeneic purified HSCs. Comparison of stem-cell dose required to achieve early hematopoietic recovery in syngeneic vs. allogeneic irradiated mice. Syngeneic or allogeneic mice were transplanted with purified Thy-1^{lo}Sca-1$^+$Lin$^{-/lo}$c-kit^+ (KTLS) cells and bled on sequential days post-transplant. The kinetics of white blood cell recovery were categorized into delayed, intermediate and rapid recovery. (Adapted from [5] with permission.)

engraftment of allogeneic HSCs might be a cell that presents MHC/peptide antigens to reactive T and NK cells without delivering a co-stimulatory signal, or induce the cells to undergo activation-induced cell death; and these same cells might be responsible for the veto of active CD4 and CD8 T cells that recognize and respond to them.

It has been known since the pioneering work of Main and Prehn that bone marrow chimeras are usually transplantation tolerant to cells tissues or organs from the hematopoietic cell donor [359]. This method of induction of transplantation tolerance has been substantiated with pure HSC transplants [352,360], either in the myeloablative or nonmyeloablative setting, and whether the transplant is concurrent with the HSC transplant or occurs months later [352,360]. Hematopoietic chimeras in humans are also usually specifically transplant tolerant of donor tissues, and new trials for inducing tolerance with bone marrow cells in a nonmyeloablative but lymphoablative setting along with organ allografts from the bone marrow donor are underway [361].

Partial or complete replacement of an autoimmune diabetes-prone hematopoietic system in mice with purified HSCs from diabetes-resistant strains of mice in the prediabetic period completely precludes progression to diabetes (see Chapter 25), whereas the same treatment of already diabetic hosts along with donor strain islet cell transplants cures the small numbers of mice undergoing this protocol [362]. This too has been accomplished in both the myeloablative and the nonmyeloablative but lymphoablative setting.

Cotransplantation of HSC and hematopoietic progenitors to protect against opportunistic infections

The bane of clinical HCT in terms of infectious disease is the often lethal infections with *Aspergillus fumigatus*, CMV and *Pseudomonas* [363,364]. Small numbers of each of these infectious organisms given to HSC transplanted mice can result in universal lethality mimicking the morbidity and mortality that occurs in patients [363,364]. With the isolation of clonal CLPs, clonal CMPs and GMPs, cellular therapies for each of these disorders has been investigated. Cotransplantation of HSCs and CLPs can completely preclude the lethality of mCMV infection in both syngeneic and allogeneic protocols [381]. Cotransplantation of HSCs and CMPs and GMPs can prevent the lethal consequences of *Aspergillus* infections if the *Aspergillus* is given on day 9, 11 or 14 after HSC transplantation, and addition of G-CSF to these HSC/CMP/GMP transplant protocols precludes *Aspergillus* infections given just 3 days after transplantation [363]. Similar CMP *plus* GMP protocols are sufficient to eliminate *Pseudomonas* infections, and in both cases these treatments work in both the syngeneic and allogeneic settings.

Origin of leukemia: leukemic stem cells

To understand the mechanisms of leukemic transformation, it is important to understand the clonogenic leukemia-initiating stem cells and their cellular origin. Malignant self-renewal might be achieved if cells can proliferate without maturation. If one views leukemia development as a series of steps in malignant progression, malignant self-renewal may be obtained through several transformation steps:
1 a block in differentiation;
2 an acquisition of self-renewing potent proliferative capacity; and
3 avoidance of programmed cell death by cell-intrinsic pathways and by immunosurveillance.

A set of early stem/progenitor cells with extensive proliferation, or with reduced programmed cell death that are not yet malignant, may form "preleukemic" clones, and these clones may receive additional oncogenic events that induce differentiation blocks at a progenitor stage to become leukemia.

Accumulation of mutations as a precondition for malignant transformation in human acute leukemias

The usefulness of molecular markers for leukemia, including oncogenic fusion proteins resulting from leukemia-specific chromosomal translocations, has disclosed the multistep nature of acute leukemia development. A typical case is chronic myelogenous leukemia (CML). CML-specific t(9;22) Philadelphia chromosome and its resultant *Bcr-Abl* fusion gene has been shown to be present in all myeloid cells, B cells and rare T cells. Additional mutation(s) and epigenetic changes in patterns of gene expression are required for blastic transformation into acute leukemia.

A similar scenario could be applied to the development of a fraction of *de novo* acute leukemias. The translocation t(8;21) is a frequent chromosomal abnormality in adult AML. AML1-ETO chimeric protein that is the product of the t(8;21) translocated genomic region is continuously detectable in t(8;21) AML patients who maintain long-term remission for more than 10 years. Although these patients are clinically "cured", AML1-ETO is expressed in various hematopoietic lineage cells including B cells, erythroid and megakaryocyte colony-forming cells [365]. A fraction of HSCs (Thy-1$^+$CD34$^+$Lin$^-$CD38$^-$) in remission marrow also are AML1-ETO transcript positive [349]. In childhood t(8;21) AML, AML1-ETO fusions are retrospectively detected in neonatal Guthrie spots [366]. A plausible explanation for these data is that AML1-ETO fusion is at the level of HSCs (in some cases *in utero*), and might persist until several secondary mutations and epigenetic events collaborate with AML1-ETO to lead to leukemic transformation. Because t(8;21) is exclusively found in AML-M2, additional transforming event(s) might occur at the level of granulocyte/macrophage-committed progenitors.

Acquisition of chromosomal translocations *in utero* is also demonstrated in infant t(4;11) and childhood t(21;21) acute leukemias. In t(4;11) acute lymphoblastic anemia (ALL), clonotypic MLL-AF4 genomic fusion sequences were demonstrated to be present in neonatal blood spots from patients who were diagnosed with ALL at ages 5 months to 2 years, and therefore cells with t(4;11) have arisen during fetal hematopoiesis *in utero*. TEL-AML1 fusions resulting from t(12;21) were shown to be present in neonatal blood spots [366–368]. TEL-AML1 was also detected in identical twins, whose genomic fusion sequence was identical [369]. In these cases, t(12;21) ALL developed at ~10 years of age, indicating that cells with TEL-AML1 persisted more than 10 years before leukemic transformation. These data suggest that MLL-AF4 and TEL-AML1 fusions must have occurred at an early stage of hematopoiesis, almost certainly at the level of self-renewing HSCs that can persist in the long term.

TEL-AML1$^+$ ALL cells in twins sometimes possess identical IgH rearrangement. Therefore, TEL-AML1$^+$ pro-B cells could be already present in fetal hematopoiesis, persist in the long term in twins, and the TEL-AML1$^+$ pro-B cells are transformed by additional mutational events after birth, although it is not clear whether the TEL-AML1 fusion is originally formed at the level of HSCs or pro-B cells in the fetus. In childhood ALL, preleukemic B or T-cell progenitors appear to persist in the long term; "leukaemic clones" possessing clonal T-cell receptor or IgH rearrangements are reported to persist more than 3 years after achieving complete remission [370]. Thus, it is reasonable to speculate that childhood ALL might develop from not fully transformed T- or B-cell committed progenitors that can persist in the long term, perhaps by acquiring the property of self-renewal at an early stage. The longevity of "preleukemic" lymphoid progenitor clones in childhood ALL may enable them to undergo additional leukemic events for final leukemic transformation.

These data strongly suggest that leukemic transformation commonly occurs by multistep processes. In mice and in humans, the only cell in the myeloid lineage that self-renews over long periods of time is the LT-HSC [1]. The preleukemic clone should exist in the long term to encounter multiple mutational events. Therefore, it appears that the accumulation of mutations occur as a precondition for leukemia development at the level of HSCs, or in progenitors that had gained the capacity of self-renewal.

Final leukemic transformation can occur at the level of myeloid progenitors

Several lines of evidence show that final myeloid leukemic transformation can only occur at the level of progenitors that have acquired the property of self-renewal. In contrast, lymphoid malignancies such as ALL and malignant lymphoma are made up of neoplastic cells with clonally rearranged T-cell receptor or immunoglobulin genes. Whereas myeloid progenitors and myelomonocytic cells are not self-renewing, lymphocytes that contribute to the memory pool are self-renewing. Thus, the final transformation to lymphatic neoplasms can occur in cells that already have regulated self-renewal capacity.

In contrast, myeloid cells lack stage-specific clonal markers. Self-renewing leukemic stem cells are present in a minor population of AML cells that possess phenotypes similar to, but distinct from normal HSCs. Long-term proliferative AML cell subsets have been examined using (non-obese diabetic) NOD-SCID reconstitution assays. AML-repopulating cells are frequently found within the CD34$^+$CD38$^-$ or CD34$^+$CD71$^-$HLA-DR$^-$ fraction, the phenotype of which is similar to that of human HSCs [371]. However, it remains unclear whether these clonogenic leukemia cells with HSC phenotype represent transformation at the level of HSCs; leukaemic stem cells may have changed their surface phenotypes into those that mimic HSC phenotypes. In fact, although a subset of CD34$^+$CD38$^-$ normal marrow cells that are HSCs are Lin$^-$ and Thy-1$^+$, a majority of MPO positive t(8;21) AML blasts are CD34$^+$CD38$^-$, but lack Thy-1 expression [349]. Thus, in this case t(8;21) AML blasts either lose CD38 expression exhibiting an unusual phenotype, or represent a stage of CD34$^+$CD38$^-$Lin$^-$Thy-1$^-$ cells [349]. Furthermore, only a fraction of CD34$^+$CD38$^-$Thy-1$^-$ AML blasts are clonogenic leukemia cells.

In some mouse AML models, transformation has been formally shown to occur at myeloid progenitor stages (Fig. 8.13). A set of mouse lines transgenic for AML-specific oncogenic fusions are established by using the promoter of small calcium-binding protein encoding genes *mrp*8. The MRP8 promotor is active at very low levels in CMPs, and higher levels in GMPs, and highest levels in granulocytes and monocytes; the MRP8 promotor is inactive in HSC, MEP or other lymphoid stages.

A mouse model of AML-M2 is established by expressing AML1/ETO driven by the MRP8 promoter. MRP8 AML1/ETO transgenic mice did not develop leukemia. After the injection of a DNA alkylating mutagen, *N*-ethyl-*N*-nitrosourea (ENU), however, almost 55% of mice develop AML-M2. Thus, AML can develop directly from myeloid progenitors [372]. Similarly, PML/RARα is a product of the t(15;17) translocation, and MRP8-PML/RARα transgenic mice develop acute promyelocytic leukemia (APL)-like disorders [373]. The frequency and rapidity of PML-RARα leukemias increases when they are crossed to MPR8 bcl-2 mice [374].

More strikingly, inhibition of apoptotic pathways alone can lead to leukemia development at progenitor stages. In these studies an antiapoptotic protein, Bcl-2 is expressed under the control of MRP8 promoter. MRP8-Bcl-2 mice display increased numbers of mature monocytes, but do not develop acute leukemia. However, an additional introduction of Fas (lpr/lpr) mutations into these mice results in transformation into

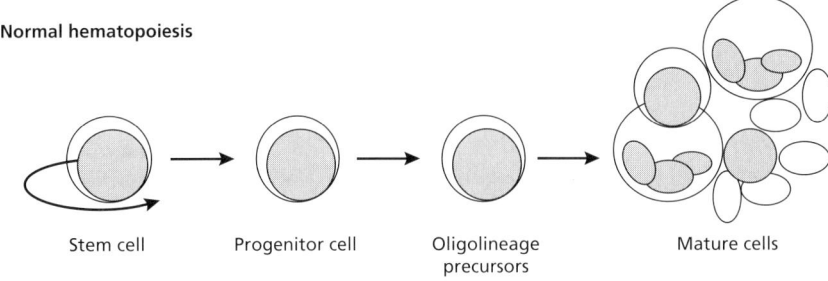
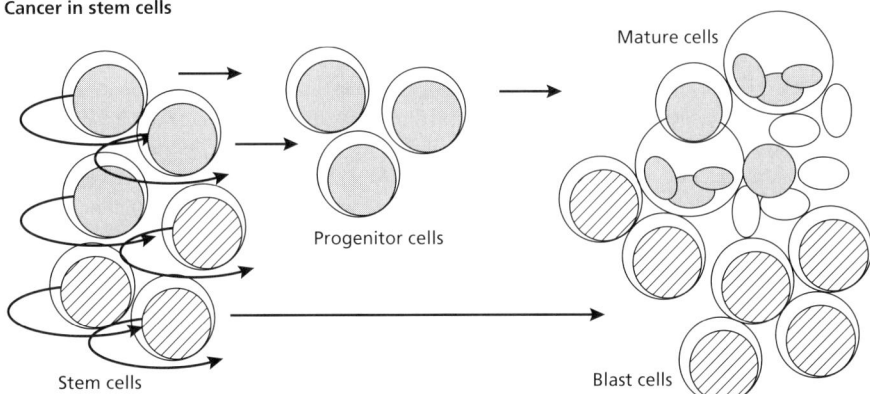
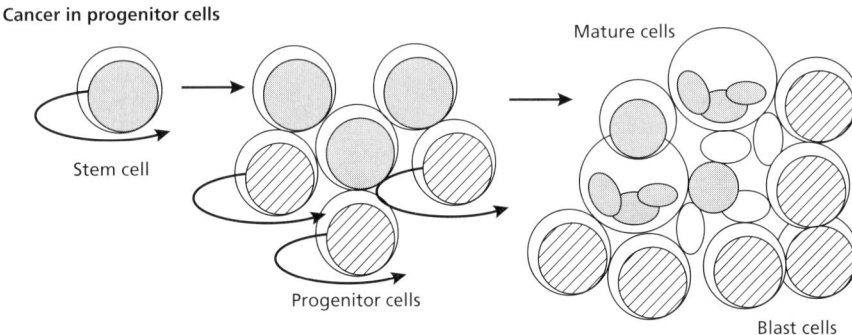

Fig. 8.13 Comparison of stem cell self-renewal during normal hematopoiesis and leukemic transformation. During normal hematopoiesis, the signaling pathways that regulate self-renewal are tightly controlled, allowing proper differentiation to each of the mature blood cell lineages (top). Dysregulation of self-renewal mechanisms in transformed cancer stem cells (hatched nuclei) leads to uncontrolled self-renewal and the production of leukemic blast cells (middle and bottom). The leukemic population capable of sustaining disease is often distinct from the blast population, and may reside in the stem cell (middle) or progenitor cell (bottom) compartment. Importantly, if the transformation event occurs in a progenitor cell, it must endow the progenitor cell with the self-renewal properties of a stem cell, because the progenitors would otherwise differentiate. (Courtesy of Julie Christensen PhD, Department of Pathology, Stanford University School of Medicine, Stanford CA94305.)

AML. We found that 15–30% of these mice 3–8 weeks following birth developed AML (M2) [375]. These leukemias are transplantable to syngeneic athymic mice, but not euthymic mice (C. Jamison, S. Jaiswal and I.L. Weissman, unpublished data). Thus, impairment of intrinsic bcl-2 inhibitable or extrinsic Fas-mediated and/or T-cell-induced apoptotic factors are critical for leukemic transformation at CMP and GMP stages. Even mpr8;bcr-abl mice have increased frequencies of conversions to acute blastic leukemias if crossed to mpr8;bcl-2 strains (S. Jaiswal, D. Traver, T. Miyamoto, in press PNAS 2003).

Impairment of differentiation machinery alone can induce accumulation of myeloid progenitors

Loss of function of myeloid transcription factors including CEBPα and PU.1 has been suggested to have a critical role in the progression of AML. C/EBPα is a key factor for granulopoiesis, and PU.1 is critical for myelomonocyte and B-cell development. A considerable fraction of AML patients harbour C/EBPα with dominant-negative mutations in one allele that inhibits normal functions of this protein [376]. It is most likely that loss of function of these transcription factors might induce a differentiation block in AML. AML1-ETO and/or oncogenic fusion proteins also can downregulate C/EBPα [376,377] and PU.1 [378].

However, differentiation block itself cannot be sufficient for leukemic transformation. In animals that are conditionally depleted of C/EBPα, granulocytes and monocytes disappear from the peripheral blood. Interestingly, the bone marrow is occupied by more than 30% immature myeloblasts, which satisfies the diagnostic criteria for AML in humans. However, the mice displayed normal levels of hemoglobin and platelets in the blood, and erythropoiesis and thrombopoiesis were intact in the bone marrow. Invasion of myeloblasts is not present in nonhematopoietic organs. These data indicate that C/EBPα$^{-/-}$ mice do not manifest some of the other characteristics usually found in human AML. In these animals, GMPs are completely eliminated, and myeloid differentiation is blocked at the transition from CMPs to GMPs.

Other "preleukemic" diseases such as chronic myeloproliferative disorders or myelodysplastic syndromes do not exhibit such accumulation of myeloblasts. In contrast, mice with loss of C/EBPα function alone mimic acute leukemia. Thus, breakage of myeloid differentiation programs, blockade of programmed cell death, escape from phagocytosis [379] and acquisition of self-renewal, as well as abnormal proliferation-stimulating signals might later trigger final leukemic transformation at the level of myeloid progenitors in at least a fraction of AML.

Potential usefulness of purified hematopoietic stem and progenitor cells for treatment of acute leukemias

Considering the multistep nature of leukemia progression, separation between self-renewing leukemic stem cells and normal HSCs in patients' bone marrow might be a potent tool in clinics, because purified HSCs are an ideal source for autologous HCT. So far, the CD34$^+$Thy1$^+$ HSC population has been purified from malignant disorders such as multiple myeloma, NHL and metastatic breast cancer, and used in autologous hematopoietic transplantation [344,345,348]. In these disorders, CD34$^+$Thy1$^+$ HSCs are intact, and the use of purified HSCs in transplantation has significant merit in that the transplanted cells are free from self-renewing malignant cells. This technique could be applied to acute leukemias because the final leukemic transformation appears to occur at progenitor stages at a considerable fraction of AML and ALL. Purified HSCs do not contain T cells, and therefore are also useful in allogeneic hematopoietic transplantation from HLA-mismatched donors.

Conclusions

With the development of a general method to isolate prospectively hematopoietic stem and progenitor cells [1,52,56] it has become possible to construct lineage pathways from LT-HSC to mature blood cells. With the exception of memory T and B lymphocytes in the entire hematopoietic lineage, only LT-HSC self-renew, and this self-renewal capacity is tightly regulated [1]. The genetic regulation of HSC self-renewal includes regulation of programmed cell death, regulation of cell-division frequency and regulation of transition to multipotent and to oligopotent progenitors. Part of this regulation appears to involve the Wnt/Fzd/β-catenin pathway, restricted to LT-HSC in the myeloid differentiation pathways. Prospectively isolated HSCs and progenitors are useful scientifically to understand the gene expression pathways in self-renewal and in lineage commitment. These same isolated HSCs and progenitors appear to be useful in clinical HCT, whether to regenerate myeloablated hematopoietic system in cancer patients, to condition allogeneic hosts for donor stain tissue or organ grafts or even to replace an autoimmune-prone hematolymphoid system with an autoimmune-resistant donor population. Finally, the concept of self-renewal as the critical regulated event limited to HSCs in normal hematopoiesis has now been extended to the hypothesis that within leukemias and cancers are relatively infrequent populations of leukemia or cancer stem cells that undergo poorly regulated self-renewal. Prospective isolation of leukemia stem cells and of cancer stem cells should allow more direct approaches to find immune and drug therapies for target molecules restricted to these malignant stem cells.

References

1 Weissman IL. Stem cells: units of development, units of regeneration, and units in evolution. *Cell* 2000; **100**: 157–68.

2 Becker A, McCulloch E, Till J. Cytological demonstration of the clonal nature of spleen colonies derived from transplanted mouse marrow cells. *Nature* 1963; **197**: 452–4.

3 Metcalf D, Moore MAS. *Hematopoietic Cells*. Amsterdam: North-Holland, 1971.

4 Smith LG, Weissman IL, Heimfeld S. Clonal analysis of hematopoietic stem-cell differentiation *in vivo*. *Proc Natl Acad Sci U S A* 1991; **88**: 2788–92.

5 Wagers AJ, Sherwood RI, Christensen JL et al. Little evidence for developmental plasticity of adult hematopoietic stem cells. *Science* 2002; **297**: 2256–9.

6 Uchida N. *Characterization of mouse hematopoietic stems cells*. PhD thesis, 1992. Stanford University.

7 Osawa M, Hanada K, Hamala H. et al. Long-term lymphohematopoietic reconstitution by a single CD34-low/negative hematopoietic stem cell. *Science* 1996; **273**: 242–5.

8 Lemischka IR, Raulet DH, Mulligan RC. Developmental potential and dynamic behavior of hematapoietic stem cells. *Cell* 1986; **45**: 917–27.

9 Brazelton TR, Rossi FM, Keshet GI et al. From marrow to brain: expression of neuronal phenotypes in adult mice. *Science* 2000; **290**: 1775–9.

10 Ferrari G, Cusella-De Angelis G, Coletta M et al. Muscle regeneration by bone marrow-derived myogenic progenitors. *Science* 1998; **279**: 1528–30.

11 Gussoni E, Soneoka Y, Strickland CD et al. Dystrophin expression in the mdx mouse restored by stem cell transplantation. *Nature* 1999; **401**: 390–4.

12 Jackson KA, Majka SM, Wang H et al. Regeneration of ischemic cardiac muscle and vascular endothelium by adult stem cells. *J Clin Invest* 2001; **107**: 1395–402.

13 Krause DS, Theise ND, Collector MI et al. Multiorgan, multi-lineage engraftment by a single bone marrow-derived stem cell. *Cell* 2001; **105**: 369–77.

14 Mezey E, Chandross KJ, Harta G et al. Turning blood into brain: cells bearing neuronal antigens generated *in vivo* from bone marrow. *Science* 2000; **290**: 1779–82.

15 Orlic D, Kajstura J, Chimenti S et al. Bone marrow cells regenerate infarcted myocardium. *Nature* 2001; **410**: 701–5.

16 Petersen BE, Bowen WC, Patrene KD et al. Bone marrow as a potential source of hepatic oval cells. *Science* 1999; **284**: 1168–70.

17 Sata M, Saiura A, Kunisato A et al. Hematopoietic stem cells differentiate into vascular cells that participate in the pathogenesis of atherosclerosis. *Nat Med* 2002; **8**: 403–9.

18 Shimizu K, Sugiyama S, Aikawa M et al. Host bone-marrow cells are a source of donor intimal smooth-muscle-like cells in murine aortic transplant arteriopathy. *Nat Med* 2001; **7**: 738–41.

19 Weissman IL. Translating stem and progenitor cell biology to the clinic: barriers and opportunities. *Science* 2000; **287**: 1442–6.

20 Kondo M, Weissman IL, Akashi K. Identification of clonogenic common lymphoid progenitors in mouse bone marrow. *Cell* 1997; **91**: 661–72.

21 Akashi K, Traver D, Miyamoto T. et al. A clonogenic common myeloid progenitor that gives rise to all myeloid lineages. *Nature* 2000; **404**: 193–7.

22 Allsopp RC, Morin G, Horner J et al. The effect of TERT overexpression on the long term transplantation capacity of hematopoietic stem cells. *Nat Med* 2003; **9**: 369–71.

23 Reya T, Morrison SJ, Clarke MF et al. Stem cells, cancer, and cancer stem cells. *Nature* 2001; **414**: 105–11.

24 Till JE, McCulloch EA. A direct measurement of the radiation sensitivity of normal mouse bone marrow cells. *Radiation Res* 1961; **14**: 1419–30.

25 McCulloch EA, Siminovitch L, Till JE. Spleen-colony formation in anemic mice of genotype W/W^v. *Science* 1964; **144**: 844–6.

26 Siminovitch L, McCulloch E, Till J. The distribution of colony-forming cells among spleen colonies. *J Cell Comp Physiol* 1963; **62**: 327–36.

27 Abramson S, Miller RG, Phillips RA. The identification in adult bone marrow of pluripotent and restricted stem cells of the myeloid and lymphoid systems. *J Exp Med* 1977; **145**: 1567–79.

28 Weissman IL, Anderson DJ, Gage F. Stem and progenitor cells: origins, phenotypes, lineage commitments, and transdifferentiations. *Annu Rev Cell Dev Biol* 2001; **17**: 387–403.

29 Anderson DJ, Gage FH, Weissman IL. Can stem cells cross lineage boundaries? *Nat Med* 2001; **7**: 393–5.

30 Lagasse E, Shizuru JA, Uchida N et al. Toward regenerative medicine. *Immunity* 2001; **14**: 425–36.

31 Jiang Y, Jahagirdar BN, Reinhardt RL, Low WC, Largaespada DA, Verfaillie CM. Pluripotency of mesenchymal stem cells derived from adult marrow. *Nature* 2002; **418**: 41–9.

32 Morrison SJ, White PM, Zock C et al. Prospective identification, isolation by flow cytometry, and *in vivo* self-renewal of multipotent mammalian neural crest stem cells. *Cell* 1999; **96**: 737–49.

33 Palmer TD, Takahashi J, Gage FH. The adult rat hippocampus contains primordial neural stem cells. *Mol Cell Neurosci* 1997; **8**: 389–404.

34 Reynolds BA, Weiss S. Generation of neurons and astrocytes from isolated cells of the adult mammalian central nervous system. *Science* 1992; **255**: 1707–10.

35 Stemple DL, Anderson DJ. Isolation of a stem cell for neurons and glia from the mammalian neural crest. *Cell* 1992; **71**: 973–85.

36 Suhonen JO, Peterson DA, Ray J, Gage FH. Differentiation of adult hippocampus-derived

progenitors into olfactory neurons *in vivo*. *Nature* 1996; **383**: 624–7.

37 Taylor G, Lehrer MS, Jensen PJ *et al*. Involvement of follicular stem cells in forming not only the follicle but also the epidermis. *Cell* 2000; **102**: 451–61.

38 Uchida N, Buck DW, He D *et al*. Direct isolation of human central nervous system stem cells. *Proc Natl Acad Sci U S A* 2000; **97**: 14720–5.

39 Jacobson LO, Marks EK, Gaston EO *et al*. Effect of spleen protection on mortality following x-irradiation. *J Lab Clin Med* 1949; **34**: 1538–43.

40 Jacobson LO, Simmons EL, Marks EK *et al*. Recovery from radiation injury. *Science* 1951; **113**: 510–11.

41 Lorenz E, Uphoff DE, Reid TR *et al*. Modification of acute irradiation injury in mice and guinea pigs by bone marrow injection. *Radiology* 1951; **58**: 863–77.

42 Gengozian N, Urso IS, Congdon CC *et al*. Thymus specificity in lethally irradiated mice treated with rat bone marrow. *Proc Soc Exp Biol* 1957; **96**: 714.

43 Ford CE, Hamerton JL, Barnes DWH *et al*. Cytological identification of radiation chimaeras. *Nature* 1956; **177**: 239–47.

44 Nowell P, Cole L, Habermeyer J *et al*. Growth and continued function of rat marrow cells in x-radiated mice. *Cancer Res* 1956; **16**: 258.

45 Wu A, Till J, Siminovitch L *et al*. Cytological evidence for a relationship between normal hematopoietic colony-forming cells and cells of the lymphoid system. *J Exp Med* 1963; **127**: 455–67.

46 Magli MC, Iscove NN, Odartchenko N. Transient nature of early haematopoietic spleen colonies. *Nature* 1982; **295**: 527–9.

47 Visser JW, Van Bekkum DW. Purification of pluripotent hemopoietic stem cells: past and present. *Exp Hematol* 1990; **18**: 248–56.

48 Na Nakorn T, Traver D, Weissman IL *et al*. Myeloerythroid-restricted progenitors are sufficient to confer radioprotection and provide the majority of day 8 CFU-S. *J Clin Invest* 2002; **109**: 1579–85.

49 Jones RJ, Wagner JE, Celano P *et al*. Separation of pluripotent haematopoietic stem cells from spleen colony-forming cells. *Nature* 1990; **347**: 188–9.

50 Morrison SJ, Weissman IL. The long-term repopulating subset of hematopoietic stem cells is deterministic and isolatable by phenotype. *Immunity* 1994; **1**: 661–73.

51 Morrison SJ, Wandycz AM, Hemmati HD *et al*. Identification of a lineage of multipotent hematopoietic progenitors. *Development* 1997; **124**: 1929–39.

52 Spangrude GJ, Heimfeld S, Weissman IL. Purification and characterization of mouse hematopoietic stem cells. *Science* 1988; **241**: 58–62.

53 Kohler G, Milstein C. Continuous cultures of fused cells secreting antibody of predefined specificity. *Nature* 1975; **256**: 495–7.

54 Hulett HR, Bonner WA, Barrett J *et al*. Cell sorting: automated separation of mammalian cells as a function of intracellular fluorescence. *Science* 1969; **166**: 747–9.

55 Ezine S, Weissman IL, Rouse RV. Bone marrow cells give rise to distinct cell clones within the thymus. *Nature* 1984; **309**: 629–31.

56 Muller-Sieburg CE, Whitlock CA, Weissman IL. Isolation of two early B lymphocyte progenitors from mouse marrow: a committed pre-pre-B cell and a clonogenic Thy-1-lo hematopoietic stem cell. *Cell* 1986; **44**: 653–62.

57 Wu AM, Till JE, Siminovitch L *et al*. A cytological study of the capacity for differentiation of normal hematopoietic colony-forming cells. *J Cell Physiol* 1967; **69**: 177–84.

58 Dexter TM, Allen TD, Lajtha LG. Conditions controlling the proliferation of haemopoietic stem cells *in vitro*. *J Cell Physiol* 1977; **91**: 335–44.

59 Weilbaecher K, Weissman I, Blume K *et al*. Culture of phenotypically defined hematopoietic stem cells and other progenitors at limiting dilution on Dexter monolayers. *Blood* 1991; **78**: 945–52.

60 Eaves C, Cashman J, Eaves A. Methodology of long-term culture of human hematopoietic cells *in vitro*. *J Tissue Culture Method* 1991; **13**: 55–62.

61 Visser JW, Bauman JG, Mulder AH *et al*. Isolation of murine pluripotent hemopoietic stem cells. *J Exp Med* 1984; **159**: 1576–90.

62 Ikuta K, Weissman IL. Evidence that hematopoietic stem cells express mouse c-*kit* but do not depend on steel factor for their generation. *Proc Natl Acad Sci U S A* 1992; **89**: 1502–6.

63 Uchida N, Weissman IL. Searching for hematopoietic stem cells: evidence that Thy-1.1^{lo}Lin$^-$Sca-1$^+$ cells are the only stem cells in C57BL/Ka-Thy-1.1 bone marrow. *J Exp Med* 1992; **175**: 175–84.

64 Baum CM, Weissman IL, Tsukamoto AS *et al*. Isolation of a candidate human hematopoietic stem-cell population. *Proc Natl Acad Sci U S A* 1992; **89**: 2804–8.

65 Civin CI, Strauss LC, Brovall C *et al*. Antigenic analysis of hematopoiesis. III. A hematopoietic progenitor cell surface antigen defined by a monoclonal antibody raised against KG-1a cells. *J Immunol* 1984; **133**: 157–65.

66 Adolfsson J, Borge OJ, Bryder D *et al*. Upregulation of Flt3 expression within the bone marrow Lin(−)Sca1(+)c-*kit*(+) stem cell compartment is accompanied by loss of self-renewal capacity. *Immunity* 2001; **15**: 659–69.

67 Christensen JL, Weissman IL. Flk-2 is a marker in hematopoietic stem cell differentiation: a simple method to isolate long-term stem cells. *Proc Natl Acad Sci U S A* 2001; **98**: 14541–6.

68 Uchida N, Sutton RE, Friera AM *et al*. HIV, but not murine leukemia virus, vectors mediate high efficiency gene transfer into freshly isolated G$_0$/G$_1$ human hematopoietic stem cells. *Proc Natl Acad Sci U S A* 1998; **95**: 11939–44.

69 Petzer AL. Hogge DE, Landsdorp PM *et al*. Self-renewal of primitive human hematopoietic cells (long-term-culture-initiating cells) *in vitro* and their expansion in defined medium. *Proc Natl Acad Sci U S A* 1996; **93**: 1470–4.

70 Larochelle A, Vormoor J, Hanenberg H *et al*. Identification of primitive human hematopoietic cells capable of repopulating NOD/SCID mouse bone marrow: implications for gene therapy. *Nat Med* 1996; **2**: 1329–37.

71 Bhatia M, Wang JC, Kapp U *et al*. Purification of primitive human hematopoietic cells capable of repopulating immune-deficient mice. *Proc Natl Acad Sci U S A* 1997; **94**: 5320–5.

72 Guenechea G, Gan OI, Dorrell C *et al*. Distinct classes of human stem cells that differ in proliferative and self-renewal potential. *Nat Immunol* 2001; **2**: 75–82.

73 DiGiusto D, Chen S, Combs J *et al*. Human fetal bone marrow early progenitors for T, B, and myeloid cells are found exclusively in the population expressing high levels of CD34. *Blood* 1994; **84**: 421–32.

74 Bhatia M, Bonnet D, Murdoch B *et al*. A newly discovered class of human hematopoietic cells with SCID-repopulating activity. *Nat Med* 1998; **4**: 1038–45.

75 Goodell MA, Rosenzweig M, Kim H *et al*. Dye efflux studies suggest that hematopoietic stem cells expressing low or undetectable levels of CD34 antigen exist in multiple species. *Nat Med* 1997; **3**: 1337–45.

76 Zanjani ED, Almeida-Porada G, Livingston AG *et al*. Human bone marrow CD34$^-$ cells engraft *in vivo* and undergo multilineage expression that includes giving rise to CD34$^+$ cells. *Exp Hematol* 1998; **26**: 353–60.

77 Allsopp RC, Cheshier S, Weissman IL. Telomere shortening accompanies increased cell cycle activity during serial transplantation of hematopoietic stem cells. *J Exp Med* 2001; **193**: 917–24.

78 Cheshier SH, Morrison SJ, Liao X *et al*. *In vivo* proliferation and cell cycle kinetics of long-term self-renewing hematopoietic stem cells. *Proc Natl Acad Sci U S A* 1999; **96**: 3120–5.

79 Fleming WH, Alpern EJ, Uchida N. *et al*. Functional heterogeneity is associated with the cell cycle status of murine hematopoietic stem cells. *J Cell Biol* 1993; **122**: 897–902.

80 Wright DE, Wagers AJ, Gulati AP *et al*. Physiological migration of hematopoietic stem and progenitor cells. *Science* 2001; **294**: 1933–6.

81 Morrison SJ, Wright DE, Weissman IL. Cyclophosphamide/granulocyte colony-stimulating factor induces hematopoietic stem cells to proliferate prior to mobilization. *Proc Natl Acad Sci U S A* 1997; **94**: 1908–13.

82 Wright DE, Cheshier SH, Wagers AJ *et al*. Cyclophosphamide/granulocyte colony-stimulating factor causes selective mobilization of bone marrow hematopoietic stem cells into the blood after M phase of the cell cycle. *Blood* 2001; **97**: 2278–85.

83 Miyamoto T, Iwasaki H, Reizis B *et al*. Myeloid or lymphoid promiscuity as a critical step in hematopoietic lineage commitment. *Dev Cell* 2002; **3**: 137–47.

84 Hayflick L. The limited lifetime of human diploid cell strains. *Exp Cell Res* 1965; **37**: 614–36.

85 Blackburn EH, Greider CW, Henderson E *et al*. Recognition and elongation of telomeres by telomerase. *Genome* 1989; **31**: 553–60.

86 Cohn M, Blackburn EH. Telomerase in yeast. *Science* 1995; **269**: 396–400.

87 Morrison SJ, Prowse KR, Ho P *et al*. Telomerase activity in hematopoietic cells is associated with self-renewal potential. *Immunity* 1996; **5**: 207–16.

88 Vaziri H, Dragowska W, Allsopp RC *et al*. Evidence for a mitotic clock in human hematopoietic stem cells: loss of telomeric DNA with age. *Proc Natl Acad Sci U S A* 1994; **91**: 9857–60.

89 Morrison SJ, Wandycz AM, Akashi K. *et al*. The aging of hematopoietic stem cells. *Nat Med* 1996; **2**: 1011–6.

90 Muller-Sieburg CE, Riblet R. Genetic control of the frequency of hematopoietic stem cells in mice: mapping of a candidate locus to chromosome 1. *J Exp Med* 1996; **183**: 1141–50.

91 Morrison SJ, Qian D, Jerabek L *et al*. A genetic determinant that specifically regulates the frequency of hematopoietic stem cells. *J Immunol* 2002; **168**: 635–42.

92 Domen J, Gandy KL, Weissman IL. Systemic overexpression of BCL-2 in the hematopoietic system protects transgenic mice from the consequences of lethal irradiation. *Blood* 1998; **91**: 2272–82.

93 Domen J, Weissman IL. Hematopoietic stem cells need two signals to prevent apoptosis; BCL-2 can provide one of these, *kitl*/c-*kit* signaling the other. *J Exp Med* 2000; **192**: 1707–18.

94 Lacaud G, Gore L, Kennedy M *et al*. Runx1 is essential for hematopoietic commitment at the hemangioblast stage of development *in vitro*. *Blood* 2002; **100**: 458–66.

95 Endoh M, Ogawa M, Orkin S *et al*. SCL/tal-1-dependent process determines a competence to select the definitive hematopoietic lineage prior to endothelial differentiation. *EMBO J* 2002; **21**: 6700–8.

96 Shalaby F, Rossant J, Yamaguchi TP *et al*. Failure of blood-island formation and vasculogenesis in Flk-1-deficient mice. *Nature* 1995; **376**: 62–6.

97 Shalaby F, Ho J, Stanford WL *et al*. A requirement for Flk1 in primitive and definitive hematopoiesis and vasculogenesis. *Cell* 1997; **89**: 981–90.

98 Weissman I, Papaioannou V, Gardner R. Differentiation of normal and neoplastic hematopoietic cells. In: Clarkson B, Mark P, Till J, eds. *Cold Spring Harbor Conferences on Cell Proliferation*, Vol. 5. New York: Cold Spring Harbor Laboratory Press, 1978.

99 Park IK, He Y, Lin F *et al*. Differential gene expression profiling of adult murine hematopoietic stem cells. *Blood* 2002; **99**: 488–98.

100 Phillips RL, Ernst RE, Brunk B *et al*. The genetic program of hematopoietic stem cells. *Science* 2000; **288**: 1635–40.

101 Terskikh AV, Easterday MC, Li L *et al*. From hematopoiesis to neuropoiesis: evidence of overlapping genetic programs. *Proc Natl Acad Sci U S A* 2001; **98**: 7934–9.

102 Bryder D, Jacobsen SE. Interleukin-3 supports expansion of long-term multilineage repopulating activity after multiple stem cell divisions *in vitro*. *Blood* 2000; **96**: 1748–55.

103 Conneally E, Cashman J, Petzer A *et al*. Expansion *in vitro* of transplantable human cord blood stem cells demonstrated using a quantitative assay of their lympho-myeloid repopulating activity in nonobese diabetic-scid/scid mice. *Proc Natl Acad Sci U S A* 1997; **94**: 9836–41.

104 Ema H, Takano H, Sudo K *et al*. In vitro self-renewal division of hematopoietic stem cells. *J Exp Med* 2000; **192**: 1281–8.

105 Fraser CC, Eaves CJ, Szilvassy SJ *et al*. Expansion *in vitro* of retrovirally marked totipotent hematopoietic stem cells. *Blood* 1990; **76**: 1071–6.

106 Glimm H, Eaves CJ. Direct evidence for multiple self-renewal divisions of human *in vivo* repopulating hematopoietic cells in short-term culture. *Blood* 1999; 94: 2161–8.

107 Miller CL, Eaves CJ. Expansion *in vitro* of adult murine hematopoietic stem cells with transplantable lympho-myeloid reconstituting ability. *Proc Natl Acad Sci U S A* 1997; **94**: 13648–53.

108 Yagi M, Ritchie KA, Sitnicka E *et al*. Sustained *ex vivo* expansion of hematopoietic stem cells mediated by thrombopoietin. *Proc Natl Acad Sci U S A* 1999; **96**: 8126–31.

109 Terskikh T, Miyamoto T, Chang C *et al*. Gene expression analysis of purified hematopoietic stem cells and committed progenitors. *Blood* 2003; **102**: 94–101.

110 McCulloch EA, Siminovitch L, Till JE *et al*. The cellular basis of the genetically determined hemopoietic defect in anemic mice of genotype Sl-Sld. *Blood* 1965; **26**: 399–410.

111 Huang E, Nocka K, Beier DR *et al*. The hematopoietic growth factor KL is encoded by the Sl locus and is the ligand of the c-*kit* receptor, the gene product of the W locus. *Cell* 1990; **63**: 225–33.

112 Sarvella PA, Russel LB. Steel, a new dominant gene in the house mouse. *J Hered* 1956; **47**: 390.

113 Williams DE, Eisenman J, Baird A *et al*. Identification of a ligand for the c-*kit* proto-oncogene. *Cell* 1990; **63**: 167–74.

114 Chabot B. Stephenson DA, Chapman VM *et al*. The proto-oncogene c-*kit* encoding a transmembrane tyrosine kinase receptor maps to the mouse W locus. *Nature* 1988; **335**: 88–9.

115 Geissler EN, Ryan MA, Housman DE. The dominant-white spotting (W) locus of the mouse encodes the c-*kit* proto-oncogene. *Cell* 1988; **55**: 185–92.

116 Karanu FN, Murdoch B, Gallacher L *et al*. The notch ligand jagged-1 represents a novel growth factor of human hematopoietic stem cells. *J Exp Med* 2000; **192**: 1365–72.

117 Varnum-Finney B, Xu L, Brashem-Stein C *et al*. Pluripotent, cytokine-dependent, hematopoietic stem cells are immortalized by constitutive Notch1 signaling. *Nat Med* 2000; **6**: 1278–81.

118 Kyba M, Perlingeiro RC, Daley GQ. *Hox*B4 confers definitive lymphoid-myeloid engraftment potential on embryonic stem cell and yolk sac hematopoietic progenitors. *Cell* 2002; **109**: 29–37.

119 Antonchuk J, Sauvageau G, Humphries RK. *Hox*B4-induced expansion of adult hematopoietic stem cells *ex vivo*. *Cell* 2002; 109: 39–45.

120 Antonchuk J, Sauvageau G, Humphries RK. *Hox*B4 overexpression mediates very rapid stem cell regeneration and competitive hematopoietic repopulation. *Exp Hematol* 2001; **29**: 1125–34.

121 Sauvageau G, Thorsteinsdottir U, Eaves CJ *et al*. Overexpression of *Hox*B4 in hematopoietic cells causes the selective expansion of more primitive populations *in vitro* and *in vivo*. *Genes Dev* 1995; **9**: 1753–65.

122 Austin TW, Solar GP, Ziegler FC *et al*. A role for the Wnt gene family in hematopoiesis: expansion of multilineage progenitor cells. *Blood* 1997; **89**: 3624–35.

123 Willert K, Brown JD, Darenberg E *et al*. Wnt proteins are lipid-modified and can act as stem cell growth factors. *Nature* 2003; **423**: 448–52.

124 Reya T, Duncan AW, Allies L. *et al*. Regulation of hematopoietic stem cells in self-renewal by the Wnt signaling pathway. *Nature* 2003; **423**: 409–14.

125 Park IK, Qian D, Kiel M *et al*. Bmi-1 is required for maintenance of adult self-renewing hematopoietic stem cells. *Nature* 2003; **423**: 302–5.

126 Jacobs JJ, Kieboom K, Marino S *et al*. The oncogene and Polycomb-group gene bmi-1 regulates cell proliferation and senescence through the ink4a locus. *Nature* 1999; **397**: 164–8.

127 Goodman J. Stem cells circulating in the blood. *Rev Eur Etudes Clin Biol* 1970; **15**: 149–50.

128 Richman CM, Weiner RS, Yankee RA. Increase in circulating stem cells following chemotherapy in man. *Blood* 1976; **47**: 1031–9.

129 Brugger W, Bross K, Frisch J *et al*. Mobilization of peripheral blood progenitor cells by sequential administration of interleukin-3 and granulocyte-macrophage colony-stimulating factor following polychemotherapy with etoposide, ifosfamide, and cisplatin. *Blood* 1992; **79**: 1193–200.

130 Duhrsen U, Villeval JL, Boyd J *et al*. Effects of recombinant human granulocyte colony-stimulating factor on hematopoietic progenitor cells in cancer patients. *Blood* 1988; **72**: 2074–81.

131 McNiece IK, Langley KE, Zsebo KM. Recombinant human stem cell factor synergises with GM-CSF, G-CSF, IL-3 and epo to stimulate human progenitor cells of the myeloid and erythroid lineages. *Exp Hematol* 1991; **19**: 226–31.

132 Siena S, Bregni M, Brando B *et al*. Circulation of CD34+ hematopoietic stem cells in the peripheral blood of high-dose cyclophosphamide-treated patients: enhancement by intravenous recombinant human granulocyte-macrophage colony-stimulating factor. *Blood* 1989; **74**: 1905–14.

133 Socinski MA, Cannistra SA, Elias A *et al*. Granulocyte-macrophage colony stimulating factor expands the circulating haemopoietic progenitor cell compartment in man. *Lancet* 1988; **1**: 1194–8.

134 Heissig B, Hattori K, Dias S *et al*. Recruitment of stem and progenitor cells from the bone marrow niche requires MMP-9 mediated release of *kit*-ligand. *Cell* 2002; **109**: 625–37.

135 Fibbe WE, Pruijt JF, Velders GA *et al*. Biology of IL-8-induced stem cell mobilization. *Ann N Y Acad Sci* 1999; **872**: 71–82.

136 Laterveer L, Lindley IJ, Hamilton MS *et al*. Interleukin-8 induces rapid mobilization of hematopoietic stem cells with radioprotective capacity and long-term myelolymphoid repopulating ability. *Blood* 1995; **85**: 2269–75.

137 Kina T, Majumdar AS, Heimfeld S *et al*. Identification of a 107-kD glycoprotein that mediates adhesion between stromal cells and hematolymphoid cells. *J Exp Med* 1991; **173**: 373–81.

138 Miyake K, Weissman IL, Greenberger JS *et al*. Evidence for a role of the integrin VLA-4 in lympho-hemopoiesis. *J Exp Med* 1991; **173**: 599–607.

139 Elices MJ, Osborn L, Takada Y *et al*. VCAM-1 on activated endothelium interacts with the leukocyte integrin VLA-4 at a site distinct from the VLA-4/fibronectin binding site. *Cell* 1990; **60**: 577–84.

140 Schweitzer KM, Drager AM, van der Valk P *et al*. Constitutive expression of E-selectin and vascular cell adhesion molecule-1 on endothelial cells of hematopoietic tissues. *Am J Pathol* 1996; **148**: 165–75.

141 Wagers AJ, Allsopp RC, Weissman IL. Changes in integrin expression are associated with altered homing properties of Lin(–/lo)Thy1.1(lo)Sca-1(+)c-*kit*(+) hematopoietic stem cells following mobilization by cyclophosphamide/granulocyte colony-stimulating factor. *Exp Hematol* 2002; **30**: 176–85.

142 Mohle R, Bautz F, Rafii S *et al*. The chemokine receptor CXCR-4 is expressed on CD34+ hematopoietic progenitors and leukemic cells and mediates transendothelial migration induced by stromal cell-derived factor-1. *Blood* 1998; **91**: 4523–30.

143 Peled A, Petit I, Kollet O *et al*. Dependence of human stem cell engraftment and repopulation of NOD/SCID mice on CXCR4. *Science* 1999; **283**: 845–8.

144 Wright DE, Bowman EP, Wagers AJ *et al*. Hematopoietic stem cells are uniquely selective in their migratory response to chemokines. *J Exp Med* 2002; **195**: 1145–54.

145 Gutman GA, Weissman IL. Homing properties of thymus-independent follicular lymphocytes. *Transplantation* 1973; **16**: 621–9.

146 Gallatin M, St John TP, Siegelman M *et al*. Lymphocyte homing receptors. *Cell* 1986; **44**: 673–80.

147 Lagasse E, Weissman IL. Enforced expression of Bcl-2 in monocytes rescues macrophages and

partially reverses osteopetrosis in op/op mice. *Cell* 1997; **89**: 1021–31.
148 Moore MA, Metcalf D. Ontogeny of the haemopoietic system: yolk sac origin of *in vivo* and *in vitro* colony forming cells in the developing mouse embryo. *Br J Haematol* 1970; **18**: 279–96.
149 Johnson GR, Moore MA. Role of stem cell migration in initiation of mouse fetal liver haemopoiesis. *Nature* 1975; **258**: 726–8.
150 Gardner RL, Lyon MF, Evans EP *et al*. Clonal analysis of X-chromosome inactivation and the origin of the germ line in the mouse embryo. *J Embryol Exp Morph* 1985; **88**: 349–63.
151 Gardner RL. The initial phase of embryonic patterning in mammals. *Int Rev Cytol* 2001; **203**: 233–90.
152 Cumano A, Godin I. Pluripotent hematopoietic stem cell development during embryogenesis. *Curr Opin Immunol* 2001; **13**: 166–71.
153 Keller G, Lacaud G, Robertson S. Development of the hematopoietic system in the mouse. *Exp Hematol* 1999; **27**: 777–87.
154 Yoder MC. Introduction: spatial origin of murine hematopoietic stem cells. *Blood* 2001; **98**: 3–5.
155 Palis J, Robertson S, Kennedy M *et al*. Development of erythroid and myeloid progenitors in the yolk sac and embryo proper of the mouse. *Development* 1999; **126**: 5073–84.
156 Carmeliet P, Ferreira V, Breier G *et al*. Abnormal blood vessel development and lethality in embryos lacking a single VEGF allele. *Nature* 1996; **380**: 435–9.
157 Williams RL, Hilton DJ, Pease S *et al*. Myeloid leukaemia inhibitory factor maintains the developmental potential of embryonic stem cells. *Nature* 1988; **336**: 684–7.
158 Haar JL, Ackerman GA. A phase and electron microscopic study of vasculogenesis and erythropoiesis in the yolk sac of the mouse. *Anat Rec* 1971; **170**: 199–223.
159 Morrison SJ, Hemmati HD, Wandycz AM *et al*. The purification and characterization of fetal liver hematopoietic stem cells. *Proc Natl Acad Sci U S A* 1995; **92**: 10302–6.
160 Rebel VI, Miller CL, Eaves CJ *et al*. The repopulation potential of fetal liver hematopoietic stem cells in mice exceeds that of their liver adult bone marrow counterparts. *Blood* 1996; **87**: 3500–7.
161 Potocnik AJ, Brakebusch C, Fassler R. Fetal and adult hematopoietic stem cells require beta1 integrin function for colonizing fetal liver, spleen, and bone marrow. *Immunity* 2000; **12**: 653–63.
162 Hirsch E, Iglesias A, Potocnik AJ *et al*. Impaired migration but not differentiation of haematopoietic stem cells in the absence of beta1 integrins. *Nature* 1996; **380**: 171–5.
163 Ikuta K, Kina T, MacNeil I *et al*. A developmental switch in thymic lymphocyte maturation potential occurs at the level of hematopoietic stem cells. *Cell* 1990; **62**: 863–74.
164 Havran WL, Allison JP. Developmentally ordered appearance of thymocytes expressing different T-cell antigen receptors. *Nature* 1988; **335**: 443–5.
165 Ying QL, Nichols J, Evans EP *et al*. Changing potency by spontaneous fusion. *Nature* 2002; **416**: 545–8.
166 Terada N, Hamazaki T, Oka M *et al*. Bone marrow cells adopt the phenotype of other cells by spontaneous cell fusion. *Nature* 2002; **416**: 542–5.
167 Bjornson CR, Rietze RL, Reynolds BA *et al*. Turning brain into blood: a hematopoietic fate adopted by adult neural stem cells *in vivo*. *Science* 1999; **283**: 534–7.
168 Lagasse E, Connors H, Al-Dhalimy M *et al*. Purified hematopoietic stem cells can differentiate into hepatocytes *in vivo*. *Nat Med* 2000; **6**: 1229–34.
169 Kawada H, Ogawa M. Bone marrow origin of hematopoietic progenitors and stem cells in murine muscle. *Blood* 2001; **98**: 2008–13.
170 McKinney-Freeman SL, Jackson KA, Camargo FD *et al*. Muscle-derived hematopoietic stem cells are hematopoietic in origin. *Proc Natl Acad Sci U S A* 2002; **99**: 1341–6.
171 Clarke D, Johansson CB, Welbertz J. *et al*. Generalized potential of adult neural stem cells. *Science* 2000; **288**: 1660–3.
172 Evans MJ, Kaufman MH. Establishment in culture of pluripotential cells from mouse embryos. *Nature* 1981; **292**: 154–6.
173 Martin GR. Isolation of a pluripotent cell line from early mouse embryos cultured in medium conditioned by teratocarcinoma stem cells. *Proc Natl Acad Sci U S A* 1981; **78**: 7634–8.
174 Thomson JA, Itskovitz-Eldor J, Shapiro SS *et al*. Embryonic stem cell lines derived from human blastocysts. *Science* 1998; **282**: 1145–7.
175 Pellegrini G, Dellambra E, Golisano O *et al*. p63 identifies keratinocyte stem cells. *Proc Natl Acad Sci U S A* 2001; **98**: 3156–61.
176 Giblett ER, Anderson JE, Cohen F *et al*. Adenosine-deaminase deficiency in two patients with severely impaired cellular immunity. *Lancet* 1972; **2**: 1067–9.
177 Ochs HD, Yount JE, Giblett ER *et al*. Adenosine-deaminase deficiency and severe combined immunodeficiency syndrome. *Lancet* 1973; **1**: 1393–4.
178 Kondo M, Takeshita T, Higuchi M *et al*. Functional participation of the IL-2 receptor gamma chain in IL-7 receptor complexes. *Science* 1994; **263**: 1453–4.
179 Noguchi M, Nakamura Y, Russell SM *et al*. Interleukin-2 receptor gamma chain: a functional component of the interleukin-7 receptor. *Science* 1993; **262**: 1877–80.
180 Hirschhorn R. Overview of biochemical abnormalities and molecular genetics of adenosine deaminase deficiency. *Pediatr Res* 1993; **33**: S35–41.
181 Georgopoulos K, Moore DD, Derfler B. Ikaros, an early lymphoid-specific transcription factor and a putative mediator for T cell commitment. *Science* 1992; **258**: 808–12.
182 Radtke F, Wilson A, Stark G *et al*. Deficient T cell fate specification in mice with an induced inactivation of Notch1. *Immunity* 1999; **10**: 547–58.
183 Weissman IL. Stem cells, clonal progenitors, and commitment to the three lymphocyte lineages: T, B, NK cells. *Immunity* 1994; **1**: 529–31 [Comment].
184 Akashi K, Shibuya T, Harada M *et al*. Acute 'bilineal-biphenotypic' leukaemia. *Br J Haematol* 1990; **74**: 402–7.
185 Akashi K, Harada M, Shibuya T *et al*. Simultaneous occurrence of myelomonocytic leukemia and multiple myeloma: involvement of common leukemic progenitors and their developmental abnormality of 'lineage infidelity'. *J Cell Physiol* 1991; **148**: 446–56.
186 Akashi K, Mizuno S, Harada M *et al*. T lymphoid/myeloid bilineal crisis in chronic myelogenous leukemia. *Exp Hematol* 1993; **21**: 743–8.
187 Akashi K, Taniguchi S, Nagafuji K *et al*. B-lymphoid/myeloid stem cell origin in Ph-positive acute leukemia with myeloid markers. *Leuk Res* 1993; **17**: 549–55.
188 al-Amin A, Lennartz K, Runde V *et al*. Frequency of clonal B lymphocytes in chronic myelogenous leukemia evaluated by fluorescence *in situ* hybridization. *Cancer Genet Cytogenet* 1998; **104**: 45–7.
189 Barlogie B, Epstein J, Selvanayagam P *et al*. Plasma cell myeloma: new biological insights and advances in therapy. *Blood* 1989; **73**: 865–79.
190 Gale RP, Ben Bassat I. Hybrid acute leukaemia. *Br J Haematol* 1987; **65**: 261–4.
191 Schmidt CA, Przybylski GK. What can we learn from leukemia as for the process of lineage commitment in hematopoiesis? *Int Rev Immunol* 2001; **20**: 107–15.
192 Takahashi N, Miura I, Saitoh K *et al*. Lineage involvement of stem cells bearing the Philadelphia chromosome in chronic myeloid leukemia in the chronic phase as shown by a combination of fluorescence-activated cell sorting and fluorescence *in situ* hybridization. *Blood* 1998; **92**: 4758–63.
193 Hirayama F, Shih JP, Awgulewitsch A *et al*. Clonal proliferation of murine lymphohemopoietic progenitors in culture. *Proc Natl Acad Sci U S A* 1992; **89**: 5907–11.
194 Hirayama F, Ogawa M. Negative regulation of early T lymphopoiesis by interleukin-3 and interleukin-1 alpha. *Blood* 1995; **86**: 4527–31.
195 Lacaud G, Carlsson L, Keller G. Identification of a fetal hematopoietic precursor with B cell, T cell, and macrophage potential. *Immunity* 1998; **9**: 827–38.
196 Ogawa M. Differentiation and proliferation of hematopoietic stem cells. *Blood* 1993; **81**: 2844–53.
197 Ogawa M. Stochastic model revisited. *Int J Hematol* 1999; **69**: 2–5.
198 Suda J, Suda T, Ogawa M. Analysis of differentiation of mouse hemopoietic stem cells in culture by sequential replating of paired progenitors. *Blood* 1984; **64**: 393–9.
199 Goodwin RG, Friend D, Ziegler SF *et al*. Cloning of the human and murine interleukin-7 receptors: demonstration of a soluble form and homology to a new receptor superfamily. *Cell* 1990; **60**: 941–51.
200 Kondo M, Takeshita T, Ishii N *et al*. Sharing of the interleukin-2 (IL-2) receptor gamma chain between receptors for IL-2 and IL-4. *Science* 1993; **262**: 1874–7.
201 Peschon JJ, Morrissey PJ, Grabstein KH *et al*. Early lymphocyte expansion is severely impaired in interleukin 7 receptor-deficient mice. *J Exp Med* 1994; **180**: 1955–60.
202 von Freeden-Jeffry U, Vieira P, Lucian LA *et al*. Lymphopenia in interleukin (IL) -7 gene-deleted mice identifies IL-7 as a nonredundant cytokine. *J Exp Med* 1995; **181**: 1519–26.
203 Cao X, Shores EW, Hu-Li J *et al*. Defective lymphoid development in mice lacking expression of the common cytokine receptor gamma chain. *Immunity* 1995; **2**: 223–38.
204 DiSanto JP, Rieux-Laucat F, Dautry-Varsat A *et al*. Defective human interleukin 2 receptor gamma chain in an atypical X chromosome-linked severe combined immunodeficiency with peripheral T cells. *Proc Natl Acad Sci U S A* 1994; **91**: 9466–70.
205 Ohbo K, Suda T, Hashiyama M *et al*. Modulation of hematopoiesis in mice with a truncated mutant of the interleukin-2 receptor gamma chain. *Blood* 1996; **87**: 956–67.
206 Lodolce JP, Boone DL, Chai S *et al*. IL-15 receptor maintains lymphoid homeostasis by supporting

207 Ogasawara K, Hida S, Azimi N et al. Requirement for IRF-1 in the microenvironment supporting development of natural killer cells. *Nature* 1998; **391**: 700–3.

208 Suzuki H, Duncan GS, Takimoto H et al. Abnormal development of intestinal intraepithelial lymphocytes and peripheral natural killer cells in mice lacking the IL-2 receptor beta chain. *J Exp Med* 1997; **185**: 499–505.

209 Miyazaki T, Kawahara A, Fujii H et al. Functional activation of Jak1 and Jak3 by selective association with IL-2 receptor subunits. *Science* 1994; **266**: 1045–7.

210 Russell SM, Johnston JA, Noguchi M et al. Interaction of IL-2R beta and gamma c chains with Jak1 and Jak3: implications for XSCID and XCID. *Science* 1994; **266**: 1042–5.

211 Nosaka T, van Deursen JM, Tripp RA et al. Defective lymphoid development in mice lacking Jak3. *Science* 1995; **270**: 800–2.

212 Park SY, Saijo K, Takahashi T, Osawa M et al. Developmental defects of lymphoid cells in Jak3 kinase-deficient mice. *Immunity* 1995; **3**: 771–82.

213 Thomis DC, Gurniak CB, Tivol E et al. Defects in B lymphocyte maturation and T lymphocyte activation in mice lacking Jak3. *Science* 1995; **270**: 794–7.

214 Macchi P, Villa A, Giliani S et al. Mutations of Jak-3 gene in patients with autosomal severe combined immune deficiency (SCID). *Nature* 1995; **377**: 65–8.

215 Russell SM, Tayebi N, Nakajima H et al. Mutation of Jak3 in a patient with SCID: essential role of Jak3 in lymphoid development. *Science* 1995; **270**: 797–800.

216 Akashi K, Kondo M, Weissman IL. Role of interleukin-7 in T-cell development from hematopoietic stem cells. *Immunol Rev* 1998; **165**: 13–28.

217 Sudo T, Nishikawa S, Ohno N et al. Expression and function of the interleukin 7 receptor in murine lymphocytes. *Proc Natl Acad Sci U S A* 1993; **90**: 9125–9.

218 Vaux DL, Cory S, Adams JM. Bcl-2 gene promotes haemopoietic cell survival and cooperates with c-myc to immortalize pre-B cells. *Nature* 1988; **335**: 440–2.

219 Akashi K, Kondo M, von Freeden-Jeffry U et al. Bcl-2 rescues T lymphopoiesis in interleukin-7 receptor-deficient mice. *Cell* 1997; **89**: 1033–41.

220 Maraskovsky E, O'Reilly LA, Teepe M et al. Bcl-2 can rescue T lymphocyte development in interleukin-7 receptor-deficient mice but not in mutant rag-1−/− mice. *Cell* 1997; **89**: 1011–9.

221 Pestano GA, Zhou Y, Trimble LA et al. Inactivation of misselected CD8 T cells by CD8 gene methylation and cell death. *Science* 1999; **283**: 1187–91.

222 Corcoran AE, Smart FM, Cowling RJ et al. The interleukin-7 receptor alpha chain transmits distinct signals for proliferation and differentiation during B lymphopoiesis. *EMBO J* 1996; **15**: 1924–32.

223 Corcoran AE, Riddell A, Krooshoop D et al. Impaired immunoglobulin gene rearrangement in mice lacking the IL-7 receptor. *Nature* 1998; **391**: 904–7.

224 Ye SK, Maki K, Kitamura T et al. Induction of germline transcription in the TCRgamma locus by Stat5: implications for accessibility control by the IL-7 receptor. *Immunity* 1999; **11**: 213–23.

225 Ye SK, Agata Y, Lee HC et al. The IL-7 receptor controls the accessibility of the TCRgamma locus by Stat5 and histone acetylation. *Immunity* 2001; **15**: 813–23.

226 Adkins B, Mueller C, Okada CY et al. Early events in T-cell maturation. *Annu Rev Immunol* 1987; **5**: 325–65.

227 Godfrey DI, Kennedy J, Suda T et al. A developmental pathway involving four phenotypically and functionally distinct subsets of CD3−CD4−CD8− triple-negative adult mouse thymocytes defined by CD44 and CD25 expression. *J Immunol* 1993; **150**: 4244–52.

228 Matsuzaki Y, Gyotoku J, Ogawa M et al. Characterization of c-kit positive intrathymic stem cells that are restricted to lymphoid differentiation. *J Exp Med* 1993; **178**: 1283–92.

229 Wu L, Scollay R, Egerton M et al. CD4 expressed on earliest T-lineage precursor cells in the adult murine thymus. *Nature* 1991; **349**: 71–4.

230 Ardavin C, Wu L, Li CL et al. Thymic dendritic cells and T cells develop simultaneously in the thymus from a common precursor population. *Nature* 1993; **362**: 761–3.

231 Antica M, Wu L, Shortman K et al. Thymic stem cells in mouse bone marrow. *Blood* 1994; **84**: 111–7.

232 Allman D, Sambandam A, Kim S et al. Thymopoiesis independent of common lymphoid progenitors. *Nat Immunol* 2003; **6**: 6.

233 Dejbakhsh-Jones S, Jerabek L, Weissman I. et al. Extrathymic maturation of αβ T cells from hematopoietic stem cells. *J Immunol* 1995; **155**: 3338–44.

234 Dejbakhsh-Jones S, Garcia-Ojeda ME, Chatterjea-Matthes D et al. Clonable progenitors committed to the T lymphocyte lineage in the mouse bone marrow: use of an extrathymic pathway. *Proc Natl Acad Sci U S A* 2001; **98**: 7455–60.

235 Allman D, Li J, Hardy RR. Commitment to the B lymphoid lineage occurs before DH-JH recombination. *J Exp Med* 1999; **189**: 735–40.

236 Hardy RR, Carmack CE, Shinton SA et al. Resolution and characterization of pro-B and pre-pro-B cell stages in normal mouse bone marrow. *J Exp Med* 1991; **173**: 1213–25.

237 Li YS, Wasserman R, Hayakawa K et al. Identification of the earliest B lineage stage in mouse bone marrow. *Immunity* 1996; **5**: 527–35.

238 Sanchez MJ, Muench MO, Roncarolo MG et al. Identification of a common T/natural killer cell progenitor in human fetal thymus. *J Exp Med* 1994; **180**: 569–76.

239 Gore SD, Kastan MB, Civin CI. Normal human bone marrow precursors that express terminal deoxynucleotidyl transferase include T-cell precursors and possible lymphoid stem cells. *Blood* 1991; **77**: 1681–90.

240 LeBien TW. Fates of human B-cell precursors. *Blood* 2000; **96**: 9–23.

241 Galy A, Travis M, Cen D et al. Natural killer, and dendritic cells arise from a common bone marrow progenitor cell subset. *Immunity* 1995; **3**: 459–73.

242 Hao QL, Zhu J, Price MA et al. Identification of a novel, human multilymphoid progenitor in cord blood. *Blood* 2001; **97**: 3683–90.

243 Prieyl JA, LeBien TW. Interleukin 7 independent development of human B cells. *Proc Natl Acad Sci U S A* 1996; **93**: 10348–53.

244 Puel A, Ziegler SF, Buckley RH et al. Defective IL7R expression in T(−)B(+)NK(+) severe combined immunodeficiency. *Nat Genet* 1998; **20**: 394–7.

245 Roifman CM, Zhang J, Chitayat D et al. A partial deficiency of interleukin-7R alpha is sufficient to abrogate T-cell development and cause severe combined immunodeficiency. *Blood* 2000; **96**: 2803–7.

246 Spits H, Blom B, Jaleco AC et al. Early stages in the development of human T, natural killer and thymic dendritic cells. *Immunol Rev* 1998; **165**: 75–86.

247 Humphries RK, Jacky PB, Dill FJ et al. CFU-S in individual erythroid colonies derived *in vitro* from adult mouse marrow. *Nature* 1979; **279**: 718–20.

248 Nakorn TN, Miyamoto T, Weissman IL. Characterization of mouse clonogenic megakaryocyte progenitors. *Proc Natl Acad Sci U S A* 2003; **100**: 205–10.

249 de Wynter EA, Heyworth CM, Mukaida N et al. CCR1 chemokine receptor expression isolates erythroid from granulocyte-macrophage progenitors. *J Leukoc Biol* 2001; **70**: 455–60.

250 Fritsch G, Buchinger P, Printz D et al. Rapid discrimination of early CD34+ myeloid progenitors using CD45-RA analysis. *Blood* 1993; **81**: 2301–9.

251 Huang S, Chen Z, Yu JF et al. Correlation between IL-3 receptor expression and growth potential of human CD34+ hematopoietic cells from different tissues. *Stem Cells* 1999; **17**: 265–72.

252 Lansdorp PM, Sutherland HJ, Eaves CJ. Selective expression of CD45 isoforms on functional subpopulations of CD34+ hemopoietic cells from human bone marrow. *J Exp Med* 1990; **172**: 363–6.

253 Olweus J, Thompson PA, Lund-Johansen F. Granulocytic and monocytic differentiation of CD34hi cells is associated with distinct changes in the expression of the PU.1-regulated molecules, CD64 and macrophage colony-stimulating factor receptor. *Blood* 1996; **88**: 3741–54.

254 Olweus J, BitMansour A, Warnke R et al. Dendritic cell ontogeny: a human dendritic cell lineage of myeloid origin. *Proc Natl Acad Sci U S A* 1997; **94**: 12551–6.

255 Rappold I, Ziegler BL, Kohler I et al. Functional and phenotypic characterization of cord blood and bone marrow subsets expressing FLT3 (CD135) receptor tyrosine kinase. *Blood* 1997; **90**: 111–25.

256 Manz MG, Miyamoto T, Akashi K et al. Prospective isolation of human clonogenic common myeloid progenitors. *Proc Natl Acad Sci U S A* 2002; **22**: 22.

257 Irie-Sasaki J, Sasaki T, Matsumoto W et al. CD45 is a JAK phosphatase and negatively regulates cytokine receptor signalling. *Nature* 2001; **409**: 349–54.

258 Kimura T, Sakabe H, Tanimukai S et al. Simultaneous activation of signals through gp130, c-kit, and interleukin-3 receptor promotes a trilineage blood cell production in the absence of terminally acting lineage-specific factors. *Blood* 1997; **90**: 4767–78.

259 Holyoake TL, Nicolini FE, Eaves CJ. Functional differences between transplantable human hematopoietic stem cells from fetal liver, cord blood, and adult marrow. *Exp Hematol* 1999; **27**: 1418–27.

260 Jordan CT, Astle CM, Zawadzki J et al. Long-term repopulating abilities of enriched fetal liver stem cells measured by competitive repopulation. *Exp Hematol* 1995; **23**: 1011–5.

261 Pawliuk R, Eaves C, Humphries RK. Evidence of both ontogeny and transplant dose-regulated expansion of hematopoietic stem cells *in vivo*. *Blood* 1996; **88**: 2852–8.

262 Hayakawa K, Hardy RR. Development and function of B-1 cells. *Curr Opin Immunol* 2000; **12**: 346–53.

263 Mebius RE, Miyamoto T, Christensen J *et al*. The fetal liver counterpart of adult common lymphoid progenitors gives rise to all lymphoid lineages, CD45$^+$CD4$^+$CD3$^-$ cells, as well as macrophages. *J Immunol* 2001; **166**: 6593–601.

264 Traver D, Miyamoto T, Christensen J *et al*. Fetal liver myelopoiesis occurs through distinct, prospectively isolatable progenitor subsets. *Blood* 2001; **98**: 627–35.

265 Adachi S, Yoshida H, Kataoka H *et al*. Three distinctive steps in Peyer's patch formation of murine embryo. *Int Immunol* 1997; **9**: 507–14.

266 Mebius RE, Streeter PR, Michie S *et al*. A developmental switch in lymphocyte homing receptor and endothelial vascular addressin expression regulates lymphocyte homing and permits CD4$^+$ CD3$^-$ cells to colonize lymph nodes. *Proc Natl Acad Sci U S A* 1996; **93**: 11019–24.

267 Mebius RE, Rennert P, Weissman IL. Developing lymph nodes collect CD4$^+$CD3$^-$ LTbeta$^+$ cells that can differentiate to APC, NK cells, and follicular cells but not T or B cells. *Immunity* 1997; **7**: 493–504.

268 Nutt SL, Heavey B, Rolink AG *et al*. Commitment to the B-lymphoid lineage depends on the transcription factor Pax5. *Nature* 1999; **401**: 556–62 [See comments].

269 Katoh S, Tominaga A, Migita M *et al*. Conversion of normal Ly-1-positive B-lineage cells into Ly-1-positive macrophages in long-term bone marrow cultures. *Dev Immunol* 1990; **1**: 113–25.

270 Klinken SP, Alexander WS, Adams JM. Hemopoietic lineage switch: v-raf oncogene converts Emu-myc transgenic B cells into macrophages. *Cell* 1988; **53**: 857–67.

271 Martin M, Strasser A, Baumgarth N *et al*. A novel cellular model (SPGM 1) of switching between the pre-B cell and myelomonocytic lineages. *J Immunol* 1993; **150**: 4395–406.

272 Kondo M, Scherer DC, Miyamoto T *et al*. Cell-fate conversion of lymphoid-committed progenitors by instructive actions of cytokines. *Nature* 2000; **407**: 383–6.

273 Cumano A, Paige CJ, Iscove NN *et al*. Bipotential precursors of B cells and macrophages in murine fetal liver. *Nature* 1992; **356**: 612–5.

274 Kawamoto H, Ohmura K, Katsura Y. Direct evidence for the commitment of hematopoietic stem cells to T, B and myeloid lineages in murine fetal liver. *Int Immunol* 1997; **9**: 1011–9.

275 Katsura Y. Redefinition of lymphoid progenitors. *Nat Rev Immunol* 2002; **2**: 127–32.

276 Montecino-Rodriguez E, Leathers H, Dorshkind K. Bipotential B-macrophage progenitors are present in adult bone marrow. *Nat Immunol* 2001; **2**: 83–8.

277 Kondo M, Akashi K, Domen J *et al*. Bcl-2 rescues T lymphopoiesis, but not B or NK cell development, in common gamma chain-deficient mice. *Immunity* 1997; **7**: 155–62.

278 Traver D, Akashi K, Manz M *et al*. Development of CD8alpha-positive dendritic cells from a common myeloid progenitor. *Science* 2000; **290**: 2152–4.

279 Banchereau J, Steinman RM. Dendritic cells and the control of immunity. *Nature* 1998; **392**: 245–52.

280 Hart DN. Dendritic cells: unique leukocyte populations which control the primary immune response. *Blood* 1997; **90**: 3245–87.

281 Steinman RM. The dendritic cell system and its role in immunogenicity. *Annu Rev Immunol* 1991; **9**: 271–96.

282 Liu YJ, Kanzler H, Soumelis V *et al*. Dendritic cell lineage, plasticity and cross-regulation. *Nat Immunol* 2001; **2**: 585–9.

283 Shortman K, Liu YJ. Mouse and human dendritic cell subtypes. *Nat Rev Immunol* 2002; **2**: 151–61.

284 Vremec D, Zorbas M, Scollay R *et al*. The surface phenotype of dendritic cells purified from mouse thymus and spleen: investigation of the CD8 expression by a subpopulation of dendritic cells. *J Exp Med* 1992; **176**: 47–58.

285 Wu L, Li CL, Shortman K. Thymic dendritic cell precursors. relationship to the T lymphocyte lineage and phenotype of the dendritic cell progeny. *J Exp Med* 1996; **184**: 903–11.

286 Wu L, D'Amico A, Winkel KD *et al*. RelB is essential for the development of myeloid-related CD8alpha$^-$ dendritic cells but not of lymphoid-related CD8alpha$^+$ dendritic cells. *Immunity* 1998; **9**: 839–47.

287 Guerriero A, Langmuir PB, Spain LM *et al*. PU.1 is required for myeloid-derived but not lymphoid-derived dendritic cells. *Blood* 2000; **95**: 879–85.

288 Wu L, Nichogiannopoulou A, Shortman K *et al*. Cell-autonomous defects in dendritic cell populations of Ikaros mutant mice point to a developmental relationship with the lymphoid lineage. *Immunity* 1997; **7**: 483–92.

289 Radtke F, Ferrero I, Wilson A *et al*. Notch1 deficiency dissociates the intrathymic development of dendritic cells and T cells. *J Exp Med* 2000; **191**: 1085–94.

290 Manz MG, Traver D, Miyamoto T *et al*. Dendritic cell potentials of early lymphoid and myeloid progenitors. *Blood* 2001; **97**: 3333–41.

291 Wu L, D'Amico A, Hochrein H *et al*. Development of thymic and splenic dendritic cell populations from different hemopoietic precursors. *Blood* 2001; **98**: 3376–82.

292 Caux C, Vanbervliet B, Massacrier C *et al*. CD34$^+$ hematopoietic progenitors from human cord blood differentiate along two independent dendritic cell pathways in response to GM–CSF+TNF alpha. *J Exp Med* 1996; **184**: 695–706.

293 Young JW, Szabolcs P, Moore MA. Identification of dendritic cell colony-forming units among normal human CD34$^+$ bone marrow progenitors that are expanded by c-*kit*-ligand and yield pure dendritic cell colonies in the presence of granulocyte/macrophage colony-stimulating factor and tumor necrosis factor alpha. *J Exp Med* 1995; **182**: 1111–9.

294 Randolph GJ, Beaulieu S, Lebecque S *et al*. Differentiation of monocytes into dendritic cells in a model of transendothelial trafficking. *Science* 1998; **282**: 480–3 [See comments].

295 Romani N, Gruner S, Brang D *et al*. Proliferating dendritic cell progenitors in human blood. *J Exp Med* 1994; **180**: 83–93.

296 Sallusto F, Lanzavecchia A. Efficient presentation of soluble antigen by cultured human dendritic cells is maintained by granulocyte/macrophage colony-stimulating factor plus interleukin 4 and downregulated by tumor necrosis factor alpha. *J Exp Med* 1994; **179**: 1109–18.

297 Grouard G, Rissoan MC, Filgueira L. The enigmatic plasmacytoid T cells develop into dendritic cells with interleukin (IL)-3 and CD40-ligand. *J Exp Med* 1997; **185**: 1101–11.

298 Cella M, Jarrossay D, Facchetti F *et al*. Plasmacytoid monocytes migrate to inflamed lymph nodes and produce large amounts of type I interferon. *Nat Med* 1999; **5**: 919–23.

299 Jarrossay D, Napolitani G, Colonna M *et al*. Specialization and complementarity in microbial molecule recognition by human myeloid and plasmacytoid dendritic cells. *Eur J Immunol* 2001; **31**: 3388–93.

300 Kadowaki N, Antonenko S, Lau JY *et al*. Natural interferon alpha/beta-producing cells link innate and adaptive immunity. *J Exp Med* 2000; **192**: 219–26.

301 Kadowaki N, Ho S, Antonenko S *et al*. Subsets of human dendritic cell precursors express different toll-like receptors and respond to different microbial antigens. *J Exp Med* 2001; **194**: 863–9.

302 Asselin-Paturel C, Boonstra A, Dalod M *et al*. Mouse type I IFN-producing cells are immature APCs with plasmacytoid morphology. *Nat Immunol* 2001; **2**: 1144–50.

303 Bjorck P. Isolation and characterization of plasmacytoid dendritic cells from Flt3 ligand and granulocyte-macrophage colony-stimulating factor-treated mice. *Blood* 2001; **98**: 3520–6.

304 Nakano H, Yanagita M, Gunn MD. CD11c(+)-B220(+)Gr-1(+) cells in mouse lymph nodes and spleen display characteristics of plasmacytoid dendritic cells. *J Exp Med* 2001; **194**: 1171–8.

305 Liu YJ. Dendritic cell subsets and lineages, and their functions in innate and adaptive immunity. *Cell* 2001; **106**: 259–62.

306 Bendriss-Vermare N, Barthelemy C, Durand I *et al*. Human thymus contains IFN-alpha-producing CD11c(–), myeloid CD11c(+), and mature interdigitating dendritic cells. *J Clin Invest* 2001; **107**: 835–44.

307 Spits H, Couwenberg F, Bakker AQ *et al*. Id2 and Id3 inhibit development of CD34(+) stem cells into predendritic cell (pre-DC) 2 but not into pre-DC1. Evidence for a lymphoid origin of pre-DC2. *J Exp Med* 2000; **192**: 1775–84.

308 Heemskerk MH, Blom B, Nolan G *et al*. Inhibition of T cell and promotion of natural killer cell development by the dominant negative helix loop helix factor Id3. *J Exp Med* 1997; **186**: 1597–602.

309 Jaleco AC, Stegmann AP, Heemskerk MH *et al*. Genetic modification of human B-cell development: B-cell development is inhibited by the dominant negative helix loop helix factor Id3. *Blood* 1999; **94**: 2637–46.

310 King AG, Kondo M, Scherer DC *et al*. Lineage infidelity in myeloid cells with TCR gene rearrangement: a latent developmental potential of proT cells revealed by ectopic cytokine receptor signaling. *Proc Natl Acad Sci U S A* 2002; **99**: 4508–13.

311 Sieweke MH, Graf T. A transcription factor party during blood cell differentiation. *Curr Opin Genet Dev* 1998; **8**: 545–51.

312 DeKoter RP, Singh H. Regulation of B lymphocyte and macrophage development by graded expression of PU.1. *Science* 2000; **288**: 1439–41.

313 Hu M, Krause D, Greaves M *et al*. Multilineage gene expression precedes commitment in the hemopoietic system. *Genes Dev* 1997; **11**: 774–85.

314 Berger SL. Molecular biology: the histone modification circus. *Science* 2001; **292**: 64–5.

315 Felsenfeld G, Boyes J, Chung J *et al*. Chromatin structure and gene expression. *Proc Natl Acad Sci U S A* 1996; **93**: 9384–8.

316 Weintraub H. High-resolution mapping of S1- and DNase I-hypersensitive sites in chromatin. *Mol Cell Biol* 1985; **5**: 1538–9.

317 Cross MA, Heyworth CM, Dexter TM. How do stem cells decide what to do? *Ciba Found Symp* 1997; 204: 3–14; discussion 14–8.

318 Skov S, Rieneck K, Bovin LF et al. Histone deacetylase inhibitors: a new class of immunosuppressors targeting a novel signal-pathway essential for CD154 expression. *Blood* 2002; **101**: 1430–8.

319 Jung M. Inhibitors of histone deacetylase as new anticancer agents. *Curr Med Chem* 2001; **8**: 1505–11.

320 Marks PA, Richon VM, Rifkind RA. Histone deacetylase inhibitors. inducers of differentiation or apoptosis of transformed cells. *J Natl Cancer Inst* 2000; **92**: 1210–6.

321 Jimenez G, Griffiths SD, Ford AM et al. Activation of the beta-globin locus control region precedes commitment to the erythroid lineage. *Proc Natl Acad Sci U S A* 1992; **89**: 10618–22.

322 Ford AM, Bennett CA, Healy LE et al. Immunoglobulin heavy-chain and CD3 delta-chain gene enhancers are DNase I-hypersensitive in hemopoietic progenitor cells. *Proc Natl Acad Sci U S A* 1992; **89**: 3424–8.

323 Zhu J, Bennett CA, MacGregor AD et al. A myeloid-lineage-specific enhancer upstream of the mouse myeloperoxidase (MPO) gene. *Leukemia* 1994; **8**: 717–23.

324 Delassus S, Titley I, Enver T. Functional and molecular analysis of hematopoietic progenitors derived from the aorta-gonad-mesonephros region of the mouse embryo. *Blood* 1999; **94**: 1495–503.

325 Porcher C, Swat W, Rockwell K et al. The T cell leukemia oncoprotein SCL/tal-1 is essential for development of all hematopoietic lineages. *Cell* 1996; **86**: 47–57.

326 Shivdasani RA, Mayer EL, Orkin SH. Absence of blood formation in mice lacking the T-cell leukemia oncoprotein tal-1/SCL. *Nature* 1995; **373**: 432–4.

327 Tsai FY, Keller G, Kuo FC et al. An early haematopoietic defect in mice lacking the transcription factor GATA-2. *Nature* 1994; **371**: 221–6.

328 Fujiwara Y, Browne CP, Cunniff K et al. Arrested development of embryonic red cell precursors in mouse embryos lacking transcription factor GATA-1. *Proc Natl Acad Sci U S A* 1996; **93**: 12355–8.

329 Shivdasani RA, Fujiwara Y, McDevitt MA et al. A lineage-selective knockout establishes the critical role of transcription factor GATA-1 in megakaryocyte growth and platelet development. *EMBO J* 1997; **16**: 3965–73.

330 Zhang DE, Zhang P, Wang ND et al. Absence of granulocyte colony-stimulating factor signaling and neutrophil development in CCAAT enhancer binding protein alpha-deficient mice. *Proc Natl Acad Sci U S A* 1997; **94**: 569–74.

331 Morgan B, Sun L, Avitahl N et al. Aiolos, a lymphoid restricted transcription factor that interacts with Ikaros to regulate lymphocyte differentiation. *EMBO J* 1997; **16**: 2004–13.

332 Klug CA, Morrison SJ, Masek M et al. Hematopoietic stem cells and lymphoid progenitors express different Ikaros isoforms, and Ikaros is localized to heterochromatin in immature lymphocytes. *Proc Natl Acad Sci U S A* 1998; **95**: 657–62.

333 Georgopoulos K, Bigby M, Wang JH et al. The Ikaros gene is required for the development of all lymphoid lineages. *Cell* 1994; **79**: 143–56.

334 Ting CN, Olson MC, Barton KP et al. Transcription factor GATA-3 is required for development of the T-cell lineage. *Nature* 1996; **384**: 474–8.

335 Enver T, Greaves M. Loops, lineage, and leukemia. *Cell* 1998; **94**: 9–12.

336 Sieweke MH, Tekotte H, Frampton J et al. MafB is an interaction partner and repressor of Ets-1 that inhibits erythroid differentiation. *Cell* 1996; **85**: 49–60.

337 Zhang P, Zhang X, Iwama A et al. PU.1 inhibits GATA-1 function and erythroid differentiation by blocking GATA-1 DNA binding. *Blood* 2000; **96**: 2641–8.

338 Kulessa H, Frampton J, Graf T. GATA-1 reprograms avian myelomonocytic cell lines into eosinophils, thromboblasts, and erythroblasts. *Genes Dev* 1995; **9**: 1250–62.

339 Chiang MY, Monroe JG. BSAP/Pax5A expression blocks survival and expansion of early myeloid cells implicating its involvement in maintaining commitment to the B-lymphocyte lineage. *Blood* 1999; **94**: 3621–32.

340 Anderson MK, Weiss AH, Hernandez-Hoyos G et al. Constitutive expression of PU.1 in fetal hematopoietic progenitors blocks T cell development at the pro-T cell stage. *Immunity* 2002; **16**: 285–96.

341 Thomas ED. A history of haemopoietic cell transplantation. *Br J Haematol* 1999; **105**: 330–9.

342 Thomas ED. Bone marrow transplantation from bench to bedside. *Ann N Y Acad Sci* 1995; **770**: 34–41.

343 Uchida N, Tsukamoto A, He D et al. High doses of purified stem cells cause early hematopoietic recovery in syngeneic and allogeneic hosts. *J Clin Invest* 1998; **101**: 961–6.

344 Negrin RS, Atkinson K, Leemhuis T et al. Transplantation of highly purified CD34+Thy-1+ hematopoietic stem cells in patients with metastatic breast cancer. *Biol Blood Marrow Transplant* 2000; **6**: 262–71.

345 Vose JM, Bierman PJ, Lynch JC et al. Transplantation of highly purified CD34+Thy-1+ hematopoietic stem cells in patients with recurrent indolent non-Hodgkin's lymphoma. *Biol Blood Marrow Transplant* 2001; **7**: 680–7.

346 Stadtmauer EA, O'Neill A, Goldstein LJ et al. Conventional-dose chemotherapy compared with high-dose chemotherapy plus autologous hematopoietic stem-cell transplantation for metastatic breast cancer. Philadelphia Bone Marrow Transplant Group. *N Engl J Med* 2000; **342**: 1069–76.

347 Gazitt Y, Tian E, Barlogie B et al. Differential mobilization of myeloma cells and normal hematopoietic stem cells in multiple myeloma after treatment with cyclophosphamide and granulocyte-macrophage colony-stimulating factor. *Blood* 1996; **87**: 805–11.

348 Michallet M, Philip T, Philip I et al. Transplantation with selected autologous peripheral blood CD34+Thy1+ hematopoietic stem cells (HSCs) in multiple myeloma: impact of HSC dose on engraftment, safety, and immune reconstitution. *Exp Hematol* 2000; **28**: 858–70.

349 Miyamoto T, Weissman IL, Akashi K. AML1/ETO-expressing nonleukemic stem cells in acute myelogenous leukemia with 8;21 chromosomal translocation. *Proc Natl Acad Sci U S A* 2000; **97**: 7521–6.

350 Ferrara JL, Levy R, Chao NJ. Pathophysiologic mechanisms of acute graft-vs.-host disease. *Biol Blood Marrow Transplant* 1999; **5**: 347–56.

351 Shizuru JA, Jerabek L, Edwards CT et al. Transplantation of purified hematopoietic stem cells: requirements for overcoming the barriers of allogeneic engraftment. *Biol Blood Marrow Transplant* 1996; **2**: 3–14.

352 Shizuru JA, Weissman IL, Kernoff R et al. Purified hematopoietic stem cell grafts induce tolerance to alloantigens and can mediate positive and negative T cell selection. *Proc Natl Acad Sci U S A* 2000; **97**: 9555–60.

353 Gandy KL, Domen J, Aguila H, Weissman IL. CD8+TCR+ and CD8+TCR− cells in whole bone marrow facilitate the engraftment of hematopoietic stem cells across allogeneic barriers. *Immunity* 1999; **11**: 579–90.

354 Kaufman CL, Colson YL, Wren SM et al. Phenotypic characterization of a novel bone marrow-derived cell that facilitates engraftment of allogeneic bone marrow stem cells. *Blood* 1994; **84**: 2436–46.

355 Martin PJ. Donor CD8 cells prevent allogeneic marrow graft rejection in mice: potential implications for marrow transplantation in humans. *J Exp Med* 1993; **178**: 703–12.

356 Heeg K, Wagner H. Induction of peripheral tolerance to class I major histocompatibility complex (MHC) alloantigens in adult mice: transfused class I MHC-incompatible splenocytes veto clonal responses of antigen-reactive Lyt-2+ T cells. *J Exp Med* 1990; **172**: 719–28.

357 Thomas JM, Verbanac KM, Carver FM et al. Veto cells in transplantation tolerance. *Clin Transplant* 1994; **8**: 195–203.

358 Steinman RM, Nussenzweig MC. Avoiding horror autotoxicus. the importance of dendritic cells in peripheral T cell tolerance. *Proc Natl Acad Sci U S A* 2002; **99**: 351–8.

359 Main JM, Prehn RT. Successful skin homografts after the administration of high dosage x-irradiation and homologous bone marrow. *J Natl Cancer Inst* 1955; **15**: 1023–9.

360 Gandy KL, Weissman IL. Tolerance of allogeneic heart grafts in mice simultaneously reconstituted with purified allogeneic hematopoietic stem cells. *Transplantation* 1998; **65**: 295–304.

361 Millan MT, Shizuru JA, Hoffmann P et al. Mixed chimerism and immunosuppressive drug withdrawal after HLA- mismatched kidney and hematopoietic progenitor transplantation. *Transplantation* 2002; **73**: 1386–91.

362 Beilhack GF, Scheffold YC, Weissman IL et al. Purified allogeneic hematopoietic stem cell transplantation blocks diabetes pathogenesis in NOD mice. *Diabetes* 2003; **52**: 59–68.

363 BitMansour A, Burns SM, Traver D et al. Myeloid progenitors protect against invasive aspergillosis and *Pseudomonas aeruginosa* infection following hematopoietic stem cell transplantation. *Blood* 2002; **100**: 4660–7.

364 Brown JM, Weissman IL, Shizuru JA. Immunity to infections following hematopoietic cell transplantation. *Curr Opin Immunol* 2001; **13**: 451–7.

365 Miyamoto T, Nagafuji K, Akashi K. et al. Persistence of multipotent progenitors expressing AML1/ETO transcripts in long-term remission patients with t(8;21) acute myelogenous leukemia. *Blood* 1996; **87**: 4789–96.

366 Wiemels JL, Xiao Z, Buffler PA et al. In utero origin of t(8;21) AML1-ETO translocations in childhood acute myeloid leukemia. *Blood* 2002; **99**: 3801–5.

367 Gale KB, Ford AM, Repp R et al. Backtracking leukemia to birth: identification of clonotypic gene

368 Hjalgrim LL, Madsen HO, Melbye M *et al.* Presence of clone-specific markers at birth in children with acute lymphoblastic leukaemia. *Br J Cancer* 2002; **87**: 994–9.

369 Ford AM, Bennett CA, Price CM *et al.* Fetal origins of the *TEL-AML1* fusion gene in identical twins with leukemia. *Proc Natl Acad Sci U S A* 1998; **95**: 4584–8.

370 Cave H, van der Werff ten Bosch J, Suciu S *et al.* Clinical significance of minimal residual disease in childhood acute lymphoblastic leukemia. European Organization for Research and Treatment of Cancer: Childhood Leukemia Cooperative Group. *N Engl J Med* 1998; **339**: 591–8.

371 Bonnet D, Dick JE. Human acute myeloid leukemia is organized as a hierarchy that originates from a primitive hematopoietic cell. *Nat Med* 1997; **3**: 730–7.

372 Yuan Y, Zhou L, Miyamoto T *et al.* AML1-ETO expression is directly involved in the development of acute myeloid leukemia in the presence of additional mutations. *Proc Natl Acad Sci U S A* 2001; **98**: 10398–403.

373 Brown D, Kogan S, Lagasse E *et al.* A PMLRARalpha transgene initiates murine acute promyelocytic leukemia. *Proc Natl Acad Sci U S A* 1997; **94**: 2551–6.

374 Kogan SC, Brown DE, Shultz DB *et al.* BCL-2 cooperates with promyelocytic leukemia retinoic acid receptor alpha chimeric protein (PMLRAlpha) to block neutrophil differentiation and initiate acute leukemia. *J Exp Med* 2001; **193**: 531–43.

375 Traver D, Akashi K, Weissman IL, Lagasse E. Mice defective in two apoptosis pathways in the myeloid lineage develop acute myeloblastic leukemia. *Immunity* 1998; **9**: 47–57.

376 Pabst T, Mueller BU, Harakawa N *et al.* AML1-ETO downregulates the granulocytic differentiation factor C/EBPalpha in t(8;21) myeloid leukemia. *Nat Med* 2001; **7**: 444–51.

377 Perrotti D, Cesi V, Trotta R *et al.* BCR-ABL suppresses C/EBPalpha expression through inhibitory action of hnRNP E2. *Nat Genet* 2002; **30**: 48–58.

378 Vangala RK, Heiss-Neumann MS, Rangatia JS. The myeloid master regulator transcription factor PU.1 is inactivated by AML1-ETO in t(8;21) myeloid leukemia. *Blood* 2003; **101**: 270–7.

379 Lagasse E, Weissman IL. bcl-2 inhibits apoptosis of neutrophils but not their engulfment by macrophages. *J Exp Med* 1994; **179**: 1047–52.

380 Ikuta K, Uchida N, Friedman J, Weissman IL. Lymphocyte development from stem cells. *Ann Review Immuno* 1992; **10**: 759–83.

381 Arber C, BitMansour A, Sparer TE *et al.* Common lymphoid progenitors rapidly engraft and protect against lethal murine cytomegalovirus infection after haematopoietic stem cell transplantation. *Blood* 2003; **102**: 421–8.

382 Karsunky H, Merad M, Cottio A *et al.* Flt3 ligand regulates dendritic cell development from Flt3-positive lymphoid and myeloid committed progenitors to Flt3-positive dendritic cells *in vivo. J Exp Med* 2003, in press.

9

Colleen Delaney, Robert Andrews & Irwin Bernstein

Expansion of Hematopoietic Stem Cells

Introduction

Hematopoietic stem cells (HSCs) have clearly proven to be useful in a variety of clinical settings, and are routinely available in sufficient numbers from a variety of sources including bone marrow (BM) and mobilized peripheral blood. However, there are instances where the number of available HSCs are insufficient for adequate and/or timely engraftment of the host, in particular when cord blood is used as the source of HSCs for transplantation or, in the case of gene therapy, where the frequency of transduced cells is too low. One potential solution to the problem of low stem cell numbers is *ex vivo* proliferation of the cells prior to transplantation. Extensive research has been done to define the optimal conditions necessary for *ex vivo* expansion of HSCs and various expansion techniques have been developed for this purpose [1–5]. However, there is still a lack of convincing data that pluripotent stem cells increase in number and retain an ability to engraft and sustain multilineage hematopoiesis in a myeloablated recipient following *ex vivo* expansion.

In order to maintain hematopoietic function throughout the life of the organism, pluripotent HSCs are thought to undergo self-renewal, where at least one, possibly identical progeny, remains undifferentiated and capable of long-term, multilineage hematopoietic repopulation, thus preserving the stem cell pool [6]. The differentiated progeny of long-term repopulating cells are thought to include pluripotent, short-term repopulating cells, which in turn generate precursors committed to lymphoid or myeloid differentiation [7,8]. Whereas maintenance of the HSC pool *in vivo* requires asymmetric division in which only one of the progeny maintains stem cell properties, HSC expansion requires symmetric divisions giving rise to two HSCs. The ability of HSCs to undergo symmetric divisions and expand in numbers has been demonstrated in transplantation studies. However, serial transplant studies have also demonstrated that HSC life span is limited and self-renewal potential diminishes with the age of the animal [9–11]. While several recent studies challenge our concepts of HSC senescence [12–14], the central tenet remains that, in the absence of transforming events, HSCs have finite, though very lengthy, life spans *in vivo* [15–17]. These "aging" or senescence processes appear to be accelerated in *ex vivo* cultures [18,19]. Nevertheless, studies suggest that HSC progeny formed after several divisions retain the ability to engraft recipients long-term, but may actually be somewhat more differentiated with less proliferative capacity that is detectable only under stress conditions. Thus, cells with HSC properties may themselves be heterogeneous, and their self-renewal capacity may depend on the source from which they are derived, with fetal liver HSCs having greater self-renewal capacity than cord blood HSCs, which in turn have greater self-renewal capacity than cells from adult marrow [16,20–22].

Substantial effort has focused on the exogenous signals that may be used to favor stem cell self-renewal vs. differentiation in order to develop optimal conditions for the *ex vivo* expansion of stem cells. Most studies have evaluated using combinations of cytokines and/or BM stroma and have met with limited success (for more details, see [1–5,23]). The effect of cytokines that support hematopoietic cell survival, proliferation and differentiation has been extensively studied *in vitro*, but a significant role for these cytokines in enhancing self-renewal has not been shown. Consequently, a stochastic model of determination has been suggested in which the fate of hematopoietic precursors is not instructed by soluble cytokines [24,25] but rather by specific interactions between stem and other cells within a particular microenvironment or "stem cell niche". These interactions are mediated by extrinsic regulators of stem cell fate and are likely to play a key role maintaining numbers of stem cells by regulating their self-renewal and differentiation [26,27]. Thus, more recent studies are aimed at identifying intrinsic and extrinsic factors that regulate HSC fate. Clinical trials, which have also mainly evaluated cytokine-driven expansion systems, have not yet provided evidence for stem cell expansion but have demonstrated the feasibility and safety of *ex vivo* culturing of stem cells (see below sections for more detail). Here, we address studies of *ex vivo* HSC expansion in animals and humans, as well as promising approaches under development.

Preclinical studies: growth factor and stroma-induced expansion

In this section, we review work in mice and large animal models designed to address the *ex vivo* expansion of HSCs. We will focus on studies that have used *in vivo* repopulating assays to evaluate stem cell expansion as *in vitro* assays have not always proven informative of HSC function. We then briefly review factors that regulate HSCs fate in *ex vivo* expansion cultures

Murine studies

The discovery of transplantable HSCs in long-term marrow cultures (LTMC) of mouse marrow cells initially described by Dexter *et al.* [28–30] suggested that HSCs might possibly expand in *ex vivo* cultures. The HSCs in these LTMC were dependent on the stromal cells for survival and their cell cycle status was influenced both positively and negatively by growth factors [31,32] as well as cellular and noncellular components of the stromal cell layers [33]. However, it was unclear whether HSCs in LTMC divided or simply remained quiescent. Subsequent studies using gene marking to follow the progeny of individual HSCs, demonstrated that HSCs were able to undergo several divisions and still maintain HSC function measured *in vivo* [34]. Evidence for a limited number of *in vitro* divisions before loss of HSC function also came from studies demonstrating that progeny of isolated HSCs, formed after one to three *in vitro* divisions, maintained *in vivo* repopulating function [35]. However, none of these and other studies [36] demonstrated net gains of HSC numbers in these cultures indicating that divisions were mainly asymmetric.

HSCs cultured for purposes of *ex vivo* expansion are altered in obvious as well as subtle ways, including the expression of various cell surface antigens such as receptors that function in cell adhesion and motility. Moreover, the impact of stem cell death, loss of homing properties [37,38] and change of cell cycle status [39–41] that occurs during *in vitro* culture of HSCs and how these influence *in vivo* repopulating ability has not yet been fully elucidated. For example, both mouse HSCs and human hematopoietic precursors appear to have diminished repopulating function if transplanted during the G_1 and S phases of the cell cycle rather than in G_0. The combination of cytokines is also critical, with specific hematopoietic growth factors involved in promoting or inhibiting HSC function during *ex vivo* expansion. Elegant single-cell manipulation studies demonstrated that interleukin 3 (IL-3) and IL-1 can abrogate the self-renewal of murine HSCs *in vitro* [42], in contrast to stem cell factor (SCF) and Flt3 ligand (Flt3L) which maintain HSCs [43]. Furthermore, the addition of exogenous thrombopoietin (TPO) to murine LTMC led to an expansion of marrow repopulating cells [44]. Members of the TGF family and cooperating factors have been demonstrated to inhibit the cell cycle progression of HSCs *in vitro* [45–47]. The type of culture medium used can also influence the *ex vivo* expansion of HSCs. Whereas numerous studies using serum-containing medium have shown maintenance or loss of HSC activity following culture with cytokines, more recent studies using serum-free medium, which allows for more careful dissection of the interaction of HSCs with defined ligands and avoids the introduction of inhibitory molecules such as transforming growth factor beta (TGF-β) have demonstrated enhanced repopulating ability with some studies documenting a few-fold expansion of murine marrow HSCs [45].

Large animal studies

To date, human trials of gene therapy and HSC manipulation have not been nearly as successful as experiments in mice might have predicted, and important differences in HSC behavior *in vivo* in large animals are beginning to be appreciated [48–50]. Thus, studies of stem cell expansion using clinically feasible procedures in larger animals to better mimic human physiology that are now being done may provide important insights needed for human clinical application. Thus far, *ex vivo* cultured cells have mainly led to an enhanced rate of engraftment, but this may have occurred at the expense of long-term repopulating cells. The possibility of enhancing short-term repopulating activity by *ex vivo* expansion was suggested by two studies of lethally irradiated baboons engrafted with *ex vivo* expanded CD34-enriched peripheral blood stem cells (PBSC) collected after granulocyte colony-stimulating factor (G-CSF) mobilization [51–53]. Significant expansion of precursor cells with *in vitro* colony-forming activities was documented in both studies and, in one study, severe combined immunodeficiency syndrome (SCID) mouse repopulating cells were also expanded twofold. Animals transplanted with *ex vivo* expanded cells experienced significantly shorter periods of post-transplant neutropenia; however, the recovery of platelet and red cell production was significantly slower, and administration of TPO had no effect on platelet recovery. Although these studies were not designed to assess effects on long-term reconstituting stem cells, the possibility that cytokine-driven expansion may deplete long-term repopulating HSCs in primate models has been suggested by gene marking studies in which prolonging the period of *in vitro* culture worsened rather than improved gene transfer efficiency [54,55].

An increase in the numbers of precursors at the expense of *in vivo* marrow reconstituting function has also been observed in cats following *ex vivo* expansion of marrow cells [56]. In dogs, HSCs and progenitors have been cultured *ex vivo* for brief periods to promote gene transfer into marrow repopulating cells. The detection of gene marked progeny *in vivo* suggests at least a limited number of cells with HSC function divided in the *ex vivo* culture [57].

Xenogeneic animal models: transplantation of human cells

Immunodeficient mouse xenogeneic transplant models

In preclinical studies, xenogeneic transplant models have been developed in which human hematopoietic cells can engraft in immunodeficient mice and then be serially passaged *in vivo* [20,21,58–64]. These engrafting cells are referred to as SCID-repopulating cells (SRC). At present, the relationship of SRC to HSCs in humans remains to be clarified. Nevertheless, human SRC expansion has been assayed in various immune deficient mouse strains. The necessity for *in vivo* assessment of *ex vivo* HSC expansion was emphasized by several studies in which *ex vivo* cultures of CD34[+] cells have resulted in the dramatic increase in numbers of colony forming cells (CFC) or even long-term culture initiating cells (LTC-IC) activity but with concomitant decrease in SRC [65–68]. In contrast, several other studies have suggested a modest increase in engraftment of immunodeficient mice following short-term culture, in which cells were cultured with multiple cytokines or in the presence of stromal cells or stroma-cell conditioned medium [1,69–74].

Quantitative studies using limiting dilution SRC assays have confirmed modest twofold to fourfold cytokine-induced increases in SRC. For example, Bhatia *et al.* [75] and Conneally *et al.* [60] have cultured CD34[+] CD38[−] cord blood cells in serum-free medium supplemented with SCF, Flt3L, G-CSF, IL-3 and IL-6, and showed expansion of SRC. The study by Bhatia *et al.* in which cells were cultured for 4 days, found a fourfold increase in CD34[+] CD38[−] cord blood cells, a 10-fold increase in CFC and a twofold to fourfold increase in SRC [75]. However, all SRC were lost after 9 days of culture, despite continued expansion in the total number of cells throughout the culture period. In a similar study, Conneally *et al.* confirmed that this culture system produced significant increases in CFC (100-fold) and LTC-IC (fourfold), as well as a modest twofold increase in SRC [60]. Similarly, studies using an IL-6/IL-6-receptor chimera induced significantly higher levels of CD34[+]CD38[−] cells and a fourfold increase in SRC by limiting dilution methods [73,76–79].

Cytokine-induced expansion systems have also utilized several cloned stromal feeders as sources of growth factors and have been shown to support long-term repopulating cells [80,81]. However, because the cultured cells are in contact with the stromal feeders in this type of culturing system, it is less advantageous to use this system for clinical application and noncontact stromal-based culture systems are also being explored as HSC expansion systems [74,82–84]. An example of this type of expansion system was reported by Shih and colleagues [82], in which a murine BM-derived stromal cell line, AC6.21, treated with leukemia inhibitory factor (LIF), secreted a factor that resulted in expansion of human HSCs when the HSCs were cultured with the conditioned medium. The expansion occurred in the absence of the stromal cells and the magnitude of expansion was dependent on the concentration of the secreted factor activity. In another example, Lewis *et al.* cultured umbilical cord blood (UCB) CD34[+] with IL-7, SCF, Flt3L, and TPO in a transwell (where stromal cells are separated from CD34[+] cells by a transmembrane) above the murine fetal liver cell stromal feeder line, AFT024, for 7 days and demonstrated the maintenance of long-term repopulating cells in culture using secondary transplants into nonobese diabetic with severe combined immunodeficiency syndrome (NOD/SCID) mice as well as secondary and tertiary transplants into fetal sheep [85]. Additionally, the use of conditioned medium from the HS-5 cell line, an immortalized stromal cell line derived from human marrow after transduction with a replication-defective retrovirus containing the human papilloma virus E6/E7 gene, has been shown to support the proliferation of hematopoietic progenitors and maintain colony-forming cells for up to 8 weeks in culture [84,86].

While the above studies documented expansion of SRCs in short-term culture conditions only, Piacibello et al. [87] reported maintenance of cord blood CD34+ cell growth for up to 12 weeks in serum-containing medium supplemented with Flt3L, SCF, and IL-6. Additionally, limiting dilution transplants demonstrated a more than 70–fold expansion of SRC. Although it is not clear whether this approach will be reproducible, Tanavde et al. [88] recently reported the ability to expand and maintain UCB SRC for up to 4 weeks using CD34+ from UCB and adult mobilized peripheral blood progenitor cells (mPBPC) cultured in serum-free medium supplemented with Flt3L, SCF and TPO with or without IL-6/IL-6R chimera. UCB cells demonstrated extensive in vitro expansion and maintained repopulating ability throughout the 4-week culture period, whereas mPBPC showed less expansion and no engrafting potential of cultured cells (only fresh cells engrafted). While the ability to maintain and expand repopulating cells in vitro for extended periods would be beneficial for gene therapy, augmentation of clinical transplantation studies with expanded cells will require shorter expansion times. Moreover, there is always the concern that long-term culture of cells may in fact induce transformation of the cultured cells.

Fetal sheep xenogeneic transplant model

When primitive hematopoietic cells isolated from both cord blood and adult BM are expanded ex vivo and transplanted into fetal sheep, only short-term engraftment of the animals is seen. In their initial study attempting ex vivo expansion of enriched adult human BM cells with in vivo engrafting capabilities, Shimizu and colleagues were able to document the maintenance of cells with engrafting capabilities in fetal sheep for up to 2 months when cultured with kit ligand, Flt3L, IL-6 and erythropoietin (EPO) with or without IL-3 [89]. Engraftment was noted in secondary recipients of fresh human cells but not in recipients of cultured cells, suggesting that the culture conditions used were unable to support or expand long-term engrafting cells. Similar results were demonstrated by McNiece et al. using a two-step culture procedure in which cord blood progenitors cultured in the presence of SCF, megakaryocyte growth and development factor (MGDF) and G-CSF for 7 or 14 days prior to transplant provided no long-term engraftment of fetal sheep [90]. While the expanded cells were capable of early rapid engraftment (three-fold over fresh), they lacked secondary and tertiary engrafting potential compared with fresh cells, again suggesting that the culture conditions described resulted in the loss of long-term repopulating cells and led to an increase of more mature short-term repopulating cells.

Overall, preclinical studies of human HSC expansion assayed based on repopulating ability in xenogeneic transplant models are encouraging but must be interpreted with caution, as human NOD/SCID or fetal sheep repopulating ability has not been correlated with nonhuman primate or human in vivo repopulating ability. In fact, studies that compared repopulation by gene-marked cells from nonhuman primates in autologous recipients and NOD/SCID mice revealed substantially greater repopulation in mice (H.P. Kiem, personal communication). Although this finding might reflect detection in mice of a more mature precursor, perhaps a short-term repopulating cell, other studies have demonstrated serial repopulation by expanded human cells in murine recipients, a function consistent with self-renewing stem cells. Furthermore, while these studies have shown in vitro expansion of SRC, the results are highly variable, and include numerous reports of loss of stem cell activity after ex vivo culture [66,90–93]. Finally, while studies of cytokine-induced expansion suggest the potential for enhancement of short- and long-term repopulating activity, only a few cell divisions at most have been observed. Thus, current efforts are now focused on identifying and exploiting other extrinsic and intrinsic regulators of stem cell fate.

Novel approaches for ex vivo HSC expansion using extrinsic and intrinsic regulators of stem cell fate

Optimization of cytokine-driven expansion systems has not led to clinically significant HSC expansion, perhaps due to a predominantly permissive, rather than directed, role in determining stem cell fate. The search for extrinsic and intrinsic regulators that act directly on human HSCs in regulating cell fate and self-renewal has suggested a role for regulatory molecules active in early development that are important in HSC maintenance and regulation. More recent studies have focused on the regulation of intrinsic signaling pathways by retrovirus-mediated transduction of HSCs, e.g. expression of homeobox genes. However, culture of cells for clinical application require use of extrinsic regulators of transcription factors as well as signaling factors including bone morphogenic proteins (BMPs), Sonic hedgehog (Shh), Wnt and Notch ligands.

Retroviral-mediated overexpression of Hox transcription factors, in particular HoxB4, has led to extensive ex vivo HSC expansion in vitro (3 logs over control cultures) without loss of full in vivo lympho-myeloid repopulating ability [94–97]. Although methods to alter homeobox gene expression in the absence of transducing cells are not available, the self-renewal induced by HoxB4 has suggested the exploration of extrinsic regulators of cell-fate involved in embryonic development such as BMP-4, a member of the TGF-β superfamily and Shh of the Hedgehog family of proteins, both having been implicated in early hematopoietic development [98,99]. In ex vivo expansion of human cord blood, soluble human BMP-4 has been shown to increase the survival of repopulating blood cells in ex vivo culture [98], while Shh has been shown to induce a few-fold increase in repopulating cells via mechanisms that are dependent on downstream BMP signals [100]. Wnt proteins, which are involved in the growth and differentiation of a variety of primitive tissues, have also been implicated in the regulation of hematopoiesis, possibly exerting their effects through stromal cells [101], and have been shown to stimulate the proliferation of hematopoietic precursor cells [102].

The most extensively studied and successfully utilized extrinsic regulators have been ligands that activate the Notch pathway. All four Notch receptors (Notch 1, 2, 3 and 4) identified in vertebrates have been detected in hematopoietic cells [103], and several investigators have reported the expression of Notch-1 and Notch-2 in human CD34+ or CD34+Lin− precursors [103–105] and of the Notch ligands, Delta-1 and Jagged-1, in human BM stromal cells and in human hematopoietic precursors [106–109]. Moreover, expression of a constitutively active, truncated form of Notch-1 in murine hematopoietic precursors inhibited differentiation and enhanced self-renewal, leading to establishment of an immortal cell line that phenotypically resembles primitive hematopoietic precursors [110]. This cell line, depending upon the cytokine context, can differentiate along the lymphoid or myeloid lineage. More recently, expression of constitutively active Notch in murine precursors transplanted in vivo led to increased stem cell numbers that was evident in secondary transplantation studies [111]. While these findings point to a role for Notch signaling in the regulation of stem cell self-renewal, expression of activated Notch-1 in human CD34+ cord blood precursors induced only a modest increase in the number of progenitors [112].

In order to affect nontransduced cells, exogenous Notch ligands have been used to induce Notch signaling in HSCs. Initial studies in mice and humans using soluble or cell-bound ligand revealed limited increases in precursor cell numbers [106,107]. However, Varnum-Finney et al. [113] recently demonstrated a requirement for ligand immobilization to induce

Notch signaling. Use of an engineered ligand immobilized on the surface of plastic culture plates achieved a several-log expansion of murine precursors with short-term repopulating ability (B. Varnum-Finney, submitted). Moreover, the use of immobilized ligand in the culture of purified UCB CD34$^+$/38$^-$ stem cells has led to a substantial increase in the human cord blood cell myeloid and B-cell-repopulating ability in NOD/SCID mice deficient in β_2-microglobulin (β_2m$^{-/-}$), as well as the generation of cells that engraft the thymus with CD3$^+$ T cells [114]. These data indicate that Notch 1-induced signaling can enhance stem cell self-renewal ex vivo and thereby increase HSC numbers for transplantation.

Despite limited evidence of *ex vivo* HSC expansion with current methodologies, including stroma and stroma-free systems, clinical trials have been conducted with autologous marrow, cytokine-mobilized peripheral blood cells or cord blood cells cultured with cytokines and their ability to shorten engraftment periods determined. Stroma-free systems provide a clear advantage for clinical use, since they are easier to standardize and maintain for cyclic guanosine monophosphate (cGMP). However, some studies have used noncontact systems in which stromal cells serve to condition the medium. These trials will be discussed in the next section.

Clinical trials of *ex vivo* expanded HSCs

The first report of a clinical trial using *in vitro* cultured hematopoietic progenitor cells (HPC) appeared in 1992. Since then, a number of trials have been carried out with the primary goal of enhancing hematopoietic recovery after high-dose chemotherapy with the infusion of expanded stem cell grafts derived from BM, mobilized peripheral blood or cord blood.

Clinical trials using BM and mobilized peripheral blood

Table 9.1 summarizes some trials with autologous BM or mPBPC cultured *ex vivo* with cytokines and/or stromal elements [115–124]. Studies of expanded mPBPC were all done in the autologous setting and included only those patients with sufficient stem cell harvests to allow the use of an aliquot of the apheresis product for expansion. This excluded "poor mobilizers" who clearly stand to benefit from expansion procedures allowing them to undergo treatment with high-dose therapy. However, it is not known whether HSCs derived from such patients are equivalent to those derived from patients with adequate mobilization of HSCs. These trials, primarily in breast cancer patients, assessed enhanced short-term repopulation as a function of decreased time to neutrophil and/or platelet engraftment. With one exception, these studies were unable to address expansion of long-term repopulating HSCs because patients received nonmyeloablative chemotherapy and/or infusion of noncultured cells.

Overall, although the safety and feasibility of stem cell expansion approaches were demonstrated, more rapid engraftment was not observed in patients receiving nonmyeloablative therapy. There have, however, been suggestions of *ex vivo* expansion of short-term repopulating cells in patients who received myeloablative therapy. For example, in a study by Holyoake et al. [118] the gain of short-term repopulating cells at the expense of long-term repopulating cells was suggested. In that study, mPBPC cultured *ex vivo* with SCF, IL-1β, IL-3, IL-6, EPO and autologous plasma for 8 days were infused in the absence of noncultured cells into patients that had received myeloablative chemotherapy. None of the four patients showed evidence of long-term hematopoietic recovery and all required infusions of unmanipulated cyropreserved autologous backup mPBPC, after which full hematopoietic recovery was seen. Three patients showed initial neutrophil engraftment that was unsustained, suggesting that short-term repopulating cells may have been generated *ex vivo* at the expense of long-term repopulating ones, possibly by inducing their differentiation. A shortening of the neutropenic period post high-

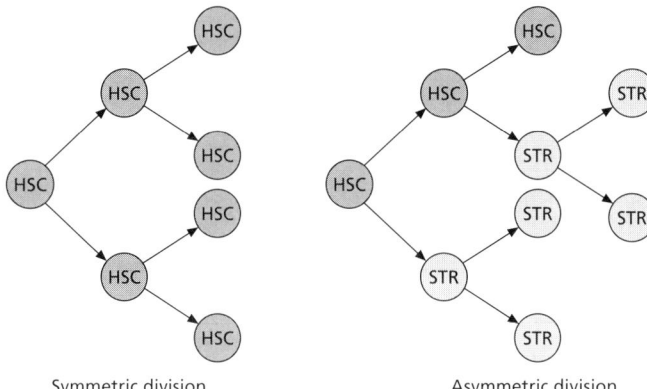

Fig. 9.1 Maintenence versus expansion of hematopoietic stem cell numbers: symmetric divisions will expand stem cell numbers, whereas assymetric divisions maintain numbers. The number of HSC generated may also be affected by cell loss due to apoptosis and, for transplantable stem cells, loss of homing properties.

dose chemotherapy in 21 patients with breast cancer was also shown in a study in which autologous mPBPC were cultured with SCF, G-CSF and MGDF for 10 days. The patients in this study were divided into two cohorts, those who received expanded cells only and those who received both expanded and unmanipulated cells in tandem [120]. Expanded PBPC resulted in a more rapid neutrophil engraftment ($p = 0.02$ for cohorts 1 and 2 vs. the historical controls) and the best predictor of time to neutrophil engraftment was the total number of cells harvested after expansion, and patients receiving >4 $\times$ 10^7 cells/kg engrafted by day 8. Reiffers et al. also reported a decreased time to neutrophil engraftment using the same culture conditions to expand autologous mPBPC for infusion with unmanipulated cells into multiple myeloma patients after myeloablative conditioning [119].

The use of continuous perfusion methods for the expansion of BM has recently been evaluated in three trials utilizing the automated perfusion bioreactor system, AastromReplicell™ [121–123]. Notably, these are the only trials that used BM (unselected for CD34$^+$) as the source of stem cells for *ex vivo* expansion, thereby perhaps including accessory or stromal cells of unclear significance in expansion cultures and perhaps enhancing the engraftment ability of this expanded cell population. In these studies, breast cancer patients underwent the same conditioning regimen, and cells derived from autologous BM were placed directly into the automated perfusion bioreactor system for expansion with Flt3L, EPO and Pixy 321 cytokines as well as fetal bovine serum and horse serum. In all trials, cultures were initiated with small amounts of harvested marrow (75–100 mL). The trials by Stiff et al. [121] and Engelhardt et al. [123] used expanded cells only, while Pecora et al. [122] also infused mPBPC in low doses. Engraftment was not enhanced but did occur, suggesting the maintenance of HSCs in the BM cultures, and all trials reported a correlation between the time to neutrophil and platelet engraftment with CD34$^+$Lin$^-$ cell dose/kg. Stiff et al. reported that only 2 $\times$ 10^5 CD34$^+$ cells/kg of the expanded cells were needed to produce optimal platelet engraftment [121]. This was lower than the number of cells required for predictable platelet engraftment by day 28 in breast cancer patients undergoing PBPC transplants in which the minimal number of CD34$^+$ cells required was reported to be 2–5 $\times$ 10^6/kg [125].

Clinical trials using UCB cells

Rationale for the use of UCB stem cells for *ex vivo* expansion

The use of UCB as an alternative source of stem cells in allogeneic transplantation has been pursued for many reasons. For those patients in need

Table 9.1 Selected bone marrow and mobilized peripheral blood clinical expansion trials.

Author/reference	Patients	Stem cell source	Cytokines/serum	Conditioning regimen	Infusion exp cells	Notes
Williams et al. (1996) [115]	n = 9 Met breast CA	MPBPC	PIXY321, Hu serum alb 1% × 12 days	NM*	Day +1	↑TNC 26 fold CD15+ post expansion average 29%
Alcorn et al. (1996) [116]	n = 10 Nonmyeloid malig	MPBPC	SCF, IL-1β, IL3, IL6, EPO +Autol plasma × 8 days	M/NM†	Day 0	↑TNC 21 fold, CFU-GM 139-fold, BFU-E 114-fold (mean) No change in engraftment compared to controls
Bertolini et al. (1997) [117]	n = 10 8 Breast CA/2NHL	MPBPC	MGDF, SCF, IL3, IL6, IL11, Flt3L, MIP-1α, × 7 days	NM‡	Day 0	Study aimed at looking at generating megakaryocytic progenitors
Holyoake et al. (1997) [118]	n = 4 2 NHL, 2 MM	MPBPC Exp cells only	SCF, IL-1β, IL3, IL6, EPO +Autol plasma × 8 days	M§	Day 0	No long term engraftment seen ↑TNC 8–27, CFU-GM 17–130
Reiffers et al. (1999) [119] (letter to editor)	n = 14 MM	MPBPC	SCF, GCSF, MGDF	M‖	Day 0	↑TNC 34.4 fold, CD34+ cells 2.6-fold, CFU-GM 14.1-fold (median)
McNiece et al. (2000) [120]	2 cohorts 1 n = 10 2 n = 11 Breast CA	MPBPC Cohort 2—exp cells only	SCF, GCSF, MGDF × 10 days	NM¶	Day 0	Cohort 1: ↑TNC 20-fold (median) ↑CD34+ cells 1.8 fold Cohort 2: ↑TNC 14-fold (median) ↑CD34+ cells 2.0 fold TNC/kg post-exp best predictor of time to neutrophil engraftment
Stiff et al. (2000) [121]	n = 19 Breast CA	BM (~75 mL)—exp cells only	AastromReplicell Bioreactor Flt3L, EPO, PIXY321 10% FBS, 10% horse sera × 12 days	NM*	Day 0	↑TNC 4.8, CFU-GM 4.2, CD34+/lin− cells 0.9, LTCIC 1.2 (median) Engraftment times similar to auto BMT Correlation: cell dose and engraftment
Pecora et al. (2001) [122]	n = 34 Breast CA	BM (50–100 mL) for expansion + low dose MPBPC	AastromReplicell Bioreactor Flt3L, EPO, PIXY321 (+TPO in seven cases) 10% FBS, 10% horse sera × 12 days	NM*	Day 0	CD34+lin− cell number and quantity of stromal progenitors contained in the expanded product correlated with engraftment outcome
Engelhardt et al. (2001) [123]	n = 10 Breast CA	BM (median 97 mL) —exp cells only 2 pts: irradiated PBPCs	AastromReplicell Bioreactor Flt3L, EPO, PIXY321 10% FBS, 10% horse sera × 12 days	NM*	Day 0	↑TNC 4.5, CFU-GM 18 (median) Correlation: CD34+ lin− cells and engraftment
Paquette et al. (2002) [124]	n = 43 Breast CA	MPBPC	GCSF, SCF, MGDF, 1% hu albumin, transferrin × 9–14 days	NM**	Day 0	Varied duration of cultures and starting cell density

*CPM/carbo/thiotepa (STAMP V)
†melphalan/TBI, BEAM, thiotepa/cyclophosphamide, carboplatin/etoposide/melphalan, Cy/TBI
‡thiotepa/melphalan (Breast Ca); Mitoxantrone/melphalan (NHL)
§Cy/TBI (NHL) and Bu/melphalan (MM)
‖Melphalan +/− TBI
¶CPM/cisplat/BCNU or taxol/CPM/cisplatin or taxotere/melphalan/carboplatin
**CPM/carmustine/Cisplatin

NM, nonmyeloablative; BM, bone marrow; M, myeloablative; MM, multiple myeloma; MPBPC, mobilized peripheral blood progenitor cells; NHL, Non-Hodgkin's lymphoma; TNC, total nucleated cells.

of an hematopoietic stem cell transplantation (HSCT) but lacking a suitable human leukocyte antigen (HLA) donor, UCB has increased the donor pool and treatment options. Moreover, data from umbilical cord blood transplantation (UCBT) results to date have revealed decreased rates of graft-vs.-host disease (GVHD) compared to BM or PBPC, despite increased HLA disparity [126–128], thought to be secondary to fewer and/or more naive T cells present in the UCB graft. However, delayed hematopoietic recovery and increased early transplant related mortality remain the most challenging issues in UCBT and have been shown to be highly correlated with cell dose [128–131]. *Ex vivo* expansion of cord blood progenitors, including short-term progenitors, could possibly produce faster engraftment rates, making UCBT a safer and more viable option for allogeneic transplantation, especially in adults and larger children.

Several lines of evidence suggest that UCB contains a higher frequency of primitive hematopoietic progenitor cells and early committed progenitors than adult BM or peripheral blood [20,63]. There is also increasing evidence that the stem cells isolated from UCB survive longer in culture [88] and may be less mature and have greater proliferative capacity [71,132–134]. Phenotypic analyzes of UCB have shown that the more primitive cell population which express the CD34 antigen, but not the CD38 antigen, is fourfold more prevalent than in BM or PBPC, and that this subpopulation has a higher *in vitro* cloning efficiency than the same population isolated from adult BM [135]. These findings correlate with data from studies using *in vitro* colony-forming assays to show that UCB contains greater numbers of immature colony forming cells compared to BM or PBPC [136–138]. Second, there are numerous reports of the increased proliferative potential of UCB cells in response to cytokine stimulation. For example, using IL-11, SF and G-CSF or granulocyte macrophage colony-stimulating factor (GM-CSF), van de Ven *et al.* demonstrated an 80-fold increase after a 14-day expansion of UCB vs. adult BM [139]. Moreover, compared with adult BM, UCB has been shown to have increased serial *in vitro* replating efficiency [132] and increased culture life span with increased progenitor cell production [87,136]. Finally, *in vivo* assays of UCB vs. BM have shown that HSCs from UCB, but not adult BM can engraft NOD/SCID mice without the use of exogenous cytokines [58]. More recently, Rosler *et al.* [21] showed that expanded cord blood had a competitive repopulating advantage as compared to expanded adult BM using an *in vivo* assay with NOD/SCID mice.

A potential contribution to the differences observed between UCB and adult HSC may arise from the differential response of HSCs from different sources in cytokine-driven expansion systems, leading to variations in cell cycle status and homing ability of the expanded cells. Other possible sources of stem cells may have even greater proliferative potential. For example, murine fetal liver cells have greater proliferation and repopulation potential than HSCs isolated from adult murine BM or peripheral blood [140,141]. Overall, these results suggest that UCB progenitor cells are functionally superior to adult BM, with greater proliferative potential and possibly greater self-renewal capacity. Thus, UCB may represent a more viable target for *ex vivo* stem cell expansion, a possibility that has led to several clinical studies on the *ex vivo* expansion of cord blood cells to augment conventional UCBT.

Clinical *ex vivo* expansion trials with UCB

UCB expansion trials (summarized in Table 9.2) [142–146] were undertaken to determine whether the delayed engraftment associated with UCBT could be overcome if a portion of the cells from the UCB unit were expanded *ex vivo*. Like the trials using PBPC and BM, these trials utilized cytokine-based expansion systems as well as newer automated perfusion systems. The choice of exogenous cytokines used for culture has varied, reflecting the still undefined optimal conditions for expansion of the stem/progenitor cell. In all of the studies, only a portion of the cord blood was used for expansion, and the expanded cells were infused in addition to unmanipulated cells since the cultured cells may have differentiated and lost HSC properties. There have been no adverse toxicities associated with infusion of the expanded cell product, nor has there been any change in engraftment kinetics. However, only two of the studies have enrolled more than a handful of patients, making it difficult to draw any definitive conclusions.

In one of the larger studies to date, Jaroscek *et al.* [146] reported preliminary data from a phase 1 trial at Duke University Medical Center undertaken to assess augmentation of UCBT with cells expanded *ex vivo* in the AastromReplicell™ Cell Production System. This trial included 28 patients with both malignant and inherited disorders who were conditioned with one of three regimens (see Table 9.2) depending on diagnosis. The patients had a median age of 4.5 years and a median weight of 17.1 kg. On day 0, a portion of the UCB from unrelated donors was expanded *ex vivo* in medium supplemented with fetal bovine serum, horse serum and the cytokines Epo, Pixy 321 and Flt3L for 12 days. The expanded cells were then infused to augment the conventional transplant on day +12. Although expansion of total nucleated cells (TNC) and CFC occurred *in vitro* in all cases, no increase in $CD34^+Lin^-$ cell number was achieved. *In vivo*, significant effects on engraftment kinetics were not observed with median time to neutrophil engraftment (absolute neutrophil count, ANC, >500) of 22 days, range 13–40. For the 16 patients who engrafted platelets, the median time to engraftment was 71 days (range 39–139). No adverse reactions were observed due to infusion of the cultured cells. This phase 1 trial is an important contribution to the concept and development of *ex vivo* expansion of UCB $CD34^+$ cells for use in the clinical setting since it demonstrates both the safety of reserving an aliquot of an already small cord blood unit for expansion and the feasibility of expansion in a clinical setting. It is also possible that, although the numbers of $CD34^+Lin^-$ and $CD3^+$ cells were not expanded with this culture system, and may have explained the failure to improve engraftment, the delayed infusion (day +10 to +12) of expanded cells may have masked or prevented the benefit of a more rapid engraftment, which was seen in a few anecdotal reports where the infusion of cultured cells on day 0 was associated with rapid neutrophil engraftment [143].

Another trial has been performed at the University of Colorado by Shpall and colleagues [145], in which patients are receiving expanded cells on day 0 ($n = 12$) or day +10 ($n = 25$) depending on whether the UCB units were frozen as a single or split fraction. Interim analysis of the first 37 patients has also shown no difference in the time to neutrophil or platelet engraftment between the two strata. All fractions of UCB (40% or 60%) used for expansion were CD34 selected and then expanded in Teflon bags containing serum-free medium supplemented with recombinant human SCF, recombinant human G-CSF, and recombinant human MGDF (100 ng/mL each). Overall, the median-fold expansion of TNC and $CD34^+$ was 56 (range 1–278) and 4 (range 0.1–20.0), respectively. Neutrophil engraftment occurred in all patients that were evaluable in a median of 28 days (35 days for adults and 25 days for pediatric patients) (range 15–49), and platelet engraftment occurred at a median of 106 days (261 days for adults and 65 days for pediatric patients) (range 38–345). No significant correlation between the TNC per kilogram (pre or postthaw) and time to neutrophil engraftment was demonstrated. Thus, although there was no appreciable clinical benefit with regard to engraftment kinetics, this trial resulted in no failures of neutrophil engraftment, despite being conducted primarily in adult patients where cell dose is lower and rates of engraftment failure are higher [128–131]. This result may suggest an effect of the cells expanded with this particular methodology. In contrast, in the previously discussed trial by Jaroscek *et al.* which enrolled primarily pediatric patients (26 out of 28 total), three of the 28 patients failed to engraft despite the infusion of expanded cells,

Table 9.2 Selected umbilical cord blood clinical expansion trials.

Author/reference	Patients	Stem cell source	Cytokines/serum	Conditioning regimen	Infusion exp cells	Notes
Stiff et al. (1998—ASH, abstract) [142]	$n = 9$ Dx: Advanced hematologic disorders	UCB (unrelated) Expanded + unmanipulated	AastromReplicell system Epo, Pixy 321, Flt3l × 12 days	Cy/TBI or Bu/Cy/ATG	Day +12	No significant change in neutrophil engraftment No infusional toxicities 2 deaths prior to engraftment
Kögler et al. (1999) [143] (case report)	$n = 1$ High risk leukemia	UCB—sibling 12.5% expanded + 87.5% unmanipulated	G-CSF, TPO, Flt3L, 10% autologous CB plasma × 10 days liquid culture system in Teflon bags	TBI/thiotepa/Cy	Day +1	ANC 310 by day +8 EFS now greater than one year
Pecora et al. (2000) [144]	$n = 2$ CML (blast crisis and accelerated phase	UCB (unrelated) 11%, 17% expanded + 89%, 83% unmanipulated cells	AastromReplicell system Epo, Pixy 321, Flt3L × 12 days	1 busulfan/ATG Cy 2 Cy/TBI/ATG	Day +12	No infusional toxicities Improved plt engraftment and same neutrophil engraftment Lin^-, $CD34^+$ cells decreased in one patient, increase 1.7 in other patient
Shpall et al. (2002) [145]	$n = 37$ (25 adult) Stratum A = 25 Stratum B = 12 (split unit) Dx: Hem Malig (34) Breast CA (3)	UCB (unrelated) Expanded fraction Cohort A = 40% Cohort B = 60% + unmanipulated cells	GCSF, SCF, MGDF expanded in Teflon bags × 10 days	Adults: HD Mel/ATG/TBI, or HD Mel/ATG/Bu Children: Cy/TBI/AraC/ATG	Stratum (a) day +10 (b) day 0	No infusional toxicities No change in engraftment seen No neutrophil engraftment failures
Jaroscak et al. (in press) [146]	$n = 28$ (26 children) Varied dx—both malignancies and inherited disorders	UCB (unrelated, one sibling) Expanded + unmanipulated cells	AastromReplicell system PIXY321, Epo, Flt3L, 10% horse serum, 10% FBS × 12 days	Hematologic malig TBI/Melph/ATG, or Bu/melph/ATG Inherited disorders Bu/Cy/ATG	Day +12	No infusional toxicities Clinically feasible No alteration in time to engraftment ↑TNC 2.4-fold, CFU-GM 82.7-fold, $CD34^+$ 0.5-fold (median)

ATG, Anti-thymocyte globulin; Cy, Cyclophosphamide; EFS, event free survival; FBS, fetal bovine serum; TBI, Total body irradiation.

and thus does not provide convincing evidence for this expansion methodology [146]. A definitive trial involving simultaneous infusion of expanded cells with unmanipulated cells on day 0 has yet to be completed.

Conclusion

Although optimal conditions for expanding HSC numbers remain undefined, the collective results of the studies outlined above suggest that enhanced short-term and long-term repopulating ability may be achievable with cytokine-induced expansion systems. However, these studies further suggest that cytokine-induced effects on HSC self-renewal and expansion are limited and clinically significant expansion has not been achieved. It is likely that we have not yet identified critical factors and combinations required to induce symmetric HSC self-renewal, and thus, current efforts are now focused on identifying and exploiting factors previously shown to regulate stem cell fate in other developing organ systems or during embryogenesis. This approach is beginning to yield promising results and improved methods for HSC expansion are anticipated. Identification of genes and regulatory elements that are responsible for preventing stem cell senescence and driving symmetric divisions of the HSC, and a better understanding of how culturing affects the homing ability of stem cells and of the complex cellular interactions in the BM microenvironment are all essential to the ultimate success of *ex vivo* expansion. These areas are discussed in more detail in Chapters 6 & 7. Clinically, *ex vivo* expansion studies of primitive cells from BM, PBPC and UCB have demonstrated the feasibility and safety of *ex vivo* expansion and have suggested the enhancement of short-term repopulating cells perhaps at the expense of long-term repopulating cells. Further development of methods using novel stem cell regulators that are shown to expand HSCs in preclinical studies is necessary and holds promise for the future of expanding HSC numbers *ex vivo*.

References

1 Verfaillie C. *Ex vivo* expansion of hematopoeitic stem cells. In: Zon L, ed. *Hematopoiesis: A Developmental Approach*. New York: Oxford University Press, 2001: 119–29.

2 McNiece I, Briddell R. *Ex vivo* expansion of hematopoietic progenitor cells and mature cells. *Exp Hematol* 2001; **29**: 3–11.

3 Scheding S, Kratz-Albers K, Meister B, Brugger W, Kanz L. *Ex vivo* expansion of hematopoietic progenitor cells for clinical use. *Semin Hematol* 1998; **35**: 232–40.

4 Hoffman R. Progress in the development of systems for *in vitro* expansion of human hematopoietic stem cells. *Curr Opin Hematol* 1999; **6**: 184–91.

5 Emerson SG. *Ex vivo* expansion of hematopoietic precursors, progenitors, and stem cells: the next generation of cellular therapeutics. *Blood* 1996; **87**: 3082–8.

6 Ogawa M. Differentiation and proliferation of hematopoietic stem cells. *Blood* 1993; **81**: 2844–53.

7 Morrison SJ, Wandycz AM, Hemmati HD, Wright DE, Weissman IL. Identification of a lineage of multipotent hematopoietic progenitors. *Development* 1997; **124**: 1929–39.

8 Weissman IL. Stem cells. Units of development, units of regeneration, and units in evolution. *Cell* 2000; **100**: 157–68.

9 Ogden DA, Mickliem HS. The fate of serially transplanted bone marrow cell populations from young and old donors. *Transplantation* 1976; **22**: 287–93.

10 Ross EA, Anderson N, Micklem HS. Serial depletion and regeneration of the murine hematopoietic system. Implications for hematopoietic organization and the study of cellular aging. *J Exp Med* 1982; **155**: 432–44.

11 Harrison DE, Astle CM. Loss of stem cell repopulating ability upon transplantation. Effects of donor age, cell number, and transplantation procedure. *J Exp Med* 1982; **156**: 1767–79.

12 Morrison SJ, Wandycz AM, Akashi K, Globerson A, Weissman IL. The aging of hematopoietic stem cells. *Nat Med* 1996; **2**: 1011–6.

13 Iscove NN, Nawa K. Hematopoietic stem cells expand during serial transplantation *in vivo* without apparent exhaustion. *Curr Biol* 1997; **7**: 805–8.

14 Sudo K, Ema H, Morita Y, Nakauchi H. Age-associated characteristics of murine hematopoietic stem cells. *J Exp Med* 2000; **192**: 1273–80.

15 Rosendahl M, Hodgson GS, Bradley TR. Organization of hematopoietic stem cell: the generation age hypothesis. *Cell Tissue Kinet* 1979; **12**: 17–29.

16 Geiger H, Van Zant G. The aging of lymphohematopoietic stem cells. *Nat Immunol* 2002; **3**: 329–33.

17 Allsopp RC, Weissman IL. Replicative senescence of hematopoietic stem cells during serial transplantation: does telomere shortening play a role? *Oncogene* 2002; **21**: 3270–3.

18 Halene S, Kohn DB. Gene therapy using hematopoietic stem cells: Sisyphus approaches the crest. *Hum Gene Ther* 2000; **11**: 1259–67.

19 Mulligan RC. The basic science of gene therapy. *Science* 1993; **260**: 926–32.

20 Holyoake TL, Nicolini FE, Eaves CJ. Functional differences between transplantable human hematopoietic stem cells from fetal liver, cord blood, and adult marrow. *Exp Hematol* 1999; **27**: 1418–27.

21 Rosler ES, Brandt JE, Chute J, Hoffman R. An *in vivo* competitive repopulation assay for various sources of human hematopoietic stem cells. *Blood* 2000; **96**: 3414–21.

22 Weekx SF, Van Bockstaele DR, Plum J *et al*. $CD34^{++}CD38^{-}$ and $CD34^{+}CD38^{+}$ human hematopoietic progenitors from fetal liver, cord blood, and adult bone marrow respond differently to hematopoietic cytokines depending on the ontogenic source. *Exp Hematol* 1998; **26**: 1034–42.

23 Verfaillie CM. Hematopoietic stem cells for transplantation. *Nat Immunol* 2002; **3**: 314–7.

24 Nakahata T, Gross AJ, Ogawa M. A stochastic model of self-renewal and commitment to differentiation of the primitive hemopoietic stem cells in culture. *J Cell Physiol* 1982; **113**: 455–8.

25 Socolovsky M, Lodish HF, Daley GQ. Control of hematopoietic differentiation: lack of specificity in signaling by cytokine receptors. *Proc Natl Acad Sci U S A* 1998; **95**: 6573–5.

26 Spradling A, Drummond-Barbosa D, Kai T. Stem cells find their niche. *Nature* 2001; **414**: 98–104.

27 Watt FM, Hogan BL. Out of Eden: stem cells and their niches. *Science* 2000; **287**: 1427–30.

28 Dexter TM, Moore MA, Sheridan AP. Maintenance of hemopoietic stem cells and production of differentiated progeny in allogeneic and semiallogeneic bone marrow chimeras *in vitro*. *J Exp Med* 1977; **145**: 1612–6.

29 Fraser CC, Eaves CJ, Szilvassy SJ, Humphries RK. Expansion *in vitro* of retrovirally marked totipotent hematopoietic stem cells. *Blood* 1990; **76**: 1071–6.

30 Miller CL, Eaves CJ. Expansion *in vitro* of adult murine hematopoietic stem cells with transplantable lympho-myeloid reconstituting ability. *Proc Natl Acad Sci U S A* 1997; **94**: 13,648–53.

31 Dexter TM, Allen TD, Lajtha LG. Conditions controlling the proliferation of haemopoietic stem cells *in vitro*. *J Cell Physiol* 1977; **91**: 335–44.

32 Roberts R, Gallagher J, Spooncer E, Allen TD, Bloomfield F, Dexter TM. Heparan sulphate bound growth factors: a mechanism for stromal cell mediated haemopoiesis. *Nature* 1988; **332**: 376–8.

33 Spooncer E, Gallagher JT, Krizsa F, Dexter TM. Regulation of haemopoiesis in long-term bone marrow cultures. IV. Glycosaminoglycan synthesis and the stimulation of haemopoiesis by β-D-xylosides. *J Cell Biol* 1983; **96**: 510–4.

34 Fraser CC, Szilvassy SJ, Eaves CJ, Humphries RK. Proliferation of totipotent hematopoietic stem cells *in vitro* with retention of long-term competitive *in vivo* reconstituting ability. *Proc Natl Acad Sci U S A* 1992; **89**: 1968–72.

35 Trevisan M, Yan XQ, Iscove NN. Cycle initiation and colony formation in culture by murine marrow cells with long-term reconstituting potential *in vivo*. *Blood* 1996; **88**: 4149–58.

36 Ema H, Takano H, Sudo K, Nakauchi H. *In vitro* self-renewal division of hematopoietic stem cells. *J Exp Med* 2000; **192**: 1281–8.

37 Giet O, Van Bockstaele DR, Di Stefano I *et al*. Increased binding and defective migration across fibronectin of cycling hematopoietic progenitor cells. *Blood* 2002; **99**: 2023–31.

38 Berrios VM, Dooner GJ, Nowakowski G *et al*. The molecular basis for the cytokine-induced defect in homing and engraftment of hematopoietic stem cells. *Exp Hematol* 2001; **29**: 1326–35.

39 Habibian HK, Peters SO, Hsieh CC *et al*. The fluctuating phenotype of the lymphohematopoietic stem cell with cell cycle transit. *J Exp Med* 1998; **188**: 393–8.

40 Gothot A, Pyatt R, McMahel J, Rice S, Srour EF. Assessment of proliferative and colony-forming capacity after successive *in vitro* divisions of single human $CD34^+$ cells initially isolated in G_0. *Exp Hematol* 1998; **26**: 562–70.

41 Gothot A, van der Loo JC, Clapp DW, Srour EF. Cell cycle-related changes in repopulating capacity of human mobilized peripheral blood CD34+ cells in nonobese diabetic/severe combined immune-deficient mice. *Blood* 1998; **92**: 2641–9.

42 Yonemura Y, Ku H, Hirayama F, Souza LM, Ogawa M. Interleukin 3 or interleukin 1 abrogates the reconstituting ability of hematopoietic stem cells. *Proc Natl Acad Sci U S A* 1996; **93**: 4040–4.

43 Yonemura Y, Ku H, Lyman SD, Ogawa M. *In vitro* expansion of hematopoietic progenitors and maintenance of stem cells: comparison between Flt3/Flk2 ligand and kit ligand. *Blood* 1997; **89**: 1915–21.

44 Yagi M, Ritchie KA, Sitnicka E, Storey C, Roth GJ, Bartelmez S. Sustained *ex vivo* expansion of hematopoietic stem cells mediated by thrombopoietin. *Proc Natl Acad Sci U S A* 1999; **96**: 8126–31.

45 Cashman JD, Eaves AC, Raines EW, Ross R, Eaves CJ. Mechanisms that regulate the cell cycle status of very primitive hematopoietic cells in long-term human marrow cultures. I. Stimulatory role of a variety of mesenchymal cell activators and inhibitory role of TGF-β. *Blood* 1990; **75**: 96–101.

46 Cashman JD, Eaves CJ, Sarris AH, Eaves AC. MCP-1, not MIP-1α, is the endogenous chemokine that cooperates with TGF-β to inhibit the cycling of primitive normal but not leukemic (CML) progenitors in long-term human marrow cultures. *Blood* 1998; **92**: 2338–44.

47 Eaves CJ, Cashman JD, Kay RJ et al. Mechanisms that regulate the cell cycle status of very primitive hematopoietic cells in long-term human marrow cultures. II. Analysis of positive and negative regulators produced by stromal cells within the adherent layer. *Blood* 1991; **78**: 110–7.

48 Abkowitz JL, Catlin SN, McCallie MT, Guttorp P. Evidence that the number of hematopoietic stem cells per animal is conserved in mammals. *Blood* 2002; **100**: 2665–7.

49 Mahmud N, Devine SM, Weller KP et al. The relative quiescence of hematopoietic stem cells in nonhuman primates. *Blood* 2001; **97**: 3061–8.

50 Chesier S, Morrison SJ, Liao X, Weissman IL. *In vivo* proliferation and cell cycle kinetics of long-term self-renewing hematopoietic stem cells. *Proc Natl Acad Sci U S A* 1999; **96**: 3120–5.

51 Andrews RG, Briddell RA, Hill R, Gough M, McNiece IK. Engraftment of primates with G-CSF mobilized peripheral blood CD34+ progenitor cells expanded in G-CSF, SCF and MGDF decreases the duration and severity of neutropenia. *Stem Cells* 1999; **17**: 210–8.

52 Norol F, Drouet M, Mathieu J et al. *Ex vivo* expanded mobilized peripheral blood CD34+ cells accelerate haematological recovery in a baboon model of autologous transplantation. *Br J Haematol* 2000; **109**: 162–72.

53 Drouet M, Herodin F, Norol F, Mourcin F, Mayol JF. Cell cycle activation of peripheral blood stem and progenitor cells expanded *ex vivo* with SCF, FLT-3 ligand, TPO, and IL-3 results in accelerated granulocyte recovery in a baboon model of autologous transplantation but G_0/G_1 and $S/G_2/M$ graft cell content does not correlate with transplantability. *Stem Cells* 2001; **19**: 436–42.

54 Kiem HP, Rasko JE, Morris J, Peterson L, Kurre P, Andrews RG. *Ex vivo* selection for oncoretrovirally transduced green fluorescent protein-expressing CD34-enriched cells increases short-term engraftment of transduced cells in baboons. *Hum Gene Ther* 2002; **13**: 891–9.

55 Tisdale JF, Hanazono Y, Sellers SE et al. *Ex vivo* expansion of genetically marked rhesus peripheral blood progenitor cells results in diminished long-term repopulating ability. *Blood* 1998; **92**: 1131–41.

56 Abkowitz JL, Taboada MR, Sabo KM, Shelton GH. The *ex vivo* expansion of feline marrow cells leads to increased numbers of BFU-E and CFU-GM but a loss of reconstituting ability. *Stem Cells* 1998; **16**: 288–93.

57 Goerner M, Horn PA, Peterson L et al. Sustained multilineage gene persistence and expression in dogs transplanted with CD34+ marrow cells transduced by RD114-pseudotype oncoretrovirus vectors. *Blood* 2001; **98**: 2065–70.

58 Vormoor J, Lapidot T, Pflumio F et al. Immature human cord blood progenitors engraft and proliferate to high levels in severe combined immunodeficient mice. *Blood* 1994; **83**: 2489–97.

59 Larochelle A, Vormoor J, Hanenberg H et al. Identification of primitive human hematopoietic cells capable of repopulating NOD/SCID mouse bone marrow: implications for gene therapy. *Nat Med* 1996; **2**: 1329–37.

60 Conneally E, Cashman J, Petzer A, Eaves C. Expansion *in vitro* of transplantable human cord blood stem cells demonstrated using a quantitative assay of their lympho-myeloid repopulating activity in nonobese diabetic-SCID/SCID mice. *Proc Natl Acad Sci U S A* 1997; **94**: 9836–41.

61 Bhatia M, Wang JC, Kapp U, Bonnet D, Dick JE. Purification of primitive human hematopoietic cells capable of repopulating immune-deficient mice. *Proc Natl Acad Sci U S A* 1997; **94**: 5320–5.

62 Bhatia M, Bonnet D, Murdoch B, Gan OI, Dick JE. A newly discovered class of human hematopoietic cells with SCID-repopulating activity. *Nat Med* 1998; **4**: 1038–45.

63 Wang JC, Doedens M, Dick JE. Primitive human hematopoietic cells are enriched in cord blood compared with adult bone marrow or mobilized peripheral blood as measured by the quantitative *in vivo* SCID-repopulating cell assay. *Blood* 1997; **89**: 3919–24.

64 Glimm H, Eisterer W, Lee K et al. Previously undetected human hematopoietic cell populations with short-term repopulating activity selectively engraft NOD/SCID-β$_2$ microglobulin-null mice. *J Clin Invest* 2001; **107**: 199–206.

65 Gan OI, Murdoch B, Larochelle A, Dick JE. Differential maintenance of primitive human SCID-repopulating cells, clonogenic progenitors, and long-term culture-initiating cells after incubation on human bone marrow stromal cells. *Blood* 1997; **90**: 641–50.

66 Mobest D, Goan SR, Junghahn I et al. Differential kinetics of primitive hematopoietic cells assayed *in vitro* and *in vivo* during serum-free suspension culture of CD34+ blood progenitor cells. *Stem Cells* 1999; **17**: 152–61.

67 Dorrell C, Gan OI, Pereira DS, Hawley RG, Dick JE. Expansion of human cord blood CD34+ CD38− cells in *ex vivo* culture during retroviral transduction without a corresponding increase in SCID repopulating cell (SRC) frequency: dissociation of SRC phenotype and function. *Blood* 2000; **95**: 102–10.

68 Danet GH, Lee HW, Luongo JL, Simon MC, Bonnet DA. Dissociation between stem cell phenotype and NOD/SCID repopulating activity in human peripheral blood CD34+ cells after *ex vivo* expansion. *Exp Hematol* 2001; **29**: 1465–73.

69 Gilmore GL, DePasquale DK, Lister J, Shadduck RK. *Ex vivo* expansion of human umbilical cord blood and peripheral blood CD34+ hematopoietic stem cells. *Exp Hematol* 2000; **28**: 1297–305.

70 Luens KM, Travis MA, Chen BP, Hill BL, Scollay R, Murray LJ. Thrombopoietin, kit ligand, and Flk2/Flt3 ligand together induce increased numbers of primitive hematopoietic progenitors from human CD34+Thy-1+Lin− cells with preserved ability to engraft SCID-hu bone. *Blood* 1998; **91**: 1206–15.

71 Piacibello W, Sanavio F, Severino A et al. Engraftment in nonobese diabetic severe combined immunodeficient mice of human CD34+ cord blood cells after *ex vivo* expansion: evidence for the amplification and self-renewal of repopulating stem cells. *Blood* 1999; **93**: 3736–49.

72 Novelli EM, Cheng L, Yang Y et al. *Ex vivo* culture of cord blood CD34+ cells expands progenitor cell numbers, preserves engraftment capacity in nonobese diabetic/severe combined immunodeficient mice, and enhances retroviral transduction efficiency. *Hum Gene Ther* 1999; **10**: 2927–40.

73 Ueda T, Tsuji K, Yoshino H et al. Expansion of human NOD/SCID-repopulating cells by stem cell factor, Flk2/Flt3 ligand, thrombopoietin, IL-6, and soluble IL-6 receptor. *J Clin Invest* 2000; **105**: 1013–21.

74 Bhatia R, McGlave PB, Miller JS, Wissink S, Lin WN, Verfaillie CM. A clinically suitable *ex vivo* expansion culture system for LTC-IC and CFC using stroma-conditioned medium. *Exp Hematol* 1997; **25**: 980–91.

75 Bhatia M, Bonnet D, Kapp U, Wang JC, Murdoch B, Dick JE. Quantitative analysis reveals expansion of human hematopoietic repopulating cells after short-term *ex vivo* culture. *J Exp Med* 1997; **186**: 619–24.

76 Kollet O, Aviram R, Chebath J et al. The soluble interleukin-6 (IL-6) receptor/IL-6 fusion protein enhances *in vitro* maintenance and proliferation of human CD34+ CD38−/low cells capable of repopulating severe combined immunodeficiency mice. *Blood* 1999; **94**: 923–31.

77 Tajima S, Tsuji K, Ebihara Y et al. Analysis of interleukin 6 receptor and GP130 expressions and proliferative capability of human CD34+ cells. *J Exp Med* 1996; **184**: 1357–64.

78 Kimura T, Sakabe H, Tanimukai S et al. Simultaneous activation of signals through GP130, c-kit, and interleukin-3 receptor promotes a trilineage blood cell production in the absence of terminally acting lineage-specific factors. *Blood* 1997; **90**: 4767–78.

79 Kimura T, Wang J, Minamiguchi H et al. Signal through GP130 activated by soluble interleukin (IL)-6 receptor (R) and IL-6 or IL-6R/IL-6 fusion protein enhances *ex vivo* expansion of human peripheral blood-derived hematopoietic progenitors. *Stem Cells* 2000; **18**: 444–52.

80 Hanania EG, Giles RE, Kavanagh J et al. Results of MDR-1 vector modification trial indicate that granulocyte/macrophage colony-forming unit cells do not contribute to posttransplant hematopoietic recovery following intensive systemic therapy. *Proc Natl Acad Sci U S A* 1996; **93**: 15,346–51.

81 Emmons RV, Doren S, Zujewski J et al. Retroviral gene transduction of adult peripheral blood or marrow-derived CD34+ cells for six hours without growth factors or on autologous stroma does not improve marking efficiency assessed *in vivo*. *Blood* 1997; **89**: 4040–6.

82. Shih C, Hu MC, Hu J *et al*. A secreted and LIF-mediated stromal cell-derived activity that promotes *ex vivo* expansion of human hematopoietic stem cells. *Blood* 2000; **95**: 1957–66.
83. Verfaillie CM, Catanzarro PM, Li WN. Macrophage inflammatory protein 1 alpha, interleukin 3 and diffusible marrow stromal factors maintain human hematopoietic stem cells for at least eight weeks *in vitro*. *J Exp Med* 1994; **179**: 643–9.
84. Roecklein B, Almaida-Porada G, Torok-Storb B *et al*. Serial xenogeneic transplantation of *ex vivo* expanded human CD34+ cells. *Blood* 1997; **90**: 1750a [Abstract].
85. Lewis ID, Almeida-Porada GJ, Du J *et al*. Umbilical cord blood cells capable of engrafting in primary, secondary, and tertiary xenogeneic hosts are preserved after *ex vivo* culture in a noncontact system. *Blood* 2001; **97**: 3441–9.
86. Roecklein BA, Torok-Storb B. Functionally distinct human marrow stromal cell lines immortalized by transduction with the human papilloma virus E6/E7 genes. *Blood* 1995; **85**: 997–1005.
87. Piacibello W, Sanavio F, Garetto L *et al*. Extensive amplification and self-renewal of human primitive hematopoietic stem cells from cord blood. *Blood* 1997; **89**: 2644–53.
88. Tanavde VM, Malehorn MT, Lumkul R *et al*. Human stem-progenitor cells from neonatal cord blood have greater hematopoietic expansion capacity than those from mobilized adult blood. *Exp Hematol* 2002; **30**: 816–23.
89. Shimizu Y, Ogawa M, Kobayashi M, Almeida-Porada G, Zanjani ED. Engraftment of cultured human hematopoietic cells in sheep. *Blood* 1998; **91**: 3688–92.
90. McNiece IK, Almeida-Porada G, Shpall EJ, Zanjani E. *Ex vivo* expanded cord blood cells provide rapid engraftment in fetal sheep but lack long-term engrafting potential. *Exp Hematol* 2002; **30**: 612–6.
91. Guenechea G, Segovia JC, Albella B *et al*. Delayed engraftment of nonobese diabetic/severe combined immunodeficient mice transplanted with *ex vivo*-expanded human CD34+ cord blood cells. *Blood* 1999; **93**: 1097–105.
92. Glimm H, Eaves CJ. Direct evidence for multiple self-renewal divisions of human *in vivo* repopulating hematopoietic cells in short-term culture. *Blood* 1999; **94**: 2161–8.
93. Ballen K, Becker PS, Greiner D *et al*. Effect of *ex vivo* cytokine treatment on human cord blood engraftment in NOD-SCID mice. *Br J Haematol* 2000; **108**: 629–40.
94. Sauvageau G, Thorsteinsdottir U, Eaves CJ *et al*. Overexpression of *Hox*B4 in hematopoietic cells causes the selective expansion of more primitive populations *in vitro* and *in vivo*. *Genes Dev* 1995; **9**: 1753–65.
95. Thorsteinsdottir U, Sauvageau G, Humphries RK. Enhanced *in vivo* regenerative potential of *Hox*B4-transduced hematopoietic stem cells with regulation of their pool size. *Blood* 1999; **94**: 2605–12.
96. Antonchuk J, Sauvageau G, Humphries RK. *Hox*B4 overexpression mediates very rapid stem cell regeneration and competitive hematopoietic repopulation. *Exp Hematol* 2001; **29**: 1125–34.
97. Antonchuk J, Sauvageau G, Humphries RK. *Hox*B4-induced expansion of adult hematopoietic stem cells *ex vivo*. *Cell* 2002; **109**: 39–45.
98. Bhatia M, Bonnet D, Wu D *et al*. Bone morphogenetic proteins regulate the developmental program of human hematopoietic stem cells. *J Exp Med* 1999; **189**: 1139–48.
99. Zon LI. Self-renewal versus differentiation, a job for the mighty morphogens. *Nat Immunol* 2001; **2**: 142–3.
100. Bhardwaj G, Murdoch B, Wu D *et al*. Sonic hedgehog induces the proliferation of primitive human hematopoietic cells via BMP regulation. *Nat Immunol* 2001; **2**: 172–80.
101. Yamane T, Kunisada T, Tsukamoto H *et al*. Wnt signaling regulates hemopoiesis through stromal cells. *J Immunol* 2001; **167**: 765–72.
102. Austin TW, Solar GP, Ziegler FC, Liem L, Matthews W. A role for the Wnt gene family in hematopoiesis: expansion of multilineage progenitor cells. *Blood* 1997; **89**: 3624–35.
103. Kojika S, Griffin JD. Notch receptors and hematopoiesis. *Exp Hematol* 2001; **29**: 1041–52.
104. Milner LA, Kopan R, Martin DI, Bernstein ID. A human homologue of the Drosophila developmental gene, Notch, is expressed in CD34+ hematopoietic precursors. *Blood* 1994; **83**: 2057–62.
105. Ohishi K, Varnum-Finney B, Flowers D, Anasetti C, Myerson D, Bernstein ID. Monocytes express high amounts of Notch and undergo cytokine specific apoptosis following interaction with the Notch ligand, Delta-1. *Blood* 2000; **95**: 2847–54.
106. Karanu FN, Murdoch B, Gallacher L *et al*. The notch ligand Jagged-1 represents a novel growth factor of human hematopoietic stem cells. *J Exp Med* 2000; **192**: 1365–72.
107. Karanu FN, Murdoch B, Miyabayashi T *et al*. Human homologues of Delta-1 and Delta-4 function as mitogenic regulators of primitive human hematopoietic cells. *Blood* 2001; **97**: 1960–7.
108. Jones P, May G, Healy L *et al*. Stromal expression of Jagged 1 promotes colony formation by fetal hematopoietic progenitor cells. *Blood* 1998; **92**: 1505–11.
109. Li L, Milner LA, Deng Y *et al*. The human homolog of rat Jagged1 expressed by marrow stroma inhibits differentiation of 32D cells through interaction with Notch1. *Immunity* 1998; **8**: 43–55.
110. Varnum-Finney B, Xu L, Brashem-Stein C *et al*. Pluripotent, cytokine-dependent, hematopoietic stem cells are immortalized by constitutive Notch1 signaling. *Nat Med* 2000; **6**: 1278–81.
111. Stier S, Cheng T, Dombkowski D, Carlesso N, Scadden DT. Notch1 activation increases hematopoietic stem cell self-renewal *in vivo* and favors lymphoid over myeloid lineage outcome. *Blood* 2002; **99**: 2369–78.
112. Carlesso N, Aster JC, Sklar J, Scadden DT. Notch1-induced delay of human hematopoietic progenitor cell differentiation is associated with altered cell cycle kinetics. *Blood* 1999; **93**: 838–48.
113. Varnum-Finney B, Wu L, Yu M *et al*. Immobilization of Notch ligand, Delta-1, is required for induction of notch signaling. *J Cell Sci* 2000; **113**(23): 4313–8.
114. Ohishi K, Varnum-Finney B, Bernstein I. Delta-1 enhances marrow and thymic repopulating ability of human CD34+CD38− cord blood cells. *J Clin Inv* 2002; **110**: 1165–74.
115. Williams SF, Lee WJ, Bender JG *et al*. Selection and expansion of peripheral blood CD34+ cells in autologous stem cell transplantation for breast cancer. *Blood* 1996; **87**: 1687–91.
116. Alcorn MJ, Holyoake TL, Richmond L *et al*. CD34-positive cells isolated from cryopreserved peripheral-blood progenitor cells can be expanded *ex vivo* and used for transplantation with little or no toxicity. *J Clin Oncol* 1996; **14**: 1839–47.
117. Bertolini F, Battaglia M, Pedrazzoli P *et al*. Megakaryocytic progenitors can be generated *ex vivo* and safely administered to autologous peripheral blood progenitor cell transplant recipients. *Blood* 1997; **89**: 2679–88.
118. Holyoake TL, Alcorn MJ, Richmond L *et al*. CD34 positive PBPC expanded *ex vivo* may not provide durable engraftment following myeloablative chemoradiotherapy regimens. *Bone Marrow Transplant* 1997; **19**: 1095–101.
119. Reiffers J, Cailliot C, Dazey B, Attal M, Caraux J, Boiron J. Abrogation of post-myeloablative chemotherapy neutropenia by *ex-vivo* expanded autologous CD34-positive cells. *Lancet* 1999; **354**: 1092–3.
120. McNiece I, Jones R, Bearman SI *et al*. *Ex vivo* expanded peripheral blood progenitor cells provide rapid neutrophil recovery after high-dose chemotherapy in patients with breast cancer. *Blood* 2000; **96**: 3001–7.
121. Stiff P, Chen B, Franklin W *et al*. Autologous transplantation of *ex vivo* expanded bone marrow cells grown from small aliquots after high-dose chemotherapy for breast cancer. *Blood* 2000; **95**: 2169–74.
122. Pecora AL, Stiff P, LeMaistre CF *et al*. A phase II trial evaluating the safety and effectiveness of the AastromReplicell™ system for augmentation of low-dose blood stem cell transplantation. *Bone Marrow Transplant* 2001; **28**: 295–303.
123. Engelhardt M, Douville J, Behringer D *et al*. Hematopoietic recovery of *ex vivo* perfusion culture expanded bone marrow and unexpanded peripheral blood progenitors after myeloablative chemotherapy. *Bone Marrow Transplant* 2001; **27**: 249–59.
124. Paquette RL, Dergham ST, Karpf E *et al*. Culture conditions affect the ability of *ex vivo* expanded peripheral blood progenitor cells to accelerate hematopoietic recovery. *Exp Hematol* 2002; **30**: 374–80.
125. Glaspy JA, Shpall EJ, LeMaistre CF *et al*. Peripheral blood progenitor cell mobilization using stem cell factor in combination with filgrastim in breast cancer patients. *Blood* 1997; **90**: 2939–51.
126. Wagner JE, Rosenthal J, Sweetman R *et al*. Successful transplantation of HLA-matched and HLA-mismatched umbilical cord blood from unrelated donors: analysis of engraftment and acute graft-versus-host disease. *Blood* 1996; **88**: 795–802.
127. Wagner JE, Barker JN, DeFor TE *et al*. Transplantation of unrelated donor umbilical cord blood in 102 patients with malignant and nonmalignant diseases: influence of CD34 cell dose and HLA disparity on treatment-related mortality and survival. *Blood* 2002; **100**: 1611–8.
128. Gluckman E. Current status of umbilical cord blood hematopoietic stem cell transplantation. *Exp Hematol* 2000; **28**: 1197–205.
129. Locatelli F, Rocha V, Chastang C *et al*. Factors associated with outcome after cord blood transplantation in children with acute leukemia. *Eurocord-Cord Blood Transplant Group Blood* 1999; **93**: 3662–71.
130. Gluckman E, Rocha V, Boyer-Chammard A *et al*. Outcome of cord-blood transplantation from related and unrelated donors. Eurocord Transplant Group and the European Blood and Marrow Transplantation Group. *N Engl J Med* 1997; **337**: 373–81.
131. Kurtzberg J, Laughlin M, Graham ML *et al*. Placental blood as a source of hematopoietic stem

131 cells for transplantation into unrelated recipients. *N Engl J Med* 1996; **335**: 157–66.
132 Lu L, Xiao M, Shen RN, Grigsby S, Broxmeyer HE. Enrichment, characterization, and responsiveness of single primitive CD34 human umbilical cord blood hematopoietic progenitors with high proliferative and replating potential. *Blood* 1993; **81**: 41–8.
133 Broxmeyer HE, Hangoc G, Cooper S *et al*. Growth characteristics and expansion of human umbilical cord blood and estimation of its potential for transplantation in adults. *Proc Natl Acad Sci U S A* 1992; **89**: 4109–13.
134 Mayani H, Dragowska W, Lansdorp PM. Characterization of functionally distinct subpopulations of CD34$^+$ cord blood cells in serum-free long-term cultures supplemented with hematopoietic cytokines. *Blood* 1993; **82**: 2664–72.
135 Hao QL, Thiemann FT, Petersen D, Smogorzewska EM, Crooks GM. Extended long-term culture reveals a highly quiescent and primitive human hematopoietic progenitor population. *Blood* 1996; **88**: 3306–13.
136 Hows JM, Bradley BA, Marsh JC *et al*. Growth of human umbilical-cord blood in long-term haematopoietic cultures. *Lancet* 1992; **340**: 73–6.
137 Mayani H, Lansdorp PM. Thy-1 expression is linked to functional properties of primitive hematopoietic progenitor cells from human umbilical cord blood. *Blood* 1994; **83**: 2410–7.
138 Steen R, Tjonnfjord GE, Egeland T. Comparison of the phenotype and clonogenicity of normal CD34$^+$ cells from umbilical cord blood, granulocyte colony-stimulating factor- mobilized peripheral blood, and adult human bone marrow. *J Hematother* 1994; **3**: 253–62.
139 van de Ven C, Ishizawa L, Law P, Cairo MS. IL-11 in combination with SLF and G-CSF or GM-CSF significantly increases expansion of isolated CD34$^+$ cell population from cord blood vs. adult bone marrow. *Exp Hematol* 1995; **23**: 1289–95.
140 Rebel VI, Miller CL, Eaves CJ, Lansdorp PM. The repopulation potential of fetal liver hematopoietic stem cells in mice exceeds that of their liver adult bone marrow counterparts. *Blood* 1996; **87**: 3500–7.
141 Szilvassy SJ, Meyerrose TE, Ragland PL, Grimes B. Differential homing and engraftment properties of hematopoietic progenitor cells from murine bone marrow, mobilized peripheral blood, and fetal liver. *Blood* 2001; **98**: 2108–15.
142 Stiff P, Pecora A, Parthasarathy M *et al*. Umbilical cord blood transplants in adults using a combination of unexpanded and *ex vivo* expanded cells: preliminary clinical observations. *Blood* 1998; **92**: 646a [Abstract].
143 Kögler G, Nurnberger W, Fisher J *et al*. Simultaneous cord blood transplantation of *ex vivo* expanded together with nonexpanded cells for high risk leukemia. *Bone Marrow Transplant* 1999; **24**: 397–403.
144 Pecora AL, Stiff P, Jennis A *et al*. Prompt and durable engraftment in two older adult patients with high risk chronic myelogenous leukemia (CML) using *ex vivo* expanded and unmanipulated unrelated umbilical cord blood. *Bone Marrow Transplant* 2000; **25**: 797–9.
145 Shpall E, Quinines R, Giller R *et al*. Transplantation of *ex vivo* expanded cord blood. *Biol Blood Marrow Transplant* 2002; **8**: 368–76.
146 Jaroscak J, Goltry K, Smith A *et al*. Augmentation of umbilical cord blood (UCB) transplantation with *ex-vivo* expanded UCB cells: results of a phase I trial using the AastromReplicell™ system. *Blood* 2003; **101**: 5061–7.

10
Thomas Moritz & David A. Williams

Methods for Gene Transfer: Genetic Manipulation of Hematopoietic Stem Cells

Introduction

As a genetic basis becomes obvious in a rapidly increasing number of diseases and many of the abnormal genes involved in the pathogenesis of these diseases have been identified and cloned, somatic gene therapy —that is the introduction of new genetic material into the cells of an organism for therapeutic purposes—has emerged as a realistic new treatment modality. Within the field of hematology, genetic manipulation of hematopoietic cells has been vigorously investigated as a way to improve therapeutic options for severe and otherwise difficult to treat diseases as diverse as genetic diseases of hematopoiesis or the immune system, leukemias and other malignancies or acquired immune deficiency syndrome (AIDS). Most efforts so far have focused on modification of long-lived hematopoietic stem cells (HSCs). This will most likely be required for any curative approach in genetic diseases. Substantial progress has recently been achieved in this field with the first therapeutically successful clinical trial for a monogenic disease. Nevertheless, HSCs remain a difficult target population to manipulate using currently available retrovirus vector-based gene transfer technology. Therefore, a number of new technologies, including novel vector systems, have recently been introduced to the field. On the other hand, gene transfer into more committed hematopoietic cells, such as clonogenic cells or lymphocytes, is readily achievable even with the existing technologies and already allows specific clinical applications.

The aims of this chapter are to provide some historic background on the development of gene transfer technology in regard to transduction of hematopoietic cells; to provide an understanding of the principles of retrovirus-based gene transfer technology; and to provide a discussion of the present status of this technology with respect to HSC transduction. In addition, alternative gene transfer systems, in particular lentiviral gene transfer but also foamy-, adeno-, adeno-associated- or herpes virus-based vectors, as well as therapeutic strategies utilizing foreign gene expression in more differentiated hematopoietic cells, are discussed.

Historical background

The long-lived nature and extensive proliferative capacity of HSCs in combination with the easy accessibility of these cells through bone marrow (BM) aspiration, cord blood stem cell (CBSC) collection or leukapheresis make them one of the most attractive target cells for manipulation for the purpose of genetic therapy. Thus, the use of these cells for genetic modification was vigorously pursued simultaneous with the development of retroviruses as gene transfer vectors. The first successful retroviral mediated gene transfer into a hematopoietic cell was described in 1983, when the dominant selectable marker neomycin phosphotransferase (NEO) was introduced into murine clonogenic cells [1]. This was followed, in 1984, by the first report of gene transfer into a transplantable cell, the colony forming unit-spleen (CFU-S)—a primitive multilineage HSC with limited self-renewal capacity in the murine system [2]. In 1985 the feasibility of successful gene transfer into a pluripotent HSC capable of long-term and multilineage reconstitution was further verified by retroviral integration pattern analysis showing clonally derived *NEO*-gene containing cells in murine BM, thymus and spleen following transplantation of transduced HSCs [3,4].

Since these early reports, a wide variety of different genes have been introduced into hematopoietic clonogenic cells from mice, humans, primates or other animals. These genes include marker genes like *NEO*, β-galactosidase or drug-resistance genes as well as a wide variety of potentially therapeutic genes. Efficient transduction of long-term repopulating HSCs in the murine system meanwhile is now well established. Efficient transduction of long-term repopulating cells in large animal models or in the clinical setting has been more problematic (for a complete review of human gene therapy trials, see Chapter 11). Although the initial gene transfer trials in children with leukemia and neuroblastoma achieved long-term gene marking in up to 15% of peripheral blood stem cell (PBSC) progeny of transduced HSCs [5,6], the experience of other investigators has been disappointing. Over the last years, however, some of the fundamental obstacles preventing efficient HSC gene transfer have become better defined and substantial progress has been made in several aspects of retroviral gene transfer technology. This includes the development of retroviral vectors specifically designed for high level gene expression in primitive hematopoietic cells [7,8], the use of retroviral particles with altered receptor specificity [9,10], incorporation of novel growth factors into the transduction protocol [11,12], as well as the use of fibronectin (FN) fragments to facilitate the initial target cell/virus interaction [13,14]. Owing to these improvements, long-lasting gene transfer and transgene expression in 10–20% of mature blood cells has recently been described in large outbred animal models as well as in clinical studies [15,16], and this has led to the first evidence of successful therapy using gene transfer methods in a monogenic disease (see also Chapter 11) [17].

Retroviral vectors

At present retrovirus based vectors are the only vector system for which substantial clinical experience is available with hematopoietic cells. These vectors are based on the genome of murine oncoretroviruses, usually Moloney murine leukemia virus (MoMuLV) or other murine leukemia viruses (MLM), which are small RNA viruses composed of an outer glycoprotein envelope and an inner RNA- and protein-containing

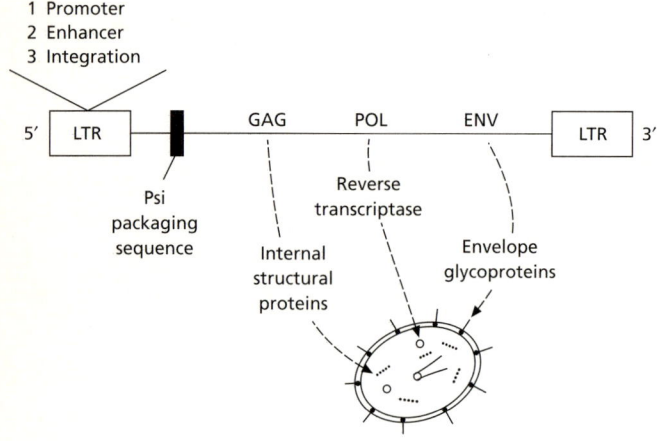

Fig. 10.1 Genomic structure of prototype oncoretrovirus. Env, envelope glycoproteins; Gag, gene-encoding core proteins; LTR, long-terminal repeats; Pol, reverse transcriptase. From: Williams [18] with permission.

core (Fig. 10.1 [18]). The retroviral genome consists of three coding regions termed *gag*, *pol* and *env*, which encode viral capsid proteins and integrase, reverse transcriptase, and the envelope proteins, respectively. The noncoding sequences include the psi region, located 5′ of the *gag* gene, which directs packaging of the viral RNA and which is required *in cis* to allow production of infectious viral particles [19]. The whole genome is contained within two repetitive elements, the long-terminal repeats (LTR), supplying promoter/enhancer elements and directing integration and replication of the viral genome and transcription of viral-encoded proteins.

Retroviral infection, integration and replication follow a specific life cycle (Fig. 10.2 [18]). After binding to receptors on the cell surface of host cells, virus particles are internalized into the cells and uncoat (lose their envelope proteins). Viral-encoded reverse transcriptase carried within the viral particle, together with host-cell DNA polymerase, produces a double-stranded DNA copy of the viral genome. The proviral DNA integrates into the host genome (in relatively random sites); subsequently, gene function depends completely on host-cell metabolism for expression. The integrated proviral DNA is transmitted within the genome to all subsequent progeny derived from this cell. Infected host cells now produce viral RNA and proteins using the 5′ LTR promotor/enhancer, whereas polyadenylation of transcribed messenger (m)RNA occurs via sequences in the 3′ LTR. Viral RNA and proteins are assembled into infectious virus particles inside the host cell and subsequently bud off from the cell membrane in a nonlytic fashion.

To create vectors for gene therapy *gag*, *pol* and *env* genes, which constitute roughly 80% of the retroviral genome, can be deleted and replaced by heterologous DNA sequences. Following proviral integration in a target cell, these inserted DNA sequences will be transcribed in place of the missing viral genes. As the essential viral genes are absent, new viral particles are not produced in the infected cell. Thus, the recombinant retrovirus is capable of only one round of infection (i.e. is replication-defective), unless the necessary viral proteins are supplied *in trans*. To achieve initial packaging of replication-defective recombinant virus, the retroviral Gag, Pol and Env proteins are supplied in special "packaging lines", which contain a psi-deleted retroviral genome. At least in theory,

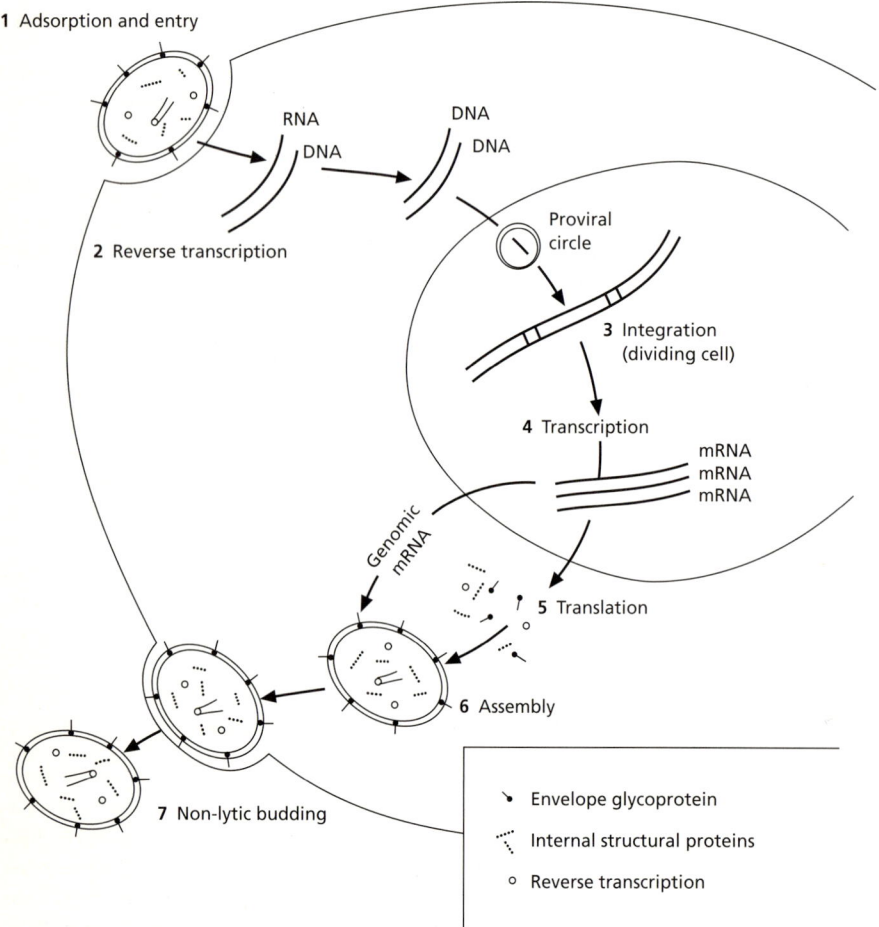

Fig. 10.2 Life cycle of prototype retrovirus. From Williams [18].

the Gag, Pol and Env proteins encoded by this genome can only be used to package the genome of the recombinant virus which contains the *psi* packaging sequence, but not the RNA of the psi-deleted wild-type virus. Several packaging lines that are able to produce high-titre recombinant retrovirus have been constructed using this approach. However, some replication-competent helper virus is generated by these cells because packaging of wild-type RNA (although reduced more than 1000-fold) is not completely blocked by deletion of the *psi* sequence and recombination events can occur in the packaging lines supplying the wild-type genome with an intact *psi* sequence. Therefore, improved packaging cell lines have been generated by making multiple additional deletions and mutations in the *psi*-deleted helper-virus genome. Since multiple independent recombination events must occur before intact helper virus can be generated, these packaging lines are considered relatively safe [20–23]. (For a review of virus producer lines, see [24].)

Though most experimental and clinical work is done utilizing these packaging lines, the generation of high-titre retroviral vector preparations for gene therapy is a long and cumbersome procedure that usually involves generating and testing a large number of individual producer clones. Recently, considerable progress has been made in the ability to generate high-titre recombinant retroviral vectors after transient transfection of packaging lines [25,26]. This approach avoids most of the time-consuming screening process that is necessary for the selection of cloned, stable producer clones. Transient transfection systems use packaging cell lines based primarily on 293 cells, an adenovirus-5 transformed human embryonic kidney cell line. These cells are more efficiently transfected than standard NIH/3T3 based packaging cell lines, thus producing high transient viral titres. For instance, following a single round of transfection using chemical agents which lead to physical uptake of DNA into cells, such as lipofection or calcium phosphate precipitation, high-titre ($= 10^6$ virions/mL) helper virus-free viral stocks can be generated.

Wild-type retroviruses express their genes from the 5' LTR promoter/enhancer, the *gag* and *pol* genes via genomic mRNA, the *env* gene via a subgenomic (spliced) message. Gene sequences introduced into the retroviral vectors may also be transcribed using the 5' LTR, or may be introduced in combination with a heterologous (internal) promoter (Fig. 10.3a). In the past most investigators have utilized vectors based on MLV, and the problems encountered in expressing transferred genes from these vectors led to a widespread use of very simple vectors, expressing only one gene from the 5' LTR or an internal promotor ("simplified vectors"). Though some of these vectors, such as those utilizing the human phosphoglycerokinase (PGK) promoter [27,28], have achieved long-lived gene expression in cells of hematopoietic origin, promoters from other viruses, such as the myeloproliferative sarcoma virus (MPSV), appear to be more reliable to express genes in hematopoietic tissues [29,30]. MPSV-derived vectors have been shown to facilitate the expression of exogenous genes in undifferentiated, totipotent embryonic stem cells [31] and have successfully been used for gene transfer into hematopoietic cells from a variety of species including human clonogenic cells [32,33]. Also, vectors that combine elements of MPSV and the spleen focus-forming virus (SFFV), to further improve gene expression in primitive hematopoietic cells, have been developed [8,34,35].

With the progress in viral backbones, there has also been a renewed interest to express multiple genes from retrovirus vectors, to allow for either selection strategies or the combination of therapeutic genes. In these constructs genes may be expressed from the 5' LTR, directly or via a spliced message, from internal promoters, or a combination thereof (Fig. 10.3b). A newer approach is the utilization of the polyoma- or encephalomyelitis-virus internal ribosome entry site (IRES). The presence of an IRES allows for the cap-independent translation of polycistronic mRNA and vectors using this design allow coexpression of multiple gene products from the same mRNA with high efficiency [36].

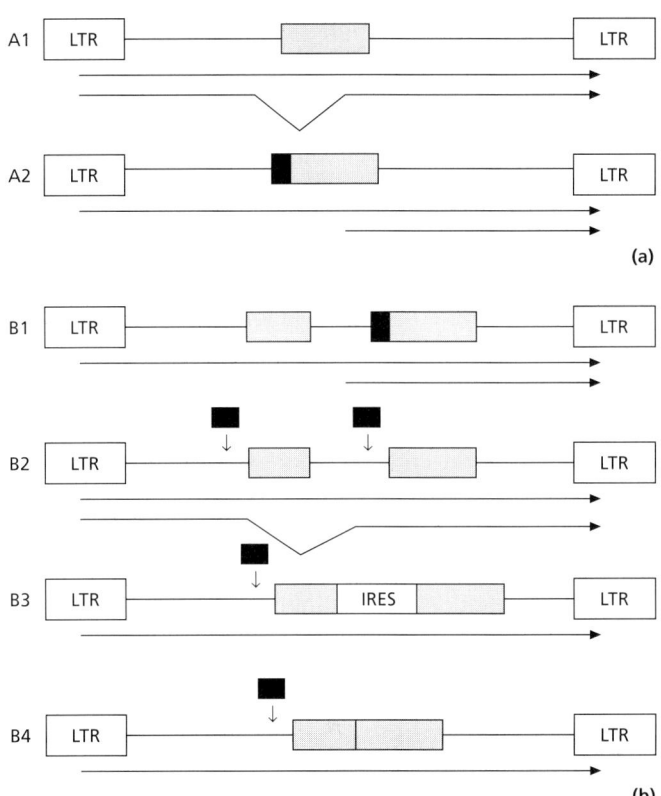

Fig. 10.3 Schematic representation of retrovirus vectors used for gene therapy. (a) Simplified vectors expressing one gene from 5' long-terminal repeats (LTR) (A1) or internal promoter (A2). (b) Vectors expressing two gene products from 5' LTR and internal promoter (B1), 5' LTR using spliced and nonspliced RNA (B2), using internal ribosome entry site (B3) or using expression of a fused protein product (B4). Versions B2–B4 may incorporate additional promoters. Gray rectangles, complementary DNA (cDNA) or gene sequence; black rectangles, promotor/enhancer sequences; arrow, expected RNA transcript; IRES, internal ribosome entry site; LTR, long-terminal repeat.

Also fusion proteins combining functional products of two different genes in one molecule have been successfully investigated *in vitro* [37] and *in vivo* [38].

Infection protocols: current improvements and remaining problems

Although the first therapeutic successes from HSC-gene transfer technology have begun to emerge, significant difficulties still hinder the broad-based application of this technology for curative options. The intense research efforts made over the last two decades, however, have helped define the areas where progress is most required before further therapeutic trials can be successful. Some of these areas relate to specific steps in the retroviral life cycle, such as the initiation of contact between virus and cell, receptor occupancy by the virus and integration of the proviral DNA into the target cell genome. Others are related to our still very rudimentary understanding of the biology of HSCs including the regulation of gene expression within these cells.

Initiating contact between virus and target cell

Retroviral transduction requires direct contact between the retroviral vector particles and the target cells and a process called adhesion strengthening, to allow subsequent specific binding of the ligand on the retrovirus and the retroviral receptor on the target cell [39]. To establish the

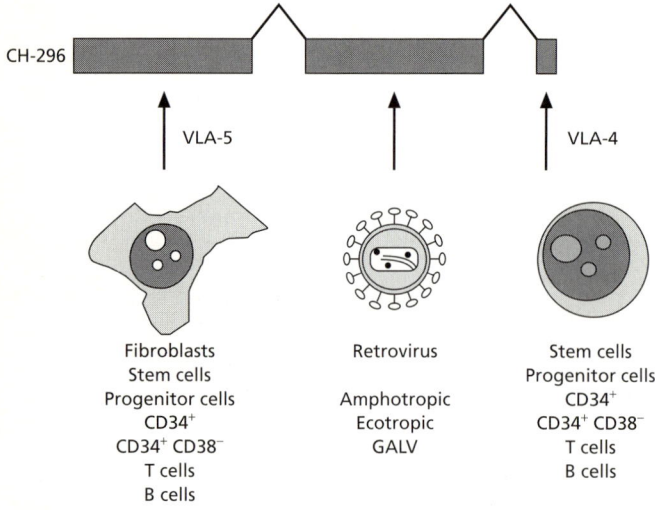

Fig. 10.4 Colocalization of retrovirus and target cells on recombinant fibronectin (FN) fragment containing central cell binding site (binds VLA-5), heparin binding domain II (binds retrovirus) and CS-I sequence (binds VLA-4).

receptor–ligand interactions different types of physicochemical forces acting between the phospholipid bilayers of retrovirus and cell have to be overcome, including van der Waals forces, electrostatic repulsion forces from the negatively charged lipid bilayers, hydration or solvation forces and steric forces due to the presence of protein on the surface of both retrovirus and cell [40]. Therefore, gene transfer efficiency is critically dependent on techniques that increase the frequency and/or duration of contact between the short lived retrovirus (extracellular half-life of 4–8 h [41,42]) and the target cell as the first step which is essential for subsequent specific receptor-mediated virus binding. Towards this aim the polycations polybrene or protamine, which reduce repulsion forces between the negative charges of both vector and target cells, have been used in retroviral transduction protocols for many years.

More recently, four additional approaches to increase the nonspecific binding of vector and target cell have been developed: manipulations to increase the titre of the virus supernatant; centrifugation of retrovirus and target cells; "flow-through technology" and colocalization of retrovirus and target cells on FN fragments. Increase of the retroviral titres can be achieved by filtration [41,43], by the use of roller bottles [43] or other cell culturing systems [44], by lyophilization and reconstitution in a smaller volume [43], or by reducing the temperature at which virus supernatant is collected from 37°C to 32°C [43]. Prolonged and high-speed centrifugation of target cells in the presence of retrovirus-containing supernatant and polybrene has also been used to increase the transduction efficiency of fibroblast and other cell lines [43,45]. However, whether these prolonged mechanical forces can be safely applied to primitive hematopoietic cells remains unknown. In addition, a method utilizing the flow of retroviral supernatant through a porous membrane holding the target cells was reported to increase the frequency of the initial nonspecific adhesion [46].

Another approach that has been employed to improve the initial adhesion step takes advantage of the physiological ability of certain target cells to specifically bind to FN via endogenous integrin receptors $\alpha_4\beta_1$ and/or $\alpha_5\beta_1$ [47,48]. As retroviral particles bind to the same FN fragment [49,50], the colocalization of retrovirus and the target cells in close proximity on the fragment allows the specific interaction of the viral surface proteins with its receptors on the target cell to occur more frequently (Fig. 10.4). Indeed it was shown that this technology allows efficient transduction of human CD34+ hematopoietic cells from BM or CBSC as well as long-lived HSCs in the murine system [13,49,51]. These protocols have been optimized further such that, at this time, factors other than the initial viral adhesion limit transduction efficiency of the hematopoietic cells [52]. Meanwhile this technology has been proven successful in a gene therapy/bone marrow transplantation (BMT) model in baboons [15] as well as in first clinical studies [16,17], and has gained wide acceptance in the field.

Receptor binding and pseudotyped vectors

Retroviruses of the Oncovidinae subfamily are grouped according to differences in their *env* gene sequence, which confers binding specificity to cellular receptors and thereby also determines host range. While ecotropic viruses only infect murine cells, amphotropic viruses infect the cells of a wide variety of species including human cells, and for a long time amphotropic viruses were the principal pseudotype used to transduce human cells. Since the cloning of the receptor for amphotropic retrovirus [53,54], it has become increasingly clear that primitive hematopoietic cells constitutively express this receptor at very low levels [55]. The low receptor density found on these cells appears to be a limiting factor for efficient retroviral transduction of HSCs. This observation is supported by murine studies, in which ecotropic retrovirus leads to transduction of long-lived HSCs with relatively high efficiency. The receptor density of the ecotropic receptor on murine HSCs appears to be considerably higher than the density of amphotropic receptors on human HSCs.

To circumvent these problems heterotypic or "pseudotyped" vectors have been generated which combine characteristics of different viruses or viral subgroups. One such pseudotype combines the MLV *gag* and *pol* genes with the envelope protein of gibbon ape leukemia virus (GALV), a closely related retrovirus. These vectors compare favorably with standard amphotropic vectors with respect to infection efficiency of monkey respiratory epithelial cells [56] and have also been shown to increase transduction efficiency of hematopoietic cells over amphotropic vectors [15]. Vectors pseudotyped with the RD114 envelope protein from the endogenous feline leukemia virus have been introduced to the field more recently [57] and have been demonstrated to efficiently transduce nonobese diabetic with severe combined immunodeficiency syndrome (NOD/SCID)-repopulating cells derived from human CBSC [58]. Another heterotypic retroviral vector system uses the vesicular stomatitis virus (VSV) envelope protein in combination with the MLV *gag/pol* genes [10]. This vector has the wide host range of VSV and, in addition, can be concentrated by density centrifugation to titres of up to 10^9 virions/mL. However, up to now this system has not led to any improvements in HSC transduction rates, most likely due to toxicity of membrane fusion that is associated with uptake of VSV or VSV-pseudotyped vectors.

Cell cycle and retroviral integration

Oncoretrovirus integration within the target cell genome requires active division of the host cell, as breakdown of the nuclear membrane that occurs during mitosis, is probably required for entry of the proviral DNA into the nucleus [59]. In steady state hematopoiesis, however, HSCs are usually quiescent and divide less frequently than more differentiated clonogenic cells. Therefore, several methods have been utilized to increase the number of HSCs in cycle at the time of infection. Chemotherapeutic agents such as 5-fluorouracil (5-FU) increase cycling of otherwise dormant HSCs during the recovery-phase from chemotherapy [60] and 5-FU pretreatment of donor animals is now a routine part of murine BMT/gene-transfer protocols [4,61]. The high gene-transfer efficiency of some HSC marking studies [6] may be attributable to increased HSC cycling rates induced by the intensive chemotherapy regimen applied to the patients prior to the transduction procedures. *In vivo* application of growth factors, such as granulocyte colony-stimulating factor (G-CSF) or stem cell factor (SCF), also can induce proliferation in BM HSCs [62]. In a primate transplant model modestly increased retroviral transduction efficiency following *in vivo* growth factor application to the donor animal has been described. Most reproducibly, exposure of target cells to hematopoietic growth factors *in vitro*, in particular interleukin 3 (IL-3), IL-6, SCF, thrombopoietin, Flt-3 ligand and G-CSF, or various combinations thereof, has been demonstrated to enhance gene transfer into HSCs and this "prestimulation" is part of most clinically applied transduction protocols. Similarly, transduction in the presence of hematopoiesis-supporting stromal cells has been reported to improve results [63–65].

Interestingly, induction of proliferation may not be the only mechanism by which growth factors or stromal support enhance gene-transfer efficiency. Growth factors have been demonstrated to improve binding of amphotropic vectors to CD34⁺ hematopoietic target cells [66] and stromal cells produce extracellular matrix molecules, including FN, and thus also may facilitate virus to cell contact. On the other hand, the widespread use of growth factors within transduction protocols may be problematic, as prolonged exposure of long-lived HSCs to growth factors *in vitro* leads to differentiation and loss of HSC characteristics. FN fragments have been demonstrated to maintain the reconstitutive abilities of HSCs during the *in vitro* incubation with growth factors [67] and similar effects were reported with the use of neutralizing antibodies to transforming growth factor beta (TGF-β) or antisense oligonucleotides to p27^{kip-1} [68]. Novel vector systems, which no longer require cell cycling for transduction (see below), may be an ultimate solution for this obstacle.

Animal xenograft models

As numerous studies in large animals as well as humans have demonstrated over the years, it is impossible to predict the efficiency of gene transfer and transgene expression in primary hematopoietic cells for any specific vector or transduction protocol from *in vitro* testing. Instead, xenograft models, which allow transplantation and long-term maintenance of human hematopoietic cells into severely immunocompromised xenogeneic host animals such as fetal sheep [69] or SCID, NOD/SCID or beige/nude/xid (bnx) mice [70–73], have become a valuable assay to assess gene-transfer efficiency into human HSCs [74–76]. Although the high transduction rates achieved for NOD/SCID-repopulating cells by several groups [58,77–79] suggest that the cells measured in these systems are not fully equivalent to long-term repopulating cells responsible in humans for reconstitution after BMT, at the moment murine xenograft models seem a suitable method to generate predictive preclinical results for the ability of specific vector constructs or transduction protocols to transduce long-lived human HSCs. Recent data, however, suggest that the data generated in a primate (r)NOD/SCID model do not predict the gene transfer in large animal autologous transplant [80].

Selection strategies

Given the low transduction efficiency for human HSCs, selection strategies to identify and expand transduced cells have been investigated for more than a decade. For the purpose of *in vitro* selection, marker genes that allow rapid sorting of transduced cells by flow cytometry appear most suitable and have, to a large extent, replaced *NEO* and other drug resistance genes. Gene coding for surface proteins normally not expressed in the targeted cells, such as murine CD24 (in human cells) or a truncated version of the human nerve growth factor receptor (NGFR) (in hematopoietic cells), have been used [81,82]. However, a recent study suggests that unanticipated side-effects may occur using truncated receptors [83]. For instance, in the case of truncated NGFR, the intracytoplasmic sequence deleted may contain a pro-apoptotic function. This truncated version has been implicated in abnormal cell proliferation in the presence of ligand (see below). Most recently, fluorescence-conferring genes, such as the green fluorescent protein (GFP) have shown excellent promise with respect to efficient selection/purification of transduced cells [84,85].

At least in the murine system, *in vivo* selection for transduced cells has been demonstrated using vectors expressing drug-resistance genes. In particular dihydrofolate reductase (DHFR), conferring resistance to methotrexate, the multidrug resistance 1 (*MDR-1*) gene, coding for the *P*-glycoprotein and conferring resistance to vinca alkaloids, taxol, anthracyclines and etoposide (VP16), or the DNA repair protein O⁶-methylguanine DNA methyltransferase (MGMT), conferring resistance to chloroethylnitrosourea type drugs have proven useful [86–90]. In addition, *in vivo* selection of *MDR-1* transduced primary human hematopoietic cells has been described in the NOD/SCID model [91]. Due to the documented mutagenic properties of most of the drugs involved, application of drug resistance genes outside the field of cancer treatment may be problematic. However, mutagenic side-effects have not been described following long-term treatment with methotrexate. Thus, the use of DHFR to enrich corrected cells within therapeutic strategies for monogenic diseases can be envisioned, especially in situations where the therapeutic gene does not confer a survival advantage *per se* to transduced cells.

Toxicities associated with integration

A theoretical risk of vector systems, which leads to integration of vector sequences into chromosomal DNA, relates to insertional mutagenesis. Toxicity would be due to disruption of a key gene or activation of a cellular oncogene, or a gene associated in some way with a survival or growth advantage. Two instances of apparent insertional mutagenesis have recently come to light. The first involved development of a mouse leukemia after integration of a truncated NGFR-expressing retrovirus in the murine *Avi-1* gene [83]. The second, not yet fully reported, was the development of leukemia in a child participating in the IL-2 common β-chain gene-therapy trial for SCID (see [92–94]). In this case, insertion of the vector sequences occurred in the *LMO-2* gene, which is commonly associated with T-cell acute lymphoblastic leukemia in children. In both cases, it appears that a complex combinatorial interaction occurred between dysregulated expression of an endogenous gene and transgene expression (for a full review of "genotoxicity" of vectors, see [95]).

Alternative gene transfer systems

A variety of new gene delivery systems are currently being evaluated for use in human gene therapy (Table 10.1 [96]). However, among virus-based systems only retroviral vectors and adenoviral vectors have been tested to any large extent in clinical studies. Only basic experimental data are available on the other systems described here. Adeno-associated viruses (AAVs), lentiviruses and foamy viruses mediate integration of the transferred gene into the host cell genome and stable transduction of cells, as required for curative therapy of genetic diseases. Adeno- and herpes-virus vectors allow only transient modification of target cells and their applications are more limited. Of the physical DNA-transfer methods, liposome mediated gene transfer [97,98] has been investigated to the greatest extent, but in general these methods are still too inefficient to be considered of clinical value for the generation of gene modified hematopoietic cells [99].

Lentivirus-based vectors

In comparison to retroviruses of the Oncovidinae subfamily, lentiviruses such as the human immunodeficiency virus 1 (HIV-1) and HIV-2 or the simian immunodeficiency virus (SIV) have a more complex genome and

Table 10.1 Properties of viral vectors.

Property	Murine retrovirus	Adeno-associated virus	Adenovirus	Herpesvirus	Lentivirus	Foamy virus
Titer	10^6–10^7/mL	10^6–10^{12}/mL	10^{11}–10^{12}/mL	10^4–10^{10}/mL	10^6–10^8/mL No stable producer lines	10^4–10^5/mL (wild type 10^9) No stable producer lines
Genome	RNA	ssDNA	dsDNA	dsDNA	RNA	RNA
Integration	Yes	Sometimes	No	No	Yes	Yes
Insert size	6–7 kb	2.0–4.5 kb	7–36 kb	10–100 kb	8–9 kb	9–10 kb
Cell proliferation	Requires mitosis	Prefers S-phase	Not required	Not required	Not required but helpful	Not required but helpful
Helper virus pathogenicity	Potentially dangerous	Not pathogenic	Mild pathogen	Varies	Probably dangerous	Not pathogenic
Host response	Complement inactivates	?	Immunogenic and inflammatory	? (latency)	?	?

Modified from Williams *et al*. [96] with permission.
ds, double-stranded; ss, single-stranded.

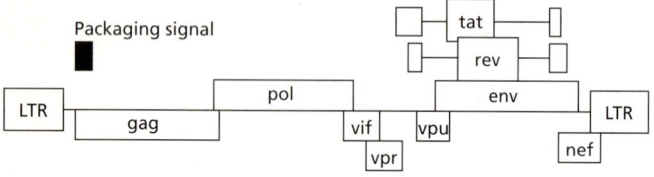

Fig. 10.5 Genomic structure of HIV-1, a prototype lentivirus. As for oncoretroviruses (see Fig. 10.1) long-terminal repeats (LTR), *gag*, *pol*, and *env* genes, as well as a packaging signal, are present. In addition, a number of accessory genes, such as *vif*, *vpr*, *vpn*, *vpu*, *tat*, *ref* and *nef*, are expressed from multiple spliced mRNAs.

a more complex life cycle (Fig. 10.5). For the purpose of gene therapy the major advantage of lentivirus over oncoretrovirus vectors is the purported capability to transduce noncycling cells [100–103]. This capacity is conferred to lentiviruses by nuclear localization sequences present within the viral integrase and Gag protein as well as by the ability of the Vpr protein to bind directly to the nuclear pore complex. However, the exact mechanism by which the viral preintegration complex passes through the intact nuclear membrane is not completely understood [104–106]. In addition, at least in some cell types progression through the cell cycle promotes lentiviral infection [107]. Meanwhile lentivirus vectors have convincingly been demonstrated to confer transgene expression to terminally differentiated cells, such as neuronal, retinal, muscle or liver cells, as well as to primitive hematopoietic cells (for review see [108]).

Currently the majority of lentivirus vectors are based on the genome of HIV-1, and initial constructs using the HIV-1 envelope protein were restricted in their tropism to CD4 positive cells. Similar to oncoretrovirus vectors, however, pseudotyped lentivirus vectors can be generated utilizing amphotropic, ecotropic, VSV, or human T-cell lymphotropic virus 1 (HTLV-1) envelope proteins extending the host range of these vectors considerably [100,101,109,110]. Substantial progress also has been made towards the generation of safe and efficient packaging systems for lentivirus vectors. In the past, this has been a significant obstacle to the development of HIV-1-based lentivirus vectors, especially as several lentivirus-encoded proteins, such as Gag, Rev and Vpr display considerable cellular toxicity. Therefore, the demonstration of stable expression of HIV-1 proteins in cells has been a significant advance in the potential generation of stable lentivirus packaging cell lines [111–113]. In addition, intense research efforts have helped to better define the minimal requirements for the propagation of lentivirus vectors. Thus, it has been possible to minimize the overlap of *cis*-acting sequences between HIV-1 vector and helper constructs and to decrease the risk of inadvertent viral recombination within producer cells [114–116]. Other steps that have been explored to produce safer lentivirus vectors have been the development of self-inactivating vectors eliminating expression from the HIV-1 LTR [115] and the generation of vectors based on less pathogenic lentiviruses such as HIV-2 and SIV, or the nonprimate feline immunodeficiency virus (FIV) and equine infectious anemia virus (EIAV) lentiviruses.

The newer generation HIV-1-based vectors have been used to transduce hematopoietic cells. Transduction rates of up to 90% have been reported for human CD34 positive hematopoietic cells [101,109,117]. Efficient gene transfer into highly purified quiescent CD34$^+$/CD38$^-$ and G$_0$/G$_1$ hematopoietic cells [118,119] and NOD/SCID-repopulating HSCs, including secondary repopulating cells, has been achieved [120–123]. Though in several of these studies lentivirus vectors compared favorably with MLV-type oncoretrovirus vectors, the data clearly need further confirmation as: (i) transduction of cells in G$_1$ or G$_2$/S/M is clearly more efficient than CD34$^+$ cells in G$_0$ [124]; (ii) in the presence of appropriate growth factors similar gene-transfer efficiency into murine reconstituting HSCs was demonstrated for MLV-type vectors compared with lentivirus vectors [125]; and (iii) up to now convincing data from large animal experiments or clinical trials for lentivirus vectors are still unavailable or limited. These issues, in addition to the considerable safety concerns, need to be addressed before lentivirus vectors will be considered for clinical studies on any larger scale.

Foamy virus-based vectors

Foamy viruses, or spumaviruses, are a class of retroviruses different from lentiviruses or Oncovidinae [126]. Though these viruses have not been associated with human diseases, they have been isolated from hematopoietic cells in primates and studies with wild-type virus have demonstrated the capacity of foamy virus to infect hematopoietic cells *in vitro* [112]. Similar to lentiviruses, foamy viruses can transduce nondividing cells and nuclear localization signals have been identified in foamy virus

Gag sequences [127]. Vectors based on the genome of human foamy virus have been constructed and efficient transduction of primary hematopoietic cells from different animal species, including humans, has been achieved with these vectors [128]. A major drawback up to this point has been the lack of high-titre helper-free packaging systems for foamy virus vectors. However, recently improved vector constructs and production systems have been generated [129,130] and foamy virus vectors have been used to efficiently transduce human CD34$^+$ clonogenic cells. In addition, mice that received transduced BM cells expressed a foamy virus vector-encoded transgene long-term in all major hematopoietic lineages in primary and secondary recipients [131]. Recent studies also demonstrate transduction of NOD/SCID repopulating human cells [132,133]. Thus, foamy virus-based vectors appear a potential new tool for hematopoietic cell gene therapy and further evaluation of this technology in clinically relevant models seems warranted.

Adeno-associated virus (AAV)-based vectors

AAV is a human DNA-containing parvovirus that has not been implicated in known human diseases. AAV is capable of infecting a wide range of host cells independent of their cycling status and integrates stably and in a site-specific manner (on chromosome 19q in human cells) into the host cell genome [134]. These features, mainly derived from experiments in cell lines, make AAV a suitable candidate virus for the development of gene-transfer vectors and AAV-derived vectors have been shown to infect several hematopoietic cell lines with high efficiency [135,136]. However, integration and long-term expression of the introduced genetic sequence via AAV-based vectors have not been consistently demonstrated. In addition, the removal of large parts of the viral genome, which are required for the construction of vectors for gene transfer, leads to loss of the site-specific integration. Other problems that are associated with AAV-based vectors are: (i) the restriction in size of the introduced sequence to less than 5 kb; (ii) the rather low integration frequency into the genome of primary cells; and (iii) the difficulties in obtaining adenovirus-free helper virus stocks (for review see [137]).

Despite these problems, efficient transduction of human CD34-positive or long-term culture initiating cells (LTC-IC) from BM, PBSC and CBSC has been demonstrated by several groups using marker or therapeutic genes [138–140]. However, unequivocally positive data on efficient transduction of long-lived HSCs is missing. Even in the well-characterized mouse system only sporadic reports of relatively inefficient gene transfer into transplantable HSCs have been published thus far [141].

Adenovirus- and herpesvirus-based vectors

Vector systems allow only transient transgene expression. Therefore, application to hematopoietic cell gene therapy is limited to strategies requiring expression of the therapeutic transgene for defined (and limited) time periods, such as modification of committed hematopoietic cells (see below) or antileukemia vaccination strategies. For adenovirus-based vectors, attractive features with respect to potential clinical utility include the capacity to efficiently infect nondividing cells, express transgenes at high levels (with no integration site-specific effects), infect a broad range of host cells, be concentrated to high titres by centrifugation and have the potential to accommodate large fragments of DNA. Adenoviral vectors have been used only sporadically for gene transfer into hematopoietic cells. These studies have shown that the major blood lineages are relatively resistant to adenovirus infection, with only CD34$^+$ clonogenic cells or glycophorin A$^+$, erythroid lineage cells being permissive. While gene transfer into clonogenic cells with up to 79% efficiency was demonstrated in some studies, adenoviral toxicity seemed to limit transduction results for more primitive hematopoietic cells such as LTC-IC [142–144].

Human herpesviruses, in particular herpes simplex virus, type 1 (HSV-1), contain a very large genome of double-stranded DNA (approximately 150 kb) which allows incorporation of up to 35 kb of heterologous DNA. These viruses are capable of infecting a wide variety of quiescent or proliferating cell types and can be used to generate high-titer virus preparations [145–147]. Safety modified recombinant HSV-vectors, HSV-mini-vectors or amplicon vectors, which are devoid of all viral genes and contain multiple copies (up to 10) of the gene of interest in their genome have been generated [147–149]. The feasibility of using HSV-derived vectors to transduce hematopoietic cells has been established and transduction efficiencies of 80–100% for normal and leukemic CD34$^+$ target cells with minimal toxicity and high expression of the marker gene for up to 2 weeks have been reported [150]. This vector system thus appears suited to situations where transient gene expression is required, such as transduction of leukemic cells for the purpose of vaccination or immunotherapy.

Sources of hematopoietic target cells

At present the CD34 surface molecule is the only widely used marker for HSC enrichment in clinical gene-therapy protocols. CD34 selection is of practical importance as it leads to a large reduction in the numbers of cells that need to be handled during the retroviral infection protocol. Indeed 0.1–5.0% of total BM mononuclear cells or PBSC leukapheresis product are selected depending on the procedure. Other markers, such as CD15, CD33, CD38, HLA-DR, or exclusion of dyes, such as rhodamine or Hoechst 33342, have been suggested but so far have not proven specific enough or have been too complicated to utilize in large-scale clinical trials.

Three different sources of hematopoietic CD34$^+$ cells are available and have been successfully used for HSC transplantation after myeloablative preparative therapy: BM, CBSC and PBSC. Efficient genetic modification using retroviral vectors has been demonstrated for CD34$^+$ cells from all three sources. It has been suggested from *in vitro* studies on clonogenic cells and LTC-IC as well as from data obtained in NOD/SCID mice that retrovirus based gene-transfer technology might allow more efficient transduction of hematopoietic cells from cord blood compared to BM or mobilized PB [151–154]. However, this has not been verified to date in clinical studies [155].

Committed clonogenic cells

Clonogenic cells, such as colony forming units-granulocyte/macrophage (CFU-GM), burst forming units-erythroid (BFU-E) or colony forming units-granulocyte/erythroid/macrophage/megakaryocyte (CFU-GEMM) have already undergone some degree of differentiation and commitment, but these cells still have the capacity to generate large numbers of mature progeny. Due to the loss of HSC characteristics, committed clonogenic cells are not suitable targets for the lifelong replacement of defective or missing gene products. A major advantage of targeting these cells is that efficient transduction can be accomplished using retrovirus vectors and relatively simple infection protocols. Similar results have been shown using adenovirus- and herpes virus-based vector systems.

At the moment the major clinical application that could be envisioned for gene transfer into committed clonogenic cells is the generation of chemotherapy-resistant hematopoietic cells to protect the hematopoietic system against therapy-induced myelosuppression. Despite the use of hematopoietic growth factors and autologous HSC support, hematopoietic toxicity is still an important obstacle to dose intensification, especially in heavily pretreated patients. The strategy suggested in this context might be the infusion of autologous hematopoietic cells that have been modified *ex vivo* to express specific drug resistance genes. A number of these genes have been identified and cloned, the most well-studied of which are *DHFR*, *MDR-1*, *MGMT*, aldehyde dehydrogenase (*ALDH*), or glutathione *S*-transferase (*GST*) conferring resistance to a wide variety of commonly used chemotherapeutic agents. While most genes are currently under preclinical investigation, several clinical studies have been reported with *MDR-1* and *MGMT*, and studies with *DHFR* are about to start (for review see [156,157]).

Similar to erythro-myeloid clonogenic cells efficient retroviral gene transfer is also achievable for lymphocytes and lymphoid precursor cells [158,159]. In clinical studies this approach has initially been evaluated for gene therapy of SCID due to adenosine deaminase (ADA) deficiency [160,161]. More recently, transduction of lymphoid precursor cells with the herpes simplex thymidine kinase gene prior to allogeneic transplantation has been successfully used to control severe graft-vs.-host disease (GVHD) by administration of ganciclovir [38,162].

Implications and outlook

With currently available technology, therapeutic results of using hematopoietic cell gene therapy may be obtained in a few well-defined settings. However, these future, more widespread uses of this technology, will most likely depend on new technologies that may incorporate developments discussed in this chapter. In this context, however, it is important to note that one of the major obstacles to efficient genetic manipulation of long-lived HSCs is our limited knowledge about HSC biology, including our lack of understanding of the complicated processes that regulate cell fate decisions, such as differentiation, apoptosis or self-renewal in these cells. Therefore, major breakthroughs in HSC biology will be necessary before the genetic manipulation of these cells may offer therapeutic strategies for many of the most devastating genetic diseases in humans.

References

1 Joyner A, Keller G, Phillips RA, Bernstein A. Retrovirus transfer of a bacterial gene into mouse haematopoietic progenitor cells. *Nature* 1983; **305**: 556–8.

2 Williams DA, Lemischka IR, Nathan DG, Mulligan RC. Introduction of new genetic material into pluripotent haematopoietic stem cells of the mouse. *Nature* 1984; **310**: 476–80.

3 Keller G, Paige C, Gilboa E, Wagner EF. Expression of a foreign gene in myeloid and lymphoid cells derived from multipotent haematopoietic precursors. *Nature* 1985; **318**: 149–54.

4 Dick JE, Magli MC, Huszar D, Phillips RA, Bernstein A. Introduction of a selectable gene into primitive stem cells capable of long-term reconstitution of the hemopoietic system of W/Wv mice. *Cell* 1985; **42**(1): 71–9.

5 Brenner MK, Rill DR, Moen RC et al. Gene-marking to trace origin of relapse after autologous bone-marrow transplantation. *Lancet* 1993; **341**: 85–6.

6 Brenner MK, Rill DR, Holladay MS et al. Gene marking to determine whether autologous marrow infusion restores long-term haemopoiesis in cancer patients. *Lancet* 1993; **342**: 1134–7.

7 Hawley RG, Lieu FH, Fong AZ, Hawley TS. Versatile retroviral vectors for potential use in gene therapy. *Gene Ther* 1994; **1**(2): 136–8.

8 Baum C, Hegewisch-Becker S, Eckert HG, Stocking C, Ostertag W. Novel retroviral vectors for efficient expression of the multidrug resistance (*MDR-1*) gene in early hematopoietic cells. *J Virol* 1995; **69**: 7541–7.

9 von Kalle C, Kiem HP, Goehle S et al. Increased gene transfer into human hematopoietic progenitor cells by extended *in vitro* exposure to a pseudotyped retroviral vector. *Blood* 1994; **84**(9): 2890–7.

10 Burns JC, Friedmann T, Driever W, Burrascano M, Yee J-K. Vesicular stomatitis virus G glycoprotein pseudotyped retroviral vectors: concentration to very high titer and efficient gene transfer into mammalian and nonmammalian cells. *Proc Natl Acad Sci U S A* 1993; **90**: 8033–7.

11 Hanenberg H, Hashino K, Konishi H, Hock RA, Kato I, Williams DA. Optimization of fibronectin-assisted retroviral gene transfer into human CD34+ hematopoietic cells. *Human Gene Ther* 1997; **8**(18): 2193–206.

12 Murray L, Luens K, Tushinski R et al. Optimization of retroviral gene transduction of mobilized primitive hematopoietic progenitors by using thrombopoietin, Flt3 and kit ligands and Retro-Nectin™ culture. *Hum Gene Ther* 1999; **10**(11): 1743–52.

13 Hanenberg H, Xiao XL, Dilloo D, Hashino K, Kato I, Williams DA. Colocalization of retrovirus and target cells on specific fibronectin fragments increases genetic transduction of mammalian cells. *Nat Med* 1996; **2**(8): 876–82.

14 Moritz T, Patel VP, Williams DA. Bone marrow extracellular matrix molecules improve gene transfer into human hematopoietic cells via retroviral vectors. *J Clin Invest* 1994; **93**(4): 1451–7.

15 Kiem H-P, Andrews RG, Morris J et al. Improved gene transfer into baboon marrow repopulating cells using recombinant human fibronectin fragment CH-296 in combination with IL-6, stem cell factor, Flt-3 ligand, and megakaryocyte growth and development factor. *Blood* 1998; **92**(6): 1878–86.

16 Abonour R, Williams DA, Einhorn L et al. Efficient retrovirus-mediated transfer of the multidrug resistance 1 gene into autologous human long-term repopulating hematopoietic stem cells. *Nat Med* 2000; **6**: 652–8.

17 Cavazzana-Calvo M, Hacein-Bey S, de Saint Basile G et al. Gene therapy of human severe combined immunodeficiency (SCID)-X1 disease [see comments]. *Science* 2000; **288**(5466): 669–72.

18 Williams DA. Gene transfer and the prospects for somatic gene therapy. *Hematol Oncol Clin North Am* 1988; **2**: 277–87.

19 Mann R, Mulligan RC, Baltimore D. Construction of a retrovirus packaging mutant and its use to produce helper-free defective retrovirus. *Cell* 1983; **33**: 153–9.

20 Miller AD, Trauber DR, Buttimore C. Factors involved in production of helper-virus free retrovirus vectors. *Somat Cell Mol Genet* 1986; **12**: 175–81.

21 Markowitz D, Goff S, Bank A. A safe packaging line for gene transfer. Separating viral genes on two different plasmids. *J Virol* 1988; **62**(4): 1120–4.

22 Danos O, Mulligan RC. Safe and efficient generation of recombinant retroviruses with amphotropic and ecotropic host ranges. *Proc Natl Acad Sci U S A* 1988; **85**: 6460–4.

23 Dougherty JP, Wisniewski R, Yang S, Rhode BW, Temin HM. New retrovirus helper cells with almost no nucleotide sequence homology to retrovirus vectors. *J Virol* 1989; **63**: 3209–12.

24 Miller AD. Retrovirus packaging cells. *Hum Gene Ther* 1990; **1**: 5–14.

25 Pear WS, Nolan GP, Scott ML, Baltimore D. Production of high-titer helper-free retroviruses by transient transfection. *Proc Natl Acad Sci U S A* 1993; **90**: 8392–6.

26 Kinsella TM, Nolan GP. Episomal vectors rapidly and stably produce high titer recombinant retrovirus. *Hum Gene Ther* 1996; **7**: 1405–13.

27 Luskey BD, Rosenblatt M, Zsebo K, Williams DA. Stem cell factor, interleukin-3, and interleukin-6 promote retroviral-mediated gene transfer into murine hematopoietic stem cells. *Blood* 1992; **80**: 396–402.

28 Lim B, Williams DA, Orkin SH. Retrovirus-mediated gene transfer of human adenosine deaminase: Expression of functional enzyme in murine hematopoietic stem cells *in vivo*. *Mol Cell Biol* 1987; **7**: 3459–65.

29 Stocking C, Kollek R, Bergholz U, Ostertag W. Long terminal repeat sequences impart hematopoietic transformation properties to the myeloproliferative sarcoma virus. *Proc Natl Acad Sci U S A* 1985; **82**: 5746–50.

30 Hawley RG, Lieu FHL, Fong AZC, Hawley TS. Versatile retroviral vectors for potential use in gene therapy. *Gene Ther* 1994; **1**: 136–8.

31 Grez M, Akgun E, Hilberg F, Ostertag W. Embryonic stem cell virus, a recombinant murine retrovirus with expression in embryonic stem cells. *Proc Natl Acad Sci U S A* 1990; **87**: 9202–6.

32 Hawley RG, Fong AZC, Ngan BY, de Lanux VM, Clark SC, Hawley TS. Progenitor cell hyperplasia with rare development of myeloid leukemia in interleukin 11 bone marrow chimeras. *J Exp Med* 1993; **178**: 1175–88.

33 Cheng LC, Lavau C et al. Sustained gene expression in retrovirally transduced, engrafting human hematopoietic stem cells and their lympho-myeloid progeny. *Blood* 1998; **92**(1): 83–92.

34 Eckert H-G, Stockschlader M, Just U et al. High-dose multidrug resistance in primary human hematopoietic progenitor cells transduced with optimized retroviral vectors. *Blood* 1996; **88**: 3407–15.

35 Hildinger M, Abel KL, Ostertag W, Baum C. Design of 5′ untranslated sequences in retroviral vectors developed for medical use. *J Virol* 1999; **73**(5): 4083–9.

36 Aran JM, Gottesman MM, Pastan I. Drug-selected coexpression of human glucocerebrosidase and

P-glycoprotein using a bicistronic vector. *Proc Natl Acad Sci U S A* 1994; **91**: 3176–80.
37. Gottesman M, Pastan I. Biochemistry of multidrug resistance mediated by the multidrug transporter. *Annu Rev Biochem* 1993; **62**: 385–427.
38. Bonini C, Ferrari G, Verzeletti S et al. HSV-TK gene transfer into donor lymphocytes for control of allogeneic graft-versus-leukemia. *Science* 1997; **276**(5319): 1719–24.
39. Haywood AM. Virus receptors. Binding, adhesion strengthening, and changes in viral structure. *J Virol* 1994; **68**: 1–5.
40. Andreadis S, Palsson BO. Coupled effects of polybrene and calf serum on the efficiency of retroviral transduction and the stability of retroviral vectors. *Hum Gene Ther* 1997; **8**: 285–91.
41. Paul RW, Morris D, Hess BW, Dunn J, Overell RW. Increased viral titers through concentration of viral harvests from retroviral packaging lines. *Hum Gene Ther* 1993; **4**: 609–15.
42. Sanes JR, Rubenstein JL, Nicolas J-F. Use of a recombinant retrovirus to study post-implantation cell lineage in mouse embryos. *EMBO J* 1986; **5**: 3133–42.
43. Kotani H, Newton PBI, Zhang S et al. Improved methods of retroviral vector transduction and production for gene therapy. *Hum Gene Ther* 1994; **5**(1): 19–28.
44. Eipers PG, Krauss JC, Palsson BO, Emerson SG, Todd RF, Clarke MF. Retroviral-mediated gene transfer in human bone marrow cells grown in continuous perfusion culture vessels. *Blood* 1995; **86**: 3754–62.
45. Bahnson AB, Dunigan JT, Baysal BE et al. Centrifugal enhancement of retroviral mediated gene transfer. *J Virol Meth* 1995; **54**: 131–43.
46. Chuck AS, Palsson BO. Consistent and high rates of gene transfer can be obtained using flow-through transduction over a wide range of retroviral titers. *Hum Gene Ther* 1996; **7**: 743–50.
47. Williams DA, Rios M, Stephens C, Patel V. Fibronectin and VLA-4 in haematopoietic stem cell–microenvironment interactions. *Nature* 1991; **352**: 438–41.
48. Yoder MC, Williams DA. Matrix molecule interactions with hematopoietic stem cells. *Exp Hematol* 1995; **23**(9): 961–7.
49. Moritz T, Dutt P, Xiao XL et al. Fibronectin improves transduction of reconstituting hematopoietic stem cells by retroviral vectors: evidence of direct viral binding to chymotryptic carboxyterminal fragments. *Blood* 1996; **88**(3): 855–62.
50. Carstanjen D, Dutt P, Moritz T. Heparin inhibits retrovirus binding to fibronectin as well as retrovirus gene transfer on fibronectin fragments. *J Virol* 2001; **75**(13): 6218–22.
51. Moritz T, Patel VP, Williams DA. Bone marrow extracellular matrix molecules improve gene transfer into human hematopoietic cells via retroviral vectors. *J Clin Invest* 1994; **93**: 1451–7.
52. MacNeill EC, Hanenberg H, Pollok KE et al. Simultaneous infection with retroviruses pseudotyped with different envelope proteins bypasses viral receptor interference associated with colocalization of gp70 and target cells on fibronectin CH-296. *J Virol* 1999; **73**(5): 3960–7.
53. Miller DG, Edwards RH, Miller AD. Cloning of the cellular receptor for amphotropic murine retroviruses reveals homology to that for gibbon ape leukemia virus. *Proc Natl Acad Sci U S A* 1994; **91**: 1178–82.
54. van Zeijl M, Johann SV, Closs E et al. A human amphotropic retrovirus receptor is a second member of the gibbon ape leukemia virus receptor family. *Proc Natl Acad Sci U S A* 1994; **91**: 1168–72.
55. Orlic D, Girard LJ, Jordan CT, Anderson SM, Cline AP, Bodine DM. The level of mRNA encoding the amphotropic retrovirus receptor in mouse and human hematopoietic stem cells is low and correlates with the efficiency of retroviral transduction. *Proc Natl Acad Sci U S A* 1996; **93**: 11,097–102.
56. Bayle J-Y, Johnson LG, St. George JA, Boucher RC, Olsen JC. High-efficiency gene transfer to primary monkey airway epithelial cells with retrovirus vectors using the gibbon ape leukemia virus receptor. *Hum Gene Ther* 1993; **4**: 161–70.
57. Porter CD, Collins MK, Tailor CS et al. Comparison of efficiency of infection of human gene therapy target cells via four different retroviral receptors. *Hum Gene Ther* 1996; **7**(8): 913–9.
58. Kelly PF, Vandergriff J, Nathwani A, Nienhuis AW, Vanin EF. Highly efficient gene transfer into cord blood NOD/SCID repopulating cells by oncoretroviral vector particles pseudotyped with the feline endogenous retrovirus (RD114) envelope protein. *Blood* 2000; **96**(4): 1206–14.
59. Roe T, Reynolds TC, Yu G, Brown PO. Integration of murine leukemia virus DNA depends on mitosis. *EMBO J* 1993; **12**: 2099–108.
60. Hodgson GS, Bradley TR. Properties of haematopoietic stem cells surviving 5-fluorouracil treatment: evidence for a pre-CFU-S cell? *Nature* 1979; **281**: 381–2.
61. Bodine DM, McDonagh KT, Seidel NE, Nienhuis AW. Survival and retrovirus infection of murine hematopoietic stem cells *in vitro*: effects of 5-FU and method of infection. *J Exp Hematol* 1991; **19**: 206–12.
62. Dunbar CE, Seidel NE, Doren S et al. Improved retroviral gene transfer into murine and rhesus peripheral blood or bone marrow repopulating cells primed *in vivo* with stem cell factor and granulocyte colony-stimulating factor. *Proc Natl Acad Sci U S A* 1996; **93**: 11,871–6.
63. Moore KA, Deisseroth AB, Reading CL, Williams DE, Belmont JW. Stromal support enhances cell-free retroviral vector transduction of human bone marrow long-term culture-initiating cells. *Blood* 1992; **79**(6): 1393–9.
64. Bodine DM, Moritz T, Donahue RE et al. Long-term *in vivo* expression of a murine adenosine deaminase gene in rhesus monkey hematopoietic cells of multiple lineages after retroviral mediated gene transfer into CD34+ bone marrow cells. *Blood* 1993; **82**: 1975–80.
65. Bienzle D, Abrams-Ogg AC, Kruth SA et al. Gene transfer into hematopoietic stem cells: long-term maintenance of *in vitro* activated progenitors without marrow ablation. *Proc Natl Acad Sci U S A* 1994; **91**(1): 350–4.
66. Crooks GM, Kohn DB. Growth factors increase amphotropic retrovirus binding to human CD34+ bone marrow progenitor cells. *Blood* 1993; **82**(11): 3290–7.
67. Dao MA, Hashino K, Kato I, Nolta JA. Adhesion to fibronectin maintains regenerative capacity during *ex vivo* culture and transduction of human hematopoietic stem and progenitor cells. *Blood* 1998; **92**(12): 4612–21.
68. Dao MA, Taylor N, Nolta JA. Reduction in levels of the cyclin-dependent kinase inhibitor p27 (kip-1) coupled with transforming growth factor beta neutralization induces cell-cycle entry and increases retroviral transduction of primitive human hematopoietic cells. *Proc Natl Acad Sci U S A* 1998; **95**(22): 13,006–11.
69. Srour EF, Zanjani ED, Cornetta K et al. Persistence of human multilineage, self-renewing lymphohematopoietic stem cells in chimeric sheep. *Blood* 1993; **82**: 3333–42.
70. Lapidot T, Pflumio F, Doedens M, Murdoch B, Williams DE, Dick JE. Cytokine stimulation of multilineage hematopoiesis from immature human cells engrafted in SCID mice. *Science* 1992; **255**: 1137–41.
71. Vormoor J, Lapidot T, Pflumio F et al. Immature human cord blood progenitors engraft and proliferate to high levels in severe combined immunodeficient mice. *Blood* 1994; **83**: 2489–97.
72. Nolta JA, Hanley MB, Kohn DB. Sustained human hematopoiesis in immunodeficient mice by cotransplantation of marrow stroma expressing human interleukin-3: analysis of gene transduction of long-lived progenitors. *Blood* 1994; **83**: 3041–51.
73. Bhatia M, Wang JC, Kapp U, Bonnet D, Dick JE. Purification of primitive human hematopoietic cells capable of repopulating immune-deficient mice. *Proc Natl Acad Sci U S A* 1997; **94**(10): 5320–5.
74. Larochelle A, Vormoor J, Hanenberg H et al. Identification of primitive human hematopoietic cells capable of repopulating NOD/SCID mouse bone marrow: implications for gene therapy. *Nat Med* 1996; **2**(12): 1329–37.
75. van Hennik PB, Verstegen MM, Bierhuizen MF et al. Highly efficient transduction of the green fluorescent protein gene in human umbilical cord blood stem cells capable of cobblestone formation in long-term cultures and multilineage engraftment of immunodeficient mice. *Blood* 1998; **92**(11): 4013–22.
76. Marandin A, Dubart A, Pflumio F et al. Retrovirus-mediated gene transfer into human CD34+38^{low} primitive cells capable of reconstituting long-term cultures *in vitro* and nonobese diabetic-severe combined immunodeficiency mice *in vivo*. *Hum Gene Ther* 1998; **9**(10): 1497–511.
77. Conneally E, Eaves CJ, Humphries RK. Efficient retroviral-mediated gene transfer to human cord blood stem cells with *in vivo* repopulating potential. *Blood* 1998; **91**(9): 3487–93.
78. Hennemann B, Oh IH, Chuo JY et al. Efficient retrovirus-mediated gene transfer to transplantable human bone marrow cells in the absence of fibronectin. *Blood* 2000; **96**(7): 2432–9.
79. Schiedlmeier B, Kühlcke K, Eckert HG, Baum C, Zeller WJ, Fruehauf S. Quantitative assessment of retroviral transfer of the human multidrug resistance 1 gene to mobilized peripheral blood progenitor cells engrafted in nonobese diabetic/severe combined immunodeficient mice. *Blood* 2000; **95**(4): 1237–48.
80. Horn PA, Morris JC, Topp MS, Peterson L, Kiem HP. Direct comparison of gene transfer efficiencies into hematopoietic repopulating cells as measured by the NOD/SCID xenotransplant system versus autologous transplantation in the baboon suggests that distinct stem/progenitor cells are assayed. *Blood* 2001; **98**(11): 816a–17a [Abstract].
81. Conneally E, Bardy P, Eaves CJ et al. Rapid and efficient selection of human hematopoietic cells expressing murine heat-stable antigen as an indicator of retroviral-mediated gene transfer. *Blood* 1996; **87**: 456–64.

82 Mavilio F, Ferrari G, Rossini S et al. Peripheral blood lymphocytes as target cells of retroviral vector-mediated gene transfer. Blood 1994; 83: 1988–96.

83 Li Z, Dullmann J, Schiedlmeier B et al. Murine leukemia induced by retroviral gene marking. Science 2002; 296(5567): 497.

84 Limon A, Briones J, Puig T et al. High-titer retroviral vectors containing the enhanced green flourescent protein gene for efficient expression in hematopoietic cells. Blood 1997; 90(9): 3316–21.

85 Bierhuizen MF, Westerman Y, Visser TP, Dimjati W, Wognum AW, Wagemaker G. Enhanced green fluorescent protein as selectable marker of retroviral-mediated gene transfer in immature hematopoietic bone marrow cells. Blood 1997; 90(9): 3304–15.

86 Sorrentino BP, Brandt SJ, Bodine D et al. Selection of drug-resistant bone marrow cells in vivo after retroviral transfer of human MDR1. Science 1992; 257: 99–103.

87 Maze R, Kapur R, Kelley MR, Hansen WK, Oh SY, Williams DA. Reversal of 1,3-bis (2-chloroethyl)-1-nitrosourea-induced severe immunodeficiency by transduction of murine long-lived hematopoietic progenitor cells using O^6-methylguanine DNA methyltransferase complementary DNA. J Immunol 1997; 158: 1006–13.

88 Allay JA, Persons DA, Galipeau J et al. In vivo selection of retrovirally transduced hematopoietic stem cells. Nature Med 1998; 4(10): 1136–43.

89 Davis BM, Koc ON, Gerson SL. Limiting numbers of G156A O^6-methylguanine-DNA methyltransferase-transduced marrow progenitors repopulate nonmyeloablated mice after drug selection. Blood 2000; 95(10): 3078–84.

90 Ragg S, Xu-Welliver M, Bailey J et al. Direct reversal of DNA damage by mutant methyltransferase protein protects mice against dose-intensified chemotherapy and leads to in vivo selection of hematopoietic stem cells. Cancer Res 2000; 60(18): 5187–95.

91 Schiedlmeier B, Schilz AJ, Kuhlcke K et al. Multidrug resistance 1 gene transfer can confer chemoprotection to human peripheral blood progenitor cells engrafted in immunodeficient mice. Hum Gene Ther 2002; 13(2): 233–42.

92 Marshall E. Gene therapy. What to do when clear success comes with an unclear risk? Science 2002; 298(5593): 510–1.

93 Check E. Gene therapy: a tragic setback. Nature 2002; 420(6912): 116–8.

94 Bonetta L. Leukemia case triggers tighter gene-therapy controls. Nat Med 2002; 8(11): 1189.

95 Baum C, Düllman J, Li X et al. Side effects of retrovirus gene transfer into hematopoietic stem cells. Blood 2003; 101: 2099–114.

96 Williams DA, Levitsky HI, Dinauer MD, Russell DW. Genetic Therapies in Hematology: Human Diseases, Mouse Models and New Approaches. In Educational Program. American Society of Hematology, Washington D.C. 1997: pp. 61–80.

97 Felgner PL, Ringold GM. Cationic liposome-mediated transfection. Nature 1989; 337: 387–8.

98 Nabel GJ. Direct gene transfer with DNA-liposome complexes in melanoma. Proc Natl Acad Sci U S A 1993; 90: 11,307–11.

99 Crystal RG. Transfer of genes to humans: early lessons and obstacles to success. Science 1995; 270: 404–10.

100 Naldini L, Blomer U, Gallay P et al. In vivo gene delivery and stable transduction of nondividing cells by a lentiviral vector [see comments]. Science 1996; 272(5259): 263–7.

101 Reiser J, Harmison G, Kluepfel-Stahl S, Brady RO, Karlson S, Schubert M. Transduction of nondividing cells using pseudotyped defective high-titer HIV type 1 particles. Proc Natl Acad Sci U S A 1996; 93: 15,266–71.

102 Lewis PF, Emerman M. Passage through mitosis is required for oncoretroviruses but not for the human immunodeficiency virus. J Virol 1994; 68(1): 510–6.

103 Poeschla EM, Wong-Staal F, Looney DJ. Efficient transduction of nondividing human cells by feline immunodeficiency virus lentiviral vectors. Nature Med 1998; 4(3): 354–7.

104 Bukrinsky MI, Haggerty S, Dempsey MP et al. A nuclear localization signal within HIV-1 matrix protein that governs infection of nondividing cells [see comments]. Nature 1993; 365(6447): 666–9.

105 Gallay P, Swingler S, Song J, Bushman F, Trono D. HIV nuclear import is governed by the phosphotyrosine-mediated binding of matrix to the core domain of integrase. Cell 1995; 83: 569–76.

106 Heinzinger NK, Bukrinsky MI, Haggerty SA et al. The VPR protein of human immunodeficiency virus type 1 influences nuclear localization of viral nucleic acids in nondividing host cells. Proc Natl Acad Sci U S A 1994; 91(15): 7311–5.

107 Korin YD, Zack JA. Progression to the G_{1b} phase of the cell cycle is required for completion of human immunodeficiency virus type 1 reverse transcription in T cells. J Virol 1998; 72(4): 3161–8.

108 Buchschacher GLJ, Wong-Staal F. Development of lentiviral vectors for gene therapy for human diseases. Blood 2000; 95(8): 2499–504.

109 Akkina RK, Walton RM, Chen ML, Li QX, Planelles V, Chen IS. High-efficiency gene transfer into $CD34^+$ cells with a human immunodeficiency virus type 1-based retroviral vector pseudotyped with vesicular stomatitis virus envelope glycoprotein G. J Virol 1996; 70: 2581–5.

110 Landau NR, Page KA, Littman DR. Pseudotyping with human T-cell leukemia virus type 1 broadens the human immunodeficiency virus host range. J Virol 1991; 65: 162–9.

111 Srinivasakumar N, Chazal N, Helga-Maria C, Prasad S, Hammarskjold ML, Rekosh D. The effect of viral regulatory protein expression on gene delivery by human immunodeficiency virus type 1 vectors produced in stable packaging cell lines. J Virol 1997; 71(8): 5841–8.

112 Yu SF, Stone J, Linial ML. Productive persistent infection of hematopoietic cells by human foamy virus. J Virol 1996; 70: 1250–4.

113 Corbeau P, Kraus G, Wong-Staal F. Efficient gene transfer by a human immunodeficiency virus type 1 (HIV-1)-derived vector utilizing a stable HIV packaging cell line. Proc Natl Acad Sci U S A 1996; 93(24): 14,070–5.

114 Zufferey R, Nagy D, Mandel RJ, Naldini L, Trono D. Multiply attenuated lentiviral vector achieves efficient gene delivery in vivo. Nat Biotechnol 1997; 15(9): 871–5.

115 Zufferey R, Dull T, Mandel RJ et al. Self-inactivating lentivirus vector for safe and efficient in vivo gene delivery. J Virol 1998; 72(12): 9873–80.

116 Kim VN, Mitrophanous K, Kingsman SM, Kingsman AJ. Minimal requirement for a lentivirus vector based on human immunodeficiency virus type 1. J Virol 1998; 72(1): 811–6.

117 Douglas J, Kelly P, Evans JT, Garcia JV. Efficient transduction of human lymphocytes and $CD34^+$ cells via human immunodeficiency virus-based gene transfer vectors. Hum Gene Ther 1999; 10(6): 935–45.

118 Uchida N, Sutton RE, Friera AM et al. HIV, but not murine leukemia virus, vectors mediate high efficiency gene transfer into freshly isolated G_0/G_1 human hematopoietic stem cells. Proc Natl Acad Sci U S A 1998; 95(20): 11,939–44.

119 Case SS, Price MA, Jordan CT et al. Stable transduction of quiescent $CD34^+CD38^-$ human hematopoietic cells by HIV-1-based lentiviral vectors. Proc Natl Acad Sci U S A 1999; 96(6): 2988–93.

120 Evans JT, Kelly PF, O'Neill E, Garcia JV. Human cord blood $CD34^+CD38^-$ cell transduction via lentivirus-based gene transfer vectors. Hum Gene Ther 1999; 10(9): 1479–89.

121 Miyoshi H, Smith KA, Mosier DE, Verma IM, Torbett BE. Transduction of human $CD34^+$ cells that mediate long-term engraftment of NOD/SCID mice by HIV vectors. Science 1999; 283(5402): 682–6.

122 Hanawa H, Kelly PF, Nathwani AC et al. Comparison of various envelope proteins for their ability to pseudotype lentiviral vectors and transduce primitive hematopoietic cells from human blood. Mol Ther 2002; 5(3): 242–51.

123 Woods NB, Fahlman C, Mikkola H et al. Lentiviral gene transfer into primary and secondary NOD/SCID repopulating cells. Blood 2000; 96(12): 3725–33.

124 Sutton RE, Reitsma MJ, Uchida N, Brown PO. Transduction of human progenitor hematopoietic stem cells by human immunodeficiency virus type 1-based vectors is cell cycle dependent. J Virol 1999; 73(5): 3649–60.

125 Barrette S, Douglas JL, Seidel NE, Bodine DM. Lentivirus-based vectors transduce mouse hematopoietic stem cells with similar efficiency to moloney murine leukemia virus-based vectors. Blood 2000; 96(10): 3385–91.

126 Flugel RM. Spumaviruses. A group of complex retroviruses. J Acquir Immune Defic Syndr 1991; 4: 739–50.

127 Schliephake AW, Rethwilm A. Nuclear localization of foamy virus Gag precursor protein. J Virol 1994; 68: 4946–54.

128 Hirata RK, Miller AD, Andrews RG, Russell DW. Transduction of hematopoietic cells by foamy virus vectors. Blood 1996; 88: 3654–61.

129 Trobridge GD, Russell DW. Helper-free foamy virus vectors. Hum Gene Ther 1998; 9(17): 2517–25.

130 Heinkelein M, Dressler M, Jarmy G et al. Improved primate foamy virus vectors and packaging constructs. J Virol 2002; 76(8): 3774–83.

131 Vassilopoulos G, Trobridge G, Josephson NC, Russell DW. Gene transfer into murine hematopoietic stem cells with helper-free foamy virus vectors. Blood 2001; 98(3): 604–9.

132 Josephson NC, Vassilopoulos G, Trobridge GD et al. Transduction of human NOD/SCID-repopulating cells with both lymphoid and myeloid potential by foamy virus vectors. Proc Natl Acad Sci U S A 2002; 99(12): 8295–300.

133 Leurs C, Jansen M, Pollok KE et al. Comparison of three retroviral vector systems for transduction of NOD/SCID mice repopulating human $CD34^+$ cord blood cells. Hum Gene Ther 2003; 14: 509–19.

134 Kotin RM, Siniscalco M, Samulski RJ. Site specific integration by adeno-associated virus. Proc Natl Acad Sci U S A 1990; 87: 2211–5.

135 Miller JL, Walsh CE, Ney PA, Samulski RJ, Nienhuis AW. Single-copy transduction and expres-

sion of human α-globin in K562 erythro-leukemia cells using recombinant adeno-associated virus vectors: the effect of mutations in NF-E2 and GATA-1 binding motifs within the hypersensitivity site 2 enhancer. *Blood* 1993; **82**: 1900–6.
136 Walsh CE, Liu JM, Xiao X, Young NS, Nienhuis AW, Samulski RJ. Regulated high level expression of a human γ-globin gene introduced into erythroid cells by an adeno-associated virus vector. *Proc Natl Acad Sci U S A* 1992; **89**: 7257–61.
137 Russell DW, Kay MA. Adeno-associated virus vectors and hematology. *Blood* 1999; **94**(3): 864–74.
138 Walsh CE, Nienhuis AW, Samulski RJ *et al.* Phenotypic correction of Fanconi anemia in human hematopoietic cells with a recombinant adeno-associated virus vector. *J Clin Invest* 1994; **94**: 1440–8.
139 Zhou SZ, Broxmeyer HE, Cooper S, Harrington MA, Srivastava A. Adeno-associated virus 2-mediated high efficiency gene transfer into immature and mature subsets of hematopoietic progenitor cells in human umbilical cord blood. *J Exp Med* 1994; **179**: 1867–73.
140 Chatterjee S, Li W, Wong CA *et al.* Transduction of primitive human marrow and cord blood-derived hematopoietic progenitor cells with adeno-associated virus vectors. *Blood* 1999; **93**(6): 1882–94.
141 Ponnazhagan S, Yoder M, Srivastava A. Adeno-associated virus type 2-mediated transduction of murine hematopoietic cells with long-term repopulating ability and sustained expression of a human globin gene *in vivo*. *J Virol* 1997; **71**: 3098–104.
142 Watanabe T, Kuszynski C, Ino K *et al.* Gene transfer into human bone marrow hematopoietic cells mediated by adenovirus vectors. *Blood* 1996; **87**: 5032–9.
143 Neering SJ, Hardy SF, Minamoto D, Spratt SK, Jordan CT. Transduction of primitive human hematopoietic cells with recombinant adenovirus vectors. *Blood* 1996; **88**: 1147–55.
144 MacKenzie KL, Hackett NR, Crystal RG, Moore MA. Adenoviral vector-mediated gene transfer to primitive human hematopoietic progenitor cells: assessment of transduction and toxicity in long-term culture. *Blood* 2000; **96**(1): 100–8.
145 Roizmann B, Sear AE. Herpes simplex viruses and their replication. In: Fields BN, Knipe DM, eds. *Fields Virology*, 2nd edn. New York: Raven Press, 1990: 1795–841.
146 Marconi P, Krisky D, Oligino R. Replication-defective HSV vectors for gene transfer *in vivo*. *Proc Natl Acad Sci U S A* 1996; **93**: 11,319–20.
147 Kwong AD, Frenkel N. Biology of herpes simplex virus (HSV) defective viruses and development of the amplicon system. In: Kaplitt MG, Lowery AD, eds. *Viral Vectors*. San Diego: Academic Press, 1995: 25–42.
148 Tung C, Federoff. HJ, Brownlee M *et al.* Rapid production of interleukin-2-secreting tumor cells by herpes simplex virus-mediated gene transfer. Implications for autologous vaccine production. *Hum Gene Ther* 1996; **7**: 2217–24.
149 Goins WF, Krisky D, Marconi P *et al.* Herpes simplex virus-based gene transfer vectors for the nervous system. *J Neuro Virol* 1997; **3**: 80–8.
150 Dilloo D, Rill D, Enwistle C, Boursnell M, Holladay M, Brenner MF. A novel herpes vector for the high efficiency transduction of normal and malignant human hematopoietic cells. *Blood* 1997; **89**(1): 199–27.
151 Moritz T, Keller DC, Williams DA. Human cord blood cells as targets for gene transfer: potential use in genetic therapies of severe combined immunodeficiency disease. *J Exp Med* 1993; **178**: 529–36.
152 Clapp DW, Williams DA. The use of umbilical cord blood as a cellular source for correction of genetic diseases affecting the hematopoietic system. *Stem Cells* 1995; **13**: 613–21.
153 Movassagh M, Desmyter C, Baillou C *et al.* High-level gene transfer to cord blood progenitors using gibbon ape leukemia virus pseudotype retroviral vectors and an improved clinically applicable protocol. *Hum Gene Ther* 1998; **9**(2): 225–34.
154 Pollok KE, van Der Loo JC, Cooper RJ *et al.* Differential transduction efficiency of SCID-repopulating cells derived from umbilical cord blood and granulocyte colony-stimulating factor-mobilized peripheral blood. *Hum Gene Ther* 2001; **12**(17): 2095–108.
155 Kohn DB, Weinberg KI, Nolta JA *et al.* Engraftment of gene-modified umbilical cord blood cells in neonates with adenosine deaminase deficiency. *Nat Med* 1995; **1**: 1017–23.
156 Moritz T, Williams DA. Marrow protection-transduction of hematopoietic cells with drug resistance genes. *Cytotherapy* 2001; **3**(2): 67–84.
157 Sorrentino BP. Gene therapy to protect haematopoietic cells from cytotoxic cancer drugs. *Nat Rev Cancer* 2002; **2**(6): 431–41.
158 Pollok K, van der Loo J, Cooper R, Kennedy L, Williams D. Costimulation of transduced T lymphocytes via T-cell receptor/CD3 complex and CD28 leads to increased transcription of integrated retrovirus. *Human Gene Ther* 1999; **10**(13): 2221–36.
159 Hacein-Bey S, Gross F, Nusbaum P *et al.* Optimization of retroviral gene transfer protocol to maintain the lymphoid potential of progenitor cells. *Hum Gene Ther* 2001; **12**(3): 291–301.
160 Blaese RM, Culver KW, Miller AD *et al.* T lymphocyte-directed gene therapy for ADA⁻ SCID. initial trial results after 4 years. *Science* 1995; **270**: 475–80.
161 Bordignon C, Notarangelo LD, Nobili N *et al.* Gene therapy in peripheral blood lymphocytes and bone marrow for ADA-immunodeficient patients. *Science* 1995; **270**: 470–5.
162 Tiberghien P, Cahn JY, Brion A *et al.* Use of donor T-lymphocytes expressing herpes-simplex thymidine kinase in allogeneic bone marrow transplantation: a phase I–II study. *Human Gene Ther* 1997; **8**: 615–24.

11

Donald B. Kohn & Gay M. Crooks

Clinical Trials of Gene Marking and Gene Therapy Using Hematopoietic Stem Cells

Introduction

Disease and cell targets

Transplantation of genetically normal, allogeneic hematopoietic stem cells (HSCs) has been used successfully to treat many of the genetic diseases that involve hematopoietic and lymphoid cells [1]. The major limitations to the application of hematopoietic stem cell transplantation (HSCT) for genetic diseases are the immunologic problems encountered with allogeneic cell transplant, including graft rejection, graft-vs.-host disease (GVHD) and the need for immunosuppressive therapy. These successes and limitations provide the rationale for consideration of gene therapy using transplantation of genetically corrected, autologous stem cells for treatment of the same conditions (Table 11.1) [2,3]. Ideally, the use of autologous cells for gene replacement may eliminate the immunologic problems of allogeneic cell transplantation but afford the same or greater benefits.

The potential for applying these techniques for genetically augmenting the properties of normal HSCs or their mature progeny for the treatment of malignant or infectious diseases has been under study in clinical trials since the early 1990s (Tables 11.2 & 11.3). In the past few years, initial undisputable clinical successes have been achieved, but significant further progress will be needed to reach the final goals of safe and effective gene therapy for each of these conditions.

The basic technical requisites for successful gene therapy using HSCs are effective gene transfer into pluripotent stem cells followed by appropriate gene expression in the mature hematopoietic or lymphoid cells, without adverse effects on the function of the stem cells or the mature cells (Chapter 10 provides a more detailed discussion of the biology of gene transfer). Pluripotent stem cells are the ideal target for gene modification, due to their abilities to produce cells of all hematopoietic and lymphoid lineages, presumably for the life of the host. Thus, genetic modification and engraftment of pluripotent stem cells should result in a permanent effect. In contrast, gene transfer into more mature and committed progenitor cells may be expected to have only a short-term effect, until the modified cells are exhausted and replaced by new progenitors derived from nonmodified stem cells.

Table 11.1 Diseases involving hematopoietic or lymphoid cells that may be candidates for gene therapy using hematopoietic stem cells (HSCs).

1 Primary immune deficiencies:
   Severe combined immunodeficiency
   Chronic granulomatous disease
   Leukocyte adhesion deficiency
   Wiskott–Aldrich syndrome
   X-linked hyper-IgM syndrome (CD40 ligand deficiency)
   X-linked agammaglobulinemia

2 Erythrocyte disorders:
   Hemoglobinopathies: sickle cell disease, thalassemia
   Red cell membrane protein defects
   Hereditary hemolytic anemias

3 Lysosomal storage/metabolic disorders:
   Gaucher's disease
   Hurler's syndrome
   Hunter's syndrome
   Adrenoleukodystrophy

4 Stem cell disorders:
   Fanconi anemia

Table 11.2 Techniques employing gene therapy for the treatment of malignant diseases.

Gene modification of HSCs for enhancement of cell properties:
Drug resistance genes to decrease chemotherapy-induced myelosuppression
Genes which block oncogenes (e.g. antisense, ribozymes)
Tumor suppressor or pro-apoptotic genes (e.g. p53, *Rb*)
Tumor-associated antigens for expression in dendritic cells for cancer immunotherapy

Gene modification of T cells or other immune effector cells:
Suicide genes into allogeneic T cells to prevent GVHD
Chimeric antibody/T-cell receptor genes to direct cytotoxic effector cells against malignant cells
Cytokine genes to augment antineoplastic cytolytic activities
Tumor-associated antigen genes to induce antineoplastic immune responses

GVHD, graft-vs.-host disease; HSCs, hematopoietic stem cells.

Table 11.3

Infectious diseases being treated with gene therapy using:
   HIV-1
   CMV
   Parvovirus B19

CMV, cytomegalovirus; HIV, human immunodeficiency virus.

Table 11.4 Thresholds of gene transfer into hematopoietic stem cells (HSCs) expected to yield clinical benefits in specific disorders.

Low-level gene transfer (0.01% of stem cells) *may* be beneficial:
  Congenital immune deficiencies
  Fanconi anemia
  HIV-1 infection

Moderate-level gene transfer (0.05–5%) likely needed:
  Lysosomal storage diseases
  Protein deficiencies: hemophilia
  Resistance to chemotherapy-induced myelosuppression

High-level gene transfer (30–100%) required:
  Hemoglobinopathies
  Malignancy: antisense, antioncogene, tumor suppressor genes

HIV, human immunodeficiency virus.

The percentage of engrafted stem cells carrying a transferred gene that will be needed for a therapeutic effect will differ for specific disease applications (Table 11.4). It is expected that progress in the field will proceed through this hierarchy with the initial successes so far seen in those diseases where low levels of gene transfer may be beneficial (e.g. severe combined immunodeficiency syndrome [SCID]).

While the pluripotent HSC remains the target for permanently curing genetic diseases of blood cells, the recent identification of lineage-restricted progenitor cells, the common lymphocyte progenitor (CLP) and the common myeloid progenitor (CMP), may provide additional useful cell targets [4–6]. The progenitor cells may be transduced more readily than pluripotent HSCs and can produce specific mature effector cells (e.g. granulocytes, T lymphocytes, dendritic cells). Although progenitor cells contribute to mature cell production for only finite time-periods, gene-corrected progenitor cells could provide the mature cells of a needed lineage for weeks or months. Neutrophils produced from gene-corrected CMP from patients with chronic granulomatous disease could allow the patient to cope with an acute, serious infection. Dendritic cells may be derived from CD34$^+$ progenitor cells that have been transduced with genes expressing tumor-associated antigens and driven to differentiate *in vitro* for use to immunize patients against the tumor antigens. A burst of lymphocytes produced from a CLP could lead to long-lasting immune effector cells, such as memory T cells. These approaches have not been widely studied in clinical trials to date.

Gene transfer

Retroviral vectors

All of the clinical studies that have attempted to stably transduce hematopoietic stem or progenitor cells have used murine retroviral vectors for the gene delivery. Stable persistence of the transferred gene, either by integration into the chromosomes or by self-replication at a pace that keeps up with cellular division, would be needed for the gene transfer effect to be permanent. Retroviral vectors stably integrate the genes they carry into the chromosomal DNA of their target cells which allows the genes to be replicated with the cellular chromosomes and passed on to all progeny cells.

A major limitation of retroviral vectors is that they will only transduce cells that are actively dividing, because the viral genome can only gain access to the cellular chromosomes during mitosis when the nuclear membrane is dissolved. Pluripotent HSCs, especially from large mammals including dogs, monkeys and humans, are largely nondividing, quiescent cells and, thus, resistant to retroviral-mediated gene transfer. Studies performed with murine bone marrow demonstrated that stimulation of cellular division with the appropriate hematopoietic growth factors (e.g. interleukins 3 and 6 [IL-3, IL-6]) increased the efficiency of gene transfer to HSCs, to levels as high as 30–90% [7]. The manipulations of HSCs that produce high levels of transduction in murine models have been far less effective when applied to stem cells from larger animal models, with most studies finding the level of transduction of engrafting stem cells to be less than 1–10% [8,9].

The known optimal conditions for facilitating retroviral-mediated gene transfer to human HSC have evolved incrementally over time, as new hematopoietic growth factors and other elements have been identified (Table 11.5). Systematic evaluations of multiple elements of the gene transduction protocols have been performed using assays of human cells in *in vitro* cultures and *in vivo* xenograft assays and in nonhuman primate transplant models. Among the beneficial elements are the use of the envelope proteins from the gibbon ape leukemia virus (GALV) or the feline RD114 virus to serve as outer component of vectors to target cellular surface receptors (pseudotype) instead of the envelope from a murine (amphotropic) retrovirus which was used earlier; the use of recombinant fibronectin fragments (retronectin) to enhance cell/vector interactions and decrease apoptosis of stem cells; the use of newer cytokines (Flt-3 ligand, thrombopoietin) to stimulate stem cell proliferation; the use of "activated bone marrow" some days after granulocyte colony-stimulating factor (G-CSF) mobilization; and manipulation of cell cycle kinetics [10–18]. Combinations of these techniques have resulted in significant increases in gene marking in primate stem cell transplant models (e.g. 10%, up from the previous ceiling of 0.1–1.0%) [8,9]. Accordingly, the use of these newer approaches in current clinical trials is leading to better gene transfer, although the efficiency still remains the major factor limiting clinical benefits.

As retroviral vectors integrate into different, random chromosomal sites in each target cell, they can serve as genetic tags for analysis of the clonality of stem cells marking and differentiation. Techniques have been developed that allow tracking of multiple retroviral vector chromosomal

Table 11.5 Typical conditions used for *ex vivo* transduction of human hematopoietic stem cell (HSC) in clinical trials.

Condition\era	1993	1995	1997	1999	Soon
Growth factors	IL-3/IL-6/c-kitL	IL-3/IL-6/c-kitL	Flt-3L/IL-6/c-kitL	Flt3L/TPO/c-kitL	Flt3L/TPO/c-kitL
Support matrix	None	Stromal cells	rFBN	rFBN	rFBN
Vector	Retroviral	Retroviral	Retroviral	Retroviral	Lentiviral
Envelope	Ampho	Ampho	Ampho	GALV	VSV-G
Other				Serum-free	Serum-free

Ampho, amphoptropic; c-kitL, c-kit ligand (a.k.a. stem-cell factor); Flt3L, flt-3 ligand; GALV, gibbon ape leukemia virus; IL-3, interleukin 3; IL-6, interleukin 6; rFBN, recombinant fibronectin fragment; TPO, thrombopoietin; VSV, vesicular stomatitis virus.

integration sites, including inverse polymerase chain reaction (PCR) and ligation-mediated PCR [19]. Studies in human cells xenografted in immune-deficient murine hosts [20,21] showed that current gene-transfer techniques with retroviral vectors do transduce long-term pluripotent stem cells, with the same vector proviral integrant seen in myeloid and lymphoid cells derived from a common HSC. In nonhuman primate HSCT models, the same vector clonal integrant has been seen at multiple times in cells of both myeloid and lymphoid lineages, consistent with gene transduction of HSC that contribute to hematopoiesis for extended times. In contrast, a retrospective analysis of the clonality of gene marking in a trial performed for adenosine deaminase (ADA)-deficient SCID using earlier gene transfer methods now believed to be less effective, showed that the gene marking was oligoclonal and mainly from lineage-specific progenitors [22].

Adenoviral vectors

Adenoviral vectors are highly efficient for gene delivery to many cell types, independent of the requirement for target cellular proliferation that limits retroviral transduction of HSCs [23]. Adenoviral vectors have relatively large capacity to carry foreign genes (≤30 kb in fully deleted vectors) and therefore can accommodate the lengths of DNA sequences that contain sufficient *cis*-elements to yield controlled gene expression, e.g. the β-globin gene locus control region, enhancers, promoters and structural gene.

Although efficient for gene delivery, adenoviral vectors do not integrate into the chromosomes of the target cells and, thus, persist only transiently in transduced cells (days to weeks). Adenoviral vectors may be directly cytotoxic at high viral multiplicities of infection. Adenoviral vectors may cause acute local or systemic inflammation and be immunogenic when they are administered *in vivo* [24]. The low levels of residual adenoviral vectors that may be present on cells following *ex vivo* transduction are not expected to cause significant toxicity, although the transduced cells may be rendered immunogenic and thereby have accelerated elimination.

Although transduction of HSCs by adenoviral vectors would be transient with the transferred gene lost upon proliferation of the stem cells, adenoviral vectors may be useful to express genes for a short time to modify the properties of stem cells. One potential application for transient gene expression in hematopoietic stem or progenitor cells is the introduction of genes encoding tumor-associated antigens to be expressed after the cells differentiate into antigen-presenting cells, such as dendritic cells. Another way in which short-term gene expression by adenoviral vectors may be useful is to express genes that facilitate stable transduction by a second vector, like a retroviral vector. Adenoviral vectors may be used to express the gene for a new receptor protein, to stimulate stem cell proliferation or expansion, or to help maintain stem cell potential during transduction.

Adenoviruses have more than 80 different serotypes. The Ad5 serotype has been used most commonly as the basis for adenoviral vectors. In general, these Ad5 serotype vectors poorly transduce human hematopoietic and lymphoid cells. Laboratory studies have shown that CD34+ cells can be transduced by Ad5 adenoviral vectors at levels sufficient to express new vector receptor proteins or to express stimulatory proteins to induce proliferation and enhance subsequent retroviral transduction [25,26]. Adenoviral vectors substituting the fibre protein from Ad35 or Ad11 serotypes show significantly better ability to transduce human hematopoietic cells [27].

Two clinical trials have used Ad5 serotype adenoviral vectors to purge tumor cells contaminating autologous HSCs by transduction with genes promoting apoptosis, either the p53 gene or a dominant-negative mutant of the *bcl-2* gene (Table 11.6). The efficient transduction of carcinoma cells coupled to the poor transduction of HSC by adenoviral vectors provides a high ratio of selectivity for delivering the pro-apoptotic genes to the tumor cells [28]. Clinical trials using adenoviral vectors of the serotypes that allow better transduction of HSC have not yet been proposed.

Table 11.6 Clinical trials of gene transfer/gene therapy using hematopoietic stem cells (HSCs) reviewed by the NIH recombinant DNA advisory committee, USA.*

Category of trial	No. of trials	Vector
Gene marking	18 (neomycin resistance gene)	Retroviral
Chemotherapy resistance	8 *MDR-1* 3 *DHFR* 2 *MGMT*	Retroviral
Genetic diseases	6 SCID (2 ADA, 3 XSCID, 1 JAK-3) 3 Gaucher's disease 3 chronic granulomatous disease 3 Fanconi anemia 1 leukocyte adhesion deficiency	Retroviral
HIV-1	5 dominant negative *rev* 4 ribozyme 3 antisense 1 RRE decoy	Retroviral
Tumor cell purging	1 Ad5/p53 1 Ad5 bcl-2 dominant negative	Adenoviral

*As of March 2002 (http://www4.od.nih.gov/oba/rac/protocol.pdf).
ADA, adenosine deaminase; DHFR, dihydrofolate reductase; JAK-3, Janus kinase 3; MDR-1, multidrug resistant 1; MGMT, O^6-methylguanine DNA methyltransferase; SCID, severe combined immunodeficiency syndrome; XSCID, X-linked severe combined immune deficiency syndrome.

Gene expression

While effective gene transfer currently remains the rate-limiting step for gene therapy using stem cells, effective control of gene expression is also essential to achieve success. Housekeeping genes, such as *ADA* or glucocerebrosidase, probably do not require tightly regulated expression for a safe and therapeutic effect. However, a number of other therapeutic genes will require greater degrees of specificity in the levels of expression and/or cell types where expression occurs.

For example, transfer of β-globin for the treatment of hemoglobinopathies will require both lineage-specificity, with β-globin expression limited to the erythroid lineage, as well as a fairly well-regulated level of expression of the transferred β-globin gene to meet the levels of endogenous α-globin [29]. There has been a great deal of work attempting to include elements of the β-globin transcriptional control sequences, such as the enhancer and locus control region in retroviral vectors. However, these elements have been found to destabilize retroviral vectors, although progress has been made towards identifying and modifying these sequences while preserving their transcriptional activity [30,31].

Other genes required to treat genetic deficiencies may pose significant risks if expression occurs in a poorly regulated manner. Examples of this include the Bruton's tyrosine kinase (*btk*), deficient in X-linked agammaglobulinemia, the gene for the CD40 ligand, defective in X–linked hyper-immunoglobulin M (hyper-IgM) syndrome, and the WASP protein, defective in Wiskott–Aldrich syndrome [32–34]. Each of these gene products affects cellular proliferation or signal transduction pathways and inappropriate expression of them could be either cytotoxic or transforming.

Other issues

Cytoreductive conditioning

Complete marrow cytoablation is used prior to most allogeneic HSCT for genetic diseases, other than SCID, both to eliminate the recipient's marrow to "make space" for the normal donor HSC as well as to immune suppress the recipient to prevent graft rejection. In contrast, most of the clinical trials of gene transfer to autologous HSC performed outside of the oncology setting have not used cytoreductive conditioning of the subject's endogenous bone marrow, to avoid the risks associated with cytoablation in the face of the unknown benefits of the experimental gene transfer. One of the attractive aspects of SCID as a candidate disorder is that the strong selective survival advantage of gene-corrected T cells or their progenitors may allow immunologic reconstitution from a few gene-corrected stem cells, obviating the need for marrow cytoreduction to make space or prevent rejection.

For most other genetic disorders to be treated by gene therapy with HSC, there will be little or no selective advantage for the gene-corrected cells, and therefore it may be necessary to use variable degrees of cytoreduction to obtain sufficient levels of transduced HSC and the needed mature cells. Several studies have shown that modest dosages of cytoreductive radiation (e.g. 200–400 cGy) or chemotherapy (e.g. low dosages of busulfan [BU]) can cause significant increases in the levels of engraftment of donor HSC in murine and canine models [35–39]. As discussed below, a clinical trial performed by Aiuti and coworkers in Milan, Italy, for ADA-deficient SCID used a moderate dosage of BU (4 mg/kg) prior to transplantation of autologous gene-corrected bone marrow $CD34^+$ cells and achieved a relatively high level of engraftment of gene-containing HSCs [40]. As further confidence is gained with the effectiveness of gene transfer and expression methods, the use of increasing levels of cytoablation will become more appropriate.

Immune responses to the product of the transferred gene

Another important consideration in the use of gene transfer and gene therapy is the potential for immune responses to the product of the transferred gene. Retroviral and lentiviral vectors usually do not encode any viral proteins and therefore do not elicit immune responses against transduced cells. However, the protein product of the normal gene can be seen as a foreign antigen, especially in patients with null mutations resulting in the complete absence of the endogenous gene product. Foreign marker, reporter or suicide gene products (e.g. neomycin phosphotransferase, green fluorescent protein or herpes simplex thymidine kinase) can certainly be immunogenic. Cells expressing the transferred gene may be eliminated by either antibodies or cytotoxic T lymphocytes induced by presentation of peptides derived from the normal protein on host cells. There has not been a clinical report of an immune response to the product of a normal human gene transferred into an HSC, although an immunologic reaction to the jellyfish-derived green fluorescent protein reporter gene has been documented to lead to the loss of engrafted cells in a non-human primate transplant model [41]. Due to their innate immune deficiency, SCID patients are not likely to develop significant immune responses to the normal gene product that would be expressed during the process of immune reconstitution. However, for most other disorders, immune responses to the normal gene product may prevent sustained persistence of gene-expressing cells.

The potential to develop immune responses to proteins expressed by transferred genes is greatest when no cytoreductive conditioning is given, but it is not known what degree of immune suppression will be needed to allow tolerance to develop. It is likely that dosages of total-body irradiation typically used for complete cytoablation in the setting of HSCT (i.e. 1000–1200 cGy) will be sufficiently immune suppressive to eliminate immune reactivity to the normal protein expressed from cells derived from transduced and transplanted HSCs. Expression of the transgene product in antigen-presenting cells of the thymus derived from the transduced HSCs may play a role in initiation of central tolerance [42]. Other specific measures to induce tolerance in association with gene therapy may involve the use of immune suppressive drugs (e.g. cyclosporin), blockage of accessory or costimulatory molecules involved in immune responses (e.g. monoclonal antibodies to the CD40 ligand protein) [43], or tolerization schema using administration of the antigen by oral or intrathymic routes.

Clinical trials of gene transfer/gene therapy using HSCs

Of the 524 protocols reviewed by the US Recombinant DNA Advisory Committee of the National Institutes of Health (NIH) as of March 2002, 62 have been in the setting of HSCT. The majority used retroviral vectors based upon the Moloney murine leukemia virus (MuMLV) for direct gene modification of HSC (Table 11.6). Two studies used adenoviral vectors to purge breast tumor cells contaminating autologous HSCs by transduction with genes promoting apoptosis (http://www4.od.nih.gov/oba/roc/protocol.pdf).

Practical issues in performing clinical trials of gene transfer

The pathway to performing a clinical trial of gene transfer may be long and tortuous (Table 11.7). As in other clinical research studies, a clinical trial protocol and informed consent document must be developed based upon sufficient preclinical data to define potential efficacy and toxicity. It is challenging to provide informed consent for gene transfer studies that fully conveys the possible benefits and risks of the complex and novel gene transfer technology and yet states them in a way that is comprehensible to a lay subject. Multiple steps of regulatory review are required and

Table 11.7 The pathway to clinical trials of gene transfer/gene therapy.

Perform basic and preclinical studies to support feasibility and safety
Develop clinical trial protocol and informed consent document
Undergo regulatory review and approval process:
    Institutional review board(s)
    Institutional biosafety committee(s)
    Recombinant DNA Advisory Committee, Office of Biotechnology Activities, NIH
    Center for Biologics Evaluation and Research, FDA for IND permit
    Possible: NIH institutes, GCRC GAC, NGVL, DSMB
Produce and certify clinical grade vector
Obtain suitable ancillary products
Develop clinical trial organization and oversight documents and mechanisms
Train/certify clinicians and laboratory personnel
Perform clinical trial using Good Clinical Practice

DSMB, Data Safety and Monitoring Board; FDA, Food and Drug Administration; GAC, General Advisory Committee; GCRC, General Clinical Research Center; IND, Investigational New Drug; NGVL, National Gene Vector Laboratory; NIH, National Institutes of Health.

some may be done in parallel, although all protocol or consent changes that are made at a subsequent step need to be resubmitted to committees that gave approval at prior steps. The first steps involve review by local Institutional Review Boards (IRB) and Institutional Biosafety Committees (IBC), which may lack expertise on the biosafety issues of recombinant viral vectors, but have the highest expertise concerning local community standards for human subjects protection. In the USA, review and approval by the Recombinant DNA Advisory Committee (RAC) of the Office of Biotechnology Activities (OBA) at the NIH is required for any studies performed at institutions receiving federal funding. As the RAC has gained experience with clinical trials involving retroviral-mediated gene transfer to HSCs, they often review and approve new studies by expedited administrative process rather than full public review at a meeting, unless the trial poses new potential biosafety risks to subjects or the public. The Center for Biologic Evaluation and Research (CBER) of the Food and Drug Administration (FDA) reviews applications for gene therapy trials, viewing the gene and vector as the Investigational New Drug (IND) and the transduced cells as clinical cellular product. The FDA CBER review covers aspects of the clinical trial itself, with detailed review of the production and characterization of the vector and cells and the preclinical toxicology data. Additional reviews of the protocol and consent documents may be required by committees of NIH providing grant funding support, the National Gene Vector Laboratory (NGVL; see below) in consideration of an application to produce the clinical-grade vector and a General Clinical Research Center (GCRC) Advisory Committee if the trial will be performed at such a site. In recent years, it has become common for a Data Safety and Monitoring Board (DSMB) to be used to provide ongoing oversight of clinical gene therapy trials to ensure patient safety.

Production of clinical grade vector may be performed using appropriate Good Manufacturing Practices (GMP) at a facility at an academic center, at a commercial facility or by the NGVL established by the NIH National Center for Research Resources to provide access to vectors for academic investigations. A typical batch of clinical grade retroviral vector supernatant consists of 10–20 L of cell culture medium collected from cells releasing retroviral vector particles; this may be sufficient to treat the cells from five to 20 patients. Production of a batch of retroviral vector at optimal titer often requires trial-and-error production runs at various cell densities, incubator temperatures, culture medium, etc. The costs for producing the vector are in the range of $10,000–$20,000. Certification of each batch of a vector involves a number of tests to determine the absence of microbial contamination, absence of replication competent retrovirus, as well as assays to evaluate and identify the potency of the vector in terms of titer, sequence and functionality. These tests may take 3–6 months to perform and can cost from $30,000–$60,000. Ancillary products, such as $CD34^+$ cell enrichment devices, recombinant hematopoietic growth factors, recombinant fibronectin and other excipients also must be obtained at a quality suitable for clinical use and this process may be frustrating and complicated, with multiple over-lapping intellectual property issues to be resolved. Finally, the clinical trial must be performed under the standards of GMP, with appropriate monitoring, quality control, and documentation. It may be difficult to marshal the necessary resources, especially the salary support for laboratory and clinical regulatory personnel, to perform even small pilot studies in the academic setting. Thus, some studies that receive approvals from some or all of the regulatory review boards are never initiated, due to inability to obtain reagents, lack of financial support, or intervening scientific or personal developments.

Clinical trials of gene marking

The first clinical trials of gene transfer with HSCs did not involve transfer of potentially therapeutic genes but, instead, used a neutral marker gene to serve as a genetic tag of the cells being transplanted. The gene marking studies had two goals. One goal was to examine whether autologous bone marrow or mobilized peripheral blood stem cell (PBSC) preparations from oncology patients contained residual tumor cells that could contribute to relapse after transplantation. If there were tumor cells in the transplant inoculum tagged by the retroviral vector that contributed to a subsequent relapse after transplantation, the progeny of those tumor cells would also contain the vector tag, identifying their origin in the transplant.

In clinical trials incorporating gene marking into autologous bone marrow transplantation (BMT) for leukemia and cancer, gene marking of tumor cells contaminating the autologous transplant grafts was documented. In studies performed by Rill and coworkers in pediatric patients with acute myeloid leukemia (AML) and neuroblastoma and by Deisseroth and colleagues in adults with chronic myeloid leukemia (CML) the marker gene sequences were identified in leukemia or tumor cells at some subsequent relapses [44–46]. These studies provide strong direct evidence of the need for purging tumor cells from these types of cell sources for autologous transplantation.

The second goal of the gene marking studies was to gain insight into the nature of the normal human HSC that reconstitute hematopoiesis after transplantation and the ability to genetically modify the HSC. Most of the marking studies were performed before 1995 when the state of the art was less developed and gene transfer techniques that were used are now known to be suboptimal for effecting gene transfer to primitive pluripotent HSC (Table 11.5). Gene marking was performed by exposing unstimulated bone marrow cells to the retroviral vector or by attempting to stimulate proliferation of bone marrow cells using hematopoietic growth factor combinations (e.g. granulocyte macrophage colony-stimulating factor [GM-CSF], IL-3) now known to act primarily on mature committed progenitor cells, rather than on HSCs.

In the first studies, performed by Brenner and coworkers with pediatric BMT subjects, the marker gene was detected in 1–5% of the nonmalignant colony-forming cells of the bone marrow, persisting for more than 5 years of follow-up [47]. These findings provided the first clinical evidence that human HSCs may be transduced using retroviral vectors. The observed levels of gene marking of the normal reconstituting hematopoietic cells observed in most other marking studies (with adult subjects) were much lower, typically less than one gene-containing cell per 10,000 (0.01%), and generally the presence of cells with the marker gene was transient. It is speculated that the combination of the high proliferative potential of HSCs from the pediatric subjects and their use during periods of hematologic recovery from intensive chemotherapy led to a relatively high percentage of HSCs that were proliferating and, thus, susceptible to retroviral-mediated transduction. Of note, the studies by Brenner targeted unfractionated bone marrow cells, rather than the mobilized peripheral blood $CD34^+$ cells targeted by the trials in adults [47].

Few clinical gene marking studies have been proposed in recent years, but the approach of gene marking continues to be used in the nonhuman primate transplant studies to guide development of more effective gene transfer techniques for clinical trials with therapeutic intent [48].

Clinical trials of gene therapy

Subsequently, many clinical trials have been performed to examine the efficacy of gene therapy using HSCs for both gene replacement and gene augmentation (Table 11.6). These trials are phase 1 studies in which the toxicities of the vectors are assessed. In a sense, they are also pilot studies, with some endpoints of efficacy being evaluated, generally in small numbers of subjects.

Drug resistance gene transfer

Among the first clinical trials targeting HSCs with potentially therapeutic genes were studies to transfer genes conferring resistance to chemotherapeutic agents. The goal of this approach is to confer increased resistance to the dose-limiting myelosuppressive effects of chemotherapy, so that additional antineoplastic treatment may be given to the patients prophylactically after transplant or, if needed, at relapse. In addition, if selection for gene-transduced stem cells can be achieved with this approach, it may be possible to use these drug resistance genes as coselectable markers in vectors also carrying a therapeutic gene (e.g. β-globin). After transduced stem cells are transplanted, moderate doses of stem cell ablative chemotherapy could be given to reduce the fraction of nontransduced cells.

Initial clinical trials examined transfer of the multidrug resistance 1 (*MDR-1* or P-glycoprotein) copy DNA (cDNA) into the HSCs of cancer patients [49–51]. These studies showed low but detectable numbers of cells containing the *MDR-1* gene in some of the patients, although the benefits of expression of the exogenous *MDR-1* gene during subsequent chemotherapy have not yet been demonstrated.

In a clinical trial performed more recently, Abonour *et al.* [52] transferred the *MDR-1* cDNA to HSCs of patients with germ cell tumors undergoing tandem cycles of high-dose chemotherapy with autologous HSC rescue. The goal was to make some HSCs relatively resistant to chemotherapy-induced myelosuppression by expression of *MDR-1* to allow administration of post-transplant oral etoposide. CD34$^+$ PBSCs were obtained from G-CSF mobilized periperal blood and used for support of two tandem transplants. In the first cycle, only nontransduced PBSCs were given and, in the second, only PBSCs transduced with a retroviral vector carrying the human *MDR-1* cDNA were given. This study was the first to use recombinant fibronectin as a support matrix for *ex vivo* transduction of CD34$^+$ cells and it achieved a relatively high level of gene-marking, with 6–12% of bone marrow colony forming units (CFU) containing the vector as detected by PCR up to 1 year after transplant. The level of marking was lower in peripheral blood cells, with 0.01% of granulocytes containing the gene. The level of gene marking increased modestly (to 0.1% of granulocytes) after the post-transplant etoposide, consistent with a relative resistance to chemotherapy for progenitor cells expressing the transferred *MDR-1* gene.

This study is notable for being the first clinical trial to give only CD34$^+$ cells that had been manipulated *ex vivo* for gene transfer after an essentially fully marrow cytoablative regimen. The engraftment kinetics using the transduced PBSC were identical to those seen in the first of the tandem transplants that gave only nontransduced PBSC. Prior studies had shown that *ex vivo* culture of HSC led to loss of reconstituting activity, either due to apoptosis or differentiation [53]. The investigators attributed the rapid recovery of hematopoiesis in this trial as being due to preservation of stem cell engraftment capacity because of the use of the recombinant fibronectin. Nevertheless, there was minimal transduction and engraftment of long-term HSC, with no detectable gene-containing cells after 1 year in most subjects.

The use of *MDR-1* as a drug resistance gene has come into question. It is a relatively large cDNA and vectors carrying it may be subject to aberrant splicing, low titres and poor expression. Eckert *et al.* [54] have developed optimized vectors using the long-terminal repeats (LTR) from the spleen focus-forming virus (SFFV) which do express at higher levels. Of some concern, Bunting and coworkers observed that transduction of murine marrow with an *MDR-1* gene vector conferred a relative proliferative advantage on cells leading to myeloproliferation [55,56]. These proliferative effects of the *MDR-1* gene were not observed in nonhuman primates transplanted with *MDR-1*-transduced CD34$^+$ cells and so its clinical relevance is unclear [57].

Other genes being studied for the purpose of augmenting HSC resistance to chemotherapy include: the dihydrofolate reductase (*DHFR*) gene conferring resistance to methotrexate [58], the O^6-methylguanine DNA methyltransferase (*MGMT*) gene conferring resistance to alkylating agents such as 1,3-bis(2-chloroethyl)-1-nitrosourea (BCNU) [59], and the aldehyde reductase (*AR*) gene conferring resistance to cyclophosphamide [60]. Sawai *et al.* and Davis *et al.* have recently completed a trial using a retroviral vector carrying the *MGMT* gene into HSC of patients undergoing autologous transplant for brain tumors. The *MGMT*/BCNU system has been developed further to be especially robust for selection at the stem cell level by using a drug (O^6-benzyl-guanine [O^6-BG]) to inactivate the wild-type *MGMT* gene in nontransduced HSC (and tumor cells) rendering them highly sensitive to BCNU-mediated cytotoxicity while over-expressing an O^6-BG-resistant mutant of the *MGMT* gene in HSC to render them highly resistant to BCNU [61,62]. Gerson and coworkers have a newly initiated trial using this approach to transfer an O^6-BG-resistant mutant of *MGMT* to CD34$^+$ cells for autologous transplantation of patients with advanced malignancies to be followed by post-transplant antitumor treatment with BCNU and O^6-BG.

It remains unknown whether selection for resistance to chemotherapy will be at the level of the stem cells, and, thus, long lasting, or only at the progenitor cell level. Selection at the progenitor cell level would be expected to be transient and may revert to preselection levels after completion of a course of chemotherapy when new progenitor cells are made from nonselected stem cells. Additionally, it remains to be proven that decreased susceptibility to myelosuppression will allow sufficient dose escalations to the next limit of toxicity to truly result in increased clinical responses compared to, for example, the use of recombinant growth factors.

Clinical trials of gene therapy for genetic diseases

Congenital immune deficiencies

The field of gene therapy using HSCs has produced two highly significant positive results in the past few years in studies for X-linked severe combined immune deficiency (XSCID) and ADA-deficient SCID. SCID was initially chosen as a candidate disease for early gene therapy efforts because of the presumed selective expansion or survival advantage of normal T lymphocytes or their progenitors compared to genetically defective cells of the SCID subjects. Experience with allogeneic BMT for SCID since 1968 had shown that a completely protective, donor-derived immune system can develop after transplantation of HLA-matched sibling bone marrow without any cytoreductive preparation [1]. The recipient's marrow continues to be responsible for hematopoiesis, with only T lymphocytes (and in some cases B cells and/or natural killer [NK] cells) being donor-derived. It is uncertain whether the selective production of lymphocytes represents restricted differentiation from engrafted donor-derived pluripotent HSCs or lymphocyte production from donor-derived common lymphoid progenitor cells. A few rare case reports of SCID subjects who had some degree of spontaneous improvement without any therapeutic intervention were shown to be the result of reversion of the disease causing allele, possibly in a single stem or progenitor cell [63–65]. Thus, it was expected that a similar selective advantage would amplify the effects from gene correction of only a small number of autologous recipient HSCs or common lymphocyte progenitor (CLP).

Initial clinical trials that targeted CD34$^+$ cells from ADA-deficient bone marrow or cord blood did show evidence for selective expansion of gene-corrected T lymphocytes, but the absolute numbers of gene-corrected cells was low [66,67]. These subjects were all treated with ADA enzyme-replacement therapy (pegylated bovine [PEG]-ADA or

ADAGEN), which by itself led to immune reconstitution; by allowing T cells lacking a functional *ADA* gene to survive, the ADA enzyme therapy may have blunted the potential selective advantage of the T cells that contained the corrective *ADA* gene [68].

X-linked severe combined immune deficiency syndrome (XSCID)

Cavazzano-Calvo *et al.* and Hacein-Bey-Abina *et al.* in Paris, France, have treated a series of infants with XSCID by retroviral-mediated transfer of the relevant common cytokine γ chain (γc) into bone marrow CD34$^+$ cells [69,70]. They used an MLV-based retroviral vector and the currently best available hematopoietic growth factors (IL-3, c-kit ligand, Flt-3 ligand and thrombopoietin) and recombinant fibronectin support. Initial results with two subjects showed that this procedure led to restoration of immunity [69]. After infusion of the transduced CD34$^+$ cells, there was development of increasing numbers of functional T cells that responded to foreign antigens, over a time-course similar to that seen in allogeneic transplant of bone marrow from an human leukocyte antigen (HLA)-matched sibling. The level of gene-containing T lymphocytes greatly exceeded that present in cells of other lineages, confirming the selective advantage of T lymphocytes expressing the γc gene.

A subsequent publication extended the observations to three additional subjects and to longer times of follow-up [70]. This report confirmed the therapeutic benefits, with persistence of essentially normal T-lymphocyte function and apparently adequate B-cell function (levels of total immunoglobulins and specific antibodies), despite only low numbers of gene-corrected B cells detected in circulation. These children are currently healthy and living at home. Unfortunately, one of these subjects suffered a serious adverse event as a result of gene transfer, as discussed below.

Gene therapy likely worked for XSCID in this trial because the selective survival advantage of the corrected T cells could manifest fully in the absence of any form of protein replacement therapy that could blunt the selective advantage. In contrast, in the prior studies for ADA-deficient SCID, the PEG-ADA enzyme replacement therapy probably reduced the selective advantage for the corrected cells.

ADA-deficient SCID

Aiuti and coworkers in Milan, Italy, have recently reported encouraging results using retroviral-mediated gene transfer to CD34$^+$ cells from the bone marrow of two children with ADA-deficient SCID [40]. They were *not* being treated with PEG-ADA enzyme replacement therapy due to financial constraints in their countries of origin. Both infants were also given relatively low dosages of BU (4 mg/kg) prior to transplantation of their transduced autologous cells, representing the first time that cytoreduction has been used in a study of gene transfer for a genetic disease.

The two infants are developing significant levels of gene-containing peripheral blood cells and are undergoing immune reconstitution with 75–100% of peripheral blood T lymphocytes containing the vector. The effective immunologic recovery from the gene transfer likely occurred because the absence of PEG-ADA enzyme therapy allowed the selective advantage of the gene-corrected T lymphocytes to be manifest. The level of gene-containing peripheral blood myeloid cells, which do not benefit from the presence of the *ADA* gene, can be used as an index of the engraftment level of transduced HSC. Seven to sixteen percent of the myeloid cells contain the inserted *ADA* gene, which is significantly higher than levels achieved in prior studies that did not apply cytoreduction. These results support the utility of partial cytoreduction to enhance engraftment of gene-modified HSC, although further studies will be needed to define the optimal degree of cytoreduction for each condition.

Chronic granulomatous disease (CGD)

CGD is another inherited immune deficiency that has been the subject of clinical gene therapy trials. CGD is characterized by the inability of granulocytes to kill bacteria they have ingested due to the genetic absence of one of the oxidase proteins that generates toxic antimicrobial oxygen moieties. CGD patients have recurrent pyogenic infections, like Staphylococcal skin infections, and can have deep-seated abscesses with fungi, such as Aspergillus.

Malech and coworkers at the NIH, Bethesda, MD, have used G-CSF mobilized PBSCs as the target for a retroviral vector carrying the normal oxidase gene (p47*phox*) that is lacking in some CGD subjects [71]. Using a sensitive fluorescence activated cell sorter (FACS)-based assay for oxidase function, they demonstrated the presence of genetically corrected neutrophils in the peripheral circulation from 2 to 12 weeks after treatment, although at a frequency of only 0.1%. After this period, the corrected neutrophils were no longer detected. Similar results have been seen in a study by Dinauer and colleagues at Indiana University for the X-linked form of CGD, with a retroviral vector carrying the gp91*phox* cDNA (J. Croop, personal communication). No selective survival advantage is expected for gene corrected granulocytes (only better function), so there was no amplification of the presumably low numbers of stem cells that were corrected. The findings are consistent with transduction and engraftment of only relatively short-lived, committed progenitors; after the transduced progenitor cells had completed their time of contribution to mature cell pools, new progenitors derived from nontransduced stem cells produced neutrophils that lacked the transferred oxidase gene. It is possible that this transient production of gene-corrected neutrophils could confer some clinical benefits for a CGD patient suffering an acute infection.

Other congenital immune deficiencies

Bauer and Hickstein have performed preclinical studies and a clinical trial for two subjects with leukocyte adhesion deficiency, due to genetic defects in the gene for CD18, a component of a family of leucocyte hetero-dimeric adhesion molecules [72]. They had shown that transfer of a normal CD18 gene into patient cells restores expression and function of the adhesion molecule. In the clinical trial targeting G-CSF mobilized PBSCs, the levels of gene transfer achieved were too low and short-lived for an appreciable effect, as in the studies for CGD.

Other primary immune deficiencies are also candidates for gene therapy, including other genetic forms of SCID (Janus kinase 3 deficiency, Zap70 kinase deficiency, rag1/2 deficiency), as well as X-linked agammaglobulinemia, X-linked hyper-IgM syndrome (CD40 ligand deficiency) and Wiskott–Aldrich syndrome. However, each specific gene defect requires extensive research to develop clinical approaches.

It will be technically more difficult to correct disorders where the transferred gene requires regulated expression. For example, Brown *et al.* [33] showed that constitutive expression of the CD40 ligand gene transferred into murine bone marrow in a model of X-linked hyper-IgM syndrome led to chronic T-lymphocyte stimulation progressing to lymphoma. It will be necessary to recapitulate the physiologic expression pattern of CD40 ligand specifically in response to T-cell activation to achieve safe and effective correction of this disorder.

Thus, until now, gene therapy has only been beneficial for two genetic forms of SCID, where the strong, unopposed selective survival advantage allowed immune function to be restored. Better methods for gene delivery to stem cells, such as vectors derived from human immunodeficiency virus (HIV)-1 or other lentiviruses, and for control of gene expression are needed for further progress to be realized.

Fanconi anemia

Fanconi anemia is characterized by progressive anemia and bone marrow failure, predisposition to leukemia and other malignancies, associated with variable congenital anomalies with an underlying hyper-sensitivity to DNA damage [73]. Multiple different genes have been identified that cause Fanconi anemia and initial gene therapy trials have been performed using retroviral vectors to carry the relevant cDNA to HSCs.

Fanconi anemia is another disorder for which a relatively low level of gene transfer may yield a clinical benefit and, thus, is a logical early candidate. Genetically corrected cells from patients with Fanconi anemia may have a selective survival advantage allowing engraftment and hematologic benefit without cytoablation. Autologous gene transfer/BMT without cytoablative conditioning would likely decrease the potential for late secondary malignancies, which poses a risk for patients with Fanconi anemia undergoing allogeneic transplant. There is a theoretical concern that, in the absence of cytoablation, residual uncorrected hematopoietic elements may retain the malignant potential that predisposes these patients to leukemia. Possibly, effective hematopoiesis by corrected stem cells may decrease the proliferative demands on the uncorrected stem cells and lessen their malignant potential.

Liu and colleagues have performed trials of retroviral-mediated transfer of the Fanconi anemia complementation group A (*FAC*) and C (*FAC*) gene [74]. CD34$^+$ cells from autologous mobilized peripheral blood were transduced and then infused without prior cytoablation. Corrected peripheral blood cells were seen in the first months after treatment but were not present after 1 year. One subject of this trial who subsequently underwent localized radiation therapy for a malignancy had the reappearance of gene-containing leukocytes, although long-term results in this subject have not been reported. This observation suggests that gene-containing cells were present at a level too low to detect until the radiation therapy caused preferential suppression of hematopoiesis from the endogenous radiation hypersensitive noncorrected marrow with a selective proliferation of the gene-corrected cells. Further incremental increases in the efficiency of gene transfer may lead to sufficient numbers of corrected cells to restore hematopoiesis in patients with Fanconi anemia.

Lysosomal storage disease

For the lysosomal storage diseases, the percentages of corrected cells needed for a clinical benefit are not known. Some of these disorders (e.g. the mucopoly saccharidoses Hurler's and Hunter's syndromes) display the phenomenon of cross-correction in which cells expressing normal levels of the relevant enzymes can serve as donors to enzyme-deficient cells through a pathway mediated by secretion and uptake of proteins modified with mannose-6-phosphate residues [75]. Therefore, a relatively small number of corrected cells, especially if they over-express the relevant enzyme, may provide enzyme *in trans* to connective and neural tissues, as has been demonstrated in murine models of mucopolysaccharidosis (MPS) VII [76].

Three studies were performed in the mid-1990s targeting stem cells from patients with Gaucher's disease. These studies yielded relatively poor transduction of the marrow or peripheral blood CD34$^+$ cells and minimal detectable gene-containing cells in the circulation of patients after treatment [77,78]. In the absence of a selective survival advantage or significant cross-correction of host cells by gene-containing cells, Gaucher's disease is likely to need relatively high levels of gene transfer to stem cells with at least partial cytoreduction for a therapeutic effect to be reached.

Gene therapy for HIV-1 infection

A few studies have been performed using HSCs from patients infected by the acquired immune deficiency syndrome (AIDS) virus, HIV-1. These studies are trying to introduce into the stem cells synthetic "anti-HIV-1 genes" that make cells incapable of supporting growth of HIV-1. Investigators exploring the potential of genetic approaches to inhibit HIV-1 replication have developed a large number of synthetic genes which can suppress HIV-1 replication ("anti-HIV-1 genes"), including: antisense, ribozymes, dominant-negative mutants, RNA decoys, intracellular antibodies to block the activity of viral proteins or cellular coreceptors, siRNA, etc. [79]. In many cases, these anti-HIV-1 genes have been shown in model systems to suppress significantly the replication of HIV-1 and, in some cases, even limit virus entry into cells.

Ideally, if essentially 100% of a patient's T lymphocytes and monocytic cells could be made incapable of supporting HIV-1 replication, it is likely that decreased viral burdens would result. Theoretically, active inhibition of HIV-1 replication in 99.9% of the susceptible cells would be required to produce a 3-log reduction in virus load, an effect often produced by highly active antiretroviral therapy. However, with the limited capabilities to effectively transduce high percentages of human HSCs, it is not currently possible to protect the majority of susceptible cells. An alternative mechanism for efficacy is based on the possibility that cells engineered to be incapable of supporting active HIV-1 replication may be protected from viral-induced cytopathicity and, thus, have a selective survival advantage compared to nonprotected cells [80]. By analogy to the selective survival achieved by genetic correction of T-lymphocyte precursors with patients with SCID, a modest number of lymphoid progenitor cells that are protected from HIV-1 may contribute an increased percentage of all T lymphocytes leading to some preservation of immune function.

Initial gene transfer studies in subjects infected by HIV-1 have been designed to determine whether HSCs from patients with HIV-1 infection can be successfully transduced, whether they will engraft and whether expression of these genes to inhibit HIV-1 will allow prolonged survival of transduced T cells. Some of the clinical trials that have been performed sought to observe whether this selective advantage does occur, by using a competitive marking approach with half of each subject's CD34$^+$ cells transduced with the anti-HIV-1 gene vector and half of the cells transduced by a neutral marker vector. Selective protection by the anti-HIV-1 gene would lead to higher levels of peripheral blood cells with the anti-HIV-1 gene than the neutral marker gene.

Most of the initial clinical trials performed targeting anti-HIV-1 genes to HSC, found low levels of gene transfer with minimal levels of gene-containing cells seen *in vivo* after transplant [81,82]. Thus, no detectable suppression of HIV-1 or selective survival advantage was seen. More recent studies have achieved somewhat higher levels of gene-containing leukocytes, and a modest preferential survival of cells with the active anti-HIV-1 gene have been seen [83,84].

Development of T lymphoproliferation in an XSCID subject after gene therapy

Two of the subjects from the clinical trial of gene therapy for XSCID performed by the Paris group discussed above [69,70] developed serious adverse events approximately two and a half years after gene therapy was performed. These infants were 1 and 3 months old at the time of gene transfer and were given 14 and 20×10^6 transduced CD34$^+$ cells/kg respectively. Both appreciated rapid immune reconstitution but, more than two years later, were noted to have monoclonal T cell proliferations, with increasing white blood cell count and organomegaly. The malignant clone in both cases contained a single intact copy of the retroviral vector with the c gene. Once specific PCR primers were developed to amplify the junction between the vector provirus and the cellular DNA in the first child, the emergence of the T cell clone could be detected retrospectively since eight months after the gene transfer.

In the malignant T cells of both patients, the vector had integrated on chromosome 11p13, in the locus of the *LM02* gene. *LM02* is a transcriptional factor normally involved in stem cell and red cell differentiation and proliferation. *LM02* is a putative proto-oncogene that is activated in some human T cell leukemia by Rag-mediated translocation [t11;14 (p13;q11)]. Thus, it is quite likely that this represents insertional oncogenesis, where the chance insertion of the vector into the *LM02* gene activated its ectopic expression, playing a causal role in transformation.

Both adverse events were promptly reported to French regulatory authorities and to gene therapy investigators world-wide. Most similar studies were placed on temporary clinical hold while the nature of the events could be assessed. Other subjects of gene transfer trials have not been found to have evidence of lymphoproliferation. It is uncertain why this lymphoproliferation occurred in these subject and no others to date. because of the subjects' young age at the time of gene transfer, there was a relatively high bone marrow cell dosage, efficient gene transduction and subsequent massive proliferation of the transduced cells during thymopoiesis. Insertional oncogenesis may represent a stochastic event that occurs randomly as a function of rare integrations of the vector in the vicinity of transforming genes. It remains unclear what the frequency of this type of problem will be using integrating vectors for stable gene delivery.

Summary

To the present time, the initial results have been most promising in clinical trials where there is a strong selective advantage for the rare transduced cells. For conditions lacking this strong selective advantage, results have been modest. In terms of safety, the technology to produce replication-incompetent vectors has been successful, with no reports of replication competent virus observed in subjects. However, the recent emergence of the serious adverse event of leukemia in one XSCID subject has engendered strong caution until the absolute rate of this complication is known better. As with all new therapies, the benefits and risks of gene therapy relative to other treatments (such as haplo-identical BM) will need to be determined through the clinical trial process and will be revealed over time

Future directions

Lentiviral vectors for transduction of HSC

Vectors based upon lentiviruses, such as HIV-1, have been developed and hold promise for being more effective than retroviral vectors for stably transducing quiescent human HSCs. Lentiviruses are a class of retroviral vectors capable of infecting nondividing cells, in contrast to the retroviruses that require their target cells to be dividing to be able to infect them. Early attempts to develop vectors based on HIV-1 showed limited results, with low titers [85,86]. Since then, HIV-1-based vectors have been produced with higher transduction capacity, by applying more recently obtained knowledge of HIV-1 virology and from using the vesicular stomatitis virus G protein (VSV-G) protein to serve as the envelope which produces virion with sufficient physical stability to allow concentration to high titers by ultracentrifugation [87].

There are numerous published reports on the use of lentiviral vectors for transduction of human hematopoietic cells, with lentiviral vectors generally showing more favorable transduction capacity than retroviral vectors. For example, Case *et al.* [88] showed that lentiviral vectors could transduce $CD34^+/CD38^-$ cells that grow in extended long-term culture, whereas retroviral vectors could not. Others have shown that lentiviral vectors can transduce $CD34^+$ cells which engraft in NOD/SCID mice in a 1 or 2 day culture period, whereas retroviral vectors require more extensive culture of $CD34^+$ cells for transduction and the prolonged culture leads to a decrease in engraftment capacity [89–91].

While these initial findings are encouraging, they do not definitively prove that lentiviral vectors can efficiently transduce high percentages of pluripotent human HSCs which are quiescent (G_0) cells, and may not be read-out even in the more sophisticated assays [92]. Korin and Zack demonstrated that HIV-1 did not infect G_0 T lymphocytes and provided evidence that reverse transcription did not proceed effectively in these quiescent cells [93]. No superior efficacy by lentiviral vectors has been shown in studies reported to date for transduction of reconstituting HSC in nonhuman primate BMT models, compared to retroviral vectors [94], although it is not clear that optimal vectors or methods were used.

Lentiviral vectors have been shown to be capable of carrying larger genetic elements than retroviral vectors, leading to improved expression control [95,96]. The probable reason that lentiviral vectors can carry intact these genomic fragments is the presence of the rev/RRE mechanism of HIV-1 that facilitate the nuclear-to-cytoplasmic export of intact, unspliced vector transcripts, which would then be packaged into virion and transferred to target cells. In contrast, retroviral vectors do not have this mechanism for RNA export and, thus, large unspliced transcripts are retained in the nucleus; only transcripts undergoing aberrant splicing are exported, leading to the transmission of vectors with deletions.

While there are significant, but not insurmountable, biosafety concerns which would need to be addressed before lentiviral-based vectors can be used in human subjects, the setting of subjects already infected by HIV-1 may overcome some of the concerns while raising others. The first clinical trials proposing to use lentiviral vectors are undergoing regulatory review.

Hemoglobinopathies

Hemoglobinopathies comprise one of the most attractive target diseases for the use of gene therapy with HSCs due to the very high prevalence of these disorders. And yet, use of gene therapy for hemoglobinopathies has also proven to be one of the most challenging disease targets.

The fraction of corrected cells needed to benefit patients with hemoglobinopathies is not known. In thalassemia syndromes, genetically corrected cells should be capable of effective erythropoiesis, providing a selective advantage at the level of relatively mature erythroid progenitors [97,98]. Thus, expression of normal levels of globin in a small number of cells may be clinically helpful. In contrast, expression of HbS in sickle cell disease does not impair erythrocyte production, so that corrected cells expressing normal β- or α-globin genes would not be expected to have a selective production advantage, although they are likely to have prolonged survival. Treatment of acute sickle cell crises by exchange transfusion is effective when approximately 40–70% of the erythrocytes are from the normal HbA donor, which may serve as a target level of genetically corrected erythrocytes needed for benefit from gene therapy [99]. Thus, these diseases are likely to require fairly high levels of gene transfer efficiency to realize benefits.

As discussed above, expression of a transferred globin gene is likely to require well-regulated control of gene expression to restrict expression to erythroid cells at appropriate levels. The genomic DNA sequences that are necessary to achieve this degree of expression control have been defined using transgenic mouse models, and include the structural gene for the globin chain, introns that may contain enhancers, as well as multiple flanking DNA sequence elements with enhancer and locus control activities. Inclusion of these sequences in retroviral vectors caused instability of the vector genomes with high rates of deletions and rearrangements, limiting vector titers.

In the past few years, lentiviral vectors have been shown to be superior to retroviral vectors for carrying the globin expression cassettes. May et al. [95] first showed correction of a murine model of β-thalassemia using a lentiviral vector and Pawliuk et al. [100] have shown efficacy in a murine model of sickle cell disease. These lentiviral vectors carrying globin genes are likely to be introduced into clinical trials within the next few years.

Gene correction

Ideally, correction of defective genes at their normal chromosomal site by homologous recombination would result in maintenance of their precise, physiologically regulated gene expression. At present, homologous recombination for gene repair is far too inefficient to be of clinical utility with primary cells, although recent advances have been reported [101,102]. Once effective gene repair can be accomplished, it may be possible to correct a few of a patient's stem cells, perform ex vivo stem cell expansion (another desired but currently nonfeasible feat), and transplant truly corrected, autologous HSCs. Obviously, there is a great distance to go to realize this vision and the initial trials described here represent only the first steps.

References

1. Parkman R. The application of bone marrow transplantation to the treatment of genetic diseases. Science 1986; 232: 1373–8.
2. Anderson WF. Prospects for human gene therapy. Science 1984; 226: 401–9.
3. Kohn DB. Gene therapy for genetic and hematological disorders and immunodeficiencies. J Int Med 2001; 249: 379–90.
4. Kondo M, Weissman IL, Akashi K. Identification of clonogenic common lymphoid progenitors in mouse bone marrow. Cell 1997; 91: 661–72.
5. Hao QL, Zhu J, Price MA, Payne KJ, Barsky LW, Crooks GM. Identification of a novel, human multilymphoid progenitor in cord blood. Blood 2001; 97: 3683–90.
6. Akashi K, Traver D, Miyamoto T, Weissman IL. A clonogenic common myeloid progenitor that gives rise to all myeloid lineages. Nature 2000; 404: 193–7.
7. Bodine DM, Karlsson S, Nienhuis AW. Combination of interleukins 3 and 6 preserves stem cell function in culture and enhances retrovirus-mediated gene transfer into hematopoietic stem cells. Proc Natl Acad Sci U S A 1989; 86: 8897–901.
8. Kiem H-P, Andrews RG, Morris J et al. Improved gene transfer into baboon marrow repopulating cells using recombinant human fibronectin fragment CH-296 in combination with interleukin 6, stem cell factor, FLT-3 ligand, and megakaryocyte growth and development factor. Blood 1998; 92: 1878–86.
9. Wu T, Kim HJ, Sellers SE et al. Prolonged high-level detection of retrovirally marked hematopoietic cells in nonhuman primates after transduction of CD34+ progenitors using clinically feasible methods. Mol Ther 2000; 1: 285–93.
10. Kiem HP, Heyward S, Winkler A et al. Gene transfer into marrow repopulating cells. Comparison between amphotropic and gibbon ape leukemia virus pseudotyped retroviral vectors in a competitive repopulation assay in baboons. Blood 1997; 90: 4638–45.
11. Kelly PF, Vandergriff J, Nathwani A, Nienhuis AW, Vanin EF. Highly efficient gene transfer into cord blood nonobese diabetic/severe combined immunodeficiency repopulating cells by oncoretroviral vector particles pseudotyped with the feline endogenous retrovirus (RD114) envelope protein. Blood 2000; 96: 1206–14.
12. Hanenberg H, Xiao XL, Dilloo D, Hashino K, Kato I, Williams DA. Colocalization of retrovirus and target cells on specific fibronectin fragments increases genetic transduction of mammalian cells. Nat Med 1996; 2: 876–82.
13. Dao MA, Hashino K, Kato I, Nolta JA. Adhesion to fibronectin maintains regenerative capacity during ex vivo culture and transduction of human hematopoietic stem and progenitor cells. Blood 1998; 92: 4612–21.
14. Shah AJ, Smogorzewska EM, Hannum C, Crooks GM. Flt3 ligand induces proliferation of quiescent human bone marrow CD34+CD38− cells and maintains progenitor cells in vitro. Blood 1996; 87: 3563–70.
15. Piacibello W, Sanavio F, Garetto L et al. Extensive amplification and self-renewal of human primitive hematopoietic stem cells from cord blood. Blood 1997; 89: 2644–53.
16. Dao MA, Hannum CH, Kohn DB, Nolta JA. Flt3 ligand preserves the ability of human CD34+ progenitors to sustain long-term hematopoiesis in immune-deficient mice after ex vivo retroviral-mediated transduction. Blood 1997; 89: 446–56.
17. Dunbar CE, Seidel NE, Doren S et al. Improved retroviral gene transfer into murine and rhesus peripheral blood or bone marrow repopulating cells primed in vivo with stem cell factor and granulocyte colony-stimulating factor. Proc Natl Acad Sci U S A 1996; 93: 11,871–6.
18. Dao MA, Taylor N, Nolta JA. Reduction in levels of the cyclin-dependent kinase inhibitor p27^{kip-1} coupled with transforming growth factor neutralization induces cell-cycle entry and increases retroviral transduction of primitive human hematopoietic cells. Proc Natl Acad Sci U S A 1998; 95: 13,006–11.
19. Schmidt M, Hoffmann G, Wissler M et al. Detection and direct genomic sequencing of multiple rare unknown flanking DNA in highly complex samples. Hum Gene Ther 2001; 12: 743–9.
20. Nolta JA, Dao MA, Wells S, Smogorzewska EM, Kohn DB. Transduction of pluripotent human hematopoietic stem cells demonstrated by clonal analysis after engraftment in immune deficient mice. Proc Natl Acad Sci U S A 1996; 93: 2414–9.
21. Guenechea G, Gan OI, Dorrell C, Dick JE. Distinct classes of human stem cells that differ in proliferative and self-renewal potential. Nat Immunol 2000; 2: 75–82.
22. Schmidt M, Carbonaro D, Speckmann C et al. Clonality analysis after retroviral-mediated gene transfer to cord blood CD34+ cells of an ADA-deficient SCID infant. Nature Medicine 2003; 9: 463–8.
23. Brenner M. Gene transfer by adenovectors. Blood 1999; 94: 3965–7.
24. Zhang Y, Chirmule N, Gao GP et al. Acute cytokine response to systemic adenoviral vectors in mice is mediated by dendritic cells and macrophages. Mol Ther 2001; 3: 697–707.
25. Neering SJ, Hardy SF, Minamoto D, Spratt SK, Jordan CT. Transduction of primitive human hematopoietic cells with recombinant adenovirus vectors. Blood 1996; 88: 1147–55.
26. Nathwani A, Persons D, Stevenson S et al. Adenovirus-mediated expresssion of the murine ecotropic receptor facilitates transduction of human hematopoietic cells with an ecotropic retroviral vector. Gene Ther 1999; 6(8): 1456–68.
27. Shayakhmetov DM, Papayannopoulou T, Stamatoyannopoulos G, Lieber A. Efficient gene transfer into human CD34+ cells by a retargeted adenovirus vector. J Virol 2000; 74: 2567–83.
28. Garcia-Sanchez F, Pizzorno G, Fu SQ et al. Cytosine deaminase adenoviral vector and 5-fluorocytosine selectively reduce breast cancer cells 1 million-fold when they contaminate hematopoietic cells: a potential purging method for autologous transplantation. Blood 1998; 92: 672–82.
29. Tisdale J, Sadelain M. Toward gene therapy for disorders of globin synthesis. Semin Hematol 2001; 38: 382–92.
30. Leboulch P, Huang GMS, Humphries RK et al. Mutagenesis of retroviral vectors transducing human β-globin gene and β-globin locus control region derivatives results in stable transmission of an active transcriptional structure. EMBO J 1994; 13: 3065–76.
31. Sadelain M, Wang CH, Antoniou M, Grosveld F, Mulligan RC. Generation of a high-titer retroviral vector capable of expressing high levels of the human β-globin gene. Proc Natl Acad Sci U S A 1995; 92: 6728–32.
32. Rawlings DJ, Witte ON. The Btk subfamily of cytoplasmic tyrosine kinases: structure, regulation and function. Semin Immunol 1995; 7: 237–46.
33. Brown MO, Topham DJ, Sangster MJ et al. Thymic lymphoproliferative disease after successful correction of CD4− ligand deficiency by gene transfer in mice. Nat Med 1998; 4: 1253–60.
34. Derry JM, Ochs HD, Francke U. Isolation of a novel gene mutated in Wiskott–Aldrich syndrome. Cell 1994; 79: 635–44.
35. Barquinero J, Kiem H-P, von Kalle C et al. Myelosuppressive conditioning improves autologous engraftment of genetically marked hematopoietic

36 Stewart FM, Zhong S, Wuu J, Hsieh C-C, Nilsson SK, Quesenbery PJ. Lymphohematopoietic engraftment in minimally myeloablated hosts. *Blood* 1998; **91**: 3681–7.
37 Huhn RD, Tisdale JF, Agricola B, Metzger ME, Donahue RE, Dunbar CE. Retroviral marking and transplantation of rhesus hematopoietic cells by nonmyeloablative conditioning. *Human Gene Ther* 1999; **10**: 1783–90.
38 Mardiney M III, Malech HL. Enhanced engraftment of hematopoietic progenitor cells in mice treated with granulocyte colony-stimulating factor before low-dose irradiation: implications for gene therapy. *Blood* 1996; **87**: 4049–58.
39 Rosenzweig M, MacVittie TJ, Harper D *et al.* Efficient and durable gene marking of hematopoietic progenitor cells in nonhuman primates after nonablative conditioning. *Blood* 1999; **94**: 2271–86.
40 Aiuti A, Slavin S, Aker M *et al.* Correction of ADA-SCID by stem cell gene therapy combined with nonmyeloablative conditioning. *Science* 2002; **296**: 2410–3.
41 Rosenzweig M, Connole M, Glickman R *et al.* Induction of cytotoxic T lymphocyte and antibody responses to enhanced green fluorescent protein following transplantation of transduced CD34+ hematopoietic cells. *Blood* 2001; **97**: 1951–9.
42 Wekerle T, Kurtz J, Ito H *et al.* Allogeneic bone marrow transplantation with co-stimulatory blockade induces macrochimerism and tolerance without cytoreductive host treatment. *Nat Med* 2000; **6**: 464–9.
43 Taylor PA, Friedman TM, Korngold R, Noelle RJ, Blazar BR. Tolerance induction of alloreactive T cells via *ex vivo* blockade of the CD40: CD40L costimulatory pathway results in the generation of a potent immune regulatory cell. *Blood* 2002; **99**: 4601–9.
44 Brenner MK, Rill DR, Moen RC *et al.* Gene-marking to trace origin of relapse after autologous bone-marrow transplantation. *Lancet* 1993; **341**: 85–6.
45 Rill DR, Santana VM, Roberts WM *et al.* Direct demonstration that autologous bone marrow transplantation for solid tumors can return a multiplicity of tumorigenic cells. *Blood* 1994; **84**: 380–3.
46 Deisseroth AB, Zu Z, Claxton D *et al.* Genetic marking shows that Ph+ cells present in autologous transplants of chronic myelogenous leukemia (CML) contribute to relapse after autologous bone marrow in CML. *Blood* 1994; **83**: 3068–76.
47 Brenner MK, Rill DR, Holladay MS *et al.* Gene marking to determine whether autologous marrow infusion restores long-term haemopoiesis in cancer patients. *Lancet* 1993; **342**: 1134–7.
48 Shi PA, Hematti P, von Kalle C, Dunbar CE. Genetic marking as an approach to studying *in vivo* hematopoiesis: progress in the non-human primate model. *Oncogene* 2002; **21**: 3274–83.
49 Hanania EG, Giles RE, Kavanagh J *et al.* Results of *MDR-1* vector modification trial indicates that granulocyte/macrophage colony-forming unit cells do not contribute to posttransplant hematopoietic recovery following intensive systemic therapy. *Proc Natl Acad Sci U S A* 1996; **93**: 15,346–51.
50 Hesdorffer C, Ayello J, Ward M *et al.* A phase I trial of retroviral-mediated transfer of the human MDR-1 gene as marrow chemoprotection in patients undergoing high-dose chemotherapy and autologous stem-cell transplantation. *J Clin Oncol* 1998; **16**: 165–72.
51 O'Shaughnessy JA, Cowan KH, Nienhuis AW *et al.* Retroviral-mediated transfer of the human multidrug resistance gene (*MDR-1*) into hematopoietic stem cells during autologous transplantation after intensive chemotherapy for metastatic breast cancer. *Hum Gene Ther* 1994; **5**: 891–911.
52 Abonour R, Williams DA, Einhorn L *et al.* Efficient retrovirus-mediated transfer of the multidrug resistance 1 gene into autologous human long-term repopulating hematopoietic stem cells. *Nat Med* 2000; **6**: 652–8.
53 Peters SO, Kittler EL, Ramshaw HS, Quesenberry PJ. *Ex vivo* expansion of murine marrow cells with interleukin 3 (IL-3), IL-6, IL-11, and stem cell factor leads to impaired engraftment in irradiated hosts. *Blood* 1996; **87**: 30–7.
54 Eckert HG, Stockschlader M, Just U *et al.* High-dose multidrug resistance in primary human hematopoietic progenitor cells transduced with optimized retroviral vectors. *Blood* 1996; **88**: 3407–15.
55 Bunting KD, Galipeau J, Topham D, Benaim E, Sorrentino BP. Transduction of murine bone marrow cells with an MDR1 vector enables *ex vivo* stem cell expansion, but these expanded grafts cause a myeloproliferative syndrome in transplanted mice. *Blood* 1998; **92**: 2269–79.
56 Bunting KD, Zhou S, Lu T, Sorrentino BP. Enforced P-glycoprotein pump function in murine bone marrow cells results in expansion of side population stem cells *in vitro* and repopulating cells *in vivo*. *Blood* 2000; **96**: 902–9.
57 Sellers SE, Tisdale JF, Agricola BA *et al.* The effect of multidrug-resistance 1 gene versus neo transduction on *ex vivo* and *in vivo* expansion of rhesus macaque hematopoietic repopulating cells. *Blood* 2001; **97**: 1888–91.
58 Allay JA, Persons DA, Galipeau J *et al.* In vivo selection of retrovirally transduced hematopoietic stem cells. *Nat Med* 1998; **4**: 1136–43.
59 Ragg S, Xu-Welliver M, Bailey J *et al.* Direct reversal of DNA damage by mutant methyltransferase protein protects mice against dose-intensified chemotherapy and leads to *in vivo* selection of hematopoietic stem cells. *Cancer Res* 2000; **60**: 5187–95.
60 Takebe N, Zhao SC, Adhikari D *et al.* Generation of dual resistance to 4-hydroperoxycyclophosphamide and methotrexate by retroviral transfer of the human aldehyde dehydrogenase class 1 gene and a mutated dihydrofolate reductase gene. *Mol Ther* 2001; **3**: 88–96.
61 Sawai N, Zhou S, Vanin EF, Houghton P, Brent TP, Sorrentino BP. Protection and *in vivo* selection of hematopoietic stem cells using temozolomide, O^6-benzylguanine, and an alkyltransferase-expressing retroviral vector. *Mol Ther* 2001; **3**: 78–87.
62 Davis BM, Reese JS, Koc ON, Lee K, Schupp JE, Gerson SL. Selection for G156A O^6-methylguanine DNA methyltransferase gene-transduced hematopoietic progenitors and protection from lethality in mice treated with O^6-benzylguanine and 1,3-bis(2-chloroethyl)-1-nitrosourea. *Cancer Res* 1997; **57**: 5093–9.
63 Stephan V, Wahn V, Le Deist F *et al.* Atypical X-linked severe combined immunodeficiency due to possible spontaneous reversion of the genetic defect in T cells. *N Eng J Med* 1996; **335**: 1563–7.
64 Hirschhorn R, Yang DR, Puck JM, Hiue ML, Jiang CK, Kurlandsky LE. Spontaneous *in vivo* reversion to normal of an inherited mutation in a patient with adenosine deaminase deficiency. *Nat Genet* 1996; **13**: 290–5.
65 Ariga T, Oda N, Yamaguchi K *et al.* T-cell lines from two patients with adenosine deaminase (ADA) deficiency showed the restoration of ADA activity resulted from the reversion of an inherited mutation. *Blood* 2001; **97**: 2896–9.
66 Bordignon C, Notarangelo LD, Nobili N *et al.* Gene therapy in peripheral blood lymphocytes and bone marrow for ADA-immunodeficient patients. *Science* 1995; **270**: 470–5.
67 Kohn DB, Hershfield MS, Carbonaro D *et al.* T lymphocytes with a normal *ADA* gene accumulate after transplantation of transduced autologous umbilical cord blood CD34+ cells in ADA-deficient SCID neonates. *Nat Med* 1998; **4**: 775–80.
68 Aiuti A, Vai S, Mortellaro A *et al.* Immune reconstitution in ADA-SCID after *PBL* gene therapy and discontinuation of enzyme replacement. *Nat Med* 2002; **8**: 423–5.
69 Cavazzana-Calvo M, Hacein-Bey S, de Saint Basile G *et al.* Gene therapy of human severe combined immunodeficiency (SCID)-X1 disease. *Science* 2000; **288**: 669–72.
70 Hacein-Bey-Abina S, Le Deist F, Carlier F *et al.* Sustained correction of X-linked severe combined immunodeficiency by *ex vivo* gene therapy. *N Engl J Med* 2002; **346**: 1185–93.
71 Malech HL, Maples PB, Whiting-Theobald N *et al.* Prolonged production of NADPH oxidase-corrected granulocytes after gene therapy of chronic granulomatous disease. *Proc Natl Acad Sci U S A* 1997; **94**: 12,133–8.
72 Bauer TR Jr, Hickstein DD. Gene therapy for leukocyte adhesion deficiency. *Curr Opin Mol Ther* 2000; **2**: 383–8.
73 Joenje H, Patel KJ. The emerging genetic and molecular basis of Fanconi anemia. *Nat Rev Genet* 2001; **2**: 446–57.
74 Liu JM, Kim S, Read EJ *et al.* Engraftment of hematopoietic progenitor cells Fanconi anemia group C gene (FANCC). *Hum Gene Ther* 1999; **10**: 2337–46.
75 Neufeld EF. Lysosomal storage diseases. *Annu Rev Biochem* 1991; **60**: 257–80.
76 Wolfe JH, Sands MS, Barker JE *et al.* Reversal of pathology in murine mucopolysaccharidosis type VII by somatic cell gene transfer. *Nature* 1992; **360**: 749–53.
77 Dunbar CE, Kohn DB, Schiffmann R *et al.* Retroviral transfer of the glucocerebrosidase gene into CD34+ cells from patients with Gaucher disease: *in vivo* detection of transduced cells without myeloablation. *Hum Gene Ther* 1998; **9**: 2629–40.
78 Schuening F, Longo WL, Atkinson ME *et al.* Retrovirus-mediated transfer of the cDNA for human glucocerebrosidase into peripheral blood repopulating cells of patients with Gaucher's disease. *Hum Gene Ther* 1997; **8**: 2143–60.
79 Engel BC, Kohn DB. Stem cell directed gene therapy. *Front Biosci* 1999; **4**: e26–33.
80 Woffendin C, Ranga U, Yang Z-Y, Nabel GJ. Expression of a protective gene prolongs survival of T cells in human immunodeficiency virus-infected patients. *Proc Natl Acad Sci U S A* 1996; **93**: 2889–94.
81 Kohn DB, Bauer GH, Valdez P *et al.* A clinical trial of retroviral-mediated transfer of an RRE Decoy gene into CD34+ cells from the bone marrow of HIV-1 infected children. *Blood* 1999; **94**: 368–71.

82 Zaia JA, Rossi JJ, Krishnan A *et al.* Autologous stem cell transplantation using retrovirus-transduced peripheral blood progenitor cells in HIV-infected persons. Comparison of gene marking post-engraftment with and without myeloablative therapy. *Blood* 1999; **94** (Suppl. 1): 642a.

83 Liu D, Conant MA, Cowan MJ *et al.* Engraftment and development of HGTV43-transduced CD34+ PBSC in HIV-1 seropositive individuals. Presented at the 5th annual meeting of the American Society of Gene Therapy, June 2002.

84 Amado RG, Mitsuyasu RT, Symonds G *et al.* A phase I trial of autologous CD34+ hematopoietic progenitor cells transduced with an anti-HIV ribozyme. *Hum Gene Ther* 1999; **10**(13): 2255–70.

85 Poznansky M, Lever A, Bergeron L, Haseltine W, Sodroski J. Gene transfer into human lymphocytes by a defective human immunodeficiency virus type 1 vector. *J Virol* 1991; **65**(532): 532–6.

86 Shimada T, Fujii H, Mitsuya H, Nienhuis AW. Targeted and highly efficient gene transfer into CD4+ cells by a recombinant human immunodeficiency virus retroviral vector. *J Clin Invest* 1991; **88**: 1043–7.

87 Naldini L, Blomer U, Gallay P *et al.* In vivo gene delivery and stable transduction of nondividing cells by a lentiviral vector. *Science* 1996; **272**: 263–7.

88 Case SS, Price MA, Jordan CT *et al.* Stable transduction of quiescent CD34+ CD38− human hematopoietic cells by HIV-1 based lentiviral vectors. *Proc Natl Acad Sci U S A* 1999; **96**: 2988–93.

89 Miyoshi H, Smith K, Mosier DE, Verma IM, Torbett BE. Efficient transduction of human CD34+ cells that mediate long-term engraftment of NOD/SCID mice by HIV vectors. *Science* 1999; **283**: 682–6.

90 Sutton RE, Wu HTM, Rigg R, Böhnlein E, Brown PO. Human immunodeficiency virus type 1 vectors efficiently transduce human hematopoietic stem cells. *J Virol* 1998; **72**: 5781–8.

91 Guenechea G, Gan OI, Inamitsu T *et al.* Transduction of human CD34+ CD38− bone marrow and cord blood-derived SCID-repopulating cells with third generation lentiviral vectors. *Mol Ther* 2000; **1**: 566–73.

92 Sutton RE, Reitsma MJ, Uchida N, Brown PO. Transduction of human progenitor hematopoietic stem cells by human immunodeficiency virus type 1-based vectors is cell cycle dependent. *J Virol* 1999; **73**: 3649–60.

93 Korin YD, Zack JA. Progression to the G_1b phase of the cell cycle is required for completion of human immunodeficiency virus type 1 reverse transcription in T cells. *J Virol* 1998; **72**: 3161–8.

94 An DS, Kung SK, Bonifacino A *et al.* Lentivirus vector-mediated hematopoietic stem cell gene transfer of common γ-chain cytokine receptor in rhesus macaques. *J Virol* 2001; **75**: 3547–55.

95 May C, Rivella S, Callegari J *et al.* Therapeutic haemoglobin synthesis in β-thalassaemic mice expressing lentivirus-encoded human β-globin. *Nature* 2000; **406**: 82–6.

96 Kowolik CM, Hu J, Yee JK. Locus control region of the human *CD2* gene in a lentivirus vector confers position-independent transgene expression. *J Virol* 2001; **75**: 4641–8.

97 Bethel CA, Murugesh D, Harrison MR, Mohandas N, Rubin EM. Selective erythroid replacement in murine β-thalassemia using fetal hematopoietic stem cells. *Proc Natl Acad Sci U S A* 1993; **90**: 10,120–4.

98 Van de Bos C, Kieboom D, Wagemaker G. Correction of murine β-thalassemia by partial bone marrow chimerism: selective advantage of normal erythropoiesis. *Bone Marrow Transplant* 1993; **12**: 9–13.

99 Vichinsky EP, Haberkern CM, Neumayr L *et al.* A comparison of conservative and aggressive transfusion regimens in the perioperative management of sickle cell disease. The Preoperative Transfusion in Sickle Cell Disease Study Group. *New Engl J Med* 1995; **333**: 206–13.

100 Pawliuk R, Westerman KA, Fabry ME *et al.* Correction of sickle cell disease in transgenic mouse models by gene therapy. *Science* 2001; **294**: 2368–71.

101 Goncz KK, Prokopishyn Chow NL, Davis BL, Davis BR, Gruenert DC. Application of SFHR to gene therapy of monogenic disorders. *Gene Ther* 2002; **9**: 691–4.

102 Liu H, Agarwal S, Kmiec E, Davis BR. Targeted β-globin gene conversion in human hematopoietic CD34+ and Lin− CD38− cells. *Gene Ther* 2002; **9**: 118–26.

12

James H. Doroshow & Timothy Synold

Pharmacologic Basis for High-Dose Chemotherapy

The feasibility of utilizing high doses of chemotherapeutic drugs, rather than ionizing radiation, as conditioning agents prior to allogeneic bone marrow transplantation (BMT) was initially demonstrated in animal models over 30 years ago [1]. Successful human trials that employed high-dose cyclophosphamide (CY) with or without total body irradiation (TBI) for patients with aplastic anemia or acute leukemia undergoing BMT were performed soon thereafter [2–5]. A decade earlier, autologous BMT for patients with hematologic malignancies following TBI or high-dose single-agent nitrogen mustard chemotherapy was reported, albeit with little success [6].

The outcome of allogeneic approaches to BMT depends, to a significant degree, on the immunosuppressive properties of the conditioning regimen. As outlined in Chapter 3, CY became a critical part of allogeneic transplant procedures 30 years ago because it combined significant antileukemic activity with profound effects on several different components of the immune system. In the course of the past 10 years, however, as the number of autologous marrow or peripheral blood hematopoietic cell (PBHC) transplants has increased, the specific therapeutic spectrum of action of the chemotherapeutic agents employed, the degree of enhanced tumor cell killing produced by the dose escalation made possible with hematopoietic cell (HC) support, and the extent to which specific drugs or drug combinations produce dose-limiting extramedullary toxicities has become as important as their immunosuppressive nature.

In this chapter, the rationale for the use of chemotherapeutic agents in higher than standard dosage is examined from both a mechanistic perspective and with regard to the general pharmacodynamic features of high-dose chemotherapy, which has a critical role in drug selection. In turn, each of the classes of antineoplastic agents currently employed in the high-dose treatment of both hematologic malignancies and solid tumors are reviewed with respect to their mechanism(s) of action and resistance, pharmacokinetics, pharmacodynamics, drug–drug interactions and dose-limiting toxicities. Structural formulas are shown in Fig. 12.1 and kinetic parameters in Table 12.1. The pharmacologic underpinnings developed in this chapter provide a basis from which to evaluate the rationale for the high-dose chemotherapy combinations described in Chapter 13.

Pharmacologic rationale for high-dose chemotherapy

Pharmacologic basis of dose intensity

Pharmacologic definition of high-dose chemotherapy

Although it has been estimated that 40,000 patients worldwide received high-dose chemotherapy with HC support in 2000, an adequate definition of the procedure in many ways remains elusive [7]. To define high-dose chemotherapy as the utilization of drug regimens that produce bone marrow ablation would not be accurate in the setting of autologous HC support; furthermore, recent studies suggest that this definition would also be inaccurate for patients receiving non-myeloablative allogeneic BMTs. Assuming that a level of drug dosage that requires HC support for safety reasons is, by itself, a sufficient definition of what constitutes "high-dose chemotherapy" is uninformative because it has no clear therapeutic implication.

For many chemotherapeutic agents, an approximate threefold increase in area-under-the-curve (AUC) can be translated *in vitro* into a 10-fold increase in cytotoxicity (probably the smallest increment in cell kill that may be associated with clinical benefit). Thus, one possible definition of the minimum dose of a chemotherapeutic agent alone or in combination that qualifies as "high-dose chemotherapy" is a dose that increases systemic exposure by a factor of 3 compared to the standard chemotherapeutic dose. Establishing a pharmacokinetic definition of high-dose chemotherapy that takes into account systemic exposure would allow much more definitive pharmacodynamic comparisons of both treatment outcomes and toxicities for both currently available and future high-dose chemotherapy programs.

Concentration–response effects in preclinical models

Abundant *in vitro* evidence exists demonstrating various drug-specific, concentration-dependent patterns of induced cytotoxicity or apoptosis, or both, in human tumor cell model systems [7–11]. In general, the alkylating agents (such as melphalan, thiotepa and bis-chloroethyl-nitrosourea [BCNU]) and platinum derivatives produce the most profound inhibition of tumor cell growth *in vitro* with the smallest increment in drug concentration. Antimetabolites (such as methotrexate and cytarabine), on the other hand, frequently demonstrate a plateau effect in which cytotoxicity ceases to be log-linear within a more narrow range of drug concentration. The anthracyclines, the taxanes and etoposide are intermediate in this regard (Fig. 12.2); however, for these latter classes of drugs, prolonged exposure *in vitro* can markedly increase tumor cell killing out of proportion to the observed concentration × time product, suggesting that both the cellular pharmacology (drug uptake) and mechanism of growth arrest for these chemotherapeutic agents involve a variety of dynamic intracellular targets [10,12].

Tumor cell heterogeneity and growth kinetics

While much has been made of the "steepness" of the slope of *in vitro* cytotoxicity curves in the selection of drugs for use in high-dose chemotherapy [13–15], it remains clear that a multiplicity of conditions, including the genotypic and phenotypic heterogeneity of tumor cells, variations in the perfusion or oxygenation of the tumor, as well as immunologic

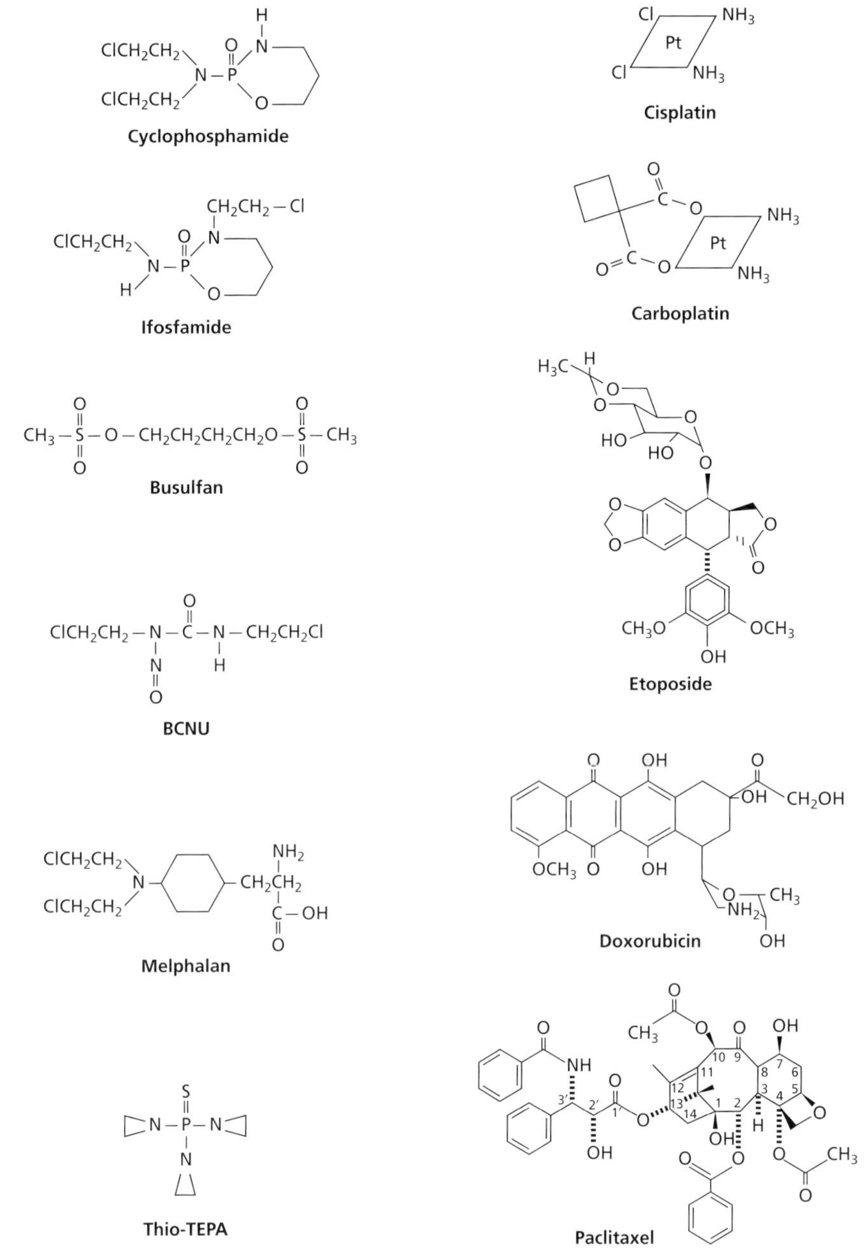

Fig. 12.1 Structural formulas for the principal drugs used in high-dose chemotherapy with hematopoietic cell support.

Table 12.1 Pharmacokinetic and pharmacodynamic features of drugs employed for high-dose chemotherapy.

Drug	Elimination	Pharmacokinetics	Dose intensity	Pharmacodynamics
Cyclophosphamide	Renal	Non-linear for active species	8×	Cardiac toxicity and low AUC
Melphalan	Hydrolysis	Linear; 30–120 min	6×	Mucositis
Thiotepa	Hepatic	Linear; 1–3 h	8–10×	Mucositis; CNS
Busulfan	Liver	Linear; 3 h	8×	VOD
BCNU	Hydrolysis/liver	Linear; 30 min	3×	Lung; VOD
Cisplatin	Renal	Linear; 30–45 min	3×	Kidney; neuropathy
Carboplatin	Renal	Linear; 7–20 h	4–5×	Ototoxicity; kidney
Etoposide	Renal	Linear; 4–8 h	3–6×	Mucositis
Doxorubicin	Hepatic/biliary	Linear; 12–20 h	3–4×	Mucositis
Paclitaxel	Hepatic/biliary	Non-linear; 15 h	5× increase in dose yields 15× AUC	Neuropathy and mucositis

AUC, area-under-the-curve; BCNU, bis-chloroethyl-nitrosourea; CNS, central nervous system; VOD, veno-occlusive disease.

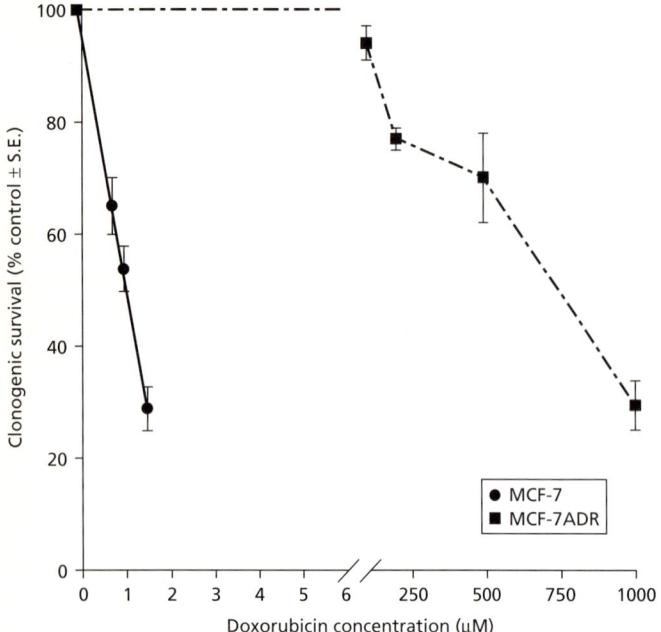

Fig. 12.2 Cytotoxicity of doxorubicin in MCF-7 and pleiotropically resistant MCF-7^{ADR} breast cancer cells *in vitro*. Tumor cells in logarithmic phase growth were exposed for 1 h to doxorubicin at the concentrations shown, washed in drug-free medium and plated on tissue culture dishes. Clonogenic survival was calculated by counting colonies of tumor cells (more than 40 cells/colony) in treated and untreated dishes and expressing the result as a percentage of control. Data represent the mean ± SE of three separate experiments. MCF-7^{ADR} cells were developed by sequential passage in increasing concentrations of doxorubicin; they express high levels of the *MDR*1 gene product as well as alterations in topoisomerase II and various antioxidant enzymes.

Table 12.2 Mechanisms of therapeutic resistance in high-dose chemotherapy.

1 Decreased drug uptake or enhanced drug efflux producing a net reduction in the intracellular concentration of the cytotoxic agent
2 Increased repair of DNA damage or damage to other critical targets
3 Development of alternative synthetic pathways for metabolites critical for tumor cell growth
4 Overexpression of the gene product targeted by the chemotherapeutic agent or the production of an aberrant target that supports tumor cell growth but is not affected by the drug utilized
5 Enhanced intracellular detoxification or metabolism of the high-dose therapy that limits tumor cell killing
6 Overexpression of cytoprotective gene products that alter tumor cell sensitivity to the drug-induced cell death program
7 Altered tumoral blood supply (oxygenation) or tissue factors that diminish drug activity or delivery

factors all come into play in determining the success or failure of intensive chemotherapy strategies *in vivo* [16–18]. None of these features can be strictly predicted by *in vitro* cytotoxicity assays; hence, *in vivo* preclinical models continue to play a critical part in the overall assessment of combination high-dose chemotherapy strategies, including those that employ high doses of alkylating agents [19–21].

Studies in murine systems established the ability of many classes of antineoplastic agents to kill tumor cells according to first-order kinetics; i.e. a given concentration of drug utilized for a particular time period will kill a fixed number of tumor cells [19]. If each treatment course at a given dose is cytotoxic for a constant fraction of cells, the curability of the particular therapy depends on the number of courses delivered, the drug concentration applied and the initial tumor burden [22]. While this concept has been unequivocally verified in many animal tumor models that undergo logarithmic tumor cell expansion, it is not clear how well it applies to more slowly growing and genetically heterogeneous tumors in humans. However, the model does, in part, form the basis for the rational use of high-dose chemotherapy in the adjuvant setting which is employed to destroy microscopic residual disease after surgical excision, radiation or standard dose chemotherapy has eradicated most or all macroscopically detectable tumor cells [23].

A major factor which underlies the efficacy of all systemic cancer treatment is the genetic heterogeneity of human tumors [18]. Although most cancers may develop initially from a single malignant clone, all malignancies demonstrate genetic instability which leads to a remarkable degree of biochemical heterogeneity that can be observed not only from metastatic site to metastatic site but from cell to cell in a single tumor mass [24,25]. Thus, the enormous inherent variation in the expression of any one of the wide range of proteins that establish the innate sensitivity of malignant cells to systemic agents is probably responsible for both the unpredictability of the efficacy of treatment (from patient to patient but not in populations of patients) as well as the regrowth of clones of malignant cells after an initial response to treatment. Thus, regrowth may represent the expansion of tumor cells that, before any systemic drug exposure, already expressed gene products capable of providing a growth advantage under the selective pressure of treatment with high-dose chemotherapy.

The demonstration of heterogeneous populations of tumor cells in humans has provided a critical rationale for the use of combinations of high-dose systemic agents with different sites of action which might circumvent at least some mechanisms of inherent drug insensitivity. Acknowledgment of the extent of human tumor cell heterogeneity provides additional support for strategies that reduce tumor cell mass prior to high-dose chemotherapy administration, because it has been predicted that the probability of a tumor possessing random mutations leading to insensitivity to systemic treatment is a function of the tumor cell burden [26]. Thus, reduction of tumor mass prior to systemic treatment may decrease not only the total body burden of cancer but also the percentage of tumor cells inherently resistant to dose-intensive treatment.

A critical kinetic issue that currently surrounds the use of high-dose chemotherapy, especially for the treatment of solid tumors, is whether a single course of high-dose treatment can produce a sufficient reduction in the total burden of cancer cells in the body, even in the adjuvant setting, to provide a survival benefit. Evaluation of the efficacy of administering multiple cycles of dose-intensive treatment with hematopoietic support will be a major future challenge.

Tumor cell resistance to high-dose chemotherapy

High-dose chemotherapy is not uniformly successful because many types of cancers in humans harbor small populations of tumor cells that are intrinsically resistant to treatment or acquire resistance during therapy. High-dose chemotherapy may also fail because the incremental increase in drug exposure possible with HC support is either insufficient to produce lethal tumor cell damage or cannot be delivered in sufficient concentration to the tumor to be cytotoxic [26]. Where sufficient drug exposure is possible, however, even highly resistant tumor cells can be killed (Fig. 12.2).

Mechanisms by which resistance to high-dose chemotherapy develops are, at least in part, specific to the mechanism of action of the class of agents being utilized. However, many different biochemical and physiologic phenomena have been observed either *in vitro* or *in vivo* to modulate the effectiveness of several different antineoplastic drug classes utilized for high-dose chemotherapy (Table 12.2):

- reduced drug uptake by the tumor cell [27];
- enhanced drug efflux [28];
- increased repair of drug-induced damage to DNA or other critical tumor cell targets [17];
- development of alternative routes for the synthesis of biologically important molecules when the primary synthetic pathway is blocked by a given drug [29];
- overexpression of the target gene product for a specific drug [30];
- production of an aberrant drug target that does not interact with a given agent, yet retains biochemical function sufficient to support tumor cell growth [31];
- enhanced intracellular metabolism or detoxification of the chemotherapeutic agent which limits tumor cell toxicity [32];
- overexpression or modification of cytoprotective gene products which alter tumor cell sensitivity to the anticancer agent [33];
- variations in the oxygenation state or blood supply of the tumor which can blunt the effectiveness of the drug directly or the delivery of the drug to the tumor itself [34]; and
- factors in the normal tissues of the host which can significantly change the concentration of drug delivered to the tumor [35].

Although the clinical relevance of each of these mechanisms is uncertain, samples of human tumors have been shown to express one or more phenotypic markers of drug resistance [36,37]. The mutations that lead to the expression of these characteristics may occur prior to the "recognition" of a tumor and can become more prominent under the selective pressure of therapy [38]. A tumor cell does not start to express a resistance phenotype in the presence of a given drug; instead, cells with a particular phenotype emerge by a process of mutation and/or evolution [39].

Certain physiologic characteristics of tumors, distinct from their genotype, can impede delivery of effective concentrations of drug to the entire tumor. A major impediment is size; large tumor masses often contain areas of poorly vascularized tissue. Consequently, delivery of cytotoxic drugs to these areas of tumor via the blood will be poor, even after high-dose chemotherapy [34,40]. For this reason, and because of the constraints of non-linear dose–response relationships and growth kinetics that exist for large heterogeneous tumors, the likelihood of benefit of high-dose chemotherapy in the clinic has regularly been shown to be greater in the presence of low-bulk disease or in the adjuvant setting [41–43].

Genetic basis for variability in response to high-dose chemotherapy

Contribution of pharmacogenomics to clinical response and toxicity

Evidence for inherited differences in response to drug therapy dates to the 1950s. Early observations relating the extent of acetylation of isoniazid to peripheral neuropathy [44] and plasma cholinesterase activity to prolonged muscle relaxation in response to suxamethonium [45] are examples of inherited determinants of the variability in the clinical response to drugs that gave rise to the modern field of "pharmacogenomics". Pharmacogenomics is the study of inherited genetic variations (polymorphisms) in the genes involved in drug metabolism, therapeutic response and toxicity, and how these polymorphisms relate to inherited differences in pharmacokinetics and drug effects.

The mechanistic basis for inherited pharmacologic traits first began to be elucidated in the 1980s with the cloning of a polymorphic human gene encoding the drug-metabolizing enzyme debrisoquin hydroxylase (*CYP2D6*) [46]. Large population studies of individuals given the antihypertensive debrisoquine, a drug that caused an unusual fainting response in some patients, revealed two distinct phenotypes ("extensive" and "poor" metabolizers), based upon the extent of urinary excretion of hydroxylated debrisoquin metabolites [47]. In 1988, the wild-type human *CYP2D6* gene was cloned from "extensive" metabolizers along with three different variant transcripts from "poor" metabolizers, and expressed in mammalian cells [46]. The variant gene products arose from mutations that resulted in alternatively spliced proteins that were not functional, thereby providing a molecular explanation for the inherited differences seen in debrisoquin pharmacokinetics and hemodynamics.

For a gene to be considered "polymorphic", the genetic variants must exist stably in the population and one or more of the variants must result in a protein with altered activity relative to the wild-type sequence. While in most cases polymorphisms are associated with decreased protein activity, there are also examples where the genetic variation results in increased protein activity, usually as a result of amplification of gene expression [48–50]. Since the initial cloning and characterization of the *CYP2D6* gene, many more polymorphic human genes involved in drug metabolism and drug response pathways have been identified.

Traditional approaches to pharmacogenomic investigations have been monogenic, focusing on the contribution of a single gene to phenotypic variability. Although in some cases the effects of alterations at a single gene locus are sufficient to produce major phenotypic changes, the clinical response to most pharmacologic agents is a polygenic process, with multiple genes playing a part in both the pharmacokinetics and the therapeutic mechanism of action of the agent. However, powerful molecular epidemiologic tools and high-throughput gene sequencing technology utilizing more than 1.4 million single nucleotide polymorphisms (SNPs) that have been demonstrated across the entire genome have generated great enthusiasm for the possibility of a genetics-based approach for assessing disease risk and individualizing drug therapy [51].

Inherited variability in drug metabolism and transport

Stable genetic variants have been identified for nearly every gene involved in drug metabolism, although such polymorphisms do not always have clear clinical significance. Depending upon the nature of the genetic change, the importance of the enzyme for the overall metabolism of a given drug and the expression of other drug-metabolizing enzymes, a genotype–phenotype relationship may not be obvious. While almost every gene is subject to genetic polymorphisms, the phenotypic consequences of the polymorphism may be subtle, such as placing an individual on one end of a normal distribution of drug metabolism phenotypes, rather than conferring a complete deficiency of the encoded enzyme. Thus, inactivating polymorphisms can be broadly categorized into two groups: those that confer complete or near-complete loss of activity, and those that confer more subtle changes in protein function.

The molecular mechanisms that inactivate genes involved in drug metabolism include splice site mutations resulting in exon skipping, microsatellite nucleotide repeats, gene duplication, point mutations resulting in early stop codons, enhanced proteolysis, altered promoter functions, critical amino acid substitutions, or large gene deletions [52]. Conversely, gene duplication has been associated with enhanced activity for some drug-metabolizing enzymes [49,50]. A number of clinically relevant polymorphisms have been identified in genes involved in both detoxification and activation of anticancer agents used in the high-dose setting. Because these genetic variants typically encode proteins with decreased enzymatic activity, the impact of these inherited differences on *in vivo* drug biotransformation are amplified as doses are increased.

Cytochrome P450 2C subfamily

The members of the CYP2C group of proteins are an important subfamily of cytochrome p450 enzymes consisting of four members, CYP2C8, CYP2C9, CYP2C18 and CYP2C19. In addition to involvement in the metabolism of arachidonic acid [53], CYP2Cs also metabolize many commonly used drugs, including the anticancer agents CY, ifosfamide and paclitaxel employed in high-dose therapy. Inactivating polymorphisms have been identified for each member of this subfamily, the best described being those found in the gene encoding CYP2C19. All of the inactivating genetic changes are single nucleotide transitions resulting in splicing defects, early stop codons and amino acid substitutions. Poor metabolizers of substrates for CYP2C19 are homozygous for the variant alleles and represent approximately 3–5% of Caucasians, a similar percentage of African-Americans and 12–100% of Asian groups [54]. Inactivating polymorphisms in CYP2C19 have been shown to affect the metabolism of mephenytoin [55], omeprazole [56], diazepam [57,58], certain antidepressants [59] and proguanil [60]. Toxic effects related to decreased rate of clearance and increased systemic exposure occur in poor metabolizers given diazepam [54]. Furthermore, the efficacy of proton pump inhibitors, such as omeprazole, may be greater in poor compared to extensive metabolizers at lower doses of these drugs [61]. Each of the CYP2C subfamily members has been shown to catalyze the activation step of ifosfamide and CY to their 4-hydroxy metabolites in the following order of affinity: CYP2C19 < CYP2C18 < CYP2C9 < CYP2C8 [62]. Inactivating polymorphisms in these enzymes may result in decreased formation of the active oxazaphosphorine 4-hydroxylated metabolites *in vivo*, leading to decreased clinical efficacy of these important anticancer agents during high-dose therapy.

CYP2C8 is present at relatively high levels in most human livers and plays a major part in the metabolism of the taxanes; CYP2C8 is the major cytochrome P450 isoform catalysing paclitaxel 6α-hydroxylation, the primary inactivating step in paclitaxel metabolism *in vivo* [63,64]. Multiple polymorphisms have been identified in the gene encoding CYP2C8, resulting in protein variants with decreased enzymatic activity compared to the wild-type sequence. The existence of at least four CYP2C8 variant alleles, including two involving non-synonymous mutations, has been confirmed [65]. The allelic frequencies in various ethnic populations have not yet been determined. Two of the genetic variants resulting from single amino acid substitutions, G416A (CYP2C8*3) and C792G (CYP2C8*4), exhibit decreased rates of paclitaxel 6α-hydroxylation *in vitro* [65,66]. As a result, patients with one or more alleles carrying inactivating polymorphisms in CYP2C8 would be expected to have a decreased rate of metabolic clearance of paclitaxel. Moreover, it is anticipated that the clinical impact of lowered enzymatic activity would become more significant as the dose of paclitaxel is increased. The relevance of inactivating polymorphisms in CYP2C8 in patients receiving high-dose paclitaxel is currently under active investigation.

Cytochrome P450 3A subfamily

Members of the CYP3A subfamily catalyze the oxidative and reductive metabolism of a structurally diverse set of exogenous and endogenous compounds [67]. The CYP3A members are the most abundant cytochrome P450s in human liver and small intestine [68,69]. Substantial interindividual differences exist in CYP3A expression, exceeding 30-fold in some populations [69,70]. The wide variation in expression contributes greatly to variation in oral bioavailability and systemic clearance of CYP3A substrates. Such variation in CYP3A can result in clinically significant differences in drug toxicities and response. Human CYP3A activities reflect the heterogeneous expression of at least three CYP3A subfamily members: CYP3A4, CYP3A5 and CYP3A7 [70]. Functional CYP3A4 is found in most adults, with a 10- to 40-fold variation in its expression [71,72]. CYP3A7 is predominantly expressed in fetal life, and its expression seems to be silenced shortly after birth; however, some individuals express CYP3A7 mRNA into adulthood. CYP3A5 can also be detected in the liver and small intestine of certain white adults [73–75].

CYP3A4, the most abundant isoform of cytochrome P450 in adult human liver, is important for the metabolism of many clinically important anticancer compounds used in high-dose therapy, including the taxanes [63,76], vinca alkaloids [77,78], epipodophyllotoxins [79] and CY [62,80]. In addition to a high constitutive expression, CYP3A4 is inducible in response to certain exogenous substrates. Although several CYP3A4 variants have been identified, including five that result in coding sequence changes, none of the polymorphisms described affect enzyme catalytic activity [81]. However, a polymorphism in the promoter region for CYP3A4 has been described that may affect the extent to which CYP3A4 is inducible, rather than altering constitutive levels of the enzyme [82].

A polymorphism has recently been discovered in intron 3 of the human *CYP3A5* gene that creates an ectopic splice site, leading to a premature stop codon [83]. This common allelic variant in CYP3A5 is the principal genetic basis for polymorphic expression of this enzyme in humans and explains why CYP3A5 expression is only detectable in a subset of the population. Because many CYP3A4 substrates are also substrates for CYP3A5, the CYP3A5 polymorphism influences overall CYP3A activity, and would be expected to shift subjects to the higher end of the phenotypic distribution for CYP3A activity. Thus, CYP3A5 should contribute significantly to the total metabolic clearance of many CYP3A substrates. Moreover, because CYP3A4 and CYP3A5 have slightly differing catalytic activities and substrate specificities, polymorphic CYP3A5 expression may also contribute to differences in metabolite profiles and in susceptibility to inhibitory drug interactions. Therefore, a polymorphism in CYP3A5 may be one important factor contributing to individual variation in overall CYP3A-mediated metabolism of drugs. For this reason, simple DNA-based tests have been developed that can be used to determine how individual differences in CYP3A5 contribute to the overall metabolic fate of CYP3A substrates, and to their pharmacokinetic and pharmacodynamic variability. Although the clinical utility of prospective determinations of polymorphisms in the *CYP3A* gene family has yet to be demonstrated, investigations are ongoing.

Glutathione S-transferases

The glutathione S-transferase (GST) family of enzymes is coded by a large supergene family located on several different chromosomes. In general, the GSTs detoxify strong electrophiles by catalysing their conjugation to glutathione. A wide variety of substrates are detoxified by GSTs either by direct conjugation with glutathione or by inactivation of the cellular byproducts of oxidative stress. As a result, the GST family of proteins plays a critical part in defense against environmental toxins (e.g. polycyclic aromatic hydrocarbons) and reactive oxygen species. Furthermore, many of the chemotherapeutic agents used in high-dose therapy are detoxified by GSTs, including busulfan (BU) [84,85], thiotepa [86], CY and ifosfamide [87,88], platinum-containing compounds and anthracyclines [89–91]. Overexpression of GSTs results in cellular resistance to the cytotoxic effects of these chemotherapeutic drugs [92]; conversely, cells that have been depleted of glutathione are further sensitized to the toxic effects of these agents [93,94].

Because several of the GST genes are polymorphic, there has been considerable interest in determining whether particular allelic variants of each are associated with altered clinical phenotypes. The preponderance of evidence suggesting a role for GSTs in detoxifying reactive compounds comes from several molecular epidemiologic studies linking GST genotype with cancer risk [95–97]. However, much less is known about the importance of GST genotype as a determinant of either the pharmacokinetics of or response to high-dose chemotherapy. Conjugation with glutathione is the major route of biotransformation for BU, and is predominantly catalyzed by the GST isozyme GSTA1 [85]. At least seven polymorphisms of GSTA1 have been identified, and haplotype analysis has revealed the existence of five unique alleles. However, there is no effect on any of the known GSTA1 polymorphisms or haplotypes on hepatic GSTA1 expression or GSTA1 function.

Multiple drug resistance gene 1 (MDR1)

Although passive diffusion accounts for the cellular distribution of some drugs and metabolites, more attention has been paid to the role of membrane transport proteins in critical physiologic functions such as oral drug absorption, biliary and renal excretion, and distribution of drugs into "therapeutic sanctuaries", such as the brain and testes. The most widely studied drug transporter is the adenosine triphosphate (ATP) binding cassette family member *MDR1*, which encodes the P-glycoprotein. While multiple SNPs resulting in single amino acid changes have been identified for *MDR1*, only one has been demonstrated to have a phenotypic effect. An SNP in exon 26 of the *MDR1* gene, C3435T, is correlated with both P-glycoprotein levels and substrate uptake. Individuals homozygous for the T allele have fourfold lower P-glycoprotein levels in their liver and intestine compared with C/C individuals. Clinical investigations have further demonstrated that the *MDR1* genotype is correlated with oral bioavailability and renal clearance of known substrates of P-glycoprotein, with T/T homozygotes, as expected, having higher bioavailability and decreased renal excretion [98,99]. Although the specific role of the *MDR1* C3435T polymorphism in the setting of high-dose chemotherapy is still under investigation, because many of the most commonly used anticancer agents are also substrates for P-glycoprotein, it is likely that *MDR1* genotype will affect both the pharmacokinetics and possibly the tumor cell pharmacodynamics of high-dose chemotherapy.

Drug metabolism, pharmacokinetics and pharmacodynamics of high-dose chemotherapy

Pharmacokinetic variability in high-dose chemotherapy

The basic pharmacokinetic features that ultimately affect systemic exposure to a drug include the processes of absorption, tissue distribution, metabolism and excretion. Although patient–patient pharmacokinetic variability is common for all of the chemotherapeutic agents in current oncologic practice, the extent of inter- and intrapatient pharmacokinetic variability is accentuated in the high-dose chemotherapy setting [100–104]. It has been reported that, as a result of interpatient differences in pharmacokinetics, the systemic clearances of many of the most commonly used cytotoxic drugs vary over three- to 10-fold [105]. The wide range in the rate of drug elimination results in a correspondingly large variation in total drug exposures (e.g. AUC and steady-state drug concentration [C_{ss}]) in patients treated with equivalent doses. For drugs with steep dose–response curves and narrow therapeutic windows, the implication of such significant pharmacokinetic variability is the unpredictable probability of either clinical response or toxicity. The degree of pharmacokinetic variability that is routinely observed during high-dose chemotherapy may be caused by pharmacogenetic variations in the population [106], by the metabolic pattern of the specific drug [107], by metabolic interactions amongst high-dose chemotherapeutic agents used in combination [108], by drug–drug interactions between the chemotherapeutic agents employed and other drugs required for symptom control or the treatment of associated infections [109,110], as well as by other physiologic or environmental factors [111–114].

Perhaps the most important aspect of the pharmacokinetic variability of high-dose chemotherapy is the recent demonstration that the metabolism of several of the most important agents is saturable, leading to potentially large, unpredictable and non-linear changes in systemic exposure with modest changes in drug dose within the high-dose chemotherapy range. As described later for CY (Fig. 12.3), there appears to be saturation of CY activation pathways when the agent is used at high dose [115]. While the clearances of high-dose doxorubicin (Fig. 12.4) and etoposide increase linearly with dose, high-dose paclitaxel (Fig. 12.5) exhibits dramatic deviations from linearity as drug dosage levels are escalated.

The implications of non-linear pharmacokinetics for agents employed in the high-dose chemotherapy setting are significant. Because the toxicities associated with high-dose chemotherapy are substantial, the margin for error (therapeutic ratio) is low. The inability to predict the pharmacokinetic behavior of a drug at high dose increases the potential risk of severe side-effects from that compound. Thus, the potential utility of therapeutic drug monitoring that will allow targeted systemic exposures in the high-dose chemotherapy setting is greatly enhanced for agents that demonstrate non-linear pharmacokinetics.

Pharmacodynamics of high-dose chemotherapy and the individualization of chemotherapeutic drug exposures

The prediction of toxicity or therapeutic outcome after high-dose chemotherapy based on pharmacokinetic parameters is in its infancy. The first evidence that modification of drug dosage based on the pharmacokinetic behavior of a chemotherapeutic agent in an individual undergoing high-dose chemotherapy could positively affect the toxicity of treatment was published in 1989. The incidence of hepatic veno-occlusive disease (VOD) after BU conditioning was demonstrated to be dramatically

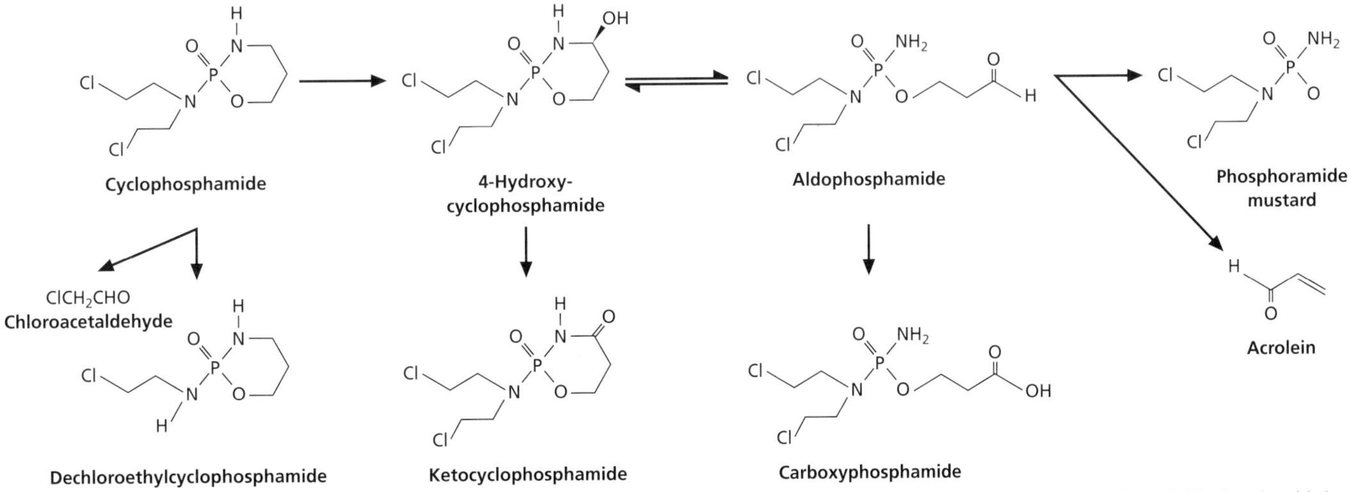

Fig. 12.3 Activation and detoxification pathway of cyclophosphamide (CY). The drug is activated to 4-hydroxycyclophosphamide (4-HC) and aldophosphamide by cytochrome P450 isoenzymes and to phosphoramide mustard by exonucleases. P450 isoenzymes appear to detoxify CY to the dechloroethyl derivative; aldehyde oxidase breaks down 4-HC to ketocyclophosphamide; and aldehyde dehydrogenases detoxify aldophosphamide [115].

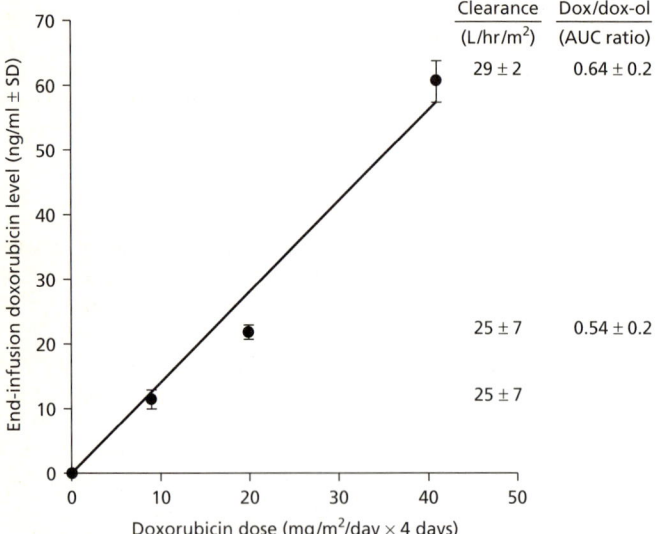

Fig. 12.4 End of infusion concentration of doxorubicin as a function of delivered dose following 96-h continuous intravenous drug dose. Linear pharmacokinetics, including linear conversion of doxorubicin to its major metabolite doxorubicinol, demonstrated for a 4.5-fold range of doxorubicin doses.

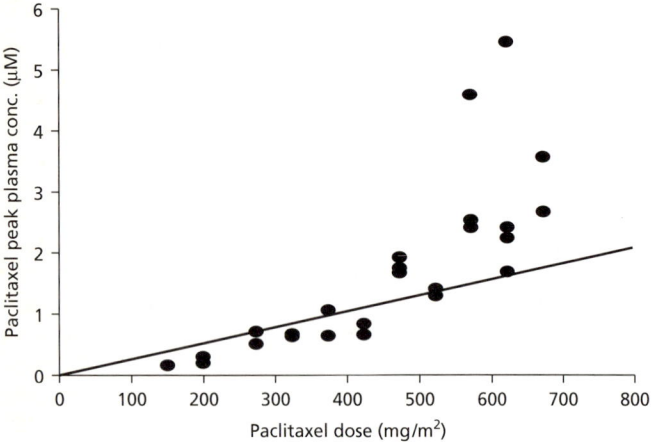

Fig. 12.5 Peak plasma concentration of paclitaxel during a 24-h continuous infusion as a function of paclitaxel dose. Non-linear pharmacokinetics of paclitaxel shown for doses greater than 450 mg/m^2.

decreased in patients undergoing allogeneic BMT by prospective monitoring of BU levels and modification of drug dosage based on a targeted "safe" AUC [116–118]. Since then, the pulmonary toxicity of breast cancer patients receiving high-dose BCNU, cisplatin and CY has been related to the AUC of BCNU [119,120], and the ototoxicity of patients treated with high-dose thiotepa, CY and carboplatin has been associated with the carboplatin AUC [121]. The application of more detailed therapeutic drug monitoring and adaptive control strategies in the high-dose chemotherapy setting may also allow the safer use of agents with saturable pharmacokinetics [122]. Ultimately, the demonstration that systemic exposure to one or more high-dose chemotherapy agents is correlated with therapeutic outcome, as has recently been shown for standard dose methotrexate in the treatment of childhood acute lymphoblastic leukemia [123], remains a critical goal for future high-dose chemotherapy trials.

The considerable time and effort spent determining the extent and causes of pharmacokinetic variability for each of the cytotoxic agents described in this chapter has been undertaken with the ultimate goal of developing predictive models for drug disposition that will allow the clinician to administer an optimal dose based on each individual's own physiologic, genetic or environmental profile. The fundamental approach to optimizing cytotoxic drug therapy in the past has been the assignment of dosage based on a measure of patient size, while more intensive methods have involved near real-time monitoring of circulating drug concentrations in individual patients with subsequent dosage adjustment to achieve a predefined target drug level. The relative merits of any approach aimed at optimizing exposure based solely on the pharmacokinetic behavior of a drug is subject to debate because of the added contributions of cellular drug disposition and pharmacodynamic effects to the variability of drug response. However, in light of the significant patient–patient differences in the measured concentrations of most cytotoxic agents used in high-dose chemotherapy, optimizing drug exposures based on all currently available information regarding potential sources of pharmacokinetic variability is an appropriate initial strategy.

Dosage adjustments based on body surface area

One of the earliest approaches to normalizing cytotoxic drug exposures was the use of body surface area (BSA) to correct for differences in individual patient size. This practice was based on the findings of Freireich et al. [124] who showed that the maximum tolerated doses of cytotoxic drugs in different animal species were most similar when scaled to surface area. During the initial stages of clinical drug development, BSA is used to guide dosage escalation to the point of defining the maximum tolerated dose. The recommended dosage of drugs that are developed in this way are ultimately assigned upon a BSA-based dosage algorithm. As a result, it has become common practice in clinical oncology to tailor anticancer drugs on the basis of a patient's BSA with the aim of reducing interindividual variability in drug exposure as a result of factors related to patient size.

The most commonly used formula to estimate BSA originates from 1916 [125], and was based on plaster of Paris models made of nine subjects ranging in weight from 25 to 90 kg. The surface area of the completed molds was calculated and a formula derived based upon the mathematical relationship between each subject's weight and height and their calculated surface area. Despite reports questioning the predictive performance of this formula [126,127], the original method of DuBois has been utilized in clinical oncologic practice for over 40 years [114]. However, during the last decade, the use of BSA-based regimens has been criticized and various alternative body-size measures have been proposed, such as lean body mass, which might be better predictors of drug clearance [128,129]. The growing skepticism of BSA as a tool to optimize drug regimens corresponds with an increased understanding of the magnitude of pharmacokinetic variability and its many sources. A relationship between BSA and physiologic measures relevant to drug elimination such as hepatic and renal function has never been demonstrated beyond the contribution of body weight alone [130,131]. Furthermore, for several cytotoxic drugs no relationship exists between the pharmacokinetic parameters of the drug and BSA [132].

That BSA cannot explain pharmacokinetic variability is not surprising because BSA varies over a fairly narrow range compared to the wider variations (three- to 10-fold) in drug clearance, volume of distribution and excretion observed for essentially all antineoplastic agents. It has recently been suggested that the practice of BSA-based regimens should be performed only for those agents where a significant relationship between BSA and drug clearance has been proven [132]. For all other cytotoxic drugs, it has been proposed that regimens be fixed or adjusted based on other more meaningful predictors of pharmacokinetics such as indices of renal or hepatic function. Perhaps the strongest rationale for abandoning BSA-based regimens is that, by eliminating the need for

BSA normalization, a significant source of dosage calculation errors could be eliminated without producing a significant impact on the probability of under- or overtreating patients based on differences in size, the net result of which might be increased patient safety [133]. Whether or not cytotoxic drug dosage based on BSA is abandoned, it is clear that better predictors of the pharmacokinetics of high-dose chemotherapy are required to optimize anticancer drug therapy.

Dosage based on indices of renal or hepatic function

In contrast to BSA, the pharmacokinetics of anticancer agents have frequently been associated with the functional indices of the major drug-clearing organs, the liver and kidneys. Depending on the major route of elimination for a particular drug, it can be reliably predicted that significant changes in either hepatic or renal function will result in corresponding changes in drug clearance. Carboplatin is associated with an increased risk of severe toxicity in patients with creatinine clearances of less than 60 mL/min because of decreased drug clearance and greater total drug exposure [134]. The rationale for reducing the dosage of cytotoxic drugs in the presence of hepatic impairment is also well documented for agents such as doxorubicin, vincristine, docetaxel and paclitaxel [135]. In the case of hepatic impairment, the guidelines for dosage adjustment are based on clinical measures of liver function such as bilirubin (e.g. doxorubicin and vincristine), aspartate aminotransferase AST (e.g. paclitaxel and docetaxel) or alkaline phosphatase (e.g. docetaxel).

The association between drug-clearing organ function and pharmacokinetics has also led to the development of cytotoxic drug regimens based on indices of renal and hepatic function in patients with organ function tests within the normal limits. The best current example of dose adjustment guidelines for a cytotoxic agent based on organ function is carboplatin. Calvert *et al.* [112] first demonstrated that carboplatin AUC could be accurately predicted using an equation that utilizes pretreatment renal function. This *a priori* method for carboplatin regimens has led to a substantial reduction in pharmacokinetic variability, such that carboplatin is currently one the few drugs of any class that is routinely given to achieve a target systemic exposure rather than on a mg/m^2 or mg/kg basis. Although the original method of carboplatin dosage adjustment relied on measurement of glomerular filtration rate (GFR) by determining ^{51}Cr-EDTA clearance, subsequent studies have shown that other measures of GFR can be substituted [136,137]. Therefore, the pharmacokinetics of carboplatin can be reliably predicted from routine clinical measurements leading to improved dosage regimens.

Routinely available clinical indices of hepatic function are less helpful in predicting cytotoxic drug metabolism than creatinine clearance in the case of kidney function. Liver function tests are not sufficiently sensitive to detect differences in drug-clearing capacity within the normal range of organ function, and are only correlated with drug clearance in the setting of clinically impaired hepatic function. As a result, the predictive value of any one clinical marker of liver function is usually limited with respect to the metabolism and transport of drugs. Composite scoring approaches based on multiple liver function tests, such as the Childs–Pugh classification [138], have been proposed as an alternative to single laboratory measures. However, as with individual liver function tests, such scoring systems have only demonstrated utility in patients with impaired hepatic function [139]. In addition, other standard clinical tests that measure the functional capacity of the liver, such as prothrombin time and albumin, are of limited value as predictors of drug clearance because of the lag time required for a change in the synthetic function of the liver to be reflected in an alteration in drug clearance.

To identify better surrogate markers of hepatic metabolic or extraction pathways, several investigators have examined the clearance of model substrates as predictors of cytotoxic drug elimination. Non-cytotoxic agents such as indocyanine green [140], lidocaine [141],
^{14}C-erythromycin [142], caffeine [143] and antipyrine [144] have been shown to correlate with the hepatic elimination of various drugs. The clearance of docetaxel can be predicted from the metabolism and renal excretion of cortisol [145]. Therefore, it may ultimately be possible to optimize the amount of cytotoxic agents that are cleared in the liver based on surrogate predictors of drug clearance.

Therapeutic drug level monitoring in high-dose chemotherapy

Therapeutic drug monitoring (TDM) has a long history of use in solid organ transplantation, as well as other areas of clinical practice. The widespread use of TDM is based on the principle of an optimal therapeutic window for the particular agent being monitored. TDM involves near real-time measurement of circulating drug levels followed by subsequent dose adjustment to achieve a predefined target drug exposure. In the case of antibiotics, the goal of TDM is to assure that the drug concentration is maintained above the minimum inhibitory concentration for the infective agent being targeted, while staying below the concentrations associated with normal organ toxicity.

The use of TDM in oncologic therapeutics, although promising, has been limited, in part because performing real-time pharmacokinetic monitoring of even a single cytotoxic agent requires dedicated laboratory personnel and resources typically available only at major medical centres. The first step in the process of developing TDM for high-dose chemotherapy is to demonstrate its value in a given clinical setting before subsequent work is done to make the process more practical. Once the role of individualization of a cytotoxic agent has been established, the use of limited pharmacokinetic sampling methods and automated assay techniques can be applied.

Recently, investigators evaluated the benefit of paclitaxel TDM in high-dose chemotherapy. Based on the initial observation of wide interpatient differences in paclitaxel exposure for patients enrolled on a phase 1 trial of high-dose chemotherapy with HC support for advanced solid tumors, Doroshow *et al.* [146] examined the feasibility of reducing pharmacokinetic variability by real-time measurement of plasma paclitaxel concentrations with subsequent adjustment of the infusion rate to achieve a target drug exposure. Starting at hour 48 of a 96-h infusion, paclitaxel doses were adjusted based on measured concentrations to achieve a targeted paclitaxel AUC equivalent to the mean AUC determined in a cohort of patients treated without dose adjustment. Using TDM, one-third of the patients required a dose increase to achieve the target, one-third required a dose decrease, while the remaining third required no change in dose. Furthermore, TDM significantly decreased the variability in paclitaxel AUC, as well as the variability in several measures of clinical outcome, including time to hematologic recovery, days of morphine-requiring mucositis and length of hospital stay.

Perhaps the most widely reported use of TDM in the area of high-dose chemotherapy is the practice of pharmacokinetic monitoring of BU in patients undergoing BMT. High-dose BU is an important component of many preparative regimens. The dose-limiting toxicity of high-dose BU is hepatic VOD, which occurs in approximately 20–40% of patients. BU is erratically absorbed after oral administration; at a given dose, there is considerable variability in its systemic exposure. Grochow *et al.* [117] first described the correlation between the AUC after the first dose of oral BU with the occurrence of VOD. Subsequently, several investigators confirmed the association between measured BU exposure and risk of VOD [147,148]. Generally, the risk of VOD has been shown to be increased with BU C_{ss} >900 µg/L and first-dose AUC >1500 µmol × min. In addition, lower rates of relapse in chronic myeloid leukemia (CML) have been reported to occur in patients with higher BU exposures without an increased risk of toxicity [149]. Furthermore, measured BU exposure has been reported to be related to the rate of engraftment in children [150,151]. Therefore, it is now widely accepted that an optimal therapeutic window exists for BU, leading many investigators to advocate the use of BU TDM to maximize the likelihood of engraftment and minimize the risk of toxicity and relapse in patients receiving the BU/CY preparative regimen.

However, for each conditioning regimen that includes BU, as well as for each of the many different diseases for which BMT is a therapeutic option, the therapeutic window for BU is likely to be different. Therefore, more data are needed to define the optimal use of BU in each specific clinical situation. Complicating the issue of BU TDM is the recent availability of an intravenous BU formulation that has led to a significant decrease in the incidence of VOD in the absence of TDM [152]. The intravenous route of BU administration avoids the hepatic first-pass effect, thereby decreasing the high local drug concentrations achieved in hepatic sinusoids with oral regimens. Furthermore, the pharmacokinetic profile of BU is greatly improved by intravenous administration with respect to decreased inter- and intrapatient variability [153]. It is possible that the use of intravenous BU may ultimately obviate the need for TDM if it can be established that the therapeutic window is sufficiently large to allow for a fixed dose of drug that will be within the optimal range of systemic exposure for all patients.

Despite the remaining questions regarding the utility of BU TDM, and because of the apparent success of BU TDM to date, a number of limited sampling approaches have been developed to simplify the procedures associated with drug level monitoring [154–156]. Growing evidence for an optimal therapeutic window, along with significant interpatient pharmacokinetic variability, has made BU TDM the standard of practice in many BMT centers with access to analytical laboratories and clinical pharmacology resources. The challenge for further optimizing the use of high-dose BU will be to better define the therapeutic range in each particular clinical setting and to simplify the actual procedures for drug level monitoring.

Therapeutic drug selection and drug development in the high-dose chemotherapy setting

Drug selection in the high-dose chemotherapy setting

Studies of new dose-escalation regimens supported by HCs, as described previously, are frequently based on concentration–response relationships developed *in vitro*. While such studies may provide important new leads, it is remarkable how frequently investigators appear to utilize such data to the exclusion of the single most important criterion of drug selection in the high-dose chemotherapy setting—the degree of activity of the agent to be escalated for the disease in question. Clinical evidence of therapeutic activity for the drug at standard dose against the disease to be treated in the high-dose chemotherapy setting should be the minimum starting point for the development of a high-dose chemotherapy program. Unfortunately, abundant evidence is available demonstrating that this first principle is frequently ignored. One example is the use of high-dose mitoxantrone for breast cancer. Despite excellent clinical data indicating that a dose–response relationship does not clearly exist for mitoxantrone in the treatment of this disease [157], it has frequently been included in high-dose chemotherapy programs because of its modest extramedullary toxicity profile [158,159].

The other important criteria that should be used for the development of high-dose chemotherapy programs include the absence of non-additive extramedullary toxicities when the agents are used in combination (such as VOD), which can dramatically decrease the safe level of dose escalation; the presence of divergent mechanisms of cytotoxicity and lack of cross-resistance for the agents being combined; and the extent of dose escalation possible for each drug in the combination with HC support. None of these individual criteria, however, is more important than optimizing the use of the most therapeutically active chemotherapeutic agents.

Conduct of drug development trials in high-dose chemotherapy

The conduct of phase 1 trials in high-dose chemotherapy is a substantial investigational challenge [160]. Although the selection of drug combinations and doses for high-dose chemotherapy has often been based on many of the same dose-escalation principles used in studies performed at standard levels of dose intensity and without HC support, the modality of allogeneic transplantation itself is associated with specific morbidities that may confound attempts to attribute adverse events to the drug being escalated. Thus, the presence of underlying graft-vs.-host disease (GVHD) and multiorgan compromise from infection can make the attribution of toxicity extraordinarily difficult. In both the allogeneic and autologous transplant setting, the tendency in the past has been to avoid formal, complete dose-escalation schemas for all of the drugs that comprise a specific combination, which leads to uncertainty about whether or not a particular regimen utilizes all of the agents at their maximally tolerated dose.

One important aspect of the development of high-dose chemotherapy programs that is seldom considered is the remarkable lack of single agent data conclusively demonstrating that a clinical dose–response actually exists for a particular agent in a specific disease. Close inspection of the data on the dose-intensive treatment of advanced breast cancer would indicate that only for the anthracyclines and perhaps CY does a definitive dose–response relationship clearly exist at the level of single-agent trials [161]. Thus, there is a critical need to examine the clinical dose–response curve of important new therapeutic agents, such as the taxanes, in the diseases that may benefit from high-dose chemotherapy.

The success of high-dose systemic therapies is also clearly linked to a number of factors specific to the host that bears the tumor including nutritional status, functional capabilities and integrity of major organ systems. The effect of these factors on the development of new high-dose chemotherapy programs cannot be overstated. Accurate assessment of organ system reserve prior to entry on novel high-dose chemotherapy treatment regimens is of fundamental importance, because the recognition of novel and potentially life-threatening side-effects produced by new high-dose chemotherapy combinations is a common event. Patients with dysfunction of an organ that is necessary for the metabolism or excretion of a high-dose cytotoxic are so likely to suffer untoward toxicity that they should not participate in early phase 1 high-dose chemotherapy trials. An outline of a recently proposed set of guidelines for the development of new high-dose chemotherapy trials is provided in Table 12.3 (adapted from [160]).

Clinical pharmacology of drugs utilized for high-dose chemotherapy and hematopoietic cell transplantation: pharmacokinetic, pharmacodynamic and mechanistic considerations

Alkylating agents

The first chemotherapeutic agents to be utilized as preparatory regimens for BMT were the alkylating agents, a large group of drugs with the ability to covalently bind DNA and other biologically significant molecules through an alkyl group consisting of one or more saturated carbon atoms [162–164]. The common feature of these compounds is that they are composed of mono- or bifunctional alkyl groups linked to a core structure that confers pharmacologic and toxicologic differences on the alkylating moieties. The simplest backbone for a bifunctional alkylating agent is that of nitrogen mustard (HN_2, mechlorethamine), which consists of a nitrogen atom (as NCH_3) linked to two chloroethyl groups. As shown in Fig. 12.1, by contrast, L-phenylalanine mustard (melphalan) consists of the same bifunctional alkylating groups attached to the L-phenylalanine

Table 12.3 Guidelines for the development of new high-dose chemotherapy trials. (Adapted from Margolin *et al.* [160].)

---

1 Preclinical and clinical support required for the selection of drugs to dose-escalate:
  • Select agents with steep dose–response curves for the tumor of interest
  • Preference for drugs with myelosuppressive dose-limiting toxicities
2 Pharmacologic basis for the dose, schedule and combination of drugs chosen:
  • Existing database supporting schedule of administration
  • Additive or synergistic antitumor activity with other agents in regimen; minimization of overlapping toxicities
  • Pharmacokinetic methodologies exist to measure plasma or serum levels of all agents employed in regimen
3 Toxicity grading scale, definition of maximally tolerated dose and assessment of late toxicities:
  • Select a scale validated for use in high-dose chemotherapy and employ it precisely to define parameters for dose escalation and for the determination of dose-limiting toxicities
  • Distinguish modality-related adverse events from dose- or exposure-related toxicities in determining the maximally tolerated dose in any new regimen
  • Provide specific guidelines for the evaluation of dose escalation in tandem cycle high-dose regimens
  • Assess late-occurring adverse effects (such as secondary leukemia) as well as persistent toxicities (peripheral neuropathy or pulmonary fibrosis)
4 Statistical considerations:
  • Select a design for dose levels and escalation procedures that will adequately characterize the dose-toxicity relationship and include pharmacologic correlates; this may require the accrual of more than the standard 3–6 patients per cohort
  • Apply the statistical plan throughout the study, avoiding exploratory or hypothesis-generating late analyses

---

molecule; CY and ifosfamide are two other clinically useful alkylating agents that have substituted other side chains for the methyl group in HN_2. The common mechanistic feature of the alkylating agents is that, upon entering cells, the alkyl groups bind to electrophilic sites in DNA and other biologically active molecules; bifunctional alkylation of DNA can result in crosslinks between strands of DNA, which impedes replication. Other biochemically important molecules are also alkylated by such agents, but the dominant effect appears to be DNA crosslinking.

Cyclophosphamide

Cyclophosphamide is a member of the oxazaphosphorine group of nitrogen mustard derivatives and is the most widely used alkylating agent in BMT preparatory regimens based, in part, on its broad range of antineoplastic activity as well as its immunomodulatory properties [165]. CY has significant activity against both Hodgkin's and non-Hodgkin's lymphoma; acute and chronic leukemia; breast, lung and ovarian cancer, and a variety of childhood solid tumors. With HC support, it can be escalated eight- to 10-fold from standard intermittent intravenous doses of 600–1000 mg/m^2 to 4000–7000 mg/m^2 when used in combination high-dose chemotherapy programs [14,166]. High-dose CY is frequently used in combination with thiotepa and carboplatin for the high-dose treatment of high-risk primary breast cancer [167], with BU as a preparatory regimen for patients with acute or chronic myelogenous leukemia (CML) [168], and with high-dose etoposide and TBI for patients with non-Hodgkin's lymphoma [169].

Mechanism of action

As described in detail in following sections, CY is a prodrug that must be activated by the hepatic cytochrome P450 system to cytotoxic alkylating intermediates (see Fig. 12.3). The presumed cytotoxic species, phosphoramide mustard, produces inter- and intrastrand DNA crosslinks that are lethal, and which can induce apoptosis [170,171].

While little is known about the cellular pharmacology of CY and its active metabolites, a great deal is understood regarding cellular resistance mechanisms for this agent. The most clearly delineated pathway of CY resistance is the development of increased intracellular pools of reduced non-protein sulfhydryls, including the tripeptide glutathione (GSH) [172]; alterations in intracellular GSH levels can significantly affect the level of phosphoramide mustard-induced DNA crosslinking [173]. Conjugation reactions between GSH, glutathione *S*-transferases (GSTs) and phosphoramide mustard provide an enzymatically enhanced detoxification pathway for CY degradation, decreasing tumor cell sensitivity [174]. In addition to GSH transferases, increased intracellular levels of aldehyde dehydrogenases (particularly the 1A1 isoform), which convert aldophosphamide to the inactive carboxyphosphamide derivative (see Fig. 12.3), lead to CY resistance [175,176]. Finally, it seems reasonable to conclude that overexpression of certain DNA repair genes capable of rendering tumor cells resistant to other nitrogen mustard derivatives is also likely to contribute to the clinical spectrum of tumor cell insensitivity to CY [177].

Metabolism, pharmacokinetics and pharmacodynamics

The complex metabolism of CY is shown in Fig. 12.3; although the pharmacokinetics of the drug have been studied by several laboratories in the high-dose chemotherapy setting [178,179], recent evidence utilizing sophisticated analytical techniques has changed the interpretation of the CY metabolic pathway [115,180]. The initial bioactivation of CY is produced by hepatic microsomal P450-dependent hydroxylation to produce 4-hydroxycyclophosphamide (4-HC), which is in equilibrium with the ring-opened aldehyde, aldophosphamide. 4-HC or aldophosphamide, or both, can be detoxified by aldehyde oxidase or aldehyde dehydrogenase, respectively, to produce the inactive metabolites ketocyclophosphamide and carboxyphosphamide, which are excreted in the urine together with the parent compound and account for the majority of a delivered dose of CY. Aldophosphamide that is not detoxified enters tumor cells and, through the process of β-elimination, produces the active alkylating species phosphoramide mustard and acrolein, the toxic species responsible for CY-induced cystitis.

Because of the multilayered metabolism of CY, it has been difficult to assign pharmacodynamic correlations for this drug. However, the incidence of CY-related cardiac toxicity after high-dose therapy has been associated with lower parental drug AUC and, presumably, increased activation to potentially toxic intermediates [181]. The effect of high-dose drug administration on the metabolism of CY has recently been extensively studied by two groups using improved analytical techniques [115,180,182,183]. It appears that while the overall pharmacokinetics of parental CY are similar over an eightfold range of drug concentration, there is substantial evidence that CY activation is saturated at a dose of 100 mg/kg. Increased renal clearance of the parent drug, and of the inactive carboxyphosphamide metabolite, parallel a decrease in the clearance of bioactivated species in the high-dose setting. These results bring into question the use of doses above 100 mg/kg which may only enhance toxicity, particularly cardiac toxicity, without improving exposure of the tumor to cytotoxic alkylating species [184]. Furthermore, it appears that with these more sensitive techniques, important drug–drug interactions between CY and thiotepa (which appears to inhibit CY metabolism), BU or phenytoin [108,185] (which may increase CY clearance), and TBI

[186] (which has no effect on the bioactivation of CY) can be defined for the first time.

The pharmacokinetics of unchanged CY in the plasma reveal considerable interpatient variability with a terminal half-life of 3–9 h; however, the usefulness of monitoring the disappearance of the parental drug is unclear based on the saturable nature of the bioactivation pathways of CY at high dose. Approximately 10% of the parental drug is excreted unchanged in the urine; recently, it has been reported that the unchanged parental molecule can be sufficiently cleared by hemodialysis to allow the use of high-dose CY in patients with end-stage renal disease [187]. In addition to the drugs described above, other authors have found that inducers of microsomal metabolism, such as phenobarbital or dexamethasone, can enhance CY clearance. However, CY dosage does not require alteration in the face of hepatic dysfunction.

The major dose-limiting toxicity of high-dose CY is cardiac injury, which occurs much more frequently at doses above 150 mg/kg [184,188]. Endothelial damage has been associated with myocardial necrosis and the development of potentially lethal congestive heart failure. The etiology of CY cardiac toxicity appears to be related to severe depletion of cardiac reduced thiol stores [172,189]. In addition, high-dose CY therapy has been associated with severe hemorrhagic cystitis; however, forced diuresis or coadministration, or both, of the thiol sodium-2-mercaptoethane sulfonate (mesna) has markedly decreased the incidence of this toxicity of acrolein. Pulmonary toxicity and VOD also occur more frequently in combination high-dose chemotherapy regimens that utilize CY. Finally, renal tubular injury may mimic the clinical picture of inappropriate antidiuretic hormone secretion [190].

Melphalan

The development of the bifunctional alkylating agent melphalan (MEL) dates to its synthesis in 1953; that synthetic effort was based on the hypothesis that substitution of phenylalanine for the methyl group of nitrogen mustard would produce an agent selectively concentrated by melanoma cells, because those cells utilize phenylalanine in several metabolic pathways [191]. MEL is actively transported into tumor cells but not specifically into melanomas; however, its activity in the treatment of multiple myeloma, neuroblastoma and breast cancer has led to the use of the drug in the high-dose chemotherapy setting [192]. The availability of an intravenous formulation in the USA in 1992 spurred the development of high-dose regimens utilizing MEL [193]. In comparison with the standard chemotherapy setting, the use of hematopoietic cell support allows the administration of MEL as a single agent in doses of 180–200 mg/m^2, approximately sixfold higher than the standard dose range [192].

Mechanism of action

As an analog of nitrogen mustard, MEL hydrolyzes intracellularly, and produces interstrand and intrastrand crosslinking of DNA by way of its two chloroethyl groups, which spontaneously lose chloride ions to form reactive intermediates [194]. While a variety of different alkylation sites exist on DNA, it remains difficult to discern which of the various base oxygens or amino groups is the critical site underlying the cytotoxic properties of MEL. However, it is clear that DNA interstrand crosslinks correlate more closely with tumor cell killing than DNA-protein crosslinking [194,195]. The cytotoxicity of melphalan *in vitro* can be correlated with total drug exposure (concentration × time); furthermore, the extent of cytotoxic DNA crosslinking increases with time, suggesting that critical bifunctional adducts develop from much more numerous monofunctional lesions [196]. The production of DNA adducts by MEL activates the poly adenosine diphosphate (ADP)-ribose polymerase system in the nucleus and may contribute to tumor cell killing through the depletion of intracellular pools of nicotinamide adenine dinucleotide [197,198].

Melphalan is transported into tumor cells by two different energy-dependent drug carriers [199–203]. A high-affinity L-amino acid transport system, which also carries leucine and glutamine, is augmented by a second less efficient transporter at low MEL concentrations. *In vitro*, and potentially *in vivo*, high concentrations of leucine can protect cells from the cytotoxic effect of MEL by decreasing drug uptake in a competitive manner [204]; on the other hand, enhanced tumor tissue uptake of MEL occurs in experimental systems *in vivo* during exposure to an amino acid-lowering diet [205].

Resistance to melphalan may occur along general lines common for the alkylating agents, which include increased intracellular thiol content [32,206,207], increased detoxification by way of the glutathione S-transferase system [208,209] and enhanced DNA repair [210]. However, because of the specific transport pathways that exist for MEL, altered drug-carrier proteins are also capable of producing significant degrees of resistance *in vivo* [211]. A specific mutation has been described in L1210 murine leukemia cells which results in lower affinity of the high-velocity transporter for melphalan with associated high level drug resistance [212].

Metabolism, pharmacokinetics and pharmacodynamics

Melphalan undergoes rapid hydrolysis in plasma to its inactive mono- and dihydroxy derivatives; it is also extensively (90%) protein-bound [213]. Of the delivered dose of MEL, 5–13% is excreted in the urine [214,215]. The penetration of MEL into tumor tissue demonstrates significant variability consistent with variations in perfusion [18].

Despite the development of the intravenous formulation, which is used for high-dose chemotherapy with MEL, inter- and intrapatient pharmacokinetic variability is substantial [101], often in excess of 10-fold with respect to systemic exposure [216]. MEL distribution follows a biexponential decay with a short distribution phase, $t_{1/2\alpha}$ 5–15 min, and subsequent $t_{1/2\beta}$ 30–120 min [217,218]. There does not appear to be any difference in the clearance of MEL in children compared to adults [219]. Because of the short β phase of elimination, marrow or PBHC reinfusion following high-dose MEL can occur safely within 12–24 h following drug treatment. The pharmacokinetics of MEL are linear over a very wide dose range [217,220]. This fact has allowed the use of a small test dose of MEL for the adaptive control of MEL exposure in individual patients. In this fashion it has been possible to predict MEL clearance prior to high-dose treatment, and to then choose a dose that produces a target AUC level with less than 15% deviation from the desired systemic exposure. Ongoing studies will determine whether adaptive control of high-dose MEL will prove essential from a pharmacodynamic perspective.

Because of the limited renal excretion of MEL, high-dose therapy has been attempted in patients with multiple myeloma and significantly compromised kidney function (creatinine clearance less than 40 mL/min); no evidence of alterations in half-life or AUC were demonstrated, although the performance status of such patients may enhance their toxicity profile [216]. The lack of any major effect of renal dysfunction on the clearance of high-dose MEL has been confirmed [221].

The dose-limiting toxicities of high-dose MEL are mucositis and VOD [192]. Gastrointestinal muscosal injury both limits the escalation of drug dose above 200 mg/m^2 as a single agent and its use at doses above 140 mg/m^2 with other agents that produce severe gastrointestinal tract toxicity. VOD has been observed especially when high-dose MEL has been combined with other high-dose alkylating agents [222]. High-dose MEL, like other alkylating agents, can produce diffuse pulmonary alveolitis [223,224]; it also can stimulate inappropriate antidiuretic hormone secretion in the high-dose chemotherapy setting [225].

The major current role of high-dose MEL therapy is in the treatment of multiple myeloma [216] and neuroblastoma [226]. Its role in combination high-dose chemotherapy programs for ovarian [227–229] or breast cancer [222,230,231] or other hematopoietic malignancies [232] is currently being defined.

Thiotepa

The role of thiotepa in high-dose chemotherapy has principally been as part of combination regimens with other alkylating agents used for patients with high-risk primary and responsive metastatic breast cancer [23,167,233,234] or for the high-dose therapy of hematopoietic malignancies [235]. The usual dose of thiotepa as part of such treatment programs is 500–800 mg/m^2, which is an 8–12-fold increase over standard dose levels.

Mechanism of action

Thiotepa (N,N′,N″-triethylenethiophosphoramide) was developed as an aziridine analog of nitrogen mustard (Cl-CH$_2$CH$_2$N[CH$_3$]CH$_2$CH$_2$-Cl) because the loss of chlorine in the decomposition reaction of nitrogen mustard leads to the formation of a reactive cyclic aziridinium intermediate which produces the initial alkylation product. Alkylation by thiotepa, producing interstrand crosslinking in DNA, occurs after opening of the aziridine rings. While it seems clear that DNA crosslinks play a critical part in the cytotoxicity of thiotepa (or the parent drug's immediate breakdown product), and that tumor cell killing is enhanced in an aerobic rather than an hypoxic environment [236], issues remain regarding the role of crosslinks vs. the production of alkali-labile sites as cytotoxic features of tepa, its major metabolite [237]. Tepa is less cytotoxic and less stable chemically than the parent molecule as well as being extensively protein-bound [238,239].

The cellular pharmacology of thiotepa, which is highly lipid soluble, is characterized by an initial rapid diffusion-mediated uptake into tumor cells [240–242] followed by irreversible binding to intracellular macromolecules. A secondary, much slower, but linear energy-dependent increase in intracellular thiotepa concentration reflects the balance between uptake and binding of a non-exchangeable pool of drug; cells lacking nuclei demonstrate a significantly reduced non-diffusion-mediated drug accumulation rate.

Tumor cell resistance to thiotepa, where it has been investigated, appears to follow typical patterns of alkylating agent resistance. Alterations in intracellular thiol (glutathione) pools and, in particular, the GST detoxification system may play an important part in the intracellular deactivation of thiotepa [86]. Thiotepa reacts directly with glutathione at neutral pH; however, the reaction to form monoglutathionyl thiotepa is significantly increased by both GST α and π but not GST μ. Tepa also reacts readily with GST α and π, suggesting that the aziridine moieties of these molecules are the functional substrates. Because increased GST isoenzyme expression has been demonstrated previously to play an important part in the development of resistance to other alkylating agents that are GST substrates [243–245], it is likely that GST-mediated detoxification could contribute to the insensitivity of malignant cells to thiotepa. Recent experiments have also demonstrated that overexpression of a member of the glycosylase family of DNA repair proteins (formamidopyrimidine-DNA glycosylase) is specifically capable of removing the aziridine alkylation products of thiotepa in DNA (N7-aminoethyl guanine and aminoethyl adenine); repair of these lesions produces resistance to both the cytotoxic and mutagenic effects of thiotepa. In addition to providing a potential resistance mechanism, these studies suggest that ring-opened guanines contribute to the mechanism of action of the drug [246]. Other base excision repair gene products may also contribute to thiotepa resistance [247].

Metabolism, pharmacokinetics and pharmacodynamics

Thiotepa is extensively metabolized in the liver [248–250]; it is oxidatively desulfurated to tepa (triethylenephosphoramide) by the hepatic microsomal P450 system, in particular by CYP2B1, the major phenobarbital-inducible P450, CYP2C11, a male-specific constitutive isoenzyme, as well as by CYP3A4 and, to a minor extent, CYP2B6 [251]. In murine species, phenobarbital pretreatment can block tumor growth delay after thiotepa treatment, consistent with increased conversion to the less cytotoxic tepa. The elimination of thiotepa occurs both by microsomal metabolism and tissue alkylation [252]. Recent experiments have demonstrated that thiotepa is a specific and potent inhibitor of CYP2B6, the P450 isoform that has an important role in the 4-hydroxylation of CY [253]. This observation is of real significance because recent clinical studies have shown that 4-HC levels are significantly diminished soon after the initiation of a thiotepa infusion if thiotepa and CY are administered concurrently [254]. Alterations in the activation of CY produced by thiotepa could substantially diminish the therapeutic benefit of high-dose CY, suggesting that thiotepa should be delivered after the completion of any CY infusion. On the other hand, no clinically important effects on thiotepa metabolism have been demonstrated for CY or carboplatin [255].

The pharmacokinetics of high-dose thiotepa have been studied in detail [256–262]. The drug is cleared following a biexponential decay pattern with $t_{1/2\alpha}$ 10 min and $t_{1/2\beta}$ 60–200 min. The apparent terminal elimination of tepa is in excess of 8 h; however, because of the extensive protein binding of tepa, the importance of this prolonged elimination is unclear. It also remains uncertain whether tepa clearance is saturable. In children, thiotepa does not appear to present the problem of non-linear pharmacokinetics; however, this observation has been reported by some laboratories in the adult population, but not others [257]. Both thiotepa and tepa have been detected in the urine after high-dose therapy; in the 48 h following drug administration, approximately 10% of the administered dose was quantified in urine as tepa or thiotepa mercapturic acid derivatives, and less than 1% as parent drug [263]. Although a potential method for the adaptive control of thiotepa dosage has been proposed, it has not yet been reduced to clinical practice [264].

The two major dose-limiting toxicities of high-dose thiotepa are in the central nervous system (CNS) and the gastrointestinal tract [265]. High-dose thiotepa (≥900 mg/m^2) as a single agent can produce somnolence, coma and confusion. At single-agent doses over 720 mg/m^2, severe oral and esophageal mucositis as well as enterocolitis become significant problems. Other important side-effects include transient elevations of hepatic enzymes (related to the total systemic exposure of thiotepa and tepa, which may contribute to the development of VOD when thiotepa is used in combination with other high-dose alkylating agents), an acute erythroderma associated with maculopapular dissemination and desquamation, interstitial pneumonitis and cardiac toxicity [239,266–268]. These side-effects are relatively specific for the high-dose setting and must be considered in the development of combination high-dose regimens, in particular with drugs that have the potential to produce overlapping extramedullary toxicities. Combinations in addition to STAMP V (thiotepa, carboplatin and CY) and thiotepa and CY that have been reported to date include thiotepa and MEL [269]; thiotepa, etoposide and carboplatin [270]; thiotepa, cisplatin and CY [271]; thiotepa, MEL and CY [101]; thiotepa, topotecan and carboplatin [272]; and thiotepa, mitoxantrone and etoposide [158].

Busulfan

Busulfan (BU), which is one of the alkylating agents in longest use, plays an important part as a myeloablative agent in combination preparative regimens for patients with hematopoietic malignancies undergoing allogeneic or autologous BMT, where the dose employed (16 mg/kg) is eight- to ninefold higher than standard dose levels [118,273].

Mechanism of action

Busulfan is an alkyl alkane sulfonate (see Fig. 12.1); unlike nitrogen mustard, the alkylation pattern of BU involves a bimolecular displacement reaction rather than the initial formation of a reactive intermediate, and is thus less rapid. This difference in reaction sequence does not, however, explain the profound effect of BU on myeloid precursors as well as CML and certain myeloproliferative disorders compared to other alkylating agents [274,275]. BU clearly produces DNA-protein crosslinks which may play a part in its mechanism of cytotoxicity; in some tumor cell models, DNA-protein crosslinking is much more prominent than DNA interstrand crosslink formation [276]. The drug is also profoundly mutagenic and can produce a wide range of chromosomal aberrations [277].

Busulfan can be conjugated with glutathione by GST α to a much greater extent than by the μ or π isoenzymes; overexpression of the α isoform may contribute to BU resistance both *in vitro* and *in vivo* [85]. Alterations in the repair of DNA crosslinks have also been associated with BU resistance, as might be expected from a member of the alkylator class [278]. Finally, BU resistance in human tumor cell xenografts has also been associated with alterations in drug transport [279].

Metabolism, pharmacokinetics and pharmacodynamics

Busulfan is highly lipophilic and demonstrates minimal protein binding; the parent molecule is eliminated principally by the liver and through tissue alkylation with less than 5% of an administered dose excreted unchanged in the urine [280]. The tissue distribution of BU has been studied in primates where drug levels are highest in liver; BU crosses the blood–brain barrier and reaches the substance of the brain at levels approximately 11% of those in the liver [281,282]. Although only a minor portion of BU is excreted into the urine, BU can be cleared in part by hemodialysis; however, multiple dialysis procedures are required to diminish systemic exposure to the drug [283].

The elimination half-life of BU in adults ranges from 1 to 7 h (mean 3 h); peak plasma levels are found after oral doses in 1–3 h [116]. Over the typical 4-day course of oral administration, however, steady state concentrations after the last dose are significantly lower than those predicted from the AUC measurements following the first dose, suggesting that BU induces its own metabolism [280]. In children [284,285], the mean elimination half-life is 2 h or less and no significant change in clearance has been demonstrated from first to last dose. Differences in the pharmacokinetics of BU in children undergoing high-dose chemotherapy compared to adults consistently include lower peak drug levels, faster elimination and clearance, and a larger apparent volume of distribution [286–288]. Wide inter- and intrapatient variability in BU disposition after oral administration has been observed in both adults and children [102,103], caused in part by age, altered hepatic function, drug interactions, circadian rhythmicity and bioavailability [109,153,289–292]. In adults, oral bioavailability varies over a twofold range; the degree of variation is up to sixfold in children. Furthermore, the acute emetic events that may occur during oral BU regimens further complicate the use of the oral route of administration [152].

Over the past decade, the importance of BU pharmacodynamics has been increasingly recognized [116,117,148,284,293]. The dose-limiting toxicity of BU in the setting of high-dose chemotherapy with HC support for the treatment of hematologic malignancies is VOD of the liver [117]. Multivariate analysis of patients in whom VOD was diagnosed demonstrated that BU AUC correlated strongly with the development of this serious complication of treatment; furthermore, adaptive control of BU regimens based on the plasma AUC of the drug after the initial dose(s) to produce a target AUC level significantly reduced the incidence of VOD. Therapeutic drug monitoring of BU in the high-dose chemotherapy setting is now a standard part of treatment [168,294], even though the etiology of VOD is complex and is likely to involve factors in addition to BU AUC [118,289]. The recent availability of intravenous BU formulations has improved the therapeutic index of the drug in HC-supported high-dose therapy [295]. In part, this improvement is due to a reduction in BU exposure to the cells of the hepatic sinusoids that are the target of BU hepatic toxicity, decreasing the incidence of VOD. However, intravenous BU administration does not eliminate the potential for significant interpatient pharmacokinetic variability. New approaches to therapeutic drug monitoring of intravenous BU utilizing limited sampling strategies promise to rationalize BU pharmacodynamics, diminishing variations in BU systemic exposure, and toxicity, even further [152,154]. Finally, in addition to the toxicologic implications of BU pharmacokinetics, BU concentration in plasma may also be an important determinant of graft survival [296,297] and the development of GVHD [298].

In addition to VOD, the dose-limiting toxicities of high-dose BU include neurotoxicity characterized by seizures, mucositis, the potential for radiation recall phenomenon, and pulmonary fibrosis. The gonadal toxicity of high-dose BU, furthermore, is extensive; essentially no return of ovarian function can be expected following typical high-dose BU/CY conditioning.

Drug–drug interactions involving BU include the observation that the antifungal agent itraconazole can decrease the clearance of BU by up to 20%, probably through hepatic microsomal cytochrome P450-mediated interactions [110]; in similar fashion, patients treated with diphenylhydantoin to prevent CNS toxicity from high-dose BU have significantly lower BU AUCs and shorter elimination half-lives. Diazepam, used for the same purpose, does not alter BU disposition [109]. Finally, administration of high-dose BU prior to high-dose CY significantly enhances the conversion of CY to 4-HC; this interaction is especially important in light of the frequency with which BU and CY are combined as conditioning agents prior to hematopoietic cell transplantation (HCT); it provides a further level of understanding for the degree of interpatient variability in the pharmacokinetics of both drugs in the high-dose chemotherapy setting [108]. Recent studies suggest that if CY administration is delayed until at least 24 h after BU, at least some of the metabolic interactions between the two drugs may be eliminated [299].

BCNU

BCNU (*bis*-chloroethyl-nitrosourea; carmustine) is a lipophilic bifunctional alkylating agent linked to a nitrosourea moiety. It was originally developed in the early 1960s because of its ability to cross the blood–brain barrier in murine species. BCNU remains in active use for the treatment of primary CNS malignancies at standard doses of 200 mg/m^2, which can be increased to 600 mg/m^2 when the drug is used in combination with high-dose CY and cisplatin and HC support for patients with high-risk primary or responsive metastatic breast cancer [14].

Mechanism of action

BCNU undergoes spontaneous hydrolysis at physiologic pH in plasma or intravenous solutions and thus must be utilized quickly after mixing. This spontaneous decomposition leads to the formation of the chloroethyl carbonium ion that is capable of alkylating macromolecules [13]. Bifunctional stepwise alkylation of DNA produces inter- and intrastrand DNA crosslinks as well as less cytotoxic DNA-protein crosslinks [300]. Breakdown products of BCNU produce isocyanates which bind sulfhydryl and amino groups on proteins inhibiting such enzymes as glutathione reductase and DNA ligase. The lipophilicity of BCNU allows it to enter tumor cells by passive diffusion.

Resistance to BCNU follows several of the known pathways for alkylating agents; in particular, enhanced intracellular thiol levels [301] and glutathione transferase activity [174] have been associated with BCNU resistance. However, most recent efforts to modulate tumor cell resistance to BCNU has focused on the mammalian enzyme O^6-alkylguanine-DNA alkyltransferase, which is the specific DNA repair protein that removes alkylated guanines produced by BCNU in DNA [302–304]. A specific inhibitor of this enzyme, O^6-benzyl guanine, has now become available for clinical testing; *in vitro* and in murine models it has been demonstrated to markedly enhance the cytotoxicity of BCNU [305].

Metabolism, pharmacokinetics and pharmacodynamics

In addition to spontaneous decomposition, BCNU may undergo denitrosation by hepatic microsomes, probably by glutathione transferases [174]. Phenobarbital-induced microsomes decrease the therapeutic effect of the nitrosoureas and increase drug clearance. BCNU undergoes a biexponential decay with $t_{1/2\alpha}$ 5–10 min and $t_{1/2\beta}$ 10–30 min; it is highly (more than 75%) protein-bound [306]. Significant interpatient variability in BCNU clearance has been observed. Approximately 80% of the administered dose is excreted in the urine as metabolites.

Both CY and cisplatin, the two drugs with which BCNU is most frequently combined in the high-dose chemotherapy setting, increase the AUC and the pharmacokinetic variability of BCNU in model systems [307]. This pharmacokinetic variability may help to explain the pulmonary toxicity of the CY, cisplatin and BCNU high-dose regimen that has been correlated in the clinic with the AUC of BCNU [119]. This potentially severe pulmonary toxicity, which may be related to the depletion of pulmonary GSH levels, frequently requires corticosteroid management and may be fatal [308–310]. In addition to pulmonary toxicity, high-dose BCNU therapy has been associated with an increased risk of VOD [311], hypotension and myocardial ischemia [312,313], delayed renal toxicity after cumulative doses above 1200 mg/m^2 [13] and, rarely, encephalopathy.

Platinating agents

Cisplatin

The serendipitous finding that platinum salts, produced by the effect of an electric current passed through a platinum electrode in growth medium, were toxic to bacteria led to the discovery that the platinum complex that was produced had significant antineoplastic activity [314]. The prototype platinum coordination complex is the drug cisplatin (*cis*-diamminedichloroplatinum II), which continues to play a critical part in the curative therapy of testicular germ cell tumors [315] and ovarian cancer [316], and the palliative care of patients with breast, lung and head and neck cancer [317–319]. Because of its therapeutic spectrum, over the past decade cisplatin has been used extensively as part of the STAMP I high-dose chemotherapy regimen (including CY, cisplatin and BCNU) for patients with either responsive metastatic or high-risk primary breast cancer [14,15,42]. High-dose cisplatin has also been combined with high-dose CY and melphalan [320], CY and thiotepa [321], and CY and etoposide [166] for a variety of solid tumors in conjunction with autologous bone marrow or stem cell support. The usual dose range for cisplatin in these treatment programs is 150–250 mg/m^2 (approximately threefold standard levels) delivered either as a 72–96 h continuous infusion or as a divided dose delivered over 1 week.

Mechanism of action

The chloride groups on cisplatin, shown in Fig. 12.1, are labile [322], reacting in solution to form an aquated species in which the chloride molecules are replaced by water. Conversion to this more reactive species is facilitated by the significantly lower intracellular chloride concentration compared to that in plasma. The reactive aquated molecule can then undergo displacement reactions analogous to the alkylating agents to produce covalent crosslinks with a variety of macromolecules including DNA [323,324]. Tumor cell killing by cisplatin can be correlated with the formation of interstrand crosslinks as well as specific intrastrand lesions. DNA binding also decreases the efficiency of specific DNA repair enzymes [322] while having a role as a transcriptional activator [325,326].

The sites on the platinum atom previously occupied by the chloride groups can be covalently linked to other biologically important macromolecules in addition to DNA. Thus, binding of the aquated platinum species to ubiquitous intracellular protein and non-protein-bound thiols, including glutathione, has been well documented; this includes the thiol groups on metallothionein [327,328]. Furthermore, cisplatin exposure has been reported to alter amino acid transport at the cell surface, as well as mitochondrial respiration and Na$^+$, K$^+$-ATPase activity; all of the proteins involved in these processes have critical thiol groups which may be targets for cisplatin binding. Finally, recent evidence implicates several different signal transduction circuits in the cisplatin cell death pathway [329,330]. In recent studies, cisplatin has been demonstrated to stimulate proliferation-dependent apoptosis that is, at least in part, p53 dependent [331,332]. The precise cytotoxic contribution of the formation of platinum adducts with macromolecules other than DNA remains an area of active investigation.

The mechanisms that have been described to explain tumor cell resistance to cisplatin fall into three broad categories: decreased drug uptake, increased intracellular binding (and thus sequestration) of activated platinum species to thiols, and altered DNA interactions with or without changes in signal transduction [333]. *In vitro*, cell lines with acquired defects in cisplatin uptake have been well described; however, no clear evidence for a specific platinum efflux pump has been developed [334]. Several laboratories have demonstrated that alterations in intracellular thiol status significantly affect platinum cytotoxicity. Overexpression of the metallothionein gene [335] as well as its upregulation by heavy metal pre-exposure decreases tumor cell sensitivity to cisplatin, probably by providing enhanced access to this sulfhydryl-rich protein. Furthermore, acquired resistance to cisplatin has been associated with enhanced glutathione synthesis in human ovarian and lung cancer cell lines [245,327] and can be at least partially reversed by glutathione depletion [32].

In addition to altered drug accumulation or enhanced thiol-dependent sequestration (both leading to diminished nuclear platinum concentrations), resistance to cisplatin may also result from decreased binding of platinum to DNA or chromatin, or enhanced repair of platinum-DNA adducts [336–338]. The steady-state level of platinum-DNA adducts in peripheral blood mononuclear cells has been correlated with response to platinum-containing chemotherapy regimens [339,340]. In addition to increased DNA repair rates, platinum resistance has also been associated with altered transcription factor activation, in particular diminished c-*jun* activation after cisplatin exposure, with a concomitant decrease in drug-related apoptosis in resistant cells [341].

Metabolism, pharmacokinetics and pharmacodynamics

The clearance of cisplatin is primarily through endogenous inactivation via binding to biologic macromolecules, including protein sulfhydryls and renal excretion. Cisplatin is extensively bound to plasma proteins. Its multiexponential clearance involves the initial disappearance of "free" or unbound drug in approximately 30–45 min, and the prolonged decay of protein-bound cisplatin over a terminal half-life in excess of 24 h [342]; interpatient pharmacokinetic variability is substantial [104]. The excretion of cisplatin is almost exclusively by a process of renal tubular filtration, secretion and reabsorption [343]; the clearance of cisplatin is proportional to the glomerular filtration rate. However, recent data demonstrate clearly that even with appropriately vigorous saline diuresis, there is extensive and long-term binding of cisplatin to renal tubules; measurable platinum species have been detected in urine for as long as 8 years after treatment with the drug [344]. Hence, the use of high-dose cisplatin requires that patients enter treatment with normal renal function.

Several interactions between cisplatin and other agents employed during high-dose chemotherapy have been described. Antiemetics used during high-dose cisplatin therapy may affect drug clearance. Ondansetron appears to decrease the AUC of cisplatin while prochlorperazine may increase plasma levels of cisplatin in the high-dose chemotherapy setting [345,346]. In preclinical model systems, prior TBI has been demonstrated to diminish cisplatin renal clearance [347]. Inhibition of cisplatin secretion by the renal tubule with probenecid appears to protect the kidney from cisplatin toxicity after high-dose (up to 160 mg/m^2) treatment [348]. High-dose cisplatin does not appear to alter the pharmacokinetics of high-dose melphalan or high-dose etoposide [349,350].

The maximally tolerated intravenous dose of cisplatin during combination high-dose chemotherapy with HC support is a total dose of 250 mg/m^2 administered in two fractions 1 week apart [166]. The dose-limiting toxicity of high-dose cisplatin is renal dysfunction including significant electrolyte wasting; hence, great care must be taken to ensure that a continuing vigorous diuresis occurs before, during and after high-dose platinum administration [351]. In addition, high-dose cisplatin is frequently associated with ototoxicity characterized by high-frequency hearing loss, especially above 2000 Hz [166,348,351]. Peripheral neuropathy, even at these high cisplatin doses, has been reversible and not dose-limiting in most studies, probably because the majority of patients treated (who had breast cancer) had little or no prior cisplatin exposure. Nausea and vomiting from high-dose cisplatin-containing regimens can be managed well with the newer 5-HT$_3$ antagonists. The ability to deliver the full 250 mg/m^2 of cisplatin during the HCT course was found to correlate favorably with relapse-free survival in women treated with high-dose cisplatin, CY, etoposide and autologous stem cells for high-risk primary breast cancer [43].

Carboplatin

Carboplatin (diammine 1,1-cyclobutanedicarboxylatoplatinum II) is an analog of cisplatin in which the two chloride ligands are replaced by the carboxylate moiety. Carboplatin has become a major component of high-dose chemotherapy regimens for the treatment of advanced testicular [352,353], ovarian [354,355] and breast cancer [233]. The DNA cross-linking species formed by carboplatin are identical to those formed with cisplatin, but the pharmacokinetics and spectrum of toxicity of this analog are different.

Metabolism, pharmacokinetics and pharmacodynamics

Carboplatin disappearance is caused, almost exclusively, by renal excretion; the drug is much less extensively protein-bound (18–30%) than cisplatin [356]. The disappearance of carboplatin from plasma is characterized by a triexponential decay with $t_{1/2\alpha}$ approximately 20 min, $t_{1/2\beta}$ about 1.5 h and $t_{1/2\gamma}$ approximately 7.5–20 h. Essentially, all unbound platinum species have been cleared from the plasma within 24 h after the completion of a high-dose carboplatin infusion [357]. Because there is minimal active tubular secretion of carboplatin, its clearance can be predicted from various formulas that utilize estimates of the glomerular filtration rate [112,358]. However, recent studies suggest that clearance estimates utilizing limited sampling schedules rather than measured creatinine clearance much more accurately reflect the actual delivered AUC of carboplatin in the setting of high-dose chemotherapy with autologous HC reinfusion [359,360]. Over a substantial range of carboplatin dosage, clearance appears to be linear (50–70 mL/min) although there is significant interpatient variability, especially when high-dose carboplatin is used in combination high-dose regimens [361]. Furthermore, the pharmacokinetic parameters defining high-dose carboplatin disappearance from plasma are similar whether the drug is administered as a short (1 h) or continuous (96 h) infusion [356]. Several studies have also demonstrated that carboplatin species can be removed from the plasma by hemodialysis [362,363].

Potential drug–drug interactions have been defined for high-dose carboplatin; however, certain conflicting reports cloud interpretation of the data. High-dose carboplatin may affect melphalan clearance [364], but not that of paclitaxel [365]; paclitaxel does not impair the clearance of carboplatin [366]. High-dose carboplatin has been reported either to have no effect [367] or to significantly decrease [368] the clearance of high-dose etoposide.

The maximally tolerated dose of carboplatin with HC support when the drug is used as a single agent is 1600–2400 mg/m^2 and 800–1200 mg/m^2 in combination high-dose chemotherapy regimens [233,369,370]. While the drug produces minimal hepatic, renal, mucosal or ototoxicity or peripheral neuropathy when used at standard dose, there is no question that dose-limiting liver toxicity, mucositis and peripheral neuropathy are observed in the high-dose chemotherapy setting [369,371,372], where the AUC of the drug is correlated with these side-effects when it is used in combination with etoposide. In combination with high-dose thiotepa and CY, cumulative carboplatin AUC has been correlated with the development of ototoxicity [121]. Furthermore, there is little doubt that when it is used at high dose, especially in patients with prior cisplatin exposure, carboplatin may produce significant nephrotoxicity. Despite these toxicities, the dose intensity of carboplatin in the setting of high-dose chemotherapy can be safely increased four- to sixfold with HC support compared to threefold for cisplatin, making it a valuable agent for the treatment of those diseases in which the therapeutic activity of carboplatin and cisplatin are equivalent.

Topoisomerase II inhibitors and agents with pleiotropic mechanisms of action

Etoposide

Podophyllotoxin derivatives from the mandrake plant have been known for many years to possess antiproliferative effects [373]. Etoposide (VP-16) is the podophyllotoxin derivative most commonly used in both standard clinical oncologic practice and as a component of many high-dose chemotherapy regimens for hematopoietic malignancies [374,375], germ cell cancer [352,353] and other solid tumors [166,376,377]. The usual dose range for etoposide in the BMT setting is approximately 25–60 mg/kg delivered in divided doses, often over 3 days, an approximate three- to sixfold increase over standard therapy. Etoposide has been utilized extensively in the high-dose chemotherapy setting both because of its therapeutic activity and its relatively modest spectrum of extramedullary side-effects.

Mechanism of action

The most thoroughly evaluated mechanism of tumor cell killing by etoposide has been its interaction with the nuclear enzyme topoisomerase II (topo II), which facilitates the uncoiling of DNA prior to DNA replication [378–380]. Topoisomerase IIα is a 170-kDa dimer that is normally responsible for producing the transient DNA single-strand breaks that are necessary for relieving torsional strain in DNA during transcription, replication and repair. This is an ATP-dependent process [381] that is inhibited by the interaction of etoposide with the enzyme, preventing re-ligation of DNA. With the formation of a cleavable complex between topo II and etoposide, the enzyme is trapped prior to DNA ligation; in the presence of protein-digesting enzymes, protein-associated DNA strand breaks become apparent. When etoposide-related cleavable complex formation is decreased through competition with other catalytic inhibitors of topo II, cytotoxicity is diminished [382,383].

Although there is little question about the formation of topo II-mediated DNA damage after etoposide exposure *in vitro*, cleavable complex formation is clearly not sufficient in itself to explain the cytotoxicity of etoposide [384]. Because topo II-mediated DNA damage from etoposide is rapidly reversible, has not yet been convincingly demonstrated *in vivo* [385] and produces mainly single- rather than more lethal double-stranded DNA scission, other mechanisms may contribute to the cytotoxic effects of etoposide. Etoposide can be metabolized to a free radical species [386] that enhances macromolecular binding of the drug [387] and may contribute to DNA damage and apoptosis [388,389]. Recently, etoposide has been demonstrated to produce caspase activation leading to programmed cell death [390–393], as well as cleavage of poly ADP ribose polymerase [394–396] that may, in part, be mediated by p53 [397]. It appears, furthermore, that binding of etoposide to topo II is not itself critical for the induction of apoptosis [398]. Thus, the etoposide–topo II interaction may be viewed as producing only potentially lethal damage to the tumor cell.

Tumor cell resistance to etoposide can be produced by several different mechanisms [399,400] including alterations in drug uptake and efflux as well as changes in either the amount or binding affinity of topo II. Etoposide is a substrate for the P-glycoprotein, and overexpression of the *MDR*1 gene product leads to both decreased uptake and enhanced efflux of etoposide [401,402]. Inhibitors of P-glycoprotein have been employed to enhance the therapeutic activity of etoposide clinically [403,404]. However, acquired etoposide resistance may also be caused by increased drug efflux that is related to the overexpression of the multidrug resistance-associated protein (MRP) rather than *MDR*1 [405–407]. In certain subclasses of acute myelogenous leukemia, MRP, rather than *MDR*1, expression has greater prognostic significance [408].

In addition to drug transport, the level of topo II protein or its specific activity significantly affect the tumor cell sensitivity of etoposide. Decreased drug-related cleavable complex formation may be caused by lower absolute levels of topo II, by mutations in the enzymes that affect drug binding or by the degree of topo II phosphorylation [31,407,409]. Furthermore, evidence for the coevolution of these resistance phenotypes (e.g. overexpression of MRP that occurs synchronously with alterations in topo II level) has been demonstrated recently [407]. Finally, etoposide exposure may initiate the programmed cell death cascade [391]; hence, intrinsic or acquired overexpression of specific genes participating in apoptosis may lead to etoposide resistance [410–412].

Metabolism, pharmacokinetics and pharmacodynamics

Etoposide is principally metabolized in the liver to its glucuronide [413]: approximately one-third of the drug is excreted by the kidney as the unchanged parent molecule and another 10–20% as etoposide-glucuronide. Because renal clearance is increased in the presence of hyperbilirubinemia or liver metastases, no adjustment of etoposide dose is required in the presence of hepatic dysfunction [413–415]. However, the systemic clearance of etoposide is closely related to creatinine clearance [416]. Because etoposide dosage must be reduced in the presence of renal dysfunction, high-dose etoposide therapy should not routinely be considered in patients suffering from even a modest degree of kidney failure. Furthermore, caution must be exercised when high-dose etoposide is delivered immediately after high-dose cisplatin, because acute cisplatin exposure can reduce the systemic clearance of etoposide by approximately 25%, leading to a substantially greater than expected etoposide area AUC and toxicity level [417]. High-dose carboplatin exposure, on the other hand, may not alter the disposition of high-dose etoposide [367].

The pharmacokinetics of etoposide have been studied over the entire range of intravenous regimens, from 0.1 to 3 g/m^2. Etoposide, which is highly protein-bound, has a biexponential decay with a mean terminal half-life after high-dose therapy of between 4 and 8 h [418]; even when delivered at high dose (30–60 mg/kg), essentially all detectable drug has disappeared from plasma in 36–48 h [374]. Changes in etoposide dosage over its entire therapeutic range produce linear changes in associated plasma AUC [367,418–420]. The linear pharmacokinetics of etoposide disposition, despite significant interpatient pharmacokinetic variability [100], make its toxicity profile predictable and potentially amenable to adaptive control strategies capable of targeting specific etoposide systemic exposures through the use of therapeutic drug level monitoring [122].

In addition to its potential pharmacodynamic interaction with cisplatin, the clearance of etoposide is increased by approximately one-third (with a concomitant decrease in AUC) in patients treated with BU and phenytoin before high-dose etoposide, compared to patients who are receiving TBI and etoposide [421]. Whether this alteration in clearance is caused by the effect of phenytoin itself on the hepatic metabolism of etoposide or the combined interaction of phenytoin and BU on liver microsomal enzyme systems is unknown. Finally, it has been shown that the emulsifying agent Cremophor-EL, used to solubilize paclitaxel, significantly decreases the total body clearance of etoposide [422]. In light of the pharmacokinetic interactions that have been demonstrated between paclitaxel and doxorubicin caused by this emulsifier [423], significant care is required in the development of schedules of high-dose chemotherapy programs combining etoposide with paclitaxel to avoid potentially severe levels of toxicity.

The toxicity profile of high-dose etoposide is, in part, related to the drugs with which it is combined in BMT [166,226,424]. However, even when etoposide is administered as a single agent [425], mucositis has clearly been demonstrated to be dose-limiting, which has an important effect on the ability to combine high-dose etoposide with other drugs whose dose-limiting extramedullary toxicity is also focused on the gastrointestinal tract [158,424].

Anthracyclines

The anthracycline antibiotic doxorubicin, isolated from *Streptomyces* species over 30 years ago [426], has a wide spectrum of antineoplastic action and is a major component of curative combination chemotherapy regimens for the hematopoietic malignancies as well as breast and ovarian cancer and many childhood solid tumors [427,428]. Doxorubicin is one of the few antineoplastic agents with significant clinical utility for which a clear dose–response relationship (including doses several-fold greater than those traditionally used) has been demonstrated in humans [161,429,430].

It has been traditional to assume that the dose-limiting cumulative cardiac toxicity of doxorubicin [431] would make it difficult to use in the high-dose chemotherapy setting [26]. However, with the understanding that the risk of doxorubicin cardiac toxicity is more closely related to peak plasma levels of the drug rather than its systemic exposure [432–435], it has recently been possible to demonstrate both the feasibility and efficacy of high-dose doxorubicin therapy when used in combination with high-dose CY or high-dose etoposide, or both, and HCT for the treatment of patients with responsive metastatic or high-risk primary breast or ovarian cancer [43,424,436–438]. These recent observations are likely to support the wider application of high-dose chemotherapy regimens that incorporate an anthracycline [439,440].

Mechanism of action

Doxorubicin interacts pleiotropically with intracellular organelles and alters the biochemistry of the cell surface, the mitochondrion, many signal transduction pathways, as well as the nuclear replication apparatus [441–446]. Many of these interactions contribute to its broad antineoplastic activity. Doxorubicin exerts its antiproliferative effects through each of the following mechanisms:

- binding to the nuclear enzyme topoisomerase II to form a cleavable complex that interferes with the ability of this enzyme to reduce the torsional strain in DNA which occurs during mitosis;
- the generation of reactive oxygen species (including the hydroxyl radical) that damage the mitochondrial electron transport chain and hinder

cellular energy production as well as producing DNA base oxidation; and
- the activation of signal transduction pathways ultimately leading to programmed cell death [441,447,448].

As might be expected from an agent with such a wide repertoire of mechanisms of cell kill, drug resistance, both *in vitro* and *in vivo*, may involve alterations in a variety of cytotoxic pathways. Prominent among the resistance pathways that have been described are alterations in doxorubicin uptake and enhanced cellular efflux modulated by the overexpression of one or more of several drug efflux pumps including the P-glycoprotein, the MRP, the lung-resistance protein or the breast cancer-resistance protein, the presence of which have all been described as conferring an adverse prognosis in anthracycline-resistant hematopoietic malignancies [37,408,449,450]. However, as shown in Fig. 12.2, even tumor cells that overexpress the P-glycoprotein or other enhanced efflux mechanisms can be killed in a log-linear fashion if doxorubicin exposure can be increased sufficiently. The same is true, in part, for the ability to overcome tumor cell resistance to doxorubicin mediated by alterations in intracellular topoisomerase II levels, antioxidant proteins, antiapoptosis genes or DNA repair enzymes. It is when tumor cells become pleiotropically resistant that the threefold changes in doxorubicin dose that are possible in the high-dose setting may not be sufficient to produce multilog tumor cell kill.

Metabolism, pharmacokinetics and pharmacodynamics
Doxorubicin is principally metabolized in the liver either by flavin dehydrogenases, which catalyze the one-electron reduction of its quinone moiety with the ultimate formation of an aglycone species that is more easily conjugated for biliary export, or by aldo-keto reductases which reduce the carbonyl side chain of the drug, leading to a less cytotoxic species [451–454]. Only about 60% of the elimination of doxorubicin can be accounted for, even when the minor amount of renal clearance is included; it is likely that much of the remaining drug is bound to DNA and lipid membranes from which it is slowly released. It is not surprising therefore that the pharmacokinetics of doxorubicin demonstrate triexponential decay with a long-terminal half-life in plasma of approximately 12–20 h for both the parent drug and its side-chain alcohol metabolite, doxorubicinol [455]. Because of the predominant hepatic metabolism of the drug, individuals with liver dysfunction may exhibit considerably enhanced anthracycline toxicity because of delayed drug clearance [456].

Of particular importance for the use of doxorubicin in high-dose chemotherapy, even doses between 150 and 165 mg/m^2 delivered over 96 h by continuous intravenous infusion (approximately threefold higher than standard treatment programs) produce steady state plasma concentrations 10-fold lower than the peak drug levels observed after bolus administration of 50–60 mg/m^2 doxorubicin [457]. Furthermore, as shown in Fig. 12.4, over a broad range of doses, the pharmacokinetics and metabolism of doxorubicin are linear, suggesting that drug activation and detoxification pathways are not exceeded when the doxorubicin dose is escalated into the high-dose chemotherapy range.

The toxicity of doxorubicin of particular relevance to the high-dose chemotherapy setting, other than cardiac toxicity, is dose-limiting damage to the oral and gastrointestinal mucosa, resulting in reversible but potentially severe stomatitis and diarrhea [424]. A reversible typhlitis, which is managed conservatively with parenteral nutrition, analgesics and careful attention to fluid and electrolyte balance, may be observed in approximately 5% of patients receiving high-dose chemotherapy combinations including doxorubicin or etoposide, or both. This syndrome is self-limited, should not require surgical intervention and resolves rapidly as hematopoietic function recovers.

The unique toxicity of doxorubicin is its cumulative dose-dependent myocardial damage. Studies that have employed either gated cardiac blood pool scanning or endomyocardial biopsy as endpoints for functional or histological confirmation of doxorubicin cardiac toxicity have demonstrated that the incidence of measurable heart damage begins to climb precipitously above a cumulative dose of 350–400 mg/m^2 (rather than the traditional figure of 450–500 mg/m^2) if the drug has been administered by short intravenous infusion. In patients for whom high-dose chemotherapy will include doxorubicin at a dose of 150 mg/m^2 or higher, administered by 96-h continuous infusion, recent studies utilizing endomyocardial biopsy suggest that the maximum prior bolus doxorubicin exposure should not exceed 200 mg/m^2 [436]. However, in individuals who have a long history of hypertensive heart disease or higher previous cumulative doxorubicin exposures, the safety of high-dose doxorubicin remains to be demonstrated. Dexrazoxane, a novel iron-chelating agent that significantly ameliorates doxorubicin cardiac toxicity, may in the future allow the use of high-dose doxorubicin in these patient populations.

Taxanes
Paclitaxel is the lead compound in the taxane class of antimicrotubule agents. Originally isolated from the bark of the Pacific yew, *Taxus brevifolia*, it is now available from semisynthetic and totally synthetic approaches [458,459]. Paclitaxel has a wide spectrum of antineoplastic activity, including breast, lung and ovarian cancer, for which it is among the most active drugs currently available [460–463].

Mechanism of action
Paclitaxel has a unique mechanism of tumor cell killing. After binding to the β subunit of tubulin, paclitaxel inhibits the dissolution of microtubules, upsetting the dynamic balance between microtubular formation and dissolution upon which many intracellular processes are dependent [464–467]. The net effect of enhanced tubulin polymerization is to produce a block in the metaphase of mitosis, leading to growth inhibition. However, paclitaxel has also been shown to diminish cell-cycle traverse in the non-mitotic phases of cell proliferation [466], which may be caused by the effects of tubulin polymerization on both the cytoskeleton and signal transduction pathways. Paclitaxel also enhances the cytotoxic effects of ionizing radiation at concentrations that are achievable in the clinic [468,469]. Other important biochemical effects of paclitaxel in tumor cell systems include the activation of the NF-κB nuclear transcription factor and the phosphorylation of *bcl-2*, both of which may affect paclitaxel-induced programmed cell death [470,471].

By a sequence of events that remains to be completely characterized, paclitaxel exposure leads to apoptosis in a wide variety of tumor cell types [472–474]. Non-apoptotic cell killing also occurs [475]. One of the characteristic features of paclitaxel-related cytotoxicity is that it is independent of p53 status, which may help to explain the broad therapeutic range of the drug [476,477].

Two distinct mechanisms of paclitaxel resistance have been described. *In vitro*, paclitaxel-resistant tumor cells overexpress specific isoforms of β-tubulin [478]; furthermore, in human ovarian tumors, increased expression of class III and IVa β-tubulin isotypes has been demonstrated in ascites tumor cells from patients clinically resistant to paclitaxel compared to untreated patient samples [479]. Paclitaxel is also a substrate for the P-glycoprotein; resistance *in vitro* mediated by enhanced drug efflux has been shown for both hematopoietic and solid tumors [467,474,480]. Similar to other known substrates for the *MDR*1 gene product, paclitaxel resistance can be modified by a variety of drug classes that decrease chemotherapeutic drug efflux [481,482]. The role of P-glycoprotein expression in modulating paclitaxel resistance in the clinic is under active investigation.

Metabolism, pharmacokinetics and pharmacodynamics
Paclitaxel is cleared primarily by the cytochrome P450 system in the liver

[483] and excreted, in part unchanged, in the bile. 6α-Hydroxypaclitaxel is the major hepatic microsomal metabolite found both in plasma and bile; it is formed through the action of the CYP2C isoform of cytochrome P450. Other, less abundant byproducts that result from hydroxylation of the lateral chain are due to metabolism by the CYP3A4 isoform of cytochrome P450. Neither cimetidine, ranitidine nor diphenylhydramine affect paclitaxel metabolism; however, induction of CYP3A isoforms by barbiturates has been shown *in vitro* to affect the biotransformation of paclitaxel to less cytotoxically active species. Because of its extensive microsomal elimination, alterations in hepatic function play a major part in the elimination of paclitaxel [484,485]. Because even modest abnormalities in liver function can alter the pharmacokinetics of paclitaxel, patients receiving high-dose chemotherapy regimens containing paclitaxel must have normal hepatic function prior to treatment.

The pharmacokinetics of paclitaxel when administered over 3 or 24 h demonstrate a bi- or triexponential elimination with a prolonged γ-phase of approximately 15 h [486]. Recent pharmacokinetic studies have detailed the saturability of paclitaxel elimination, which is most prominent with short administration times or with increasing dose levels [107,440,487]. Whether or not the saturable distribution and elimination of paclitaxel is caused by the affect of the Cremophor-EL vehicle in which paclitaxel is solubilized [423,488], the non-linear pharmacokinetic profile of paclitaxel has important clinical ramifications. As shown in Fig. 12.5, for patients receiving high-dose paclitaxel over 24 h, peak plasma concentrations clearly become non-linear at doses above 450 mg/m^2; furthermore, the range of peak plasma concentrations observed at individual dose levels also widens. Thus, a threefold increase in dose from 250 to 750 mg/m^2 leads to a 15-fold increase in peak plasma concentration and AUC. The disproportionate change in observed systemic exposure may lead to an unexpected degree of toxicity if it is not anticipated. Thus, while high-dose paclitaxel regimens produce peak plasma concentrations greater than 50-fold higher than those observed with standard paclitaxel doses (2.5–5 vs. 0.05 μmol), which may be therapeutically beneficial [10], current trials of high-dose paclitaxel are evaluating the role of adaptive control techniques aimed at minimizing interpatient variability in paclitaxel exposure with the goal of reducing large potential variations in toxicity [489].

The major dose-limiting features of high-dose paclitaxel therapy are the development of significant peripheral neuropathy [490] and mucositis [491,492], the severity of which has been correlated with the observed paclitaxel AUC [491]. At paclitaxel doses of 725–750 mg/m^2 administered over 24 h, however, in combination with either high-dose CY and cisplatin or high-dose CY and doxorubicin and HC support, the level of these toxicities has been acceptable [437,491].

Conclusions

Because the toxicity profile and pharmacokinetic properties of the commonly used antineoplastic agents frequently change when these drugs are used for high-dose chemotherapy, the development of novel treatment programs that utilize HC support depends on an intimate familiarity with the pharmacologic properties of the drugs employed in this setting. It is likely that better utilization of both currently available and investigational chemotherapeutic agents through therapeutic drug monitoring with adaptive control of drug exposure will both increase the efficacy and decrease the risks of high-dose chemotherapy, as well as improve our ability to combine drugs and overcome inherent or acquired resistance. A renewed focus on the therapeutic effects of the drugs employed with a special emphasis on disease-specific tumor cell killing and the critical part played by pharmacogenetically related variations in drug exposure is likely to enhance the outcome of high-dose chemotherapy in the future for patients with both hematologic malignancies and solid tumors.

References

1 Santos GW, Owens AH Jr. Allogeneic marrow transplants in cyclophosphamide treated mice. *Transplant Proc* 1969; **1**: 44–6.

2 Santos GW, Sensenbrenner LL, Burke PJ et al. Marrow transplanation in man following cyclophosphamide. *Transplant Proc* 1971; **3**: 400–4.

3 Thomas ED, Storb R, Fefer A et al. Aplastic anaemia treated by marrow transplantation. *Lancet* 1972; **1**: 284–9.

4 Buckner CD, Clift RA, Fefer A et al. Marrow transplantation for the treatment of acute leukemia using HL-A-identical siblings. *Transplant Proc* 1974; **6**: 365–6.

5 Storb R, Buckner CD, Fefer A et al. Marrow transplantation in aplastic anemia. *Transplant Proc* 1974; **6**: 355–8.

6 Haurani FI, Repplinger E, Tocantins LM. Attempts at transplantation of human bone marrow in patients with acute leukemia and other marrow depletion disorders. *Am J Med* 1960; **28**: 794–806.

7 Saijo N. Chemotherapy: the more the better? Overview. *Cancer Chemother Pharmacol* 1997; **40** (Suppl.): S100–S106.

8 Frei EI, Canellos GP. Dose: a critical factor in cancer chemotherapy. *Am J Med* 1980; **69**: 585–94.

9 Frei E III. Pharmacologic strategies for high-dose chemotherapy. In: Armitage JO, Antman KH, eds. *High-Dose Cancer Therapy: Pharmacology, Hematopoietins, Stem Cells*. Baltimore: Williams & Wilkins, 1995: 3–16.

10 Kelland LR, Abel G. Comparative *in vitro* cytotoxicity of taxol and Taxotere against cisplatin-sensitive and -resistant human ovarian carcinoma cell lines. *Cancer Chemother Pharmacol* 1992; **30**: 444–50.

11 Porrata LF, Adjei AA. The pharmacologic basis of high dose chemotherapy with haematopoietic stem cell support for solid tumours. *Br J Cancer* 2001; **85**: 484–9.

12 Long BH, Brattain MG. The activity of etoposide (VP-16–213) and teniposide (VM-26) against human lung tumor cells *in vitro*: cytotoxicity and DNA breakage. In: Issell BF, Muggia FM, Carter SK, eds. *Etoposide (VP-16): Current Status and New Developments*. New York: Academic Press, 1984: 63–86.

13 Jones RB, Matthes S, Dufton C. Pharmacokinetics. In: Armitage JO, Antman KH, eds. *High-Dose Cancer Therapy: Pharmacology, Hematopoietins, Stem Cells*. Baltimore: Williams & Wilkins, 1995: 49–6.

14 Antman K, Eder JP, Elias A et al. High-dose combination alkylating agent preparative regimen with autologous bone marrow support: The Dana-Farber Cancer Institute/Beth Israel Hospital experience. *Cancer Treat Rep* 1987; **71**: 119–25.

15 Peters WP. High-dose chemotherapy and autologous bone marrow support for breast cancer. In: DeVita VT Jr, Hellman S, Rosenberg SA, eds. *Important Advances in Oncology*. Philadelphia: J.B. Lippincott, 1991: 135–50.

16 Dexter DL, Spremulli EN, Fligiel Z et al. Heterogeneity of cancer cells from a single human colon carcinoma. *Am J Med* 1981; **71**: 949–56.

17 Harris AL. DNA repair: relationship to drug and radiation resistance, metastasis and growth factors. *Int J Radiat Biol Relat Stud Phys Chem Med* 1985; **48**: 675–90.

18 Simpson-Herren L, Noker PE, Wagoner SD. Variability of tumor response to chemotherapy. II. Contribution of tumor heterogeneity. *Cancer Chemother Pharmacol* 1988; **22**: 131–6.

19 Schabel FM Jr, Trader MW, Laster WR Jr, Wheeler GP, Witt MH. Patterns of resistance and therapeutic synergism among alkylating agents. *Antibiot Chemother* 1978; **23**: 200–15.

20 Schabel FM Jr, Corbett TH. Cell kinetics and the chemotherapy of murine solid tumors. *Antibiot Chemother* 1980; **28**: 28–34.

21 Corbett TH, Griswold DP, Mayo JG, Laster WR, Schabel FM Jr. Cyclophosphamide–adriamycin combination chemotherapy of transplantable murine tumors. *Cancer Res* 1975; **35**: 1568–73.

22 Ozols RF, Grotzinger KR, Fisher RI, Myers CE, Young RC. Kinetic characterization and response to chemotherapy in a transplantable murine ovarian cancer. *Cancer Res* 1979; **39**: 3202–8.

23 Antman KH, Rowlings PA, Vaughan WP et al. High-dose chemotherapy with autologous hematopoietic stem-cell support for breast cancer in North America. *J Clin Oncol* 1997; **15**: 1870–9.

24 Lee FY, Vessey A, Rofstad E, Siemann DW, Sutherland RM. Heterogeneity of glutathione content in human ovarian cancer. *Cancer Res* 1989; **49**: 5244–8.

25 Oberley TD, Sempf JM, Oberley MJ, McCormick

ML, Muse KE, Oberley LW. Immunogold analysis of antioxidant enzymes in human renal cell carcinoma. *Virchows Arch* 1994; **424**: 155–64.
26 Doroshow JH. Principles of medical oncology. In: Pollock RE, Doroshow JH, Geraghty JG, Khayat D, Kim J-P, O'Sullivan B, eds. *Manual of Clinical Oncology*. New York: John Wiley & Sons, 1999: 275–92.
27 Politi PM, Sinha BK. Role of differential drug uptake, efflux, and binding of etoposide in sensitive and resistant human tumor cell lines: implications for the mechanisms of drug resistance. *Mol Pharmacol* 1989; **35**: 271–8.
28 Brophy NA, Marie JP, Rojas VA et al. Mdr1 gene expression in childhood acute lymphoblastic leukemias and lymphomas: a critical evaluation by four techniques. *Leukemia* 1994; **8**: 327–35.
29 Bertino JR. Toward improved selectivity in cancer chemotherapy. The Richard and Hinda Rosenthal Foundation Award Lecture. *Cancer Res* 1979; **39**: 293–304.
30 Cowan KH, Goldsmith ME, Levine RM et al. Dihydrofolate reductase gene amplification and possible rearrangement in estrogen-responsive methotrexate-resistant human breast cancer cells. *J Biol Chem* 1982; **257**: 15079–86.
31 Ganapathi R, Zwelling L, Constantinou A, Ford J, Grabowski D. Altered phosphorylation, biosynthesis and degradation of the 170 kDa isoform of topoisomerase II in amsacrine-resistant human leukemia cells. *Biochem Biophys Res Commun* 1993; **192**: 1274–80.
32 Hamilton TC, Winker MA, Louie KG et al. Augmentation of adriamycin, melphalan, and cisplatin cytotoxicity in drug-resistant and -sensitive human ovarian carcinoma cell lines by buthionine sulfoximine mediated glutathione depletion. *Biochem Pharmacol* 1985; **34**: 2583–6.
33 Manome Y, Weichselbaum RR, Kufe DW, Fine HA. Effect of Bcl-2 on ionizing radiation and 1-beta-D arabinofuranosylcytosine-induced internucleosomal DNA fragmentation and cell survival in human myeloid leukemia cells. *Oncol Res* 1993; **5**: 139–44.
34 Vaupel P, Kallinowski F, Okunieff P. Blood flow, oxygen and nutrient supply, and metabolic microenvironment of human tumors: a review. *Cancer Res* 1989; **49**: 6449–65.
35 Vaupel PW, Frinak S, Bicher HI. Heterogeneous oxygen partial pressure and pH distribution in C3H mouse mammary adenocarcinoma. *Cancer Res* 1981; **41**: 2008–13.
36 Marie J-P, Zittoun R, Sikic BI. Multidrug resistance (*mdr*1) gene expression in adult acute leukemias: correlations with treatment outcome and invitro drug sensitivity. *Blood* 1991; **78**: 586–92.
37 List AF. The role of multidrug resistance and its pharmacological modulation in acute myeloid leukemia. *Leukemia* 1996; **10** (Suppl. 1): S36–8.
38 Scheider J, Bak M, Efferth T. P-glycoprotein expression in treated and untreated human breast cancer. *Br J Cancer* 1989; **61**: 815–7.
39 Lonn U, Lonn S, Nylen U, Stenkvist B. Appearance and detection of multiple copies of the *mdr*-1 gene in clinical samples of mammary carcinoma. *Int J Cancer* 1992; **51**: 682–6.
40 Sartorelli AC. Therapeutic attack of hypoxic cells of solid tumors: presidential address. *Cancer Res* 1988; **48**: 775–8.
41 Antman K, Gale RP. Advanced breast cancer: high dose chemotherapy and bone marrow autotransplants. *Ann Intern Med* 1988; **108**: 570–4.
42 Peters WP, Ross M, Vredenburgh JJ et al. High-dose chemotherapy and autologous bone marrow support as consolidation after standard-dose adjuvant therapy for high-risk primary breast cancer. *J Clin Oncol* 1993; **11**: 1132–43.
43 Somlo G, Doroshow JH, Forman SJ et al. High-dose chemotherapy and stem-cell rescue in the treatment of high-risk breast cancer: prognostic indicators of progression-free and overall survival. *J Clin Oncol* 1997; **15**: 2882–93.
44 Hughes HB, Biehl JP, Jones AP, Schmidt LH. Metabolism of isoniazid in man as related to occurrence of peripheral neuritis. *Am J Tuberc* 1954; **70**: 266–73.
45 Kalow W. Familial incidence of low pseudocholinesterase level. *Lancet* 1956; **211**: 576–7.
46 Gonzalez FJ, Skoda RC, Kimura S et al. Characterization of the common genetic defect in humans deficient in debrisoquine metabolism. *Nature* 1988; **331**: 442–6.
47 Mahgoub A, Idle JR, Dring LG, Lancaster R, Smith RL. Polymorphic hydroxylation of debrisoquine in man. *Lancet* 1977; **2**: 584–6.
48 Ingelman-Sundberg M. Duplication, multiduplication, and amplification of genes encoding drug-metabolizing enzymes: evolutionary, toxicological, and clinical pharmacological aspects. *Drug Metab Rev* 1999; **31**: 449–59.
49 Lundqvist E, Johansson I, Ingelman-Sundberg M. Genetic mechanisms for duplication and multiduplication of the human *CYP2D6* gene and methods for detection of duplicated *CYP2D6* genes. *Gene* 1999; **226**: 327–38.
50 Marsh S, Ameyaw MM, Githang'a J, Indalo A, Ofori-Adjei D, McLeod HL. Novel thymidylate synthase enhancer region alleles in African populations. *Hum Mutat* 2000; **16**: 528.
51 Sachidanandam R, Weissman D, Schmidt SC et al. A map of human genome sequence variation containing 1.42 million single nucleotide polymorphisms. *Nature* 2001; **409**: 928–33.
52 Evans WE, Johnson JA. Pharmacogenomics: the inherited basis for interindividual differences in drug response. *Annu Rev Genomics Hum Genet* 2001; **2**: 9–39.
53 Rifkind AB, Lee C, Chang TK, Waxman DJ. Arachidonic acid metabolism by human cytochrome P450s 2C8, 2C9, 2E1, and 1A2. regioselective oxygenation and evidence for a role for CYP2C enzymes in arachidonic acid epoxygenation in human liver microsomes. *Arch Biochem Biophys* 1995; **320**: 380–9.
54 Goldstein JA. Clinical relevance of genetic polymorphisms in the human CYP2C subfamily. *Br J Clin Pharmacol* 2001; **52**: 349–55.
55 de Morais SM, Wilkinson GR, Blaisdell J, Nakamura K, Meyer UA, Goldstein JA. The major genetic defect responsible for the polymorphism of S-mephenytoin metabolism in humans. *J Biol Chem* 1994; **269**: 15419–22.
56 Balian JD, Sukhova N, Harris JW et al. The hydroxylation of omeprazole correlates with S-mephenytoin metabolism: a population study. *Clin Pharmacol Ther* 1995; **57**: 662–9.
57 Jung F, Richardson TH, Raucy JL, Johnson EF. Diazepam metabolism by cDNA-expressed human 2C P450s: identification of P4502C18 and P4502C19 as low K (M) diazepam N-demethylases. *Drug Metab Dispos* 1997; **25**: 133–9.
58 Wan J, Xia H, He N, Lu YQ, Zhou HH. The elimination of diazepam in Chinese subjects is dependent on the mephenytoin oxidation phenotype. *Br J Clin Pharmacol* 1996; **42**: 471–4.
59 Skjelbo E, Gram LF, Brosen K. The N-demethylation of imipramine correlates with the oxidation of S-mephenytoin (S/R-ratio): a population study. *Br J Clin Pharmacol* 1993; **35**: 331–4.
60 Birkett DJ, Rees D, Andersson T, Gonzalez FJ, Miners JO, Veronese ME. *In vitro* proguanil activation to cycloguanil by human liver microsomes is mediated by CYP3A isoforms as well as by S-mephenytoin hydroxylase. *Br J Clin Pharmacol* 1994; **37**: 413–20.
61 Furuta T, Ohashi K, Kamata T et al. Effect of genetic differences in omeprazole metabolism on cure rates for *Helicobacter pylori* infection and peptic ulcer. *Ann Intern Med* 1998; **129**: 1027–30.
62 Chang TK, Weber GF, Crespi CL, Waxman DJ. Differential activation of cyclophosphamide and ifosphamide by cytochromes P-450 2B and 3A in human liver microsomes. *Cancer Res* 1993; **53**: 5629–37.
63 Cresteil T, Monsarrat B, Alvinerie P, Treluyer JM, Vieira I, Wright M. Taxol metabolism by human liver microsomes: identification of cytochrome P450 isozymes involved in its biotransformation. *Cancer Res* 1994; **54**: 386–92.
64 Rahman A, Korzekwa KR, Grogan J, Gonzalez FJ, Harris JW. Selective biotransformation of taxol to 6 alpha-hydroxytaxol by human cytochrome P450 2C8. *Cancer Res* 1994; **54**: 5543–6.
65 Soyama A, Saito Y, Hanioka N et al. Non-synonymous single nucleotide alterations found in the CYP2C8 gene result in reduced *in vitro* paclitaxel metabolism. *Biol Pharm Bull* 2001; **24**: 1427–30.
66 Dai D, Zeldin DC, Blaisdell JA et al. Polymorphisms in human CYP2C8 decrease metabolism of the anticancer drug paclitaxel and arachidonic acid. *Pharmacogenetics* 2001; **11**: 597–607.
67 Rendic S, Di Carlo FJ. Human cytochrome P450 enzymes: a status report summarizing their reactions, substrates, inducers, and inhibitors. *Drug Metab Rev* 1997; **29**: 413–580.
68 Cholerton S, Daly AK, Idle JR. The role of individual human cytochromes P450 in drug metabolism and clinical response. *Trends Pharmacol Sci* 1992; **13**: 434–9.
69 Shimada T, Yamazaki H, Mimura M, Inui Y, Guengerich FP. Interindividual variations in human liver cytochrome P-450 enzymes involved in the oxidation of drugs, carcinogens and toxic chemicals: studies with liver microsomes of 30 Japanese and 30 Caucasians. *J Pharmacol Exp Ther* 1994; **270**: 414–23.
70 Koch I, Weil R, Wolbold R. et al. Interindividual variability and tissue-specificity in the expression of cytochrome p450, 3A mRNA. *Drug Metab Dispos* 2002; **30**: 1108–14.
71 Watkins PB. Cyclosporine and liver transplantation: will the midazolam test make blood level monitoring obsolete? *Hepatology* 1995; **22**: 994–6.
72 Hirth J, Watkins PB, Strawderman M, Schott A, Bruno R, Baker LH. The effect of an individual's cytochrome CYP3A4 activity on docetaxel clearance. *Clin Cancer Res* 2000; **6**: 1255–8.
73 Schuetz JD, Molowa DT, Guzelian PS. Characterization of a cDNA encoding a new member of the glucocorticoid-responsive cytochromes P450 in human liver. *Arch Biochem Biophys* 1989; **274**: 355–65.
74 Paine MF, Khalighi M, Fisher JM et al. Characterization of interintestinal and intraintestinal variations in human CYP3A-dependent metabolism. *J Pharmacol Exp Ther* 1997; **283**: 1552–62.

75 Wrighton SA, Ring BJ, Watkins PB, Vanden-Branden M. Identification of a polymorphically expressed member of the human cytochrome P-450III family. *Mol Pharmacol* 1989; **36**: 97–105.

76 Shou M, Martinet M, Korzekwa KR, Krausz KW, Gonzalez FJ, Gelboin HV. Role of human cytochrome P450 3A4 and 3A5 in the metabolism of taxotere and its derivatives: enzyme specificity, interindividual distribution and metabolic contribution in human liver. *Pharmacogenetics* 1998; **8**: 391–401.

77 Kajita J, Kuwabara T, Kobayashi H, Kobayashi S. CYP3A4 is mainly responsible for the metabolism of a new vinca alkaloid, vinorelbine, in human liver microsomes. *Drug Metab Dispos* 2000; **28**: 1121–7.

78 Zhou-Pan XR, Seree E, Zhou XJ. *et al*. Involvement of human liver cytochrome P450, 3A in vinblastine metabolism: drug interactions. *Cancer Res* 1993; **53**: 5121–6.

79 Relling MV, Nemec J, Schuetz EG, Schuetz JD, Gonzalez FJ, Korzekwa KR. O-demethylation of epipodophyllotoxins is catalyzed by human cytochrome P450 3A4. *Mol Pharmacol* 1994; **45**: 352–8.

80 Ren S, Yang JS, Kalhorn TF, Slattery JT. Oxidation of cyclophosphamide to 4-hydroxycyclophosphamide and deschloroethylcyclophosphamide in human liver microsomes. *Cancer Res* 1997; **57**: 4229–35.

81 Lamba JK, Lin YS, Thummel K *et al*. Common allelic variants of cytochrome P4503A4 and their prevalence in different populations. *Pharmacogenetics* 2002; **12**: 121–32.

82 Westlind A, Lofberg L, Tindberg N, Andersson TB, Ingelman-Sundberg M. Interindividual differences in hepatic expression of CYP3A4: relationship to genetic polymorphism in the 5′-upstream regulatory region. *Biochem Biophys Res Commun* 1999; **259**: 201–5.

83 Kuehl P, Zhang J, Lin Y *et al*. Sequence diversity in CYP3A promoters and characterization of the genetic basis of polymorphic CYP3A5 expression. *Nat Genet* 2001; **27**: 383–91.

84 Gibbs JP, Czerwinski M, Slattery JT. Busulfan–glutathione conjugation catalyzed by human liver cytosolic glutathione S-transferases. *Cancer Res* 1996; **56**: 3678–81.

85 Czerwinski M, Gibbs JP, Slattery JT. Busulfan conjugation by glutathione S-transferases alpha, mu, and pi. *Drug Metab Dispos* 1996; **24**: 1015–9.

86 Dirven HA, Dictus EL, Broeders NL, Van Ommen B, Van Bladeren PJ. The role of human glutathione S-transferase isoenzymes in the formation of glutathione conjugates of the alkylating cytostatic drug thiotepa. *Cancer Res* 1995; **55**: 1701–6.

87 Dirven HA, Megens L, Oudshoorn MJ, Dingemanse MA, Van Ommen B, Van Bladeren PJ. Glutathione conjugation of the cytostatic drug ifosfamide and the role of human glutathione S-transferases. *Chem Res Toxicol* 1995; **8**: 979–86.

88 Dirven HA, Van Ommen B, Van Bladeren PJ. Involvement of human glutathione S-transferase isoenzymes in the conjugation of cyclophosphamide metabolites with glutathione. *Cancer Res* 1994; **54**: 6215–20.

89 Nakagawa K, Saijo N, Tsuchida S *et al*. Glutathione-S-transferase pi as a determinant of drug resistance in transfectant cell lines. *J Biol Chem* 1990; **265**: 4296–301.

90 Goto S, Ihara Y, Urata Y *et al*. Doxorubicin-induced DNA intercalation and scavenging by nuclear glutathione S-transferase pi. *FASEB J* 2001; **15**: 2702–14.

91 Beaumont PO, Moore MJ, Ahmad K, Payne MM, Lee C, Riddick DS. Role of glutathione S-transferases in the resistance of human colon cancer cell lines to doxorubicin. *Cancer Res* 1998; **58**: 947–55.

92 Tew KD, Ronai Z. GST function in drug and stress response. *Drug Resist Updat* 1999; **2**: 143–7.

93 Siemann DW, Beyers KL. In vivo therapeutic potential of combination thiol depletion and alkylating chemotherapy. *Br J Cancer* 1993; **68**: 1071–9.

94 Peters RH, Jollow DJ, Stuart RK. Role of glutathione in the *in vitro* synergism between 4-hydroperoxy-cyclophosphamide and cisplatin in leukemia cell lines. *Cancer Res* 1991; **51**: 2536–41.

95 Rebbeck TR, Walker AH, Jaffe JM, White DL, Wein AJ, Malkowicz SB. Glutathione S-transferase-mu (GSTM1) and -theta (GSTT1) genotypes in the etiology of prostate cancer. *Cancer Epidemiol Biomarkers Prev* 1999; **8**: 283–7.

96 Stucker I, de Hirvonen AW, I *et al*. Genetic polymorphisms of glutathione S-transferases as modulators of lung cancer susceptibility. *Carcinogenesis* 2002; **23**: 1475–81.

97 Lewis SJ, Cherry NM, Niven RM, Barber PV, Povey AC. GSTM1, GSTT1 and GSTP1 polymorphisms and lung cancer risk. *Cancer Lett* 2002; **180**: 165–71.

98 Hoffmeyer S, Burk O, von Richter O *et al*. Functional polymorphisms of the human multidrug-resistance gene: multiple sequence variations and correlation of one allele with P-glycoprotein expression and activity *in vivo*. *Proc Natl Acad Sci U S A* 2000; **97**: 3473–8.

99 Kurata Y, Ieiri I, Kimura M *et al*. Role of human MDR1 gene polymorphism in bioavailability and interaction of digoxin, a substrate of P-glycoprotein. *Clin Pharmacol Ther* 2002; **72**: 209–19.

100 Mick R, Ratain MJ. Modeling interpatient pharmacodynamic variability of etoposide. *J Natl Cancer Inst* 1991; **83**: 1560–4.

101 Choi KE, Ratain MJ, Williams SF *et al*. Plasma pharmacokinetics of high-dose oral melphalan in patients treated with trialkylator chemotherapy and autologous bone marrow reinfusion. *Cancer Res* 1989; **49**: 1318–21.

102 Hassan M, Ljungman P, Bolme P *et al*. Busulfan bioavailability. *Blood* 1994; **84**: 2144–50.

103 Hassan M, Ehrsson H, Ljungman P. Aspects concerning busulfan pharmacokinetics and bioavailability. *Leuk Lymphoma* 1996; **22**: 395–407.

104 Gamelin E, Allain P, Maillart P *et al*. Long-term pharmacokinetic behavior of platinum after cisplatin administration. *Cancer Chemother Pharmacol* 1995; **37**: 97–102.

105 Evans WE, Relling MV. Clinical pharmacokinetics–pharmacodynamics of anticancer drugs. *Clin Pharmacokinet* 1989; **16**: 327–36.

106 Relling MV, Dervieux T. Pharmacogenetics and cancer therapy. *Nature Rev Cancer* 2001; **1**: 99–108.

107 Sonnichsen DS, Hurwitz CA, Pratt CB, Shuster JJ, Relling MV. Saturable pharmacokinetics and paclitaxel pharmacodynamics in children with solid tumors. *J Clin Oncol* 1994; **12**: 532–8.

108 Slattery JT, Kalhorn TF, McDonald GB *et al*. Conditioning regimen-dependent disposition of cyclophosphamide and hydroxycyclophosphamide in human marrow transplantation patients. *J Clin Oncol* 1996; **14**: 1484–94.

109 Hassan M, Oberg G, Bjorkholm M, Wallin I, Lindgren M. Influence of prophylactic anticonvulsant therapy on high-dose busulphan kinetics. *Cancer Chemother Pharmacol* 1993; **33**: 181–6.

110 Buggia I, Zecca M, Alessandrino EP *et al*. Itraconazole can increase systemic exposure to busulfan in patients given bone marrow transplantation. Gruppo Italiano Trapianto di Midollo Osseo (GITMO). *Anticancer Res* 1996; **16**: 2083–8.

111 Bruno R, Vivier N, Veyrat-Follet C, Montay G, Rhodes GR. Population pharmacokinetics and pharmacokinetic–pharmacodynamic relationships for docetaxel. *Invest New Drugs* 2001; **19**: 163–9.

112 Calvert AH, Newell DR, Gumbrell LA *et al*. Carboplatin dosage: prospective evaluation of a simple formula based on renal function. *J Clin Oncol* 1989; **7**: 1748–56.

113 Lichtman SM, Etcubanas E, Budman DR *et al*. The pharmacokinetics and pharmacodynamics of fludarabine phosphate in patients with renal impairment: a prospective dose adjustment study. *Cancer Invest* 2002; **20**: 904–13.

114 Sawyer M, Ratain MJ. Body surface area as a determinant of pharmacokinetics and drug dosing. *Invest New Drugs* 2001; **19**: 171–7.

115 Busse D, Busch FW, Bohnenstengel F *et al*. Dose escalation of cyclophosphamide in patients with breast cancer: consequences for pharmacokinetics and metabolism. *J Clin Oncol* 1997; **15**: 1885–96.

116 Grochow LB, Jones RJ, Brundrett RB *et al*. Pharmacokinetics of busulfan: correlation with veno-occlusive disease in patients undergoing bone marrow transplantation. *Cancer Chemother Pharmacol* 1989; **25**: 55–61.

117 Grochow LB. Busulfan disposition. the role of therapeutic monitoring in bone marrow transplantation induction regimens. *Semin Oncol* 1993; **20**: 18–25.

118 Jones RJ, Grochow LB. Pharmacology of bone marrow transplantation conditioning regimens. *Ann N Y Acad Sci* 1995; **770**: 237–41.

119 Jones RB, Matthes S, Shpall EJ *et al*. Acute lung injury following treatment with high-dose cyclophosphamide, cisplatin, and carmustine: pharmacodynamic evaluation of carmustine. *J Natl Cancer Inst* 1993; **85**: 640–7.

120 Nieto Y. Pharmacodynamics of high-dose chemotherapy. *Curr Drug Metab* 2001; **2**: 53–66.

121 van Warmerdam LJ, Rodenhuis S, van der Wall E, Maes RA, Beijnen JH. Pharmacokinetics and pharmacodynamics of carboplatin administered in a high-dose combination regimen with thiotepa, cyclophosphamide and peripheral stem cell support. *Br J Cancer* 1996; **73**: 979–84.

122 Sanathanan LP, Peck CC. The randomized concentration-controlled trial: an evaluation of its sample size efficiency. *Control Clin Trials* 1991; **12**: 780–94.

123 Evans WE, Relling MV, Rodman JH, Crom WR, Boyett JM, Pui CH. Conventional compared with individualized chemotherapy for childhood acute lymphoblastic leukemia. *N Engl J Med* 1998; **338**: 499–505.

124 Freireich EJ, Gehan EA, Rall DP, Schmidt LH, Skipper HE. Quantitative comparison of toxicity of anticancer agents in mouse, rat, hamster, dog, monkey, and man. *Cancer Chemother Rep* 1966; **50**: 219–44.

125 Du Bois D, Du Bois EF. A formula to estimate the approximate surface area if height and weight be known. *Arch Intern Med* 1916; **17**: 863–71.

126 Mitchell D, Strydom NB, van Graan CH, van der Walt WH. Human surface area: comparison of the Du Bois formula with direct photometric measurement. *Pflügers Arch* 1971; **325**: 188–90.

127 Gehan EA, George SL. Estimation of human body surface area from height and weight. *Cancer Chemother Rep* 1970; **54**: 225–35.

128 Cosolo WC, Morgan DJ, Seeman E, Zimet AS, McKendrick JJ, Zalcberg JR. Lean body mass, body surface area and epirubicin kinetics. *Anticancer Drugs* 1994; **5**: 293–7.

129 Morgan DJ, Bray KM. Lean body mass as a predictor of drug dosage: implications for drug therapy. *Clin Pharmacokinet* 1994; **26**: 292–307.

130 Murry DJ, Crom WR, Reddick WE, Bhargava R, Evans WE. Liver volume as a determinant of drug clearance in children and adolescents. *Drug Metab Dispos* 1995; **23**: 1110–16.

131 Nawaratne S, Brien JE, Seeman E et al. Relationships among liver and kidney volumes, lean body mass and drug clearance. *Br J Clin Pharmacol* 1998; **46**: 447–52.

132 Baker SD, Verweij J, Rowinsky EK et al. Role of body surface area in dosing of investigational anticancer agents in adults, 1991–2001. *J Natl Cancer Inst* 2002; **94**: 1883–8.

133 Gurney H. How to calculate the dose of chemotherapy. *Br J Cancer* 2002; **86**: 1297–302.

134 Alberts DS. Clinical pharmacology of carboplatin. *Semin Oncol* 1990; **17**: 6–8.

135 Donelli MG, Zucchetti M, Munzone E, D'Incalci M, Crosignani A. Pharmacokinetics of anticancer agents in patients with impaired liver function. *Eur J Cancer* 1998; **34**: 33–46.

136 Donahue A, McCune JS, Faucette S et al. Measured versus estimated glomerular filtration rate in the Calvert equation: influence on carboplatin dosing. *Cancer Chemother Pharmacol* 2001; **47**: 373–9.

137 Wright JG, Boddy AV, Highley M, Fenwick J, McGill A, Calvert AH. Estimation of glomerular filtration rate in cancer patients. *Br J Cancer* 2001; **84**: 452–9.

138 Pugh RN, Murray-Lyon IM, Dawson JL, Pietroni MC, Williams R. Transection of the oesophagus for bleeding oesophageal varices. *Br J Surg* 1973; **60**: 646–9.

139 Twelves C, Glynne-Jones R, Cassidy J et al. Effect of hepatic dysfunction due to liver metastases on the pharmacokinetics of capecitabine and its metabolites. *Clin Cancer Res* 1999; **5**: 1696–702.

140 Twelves CJ, Dobbs NA, Gillies HC, James CA, Rubens RD, Harper PG. Doxorubicin pharmacokinetics: the effect of abnormal liver biochemistry tests. *Cancer Chemother Pharmacol* 1998; **42**: 229–34.

141 Robieux I, Sorio R, Borsatti E et al. Pharmacokinetics of vinorelbine in patients with liver metastases. *Clin Pharmacol Ther* 1996; **59**: 32–40.

142 Rivory LP, Slaviero K, Seale JP et al. Optimizing the erythromycin breath test for use in cancer patients. *Clin Cancer Res* 2000; **6**: 3480–5.

143 Evans WE, Relling MV, Petros WP, Meyer WH, Mirro J Jr, Crom WR. Dextromethorphan and caffeine as probes for simultaneous determination of debrisoquin-oxidation and N-acetylation phenotypes in children. *Clin Pharmacol Ther* 1989; **45**: 568–73.

144 Crom WR, Webster SL, Bobo L, Teresi ME, Relling MV, Evans WE. Simultaneous administration of multiple model substrates to assess hepatic drug clearance. *Clin Pharmacol Ther* 1987; **41**: 645–50.

145 Yamamoto N, Tamura T, Kamiya Y, Sekine I, Kunitoh H, Saijo N. Correlation between docetaxel clearance and estimated cytochrome P450 activity by urinary metabolite of exogenous cortisol. *J Clin Oncol* 2000; **18**: 2301–8.

146 Doroshow JH, Synold T, Somlo G et al. Adaptive control (AC) of paclitaxel (P) systemic exposure during high-dose chemotherapy (HDCT) with P, cisplatin (DDP), cyclophosphamide (CY) and cyclosporine A (CSA) followed by stem cell rescue significantly decreases variation in hematologic recovery (HR), mucositis, and hospital stay (HS). *Proc Am Soc Clin Oncol* 1999; **18**: 200a.

147 Vassal G, Koscielny S, Challine D et al. Busulfan disposition and hepatic veno-occlusive disease in children undergoing bone marrow transplantation. *Cancer Chemother Pharmacol* 1996; **37**: 247–53.

148 Copelan EA, Bechtel TP, Avalos BR et al. Busulfan levels are influenced by prior treatment and are associated with hepatic veno-occlusive disease and early mortality but not with delayed complications following marrow transplantation. *Bone Marrow Transplant* 2001; **27**: 1121–4.

149 Slattery JT, Clift RA, Buckner CD et al. Marrow transplantation for chronic myeloid leukemia: the influence of plasma busulfan levels on the outcome of transplantation. *Blood* 1997; **89**: 3055–60.

150 Bleyzac N, Souillet G, Magron P et al. Improved clinical outcome of paediatric bone marrow recipients using a test dose and Bayesian pharmacokinetic individualization of busulfan dosage regimens. *Bone Marrow Transplant* 2001; **28**: 743–51.

151 McCune JS, Gooley T, Gibbs JP et al. Busulfan concentration and graft rejection in pediatric patients undergoing hematopoietic stem cell transplantation. *Bone Marrow Transplant* 2002; **30**: 167–73.

152 Grochow LB. Parenteral busulfan: is therapeutic monitoring still warranted? *Biol Blood Marrow Transplant* 2002; **8**: 465–7.

153 Cremers S, Schoemaker R, Bredius R et al. Pharmacokinetics of intravenous busulfan in children prior to stem cell transplantation. *Br J Clin Pharmacol* 2002; **53**: 386–9.

154 Vaughan WP, Carey D, Perry S, Westfall AO, Salzman DE. A limited sampling strategy for pharmacokinetic directed therapy with intravenous busulfan. *Biol Blood Marrow Transplant* 2002; **8**: 619–24.

155 Tabak A, Hoffer E, Rowe JM, Krivoy N. Monitoring of busulfan area under the curve: estimation by a single measurement. *Ther Drug Monit* 2001; **23**: 526–8.

156 Balasubramanian P, Chandy M, Krishnamoorthy R, Srivastava A. Evaluation of existing limited sampling models for busulfan kinetics in children with beta thalassaemia major undergoing bone marrow transplantation. *Bone Marrow Transplant* 2001; **28**: 821–5.

157 Shpall EJ, Jones RB, Holland JF et al. Intensive single-agent mitoxantrone for metastatic breast cancer. *J Natl Cancer Inst* 1988; **80**: 204–8.

158 Wallerstein R, JrSpitzer G, Dunphy F et al. A phase 2 study of mitoxantrone, etoposide, and thiotepa with autologous marrow support for patients with relapsed breast cancer. *J Clin Oncol* 1990; **8**: 1782–5.

159 Broun ER, Sledge GW, Einhorn LH, Tricot GJK. High-dose carboplatin and mitoxantrone with autologous bone marrow support in the treatment of advanced breast cancer. *Am J Clin Oncol* 1993; **16**: 9–13.

160 Margolin K, Synold T, Longmate J, Doroshow JH. Methodologic guidelines for the design of high-dose chemotherapy regimens. *Biol Blood Marrow Transplant* 2001; **7**: 414–32.

161 Jones RB, Holland JF, Bhardwaj S, Norton L, Wilfinger C, Strashun A. A phase 1–2 study of intensive-dose adriamycin for advanced breast cancer. *J Clin Oncol* 1987; **5**: 172–7.

162 Bender RA, Zwelling LA, Doroshow JH et al. Antineoplastic drugs: clinical pharmacology and therapeutic use. *Drugs* 1978; **16**: 46–87.

163 Shulman LN. The biology of alkylating-agent cellular injury. *Hematol Oncol Clin North Am* 1993; **7**: 325–35.

164 Haurani FI. Thirty-one-year survival following chemotherapy and autologous bone marrow in malignant lymphoma. *Am J Hematol* 1997; **55**: 35–8.

165 Chabner BA, Myers CE, Coleman CN, Johns DG. The clinical pharmacology of antineoplastic agents (second of two parts). *N Engl J Med* 1975; **292**: 1159–68.

166 Somlo G, Doroshow JH, Forman SJ et al. High-dose cisplatin, etoposide, and cyclophosphamide with autologous stem cell reinfusion in patients with responsive metastatic or high-risk primary breast cancer. *Cancer* 1994; **73**: 125–34.

167 Antman K, Ayash L, Elias A et al. A phase II study of high-dose cyclophosphamide, thiotepa, and carboplatin with autologous marrow support in women with measurable advanced breast cancer responding to standard-dose therapy. *J Clin Oncol* 1992; **10**: 102–10.

168 Demirer T, Buckner CD, Appelbaum FR et al. Busulfan, cyclophosphamide and fractionated total body irradiation for autologous or syngeneic marrow transplantation for acute and chronic myelogenous leukemia: Phase 1 dose escalation of busulfan based on targeted plasma levels. *Bone Marrow Transplant* 1996; **17**: 491–5.

169 Nademanee A, Sniecinski I, Schmidt GM et al. High-dose therapy followed by autologous peripheral-blood stem-cell transplantation for patients with Hodgkin's disease and non-Hodgkin's lymphoma using unprimed and granulocyte colony-stimulating factor-mobilized peripheral-blood stem cells. *J Clin Oncol* 1994; **12**: 2176–86.

170 Dong Q, Barsky D, Colvin ME et al. A structural basis for a phosphoramide mustard-induced DNA interstrand cross-link at 5′-d (GAC). *Proc Natl Acad Sci U S A* 1995; **92**: 12170–4.

171 Schwartz PS, Waxman DJ. Cyclophosphamide induces caspase 9-dependent apoptosis in 9L tumor cells. *Mol Pharmacol* 2001; **60**: 1268–79.

172 Friedman HS, Colvin OM, Aisaka K et al. Glutathione protects cardiac and skeletal muscle from cyclophosphamide-induced toxicity. *Cancer Res* 1990; **50**: 2455–62.

173 Chresta CM, Crook TR, Souhami RL. Depletion of cellular glutathione by N,N′-bis (trans-4-hydroxycyclohexyl)-N′-nitrosourea as a determinant of sensitivity of K562 human leukemia cells to 4-hydroperoxycyclophosphamide. *Cancer Res* 1990; **50**: 4067–71.

174 Tew KD. Glutathione-associated enzymes in anticancer drug resistance. *Cancer Res* 1994; **54**: 4313–20.

175 Magni M, Shammah S, Schiro R, Mellado W, Dalla-Favera R, Gianni AM. Induction of

cyclophosphamide-resistance by aldehyde–dehydrogenase gene transfer. *Blood* 1996; **87**: 1097–103.

176. Sladek NE, Kollander R, Sreerama L, Kiang DT. Cellular levels of aldehyde dehydrogenases (ALDH1A1 and ALDH3A1) as predictors of therapeutic responses to cyclophosphamide-based chemotherapy of breast cancer: a retrospective study. Rational individualization of oxazaphosphorine-based cancer chemotherapeutic regimens. *Cancer Chemother Pharmacol* 2002; **49**: 309–21.

177. Chaney SG, Sancar A. DNA repair: enzymatic mechanisms and relevance to drug response. *J Natl Cancer Inst* 1996; **88**: 1346–60.

178. Fasola G, Lo Greco P, Calori E et al. Pharmacokinetics of high-dose cyclophosphamide for bone marrow transplantation. *Haematologica* 1991; **76**: 120–5.

179. Cunningham D, Cummings J, Blackie RB et al. The pharmacokinetics of high-dose cyclophosphamide and high dose etoposide. *Med Oncol Tumor Pharmacother* 1988; **5**: 117–23.

180. Chen TL, Kennedy MJ, Anderson LW et al. Nonlinear pharmacokinetics of cyclophosphamide and 4-hydroxycyclophosphamide/aldophosphamide in patients with metastatic breast cancer receiving high-dose chemotherapy followed by autologous bone marrow transplantation. *Drug Metab Dispos* 1997; **25**: 544–51.

181. Ayash LJ, Wright JE, Tretyakov O et al. Cyclophosphamide pharmacokinetics: correlation with cardiac toxicity and tumor response. *J Clin Oncol* 1992; **10**: 995–1000.

182. Anderson LW, Chen TL, Colvin OM et al. Cyclophosphamide and 4-hydroxycyclophosphamide/aldophosphamide kinetics in patients receiving high-dose cyclophosphamide chemotherapy. *Clin Cancer Res* 1996; **2**: 1481–7.

183. Chen TL, Passos-Coelho JL. Noe DA et al. Nonlinear pharmacokinetics of cyclophosphamide in patients with metastatic breast cancer receiving high-dose chemotherapy followed by autologous bone marrow transplantation. *Cancer Res* 1995; **55**: 810–6.

184. Braverman AC, Antin JH, Plappert MT, Cook EF, Lee RT. Cyclophosphamide cardiotoxicity in bone marrow transplantation: a prospective evaluation of new drug dosing regimens. *J Clin Oncol* 1991; **9**: 1215–23.

185. Huitema AD, Mathot RA, Tibben MM, Rodenhuis S, Beijnen JH. A mechanism-based pharmacokinetic model for the cytochrome P450 drug–drug interaction between cyclophosphamide and thiotepa and the autoinduction of cyclophosphamide. *J Pharmacokinet Pharmacodyn* 2001; **28**: 211–30.

186. Mentre F, Mallet A, Steimer JL, Lokiec F. An application of population pharmacokinetics to the clinical use of cyclosporine in bone marrow transplant patients. *Transplant Proc* 1988; **20**: 466–70.

187. Perry JJ, Fleming RA, Rocco MV et al. Administration and pharmacokinetics of high-dose cyclophosphamide with hemodialysis support for allogeneic bone marrow transplantation in acute leukemia and end-stage renal disease. *Bone Marrow Transplant* 1999; **23**: 839–42.

188. Murdych T, Weisdorf DJ. Serious cardiac complications during bone marrow transplantation at the University of Minnesota, 1977–97. *Bone Marrow Transplant* 2001; **28**: 283–7.

189. Newell DR, Gore ME. Toxicity of alkylating agents: clinical characteristics and pharmacokinetic determinants. *The Toxicity of Anticancer Drugs.* Powis G, Hacker MP, eds. New York: Pergamon Press, 1991: 44–62.

190. van der Wall E, Beijnen JH, Rodenhuis S. High-dose chemotherapy regimens for solid tumors. *Cancer Treat Rev* 1995; **21**: 105–32.

191. Bergel F, Stock JA. Cytotoxic alpha amino acids and endopeptidase. *Br Emp Cancer Comp Annu* 1953; **31**: 6–21.

192. Samuels BL, Bitran JD. High-dose intravenous melphalan: a review. *J Clin Oncol* 1995; **13**: 1786–99.

193. Sarosy G, Leyland-Jones B, Soochan P, Cheson BD. The systemic administration of intravenous melphalan. *J Clin Oncol* 1988; **6**: 1768–82.

194. Ducore JM, Erickson LC, Zwelling LA, Laurent G, Kohn KW. Comparative studies of DNA cross-linking and cytotoxicity in Burkitt's lymphoma cell lines treated with *cis*-diamminedichloroplatinum (II) and L-phenylalanine mustard. *Cancer Res* 1982; **42**: 897–902.

195. Zwelling LA, Michaels S, Schwartz H, Dobson PP, Kohn KW. DNA cross-linking as an indicator of sensitivity and resistance of mouse L1210 leukemia to *cis*-diamminedichloroplatinum (II) and L-phenylalanine mustard. *Cancer Res* 1981; **41**: 640–9.

196. Ross WE, Ewig RA, Kohn KW. Differences between melphalan and nitrogen mustard in the formation and removal of DNA cross-links. *Cancer Res* 1978; **38**: 1502–6.

197. Chatterjee S, Cheng MF, Berger NA. Hypersensitivity to clinically useful alkylating agents and radiation in poly (ADP-ribose) polymerase-deficient cell lines. *Cancer Commun* 1990; **2**: 401–7.

198. Berger NA. Poly (ADP-ribose) in the cellular response to DNA damage. *Radiat Res* 1985; **101**: 4–15.

199. Begleiter A, Grover J, Froese E, Goldenberg GJ. Membrane transport, sulfhydryl levels and DNA cross-linking in Chinese hamster ovary cell mutants sensitive and resistant to melphalan. *Biochem Pharmacol* 1983; **32**: 293–300.

200. Goldenberg GJ, Begleiter A. Membrane transport of alkylating agents. *Pharmacol Ther* 1980; **8**: 237–74.

201. Begleiter A, Froese EK, Goldenberg GJ. A comparison of melphalan transport in human breast cancer cells and lymphocytes *in vitro*. *Cancer Lett* 1980; **10**: 243–51.

202. Begleiter A, Grover J, Goldenberg GJ. Mechanism of efflux of melphalan from L5178Y lymphoblasts *in vitro*. *Cancer Res* 1982; **42**: 987–91.

203. Begleiter A, Lam HY, Grover J, Froese E, Goldenberg GJ. Evidence for active transport of melphalan by two amino acid carriers in L5178Y lymphoblasts *in vitro*. *Cancer Res* 1979; **39**: 353–9.

204. Vistica DT, Toal JN, Rabinovitz M. Amino acid conferred protection against melphalan. interference with leucine protection of melphalan cytotoxicity by the basic amino acids in cultured murine L1210 leukemia cells. *Mol Pharmacol* 1978; **14**: 1136–42.

205. Groothuis DR, Lippitz BE, Fekete I et al. The effect of an amino acid-lowering diet on the rate of melphalan entry into brain and xenotransplanted glioma. *Cancer Res* 1992; **52**: 5590–6.

206. Fernandes RS, Cotter TG. Apoptosis or necrosis: intracellular levels of glutathione influence mode of cell death. *Biochem Pharmacol* 1994; **48**: 675–81.

207. Rothbarth J, Vahrmeijer AL, Mulder GJ. Modulation of cytostatic efficacy of melphalan by glutathione: mechanisms and efficacy. *Chem Biol Interact* 2002; **140**: 93–107.

208. Schecter RL, Woo A, Duong M, Batist G. In vivo and in vitro mechanisms of drug resistance in a rat mammary carcinoma model. *Cancer Res* 1991; **51**: 1434–42.

209. Yokomizo A, Kohno K, Wada M et al. Markedly decreased expression of glutathione S-transferase pi gene in human cancer cell lines resistant to buthionine sulfoximine, an inhibitor of cellular glutathione synthesis. *J Biol Chem* 1995; **270**: 19451–7.

210. Spanswick VJ, Craddock C, Sekhar M et al. Repair of DNA interstrand crosslinks as a mechanism of clinical resistance to melphalan in multiple myeloma. *Blood* 2002; **100**: 224–9.

211. Moscow JA, Swanson CA, Cowan KH. Decreased melphalan accumulation in a human breast cancer cell line selected for resistance to melphalan. *Br J Cancer* 1993; **68**: 732–7.

212. Redwood WR, Colvin OM. Transport of melphalan by sensitive and resistant L1210 cells. *Cancer Res* 1980; **40**: 1144–9.

213. Reece PA, Hill HS, Green RM et al. Renal clearance and protein binding of melphalan in patients with cancer. *Cancer Chemother Pharmacol* 1988; **22**: 348–52.

214. Ninane J, Baurain R, de Selys A, Trouet A, Cornu G. High-dose melphalan in children with advanced malignant disease: a pharmacokinetic study. *Cancer Chemother Pharmacol* 1985; **15**: 263–7.

215. Alberts DS, Chang SY, Chen HS et al. Kinetics of intravenous melphalan. *Clin Pharmacol Ther* 1979; **26**: 73–80.

216. Tricot G, Alberts DS, Johnson C et al. Safety of autotransplants with high-dose melphalan in renal failure: a pharmacokinetic and toxicity study. *Clin Cancer Res* 1996; **2**: 947–52.

217. Ploin DY, Tranchand B, Guastalla JP et al. Pharmacokinetically guided dosing for intravenous melphalan: a pilot study in patients with advanced ovarian adenocarcinoma. *Eur J Cancer* 1992; **28A**: 1311–15.

218. Pinguet F, Martel P, Fabbro M et al. Pharmacokinetics of high-dose intravenous melphalan in patients undergoing peripheral blood hematopoietic progenitor-cell transplantation. *Anticancer Res* 1997; **17**: 605–11.

219. Ardiet C, Tranchand B, Biron P, Rebattu P, Philip T. Pharmacokinetics of high-dose intravenous melphalan in children and adults with forced diuresis: report in 26 cases. *Cancer Chemother Pharmacol* 1986; **16**: 300–5.

220. Tranchand B, Ploin YD, Minuit MP et al. High-dose melphalan dosage adjustment: possibility of using a test-dose. *Cancer Chemother Pharmacol* 1989; **23**: 95–100.

221. Kergueris MF, Milpied N, Moreau P, Harousseau JL, Larousse C. Pharmacokinetics of high-dose melphalan in adults: influence of renal function. *Anticancer Res* 1994; **14**: 2379–82.

222. Ayash LJ, Elias A, Schwartz G et al. Double dose-intensive chemotherapy with autologous stem-cell support for metastatic breast cancer: no improvement in progression-free survival by the sequence of high-dose melphalan followed by cyclophosphamide, thiotepa, and carboplatin. *J Clin Oncol* 1996; **14**: 2984–92.

223. Westerfield BT, Michalski JP, McCombs C, Light

RW. Reversible melphalan-induced lung damage. *Am J Med* 1980; 68: 767–71.
224 Akasheh MS, Freytes CO, Vesole DH. Melphalan-associated pulmonary toxicity following high-dose therapy with autologous hematopoietic stem cell transplantation. *Bone Marrow Transplant* 2000; 26: 1107–9.
225 Greenbaum-Lefkoe B, Rosenstock JG, Belasco JB, Rohrbaugh TM, Meadows AT. Syndrome of inappropriate antidiuretic hormone secretion: a complication of high-dose intravenous melphalan. *Cancer* 1985; 55: 44–6.
226 Valteau-Couanet D, Vassal G, Pondarre C et al. Phase 1 study of high-dose continuous intravenous infusion of VP-16 in combination with high-dose melphalan followed by autologous bone marrow transplantation in children with stage IV neuroblastoma. *Bone Marrow Transplant* 1996; 17: 485–9.
227 Dauplat J, Legros M, Condat P, Ferriere JP, Ben Ahmed S, Plagne R. High-dose melphalan and autologous bone marrow support for treatment of ovarian carcinoma with positive second-look operation. *Gynecol Oncol* 1989; 34: 294–8.
228 Viens P, Maraninchi D, Legros M et al. High dose melphalan and autologous marrow rescue in advanced epithelial ovarian carcinomas: a retrospective analysis of 35 patients treated in France. *Bone Marrow Transplant* 1990; 5: 227–33.
229 Donato ML, Gershenson DM, Wharton JT et al. High-dose topotecan, melphalan, and cyclophosphamide (TMC) with stem cell support: a new regimen for the treatment of advanced ovarian cancer. *Gynecol Oncol* 2001; 82: 420–6.
230 Somlo G, Chow W, Hamasaki V et al. Tandem-cycle high-dose melphalan and cisplatin with peripheral blood progenitor cell support in patients with breast cancer and other malignancies. *Biol Blood Marrow Transplant* 2001; 7: 284–93.
231 Gutierrez-Delgado F, Holmberg LA, Hooper H et al. High-dose busulfan, melphalan and thiotepa as consolidation for non-inflammatory high-risk breast cancer. *Bone Marrow Transplant* 2000; 26: 51–9.
232 Moreau P, Kergueris MF, Milpied N et al. A pilot study of 220 mg/m2 melphalan followed by autologous stem cell transplantation in patients with advanced haematological malignancies: Pharmacokinetics and toxicity. *Br J Haematol* 1996; 95: 527–30.
233 Antman K, Eder JP, Elias A et al. High-dose thiotepa alone and in combination regimens with bone marrow support. *Semin Oncol* 1990; 17: 33–8.
234 Prince HM, Rischin D, Toner GC et al. Repetitive high-dose therapy with cyclophosphamide, thiotepa and docetaxel with peripheral blood progenitor cell and filgrastim support for metastatic and locally advanced breast cancer: results of a phase I study. *Bone Marrow Transplant* 2000; 26: 955–61.
235 Bibawi S, Abi-Said D, Fayad L et al. Thiotepa, busulfan, and cyclophosphamide as a preparative regimen for allogeneic transplantation for advanced myelodysplastic syndrome and acute myelogenous leukemia. *Am J Hematol* 2001; 67: 227–33.
236 Teicher BA, Waxman DJ, Holden SA et al. Evidence for enzymatic activation and oxygen involvement in cytotoxicity and antitumor activity of N,N′,N″-triethylenethiophosphoramide. *Cancer Res* 1989; 49: 4996–5001.
237 Cohen NA, Egorin MJ, Snyder SW et al. Interaction of N,N′,N″-triethylenethiophosphoramide and N,N′,N″-triethylenephosphoramide with cellular DNA. *Cancer Res* 1991; 51: 4360–6.
238 Miller B, Tenenholz T, Egorin MJ, Sosnovsky G, Rao NU, Gutierrez PL. Cellular pharmacology of N,N′,N″-triethylene thiophosphoramide. *Cancer Lett* 1988; 41: 157–68.
239 Maanen MJ, Smeets CJ, Beijnen JH. Chemistry, pharmacology and pharmacokinetics of N,N′,N″-triethylenethiophosphoramide (thiotepa). *Cancer Treat Rev* 2000; 26: 257–68.
240 Egorin MJ, Snyder SW, Pan S-S, Daly C. Cellular transport and accumulation of thiotepa in murine, human, and avian cells. *Cancer Res* 1989; 49: 5611–17.
241 Egorin MJ, Snyder SW, Pan SS, Daly C. Cellular transport and accumulation of thiotepa. *Semin Oncol* 1990; 17: 7–17.
242 Egorin MJ, Snyder SW, Wietharn BE. Effects of ethanolamine and choline on thiotepa cellular accumulation and cytotoxicity in L1210 cells. *Cancer Res* 1990; 50: 4322–7.
243 Buller AL, Clapper ML, Tew KD. Glutathione S-transferases in nitrogen mustard-resistant and—sensitive cell lines. *Molec Pharmacol* 1987; 31: 575–8.
244 Ciaccio PJ, Tew KD, LaCreta FP. Enzymatic conjugation of chlorambucil with glutathione by human glutathione S-transferases and inhibition by ethacrynic acid. *Biochem Pharmacol* 1991; 42: 1504–7.
245 O'Dwyer PJ, Hamilton TC, Yao KS, Tew KD, Ozols RF. Modulation of glutathione and related enzymes in reversal of resistance to anticancer drugs. *Hematol Oncol Clin North Am* 1995; 9: 383–96.
246 Gill RD, Cussac C, Souhami RL, Laval F. Increased resistance to N,N′,N″-triethylenethiophosphoramide (thiotepa) in cells expressing the *Escherichia coli* formamidopyrimidine-DNA glycosylase. *Cancer Res* 1996; 56: 3721–4.
247 Xu Y, Hansen WK, Rosenquist TA, Williams DA, Limp-Foster M, Kelley MR. Protection of mammalian cells against chemotherapeutic agents thiotepa, 1,3-N,N′-*bis* (2-chloroethyl) -N-nitrosourea, and mafosfamide using the DNA base excision repair genes Fpg and alpha-hOgg1: implications for protective gene therapy applications. *J Pharmacol Exp Ther* 2001; 296: 825–31.
248 Ng SF, Waxman DJ. N,N′,N″-triethylenethiophosphoramide (thiotepa) oxygenation by constitutive hepatic P450 enzymes and modulation of drug metabolism and clearance *in vivo* by P450-inducing agents. *Cancer Res* 1991; 51: 2340–7.
249 Hagen B, Dale O, Neverdal G, Azri S, Nilsen OG. Metabolism and alkylating activity of thiotepa in rat liver slice incubation. *Cancer Chemother Pharmacol* 1991; 28: 441–7.
250 Chang TK, Chen G, Waxman DJ. Modulation of thiotepa antitumor activity *in vivo* by alteration of liver cytochrome P450-catalyzed drug metabolism. *J Pharmacol Exp Ther* 1995; 274: 270–5.
251 Jacobson PA, Green K, Birnbaum A, Remmel RP. Cytochrome P450 isozymes 3A4 and 2B6 are involved in the *in vitro* human metabolism of thiotepa to TEPA. *Cancer Chemother Pharmacol* 2002; 49: 461–7.
252 Bibby MC, McDermott BJ, Double JA, Phillips RM, Loadman PM, Burgess L. Influence of the tissue distribution of Thiotepa and its metabolite, TEPA, on the response of murine colon tumours. *Cancer Chemother Pharmacol* 1987; 20: 203–6.
253 Rae JM, Soukhova NV, Flockhart DA, Desta Z. Triethylenethiophosphoramide is a specific inhibitor of cytochrome P450 2B6: implications for cyclophosphamide metabolism. *Drug Metab Dispos* 2002; 30: 525–30.
254 Huitema AD, Kerbusch T, Tibben MM, Rodenhuis S, Beijnen JH. Reduction of cyclophosphamide bioactivation by thiotepa: critical sequence-dependency in high-dose chemotherapy regimens. *Cancer Chemother Pharmacol* 2000; 46: 119–27.
255 van Maanen MJ, Huitema AD, Beijen JH. Influence of co-medicated drugs on the biotransformation of thiotepa to TEPA and thiotepa-mercapturate. *Anticancer Res* 2000; 20: 1711–6.
256 Henner WD, Shea TC, Furlong EA et al. Pharmacokinetics of continuous-infusion high-dose thiotepa. *Cancer Treat Rep* 1987; 71: 1043–7.
257 Ackland SP, Choi KE, Ratain MJ et al. Human plasma pharmacokinetics of thiotepa following administration of high-dose thiotepa and cyclophosphamide. *J Clin Oncol* 1988; 6: 1192–6.
258 O'Dwyer PJ, LaCreta F, Engstrom PF et al. Phase 1/pharmacokinetic reevaluation of thiotepa. *Cancer Res* 1991; 51: 3171–6.
259 Kletzel M, Kearns GL, Wells TG, Thompson HC Jr. Pharmacokinetics of high dose thiotepa in children undergoing autologous bone marrow transplantation. *Bone Marrow Transplant* 1992; 10: 171–5.
260 O'Dwyer PJ, LaCreta FP, Schilder R et al. Phase 1 trial of thiotepa in combination with recombinant human granulocyte-macrophage colony-stimulating factor. *J Clin Oncol* 1992; 10: 1352–8.
261 Przepiorka D, Madden T, Ippoliti C, Estrov Z, Dimopoulos M. Dosing of thiotepa for myeloablative therapy. *Cancer Chemother Pharmacol* 1995; 37: 155–60.
262 Chen TL, Kennedy MJ, Kiraly SB, Manos AS, Goodman SN, Grochow LB. Pharmacokinetics and urinary excretion of thiotepa and tepa in patients with metastatic breast cancer receiving high-dose chemotherapy followed by autologous bone marrow transplantation. *Proc Am Assoc Cancer Res* 1997; 38: A7.
263 van Maanen MJ, Huitema AD, Rodenhuis S, Beijnen JH. Urinary excretion of thiotepa and its metabolites in patients treated with high-dose cyclophosphamide, thiotepa and carboplatin. *Anticancer Drugs* 2001; 12: 519–24.
264 Huitema AD, Mathot RA, Tibben MM, Rodenhuis S, Beijnen JH. Validation of a therapeutic drug monitoring strategy for thiotepa in a high-dose chemotherapy regimen. *Ther Drug Monit* 2001; 23: 650–7.
265 Wolff SN, Herzig RH, Fay JW et al. High-dose N,N′,N″-triethylenethiophosphoramide (thiotepa) with autologous bone marrow transplantation: phase 1 studies. *Semin Oncol* 1990; 17: 2–6.
266 Huitema AD, Spaander M, Mathjt RA et al. Relationship between exposure and toxicity in high-dose chemotherapy with cyclophosphamide, thiotepa and carboplatin. *Ann Oncol* 2002; 13: 374–84.
267 Mileshkin L, Prince HM, Rischin D, Zimet A. Severe interstitial pneumonitis following high-dose cyclophosphamide, thiotepa and docetaxel: two case reports and a review of the literature. *Bone Marrow Transplant* 2001; 27: 559–63.
268 Alidina A, Lawrence D, Ford LA et al. Thiotepa-associated cardiomyopathy during blood or marrow transplantation: association with the female sex and cardiac risk factors. *Biol Blood Marrow Transplant* 1999; 5: 322–7.
269 Bengala C, Tibaldi C, Pazzagli I et al. High-dose (HD) thiotepa and melphalan (L-PAM) with

hemopoietic progenitor support as consolidation treatment following paclitaxel (TXL) -containing chemotherapy in metastatic breast cancer (MBC): a phase 2 study with pharmacokinetic profile analysis. *Proc Am Soc Clin Oncol* 1997; **16**: A343.

270 Small EJ, Damon LE, Frye J et al. Thiotepa, VP-16 and dose-adjusted carboplatin (TVCA) with autologous bone marrow (ABM) or peripheral blood stem cell (PBSC) rescue for treatment of refractory germ cell tumors: efficacy and pharmacokinetic data. *Proc Am Soc Clin Oncol* 1995; **14**: A1507.

271 Shpall EJ, Jones RB, Bearman SI, Purdy MP. Future strategies for the treatment of advanced epithelial ovarian cancer using high-dose chemotherapy and autologous bone marrow support. *Gynecol Oncol* 1994; **54**: 357–61.

272 Kushner BH, Cheung NK, Kramer K, Dunkel IJ, Calleja E, Boulad F. Topotecan combined with myeloablative doses of thiotepa and carboplatin for neuroblastoma, brain tumors, and other poor-risk solid tumors in children and young adults. *Bone Marrow Transplant* 2001; **28**: 551–6.

273 Buggia I, Locatelli F, Regazzi MB, Zecca M. Busulfan. *Ann Pharmacother* 1994; **28**: 1055–62.

274 Marsh JC. The effects of cancer chemotherapeutic agents on normal hematopoietic precursor cells: a review. *Cancer Res* 1976; **36**: 1853–82.

275 Tohda S, Nagata K, Suzuki T, Nara N. Comparative effects of busulfan, cytosine arabinoside and adriamycin on different maturation stages of normal human bone marrow cells. *Acta Haematol* 1990; **83**: 16–21.

276 Pacheco DY, Stratton NK, Gibson NW. Comparison of the mechanism of action of busulfan with hepsulfam, a new antileukemic agent, in the L1210 cell line. *Cancer Res* 1989; **49**: 5108–10.

277 Miltenburger HG, Metzger P, Krause C. Busulphan-induced chromosomal aberrations in intestinal cells of Chinese hamster. *Mutat Res* 1980; **79**: 257–62.

278 Bedford P, Fox BW. Repair of DNA interstrand crosslinks after busulphan: a possible mode of resistance. *Cancer Chemother Pharmacol* 1982; **8**: 3–7.

279 Hare CB, Elion GB, Colvin OM et al. Characterization of the mechanisms of busulfan resistance in a human glioblastoma multiforme xenograft. *Cancer Chemother Pharmacol* 1997; **40**: 409–14.

280 Hassan M, Oberg G, Ehrsson H et al. Pharmacokinetic and metabolic studies of high-dose busulphan in adults. *Eur J Clin Pharmacol* 1989; **36**: 525–30.

281 Hassan M, Oberg G, Ericson K et al. In vivo distribution of [^{11}C]-busulfan in cynomolgus monkey and in the brain of a human patient. *Cancer Chemother Pharmacol* 1992; **30**: 81–5.

282 Hassan M, Ehrsson H, Smedmyr B et al. Cerebrospinal fluid and plasma concentrations of busulfan during high-dose therapy. *Bone Marrow Transplant* 1989; **4**: 113–4.

283 Ullery LL, Gibbs JP, Ames GW, Senecal FM, Slattery JT. Busulfan clearance in renal failure and hemodialysis. *Bone Marrow Transplant* 2000; **25**: 201–3.

284 Vassal G, Gouyette A, Hartmann O, Pico JL, Lemerle J. Pharmacokinetics of high-dose busulfan in children. *Cancer Chemother Pharmacol* 1989; **24**: 386–90.

285 Hassan M, Fasth A, Gerritsen B et al. Busulphan kinetics and limited sampling model in children with leukemia and inherited disorders. *Bone Marrow Transplant* 1996; **18**: 843–50.

286 Grochow LB, Krivit W, Whitley CB, Blazar B. Busulfan disposition in children. *Blood* 1990; **75**: 1723–7.

287 Hassan M, Oberg G, Bekassy AN et al. Pharmacokinetics of high-dose busulphan in relation to age and chronopharmacology. *Cancer Chemother Pharmacol* 1991; **28**: 130–4.

288 Regazzi MB, Locatelli F, Buggia I et al. Disposition of high-dose busulfan in pediatric patients undergoing bone marrow transplantation. *Clin Pharmacol Ther* 1993; **54**: 45–52.

289 Vassal G. Pharmacologically-guided dose adjustment of busulfan in high-dose chemotherapy regimens: rationale and pitfalls. *Anticancer Res* 1994; **14**: 2363–70.

290 Vassal G, Challine D, Koscielny S et al. Chronopharmacology of high-dose busulfan in children. *Cancer Res* 1993; **53**: 1534–7.

291 Shaw PJ, Scharping CE, Brian RJ, Earl JW. Busulfan pharmacokinetics using a single daily high-dose regimen in children with acute leukemia. *Blood* 1994; **84**: 2357–62.

292 Baker KS, Bostrom B, DeFor T, Ramsay NK, Woods WG, Blazar BR. Busulfan pharmacokinetics do not predict relapse in acute myeloid leukemia. *Bone Marrow Transplant* 2000; **26**: 607–14.

293 Kashyap A, Wingard J, Cagnoni P et al. Intravenous versus oral busulfan as part of a busulfan/cyclophosphamide preparative regimen for allogeneic hematopoietic stem cell transplantation: decreased incidence of hepatic veno-occlusive disease (HVOD), HVOD-related mortality, and overall 100-day mortality. *Biol Blood Marrow Transplant* 2002; **8**: 493–500.

294 Dix SP, Wingard JR, Mullins RE et al. Association of busulfan area under the curve with venoocclusive disease following BMT. *Bone Marrow Transplant* 1996; **17**: 225–30.

295 Russell JA, Tran HT, Quinlan D et al. Once-daily intravenous busulfan given with fludarabine as conditioning for allogeneic stem cell transplantation: study of pharmacokinetics and early clinical outcomes. *Biol Blood Marrow Transplant* 2002; **8**: 468–76.

296 Slattery JT, Sanders JE, Buckner CD et al. Graft-rejection and toxicity following bone marrow transplantation in relation to busulfan pharmacokinetics. *Bone Marrow Transplant* 1995; **16**: 31–42.

297 Bolinger AM, Zangwill AB, Slattery JT et al. Target dose adjustment of busulfan in pediatric patients undergoing bone marrow transplantation. *Bone Marrow Transplant* 2001; **28**: 1013–8.

298 Andersson BS, Thall PF, Madden T et al. Busulfan systemic exposure relative to regimen-related toxicity and acute graft-versus-host disease: defining a therapeutic window for i.v. BUCY2 in chronic myelogenous leukemia. *Biol Blood Marrow Transplant* 2002; **8**: 477–85.

299 Hassan M, Ljungman P, Ringden O et al. The effect of busulphan on the pharmacokinetics of cyclophosphamide and its 4-hydroxy metabolite: Time interval influence on therapeutic efficacy and therapy-related toxicity. *Bone Marrow Transplant* 2000; **25**: 915–24.

300 Kohn KW, Ewig RAG, Erickson LC, Zwelling LA. Measurement of strand breaks and cross-links by alkaline elution. In: Friedberg EC, Hanawalt PC, eds. *DNA Repair: A Laboratory Manual of Research Procedures*. New York: Marcel Dekker, 1981: 379–401.

301 Frischer H, Kennedy EJ, Chigurupati R, Sivarajan M. Glutathione, cell proliferation, and 1,3–(2-chloroethyl)-1-nitrosourea in K562 leukemia. *J Clin Invest* 1993; **92**: 2761–7.

302 Dolan ME, Chae MY, Pegg AE, Mullen JH, Friedman HS, Moschel RC. Metabolism of O6-benzylguanine, an inactivator of O6-alkylguanine-DNA alkyltransferase. *Cancer Res* 1994; **54**: 5123–30.

303 He XM, Ostrowski LE, von Wronski MA et al. Expression of O6-methylguanine-DNA methyltransferase in six human medulloblastoma cell lines. *Cancer Res* 1992; **52**: 1144–8.

304 Gerson SL, Willson JK. O6-alkylguanine-DNA alkyltransferase: a target for the modulation of drug resistance. *Hematol Oncol Clin North Am* 1995; **9**: 431–50.

305 Kurpad SN, Dolan ME, McLendon RE et al. Intra-arterial O6-benzylguanine enables the specific therapy of nitrosourea-resistant intracranial human glioma xenografts in athymic rats with 1,3-bis (2-chloroethyl)-1-nitrosourea. *Cancer Chemother Pharmacol* 1997; **39**: 307–16.

306 Henner WD, Peters WP, Eder JP et al. Pharmacokinetics and immediate effects of high-dose carmustine in man. *Cancer Treat Rep* 1986; **70**: 877–80.

307 Jones RB, Matthes S, Kemme D, Dufton C, Kernan S. Cyclophosphamide, cisplatin, and carmustine: pharmacokinetics of carmustine following multiple alkylating-agent interactions. *Cancer Chemother Pharmacol* 1994; **35**: 59–63.

308 Abushamaa AM, Sporn TA, Folz RJ. Oxidative stress and inflammation contribute to lung toxicity after a common breast cancer chemotherapy regimen. *Am J Physiol Lung Cell Mol Physiol* 2002; **283**: L336–L345.

309 Todd NW, Peters WP, Ost AH, Roggli VL, Piantadosi CA. Pulmonary drug toxicity in patients with primary breast cancer treated with high-dose combination chemotherapy and autologous bone marrow transplantation. *Am Rev Respir Dis* 1993; **147**: 1264–70.

310 Cao TM, Negrin RS, Stockerl-Goldstein KE et al. Pulmonary toxicity syndrome in breast cancer patients undergoing BCNU-containing high-dose chemotherapy and autologous hematopoietic cell transplantation. *Biol Blood Marrow Transplant* 2000; **6**: 387–94.

311 Ayash LJ, Hunt M, Antman K et al. Hepatic venooclusive disease in autologous bone marrow tranplantation of solid tumors and lymphomas. *J Clin Oncol* 1990; **8**: 1699–706.

312 Kanj SS, Sharara AI, Shpall EJ, Jones RB, Peters WP. Myocardial ischemia associated with high-dose carmustine infusion. *Cancer* 1991; **68**: 1910–2.

313 Nieto Y, Cagnoni PJ, Bearman SI, Shpall EJ, Matthes S, Jones RB. Cardiac toxicity following high-dose cyclophosphamide, cisplatin, and BCNU (STAMP-I) for breast cancer. *Biol Blood Marrow Transplant* 2000; **6**: 198–203.

314 Rosenberg B, VanCamp L, Trosko JE, Mansour VH. Platinum compounds: a new class of potent antitumour agents. *Nature* 1969; **222**: 385–6.

315 Motzer RJ, Bajorin DF, Bosl GJ. 'Poor-risk' germ cell tumors: current progress and future directions. *Semin Oncol* 1992; **19**: 206–14.

316 McGuire WP, Hoskins WJ, Brady MF et al. Taxol and cisplatin (TP) improves outcome in advanced ovarian cancer (AOC) as compared to cytoxan and cisplatin (CP). *Proc Am Soc Clin Oncol* 1995; **14**: 275.

317 Sledge GW Jr, Loehrer PJSr, Roth BJ, Einhorn LH.

Cisplatin as first-line therapy for metastatic breast cancer. *J Clin Oncol* 1988; **6**: 1811–4.
318 Gandara DR, Wold H, Perez EA *et al*. Cisplatin dose intensity in non-small cell lung cancer: phase 2 results of a day 1 and day 8 high-dose regimen. *J Natl Cancer Inst* 1989; **81**: 790–4.
319 Vokes EE, Moormeier JA, Ratain MJ *et al*. 5-Fluorouracil, leucovorin, hydroxyurea, and escalating doses of continuous-infusion cisplatin with concomitant radiotherapy: a clinical and pharmacologic study. *Cancer Chemother Pharmacol* 1992; **29**: 178–84.
320 Peters WP, Stuart A, Klotman M *et al*. High-dose combination cyclophosphamide, cisplatin, and melphalan with autologous bone marrow support: a clinical and pharmacologic study. *Cancer Chemother Pharmacol* 1989; **23**: 377–83.
321 Hussein AM, Petros WP, Ross M *et al*. A phase 1/2 study of high-dose cyclophosphamide, cisplatin, and thioTEPA followed by autologous bone marrow and granulocyte colony-stimulating factor-primed peripheral-blood progenitor cells in patients with advanced malignancies. *Cancer Chemother Pharmacol* 1996; **37**: 561–8.
322 Farrell N. Non-classical platinum antitumor agents: perspectives for design and development of new drugs complementary to cisplatin. *Cancer Invest* 1993; **11**: 578–89.
323 Zwelling LA, Kohn KW, Ross WE, Ewig RA, Anderson T. Kinetics of formation and disappearance of a DNA cross-linking effect in mouse leukemia L1210 cells treated with *cis*- and *trans*-diamminedichloroplatinum (II). *Cancer Res* 1978; **38**: 1762–8.
324 Zwelling LA, Kohn KW. Mechanism of action of *cis*-dichlorodiammineplatinum (II). *Cancer Treat Rep* 1979; **63**: 1439–44.
325 Aghajanian C, Zhuo Y, Rosales SN, Schwartz GK, Spriggs DR. Transcriptional activators involved in cellular resistance to cisplatin. *Proc Am Assoc Cancer Res* 1996; **37**: A2750.
326 Kaneko T, Sakaguchi Y, Matsuda H *et al*. Induction of p53 protein and apoptosis following treatment with chemotherapeutic agents alone and combined with hyperthermia in a rat mammary adenocarcinoma cell line. *Proc Am Assoc Cancer Res* 1995; **36**: A2475.
327 Meijer C, Mulder NH, Timmer-Bosscha H, Sluiter WJ, Meersma GJ, de Vries EGE. Relationship of cellular glutathione to the cytotoxicity and resistance of seven platinum compounds. *Cancer Res* 1992; **52**: 6885–9.
328 de Graeff A, Slebos RJC, Rodenhuis S. Resistance to cisplatin and analogues: mechanisms and potential clinical implications. *Cancer Chemother Pharmacol* 1988; **22**: 325–32.
329 Bose RN. Biomolecular targets for platinum antitumor drugs. *Mini Rev Med Chem* 2002; **2**: 103–11.
330 Levresse V, Marek L, Blumberg D, Heasley LE. Regulation of platinum-compound cytotoxicity by the c-Jun *N*-terminal kinase and c-Jun signaling pathway in small-cell lung cancer cells. *Mol Pharmacol* 2002; **62**: 689–97.
331 Evans DL, Tilby M, Dive C. Differential sensitivity to the induction of apoptosis by cisplatin in proliferating and quiescent immature rat thymocytes is independent of the levels of drug accumulation and DNA adduct formation. *Cancer Res* 1994; **54**: 1596–603.
332 Brown R, Anthoney A, Gallagher W, McIlwrath A, Jones N, Dive C. p53 Dependent signal pathways as drug targets. *EORTC Early Drug Development Meeting*. 1995: 29–30.
333 Gosland M, Lum B, Schimmelpfennig J, Baker J, Doukas M. Insights into mechanisms of cisplatin resistance and potential for its clinical reversal. *Pharmacotherapy* 1996; **16**: 16–39.
334 Parker RJ, Eastman A, Bostick-Bruton F, Reed E. Acquired cisplatin resistance in human ovarian cancer cells is associated with enhanced repair of cisplatin-DNA lesions and reduced drug accumulation. *J Clin Invest* 1991; **87**: 772–7.
335 Kelley SL, Basu A, Teicher BA, Hacker MP, Hamer DH, Lazo J. Overexpression of metallothionein confers resistance to anticancer drugs. *Science* 1988; **241**: 1813–5.
336 Dabholkar M, Vionnet J, Bostick-Bruton FYuJJ, Reed E. Messenger RNA levels of XPAC and ERCC1 in ovarian cancer tissue correlate with response to platinum-based chemotherapy. *J Clin Invest* 1994; **94**: 703–8.
337 States JC, Reed E. Enhanced XPA mRNA levels in cisplatin-resistant human ovarian cancer are not associated with XPA mutations or gene amplification. *Cancer Lett* 1996; **108**: 233–7.
338 Shirota Y, Stoehlmacher J, Brabender J *et al*. ERCC1 and thymidylate synthase mRNA levels predict survival for colorectal cancer patients receiving combination oxaliplatin and fluorouracil chemotherapy. *J Clin Oncol* 2001; **19**: 4298–304.
339 Poirier MC, Reed E, Zwelling LA, Ozols RF, Litterst CL, Yuspa SH. Polyclonal antibodies to quantitate *cis*-diamminedichloroplatinum (II): DNA adducts in cancer patients and animal models. *Environ Health Perspect* 1985; **62**: 89–94.
340 Reed E, Yuspa SH, Zwelling LA, Ozols RF, Poirier MC. Quantitation of *cis*-diamminedichloroplatinum II (cisplatin): DNA-intrastrand adducts in testicular and ovarian cancer patients receiving cisplatin chemotherapy. *J Clin Invest* 1986; **77**: 545–50.
341 Zhao R, Rabo YB, Egyhazi S *et al*. Apoptosis and c-jun induction by cisplatin in a human melanoma cell line and a drug-resistant daughter cell line. *Anticancer Drugs* 1995; **6**: 657–68.
342 Ribrag V, Droz JP, Morizet J, Leclercq B, Gouyette A, Chabot GG. Test dose-guided administration of cisplatin in an anephric patient: a case report. *Ann Oncol* 1993; **4**: 679–82.
343 Osman NM, Litterst CL. Effect of probenecid and N′-methylnicotinamide on renal handling of cis-dichlorodiammineplatinum-II in rats. *Cancer Lett* 1983; **19**: 107–11.
344 Schierl R, Rohrer B, Hohnloser J. Long-term platinum excretion in patients treated with cisplatin. *Cancer Chemother Pharmacol* 1995; **36**: 75–8.
345 Cagnoni PJ, Matthes S, Dufton C *et al*. Ondansetron significantly reduces the area under the curve (AUC) of cyclophosphamide (CPA) and cisplatin (CDDP). *Proc Am Soc Clin Oncol* 1995; **14**: A1489.
346 Petros W, Gilbert C, Fehdrau R, Ohly K, Peters W. The effect of prochlorperazine vs. metoclopramide on cisplatin pharmacokinetics/pharmacodynamics. *Proc Am Assoc Cancer Res* 1996; **37**: A1219.
347 Moulder JE, Fish BL, Holcenberg JS, Sun GX. Hepatic function and drug pharmacokinetics after total body irradiation plus bone marrow transplant. *Int J Radiat Oncol Biol Phys* 1990; **19**: 1389–96.
348 Jacobs C, Kaubisch S, Halsey J *et al*. The use of probenecid as a chemoprotector against cisplatin nephrotoxicity. *Cancer* 1991; **67**: 1518–24.
349 Zucchetti M, D'Incalci M, Willems Y, Cavalli F, Sessa C. Lack of effect of cisplatin on i.v. L-PAM plasma pharmacokinetics in ovarian cancer patients. *Cancer Chemother Pharmacol* 1988; **22**: 87–9.
350 Thomas HD, Porter DJ, Bartelink I *et al*. Randomized cross-over clinical trial to study potential pharmacokinetic interactions between cisplatin or carboplatin and etoposide. *Br J Clin Pharmacol* 2002; **53**: 83–91.
351 Somlo G, Doroshow JH, Lev-Ran A *et al*. Effect of low-dose prophylactic dopamine on high-dose cisplatin-induced electrolyte wasting, ototoxicity, and epidermal growth factor excretion: a randomized, placebo-controlled, double-blind trial. *J Clin Oncol* 1995; **13**: 1231–7.
352 Motzer RJ, Gulati SC, Tong WP *et al*. Phase 1 trial with pharmacokinetic analyses of high-dose carboplatin, etoposide, and cyclophosphamide with autologous bone marrow transplantation inpatients with refractory germ cell tumors. *Cancer Res* 1993; **53**: 3730–5.
353 Margolin K, Doroshow JH, Hamasaki V *et al*. Treatment of relapsed germ cell cancer with two cycles of high-dose ifosfamide, carboplatin, and etoposide with autologous stem cell support. *J Clin Oncol* 1996; **14**: 2631–7.
354 Stiff PJ, McKenzie RS, Alberts DS *et al*. Phase 1 clinical and pharmacokinetic study of high-dose mitoxantrone combined with carboplatin, cyclophosphamide, and autologous bone marrow rescue: high response rate for refractory ovarian carcinoma. *J Clin Oncol* 1994; **12**: 176–83.
355 O'Reilly S, Walczak J, Egorin M *et al*. A phase 1 trial of high dose chemotherapy (HDC) with cyclophosphamide (CY) and AUC dosed carboplatin (CBDCA) in advanced ovarian cancer using a continuous reassessment method for dose escalation. *Proc Am Soc Clin Oncol* 1996; **15**: A802.
356 Murry DJ, Sandlund JT, Stricklin LM, Rodman JH. Pharmacokinetics and acute renal effects of continuously infused carboplatin. *Clin Pharmacol Ther* 1993; **54**: 374–80.
357 van Warmerdam LJ, van der Wall E, ten Bokkel Huinink WW, Schornagel JH, Beijnen JH, Rodenhuis S. Pharmacokinetics and pharmacodynamics of carboplatin administered in a high-dose combination regimen with thiotepa, cyclophosphamide and peripheral stem cell support (PSCS). *Proc Am Soc Clin Oncol* 1995; **14**: A1503.
358 Egorin MJ, Van Echo DA, Olman EA, Whitacre MY, Forrest A, Aisner J. Prospective validation of a pharmacologically based dosing scheme for the *cis*-diamminedichloroplatinum (II) analogue diamminecyclobutanedicarboxylatoplatinum. *Cancer Res* 1985; **45**: 6502–6.
359 Johansen MJ, Madden T, Mehra RC *et al*. Phase I pharmacokinetic study of multicycle high-dose carboplatin followed by peripheral-blood stem-cell infusion in patients with cancer. *J Clin Oncol* 1997; **15**: 1481–91.
360 Colby C, Koziol S, McAfee SL, Yeap B, Spitzer TR. High-dose carboplatin and regimen-related toxicity following autologous bone marrow transplant. *Bone Marrow Transplant* 2002; **29**: 467–72.
361 Wright JE, Antman KH, Willinghurst LA *et al*. Carboplatin infusion pharmacokinetics in the autologous bone marrow transplant setting. *Proc Am Assoc Cancer Res* 1990; **31**: A1080.
362 Motzer RJ, Niedzwiecki D, Isaacs M *et al*. Carboplatin-based chemotherapy with pharma-

363 Suzuki S, Koide M, Sakamoto S, Matsuo T. Pharmacokinetics of carboplatin and etoposide in a haemodialysis patient with Merkel-cell carcinoma. *Nephrol Dial Transplant* 1997; **12**: 137–40.

364 Tranchand B, Ardiet C, Bouffet E *et al*. Effect of carboplatin on the pharmacokinetics of melphalan administered intravenously. *Bull Cancer (Paris)* 1994; **81**: 43–6.

365 Shea T, Graham M, Bernard S *et al*. A clinical and pharmacokinetic study of high-dose carboplatin, paclitaxel, granulocyte colony-stimulating factor, and peripheral blood stem cells in patients with unresectable or metastatic cancer. *Semin Oncol* 1995; **22**: 80–5.

366 Obasaju CK, Johnson SW, Rogatko A *et al*. Evaluation of carboplatin pharmacokinetics in the absence and presence of paclitaxel. *Clin Cancer Res* 1996; **2**: 549–52.

367 Kohl P, Koppler H, Schmidt L *et al*. Pharmacokinetics of high-dose etoposide after short-term infusion. *Cancer Chemother Pharmacol* 1992; **29**: 316–20.

368 Rodman JH, Murry DJ, Madden T, Santana VM. Altered etoposide pharmacokinetics and time to engraftment in pediatric patients undergoing autologous bone marrow transplantation. *J Clin Oncol* 1994; **12**: 2390–7.

369 Shea TC, Flaherty M, Elias A *et al*. A phase 1 clinical and pharmacokinetic study of carboplatin and autologous bone marrow support. *J Clin Oncol* 1989; **7**: 651–61.

370 Wright JE, Elias A, Tretyakov O *et al*. High-dose ifosfamide, carboplatin, and etoposide pharmacokinetics: correlation of plasma drug levels with renal toxicity. *Cancer Chemother Pharmacol* 1995; **36**: 345–51.

371 Shea TC, Mason JR, Storniolo AM *et al*. Sequential cycles of high-dose carboplatin administered with recombinant human granulocyte-macrophage colony-stimulating factor and repeated infusions of autologous peripheral-blood progenitor cells: a novel and effective method for delivering multiple courses of dose-intensive therapy. *J Clin Oncol* 1992; **10**: 464–73.

372 Broun ER, Gonin R, Nichols CR, Einhorn LH. A retrospective analysis of carboplatin (CBDCA) area under the curve (AUC) in relation to toxicity and survival in testis cancer patients undergoing high dose therapy (HDT) with autologous bone marrow transplant (ABMT). *Proc Am Soc Clin Oncol* 1996; **15**: A703.

373 Vogelzang NJ, Raghavan D, Kennedy BJ. VP-16–213 (etoposide): the mandrake root from Issyk-Kul. *Am J Med* 1982; **72**: 136–44.

374 Blume KG, Forman SJO, Donnell MR *et al*. Total body irradiation and high-dose etoposide: a new preparatory regimen for bone marrow transplantation in patients with advanced hematologic malignancies. *Blood* 1987; **69**: 1015–20.

375 Schmitz N, Gassmann W, Rister M *et al*. Fractionated total body irradiation and high-dose VP-16–213 followed by allogeneic bone marrow transplantation in advanced leukemias. *Blood* 1988; **72**: 1567–73.

376 Neidhart JA, Kohler W, Stidley C *et al*. Phase 1 study of repeated cycles of high-dose cyclophosphamide, etoposide, and cisplatin administered without bone marrow transplantation. *J Clin Oncol* 1990; **8**: 1728–38.

377 Wilson WH, Jain V, Bryant G. Phase 1 and 2 study of high-dose ifosfamide, carboplatin, and etoposide with autologous bone marrow rescue in lymphomas and solid tumors. *J Clin Oncol* 1992; **10**: 1712–22.

378 Pommier Y, Leteurtre F, Fesen MR *et al*. Cellular determinants of sensitivity and resistance to DNA topoisomerase inhibitors. *Cancer Invest* 1994; **12**: 530–42.

379 Pommier Y. DNA topoisomerase I and II in cancer chemotherapy: update and perspectives. *Cancer Chemother Pharmacol* 1993; **32**: 103–8.

380 Zwelling LA. DNA topoisomerase II as a target of antineoplastic drug therapy. *Cancer Metastasis Rev* 1985; **4**: 263–76.

381 Kupfer G, Bodley AL, Liu LF. Involvement of intracellular ATP in cytotoxicity of topoisomerase II-targetting antitumor drugs. *NCI Monogr* 1987; **4**: 37–40.

382 Sehested M, Jensen PB, Sorenson BS, Holm B, Friche E, Demant EJF. Antagonistic effect of the cardioprotector (+)-1,2-*bis* (3,5-dioxopiperazinyl-1-yl) propane (ICRF-187) on DNA breaks and cytotoxicity induced by the topoisomerase II directed drugs daunorubicin and etoposide (VP-16). *Biochem Pharmacol* 1993; **46**: 389–93.

383 Holm B, Jensen PB, Sehested M, Hansen HH. *In vivo* inhibition of etoposide-mediated apoptosis, toxicity, and antitumor effect by the topoisomerase II-uncoupling anthracycline aclarubicin. *Cancer Chemother Pharmacol* 1994; **34**: 503–8.

384 Bertrand R, Kerrigan D, Sarang M, Pommier Y. Cell death induced by topoisomerase inhibitors: role of calcium in mammalian cells. *Biochem Pharmacol* 1991; **42**: 77–85.

385 Kaufman SH, Karp JE, Jones RJ *et al*. Topoisomerase II levels and drug sensitivity in adult acute myelogenous leukemia. *Blood* 1994; **83**: 517–30.

386 Kalyanaraman B, Nemec J, Sinha BK. Characterization of free radicals produced during oxidation of etoposide (VP-16) and its catechol and quinone derivatives: an ESR Study. *Biochemistry* 1989; **28**: 4839–46.

387 Katki AG, Kalyanaraman B, Sinha BK. Interactions of the antitumor drug, etoposide, with reduced thiols *in vitro* and *in vivo*. *Chem Biol Interact* 1987; **62**: 237–47.

388 Sinha BK, Eliot HM, Kalyanaraman B. Iron-dependent hydroxyl radical formation and DNA damage from a novel metabolite of the clinically active antitumor drug VP-16. *FEBS Lett* 1988; **227**: 240–4.

389 Custodio JB, Cardoso CM, Almeida LM. Thiol protecting agents and antioxidants inhibit the mitochondrial permeability transition promoted by etoposide: implications in the prevention of etoposide-induced apoptosis. *Chem Biol Interact* 2002; **140**: 169–84.

390 Kaufman SH. Induction of endonucleolytic DNA cleavage in human acute myelogenous leukemia cells by etoposide, camptothecin, and other cytotoxic anticancer drugs: a cautionary note. *Cancer Res* 1989; **49**: 5870–8.

391 Walker PR, Smith C, Youdale T, Leblanc J, Whitfield JF, Sikorska M. Topoisomerase II-reactive chemotherapeutic drugs induce apoptosis in thymocytes. *Cancer Res* 1991; **51**: 1078–85.

392 Lassus P, Opitz-Araya X, Lazebnik Y. Requirement for caspase-2 in stress-induced apoptosis before mitochondrial permeabilization. *Science* 2002; **297**: 1352–4.

393 Robertson JD, Enoksson M, Suomela M, Zhivotovsky B, Orrenius S. Caspase-2 acts upstream of mitochondria to promote cytochrome c release during etoposide-induced apoptosis. *J Biol Chem* 2002; **277**: 29803–9.

394 Tanizawa A, Kubota M, Hashimoto H *et al*. VP-16-induced nucleotide pool changes and poly (ADP-ribose) synthesis: the role of VP-16 in interphase death. *Exp Cell Res* 1989; **185**: 237–46.

395 Kubota M, Tanizawa A, Hashimoto H *et al*. Cell type dependent activation of poly (ADP-ribose) synthesis following treatment with etoposide. *Leuk Res* 1990; **14**: 371–5.

396 Kaufmann SH, Desnoyers S, Ottaviano Y, Davidson NE, Poirier GG. Specific proteolytic cleavage of poly (ADP-ribose) polymerase: an early marker of chemotherapy-induced apoptosis. *Cancer Res* 1993; **53**: 3976–85.

397 Lowe SW, Ruley HE, Jacks T, Housman DE. p53-dependent apoptosis modulates the cytotoxicity of anticancer agents. *Cell* 1993; **74**: 957–67.

398 Beere HM, Chresta CM, Hickman JA. Selective inhibition of topoisomerase II by ICRF-193 does not support a role for topoisomerase II activity in the fragmentation of chromatin during apoptosis of human leukemia cells. *Mol Pharmacol* 1996; **49**: 842–51.

399 Sinha BK, Haim N, Dusre L, Kerrigan D, Pommier Y. DNA strand breaks produced by etoposide (VP-16-213) in sensitive and resistant human breast tumor cells: implications for the mechanism of action. *Cancer Res* 1988; **48**: 5096–100.

400 Spiridonidis CA, Chatterjee S, Petzold SJ, Berger NA. Topoisomerase II-dependent and -independent mechanisms of etoposide resistance in chinese hamster cell lines. *Cancer Res* 1989; **49**: 644–50.

401 Hait WN, Choudhury S, Srimatkandada S, Murren JR. Sensitivity of K562 human chronic myelogenous leukemia blast cells transfected with a human multidrug resistance cDNA to cytotoxic drugs and differentiating agents. *J Clin Invest* 1993; **91**: 2207–15.

402 Mickisch GH, Merlino GT, Galski H, Gottesman MM, Pastan I. Transgenic mice that express the human multidrug-resistance gene in bone marrow enable a rapid identification of agents that reverse drug resistance. *Proc Natl Acad Sci U S A* 1991; **88**: 547–51.

403 Lum BL, Kaubisch S, Yahanda AM *et al*. Alteration of etoposide pharmacokinetics and pharmacodynamics by cyclosporine in a phase 1 trial to modulate multidrug resistance. *J Clin Oncol* 1992; **10**: 1635–42.

404 Kornblau SM, Estey E, Madden T *et al*. Phase 1 study of mitoxantrone plus etoposide with multidrug blockade by SDZ PSC-833 in relapsed or refractory acute myelogenous leukemia. *J Clin Oncol* 1997; **15**: 1796–802.

405 Schneider E, Yamazaki H, Sinha BK, Cowan KH. Buthionine sulphoximine-mediated sensitisation of etoposide-resistant human breast cancer MCF7 cells overexpressing the multidrug resistance-associated protein involves increased drug accumulation. *Br J Cancer* 1995; **71**: 738–43.

406 Grant CE, Valdimarsson G, Hipfner DR, Almquist KC, Cole SPC, Deeley RG. Overexpression of multidrug resistance-associated protein (MRP) increases resistance to natural product drugs. *Cancer Res* 1994; **54**: 357–61.

407 Schneider E, Horton JK, Yang CH, Nakagawa M, Cowan KH. Multidrug resistance-associated

protein gene overexpression and reduced drug sensitivity of topoisomerase II in a human breast carcinoma MCF7 cell line selected for etoposide resistance. *Cancer Res* 1994; **54**: 152–8.

408 Schneider E, Cowan KH, Bader H *et al.* Increased expression of the multidrug resistance-associated protein gene in relapsed acute leukemia. *Blood* 1995; **85**: 186–93.

409 Zwelling LA, Hinds M, Chan D *et al.* Characterization of an amsacrine-resistant line of human leukemia cells: evidence for a drug-resistant form of topoisomerase II. *J Biol Chem* 1989; **264**: 16411–20.

410 Miyashita T, Reed JC. Bcl-2 oncoprotein blocks chemotherapy-induced apoptosis in a human leukemia cell line. *Blood* 1993; **81**: 151–7.

411 Kondo S, Yin D, Morimura T, Oda Y, Kikuchi H, Takeuchi J. Transfection with a *bcl-2* expression vector protects transplanted bone marrow from chemotherapy-induced myelosuppression. *Cancer Res* 1994; **54**: 2928–33.

412 Kuhl JS, Krajewski S, Duran GE, Reed JC, Sikic BI. Spontaneous overexpression of the long form of the Bcl-X protein in a highly resistant P388 leukaemia. *Br J Cancer* 1997; **75**: 268–74.

413 Hande KR, Wolff SN, Greco FA, Hainsworth JD, Reed G, Johnson DH. Etoposide kinetics in patients with obstructive jaundice. *J Clin Oncol* 1990; **8**: 1101–7.

414 Arbuck SG, Douglass HO, Crom WR *et al.* Etoposide pharmacokinetics in patients with normal and abnormal organ function. *J Clin Oncol* 1986; **4**: 1690–5.

415 Stewart CF, Arbuck SG, Fleming RA, Evans WE. Changes in the clearance of total and unbound etoposide in patients with liver dysfunction. *J Clin Oncol* 1990; **8**: 1874–9.

416 Joel SP, Shah R, Clark PI, Slevin ML. Predicting etoposide toxicity: relationship to organ function and protein binding. *J Clin Oncol* 1996; **14**: 257–67.

417 Relling MV, McLeod HL, Bowman LC, Santana VM. Etoposide pharmacokinetics and pharmacodynamics after acute and chronic exposure to cisplatin. *Clin Pharmacol Ther* 1994; **56**: 503–11.

418 Newman EM, Doroshow JH, Forman SJ, Blume KG. Pharmacokinetics of high-dose etoposide. *Clin Pharmacol Ther* 1988; **43**: 561–4.

419 Green JA, Tarpey AW, Warenius HM. Pharmacokinetic study of high dose etoposide infusion in patients with small cell lung cancer. *Acta Oncol* 1988; **27**: 819–22.

420 Schwinghammer TL, Fleming RA, Rosenfeld CS *et al.* Disposition of total and unbound etoposide following high-dose therapy. *Cancer Chemother Pharmacol* 1993; **32**: 273–8.

421 Mross K, Bewermeier P, Kruger W, Stockschlader M, Zander A, Hossfeld DK. Pharmacokinetics of undiluted or diluted high-dose etoposide with or without busulfan administered to patients with hematologic malignancies. *J Clin Oncol* 1994; **12**: 1468–74.

422 Ellis AG, Crinis NA, Webster LK. Inhibition of etoposide elimination in the isolated perfused rat liver by Cremophor EL and Tween 80. *Cancer Chemother Pharmacol* 1996; **38**: 81–7.

423 Gianni L, Vigano L, Locatelli A *et al.* Human pharmacokinetic characterization and *in vitro* study of the interaction between doxorubicin and paclitaxel in patients with breast cancer. *J Clin Oncol* 1997; **15**: 1906–15.

424 Somlo G, Doroshow JH, Forman SJ *et al.* High-dose doxorubicin, etoposide, and cyclophosphamide with autologous stem cell reinfusion in patients with responsive metastatic or high-risk primary breast cancer. *Cancer* 1994; **73**: 1678–85.

425 Wolff SN, Fer MF, McKay CM, Hande KR, Hainsworth JD, Greco FA. High-dose VP-16–213 and autologous bone marrow transplantation for refractory malignancies: a phase I study. *J Clin Oncol* 1983; **1**: 701–5.

426 Arcamone F, Cassinelli G, Fantini G *et al.* Adriamycin, 14-hydroxydaunomycin, a new antitumor antibiotic from *S. peucetius* var. *caesius*. *Biotechnol Bioeng* 1969; **11**: 1101–10.

427 Young RC, Ozols RF, Myers CE. The anthracycline antineoplastic drugs. *N Engl J Med* 1981; **305**: 139–53.

428 Weiss RB. The anthracyclines: will we ever find a better doxorubicin. *Semin Oncol* 1992; **19**: 670–86.

429 Bronchud MH, Howell A, Crowther D, Hopwood P, Souza L, Dexter TM. The use of granulocyte colony-stimulating factor to increase the intensity of treatment with doxorubicin in patients with advanced breast and ovarian cancer. *Br J Cancer* 1989; **60**: 121–5.

430 Launchbury AP, Habboubi N. Epirubicin and doxorubicin: a comparison of their characteristics, therapeutic activity and toxicity. *Cancer Treat Rev* 1993; **19**: 197–228.

431 Doroshow JH. Doxorubicin-induced cardiac toxicity. *N Engl J Med* 1991; **324**: 843–5.

432 Legha SS, Benjamin RS, Mackay B *et al.* Reduction of doxorubicin cardiotoxicity by prolonged continuous intravenous infusion. *Ann Intern Med* 1982; **96**: 133–9.

433 Legha SS, Benjamin RS, Mackay B *et al.* Adriamycin therapy by continuous intravenous infusion in patients with metastatic breast cancer. *Cancer* 1982; **49**: 1762–6.

434 Legha SS, Wang YM, Mackay B *et al.* Clinical and pharmacologic investigation of the effects of alpha-tocopherol on adriamycin cardiotoxicity. *Ann N Y Acad Sci* 1982; **393**: 411–8.

435 Legha SS. The anthracyclines and mitoxantrone. In: Lokich JJ, ed. *Cancer Chemotherapy by Infusion*, 2nd edn. Chicago, IL: Precept Press, 1990: 197–217.

436 Morgan RJ Jr, Doroshow JH, Venkataraman K *et al.* High-dose infusional doxorubicin and cyclophosphamide: a feasibility study of tandem high-dose chemotherapy cycles without stem cell support. *Clin Cancer Res* 1997; **3**: 2337–45.

437 Somlo G, Simpson JF, Frankel P *et al.* Predictors of long-term outcome following high-dose chemotherapy in high-risk primary breast cancer. *Br J Cancer* 2002; **87**: 281–8.

438 Morgan RJ, Doroshow JH, Leong L *et al.* Phase 2 trial of high-dose intravenous doxorubicin, etoposide, and cyclophosphamide with autologous stem cell support in patients with residual or responding recurrent ovarian cancer. *Bone Marrow Transplant* 2001; **28**: 859–63.

439 Basser RL, To LB, Begley CG *et al.* Adjuvant treatment of high-risk breast cancer using multicycle high-dose chemotherapy and filgastim-mobilized peripheral blood progenitor cells. *Clin Cancer Res* 1995; **1**: 715–21.

440 Somlo G, Doroshow JH, Synold T *et al.* High-dose paclitaxel in combination with doxorubicin, cyclophosphamide and peripheral blood progenitor cell rescue in patients with high-risk primary and responding metastatic breast carcinoma: toxicity profile, relationship to paclitaxel pharmacokinetics and short-term outcome. *Br J Cancer* 2001; **84**: 1591–8.

441 Doroshow JH. Anthracyclines and anthracenediones. In: Chabner BA, Longo DL, eds. *Cancer Chemotherapy and Biotherapy: Principles and Practice*. Philadelphia: Lippincott, Williams, and Wilkins, 2001: 500–37.

442 Tritton TR. Cell death in cancer chemotherapy: the case of Adriamycin. In: Tomei LD, Cope, FO, eds. *Apoptosis: the Molecular Basis of Cell Death*. Cold Spring Harbor: Cold Spring Harbor Laboratory Press, 1991: 121–37.

443 Jensen PB, Sorensen BS, Sehested M *et al.* Different modes of anthracycline interaction with topoisomerase II. Separate structures critical for DNA-cleavage and for overcoming topoisomerase II-related drug resistance. *Proc Am Assoc Cancer Res* 1993; **34**: A1968.

444 Tepper CG. Integrity of mitochondrial DNA during cell death. *Diss Abstract Int [B]* 1993; **54**: 2910.

445 Azmi S, Bhatia L, Khanna N, Dhawan D, Singh N. Adriamycin induces apoptosis in rat thymocytes. *Cancer Lett* 1997; **111**: 225–31.

446 Zwelling LA, Bales E, Altschuler E, Mayes J. Circumvention of resistance by doxorubicin, but not by idarubicin, in a human leukemia cell line containing an intercalator-resistant form of topoisomerase II. Evidence for a non-topoisomerase II-mediated mechanism of doxorubicin cytotoxicity. *Biochem Pharmacol* 1993; **45**: 516–20.

447 Doroshow JH, Synold TW, Somlo G, Akman SA, Gajewski E. Oxidative DNA base modifications in peripheral blood mononuclear cells of patients treated with high-dose infusional doxorubicin. *Blood* 2001; **97**: 2839–45.

448 Bertheau P, Plassa F, Espie M *et al.* Effect of mutated TP53 on response of advanced breast cancers to high-dose chemotherapy. *Lancet* 2002; **360**: 852–4.

449 Hunault M, Zhou D, Delmer A *et al.* Multidrug resistance gene expression in acute myeloid leukemia: major prognosis significance for in vivo drug resistance to induction treatment. *Ann Hematol* 1997; **74**: 65–71.

450 Allen JD, Jackson SC, Schinkel AH. A mutation hot spot in the Bcrp1 (Abcg2) multidrug transporter in mouse cell lines selected for Doxorubicin resistance. *Cancer Res* 2002; **62**: 2294–9.

451 Bachur NR, Hildebrand RC, Jaenke RS. Adriamycin and daunorubicin disposition in the rabbit. *J Pharmacol Exp Ther* 1974; **191**: 331–40.

452 Ahmed NK, Felsted RL, Bachur NR. Heterogeneity of anthracycline antibiotic carbonyl reductases in mammalian livers. *Biochem Pharmacol* 1978; **27**: 2713–9.

453 Lovless H, Arena E, Felsted RL, Bachur NR. Comparative mammalian metabolism of adriamycin and daunorubicin. *Cancer Res* 1978; **38**: 593–8.

454 Bachur NR, Gordon SL, Gee MV, Kon H. NADPH cytochrome P-450 reductase activation of quinone anticancer agents to free radicals. *Proc Natl Acad Sci USA* 1979; **76**: 954–7.

455 Andrews PA, Brenner DE, Chou FT, Kubo H, Bachur NR. Facile and definitive determination of human adriamycin and daunoribicin metabolites by high-pressure liquid chromatography. *Drug Metab Dispos* 1980; **8**: 152–6.

456 Ackland SP, Ratain MJ, Vogelzang NJ, Choi KE, Ruane M, Sinkule JA. Pharmacokinetics and pharmacodynamics of long-term continuous-infusion doxorubicin. *Clin Pharmacol Ther* 1989; **45**: 340–7.

457 Synold T, Doroshow JH. Anthracycline dose intensity: clinical pharmacology and pharmacokinetics of high-dose doxorubicin administered as a 96-hour continuous intravenous infusion. *J Infus Chemother* 1996; **6**: 69–73.

458 Rowinsky EK, Onetto N, Canetta RM, Arbuck SG. Taxol: the first of the taxanes, an important new class of antitumor agents. *Semin Oncol* 1992; **19**: 646–62.

459 Nicolaou KC, Yang Z, Liu JJ *et al*. Total synthesis of taxol. *Nature* 1994; **367**: 630–4.

460 Holmes FA, Walters RS, Theriault RL *et al*. Phase 2 trial of taxol, an active drug in the treatment of metastatic breast cancer. *J Natl Cancer Inst* 1991; **83**: 1797–805.

461 Gianni L, Munzone E, Capri G *et al*. Paclitaxel in metastatic breast cancer: a trial of two doses by a 3-hour infusion in patients with disease recurrence after prior therapy with anthracyclines. *J Natl Cancer Inst* 1995; **87**: 1169–75.

462 McGuire WP, Rowinsky EK, Rosenshein NB. Taxol: a unique antineoplastic agent with significant activity in advanced ovarian epithelial neoplasms. *Ann Intern Med* 1989; **111**: 273–9.

463 Lau D, Leigh B, Gandara D *et al*. Twice-weekly paclitaxel and weekly carboplatin with concurrent thoracic radiation followed by carboplatin/paclitaxel consolidation for stage III non-small-cell lung cancer: a California Cancer Consortium phase 2 trial. *J Clin Oncol* 2001; **19**: 442–7.

464 Schiff PB, Fant J, Horwitz SB. Promotion of microtubule assembly *in vitro* by taxol. *Nature* 1979; **277**: 665–7.

465 Rowinsky EK, Donehower RC. The clinical pharmacology and use of antimicrotubule agents in cancer chemotherapeutics. *Pharmacol Ther* 1991; **52**: 35–84.

466 Rowinsky EK, Donehower RC, Jones RJ, Tucker RW. Microtubule changes and cytotoxicity in leukemic cell lines treated with taxol. *Cancer Res* 1988; **48**: 4093–100.

467 Horwitz SB, Cohen D, Rao S, Ringel I, Shen H-J, Yang C-PH. Taxol: mechanisms of action and resistance. *J Natl Cancer Inst Monogr* 1993; **15**: 55–61.

468 Tishler RB, Schiff PB, Geard CR. Taxol: a novel radiation sensitizer. *Int J Radiat Oncol Biol Phys* 1992; **22**: 613–7.

469 Choy H, Akerley W, Safran H *et al*. Phase 1 trial of outpatient weekly paclitaxel and concurrent radiation therapy for advanced non-small-cell lung cancer. *J Clin Oncol* 1994; **12**: 2682–6.

470 Das KC, White CW. Activation of NF-kappaB by antineoplastic agents: role of protein kinase C. *J Biol Chem* 1997; **272**: 14914–20.

471 Haldar S, Chintapalli J, Croce CM. Taxol induces bcl-2 phosphorylation and death of prostate cancer cells. *Cancer Res* 1996; **56**: 1253–5.

472 Ibrado AM, Liu L, Bhalla K. Bcl-xL overexpression inhibits progression of molecular events leading to paclitaxel-induced apoptosis of human acute myeloid leukemia HL-60 cells. *Cancer Res* 1997; **57**: 1109–15.

473 Saunders DE, Lawrence WD, Christensen C, Wappler NL, Ruan H, Deppe G. Paclitaxel-induced apoptosis in MCF-7 breast-cancer cells. *Int J Cancer* 1997; **70**: 214–20.

474 Bhalla K, Huang Y, Tang C *et al*. Characterization of a human myeloid leukemia cell line highly resistant to taxol. *Leukemia* 1994; **8**: 465–75.

475 Milas L, Hunter NR, Kurdoglu B *et al*. Kinetics of mitotic arrest and apoptosis in murine mammary and ovarian tumors treated with taxol. *Cancer Chemother Pharmacol* 1995; **35**: 297–303.

476 Strobel T, Swanson L, Korsmeyer S, Cannistra SA. BAX enhances paclitaxel-induced apoptosis through a p53-independent pathway. *Proc Natl Acad Sci U S A* 1996; **93**: 14094–9.

477 Alesse E, Ricevuto E, Ficorella C *et al*. p53-independent apoptosis induced by taxanes and doxorubicin. *Anti-Cancer Treatment, Sixth International Congress*. 1996: 141.

478 Haber M, Burkhart CA, Regl DL, Madafiglio J, Norris MD, Horwitz SB. Altered expression of M beta 2, the class II beta-tubulin isotype, in a murine J774.2 cell line with a high level of taxol resistance. *J Biol Chem* 1995; **270**: 31269–75.

479 Kavallaris M, Kuo DYS, Burkhart CA *et al*. Taxol-resistant epithelial ovarian tumors are associated with altered expression of specific beta-tubulin isotypes. *J Clin Invest* 1997; **100**: 1282–93.

480 Parekh H, Wiesen K, Simpkins H. Acquisition of taxol resistance via P-glycoprotein- and non-P-glycoprotein-mediated mechanisms in human ovarian carcinoma cells. *Biochem Pharmacol* 1997; **53**: 461–70.

481 Yang JM, Sommer S, Hait WN. Reversal of Taxol resistance *in vitro* and *in vivo* by trans-flupenthixol and cyclosporin A. *Proc Am Assoc Cancer Res* 1994; **35**: 355.

482 Lehnert M, Emerson S, Dalton WS, de Giuli R, Salmon SE. *In vitro* evaluation of chemosensitizers for clinical reversal of P-glycoprotein-associated Taxol resistance. *J Natl Cancer Inst Monogr* 1993; **15**: 63–7.

483 Monsarrat B, Royer I, Wright M, Cresteil T. Biotransformation of taxoids by human cytochromes P450: structure–activity relationship. *Bull Cancer* 1997; **84**: 125–33.

484 Venook AP, Egorin MJ, Rosner GL *et al*. Phase 1 and pharmacokinetic trial of paclitaxel in patients with hepatic dysfunction: cancer and leukemia group B 9264. *J Clin Oncol* 1998; **16**: 1811–9.

485 Panday VR, Huizing MT, Willemse PH *et al*. Hepatic metabolism of paclitaxel and its impact in patients with altered hepatic function. *Semin Oncol* 1997; **24**: S11–38.

486 Gianni L, Kearns KM, Giani A *et al*. Non-linear pharmacokinetics and metabolism of paclitaxel and pharmacokinetic–pharmacodynamic relationships in humans. *J Clin Oncol* 1995; **13**: 180–90.

487 Papadopoulos KP, Egorin MJ, Huang M *et al*. The pharmacokinetics and pharmacodynamics of high-dose paclitaxel monotherapy (825 mg/m^2 continuous infusion over 24 h) with hematopoietic support in women with metastatic breast cancer. *Cancer Chemother Pharmacol* 2001; **47**: 45–50.

488 Sparreboom A, van Tellingen O, Nooijen WJ, Beijnen JH. Non-linear pharmacokinetics of paclitaxel in mice results from the pharmaceutical vehicle Cremophor EL. *Cancer Res* 1996; **56**: 2112–5.

489 Doroshow JH, Synold T, Somlo G *et al*. High-dose infusional paclitaxel (P), platinum (DDP), cyclophosphamide (CY), and cyclosporine A (CSA) with peripheral blood progenitor cell rescue for high-risk primary and responsive metastatic breast cancer (BC). *Proc Am Soc Clin Oncol* 1997; **16**: 235a.

490 Einzig AI, Wiernik PH, Wadler S *et al*. Phase 1 study of paclitaxel (Taxol) and granulocyte colony stimulating factor (G-CSF) in patients with unresectable malignancy. *Invest New Drugs* 1998; **16**: 29–36.

491 Stemmer SM, Cagnoni PJ, Shpall EJ *et al*. High-dose paclitaxel, cyclophosphamide, and cisplatin with autologous hematopoietic progenitor-cell support: a phase 1 trial. *J Clin Oncol* 1996; **14**: 1463–72.

492 Pestalozzi BC, Sotos GA, Choyke PL, Fisherman JS, Cowan KH, O'Shaughnessy JA. Typhlitis resulting from treatment with taxol and doxorubicin in patients with metastatic breast cancer. *Cancer* 1993; **71**: 1797–800.

13

William I. Bensinger & Ricardo Spielberger

Preparative Regimens and Modification of Regimen-Related Toxicities

Introduction

Treatment regimens used for hematopoietic cell transplantation (HCT) must accomplish two goals, depending on the patient's disease and the source of the graft. Since the majority of autologous and allogeneic transplant procedures are performed for the treatment of malignant diseases, the regimens must provide tumor cytoreduction and ideally disease eradication. The pharmacologic basis for this is discussed in Chapter 12. In the case of allogeneic transplants, the regimen must be sufficiently immunosuppressive to overcome host rejection of the graft. This second goal is discussed in detail in Chapter 3. This chapter will review high-dose chemotherapy and chemo-radiotherapy regimens administered prior to autologous, syngeneic or allogeneic hematopoietic cell infusion as well as efforts to reduce toxicities associated with these regimens. Most of the high-dose regimens described have been utilized for patients with hematologic malignancies. Some high-dose regimens, however, have been developed specifically for patients with solid tumors, especially breast cancer. The overall results of HCT utilizing these high-dose treatment regimens are discussed in more detail in chapters dealing with specific diseases.

The success of HCT as curative therapy for patients with malignancy is limited, in part, by transplant-related morbidity and mortality. Even if all transplant-related problems were solved, however, about one-half (range 10–90%) of patients receiving transplants for various stages of malignant diseases would die due to the inability of high-dose regimens to eradicate malignancy. This has led to intensive efforts to develop more effective high-dose regimens.

Evaluation of new treatment regimens

The development of new treatment regimens has, in general, been empirical with the evaluation of a variety of drugs and radiation doses and schedules. Attempts have been made to systematize the development of new treatment regimens by performing phase I dose escalation trials followed by phase II potential efficacy trials. Promising new regimens are then compared to established treatment regimens in randomized phase III trials. The methodology for trial design is discussed in more detail in Chapter 31.

Phase I trials

Dose escalation trials to define maximum tolerated dose (MTD) and phase II trials to define potential efficacy are, in general, performed on patients with advanced disease incurable by conventional therapy. Once a tolerable regimen is developed it can be evaluated in phase II and III trials in patients with less-advanced disease. Conventional phase I trials of chemotherapeutic agents have beginning doses that are known to be nontoxic and are escalated to mild or moderate toxicity, which is usually hematologic. In the transplant setting this is not a useful strategy as only nonhematologic toxicities are considered. An alternative approach is to make an estimate of the likely MTD, based on nonhematologic toxicities, for a combination of agents given in high doses [1,2]. This estimated MTD is then used as the starting dose with escalation and de-escalation depending on observed toxicities. The regimen-related toxicity (RRT) grading system, described below, is used to determine escalation or de-escalation of doses. In phase I studies, attempts are made to keep observed grade 3–4 toxicities to <25%, and patients are studied in groups of four as shown in Table 13.1.

With this Fibonacci scheme, a maximum of 16–20 patients are required to make a first estimation of the MTD of most new treatment regimens. Using the above methodology, several phase I trials have been successfully performed in the transplant community [3–8].

RRT grading system

In order to carry out meaningful phase I and II studies of new high-dose treatment regimens in transplant patients, a new toxicity grading system, excluding hematologic toxicities, has been designed. This grading system estimates the nonhematologic toxicities directly caused by a given transplant treatment regimen [9]. Morbidity is assessed in nine organ systems: heart, bladder, kidneys, lungs, liver, mucosa, central nervous system (CNS), gastrointestinal (GI) tract and skin. Toxicity is graded on a 0–4 scale with grade 4 being fatal and grade 3 being life-threatening. Toxicities due to graft-vs.-host-disease (GVHD), infection and drugs administered post-transplant are excluded from this grading system. Utilizing this grading system, one can begin to estimate the specific contribution that the treatment regimen makes to overall morbidity and mortality of the transplant procedure [10–12].

Table 13.1 Schema for conduct of phase I trials in HCT.

Severe RRT/total	Dose level for next four patients
0/4	Next higher
1/4	Same
2/4	Next lower

RRT, regimen-related toxicity; HCT, hematopoietic cell transplantation.

Marrow ablative agents—MTD when administered with HCT (Table 13.2)

Total body irradiation (Tables 13.2–13.5)

Total body irradiation (TBI) has been the primary therapeutic modality for autologous and allogeneic HCT for patients with hematologic malignancies. TBI has retained wide usage over the past 30 years because of excellent immunosuppressive properties, activity against a wide variety of malignancies even if resistant to chemotherapy, penetration of sanctuary sites, such as the CNS and testicles, and the relative lack of nonmarrow toxicities when given at high doses.

Only one single study has evaluated TBI alone [13] while other trials have involved the concomitant administration of cytotoxic agents, usually cyclophosphamide (CY). Extensive experience has been accumulated with 10–16 Gy of TBI given as a single dose or fractionated, following or preceding high doses of CY (Tables 13.2–13.4).

A large body of experimental data has been developed concerning methods to improve the therapeutic index of TBI [14,15]. Larger doses of TBI that might reduce the likelihood of relapse are limited by GI and pulmonary toxicity and long-term by impaired growth and development, chronic pulmonary insufficiency, and second malignancies. In addition to the total dose, many factors, including radiation exposure rate, dose per fraction, interval between fractions, and radiation source (cobalt-60 [^{60}Co] or linear accelerator) have effects on efficacy and toxicity [14] (see Chapter 14). Many of the techniques of hyperfractionation were developed at the Memorial Sloan Kettering Cancer Center [16–18]. Experimental studies and clinical trials indicate that TBI administered in fractions is more tolerable than single dose administration and that fractionation, if compensated for by increased total dose, can be given without compromising antitumor effects. Based on this principle the use of

Table 13.2 MTD of single agent therapies used with HCT.

Ref.	Agent	MTD	Dose-limiting toxicities
Marrow ablative single agents used in high-dose regimens with stem cell support			
[14]	TBI	10–16 Gy	GI, hepatic, pul
[34]	BU	20 mg/kg	GI, hepatic, pul
[73]	Carmustine	1200 mg/m^2	Pul, hepatic
[98]	MEL	200 mg/kg	GI
[105]	TT	1135 mg/m^2	CNS, GI
Nonmarrow ablative single agents used in high-dose regimens with stem cell support			
[109]	CY	200 mg/kg	Cardiac
[110]	Ifosfamide	18–20 g/m^2	Renal, bladder and neurologic
[112]	VP16	2400 mg/m^2	GI
Agents used in high-dose regimens without determination of MTD with stem cell support			
[116]	Mitoxantrone	90 mg/m^2*	Cardiac
[33]	Cisplatin	250 mg/m^2*	Renal
[118]	Carboplatin	2000 mg/m^2	Hepatic, renal
[124]	Cytarabine	36 g/m^2*	CNS

BU, busulfan; CNS, central nervous system; CY, cyclophosphamide; GI, gastrointestinal; MEL, melphalan; MTD, maximum tolerated dose; pul, pulmonary; TBI, total body irradiation; TT, thiotepa; VP16, etoposide; HCT, hematopoietic cell transplantation.
*Maximum dose given with other agents with stem cell support.

Table 13.3 Maximum tolerated doses (MTDs) of total body irradiation (TBI) given with cyclophosphamide 120 mg/kg.

Ref.	Total dose (Gy)	Fraction size (Gy)	Fractionation interval (h)	Fraction number	Days TBI
[19]	10.00	10.0	—	1	1
[23]	15.75	2.25	24	7	7
[242]	16.00	2.0	24	8	8
[3]	16.00	2.0	6–8	8	4
[25]	14.40 (children)	1.2	4–6	12	4
[4]	13.20 (adults)	1.2	4–6	11	4

Table 13.4 Randomized trials of total body irradiation (TBI) regimens given with cyclophosphamide 120 mg/kg.

Diagnosis [Ref.]	No. patients	Fraction size (Gy)	No. fractions	Total dose (Gy)	Probability of relapse	Probability of EFS
AML: first remission [19]	27	10.0	1	10.0	0.55	0.33
	26	2.0	6	12.0	0.20	0.54
AML: first remission [23]	34	2.0	6	12.0	0.35	0.60
	37	2.25	7	15.75	0.12	0.60
CML: chronic phase [24]	57	2.0	6	12.0	0.19	0.73
	59	2.25	7	15.75	0.00	0.66
Hematologic malignancies [20]	73	10.0	1	10.0	0.37	0.38
	74	1.35	11	14.85	0.23	0.45

AML, acute myeloid leukemia; CML, chronic myeloid leukemia; EFS, event-free survival.

Table 13.5 Chemotherapeutic agents given with total body irradiation (TBI) and with or without cyclophosphamide (CY).

Ref.	CY (mg/kg)	Total dose TBI (Gy)	Chemotherapy	Total dose
[124]	—	10–12	Cytarabine	36 g/m^2
[113]	—	13.2	VP16	60 mg/kg
[102,103,130]	—	9.5–11.5	MEL	110–140 mg/m^2
[243]	—	5 or 12*	MEL	140–180 mg/m^2
	—		VP16	60 mg/kg
[129]	60–120	5–12	Cytarabine	36 g/m^2
[2]	50	12	BU	7 mg/kg (allo)
	60	12		8 mg/kg (auto)
[132]	100	12	VP16	60 mg/kg × 1

BU, busulfan; MEL, melphalan; VP16, etoposide.
*5 Gy at 50 cGy/min × 1 or 12 Gy in six fractions.

fractionated TBI regimens has been explored in several centers, but there is a paucity of controlled studies of acute and delayed toxicities or of clinical efficacy as compared to single dose TBI. Two prospective randomized studies of fractionation vs. single dose TBI have been performed. One demonstrated clear superiority in event-free survival (EFS) following a fractionated regimen in patients with acute myeloid leukemia (AML) transplanted in first remission [19] (Table 13.4).

The second trial was performed in patients with a variety of hematologic malignancies autologous or allogenic HCT. Although the patients who received hyperfractionated TBI had trends toward better survival and a lower rate of relapse than patients receiving single fraction TBI, these differences were not statistically significant [19–21]. Other studies suggest that fractionation decreases the incidence of idiopathic interstitial pneumonia syndrome (IPS) (see Chapter 64) and cataracts [22] (see Chapter 69). A 1990 survey of TBI administration at 15 transplant centers found that 13 utilized some form of fractionation [14]. It is likely that almost all centers now utilize fractionated TBI, due to the decreased acute and delayed toxicities [21].

Studies suggest that both the antileukemic effects and normal tissue toxicities of TBI have a relatively steep dose–response curve. In a study in patients with AML in first remission, patients receiving 15.75 Gy had a markedly decreased actuarial incidence of relapse compared to patients given 12 Gy. Survival was not improved, however, due to an increase in fatal toxicities to the lung and liver [23]. Another study comparing 12.0 Gy vs. 15.75 Gy TBI in patients with CML in chronic phase demonstrated a markedly reduced relapse rate among patients receiving the higher TBI dose but, again, a markedly increased transplant-related mortality that actually reduced relapse free survival (RFS) compared to patients receiving 12 Gy of TBI [24].

In studies examining the effect of escalating doses of hyper-fractionated TBI at 2.0 Gy given twice daily, the MTD was 16.0 Gy [3]. When 1.2 Gy was given three times a day, however, the MTD was only 14.4 Gy [4], suggesting that the shorter interval between doses of TBI prevented DNA repair in normal tissues.

In the past, most of the TBI regimens used in the Seattle Marrow Transplant Team have utilized dual opposing ^{60}Co sources [22]. This approach has the advantage of providing highly homogenous radiation exposure and allows the patient some freedom of movement. However, it is difficult to shield organs and radiation can be delivered only at relatively low exposure rates (8 cGy/min). The majority of marrow transplant teams use linear accelerators to deliver TBI (see Chapter 14). With a linear accelerator, dose rates of 40 cGy/min or higher can be administered. The use of linear accelerators may have additional benefits as the radiation field can be shaped with the use of lung shielding to reduce pulmonary toxicity [25]. Electron beam radiation can also be delivered to the chest wall and spine to compensate for the lower dose of TBI to these shielded areas [25,26]. Shielding of other organs, such as the liver, may be useful if specific organ toxicity limits further increase in TBI dose [26]. Delivery of TBI with shielding of both lung and liver may be useful in patients with disease limited to bone, such as multiple myeloma (MM), breast cancer and Ewing's sarcoma [26–28].

High-dose chemotherapy regimens (Tables 13.6–13.10)

There have been extensive efforts to develop non-TBI containing transplant regimens. There are several reasons for pursuing this line of research. Many patients with Hodgkin's disease or lymphoma have received prior dose-limiting radiotherapy, especially to the mediastinum, which results in a high incidence of fatal IPS following TBI [29]. Chemotherapy regimens may also avoid the long-term sequelae of TBI including cataracts, sterility, second malignancies, and growth and

Table 13.6 Busulfan-based regimens.

Ref.	Regimen	Chemotherapy	Total dose
[55]	BU/CY	BU	16 mg/kg
		CY	120–200 mg/kg
[56]	BU/CY	BU	16 mg/kg
		CY	120 mg/kg
[37]	BU/CY	BU	14 mg/kg
		CY	150 mg/kg
[64]	BU/MEL	BU	16 mg/kg
		MEL	140 mg/m^2
[8]	BU/MEL/TT	BU	12 mg/kg
		MEL	100 mg/m^2
		TT	500 mg/m^2
[244]	BU/CY/MEL	BU	16 mg/kg
[245]		CY	120 mg/kg
		MEL	90–140 mg/m^2
[70]	BU/CY/TT (autografts)	BU	10 mg/kg
		CY	120 mg/kg
		TT	750 mg/m^2
[71]	BU/CY/TT (allografts)	BU	12 mg/kg
		CY	120 mg/kg
		TT	750 mg/m^2
[59,246]	BU/VP16	BU	16 mg/kg
[61]		VP16	60 mg/kg
[72]	BU/CY/VP16	BU	16 mg/kg
		CY	150 mg/kg
		VP16	30 mg/kg
[247]	BU/CY/VP16	BU	16 mg/kg
		CY	120 mg/kg
		VP16	5–40 mg/kg

BU, busulfan; CY, cyclophosphamide; MEL, melphalan; TT, thiotepa; VP16, etoposide.

Table 13.7 Nitrosourea-based high-dose chemotherapy regimens.

Ref.	Regimen	Chemotherapy	Total dose
[248]	CBV*	Carmustine	300–600 mg/m^2
[80]		CY	6.0–7.2 g/m^2
[79]		VP16	600–2400 mg/m^2
[132]	CBV†	Carmustine	15 mg/kg
		CY	100 mg/kg
		VP16	60 mg/kg
[86]	CBV ± CPPD	Carmustine	500 mg/m^2
		CY	7.2 g/m^2
		VP16	2.4 g/m^2
		Cisplatin	150 mg/m^2
[88]		Lomustine	15 mg/kg
		CY	100 mg/kg
		VP16	60 mg/kg
[92]	BEAM	Carmustine	300–600 mg/m^2
[93]		VP16	400–800 mg/m^2
[94]		Cytarabine	800–1600 mg/m^2
[67]		MEL	140 mg/m^2
[90]	BEAC	Carmustine	300 mg/m^2
[91]		VP16	300 mg/m^2
		Cytarabine	800 mg/m^2
		CY	6 g/m^2
[75]	STAMP-I	Carmustine	600 mg/m^2
		CY	5.6 g/m^2
		Cisplatin	165 mg/m^2
[249]	BAVC	Carmustine	800 mg/m^2
		AMSA	450 mg/m^2
		Cytarabine	900 mg/m^2
		VP16	450 mg/m^2
[250]		Carmustine	500 mg/m^2
		MEL	80–140 mg/m^2
		VP16	300 mg/m^2
[250]		Carmustine	500 mg/m^2
		MEL	140 mg/m^2
[251]		Carmustine	60–100 mg/m^2
		VP16	2400–3000 mg/m^2
		Cisplatin	200 mg/m^2

AMSA, amsacrine; BAVC, BCNU, amsacrine and etoposide; BEAC, BCNU, etoposide, cytosine arabinoside and cyclophosphamide; BEAM, BCNU, etoposide, cytosine arabinoside and melphalan; CBV, cyclophosphamide, BCNU and etoposide; CPPD, cisplatin; CY, cyclophosphamide; MEL, melphalan; STAMP-I, carmustine, cisplatin and cyclophosphamide; TT, thiotepa; VP16, etoposide.
*Drugs given simultaneously over 3 days.
†Each drug given on a separate day with a day's rest in between.

Table 13.8 Melphalan-based high-dose regimens.

Ref.	Regimen	Chemotherapy	Total dose
[85]	MEL/VP16	MEL	140–180 mg/m^2
		VP16	60 mg/kg
[125]	MEL/Cytarabine	MEL	140 mg/m^2
		Cytarabine	12 g/m^2
[117]	MEL/Mit	MEL	180 mg/m^2
		Mitoxantrone	60 mg/m^2
[120]	MEL/Mit/Carboplatin	MEL	160 mg/m^2
		Mitoxantrone	50 mg/m^2
		Carboplatin	1400 mg/m^2
[252]	MEL/CY/Cisplatin	MEL	80 mg/m^2
		CY	5.6 g/m^2
		Cisplatin	180 mg/m^2
[127]	MEL/Mit/Paclitaxel	MEL	180 mg/m^2
		Mitoxantrone	60–90 mg/m^2
		Paclitaxel	500–700 mg/m^2

CY, cyclophosphamide; MEL, melphalan; Mit, mitoxantrone; VP16, etoposide.

Table 13.9 Thiotepa-based high-dose regimens.

Ref.	Regimen	Chemotherapy	Total dose
[106]	STAMP-V (CTCb)	TT	500 mg/m^2
		CY	6 g/m^2
		Carboplatin	800 mg/m^2
[253]	TT/CY/Mit	TT	675 mg/m^2
		CY	7.5 g/m^2
		Mitoxantrone	60 mg/m^2
[116]	TT/Mit	TT	1.2 g/m^2
		Mitoxantrone	90 mg/m^2
[254]	CY/TT	TT	700 mg/m^2
		CY	7 g/m^2
[255]	CY/TT/Cisplatin	TT	600 mg/m^2
[127]		Cisplatin	40 mg/m^2
		CY	3.75 g/m^2

CTCb, STAMP-V; CY, cyclophosphamide; Mit, mitoxantrone; STAMP-V, thiotepa, cyclophosphamide and carboplatin; TT, thiotepa.

development problems in children. There has recently been concern about the development of myelodysplasia [30,31].

There are potential advantages in the convenience and in the expense of moving away from TBI, in that TBI utilizes already overextended radiation resources, often for prolonged periods of time, and requires the skills of physicists and radiotherapists. Finally, it may be possible to develop chemotherapy regimens that are more effective than those containing TBI. It is unfortunate that, at present, few studies exist on outcomes following HCT which compare specific regimens.

Alkylating agents

Alkylating agents are the major class of drugs used in high-dose regimens with HCT support because they have several desirable characteristics. Many alkylating agents have marrow toxicity as the major dose-limiting factor, which allows for dose escalation when stem cells are utilized.

Table 13.10 Etoposide (VP16)-based high-dose regimens.

Ref.	Regimen	Chemotherapy	Total dose
[256]	ICE	Ifosfamide	16 g/m^2
		Carboplatin	1.8 g/m^2
		VP16	1.5 g/m^2
[116]	ICE	Ifosfamide	20 g/m^2
		Carboplatin	1.8 g/m^2
		VP16	3 g/m^2
[257]		VP16	650 mg/m^2
		Cisplatin	100 mg/m^2
		Carboplatin	1.8 g/m^2
[33]	CEP	VP16	30 mg/kg
		CY	100 mg/kg
		Cisplatin	250 mg/m^2
[258]	CEP	CY	4.5–5.25 g/m^2
		VP16	750–1200 mg/m^2
		Cisplatin	120–180 mg/m^2
[101]		VP16	2250 mg/m^2
		Carboplatin	2100 mg/m^2
[33]		Doxorubicin	165 mg/m^2
		VP16	60 mg/kg
		CY	100 mg/kg
[101]		CY	6 g/m^2
		Carboplatin	2 g/m^2
		VP16	625 mg/m^2

CEP, cyclophosphamide, etoposide, cisplatin; CY, cyclophosphamide; ICE, ifosphomide, carboplatin, etoposide; VP16, etoposide.

Alkylators are not cell cycle specific, making them capable of killing nondividing, resting tumor cells. In *in vitro* testing, alkylators do not generally exhibit cross-resistance and have relatively steep log-linear dose–response curves [32]. Although it is not possible to combine alkylating agents at full dose when used alone, between 50 and 70% of the single agent MTD can be used in two to three drug combinations.

Increasingly, as regimens for the treatment of solid tumors evolve, there has been movement to incorporate tumor-specific drugs into the high-dose therapy setting [33]. It is important to point out, however, that drugs such as mitoxantrone or paclitaxel, which are highly active against tumors such as breast or ovarian cancer at conventional doses, are more difficult to deliver at higher doses due to nonhematologic toxicities, i.e. cardiac or neurologic. These characteristics limit the usefulness of such drugs in high-dose therapy regimens and their value in comparison to alkylator-based regimens remains to be proven.

Busulfan (Tables 13.2 & 13.6)

Busulfan (BU) is an alkylating agent with profound myeloablative properties, marked activity against nondividing marrow cells and possibly nondividing malignant cells as well. The MTD of BU, given as a single agent over 4 days followed by stem-cell support is approximately 20 mg/kg [34]. Single agent testing to determine the spectrum of activity in patients with malignant disease has not been extensive [34–36]. However, BU is probably active in a variety of malignancies including MM [35,37], lymphoma [38], acute lymphoblastic leukemia (ALL) [38], myeloid metaplasia [39], testicular tumors [40], Ewing's sarcoma [40] and breast cancer [41]. Although generally combined with other drugs, BU alone has been used as the conditioning regimen prior to first autologous transplants and for second allogeneic transplants in patients with CML [42].

One of the former problems with optimal utilization of BU had been the availability of only the oral form. Pharmacokinetic variability between patients is high with a two- to threefold difference in plasma levels between patients [43]. Children have lower mean plasma levels of BU (650 ng/mL) than adults (1050 ng/mL) [44,45], which may be partially compensated for by dosing children by body surface area rather than weight [45]. Variation in BU plasma levels between individuals probably contributes to the significant differences observed in toxicity and clinical response in patients receiving the same mg/kg or mg/m^2 dose. Slattery *et al.* [45] have demonstrated a relationship between low BU steady-state plasma concentrations and graft rejection in children. There are also data suggesting a direct relationship between the severity of RRT, especially sinusoidal obstruction syndrome (SOS) of the liver, and high BU plasma levels [43,46]. This is discussed in more detail in Chapter 58. In a patient accidentally overdosed with BU, hemodialysis resulted in accelerated clearance of the drug [47].

More recently it has been shown that the steady-state BU concentration correlates with relapse in patients receiving human leukocyte antigen (HLA) compatible transplants for chronic myeloid leukemia (CML) in chronic phase [48]. Seven relapses occurred among the 22 patients with BU state concentrations below the median of 918 ng/mL compared to none among the 23 patients at or above the median ($p = 0.0003$).

Thus, the average steady-state concentration of BU over a 4-day period may be a more important determinant of toxicity and efficacy than the exact mg/kg or mg/m^2 dose administered to any given patient [45,48]. Fortunately, within a given patient, BU is a pharmacokinetically predictable drug, and its absorption and elimination rate remain linear over a wide dose range and constant with time [45]. With repeated oral administration, steady-state BU plasma concentrations are achieved rapidly and can be predicted from first dose kinetics. Following determination of first dose kinetics, oral doses can be adjusted up or down to achieve the desired plasma levels. The strategy of targeted steady-state BU dosing has been used successfully to perform a dose escalation trial in patients receiving fixed doses of CY and TBI [49]. Theoretically, targeting of the steady-state plasma level of BU should increase the therapeutic index; a prospective trial for patients with CML is currently being carried out to confirm this hypothesis. Preliminary results of a phase II study indicate that targeting oral BU in patients with CML results in low transplant-related toxicity and a low relapse rate [50].

Recently, an intravenous preparation of BU has become available and initial phamacokinetic data indicate considerably less individual variation in area under the curve (AUC) values than seen with the oral preparation [51]. In preliminary studies, intravenous BU could be given as a single daily dose over 3 h or twice daily rather than the usual four oral doses per day [52,53]. Retrospective comparisons of intravenous BU with oral BU suggest less hepatic toxicity in patients receiving the intravenous form [54].

A regimen of BU combined with CY has been developed which has had a wide application for treatment of a variety of malignant and non-malignant diseases using autologous and allogeneic stem-cell support [55]. The original regimen included BU 4 mg/kg/day for 4 days followed by CY 50 mg/kg/day for 4 days [55]. This regimen was subsequently modified by lowering the dose of CY to 120 mg/kg with an apparent decrease in toxicity without an increase in relapses [56]. It has been reported that 16 mg/kg combined with 120 mg/kg of CY results in prohibitive toxicity in older patients with MM and breast cancer undergoing autologous or allogeneic transplantation [28,37,41]. Although these reports could be due to small numbers of patients with advanced disease, lowering the dose of BU to 14 mg/kg decreased toxicity and allowed for an increase in the dose of CY to 150 mg/kg [37]. It has also been more recently shown that older patients with CML or myelodysplastic syndrome tolerate targeted BU and CY 120 mg/kg quite well [50,57]. In patients with thalassemia, BU 14 mg/kg followed by CY 120–200 mg/kg has been a well-tolerated and effective regimen for allografting [58].

Etoposide (VP16) (60 mg/kg) has been substituted for CY for the treatment of patients with AML undergoing autologous bone marrow transplantation with an encouraging disease-free survival (DFS) [59–62]. The major toxicities, veno-occlusive disease, mucositis and skin breakdown, are similar to those described with BU + CY or BU + melphalan.

BU (16 mg/kg) and melphalan (140 mg/m^2) have been combined and evaluated in patients undergoing autologous or allogeneic HCT for a variety of hematologic malignancies [63–68].

A regimen of BU (12 mg/kg), melphalan (100 mg/m^2) and thiotepa (500 mg/m^2) followed by autologous HCT has been evaluated in patients with a variety of malignant diseases [8,69]. This regimen produces profound marrow ablation with significant mucositis and is associated with an approximate 5% treatment-related mortality due to IPS. Regimens involving BU, thiotepa and CY have been utilized for auto [70] and allografting [71]. A regimen involving BU, CY and VP16 has been utilized prior to an autologous and allogeneic HCT [72].

Nitrosoureas (Tables 13.2 & 13.7)

Carmustine (1,3-bis(2-chloroethyl)-1-nitrosourea [BCNU]) is a nitrosourea commonly used as a marrow ablative agent because it is active against a variety of tumors [73]. The active metabolite of BCNU is a chloroethyl carbonium ion produced by hydrolysis. It is highly lipid soluble and has been used extensively for the treatment of malignant brain tumors. In conventional doses BCNU is limited by delayed marrow toxicity, pulmonary fibrosis and renal dysfunction. The MTD, as a single agent, is 1200 mg/m^2 when given with autologous stem-cell infusions. The dose-limiting toxicities are pulmonary and hepatic [73]. When carmustine is used in combinations that include cisplatin and CY there is a substantial increase in the risk of lung injury [74–76]. When carboplatin and CY are added to carmustine, a high rate of veno-occlusive disease has been reported [77].

BCNU and CY are often combined and may have synergistic activity. The first multidrug transplant regimen consisted of a combination of BCNU, cytarabine, CY, and thioguanine (BACT) [78]. Variations of these drugs have evolved into the three and four drug combinations in common use today involving BCNU.

Regimens containing CY, BCNU and VP16 (CBV) have been evaluated extensively in patients with malignant lymphoma receiving autologous transplants [79–82]. The doses of drugs and the schedules are shown in Table 13.6. These regimens are often used as substitutes for TBI-based regimens for patients with lymphoma who have received prior dose-limiting irradiation [83]. Doses of BCNU exceeding 450 mg/m^2 are associated with unacceptable pulmonary toxicity [84]. Less frequent severe toxicities include SOS, hemorrhagic cystitis and nephrotoxicity. Although not extensively evaluated, all of these combinations are probably sufficiently immunosuppressive to achieve allogeneic engraftment [85]. These regimens, which involve BCNU doses above 400–500 mg/m^2, are associated with excessive pulmonary toxicity. Early institution of steroid therapy at the first sign of dyspnea may prevent the more serious and often fatal complication of pulmonary fibrosis [74,86]. Patients who receive high-dose BCNU should receive close long-term followup for pulmonary complications that have been noted in adults who received large doses of BCNU as children [87]. Lomustine has been substituted for carmustine in an attempt to decrease pulmonary toxicities [88] but without a clear reduction in lung complications [89].

BCNU, etoposide, cytarabine and CY (BEAC), have been extensively evaluated for patients with malignant lymphoma [90,91]. Melphalan has been substituted for CY in the BEAC regimen to create BEAM and has also been extensively evaluated in patients with malignant lymphoma [67,92–94]. Since most patients with malignant lymphoma have peripheral blood stem cell (PBSC) collected after CY containing regimens, the BEAM regimen may be more attractive than the BEAC regimen. Furthermore, the substitution of melphalan for CY obviates the problem of cystitis and the need for mesna and/or bladder irrigation making this a preferred outpatient regimen for patients with malignant lymphoma. More recently, allogeneic marrow transplants have been performed following administration of BEAM [95].

A regimen of carmustine, cisplatin and CY (STAMP-I) has been commonly used for patients with breast cancer [75]. However, even in patients with stage II-III breast cancer, treatment-related mortality has been reported to be 12%, predominantly due to pulmonary toxicities associated with the high-dose of carmustine (600 mg/m^2) [76]. The increase of pulmonary toxicities associated with this dose of carmustine has been reported to be as high as 59%, but appears to respond to early intervention with corticosteroids [96].

Melphalan (Tables 13.2 and 13.8)

One of the earliest chemotherapeutic agents developed, melphalan is a bifunctional alkylating agent whose structure incorporates nitrogen mustard and phenylalanine [97]. Single doses of melphalan, 150–240 mg/m^2, followed by autologous stem-cell infusion have been evaluated in patients with MM and breast cancer with the dose-limiting toxicities being GI and hepatic [98]. Melphalan, 240 mg/m^2 has been utilized alone as a conditioning regimen for patients with hematologic malignancies receiving allogeneic transplants from HLA-matched siblings [99]. Melphalan has been widely used in high-dose regimens for patients with breast and ovarian cancer, MM or lymphoma. Melphalan 100 mg/m^2 has been used as a reduced intensity-conditioning regimen prior to allogeneic stem-cell transplantation in patients with MM [100].

Melphalan is included in several of the BU and carmustine based regimens in Tables 13.6 and 13.7, and Table 13.8 summarizes additional regimens that have included melphalan for myeloablation.

Melphalan is frequently combined with carmustine (BEAM), a regimen utilized for patients with malignant lymphoma [92–94]. It is frequently utilized alone or with TBI to treat patients with MM [101,102] or leukemia [103].

Thiotepa (Tables 13.2 & 13.9)

Thiotepa was first recognized for its antitumor properties in the 1950s but, because of severe myelosuppression, saw only limited use in breast and ovarian cancer. Both thiotepa and its major metabolite tepa are active against tumor cell lines, *in vitro*. The plasma half-life of tepa is much longer than that of thiotepa and accounts for much of the clinical toxicity [104]. The MTD for thiotepa, as a single agent with stem-cell support, is approximately 1100 mg/m^2. Dose-limiting toxicities are CNS, GI, hepatic and skin [105].

Thiotepa is included in several of the above BU, carmustine and melphalan based regimens outlined in Tables 13.6–13.8 and Table 13.9 summarizes additional regimens that include high-doses of thiotepa. The most frequently used regimen for women with breast cancer is the combination of thiotepa, CY and carboplatin (STAMP-V) [106]. When breast cancer was the most commonly treated disease with stem-cell support, STAMP-V was likely the most widely used of all regimens. This is no longer the case, however, since there has been a marked decline in transplantation for breast cancer. Some investigators administer all three drugs by continuous infusion over 3 days [106], others by bolus on 3 consecutive days [107] and others give CY and thiotepa by bolus and carboplatin by continuous infusion. The superiority of any one of these methods of administration has not been documented.

Nonmarrow ablative agents and agents where MTD with stem-cell support is not known

Cyclophosphamide (Table 13.2)

Cyclophosphamide (CY) alone was originally used to achieve allogeneic engraftment in patients with aplastic anaemia and hematologic malignancies but was abandoned in patients with malignant disease in favor of TBI-based regimens or combinations of chemotherapeutic agents. However, CY, with or without antithymocyte globulin, is still the most commonly used regimen for immunosuppression of patients with aplastic anaemia prior to allogeneic transplantation [22]. CY is very immunosuppressive but is not marrow ablative as the dose-limiting toxicity is hemorrhagic myocarditis [108]. The MTD, as a single agent, is approximately 200 mg/kg and infusion of marrow has no impact on survival at this or higher doses [109]. The major side-effect, at doses of 120–200 mg/kg, is hemorrhagic cystitis which can be diminished by bladder irrigation or the administration of mesna. Both CY and its isomer, ifosfamide have been extensively utilized with high-dose chemotherapy regimens for most tumor types treated with HCT.

Ifosfamide (Table 13.2)

Ifosfamide, a structural isomer of CY, has been evaluated in high-dose regimens followed by autologous stem cells as a substitute for CY. However, similar to CY, hematopoietic toxicity is not dose-limiting even when high doses of ifosfamide are administered [110]. The MTD is 18–20 g/m^2 with the dose-limiting toxicities being renal, bladder and neurologic with lethargy, confusion and seizures. Ifosfamide is always given with mesna for bladder protection. Ifosfamide is frequently combined with VP16 and carboplatin for the treatment of lymphoma [111].

Etoposide (Tables 13.2 & 13.10)

Etoposide (VP16) is a semisynthetic derivative of podophyllin. It appears to act by stabilization of the topoisomerase II-DNA complex with subsequent DNA breaks and cell-cycle arrest. This mechanism of action may promote synergistic cell killing when combined with alkylators [85]. The MTD for VP16, as a single agent with stem-cell support, is approximately 2400 mg/m^2. Although VP16 has substantial myelotoxicity, the dose-limiting toxicity is GI. In a phase I study with marrow support, the tempo of recovery of peripheral counts was not related to the dose of VP16 and was more rapid than recovery after TBI regimens with marrow support [112].

The use of VP16 in high-dose regimens has been reviewed [85]. VP16 is commonly used with TBI [113] in the regimens listed in Tables 13.7 and 13.8, and additional regimens are outlined in Table 13.10. It is not clear whether any of the regimens in Table 13.10 require HCT. BU has been combined with VP16 (Table 13.6) resulting in a unique high dose therapy regimen that is particularly active in patients with acute leukemias [59,60]. The major dose-limiting toxicities of this regimen are GI and pulmonary.

Mitoxantrone (Tables 13.2 & 13.8) and doxorubicin (Table 13.10)

Mitoxantrone has been utilized in a variety of high-dose regimens; however, the MTD as a single agent with stem-cell support has not been reported [114]. Single agent dose escalation trials in patients with metastatic breast cancer were limited by cardiac toxicity and were disappointing in terms of response rates [115]. The highest dose of mitoxantrone administered in a high-dose combination regimen has been 90 mg/m^2 given with 1200 mg/m^2 of thiotepa [116].

Regimens including mitoxantrone are included in Tables 13.8 and 13.9. In one study, CY, 7 g/m^2 and escalating doses of mitoxantrone led to unacceptable hemorrhagic cystitis despite mesna leading the investigator to substitute melphalan for CY [117].

In a similar fashion doxorubicin, a compound structurally related to mitoxantrone, has been combined with VP16 and CY as a high-dose regimen for patients with breast cancer [33]. The MTD of doxorubicin was 165 mg/m^2 with the dose-limiting toxicity being mucositis. It is not clear that the use of mitoxantrone or doxorubicin in high-dose regimens requires stem-cell support and it remains to be determined whether such anthracycline-based regimens are more efficacious than alkylator-based combinations.

Cisplatin (Table 13.2)

The MTD for cisplatin as a single agent with HCT has not been reported and the highest dose given in combination regimens has been 250 mg/m^2 given with VP16 60 mg/kg and CY 100 mg/kg [33].

Regimens including cisplatin are outlined in Tables 13.7–13.10. Although limited by nephrotoxicity when utilized as a single agent, when used with other drugs the doses of cisplatin do not exceed 200 mg/m^2 and, with adequate hydration, renal dysfunction is generally avoidable.

Carboplatin (Table 13.2)

The MTD for carboplatin with HCT is approximately 2000 mg/m^2 with the dose-limiting toxicities being hepatic and renal [118]. Carboplatin, in conventional doses is usually given on a formula based on renal function [119]. However, Shea et al. [118] administered carboplatin in doses of 375–2400 mg/m^2 and found a direct correlation between mg/m^2 and the measured AUC suggesting that high doses could be based on body surface area. In one study, carboplatin was administered at doses of 1000–1600 mg/m^2 in conjunction with high doses of melphalan and mitoxantrone [120]. In a retrospective analysis of this study, dosing by the Calvert formula was more predictive of grade 3–4 toxicities than dosing by body surface area [120]. These data suggested that dosing of carboplatin to an AUC of 20 mg/mL/min rather than 1400 mg/m^2 would decrease grade 3–4 RRT in patients receiving melphalan (160 mg/m^2) and mitoxantrone (50 mg/m^2) followed by autologous PBSC infusion [120].

High-dose combination alkylating agent chemotherapy with carboplatin has been reviewed [121]. High-dose chemotherapy regimens including carboplatin are outlined in Tables 13.8–13.10. A phase I–II trial determined that the MTD of carboplatin and CY administered together are 1.8 and 6.0 g/m^2, respectively [122]. Carboplatin (1500 mg/m^2) with CY (120 mg/m^2) and mitoxantrone (75 mg/m^2) appears to be an active regimen for the treatment of patients with ovarian cancer [123].

Cytarabine (Table 13.2)

Cytarabine is a cell cycle specific antineoplastic agent that affects cells only in S-phase. Although its mechanism of action is not fully understood, it metabolite cytarabine-triphosphate is believed to inhibit the action of DNA polymerase. It may also function as a false substrate when incorporated into DNA. The MTD of cytarabine when administered as a single agent with HCT has not been determined. However, in combination with other agents given in high doses, cytarabine is usually administered in doses of 3 g/m^2 for 4–12 doses at 12 h intervals [124,125]. Cytarabine, 12–36 g/m^2 is included in several regimens utilized for the treatment of patients with hematologic malignancies as outlined in Tables 13.7 and 13.8.

Paclitaxel

Paclitaxel is an antimicrotubule drug that facilitates microtubule assembly from tubulin dimers and stabilizes microtubules by preventing depolymerization. This stabilization inhibits microtubule reorganization, preventing progression to mitosis. Paclitaxel, 775 mg/m^2, has been substituted for carmustine in a regimen including 5.6 mg/m^2 of CY and 165 mg/m^2 of cisplatin [126]. Paclitaxel, 500–700 mg/m^2 has been administered with melphalan (180 mg/m^2) and mitoxantrone (60–90 mg/m^2) to patients with advanced ovarian cancer (Table 13.8) [127].

High-dose regimens with TBI

TBI with CY (Table 13.3)

The use of CY with TBI is based on empirical observations. CY (120 mg/kg) was originally given prior to TBI to a patient undergoing a syngeneic marrow transplant for advanced lymphoma in 1970 [128], in order to avoid tumor lysis and acute renal failure which had been previously observed with TBI given in a single dose of 10 Gy. This patient is alive without disease more than 30 years post-transplant [E.D. Thomas unpublished data]. After this initial patient, CY was regularly given prior to TBI in patients receiving allogeneic or syngeneic marrow transplants with no apparent excess toxicity over that observed following TBI alone and thus became a "standard regimen" widely used in many transplant centers. Although several agents have been added to or substituted for CY (Table 13.5), most of the TBI regimens tested over the past 20 years have included CY before or after TBI. A variety of TBI regimens have been evaluated in attempts to define an optimal dose and schedule. Table 13.3 summarizes the MTD for several different schedules of TBI (delivered by ^{60}Co sources at dose rates of 5–10 cGy/min) given after CY 120 mg/kg [21,23,24].

Randomized trials involving different TBI regimens (Table 13.4)

There has been a paucity of randomized controlled trials evaluating different TBI regimens (see Chapter 14). Three trials reported by the Seattle Marrow Transplant Team are summarized in Table 13.4 [19,21,23,24]. The first study demonstrated that 12.0 Gy of TBI given in 2.0 Gy daily fractions was superior to 10.0 Gy TBI delivered as a single dose [19,21]. The second and third trials evaluated a higher dose of TBI (15.75 Gy) in patients with AML in first remission or CML in chronic phase [23,24]. Both studies showed a decrease in the probability of relapse following the higher dose of TBI but no improvement in survival due to increased transplant-related mortality. Methods to decrease the toxicity of TBI or the use of an intermediate dose of TBI could possibly improve survival in these patients.

TBI with drugs other than CY (Table 13.5)

Drugs other than CY have been administered with TBI, as shown in Table 13.5 [6,103,113,124,129–131]. At the present time there is no evidence that any of these agents are superior to CY when given with TBI since randomized, controlled trials have not been performed.

CY and TBI with other drugs (Table 13.5)

Other agents have been combined with CY and TBI, as shown in Table 13.5 [2,129,132]. Phase II trials suggest that many of these combinations may have better therapeutic efficacy than CY/TBI; however, none of these regimens has been subjected to randomized comparison studies.

Table 13.11 Randomized trials of busulfan/cyclophosphamide (BU/CY) vs. total body irradiation (TBI) ± etoposide (VP16) ± CY.

Ref.	Diagnosis	Regimen	No.	Survival	Relapse	EFS
[135]	AML	BU/CY	51	0.51	0.34	0.47
		CY/TBI	50	0.75	0.14	0.72
[134]	CML	BU/CY	65	0.61	0.44	0.59
		CY/TBI	55	0.63	0.11	0.55
[133]	CML	BU/CY	73	0.80	0.13	0.68
		CY/TBI	69	0.80	0.13	0.71
[131]	"Advanced" leukemias	BU/CY	61	0.30	NR	0.20
		VP16/TBI	61	0.30	NR	0.20

AML, acute myeloid leukemia; BU, busulfan; CY, cyclophosphamide; EFS, event-free survival; NR, not reported; TBI, total body irradiation; VP16, etoposide.

High-dose chemotherapy vs. high-dose chemoradiotherapy (Table 13.11)

Two randomized trials have demonstrated equivalency of BU/CY and CY/TBI in patients with CML in chronic phase receiving HLA-matched allografts [133,134]. One study of patients receiving HLA-compatible transplants for AML showed superiority for the CY/TBI regimen due to a lower relapse rate [135]. The South-west Oncology Group compared BU/CY to VP16/TBI in 122 patients with advanced acute leukemias or CML beyond first chronic phase undergoing matched allogeneic transplantation. There were no significant differences in toxicity, acute GVHD, survival or DFS in patients entered on either regimen [131]. An analysis of nonrandomized trials reported by Horning et al. [132] have suggested equivalency between patients with lymphoma receiving TBI and VP16 or CBV given prior to autologous transplant.

Marrow ablation using radioisotopes

Alternatives to external beam delivery of radiation have been reviewed and are discussed in more detail in Chapter 15 [15]. One approach to improving the cure rate of transplant conditioning regimens while simultaneously decreasing toxicities to normal organs is to replace or augment nonspecific external-beam TBI with targeted radiotherapy. Radiolabeled monoclonal antibodies have the potential to focus higher doses of radiation on tumor sites than is possible with external-beam TBI and expose normal organs to lower doses of radiation. Recent evaluations of these techniques have been performed in patients with MM, malignant lymphoma and AML [136–144].

Bone-seeking radioisotopes

Isotopes that selectively bind to bone by themselves (Yttrium-90 [^{90}Y]) [145] or when complexed to bone seeking compounds are an attractive way to target radiation for patients with malignancies in which bone or bone marrow is the primary site of disease. Few studies have utilized radioisotopes alone for marrow ablation. Bayouth et al. [141] performed a phase I trial of Holmium-166 complexed to the bone seeking isotope-1,4,7,10 tetraazacyclododecane-1,4,7,10-tetramethylene-phosphonic acid (DOTMP) in patients with MM. The total radiation adsorbed dose delivered to the BM for six patients ranged from 7.9 to 41.4 Gy, and marrow ablation requiring the infusion of stem cells was achieved in two patients.

The role of bone-seeking isotopes should be expanded over the next several years and may become a major therapeutic approach to the treatment of malignancies involving the BM.

Radiolabeled monoclonal-antibody studies

Twelve patients with advanced Hodgkin's disease were treated with ^{90}Y-labeled antiferritin monoclonal antibody followed by a CBV regimen and autologous BM transplantation [139]. Three of the 12 patients were alive and disease-free at 24–28 months.

Iodine-131 (^{131}I)-tositumomab (anti-CD20) was evaluated as the sole therapy in 25 patients with relapsed B-cell lymphomas [146]. Twenty-two patients had a biodistribution where more radiation to tumor than normal organs was achieved. Twenty-one received therapeutic infusions with autologous stem-cell support. Sixteen patients achieved complete responses. Subsequently, ^{131}I-tositumomab (anti-CD20) was given with VP16 and CY to 52 patients with relapsed B-cell lymphomas, escalating the doses of isotope, followed by autologous stem-cell transplantation [147]. The maximum tolerable dose to critical normal organs (nonmarrow) was 25 Gy. At 2 years the estimated overall survival and EFS were 83% and 68%, respectively, which compared favorably to a historical control group receiving external beam TBI. This approach was used to treat 16 patients with relapsed mantle cell lymphoma [148]. Estimated survival and progression-free survival at 3 years were 93% and 61%, respectively, a result that may be considerably improved over standard high-dose regimens for this disease.

Anti-CD33 monoclonal antibody therapy for patients with AML has been reviewed [144]. Initial studies utilizing an ^{131}I-labeled anti-CD33 monoclonal antibody, p67, were relatively unsuccessful with only four of nine patients achieving a favorable biodistribution [137]. Scheinberg *et al.* [136] has reported better biodistribution, with longer marrow retention, of an ^{131}I-labeled anti-CD33 monoclonal antibody, M195, in patients with AML. In other studies, antibody M195, complexed to ^{131}I has been given to patients with advanced AML before undergoing conditioning for allogeneic transplantation with a BU/CY regimen [140]. The delivery of up to 160 mCi/m^2 of ^{131}I with BU/CY was well tolerated.

^{131}I-labeled anti-CD45 antibody achieved a favorable biodistribution in 37 of 44 patients with advanced AML or myelodysplasia [149]. In that study 34 patients received ^{131}I-labeled anti-CD45 monoclonal antibody prior to receiving CY and TBI. Patients received up to 12.3 Gy to the liver and 24–28 Gy to bone marrow in addition to the 12.0 Gy of TBI. Seven of 25 patients with AML or refractory anemia with excess blasts were alive and disease-free at 15–89 months. Preliminary studies suggest that the same approach can be utilized in patients with AML in first complete remission (CR) receiving a BU/CY regimen [150].

The above studies are exciting and promise to add a new approach to the eradication of malignancy in selected patients with AML or lymphoma. However, these studies are labor intensive, involve a few, highly selected patients (less than one patient per month being treated in most studies) and have been carried out only in large research institutions. Recently, a low-dose ^{90}Y-CD20 antibody (ibritumomab) which has been approved by the Food and Drug Administration (FDA) [151,152], has been utilized as part of a high-dose regimen (40–100 mCi) with VP16 and CY to treat 18 patients with advanced lymphomas [153]. Excellent response rates with no transplant-related mortality were observed. This topic is reviewed more thoroughly in Chapter 15.

Sequential regimens with peripheral blood hematopoietic cell support

The concept of administering tandem high-dose cycles or multiple, less intensive treatments more frequently as an alternative to single high-dose marrow ablative therapy has only recently been explored [101,154–157]. Sequential cycles of high-dose carboplatin have been administered with growth factor and repeated PBSC infusions [154]. In a similar fashion some groups have utilized tandem cycles of high-dose melphalan 200 mg/m^2 or melphalan and TBI, followed by autologous stem-cell infusion for the treatment of patients with MM [156] or double transplants for breast cancer [101,157]. Tandem cycles of melphalan produced complete response rates of 44% in patients with myeloma. Several prospective, randomized trials of single vs. double-intensive therapy for patients with MM are underway. Tandem cycles of CY, carboplatin and VP16 used to treat 28 patients with untreated metastatic breast cancer resulted in a 50% CR rate and a 30% RFS at 24 months [101]. In another study, patients with stage IV breast cancer treated with a cycle of high-dose melphalan followed by the STAMP-V regimen did not have a better outcome than a single cycle of STAMP-V [157]. It remains to be determined whether or not this approach will be superior to single high-dose ablative regimens.

Allogeneic transplantation with nonmarrow ablative regimens

There is increasing evidence that stable donor chimerism can be achieved with sublethal doses of TBI and immunosuppressive drugs [158]. Partial, but stable grafts, would be of benefit for patients with nonmalignant diseases, such as thalassemia or sickle cell anaemia if they could be achieved without transplant-related mortality [159]. Patients with malignancies are often considered too old for high-dose regimens or when young enough, have organ dysfunction that precludes administration of intensive regimens prior to allografting. In contrast to nonmalignant diseases, however, successful treatment of cancers with allogeneic transplant almost certainly requires full donor engraftment in order utilize the "graft-vs.-leukemia" effects. It is of major interest to develop nontoxic methods of achieving donor chimerism thus allowing the evaluation of post-transplant immunotherapy with donor lymphocytes, which would then be relied on to produce the bulk of the antileukemic therapy [160]. Nonablative allografting strategies are discussed in detail in Chapters 85 and 86.

Preparative regimens—Conclusions

Because of the relatively high probability of relapse in many patients receiving HCT, further development of new treatment regimens is warranted. However, one can predict that it will continue to be difficult to identify more effective treatment regimens. Incremental improvements in treatment regimens are expected to be small, difficult to measure and will require the study of large numbers of patients. As HCT becomes more widely used, there will be a great need for controlled trials to evaluate the effectiveness of specific treatment regimens for specific groups of patients. Only centers with large numbers of patients or cooperative study groups can successfully perform the trials necessary to substantiate the effectiveness of a given treatment regimen. In order to make high-dose therapies and PBSC support generally available the procedure will have to be performed with low mortality and minimal morbidity in an outpatient setting. To achieve this goal without sacrificing efficacy, agents that protect normal, nonhematopoietic tissues from RRT may have to be utilized.

Modification of RRT

As noted above dose intensity may be related to clinical outcome [161], thus, chemotherapy and radiotherapy-associated toxicity may affect the morbidity and mortality and the overall treatment outcome of HCT. Currently, myeloablative conditioning regimens in autologous and allogeneic

Table 13.12 Classification of cytoprotective agents.

	Type of agent	Examples
I	Local agents for local cytoprotection	Cryotherapy, oral rinses?, bladder irrigation
II	Systemic agents for local cytoprotection	Mesna, ursodeoxycolic acid, dexrazoxane
III	Systemic agents for systemic cytoprotection	Amifostine, KGF, lysofylline?, IL-11

IL-11, interleukin 11; KGF, keratinocyte growth factor.

HCT use agents at their MTD and their antitumor efficacy is influenced by the status of the disease at the time of HCT (first CR vs. refractory relapse, chronic phase vs. blast phase, etc.) as well as by the age of the patient and other comorbidities. Hence, agents that may prevent, modify or decrease the toxicities of these regimens would potentially allow their use for: (a) patients earlier in their disease course; (b) broader groups of patients such as older patients or those with other comorbidities; (c) further dose-intensification or combination with other agents for patients with more advanced malignancies; (d) improving the short-term and long-term quality of life of patients; and (e) decreasing the costs of HCT. The agents should have a low toxicity profile while providing protection to normal tissues without decreasing the cytotoxic properties of the conditioning regimen. These properties form the basis for the concept of cytoprotection [162].

Cytoprotective strategies need to be based on a clear understanding of the mechanisms by which chemotherapeutic and radiotherapeutic agents can lead to damage of normal cells and tissues. These strategies can range from local agents or measures for cytoprotection; for example, the use of cryotherapy to try to prevent or decrease mucositis, to the use of agents administered systemically for cytoprotection. The latter may provide mostly local or regional cytoprotection like the use of mesna for the protection of the uro-epithelium from the metabolite acrolein derived from ifosfamide and CY. Other systemic agents may provide cytoprotection or decrease regimen-related toxicities in multiple sites. A classification of cytoprotective agents is provided in Table 13.12.

As stated earlier in this chapter, clinical trials of new anticancer agents usually proceed through a sequence of studies in which the objectives vary, i.e. phase I studies to identify the toxicity/safety profile as well as possible dose and schedule, phase II studies to determine biologic/therapeutic activity and, if justified, phase III trials to compare the new agent with the current standard therapy. However, in the case of studies of new agents that may modify RRT the design is different [163]. Dose-finding studies for these agents should take into consideration the biologic data from animal studies and proof that when used alone their biological effects occur at doses below those that cause significant toxicity. Thus, phase I and II studies of these agents should be done in combination with chemotherapy and be able to determine the safety profile, dose and schedule at which protective effects are obtained (if any). In this way enough information should be available to determine the usefulness of performing a phase III trial where the goals are clear in terms of comparison of clinically important outcomes when compared to standard therapy [163].

Before discussing more specific agents in use and under investigation for the reduction of RRT, it is important to point out other strategies that do not involve cytoprotective agents that have been shown to decrease RRT. They are discussed in other chapters of this textbook and include: (a) improvements in the physiologic and risk assessment evaluation of candidates for HCT (see Chapter 33); (b) the optimization of the pharmacokinetic understanding of high-dose cancer chemotherapy (see Chapter 12) [164,165]; (c) the use of pharmacogenomics and pharmacogenetics to better identify patients at greater risk of toxicity or greater likelihood of response to cytotoxic agents [166]; (d) the optimization of the mobilization and the number of peripheral blood progenitor cells to be collected (see Chapters 45 & 46) [167,168]; (e) the use of more targeted chemo and/or radiotherapeutic agents (discussed above and Chapter 15); and (f) in the case of allogeneic HCT the use of nonmyeloablative or "intensity-reduced" regimens (discussed above and in Chapters 85 & 86).

Agents used locally for local cytoprotection

Local measures and agents have been mainly employed in the setting of high-dose HCT to the prevention of hemorrhagic cystitis and oral mucositis. Oral mucositis can be defined as the inflammation and later ulceration of the oral mucosa; however, it can be argued that in the case of the use of systemic chemo-radiotherapy this process can take place throughout the GI mucosa and, thus, the term mucosal barrier injury would be more precise [169]. It is one of the most common toxicities and most-frequent dose-limiting toxicities affecting about 70–80% of patients. It not only affects quality of life but also because of the breakdown of natural barriers increases the risk of local and systemic infections. Its development may increase length of hospitalization, use of parenteral narcotics, nutrition and costs. At this time there are no definitive approved methods/agents that can prevent and/or reduce the severity, incidence and duration of oral mucositis. Several have been and are currently under study and will be discussed below (Table 13.13).

Cryotherapy

The use of local ice chips or popsicles is based on the local vasoconstrictive effect of cold which would then potentially reduce temporarily the exposure of the local mucosa to the peak levels of systemic chemotherapy. This method has shown some utility with agents with a short plasma half-life like 5-fluorouracil (5-FU) [169,170], but its benefit in HCT has not been clearly shown in randomized trials.

Antimicrobials

In the setting of a damaged mucosal barrier and neutropenia, local secondary infections, that can become systemic, may develop. These secondary infections lead to a greater release of cytokines, such as tumor necrosis factor alpha (TNF-α) and interleukin 1beta (IL-1β), which cause more oedema and inflammation: this tends to occur during the third or ulcerative phase of oral mucositis [170,171]. In an early effort to reduce infections following HCT, high-level protective isolation and GI decontamination with nonabsorbable antibiotics were frequently utilized [172–174]. These measures may not only have reduced infectious complications but may have also reduced noninfectious RRT by reducing the systemic absorption of endotoxins or other bacterial inflammatory cytokines. With the development of more potent antimicrobials, including quinolones, the use of gut decontamination has been markedly reduced. One approach to modify this RRT has been to try to use local antimicrobial/disinfectant agents (Table 13.14). Currently approved agents have not, in general, led to a significant improvement in mucositis [175]. They also do not have an effect on the initial insult to the GI mucosa caused by the

Table 13.13 Local agents/methods to reduce local regimen-related toxicity (RRT).

Agents for oral mucositis	Ref.	Comments
Cryotherapy	[169,170]	No definitive benefit in HCT
Antimicrobials	See Table 13.14	
Local anesthetics	[186]	No benefit prophylactically. Limited benefit used alone or in combination
Cytokines		
TGF-β_3	[180,181,260]	No benefit
GM-CSF	[175,179,182]	No benefit topically. Potential benefit systemically
G-CSF	[183]	Potential benefit but small trial
Nutritional supplements		
Glutamine	[261,262]	Oral glutamine may decrease pain in a subgroup of patients [182]. Potential benefit of IV glutamine
Anti-inflammatory or protectant agents		
Sucralfate, prostagladin E_2, retinoids, vitamin E, topical corticosteroids	[263,264]	Studies with limitations that show some or no benefit
Other agents		
Allopurinol mouthwash	[265]	No benefit
Other methods		
Low-energy laser	[266]	Potential benefit
Radiation shields	[267]	More studies needed
Agents for hemorrhagic cystitis		
Continuous bladder irrigation	[184,185]	Not better than mesna or vigorous IV fluids

G-CSF, granulocyte colony-stimulating factor; GM-CSF, granulocyte macrophage colony-stimulating factor; HCT, hematopoietic cell transplantation; IV, intravenous; TGF, transforming growth factor.

Table 13.14 Local antimicrobials used/studied to reduce local regimen-related toxicity (RRT).

	Ref.	Comments
Chlorhexidine MW	[268]	No benefit
Hydrogen peroxide MW	[269]	No benefit
Topical antifungals	[270,271]	Frequently used but without definitive proven benefit
Multiagent MW	[177]	Potential benefit
Immunol MW (triclosan)	[178]	Phase II study, potential benefit

MW, mouthwash.

conditioning regimen, although newer agents may be effective in decreasing the complications of secondary infections both locally and systemically. Agents under investigation like iseganan (protegrin IB-367) and immunol (triclosan-based mouth wash) have shown promising results in phase II trials of patients undergoing high-dose HCT [176–178] but were ineffective in phase III trials.

Cytokines

Transforming growth factor beta 3 (TGF-β3) can decrease the proliferation of mucosal epithelium and, when tested in animal (hamster) models [179] and later in a phase I trial [180], encouraging results were seen. However, in a multicenter, randomized, double-blind, placebo-controlled study no clear benefit was found [181].

Granulocyte macrophage colony-stimulating factor (GM-CSF) and granulocyte colony-stimulating factor (G-CSF) have also been tested topically. For GM-CSF there is no benefit when used locally [182] and for G-CSF a small trial showed a benefit that needs to be confirmed in a larger, randomized, double-blind study [183].

Other agents or methods that have been used and/or tested are listed in Table 13.13. In various studies, none of them have proven to be of definite benefit. Some require further rigorous testing, and some of them despite no proven benefit continue to be used.

Agents used systemically for local cytoprotection

Mesna

Both ifosfamide and CY are prodrugs that undergo metabolic activation via the hepatic P-450 system. One of their metabolites, acrolein, is implicated as the major cause of oxazaphosphorine urothelial toxicity. With CY, hemorrhagic cystitis is seen more frequently when used at the high doses for HCT. Mesna is a thiol compound that undergoes rapid oxidation in the plasma to dimesna [184]. Both mesna and dimesna are hydrophilic and are rapidly cleared by the kidneys. Thus, urinary mesna concentrations exceed those in the plasma and this is why its beneficial effects are loco-regional and why mesna does not protect from the other systemic toxicities of ifosfamide and CY. This is also why it does not interfere with their cytotoxic activity. The free thiol groups of mesna combine directly with acrolein and other oxazaphosphorine metabolites and stable nontoxic compounds are formed [185].

The current guidelines of the American Society of Clinical Oncology [186] recommend mesna along with saline diuresis or forced saline diuresis when high-dose CY is used. However, in the case of high-dose ifosfamide (doses >2.5 g/m^2/day) the evidence of benefit is insufficient, although more frequent and prolonged administration of mesna should be considered [186]. An oral from of mesna was also recently approved for use in the USA.

Desrazoxane

Doxorubicin and daunorubicin are anthracycline antibiotics that have been used, but not frequently, as part of the conditioning regimens of HCT [33]. Nevertheless, doxorubicin in particular has a major role in the treatment of numerous solid tumors and hematologic malignancies in adults and children. Unfortunately, its use in short infusion is limited by cumulative dose-dependent cardiotoxicity [187] and, despite limiting its cumulative dose, late cardiotoxicity has recently been reported in patients treated with an anthracycline for a malignancy during childhood [188] and in women with operable breast cancer that received doxorubicin in the adjuvant setting [189]. Agents that could then offer cardioprotection from anthracyclines would be extremely important.

Desrazoxane is a bis-dioxopiperazine compound that is hydrolyzed intracellularly to form a chelating agent analogous to ethylene diamine tetracetic acid. Its use prior to short-infusion doxorubicin has been shown to decrease the incidence of anthracycline-associated cardiomyopathy. The proposed mechanism of cardiac protection is explained by its chelation to unbound transition metals like iron, which leads to a decrease in free-radical generation [190].

For patients receiving high-dose anthracycline therapy or for those patients with cardiac risk factors or underlying cardiac disease the recent guidelines do not formally recommend the use of dexrazoxane [186]. Newer ways of administering dexrazoxane in a prolonged intravenous form are being studied that have shown its own cytotoxic effects [191] but may also be useful as a cardiac protectant in the setting of prolonged infusion high-dose doxorubicin regimens [192].

Ursodeoxycholic acid

Sinusoidal obstruction syndrome (SOS) and other liver problems related to the conditioning regimen are a common RRT in patients undergoing high-dose conditioning HCT. They are discussed in detail in Chapter 58. The reported incidence of hepatic SOS varies broadly from 1% to 70% of patients [193–195] and this may be related to the patient population, definition of SOS, as well as the conditioning regimen utilized. The treatment of established SOS has not been very effective; thus, agents that may prevent SOS and/or decrease its severity are important.

Ursodeoxycholic acid is a naturally occurring hydrophilic bile acid (5% of bile acids in normal bile) that has been shown to be nontoxic to the liver parenchyma (while hydrophobic bile acids are). It has been used for patients with primary biliary cirrhosis and in patients after liver transplantation [196], and generally is not associated with major side-effects. Studies over the last 5 years have shown mixed results in terms of its effectiveness for reducing the incidence and severity of hepatic SOS either when used alone [197–199] or in combination with heparin [200].

The study from Ruutu et al. [199], which was a randomized, open-label study in an allogeneic HCT population, did not show significant difference in the incidence of SOS, but it did show a statistical difference in the elevation of bilirubin and alanine aminotransferase, as well as severe acute GVHD and 1-year overall survival in favor of the patients receiving ursodeoxycolic acid. A double-blind, placebo-controlled study is needed to confirm these findings.

Systemic agents for systemic cytoprotection

Lysofylline

In the setting of cytotoxic therapy there is the release of proinflammatory molecules as well as hematopoietic inhibitory cytokines. These may further alter the integrity and decrease the rate of recovery of the mucosa and other tissues leading to greater RRT. Lisofylline, one of the metabolites of pentoxyfilline, is a methylxanthine that in the laboratory and preclinical models has shown antiinflammatory properties [201,202], thus potentially decreasing disruption of the mucosa and the incidence of infections. A published randomized placebo-controlled trial of lisofylline at two different doses in the allogeneic HCT setting reported an improved 100-day survival and lower incidence of infections in the subgroup that received the higher dose of lisofylline compared the subgroups that received placebo or the lower dose. Nevertheless, 25% of randomized patients did not complete the double-blind treatment period; 14% of patients were withdrawn early from study because of nausea and vomiting, and not all subgroups were well-balanced by risk factors [203]. A phase III trial would be needed to confirm these findings before lisofylline could be recommended as an agent that can reduce RRT in the setting of high-dose regimen HCT.

Interleukin-11

Interleukin-11 (IL-11) is a cytokine member of the IL-6 family and it has multiple functions besides its effect on the hematopoietic tissues. In *in vitro* and *in vivo* animal models it has been shown to increase the proliferation of stem cells in the base of intestinal crypts, enhance mucosal regeneration, decrease apoptosis and, by doing so, potentially protect from the toxicity of therapy [204,205]. Despite these results clinical trials have not been so encouraging. In a phase I, double-blind, placebo-controlled trial in patients undergoing HCT using BU, melphalan and thiotepa as the conditioning regimen, IL-11 was shown to reduce the severity, incidence and duration of severe mucositis when used at doses that are more frequently associated with potential toxicities like fluid retention [206]. In another phase I–II double-blind, placebo-controlled study using recombinant IL-11 for patients undergoing allogeneic HCT where the main endpoint was related to prevention of GVHD there was no improvement in the degree of oral mucositis for those patients receiving IL-11 compared to those on placebo [207]. Thus, unless a new schedule of administration is developed where a benefit can be seen with no added serious toxicity, IL-11 can not at this time be recommended to reduce RRT in the setting of high-dose conditioning HCT.

Keratinocyte growth factor

Keratinocyte growth factor (KGF), also termed fibroblast growth factor 7 (FGF-7), is a member of the heparin-binding fibroblast growth factor family. It was initially described by Rubin and coworkers in 1989 who isolated it from conditioned medium from human embryonic lung fibroblasts [208]. The 2.4 kb transcript of KGF has been detected in a variety of mesenchymal cells adjacent to epithelial cells like those from the lung, salivary gland, gut and dermis [209]. Whereas other FGF's affect the various cell types, KGF binds to its receptor (which is a transmembrane tyrosine kinase receptor) specifically on epithelial cells where it stimulates proliferation and differentiation. Cytoprotective functions of KGF that have been described in various *in vitro* as well as animal models include injury repair in skin, alveolar type II cells, GI tract, liver and urothelial epithelium [210–215]. KGF may also protect tissues from oxygen radicals generated during inflammation by inducing an increase in glutathione peroxidase activity [216].

The initial safety studies using KGF, done in healthy volunteers, showed a proliferation of oral epithelial cells with no major side-effects [217]. These studies were followed by two other phase I trials. One examining safety, dose and schedule in patients with metastatic colorectal cancer receiving a 5-FU and leucovorin regimen [218] and the other was a placebo-controlled, dose-escalation trial of KGF in patients with lymphoma who received conditioning with BEAM and autologous HCT [219]. In the latter study 234 patients were randomized in eight sequential dose level cohorts to receive intravenous KGF or placebo starting 3 days before conditioning with BEAM and 3 days after BEAM. With safety of KGF as the major endpoint this study, KGF administration was shown to be safe using these schedules. The study also showed that severe oral mucositis (grades 3–4 by the World Health Organization) was decreased in the KGF group (at the optimal therapeutic doses) compared to placebo. This study led to a phase II multiinstitutional, double-blind, placebo-controlled trial comparing KGF to placebo in patients with hematologic malignancies undergoing autologous HCT [220]. The conditioning regimen used in this trial was highly mucotoxic (fractionated TBI, VP16 and CY) and patients were randomized to one of three possible regimens using six doses of study drug: three daily doses were given before the start of conditioning and three doses after HCT (days 0, +1, +2). Three study drug treatment arms were thus created: one arm of placebo only, one arm of patients that received KGF preradiation and placebo post-HCT, and in the third arm KGF was administered both before conditioning and after HCT. The dose of KGF was 60 µg/kg/day, which was derived from the phase I study discussed above. The primary endpoint of the study was to establish the impact of KGF on the duration of severe oral mucositis.

One hundred and twenty-nine patients completed the study period and there was a reduction in the mean duration of severe oral mucositis for the group of patients that received KGF. For the group that received placebo only the mean duration was 7.7 days, for the group that received KGF only preconditioning it was 5 days (35% reduction, $p = 0.04$) and for the group that received KGF pre and postconditioning the mean duration was 4 days (48% reduction compared to placebo only, $p = 0.001$) [220]. These encouraging results have lead to a larger phase III trial comparing placebo to the 60 µg/kg/day dose of KGF given three daily doses before conditioning and three daily doses post-HCT (days 0, +1 and +2).

Besides its cytoprotectant benefit KGF may have other immunomodulatory effects by protecting thymic function from injury during conditioning [221] and accelerate GI repair after injury from acute GVHD [222]. In addition, KGF by protecting the integrity of the GI tract may play an important role in the prevention of acute GVHD [223].

Amifostine

Amifostine (WR-2721, ethyol) is a naturally occurring phosphorylated thiol that is metabolized after rapidly being cleared from the plasma into an active dephosphorilated thiol metabolite (WR-1065) which is taken into cells [224,225]. In animal models amifostine was evaluated and shown to protect normal tissues (except the CNS) from the effects of radiation therapy and from the toxicity of alkylating and platinum chemotherapeutic agents [226]. Amifostine's active metabolite is WR-1065 and its cytoprotective effect has been shown to be due to its oxygen-free radical scavenger activity as well as its ability to detoxify reactive molecules formed by alkylating and platinum agents [227–229]. It selectively protects normal tissues over tumor tissues for reasons that include differences in levels of tissue alkaline phosphatase, tissue pH and capillary permeability [230,231]. Also, clinically there is no evidence that amifostine use leads to tumor protection.

Amifostine has been evaluated in a number of trials since the 1980s. It is generally well-tolerated and its major side-effects include hypotension (not frequent but most significant), nausea, vomiting, metallic taste during infusion, flushing, sneezing, mild somnolence and occasional allergic reactions [185].

In the transplant setting amifostine has been tested in several scenarios. Based on the understanding that amifostine may protect hematopoietic progenitors from the toxicity of chemotherapy as well as increase the recovery of colony forming units-granulocyte/erythroid/macrophage/megakaryocyte (CFU-GEMM) and burst forming units-erythroid (BFU-E) [232] amifostine has been used to be protect the normal marrow and peripheral blood derived progenitors from the *in vitro* purging effects of 4-hydroperoxycyclophosphamide (4-HC) [233,234]. Shpall *et al.* [233] compared bone marrow from patients with breast cancer used for HCT after marrow was purged with 4-HC with or without amifostine. After the marrow transplant they observed a faster leucocyte engraftment, a decrease in the number of platelet transfusions and fewer days of antibiotic therapy in patients whose marrows were treated with 4-HC plus amifostine. In another study, patients with non-Hodgkin's lymphoma were randomized to receive (or not) amifostine *in vivo* as part of their salvage chemotherapy regimen prior to stem-cell collection [235]. Although the study had a small number of patients, the authors report that amifostine was well-tolerated and its use was associated with a higher stem-cell collection. However, this did not translate into a shortened time to engraftment or to a decrease in the RRT between the two groups.

Amifostine has also been used is as a cytoprotectant during the conditioning regimen prior to HCT. The studies published vary in the study design, number and characteristics of patients enrolled as well as in the conditioning regimen used, dose of amifostine being employed and outcomes measured. Thus, firm conclusions of the potential benefit of amifostine as an effective cytoprotectant agent in HCT cannot be established [236–241].

Summary

As presented above, limitations exist in further dose escalation of the currently available chemotherapeutic agents. The limitations are usually related to the nonhematologic toxicities when these agents are given at MTD. The development of cytoprotectant drugs that modify the morbidity and mortality risks is, thus, important for the further applicability of HCT options to a broader patient population both in age and at an earlier stage of their disease. Some agents have not been able to keep their promise when moved from the laboratory to the bedside; others, however, appear to be based on randomized clinical trials. The data are too preliminary to recommend their use outside of a clinical trial. It is likely though that in the next few years, with a greater understanding of the pharmacokinetics and pharmacogenomics of the agents currently in use, as well as the use of more targeted treatment and cytoprotective approaches, RRT will be reduced. This will allow HCT to be applied to a broader population of patients, reduce costs and improve patients' quality of life in the immediate and late post-HCT period.

References

1. Etzioni R, Pepe MS. Monitoring of a pilot toxicity study with two adverse outcomes. *Stat Med* 1994; **13**: 2311–21.
2. Petersen FB, Buckner CD, Appelbaum FR *et al.* Busulfan, cyclophosphamide and fractionated total body irradiation as a preparatory regimen for marrow transplantation in patients with advanced hematological malignancies: a phase I study. *Bone Marrow Transplant* 1989; **4**: 617–23.
3. Petersen FB, Deeg HJ, Buckner CD *et al.* Marrow transplantation following escalating doses of fractionated total body irradiation and cyclophosphamide. A phase I trial. *Int J Radiat Oncol Biol Phys* 1992; **23**: 1027–32.
4. Demirer T, Petersen FB, Appelbaum FR *et al.* Allogeneic marrow transplantation following cyclophosphamide and escalating doses of hyperfractionated total body irradiation in patients with advanced lymphoid malignancies: a phase I/II trial. *Int J Radiat Oncol Biol Phys* 1995; **32**: 1103–9.
5. Petersen FB, Appelbaum FR, Bigelow CL *et al.* High-dose cytarabine, total body irradiation and marrow transplantation for advanced malignant lymphoma. *Bone Marrow Transplant* 1989; **4**: 483–8.
6. Petersen FB, Buckner CD, Appelbaum FR *et al.* Etoposide, cyclophosphamide and fractionated total body irradiation as a preparatory regimen for marrow transplantation in patients with advanced hematological malignancies: a phase I study. *Bone Marrow Transplant* 1992; **10**: 83–8.
7. Petersen FB, Appelbaum FR, Buckner CD *et al.* Simultaneous infusion of high-dose cytarabine with cyclophosphamide followed by total body irradiation and marrow infusion for the treatment of patients with advanced hematological malignancy. *Bone Marrow Transplant* 1988; **3**: 619–24.
8. Weaver CH, Bensinger WI, Appelbaum FR *et al.* Phase I study of high-dose busulfan, melphalan and thiotepa with autologous stem cell support in patients with refractory malignancies. *Bone Marrow Transplant* 1994; **14**: 813–9.
9. Bearman SI, Appelbaum FR, Buckner CD *et al.* Regimen-related toxicity in patients undergoing bone marrow transplantation. *J Clin Oncol* 1988; **6**: 1562–8.
10. Bearman SI, Appelbaum FR, Back A *et al.* Regimen-related toxicity and early post-transplant survival in patients undergoing marrow transplantation for lymphoma. *J Clin Oncol* 1989; **7**: 1288–94.
11. Bearman SI, Mori M, Beatty PG *et al.* Comparison of morbidity and mortality after marrow transplantation from HLA-genotypically identical siblings and HLA-phenotypically identical unrelated donors. *Bone Marrow Transplant* 1994; **13**: 31–5.
12. Petersen FB, Bearman SI. Preparative regimens and their toxicity. In: Forman SJ, Blume KG, Thomas ED, eds. *Bone Marrow Transplantation*. Boston, MA: Blackwell Scientific Publications, 1994: 79–95.
13. Thomas ED, Bryant JI, Buckner CD *et al.* Allogeneic marrow grafting using HL-A matched donor-recipient sibling pairs. *Trans Assoc Am Physicians* 1971; **84**: 248–61.
14. Vriesendorp HM. Radiobiological speculations on therapeutic total body irradiation. *Critical Review Oncol Hematol* 1990; **10**: 211–24.
15. Appelbaum FR, Badger CC, Bernstein ID *et al.* Is there a better way to deliver total body irradiation? *Bone Marrow Transplant* 1992; **10**: 77–81.
16. Shank B. Total body irradiation for marrow or stem-cell transplantation (Review). *Cancer Invest* 1998; **16**: 397–404.
17. Shank B, Chu FC, Dinsmore R *et al.* Hyperfractionated total body irradiation for bone marrow transplantation. Results in seventy leukemia patients with allogeneic transplants. *Int J Radiat Oncol Biol Phys* 1983; **9**: 1607–11.
18. Shank B. Hyperfractionation versus single dose irradiation in human acute lymphocytic leukemia cells: application to TBI for marrow transplantation. *Radiother Oncol* 1993; **27**: 30–5.
19. Thomas ED, Clift RA, Hersman J *et al.* Marrow transplantation for acute nonlymphoblastic leukemia in first remission using fractionated or single-dose irradiation. *Int J Radiat Oncol Biol Phys* 1982; **8**: 817–21.
20. Girinsky T, Benhamou E, Bourhis J-H *et al.* Prospective randomized comparison of single-dose versus hyperfractionated total-body irradiation in patients with hematologic malignancies. *J Clin Oncol* 2000; **18**: 981–6.
21. Deeg HJ, Sullivan KM, Buckner CD *et al.* Marrow transplantation for acute nonlymphoblastic leukemia in first remission: Toxicity and long-term follow-up of patients conditioned with single dose or fractionated total body irradiation. *Bone Marrow Transplant* 1986; **1**: 151–7.
22. Storb R. Preparative regimens for patients with leukemias and severe aplastic anemia (overview): biological basis, experimental animal studies and clinical trials at the Fred Hutchinson Cancer Research Center (Review). *Bone Marrow Transplant* 1994; **14** (Suppl.): S1–S3.
23. Clift RA, Buckner CD, Appelbaum FR *et al.* Allogeneic marrow transplantation in patients with acute myeloid leukemia in first remission: a randomized trial of two irradiation regimens. *Blood* 1990; **76**: 1867–71.
24. Clift RA, Buckner CD, Appelbaum FR *et al.* Allogeneic marrow transplantation in patients with chronic myeloid leukemia in the chronic phase: a randomized trial of two irradiation regimens. *Blood* 1991; **77**: 1660–5.
25. Brochstein JA, Kernan NA, Groshen S *et al.* Allogeneic bone marrow transplantation after hyperfractionated total-body irradiation and cyclophosphamide in children with acute leukemia. *N Engl J Med* 1987; **317**: 1618–24.
26. Bensinger W, Tesh D, Appelbaum F *et al.* A phase I study of total body irradiation with liver and lung shielding, busulfan (BU) and cyclophosphamide (CY), in preparation for marrow transplant for multiple myeloma (MM). *Exp Hematol* 1993; **21**: 1110 [Abstract].
27. Bensinger WI, Buckner CD, Anasetti C *et al.* Allogeneic marrow transplantation for multiple myeloma: an analysis of risk factors on outcome. *Blood* 1996; **88**: 2787–93.
28. Bensinger WI, Rowley SD, Demirer T *et al.* High-dose therapy followed by autologous hematopoietic stem-cell infusion for patients with multiple myeloma. *J Clin Oncol* 1996; **14**: 1447–56.
29. Pecego R, Hill R, Appelbaum FR *et al.* Interstitial pneumonitis following autologous bone marrow transplantation. *Transplantation* 1986; **42**: 515–7.
30. Metayer C, Curtis RE, Vose J *et al.* Myelodysplastic syndrome and acute myeloid leukemia after autotransplantation for lymphoma: a multicenter case-control study. *Blood* 2003; **101**: 2015–23.
31. Friedberg JW, Neuberg D, Stone RM *et al.* Outcome in patients with myelodysplastic syndrome after autologous bone marrow transplantation for non-Hodgkin's lymphoma. *J Clin Oncol* 1999; **17**: 3128–35.
32. Frei E, Holden SA, Gonin R, Waxman DJ, Teicher BA. Antitumor alkylating agents. *In vitro* cross-resistance and collateral sensitivity studies. *Cancer Chemother Pharmacol* 1993; **33**: 113–22.
33. Somlo G, Doroshow JH, Forman SJ *et al.* High-dose doxorubicin, etoposide, and cyclophosphamide with stem cell reinfusion in patients with metastatic or high-risk primary breast cancer. City of Hope Bone Marrow Oncology Team. *Cancer* 1994; **73**: 1678–85.
34. Peters WP, Henner WD, Grochow LB. Clinical and pharmacologic effects of high dose single agent busulfan with autologous marrow support in the treatment of solid tumors. *Cancer Res* 1987; **47**: 6402–6.
35. Mansi J, da Costa F, Viner C, Judson I, Gore M, Cunningham D. High-dose busulfan in patients with myeloma. *J Clin Oncol* 1992; **10**: 1569–73.
36. Kanfer EJ, Petersen FB, Buckner CD *et al.* Phase I study of high-dose dimethylbusulfan followed by autologous bone marrow transplantation in patients with advanced malignancy. *Cancer Treat Rep* 1987; **71**: 101–2.
37. Bensinger WI, Buckner CD, Clift RA *et al.* Phase I study of busulfan and cyclophosphamide in preparation for allogeneic marrow transplant for patients with multiple myeloma. *J Clin Oncol* 1992; **10**: 1492–7.
38. Copelan EA, Deeg HJ. Conditioning for allogeneic marrow transplantation in patients with lymphohematopoietic malignancies without the use of total body irradiation. *Blood* 1992; **80**: 1648–58.
39. Anderson JE, Tefferi A, Craig F *et al.* Myeloablation and autologous peripheral blood stem cell rescue results in hematologic and clinical responses in patients with myeloid metaplasia with myelofibrosis. *Blood* 2001; **98**: 586–93.
40. Kanfer EJ, Buckner CD, Fefer A *et al.* Allogeneic and syngeneic marrow transplantation following high dose dimethylbusulfan, cyclophosphamide and total body irradiation. *Bone Marrow Transplant* 1987; **1**: 339–46.
41. Demirer T, Buckner CD, Appelbaum FR *et al.* High-dose busulfan and cyclophosphamide followed by autologous transplantation in patients with advanced breast cancer. *Bone Marrow Transplant* 1996; **17**: 769–74.
42. Olavarria E, Hassan M, Eades A *et al.* A phase I/II study of multiple-dose intravenous busulfan as myeloablation prior to stem cell transplantation. *Leukemia* 2000; **14**: 1954–9.
43. Grochow LB. Busulfan disposition. The role of therapeutic monitoring in bone marrow transplantation induction regimens. *Semin Oncol* 1993; **20**: 18–25.
44. Grochow LB, Krivit W, Whitley CB, Blazar B. Busulfan disposition in children. *Blood* 1990; **75**: 1723–7.
45. Slattery JT, Sanders JE, Buckner CD *et al.*

Graft-rejection and toxicity following bone marrow transplantation in relation to busulfan pharmacokinetics. *Bone Marrow Transplant* 1995; **16**: 31–42.

46 Grochow LB, Jones RJ, Brundrett RB et al. Pharmacokinetics of busulfan: correlation with veno-occlusive disease in patients undergoing bone marrow transplantation. *Cancer Chemother Pharmacol* 1989; **25**: 55–61.

47 Stein J, Davidovitz M, Yaniv I et al. Accidental busulfan overdose: enhanced drug clearance with hemodialysis in a child with Wiskott–Aldrich syndrome. *Bone Marrow Transplant* 2001; **27**: 551–3.

48 Slattery JT, Clift RA, Buckner CD et al. Marrow transplantation for chronic myeloid leukemia: the influence of plasma busulfan levels on the outcome of transplantation. *Blood* 1997; **89**: 3055–60.

49 Demirer T, Buckner CD, Appelbaum FR et al. Busulfan, cyclophosphamide and fractionated total body irradiation for allogeneic marrow transplantation in advanced acute and chronic myelogenous leukemia: phase I dose escalation of busulfan based on targeted plasma levels. *Bone Marrow Transplant* 1996; **17**: 341–6.

50 Radich JP, Gooley T, Clift R, Bryant E, Flowers MED, Appelbaum FR. Allogeneic-related transplantation for chronic phase chronic myeloid leukemia (CML) using a targeted busulfan and cytoxan preparative regimen. *Blood* 2001; **98**(1): 778a [Abstract].

51 Andersson BS, Madden T, Tran HT et al. Acute safety and pharmacokinetics of intravenous busulfan when used with oral busulfan and cyclophosphamide as pretransplantation conditioning therapy: a phase I study. *Biol Blood Marrow Transplant* 2000; **6**: 548–54.

52 Fernandez HF, Tran HT, Albrecht F, Lennon S, Caldera H, Goodman MS. Evaluation of safety and pharmacokinetics of administering intravenous busulfan in a twice-daily or daily schedule to patients with advanced hematologic malignant disease undergoing stem cell transplantation. *Biol Blood Marrow Transplant* 2002; **8**: 486–92.

53 Russell JA, Tran HT, Quinlan D et al. Once-daily intravenous busulfan given with fludarabine as conditioning for allogeneic stem cell transplantation: study of pharmacokinetics and early clinical outcomes. *Biol Blood Marrow Transplant* 2002; **8**: 468–76.

54 Kashyap A, Wingard J, Cagnoni P et al. Intravenous versus oral busulfan as part of a busulfan/cyclophosphamide preparative regimen for allogeneic hematopoietic stem cell transplantation: decreased incidence of hepatic venoocclusive disease (HVOD), HVOD-related mortality, and overall 100-day mortality. *Biol Blood Marrow Transplant* 2002; **8**: 493–500.

55 Santos GW, Tutschka PJ, Brookmeyer R et al. Marrow transplantation for acute nonlymphocytic leukemia after treatment with busulfan and cyclophosphamide. *N Engl J Med* 1983; **309**: 1347–53.

56 Tutschka PJ, Copelan EA, Klein JP. Bone marrow transplantation for leukemia following a new busulfan and cyclophosphamide regimen. *Blood* 1987; **70**: 1382–8.

57 Deeg HJ, Storer B, Slattery JT et al. Conditioning with targeted busulfan and cyclophosphamide for hemopoietic stem cell transplantation from related and unrelated donors in patients with myelodysplastic syndrome. *Blood* 2002; **100**: 1201–7.

58 Lucarelli G, Galimberti M, Polchi P et al. Marrow transplantation in patients with thalassemia responsive to iron chelation therapy. *N Engl J Med* 1993; **329**: 840–4.

59 Chao NJ, Stein AS, Long GD et al. Busulfan/etoposide: initial experience with a new preparatory regimen for autologous bone marrow transplantation in patients with acute nonlymphoblastic leukemia. *Blood* 1993; **81**(2): 319–23.

60 Linker CA, Ries CA, Damon LE, Rugo HS, Wolf JL. Autologous bone marrow transplantation for acute myeloid leukemia using busulfan plus etoposide as a preparative regimen. *Blood* 1993; **81**: 311–8.

61 Linker CA, Damon LE, Ries CA, Rugo HS, Wolf JL. Busulfan plus etoposide as a preparative regimen for autologous bone marrow transplantation for acute myelogenous leukemia: an update. *Semin Hematol* 1993; **20** (Suppl. 4): 40–8.

62 Linker CA, Ries CA, Damon LE et al. Autologous stem cell transplantation for acute myeloid leukemia in first remission. *Blood* 1995; **86**: 384 [Abstract].

63 Srivastava A, Bradstock KF, Szer J, de Bortoli L, Gottlieb DJ. Busulphan and melphalan prior to autologous bone marrow transplantation. *Bone Marrow Transplant* 1993; **12**: 323–9.

64 Martino R, Badell I, Brunet S et al. High-dose busulfan and melphalan before bone marrow transplantation for acute nonlymphoblastic leukemia. *Bone Marrow Transplant* 1995; **16**: 209–12.

65 Cony-Makhoul P, Marit G, Boiron JM, Puntous M, Reiffers J. Busulphan and melphalan prior to autologous transplantation for myeloid malignancies. *Bone Marrow Transplant* 1995; **16**: 69–70.

66 Alegre A, Lamana M, Arranz R et al. Busulfan and melphalan as conditioning regimen for autologous peripheral blood stem cell transplantation in multiple myeloma. *Br J Haematol* 1995; **91**: 380–6.

67 van Besien K, Demuynck H, LeMaistre CF, Bogaerts MA, Champlin R. High-dose melphalan allows durable engraftment of allogeneic bone marrow. *Bone Marrow Transplant* 1995; **15**: 321–3.

68 Vey N, De Prijck B, Faucher C et al. A pilot study of busulfan and melphalan as preparatory regimen prior to allogeneic bone marrow transplantation in refractory or relapsed hematological malignancies. *Bone Marrow Transplant* 1996; **18**: 495–9.

69 Schiffman KS, Bensinger WI, Appelbaum FR et al. Phase II study of high-dose busulfan, melphalan and thiotepa with autologous peripheral blood stem cell support in patients with malignant disease. *Bone Marrow Transplant* 1996; **17**: 943–50.

70 Dimopoulos MA, Alexanian R, Przepiorka D et al. Thiotepa, busulfan, and cyclophosphamide: a new preparative regimen for autologous marrow or blood stem cell transplantation in high-risk multiple myeloma. *Blood* 1993; **82**: 2324–8.

71 Przepiorka D, Nath R, Ippoliti C et al. A phase I–II study of high-dose thiotepa, busulfan and cyclophosphamide as a preparative regimen for autologous transplantation for malignant lymphoma. *Leukemia Lymphoma* 1995; **17**: 427–33.

72 Jones RJ, Santos GW. New conditioning regimens for high-risk marrow transplants. *Bone Marrow Transplant* 1989; **4** (Suppl. 4): 15–7.

73 Phillips GL, Wolff SN, Fay JW et al. Intensive 1,3-bis(2-chloroethyl)-1-nitrosourea (BCNU) monochemotherapy and autologous marrow transplantation for malignant glioma. *J Clin Oncol* 1986; **4**: 639–45.

74 Jones RB, Matthes S, Shpall EJ et al. Acute lung injury following treatment with high-dose cyclophosphamide, cisplatin, and carmustine: pharmacodynamic evaluation of carmustine. *J Natl Cancer Inst* 1993; **85**: 640–7.

75 Peters WP, Shpall EJ, Jones RB et al. High-dose combination alkylating agents with bone marrow support as initial treatment for metastatic breast cancer. *J Clin Oncol* 1988; **6**: 1368–76.

76 Peters WP, Ross M, Vredenburgh JJ et al. High-dose chemotherapy and autologous bone marrow support as consolidation after standard-dose adjuvant therapy for high-risk primary breast cancer. *J Clin Oncol* 1993; **11**: 1132–43.

77 Jones RB, Shpall EJ, Ross M, Coniglio D, Affronti ML, Peters WP. High-dose carboplatin, cyclophosphamide, and BCNU with autologous bone marrow support: excessive hepatic toxicity. *Cancer Chemother Pharmacol* 1990; **26**: 155–6.

78 Graw RG Jr, Lohrmann H-P, Bull MI et al. Bone-marrow transplantation following combination chemotherapy imunosuppression (BACT) in patients with acute leukemia. *Transplant Proc* 1974; **6**: 349–54.

79 Jagannath S, Dicke KA, Armitage JO et al. High-dose cyclophosphamide, carmustine, and etoposide and autologous bone marrow transplantation for relapsed Hodgkin's disease. *Ann Intern Med* 1986; **104**: 163–8.

80 Ahmed T, Ciavarella D, Feldman E et al. High-dose, potentially myeloablative chemotherapy and autologous bone marrow transplantation for patients with advanced Hodgkin's disease. *Leukemia* 1989; **3**: 19–22.

81 Gribben JG, Linch DC, Singer CRJ, McMillan AK, Jarrett M, Goldstone AH. Successful treatment of refractory Hodgkin's disease by high-dose combination chemotherapy and autologous bone marrow transplantation. *Blood* 1989; **73**: 340–4.

82 Phillips GL, Reece DE. Clinical studies of autologous bone marrow transplantation in Hodgkin's disease. In: Goldstone AH, ed. *Clinics in Haematology. Autologous Bone Marrow Transplantation.* Philadelphia: WB Saunders, 1986: 151–66.

83 Weaver CH, Appelbaum FR, Petersen FB et al. High-dose cyclophosphamide, carmustine and etoposide followed by autologous bone marrow transplantation in patients with lymphoid malignancies who have received dose-limiting radiation therapy. *J Clin Oncol* 1993; **11**: 1329–35.

84 Schmitz N, Diehl V. Carmustine and the lungs. *Lancet* 1997; **349**: 1712–3.

85 Blume K, Buckner D. Workshop: high dose etoposide containing regimens. *Bone Marrow Transplant* 1995; **15** (Suppl. 1): S207–S12.

86 Reece DE, Connors JM, Spinelli JJ et al. Intensive therapy with cyclophosphamide, carmustine, etoposide ± cisplatin, and autologous bone marrow transplantation for Hodgkin's disease in first relapse after combination chemotherapy. *Blood* 1994; **83**: 1193–9.

87 O'Driscoll BR, Hasleton PS, Taylor PM, Poulter LW, Gattameneni HR, Woodcock AA. Active lung fibrosis up to 17 years after chemotherapy with carmustine (BCNU) in childhood. *N Engl J Med* 1990; **323**: 378–82.

88 Chao NJ, Kastrissios H, Long GD et al. A new preparatory regimen for autologous bone marrow transplantation for patients with lymphoma. *Cancer* 1995; **75**: 1354–9.

89 Stuart MJ, Chao NS, Horning SJ et al. Efficacy and toxicity of a CCNU-containing high-dose chemotherapy regimen followed by autologous

89. hematopoietic cell transplantation in relapsed or refractory Hodgkin's disease. *Biol Blood Marrow Transplant* 2001; **7**: 552–60.
90. Philip T, Dumont J, Teillet F et al. High dose chemotherapy and autologous bone marrow transplantation in refractory Hodgkin's disease. *Br J Cancer* 1986; **53**: 737–42.
91. Philip T, Guglielmi C, Hagenbeek A et al. Autologous bone marrow transplantation as compared with salvage chemotherapy in relapses of chemotherapy-sensitive non-Hodgkin's lymphoma. *N Engl J Med* 1995; **333**: 1540–5.
92. Gaspard MH, Maraninchi D, Stoppa AM et al. Intensive chemotherapy with high doses of BCNU, etoposide, cytarabine, and melphalan (BEAM) followed by autologous bone marrow transplantation: toxicity and antitumor activity in 26 patients with poor-risk malignancies. *Cancer Chemother Pharmacol* 1988; **22**: 256–62.
93. Chopra R, Goldstone AH, Pearce R et al. Autologous versus allogeneic bone marrow transplantation for non-Hodgkin's lymphoma: a case-controlled analysis of the European bone marrow transplant group registry data. *J Clin Oncol* 1992; **10**: 1690–5.
94. Mills W, Chopra R, McMillan A, Pearce R, Linch DC, Goldstone AH. BEAM chemotherapy and autologous bone marrow transplantation for patients with relapsed or refractory non-Hodgkin's lymphoma. *J Clin Oncol* 1995; **13**: 588–95.
95. Przepiorka D, van Besien K, Khouri I et al. Carmustine, etoposide, cytarabine and melphalan as a preparative regimen for allogeneic transplantation for high-risk malignant lymphoma. *Ann Oncol* 1999; **10**: 527–32.
96. Cao TM, Negrin RS, Stockerl-Goldstein KE et al. Pulmonary toxicity syndrome in breast cancer patients undergoing BCNU-containing high-dose chemotherapy and autologous hematopoietic cell transplantation. *Biol Blood Marrow Transplant* 2000; **6**: 387–94.
97. Sarosy G, Leyland-Jones B, Soochan P, Cheson BD. The systemic administration of intravenous melphalan. *J Clin Oncol* 1988; **6**: 1768–82.
98. Corringham R, Gilmore M, Prentice H et al. High-dose melphalan with autologous bone marrow transplant: treatment of poor prognosis tumors. *Cancer* 1983; **52**: 1783–7.
99. Singhal S, Powles R, Treleaven J, Horton C, Swansbury GJ, Mehta J. Melphalan alone prior to allogeneic bone marrow transplantation from HLA-identical sibling donors for hematologic malignancies. Alloengraftment with potential preservation of fertility in women. *Bone Marrow Transplant* 1996; **18**: 1049–55.
100. Badros A, Barlogie B, Siegel E et al. Improved outcome of allogeneic transplantation in high-risk multiple myeloma patients after nonmyeloablative conditioning. *J Clin Oncol* 2002; **20**: 1295–303.
101. Broun ER, Sridhara R, Sledge GW et al. Tandem autotransplantation for the treatment of metastatic breast cancer. *J Clin Oncol* 1995; **13**: 2050–5.
102. Gore ME, Viner C, Meldrum M et al. Intensive treatment of multiple myeloma and criteria for complete remission. *Lancet* 1989; **2**: 879–82.
103. Powles RL, Milliken S, Helenglass G. The use of melphalan in conjunction with total body irradiation as treatment for acute leukaemia. *Transplant Proc* 1989; **21**: 2955–7.
104. Cole DE, Johnson G, Tartaglia RL, O'Dwyer P, Balis F, Poplack DG. Correlation between plasma pharmacokinetics and *in vitro* cytotoxicity of thiotepa (TT) and tepa (TP). *Proc ASCO* 1989; **8**: 72 [Abstract].
105. Wolff SN, Herzig RH, Fay JW et al. High-dose N,'N"triethylenethiophosphoramide (thiotepa) with autologous bone marrow transplantation: phase I studies. *Semin Oncol* 1990; **17**: 2–6.
106. Antman K, Ayash L, Elias A et al. A phase II study of high-dose cyclophosphamide, thiotepa, and carboplatin with autologous marrow support in women with measurable advanced breast cancer responding to standard-dose therapy. *J Clin Oncol* 1992; **10**: 102–10.
107. Weaver CH, West WH, Schwartzberg LS et al. Induction, mobilization of peripheral blood stem cells (PBSC), high-dose chemotherapy and PBSC infusion in patients with untreated stage IV breast cancer: outcomes by intent to treat analyses. *Bone Marrow Transplant* 1997; **19**: 661–70.
108. Storb R, Buckner CD, Dillingham LA, Thomas ED. Cyclophosphamide regimens in rhesus monkeys with and without marrow infusion. *Cancer Res* 1970; **30**: 2195–203.
109. Buckner CD, Rudolph RH, Fefer A et al. High-dose cyclophosphamide therapy for malignant disease. Toxicity, tumor response, and the effects of stored autologous marrow. *Cancer* 1972; **29**: 357–65.
110. Elias AD, Eder JP, Shea T, Begg CB, Frei E, Antman KH. High-dose ifosfamide with mesna uroprotection: a phase I study. *J Clin Oncol* 1990; **8**: 170–8.
111. Moskowitz CH, Bertino JR, Glassman JR et al. Isofamide, carboplatin, and etoposide: a highly effective cytoreduction and peripheral-blood progenitor-cell mobilization regimen for transplant-eligible patients with non-Hodgkin's lymphoma. *J Clin Oncol* 1999; **17**: 3776–85.
112. Wolff SN, Fer MF, McKay CM, Hande KR, Hainsworth JD, Greco FA. High-dose VP-16–213 and autologous bone marrow transplantation for refractory malignancies: a phase I study. *J Clin Oncol* 1983; **1**: 701–5.
113. Blume KG, Forman SJ, O'Donnell MR et al. Total body irradiation and high-dose etoposide: a new preparatory regimen for bone marrow transplantation in patients with advanced hematologic malignancies. *Blood* 1987; **69**: 1015–20.
114. LeMaistre CF, Herzig R. Mitoxantrone: potential for use in intensive therapy (Review). *Semin Oncol* 1990; **17**: 43–8.
115. Shpall EJ, Jones RB, Holland JF et al. Intensive single-agent mitoxantrone for metastatic breast cancer. *J Natl Cancer Inst* 1988; **80**: 204–8.
116. Fields KK, Elfenbein GJ, Perkins JB et al. Two novel high-dose treatment regimens for metastatic breast cancer: ifosfamide, carboplatin, plus etoposide and mitoxantrone plus thiotepa: outcomes and toxicities. *Semin Oncol* 1993; **20**: 59–66.
117. Mulder PO, Sleijfer DT, Willemse PH, de Vries EG, Uges DR, Mulder NH. High-dose cyclophosphamide or melphalan with escalating doses of mitoxantrone and autologous bone marrow transplantation for refractory solid tumors. *Cancer Res* 1989; **49**: 4654–8.
118. Shea TC, Mason JR, Storniolo AM et al. Sequential cycles of high-dose carboplatin administered with recombinant human granulocyte-macrophage colony-stimulating factor and repeated infusions of autologous peripheral-blood progenitor cells: a novel and effective method for delivering multiple courses of dose-intensive therapy. *J Clin Oncol* 1992; **10**: 464–73.
119. Calvert AH, Newell DR, Gumbrell LA et al. Carboplatin dosage: prospective evaluation of a simple formula based on renal function. *J Clin Oncol* 1989; **7**: 1748–56.
120. Weaver CH, Greco FA, Hainsworth JD et al. A phase I–II study of high-dose melphalan, mitoxantrone and carboplatin with peripheral blood stem cell support in patients with advanced ovarian or breast carcinoma. *Bone Marrow Transplant* 1997; **20**: 847–53.
121. Eder JP, Shea TC, Henner WD et al. High-dose combination alkylating agent therapy with carboplatin and autologous bone marrow transplantation in solid tumors. In: Bunn PA Jr, Canetta R, Ozols RF, Rozencweig M, eds. *Carboplatin (JM-8) Current Perspectives and Future Directions*. Philadelphia: WB Saunders, 1990: 353–62.
122. Spitzer TR, Cirenza E, McAfee S et al. Phase I–II trial of high-dose cyclophosphamide, carboplatin and autologous bone marrow or peripheral blood stem cell rescue. *Bone Marrow Transplant* 1995; **15**: 537–42.
123. Stiff PJ, McKenzie RS, Alberts DS et al. Phase I clinical and pharmacokinetic study of high-dose mitoxantrone combined with carboplatin, cyclophosphamide, and autologous bone marrow rescue: high response rate for refractory ovarian carcinoma. *J Clin Oncol* 1994; **12**: 176–83.
124. Coccia PF, Strandjord SE, Warkentin PI et al. High-dose cytarabine and fractionated total-body irradiation: An improved preparative regimen for bone marrow transplantation of children with acute lymphoblastic leukemia in remission. *Blood* 1988; **71**: 888–93.
125. Matulonis UA, Griffin JD, Canellos GP. Autologous peripheral blood stem cell transplantation of the blastic phase of chronic myeloid leukemia following sequential high-dose cytarabine and melphalan. *Am J Hematol* 1994; **45**: 283–7.
126. Cagnoni PJ, Shpall EJ, Bearman SI et al. Paclitaxel-containing high-dose chemotherapy: the University of Colorado experience. *Semin Oncol* 1996; **23**: 43–8.
127. Stiff PJ, Bayer R, Kerger C et al. High-dose chemotherapy with autologous transplantation for persistent/relapsed ovarian cancer: a multivariate analysis of survival for 100 consecutively treated patients. *J Clin Oncol* 1997; **15**: 1309–17.
128. Fefer A, Einstein AB, Thomas ED et al. Bone-marrow transplantation for hematologic neoplasia in 16 patients with identical twins. *N Engl J Med* 1974; **290**: 1389–93.
129. Riddell S, Appelbaum FR, Buckner CD et al. High-dose cytarabine and total body irradiation with or without cyclophosphamide as a preparative regimen for marrow transplantation for acute leukemia. *J Clin Oncol* 1988; **6**: 576–82.
130. Mehta J, Powles R, Singhal S, Horton C, Tait D, Treleaven J. Melphalan: total body irradiation and autologous bone marrow transplantation for adult acute leukemia beyond first remission. *Bone Marrow Transplant* 1996; **18**: 119–23.
131. Blume KG, Kopecky KJ, Henslee-Downey JP et al. A prospective randomized comparison of total body irradiation: etoposide versus busulfan–cyclophosphamide as preparatory regimens for bone marrow transplantation in patients with recurrent leukemia: a Southwest Oncology Group Study. *Blood* 1993; **81**: 2187–93.

132 Horning S, Chao N, Negrin R et al. The Stanford experience with high-dose etoposide cytoreductive regimens and autologous bone marrow transplantation in Hodgkin's disease and non-Hodgkin's lymphoma: preliminary data. Ann Oncol 1991; 2: 47–50.

133 Clift RA, Buckner CD, Thomas ED et al. Marrow transplantation for chronic myeloid leukemia: a randomized study comparing cyclophosphamide and total body irradiation with busulfan and cyclophosphamide. Blood 1994; 84: 2036–43.

134 Devergie A, Blaise D, Attal M et al. Allogeneic bone marrow transplantation for chronic myeloid leukemia in first chronic phase: a randomized trial of busulfan–cytoxan versus cytoxan–total body irradiation as preparative regimen: a report from the French Society of Bone Marrow Graft (SFGM). Blood 1995; 85: 2263–8.

135 Blaise D, Maraninchi D, Archimbaud E et al. Allogeneic bone marrow transplantation for acute myeloid leukemia in first remission: a randomized trial of a busulfan–cytoxan versus cytoxan–total body irradiation as preparative regimen: a report from the Groupe d'Etudes de la Greffe de Moelle Osseuse. Blood 1992; 79: 2578–82.

136 Scheinberg DA, Lovett D, Divgi CR et al. A phase I trial of monoclonal antibody M195 in acute myelogenous leukemia: specific bone marrow targeting and internalization of radionuclide. J Clin Oncol 1991; 9: 478–90.

137 Appelbaum FR, Matthews DC, Eary JF et al. Use of radiolabeled anti-CD33 antibody to augment marrow irradiation prior to marrow transplantation for acute myelogenous leukemia. Transplantation 1992; 54: 829–33.

138 Press OW, Eary JF, Appelbaum FR et al. Radiolabeled-antibody therapy of B-cell lymphoma with autologous bone marrow support. N Engl J Med 1993; 329: 1219–24.

139 Bierman PJ, Vose JM, Leichner PK et al. Yttrium 90-labeled antiferritin followed by high-dose chemotherapy and autologous bone marrow transplantation for poor-prognosis Hodgkin's disease. J Clin Oncol 1993; 11: 698–703.

140 Papadopoulos EB, Caron P, Castro-Malaspina H et al. Results of allogeneic bone marrow transplant following ^{131}I-M195/busulfan/cyclophosphamide (BU/CY) in patients with advanced/refractory myeloid malignancies. Blood 1993; 82 (Suppl. 1): 80a [Abstract].

141 Bayouth JE, Macey DJ, Kasi LP et al. Pharmacokinetics, dosimetry and toxicity of holmium-166-DOTMP for bone marrow ablation in multiple myeloma. J Nucl Med 1995; 36: 730–7.

142 Press OW, Eary JF, Appelbaum FR, Bernstein ID. Myeloablative radiolabeled antibody therapy with autologous bone marrow transplantation for relapsed B cell lymphomas. In: Buckner CD, Clift R, eds. Technical and Biological Components of Marrow Transplantation. Boston: Academic Publishers, 1995: 281–97.

143 Matthews DC, Appelbaum FR, Eary JF et al. Development of a marrow transplant regimen for acute leukemia using targeted hematopoietic irradiation delivered by ^{131}I-labeled anti-CD45 antibody, combined with cyclophosphamide and total body irradiation. Blood 1995; 85: 1122–31.

144 Jurcic JG, Caron PC, Nikula TK et al. Radiolabeled anti-CD33 monoclonal antibody M195 for myeloid leukemias. Cancer Res 1995; 55 (Suppl. 23): S5908–S10.

145 Rösch F, Herzog H, Plag C et al. Radiation doses of yttrium-90 citrate and yttrium-90 EDTMP as determined via analogous yttrium-86 complexes and position emission tomography. Eur J Nucl Med 1996; 23: 958–66.

146 Press OW, Eary JF, Appelbaum FR et al. Phase II trial of ^{131}I-B1 (anti-CD20) antibody therapy with autologous stem cell transplantation for relapsed B cell lymphomas. Lancet 1995; 346: 336–40.

147 Press OW, Eary JF, Gooley T et al. A phase I/II trial of iodine-131-tositumomab (anti-CD20), etoposide, cyclophosphamide, and autologous stem cell transplantation for relapsed B-cell lymphomas (Plenary paper). Blood 2000; 96: 2934–42.

148 Gopal AK, Rajendran JG, Petersdorf SH et al. High-dose chemo-radioimmunotherapy with autologous stem cell support for relapsed mantle cell lymphoma. Blood 2002; 99: 3158–62.

149 Matthews DC, Appelbaum FR, Eary JF et al. Phase I study of ^{131}I-Anti-CD45 antibody plus cyclophosphamide and total body irradiation for advanced acute leukemia and myelodysplastic syndrome. Blood 1999; 94: 1237–47.

150 Matthews DC, Appelbaum FR, Eary JF, Mitchell D, Press OW, Bernstein ID. ^{131}I-anti-CD45 antibody plus busulfan/cyclophosphamide in matched related transplants for AML in first remission. Blood 1996; 88: 142a [Abstract].

151 Wiseman GA, Gordon LI, Multani PS et al. Ibritumomab tiuxetan radioimmunotherapy for patients with relapsed or refractory non-Hodgkin lymphoma and mild thrombocytopenia: a phase II multicenter trial. Blood 2002; 99: 4336–42.

152 Witzig TE, Flinn IW, Gordon LI et al. Treatment with ibritumomab tiuxetan radioimmunotherapy in patients with rituximab-refractory follicular non-Hodgkin's lymphoma. J Clin Oncol 2002; 20: 3262–9.

153 Nademanee A, Molina A, Forman SJ et al. A phase I/II trial of high-dose radioimmunotherapy (RIT) with zevalin in combination with high-dose etoposide (VP-16) and cyclophosphamide (CY) followed by autologous stem cell transplant (ASCT) in patients with poor-risk or relapsed B-cell non-Hodgkin's lymphoma (NHL). Blood 2002; 100(1): 182a [Abstract].

154 Shea TC, Flaherty M, Elias A et al. A phase I clinical and pharmacokinetic study of carboplatin and autologous bone marrow support. J Clin Oncol 1989; 7: 651–61. Erratum: J Clin Oncol 1989; 7: 1177.

155 Fennelly D, Wasserheit C, Schneider J et al. Simultaneous dose escalation and schedule intensification of carboplatin-based chemotherapy using peripheral blood progenitor cells and filgrastim: a phase I trial. Cancer Res 1994; 54: 6137–42.

156 Vesole DH, Jagannath S, Glenn LD, Barlogie B. Allogeneic bone marrow transplantation (AlloBMT) in multiple myeloma (MM). Proc Am Soc Clin Oncol 1993; 12: 405 [Abstract].

157 Ayash LJ, Elias A, Wheeler C et al. Double dose-intensive chemotherapy with autologous marrow and peripheral-blood progenitor-cell support for metastatic breast cancer: a feasibility study. J Clin Oncol 1994; 12: 37–44.

158 Storb RYuC, Wagner JL et al. Stable mixed hematopoietic chimerism in DLA-identical littermate dogs given sublethal total body irradiation before and pharmacological immunosuppression after marrow transplantation. Blood 1997; 89: 3048–54.

159 McSweeney PA, Niederwieser D, Shizuru JA et al. Hematopoietic cell transplantation in older patients with hematologic malignancies: replacing high-dose cytotoxic therapy with graft-versus-tumor effects. Blood 2001; 97: 3390–400.

160 Mackinnon S, Papadopoulos EB, Carabasi MH et al. Adoptive immunotherapy evaluating escalating doses of donor leukocytes for relapse of chronic myeloid leukemia after bone marrow transplantation: separation of graft-versus-leukemia responses from graft-versus-host disease. Blood 1995; 86: 1261–8.

161 Hryniuk WM, Figueredo A, Goodyear M. Applications of dose intensity to problems in chemotherapy of breast and colorectal cancer. Semin Oncol 1987; 14: 3–11.

162 Bukowski RM. The need for cytoprotection (Review). Eur J Cancer 1996; 32(A) (Suppl. 4): S2–S4.

163 Phillips KA, Tannock IF. Design and interpretation of clinical trials that evaluate agents that may offer protection from the toxic effects of cancer chemotherapy (Review). J Clin Oncol 1998; 16: 3179–90.

164 Rousseau A, Marquet P, Debord J, Sabot C, Lachatre G. Adaptive control methods for the dose individualisation of anticancer agents (Review). Clin Pharmacokinetics 2000; 38: 315–53.

165 Masson E, Zamboni WC. Pharmacokinetic optimisation of cancer chemotherapy. Effect on outcomes (Review). Clin Pharmacokinetics 1997; 32: 324–43.

166 Chabner BA. Cytotoxic agents in the era of molecular targets and genomics. Oncologist 2002; 7 (Suppl. 2): 34–41.

167 Scheid C, Draube A, Reiser M et al. Using at least $5 \times 10(6)$/kg CD34$^+$ cells for autologous stem cell transplantation significantly reduces febrile complications and use of antibiotics after transplantation. Bone Marrow Transplant 1999; 23: 1177–81.

168 Bociek RG, Lynch JC, Yee GC et al. Outcome and factors associated with slow mobilization of peripheral blood progenitor cells (PBPC) in patients undergoing autologous transplantation for non-Hodgkin's lymphoma (NHL). Blood 2001; 98: 861a [Abstract].

169 Blijlevens NM, Donnelly JP, De Pauw BE. Mucosal barrier injury: biology, pathology, clinical counterparts and consequences of intensive treatment for haematological malignancy: an overview (Review). Bone Marrow Transplant 2000; 25: 1269–78.

170 Rocke LK, Loprinzi CL, Lee JK et al. A randomized clinical trial of two different durations of oral cryotherapy for prevention of 5-fluorouracil-related stomatitis. Cancer 1993; 72: 2234–8.

171 Sonis ST. Mucositis as a biological process. A new hypothesis for the development of chemotherapy-induced stomatotoxicity (Review). Oral Oncol 1998; 34: 39–43.

172 Buckner CD, Clift RA, Thomas ED et al. Early infectious complications in allogeneic marrow transplant recipients with acute leukemia: effects of prophylactic measures. Infection 1983; 11: 243–50.

173 Buckner CD. Gnotobiotics and human marrow transplantation. In: Wostmann BS, ed. Germfree Research: Microflora Control and its Application to the Biomedical Sciences. New York: Alan R Liss, 1985: 423–7.

174 Buckner CD, Clift RA, Sanders JE et al. Protective environment for marrow transplant recipients. A

prospective study. *Ann Intern Med* 1978; **89**: 893–901.
175 Stiff P. Mucositis associated with stem cell transplantation. Current status and innovative approaches to management (Review). *Bone Marrow Transplant* 2001; **27** (Suppl. 2): S3–S11.
176 Giles FJ, Redman R, Yazji S, Bellm L. Iseganan HCl: a novel antimicrobial agent. *Expert Opinion Invest Drugs* 2002; **11**: 1161–70.
177 Spijkervet FK, Van Saene HK, Van Saene JJ *et al.* Effect of selective elimination of the oral flora on mucositis in irradiated head and neck cancer patients. *J Surg Oncol* 1991; **46** (Suppl.): 167–73.
178 Goldberg SL, Pineiro L, Schuster MW *et al.* Randomized, vehicle controlled study of immunol oral rinse for the prevention of oral mucositis in bone marrow transplant patients undergoing intensive chemotherapy and/or radiotherapy. *Blood* 2001; **98**(1): 854a [Abstract].
179 Carnel SB, Blakeslee DB, Oswald SG, Barnes M. Treatment of radiation- and chemotherapy-induced stomatitis. *Otolaryngol Head Neck Surg* 1990; **102**: 326–30.
180 Sonis ST, Lindquist L, Van Vugt A *et al.* Prevention of chemotherapy-induced ulcerative mucositis by transforming growth factor β3. *Cancer Res* 1994; **54**: 1135–8.
181 Wymenga AN, van der Graaf WT, Hofstra LS *et al.* Phase I study of transforming growth factor-β_3 mouthwashes for prevention of chemotherapy-induced mucositis. *Clin Cancer Res* 1999; **5**: 1363–8.
182 Valcarcel D, Sanz MA Jr, Sureda A *et al.* Mouth-washings with recombinant human granulocyte-macrophage colony stimulating factor (rhGM-CSF) do not improve grade III–IV oropharyngeal mucositis (OM) in patients with hematological malignancies undergoing stem cell transplantation. Results of a randomized double-blind placebo-controlled study. *Bone Marrow Transplant* 2002; **29**: 783–7.
183 Karthaus M, Rosenthal C, Huebner G *et al.* Effect of topical oral G-CSF on oral mucositis: a randomised placebo-controlled trial. *Bone Marrow Transplant* 1998; **22**: 781–5.
184 Brock N, Pohl J, Stekar J, Scheef W. Studies on the urotoxicity of oxazaphosphorine cytostatics and its prevention. III. Profile of action of sodium 2-mercaptoethane sulfonate (mesna). *Eur J Cancer Clin Oncol* 1982; **18**: 1377–87.
185 Hensley ML, Schuchter LM, Lindley C *et al.* American Society of Clinical Oncology clinical practice guidelines for the use of chemotherapy and radiotherapy protectants. *J Clin Oncol* 1999; **17**: 3333–55.
186 Schuchter LM, Hensley ML, Meropol NJ, Winer EP. American Society of Clinical Oncology Chemotherapy and Radiotherapy Expert Panel 2002 update of recommendations for the use of chemotherapy and radiotherapy protectants: clinical practice guidelines of the American Society of Clinical Oncology. *J Clin Oncol* 2002; **20**: 2895–903.
187 Von Hoff DD, Layard MW, Basa P *et al.* Risk factors for doxorubicin-induced congestive heart failure. *Ann Intern Med* 1979; **91**: 710–7.
188 Kremer LC, van Dalen EC, Offringa M, Ottenkamp J, Voute PA. Anthracycline-induced clinical heart failure in a cohort of 607 children: long-term follow-up study. *J Clin Oncol* 2001; **19**: 191–6.
189 Zambetti M, Moliterni A, Materazzo C *et al.* Long-term cardiac sequelae in operable breast cancer patients given adjuvant chemotherapy with or without doxorubicin and breast irradiation. *J Clin Oncol* 2001; **19**: 37–43.
190 Speyer JL, Green MD, Kramer E *et al.* Protective effect of the bispiperazinedione ICRF-187 against doxorubicin-induced cardiac toxicity in women with advanced breast cancer. *N Engl J Med* 1988; **319**: 745–52.
191 Tetef ML, Synold TW, Chow W *et al.* Phase I trial of 96-hour continuous infusion of dexrazoxane in patients with advanced malignancies. *Clin Cancer Res* 2001; **7**: 1569–76.
192 Morgan RJJ, Doroshow JH, Venkataraman K *et al.* High-dose infusional doxorubicin and cyclophosphamide: a feasibility study of tandem high-dose chemotherapy cycles without stem cell support. *Clin Cancer Res* 1997; **3**: 2337–45.
193 Bearman SI, Anderson GL, Mori M, Hinds MS, Shulman HM, McDonald GB. Venoocclusive disease of the liver: development of a model for predicting fatal outcome after marrow transplantation. *J Clin Oncol* 1993; **11**: 1729–36.
194 Bearman SI. The syndrome of hepatic veno-occlusive disease after marrow transplantation. *Blood* 1995; **85**: 3005–20.
195 Carreras E, Bertz H, Arcese W *et al.* Incidence and outcome of hepatic veno-occlusive disease after blood or marrow transplantation: a prospective cohort study of the European Group for Blood and Marrow Transplantation. European Group for Blood and Marrow Transplantation Chronic Leukemia Working Party. *Blood* 1998; **92**: 3599–604.
196 Barnes D, Talenti D, Cammell G *et al.* A randomized clinical trial of ursodeoxycholic acid as adjuvant treatment to prevent liver transplant rejection. *Hepatology* 1997; **26**: 853–7.
197 Essell JH, Schroeder MT, Harman GS *et al.* Ursodiol prophylaxis against hepatic complications of allogeneic bone marrow transplantation. A randomized, double-blind, placebo-controlled trial. *Ann Intern Med* 1998; **128**: 975–81.
198 Ohashi K, Tanabe J, Watanabe R *et al.* The Japanese multicenter open randomized trial of ursodeoxycholic acid prophylaxis for hepatic veno-occlusive disease after stem cell transplantation. *Am J Hematol* 2000; **64**: 32–8.
199 Ruutu T, Eriksson B, Remes K *et al.* Ursodeoxycholic acid for the prevention of hepatic complications in allogeneic stem cell transplantation. *Blood* 2002; **100**: 1977–83.
200 Park SH, Lee MH, Lee H *et al.* A randomized trial of heparin plus ursodiol vs. heparin alone to prevent hepatic veno-occlusive disease after hematopoietic stem cell transplantation. *Bone Marrow Transplant* 2002; **29**: 137–43.
201 Rice GC, Rosen JW, Weeks R, Michnick J, Bianco JA, Singer JW. CT-1501R selectively inhibits induced inflammatory monokines in human whole blood *ex vivo*. *Shock* 1994; **1**: 254–66.
202 de Vries P, Xu Z, Rice GC, Singer JW. *In vivo* therapy with lisofylline (LSF) in mice suppresses the *ex vivo* release of multi-lineage hematopoietic inhibitory activity induced by cancer chemotherapeutic agents (chemo) from murine splenocytes. *Blood* 1996; **88**: 114b [Abstract].
203 List AF, Maziarz R, Stiff P *et al.* A randomized placebo-controlled trial of lisofylline in HLA-identical, sibling-donor, allogeneic bone marrow transplant recipients. The Lisofylline Marrow Transplant Study Group. *Bone Marrow Transplant* 2000; **25**: 283–91.
204 Potten CS. Protection of the small intestinal clonogenic stem cells from radiation-induced damage by pretreatment with interleukin 11 also increases murine survival time. *Stem Cells* 1996; **14**: 452–9.
205 Sonis S, Edwards L, Lucey C. The biological basis for the attenuation of mucositis: the example of interleukin-11 (Review). *Leukemia* 1999; **13**: 831–4.
206 Schwerkoske J, Schwartzberg L, Weaver C, Schwertschlag U, Goodfellow J, Bedrosian C. A phase 1 double-masked, placebo-controlled study to evaluate tolerability of Neumega (rhIL-11; oprelvekin) to reduce mucositis in patients with solid tumors or lymphoma receiving high-dose chemotherapy (CT) with autologous peripheral blood stem cell reinfusion (PBSCT). *Proc Am Soc Clin Oncol* 1999: 584a [Abstract].
207 Antin JH, Lee SJ, Neuberg D *et al.* A phase I/II double-blind, placebo-controlled study of recombinant human interleukin-11 for mucositis and acute GVHD prevention in allogeneic stem cell transplantation. *Bone Marrow Transplant* 2002; **29**: 373–7.
208 Rubin JS, Osada H, Finch PW, Taylor WG, Rudikoff S, Aaronson SA. Purification and characterization of a newly identified growth factor specific for epithelial cells. *Proc Natl Acad Sci U S A* 1989; **86**: 802–6.
209 Wirth K, Mertelsmann R. Cytoprotective function of keratinocyte growth factor in tumour therapy-induced tissue damage (Review). *Br J Haematol* 2002; **116**: 505–10.
210 Werner S. Keratinocyte growth factor: a unique player in epithelial repair processes (Review). *Cytokine Growth Factor Rev* 1998; **9**: 153–65.
211 Yi ES, Williams ST, Lee H *et al.* Keratinocyte growth factor ameliorates radiation- and bleomycin-induced lung injury and mortality. *Am J Pathol* 1996; **149**: 1963–70.
212 Farrell CL, Bready JV, Rex KL *et al.* Keratinocyte growth factor protects mice from chemotherapy and radiation-induced gastrointestinal injury and mortality. *Cancer Res* 1998; **58**: 933–9.
213 Farrell CL, Rex KL, Chen JN *et al.* The effects of keratinocyte growth factor in preclinical models of mucositis (Review). *Cell Prolif* 2002; **35** (Suppl. 1): 78–85.
214 Senaldi G, Shaklee CL, Simon B, Rowan CG, Lacey DL, Hartung T. Keratinocyte growth factor protects murine hepatocytes from tumor necrosis factor-induced apoptosis *in vivo* and *in vitro*. *Hepatology* 1998; **27**: 1584–91.
215 Ulich TR, Whitcomb L, Tang W *et al.* Keratinocyte growth factor ameliorates cyclophosphamide-induced ulcerative hemorrhagic cystitis. *Cancer Res* 1997; **57**: 472–5.
216 Frank S, Munz B, Werner S. The human homologue of a bovine non-selenium glutathione peroxidase is a novel keratinocyte growth factor-regulated gene. *Oncogene* 1997; **14**: 915–21.
217 Serdar CM, Heard R, Prathikanti R *et al.* Safety, pharmacokinetics and biologic activity of rHuKGF in normal volunteers: results of a placebo-controlled randomized double-blind phase I study. *Blood* 1997; **90**: 172a [Abstract].
218 Meropol N, Gutheil J, Pelley R *et al.* Keratinocyte growth factor (KGF) as a mucositis protectant: a randomized phase I trial. *Proc Am Soc Clin Oncol* 2000; **603**(A): 2374 [Abstract].

219 Durrant S, Pico JL, Schmitz N et al. A phase 1 study of recombinant human keratinocyte growth factor (RHUKGF) in lymphoma patients receiving high-dose chemotherapy (HDC) with autologous peripheral blood progenitor cell transplantation (autoPBCT). *Blood* 1999; **94**: 708a [Abstract].

220 Spielberger RT, Stiff P, Emmanouilides C et al. Efficacy of recombinant human keratinocyte growth factor (rHuKGF) in reducing mucositis in patients with hematologic malignancies undergoing autologous peripheral blood progenitor cell transplantation (auto-PBPCT) after radiation-based conditioning: results of a phase 2 trial. *Proc ASCO* 2001; **20**(1): 7a [Abstract].

221 Min D, Taylor PA, Panoskaltsis-Mortari A et al. Protection from thymic epithelial cell injury by keratinocyte growth factor: a new approach to improve thymic and peripheral T-cell reconstitution after bone marrow transplantation. *Blood* 2002; **99**: 4592–600.

222 Rossi S, Blazar BR, Farrell CL et al. Keratinocyte growth factor preserves normal thymopoiesis and thymic microenvironment during experimental graft-versus-host disease. *Blood* 2002; **100**: 682–91.

223 Hill GR, Ferrara JL. The primacy of the gastrointestinal tract as a target organ of acute graft-versus-host disease: rationale for the use of cytokine shields in allogeneic bone marrow transplantation. [Review]. *Blood* 2000; **95**: 2754–9.

224 Capizzi RL. The preclinical basis for broad-spectrum selective cytoprotection of normal tissues from cytotoxic therapies by amifostine (Review). *Semin Oncol* 1999; **26**: 3–21.

225 Shaw LM, Glover D, Turrisi A et al. Pharmacokinetics of WR-2721 (Review). *Pharmacol Therapeutics* 1988; **39**: 195–201.

226 Schuchter LM, Glick J. The current status of WR-2721 (Amifostine): a chemotherapy and radiation therapy protector. *Biologic Ther Cancer* 1993; **3**: 1–10.

227 Smoluk GD, Fahey RC, Calabro-Jones PM, Aguilera JA, Ward JF. Radioprotection of cells in culture by WR-2721 and derivatives: form of the drug responsible for protection. *Cancer Res* 1988; **48**: 3641–7.

228 DeNeve WJ, Everett CK, Suminski JE, Valeriote FA. Influence of WR2721 on DNA cross-linking by nitrogen mustard in normal mouse bone marrow and leukemia cells in vivo. *Cancer Res* 1988; **48**: 6002–5.

229 Treskes M, Nijtmans LG, Fichtinger-Schepman AM, Van der Vijgh WJ. Effects of the modulating agent WR2721 and its main metabolites on the formation and stability of cisplatin-DNA adducts in vitro in comparison to the effects of thiosulphate and diethyldithiocarbamate. *Biochem Pharmacol* 1992; **43**: 1013–9.

230 Calabro-Jones PM, Fahey RC, Smoluk GD, Ward JF. Alkaline phosphatase promotes radioprotection and accumulation of WR-1065 in V79-171 cells incubated in medium containing WR-2721. *Int J Radiat Biol Related Studies Phys Chem Med* 1985; **47**: 23–7.

231 Utley JF, Marlowe C, Waddell WJ. Distribution of ^{35}S-labeled WR-2721 in normal and malignant tissues of the mouse1,2. *Radiat Res* 1976; **68**: 284–91.

232 List AF, Heaton R, Glinsmann-Gibson B, Capizzi RL. Amifostine protects primitive hematopoietic progenitors against chemotherapy cytotoxicity. *Semin Oncol* 1996; **23**: 58–63.

233 Shpall EJ, Stemmer SM, Hami L et al. Amifostine (WR-2721) shortens the engraftment period of 4-hydroperoxycyclophosphamide-purged bone marrow in breast cancer patients receiving high-dose chemotherapy with autologous bone marrow support. *Blood* 1994; **83**: 3132–7.

234 Fauth F, Martin H, Sonnhoff S et al. Purging of G-CSF-mobilized peripheral autografts in acute leukemia with mafosfamide and amifostine to protect normal progenitor cells. *Bone Marrow Transplant* 2000; **25**: 831–6.

235 Emmanouilides C, Territo M, Andrey J, Mason J. A randomized phase II study of amifostine used as stem cell protectant in non-Hodgkin lymphoma patients receiving cisplatin-based salvage chemotherapy prior to stem cell transplant. *J Hematother Stem Cell Res* 2001; **10**: 887–93.

236 Gabriel D, Shea T, Wiley J et al. Use of amifostine to reduce mucositis following total body irradiation (TBI)-based autotransplants for lymphoma. *Proc Am Soc Clin Oncol* 2000; **69**(A): 268a [Abstract].

237 Rick O, Beyer J, Schwella N, Schubart H, Schleicher J, Siegert W. Assessment of amifostine as protection from chemotherapy-induced toxicities after conventional-dose and high-dose chemotherapy in patients with germ cell tumor. *Ann Oncol* 2001; **12**: 1151–5.

238 Capelli D, Santini G, De Souza C et al. Amifostine can reduce mucosal damage after high-dose melphalan conditioning for peripheral blood progenitor cellautotransplant: a retrospective study. *Br J Haematol* 2000; **110**: 300–7.

239 Phillips G, Hale G, Howard D et al. Amifostine (AMI) cytoprotection (CP) of escalating doses of melphalan (MEL) and autologous hematopoietic stem cell transplantation (AHSCT): a phase I–II study. *Proc Am Soc Clin Oncol* 2000; **49**(A): 189 [Abstract].

240 Hartmann JT, von Vangerow A, Fels LM et al. A randomized trial of amifostine in patients with high-dose VIC chemotherapy plus autologous blood stem cell transplantation. *Br J Cancer* 2001; **84**: 313–20.

241 Chauncey TR, Gooley TA, Lloid ME et al. Pilot trial of cytoprotection with amifostine given with high-dose chemotherpay and autologous peripheral blood stem cell transplantation. *Am J Clin Oncol* 2000; **23**: 406–11.

242 Buckner CD, Clift RA, Thomas ED et al. Allogeneic marrow transplantation for acute non-lymphoblastic leukemia in relapse using fractionated total body irradiation. *Leuk Res* 1982; **6**: 389–94.

243 Keating A, Brandwein J. Autologous marrow transplantation for non-Hodgkin's lymphoma. High dose etoposide and melphalan with or without total body irradiation. In: Dicke KA, Armitage JO, Dicke-Evinger MJ, eds. *Autologous Bone Marrow Transplantation, Proceedings of the Fifth International Symposium.* Omaha: The University of Nebraska Medical Center, 1991: 427–31.

244 Phillips GL, Shepherd JD, Barnett MJ et al. Busulfan, cyclophosphamide, and melphalan conditioning for autologous bone marrow transplantation in hematologic malignancy. *J Clin Oncol* 1991; **9**: 1880–8.

245 Locatelli F, Pession A, Bonetti F et al. Busulfan, cyclophosphamide and melphalan as conditioning regimen for bone marrow transplantation in children with myelodysplastic syndromes. *Leukemia* 1994; **8**: 844–9.

246 Blume KG, Forman SJ. High dose busulfan/etoposide as a preparatory regimen for second bone marrow transplants in hematologic malignancies. *Blut* 1987; **55**: 49–53.

247 Crilley P, Lazarus H, Topolsky D et al. Comparison of preparative transplantation regimens using carmustine/etoposide/cisplatin or busulfan/etoposide/cyclophosphamide in lymphoid malignancies. *Semin Oncol* 1993; **20**: 50–4.

248 Gulati SC, Shank B, Black P et al. Autologous bone marrow transplantation for patients with poor-prognosis lymphoma. *J Clin Oncol* 1988; **6**: 1303–13.

249 Meloni G, De Fabritiis P, Petti MC, Mandelli F. BAVC regimen and autologous bone marrow transplantation in patients with acute myelogenous leukemia in second remission. *Blood* 1990; **75**: 2282–5.

250 Zulian GB, Selby P, Milan S et al. High dose melphalan, BCNU and etoposide with autologous bone marrow transplantation for Hodgkin's disease. *Br J Cancer* 1989; **59**: 631–5.

251 Lazarus HM, Crilley P, Ciobanu N et al. High-dose carmustine, etoposide, and cisplatin and autologous bone marrow transplantation for relapsed and refractory lymphoma. *J Clin Oncol* 1992; **10**: 1682–9.

252 Peters WP, Stuart A, Klotman M et al. High-dose combination cyclophosphamide, cisplatin, and melphalan with autologous bone marrow support. A clinical and pharmacologic study. *Cancer Chemother Pharmacol* 1989; **23**: 377–83.

253 Ellis ED, Williams SF, Moormeier JA, Kaminer LS, Bitran JD. A phase I–II study of high-dose cyclophosphamide, thiotepa and escalating doses of mitoxantrone with autologous stem cell rescue in patients with refractory malignancies. *Bone Marrow Transplant* 1990; **6**: 439–42.

254 Williams SF, Bitran JD, Kaminer L et al. A phase I–II study of bialkylator chemotherapy, high-dose thiotepa, and cyclophosphamide with autologous bone marrow reinfusion in patients with advanced cancer. *J Clin Oncol* 1987; **5**: 260–5.

255 Shpall EJ, Clarke-Pearson D, Soper JT et al. High-dose alkylating agent chemotherapy with autologous bone marrow support in patients with stage III/IV epithelial ovarian cancer. *Gynecol Oncol* 1990; **38**: 386–91.

256 Wilson WH, Jain V, Bryant G et al. Phase I and II study of high-dose ifosfamide, carboplatin, and etoposide with autologous bone marrow rescue in lymphomas and solid tumors. *J Clin Oncol* 1992; **10**: 1712–22.

257 Pierelli L, Menichella G, Foddai ML et al. High dose chemotherapy with cisplatin, VP16 and carboplatin with stem cell support in patients with advanced ovarian cancer. *Haematologica* 1991; **76** (Suppl. 1): 63–5.

258 Dunphy FR, Spitzer G, Buzdar AU et al. Treatment of estrogen receptor-negative or hormonally refractory breast cancer with double high-dose chemotherapy intensification and bone marrow support. *J Clin Oncol* 1990; **8**: 1207–16.

259 Hennekens CH, Buring JE. Measures of disease frequency and association. In: Mayrent SL, ed. *Epidemiology in Medicine*. Boston: Little Brown, 1987: 54–98.

260 Foncuberta MC, Cagnoni PJ, Brandts CH et al. Topical transforming growth factor-β3 in the prevention or alleviation of chemotherapy-induced oral mucositis in patients with lymphomas or solid tumors. *J Immunotherapy* 2001; **24**: 384–8.

261 Schloerb PR, Skikne BS. Oral and parenteral glutamine in bone marrow transplantation: a randomized, double-blind study. *JPEN* 1999; **23**: 117–22.

262 Anderson PM, Ramsay NK, Shu XO *et al*. Effect of low-dose oral glutamine on painful stomatitis during bone marrow transplantation. *Bone Marrow Transplant* 1998; **22**: 339–44.

263 Chiara S, Nobile MT, Vincenti M *et al*. Sucralfate in the treatment of chemotherapy-induced stomatitis: a double-blind, placebo-controlled pilot study. *Anticancer Res* 2001; **21**: 3707–10.

264 Labar B, Mrsic M, Pavletic Z *et al*. Prostaglandin E2 for prophylaxis of oral mucositis following BMT. *Bone Marrow Transplant* 1993; **11**: 379–82.

265 Loprinzi CL, Cianflone SG, Dose AM *et al*. A controlled evaluation of an allopurinol mouthwash as prophylaxis against 5-fluorouracil-induced stomatitis. *Cancer* 1990; **65**: 1879–82.

266 Cowen D, Tardieu C, Schubert M *et al*. Low energy helium-neon laser in the prevention of oral mucositis in patients undergoing bone marrow transplant: results of a double blind randomized trial. *Int J Radiat Oncol Biol Phys* 1997; **38**: 697–703.

267 Perch SJ, Machtay M, Markiewicz DA, Kligerman MM. Decreased acute toxicity by using midline mucosa-sparing blocks during radiation therapy for carcinoma of the oral cavity, oropharynx, and nasopharynx. *Radiology* 1995; **197**: 863–6.

268 Weisdorf DJ, Bostrom B, Raether D *et al*. Oropharyngeal mucositis complicating bone marrow transplantation: prognostic factors and the effect of chlorhexidine mouth rinse. *Bone Marrow Transplant* 1989; **4**: 89–95.

269 Feber T. Management of mucositis in oral irradiation. *Clin Oncol (R Coll Radiol)* 1996; **8**: 106–11.

270 Barrett AP. Evaluation of nystatin in prevention and elimination of oropharyngeal Candida in immunosuppressed patients. *Oral Surg Oral Med Oral Pathol* 1984; **58**: 148–51.

271 Aviles A. Clotrimazole treatment for prevention of oral candidiasis in patients with acute leukemia undergoing chemotherapy. *Am J Med* 1987; **82**: 867–8.

Brenda Shank & Richard T. Hoppe

Radiotherapeutic Principles of Hematopoietic Cell Transplantation

Introduction

For hematopoietic cell transplantation (HCT), irradiation is used primarily as a systemic agent in the form of total body irradiation (TBI), total lymphoid irradiation (TLI), or thoracoabdominal irradiation (TAI). In addition, localized irradiation may be used as "boost" treatment for areas of presumed higher concentrations of malignant cells. The main roles for irradiation as a systemic agent are for immunosuppression and malignant cell eradication.

There are many advantages of irradiation as a systemic agent when compared with chemotherapy: (i) it is not crossreactive with any other agent; (ii) a given dose of irradiation may be quite homogeneous regardless of blood supply; (iii) there is no sanctuary sparing such as of the testes; (iv) after the radiation is given, there is no detoxification or excretion required; and (v) the dose distribution may be tailored within the body by means of shielding of areas of greater sensitivity or "boosting" areas which may contain more than microscopic amounts of malignant cells. The ultimate tailoring of dose distribution may prove to be best achieved in the future by means of radiolabeled antibodies against leukemias and lymphomas, with or without TBI and/or chemotherapy; these techniques are under active investigation at several centers [1–5].

Irradiation, however, does have deleterious effects on normal tissues, as does chemotherapy. For example, the gastrointestinal tract is particularly sensitive to radiation acutely; lung and lens are at risk for late complications.

The delivery of radiation may be optimized by varying the time, dose, and fractionation according to radiobiological principles in order to minimize the toxicity to normal tissues, to increase malignant cell kill, and to increase immunosuppression by greater lymphocyte destruction. Radiation delivery may also be optimized by manipulating physical parameters, such as beam energy, dose rate and patient position, to increase accuracy, dose homogeneity and comfort of the patient. The goals of this chapter are to explain the radiobiological principles involved in magnafield irradiation with TBI as the prototype, to review the physical principles and to examine the clinical evidence favoring various TBI regimens. Finally, the use of TLI and TAI is briefly discussed.

Radiobiological principles

Basic principles

All of radiotherapy is considered to be based on what has been described as the four "R's": repair, reoxygenation, redistribution and repopulation [6]. Repair is the process in which cells are able to repair at least a portion of the damage caused by irradiation. The amount of repair that is going to occur usually is complete in a period of 6 h in most cells. Reoxygenation has been considered important in solid tumors that have become anoxic through growth beyond their blood supply, but probably is not important in well-oxygenated leukemic cells. Reoxygenation occurs as tumor cells are destroyed by irradiation and dead cells are lost from the tumor, so that the remaining tumor cells become closer to the blood supply in capillaries. Redistribution is the process whereby cells become distributed nonhomogeneously throughout the cell cycle as a result of irradiation, which can destroy more cells in mitosis or in S-phase than in the other phases of the cell cycle. During an interval between two radiation fractions, cells may advance through the cell cycle to be in either a more or less sensitive phase of the cell cycle by the time the second dose is given [7]. Repopulation is the process whereby cells continue to grow if the interval of time between two doses of irradiation is large relative to the cell cycle time. Two widely spaced radiation doses appear to result in less cell kill in dividing cells than do doses given a short time apart.

The radiation sensitivity of any given cell type is described by a cell survival curve (Fig. 14.1 [8]), which is a plot of the percentage or fraction of surviving cells vs. the dose of irradiation. This relationship may yield a straight line when plotted on logarithmic paper (exponential cell kill) if there is no repair. In contrast, if repair takes place, there is a shoulder to the survival curve reflecting the extent of repair. There are two formulations to describe these cell survival curves. One is the multihit multitarget model, which allows description of the fraction of cells surviving, S, as a function of the dose per fraction, D, in terms of D_0, which represents the slope of the survival curve beyond the initial shoulder, and n, the extrapolation number, which is the fraction on the y-axis through which the straight line portion of the survival curve can be extrapolated (see Fig. 14.1). This relationship is:

$$S = [1 - (1 - e^{-D/D_0})^n]^f$$

where f is the number of fractions of irradiation.

Another formulation that has come into increasing use is the linear-quadratic or LQ model [9]. This formulation is simply an expression of S as a function of two terms, a linear function of D and a function of D^2:

$$-\ln S = f(\alpha D + \beta D^2).$$

By dividing this equation through by β, one has a term, α/β, which is characteristic of the type of effects in either tumor or normal tissue. There is a consistent finding of low values of α/β (<5 Gy) for late effects and higher values (~10 Gy), for early reactions. Tumor effects generally fall in the range of early reactions with an α/β of approximately 10 Gy.

For radiation to be of benefit in treating any malignancy, there must be a therapeutic ratio greater than one. This therapeutic ratio is the dose required to achieve a given effect (e.g. cell kill) in normal tissue divided

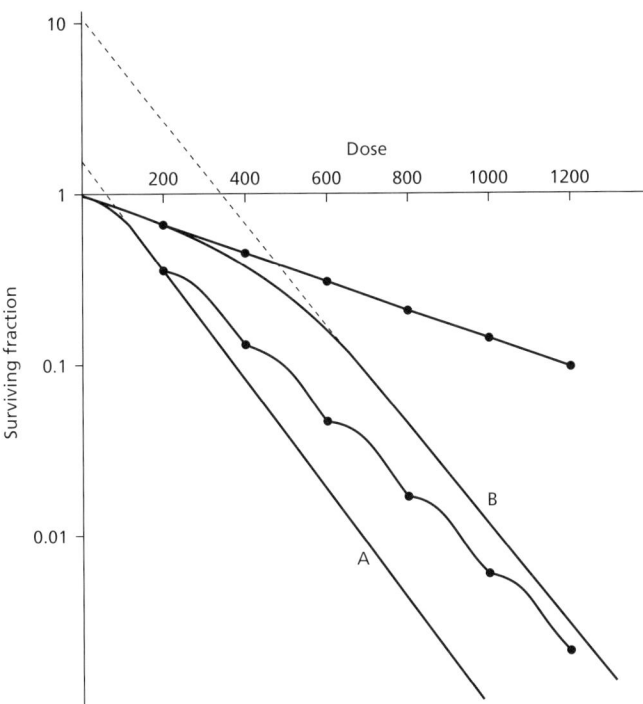

Fig. 14.1 Representation of the effect of fractionation on survival of two cell populations, using 2 Gy fractions. Cell population A has only a minimal capacity to repair radiation injury (typical of many leukemic cells) compared with population B, which has a large repair capacity (similar to many normal tissues, such as lung). Reproduced with permission from Peters *et al.* [8].

by the dose required to achieve the same effect (cell kill) in the malignancy. With TBI, there are a multiplicity of normal tissues to consider that are likely to be affected by irradiation. The remainder of this section on radiobiology describes what is known about the effect of radiation on lymphocytes (the target tissue for immunosuppression), leukemic cells (the malignancy most frequently treated with TBI) and the normal organ of most concern, the lungs.

Immunosuppression (normal lymphocytes)

It has been argued that the most important benefit of TBI is immunosuppression but this argument is not widely accepted [10]. It has been shown in dogs that increasing doses of radiation allowed increasing engraftment [11,12]. Storb *et al.* [12] also showed that single-dose irradiation was more immunosuppressive than the same total doses when fractionated. Terenzi and associates verified this observation in mice as measured by splenic lymphocyte cell kill but demonstrated that there was greater bone marrow myeloid eradication with hyperfractionation (total dose of 14.4 Gy) compared with single-dose TBI [13]. They suggested that in T-cell-depleted bone marrow transplantation (BMT) for chronic myeloid leukemia (CML), where relapse is the major cause of failure, a hyperfractionated TBI regimen would be preferable. Other data from studies in dogs, rats and monkeys show similarly that there is a dose fractionation relationship with rejection [10]. When treatment is split into multiple fractions given over several days, higher doses of irradiation (e.g. 15 Gy in 4–5 days compared with 8 Gy in a single dose) are necessary for engraftment in these animals.

Down and colleagues, in a mouse marrow chimera model, showed a steep increase in engraftment of H-2 compatible allogeneic marrow from LP mice into standard B6 recipients, with increasing TBI dose (without cyclophosphamide [CY]) when given as a single dose at a high-dose rate

(1 Gy/min) [14]. Low-dose rate (0.05 Gy/min) and fractionated TBI required higher total doses for equivalent engraftment, and increasing the interval between fractions from 6 to 24 h required a further increase in dose. These data were considered by the authors to be consistent with appreciable sublethal damage repair in the self-renewing stem cell population of the host. In another study in mice, engraftment was also shown to be critically dependent upon TBI dose, and the dose necessary for engraftment increased as the genetic disparity between donor and host increased [15]. In a murine study from the Institut Gustave Roussy, a fractionated schedule of 1.25 Gy three times a day to a total dose of 7.5 Gy (0.25 Gy/min) had the same effect on the hemopoietic system as 7.5 Gy in a single dose at a low-dose rate (0.04 Gy/min) [16]. There was no significant repopulation seen with the fractionated course.

In humans undergoing allogeneic BMT using non-T-cell-depleted marrow from matched sibling donors, none of the typical high-dose myeloablative TBI regimens show any difference in engraftment; essentially there is 100% engraftment with all. In non-T-cell-depleted grafts from related, nonsibling donors, graft failure has been shown to increase with increasing degree of donor incompatibility [17]. When allogeneic bone marrow depleted of T lymphocytes to prevent graft-vs.-host disease (GVHD) was given, there also were difficulties in sustaining engraftment. Studies in animals [18] and humans [19–27] showed that it is possible to increase engraftment either by increasing the TBI dose or by adding TLI to TBI. TLI irradiates the sites along the central axis in which there is a higher concentration of T lymphocytes in lymph nodes and the thoracic duct. Many studies have shown the importance of T lymphocytes in the process of graft rejection [28,29]. One author calculated that the addition of a single 2 Gy TBI fraction may be sufficient to decrease host T cells by 1 log, which could be enough to prevent graft failures in T-cell-depleted transplants but this has not been proved experimentally [30].

When looking at either cell culture or lymphocyte survival *in vivo*, it would appear that lymphocytes have either no, or a very small, shoulder to the survival curve (curve A in Fig. 14.1). In a study from the Institut Gustave Roussy, it was found that the D_0 of lymphocytes was 1.2 Gy and there was a half-time for cell loss of 30 h after a single fraction of TBI [31]. During fractionated irradiation, the half-time also appeared to be 30 h. When lymphocyte subsets were examined, there did not appear to be a different radiosensitivity either *in vivo* or with the same patient cells *in vitro* between B and T cells or between helper (OKT4) and suppressor/cytotoxic (OKT8) T cells.

A later study by the same group of investigators of a patient who received only 3.85 Gy in three TBI fractions without a BMT because of patient refusal to continue, showed similar radiosensitivities again between the T-lymphocytes, B-lymphocytes and the T-cell subsets CD4 and CD8 [32]. Lymphocytes reached their nadir 48 h after the last fraction of irradiation and, although the lymphocytes increased again at approximately 2 months, there was still a lymphopenia 3 months later. The D_0 obtained in this patient from the multihit multitarget equation was 1.75 Gy. In a study from the Memorial Sloan Kettering Cancer Center (MSKCC), two patients who received only a single dose of TBI (1.25 Gy), out of a planned hyperfractionated course, had similar lymphocyte decrements, yielding a D_0 of 1.35 Gy for one patient and 1.75 Gy for the other [33].

Leukemic cells

For the purposes of this discussion the only malignant cells considered are leukemic cells since the majority of cytoreductive procedures utilizing TBI are for leukemia. Leukemic cells, like normal lymphocytes, have generally been considered to have either no shoulder or a very minimal shoulder on the cell survival curve. Most analyses utilized the multihit multitarget model and cited D_0 and *n*-values. Many authors studied the radiation survival curve parameters for leukemic cells *in vitro* [34–38]. It is clear from these studies that D_0 and n-values vary considerably for different cell types and even different cell lines from the same type of leukemia. In some of these cell lines there appears to be no repair at all, whereas in others there appears to be a repair component [39,40].

In one leukemic line (Reh) from a patient with acute lymphoblastic leukemia (ALL) studied in detail, cell survival fit the LQ model with a continuously downward-curving cell survival plot [41]. Repair between fractions of a hyperfractionation TBI regimen (three times/day) could explain completely the overall cell survival curve obtained when these cells were irradiated on that schedule. However, because of the relatively small amount of repair in most leukemic cells and the large amount of repair seen in most normal tissues (see discussion below), fractionation of a given total dose of TBI should have a better therapeutic ratio than the same total dose given as a single dose: leukemic cell kill should be similar, providing that there is no or minimal cell growth between fractions, but normal-tissue damage should be less since these cells will repair themselves to a greater degree than the leukemic cells.

Normal tissues

Many normal organs are affected by TBI (Fig. 14.2 [42]), the most critical being the lungs, gastrointestinal tract, and lenses. Lung tissue is the focus of this section, since it has been the principal dose-limiting tissue of concern in TBI. Within some early single-dose series, some form of interstitial pneumonia (IP) developed in 50–100% of patients [43–45]. Approximately two-thirds of the affected patients died from this complication [43]. Wara and colleagues determined, from the concept of effective dose to lung tissue, that increasing the number of fractions contributed more to reducing lung damage than did increasing the overall treatment time [46].

Thus, the use of hyperfractionated regimens, in which relatively small doses per fraction are given two to three times a day over a few days to minimize leukemia regrowth, may be of great value in reducing lung toxicity. This type of schedule allows achievement of a higher total dose, thereby increasing leukemic cell kill. Peters *et al.* [8,47] suggested in 1979 that the use of fractionated irradiation would be better than single-dose TBI in reducing toxicity to normal tissue.

Various clinical studies have shown that a fractionated regimen, either daily fractionation or hyperfractionation (multiple fractions/day) decrease overall lung toxicity. These studies are discussed in the Clinical results section below.

Vriesendorp [10,48] took the approach of modeling the surviving fraction of cells, which determines normal tissue damage and organ function for various TBI fractionation schemes. He used published clinical data from different fractionation regimens to attempt to determine which values of D_0 and n best fit the ultimate clinical results. Using the values of n and D_0 that he deduced for different tissues, he created a table of surviving target cells, lungs, intestines, bone marrow and immune system (i.e. lymphocytes) for a variety of different TBI schedules in the literature. The results show the impressive sparing of the lungs and intestines to be expected with more fractionated regimens (Table 14.1 [10,48]). The immune system survival results were in error; when corrected (as was done in Table 14.1) and when similar calculations for high-total-dose hyperfractionated regimens were added, immunosuppression is also predicted to be excellent with these high-total-dose (15 Gy) hyperfractionated regimens. Malignant lymphocytes may be expected to respond similarly because they have similar cell-survival parameters.

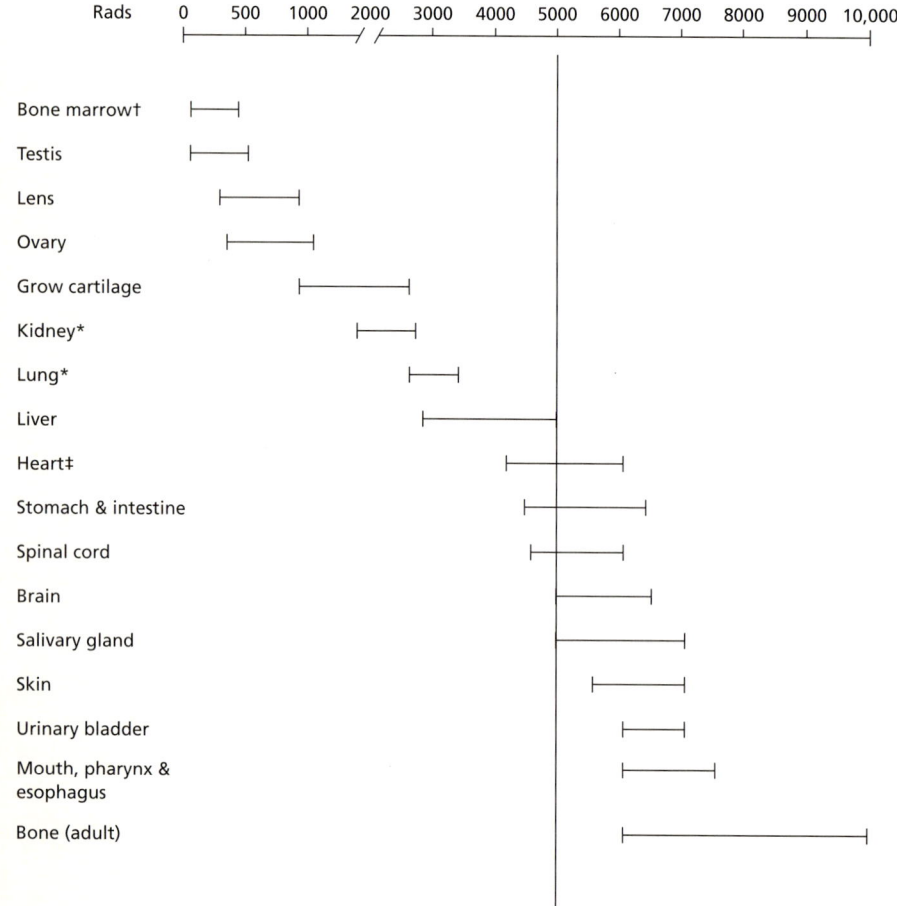

Fig. 14.2 Sensitivity of various organs to radiation complications, expressed as a range, from the dose (rad = cGy) that causes 5% complications, to the dose that causes 50% complications within 5 years, assuming 2 Gy fractions 5 days per week. †Indicates acute injury to bone marrow. *Bilateral irradiation. ‡Irradiation of 60% of the heart. Reproduced with permission from Fajardo [42].

Table 14.1 Surviving target cells after different total body irradiation (TBI) schedules*. Adapted with permission from Vriesendorp [10,48].

	A	B	C	D	E	F	G	H	I	J	K
									Lymphocytes Lung		
	1×9.0[†]	2×5.0	5×2.25	2×6.0	3×4.0	4×3.0	6×2.0	11×1.2	8×1.8	12×1.25	10×1.5
Lung	**7.61×10^{-3}** **(100)**[‡]	**19.3×10^{-3}** (254)	187×10^{-3} (2460)	**4.68×10^{-3}** **(61)**	20.3×10^{-3} (267)	61.3×10^{-3} (806)	238×10^{-3} (3130)	626×10^{-3} (8230)	249×10^{-3} (3270)	551×10^{-3} (7240)	385×10^{-3} (5060)
Immune system	**3.10×10^{-3}** **(100)**	**1.97×10^{-3}** **(64)**	1.45×10^{-3} (48)	0.522×10^{-3} (17)	0.638×10^{-3} (21)	0.763×10^{-3} (25)	1.03×10^{-3} (33)	0.846×10^{-3} (27)	0.289×10^{-3} (9)	0.308×10^{-3} (10)	0.25×10^{-3} (8)

	n	D_0
	1.25	1.50
	6.0	1.35

*Model (see text): $S = [1 - (1 - e^{-D/D_0})^n]^f$.
[†]No. fractions (f) × dose/fraction (D) in Grays.
[‡]Surviving fraction (S for indicated schedule as a percentage of S for Schedule A).
Numbers in bold type are considered unacceptable.

Table 14.2 Relative effectiveness of different dose rates and fractionation schemes for lung and leukemia. Reproduced with permission from Vitale et al. [50].

Total dose (Gy/No. fractions)	Tissue type	Dose rate (Gy/min)			
		0.01	0.05	0.10	0.25
9.9/3.0	Lung	0.80	1.00*	1.04	1.06
	Leukemia	0.94	1.00*	1.01	1.02
10/1	Lung	0.91	1.62	1.89	2.09
	Leukemia	0.98	1.21	1.29	1.36
12/6	Lung	0.89	1.00	1.02	1.03
	Leukemia	1.11	1.14	1.15	1.15
15/12	Lung	1.02	1.09	1.10	1.10
	Leukemia	1.35	1.38	1.38	1.38

*Reference values.

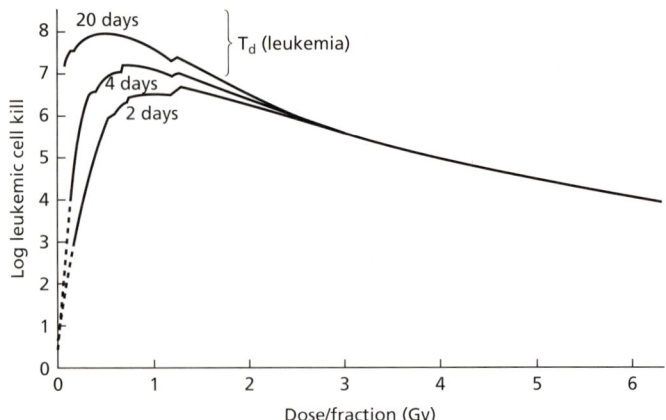

Fig. 14.3 Leukemic cell kill as a function of dose/fraction, assuming two fractions per day, no weekend treatments and total doses that would yield lung damage equivalent (isoeffective) to six fractions of 2 Gy. Curves are shown for three possible cell doubling times (Td). Reproduced with minor changes by permission from O'Donoghue et al. [51].

Evans performed mouse experiments that also support the concept that increasing fractionation is very important in decreasing lung toxicity as measured by the dose that would be lethal for 50% of the animals in 30 days ($LD_{50/30}$) [49]. He obtained a 21% increase in the $LD_{50/30}$ after increasing the number of fractions from one to six, with a dose rate of 0.25 Gy/min. With a lower dose rate (0.08 Gy/min) there was still an effect of fractionation but the $LD_{50/30}$ was increased by only 14% for development of pneumonitis in these mouse studies.

Many investigators attempted to do some form of modeling of the impact of fractionation and dose rate to predict an optimum TBI regimen. Vitale and coworkers performed calculations for four fractionation regimens varying from 10 Gy in a single dose, up to 15 Gy in 12 fractions in 4 days, the regimen initiated at MSKCC (Table 14.2) [50]. They used the concept of biologically effective dose based on the LQ model of cell survival. Targets considered were lung and leukemic cells. They compared the relative effectiveness of these different fractionation schemes for lung and leukemic cells based on the reference value of their own regimen of 9.9 Gy in three fractions at a dose rate of 0.05 Gy/min. The dose rate effect was more pronounced in lung than in leukemic cells in their model but became insignificant in highly fractionated schemes, such as 15 Gy in 12 fractions. At any dose rate, the antileukemic effect relative to the effect on lung cells was greatest with the fractionation regimen that allowed a greater total dose to be given.

O'Donoghue and colleagues also used a mathematical model for optimal scheduling of TBI. They suggested that TBI schedules of the "accelerated hyperfractionation" type are optimal, based on their comparison of schedules that were considered isoeffective for lung damage [51]. They recognized in their calculations that, in a hyperfractionated regimen, there is a requirement for at least 6 h between fractions to get maximum repair of normal tissues. Therefore, they suggested that two fractions per day would be optimal. With this constraint, they looked at leukemic cell kill as a function of dose/fraction for twice-daily schedules, assuming no treatment over the weekend (a reality in most radiation oncology departments). They concluded that a schedule of 10 fractions (in 5 days) of 1.37 Gy would be close to optimal for leukemic cells with a presumed doubling time of 2 or 4 days (Fig. 14.3 [51]). For longer doubling times, a smaller fraction size would be optimal, but doubling times of 2–4 days are probably most appropriate for leukemias [52]. They suggested that a practical schedule of 10 fractions of between 1.3 and 1.5 Gy in 5 days would be worth considering and should be tested clinically. This schedule (1.5 Gy twice a day for 5 days to a total dose of 15 Gy) has been used at The Mount Sinai Medical Center in New York since 1990 with no untoward acute toxicity and excellent clinical results in patients with CML but no randomized trial has been done to evaluate this regimen [53].

Another publication by O'Donoghue [54] suggested that, with the appropriate choice of a low-dose rate, single-dose TBI in principle could be radiobiologically equivalent to fractionated TBI. However, he noted that such low-dose rates would necessitate extremely long treatment times (on the order of 24 h), which would be not only uncomfortable for patients but also impractical for most centers. Therefore, they again concluded that fractionated TBI (with high-dose rates) is preferable to low-dose-rate therapy for leukemias and other rapidly growing tumors, such as neuroblastoma.

G.W. Jones and T. Farrell from Hamilton Regional Cancer Center, Ontario, Canada (personal communication) compared in 1992 published clinical results from a variety of regimens in a three-dimensional graphic form, with mortality plotted against total dose and dose per fraction. This presentation shows that the highly fractionated regimens, which achieve total doses of 14–15 Gy, result in a minimum mortality and thus appear optimal by this endpoint.

Studies on sequencing of CY and TBI in mice have shown that there is less lung damage when CY is given 12–24 h after TBI than when given 24–48 h before TBI [55,56]. In contrast, bone marrow damage is greater when TBI is given first [55]. Other murine studies indicated that CY may actually be marrow protective when given prior to TBI [57]. This finding suggests that TBI should be given prior to CY for normal-tissue protection. In contrast, Okunewick et al. [58] showed that in mice, when the bulk of radiation was given before chemotherapy, there was a high incidence of early deaths due to regimen-related toxicity. In humans, TBI has been given either before or after CY, at different institutions. No obvious differences have been noted other than anecdotal evidence of improved acute tolerance of irradiation when CY was given after TBI; no randomized studies have been done. There was a nonsignificant trend toward a shorter half-life of CY after TBI (and etoposide [VP16]) in humans in one study when compared with the half-life of CY when given prior to TBI in a separate study by the same authors [59].

Physical considerations

When TBI or any other magnafield irradiation is performed, physical parameters to be selected include: energy, total dose, number of fractions, dose per fraction, total treatment time, dose rate, patient position, distance of the patient from the source, dose homogeneity, shielding (deliberate inhomogeneity) and "boost" irradiation. Many of these parameters, such as those dealing with dose, time and fractionation depend on radiobiology and have already been considered in the previous section. For an overall discussion of these technical factors at various centers, readers are directed to two clinical reviews [60,61]. For discussions of dose measurements (dosimetry) and dose calibration, which are outside of the range of this chapter, there are several good references [62–65]. Large fields have very special problems associated with dosimetry because of the large amount of internal scatter within the patient, the scatter of the wall behind the patient and the angled gantry over large treatment distances, among others. The references cited are particularly informative sources with regard to these problems.

Energy

Centers engaged in HCT in this country have primarily used energies ranging from 1.25 MV (cobalt-60 [^{60}Co]) to 10 MV using a linear accelerator. Occasionally, higher energies up to 25 MV have been used, especially in Europe. When energies higher than ^{60}Co energy are used, one must use a tissue-equivalent material in front of the patient (beam spoiler) such as 1 cm of polycarbonate resin (Lexan®) for 10 MV photons. This allows for adequate buildup of dose at the patient's surface and prevents skin underdosage. Examples of typical techniques are shown in Fig. 14.4 [60]. The technique from MSKCC (lower right in Fig. 14.4) demonstrates the use of a beam spoiler in front of the patient.

Dose rate and distance from the source rate and distance from the source

High-dose TBI given in a single dose requires a low-dose rate (≤0.05 Gy/min) to prevent IP, according to both animal [66–68] and human data [69,70]. Low-dose rates may still be needed for fractionated irradiation schemes that employ 2 Gy or more per fraction, as mouse experiments have shown that fractionation regimens that employ fractions of 2 Gy still have a dose rate effect [71]. When a high-dose rate has been used, total dose has been limited [72,73]; one group reported a high relapse rate (62%) in patients with other than first-remission ALL or acute myeloid leukemia (AML), or in the first chronic phase of CML, when a 5 Gy total dose was used at a dose rate of 0.4–0.9 Gy/min [73].

To fit the entire body in the TBI field with minimum contortion of the patient, it is necessary to increase the distance from the source because the field size increases linearly with the distance from the source. The necessary distance to allow the patient to stand or lie in an unflexed position is a function of the patient's height and the collimator opening of the particular machine used. This collimator opening differs on machines made by different manufacturers. Some treatment rooms are not long enough to allow extended distances sufficient to fit a fully extended patient within the field. Rotating the collimator to the diagonal of the square field can help, provided there is not a primary circular collimator, which limits this diagonal length.

Patient position

The many patient positions that have been used are shown in Fig. 14.4. Patient positioning at various HCT centers has been a function of the room size and the resultant distance achievable from the source, the type of lung shielding desired, concerns over reproducibility and attempts to achieve homogeneity and patient comfort.

If the patient is sitting and/or lying down and is treated laterally, the patient is comfortable but inhomogeneity becomes a problem and lung

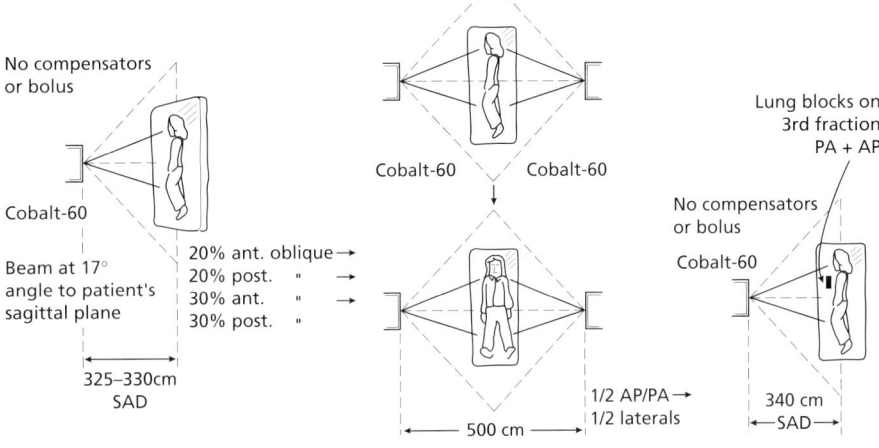

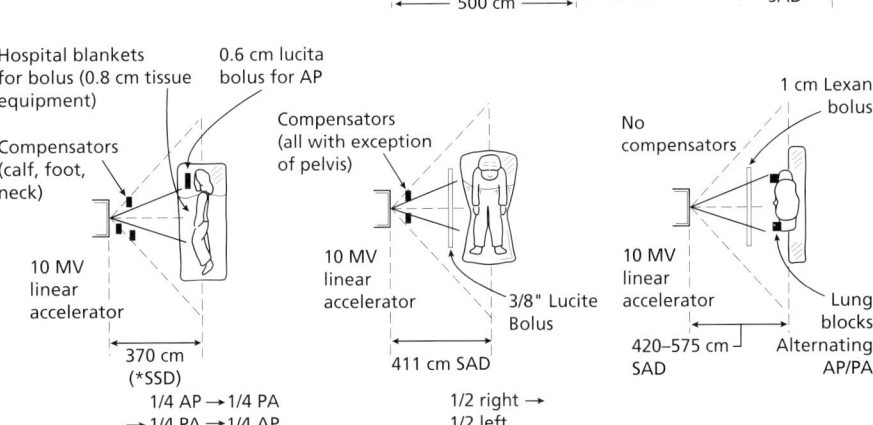

Fig. 14.4 Diagram of six different patient set-ups for total body irradiation (TBI) from different institutions. The middle top example utilized two positions during the course of treatment (note arrow between the positions). Bolus and/or compensators are indicated, as well as source-axis-distance (SAD) or source-skin-distance (SSD). The lower right example shows the lung blocks used at Memorial Sloan Kettering Cancer Center (MSKCC). AP, anterior posterior; PA, posterior anterior. Reproduced with permission from Shank [60].

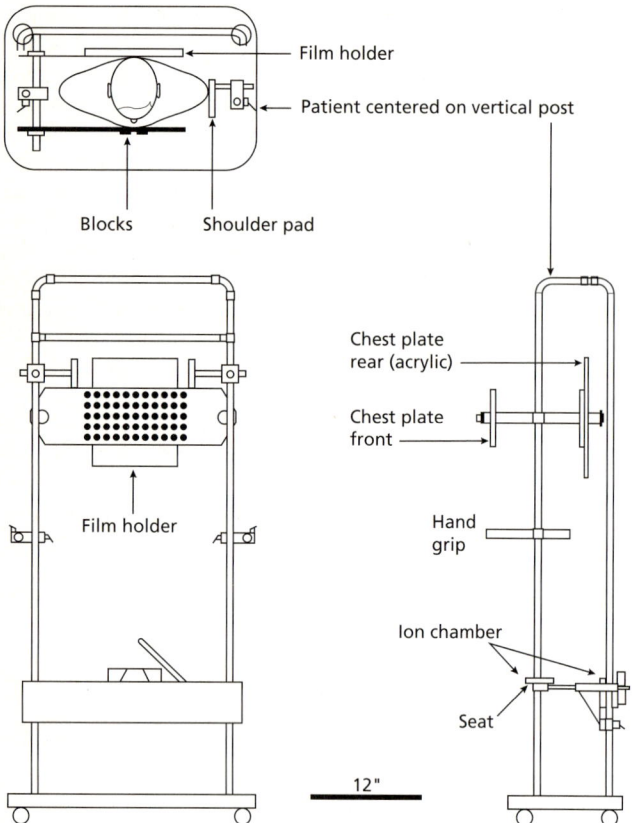

Fig. 14.5 Example of total body irradiation (TBI) stand originally constructed at Memorial Sloan Kettering Cancer Center (MSKCC). Top: superior view; bottom left: anterior view; bottom right: lateral view.

shielding is difficult. Better homogeneity is achieved and lung shielding is easier with the patient lying on his or her side using anterior-posterior/posterior-anterior fields, but accurate positioning is difficult and time-consuming [74]. Many centers have treated patients in the standing position, utilizing special treatment stands. An example of this is the stand used at MSKCC, which evolved over several years of use (Fig. 14.5) and incorporates a bicycle seat for patient comfort; the patient is still in the standing position. Special port film holders and supporting devices, which can be individualized and accurately reproduced day to day, are part of the device.

Some of the special stands that have been used have been described in the literature [75–78]. Another treatment device includes a plaster vest used as a lung block support [79].

Shielding

Many institutions have used lung shielding either (i) on all fractions whether anterior or posterior, (ii) on some fractions, or (iii) on only one lung. An example of these are the one-half-value-layer lung blocks used at MSKCC, which have been incorporated into the techniques of many other centers [43]. Some institutions have treated patients laterally and used the patient's arms to shield the lungs partially. This may be simple to do, but arm position is not very reproducible and, therefore, the lung dose distribution is variable from fraction to fraction.

One institution has used shielding of the liver with a 10% block in an attempt to decrease the incidence of veno-occlusive disease (VOD) of the liver [80]. The same institution also used partial renal shielding. Liver shielding could create a problem of potential leukemic relapse, but long-term results addressing this issue are not yet available. Furthermore, VOD has been more frequently correlated with patient age, GVHD, prior hepatitis, and chemotherapy agents (e.g. busulfan [BU] or cytarabine] than with TBI *per se* [81,82].

In protocols for some diseases it is possible to use eye shielding; for example, at MSKCC, when TBI was used for immunosuppression for patients with aplastic anemia, the eyes were shielded during the anterior treatment [83]. Regimens for these benign diseases frequently employ TLI or TAI instead of TBI so that the eyes are outside of the field and such blocking becomes unnecessary. Eye shields generally should not be used for leukemic patients due to the potential for recurrence in the eye or orbit. One report described the use of eye shields in a leukemic patient who was an airline pilot; his livelihood depended upon excellent vision. Long-term follow-up of the patient was not provided [84].

Homogeneity

The use of a tissue-equivalent screen for homogeneity at the skin surface has been discussed. Some centers have also used compensators in very thin body areas such as the neck or calf and foot. Some institutions have even used tissue compensators for the entire patient with thinner areas having a larger amount of compensation than somewhat thicker areas such as the head or the thigh. When questioned, investigators from seven major transplant institutions indicated that there was a 30% variation in different areas of the patient when compensators were not used (i.e. doses varied either from 80% to 110% or from 90% to 120%) [60]. When compensators and bolus were used, there was only an 8% variation in dose throughout the patient (from 94% to 102%). Generally a variation in dose throughout the body of ±5% is considered excellent and ±10% is acceptable [62].

"Boosting"

The term *boosting* describes the process of giving an additional dose of radiation by means of decreasing the original field size to give a greater dose to a local region considered to have a higher concentration of residual malignant cells. This dose may be given either before or after the larger area (e.g. TBI) has been treated. Many areas of the body have received boost irradiation as part of various treatment regimens.

Chest wall boost

The regimen initiated at MSKCC has used lung shields on each fraction. The chest wall in the area of the lung blocks were boosted with electrons, which do not penetrate deeply into lung, to deliver to the marrow in the ribs a radiation dose equivalent to that in marrow in other sites of the body [43]. Radiobiologic theory [85] and results from the Institut Gustave Roussy without chest wall boosts [86] suggest no increased leukemic relapse when these boosts are not given as part of a similar hyperfractionated regimen (14.85 Gy in 11 fractions).

Testicular boost

A high relapse rate was noted in early studies at MSKCC in the testes in leukemic patients (four of 28 males—two with ALL, two with AML and one with acute myelomonocytic leukemia), which was in some patients an isolated relapse [87]. As a result of this high relapse rate, an electron boost was added to the testes (4 Gy). Following the addition of this boost, there were no further relapses in the testes in more than 300 males subsequently treated. Another report has also described an isolated testicular relapse, occurring 5 years after BMT, when testicular irradiation was not given during cytoreduction utilizing BU and CY [88].

Splenic boost

In CML, the spleen may harbor a high leukemic cell burden. Some investigators have chosen to give a splenic boost prior to cytoreduction in CML patients, usually 10 Gy in three fractions [53]. This treatment is planned by shaping the field with the aid of the posterior image of the spleen from a liver/spleen radionuclide scan.

Boosts to bulky or gross disease (consolidative irradiation)

For some diseases, it has been considered desirable to boost sites of initial involvement of bulky disease, residual disease after induction chemotherapy, bulky sites of relapse, all sites of relapse, or even more extensive treatment, such as TLI. In lymphoma, for example, 12- to 40-Gy boost treatments have been added to TBI-containing or to chemotherapy-only regimens [89–94].

Clinical results

Total body irradiation

Acute side-effects

In all TBI regimens, nausea and vomiting have been the most noticeable acute side-effects. The hyperfractionated regimen instituted at MSKCC was found to be considerably more tolerable for the patient when compared with the original single-dose regimen [33]. One report showed that emesis was universal after one dose of 1.2 Gy in a fractionated regimen, but showed a statistically significant decline over the 4 days of a hyperfractionated course of irradiation ($p = 0.046$) [95]. Both ondansetron [96–98] and granisetron [97,99,100] were effective in decreasing the incidence and number of emetic episodes during TBI in randomized trials.

Other acute side-effects include occasional syncope in some patients when treated in the standing position; this has been found to be aggravated by the use of phenothiazines, which cause orthostatic hypotension, or by a low hemoglobin concentration in patients with aplastic anaemia. Another problem is salivary gland swelling and discomfort, which are usually transient at the end of the TBI course, lasting a few days. One study found that when fractionated irradiation was used (12 Gy in six fractions), there was no parotiditis, compared with single-dose irradiation (10 Gy), after which a 40% incidence of parotiditis was seen [101]. In one study using 12 Gy in six fractions given over 3 days (twice a day), 49% of women and 28% of men experienced a fatigue syndrome [102].

In a study that randomized TBI dose rates, both single-dose and hyperfractionated twice-a-day regimens were used, although fractionation was not randomized [103,104]. It was found that acute reactions (nausea and vomiting, mucositis, diarrhea, and parotiditis) were all less with the hyperfractionated schedule than with single-dose TBI.

Immunosuppression

With conventional allografts (i.e. without T-cell depletion), graft failures have rarely occurred regardless of the TBI regimen used. However, when T-cell-depleted marrow transplants are used, graft failures are frequent. It has been suggested that there are more graft failures with fractionated irradiation than with single-dose irradiation. Many reports have indicated that higher doses of TBI [23–25,105] or the addition of TLI [19–22,26,27] may overcome such rejection in a large proportion of patients. However, decreased numbers of graft failures have not been consistently reported with either increased TBI dose [106,107] or with the addition of TLI [108].

Single fraction low-dose TBI has been used as immunosuppressive therapy prior to HCT and allogeneic donor lymphocyte infusion (DLI) [109,110]. In a multiinstitutional study, 45 patients with human leukocyte antigen (HLA)-identical sibling donors, who were ineligible for conventional HCT because of age or medical contraindications, were treated with 2 Gy single-fraction TBI prior to HCT, with cyclosporine and mycophenylate mofetil given concurrently and after HCT for additional immunosuppression and GVHD prevention [109]. DLI was given based on the presence of stable mixed chimerism and absence of GVHD, or for persistent or progressive disease. Although approximately 80% achieved an early mixed chimerism, it was usually unstable. Acute and chronic GVHD were appreciable. Of the patients with sustained engraftment, 53% were in complete remission (CR), including eight with molecular remissions (five CML, three chronic lymphocytic leukemia [CLL]), demonstrating the feasibility and potential of such an approach. In another study of 11 patients with refractory hematologic malignancies, who were treated with 1 Gy single-fraction TBI and sibling donor cells, nine achieved donor chimerism and four had a sustained CR of their cancers [110].

Relapse

Leukemic relapse as a function of dose, dose rate, or fractionation has been studied in several institutions. An early twin BMT study with solely single-dose TBI (10 Gy) for cytoreduction demonstrated that, although engraftment was prompt, irradiation alone at this dose was insufficient in itself to destroy all leukemic cells in these patients with far advanced disease; relapses occurred within 3 months in both patients. TBI regimens now are always combined with CY or other chemotherapeutic agents [111].

Three randomized studies of different TBI schemes in combination with CY have been reported in the literature [112–117]. In two studies from Seattle, two fractionation schemes were used (12 Gy in 2 Gy fractions for 6 days vs. 15.75 Gy in 2.25 Gy fractions for 7 days) for conventional marrow grafts. In the study involving patients with CML, the relapse rate was lower in the regimen in which patients received the higher dose of 15.75 Gy; however, there was an increase in nonrelapse mortality, which resulted in a decreased overall survival (OS) rate with the higher-dose regimen [112,115]. However, a later retrospective study from New York, using a similar high total dose (15 Gy) in 1.5 Gy fractions twice a day for 5 days, with potentially improved supportive care, achieved a Kaplan–Meier event-free survival (EFS) at 3 years of 62% ± 7% for 44 CML patients in chronic phase [118]. Relapse rate was only 9% (4 patients).

Patients with CML are, on average, older than patients with AML, who have had a somewhat different outcome in randomized studies. In the study in patients with AML, again there was a decrease in relapse in the higher-total-dose regimen [114,115]. For these patients, although there was also an increase in nonrelapse mortality, it did not translate into a lower survival rate. An earlier randomized trial from Seattle compared single-dose irradiation (10 Gy) with fractionated irradiation (12 Gy in 6 daily fractions) in patients with AML [113,116]. In this study, there was a higher relapse rate (22%) in the single-dose regimen than in the fractionated regimen (12%). One trial, with patients receiving single-dose or hyperfractionated TBI according to physician preference, randomized patients to a high or low instantaneous dose rate within the fractionation groups [103]. There was no difference in relapse between any of the groups.

Other studies were either single-arm studies or comparisons within institutions in different eras of their experience as they shifted from one regimen to another [86,119–121]. In many of the studies it is difficult to separate the effects of fractionation from that of total dose, as both changed in the regimens used.

In a study from Italy that provides a good comparison of total dose, Frassoni and associates reported on patients with AML and CML who were ostensibly treated with a regimen of three fractions of 3.3 Gy each, to a 9.9 Gy total dose [122]. However, this was only a nominal planned dose; the actual doses received were calculated retrospectively based on actual *in vivo* physics measurements. The authors found that the incidence of relapse at 7 years was 55% in patients who received less than

9.9 Gy, compared with only 11% in patients who received more than 9.9 Gy ($p = 0.0005$). This difference ultimately had a major impact on survival rate: 74% at 8 years for the group who received more than 9.9 Gy, compared with only 38% for the group who received less than 9.9 Gy ($p = 0.005$). Further analysis of these patients by Scarpati *et al.* [123] showed that total dose was the most significant factor affecting relapse.

A publication from France described a large nonrandomized multiinstitutional study in which there was an increase in relapse rate with fractionated TBI (10.0–13.2 Gy) when compared with a single-dose regimen (10 Gy) [124]. The 126 patients in the single-dose group had a relapse rate of 16%, whereas the 54 patients in the fractionated group had a relapse rate of 29%. In contrast, a study from the Children's Cancer Study Group showed that there was an increased relapse rate associated with the single-dose regimens (7.5–10.0 Gy) given at different institutions when compared with fractionated regimens at other institutions (2 Gy for six fractions over 6 days or 1.2 Gy 3 times a day for 4 days for a total dose of 13.2 Gy) [125]. The 2-year relapse risk was 23% (10/51) in the single-dose group vs. 0% (0/15) in the fractionated groups ($p = 0.07$).

A large European study also demonstrated that greater fractionation decreased the relapse rate, although the study was not designed to compare regimens [126]. Patients who achieved a CR after a common intensive consolidation and were not eligible for an allogeneic BMT were randomized to undergo autologous BMT or a second intensive consolidation course. The analysis of the 105 allograft patients who were treated with a TBI-containing regimen showed that the relapse risk at 3 years was less (12%) when TBI was given in more than three fractions compared with single-dose TBI (32%). The disease-free survival (DFS) rate at 3 years was also superior with higher fractionation: 70% for TBI in more than three fractions, 63% for two or three fractions and only 41% for single-dose TBI. The choice of regimen was left to the discretion of the clinicians at the various institutions.

There have been some attempts to escalate the total TBI dose to levels above 15 Gy [127,128]. In patients with advanced hematologic malignancies, the maximum tolerated dose in one study was 16 Gy when given in fractions of 2 Gy twice a day 6 h apart (instantaneous dose rate of 8 cGy/min) [127]. A recent dose escalation phase I–II study, with nine patients receiving autologous peripheral blood HCT, employed three dose levels: 16, 18 and 20 Gy, at 2 Gy per fraction twice a day, with three patients at each dose level [128]. Fifty percent lung transmission blocks were used with electron chest wall boost irradiation to those areas and the kidneys were shielded to a maximum of 16 Gy. Toxicity was moderate, and four patients achieved CR, with one remaining disease-free 5 years post-transplant.

In summary, in non-T-cell-depleted marrow transplants, leukemic relapse is generally less with higher total doses of TBI when various fractionated regimens are compared. This gain is often achieved at the expense of a higher treatment-related morbidity, so that survival advantages are not seen in every study. Comparisons of single-dose regimens with fractionated regimens show no consistent difference with regard to relapse. Nonrandomized studies showed a low relapse rate with hyperfractionation to high-doses (13.2–15.0 Gy), but no randomized studies comparing such regimens to a daily fractionation scheme have been done [53,119].

In T-cell-depleted BMT, however, several studies found an increase in relapse rate in patients with CML when fractionated schedules were used in comparison to single-dose fractionation schedules [129–132]. MSKCC performed a study randomizing 45 patients with ALL or AML to receive either T-cell-depleted or conventional transplants; there was no difference in relapse rates, using 15 Gy TBI and CY for preparation [133]. Other authors reported increased relapse rates with T-cell-depleted transplants [108,134,135].

Champlin *et al.* [22] found a decrease in relapse rate in recipients of T-cell-depleted transplants when they switched from a protocol of 11.25 Gy in five fractions to a protocol of 13.5 Gy in six fractions. In the latter protocol, they also added one treatment with TLI (2.25 Gy). Their actuarial relapse rate dropped from 82% to 15%.

The amount of lung shielding may also prove to be critical in the prevention of relapse. A study from France demonstrated that when patients were randomized to one of two different total lung doses by means of different amounts of lung shielding, there was an unexpected increase in relapse to 25% when the lung dose was only 6 Gy, compared with no relapses when the lung dose was 8 Gy [136].

The addition of splenic irradiation may also have an impact on relapse in some CML patients. Although a European randomized study of splenic irradiation to 10 Gy in 3 days did not demonstrate a difference in DFS at 2 years [137], one subset of patients did benefit, as described in an update of that study [138]. Patients in an intermediate-risk group, defined by having peripheral blood basophil levels higher than 3% prior to transplantation and by not having a T-cell-depleted BMT, fared better with splenic irradiation. The relapse rate at 8 years was only 8% in this group when splenic irradiation was performed, compared with 30% when no irradiation was used ($p < 0.05$). This boost schedule has been used in CML patients just prior to TBI in the cytoreduction regimen used at Mount Sinai Medical Center; an excellent DFS rate (92% in patients with chronic-phase CML) has been observed but the follow-up time is still short [53].

In patients with lymphoma, the value of adding involved-field (IF) boost irradiation to sites of residual disease or to areas with gross disease prior to chemotherapy is still unclear. Nonrandomized studies showed either a decreased relapse rate in the area of the IF irradiation [90] or an improvement in progression-free or EFS [91,94,139]. For further discussion of this issue, see the Consolidative irradiation in high-dose therapy regimens section, below.

Normal-tissue toxicity

There are many normal-tissue toxicities to consider when TBI is administered. Some authors analyzed factors of transplantation that affect all of the toxicities grouped together, termed regimen-related toxicity [140]. One major factor was TBI dose. Two regimens were used: 12 Gy in six daily fractions of 2 Gy and 15.75 Gy in seven daily fractions of 2.25 Gy. The only factor among the allogeneic marrow recipients that was significantly associated with less toxicity was the lower TBI dose. The results are somewhat confounded by the probability that other variables act in concert. For example, the higher-dose TBI was more commonly administered to relapsed patients and to patients receiving mismatched grafts. However, even in the multivariate analysis, patients receiving a higher TBI dose had a higher incidence of severe toxicity. Whether the marrow was autologous or allogeneic was the only other significant variable that emerged in this multivariate analysis.

Lung

Radiation pneumonopathy is a two-phase process with the occurrence and intensity of these phases independent of each other. The first phase is an acute IP involving inflammation and edema of the alveolar lining cells. It appears clinically usually 1–4 months after the initiation of irradiation. Clinically, there may be dyspnea, cough, fever, pleuritic pain and rales. Chest radiographs demonstrate diffuse bilateral lung infiltrates, often described as a "ground-glass" appearance. The second phase is a chronic progressive irreversible pulmonary fibrosis, often asymptomatic, occurring most often from 4 months to 1 year after irradiation. Lung volumes and compliance may decrease, along with a reduction in maximum breathing capacity. Radiographically, there is often a streaky, fibrous-appearing pattern with notable lung volume loss.

Table 14.3 Comparison of interstitial pneumonitis (IP) incidence in single-dose and fractionated regimens.

Study	Single-dose regimen		Fractionated regimen	
	Total dose (Gy)	%IP (%Fatal IP)	Total dose (Gy)	%IP (%Fatal IP)
MSKCC [87]	10	70 (50)	13.2/11.0*	24 (18)
Seattle [113] (randomized study)	10	26 (26)	12/6	15 (15)
Inst. Gustave-Roussy [86]	10*	45 (26)	13.2/11.0*	13 (4)
City of Hope [121]	10	28 (–)	13.2/11.0*	10 (–)
Johns Hopkins [44]	8–10	70 (–)	8–12/2–4*	37 (–)
French Multiinstitute Study [124]	10*	38† (26)	12.0–13.2/3–11*	18 (11)
Univ. Minnesota [120]	7.5	25 (8)	13.2/8.0	23 (13)
Genoa [50]	10	60 (–)	9.9/3.0	5 (–)
Royal Marsden Hospital [142]	9.5–10.5‡	10 (5)	—	—
Montréal [143]	7.5–9.0	56 (41)	12/6	25 (21)
Hôpital Tenon, Paris	10* (0.15 Gy/m)	45	12/6* (0.06 Gy/m)	29
Randomized Dose Rate Study [103]	10* (0.06 Gy/m)	25	12/6* (0.03 Gy/m)	31
Non-randomized ABMT Study [141]	10*	16	12/6*	18
Perugia [144]	—	—	14.4/12.0 }±*	4 (–)
			15.0–15.6/12–13	18 (–)
GEGMO [145]	10*	23	11–14/5–11*	12

*Lung blocks also used.
†Five-year actuarial projected incidence.
‡Lung dose: nominal dose rate = 0.025 Gy/min.
ABMT, autologous bone marrow transplantation; GEGMO, Group d'Etudes de la Greffe de Moelle Osseuse; MSKCC, Memorial Sloan Kettering Cancer Center.

Comparison between institutions of the incidence of any pneumonitis or fatal pneumonitis in TBI studies has been difficult because often the definition of IP differs; some authors include IP of known infectious etiology and others consider it to be only idiopathic IP. There is good reason to report both in studies that examine IP. Although idiopathic IP is most likely attributable to irradiation, other factors such as chemotherapy (BU, CY, 1,3-bis(2-chloroethyl)-1-nitrosourea [BCNU], bleomycin and adriamycin) and GVHD may have a role, and the incidence depends on how aggressively one pursues other causes. Furthermore, although infectious IP may not be directly attributable to irradiation, TBI may have a role (e.g. in increased intestinal toxicity allowing a port of entry to infectious agents).

The time frame between studies in different institutions has often been quite different; some institutions have considered only IP developing within 100 days of the transplantation, whereas others consider IP as late as 1 or 2 years following BMT. There are a few comparison studies within institutions but they are generally comparisons between sequential methods of treatment.

IP was one of the endpoints examined in the randomized study from Seattle, comparing single dose with fractionated irradiation in patients with AML in first remission [113,116]. Single-dose TBI (10 Gy) and TBI fractionated daily with fractions of 2 Gy for 6 days were the regimens used. The incidence of IP was less with the fractionated regimen (15%) when compared with the single-dose regimen (26%). In this study, in which patients were followed for 9 years, there was a significant overall difference in survival rate between the two regimens: 30% in the single-dose group compared with 54% in the fractionated group [112]. The difference in the survival curves is primarily a result of the difference in early mortality, suggesting that the improvement with fractionation is primarily a result of reduced toxicity, not decreased relapse.

A French study with single-dose (10 Gy) and hyperfractionated TBI (2 Gy twice daily for 3 days) treatment groups randomized patients within each group to receive either high- or low-instantaneous-dose-rate TBI [103]. Instantaneous dose rate means the dose rate while the beam is on (i.e. not averaging in any interruptions in treatment). Although the high-dose-rate single-dose group had a 45% incidence of IP compared with only 25% in the low-dose-rate single-dose group, only 57 patients received single-dose TBI; this difference was, therefore, not significant ($p = 0.18$). A retrospective analysis of the effects of instantaneous dose rate in a nonrandomized study by the same investigators [141] in 186 patients who had an autologous BMT did show a statistically significant difference in IP as a function of dose rate. There was a 5-year IP incidence of 56% with a high-dose rate (>0.09 Gy/min), 13% with a medium dose rate (>0.048 Gy/min and ≤0.09 Gy/min) and 20% with a low-dose rate (≤0.048 Gy/min). This analysis was highly significant for the comparison between high and medium dose rates ($p = 0.002$). The 56% incidence of IP in the high-dose-rate group is especially notable, because it occurred in patients who received autologous transplants, in which the IP rate is usually very low (<20%).

Other studies within single institutions are listed along with the above-mentioned studies in Table 14.3 [44,50,86,87,113,120,103,121,124,141–145], and it can be seen that almost any fractionated regimen is associated with both a lower incidence of and fewer fatalities due to IP when compared with single-dose regimens. Differences are often striking; for example, there was only an 18% incidence of fatal IP when the dose was hyperfractionated, compared with a 50% incidence of fatal IP in the single-dose group at MSKCC. However, lung blocks were also utilized in the fractionated group but not in the single-dose group, which confounds the effect of fractionation. When comparisons were made between single-dose and hyperfractionated groups at an institution where blocks were used in both regimens and the lung dose was similar, there was still a decrease in the incidence of IP, as seen in the data from the Institut Gustave Roussy [86]. This group found a 45% incidence of IP (26% fatal) in the single-dose group but only a 13% incidence of IP (4% fatal) in the fractionated group.

With single-dose TBI, very low-dose rates (0.025 Gy/min) led to a low incidence of IP (10%) and fatal IP (5%), but treatment times were as long as 7 h [142]. In contrast, a study from Montreal showed that single-dose TBI (9 Gy), with a high instantaneous dose rate using a sweeping beam technique (0.210–0.235 Gy/min) resulted in a high incidence of severe IP (8/11, with 4 fatal), when compared with the same dose given with ^{60}Co at a constant dose rate of 0.047–0.063 Gy/min (6/11 IP cases, mild in 3 and fatal in none) [143]. A summary of the experience from several institutions that used low-dose-rate single-dose TBI demonstrated that the crude incidence of idiopathic IP increased with absolute dose to lung [146]. The best-fit curve was sigmoidal (probit regression analysis); a 50% incidence of IP occurred at approximately 11.5 Gy.

All these studies were done in patients who received conventional transplants, with the exception of the study from Perugia [144,147], which was done in patients who received T-cell-depleted marrow transplants. In a comparison of this study with the others, there was even a lower incidence of IP with T-cell-depletion, presumably as a result of the abrogation of GVHD. Only fractionated regimens were used, but total doses differed. The incidence of IP was only 4% in the group receiving 14.4 Gy and 18% when the dose was increased by one fraction to 15.6 Gy, but patient numbers were low in each group.

At MSKCC, in 67 adult patients with CML who received T-cell-depleted transplants, a group that historically had had a high incidence of GVHD and IP, only 11 of 67 patients (16%) had IP, which was fatal in five (7%) [33]. In the historical adult CML conventional transplant group, 40% (6/15) IP cases had been fatal, which was associated with a 73% incidence of GVHD.

In a retrospective review of 339 patients who had undergone SCT for hematologic disorders, investigators from Boston found that T-cell depletion as GVHD prophylaxis was significantly better than the use of cyclosporine and methotrexate in decreasing the incidence of severe pulmonary complications (8% vs. 33%) [148]. These complications were defined as diffuse alveolar hemorrhage, need for a respirator, or death from respiratory failure.

A study from Glasgow assessed two types of regimens with respect to their effect on pulmonary function tests at various times after the BMT [149]. One was a single-dose regimen of 9.5 Gy with a lung dose of 8 Gy, and the others were fractionated regimens, which varied from 12.0 to 14.4 Gy in six to eight fractions, with lung doses from 11.0 to 13.5 Gy. In all instances, there was impairment of pulmonary function after transplantation, but it gradually returned to normal. The most significantly altered findings were those for gas exchange: diffusion capacity and transfer coefficient. With the fractionated regimens, the authors found a significantly less marked impairment of gas exchange compared with the single-dose regimen. Furthermore, patients who had received single-dose TBI had a slower and less complete recovery of gas exchange than did those who had been treated with the fractionated regimens.

The effect of lung shielding was compared in a very small nonrandomized study from Croatia [150]. In patients for whom lung shields were used during TBI, there was only an 8% (1/13) incidence of IP, compared to 27% (4/15) in those without lung shields.

Lens

Many studies have now reported a decrease in the incidence of cataract development by use of fractionated courses of TBI compared with single-dose irradiation. The first study to report this finding was that of Deeg et al. [151] in 1984. They found only an 18% incidence of cataract development in the group of patients who received a fractionated course of irradiation (either 12 Gy in six fractions or 15.75 Gy in seven fractions), compared with an incidence of 80% in patients who received 10 Gy single-dose TBI. In a later study from the same institution, Benyunes et al. [152] compared the incidence of cataracts and the need for surgery, between single-dose TBI (10 Gy) and two dose ranges of fractionated TBI. There was an 85% incidence of cataracts in the single-dose group, compared with 50% for the >12 Gy and 34% for the <12 Gy fractionated TBI groups. In the single-dose group, 59% required surgery, compared with only 33% in the >12 Gy fractionated group and 22% in the <12 Gy group.

Deeg et al. [151] also noted that steroids and GVHD enhanced the development of cataracts. Dunn and associates also described an increased incidence of cataracts with steroid use after fractionated TBI, an 18% incidence in patients who had received steroids compared with 4% in those without steroids [153]. In their study, patients who did not receive TBI in their preparative regimen had a 12% incidence of cataracts.

Two groups reported a high incidence of cataracts in a single-dose TBI group (83% in one and 100% in the other study) compared with none in a fractionated TBI group [154,155]. Calissendorff et al. [156] compared children who had received 10 Gy TBI in a single dose for hematologic malignancies with children with severe aplastic anemia who received no TBI or only 8 Gy TBI plus eye shielding. In the single-dose group, lens opacification developed in all children after 3 years, whereas none developed in the group with no TBI or eye-shielded TBI.

Kim et al. [120] also noted a decreased incidence of cataracts with hyperfractionated irradiation (1.65 Gy twice daily for 4 days at a dose rate of 0.1 Gy/min) when compared with high-dose-rate (0.26 Gy/min) single-dose irradiation of 7.5 Gy. Although the difference was not significant, the 3-year estimated incidence of cataracts was 27% in the single-dose TBI group and only 12% in the fractionated group. The median age for the single-dose group was 15 years, compared with 25 years for the fractionated group. Because risk for cataract development increases with age, a higher incidence in the fractionated group on the basis of age would have been expected [157].

In a randomized study of high- and low-dose rates in single-dose (10 Gy) and hyperfractionated TBI (2 Gy/fraction twice daily for 3 days), there was a statistically significant difference between dose rates ($p = 0.049$) only in the single-dose groups [103]. In the low-dose-rate group (0.06 Gy/min), cataracts developed in three of 28 patients (11%) compared with seven of 29 (24%) in the high-dose-rate group (0.15 Gy/min), with 5-year estimated incidences of 24% and 53%, respectively. In the hyperfractionated groups with dose rates of 0.03 and 0.06 Gy/min, cataracts developed in 2% vs. 10%, respectively. The difference in 5-year estimated incidences for single-dose (18%) and fractionated TBI (6%) was statistically significant, but fractionation was not a randomized parameter. When patients who received single-dose and fractionated TBI were combined, low instantaneous dose rates resulted in a lower 5-year incidence of cataracts (12%) than did the high-dose rates (34%).

In patients with malignancies treated with rapidly fractionated TBI regimens (10.5–12.0 Gy in 3–6 fractions over 36 h to 3 days), Bray et al. [158] demonstrated a 63% incidence of cataracts compared with patients who received no TBI (only melphalan), who had only a 9% incidence of cataracts.

In one study, T-cell depletion, presumably through its role in decreasing GVHD, appeared to reduce cataract incidence in patients who received single-dose TBI [159]. At 9 years, the T-cell-depleted group had a 72% incidence of cataracts, compared to 100% in the non-T-cell-depleted group. A multivariate analysis of patients who had received single-dose TBI (9–12 Gy) in a nonrandomized study revealed other risk factors for cataract development related to radiation: cranial irradiation prior to TBI (relative risk [RR] = 4.3), skull dose higher than 10 Gy (RR = 2.2), and a TBI dose rate of 0.035 Gy/min or greater (RR = 2.1) [160].

The increase in cataracts after prior cranial irradiation was suggested also in a retrospective study of 260 patients who received hyperfractionated TBI, although the difference was not statistically significant (Chi-square, $p > 0.05$) [161]. Cataract patients had received whole brain irradiation more often (14%) than those without cataracts (11%). In contrast, another nonrandomized study did not demonstrate an influence of prior cranial irradiation in children, but multivariate analysis showed a statistically significant increase in cataract incidence with higher dose rates [162]. The 5-year incidence of cataracts was 54% for high-dose rates (≥0.09 Gy/min), 30% for medium-dose rates (≥0.048 Gy/min and <0.09 Gy/min) and 3.5% for low-dose rates (<0.048 Gy/min). All possible dose rate comparisons between these groups were statistically significant.

A retrospective analysis of 1063 patients from centers participating in the European Bone Marrow Transplant Group showed an advantage for fractionation over single-dose TBI, and multivariate analysis within each of these two groups revealed favorable independent factors to include low-dose rate (<0.048 Gy/min) for both groups, and more than six fractions for the fractionated TBI group [163]. The use of heparin and avoidance of steroids played a role in the single-dose group. Heparin, used as prophylaxis against VOD, had protected against cataract formation in the study reported by Belkacemi *et al.* [162]. At 5 years, the estimated incidence of cataracts was 16% when heparin was used, compared with 28% when it was not ($p = 0.01$).

Other organs and systems

There are many more normal tissues and physiological functions of importance affected by TBI, including the endocrine system, bone growth and fertility. Decreased morbidity has been noted with fractionated courses of irradiation compared with single-dose irradiation. Several good reviews on this subject exist [164,165]. In addition, Sanders [166] published an excellent review on endocrine problems and effects on growth and development (see also Chapter 68). In the studies from Seattle, after 10 Gy single-dose TBI, there was a much higher incidence of compensated hypothyroidism as well as overt hypothyroidism in children when compared with fractionated TBI (12.00–15.75 Gy over 4–7 days) [164]. Two studies have shown significant deleterious effects on growth from single-dose TBI and a significant reduction of this negative effect with fractionated TBI [167,168]. Significant effects on height were also seen after the use of TAI in children, suggesting that the deleterious effects of irradiation are probably related to effects on bone epiphyses, thyroid and/or gonads rather than cranial neuroendocrine structures alone [169].

One other important area that should be studied in more detail after TBI is brain function. Children with ALL who have more than one course of cranial irradiation have increased toxicity, with larger decrements in IQ and achievement than children who did not have such treatment [170]. A case report described somnolence syndrome 8 weeks after irradiation in an adult with AML who received CY and a rapid course of TBI (2.2 Gy twice daily for 3 days, for a total dose of 13.2 Gy) [171]. One study of TBI patients demonstrated an increasing cognitive dysfunction with increasing dose of TBI, by both univariate and multivariate analysis [172]. The role of fractionation or prior cranial irradiation was not studied. It would be of value to study cognitive function using the same total doses with different fractionations and to compare patients who have had TBI with and without prior prophylactic cranial irradiation.

One study suggests that, in patients who had received an autologous BMT after hyperfractionated TBI and CY, behavioral function improved to premorbid levels after 10 years from the onset of their disease if they had received no pretreatment brain irradiation or intrathecal methotrexate [173]. A prospective study of 58 patients who had received hyperfractionated TBI showed no deterioration in cognitive testing in the 21 recurrence-free survivors who were examined at 6–30 months after TBI completion [174].

VOD also occurs less frequently with fractionated or hyperfractionated TBI regimens compared with single-dose TBI [82,86,116,175,176]; in two other studies, however, neither TBI fractionation or dose rate influenced the incidence of VOD [103,177]. In neither of these two studies was fractionation randomized but the dose rate was randomized in one [103]. Renal dysfunction was strongly correlated with total TBI dose and dose/fraction in two studies [178,179].

From the studies on normal-tissue toxicity, it is clear that fractionation allows higher doses of irradiation to be given with less toxicity than single-dose irradiation.

Can chemotherapy-only regimens replace TBI?

It has been suggested that TBI may be replaced with BU as part of the conditioning regimen of patients with leukemia for allogeneic marrow transplantation [180]. However, the alternative of BU with CY is not without risk [181–184].

The toxicity of the BU/CY regimen was compared with the TBI/CY regimen in sequential patient populations by Morgan and associates [185]. They found a high incidence of VOD in the BU/CY group (19%) compared with only 1% in the TBI/CY group. Hemorrhagic cystitis developed in 30% of the patients with BU/CY compared with 14% in the group with TBI/CY. The IP incidence and fatalities were similar in both groups. In an International Bone Marrow Transplant Registry (IBMTR) analysis, transplant conditioning that included single-dose TBI was significantly less toxic to the liver (3% VOD incidence) than was BU/CY (12% VOD incidence) [186]. A retrospective study of Japanese BMT registry patients, that compared TBI-containing regimens with cytoreduction without TBI, showed no significant difference in IP incidence between the two groups [187]. A meta-analysis of adverse effects of BU/CY vs. TBI-containing regimens demonstrated that VOD was more common among patients treated utilizing BU/CY than among those using TBI [188]. There was little difference between the regimens in the incidence of IP.

We have the results of several randomized trials of BU/CY vs. CY/TBI, as well as several large registry analyses (Fig. 14.6). The French Multiinstitutional Group for the Study of Bone Marrow Transplantation (Group d'Etudes de la Greffe de Moelle Osseuse [GEGMO]) found that, in a randomized study in patients with AML in first remission, CY/TBI resulted in a statistically significant improvement in DFS (72% vs. 47%; $p < 0.01$) and survival (75% vs. 51%; $p < 0.02$) [189]. Relapse was less in the CY/TBI group (14% vs. 34%; $p < 0.04$), as was transplant-related mortality (8% vs. 27%; $p < 0.06$).

In a retrospective review of patients with acute leukemia in the European BMT database, there was no significant difference in relapse incidence, leukemia-free survival rate or transplant-related mortality between the preparative regimens in any allogenic group receiving BMT [190]. However, for patients who received an autologous BMT, who were in a second or later remission or in a first relapse ("intermediate disease") of ALL, the incidence of relapse was significantly higher ($p = 0.002$) after BU/CY treatment (82%) than after CY/TBI (62%), and the 2-year leukemia-free survival was significantly lower ($p = 0.002$) with BU/CY than with CY/TBI (14% vs. 34%). VOD and hemorrhagic cystitis were more common with the BU/CY regimen in both the autologous and allogeneic groups.

In a retrospective study of BMT for acute leukemia in children from registry data of the Pediatric Hematology Oncology Italian Association, there were no significant differences seen in DFS after allogeneic BMT [191]. However, DFS was better after autologous BMT when TBI was used for patients with ALL in second or subsequent CR ($p = 0.0003$), including those in CR after extramedullary relapse ($p = 0.002$) or in patients with AML in first CR ($p = 0.001$).

There were no significant differences found between BU/CY and CY/TBI regimens for OS in any of the randomized studies in chronic-phase CML patients (Fig. 14.6) [192–197]. In the GEGMO study, however, there was a higher relapse rate ($p = 0.04$) in the TBI arms (11% for

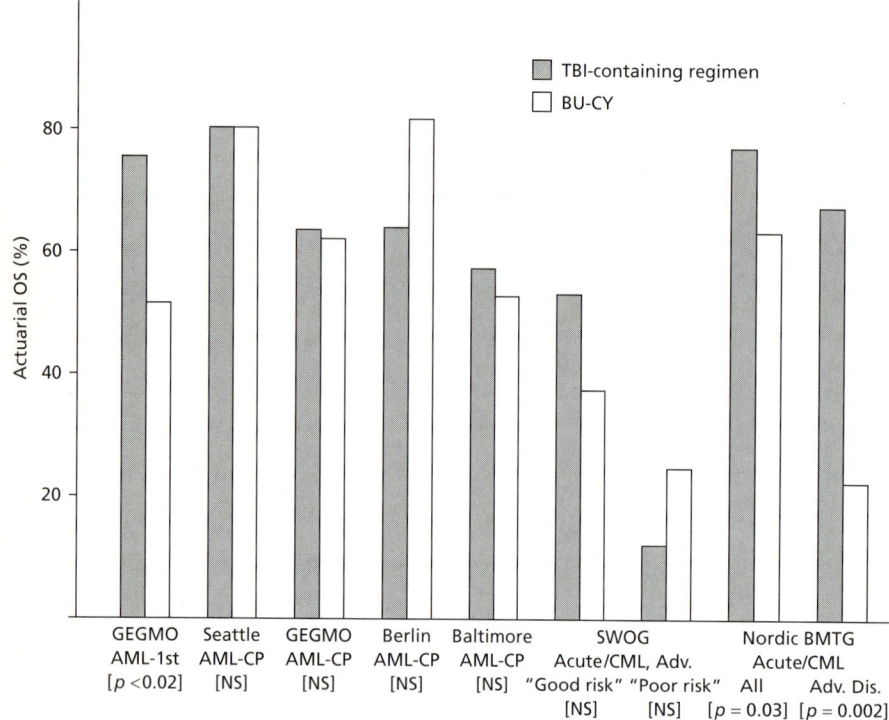

Fig. 14.6 Comparison of actuarial percent overall survival (OS) for randomized trials of busulfan and cyclophosphamide (BU-CY) vs. total body irradiation (TBI)-containing regimens. TBI regimens were all CY and TBI with the exception of the South-west Oncology Group (SWOG) regimen, which was TBI and etoposide (VP16). Adv. Dis., advanced disease; AML, acute myeloid leukemia; BMTG, Bone Marrow Transplantation Group; CML, chronic myeloid leukemia; CP, chronic phase; GEGMO, Group d'Etudes de la Greffe de Moelle Osseuse; NS, not significant.

single-dose TBI and 31% for fractionated TBI) when compared with the BU/CY arm (4%), which was not reflected in either DFS or OS rates [194]. There was a trend toward a better engraftment rate in the TBI/CY arm.

Two of the randomized studies mixed patients with acute leukemias and those with CML [198,199]. The Southwest Oncology Group study [198], which compared TBI/VP16 to BU/CY, showed no significant differences, but the Nordic study [199] favored the TBI/CY regimen over the BU/CY regimen, with highly significant differences in both OS and DFS rates for the advanced disease patients. In an update at 7 years, these results were still highly significant in patients with advanced disease [200]. BU/CY was more toxic in the entire group, with significantly increased VOD, chronic GVHD, obstructive bronchiolitis and hemorrhagic cystitis. A long-term follow-up of four of the randomized studies for myeloid leukemia concluded that BU/CY and CY/TBI provided similar probabilities for cure for patients with CML, but for AML, there was a 10% lower survival rate after BU/CY (not statistically significant) [201]. Late complications were similar in each regimen, except for an increased cataract risk with CY/TBI and increased alopecia with BU/CY. It is important to have long follow-up in all of these studies.

A retrospective study in children 16 years or younger with AML in first CR emphasized the importance of CY dose [202]. The study concluded that the combination of BU/CY (200 mg/kg) was equivalent to TBI/CY for relapse (13% and 10%, respectively) and EFS (82% and 80%), but that BU with CY at a lower dose (120 mg/kg) was inferior, with a 54% relapse rate and 46% EFS rate.

For autologous purged marrow transplantation, a randomized study of TBI/CY vs. BU/CY was done in AML patients [203]. TBI/CY was found to be equivalent to BU/CY, or better, for all endpoints studied, but there were too few patients to achieve statistical significance. The endpoints were relapse, relapse-free survival, OS and VOD incidence. When these randomized patients were combined with 40 nonrandomized AML patients, there was a statistically significant improvement ($p = 0.04$) in DFS at 2 years in the TBI/CY subset of patients who were in second or later remission (38% vs. 7%) [204].

Consolidative irradiation in high-dose therapy regimens
Rationale

Radiation therapy is an extremely effective agent in the treatment of lymphoma. When employed as a single agent, radiation therapy is curative for many patients with early stage Hodgkin's disease, follicular lymphoma and even selected patients with early stage diffuse large B-cell lymphoma. Patients who are candidates for high-dose therapy and HCT generally have systemic disease; however, locoregional disease may often contribute to relapse in these patients.

Several investigators have analyzed sites of failure after high-dose therapy for relapsed Hodgkin's disease. A Vancouver group reported that among 56 transplanted patients, progression or failure occurred in previous sites of disease in 16 of the 17 patients who relapsed [205]. A Seattle report on 127 patients demonstrated that 33 of the 49 patients who relapsed failed exclusively in sites of previous disease [206].

Investigators from Genoa reported on sites of progression in 50 transplanted patients [207]. Eighty-two percent had progression of disease primarily at initial sites of involvement. Results from Stanford in 100 patients showed that 22 of the 32 patients who relapsed after transplantation relapsed in sites involved immediately prior to transplantation, and an additional three patients relapsed in sites that had been remotely involved [92].

In a similar analysis of patients with Hodgkin's disease treated with high-dose chemotherapy at the University of Chicago, 38% of 13 patients who relapsed failed exclusively in sites previously involved, 54% failed in both previously involved and new sites, and only 8% failed exclusively in new sites [91].

In a collaborative study from St. Bartholomew's and Royal London Hospitals, Queen Mary and Westfield College, Smithfield, London, 100 patients underwent autologous transplantation for relapsed or refractory Hodgkin's disease [208]. The 37 patients who relapsed recurred at previous sites of disease in 81%.

Similar observations have been made in series reporting transplantation results for the non-Hodgkin's lymphomas. Mundt *et al.* [209] from the University of Chicago evaluated sites of failure after high-dose therapy for aggressive non-Hodgkin's lymphoma. Pre or post-transplant local irradiation was administered to 13% of the patients in this series because of initial bulky disease, persistent disease or to consolidate a complete response. Among the 21 patients treated with high-dose chemotherapy who relapsed, 48% failed exclusively in sites previously involved, 29% failed in both previously involved and new sites and 24% failed exclusively in new sites.

In a report from Seattle, sites of relapse were evaluated among 101 patients transplanted for lymphoma (80% non-Hodgkin's lymphoma) [210]. Among 62 patients who experienced a relapse, 59 (95%) experienced a relapse in sites involved by disease pretransplant. In an analysis of the outcome of 78 patients autotransplanted for intermediate- or high-grade lymphoma, 39 patients relapsed; in 33 of these (84.6%), the initial relapse occurred in sites of prior disease [211]. In a collaborative study of 100 patients with intermediate- or high-grade lymphoma by Philip et al. [212] 76.5% of patients who relapsed had a component of relapse in prior disease sites.

Since the reason for failure of the transplant procedure is frequently related to recurrence of lymphoma in the initial sites of involvement, it is easy to understand the rationale for inclusion of locoregional radiation therapy for these salvage programs. If radiation therapy is included, parameters to be addressed include timing (pre or post-transplant), extent of radiation fields and dose.

The advantages of utilizing radiation therapy as cytoreductive treatment prior to high-dose therapy are that it can effectively reduce the tumor burden before high-dose treatment, and the risk of interruption or delay of the locoregional radiation therapy is minimal. The primary disadvantages include potential delay of the high-dose therapy and the potential overlapping toxicities of the locoregional irradiation and high-dose therapy, including mucositis and pneumonitis [213]. Cytoreductive radiation treatment may include all sites of relapse, the bulky sites of relapse, sites with an incomplete response, or even more extensive treatment, such as TLI.

Given the logical rationale for locoregional irradiation, it is not surprising that most large published series of high-dose therapy for Hodgkin's disease and other lymphomas have included locoregional irradiation in at least selected patients. However, there has been wide variation in exactly how to employ it. In some series, radiation is given pretransplant [214–217], although in the majority, it is given after transplant [139,218–226]. The range of intervals from transplant to irradiation varies from 1 to 4 months.

Often, the fields treated include sites of bulky disease (variably defined) at the time of relapse [215–218,222,223,225] or areas of residual disease after high-dose therapy has been administered [139,219,221,223,225]. Some have included all sites involved at the time of relapse [139,224]. Others include TLI but with a differential dose, depending upon disease status [214].

The range of radiation doses employed varies substantially in these series, from 18 to 40 Gy. In general, lower doses are employed in situations where initially nonbulky disease is included in the treatment, or if there has been a complete response to high-dose therapy.

Outcome

The use of locoregional irradiation in high-dose therapy programs has the potential for altering the patterns of failure and perhaps reducing the risk of failure. For example, in the Stanford series of patients who underwent high-dose therapy for relapse of Hodgkin's disease, 49 patients with relapsed Stage I–III disease, who had involved field irradiation as a component of their salvage treatment, had 3-year freedom-from-relapse, survival and EFS rates of 100%, 85% and 85%, respectively, compared with only 67%, 60% and 54%, respectively, for the 13 patients who received high-dose chemotherapy alone [92]. The difference in freedom from relapse was statistically significant ($p = 0.04$).

In a similar analysis of patients with Hodgkin's disease reported from the University of Chicago, the 5-year local control in involved sites was 94% among patients who received irradiation as a component of therapy vs. 73% when the sites were not irradiated ($p = 0.008$) [91]. At the University of Rochester, the EFS for irradiated patients was 44%, compared to only 28% for patients treated with high-dose chemotherapy alone ($p = 0.03$) [224].

Moskowitz et al. [214] at MSKCC reported the use of more extensive cytoreductive radiation therapy for patients with refractory or relapsed Hodgkin's disease. Patients were treated with a second line chemotherapy program. This was followed by high-dose chemotherapy with a combination of VP16 and CY as preparation for autologous transplantation. Prior to high-dose chemotherapy and peripheral stem cell transplant, patients who had not received previous irradiation were treated with involved field irradiation to 18 Gy and TLI to 18 Gy (both with twice-daily fractionation). Patients who had prior irradiation were treated with involved field irradiation, if organ tolerance would not be exceeded, to a dose of 18–36 Gy in 5–10 days (twice-daily fractionation) depending on the prior doses received by the involved sites. The EFS rate was 68% and the OS rate was 81% for the 56 patients who underwent transplantation. Only three (18%) treatment failures occurred in a site that was irradiated during the salvage program.

Similar observations have been made in series reporting transplantation results for the non-Hodgkin's lymphomas. The University of Chicago group evaluated sites of failure after high-dose therapy for aggressive non-Hodgkin's lymphoma [209]. Among patients who received local irradiation as a component of therapy there were no relapses in the irradiated sites ($p = 0.04$). A series of 120 patients who underwent autologous HCT for non-Hodgkin's lymphoma was reported from the Hôpital Saint-Antoine in Paris, France [227]. Following transplantation, 45 of the 120 patients received radiation therapy (median dose: 20 Gy) to previous sites of lymphoma. The addition of irradiation was associated with an improved EFS in both univariate ($p = 0.03$) and multivariate ($p = 0.02$, RR = 0.021) analyses. In the well-publicized "Parma" trial, patients who received local radiation therapy in addition to high-dose salvage chemotherapy had a relapse risk of only 36% compared to a risk of 55% for patients on the high-dose therapy arm who received no radiation ($p = 0.19$), even though patients were selected to receive radiation therapy because of the presence of bulky disease [216].

There is mounting evidence that locoregional irradiation may be a beneficial component of high-dose therapy programs. As noted, many series reported an improvement in outcome in irradiated patients, although none of the trials were randomized and patients were often selected for radiation because of adverse risk factors such as bulk of disease or incomplete response to systemic therapy. The diversity of ways in which irradiation was incorporated into these studies makes interpretation difficult, making this an area ripe for clinical investigation. Recently, the Australasian Leukemia and Lymphoma Group initiated a clinical trial to test the feasibility of pre or post-transplant radiation therapy for all patients undergoing high-dose salvage therapy for Hodgkin's disease and the non-Hodgkin's lymphomas [228].

Total lymphoid irradiation

For marrow transplantation, TLI has been used alone when only immunosuppression was needed (e.g. in patients with aplastic anemia). It has been used in either a single dose, as at the University of Minnesota [229,230], or in a fractionated regimen, as at MSKCC [83]. The fields used evolved from studies in patients with Hodgkin's disease, which demonstrated the extensive immunosuppression attained with TLI [231].

For transplantation, the mantle and inverted-Y fields, which cover the entire central lymphoid axis, are treated in the same treatment session. The advantage of using TLI for immunosuppression is that one can spare many normal tissues outside of the field, such as the brain, eyes, kidneys, much of the small bowel and lungs. In planning TLI regimens for immunosuppression purposes, Shank et al. [83] determined the relative dose equivalence of TLI to TBI for immunosuppression as measured by the percent of lymphocytes remaining after each technique. For 1 log lymphocyte loss, 6 Gy TBI was equivalent to 10 Gy TLI when fractionated, as done at MSKCC in patients with aplastic anemia (TBI given in 2 Gy daily fractions and TLI given in 1 Gy fractions three times a day for 2 days). To prevent rejection in patients with aplastic anemia receiving T-cell-depleted grafts, Slavin and associates increased the TLI dose to 18 Gy with twice-daily fractionation [26,27]. Early reports showed no GVHD and no rejection, with relatively short follow-up.

The uses of TLI in BMT include the addition of TLI to TBI regimens, which increases engraftment when T-cell-depleted marrows are utilized (as described in the Immunosuppression section under Clinical results). TLI combined with VP16 and CY has also been used successfully as disease treatment rather than immunosuppression in autologous BMT in Hodgkin's disease patients who had either relapsed or had refractory disease [232], as expanded upon in the Consolidative irradiation in high-dose therapy regimens section above.

Thoracoabdominal irradiation

TAI in combination with CY has been used successfully primarily for transplantation of patients with Fanconi anemia and also severe aplastic anemia [233,234]. These fields treat more than just the abdomen, but they spare the brain, eyes and lungs. It is a somewhat easier regimen to use in small children, because the field does not have as complicated a block arrangement as the more complex TLI fields [83]. There are no data available that directly compare TLI with TAI for aplastic anemia. One study [235] implicated TAI as a contributing factor to a high rate of secondary malignancies (22% at 8 years) in patients with aplastic anemia and Fanconi anemia, which was not found in another study [236] when CY was used alone, with antithymocyte globulin, or with chemotherapeutic agents. There is an association of squamous cell carcinomas in patients with Fanconi anemia, even without irradiation [237].

Summary

Many regimens utilizing large field irradiation have been used clinically in preparation for HCT. For leukemias, when non-T-cell-depleted transplantation is performed, leukemic relapse is usually less with fractionated daily TBI regimens when high total doses (315 Gy) are used, but morbidity may also be high. Relapse rates for single-dose regimens are similar to those for fractionated daily regimens. Although hyperfractionation of TBI to high doses (13.2–15.0 Gy) has theoretical radiobiological advantages and did result in low relapse rates and low morbidity in nonrandomized studies, randomized studies to test this potential advantage against daily fractionation have not been done and should be encouraged.

For lymphoma, although nonrandomized studies suggest that IF irradiation may be of value when given to sites of residual or bulky disease, randomized studies are necessary to definitively prove the value of IF irradiation for lymphomas.

References

1 Matthews DC, Appelbaum FR, Eary JF et al. Development of a marrow transplant regimen for acute leukemia using targeted hematopoietic irradiation delivered by ^{131}I-labeled anti-CD45 antibody, combined with cyclophosphamide and total body irradiation. Blood 1995; 85: 1122–31.

2 Bunjes D, Buchmann I, Duncker C et al. Rhenium 188-labeled anti-CD66 (a, b, c, e) monoclonal antibody to intensify the conditioning regimen prior to stem cell transplantation for patients with high-risk acute myeloid leukemia or myelodysplastic syndrome: results of a phase I–II study. Blood 2001; 98: 565–72.

3 Press OW, Eary JE, Appelbaum FR et al. Phase II trial of ^{131}I-B1 (anti-CD20) antibody therapy with autologous stem cell transplantation for relapsed B cell lymphomas. Lancet 1995; 346: 336–40.

4 Knox SJ, Goris ML, Trisler KD et al. ^{90}Y-anti-CD20 monoclonal antibody therapy of recurrent B-cell lymphoma. Clin Cancer Res 1996; 2: 457–70.

5 Matthews DC, Appelbaum FR, Eary JE et al. Phase I study of ^{131}I-anti-CD45 antibody plus cyclophosphamide and total body irradiation for advanced leukemia and myelodysplastic syndrome. Blood 1999; 94: 1237–47.

6 Withers HR. The four R's of radiotherapy. Adv Rad Biol 1975; 5: 241–71.

7 Caldwell WL, Lamerton LF. Increased sensitivity of in vitro murine leukemia cells to fractionated X-rays and fast neutrons. Nature 1965; 208: 168–70.

8 Peters LJ, Withers HR, Cundiff JH, Dicke KA. Radiobiological considerations in the use of total-body irradiation for bone-marrow transplantation. Radiology 1979; 131: 243–7.

9 Fowler JF. The linear-quadratic formula and progress in fractionated radiotherapy. Br J Radiol 1989; 62: 679–94.

10 Vriesendorp HM. Radiobiological speculations on therapeutic total body irradiation. Crit Rev Oncol Hematol 1990; 10: 211–24.

11 Vriesendorp HM, Johnson PM, Fey TA, McDonough CM, Zoetelief J, van Bekkum DW. Optimal dose of total body irradiation for allogeneic bone marrow transplantation. Transplant Proc 1985; 17: 517–20.

12 Storb R, Raff RF, Appelbaum FR et al. Comparison of fractionated to single-dose total body irradiation in conditioning canine littermates for DLA-identical marrow grafts. Blood 1989; 74: 1139–43.

13 Terenzi A, Aristei C, Aversa F et al. Comparison of immunosuppressive effects of single-dose and hyperfractionated total body irradiation. Transplant Proc 1994; 26: 3217.

14 Down JD, Tarbell NJ, Thames HD, Mauch PM. Syngeneic and allogeneic bone marrow engraftment after total body irradiation: dependence on dose, dose rate, and fractionation. Blood 1991; 77: 661–9.

15 Van Os R, Konings AWT, Down JD. Radiation dose as a factor in host preparation for bone marrow transplantation across different genetic barriers. Int J Radiat Biol 1992; 61: 501–10.

16 Girinski T, Socie G, Cosset JM, Dutreix J, Chassagne D. Similar effects on murine haemopoietic compartment of low dose rate single dose and high dose rate fractionated total body irradiation. Preliminary results after a unique dose of 750 cGy. Br J Radiol 1990; 61: 797–800.

17 Anasetti C, Amos D, Beatty PG et al. Effect of HLA compatibility on engraftment of bone marrow transplants in patients with leukemia or lymphoma. N Engl J Med 1989; 320: 197–204.

18 Soderling CCB, Song CH, Blazar BR, Vallera DA. A correlation between conditioning and engraftment in recipients of MHC-mismatched T cell-depleted murine bone marrow transplants. J Immunol 1985; 135: 941–6.

19 Soiffer RJ, Mauch P, Tarbell NJ et al. Total lymphoid irradiation to prevent graft rejection in recipients of HLA non-identical T cell-depleted allogeneic marrow. Bone Marrow Transplant 1991; 7: 23–33.

20 James ND, Apperley JF, Kam KC et al. Total lymphoid irradiation preceding bone marrow transplantation for chronic myeloid leukemia. Clin Radiol 1989; 40: 195–8.

21 Pipard G, Stepanian E, Chapuis B et al. Total lymphoid irradiation (TLI), chemotherapy (CT) and total body irradiation (TBI) before T-cell depleted bone marrow allografts. ESTRO, 7th annual meeting, Den Haag, The Netherlands 1988: 36 [Abstract].

22 Champlin R, Ho WG, Mitsuyasu R et al. Graft failure and leukemia relapse following T-lymphocyte depleted bone marrow transplantation; effect of intensification of immunosuppressive conditioning. Transplant Proc 1987; 19: 2616–9.

23 Burnett AK, Robertson AG, Hann IM, Alcorn M, Gibson BE, McKinnon S. In vitro T-cell depletion of allogeneic bone marrow: prevention of rejection in HLA-matched transplants by increased TBI. Bone Marrow Transplant 1986; 1 (Suppl. 1): 121.

24 Martin PJ, Hansen JA, Buckner CD et al. Effects of

in vitro depletion of T cells in HLA-identical allogeneic marrow grafts. *Blood* 1985; **66**: 664–72.

25 Racadot E, Herve P, Beaujean F *et al.* Prevention of graft-versus-host disease in HLA-matched bone marrow transplantation for malignant diseases: multicentric study of 62 patients using 3-pan-T monoclonal antibodies and rabbit complement. *J Clin Oncol* 1987; **5**: 426–35.

26 Slavin S, Or R, Naparstek E *et al.* New approaches for the prevention of rejection and graft-versus-host disease in clinical bone marrow transplantation. *Israel J Med Sci* 1986; **22**: 264–7.

27 Slavin S, Or R, Weshler Z, Hale G, Waldmann H. The use of total lymphoid irradiation for abrogation of host resistance to T-cell depleted marrow allografts. *Bone Marrow Transplant* 1986; **1** (Suppl. 1): 98.

28 Bordignon C, Kernan NA, Keever CA *et al.* The role of residual host immunity in graft failures following T-cell-depleted marrow transplants for leukemia. *Ann N Y Acad Sci* 1987; **511**: 442–6.

29 Kernan NA, Bordignon C, Keever CA *et al.* Graft failures after T cell depleted marrow transplants for leukemia: clinical and *in vitro* characteristics. *Transplant Proc* 1987; **19** (Suppl. 7): 29–32.

30 van Bekkum DW, Wielenga JJ, van Gils F, Wagemaker G. Factors influencing reconstitution by bone marrow transplantation. In: Dainiak N, Cronkite EP, McCaffrey R, Shadduck RK, eds. *The Biology of Hematopoiesis*. New York: Wiley-Liss, 1990: 479–91.

31 Dutreix J, Girinski T, Cosset JM *et al.* Blood cell kinetics and total body irradiation. *Radiother Oncol* 1987; **9**: 119–29.

32 Girinsky T, Baume D, Socie G, Pico JL, Malaise E, Cosset JM. Blood cell kinetics after a 385 cGy total body irradiation given to a CML patient for bone marrow transplantation. *Bone Marrow Transplant* 1991; **7**: 317–20.

33 Shank B, O'Reilly RJ, Cunningham I *et al.* Total body irradiation for bone marrow transplantation: the Memorial Sloan-Kettering Cancer Center experience. *Radiother Oncol* 1990; **1** (Suppl.): 68–81.

34 Weichselbaum RR, Greenberger JS, Schmidt A, Karpas A, Moloney WC, Little JB. *In vitro* radiosensitivity of human leukemia cell lines. *Radiology* 1981; **139**: 485–7.

35 Kimler BF, Park CH, Yakar D, Mies RM. Radiation response of human normal and leukemic hemopoietic cells assayed by *in vitro* colony formation. *Int J Radiat Oncol Biol Phys* 1985; **11**: 809–16.

36 Ozawa K, Miura Y, Suda T, Motoyoshi K, Takaku F. Radiation sensitivity of leukemic progenitor cells in acute nonlymphocytic leukemia. *Clin Radiol* 1983; **43**: 2339–41.

37 Fitzgerald TJ, McKenna M, Kase K, Daugherty C, Rothstein L, Greenberger JS. Effect of X-irradiation dose rate on the clonogenic survival of human and experimental animal hematopoietic tumor cell lines: evidence for heterogeneity. *Int J Radiat Oncol Biol Phys* 1986; **12**: 69–73.

38 Lehnert S, Rybka WB, Suissa S, Giambattisto D. Radiation response of haematopoietic cell lines of human origin. *Int J Radiat Biol* 1986; **49**: 423–31.

39 Song CW, Kim TH, Khan FM, Kersey JH, Levitt SH. Radiobiological basis of total body irradiation with different dose rate and fractionation: repair capacity of hemopoietic cells. *Int J Radiat Oncol Biol Phys* 1981; **7**: 1695–701.

40 Rhee JG, Song CW, Kim TH, Levitt SH. Effect of fractionation and rate of radiation dose on human leukemic cells, HL-60. *Radiat Res* 1985; **101**: 519–27.

41 Shank B. Hyperfractionation (TID) vs. single dose irradiation in human acute lymphocytic leukemia cells: application to TBI for marrow transplantation. *Radiother Oncol* 1993; **27**: 30–5.

42 Fajardo L-G. *Pathology of Radiation Injury*. New York: Raven, l982: 4.

43 Shank B, Hopfan S, Kim JH *et al.* Hyperfractionated total body irradiation for bone marrow transplantation. I. Early results in leukemia patients. *Int J Radiat Oncol Biol Phys* 1981; **7**: 1109–15.

44 Pino y Torres JL, Bross DS, Lam W-C, Wharam MD, Santos GW, Order SE. Risk factors in interstitial pneumonitis following allogenic bone marrow transplantation. *Int J Radiat Oncol Biol Phys* 1982; **8**: 1301–7.

45 Lichter AS, Tracy D, Lam W-C, Order SE. Total body irradiation in bone marrow transplantation. The influence of fractionation and delay of marrow infusion. *Int J Radiat Oncol Biol Phys* 1980; **6**: 301–9.

46 Wara WM, Phillips TL, Margolis LW, Smith V. Radiation pneumonitis. A new approach to the derivation of time-dose factors. *Cancer* 1973; **32**: 547–52.

47 Peters L. Discussion. The radiobiological bases of TBI. *Int J Radiat Oncol Biol Phys* 1980; **6**: 785–7.

48 Vriesendorp HM. Prediction of effects of therapeutic total body irradiation in man. *Radiother Oncol* 1990; **1** (Suppl.): 37–50.

49 Evans RG. Radiobiological considerations in magna-field irradiation. *Int J Radiat Oncol Biol Phys* 1983; **9**: 1907–11.

50 Vitale V, Scarpati D, Frassoni F, Corvo R. Total-body irradiation: single dose, fractions, dose rate. *Bone Marrow Transplant* 1989; **4** (Suppl. 1): 233–5.

51 O'Donoghue JA, Wheldon TE, Gregor A. The implications of *in-vitro* radiation-survival curves for the optimal scheduling of total-body irradiation with bone marrow rescue in the treatment of leukaemia. *Br J Radiol* 1987; **60**: 279–83.

52 Steel GG. *Growth Kinetics of Tumours*. Oxford: Clarendon Press, 1977.

53 Fruchtman S, Scigliano E, Isola L, Vlachos A, Mandell L, Shank B. Hyperfractionated total body irradiation (HF-TBI) and whole allogeneic marrow grafts: an intensive, safe, and highly efficacious approach to the cure of leukemia. *Blood* 1995; **86** (Suppl. 1): 945a [Abstract].

54 O'Donoghue JA. Fractionated versus low dose-rate total-body irradiation. Radiobiological considerations in the selection of regimes. *Radiother Oncol* 1986; **7**: 241–7.

55 Yan R, Peters LJ, Travis EL. Cyclophosphamide 24 hours before or after total body irradiation. Effects on lung and bone marrow. *Radiother Oncol* 1991; **21**: 149–56.

56 Collis CH, Steel GG. Lung damage in mice from cyclophosphamide and thoracic irradiation: the effect of timing. *Int J Radiat Oncol Biol Phys* 1983; **9**: 685–9.

57 Blackett NM, Aguado M. The enhancement of haemopoietic stem cell recovery in irradiated mice by prior treatment with cyclophosphamide. *Cell Tissue Kinet* 1979; **12**: 291–8.

58 Okunewick JP, Kociban DL, Young CK, Buffo MJ. Effect of radiation and drug order in preparatory regimens for bone marrow transplantation. Radiation Research Society, 36th Annual Mtg. 1988: 157 [Abstract].

59 Schueler U, Waidelich P, Kolb H, Wagner T, Ehninger G. Pharmacokinetics and metabolism of cyclophosphamide administered after total body irradiation of bone marrow transplant recipients. *Eur J Clin Pharmacol* 1991; **40**: 521–3.

60 Shank B. Techniques of magna-field irradiation. *Int J Radiat Oncol Biol Phys* 1983; **9**: 1925–31.

61 Kim TH, Khan FM, Galvin JM. A report of the work party: comparison of total body irradiation techniques for bone marrow transplantation. *Int J Radiat Oncol Biol Phys* 1980; **6**: 779–84.

62 Rider WD, Van Dyk J. Total and partial body irradiation. In: Bleehen NM, Glatstein E, Haybittle JL, eds. *Radiation Therapy Planning*. New York: Marcel Dekker, 1983: 559–94.

63 Briot E, Dutreix A, Bridier A. Dosimetry for total body irradiation. *Radiother Oncol* 1990; **1** (Suppl.): 16–29.

64 Van Dyk J. Dosimetry for total body irradiation. *Radiother Oncol* 1987; **9**: 107–18.

65 Van Dyk J, Galvin JM, Glasgow GP, Podgorsak EB. *The Physical Aspects of Total and Half Body Photon Irradiation* (AAPM Report no. 17). New York: American Institute of Physics, 1986.

66 Sherman DM, Carabell SC, Belli JA, Hellman S. The effect of dose rate and adriamycin on the tolerance of thoracic radiation in mice. *Int J Radiat Oncol Biol Phys* 1982; **8**: 45–51.

67 Travis EL, Peters LJ, McNeill J, Thames HD Jr, Karolis C. Effect of dose-rate on total body irradiation: lethality and pathologic findings. *Radiother Oncol* 1985; **4**: 341–51.

68 Down JD, Easton DF, Steel GG. Repair in the mouse lung during low dose-rate irradiation. *Radiother Oncol* 1986; **6**: 29–42.

69 Bortin MM. Pathogenesis of interstitial pneumonitis following allogeneic bone marrow transplantation for acute leukemia. In: Gale RP, ed. *Recent Advances in Bone Marrow Transplantation*. New York: Alan R Liss, 1983: 445–60.

70 Fryer CJH, Fitzpatrick PJ, Rider WD, Poon P. Radiation pneumonitis. Experience following a large single dose of radiation. *Int J Radiat Oncol Biol Phys* 1978; **4**: 931–6.

71 Tarbell NJ, Amato DA, Down JD, Mauch P, Hellman S. Fractionation and dose rate effects in mice: a model for bone marrow transplantation in man. *Int J Radiat Oncol Biol Phys* 1987; **13**: 1065–9.

72 Kim TH, Kersey JH, Sewchand W, Nesbit ME, Krivit W, Levitt SH. Total body irradiation with a high-dose-rate linear accelerator for bone-marrow transplantation in aplastic anemia and neoplastic disease. *Radiology* 1977; **122**: 523–5.

73 Fyles GM, Messner HA, Lockwood G *et al.* Long-term results of bone marrow transplantation for patients with AML, ALL, and CML prepared with single dose total body irradiation of 500 cGy delivered with a high dose rate. *Bone Marrow Transplant* 1991; **8**: 453–63.

74 Leer JWH, Broerse JJ, DeVroome H, Chin A, Noordijk EM, Dutreix A. Techniques applied for total body irradiation. *Radiother Oncol* 1990; **18** (Suppl. 1): 10–5.

75 Glasgow GP, Wang S, Stanton J. A total body irradiation stand for bone marrow transplant patients. *Int J Radiat Oncol Biol Phys* 1989; **16**: 875–7.

76 Kutcher GJ, Bonfiglio P, Shank B, Masterson ME. Combined photon and electron technique for total

body irradiation. *ESTRO*, 7th annual meeting, Den Haag, The Netherlands 1988: 31 [Abstract].
77 Miralbell R, Rouzaud M, Grob E et al. Can a total body irradiation technique be fast and reproducible? *Int J Radiat Oncol Biol Phys* 1994; **29**: 1167–73.
78 Gerbi BJ, Dusenbery KE. Design specifications for a treatment stand used for total body photon irradiation with patients in a standing position. *Med Dosim* 1995; **20**: 25–30.
79 Breneman JC, Elson HR, Little R, Lamba M, Foster AE, Aron BS. A technique for delivery of total body irradiation for bone marrow transplantation in adults and adolescents. *Int J Radiat Oncol Biol Phys* 1990; **18**: 1233–6.
80 Lawton CA, Barber-Derus S, Murray KJ et al. Technical modifications in hyperfractionated total body irradiation for T-lymphocyte deplete bone marrow transplant. *Int J Radiat Oncol Biol Phys* 1989; **17**: 319–22.
81 Berk PD, Popper H, Krueger GRF, Decter J, Herzig G, Graw RG Jr. Veno-occlusive disease of the liver after allogeneic bone marrow transplantation. *Ann Intern Med* 1979; **90**: 158–64.
82 McDonald GB, Sharma P, Matthews DE, Shulman HM, Thomas ED. Venocclusive disease of the liver after bone marrow transplantation: diagnosis, incidence, and predisposing factors. *Hepatology* 1984; **4**: 116–22.
83 Shank B, Brochstein JA, Castro-Malaspina H, Yahalom J, Bonfiglio P, O'Reilly RJ. Immunosuppression prior to marrow transplantation for sensitized aplastic anemia patients. Comparison of TLI with TBI. *Int J Radiat Oncol Biol Phys* 1988; **14**: 1133–41.
84 Reft C, Rash C, Dabrowski J, Roeske JC, Hallahan D. Eye shielding for patients treated with total body irradiation *Med Dosim* 1996; **21**: 73–8.
85 Dutreix J, Janoray P, Bridier A, Houlard J-P, Cosset JM. Biologic and anatomic problems of lung shielding in whole-body irradiation. *JNCI* 1986; **76**: 1333–5.
86 Cosset JM, Baume D, Pico JL et al. Single dose versus hyperfractionated total body irradiation before allogeneic bone marrow transplantation: a non-randomized comparative study of 54 patients at the Institut Gustave-Roussy. *Radiother Oncol* 1989; **15**: 151–60.
87 Shank B, Chu FCH, Dinsmore R et al. Hyperfractionated total body irradiation for bone marrow transplantation. Results in seventy leukemia patients with allogeneic transplants. *Int J Radiat Oncol Biol Phys* 1983; **9**: 1607–11.
88 Lehmann LE, Guinan EC, Halpern SL, Donovan MJ, Bierer BE, Parsons SK. Isolated testicular relapse in an adolescent 5 years following allogeneic bone marrow transplantation for acute myelogenous leukemia. *Bone Marrow Transplant* 1997; **19**: 849–51.
89 Chadha M, Shank B, Fuks Z et al. Improved survival of poor prognosis diffuse histiocytic (large cell) lymphoma managed with sequential induction chemotherapy, "boost" radiation therapy, and autologous bone marrow transplantation. *Int J Radiat Oncol Biol Phys* 1988; **14**: 407–15.
90 Pezner RD, Nademanee A, Niland JC, Vora N, Forman SJ. Involved field radiation therapy for Hodgkin's disease autologous bone marrow transplantation regimens. *Radiother Oncol* 1995; **34**: 23–9.
91 Mundt AJ, Sibley G, Williams S, Hallahan D, Nautiyal J, Weichselbaum RR. Patterns of failure following high-dose chemotherapy and autologous bone marrow transplantation with involved field radiotherapy for relapsed/refractory Hodgkin's disease. *Int J Radiat Oncol Biol Phys* 1995; **33**: 261–70.
92 Poen JP, Hoppe RT, Horning SJ. High-dose therapy and autologous bone marrow transplantation for relapsed/refractory Hodgkin's disease: the impact of involved field radiotherapy on patterns of failure and survival. *Int J Radiat Oncol Biol Phys* 1996; **36**: 3–12.
93 Phillips GL, Fay JW, Herzig RH et al. The treatment of progressive non-Hodgkin's lymphoma with intensive chemoradiotherapy and autologous marrow transplantation. *Blood* 1990; **75**: 831–8.
94 Rapoport AP, Rowe JM, Kouides PA et al. One hundred autotransplants for relapsed or refractory Hodgkin's disease and lymphoma: value of pre-transplant disease status for predicting outcome. *J Clin Oncol* 1993; **11**: 2351–61.
95 Spitzer TR, Deeg HJ, Torrisi J et al. Total body irradiation (TBI) induced emesis is universal after small dose fractions (120 cGy) and is not cumulative dose related. *Proc Am Soc Clin Oncol* 1990; **9**: 14 [Abstract].
96 Spitzer TR, Bryson JC, Cirenza E et al. Randomized double-blind, placebo-controlled evaluation of oral ondansetron in the prevention of nausea and vomiting associated with fractionated total-body irradiation. *J Clin Oncol* 1994; **12**: 2432–8.
97 Spitzer TR, Friedman CJ, Bushnell W, Frankel SR, Raschko J. Double-blind, randomized, parallel-group study on the efficacy and safety of oral granisetron and oral ondansetron in the prophylaxis of nausea and vomiting in patients receiving hyperfractionated total body irradiation. *Bone Marrow Transplant* 2000; **26**: 203–10.
98 Tiley C, Powles R, Catalano J et al. Results of a double blind placebo controlled study of ondansetron as an antiemetic during total body irradiation in patients undergoing bone marrow transplantation. *Leuk Lymphoma* 1992; **7**: 317–21.
99 Prentice HG, Cunningham S, Gandhi L, Cunningham J, Collis C, Hamon MD. Granisetron in the prevention of irradiation-induced emesis. *Bone Marrow Transplant* 1995; **15**: 445–8.
100 Okamoto S, Takahashi S, Tanosaki R et al. Granisetron in the prevention of vomiting induced by conditioning for stem cell transplantation: a prospective randomized study. *Bone Marrow Transplant* 1996; **17**: 679–83.
101 Valls A, Granena A, Carreras E, Ferrer E, Algara M. Total-body irradiation in bone marrow transplantation: fractionated vs. single dose. Acute toxicity and preliminary results. *Bull Cancer* 1989; **76**: 797–804.
102 Buchali A, Feyer P, Groll J, Massenkeil G, Arnold R, Budach V. Immediate toxicity during fractionated total body irradiation as conditioning for bone marrow transplantation. *Radiother Oncol* 2000; **54**: 157–62.
103 Ozsahin M, Pene F, Touboul E et al. Total-body irradiation before bone marrow transplantation: results of two randomized instantaneous dose rates in 157 patients. *Cancer* 1992; **69**: 2853–65.
104 Belkacemi Y, Pene F, Touboul E et al. Total-body irradiation before bone marrow transplantation for acute leukemia in first or second complete remission: results and prognostic factors in 326 consecutive patients. *Strahlenther Onkol* 1998; **174**: 92–104.
105 Iriondo A, Hermosa V, Richard C et al. Graft rejection following T lymphocyte depleted bone marrow transplantation with two different TBI regimens. *Br J Haematol* 1987; **65**: 246–8.
106 Kernan NA, Bordignon C, Heller G et al. Graft failure after T-cell-depleted human leukocyte antigen identical marrow transplants for leukemia: I. Analysis of risk factors and results of secondary transplants. *Blood* 1989; **74**: 2227–36.
107 Poynton CH, MacDonald D, Byrom NA, Barrett AJ. Rejection after T cell depletion of donor bone marrow. *Bone Marrow Transplant* 1987; **2** (Suppl. 1): 153.
108 Ganem G, Kuentz M, Beaujean F, LeBourgeois JP, Vinci G, Cordonnier C, Vernant JP. Additional total-lymphoid irradiation in preventing graft failure of T-cell-depleted bone marrow transplantation (BMT) from HLA-identical siblings. Results of a prospective randomized study. *Bone Marrow Transplantation* 1988; **45**: 244–8.
109 McSweeney PA, Niederwieser D, Shizuru JA et al. Hematopoietic cell transplantation in older patients with hematologic malignancies: replacing high-dose cytotoxic therapy with graft-versus-tumor effects. *Blood* 2001; **97**: 3390–400.
110 Ballen KK, Becker PS, Emmons RV et al. Low-dose total body irradiation followed by allogeneic lymphocyte infusion may induce remission in patients with refractory hematologic malignancy. *Blood* 2002; **100**: 442–50.
111 Thomas ED, Lochte HL Jr, Cannon JH, Sahler OD, Ferrebee JW. Supralethal whole body irradiation and isologous marrow transplantation in man. *J Clin Invest* 1959; **38**: 1709–16.
112 Thomas ED. Total body irradiation regimens for marrow grafting. *Int J Radiat Oncol Biol Phys* 1990; **19**: 1285–8.
113 Thomas ED, Clift RA, Hersman J et al. Marrow transplantation for acute nonlymphoblastic leukemia in first remission using fractionated or single-dose irradiation. *Int J Radiat Oncol Biol Phys* 1982; **8**: 817–21.
114 Clift RA, Buckner CD, Appelbaum FR et al. Allogeneic marrow transplantation in patients with acute myeloid leukemia in first remission: a randomized trial of two irradiation regimens. *Blood* 1990; **76**: 1867–71.
115 Clift RA, Buckner CD, Appelbaum FR et al. Allogeneic marrow transplantation in patients with chronic myeloid leukemia in the chronic phase: a randomized trial of two irradiation regimens. *Blood* 1991; **77**: 1660–5.
116 Deeg HJ, Sullivan KM, Buckner CD et al. Marrow transplantation for acute non lymphoblastic leukemia in first remission: toxicity and long-term follow-up of patients conditioned with single dose or fractionated total body irradiation. *Bone Marrow Transplant* 1986; **1**: 151–7.
117 Clift R, Buckner CD, Bianco J, Petersen F, Appelbaum F. Marrow transplantation in patients with acute myeloid leukemia. *Leukemia* 1992; **6** (Suppl. 2): 104–9.
118 Singh H, Isola L, Richards S, Scigliano E, Fruchtman SM. Higher dose total body irradiation with allogeneic BMT for CML-CP results in fewer relapses. *Blood* 2000; **96**: 358b [Abstract].
119 Brochstein JA, Kernan NA, Groshen S et al. Allogeneic bone marrow transplantation after hyperfractionated total-body irradiation and cyclophosphamide in children with acute leukemia. *N Engl J Med* 1987; **317**: 1618–24.

120 Kim TH, McGlave PB, Ramsay N et al. Comparison of two total body irradiation regimens in allogeneic bone marrow transplantation for acute non-lymphoblastic leukemia in first remission. Int J Radiat Oncol Biol Phys 1990; 19: 889–97.

121 Blume KG, Forman SJ, Snyder DS et al. Allogeneic bone marrow transplantation for acute lymphoblastic leukemia during first complete remission. Transplantation 1987; 43: 389–92.

122 Frassoni F, Scarpati D, Bacigalupo A et al. The effect of total body irradiation dose and chronic graft-versus-host disease on leukaemic relapse after allogeneic bone marrow transplantation. Br J Haematol 1989; 73: 211–6.

123 Scarpati D, Frassoni F, Vitale V et al. Total body irradiation in acute myeloid leukemia and chronic myelogenous leukemia: influence of dose and dose-rate on leukemia relapse. Int J Radiat Oncol Biol Phys 1989; 17: 547–52.

124 Socie G, Devergie A, Girinsky T et al. Influence of the fractionation of total body irradiation on complications and relapse rate for chronic myelogenous leukemia. Int J Radiat Oncol Biol Phys 1991; 20: 397–404.

125 Feig SA, Nesbit ME, Buckley J et al. Bone marrow transplantation for acute non-lymphocytic leukemia: a report from the Childrens Cancer Study Group of sixty-seven children transplanted in first remission. Bone Marrow Transplant 1987; 2: 365–74.

126 Keating S, Suciu S, de Witte T et al. Prognostic factors of patients with acute myeloid leukemia (AML) allografted in first complete remission: An analysis of the EORTC-GIMEMA AML 8A trial. Bone Marrow Transplant 1996; 17: 993–1001.

127 Petersen FB, Deeg HJ, Buckner CD et al. Marrow transplantation following escalating doses of fractionated total body irradiation and cyclophosphamide—a phase I trial. Int J Radiat Oncol Biol Phys 1992; 23: 1027–32.

128 McAfee SL, Powell SN, Colby C, Spitzer TR. Dose-escalated total body irradiation and autologous stem cell transplantation for refractory hematologic malignancy. Int J Radiat Oncol Biol Phys 2002; 53: 151–6.

129 Apperley JF, Arthur C, Jones L et al. Risk factors for relapse after T cell depleted allogeneic BMT for CML in chronic phase. Bone Marrow Transplant 1987; 2 (Suppl. 1): 140.

130 Devergie A, Gluckman E, Reiffers J et al. Bone marrow transplantation for patients with chronic granulocytic leukemia in France 1979–86. Bone Marrow Transplant 1987; 2 (Suppl. 1): 24.

131 Papa G, Arcese W, Bianchi A et al. T cell depleted bone marrow transplantation in Ph+ myeloid leukemia. Bone Marrow Transplant 1987; 2 (Suppl. 1): 39.

132 Goldman JM, Gale RP, Horowitz MM et al. Bone marrow transplantation for chronic myelogenous leukemia in chronic phase. Ann Intern Med 1988; 108: 806–14.

133 Childs B, Castro-Malaspina H, Kernan N et al. Conventional versus T-cell depleted allogeneic bone marrow transplantation for early remission acute leukemia. J Cell Biochem 1992; 16(A) (Suppl.): 194 [Abstract].

134 Marmont A, Bacigalupo A, van Lint MT et al. T cell depletion in allogeneic BMT for leukemia: the Genoa experience. Bone Marrow Transplant 1987; 2 (Suppl. 1): 139.

135 Mitsuyasu RT, Champlin RE, Gale RP et al. Treatment of donor marrow with monoclonal anti-T-cell antibody and complement for the prevention of graft-versus-host disease: a prospective, randomised double-blind trial. Ann Intern Med 1986; 105: 20–6.

136 Girinsky T, Socie G, Ammarguellat H et al. Consequences of two different doses to the lungs during a single dose of total body irradiation: results of a randomized study on 85 patients. Int J Radiat Oncol Biol Phys 1994; 30: 821–4.

137 Gratwohl A, Hermans J, Biezen AV et al. No advantage for patients who receive splenic irradiation before bone marrow transplantation for chronic myeloid leukemia. Bone Marrow Transplant 1992; 10: 147–52.

138 Gratwohl A, Hermans J, Biezen AV et al. Splenic irradiation before bone marrow transplantation for chronic myeloid leukaemia. Br J Haematol 1996; 95: 494–500.

139 Rapoport AP, Lifton R, Constine LS et al. Autotransplantation for relapsed or refractory non-Hodgkin's lymphoma (NHL): long-term follow-up and analysis of prognostic factors. Bone Marrow Transplant 1997; 19: 883–90.

140 Bearman SI, Appelbaum FR, Buckner CD et al. Regimen-related toxicity in patients undergoing bone marrow transplantation. J Clin Oncol 1988; 6: 1562–8.

141 Ozsahin M, Belkacemi Y, Pene F et al. Interstitial pneumonitis following autologous bone-marrow transplantation conditioned with cyclophosphamide and total-body irradiation. Int J Radiat Oncol Biol Phys 1996; 34: 71–7.

142 Barrett A, Depledge MH, Powles RL. Interstitial pneumonitis following bone marrow transplantation after low dose rate total body irradiation. Int J Radiat Oncol Biol Phys 1983; 9: 1029–33.

143 Kim TH, Rybka WB, Lehnert S, Podgorsak EB, Freeman CR. Interstitial pneumonitis following total body irradiation for bone marrow transplantation using two different dose rates. Int J Radiat Oncol Biol Phys 1985; 11: 1285–91.

144 Latini P, Aristei C, Aversa F et al. Lung damage following bone marrow transplantation after hyperfractionated total body irradiation. Radiother Oncol 1991; 22: 127–32.

145 Sutton L, Kuentz M, Cordonnier C et al. Allogeneic bone marrow transplantation for adult acute lymphoblastic leukemia in first complete remission: factors predictive of transplant-related mortality and influence of total body irradiation modalities. Bone Marrow Transplant 1993; 12: 583–9.

146 Keane TJ, Van Dyk J, Rider WD. Idiopathic interstitial pneumonia following bone marrow transplantation: the relationship with total body irradiation. Int J Radiat Oncol Biol Phys 1981; 7: 1365–70.

147 Latini P, Aristei C, Aversa F et al. Interstitial pneumonitis after hyperfractionated total body irradiation in HLA-matched T-depleted bone marrow transplantation. Int J Radiat Oncol Biol Phys 1992; 23: 401–5.

148 Ho VT, Weller E, Lee SJ, Alyea EP, Antin JH, Soiffer RJ. Prognostic factors for early severe pulmonary complications after hematopoietic stem cell transplantation. Biol Blood Marrow Transplant 2001; 7: 223–9.

149 Tait RC, Burnett AK, Robertson AG et al. Subclinical pulmonary function defects following autologous and allogeneic bone marrow transplantation: relationship to total body irradiation and graft-versus-host disease. Int J Radiat Oncol Biol Phys 1991; 20: 1219–27.

150 Labar B, Bogdanic V, Nemet D et al. Total body irradiation with or without lung shielding for allogeneic bone marrow transplantation. Bone Marrow Transplant 1992; 9: 343–7.

151 Deeg HJ, Flournoy N, Sullivan KM et al. Cataracts after total body irradiation and marrow transplantation: a sparing effect of dose fractionation. Int J Radiat Oncol Biol Phys 1984; 10: 957–64.

152 Benyunes MC, Sullivan KM, Deeg HJ et al. Cataracts after bone marrow transplantation: long-term follow-up of adults treated with fractionated total body irradiation. Int J Radiat Oncol Biol Phys 1995; 32: 661–70.

153 Dunn JP, Jabs DA, Wingard J, Enger C, Vogelsang G, Santos G. Bone marrow transplantation and cataract development. Arch Ophthalmol 1993; 111: 1367–73.

154 Livesey SJ, Holmes JA, Whittaker JA. Ocular complications of bone marrow transplantation. Eye 1989; 3: 271–6.

155 Lappi M, Rajantie J, Uusitalo RJ. Irradiation cataract in children after bone marrow transplantation. Graefes Arch Clin Exp Ophthalmol 1990; 228: 218–21.

156 Calissendorff B, Bolme P, el Azazi M. The development of cataract in children as a late side-effect of bone marrow transplantation. Bone Marrow Transplant 1991; 7: 427–9.

157 Choshi K, Takaku I, Mishima H et al. Ophthalmologic changes related to radiation exposure and age in adult health study sample, Hiroshima and Nagasaki. Radiat Res 1983; 96: 560–79.

158 Bray LC, Carey PJ, Proctor SJ, Evans RGB, Hamilton PJ. Ocular complications of bone marrow transplantation. Br J Ophthalmol 1991; 75: 611–4.

159 Hamon MD, Gale RP, MacDonald ID et al. Incidence of cataracts after single fraction total body irradiation: the role of steroids and graft-versus-host disease. Bone Marrow Transplant 1993; 12: 233–6.

160 Fife K, Milan S, Westbrook K, Powles R, Tait D. Risk factors for requiring cataract surgery following total body irradiation. Radiother Oncol 1994; 33: 93–8.

161 Zierhut D, Lohr F, Schraube P et al. Cataract incidence after total-body irradiation. Int J Radiat Oncol Biol Phys 2000; 46: 131–5.

162 Belkacemi Y, Ozsahin M, Pene F et al. Cataractogenesis after total body irradiation. Int J Radiat Oncol Biol Phys 1996; 35: 53–60.

163 Belkacemi Y, Labopin M, Vernant JP et al. Cataracts after total body irradiation and bone marrow transplantation in patients with acute leukemia in complete remission: a study of the European Group for Blood and Bone Marrow Transplantation. Int J Radiat Oncol Biol Phys 1998; 41: 659–68.

164 Sanders JE. Late effects in children receiving total body irradiation for bone marrow transplantation. Radiother Oncol 1990; 1 (Suppl.): 82–7.

165 Deeg HJ. Delayed complications and long-term effects after bone marrow transplantation. Bone Marrow Transplant 1990; 4: 641–57.

166 Sanders JE. Long-term Follow-up Team. Endocrine problems in children after bone marrow transplant for hematologic malignancies. Bone Marrow Transplant 1991; 8 (Suppl. 1): 2–4.

167 Hovi L, Saarinen UM, Siimes MA. Growth failure in children after total body irradiation preparative

for bone marrow transplantation. *Bone Marrow Transplant* 1991; **8** (Suppl. 1): 10–3.
168 Cohen A, Rovelli A, Bakker B *et al*. Final height of patients who underwent bone marrow transplantation for hematological disorders during childhood: a study by the Working Party for Late Effects, EBMT. *Blood* 1999; **93**: 4109–15.
169 Cohen A, Duell T, Socie G *et al*. Nutritional status and growth after bone marrow transplantation (BMT) during childhood: EBMT Late-Effects Working Party retrospective data. European Group for Blood and Marrow Transplantation. *Bone Marrow Transplant* 1999; **23**: 1043–7.
170 Mulhern RK, Ochs J, Fairclough D, Wasserman AL, Davis KS, Williams JM. Intellectual and academic achievement status after CNS relapse: a retrospective analysis of 40 children treated for acute lymphoblastic leukaemia. *J Clin Oncol* 1987; **5**: 933–40.
171 Goldberg SL, Tefferi A, Rummans TA, Chen MG, Solberg LA, Noel P. Post-irradiation somnolence syndrome in an adult patient following allogeneic bone marrow transplantation. *Bone Marrow Transplant* 1992; **9**: 499–501.
172 Andrykowski MA, Altmaier EM, Barnett RL, Burish TG, Gingrich R, Henslee-Downey PJ. Cognitive dysfunction in adult survivors of allogeneic marrow transplantation: relationship to dose of total body irradiation. *Bone Marrow Transplant* 1990; **6**: 269–76.
173 Peper M, Steinvorth S, Schraube P *et al*. Neurobehavioral toxicity of total body irradiation: a follow-up in long-term survivors. *Int J Radiat Oncol Biol Phys* 2000; **46**: 303–11.
174 Wenz F, Steinvorth S, Lohr F *et al*. Prospective evaluation of delayed central nervous system (CNS) toxicity of hyperfractionated total body irradiation (TBI). *Int J Radiat Oncol Biol Phys* 2000; **48**: 1497–501.
175 Resbeut M, Cowen D, Blaise D *et al*. Fractionated or single-dose total body irradiation in 171 acute myeloblastic leukemias in first complete remission: is there a best choice? *Int J Radiat Oncol Biol Phys* 1995; **31**: 509–17.
176 Girinsky T, Benhamou E, Bourhis J-H *et al*. Prospective randomized comparison of single-dose versus hyperfractionated total-body irradiation in patients with hematologic malignancies. *J Clin Oncol* 2000; **18**: 981–6.
177 Belkacemi Y, Ozsahin M, Rio B *et al*. Is veno-occlusive disease incidence influenced by the total-body irradiation technique? *Semin Oncol* 1995; **171**: 694–7.
178 Rhoades JL, Lawson CA, Cohen EP *et al*. Incidence of bone marrow transplant nephropathy (BMT-Np) after twice-daily hyperfractionated total body irradiation. *Cancer J Sci Am* 1997; **3**: 116 [Abstract].
179 Miralbell R, Bieri S, Mermillod B *et al*. Renal toxicity after allogeneic bone marrow transplantaion. The combined effects of total-body irradiation and graft-versus-host disease. *J Clin Oncol* 1996; **14**: 579–85.
180 Tutschka PJ, Copelan EA, Kapoor N. Replacing total-body irradiation with busulfan as conditioning of patients with leukemia for allogeneic marrow transplantation. *Transplant Proc* 1989; **21**: 2952–4.
181 Nevill TJ, Barnett MJ, Klingemann H-G, Reece DE, Shepherd JD, Phillips GL. Regimen-related toxicity of a busulfan–cyclophosphamide conditioning regimen in 70 patients undergoing allogeneic bone marrow transplantation. *J Clin Oncol* 1991; **9**: 1224–32.
182 Ozkaynak MF, Weinberg K, Kohn D, Sender L, Parkman R, Lenarsky C. Hepatic veno-occlusive disease post-bone marrow transplantation in children conditioned with busulfan and cyclophosphamide: incidence, risk factors, and clinical outcome. *Bone Marrow Transplant* 1991; **7**: 467–74.
183 DeLaCamara R, Tomas JF, Figuera A, Berberana M, Fernandez-Ranada JM. High dose busulfan and seizures. *Bone Marrow Transplant* 1991; **7**: 363–4.
184 Santos GW. Busulfan and cyclophosphamide for marrow transplantation. *Bone Marrow Transplant* 1989; **4** (Suppl. 1): 236–9.
185 Morgan M, Dodds A, Atkinson K, Szer J, Downs K, Biggs J. The toxicity of busulphan and cyclophosphamide as the preparative regimen for bone marrow transplantation. *Br J Haematol* 1991; **77**: 529–34.
186 Rozman C, Carreras E, Qian C *et al*. Risk factors for hepatic veno-occlusive disease following HLA-identical sibling bone marrow transplants for leukemia. *Bone Marrow Transplant* 1996; **17**: 75–80.
187 Inoue T, Ikeda H, Yamazaki H *et al*. Role of total body irradiation as based on the comparison of preparation regimens for allogeneic bone marrow transplantation for acute leukemia in first complete remission. *Strahlenther Onkol* 1993; **169**: 250–5.
188 Hartman AR, Williams SF, Dillon JJ. Survival, disease-free survival and adverse effects of conditioning for allogeneic bone marrow transplantation with busulfan/cyclophosphamide vs. total body irradiation: a meta-analysis. *Bone Marrow Transplant* 1998; **22**: 439–43.
189 Blaise D, Maraninchi D, Archimbaud E *et al*. Allogeneic bone marrow transplantation for acute myeloid leukemia in first remission: a randomized trial of a busulfan–cytoxan versus cytoxan–total body irradiation as preparative regimen: a report from the Groupe d'Etudes de la Greffe de Moelle Osseuse. *Blood* 1993; **79**: 2578–82.
190 Ringden O, Labopin M, Tura S *et al*. A comparison of busulphan versus total body irradiation combined with cyclophosphamide as conditioning for autograft or allograft bone marrow transplantation in patients with acute leukemia. *Br J Haematol* 1996; **93**: 637–45.
191 Favre C, Nardi M, Dini G *et al*. The role of total body irradiation (TBI). *Bone Marrow Transplant* 1996; **18**: 71–4.
192 Schwerdtfeger R, Kirsch A, Sonntag S, Sauberlich S, Siegert W. Allogeneic bone marrow transplantation in chronic myeloid leukemia. What is the best conditioning regime? *Bone Marrow Transplant* 1993; **12** (Suppl. 2): 13.
193 Miller G, Wagner JE, Vogelsang GB, Santos GW. A randomized trial of busulfan–cyclophosphamide (Bu–Cy) versus cyclophosphamide–total body irradiation (Cy–TBI) as preparative regimen for patients with chronic myelogenous leukemia (CML). *Blood* 1991; **78** (Suppl. 1): 291a [Abstract].
194 Devergie A, Blaise D, Attal M *et al*. Allogeneic bone marrow transplantation for chronic myeloid leukemia in first chronic phase: a randomized trial of busulfan–cytoxan versus cytoxan–total body irradiation as preparative regimen: a report from the French Society of Bone Marrow Graft (SFGM). *Blood* 1995; **85**: 2263–8.
195 Clift RA, Buckner CD, Thomas ED *et al*. Marrow transplantation for chronic myeloid leukemia: a randomized study comparing cyclophosphamide and total body irradiation with busulfan and cyclophosphamide. *Blood* 1994; **84**: 2036–43.
196 Clift RA, Storb R. Marrow transplantation for CML. The Seattle experience. *Bone Marrow Transplant* 1996; **17** (Suppl. 3): S1–S3.
197 Clift RA, Radich J, Appelbaum FR *et al*. Long-term follow-up of a randomized study comparing cyclophosphamide and total body irradiation with busulfan and cyclophosphamide for patients receiving allogeneic marrow transplants during chronic phase of chronic myeloid leukemia. *Blood* 1999; **94**: 3960–2.
198 Blume KG, Kopecky KJ, Henslee-Downey JP *et al*. A prospective randomized comparison of total body irradiation: VP16 versus busulfan–cyclophosphamide as preparatory regimens for bone marrow transplantation in patients with leukemia who were not in first remission. *Blood* 1993; **81**: 2187–93.
199 Ringden O, Ruutu T, Remberger M *et al*. A randomized trial comparing busulfan with total body irradiation as conditioning in allogeneic marrow transplant recipients with leukemia: a report from the Nordic Bone Marrow Transplant Group. *Blood* 1994; **83**: 2723–30.
200 Ringden O, Remberger M, Ruutu T *et al*. Increased risk of chronic graft-versus-host disease, obstructive bronchiolitis, and alopecia with busulfan versus total body irradiation: long-term results of a randomized trial in allogeneic marrow recipients with leukemia. *Blood* 1999; **93**: 2196–201.
201 Socie G, Clift RA, Blaise D *et al*. Busulfan plus cyclophosphamide compared with total-body irradiation plus cyclophosphamide before marrow transplantation for myeloid leukemia: long-term follow-up of four randomized studies. *Blood* 2001; **98**: 3569–74.
202 Michel G, Gluckman E, Esperou-Bourdeau H *et al*. Allogeneic bone marrow transplantation for children with acute myeloblastic leukemia in first complete remission: impact of conditioning regimen without total-body irradiation: a report from the Societe Francaise de Greffe de Moelle. *J Clin Oncol* 1994; **12**: 1217–22.
203 Dusenbery KE, Daniels KA, McClure JS *et al*. Randomized comparison of cyclophosphamide–total body irradiation vs. busulfan–cyclophosphamide conditioning in autologous bone marrow transplantation for acute myeloid leukemia. *Int J Radiat Oncol Biol Phys* 1995; **31**: 119–28.
204 Dusenbery KE, Steinbuch M, McGlave PB *et al*. Autologous bone marrow transplantation in acute myeloid leukemia: the University of Minnesota experience. *Int J Radiat Oncol Biol Phys* 1996; **36**: 335–43.
205 Reece D, Barnett M, Connors J *et al*. Intensive chemotherapy with cyclophosphamide, carmustine, and VP16 followed by autologous bone marrow transplantation for relapsed Hodgkin's disease. *J Clin Oncol* 1991; **9**: 1871–9.
206 Anderson JE, Litzow MR, Appelbaum FR *et al*. Allogeneic, syngeneic, and autologous marrow transplantation for Hodgkin's disease: the 21-year Seattle experience. *J Clin Oncol* 1993; **11**: 2342–50.
207 Carella AM, Congiu AM, Gaozza E *et al*. High-dose chemotherapy with autologous bone marrow transplantation in 50 advanced resistant Hodgkin's

208. Shamash J, Lee SM, Radford JA *et al.* Patterns of relapse and subsequent management following high-dose chemotherapy with autologous haematopoietic support in relapsed or refractory Hodgkin's lymphoma: a two center study. *Ann Oncol* 2000; **11**: 715–9.
209. Mundt AJ, Williams SF, Hallahan D. High dose chemotherapy and stem cell rescue for aggressive non-Hodgkin's lymphoma: pattern of failure and implications for involved-field radiotherapy. *Int J Radiat Oncol Biol Phys* 1997; **39**: 617–25.
210. Petersen FB, Appelbaum FR, Hill R *et al.* Autologous marrow transplantation for malignant lymphoma: a report of 101 cases from Seattle. *J Clin Oncol* 1990; **8**: 638–47.
211. Wheeler C, Strawderman M, Ayash L *et al.* Prognostic factors for treatment outcome in autotransplantation of intermediate-grade and high-grade non-Hodgkin's lymphoma with cyclophosphamide, carmustine, and VP16. *J Clin Oncol* 1993; **11**: 1085–91.
212. Philip T, Armitage JO, Spitzer G *et al.* High-dose therapy and autologous bone marrow transplantation after failure of conventional chemotherapy in adults with intermediate-grade or high-grade non-Hodgkin's lymphoma. *N Engl J Med* 1987; **316**: 1493–8.
213. Tsang RW, Gospodarowicz MK, Sutcliffe S, Crump M, Keating A. Thoracic radiation therapy before autologous bone marrow transplantation in relapsed or refractory Hodgkin's disease. *Eur J Cancer* 1999; **35**: 73–8.
214. Moskowitz CH, Nimer SD, Zelenetz AD *et al.* A two-step comprehensive high-dose chemoradiotherapy second-line program for relapsed and refractory Hodgkin disease: analysis by intent to treat and development of a prognostic model. *Blood* 2001; **97**: 616–23.
215. Reece DE, Barnett MJ, Shepherd JD *et al.* High-dose cyclophosphamide, carmustine (BCNU), and etoposide (VP16-213) with or without cisplatin (CBV ± P) and autologous transplantation for patients with Hodgkin's disease who fail to enter a complete remission after combination chemotherapy. *Blood* 1995; **86**: 451–6.
216. Philip T, Guglielmi C, Hagenbeek A *et al.* Autologous bone marrow transplantation as compared with salvage chemotherapy in relapses of chemotherapy-sensitive non-Hodgkin's lymphoma. *N Engl J Med* 1995; **333**: 1540–5.
217. Reece DE, Connors JM, Spinelli JJ *et al.* Intensive therapy with cyclophosphamide, carmustine, etoposide ± cisplatin and autologous bone marrow transplantation for Hodgkin's disease in first relapse after combination chemotherapy. *Blood* 1994; **83**: 1193–9.
218. Rapoport AP, Meisenberg B, Sarkodee-Adoo C *et al.* Autotransplantation for advanced lymphoma and Hodgkin's disease followed by post-transplant rituxan/GM-CSF or radiotherapy and consolidation chemotherapy. *Bone Marrow Transplant* 2002; **29**: 303–12.
219. Ferme C, Mounier N, Divine M *et al.* Intensive salvage therapy with high-dose chemotherapy for patients with advanced Hodgkin's disease in relapse or failure after initial chemotherapy: results of the Groupe d'Etudes des Lymphomes de l'Adulte H89 Trial. *J Clin Oncol* 2002; **20**: 467–75.
220. Kluin-Nelemans HC, Zagonel V, Anastasopoulou A *et al.* Standard chemotherapy with or without high-dose chemotherapy for aggressive non-Hodgkin's lymphoma: randomized phase III EORTC study. *J Natl Cancer Inst* 2001; **93**: 22–30.
221. Argiris A, Seropian S, Cooper DL. High-dose BEAM chemotherapy with autologous peripheral blood progenitor-cell transplantation for unselected patients with primary refractory or relapsed Hodgkin's disease. *Ann Oncol* 2000; **11**: 665–72.
222. Perry AR, Peniket AJ, Watts MJ, Leverett D, Goldstone AH, Linch DC. Peripheral blood stem cell versus autologous bone marrow transplantation for Hodgkin's disease equivalent survival outcome in a single-centre matched-pair analysis. *Br J Haematol* 1999; **105**: 280–7.
223. Cortelazzo S, Rossi A, Bellavita P *et al.* Clinical outcome after autologous transplantation in non-Hodgkin's lymphoma patients with high international prognostic index (IPI). *Ann Oncol* 1999; **10**: 427–32.
224. Lancet JE, Rapoport AP, Brasacchio R *et al.* Autotransplantation for relapsed or refractory Hodgkin's disease: long-term follow-up and analysis of prognostic factors. *Bone Marrow Transplant* 1998; **22**: 265–71.
225. Gianni AM, Bregni M, Siena S *et al.* High-dose chemotherapy and autologous bone marrow transplantation compared with MACOP-B in aggressive B-cell lymphoma. *N Engl J Med* 1997; **336**: 1290–7.
226. Bierman PJ, Anderson JR, Freeman MB *et al.* High-dose chemotherapy followed by autologous hematopoietic rescue for Hodgkin's disease patients following first relapse after chemotherapy. *Ann Oncol* 1996; **7**: 151–6.
227. Fouillard L, Laporte JP, Labopin M *et al.* Autologous stem-cell transplantation for non-Hodgkin's lymphomas: the role of graft purging and radiotherapy post-transplantation: results of a retrospective analysis on 120 patients autografted in a single institution. *J Clin Oncol* 1998; **16**: 2803–16.
228. Wirth A, Prince HM, Wolf M *et al.* Optimal timing to reduce morbidity of involved-field radiotherapy (IFRT) with transplantation for lymphomas: a prospective Australasian Leukemia and Lymphoma Group study. *Ann Oncol* 2002; **13** (Suppl. 2): 75 [Abstract].
229. Ramsay NKC, Kim TH, McGlave P *et al.* Bone marrow transplantation for severe aplastic anemia following preparation with cyclophosphamide and total lymphoid irradiation. In: *Aplastic Anemia: Stem Cell Biology and Advances in Treatment*. New York: Alan R Liss, 1984: 315–24.
230. Kim TH, Kersey JH, Khan FM *et al.* Single dose total lymphoid irradiation combined with cyclophosphamide as immunosuppression for human marrow transplantation in aplastic anemia. *Int J Radiat Oncol Biol Phys* 1979; **5**: 993–6.
231. Fuks Z, Strober S, Bobrove AM, Sasazuki T, McMichael A, Kaplan HS. Long term effects of radiation of T and B lymphocytes in peripheral blood of patients with Hodgkin's disease. *J Clin Invest* 1976; **58**: 803–14.
232. Yahalom J, Gulati S, Shank B, Clarkson B, Fuks Z. Total lymphoid irradiation, high-dose chemotherapy and autologous bone marrow transplantation for chemotherapy-resistant Hodgkin's disease. *Int J Radiat Oncol Biol Phys* 1989; **17**: 915–22.
233. Vitale V, Barra S, Corvo R, Bacigalupo A, van Lint MT, Locatelli F. The role of thoraco-abdominal irradiation before marrow transplantation. *Bone Marrow Transplant* 1991; **7** (Suppl. 3): 35–6.
234. Gluckman E. Radiosensitivity in Fanconi anemia: application to the conditioning for bone marrow transplantation. *Radiother Oncol* 1990; **18** (Suppl. 1): 88–93.
235. Socie G, Henry-Amar M, Cosset JM, Devergie A, Girinsky T, Gluckman E. Increased incidence of solid malignant tumors after bone marrow transplantation for severe aplastic anemia. *Blood* 1991; **78**: 277–9.
236. Witherspoon RP, Storb R, Pepe M, Longton G, Sullivan KM. Cumulative incidence of secondary solid malignant tumors in aplastic anemia. *Blood* 1992; **79**: 289–90.
237. Reed K, Ravikumar TS, Gifford RRM, Grage TB. The association of Fanconi's anemia and squamous cell carcinoma. *Cancer* 1983; **52**: 926–8.

15

Dana C. Matthews & Frederick R. Appelbaum

Radioimmunotherapy and Hematopoietic Cell Transplantation

Historical background

Radioimmunotherapy (RAIT) involves the use of antibodies to deliver locally acting radionuclides specifically to target sites. An important first step in the development of RAIT was made in the late 1940s with the report of a method to link radioactive iodine to antibodies without significantly altering the immunologic specificity of the antibody [1]. Using this labeling technique, Pressman and Korngold [2] first showed that antisera developed against a specific tumor and then labeled with iodine-131 (^{131}I) would, after intravenous administration, accumulate to a greater degree in the tumor than in normal tissue, whereas nonimmune serum failed to do so [3]. Based on these experiments and the concept that radiolabeled antisera might deliver significant systemic radiotherapy to tumor sites without undue toxicity, clinical trials of RAIT were begun in the late 1950s. In one of the earliest trials, Beierwaltes [4] treated 14 patients for metastatic melanoma using an ^{131}I-labeled rabbit antisera and noted a complete response in one of the patients. Radioiodinated antifibrinogen antiserum was tested as a therapeutic agent for a variety of cancers in the 1960s with symptomatic improvement in some patients noted [5]. In the late 1960s, investigators began testing radiolabeled polyclonal antibodies developed against tumor associated antigens such as carcinoembryonic antigen (CEA) and in the 1970s, Ettinger *et al*. [6] reported significant responses in patients with hepatoma treated with ^{131}I-anti-CEA antibodies or ^{131}I-antiferritin antibodies in combination with external beam radiation and doxorubicin chemotherapy.

In 1975, the field of RAIT (and many other fields of research, as well) were aided considerably with the development of a technique for the development of monoclonal antibodies by Köhler and Milstein [7]. The availability of large quantities of monoclonal antibodies with defined and reproducible specificity was of great benefit to investigators attempting to better understand the biologic principles of RAIT and made the development of a practical pharmaceutical a realistic possibility. When monoclonal antibodies first became available, there was hope that even unlabeled antibodies would have important therapeutic effects. However, with the exceptions of treatment of low-grade non-Hodgkin's lymphoma (NHL) with anti-CD20 antibody [8,9] and breast cancer with anti-*HER-2/neu* antibody [10,11], clinical trials have generally shown that unconjugated antibodies are incapable of either eliminating substantial amounts of tumor or altering the tumor's growth sufficiently to affect the patient's clinical course. These results were, for the most part, predictable from animal experiments, which defined some of the reasons for the lack of effectiveness of unmodified monoclonal antibodies.

The first and most important limitation demonstrated by these studies is the lack of effective host effector mechanisms. Even though tumor cells bind antibody to their surface, they often continue to survive and replicate. The second limitation of unmodified antibody is antigenic modulation, or disappearance of the target by shedding or internalization following antibody binding. The third limitation is the heterogeneity of antigen expression among tumor cells with the existence of antigen-negative variants within most tumors. Finally, the ability of antibody to reach all target cells may be limited in very large tumors. A major impetus for studies of RAIT was the realization that all of these limitations, with the potential exception of poor antibody diffusion in large tumor masses, might be addressed by adding a radiolabel to the monoclonal antibody. Antibodies would be provided with an effector mechanism rather than having to rely on those of the host. Antigen modulation might be less of a problem if the radionuclides were internalized and retained intracellularly, and, finally, radionuclides which deposit their energy over several cell diameters should kill not only the targeted cell but neighboring antigen-negative variants as well.

Accordingly, beginning in the late 1970s and continuing to the early 1980s, preclinical studies of radiolabeled monoclonal antibodies as antitumor agents were conducted. Underlying these studies was the general understanding that the effectiveness of RAIT as a treatment for malignant disease depends both on the relative specificity achieved in the delivery of radiation to sites of disease as well as the ability of radiation to destroy tumor cells following its delivery. Thus, many of these studies had as their goal a better understanding of those factors that influence the biodistribution of administered immunoconjugates, while other studies pursued the ability of RAIT to eradicate tumor in these experimental models. As outlined in the next section, these studies uncovered a number of principles concerning the biodistribution of radiolabeled monoclonal antibodies. In addition, these studies demonstrated that radiolabeled monoclonal antibody could deliver considerably more radiation to the tumor than to normal organs, often four to 10-fold more, and that significant antitumor responses could be achieved, but that marrow toxicity prevented the administration of curative doses of radionuclides in most model systems [12,13]. These approaches thus encouraged experiments of RAIT with hematopoietic cell (HC) support.

Another series of observations which encouraged experiments of RAIT with HC support came from clinical trials of bone marrow transplantation (BMT) for leukemia. In the early 1970s, Thomas and colleagues at Seattle demonstrated the effectiveness of total body irradiation (TBI) as an antileukemic agent when used in the context of BMT [14]. Several studies have since documented the importance of TBI dose in affecting outcome. Two randomized trials, one in acute myeloid leukemia (AML) and a second in chronic myeloid leukemia (CML), compared cyclophosphamide (CY) and either 12 Gy or 15.75 Gy TBI as preparative regimens for patients undergoing allogeneic BMT from matched siblings [15,16]. In both cases, the higher TBI dose was associated with a reduction in the probability of post-transplant relapse, from 35% to 13% in AML and from 30% to 7% in CML. However, the higher dose regimens were also associated with an increased incidence of severe or fatal toxicities, principally involving the lung, liver or mucous membranes. Thus, the increased doses of TBI did not improve overall survival (OS). These studies did, however, demonstrate the steep dose–response of leukemia to radiation and, thus, provided additional reasons to develop methods to increase the dose of radiation that could be delivered to sites of malignant disease while sparing normal organs.

Subsequent studies in animal models demonstrated that it was possible to ablate the hematopoietic system using radiolabeled monoclonal antibodies directed at marrow cells and that the myeloablative effects of radiolabeled antibodies could be overcome with subsequent BMT [17]. With this background, clinical trials of high-dose RAIT with HC support began in earnest in the early 1990s.

Elements of RAIT

Most studies of RAIT involve the intravenous administration of a radiolabeled monoclonal antibody. Following infusion, a portion of the immunoconjugate distributes relatively nonspecifically, contributing to nonspecific TBI, while a second proportion of the immunoconjugate binds specifically to its target antigen (Fig. 15.1). Both the bound and unbound fractions of the immunoconjugate are cleared from the body over time. The relative distribution of radionuclide throughout the body over this period is termed its *biodistribution*. In murine models, the biodistribution of a radiolabeled antibody is determined by infusing the immunoconjugate to a number of animals, sacrificing a fraction of the animals at set time points after infusion and determining the actual content of radionuclide per gram of tissue in each organ [12]. Usually an irrelevant antibody labeled with a second radionuclide that can be measured separately is included as a control. In larger animal studies and in

Table 15.1 Factors that influence biodistribution of radiolabeled antibodies.

I. *Nature of the targeted antigen*
a. Tissue distribution
b. Cell surface stability

II. *Antibody*
a. Specificity
b. Immunoreactivity
c. Form
d. Isotype

III. *Antibody pharmacology*
a. Dose
b. Infusion schedule
c. Route

IV. *Labeling procedure*
a. Choice of radionuclide
b. Labeling chemistry

humans, the biodistribution of a radiolabeled antibody is usually determined by infusing the radiolabeled antibody and then obtaining serial quantitative gamma camera images over several days [18]. Representative areas over the liver, lung, kidney, spleen, marrow and other organs of interest are identified and, using the serial scans, activity curves representing the counts per pixel are generated. A correlation between these activity curves and actual radionuclide content is determined by blood sampling and actual tissue biopsy. This biodistribution information can be used to calculate the corresponding radiation dosimetry associated with the use of the antibody conjugate using methods recommended by the Society of Nuclear Medicine Special Committee on medical internal radiation dose (MIRD) [19].

Using these techniques, through careful murine, canine and human studies, a number of factors have been demonstrated to have major effects on the biodistribution of radiolabeled antibodies (Table 15.1).

Target antigen

The nature of the antigen chosen as the target for RAIT plays a major role in determining biodistribution. A first issue is the tissue distribution of the antigen. While a target antigen with expression limited to tumor would theoretically be optimal, in practice such antigens are uncommon. However, when RAIT is considered in the context of hematopoietic cell transplantation (HCT) and, in particular, when the disease being treated is leukemia, the presence of the antigen on normal marrow elements as well as the tumor is not a problem and may, in fact, be preferred because it allows for the killing of rare leukemic cells within remission marrow. The number of antigen sites per target cell is an important consideration. In a xenograft model of human melanoma, accumulation of antibody at the tumor directly correlated with the level of antigenic expression [20]. In general, if the number of antigenic targets per cell is low (<10,000), the relative concentration of radionuclide at the tumor site compared to background is lessened. Also, the maximum dose of antibody that can be given without saturating tumor sites is limited. Since each antibody molecule can only be labeled with a certain amount of radionuclide before its immunoreactivity is impaired, if the number of antigenic sites per cell is limited, depending on the radionuclide used, it may be impossible to administer a therapeutic dose of radiation to the target. A third feature of importance is the behavior of the antigen after antibody binding. Some antigens remain on the cell surface. Others undergo a process of internalization which involves endocytosis following which the

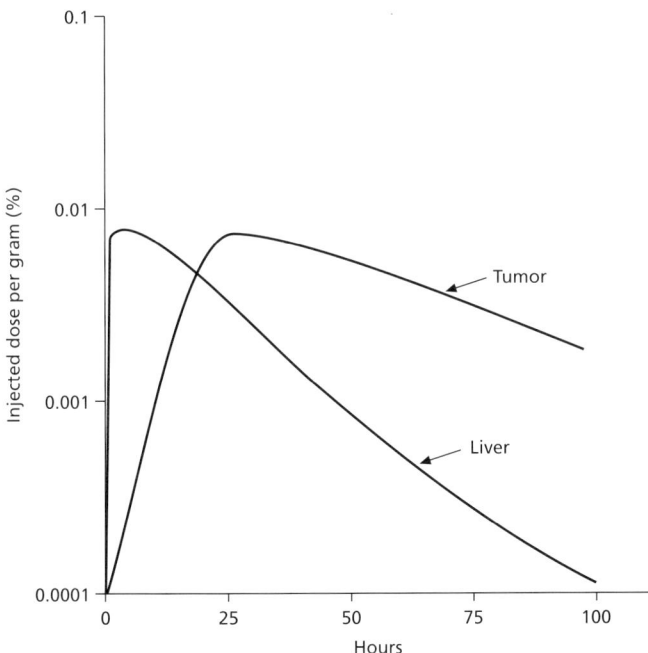

Fig. 15.1 The curves represent the concentration of iodine-131 (^{131}I) in the liver and in a lymphomatous mass following injection of a radioiodinated anti-B-cell antibody to a patient with a B-cell lymphoma. A portion of the antibody distributes nonspecifically throughout the body including the liver and is subsequently cleared. An additional fraction localizes to the tumor where it is more stably retained.

antigen-immunoconjugate complexes are routed to lysosomes where they are proteolytically degraded. Following internalization, the amount of antigen on the cell surface may diminish for several days. The impact of internalization of the targeted antigen depends on other features of the radiolabeled antibody and the infusion schedule. If, for example, the antibody is conventionally labeled with ^{131}I and the antigen-antibody complex internalizes, the result is the rapid lysosomal metabolism of the conjugate with the subsequent rapid excretion of ^{131}I-monoiodotyrosine from the cell, a process that substantially shortens the residence time of the radionuclide at the target site. If, on the other hand, similar antibodies are labeled instead with indium-111 (^{111}In) or yttrium-90 (^{90}Y), small molecular weight ^{111}In or ^{90}Y metabolites remain trapped in the lysosomes and, thus, stay within the cell [21]. In contrast, there is little difference in cellular retention among antibodies labeled with ^{131}I, ^{111}In or ^{90}Y when the targeted antigen is one that remains relatively cell surface stable [21,22].

Antibody

The specificity of the antibody is another important consideration. If RAIT is planned without HC support, cross reactivity with marrow elements is a primary concern because of potential myelosuppression. In the setting where RAIT is used with marrow support, cross reactivity with organs known to be particularly radiosensitive can be problematic, especially, the lung and liver. Given a particular antigen-antibody system, the immunoreactivity of the antibody can dramatically alter its biodistribution. For example, if antibodies are damaged or agglutinated during the labeling procedure, they will be largely taken up by the liver. Antibodies with low immunoreactivity behave more like irrelevant antibodies and distribute relatively nonspecifically. Even relatively minor changes in the binding characteristics of an antibody can alter its biodistribution. For example, CD45 is an antigen expressed by most lymphohematopoietic tissues. When two different anti-CD45 antibodies were studied in an animal model, the one with a slightly higher avidity bound preferentially to the most accessible antigen-positive cells, particularly those in the circulation, in the spleen and in the marrow, and by 2 h was largely cleared from the circulation [23]. A second anti-CD45 antibody with a lower avidity stayed in the circulation longer and ultimately concentrated to a higher degree in lymph nodes which are, in general, less accessible to antibody than cells in the circulation, the marrow or spleen. Use of antibody fragments (Fab or F(ab')$_2$) has been studied with the hope that these lower molecular weight molecules would penetrate into tumors more rapidly and more completely. While more rapid penetration has been documented, the fragments also clear out of the tumor and circulation faster and often have decreased binding affinity, and have not generally resulted in improved biodistribution compared to whole antibody [24,25]. Most monoclonal antibodies studied so far in RAIT trials have been murine in origin. Thus, patients often generate a human antimouse antibody (HAMA) response, usually 4–8 weeks after exposure. The presence of HAMA in the circulation alters the biodistribution of murine antibodies resulting in their rapid clearance from the circulation and increased uptake in the liver. Thus, if repetitive treatments are being considered, the use of murine antibodies can be problematic. However, if RAIT is being used in the context of HCT where the exposure will be limited to several weeks, development of HAMA usually poses no problem. If repetitive lower dose therapy is planned, the use of potentially less immunogenic antibodies, for example, chimeric or humanized antibodies, should be considered.

Antibody pharmacology

Both murine and human studies have demonstrated the important influence of antibody dose on biodistribution [12,13,26]. For each antibody-antigen system, there appears to be a specific dose range that results in optimal biodistribution. These doses appear to approximate the minimum dose that results in saturation of antigen sites at the target tissue. Because the antibody must first disperse throughout the body, very low doses distribute relatively nonspecifically. Very high doses that exceed those that saturate antigen sites result in an increase in the percent of dose that circulates nonspecifically.

In most clinical trials of RAIT, the immunoconjugate has been given as a single infusion over several hours. The infusion rate has been determined largely by the development of febrile or other reactions such as dyspnea or hypotension when antibodies are administered more rapidly. Alternative infusion schedules have been explored in the setting of RAIT for leukemia. Where the antibody reacts with circulating cells, there have been concerns that a portion of the radiolabeled antibody would bind to circulating cells and be cleared by the liver leading to increased hepatic uptake. In animal studies, it was shown by first administering a small dose of unlabeled antibody that circulating cells could be cleared, leading to improved biodistribution of the subsequently administered labeled dose [27]. However, preliminary experiments have not been able to demonstrate a clear benefit of this strategy for patients [18]. In the setting where an antigen that is known to modulate is the target, attempts have been made to improve biodistribution and to deliver an adequate dose by giving the dose in two or three fractions, each separated by 48–72 h in order to allow antigen reexpression [28].

The vast majority of studies of RAIT have involved intravenous administration of the drug. However, there have been a limited number of trials exploring intracavitary or intrathecal administration as therapy for malignant ascites or central nervous system disease.

Labeling procedure

The characteristics of the radionuclide that are important in RAIT include its emission characteristics, half-life, ability to be conjugated easily to proteins, availability and cost, among others. ^{131}I has been the radionuclide used most often in RAIT trials because its 0.6 MeV beta emission is suitable for therapy, it has a high energy gamma emission that allows for imaging so that biodistribution studies can be conducted with the same reagent, the chemistry of labeling proteins with iodine has been well worked out, and ^{131}I is readily available and relatively inexpensive. One major disadvantage of ^{131}I is that if an antibody is conventionally labeled with iodine and used to target an internalizing antigen, following internalization the radionuclide is rapidly metabolized and released from the cell, markedly diminishing the residence time of the radionuclide at its target. Another concern with the use of ^{131}I is that the gamma rays emitted, while useful for performing dosimetry, are relatively high energy (364 KeV) and, thus, are a hazard to health care workers and require that the patient be treated in radiation isolation. A number of other radionuclides have been explored (Table 15.2). ^{90}Y is an attractive alternative to ^{131}I because of its higher beta energy, because its half-life is appropriate for use with antibodies that may take from 1 to 3 days to reach peak concentrations at their target site, and because, after internalization, the small molecular weight metabolites of ^{90}Y tend to remain trapped in lysosomes and therefore stay within the cell. ^{90}Y lacks a gamma emission and thus cannot be detected by external scanning, making dosimetry estimates problematic. Accordingly, ^{111}In-labeled antibodies have been used as a tracer for ^{90}Y-labeled antibodies, but some experiments have found that the biodistribution of ^{90}Y- and ^{111}In-labeled antibodies may differ somewhat. Both rhenium-186 (^{186}Re) and rhenium-188 (^{188}Re) have certain attractive features in that they have both beta and gamma emissions, and chelation chemistries have been developed. The short half-life of ^{188}Re is a relative disadvantage. Copper-67 (^{67}Cu), like ^{131}I and ^{186}Re, has both a beta and gamma emission and has a sufficiently long half-life for use with

Table 15.2 Radionuclides for radioimmunotherapy (RAIT).

Radionuclide	Physical half-life	Particulate energy (MeV)	Path length (mm)	Comments
β-emitters				
Iodine-131	8.1 days	0.6	0.8	Inexpensive; well-defined chemistry, γ and β emissions, dehalogenation a problem
Yttrium-90	2.5 days	2.2	5.3	High-energy β, no γ, accumulates in bone
Rhenium-188	17 h	2.1	4.4	Labeling chemistry similar to technetium, γ and β emissions
Rhenium-186	89 h	1.1	1.8	Like rhenium-188, but longer half-life and less energetic β emissions
α-emitters				
Bismuth-213	46 min	8.0	0.04–0.08	High energy, short path length, very short half-life a problem
Astatine-211	7.2 h	5.9	0.04–0.08	Requires cyclotron for production

intact antibodies. Like ^{90}Y, it appears to be retained intracellularly after internalization, a characteristic which may offer an advantage over ^{131}I. However, ^{67}Cu is not regularly available.

Alpha emitters deposit energy over a much shorter range than beta particles. There is interest in their use in RAIT because they may have the ability to kill only the targeted cell and spare neighboring normal cells, an obvious advantage if avoidance of marrow toxicity is a goal. In general, the very short half-lives of the currently available alpha emitters make them impractical for clinical trials. However, as leukemic cells can be rapidly targeted by circulating antibody, leukemia may be the optimum disease in which to apply radiolabeled antibody labeled with alpha emitters of short half-life.

The actual labeling of antibodies with radionuclides requires considerable care and experience. The immunoreactivity of an antibody must be retained, the procedure must be conducted sterily, and the safety of the technologist must be assured. Some radioisotopes, like ^{131}I, can be covalently bound to antibodies, usually on a tyrosine residue. This form of labeling is probably the most commonly used but, as noted earlier, following internalization, radioiodine bound in this way can be rapidly metabolized and released from the cell. Thus, alternative techniques to label antibodies with radioiodine have been developed, including one termed *tyramine cellobiose* where a polysaccharide bridge between the antigen and the halogen radionuclide leads to trapping of the radioligand intracellularly following lysosomal catabolism [29]. Most nonhalogen radionuclides, including ^{90}Y, ^{186}Re and ^{67}Cu, cannot be firmly attached to antibodies by direct binding. Instead, these radionuclides are attached to the antibody by an intermediary molecule termed a *chelate*. A commonly used chelate in the past was the cyclic anhydride of diethylenetriaminepentaacetic acid (DTPA) which bound the radiometal and also attached to the antibody [30]. More recent studies using newer chelation techniques including isothiocyanotobenzyl DTPA, or 1, 4, 7, 10-tetra-azacyclododecane-N, N^1, N^{11} N^{111}-tetraacetic acid (DOTA), suggest that more stable and more reliable labeling chemistries are possible [31].

Dosimetry

An accurate assessment of the dose delivered by radiolabeled antibodies is necessary both for treatment planning and to assess results. Accurate dosimetry requires an accurate prediction of the biodistribution of the radioimmunoconjugate. As noted earlier, in clinical settings this goal is usually accomplished by exposing the patient to a trace-labeled dose of antibody and following the distribution of the radiolabel by serial external planar imaging using a gamma camera and fixing the activity curves over specific regions of interest to actual tissue content of radionuclide by tissue biopsies. While this technique has been validated in animal models [32], it is not especially good for determining the dose delivered to deep seated tumors that cannot be biopsied. Experiments using single-photon emission computed tomography or positron emission tomography suggest that they may, in the future, offer a method to more reliably determine biodistribution. Any scanning method tends to average the radionuclide content of an organ over its entire volume. On a cellular level, however, antibodies tend to be distributed heterogenously within the tumor. This heterogeneity is more pronounced in larger tumors, tumors with poorly perfused areas, and with the use of antibodies with very high affinity, which tend to bind close to the vascular supply. The use of more powerful beta emitters would tend to reduce the impact of this heterogeneity.

With a given biodistribution, MIRD tables can be used to determine the dosimetry associated with a given radionuclide dose. The calculations take into account the direct effect of radionuclide deposited at that target site, the effects of radiation delivered by the radionuclide in the blood stream and the radiation delivered from neighboring organs (i.e. the radionuclide deposited in the liver would radiate, to some extent, the kidney, and vice versa). By determining the biodistribution of the radioimmunoconjugate and then performing these calculations, the dose of radiation delivered to each organ and to tumor can be determined for any given amount of radionuclide administered.

Radiation effects

The external beam TBI used in HCT is usually delivered in fractionated doses of 1–2 Gy at 7–25 cGy/min to a total dose of 10–15 Gy. With RAIT, the radiation is delivered continuously at a low-dose rate that initially increases as the radiolabel accumulates at the target and then decreases as a result of clearance of the radionuclide and its physical decay. Differences in the relative biologic effects of radiation delivered in these two very different ways have not been systematically explored. For the purposes of HCT, the three effects of greatest interest are the relative antitumor effects, immunosuppressive effects and nonhematopoietic toxicities of the radiation. With external beam TBI, the antileukemic effects are clearly related to total dose but are also likely influenced by dose rate with greater antileukemic effects seen at high-dose rates, and possibly by dose fractionation [33]. Very little is known about the relative antileukemic effect of radiation delivered by RAIT. While it seems likely that the antileukemic effects of RAIT on a Gray per Gray basis would be less than the more rapidly administered external beam TBI, several human tumor xenograft experiments involving nonhematopoietic tumors have suggested that radiolabeled antibodies may have equivalent or even greater antitumor activity than external beam radiation [34–36]. The immunosuppressive effects of external beam radiation are also dose dependent and there is compelling evidence that they are also influenced by dose fractionation [37,38]. The immunosuppressive effects of RAIT are only beginning to be explored. In two sets of murine experiments, we found that ^{131}I-labeled anti-CD45 antibodies could substitute for TBI in T-cell-depleted transplants from H2-matched, minor-antigen mismatched donors, and when added to an otherwise ineffective dose of external beam TBI, could allow for T-cell-depleted transplants across H2 barriers [39,40]. A recent study in a canine transplant model of nonmyeloablative transplantation suggested that anti-CD45 antibody labeled with the alpha emitter Bismuth-213 (^{213}Bi) could substitute for 2 Gy TBI [41]. Like the antitumor and immunosuppressive effects of external beam TBI, the toxic effects of TBI are also influenced by total dose, dose rate and dose fractionation [42,43]. One would anticipate a similar trend with RAIT. In addition to diminished toxicities due to lower dose rates, the real attraction of RAIT is the ability to redistribute the radiation dose to sites of disease and away from critical normal organs.

Clinical trials

Leukemia

Initial studies of the use of RAIT as a component of a HCT preparative regimen in leukemia explored the use of an anti-CD33-antibody labeled with ^{131}I. CD33 is a myeloid-associated glycoprotein expressed on AML cells in over 90% of patients and on normal myeloid cells from the myeloblast to the myelocyte/metamyelocyte stage. It is not expressed by nonhematopoietic tissues. In an initial study, patients with AML were first given a trace labeled dose of antibody and, if it was found that more radiation would be delivered to marrow and spleen than to any normal organ, a situation termed *favorable biodistribution*, then patients were treated with escalating doses of ^{131}I conjugated to the antibody followed by a standard preparative regimen of CY plus 12 Gy TBI [44]. The protocol design was chosen because the immunosuppressive effects of RAIT are largely unknown. By retaining a standard preparative regimen, albeit one at the lower side of the standard dose range, provision of adequate immunosuppression to insure engraftment was not an issue while, at the same time, the lower dose regimen allowed for some dose escalation. Favorable biodistribution was found in only four of the nine patients studied. The residence time of the radionuclide in the marrow was brief, ranging from 9 to 41 h, presumably due to modulation of the antibody-antigen complex with subsequent digestion and release of ^{131}I from the marrow space. In addition, marrow antigenic sites were saturated at doses above 5 mg/m^2 of antibody, a reflection of the relatively low copy numbers of CD33 per cell. The four patients with favorable biodistribution went on to transplantation and tolerated the procedure well, but three of the four subsequently relapsed. The short residence time of the radionuclide in the marrow and the limitation in the dose of antibody that could be given without exceeding saturation of marrow sites made it impossible to continue the dose escalation trial and so this study was stopped. While the study showed the overall feasibility of this approach, it also highlighted the limitations of conventionally labeled anti-CD33 antibody.

At the same time that these studies at the Fred Hutchinson Cancer Research Center (FHCRC) of the p67 anti-CD33 antibody were being conducted, the group from the Memorial Sloan Kettering Cancer Center (MSKCC) was studying another anti-CD33 antibody, M195, also labeled with ^{131}I. In an initial study examining the biodistribution of M195, they found the biodistribution to be similar to that of the radiolabeled p67 anti-CD33 antibody, with saturation of antigenic sites seen at doses above 5 mg/m^2. However, in some cases the half-life of the radionuclide in marrow with M195 antibody was reported to be somewhat longer than in the FHCRC experience [45]. In their initial treatment trials, 24 patients with myeloid malignancies were given M195 labeled with increasing doses of ^{131}I [46]. The ^{131}I-M195 was given in divided doses to allow reexpression of CD33 and HCT was not at first a planned part of the regimen. Administration of the radiolabeled antibody was associated with a marked decrease in peripheral and marrow blasts in 90% of cases. At a dose of ^{131}I of ≥5 GBq (135 mCi)/m^2, pancytopenia was profound and lasted more than 2 weeks. However, no complete remissions (CRs) were achieved at doses <5.9 GBq (160 mCi)/m^2. Eight patients treated with 5.9 GBq (160 mCi)/m^2 or more went on to receive an autologous or allogeneic transplant, one of whom was reported to be in remission at the time of their report. These investigators have also investigated a transplant preparative regimen combining ^{131}I-M195 labeled with 4.4–8.5 GBq (120–230 mCi)/m^2 with busulfan (BU) and CY followed by allogeneic HCT. All 19 patients with relapsed or refractory myeloid leukemia receiving this regimen engrafted, and all but one achieved a remission. Three patients were surviving disease-free 18–29 months post-transplant, with 10 patients experiencing transplant-related mortality and six relapsing after transplant [28].

The problem of a short residence time for radioisotope in marrow because of rapid dehalogenation of internalized ^{131}I-anti-CD33 antibody could be avoided with the use of an isotope that is retained within the cell once internalized. The investigators at MSKCC have recently studied a humanized version of their anti-CD33 antibody, Hu-M195, labeled with ^{90}Y in a non-HCT study of patients with advanced AML [47,48]. Nineteen patients received a single dose of 3.7 MBq (0.1 mCi)–11.1 MBq (0.3 mCi) ^{90}Y/kg, with dose-limiting neutropenia seen at 11.1 MBq/kg, the maximum tolerated dose (MTD). Of the 10 patients treated at the highest dose levels (10.2–11.1 MBq [0.275–0.300 mCi]/kg), five had hypocellular marrows without obvious leukemia 2–4 weeks after treatment, with one CR of 5 months duration. This group of investigators is currently studying this radioimmunoconjugate in the HCT setting.

The MSKCC group has also published the first experience using an alpha emitter, ^{213}Bi, as a radiolabel to treat leukemia [49]. The same humanized anti-CD33 antibody Hu-M195 was administered labeled with escalating doses (10.36–37.00 MBq [0.28–1.00 mCi]/kg) of ^{213}Bi in a phase I, non-HCT, dose-escalation study in patients with advanced AML. The MTD was not reached, as the escalation of ^{213}Bi dose was limited by the cost and availability of the actinium-225 generator. Localization of ^{213}Bi in the marrow, liver, and spleen was demonstrated by gamma camera imaging in all 17 patients. Estimated radiation doses delivered to these organs and to the blood were much higher than estimated doses to lung, kidney, heart, or whole body. All evaluable patients experienced myelosuppression, but extramedullary toxicities were limited to grade I or II hepatic abnormalities. Transient reductions in leukemic cell percentages in marrow were seen in 78% of patients.

In an effort to overcome some of the limitations of radiolabeled CD33 antibody, the group at FHCRC has studied radiolabeled anti-CD45 antibody. CD45 is an antigen expressed on virtually all HCs with the exception of mature red cells and platelets, and is expressed by 85–95% of acute myeloid and lymphocytic leukemias. The number of CD45 antigenic sites per leukemic cell is, on average, approximately 1 log higher than CD33 (100–200,000 vs. 10–20,000) and, unlike CD33, CD45 is maintained on the cell surface after ligand binding. Studies in rodents and macaques demonstrated that radioiodinated anti-CD45 antibody was capable of delivering approximately two to four times more radiation to marrow and four times more to spleen than to lung, liver or kidneys [23,25]. Based on these experiments, a clinical trial of an ^{131}I-labeled CD45 antibody (BC8) in patients with AML or acute lymphoblastic leukemia (ALL) was conducted using a design identical to that described earlier for the anti-CD33 antibody [18,50]. The initial uptake of ^{131}I-BC8 in marrow was higher than seen with ^{131}I-anti-CD33, presumably reflecting the increased number of antigenic sites, and the radionuclide was retained within the marrow approximately twice as long as the anti-CD33 antibody ($t^{1/2}$ = 44.2 h. vs. $t^{1/2}$ of 21.4 h). These differences resulted in overall improvement in the biodistribution with 37 of 44 patients (84%) having favorable biodistribution with, on average, approximately 2.3-fold

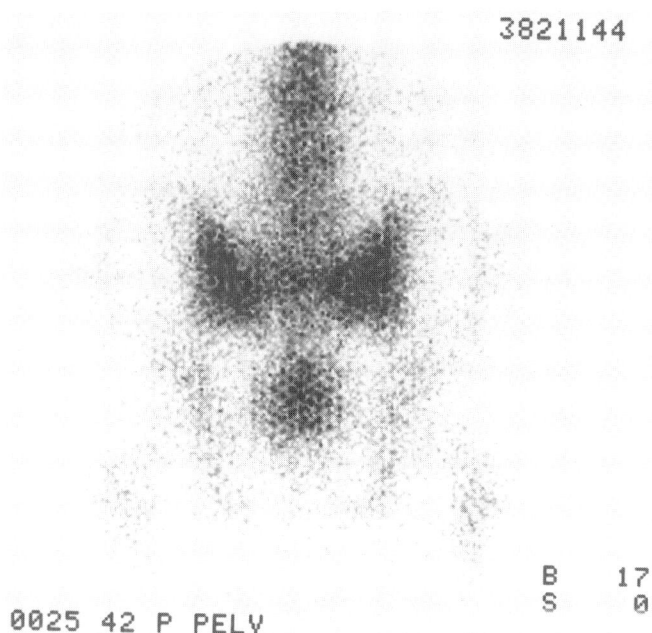

Fig. 15.2 This posterior gamma camera image shows accumulations of iodine-131 (^{131}I) in the marrow in the lower lumbar vertebrae and the pelvic axial skeleton in a patient with acute myeloid leukemia (AML) 42 h following infusion of a trace-labeled anti-CD45 antibody.

more radiation being delivered to the marrow than to the liver, the normal organ with the highest average radiation dose (Fig. 15.2). This ratio was somewhat higher for patients in relapse with hypercellular marrows than in remission patients.

Thirty-four of the patients with favorable biodistribution went on to the treatment phase of the study, which was a phase I dose escalation design in which increasing doses of ^{131}I-BC8 antibody were added to a standard CY/TBI preparative regimen. The doses of ^{131}I-BC8 antibody at each dose level were adjusted to deliver a predetermined dose of radiation to the normal organ receiving the highest dose, usually the liver. The MTD was estimated to be 10.5 Gy to liver, at which average estimated radiation doses of 24 Gy to marrow and 50 Gy to spleen can be delivered. The dose-limiting toxicity was life-threatening mucositis. Of the 25 patients with advanced AML or myelodysplastic syndrome (MDS), six remain in remission from 5 to 11 years post-transplant, as do three of the nine patients with advanced ALL. A phase II clinical trial using this transplant preparative regimen has been initiated for patients with advanced AML with human leukocyte antigen (HLA)-matched related or unrelated donors [51].

Based on these encouraging results, the Seattle group initiated a similar study for patients with AML in first CR with supplemental radiation delivered by ^{131}I-BC8 antibody combined with a standard preparative regimen of BU 16 mg/kg and CY 120 mg/kg [52]. Favorable biodistribution of trace-labeled antibody was seen in 89% of patients studied. Forty-one patients have been treated with ^{131}I-BC8 antibody combined with BU/CY, with all but three receiving estimated radiation doses of 5.25 Gy to the liver and average estimated radiation absorbed doses of 11 Gy to bone marrow. Overall, 61% of patients are surviving disease-free a median of 78 months post-transplant, with eight transplant-related deaths and eight relapses.

An alternative approach to delivering radiation to marrow by radiolabeled antibody for patients with AML or MDS has been to target the CD66 (a, b, c, e) antigen with an antibody labeled with ^{188}Re [53]. This antigen is expressed at high levels (2×10^5 molecules/cell) on myelocytic cells at or beyond the promyelocyte stage, and is not appreciably internalized or shed from the cell surface. However, as it is not expressed by AML cells, this approach relies entirely upon "by-stander" radiation from radioimmunoconjugate bound to nonleukemic cells in marrow. Thirty-six patients with AML or MDS judged to be at high risk of relapse with conventional HCT, in remission or good partial remission (PR), received a biodistribution dose of 1–2 mg of anti-CD66 antibody in a phase I/II clinical trial. All patients had favorable biodistribution of antibody, with average estimated radiation absorbed doses (Gy/GBq ^{188}Re) of 1.5 ± 0.6 to the marrow, 1.6 ± 1.3 to the spleen, 0.7 ± 0.2 to the kidney and 0.5 ± 0.2 to the liver. All patients received a therapy dose of ^{188}Re-anti-CD66 antibody delivering an average of 15.3 ± 4.8 Gy to marrow, followed by varying standard full-dose preparative regimens. Most patients received granulocyte colony-stimulating factor (G-CSF)-stimulated peripheral blood hematopoietic cells (PBHCs), with T-cell-depletion for HLA-matched related ($n = 15$) or alternative donors ($n = 17$). While generally well-tolerated with no increase in early transplant-related mortality, there was a 17% incidence of late renal toxicity, which was most likely to occur in patients receiving more than 12 Gy to the kidney. Overall disease-free survival was 45% at 2 years, with the expected improved outcome in patients transplanted in remission (67%) as compared to relapse (31%).

In contrast, a separate study combining ^{188}Re-anti-CD66 antibody with conventional preparative regimens for patients with high-risk AML or ALL receiving primarily non-T-cell-depleted PBHC grafts from HLA-matched related or unrelated donors had a much higher incidence of transplant-related toxicity and acute graft-vs.-host disease (GVHD), with transplant-related mortality in nine of 19 patients treated [54]. These studies demonstrate the challenges inherent in evaluating the outcome of individual clinical trials in the complex setting of HCT, where many factors, including patient selection, degree of donor match, T-cell depletion, therapies administered in addition to the radioimmunoconjugate and post-transplant interventions can influence outcome.

Other investigators have begun to explore the application of RAIT for leukemia, including studies of a radiolabeled anti-interleukin (IL)-2 receptor for the treatment of acute T-cell leukemia and the use of a radiolabeled antibody termed LYM-1 to treat chronic lymphocytic leukemia, but none of these other studies have explored the use of high-dose therapy requiring stem cell support.

Non-Hodgkin's lymphoma

A series of studies exploring the use of RAIT in the treatment of NHL has been conducted in Seattle. The initial study involved 43 patients and had three major goals: to compare the relative biodistribution of several different B-cell antibodies in patients with recurrent NHL, to determine the effect of antibody dose on biodistribution, and to evaluate the toxicity and potential efficacy of increasing doses of ^{131}I conjugated to the B-cell antibodies [26,55]. The antibodies studied included two reactive with CD20 (B1 and 1F5), one reactive with CD37 (MB1) and, in several patients, tailor made anti-idiotypic antibodies. On successive weeks, patients were infused with trace-labeled antibodies at various doses, usually 0.5, 2.5 and 10.0 mg/kg, and the relative biodistribution was measured. If favorable biodistribution was demonstrated, patients received therapy using increasing amounts of ^{131}I conjugated to the antibody and protein dose found optimal in the trace labeled studies. Unlike many of the leukemia studies mentioned earlier, this study was conducted using only autologous rather than allogeneic marrow support. Therefore, there was no concern about providing sufficient immunosuppression to ensure engraftment, allowing for the study of the immunoconjugate as a single agent without additional immunosuppression. The biodistribution studies demonstrated, first, that favorable biodistribution could be achieved in the majority of patients. Use of anti-idiotypic antibodies, while attractive because of their unique specificities, did not result in superior biodistribution, in part because of binding to circulating id protein. Few patients with splenomegaly or large tumor burdens (>500 g of tumor) displayed favorable biodistribution, presumably because of antibody binding to accessible sites in the spleen and the margins of the tumor with limited penetration and binding in the middle of large tumor masses. The antibody dose also influenced biodistribution and, for each antibody studied, a different dose seemed optimal. As an example, for the anti-CD37 antibody MB1, favorable biodistribution was most often seen with the highest dose tested (10 mg/kg) whereas for the anti-CD20 antibody B1, favorable biodistribution was more often seen at 2.5 mg/kg than at higher or lower doses.

Nineteen patients with favorable biodistribution were treated with escalating doses of ^{131}I-labeled anti-B-cell antibodies delivering from 10 Gy to 30.75 Gy to the normal organ receiving the highest radiation dose, usually the lung. This dose of ^{131}I (8.7–28.8 GBq [234–777 mCi]) was estimated to deliver from 10.1 Gy to 92.0 Gy to tumor. The immunoconjugate infusions were well-tolerated and were followed by the expected pancytopenia and subsequent hematopoietic recovery following infusion of autologous marrow. Nausea, vomiting, mucositis and alopecia, although seen in some patients, were markedly less than with standard transplant preparative regimens. Life-threatening cardio-pulmonary toxicities occurred in two patients who received 27 Gy and 31 Gy to the lung and defined the MTD as approximately 25 Gy. CRs were seen in 16 of 19 patients with two partial responses and one minor response.

Following completion of this phase I trial, a phase II study in patients with recurrent NHL was conducted using the antibody, B1 (tositumomab) and protein dose, 2.5 mg/kg, that gave the best biodistribution results in the phase I trial [56]. The high rate of favorable biodistribution seen, 22 of the 25 patients studied, probably reflects both the use of only B1 and perhaps selection of patients with lower tumor burden. Of interest, three patients with initially unfavorably biodistribution were given "debulking" chemotherapy and, on subsequent study, were found to have favorable biodistribution. Twenty-one patients were treated with ^{131}I-tositumomab at a dose designed to deliver 25–27 Gy to the normal organ receiving the highest dose, with complete responses in 17 patients. Combining data from both the phase I and phase II studies for the 29 patients treated with ^{131}I-tositumomab, 25 patients (86%) had major responses, with 23 complete responses [57]. The quality of response appears to be dose-related, with an apparent correlation between duration of progression-free survival and the estimated radiation dose. The estimated overall and progression-free survival at a median follow-up of 42 months were 68% and 42%, respectively, and when last published, eleven of 29 patients remained in unmaintained remissions of 5–10 years [58]. Sixty percent developed hypothyroidism and two developed secondary malignancies, but none have developed myelodysplasia.

While ^{131}I-tositumomab was well-tolerated as a single agent and had encouraging and often long-lasting antitumor effect, the fact that more than half of patients treated ultimately went on to relapse suggested that further intensification of treatment was required. ^{131}I-tositumomab was thus subsequently combined with conventional transplant doses of etoposide (VP16) and CY in a phase I/II study [58]. Fifty-two patients with relapsed NHL were treated with ^{131}I-tositumomab at 20–27 Gy, combined with 100 mg/kg CY and 60 mg/kg VP16 (60 mg/kg CY and 30 mg/kg VP16 in patients over the age of 55). The MTD was estimated to be 25 Gy, and toxicities more closely approximated those seen with conventional transplant preparative regimens. Grade III/IV (life-threatening/fatal) toxic effects were seen in 8 patients (15%). Of the 31 patients evaluable for response to treatment, 24 (77%) had a complete response, three had a partial response, two had stable disease and one had progressive disease. When compared to a concurrent, nonrandomized group of 105 patients treated at FHCRC with CY/VP16 and 12 Gy TBI for relapsed NHL, the group of patients treated with ^{131}I-tositumomab/CY/VP16 had superior progression-free and OS.

Of interest, ^{131}I-tositumomab has been effective in mantle cell lymphoma, a typically aggressive lymphoma with a median survival of less than three years with conventional therapy. Sixteen patients with mantle cell lymphoma received ^{131}I-tositumomab with CY/VP16, with a complete response in eight of 11 patients with evaluable disease and an estimated 3 years overall and progression-free survival of 93% and 61%, respectively [59]. Behr et al. [60] reported a complete response in six of seven mantle cell patients treated with ^{131}I-rituximab anti-CD20 antibody at lung doses not exceeding 27 Gy. Two have relapsed and five remained in remission 11+ to 38+ months after treatment.

Few other published studies have described the use of ablative doses of RAIT. Nademanee et al. [61] recently reported preliminary results of a phase I/II trial of ^{90}Y-ibritumomab tiuxetan (anti-CD20) combined with VP16 and CY followed by autologous HCT in patients with poor-risk or relapsed NHL. ^{90}Y doses of 1.3–3.9 GBq (34–105 mCi) were selected to deliver an estimated dose of 10 Gy to the normal organ receiving the highest dose. Eighteen patients were treated, and a CR was achieved by the seven patients with active disease at the time of transplant. There were no transplant-related deaths and 17 patients were in remission at a median follow up of 8 months (range 1–24 months). Vose et al. [62] conducted a phase I/II trial combining conventional, nonmyeloablative doses of ^{131}I-tositumomab with the BCNU, etoposide, cytosine arabinoside and melphalan (BEAM) high-dose chemotherapy transplant regimen followed by autologous HCT in 23 patients with aggressive, chemo-refractory NHL. The overall response rate was 66%, with an estimated 1-year event-free and OS of 60% and 78%, respectively.

Juweid et al. [63] treated three patients with high-dose ^{131}I anti-CD22 antibody followed by autologous marrow transplantation and reported partial responses in two, lasting 3 and 8 months. Behr et al. [64] treated seven patients with potentially myeloablative doses of ^{131}I delivered via chimeric anti-CD20 antibody (five patients) or humanized LL2 (anti-CD22) antibody (two patients), with the achievement of a CR in five patients. Vose et al. [65] reported a phase I/II trial of multiple dose ^{131}I-LL2 antibody in 21 patients, five of whom required reinfusion of autologous stem cells because of prolonged cytopenias, with a CR rate of 24%.

Not surprisingly, the use of HC support to allow delivery of maximum radiation doses to tumor has generally resulted in higher rates of complete response and longer-lasting remissions compared to those seen with ^{131}I-tositumomab at nonablative doses. For example, of 53 patients receiving ^{131}I-tositumomab at total body radiation doses of 0.45–0.75 Gy, the 20 patients (34%) with a complete response had a median progression-free survival of 20.3 months [66]. Similar response rates of 30%, with median duration of 14.2 months, were seen in patients treated at non-myeloablative doses with ^{90}Y-ibritumomab tiuxetan (anti-CD20), the only Food and Drug Administration-approved radioimmunoconjugate [67].

Hodgkin's disease

Studies of RAIT for Hodgkin's disease have largely employed polyclonal antibodies reactive with ferritin, a protein that is widely expressed throughout the body but present in higher concentrations in Hodgkin's tissues. Following initial studies using ^{131}I-antiferritin at nonmyeloablative doses, the group at Johns Hopkins University studied 45 patients with advanced Hodgkin's disease, first, with a dose of ^{111}In-labeled antiferritin to determine biodistribution and, if uptake of the radiolabel was seen in the tumor, with a therapeutic dose of immunoglobulin labeled with 0.74–1.85 GBq (20–50 mCi) of ^{90}Y [68]. Among 39 patients receiving treatment doses, the overall response rate was 51%, and 10 patients (36%)

achieved complete responses. Responses were most commonly achieved in patients with smaller tumors (<30 cm^3 vs. >500 cm^3), a longer disease history and higher blood radioactivity levels at 1 h after infusion. Five of the patients were alive at the time of the report, but all had suffered a disease recurrence. Bierman et al. [69] evaluated the use of ^{90}Y-antiferritin combined with high-dose chemotherapy and autologous transplantation for recurrent Hodgkin's disease. Twelve patients received ^{90}Y-antiferritin (0.67–1.22 GBq [0.67–1.22 mCi]) followed by a standard CY, carmustine and VP16 preparation regimen and autologous marrow reinfusion. Four patients died of early transplant complications, while three achieved and remained in CR beyond 2 years from treatment.

More recently, ^{131}I-anti-CD30 antibody has been used at nonmyeloablative doses in patients with refractory Hodgkin's disease, with six of 21 patients experiencing a CR or PR after one treatment [70].

Solid tumors

The majority of studies of RAIT in solid tumors have involved nonmyeloablative doses of radionuclides. However, several studies have begun to examine the use of escalating doses of targeted radiotherapy to treat metastatic breast cancer. Richman and DeNardo initiated a trial of ^{131}I-labeled L6, a chimeric antibody reactive with a nonmodulating antigen associated with various adenocarcinomas [71]. Three patients have been treated with doses of ^{131}I presumed to cause myeloablation (or severe myelosuppression) and autologous marrow reinfusion, with a minimal response in one. Schrier et al. [72] have initiated a phase I dose escalation trial with marrow support using high-dose ^{90}Y conjugated to BrE-3, a monoclonal antibody reactive with a human milk fat-associated antigen. Nine patients were treated with 0.56 GBq (15 mCi)/m^2–0.74 GBq (20 mCi)/m^2 ^{90}Y together with a trace amount of ^{111}In-BrE-3. The ^{111}In-BrE-3 visualized 89% of known tumor sites, and four of the eight patients with measurable tumors achieved partial responses. As most patients developed HAMA to that murine antibody, a humanized BrE-3 was subsequently developed and used in a phase I/II study employing G-CSF-mobilized PBHCs [73,74]. Eleven patients received doses of ^{90}Y ranging from 0.37 to 1.85 GBq (10–50 mCi)/m^2 without nonhematologic toxicities and the MTD was not reached. An alternate antibody reactive with a different epitope on this MUC-1 target peptide, 170H.82, has been labeled with ^{90}Y and administered to three patients with metastatic breast cancer followed by autologous PBHC support, with one partial response [75]. Wong et al. [76] reported tumor imaging in six of seven patients receiving a biodistribution dose of ^{111}In-labeled chimeric T84.66 anti-CEA antibody in patients with CEA-producing refractory breast cancer. Three of six patients treated with 0.56 or 0.83 GBq (15 or 22.5 mCi)/kg ^{90}Y-labeled antibody followed by autologous HC reinfusion had stable disease for 3–14 months, and no dose-limiting toxicities were observed.

Cheung et al. [77] included ^{131}I-labeled 3F8 anti-GD2 antibody followed by autologous PBHC support as part of consolidation therapy in children with high-risk neuroblastoma. Autologous HC have also been used to allow dose escalation of ^{131}I-anti-CEA antibody in patients with progressive metastatic medullary thyroid cancer [78].

Toxicities

Two general categories of toxicities have been seen in these clinical trials, those that are acute infusion-related and those associated with the delivered radiotherapy. The extent of acute infusion-related toxicities is related to the specific antibody, the antibody dose and the speed of infusion. Some antibodies, for example, the anti-CD20-B1 antibody, are very well-tolerated and only rarely associated with infusion reactions. Others, like the anti-CD45-BC8, are almost always accompanied by fever, chills and, if given too rapidly, hypotension. These reactions are usually short-lived and premedication with diphenhydramine, meperidine hydrochloride or hydrocortisone appears to lessen their severity. The major toxicity associated with the delivered radiotherapy is pancytopenia, which usually is seen within 2 weeks of the radiotherapy and is readily reversed with HCT. Because residual radionuclide in the marrow space could irradiate and, therefore, damage transplanted marrow, transplants are usually delayed until the amount of residual radiation in the marrow space has fallen to very low levels. The dose-limiting nonhematopoietic toxicities of radiolabeled antibody as a single agent have been defined only in a single study and, in that study, a calculated dose of 27 Gy to the lung was dose-limiting [55]. This report contrasts with results of external beam TBI where doses above 16 Gy have not been tolerated. This difference most likely reflects differences in the biologic effects of radiation delivered at the markedly different dose rates of RAIT vs. external beam TBI. Other toxicities seen with RAIT include those normally associated with TBI including mucositis, alopecia and nausea and vomiting. Hypothyroidism is a common late toxicity seen after high-dose ^{131}I therapy, even with administration of cold I to block thyroid uptake.

Taken together, the published clinical trials of high-dose RAIT with HCT demonstrate several general principles. First, using currently available antibody radionuclide conjugates conventionally labeled with ^{131}I or ^{90}Y, it is possible to deliver from two- to fourfold more radiation to sites of disease than to surrounding normal tissues. At maximally tolerated doses, RAIT appears capable of regularly inducing enduring CRs in NHL and, when combined with high-dose therapy, RAIT appears effective in treating acute leukemia. Results in other diseases, particularly solid tumors, are, as yet, much less encouraging. Using external beam radiation as a judge, it requires in excess of 60 Gy to eradicate, for example, a breast cancer mass. The doses delivered with current RAIT techniques are somewhat less than this level, and it is unclear if a Gray delivered by RAIT is as effective as a Gray delivered by external beam radiation therapy. At least on the basis of the maximally tolerated dose of radiation to lung (28 Gy with RAIT vs. 16 Gy with TBI) a Gray delivered by RAIT can be thought of as perhaps 0.6 times as potent as a Gray delivered by external beam radiation. Thus, in order to make RAIT applicable to a broader range of tumors, substantial improvement in the doses of radiotherapy that can be delivered safely to a tumor is needed.

Future directions

Many approaches are being taken to improve the outcome of RAIT. Continued efforts are being made to identify antigenic targets that are expressed more specifically or in greater abundance at the target site. Attempts are also being made to optimize the pairings of antibody and the radionuclide conjugate. For example, experiments have been conducted using models of human tumor grown in immunodeficient mice in which the biodistribution of a combination of an antibody directed at a cell surface stable antigen labeled with ^{131}I have been compared to those achieved using an antibody against an internalizing antigen labeled with a radiometal. Studies of antibody dose and dose scheduling are also being performed. Optimizing each of these variables likely will result in some improvement in biodistribution. Novel approaches to the use of alpha-emitters include the labeling of antibody with actinium-225, which decays to three daughter atoms via alpha decay over a 10-day half-life, thus avoiding the problems associated with the very short half-life of the alpha emitters used previously [79].

Other studies using preclinical models have suggested several novel techniques that may allow substantially greater improvements in the relative specificity of RAIT. A limitation of currently employed techniques of RAIT is that a sizable proportion of radiation is delivered nonspecifically by the radioimmunoconjugate as it circulates in the bloodstream prior to binding to its target antigen and by the proportion of the radioimmunoconjugate that never binds to the target. One potentially effective but involved approach to improving this situation is a technique termed *pretargeting* [80]. In this approach, the patient is first treated with a tumor-reactive antibody that has been conjugated to a nonradioactive streptavidin label. This antibody is allowed to bind to the target tumor and that proportion which does not bind is cleared from the circulation with a small dose of a biotin-clearing agent. The patient is then treated with a low molecular weight radiolabeled biotin compound. Because the antibody is already at the tumor site and the radiolabeled biotin compound is of low molecular weight, the radiolabel rapidly binds to the tumor and that which does not bind is promptly cleared by the kidneys. In animal models, this approach can improve the tumor to background radiation ratios of RAIT to greater than 10 : 1, and has achieved cure of tumor xenografts without requiring HC support [80,81]. While early studies in humans have demonstrated the challenge in establishing the optimum conditions for this complex treatment, initial clinical studies in patients with NHL, including one using streptavidin-rituximab and a second using a single-chain anti-CD20 streptavidin fusion protein, have demonstrated the ability to markedly decrease the level of circulating antibody with administration of the clearing agent, and impressive tumor to whole body ratios in most patients studied [82,83]. If high tumor to normal organ ratios could be achieved reliably in humans using pretargeting, RAIT delivered in this fashion with stem cell support might provide doses of radiotherapy sufficiently high to completely eliminate some solid tumors such as breast cancer, small cell lung cancer or other relatively radiosensitive tumors.

References

1 Eisen HN, Keston AS. The immunologic reactivity of bovine serum albumin labeled with trace-amounts of radioactive iodine (I-131). *J Immunol* 1950; **63**: 71–80.

2 Pressman D, Korngold L. The *in vivo* localization of anti-Wagner-osteogenic sarcoma antibodies. *Cancer* 1953; **6**: 619–23.

3 Pressman D, Day ED, Blau M. The use of paired labeling in the determination of tumor-localizing antibodies. *Cancer Res* 1957; **17**: 845–50.

4 Beierwaltes WH. Radioiodine-labeled compounds previously or currently used for tumor localization. In: Agency IAE, ed. *Proceedings of an Advisory Group Meeting on Tumour Localization with Radioactive Agents. Panel Proceedings.* Vienna, Austria: International Atomic Energy Agency, 1950: 47–56.

5 Spar IL, Bale WF, Marrack D, Dewey WC, McCardle RJ, Harper PV. ^{131}I-labeled antibodies to human fibrinogen. Diagnostic studies and therapeutic trials. *Cancer* 1967; **20**: 865–70.

6 Ettinger DS, Order SE, Wharam MD, Parker MK, Klein JL, Leichner PK. Phase I–II study of isotope immunoglobulin therapy for primary liver cancer. *Cancer Treat Rep* 1982; **66**: 289–97.

7 Köhler G, Milstein C. Continuous cultures of fused cells secreting antibody of pre-defined specificity. *Nature* 1975; **256**: 495–7.

8 Press OW, Appelbaum F, Ledbetter JA *et al.* Monoclonal antibody 1F5 (anti-CD20) serotherapy of human B cell lymphomas. *Blood* 1987; **69**: 584–91.

9 McLaughlin P, Grillo-Lopez A, Link BK *et al.* Rituximab chimeric anti-CD20 monoclonal antibody therapy for relapsed indolent lymphoma: half of patients respond to a four-dose treatment program. *J Clin Oncol* 1998; **16**: 2825–33.

10 Cobleigh MA, Vogel CL, Tripathy D *et al.* Multinational study of the efficacy and safety of humanized anti-HER2 monoclonal antibody in women who have HER2-overexpressing metastatic breast cancer that has progressed after chemotherapy for metastatic disease. *J Clin Oncol* 1999; **17**: 2639–48.

11 Slamon DJ, Leyland-Jones B, Shak S *et al.* Use of chemotherapy plus a monoclonal antibody against HER2 for metastatic breast cancer that overexpresses HER2. *N Engl J Med* 2001; **344**: 783–92.

12 Badger CC, Krohn KA, Peterson AB, Shulman H, Bernstein ID. Experimental radiotherapy of murine lymphoma with ^{131}I-labeled anti-Thy-1.1 monoclonal antibody. *Cancer Res* 1985; **45**: 1536–44.

13 Badger CC, Krohn KA, Shulman H, Flournoy N, Bernstein ID. Experimental radioimmunotherapy of lymphoma with ^{131}I-labeled anti-T-cell antibodies. *Cancer Res* 1986; **46**: 6223–8.

14 Thomas ED, Storb R, Clift RA *et al.* Bone-marrow transplantation. *N Engl J Med* 1975; **292**: 832–43.

15 Clift RA, Buckner CD, Appelbaum FR *et al.* Allogeneic marrow transplantation in patients with acute myeloid leukemia in first remission. A randomized trial of two irradiation regimens. *Blood* 1990; **76**: 1867–71.

16 Clift RA, Buckner CD, Appelbaum FR *et al.* Allogeneic marrow transplantation in patients with chronic myeloid leukemia in the chronic phase: a randomized trial of two irradiation regimens. *Blood* 1991; **77**: 1660–5.

17 Appelbaum FR, Brown P, Sandmaier B *et al.* Antibody-radionuclide conjugates as part of a myeloablative preparative regimen for marrow transplantation. *Blood* 1989; **73**: 2202–8.

18 Matthews DC, Appelbaum FR, Eary JF *et al.* Development of a marrow transplant regimen for acute leukemia using targeted hematopoietic irradiation delivered by ^{131}I-labeled anti-CD45 antibody, combined with cyclophosphamide and total body irradiation. *Blood* 1995; **85**: 1122–31.

19 Society of Nuclear Medicine. *MIRD Primer for Absorbed Dose Calculations.* New York: Society of Nuclear Medicine, 1988.

20 Shockley TR, Lin K, Sung C *et al.* A quantitative analysis of tumor specific monoclonal antibody uptake by human melanoma xenografts: Effects of antibody immunological properties and tumor antigen expression levels. *Cancer Res* 1992; **52**: 357–66.

21 van der Jagt RH, Badger CC, Appelbaum FR *et al.* Localization of radiolabeled antimyeloid antibodies in a human acute leukemia xenograft tumor model. *Cancer Res* 1992; **52**: 89–94.

22 Press OW, Shan D, Howell-Clark J *et al.* Comparative metabolism and retention of iodine-125, yttrium-90 and indium-111 radioimmunoconjugates by cancer cells. *Cancer Res* 1996; **56**: 2123–9.

23 Matthews DC, Appelbaum FR, Eary JF *et al.* Radiolabeled anti-CD45 monoclonal antibodies target lymphohematopoietic tissue in the macaque. *Blood* 1991; **78**: 1864–74.

24 Yokota T, Milenic DE, Whitlow M, Schlom J. Rapid tumor penetration of single-chain Fv and comparison with other immunoglobulin forms. *Cancer Res* 1992; **52**: 3402–8.

25 Matthews DC, Badger CC, Fisher DR *et al.* Selective radiation of hematolymphoid tissue delivered by anti-CD45 antibody. *Cancer Res* 1992; **52**: 1228–34.

26 Press OW, Eary JF, Badger CC *et al.* Treatment of refractory non-Hodgkin's lymphoma with radiolabeled MB-1 (anti-CD37) antibody. *J Clin Oncol* 1989; **7**: 1027–38.

27 Bianco JA, Sandmaier B, Brown PA *et al.* Specific marrow localization of an ^{131}I-labeled anti-myeloid antibody in normal dogs: effects of a "cold" antibody pretreatment dose of marrow localization. *Exp Hematol* 1989; **17**: 929–34.

28 Papadopoulos EB, Caron P, Castro-Malaspina H *et al.* Results of allogeneic bone marrow transplant following ^{131}I-M195/busulfan/cyclophosphamide (BU/CY) in patients with advanced/refractory myeloid malignancies. *Blood* 1993; **82**: 80a [Abstract].

29 Ali S, Warren S, Richter K *et al.* Improving the tumor retention of radiolabeled antibody: aryl carbohydrate adducts. *Cancer Res* 1990; **50**: S783–8.

30 Hnatowich DJ, McGann J. DTPA-coupled proteins: procedures and precautions. *Int J Radiat Appl Instrum Part B Nucl Med Biol* 1987; **14**: 563–8.

31 Kosmas C, Snook D, Gooden CS *et al.* Development of humoral immune responses against a macrocyclic chelating agent (DOTA) in cancer patients receiving radioimmunoconjugates for imaging and therapy. *Cancer Res* 1992; **52**: 904–11.

32 Eary JF, Appelbaum FR, Durack L, Brown P. Preliminary validation of the opposing view method for quantitative gamma camera imaging. *Med Phys* 1989; **16**: 382–7.

33 Fyles GM, Messner HA, Lockwood G *et al.* Long-term results of bone marrow transplantation for patients with AML, ALL and CML prepared with single dose total body irradiation of 500 cGy delivered with a high dose rate. *Bone Marrow Transplant* 1991; **8**: 453–63.

34 Knox SJ, Levy R, Miller Ra *et al.* Determinants of the antitumor effect of radiolabeled monoclonal antibodies. *Cancer Res* 1990; **50**: 4935–40.

35 Neacy W, Wessels BW, Bradley E *et al.* Comparison of radioimmunotherapy (RIT) and 4 mV external beam radiotherapy of human tumor xenografts in athymic mice. *J Nucl Med* 1986; **27**: 902–3.

36 Wessels BW, Vessella RL, Palme DF, Berkopec JM, Smith GK, Bradley EW. Radiobiological comparison of external beam irradiation and radioimmunotherapy in renal cell carcinoma xenografts. *Int J Radiat Oncol Biol Phys* 1989; **17**: 1257–63.

37 Storb R, Raff RF, Appelbaum FR *et al.* What radiation dose for DLA-identical canine marrow grafts? *Blood* 1988; **72**: 1300–4.

38. Storb R, Raff RF, Appelbaum FR et al. Comparison of fractionated to single-dose total body irradiation in conditioning canine littermates for DLA-identical marrow grafts. Blood 1989; **74**: 1139–43.
39. Ruffner KL, Martin PJ, Hussell S et al. Immunosuppressive effects of ^{131}I-anti-CD45 antibody in unsensitized and donor antigen-presensitized H2-matched, minor antigen-mismatched murine transplant models. Cancer Res 2001; **61**: 5126–31.
40. Matthews DC, Martin PJ, Nourigat C, Appelbaum FR, Fisher DR, Bernstein ID. Marrow ablative and immunosuppressive effects of ^{131}I-anti-CD45 antibody in congenic and H2-mismatched murine transplant models. Blood 1999; **93**: 737–45.
41. Sandmaier BM, Bethge WA, Wilbur DS et al. Bismuth 213-labeled anti-CD45 radioimmunoconjugate to condition dogs for nonmyeloablative allogeneic marrow grafts. Blood 2002; **100**: 318–26.
42. Deeg HJ, Storb R, Longton G et al. Single dose or fractionated total body irradiation and autologous marrow transplantation in dogs: effects of exposure rate, fraction size, and fractionation interval on acute and delayed toxicity. Int J Radiat Oncol Biol Phys 1988; **15**: 647–53.
43. Deeg HJ, Storb R, Weiden PL et al. High-dose total-body irradiation and autologous marrow reconstitution in dogs: dose-rate-related acute toxicity and fractionation-dependent long-term survival. Radiat Res 1981; **88**: 385–91.
44. Appelbaum FR, Matthews DC, Eary JF et al. The use of radiolabeled anti-CD33 antibody to augment marrow irradiation prior to marrow transplantation for acute myelogenous leukemia. Transplantation 1992; **54**: 829–33.
45. Scheinberg DA, Lovett D, Divgi CR et al. A phase I trial of monoclonal antibody M195 in acute myelogenous leukemia: specific bone marrow targeting and internalization of radionuclide. J Clin Oncol 1991; **9**: 478–90.
46. Schwartz MA, Lovett DR, Redner A et al. Dose-escalation trial of M195 labeled with iodine 131 for cytoreduction and marrow ablation in relapsed or refractory myeloid leukemias. J Clin Oncol 1993; **11**: 294–303.
47. Jurcic JG, Divgi CR, McDevitt MR et al. Potential for myeloablation with yttrium-90-HuM195 (anti-CD33) in myeloid leukemia. J Clin Oncol 2000; **19**: 8a [Abstract].
48. Jurcic JG. Antibody therapy of acute myelogenous leukemia. Cancer Biother Radio 2000; **15**: 319–26.
49. Jurcic JG, Larson SM, Sgouros G et al. Targeted alpha particle immunotherapy for myeloid leukemia. Blood 2002; **100**: 1233–9.
50. Matthews DC, Appelbaum FR, Eary JF et al. Phase I study of ^{131}I-anti-CD45 antibody plus cyclophosphamide and total body irradiation for advanced acute leukemia and myelodysplastic syndrome. Blood 1999; **94**: 1237–47.
51. Rosario E, Rajendran J, Ruffner KL et al. Radiolabeled anti-CD45 antibody with cyclophosphamide (CY) and total body irradiation (TBI) followed by allogeneic hematopoietic stem cell transplantation (HSCT) for patients with advanced acute myeloid leukemia (AML) or myelodysplastic syndrome. Blood 2001; **98**: 857a [Abstract].
52. Matthews DC, Appelbaum FR, Eary JF, Mitchell D, Press OW, Bernstein ID. ^{131}I-anti-CD45 antibody plus busulfan/cyclophosphamide in matched related transplants for AML in first remission. Blood 1996; **88** (Suppl. 1): 142a [Abstract].

53. Bunjes D, Buchmann I, Duncker C et al. Rhenium 188-labeled anti-CD66 (a, b, c, e) monoclonal antibody to intensify the conditioning regimen prior to stem cell transplantation for patients with high-risk acute myeloid leukemia or myelodysplastic syndrome: results of a phase I–II study. Blood 2001; **98**: 565–72.
54. Klein SA, Hermann S, Dietrich JW, Hoelzer D, Martin H. Transplantation-related toxicity and acute intestinal graft-versus-host disease after conditioning regimens intensified with rhenium 188-labeled anti-CD66 monoclonal antibodies (Letter). Blood 2002; **99**: 2270–1.
55. Press OW, Eary JF, Appelbaum FR et al. Radiolabeled antibody therapy of B cell lymphomas with autologous bone marrow support. N Engl J Med 1993; **329**: 1219–24.
56. Press OW, Eary JF, Appelbaum FR et al. Phase II trial of ^{131}I-B1 (anti-CD20) antibody therapy with autologous stem cell transplantation for relapsed B cell lymphomas. Lancet 1995; **346**: 336–40.
57. Liu SY, Eary JF, Petersdorf SH et al. Follow-up of relapsed B-cell lymphoma patients treated with iodine-131-labeled anti-CD20 antibody and autologous stem-cell rescue. J Clin Oncol 1998; **16**: 3270–8.
58. Press OW, Eary JF, Gooley T et al. A phase I/II trial of iodine-131-tositumomab (anti-CD20), etoposide, cyclophosphamide, and autologous stem cell transplantation for relapsed B-cell lymphomas. Blood 2000; **96**: 2934–42.
59. Gopal AK, Rajendran JG, Petersdorf SH et al. High-dose chemo-radioimmunotherapy with autologous stem cell support for relapsed mantle cell lymphoma. Blood 2002; **99**: 3158–62.
60. Behr TM, Griesinger F, Riggert J et al. High-dose myeloablative radioimmunotherapy of mantle cell non-Hodgkin lymphoma with the iodine-131-labeled chimeric anti-CD20 antibody C2B8 and autologous stem cell support. Results of a pilot study. Cancer 2002; **94**: 1363–72.
61. Nademanee A, Molina A, Forman SJ et al. A phase I/II trial of high-dose radioimmunotherapy (RIT) with Zevalin in combination with high-dose etoposide (VP16) and cyclophosphamide (CY) followed by autologous stem cell transplant (ASCT) in patients with poor-risk or relapsed B-cell non-Hodgkin's lymphoma (NHL). Blood 2002; **100**: 182a [Abstract].
62. Vose JM, Bierman PJ, Lynch JC et al. Radioimmunotherapy with Bexxar combined with high-dose chemotherapy (HDC) followed by autologous hematopoietic stem cell transplantation (ASCT) for refractory non-Hodgkin's lymphoma (NHL): synergistic results with no added toxicity. J Clin Oncol 2001; **20**: 6a [Abstract].
63. Juweid M, Sharkey RM, Markowitz A et al. Treatment of non-Hodgkin's lymphoma with radiolabeled murine, chimeric, or humanized LL2, an anti-CD22 monoclonal antibody. Cancer Res 1995; **55**: S5899–907.
64. Behr TM, Wormann B, Gramatzki M et al. Low- versus high-dose radioimmunotherapy with humanized anti-CD22 or chimeric anti-CD20 antibodies in a broad spectrum of B cell-associated malignancies. Clin Cancer Res 1999; **5**: S3304–14.
65. Vose JM, Colcher D, Gobar L et al. Phase I/II trial of multiple dose [131]iodine-MAb LL2 (CD22) in patients with recurrent non-Hodgkin's lymphoma. Leuk Lymphoma 2000; **38**: 91–101.
66. Kaminski MS, Estes J, Zasadny KR et al. Radioimmunotherapy with iodine ^{131}I tositumomab for relapsed or refractory B-cell non-Hodgkin lymphoma: updated results and long-term follow-up of the University of Michigan experience. Blood 2000; **96**: 1259–66.
67. Witzig TE, Gordon LI, Cabanillas F et al. Randomized controlled trial of yttrium-90-labeled ibritumomab tiuxetan radioimmunotherapy versus rituximab immunotherapy for patients with relapsed or refractory low-grade, follicular, or transformed B-cell non-Hodgkin's lymphoma. J Clin Oncol 2002; **20**: 2453–63.
68. Herpst JM, Klein JL, Leichner PK, Quadri SM, Vriesendorp HM. Survival of patients with resistant Hodgkin's disease after polyclonal yttrium 90-labeled antiferritin treatment. J Clin Oncol 1995; **13**: 2394–400.
69. Bierman PJ, Vose JM, Leichner PK et al. Yttrium 90-labeled antiferritin followed by high-dose chemotherapy and autologous bone marrow transplantation for poor-prognosis Hodgkin's disease. J Clin Oncol 1993; **11**: 698–703.
70. Schnell R, Dietlein M, Staak O et al. Non-myeloablative radioimmunotherapy with an iodine-131-tagged anti-CD30 antibody (^{131}I-Ki-4) in patients with refractory Hodgkin's lymphoma. Blood 2002; **100**: 203a [Abstract].
71. Richman CM, DeNardo SJ. Systemic radiotherapy in metastatic breast cancer using ^{90}Y-linked monoclonal MUC-1 antibodies. Crit Rev Oncol Hemat 2001; **38**: 25–35.
72. Schrier DM, Stemmer SM, Johnson T et al. High-dose [90]Y Mx-diethylenetriaminepentaacetic acid (DTPA)-BrE-3 and autologous hematopoietic stem cell support (AHSCS) for the treatment of advanced breast cancer: a phase I trial. Cancer Res 1995; **55**: S5921–4.
73. Cagnoni PJ, Ceriani RL, Cole WC et al. Phase I study of high-dose radioimmunotherapy with ^{90}Y-hu-BrE-3 followed by autologous stem cell support (ASCS) in patients with metastatic breast cancer. Cancer Biother Radio 1998; **13**: 328a [Abstract].
74. Cagnoni PJ, Ceriani RL, Cole WC et al. High-dose radioimmunotherapy with ^{90}Y-hu-BrE-3 followed by autologous hematopoietic stem cell support (AHSCS) in patients with metastatic breast cancer. Cancer Biother Radio 1999; **14**: 318a [Abstract].
75. Richman CM, DeNardo SJ, O'Donnell RT et al. Dosimetry-based therapy in metastatic breast cancer patients using ^{90}Y monoclonal antibody 170H.82 with autologous stem cell support and cyclosporin A. Clin Cancer Res 1999; **5**: S3243–8.
76. Wong JY, Somlo G, Odom-Maryon T et al. Initial clinical experience evaluating yttrium-90-chimeric T84.66 anticarcinoembryonic antigen antibody and autologous hematopoietic stem cell support in patients with carcinoembryonic antigen-producing metastatic breast cancer. Clin Cancer Res 1999; **5**: S3224–31.
77. Cheung NK, Kushner BH, LaQuaglia M et al. N7: a novel multi-modality therapy of high-risk neuroblastoma (NB) in children diagnosed over 1 year of age. Med Ped Oncol 2001; **36**: 227–30.
78. Juweid ME, Hajjar G, Stein R et al. Initial experience with high-dose radioimmunotherapy of metastatic medullary thyroid cancer using ^{131}I-MN-14 F(ab')$_2$ anti-carcinoembryonic antigen MAb and AHSCR. J Nucl Med 2000; **41**: 93–103.
79. McDevitt MR, Ma D, Lai LT et al. Tumor therapy with targeted atomic nanogenerators. Science 2001; **294**: 1537–40.

80 Axworthy DB, Reno JM, Hylarides MD *et al.* Cure of human carcinoma xenografts by a single dose of pretargeted yttrium-90 with negligible toxicity. *Proc Natl Acad Sci U S A* 2000; **97**: 1802–7.

81 Press OW, Corcoran M, Subbiah K *et al.* A comparative evaluation of conventional and pretargeted radioimmunotherapy of CD20-expressing lymphoma xenografts. *Blood* 2001; **98**: 2535–43.

82 Weiden PL, Breitz HB. Pretargeted radioimmunotherapy (PRIT) for treatment of non-Hodgkin's lymphoma (NHL). *Crit Rev Oncol Hemat* 2001; **40**: 37–51.

83 Knox SJ, Forero-Torres A, Vose JM, Picozzi VJ, Breitz H, Sims RB. A phase I dose optimization study of anti-CD20 pretarget radioimmunotherapy in patients with relapsed or refractory NHL. *Blood* 2002; **100**: 162a [Abstract].

16

Nelson J. Chao

Pharmacology and the Use of Immunosuppressive Agents after Hematopoietic Cell Transplantation

Graft-vs.-host disease (GVHD) is the result of an intricate immune response to foreign allogeneic stimuli. This disease, which can be acute or chronic, is caused by donor T-cell recognition of histocompatibility antigens that differ between the host and the donor. The amplification of this T-cell recognition process contributes to the occurrence of GVHD. The proliferation of activated T cells leads to the production and secretion of a variety of cytokines that are responsible for the inflammatory effects and tissue damage [1]. Much of the damage is caused by inflammatory cytokines, such as interleukin 1 (IL-1), IL-2, tumor necrosis factor (TNF) and interferon-gamma (IFN-γ) [2]. Awareness of the critical events that lead to the activation of these alloreactive T cells and the subsequent amplification of the signals involved in T-cell proliferation has led to an understanding of the mechanisms of action of specific immunosuppressants. This understanding will allow for the development and testing of novel immunosuppressive agents. This chapter will focus on the most commonly used commercially available immunosuppressive drugs and discuss some of the newer drugs that have or may soon become available.

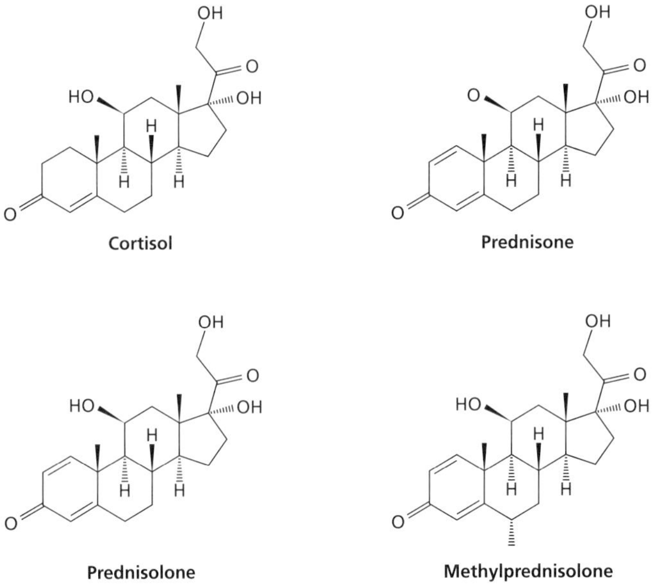

Nonspecific immunosuppressive drugs

Corticosteroids

Corticosteroids are the most widely used "front-line" therapy for the treatment of clinical GVHD. This class of drug has been combined with other immunosuppressants in the prophylaxis against GVHD. However, we still do not fully understand their mechanism of action.

Pharmacology

The most commonly utilized corticosteroid is methylprednisolone (MP), which differs from prednisolone and prednisone only by the addition of 6-α-methyl group (Fig. 16.1). The 6-α-methyl group blocks the specific binding of this corticosteroid to transcortin, the plasma protein that carries steroids. Instead, MP is primarily bound to albumin. The frequent side-effects from MP may be dependent on the albumin level in the host. The lack of transcortin-binding leads to a larger partition coefficient and the result is a significantly greater penetration into bronchial alveolar fluids, which may provide a therapeutic advantage for treatment of pulmonary inflammatory states.

Signaling by the steroid molecules is achieved through binding to a specific cytosolic receptor thereby initiating its pharmacologic effects (Fig. 16.2). This binding of steroid to receptor activates the complex enabling it to translocate rapidly into the nucleus. There it is associated with specific sequences known as the glucocorticoid response elements (GRE). These response elements regulate the mRNA expression of certain proteins, leading to the known biological effects. Generally, larger

Fig. 16.1 Structure of corticosteroids.

doses produce greater intensity and duration of effects. The utility of corticosteroids in GVHD is thought to be related to its lympholytic activity [3]. The presumed activity is that corticosteroids destroy the lymphoid cells, which it certainly does *in vitro* and *in vivo*. However, there are cells that survive both in murine and human studies which can mount an immune response [3]. Thus, other mechanisms, such as down modulation of cytokines, are likely to be responsible as well [2]. There are data to suggest that the major effect of corticosteroids is the suppression of pro-inflammatory cytokines rather than direct cellular cytotoxicity of lymphocytes [4]. In clinical trials that measured cytokines, the levels of TNF-α decreased after the initiation of corticosteroids used for the therapy of GVHD [5].

Toxicity

There are many adverse effects associated with corticosteroids. In addition to their immunosuppressive effects, which set the stage for infectious complications, most of the adverse effects are related to Cushingoid features, hyperglycemia, occasional psychosis or neurotoxicity as well as myopathy. Other chronic effects such as osteoporosis, cataract formation and aseptic necrosis also occur. Corticosteroids are sensitive to a variety of drug interactions, specifically anticonvulsants, which may increase the total clearance of unbound corticosteroids.

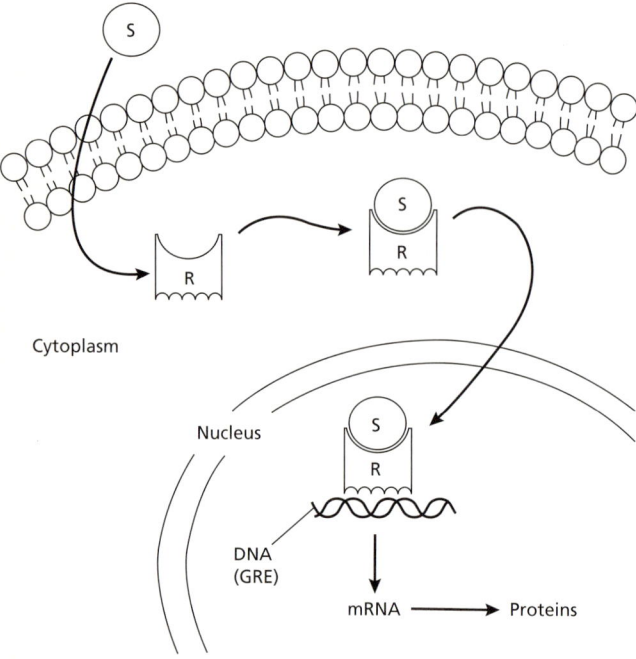

Fig. 16.2 Diagram of the mechanisms of action of steroids and the intracellular receptor. The complex of the drug and receptor translocates efficiently into the nucleus where it interacts with glucocorticoid response elements (GREs) leading to the generation of messenger RNA and protein synthesis.

Clinical use

Corticosteroids are given intravenously (IV) when used as prophylaxis or therapy of acute GVHD. The drug of choice has been MP followed by oral prednisone when patients are able to eat sufficiently or when a patient's diarrhea has resolved so that one can be confident that they will absorb the medication without difficulty. One regimen which combines cyclosporine (CSP), methotrexate (MTX) and prednisone (beginning after all MTX doses have been administered), is among the most potent combination for the prevention of acute GVHD, resulting in only 9% grade II–IV acute GVHD in the best candidates (first remission of acute leukemia or first chronic phase of chronic myeloid leukemia) for allogeneic bone marrow transplantation (BMT) [6]. The doses of MP given for prophylaxis have varied and most GVHD prevention regimens do not include corticosteroids. In support of the delayed use of corticosteroids are the results noted in a prospective randomized study comparing CSP, MTX, and MP vs. CSP and MTX in patients receiving BMT from an HLA-identical sibling [7]. MTX was given in four doses (days 1, 3, 6 and 11), and MP was not begun until day 14. Acute GVHD was more common in the patients treated without MP. However, a second randomized study found no difference between these two regimens in preventing either acute or chronic GVHD [8]. Based on these data, our current recommendation is to save the use of corticosteroids for the treatment of acute GVHD.

Most regimens taper the steroid dose to zero by +180 days. The usual corticosteroid dose for acute GVHD is 1–2 mg/kg administered in divided doses with a tapering schedule after about 2 weeks of 10% every 3–5 days. Occasionally higher pulse doses up to 10 mg/kg have been used. Chronic GVHD treatment dose is started in the range of 1 mg/kg on a daily basis. The goal thereafter is to switch patients to an alternating day regimen to spare side-effects of corticosteroids. For those patients in the older age range, a small dose of prednisone, similar to those used in autoimmune diseases, may be necessary to suppress reactivation of GVHD.

Corticosteroids have also been used as local treatment for GVHD. Beclomethasone 17, 21-dipropionate (BDP) is a synthetic diester of beclomethasone, a corticosteroid analog that has appeal in the treatment of gastrointestinal (GI) GVHD by virtue of its ability to direct therapy to inflamed GI mucosa. A randomized, placebo-controlled, double-blind study evaluating BDP in the treatment of grade II GVHD with GI symptoms has been performed [9]. Patients were randomized to receive prednisone 1 mg/kg/day plus either BDP (8 mg/day) or placebo for 10 days. The results of this study demonstrated that oral BDP was more effective than placebo in restoring oral intake in patients with grade II GVHD with GI symptoms, and allows prednisone to be rapidly tapered without a flare of intestinal symptoms. Oral BDP was well tolerated; no patients on BDP alone became Cushingoid or developed evidence of bacterial or fungal overgrowth on surveillance cultures. A larger phase III study is ongoing.

Methotrexate (MTX)

MTX is an analog of aminopterin, the folic acid antagonist introduced in 1948 for the treatment of acute leukemia [10]. As one of the antimetabolites, it functions as a decoy substrate for critical biochemical reactions leading to cell death. The amino group substitution found in MTX results in a less potent antifolate but a drug with more predictable toxicity profile and equivalent clinical results. The precise mechanism by which MTX prevents GVHD is not understood; however, it is likely related to MTX's ability to inhibit cellular growth and division. Therefore, antigen activated T cells that are rapidly proliferating would be particularly sensitive to this antimetabolite.

MTX can induce tolerance following marrow transplantation. In canine transplantation, MTX given after the graft was effective in controlling GVHD and in inducing tolerance when donor and recipient were matched for the dog leukocyte antigen system [11].

Pharmacology

MTX was one of the first chemotherapy agents introduced for the therapy of malignancies. Studies have detailed its pharmacokinetics and mechanisms of action at the intracellular level. How these mechanisms translate to its *in vivo* effects and how it functions in the prevention of GVHD, facilitation of engraftment, and induction of tolerance are not well understood. At the cellular level, MTX exerts its cytotoxic effect by inhibiting dihydrofolate reductase (DHFR). DHFR is the intracellular enzyme responsible for converting folic acid to reduced folate cofactors. The reduced state of the folates, namely the tetrahydrofolates are responsible for the transport of single carbon groups that are required for purine and thymidylate synthesis [12]. Once the single carbon group is delivered, the oxidized folates must be converted back to tetrahydrofolates by DHFR. MTX binds to DHFR, thereby preventing its ability to reduce the oxidized folates to tetrahydrofolate and blocking further purine or thymidylate synthesis [13].

Following the administration of MTX approximately 50% is bound to plasma proteins, especially albumin, with the highest tissue-plasma equilibrium reported in the kidney, liver, GI tract and muscle [14]. The GI tract is an important site of distribution and metabolism of MTX, perhaps accounting for one of the primary sites of toxicity. One concern in using MTX is its clearance in those patients who have pleural or ascitic fluid since these reservoir spaces can have a substantial impact on the disposition of MTX. These spaces can be a reservoir from which MTX can be continuously released, leading to severe toxicity. At the low IV doses, MTX clearance correlates with glomerular filtration, and renal excretion of unmetabolized drug is the major route for elimination.

Polyglutamate formation is also important to MTX metabolism [15]. The formation of MTX polyglutamates intracellularly may account for its retention within the cell and its cytotoxic effects. The enzyme folyl

Table 16.1 Outline of a regimen used for graft-vs.-host disease (GVHD) prophylaxis.

CSP			MTX		
Day	Dose	Route	Day	Dose	Route
−2 to +3	5 mg/kg	IV QD over 20 h	+1	15 mg/m^2	IV
+4 to +14	3 mg/kg	IV QD over 20 h	+3	10 mg/m^2	IV
+15 to +35	3.75 mg/kg	IV QD over 20 h	+6	10 mg/m^2	IV
+36 to +83	5 mg/kg	po BID	+11	10 mg/m^2	IV
+84 to +97	4 mg/kg	po BID			
+98 to +119	3 mg/kg	po BID			
+120 to +180	2 mg/kg	po BID			
+181	Off				

BID, twice a day; IV, intravenous; po, taken orally; QD, four times daily.

Table 16.2 Suggested dose adjustments for methotrexate (MTX).

	Dose (%)
Bilirubin mg/dL	
<2.0	100
2.1–3.0	50
3.1–5.0	25
>5.0	Hold dose
Creatinine mg/dL	
<1.5	100
1.5–1.7	75
1.8–2.0	50
>2.0	Hold dose

polyglutamate synthetase adds glutamate residues to folates or antifolates such as MTX. These polyglutamate moieties are then retained inside the cell leading to prolonged antifolate activity. The polyglutamate derivatives of MTX appear to be as toxic to DHFR as the native compound. If the retained MTX polyglutamates are produced differentially in lymphocytes compared to other normal cells, the effective concentrations of the drug would differ. For example, these differences in intracellular concentrations may account for selective toxicities and may selectively inhibit certain subpopulations of cells [16].

Toxicity

The most common adverse effects of MTX when used for GVHD prophylaxis are renal, hepatic, and GI toxicity. Patients may have an elevation in creatinine and elevation of bilirubin levels following the administration of MTX. As these are also the side-effects of CSP or tacrolimus, dose attenuation of MTX and CSP or tacrolimus may be necessary. Full target doses may not be achievable in patients with grade III–IV mucositis resulting from the preparatory regimen because of airway obstruction and severe oropharyngeal bleeding.

Clinical use

The use of MTX following allogeneic BMT has been exclusively with the IV formulation. The drug doses administered have been relatively small given the inability to dose escalate MTX significantly (Table 16.1). Initial studies in Seattle tested MTX as a single agent on a weekly basis up to day +100 but, because of the toxicity of weekly administration of MTX, the dose was changed to four doses and combined with CSP [17]. MTX, when used with CSP or tacrolimus, generally is injected IV on days +1, +3, +6 and +11 following BMT. This schema is the most commonly utilized regimen today. Another schema that is commonly used following unrelated stem cell transplantation has been named "mini-dose MTX", usually used in conjunction with tacrolimus [18]. In this regimen, MTX is given on days 1, 3, 6 and 11 at 5 mg/m^2. The overall prevention of GVHD was similar with lower systemic toxicities. In general, patients should be very well hydrated, have their urine alkalinized with sodium bicarbonate, and MTX should not be administered until the urine pH is 8 or greater. Moreover, dose attenuation should be considered for elevations of the creatinine, bilirubin and grade III–IV mucositis. One suggested schema for dose attenuation of MTX is shown in Table 16.2. There has been one report of leucovorin rescue after MTX [19]. In this small series, use of leucovorin was not associated with an adverse outcome, although this practice is not commonly used. Leucovorin circumvents the blocked tetrahydrofolate synthesis by supplying reduced folates directly therefore bypassing the blocked DHFR.

Specific T-cell immunosuppressive drugs

Cyclosporine (CSP)

CSP, also known as cyclosporin A, has led to a considerable expansion of the field of allogeneic transplantation given its potent immunosuppressive activity. CSP is a cyclic peptide extracted in 1969 from two strains of fungi isolated from soil samples. CSP was tested as an antifungal agent and demonstrated only limited effects, but it was highly effective as an immunosuppressive agent. These studies led to it being administered to patients in 1978 [20].

Pharmacology

CSP is a neutral hydrophobic cyclic peptide composed of 11 amino acids (Fig. 16.3). Over the past decade, much work has been devoted to understanding the mechanism of CSP's activity. Moreover, CSP, as well as tacrolimus, has been used as a chemical probe to dissect the pathways of T-cell activation. This understanding will lead to novel immunosuppressants that may be more specific and potentially less toxic. While CSP and tacrolimus are distinct in their molecular structure (Fig. 16.3), their mechanism of action will be discussed together since they are almost indistinguishable in their cellular functions. What is known thus far is that CSP (and tacrolimus) block the calcium-dependent signal transduction pathways distal to engagement of the T-cell receptor (TCR) (Fig. 16.4). This block interrupts the activation of T cells since the signaling from the TCR is prevented. In dissecting the signaling pathway, several critical intracellular molecules have been identified and include calmodulin, calcineurin and the nuclear factor of activated T cells (NF-AT). The activation cascade includes calcium binding to calmodulin, which leads to binding calcineurin. The activated calcineurin may dephosphorylate the cytoplasmic unit of NF-AT, which allows translocation of the NF-AT from the cytoplasm into the nucleus to form a competent transcriptional activator of the *IL-2* gene [21].

The cytosolic binding protein for CSP was isolated in 1984 from lymphocytes and named cyclophilin for its high affinity for CSP [22]. The analogous major isoform for the binding protein for tacrolimus has been termed tacrolimus binding protein (FKBP). Both cyclophilin and FKBP are highly basic and very abundant in the cytoplasm. Although these two proteins do not have sequence homology, they both function as the enzyme prolyl *cis-trans* isomerase (or rotamase) [23]. Rotamase accelerates the conversion of *cis* and *trans* rotamers of proline containing

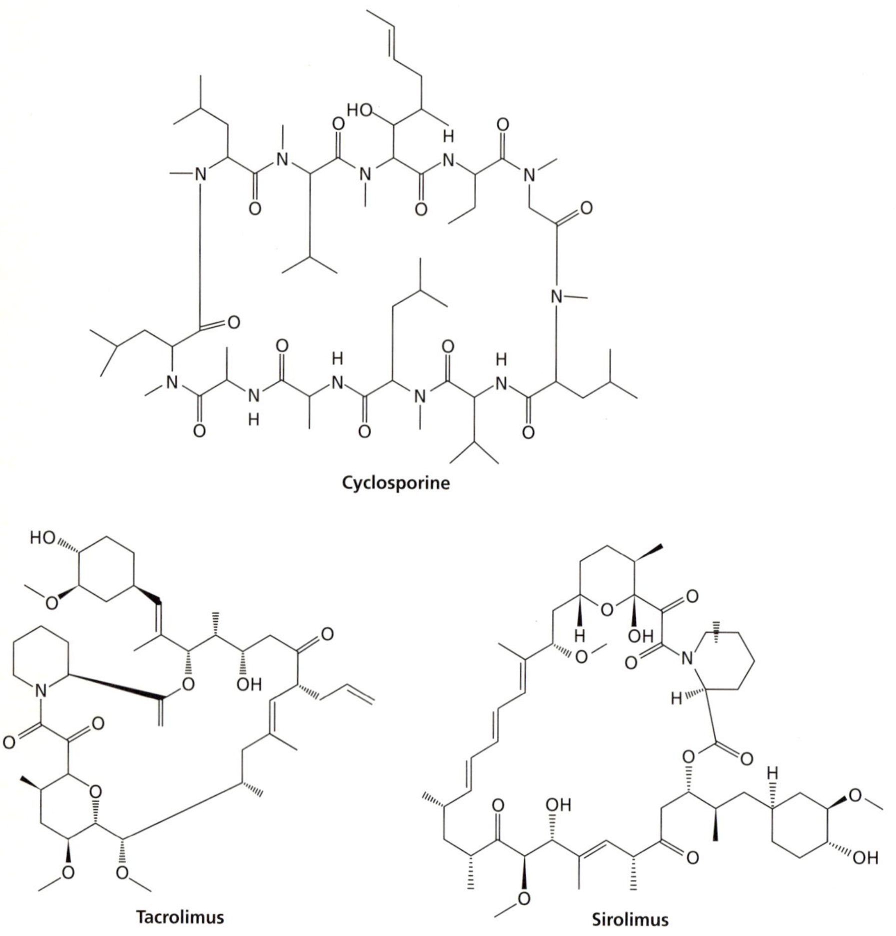

Fig. 16.3 Structure of cyclosporine (CSP), tacrolimus and sirolimus.

peptides or proteins. This conversion step is thought to be the rate-limiting step during normal protein folding. Both of these molecules are potent inhibitors of rotamase activity. The binding of CSP or tacrolimus to these rotamases suggests that inhibition of this enzyme may be an important step leading to immunosuppression. The mechanism of action of CSP is exerted through binding to cyclophilin (as tacrolimus is bound to FKBP). This complex of drug and binding protein interrupts the activation cascade at the level of NF-AT dephosphorylation, and therefore, NF-AT is not able to enter the nuclear domain and activate IL-2 (Fig. 16.4).

CSP is a highly lipophilic drug which is extensively metabolized with subsequent biliary and, to a lesser extent, urinary secretion. Over 15 metabolites have been isolated and identified. Some metabolites also have immunosuppressive activity while others are nephrotoxic. Thus, the clinical efficacy and interactions between CSP and the other drugs may be confounded by its metabolites. However, the most commonly reported inhibition or induction of CSP metabolism is by cytochrome p450 enzymes, specifically, HLp and PCN1 enzymes that are members of the cytochrome P450 IIIA gene family [24].

Toxicity

The major clinical toxicities that need to be monitored with CSP administration are renal insufficiency and elevation of bilirubin levels. Both of these complications appear to be dose related [25]. The acute nephrotoxicity is due to vasoconstriction and ischemia of the afferent arterioles in the kidney [26]. These acute changes are reversible but if present for too long can lead to an irreversible interstitial injury with glomerular thrombosis resulting in permanent azotemia. A major difficulty clinically is to differentiate specific side-effects of CSP from those of other drugs such as amphotericin, MTX, aminoglycoside or from an underlying disease process such as GVHD. Other side-effects that are commonly encountered are hypertension, hyperglycemia, headaches and hirsutism. Rarer events include gum hypertrophy, brittle nails, acne, nausea and vomiting. One specific clinical concern is the apparent association of hypomagnesemia and seizures in patients on CSP. Many patients who have a seizure while on CSP may also have concurrent hypomagnesemia and hypertension. Correction of these two abnormal findings are important in the management of patients. Hypertension alone can occasionally become a significant problem. Usually nifedipine is the drug of choice since it is an effective antihypertensive, and it has not been associated with changes in the CSP levels. Another rare but important toxicity of CSP (and tacrolimus) is the induction of an hemolytic uremic syndrome (HUS)/thrombotic thrombocytopenic purpura (TTP) syndrome. Patients will present with schistocytes and an elevated creatinine with or without mental status changes. In some circumstances, this toxicity will abate if one calcineurin inhibitor is substituted for the other.

Clinical use

CSP can be administered IV or orally. It is initially administered IV since in the early phase following transplantation many patients develop mucositis and GI damage from the preparatory regimen as well as from MTX given for GVHD prophylaxis. Once the patient is eating and drinking without significant difficulties CSP may be switched to an oral preparation. CSP is available as an olive oil solution and as soft gelatin capsules as well as in the microencapsulated form. CSP is erratically and incompletely absorbed after oral administration with many factors reported to influence oral CSP bioavailability. For example, food intake may impact its absorption, especially if the meal is high in fat content. Absorption kinetics of CSP have been described as either zero order or a

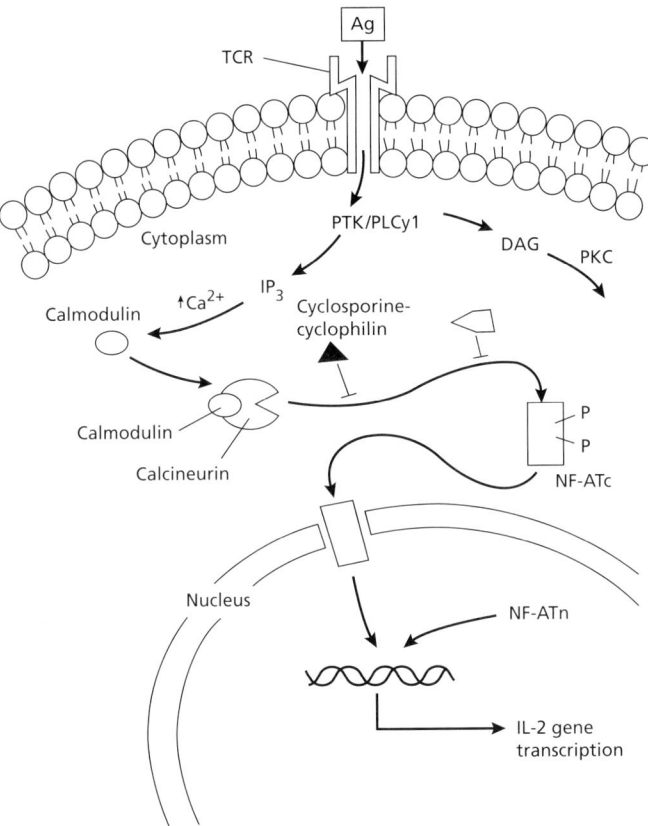

Fig. 16.4 A simplified diagram of the signal transduction found in the activation of a T cell through the T-cell receptor (TCR) and the point where cyclosporine (CSP) and tacrolimus interact with its binding proteins to block the generation of nuclear factor of activated T cells (NF-AT) and its subsequent generation of interleukin 2 (IL-2). Sirolimus, while similar to tacrolimus in structure, does not inhibit the signaling through the TCR but rather inhibits signaling through the CD28/B7 family of molecules and prevents the egress of cells from the G_1 phase. DAG, diacylglycerol; IP3, inositol triphosphate; PKC, protein kinase C; PLC, phospholipase C; PTK, protein tyrosine kinase.

Table 16.3 Cyclosporine (CSP) drug interactions [30,31].

Decrease CSP levels	Increase CSP levels
Phenytoin	Erythromycin*
Phenobarbital	Ketoconazole
Carbamazepine	Itraconazole
Primidone	Fluconazole
Rifampicin	Diltiazem
Nafcillin	Verapamil
Octreotide	Nicardipine
Sulfonamides	Acetozolamide
Trimethoprim	Alcohol
	Colchicine
	Fluoroquinolones
	Imipenim

*Not all macrolides are identical in effects because some do not form stable complexes with cytochrome P450 enzymes.

series of first order processes. CSP dosage usually is governed by research protocols, beginning the drug at a higher dose as a "loading dose", with a gradual taper over time. However there are several variations of dosing schedules. An example of a CSP regimen in given in Table 16.1.

There have been several studies attempting to correlate the efficacy of prophylactic CSP with its level in either whole blood, plasma or serum. The only assay that is completely specific for the parent compound is high-pressure liquid chromatography (HPLC). Other assays such as polyclonal or monoclonal antibodies immunoassays measure varying amounts of CSP metabolites. The target level that one uses will vary depending on which assay the diagnostic laboratory utilizes for measuring CSP levels. While the specific analytic methods are clearly more precise and preferable to the nonspecific methods for therapeutic drug monitoring, the technical difficulties in current HPLC methods make it less practical to utilize it widely. Moreover, there are limited data to suggest that there is a correlation between CSP levels and clinical outcome. The results from these studies suggest that there may be a complex relationship between dose, blood level and occurrence of GVHD [27–29]. These studies failed to demonstrate a clear direct correlation between drug level and occurrence of GVHD. The results did confirm the intricate interactions and balance of the immune responses in the host.

From a practical standpoint, CSP is administered to achieve a "therapeutic level", but, beyond that, it is important to deliver the planned dose per protocol. It is also important to be certain that the level drawn is a trough level in steady state, otherwise the values will not be interpretable. CSP levels are used to increase the dose if it is below the therapeutic threshold. In general, the dose is not decreased for elevated levels if no toxicity is present, but if the level is above two times the upper limit of the therapeutic range, then it is reasonable to decrease the dose to avoid potential neurotoxicity (i.e., seizures). Therefore, there is a range (up to two times normal) where CSP levels do not result in any change in clinical management. There are also concerns about the possible interactions between CSP and other medications. Many different drugs have been implicated in increasing or decreasing CSP levels in patients. Such medications and their effects are listed in Table 16.3 [30,31].

Tacrolimus (FK506)

Tacrolimus is a macrolide antibiotic extracted from the soil fungus *Streptomyces tsukubaensis* [32]. It is completely different from the cyclic peptide CSP, but it does exhibit a very similar selective immunosuppressive activity (Fig. 16.3). Its mechanism of action is also through the inhibition of signaling through the TCR (Fig. 16.4).

Pharmacology

Tacrolimus is highly lipophilic, and its method of administration is similar to that of CSP. Its mechanism of action has been reviewed above in conjunction with CSP. It is generally given IV in the early phases following allogeneic transplantation and then switched to the oral formulation. There is rapid distribution of the drug to the central compartment after a short IV infusion. Following oral administration, tacrolimus is erratically and incompletely absorbed [33,34]. The major difference to CSP is that the absorption of tacrolimus does not seem to depend on the presence of bile salts. Tacrolimus undergoes extensive distribution with highest levels found in the lung, kidney, heart and spleen. While in the blood, it is distributed into red blood cells. Less than 1% of the IV or oral dose appears unchanged in the urine indicating that the drug is almost completely metabolized in the liver prior to its elimination. It is eliminated primarily through monodemethylation, dimethylation, and hydroxylation. The half-life of tacrolimus is approximately 9 h and longer in those patients who have hepatic dysfunction. Tacrolimus is monitored in a similar fashion to CSP. Appropriate doses and levels of tacrolimus have not yet been clearly defined in patients undergoing allogeneic BMT, but the general target doses have been 10–20 ng/dL.

Toxicities

Tacrolimus is moderately well tolerated in humans. Most of the data on adverse events can be categorized into neurotoxicity, renal toxicity, and hyperglycemia and generally have been reported in solid organ transplantation recipients. Tacrolimus can cause an increase in serum creatinine concentration similar to that of CSP probably secondary to decrease in glomerular filtration. Hypertension in previously normotensive patients has also been described. Occasionally hypertension can be quite refractory to antihypertensive medication. The most commonly utilized antihypertensives have included the calcium channel blockers. Central nervous system (CNS) effects have also been found, including headaches, tremors, parathesias, photophobia and mental status changes. Seizure and coma have also been reported. Other findings include pulmonary symptoms such as dyspnea, musculoskeletal pain, itching, GI complaints (including anorexia, nausea, vomiting, abdominal pains) and fatigue. While the adverse effects of CSP and tacrolimus appear to be similar, there may be some advantage of tacrolimus in hypertensive patients. Hyperkalemia has also been observed following tacrolimus administration.

Clinical use

Tacrolimus has been evaluated in combination with MTX for the prevention of GVHD. In a multicenter trial, 329 recipients of HLA-identical marrow transplants were randomized to receive a short course of MTX plus either tacrolimus or CSP [35]. The incidence of grade II–IV acute GVHD was significantly lower in patients who received tacrolimus (32% vs. 44% with CSP), even though more unfavorable patients were enrolled in the tacrolimus group. This difference was largely due to a reduction in grade II disease. The incidence of chronic GVHD was similar in the two groups (56% and 49%), but severe chronic disease was more likely with CSP. There were, however, surprising adverse findings in the tacrolimus group:

1 There was lower rate of 2-year survival (41% vs. 50% with CSP) and overall survival (47% vs. 57% with CSP) that was largely due to poorer survival of patients with advanced disease (25% vs. 42%).
2 There was a higher incidence of regimen-related adverse events which predominantly occurred in patients with advanced disease.

The conclusion of the study was that in patients without advanced disease, tacrolimus plus MTX was more effective than CSP plus MTX in the prevention of acute GVHD with no difference in disease-free or overall survival. The survival disadvantage in patients with advanced disease warrants further study.

Another randomized trial also compared tacrolimus and MTX to CSP and MTX [36]. Tacrolimus was more effective than CSP for the prophylaxis of acute GVHD but there was no difference in patient survival or relapse. Although these trials were performed in patients with HLA-identical marrow transplants, uncontrolled [37,38] and controlled [39] observations indicate that tacrolimus also has activity against acute GVHD in recipients of matched unrelated donor transplants. The doses used in GVHD prophylaxis trials begin at 0.03–0.04 mg/kg/day as a continuous infusion. When patients are able to sustain near normal oral food and fluid intake, the drug is given orally at a dose of 0.15 mg/kg/day administered in two divided doses.

Sirolimus (rapamycin)

Sirolimus is a lipophilic macrolide which was identified more than 20 years ago during an antibiotic screening at Ayerst Research Laboratories [40]. This molecule is produced by a strain of *Streptomyces hygroscopicus* isolated from a soil sample from Easter Island (Rapa Nui). Although lacking antibacterial activity, it inhibited yeast growth and growth of filamentous fungi. The first demonstration of sirolimus' immunosuppressive activity was obtained from studies demonstrating the inhibition of immunoglobulin E (IgE) production as well as its efficacy in experimental allergic encephalomyelitis and adjuvant arthritis [41]. The interest in sirolimus as an immunosuppressive agent coincided with a discovery of the immunosuppressive activity of tacrolimus since the structure of both of these molecules contained a distinctive hemiketal-masked αβ-diketopipecolic acid amidic component (Fig. 16.3) [42].

Pharmacology

Sirolimus binds to the same family of intracellular receptors as tacrolimus, termed tacrolimus binding proteins (FKBPs). In a similar fashion to tacrolimus, sirolimus has two domains, a domain bound by FKBP and an effector domain forming a composite surface that interacts with the mammalian target of sirolimus [43]. The intracellular target of sirolimus (termed the mammalian target of rapamycin [mTOR]) is ubiquitously expressed in human tissue with the highest level found in the testes and skeletal muscle.

While sirolimus and tacrolimus bind to the same family of intracellular binding proteins, the mechanisms of immunosuppression are clearly distinct. Sirolimus inhibits the growth of hematopoietic and lymphoid cells *in vitro*. The most striking observation is that it suppresses cytokine-driven growth of these cells. The data demonstrate a significant increase in the proportion of G_1 phase cells when sirolimus is added [44]. The mechanism of action of sirolimus is to inhibit specifically the progression of cells from G_1 into the S phase, suggesting that it may interfere with the signaling that is critical for the cyclin/cyclin dependent kinase (CDK) complex required for cellular proliferation. Recent data using human peripheral blood T cells demonstrate that the block of G_1 may be related to an increase in a species of titratable inhibitor of G_1 cyclin/CDK [45]. In addition to regulation of the cell cycle, sirolimus may also exert an effect in signal transduction pathways which mediates specific cytokine responses. For example, sirolimus has been shown to inhibit IL-1 driven IFN-γ production [46]. Moreover, the secondary signals required for T-cell activation and proliferation are dependent on ligation of the B7 family with CD28. Lack of the secondary signal has been shown to result in anergy in the responding T cell. While the signaling through the TCR is not affected by sirolimus, the signaling through CD28 is inhibited by sirolimus [47]. CD28 signaling leads to a sustained down regulation of the inhibitor I kappa B (IκB). CD28 mediated down regulation of IκB-α is prevented by sirolimus. These data suggest that sirolimus affects the CD28 signaling pathway which may be a significant mechanism of its action and distinct from either CSP or tacrolimus.

Toxicity

There have not yet been any large clinical studies with this agent in BMT recipients. Its use has been primarily centered on a second or third line regimen for patients developing acute or chronic GVHD. Most of these reports have been abstracts presented at meetings. What is currently known is based on animal observations as well as studies in the field of solid organ transplantation. These data suggest that sirolimus is toxic to the GI system including elevation of liver function tests and diarrhea. In contrast to the renal side-effects which are common with CSP and tacrolimus, nephrotoxicity is rarely encountered with sirolimus. However, sirolimus may potentiate the nephrotoxicity of CSP [48,49]. Other toxicities of sirolimus include hypertriglyceridemia, a decrease in platelets and leukocytes, epistaxis, blood pressure changes, headaches, nausea, mucous membrane irritation and infections. Adverse reactions previously observed with other macrolide antibiotics are also of concern. Testicular atrophy has been observed in both mice and nonhuman primates. These early observations suggest that liver function abnormalities, thrombocytopenia, and neutropenia may be its dose limiting toxicity.

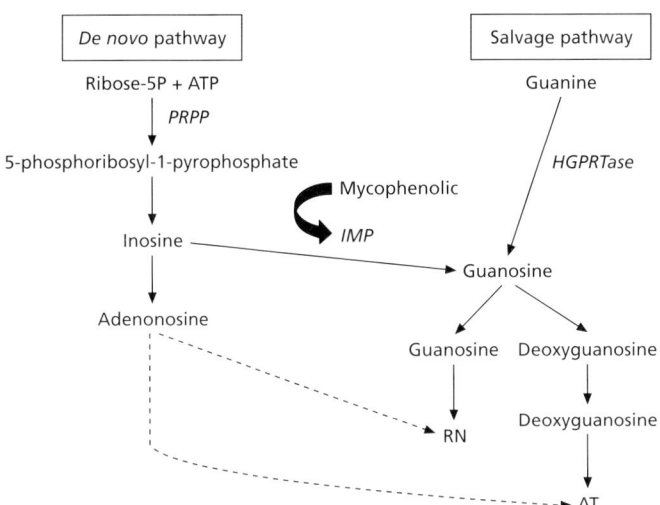

Fig. 16.5 The salvage and *de novo* pathway of purine synthesis. Inositol monophosphate (IMP) is at a central position and mycophenolate mofetil (MMF) inhibits IMP dehydrogenase. HGPRTase, hypoxanthine-guanine phosphoryboxyltransferase; PRPP, 5-phosphoriboxyl-1-pyrophosphate.

Mycophenolate mofetil (MMF)

MMF is a morpholinoethyl ester of mycophenolic acid (MPA). MPA is produced by several species of *Penicillium* molds and this agent possesses antibacterial, antifungal, antiviral, antitumor and immunosuppressive properties [50]. MMF's immunosuppressive activity occurs after hydrolysis to MPA. Therefore, MPA is the active moiety but it is formulated as MMF to enhance its bioavailability. MMF inhibits the proliferation of T and B cells and the production of antibodies [51,52]. Most of the clinical data are in the solid organ literature. The developmental work on MMF has utilized the dog model in BMT. Studies in the dog model of allogeneic transplantation by Storb *et al.* [53] demonstrated that the combination of MMF/CSP was highly effective at the prevention of host-vs.-graft rejection and graft-vs.-host reaction following a nonmyeloablative regimen. These studies have led to the marked increase in this form of transplantation worldwide. The contribution of MMF to the development of this approach was significant.

Pharmacology

Purines are essential for the growth and survival of cells. Cells have two pathways to produce purines: *de novo* and salvage pathways. Lymphocytes are highly dependent on the *de novo* synthesis while other cells can utilize both (Fig. 16.5). In the *de novo* pathway, the ribose-phosphate portion of the purine nucleotide is derived from 5-phosphoribosyl-1-pyrophosphate which is derived from adenosine triphosphate and the sugar ribose-5-phosphate. Therefore, 5-phosphoribosyl-1-pyrophosphate is an essential intermediary in the synthesis of purines. Following T-cell stimulation, there is a brisk and sustained increase in 5-phosphoribosyl-1-pyrophosphate and guanosines and deoxyguanosines activate 5-phosphoribosyl-1-pyrophosphate synthetase [54]. Therefore, depletion of guanosines would lead to a decrease in 5-phosphoribosyl-1-pyrophosphate synthetase and inhibition of purine synthesis which is required for T-cell activation. MPA action is through the inhibition of inosine monophosphate dehydrogenase (IMPDH). This enzyme catalyzes oxidation of inosine monophosphate to xanthine monophosphate. Xanthine monophosphate is a required intermediate metabolite in the synthesis of guanosine triphosphate. The enzyme IMPDH is a critical enzyme for the *de novo* biosynthesis of purine nucleotides, specifically guanosine monophosphate (GMP). Blockade of GMP synthesis leads to a negative feedback inhibition of 5-phosphoribosyl-1-pyrophosphate and prevention of T-cell activation. The therapeutic index of MMF depends on the lymphocytes reliance on *de novo* synthesis of purines, allowing for greater immunosuppressive activity with less toxicity.

Toxicity

Most of the trials in humans have demonstrated the efficacy of the drug in preventing early acute rejection in the first 6 months following renal transplantation [55–57]. MMF has been administered in the allograft setting using 15 mg/kg IV every 8 h or orally twice daily. The side-effects of the drug at this dose have been quite minimal. The major effect has been suppression of the hematopoietic system with neutropenia as an important side-effect. GI side-effects have also been reported occasionally. The optimal dose of MMF has not been determined but doses as high as 15 mg/kg four times daily have been reported to be tolerable. Of note, MMF does not seem to deplete GTP in neutrophils in contrast to lymphocytes and monocytes. Its selective action on lymphocytes seems to spare the higher risk of acute infections. Doses up to 1.5 g twice daily had no nephrotoxicity, myelosuppression or other serious side-effects in patients with rheumatoid arthritis [58]. Methods to monitor drug levels of MMF are being developed.

Antibodies

Many antibodies have been used for the prevention and treatment of GVHD. Most of the promising data have come from studies using selected monoclonal antibodies directed at specific epitopes. However, these antibodies are not generally available and most of the studies have involved small groups of patients. Several antibodies will be discussed, namely intravenous immunoglobulin (IVIg), anti-CD3, antithymocyte globulin (ATG), daclizumab or basiliximab (anti-IL-2 receptor) and infliximab (anti-TNF-α receptor).

Anti CD-3

OKT3 is an anti CD-3 monoclonal antibody that is commercially available. This antibody has been used to treat GVHD, but because it is a stimulatory antibody to the T cell, the results have not been uniformly successful [59,60]. Carpenter and colleagues have shown that soluble antihuman CD3 monoclonal antibodies induce apoptosis of activated T cells. They evaluated different anti-CD3 antibodies and demonstrated that the ability to induce apoptosis varied among them. Compared with OKT3, one monoclonal termed HuM291 induced more sustained phosphorylation of ERK-2, greater release of IFN-γ, and more activation-induced T-cell death [61]. The use of HuM291 (visilizumab) in a phase I study in patients with steroid refractory acute GVHD was highly encouraging and this agent is currently undergoing clinical trials for the treatment of steroid refractory acute GVHD as well as front line therapy for those who develop grade II–IV acute GVHD. This antibody is not capable of crosslinking with Fc receptors on accessory cells and therefore does not activate proliferation of T cells. In one study, of the 17 enrolled patients, five achieved a complete resolution of GVHD, eight had partial improvement, two showed no change, and two progressed [61]. Eight of the 13 responders had sustained responses, but the estimated one-year survival was only 24%.

Intravenous immunoglobulin (IVIg)

Polyclonal human immunoglobulins purified and sterilized from serum pooled from many donors have been used to manipulate the immune system [62]. There are many preparations of IVIg with different titres of anti-cytomegalovirus activity. To date there are no known clinical differences with the use of any of these commercial preparations. Occasionally, one preparation may be preferable to another based on the need to conserve on the volume that a patient receives. The initial studies focused on its use to prevent infectious complications following BMT [63,64]. However, in a large randomized trial of IVIg, this product was also associated with a decrease in the incidence of GVHD, especially in BMT recipients under the age of 20 years. Moreover, there was a decrease in the overall mortality in favor of those who had received IVIg [63]. While this agent is effective in the early phase following BMT, its prolonged use, in the absence of hypogammaglobulinemia after day +100, does not reduce late complications or chronic GVHD and may be associated with impairment of humoral immune recovery [65]. Moreover, serious issues such as the extremely high costs of these products and occasional limited availability have led to a drop in their use.

Antithymocyte globulin (ATG)

ATG is a polyclonal immunoglobulin prepared by injecting horses or rabbits with human thymocytes. These antibodies are capable of destroying human leukocytes. Since the process of generating this product is inconsistent (i.e. different animals, different pooled lymphocytes, different dominant responses), it is difficult to determine pharmacokinetics and efficacy because there is significant lot-to-lot and animal-to-animal variabilities. The half-life of these antibodies also vary significantly between the horse vs. rabbit ATG and the functional half-life of these antibodies is not well defined, although rabbit ATG is more potent than horse ATG. ATG has been used as part of the preparatory regimen prior to infusion of donor cells to decrease the incidence of graft rejection or following BMT to prevent GVHD. In two prospective studies using ATG as part of GVHD prophylaxis, ATG was not effective [66,67]. Its use as therapy of GVHD has also been tested. The response rates are encouraging but the overall survival remains poor [68]. The doses varied widely, but were generally in the range of 10–30 mg/kg/day (for horse ATG). Since ATG is a foreign xenogeneic protein and an antibody, serum sickness can occur. Corticosteroids, acetaminophen, H1 and H2 blockers are frequently used to prevent or treat the symptoms associated with the infusion of ATG. The use of ATG after BMT has been associated with an increase in lymphoproliferative disorders [69].

Anticytokine therapy

Several cytokines have been implicated in GVHD. IL-2 is a critical molecule in T-cell survival and stimulation. There are two monoclonal antibodies in clinical use directed against the IL-2 α receptor (daclizumab) as well as a chimeric anti-IL-2 monoclonal antibody (basiliximab) [70]. The bulk of the data have been obtained from solid organ allograft rejection studies. The use of anticytokine agents in stem cell transplantation is limited. The initial results of the use of dacluzimab are encouraging, although these are phase II data and further studies are necessary to confirm these encouraging results. As with all antibodies, toxicities associated with such proteins are common and include myalgia, fevers, rash, pruritus, arthritis, and headaches.

TNF is another cytokine that has been implicated in acute GVHD. Use of a polyclonal neutralizing antibody against TNF-α resulted in a 70% reduction in GVHD-associated mortality and also in diminished lesions in the skin and the intestines in an experimental model [71]. Similar findings were observed using a neutralizing antibody against murine TNF with reduction of splenomegaly in GVHD models [72]. Higher TNF levels have also been described in those patients who develop GVHD, although this finding has not been universally observed [73]. There are two anti-TNF molecules. Infliximab is a chimeric monoclonal antibody that binds to TNF. There is also a fusion molecule, etanercept, that consists of the soluble TNF receptor (p75) linked to the Fc portion of human IgG_1 (TNFR : Fc) [74,75]. These molecules are successful in the therapy of Crohn's disease and rheumatoid arthritis and could be equally useful following allogeneic BMT, but well designed studies will be necessary. There are preliminary data for the use of infliximab in the therapy of acute GVHD, but these data have not been reported in the peer-reviewed literature. Given the known importance of cytokines such as TNF in the genesis of GVHD, the use of such agents will be explored further both for therapy and prevention.

Other agents

Thalidomide

Thalidomide was first synthesized in March 1954 by W.H. Kunz, a chemist working for Chemie Gruenenthal, in Germany. The antihistaminic properties for which it was initially synthesized were weak, but it produced significant sedation in animals leading to its clinical use as a sedative. Its use was widespread until the observation of increased limb malformations was reported in Germany and neighboring countries, which led to the withdrawal of the drug from the market.

The first new indication for the use of thalidomide following BMT came from animal studies done in 1966 in which allogeneic BMT recipients treated with thalidomide had a splenic weight that was lower than those who received placebo, demonstrating that GVHD activity was decreased by the addition of thalidomide [76]. It is important to note that thalidomide should be considered more as an "immunomodulator" since it lacks a global inhibitory effect upon lymphocyte proliferation and does not impair delayed type hypersensitivity [77].

Pharmacology

Thalidomide (2-(2,6-dioxo-piperidine-3-yl)-iso-indole-1,3-dione) is a racemic mixture in which both enantiomers undergo racemization with a relatively fast velocity under physiologic conditions. There are data to suggest that the S-form may be the major enantiomer associated with the immune effects [77]. Thalidomide is poorly water soluble and is not well absorbed when given orally. Thalidomide is degraded into 12 breakdown products. About 40% of the oral dose is excreted renally as hydrolysis products. The intracellular activities of thalidomide are not well understood. The observation of its teratogenic effect led to the suggestion that inhibition of angiogenesis led to the defect of limb bud formation. There has been keen interest to understand thalidomide's interaction with angiogenesis as well as its interaction with vascular or endothelial adhesion molecules. For example, up-regulation of the adhesion molecules E-selectin and vascular cell adhesion molecule (VCAM) is inhibited by high concentrations of thalidomide [78]. Effects on these molecules may be one mechanism of action by which thalidomide leads to immunosuppression. For example, interference with adhesion of T cells to antigen-presenting cells or proper T-cell migration and trafficking may result in a delay or prevention of T-cell responses. There have been some suggestions that thalidomide analogs may bind with high avidity to macrophages as well as CD4 and CD8 cells [77]. While the mechanistic effects of thalidomide are not known, its effects are clearly distinct from those of steroids and CSP or the macrolide immunosuppressants. They also differ from phosphodiesterase inhibitors such as pentoxyfiline, inhibitors of arachidonic acid synthesis, nucleotide analogs or natural products such as MPA.

Toxicity

The major side-effects of thalidomide in its use following BMT are its sedative effects and constipation. These are dose related. Many of these side-effects may improve with continued use of the drug [79]. In the study of 80 patients with steroid resistant chronic GVHD at Stanford

University and the City of Hope National Medical Center, the toxicities of thalidomide were: sedation (40%), constipation/nausea (30%), neutropenia or thrombocytopenia (18%), new skin rash (16%) and neuropathy (5%) [80]. The primary reasons for discontinuation of the drug were the neuropathy and neutropenia, although occasionally sedation and the GI symptoms were severe enough to warrant stoppage. Infectious complications were not a common finding in this group of patients.

Clinical use

Thalidomide has primarily been used for the treatment of chronic GVHD with a response rate ranging from 20% to 60% depending on the timing and the patient population [79,80]. Because the drug is available only as an oral formulation it has not been tried systematically in the therapy of acute GVHD. The dose of the drug has not been well defined. Correlative studies have suggested that up to 1.6 g of thalidomide in divided doses are necessary to achieve the equivalent serum levels found in the rodent system to obtain an effect on GVHD [81]. Thalidomide is usually started at a dose of 100 mg twice a day and escalated gradually by doubling the dose every 4–7 days to achieve a dose of 800–1600 mg based on patient tolerability and acceptance. The median dose of thalidomide was 800 mg/day in divided doses in one study [80]. If the patient responded and improved, the drug was maintained for 6–12 months and then gradually tapered. If a patient's GVHD flared, the drug was increased back to the prior level. Use of a laxative is helpful and often one dose of thalidomide can be taken prior to bedtime to take advantage of its sedative effects.

Thalidomide has also been tested for prevention of chronic GVHD [82]. The rationale was that perhaps a lower dose of a drug that was effective in the treatment of chronic GVHD would be effective in preventing the occurrence of chronic GVHD. Patients were randomized to receive either placebo or thalidomide (200 mg orally twice a day) beginning 80 days following allogeneic BMT. Fifty-three evaluable patients were analyzed, 26 patients received placebo and 27 patients received thalidomide. Following the first interim analysis using intent to treat parameters, there was a statistically significant difference in the incidence of chronic GVHD. Surprisingly, patients receiving thalidomide developed more chronic GVHD compared to patients receiving placebo ($p = 0.05$). Moreover, there was an advantage of overall survival for patients receiving placebo compared to those receiving thalidomide ($p = 0.005$). These results demonstrated that while thalidomide might be of some benefit in the therapy of chronic GVHD, its use at these doses for the prophylaxis of chronic GVHD resulted in a paradoxical outcome with a higher incidence of chronic GVHD and a lower overall survival. Thalidomide treatment appeared to effect a shift in the balance between GVHD and induction of tolerance. These data demonstrate again the importance of phase III double-blind controlled randomized studies.

Clofazimine

Clofazimine is another drug that, like thalidomide, has been used to treat leprosy. Clofazimine is a substituted, phendimetrazine tartrate-derived, iminophenazine dye, which becomes sequestered in macrophages and possibly neutrophils. The drug inhibits mycobacterial growth by binding to bacterial DNA. Of interest, this drug not only was successful in treating the mycobacterium, but it was also able to treat the skin inflammation associated with leprosy as well as other autoimmune skin disorders. The mechanism of action of this drug in GVHD is not known. Patients were treated with a dose of 300 mg orally daily for 90 days and then the dose was lowered to 100 mg daily indefinitely [83]. The patients tolerated this regimen well with GI and hyperpigmentation being the most common side-effect. The preliminary results have been encouraging but again, the overall experience is limited.

Hydroxychloroquine

Hydroxychloroquine is a 4-aminoquinoline antimalarial drug used for the treatment of autoimmune diseases. Laboratory observations demonstrated that hydroxychloroquine blocks antigen processing and presentation. Hydroxychloroquine appears to prevent the function of transporter associated with antigen processing (TAP) proteins, which are essential for the proper transport of peptides with the major histocompatibility complex (MHC) molecules to the cell surface [84]. This block in antigen presentation leads to a drop in cytokine production, and cytotoxicity. Moreover, in laboratory experiments, this drug is synergistic with CSP and tacrolimus. Hydroxychloroquine (800 mg or 12 mg/kg) has been used clinically for patients with steroid refractory chronic GVHD in a phase II study [85]. Forty patients were studied. There were three complete responses and 14 partial responses in 32 evaluable patients (53% response rate). Of note, all patients who responded were able to have their steroid dose attenuated. There was no significant toxicity attributed to hydroxychloroquine. A prospective randomized study for the treatment of chronic GVHD is ongoing.

Novel agents

Peptides/polymers

With the improved understanding of the mechanisms of T-cell antigen recognition and the pathways of T-cell activation, novel approaches have been developed in laboratory models to specifically target one or more of the signaling pathways to prevent or decrease T-cell responses. When the BMT recipient and donor are identical at the MHC, GVHD occurs through recognition by the T cell and its receptor of different peptides bound to the MHC, the so-called minor histocompatibility antigens. Because the manner by which a protein is processed is dependent on genes outside of the MHC, two siblings will have many different peptides in the MHC groove. Therefore, one potential area to interfere with signal recognition is at the level of MHC–peptide–TCR interaction. Administration of peptides with high affinity binding for their respective MHC class II molecules prevented GVHD in two different murine models [86]. This prevention of GVHD was also confirmed by using a random copolymer consisting of l-amino acids: glutamic acid, lysine, alanine and tyrosine. This polymer binds ubiquitously to class II MHC molecules in mice and in humans. Use of this polymer in a murine model of GVHD demonstrated that it is capable of preventing GVHD and is associated with a significant survival difference [87]. A feasibility study in 12 patients at Stanford and Duke University with severe acute GVHD demonstrated no clear toxicity with some encouraging responses. A larger phase II trial is planned. Another approach has been developed using a peptide derived from the D1 immunoglobulin-like domain of the CD4 molecule [88]. This D1 region is involved in binding to nonpolymorphic sites of the class II molecule. Use of a peptide analog that mimicked the surface of the CDR3-like region of the CD4-D1 domain was very effective in the prevention of the mixed lymphocyte reaction and GVHD. This peptide appears to inhibit only antigen specific responses and may be effective by binding to either donor or host cells.

Induction of anergy

Data generated from studies of T-cell activation have clearly demonstrated that there is a critical need for a second costimulatory signal for a positive immune response. Lack of secondary signals results in specific T-cell anergy. CTLA-4-Ig is a fusion protein designed in an attempt to prevent costimulation signals. Variable results have been observed using the CTLA-4-Ig fusion protein to block GVHD across major

Drug	Target	Mechanism(s) of action
Corticosteroids	Steroid receptor	Multiple, including cytokine expression, lymphocyte activation and cell depletion
MTX	DHFR	Blocks DNA synthesis
CSP	Calcineurin	Blocks lymphocyte activation
Tacrolimus	Calcineurin	Blocks lymphocyte activation
Sirolimus	mTOR	Blocks costimulatory signal and cell division
MPA	IMPD	Blocks DNA synthesis
Dacluzimab/basiliximab	IL-2 receptor	Blocks lymphocyte activation
IVIg	Multiple	Unknown
ATG	Multiple	Blocks lymphocyte activation
Infliximab	TNF receptor	Blocks lymphocyte activation
Etanercept	TNF	Blocks lymphocyte activation
Thalidomide	Unknown	Unknown
Clofazimine	Unknown	Unknown
Hydroxychloroquine	TAP proteins	Blocks lymphocyte activation
GLAT polymer	MHC class II	Blocks lymphocyte activation
CD4-D1 peptide	CD4	Blocks lymphocyte activation
CTLA-4-Ig	CD28	Blocks lymphocyte activation

Table 16.4 Immunosuppressive drugs, target and mechanism of action discussed in this chapter.

ATG, antithymocyte globulin; CSP, cyclosporine; DHFR, dihydrofolate reductase; IL, interleukin; IMPD, inosine monophosphate dehydrogenase; IVIG, intravenous immunoglobulin; MHC, major histocompatibility complex; MPA, mycophenolic acid; MTA, mycophenolic acid; MTX, methotrexate; TAP, transporter associated with antigen processing; TNF, tumor necrosis factor.

histocompatibility barriers [89]. These results may be variable according to the model of GVHD selected (i.e. major histocompatibility differences) or the activation state of T cells. Methods to block costimulation hold significant promise in achieving antigen specific unresponsiveness or anergy and therefore a state of tolerance [90,91]. In a clinical trial of tolerance induction, haplo-identical bone marrow was treated *ex vivo* with CTLA-4-Ig in the presence of recipient peripheral blood [92]. The laboratory parameters such as T-cell precursor frequency against allogeneic targets were markedly reduced. The preliminary clinical data were encouraging with low incidence of GVHD and encouraging overall survival. Such new approaches may circumvent the need for prolonged immunosuppression after BMT and may be clinically beneficial for patients who require an allogeneic BMT.

Conclusion

This chapter has focused primarily on the most frequently used drugs for immunosuppression or immunomodulation for GVHD (Table 16.4). Other drugs or nonpharmacological treatment options which appear to be promising are psoralen and ultraviolet light A (PUVA), radiation therapy for chronic GVHD and other novel molecules such as a fusion immunotoxins directed against CD3 [93]. Because GVHD and solid organ rejection remain such a difficult clinical problem, there is a need for continued efforts to develop novel immunosuppressive or immunomodulatory agents.

References

1 Ferrara JLM, Deeg HJ. Graft-versus-host disease. *N Engl J Med* 1997; **324**: 667–74.
2 Antin JH, Ferrara JLM. Cytokine dysregulation and acute graft-versus-host disease. *Blood* 1992; **80**: 2964–9.
3 Cohen JJ, Fischbach M, Claman HN. Hydrocortisone resistance of graft vs. host activity in mouse thymus, spleen and bone marrow. *J Immunol* 1970; **105**: 1146–50.
4 Almawi WY, Lipman ML, Stevens AC, Zanker B, Hadro ET, Strom TB. Abrogation of glucocorticoid-mediated inhibition of T cell proliferation by the synergistic action of IL-1, IL-6 and IFN gamma. *J Immunol* 1991; **146**: 3523–7.
5 Holler E, Kolb HJ, Wilmanns W. Treatment of GVHD-TNF antibodies and related antagonists. *Bone Marrow Transplant* 1993; **3**: 29–31.
6 Chao NJ, Schmidt GM, Niland JC *et al*. Cyclosporine, methotrexate, and prednisone compared with cyclosporine and prednisone for prophylaxis of acute graft-versus-host disease. *N Eng J Med* 1993; **327**: 1225–30.
7 Ruutu T, Volin L, Parkkali T *et al*. Cyclosporine, methotrexate, and methylprednisolone compared with cyclosporine and methotrexate for the prevention of graft-versus-host disease in bone marrow transplantation from HLA-identical sibling donor: a prospective randomized study. *Blood* 2000; **96**: 2391–8.
8 Chao NJ, Snyder DS, Jain M *et al*. Equivalence of two effective graft-versus-host disease prophylaxis regimens: results of a prospective double-blind randomized trial. *Biol Blood Marrow Transplant* 2000; **6**: 254–61.
9 McDonald GB, Bouvier M, Hockenbery DM *et al*. Oral beclomethasone dipropionate for treatment of intestinal graft-versus-host disease: a randomized, controlled trial. *Gastroenterology* 1998; **115**: 28–35.
10 Bleyer WA. Methotrexate. clinical pharmacology, current status and therapeutic guidelines. *Cancer Treat Rev* 1977; **4**: 87–94.
11 Storb R, Epstein RB, Graham TC, Thomas ED. Methotrexate regimens for control of graft-versus-host disease in dogs with allogeneic marrow grafts. *Transplantation* 1970; **9**: 240–6.
12 Zaharko DS, Fung W-P, Yang F-H. Relative biochemical aspects of low and high doses of methotrexate in mice. *Cancer Res* 1977; **37**: 1602–7.
13 Bertino JR. Karnofsky memorial lecture. Ode to methotrexate. *J Clin Oncol* 1993; **11**: 5–14.
14 Henderson ES, Adamson RH, Denham C, Oliverio VT. The metabolic fate of tritiated methotrexate. II. Absorption and excretion in man. *Cancer Res* 1965; **25**: 1018–23.
15 Schilsky RL, Bailey BD, Chabner BA *et al*. Methotrexate polyglutamate synthesis by cultured human breast cancer cells. *Proc Natl Acad Sci* 1980; **77**: 2919–24.

16 Fabre G, Goldman ID. Formation of 7-hydroxy-methotrexate polyglutamyl derivatives and their cytotoxicity in human chronic myelogenous leukemia cells, *in vitro*. *Cancer Res* 1985; **25**: 1227–32.

17 Storb R, Deeg HJ, Whitehead J et al. Methotrexate and cyclosporine versus cyclosporine alone for prophylaxis of acute graft-versus-host disease after marrow transplantation for leukemia. *N Engl J Med* 1986; **314**: 729–35.

18 Przepiorka D, Ippoliti C, Khouri I et al. Tacrolimus and minidose methotrexate for prevention of acute graft-versus-host disease after matched unrelated donor marrow transplantation. *Blood* 1996; **88**: 4383–9.

19 Nevill TJ, Tirgan MH, Deeg HJ et al. Influence of post-methotrexate folinic acid rescue on regimen-related toxicity and graft-versus-host disease after allogeneic bone marrow transplantation. *Bone Marrow Transplant* 1993; **11**: 251–6.

20 Borel JF. The history of cyclosporin A and its significance. In: White DJG, ed. *Cyclosporin A*. New York: Elsevier, 1982; 5–18.

21 Bierer BE. Advances in therapeutic immunosuppression. biology, molecular actions and clinical implications. *Curr Opin Hematol* 1993; **1**: 149–59.

22 Bram RJ, Hung DT, Martin PK, Schreiber SL, Crabtree GR. Identification of the immunophilins capable of mediating inhibition of signal transduction by cyclosporin A and tacrolimus: roles of calcineurin and cellular location. *Mol Cell Biol* 1993; **13**: 4760–9.

23 Gething M-J, Sambrook J. Protein folding in the cell. *Nature* 1992; **355**: 33–45.

24 Nebert DW, Nelson DR, Adesnik M et al. The P450 superfamily: update listing of all genes and recommended nomenclature for the chromosomal loci. *DNA* 1989; **8**: 1–13.

25 Bennett WM, Pulliam JP. Cyclosporine nephrotoxicity. *Ann Int Med* 1983; **99**: 851–4.

26 Petric R, Freeman DJ, Wallace C, McDonald J, Stiller C, Keown P. Effect of cyclosporine on urinary prostanoic excretion, renal blood flow and glomerulotubular function. *Transplantation* 1988; **45**: 883–9.

27 Gluckman E, Lokeic F, Devergie A. Pharmacokinetic monitoring of cyclosporine in allogeneic bone marrow transplants. *Transplant Proc* 1980; **20**: 122–30.

28 Santos GW, Tutschka PJ, Brookmeyer R et al. Cyclosporine plus methylprednisolone versus cyclophosphamide plus methylprednisolone as prophylaxis for graft-versus-host disease: a randomized double-blind study in patients undergoing allogeneic marrow transplantation. *Clin Transplant* 1987; **1**: 21–8.

29 Yee GC, Self SG, McGuire TR, Carlin J, Sanders JE, Deeg HJ. Serum cyclosporine concentrations and risk of acute graft-versus-host disease after allogeneic marrow transplantation. *N Engl J Med* 1988; **99**: 851–4.

30 Yee GV, McGuire R. Pharmacokinetic drug interactions with cyclosporin (Part I). *Clin Pharmacokinet* 1990; **19**: 319–32.

31 Yee GV, McGuire R. Pharmacokinetic drug interactions with cyclosporin (Part II). *Clin Pharmacokinet* 1990; **19**: 400–15.

32 Kino T, Hatanaka H, Miyata S et al. FK506, a novel immunosuppressant isolated from a Streptomyces. II. Immunosuppressive effects of FK506 *in vitro*. *J Antibiot* 1987; **40**: 1256–65.

33 Lee C, Jusko W, Shaefer M et al. Pharmacokinetics of tacrolimus (FK506) in liver transplant patients. *Clin Pharmacol Ther* 1993; **53**: 181–6.

34 Mekki Q, Lee C, Aweeka F et al. Pharmacokinetics of tacrolimus (FK506) in kidney transplant patients. *Clin Pharmacol Ther* 1993; **53**: 238–42.

35 Ratanatharathorn V, Nash RA, Przepiorka D et al. Phase III study comparing methotrexate and tacrolimus (Prograf®, FK506) with methotrexate and cyclosporine for graft-versus-host disease prophylaxis after HLA-identical sibling bone marrow transplantation. *Blood* 1998; **92**: 2303–14.

36 Hiraoka A, Ohashi Y, Okamoto S et al. The Japanese FK506 BMT (Bone Marrow Transplantation) Study Group. Phase III study comparing tacrolimus (FK506) with cyclosporine for graft-versus-host disease prophylaxis after allogeneic bone marrow transplantation. *Bone Marrow Transplant* 2001; **28**: 181–5.

37 Nash RA, Pineiro LA, Storb R et al. FK506 in combination with methotrexate for the prevention of graft-versus-host disease after marrow transplantation from matched unrelated donors. *Blood* 1996; **88**: 3634–41.

38 Przepiorka D, Ippoliti C, Khouri I et al. Tacrolimus and minidose methotrexate for prevention of acute graft-versus-host disease after matched unrelated donor marrow transplantation. *Blood* 1996; **88**: 4383–9.

39 Nash RA, Antin JH, Karanes C et al. Phase 3 study comparing methotrexate and tacrolimus with methotrexate and cyclosporine for prophylaxis of acute graft-versus-host disease after marrow transplantation from unrelated donors. *Blood* 2000; **96**: 2062–8.

40 Vezina C, Kudelski A, Sehgal SN. Rapamycin (AY-22,989), a new antifungal antibiotic. I. Taxonomy of the producing streptocycete and isolation of the active principle. *J Antibiot* 1975; **28**: 721–6.

41 Martel RR, Klicius J, Galet S. Inhibition of the immune response by rapamycin, a new antifungal antibiotic. *Can J Physiol* 1977; **55**: 48–51.

42 Morris RE, Meiser BM. Identification of a new pharmacologic action for an old compound. *Med Sci Res* 1989; **17**: 609–10.

43 Griffith JP, Kim JL, Sintchak MD et al. X-ray structure of calcineurin inhibited by the immunophilin-immunosuppressant FKBP-FK506 complex. *Cell* 1995; **82**: 507–22.

44 Morice W, Brunn G, Wiederrecht G, Siekierka J, Abraham R. Rapamycin-induced inhibition of p34^{cdc2} kinase activation is associated with G_1/S-phase growth arrest in T lymphocytes. *J Biol Chem* 1993; **268**: 3734–8.

45 Nourse J, Firpo E, Flanagan W et al. Interleukin-2-mediated elimination of the p27^{Kip1} cyclin-dependent kinase inhibitor prevented by rapamycin. *Nature* 1994; **372**: 570–3.

46 Altmeyer A, Dumont F. Rapamycin inhibits IL-1-mediated interferon-γ production in the YAC-1 T cell lymphoma. *Cytokine* 1993; **5**: 133–43.

47 Lai J-H, Tan T-H. CD28 signaling causes a sustained down-regulation of IκB-α which can be prevented by the immunosuppressant rapamycin. *J Biol Chem* 1994; **30**: 77–80.

48 Halloran PF. Sirolimus and cyclosporin for renal transplantation. *Lancet* 2000; **356**: 179–80.

49 McAlister VC, Gao Z, Peltekian K et al. Sirolimus-tracrolimus combination immunosuppression. *Lancet* 2000; **355**: 376–7.

50 Franklin TJ, Cook JM. The inhibition of nucleic acid synthesis by mycophenolic acid. *Biochem J* 1969; **113**: 515–24.

51 Halloran P, Mathew T, Tomlanovich S et al. Mycophenolate mofetil in renal allograft recipients: a pooled efficacy analysis of three randomized, double blind, clinical studies in prevention of rejection. *Transplantation* 1997; **63**: 39–47.

52 Suthanthiran M, Morris RE, Strom TB. Immunosuppressants: cellular and molecular mechanisms of action. *Am J Kidney Dis* 1996; **28**: 159–72.

53 Storb R, Yu C, Wagner JL et al. Stable mixed hematopoietic chimerism in DLA-identical littermate dogs given sublethal total body irradiation before and pharmacological immunosuppression after marrow transplantation. *Blood* 1997; **89**: 3048–54.

54 Hovi T, Allison AC, Allsop J. Rapid increase of phosphorybosil pyrophosphate concentration after mitogenic stimulation of lymphocytes. *FEBS Lett* 1975; **55**: 291–3.

55 Sollinger HW, Deierhoi MH, Belzer FO, Dielthelm A, Kauffman RS. RS-61443. A phase I clinical trial and pilot rescue study. *Transplantation* 1992; **53**: 428–32.

56 Sollinger HW, Belzer FO, Deierhoi MH et al. RS-61443 (mycophenolate mofetil). A multicenter study for refractory kidney transplant rejection. *Am Surg* 1993; **216**: 513–6.

57 Freise CE, Hebert M, Osorio RW et al. Maintenance immunosuppression with prednisolone and RS-61443 alone following liver transplantation. *Transplant Proc* 1993; **25**: 1758–9.

58 Schiff MH, Goldblum R, Rees MMC. 2-Morpholino-ethyl mycophenolic acid (ME-MPA) in the treatment of refractory rheumatoid arthritis. *Arthritis Rheum* 1990; **33**: s1–5.

59 Martin PJ, Hansen JA, Anasetti C et al. Treatment of acute graft-versus-host disease with anti-CD3 monoclonal antibodies. *Am J Kidney Dis* 1988; **11**: 149–52.

60 Anasetti C, Martin PJ, Storb R et al. Treatment of acute graft-versus-host disease with a nonmitogenic anti-CD3 monoclonal antibody. *Transplantation* 1992; **54**: 844–51.

61 Carpenter PA, Appelbaum FR, Corey L et al. A humanized non-FcR-binding anti-CD3 antibody, visilizumab, for treatment of steroid-refractory acute graft-versus-host disease. *Blood* 2002; **99**: 2712–9.

62 Dwyer JM. Manipulating the immune system with immune globulin. *N Engl J Med* 1992; **326**: 107–116.

63 Winston DJ, Ho WG, Lin C-H et al. Intravenous immune globulin for prevention of cytomegalovirus infection and interstitial pneumonia after bone marrow transplantation. *Ann Intern Med* 1987; **106**: 2–18.

64 Sullivan KM, Kopecky KJ, Jocom J et al. Immunomodulatory and antimicrobial efficacy of intravenous immunoglobulin in bone marrow transplantation. *N Engl J Med* 1990; **323**: 705–12.

65 Sullivan KM, Storek J, Kopecky KJ et al. A controlled trial of long-term administration of intravenous immunoglobulin to prevent late infection and chronic graft-vs.-host disease after marrow transplantation: Clinical outcome and effect on subsequent immune recovery. *Biol Blood Marrow Transplant* 1996; **2**: 44–53.

66 Weiden PL, Doney K, Storb R, Thomas ED. Anti-human thymocyte globulin for prophylaxis of graft-versus-host disease. A randomized trial in patients with leukemia treated with HLA-identical sibling marrow grafts. *Transplantation* 1979; **27**: 227–30.

67 Doney KC, Weiden PL, Storb R, Thomas ED. Failure of early administration of antithymocyte globulin to lessen graft-versus-host disease in human allogeneic marrow transplant recipients. *Transplantation* 1981; **31**: 141–3.

68 Dugan MJ, DeFor TE, Steinbuch M *et al.* ATG plus corticosteroid therapy for acute graft-versus-host disease: predictors of response and survival. *Ann Hematol* 1997; **75**: 41–6.

69 Bhatia S, Ramsay NK, Steinbuch M *et al.* Malignant neoplasms following bone marrow transplantation. *Blood* 1996; **87**: 3633–9.

70 Przepiorka D, Kernan NA, Ippoliti C *et al.* Daclizumab, a humanized anti-interleukin-2 receptor alpha chain antibody, for treatment of acute graft-versus-host disease. *Blood* 2000; **95**(1): 83–9.

71 Piguet P, Grau GE, Allet B, Vassalli P. Tumor necrosis factor/cachectin is an effector of skin and gut lesions of the acute phase of graft-vs.-host disease. *Blood* 1987; **166**: 1280–8.

72 Shalaby M, Fendly B, Sheehan K, Schreiber RD, Ammann AJ. Prevention of graft-versus-host reaction in newborn mice by antibodies to tumor necrosis alpha. *Transplantation* 1989; **47**: 1057–62.

73 Holler E, Kolb HJ, Møller A *et al.* Increased serum levels of tumor necrosis factor α precede major complications of bone marrow transplantation. *Blood* 1990; **75**: 1011–9.

74 Moreland LW, Baumgartner SW, Schiff MH *et al.* The treatment of rheumatoid arthritis with a recombinant human tumor necrosis factor receptor (p75)-Fc fusion protein. *N Engl J Med* 1997; **337**: 141–7.

75 Targan SR, Hanauer SB, van Deventer SJ *et al.* A short-term study of chimeric monoclonal antibody cA2 to tumor necrosis factor alpha for Crohn's disease. Crohn's Disease cA2 Study Group. *N Engl J Med* 1997; **337**: 1029–35.

76 Fields EO, Gibbs JE, Tucker DF, Hellmann K. Effect of thalidomide on graft-versus-host reaction. *Nature* 1966; **211**: 1308–10.

77 Zwingenberger K, Wendt S. Immunomodulation by thalidomide. Systematic review of the literature and of unpublished observations. *J Inflam* 1996; **46**: 77–211.

78 Nogeira AC, Neubert R, Neubert D. Thalidomide and the immune system. 3. Simultaneous up- and down-regulation of different integrin receptors on human white blood cells. *Life Sci* 1994; **55**: 77–92.

79 Vogelsang GB, Evan MD, Farmer ER *et al.* Thalidomide for the treatment of chronic graft-versus-host disease. *N Engl J Med* 1992; **326**: 1055–60.

80 Parker PM, Chao N, Nademanee A *et al.* Thalidomide as salvage therapy for chronic graft-versus-host disease. *Blood* 1995; **86**: 3604–9.

81 Vogelsang GB, Hess AD, Friedman KJ, Santos GW. Therapy of chronic graft-v-host disease in a rat model. *Blood* 1989; **74**: 507–12.

82 Chao NJ, Parker PM, Niland JC *et al.* Paradoxical effect of thalidomide prophylaxis on chronic graft-vs.-host disease. *Biol Blood Marrow Transplant* 1996; **2**: 86–92.

83 Lee SJ, Wegner SA, McGarigle CJ *et al.* Treatment of chronic graft-versus-host disease with clofazimine. *Blood* 1997; **89**: 2298–302.

84 Schultz KR, Bader S, Paquet J, Li W. Chloroquine treatment affects T cell priming to minor histocompatibility antigens and graft-versus-host disease. *Blood* 1995; **86**: 4344–52.

85 Gilman AL, Chan KW, Mogul A *et al.* Hydroxychloroquine for the treatment of chronic graft-versus-host disease. *Biol Blood Marrow Transplant* 2000; **6**: 327–34.

86 Schlegel PG, Aharoni R, Smilek DE *et al.* Prevention of graft-versus-host disease by peptides binding to class II major histocompatibility complex molecules. *Blood* 1994; **84**: 2902–9.

87 Schlegel PG, Aharoni R, Chen Y *et al.* A synthetic random basic copolymer with promiscuous binding to class II major histocompatibility complex molecules inhibits T cell proliferative responses to major and minor histocompatibility antigens *in vitro* and confers the capacity to prevent murine graft-versus-host disease *in vivo*. *Proc Natl Acad Sci* 1996; **93**: 5061–6.

88 Townsend RM, Briggs C, Marini JC, Murphy GF, Korngold R. Inhibitory effect of a CD4-CDR3 peptide analog on graft-versus-host disease across a major histocompatibility complex–haploidentical barrier. *Blood* 1996; **88**: 3038–47.

89 Wallace P, Johnson JS, MacMaster JF, Kennedy KA, Gladstone P, Linsley PS. CTLA4Ig treatment ameliorates the lethality of murine graft-versus-host disease across major histocompatibility complex barrier. *Transplantation* 1994; **58**: 602–9.

90 Gribben JG, Guinan EC, Boussiotis VA *et al.* Complete blockade of B7 family-mediated costimulation is necessary to induce human alloantigen-specific anergy: a method to ameliorate graft-versus-host disease and extend the donor pool. *Blood* 1996; **87**: 4887–93.

91 Blazar BR, Taylor PA, Panoskaltsis-Mortari A, Gray GS, Vallera DA. Coblockade of the LFA1: ICAM and CD28/CTLA4: B7 pathways is a highly effective means of preventing acute lethal graft-versus-host disease induced by fully major histocompatibility complex-disparate donor grafts. *Blood* 1995; **85**: 2607–18.

92 Guinan EC, Boussiotis VA, Neuberg D *et al.* Transplantation of anergic histoincompatible bone marrow allografts. *N Engl J Med* 1999; **340**: 1704–14.

93 Vallera DA, Panoskaltsis-Mortari A, Jost C *et al.* Anti-graft-versus-host disease effect of DT390-anti-CD3sFv, a single-chain Fv fusion immunotoxin specifically targeting the CD3 epsilon moiety of the T cell receptor. *Blood* 1996; **88**: 2342–53.

17

Robert J. Soiffer

T-Cell Depletion to Prevent Graft-vs.-Host Disease

Introduction

Graft-vs.-host disease (GVHD) is the most significant complication of allogeneic hematopoietic cell transplantation (HCT). Morbidity and mortality result as a consequence of direct organ damage and as sequelae of opportunistic infections promoted by the use of immune suppressive medications employed to prevent or treat GVHD [1–4]. Based on preclinical evidence implicating donor T cells in GVHD pathogenesis, numerous studies evaluating the effect of donor T-cell depletion (TCD) were undertaken in the 1980s. It was hoped that TCD could prevent GVHD and improve disease-free survival after allogeneic HCT [5]. Most early trials documented that TCD could substantially limit acute GVHD. However, these decreases in the incidence of severe GVHD were counterbalanced by unexpectedly high rates of graft failure, Epstein–Barr virus-associated lympoproliferative disorders (EBV-LPD), and disease recurrence. Efforts to reduce these complications of TCD by increasing the specificity of depletion, optimizing stem-cell number and adding safe and effective post-transplant immune modulation offer the hope that overall outcome of allogeneic HCT can be substantially improved.

T cells and GVHD

In the 1950s, experiments demonstrated that irradiated animals infused with inoculations of allogeneic marrow would develop a fatal wasting condition called "secondary phase of irradiation syndrome" [6]. It was subsequently demonstrated that this GVHD did not occur if the animals were infused with cells from fetal splenic tissue that lacked mature T lymphocytes [7]. These observations established the critical link between mature donor T lymphocytes and GVHD, and suggested the potential benefits of removing T cells from the allograft.

Animal models of TCD

The development of physical separation techniques to remove alloreactive lymphocytes from donor hematopoietic precursors permitted the first opportunity to assess the effect of graft engineering on GVHD. Irradiated mice infused with splenic cells that had undergone differential centrifugation on a discontinuous albumin gradient to remove lymphocytes experienced hematopoietic recovery with a low incidence of GVHD [8]. As well, treatment of mouse bone marrow and spleen cell suspensions with soybean and/or peanut agglutinin resulted in a fraction of hematopoietic precursors depleted of T cells that did not induce GVHD [9].

The application of anti-T-cell antibodies to experimental transplantation confirmed the power of TCD as a strategy for GVHD prophylaxis. *Ex vivo* TCD with antilymphocyte serum (ALS), antithymocyte globulin (ATG) or monoclonal antibody permitted transplantation across major histocompatibility barriers in several animal systems [10–15]. Overall survival was superior in animals receiving bone marrow or splenic suspensions depleted of T cells.

Methods of TCD

There are three major TCD strategies actively in use: (i) *ex vivo* negative selection of T cells; (ii) *ex vivo* positive selection of CD34$^+$ stem cells; and (iii) *in vivo* anti-T-cell antibody administration. Most of the studies conducted in the 1980s and in the early 1990s utilized *ex vivo* negative selection TCD whereby the targeted cell population is removed from the bone marrow or apheresis product by physical separation or antibody based purging (Table 17.1). Examples of physical separation techniques include differential agglutination with lectins followed by rosetting with sheep red blood cells [16,17], counterflow centrifugal elutriation [18–20] and fractionation on density gradients [21]. Monoclonal antibodies have been used alone [22–24], in conjunction with homologous, heterologous or rabbit complements [25–34], as immunotoxins [35–38] or as immunomagnetic beads [39]. The antigenic targets of these antibodies can vary (Table 17.2) and some methods may deplete cells other than T lymphocytes.

Table 17.1 T-cell-depletion techniques.

Negative selection

Physical methods
Density gradient fractionation
Soybean lectin agglutination + E-rosette depletion
Counterflow centrifugal elutriation
Photoinactivation

Immunological methods
Ex vivo depletion:
   Monoclonal antibody alone
   Monoclonal antibody + rabbit complement
   Immunotoxins
   Immunomagnetic beads
In vivo depletion:
   Monoclonal antibody (e.g. Campath-1H/alemtuzumab)
   Antithymocyte globulin

Positive selection

CD34$^+$ stem cell selection via immunoadsorption columns ± negative selection with monoclonal antibody

Table 17.2 Advantages and disadvantages of T-cell depletion (TCD).

Advantages	Disadvantages
Low incidence of acute and chronic GVHD	Higher incidence of graft failure
Reduced or no requirement for post-transplant immune suppression as GVHD prophylaxis	Loss of GVL activity (higher incidence of disease relapse, especially with CML)
Decreased pulmonary and hepatic toxicity early after BMT	Delayed immune reconstitution
Decreased early transplant-related mortality	Increased risk for post-transplant EBV associated lymphoproliferative disorder
?Shorter time to engraftment in the absence of methotrexate	Higher incidence of CMV reactivation
?Decreased cost due to decreased complications	Overall survival not improved compared to non-TCD BMT

BMT, bone marrow transplantation; CML, chronic myeloid leukemia; EBV, Epstein–Barr virus; GVHD, graft-vs.-host disease; GVL, graft-vs.-leukemia.

The development of anti-CD34 antibody-coated columns to select hematopoietic progenitors has provided an alternative to traditional negative selection strategies of TCD. By positively selecting CD34+ stem cells, this technique can reduce the lymphocyte content in the infused product by as much as 4–5 log [40–44]. Moreover, it may offer practical advantages over traditional negative selection methods for the depletion of peripheral blood hematopoietic cells (PBHC) given the larger volume and 10-fold excess lymphocyte content in mobilized peripheral blood compared to bone marrow. Positive stem-cell selection techniques can be followed by antibody based negative selection to further deplete specific undesired T cell populations.

The development of commercially available humanized anti-T-cell antibodies may permit effective TCD without cumbersome and time consuming *ex vivo* manipulations. *In vivo* TCD with either ATG preparations or humanized anti-T-cell antibodies such as Campath-1H (which targets the broadly expressed CDw52 antigen and which can fix human complement) is being used with increasing frequency as a primary or adjunctive method of GVHD prophylaxis [45,46]. These antibodies have been administered pre- and post-graft infusion both to target recipient T cells that could mediate graft rejection and to delay recovery of donor T cells that might induce GVHD.

The impact of T-cell dose

The extent of protection against GVHD has varied in different TCD studies and depends upon the approach utilized for purging. TCD techniques differ in the extent and specificity of T-cell removal. The range of TCD may vary from 2 to 5 log. The precise extent of TCD needed to prevent GVHD is not clear. It is unlikely that the relationship between T-cell number and the incidence of acute GVHD is linear. Most studies suggest that a minimum of 2 log-depletion of functional T cells from the marrow is necessary for effective GVHD prophylaxis with reduced or no post-transplant immune suppression. Limiting dilution analyses have suggested a threshold of approximately $1–3 \times 10^5$ T cells/kg for development of GVHD in recipients of human leukocyte antigen (HLA)-identical, related bone marrow [47,48]. It is less clear what that threshold would be in recipients of peripheral blood cell transplants. In general, however, the more exhaustive the TCD, the lower the risk of GVHD.

It may be that the degree of TCD necessary to prevent GVHD is greater for unrelated and HLA mismatched transplants than for HLA-matched siblings. In a comparative analysis of CD6+ TCD allogeneic transplantation, the incidence of GVHD for recipients of unrelated marrow was more than twice as great as that observed in related marrow recipients (42% vs. 20%, $p = 0.004$) [49]. In trials of patients receiving PBHCs, acute GVHD rates in the absence of pharmacologic immune suppression were low when the number of infused T cells was below $2–3 \times 10^4$ T cells/kg, a log lower than the threshold for recipients of HLA-matched bone marrow [50]. There is likely to be significant variability in the threshold T-cell GVHD dose between donor/recipient pairs depending on the degree of minor HLA antigen disparity and other potential polymorphisms [51].

Specificity of TCD

Methods of TCD differ, not only in the extent of T-cell removal, but also in the specificity of depletion. Some approaches (e.g. positive selection with CD34 columns or negative selection by soybean lectin agglutination or counterflow centrifugal elutriation) may indiscriminately eliminate natural killer (NK) cells, immature thymocytes, B cells and dendritic cells in addition to T cells. If these other cellular elements contribute to processes such as immune surveillance, promotion of engraftment, or elimination of minimal residual disease, then the specificity of the TCD technique used could have a profound effect on outcome.

Ex vivo antibody-based purging techniques may have narrow or broad spectra of reactivity. Often those with narrow specificities, targeting mature T cells (e.g. $T_{10}B_9$—anti-TCR, anti-CD6, anti-CD5), have not been associated with the same degree of complications (e.g. graft failure) noted with broad specificity approaches (e.g. Campath, multiple antibody combinations) [34,36–38,52]. An International Bone Marrow Transplant Registry (IBMTR) study of unrelated donor transplantation demonstrated that the use of narrow specificity anti-T-cell antibodies was associated with better leukemia-free survival than the use of broad specificity approaches, such as Campath antibodies, counterflow centrifugal elutriation and soybean lectin agglutination [53].

It is not clear what contributions distinct T-cell subsets make to the pathogenesis of GVHD and the development of graft-vs.-leukemia (GVL) activity. Our current ability to distinguish and separate the T-cell compartment into subgroups with specific functional capacities is crude. Investigators still rely on anatomic subsets defined by differential surface antigen expression. The most accessible T-cell subsets to examine have been CD4$^+$ and CD8$^+$ cells. However, the role of CD4$^+$ or CD8$^+$ T cells in human GVHD pathogenesis has been difficult to determine from animal models. Interpretation of murine studies is complicated by the use of varied genetic strain combinations that rely on different major or minor histocompatibility discrepancies to drive GVH reactions. In addition, these antigenic surface markers are not confined to T cells with one defined functional role, but can be present on dendritic cells, NK cells and T cells with different regulatory capacities.

Human trials of TCD

Acute GVHD

Transplantation from matched sibling donors

Studies in humans throughout the 1980s and 1990s confirmed that TCD methods (counterflow centrifugal elutriation, E-rosetting with soybean lectin agglutination and various monoclonal antibody approaches) that removed at least 2 log of T cells decreased the incidence of clinically significant acute GVHD to 0–25% after matched sibling transplantation [17,18,26,29–38,54–56]. In many of these studies, the low incidence of GVHD was achieved in the absence of immunosuppression post-transplantation.

The use of *in vivo* TCD using ATG preparations or humanized antibodies, such as Campath-1H, has also been successful in reducing the incidence of acute GVHD [45,46]. These *in vivo* TCD approaches have particularly been explored in nonmyeloablative transplantation [57,58]. The reported incidence of GVHD after nonmyeloablative transplantation with *in vivo* Campath has been lower that that associated with regimens that do not include any form of TCD [58]. Infusion of anti-T-cell antibodies directly to the patient prior to graft infusion can facilitate engraftment by preventing host T-cell-mediated donor stem-cell destruction. As well, these antibody preparations also deplete T cells from the infused inoculum. T-cell antibodies with long half-lives can persist for weeks and may interfere with early T-cell reconstitution.

Studies of HLA-identical sibling peripheral blood HCT using CD34$^+$ positive selection of mobilized peripheral blood have reported a wide variation in acute GVHD incidence [40–44]. This variability was likely influenced by factors such as the number of CD3$^+$ cells infused, immune suppressive agents given post-transplant and type of CD34$^+$ selection devices used. Recent reports have suggested that the number of CD34$^+$ cells infused may profoundly influence subsequent GVHD development in recipients of CD34 selected or unmanipulated peripheral hematopoietic blood cell transplants [59,60]. The mechanism underlying the association between CD34 count and GVHD is unclear, but investigation of this observation may improve our understanding of GVHD pathogenesis. As more efficient CD34$^+$ selection techniques are developed, the incidence of GVHD after peripheral blood HCT is declining and the need for post-transplant GVHD prophylaxis may be eliminated altogether.

Alternative donor transplantation

Because marrow transplant from donors other than HLA-identical sibling donors carries a higher risk of GVHD, it has been thought that TCD may be particularly beneficial in this setting. Reports from the National Marrow Donor Program (NMDP) and other sources have suggested that the incidence of acute GVHD after unrelated T-cell-depleted bone marrow transplantation (BMT) is 15–50% [53,61–63], which compares favorably to the >50% incidence of acute GVHD observed in many series of unrelated marrow transplantation where TCD is not employed. The incidence of acute GVHD, however, is not as low as that observed after related donor transplantation. Analysis of transplants performed with anti-CD6 monoclonal antibody as the sole form of GVHD prophylaxis revealed an incidence of grades II–IV acute GVHD of 20% for related vs. 42% for unrelated marrow recipients ($p = 0.004$) [49]. In 1993, multicenter data from the NMDP involving 462 unrelated transplants (92 TCD, 367 non-TCD) indicated that the absence of TCD was the most significant predictor for the development of severe (grades III–IV) acute GVHD [61]. In an analysis from the IBMTR of 1868 leukemia patients who received allogeneic marrow transplants from donors other than HLA-identical siblings, the incidence of grade II–IV GVHD was between 34% and 38% in the TCD group, as compared to 57% in the non-TCD group ($p <0.0001$) [53]. Preliminary results from the first large prospective randomized trial of TCD were reported in 2002. A total of 410 patients were randomized to receive either TCD with monoclonal antibody $T_{10}B_9$ or soybean lectin agglutination or immune suppression with cyclosporine (CSP)/methotrexate (MTX). Patients receiving TCD marrow plus CSP experienced less grade III–IV acute GVHD than those receiving CSP/MTX (15% vs. 27%, $p <0.01$) [64].

Early studies of TCD in HLA-mismatched related marrow transplants were plagued by high incidences of graft failure and GVHD [65]. However, recent series have yielded better results. In single institution studies, grade II–IV GVHD incidence has ranged from 18% to 40% in recipients of HLA-mismatched BMT after TCD using monoclonal antibody or *in vivo* TCD [66,67]. Rigorous CD34 selection resulting in infused T-cell numbers in the range of 1×10^4/kg appears to allow haplomismatched transplantation to be conducted with a low incidence of GVHD in the absence of immune suppression [50].

Chronic GVHD

It is more difficult to gauge the effect of TCD upon chronic GVHD than acute GVHD. There are inconsistencies in the uniformity of scoring of chronic GVHD in many transplant series. Many reports of the effect of acute GVHD prophylactic regimens, like TCD, do not include sufficient follow-up to determine whether chronic GVHD has developed. Several approaches under clinical study for over 10 years (e.g. soybean lectin agglutination, Campath antibodies and anti-CD6 antibody + complement) have reported very low rates of chronic GVHD (<15%) in matched sibling transplantation. In a cohort study of nonmyeloablative transplantation, the use of *in vivo* alemtuzumab (Campath-1H) was associated with a reduced incidence of chronic GVHD (5% vs. 66%, $p <0.001$) [58]. The results in unrelated transplantation are less clear. In the recently reported randomized trial of TCD (using $T_{10}B_9$ or soybean lectin agglutination) plus CSP vs. CSP/MTX, no significant difference in the reported incidence of chronic GVHD at 2 years was observed (24% vs. 29%) [64]. However, the incidence of chronic GVHD in either arm appears substantially lower than that reported in previous studies and may underrepresent the true rate.

Organ dysfunction after T-cell-depleted BMT

In several series, TCD has been associated with less organ toxicity compared to conventional BMT. A likely explanation for this reduction in organ toxicity is the elimination or reduction in the use of GVHD prophylactic agents, such as MTX and CSP/tacrolimus. It is also possible that decreases in alloreactivity after T-cell-depleted BMT result in lower levels of circulating cytokines that might be damaging to hepatic, renal, or pulmonary parenchyma. The incidence of hepatic veno-occlusive disease (VOD) has been reported to be quite low after T-cell-depleted BMT, 3.1% overall and 1.2% in patients receiving TBI as part of their conditioning [68]. As well, the risk of severe renal insufficiency requiring dialysis is clearly less when TCD is utilized in the absence of additional nephrotoxic immune suppressive medications.

TCD has also been associated with decreased pulmonary complications after BMT [69]. In a recent analysis of 199 allogeneic transplants at a single institution, the incidence of life-threatening pulmonary complications within the first 60 days of BMT was 8% among those who received TCD as the sole form of GVHD prophylaxis, but 33% among those who received CSP and MTX ($p <0.0001$) [70]. In this study, the protective effect of TCD against pulmonary complications was independent of the diagnosis of acute GVHD, perhaps implicating immune suppressive medications as mediators of tissue injury. These observations have been supported by the preliminary results of the randomized trial of TCD/CSP vs. CSP/MTX in which assessment of pulmonary, hepatic, renal, central nervous system and mucosal toxicity by the Bearman toxicity scale revealed a significantly lower incidence and severity of organ damage in the TCD cohort [64].

Transplant-related mortality

Since TCD protects against GVHD and reduces organ dysfunction after BMT, one would expect these benefits to translate into lower transplant-related mortality. Indeed, in a number of series, transplant-related mortality after T-cell-depleted BMT has been quite low. Some matched sibling T-cell-depleted transplant series have reported the incidence of transplant-related mortality to be between 2% and 15% [34,70–73]. However, other TCD studies have reported transplant-related mortality rates from 20% to 40% even after matched sibling transplants, with many deaths being secondary to infection and EBV post-transplant lymphoproliferative disease (PTLD) [38,74–76]. This variability highlights the fact that factors other than GVHD, such as the intensity of conditioning, use of post-transplant immune suppression, rate of graft failure and pace of immune reconstitution, also contribute significantly to transplant-related mortality. It further reinforces the point that for a TCD regimen to be successful, it must do more than just protect against GVHD. It must also preserve GVL, engraftment potential and spare patients from excessive transplant-related toxicity.

Costs and quality of life

If TCD can limit morbidity by decreasing GVHD and organ toxicity, then it might also improve the quality of life (QOL) in patients after transplant. In addition, diminished toxicity could also lead to decreased costs [76]. These endpoints were assessed in a comparative single institution study in which patients who had received TCD or unmanipulated unrelated bone marrow were compared [77]. No major difference in parameters of QOL could be ascertained by questionnaire. Costs through the first 6 months post-transplant were significantly less, however, in recipients of T-cell-depleted marrow. Future trials comparing TCD and unmanipulated grafts should examine these issues in a prospective fashion.

Disadvantages of TCD

Graft failure after T-cell-depleted BMT

Prior to the use of TCD, graft failure after HLA-identical sibling BMT was a rare event, and was often restricted to patients with aplastic anaemia who had received multiple blood transfusions [78]. For leukemia patients conditioned with cyclophosphamide and total body irradiation (TBI), the incidence of graft failure after non-T-cell-depleted BMT is less than 1% for HLA-matched transplants and 5% for HLA-mismatched related marrow [79,80]. In contrast, most T-cell-depleted BMT series in the 1980s and early 1990s reported higher incidences of graft failure [20,21,27,28,31,35,36,54,81–85]. In an analysis from the IBMTR of more than 3000 patients who received T-cell-depleted or non-T-cell-depleted BMT for leukemia, TCD was associated with a ninefold increased risk for graft failure compared to unmanipulated marrow transplantation ($p <0.0001$) [86]. Yet in the more recent prospective randomized trial of T-cell-depleted vs. unmanipulated marrow grafts, the rates of neutrophil and platelet engraftment were equivalent in each cohort [64].

Graft failure after T-cell-depleted BMT can occur either as failure of primary engraftment, initial engraftment followed by graft rejection within several weeks of BMT, or delayed graft failure months following transplant. The pathophysiologic mechanisms behind these different patterns are not well understood, although there is evidence that early graft failure after T-cell-depleted transplantation results primarily from immunologic rejection of donor hematopoietic elements by host lymphoid elements that have survived the conditioning process. Direct evidence for the role of the host immune system has come from the identification of host T lymphocytes from patients at the time of graft rejection which exhibit donor specific cytotoxic activity, and which suppress proliferation of donor lineage specific colony forming units *in vitro* [82,87–96].

In most circumstances, it is unlikely that failure of initial engraftment is caused by injury to hematopoietic progenitors or auxiliary cells during marrow manipulation, since autologous marrow processed with monoclonal antibodies and complement engraft without significant difficulty [97–99]. It is possible that viral infections, such as cytomegalovirus (CMV) or human herpes virus 6 (HHV-6), may contribute to late graft failure after BMT [100–103]. However, although T-cell-depleted BMT patients may have a higher risk of CMV reactivation after transplant [104–106], direct clinical evidence implicating this and other viruses to graft failure after T-cell-depleted transplantation is lacking.

Mixed lymphoid and myeloid chimerism is more common after T-cell-depleted BMT and appears to be associated with graft failure [107–111]. Viable host derived hematopoietic cells can often be recovered from patients after T-cell-depleted marrow transplantation [112,113], and their coexistence with the donor graft implies a state of immune tolerance between the graft and host. Graft failure could result when host lymphoid tolerance of the graft is broken.

As yet, it remains unknown what cells promote engraftment after transplantation. Some murine models have suggested that donor NK cells are critical to engraftment [114], while others have implicated donor CD8$^+$ T cells [115]. There are no direct data in human studies that implicate NK cells in hemaopoietic engraftment. However, donor T cells that recognize alloantigens on recipient immune effector cells may have potent effects in preventing marrow graft rejection. In a recent human trial using donor grafts with graded dose of CD4$^+$ and CD8$^+$ cells, it was suggested that depletion of donor CD8$^+$ cells, but not CD4$^+$ cells, was associated with increased graft rejection. Of note, while CD4$^+$ depletion did not adversely affect engraftment, it also did not provide adequate protection against GVHD [116].

Several approaches have been used to address the increased risk of graft failure associated with TCD. These strategies have included increased myeloablation, increased host directed immune suppression, adjustment of the extent of TCD, narrowing of the breadth of TCD and infusion of increased numbers of hematopoietic precursors. It has been suggested that intensifying the myeloablative regimen can empty out the host marrow more effectively and thus increase "hematopoietic space" for the incoming donor graft. It should be noted that these myelosuppressive agents have potent immune suppressive properties as well. High doses of cytarabine, thiotepa and anthracyclines have been incorporated into standard myeloablative regimens and shown to reduce the rate of graft failure after T-cell-depleted BMT but the benefit of decreased graft failure may be offset by increased regimen-related toxicity [74,117–122]. Increased immunosuppression with total lymphoid irradiation, augmentation of TBI, corticosteroids or *in vivo* anti-T-cell antibodies to target host alloreactive T cells with antidonor cytotoxic potential have been used with success as suggested in phase 2 trials [46,75,84,107,123–126].

Adjustment of the T-cell content after TCD has been investigated as a way to reduce graft rejection. In one study following centrifugal elutriation for T-cell separation, the reintroduction of T lymphocytes to a final dose of 0.5×10^6 cells/kg protected against GVHD while maintaining engraftment at over 95% of patients [56]. Similar strategies have been studied after *ex vivo* treatment with Campath antibodies and CD34 selection. Unfortunately, this strategy can be problematic because of the potential for precipitation of severe GVHD as the number of T cells added back is increased [127,128].

Selective removal of T cells appears to result in decreased graft failure rates when compared to broader more nonspecific methods. Studies using anti-CD5 immunotoxins, anti-CD6, and anti-T-cell receptor (TCR)-$\alpha\beta$ ($T_{10}B_9$) antibodies have all demonstrated low graft failure rates without compromising GVHD prophylaxis, with risks of graft failure as low as 1–2% with a 15–20% risk of clinically significant GVHD [34,36–38,52,70]. The randomized trial of TCD (in which $T_{10}B_9$ antibody was the predominant method used) vs. CSP/MTX found no significant differences between groups with respect to the incidence of neutrophil or platelet engraftment [64].

Dose escalation of $CD34^+$ stem cells may be another effective way to overcome graft failure after T-cell-depleted BMT. Preclinical models have shown that mice given "megadoses" of T-cell-depleted marrow could engraft despite sublethal doses of conditioning irradiation [129]. In human studies, the addition of $CD34^+$ cells to T-cell-depleted marrow to augment stem-cell dose has permitted reliable engraftment in leukemia patients despite full HLA haplotype mismatches [50,130]. It is postulated that a subset of progenitor cells, so-called "veto" cells, may be responsible for the induction of tolerance in high stem-cell dose transplants [131]. It is possible that *ex vivo* TCD of mobilized peripheral blood progenitor cells may not carry the same risk of graft failure because of the increased number of CD34 cells infused with peripheral blood compared to BMTs. Recent experience with CD8 depletion of mobilized peripheral blood has been associated with no episodes of graft rejection [132].

Delayed immune reconstitution and EBV lymphoproliferative disease after T-cell-depleted BMT

Because T-cell-depleted marrow contain significantly fewer T cells compared to unmanipulated marrow grafts, delayed T-cell immune reconstitution is a concern after T-cell-depleted BMT. Immune recovery after T-cell-depleted BMT has been studied in a number of transplant centers using various methods of TCD [133–143]. Regardless of the type of transplant, NK cells appear to be the first lymphoid subset to emerge, usually within 2–3 weeks after transplant, followed by B cells (3–6 months), and T cells (3–12 months). Phenotypic analyses reveal that total lymphocyte numbers are usually higher early after BMT in recipients of conventional marrow transplants compared to those who receive T-cell-depleted grafts. Furthermore, the reconstituted T-cell compartment is predominantly of the $CD8^+$ subset, and most T-cell-depleted BMT patients will have a deficit in $CD4^+$ cells, with an inverted $CD4^+$ to $CD8^+$ ratio for up to 2 years [134]. The number of $CD4^+$ cells normalizes at 7–9 months after conventional BMT, but this process is further delayed after T-cell-depleted BMT [135].

Functional recovery of T cells appears to be impaired after T-cell-depleted BMT as well. The proliferative response of peripheral blood mononuclear cells to exogenous interleukin 2 (IL-2) stimulation is abnormal for up to 6 months, compared to only 1 month for recipients of conventional BMTs [133]. Similarly, the proliferative response of T cells to mitogenic stimulation can be impaired for over 18 months post-BMT in recipients of T-cell-depleted marrow [134]. The T-cell compartment after transplantation is largely expanded from lymphocytes cotransfused with the marrow and, therefore, recipients of T-cell-depleted transplants would have much fewer precursors with which to reconstitute their repertoire than recipients of conventional BMT. T lymphocytes from recipients of T-cell-depleted BMT have restricted variability in their TCR repertoires [138,140]. CDR3 spectratyping has revealed that patients with persistent mixed chimerism after T-cell-depleted BMT have markedly abnormal TCR repertoires, while others who had converted to full donor hematopoiesis possess a normal spectrum of TCR variability [140]. Analysis of T-cell neogenesis through T-cell receptor excision circles after transplantation has revealed impairment of T-cell receptor excision circles generation after T-cell-depleted BMT, which has correlated to an increased risk of infection [142,143].

The delayed reconstitution in numbers and functional activity of T cells have led many to speculate that T-cell-depleted BMT recipients may be at higher risk for opportunistic infections. Although there is little reported evidence to suggest an increased risk of bacterial or fungal infections after T-cell-depleted transplantation, a number of studies have demonstrated a higher probability of reactivation for viruses such as CMV [104–106,144,145]. It is likely that the removal of CMV-specific $CD8^+$ T cells from the donor graft hinders surveillance against reactivation of CMV in the recipient, though less exhaustive TCD methods may not compromise anti-CMV immunity [146]. A higher incidence of CMV infection after T-cell-depleted BMT was observed in the randomized trial of TCD/CSP vs. CSP/MTX in unrelated transplant recipients [64].

EBV-PTLD is known to occur in immunosuppressed patients after solid organ transplantation, but is surprisingly uncommon after BMT except in the TCD setting, where its incidence have been reported to be between 3% and 30% (see Chapter 56) [147,148]. Recipients of T-cell-depleted transplants using HLA-mismatched or unrelated donor marrow appear to be at particularly high risk [117,147,148], as are patients with severe GVHD and those treated with certain anti-T-cell monoclonal antibodies [147,149]. EBV-PTLD is felt to primarily arise from infected donor B cells that have been cotransplanted with the allograft. However, there have been cases of EBV lymphoma in B cells from EBV seronegative donors, suggesting that *de novo* infection in transplant recipients or reactivation of EBV in recipient cells can occur.

A potential strategy for the treatment of EBV-PTLD has been adoptive immunotherapy using donor lymphocyte infusion (DLI) [150]. Administration of EBV-specific cytotoxic T lymphocytes (CTLs) cultivated *in vitro* from donor lymphocytes is effective treatment of EBV-PTLD [151–153]. Case series have reported promising responses with the use of anti-B cell antibodies, including the anti-CD20 monoclonal antibody rituximab [154–156]. Rituximab is relatively safe and has become the preferred first-line approach to EBV-PTLD. Strategies to prevent development of EBV-PTLD have included B cell depletion of the donor graft [157,158], prophylactic administration of EBV-specific CTLs [153] and the use of polymerase chain reaction (PCR) methods to detect rising EBV DNA levels which could signal the onset of clinically evident disease [159,160].

Increased leukaemic relapse after T-cell-depleted BMT

The higher incidence of leukemic relapse associated with T-cell-depleted BMT was first suggested in a prospective randomized trial, which included 40 patients with acute and chronic leukemia [31]. Of the 20 patients randomized to the T-cell-depleted arm, seven had clinically apparent relapse, compared to only two in the control (non-T-cell-depleted) arm. Multiple retrospective studies have subsequently demonstrated that disease relapse is indeed more frequent after T-cell-depleted BMT, especially for chronic myeloid leukemia (CML) [81,161–166].

The increased rate of leukemic relapse after T-cell-depleted BMT has been linked, as least in part, to the reduction in GVHD and concomitant loss of the GVL activity. In recipients of T-cell replete marrow, patients who develop clinically significant GVHD generally have lower incidence of leukemic relapse compared to those who do not develop GVHD [167–169]. More convincing evidence linking T cells and GVL comes from studies using DLI in patients with CML who have relapsed after BMT, where complete response rates of 70–80% are achieved [170,171].

An increased rate of relapse has been observed in virtually all studies using TCD of HLA-identical sibling bone marrow on patients with CML [86,161–166]. This increase in CML relapse has not been as apparent after T-cell-depleted transplantation using matched unrelated marrow [61,62,172–174]. In an European analysis of CML patients who received unrelated donor BMT, TCD was associated with a significantly higher incidence of relapse in the univariate analysis, but the difference was not significant in the multivariate analysis [175]. However, in a prospective randomized trial of TCD vs. CSP/MTX as GVHD prophylaxis, relapse of CML was higher (16% vs. 6%, $p = 0.02$) in the T-cell-depleted arm [64].

Unlike CML, TCD appears to have only a modest effect in the relapse rates of patients transplanted for acute leukemia. Reported rates of relapse after T-cell-depleted BMT for acute myeloid leukemia (AML) in first remission have ranged from 0% to 31% in different centers [71,74,176–179]. Retrospective data from the IBMTR, which included 731 T-cell-depleted and 2480 non-T-cell-depleted marrow transplants for leukemia from 137 institutions, have shown that TCD is associated with a slightly increased risk of recurrence in patients with acute lymphoblastic leukemia (ALL) in any phase and in patients with AML who are transplanted in relapse or in first complete remission (CR) [86]. Surprisingly, in this same analysis, AML patients transplanted in second CR actually had a lower risk of relapse with TCD. In a small randomized trial comparing TCD with MTX/CSP as GVHD prophylaxis for leukemia patients undergoing HLA-matched related BMT, a higher relapse rate was observed after T-cell-depleted BMT only in patients with CML, but not in patients with acute leukemia [180]. No differences in acute leukemia relapse rates were noted in the recently reported large unrelated donor randomized trial (26% vs. 24%) [64].

The specificity of TCD may influence relapse rates. An IBMTR analysis from 870 patients who underwent T-cell-depleted unrelated- or mismatched-donor BMT for leukemia demonstrated that the relapse rates for patients whose grafts were T-cell-depleted with "narrow specificity" antibodies (e.g. anti-CD5, CD6, anti-TCRαβ, etc.) were significantly lower than those whose grafts had been T-cell-depleted with "broad specificity" antibodies (e.g. anti-CD2, ATG, Campath antibodies, elutriation or lectin/sheep red blood cell agglutination). The 5-year probability of leukemia relapse was 28% for recipients of narrow-specificity T-cell-depleted BMT vs. 51% for recipients T-cell-depleted by other techniques ($p < 0.001$) [53]. The 5-year relapse rate in recipients of "narrow specificity" T-cell-depleted BMT was similar to that observed in recipients of unmanipulated BMT. These important results may suggest that, at least in the setting of unrelated or mismatched BMT, T-cell-depleted using "narrow specificity" antibodies is not associated with substantial loss of GVL activity.

Efforts to reduce leukemic relapse after T-cell-depleted BMT have included selective purging of T-lymphocyte subsets which may preferentially mediate GVHD over GVL, addition of cytokines post-transplant to stimulate effectors other than T lymphocytes which contribute to the antileukemic effect, and reintroduction of donor T lymphocytes after transplantation to restore GVL activity. While both GVL and GVHD are initiated by T cells in the donor graft, it has been suggested that specific subsets of T lymphocytes may be involved in these processes and that GVL activity could exist in the absence of GVHD [52,181,182]. In animal models, both donor CD4$^+$ and CD8$^+$ cells play a significant role in GVHD, but donor CD4$^+$ cells in the absence of CD8$^+$ cells can still mediate GVL [183]. In humans, CD8$^+$ T cells have clearly been implicated in GVHD development. Infiltrates of CD8$^+$ T cells are often found in target organs of patients with GVHD. As well, the presence of high numbers of CD8$^+$ T cells in peripheral blood early post-BMT has been associated with the subsequent development of GVHD [184]. In an early trial of CD8$^+$ depletion followed by post-transplant CSP, a reduced incidence and severity of GVHD was noted with only 11% of patients suffering leukemic relapse [55]. In a follow-up double-blind randomized trial, the CSP plus CD8$^+$ depletion arm experienced significantly less grade II–IV GVHD compared to the control arm receiving CSP alone (20% vs. 80%, $p < 0.004$). The leukemia relapse rate was similar between the two groups, suggesting that CD8$^+$ depletion reduced GVHD without abolishing GVL [76].

More direct evidence to suggest that GVL can be separated from GVHD comes from studies of DLI in patients who have relapsed post-BMT. Although many of these studies have demonstrated an association between development of GVHD and antileukemic response, it is clear that a number of patients have experienced remission in the absence of GVHD. This separation between GVHD and GVL is further evidenced in DLI studies using CD8$^+$ depletion. CD8$^+$ depleted DLI has been shown to significantly reduce the incidence of GVHD, but retain important GVL activity with preserved clinical responses in patients with relapsed CML [185,186]. A randomized study of CD8 depletion in patients receiving DLI demonstrated a reduction in acute GVHD from 66% to 0% without loss of GVL activity [187]. In this study, both CD8 depleted and unmanipulated DLI were equally capable of converting from mixed to full donor hematopoietic chimerism, restoring T-cell repertoire diversity and increasing T-cell neogenesis as measured by T-cell receptor excision circles activity. Although studies with CD8 depletion have been encouraging, separating GVH from GVL is likely to be far more complicated. It is possible that CD4 cells induce GVL activity by providing help to endogenous CD8 cytotoxic CD8$^+$ T cells to kill leukemic targets [188]. It is also possible that, in different donor/recipient pairs, the role of CD4 and CD8 cells with respect to GVH and GVL activity depends upon the specific minor histocompatibility disparities which drive the alloreaction. Definitive dissection of the anatomic subsets responsible for GVHD and GVL remains a crucial but elusive goal for investigators hoping to reduce disease relapse after T-cell-depleted BMT.

NK cells may be important mediators of antileukemic activity. Addition of IL-2 to peripheral blood lymphocytes collected from CML patients after allogeneic BMT has been shown to induce an NK cell cytolytic response against cryopreserved leukemic cell targets [189,190]. IL-2 is known to stimulate both NK cells and activated T cells at high concentrations. However, IL-2 at low doses appears to stimulate NK cells preferentially. As such, it has been postulated that administration of low doses of IL-2 may enhance GVL activity through NK cell stimulation without inducing GVHD since T cells remain unaffected. Prolonged infusion of low-dose recombinant interleukin-2 (rIL-2) following T-cell-depleted allogeneic BMT has been shown to be well tolerated and results in a marked increase in cytotoxic NK cells with a suggestion that such treatment lower the incidence of disease relapse relative to historical controls [191,192].

The role of NK cells in human transplantation has recently undergone additional scrutiny. Killer immunoglobulin-like receptors (KIR) on NK cells recognize groups of HLA class I (particularly *HLA-Bx4* and *HLA-C*) alleles and can inhibit NK reactivity. Absence of recognition of these alleles on a cell can trigger NK cell destruction of that target. In an analysis of patients who received allografts mismatched at the *HLA-C* or

Bw4 allele in the direction of GVHD, donor vs. recipient alloreactive NK cell clones could be isolated post-transplant in patients without evidence of GVHD [193]. These alloreactive NK cell clones could lyse pretransplant cryopreserved leukemia cells *in vitro*, suggesting that GVL activity mediated by NK cells exists in these patients without GVHD. In the setting of haploidentical transplantation under conditions of exhaustive TCD, donor NK activity appears to protect against relapse of AML without inducing GVHD, perhaps in part by eliminating host antigen presenting cells [194,195]. Such a role for NK cells may be limited to conditions of haploidentical transplantation and extensive TCD, as one analysis of KIR incompatibility as assessed by *HLA-Bw4* and -*C* discrepancies in matched unrelated transplants showed no advantage in terms of relapse or GVHD [196].

Adoptive immunotherapy using DLI has also emerged as a potential approach to compensate for the higher rate of leukemic relapse after T-cell-depleted BMT. In 86 CML patients who underwent T-cell-depleted (with anti-CD6) or non-T-cell-depleted BMT, the TCD group, as expected, had a lower incidence of GVHD and treatment-related mortality, but a higher probability of hematologic or molecular relapse compared to the non-T-cell-depleted group. However, most of the relapsed patients were successfully salvaged with DLI, compensating for the initial higher relapse rate associated with TCD [197]. Similarly, in patients undergoing T-cell-depleted ($T_{10}B_9$) BMT, the 5-year overall survival was 80% despite a high cumulative incidence of CML relapse (49%) because most relapsed patients achieved durable remissions with DLI therapy [72]. A retrospective analysis of CML patients receiving CD34+ peripheral blood cells with T cell add-back demonstrated a lower rate of GVHD and superior 3-year survival (90%) compared with recipients of unmanipulated mobilized peripheral blood (68%, $p < 0.03$) or bone marrow (63%, $p < 0.01$) [198]. Taken together, these results suggest that T-cell-depleted BMT followed by post-transplant DLI at, or even before, disease relapse could be a reasonable option for patients with CML, especially for those with concurrent comorbidity or advanced age who would otherwise be suboptimal candidates for conventional (non-T-cell-depleted) marrow transplantation.

The success of DLI in salvaging CML patients after BMT has led to further investigation of T-cell infusions after T-cell-depleted BMT. This approach potentially combines the benefits of TCD early after BMT (i.e. decreased GVHD and transplant-related toxicity) with restoration of the GVL effect at a later time with DLI. This conceptual framework is not unlike that which underlies the strategy of DLI following nonmyeloablative HCT for patients with persistent mixed chimerism and residual disease [199]. This approach has been tested in multiple myeloma. Twenty-four patients with myeloma who underwent a T-cell-depleted BMT were given DLI 6 months post-BMT. Of the 11 patients in that series who had persistent myeloma 6 months after transplant, 10 responses (six CR, four partial remission) were observed after DLI. The 2-year progression free survival for all 14 patients who received DLI was significantly improved compared to a comparable historical cohort who received T-cell-depleted BMT without DLI [200]. It must be noted that 10 of the 24 patients did not receive DLI in this study, either because of early relapse, GVHD, infection, PTLD or refusal. For this strategy to be optimally effective, the T-cell-depleted transplant itself must be of sufficiently low morbidity that patients are stable enough to receive DLI. As well, even though DLI is performed when the patient is removed from the damaging effects of conditioning therapy and away from an active inflammatory cytokine milieu, GVHD remains a major complication of this treatment modality. For prophylactic DLI to be viable, it must reduce relapse rates without inducing GVHD, perhaps by lowering the dose of lymphocytes infused [201], fractionating infusions [202], selectively depleting CD8+ cells from the lymphocyte pool [185,186] or by suicide gene insertion [203–205].

Future directions in T-cell-depleted transplantation

Functional TCD

Rather than focusing upon removal of anatomic subsets of T cells, some investigators have turned their attention to TCD techniques in which only alloreactive T cells are removed from the graft either through photoinactivation [206] or immunologic purging. After donor T cells are stimulated by recipient mononuclear cells *in vitro*, alloreactive cells can be identified by expression of activation markers, such as CD25, CD69, CD71 or HLA-DR, and separated from the remaining cells by immunomagnetic cell sorting [207–209]. In one study, approximately 90% of the alloreactive component could be purged while preserving >70% residual immunity as measured by third party alloantigen response [208]. It is postulated that this method would preferentially purge alloreactive lymphoctyes from the graft that are responsible for GVHD, but retain "nonreactive" T cells which may improve post-transplant immune reconstitution, and enhance engraftment by exerting a potential veto effect on host CTLs.

Induction of T-cell anergy to prevent GVHD

Induction of anergy in donor T cells prior to transplantation as a means of reducing GVHD has also been investigated. Murine marrow transplant studies have shown that GVHD could be reduced even across major genetic barriers by treating the recipient with CTLA4-Ig, an agent that blocks the CTLA4-BB1 (a.k.a. CD28-B7) interaction between T lymphocytes and antigen-presenting cells. Blockade of this and other costimulatory pathways (LFA-1/ICAM, CD40-CD40L) has since been shown to deactivate T cells and induce a state of alloimmune tolerance after BMT [210–212]. In the first series of human patients transplanted with HLA-mismatched marrow allografts that had been treated *in vitro* with CTLA4-Ig as a method of T-anergy induction, all engrafted normally and only three of 11 were reported to have experienced GVHD [213]. These results suggest that CTL4-Ig or other agents of costimulatory signal blockade may be effective for inducing specific donor T-cell anergy after BMT. If differential targets for GVHD and GVL can be identified, it may be possible to expose donor marrow *in vitro* to GVHD targets in the presence of CTLA4-Ig to induce GVHD specific anergy, while preserving the T-cell response to tumor antigens for a full GVL effect.

T-cell modification to facilitate elimination

In recent years, researchers have introduced the herpes simplex thymidine kinase (*HS-TK*) gene into donor T cells as a novel approach for controlling GVHD after DLI. The insertion of this "suicide" gene into donor T lymphocytes renders them susceptible to destruction with ganciclovir and, therefore, provides a reliable means of eliminating these cells should severe GVHD develop after the infusion [203–205]. The use of "suicide" gene therapy may also be applicable in conjunction with T-cell-depleted BMT. *HS-TK* gene modified T lymphocytes infused along with T-cell-depleted marrow at the time of transplantation do not appear to interfere with engraftment [204]. More significantly, long-lasting circulation of the gene-modified cells post-transplant can be detected. In two of three patients who developed GVHD, a complete response was observed upon treatment with ganciclovir. A case of chronic cutaneous GVHD responsive to ganciclovir has also been recently reported in a patient who had received T cells bearing the *HS-TK* gene at the time of BMT [214].

Vaccine strategies to reduce relapse

As new leukemia antigens are identified that are potential targets for the GVL response, allogeneic tumor vaccines may be developed to stimulate specific antitumor activity without GVHD after TCD. Vaccinations with tumor specific antigens, like the recently identified serine proteinase PR-1, may provide avenues to reduce relapse rates after transplantation [215]. Still unanswered is whether TCD will render human subjects sufficiently immune incompetent so that they cannot respond to vaccine. However, in a murine model, animals that had undergone T-cell-depleted marrow transplantation could mount a donor cell mediated antitumor response without GVHD after vaccination with irradiated tumor cells genetically engineered to secrete granulocyte macrophage colony-stimulating factor (GM-CSF) [216].

Conclusions

Although outcomes after T-cell-depleted transplantation have improved over the past decade from the use of selective TCD and adoptive immunotherapy, the role of TCD in transplantation remains undefined. Reasonable applications for TCD may include those patients at high risk for GVHD (unrelated or mismatched grafts) or patients with comorbid medical conditions who are suboptimal candidates for conventional BMT. TCD may be ideal for patients with diseases where the GVL effect is less critical, such as acute leukemia in remission. Nonetheless, the only randomized trial of TCD (in an unrelated setting) could demonstrate no benefit for TCD. There still remain many unanswered questions including: (i) who should receive a T-cell-depleted transplant; (ii) how marrow or stem cells should be purged; and (iii) what is the optimal number of T cells to include in the graft. It remains unclear whether additional medications are needed to promote engraftment or control GVHD, or what the nature and timing of immunomodulating manipulations to reduce the risk of relapse should be. These questions will not be fully resolved until there is a better understanding of the pathogenesis of GVHD. Hopefully, the role of minor HLA antigens can soon be defined and antigen targets for GVHD and GVL can potentially be exploited through graft engineering. It would be ideal to be able to manipulate different cellular subgroups responsible for GVHD and GVL. Being able to do so will be critical to the future success of allogeneic stem-cell transplantation.

References

1 Ferrara JL, Levy R, Chao NJ. Pathophysiologic mechanisms of acute graft-versus-host disease. *Biol Blood Marrow Transplant* 1999; **5**: 347–56.

2 Sullivan KM, Shulman HM, Storb R *et al*. Chronic graft versus host disease in 52 patients: adverse natural course and successful treatment with combination immunosuppression. *Blood* 1981; **57**: 267–76.

3 Martin PJ, Schoch G, Fisher L *et al*. A retrospective analysis of therapy for acute graft-versus-host disease: initial treatment. *Blood* 1990; **76**: 1464–72.

4 Weisdorf D, Haake R, Blazar B *et al*. Treatment of moderate/severe acute graft-versus-host disease after allogeneic bone marrow transplantation: an analysis of clinical risk features and outcome. *Blood* 1990; **75**: 1024–30.

5 Ho VY, Soiffer RJ. The history and future of T-cell depletion as graft-versus-host disease prophylaxis for allogeneic hematopoietic stem cell transplantation. *Blood* 2001; **98**: 3192–204.

6 Barnes DWH, Loutit JF. The immunological and histological responses following spleen treatment in irradiated mice. In: Mitchel JS, Holmes BE, eds. *Progress in Radiobiology*. Edinburgh: Oliver and Boyd, 1954: 291–300.

7 Uphoff DE. Preclusion of secondary phase of irradiation syndrome by innoculation of hematopoietic tissue following lethal total body X-irradiation. *J Natl Cancer Inst* 1958; **20**: 625–31.

8 Dicke KA, van Hoot JIM, van Bekkum DW. The selective elimination of immunologically competent cells from bone marrow and lymphatic cell mixtures. II. Mouse spleen cell fractionation: a discontinuous albumin gradient. *Transplantation* 1968; **6**: 562–8.

9 Reisner Y, Itzicovitch L, Meshorer A, Sharon N. Hematopoietic stem cell transplantation using mouse bone marrow and spleen cells fractionated by lectins. *Proc Natl Acad Sci U S A* 1978; **75**: 2933–6.

10 Trentin JJ, Judd KP. Prevention of acute graft-versus-host (GVH) mortality with spleen-absorbed antithymocyte globulin (ATG). *Transplant Proc* 1973; **5**: 865–8.

11 Rodt H, Kolb HJ, Netzel B *et al*. GVHD suppression by incubation of bone marrow grafts with anti-T-cell globulin: effect in canine model and application to clinical bone marrow transplantation. *Transplant Proc* 1979; **11**: 962–6.

12 Korngold R, Sprent J. Lethal graft-versus-host disease after bone marrow transplantation across minor histocompatibility barriers in mice. Prevention by removing mature T cells from marrow. *J Exp Med* 1978; **148**: 1687–98.

13 Rodt H, Theirfelder S, Eulitz M. Antilymphocyte antibodies and marrow transplantation. III. Effect of heterologous anti-brain antibodies on acute secondary disease in mice. *Eur J Immunol* 1974; **4**: 15–9.

14 Kolb HJ, Rieder I, Rodt H *et al*. Antilymphocyte antibodies and marrow transplantation. VI. Graft-versus-host tolerance in DLA-incompatible dogs after *in vitro* treatment of donor marrow absorbed with antithymocyte globulin. *Transplantation* 1979; **27**: 242–5.

15 Vallera DA, Soderling CC, Carlson GJ, Kersey JH. Bone marrow transplantation across major histocompatibility barriers in mice. *Transplantation* 1981; **31**: 218–22.

16 Reisner Y, Kapoor N, Kirkpatrick D *et al*. Transplantation for acute leukemia with HLA-A and B nonidentical parental marrow cells fractionated with soybean agglutinin and sheep red blood cells. *Lancet* 1981; **2**(8242): 327–31.

17 Reisner Y, Kapoor N, Kirkpatrick D *et al*. Transplantation for severe combined immunodeficiency with HLA-A, B, D, DR incompatibility parental marrow cells fractionated by soybean agglutinin and sheep red blood cells. *Blood* 1983; **161**: 341–8.

18 De Witte T, Hoogenhout J, de Pauw B *et al*. Depletion of donor lymphocytes by counterflow centrifugation successfully prevents acute graft-versus-host disease in matched allogeneic marrow transplantation. *Blood* 1986; **67**: 1302–8.

19 Noga SJ, Donnenberg AD, Schwartz CL *et al*. Development of a simplified counterflow centrifugation elutriation procedure for depletion of lymphocytes from human bone marrow. *Transplantation* 1986; **41**: 220–5.

20 Wagner JE, Donnenberg AD, Noga SJ *et al*. Lymphocyte depletion of donor bone marrow by counterflow centrifugal elutriation: results of a phase I clinical trial. *Blood* 1988; **72**: 1168–76.

21 Lowenberg B, Wagemaker E, van Bekkum DW *et al*. Graft-versus-host disease following transplantation of 'one log' versus 'two log' T-lymphocyte depleted bone marrow from HLA-identical donors. *Bone Marrow Transplant* 1986; **1**: 133–40.

22 Prentice HG, Blacklock HA, Janossy G *et al*. Use of anti-T-cell monoclonal antibody OKT3 to prevent acute graft versus host disease in allogeneic bone marrow transplantation for acute leukemia. *Lancet* 1982; **1**(8274): 700–3.

23 Filipovich AH, McGlave PB, Ramsay NKC *et al*. Pretreatment of donor bone marrow with monoclonal antibody OKT3 for prevention of acute graft versus host disease in allogeneic histocompatible bone marrow transplantation. *Lancet* 1982; **1**(8284): 1266–9.

24 Martin PJ, Hansen JA, Thomas ED. Preincubation of donor bone marrow cells with a combination of murine monoclonal anti-T-cell antibodies without complement does not prevent graft-versus-host disease after allogeneic marrow transplantation. *J Clin Immunol* 1984; **4**: 18–22.

25 Reinherz EL, Geha R, Rappeport JM *et al*. Reconstitution after transplantation with T-lymphocyte-depleted HLA haplotype-mismatched bonz marrow for severe combined immunodeficiency. *Proc Natl Acad Sci U S A* 1982; **79**: 6047–51.

26 Prentice HG, Janossy G, Price-Jones L *et al*. Depletion of T lymphocytes in donor marrow prevents significant graft-versus-host disease in matched allogeneic leukemic marrow transplant recipients. *Lancet* 1984; **1**(8375): 472–6.

27 Waldmann HG, Polliak A, Hale G *et al*. Elimination of graft-versus-host disease by *in vitro* depletion of alloreactive lymphocytes with a monoclonal rat anti-human lymphocyte antibody (Campath-1). *Lancet* 1984; **2**(8401): 483–6.

28 Martin PJ, Hansen JA, Buckner CD *et al*. Effects of *in vitro* depletion of T cells in HLA-identical allogeneic marrow grafts. *Blood* 1985; **66**: 664–72.

29 Herve P, Flesch M, Cahn JY *et al*. Removal of marrow T cells with OKT3-OKT11 monoclonal antibodies and complement to prevent graft-versus-host disease. *Transplantation* 1985; **39**: 138–43.

30 Trigg ME, Billing R, Sondel PM *et al*. Clinical trial depleting T lymphocytes from donor marrow for

matched and mismatched allogeneic bone marrow transplants. *Canc Treat Rep* 1985; **69**: 377–86.
31. Mitsuyasu RT, Champlin RE, Gale RP *et al.* Treatment of donor bone marrow with monoclonal anti-T-cell antibody and complement for the prevention of graft versus host disease. *Ann Int Med* 1986; **105**: 20–6.
32. Maraninchi D, Gluckman E, Blaise D *et al.* Impact of T-cell depletion on outcome of allogeneic bone-marrow transplantation for standard-risk leukaemia. *Lancet* 1987; **2**(8552): 175–8.
33. Cahn JY, Herve P, Flesch M *et al.* Marrow transplantation from HLA non-identical family donors for the treatment of leukaemias: a pilot study of 15 patients using additional immunosuppression and T-cell depletion. *Br J Haematol* 1988; **69**: 345–9.
34. Soiffer RJ, Murray C, Mauch P *et al.* Prevention of graft-versus-host disease by selective depletion of CD6-positive T lymphocytes from donor bone marrow. *J Clin Oncol* 1992; **10**: 1191–200.
35. Filipovich AH, Vallera DA, Youle RJ *et al.* Graft-versus-host disease prevention in allogeneic bone marrow transplantation from histocompatible siblings. *Transplantation* 1987; **44**: 62–6.
36. Laurent G, Maraninchi D, Gluckman E *et al.* Donor bone marrow treatment with T101 Fab fragment-ricin A-chain immunotoxin prevents graft-versus-host disease. *Bone Marrow Transplant* 1989; **4**: 367–72.
37. Filipovich AH, Vallera D, McGlave P *et al.* T cell depletion with anti-CD5 immunotoxin in histocompatible bone marrow transplantation. *Transplantation* 1990; **50**: 410–4.
38. Antin JH, Bierer BE, Smith BR *et al.* Selective depletion of bone marrow T lymphocytes with anti-CD5 monoclonal antibodies: effective prophylaxis for graft-versus-host disease in patients with hematologic malignancies. *Blood* 1991; **78**: 2139–44.
39. Vartdal F, Albrechtsen D, Ringden O *et al.* Immunomagnetic treatment of bone marrow allografts. *Bone Marrow Transplant* 1987; **2**: 94–8.
40. Bensinger WI, Buckner CD, Shannon-Dorcy K *et al.* Transplantation of allogeneic $CD34^+$ peripheral blood stem cells in patients with advanced hematologic malignancy. *Blood* 1996; **88**: 4132–7.
41. Finke J, Brugger W, Bertz H *et al.* Allogeneic transplantation of positively selected peripheral blood $CD34^+$ progenitor cells from matched related donors. *Bone Marrow Transplant* 1996; **18**: 1081–5.
42. Link H, Arseniev L, Bahre O *et al.* Transplantation of allogeneic $CD34^+$ blood cells. *Blood* 1996; **87**: 4903–8.
43. Urbano-Ispizua A, Solano C, Brunet S *et al.* Allogeneic transplantation of selected $CD34^+$ cells from peripheral blood: experience of 62 cases using immunoabsorption or immunomagnetic technique. *Bone Marrow Transplant* 1998; **22**: 519–24.
44. Vij R, Brown R, Shenoy S *et al.* Allogeneic peripheral blood stem cell transplantation following $CD34^+$ enrichment by density gradient separation. *Bone Marrow Transplant* 2000; **25**: 1223–8.
45. Hale G, Jacobs P, Wood L *et al.* CD52 antibodies for prevention of graft-versus-host disease and graft rejection following transplantation of allogeneic peripheral blood stem cells. *Bone Marrow Transplant* 2000; **26**: 69–75.
46. Henslee-Downey PJ, Parrish RS, MacDonald JS *et al.* Combined *in vitro* and *in vivo* T lymphocyte depletion for the control of graft-versus-host disease following haploidentical marrow transplant. *Transplantation* 1996; **61**: 738–43.
47. Kernan NA, Collins NM, Juliano L *et al.* Clonable T lymphocytes in T cell-depleted bone marrow transplants correlate with development of graft-v-host disease. *Blood* 1986; **68**: 770–5.
48. Martin PJ, Hansen JA. Quantitative assays for detection of residual T cells in T-depleted human marrow. *Blood* 1985; **65**: 1134–9.
49. Alyea EP, Weller E, Fisher DC *et al.* Comparable outcome with T cell depleted unrelated donor versus related donor allogeneic bone marrow transplantation. *Biol Blood Marrow Transplant* 2002; **8**: 601–7.
50. Aversa F, Tabilio A, Velardi A *et al.* Treatment of high-risk acute leukemia with T-cell-depleted stem cells from related donors with one fully mismatched HLA haplotype. *N Engl J Med* 1998; **339**: 1186–91.
51. Goulmy E, Schipper R, Pool J *et al.* Mismatches of minor histocompatibilitiy antigens between HLA-identical donors and recipients and development of graft-versus-host disease after bone marrow transplantation. *N Engl J Med* 1996; **334**: 281–7.
52. Kawanishi Y, Passweg J, Drobyski WR *et al.* Effect of T cell subset dose on outcome of T cell-depleted bone marrow transplantation. *Bone Marrow Transplant* 1997; **19**: 1069–74.
53. Champlin RE, Passweg JR, Zhang MJ *et al.* T-cell depletion of bone marrow transplants for leukemia from donors other than HLA-identical siblings: advantage of T-cell antibodies with narrow specificities. *Blood* 2000; **95**: 3996–4002.
54. Hale G, Cobbold S, Waldmann H. T-cell depletion with Campath-1 in allogeneic bone marrow transplantation. *Transplantation* 1988; **45**: 753–9.
55. Champlin R, Ho W, Gajewski J *et al.* Selective depletion of $CD8^+$ T lymphocytes for prevention of graft-versus-host disease after allogeneic bone marrow transplantation. *Blood* 1990; **76**: 418–23.
56. Wagner JE, Santos GW, Noga SJ *et al.* Bone marrow graft engineering by counterflow elutriation: results of a phase I–II clinical trial. *Blood* 1990; **75**: 1370–5.
57. Spitzer TR, McAfee S, Sackstein R *et al.* Intentional induction of mixed chimerism and achievement of antitumor responses after nonmyeloablative conditioning therapy and HLA-matched donor bone marrow transplantation for refractory hematologic malignancies. *Biol Blood Marrow Transplant* 2002; **6**: 309–15.
58. Perez-Simon JA, Kottaridis PD, Martino R *et al.* Nonmyeloablative transplantation with or without alemtuzumab: comparison between two prospective studies in patients with lymphoproliferative disorders. *Blood* 2002; **100**: 3121–7.
59. Urbano-Ispizua A, Rozman C, Pimentel P *et al.* Risk factors for acute graft-versus-host disease in patients undergoing transplantation with $CD34^+$ selected blood cells from HLA-identical siblings. *Blood* 2002; **100**: 724–7.
60. Przepiorka D, Smith TL, Folloder J *et al.* Risk factors for acute graft-versus-host disease after allogeneic blood stem cell transplantation. *Blood* 1999; **94**: 1465–70.
61. Kernan NA, Bartsch G, Ash RC *et al.* Analysis of 462 transplantations from unrelated donors facilitated by the National Marrow Donor Program. *N Engl J Med* 1993; **328**: 593–9.
62. Soiffer RJ, Weller E, Alyea EP *et al.* $CD6^+$ donor marrow T-cell depletion as the sole form of graft-versus-host disease prophylaxis in patients undergoing allogeneic bone marrow transplant from unrelated donors. *J Clin Oncol* 2001; **19**: 1152–9.
63. Drobyski WR, Ash RC, Casper JT *et al.* Effect of T-cell depletion as graft-versus-host disease prophylaxis on engraftment, relapse, and disease-free survival in unrelated marrow transplantation for chronic myelogenous leukemia. *Blood* 1994; **83**: 1980–6.
64. Wagner JE, Thompson JS, Carter S *et al.* Impact of graft-versus-host disease (GVHD) prophylaxis on 3-year disease-free survival (DFS): results of a multi-center, randomized phase II–III trial comparing T cell depletion (TCD)/cyclosporine and methotrexate/cyclosporine (M/C) in 410 recipients of unrelated donor bone marrow (BM). *Blood* 2002; **100**: 75a.
65. Ash RC, Horowitz MM, Gale RP *et al.* Bone marrow transplantation from related donors other than HLA-identical siblings: effect of T cell depletion. *Bone Marrow Transplant* 1991; **7**: 443–7.
66. Soiffer RJ, Mauch P, Fairclough D *et al.* $CD6^+$ T cell depleted allogeneic bone marrow transplantation from genotypically HLA nonidentical related donors. *Biol Blood Marrow Transplant* 1997; **3**: 11–7.
67. Henslee-Downey PJ, Abhyankar SH, Parrish RS *et al.* Use of partially mismatched related donors extends access to allogeneic marrow transplant. *Blood* 1997; **89**: 3864–1.
68. Soiffer RJ, Dear K, Rabinowe SN *et al.* Hepatic dysfunction following T-cell-depleted allogeneic bone marrow transplantation. *Transplantation* 1991; **52**: 1014–9.
69. Breuer R, Or R, Lijovetzky G *et al.* Interstitial pneumonitis in T cell-depleted bone marrow transplantation. *Bone Marrow Transplant* 1988; **3**: 625–30.
70. Ho VT, Weller E, Lee SJ *et al.* Prognostic factors for early severe pulmonary complications after hematopoietic stem cell transplantation. *Biol Blood Marrow Transplant* 2001; **7**: 223–9.
71. Soiffer RJ, Fairclough D, Robertson M *et al.* CD6-depleted allogeneic bone marrow transplantation for acute leukemia in first complete remission. *Blood* 1997; **89**: 3039–47.
72. Drobyski WR, Hessner MJ, Klein JP *et al.* T-cell depletion plus salvage immunotherapy with donor leukocyte infusions as a strategy to treat chronic-phase chronic myelogenous leukemia patients undergoing HLA-identical sibling marrow transplantation. *Blood* 1999; **94**: 434–9.
73. Hale G, Zhang MJ, Bunjes D *et al.* Improving the outcome of bone marrow transplantation by using CD52 monoclonal antibodies to prevent graft-versus-host disease and graft rejection. *Blood* 1998; **92**: 4581–7.
74. Papadopoulos EB, Carabasi MH, Castro-Malaspina H *et al.* T-cell-depleted allogeneic bone marrow transplantation as postremission therapy for acute myelogenous leukemia: freedom from relapse in the absence of graft-versus-host disease. *Blood* 1998; **91**: 1083–8.
75. Hale G, Waldmann H. Control of graft-versus-host disease and graft rejection by T cell depletion of donor and recipient with Campath-1 antibodies. Results of matched sibling transplants for malignant diseases. *Bone Marrow Transplant* 1994; **13**: 597–602.
76. Nimer SD, Giorgi J, Gajewski JL *et al.* Selective depletion of $CD8^+$ cells for prevention of graft-versus-host disease after bone marrow transplantation.

A randomized controlled trial. *Transplantation* 1994; **57**: 82–9.
77 Lee SJ, Zahrieh D, Alyea EP *et al.* Comparison of T-cell-depleted and non-T-cell-depleted unrelated donor transplantation for hematologic diseases: clinical outcomes, quality of life, and costs. *Blood* 2002; **100**: 2697–702.
78 Champlin RE, Horowitz MM, van Bekkum DW *et al.* Graft failure following bone marrow transplantation for severe aplastic anemia: risk factors and treatment results. *Blood* 1989; **73**: 606–11.
79 Beatty PG, Clift RA, Mickelson EM *et al.* Marrow transplantation for related donors other than HLA-identical siblings. *New Engl J Med* 1985; **313**: 765–70.
80 Powles RL, Kay HEM, Clink HM *et al.* Mismatched family donors for bone marrow transplantation as treatment for acute leukemia. *Lancet* 1983; **1**: 612–5.
81 Patterson J, Prentice HG, Brenner MK *et al.* Graft rejection following HLA matched T-lymphocyte depleted bone marrow transplantation. *Br J Haematol* 1986; **63**: 221–5.
82 O'Reilly R, Collins NH, Kernan N *et al.* Transplantation of marrow-depleted T cells by soybean lectin agglutination and E-rosette depletion: major histocompatibility complex-related graft resistance in leukemic transplant patients. *Transplant Proc* 1985; **17**: 455–62.
83 Martin PJ, Hansen JA, Torok-Storb B *et al.* Graft failure in patients receiving T cell-depleted HLA-identical allogeneic marrow transplants. *Bone Marrow Transplant* 1988; **3**: 445–52.
84 Delain M, Cahn JY, Racadot E *et al.* Graft failure after T cell depleted HLA identical allogeneic bone marrow transplantation: risk factors in leukemic patients. *Leuk Lymph* 1993; **11**: 359–64.
85 Kernan NA, Bordignon C, Heller G *et al.* Graft failure after T-cell-depleted leukocyte antigen identical marrow transplants for leukemia: I. analysis of risk factors and results of secondary transplants. *Blood* 1989; **74**: 2227–33.
86 Marmont A, Horowitz MM, Gale RP *et al.* T-cell depletion of HLA-identical transplants in leukemia. *Blood* 1991; **78**: 2120–6.
87 Sondel PM, Hank JA, Trigg ME *et al.* Transplantation of HLA-haploidentical T cell-depleted marrow for leukemia: autologous marrow recovery with specific immune sensitization to donor antigens. *Exp Hematol* 1986; **14**: 278–83.
88 Bunjes D, Heit W, Arnold R *et al.* Evidence for the involvement of host derived OKT8-positive T cells in the rejection of T-depleted, HLA-identical bone marrow grafts. *Transplantation* 1987; **43**: 501–7.
89 Bunjes D, Theobald M, Wiesneth M *et al.* Graft rejection by a population of primed CDw52-host T cells after *in vivo/ex vivo* T-depleted bone marrow transplantation. *Bone Marrow Transplant* 1993; **12**: 209–14.
90 Kernan NA, Flomenberg N, Dupont B, O'Reilly RJ. Graft rejection in recipients of T cell depleted HLA-nonidentical marrow transplants for leukemia. *Transplantation* 1987; **43**: 842–7.
91 Bierer BE, Emerson SG, Antin J *et al.* Regulation of cytotoxic T lymphocyte-mediated graft rejection following bone marrow transplantation. *Transplantation* 1990; **49**: 714–8.
92 Bordignon C, Keever CA, Small TN *et al.* Graft failure after T-cell-depleted leukocyte antigen identical marrow transplants for leukemia: II. *in vitro* analysis of host effector mechanisms. *Blood* 1989; **74**: 2237–42.
93 Bosserman L, Murray C, Takvorian T *et al.* Mechanism of graft failure in HLA-matched and HLA-mismatched bone marrow transplant recipients. *Bone Marrow Transplant* 1989; **4**: 239–44.
94 Voogt PJ, Fibbe WE, Marjit WA *et al.* Rejection of bone marrow graft by recipient derived cytotoxic T lymphocytes against minor histocompatibility antigens. *Lancet* 1990; **335**: 135–9.
95 Fleischauer K, Kernan NA, O'Reilly RJ *et al.* Bone marrow-allograft rejection by T lymphocytes recognizing a single amino acid difference on HLA-B44. *New Engl J Med* 1990; **323**: 1818–25.
96 Donohue J, Homge M, Kernan NA. Characterization of cells emerging at the time of graft failure after bone marrow transplantation from an unrelated bone marrow donor. *Blood* 1993; **82**: 1023–9.
97 Gerritsen WR, Wagemaker G, Jonker M *et al.* The repopulation capacity of bone marrow grafts following pretreatment with monoclonal antibodies against T lymphocytes in rhesus monkeys. *Transplantation* 1988; **45**: 301–7.
98 Anderson KC, Barut BA, Ritz J *et al.* Monoclonal antibody-purged autologous bone marrow transplantation therapy for multiple myeloma. *Blood* 1991; **77**: 712–20.
99 Soiffer RJ, Roy DC, Gonin R *et al.* Monoclonal antibody-purged autologous bone marrow transplantation in adults with acute lymphoblastic leukemia at high risk of relapse. *Bone Marrow Transplant* 1993; **12**: 243–51.
100 Mutter W, Reddehase MJ, Busch FW *et al.* Failure in generating hemopoietic stem cells is the primary cause of death from cytomegalovirus disease in the immunocompromised host. *J Exp Med* 1988; **167**: 1645–50.
101 Steffens HP, Podlech J, Kurz S *et al.* Cytomegalovirus inhibits the engraftment of donor bone marrow cells by downregulation of hemopoietin gene expression in recipient stroma. *J Virol* 1998; **72**: 5006–11.
102 Johnston RE, Geretti AM, Prentice HG *et al.* HHV-6-related secondary graft failure following allogeneic bone marrow transplantation. *Br J Haematol* 1999; **105**: 1041–6.
103 Rosenfeld CS, Rybka WB, Weinbaum D *et al.* Late graft failure due to dual bone marrow infection with variants A and B of human herpesvirus-6. *Exp Hematol* 1995; **23**: 626–30.
104 Couriel D, Canosa J, Engler H *et al.* Early reactivation of cytomegalovirus and high risk of interstitial pneumonitis following T-depleted BMT for adults with hematological malignancies. *Bone Marrow Transplant* 1996; **18**: 347–51.
105 Hertenstein B, Hampl W, Bunjes D *et al. In vivo/ex vivo* T cell depletion for GVHD prophylaxis influences onset and course of active cytomegalovirus infection and disease after BMT. *Bone Marrow Transplant* 1995; **15**: 387–91.
106 Broers AEC, van der Holt R, van Esser JWJ *et al.* Increased transplant-related morbidity and mortality in CMV-seropositive patients despite highly effective prevention of CMV disease after allogeneic T-cell-depleted stem cell transplantation. *Blood* 2000; **95**: 224–9.
107 Burnett AK, Hann IM, Robertson AG *et al.* Prevention of graft-versus-host disease by *ex vivo* T cell depletion: reduction in raft failure with augmented total body irradiation. *Leukemia* 1988; **2**: 300–6.
108 Bertheas MF, Lafage M, Levy P *et al.* Influence of mixed chimerism on the results of allogeneic bone marrow transplantation for leukemia. *Blood* 1991; **78**: 3103–8.
109 Offit K, Burns JP, Cunningham I *et al.* Cytogenetic analysis of chimerism and leukemia relapse in chronic myelogenous leukemia patients after T cell-depleted bone marrow transplantation. *Blood* 1990; **75**: 1346–51.
110 Mackinnon S, Barnett L, O'Reilly RJ. Minimal residual disease is more common in patients who have mixed T-cell chimerism after bone marrow transplantation for chronic myelogenous leukemia. *Blood* 1994; **83**: 3409–15.
111 van Leeuwen JEM, van Tol MJD, Joosten AM *et al.* Mixed T-lymphoid chimerism after allogeneic bone marrow transplantation for hematologic malignancies of children is not correlated with relapse. *Blood* 1993; **82**: 1921–7.
112 Butturini A, Seeger RC, Gale RP. Recipient immune-competent T lymphocytes can survive intensive conditioning for bone marrow transplantation. *Blood* 1986; **68**: 954–9.
113 Kedar E, Or R, Naparstek E *et al.* Preliminary characterization of functional residual host-type T lymphocytes following conditioning for allogeneic HLA-matched bone marrow transplantation (BMT). *Bone Marrow Transplant* 1988; **3**: 129–34.
114 Manilay JO, Sykes M. Natural killer cells and their role in graft rejection. *Curr Opin Immunol* 1988; **10**: 532–9.
115 Martin PJ. Donor CD8 cells prevent allogeneic marrow graft rejection in mice: potential implications for marrow transplantation in humans. *J Exp Med* 1993; **178**: 703–9.
116 Martin PJ, Rowley SD, Anasetti C *et al.* A phase I–II clinical trial to evaluate removal of CD4 cells and partial depletion of CD8 cells from donor marrow for HLA-mismatched unrelated recipients. *Blood* 1999; **94**: 2192–9.
117 Ash RC, Casper JT, Chitambar CR *et al.* Successful allogeneic transplantation of T-cell-depleted bone marrow from closely HLA-matched unrelated donors. *New Engl J Med* 1990; **322**: 485–91.
118 Aversa F, Pelicci PG, Terenzi A *et al.* Results of T-depleted BMT in chronic myelogenous leukaemia after a conditioning regimen that included thiotepa. *Bone Marrow Transplant* 1991; **7** (Suppl. 2): 24–6.
119 Schaap N, Schattenberg A, Bar B *et al.* Outcome of transplantation for standard-risk leukaemia with grafts depleted of lymphocytes after conditioning with an intensified regimen. *Br J Haematol* 1997; **98**: 750–6.
120 Schattenberg A, Schaap N, Preijers F *et al.* Outcome of T cell-depleted transplantation after conditioning with an intensified regimen in patients aged 50 years or more is comparable with that in younger patients. *Bone Marrow Transplant* 2000; **26**: 17–22.
121 Guyotat D, Dutou L, Erhsam A *et al.* Graft rejection after T cell-depleted marrow transplantation: role of fractionated irradiation. *Br J Haematol* 1987; **65**: 499–504.
122 Bozdech MJ, Sondel PM, Trigg ME *et al.* Transplantation of HLA-haploidentical T-cell-depleted marrow for leukemia: addition of cytosine arabinoside to the pretransplant conditioning prevents rejection. *Exp Hematol* 1985; **13**: 1201–6.
123 Soiffer RJ, Mauch P, Tarbell NJ *et al.* Total lymphoid irradiation to prevent graft rejection in recipients of HLA non-identical T cell-depleted allogeneic marrow. *Bone Marrow Transplant* 1991; **7**: 23–33.
124 Ganem G, Kuentz M, Beaujean F *et al.* Additional total lymphoid irradiation in preventing graft fail-

ure of T-cell depleted bone marrow transplantation from HLA-identical siblings. *Transplantation* 1987; **45**: 244–9.
125. Cobbold S, Martin G, Waldmann H. Monoclonal antibodies for the prevention of graft-versus-host disease and marrow graft rejection. The depletion of T cell subsets *in vitro* and *in vivo*. *Transplantation* 1986; **42**: 239–44.
126. Castro-Malaspina H, Childs B, Laver J *et al*. Hyperfractionated total lymphoid irradiation and cyclophosphamide for preparation of previously transfused patients undergoing HLA-identical marrow transplantation for severe aplastic anemia. *Int J Radiat Oncol Biol Phys* 1994; **29**: 847–52.
127. Barrett AJ, Mavroudis D, Tisdale J *et al*. T cell-depleted bone marrow transplantation and delayed T cell add-back to control acute GVHD and conserve a graft-versus-leukemia effect. *Bone Marrow Transplant* 1998; **21**: 543–51.
128. Potter MN, Pamphilon DH, Cornish JM, Oakhill A. Graft-versus-host disease in children receiving HLA-identical allogeneic bone marrow transplants with a low adjusted T lymphocyte dose. *Bone Marrow Transplant* 1991; **8**: 357–62.
129. Bachar-Lustig E, Rachamim N, Li HW *et al*. Megadose of T cell-depleted bone marrow overcomes MHC barriers in sublethally irradiated mice. *Nat Med* 1995; **1**: 1268–72.
130. Aversa F, Tabilio A, Terenzi A *et al*. Successful engraftment of T-cell-depleted haploidentical transplants in leukemia patients by addition of recombinant human granulocyte colony-stimulating factor-mobilized peripheral blood progenitor cells to bone marrow inoculum. *Blood* 1994; **84**: 3948–53.
131. Reisner Y, Martelli MF. Tolerance induction by 'megadose' transplants of $CD34^+$ stem cells: a new option for leukemia patients without an HLA-matched donor. *Curr Opin Immunol* 2000; **12**: 536–41.
132. Soiffer RJ, Alyea EP, Kim H *et al*. Engraftment, graft-vs.-host disease (GVHD), and survival after $CD8^+$ T cell depleted allogeneic peripheral blood stem cell transplantation (PBSCT). *Blood* 2002; **100**: 418a [Abstract].
133. Welte K, Keever CA, Levick J *et al*. Interleukin-2 production and response to interleukin-2 by peripheral blood mononuclear cells from patients after bone marrow transplantation. II. Patients receiving soybean lectin-separated and T cell-depleted bone marrow. *Blood* 1987; **70**: 1595–60.
134. Soiffer RJ, Bosserman L, Murray C *et al*. Reconstitution of T-cell function after CD6-depleted allogeneic bone marrow transplantation. *Blood* 1990; **75**: 2076–84.
135. Keever CA, Small TN, Flomenberg N *et al*. Immune reconstitution following bone marrow transplantation: comparison of recipients of T-cell depleted marrow with recipients of conventional marrow grafts. *Blood* 1989; **73**: 1340–5.
136. Ault KA, Antin JH, Ginsburg D *et al*. Phenotype of recovering lymphoid cell populations after marrow transplantation. *J Exp Med* 1985; **161**: 1483–7.
137. Parreira A, Smith J, Hows JM *et al*. Immunological reconstitution after bone marrow transplant with Campath-1 treated bone marrow. *Clin Exp Immunol* 1987; **67**: 142–8.
138. Roux E, Helg C, Dumont-Girard F *et al*. Analysis of T-cell repopulation after allogeneic bone marrow transplantation: significant differences between recipients of T-cell depleted and unmanipulated grafts. *Blood* 1996; **87**: 3984–9.
139. Roux E, Dumont-Girard F, Starobinski M *et al*. Recovery of immune reactivity after T-cell-depleted bone marrow transplantation depends on thymic activity. *Blood* 2000; **96**: 2299–305.
140. Wu CJ, Chillemi A, Alyea EP *et al*. Reconstitution of T-cell receptor repertoire diversity following T-cell depleted allogeneic bone marrow transplantation is related to hematopoietic chimerism. *Blood* 2000; **95**: 352–9.
141. Small TN, Papadopoulos EB, Boulad F *et al*. Comparison of immune reconstitution after unrelated and related T-cell-depleted bone marrow transplantation: effect of patient age and donor leukocyte infusions. *Blood* 1999; **93**: 467–80.
142. Hochberg EP, Chillemi AC, Wu CJ *et al*. Quantitation of T-cell neogenesis *in vivo* after allogeneic bone marrow transplantation in adults. *Blood* 2001; **98**: 2116–21.
143. Lewin SR, Heller G, Zhang L *et al*. Direct evidence for new T-cell generation by patients after either T-cell-depleted or unmodified allogeneic hematopoietic stem cell transplantations. *Blood* 2002; **100**: 2235–42.
144. Engelhard D, Or R, Strauss N *et al*. Cytomegalovirus infection and disease after T cell depleted allogeneic bone marrow transplantation for malignant hematologic diseases. *Transplant Proc* 1989; **21**: 3101–5.
145. Martino R, Rovira M, Carreras E *et al*. Severe infections after allogeneic peripheral blood stem cell transplantation: a matched-pair comparison of unmanipulated and $CD34^+$ cell-selected transplantation. *Haematologica* 2001; **86**: 1075–9.
146. Lin TS, Zahrieh D, Weller E, Alyea EP, Antin JH, Soiffer RJ. Risk factors for cytomegalovirus reactivation after $CD6^+$ T-cell-depleted allogeneic bone marrow transplantation. *Transplantation* 2002; **74**: 49–54.
147. Zutter MM, Martin PJ, Sale GE *et al*. Epstein–Barr virus lymphoproliferation after bone marrow transplantation. *Blood* 1988; **72**: 520–6.
148. Gerritsen EJ, Stam ED, Hermans J *et al*. Risk factors for developing EBV-related B cell lymphoproliferative disorders (BLPD) after non-HLA-identical BMT in children. *Bone Marrow Transplant* 1996; **18**: 377–81.
149. Martin P, Schulman H, Schubach W *et al*. Fatal Epstein–Barr virus associated proliferation of donor B-cells after treatment of acute graft-versus-host disease with a murine anti-T-cell antibody. *Ann Int Med* 1984; **101**: 310–4.
150. Papadopoulos EB, Ladanyi M, Emmanuel D *et al*. Infusions of donor leukocytes to treat Epstein–Barr-associated lymphoproliferative disorders after allogeneic bone marrow transplantation. *New Engl J Med* 1994; **330**: 1185–90.
151. Heslop HE, Brenner MK, Rooney C *et al*. Administration of neomycin-resistance-gene-marked EBV-specific cytotoxic T lymphocytes to recipients of mismatched-related or phenotypically similar unrelated donor marrow grafts. *Hum Gene Ther* 1994; **5**: 381–5.
152. Rooney CM, Smith CA, Ng CY *et al*. Use of gene-modified virus-specific T lymphocytes to control Epstein–Barr-virus-related lymphoproliferation. *Lancet* 1995; **345**: 9–12.
153. Rooney CM, Smith CA, Ng CY *et al*. Infusion of cytotoxic T cells for the prevention and treatment of Epstein–Barr virus-induced lymphoma in allogeneic transplant recipients. *Blood* 1998; **92**: 1549–55.
154. Fischer A, Blanche S, Le Bidois J *et al*. Anti-B-cell monoclonal antibodies in the treatment of severe B-cell lymphoproliferative syndrome following bone marrow and organ transplantation. *N Engl J Med* 1991; **324**: 1451–6.
155. McGuirk JP, Seropian S, Howe G *et al*. Use of rituximab and irradiated donor-derived lymphocytes to control Epstein–Barr virus-associated lymphoproliferation in patients undergoing related haploidentical stem cell transplantation. *Bone Marrow Transplant* 1999; **24**: 1253–7.
156. Kuehnle I, Huls MH, Liu Z *et al*. CD20 monoclonal antibody (rituximab) for therapy of Epstein–Barr virus lymphoma after hemopoietic stem-cell transplantation. *Blood* 2000; **95**: 1502–6.
157. Cavazzana-Calvo M, Bensoussan D, Jabado N *et al*. Prevention of EBV-induced B-lymphoproliferative disorder by *ex vivo* marrow B-cell depletion in HLA-phenoidentical or non-identical T-depleted bone marrow transplantation. *Br J Haematol* 1998; **103**: 543–7.
158. Hale G, Waldmann H. Risks of developing Epstein–Barr virus-related lymphoproliferative disorders after T-cell-depleted marrow transplants. *Blood* 1998; **91**: 3079–84.
159. Gustafsson A, Levitsky V, Zou JZ *et al*. Epstein–Barr virus (EBV) load in bone marrow transplant recipients at risk to develop posttransplant lymphoproliferative disease: prophylactic infusion of EBV-specific cytotoxic T cells. *Blood* 2000; **95**: 807–13.
160. Rooney CM, Loftin SK, Holladay MS *et al*. Early identification of Epstein–Barr virus-associated post-transplantation lymphoproliferative disease. *Br J Haematol* 1995; **89**: 98–102.
161. Goldman JM, Gale RP, Horowitz MM *et al*. Bone marrow transplantation for chronic myelogenous leukemia in chronic phase. Increased risk for relapse associated with T-cell depletion. *Ann Int Med* 1988; **108**: 806–10.
162. Martin P, Clift RA, Fisher LD *et al*. HLA-identical marrow transplantation during accelerated-phase chronic myelogenous leukemia: analysis of survival and remission duration. *Blood* 1988; **72**: 1978–83.
163. Marks DI, Hughes TP, Szydlo R *et al*. HLA-identical sibling donor bone marrow transplantation for chronic myeloid leukaemia in first chronic phase: influence of GVHD prophylaxis on outcome. *Br J Haematol* 1992; **81**: 383–6.
164. Wagner JE, Zahurak M, Piantadosi S *et al*. Bone marrow transplantation of chronic myelogenous leukemia in chronic phase: evaluation of risks and benefits. *J Clin Oncol* 1992; **10**: 779–84.
165. Gratwohl A, Hermans J, Niderwieser D *et al*. Bone marrow transplantation for chronic myeloid leukemia: long-term results. *Bone Marrow Transplant* 1993; **12**: 509–14.
166. Apperley JF, Mauro FR, Goldman JM *et al*. Bone marrow transplantation for chronic myeloid leukaemia in first chronic phase: importance of a graft-versus-leukaemia effect. *Br J Haematol* 1988; **69**: 239–43.
167. Weiden PL, Flournoy N, Thomas ED *et al*. Antileukemic effect of graft-versus-host disease in recipients of allogeneic-marrow grafts. *New Engl J Med* 1979; **300**: 1068–72.
168. Sullivan KM, Weiden PL, Storb R *et al*. Influence of acute and chronic graft-versus-host disease on relapse and survival after bone marrow transplantation from HLA-identical siblings as treatment of acute and chronic leukemia. *Blood* 1989; **73**: 1720–6.
169. Horowitz MM, Gale RP, Sondel PM *et al*.

Graft-versus-leukemia reactions after bone marrow transplantation. *Blood* 1990; **75**: 555–61.

170 Kolb HJ, Schattenberg A, Goldman JM et al. Graft-versus-leukemia effect of donor lymphocyte transfusions in marrow grafted patients. *Blood* 1995; **86**: 2041–6.

171 Collins R, Shpilberg O, Drobyski W et al. Donor leukocyte infusions in 140 patients with relapsed malignancy after allogeneic bone marrow transplantation. *J Clin Oncol* 1997; **15**: 433–8.

172 Enright H, Davies SM, DeFor T et al. Relapse after non-T-cell-depleted allogeneic bone marrow transplantation for chronic myelogenous leukemia: early transplantation, use of an unrelated donor, and chronic graft-versus-host disease are protective. *Blood* 1996; **88**: 714–9.

173 McGlave P, Bartsch G, Anasetti C et al. Unrelated donor marrow transplantation therapy for chronic myelogenous leukemia: initial experience of the National Marrow Donor Program. *Blood* 1993; **81**: 543–8.

174 Hessner MJ, Endean DJ, Casper JT et al. Use of unrelated marrow grafts compensates for reduced graft-versus-leukemia reactivity after T-cell-depleted allogeneic marrow transplantation for chronic myelogenous leukemia. *Blood* 1995; **86**: 3987–92.

175 Devergie A, Apperley JF, Labopin M et al. European results of matched unrelated donor bone marrow transplantation for chronic myeloid leukemia. Impact of HLA class II matching. Chronic Leukemia Working Party of the European Group for Blood and Marrow Transplantation. *Bone Marrow Transplant* 1997; **20**: 11–7.

176 Young JW, Papadopoulos EB, Cunningham I et al. T-cell-depleted allogeneic bone marrow transplantation in adults with acute nonlymphocytic leukemia in first remission. *Blood* 1992; **79**: 3380–5.

177 Bunjes D, Hertenstein B, Wiesneth M et al. *In vivo/ex vivo* T cell depletion reduces the morbidity of allogeneic bone marrow transplantation in patients with acute leukaemias in first remission without increasing the risk of treatment failure: comparison with cyclosporin/methotrexate. *Bone Marrow Transplant* 1995; **15**: 563–8.

178 Aversa F, Terenzi A, Carotti A et al. Improved outcome with T-cell-depleted bone marrow transplantation for acute leukemia. *J Clin Oncol* 1999; **17**: 1545–50.

179 Novitzky N, Thomas V, Hale G, Waldmann H. *Ex vivo* depletion of T cells from bone marrow grafts with Campath-1 in acute leukemia: graft-versus-host disease and graft-versus-leukemia effect. *Transplantation* 1999; **67**: 620–5.

180 Remberger M, Ringden O, Aschan J et al. Long-term follow-up of a randomized trial comparing T-cell depletion with a combination of methotrexate and cyclosporine in adult leukemic marrow transplant recipients. *Transplant Proc* 1994; **26**: 1829–33.

181 Korngold R, Sprent J. T cell subsets and graft versus host disease. *Transplantation* 1987; **44**: 335–43.

182 Baker J, Verneris MR, Ito M et al. Expansion of cytolytic $CD8^+$ natural killer T cells with limited capacity for graft-versus-host disease induction due to interferon gamma production. *Blood* 2001; **97**: 2923–8.

183 Jiang YZ, Barrett J. The allogeneic $CD4^+$ T-cell-mediated graft-versus-leukemia effect. *Leuk Lymph* 1997; **28**: 33–8.

184 Soiffer RJ, Gonin R, Murray C et al. Prediction of graft-versus-host disease by phenotypic analysis of early immune reconstitution after CD6-depleted allogeneic bone marrow transplantation. *Blood* 1993; **82**: 2216–23.

185 Giralt S, Hester J, Huh Y et al. CD8-depleted donor lymphocyte infusion as treatment for relapsed chronic myelogenous leukemia after allogeneic bone marrow transplantation. *Blood* 1995; **86**: 4337–42.

186 Alyea EP, Soiffer RJ, Canning C et al. Toxicity and efficacy of defined doses of $CD4^+$ donor lymphocytes for treatment of relapse after allogeneic bone marrow transplant. *Blood* 1998; **91**: 3671–80.

187 Soiffer RJ, Alyea EP, Hochberg E et al. Randomized trial of $CD8^+$ T-cell depletion in the prevention of graft-versus-host disease associated with donor lymphocyte infusion. *Biol Blood Marrow Transplant* 2002; **8**: 625–32.

188 Zorn E, Wang KS, Hochberg EP et al. Infusion of $CD4^+$ donor lymphocytes induces the expansion of $CD8^+$ donor T cells with cytolytic activity directed against recipient hematopoietic cells. *Clin Canc Res* 2002; **8**: 2052–60.

189 Mackinnon S, Hows JM, Goldman JM. Induction of *in vitro* graft-versus-leukemia activity following bone marrow transplantation for chronic myeloid leukemia. *Blood* 1990; **76**: 2037–43.

190 Hauch M, Gazzola MV, Small T et al. Antileukemia potential of interleukin-2 activated natural killer cells after bone marrow transplantation for chronic myelogenous leukemia. *Blood* 1990; **75**: 2250–5.

191 Soiffer RJ, Murray C, Cochran K et al. Clinical and immunologic effects of prolonged infusion of low-dose recombinant interleukin-2 after autologous and T-cell-depleted allogeneic bone marrow transplantation. *Blood* 1992; **79**: 517–26.

192 Soiffer RJ, Murray C, Gonin R, Ritz J. Effect of low-dose interleukin-2 on disease relapse after T-cell-depleted allogeneic bone marrow transplantation. *Blood* 1994; **84**: 964–7.

193 Ruggeri L, Capanni M, Casucci M et al. Role of natural killer cell alloreactivity in HLA-mismatched hematopoietic stem cell transplantation. *Blood* 1999; **94**: 333–8.

194 Ruggeri L, Capanni M, Urbani E et al. Effectiveness of donor natural killer cell alloreactivity in mismatched hematopoietic transplants. *Science* 2002; **295**: 2097–100.

195 Schlomchik WD, Couzens MS, Tang CB et al. Prevention of graft-versus-host disease by inactivation of host antigen presenting cells. *Science* 1999; **285**: 412–5.

196 Davies SM, Ruggieri L, DeFor T et al. Evaluation of KIR ligand incompatibility in mismatched unrelated donor hematopoietic transplants. Killer immunoglobulin-like receptor. *Blood* 2002; **100**: 3825–31.

197 Sehn LH, Alyea EP, Weller E et al. Comparative outcomes of T-cell-depleted and non-T-cell-depleted allogeneic bone marrow transplantation for chronic myelogenous leukemia: impact of donor lymphocyte infusion. *J Clin Oncol* 1999; **17**: 561–8.

198 Elmaagacli AH, Peceny R, Steckel N et al. Outcome of transplantation of highly purified peripheral blood $CD34^+$ cells with T-cell ad-back compared with unmanipulated bone marrow or peripheral blood stem cells from HLA-identical sibling donors in patients with first chronic phase chronic myeloid leukemia. *Blood* 2000; **101**: 446–53.

199 Slavin S, Nagler A, Naparstek E et al. Nonmyeloablative stem cell transplantation and cell therapy as an alternative to conventional bone marrow transplantation with lethal cytoreduction for the treatment of malignant and nonmalignant hematologic diseases. *Blood* 1998; **91**: 756–61.

200 Alyea E, Weller E, Schlossman R et al. T cell depleted allogeneic bone marrow transplantation followed by donor lymphocyte infusion in patients with multiple myeloma: induction of graft versus myeloma effect. *Blood* 2001; **8**: 934–9.

201 Mackinnon S, Papadapoulos EB, Carabasi MH et al. Adoptive immunotherapy evaluating escalating doses of donor leukocytes for relapse of chronic myeloid leukemia after bone marrow transplantation: separation of graft-versus-leukemia responses from graft-versus-host disease. *Blood* 1995; **86**: 1261–6.

202 Dazzi F, Szydlo RM, Craddock C et al. Comparison of single-dose and escalating-dose regimens of donor lymphocyte infusion for relapse after allografting for chronic myeloid leukemia. *Blood*, 2000; **95**: 67–71.

203 Munshi NC, Govindarajan R, Drake R et al. Thymidine kinase (*TK*) gene-transduced human lymphocytes can be highly purified, remain fully functional, and are killed efficiently with ganciclovir. *Blood* 1997; **89**: 1334–9.

204 Tiberghien P, Ferrand C, Lioure B et al. Administration of herpes simplex-thymidine kinase-expressing donor T cells with a T-cell-depleted allogeneic marrow graft. *Blood* 2001; **97**: 63–9.

205 Link CJ, Burt RK, Traynor AE et al. Adoptive immunotherapy for leukemia: donor lymphocytes transduced with the herpes simplex thymidine kinase gene for remission induction. HGTRI 0103. *Hum Gene Ther* 1998; **9**: 115–20.

206 Chen BJ, Cui X, Liu C, Chao NJ. Prevention of graft-versus-host disease while preserving graft-versus-leukemia effect after selective depletion of host-reactive T cells by photodynamic cell purging process. *Blood* 2002; **99**: 3083–8.

207 Koh MB, Prentice HG, Lowdell MW. Selective removal of alloreactive cells from haematopoietic stem cell grafts: graft engineering for GVHD prophylaxis. *Bone Marrow Transplant* 1999; **23**: 1071–9.

208 Gaderet L, Snell V, Przepiorka D et al. Effective depletion of alloreactive lymphocytes from peripheral blood mononuclear cell preparations. *Transplantation* 1999; **67**: 124–30.

209 Harris DT, Sakiestewa D, Lyons C, Kreitman RJ, Pastan I. Prevention of graft-versus-host disease (GVHD) by elimination of recipient-reactive donor T cells with recombinant toxins that target the interleukin 2 (IL-2) receptor. *Bone Marrow Transplant* 1999; **23**: 137–44.

210 Blazar BR, Taylor PA, Linsley PS, Vallera DA. *In vivo* blockade of CD28/CTLA4: B7/BB1 interaction with CTLA4-Ig reduces lethal murine graft-versus-host disease across the major histocompatibility complex barrier in mice. *Blood* 1994; **83**: 3815–25.

211 Blazar BR, Taylor PA, Panoskaltsis-Mortari A et al. Coblockade of the LFA1: ICAM and CD28/CTLA4: B7 pathways is a highly effective means of preventing acute lethal graft-versus-host disease induced by fully major histocompatibility complex-disparate donor grafts. *Blood* 1995; **85**: 2607–18.

212 Blazar BR, Taylor PA, Panoskaltsis-Mortari A et al. Blockade of CD40 ligand–CD40 interaction impairs $CD4^+$ T cell-mediated alloreactivity by

inhibiting mature donor T cell expansion and function after bone marrow transplantation. *J Immunol* 1997; **158**: 29–39.
213 Guinan EC, Boussiotis VA, Neuberg D *et al.* Transplantation of anergic histoincompatible bone marrow allografts [see comments]. *N Engl J Med* 1999; **340**: 1704–14.
214 Aubin F, Cahn JY, Ferrand C *et al.* Extensive vitiligo after ganciclovir treatment of GVHD in a patient who had received donor T cells expressing herpes simplex virus thymidine kinase. *Lancet* 2000; **355**(9204): 626–7.
215 Molldrem JJ, Lee PP, Wang C *et al.* Evidence that specific T lymphocytes may participate in the elimination of chronic myelogenous leukemia. *Nat Med* 2000; **6**: 1018–21.
216 Teshima T, Mach N, Hill GR *et al.* Tumor cell vaccine elicits potent antitumor immunity after allogeneic T-cell-depleted bone marrow transplantation. *Canc Res* 2001; **61**: 162–6.

18

Eileen Bryant & Paul J. Martin

Documentation of Engraftment and Characterization of Chimerism Following Hematopoietic Cell Transplantation

Genetic markers in hematopoietic cell transplantation

Marrow, growth factor-mobilized peripheral blood cells, and cord blood cells used for hematopoietic cell transplantation (HCT) contain a wide variety of cell types that differ in function and life span. Hematopoietic stem cells (HSCs) in the graft are of central importance for recovery of marrow function after HCT. With the use of genetic markers, the survival, distribution and differentiation of engrafted donor cells can be traced throughout the entire life of the recipient. When HSCs are obtained from a syngeneic donor, the only markers that might distinguish donor and recipient cells after HCT are those related to the underlying disease in the recipient. When autologous HSCs are used, genetic markers have sometimes been introduced into the graft in order to demonstrate that the graft contributes to long-term marrow function [1] and to determine whether recurrent malignancy after transplantation originated from neoplastic cells that survived the pretransplant preparative regimen or from neoplastic cells infused with the graft (see Chapter 11) [2,3]. In allogeneic HCT, donor and recipient cells can be distinguished by testing informative genetic markers.

Informative genetic markers in allogeneic HCT are those that distinguish cells of the donor from those of the recipient and those that distinguish cells of the recipient from those of the donor. In many cases, the donor and recipient alleles at a single genetic locus will be informative in both directions. For a heterozygous donor with alleles "*a*" and "*b*" and a heterozygous recipient with alleles "*a*" and "*c*", the "*b*" allele is informative for donor-derived cells, while the "*c*" allele is informative for recipient-derived cells. In some cases, the alleles at a single locus will not be informative in both directions. For a homozygous donor with the "*a*" allele and a heterozygous recipient with alleles "*a*" and "*c*", the "*c*" allele is informative for recipient cells, but there is no informative donor allele at this locus. Evaluation of genetic markers in the donor and recipient before HCT allows loci that are informative to be identified for testing after the transplant.

The probability of finding informative markers depends on the number of loci tested, the number of alleles at each locus, the allele distribution and the relationship between the donor and recipient. Within members of a family, no more than four alleles can be defined at any single locus, while the number of alleles at any given locus in the population can be much larger. For this reason, it is easier to find informative genetic markers with unrelated donors and recipients than with siblings.

Methods for evaluating chimerism

Historical perspective

In ancient Greek mythology, Chimera was a fearsome three-headed creature, lion at the front, goat in the middle and serpent at the rear. In today's medical parlance, the term "chimerism" has been used to describe the presence of allogeneic hematopoietic or lymphoid cells in a transplant recipient. HCT recipients are sometimes described as having "full chimerism" when all hematopoietic cells and lymphoid cells are derived from an allogeneic donor. The terms "partial chimerism" and "mixed chimerism" are sometimes used when recipient hematopoietic or lymphoid cells persist together with donor cells after HCT. The term "split chimerism" is sometimes used when donor cells are present within some hematopoietic or lymphoid lineages but not in others. The claim that full chimerism has been established must always be qualified by understanding the limits of detection in the assay used to measure chimerism and by defining the hematopoietic and lymphoid lineages encompassed in the test. During the first few weeks after HCT, recipient-derived cells can be found in the blood or marrow of virtually all patients when sensitive tests are used [4–6].

The genetic markers and laboratory methods used for testing chimerism have evolved considerably during the history of HCT. Erythrocyte antigens were among the first markers widely used for confirmation of donor cell engraftment in HCT recipients [7–9]. Antigens tested for analysis of chimerism after HCT have included those of the ABO, MN and Rh systems and those of the Kell, Kidd, Duffy, Lutheran, Ss and P systems. With assays for a wide variety of erythrocyte antigens, informative donor and recipient markers can be identified in more than 80% of sibling pairs [10]. Mixed agglutination and flow cytometry assays can detect admixtures with a sensitivity of 0.1–0.5% [11,12]. Because erythrocytes have a relatively long life span in circulation, assay results can be confounded by transfusions before or after HCT unless precautions are taken to ensure that the HCT donor has a marker distinctive from those of the recipient and all transfusion donors. Although the long life span of erythrocytes makes it difficult to assess the function of the graft in an ongoing manner, this shortcoming can be circumvented by assays that define antigens on reticulocytes [12,13]. Finally, hemolysis caused by ABO incompatibility can delay the appearance of donor erythrocytes in patients who are well engrafted with donor myeloid cells, and results of chimerism studies limited to the erythroid lineage could be misleading.

Conventional cytogenetic analysis of metaphase chromosomes was historically well established as a method for evaluating chimerism in the blood and marrow after allogeneic HCT. Gender disparity between the donor and recipient allows sex chromosomes to be used as convenient

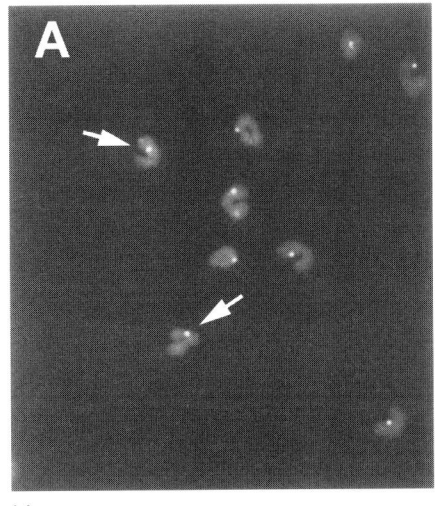 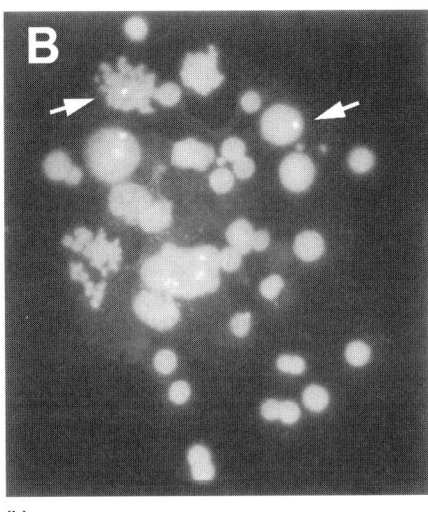

Fig. 18.1 Assessment of chimerism in sorted granulocytes (a) and leukemic blasts (b) by dual-color fluorescence *in situ* hybridization (FISH). Hybridization was carried out with a biotin-labeled Y chromosome-specific DNA probe and a digoxigenin-labeled X chromosome-specific DNA probe. Hybridization was detected with Texas Red-conjugated avidin and fluorescein-conjugated antibody against digoxigenin. Cells were counterstained with 4',6-diamidino-2-phenylindole API. Male cells contain a single red fluorescent spot and a single green fluorescent spot, while female cells contain two green fluorescent spots and no red fluorescent spots. In this case, granulocytes were derived from a male donor and leukemic blasts were derived from the female recipient. (*See also Plate 18.1, facing p. 296*)

genetic markers [9,14,15]. In some cases, a constitutional structural rearrangement or heteromorphism can be used as a genetic marker in same sex pairs [16,17]. Four major problems limit the applicability of cytogenetic assays for assessment of chimerism after HCT. First, informative markers are generally not available for same-sex pairs except in cases where a disease-specific cytogenetic abnormality is present in the recipient. Second, techniques for cytogenetic analysis are highly labor-intensive and cumbersome. Third, results are limited to cells in metaphase at the time of harvest. Finally, the number of metaphase cells that can be evaluated in any single assay is limited.

During the late 1980s, techniques of molecular biology revolutionized the use of genetic markers in HCT [4,18–28]. The two tests most widely used today are *in situ* hybridization with sex chromosome-specific probes [4,25–28] and typing of variable number of tandem repeat (VNTR) or short tandem repeat (STR) polymorphisms by DNA amplification [21–24]. *In situ* hybridization permits examination at the level of single cells, but this method is applicable only when the donor and recipient are of opposite sex or when an informative autosomal marker is present [29]. Informative VNTR/STR polymorphisms can be identified in virtually all allogeneic donor/recipient pairs, but testing at the level of single cells is not possible. Both methods have high sensitivity and specificity, and both methods can provide quantitative results. Both methods can be adapted easily for use in clinical laboratories, and both can be used for evaluating archival specimens.

Molecular cytogenetics

Molecular cytogenetic techniques have many advantages over conventional cytogenetic analysis of metaphase chromosomes. Techniques for *in situ* hybridization are simple and highly time-efficient, and the analysis can be applied equivalently for interphase and metaphase cells [30]. Techniques are sufficiently flexible to allow simultaneous determination of genotype and morphology or surface marker expression in single cells [31–33]. Large numbers of cells can be analyzed, allowing high precision and sensitivity.

Initial reports of molecular cytogenetic techniques for chimerism testing described the use of a human Y chromosome-specific repetitive DNA sequence probe for fluorescence *in situ* hybridization (FISH) [4,25–28]. The upper limit of false-negatives in males was 5.6% and the upper limit of false-positives in females was 2.7% [4]. Age-associated loss of the Y chromosome in cells from older males [34], Y chromosome loss associated with the tumor cell karyotype and constitutional variation in the Y chromosome DNA probe target sequences are potential limitations of the assay. These limitations make it essential to test specimens either by conventional cytogenetics or by *in situ* hybridization before the transplant to ensure Y chromosome integrity. Cells that show no signal with the use of a Y chromosome-specific probe are inferred to be of female origin. The absence of signal with a Y chromosome-specific probe could result from technical errors that prevent hybridization. This potential problem can be avoided by the use of a mixture of X and Y chromosome-specific probes each labeled with a different chromophor to allow dual color detection (Fig. 18.1; *see also Plate 18.1, facing p. 296*). With these reagents the upper limit of false-positive XX cells in males was 0.63% and the upper limit of false-positive XY cells in females was 0.30% [35].

VNTR and STR polymorphisms

Certain core DNA sequences are tandemly repeated in the genome, and the number of such tandem repeats at any given locus varies among different individuals (Figs 18.2 & 18.3 [36,37]). VNTR sequences are comprised of "minisatellite" cores 8–50 base pairs in length [38], while STR sequences are comprised of "microsatellite" cores 2–8 base pairs in length (e.g. CACACA and complementary GTGTGT) [39]. Polymorphisms in the number of tandemly repeated core sequences within a locus are inherited as codominant Mendelian traits. A large number of loci are available for testing, and certain loci have more than 25 alleles [40,41]. Informative donor and recipient markers can be identified in virtually all allogeneic sibling pairs with a panel of as few as six loci.

VNTR/STR polymorphisms can be identified most conveniently by using the polymerase chain reaction to amplify defined segments of DNA [42]. In these assays, oligonucleotides complementary to nonpolymorphic 5' and 3' sequences on opposite strands flanking the polymorphic VNTR/STR core (Fig. 18.2) are used to prime DNA synthesis through repeated cycles of denaturing, primer annealing and heat stable polymerase-mediated extension. When the two primer binding sites are spaced within a short distance of each other, each cycle of extension creates a primer-binding site for initiation of opposite strand synthesis in the

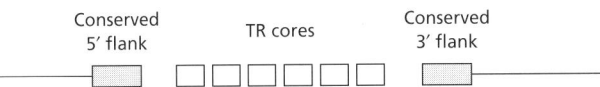

Fig. 18.2 Variable number of tandem repeat (VNTR)/short tandem repeat (STR) structure. Alleles reflecting differences in the number of tandem repeats can be distinguished by the length of fragments generated after DNA amplification with 5' and 3' primers specific for conserved sequences flanking the tandem repeat (TR) core region.

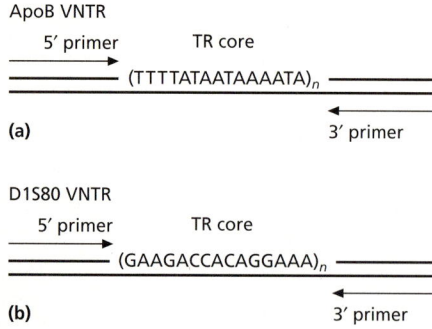

Fig. 18.3 Representative tandem repeat (TR) core sequences for (a) the D1S80 locus [36] and (b) the apoB locus [37]. Arrows show position of primers complementary to conserved sequences flanking the tandem repeat regions. Core sequences at each locus show some heterogeneity resulting from base substitutions, insertions, or deletions.

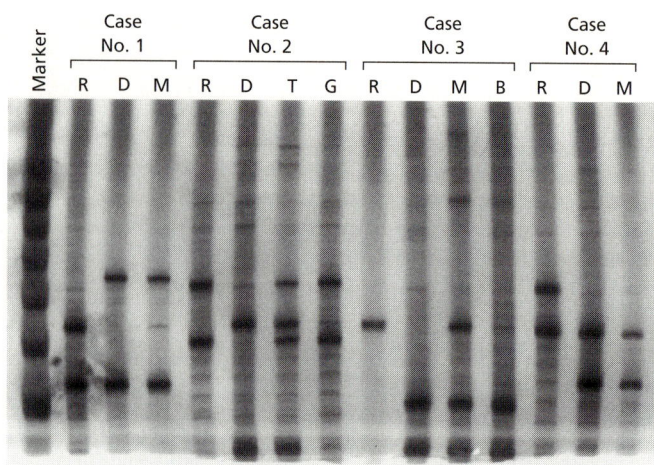

Fig. 18.4 Assessment of chimerism by testing variable number of tandem repeat (VNTR) polymorphisms. DNA segments containing tandem repeat sequences amplified from the 33.6 locus [38] were electrophoresed in a polyacrylamide gel and stained with silver. The figure shows results with samples from four donor/recipient pairs. Lanes are labeled R (recipient before transplantation), D (donor), and M (marrow), T (T cells), G (granulocytes) or B (blood) from the patient after transplantation. The marrow samples from Case No. 1 on day 28 after transplantation was estimated to contain approximately 95–99% donor cells and 1–5% recipient cells. Cytogenetic analysis of the same sample showed leukemia-specific abnormalities in two of 20 metaphases. The T-cell-enriched sample from Case No. 2 on day 287 after transplantation was estimated to contain approximately 50% donor-derived cells and 50% recipient-derived cells, but the granulocyte-enriched fraction was derived almost entirely from the recipient. Molecular studies 2.5 months earlier showed evidence of BCR-ABL rearrangement in the blood and marrow indicating recurrent chronic myeloid leukemia (CML) after the transplant. The marrow sample from Case No. 3 on day 320 after transplantation was estimated to contain approximately 50% donor-derived cells and 50% recipient-derived cells, but the blood cells were predominantly of donor origin. A marrow sample obtained 25 days earlier showed leukemic abnormalities in 12 of 24 metaphases. The marrow sample from Case No. 4 on day 28 after transplantation was estimated to contain approximately 95–99% donor cells and approximately 1–5% recipient cells. The recipient-specific 33.6 allele in this sample was not well amplified in the presence of shorter donor-derived alleles. The presence of recipient-specific DNA was more apparent from testing another marker. Cytogenetic studies with this marrow sample did not show evidence of recurrent leukemia.

next cycle. The 10^6–10^9-fold amplification of donor and recipient-derived DNA during the reaction allows fragment length to be analyzed directly by staining with ethidium bromide staining or silver (Fig. 18.4 [38]). With the use of fluorescent primers, reaction products can be visualized by a DNA sequencer or by capillary gel electrophoresis [43–47] (Fig. 18.5 [48]). Efficiency can be improved by simultaneous amplification of different loci in a single "multiplex" reaction [44,45,49].

The use of DNA amplification enables chimerism testing with extremely small amounts of starting material, a major advantage when attempting to analyze samples from patients with graft failure and severe leukopenia. Depending on fragment length and the efficiency of amplification, the sensitivity for detecting admixtures is 1–5% and can approach 0.1% in certain cases. With amplification of certain Y chromosome-specific sequences, sensitivity can approach 0.01% [50,51]. Methods involving DNA amplification can be confounded by contamination, which can be recognized when the DNA has originated from an individual other than the donor or recipient. Concurrent amplification of pretransplant samples from the donor and recipient together with the post-transplant sample generally allows unambiguous identification of donor-specific and recipient-specific reaction products and avoids confusion that could be caused by background bands (Fig. 18.4). With the inclusion of standards, assays can be adapted for quantitative determination.

DNA amplification of other loci for assessment of chimerism

Loci with biallelic polymorphism not involving VNTR/STR have also been used for quantitative and highly sensitive measurement of chimerism [48]. Unlike assays with VNTR/STR loci in which amplification products from both donor and recipient DNA are measured simultaneously at the end of the reaction, assays with these loci measure amplification products from DNA of either the donor or the recipient in real-time as they accumulate during the reaction. The real-time assay had 0.1% sensitivity (Fig. 18.4) and showed better linearity than assays with VNTR/STR loci. Informative markers were identified for more than 90% of related donors/recipient pairs by testing 11 biallelic loci on nine different chromosomes.

Clinical application of chimerism tests

Samples used for chimerism testing

Alleles that are informative for the donor and recipient must be identified before post-transplant samples from the recipient can be tested for chimerism. This identification can be easily accomplished by testing blood cells from the donor and recipient before the transplant. When a pretransplant recipient sample is not available, material from a buccal scraping can be used after the transplant to identify recipient alleles [52]. Mouthwash specimens contain large numbers of cells that originate from the blood and cannot reliably be used to identify recipient alleles after the transplant [53].

Cells from blood or marrow are most frequently used for clinical chimerism testing. Under most circumstances, results from testing blood cells can provide the necessary clinical information. One exception is the detection of minimal residual disease when malignant cells infiltrate the marrow but are not found in the circulation. Selected lineage-specific populations of interest can be isolated by flow cytometry in order to improve diagnostic accuracy and sensitivity for detecting small numbers of recipient or donor-derived cells [54–56]. For example, separation of blood samples into T lymphocyte and granulocyte fractions can be very helpful in the interpretation of results in patients who have received a nonmyeloablative conditioning regimen [54–56]. Likewise, the diagnosis of recurrent malignancy can be confirmed by demonstrating that a small population of cells with an aberrant phenotype originated from the

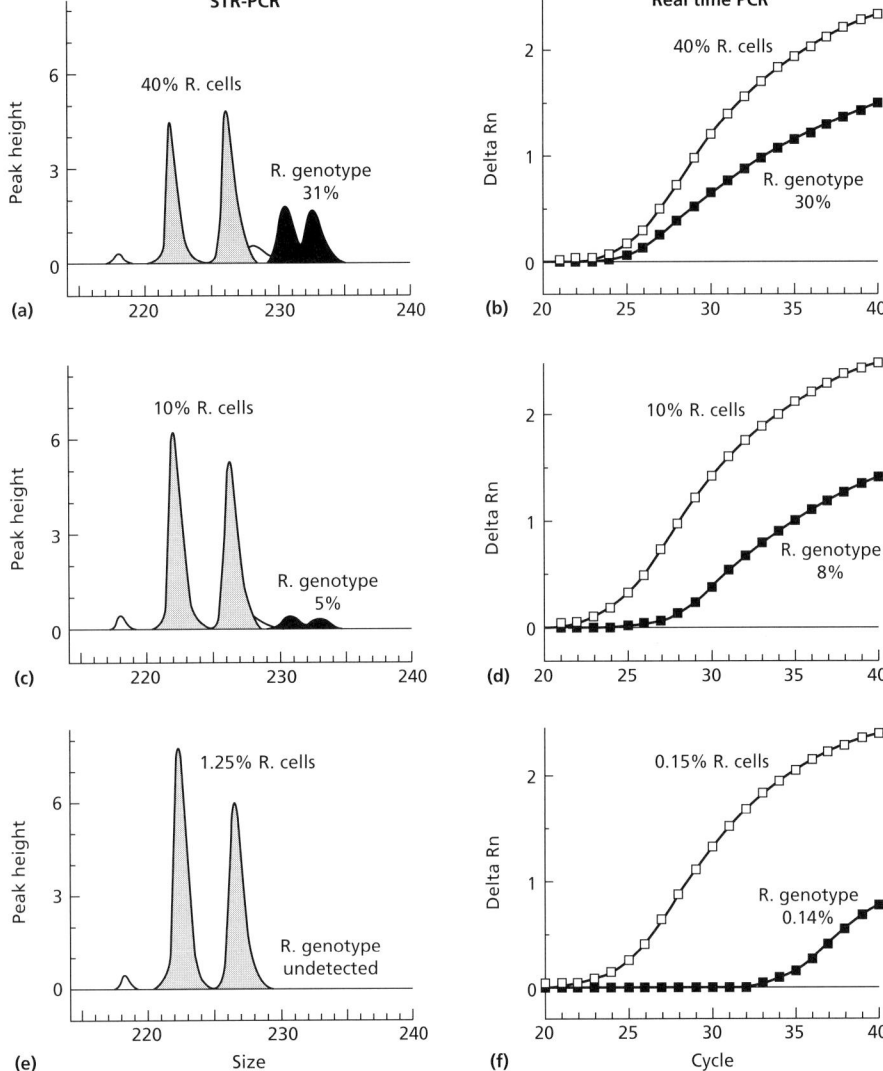

Fig. 18.5 Comparison of short tandem repeat polymerase chain reaction (STR-PCR) and real-time PCR chimerism assays. Mixtures contained 40% (a and b), 10% (c and d) 1.25% (e) or 0.15% (f) "recipient" cells. In this case, the D21S11 STR alleles of the recipient (black peaks) were longer than those of the recipient (gray peaks) (a and c). This STR-PCR assay was able to detect the presence of 40% or 10% recipient cells (a and c), but 1.25% recipient cells could not be detected (e). Preferential amplification of shorter alleles is characteristic of STR-PCR assays, which explains the under-representation of recipient alleles in A and C. Donor (□) and recipient (■) alleles were tested individually in separate real-time assays (b, d and f). The increase in fluorescence indicates the accumulation of amplification products as the reaction progresses from one cycle to the next. With decreasing amounts of the recipient S09a allele, fluorescence exceeds the threshold of detection (horizontal line) at progressively later cycles, shifting the curve to the right (■). With increasing amounts of the donor S 09b allele, fluorescence exceeds the threshold of detection earlier, shifting the curve slightly to the left (□). The real-time assay was easily able to detect 0.15% recipient DNA (f). Reproduced with permission from Alizadeh et al. [48]. Copyright, American Society of Hematology.

recipient [57–60]. Chimerism testing with isolated cell populations is particularly helpful in confirming the diagnosis of recurrent malignancy when the aberrant population represents <1% of the sample and when the aberrant phenotype detected after the transplant resembles a normal pattern of hematopoietic regeneration or differs from the pretransplant malignant phenotype.

General principles

Chimerism tests have been used for a variety of purposes in human HCT (Table 18.1). With sufficiently sensitive assays, recipient cells have been shown to persist for longer than 2 years in most patients after treatment with a myeloablative conditioning regimen [6]. A complex interplay between the pretransplant conditioning regimen, the post-transplant immunosuppressive regimen and the effects of donor T cells in the graft governs the ability of recipient-derived lymphoid and hematopoietic cells to survive after HCT (see Chapter 3). In general, more intensive conditioning regimens would be expected to decrease the persistence of recipient cells after transplantation [28,61–69]. Given the critical role of donor T cells in helping to eliminate recipient lymphoid and hematopoietic cells that survive the conditioning regimen, depletion of donor T cells would generally be expected to increase the incidence of mixed chimerism after transplantation [4,17,40,69–73].

Table 18.1 Clinical applications of chimerism tests in marrow transplantation.

1 Routine documentation of donor cell engraftment
2 Evaluate the persistence of donor cells in:
  (a) Patients with inadequate marrow function
  (b) Patients who are candidates for donor lymphocyte infusion
  (c) Patients who are candidates for a second allogeneic transplant
  (d) Long-term follow-up patients who are at increased risk of occult rejection
3 Assess the prognostic risks of graft-vs.-host disease (GVHD), rejection or recurrent malignancy
4 Define whether recurrent malignancy or lymphoproliferative syndrome has originated from donor or recipient cells
5 Identify maternal cells in pretransplant patients with severe combined immunodeficiency
6 Correlate immune reconstitution with engraftment after transplantation for treatment of severe combined immunodeficiency
7 Determine whether cells from a transfusion donor can be implicated in causing GVHD
8 Verify the genetic identity of twins

General recommendations for chimerism testing after allogeneic HSC transplantation have been published [56]. Before discussing individual applications of chimerism testing in detail, several points should be emphasized:

1 The clinical context weighs heavily in the interpretation of chimerism test results. For example, the absence of donor cells in patients with marrow aplasia could indicate rejection, but a similar absence of detectable donor cells in nonfractionated marrow or blood of a patient with florid leukemia relapse could be caused by an overwhelming preponderance of recipient cells.
2 Test results are reported as a ratio where changes in the numbers of donor and recipient cells can occur independently. Thus an increase in the proportion of donor cells can be caused both by an increase in the number of donor cells and by a decrease in the number of recipient cells.
3 The interpretation of results depends on awareness of the types of cells tested in the assay. For example, peripheral blood mononuclear cells can include T and B lymphocytes, monocytes, immature myeloid precursors and leukemic blasts. More informative results can be obtained by analysing purified cell populations.
4 The presence of a particular cell population does not allow direct inferences concerning its functional capabilities or effects. For example, the detection of recipient T cells after HCT does not necessarily indicate that rejection is likely to occur.
5 The inability to detect a particular cell population does not necessarily indicate its absence. The interpretation of test results must always be made with an understanding of the assay sensitivity.
6 Time trends are often more informative than test results at single time point. For example, the presence of 5% recipient cells at day 28 after HCT might have no clinical significance in and of itself, but a progressive increase in the proportion of recipient cells could herald rejection or recurrent leukemia.
7 Abnormalities within a single patient can have multiple causes. Thus the inability to detect donor cells after HCT could indicate the occurrence of both rejection and recurrent malignancy.

Chimerism testing in patients with graft failure

Although chimerism tests can be done for routine monitoring of donor cell engraftment after HCT [74,75], the results are of greatest importance in patients who have inadequate marrow function and in patients who might be candidates for donor lymphocyte infusion or for a second transplant from the same donor. Marrow graft rejection is usually defined by the absence of donor cells in a patient with pancytopenia and reduced marrow cellularity, but "occult" rejection and complete reconstitution with recipient cells can occur, especially in patients who have received a nonmyeloablative conditioning regimen [76] and in patients with a pre-transplant diagnosis of chronic myeloid leukemia (CML) [77]. As noted, the presence of donor cells can be obscured by florid leukemia relapse or by a myelosuppressive malignant population. Testing the origin of mature T cells can be helpful to exclude rejection in this situation since these cells are not usually affected by recurrent malignancy.

Diagnostic assessments of chimerism test results are especially difficult in patients with poor marrow function. The presence of recipient cells in the blood or marrow does not necessarily indicate that rejection is the cause of poor marrow function since recipient cells are frequently identified early after HCT in patients with normal marrow function [4–6]. Thus a patient with "benign" mixed chimerism [14,51] could have poor marrow function because of drug toxicity, viral infection or a possible marrow stromal defect. Likewise, the inability to detect recipient cells in any single test does not eliminate rejection or occult recurrent malignancy as possible causes of poor marrow function. In these situations, serial testing can be highly informative.

Table 18.2 Testing of isolated cell populations by single-color or dual-color fluorescence *in situ* hybridization (FISH) to detect recurrent leukemia.

Sample	Percent in original sample	Genotype (%)			
		Y	XY	XX	X
Unsorted marrow		98.5			
Granulocytes	89.0		100.0	0.0	
Lymphocytes	1.6		97.7	0.3	
Blasts	0.2		2.0	86.9	11.1

Single-color FISH with a Y chromosome-specific probe on day 45 after the transplant did not detect an appreciable population of female recipient cells in unsorted marrow from this patient. Granulocytes were isolated by flow sorting of cells with high side scatter characteristics and low expression of CD45, and lymphocytes were isolated by sorting cells with low side scatter characteristics and high expression of CD45. A small population of blasts was isolated by sorting cells with high expression of CD34 and low expression of CD45. Two-color FISH demonstrated that the granulocyte and lymphocyte populations were derived from the male donor, while the blasts with aberrant antigen expression were derived from the female recipient. Some of the malignant cells in this patient had a single X chromosome.

In patients who are candidates for donor lymphocyte infusions as treatment for recurrent malignancy (see Chapter 84) [78,79], the detection of persisting donor cells by chimerism tests offers reassurance that rejection has not occurred. In addition, the risk of transient or irreversible aplasia after donor lymphocyte infusion may be much higher in patients with a low proportion of donor cells in the blood or marrow as compared to those with a high proportion of donor cells in the blood or marrow [80,81]. In patients who are candidates for a second transplant from the original donor [82], the persistence of donor cells indicates that the recipient is still tolerant of donor cells. In this situation, the risk of rejection after a second transplant is negligible, and the preparative regimen can be designed for the sole purpose of eliminating malignant cells.

Late "occult" rejection and complete hematopoietic reconstitution with recipient cells has been observed in long-term follow-up after HCT for treatment of aplastic anaemia [76,83]. This distinctly unusual outcome is of biologic interest but probably has no medical significance except for theoretical concerns that aplastic anaemia might recur or that myelodysplasia might develop in the future.

Chimerism testing in patients at risk of recurrent malignancy

Under certain circumstances, chimerism tests can be useful in predicting recurrent malignancy after HCT. Findings that demonstrate an increasing proportion of recipient-derived cells in the blood or marrow after HCT can unquestionably herald relapse [40,84–92]. By itself, stable mixed chimerism in nonfractionated blood or marrow cells does not predict recurrent malignancy [14,88,93–96], although persistence of recipient cells within the CD19-positive population has been correlated with an increased risk of relapse in patients with pre-B lineage acute lymphoblastic leukemia [97]. Testing of isolated cell populations with aberrant expression of cell surface antigens can facilitate early detection of recurrent leukemia [57–60] (Table 18.2). Serial chimerism testing has been useful for early detection of recurrent malignancy in patients with less rapidly progressive diseases such as CML [90,98,99]. Highly sensitive tests and very frequent monitoring would likely be necessary to gain early warning of impending relapse in patients with rapidly progressive diseases such as acute leukemia [60,75,100].

A correlation between persistence of recipient T cells after HCT and an increased risk of recurrent malignancy has been found in patients who received T-cell-depleted marrow for treatment of CML [101]. The absence of donor T cells in the graft presumably allowed both T cells and malignant HSCs of the recipient to survive after HCT. With the use of a more intensive pretransplant conditioning regimen, persistence of recipient lymphocytes after T-cell-depleted HCT was not associated with an increased risk of recurrent CML [102]. The persistence of recipient cells in the blood or marrow during the first 3 months after HCT has not been associated with an increased risk of relapse in patients who received unmodified (T-cell-replete) marrow for treatment of CML [83]. This result is consistent with earlier findings that the detection of BCR-ABL rearrangements in the blood or marrow during the first 3 months after HCT is not associated with an increased risk of relapse [103].

Chimerism testing after a nonmyeloablative conditioning regimen

A new two-stage strategy for HCT involves the initial establishment of mixed chimerism with the use of a reduced intensity, nonmyeloablative pretransplant conditioning regimen, combined with potent post-transplant immunosuppression to prevent rejection and graft-vs.-host disease (GVHD). After engraftment has been established, immunosuppression is withdrawn, allowing donor T cells to eliminate residual hematopoietic cells or malignant cells in the recipient through immunological mechanisms (see Chapters 85 & 86). In some situations, donor lymphocytes may be infused if withdrawal of immunosuppression does not have the desired clinical effect.

Genetic marker studies and state-of-the-art chimerism tests play an essential part in the clinical management with this approach to HCT and in the evaluation of results from these clinical trials. Results of preliminary studies have suggested that full donor T-cell engraftment precedes the development of full donor myeloid engraftment, GVHD and antitumor effects [56,104]. Chimerism tests showing low levels of donor T-cell engraftment at early time points after the transplant have been associated with an increased risk of rejection and the absence of antitumor effects, while high levels of donor T-cell engraftment have been associated with an increased risk of GVHD [56]. In some cases, incipient rejection has been reversed by administration of donor lymphocytes [56].

Other applications for genetic marker studies

Genetic marker studies have found a variety of other useful applications in HCT. In rare cases, for example, it has been possible to demonstrate that hematologic malignancy after HCT originated in donor cells rather than recipient cells [105–107]. Chimerism tests allow these unusual cases to be identified for further intensive study, although the mechanisms involved in malignant transformation of donor cells remain obscure. With chimerism tests it has likewise been possible to assess the involvement of donor or recipient-derived B lymphocytes in lymphoproliferative disorders caused by Epstein–Barr virus infection (see Chapter 56) [108,109].

In rare cases, genetic marker studies have demonstrated that GVHD in a transplant recipient was caused by the inadvertent administration of nonirradiated blood product transfusions [110]. Evidence implicating cells of the blood transfusion donor came from tests demonstrating the presence of genetic markers different from those of either the donor or the recipient. In some cases, it has been possible to trace the donor through further testing. The universal practice of irradiating all blood product transfusions should eliminate any risk of transfusion-induced GVHD in HCT recipients.

An extremely useful clinical application of genetic marker studies in HCT is the assessment of monozygosity in twins. With an identical twin donor there is no risk of rejection or GVHD and hence no need for immunosuppressive treatment before or after HCT. In this situation, the pretransplant conditioning regimen is designed solely to eliminate malignant cells. The alleles of a genetic locus are fully informative in a family study when they allow unambiguous assessment of inheritance, which requires parental heteozygosity and the absence of allele matching between the parents. With human leukocyte antigen (HLA)-identical twins of the same sex and with identity at three additional unlinked fully informative genetic loci there is a less than 1 : 100 chance that the twins are not genetically identical. With identity at four unlinked fully informative loci in addition to HLA, there is a less than 1 : 500 chance that the twins are not genetically identical, and with identity at five unlinked fully informative loci in addition to HLA there is a less than 1 : 1000 chance that the twins are not genetically identical [111].

Biologic insights from genetic marker studies

Beyond the clinical applications described above, genetic marker studies have contributed valuable information towards understanding the biology of HCT. Genetic marker studies have recently emerged as powerful tools in studies of HCT for treatment of congenital immunodeficiency. Infants with severe combined immunodeficiency syndromes (SCIDs) often have occult maternal T cells in the circulation. The presence of these cells might require immunosuppression to avoid rejection (see Chapter 105) [112,113]. Important information for understanding immune reconstitution after transplantation for treatment of SCID has been obtained by analysing the lineage-specific patterns of donor cell engraftment [114,115].

Results of genetic marker studies have made it clear that clinical resolution of nonmalignant diseases often can be achieved without complete donor replacement of the defective recipient lymphohematopoietic system [115–119]. For example, the need for red cell transfusions in patients with thalassemia can be averted by establishing mixed hematopoietic chimerism with only 25% normal donor cells in the marrow [117–119].

Genetic marker studies after HCT have been used to characterize the diversity of marrow-derived cells throughout the body. From these studies, it is now recognized that marrow-derived cells include not only hematopoietic and lymphoid populations, but also tissue macrophages, Kupffer cells in the liver, Langerhan cells in the skin, dendritic cells in the blood and microglial cells in the brain [120–126]. The donor origin of tissue macrophages and microglial cells has given impetus to the application of HCT for treatment of certain congenital enzyme deficiency diseases (see Chapter 107). Most investigators agree that stromal cells in the marrow after transplantation are derived from the recipient, even when tested as long as 27 years after the transplant [127–132]. Some investigators have reported that marrow-derived cells can differentiate into mature hepatocytes and epithelial cells of the skin and gastrointestinal tract [133–135], although further work will be needed to confirm these findings [136].

Summary

The origin of marrow and blood cells after HCT can be identified by testing informative genetic markers that distinguish the donor and recipient. Molecular methods for *in situ* hybridization and DNA amplification have made chimerism tests widely accessible for a variety of clinical applications after HCT. Further work will be needed to develop standardized testing procedures for application to routine practice. Biologic insights gained from testing genetic markers will continue to guide future progress as new approaches are developed in using HCT for treatment of malignant and nonmalignant diseases.

References

1 Brenner MK, Rill DR, Holladay MS et al. Gene marking to determine whether autologous marrow infusion restores long-term haematopoiesis in cancer patients. *Lancet* 1993; **342**: 1134–7.

2 Brenner MK, Rill DR, Moen RC et al. Gene-marking to trace origin of relapse after autologous bone-marrow transplantation. *Lancet* 1993; **341**: 85–6.

3 Rill DR, Santana VM, Roberts WM et al. Direct demonstration that autologous bone marrow transplantation for solid tumors can return a multiplicity of tumorigenic cells. *Blood* 1994; **84**: 380–3.

4 Durnam DM, Anders KR, Fisher L, O'Quigley J, Bryant EM, Thomas ED. Analysis of the origin of marrow cells in bone marrow transplant recipients using a Y-chromosome-specific in situ hybridization assay. *Blood* 1989; **74**: 2220–6.

5 Lapointe C, Forest L, Lussier P et al. Sequential analysis of early hematopoietic reconstitution following allogeneic bone marrow transplantation with fluorescence in situ hybridization (FISH). *Bone Marrow Transplant* 1996; **17**: 1143–8.

6 Mangioni S, Balduzzi A, Rivolta A et al. Long-term persistence of hemopoietic chimerism following sex-mismatched bone marrow transplantation. *Bone Marrow Transplant* 1997; **20**: 969–73.

7 Thomas ED, Lochte HL, Lu WC, Ferrebee JW. Intravenous infusion of bone marrow in patients receiving radiation and chemotherapy. *N Engl J Med* 1957; **257**: 491–6.

8 Sparkes MC, Crist ML, Sparkes RS, Gale RP, Feig SA. The UCLA Transplantation Group. Gene markers in human bone marrow transplantation. *Vox Sang* 1977; **33**: 202–5.

9 Blume KG, Beutler KJ, Bross KJ, Schmidt GM, Spruce WE, Teplitz RL. Genetic markers in human bone marrow transplantation. *Am J Hum Genet* 1980; **32**: 414–9.

10 Schouten HC, Sizoo W, van Veer MB, Hagenbeek A, Lowenberg B. Incomplete chimerism in erythroid, myeloid and B lymphocyte lineage after T cell-depleted allogeneic bone marrow transplantation. *Bone Marrow Transplant* 1988; **3**: 407–12.

11 Gemke RJBJ, Kanhai HHH, Overbeeke MAM et al. ABO and rhesus phenotyping of fetal erythrocytes in the first trimester of pregnancy. *Br J Haematol* 1986; **64**: 689–97.

12 David B, Bernard D, Navenot JM, Muller JY, Blanchard D. Flow cytometric monitoring of red blood cell chimerism after bone marrow transplantation. *Transfusion Med* 1999; **9**(3): 209–17.

13 Zuazu J, Duran-Suarez JR, Julia A, Martin VC, Massague I, Massuet L. Demonstration of chimerism after bone marrow transplantation by reticulocyte blood group typing. *Bone Marrow Transplant* 1988; **3**: 521–2.

14 Petz LD, Yam P, Wallace RB et al. Mixed hematopoietic chimerism following bone marrow transplantation for hematologic malignancies. *Blood* 1987; **70**: 1331–7.

15 Lawler SD, Baker MC, Harris H, Morgenstern GR. Cytogenetic studies on recipients of allogeneic bone marrow using the sex chromosomes as markers of cellular origin. *Br J Haematol* 1984; **56**: 431–43.

16 Olson SB, Magenis RE, Lovrien EW. Human chromosome variation. The discriminatory power of Q-band heteromorphism (variant) analysis in distinguishing between individuals with specific application to cases of questionable paternity. *Am J Hum Genet* 1986; **38**: 235–52.

17 Offit K, Burns JP, Cunningham I et al. Cytogenetic analysis of chimerism and leukemia relapse in chronic myelogenous leukemia patients after T-cell-depleted bone marrow transplantation. *Blood* 1990; **75**: 1346–55.

18 Blazar BR, Orr HT, Arthur DC, Kersey JH, Filipovich AH. Restriction fragment length polymorphisms as markers of engraftment in allogeneic marrow transplantation. *Blood* 1985; **66**: 1436–44.

19 Ginsburg D, Antin JH, Smith BR, Orkin SH, Rappeport JM. Origin of cell populations after bone marrow transplantation. Analysis using DNA sequence polymorphisms. *J Clin Invest* 1985; **75**: 596–603.

20 Minden MD, Messner HA, Belch A. Origin of leukemic relapse after bone marrow transplantation detected by restriction fragment length polymorphism. *J Clin Invest* 1985; **75**: 91–3.

21 Min GL, Hibbin J, Arthur C, Apperley J, Jeffreys A, Goldman J. Use of minisatellite DNA probes for recognition and characterization of relapse after allogeneic bone marrow transplantation. *Br J Haematol* 1988; **68**: 195–201.

22 Weitzel JN, Hows J, Jeffreys AJ, Gao Long M, Goldman JM. Use of a hypervariable minisatellite DNA probe (33.15) for evaluating engraftment 2 or more years after bone marrow transplantation for aplastic anaemia. *Br J Haematol* 1988; **70**: 91–7.

23 Hutchinson RM, Pringle JH, Potter L, Patel I, Jeffreys AJ. Rapid identification of donor and recipient cells after allogeneic bone marrow transplantation using specific genetic markers. *Br J Haematol* 1989; **72**: 133–40.

24 Lawler M, McCann SR, Conneally E, Humphries P. Chimaerism following allogeneic bone marrow transplantation. Detection of residual host cells using the polymerase chain reaction. *Br J Haematol* 1989; **73**: 205–10.

25 Morisaki H, Morisaki T, Nakahori Y et al. Genotypic analysis using a Y-chromosome-specific probe following bone marrow transplantation. *Am J Hematol* 1988; **27**: 30–3.

26 Przepiorka D, Ramberg R, Thomas ED. Host metaphases after chemoradiotherapy and allogeneic bone marrow transplantation for acute nonlymphoblastic leukemia. *Leuk Res* 1989; **13**: 661–5.

27 Van Dekken H, Hagenbeek A, Bauman JGL. Marrow transplantation by fluorescent in situ hybridization with a Y chromosome specific probe. *Leukemia* 1989; **3**: 724–8.

28 Przepiorka D, Thomas ED, Durnam DM, Fisher L. Use of a probe to repeat sequence of the Y chromosome for detection of host cells in peripheral blood of bone marrow transplant recipients. *Am J Clin Pathol* 1991; **95**: 201–6.

29 Buno I, Diez-Martin JL, Lopez-Fernandez C. Polymorphisms for the size of heterochromatic regions allow sex-independent quantification of post-BMT chimerism targeting metaphase and interphase cells. *Haematologica* 1999; **84**: 138–41.

30 Pinkel D, Straume T, Gray JW. Cytogenetic analysis using quantitative, high sensitivity, fluorescence in situ Y hybridization. *Proc Natl Acad Sci U S A* 1986; **83**: 2934–6.

31 Anastasi J, Vardiman JW, Rudinsky R et al. Direct correlation of cytogenetic findings with cell morphology using in situ hybridization: an analysis of suspicious cells in bone marrow specimens of two patients completing therapy for acute lymphoblastic leukemia. *Blood* 1991; **77**: 2456–2.

32 Van den Berg H, Vossen JM, Van den Berg RL, Bayer J, Van Tol MJ. Detection of Y chromosome in situ hybridization in combination with membrane antigens by two-color immunofluorescence. *Laboratory Invest* 1991; **64**: 623–49.

33 Weber-Matthiesen K, Deerberg J, Muller-Hermelink B, Schlegeberger B, Grote W. Rapid immunophenotypic characterization of chromosomally aberrant cells by the new FICTION method. *Cytogenet Cell Genet* 1993; **63**: 123–5.

34 Pierre RV, Hoagland HC. Age-associated aneuploidy-loss of Y chromosome from human bone marrow cells with aging. *Cancer* 1972; **30**: 889–94.

35 Dewald GW, Schad CR, Christensen ER et al. Fluorescence in situ hybridization with X and Y chromosome probes for cytogenetic studies on bone marrow cells after opposite sex transplantation. *Bone Marrow Transplant* 1993; **12**: 149–54.

36 Sharf S. PCR amplification of VNTRs. In: Innis MA, Gelfand DH, Sminsky JJ, eds. *PCR Strategies*. San Diego, CA: Academic Press, 1995: 161–75.

37 Boerwinkle E, Xiong W, Fourest E, Chan L. Rapid typing of tandemly repeated hypervariable loci by the polymerase chain reaction: Application to the apolipoprotein B 3′ hypervariable region. *Proc Natl Acad Sci U S A* 1989; **86**: 212–6.

38 Jeffreys AJ, Wilson V, Neumann R, Keyte J. Amplification of human minisatellites by the polymerase chain reaction: towards DNA fingerprinting of single cells. *Nucl Acids Res* 1988; **16**: 10,953–71.

39 Weber JL, May PE. Abundant class of DNA polymorphism which may be typed using the polymerase chain reaction. *Am J Hum Genet* 1989; **44**: 388–96.

40 Lawler M, Humphries P, McCann SR. Evaluation of mixed chimerism by in vitro amplification of dinucleotide repeat sequences using the polymerase chain reaction. *Blood* 1991; **77**: 2504–14.

41 Scharf SJ, Horn GT, Erlich HA. Direct cloning and sequence analysis of enzymatically amplified genomic sequences. *Science* 1986; **233**: 1076–8.

42 Ugozolli L, Yam P, Petz LD et al. Amplification by the polymerase chain reaction of hypervariable regions of the human genome for evaluation of chimerism after bone marrow transplantation. *Blood* 1991; **77**: 1607–15.

43 Scharf SJ, Smith AG, Hansen JA, McFarland C, Erlich HA. Quantitative determination of bone marrow transplant engraftment using fluorescent polymerase chain reaction primers for human identity markers. *Blood* 1995; **85**: 1954–63.

44 Pindolia K, Janakiraman N, Kasten-Sportes C. Enhanced assessment of allogeneic bone marrow transplant engraftment using automated fluorescent-based typing. *Bone Marrow Transplant* 1999; **24**: 1235–41.

45 Millson AS, Spangler FL, Wittwer CT, Lyon E. Comparison of automated short tandem repeat and manual variable number of tandem repeat analysis of chimerism in bone marrow transplant patients. *Diagn Mol Pathol* 2000; **9**: 91–7.

46 Jone CM, Akel N, Killeen AA. Evaluation of chimerism in DNA samples by PCR amplification of D1S80 with detection by capillary electrophoresis. *Mol Diagn* 2000; **5**: 101–5.

47. Luhm RA, Bellissimo DB, Uzgiris AJ, Drobyski WR, Hessner MJ. Quantitative evaluation of post-bone marrow transplant engraftment status using fluorescent-labeled variable number of tandem repeats. *Mol Diagn* 2000; **5**: 129–38.
48. Alizadeh M, Bernard M, Danic B *et al*. Quantitative assessment of hematopoietic chimerism after bone marrow transplantation by real-time quantitative polymerase chain reaction. *Blood* 2002; **99**: 4618–25.
49. Thiede C, Florek M, Bornhauser M *et al*. Rapid quantification of mixed chimerism using multiplex amplification of short tandem repeat markers and fluorescence detection. *Bone Marrow Transplant* 1999; **23**: 1055–60.
50. Landman-Parker J, Socie G, Petit T *et al*. Detection of recipient cells after non T-cell depleted bone marrow transplantation for leukemia by PCR amplification of minisatellites or of a Y chromosome marker that has a different prognostic value. *Leukemia* 1994; **8**: 1989–94.
51. Petit T, Raynal B, Socie G *et al*. Highly sensitive polymerase chain reaction methods show the frequent survival of residual recipient multipotent progenitors after non T-cell depleted bone marrow transplantation. *Blood* 1994; **84**: 3575–83.
52. Thiede C, Prange-Krex G, Freiberg-Richter J, Mornhauser M, Ehninger G. Buccal swabs but not mouthwash samples can be used to obtain pretransplant DNA fingerprints from recipients of allogeneic bone marrow transplants. *Bone Marrow Transplant* 2000; **25**: 575–7.
53. Endler G, Greinix H, Winkler K, Mitterbauer G, Mannhalter C. Genetic fingerprinting in mouthwashes of patients after allogeneic bone marrow transplantation. *Bone Marrow Transplant* 1999; **24**: 95–8.
54. Winiarski J, Mattsson J, Gustafsson A *et al*. Engraftment and chimerism, particularly of T- and B-cells, in children undergoing allogeneic bone marrow transplantation. *Ped Transplant* 1998; **2**: 150–6.
55. Winiarski J, Gustafsson A, Wester D, Dalianis T. Follow-up chimerism, including T- and B-lymphocytes and granulocytes in children more than 1 year after allogeneic bone marrow transplantation. *Ped Transplant* 2000; **4**: 132–9.
56. Antin JH, Childs R, Filipovich AH *et al*. Establishment of complete and mixed donor chimerism after allogeneic lymphohematopoietic transplantation: recommendations from a workshop at the 2001 Tandem meetings. *Biol Blood Marrow Transplant* 2001; **7**: 473–85.
57. Cotteret S, Belloc F, Boiron JM *et al*. Fluorescent *in situ* hybridization on flow-sorted cells as a tool for evaluating minimal residual disease or chimerism after allogeneic bone marrow transplantation. *Cytometry (Comm Clin Cytometry)* 1998; **34**: 216–22.
58. Shulman HM, Wells D, Gooley T, Myerson D, Bryant E, Loken M. The biologic significance of rare peripheral blasts after hematopoietic cell transplantation is predicted by multidimensional flow cytometry. *Hematopathology* 1999; **112**: 513–23.
59. Lion T, Daxberger H, Dubovsky J *et al*. Analysis of chimerism within specific leukocyte subsets for detection of residual or recurrent leukemia in pediatric patients after allogeneic stem cell transplantation. *Leukemia* 2001; **15**: 307–10.
60. Mattsson J, Uzunel M, Tammik L, Aschan J, Ringden O. Leukemia-specific chimerism analysis is a sensitive predictor of relapse in patients with acute myeloid leukemia and myelodysplastic syndrome after allogeneic stem cell transplantation. *Leukemia* 2001; **15**: 1976–85.
61. Champlin RE, Horowitz MM, Van Beckum DW *et al*. Severe aplastic anemia: a prospective study on the effect of early marrow transplantation on acute mortality. *Blood* 1989; **73**: 606–13.
62. Frassoni F, Strada P, Sessarego M *et al*. Mixed chimerism after allogeneic marrow transplantation for leukaemia: correlation with dose of total body irradiation and graft-versus-host disease. *Bone Marrow Transplant* 1990; **5**: 235–40.
63. Chalmers EA, Sproul AM, Mills KI *et al*. Effect of radiation dose on the development of mixed haemopoietic chimerism following T-cell-depleted allogeneic bone marrow transplantation. *Bone Marrow Transplant* 1992; **10**: 425–30.
64. Fishleder AJ, Bolwell B, Lichten AE. Incidence of mixed chimerism using busulfan/cyclophosphamide containing regimens in allogeneic bone marrow transplantation. *Bone Marrow Transplant* 1992; **9**: 293–7.
65. Mackinnon S, Barnett L, Bourhis JH, Black P, Heller G, O'Reilly RJ. Myeloid and lymphoid chimerism after T-cell-depleted bone marrow transplantation: evaluation of conditioning regimens using the polymerase chain reaction to amplify human minisatellite regions of genomic DNA. *Blood* 1992; **80**: 3235–41.
66. Bar BM, Schattenberg A, DeMan AJ *et al*. Influence of the conditioning regimen on erythrocyte chimerism, graft-versus-host disease and relapse after allogeneic transplantation with lymphocyte depleted marrow. *Bone Marrow Transplant* 1992; **10**: 45–52.
67. Nesci S, Manna M, Andreani M, Fattorini P, Graziosi G, Lucarelli G. Mixed chimerism in thalassemic patients after bone marrow transplantation. *Bone Marrow Transplant* 1992; **10**: 143–6.
68. Miralbell R, Chapuis B, Nouet P *et al*. Conditioning the leukemic patient before allogeneic BMT. Value of intensifying immunosuppression in the context of different levels of T lymphocyte depletion of the graft. *Bone Marrow Transplant* 1993; **11**: 447–51.
69. van Leeuwen JEM, van Tol MJ, Joosten AM *et al*. Persistence of host-type hematopoiesis after allogeneic bone marrow transplantation for leukemia is significantly related to the recipient's age and/or the conditioning regimen, but it is not associated with an increased risk of relapse. *Blood* 1994; **83**: 3059–67.
70. Bretagne S, Vidaud M, Kuentz M *et al*. Mixed blood chimerism in T-cell-depleted bone marrow transplant recipients: evaluation using DNA polymorphisms. *Blood* 1987; **70**: 1692–5.
71. Arthur CK, Apperley JF, Guo AP, Rassool F, Gao LM, Goldman JM. Cytogenetic events after bone marrow transplantation for chronic myeloid leukemia in chronic phase. *Blood* 1988; **71**: 1179–86.
72. Berthesa MF, Maraninchi D, Lafage M *et al*. Partial chimerism after T-cell-depleted allogeneic bone marrow transplantation in leukemic HLA-matched patients: a cytogenetic documentation. *Blood* 1988; **72**: 89–93.
73. Roux E, Helg C, Chapuis B *et al*. Evolution of mixed chimerism after allogeneic bone marrow transplantation as determined on granulocytes and mononuclear cells by the polymerase chain reaction. *Blood* 1992; **79**: 2775–83.
74. Gyger M, Baron C, Forest L *et al*. Quantitative assessment of hematopoietic chimerism after allogeneic bone marrow transplantation has predictive value for the occurrence of irreversible graft failure and graft-vs.-host disease. *Exp Hematol* 1998; **26**: 426–34.
75. Dubovsky J, Daxberger H, Fritsch G. Kinetics of chimerism during the early post-transplant period in pediatric patients with malignant and non-malignant hematologic disorders: implications for timely detection of engraftment, graft failure and rejection. *Leukemia* 1999; **13**: 2059–69.
76. Hill RS, Petersen FB, Storb R *et al*. Mixed hematologic chimerism after allogeneic marrow transplantation for severe aplastic anemia is associated with a higher risk of graft rejection and a lessened incidence of acute graft-versus-host disease. *Blood* 1986; **67**: 811–6.
77. Sill H, Rule SA, Joske DJ *et al*. Reconstitution with Philadelphia chromosome-negative recipient hematopoiesis early after allogeneic BMT for CML. *Bone Marrow Transplant* 1996; **17**: 453–5.
78. Kolb HJ, Schattenberg A, Goldman JM *et al*. Graft-versus-leukemia effect of donor lymphocyte transfusions in marrow grafted patients. *Blood* 1995; **86**: 2041–50.
79. Collins RHJ, Shpilberg O, Drobyski WR *et al*. Donor leukocyte infusions in 140 patients with relapsed malignancy after allogeneic bone marrow transplantation. *J Clin Oncol* 1997; **15**: 433–44.
80. Keil F, Haas OA, Fritsch G *et al*. Donor leukocyte infusion for leukemic relapse after allogeneic marrow transplantation: lack of residual donor hematopoiesis predicts aplasia. *Blood* 1997; **89**: 3113–7.
81. Rapanotti MC, Arcese W, Buffolino S *et al*. Sequential molecular monitoring of chimerism in chronic myeloid leukemia patients receiving donor lymphocyte transfusion for relapse after bone marrow transplantation. *Bone Marrow Transplant* 1997; **19**: 703–7.
82. Radich JP, Sanders JE, Buckner CD *et al*. Second allogeneic marrow transplantation for patients with recurrent leukemia after initial transplant with total-body irradiation-containing regimens. *J Clin Oncol* 1993; **11**: 304–13.
83. Huss R, Deeg HJ, Gooley T *et al*. Effect of mixed chimerism on graft-versus-host disease, disease recurrence and survival after HLA-identical marrow transplantation for aplastic anemia or chronic myelogenous leukemia. *Bone Marrow Transplant* 1996; **18**: 767–76.
84. Palka G, Stuppia L, DiBartolomeo P *et al*. FISH detection of mixed chimerism in 33 patients, submitted to bone marrow transplantation. *Bone Marrow Transplant* 1996; **17**: 231–6.
85. Molloy K, Goulden N, Lawler M *et al*. Patterns of hematopoietic chimerism following bone marrow transplantation for childhood acute lymphoblastic leukemia from volunteer unrelated donors. *Blood* 1996; **87**: 3027–31.
86. Bader P, Beck J, Schlegel PG, Handgretinger R, Niethammer D, Klingebiel T. Additional immunotherapy on the basis of increasing mixed hematopoietic chimerism after allogeneic BMT in children with acute leukemia: is there an option to prevent relapse? *Bone Marrow Transplant* 1997; **20**: 79–81.
87. Bader P, Beck J, Frey A *et al*. Serial and quantitative analysis of mixed hematopoietic chimerism by PCR in patients with acute leukemias allows the prediction of relapse after allogeneic BMT. *Bone Marrow Transplant* 1998; **21**: 487–95.

88 Ortega M, Escudero T, Caballin MR, Olive T, Ortega JJ, Coll MD. Follow-up of chimerism in children with hematological diseases after allogeneic hematopoietic progenitor cell transplants. *Bone Marrow Transplant* 1999; **24**: 81–7.

89 Miflin G, Stainer CJ, Carter GI, Byrne JL, Haynes AP, Russell NH. Comparative serial quantitative measurements of chimaerism following unmanipulated allogeneic transplantation of peripheral blood stem cells and bone marrow. *Br J Haematol* 1999; **107**: 429–40.

90 Formankova R, Honzatkova L, Moravcova J *et al.* Prediction and reversion of post-transplant relapse in patients with chronic myeloid leukemia using mixed chimerism and residual disease detection and adoptive immunotherapy. *Leuk Res* 2000; **24**: 339–47.

91 Thiede C, Bornhauser M, Oelschlagel U *et al.* Sequential monitoring of chimerism and detection of minimal residual disease after allogeneic blood stem cell transplantation (BSCT) using multiplex PCR amplification of short tandem repeat-markers. *Leukemia* 2001; **15**: 293–302.

92 Klingebeil T, Niethammer D, Dietz K, Bader P. Progress in chimerism analysis in childhood malignancies—the dilemma of biostatistical considerations and ethical implications. *Leukemia* 2001; **15**: 1989–91.

93 Schattenberg A, DeWitte T, Salden M *et al.* Mixed hematopoietic chimerism after allogeneic transplantation with lymphocyte-depleted bone marrow is not associated with a higher incidence of relapse. *Blood* 1989; **73**: 1367–72.

94 Roy DC, Tantravahi R, Murray C *et al.* Natural history of mixed chimerism after bone marrow transplantation with CD6-depleted allogeneic marrow: a stable equilibrium. *Blood* 1990; **75**: 296–304.

95 van Leeuwen JEM, van Tol MJ, Joosten AM *et al.* Mixed T-lymphoid chimerism after allogeneic bone marrow transplantation for hematologic malignancies of children is not correlated with relapse. *Blood* 1993; **82**: 1921–8.

96 Choi SJ, Lee KH, Lee JH *et al.* Prognostic value of hematopoietic chimerism in patients with acute leukemia after allogeneic bone marrow transplantation: a prospective study. *Bone Marrow Transplant* 2000; **26**: 327–32.

97 Zetterquist H, Mattsson J, Uzunel M *et al.* Mixed chimerism in the B cell lineage is a rapid and sensitive indicator of minimal residual disease in bone marrow transplant recipients with pre-B cell acute lymphoblastic leukemia. *Bone Marrow Transplant* 2000; **25**: 843–51.

98 Serrano J, Roman J, Sanchez J *et al.* Molecular analysis of lineage-specific chimerism and minimal residual disease by RT-PCR of p210 (BCR-ABL) and p190 (BCR-ABL) after allogeneic bone marrow transplantation for chronic myeloid leukemia: increasing mixed myeloid chimerism and p190 (BCR-ABL) detection precede cytogenetic relapse. *Blood* 2000; **95**: 2659–65.

99 Roman J, Serrano J, Jimenez A *et al.* Myeloid mixed chimerism is associated with relapse in bcr-abl positive patients after unmanipulated allogeneic bone marrow transplantation for chronic myelogenous leukemia. *Haematologica* 2000; **85**: 173–80.

100 Bader P, Holle W, Klingebiel T *et al.* Mixed hematopoietic chimerism after allogeneic bone marrow transplantation: the impact of quantitative PCR analysis for prediction of relapse and graft rejection in children. *Bone Marrow Transplant* 1997; **19**: 697–702.

101 Mackinnon S, Barnett L, Heller G, O'Reilly RJ. Minimal residual disease is more common in patients who have mixed T-cell chimerism after bone marrow transplantation for chronic myelogenous leukemia. *Blood* 1994; **83**: 3409–16.

102 Weisneth M, Schreiner T, Bunjes D *et al.* Comparison of T-cell-depleted BMT and PBPCT with respect to chimerism, graft rejection, and leukemic relapse. *J Hematother* 1999; **8**: 269–74.

103 Radich JP, Gehly G, Gooley T *et al.* Polymerase chain reaction detection of the BCR-ABL fusion transcript after allogeneic marrow transplantation for chronic myeloid leukemia: results and implications in 346 patients. *Blood* 1995; **85**: 2632–8.

104 Childs R, Clave E, Contentin N *et al.* Engraftment kinetics after nonmyeloablative allogeneic peripheral blood stem cell transplantation: full donor T-cell chimerism precedes alloimmune responses. *Blood* 1999; **94**: 3234–41.

105 Thomas ED, Bryant JI, Buckner CD *et al.* Leukaemic transformation of engrafted human marrow cells *in vivo*. *Lancet* 1972; **1**: 1310–3.

106 Cooley LD, Sears DA, Udden MM, Harrison WR, Baker KR. Donor cell leukemia: report of a case occurring 11 years after allogeneic bone marrow transplantation and review of the literature. *Am J Hematol* 2000; **63**: 46–53.

107 Hambach L, Eder M, Dammann E *et al.* Donor cell-derived acute myeloid leukemia developing 14 months after matched unrelated bone marrow transplantation for chronic myeloid leukemia. *Bone Marrow Transplant* 2001; **28**: 705–7.

108 Shapiro RS, McClain K, Frizzera G *et al.* Epstein–Barr virus associated B cell lymphoproliferative disorders following bone marrow transplantation. *Blood* 1988; **71**: 1234–43.

109 Zutter MM, Martin PJ, Sales GE *et al.* Epstein–Barr virus lymphoproliferation after bone marrow transplantation. *Blood* 1988; **72**: 520–9.

110 Drobyski W, Thibodeau S, Truitt RL *et al.* Third-party-mediated graft rejection and graft-versus-host disease after T-cell-depleted bone marrow transplantation, as demonstrated by hypervariable DNA probes and HLA-DR polymorphism. *Blood* 1989; **74**: 2285–94.

111 Maynard Smith S, Penrose LS. Monozygotic and dizygotic twin diagnosis. *Ann Hum Genetics* 1955; **18**: 273–89.

112 O'Reilly RJ, Brochstein J, Dinsmore R, Kirkpatrick D. Marrow transplantation for congenital disorders. *Semin Hematol* 1984; **21**: 188–221.

113 O'Reilly RJ, Keever CA, Small TN, Brochstein J. The use of HLA-non-identical T-cell-depleted marrow transplants for correction of severe combined immunodeficiency disease. *Immunodeficiency Rev* 1989; **1**: 273–309.

114 van Leeuwen JEM, van Tol MJD, Joosten AM *et al.* Relationship between patterns of engraftment in peripheral blood and immune reconstitution after allogeneic bone marrow transplantation for (severe) combined immunodeficiency. *Blood* 1994; **84**: 3936–47.

115 Haddad E, Le Deist F, Aucouturier P *et al.* Long-term chimerism and B-cell function after bone marrow transplantation in patients with severe combined immunodeficiency: a single-center study of 22 patients. *Blood* 1999; **94**: 2923–30.

116 Mottonen M, Lanning M, Saarinen UM. Allogeneic bone marrow transplantation in Chediak–Higashi syndrome. *Pediatr Hematol Oncol* 1995; **12**: 55–9.

117 Kapelushnik J, Or R, Filon D *et al.* Analysis of β-globin mutations shows stable mixed chimerism in patients with thalassemia after bone marrow transplantation. *Blood* 1995; **86**: 3241–6.

118 Andreani M, Manna M, Lucarelli G *et al.* Persistence of mixed chimerism in patients transplanted for the treatment of thalassemia. *Blood* 1996; **87**: 3494–9.

119 Andreani M, Nesci S, Lucarelli G *et al.* Long-term survival of ex-thalassemic patients with persistent mixed chimerism after bone marrow transplantation. *Bone Marrow Transplant* 2000; **25**: 401–13.

120 Thomas ED, Ramberg RE, Sale GE, Sparkes RS, Golde DW. Direct evidence for a bone marrow origin of the alveolar macrophage in man. *Science* 1976; **192**: 1016–8.

121 Gale RP, Sparkes RS, Golde DW. Bone marrow origin of hepatic macrophages (Kupffer cells) in humans. *Science* 1978; **201**: 937–8.

122 Volc-Platzer B, Stingl G, Wolff K *et al.* Cytogenetic identification of allogeneic epidermal Langerhans cells in a bone marrow graft recipient. *N Engl J Med* 1984; **310**: 1123–4.

123 Krall WJ, Challita PM, Perlmutter LS, Skelton DC, Kohn DB. Cells expressing human glucocerebrosidase from a retroviral vector repopulate macrophages and central nervous system microglia after murine bone marrow transplantation. *Blood* 1994; **83**: 2737–48.

124 Hessel H, Mittermuller J, Zitzelsberger H, Weier HU, Bauchinger M. Combined immunophenotyping and FISH with sex chromosome-specific DNA probes for the detection of chimerism in epidermal Langerhans cells after sex-mismatched bone marrow transplantation. *Histochem Cell Biol* 1996; **106**: 481–5.

125 Kennedy DW, Abkowitz JL. Kinetics of central nervous system microglial and macrophage engraftment: analysis using a transgenic bone marrow transplantation model. *Blood* 1997; **90**: 986–93.

126 Auffermann-Gretzinger S, Lossos IS, Vayntrub TA *et al.* Rapid establishment of dendritic cell chimerism in allogeneic hematopoietic cell transplant recipients. *Blood* 2002; **99**: 1441–8.

127 Golde DW, Hocking WG, Quan SG, Sparkes RS, Gale RP. Origin of human bone marrow fibroblasts. *Br J Haematol* 1980; **44**: 183–7.

128 Keating A, Singer JW, Killen PD *et al.* Donor origin of the *in vitro* haematopoietic microenvironment after marrow transplantation in man. *Nature* 1982; **298**: 280–3.

129 Lim B, Izaguirre CA, Aye MT *et al.* Characterization of reticulofibroblastoid colonies (CFU-RF) derived from bone marrow and long-term marrow culture monolayers. *J Cell Physiol* 1986; **127**: 45–54.

130 Laver J, Jhanwar SC, O'Reilly RJ, Castro-Malaspina H. Host origin of the human hematopoietic microenvironment following allogeneic bone marrow transplantation. *Blood* 1987; **70**: 1966–8.

131 Simmons PJ, Przepiorka D, Thomas ED, Torok-Storb B. Host origin of marrow stromal cells following allogeneic bone marrow transplantation. *Nature* 1987; **328**: 429–32.

132 Awaya N, Rupert K, Bryant E, Torok-Storb B. Failure of adult marrow-derived stem cells to generate marrow stroma after successful hematopoietic

stem cell transplantation. *Exp Hematol* 2002; **30**: 937–42.
133 Alison MR, Poulsom R, Jeffrey R *et al.* Hepatocytes from nonhepatic adult stem cells. *Nature* 2000; **406**: 257.
134 Thiese ND, Nimmakayalu M, Gardner R *et al.* Liver from bone marrow in humans. *Hepatology* 2000; **32**: 11–6.
135 Körbling M, Katz RL, Khanna A *et al.* Hepatocytes and epithelial cells of donor origin in recipients of peripheral-blood stem cells. *N Engl J Med* 2002; **346**: 738–46.
136 Hematti P, Sloand EM, Carvallo CA *et al.* Absence of donor-derived keratinocyte stem cells in skin tissues cultured from patients after mobilized peripheral blood hematopoietic stem cell transplantation. *Exp Hematol* 2002; **30**: 943–9.

19

John G. Gribben

Antibody Mediated Purging

Despite the success of the use of combination chemotherapy for the treatment of advanced stage malignancies, the majority of these patients die of their disease. In an attempt to overcome drug resistance, high-dose chemotherapy is used with curative attempt both in patients with previously relapsed disease and, increasingly, as consolidation therapy in high-risk patients in first complete remission (CR). The myeloablation induced by high-dose therapy can be reversed by autologous or allogeneic hematopoietic cell transplantation (HCT). Autologous cells have several potential advantages over allogeneic cells for HCT. Autologous HCT overcomes the need for a human leukocyte antigen (HLA)-identical donor, eliminates the risk of graft-vs.-host disease (GVHD) and enables the use of chemotherapy dose escalation for a large number of patients with hematologic and solid tumors [1–4].

One of the major obstacles to the use of autologous HCT after high-dose chemotherapy is that contaminating tumor cells might be infused back to the patient and would then contribute to subsequent relapse. To enable the use of autologous HCT, a variety of methods have been developed to "purge" malignant cells. The aim of purging is to eliminate any contaminating malignant cells and leave intact the hematopoietic cells that are necessary for engraftment. The development of purging techniques has led subsequently to a number of studies of autologous HCT in patients with either a previous history of peripheral blood or bone marrow (BM) involvement or even overt peripheral blood or BM involvement at the time of stem cell collection [2,5–7]. These clinical studies have demonstrated that purging can result in depletion of malignant cells *in vitro* without significant impairment of hematologic reconstitution. The rationale for removing tumor cells from hematopoietic cells might appear compelling, yet the issue of purging remains controversial. The finding that the majority of patients who relapse after autologous bone marrow transplantation (BMT) do so at sites of prior disease has led to the widespread view that purging of autologous marrow cannot contribute to outcome in those patients who are destined to relapse from their endogenous disease. In addition, the few clinical trials reported to date testing the efficacy of purging by comparison of infusion of purged vs. unpurged autologous hematopoietic cells have not demonstrated a survival advantage for the use of purged stem cells. These issues, in addition to the lack of availability of effective purging strategies that are approved for widespread use, have made it difficult to design and perform definitive studies to address the contribution of purging.

In assessing the potential value of purging, three basic questions have to be addressed. First, what is the evidence that residual malignant cells are contained within autologous BM or peripheral blood mononuclear cell (PBMC) collections? Second, can these tumor cells be purged using currently available techniques? Third, do reinfused tumor cells contribute to relapse and does removal of these cells lead to improved outcome after treatment?

Detection of residual disease in autologous hematopoietic cells

The likelihood that autologous hematopoietic cells are contaminated with neoplastic cells is determined by a number of clinical variables. BM and peripheral blood involvement is extremely rare in some tumors such as testicular or ovarian cancers, more common in non-Hodgkin's lymphoma (NHL) and in solid tumors such as small cell lung cancer, neuroblastoma and breast cancer, and invariable in the leukemias. Generally, the higher the stage of the tumor the more likely it is that the BM and peripheral blood are involved. In addition, the ability to detect malignant cells within the circulation is dependent upon the sensitivity of the assay used (Table 19.1).

Since the limit of detection of marrow infiltration by histologic examination is 5% and approximately 10^{11} cells are collected at the time of BM harvest, a BM harvest that is judged to be normal by histologic examination may still contain as many as 5×10^8 malignant cells. Although the level of tumor contamination may be at a lower concentration in peripheral blood cell collections, the total number of cells collected is also greater so that the number of tumor cells collected may be of the same order of magnitude. More sensitive assays to detect the presence of malignant infiltration such as immunocytochemistry, flow cytometric analysis, molecular biologic techniques and clonogenic assays have greatly increased the sensitivity of detection of malignant cells beyond that possible by histology. These techniques have all demonstrated the presence of minimal residual disease (MRD) in patients in whom there is

Table 19.1 Sensitivity of tumor cell detection.

Method	Sensitivity
Light microscopy	1 in 10^1–10^2
Southern Blot analysis	1 in 10^2
FISH	1 in 10^2
Flow cytometry	1 in 10^4–$\geq 10^4$
Immunocytochemistry (APAAP)	1 in 10^4–10^6
Clonogenic assays	1 in 10^4–10^6
PCR	1 in 10^5–10^6

FISH, fluorescence *in situ* hybridization; PCR, polymerase chain reaction.

no morphologic evidence of tumor infiltration in PBMC collections, as outlined in detail in Chapter 22.

Immunocytochemistry

Immunocytochemical techniques have been most widely used to detect MRD in solid tumors. Detection rates and levels of sensitivity vary widely depending upon the tumor type, the stage of disease in the patient population being studied, and also the methodology used to detect the tumor cells. The use of monoclonal antibodies (MABs) that recognize cytokeratins is one of the most widely used methods, particularly in breast cancer [8]. Since there are no true tumor antigens that are recognized using these techniques, great care must be taken in interpretation of data to ensure that normal cells that express these antigens are not also scored as tumor cells. It is one great advantage of immunocytochemical techniques that it allows morphologic examination of the positively stained cells, although it is not always possible to determine whether a stained cell is malignant. Additional markers that stain cycling cells, such as Ki-67, may improve the ability to discern malignant cells from background normal cells.

Molecular biologic techniques

The underlying principle for the application of molecular biological techniques to the diagnosis of human malignancies lies in the detection of clonal proliferation of tumor specific chromosomal translocations or gene rearrangements. These have been studied most widely in the lymphoproliferative malignancies because of the specific nature of gene rearrangements occurring at the antigen receptors. The use of the polymerase chain reaction (PCR) has greatly increased the sensitivity of detection of MRD. Nonrandom chromosomal translocations are ideal candidates for PCR amplification if the DNA sequences at the chromosomal breakpoints are known. For example, cloning of the t(14;18) breakpoints involving the *bcl-2* protooncogene on chromosome 18 and the immunoglobulin (Ig) heavy chain locus on chromosome 14 has made it possible to use PCR amplification to detect lymphoma cells containing this translocation [9]. Using this technique residual lymphoma cells were detected in the BM at the time of initial assessment and following induction or salvage therapy of all patients with advanced stage NHL containing the *bcl-2* translocation [9–11]. Although a number of leukemias and lymphomas are characterized by nonrandom chromosomal translocations, the majority of malignancies, especially the solid tumors, do not demonstrate such nonrandom chromosomal translocations and are less suitable for detection by PCR amplification. PCR techniques can still be used to detect genes expressed within tumor cells that should not normally be detected within peripheral blood and can act as a surrogate marker for tumor detection as described in more detail below.

Cell culture techniques

The biggest disadvantage of molecular and immunocytochemical techniques in detection of MRD is that these techniques do not differentiate between clonogenic tumor cells and cells that have lost the potential to proliferate. Clonogenic tumor assays have the capacity to detect the tumor cells that may be most relevant for subsequent relapse. However, the precise nature of the clonogenic tumor cell that can grow in the host and contribute to subsequent relapse has still to be defined. The cell capable of initiating human disease must have the potential for self-renewal and be capable of proliferating. In a model in nonobese diabetic mice with severe combined immunodeficiency disease (NOD-SCID mice), in all subtypes of human acute myeloid leukemia (AML) analyzed, cells capable of expanding in the NOD-SCID mice were exclusively $CD34^+ + CD38^-$, which are found at a low frequency with the leukemic blast population [12]. Unfortunately, the conditions for clonogenic tumor growth and the characteristics of the tumor stem cell have not been well characterized in the majority of tumors. Sensitive culture techniques have demonstrated clearly that clonogenic malignant cells can be grown from BM with no morphologic evidence of infiltration [13–18]. At least for breast cancer, there appears to be a good association between immunocytochemical and clonogenic assays for detection of MRD [17,18].

Residual tumor cells in peripheral blood mononuclear cell (PBMC) collections

Recently, PBMC collections have been preferred over autologous BM harvests due to reduced engraftment time and ease of attainment. This issue is discussed in more detail in Chapter 45. Although it is widely assumed that PBMC provided a source of stem cells that contains fewer tumor cells than harvested BM, this has not been extensively studied. A number of studies have now demonstrated that PBMC are often contaminated with tumor cells so that this source of hematopoietic cells may also require further processing to separate the hematopoietic cells from tumor cells.

In a multi-institutional study of PBMC transplantation in patients with advanced multiple myeloma (MM) receiving myeloablative chemotherapy, tumor cells were detected in leukapheresis products from eight of 14 unselected patients and ranged from 1.13×10^4–2.14×10^6 malignant cells/kg [19]. After CD34 selection, residual tumor was detected in only three patients' products. Overall, a greater than 2.7–4.5-log reduction in contaminating MM cells was achieved. In a retrospective analysis cryopreserved BM aspirates from 83 patients with high-risk stage II, III, and IV breast cancer were obtained after induction chemotherapy but before stem cell harvest. All samples had no evidence of BM infiltration by morphologic assessment. PCR for cytokeratin 19 was performed and results correlated with the probability of relapse following high-dose therapy and autologous HCT. The incidence of detection of cytokeratin 19 positivity assessed by PCR analysis in BM increased significantly with advancing stage: 52% for 19 stage II, 57% for 14 stage III and 82% for 50 stage IV patients ($p = 0.0075$) [20].

In one study, paired PBMC and BM samples from 48 patients were analyzed using immunocytochemical and clonogenic tumor colony techniques [17]. Immunocytochemistry detected tumor cells at a significantly higher rate in BM than in PBMC ($p < 0.005$). Tumor cells were detected in 13 of 133 PBMC specimens (9.8%) from nine of 48 patients (18.7%) and in 38 of 61 BM specimens (62.3%) from 32 of these 48 patients (66.7%). Clonogenic tumor colonies grew in 21 of 26 specimens positive by immunocytochemistry. No tumor colony growth was detected in 30 of 32 specimens that were negative by immunocytochemistry. Immunocytochemical detection of tumor involvement in BM and PBMC was correlated significantly with *in vitro* clonogenic growth ($p < 0.0001$). PBMCs appear to contain fewer tumor cells than paired BM specimens from patients with advanced breast cancer, but these tumor cells appear to be capable of clonogenic growth *in vitro* [17]. Although is seems clear that in the resting state PB contains fewer tumor cells than BM in some malignancies, a number of factors must be taken into account. First, there is now considerable evidence that mobilization with chemotherapy and growth factors mobilizes tumor cells as well as stem cells [21]. Second, a greater number of PBMC than BM cells must be collected so that the cell dose infused becomes an important determinant, in that the total number of tumor cells, rather than the concentration of such cells is likely to be more relevant. This issue was addressed in a study in patients with MM [22]. Quantitative PCR analysis of the Ig heavy chain variable region sequence of the patient's myeloma cells was performed to assess tumor burden in samples from PBMC collections and BM harvests from 13 patients with MM. As expected, the percentage of tumor cells contaminating the BM harvest (median, 0.74%) was higher than in the PBMC specimens (median, 0.0024%). Because of the increased total number of cells used for PBMC transplantation, the increase in total number of contaminating cells in the BM vs. PBMC autografts was less pronounced (BM vs. PBMC tumor contamination ratios ranging from 0.9 to >4500; median, 14) [22]. In patients with NHL, although the concentration of tumor cells was also higher in BM than in PBSC, there was less than 1 log difference. When allowance was made for the greater number of PBMC used there was no difference in the total number of tumor cells within the collected products [23].

Taken together, these data demonstrate that it is naive to assume that PBMC collections are free from contaminating tumor cells. Clinical trials examining the question of tumor contamination and its clinical significance for subsequent outcome after HCT using PBMCs are ongoing.

Immunologic purging of malignant cells

At the same time that techniques were being developed to demonstrate the existence of MRD, attempts were being made to develop methodologies to deplete contaminating malignant cells without impairing hematopoietic progenitor cells (Table 19.2). Most studies performed have utilized immunologic maneuvers to remove malignant cells from the autologous marrow by a process of negative selection. An alternative and highly attractive strategy would be to select positively the hematopoietic stem cells (HSCs) based upon expression of surface antigens such as CD34. These studies are described in detail in Chapter 8. These studies have been hampered largely by the relative inefficiency of CD34 selection techniques [24]. Preclinical studies are underway in many centers examining the potential role of positive selection of CD34 cells followed by negative depletion steps to remove residual contaminating tumor cells [25–28].

Characteristics of ideal monoclonal antibodies (MABs) for purging

Because of their specificity, MABs make ideal agents to identify and target such malignant cells. A number of mouse antihuman MABs have

Table 19.2 Methodologies for purging of tumor cells.

Physical separation
Size
Density
Osmotic lysis
Lectin agglutination
Hyperthermia

Pharmacologic
4-hydroperoxycyclophosphamide
Asta-Z

Immunologic
Uncoupled monoclonal antibodies
   Complement mediated lysis
   Immunomagnetic beads
Directly coupled
   Chemotherapeutic agent
   Toxins
   Magnetic beads
   Radionuclide

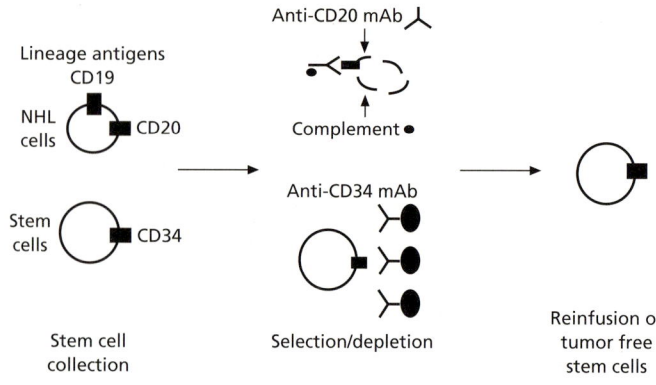

Fig. 19.1 Principles of immunologic purging. Targeted antigens are present on the surface of malignant cells but are not expressed on hematopoietic progenitors. Malignant cells escaping the purging procedure are likely not to express or express only weakly the targeted antigens.

Table 19.3 Ideal target antigens for tumor cell purging.

Not expressed on hematopoietic progenitors
Expressed on clonogenic tumor cell
High density of expression on malignant cell
Limited heterogeneity of expression on tumor cell
Lineage restriction
Depending on strategy for purging—ability to modulate

been generated with specificity for human cell surface antigens by immunizing mice with human malignant cells or malignant cell membranes. Despite the hope that unique tumor specific cell surface proteins would be recognized, all of the cell surface antigens identified to date on neoplastic cells of the hematopoietic or solid tumor malignancies represent normal differentiation antigens, and true leukemia, lymphoma or cancer specific antigens have not been identified. The most important factor to be determined is that the MAB targets the malignant cell as specifically as possible but have no effect on HSCs necessary for marrow engraftment. The principle for the selective depletion of contaminating residual tumor cells from HSCs is illustrated in Fig. 19.1. Likely mechanisms of failure of immunologic purging include antigenic heterogeneity whereby not all tumor cells express the targeted antigen and the relative inefficiency of the purging methodology employed to "purge" the targeted cells.

The ideal characteristics of MABs for purging are shown in Table 19.3. The targeted antigen should be present at high density on the cell surface to increase the efficiency of subsequent cell killing or removal. To limit the effect of antigenic heterogeneity of expression on the target cell, multiple MAB cocktails are employed targeting multiple antigens.

Selection of purging methods

Since MAB are not by themselves toxic, they must be used in combination with other agents to kill the targeted cell. The most widely studied methods of immunologic purging are complement-mediated lysis, immunomagnetic bead depletion and immunotoxins. The potential advantages and disadvantages of each of these techniques are shown in Table 19.4.

If MABs are used with complement, complement fixing isotypes must be used, the most efficient being immunoglobulin M (IgM). The earliest preclinical studies involved the addition of complement to MAB coated cells which were then eliminated by complement-mediated cytotoxicity. For immunologic purging using complement-mediated lysis or immunomagnetic bead separation it is important that the antigen–antibody

Table 19.4 Comparison of methods of immunological purging.

Method of tumor depletion	Nature of antibody/antigen interaction	Technical issues	Resistance to tumor cell	Expense
Complement mediated lysis	Antibody must fix complement High antigen density expression Antigen should not modulate	Screen complement lots for toxicity Multiple cycles are required Multiple antibodies additive	Antigen heterogeneity Resistance to complement lysis	Low
Immunotoxins	Antibody/antigen complex must internalize High antigen density expression	Nonspecific cell loss Longer incubation time More easy to standardize Difficult to assess efficacy of purge	Antigen heterogeneity Few antigen targets internalize Resistance to toxin mechanism	Intermediate
Immunomagnetic bead depletion	All antibodies are candidate targets High antigen density expression	Nonspecific cell loss Easy to standardize Simple and rapid Fewer cycles required	Antigen heterogeneity Antigen shedding	High

complex remains on the cell surface and is not internalized. In contrast, if immunotoxins are used then the targeted antigen–antibody complex should be internalized to ensure intracellular delivery of the cellular toxin.

Complement-mediated lysis

The earliest preclinical studies utilized the ability of MAB to fix complement to the MAB-coated cells that were then eliminated by complement-mediated cytotoxicity. Complement-mediated cytolysis was previously the most commonly employed method for immunologic purging, due in part to its efficiency, specificity and relatively low cost. In most studies, rabbit complement has been used to circumvent the problem of homologous species restriction, the process whereby cells are generally resistant to lysis by complement from the same species. The ideal complement source must be toxic to cells coated with MAB but not toxic to cells that have not been coated with antibody. There are major disadvantages of using complement. There is considerable variability among different lots of complement so that each new lot must be tested for nonspecific toxicity. There are nonspecific cell losses that occur because of the need for cell washing steps. In addition, complement-mediated lysis is inefficient when the neoplastic cells only weakly express the targeted antigen. In addition, regulatory issues in the USA related to the use of nonhuman sources of protein for human cell manipulation have markedly decreased the use of complement mediated lysis for clinical purging.

Among the factors that may influence the efficiency of complement-mediated lysis are the density of surface antigen expression, antigen modulation and resistance to complement lysis. Failure of immunologic purging using complement-mediated lysis could be attributed to three possible mechanisms. First, the clonogenic tumor cells might not express, or only express weakly, the surface antigens expressed by the majority of tumor cells. Second, modulation of one or more of the surface antigens following attachment of the MAB to its ligand might limit complement-mediated lysis. Third, a subgroup of patients may have malignancies which are intrinsically more resistant to complement-mediated lysis.

Tumor cell killing by antibody-mediated complement activation most likely results from osmotic cell lysis following disruption of the semipermeable properties of the cell membrane. An actively metabolizing cell is capable of turning over its cell membrane. This phenomenon may result not only in antigen modulation but also in neutralization of the lytic effects of the complement. Previous studies have shown associations between biochemical events in the cell and sensitivity to complement-mediated lysis [29,30]. In addition, an anticomplementary factor has been described in normal BM cells that limits complement activation, not only on the cells that produce the factor, but also on antibody-coated cells within the normal marrow [31]. These anticomplementary effects may be overcome by repeated treatments with complement and previous studies have suggested that the use of repeated treatment cycles is more efficient in removing contaminating tumor cells than single treatment cycles. This approach is time consuming, increases the expense of the procedure in both reagents and in laboratory staff effort, and may increase the nonspecific loss of HSCs. The continuous infusion of fresh complement while removing media containing the used complement may increase the efficiency and time taken to perform the procedure [32]. Studies have been reported that address whether these mechanisms of complement resistance can be overcome by chemical engineering of MABs [33] or by neutralization of CD59 activity [34]. Expression of membrane-bound regulators of complement activation including CD46, CD55, and CD59 protect nucleated cells from complement-mediated injury. Increased expression of these molecules may be a mechanism by which tumor cells protect themselves from inflammatory responses and complement-mediated injury.

Populations of cells that survive following MAB purging appear to be more resistant to subsequent treatments with the same MAB and complement, presumably because of the emergence of subpopulations of cells with a relative decrease in the surface expression of the targeted antigens [35]. Such changes in relative expression of antigen density have also been observed following treatment with chemotherapy. It is important to demonstrate that the tumor to be purged expresses the targeted antigen, not only at the time of diagnosis, but also at the time of HSC harvest. This is increasingly the case now that humanized MABs are in routine use in the treatment of patients with a variety of malignances. Although the emergence of target antigen negative tumor cells is relatively rare, this has been observed [36–39].

The combination of immunologic and pharmacologic purging appears to be more efficient than either method alone in eliminating clonogenic Burkitt cell lines from human BM [40]. The effectiveness of purging small cell lung cancer cell lines was also significantly increased when MAB and complement-mediated lysis was used in combination with the cyclophosphamide derivative Asta-Z 7557 although there was significant reduction in myeloid colony growth [41]. In T-cell malignancies, 2′deoxycoformycin has been used in combination with anti-T-cell MABs to eliminate clonogenic malignant human T cells [42]. A combined approach was taken to attempt to eliminate multidrug-resistant (MDR) leukemic cell lines from BM using a MAB directed against the cell surface product of the *MDR* gene [43]. This treatment did not affect normal committed precursors. Following antibody purging the addition of etoposide (VP16) enhanced the purging efficacy and resulted in a 4.6-log reduction of malignant cells. Furthermore, this antibody was effective when used against the patients' leukemic blasts, suggesting that this approach was effective and selective for removal of MDR expressing cells from HSC transplantation.

Magnetic bead depletion

The use of immunomagnetic beads has the advantage that there is no biologic variability between lots as has been observed with complement. Most studies have utilized magnetic microspheres coated with affinity-purified sheep antimouse antibodies directed against the Fc portion of the MAB (Dynabeads®, Dynal, Oslo, Norway). More recently, a number of particles have been developed that are directly attached to the primary MABs used for purging. These reagents have the advantage of allowing more rapid and simpler purging procedures. Instruments to remove the immunomagnetic beads are now available commercially.

Immunomagnetic bead depletion is used increasingly as a method of eliminating malignant cells for HCT. The use of immunomagnetic beads was originally developed to facilitate depletion of neuroblastoma cells since the available MAB did not fix complement [44]. The majority of clinical studies of marrow purging using immunomagnetic beads have been performed in children with neuroblastoma. More recently, a number of studies have been performed for a variety of other malignancies, including small-cell lung cancer, breast cancer, acute lymphoblastic leukemia (ALL), myeloma and lymphomas as described below. The efficacy of MABs and immunomagnetic beads in removing Burkitt lymphoma cells from normal BM has been demonstrated in a number of studies. Clonogenic lymphoma cell assays have demonstrated that different anti-B-cell MABs differ in their efficiency of depleting lymphoma cells from 1.9 to 2.8 logs in one cycle. When three MAB were used in a cocktail, the efficiency of purging increased to 3.3 logs following a single cycle of treatment and 5 logs after two cycles. Treatment of the BM with beads alone or with the MAB did not significantly reduce the number of HSC as assessed by colony assays [45]. A cocktail of two MAB was used to assess the relative efficiency of purging of two different immunomagnetic particles [46]. The efficacy of purging the cell line Nalm 6 was assessed using immunofluorescence or colony assays. Log tumor cell kill was significantly better using BioMag® particles (3.1 logs) vs. Dynabeads® (1.8 logs) following a single cycle of treatment. These beads differ in size, and the smaller particles appeared to remove cells more efficiently. There was no significant difference in the efficiency of purging after two treatment cycles and >4.5 logs of tumor cell depletion was obtained using either immunomagnetic bead.

In preclinical experiments, treatment of BM samples from patients with follicular lymphoma that were contaminated with up to 20% lymphoma cells were purged with either a three or a four MABs cocktail followed by immunomagnetic bead depletion. This resulted in the loss of all PCR detectable cells after three cycles of treatment in all 25 patients studied [47]. After two treatment cycles of immunomagnetic bead depletion, four MAB were more efficient than three MABs for purging. In these same patient samples, treatment with three MABs and complement depleted all PCR detectable lymphoma cells in only 44% of samples. The addition of a fourth MAB to this cocktail followed by complement lysis successfully purged the BM of only 64% of marrow samples. In this study, immunomagnetic bead depletion had no significant effect on myeloid colony forming assays, suggesting that repeated cycles of immunomagnetic bead depletion might be performed safely. The results of this study suggest that immunomagnetic bead depletion is significantly more efficient than complement-mediated lysis in depleting lymphoma cells and that four MABs are more efficient than three MABs. The results also demonstrate that multiple cycles of immunomagnetic bead depletion may still be required to remove PCR detectable lymphoma cells. Theoretically, attachment of a single magnetic particle may be sufficient to allow removal of the targeted cell in a magnetic field and some lymphoma cells may have sufficiently low density of expression of the targeted antigens to allow elimination with immunomagnetic beads but not to allow complement-mediated lysis.

Immunotoxins

Purging of autologous marrow *in vitro* using immunotoxins is a particularly promising approach. Several exquisitely effective candidate toxins have been identified that mediate their cytotoxic function by inhibiting cellular protein synthesis. Because the mechanism of killing by toxins is different from that of chemotherapeutic agents, they are capable of killing cells that are resistant to chemotherapy [48]. These toxins are cytotoxic to both normal and malignant cells and must be targeted to the malignant cell to demonstrate specificity. The combination of these toxins with a MAB to target delivery specifically to the neoplastic cells is a theoretically attractive proposition [49]. If native toxins were to be conjugated to MAB, the resultant immunotoxin would still be capable of binding to nonspecific targets by binding to the toxin-binding site on normal cells. This nonspecific binding is overcome by modification of the toxin moiety to delete the binding site but leave the toxin domains intact. The most widely studied toxins have been ricin, *Pseudomonas exotoxin* and diphtheria toxin. Most experience of *in vitro* marrow purging has been with ricin. Multiple anti-T-cell intact ricin immunotoxins have been evaluated as potential purging agents [50]. The cocktail containing all four immunotoxins in equimolar concentrations eliminated more than 4 logs of clonogenic leukemic cells at a dose that spared more than 70% of the pluripotent HSCs.

Assessment of the efficacy of purging

The identical techniques that can be used to assess whether a hematopoietic cell collection contains residual tumor cells can be used to assess whether tumor cells remain present after immunologic purging, including culture systems, clonogenic assays and PCR analysis. These studies have demonstrated that different anti-B-cell MABs differ in their efficiency to deplete lymphoma cells [45]. Multiple rounds of treatments were more efficient than single treatments and the combination of two or more antibodies was more efficient than a single MAB to eliminate tumor cells [51,52]. PCR has been used to assess the efficacy of immunologic purging both in models using cell lines [53] and patient samples [11,47]. The efficacy of MAB and immunomagnetic beads has also been demonstrated in a number of studies [25,45,47]. Clonogenic lymphoma cell assays have demonstrated that the efficiency of purging increased significantly when three MABs were used in a cocktail. A cocktail of two MABs was used to assess the relative efficiency of purging of two different immuno-magnetic particles [54]. Log tumor cell kill was significantly better using BioMag® particles (3.1 logs) vs. Dynabeads® (1.8 logs) following a single cycle of treatment. There was no significant difference in the efficiency of purging after two treatment cycles and >4.5 logs of tumor cell depletion was obtained using either immunomagnetic bead. Treatment of harvested BM samples from lymphoma patients with either a three or a four MAB cocktail followed by immunomagnetic bead depletion resulted in the loss of all PCR detectable cells after three cycles of treatment in all patients studied [47]. This study suggests that immunomagnetic bead depletion is significantly more efficient than complement-mediated lysis in depleting lymphoma cells but that multiple cycles of immunomagnetic bead depletion may still be required to remove PCR detectable lymphoma cells.

Table 19.5 Impact of immunological purging on engraftment.

Disease	No. of pts	Antigen/MAB	Days to neutrophils >500	Days to platelets >20,000	Reference
Complement					
AML	138	CD14, CD15	27 (1st CR)	38	[3]
AML	12	CD33	30	45	[60]
ALL	54	CD10, CD19, CD7	24	40	[69]
NHL	100	CD10, CD20, B5	27	29	[7]
Immunomagnetic beads					
Neuroblastoma	91	UJ13A, Thy 1, UJ127.11, UJ181.4	28	42	[61]
ALL	8	CD10, CD9	15	27	[62]
Immunotoxins					
ALL	13	CD7	17	40	[63]
ALL	14	CD5, CD7	27	NS	[64]

ALL, acute lymphoblastic leukemia; AML, acute myeloid leukemia; CR, complete remission; MAB, monoclonal antibody; NHL, non-Hodgkin's lymphoma.

Using a single cycle of treatment with multiple MABs and beads, approximately 2.5 logs of small cell lung cancer lines could be depleted, although there was variability in the efficiency of purging different cell lines [55]. In parallel studies, there was no significant toxicity noted to myeloid progenitors. Using two small-cell lung cancer lines, immunomagnetic bead depletion was shown to result in a 4–5-log reduction of cancer cells and did not adversely affect BM colony growth [56]. Anti-CD15 MAB, expressed on a variety of human cancer cell lines, was capable of depleting up to 3 logs of breast cancer cells from normal contaminated marrow using immunomagnetic bead depletion but minimally affected normal hematopoietic progenitors [57]. The combination of 4-hydroperoxycyclophosphamide and immunomagnetic bead depletion removed 4–5 logs of clonogenic breast cancer cells [58].

Evaluation of the purging efficiency of an immunotoxin prepared by conjugating anti-CD7 with pokeweed antiviral protein revealed that approximately 3 logs of clonogenic T cells could be eliminated. The addition of 2'deoxycoformycin and deoxyadenosine to the immunotoxin resulted in the elimination of up to 6 logs of the T-cell line but also resulted in decreased myeloid progenitor colony assay growth [59].

Contribution of infused tumor cells to relapse

The finding that the majority of patients who relapse after autologous HCT do so at sites of prior disease has led to the widespread view that purging of autologous marrow could contribute little to subsequent outcome after autologous HCT. Although no direct study has been made comparing the infusion of purged vs. unpurged marrow, indirect approaches can be made to assess the clinical significance of immunologic purging. Methods to assess the clinical utility of purging are shown in Table 19.5 [3,7,60–64,69].

Clinical studies of immunologic purging

Immunologic purging was first performed in NHL and has been most widely studied in this disease [5,7,11,65,66]. Additional studies have been performed in MM [24,67,68], ALL [69,70], AML [3,60], breast cancer [71], small cell lung cancer [41] and neuroblastoma [62,72] among others. These studies have confirmed that immunologic purging can be performed safely and that subsequent hematopoietic engraftment is not significantly delayed. No randomized prospective study has

Table 19.6 Approaches to demonstrate clinical efficacy of purging.

Surrogate endpoints
   Depletion of PCR detectable cell
   Depletion of clonogenic tumor cells

Gene transfer of marker gene

Randomized trial
   Purged vs. unpurged autologous hematopoietic cells

PCR, polymerase chain reaction.

demonstrated whether the removal of occult or overt neoplastic cells resulted in improved disease-free survival [24,68]. Whether the failure to demonstrate an advantage of purging is due to the relative inefficiency of the purging technique or the intrinsic resistance of the tumor cells to the high-dose chemotherapy approach used is not clear. The results obtained in the larger reported trials using immunologic purging are shown in Table 19.6.

Complement-mediated lysis

In a clinical trial of 138 patients with AML, BM purging was performed using two MABs and complement-mediated lysis [3]. One-hundred-and-ten patients were in CR at the time of transplantation (23 in first CR, 87 in second or third CR). Engraftment was prompt in most patients, and only one very heavily pretreated patient in third CR failed to engraft. Engraftment was faster in those patients infused with larger numbers of colony forming units (CFUs). This study did not compare results obtained using purged vs. unpurged marrow, but the relapse-free survival of the patients in second and third remission appears to be comparable to that obtained following allogeneic transplantation in similar risk patients. Anti-CD33 MAB and complement-mediated lysis was used to purge the BM of 12 patients with AML [60]. Patients had durable but delayed engraftment and platelet engraftment was particularly delayed in some patients. Of note, colony forming unit-granulocyte macrophage (CFU-GM) colony growth was markedly reduced following purging. In a multicenter study, autologous HCT was used in 54 patients with ALL [69]. The BM was purged using as anti-CD10, anti-CD19 and anti-CD7 MABs and rabbit complement. The transplant related mortality was 5% and engraftment was rapid. Of note, this study was not designed to demonstrate efficacy.

One-hundred patients with B-cell NHL were treated at the Dana-Farber Cancer Institute with purged autologous BMT when they were in CR or minimal disease state [7]. Notably, 69 patients had prior history of histologic marrow involvement and 37 patients had overt marrow disease at the time of BM harvest. This study was associated with low treatment-related mortality. Engraftment was rapid in all cases. The results of the use of HCT in patients with follicular lymphoma in first complete or partial remission have also been reported [5,73]. These studies address not only the outcome for those patients receiving autologous HCT but enrolled patients on an "intent-to-treat basis" and suggested that virtually all patients with follicular lymphoma can achieve minimal disease state before proceeding to autologous HCT. Long-term follow up of patients treated at the Dana-Farber Cancer Institute was reported on 153 patients with B-cell NHL with purged autologous BMT when they were in CR or minimal disease state [2]. Notably, 47% of patients had overt marrow disease at the time of BM harvest. This study was associated with low treatment-related mortality and engraftment was rapid in all cases.

Immunomagnetic bead depletion

The first clinical studies of purging using immunomagnetic beads were performed for children with neuroblastoma [62]. Immunomagnetic bead depletion was used to purge 123 BMs before autologous stem cell transplantation in 91 cases of neuroblastoma [61]. In this study, 59 patients received a single graft and 32 patients received two sequential procedures. Although the procedure resulted in a significant loss of mononuclear cells, there was little evidence of additional toxic effects on myeloid progenitors. Immunomagnetic beads were used to deplete leukemic cells from the marrows of patients with common ALL [62]. In this study, the marrows of 18 patients were purged using a cocktail of three MABs, although only eight of these patients were subsequently treated with high-dose therapy and autologous HCT. Engraftment was rapid in all cases although slower than that observed in patients with neuroblastoma.

A novel approach for the separation of malignant cells was reported for 16 patients with B-cell malignancies using floating immunobeads [74]. Here low-density polypropylene beads precoated with rat antimouse MAB were added to the harvested autologous BM following incubation with anti-B-cell MAB. A 75% recovery of mononuclear cells was achieved with an 83% recovery of myeloid progenitors.

Immunotoxins

Fewer clinical trials have been reported using immunotoxins for purging. Seven patients with high-risk T-cell ALL and six patients with T-cell lymphoma were treated by autologous BMT following purging with anti-CD7 ricin A immunotoxin (WT1-ricin A) [63]. Incubation of the marrow with up to 10^{-8} mol/L had no significant effect on HSC progenitors as assessed by colony assay growth or by subsequent delay of engraftment. Using a different approach, autologous marrow from 14 consecutive patients with T-cell ALL was purged with a combination of two immunotoxins, anti-CD5 and anti-CD7 linked to intact ricin, plus 4-hydroperoxycyclophosphamide [64]. The efficacy of purging was assessed using multiparameter flow analysis, cell sorting and leukemic progenitor cell colony assay. Following purging, no blast colonies were observed in the marrows of 11 of 13 evaluable patients. Engraftment occurred in 13 of the 14 patients and the median time to reach an absolute neutrophil count greater than 500/μL was 27 days. Despite the apparent efficiency of purging, nine patients relapsed, the majority of them shortly after transplantation. In this study, relapse after transplantation was most likely due to failure of the high-dose therapy to ablate endogenous disease in these high-risk patients.

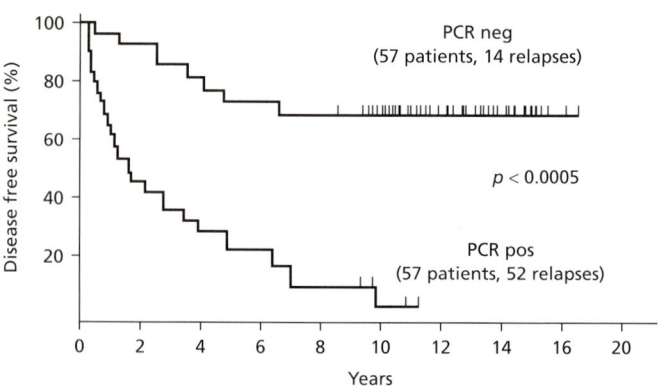

Fig. 19.2 The disease-free survival of lymphoma patients who were infused with autologous bone marrow (BM) with no polymerase chain reaction (PCR) detectable lymphoma cells (PCR negative) was significantly improved compared to those infused with a BM containing residual PCR detectable lymphoma (PCR positive). All patients had PCR detectable lymphoma cells in the BM before immunologic purging.

Outcome after successful immunologic purging

In studies at the Dana-Farber Cancer Institute, PCR amplification of the t(14;18) was used to detect residual lymphoma cells in the BM before and after purging to assess whether efficient purging had any impact on disease-free survival [11]. In this study 114 patients with B-cell NHL and the *bcl-2* translocation were studied. Residual lymphoma cells were detected in all patients in the harvested autologous BM. Following three cycles of immunologic purging using the anti-B-cell MAB J5 (anti-CD10), B1 (anti-CD20) and B5 and complement-mediated lysis, PCR amplification detected residual lymphoma cells in 57 of these patients. The incidence of relapse was significantly increased in patients who had residual detectable lymphoma cells compared to those in whom no lymphoma cells were detectable. The long-term follow up results of this patient cohort by the result obtained after purging is shown in Fig. 19.2. This demonstrates that patients who were infused with a source of hematopoietic cells that was free of detectable lymphoma cells had improved outcome compared to those who had residual detectable lymphoma. This finding was independent of the histology of the lymphoma, the degree of BM infiltration at the time of BM harvest, or remission status at the time of autologous BMT. These findings suggest that the detection of residual lymphoma cells is associated with or provides a surrogate marker for subsequent relapse. A major problem with this finding is that the majority of patients who relapse do so at sites of previous disease, suggesting that the major contribution to subsequent relapse came from endogenous disease. In 60 consecutive patients with a PCR detectable *bcl-2* translocation who had undergone immunologic purging and autologous BMT, there was also an association between the presence of residual lymphoma cells after purging, and the presence of circulating lymphoma cells that could be detected as little as 2 h after infusion of autologous BM. It is possible that these circulating lymphoma cells are capable of homing back to the sites of previous disease and that these sites that provide the microenvironmental conditions conducive for cell growth.

Additional studies have provided further indirect evidence that the use of sources of hematopoietic cells that are contaminated with malignant cells is associated with poorer outcome after HCT. In NHL, two additional studies have demonstrated that the presence of residual lymphoma cells within the stem cell product was associated with poorer outcome [16,75]. Studies at the University of Nebraska have demonstrated that those patients who are infused with morphologically normal BM containing clonogenic lymphoma cells have an increased incidence of relapse after HCT [15,16]. Even in metastatic breast cancer, under circumstances where it is likely that endogenous disease in the patient contributes highly to subsequent failure the presence of contaminating breast cancer cells may be associated with poor outcome after high-dose therapy. In a retrospective analysis cryopreserved BM aspirates from 83 patients with high-risk stage II, III, and IV breast cancer were obtained after induction chemotherapy but before BM harvest [20]. All samples had no evidence of BM infiltration by morphologic assessment. PCR for cytokeratin 19 was performed and results correlated with the probability of relapse following high-dose therapy and autologous BMT. The incidence of detection of cytokeratin 19 positivity assessed by PCR analysis in BM increased significantly with advancing stage [19]. Furthermore, in patients with advanced stage breast cancer detection of message for cytokeratin 19 in BM was associated with a significantly higher ($P = 0.0002$) incidence of subsequent relapse. The probability of relapse at 3 years after autologous BMT for PCR-positive patients was 32% for stage II/III and 94% and stage IV patients, respectively. Patients with no PCR detectable disease had better outcome, with having probability of relapse of 10% for stage II/III and 14% for stage IV patients [20].

None of the studies listed above provide definitive proof that infusion of residual cells at the time of autologous HCT contributes to relapse since it is possible that the detection of residual cancer cells at the time of HCT is associated with inherently worse prognosis in these patients. This could be due to the fact that patients who are not purged could have a higher tumor burden than patients who are not purged successfully. Patients who purge successfully could have a higher level of expression of the target antigen on the cell surface of the clonogenic tumor cell or be more sensitive to complement mediated lysis and this could be associated with an inherently different outcome. Irrespective of the mechanism, the finding of residual malignant cells in autologous hematopoietic cells does appear to provide a powerful prognostic surrogate marker for relapse, independent of other clinical parameters.

A retrospective analysis of the European Blood and Marrow Transplant Lymphoma Registry compared the outcome of 270 patients whose BM had been purged and compared the outcome with 270 case-matched control patients [76]. A variety of purging methodologies was used. In this study there was no advantage in outcome if patients received purged BM. Patients with low-grade lymphoma did not have a significantly improved progression free survival if the BM was purged ($p = 0.1757$), but they did have a significantly improved overall survival ($p = 0.00184$). In this study time to hematologic engraftment, response to autologous BMT and number of procedure-related deaths were similar in purged and unpurged patients.

Marker gene studies demonstrate that infused cells contribute to relapse

Transfection of a marker gene into clonogenic malignant cells *ex vivo* provides a method to assess the fate of malignant cells within the autologous hematopoietic cells, as described in more detail in Chapter 10. If the majority of cells at the site of relapse expressed the marker gene, this would provide compelling evidence that infused malignant cells contribute to relapse. Since the efficiency of transfection is low using existing technology, a negative result would still not be definitive. Results published to date have demonstrated that when relapse occurs there is evidence of malignant cells with the marker gene suggesting strongly that the reinfused malignant cells contributed to relapse [77–80]. In these studies, the neomycin-resistance gene was retrovirally transferred to mark BM harvested from eight patients with childhood tumors, including leukemia and neuroblastoma. The marked marrow cells were subsequently reinfused as part of an autologous HCT. The marker gene could be identified in the malignant cell populations in the majority of patients at relapse. Analysis of tumor cell DNA for discrete marker gene integration sites suggested that at least 200 malignant cells, each capable of tumor formation, were introduced at HCT and contributed to relapse [80]. The authors concluded that autologous BM may contain a multiplicity of malignant cells that subsequently contribute to relapse.

In vivo purging

The availability of humanized antibodies allows the use of MABs to be given *in vivo* unlike the murine MABs that could only be used for *ex-vivo* manipulations. Humanized MAB have been given as additional systemic therapy to eliminate tumor cells from the PBSC collection as an *in-vivo* purging approach [81–83]. This clearly has the advantages that it is easier to perform, does not require a cell manipulation laboratory and allows treatment not only of the collected stem cells, but also of the whole patients. Moreover, this approach can be repeated following infusion of the autologous stem cells. A disadvantage at present is the limited availability of suitable antibodies such that only one antigen is being targeted. Ongoing clinical trials are assessing the efficacy of this approach to obtain tumor-free sources of stem cells.

Design of randomized clinical trial

A randomized trial using purged vs. unpurged autologous marrow would likely provide a definitive answer that would require a multicenter study of several hundred patients. In MM a randomized phase III trial using purged vs. unpurged autologous PBMC was performed using CD34 selection [24]. After CD34 selection tumor burden was reduced by a median of 3.1 logs with 54% of CD34 selected products having no detectable tumor. In this study there was no improvement in disease free or overall survival. Short-term and long-term engraftment were equivalent in the two arms of the study. Immune resconstitution including lymphocyte subset recovery, Ig levels were identical in both arms at 1 year. There was no difference in infection rates at all time points. Therefore, although purging appears to have no significant toxicity, it is expensive and there are no definitive data that unpurged marrow contributes to relapse. The expense of purging would increase the cost of autologous HCT considerably for those patients who may not require purging. Although data do not prove that purging is essential, they are consistent with the interpretation that MRD in the marrow may contribute to relapse. Lastly, data suggest that even if purging is performed, it is likely to have benefit only if it is successful in eradicating residual tumor cells. Many studies performed to date have not analyzed whether the purging procedure performed has successfully eradicated detectable tumor. While purging procedures remain suboptimal, it may not be possible to perform adequate studies to resolve fully whether purging has any benefit.

Summary

Immunologic methods exist that are capable of eradicating minimal and overt disease from autologous hematopoietic cells. The evidence that such eradication of tumor cells results in improved disease free or overall survival is circumspect at best. Techniques are now available to assess whether purging techniques have successfully eradicated tumor cells from the autologous HSCs from a variety of tumor types. It is important to continue to assess whether successful eradication of detectable tumor from the source of autologous HSCs results in improved outcome. *Ex vivo* manipulation of human cells is now federally regulated in the USA, limiting the applicability of methodologies and devices used for purging clinical samples. Such procedures should be continued only in the clinical trial setting since it is under these circumstances that it will eventually be possible to determine the clinical impact of immunologic purging.

References

1 Craddock C. Hemopoietic stem-cell transplantation. Recent progress and future promise. *Lancet Oncol* 2000; **1**: 227–34.
2 Freedman AS, Neuberg D, Mauch P et al. Long-term follow-up of autologous bone marrow transplantation in patients with relapsed follicular lymphoma. *Blood* 1999; **94**: 3325–33.
3 Ball ED, Wilson J, Phelps V, Neudorf S. Autologous bone marrow transplantation for acute myeloid leukemia in remission or first relapse using monoclonal antibody-purged marrow. Results of phase II studies with long-term follow-up. *Bone Marrow Transplant* 2000; **25**: 823–9.
4 Nieto Y, Champlin RE, Wingard JR et al. Status of high-dose chemotherapy for breast cancer: a review. *Biol Blood Marrow Transplant* 2000; **6**: 476–95.
5 Freedman AS, Gribben JG, Neuberg D et al. High dose therapy and autologous bone marrow transplantation in patients with follicular lymphoma during first remission. *Blood* 1996; **88**: 2780–6.
6 Hurd DD, LeBien TW, Lasky LC et al. Autologous bone marrow transplantation in non-Hodgkin's lymphoma: monoclonal antibodies plus complement for ex vivo marrow treatment. *Am J Med* 1988; **85**: 829–34.
7 Freedman AS, Takvorian T, Anderson KC et al. Autologous bone marrow transplantation in B-cell non-Hodgkin's lymphoma: very low treatment-related mortality in 100 patients in sensitive relapse. *J Clin Oncol* 1990; **8**: 784–91.
8 Braun S, Pantel K, Muller P et al. Cytokeratin-positive cells in the bone marrow and survival of patients with stage I, II, or III breast cancer. *N Engl J Med* 2000; **342**: 525–33.
9 Gribben JG, Neuberg D, Freedman AS et al. Detection by polymerase chain reaction of residual cells with the *bcl-2* translocation is associated with increased risk of relapse after autologous bone marrow transplantation for B-cell lymphoma. *Blood* 1993; **81**: 3449–57.
10 Gribben JG, Freedman A, Woo SD et al. ALL advanced stage non-Hodgkin's lymphomas with a polymerase chain reaction amplifiable breakpoint of *bcl-2* have residual cells containing the *bcl-2* rearrangement at evaluation and after treatment. *Blood* 1991; **78**: 3275–80.
11 Gribben JG, Freedman AS, Neuberg D et al. Immunologic purging of marrow assessed by PCR before autologous bone marrow transplantation for B-cell lymphoma. *N Engl J Med* 1991; **325**: 1525–33.
12 Bonnet D, Dick JE. Human acute myeloid leukemia is organized as a hierarchy that originates from a primitive hematopoietic cell. *Nat Med* 1997; **3**: 730–7.
13 Benjamin D, Magrath IT, Douglass EC, Corash LM. Derivation of lymphoma cell lines from microscopically normal bone marrow in patients with undifferentiated lymphoma: evidence of occult bone marrow involvement. *Blood* 1983; **61**: 1017–9.
14 Estrov Z, Grunberger T, Dube ID. Detection of residual acute lymphoblastic leukemia cells in cultures of bone marrow obtained during remission. *N Engl J Med* 1986; **315**: 538–42.

15 Sharp JG, Joshi SS, Armitage JO et al. Significance of detection of occult non-Hodgkin's lymphoma in histologically uninvolved bone marrow by culture technique. *Blood* 1992; **79**: 1074–80.
16 Sharp JG, Kessinger A, Mann S et al. Outcome of high dose therapy and autologous transplantation in non-Hodgkin's lymphoma based on the presence of tumor in the marrow or infused hematopoietic harvest. *J Clin Oncol* 1996; **14**: 214–9.
17 Ross AA, Cooper BW, Lazarus HM et al. Detection and viability of tumor cells in peripheral blood stem cell collections from breast cancer patients using immunocytochemical and clonogenic assay techniques. *Blood* 1993; **82**: 2605–10.
18 Ross RE, Jeter EK, Gazitt Y, Laver J. Predictive factors for the rate of engraftment of neuroblastoma patients autotransplanted with purged marrow. *Prog Clin Biol Res* 1994; **389**: 139–43.
19 Schiller G, Vescio R, Freytes C et al. Transplantation of CD34+ peripheral blood progenitor cells after high-dose chemotherapy for patients with advanced multiple myeloma. *Blood* 1995; **86**: 390–7.
20 Fields KK, Elfenbein GJ, Trudeau WL et al. Clinical significance of bone marrow metastases as detected using the polymerase chain reaction in patients with breast cancer undergoing high-dose chemotherapy and autologous bone marrow transplantation. *J Clin Oncol* 1996; **14**: 1868–76.
21 Brugger W, Bross KJ, Glatt M et al. Mobilization of tumor cells and hematopoietic progenitor cells into peripheral blood of patients with solid tumors. *Blood* 1994; **83**: 636–40.
22 Vescio RA, Han EJ, Schiller GJ et al. Quantitative comparison of multiple myeloma tumor contamination in bone marrow harvest and leukapheresis autografts. *Bone Marrow Transplant* 1996; **18**: 103–10.
23 Leonard BM, Hetu F, Busque L et al. Lymphoma cell burden in progenitor cell grafts measured by competitive polymerase chain reaction: less than one log difference between bone marrow and peripheral blood sources. *Blood* 1998; **91**: 331–9.
24 Stewart AK, Vescio R, Schiller G et al. Purging of autologous peripheral-blood stem cells using CD34 selection does not improve overall or progression-free survival after high-dose chemotherapy for multiple myeloma: results of a multicenter randomized controlled trial. *J Clin Oncol* 2001; **19**: 3771–9.
25 Kvalheim G, Wang MY, Pharo A et al. Purging of tumor cells from leukapheresis products: experimental and clinical aspects. *J Hematotherapy* 1996; **4**: 427–36.
26 Mohr M, Hilgenfeld E, Fietz T et al. Efficacy and safety of simultaneous immunomagnetic CD34+ cell selection and breast cancer cell purging in peripheral blood progenitor cell samples used for hematopoietic rescue after high-dose therapy. *Clin Cancer Res* 1999; **5**: 1035–40.
27 Mohr M, Dalmis F, Hilgenfeld E et al. Simultaneous immunomagnetic CD34+ cell selection and B-cell depletion in peripheral blood progenitor cell samples of patients suffering from B-cell non-Hodgkin's lymphoma. *Clin Cancer Res* 2001; **7**: 51–7.

28 Rasmussen T, Bjorkstrand B, Andersen H, Gaarsdal E, Johnsen HE. Efficacy and safety of CD34-selected and CD19-depleted autografting in multiple myeloma patients: a pilot study. *Exp Hematol* 2002; **30**: 82–8.
29 Schlager SI, Boyle MDP, Ohanian SH, Borsos T. Effect of inhibiting DNA, RNA and protein synthesis of tumor cells on their susceptibility to killing by antibody and complement. *Cancer Res* 1977; **37**: 1432–7.
30 Schlager SI, Ohanian SH, Borsos T. Identification of lipids associated with the ability of tumor cells to resist humoral immune attack. *J Immunol* 1978; **120**: 472–80.
31 Gee AP, Bruce KM, Morris TD, Boyle MD. Evidence for an anticomplementary factor associated with human bone marrow cells. *J Natl Cancer Inst* 1985; **75**: 441–5.
32 Howell AL, Fogg LM, Davis BH, Ball ED. Continuous infusion of complement by an automated cell processor enhances cytotoxicity of monoclonal antibody sensitized leukemia cells. *Bone Marrow Transplant* 1989; **4**: 317–22.
33 Harris CL, Kan KS, Stevenson GT, Morgan BP. Tumor cell killing using chemically engineered antibody constructs specific for tumor cells and the complement inhibitor CD59. *Clin Exp Immunol* 1997; **107**: 364–71.
34 Junnikkala S, Hakulinen J, Meri S. Targeted neutralization of the complement membrane attack complex inhibitor CD59 on the surface of human melanoma cells. *Eur J Immunol* 1994; **24**: 611–5.
35 Gee AP, Boyle MDP. Purging tumor cells from bone marrows by use of antibody and complement: a critical appraisal. *J Natl Cancer Inst* 1988; **80**: 154–9.
36 Lee R, Braylan RC. Regarding the loss of CD20 after rituximab therapy. *Br J Haematol* 2002; **118**: 927.
37 Maloney DG, Smith B, Rose A. Rituximab. Mechanism of action and resistance. *Semin Oncol* 2002; **29**: 2–9.
38 Foran JM, Norton AJ, Micallef IN et al. Loss of CD20 expression following treatment with rituximab (chimaeric monoclonal anti-CD20): a retrospective cohort analysis. *Br J Haematol* 2001; **114**: 881–3.
39 Davis TA, Czerwinski DK, Levy R. Therapy of B-cell lymphoma with anti-CD20 antibodies can result in the loss of CD20 antigen expression. *Clin Cancer Res* 1999; **5**: 611–5.
40 De Fabritiis P, Bregni M, Lipton J et al. Elimination of clonogenic Burkitt's lymphoma cells from human bone marrow using 4-hydroperoxycyclophosphamide in combination with monoclonal antibodies and complement. *Blood* 1985; **65**: 1064–70.
41 Humblet Y, Feyens AM, Sekhavat M et al. Immunological and pharmacological removal of small cell lung cancer cells from bone marrow autografts. *Cancer Res* 1989; **49**: 5058–61.
42 Schwartz CL, Minniti CP, Harwood P et al. Elimination of clonogenic malignant human T cells using monoclonal antibodies in combination with 2′-deoxycoformycin. *J Clin Oncol* 1987; **5**: 1900–11.
43 Aihara M, Aihara Y, Schmidt-Wolf G et al. A combined approach for purging multidrug-resistant leukemic cell lines in bone marrow using a mono-

clonal antibody and chemotherapy. *Blood* 1991; **77**: 2079–84.
44. Treleaven J, Gibson F, Udelstad J. Removal of neuroblastoma cells from bone marrow with monoclonal antibodies conjugated to magnetic microsphere. *Lancet* 1984; ii: 70–6.
45. Kvalheim G, Sorensen O, Fodstad O et al. Immunomagnetic removal of B-lymphoma cells from human bone marrow: a procedure for clinical use. *Bone Marrow Transplant* 1988; **3**: 31–41.
46. Trickett AE, Ford DJ, Lam-Po-Tang PRL, Vowels MR. Immunomagnetic bone marrow purging of common acute lymphoblastic leukemia cells: suitability of BioMag particles. *Bone Marrow Transplant* 1991; **7**: 199–203.
47. Gribben JG, Saporito L, Barber M et al. Bone marrows of non-Hodgkin's lymphoma patients with a bcl-2 translocation can be purged of polymerase chain reaction-detectable lymphoma cells using monoclonal antibodies and immunomagnetic bead depletion. *Blood* 1992; **80**: 1083–9.
48. Fitzgerald DJ, Willingham MC, Cardarelli CO et al. A monoclonal antibody-pseudomonas toxin conjugate that specifically kills multidrug-resistant cells. *Proc Natl Acad Sci U S A* 1987; **84**: 4288–92.
49. Grossbard ML, Nadler LM. Immunotoxin therapy of malignancy. In: DeVita VT, Hellamn S, Rosenberg SA, eds. *Important Advances in Oncology*. Philadelphia: Lippincott JB, 1992: 111–35.
50. Strong RC, Uckun F, Youle RJ, Kersey J, Vallera DA. Use of multiple T cell-directed intact ricin immunotoxins for autologous bone marrow transplantation. *Blood* 1985; **66**: 627–35.
51. LeBien TW, Stepan DE, Bartholomew RM, Strong RC, Anderson JM. Utilization of a colony assay to assess the variables influencing elimination of leukemic cells from human bone marrow with monoclonal antibodies and complement. *Blood* 1985; **65**: 945–50.
52. Bast RC, De Fabritiis P, Lipton J et al. Elimination of malignant clonogenic cells from human bone marrows using multiple monoclonal antibodies and complement. *Cancer Res* 1985; **45**: 499–503.
53. Negrin RS, Kiem HP, Schmidt WI, Blume KG, Cleary ML. Use of the polymerase chain reaction to monitor the effectiveness of *ex vivo* tumor cell purging. *Blood* 1991; **77**: 654–60.
54. Trickett AE. Tumor cell purging for autologous bone marrow transplantation. *Med Laboratory Sci* 1990; **47**: 120–31.
55. Elias AD, Pap SA, Bernal SD. Purging of small cell lung cancer-contaminated bone marrow by monoclonal antibodies and magnetic beads. *Prog Clin Biol Res* 1990; **333**: 263–75.
56. Vrendenburgh JJ, Ball ED. Elimination of small cell carcinoma of the lung from human bone marrow by monoclonal antibodies and immunomagnetic beads. *Cancer Res* 1990; **50**: 7216–120.
57. Vrendenburgh JJ, Simpson W, Memoli VA, Ball ED. Reactivity of anti-CD15 monoclonal antibody PM-81 with breast cancer and elimination of breast cancer cell lines from human bone marrow by PM-81 and immunomagnetic beads. *Cancer Res* 1991; **51**: 2451–5.
58. Schpall EJ, Bast RC, Jones WT et al. Immunomagnetic purging of breast cancer from bone marrow for autologous transplantation. *Bone Marrow Transplant* 1991; **7**: 145–51.
59. Montgomery RB, Kurtzberg J, Rhinehardt-Clark A et al. Elimination of malignant clonogenic T cells from human bone marrow using chemoimmunoseparation with 2′-deoxycoformycin, deoxyadenosine and an immunotoxin. *Bone Marrow Transplant* 1990; **5**: 395–402.
60. Robertson MJ, Soiffer RJ, Freedman AS et al. Human bone marrow depleted of CD33-positive cells mediates delayed but durable reconstitution of hematopoiesis: clinical trial of My9 monoclonal antibody-purged autografts for the treatment of acute myeloid leukemia. *Blood* 1992; **79**: 2229–36.
61. Combaret V, Favrot MC, Chauvin F et al. Immunomagnetic depletion of malignant cells from autologous bone marrow graft: from experimental models to clinical trials. *J Immunogenet* 1989; **16**: 125–36.
62. Kemshead JT, Treleaven J, Heath L et al. Monoclonal antibodies and magnetic microspheres for the depletion of leukemic cells from bone marrow harvested for autologous transplantation. *Bone Marrow Transplant* 1987; **2**: 133–9.
63. Preijers FWMB, De Witte T, Wessels JMC et al. Autologous transplantation of bone marrow purged *in vitro* with anti-CD7-(WT1-) ricin A immunotyoxin in T-cell lymphoblastic leukemia and lymphoma. *Blood* 1989; **74**: 1152–8.
64. Uckun F, Kersey JH, Vallera DA et al. Autologous bone marrow transplantation in high risk remission T-lineage acute lymphoblastic leukemia using immunotoxins plus 4-hydroperoxycyclophosphamide for marrow purging. *Blood* 1990; **76**: 1723–33.
65. Freedman AS, Takvorian T, Neuberg D et al. Autologous bone marrow transplantation in poor-prognosis intermediate-grade and high-grade B-cell non-Hodgkin's lymphoma in first remission: a pilot study. *J Clin Oncol* 1993; **11**: 931–6.
66. Freedman AS, Neuberg D, Gribben JG et al. High-dose chemoradiotherapy and anti-B-cell monoclonal antibody-purged autologous bone marrow transplantation in mantle-cell lymphoma: no evidence for long-term remission [see comments]. *J Clin Oncol* 1998; **16**: 13–8.
67. Anderson KC, Andersen J, Soiffer R et al. Monoclonal antibody-purged bone marrow transplantation therapy for multiple myeloma. *Blood* 1993; **82**: 2568–76.
68. Vescio R, Schiller G, Stewart AK et al. Multicenter phase III trial to evaluate CD34+ selected versus unselected autologous peripheral blood progenitor cell transplantation in multiple myeloma. *Blood* 1999; **93**: 1858–68.
69. Simonsson B, Burnett AK, Prentice HG et al. Autologous bone marrow transplantation with monoclonal antibody purged marrow for high-risk acute lymphoblastic leukemia. *Leukemia* 1989; **3**: 631–6.
70. Billett AL, Kornmehl E, Tarbell NJ et al. Autologous bone marrow transplantation after a long first remission for children with recurrent acute lymphoblastic leukemia. *Blood* 1993; **81**: 1651–7.
71. Shpall EJ, Jones RB, Bearman S. High-dose therapy with autologous bone marrow transplantation for the treatment of solid tumors [review]. *Current Opinion Oncol* 1994; **6**: 135–8.
72. Kemshead JT, Heath L, Gibson FM et al. Magnetic microspheres and monoclonal antibodies for the depletion of neuroblastoma cells from bone marrow: experiences, improvements and observations. *Br J Cancer* 1986; **54**: 771–8.
73. Horning SJ, Negrin RS, Hoppe RT et al. High-dose therapy and autologous bone marrow transplantation for follicular lymphoma in first complete or partial remission: results of a phase II clinical trial. *Blood* 2001; **97**: 404–9.
74. Stoppa AM, Hirn J, Blaise D et al. Autologous bone marrow transplantation for B cell malignancies after *in vitro* purging with floating immunobeads. *Bone Marrow Transplant* 1990; **6**: 301–7.
75. Corradini P, Astolfi M, Cherasco C et al. Molecular monitoring of minimal residual disease in follicular and mantle cell non-Hodgkin's lymphomas treated with high dose chemotherapy and peripheral blood progenitor cell autografting. *Blood* 1997; **89**: 724–31.
76. Williams CD, Goldstone AH, Pearce RM et al. Purging of bone marrow in autologous bone marrow transplantation for non-Hodgkin's lymphoma: a case-matched comparison with unpurged cases by the European Blood and Marrow Transplant Lymphoma Registry. *J Clin Oncol* 1996; **14**: 2454–64.
77. Brenner MK, Rill DR, Holladay MS et al. Gene marking to determine whether autologous marrow infusion restores long-term haemopoiesis in cancer patients. *Lancet* 1993; **342**: 1134–7.
78. Rill DR, Buschle M, Foreman NK et al. Retrovirus-mediated gene transfer as an approach to analyze neuroblastoma relapse after autologous bone marrow transplantation. *Human Gene Ther* 1992; **3**: 129–36.
79. Rill DR, Moen RC, Buschle M et al. An approach for the analysis of relapse and marrow reconstitution after autologous marrow transplantation using retrovirus-mediated gene transfer. *Blood* 1992; **79**: 2694–700.
80. Rill DR, Santana VM, Roberts WM et al. Direct demonstration that autologous bone marrow transplantation for solid tumors can return a multiplicity of tumorigenic cells. *Blood* 1994; **84**: 380–3.
81. Flinn IW, O'Donnell PV, Goodrich A et al. Immunotherapy with rituximab during peripheral blood stem cell transplantation for non-Hodgkin's lymphoma. *Biol Blood Marrow Transplant* 2000; **6**: 628–32.
82. Ladetto M, Zallio F, Vallet S et al. Concurrent administration of high-dose chemotherapy and rituximab is a feasible and effective chemo/immunotherapy for patients with high-risk non-Hodgkin's lymphoma. *Leukemia* 2001; **15**: 1941–9.
83. Magni M, Di Nicola M, Devizzi L et al. Successful *in vivo* purging of CD34-containing peripheral blood harvests in mantle cell and indolent lymphoma: evidence for a role of both chemotherapy and rituximab infusion. *Blood* 2000; **96**: 864–9.

20

O. Michael Colvin

Pharmacologic Purging of Bone Marrow

The initial use of autologous bone marrow transplantation (BMT) was for the treatment of leukemia and lymphoma, with the concept of eradication of the tumor by the use of total body irradiation (TBI) and/or drugs and replacement of the bone marrow with autologous marrow from the patient [1,2]. The importance of an immunological reaction against the malignancy by an allogeneic graft was demonstrated by the earlier studies of Thomas and colleagues [3]. After the problem of graft-vs.-host disease (GVHD) had been addressed with the use of human leukocyte antigen (HLA)-matched sibling marrow and appropriate immunosuppression, it was possible to demonstrate by the mid-1970s that long-term remissions of acute leukemia could be achieved with allogeneic BMT without intolerable toxicity.

By the end of the 1970s, the feasibility and therapeutic value of autologous BMT for lymphoma were demonstrated [4,5]. Autologous BMT was attempted in patients with relapsed leukemia using marrow collected while the patients were in complete remissions, but all these patients relapsed [6,7]. This experience increased concern about reinfusing leukemic cells from even a remission marrow. Recognition of this problem stimulated interest in developing approaches to eradicating tumor cells from autologous bone marrow *in vitro* ("bone marrow purging").

This chapter will discuss pharmacological and related approaches to the eradication of tumor cells from autologous bone marrow preparations. Antibodies, viral vectors and mechanical methods, such as immunomagnetic beads, are also utilized and are discussed in Chapters 19 and 21. Although a number of antitumor agents have been utilized for *in vitro* elimination of tumor cells from bone marrow, the first and most widely used agents have been the *in vitro* active analogs of the oxazophosphorines cyclophosphamide (CY) and ifosfamide (Fig. 20.1). Other agents have been used in bone marrow purging and are discussed below. However, the experience has been much less with pharmacologic agents other than the oxazophosphorines, and there is little reported information on the effects of these purging agents on bone marrow recovery time.

The initial pharmacological approach to the elimination of tumor cells from autologous bone marrow was based on the demonstrated relative sparing of HSCs by CY *in vivo* [8] and by activated derivatives of CY in *in vitro* studies. This sparing was demonstrated to be due to the high expression of the enzyme aldehyde dehydrogenase (ALDH) in stem cells and the ability of this enzyme to inactivate the active metabolites of CY. Studies by Sensenbrenner and colleagues demonstrated that the initial hydroxylation product of CY, 4-hydroxycyclophosphamide, is metabolized and inactivated by ALDH and the reactive alkylating agent, phosphoramide mustard, is not produced (Fig. 20.1) [9]. These findings also explained previous clinical observations that CY was less toxic to the bone marrow that other antitumor agents. These findings were confirmed and extended by Kohn and colleagues [10].

In 1980, Sharkis *et al.* [11] demonstrated in a rat model of acute

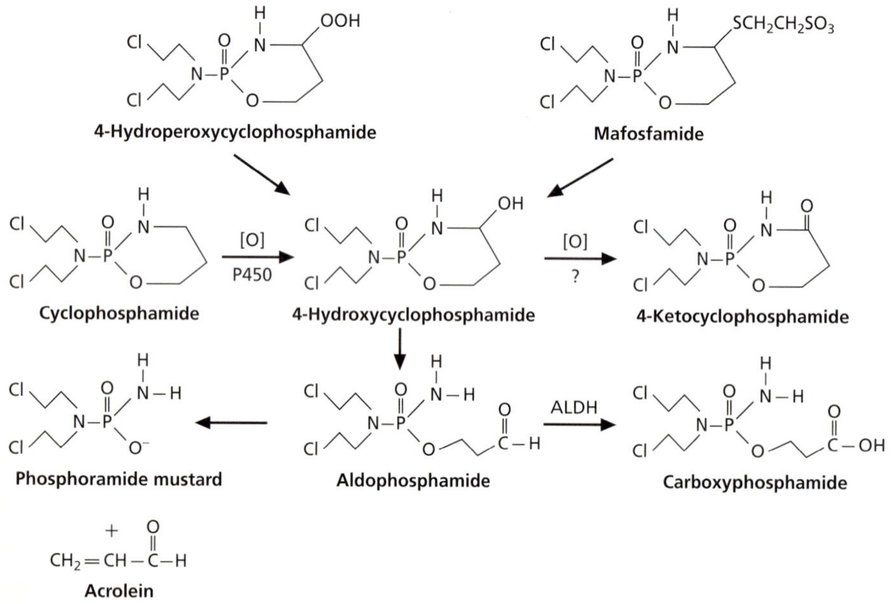

Fig. 20.1 Generation of 4-hydroxycyclophosphamide from cyclophosphamide (CY), 4-hydroperoxycyclophosphamide (4-HC) and mafosfamide.

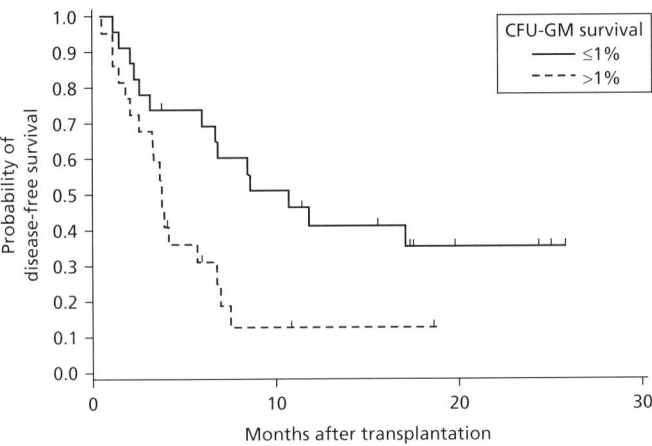

Fig. 20.2 Probability of disease-free survival (DFS) for patients stratified by percentage of colony forming units-granulocyte/macrophage (CFU-GM) survival. Tick marks represent patients alive and disease-free at time of analysis ($p = 0.006$, log rank). Reproduced with permission from [36].

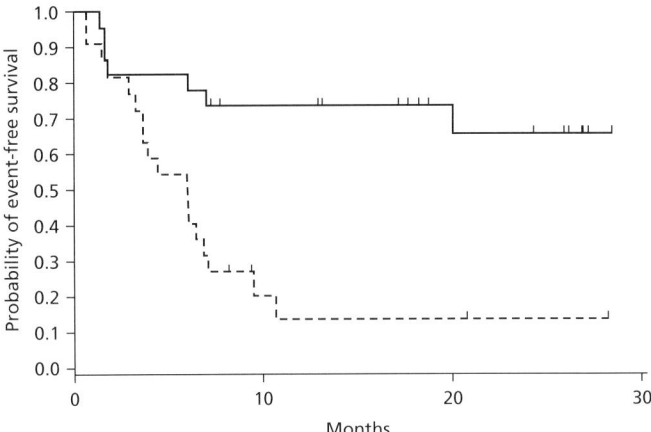

Fig. 20.3 Actuarial probability of event-free survival after autologous bone marrow transplantation (BMT) in 23 patients whose colony forming units-leukemia (CFU-L) were sensitive to 4-HC (solid line) and the 22 patients whose CFU-L were resistant (dashed line). The proportions that are event-free are 67% (38–85%) and 13% (3–32%) respectively. Reproduced with permission from Miller and Zehnbauer [23].

myeloid leukemia (AML) that rat leukemic cells mixed with normal rat marrow could be eradicated by *ex vivo* incubation with 4-hydroperoxycyclophosphamide (4-HC) with sufficient sparing of normal HSCs (HSCs) to repopulate the marrow and allow disease-free survival (DFS) of the rats. This observation was rapidly translated to the clinic, and it was demonstrated that autologous BMT with marrow treated *ex vivo* with 4-HC was feasible and produced prolonged survival in up to 35% of relapsed AML patients (Fig. 20.2) [12,13]. Gorin and colleagues in Europe have published on their extensive and promising experience with autologous marrow purging with mafosfamide, another *in vitro* active analog of CY (Fig. 20.1), in the treatment of AML [14–18]. Chao et al. [19], after a median follow-up of 31 months, found an actuarial DFS of 28% for the first 20 patients who received untreated marrow compared to 57% for the subsequent 28 patients who received 4-HC purged marrow.

The major complication of pharmacologic *in vitro* purging of autologous marrow has been a delay in engraftment time. Chopra and colleagues, in a study of AML patients utilizing unpurged marrow, reported a mean time to return of 500 neutrophils/μL of 22 days (range 22–101) and of 62 days to return to 50,000 platelets/μL [20]. This can be contrasted to a study by Rowley et al. [21], with a median time to return of 40 days for 500 neutrophils/μL and of 70 days to independence from platelet transfusions, in patients whose marrow was purged *in vitro* with 4-HC. These results are similar to the experiences of other investigators using oxazaphosphorine-purged autografts.

The Cancer Drugs Review Committee of the Food and Drug Administration (FDA) considered the approval of perfosfamide (4-HC) for the pharmacologic treatment of autologous bone marrow, but did not approve it because of the lack of a randomized controlled trial of the efficacy of purged vs. nonpurged autologous marrow. This decision was influenced by the well-established delay in engraftment associated with the *in vitro* treatment of bone marrow.

While a randomized trial of perfosfamide purged vs. nonpurged autologous BMT has still not been carried out, Miller et al. [22] studied the records of 294 patients from the Autologous Blood and Bone Marrow Registry who had been treated for AML in first or second remission with either 4-HC purged or unpurged bone marrow, all transplanted less than 6 months after remission. While the patients receiving the 4-HC treated grafts had a longer time to marrow recovery, as described above, the transplant-related mortality was similar in the two groups. Multivariate analysis demonstrated that patients receiving 4-HC purged transplants had lower risks of treatment failure than those receiving unpurged transplants (relative risk, 0.69, $p = 0.12$, in the 1st post-transplant year; relative risk, 0.28, $p <0.0001$ thereafter). Adjusted 3-year probabilities of leukemia-free survival (95% confidence interval) were 56% (47–64%) and 31% (18–45%) after 4-HC purged and unpurged transplants in first remission, respectively. Corresponding probabilities in second remission were 39% (25–53%) and 10% (1–29%). The conclusion of this study was that grafts purged with 4-HC are associated with higher leukemia-free survival after autologous BMTs for AML. These data were presented to the FDA but 4-HC was still not approved for marrow purging. While clinical grade 4-HC (perfosfamide) is not available at present for purging studies for clinical trials, mafosfamide is manufactured by the Asta-Werke Company and is currently being used by investigators for bone marrow purging in clinical trials with what appears to be similar effects to 4-HC (see publications of Gorin and colleagues [14–18]).

The problem of drug resistance in autologous BMT, for both the preparative chemotherapy regimen and the purging regimen, was demonstrated in a study by Miller et al. [23]. Colony forming units-leukemia (CFU-L) were cultured from the marrow and their sensitivity to 4-HC determined (Fig. 20.3) [23]. Of the patients whose CFU-L were relatively resistant to 4-HC, only 13% remained in remission at 15 months, while 67% of those patients whose CFU-Ls were more sensitive were free of disease at that time.

The evidence discussed above indicates that pharmacologic purging of bone marrow with the oxazophosphorine agents can reduce the chance of tumor recurrence, or at least delay recurrence, but at the cost of delayed engraftment with risks of infection to the patient. The overall risk–benefit ratio is still in question, but it is clear that finding even more selective agents will be important.

Mutagenesis

In vitro treatment of hematopoietic precursors raises the concern of mutagenesis of these early cells. A study by Shah et al. [24] addressed this concern. Fifty-five patients from the Johns Hopkins program had cytogenetic studies after systemic treatment with CY and TBI or CY and busulfan. Fourteen were found to have cytogenetic abnormalities. Of these, seven were clonal, and all of these patients were in leukemic relapse. Of the seven with nonclonal abnormalities, three subsequently relapsed. No clonal abnormalities of chromosome one were seen and it was concluded that the cytogenetic abnormalities were related to leukemic relapse and unlikely to be related to the chemical purging.

Other pharmacologic agents

Kushner et al. [25] reported that etoposide [VP16] spared early marrow precursors and stromal cells relative to lymphoma cells and HL-60 myeloid leukemic cells. These investigators also reported that the use of the combination of 4-HC and VP16 was synergistically toxic against tumor cells but not marrow stem cells. This combination was studied in a clinical trial [26] in 1989, but further studies have not been reported.

In 1984, Glasser et al. [27] reported the use of an alkylysolipid compound to eradicate cells of a b-cell human tumor line (WEHI) tumor cells from murine marrow without compromising the ability of the marrow to engraft. Subsequently, a clinical trial was reported in 29 patients [28], but no further reports have appeared.

Several preclinical studies have demonstrated that the photosensitizing agent merocycanine 540 with light exposure will produce selective killing of tumor cells, with sparing of HSCs [29]. However, clinical trials have not been reported.

Kurtzberg [30] demonstrated that guanine arabinoside (ARA-G) is an effective agent to use for the selective ablation of malignant T leukemic cells from human marrow. With exposure to 100 μmol ARA-G for 18 h, up to 6 log of clonogenic T cells were eliminated without apparent toxicity to normal hematopoietic cells. A study in a murine model of acute lymphoblastic leukemia demonstrated that marrow contaminated with malignant T cells and purged *ex vivo* with ARA-G reconstituted both the lymphoid and myeloid lines with no evidence of leukemic cells.

Ribizzi et al. [31] have recently reported that the compound taurolidine is highly toxic to tumor cells, but not to normal hematopoietic precursors, but clinical studies have not been reported. Hatta and colleagues have reported that the combination of 2 mM adenosine triphosphate and 2 μg/mL of 4-HC was quite effective for the elimination of leukemic cells, with a minimal effect on normal stem cells, but this combination has also not been investigated clinically [32].

A very attractive approach to marrow purging is the use of antisense oligonucleotides, because of the inherent specificity of these compounds and that high concentrations can be achieved *in vitro*. Luger and colleagues used an oligodeoxynucleotide (ODN) targeted to the c-*myb* protooncogene to purge marrow autografts administered to allograft-ineligible chronic myeloid leukemia patients [33]. CD34+ marrow cells were purged with ODN for either 24 h (n = 19) or 72 h (n = 5). After purging, Myb messenger RNA (mRNA) levels declined substantially in approximately 50% of patients. Analysis of bcr-abl expression in long-term culture-initiating cells suggested that purging had been accomplished at a primitive cell level in more than 50% of patients and was ODN dependent. Day 100 cytogenetics were evaluated in surviving patients who engrafted without infusion of unmanipulated "back-up" marrow (n = 14). Whereas all patients were approximately 100% Philadelphia chromosome positive (Ph+) before transplantation, two patients had complete cytogenetic remissions, three patients had fewer than 33% Ph+ metaphases and eight remained 100% Ph+. Thus it appears that this highly specific technology has promise for marrow purging and should be further studied.

Our work at Duke University with CY analogs has led to an alternative approach to the elimination of malignant cells from autologous bone marrow by the selective positive selection of stem cells from marrow or blood. Storms and colleagues reported in 1999 the selective isolation of hematopoietic precursor cells from harvested bone marrow and umbilical cord blood by the use of flow cytometry [34]. The technique depends on the presence of high activity of the enzyme ALDH in early hematopoietic precursors to generate an anionic fluorescent dye that is retained in the hematopoietic precursor. After isolation the fluorescent dye is exported from the cell by MdR and related transporters. Thus the isolated cells contain no foreign compound or attached antibodies. This approach rejects tumor cells on the basis of both size and lack of ALDH. The selected hematopoietic cells are expandable in culture with preservation of pluripotent cells (A. Balber & J. Kurtzberg, unpublished data, 2002) and the expanded cells consist of a greater variety of cell types than are produced from expanded CD34+ cells. Clinical trials with this technique have not yet been initiated.

The expandability of ALDH+ cells is consistent with the observations of Roecklein and colleagues who reported that bone marrow purged with 4-HC could be expanded to produce progenitor hematopoietic cells [35]. Thus, the ALDH+ selection approach to isolating hematopoietic precursors promises to obtain tumor-free autologous hematopoietic grafts without toxicity to pluripotent hematopoietic cells for lymphomas and solid tumors as well as leukemia.

References

1 Appelbaum FR, Herzig GP, Zeigler JL *et al.* Successful engraftment of cryopreserved autologous bone marrow in patients with malignant lymphoma. *Blood* 1978; **52**: 85–95.

2 Kaizer H, Leventhal BG, Wharam MD *et al.* Cryopreserved autologous bone marrow transplantation in the treatment of selected pediatric malignancies: a preliminary report. *Transplantation Proc* 1979; **11**: 208–11.

3 Thomas ED, Storb R, Clift RA *et al.* Bone marrow transplantation. *N Engl J Med* 1975; **292**: 832–43 and 895–902.

4 Appelbaum FR, Herzig GP, Ziegler JL *et al.* Successful engraftment of cryopreserved autologous bone marrow in patients with malignant lymphoma. *Blood* 1978; **52**: 85–95.

5 Kaizer H, Leventhal BG, Wharam MD *et al.* Cryopreserved autologous bone marrow transplantation in the treatment of selected pediatric malignancies: a preliminary report. *Transplant Proc* 1979; **11**: 208–11.

6 Gorin NC, Najman A, Salmon C *et al.* High dose combination chemotherapy with and without autologous bone marrow transplantation for the treatment of acute leukemia and other malignant diseases. *Eur J Cancer* 1979; **15**: 1113–9.

7 Gorin NC. Autologous bone marrow transplantation in acute leukemia. *J Natl Cancer Inst* 1986; **76**: 1281–7.

8 Nissen-Meyer R, Host H. A comparison between the hematological side effects of cyclophosphamide and nitrogen mustard. *Cancer Chemother Rep* 1960; 951–5.

9 Sensenbrenner LL, Marini JJ, Colvin OM. Comparative effects of cyclophosphamide, isophosphamide, 4-methylcyclophosphamide, and phosphoramide mustard on murine hematopoietic and immunocompetent cells. *J Natl Cancer Inst* 1979; **62**: 975–81.

10 Kohn FR, Landkammer GJ, Manthey CL, Ransay NKC, Sladek NE. Effect of aldehyde dehydrogenase inhibitors on the *ex vivo* sensitivity of human multipotent and committed hematopoietic progenitor cells and malignant blood cells to oxazophosphorines. *Cancer Res* 1987; **47**: 3180–5.

11 Sharkis SJ, Santos GW, Colvin M. Elimination of acute myelogenous leukemic cells from marrow and tumor suspensions in the rat with 4-hydroperoxycyclophosphamide. *Blood* 1980; **55**: 521–3.

12 Yeager AM, Kaizer H, Santos GW *et al.* Autologous bone marrow transplantation in patients with acute nonlymphocytic leukemia using *ex vivo* marrow treatment with 4-hydroperoxycyclophosphamide. *N Engl J Med* 1986; **315**: 141–7.

13 Rosenfeld C, Shadduck RK, Przepiorka D, Mangan KF, Colvin OM. Autologous bone marrow transplantation with 4-hydroperoxycyclophosphamide purged marrows for acute non-lymphoblastic leukemia in second remission. *Bone Marrow Transplant* 1990; **6**: 425–9.

14 Isnard F, Guiguet M, Laporte JP *et al.* Improved efficiency of remission-induction facilitates autologous BMT harvesting and improves overall survival in adults with AML: 108 patients treated at a single institution. *Bone Marrow Transplant* 2001; **27**: 1045–52.

15 Gorin NC, Herve P, Aegerter A *et al.* Autologous bone marrow transplantation for acute leukaemia in remission. *Br J Haematol* 1986; **64**: 385–95.

16 Gorin NC, Aegerter P, Auvert B *et al.* Autologous

bone marrow transplantation for acute myelocyticleukemia in first remission: a European survey of the role of marrow purging. *Blood* 1990; **75**: 1606–14.

17 LaPorte JP, Duay L, Lopez M *et al*. One hundred and twenty-five adult patients with primary acute leukemia autografted with marrow purged by mafosfamide: a 10-year single institution experience. *Blood* 1994; **84**: 3810–8.

18 Douay L, Laporte JP, Mary JY *et al*. Difference in kinetics of hematopoietic reconstitution after autologous bone marrow transplantation with marrow treated *in vitro* with mafosfamide. *Bone Marrow Transplant* 1987; **187**(2): 33–43.

19 Chao NJ, Stein AS, Long GD *et al*. Busulfan/etoposide: initial experience with a new preparatory regimen for autologous bone marrow transplantation in patients with acute nonlymphoblastic leukemia. *Blood* 1993; **81**: 319–23.

20 Chopra R, Goldstone AH, McMillan AK *et al*. Successful treatment of actue myeloid leukemia beyond first remission with autologous bone marrow transplantation using busulfan/cyclophosphamide and unpurged marrow: The British autograft group experience. *J Clin Oncol* 1991; **9**: 1840–7.

21 Rowley SD, Jones RJ, Piantidosi S *et al*. Efficacy of *ex vivo* purging for autologous bone marrow transplantation for acute myelogenous leukemia. *Exp Hematol* 2001; **29**(11): 1336–46.

22 Miller CB, Rowlings PA, Zhang MJ *et al*. The effect of graft purging with 4-hydroperoxycyclophosphamide in autologous bone marrow transplantation for acute myelogenous leukemia. *Exp Hematol* 2001; **29**(11): 1336–46.

23 Miller CB, Zehnbauer BA, Piantadosi S *et al*. Correlation of occult clonogenic leukemia drug sensitivity with relapse after autologous bone marrow transplantation. *Blood* 1991; **78**: 1125–31.

24 Shah NK, Wingard JR, Piantidosi S, Rowley S, Santos GW, Griffin CA. Chromosomal abnormalities in patients treated with 4-hyroperoxycyclophosphamide-purged bone marrow transplantation. *Cancer Genet Cytogenet* 1993; **65**: 135–40.

25 Kushner BH, Kwon JH, Gulati SC, Castro-Malaspina H. Preclinical assessment of purging with VP-16-213: key role for long-term marrow cultures. *Blood* 1987; **69**: 65–71.

26 Gulati SC, Shank B, Sarris A *et al*. Autologous bone marrow transplant using 4-HC, VP-16 purged bone marrow for acute non-lymphoblastic leukemia. *Bone Marrow Transplant* 1989; **4** (Suppl. 1): 116–8.

27 Glasser L, Somberg LB, Vogler WR. Purging murine leukemic marrow with alkyl-lysophospholipids—a new family of anticancer drugs. *Blood* 1984; **64**: 1288–91.

28 Vogler WR. Bone marrow purging in acute leukemia with alkyl-lysophospholipids—a new family of anticancer drugs. *Leuk Lymphoma* 1994; **13**: 53–60.

29 Itoh T, Messner HA, Jamal N, Tweeddale M, Sieber F. Merocyanine540-sensitized photoinactivation of high grade non-Hodgkin's lymphoma cells: potential application in autologous BMT. *Bone Marrow Transplant* 1993; **12**: 191–6.

30 Kurtzberg J. Guanine arabinoside as a bone marrow purging agent. *Ann NY Acad Sci* 1993; **685**: 225–36.

31 Ribizzi I, Darnowski JW, Goulette FA, Akhtar MS, Chatterjee D, Calabresi P. Taurolidine. Preclinical evaluation of a novel, highly selective, agent for bone marrow purging. *Bone Marrow Transplant* 2002; **29**(4): 313–9.

32 Hatta Y, Itoh T, Baba M *et al*. Purging in autologous hematopoietic stem cell transplantation using adenosine triphosphate (ATP) and 4-hydroperoxycyclophosphamide (4-HC). *Leukemia Res* 2002; **26**(5): 477–82.

33 Luger SM, O'Brien SG, Ratajczak J *et al*. Oligodeoxynucleotide-mediated inhibition of *c-myb* gene expression in autografted bone marrow: a pilot study. *Blood* 2002; **99**(4): 1150–8.

34 Storms R, Trujillo AP, Springer JB *et al*. Isolation of primitive human hematopoietic progenitors on the basis of aldehyde dehydrogenase activity. *Proc Natl Acad Sci U S A* 1999; **96**(16): 9118–23.

35 Roecklein BA, Reems J, Rowley S, Torok-Storb B. *Ex vivo* expansion of immature 4-hydroperoxycyclophosphamide-resistant progenitor cells from G-CSF-mobilized peripheral blood. *Biol Blood Marrow Transplant* 1998; **4**(2): 61–8.

36 Rowley SD, Jones RJ, Piantidosi S *et al*. Efficacy of *ex vivo* purging for autologous bone marrow transplantation in the treatment of AML. *Blood* 1989; **74**: 501–6.

21

Joanna B. Opalinska & Alan M. Gewirtz

Molecular Inhibition of Gene Expression in Hematopoietic Cells

Introduction

Our present approaches to treating hematologic malignancies are grounded in the use of chemotherapeutic agents and radiation. While clearly effective, these agents are largely nonspecific in their action. Accordingly, they are associated with highly predictable, dose dependent cytotoxicity which is the cause of significant morbidity and, not infrequently, mortality. For obvious reasons, the last decade has been characterized by a rush to develop "targeted therapies" that focus on ways of defeating malignant cells based on their immunochemical, biochemical or molecular signatures. Successful examples of the first two approaches include the anti-CD20 monoclonal antibody rituximab for the treatment of various lymphomas [1] and the small molecule abl tyrosine kinase inhibitor imatinib mesylate (STI571; Gleevec®) for chronic myeloid leukemia (CML) [2]. While these approaches continue to develop, a parallel effort [3] has also gone into the development of molecularly targeted therapies. With their promise of high specificity and low toxicity, many believe that gene targeted therapies will lead to a revolution in cancer therapeutics [4–6]. The goal of this chapter is to review the development and to discuss the ultimate potential of nucleic acid based pharmaceuticals whose goal is to silence the expression of specific genes with therapeutic intent. Nucleic acid based therapies ultimately work by hybridizing to their intended gene target, or messenger RNA (mRNA). Accordingly, they may inhibit gene expression at either the transcriptional, or post-transcriptional levels [7]. With the successful initial sequencing of the human genome [8], and the concurrent revolution in molecular biology, the identification of many genes responsible for initiation and/or maintenance of hematologic malignancies is being accomplished [9–15]. These genes, and those that have yet to be described, have become legitimate targets for therapeutically motivated attempts to silence their expression. By targeting genes that are absolutely or relatively tumor specific, it is hoped that more effective, less toxic cancer treatments will result.

Gene silencing with nucleic acids

The hypothesis that gene expression could be modified through use of exogenous nucleic acids derives from studies by Paterson et al. [16] who first used a complementary (antisense) single stranded DNA to inhibit RNA translation in a cell free system in 1977. Stephenson and Zamecnik demonstrated shortly thereafter that a short (13mer) DNA oligodeoxynucleotide (ODN) antisense to the Rous sarcoma virus could inhibit viral replication in culture [17]. As a result of this work, Zamecnik and Stephenson are often credited with having first suggested the therapeutic utility of antisense nucleic acids (for which Zamecnik was ultimately given a Lasker Special Achievement Award in 1996). In the mid-1980s, the existence of naturally occurring antisense RNAs and their role in regulating gene expression was reported by several groups [18–20]. These observations were particularly important because they lent support to the idea that "antisense" was more than a laboratory phenomenon and encouraged belief in the hypothesis that antisense nucleic acids could be utilized in living cells to manipulate gene expression. These seminal papers, and the many thousands that have followed, have driven the development of gene silencing technologies and the field of nucleic acid therapeutics.

Targeting genes and transcription

Strategies for silencing gene expression may be categorized as being either "antigene" or anti-mRNA (see below, reviewed in [7]). Antigene strategies focus primarily on gene targeting by homologous recombination [21,22], or by triple-helix forming ODNs (TFOs) [23]. Since homologous recombination is primarily a laboratory based technique it will not be considered further in this discussion. TFOs bind in the major groove of duplex DNA in a sequence specific manner (Fig. 21.1; see also Plate 21.1, facing p. 296) [24]. Gene targeting with these molecules is constrained by the fact that TFOs require runs of purines on one strand and pyrimidines on the other (~10–30 nucleotides in length) for stable hybridization. The TFO can be composed of either polypurine or polypyrimidine bases but hybridization always occurs on the purine strand of the duplex through formation of Hoogsteen hydrogen bonds, after the individual who first described them. They may form in the parallel or antiparallel (reverse Hoogsteen) orientation relative to the 5′-3′ orientation of the purine strand, depending on the thermodynamics of the specific base interactions involved. An A or a T in the TFO can bond with the A of an AT pair in the DNA duplex, while G can bond with the G of a GC pair. C can also bond with the G of a GC pair if protonated (C^+). Accordingly, TFOs containing C form stable hybrids under acidic conditions. Though this tendency can be modified somewhat by methylation of the cytosine at the C-5 position [25], C containing TFOs are expected to be less active at physiologic pH. In contrast, G and T containing TFOs can form stable hybrids at physiologic pH [26]. However, these TFOs are plagued by the fact that physiologic concentrations of potassium inhibit triple-helix formation though some very recent studies suggest that TFOs substituted with 7-deazaxanthine can hybridize efficiently with their target even in the presence of 140 mM K^+ [27]. G containing TFOs also require divalent cations such as Mg^{++} for stability, while A containing TFOs appear to require Zn^{++}.

The problems discussed above have led to a number of solutions for optimizing the activity of the TFO. One is to use an oligonucleotide that

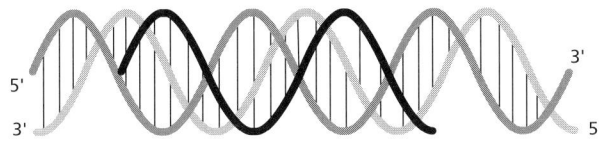

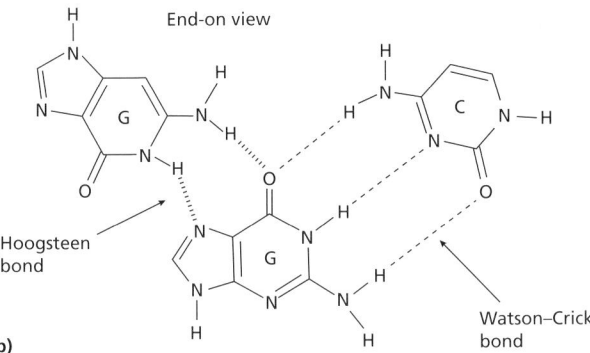

Fig. 21.1 Triple-helix formation. (a) DNA strands (green and red) with triple helix forming oligonucleotice (TFO) (yellow) in major groove. (b) Biochemical representation of Watson–Crick and Hoogsteen bonds formed between the TFO and the DNA backbone at the single nucleotide level. (*See also Plate 21.1, facing p. 296.*)

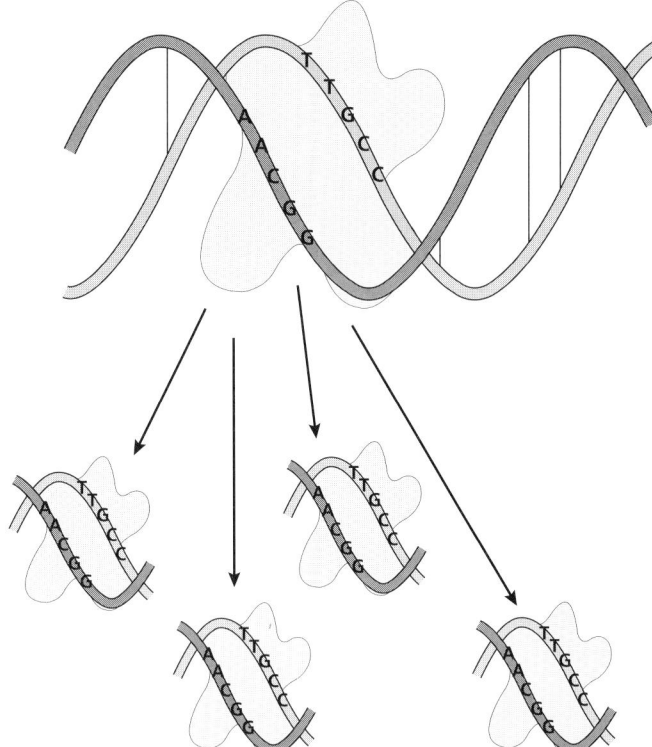

Fig. 21.2 Decoy oligonucleotide. Transcription factor (light yellow) shown binding its recognition sequence in DNA double strand (green and red). Decoy molecules (small green and red double strands with black spots) are shown attracting away (arrows) the transcription factor from its authentic binding site. (*See also Plate 21.2, facing p. 296.*)

binds to alternate strands of the duplexed DNA [28], a maneuver that obviates the requirement for polypurine–polypyrimidine sequence in the target DNA. Another is to increase the binding affinity of the TFO by covalently linking the DNA to intercalating groups such as acridine [29,30] and psoralens [31,32]. Incorporation of strand cleaving moieties may also increase efficiency of TFOs [33]. Finally, work on expanding the third strand binding code may also enhance the utility of this approach. Recent experiments from Wang *et al.* [34] and from Kochetkova *et al.* [35,36] have provided evidence that triple-helix formation can occur in living cells suggesting that these difficulties may ultimately be overcome. If shown practical, it has also been postulated that TFOs may prove useful in the treatment of certain genetic disorders such as sickle cell anaemia and hemophilia B, where their ability to induce mutations might be used to correct single base pair mistakes responsible for the disease [34,37,38]. Since this method may also inadvertently introduce undesired mutations into the genome by the same mechanism, concerns have been raised about using this approach in patients.

While successful use of this strategy for blocking transcription, and inducing specific mutations, *in vitro*, and *in vivo*, has been reported (reviewed in [24]), the frequency of such events is considerably <1%. Clearly, application of this technique to clinical problems would be rather doubtful at this frequency and will require considerable increase in efficiency of the process. A correlative approach would be to induce mutations that result in repair of a gene made defective by inherited or acquired point mutation. Work supporting this concept using chimeric DNA/RNA oligonucleotides (chimeraplasts) has been reported to occur at frequencies of >40%, but the reproducibility of such reports has recently been called into question [39]. In the hands of most researchers, the frequency of such repairs is also far too low to be of clinical use at this time [40–43].

Nucleic-acid double strands with sequences corresponding to the recognition sites of various transcription factors have also been employed to disrupt gene expression at the level of transcription [44]. Such double strands are thought to act as "decoys" that, when present in sufficient amounts, attract transcription factors away from their normal promoter binding sites thereby preventing gene transcription (Fig. 21.2; see also Plate 21.2, *facing p. 296*). They may be DNA or RNA and do not necessarily require a specific nucleotide sequence for activity. For example, nucleic acid molecules adopt physical structures that are dictated by their nucleotide content. Such structures, called aptamers, may coincidently bind specific transcription factors, or in fact, may bind to DNA or RNA directly when the structures find ways to "fit" [45–47]. For many technical reasons, including limited accessibility within the nuclear/chromosomal structure, the clinical application of these methods has not progressed at a very rapid rate.

An alternative approach, using polyamides, or lexitropsins, has been described by Kielkopf and colleagues [48–50]. Polyamide ligands contain the aromatic amino acids pyrrole (Py), hydroxypyrrole (Hp) and imidazole (Im). These small molecules have the ability to diffuse into the nucleus where they can then contact double stranded DNA in the minor groove (Fig. 21.3; see also Plate 21.3, *facing p. 296* [51]). Once bound, transcription is prevented by inhibition of duplex unwinding, or by the inhibition of binding of transcription factors to their promoters. These amino acids can be synthesized in a manner that will allow them to recognize specific Watson–Crick base pairs. It is theoretically possible then to construct polyamides that will function to suppress transcription in a manner analogous to TFOs. However, these molecules also share problems in common with TFOs. Included among these is the fact that recognition of longer sequences, as would be required for gene specific recognition, require larger molecules which are likely to have trouble gaining access to the nucleosome. In addition, maintaining the appropriate amino acid register for accurate sequence recognition is also a

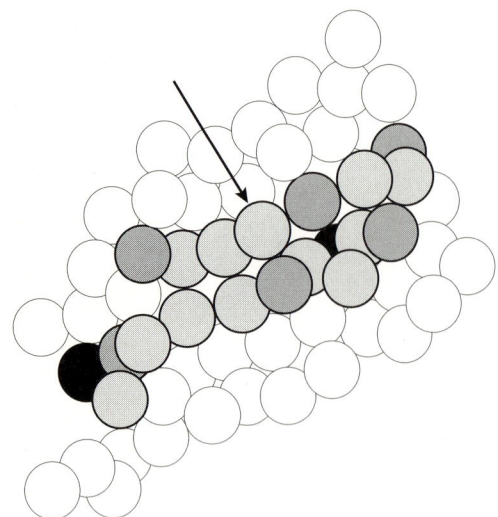

Fig. 21.3 Polyamide molecule (green and red spheres) binding in minor groove of DNA (arrow). Reproduced with permission from Goodsell [51]. (*See also Plate 21.3, facing p. 296.*)

significant issue [52]. Accordingly, much remains to be accomplished by the scientists interested in this approach before attempts at clinical use can be contemplated [53,54].

Targeting mRNA and translation

A larger body of work has focused on destabilizing mRNA. When compared to gene targeting, this approach has the theoretical disadvantage of having to hybridize with many more targets (transcribed mRNAs), but it has a physical advantage since mRNA, unlike a given gene's DNA is, theoretically, accessible to attack while being transcribed, transported from the nucleus, and translated. Two nucleic acid based strategies have emerged for blocking translation. One is the use of decoy sequences to attract away mRNA stabilizing proteins, the other to destroy mRNA as a result of hybridization between the targeting "vector" and the mRNA strand.

By attracting away mRNA stabilizing proteins, nucleic acid decoy molecules disrupt translation since an unstable mRNA is not efficiently translated and is ultimately destroyed [55,56]. The use of decoy RNAs for therapeutic purposes was initially suggested by Baltimore in 1988 [57]. The approach has gained credibility since the molecules are non-toxic, and appear to have been successful for control of viral gene expression, including human immunodeficiency virus (HIV), *in vitro* [58,59]. It is assumed in these studies that the decoy is directly interfering with HIV replication by sequestering reverse transcriptase but this was not formally proven [58]. Their mechanism of action is, therefore, uncertain. Recent studies on human α-globin mRNA are of interest in this regard. Stability determinants for this mRNA species have been defined in sufficient detail so that it can be used as a model system for testing the hypothesis that altering mRNA stability with decoys will be a useful form of therapy [60–62].

The other strategy for destabilizing mRNA is the more widely applied "antisense" strategy (Fig. 21.4) [7,63,64]. Simply stated, delivering a reverse complementary, i.e. "antisense", nucleic acid into a cell where the gene of interest is expressed, should lead to hybridization between the antisense sequence and the targeted gene's mRNA. Stable mRNA-antisense duplexes can interfere with splicing of heteronuclear RNA into mature mRNA [65,66], block translation of completed message [67,68] and, depending on the chemical composition of the antisense molecule, can lead to the destruction of the mRNA by binding of endogenous nucleases, such as ribonuclease H (RNase H) [69,70], or

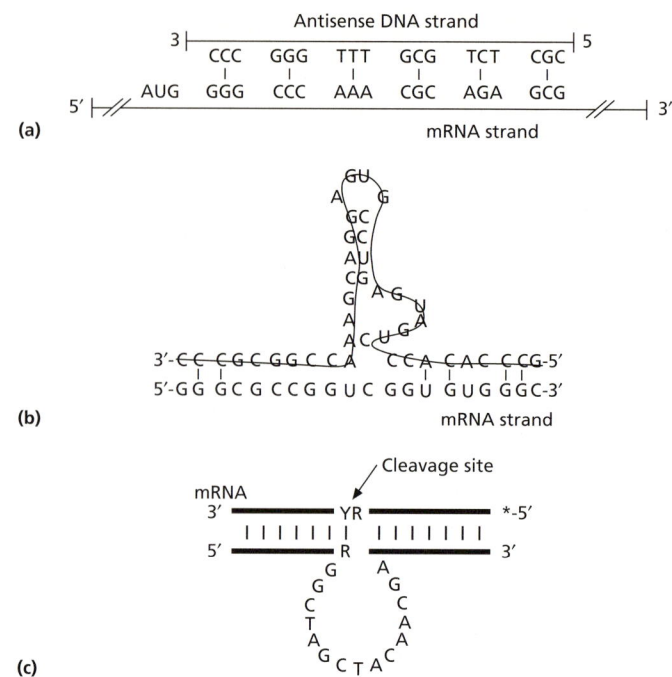

Fig. 21.4 Strategies for inhibiting translation with single stranded nucleic acid molecules. All molecules are shown hybridized to their mRNA target. (a) Simple oligodeoxynucleotide. Cleavage of mRNA is dependent on RNase H. (b) Hammerhead ribozyme. RNA molecule with inherent enzymatic activity due to presence of catalytic loop. (c) DNAzyme. DNA molecule with inherent enzymatic activity conferred by catalytic loop structure.

by intrinsic enzymatic activity engineered into the sequence as is the case with ribozymes [71,72] and DNAzymes [73,74]. Most recently, RNA interference (RNAi) has emerged as a very exciting methodology for silencing gene expression at the mRNA level [75]. Each of these approaches is discussed below.

Antisense DNA

Initial work with antisense DNA was carried out with unmodified, natural molecules. It soon became clear, however, that native DNA was subject to relatively rapid degradation, primarily through the action of 3′-exonucleases, but as a result of endonuclease attack as well [76,77]. Molecules destined for the clinic, and those used for experimental purposes, are now routinely modified to enhance their stability, as well as the strength of their hybridization with RNA. The interested reader is referred to the following articles for more details on chemical modification of oligonucleotide molecules [78,79]. Briefly, oligonucleotide drugs need to meet certain physical requirements in order to make them useful. First, they need to be able to cross cell membranes and then to hybridize with their intended target. The ability of an oligonucleotide to form a stable hybrid is minimally a function of the oligonucleotide's binding affinity and sequence specificity. Binding affinity is a function of the number of hydrogen bonds formed between the oligonucleotide and the sequence to which it is targeted. The binding affinity is measured by determining the temperature at which 50% of the double stranded material is dissociated into single strands and is known as the melting temperature, or Tm. The Tm depends on the concentration of the oligonucleotide, the nature of the base pairs and the ionic strength of the solvent in which hybridization occurs. It is worth noting that a single base mismatch, depending on its location, type, and surrounding sequence, can decrease binding affinity as much as 500-fold. mRNA associated proteins and tertiary structure also govern the ability of an oligonucleotide to hybridize with its target by physically blocking access to the region being targeted by the oligonucleotide [80,81]. Finally, it is also clear that oligonucleotides should exert little in the way of nonsequence related toxicity [82], and should remain stable in the extracellular and intracellular milieu in which they are situated. Meeting all these requirements in any one molecule has turned out to be a demanding task because, as might be expected, satisfying one criterion is often accomplished at the expense of another. It is also worth noting that the more complex the molecule, the more expensive its synthesis. In an age of increasing cost consciousness, the economics of any drug's synthesis becomes an important consideration.

First generation antisense molecules were designed to make the internucleotide linkages, the backbone on which the nucleosides are hung, more resistant to nuclease attack. This was accomplished primarily by replacing one of the nonbridging oxygen atoms in the phosphate group with either a sulfur or a methyl group. The former modification, called a phosphorothioate ODN, proved highly successful because these molecules are relatively nuclease resistant, charged and, therefore, water soluble and, finally, activate RNase H [83]. All of these properties are desirable, and virtually all of the clinical trials conducted to date have been carried out with this chemistry, although trials using so-called second generation molecules (mixed backbone/chimeric oligonucleotides) are in the planning phase. Nevertheless, the polyanionic nature of oligonucleotide molecules impairs cellular uptake and also results in unintended biologic effects due to nonspecific protein binding [84–86]. Phosphorothioates have also been reported to bind DNA polymerases, numerous members of the protein kinase C family, and transcription factors. In addition to these considerations, phosphorothioates are known to activate complement and may impair clotting by binding to factors such as thrombin [87,88]. Finally, high concentrations of phosphorothioates inhibit RNase H thereby decreasing their effectiveness [89]. The second-generation molecules mentioned briefly above were developed to overcome the disadvantageous properties of the phosphorothioates. The primary strategy employed was to decrease the number of thioate linkages in the molecules by flanking an RNase H activating phosphorothioate core, with nucleosides containing 2′-sugar modifications. These conferred increased nuclease stability, and an RNA-like structure that elevated Tm of binding. These molecules have not been evaluated in the clinic so their ultimate utility is unknown at this time.

Many chemical modifications to the phosphodiester linkage have been made. Two of the more interesting modifications currently under development are the peptide nucleic acids (PNAs) [90], and the morpholino ODNs [67]. These compounds are all but nuclease resistant. PNAs represent a more radical approach to the nuclease resistance problem as the phosphodiester linkage is completely replaced with a polyamide (peptide) backbone. They both form extremely tight bonds with their RNA targets and are likely to exert their effects by blocking translation, since neither molecule effectively activates RNase H. Whether it is necessary to preserve the ability of these molecules to activate RNase H is somewhat controversial [68], but many workers in the field still believe that molecules with this capability are likely to be more effective, at least in the clinical settings. Neither molecule moves freely across cell membranes and they must be injected or transfected into cells. Finally, PNAs are also sensitive to local ionic concentration and do not hybridize as well under physiologic conditions.

In addition to modifications to the internucleoside bridge, examples of sugar and base alterations have also been attempted. Changing the sugar's glycosidic linkage from the naturally occurring β form to the α anomeric form, where the base is projected in the opposite direction has been found to increase nuclease stability significantly. However, these structural changes compromise stability of the resulting duplexes and impair the activation of RNase H [91]. The loss of these properties might appear to be fatal flaws but Lavignon et al. [92] have reported that a 20 nt (nucleotide) α-oligonucleotide targeted to the primer binding site (PBS) of a murine retrovirus inhibited viral spreading if cells were first permeabilized in the presence of the oligonucleotide. They speculated that antisense activity resulted from a decrease in initiation or inhibition of extension of the minus or plus DNA strands. Chimeric α, β anomeric ODN have also been reported to be effective antisense compounds, as judged by their ability to inhibit in vitro translation of the pim-1 proto-oncogene because of restoration of the ability of the molecules to activate RNase H [93].

Sugars are also typically modified at the 2′ position with O-methyl, fluoro, O-propyl, O-allyl or methoxyethoxy groups. These modifications increase affinity for RNA and impart some nuclease resistance. Nevertheless, these molecules do not support RNase H activity and, for this reason, do not appear to have significant activity in some assays [94]. A number of groups have therefore used the 2′-O-methyl modification to flank natural diesters [94,95]. Such chimeric molecules do activate RNase H if there are at least five internal natural nucleotides [94]. Alteration of the C5 position of the pyrimidine bases producing the C5 propynyl substitutions have attracted notice because of their affinity for RNA, the stability of the hybrids formed and their ability to activate RNase H [96]. Whether the latter property is critical for their activity is in fact uncertain since some have reported that the tight hybrids formed by these compounds are very efficient at blocking translation [97]. Since base modifications do not protect against destruction by nucleases, which attack the phosphodiester bridges, backbones altered to confer stability (e.g. phosphorothioates) must be employed with modifications like the C5 propynyl substitution. In addition, a carrier of some type is required to move the molecules across cell membranes [98]. Finally, locked nucleic acids (LNAs) are an RNA derivative in which the ribose ring is constrained by a methylene linkage between the 2′-oxygen and the 4′-carbon. This conformation restriction increases binding affinity for complementary sequences by forcing the base into a "North up" RNA like conformation [99]. The extremely high affinity of the hybrids formed has led some to suggest that LNAs have advantages for targeting cellular nucleic acids and, for this reason, may provide a more certain route to the development of nucleic acid-based anticancer drugs [100].

Ribozymes

Naturally occurring ribozymes are catalytic RNA molecules that have the ability to cleave phosphodiester linkages without the aid of protein enzymes. This property has been exploited to specifically inhibit gene expression by targeting mRNA for catalytic cleavage especially in viral, cancer and genetic disease therapeutics (reviewed in [72,101]). Like antisense DNA, ribozymes bind to substrate RNA through Watson–Crick base pairing, thereby bringing about sequence specific cleavage of transcripts. In theory, these agents should trigger enhanced transcript turnover when compared to RNase H mediated antisense DNA degradation of transcripts because ribozymes act through bimolecular kinetics (association of ribozyme and target transcript) whereas antisense DNAs rely on trimolecular kinetics (association of antisense DNA, target transcript and RNase H). Since ribozymes are RNase H independent, 2′-modifications to increase stability do not diminish antisense effects and experiments have shown some modifications do not attenuate catalytic ability [102].

If ribozymes are to perform effectively as "enzymes", they must not only bind substrate RNA but also dissociate from the cleavage product in order to act on additional substrates. Studies suggest that, in some cases, dissociation of cleavage product may be the rate-limiting step [103,104]. Furthermore, some ribozymes require high divalent metal ion concentrations for efficient substrate cleavage, which may limit their use in intracellular environments [105]. Finally, colocalization of the ribozyme with its target is also quite important [106]. All of these concerns need to be addressed and overcome in order for ribozymes to have a future in medical therapy. Two ribozymes, the hammerhead ribozyme and the hairpin ribozyme, have been extensively studied due to their small size and rapid kinetics. Their application has been recently reviewed in several publications (reviewed in [107–110]). A more recent review classifies ribozymes as *cis* or *trans*-acting [101].

Hammerhead ribozymes

The hammerhead ribozyme consists of a highly conserved catalytic core, which was originally thought to specifically cleave substrate RNA at NUH triplets 3′ to the H, where N is any nucleotide, U is uracil and H is any nucleotide but guanidine (Fig. 21.4) [111]. More detailed study revealed, however, that hammerhead ribozymes may cleave RNA in a less restricted manner as cleavage can actually occur 3′ to any NHH triplet [112]. *In vitro* selection protocols have made it possible to screen for ribozymes with various cleavage specificities including one that cleaves at AUG sites [113]. Thus, the limitations for sequence specificity of triplet cleavage sites on the target RNA are less than previously thought. Specificity of cleavage is effected by synthesizing the sequence flanking the catalytic core so that it is complementary to the site one wishes to target.

The catalytic ability of hammerhead ribozymes is dependent on the presence of divalent metal ions, of which magnesium is most often used *in vitro*. It is postulated that the ions not only participate in RNA folding but also in the cleavage step itself [105]. As mentioned previously, studies indicate that catalytic activity requires relatively high Mg^{2+} concentrations compared to the intracellular environment. This characteristic could be problematic in applying the hammerhead ribozyme to an *in vivo* setting where intracellular Mg^{2+} concentrations are five to 10-fold lower than optimal *in vitro* conditions.

Experimental evidence supports the contention that cells treated with ribozymes exhibit diminished target mRNA levels as a direct result of the ribozyme's activity. For example, studies using very sensitive methods for detecting mRNA, such as those based on reverse transcription-polymerase chain reaction (RT-PCR), show that in cellular extracts, ribozymes will cleave the targeted mRNA at the predicted position [114,115]. Recently, more potent ribozyme-mediated effect on viral and cancer cell growth as compared to noncatalytic RNAs was reported [116,117]. However, in some instances, hammerhead ribozymes have not proven to be more effective than antisense DNA molecules. Likewise, inactive control ribozymes where antisense binding can occur but catalytic ability has been abolished give similar levels of gene inhibition when compared to fully catalytic hammerhead ribozymes, suggesting that the catalytic core, in some instances, plays little role in enhancing antisense effects [118]. Only further detailed studies will reveal the true utility of hammerhead ribozymes.

Hairpin ribozymes

The natural hairpin ribozyme is derived from a negative strand of the tobacco ringspot virus satellite RNA. Work on engineered hairpin ribozymes have resulted in broader range of cleavage sequence specificity. In general, a phosphodiester cleavage takes place 5′ to the G in the sequence NGUC where N is any nucleotide [119], although recent studies have shown even less restriction on sequence requirements for cleavage [120].

The overall structure of the hairpin ribozyme consists of two domains connected by a hinge section. One domain binds the substrate RNA to form two helical regions separated by a pair of single stranded loops. Cleavage occurs within the single stranded area of the substrate RNA. The other domain is similar in structure except the helixes are formed from the ribozyme folding back onto itself. The most important sequences for cleavage activity are those within the single stranded regions where almost every nucleotide is conserved, while the helical portions can be almost any sequence as long as there is double helix formation [110]. The hinge allows the two domains to be flexible relative to one another in space so that the two can dock together in an antiparallel orientation required for cleavage catalysis [121,122].

Both the hairpin ribozyme and the hammerhead ribozyme require metal ions for cleavage catalysis. In the hammerhead ribozyme, metal ions are believed to be involved directly in the cleavage step [123] whereas metal ions have not been implicated as directly involved with cleavage for the hairpin ribozyme [124]. The metal ions in hairpin ribozymes may instead play an important role in ribozyme structure [125]. Fluorescence resonance energy transfer (FRET) studies on docking of the two domains show that docking is metal dependent but that almost any metal will suffice even though they may not support cleavage [126]. In addition, docking is not the rate-limiting step and, since metal ions are not thought to be involved in the chemical cleavage step, it can only be assumed that there is a slower step in between docking and chemical cleavage.

One of the advantages offered by hairpin ribozymes is its unique ion dependence for catalytic action. One group has shown that aminoglycoside antibiotics with at least four amino groups are able to both support and inhibit hairpin ribozyme cleavage depending on metal ion conditions [127]. In the presence of magnesium, aminoglycoside antibiotics inhibit ribozyme cleavage with the degree of inhibition depending on the binding affinity of the antibiotic to the ribozyme. However, in the absence of metal ions, aminoglycoside antibiotics prove to assist cleavage with an optimum reaction condition at pH 5.5 and poorer kinetics as the pH is increased, exactly opposite to trends observed for magnesium. In this case, the metal ions are most likely being replaced by the amino groups of these antibiotics.

Polyamines such as spermidine and spermine have also been reported to support hairpin ribozyme cleavage ability. In the absence of magnesium, spermidine allows the cleavage reaction to persist at very slow kinetics compared to magnesium alone [125]. However, spermine alone gives very efficient cleavage of RNA comparable to that of magnesium and, when in the presence of low magnesium concentrations similar to intracellular conditions, spermine displays considerable increase in cleavage rates [127]. The fact that spermine is the major polyamine in eukaryotic cells may explain why the hairpin ribozyme has shown remarkable intracellular cleavage activity in mammalian cells and may make future therapeutic endeavors with the hairpin ribozyme much easier [128].

DNAzymes

While investigating ways to improve the function of ribozymes, Breaker and Joyce made the assumption that because RNA and DNA are very similar chemical compounds, DNA molecules with enzymatic activity could also be developed [129]. This assumption proved correct and led to the development of a "general-purpose" RNA-cleaving DNA enzyme [73]. The molecule was identified from a library of >1000 different DNA molecules by successive rounds of *in vitro* selective amplification based on the ability of individual molecules to promote $Mg^{2\pm}$ dependent, multi-turnover, cleavage of an RNA target.

The selected molecule was named the "10–23 DNA enzyme", because it was derived from the 23rd clone obtained after the 10th round of selective amplification [73]. The "10–23 DNA enzyme" is composed of a catalytic domain of 15 deoxynucleotides, flanked by two substrate-recognition domains of ~8 nt each (Fig. 21.4). The recognition domains provide the sequence information required for specific binding to an RNA substrate. They also supply the binding energy required to hold the RNA substrate within the active site of the enzyme. It is straightforward that by appropriately designing the flanking sequences the DNAzyme can be made to cleave virtually any RNA that contains a purine-pyrimidine junction.

The attraction of DNAzymes over ribozymes is that they are very inexpensive to make and they are inherently more stable than ribozymes. Nevertheless, DNAzymes must ultimately overcome the same problems faced by ribozymes and oligonucleotides if they are to be effective in cellular systems (see below). These problems are stability, as well as the ability to be targeted to the cell of interest, and to hybridize with their mRNA target. They must also be nontoxic. In this regard, many of the chemical modifications employed to stabilize ODNs can be incorporated into the 10–23 DNA enzyme without loss of activity. There is a suggestion from recent reports that issues of intracellular concentration and target hybridization may also be solvable [74,130]. Experience with these molecules as potential therapeutic agents is limited [74] but these molecules may also prove worthy in the clinical setting.

As of this writing, several phase I/II clinical trials with exogenously delivered synthetic ribozymes are in early phase clinical evaluation. For example, a ribozyme targeting the vascular endothelial growth factor-1 (VEGF1) receptor as an antiangiogenic agent is being evaluated in patients with metastatic breast and colon cancer, alone or in combination with chemotherapy. Two other trials are also in progress. One is a phase I study of a ribozyme directed against the Her2 protooncogene (encoding human epidermal growth factor receptor-2) in patients with advanced ovarian and breast cancer; the other is with a ribozyme directed against the hepatitis C virus which is currently in a phase II clinical trial. Results of these clinical investigations have not yet been reported.

RNA interference

A new, and rapidly developing, approach for targeting mRNA is called post-transcriptional gene silencing, or RNA interference (RNAi) (Fig. 21.5; see also Plate 21.4, *facing p. 296*) [75,131–133]. RNAi is the process by which double stranded (ds) RNA targets mRNA for destruction in a sequence dependent manner. The mechanism of RNAi involves processing of dsRNA into 21–23 basepair (bp) fragments that hybridize with the target mRNA and initiate its destruction (Fig. 21.5). The mechanism for RNAi is fast being elucidated, although many intriguing questions remain to be answered [75]. At this time, it appears likely that long dsRNA is processed by an ribonuclease called "Dicer" [134–136] into ~21–22 nt long double strands. These small cleavage products are then incorporated into a larger ribonucleoprotein complex called the RISC complex (RNAi induced silencing complex) [137,138] which simultaneously scans the complementary mRNA sequence for homology to the small, now unwound, RNA fragment and then promotes its destruction through enzymes integral to the complex [138–140].

While RNAi has been employed successfully for gene silencing in a variety of experimental systems including petunias, tobacco plants, neurospora, *Caenorhabditis elegans*, insects, planaria, hydra, zebrafish, the application of long dsRNA to silence expression in mammalian cells has been largely unsuccessful [141]. It has been suggested that mammalian cells recognize these long dsRNAs as invading pathogens that triggers an interferon response which leads to apoptosis and cell death [142]. However, a number of recent reports suggest that RNA double strands of ~21–22 nt in length, called short interfering RNA (siRNA), may be able to silence expression in mammalian somatic cells. Of particular interest to hematologists, one of these reports involves suppression of *bcr-abl* in CML cells [143]. Success with this technique depends on appropriate design and synthesis of the siRNA molecules [144,145]. They are most efficient when composed of 21–22 nt sense and 21–22 nt antisense strands paired in a manner to have 2–3 nt overhang at the 3' end. This mimics the natural cleavage of dsRNA by Dicer. The molecules must also be modified to contain 3'-hydroxy and 5'-phosphate groups since a 5'-phosphate is required for RISC activity [75,146–148]. Fortunately, synthetic siRNA duplexes with free 5'-hydroxyls are rapidly

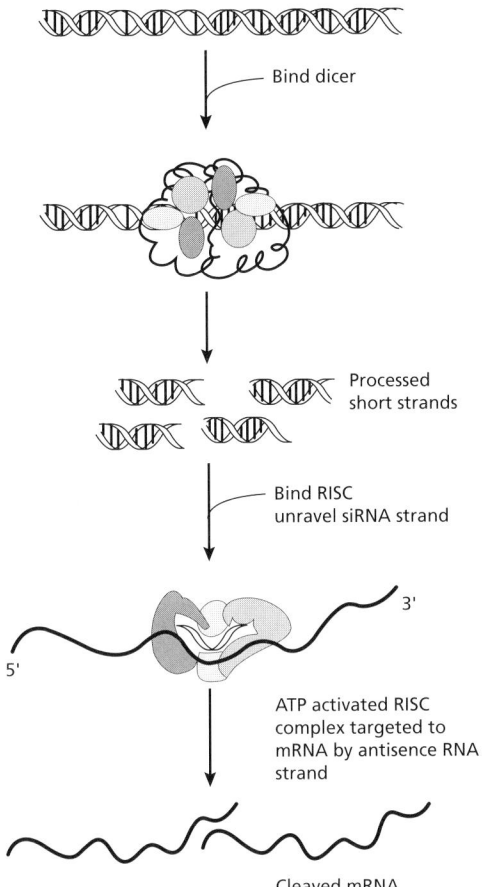

Fig. 21.5 RNA interference (RNAi). RNAi is initiated by the Dicer enzyme which processes double-stranded RNA into ~22-nucleotide small interfering RNAs (siRNA). The siRNAs are incorporated into a multicomponent nuclease, RISC (green). RISC must be activated from a latent form, containing a double-stranded siRNA to an active form, RISC*, by unwinding of siRNA. RISC* then uses the antisense strand of the unwound siRNA as a guide to substrate selection. (*See also Plate 21.4, facing p. 296.*)

phosphorylated in at least some cells [140]. Studies on the specificity of target recognition by siRNA duplexes indicate that a single point mutation located in the center of paired region of an siRNA duplex is sufficient to abolish target mRNA degradation.

Mechanistic studies of RNAi in the human system are just beginning. It appears that, unlike antisense molecules, the silencing effect is restricted to the cytoplasm [149]. This might be expected because of the location of the RISC. Tuschl and colleagues recently reported that, by using affinity-tagged siRNAs, they were able to demonstrate that a single-stranded siRNA resides in the RISC complex together with eIF2C1 and/or eIF2C2 (human GERp95) Argonaute proteins [140]. In HeLa cell cytoplasmic extracts supplemented with 21 nt siRNA duplexes, a RISC complex was rapidly formed. Interestingly, by adding single-stranded antisense RNAs, in the size range of 19–29 nt effective silencing of HeLa genes was also detected, especially when the strand was 5'-phosphorylated [140].

Given the cost of chemical synthesis of siRNAs, and the fact that exogenously administered material can have only transient effects, many investigators have tried to induce RNAi with hairpin molecules expressed from viral vectors [150–153]. At present, these methods utilize a vector containing mouse or human U6 promoter. In the approach used by Sui *et al.* [154], for example, the 22 nt selected coding sequence starting with GG (5' end) is ligated with its inverted repeat by 6 nt spacer. The inverted repeat contains 4–5 T_s at 3' end for transcription termination.

The whole cassette is subcloned into the vector down-stream from U6 promoter. RNA polymerase III transcribes the DNA into RNA and terminates at a run of T_s making it possible to create RNA with defined ends. The resulting RNA is composed of two identical 21 nt sequence motifs in an inverted orientation separated by a 6 nt spacer of nonhomologous sequence. This RNA is predicted to fold back to form a hairpin [154]. Although the T_s overhang is longer then suggested by Tuschl, the hairpin RNAs, as noted above, have been demonstrated to function effectively and inhibited expression of several genes in mammalian cells.

While reports about the utility of this method for silencing mammalian genes continue to accumulate [150,154–157], the ability to apply this method to all types of mammalian cells still remains uncertain. As is true for traditional antisense experiments, the possibility of experimental artifacts being misinterpreted as specific gene targeting is being increasingly recognized [158]. Accordingly, it is highly likely that many technical issues related to employing nucleic acid therapeutics in general will also apply to siRNA, including the need to identify mRNA accessible sequence in a predictable way [159].

Pertubation of mRNA processing

Finally, the strategy of manipulating gene expression by altering RNA processing, as opposed to mRNA destruction, is also worth mentioning as significant progress appears to have been made in this area. Kole and colleagues developed this approach using a very useful model system based on human thalassemia [160,161]. Thalassemias are highly prevalent human blood disorders characterized by faulty hemoglobin production and concomitant red cell destruction that results in anaemia. The genetic mutations responsible for these diseases are well characterized. For example, beta-thalassemia results from a mutation in intron 2 of the β-globin gene (IVS2-654) which causes aberrant splicing of β-globin premessenger RNA (premRNA) and, consequently, β-globin deficiency. Kole's group was able to show that treatment of mammalian cells stably expressing the IVS2-654 human β-globin gene with antisense oligonucleotides targeted at the aberrant splice sites blocked abnormal splicing thereby allowing the normal splice site to be used. Correction of splicing was oligo dose-dependent and, importantly, led to accumulation of normal human β-globin mRNA and polypeptide in cells [160]. Most recently, correction has been accomplished in blood cells derived from thalassemic patients [162]. In this intriguing study, peripheral blood mononuclear cells were treated with morpholino oligonucleotides antisense to several aberrant splice sites in the premRNA. The oligonucleotides restored correct splicing and synthesis of β-globin mRNA synthesis in erythroid cells from patients with IVS2-654/β(E), IVS2-745/IVS2-745 and IVS2-745/IVS2-1 genotypes. As a result, normal adult hemoglobin (hemoglobin A [HbA]) production in the red cells increased as well. The maximal HbA level for repaired IVS2-745 mutation was approximately 30% of normal. It was of great interest that HbA was still detectable 9 days after a single treatment with the oligonucleotide. This result would clearly have important clinical consequences if such treatment could be made effective at the level of the hematopoietic stem cell. These same workers suggest that this approach might have utility in the treatment of cancer as well [163].

Nucleic acid drugs in the hematology clinic

Hematologic diseases are particularly attractive candidates for the gene silencing or repair strategies, because many of the malignancies are the result of increasingly well characterized genetic lesions and the hemoglobinopathies, for example, of mutations that might be repaired. To date, however, there is very little clinical experience with any of the molecules discussed above except for phosphorothioate antisense DNAs. Accordingly, the following sections apply largely to these molecules.

During their preclinical development, there were some concerns that phosphorothioate compounds might be toxic because, when infused into primates, several of the animals died. Investigation of these occurrences revealed that they took place after rapid bolus intravenous infusions at concentrations exceeding 5–10 µg/mL, and that they were most likely due to complement activation and vascular collapse [164]. In fact, slow infusions were well tolerated by the test subjects. This experience was therefore a useful reminder that in addition to side-effects resulting from the suppression of the targeted gene, side-effects related to the chemical backbone of the oligonucleotide might also be anticipated. In actual use in the clinic, phosphorothioates have proven to be remarkably well tolerated. Abnormalities felt related to the backbone include transient fever, fatigue, nausea and vomiting, mild to moderate thrombocytopenia and transient, but clinically insignificant, prolongation of partial thromboplastin time [165–168]. As of this writing several clinical studies have been conducted utilizing a number of ODNs to different disease targets. Below we review some of those recently reported (summarized in Table 21.1 [165–179]).

Bcl-2: targeting apoptosis

Bcl-2 protein is an important regulator of programmed cell death (apoptosis) and overexpression has been implicated in the pathogenesis of some lymphomas [180]. Resistance to chemotherapy, at least *in vitro*, may also be related to Bcl-2 overexpression [181,182]. Laboratory studies have shown convincingly that exposing cells to an oligonucleotide targeted to *bcl-2* will specifically decrease the targeted mRNA and protein [6–8]. For all these reasons then, there is a great deal of interest in targeting Bcl-2 for therapeutic purposes [183]. The first clinical study to employ this strategy was carried out with a phosphorothioate compound on 9 patients with refractory lymphoma [184]. The drug was delivered as daily subcutaneous infusion and, save for local inflammation at the site of infusion, no treatment related toxicity occurred. In two patients computed tomography scans showed a decrease in tumor size. One of these was classified as minor, the other complete. In two patients the number of circulating lymphoma cells decreased during treatment. In four patients, serum concentrations of lactate dehydrogenase fell and in two of these patients symptoms improved. BCL-2 levels were measured by flow cytometry in peripheral blood of five patients, two of whom had reduced levels of BCL-2 protein. A follow-up trial was conducted on a larger number of patients. Waters *et al.* [166] administered an 18-mer ODN to 21 patients with refractory lymphomas and *bcl-2* overexpression. The material was infused subcutaneously over 14 days in doses ranging from 4.6 to 195.8 mg/m²/day. In general, treatment was well tolerated. Minor toxicities included mild thrombocytopenia, lymphopenia, nonfasting hyperglycemia, increases in aminotransferases and alkaline phosphatase. All resolved spontaneously after completion of treatment. Mild inflammation, which was easily treatable, was noted at the site of injection. More significant toxicities occurred with doses ≥147.2 mg/m²/day and included circulatory disturbances with edema, fever associated with hypotension, and grade 3 thrombocytopenia. There was one complete response, two minor responses and nine cases of stable disease. Nine patients had progressive disease despite the treatment. Keeping in mind that it was a single course of 2 weeks treatment these results appear to be promising.

c-*myb*: transcription factor targeting

The c-*myb* protooncogene encodes a transcription factor required for hematopoiesis [185–187]. Its encoded protein, MYB, regulates the expression of genes required for cell cycle progression and for maturation [188]. The protein and its mRNA both have very short half-lives [189].

Table 21.1 Summary of recently published clinical trials with antisense oligodeoxynucleotide (ODN).

Ref.	Drug/target	Type of study	No. of patients	Diagnosis	Treatment duration	Administration	Remissions
[169]	ISIS2302 ICAM-1	Multicenter Placebo-controlled Double blind	75	CD	2 days to 4 weeks	SC	NS
[170]		Placebo-controlled Double blind	20	CD	26 days	2 h IV infusion	47% steroid-free remissions
[165]	ISIS3521 PKC-α	Phase I	36	Advanced cancer	3 days/week for 3 weeks every 4 weeks	2 h IV infusion	2CR
[168]		Phase I	21	Advanced cancer	21 days every 4 weeks	21-days continuous IV infusion	3 responses
[166]	G3139 Bcl-2	Phase I	21	Relapsed NHL	14 days	Continuous SC infusion	1 CR 2 minor responses
[171]	G3131 with decarbazine	Phase I/II	14	Advanced malignant melanoma	14 days every 4 weeks	Continuous IV infusion	1 CR 2 PR 3 minor responses
[167]	G3139 with mitoxantrone	Phase I/II	26	Metastatic prostate cancer	14 days every 28 days	Continuous IV infusion	2 decreases in PSA
[172]	**Fomivirsen** CMV	Multicenter Randomized prospective	29	CMV retinitis in AIDS patients	Once a week	Intravitreously	Time to progression 71 vs. 13 days
[173]	ISIS2503 H-ras	Phase I	23	Advanced cancer	14 days every 3 weeks	Continuous IV infusion	4 stable diseases
[174]	ISIS5132 c-Raf kinase	Phase I	34	Advanced cancer	21 days every 4 weeks	Continuous IV infusion	2 stable diseases
[175]		Multicenter phase II	22	Small-cell and non-small-cell lung cancer	21 days every 4 weeks	Continuous IV infusion	No responses
[176]		Phase I	22	Advanced cancer	Weekly	24 h IV infusion	No responses
[177]	LR3s280 c-myc	Multicenter placebo controlled	78	After PTCA	Single dose	Intracoronary	No responses
[178]		Placebo controlled	85	After coronary stent implantation	Single dose	Intracoronary	No responses
[179]	**IGF-IR AS ODN** ILGF type 1 receptor	Pilot study	12	Malignant astrocytoma	6 h	*Ex vivo*	2 CR 6 PR

AIDS, acquired immune deficiency syndrome; CD, Crohn's disease; CMV, cytomegalovirus; CR, complete remission; ILGF, insulin-like growth factor; IV, intravenously; NHL, non-Hodgkin's lymphoma; NS, not significant; PKC, protein kinase C; PR, partial remission; PSA, prostate specific antigen; PTCA, percutaneous transluminal coronary angioplasty; SC, subcutaneous.

These facts in aggregate make MYB an attractive therapeutic target [190] and a recently published study from our laboratory appears to support this concept [191]. In this study, an ODN targeted to the c-*myb* protooncogene was employed to purge marrow autografts administered to allograft ineligible CML patients. CD34$^+$ marrow cells were purged with ODN for either 24 h ($n = 19$) or 72 h ($n = 5$). Post-purging, Myb mRNA levels declined substantially in ~50% of patients. Analysis of *bcr-abl* expression in a surrogate stem cell assay suggested that purging had been accomplished at a primitive cell level in >50% of patients. Day 100 cytogenetics were evaluated in surviving patients who engrafted without infusion of unmanipulated "back-up" marrow ($n = 14$). Whereas all patients were ~100% Philadelphia positive (Ph$^+$) pretransplant, two patients had complete cytogenetic remissions, three patients had <33% Ph$^+$ metaphases and eight remained 100% Ph$^+$. One patient's marrow yielded no metaphases but fluorescence *in situ* hybridization (FISH) evaluation ~18 months post-transplant revealed ~45% Bcr-Abl$^+$ cells suggesting that six of 14 patients had originally obtained a "major" cytogenetic response. Conclusions regarding clinical efficacy of ODN marrow purging could not be drawn from this small pilot study. Nevertheless, these results lead the authors to speculate that enhanced delivery of ODN, targeted to critical proteins of short half-life, might lead to the development of more effective nucleic acid drugs and enhanced clinical utility of these compounds in the future.

Targeting signal transduction molecules

Protein kinase C-α

Protein kinase C (PKC) comprises a family of biochemically and functionally distinct phospholipid dependent cytoplasmic serine threonine kinases. These proteins play a critical role in transducing the signals that regulate cell proliferation and differentiation. PKC is overexpressed in a number of tumors and antisense inhibitors of these enzymes have demonstrated some antitumor activity *in vitro* [165,192,193] and in animal models [194]. Results of two studies employing the identical 20-mer phosphorothioate ODN against PKC-α are published. Nemunaitis *et al.* [165] reported toxicity and response in 36 patients with a variety of advanced cancers. The drug was administered intravenously over 2 h, three times a week for 3 weeks of a 4-week cycle. Toxicity was mild and included hematologic changes (thrombocytopenia), transient increases in partial thromboplastin time, nausea, fever, chills and fatigue. Two patients with non-Hodgkin's lymphoma (NHL) achieved a complete remission after administration of nine and 17 cycles, respectively. Ten patients had stabilization of disease.

H-*ras*

H-*ras* is a powerful regulator of multiple interconnected receptor signaling pathways. The gene is constitutively active and promotes proliferation and malignant transformation in many human tumors. Cunningham *et al.* [173] reported results from a study carried out on 23 patients with various malignancies. The anti-Ras oligonucleotide was delivered as a continuous intravenous infusion over 14 days, and repeated every 3 weeks. As in other studies with phosphorothioate oligonucleotides only mild toxicities were observed. No complete or partial responses were achieved. Four patients had stabilized disease for 6–10 cycles.

Oligonucleotides as immunologic adjuvants

Over the last several years it has become increasingly appreciated that several types of immune cells possess pattern recognition receptors that can distinguish prokaryotic DNA from vertebrate DNA [195]. Recognition is accomplished by the ability of these receptors to distinguish unmethylated CpG dinucleotides within particular base contexts (CpG motifs) [196]. Bacterial DNA, or even synthetic ODN containing CpG motifs, can activate immune responses that have evolved to protect the host against intracellular infections. Responses of this type are T-helper type 1 subset (T$_H$1)-like in type and lead to activation of natural killer (NK) cells, dendritic cells, macrophages and B cells [197,198]. CpG DNA-induced immune activation has been shown capable of protecting certain hosts against infection alone, or in combination with vaccines. It is reasonably hypothesized then that CpG containing oligonucleotides might well prove to be effective adjuvants for immunotherapy of cancer and for boosting immune responses to antigens that are less efficient in this regard but to which one would like to immunize a host [199,200].

The most recent application of this principle was reported in abstract form at the December 2001 meeting of the American Society of Hematology where preliminary results from a clinical trial in which the safety and efficacy of a CpG adjuvant were investigated [201]. In this study, the CpG ODN was administered three times a week in 2 h infusion to 16 patients with refractory or relapsed NHL. Analysis of data accrued at the time of submission suggested that the oligonucleotide increased the number and activity of NK cells in treated patients. Antibody mediated cytotoxic effects of peripheral blood mononuclear cells were also demonstrable. Two of the 16 treated patients achieved a partial remission. The study is still ongoing and a follow-up trial of the CpG ODN in combination with rituximab is being planned.

Conclusions

Gene silencing methodologies of various types have been used with great success in the laboratory [202–213]. Several pilot or phase I studies employing this approach for therapeutic purposes have generated some encouraging results in the clinic as well [173,174,179,184,191]. Nevertheless, it is widely appreciated that the ability of nucleic acid molecules to modify gene expression *in vivo* is quite variable, in terms of both efficiency and effectiveness [81,86,214]. Several issues have been implicated as root cause of this problem, including molecule delivery to targeted cells, specific compartments within cells and identification of hybridization accessible sequence within the genomic DNA or RNA [7]. Intuitively, DNA accessibility is limited by compaction of nuclear material and transcription activity of the gene target. Formal approaches for solving this problem are not widely discussed. In mRNA sequence accessibility is dictated by internal base pairing and the proteins that associate with the RNA in a living cell. Attempts to accurately predict the *in vivo* structure of RNA have been fraught with difficulty [215]. Accordingly, mRNA targeting is largely a random process, accounting for many experiments where the addition of an antisense nucleic acid yields no effect on expression. Several approaches to this problem have been tried including trial and error oligonucleotide "walks", i.e. construction of overlapping molecules in a 5′ to 3′ direction down the target mRNA sequence [216]. Computer-assisted modeling of RNA structure [217], hybridization of RNA to random oligonucleotides arrayed on glass slides [218,219] and variations on the theme of using random oligonucleotide libraries to identify RNase H cleavable sites, in the absence or presence of crude cellular extracts [220,221], have also been utilized to address this problem. Developers of these various methodologies state that they are highly predictive and easy to carry out [222], but one could speculate that their failure to become widely adapted routines argues against these assertions. Recent work from this laboratory suggests that the self-quenching reporter molecules may be useful for solving *in vivo* RNA structure [223] but the reliability and utility of this approach also remains to be proven.

Another significant problem in this field is the limited ability to deliver nucleic acids into cells and have them reach their target [81]. Without this ability, it is clear that even an appropriately targeted sequence is not likely to be efficient. As a general rule, oligonucleotides are taken up primarily through a combination of adsorptive and fluid phase endocytosis [224–227]. After internalization, confocal and electron microscopy studies have indicated that the bulk of the oligonucleotides enter the endosome/lysosome compartment where most of the material either becomes trapped or degraded. Biologic inactivity is the predictable result of these events. Nevertheless, oligonucleotides can escape from the vesicles intact, enter the cytoplasm, and then diffuse into the nucleus where they presumably acquire their mRNA, or in the case of decoys, protein target [225,228–230]. Delivery technologies continue to improve, so it is likely that present methods and/or other newly evolving technologies will be successfully employed to delivery optimized nucleic acids to their cellular targets [231,232]. Indeed, it is our hypothesis that development of effectively targeted, and efficiently delivered, nucleic acid molecules will lead to important advances in the diagnosis and treatment of human malignancies [191] and other diseases for which this class of molecules has been proposed to be effective.

In addition to delivery, and targeting oligonucleotides within the mRNA, we believe that other considerations might improve the efficacy

Table 21.2 Ongoing and planned trials with antisense (AS) oligodeoxynucleotide (ODN) and ribozymes (RBZ).

Target	Disease
c-myc AS	Cardiovascular restenosis, phase II
Adenosine 1 receptor AS	Asthma, phase II
bcl-2 AS	Hematological malignancies
	Solid tumors, phase III
Ribonucleotide reductase AS	Solid tumors, phase I and II
HIV AS, RBZ	HIV, phase II
CpG molecules AS	Solid tumors
	Infectious diseases, phase I/II
VGFR1 RBZ	Breast, colon cancer, phase II
HCV RBZ	HCV, phase I
Her2 RBZ	Breast, ovarian cancer, phase I
PKC-α AS	Lung cancer, NHL, phase III
c-raf AS	Solid tumors, phase II
H-ras AS	Lung cancer, phase II
bcl-2 AS	NHL, phase II/III
PKA AS	Cancer, phase I

HCV, hepatitis C virus; HIV, human immunodeficiency virus; NHL, non-Hodgkin's lymphoma.

of this strategy. In particular, target mRNA abundance and half-life are also likely to be important considerations when selecting a gene target. For example, the c-myb mRNA, as well as its encoded protein, have an estimated half-life of ~30–50 min [233,234] and this could be an important factor in the apparent efficiency of mRNA targeting in one reported clinical study [191]. In contrast to Myb protein, Bcl-2 protein, for example, has a half-life that has been estimated to be ~14 h [235], and Raf and Ras proteins have half-lives estimated to be >24 h [236,237]. Attempts to eliminate these proteins from cells using exogenously delivered nucleic acid molecules may prove more difficult. Whether these considerations will apply to extremely long lived, or endogenously expressed antisense vectors remains to be seen. The latter in particular will also be subject to the many problems associated with vector delivery and expression. Finally, as the efficiency of gene silencing improves, specificity of tumor cell expression will likely become an important consideration in target selection. A possible way to expand the universe of such targets will be the development of mechanisms to target genetic polymorphisms in tumor cells affected by loss of heterozygosity [238]. In the absence of molecules that address all these issues, interim solutions are being evolved. One with obvious appeal is to combine gene-silencing approaches with traditional therapeutic modalities [239]. While this may well prove useful in the near term, one can hope that continued improvement in gene silencing methodologies will allow us to abandon these more aggressive treatment paradigms.

The concept of inhibiting gene expression with antisense nucleic acids developed from studies initiated almost a quarter of a century ago [16,17]. Clinical development of antisense compounds has proceeded to the point where a number of nucleic acid drugs have entered phase I/II and, in a few cases, phase III trials. Others are about to begin or are in late planning stages (Table 21.2). The original motivation for developing these molecules remains strong. Recent experience demonstrating the development of leukemia cells resistant to the small molecule inhibitor Gleevec® provides another [240]. While a cell might be able to evolve mutated proteins that evade inhibitors targeted to proteins, this cannot happen if the mRNA encoding that protein is no longer made. Accordingly, while only one antisense nucleic acid drug has received Food and Drug Administration approval to date [241], one can hope that others will shortly be forthcoming.

Acknowledgments

This work was supported in part by grants from the National Institutes of Health and the Doris Duke Charitable Foundation.

References

1 Cheson BD. Rituximab. Clinical development and future directions. *Expert Opin Biol Ther* 2002; **2**(1): 97–110.
2 Druker BJ. STI571 (Gleevec®) as a paradigm for cancer therapy. *Trends Mol Med* 2002; **8**(4): S14–8.
3 Cheson BD. Hematologic malignancies. New developments and future treatments. *Semin Oncol* 2002; **29**(4) (Suppl. 13): 33–45.
4 Hermiston T. Gene delivery from replication-selective viruses: arming guided missiles in the war against cancer. *J Clin Invest* 2000; **105**(9): 1169–72.
5 Nettelbeck DM, Jerome V, Muller R. Gene therapy: designer promoters for tumour targeting. *Trends Genet* 2000; **16**(4): 174–81.
6 Vile RG, Russell SJ, Lemoine NR. Cancer gene therapy. Hard lessons and new courses. *Gene Ther* 2000; **7**(1): 2–8.
7 Gewirtz AM, Sokol DL, Ratajczak MZ. Nucleic acid therapeutics. State of the art and future prospects. *Blood* 1998; **92**(3): 712–36.
8 Olivier M, Aggarwal A, Allen J et al. A high-resolution radiation hybrid map of the human genome draft sequence. *Science* 2001; **291**(5507): 1298–302.
9 Hahn WC, Counter CM, Lundberg AS, Beijersbergen RL, Brooks MW, Weinberg RA. Creation of human tumour cells with defined genetic elements [see comments]. *Nature* 1999; **400**(6743): 464–8.
10 Ma C, Staudt LM. Molecular definition of the germinal centre stage of B-cell differentiation. *Philos Trans R Soc Lond B Biol Sci* 2001; **356**(1405): 83–9.
11 Moos PJ, Raetz EA, Carlson MA et al. Identification of gene expression profiles that segregate patients with childhood leukemia. *Clin Cancer Res* 2002; **8**(10): 3118–30.
12 Walker J, Flower D, Rigley K. Microarrays in hematology. *Curr Opin Hematol* 2002; **9**(1): 23–9.
13 Golub TR. Genomic approaches to the pathogenesis of hematologic malignancy. *Curr Opin Hematol* 2001; **8**(4): 252–61.
14 Tamayo P, Slonim D, Mesirov J et al. Interpreting patterns of gene expression with self-organizing maps: methods and application to hematopoietic differentiation. *Proc Natl Acad Sci U S A* 1999; **96**(6): 2907–12.
15 Golub TR, Slonim DK, Tamayo P et al. Molecular classification of cancer: class discovery and class prediction by gene expression monitoring. *Science* 1999; **286**(5439): 531–7.
16 Paterson BM, Roberts BE, Kuff EL. Structural gene identification and mapping by DNA-mRNA hybrid-arrested cell-free translation. *Proc Natl Acad Sci U S A* 1977; **74**(10): 4370–4.
17 Stephenson ML, Zamecnik PC. Inhibition of Rous sarcoma viral RNA translation by a specific oligodeoxyribonucleotide. *Proc Natl Acad Sci U S A* 1978; **75**(1): 285–8.
18 Simons RW, Kleckner N. Translational control of IS10 transposition. *Cell* 1983; **34**(2): 683–91.
19 Izant JG, Weintraub H. Inhibition of thymidine kinase gene expression by anti-sense RNA. a molecular approach to genetic analysis. *Cell* 1984; **36**(4): 1007–15.
20 Mizuno T, Chou MY, Inouye M. A unique mechanism regulating gene expression: translational inhibition by a complementary RNA transcript (micRNA). *Proc Natl Acad Sci U S A* 1984; **81**(7): 1966–70.
21 Melton DW. Gene targeting in the mouse. *Bioessays* 1994; **16**(9): 633–8.
22 Stasiak A. Getting down to the core of homologous recombination [comment]. *Science* 1996; **272**(5263): 828–9.
23 Helene C. Control of oncogene expression by antisense nucleic acids. *Eur J Cancer* 1994; **30**A(11): 1721–6.
24 Knauert MP, Glazer PM. Triplex forming oligonucleotides: sequence-specific tools for gene targeting. *Hum Mol Genet* 2001; **10**(20): 2243–51.
25 Xodo LE, Alunni-Fabbroni M, Manzini G. Effect of 5-methylcytosine on the structure and stability

of DNA. Formation of triple-stranded concatenamers by overlapping oligonucleotides. *J Biomol Struct Dyn* 1994; **11**(4): 703–20.

26 Faucon B, Mergny JL, Helene C. Effect of third strand composition on the triple helix formation: purine versus pyrimidine oligodeoxynucleotides. *Nucl Acids Res* 1996; **24**(16): 3181–8.

27 Faruqi AF, Krawczyk SH, Matteucci MD, Glazer PM. Potassium-resistant triple helix formation and improved intracellular gene targeting by oligodeoxyribonucleotides containing 7-deazaxanthine. *Nucl Acids Res* 1997; **25**(3): 633–40.

28 de Bizemont T, Duval-Valentin G, Sun JS, Bisagni E, Garestier T, Helene C. Alternate strand recognition of double-helical DNA by (T,G)-containing oligonucleotides in the presence of a triple helix-specific ligand. *Nucl Acids Res* 1996; **24**(6): 1136–43.

29 Washbrook E, Fox KR. Alternate-strand DNA triple-helix formation using short acridine-linked oligonucleotides. *Biochem J* 1994; **301**(2): 569–75.

30 Lacoste J, Francois JC, Helene C. Triple helix formation with purine-rich phosphorothioate-containing oligonucleotides covalently linked to an acridine derivative. *Nucl Acids Res* 1997; **25**(10): 1991–8.

31 Kane SA, Hecht SM, Sun JS, Garestier T, Helene C. Specific cleavage of a DNA triple helix by FeII. Bleomycin *Biochem* 1995; **34**(51): 16715–24.

32 Gasparro FP, Havre PA, Olack GA, Gunther EJ, Glazer PM. Site-specific targeting of psoralen photoadducts with a triple helix-forming oligonucleotide: characterization of psoralen monoadduct and crosslink formation. *Nucl Acids Res* 1994; **22**(14): 2845–52.

33 Grant KB, Dervan PB. Sequence-specific alkylation and cleavage of DNA mediated by purine motif triple helix formation. *Biochemistry* 1996; **35**(38): 12,313–9.

34 Wang G, Seidman MM, Glazer PM. Mutagenesis in mammalian cells induced by triple helix formation and transcription-coupled repair. *Science* 1996; **271**(5250): 802–5.

35 Kochetkova M, Shannon MF. DNA triplex formation selectively inhibits granulocyte-macrophage colony-stimulating factor gene expression in human T cells. *J Biol Chem* 1996; **271**(24): 14,438–44.

36 Kochetkova M, Iversen PO, Lopez AF, Shannon MF. Deoxyribonucleic acid triplex formation inhibits granulocyte macrophage colony-stimulating factor gene expression and suppresses growth in juvenile myelomonocytic leukemic cells. *J Clin Invest* 1997; **99**(12): 3000–8.

37 Wang G, Levy DD, Seidman MM, Glazer PM. Targeted mutagenesis in mammalian cells mediated by intracellular triple helix formation. *Mol Cell Biol* 1995; **15**(3): 1759–68.

38 Kren BT, Bandyopadhyay P, Steer CJ. In vivo site-directed mutagenesis of the factor IX gene by chimeric RNA/DNA oligonucleotides [see comments]. *Nat Med* 1998; **4**(3): 285–90.

39 Taubes G. Gene therapy. The strange case of chimeraplasty. *Science* 2002; **298**(5601): 2116–20.

40 Gamper HB, Parekh H, Rice MC, Bruner M, Youkey H, Kmiec EB. The DNA strand of chimeric RNA/DNA oligonucleotides can direct gene repair/conversion activity in mammalian and plant cell-free extracts. *Nucl Acids Res* 2000; **28**(21): 4332–9.

41 Igoucheva O, Alexeev V, Yoon K. Nuclear extracts promote gene correction and strand pairing of oligonucleotides to the homologous plasmid. *Antisense Nucl Acid Drug Dev* 2002; **12**(4): 235–46.

42 Igoucheva O, Alexeev V, Yoon K. Targeted gene correction by small single-stranded oligonucleotides in mammalian cells. *Gene Ther* 2001; **8**(5): 391–9.

43 Yoon K, Igoucheva O, Alexeev V. Expectations and reality in gene repair. *Nat Biotechnol* 2002; **20**(12): 1197–8.

44 Sharma HW, Perez JR, Higgins-Sochaski K, Hsiao R, Narayanan R. Transcription factor decoy approach to decipher the role of NF-kappa B in oncogenesis. *Anticancer Res* 1996; **16**(1): 61–9.

45 Stull RA, Szoka FC Jr. Antigene, ribozyme and aptamer nucleic acid drugs: progress and prospects. *Pharm Res* 1995; **12**(4): 465–83.

46 Kiga D, Futamura Y, Sakamoto K, Yokoyama S. An RNA aptamer to the xanthine/guanine base with a distinctive mode of purine recognition. *Nucl Acids Res* 1998; **26**(7): 1755–60.

47 Toulme JJ, Di Primo C, Moreau S. Modulation of RNA function by oligonucleotides recognizing RNA structure. *Prog Nucl Acid Res Mol Biol* 2001; **69**: 1–46.

48 Kielkopf CL, Baird EE, Dervan PB, Rees DC. Structural basis for GC recognition in the DNA minor groove. *Nat Struct Biol* 1998; **5**(2): 104–9.

49 Kielkopf CL, White S, Szewczyk JW *et al*. A structural basis for recognition of AT and TA base pairs in the minor groove of B-DNA. *Science* 1998; **282**(5386): 111–5.

50 Kielkopf CL, Bremer RE, White S *et al*. Structural effects of DNA sequence on TA recognition by hydroxypyrrole/pyrrole pairs in the minor groove. *J Mol Biol* 2000; **295**(3): 557–67.

51 Goodsell DS. The molecular perspective. *DNA Stem Cells* 2000; **18**(2): 148–9.

52 Urbach AR, Dervan PB. Toward rules for 1 : 1 polyamide: DNA recognition. *Proc Natl Acad Sci U S A* 2001; **98**(8): 4343–8.

53 Goodsell DS. Sequence recognition of DNA by lexitropsins. *Curr Med Chem* 2001; **8**(5): 509–16.

54 Reddy BS, Sharma SK, Lown JW. Recent developments in sequence selective minor groove DNA effectors. *Curr Med Chem* 2001; **8**(5): 475–508.

55 Beelman CA, Parker R. Degradation of mRNA in eukaryotes. *Cell* 1995; **81**(2): 179–83.

56 Liebhaber SA. mRNA stability and the control of gene expression. *Nucl Acids Symp Series* 1997; **36**: 29–32.

57 Baltimore D. Gene therapy. Intracellular immunization [news]. *Nature* 1988; **335**(6189): 395–6.

58 Sullenger BA, Gallardo HF, Ungers GE, Gilboa E. Analysis of trans-acting response decoy RNA-mediated inhibition of human immunodeficiency virus type 1 transactivation. *J Virol* 1991; **65**(12): 6811–6.

59 Bevec D, Volc-Platzer B, Zimmermann K *et al*. Constitutive expression of chimeric neo-Rev response element transcripts suppresses HIV-1 replication in human CD4+ T lymphocytes. *Hum Gene Ther* 1994; **5**(2): 193–201.

60 Weiss IM, Liebhaber SA. Erythroid cell-specific mRNA stability elements in the α_2-globin 3′ non-translated region. *Mol Cell Biol* 1995; **15**(5): 2457–65.

61 Wang X, Kiledjian M, Weiss IM, Liebhaber SA. Detection and characterization of a 3′ untranslated region ribonucleoprotein complex associated with human α-globin mRNA stability. *Mol Cell Biol* 1995; **15**(3): 1769–77. Erratum: *Mol Cell Biol* 1995; **15**(4): 2331.

62 Thisted T, Lyakhov DL, Liebhaber SA. Optimized RNA targets of two closely related triple KH domain proteins, heterogeneous nuclear ribonucleoprotein K and αCP-2KL, suggest distinct modes of RNA recognition. PG-17484-96. *J Biol Chem* 2001; **276**(20): 17,484–96.

63 Scanlon KJ, Ohta Y, Ishida H *et al*. Oligonucleotide-mediated modulation of mammalian gene expression. *Faseb J* 1995; **9**(13): 1288–96.

64 Stein CA. How to design an antisense oligodeoxynucleotide experiment: a consensus approach. *Antisense Nucl Acid Drug Dev* 1998; **8**(2): 129–32.

65 Kole R, Sazani P. Antisense effects in the cell nucleus. modification of splicing. *Curr Opin Mol Ther* 2001; **3**(3): 229–34.

66 Dominski Z, Kole R. Identification and characterization by antisense oligonucleotides of exon and intron sequences required for splicing. *Mol Cell Biol* 1994; **14**(11): 7445–54.

67 Summerton J, Weller D. Morpholino antisense oligomers. Design, preparation, properties. *Antisense Nucl Acid Drug Dev* 1997; **7**(3): 187–95.

68 Iversen PL. Phosphorodiamidate morpholino oligomers: favorable properties for sequence-specific gene inactivation. *Curr Opin Mol Ther* 2001; **3**(3): 235–8.

69 Zamaratski E, Pradeepkumar PI, Chattopadhyaya J. A critical survey of the structure-function of the antisense oligo/RNA heteroduplex as substrate for RNase H. *J Biochem Biophys Meth* 2001; **48**(3): 189–208.

70 Crooke ST. Molecular mechanisms of antisense drugs. RNase H. *Antisense Nucl Acid Drug Dev* 1998; **8**(2): 133–4.

71 Castanotto D, Scherr M, Rossi JJ. Intracellular expression and function of antisense catalytic RNAs. *Meth Enzymol* 2000; **313**: 401–20.

72 Rossi JJ. Ribozymes, genomics and therapeutics. *Chem Biol* 1999; **6**(2): R33–7.

73 Santoro SW, Joyce GF. A general purpose RNA-cleaving DNA enzyme. *Proc Natl Acad Sci U S A* 1997; **94**(9): 4262–6.

74 Wu YYuL, McMahon R, Rossi JJ, Forman SJ, Snyder DS. Inhibition of *bcr-abl* oncogene expression by novel deoxyribozymes (DNAzymes). *Hum Gene Ther* 1999; **10**(17): 2847–57.

75 Hannon GJ. RNA interference. *Nature* 2002; **418**(6894): 244–51.

76 Akhtar S, Kole R, Juliano RL. Stability of antisense DNA oligodeoxynucleotide analogs in cellular extracts and sera. *Life Sci* 1991; **49**(24): 1793–801.

77 Crooke RM, Graham MJ, Cooke ME, Crooke ST. In vitro pharmacokinetics of phosphorothioate antisense oligonucleotides. *J Pharmacol Exp Ther* 1995; **275**(1): 462–73.

78 Agrawal S, Zhao Q. Mixed backbone oligonucleotides: improvement in oligonucleotide-induced toxicity *in vivo*. *Antisense Nucl Acid Drug Dev* 1998; **8**(2): 135–9.

79 Crooke ST. Molecular mechanisms of action of antisense drugs. *Biochim Biophys Acta* 1999; **1489**(1): 31–44.

80 Dewanjee MK, Ghafouripour AK, Kapadvanjwala M *et al*. Noninvasive imaging of *c-myc* oncogene messenger RNA with indium-111-antisense probes in a mammary tumor-bearing mouse model [see comments]. *J Nucl Med* 1994; **35**(6): 1054–63.

81. Gewirtz AM, Stein CA, Glazer PM. Facilitating oligonucleotide delivery. helping antisense deliver on its promise. *Proc Natl Acad Sci U S A* 1996; **93**(8): 3161–3.
82. Stein CA. Is irrelevant cleavage the price of antisense efficacy? *Pharmacol Ther* 2000; **85**(3): 231–6.
83. Zon G. Antisense phosphorothioate oligodeoxynucleotides. Introductory concepts and possible molecular mechanisms of toxicity. *Toxicol Lett* 1995; **82–83**: 419–24.
84. Stein CA, Krieg AM. Problems in interpretation of data derived from *in vitro* and *in vivo* use of antisense oligodeoxynucleotides [editorial]. *Antisense Res Dev* 1994; **4**(2): 67–9.
85. Stein CA. Does antisense exist? *Nat Med* 1995; **1**(11): 1119–21.
86. Wagner RW, Flanagan WM. Antisense technology and prospects for therapy of viral infections and cancer. *Mol Med Today* 1997; **3**(1): 31–8.
87. Iversen PL, Copple BL, Tewary HK. Pharmacology and toxicology of phosphorothioate oligonucleotides in the mouse, rat, monkey and man. *Toxicol Lett* 1995; **82–83**: 425–30.
88. Shaw DR, Rustagi PK, Kandimalla ER, Manning AN, Jiang Z, Agrawal S. Effects of synthetic oligonucleotides on human complement and coagulation. *Biochem Pharmacol* 1997; **53**(8): 1123–32.
89. Gao WY, Han FS, Storm C, Egan W, Cheng YC. Phosphorothioate oligonucleotides are inhibitors of human DNA polymerases and RNase H. Implications for antisense technology. *Mol Pharmacol* 1992; **41**(2): 223–9.
90. Nielsen PE. DNA analogues with nonphosphodiester backbones. *Annu Rev Biophys Biomol Struct* 1995; **24**: 167–83.
91. Morvan F, Porumb H, Degols G et al. Comparative evaluation of seven oligonucleotide analogues as potential antisense agents. *J Med Chem* 1993; **36**(2): 280–7.
92. Lavignon M, Tounekti N, Rayner B et al. Inhibition of murine leukemia viruses by nuclease-resistant alpha-oligonucleotides. *Antisense Res Dev* 1992; **2**(4): 315–24.
93. Gottikh M, Baud-Demattei MV, Lescot E et al. In vitro inhibition of the *pim*-1 protooncogene by chimeric oligodeoxyribonucleotides composed of α- and β-anomeric fragments. *Gene* 1994; **149**(1): 5–12.
94. Monia BP, Lesnik EA, Gonzalez C et al. Evaluation of 2′-modified oligonucleotides containing 2′-deoxy gaps as antisense inhibitors of gene expression. *J Biol Chem* 1993; **268**(19): 14,514–22.
95. Agrawal S, Zhang X, Lu Z et al. Absorption, tissue distribution and *in vivo* stability in rats of a hybrid antisense oligonucleotide following oral administration. *Biochem Pharmacol* 1995; **50**(4): 571–6.
96. Gutierrez AJ, Matteucci MD, Grant D, Matsumura S, Wagner RW, Froehler BC. Antisense gene inhibition by C-5-substituted deoxyuridine-containing oligodeoxynucleotides. *Biochemistry* 1997; **36**(4): 743–8.
97. Moulds C, Lewis JG, Froehler BC et al. Site and mechanism of antisense inhibition by C-5 propyne oligonucleotides. *Biochemistry* 1995; **34**(15): 5044–53.
98. Lewis JG, Lin KY, Kothavale A et al. A serum-resistant cytofectin for cellular delivery of antisense oligodeoxynucleotides and plasmid DNA. *Proc Natl Acad Sci U S A* 1996; **93**(8): 3176–81.
99. Braasch DA, Corey DR. Locked nucleic acid (LNA): fine-tuning the recognition of DNA and RNA. *Chem Biol* 2001; **8**(1): 1–7.
100. Elayadi AN, Corey DR. Application of PNA and LNA oligomers to chemotherapy. *Curr Opin Invest Drugs* 2001; **2**(4): 558–61.
101. Sullenger BA, Gilboa E. Emerging clinical applications of RNA. *Nature* 2002; **418**(6894): 252–8.
102. Pieken WA, Olsen DB, Benseler F, Aurup H, Eckstein F. Kinetic characterization of ribonuclease-resistant 2′-modified hammerhead ribozymes. *Science* 1991; **253**(5017): 314–7.
103. Hertel KJ, Herschlag D, Uhlenbeck OC. A kinetic and thermodynamic framework for the hammerhead ribozyme reaction. *Biochemistry* 1994; **33**(11): 3374–85.
104. Hegg LA, Fedor MJ. Kinetics and thermodynamics of intermolecular catalysis by hairpin ribozymes. *Biochemistry* 1995; **34**(48): 15,813–28.
105. Dahm SC, Uhlenbeck OC. Role of divalent metal ions in the hammerhead RNA cleavage reaction. *Biochemistry* 1991; **30**(39): 9464–9.
106. Rossi JJ. Ribozymes in the nucleolus. *Science* 1999; **285**(5434): 1685.
107. Vaish NK, Kore AR, Eckstein F. Recent developments in the hammerhead ribozyme field. *Nucl Acids Res* 1998; **26**(23): 5237–42.
108. Hampel A. The hairpin ribozyme. Discovery, two-dimensional model, and development for gene therapy. *Prog Nucl Acid Res Mol Biol* 1998; **58**: 1–39.
109. Birikh KR, Heaton PA, Eckstein F. The structure, function and application of the hammerhead ribozyme. *Eur J Biochem* 1997; **245**(1): 1–16.
110. Earnshaw DJ, Gait MJ. Progress toward the structure and therapeutic use of the hairpin ribozyme. *Antisense Nucl Acid Drug Dev* 1997; **7**(4): 403–11.
111. Eckstein F. The hammerhead ribozyme. *Biochem Soc Trans* 1996; **24**(3): 601–4.
112. Kore AR, Eckstein F. Hammerhead ribozyme mechanism: a ribonucleotide 5′ to the substrate cleavage site is not essential. *Biochemistry* 1999; **38**(34): 10,915–8.
113. Vaish NK, Heaton PA, Fedorova O, Eckstein F. In vitro selection of a purine nucleotide-specific hammerheadlike ribozyme. *Proc Natl Acad Sci U S A* 1998; **95**(5): 2158–62.
114. Ferbeyre G, Smith JM, Cedergren R. Schistosome satellite DNA encodes active hammerhead ribozymes. *Mol Cell Biol* 1998; **18**(7): 3880–8.
115. Perriman R, de Feyter R. tRNA delivery systems for ribozymes. *Meth Mol Biol* 1997; **74**: 393–402.
116. Albuquerque-Silva J, Milican F, Bollen A, Houard S. Ribozyme-mediated decrease in mumps virus nucleocapsid mRNA level and progeny in infected vero cells. *Antisense Nucl Acid Drug Dev* 1999; **9**(3): 279–88.
117. Giannini CD, Roth WK, Piiper A, Zeuzem S. Enzymatic and antisense effects of a specific anti-Ki-ras ribozyme *in vitro* and in cell culture. *Nucl Acids Res* 1999; **27**(13): 2737–44.
118. Bramlage B, Alefelder S, Marschall P, Eckstein F. Inhibition of luciferase expression by synthetic hammerhead ribozymes and their cellular uptake. *Nucl Acids Res* 1999; **27**(15): 3159–67.
119. Anderson P, Monforte J, Tritz R, Nesbitt S, Hearst J, Hampel A. Mutagenesis of the hairpin ribozyme. *Nucl Acids Res* 1994; **22**(6): 1096–100.
120. Perez-Ruiz M, Barroso-De I, Jesus A, Berzal-Herranz A. Specificity of the hairpin ribozyme. Sequence requirements surrounding the cleavage site. *J Biol Chem* 1999; **274**(41): 29,376–80.
121. Feldstein PA, Bruening G. Catalytically active geometry in the reversible circularization of 'minimonomer' RNAs derived from the complementary strand of tobacco ringspot virus satellite RNA. *Nucl Acids Res* 1993; **21**(8): 1991–8.
122. Komatsu Y, Koizumi M, Sekiguchi A, Ohtsuka E. Cross-ligation and exchange reactions catalyzed by hairpin ribozymes. *Nucl Acids Res* 1993; **21**(2): 185–90.
123. Dahm SC, Derrick WB, Uhlenbeck OC. Evidence for the role of solvated metal hydroxide in the hammerhead cleavage mechanism. *Biochemistry* 1993; **32**(48): 13,040–5.
124. Young KJ, Gill F, Grasby JA. Metal ions play a passive role in the hairpin ribozyme catalysed reaction. *Nucl Acids Res* 1997; **25**(19): 3760–6.
125. Chowrira BM, Berzal-Herranz A, Burke JM. Ionic requirements for RNA binding, cleavage, and ligation by the hairpin ribozyme. *Biochemistry* 1993; **32**(4): 1088–95.
126. Walter NG, Hampel KJ, Brown KM, Burke JM. Tertiary structure formation in the hairpin ribozyme monitored by fluorescence resonance energy transfer. *Embo J* 1998; **17**(8): 2378–91.
127. Earnshaw DJ, Gait MJ. Hairpin ribozyme cleavage catalyzed by aminoglycoside antibiotics and the polyamine spermine in the absence of metal ions. *Nucl Acids Res* 1998; **26**(24): 5551–61.
128. Seyhan AA, Amaral J, Burke JM. Intracellular RNA cleavage by the hairpin ribozyme. *Nucl Acids Res* 1998; **26**(15): 3494–504.
129. Breaker RR, Joyce GF. A DNA enzyme that cleaves RNA. *Chem Biol* 1994; **1**(4): 223–9.
130. Zhang X, Xu Y, Ling H, Hattori T. Inhibition of infection of incoming HIV-1 virus by RNA-cleaving DNA enzyme. *FEBS Lett* 1999; **458**(2): 151–6.
131. Sharp PA. RNAi and double-strand RNA. *Genes Dev* 1999; **13**(2): 139–41.
132. Nishikura K. A short primer on RNAi: RNA-directed RNA polymerase acts as a key catalyst. *Cell* 2001; **107**(4): 415–8.
133. Agami R. RNAi and related mechanisms and their potential use for therapy. *Curr Opin Chem Biol* 2002; **6**(6): 829–34.
134. Hutvagner G, McLachlan J, Pasquinelli AE, Balint E, Tuschl T, Zamore PD. A cellular function for the RNA-interference enzyme Dicer in the maturation of the let-7 small temporal RNA. *Science* 2001; **293**(5531): 834–8.
135. Ketting RF, Fischer SE, Bernstein E, Sijen T, Hannon GJ, Plasterk RH. Dicer functions in RNA interference and in synthesis of small RNA involved in developmental timing in C. Elegans. *Genes Dev* 2001; **15**(20): 2654–9.
136. Nicholson RH, Nicholson AW. Molecular characterization of a mouse cDNA encoding Dicer, a ribonuclease III ortholog involved in RNA interference. *Mamm Genome* 2002; **13**(2): 67–73.
137. Bernstein E, Caudy AA, Hammond SM, Hannon GJ. Role for a bidentate ribonuclease in the initiation step of RNA interference. *Nature* 2001; **409**(6818): 363–6.
138. Hammond SM, Boettcher S, Caudy AA, Kobayashi R, Hannon GJ. Argonaute 2, a link between genetic and biochemical analyses of RNAi. *Science* 2001; **293**(5532): 1146–50.
139. Williams RW, Rubin GM. ARGONAUTE1 is required for efficient RNA interference in

140 Drosophila embryos. *Proc Natl Acad Sci U S A* 2002; **99**(10): 6889–94.
141 Martinez J, Patkaniowska A, Urlaub H, Luhrmann R, Tuschl T. Single-stranded antisense siRNAs guide target RNA cleavage in RNAi. *Cell* 2002; **110**(5): 563–74.
142 Yang S, Tutton S, Pierce E, Yoon K. Specific double-stranded RNA interference in undifferentiated mouse embryonic stem cells. *Mol Cell Biol* 2001; **21**(22): 7807–16.
143 Bernstein E, Denli AM, Hannon GJ. The rest is silence. *RNA* 2001; **7**(11): 1509–21.
144 Wilda M, Fuchs U, Wossmann W, Borkhardt A. Killing of leukemic cells with a BCR/ABL fusion gene by RNA interference (RNAi). *Oncogene* 2002; **21**(37): 5716–24.
145 McCaffrey AP, Meuse L, Pham TT, Conklin DS, Hannon GJ, Kay MA. RNA interference in adult mice. *Nature* 2002; **418**(6893): 38–9.
146 Lewis DL, Hagstrom JE, Loomis AG, Wolff JA, Herweijer H. Efficient delivery of siRNA for inhibition of gene expression in postnatal mice. *Nat Genet* 2002; **32**(1): 107–8.
147 Yang D, Lu H, Erickson JW. Evidence that processed small dsRNAs may mediate sequence-specific mRNA degradation during RNAi in Drosophila embryos. *Curr Biol* 2000; **10**(19): 1191–200.
148 Zamore PD, Tuschl T, Sharp PA, Bartel DP. RNAi: double-stranded RNA directs the ATP-dependent cleavage of mRNA at 21–23 nucleotide intervals. *Cell* 2000; **101**(1): 25–33.
149 Elbashir SM, Martinez J, Patkaniowska A, Lendeckel W, Tuschl T. Functional anatomy of siRNAs for mediating efficient RNAi in Drosophila melanogaster embryo lysate. *Embo J* 2001; **20**(23): 6877–88.
150 Zeng Y, Cullen BR. RNA interference in human cells is restricted to the cytoplasm. *RNA* 2002; **8**(7): 855–60.
151 Paddison PJ, Caudy AA, Bernstein E, Hannon GJ, Conklin DS. Short hairpin RNAs (shRNAs) induce sequence-specific silencing in mammalian cells. *Genes Dev* 2002; **16**(8): 948–58.
152 McManus MT, Petersen CP, Haines BB, Chen J, Sharp PA. Gene silencing using micro-RNA designed hairpins. *RNA* 2002; **8**(6): 842–50.
153 Miyagishi M, Taira K. U6 promoter driven siRNAs with four uridine 3′ overhangs efficiently suppress targeted gene expression in mammalian cells. *Nat Biotechnol* 2002; **20**(5): 497–500.
154 Paul CP, Good PD, Winer I, Engelke DR. Effective expression of small interfering RNA in human cells. *Nat Biotechnol* 2002; **20**(5): 505–8.
155 Sui G, Soohoo C, Affar el B, Gay F, Shi Y, Forrester WC. A DNA vector-based RNAi technology to suppress gene expression in mammalian cells. *Proc Natl Acad Sci U S A* 2002; **99**(8): 5515–20.
156 Yu JY, DeRuiter SL, Turner DL. RNA interference by expression of short-interfering RNAs and hairpin RNAs in mammalian cells. *Proc Natl Acad Sci U S A* 2002; **99**(9): 6047–52.
157 Donze O, Picard D. RNA interference in mammalian cells using siRNAs synthesized with T7 RNA polymerase. *Nucl Acids Res* 2002; **30**(10): e46.
158 Novina CD, Murray MF, Dykxhoorn DM *et al.* siRNA-directed inhibition of HIV-1 infection. *Nat Med* 2002; **8**(7): 681–6.
159 Lassus P, Rodriguez J, Lazebnik Y. Confirming specificity of RNAi in mammalian cells. *Sci STKE* 2002; **147**: PL13.
160 Holen T, Amarzguioui M, Wiiger MT, Babaie E, Prydz H. Positional effects of short interfering RNAs targeting the human coagulation trigger tissue factor. *Nucl Acids Res* 2002; **30**(8): 1757–66.
161 Sierakowska H, Sambade MJ, Agrawal S, Kole R. Repair of thalassemic human β-globin mRNA in mammalian cells by antisense oligonucleotides. *Proc Natl Acad Sci U S A* 1996; **93**(23): 12,840–4.
162 Sierakowska H, Agrawal S, Kole R. Antisense oligonucleotides as modulators of pre-mRNA splicing. *Meth Mol Biol* 2000; **133**: 223–33.
163 Lacerra G, Sierakowska H, Carestia C *et al.* Restoration of hemoglobin A synthesis in erythroid cells from peripheral blood of thalassemic patients. *Proc Natl Acad Sci U S A* 2000; **97**(17): 9591–6.
164 Mercatante DR, Bortner CD, Cidlowski JA, Kole R. Modification of alternative splicing of Bcl-x pre-mRNA in prostate and breast cancer cells. Analysis of apoptosis and cell death. *J Biol Chem* 2001; **276**(19): 16,411–7.
165 Galbraith WM, Hobson WC, Giclas PC, Schechter PJ, Agrawal S. Complement activation and hemodynamic changes following intravenous administration of phosphorothioate oligonucleotides in the monkey. *Antisense Res Dev* 1994; **4**(3): 201–6.
166 Nemunaitis J, Holmlund JT, Kraynak M *et al.* Phase I evaluation of ISIS 3521, an antisense oligodeoxynucleotide to protein kinase C-α, in patients with advanced cancer. *J Clin Oncol* 1999; **17**(11): 3586–95.
167 Waters JS, Webb A, Cunningham D *et al.* Phase I clinical and pharmacokinetic study of Bcl-2 antisense oligonucleotide therapy in patients with non-Hodgkin's lymphoma [see comments]. *J Clin Oncol* 2000; **18**(9): 1812–23.
168 Chi KN, Gleave ME, Klasa R *et al.* A phase I dose-finding study of combined treatment with an antisense Bcl-2 oligonucleotide (Genasense) and mitoxantrone in patients with metastatic hormone-refractory prostate cancer. *Clin Cancer Res* 2001; **7**(12): 3920–7.
169 Yuen AR, Halsey J, Fisher GA *et al.* Phase I study of an antisense oligonucleotide to protein kinase C-α (ISIS 3521/CGP 64128A) in patients with cancer. *Clin Cancer Res* 1999; **5**(11): 3357–63.
170 Schreiber S, Nikolaus S, Malchow H *et al.* Absence of efficacy of subcutaneous antisense ICAM-1 treatment of chronic active Crohn's disease. *Gastroenterology* 2001; **120**(6): 1339–46.
171 Yacyshyn BR, Bowen-Yacyshyn MB, Jewell L *et al.* A placebo-controlled trial of ICAM-1 antisense oligonucleotide in the treatment of Crohn's disease. *Gastroenterology* 1998; **114**(6): 1133–42.
172 Jansen B, Wacheck V, Heere-Ress E *et al.* Chemosensitisation of malignant melanoma by BCL2 antisense therapy. *Lancet* 2000; **356**(9243): 1728–33.
173 A randomized controlled clinical trial of intravitreous fomivirsen for treatment of newly diagnosed peripheral cytomegalovirus retinitis in patients with aids (1). *Am J Ophthalmol* 2002; **133**(4): 467–74.
174 Cunningham CC, Holmlund JT, Geary RS *et al.* A phase I trial of H-ras antisense oligonucleotide ISIS 2503 administered as a continuous intravenous infusion in patients with advanced carcinoma. *Cancer* 2001; **92**(5): 1265–71.
175 Cunningham CC, Holmlund JT, Schiller JH *et al.* A phase I trial of c-Raf kinase antisense oligonucleotide ISIS 5132 administered as a continuous intravenous infusion in patients with advanced cancer [see comments]. *Clin Cancer Res* 2000; **6**(5): 1626–31.
175 Coudert B, Anthoney A, Fiedler W *et al.* Phase II trial with ISIS 5132 in patients with small-cell (SCLC) and non-small cell (NSCLC) lung cancer. A European Organization for Research and Treatment of Cancer (EORTC) Early Clinical Studies Group report. *Eur J Cancer* 2001; **37**(17): 2194–8.
176 Rudin CM, Holmlund J, Fleming GF *et al.* Phase I Trial of ISIS 5132, an antisense oligonucleotide inhibitor of c-*raf*-1, administered by 24-h weekly infusion to patients with advanced cancer. *Clin Cancer Res* 2001; **7**(5): 1214–20.
177 Roque F, Mon G, Belardi J *et al.* Safety of intracoronary administration of c-*myc* antisense oligomers after percutaneous transluminal coronary angioplasty (PTCA). *Antisense Nucl Acid Drug Dev* 2001; **11**(2): 99–106.
178 Kutryk MJ, Foley DP, van den Brand M *et al.* Local intracoronary administration of antisense oligonucleotide against c-*myc* for the prevention of in-stent restenosis: results of the randomized investigation by the Thoraxcenter of antisense DNA using local delivery and IVUS after coronary stenting (ITALICS) trial. *J Am Coll Cardiol* 2002; **39**(2): 281–7.
179 Andrews DW, Resnicoff M, Flanders AE *et al.* Results of a pilot study involving the use of an antisense oligodeoxynucleotide directed against the insulin-like growth factor type I receptor in malignant astrocytomas. *J Clin Oncol* 2001; **19**(8): 2189–200.
180 Yang E, Korsmeyer SJ. Molecular thanatopsis. A discourse on the BCL2 family and cell death. *Blood* 1996; **88**(2): 386–401.
181 Reed JC. Bcl-2 family proteins. Regulators of chemoresistance in cancer. *Toxicol Lett* 1995; **82–83**: 155–8.
182 Gazitt Y, Rothenberg ML, Hilsenbeck SG, Fey V, Thomas C, Montegomrey W. Bcl-2 overexpression is associated with resistance to paclitaxel, but not gemcitabine, in multiple myeloma cells. *Int J Oncol* 1998; **13**(4): 839–48.
183 Reed JC, Stein C, Subasinghe C *et al.* Antisense-mediated inhibition of BCL2 protooncogene expression and leukemic cell growth and survival: comparisons of phosphodiester and phosphorothioate oligodeoxynucleotides. *Cancer Res* 1990; **50**(20): 6565–70.
184 Webb A, Cunningham D, Cotter F *et al.* BCL-2 antisense therapy in patients with non-Hodgkin lymphoma. *Lancet* 1997; **349**(9059): 1137–41.
185 Mucenski ML, McLain K, Kier AB *et al.* A functional c-*myb* gene is required for normal murine fetal hepatic hematopoiesis. *Cell* 1991; **65**(4): 677–89.
186 Gewirtz AM, Anfossi G, Venturelli D, Valpreda S, Sims R, Calabretta B. G1/S transition in normal human T-lymphocytes requires the nuclear protein encoded by c-*myb*. *Science* 1989; **245**(4914): 180–3.
187 Gewirtz AM, Calabretta B. A c-*myb* antisense oligodeoxynucleotide inhibits normal human hematopoiesis *in vitro*. *Science* 1988; **242**(4883): 1303–6.
188 Lipsick JS. One billion years of Myb. *Oncogene* 1996; **13**(2): 223–35.
189 Bies J, Nazarov V, Wolff L. Identification of protein instability determinants in the carboxy-terminal region of c-Myb removed as a result of retroviral integration in murine monocytic leukemias. *J Virol* 1999; **73**(3): 2038–44.
190 Gewirtz AM. Myb targeted therapeutics for the treatment of human malignancies. *Oncogene* 1999; **18**(19): 3056–62.

191 Luger SM, O'Brien SG, Ratajczak J et al. Oligodeoxynucleotide-mediated inhibition of c-myb gene expression in autografted bone marrow: a pilot study. Blood 2002; 99(4): 1150–8.

192 Dean NM, McKay R, Condon TP, Bennett CF. Inhibition of protein kinase C-α expression in human A549 cells by antisense oligonucleotides inhibits induction of intercellular adhesion molecule 1 (ICAM-1) mRNA by phorbol esters. J Biol Chem 1994; 269(23): 16,416–24.

193 Dean NM, McKay R, Miraglia L et al. Antisense oligonucleotides as inhibitors of signal transduction: development from research tools to therapeutic agents. Biochem Soc Trans 1996; 24(3): 623–9.

194 Dean N, McKay R, Miraglia L et al. Inhibition of growth of human tumor cell lines in nude mice by an antisense oligonucleotide inhibitor of protein kinase C-α expression. Cancer Res 1996; 56(15): 3499–507.

195 Krieg AM, Yi AK, Matson S et al. CpG motifs in bacterial DNA trigger direct B-cell activation. Nature 1995; 374(6522): 546–9.

196 Krug A, Towarowski A, Britsch S et al. Toll-like receptor expression reveals CpG DNA as a unique microbial stimulus for plasmacytoid dendritic cells which synergizes with CD40 ligand to induce high amounts of IL-12. Eur J Immunol 2001; 31(10): 3026–37.

197 Brazolot Millan CL, Weeratna R, Krieg AM, Siegrist CA, Davis HL. CpG DNA can induce strong TH1 humoral and cell-mediated immune responses against hepatitis B surface antigen in young mice. Proc Natl Acad Sci U S A 1998; 95(26): 15553–8.

198 Krieg AM. From bugs to drugs: therapeutic immunomodulation with oligodeoxynucleotides containing CpG sequences from bacterial DNA. Antisense Nucl Acid Drug Dev 2001; 11(3): 181–8.

199 Krieg AM, Yi AK, Schorr J, Davis HL. The role of CpG dinucleotides in DNA vaccines. Trends Microbiol 1998; 6(1): 23–7.

200 Miconnet I, Koenig S, Speiser D et al. CpG are efficient adjuvants for specific CTL induction against tumor antigen-derived peptide. J Immunol 2002; 168(3): 1212–8.

201 Jahrsdorfer B, Hartmann G, Racila E et al. CpG DNA increases primary malignant B cell expression of costimulatory molecules and target antigens. J Leukoc Biol 2001; 69(1): 81–8.

202 Methia N, Louache F, Vainchenker W, Wendling F. Oligodeoxynucleotides antisense to the proto-oncogene c-mpl specifically inhibit in vitro megakaryocytopoiesis. Blood 1993; 82(5): 1395–401.

203 Lamb RF, Hennigan RF, Turnbull K et al. AP-1-mediated invasion requires increased expression of the hyaluronan receptor CD44. Mol Cell Biol 1997; 17(2): 963–76.

204 Stumpf G, Goppelt A, Domdey H. Pre-mRNA topology is important for 3'-end formation in Saccharomyces cerevisiae and mammals. Mol Cell Biol 1996; 16(5): 2204–13.

205 Schreibmayer W, Dessauer CW, Vorobiov D et al. Inhibition of an inwardly rectifying K+ channel by G-protein α-subunits. Nature 1996; 380(6575): 624–7.

206 Duchosal MA, Rothermel AL, McConahey PJ, Dixon FJ, Altieri DC. In vivo immunosuppression by targeting a novel protease receptor [see comments]. Nature 1996; 380(6572): 352–6.

207 Wahlestedt C, Golanov E, Yamamoto S et al. Antisense oligodeoxynucleotides to NMDA-R1 receptor channel protect cortical neurons from excitotoxicity and reduce focal ischaemic infarctions. Nature 1993; 363(6426): 260–3.

208 Mani SK, Fienberg AA, O'Callaghan JP et al. Requirement for DARPP-32 in progesterone-facilitated sexual receptivity in female rats and mice. Science 2000; 287(5455): 1053–6.

209 McMahon SB, Van Buskirk HA, Dugan KA, Copeland TD, Cole MD. The novel ATM-related protein TRRAP is an essential cofactor for the c-Myc and E2F oncoproteins. Cell 1998; 94(3): 363–74.

210 Wraight CJ, White PJ, McKean SC et al. Reversal of epidermal hyperproliferation in psoriasis by insulin-like growth factor I receptor antisense oligonucleotides. Nat Biotechnol 2000; 18(5): 521–6.

211 Dhoot GK, Gustafsson MK, Ai X, Sun W, Standiford DM, Emerson CP Jr. Regulation of Wnt signaling and embryo patterning by an extracellular sulfatase. Science 2001; 293(5535): 1663–6.

212 Good L, Awasthi SK, Dryselius R, Larsson O, Nielsen PE. Bactericidal antisense effects of peptide-PNA conjugates. Nat Biotechnol 2001; 19(4): 360–4.

213 Meshorer E, Erb C, Gazit R et al. Alternative splicing and neuritic mRNA translocation under long-term neuronal hypersensitivity. Science 2002; 295(5554): 508–12.

214 Lebedeva I, Stein CA. Antisense oligonucleotides. Promise and reality. Annu Rev Pharmacol Toxicol 2001; 41: 403–19.

215 Baskerville S, Ellington AD. RNA structure. Describing the elephant. Curr Biol 1995; 5(2): 120–3.

216 Monia BP, Sasmor H, Johnston JF et al. Sequence-specific antitumor activity of a phosphorothioate oligodeoxyribonucleotide targeted to human C-raf kinase supports an antisense mechanism of action in vivo. Proc Natl Acad Sci U S A 1996; 93(26): 15481–4.

217 Sczakiel G, Homann M, Rittner K. Computer-aided search for effective antisense RNA target sequences of the human immunodeficiency virus type 1. Antisense Res Dev 1993; 3(1): 45–52.

218 Milner N, Mir KU, Southern EM. Selecting effective antisense reagents on combinatorial oligonucleotide arrays [see comments]. Nat Biotechnol 1997; 15(6): 537–41.

219 Sohail M, Southern EM. Selecting optimal antisense reagents. Adv Drug Deliv Rev 2000; 44(1): 23–34.

220 Ho SP, Bao Y, Lesher T et al. Mapping of RNA accessible sites for antisense experiments with oligonucleotide libraries [see comments]. Nat Biotechnol 1998; 16(1): 59–63.

221 Scherr M, Rossi JJ, Sczakiel G, Patzel V. RNA accessibility prediction: a theoretical approach is consistent with experimental studies in cell extracts. Nucl Acids Res 2000; 28(13): 2455–61.

222 Ho SP, Britton DH, Bao Y, Scully MS. RNA mapping. Selection of potent oligonucleotide sequences for antisense experiments. Meth Enzymol 2000; 314: 168–83.

223 Sokol DL, Zhang X, Lu P, Gewirtz AM. Real time detection of DNA. RNA hybridization in living cells. Proc Natl Acad Sci U S A 1998; 95(20): 11,538–43.

224 Yakubov LA, Deeva EA, Zarytova VF et al. Mechanism of oligonucleotide uptake by cells: involvement of specific receptors? Proc Natl Acad Sci U S A 1989; 86(17): 6454–8.

225 Beltinger C, Saragovi HU, Smith RM et al. Binding, uptake, and intracellular trafficking of phosphorothioate-modified oligodeoxynucleotides. J Clin Invest 1995; 95(4): 1814–23.

226 Arima H, Aramaki Y, Tsuchiya S. Effects of oligodeoxynucleotides on the physicochemical characteristics and cellular uptake of liposomes. J Pharm Sci 1997; 86(4): 438–42.

227 Laktionov PP, Dazard JE, Vives E et al. Characterisation of membrane oligonucleotide-binding proteins and oligonucleotide uptake in keratinocytes. Nucl Acids Res 1999; 27(11): 2315–24.

228 Laktionov P, Dazard JE, Piette J et al. Uptake of oligonucleotides by keratinocytes. Nucleosides Nucleotides 1999; 18(6–7): 1697–9.

229 Mechti N, Leonetti JP, Clarenc JP, Degols G, Lebleu B. Nuclear location of synthetic oligonucleotides microinjected somatic cells: its implication in an antisense strategy. Nucl Acids Symp Series 1991; 24: 147–50.

230 Clarenc JP, Lebleu B, Leonetti JP. Characterization of the nuclear binding sites of oligodeoxyribonucleotides and their analogs. J Biol Chem 1993; 268(8): 5600–4.

231 Juliano RL, Alahari S, Yoo H, Kole R, Cho M. Antisense pharmacodynamics. Critical issues in the transport and delivery of antisense oligonucleotides. Pharm Res 1999; 16(4): 494–502.

232 DeLong RK, Yoo H, Alahari SK et al. Novel cationic amphiphiles as delivery agents for antisense oligonucleotides. Nucl Acids Res 1999; 27(16): 3334–41.

233 Baer MR, Augustinos P, Kinniburgh AJ. Defective c-myc and c-myb RNA turnover in acute myeloid leukemia cells. Blood 1992; 79(5): 1319–26.

234 Bies J, Nazarov V, Wolff L. Alteration of proteolytic processing of c-Myb as a consequence of its truncation in murine myeloid leukemia. Leukemia 1999; 13(Suppl. 1): S116–7.

235 Kitada S, Miyashita T, Tanaka S, Reed JC. Investigations of antisense oligonucleotides targeted against bcl-2 RNAs. Antisense Res Dev 1993; 3(2): 157–69.

236 Mandiyan S, Schumacher C, Cioffi C et al. Molecular and cellular characterization of baboon C-Raf as a target for antiproliferative effects of antisense oligonucleotides. Antisense Nucl Acid Drug Dev 1997; 7(6): 539–48.

237 Haklai R, Weisz MG, Elad G et al. Dislodgment and accelerated degradation of Ras. Biochemistry 1998; 37(5): 1306–14.

238 Basilion JP, Schievella AR, Burns E et al. Selective killing of cancer cells based on loss of heterozygosity and normal variation in the human genome: a new paradigm for anticancer drug therapy. Mol Pharmacol 1999; 56(2): 359–69.

239 Gewirtz AM. Oligonucleotide therapeutics: a step forward [editorial; comment]. J Clin Oncol 2000; 18(9): 1809–11.

240 Sawyers CL. Research on resistance to cancer drug Gleevec®. Science 2001; 294(5548): 1834.

241 de Smet MD, Meenken CJ, van den Horn GJ. Fomivirsen: a phosphorothioate oligonucleotide for the treatment of CMV retinitis. Ocul Immunol Inflamm 1999; 7(3–4): 189–98.

22

Jerald P. Radich & Marilyn L. Slovak

The Detection and Significance of Minimal Residual Disease

Introduction

Relapse is the nemesis of patients and oncologists alike. Even after the antileukemia assault of the preparative regimen and the immunological effect of the allograft, relapse still is the major obstacle to cure after hematopoietic cell transplantation (HCT). However, sensitive laboratory methods can now identify patients that harbor minimal residual disease (MRD) while appearing in morphological remission. Thus, the detection of MRD can potentially anticipate relapse in these patients. Once identified, patients with a high risk of relapse could potentially undergo additional, pre-emptive therapy to prevent relapse.

The problem of defining remission and relapse is illustrated in Fig. 22.1. At diagnosis patients may have a leukemia burden of up to 10^{10}–10^{12} cells. Thus, even a 3 log depletion of leukemia following therapy would potentially leave up to 10^7–10^9 cells despite the appearance of morphologic remission. Further therapy might decrease the burden of disease even greater, but the depth of this decrease will be unevaluable by conventional pathologic examination. The study of MRD aims to detect and quantify the burden of disease that lies below the threshold of disease monitoring provided by conventional pathological examination. Determining which patients have decreasing disease burden, and those patients in which the kinetics of disease level portends relapse, will better allow physicians to choose the appropriate therapeutic approach.

Methods of MRD detection

The standard approach to evaluate residual leukemia by routine pathologic examination of bone marrow is limited by the sometimes-subtle morphologic differences between malignant and normal cells. Thus, it is not surprising that many patients who have achieved morphological remission eventually relapse. Clearly, more sensitive methods that detect MRD in the face of normal morphology are needed to predict relapse.

Several techniques can define residual disease below the threshold of conventional pathological evaluation. These include "classic" metaphase and molecular cytogenetics, cell "flow" cytometry studies and the polymerase chain reaction (PCR) detection of specific genetic targets (Table 22.1). Each method takes advantage of differences in phenotypic and genotypic characteristics of the tumor cell compared to the normal cell and each has relative advantages, disadvantages and differences in sensitivity.

Conventional metaphase classic cytogenetics can detect approximately one leukemia cell in 10–100 normal cells (denoted in this chapter as "10^{-1}" sensitivity) if 20–50 metaphases are analyzed [1,2]. Cytogenetics remain the method of choice to detect clonal evolution consistent with acceleration of disease in chronic myeloid leukemia (CML), a suspected or evolving secondary hematopoietic disorder, or the emergence of new or minor clonal aberrations not identified at diagnosis (such as structural chromosomal abnormalities including the del(5q), del(6q), del(7q), inv(3q), or del(20q) leukemia post-bone marrow transplantation [BMT]). However, cytogenetics is limited by sampling only those few cells that divide in culture.

Molecular cytogenetics or fluorescence *in situ* hybridization (FISH) is the term to describe the detection of genomic alterations using fluorescent-labeled DNA probes. FISH utilizes chromosome-specific or locus-specific probes to target tumor specific genetic aberrations in metaphase or interphase cells (see Table 22.2 for commonly used DNA FISH probes in hematology/oncology). Widespread clinical applications of FISH techniques include: (a) gains and losses of whole chromosomes or specific chromosomal regions in tumors; (b) detection of deletion or rearrangement

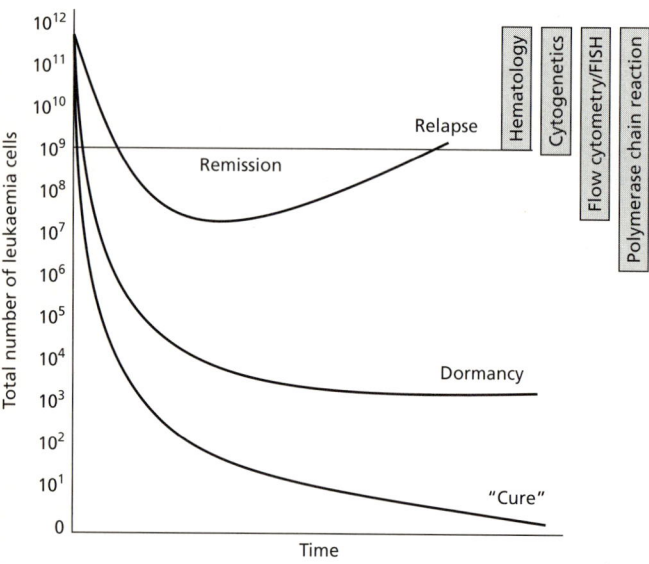

Fig. 22.1 The kinetics of remission induction, relapse, and the detection of minimal residual disease (MRD). Up to 10^{12} leukemia cells may be present in a patient at diagnosis. At remission up to 10^9 leukemia cells may remain, yet be undetected by conventional morphologic examination. More sensitive diagnostic methods such as fluorescence *in situ* hybridization (FISH), flow cytometry and polymerase chain reaction (PCR) based techniques can detect MRD in patients in morphological remission. The goal of MRD studies is to define which patients will have stable or declining MRD vs. those with an increasing burden of disease and who are bound to relapse. As discussed in this chapter, some patients in continued remission nonetheless have persisting low levels of MRD ("dormancy").

Table 22.1 Methods to detect minimal residual disease (MRD).

Method	Target	Sensitivity	Advantages	Disadvantages
Morphology	Cellular morphology	5%	Standard	Poor sensitivity
Cytogenetics	Chromosome structure	1–5%	Widely available	Low sensitivity
FISH	Specific genetic marker(s)	0.08–5.00%*	Fast (1–2 days)	Limited by probe availability
Flow cytometry	Surface antigen expression	0.1–1.0%	Fast (1–2 days) Widely applicable	Limited sensitivity Phenotypic shifts
PCR	DNA or RNA sequence	0.0001–0.1%	Very sensitive	Specific target needed

*Depends on disease, number of probes used and number of nuclei scored.
FISH, fluorescence *in situ* hybridization; PCR, polymerase chain reaction.

Table 22.2 DNA fluorescence *in situ* hybridization (FISH) probes commonly used in hematology/oncology.

DNA probe	Chromosomal location(s)	Common cytogenetic abnormality	Disease/utility
DXZ1-DYZ3	Xcen and Yα sat	Sex mismatch HCT	Any sex mismatched HCT
MYCN	2p24.1	Double minutes/HSR	Neuroblastoma
ALK	2p23	t(2;5)(p23;q35)	ALK lymphoma
D3Z1	3cen	+3	MM
BCL-6	3q27	t(3q27)	NHL
EGR-1-D5S721,D5S23	5q31	−5/del(5)(q31)	MDS/AML
D7Z1	7cen	+7	MM
D7S522-D7Z1	7q31/7cen	−7/del(7)(q22)	MDS/AML
D8Z2	8cen	+8	AML, CML, MDS, MPD, ALL
MYC-IGH	8q24/14q32	t(8;14)(q24;q32)	AML, NHL
MYCC	8q24	t(8;14)(q24;q32) t(2;8)(p11;q24) t(8;22)(q24;q11)	AML, NHL
AML1-ETO	21q22/8q22	t(8;21)(q22;q22)	AML
p16-CEP9	9p21/9cen	del(9p)	ALL, many tumors
BCR-ABL-ASS	9q34/22q11.2	t(9;22)(q34.1;q11.2) & variant translocations	CML, AML, ALL
D11Z1	11cen	+11	MM
ATM	11q22.3	del(11q)	CLL
MLL	11q23	t(4;11) or t(11; *)	MDS/AML, ALL
D12Z3	12cen	+12	CLL
TEL-AML1	12p13/21q22	t(12;21)(p13;q22)	ALL
D13S25	13q14.3	del(13q)	CLL
D13S319-12q34	13q14.3	−13/del(13q)	MM, CLL, MDS, MPD
RB-1	13q14	del(13q)	MDS, MPD
IGH5′-IGH3′	14q32.3	t(14q32)	NHL, CLL, MM, ALL
IGH-CCND1(BCL1)	14q32/11q13	t(11;14)(q13;q32)	Mantle cell lymphoma, MM
IGH-BCL2	14q32/18q22	t(14;18)(q32;q22)	NHL, ALL
PML-RARα	15q22/17q12.1	t(15;17)(q22;q12.1)	AML-M3
CBFβ or MYH11-CBFβ	16p13/16q22	inv(16)(p13;q22) (p13;q22) or t(16;16)	AML-M4Eo
TP53	17p13.1	del(17)(p13.1)	CML, CLL, AML, many tumors
HER-2/neu	17q11.2-q12	Double minutes/HSR	Breast
RARα	17q12.1	Variant t(17q12.1)	AML-M3
API1-MALT1	11q21/18q21	t(11;18)(q21;q21)	MALT lymphoma
D20S108	20q12	del(20q)	MDS, AML, MPD
AML1	21q22	+21 and del or t(21q)	AML, ALL

ALK, anaplastic lymphoma kinase; ALL, acute lymphoblastic leukemia; AML, acute myeloid leukemia; CLL, chronic lymphocytic leukemia; CML, chronic myeloid leukemia; HCT, hematopoietic cell transplantation; HSR, homogeneously staining region; MALT, mucosa associated lymphoid disease; MDS, myelodysplastic syndrome; MM, multiple myeloma; MPD, myeloproliferative disorder; NHL, non-Hodgkin's lymphoma.

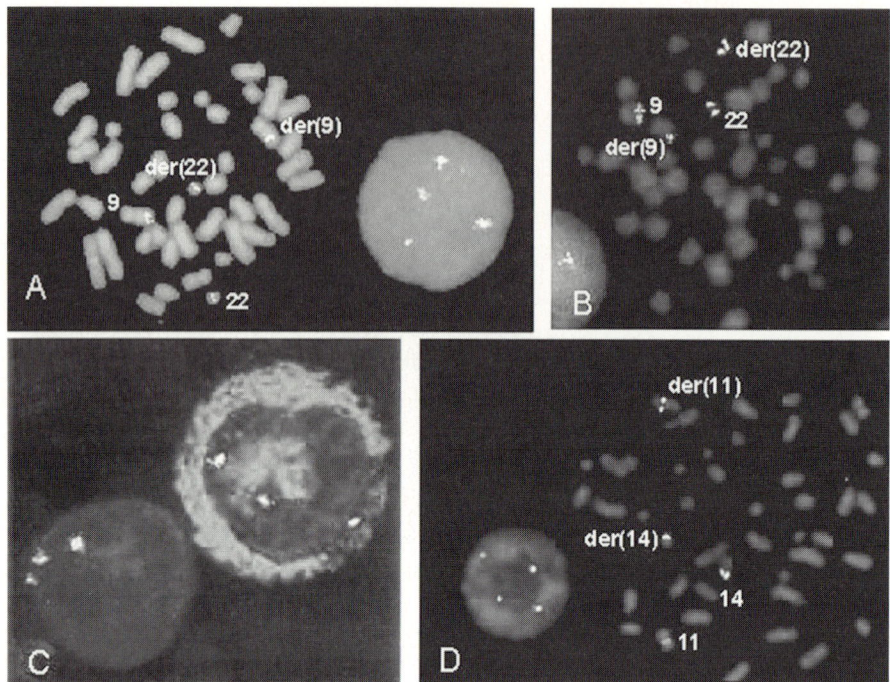

Fig. 22.2 Examples of molecular cytogenetics or fluorescence *in situ* hybridization (FISH) techniques commonly used to monitor minimal residual disease. (a) Triple probe/triple color FISH for the detection of the *BCR-ABL* gene rearrangement. Fluorescence signals from a Philadelphia chromosome positive (Ph+) metaphase and interphase cell, *ABL* (red on 9q34.1), *BCR* (green on 22q11.2) and *ASS* (aqua, 9q34.1 flanking region proximal to ABL). The der(22)t(9,22) is observed as a red/green/yellow fusion signal. The red/blue signal indicates normal chromosome 9 homologue; the green signal indicates normal chromosome 22 homologue. Chromosome with the single aqua signal is the derivative chromosome 9. The aqua signal on the der(9) indicates the *ASS* or arginine succinate synthese gene which flanks the *ABL* gene is not deleted. (b) Hypermetaphase spread hybridized with the triple probe/triple color FISH for the detection of the *BCR-ABL* gene rearrangement. Note the chromosomes are highly contracted in comparison with the conventional cytogenetic spread observed in panel (a). (c) FICTION (Fluorescent Immunophenotyping and Interphase Cytogenetics as a Tool for Investigation of Neoplasms) detecting both immunophenotype and genotype simultaneously. Trisomy 8 (three blue-green signals) was detected in a CD15 positive cell (upper right) as well as the CD15 negative cell (lower left). (d) Dual color, dual fusion LSI IgH/CCND1 (Vysis, Inc., Downers Grove, IL) detects the t(11,14)(q13;q32) observed in mantle cell lymphoma and multiple myeloma. The signal pattern shows two orange/green (yellow) fusion signals (arrows), one on each abnormal chromosome 11 and 14, in addition to the single orange and green signal identifying the normal chromosome 11 and 14, respectively, in both the interphase nucleus (right) and the metaphase (left) cell (*see also Plate 22.1, facing p. 296*).

of a single gene; (c) defining "cryptic" chromosome translocations not identified by conventional cytogenetics; (d) refining or revealing specific aberrations of complex karyotypes; (e) assessing the gene copy number of oncogenes or tumor suppressor genes (e.g. *HER2/neu* amplification in breast cancer or loss of *TP53* in leukemia); and (f) monitoring a patient's clinical course (e.g. engraftment of a sex-mismatched HCT) (Fig. 22.2; see also Plates 22.1 & 22.2, *facing p. 296*). FISH allows for a rapid screening of 200–10,000 cells for numerical chromosomal aberrations, even in samples insufficient for conventional cytogenetic analysis, and has the ability to identify minor abnormal clones undetected by karyotypic study [3]. Compared to conventional cytogenetic analysis, the sensitivity of FISH technology alone is between 10^{-1} and 10^{-3}, depending on the number of probes and number of nuclei scored. In general, FISH at disease presentation is recommended to determine baseline data, the signal pattern associated with complex and variant forms of common translocations and, perhaps, to detect clonal flanking region deletions as observed in 10–15% Philadelphia chromosome-positive (Ph+) CML [4,5]. The sensitivity of FISH may be increased by special techniques, such as "hypermetaphase" preparations [6] (Fig. 22.2b), in combination with morphology [7], immunophenotyping (Fig. 22.2c), by flow-sorted cell populations or by the simultaneous use of multiple DNA probes, the latter increasing sensitivity of the FISH assay to 10^{-3}–10^{-4} (Plate 22.1, *facing p. 296*) [8]. The main technical limitations of FISH are probe availability, false negative results due to inefficiencies of hybridization, loss of cells, subjective scoring, and false positive results due to nonspecific probe hybridization or chance colocalization of signals in interphase nuclei mimicking a translocation event. The recent introduction of automated hybridization and scoring will soon lessen the labor and time-intensive aspects of scoring large numbers of cells for MRD.

Hypermetaphase FISH is a simple extension of FISH whereby cells are cultured for 12 h in the presence of a high concentration of colcemid, a mitotic spindle poison. This prolonged exposure to colcemid allows for the visualization and quantification of chromosomal aberrations in 500–>2000 overly contracted mitotic cells, with high reliability, increased sensitivity and rapid analysis time (Fig. 22.2b; see also Plate 22.1, *facing p. 296*) [9–11]. Although less sensitive than PCR for the detection of MRD, the analysis of 1000 mitotic cells for a tumor specific marker may allow for the quantification of *proliferating* residual tumor cells. Hypermetaphase-FISH is most useful to monitor leukemias characterized by a translocation, trisomy or large deletions for which a FISH probe is available. However, only cells that enter cell division are evaluable and, due to overly contracted chromosomes and poorly spread metaphases, this assay is not suitable for MRD detection of monosomy, subtle deletions, or for identifying clonal evolution of disease.

Cell surface antigen expression can distinguish malignant from normal cells. While truly tumor-specific antigens are rare, malignant cells often express cell surface antigens in subtly different patterns than normal cells [3,6]. By using combinations of multiple antibodies, "multiparametric"

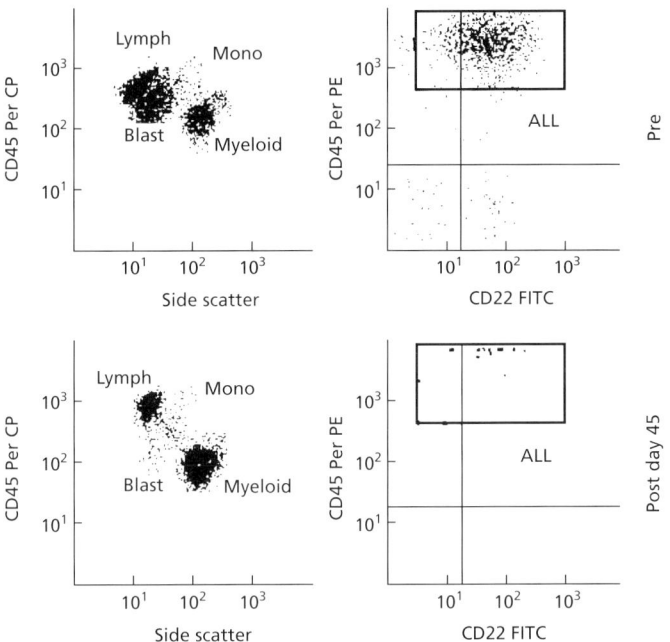

Fig. 22.3 Flow cytometric analysis of a female patient with acute lymphoblastic leukemia (ALL) at presentation (top panels) and during morphological remission following marrow transplantation from a male donor (bottom panels). At diagnosis the blasts were characterized by expression of increased CD45, CD34 and CD22 (top panels). A specimen obtained at day 45 post-transplant was in morphologic remission; however, a residual population of blasts with the same expression signature was identified at 0.2% of total nucleated cells. These suspicious cells were isolated and interrogated by fluorescence *in situ* hybridization (FISH) for the presence of X and Y chromosomes. The abnormal cells identified post-HCT were found to be 97% female while the control population of lymphocytes and neutrophils were 99% male. Figure courtesy of Dr Mike Loken. (*See also Plate 22.3, facing p. 296.*)

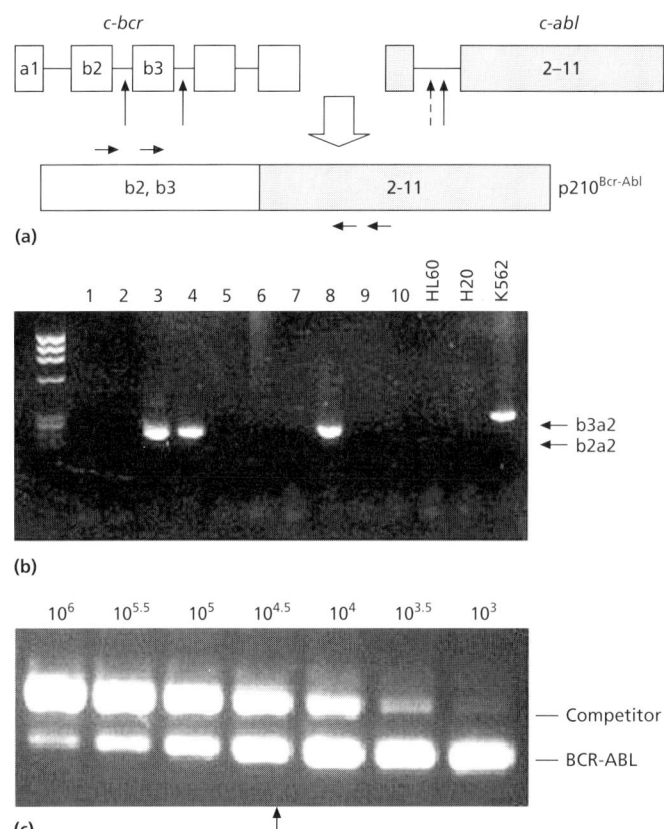

Fig. 22.4 The chimeric *bcr-abl* transcript in chronic myeloid leukemia (CML). Panel a shows the breakpoint in the bcr region of the *BCR* gene, which joins head-to-tail with the downstream *ABL* gene domains. This unique fusion gene causes the expression of the chimeric *bcr-abl* messenger RNA (mRNA), which is the template for sensitive reverse transcription-polymerase chain reaction (RT-PCR) reactions, shown in panel b. Semiquantitative RT-PCR can be achieved by "spiking" a reaction with serial dilutions of a known, engineered competitor molecule (panel c). The point at which the PCR end product of the unknown is equal in intensity to the known competitor is used as an estimate of the starting material of the unknown (arrow). Figure courtesy of Dr N. Cross and Dr J. Goldman.

flow cytometric assays uses aberrant antigen expression patterns to "fingerprint" the malignant clone (Fig. 22.3; see also Plate 22.3, *facing p. 296*). If combinations of several antibodies are used to define the aberrant antigen expression, the sensitivity can reach as low as 10^{-2}–10^{-4} in experienced hands [12,13]. This technique has been very useful in acute myeloid leukemia (AML) and acute lymphoblastic leukemia (ALL), where leukemia blasts often have evidence of abnormal antigen expression compared to normal hematopoietic cells [13,14]. In some diseases (e.g. chronic phase CML) flow cytometry is not particularly useful, since the leukemia does not display a clearly aberrant phenotype compared to normal mature granulocytes. The advantage of flow cytometry is that is relatively fast and is applicable in many cases, particularly in the acute leukemias. The disadvantages include a decreased sensitivity compared to PCR (see below) and the possibility of false negative studies due to immunophenotypic shifts that may occur in some leukemic cases, whereby the relapsed sample has a different immunophenotype than the initial diagnostic sample [15,16].

The most sensitive approach to detect MRD involves nucleic acid amplification using the PCR [17]. Unlike conventional cytogenetics or flow cytometry, a specific genetic lesion is the "fingerprint" of the malignancy in order for PCR-driven reactions to have the desired sensitivity and specificity. The power of PCR results from the exponential amplification of the specific target nucleic acid sequence; after 30 cycles of amplification, the target sequence is amplified greater than a million-fold. Gene translocations, such as t(9;22) in CML (Fig. 22.4) and t(15;17),t(8;21) and inv(16)/t(16;16) found in AML, are straightforward leukemia-specific markers for the detection of MRD [18–24]. However, given the progress in identifying disease-specific translocations, translocations can be detected and amplified in 40–50% of AML and ALL [25]. In addition, leukemia-specific "fingerprints" generated by the rearrangement of the immunoglobulin heavy chain (IgH) and T-cell receptor (TCR) can be used to monitor MRD in lymphoid malignancies [26,27]. In general, the advantages of PCR are the excellent sensitivity and specificity. Disadvantages include the potential of false positive results from contamination of the amplified product and false negatives due to RNA degradation, and the inability to detect translocations in cases where the breakpoint is highly variable and spans large DNA sequences, for example, t(11;14)(q13;q32) in mantle cell lymphoma (Fig. 22.2d; see also Plate 22.1, *facing p. 296*).

A qualitative PCR reaction (where the end product of the PCR reaction is visualized after gel electrophoresis) is poorly suited for quantification given the robust amplification of the PCR reaction (Fig. 22.4). However, at higher target concentrations the reaction eventually reaches a "plateau phase", where exponential amplification can no longer occur. This plateau may not occur in reactions beginning with very few target genes. Thus, a reaction that starts with a few copies of a target gene may at the end of the PCR have an amount of amplified products similar to the amplification product from a reaction starting with an abundance of a

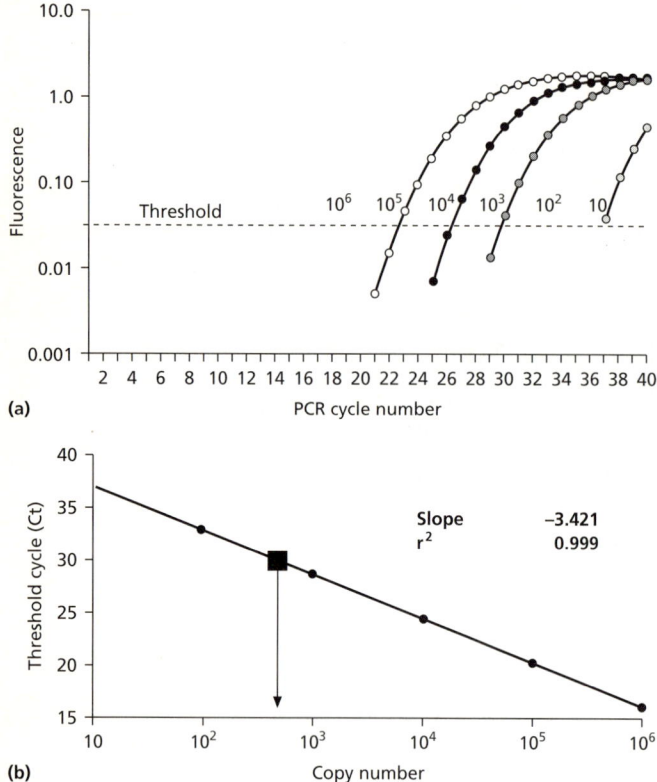

Fig. 22.5 Quantitative reverse transcription-polymerase chain reaction (RT-PCR) of the *bcr-abl* messanger RNA (mRNA) using the 5′exonuclease fluorogenic assay ("Taqman™"). Serial dilutions of a known control are first performed (a). From this control series one defines an arbitrary fluorescent threshold and, next, the starting copy number of template is plotted against the cycle number that each target reaction reached the threshold value (b). Unknowns are run and the cycle number needed to reach the threshold determined. Once this is known, the initial target amount of the unknown is back-calculated from the standard curve (arrow). Figure courtesy of Dr T. Hughes.

target gene. Several strategies for quantification have evolved. Earliest attempts used a synthetic competitor gene added to the sample that was to be quantified (Fig. 22.4). Typically the sample needs to be run in series with varying known dilutions of the competitor. The starting amount of the target gene is estimated when the intensity of the PCR product run on the gel is the same as the competitor target. This semiquantitative approach is difficult for many reasons: Competitor targets must be engineered; each assay requires several PCR reactions; the kinetics of amplification must be similar between the target and the competitor; and the determination of the PCR product (usually from dosimetric density analysis of the gel) must be accurate. Fortunately several manufacturers have developed "real time" PCR reactions that analyze the accumulation of PCR products by laser excitation of fluorochromes that accumulate during the PCR (Fig. 22.5). For example, in the "Taqman™" system [28] the PCR takes place with the addition of an internal probe that includes a 5′ fluorescent reporter molecule and a 3′ quencher molecule. As polymerization takes place from the upstream PCR primer the Taq polymerase encounters the probe and cleaves of the 5′ reporter secondary to the enzymes intrinsic 5′ exonuclease activity. The liberated reporter is excited by a laser that assays the PCR reaction several times per cycle. As PCR proceeds, reporter is continually released and its accumulation is recorded over each PCR cycle. A series of positive control dilutions are run to generate a standard curve describing the cycle number needed to reach an arbitrary fluorescent "threshold." From this standard curve the initial starting amount of target gene in the "unknowns" can be inferred by observing the cycle number taken to reach the defined threshold, then "back-calculating" to the starting target number from the standard curve. Such real-time PCR reactions have now become the standard of quantitative PCR (Q-PCR) because of their relative ease and reproducibility.

MRD detection in conventional therapy

Over the past several years, numerous studies of MRD detection in patients treated with conventional chemotherapy have been reported. The clinical import of these studies is to define the optimal timing and identify those patients who would clearly benefit from transplantation therapy, with the expectation that transplantation would lead to a higher cure rate.

In ALL, the detection of clonal IgH or TCR genes (Fig. 22.6 [29]), or the detection of aberrant blasts by multicolor flow cytometry, is associated with a high risk of subsequent relapse [26,27,30]. The relative risk of relapse in patients with MRD compared to those without MRD ranges from three to 10-fold. Cave *et al.* [26] recently reported an analysis of 246 pediatric patients enrolled in a multicenter ALL trial using junctional sequences of TCR or immunoglobulin variable-diversity-junctional (VDJ) gene rearrangements as clonal markers of leukemic cells. Residual disease detection was performed in a semiquantitative manner using a limiting dilution technique. Detection of MRD at levels $>10^{-2}$ after induction therapy was associated with a high relative risk of subsequent relapse compared to patients without MRD (relative risk = 16), whereas after consolidation and interval therapy the breakpoint of MRD burden $>10^{-3}$ was associated with a relative risk of seven and nine, respectively. Presence of MRD continued to be strongly associated with subsequent relapse even after other known risk factors for relapse such as age, white count and immunophenotype were factored into a multivariate model. In a similar patient population, van Dongen *et al.* [31] used MRD results from two separate time points (after receipt of induction chemotherapy and before consolidation chemotherapy) to classify patients into three separate risk groups for subsequent relapse. Patients with levels of MRD $>10^{-3}$ at both time points had a poor outcome, with a relapse rate of 79%. On the other end of the spectrum, patients who were MRD negative at both time points had a relapse rate of only 2%. Patients with MRD between these levels had an intermediate relapse rate of 23%. Taken together, both studies suggest that detection of MRD can distinguish a population of patients with a substantially higher risk of relapse from remaining patients.

Two additional groups also recently investigated MRD detection by PCR in pediatric ALL. In a retrospective study of 66 children, the presence of MRD was determined in cases that remained in complete remission (CR), vs. those that eventually went on to relapse. In those patients that remained in CR, the proportion who had evidence of MRD was 32%, 10% and 0% at 1, 3 and 5 months into therapy, respectively, compared with 82%, 60% and 41%, respectively, amongst the cohort who eventually experienced relapse [32]. MRD-positive patients had a 10-fold greater risk of subsequent relapse than those lacking detectable leukemia in CR. Similarly, Evans *et al.* [33] evaluated bone marrow specimens from 42 pediatric ALL patients before their second course of intensification chemotherapy at week 20. To simplify the analysis, consensus fluorescent IgH primers were used to detect patient-specific gene rearrangements. While the assay was considerably less sensitive (10^{-3} sensitivity) than a radioactive probe assay, it was performed with greater ease and less cost, since patient-specific primers were not used. Nine of the 30 evaluable patients had detectable MRD and eight of nine subsequently experienced relapse. Unfortunately, a significant portion (29%) of the other 21 patients without detectable MRD also had recurrent disease. Despite the fact that the assay did not accurately predict relapse in all patients, the 5-year disease-free survival (DFS) was 10% vs. 80% for the

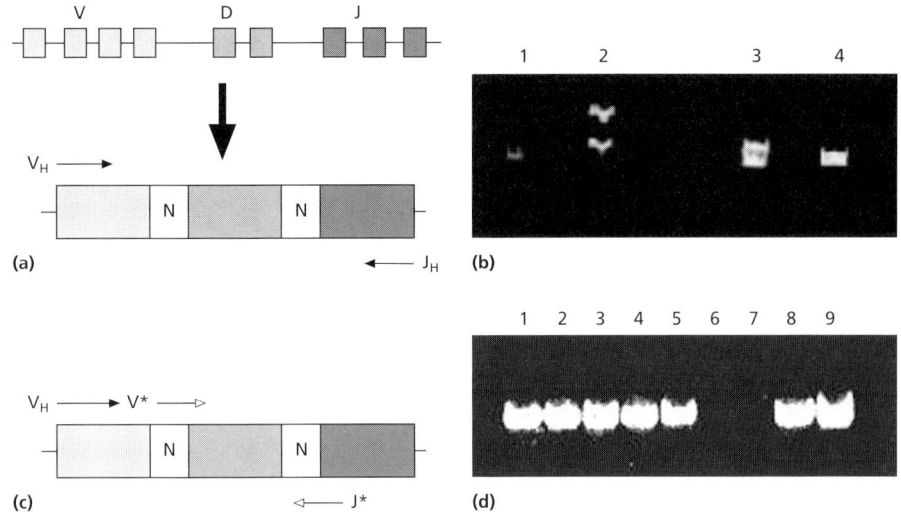

Fig. 22.6 The amplification of immunoglobulin heavy chain (IgH) variable, diversity, and junctional gene rearrangements in acute lymphoblastic leukemia (ALL). (a) The *HgH* genes rearrange from the germline configuration to form a B-cell specific IgH *V-D-J* gene rearrangement. Variable and junction consensus primers (shown as V_H and J_H) are used to amplify diagnostic ALL samples, which show single or multiple bands indicative of a predominance of clonal B cells, each cell having the same IgH *V-D-J* rearrangement. Panel b shows the amplification of four diagnostic ALL samples. The clonal rearrangements can be extracted from the gel and their sequences determined by direct nucleotide sequencing. With this data leukemia-specific primers can be made (V^* and J^* in panel C). The leukemia-specific primers are used to amplify remission samples in order to detect minimal residual disease (MRD). Lanes 1–5 in panel d are a log dilution series from 100% ALL to 10^{-5}, with lanes 6 and 7 the amplification of normal bone marrow and water, respectively. Lanes 8 and 9 are duplicates of a bone marrow in a patient in remission by conventional morphology; amplification with leukemia-specific primers demonstrates the persistence of MRD. Reproduced with permission from Radich *et al.* [29].

MRD-positive and MRD-negative patients, respectively. Taken together, the data suggest that detection of MRD is associated with relapse at either the end of induction, or later during consolidation.

It should be noted, however, that false negatives occur (that is, relapse in a patient who was previously MRD negative) because of clonal evolution of the leukemia, whereby a leukemia with a new gene rearrangement emerges at relapse [34,35]. This is a relatively infrequent occurrence and is generally seen in patients with late relapse rather than those patients who relapse relatively quickly. To prevent against this type of false negative results, some investigators recommend using two different patient-specific markers (for example, an IgH VDJ marker and a TCR marker), as clonal evolution of both markers appears unusual [36].

In AML, translocations such as t(15;17),t(8;21) and inv(16) occur with sufficient frequency to perform PCR-based studies of MRD detection and outcome, but they only account for approximately 20–30% of AML cases as characterized by conventional cytogenetics. Persistence of RNA for PML/RARα in patients in CR has previously been shown to be associated with a high risk of subsequent relapse. This observation has been confirmed in a large prospective study of 163 acute promyelocytic leukemia (APL) patients who received all *trans* retinoic acid (ATRA), idarubicin induction and three courses of consolidation therapy [37]. Because patients were excluded from the analysis if less than two PCR assays were performed, those patients who relapsed before their second test were not included. This exclusion might have introduced a bias favoring the capability of the PCR test to predict relapse in the remaining patients on study. Of the 163 patients, 21 subsequently became positive for MRD and 20 out of 21 patients experienced relapse at a median time of 3 months from the first positive assay. Conversely, only eight of 142 patients without evidence of MRD detected during CR experienced relapse. Hence, patients harboring MRD detected by PCR were 32 times more likely to subsequently experience relapse than those without MRD were. Thus, even with the possible introduction of bias, MRD detection by PCR was a powerful tool to identify patients at an especially high risk of relapse.

In small pilot studies, PCR quantification has been used to monitor the number of chimeric transcripts present in bone marrow specimens at various timepoints during therapy. Tobal *et al.* [81] used this technique in six adults with AML characterized by inv(16) and showed a decline in the number of abnormal CBFβ/MYH11 transcripts in patients who achieved a CR, compared to a slow disappearance and subsequent reemergence in a patient who eventually experienced relapse. In support of the graft-vs.-leukemia (GVL) effect known to occur after allogeneic transplants, CBFβ/MYH11 transcript levels decreased two to three orders of magnitude in two patients when they developed graft-vs.-host disease (GVHD). Similarly, Marcucci *et al.* [39] developed a "real time" Q-PCR assay for the AML1/ETO fusion transcript seen in patients with t(8;21) AML. A 2–4 log reduction of abnormal transcript number after induction therapy was observed in all five patients who had diagnostic and post-therapy samples available. Two patients experienced subsequent recurrence after serially increasing numbers of AML1/ETO copy number. However, one patient experienced relapse despite a stable AML1/ETO fusion transcript number in comparison with the remission value. Hence increasing copy number predicted relapse in only a portion of patients with t(8;21).

In CML, Q-PCR for the *bcr-abl* can help define a population of patients in cytogenetic remission who have a prolonged course of remission (Fig. 22.6). Quantitative detection of CML patients treated with the tyrosine kinase inhibitor imatinib mesylate (STI571, Gleevec®) may help in guiding therapy in regards to the depth of cytogenetic remission. Furthermore, FISH analysis has confirmed ~10–15% of Ph+ rearrangements have large deletions adjacent to the translocation breakpoint on the derivative nine chromosome, on the additional partner chromosome, or on both [40–42]. Early evidence suggests CML with derivative nine deletions is associated with a more rapid onset of blast crisis and resistance to interferon therapy [4,40]. Patients with a relatively high burden of MRD, increasing levels of *bcr-abl*, or der(9) deletions may be offered transplantation.

MRD detection in CML post-HCT

CML is the most powerful example of using MRD detection to shape therapy and potentially prevent relapse. Molecular detection and quanti-

Table 22.3 Minimal residual disease (MRD) detection post-hematopoietic cell transplantation (HCT).

Disease	Genetic target	Associated with relapse?	Comments
ALL	IgH VDJ	Yes	Detection before and after HCT is meaningful
Ph+	bcr-abl	Yes	p190 bcr-abl may be worse than p210
AML t(15;17)	PML-RARα	Yes	Levels $>10^{-3}$ associated with relapse after conventional therapy
t(8;21)	AML1-ETO	Maybe	Even "cured" patients are often PCR+; quantification will likely help
inv(16)/t(16;16)	CFBF-MYH11	Maybe	Unclear association
CML	bcr-abl	Yes	Relapse risk higher in T depleted. Quantification helps define relapse risk
NHL	Bcl2-IgH IgH V-D-J	Yes	
Myeloma	IgH VDJ/t(14q) −13/del(13q)	Probably	Very few studies
CLL	IgH VDJ 11q abn/17p del	Yes	Association stronger after autologous compared to allogeneic transplant

ALL, acute lymphoblastic leukemia; AML, acute myeloid leukemia; CLL, chronic lymphocytic leukemia; CML, chronic myeloid leukemia; HCT, hematopoietic cell transplantation; NHL, non-Hodgkin's lymphoma; PCR, polymerase chain reaction; Ph+, Philadelphia chromosome positive.

fication of bcr-abl may be performed on either peripheral blood or bone marrow specimens [43]. The qualitative detection of bcr-abl post-HCT is associated with relapse, but the strength of the effect varies according to the type of transplant and the time from transplant [43–49]. In CML, Q-PCR and FISH methods are the methods of choice in monitoring MRD. Q-FISH is favored by some centers due to the improved overall sensitivity of the second generation Bcr-Abl FISH probes, its ability to detect persistent or increasing number of abnormal cells in sequential samples, the detection of der(9) deletions and for those rare cases with variant Ph+ breakpoints falling outside the PCR primer regions. However, Q-PCR of the bcr-abl burden has been more widely studied and holds more immediate promise in refining and strengthening the predictive value of residual disease detection. Note that in the following sections, it is implied that the detection of MRD occurs in patients who appear to be in remission by conventional pathological techniques.

Risk of relapse and time from transplant

The highest risk of relapse associated with bcr-abl detection appears to be associated "early" (≤12 months) after transplant [43,45,49]. In a study of 346 patients post-HCT a single positive qualitative PCR assay for bcr-abl was associated with an elevated risk of relapse [43,45,49]. The predictive value of bcr-abl detection was strongest at 6–12 months post-BMT, where the presence of bcr-abl was associated with a 42% risk of relapse at a median of 200 days from the first PCR-positive result, as opposed to a 3% risk of relapse in PCR-negative patients. Tests earlier than 3 months post-HCT were not strongly associated with relapse. The relative risk of relapse associated with MRD was approximately 30 even after controlling for clinical variables associated with relapse, such as phase of disease and GVHD status. A study of nearly 400 patients has shown that if studied between 18 and 30 months post-HCT, 25% of patients will have at least one bcr-abl positive assay, but only 16% will relapse, compared to 1% in bcr-abl-negative patients [50]. In addition, studies at the Hammersmith Hospital in London, England, have shown that patients can be divided into patients continuously bcr-abl negative post-HCT, those with only one low level bcr-abl result and those that fulfilled their criteria for relapse [51]. In the patients with no or low level MRD, there was only one relapse among 63 patients with no history of MRD and eight of 20 patients (an estimated cumulative incidence of relapse of 54%) with low level disease.

MRD can be detected by Q-PCR for years post-HCT. Bcr-abl has been detected in 25–50% of patients ≥3 years post-transplant, with subsequent relapse rates of ~10–20% [43,44,50,52]. Costello et al. [52] found that 66 out of 117 (56%) CML patients were positive ≥3 years post-BMT but only 8% subsequently relapsed. Van Rhee et al. [53] reported 19 patients in CR for more that 10 years post-BMT, two of whom were still positive for bcr-abl. A semiquantitative assay demonstrated that bcr-abl transcript levels were very low in these patients. These data suggest that MRD in CML patient years post-HCT may not be an absolute harbinger of relapse. These patients are only candidates for intervention trials of treating molecular relapse if quantitative bcr-abl levels suggest an increasing disease burden.

Risk of relapse and donor status

The immunologic effect associated with an allograft (GVL effect) may influence the risk of relapse associated with bcr-abl detection. Unrelated donor (URD) transplants, which have a lower risk of relapse after HCT compared to matched-related transplants (presumably owing to an increased GVL effect) had a similar prevalence of bcr-abl-positivity at 6–12 months post-HCT compared to related HCT patients (25% vs. 30%), but the subsequent relapse rate was much greater in the bcr-abl-positive related donor group compared to the bcr-abl-positive URD recipients (~60% vs. 10%) [43]. This observation suggests the GVL effect may be working to control the leukemic clones that have escaped the conditioning regimen in the URD transplants. The subsequent study of "late" bcr-abl positivity showed no difference of relapse rate of URD compared to matched-related transplants [54]. This finding may reflect the immune tolerance that occurs in URD patients as time elapses, ameliorating the GVL effect.

Pichert and colleagues described the immunologic effect in controlling relapse by studying 48 T-cell-depleted and 44 recipients of untreated marrow grafts [44]. They found that over 80% of patients receiving T-cell-depleted marrow were bcr-abl positive 6–24 months post-transplant,

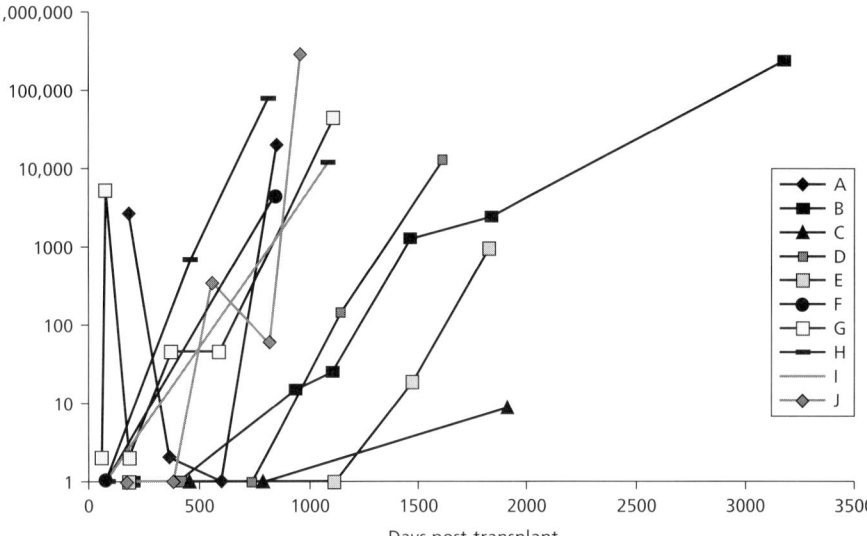

Fig. 22.7 The kinetics of *bcr-abl* emergence in CML patients who eventually relapsed after HCT. The figure shows the increase of *bcr-abl* copy number in 11 cases that eventually relapsed after HCT. Reproduced with permission from Radich et al. [50].

compared to 25% of patients receiving unmanipulated marrow. *Bcr-abl* detection was highly associated with relapse, which occurred predominately in the recipients of T-cell-depleted grafts. Furthermore, Mackinnon et al. [55] studied 36 patients following T-cell-depleted marrow HCT. Thirty of 36 patients (83%) were positive for *bcr-abl* post-HCT, and 60% of these MRD-positive patients relapsed. Of the 20 patients who became MRD positive within 6 months post-transplant, 15 (84%) eventually relapsed. Thus, while T-cell depletion limits the morbidity of GVHD, the burden of relapse is greater and may necessitate donor T-cell infusions in those patients who have MRD post-transplant. In addition, anecdotal reports of low levels of cytogenetic relapse disappearing with the removal of immunosuppression suggest the power of the GVL effect on low tumor burdens.

Quantitative studies for *bcr-abl* in CML

The predictive value of MRD detection in CML is strengthened by *bcr-abl* quantification (so-called "quantitative PCR" [Q-PCR or Q-FISH]) [50,51,56–60]. The use of Q-PCR has been pioneered in the study of MRD in CML. Lin and colleagues studied 69 patients with a competitive Q-PCR and demonstrated that the kinetics of *bcr-abl* level over time described both impending relapse and response to donor leukocyte infusion after relapse [56]. Low (or no) residual *bcr-abl* was associated with a very low risk of relapse (1%), compared to 75% relapse rate in patients with increasing or persistently high *bcr-abl* levels. Patients who relapsed had doubling times of the *bcr-abl* transcript level twice that of patients who did not relapse (15 vs. 25 days). Recently, Olavarria et al. [59] studied 138 CML patients "early" (3–5 months) post-transplant and showed that the *bcr-abl* level was highly correlated with relapse. Patients with no evidence of *bcr-abl* transcripts had a 9% risk of subsequent cytogenetic or hematologic relapse, whereas patients defined as having a "low" burden of disease (<100 *bcr-abl* transcripts/µg RNA) or "high" level of transcripts (>100 copies/µg) had a cumulative relapse rate of 30% and 74%, respectively. These results are consistent with the high risk of relapse associated with early qualitative *bcr-abl* positivity at 6 months post-BMT formerly reported [43,46]. In addition, we evaluated the qualitative and quantitative assessment of MRD in 379 CML patients "late" (>18 months) post-HCT [50]. Ninety patients (24%) had at least one assay positive for *bcr-abl and* 13 of the 90 (14%) relapsed. Conversely, three of 289 patients who were persistent *bcr-abl* negative relapsed (hazard ratio of relapse = 19). Quantification of *bcr-abl* level was performed on 344 samples from 85 patients and a rising *bcr-abl* heralded eventual relapse (Fig. 22.7 [50]). Alternatively, El-Rifai and colleagues followed 25 patients in clinical remission post-HCT by hypermetaphase Q-FISH, usually analyzing 1000 mitotic cells per sample [61]. In this study, eight patients (32%) had detectable residual CML cells at a median of 17 months post-HCT. Hematologic relapse occurred in three patients, including two patients with residual Ph+ cells detected at 2 and 8 months prior to relapse with an increase in the number of Ph+ cells in subsequent studies. The absence of Ph+ cells predicted continuing remission and Ph+ studies that remained stable over 1 year did not predict relapse. Q-FISH detects MRD in nearly 25% of CML cases within the first 6 months of HCT compared ~25–70% with qualitative PCR [43,45,47,62]. This discrepancy results from the increased sensitivity of PCR, which detects transcripts regardless of proliferative status, whereas hypermetaphase FISH quantifys only proliferating residual CML cells, which may be more relevant in predicting relapse in CML. Taken together, a simple qualitative reverse transcription-polymerase chain reaction (RT-PCR) assay for *bcr-abl* can identify patients who need close follow-up, while quantification can indicate those who might benefit from early therapeutic intervention.

Relapses are rare among patients who are *bcr-abl* negative post-HCT [43,44,47,50,52]. Does this mean that there are no, or very few, residual CML cells in these patients, or that there could be a pool of slowly proliferating CML cells that express little or no *bcr-abl* messenger RNA (mRNA) and thus escape detection? Cases where the *Bcr-Abl* gene is detected without *bcr-abl* mRNA expression are unusual [63–67] and suggest that patients who are PCR negative for *bcr-abl* mRNA do not commonly have a reservoir of cells that might become positive at a later time. Thus, it is unlikely that there is a large pool of *bcr-abl*-negative patients at risk for relapse.

In summary, MRD data in CML show that "molecular relapse" of *bcr-abl* is common in CML patients following transplantation. A qualitative *bcr-abl* result has prognostic importance and further refinement by quantitative assays detects patients who would benefit from early intervention.

MRD detection in acute leukemia post-HCT

In CML the detection of MRD is simplified by the near-universal prevalence of the t(9;22) or Philadelphia (Ph) chromosome rearrangement. Such is not the case in the acute leukemias, where multiple genetic abnormalities have been described, so that approximately 40% of cases will have some variety of genetic fingerprint [25]. The detection of MRD is made more difficult since the acute leukemias progress more quickly than CML, increasing the likelihood of tumor evading detection if the testing intervals are not sufficiently frequent.

MRD in ALL post-transplant

The detection of MRD in patients who are in CR after conventional chemotherapy may be associated with outcome after transplantation. Knechtli et al. [68] studied 71 pediatric patients who underwent allogeneic HCT. Using a semiquantitative assay to categorize patients of having no, low or high MRD burden, the level of MRD in "remission" patients was strongly associated with subsequent outcome after HCT, with the 2-year event-free survival (EFS) for no, low and high MRD disease being 73%, 36% and 0%, respectively. A subsequent study [69] also demonstrated the effect of pretransplant MRD testing in remission patients. Of the 15 patients with pretransplant positive assays for MRD, seven relapsed, compared to three relapses in the 17 patients without MRD. The association of MRD and relapse was stronger in the autologous group, where all patients with pretransplant MRD subsequently relapsed. Flow cytometry has also been used to detect MRD in remission patients. In a study of remission patients, six of the 24 had MRD prior to transplant, while 18 of the 24 were MRD negative [70]. DFS after HCT for these two groups were 33% and 74%, respectively. The burden of disease prior to transplant has also been seen in Ph+ ALL, as the 3-year DFS post-HCT for patients in relapse, patients in remission but with detectable MRD by RT-PCR of bcr-abl, and with patients in remission and free of MRD, was approximately 20%, 40% and 60%, respectively [71]. Thus, the detection of MRD at the time of transplantation is likely associated with worse outcomes compared to patients with a leukemia burden below the level of MRD detection.

The data for the detection of MRD and outcome is limited for ALL, although it appears that MRD detection prior to transplant (as noted above) and following transplantation both are strongly predictive of outcome. Studies have examined MRD detection following transplant and have also found it predictive of outcome. IgH V-D-J detection was used in 20 allogeneic transplant recipients to detect MRD, and it was found that the presence of MRD within the first 100 days after HCT was associated with a sixfold increase in relapse rate compared to PCR-negative patients [29]. Indeed, all patients who were PCR positive died after transplant; the median time from first PCR-positive assay to relapse was 30 days (median, 6–250 days). A subsequent study of 71 pediatric ALL patients after allogeneic HCT demonstrated that MRD detection at any time after transplant was a poor prognostic sign [72]. Of the 32 patients who relapsed, 16 were persistently positive for MRD, while 12 became positive at a median of 3 months prior to frank relapse. Of the 36 patients who remained in remission, only eight were MRD positive at any time post-HCT. The odds ratio for relapse associated with MRD detection in the first 3 months following transplantation was ninefold. Other studies have found MRD equally predictive of relapse, with DFS in patients without MRD >70%, compared to DFS rates of <30% in patients with MRD following transplant [69].

The Ph chromosome can be found in 5–25% of pediatric and adult ALL patients and is the MRD marker of choice in these patients. In Ph+ ALL, however, PCR must be performed on both variants of the bcr-abl chimeric mRNA, the "p210" bcr-abl variant (found in CML and some cases of ALL) and the "p190" bcr-abl (found only rarely in CML but common in ALL). Miyamura et al. [73] studied 13 patients after allogeneic ($n = 8$) and autologous ($n = 5$) transplant and found that a positive PCR assay for bcr-abl in the first 12 months following transplant was predictive of relapse. All seven patients who were PCR positive relapsed, whereas only one of six MRD-negative patients relapsed. A later study of 37 Ph+ ALL patients [74] showed the clinical utility of bcr-abl detection and fundamental differences in p190 and p210 Ph+ ALL. The relative risk of relapse of patients with a positive PCR (either p210 or p190) post-BMT compared to PCR-negative patients was approximately sixfold. Those patients with p190 bcr-abl had an 88% relapse rate in comparison to 12% for patients who expressed the p210 bcr-abl transcript. A follow-up study of 90 Ph+ ALL cases confirmed the high risk of relapse associated with the detection of bcr-abl post-HCT, with the presence of the p190 variant carrying a relative risk of relapse of ninefold compared to bcr-abl undetectable patients [71]. Similarly, hypermetaphase Q-FISH analyzing ~1000 cells for the Ph+ chromosome translocation or trisomy in 13 ALL patients treated by HCT indicated that the detection of more than 1% abnormal cells predicted relapse whereas lower levels of detection were consistent with continued clinical and hematologic remission [11].

MRD in AML post-transplant

There are few studies documenting the prevalence and significance of MRD in AML following HCT. This is due largely to the fact that the most common translocations found in AML (the t(15;17), t(8;21) and inv(16)/t(16;16) gene rearrangements), while occurring in aggregate in 20–30% of AML cases, are associated with intermediate or good outcomes with conventional chemotherapy and thus are under-represented in the transplant population. The significance of MRD depends on the specific genetic subtype of AML. In t(15;17) AML, the detection of the PML/RARα transcript following HCT is highly correlated with relapse [75,76] and follows the conventional chemotherapy MRD data, where the molecular detection of PML/RARα is highly correlated with relapse [37,77]. In t(8;21), conversely, the detection of AM1/ETO by RT-PCR is often found in patients for years following conventional chemotherapy and thus is not tightly linked to outcome [23,78]. Remarkably, the persistence of MRD occurs even after allogeneic transplant, where many patients remain with evidence of MRD, yet do not relapse [39,79,80]. In the largest study of t(8;21) AML, nine of 10 patients examined after an allogeneic HCT were positive from 7 to 83 months post-BMT and none relapsed [80]. There are few cases of inv(16)/t(16;16) detection described and it is difficult to make a conclusion as to the significance of MRD [38,81,82]. In one study of 10 patients receiving an autologous ($n = 2$) or an allogeneic ($n = 8$) transplant, three of the four patients with MRD after transplant relapsed, compared to none of the six patients without MRD [82]. In contrast, Q-FISH has proven to be a reliable technique to detect residual trisomy 8, t(8;21), t(15;17) and 7q deletions in AML [11]. For example, all four t(8;21) AML patients who received HCT were found to be negative by Q-FISH yet positive by RT-PCR for all sequential samples tested 18–108 months post-HCT. Of the four patients with chromosome 7 aberrations, the sole HCT patient did not show any abnormal cells post-HCT and remained in CR 30 months post-HCT whereas the three patients who received chemotherapy only showed MRD in follow-up samples and died of relapse. Although additional confirmatory studies are needed, in general, patients in CR who showed a persistent or increasing number of abnormal cells in two or more subsequent samples, or whose initial samples contained more than 1% abnormal cells, relapsed. Regardless, the above reports suggest that the risk of relapse associated with the absence of MRD is quite low.

The use of the tumor suppressor gene WT1 has been used as a marker of MRD following HCT [83]. The expression of this gene is found to be elevated in AML and ALL compared to bone marrow and peripheral blood and, thus, has some potential for a marker of MRD. Elmaagacli et al. [83] studied 38 patients post-HCT and fourteen of the 38 were positive for elevated WT1 at least once post-transplant. Of the 14 patients positive for MRD, seven relapsed, compared to five relapses in the 34 patients without MRD. In 17 of these patients, translocation markers were available and the authors were able to test the concordance of the leukemia-specific translocation and WT1 expression. These assays were concordant 70% of the time; in the discordant 30% roughly one-half were positive for the leukemia-specific marker and negative of WT1. Thus, while not absolutely predictive of relapse, the WT1 assay may be a useful tool for assessing risk of relapse.

MRD in other malignancies post-HCT

Other B-lineage hematologic malignancies, such as multiple myeloma, chronic lymphocytic leukemia (CLL) and non-Hodgkin's lymphoma (NHL), can be studied by similar strategies employed to study MRD in ALL, using IgH *V-D-J* rearrangements as a patient-specific disease marker. Two studies in multiple myeloma have shown that approximately one-half of patients will become MRD negative following transplantation, but the relapse rate appears similar in the MRD-positive and MRD-negative group [84,85]. Most myeloma patients who achieved a CR after allogeneic transplant became MRD negative after 6 months, but in many in took >2 years to become free of measurable MRD, with one case taking 6 years to achieve MRD negativity.

In CLL it appears that the detection of MRD by PCR or flow cytometry is predictive of subsequent relapse, especially in the context of autologous transplants [86–88]. Using a flow cytometry technique capable of detecting CLL cells at a 10^{-4} level, Rawstron *et al.* [88] found a strong correlation of quantitative level of CLL in peripheral blood and bone marrow. In 25 cases who achieved a CR after CAMPATH-1H antibody or autologous transplant, 19 were MRD-free at the time of CR and their EFS was >90%; in contrast, all six patients with MRD at the time of CR subsequently relapsed. Similar results were reported by Esteve *et al.* [86] who found that four of the five patients who had MRD while in CR following autologous transplant eventually relapsed, compared to two of the nine patients without MRD. Of the 12 patients who had an allogeneic transplant, only one of the eight cases had MRD at last contact. Some cases took up to 4 years to clear MRD following the allogeneic transplant and these patients stayed MRD-free for another year of follow-up. The slow clearance of MRD has been observed in other studies following allogeneic transplant, as well as after nonmyeloablative transplants, as some patients became MRD negative >6 months post-transplant [54,86]. Taken in whole, these studies suggest that the detection of MRD is strongly associated with relapse following autologous transplant, but MRD is tolerated and indeed slowly cleared following allogeneic transplant.

Risk-assessment to define good and poor prognostic groups are facilitated by molecular diagnostics, particularly FISH analyzes for specific cytogenetic abnormalities. Large prospective trials are needed in multiple myeloma to better define the exact prognostic value of 14q32 rearrangements and chromosome 13 changes which are frequently detected by Q-FISH. Early clinical trials suggest that patients with 14q32 rearrangements, in particular the t(4;14), t(11;14) and/or chromosome 13 aberrations, benefit from intensive chemotherapy strategies. However, the number of patients with molecular genetic studies at presentation and sequential follow-up studies post-allogeneic HCT are few [89]. Because aberrations of chromosome 13 and 14q32 are associated with poor progression-free and overall survival in multiple myeloma, interphase FISH is now recommended to monitor the new tandem transplant regimens utilizing monoclonal antibodies and nonmyeloablative HCT [90].

In addition, MRD detection by interphase FISH in CLL may play an important role in the selection and monitoring of patients receiving nonmyeloablative HCT. Analyzing mononuclear cells from 325 CLL patients using a panel of FISH DNA probes, Dohner *et al.* [91] identified chromosomal aberrations in 82% of cases allowing for the definition of five major prognostic categories: 17p/TP53 deletions, 11q/ATM deletions, trisomy 12, normal karyotype and 13q deletion as the sole anomaly. The 17p/TP53 and 11q/ATM deleted subgroups were associated with nonmutated immunoglobulin V genes and had more advanced disease ($p <0.001$) compared to the other genetic groups, with a 1 year median treatment-free interval [91,92]. In contrast, CLL patients with trisomy 12 had a reported 114 month median survival, a finding comparable to those CLL patients with normal karyotypes (median, 111 months) and patients with 13q abnormalities had a benign clinical course, surviving as long as age- and sex-matched controls (median, 133 months). These data provide the clinical framework for MRD detection and monitoring in CLL "proposed" risk-adapted prognostic groups; namely, younger B-CLL patients with 17p/TP53 and 11q/ATM deletions potentially benefiting from conventional HCT approaches, whereas nonmyeloablative transplantation may provide potentially curative options for elderly CLL patients with aggressive disease.

In NHL MRD studies have been principally employed to study the issue of purging in autologous transplants (the method and results of stem cell purging are discussed in detail in Chapters 19 & 20). Gribben *et al.* [93,94] demonstrated that the detection of MRD (using PCR to detect the *bcl2/IgH* gene rearrangement) after antibody purging of the bone marrow stem cell product prior to autologous transplant for low-grade follicular lymphoma was associated with an inferior outcome and higher relapse rates. Relapse tended to occur at the primary site of disease rather than disseminated relapse, suggesting that infusion of stem cells was not the primary cause of relapse. A more recent study in NHL also suggested a correlation of MRD in stem cell product and subsequent relapse [95]. In a study of 105 patients undergoing autologous transplant, 19 of the 46 patients randomized to a BMT were analyzed for MRD, while 22 of the 47 patients entering the peripheral blood stem cell (PBSC) transplant had MRD assays. Ten of the 19 bone marrow and 15 of the 22 PBSC products were positive for MRD. In both transplant groups, patients with no MRD enjoyed better survival than those with MRD, although the effect achieved statistical significance in the bone marrow group (EFS 68% vs. 30% in bone marrow, 42% vs. 28% in PBSC group, for MRD-negative and MRD-positive patients, respectively). In sum, the data suggests that MRD level in the stem cell product is associated with outcome, mostly as a "biosensor" of disease burden and sensitivity, rather than as the source of relapse.

Potential limitations of MRD research

While the results of many studies support the strong association of MRD and relapse, there are several limitations to applying this work prospectively. First, the association of MRD and relapse may be treatment dependent; that is, the risk of relapse may vary with treatment protocols that use different drugs and treatment schedules. Secondly, in many studies, the testing intervals for MRD are not rigidly enforced and this confounds assigning risk of relapse based on a series of MRD tests. For example, the clinical significance of two positive tests at 1 and 12 months post-transplant is likely different than at 1 and 2 months post-transplant. Q-PCR may make prediction of relapse more accurate, but interpretation of Q-PCR is also not entirely straightforward. For example, a finding of 1000 copies of the target MRD transcript can either occur if one cell produced 1000 copies of target mRNA or if 1000 leukemic cells each produced a single copy. The implications on relapse of these two situations are likely quite different. Moreover, attempts to judge relapse by the rates of increase of MRD are limited by the assumption that increases are steady and limited. For example, the rate of MRD change calculated from two Q-PCR measurements at 6 to 12 months post-transplant will give the same result in a case with a steady increase from 6 to 12 months vs. a disease that is steady from 6 to 11 months and then jumps to the same 12 month level. Because of these considerations, it should be emphasized that definitions of "molecular relapse" determined by retrospective studies should be prospectively validated in another study before being used in studies using MRD to drive new therapeutic interventions.

Even with the appeal of Q-PCR, it remains uncertain whether quantification will provide more relevant and predictive data than a less expensive qualitative test performed at frequent time intervals. Indeed, although multiparameter flow cytometry and FISH may not be as sensitive as PCR, it may eventually be shown that they predict relapse equally well. Head-to-head studies comparing the various methods of MRD are lacking, but would be greatly welcomed.

Dormancy

One of the more fascinating sidelights of MRD studies is the discovery that many patients who are "cured" have persistence of molecular disease. This has been noted after hematopoietic stem cell transplantation in CML [43,52,96] as well as in acute leukemia following conventional chemotherapy. For example, in t(8;21) AML molecular evidence of the AML1/ETO fusion mRNA is found in most patients years into continued remission. The AML1/ETO mRNA can be found in a minority of lymphoid and erythroid colonies taken from remission samples [97], implying that (a) the disease may be of "stem cell" origin and (b) that MRD detection may sometimes detect nonmyeloid cells bearing the translocation. Of additional interest is the observation that pediatric ALL patients who relapsed after 10 continuous years of remission following conventional chemotherapy present with a leukemia possessing the same clonal IgH V-D-J gene rearrangement as initially present at diagnosis [98]. The apparent "dormancy" of a leukemic clone in a disease as aggressive as ALL is quite provocative.

Why do not all patients with MRD eventually relapse? There are several potential mechanisms of dormancy (which are not mutually exclusive): (i) Prolonged immune surveillance, especially in the transplant setting; (ii) the detection of cells whose lineage is not principally involved (for unknown reasons) with the leukemia; (iii) the persistence of "preleukemic" clonal disease without the full complement of genetic lesions required for the development of frank malignancy; or (iv) the presence of a secondary genetic lesion that may render the leukemic progenitor cells relatively quiescent. Regardless, it appears that a functional "cure" of leukemia is not equivalent to the total eradication of all leukemic or preleukemic cells. The discovery of the mechanisms of dormancy may lead to inroads in defining what it takes to "cure" leukemia.

Translocations in "normals"

A common assumption in MRD is that translocation targets (e.g. bcr-abl) are "disease-specific": that is, only found in leukemic, not normal, cells. It has become clear that the reality is not so simple. Several studies have found "disease-specific" translocations in normal people. Both the BCL2/IgH rearrangement found in follicular lymphoma and the bcr-abl chimeric mRNA of CML have been found in nearly 40% of adults [99–102]. These studies have used modified PCR assays to effectively increase the sensitivity of detection more than a log over that of conventional assays employed in MRD studies. The frequency of these translocations in normal people increased with age and semiquantitative PCR assays suggest that positive cells were very rare beneath the threshold of PCR detection used in routine PCR assays. Thus, the presence of translocations in normal individuals may have little consequence towards generating false positive assays in MRD studies. Rather, the interesting question is *why* translocations occur in normal individuals. The increasing prevalence of translocation with increasing age begs the question if these genetic events represent a biomarker of increasing damage from environmental sources with years and/or decreased genetic repair occurring with increasing patient age.

The treatment of MRD

The promise of MRD detection is the potential use of early therapy to prevent relapse. Is there any evidence that the treatment of MRD works? Van Rhee et al. [103] treated 14 CML patients in hematologic, cytogenetic or molecular (i.e. bcr-abl positive) relapse with donor leukocyte infusions. Of the seven patients with hematologic relapse, three had a complete cytogenetic response to donor leukocyte infusions; however, two of these patients developed aplasia. Three patients with cytogenetic relapse and two patients with only *bcr-abl* molecular positivity were treated; all had a complete response and there were no aplastic events. There was no clear difference in the incidence of severe GVHD among the three groups. Thus, patients treated earlier in the course of relapse had improved response and fewer complications. Further studies of donor-leukocyte-infusion administration post-HCT have also suggested the potentially increased efficacy of treating a lower disease burden afforded by MRD testing [53,104–106]. In the previously cited study by the Hammersmith group [51], 20 patients who fit their definition of "molecular relapse" were treated with donor leukocyte infusions and all remained in molecular remission for 5 years of follow-up. Lastly, single patient reports exist showing the resolution of MRD as detected by WT1 or inv(16)/t(16;16) detection in AML post-HCT [107]. Both reports note the resolution of MRD after donor leukocyte infusion given for MRD up to 21 and 16 months of follow-up, respectively.

In the near future, novel therapeutic approaches may be used to treat MRD in the post-HCT setting. For example, the tyrosine kinase inhibitor, imatinib mesylate (STI571, Gleevec®), has shown remarkable promise in the treatment of interferon-resistant CML and, given its low toxicity profile, seems a logical choice for the treatment of MRD in CML patients. Indeed, a recent study showed that imatinib mesylate given to transplant patients suffering a cytogenetic relapse was effective in promoting a cytogenetic response in some patients [107]. Thus in 28 cases of relapsed CML following HCT, a complete cytogenetic response occurred in nine of the 28 (35%) and the cytogenetic response rate was greater for patients who relapsed in chronic phase rather than in progressive disease. In the future the effectiveness of imatinib for post-HCT relapse may be greater if the drug is directed at treating molecular relapse as determined by sensitive PCR techniques.

Conclusion

In sum, the studies of MRD suggest that (i) the detection of MRD is strongly associated with relapse; (ii) quantification of MRD by Q-PCR, Q-FISH, or flow cytometric techniques further defines the patients at risk of relapse; and (iii) not all patients with MRD relapse, particularly in the allogeneic setting, but even following conventional chemotherapy. Lastly, the recognition of "dormancy" suggests that "cure" does not equal the elimination of all leukemic or preleukemic cells. Understanding the mechanism of "dormancy" may allow us to adopt therapies to achieve that state, rather than persist in high-dose therapy designed to eliminate leukemia, which may be impossible.

The detection of MRD should play a pivotal role in how we manage patients with hematologic malignancies. Studies of MRD in CML patients receiving imatinib, and in acute leukemia patients receiving chemotherapy, can indicate those patients with measurable residual disease burden that need more aggressive therapy with transplantation. The importance of large clinical studies aimed at clarifying the clinical utility of MRD detection cannot be overemphasized, and all clinicians should enroll patients onto these trials, for only then can we translate what is still predominantly bench research to relevance at the bedside.

References

1 Hook EB. Exclusion of chromosomal mosaicism: tables of 90%, 95% and 99% confidence limits and comments on use. *Am J Hum Genet* 1977; **29**(1): 94–7.

2 Arthur CK, Apperley JF, Guo AP, Rassool F, Gao LM, Goldman JM. Cytogenetic events after bone marrow transplantation for chronic myeloid leukemia in chronic phase. *Blood* 1988; **71**(5): 1179–86.

3 Brizard F, Brizard A, Guilhot F, Tanzer J, Berger R. Detection of monosomy 7 and trisomies 8 and 11 in myelodysplastic disorders by interphase fluorescent *in situ* hybridization. Comparison with acute non-lymphocytic leukemias. *Leukemia* 1994; **8**(6): 1005–11.

4 Huntly BJ, Reid AG, Bench AJ et al. Deletions of the derivative chromosome 9 occur at the time of the Philadelphia translocation and provide a powerful and independent prognostic indicator in chronic myeloid leukemia. *Blood* 2001; **98**(6): 1732–8.

5 Sinclair PB, Nacheva EP, Leversha M et al. Large deletions at the t(9;22) breakpoint are common and may identify a poor–prognosis subgroup of patients with chronic myeloid leukemia. *Blood* 2000; **95**(3): 738–43.

6 Nylund SJ, Ruutu T, Saarinen U, Knuutila S. Metaphase fluorescence *in situ* hybridization (FISH) in the follow-up of 60 patients with haemopoietic malignancies. *Br J Haematol* 1994; **88**(4): 778–83.

7 Bernell P, Arvidsson I, Jacobsson B, Hast R. Fluorescence *in situ* hybridization in combination with morphology detects minimal residual disease in remission and heralds relapse in acute leukaemia. *Br J Haematol* 1996; **95**(4): 666–72.

8 Slovak ML, Zhang F, Tcheurekdjian L et al. Targeting multiple genetic aberrations in isolated tumor cells by spectral fluorescence *in situ* hybridization. *Cancer Detect Prev* 2002; **26**(3): 171–9.

9 Seong D, Giralt S, Fischer H et al. Usefulness of detection of minimal residual disease by "hypermetaphase" fluorescent *in situ* hybridization after allogeneic BMT for chronic myelogenous leukemia. *Bone Marrow Transplant* 1997; **19**(6): 565–70.

10 El-Rifai W, Ruutu T, Elonen E, Volin L, Knuutila S. Prognostic value of metaphase-fluorescence *in situ* hybridization in follow-up of patients with acute myeloid leukemia in remission. *Blood* 1997; **89**(9): 3330–4.

11 El-Rifai W, Ruutu T, Vettenranta K et al. Follow-up of residual disease using metaphase-FISH in patients with acute lymphoblastic leukemia in remission. *Leukemia* 1997; **11**(5): 633–8.

12 Neale GA, Coustan-Smith E, Pan Q et al. Tandem application of flow cytometry and polymerase chain reaction for comprehensive detection of minimal residual disease in childhood acute lymphoblastic leukemia. *Leukemia* 1999; **13**(8): 1221–6.

13 Coustan-Smith E, Behm FG, Sanchez J et al. Immunological detection of minimal residual disease in children with acute lymphoblastic leukaemia. *Lancet* 1998; **351**(9102): 550–4.

14 Sievers EL, Lange BJ, Buckley JD et al. Prediction of relapse of pediatric acute myeloid leukemia by use of multidimensional flow cytometry. *J Natl Cancer Inst* 1996; **88**(20): 1483–8.

15 Szczepanski T, Orfao A, van der Velden VH, San Miguel JF, van Dongen JJ. Minimal residual disease in leukaemia patients. *Lancet Oncol* 2001; **2**(7): 409–17.

16 Campana D, Coustan-Smith E. Advances in the immunological monitoring of childhood acute lymphoblastic leukaemia. *Best Pract Res Clin Haematol* 2002; **15**(1): 1–19.

17 Saiki RK, Gelfand DH, Stoffel S et al. Primer-directed enzymatic amplification of DNA with a thermostable DNA polymerase. *Science* 1988; **239**(4839): 487–91.

18 Claxton DF, Liu P, Hsu HB et al. Detection of fusion transcripts generated by the inversion 16 chromosome in acute myelogenous leukemia. *Blood* 1994; **83**(7): 1750–6.

19 Kawasaki ES, Clark SS, Coyne MY et al. Diagnosis of chronic myeloid and acute lymphocytic leukemias by detection of leukemia-specific mRNA sequences amplified *in vitro*. *Proc Natl Acad Sci U S A* 1988; **85**(15): 5698–702.

20 Lee MS, Chang KS, Cabanillas F, Freireich EJ, Trujillo JM, Stass SA. Detection of minimal residual cells carrying the t(14;18) by DNA sequence amplification. *Science* 1987; **237**(4811): 175–8.

21 Miller WH Jr, Levine K, DeBlasio A, Frankel SR, Dmitrovsky E, Warrell RP Jr. Detection of minimal residual disease in acute promyelocytic leukemia by a reverse transcription polymerase chain reaction assay for the PML/RAR-α fusion mRNA. *Blood* 1993; **82**(6): 1689–94.

22 Hebert J, Cayuela JM, Daniel MT, Berger R, Sigaux F. Detection of minimal residual disease in acute myelomonocytic leukemia with abnormal marrow eosinophils by nested polymerase chain reaction with allele specific amplification. *Blood* 1994; **84**(7): 2291–6.

23 Kusec R, Laczika K, Knobl P et al. AML1/ETO fusion mRNA can be detected in remission blood samples of all patients with t(8;21) acute myeloid leukemia after chemotherapy or autologous bone marrow transplantation. *Leukemia* 1994; **8**(5): 735–9.

24 Maruyama F, Stass SA, Estey EH et al. Detection of AML1/ETO fusion transcript as a tool for diagnosing t(8;21) positive acute myelogenous leukemia. *Leukemia* 1994; **8**(1): 40–5.

25 Pallisgaard N, Hokland P, Riishoj DC, Pedersen B, Jorgensen P. Multiplex reverse transcription-polymerase chain reaction for simultaneous screening of 29 translocations and chromosomal aberrations in acute leukemia. *Blood* 1998; **92**(2): 574–88.

26 Cave H, van der Werff ten Bosch J, Suciu S et al. Clinical significance of minimal residual disease in childhood acute lymphoblastic leukemia. European Organization for Research and Treatment of Cancer: Childhood Leukemia Cooperative Group. *N Engl J Med* 1998; **339**(9): 591–8.

27 Roberts WM, Estrov Z, Ouspenskaia MV, Johnston DA, McClain KL, Zipf TF. Measurement of residual leukemia during remission in childhood acute lymphoblastic leukemia. *N Engl J Med* 1997; **336**(5): 317–23.

28 Heid CA, Stevens J, Livak KJ, Williams PM. Real time quantitative PCR. *Genome Res* 1996; **6**(10): 986–94.

29 Radich J, Ladne P, Gooley T. Polymerase chain reaction-based detection of minimal residual disease in acute lymphoblastic leukemia predicts relapse after allogeneic BMT. *Biol Blood Marrow Transplant* 1995; **1**(1): 24–31.

30 Campana D, Coustan-Smith E, Janossy G. The immunologic detection of minimal residual disease in acute leukemia. *Blood* 1990; **76**(1): 163–71.

31 van Dongen JJ, Seriu T, Panzer-Grumayer ER et al. Prognostic value of minimal residual disease in acute lymphoblastic leukaemia in childhood. *Lancet* 1998; **352**(9142): 1731–8.

32 Goulden NJ, Knechtli CJ, Garland RJ et al. Minimal residual disease analysis for the prediction of relapse in children with standard-risk acute lymphoblastic leukaemia. *Br J Haematol* 1998; **100**(1): 235–44.

33 Evans PA, Short MA, Owen RG et al. Residual disease detection using fluorescent polymerase chain reaction at 20 weeks of therapy predicts clinical outcome in childhood acute lymphoblastic leukemia. *J Clin Oncol* 1998; **16**(11): 3616–27.

34 Beishuizen A, Verhoeven MA, van Wering ER, Hahlen K, Hooijkaas H, van Dongen JJ. Analysis of Ig and T-cell receptor genes in 40 childhood acute lymphoblastic leukemias at diagnosis and subsequent relapse: implications for the detection of minimal residual disease by polymerase chain reaction analysis. *Blood* 1994; **83**(8): 2238–47.

35 Steward CG, Goulden NJ, Katz F et al. A polymerase chain reaction study of the stability of Ig heavy-chain and T-cell receptor delta gene rearrangements between presentation and relapse of childhood B-lineage acute lymphoblastic leukemia. *Blood* 1994; **83**(5): 1355–62.

36 Szczepanski T, Willemse MJ, Brinkhof B, van Wering ER, van der Burg M, van Dongen JJ. Comparative analysis of Ig and TCR gene rearrangements at diagnosis and at relapse of childhood precursor-B-ALL provides improved strategies for selection of stable PCR targets for monitoring of minimal residual disease. *Blood* 2002; **99**(7): 2315–23.

37 Diverio D, Rossi V, Avvisati G et al. Early detection of relapse by prospective reverse transcriptase-polymerase chain reaction analysis of the *PML/RARα* fusion gene in patients with acute promyelocytic leukemia enrolled in the GIMEMA-AIEOP multicenter "AIDA" trial. GIMEMA-AIEOP multicenter "Aida" trial. *Blood* 1998; **92**(3): 784–9.

38 Laczika K, Novak M, Hilgarth B et al. Competitive CBFβ/MYH11 reverse-transcriptase polymerase chain reaction for quantitative assessment of minimal residual disease during postremission therapy in acute myeloid leukemia with inversion (16): a pilot study. *J Clin Oncol* 1998; **16**(4): 1519–25.

39 Marcucci G, Livak KJ, Bi W, Strout MP, Bloomfield CD, Caligiuri MA. Detection of minimal residual disease in patients with AML1/ETO-associated acute myeloid leukemia using a novel quantitative reverse transcription polymerase chain reaction assay. *Leukemia* 1998; **12**(9): 1482–9.

40 Cohen N, Rozenfeld-Granot G, Hardan I et al. Subgroup of patients with Philadelphia-positive chronic myelogenous leukemia characterized by a deletion of 9q proximal to *ABL* gene: expression profiling, resistance to interferon therapy, and poor prognosis. *Cancer Genet Cytogenet* 2001; **128**(2): 114–9.

41 Sinclair PB, Green AR, Grace C, Nacheva EP. Improved sensitivity of *BCR-ABL* detection: a triple-probe three-color fluorescence *in situ* hybridization system. *Blood* 1997; **90**(4): 1395–402.

42 Dewald GW, Wyatt WA, Juneau AL et al. Highly

sensitive fluorescence *in situ* hybridization method to detect double *BCR/ABL* fusion and monitor response to therapy in chronic myeloid leukemia. *Blood* 1998; **91**(9): 3357–65.

43 Radich JP, Gehly G, Gooley T *et al.* Polymerase chain reaction detection of the *BCR-ABL* fusion transcript after allogeneic marrow transplantation for chronic myeloid leukemia: results and implications in 346 patients. *Blood* 1995; **85**(9): 2632–8.

44 Pichert G, Roy DC, Gonin R *et al.* Distinct patterns of minimal residual disease associated with graft-versus-host disease after allogeneic bone marrow transplantation for chronic myelogenous leukemia. *J Clin Oncol* 1995; **13**(7): 1704–13.

45 Roth MS, Antin JH, Ash R *et al.* Prognostic significance of Philadelphia chromosome-positive cells detected by the polymerase chain reaction after allogeneic bone marrow transplant for chronic myelogenous leukemia. *Blood* 1992; **79**(1): 276–82.

46 Sawyers CL, Timson L, Kawasaki ES, Clark SS, Witte ON, Champlin R. Molecular relapse in chronic myelogenous leukemia patients after bone marrow transplantation detected by polymerase chain reaction. *Proc Natl Acad Sci U S A* 1990; **87**(2): 563–7.

47 Miyamura K, Tahara T, Tanimoto M *et al.* Long persistent bcr-abl positive transcript detected by polymerase chain reaction after marrow transplant for chronic myelogenous leukemia without clinical relapse: a study of 64 patients. *Blood* 1993; **81**(4): 1089–93.

48 Lion T, Henn T, Gaiger A, Kalhs P, Gadner H. Early detection of relapse after bone marrow transplantation in patients with chronic myelogenous leukaemia. *Lancet* 1993; **341**(8840): 275–6.

49 Hughes TP, Morgan GJ, Martiat P, Goldman JM. Detection of residual leukemia after bone marrow transplant for chronic myeloid leukemia: role of polymerase chain reaction in predicting relapse. *Blood* 1991; **77**(4): 874–8.

50 Radich JP, Gooley T, Bryant E *et al.* The significance of bcr-abl molecular detection in chronic myeloid leukemia patients "late", 18 months or more after transplantation. *Blood* 2001; **98**(6): 1701–7.

51 Mughal TI, Yong A, Szydlo RM *et al.* Molecular studies in patients with chronic myeloid leukaemia in remission 5 years after allogeneic stem cell transplant define the risk of subsequent relapse. *Br J Haematol* 2001; **115**(3): 569–74.

52 Costello RT, Kirk J, Gabert J. Value of PCR analysis for long term survivors after allogeneic bone marrow transplant for chronic myelogenous leukemia: a comparative study. *Leuk Lymphoma* 1996; **20**(3–4): 239–43.

53 van Rhee F, Lin F, Cross NC *et al.* Detection of residual leukaemia more than 10 years after allogeneic bone marrow transplantation for chronic myelogenous leukaemia. *Bone Marrow Transplant* 1994; **14**(4): 609–12.

54 McSweeney PA, Niederwieser D, Shizuru JA *et al.* Hematopoietic cell transplantation in older patients with hematologic malignancies: replacing high-dose cytotoxic therapy with graft-versus-tumor effects. *Blood* 2001; **97**(11): 3390–400.

55 Mackinnon S, Barnett L, Heller G. Polymerase chain reaction is highly predictive of relapse in patients following T cell-depleted allogeneic bone marrow transplantation for chronic myeloid leukemia. *Bone Marrow Transplant* 1996; **17**(4): 643–7.

56 Lin F, van Rhee F, Goldman JM, Cross NC. Kinetics of increasing *BCR-ABL* transcript numbers in chronic myeloid leukemia patients who relapse after bone marrow transplantation. *Blood* 1996; **87**(10): 4473–8.

57 Mensink E, van de Locht A, Schattenberg A *et al.* Quantitation of minimal residual disease in Philadelphia chromosome positive chronic myeloid leukaemia patients using real-time quantitative RT-PCR. *Br J Haematol* 1998; **102**(3): 768–74.

58 Preudhomme C, Chams-Eddine L, Roumier C *et al.* Detection of *BCR-ABL* transcripts in chronic myeloid leukemia (CML) using an *in situ* RT-PCR assay. *Leukemia* 1999; **13**(5): 818–23.

59 Olavarria E, Kanfer E, Szydlo R *et al.* Early detection of *BCR-ABL* transcripts by quantitative reverse transcriptase-polymerase chain reaction predicts outcome after allogeneic stem cell transplantation for chronic myeloid leukemia. *Blood* 2001; **97**(6): 1560–5.

60 Branford S, Hughes TP, Rudzki Z. Monitoring chronic myeloid leukaemia therapy by real-time quantitative PCR in blood is a reliable alternative to bone marrow cytogenetics. *Br J Haematol* 1999; **107**(3): 587–99.

61 El-Rifai W, Ruutu T, Vettenranta K, Temtamy S, Knuutila S. Minimal residual disease after allogeneic bone marrow transplantation for chronic myeloid leukaemia: a metaphase-FISH study. *Br J Haematol* 1996; **92**(2): 365–9.

62 Cross NC. Minimal residual disease in chronic myeloid leukaemia. *Hematol Cell Ther* 1998; **40**(5): 224–8.

63 Deininger M, Lehmann T, Krahl R, Hennig E, Muller C, Niederwieser D. No evidence for persistence of *BCR-ABL*-positive cells in patients in molecular remission after conventional allogeneic transplantation for chronic myeloid leukemia. *Blood* 2000; **96**(2): 779–80.

64 Chase A, Parker S, Kaeda J, Sivalingam R, Cross NC, Goldman JM. Absence of host-derived cells in the blood of patients in remission after allografting for chronic myeloid leukemia. *Blood* 2000; **96**(2): 777–8.

65 Chomel JC, Brizard F, Veinstein A *et al.* Persistence of *BCR-ABL* genomic rearrangement in chronic myeloid leukemia patients in complete and sustained cytogenetic remission after interferon-α therapy or allogeneic bone marrow transplantation. *Blood* 2000; **95**(2): 404–8.

66 Zhang JG, Goldman JM, Cross NC. Characterization of genomic *BCR-ABL* breakpoints in chronic myeloid leukaemia by PCR. *Br J Haematol* 1995; **90**(1): 138–46.

67 Zhang JG, Lin F, Chase A, Goldman JM, Cross NC. Comparison of genomic DNA and cDNA for detection of residual disease after treatment of chronic myeloid leukemia with allogeneic bone marrow transplantation. *Blood* 1996; **87**(6): 2588–93.

68 Knechtli CJ, Goulden NJ, Hancock JP *et al.* Minimal residual disease status before allogeneic bone marrow transplantation is an important determinant of successful outcome for children and adolescents with acute lymphoblastic leukaemia. *Blood* 1998; **92**(11): 4072–9.

69 Mortuza FY, Papaioannou M, Moreira IM *et al.* Minimal residual disease tests provide an independent predictor of clinical outcome in adult acute lymphoblastic leukemia. *J Clin Oncol* 2002; **20**(4): 1094–104.

70 Sanchez J, Serrano J, Gomez P *et al.* Clinical value of immunological monitoring of minimal residual disease in acute lymphoblastic leukaemia after allogeneic transplantation. *Br J Haematol* 2002; **116**(3): 686–94.

71 Stirewalt DL, Guthrie KA, Beppu L *et al.* Predictors of relapse and overall survival in Philadelphia chromosome-positive acute lymphoblastic leukemia after transplantation. *Biol Blood Marrow Transplant* 2003; **9**: 206–12.

72 Knechtli CJ, Goulden NJ, Hancock JP *et al.* Minimal residual disease status as a predictor of relapse after allogeneic bone marrow transplantation for children with acute lymphoblastic leukaemia. *Br J Haematol* 1998; **102**(3): 860–71.

73 Miyamura K, Tanimoto M, Morishima Y *et al.* Detection of Philadelphia chromosome-positive acute lymphoblastic leukemia by polymerase chain reaction: possible eradication of minimal residual disease by marrow transplantation. *Blood* 1992; **79**(5): 1366–70.

74 Radich J, Gehly G, Lee A *et al.* Detection of bcr-abl transcripts in Philadelphia chromosome-positive acute lymphoblastic leukemia after marrow transplantation. *Blood* 1997; **89**(7): 2602–9.

75 Roman J, Martin C, Torres A *et al.* Absence of detectable PML-RARα fusion transcripts in long-term remission patients after BMT for acute promyelocytic leukemia. *Bone Marrow Transplant* 1997; **19**(7): 679–83.

76 Perego RA, Marenco P, Bianchi C *et al.* PML/RARα transcripts monitored by polymerase chain reaction in acute promyelocytic leukemia during complete remission, relapse and after bone marrow transplantation. *Leukemia* 1996; **10**(2): 207–12.

77 Mandelli F, Diverio D, Avvisati G *et al.* Molecular remission in PML/RARα-positive acute promyelocytic leukemia by combined all-*trans* retinoic acid and idarubicin (AIDA) therapy. Gruppo Italiano-Malattie Ematologiche Maligne dell'Adulto and Associazione Italiana di Ematologia ed Oncologia Pediatrica Cooperative Groups. *Blood* 1997; **90**(3): 1014–21.

78 Miyamoto T, Nagafuji K, Harada M *et al.* Quantitative analysis of AML1/ETO transcripts in peripheral blood stem cell harvests from patients with t(8;21) acute myelogenous leukaemia. *Br J Haematol* 1995; **91**(1): 132–8.

79 Sugimoto T, Das H, Imoto S *et al.* Quantitation of minimal residual disease in t(8;21)-positive acute myelogenous leukemia patients using real-time quantitative RT-PCR. *Am J Hematol* 2000; **64**(2): 101–6.

80 Jurlander J, Caligiuri MA, Ruutu T *et al.* Persistence of the AML1/ETO fusion transcript in patients treated with allogeneic bone marrow transplantation for t(8;21) leukemia. *Blood* 1996; **88**(6): 2183–91.

81 Tobal K, Johnson PRE, Saunders MJ, Liu Yin JA. Detection of CBFB/MYH11 transcripts in patients with inversion and other abnormalities of chromosome 16 at presentation and remission. *Br J Haematol* 1995; **91**: 104–8.

82 Elmaagcli AH, Beelen DW, Kroll M, Trzensky S, Stein C, Schaefer UW. Detection of CBFβ/MYH11 fusion transcripts in patients with inv (16) acute myeloid leukemia after allogeneic bone marrow or peripheral blood progenitor cell transplantation. *Bone Marrow Transplant* 1998; **21**(2): 159–66.

83 Elmaagcli AH, Beelen DW, Trenschel R, Schaefer

UW. The detection of wt-1 transcripts is not associated with an increased leukemic relapse rate in patients with acute leukemia after allogeneic bone marrow or peripheral blood stem cell transplantation. *Bone Marrow Transplant* 2000; **25**(1): 91–6.
84. Corradini P, Voena C, Tarella C et al. Molecular and clinical remissions in multiple myeloma: role of autologous and allogeneic transplantation of hematopoietic cells. *J Clin Oncol* 1999; **17**(1): 208–15.
85. Cavo M, Terragna C, Martinelli G et al. Molecular monitoring of minimal residual disease in patients in long-term complete remission after allogeneic stem cell transplantation for multiple myeloma. *Blood* 2000; **96**(1): 355–7.
86. Esteve J, Villamor N, Colomer D et al. Stem cell transplantation for chronic lymphocytic leukemia: different outcome after autologous and allogeneic transplantation and correlation with minimal residual disease status. *Leukemia* 2001; **15**(3): 445–51.
87. Mattsson J, Uzunel M, Remberger M et al. Minimal residual disease is common after allogeneic stem cell transplantation in patients with B cell chronic lymphocytic leukemia and may be controlled by graft-versus-host disease. *Leukemia* 2000; **14**(2): 247–54.
88. Rawstron AC, Kennedy B, Evans PA et al. Quantitation of minimal disease levels in chronic lymphocytic leukemia using a sensitive flow cytometric assay improves the prediction of outcome and can be used to optimize therapy. *Blood* 2001; **98**(1): 29–35.
89. Moreau P, Facon T, Leleu X et al. Recurrent 14q32 translocations determine the prognosis of multiple myeloma, especially in patients receiving intensive chemotherapy. *Blood* 2002; **100**(5): 1579–83.
90. Facon T, Avet-Loiseau H, Guillerm G et al. Chromosome 13 abnormalities identified by FISH analysis and serum β_2-microglobulin produce a powerful myeloma staging system for patients receiving high-dose therapy. *Blood* 2001; **97**(6): 1566–71.
91. Dohner H, Stilgenbauer S, Dohner K, Bentz M, Lichter P. Chromosome aberrations in B-cell chronic lymphocytic leukemia. Reassessment based on molecular cytogenetic analysis. *J Mol Med* 1999; **77**(2): 266–81.
92. Stilgenbauer S, Lichter P, Dohner H. Genetic features of B-cell chronic lymphocytic leukemia. *Rev Clin Exp Hematol* 2000; **4**(1): 48–72.
93. Gribben JG, Neuberg D, Barber M et al. Detection of residual lymphoma cells by polymerase chain reaction in peripheral blood is significantly less predictive for relapse than detection in bone marrow. *Blood* 1994; **83**(12): 3800–7.
94. Gribben JG, Freedman AS, Neuberg D et al. Immunologic purging of marrow assessed by PCR before autologous bone marrow transplantation for B-cell lymphoma. *N Engl J Med* 1991; **325**(22): 1525–33.
95. Vose JM, Sharp G, Chan WC et al. Autologous transplantation for aggressive non-Hodgkin's lymphoma: results of a randomized trial evaluating graft source and minimal residual disease. *J Clin Oncol* 2002; **20**(9): 2344–52.
96. Radich JP. The detection and significance of minimal residual disease in chronic myeloid leukemia. *Medicina (B Aires)* 2000; **60** (Suppl. 2): 66–70.
97. Miyamoto T, Nagafuji K, Akashi K et al. Persistence of multipotent progenitors expressing AML1/ETO transcripts in long-term remission patients with t(8;21) acute myelogenous leukemia. *Blood* 1996; **87**(11): 4789–96.
98. Vora A, Frost L, Goodeve A et al. Late relapsing childhood lymphoblastic leukemia. *Blood* 1998; **92**(7): 2334–7.
99. Bose S, Deininger M, Gora-Tybor J, Goldman JM, Melo JV. The presence of typical and atypical BCR-ABL fusion genes in leukocytes of normal individuals: biologic significance and implications for the assessment of minimal residual disease. *Blood* 1998; **92**(9): 3362–7.
100. Biernaux C, Loos M, Sels A, Huez G, Stryckmans P. Detection of major bcr-abl gene expression at a very low level in blood cells of some healthy individuals. *Blood* 1995; **86**(8): 3118–22.
101. Ji W, Qu GZYEP, Zhang XY, Halabi S, Ehrlich M. Frequent detection of bcl-2/JH translocations in human blood and organ samples by a quantitative polymerase chain reaction assay. *Cancer Res* 1995; **55**(13): 2876–82.
102. Liu Y, Hernandez AM, Shibata D, Cortopassi GA. BCL2 translocation frequency rises with age in humans. *Proc Natl Acad Sci U S A* 1994; **91**(19): 8910–4.
103. Van Rhee F, Lin F, Cullis JO et al. Relapse of chronic myeloid leukemia after allogenic bone marrow transplant: The case for giving donor leukocyte transfusions before the onset of hematologic relapse. *Blood* 1994; **83**: 3377–83.
104. Au WY, Lie AK, Lee CK, Liang R, Kwong YL. Donor lymphocyte infusion induced molecular remission in relapse of acute myeloid leukaemia after allogeneic bone marrow transplantation. *Bone Marrow Transplant* 1999; **23**(11): 1201–3.
105. Dazzi F, Szydlo RM, Cross NC et al. Durability of responses following donor lymphocyte infusions for patients who relapse after allogeneic stem cell transplantation for chronic myeloid leukemia. *Blood* 2000; **96**(8): 2712–6.
106. Formankova R, Honzatkova L, Moravcova J et al. Prediction and reversion of post-transplant relapse in patients with chronic myeloid leukemia using mixed chimerism and residual disease detection and adoptive immunotherapy. *Leuk Res* 2000; **24**(4): 339–47.
107. Ogawa H, Tsuboi A, Oji Y et al. Successful donor leukocyte transfusion at molecular relapse for a patient with acute myeloid leukemia who was treated with allogenic bone marrow transplantation: importance of the monitoring of minimal residual disease by WT1 assay. *Bone Marrow Transplant* 1998; **21**(5): 525–7.
108. Kantarjian HM, O'Brien S, Cortes JE et al. Imatinib mesylate therapy for relapse after allogeneic stem cell transplantation for chronic myelogenous leukemia. *Blood* 2002; **100**(5): 1590–5.

23

George E. Sale, Howard M. Shulman & Robert C. Hackman

Pathology of Hematopoietic Cell Transplantation

Introduction

Pathologists encounter four major groups of complications in patients undergoing bone marrow and hematopoietic cell transplantation (HCT). Toxicities result from cytoreductive regimens, immunological problems (rejection or graft-vs.-host disease [GVHD]), infections and relapse [1]. The early post-HCT period includes the risks of infection, bleeding and toxicity of chemotherapy and/or irradiation. During the later period GVHD, relapse, late infections and late complications of radiation and chemotherapy may develop. The advances in HCT detailed in this edition have shifted the pathologists' perspective on these patients. Chief among these advances are peripheral blood hematopoietic cell technology, the expanded use of unrelated donors and the new nonmyeloablative protocols that use mixed chimerism to promote tolerance, manipulate the graft-vs.-tumor effect and dramatically decrease early toxicity. New drugs that affect the hematopoietic and other systems have altered the timing, severity and, accordingly, the interpretation of transplant complications. A broader spectrum of diseases is now being treated by HCT. New technological developments, including multiparameter flow cytometry, fluorescence *in situ* hybridization, polymerase chain reaction (PCR), and diagnostic DNA array chips have substantially improved the diagnostic monitoring of HCT recipients.

Pretransplant evaluation

The referral evaluation for HCT is crucial and complex, especially as indications for HCT have broadened. Primary diagnostic material, relapse and remission data, and knowledge of recent treatment all are needed for accurate appraisal [2]. For leukemia, the primary morphology, the immunophenotype and cytogenetics must be reviewed, and a current marrow aspiration and/or biopsy must be examined for relapse.

The pretransplant stratification of myelodysplastic syndromes into aggressive vs. milder forms (e.g. refractory anemia with excess blasts vs. refractive anemia) is based largely on the marrow blast count according to the World Health Organization classification. Outcome analysis is based on the international grading system, which includes cytogenetic and clinical data. Multiparameter flow cytometry can detect as few as 0.2% blasts and distinguish benign blasts from aberrant or malignant cells [3]. This technology is therefore helpful in the diagnosis and monitoring of hematologic malignancies and myelodysplastic syndromes, as well as in the recognition and staging of minimal residual disease [4,5]. Aplastic anemia requires very precise evaluation of bone marrow to classify the severity, and also to rule out myelodysplasia or disorders such as hairy cell leukemia insidiously simulating primary aplasia. The diagnosis of aplastic anemia should be prompt in order to avoid transfusions and thereby decrease the risks of allosensitization and post-transplant graft rejection. Lymphomas require comparison of previous diagnostic lymph nodes and current marrow material since tumor cells in the marrow might preclude an autologous HCT procedure. A lengthening list of solid tumors such as Ewing's sarcoma and neuroblastoma are now being treated with HCT and call for accurate pretransplant staging, often including immunohistochemistry. The diagnosis of marrow invasion by breast cancer may require cytokeratin immunohistochemistry to identify bland single tumor cells [6]. Evaluation of myelofibrosis is important in chronic myeloid leukemia (CML), acute myelofibrosis, myelodysplastic syndromes and metastatic disease, and repeated biopsies with reticulin and trichrome staining may be needed [7,8].

Magnetic resonance imaging of the pelvis and femur helps assess the extent and distribution of myelofibrosis and other disease. Apart from its staging utility, a liver biopsy may be necessary to evaluate the risk of developing liver toxicity syndrome after receiving myeloablative cytoreductive regimens. Inflammatory liver disorders, particularly those associated with sinusoidal fibrosis, bridging fibrosis or cirrhosis, portend a high risk of developing severe liver toxicity syndrome. Several new agents have affected pretransplant evaluation. Imatinib mesylate (STI571, Gleevec®), a drug effective in producing clinical or cytogenetic remissions in chronic phase CML, delays HCT in many cases. After this therapy patients' marrows may revert to display a normal myeloid : erythroid ratio and a low blast count for many months, presenting with a nearly normal marrow morphology. Granulocyte macrophage colony-stimulating factor, granulocyte colony-stimulating factor and other cytokines may cause confusing left shifts in hematopoietic cells that may mislead the unaware observer. Bisphosphonates given for multiple myeloma may thicken trabecular bone in pretransplant marrow biopsies.

Post-transplant evaluation

Massive destruction of the host marrow by radiation and/or chemotherapy produces acute marrow damage with features of acute serous myelitis. These features include edema, hemorrhage into the interstitium, loss of most marrow elements, except plasma and mast cells, and relative predominance of damaged fat and iron-rich macrophages. Fat necrosis is frequent. This damage gradually resolves over the first 4–6 weeks as colonies of donor marrow myeloid, megakaryocytic and erythroid precursors develop. Lymphoid cells are diffuse and sparse. Engraftment is usually simultaneous in the three major cell lines, but the anemia is usually the last to normalize. Failure to engraft is diagnosed by the absence of both peripheral and marrow myeloid, erythroid and thrombocytic cells. Rare cases may suggest apparent lymphoid engraftment only (in some instances associated with GVHD). Graft rejection has no specific his-

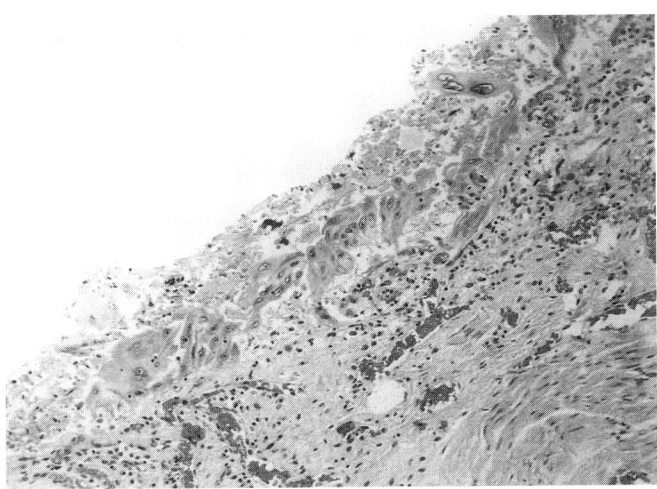

Fig. 23.1 Esophagus, conditioning toxicity, day 5. The squamous mucosa displays widespread dyspolarity and ulceration. Nuclei are enlarged, irregular and hyperchromatic, H&E.

tologic features but may be defined as transient engraftment with proliferation of at least one cell line followed by its loss. Rejection occasionally is heralded by loss of a single line analogous to pure red cell aplasia. Its elusive mechanisms are discussed in Chapter 3. Relapse of leukemia is infrequent before day 100 unless the patient has shown persistence of marrow tumor cells between day 7 and day 21 after transplantation. In the case of CML, cytogenetic evidence of relapse may predate morphologic evidence by many months. Cytogenetics, restriction fragment length polymorphism analysis, PCR for *bcr-abl* and Y chromosome DNA detection may help greatly in assessing chimerism and relapse status [9]. Other than the post-transplant lymphoproliferative disorder, known as Epstein–Barr virus (EBV)-induced lymphoma, second tumors usually occur late. EBV-associated lymphoma should be suspected in the setting of adenopathy or worsening of gastrointestinal (GI) symptoms despite treatment for acute GVHD [10]. Serial PCR measurements of plasma EBV DNA may demonstrate increasing copy numbers and, thus, allow intervention. Early use of rituximab can prevent clinically symptomatic progressive disease (see Chapter 56) [11].

Toxicity from pretransplant cytoreductive therapy

The cytoreductive therapy given for treatment of underlying malignancy, marrow ablation and immune suppression may cause widespread multi-organ dysfunction [12]. The frequency, the organ systems involved and the time of onset are related to both the type and overall intensity of the conditioning protocol. The histopathology within some affected organs, such as the heart, may be disease "nonspecific" (edema, hemorrhage, necrosis of myocytes and interstitial fibrosis), yet the associated clinico-pathologic entity may be highly characteristic of toxicity. Other changes due to toxicity, particularly those in the mucous membranes, skin, GI tract and lung, may cause diagnostic difficulties because of their clinical or histological overlap with GVHD and infection (see Plates 23.1, 23.2, 23.3, 23.9 & 23.10, *facing p. 296*). Several studies of these organs demonstrate the diffuse distribution of conditioning injury and marked lessening of these changes with time (Fig. 23.1; see also Plate 23.11, *facing p. 296*) [13]. Neither the cytological features of atypia and inflammation, nor the extent of such changes, clearly separate immunologically mediated vs. toxic injury to the epithelium.

Hepatic sinusoidal obstructive syndrome (veno-occlusive disease)

The most frequent life threatening regimen-related toxicity involves a clinical syndrome of jaundice, weight gain, ascites and painful hepatomegaly that typically develops in the first few weeks after HCT. In the earlier editions, the authors called this syndrome hepatic veno-occlusive disease (VOD), referring specifically to the occlusive lesions within the small hepatic venules [14]. However, histologic data do not define the primary site of injury or molecular events that occur in the sinusoids before clinical signs appear. Based on more recent experimental and molecular studies the authors have proposed renaming the syndrome to sinusoidal obstructive syndrome (SOS). The term SOS reflects the proximate cause, toxic injury to the zone 3 sinusoidal and venular endothelium related to specific drug metabolites and to intracellular depletion of glutathione stores [15]. Secondary events are a decrease in nitric oxide associated with vasoconstriction [16]. Deposition of coagulants evinced by factor VIII immunohistochemical staining of widened subendothelial zone and the perivenular zone corresponding to the pores that drain the sinusoids into the small venules (see Plate 23.6, *facing p. 296*) is followed by the deposition of extracellular matrix and collagens (see Chapter 58) [17].

Liver biopsy and autopsy specimens reveal that the histology of injury to the sinusoids, hepatocytes and venules may be rapidly progressive. The trichrome stain, which illuminates both parenchymal and connective tissue liver components, is critical for recognizing the diagnostic sinusoidal and venular injuries, while other connective tissue stains (e.g. Verhoeff–van Gieson and reticulin) are complementary. Examination of serial sections may be needed to identify characteristic histologic changes that may not be present in all levels. The earliest changes, occurring 6–8 days following cytoreductive conditioning, consist of venular luminal narrowing by an edematous subendothelial zone containing red cells and cellular debris between the adventitia and basement membrane of small central venules. Accompanying these changes are sinusoidal dilation with engorgement by red cells and hemorrhage into the space of Disse (see Plates 23.4 & 23.5, *facing p. 296*). Frank necrosis of perivenular hepatocytes, accentuated by anticytokeratin immunostaining, is often more widespread and severe than the extent of venular injury. A consequence of the sinusoidal obstruction, elevated sinusoidal pressure, ischemia and fragmentation of hepatocyte cords is dislodgement of clusters of liver cells, including hepatocytes, that may flow retrograde into portal veins or embolize through disrupted pores into the damaged central venules. Embolization of detached cells, including hepatocytes, into the subendothelium of venules develops. Immunohistochemical staining with CD31 demonstrates a loss of endothelium in the perivenular sinusoids around the venules and increases in monocytes/Kupffer cells in areas of ischemic hepatocyte necrosis (H.M. Shulman, personal communication). Later changes include collagenous obliteration of the venules, thickening of the outer wall of the hepatic venules (phlebosclerosis) and fibrosis in the sinusoids adjacent to the terminal hepatic venules (zone 3 of the liver acinus) associated with a marked increase in hepatic stellate cells colocalized to the areas of extracellular matrix (Fig. 23.2; see also Plate 23.8, *facing p. 296*) [18–20].

Correlation of histologic findings with clinical signs

We have found that several pericentral (zone 3) lesions that follow cytoreductive therapy are associated with the clinical syndrome. Two studies have demonstrated that zone 3 sinusoidal fibrosis and phlebosclerosis, a nonocclusive perivenular fibrosis, are also associated with the same clinical features as VOD [14,18,21]. An example of the histologic spectrum is a rapidly developing syndrome of SOS that has developed among

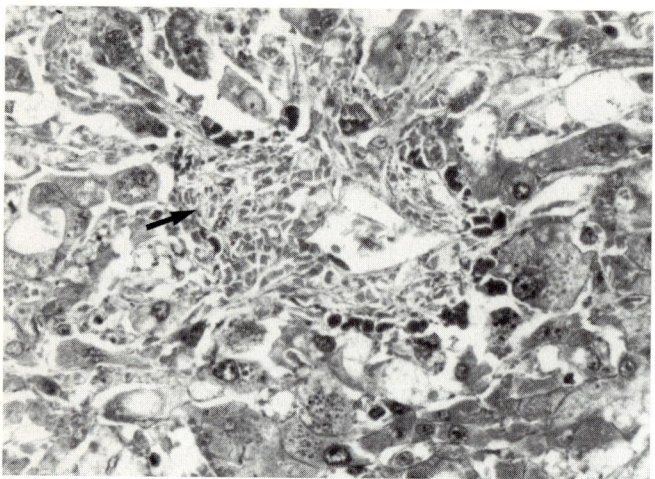

Fig. 23.2 Liver, veno-occlusive disease, day 34. Sublobular vein has nearly complete luminal obliteration by a mixture of connective tissue and entrapped blood cells (arrow). Surrounding the vein is extensive hepatocyte damage and sinusoidal congestion, trichrome.

some HCT patients treated with gemtuzumab ozogamicin (Mylotarg™), a humanized anti-CD33 monoclonal antibody conjugated to calicheamicin [22,23]. The associated histology of gemtuzumab ozogamicin-associated SOS differs slightly from SOS occurring after myeloablative cytoreductive conditioning by resulting in more sinusoidal fibrosis than venular occlusion.

Several other conditions which may result in an SOS-like picture are viral hepatitis with bridging fibrosis and alcohol related and nonalcohol-related steatohepatitis. The respective pre-existent histologic findings of bridging fibrosis or pericellular sinusoidal fibrosis may result in a loss of sinusoidal plasticity or diminished sinusoidal blood flow from increased hepatic stellate cells. Another zone 3 lesion reported to produce symptoms that resemble those of VOD is nodular regenerative hyperplasia, a change best seen on reticulin stains as localized atrophy and compression of hepatocytes with regeneration and expansion of adjacent hepatocyte cord regions creating a nonfibrotic nodularity [24]. In the authors' experience, however, nodular hyperplastic hepatocyte alterations appear infrequently (in only 8% of all autopsies in a 1-year period) and are unassociated with symptoms of early liver toxicity. Nodular hepatic lesions developing later post-HCT, are most likely secondary to disturbances in hemodynamics and serve as an indicator of compensatory repair and regeneration of hepatocytes in different zones of the liver acinus [25].

Graft-vs.-host disease

Heymer and colleagues recently published a lucid and thorough monograph on GVHD pathology, which provides a balanced discussion of the major issues in this field [26]. Pathogenetically, GVHD is usually divided into afferent and efferent stages. The afferent stage involves recognition of minor or major histoincompatibilities by donor T cells [27]. A classical concept for the efferent stage in GVHD is that donor cytotoxic lymphocytes attack host cells including some epithelial cells of skin, intrahepatic bile ducts and gut. Electron microscopic and immunohistologic data demonstrate lymphocyte epithelial attachments and activation of infiltrating cytotoxic lymphocytes in human biopsy material. CD8 positive T cells with cytotoxic marking by TIA-1 antigen, which marks cytotoxic lymphocytes, have been found in the skin and lip lesions [28]. Natural killer cells have been found less consistently in some animal and human studies. Although T cells are universally agreed to be critical initially, alternative views in this complex field suggest that there may be shifts between the T-helper type 1 subset (Th1) and T-helper type 2 subset (Th2) cell pathways of immune response mediated by cytokines such as interleukin (IL) 1, 2, 4, 10 and 12, as well as tumor necrosis factor alpha (TNF-α), which are also important determinants of subsequent events, especially in acute GVHD [29–31]. The experimental work of Baker *et al.* and Gilliam *et al.* [32–34] suggests that the cytotoxic lymphocyte-induced apoptosis, in fact, does have a major pathogenetic role in GVHD. Target cells seem to be in subregions of epithelium where epithelial stem cells or their early progeny are located (e.g. rete ridges of skin, crypt cells of gut and the parafollicular bulge of the hair follicle) (see Plates 23.18, 23.19 & 23.25, *facing p. 296*) [35]. The precise combination of surface expression of proliferation markers, receptors, cytokine signals or of human leukocyte antigen (HLA) class I or II expression which renders these cells targets has not yet been clarified [31].

Skin

The histopathologic interpretation of skin soon after HCT is a difficult differential diagnostic exercise because of competing causes of the reactions and controversy in the field [1,36,37]. The histologic grading system of Lerner and colleagues is a useful descriptor where grade I is nonspecific epidermal basal cell vacuolization, grade II is epidermal basal cell death or apoptosis with lymphoid infiltration and satellitosis, grade III is bulla formation and grade IV is ulceration of the skin. In practice, the useful dividing line is at grade II and both lymphocytes and basal apoptosis are usually required for this classification (Fig. 23.3; see also Plate 23.18, *facing p. 296*), although the lymphocytes may be sparse. The timing of the biopsy heavily influences the interpretation because direct cytotoxic effects of radiation and chemotherapy occur primarily in the first 3 weeks after HCT and produce epidermal damage overlapping with that of GVHD (see Plate 23.1, *facing p. 296*) [36]. The central feature of a lichenoid reaction with necrosis of basal cells has to be interpreted in the context of whether conditioning is myeloablative, the time following chemoradiation, the presence of a marrow graft, the degree of HLA match and the drugs used to prevent or to treat GVHD. The effects of chemo/radiotherapy usually wear off in 2–3 weeks. At that point, the difficulties are fewer, the probability of true GVHD higher, and the epithelial atypia less. Therefore, one's diagnostic confidence may be somewhat greater. Recipients of matched unrelated transplants may show earlier, more severe GVHD than those who received grafts from matched sibling donors. Nonmyeloablative transplants, although designed to induce tolerance, may also show earlier GVHD if patients are older, less well matched, or achieve less immunoprophylaxis. The diagnostic threshold may also be lower in early chronic GVHD (e.g. days 80–100) which may be subtle and focal. Serial skin biopsies are often helpful in interpreting the early skin changes and providing a guide to clinical management.

Gastrointestinal

In practice, because of greater diagnostic sensitivity, endoscopic evaluation has largely supplanted rectal biopsy and provides a wealth of data on gastric, esophageal and duodenal disease. Biopsies are typically taken from the gastric fundus and antrum [38]. For safety reasons, duodenal biopsies are avoided because of potential severe bleeding complications [39]. Diarrhea volume correlates well with rectal biopsy histology [40]. Rectal biopsies may be preferable in patients with diarrhea who lack upper gut symptoms or loss of appetite as well as in small children requiring anesthesia for upper gut endoscopy. Colonoscopic and ileal biopsies are also obtained to assess response to treatment for severe GVHD of the lower gut. Biopsies from endoscopically unremarkable mucosa may provide a histological diagnosis of GVHD [41].

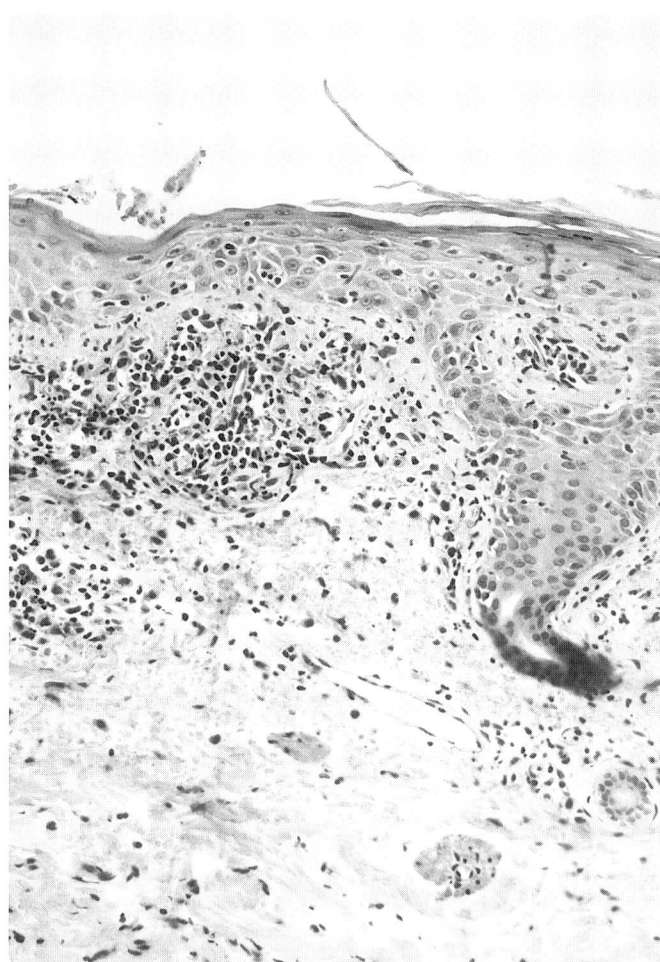

Fig. 23.3 Skin, acute graft-vs.-host disease (GVHD), day 30. Marked lichenoid reaction involving the epidermis and acrosyringium with intraepidermal lymphocytes, apoptosis and destruction of rete ridges, H&E.

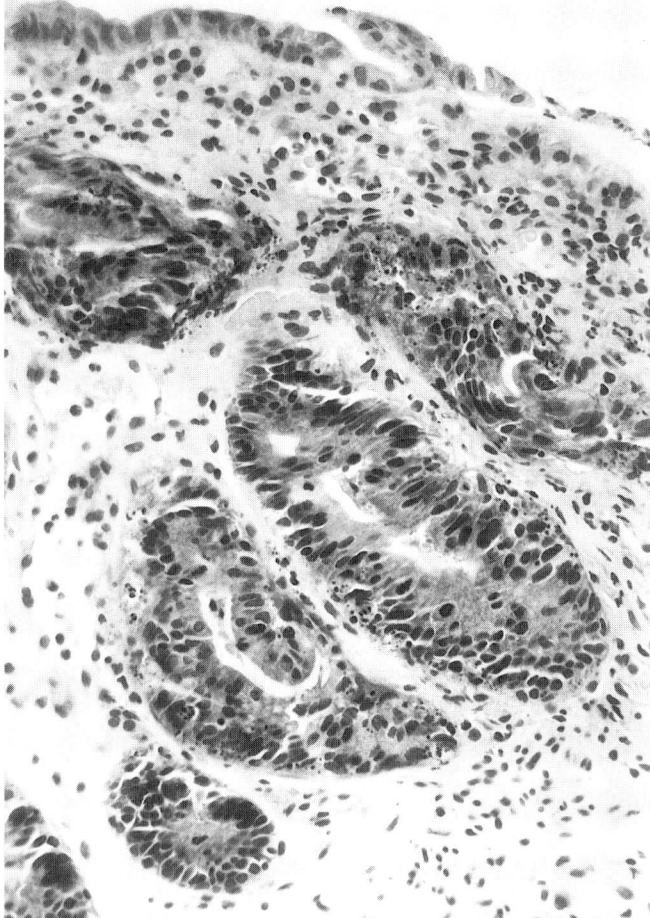

Fig. 23.4 Colonic graft-vs.-host disease (GVHD), day 36. Extensive apoptosis of enterocytes seen as nuclear dust along periphery of crypts.

Histology of GI acute GVHD

The sequence of damage in GVHD appears at four levels:

1 *Grade I*: Individual cell necrosis in basal and lateral crypts, with sparse lymphocytic infiltrate (Fig. 23.4; see also Plates 23.25, 23.26 & 23.27, *facing p. 296*). These alterations may involve only a few scattered crypts and can be easily overlooked, especially in formalin-fixed biopsies. Apoptotic crypt epithelial cells are more prominent following B5, Bouin's or Hollandes' fixation [41].

2 *Grade II*: Crypt abscess, in which polymorphonuclear leukocytes and eosinophils may participate.

3 *Grade III*: Crypt loss. (See Plate 23.31, *facing p. 296*.)

4 *Grade IV*: Mucosal denudation.

The initial sites of injury in the gut are focused on the regenerative or stem cell areas, i.e. the neck region of the gastric glands and the basal layer of esophagus and the lower portion of the crypts in the small and large bowel. Two sets of data suggest that the disease in humans involves the gut diffusely. First, the authors' autopsy study of GI GVHD showed that sections from the ileal and rectal regions were within one histological grade of each other in most cases, and that the stomach and the duodenum were frequently involved [40]. Second, gross and radiographic studies of GI GVHD show that the diffuse changes of mucosal edema with effacement of the normal mucosal folds involve the entire small and large bowel simultaneously, and sometimes include the stomach [42]. In several studies of upper endoscopic biopsies, epithelial necrosis and crypt abscesses from the small intestines were always associated with diarrhea and, usually, with similar histological changes in the rectal biopsy [43]. On the other hand, some patients with positive gastric biopsies may present with only nausea and vomiting [44].

These studies reemphasize that a diagnosis of GVHD often requires both clinical and histopathological criteria. This is particularly true when there is: (i) an isolated positive gastric biopsy; (ii) the finding of only rare grade I apoptotic bodies seen on high magnification in a small bowel biopsy; or (iii) evidence of upper GI infection with cytomegalovirus (CMV) associated with crypt abscesses or apoptotic bodies. In related studies, Nakhleh *et al.* [45] and Washington *et al.* [46] found that CMV colitis and severe T-cell deficiency have been found to produce mucosal damage which simulates GVHD. However, the presence of CMV in a gut biopsy does not preclude a diagnosis of GVHD if immunoautochemistry or in situ hybridization studies show that viral involvement is scanty and clusters of apoptotic crypt epithelial cells characteristic of GVHD are present. Histologically, protracted GVHD may show either diffuse or segmental intestinal ulceration with mucosal granulation tissue and fibrosis confined to the mucosa and submucosa (see Plate 23.29, *facing p. 296*). Transmural fibrosis and granulomatous inflammation, such as that seen in Crohn's disease, are absent. Severe GI GVHD is life threatening; even aggressive surgical management of obstruction may fail to save the patient [47].

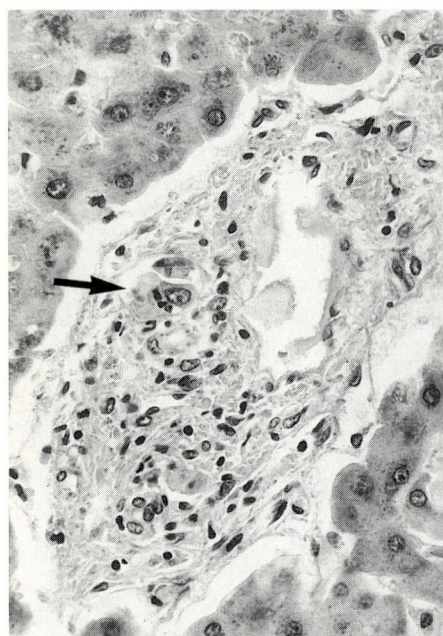
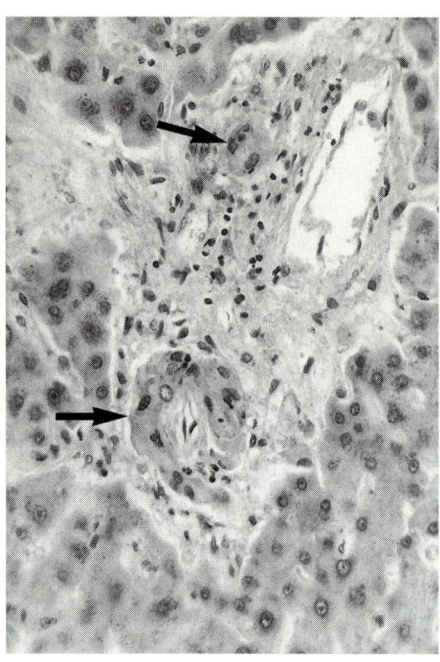

Fig. 23.5 Hepatic graft-vs.-host disease (GVHD), day 53. Despite the minimal inflammation within the portal space the bile ducts (arrow) are reduced to degenerative cytoplasmic masses with a few remaining hyperchromatic nuclei.

Like most squamous epithelia, that of the esophagus may be involved with GVHD. The diagnosis of acute GVHD presents considerable diagnostic difficulty since peptic acid reflux esophagitis is common early after grafting. Esophagitis may also be due to infection with fungi, bacteria, herpes simplex, CMV (see Plates 23.34 & 23.35, *facing p. 296*), or any combination of these organisms. Accurate diagnosis requires hematoxylin and eosin (H&E) histology, special stains for microorganisms and, frequently, immunocytochemistry studies for virus identification. Bacterial, viral and fungal cultures should be obtained from lesions endoscopically suggestive of infection.

Pathogenetic mechanisms resulting in the destruction of enteric mucosa after HCT and GVHD have been reviewed by Hill and Ferrara [48]. Cell mediated cytotoxicity with close contact to target enterocytes has been described in ultrastructural studies of human rectal biopsies of GVHD [49]. A recent study showed that activated lamina propria eosinophils are found in acute cases and flares of chronic GI GVHD [50]. The ulcerated gut is a prime target for superinfection by CMV, gram-negative bacteria and, less frequently, herpes simplex (see Plate 23.36, *facing p. 296*), adenovirus (ADV) and fungi such as *Candida*, *Aspergillus* or *Torula* [51]. Beschorner *et al.* [52], by using the immunoperoxidase technique on sections of intestine and colon, found a marked reduction in immunoglobulin A (IgA) and IgM-bearing plasma cells in the lamina propria of patients with GVHD. This observation implies a local immunodeficiency to infection by enteric flora. The summation of these different injuries may result in depletion or loss of the mucosal stem cells with a chronically ulcerated and fibrotic gut. Recently, the problem of autologous GVHD-like reactions has reappeared in the stomach biopsies of patients treated with busulfan, melphalan and thiotepa who develop protracted GI toxicity which histologically resembles GVHD (see Plate 23.28, *facing p. 296*). These lesions may persist up to several weeks following transplantation. This phenomenon reemphasizes the poorly understood, potentially autoimmune mechanism of the GVHD-like syndromes occurring in autologous and syngeneic patients, as well as the cyclosporine-mediated animal models of Hess and colleagues (see Chapter 30) [53].

Liver

The liver is a major target of both acute and chronic GVHD after allogeneic HCT and, occasionally, after autologous HCT [54]. In both the experimental and clinical settings, histopathologic and ultrastructural studies demonstrate that the small interlobular and marginal bile ducts at the periphery of the portal spaces are the preferential target of the alloimmune reaction (Fig. 23.5; see also Plate 23.33, *facing p. 296*). Experimental GVHD studies in congenic mice indicate that the cells penetrating the damaged bile ducts are CD4 T cells, that these T cells are specific for bile duct antigens, and that bile duct destruction does not require concurrent injury to the endothelium of the peribiliary capillary plexus that surround the ducts [55,56]. The principal histologic consequences of this immunological attack are a characteristic spectrum of destructive bile duct lesions, variable inflammation of the portal spaces, hepatic acinus and hepatocellular-cholangiolar cholestasis that is often marked (see Plates 23.32 & 23.33, *facing p. 296*). In both controlled experimental studies and coded histopathological studies, the histologic criteria that are most useful in discriminating between the etiologic possibilities involve cytological and destructive changes in the bile ducts [57–59]. These changes may progress from

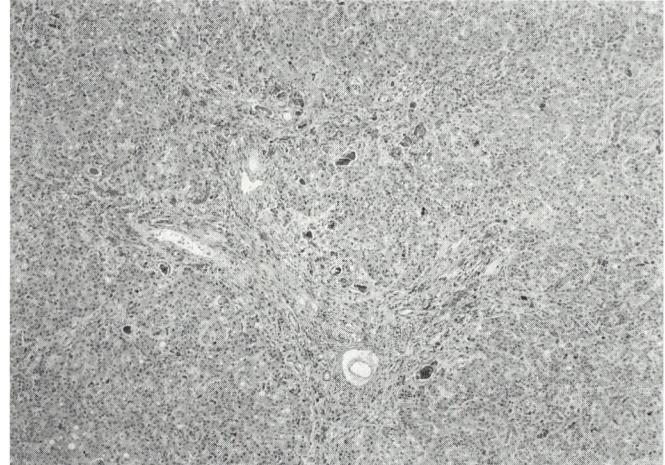

Fig. 23.6 Hepatic graft-vs.-host disease (GVHD), day 56. Pronounced hepatocellular and cholangiolar cholestasis with portal to portal bridging and parenchymal collapse. Proliferation of cholangioles along limiting plate.

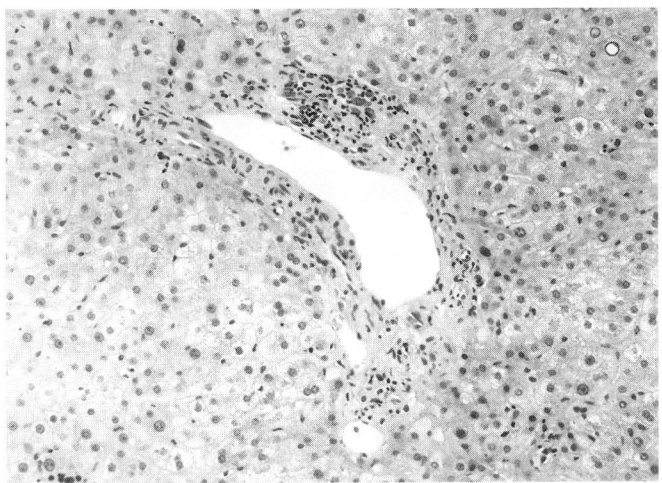

Fig. 23.7 Chronic hepatic graft-vs.-host disease (GVHD), 11 months. Destruction of small bile ducts and some portal space fibrosis with bridging or piecemeal necrosis.

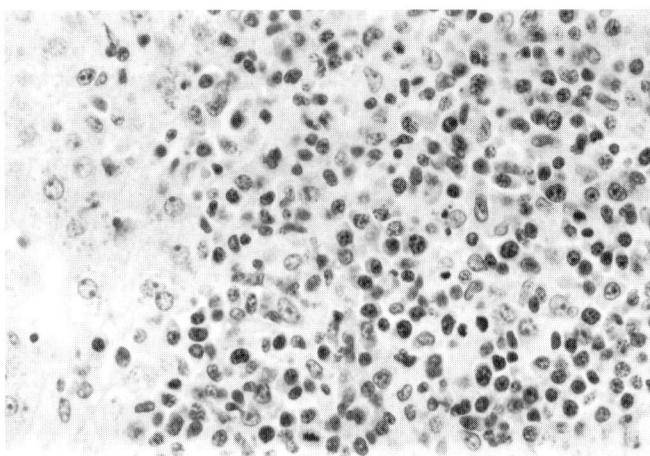

Fig. 23.8 Post-transplant lymphoproliferative disease in the liver: medium power view of a portal space that is effaced by dense infiltrate of plasmacytic to immunoblastic cells.

early cytotoxic lymphocyte attack on the ducts to a picture made up of marked cholestasis with zone 3 ballooning and dropout of hepatocytes and bizarre, dilated bile-filled periportal cholangioles seen in protracted acute GVHD of some weeks' duration (Fig. 23.6). Cholestasis and bile ductule proliferation, features often seen in long-standing GVHD, may reflect the consequences of the alloimmune segmental destruction of marginal bile ducts, an area of ductal progenitor cells [60]. Ductule proliferation may also result from the coexisting influence of gut GVHD, showering the liver with endotoxin which in turn stimulates TNF-α, a promoter of bile ductule proliferation experimentally [61,62]. Later, marked loss of bile ducts may occur. The bile duct changes that typify GVHD are illustrated in Fig. 23.5 and Plate 23.33, *facing p. 296*. The bile ducts are irregular in outline. Individual or segments of epithelial cells are flattened and missing nuclei creating a hypereosinophilic cytoplasmic syncytium. Remaining nuclei are often enlarged, hyperchromatic, irregular in shape and pseudostratified. Intraepithelial lymphocytes, the presumptive efferent cytotoxic T cells, may be present though lymphocytes are also found in other inflammatory liver diseases. Apoptosis is usually difficult to de-monstrate. The typical GVHD damaged bile ducts/ductules with withered, anucleate, focally vacuolated eosinophilic cytoplasms are sometimes best appreciated by other stains, i.e. cytokeratins, trichrome, or periodic-acid Schiff (PAS). The inflammatory component in liver GVHD, predominately in the portal spaces, is lymphocytic but may include a minor component of loosely scattered neutrophils, monocytes and plasma cells. The extent of this inflammatory infiltrate varies with duration, being less in acute than chronic GVHD (see Plate 23.59, *facing p. 296*). The most important other determinant is the concurrent use of immunosuppressive agents. Since most liver biopsies are performed while patients are receiving immunosuppressive treatment, the portal space inflammation is mild to absent, allowing much easier assessment of the bile duct changes. A notable exception occurs several months or more after transplantation when patients have been tapered or withdrawn from immunosuppressive therapy. In such patients, chronic GVHD may present with marked elevation of serum aminotransferases. In addition to characteristic bile duct features of GVHD, liver histology included a marked lobular hepatitis with intense portal sinusoidal and perivenular inflammation with many acidophilic bodies [63,64]. The distinction between chronic and acute GVHD may be difficult because flares of chronic GVHD resemble early acute GVHD. Yet, acute GVHD of 4–6 weeks' duration may have stellate portal fibrosis, bridging collapse or fibrosis (Fig. 23.6) and even loss of bile ducts

(see Fig. 6.4 in Heymer's monograph [26]). Dense portal fibrosis and loss of bile ducts, however, do correlate with chronicity (Fig. 23.7) [58]. In contrast to the unrelated donor organs used in the setting of orthotopic liver allografting, coded histopathological studies of matched sibling marrow allogeneic HCT recipients with GVHD indicate that endothelialitis is so infrequent as to be of little practical use.

Differential diagnosis

The timing of liver test abnormalities provides a good indicator as to the likely diagnostic possibilities (see Chapter 58). Based on our experience reviewing hundreds of liver biopsies from the Fred Hutchinson Cancer Research Center, and in consultation, the two greatest impediments to establishing a firm diagnosis of GVHD relate to the adequacy of the sample and quality of the histology. At least three evaluable portal spaces are recommended to evaluate for GVHD [59]. Thin core needle biopsies tend to distort portal structures. The forceps type of transvenous biopsy produces small compressed fragments. While quite adequate for diagnosing SOS (VOD), these are less suitable for the diagnosis of GVHD due to the crush artifact and the paucity of portal spaces obtained by the transvenous forceps biopsy technique. B5 and Bouins fixatives provide superior cytologic detail of GVHD-damaged bile ducts compared to formalin. Much improved histology can result by processing the formalin-fixed liver biopsies in a shortened 2-h cycle. In addition to the H&E stain, PAS with diastase and trichrome stains are very helpful, especially when there is a paucity of bile ducts.

The histologic differential diagnosis of liver GVHD includes drug liver injury and infections, especially those of viral etiologies [65,66]. However, CMV is an unlikely consideration since it results in mild anicteric hepatitis whose principle histologic findings in immunosuppressed patients are microabscesses that contain some neutrophils [67]. Hepatocyte apoptosis (acidophilic bodies) does occur in GVHD as an innocent bystander consequence of cytokine induced up-regulation of APO-1/FAS on hepatocyte membranes [68]. Following infusion of donor lymphocytes, GVHD may present as acute hepatitis with marked lobular hepatitis with elevations of serum aminotransferase greater than 10 times the upper limits of normal [69]. If the portal spaces are greatly expanded by an infiltrate rich in plasma cells, the differential diagnosis should include a post-transplant EBV-driven lymphoproliferative syndrome (Fig. 23.8) (see Chapter 56), the hepatitic onset of chronic GVHD [63] and, rarely, autoimmune hepatitis [70]. Immunohistologic markers for EBV, LMP-1 and Eber and/or the characteristic autoantibody profile are needed to establish these other entities. The development of accurate and sensitive serologic tests and immunohistologic stains for hepatitis B and C viruses does not exclude the coexistence of GVHD. In cases of severe reactivation hepatitis, it may be difficult to determine the etiology of bile duct changes.

The situation with hepatitis C virus infection, the primary cause of non-A non-B hepatitis, is more complex. Two studies indicate that post-transplantation seroconversion from negative to positive serology for hepatitis C was often accompanied by abnormal liver tests along with histologic features of chronic hepatitis [71,72]. While portal and lobular inflammation may be considerable in the hepatic onset of chronic GVHD [63], discrete portal lymphoid aggregates typical of chronic hepatitis C are not. Using the PCR, Shuhart *et al.* [73,74] followed the development of post-transplant hepatitis C infection in hepatitis C negative recipients who received blood components and/or marrow from hepatitis C viremic donors. The clinical course in their first 2 months post-HCT indicated acquisition of subclinical hepatitis C viremia. Histologic features did not overlap with those of acute GVHD. The authors previously have found that the distinction between chronic GVHD and chronic non-A non-B viral hepatitis (presumably hepatitis C) was difficult when peri-portal inflammation and bile ductule proliferation were the predominant features [58]. Moreover, immunostains for hepatitis C are much less reliable than those for hepatitis B. While liver biopsies with chronic hepatitis C have nondestructive reactive bile duct changes that might raise the possibility of liver GVHD [75,76], an international conference concluded that the bile duct lesions of rejection, a condition which closely resembles GVHD, are quantitatively and qualitatively different from hepatitis C [77]. Development of cirrhosis following chronic GVHD of the liver is extremely rare and usually occurs with the coexistence of hepatitis C. A study of long-term survivors of HCT developing cirrhosis more than 10 years after marrow transplantation demonstrated hepatitis C was the predominant etiology [68].

Immunohistology

A number of immunohistological studies have provided useful data on GVHD pathogenesis. In general, T-cell infiltrates, usually CD8 predominating, have been found in immunohistological studies of skin biopsies. Those few studies that have studied blood and tissue ratios of T-cell subsets simultaneously have found parallel CD4/8 ratios [78–80]. The routine diagnostic value of such studies seems somewhat limited, but the clear demonstration of T lymphocytes in epidermis can be helpful in deciding a borderline case. The pan-T-cell antibody UCHL-1 may be useful in paraffin-embedded tissues for this purpose. Tia-1 antibody has been proven of value in localizing cytotoxic T cells in lesions of acute and chronic GVHD and solid organ graft rejection [28]. Perforin antigen-positive lymphocytes have been reported to be demonstrable in acute skin GVHD [81]. Similarly, DR-positivity in the keratinocytes of a lesion tends to favor GVHD, although it is by no means specific [82,83]. Tunel staining for apoptosis in target cells has been reported in both animal and human GVHD and is of pathogenetic interest.

Chronic GVHD

Clinical and histopathologic manifestations of late onset or persistent GVHD are so different from those of the earlier acute period that they are separated as a group into chronic GVHD. However, the histologic changes may not always correspond to the operational definition of chronic GVHD using day 100 screening [84]. From the pathologist's viewpoint, chronic GVHD is a multiorgan inflammatory disorder that resembles a mixture of GVHD and several autoimmune diseases. Histopathological studies of chronic GVHD are vital for several reasons:

(i) Biopsies are essential to correctly diagnose chronic GVHD and indicate whether the process is active. (ii) Biopsies may exclude diagnoses and allow discontinuation of potentially toxic therapies [85]. (iii) Prognostically, histological changes of extensive chronic GVHD in certain organs may predict decreased survival [86]. (iv) Histologic studies of chronic GVHD have provided observations that suggest some of the immunologic targets and mechanisms of generalized fibrosis [84,87].

The biopsies obtained for assessment of chronic GVHD come mainly from skin, lip and liver, with fewer biopsies from the lung, muscle, vulva or synovium. In the interval since our last edition, new data have modified the use of tissue biopsies to diagnose and monitor chronic GVHD. These include recognition of the importance of the graft-vs.-tumor effect and an emphasis on survival rather than simply the presence of GVHD. A retrospective assessment of day 100 screening tests for chronic GVHD in 241 patients in a multivariant analysis of mortality found that only thrombocytopenia, elevation of serum alkaline phosphatase and a positive Schirmer's test for dry eyes predicted increased mortality. In contrast, positive oral exam, lip biopsy and skin biopsy for chronic GVHD did not demonstrate an increased likelihood of mortality [88]. Investigators at Johns Hopkins University have developed a new prognostic model for grading chronic GVHD. Based on a multivariate analysis of 23 variables, they found that survival was significantly influenced by extensive skin involvement (more than 50% of body surface area), thrombocytopenia (<100,000 µ/L), progressive onset and Karnofsky performance score <50% at time of primary treatment failure [86,89]. Accordingly, there is a wide spectrum of opinion concerning the need for oral, labial and liver biopsies in the diagnosis and management of chronic GVHD [90].

The interpretation of biopsies has also been affected by the availability of several newer immunosuppressive agents, such as phototherapy, which are often used in combination. As a result, the inflammatory lichenoid changes that typify classic extensive chronic GVHD give way to biopsies that have only small numbers of apoptotic epithelial cells with subepithelial fibrosis and little or no inflammation. Furthermore, flares that occur when immunosuppressive therapy is tapered or stopped often resemble acute GVHD. As a result, the principal question raised is "Is GVHD active and can it be distinguished from prior changes, particularly fibrosis and atrophy of the affected structures?" The pathologist should be mindful of several caveats pertinent to the histopathology of chronic GVHD:

1 The histopathology changes over time. In the early phase the predominant features are lymphoplasmacytic infiltration involving the epithelium and glands (Fig. 23.9).
2 These early inflammatory changes may in time cause widespread fibrosis, stenosis, obliteration, or atrophy of the involved tissues (Figs 23.10–12; see also Plates 23.52 & 23.61, *facing p. 296*).
3 Following a flare of chronic GVHD, the histologic changes, particularly those in the epidermis and the liver, may be more closely akin to those of acute GVHD. Further, in the absence of chronic inflammation, it may not be possible to distinguish active disease from residual late fibrotic damage (Fig. 23.11).
4 Unlike acute GVHD, chronic GVHD shows a rather extensive destruction of tubulo-alveolar glands and ducts and a corresponding clinical sicca syndrome (Figs 23.11 & 23.12).
5 Several infrequent manifestations of chronic GVHD mimic the naturally occurring autoimmune collagen vascular diseases, such as myositis (see Plate 23.58, *facing p. 296*), serositis and arthritis, and some suggest that GVHD may even rarely involve the central nervous system [91].
6 Some changes of chronic GVHD appear to be largely the consequence of damage incurred during acute GVHD such as segmental intestinal ulceration, fibrosis and stenosis. Persistent liver test abnormalities such as elevations of alkaline phosphatase and hyperbilirubinemia may also reflect damage to small bile ducts incurred mainly during acute rather than chronic GVHD.

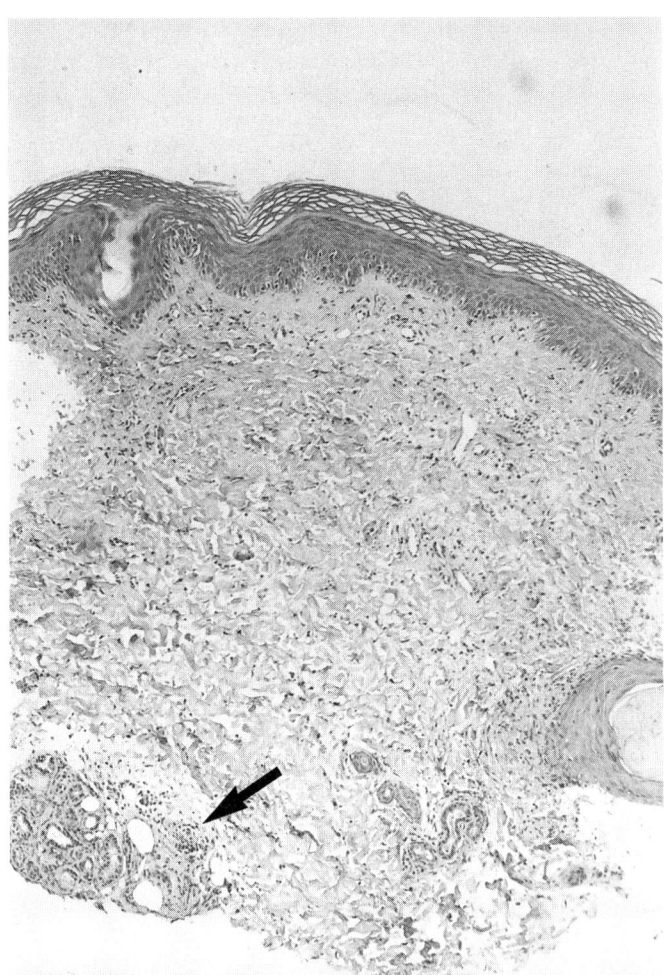

Fig. 23.9 Skin, early chronic graft-vs.-host disease (GVHD), day 314. Extensive or generalized type. The so-called lichen planus-like chronic GVHD refers to the acanthotic and hyperkeratotic epidermis that has inflammatory and destructive changes along the dermal-epidermal junction. An eccrine unit at the base of the dermis (arrow) and a follicle deep in the dermis are also being destroyed. The dermal collagen is unaltered.

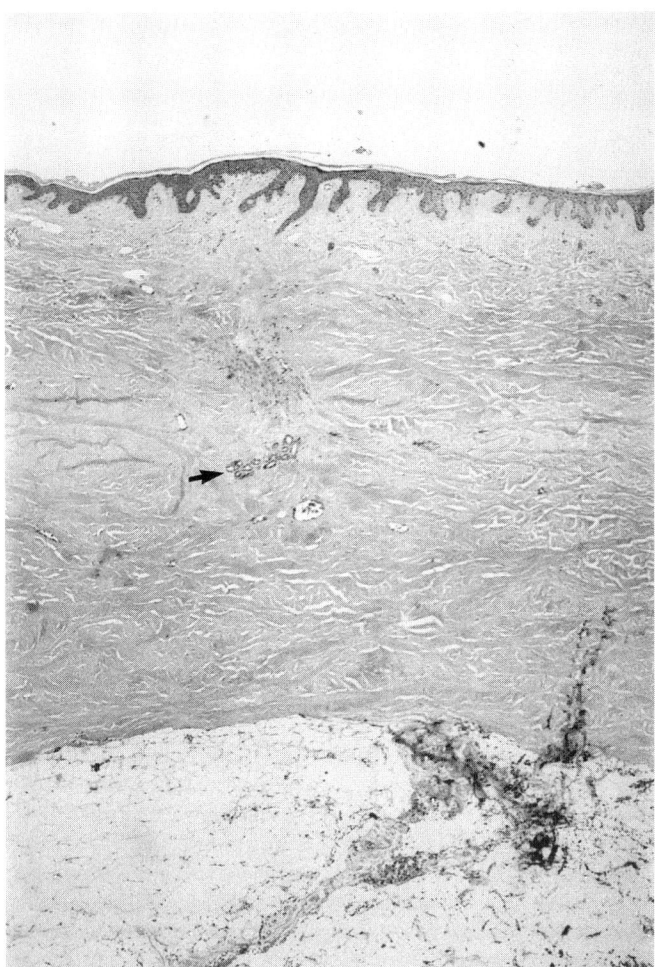

Fig. 23.10 Late sclerodermatous chronic graft-vs.-host disease (GVHD), day 910. The epidermis is atrophic. The dermal collagen is diffusely sclerotic with homogenization of the collagen and the dermal-subcutis border is straightened. The dermis below the entrapped eccrine unit (arrow) represents acquired fibrous tissue resulting from chronic GVHD.

7 The etiology of some late changes associated with chronic GVHD, such as myasthenia gravis, bullous pemphigoid, arthritis and vasculitic neuropathy, has not been fully resolved and could include GVHD, infection and true autoimmunity.

Extensive chronic GVHD of the skin is a biphasic inflammatory dermatitis, which histologically resembles a combination of lichen planus and lupus profundus in its early stages (Fig. 23.9; see also Plate 23.47, *facing p. 296*). When untreated or refractory, it resembles diffuse scleroderma with a component of fasciitis (Fig. 23.10; see also Plate 23.51, *facing p. 296*) [92]. The criterion for skin involvement is focal lichenoid inflammation as in acute GVHD. This "lichenoid" pattern of hyperkeratosis, hypergranulosis, irregular acanthosis and basal layer injury with apoptosis is associated with a decreased survival (hazard ratio of 2.2, 95% CI = 1.1–4.3) [86,93]. The irregular epidermal acanthosis in the early chronic phase is presumably a reflection of local secretion of growth factors, such as IL-3 [94] and transforming growth factor (TGF)-β_1 [95].

Additional criteria based on serial biopsies include progressive homogenization and reorganization of the dermal collagen (Fig. 23.10; Plate 23.51, *facing p. 296*), fibrous straightening of the dermal-epidermal border, inflammation about eccrine coils and, occasionally, deep panniculitis. Full thickness biopsies from recently dyspigmented or hyperkera-

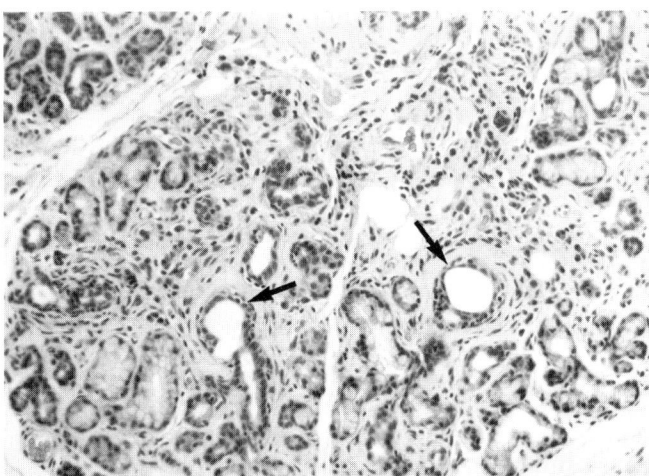

Fig. 23.11 Lip biopsy, minor salivary gland. The lymphoplasmacytic inflammatory cells are centered around small ducts. Signs of ductal epithelial cell destruction, irregularity of outline, nuclear stratification and hyperchromatism, and apoptosis (arrow) are similar to GVHD changes in small bile ducts. The glandular interstitium is becoming fibrotic and the acini atrophic resulting in a sicca syndrome.

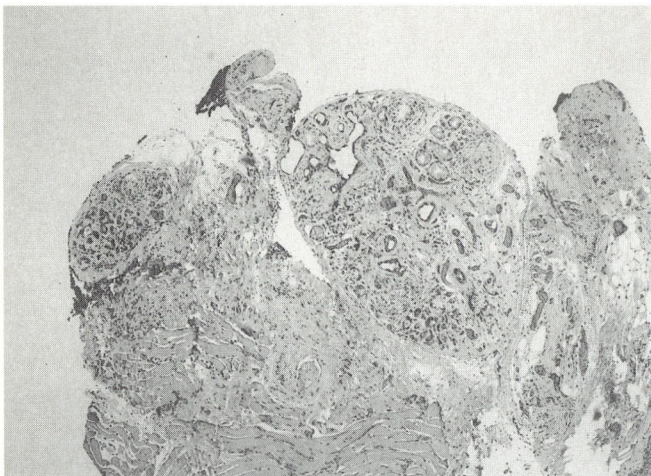

Fig. 23.12 Lip biopsy, day 376. Fibrotic and destroyed minor salivary gland contains only ectatic ducts. These changes reflect previous chronic graft-vs.-host disease (GVHD) damage. Unless they are accompanied by some inflammatory component in other glands or in the mucosa, they should not be taken as a sign of active chronic GVHD.

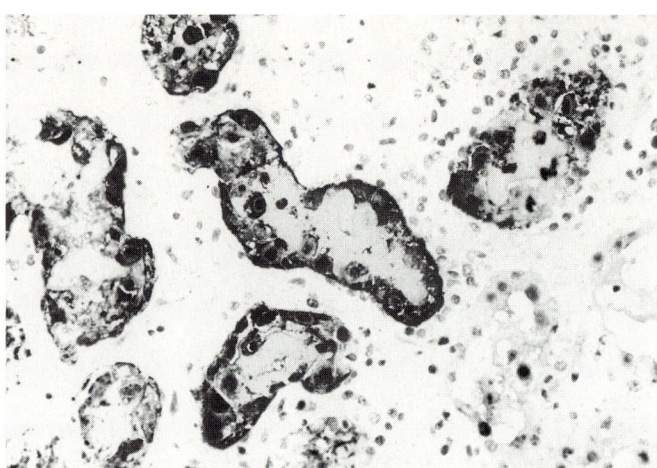

Fig. 23.13 Kidney, adenovirus (ADV) nephritis, day 77. Tubules lined by degenerating epithelial cells are strongly reactive for ADV antigen by indirect immunoperoxidase staining using a monoclonal antibody to the adenovirus hexon protein (Chemicon International, Inc., Temecula, CA). Adenovirus species 11 was isolated in culture.

totic areas should be chosen for biopsies since the chronic GVHD is not uniform in its progression or involvement. Practically speaking, the most important job of the pathologist is to distinguish residual or past damage from ongoing disease activity. Since patients often are receiving or have recently finished immunosuppressive treatment, the inflammatory changes may be quite minimal to absent. Evidence of active GVHD may be limited to epithelial vacuolar degeneration or apoptosis in the basilar layers of the skin and its appendages, oral mucosa or minor salivary glands of the lip or bile ducts.

Limited or localized chronic GVHD of the skin begins as innocent looking, dyspigmented macules with variable degrees of induration. Sampling of such areas demonstrates fibrous remodeling in the deeper reticular dermis. A small amount of epidermal degeneration or apoptosis may be present. The difference between the two types of GVHD involvement may simply depend on where in the dermis the fibrosis begins (deep with the limited form vs. subepithelial in the extensive form). Hence, it is important that biopsies be of adequate size and full thickness to include the dermis and even some subcutaneous fat.

Oral chronic GVHD has epithelial changes of GVHD in both the mucosa and minor salivary ducts as well as a fibrosing sialadenitis (see Plate 23.57, *facing p. 296*). The oral biopsies often have a background of mild inflammatory change in the mucosa and the periductal interstitium of the minor salivary glands. The histologic grading system, which the authors developed when myeloablative conditioning regimens were the norm, distinguishes between grade I inflammation which has a 50% specificity, and grade II inflammation (with apoptosis) which has a 75% specificity [96]. In the current milieu, when increasing numbers of patients receive nonmyeloablative conditioning, the specificity, particularly of grade I lesions, may be even greater. Nakhleh *et al.* [45] have utilized a modification of this threshold grading system by requiring three or more apoptotic bodies in the mucosa and at least a 10% loss of acinar tissue by inflammation before biopsies are considered positive for GVHD.

Infection

Infection is a frequent complication of HCT and the involvement of specific microorganisms has been extensively discussed in Chapters 51–57. Biopsies are valuable, not only in providing the rapid and specific diagnoses required for effective treatment, but also in providing salvage archival tissue for retrospective studies to detect organisms.

The histological demonstration of fungi in tissue (see Plate 23.45, *facing p. 296*) is often crucial to the diagnosis of invasive infection since culture isolation is slow and insensitive, fungemia is sporadic and dependable assays for antigenemia are not generally available. *Toxoplasma gondii* (see Plates 23.38 & 23.39, *facing p. 296*), *Pneumocystis carinii*, mycobacteria, Nocardia and Legionella are also organisms that may be diagnosed rapidly by histological or immunocytochemical staining and then specifically treated [97–99]. Although in most patient populations these organisms are unusual, their identification can save lives. The incidence of toxoplasmosis over a 20-year period in Seattle has been 0.3% [97], of nocardiosis over 25 years 0.2% [98] and legionellosis over 12 years has been 0.6% [99].

HCT recipients are at high risk for acquiring potentially fatal respiratory virus infections when the community prevalence of agents such as respiratory syncytial virus (RSV) is high. Because many conditioning regimens largely ablate virus-specific immunity, and because GVHD as well as its prophylaxis and treatment are broadly immunosuppressive, there is a very high rate of reactivation of latent viruses, especially members of the herpes and ADV groups [100–102]. Occasionally, viral infection of a single organ will produce an ambiguous clinical presentation best resolved by prompt biopsy and rapid tissue evaluation. For example, severe abdominal pain may suggest impending bowel infarction from reactivation of gut GVHD but may actually represent acute herpes simplex virus (HSV), varicella-zoster virus (VZV) (see Plate 23.44, *facing p. 296*) or ADV hepatitis (see Plate 23.43, *facing p. 296*), which can be diagnosed within a few hours by histological and immunocytochemical studies of a transjugular hepatic biopsy. Hematuria and costovertebral angle tenderness may result from ADV nephritis (Fig. 23.13), which we have identified by viral culture and immunocytochemical analysis of kidney tissue from 21 patients. ADV infection and disease are increasing in HCT patients. The severity of lymphopenia has been identified as a risk factor [103]. We have noted that the risk of ADV infection is decreased in patients receiving ganciclovir as prophylactic or pre-emptive therapy for CMV.

Antiviral prophylaxis has led to a significant decrease in the early incidence of CMV and the overall level of HSV infection. However, the pathologist must still remain alert to the presence of these organisms

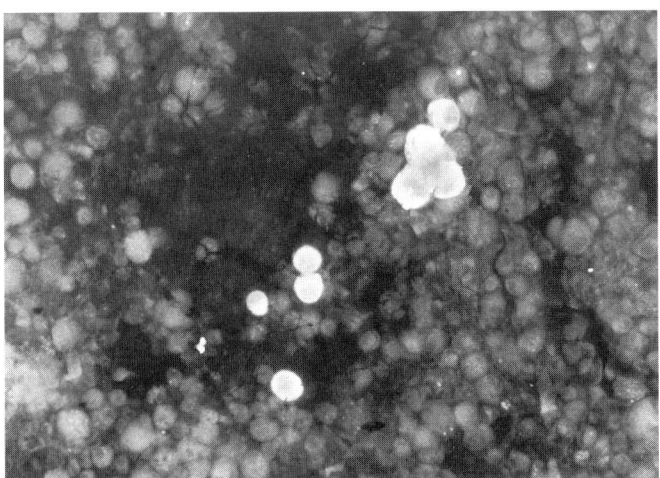

Fig. 23.14 Bronchoalveolar lavage cytospin, cytomegalovirus (CMV), day 64. Late CMV antigen is demonstrated in eight cells by indirect immunofluorescence with a monoclonal antibody primary (Genetic Systems, Seattle, WA; Syva Corp., Palo Alto, CA).

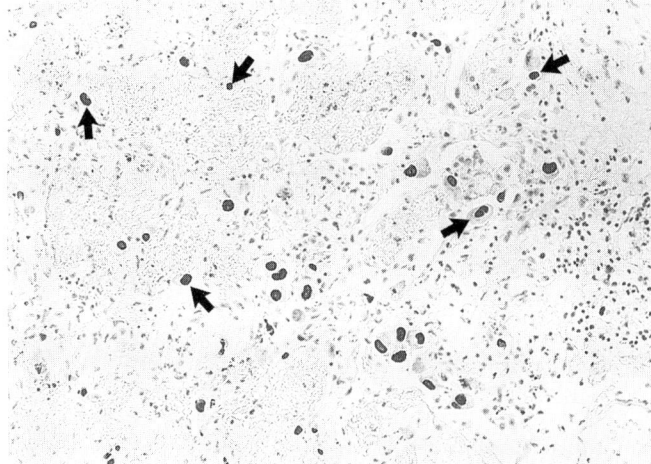

Fig. 23.16 Lung, cytomegalovirus (CMV) pneumonia, day 54. Large numbers of infected cells display nuclear reactivity (some positive cells marked by arrows) for an early CMV antigen by monoclonal antibody indirect immunoperoxidase staining (Genetic Systems, Seattle, WA; Syva Corp., Palo Alto, CA).

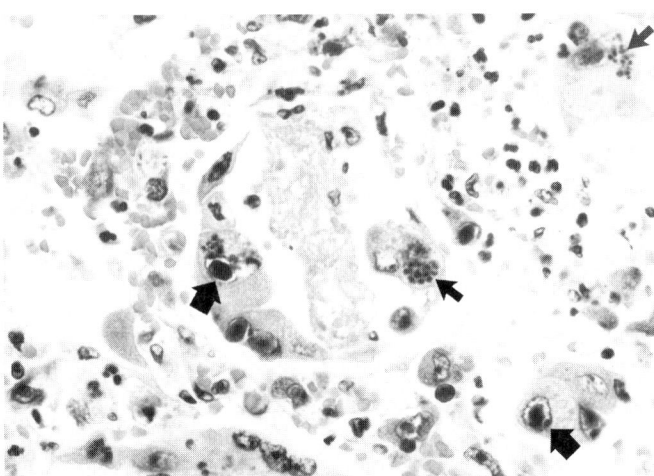

Fig. 23.15 Lung, cytomegalovirus (CMV) pneumonia, day 68. Several large cells contain Cowdry type A nuclear inclusions (large arrows) as well as six to twelve smaller cytoplasmic inclusions (small arrows) diagnostic for CMV infection, H&E.

even though they are seen less frequently. In addition, late CMV pneumonia (see Plate 23.41, *facing p. 296*) occurring at a median of approximately 24 weeks post-transplant is increasing in association with the early use of prophylactic and pre-emptive therapy [104]. The availability of more effective antiviral drugs has increased the importance of rapid and specific viral diagnosis. Demonstration of CMV by culture, cytology, immunocytochemistry (Figs 23.14–16), hybridization or PCR techniques in bronchoalveolar lavage material from a patient with pneumonia is now adequate for institution of anti-CMV therapy. However, lung biopsy may still be necessary when knowledge of the histologic pattern is needed or if the interpretation of the lavage findings is uncertain [102].

Pulmonary disease

The lung is susceptible to damage by varied and sometimes interacting mechanisms including infection, chemical toxicity, irradiation damage, immune reaction and malignant infiltration. Pathologists are appropriately reluctant to classify the pneumonia in an immunocompromised patient as definitely noninfectious since microorganisms in any of the following categories may be present:

1 Previously uncharacterized (as were Legionella and human herpes viruses 6, 7 and 8) [99].
2 Capable of causing pneumonia but usually requiring special detection techniques (*Mycoplasma*, *Chlamydia* spp.).
3 Present in other organs but of uncertain significance as a pulmonary pathogen (*Cryptosporidia*, *Campylobacter* spp.).
4 Visible by routine histology but subtle and not likely to be cultured (*Toxoplasma* spp.) [97].

In contrast, the mere presence of an infectious agent is not always sufficient evidence that it is the sole or even the major cause of pulmonary disease. Damage from chemotherapy, irradiation or GVHD may also be present but manifest only by nonspecific inflammatory alterations.

Approximately 15–20% of patients receiving allogeneic HCT for leukemia develop nonbacterial pneumonia, a clinical syndrome loosely referred to as "interstitial pneumonia" (IP), which has become approximately half as frequent over the past two decades [100]. This is a generally severe, acute process in contrast to the insidious chronic course of disorders such as usual IP of Liebow. Slightly fewer than half of these pneumonias were formerly associated with CMV, 8% with other viruses (HSV, VZV, ADV and RSV) and 4% with *Pneumocystis carinii* [100]. Pneumocystis is now much less common, developing usually in the absence of prophylactic therapy. We now rarely see CMV or HSV in bronchoalveolar lavage cells or gut biopsies because seropositive patients receive antiviral prophylaxis and antigenemia is often treated preemptively. However, these viruses are not eradicated, so late infection may develop after treatment is stopped. Human herpes virus 6 may be involved in some cases of IP [105].

The remainder of IPs, approximately one-third of the total, are noninfectious. They are part of the interstitial pneumonia syndrome (IPS), in which there are multilobar infiltrates by X-ray or scan, symptoms and signs of pneumonia with evidence of abnormal physiology, and absence of active lower respiratory tract infection [106,107]. These cases probably have a multifactorial etiology, with toxicity from chemotherapy and irradiation high on the list [108,109]. Alkylating agents such as cyclophosphamide and busulfan have long been implicated in pulmonary toxicity. There is now increasing evidence that high-dose melphalan may also cause lung damage [110].

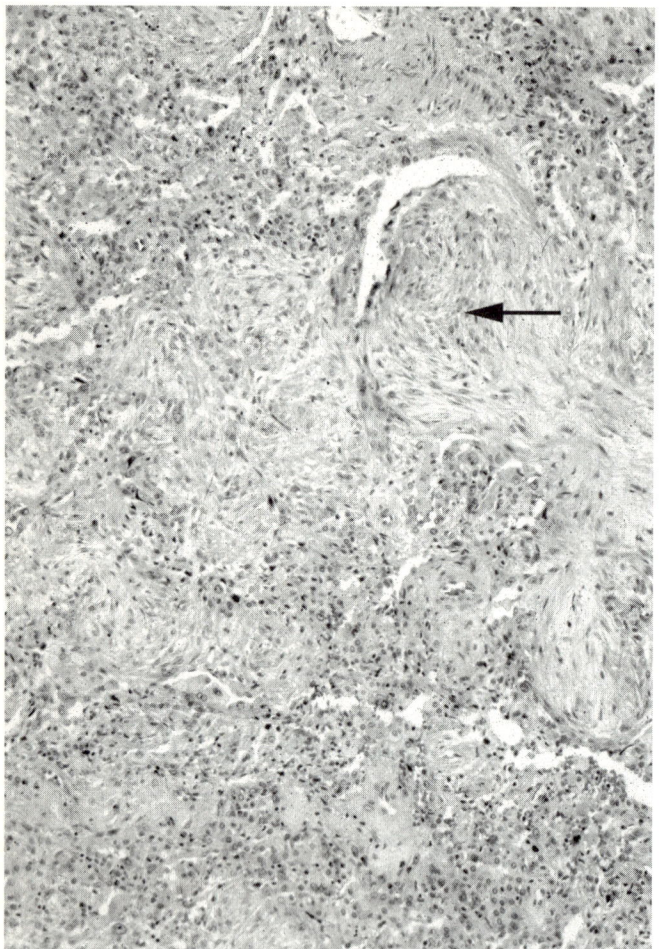

Fig. 23.17 Lung, bronchiolitis obliterans organizing pneumonia (BOOP), day 120 following marrow allograft transplantation. The patient developed dyspnea and a cough following tapering of corticosteroid therapy for chronic graft-vs.-host disease (GVHD). A chest X-ray showed multifocal alveolar opacities clinically suggestive of fungal or viral pneumonia. The biopsy demonstrated areas of consolidation in which bronchioles are blocked by granulation tissue (arrow) which also extends into nearby alveoli and is associated with interstitial and alveolar infiltration by mononuclear inflammatory cells. In hematopoietic stem cell recipients, BOOP is usually unassociated with infection, although this must be ruled out. There is increasing evidence that it often reflects pulmonary graft-vs.-host (GVH) activity. However, as is true for GVHD of skin, liver and gut, the histological changes are not pathognomonic and must be correlated with the clinical findings, H&E.

Acute GVHD is a risk factor for IPS [106,111]. IPS has not been ascribed to an allogeneic reaction in humans, although there is evidence in mice that nonbacterial pneumonia is a combined effect of GVHD and radiation [112]. Multivariate analysis of more than 180 nonmyeloablative transplant patients indicates that their risk of IPS is significantly lower than that of patients who receive myeloablative conditioning. Since the incidence of acute GVHD is the same, it appears that the major cause of early IPS is conditioning toxicity.

The spectrum of severity of IP varies from barely perceptible abnormalities to end-stage honeycomb lung. Although the pattern and severity are influenced by the timing of the biopsy, the degree of hypoxic damage and the extent of toxicity secondary to oxygen therapy, these factors cannot be separated from one another morphologically. Some cases progress to diffuse consolidation in a few days and fibrosis sufficient to produce an end-stage honeycomb picture may develop in as little as 2 weeks. Thrombocytopenia may lead to intrapulmonary oozing and a variable degree of hemorrhage associated with iron-laden macrophages. Pulmonary hemorrhage is usually present in association with other characteristics of diffuse alveolar damage such as hyaline membranes. The authors have identified two patients with symptomatic pulmonary hypertension documented by right heart catheterization. An open lung biopsy of one demonstrated pulmonary VOD (see Plate 23.13, *facing p. 296*) [113]. This unusual complication has been described after chemotherapy in several settings and may be associated with both hepatic VOD and IP [114,115].

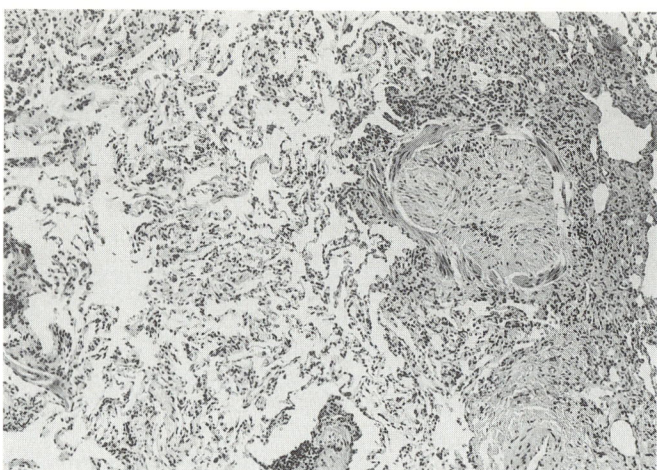

Fig. 23.18 Lung, bronchiolitis obliterans, day 395. A bronchiole displays fibrous obliteration of the lumen associated with a mild peribronchial lymphocytic infiltrate. The patient had chronic graft-vs.-host disease (GVHD) and experienced severe pulmonary obstruction, H&E.

Pulmonary GVHD

Although the existence of an acute pulmonary graft-vs.-host (GVH) reaction is conceptually appealing, its histological appearance is unclear. Where open lung biopsies are used to study the pulmonary decompensation, which sometimes coincides temporally with acute GVHD in skin, liver and gut, the histological alterations are nonspecific and can usually be classified as diffuse alveolar damage (see Plate 23.12, *facing p. 296*) or idiopathic IP. Occasionally, CMV pneumonia is present. It is possible that acute GVHD of the lung cannot be recognized in this setting because the repertoire of pulmonary responses is limited.

On the basis of a histological study of the large airways in a selected group of human autopsies, a strong correlation was described between "lymphocytic bronchitis" (i.e. mononuclear inflammatory infiltration of bronchial mucosa associated with necrosis of individual epithelial cells) and acute GVHD in other organs [116]. Because most open lung biopsies do not sample bronchi with cartilage and because studies of bronchial biopsies at several centers produced largely negative results, the entity has remained an autopsy diagnosis. Another conceptual problem is that this large airway inflammation was said to produce bronchopneumonia through impairment of the bronchociliary escalator, a pathogenetic mechanism not readily applicable to the vast majority of post-transplant pneumonias, which are interstitial. The major obstacle to acceptance of lymphocytic bronchitis as acute pulmonary GVHD has been its lack of association with GVHD in the classical target organs of skin, liver and gut either in humans or in the canine HCT model [117]. An additional problem is that lymphocytic bronchitis is a nonspecific entity, being present in untransplanted children dying with viral infections and in trauma victims.

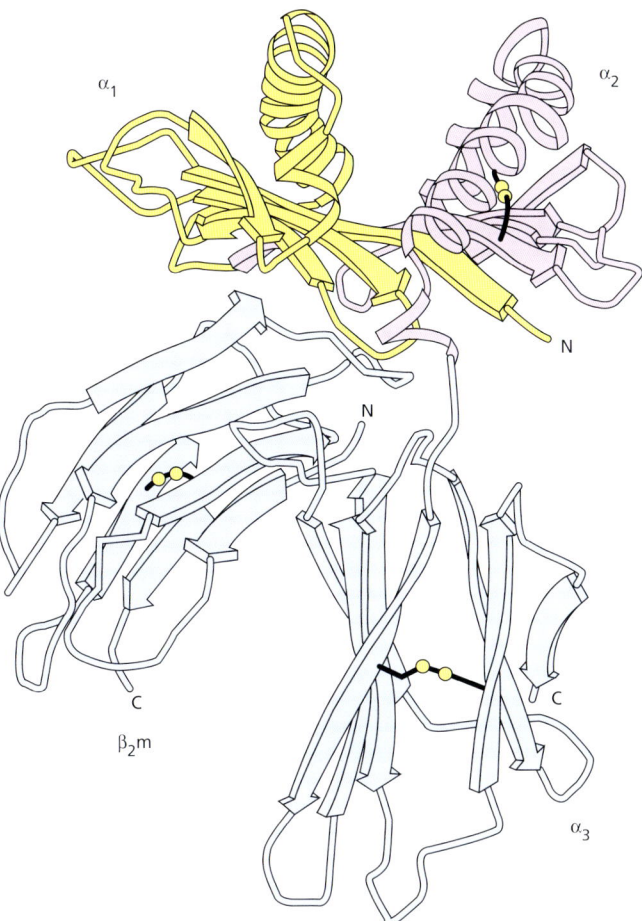

Plate 4.1 Schematic representation of an HLA class I molecule. Ribbon diagram of a class I molecule showing the four domains. The α_3 and β_2 microglobulin domains proximal to the cell membrane are shown at the bottom and the polymorphic α_1 and α_2 domains are shown at the top. The β-strands are indicated as wide arrows while α-helical portions are shown as coiled ribbons. (*See also Fig. 4.2, p. 34.*)

Plate 5.1 Localization and organization of HLA class I and class II genes on the short arm of chromosome 6 (6p21.31). Selected class I and class II genes are shown not to scale from (HLA-F) telomere towards centromere (tapasin). (*See also Fig. 5.1, p. 44.*)

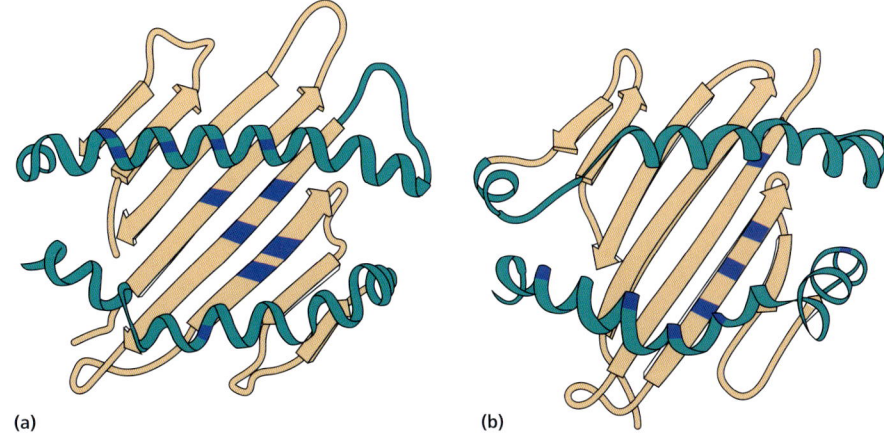

Plate 4.2 The location of polymorphic sites in the antigen-binding cleft of HLA class I and class II molecules. Schematic representation of an HLA class I molecule (a) and an HLA class II molecule (b) as seen from the top surface. The α_1 and α_2 domains (class I) and α_1 and β_1 domains (class II) form the sides of the antigen-binding cleft. Polymorphic sites with maximum amino acid variation from allele to allele are shown as colored bars. (*See also Fig. 4.3, p. 34.*)

DRB1 allelic groups	DRB2	DRB3	DRB4	DRB5	DRB6	DRB7	DRB8	DRB9
DR3, 11, 12, 13 & 14	X	X						X
DR4, 7, & 9			X			X	X	X
DR1*, 15 & 16				X	X			X
DR1, 10					X			X
DR8								X

Plate 5.2 Organization of *DRB* haplotypes. (*See also Table 5.1, p. 45.*)

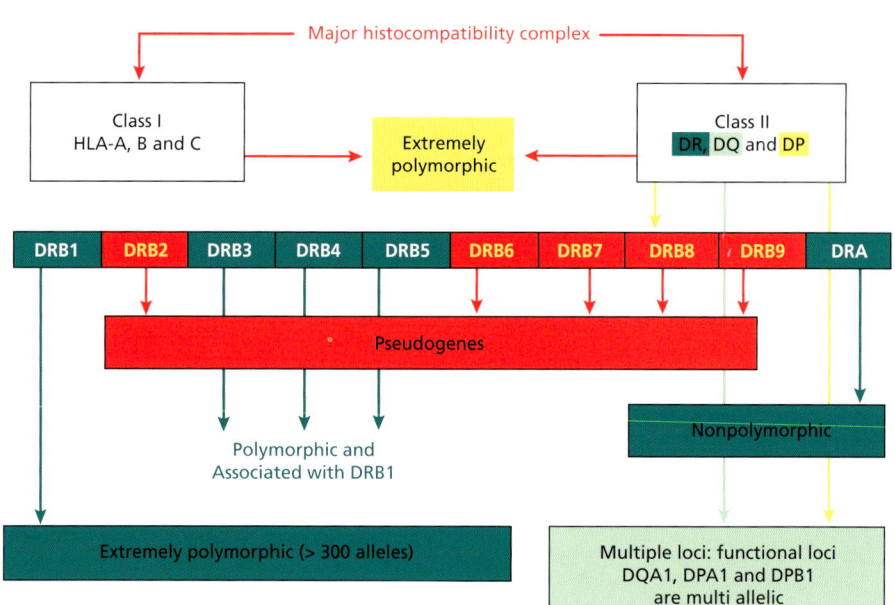

Plate 5.3 Two layer polymorphism of the major histocompatibility loci: multiple loci and multiple alleles. DR region with a variation in the number of DRB genes compared to the conserved number of DQ and DP genes is intriguing. The duplication and recombination events have affected other class II genes differently. DP and DQ clusters present a possibility of combinatorial dimers since polymorphism occurs both in α and β chain encoding genes. (*See also Fig. 5.2, p. 45.*)

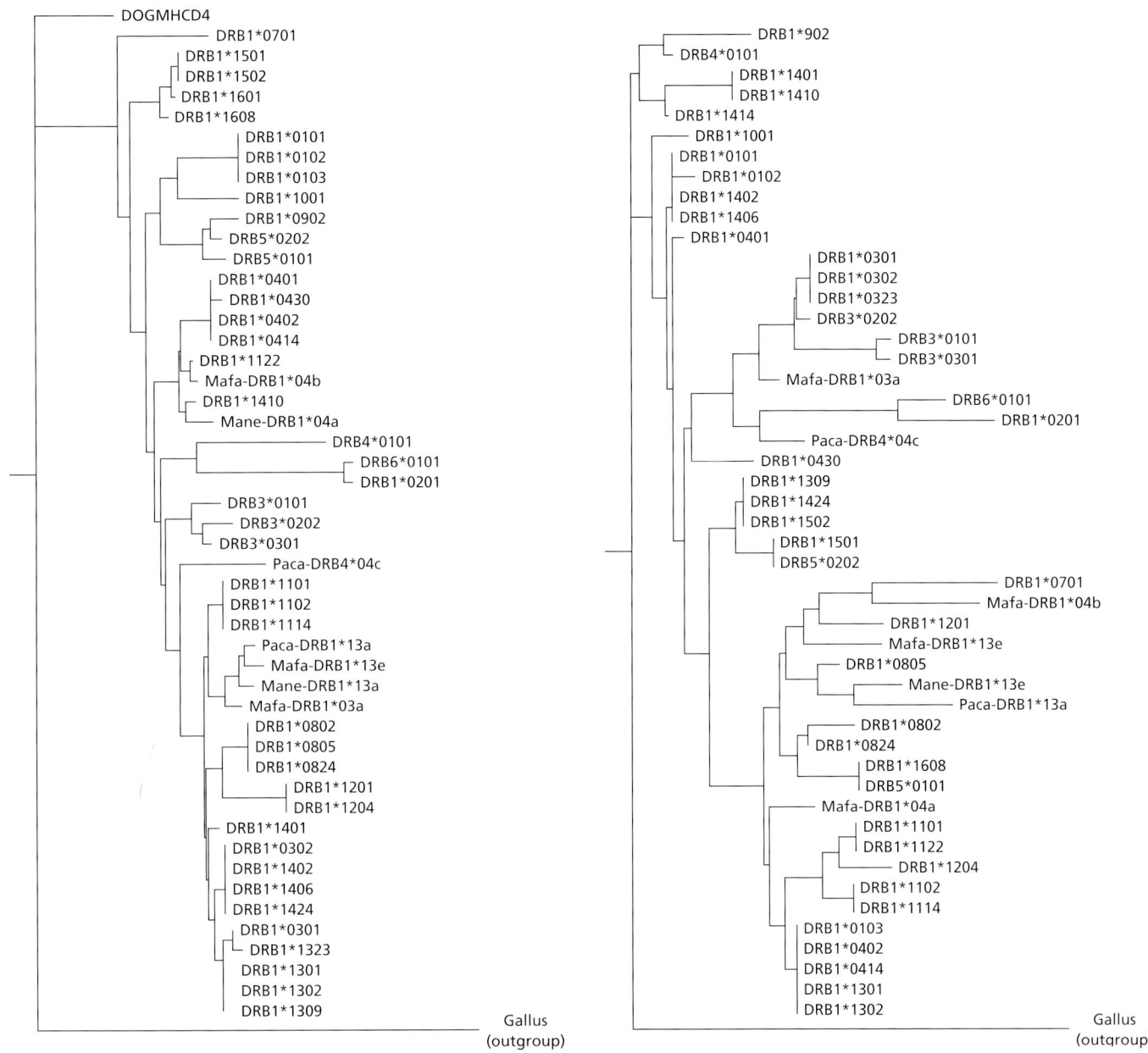

Plate 5.4 Parsimony trees showing relationships between nucleotide sequences of the second exons of human DRB (denoted simply as DRB followed by the corresponding locus number) and for nonhuman DRB alleles (species designations in the prefix) from a set of closely related primates. Sequences for residues 6–53, encoding the β-pleated sheet (a) and residues 54–78, encoding the α-helix (b) were analyzed separately. One or more allelic variants from each major allelic group were selected and phylogentic trees were created using PHYLIP (the PHYLogeny Inference Package) program neighboring joining/UPGMA method to construct the trees on the website http://hiv-web.lanl.gov/content/hiv-db/CONTAM/TreeMaker/TreeMaker.html [16: Chapter 5]. Sequence motifs in the β-pleated sheet appear to reflect a common ancestry while shared sequences encoding α-helix segments may have recombined into the framework of different alleles by segmental transfer after the divergence of ancestral allelic lineages. These results indicate that two segments of the second exon have different evolutionary histories. Included are sequences from nonhuman primate species (Mane, *Macaca nemestrina*; Mafa, *M. fascicularis*; Paca, *Papio cynocephalus anubis*. Bird, *Gallus* MHC sequence was used as outgroup). Interestingly, the old world monkey (OWM) sequences cluster with several HLA alleles, suggesting both sequence and motif conservation. (*See also Fig. 5.3, p. 46.*)

```
               7            20        30          40          50          60          70        80    86
               |            |         |           |           |           |           |         |     |
HLA-DRB1*0101  FLWQLKFECHFFNGTERVRLLERC IYNQEESVRFDSDVGEYRAVTELG RPDAEYWNSQKDLLEQRRAAVDTYRRHNYGVGE
HLA-DRB1*0402  --E-V-H------------F-D-Y F-H---Y----------------- ------------I--DE--------------V-
HLA-DRB1*0412  --E-V-H------------F-D-Y F-H---Y----------------- --S---------I--D---L-----------V-
Mane-DRB1*04a  --E-V-H------------F-D-Y FH----Y----------------- -----S------I--DA---------Y----V-
Mafa-DRB1*04c  --E-V-H------------Y-I-Y -H----NA---------------- --------G------R---Q------Y----V-
Mane-DRB1*04d  --E-V-H------------F-D-Y F-----Y----------------- ------------I---K-GQ--N--------A-
Paca-DRB1*13b  --EYSTS------------Y-D-Y F-----Y----------------- ----------------K-GQ--N----------
HLA-DRB1*1101  --EYSTS------------F-D-Y F-----Y---------F------- ---E--------F--D-----------------
HLA-DRB1*1301  --EYSTS------------F-D-Y FH----N---------F------- ------------I--DE--------------V-
Mane-DRB1*13e  --EYSTS------------F-D-Y F-----Y-------------S--- -RS-----G---F--D----S----------V-
HLA-DRB1*0301  --EYSTS------------Y-D-Y FH----N---------F------- ----------------K-GR--N--------V-
Mane-DRB1*03b  --EYSTS------------Y-D-Y F-----N----------------- ------------I---K--R--N--------F-
Mane-DRB1*03e  --EYSTS------------F-D-Y F-----NL--------F---S--- ------------F-------------Y--R---
```

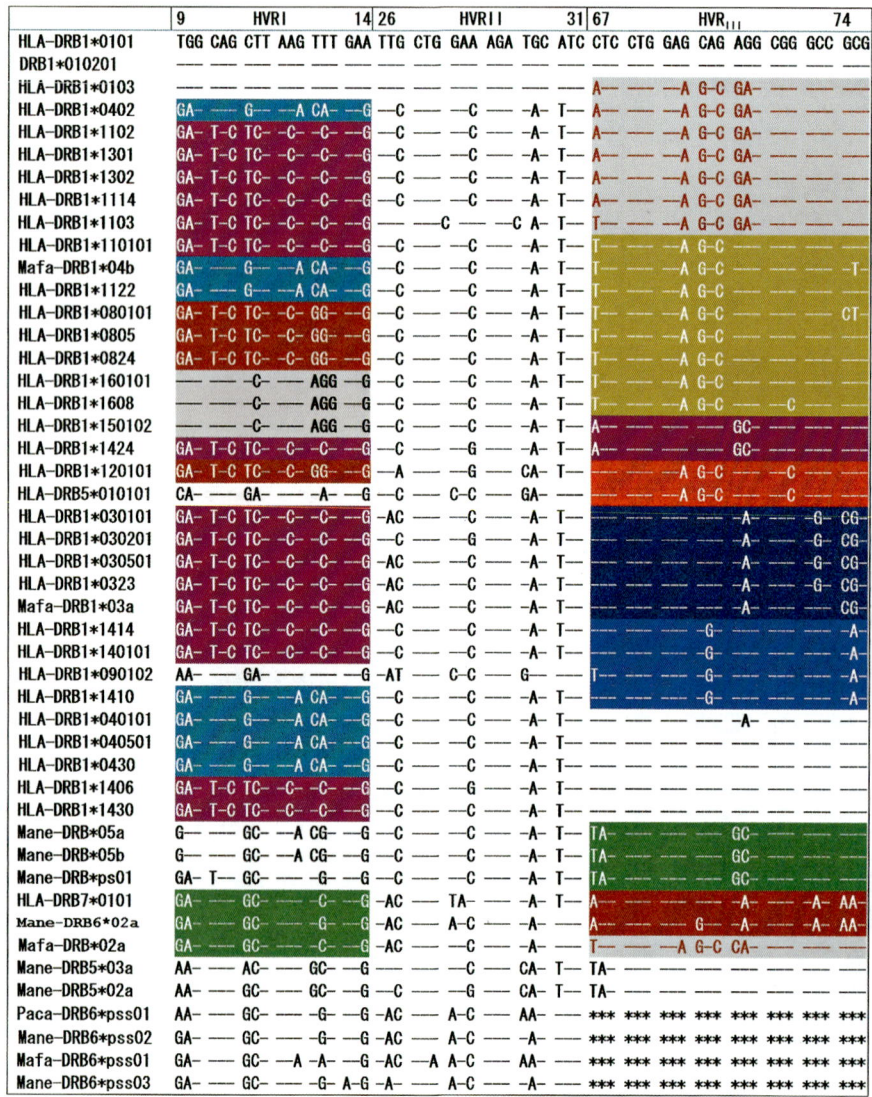

Plate 5.5 DRB second exon sequence alignment to demonstrate allelic lineages predate speciation. DRB1*04 and DRB1*13 alleles from macaques (Mane, *Macaca nemestrina*; Mafa, *M. fascicularis*) and a baboon (Paca, *Papio cynocephalus anubis*) were aligned with human contemporary human alleles. More examples from published literature see [14,15,20,23: Chapter 5]. (*See also Fig. 5.4, p. 47.*)

	9		HVRI			14	26		HVRII			31	67			HVR_{III}				74
HLA-DRB1*0101	TGG	CAG	CTT	AAG	TTT	GAA	TTG	CTG	GAA	AGA	TGC	ATC	CTC	CTG	GAG	CAG	AGG	CGG	GCC	GCG
DRB1*010201	—	—	—	—	—	—	—	—	—	—	—	—	—	—	—	—	—	—	—	—
HLA-DRB1*0103	—	—	—	—	—	—	—	—	—	—	—	—	A—	—	—A	G-C	GA-	—	—	—
HLA-DRB1*0402	GA-	—	G—	—A	CA-	—G	—C	—	—C	—	-A-	T—	A—	—	—A	G-C	GA-	—	—	—
HLA-DRB1*1102	GA-	T-C	TC-	-C-	-C-	—G	—C	—	—C	—	-A-	T—	A—	—	—A	G-C	GA-	—	—	—
HLA-DRB1*1301	GA-	T-C	TC-	-C-	-C-	—G	—C	—	—C	—	-A-	T—	A—	—	—A	G-C	GA-	—	—	—
HLA-DRB1*1302	GA-	T-C	TC-	-C-	-C-	—G	—C	—	—C	—	-A-	T—	A—	—	—A	G-C	GA-	—	—	—
HLA-DRB1*1114	GA-	T-C	TC-	-C-	-C-	—G	—C	—	—C	—	-A-	T—	A—	—	—A	G-C	GA-	—	—	—
HLA-DRB1*1103	GA-	T-C	TC-	-C-	-C-	—G	—	—C	—	—C	A-	T—	T—	—	—A	G-C	GA-	—	—	—
HLA-DRB1*110101	GA-	T-C	TC-	-C-	-C-	—G	—C	—	—C	—	-A-	T—	T—	—	—A	G-C	—	—	—	—
Mafa-DRB1*04b	GA-	—	G—	—A	CA-	—G	—C	—	—C	—	-A-	T—	T—	—	—A	G-C	—	—	—	-T-
HLA-DRB1*1122	GA-	—	G—	—A	CA-	—G	—C	—	—C	—	-A-	T—	T—	—	—A	G-C	—	—	—	—
HLA-DRB1*080101	GA-	T-C	TC-	-C-	GG-	—G	—C	—	—C	—	-A-	T—	T—	—	—A	G-C	—	—	—	CT-
HLA-DRB1*0805	GA-	T-C	TC-	-C-	GG-	—G	—C	—	—C	—	-A-	T—	T—	—	—A	G-C	—	—	—	—
HLA-DRB1*0824	GA-	T-C	TC-	-C-	GG-	—G	—C	—	—C	—	-A-	T—	T—	—	—A	G-C	—	—	—	—
HLA-DRB1*160101	—	—	-C-	—	AGG	—G	—C	—	—C	—	-A-	T—	T—	—	—A	G-C	—	—	—	—
HLA-DRB1*1608	—	—	-C-	—	AGG	—G	—C	—	—C	—	-A-	T—	T—	—	—A	G-C	—	—C	—	—
HLA-DRB1*150102	—	—	-C-	—	AGG	—G	—C	—	—C	—	-A-	T—	A—	—	—	—	GC-	—	—	—
HLA-DRB1*1424	GA-	T-C	TC-	-C-	-C-	—G	—C	—	—G	—	-A-	T—	A—	—	—	—	GC-	—	—	—
HLA-DRB1*120101	GA-	T-C	TC-	-C-	GG-	—G	—A	—	—G	—	CA-	T—	—	—	—A	G-C	—	—C	—	—
HLA-DRB5*010101	CA-	—	GA-	—	-A-	—G	—C	—	C-C	—	GA-	—	—	—	—A	G-C	—	—C	—	—
HLA-DRB1*030101	GA-	T-C	TC-	-C-	-C-	—G	-AC	—	—C	—	-A-	T—	—	—	—	—	-A-	—	-G-	CG-
HLA-DRB1*030201	GA-	T-C	TC-	-C-	-C-	—G	—C	—	—G	—	-A-	T—	—	—	—	—	-A-	—	-G-	CG-
HLA-DRB1*030501	GA-	T-C	TC-	-C-	-C-	—G	-AC	—	—C	—	-A-	T—	—	—	—	—	-A-	—	-G-	CG-
HLA-DRB1*0323	GA-	T-C	TC-	-C-	-C-	—G	-AC	—	—C	—	-A-	T—	—	—	—	—	-A-	—	-G-	CG-
Mafa-DRB1*03a	GA-	T-C	TC-	-C-	-C-	—G	-AC	—	—C	—	-A-	T—	—	—	—	—	-A-	—	—	CG-
HLA-DRB1*1414	GA-	T-C	TC-	-C-	-C-	—G	—C	—	—C	—	-A-	T—	—	—	—	-G-	—	—	—	-A-
HLA-DRB1*140101	GA-	T-C	TC-	-C-	-C-	—G	—C	—	—C	—	-A-	T—	—	—	—	-G-	—	—	—	-A-
HLA-DRB1*090102	AA-	—	GA-	—	—	—G	-AT	—	C-C	—	G—	—	T—	—	—	-G-	—	—	—	-A-
HLA-DRB1*1410	GA-	—	G—	—A	CA-	—G	—C	—	—C	—	-A-	T—	—	—	—	-G-	—	—	—	-A-
HLA-DRB1*040101	GA-	—	G—	—A	CA-	—G	—C	—	—C	—	-A-	T—	—	—	—	—	-A-	—	—	—
HLA-DRB1*040501	GA-	—	G—	—A	CA-	—G	—C	—	—C	—	-A-	T—	—	—	—	—	—	—	—	—
HLA-DRB1*0430	GA-	—	G—	—A	CA-	—G	—C	—	—C	—	-A-	T—	—	—	—	—	—	—	—	—
HLA-DRB1*1406	GA-	T-C	TC-	-C-	-C-	—G	—C	—	—G	—	-A-	T—	—	—	—	—	—	—	—	—
HLA-DRB1*1430	GA-	T-C	TC-	-C-	-C-	—G	—C	—	—C	—	-A-	T—	—	—	—	—	—	—	—	—
Mane-DRB*05a	G—	—	GC-	—A	CG-	—G	—C	—	—C	—	-A-	T—	TA-	—	—	—	GC-	—	—	—
Mane-DRB*05b	G—	—	GC-	—A	CG-	—G	—C	—	—C	—	-A-	T—	TA-	—	—	—	GC-	—	—	—
Mane-DRB*ps01	GA-	T—	GC-	—	-G-	—G	—C	—	—C	—	-A-	T—	TA-	—	—	—	GC-	—	—	—
HLA-DRB7*0101	GA-	—	GC-	—	-C-	—G	-AC	—	TA-	—	-A-	T—	A—	—	—	—	-A-	—	-A-	AA-
Mane-DRB6*02a	GA-	—	GC-	—	-G-	—G	-AC	—	A-C	—	-A-	—	A—	—	—	G—	-A-	—	-A-	AA-
Mafa-DRB*02a	GA-	—	GC-	—	-C-	—G	-AC	—	—C	—	-A-	—	T—	—	—A	G-C	CA-	—	—	—
Mane-DRB5*03a	AA-	—	AC-	—	GC-	—G	—	—	—C	—	CA-	T—	TA-	—	—	—	—	—	—	—
Mane-DRB5*02a	AA-	—	GC-	—	GC-	—G	—C	—	—G	—	CA-	T—	TA-	—	—	—	—	—	—	—
Paca-DRB6*pss01	AA-	—	GC-	—	-G-	—G	-AC	—	A-C	—	AA-	—	***	***	***	***	***	***	***	***
Mane-DRB6*pss02	GA-	—	GC-	—	-G-	—G	-AC	—	A-C	—	-A-	—	***	***	***	***	***	***	***	***
Mafa-DRB6*pss01	GA-	—	GC-	—A	-A-	—G	-AC	—A	A-C	—	AA-	—	***	***	***	***	***	***	***	***
Mane-DRB6*pss03	GA-	—	GC-	—	-G-	A-G	-A-	—	A-C	—	-A-	—	***	***	***	***	***	***	***	***

Plate 5.6 Selected human leukocyte antigen (*HLA*), macaque (*Macaca nemestrina* and *M. fascicularis*) and baboon (*Papio cynocephalus anubis*) sequence alignment representing the three hypervariable regions with the DRB second exon. The allelic designation for the primates is provisional; allelic designation "ps" indicates a pseudogene with a stop codon and "pss" indicates pseudogenes with a short sequence due to the 62-bp gap in the α-helical region. Alignment of sequence motifs from *HLA-DRB1* second exon sequences suggests shuffling of sequences generating combinations of alleles. Recurrent hypervariable region motifs are illustrated which intermix to form numerous major histocompatibility complex (MHC) allelic patterns. HVR_{III} motifs (with one or two substitutions), shown in different colors in HVR_{III}, occur almost in all lineages. Such perpetuation of successful motifs reflects strong selection for and functional importance of the motifs involved. Polymorphism among DRB genes can be viewed as a patchwork of distinct clusters of variable sequence elements (HVR) that occur in three sites including the HVR_{III} cluster encoding residues 67–74 within the α-helical loop region. Conserved sequence motifs from this region occur interspersed among loci, alleles and even between species as highlighted in this figure. Lost HVR_{III} among the NHP sequences is denoted by an asterix. Perhaps these constitute donor sequences. (*See also Chapter 5, pp. 46–8.*)

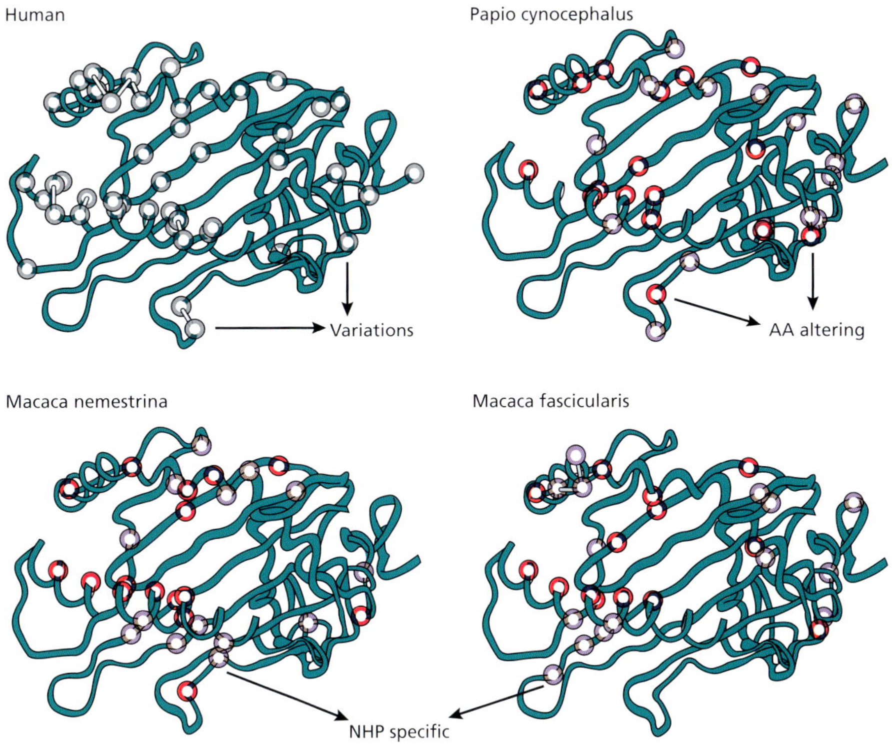

Plate 5.7 Comparison of class I molecular modeling representation from the old world monkey (OWM) species and humans highlighting the pattern of substitution in three species of old world monkeys. The human HLA class I A2 crystalline structure [63: Chapter 5] has all amino acid backbones with known variation marked on its ribbon structure with the white color balls. The other three molecules are models of a baboon (*Papio cynocephalus anubis*), pigtailed (*Macaca nemestrina*) and cynomolgus (*M. fascicularis*) macaques. The dark pink (red) points on the models indicate amino acid identities within the nonhuman primate species that are different from any known human sequence at points where polymorphism is known to occur. The light pink points in the ribbon structures indicate novel amino acids at points that are conserved in humans. (*See also Fig. 5.5, p. 49.*)

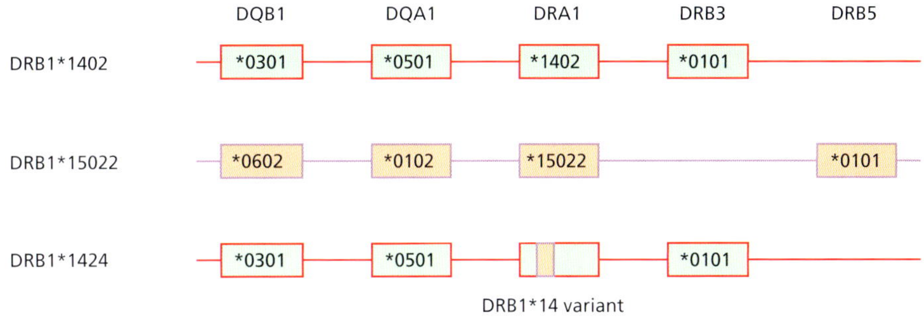

Plate 5.8 An example of segmental exchange: a DR14-DR15 recombinant on DR14 background. Donor sequence most likely is from DR15022. Other alternative donor sequence would be DRB5*0202. (*See also Fig. 5.6, p. 49.*)

Plate 5.9 Representation of conserved, polymorphic major histocompatibility complex (MHC) residues determining the specificity of amino acids bound in the key structural pockets of class II molecules. Pockets 4, 7 and 9 are represented. Macaque (*Macaca nemestrina* and *M. fascicularis*), baboon (*Papio cynocephalus anubis*) and red wolf (*Canis latrans*) *DRB* motifs were compared to human. Three pocket-9 sequence motifs were selected and comparisons were made among various sequences derived from HLA and nonhuman-specific DRB alleles. One of the nonhuman primate sequences, MafaDRB1*03, is identical to the HLA-DRB1*0301 in all three pockets. The sequence motif EYDYW is also conserved in red wolves (CalaDRB1*03). A, alanine; C, cysteine; D, aspartic acid; E, glutamic acid; F, phenylalanine; G, glycine; H, histidine; I, isoleucine; K, lysine; L, leucine; N, asparagine; Q, glutamine; R, arginine; S, serine; T, threonine; V, valine; W, tryptophan; Y, tyrosine. (*See also Chapter 5, pp. 49–50.*)

Allelic designations	Pocket 4					Pocket 7						Pocket 9				
	13	70	71	74	78	28	30	47	61	67	71	9	37	57	60	61
ManeDRB1*03e	S	Q	R	A	Y	D	Y	F	W	F	R	E	N	D	Y	W
HlaDRB1*1301	S	D	E	A	Y	D	Y	F	W	I	E	E	N	D	Y	W
HlaDRB1*0301	S	Q	K	R	Y	D	Y	F	W	L	K	E	N	D	Y	W
MafaDRB1*03	S	Q	K	R	Y	D	Y	F	W	L	K	E	N	D	Y	W
MafaDRB1*03a	S	Q	K	R	Y	D	Y	Y	W	I	K	E	N	D	Y	W
ManeDRB1*03b	S	Q	K	R	Y	D	Y	Y	W	I	K	E	N	D	Y	W
ManeDRB1*03c	S	Q	K	R	Y	E	Y	Y	W	I	K	E	N	D	Y	W
MafaDRB1*04c	H	R	R	Q	Y	I	Y	Y	W	L	R	E	N	D	Y	W
HlaDRB1*1101	S	D	R	A	Y	D	Y	F	W	F	R	E	Y	D	Y	W
MafaDRB1*13d	S	Q	R	A	Y	D	Y	F	W	F	R	E	Y	D	Y	W
DRB1*0401	L	Q	K	A	Y	D	Y	Y	W	L	K	E	Y	D	Y	W
PacaDRB1*13b	S	Q	K	Q	Y	D	Y	Y	W	L	K	E	Y	D	Y	W
DRB1*0403	L	Q	R	E	Y	D	Y	Y	W	L	R	E	Y	D	Y	W
MafaDRB1*10a	F	D	R	S	Y	E	R	Y	W	L	R	E	Y	D	Y	W
HlaDRB1*1001	F	R	R	A	Y	E	R	Y	W	L	R	E	Y	D	Y	W
MafaDRB4*05d	F	E	K	A	Y	I	V	F	W	F	K	E	Y	D	Y	W
MafaDRB4*05b	F	Q	K	R	Y	I	V	F	W	I	K	E	Y	D	Y	W
HlaDRB4*0101	C	R	R	E	Y	I	Y	Y	W	L	R	E	Y	D	Y	W
CalaDRB*13	A	R	R	E	V	V	S	Y	W	L	R	E	Y	D	Y	W
MafaDRB1*04b	H	D	R	V	V	D	Y	F	W	F	R	E	Y	S	Y	W
PacaDRB1*13a	S	D	E	A	Y	D	Y	F	W	Y	E	E	Y	S	Y	W
MafaDRB1*13c	S	D	R	A	Y	D	Y	Y	W	F	R	E	Y	S	Y	W
ManeDRB1*13e	S	D	R	S	Y	D	Y	Y	W	F	R	E	Y	S	Y	W
ManeDRB1*04b	H	D	R	V	Y	D	Y	Y	W	I	R	E	Y	S	Y	W
PacaDRB4*05a	F	Q	K	T	Y	I	V	F	W	F	K	E	Y	S	Y	W

HSC-derived non-hematopoietic cells in single HSC transplanted mice

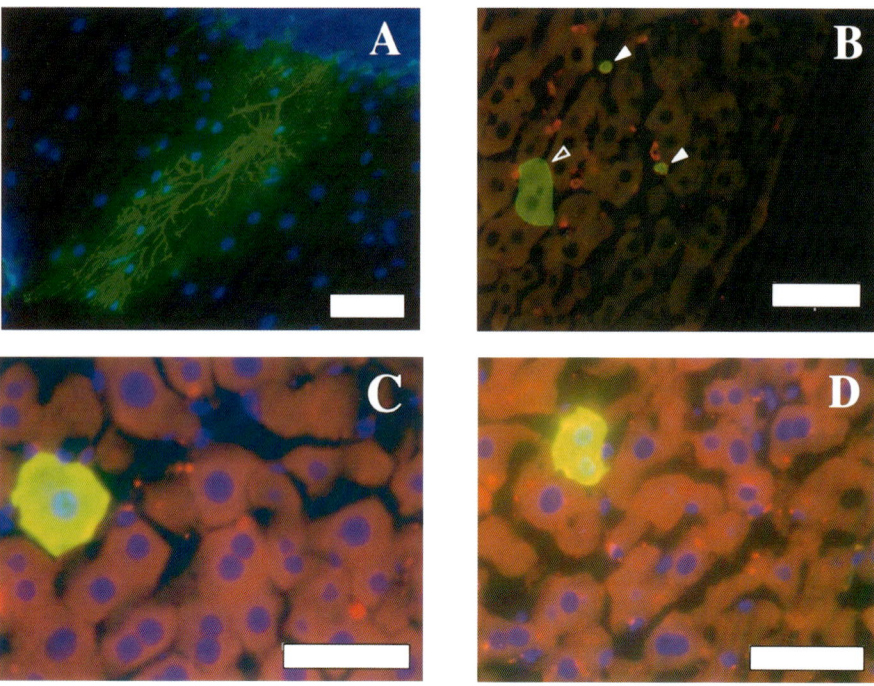

Plate 8.1 Hematopoietic stem cell (HSC) derived nonhematopoietic cells in single HSC-transplanted mice. (a) GFP$^+$ Purkinje cell in the brain of a nontransgenic recipient of a single GFP$^+$ HSC. Nuclear labeling with Hoechst dye is shown in blue and GFP expression is shown in green (bar, 50 μm). Only one GFP$^+$ neuronal cell was observed in three independently transplanted mice. (b–d) GFP$^+$ hepatocytes in the liver of nontransgenic recipients of a single GFP$^+$ HSC. (b) GFP$^+$ CD45$^-$ hepatocyte (open arrowhead) and two GFP$^+$ CD45$^+$ hematopoietic cells (closed arrowheads) are noted. GFP expression is shown in green and anti-CD45 staining is shown in red (bar, 50 μm). (c,d) Nuclear labeling with Hoechst dye is shown in blue, GFP expression in green and antialbumin reactivity is in red. Yellow color indicates colocalization of GFP and albumin (bar, 50 μm). Seven GFP$^+$ hepatocytes were observed in two independently transplanted mice. (Adapted from [5: Chapter 8].) (*See also Chapter 8, p. 69.*)

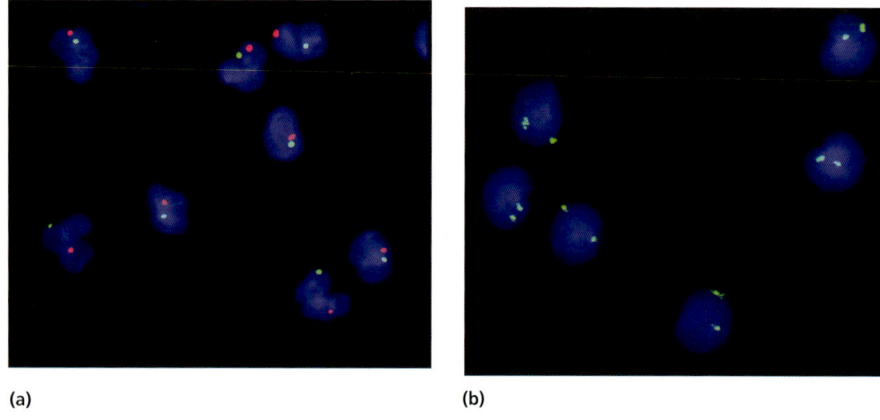

Plate 18.1 Assessment of chimerism in sorted granulocytes (a) and leukemic blasts (b) by dual-color fluorescence *in situ* hybridization (FISH). Hybridization was carried out with a biotin-labeled Y chromosome-specific DNA probe and a digoxigenin-labeled X chromosome-specific DNA probe. Hybridization was detected; Texas Red-conjugated avidin and fluorescein-conjugated antibody against digoxigenin. Cells were counterstained with DAPI. Male cells contain a single red fluorescent spot and a single green fluorescent spot, while female cells contain two green fluorescent spots and no red fluorescent spots. In this case, granulocytes were derived from a male donor and leukemic blasts were derived from the female recipient. (*See also Fig. 18.1, p. 235.*)

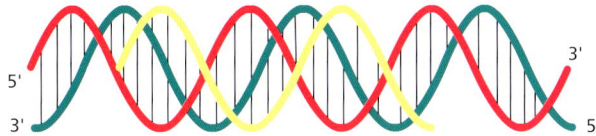

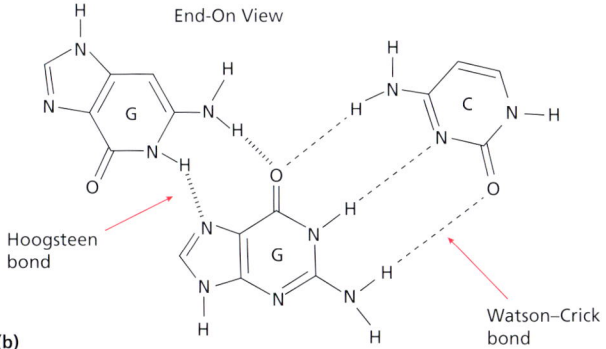

Plate 21.1 Triple-helix formation. (a) DNA strands (green and red) with triple helix forming oligonucleotice (TFO) (yellow) in major groove. (b) Biochemical representation of Watson–Crick and Hoogsteen bonds formed between the TFO and the DNA backbone at the single nucleotide level. (*See also Fig. 21.1, p. 259.*)

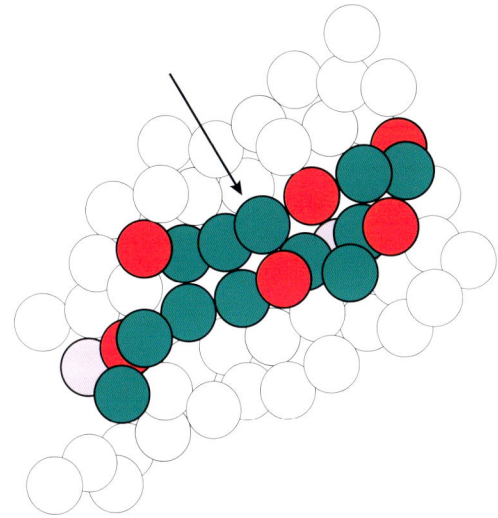

Plate 21.3 Polyamide molecule (green and red spheres) binding in minor groove of DNA (arrow). Reproduced with permission from Goodsell [51: Chapter 21]. (*See also Fig. 21.3, p. 260.*)

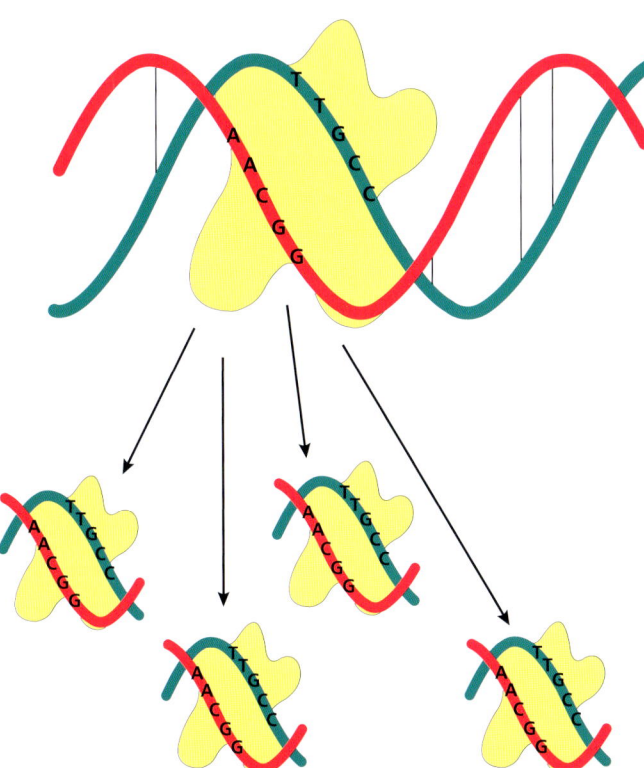

Plate 21.2 Decoy oligonucleotide. Transcription factor (light yellow) shown binding its recognition sequence in DNA double strand (green and red). Decoy molecules (small green and red double strands with black spots) are shown attracting away (arrows) the transcription factor from its authentic binding site. (*See also Fig. 21.2, p. 259.*)

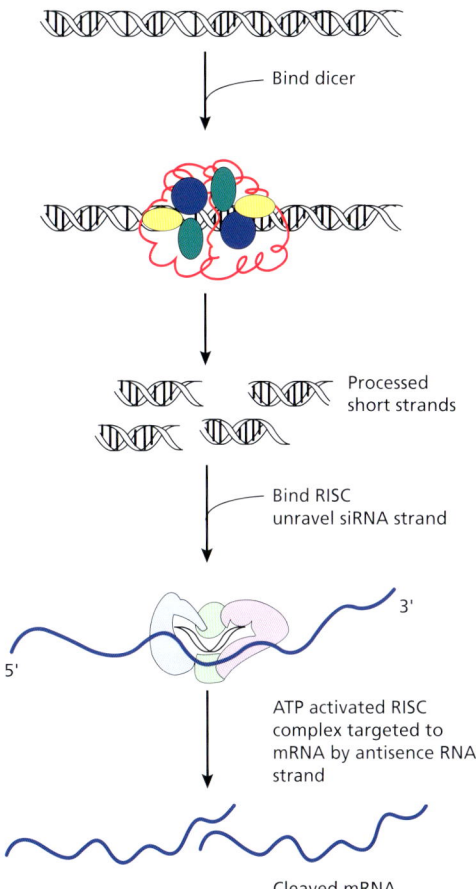

Plate 21.4 RNA interference (RNAi). RNAi is initiated by the Dicer enzyme which processes double-stranded RNA into ~22-nucleotide small interfering RNAs (siRNA). The siRNAs are incorporated into a multicomponent nuclease, RISC (green). RISC must be activated from a latent form, containing a double-stranded siRNA to an active form, RISC*, by unwinding of siRNA. RISC* then uses the antisense strand of the unwound siRNA as a guide to substrate selection. (*See also Fig. 21.5, p. 263.*)

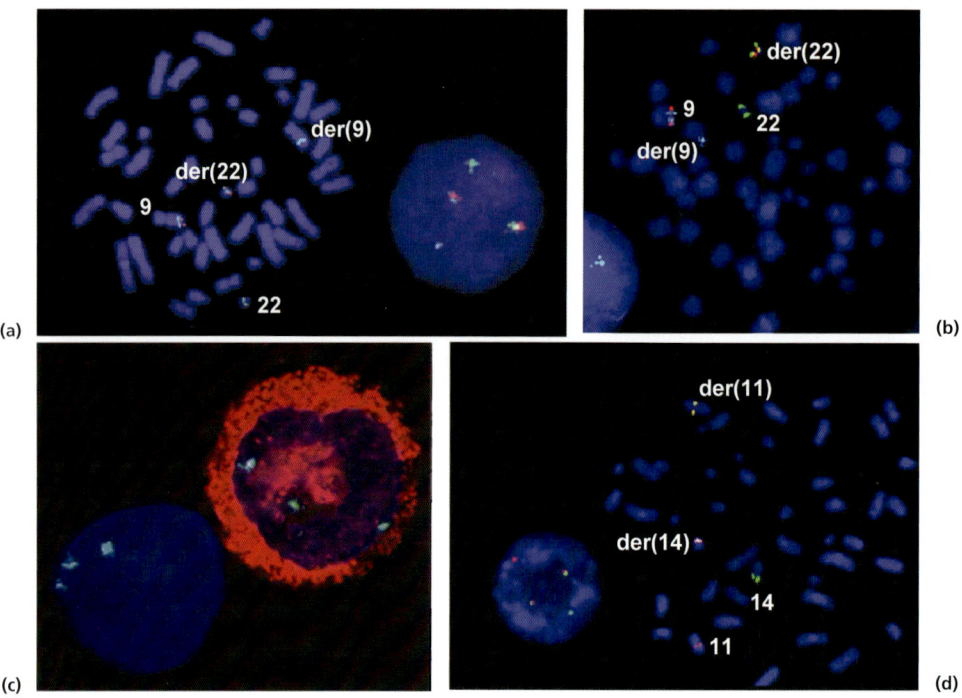

Plate 22.1 Examples of molecular cytogenetics or fluorescence *in situ* hybridization (FISH) techniques commonly used to monitor minimal residual disease. (a) Triple probe/triple color FISH for the detection of the *BCR-ABL* gene rearrangement. Fluorescence signals from a Philadelphia chromosome positive (Ph+) metaphase and interphase cell, *ABL* (red on 9q34.1), *BCR* (green on 22q11.2) and *ASS* (aqua, 9q34.1 flanking region proximal to ABL). The der(22)t(9,22) is observed as a red/green/yellow fusion signal. The red/blue signal indicates normal chromosome 9 homologue; the green signal indicates normal chromosome 22 homologue. Chromosome with the single aqua signal is the derivative chromosome 9. The aqua signal on the der(9) indicates the *ASS* or arginine succinate synthease gene which flanks the *ABL* gene is not deleted. (b) Hypermetaphase spread hybridized with the triple probe/triple color FISH for the detection of the *BCR-ABL* gene rearrangement. Note the chromosomes are highly contracted in comparison with the conventional cytogenetic spread observed in panel a. (c) FICTION detecting both immunophenotype and genotype simultaneously. Trisomy 8 (three blue-green signals) was detected in a CD15 positive cell (upper right) as well as the CD15 negative cell (lower left). (d) Dual color, dual fusion LSI IgH/CCND1 (Vysis, Inc., Downers Grove, IL) detects the t(11,14)(q13;q32) observed in mantle cell lymphoma and multiple myeloma. The signal pattern shows two orange/green (yellow) fusion signals (arrows), one on each abnormal chromosome 11 and 14, in addition to the single orange and green signal identifying the normal chromosome 11 and 14, respectively, in both the interphase nucleus (right) and the metaphase (left) cell. (*See also Fig. 22.2, p. 274.*)

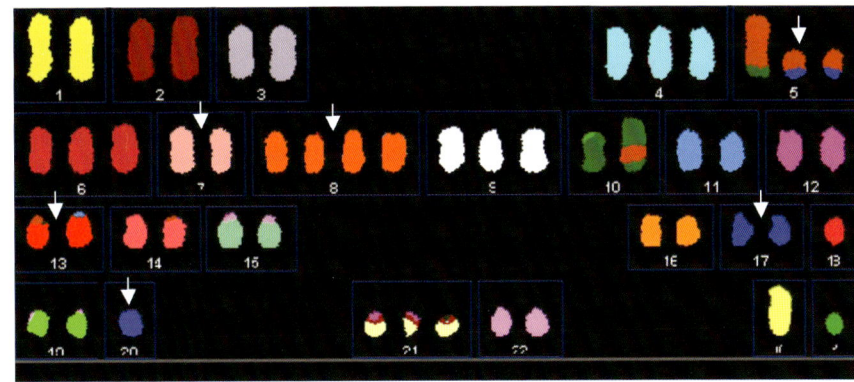

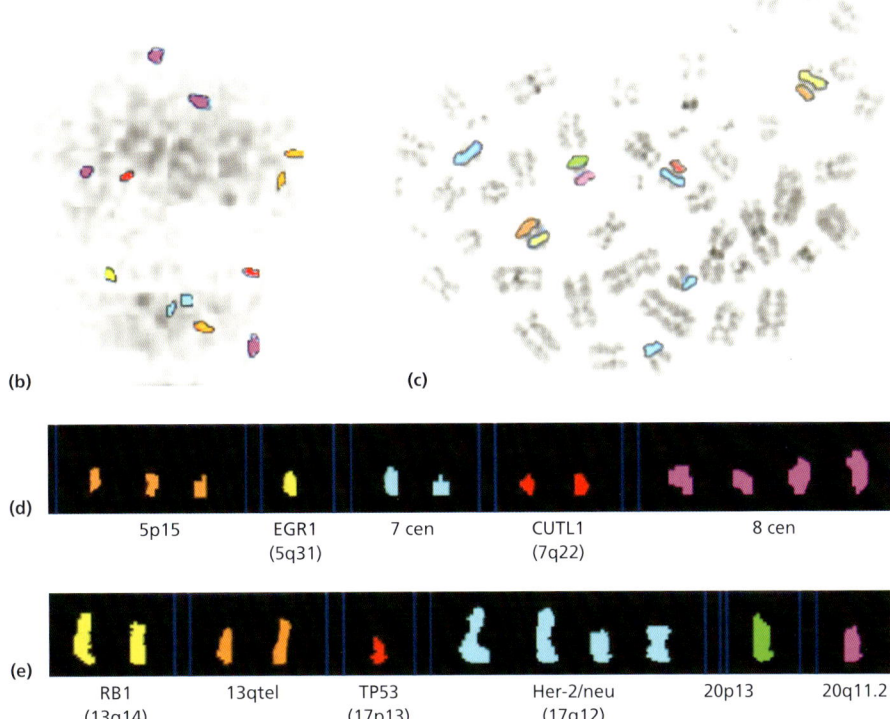

Plate 22.2 (a) 24-color karyotyping in an acute myeloid leukemia (AML) case evolving from myelodysplastic syndrome (MDS). The karyotypic designation for this hyperdiploid clone was 51, XY,+4,der(5)t(5,17)(q11.2;q12)×2,+der(5)t(5,10)(q3?5;?),+6,+8,+8,+9,ins(5,10)(q?24;?), −18, −20, +21. Compare 24-color karyotyping with the spectral fluorescence *in situ* hybridization (S-FISH) results presented in panels b–e. This clone has no normal chromosome 5, two copies of the der(5)t(5,17)×2, tetrasomy 8, two apparently normal copies of chromosome 17s, and monosomy 20.
(b–d) Example of spectral FISH for the AML case presented in panel a. S-FISH is a molecular cytogenetic approach that targets multiple chromosomal sites in interphase and metaphase cells in a single hybridization, using combinatorial fluorescence and digital imaging microscopy. (b) S-FISH of an interphase nucleus showing the signal pattern for the various DNA probes listed in panel d. In comparison with the 24-color karyotype, S-FISH confirms the presence of three 5p15 signals, one 5q31 signal, disomy 7 and tetrasomy 8.
(c) Panel c shows a metaphase of the same clone using the DNA probes listed in panel e. S-FISH recognized monosomy 20 and revealed one TP53/17p13 signal with four HER2/neu/17q12 signals. The 17q12 signals were localized to the der(5)t(5,17)s, a normal chromosome 17 and an apparently del(17p), the latter not recognized as a deletion by 24-color karyotyping. As revealed by 24-color karyotyping, a normal (disomy) 13 chromosome content was confirmed using a 13q14/13qtel probe combination. (*See also Chapter 22, p. 274.*)

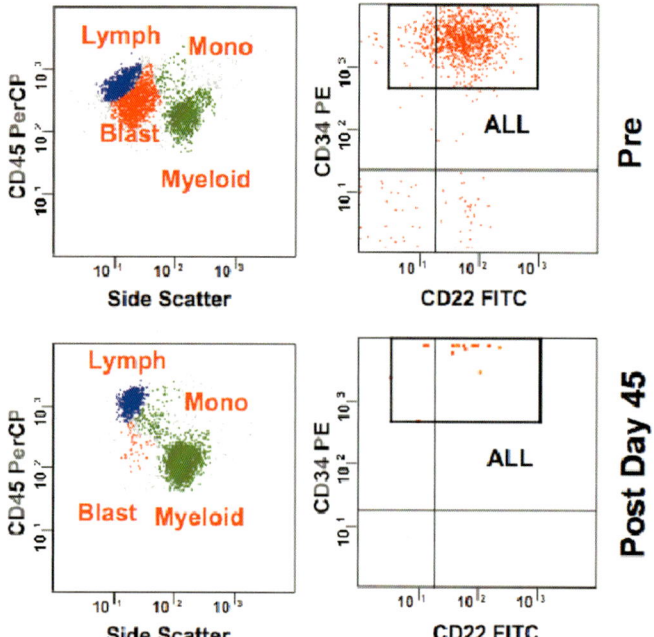

Plate 22.3 Flow cytometric analysis of a female patient with acute lymphoblastic leukemia (ALL) at presentation (top panels) and during morphological remission following marrow transplantation from a male donor (bottom panels). At diagnosis the blasts were characterized by expression of increased CD45, CD34 and CD22 (top panels). A specimen obtained at day 45 post-transplant was in morphologic remission; however, a residual population of blasts with the same expression signature was identified at 0.2% of total nucleated cells. These suspicious cells were isolated and interrogated by fluorescence *in situ* hybridization (FISH) for the presence of X and Y chromosomes. The abnormal cells identified post-HCT were found to be 97% female while the control population of lymphocytes and neutrophils were 99% male. Figure courtesy of Dr Mike Loken. (*See also Fig. 22.3, p. 275.*)

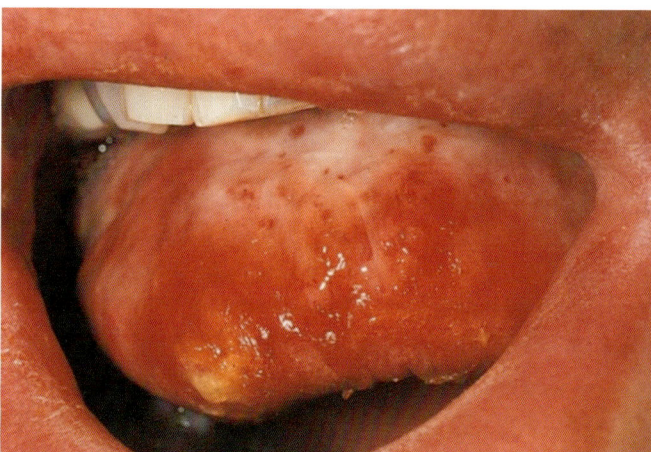

Plate 23.2 Acute glossitis 1 day post BMT after conditioning regimen of 60 mg/kg of CY followed by 12 Gy of fractionated TBI. There is early mucosal damage with severe erythema and focal atrophy. (*See also Chapter 23, p. 287.*)

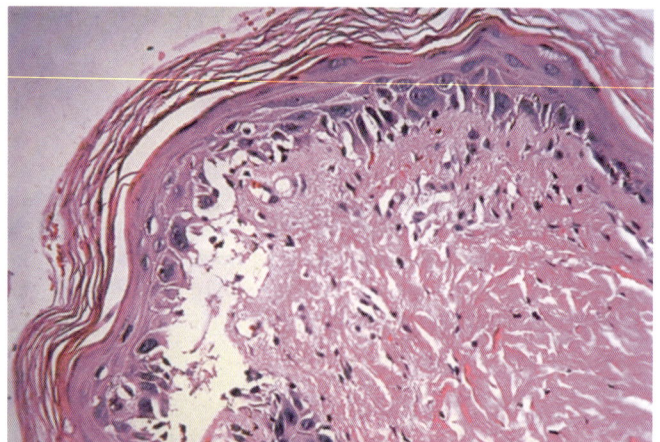

Plate 23.1 Skin biopsy from recipient of identical twin marrow who had received a single 15 mg/kg dose of dimethylbusulfan 15 days previously. The epidermal separation, keratinocyte atypia, and scanty lymphoid dermal infiltrate can also be seen in GVHD. (*See also Chapter 23, pp. 287–8.*)

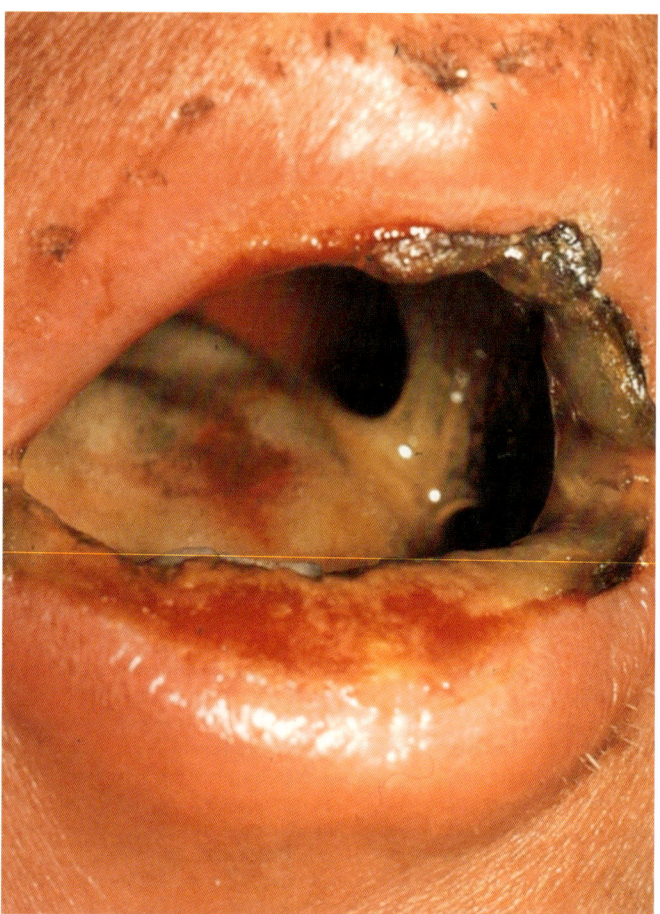

Plate 23.3 Severe mucositis of lips and tongue with pseudomembranous exudate 20 days after BMT following conditioning with TBI and chemotherapy. Similar changes may be present with severe acute GVHD or herpetic infection. (*See also Chapter 23, p. 287.*)

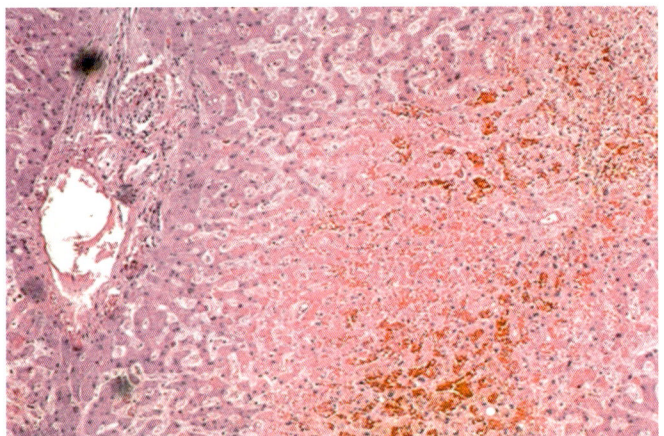

Plate 23.4 Fatal hepatic VOD at autopsy 12 days post BMT for leukemia. At this low magnification, the H&E-stained section demonstrates striking congestion, hemorrhage, and hepatocyte disruption in zone 3 (centrilobular) of the liver acinus toward the right. The portal space and surrounding acinar zone 1 on the left are well preserved. These early severe hepatic VOD lesions at times can be identified with the H&E stain after tissue fixation with B5 or methyl Carnoy's. However, stains for connective tissue are more effective. (See also Chapter 23, p. 287.)

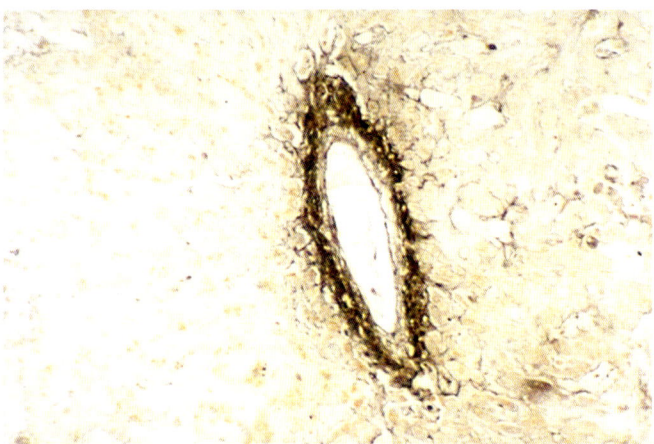

Plate 23.6 Early hepatic VOD showing perivenular staining for procoagulants. Immunohistochemical staining for factor VIII (von Willebrand) demonstrates post-sinusoidal obstruction corresponding to the endothelium-lined pores through which the sinusoids drain into the venules. Immunostaining for fibrin localizes in the same regions. These observations provide some of the rationale for using anticoagulation and anti-thrombotic therapy for hepatic VOD. (See also Chapter 23, p. 287.)

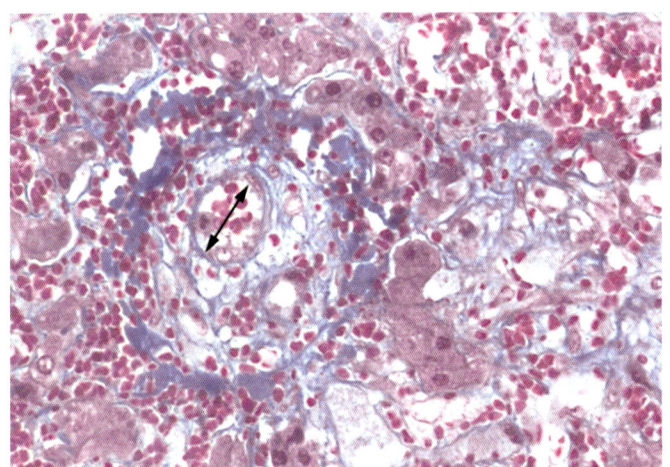

Plate 23.5 Hepatic VOD 95 days post BMT for malignancy. The trichrome stain shows the blue outline of an hepatic venule with marked luminal narrowing (arrow shows lumen diameter) caused by subendothelial trapping of red cells. The hepatocytes of acinar zone 3 are severely disrupted. When the clinical diagnosis of hepatic VOD is uncertain, it may be confirmed by a transvenous liver biopsy with measurement of an elevated gradient between wedged and free hepatic venous pressures. (See also Chapter 23, p. 287.)

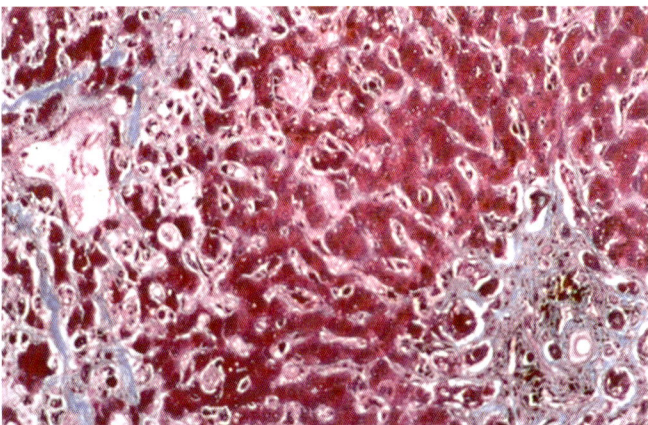

Plate 23.7 Hepatic VOD and coexistent GVHD, day 26. On this trichrome stain, the two most common liver problems after BMT can be differentiated by the zone of the liver acinus they affect. The expanded portal space in the lower right demonstrates changes from GVHD, including fibrosis, proliferation of atypical cholangioles along the limiting plate and destruction of small interlobular bile ducts. The VOD lesion along the left margin shows striking collections of embolized hepatocytes beneath the endothelial basement membrane. (See also Chapter 23, p. 290.)

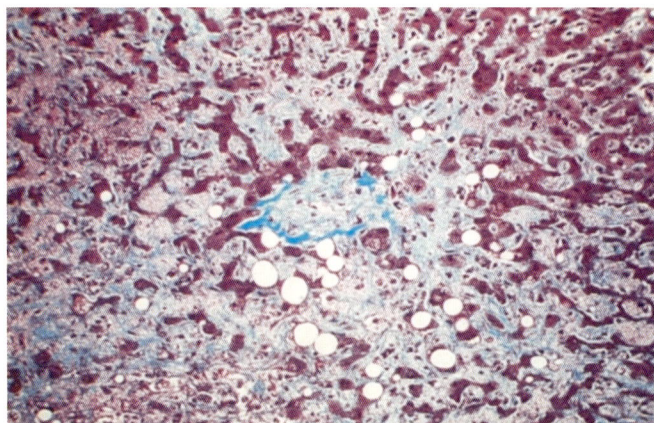

Plate 23.8 Late hepatic VOD, day 63. The trichrome stain demonstrates fibrotic obliteration of the venous lumen with extensive fibrosis in surrounding sinusoids. The resulting vascular obstruction produced intractable ascites. Immunohistochemical stains at this stage reveal extensive deposition of collagen, while fibrin and other blood procoagulants are no longer identifiable. (*See also Chapter 23, p. 287.*)

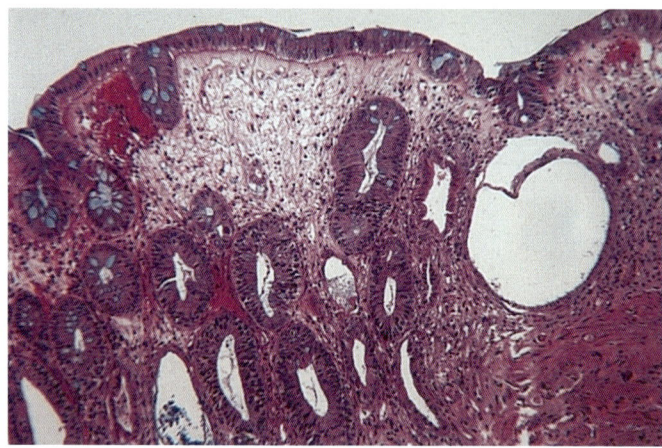

Plate 23.11 Recovery from the effects of cytoreduction therapy on colonic mucosa, day 16. This repeat biopsy from the same patient as in Plate 23.10 indicates that regeneration is occurring, although some cystic crypts remain. (H&E with alcian blue counterstain.) (*See also Chapter 23, p. 287.*)

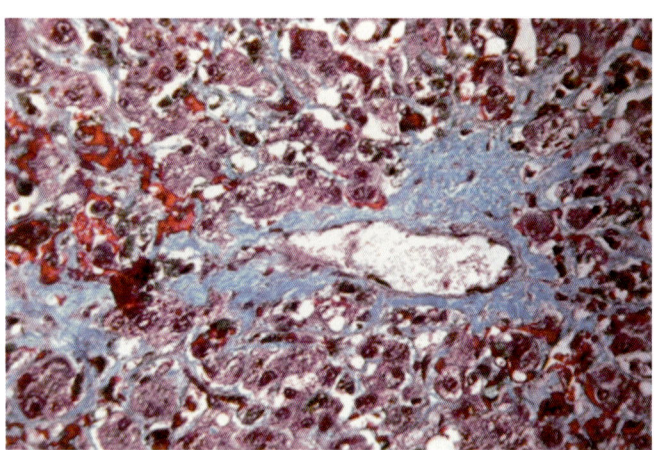

Plate 23.9 Hepatic phlebosclerosis, day 96. Eccentric thickening of the venular wall without striking luminal narrowing was associated with an early liver toxicity syndrome. The patient had received a 5-day infusion of high-dose Ara-C followed by CY and TBI. Liver function abnormalities developed prior to the infusion of marrow. Changes of phlebosclerosis were widespread, but there were no identifiable hepatic VOD lesions at autopsy. (Trichrome stain.) (*See also Chapter 23, p. 287.*)

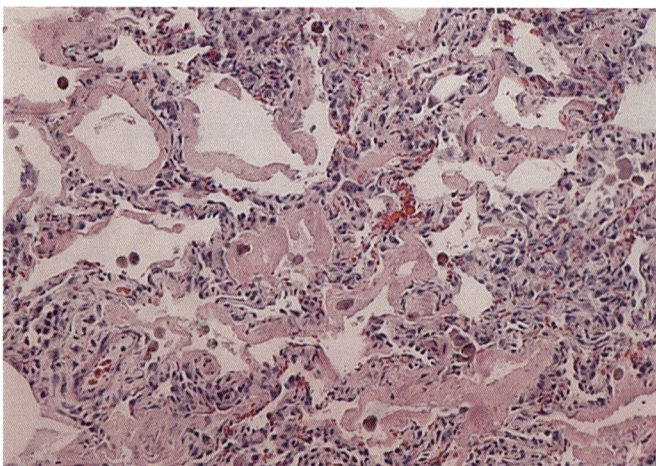

Plate 23.12 Severe diffuse alveolar damage (DAD) in a lung biopsy, day 56. Alveoli and terminal bronchioles are lined by hyaline membranes composed of degenerating cells. This nonspecific pattern of severe injury may be associated with shock, infection, chemotherapy, and other possible causes. DAD after BMT is often accompanied by renal and hepatic failure. (*See also Chapter 23, p. 296.*)

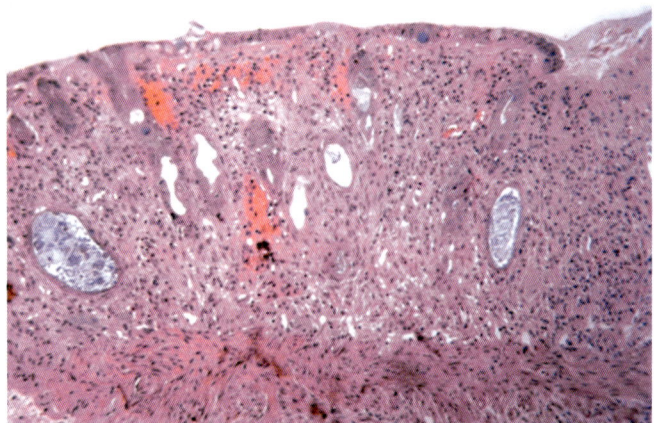

Plate 23.10 Effect of cytoreductive therapy on colonic mucosa, day 7. This biopsy specimen was taken following therapy with BU, CY, and TBI (12 Gy). There has been obliteration of almost all epithelial cells, leaving cystic crypt remnants. (H&E with alcian blue counterstain.) (*See also Chapter 23, p. 287.*)

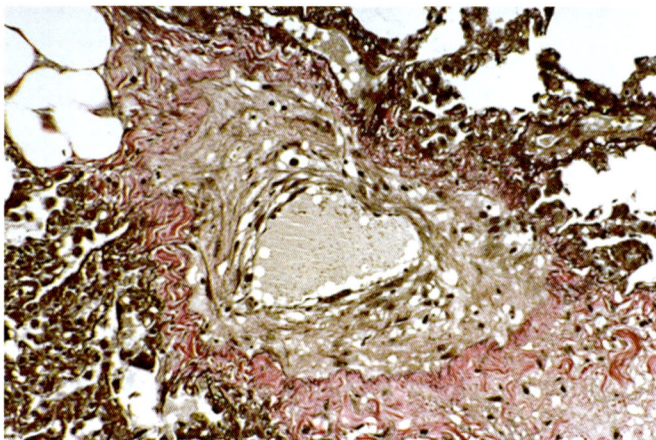

Plate 23.13 Pulmonary VOD in a lung biopsy from a patient with pulmonary hypertension 48 days post second allogeneic BMT for ALL. Loose intimal fibrosis partially occludes the interlobular vein. This complication probably results from chemotherapy and may be more frequent than previously suspected. (Verhoff–Van Gieson elastin stain.) (*See also Chapter 23, p. 296.*)

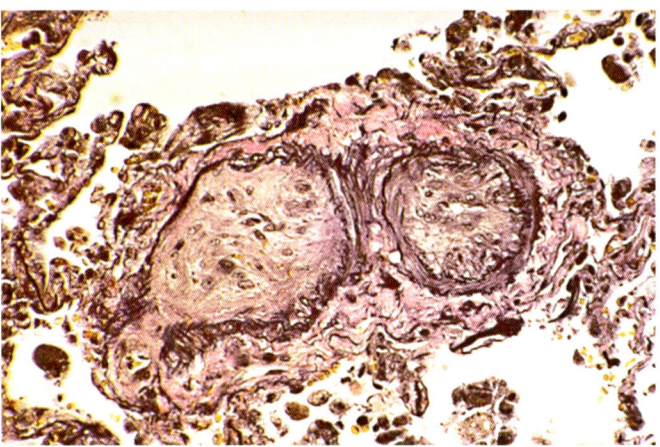

Plate 23.14 Pulmonary arterioles with severe concentric intimal fibrosis producing virtually complete luminal occlusion at autopsy 37 days post second allogeneic BMT for ALL. Severe hepatic VOD was also present. (Verhoff–Van Gieson elastin stain.) (*See also Chapter 23, p. 295.*)

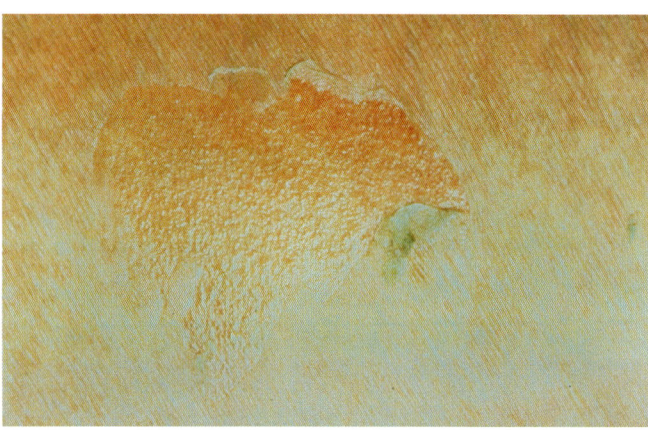

Plate 23.17 Epidermal separation of grade IV acute GVHD resembling toxic epidermal necrolysis, day 36 after an HLA-identical sibling BMT. (*See also Chapter 23, p. 288; Chapter 50, p. 638.*)

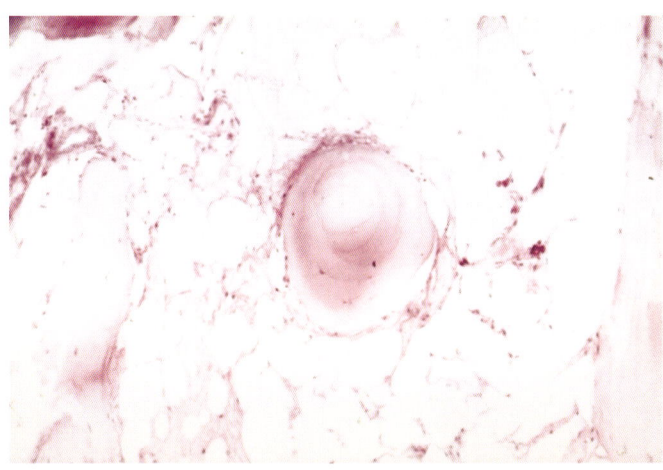

Plate 23.15 Markedly hypocellular marrow without evidence of engraftment, day 7. Subtle interstitial fluid accumulation, fat necrosis, and iron deposition are consistent with chemoirradiation damage. (*See also Chapter 23, p. 287.*)

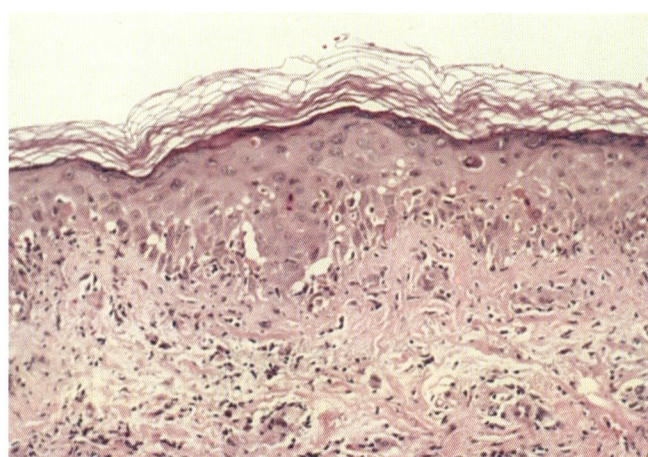

Plate 23.18 Acute skin GVHD, day 28 post mismatched allogeneic BMT. The epidermis demonstrates a prominent lichenoid reaction involving the tip of the rete ridge in the center of the specimen, a location of epithelial stem cells within the epidermis. (*See also Chapter 23, p. 288; Chapter 50, p. 638.*)

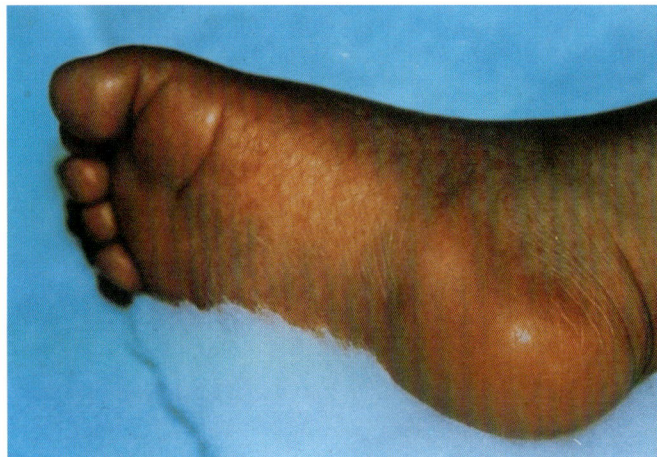

Plate 23.16 Painful red to violaceous maculopapular rash consistent with acute GVHD in a 2-year-old girl involving the sole of the foot 11 days after HLA-nonidentical BMT. (*See also Chapter 23, p. 288; Chapter 50, p. 638.*)

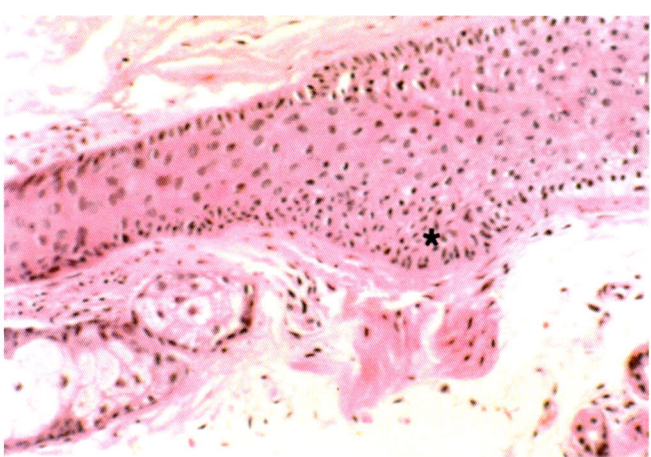

Plate 23.19 Early skin GVHD involving the parafollicular bulge region of the pilar unit. Note the small numbers of mononuclear inflammatory cells which infiltrate the parafollicular bulge area (*) near the arrector pilorum muscle in association with apoptotic bodies. (*See also Chapter 23, p. 288.*)

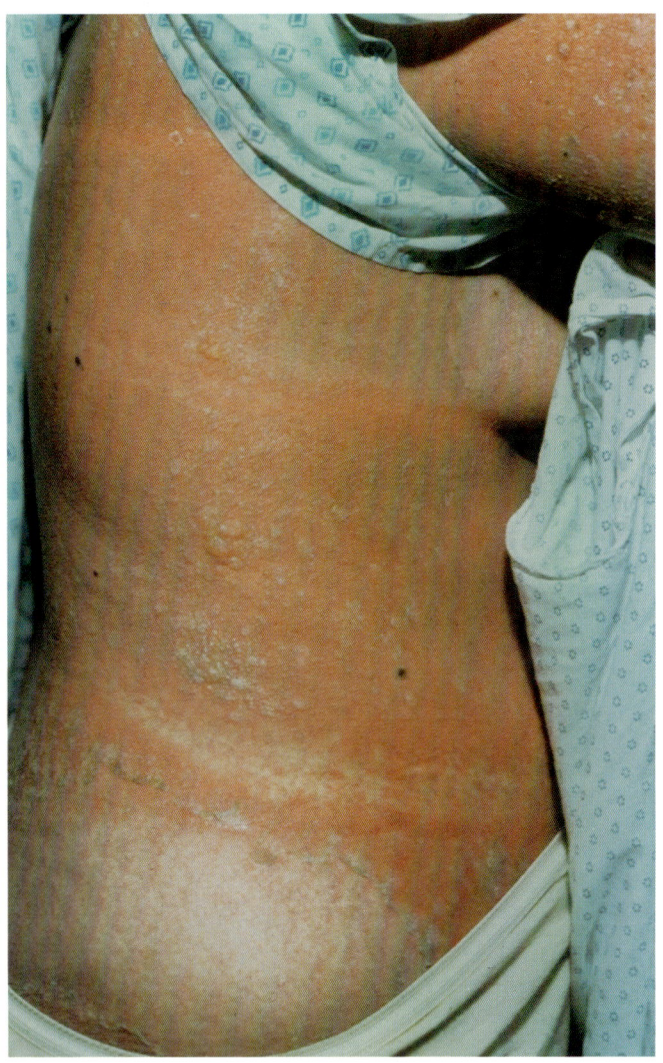

Plate 23.20 Erythema and desquamation before treatment for acute GVHD, day 27 (see Plate 23.21). (*See also Chapter 23, p. 288; Chapter 50, p. 644.*)

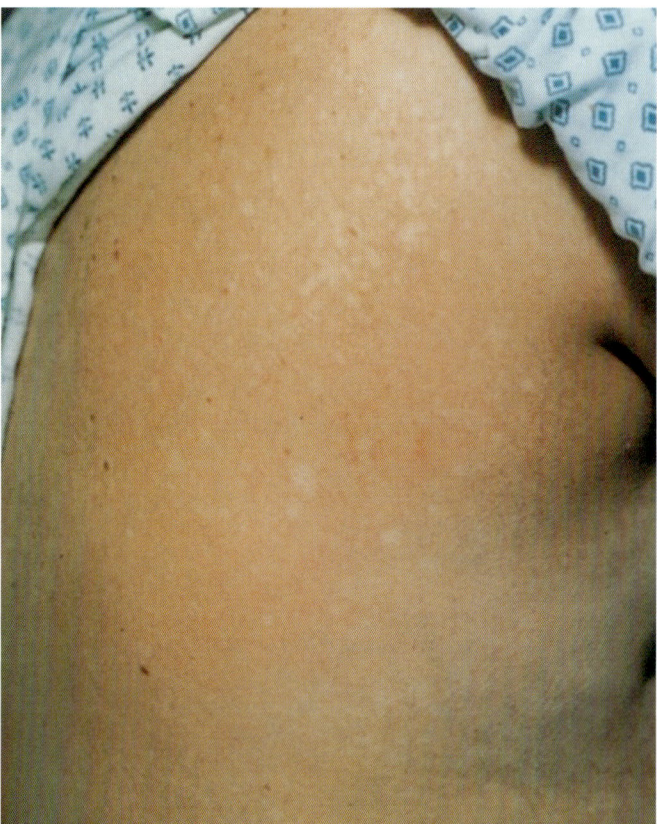

Plate 23.21 Virtually normal skin with focal depigmentation after treatment for acute GVHD, day 74 (same patient shown in Plate 23.20). (*See also Chapter 23, p. 288; Chapter 50, p. 644.*)

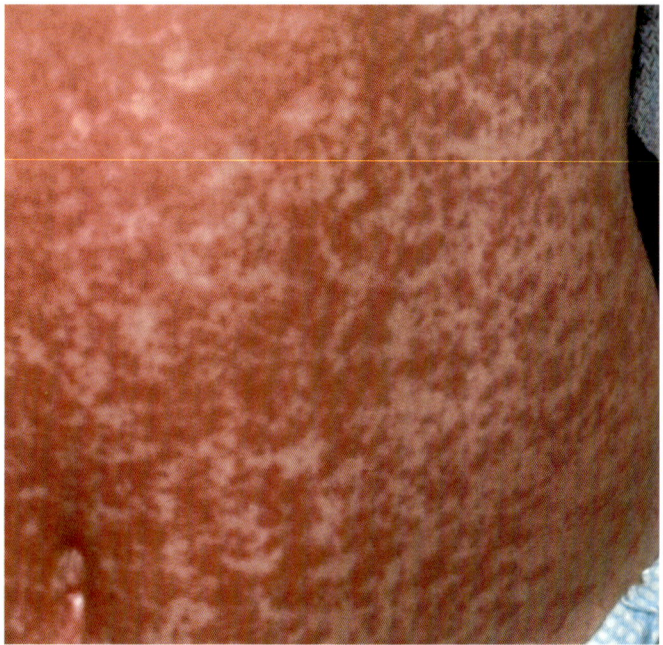

Plate 23.22 Maculopapular rash of skin GVHD without notable decrease in inflammation, 1 week after institution of PUVA therapy (see Plate 23.23). (*See also Chapter 50, pp. 638, 645, 652.*)

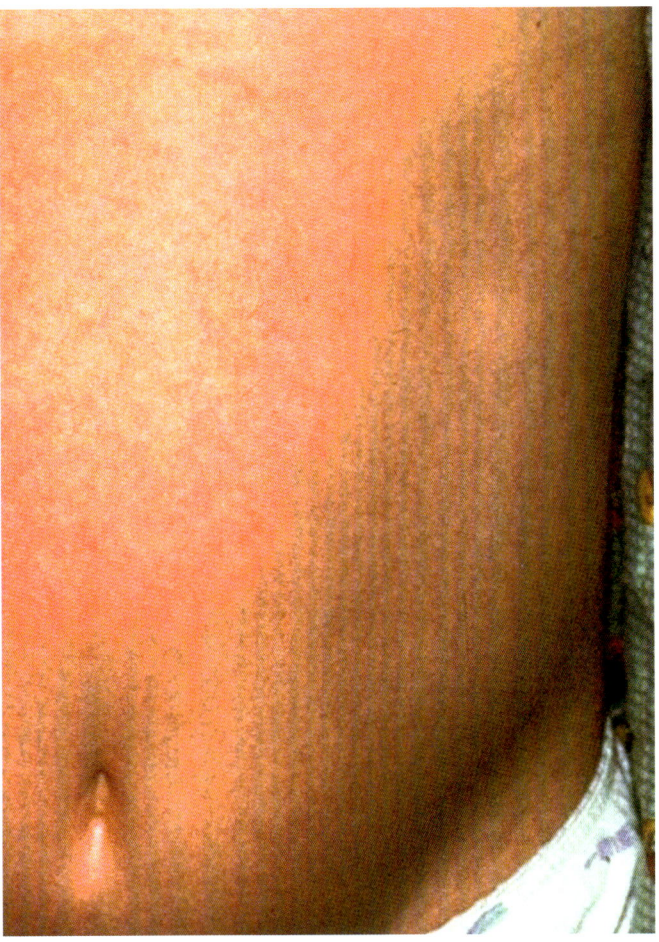

Plate 23.23 Marked improvement in skin GVHD following 6 weeks of PUVA treatment (same patient shown in Plate 23.22). (*See also Chapter 50, pp. 645, 652.*)

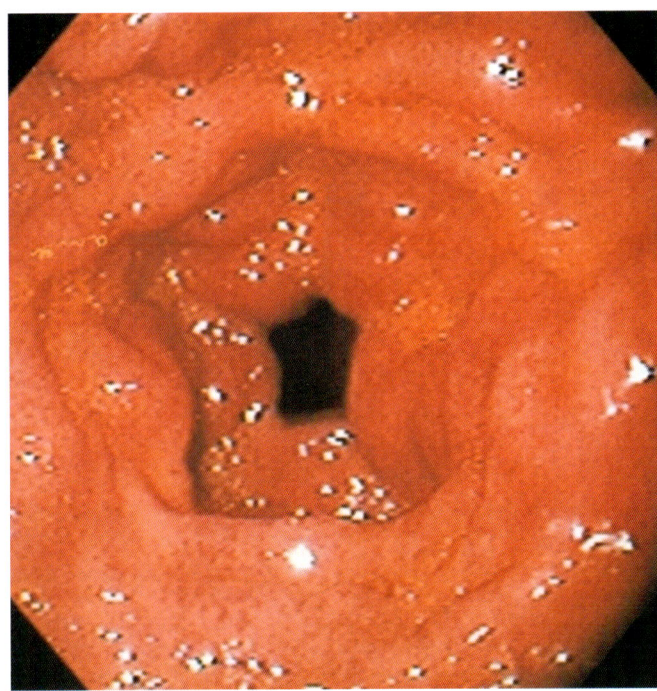

Plate 23.24 Endoscopic appearance of acute GVHD in stomach, day 32. The pyloric channel is in the center of the picture. The mucosa of the gastric antrum is edematous, reddened, and friable. (*See also Chapter 23, p. 289; Chapter 50, p. 639.*)

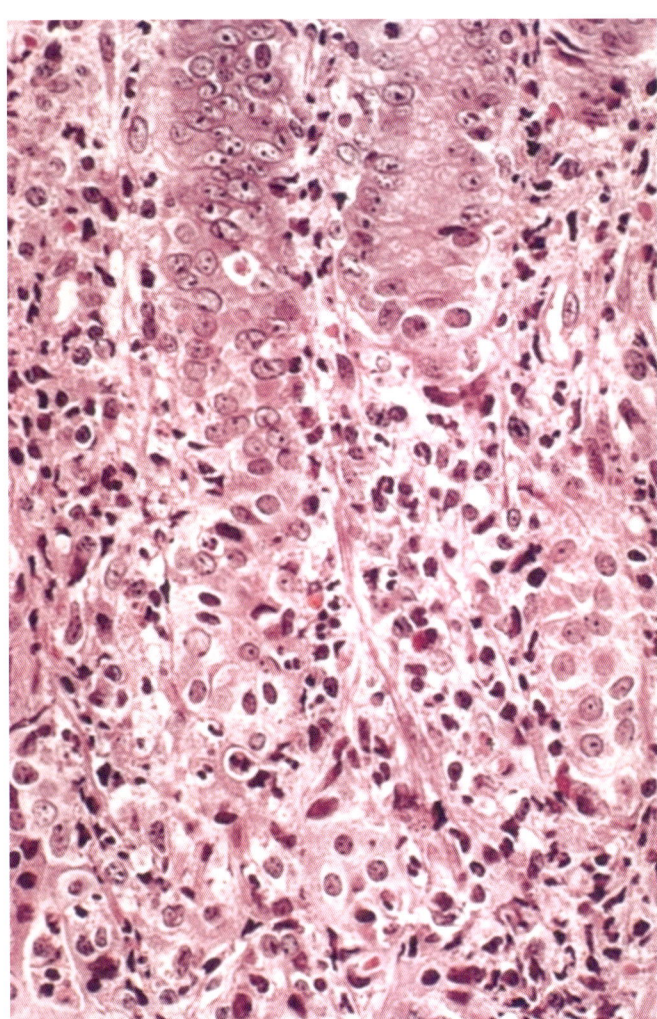

Plate 23.25 Gastric biopsy with GVHD, day 35. Of all upper endoscopic biopsy sites, that most frequently showing histologic changes of GVHD is the stomach. In the area shown here, large numbers of lymphocytes infiltrate the lamina propria and the basilar portions of the gastric crypts. There is apoptosis of crypt epithelial cells and frank early crypt destruction. Inflammation and apoptosis of this intensity are not required for the diagnosis of gastric GVHD. More subtle yet still diagnostic alterations are illustrated in Plates 23.26 & 23.27. (*See also Chapter 23, p. 289; Chapter 50, pp. 638, 639.*)

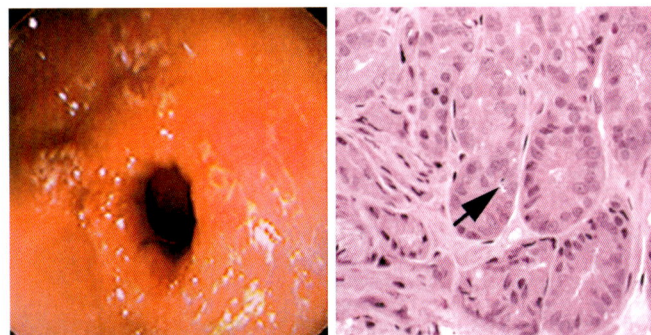

Plate 23.26 Gastric GVHD in which the severe mucosal erythema, edema, and erosion seen endoscopically on the left are more striking than the focal, mild, epithelial cell apoptosis (arrow) in the histological section on the right. Although a lymphocytic infiltrate is absent, apoptosis in multiple crypts is consistent with GVH activity. Inflammation may have been partially controlled by immunosuppressive therapy. (Reproduced from [41(Chapter 23)] with permission.) (*See also Chapter 23, p. 289; Chapter 50, p. 639.*)

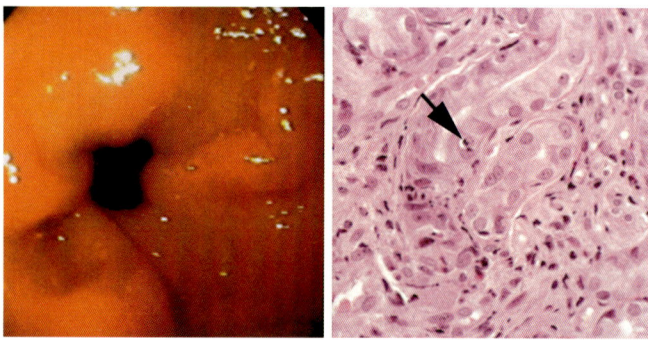

Plate 23.27 Gastric GVHD in which the antral mucosa is endoscopically normal aside from edema (left). With air insufflation through the endoscope, the antrum did not distend and there was no motor activity. Biopsy of such a bland area can be diagnostic. In this case, as shown in the photomicrograph on the right, there was epithelial cell apoptosis (arrow) and moderate lymphocytic infiltration diagnostic for GVHD. (Reproduced from [41(Chapter 23)] with permission.) (*See also Chapter 23, p. 289; Chapter 50, p. 639.*)

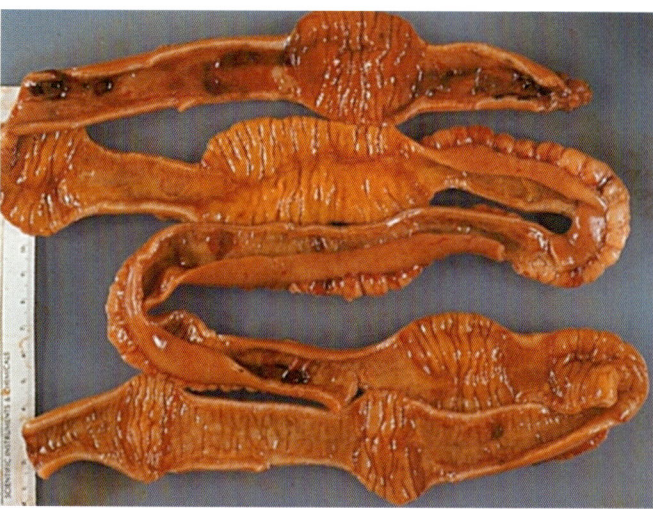

Plate 23.29 Surgical resection of severe long-standing intestinal GVHD, day 207. Scarred, ulcerated mucosa alternates with dilated areas of mucosal regeneration. The ulcerated portions demonstrate complete loss of epithelium and severe submucosal fibrosis. There is very high risk of invasive fungal or bacterial infection. Some patients have responded well to intestinal resection for localized GVHD. (*See also Chapter 23, p. 289.*)

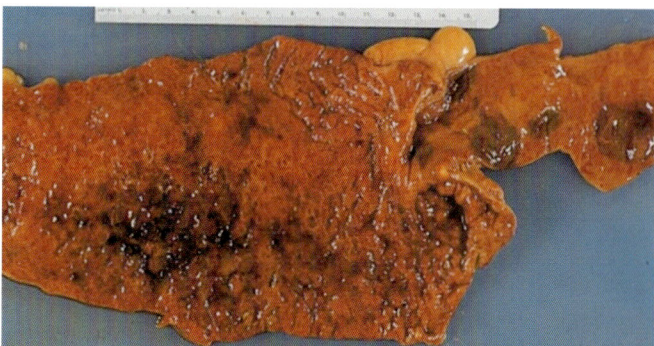

Plate 23.30 Severe GVHD of ileum and cecum, day 80. The mucosal lining and folds are replaced by a friable, beefy red, diffusely ulcerated lamina propria. The numerous exposed capillaries ooze blood and serum, a major cause of morbidity from intestinal GVHD. The endothelial cells and fibroblasts within the lamina propria are often infected with CMV, as was true in this patient (see Plate 23.42). (*See also Chapter 23, p. 289; Chapter 50, p. 639.*)

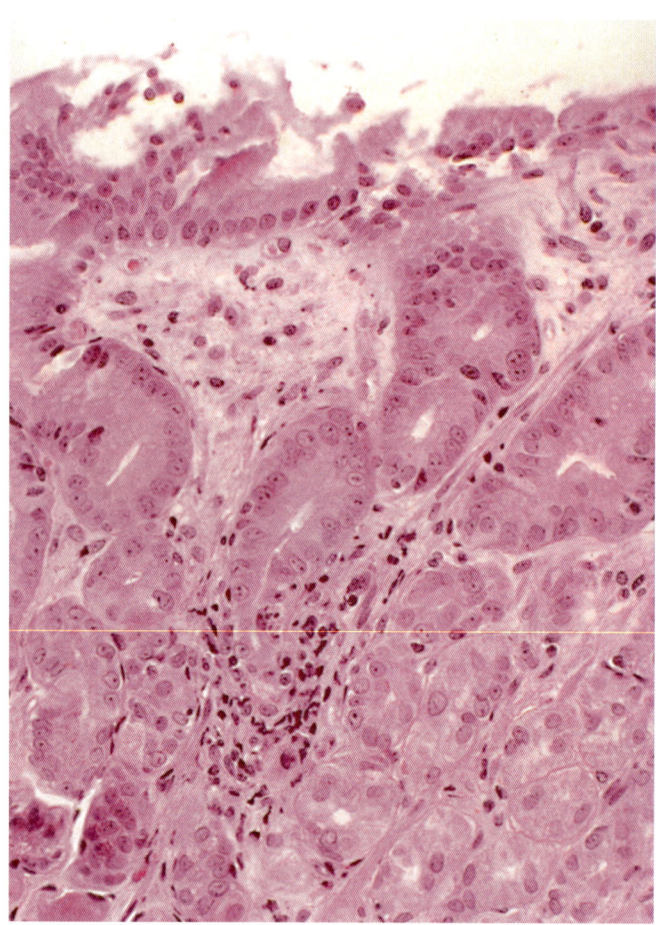

Plate 23.28 Autologous gastric GVHD or lymphocytic gastritis. The focal mononuclear inflammatory cell infiltration of the lamina propria and mucosal crypt associated with crypt epithelial cell apoptosis is histologically indistinguishable from GVHD in an allograft recipient. This inflammation may develop after autologous or syngeneic BMT if tolerance to self-MHC antigens is not reestablished and autoreactive cells are allowed to persist. (*See also Chapter 23, p. 290; Chapter 50, p. 636.*)

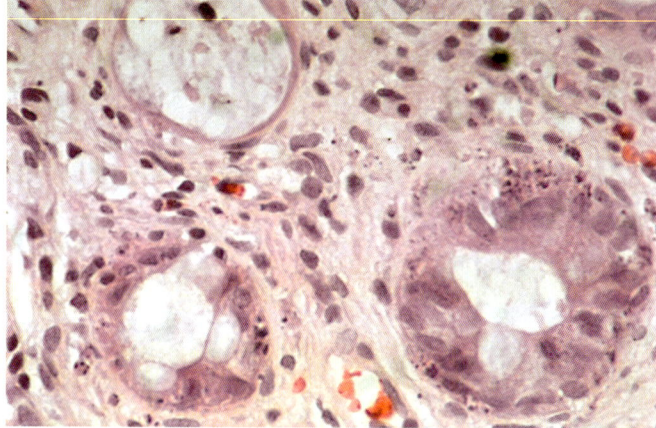

Plate 23.31 Rectal biopsy with GVHD, day 53. Three mucosal crypts display varying degrees of damage. The crypt on the right shows many apoptotic cells. More extensive cell damage is present in the crypt on the lower left. The upper crypt has lost all enterocytes. Note infiltrating lymphocytes in the lower left crypt associated with nuclear debris characteristic of apoptosis. (*See also Chapter 23, p. 289; Chapter 50, p. 639.*)

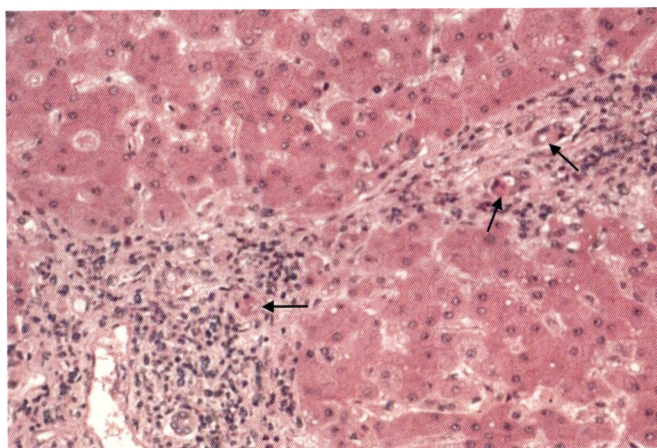

Plate 23.32 Hepatic GVHD, day 35. Portal spaces have extensively damaged bile ducts (arrows) with focally necrotic epithelium, nuclei of irregular size and shape, segmental loss of nuclei, shrinkage of ductular lumens, and an eosinophilic syncytium of cytoplasm. The cellular infiltrate associated with GVHD is typically mononuclear but may include a few eosinophils and neutrophils. The number of infiltrating cells is usually more sparse than shown here. (*See also Chapter 23, p. 290; Chapter 50, p. 638.*)

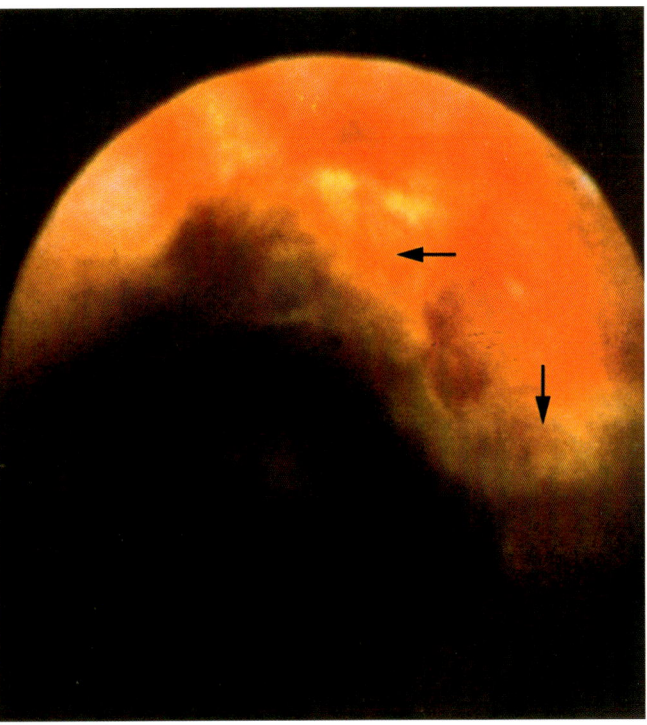

Plate 23.34 Endoscopic appearance of CMV esophagitis, day 61. A large shallow ulcer with serpiginous, reddened borders is seen in the distal esophagus. The ulcer base (arrows) has a yellow, reticulated appearance. (*See also Chapter 23, p. 290.*)

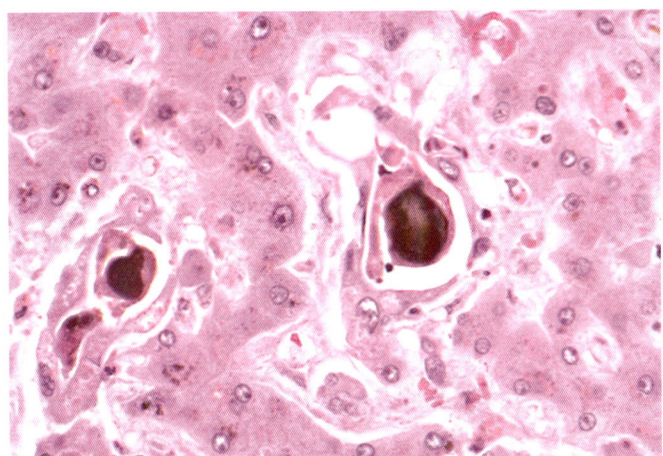

Plate 23.33 Hepatic GVHD with severe cholangiolarhepatocellular cholestasis, day 68. Accompanying the damage to the small interlobular bile ducts are proliferations of large bile-filled cholangioles along the marginal zone of the irregularly expanded and often fibrotic portal space. The full extent of this ductular proliferation is best appreciated with the use of an anticytokeratin stain. This type of cholangiolar proliferation occurs in long-standing cases of GVHD. (*See also Chapter 23, p. 290; Chapter 50, p. 639.*)

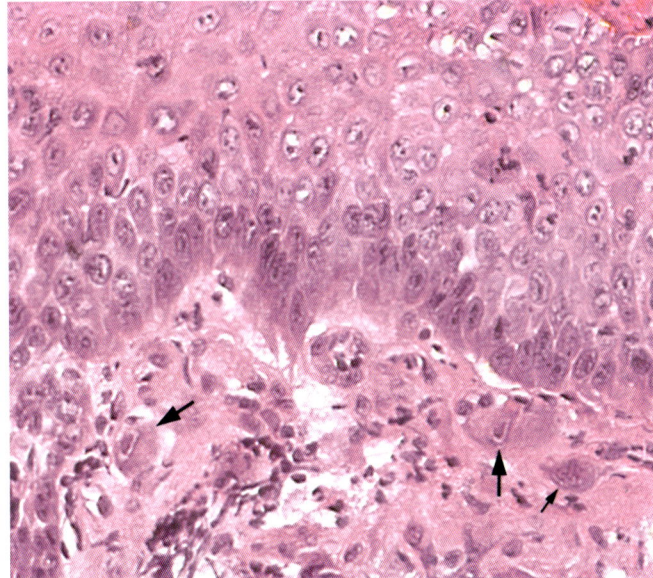

Plate 23.35 Esophageal biopsy showing CMV infection, day 61. Beneath the epithelium are two cytomegalic cells (large arrows), each containing a single, large, oval intranuclear inclusion surrounded by a clear halo (Cowdry type A). A third cell (small arrow) is probably also infected but is morphologically nondiagnostic. It would presumably be positive by immunocytochemistry and *in situ* hybridization techniques. Studies of cell morphology as well as viral DNA and antigen expression indicate that the esophageal squamous epithelium is never infected with CMV. (*See also Chapter 23, p. 290.*)

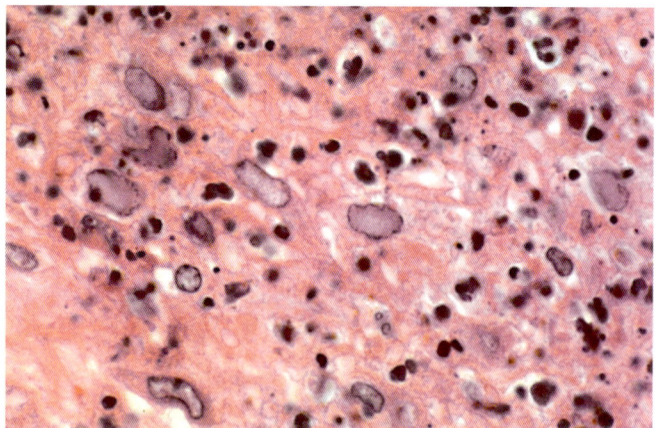

Plate 23.36 HSV infecting the lamina propria of the small intestine. Many cells display nuclear enlargement, chromatin margination, and ground-glass nuclear inclusions. Heavy involvement of the lamina propria is unusual in HSV infection of the intestine. (*See also Chapter 23, p. 290.*)

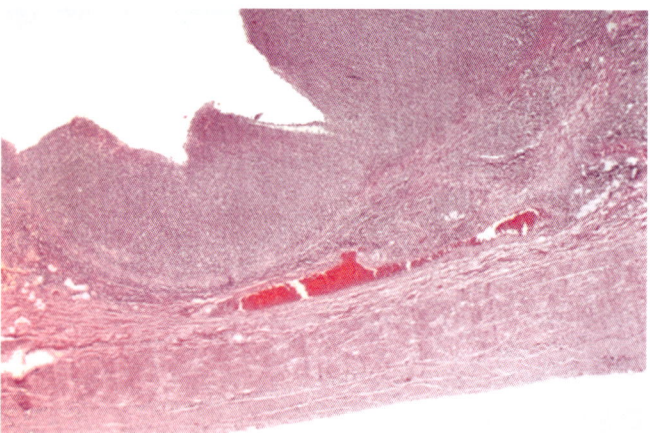

Plate 23.37 EBV-associated lymphoma infiltrating the intestinal mucosa in a boy treated for GVHD with CSP and a monoclonal antibody to T lymphocytes. Although the GVHD improved, large bizarre cells with atypical nuclei characteristic of B-cell immunoblastic sarcoma rapidly formed tumor nodules in liver, spleen, lymph nodes, and mesentery. (*See also Chapter 23, p. 291.*)

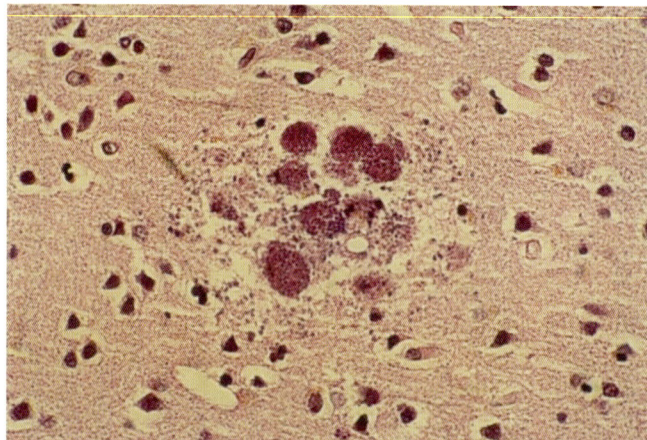

Plate 23.38 Focal *Toxoplasma* encephalitis at autopsy, day 59. The large tissue cysts have released tachyzoites, which are proliferating and destroying cells. Toxoplasmosis following BMT usually results from reactivation in seropositive patients who were chronically infected prior to transplantation. It is associated with GVHD. (*See also Chapter 23, p. 294.*)

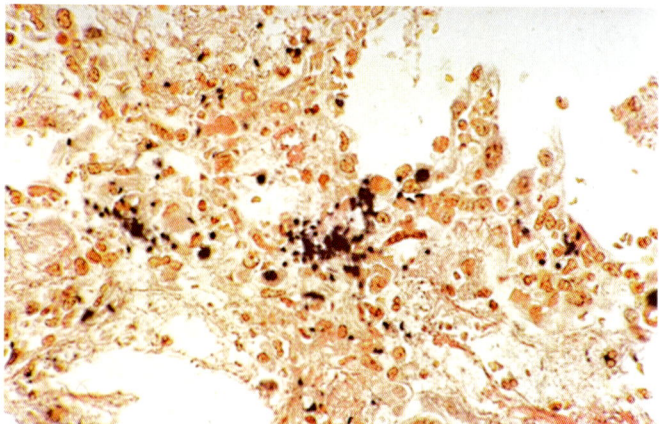

Plate 23.39 *Toxoplasma* pneumonia with immunocytochemical staining of tachyzoites, which appear as small, dark, circular, and curved forms. Disseminated infection in the lungs and other organs may be documented only at autopsy, because immunocompromised marrow recipients produce a weak or negative serological response. As a result, demonstration of parasites in tissue is usually necessary for diagnosis. (*See also Chapter 23, p. 294.*)

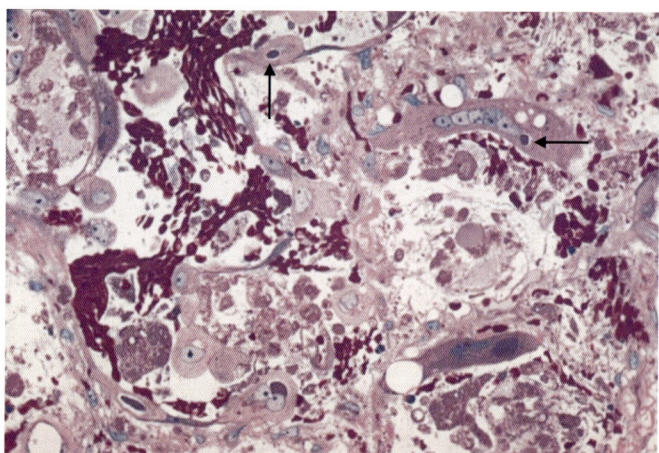

Plate 23.40 Respiratory syncytial virus (RSV) pneumonia in a lung biopsy, day 48. The presence of dark purple cytoplasmic inclusions in multinucleated epithelial cells (arrows) suggests the diagnosis but may be found with other viruses such as parainfluenza. During severe community outbreaks, infections may spread to hospitalized marrow recipients. (*See also Chapter 23, p. 294.*)

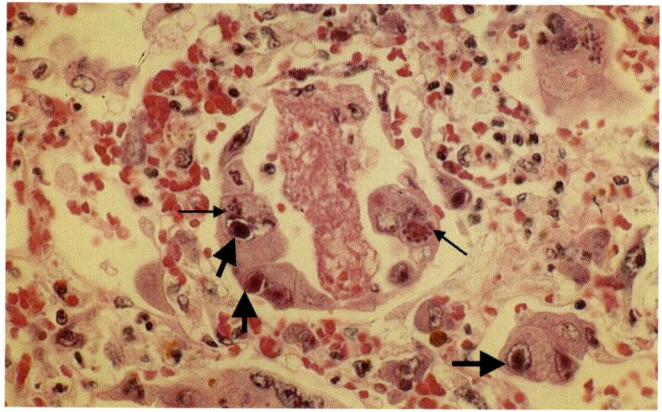

Plate 23.41 Severe CMV pneumonia at autopsy, day 81. Large oval nuclear inclusions (Cowdry type A) (large arrows) as well as small, clustered cytoplasmic inclusions (small arrows) are present. (*See also Chapter 23, p. 294.*)

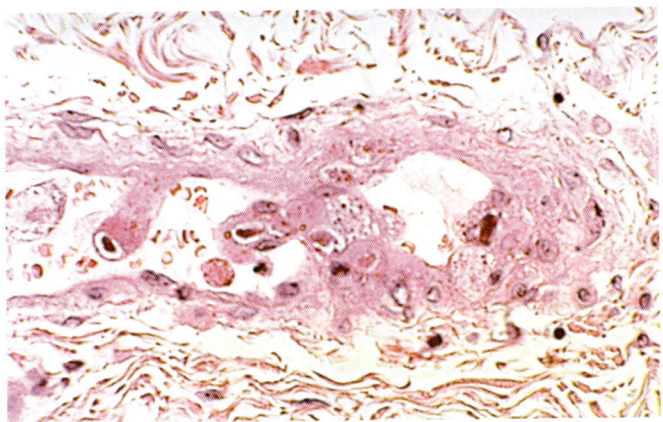

Plate 23.42 Disseminated CMV with cutaneous vasculitis, day 71. Abdominal skin from autopsy shows a venule with microthrombosis and heavy CMV infection of the endothelium. Note the Cowdry type A nuclear inclusions. Four days before death, the patient developed fever, jaundice, rising transaminases, and shock. There was extensive CMV infection of lungs, liver, pancreas, adrenals, and kidney glomeruli, as well as hemorrhagic necrosis of subcutaneous fat. Despite the frequency of CMV dissemination after BMT, cutaneous involvement is rare. (*See also Chapter 23, p. 294.*)

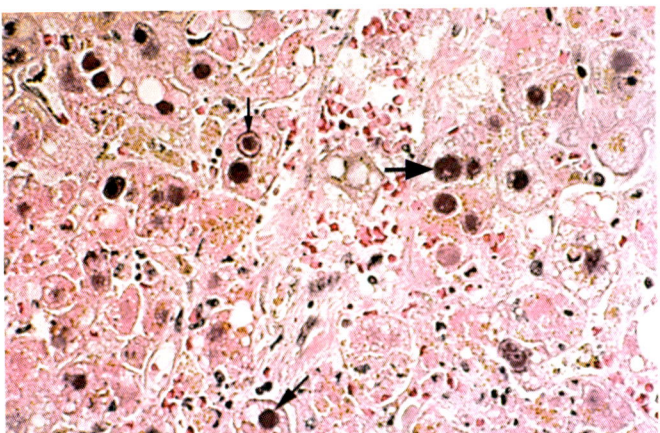

Plate 23.43 Overwhelming adenovirus hepatitis at autopsy 92 days after allogeneic BMT for AML. Dark basophilic nuclear inclusions produce "smudge cells" (large arrows) with blurred nuclear margins. Occasional cells with a halo around the inclusion (small arrow) suggest a combined infection with CMV, which was confirmed by isolation of both viruses. (*See also Chapter 23, p. 294.*)

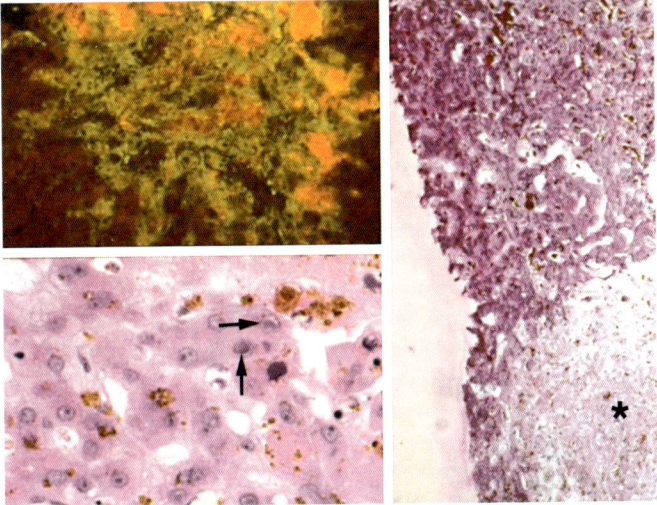

Plate 23.44 Varicella-zoster virus (VZV) hepatitis in a percutaneous needle biopsy, day 79. On the right, a PAS stain demonstrates a pale necrotic area (*) bordered by cells containing nuclear inclusions (large arrows) visible by H&E stain on the lower left. Immunofluorescence confirmed the presence of VZV (upper left), and intravenous acyclovir was begun within hours of the biopsy. (*See also Chapter 23, p. 294.*)

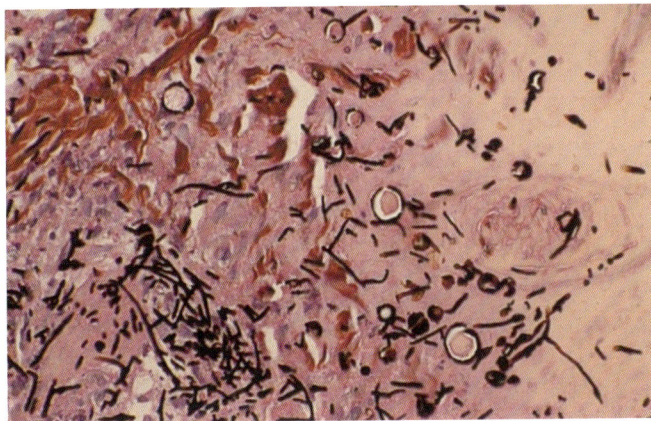

Plate 23.45 *Fusarium* hyphae invade the dermis in pretransplant skin biopsy. (*See also Chapter 23, p. 294.*)

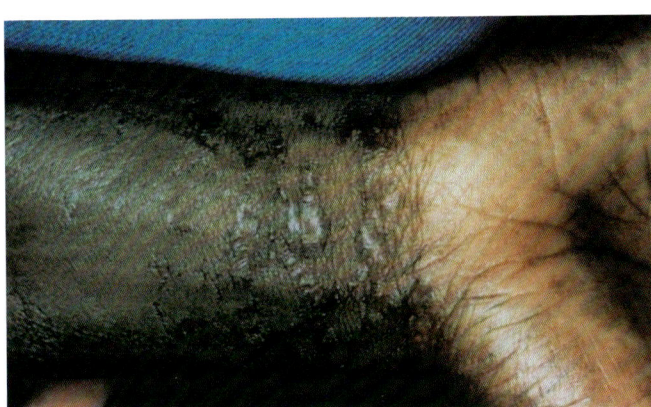

Plate 23.46 Lichen planus-like chronic GVHD of the forearm of a 24-year-old African American male 220 days after BMT of HLA-identical marrow. (*See also Chapter 23, p. 293; Chapter 50, p. 647.*)

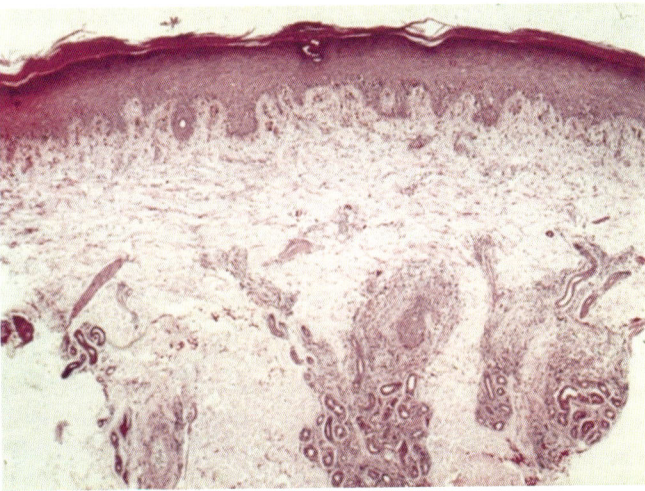

Plate 23.47 Lichen planus-like early chronic GVHD of skin, day 233. Biopsy of a papulosquamous lesion from the posterior neck demonstrates the characteristic features of the generalized or inflammatory type of chronic cutaneous GVHD. The thickened epidermis displays hyper- and parakeratosis, hyper-granulosis, and acanthosis. The extensive destruction along the dermal–epidermal junction results in sawtooth-like changes of the rete ridges, mimicking lichen planus. The papillary dermis has considerable perivascular inflammation. The lichenoid reaction also involves the hair follicles and eccrine glands seen deep in the reticular dermis. At this stage, treatment can prevent progression to fibrosis (see Plate 23.52). (*See also Chapter 23, p. 293; Chapter 50, p. 647.*)

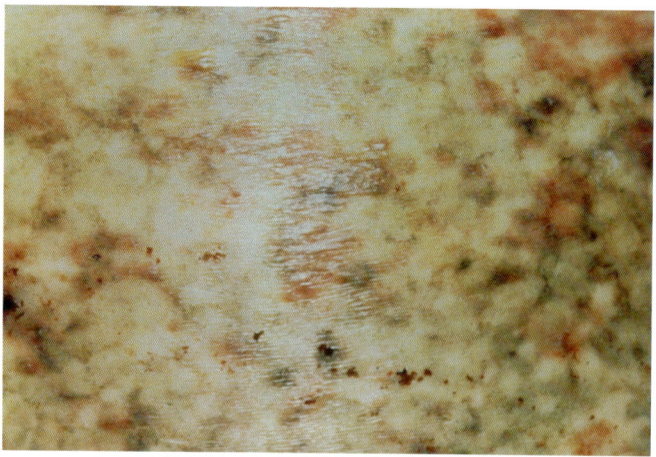

Plate 23.48 Poikiloderma in late chronic GVHD in a 2-year-old girl, day 450. Thinning of the epidermis and dermis are present along with telangiectasia and reticulated pigmentation. (*See also Chapter 23, p. 292; Chapter 50, p. 647.*)

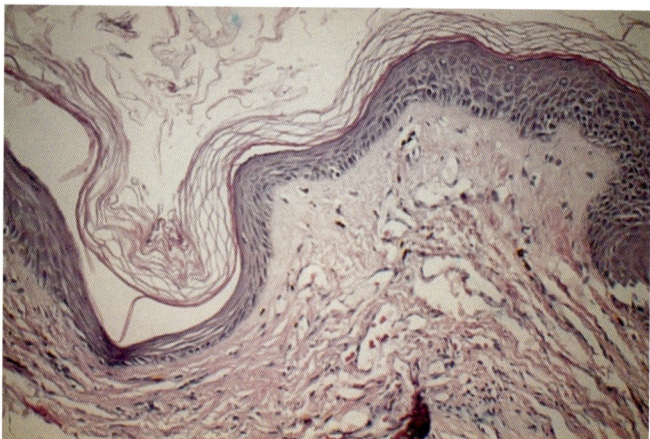

Plate 23.49 Poikiloderma, day 719. The patient was treated vigorously for extensive chronic GVHD with corticosteroids plus several other immunosuppressive agents. Though he had extensive dyspigmentation, telangiectasia, and atrophy of the skin, there were no contractures or scleroderma. Histologically, the epidermis is atrophic, with loss of rete ridges. The fibrotic papillary dermis contains many telangiectatic vessels, and there is intracellular melanin pigment. The deep dermal sweat glands remain despite earlier inflammatory involvement, and the reticular dermal collagen is normal. (*See also Chapter 23, p. 293; Chapter 50, p. 647.*)

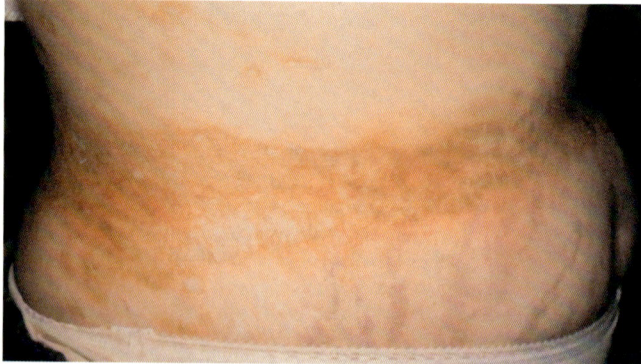

Plate 23.50 Localized late phase of chronic GVHD resembling morphea with atrophic plaque formation, induration, and peripheral hyperpigmentation, day 684. (*See also Chapter 23, p. 293; Chapter 50, p. 647.*)

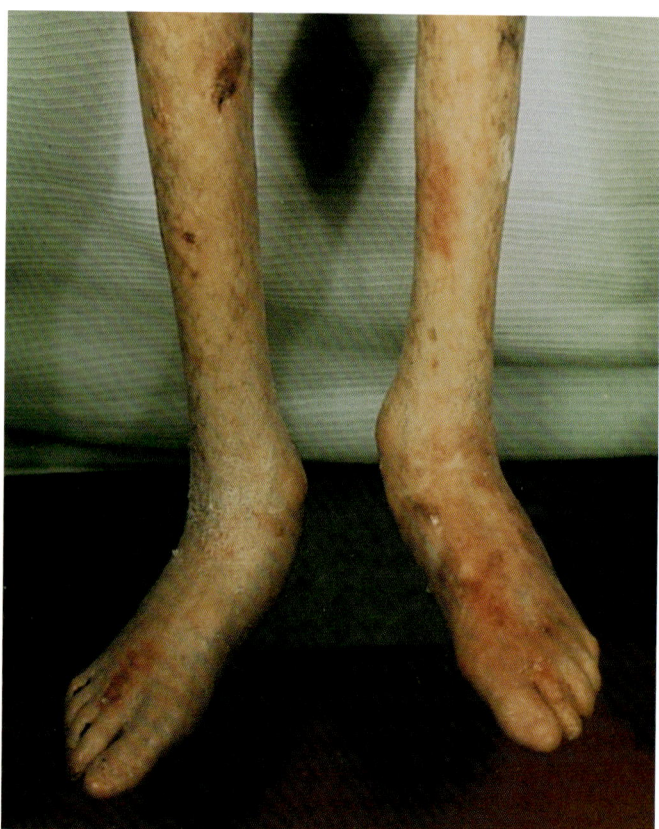

Plate 23.51 Generalized scleroderma with atrophy, sclerodactyly, and joint contracture, day 540 after HLA-identical BMT. (*See also Chapter 23, p. 293; Chapter 50, p. 647.*)

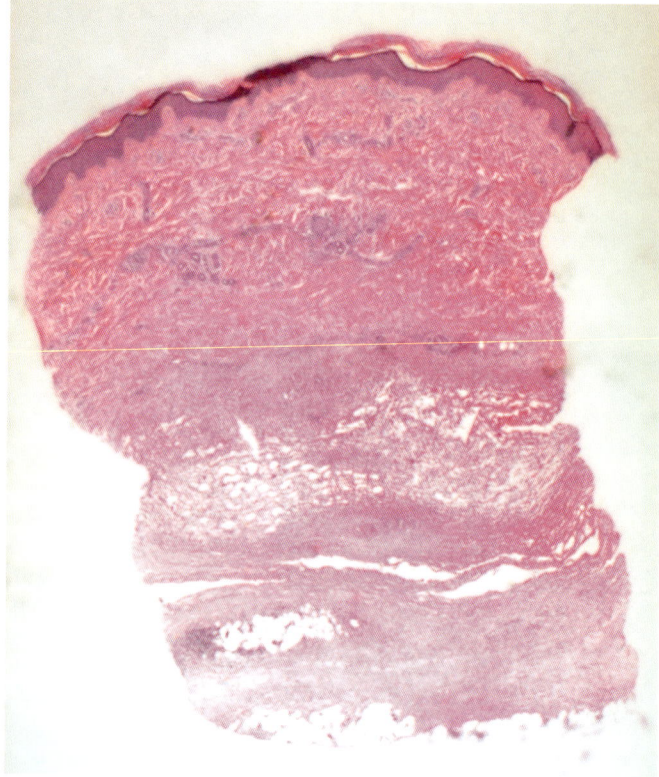

Plate 23.52 Late chronic GVHD of skin, day 959. As this patient's GVHD progressed, the epidermis became atrophic, with straightening of the dermal–epidermal junction. All dermal appendages were destroyed. The reticular dermal collagen became increasingly sclerotic. A panniculitis seen at the base of the specimen resulted in fibrosis of the subcutaneous fat and large vessels. This histological picture corresponds to the dense hidebound and sclerodermatous changes of late chronic GVHD. (*See also Chapter 23, p. 292; Chapter 50, p. 647.*)

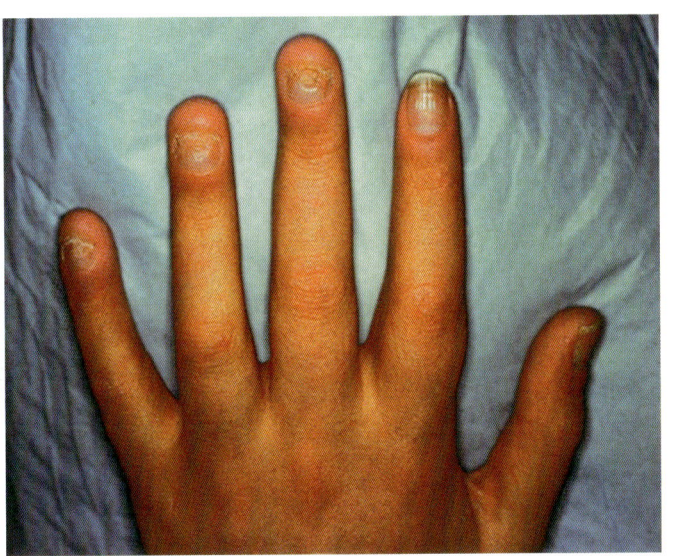

Plate 23.53 Periungual erythema and onychodystrophy 100 days after allogeneic BMT in a patient with ocular sicca and oral lesions of chronic GVHD. (*See also Chapter 23, p. 294; Chapter 50, p. 647.*)

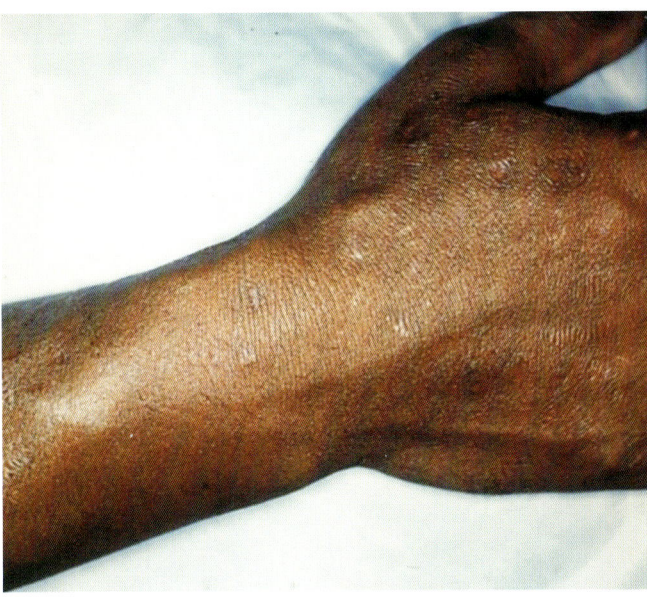

Plate 23.55 Same patient shown in Plates 23.46 & 23.54 after treatment, day 770. (*See also Chapter 23, p. 293; Chapter 50, p. 650.*)

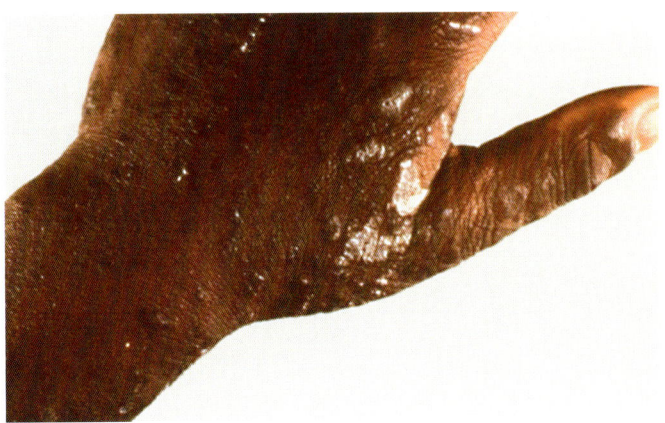

Plate 23.54 Lichen planus-like chronic GVHD before treatment, day 220. (*See also Chapter 23, p. 293; Chapter 50, p. 650.*)

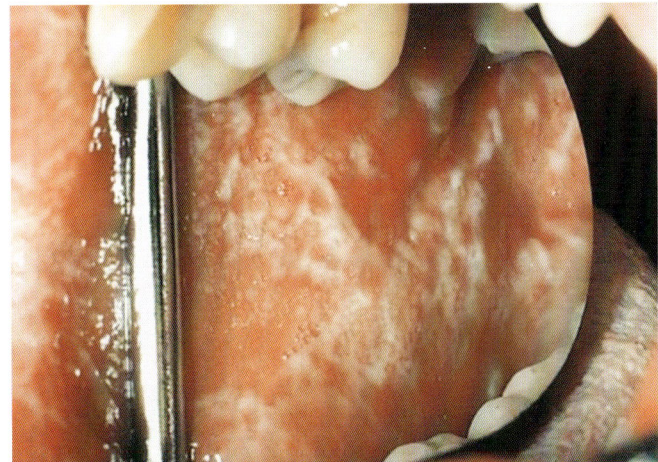

Plate 23.56 Lichenoid lesions of oral chronic GVHD showing erythema, white striae, plaque, and ulcer formation, day 394. (*See also Chapter 23, p. 294; Chapter 50, p. 647; Chapter 67, pp. 920, 922, 923.*)

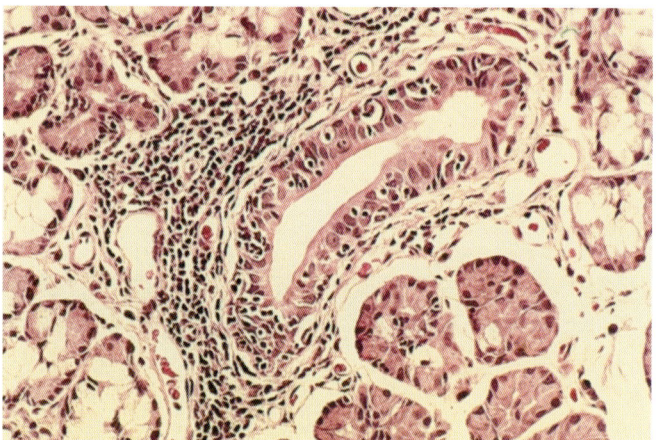

Plate 23.57 Oral labial biopsy with early chronic GVHD, day 92. The minor salivary gland exhibits a periductal mononuclear inflammatory infiltrate involving the duct epithelium, in which there is focal epithelial apoptosis. There is inflammation of adjacent acini. This process leads to fibrosis with acinar atrophy in lobules drained by the affected ducts. The squamous surface epithelium (not present here) showed grade II lesions similar to those previously illustrated in skin (see Plate 23.18). The lip biopsy is valuable in the diagnosis and staging of chronic GVHD because it frequently mirrors destructive inflammatory changes in lacrimal, tracheal, and esophageal glands as well as bile ducts. (*See also Chapter 23, p. 294; Chapter 67, pp. 921, 922.*)

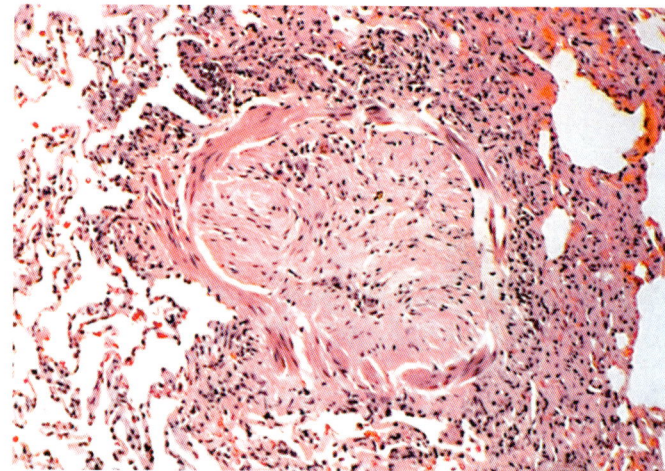

Plate 23.60 Bronchiolitis obliterans in a lung biopsy, day 396. The patient had chronic GVHD with severe obstructive pulmonary disease. Similar small airway inflammation with fibrosis is seen in lung allograft rejection. (*See also Chapter 23, p. 297; Chapter 50, p. 647.*)

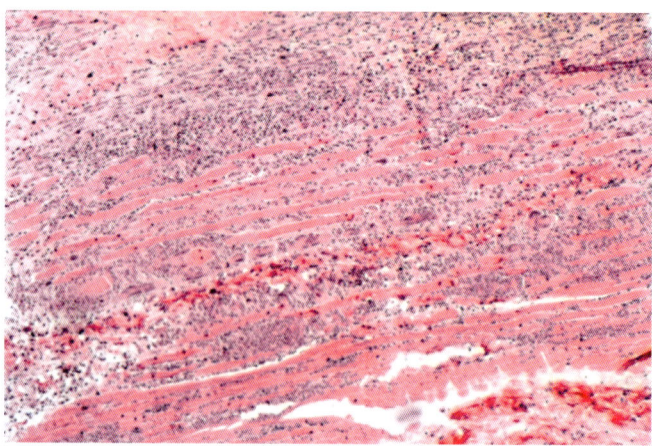

Plate 23.58 Polymyositis in deltoid muscle biopsy associated with chronic GVHD, day 1129. There is extensive endomysial chronic inflammation associated with myocyte destruction. The condition responded to immunosuppressive therapy. (*See also Chapter 23, p. 292; Chapter 50, p. 648.*)

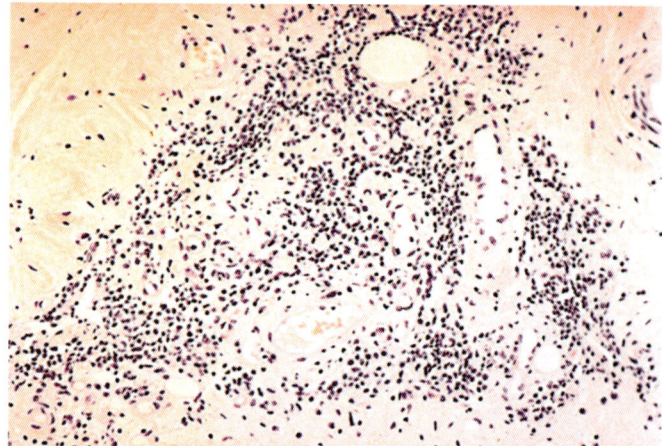

Plate 23.61 Atrophy and fibrosis of thymus associated with chronic GVHD in a 13-year-old, day 350. The patient had not received immunosuppressive drugs, so the destruction was presumably the result of chronic GVHD activity. (*See also Chapter 23, p. 292; Chapter 50, p. 646.*)

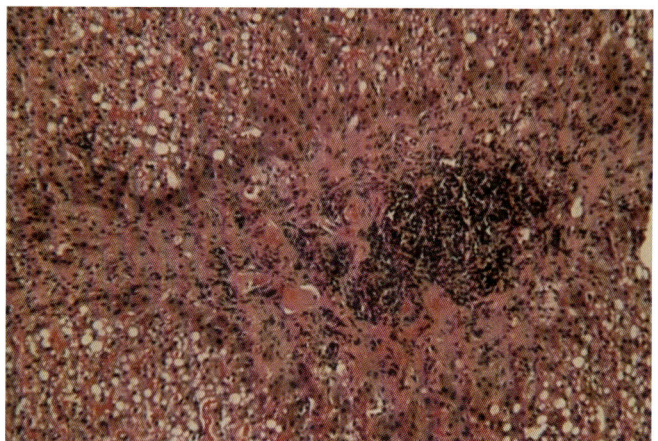

Plate 23.59 (*left*) Chronic GVHD of liver, day 166. This biopsy shows a prominent plasmacytic infiltrate in the portal area and a paucity of interlobular bile ducts. The histological dichotomy between acute and chronic GVHD is less clear in liver than in skin. However, increased portal inflammation and loss of bile ducts are more common in chronic GVHD. Despite the frequency of chronic hepatic GVHD, cirrhosis and liver failure are rare and may reflect superinfection with hepatitis C virus. (*See also Chapter 23, p. 292.*)

Acute Syngeneic GVHD **Chronic Syngeneic GVHD**

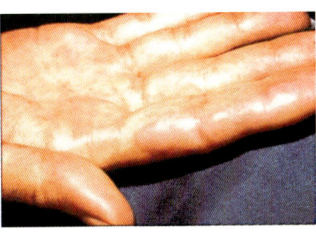

Plate 30.1 Syngeneic graft-vs.-host disease (GVHD). The initial onset of syngeneic GVHD is characterized by erythroderma and dermatitis. Histological evaluation of the tongue reveals a marked lymphocyte infiltrate into the mucosa along with epithelial cell destruction and dyskeratosis. The autoaggressive disease can progress to a chronic GVHD with significant alopecia. Histological evaluation of the skin shows a thickening of the epidermis and dermal fibrosis along with a sparse lymphocyte infiltrate. (See also Chapter 30, p. 405.)

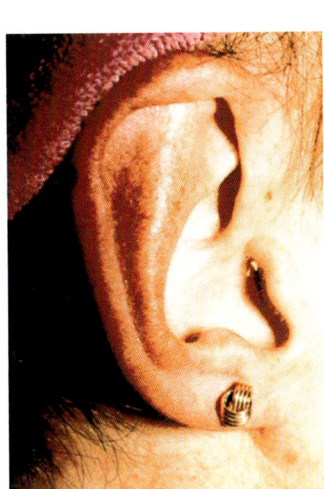

Plate 30.2 Clinical autologous graft-vs.-host disease (GVHD). The onset of clinical autologous GVHD coincides with the initial phases of engraftment and is characterized by an erythematous maculopapular rash affecting the ears, face, trunk, hands and feet. Histological analysis of skin reveals a lymphocyte infiltrate and pathology consistent with acute GVHD. Administration of interferon-gamma (IFN-γ) increases the severity of autologous GVHD. Note the necrotic area on the abdomen at the site of IFN-γ administration. (See also Chapter 30, p. 408.)

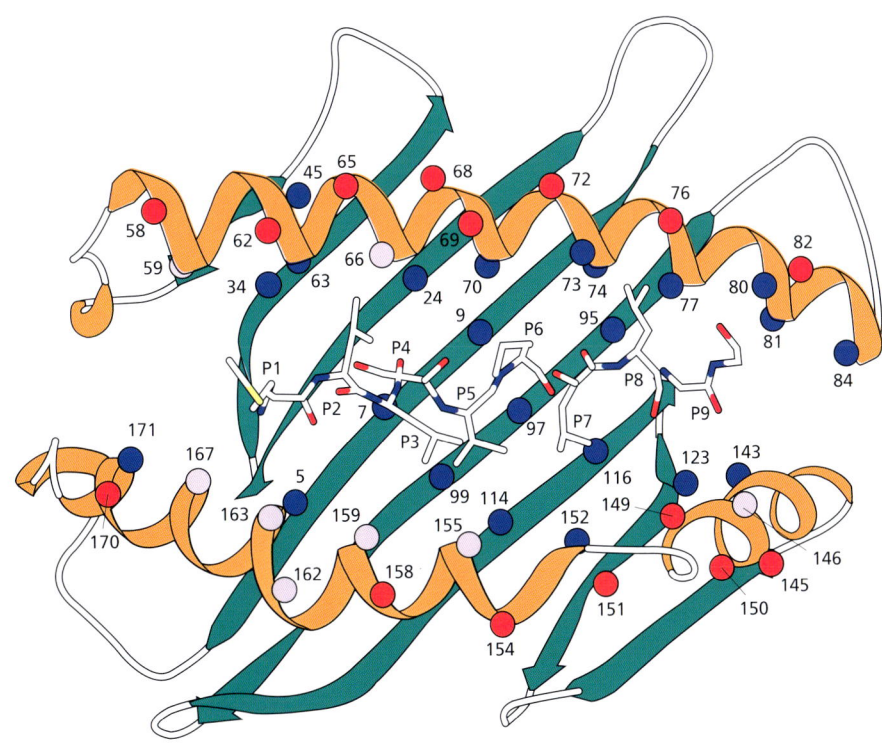

Plate 83.1 Ribbon diagram of the HLA-A2 molecule showing α-carbon backbone of the α1 and α2 domains and the β-pleated sheet. Residues are colored according to their putative role in peptide repertoire (red), TCR contact (blue) or both (lilac) [174,175]. The bound peptide is labeled (P1–P9). Residues implicated in peptide-binding are: 5,7,9,24,25,34,45,63,67,70, 73,74,77,80,81,84,95,97,99,113,114,116,123,143, 147,152,156,160, and 171. Residues implicated in TCR contact are: 58,62,65,68,69,72,76,82,145, 149,150,151,154,158,166, and 170. Residues involved in both peptide and TCR contact are: 59,66,146,155,159,162,163 and 167.

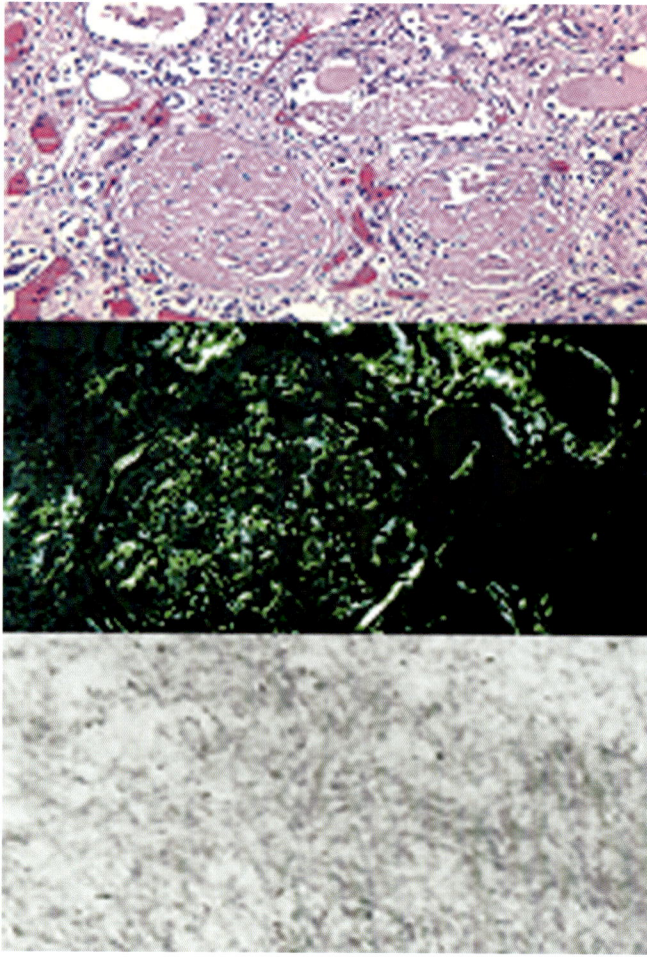

Plate 93.1 Renal biopsy showing amyloidosis. These images show three views of a renal biopsy: with periodic-acid Schiff (PAS) staining showing amorphous material in glomeruli (top), Congo red staining showing apple-green birefringence in polarized light (middle) and electron microscopy showing nonbranched linear fibrils about 10 nM in length. (*See also Chapter 93, p. 1283.*)

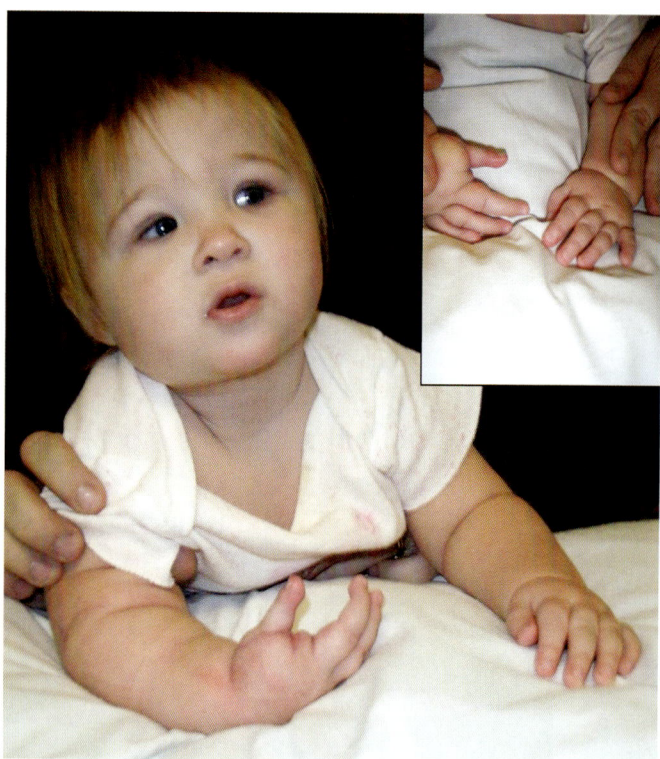

Plate 109.1 A 1¹/₁₂-year-old female who demonstrates many of the physical features associated with FA. Before policization of the right index finger, the right hand exhibited a hypoplastic radius and absent thumb; the left hand had a hypoplastic thumb only. The patient exhibits growth retardation, microophthalmia, microencephaly and café au lait spots; she also has kidney abnormality. (*See also Chapter 109, p. 1485.*)

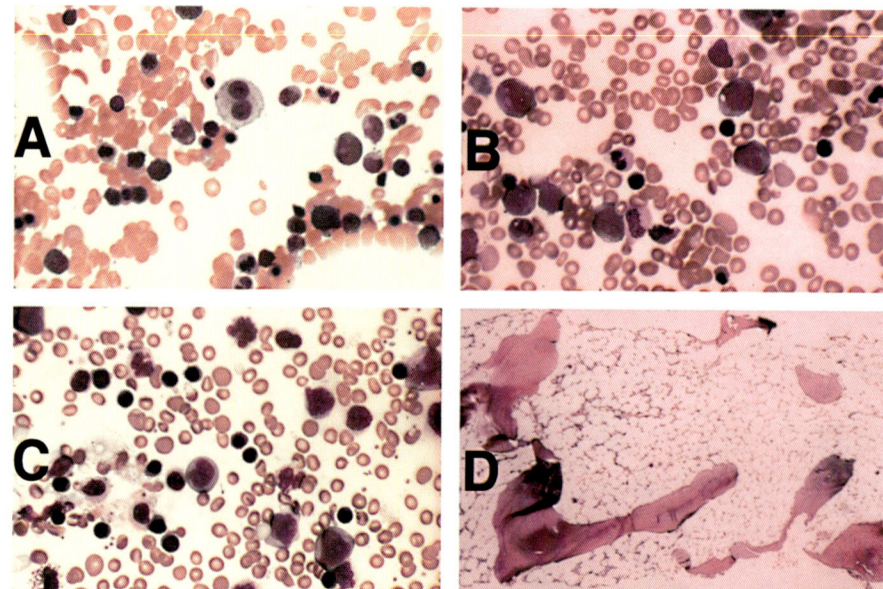

Plate 109.2 Progression of hematological abnormalities in a single patient with FA. (A) Marrow aspirate on 02-21-96 demonstrating pancytopenia and early signs of dysplastic changes in neutrophils; (B) marrow aspirate on 07-03-96 demonstrating progressive dysplasia and 3% blasts; (C) marrow aspirate on 09-24-96 demonstrating progressive dysplasia and 12% blasts; and (D) marrow biopsy on 09-24-96 demonstrating severity of marrow failure. (*See also Chapter 109, p. 1484.*)

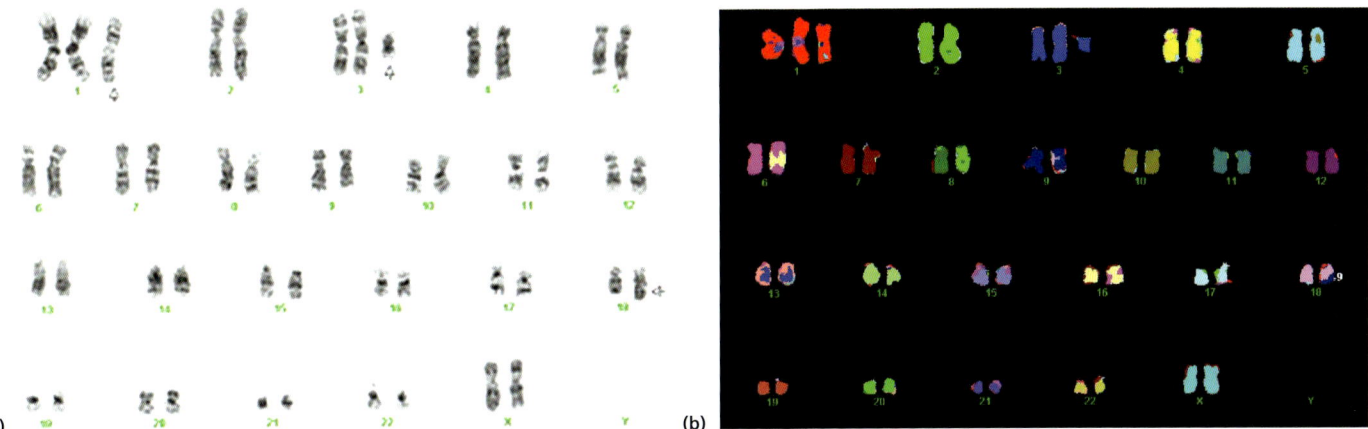

Plate 109.3 (a) G-banded karyotype from an abnormal clone in the marrow of an FA patient. This is a hyperdiploid metaphase cell with 48 chromosomes including two extra derivative chromosomes (designated by arrows): one derivative chromosome is composed of two copies of the long arm of chromosome 1, and the other contains two copies of a small portion of the long arm of chromosome 3. Thus this cell contains a total of four copies of portions of chromosomes 1 and 3. (b) A karyotype of the same abnormal clone as (a) above, as characterized by fluorescence *in situ* hybridization (FISH) using a multicolor paint probe (Vysis spectral vision M-FISH). M-FISH confirmed that the two derivative chromosomes detected by G-banding represented extra copies of portions of chromosomes 1 and 3. (Courtesy of Betsy Hirsch, PhD, Director of the Cytogenetics Laboratory of the Fairview University Medical Center, Minneapolis, MN.) (*See also Chapter 109, p. 1490.*)

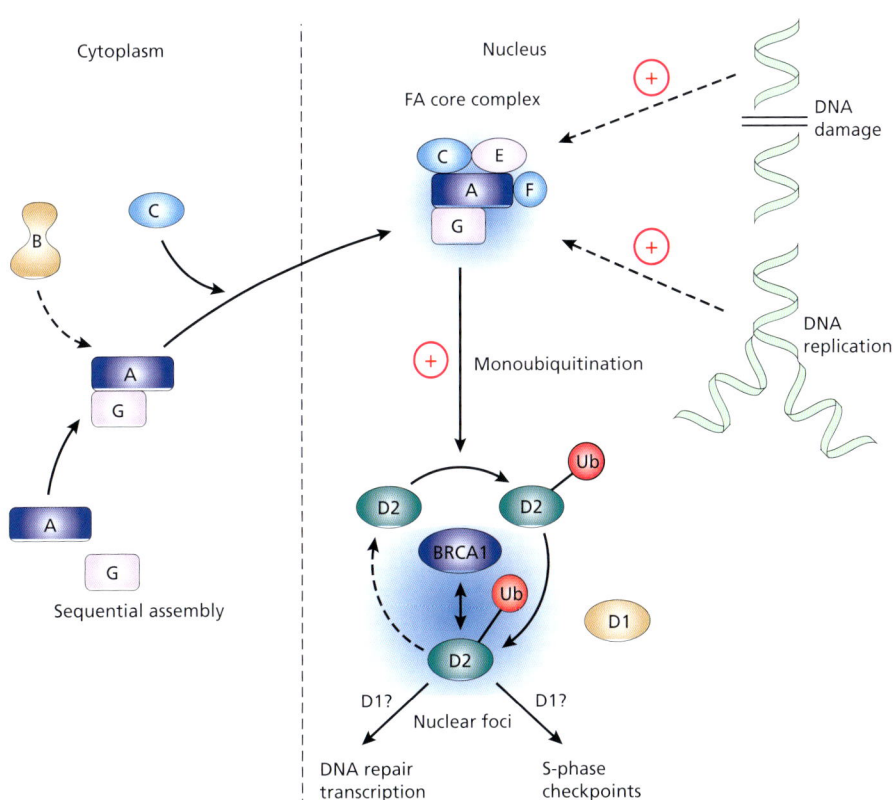

Plate 109.4 Model of the FA pathway. The model shows the sequential assembly of the FA core complex in the cytoplasm and nucleus. The defect in FA-B cells indicates that FANCB might function in an early stage of this assembly process. DNA replication or DNA damage might activate the complex, either directly or indirectly, leading to the activation of FANCD2 by monoubiquination [68; Chapter 109] and its targeting to nuclear foci. The FANCD1 protein might participate at this point. The association of BRCA1 at these sites could lead to as yet undefined downstream events, such as DNA repair or the activation of DNA synthesis (S) checkpoints. In this model, the core complex, which consists of FANCA, FANCC, FANCF, FANCG and FANCE, is the sensor for DNA damage and participates by activating FANCD2 through ubiquination. FANCD2 then facilitates repair. (Reproduced with permission. *Nature Reviews Genetics* 2001; 2: 446–59. DOI: 10.1038/3507/6590.) (*See also Chapter 109, p. 1500.*)

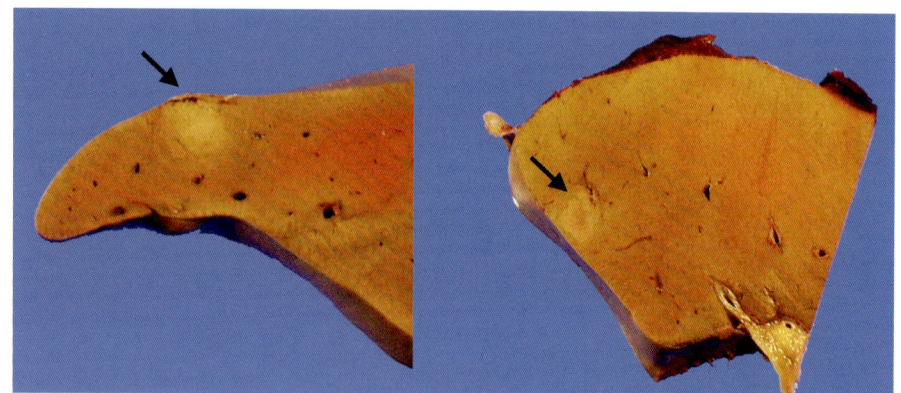

Plate 109.5 Hepatic adenomata. Pathological specimen obtained at autopsy from a patient with FA with multiple hepatic adenomata not revealed by ultrasound prior to HCT. Patient died from intrahepatic hemorrhage into an adenomatous lesion. (*See also Chapter 109.*)

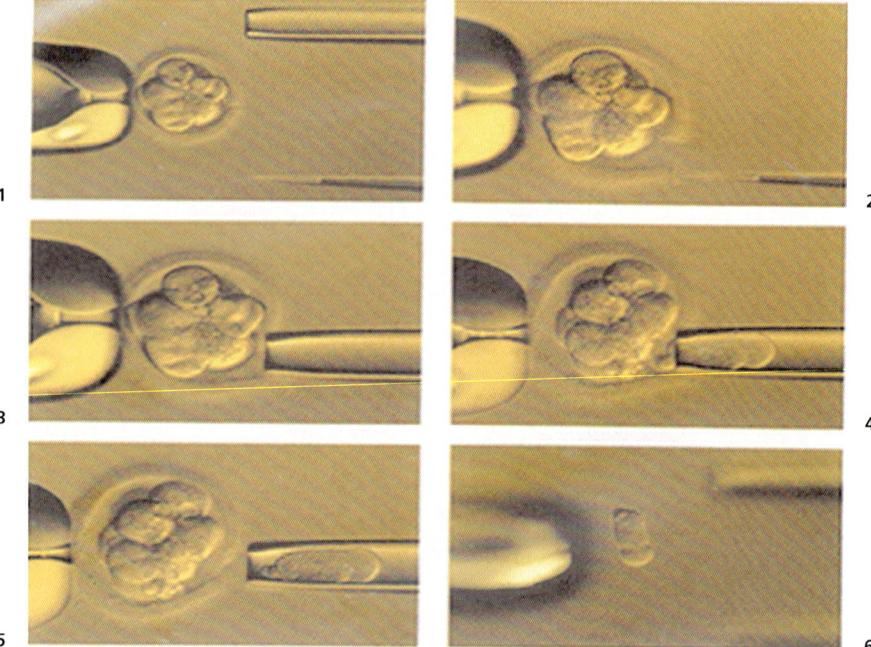

Plate 109.6 Blastomere biopsy. **1** Blastomere is held in place. **2** An opening is made in the zona pellucida using a microneedle at the 3 O'clock position. **3** The blastomere biopsy needle is passed through the opening towards the nearest blastomere. **4** The blastomere is slowly aspirated into the pipette. **5** The micropipette containing the blastomere is withdrawn from the perivitelline space. **6** The embryo is released from the holding pipette and the micropipette containing the blastomere is lowered and expelled into the drop of medium. Reproduced with permission: An atlas of Preimplantation Genetic Diagnosis (Verlinsky Y and Kuliev A, eds) Parthenon Publishing Group, New York, 2000, p. 91. (*See also Chapter 109.*)

One response to the difficulties in characterizing pulmonary GVHD has been to arbitrarily apply that designation to virtually all histological lung injury patterns including diffuse alveolar damage, IP and bronchiolitis obliterans organizing pneumonia (BOOP) [118]. In terms of patient care, the liberal diagnosis of pulmonary GVHD without strict and reproducible criteria could encourage overly aggressive medical immunosuppression and thereby increase infection. Studies of sufficient size, which focus on individual histological patterns such as BOOP, are beginning to appear. In a study of 49 patients with BOOP and a large control group, this abnormality was found to be strongly associated with both acute and chronic GVHD suggesting that it may result from pulmonary GVH activity (Fig. 23.17) [119].

Animal models of acute GVHD indicate that vascular inflammation may be an early morphological feature, one that could be obscured by later changes in biopsy or autopsy tissue from human patients. There is increasing experimental evidence that GVH reactions involve the production of cytokines such as TNF-α, IL-1 and interferon-γ with up-regulation of histocompatibility antigen expression along with the endothelial expression of cellular adhesion molecules [120].

It is well established that chronic pulmonary GVH activity is a major contributor to bronchiolar inflammation culminating in bronchiolitis obliterans (Fig. 23.18 [68]). This relationship is supported by published reports of more than 36 patients with bronchiolitis obliterans (Fig. 23.18; see also Plate 23.60, *facing p. 296*) and chronic GVHD, the strong association of airflow obstruction with chronic GVHD and the symptomatic response to immunosuppressive therapy [121,122]. Furthermore, bronchiolitis obliterans is strongly associated with lung allograft rejection in both humans and animals [123,124]. Secondary infection may have a major role in chronic GVHD because patients have important deficiencies of immunoglobulins [125].

Summary

HCT has ushered in a new group of complications, particularly GVHD, and has produced new combinations of the previously known complications of radiation, chemotherapy, immune deficiency and transplantation immunopathology. This process evolves as the success and side-effects of new treatments for tumors, GVHD and infections mandate continuous revision of the practical tenets of diagnosis.

References

1 Sale GE. Pathology of bone marrow and thymic transplantation. In: Sale GE, ed. *The Pathology of Organ Transplantation*. Stoneham, London: Butterworth Publishers, Inc., 1990: 229–59.

2 Sale GE, Buckner CD. Pathology of bone marrow in transplant recipients. *Hem Onc Clin North Am* 1988; **2**: 735–56.

3 Shulman HM, Wells D, Gooley T *et al.* The biologic significance of rare peripheral blasts after hematopoietic cell transplant is predicted by multidimensional flow cytometry. *Am J Clin Pathol* 1999; **112**: 513–23.

4 Sievers EL, Lange BJ, Buckley JD *et al.* Prediction of relapse of pediatric acute myeloid leukemia by use of multidimensional flow cytometry. *J Natl Cancer Inst* 1996; **88**: 1483–8.

5 Wells DA, Sale G, Shulman H, Bryant EM, Gooley T, Loken MR. Multidimensional flow cytometry of marrow can differentiate leukemic lymphoblasts from normal lymphoblasts and myeloblasts following chemotherapy and/or bone marrow transplant. *Am J Clini Path* 1998; **110**: 84–94.

6 Diel IJ, Kaufmann M, Costa SD, Bastert G. Monoclonal antibodies to detect breast cancer cells in bone marrow. *Important Adv Oncol* 1994; **9**: 143–64.

7 Soll E, Massumoto C, Clift RA *et al.* Relevance of marrow fibrosis in bone marrow transplantation: a retrospective analysis of engraftment. *Blood* 1995; **86**: 4667–73.

8 Rajantie J, Sale GE, Deeg HJ *et al.* Adverse effect of severe marrow fibrosis on hematological recovery after chemoradiotherapy and allogeneic bone marrow transplantation. *Blood* 1986; **67**: 1693–7.

9 Radich J, Appelbaum F, Bryant E *et al.* PCR detection of the Bcr-Abl fusion transcript after bone marrow transplant for chronic myeloid leukemia predicts subsequent relapse: a multivariate model of 356 patients. *Blood* 1995; **85**: 2632–8.

10 Zutter MM, Martin PJ, Sale GE *et al.* Epstein–Barr virus lymphoproliferation after bone marrow transplantation. *Blood* 1988; **72**: 520–9.

11 Carpenter PA, Appelbaum FR, Corey L *et al.* A humanized non-FcR-binding anti-CD3 antibody, visilizumab, for treatment of steroid-refractory acute graft-versus-host disease. *Blood* 2002; **99**: 2712–9.

12 Bearman SI, Appelbaum FR, Buckner CD *et al.* Regimen-related toxicity in patients undergoing bone marrow transplantation. *J Clin Oncol* 1988; **6**: 1562–8.

13 Epstein RJ, McDonald GB, Sale GE *et al.* The diagnostic accuracy of the rectal biopsy in acute graft-versus-host disease: a prospective study of thirteen patients. *Gastroenterology* 1980; **78**: 764–71.

14 Shulman HM, McDonald GB, Matthews D *et al.* An analysis of hepatic venoocclusive disease and centrilobular hepatic degeneration following bone marrow transplantation. *Gastroenterology* 1980; **79**: 1178–91.

15 DeLeve LD, Shulman HM, McDonald GB. *Toxic Injury to Hepatic Sinusoids: Sinusoidal Obstruction (Veno-Occlusive Disease). Seminars in Liver Disease*. New York: Thieme Medical Publishers, Inc., 2002, vol. 22: 27–41.

16 DeLeve LD, Wang X, Kanel GC *et al.* Decreased hepatic nitric oxide production contributes to the development of rat sinusoidal obstruction syndrome. *Hepatology* 2003; **38**: 900–8.

17 Shulman HM, Gown AM, Nugent DJ. Hepatic veno-occlusive disease after bone marrow transplantation. Immunohistochemical identification of the material within occluded central venules. *Am J Pathol* 1987; **127**: 549–58.

18 Shulman HM, Fisher LB, Schoch HG *et al.* Veno-occlusive disease of the liver after marrow transplantation: histological correlates of clinical signs and symptoms. *Hepatology* 1994; **19**: 1171–81.

19 Watanabe K, Iwaki H, Satoh M *et al.* Veno-occlusive disease of the liver following bone marrow transplantation: a clinical-pathological study of autopsy cases. *Artif Organs* 1996; **20**: 1145–50.

20 Sato Y, Asada Y, Hara S *et al.* Hepatic stellate cells (Ito cells) in veno-occlusive disease of the liver after allogeneic bone marrow transplantation. *Histopathology* 1999; **34**: 66–70.

21 Jones RJ, Lee KSK, Beschorner WF *et al.* Veno-occlusive disease of the liver following bone marrow transplantation. *Transplantation* 1987; **44**: 778–83.

22 Rajvanshi P, Shulman HM, Sievers EL, McDonald GB. Hepatic sinusoidal obstruction after gemtuzumab ozogamicin (Mylotarg) therapy. *Blood* 2002; **99**: 2310–1.

23 Giles FJ, Kantarjian HM, Kornblau SM *et al.* Mylotarg (gemtuzumab ozogamicin) therapy is associated with hepatic veno-occlusive disease in patients who have not received stem cell transplantation. *Cancer* 2001; **92**: 406–13.

24 Snover DC, Weisdorf S, Bloomer J *et al.* Nodular regenerative hyperplasia of the liver following bone marrow transplantation. *Hepatology* 1989; **9**: 443–8.

25 Wanless IR. Micronodular transformation (nodular regenerative hyperplasia) of the liver: a report of 64 cases among 2500 autopsies and a new classification of benign hepatocellular nodules. *Hepatology* 1990; **11**: 787–97.

26 Heymer B, Bunjes D, Friedrich W. *Clinical and Diagnostic Pathology of Graft-Versus-Host Disease*. Berlin and Heidelberg: Springer-Verlag, 2002.

27 Martin PJ. Increased disparity for minor histocompatibility antigens as a potential cause of increased GVHD risk in marrow transplantation from unrelated donors compared with related donors. *Bone Marrow Transplant* 1991; **8**: 217–23.

28 Sale GE, Anderson P, Browne M *et al.* Evidence of cytotoxic T-cell destruction of epidermal cells in human graft-versus-host disease: Immunohistology with monoclonal antibody TIA-1. *Arch Path Laboratory Med* 1992; **116**: 622–5.

29 Piguet PF. Tumor necrosis factor and graft-versus-host disease. In: Burakoff S, Deeg HJ, eds. *Graft-Versus-Host Disease*. New York and Basel: Marcel Dekker, Inc., 1990: 225–76.

30 Ferrara JLM, Cooke KR, Pan L *et al.* The immunopathophysiology of acute graft versus host disease. *Stem Cells* 1996; **14**: 473–89.

31 Teshima T, Ordemann R, Reddy P *et al.* Acute graft-versus-host disease does not require alloantigen expression in host epithelium. *Nature Med* 2002; **8**: 575–81.

32 Baker M, Altman NY, Podack ER et al. The role of cell mediated cytotoxicity in acute GVHD after MHC matched allogeneic bone marrow transplantation in mice. J Exp Med 1996; 183: 2645–56.

33 Gilliam AC, Whitaker-Mehnezes D, Korngold R, Murphy GF. Apoptosis is the predominant form of epithelial target cell injury in acute experimental graft versus host disease. J Invest Dermatol 1996; 107: 377–83.

34 Gilliam AC, Murphy GF. Cellular pathology of cutaneous graft-versus-host disease. In: Ferrara JL, Deeg HJ, Burakoff SJ, eds. Graft-Versus-Host Disease, 2nd edn. New York and Basel: Marcel Dekker, Inc., 1996: 291–313.

35 Sale GE. Does graft-versus-host disease attack epithelial stem cells? (Review) Mol Med Today 1996; 2: 114–9.

36 Sale GE, Lerner KG, Barker EA et al. The skin biopsy in the diagnosis of acute graft-versus-host disease in man. Am J Pathol 1977; 89: 621–35.

37 Lerner KG, Kao GF, Storb R et al. Histopathology of graft-versus-host reaction (GVHR) in human recipients of marrow from HLA matched sibling donors. Transplant Proc 1974; 6: 389–93.

38 Cox GJ, Matsui SM, Lo RS et al. Etiology and outcome of diarrhea after marrow transplantation: a prospective study. Gastroenterology 1994; 107: 1398–407.

39 Schwartz JM, Wolford JL, Thornquist MD et al. Severe gastrointestinal bleeding after hematopoietic cell transplantation, 1987–97: incidence, causes and outcome. Am J Gastroenterol 2001; 96: 385–93.

40 Sale GE, Shulman HM, McDonald GB, Thomas ED. Gastrointestinal graft-versus-host disease in man. A clinicopathologic study of the rectal biopsy. Am J Surg Pathol 1979; 3: 291–9.

41 Ponec RJ, Hackman RC, McDonald GB. Endoscopic and histologic diagnosis of intestinal graft-versus-host disease after marrow transplantation. Gastrointest Endosc 1999; 49: 612–21.

42 Fisk JD, Shulman HM, Greening RR et al. Gastrointestinal radiographic features of human graft-versus-host disease. Am J Roentgenol 1981; 136: 329–36.

43 Snover DC, Weisdorf SA, Vercellotti GM et al. A histopathologic study of gastric and small intestinal graft-versus-host disease following allogeneic bone marrow transplantation. Hum Pathol 1985; 16: 387–92.

44 Spencer GD, Hackman RC, McDonald GB et al. A prospective study of unexplained nausea and vomiting after marrow transplantation. Transplantation 1986; 42: 602–7.

45 Nakhleh RE, Miller W, Snover DC. Significance of mucosal versus salivary gland changes in lip biopsies in the diagnosis of chronic graft-versus-host disease. Arch Pathol Laboratory Med 1989; 113: 932–4.

46 Washington K, Bentley RC, Green A et al. Gastric graft-versus-host disease: a blinded histologic study. Am J Surg Pathol 1997; 21: 1037–46.

47 Spencer GD, Shulman HM, Myerson D et al. Diffuse intestinal ulceration after marrow transplantation: a clinicopathological study of 13 patients. Hum Pathol 1986; 17: 621–33.

48 Hill GR, Ferrara JL. The primacy of the gastrointestinal tract as a target organ of acute graft-versus-host disease: rationale for the use of cytokine shields in allogeneic bone marrow transplantation. Blood 2000; 95: 2754–9.

49 Gallucci BB, Sale GE, McDonald GB et al. The fine structure of human rectal epithelium in acute graft-versus-host disease. Am J Surg Pathol 1982; 6: 293–305.

50 Daneshpouy M, Socie G, Lemann M et al. Activated eosinophils in upper gastrointestinal tract of patients with graft-versus-host disease. Blood 2002; 99: 3033–40.

51 McDonald GB, Shulman HM, Sullivan KM et al. Intestinal and hepatic complications of human bone marrow transplantation. Gastroenterology 1986; 90: 460–7 & 770–84.

52 Beschorner WE, Yardley JH, Tutschka P et al. Deficiency of intestinal immunity with graft-versus-host disease in humans. J Infect Dis 1981; 144: 38–46.

53 Hess AD. Syngeneic graft-versus-host disease. In: Burakoff SJ, Deeg HJ, Ferrara J, Atkinson K, eds. Graft-Versus-Host Disease: Immunology, Pathophysiology, and Treatment. New York: Marcel Dekker, Inc., 1990: 95–107.

54 Saunders MD, Shulman HM, Murakami CS et al. Bile duct apoptosis and cholestasis resembling acute graft-versus-host disease after autologous hematopoietic cell transplantation. Am J Surg Path 2000; 24: 1004–8.

55 Peters M, Vierling J, Gershwin ME et al. Immunology and the liver. Hepatology 1991; 13: 977–93.

56 Li J, Helm K, Howell CD. Contributions of donor CD4 and CD8 cells to liver injury during murine graft-versus-host disease. Transplantation 1996; 62: 1621–8.

57 Sale GE, Storb R, Kolb H. Histopathology of hepatic acute graft-versus-host disease in the dog. A double blind study confirms the specificity of small bile duct lesions. Transplantation 1978; 26: 103–6.

58 Shulman HM, Sharma P, Amos D et al. A coded histologic study of hepatic graft-versus-host disease after human bone marrow transplantation. Hepatology 1988; 8: 463–70.

59 Snover DC, Weisdorf SA, Ramsay NK et al. Hepatic graft-versus-host disease: a study of the predictive value of liver biopsy in diagnosis. Hepatology 1984; 4: 123–30.

60 Fausto N, Mead JE. Biology of disease. Regulation of liver growth: Proto-oncogenes and transforming growth factors. Laboratory Invest 1989; 60: 4–13.

61 Fox ES, Broitman SA, Thomas P. Biology of disease. Bacterial endotoxins and the liver. Laboratory Invest 1990; 63: 733–41.

62 Tracey KJ, Wei H, Manogue KR et al. Cachectin/tumor necrosis factor induces cachexia, anemia and inflammation. J Exp Med 1988; 167: 1211–27.

63 Strasser SI, Shulman HM, Flowers ME et al. Chronic graft-versus-host disease of the liver: presentation as an acute hepatitis. Hepatology 2000; 32: 1265–71.

64 Fujii N, Takenaka K, Shinagawa K et al. Hepatic graft-versus-host disease presenting as an acute hepatitis after allogeneic peripheral blood stem cell transplantation. Bone Marrow Transplant 2001; 27: 1007–10.

65 Reed EC, Myerson D, Corey L et al. Allogeneic marrow transplantation in patients positive for hepatitis B surface antigen. Blood 1991; 77: 195–200.

66 Locasciulli A, Bacigalupo A, Van Lint MT et al. Hepatitis B virus (HBV) infection and liver disease after allogeneic bone marrow transplantation: a report of 30 cases. Bone Marrow Transplant 1990; 6: 25–9.

67 Snover DC, Hutton S, Balfour HH et al. Cytomegalovirus infection of the liver in transplant recipients. J Clin Gastroenterol 1987; 9: 659–65.

68 Galle PR, Hofmann WJ, Walczak H et al. Involvement of the CD95 (AP0-1/Fas) receptor and ligand in liver damage. J Exp Med 1995; 182: 1223–30.

69 Akpek G, Boitnott JK, Lee LA et al. Hepatitic variant of graft-versus-host disease after donor lymphocyte infusion. Blood 2002; 100: 3903–7.

70 Strasser SI, Sullivan KM, Myerson D et al. Cirrhosis of the liver in long-term marrow transplant survivors. Blood 1999; 93: 3259–66.

71 Taniguchi D, McDonald GB. Viral hepatitis in marrow and stem cell transplant patients. In: Willson RA, ed. Viral Hepatitis. New York: Marcel Dekker, Inc., 1997: 425–70.

72 Locasciulli A, Bacigalupo A, Van Lint MT et al. Hepatitis C virus infection in patients undergoing allogeneic bone marrow transplantation. Transplantation 1991; 52: 315–8.

73 Shuhart MC, Myerson D, Childs BH et al. Marrow transplantation from hepatitis C virus seropositive donors: transmission rate and clinical course. Blood 1994; 84: 3229–35.

74 Shuhart MC, Myerson D, Spurgeon CL et al. Hepatitis C virus (HCV) infection in bone marrow transplant patients after transfusions from anti-HCV-positive blood donors. Bone Marrow Transplant 1996; 17: 601–6.

75 Bach N, Thung SN, Schaffner F. The histological features of chronic hepatitis C and autoimmune chronic hepatitis: a comparative analysis. Hepatology 1991; 15: 572–7.

76 Danque POV, Bach N, Shaffner F et al. HLA-DR expression in bile duct damage in hepatitis C. Mod Pathol 1993; 6: 327–32.

77 Demitris AJ, Batts KP, Dhillon AP et al. An international panel. Banff schema for grading liver allograft rejection: an international consensus document. Hepatology 1997; 25: 658–63.

78 Sviland L, Pearson ADJ, Green MA et al. Immunopathology of early graft-versus-host disease: a prospective study of skin, rectum, and peripheral blood in allogeneic and autologous bone marrow transplant recipients. Transplantation 1991; 52: 1029–36.

79 Ben-Ezra JM, Stroup RM. Phenotype of bile ducts and infiltrating lymphocytes in graft-versus-host disease. Transplantation 1993; 56: 162–5.

80 Synovec MS, Braddock SW, Jones J et al. LN-3: a diagnostic adjunct in cutaneous graft-versus-host disease. Mod Path 1990; 3: 643–7.

81 Takata M. Immunohistochemical identification of perforin positive cytotoxic lymphocytes in graft versus host disease. Am J Clin Pathol 1995; 103: 324–9.

82 Beschorner WE, Farmer ER, Saral R et al. Epithelial class II antigen expression in cutaneous graft-versus-host disease. Transplantation 1987; 44: 237–42.

83 Sviland L, Pearson ADJ, Eastham EJ et al. Class II antigen by keratinocytes and enterocytes: an early feature of graft-versus-host disease. Transplantation 1988; 46: 402–6.

84 Loughran TP, Sullivan KM, Morton T et al. Value of day 100 screening studies for predicting the development of chronic graft-versus-host disease after allogeneic bone marrow transplantation. Blood 1990; 76: 228–34.

85 Jacobson DA, Monross S, Anders V et al. Clinical importance of confirming or excluding the diagnosis of chronic graft-versus-host disease. Bone Marrow Transplant 2001; 28: 1047–51.

86 Akpek G, Zahurak ML, Piantadosi S et al. Development of a prognostic model for grading chronic graft-versus-host disease. Blood 2001; 97: 1219–26.

87 Shulman HM. Pathology of chronic graft-vs.-host disease. In: Burakoff SJ, Deeg HJ, Ferrara J, Atkinson K, eds. *Graft-Vs.-Host Disease: Immunology, Pathophysiology, and Treatment*. New York: Marcel Dekker, Inc., 1990: 587–614.

88 Wagner JL, Flowers MED, Longton G et al. Use of screening studies to predict survival among patients who do not have chronic graft-versus-host disease at day 100 after bone marrow transplantation. [Letter to the editor] *Biol Blood Marrow Transplant* 2001; **7**: 239–40.

89 Vogelsang GB. How I treat chronic graft-versus-host disease. *Blood* 2001; **97**: 1196–201.

90 Lee SJ, Vogelsang G, Gilman A et al. A survey of diagnosis, management, and grading of chronic GVHD. *Biol Blood Marrow Transplant* 2002; **8**: 32–9.

91 Rouah E, Gruber R, Shear W et al. GVHD in the central nervous system: a real entity? *Am J Clin Pathol* 1988; **4**: 543–6.

92 Janin-Mercier A, Socie G, Devergie A et al. Fasciitis in chronic graft-versus-host disease. *Ann Intern Med* 1994; **120**: 993–8.

93 Wingard JR, Piantadosi S, Vogelsang GB et al. Predictors of death from chronic graft-versus-host disease after bone marrow transplantation. *Blood* 1989; **74**: 1428–35.

94 Volc-Platzer B, Valent P, Radaszkiewicz T et al. Recombinant human interleukin 3 induces proliferation of inflammatory cells and keratinocytes *in vivo*. *Laboratory Invest* 1991; **64**: 557–66.

95 Zhang Y, McCormick LL, Desai SR et al. Murine sclerodermatous graft-versus-host disease, a model for human scleroderma: cutaneous cytokines, chemokines and immune cell activation. *J Immunol* 2002; **168**: 3088–98.

96 Sale GE, Shulman HM, Schubert MM et al. Oral and ophthalmic pathology of graft-versus-host disease in man: predictive value of the lip biopsy. *Hum Pathol* 1981; **12**: 1022–30.

97 Slavin MA, Meyers JD, Remington JS et al. *Toxoplasma gondii* infection in marrow transplant recipients: a 20-year experience. *Bone Marrow Transplant* 1994; **13**: 549–57.

98 VanBurik J-A, Hackman RC, Nadeem SQ et al. Nocardiosis after bone marrow transplantation. *Clin Infect Dis* 1997; **24**: 1154–60.

99 Harrington RD, Woolfrey AE, Bowden R et al. Legionellosis in a bone marrow transplant center. *Bone Marrow Transplant* 1996; **18**: 361–8.

100 Meyers JD, Flournoy N, Thomas ED. Nonbacterial pneumonia after allogeneic marrow transplantation. A review of 10-years' experience. *Rev Infect Dis* 1982; **4**: 1119–32.

101 Shields AF, Hackman RC, Fife KH et al. Adenovirus infections in patients undergoing bone marrow transplantation. *N Engl J Med* 1985; **312**: 529–33.

102 Ruutu P, Ruutu T, Volin L et al. Cytomegalovirus is frequently isolated in bronchoalveolar lavage fluid of bone marrow transplant recipients without pneumonia. *Ann Intern Med* 1990; **112**: 913–6.

103 Chakrabarti S, Mautner V, Osman H et al. Adenovirus infections following allogeneic stem cell transplantation: incidence and outcome in relation to graft manipulation, immunosuppression and immune recovery. *Blood* 2002; **100**: 1619–27.

104 Boeckh M, Leisenring W, Riddell SR et al. Late cytomegalovirus disease and mortality in allogeneic hematopoietic stem cell transplant recipients: importance of viral load and T cell immunity. *Blood* 2003; **101**: 407–14.

105 Cone RW, Hackman RC, Huang M-L et al. Human herpes virus 6 in lung tissue from bone marrow transplant patients with pneumonia. *N Engl J Med* 1993; **329**: 156–61.

106 Clark JG, Hansen JA, Hertz MI et al. Idiopathic pneumonia syndrome after bone marrow transplantation. NHLBI workshop summary. *Am Rev Resp Dis* 1993; **147**: 1601–6.

107 Kantrow SP, Hackman RC, Boeckh M et al. Idiopathic pneumonia syndrome. *Transplantation* 1997; **63**: 1079–86.

108 Wingard JR, Mellits ED, Jones RJ et al. Association of hepatic veno-occlusive disease with interstitial pneumonitis in bone marrow transplant recipients. *Bone Marrow Transplant* 1989; **4**: 685–9.

109 Appelbaum FR, Meyers JD, Fefer A et al. Nonbacterial nonfungal pneumonia following marrow transplantation in 100 identical twins. *Transplantation* 1982; **33**: 265–8.

110 Akasheh MS, Freytes CO, Vesole DH. Melphalan-associated pulmonary toxicity following high-dose therapy with autologous hematopoietic cell transplantation. *Bone Marrow Transplant* 2000; **26**: 1107–9.

111 Crawford SW, Longton G, Storb R. Acute graft-versus-host disease and the risks for idiopathic pneumonia after marrow transplantation for severe aplastic anemia. *Bone Marrow Transplant* 1993; **12**: 225–31.

112 Lehnert S, Rybka WB, Seemayer TA. Amplification of the graft-versus-host reaction by partial body irradiation. *Transplantation* 1986; **41**: 675–9.

113 Hackman RC, Madtes DK, Petersen FB et al. Pulmonary veno-occlusive disease following bone marrow transplantation. *Transplantation* 1989; **47**: 989–92.

114 Lombard CM, Churg A, Winokur S. Pulmonary veno-occlusive disease following therapy for malignant neoplasms. *Chest* 1987; **92**: 871–6.

115 Troussard X, Bernaudin JF, Cordonnier C et al. Pulmonary veno-occlusive disease after bone marrow transplantation. *Thorax* 1984; **39**: 956–7.

116 Beschorner WE, Saral R, Hutchins GM et al. Lymphocytic bronchitis associated with graft-versus-host disease in recipients of bone marrow transplants. *N Engl J Med* 1978; **299**: 1030–6.

117 O'Brien KD, Hackman RC, Sale GE et al. Lymphocytic bronchitis unrelated to acute graft-versus-host disease in canine marrow graft recipients. *Transplantation* 1984; **37**: 233–8.

118 Yousem SA. The histological spectrum of pulmonary graft-versus-host disease in bone marrow transplant recipients. *Hum Pathol* 1995; **26**: 668–75.

119 Freudenberger TD, Madtes DK, Curtis JR et al. Association between acute and chronic graft-versus-host disease and bronchiolitis obliterans organizing pneumonia in recipients of hematopoietic stem cell transplant. *Blood*, in press.

120 Madtes DK, Crawford SW. Lung injuries associated with graft-versus-host reactions. In: Ferrara JL, Deeg HJ, Burakoff SJ, eds. *Graft-Versus-Host Disease*. New York and Basel: Marcel Dekker, Inc., 1996: 425–46.

121 Urbanski SJ, Kossakowska AE, Curtis J et al. Idiopathic small airways pathology in patients with graft-versus-host disease following allogeneic bone marrow transplantation. *Am J Surg Pathol* 1987; **11**: 965–71.

122 Clark JG, Crawford SW. Diagnostic approaches to pulmonary complications of marrow transplantation. *Chest* 1987; **91**: 477–9.

123 Yousem SA, Burke CM, Billingham ME. Pathologic pulmonary alterations in long-term human heart–lung transplantation. *Hum Pathol* 1985; **16**: 911–23.

124 Tazelaar HD, Prop J, Nieuwenhuis P et al. Airway pathology in the transplanted rat lung. *Transplantation* 1988; **45**: 864–9.

125 Sullivan KM. Intravenous immune globulin prophylaxis in recipients of a marrow transplant. *J Allergy Clin Immunol* 1989; **84**: 632–9.

24

Megan Sykes

Mechanisms of Tolerance

Introduction

In allogeneic hematopoietic cell transplantation (HCT), persistent graft survival and the absence of graft-vs.-host disease (GVHD) depend on a state of mutual tolerance of the donor to the host (graft-vs.-host, or GVH tolerance) and of the host to the donor (host-vs.-graft [HVG] tolerance). Unfortunately, this state is not always achieved and failure of engraftment or GVHD ensues. Development of tolerance in the HVG direction requires host conditioning that either eliminates mature host immune cells, creating an immunological "clean slate" or that permits pre-existing T cells to be rendered tolerant by the donor hematopoietic cells. Since newly developing T and B lymphocytes have a unique capacity to be rendered tolerant by antigens they encounter during their maturation, especially on hematopoietic cells, these lymphocytes can be educated to recognize an engrafted donor and the host as "self", and a state of donor- and host-specific tolerance results. The ability of hematopoietic stem cells (HSC) to induce a state of donor-specific tolerance suggests an additional potential application for HCT, namely the induction of organ allograft acceptance without the need for chronic immunosuppressive therapy. Reliable, nontoxic methods of achieving allogeneic HSC engraftment across major histocompatibility complex (MHC) barriers will be required before this additional application of HCT becomes clinically feasible, and recent progress in experimental systems has brought this approach close to clinical application. However, a shortage of allogeneic donors has become a major limitation to solid organ transplantation, resulting in considerable interest in xenotransplantation (i.e. transplantation of organs from other species) among transplantation researchers. It has become increasingly clear that the immunologic barriers to xenografts are even stronger than those resisting allografts, making it unlikely that an acceptable amount of nonspecific immunosuppressive therapy could be used to prevent xenograft rejection. Thus, it will be especially critical to develop methods of inducing donor-specific tolerance across xenogeneic barriers in order to make xenotransplantation routinely practicable. Because of its demonstrated potency and because of recent developments in our understanding of the mechanisms by which HCT can induce allo- and xeno-tolerance, this approach may have the greatest potential to make tolerance induction a routine part of clinical organ transplantation. This chapter will first provide a general discussion of mechanisms of T-cell tolerance, and then discuss these mechanisms in the context of specific models associated with induction of HVG tolerance in the absence or presence of HCT. The mechanisms by which both mature T cells pre-existing in allogeneic HCT inocula, as well as T cells developing *de novo* from donor hematopoietic cells can be rendered tolerant of host antigens will also be reviewed.

Mechanisms of T-cell tolerance

Three major mechanisms have been proposed to explain induction and/or maintenance of T-cell tolerance to self-or alloantigens: clonal deletion, clonal anergy, and active suppression. For developing T cells, these processes take place in the thymus, which is the central organ for T-cell development. Hence, induction of tolerance among developing thymocytes is referred to as "central", as distinguished from the "peripheral" tolerance that may develop among already mature T cells when they encounter antigen in the peripheral tissues. It will become apparent to the reader, from the discussion that follows, that many of the same mechanisms have been implicated in models involving both central and peripheral tolerance induction.

Clonal deletion

T-cell receptors (TCR) consisting of uniquely rearranged α and β chains, known as αβTCR, are the cell surface heterodimers that recognize complexes of MHC antigens plus peptide. The thymus plays a critical role in the development of tolerance by a clonal deletion mechanism. Deletion occurs during T-cell maturation when the avidity of an interaction between an immature thymocyte and an antigen-presenting cell (APC) in the thymus is sufficiently high to induce apoptotic cell death [1,2]. The concept of avidity includes variations in the intensity of T-cell signaling resulting from variations in TCR and ligand density, and from interactions of accessory molecules with their ligands on APC. High avidity of the overall T-cell/APC interreaction is due, at least in part, to a relatively high affinity interaction between a rearranged αβTCR and a self-peptide/MHC complex presented by an APC in the thymus. Several marrow-derived cell types, including dendritic cells (DCs), B cells, and thymocytes, as well as nonhematopoietic cells of the thymic stroma (reviewed in [3,4]), have the capacity to induce intrathymic tolerance by both deletional and nondeletional mechanisms, but DCs may be the most potent deletional APC in the thymus [5].

Evidence for clonal deletion as a mechanism of tolerance was originally obtained by using monoclonal antibodies (MABs) that are specific for certain V gene products contributing to the β chain of the αβTCR [6]. Certain Vβ gene products are sufficient to selectively recognize particular antigens termed "superantigens" [7], almost independently of the composition of the remainder of the αβTCR heterodimer. These superantigens bind to a unique site on the class II molecule, which is quite distinct from the peptide binding groove where classical peptide antigens bind to MHC molecules. Thus, if a particular Vβ is capable of recognizing a superantigen, a measurable proportion of all possible T cells will be activated by that superantigen. A similar phenomenon occurs when T cells develop in the thymus. Some superantigens are encoded by endogenous retroviruses that have incorporated themselves into the genome of mammalian species, such as mice. T cells bearing TCR which include $V\beta$ regions recognizing these superantigens undergo deletion in a similar fashion to that of developing thymocytes that recognize a complex of self-peptide and MHC in the thymus. Thymocytes using particular $V\beta$ are deleted from the thymi of mice that express the relevant superantigens [6]. The presence of these $V\beta$ can serve as physical markers for the presence of T-cell clones that recognize the particular superantigens. These observations allowed the original demonstration to be made that self-tolerance occurs largely through an intrathymic deletional mechanism, and that tolerance to marrow donors also occurs through a similar mechanism when allogeneic bone marrow transplantation (BMT) is performed in mice [6]. However, recognition of peptide/MHC complexes is dependent on other components of the TCR besides $V\beta$. Data supporting clonal deletion as a major mechanism for induction of self-tolerance have also been obtained from studies of TCR transgenic mice expressing TCR specific for a "self" class I MHC-restricted peptide (H-Y plus D^b) or for a class I MHC antigen (L^d). These animals show marked intrathymic deletion of $CD8^+$ T cells bearing the self-reactive TCR, consistent with the existence of similar mechanisms for the deletion during normal development of T cells recognizing conventional transplantation antigens [8–10].

Deletion is not unique to immature stages of T-cell development. Peripheral deletion has been described for mature T cells upon exposure to antigen *in vivo* [11–13]. However, the circumstances and mechanisms that drive this peripheral deletion have not been fully delineated, and the role of activation-induced cell death (AICD), which appears to be a normal physiologic consequence of high levels of T-cell activation [14,15], further complicates the picture. As is discussed below, exposure to alloantigens in the presence of costimulatory blockade can lead to peripheral deletion of donor-reactive T cells. In addition, veto cells (see below) can delete alloreactive cytotoxic lymphocytes (CTL) precursors in the peripheral tissues.

T-cell anergy

Studies on mechanisms of tolerance often include functional data, such as limiting dilution analyzes to quantify CTL, helper T cells, or T cells proliferating in response to antigen. However, the failure to detect T cells with a particular allospecificity using this approach does not distinguish between clonal deletion and functional inactivation, or so-called "anergy". Anergy may result when T cells encounter antigens without receiving adequate accessory or costimulatory signals. Anergic lymphocytes cannot be fully activated by encounter with the antigen which its clonally distributed surface receptor (surface immunoglobulin [Ig] in the case of the B cell and TCR in the case of the T cell) specifically recognizes. Frequently (but not always [16]) in the case of T cells, anergy is associated with a lack of interleukin 2 (IL-2) production, and can be overcome by providing exogenous IL-2 [17]. T-cell anergy is associated with altered signaling and tyrosine phosphorylation patterns [18,19]. Numerous methods of inducing T-cell anergy *in vitro* have been described, many of which involve blocking of molecular interactions between T-cell surface molecules and their ligands on APC [18]. Some of these interactions are termed "costimulatory signals", because they provide signals to the responding T cell, other than those transmitted through the TCR/CD3 complex, that are essential to obtaining a full state of activation [20–22]. These molecules, including CD28, ICOS, and additional newly discovered costimulatory pathways, have been targets of attempts to induce tolerance by presenting allo- or xeno-antigens without adequate costimulation [23]. T-cell anergy has, in some instances, been associated with TCR down-regulation [13,24,25], and a similar phenomenon has been associated with B-cell anergy [26]. In addition to the encounter of antigen without costimulation, T cells may also be rendered anergic by an encounter with peptide ligands for which they have low affinity [1,2]. An overall low avidity interaction between a T cell and an APC may also result in anergy [27]. It appears that, in addition to mature peripheral T cells, thymocytes are also susceptible to anergy induction and that this can be induced by antigens presented on both hematopoietic and non-hematopoietic stromal [28–30] cells. Anergy can be reversed *in vivo*, and can be overcome by infection [31] or by removal of antigen [32–35].

Anergy can be induced *in vivo* by nonhematopoietic cells. In hematopoietic chimeras prepared with recipient myeloablation followed by allogeneic BMT, all marrow-derived cells are of donor origin, so that clonal deletion of T cells recognizing host-specific antigens is incomplete [28,36]. T cells bearing these host-reactive TCR can be anergized by thymic epithelial cells [37], or by antigens encountered extrathymically [38–40]. Studies have shown that T-cell clones with specificity for particular alloantigens can exist without causing destruction of tissue bearing those antigens [27,37,38,40]. In some instances, T cells with receptors specific for the *in vivo* tolerated antigen can be stimulated to respond to the antigen *in vitro* [37,38,41], or may even induce a state of inflammation that does not lead to organ destruction in the absence of additional stimuli [27]. In other systems, the T cells are fully or partially refractory to stimulation through their TCR, and this may be considered to be a true state of anergy [27,38,42].

However, anergy is not the only mechanism that can account for the failure of T cells with self-reactive or graft-donor reactive TCR to cause rejection *in vivo*. In the situation where T cells respond to antigens *in vitro* but not *in vivo*, they seem to be able simply to ignore antigens presented in the periphery [25,43]. This may be due to the presentation of these antigens by "nonprofessional APC" which are unable to activate T cells, or it may reflect a failure of recipient T cells to migrate to the antigen-bearing tissue. The level of peripheral antigen expression, how recently the responding T cell has emerged from the thymus [25,44], and the presence of proinflammatory cytokines [45,46] and up-regulated costimulatory molecules within peripheral tissues [47] may all influence the decision of a T cell to ignore or respond to peripheral antigens. T-cell activation may even occur within a tissue without initiating the whole cascade of organ damage [27]. However, proinflammatory stimuli, as may be present due to infection, may overcome such precarious states [25,46].

Some experimental models in which transplantation tolerance has been induced may include T-cell anergy among their mechanisms. However, in most of these models, including those involving costimulatory blockade and other approaches designed to render APC non-costimulatory, anergy has not been directly shown to be a mechanism of tolerance *in vivo*.

Suppression

A third mechanism, active suppression, has also been implicated in the induction and maintenance of self- and allo-tolerance. Suppressive activity has been attributed to both T cells and non-T cells, and may be antigen-specific or nonspecific. In general, the models in which suppressor T cells have been implicated involve exposure to antigen in the presence of a pre-existing immune response to the antigen. When, on the other hand, all mature lymphocytes are eliminated prior to administration of the antigen, tolerance may be due mainly to clonal deletion or anergy mechanisms and not to active suppression. In the ensuing discussion, we categorize mechanisms of suppression in terms of the degree of specificity of their ability to suppress immune responses.

Specific suppression

While functional evidence for the existence of specific suppressor cells had been obtained in several transplantation models [48–51], until recently there had been very few successes in cloning suppressive cells, or in identifying their cell surface phenotype or mechanisms by which they suppress. In some instances, anti-idiotypic recognition, which is the recognition of determinants specifically expressed by a rearranged T-cell or Ig receptor, has been implicated [48,51]. Class I MHC-restricted human T cells with specificity for the idiotype of alloreactive CD4$^+$ T cells have been cloned and are reported to suppress by noncytotoxic mechanisms [52]. However, the mechanisms of anti-idiotypic recognition and the mechanism of suppressive effector function have not been well characterized, and apparent idiotypic specificity can be difficult to distinguish from suppression by T cells with the same specificity as the T cell being suppressed, particularly if they are both of the same CD4 or CD8 subset.

It is tempting to speculate that some antigen-specific suppressive phenomena might be explained by the dichotomy of T-helper (TH)-cell function, in which fully differentiated CD4$^+$ TH cells polarize their cytokine secretion patterns to that of the T-helper type 1 (TH1) subset, which secretes IL-2 and interferon-gamma (IFN-γ), and the T-helper type 2 (TH2) subset which secretes IL-4 and IL-10 [53]. The TH1 subset induces antibody responses of some isotypes and the generation of cytolytic CD8$^+$ T cells, and the TH2 subset helps antibody responses of other isotypes but not cytotoxic T-cell responses [53]. A similar polarization of the pattern of cytokine secretion occurs in CD8$^+$ cytotoxic T cells (Tc), and the two corresponding subsets are termed Tc1 and Tc2 [54,55]. A shift to the IL-4- and IL-10-producing TH2 type of response from a proinflammatory TH1 (IL-2- and IFN-γ-producing) response has been associated with allograft acceptance [56]. Since TH1 and TH2 responses mutually down-regulate one another, these observations led to the hypothesis that TH2 responses are tolerogenic.

For practical purposes, an immune response that is itself nondestructive and inhibits the development of destructive responses could provide a powerful means of ensuring graft acceptance. However, most data merely demonstrate an association of TH2-dominant responses with graft acceptance, and only limited data exist to implicate an active role for TH2 cells in tolerance induction [57,58]. It is clear that TH2 responses are not always benign, as TH2 cells and TH2-associated cytokines can mediate or contribute to allograft rejection [59–61]. The TH1/TH2 dichotomy of cytokine production is not always clear-cut, and additional studies are needed to clarify better the conditions under which individual cytokines promote graft acceptance and rejection.

More recently, additional subsets of regulatory T cells have been characterized. Some of the *in vivo* data discussed later in the chapter are so compelling that it is difficult to deny the importance of regulatory phenomena in self-tolerance and regulation of autoimmunity, and in certain transplantation models. Some of these suppressive cell types are briefly described in the ensuing paragraphs.

A subset of murine and human CD4 cells induced by chronic antigenic stimulation in the presence of IL-10 has been reported to be capable of suppressing antigen-specific responses *in vitro*. They have also been found to be capable of suppressing an inflammatory bowel disease syndrome induced by naive CD4 cells in the mouse model. Since they produce high levels of IL-10 without making IL-4, while producing low amounts of IL-2, these cells cannot be classified as TH1 or TH2 and have been termed "T-regulatory cells 1" (Tr1) [62]. Immature DCs can support the *in vitro* development of IL-10-producing human CD4$^+$ regulatory T cells [63].

Human, mouse and rat CD4 T cells that constitutively expresses CD25 and CTLA4 have been shown to regulate the development of inflammatory colitis, a variety of autoimmune phenomena and *in vitro* allo-sponses [62,64,65]. The regulatory cells are themselves hyporesponsive to TCR-mediated stimulation but, like "Tr1", can be grown slowly *in vitro* in the presence of certain cytokines, including IL-2. The roles of IL-4, IL-10 and transforming growth factor beta (TGF-β) and of CTLA4 in suppression by these cells are controversial and the relationship, if any, with Tr1, is unclear. Suppression seems to require cell-to-cell contact [64]. CD25$^+$CD4$^+$Treg express the memory T-cell-associated CD45 isoform (CD45RC$^+$ in the rat, CD45RB^{low} in the mouse). Although CD4 cells have been the most well-studied targets of regulation by these cells, they can also suppress CD8 T-cell reactivity [66]. While the regulatory T cells show specificity for the antigen to which they are inducing suppression, the effector mechanism of suppression is non-antigen specific [64].

Treg are generated in the postnatal thymus [64,65], and a deficiency in their numbers in neonatally thymectomized mice permits the development of multiorgan autoimmune disease in susceptible strains [64]. CD4$^+$ regulatory cells mediate tolerance induced by allogeneic thymic epithelial grafts placed in nude mice [67]. Treg may require an intermediate affinity ligand (too low for negative selection) expressed on cortical epithelial cells of the thymus for their positive selection [64,68,69].

T/NK cells (T cells that express natural killer cell-associated markers and may utilize an invariant TCR α chain) are another subset of T cells with regulatory activity, which may be mediated in part by TH2-type cytokines. These cells have been reported to suppress autoimmune diseases, apparently by suppressing IFN-γ production via an IL-4-independent mechanism [70]. The role of these cells in various transplantation models is discussed below. A double negative, NK1.1$^-$ T-cell population that suppresses skin graft rejection by CD8 T cells with the same TCR has been described in a TCR transgenic mouse model [71], and the importance of this cell population in the setting of polyclonal T-cell responses remains to be determined. Suppressive human CD8$^+$CD28$^-$ T cells have also been described [72]. Thus, while a plethora of phenotypes and activities for regulatory T cells has been described in recent years, much remains to be learned about the relative importance of each of these, and the circumstances under which they can be optimally generated.

In some instances, the phenomena of anergy and suppression may be related. It has been hypothesized that anergic cells, by consuming cytokines or blocking helper T cells, could lead to the unavailability of lymphokines needed to costimulate naive responding T cells, resulting in anergy of these naive T cells [41]. In an *in vitro* model, anergic T cells have been found to be capable of suppressing T-cell responses, provided their ligands were presented on the same APC, consistent with the above hypothesis [73]. Alternatively, recognition of antigen on APC by anergic T cells could block activation of APC and their ability to produce signals needed to costimulate naive T cells, resulting in anergy of the naive T cells [74]. A phenomenon of this nature could explain the "infectious tolerance" that is observed in mice receiving minor antigen-disparate skin allografts under cover of nondepleting anti-T-cell MABs [75].

Suppressor cells have been implicated in the maintenance of self-tolerance by rodent studies involving lethal total body irradiation (TBI), reconstitution with T-cell-depleted syngeneic marrow, and treatment with cyclosporine (CSP) during the post-BMT period of T-cell recovery. Such animals develop an autoimmune syndrome resembling GVHD when CSP is withdrawn [51,76]. Both CD4$^+$ T cells and CD8$^+$ cells with reactivity to monomorphic determinants on class II MHC molecules have been implicated in the development of this syndrome. A mixture of CD4$^+$ and CD8$^+$ cells from normal animals can protect against syngeneic GVHD, suggesting that suppressor cells normally exist to protect against autoimmunity and that such suppressive cells fail to develop in the presence of CSP. These phenomena may by due to CSP-induced abnormalities of the thymic environment.

Veto cells

Alloresponses can be down-regulated by "veto" activity, which may be mediated by several different T-cell types. "Veto" cells inactivate CTL recognizing antigens expressed on the veto cell surface [77], resulting in a pattern of apparent suppression that inactivates CTL responding to antigens shared by the veto cells. Several types of cells have been reported to have veto activity, including CTL [77] and various bone marrow subpopulations, such as CD34+ cells [78] and their progeny [79], and marrow cells with characteristics of natural killer (NK) or lymphokine-activated killer (LAK) cells [80]. Veto cells have been suggested to induce GVH tolerance [81] and facilitate allogeneic marrow engraftment [81,82] in murine BMT models. Murine studies also suggest that veto cells might contribute to the donor-specific transfusion effect [83,84], wherein prior administration of donor blood induces subsequent hyporesponsiveness to that donor. One suggested mechanism for the veto effect involves triggering of a CTL through a surface class I MHC molecule while it is also activated through its TCR, which results in programmed cell death (apoptosis) of the responding CTL [85,86]. This class I-mediated signal could result from binding of a T-cell's class I molecules to CD8 molecules on the veto cell. However, not all veto cells express CD8, so this mechanism cannot explain all veto phenomena. Veto activity has been suggested to involve the immunosuppressive cytokine TGF-β [87].

Natural suppressor (NS) cells

Another type of suppressive activity is mediated by NS cells, which suppress in an antigen-nonspecific, non-MHC-restricted manner [88,89]. These cells have been detected in sites of active hematopoiesis [88–90] and in the setting of GVHD [88]. NS cells have been detected in normal bone marrow of several species [89,90], including humans [91]. These suppressive cells copurify with hematopoietic progenitors [92], but do not express the Sca-1 pluripotent HSC marker in mice [90]. They have been reported to suppress mitogen responses, antibody responses, and T-cell responses. NS cells were originally reported to lack surface markers of T cells, B cells, or macrophages, but subsets of T cells (T/NK cells) with nonspecific suppressive activity have been described [93,94]. Soluble factors with widely varying physical characteristics have been reported to mediate NS activity, including TGF-β [95]. Other soluble molecules, such as nitric oxide [96] and prostaglandins [97], which downmodulate immune function, may also play a role. In the absence of mechanisms for ensuring specific tolerance, nonspecific suppressive cells offer no advantage over other nonspecific immunosuppressive therapies. Facilitation of specific suppressor cell development by nonspecific, phenotypically "null" NS cells has been described [98].

Mechanisms of B-cell tolerance

The above discussion has focused mainly on the induction of T-cell tolerance. If T-cell tolerance is achieved, T-cell-dependent antibody responses do not occur. However, the induction of T-cell-independent B-cell tolerance is also of importance in some situations, especially those involving natural ABO blood group-mismatched transplantation, and xenotransplantation. Several mechanisms of B-cell tolerance have been described. Newly developing B cells are tolerized during development in the bone marrow by receptor editing or clonal deletion through receptor (surface Ig) cross-linking [99–101]. Anergy can occur upon recognition of autoantigen during B-cell development [26,102,103]. Soluble antigen expressed at low levels may tolerize immature B cells via anergy, whereas membrane-bound antigen may cause deletion [26]. In some cases anergy has been associated with surface Ig receptor down-regulation [26]. Mature follicular B cells undergo a nondeletional form of tolerance involving Ig receptor down-modulation in response to soluble self-antigen [26], but interaction with membrane-bound self-antigen can break tolerance [104]. The induction of B-cell anergy vs. activation may be dependent on antigen concentration [26]. Antigen expressed only on cell membranes in the periphery has, in some instances, been associated with deletion of B cells [26,99]. Less is known about B-1 cells, the major producers of IgM natural antibodies [105], but high-density membrane-bound antigens may lead to their deletion [106].

Approaches to inducing HVG transplantation tolerance

Clinical solid organ and islet transplantation is currently limited by three major factors: (i) the need for lifelong nonspecific immunosuppressive therapy, with its toxic side-effects; (ii) late graft loss, which is usually immunologically driven, and occurs despite the use of chronic immunosuppressive therapy; (iii) the grossly inadequate solid organ and islet supply. The first two limitations could be overcome by a state of transplantation tolerance, in which the donor would be regarded as "self", so that nonspecific immunosuppressive therapy would not be required. A solution to the third limitation would be the use of xenogeneic (i.e. from other species) organ and tissue sources, such as the pig. However, it is likely that a state of tolerance will be required to achieve successful clinical xenotransplantation, since the increased immunologic barriers to xenografts would otherwise necessitate excessively toxic amounts of nonspecific immunosuppressive therapy. Thus, induction of HVG tolerance has become a major goal of research in transplantation. We will discuss some experimental approaches to inducing tolerance and will divide the discussion into efforts to induce peripheral tolerance vs. those aimed at achieving HSC engraftment and central T-cell tolerance. However, it should become apparent by the end of the discussion that tolerance cannot always be readily characterized as peripheral vs. central, and that a combination of central and peripheral tolerance mechanisms may ultimately prove to be most practical and effective for the induction of HVG tolerance.

Approaches to peripheral tolerance induction

Tolerance of pre-existing, peripheral T cells has been induced in numerous animal models, generally by mechanisms that are not fully understood. Evidence for anergy has been obtained in a few models [107–109] and, recently, a role for regulatory cells has been found in many (see below). It is important to note that many of the strategies for inducing tolerance to primarily vascularized rodent allografts such as hearts and kidneys rely heavily on the capacity of the organ graft itself to induce tolerance, and that the tolerance thereby achieved is not systemic. Most of these tolerance protocols are not effective when tested with less "tolerogenic" grafts, such as primary skin allografts across full MHC barriers. Strategies that are effective for primarily vascularized allografts in rodents are often ineffective in large animals and humans. Thus, a thorough understanding of the mechanisms involved in tolerance induction and successful extension to large animal models are important criteria to fulfill before these approaches can be attempted in humans as a substitute for chronic immunosuppressive therapy. Some experimental approaches to tolerance induction are summarized below.

Donor-specific transfusion (DST), modified APCs, or administration of autologous cells transduced with allogeneic MHC genes

DST and donor antigen-transduced recipient cells can contribute to tolerance induction to cardiac allografts across certain histocompatibility barriers in rodents [110,111]. B cells and T cells in DST, both of which can present antigen in a noncostimulatory manner, may contribute to this effect [112,113]. Administration of autologous bone marrow transduced with a single donor MHC antigen appears to allow induction of tolerance to other antigens expressed by the cardiac or renal allograft donor in mice [111] and miniature swine models, respectively [114]. Several mechanisms of tolerance have been implicated in murine DST recipients, including veto activity [84], regulatory CD4 cells [115], and a role for

TH2 cytokines IL-4 [116] and IL-10 [115]. The extension of tolerance in these models from the antigens transduced into autologous cells to additional antigens expressed on the donor organ is a form of "linked suppression" (see below).

Depletion of "professional APC" from donor organs has long interested transplantation researchers as an approach to tolerance induction [20]. In this setting, graft parenchymal cells may present donor antigens in a manner that is noncostimulatory. However, grafts are eventually populated by recipient-derived APC, which can pick up donor antigens and present them to recipient T cells.

The introduction of alloantigen on tolerogenic APC, for example by treating APC with ultraviolet irradiation [117], can contribute to T-cell unresponsiveness to donor grafts. Stimulation with immature DCs, or with DCs modified in certain ways, can lead to the development of regulatory T cells (reviewed in [118]). Attempts to intentionally immunize with "tolerogenic" DCs have been associated with prolonged survival of heart, islet and kidney allograft survival in rodent models, usually without permanent survival [118]. Strategies included the administration of immature DCs lacking costimulatory molecule expression, DCs genetically engineered to inhibit NFκB activity, viral IL-10 and TGF-β-transfected DCs, CTLA4Ig-transfected DCs, and administration of $CD8^+$ "lymphoid" DCs. While success with these approaches has thus far been limited, future studies may lead to further improvements.

Costimulatory blockade, with or without infusion of donor lymphocytes

Efforts to induce tolerance by blocking the B7/CD28 costimulatory pathway have enjoyed success in animals receiving vascularized allografts [119] under cover of CTLA4Ig, a fusion protein containing the B7-binding portion of CTLA4, one of the T-cell ligands of B7. CTLA4Ig blocks CD28 binding to both B7 molecules, B7-1 and B7-2, and this blockade, combined with the tolerogenic capacity of primarily vascularized organ allografts in rodents, can lead to long-term graft acceptance.

Signaling through the interaction of CD40 on APC and B cells with its T-cell ligand (CD40L, CD154, which is expressed transiently on activated $CD4^+$ cells) plays an important role in activating APC so that they can optimally costimulate T cells. Signaling through CD40 leads to up-regulation of B7 expression, as well as other costimulatory molecules, class II MHC, and cytokines such as IL-12, and induces Ig class switching by B cells. This APC activation via CD40 is a major facet of CD4 T-cell-mediated "help" for CTL generation [120]. Administration of DST under cover of blocking anti-CD40L MAB leads to prevention of islet allograft rejection [121]. In thymectomized mice, the combination of DST and anti-CD40L leads to long-term skin graft survival in fully MHC-mismatched recipients, but this approach is less successful in euthymic mice [122]. DST in this model leads to deletion of donor-reactive CD8 T cells [123], and a $CD4^+$ regulatory cell population has been implicated [124]. Xenogeneic skin graft prolongation is also observed with DST and anti-CD40L [125]. Cardiac allograft survival is markedly prolonged in the presence of anti-CD40L [126] but chronic graft arteriosclerosis can still take place in the presence of such treatment [127]. Graft prolongation with anti-CD40L or CD28 blockade has been associated with a TH2-dominant immune response [128], which may play a role in the development of graft arteriosclerosis [127].

The combination of CTLA4Ig and anti-CD40L antibody can markedly prolong the survival of primary skin allografts [129], renal allografts in large animals [130] and xenografts [131], but without inducing tolerance. Functional tolerance has been achieved with this combination only in rodent models of cardiac or islet allografts [132] or islet xenografts [133], but not in the more stringent models of primary skin grafting or large animal vascularized organ or islet allografts [134–136]. Costimulatory blockade more effectively suppresses CD4-mediated than CD8 cell-mediated alloreactivity [134,137], and the extent of CD8 cell-mediated resistance is genetically determined [138]. A short course of rapamycin with anti-CD40L and CTLA4Ig, has, quite remarkably, permitted long-term acceptance of primary skin allografts across full MHC barriers in mice in certain strain combinations [139]. However, none of these approaches has been shown to lead to systemic tolerance.

The mechanisms of hyporesponsiveness induced by organ transplantation with costimulatory blockade are only partly understood. Calcineurin inhibitors such as CSP and FK506 can block graft prolongation induced by costimulatory blockade [129], apparently by preventing IL-2-induced priming for AICD [139]. Consistently, IL-2 has been shown to play an essential role in the induction of tolerance with CTLA4Ig and cardiac allografts [140]. However, Fas and tumor necrosis factor alpha (TNF-α) receptors do not appear to be required for tolerance induction with this method [141,142].

Despite the observation that TH1-associated cytokines are associated with graft rejection, IFN-γ plays a critical role in graft prolongation induced with combined CD40/CD28 costimulatory blockade [140], DST with CD28 blockade [143] and DST with CD40 blockade [124]. IFN-γ has several known mechanisms for down-modulating T-cell responses, but the relevant mechanisms in the costimulatory blockade models are unclear.

Linked suppression and "infectious tolerance" (see below) have been demonstrated in several models involving costimulatory blockade [144–146]. Tolerance is not achieved in euthymic mice [144] in the most difficult models (e.g. primary, fully MHC-mismatched skin allografts in "difficult" strain combinations).

The greater success in achieving acceptance of primarily vascularized allografts in rodents using a short course of costimulatory blockade or any of a number of different immunosuppressive agents suggests that these types of grafts are highly tolerogenic. As noted above, comparable results usually have not been achieved in large animal models of organ grafting, making the clinical applicability of these approaches difficult to test. This disparity between results in large and small animals may, in part, reflect the constitutive class II antigen expression on vascular endothelial cells of large animals and humans [147], but not of rodents [147,148]. Consistent with this interpretation, the use of a short course of CSP can facilitate the ability of renal allografts to induce tolerance in rodents [149] across full MHC barriers, but tolerance induction in swine requires class II matching between donor and recipient for uniform success [150]. Pigs accepting such allografts became systemically tolerant to the donor's class I and minor antigens [151].

Antibodies to T cells and adhesion molecules

Nondepleting anti-T-cell MABs, with or without T-cell-depleting MABs, have been used to induce skin graft tolerance across minor or certain MHC barriers, and this has led to "infectious tolerance", in which $CD4^+$ T cells, rendered incapable of rejecting the allograft in the original recipients, can render naive T cells unresponsive in secondary recipients [75]. These tolerant T cells can, in turn, tolerize naive T cells in tertiary recipients. $CD4^+$ regulatory cells and TH2 cytokines have been implicated in the tolerance induced in this model [75].

Tolerance has also been induced in transplantation models by the administration of MABs that block adhesion molecules (reviewed in [152]). Molecular targets include the integrin adhesion molecule LFA-1 and its endothelial cell ligand ICAM-1. Murine cardiac allograft acceptance with such blockade has been attributed to insufficient T-cell help leading to anergy of CD8 cells [153], and has also been attributed to TH2 cytokines [154]. However, less success has been achieved with primary skin allografts [155]. The LFA-1/ICAM interaction appears to have costimulatory in addition to adhesive activity [156], making the mechanisms involved in this model potentially complex. Blockade of VLA-4/VCAM-1 interaction, alone or in combination with LFA-1/ICAM blockade, has also been reported to lead to cardiac allograft prolongation or long-term acceptance [157].

Other MABs that have been used in rodent heart graft models include combinations of anti-CD2 and anti-CD3 MABs [158], anti-CD2 alone [159], and anti-CD2 plus anti-CD28 [160]. Various mechanisms, including T$_H$2 deviation, have been implicated. Anti-CD45RB antibodies, especially in combination with anti-CD40L, lead to skin graft prolongation and tolerance to islet allografts [161]. T$_H$2 cytokine deviation and regulatory cells have been suggested as possible mechanisms [161].

Total lymphoid irradiation (TLI)

TLI has also been evaluated as immunosuppression for organ transplantation, and has been successful in about one-third of baboons [162]. In clinical transplantation, TLI has been reported to be beneficial, although it is cumbersome and toxic, especially in the case of cadaver-donor transplantation [162–164]. Donor-specific tolerance has been demonstrated in a small number of patients in whom immunosuppressive therapy was terminated following kidney transplantation under cover of TLI [165]. One of these patients was studied 12 years after immunosuppression withdrawal, and shown to have an active antidonor mixed lymphocyte reaction (MLR) and no evidence for microchimerism [165]. TLI used in conjunction with antithymocyte globulin (ATG) has been shown to induce tolerance to organs in several large animal models [166,167].

The relationship between peripheral T-cell tolerance and central tolerance

The distinction between central and peripheral tolerance may not always be clear. For example, passenger leukocytes might emigrate from the graft to the host thymus and tolerize subsequently developing thymocytes. In addition, the thymus may be capable of tolerizing T cells that were already in the periphery at the time of organ grafting. In a pig model in which class I MHC-mismatched kidneys are accepted under cover of a short course of CSP [151], the thymus appears to play a role in the induction of tolerance among pre-existing peripheral T cells [168]. It is possible that: (i) T cells that are activated in the periphery by the organ allograft recirculate to the thymus as has been described [169], and encounter donor antigen there, perhaps on passenger leukocytes, which then inactivate the T cells. This process could be a mechanism for ensuring that T cells activated in the periphery are switched off if the same antigens are present on intrathymic leukocytes; (ii) The migration of donor antigens to the thymus may result in the development of T cells that specifically recognize the donor antigens and down-regulate the activity of destructive alloreactive T cells [170] when they enter the periphery. The role of the thymus in the development of Treg has already been discussed above; (iii) Recent thymic emigrants that encounter antigen in the periphery differentiate into suppressive rather than rejecting T cells.

A second situation in which the boundary between central and peripheral tolerance is blurred arises when donor antigens are injected intrathymically to induce tolerance. The initial idea underlying this approach was to use antibody treatment to deplete peripheral T cells and to induce central tolerance among recovering T cells by direct introduction of antigen into the thymus. However, more recent studies have shown that tolerance to soluble alloantigens can be induced by intrathymic injection without peripheral T-cell depletion (TCD) [171]. Since removal of the thymus before or within the first few days of allografting results in rejection of the allograft [172], the thymus must play an active role in tolerizing pre-existing peripheral T cells, possibly by one of the mechanisms proposed in the preceding paragraph. Recent evidence suggests that donor-reactive T cells must recirculate to the recipient thymus to induce tolerance in this model [173]. Active regulatory cell populations have been reported in rats receiving intrathymic injections of allogeneic marrow cells [174].

The role that the allograft may play in inducing tolerance in animals receiving intrathymic injection, and in other models in which a pre-existing peripheral T-cell repertoire must be rendered tolerant should not be ignored. Transferable tolerance is not induced by intrathymic marrow injection alone without an organ allograft in rats [174], suggesting that the graft itself helps to render the pre-existing T-cell repertoire tolerant, perhaps by presenting antigen without adequate costimulation or by inducing regulatory cell populations. In contrast to models involving intrathymic injection (or short-term immunosuppressive treatments) and immediate solid organ transplantation, pure intrathymic deletional tolerance induced by mixed allogeneic chimerism (discussed below) is not dependent on the continued presence of an organ allograft [109,175]. In fact, this tolerance does not depend on the continual presence of any donor antigen in the periphery, as long as there is a continuous supply of donor antigen in the thymus [176].

Achieving HVG tolerance with HCT

Resistance to engraftment of HSCs

Two major factors influence the engraftment of HSCs. The first is sometimes referred to as "space" in the hematopoietic system. The mechanism by which myelosuppressive host treatment promotes marrow engraftment is not fully understood, and could include both the creation of physical niches due to the destruction of host HSCs and the up-regulation of cytokines and other molecules that transmit signals to promote hematopoiesis. It is probably the species specificity of some of these interactions that accounts for the competitive advantage enjoyed by recipient marrow over xenogeneic marrow, and which becomes increasingly evident as recovery of the host from low-dose TBI occurs [177]. An understanding of these physiologic barriers is likely to be critical to the success of the approach of using xenogeneic HCT to induce xenotolerance. Once these are understood, genetically modified donors of other species, such as pigs, could be engineered such that their HSCs would be better able to compete for hematopoietic function in a human marrow microenvironment.

In syngeneic BMT recipients, a low dose of TBI is required to make physiologic "space" for engraftment of marrow cells given in numbers similar to those which could be obtained from marrow of living human allogeneic marrow donors [178]. However, this requirement can be overcome by the administration of very high doses of marrow [179,180]. Furthermore, engraftment of high doses of allogeneic marrow can be achieved without myelosuppressive treatment in mice that receive T-cell-depleting [181] or costimulatory blocking [182] MABs.

The second factor limiting alloengraftment is the host immune system. Because of this immune resistance, allogeneic HCT can be performed successfully only in immunosuppressed recipients. The role of T cells in resisting engraftment of allogeneic HSC is discussed elsewhere in this book (see Chapter 3). Not surprisingly, T cells of the CD4 and CD8 subsets resist engraftment of class II and class I-mismatched marrow grafts, respectively. It is also noteworthy that CD4 cells weakly resist engraftment of class I-disparate marrow and that CD8 cells quite markedly resist class II-disparate marrow grafts in mice [183–185].

Apparent exceptions to the requirement to create "space" (or give high hematopoietic cell doses) in the recipient and to overcome immune resistance have been observed in the case of intraportal infusion in rodents of allogeneic BMC [186] or cells with properties of embryonic stem cells [187]. The mechanisms underlying these surprising results have not been delineated. However, subsequent studies in the infra portal BMT model indicated that the reliable induction of tolerance required the addition of a substantial dose (7 Gy) of TBI [188].

NK cells, which may kill target cells due to the absence of self-MHC molecules on allogeneic marrow cells [189], resist allogeneic marrow engraftment in mice [190] and are responsible for the ability of AxB F1 recipients to resist engraftment of AA or BB parental marrow [190]. NK cells of both humans and mice express clonally distributed surface receptors that recognize specific class I molecules. This recognition transmits an inhibitory signal to the NK cell, thereby preventing the NK cell from killing "self" class I-bearing targets [189]. While the ability of NK cells to resist engraftment of allogeneic pluripotent HSCs in mice is rather limited [191,192], NK cells might pose a more significant barrier to human leukocyte antigen (HLA)-mismatched human marrow engraftment, in which stem cell and progenitor cell numbers in the donor inoculum may be more limited. A clear role for NK cells in resisting alloengraftment has not been established for large animals or humans. In a nonhuman primate model of simultaneous kidney and marrow transplantation, however, depletion of recipient NK cells by preconditioning correlated with the achievement of chimerism and tolerance [193]. Furthermore, GVH-reactive NK cells have been reported to promote donor engraftment in mice and to mediate graft-vs.-leukemia effect (GVLE) against myeloid leukemias in humans [194], and it has been suggested that the presence or absence of NK cells in patients with severe combined immunodeficiency determines whether or not cytotoxic host conditioning is needed in order to achieve engraftment of haploidentical HCT [195].

The question of whether or not NK cells are tolerized by the induction of mixed chimerism is relevant to the long-term stability of the chimerism. Such tolerance might require that each individual NK cell expresses inhibitory receptors for two completely disparate sets of MHC molecules on donor and host cells. However, the observed changes in the expression of inhibitory (Ly-49) receptors among donor and host NK cells of mixed chimeras are not consistent with such a mechanism, and suggest that inhibitory Ly-49 receptors are simply down-modulated by interactions with their ligand [196–198]. Discrepancies between *in vitro* cytolytic assays [197] and *in vivo* studies providing clear evidence of NK cell tolerance have been noted in mixed hematopoietic chimeras [199] and other models [200,201].

Humoral mechanisms can also mediate resistance to marrow engraftment. Antibodies that inhibit engraftment can exist without prior immunization (so-called "natural antibodies" [NAB]). For example, NAB that recognize ABO blood group determinants [202,203] or xenoantigens and that exist in normal human sera [204,205] can resist the engraftment of hematopoietic cells that express the determinants recognized by the NAB. Antibodies against donors can also develop as a result of presensitization, usually from blood products. Animal studies suggest that the effect of NAB on engraftment can be overcome by administration of sufficiently high marrow doses [205–209], and in humans, consequences of ABO-incompatible BMT can usually be avoided with adequate red blood cell (RBC) depletion from the marrow product. Occasionally, plasmapheresis may be needed to remove such antibodies if they are present at particularly high titre. The presence of antibodies resulting from presensitization to donor antigens, on the other hand, is associated with a high incidence of marrow graft failure in humans [210].

A permissive environment for engraftment of allogeneic marrow can exist under several physiologic and artificially induced conditions, as outlined below. The mechanisms by which HCT induces tolerance in each of these models is discussed.

HCT to developmentally or congenitally immunodeficient recipients

HCT is widely used, with considerable success, for the treatment of severe combined immunodeficiency syndrome (SCID) (Chapter 105). Although it is not necessary to treat these recipients to create hematopoietic "space" to achieve engraftment, BMT in this setting often leads to the development of "split chimerism", in which mainly lymphocytes, but not other lineages, are reconstituted by the donor. A similar phenomenon has been observed in unconditioned SCID mice [211], indicating that hematopoietic "space" must be induced if multilineage donor reconstitution is desired. In addition to these congenitally immunodeficient recipients, hematopoietic engraftment has been achieved without conditioning in developmentally immunoincompetent recipients. This was first observed in Freemartin cattle (fraternal twins sharing a placental circulation) by Ray Owen [212]. The ability to intentionally induce immunologic tolerance to alloantigens was first demonstrated in mice that received *in utero* injections of allogeneic HSCs [213]. Since prenatal diagnosis of a number of congenital diseases has become possible, the injection of allogeneic or xenogeneic HSC to preimmune fetuses has generated renewed interest for its potential clinical applicability (Chapters 44 and 105), and some successes have been achieved [214]. However, chimerism was only detected in the lymphocyte compartment afflicted by the congenital deficiency, not in other hematopoietic lineages. In view of this result and the observation of only low levels of chimerism in preimmune nondeficient mice and sheep receiving *in utero* transplants [215], the concept that hematopoietic "space" is present in preimmune fetuses is open to question. Since the ability of *in utero* HCT to induce tolerance is somewhat unpredictable [215,216], the potential of this approach to induce tolerance for subsequent parental organ allografts in, for example, fetuses diagnosed with congenital renal or hepatic disorders, is unknown.

The importance of antigen on marrow-derived cells for the induction of tolerance among newly developing T cells in humans is illustrated by studies in SCID patients receiving HLA-mismatched BMT, and in whom donor T cell, but not B cell or myeloid engraftment, develops initially. Newly developing donor T cells from these patients exhibit reactivity toward donor class II MHC antigens. This reactivity disappears if engraftment of donor class II-bearing cells later occurs [217].

In animals rendered tolerant by injection of alloantigens shortly after birth, several mechanisms have been invoked to explain the observed HVG tolerance. Lasting microchimerism has been detected in some studies, and some findings suggest that lymphohematopoietic chimerism is essential for the maintenance of tolerance [48,218]. Evidence to support an intrathymic deletional mechanism has been obtained in some, but not other, strain combinations [219,220]. Additionally, the presence of microchimerism does not always predict skin graft tolerance in recipients of allogeneic lymphocytes perinatally and nontolerant animals can still maintain microchimerism following rejection of donor skin grafts [221,222]. Thus, it is not surprising that several additional mechanisms have been implicated in rodents in which neonatal tolerance has been induced. These include:

1 Specific suppressor T cells [219]. Tolerance cannot be easily broken by the infusion of nontolerant host-type lymphocytes in animals rendered tolerant at birth [48,218,219] and this has been attributed to the presence of suppressive T-cell populations [48]. Specific suppressor T cells (reviewed in [48,219]) have been detected. One prerequisite for the development of suppressive activity may be that alloreactivity be present. This condition may prevail in neonatally tolerized animals, since a small number of mature T cells already exist in the periphery at the time of birth. The observed difficulty in breaking tolerance by infusion of nontolerant host-type lymphocytes to neonatally tolerized mice [48,218,223–225] suggests that a potent suppressive mechanism may indeed be present in such mice. In contrast to these results, when "pure" deletional tolerance is induced in animals in which the pre-existing peripheral T-cell response has been fully ablated, the absence of suppressive cell populations makes it easy to abolish tolerance by the infusion of nontolerant host-type lymphocytes [176,226];

2 Neonatal mice have a tendency to produce TH2 responses, which have

been implicated in donor-specific skin graft acceptance [57,227]. However, neonatal mice are clearly capable of generating T$_H$1 responses under certain conditions [228,229];
3 The ability of allogeneic spleen cell infusions to induce tolerance may reflect the high ratio of noncostimulatory APCs (resting T and B cells) in donor inocula to recipient T cells in the neonate, rather than any particular susceptibility to tolerance induction at this time of life [230].

HCT in adult recipients following myeloablative conditioning

Marrow chimerism and tolerance can be achieved in otherwise normal, adult animals if immunodeficiency and "space" are artificially created by lethal TBI. Hematopoietic rescue is achieved with allogeneic BMT. In murine recipients of T-cell-depleted allogeneic BMT, lymphoid repopulation is largely (95–99%) allogeneic: a small population of host cells (mainly T cells) survives permanently in such animals [231]. If T-cell-depleted allogeneic and T-cell-depleted syngeneic marrow are coadministered, mixed allogeneic chimerism ensues; i.e. lymphohematopoietic cells of both donor and recipient type coexist permanently in the survivors [232]. These mixed chimeras show no evidence of GVHD and show specific tolerance, both *in vivo* and *in vitro*, to donor antigens [232,233]. Animals reconstituted with T-cell-depleted allogeneic marrow alone demonstrate a similar pattern of specific unresponsiveness but tend to show poorer immunocompetence both *in vivo* and *in vitro*, possibly due to a mismatch between the MHC restriction imposed by the host thymus and the MHC of donor-type APCs in full chimeras across complete MHC barriers (reviewed in [234]). However, the clinical significance of experimental results showing this incompatibility is questionable, since MHC-mismatched and, even xenogeneic, thymic transplantation can restore excellent immune function in humans and mice, respectively [235,236].

Another early approach to achieving mixed hematopoietic chimerism and donor-specific tolerance involved the use of TLI plus BMT. This approach has been very successful in rodents (reviewed in [237]). The long bones are shielded during the radiation preparative regimen, so BMT results in mixed chimerism rather than full donor reconstitution. Large numbers of allogeneic T-cell-containing marrow cells are usually required to achieve engraftment [237], possibly because some host T cells survive irradiation due to shielding of bones. Mice treated in this way have been shown to be both resistant to GVHD and tolerant to donor skin grafts. The success of this approach varies depending on the species involved. In rodent models, T$_H$2-type responses predominate following TLI, and this T$_H$1 to T$_H$2 shift may play a role in permitting graft acceptance [238,239]. This cytokine shift may be facilitated by the predominance of NK/T cells (previously referred to as NS cells) detected in the lymphoid tissues of TLI-treated mice [240].

While organ allograft tolerance has sometimes been achieved, TLI as the sole conditioning modality for BMT has only variably permitted the induction of mixed chimerism and tolerance in large animals, and this has often been associated with considerable toxicity [241–243]. A trial of donor BMT with fractionated TLI in high-risk patients receiving renal allografts was not associated with chimerism, and significant toxicity was also observed [163]. A recent trial of allogeneic HCT in patients conditioned with TLI and ATG has demonstrated transient chimerism induction, but it is too early to assess long-term tolerance [244].

Another potential advantage of mixed chimerism over allogeneic chimerism is that hematopoietic cells are most efficient at inducing clonal deletion of T cells in the thymus [6]; thus, a continuous source of host-type hematopoietic cells provides additional assurance that host-reactive T-cell clones will not emerge from the thymus [109], as can occur in animals reconstituted with T-cell-depleted allogeneic marrow alone [28].

Clonal deletion appears to be the predominant mechanism of HVG tolerance in lethal TBI-treated recipients of T-cell-depleted allogeneic BMT. Using $V\beta$-specific MABs, evidence for clonal deletion has been obtained by several groups [6,28]. *In vivo* evidence suggests that suppressor cells are not involved in the maintenance of tolerance to donor antigens, regardless of whether T-cell-depleted allogeneic marrow cells are given alone or with T-cell-depleted syngeneic cells. Tolerance can be readily broken in such chimeras by administering a relatively small number of nontolerant recipient-type spleen cells [226], indicating the absence of any potent suppressive activity. Results of *in vitro* coculture studies supported this conclusion [245]. As discussed earlier, one important difference between TBI/BMT recipients and neonatally tolerized animals is that TBI leads to elimination of most pre-existing T cells. Thus, the number of host alloreactive T cells may be too small to provide an adequate stimulus for the expansion of suppressive T-cell populations.

In contrast to chimeras reconstituted with unmanipulated allogeneic marrow, animals receiving non-T-cell-depleted allogeneic cells are highly resistant to the breaking of tolerance by administration of nontolerant host-type lymphocytes [226]. The resistance to breaking of tolerance conferred by T cells in the original reconstituting allogeneic marrow inoculum was shown, by genetic analyzes, to be dependent upon the GVH reactivity of those T cells [226]. The simplest interpretation of this finding is that GVH-reactive T cells persist long-term in these chimeras and eliminate administered nontolerant host-type lymphocytes before they can "take" and eliminate donor cells.

Studies in animal models have addressed the possibility that, following lethal irradiation and reconstitution with exhaustively T-cell-depleted autologous marrow, tolerance might be induced by expression of antigen on nonhematopoietic organs grafted simultaneously with the T-cell-depleted autologous marrow. This approach met with some limited success [246], but was insufficient to induce tolerance to MHC mismatched skin allografts in rodents or to MHC-mismatched vascularized grafts in large animal studies [247,248]. Similarly, *in vivo* treatment with depleting anti-T-cell MABs does not permit induction of skin allograft tolerance across MHC barriers in mice [41]. Thus, alloantigen seems to be required within the lymphohematopoietic system for the most complete tolerization of newly developing T cells, probably reflecting the unique ability of alloantigen expressed on marrow-derived cells to induce clonal deletion in the thymus. In murine radiation chimeras in which the host is thymectomized prior to transplantation of an allogeneic thymus, allogeneic marrow cells, and allogeneic lymphocytes, tolerance toward host antigens is not observed *in vitro* [249]. These results also suggest that extrathymic nonhematopoietic cells are incapable of fully tolerizing T cells. In transgenic mice, on the other hand, T cells may demonstrate anergy towards antigens which are only detectable on peripheral nonhematopoietic organs [25]. As is discussed later in this chapter, it seems likely that the inflammation in parenchymal tissues that is induced by conditioning such as TBI overrides the ability to tolerize T cells seeing antigens only in those locations.

An alternative to the induction of mixed chimerism in lethally irradiated recipients has been to reinfuse autologous marrow that is genetically modified to express an allogeneic MHC gene. The induction of donor-specific hyporesponsiveness achieved with this approach in a class I-mismatched mouse model [250] and with class II gene transduction in a pig model [114] is promising. While it would be technically cumbersome to modify each individual transplant recipient's marrow with all of the MHC genes of any given cadaveric organ donor, data in the porcine model suggest that the tolerance-inducing capacity of the organ graft itself can induce spreading to other graft antigens of the tolerance that is induced by a single donor class II gene introduced into the recipient marrow [114].

The discussion so far would suggest that induction of mixed chimerism may be the most straightforward way of ensuring donor- and host-specific tolerance across MHC barriers. However, the original methods for producing mixed allogeneic chimeras in mice were not directly applicable to humans, because of the toxicity of lethal TBI, the lack of success and toxicity of high-dose TLI in large animals and humans (see above) and the high risk of GVHD [251] and graft failure [210] encountered when BMT is attempted across MHC barriers in humans. BMT following lethal TBI or high-dose TLI would not be justifiable as a means of inducing tolerance for the purpose of organ transplantation, for which less toxic chronic immunosuppressive therapy is available.

Therefore, if BMT is to be used as a means of inducing donor-specific organ allograft or xenograft tolerance, it will be essential to develop methods of rendering recipients permissive for engraftment which are less toxic and more reliably effective than those which are currently available. Conditioning regimens are needed which specifically eliminate the host elements that resist alloengraftment without producing generalized toxic effects. Some newer approaches to achieving this goal are discussed later in this chapter. Another approach would involve the identification of donor cell subpopulations distinct from GVHD-producing T cells which could improve alloengraftment. The existence of such cell types has been suggested by several murine studies [231,252–256].

HCT in adult recipients following conditioning with immunosuppressive but nonmyeloablative protocols

Recently, several HCT protocols have been developed that involve myelotoxic and/or immunosuppressive but not myeloablative, conditioning regimens. Since host HSCs survive, mixed chimerism develops when allogeneic marrow is administered. Such regimens include TLI [237], sublethal TBI [257], administration of cyclophosphamide following sensitization with allogeneic donor antigens [258], and the use of MABs against host T cells in combination with other modalities [259]. HCT has also been performed in unconditioned patients receiving organ transplantation under conventional immunosuppressive drug therapy. Low levels of chimerism have been achieved but immunosuppressive therapy withdrawal has not been made possible with this approach [260,261]. However, the incidence of chronic rejection may be decreased in this setting [261]. A brief description of some nonmyeloablative conditioning approaches follows.

Sublethal TBI

Induction of mixed chimerism using fractionated sublethal TBI and allogeneic BMT has recently been shown to be associated with donor-specific tolerance across complete MHC barriers in mice [257]. Donor T cells which need not have alloreactivity against the recipient promote alloengraftment in this model and donor T cells have been shown to maintain tolerance [257]. In dogs, a low dose of TBI, in combination with post-transplant CSP and mycophenolate mofetil, has been associated with mixed chimerism and tolerance across minor, but not major, histocompatibility barriers [262].

Cyclophosphamide (CY)

High doses of CY administered several days following inoculation with large numbers of allogeneic marrow and/or spleen cells induce microchimerism and donor-specific tolerance across multiple minor histoincompatibilities and selected MHC disparities [258]. Additional host treatment with a monoclonal anti-T-cell antibody [259], with sublethal TBI [263] or with fludarabine and low-dose TBI [264] permits the induction of tolerance across complete MHC barriers. Sensitization followed by administration of CY causes selective destruction of host T cells driven into cell cycle in response to alloantigen, so that pre-existing donor-reactive T-cell clones are eliminated [259] and newly developing T cells can mature in the presence of donor marrow-derived antigen in the thymus. While thymic and peripheral chimerism can be demonstrated in animals receiving the regimen involving CY alone, the levels of such chimerism are extremely low, reflecting the fact that CY is relatively ineffective at producing marrow "space". In the model involving tolerance across minor histocompatibility barriers, evidence was obtained for intrathymic clonal deletion of T-cells bearing TCR that recognize donor superantigens [258]. Deletion of peripheral $V\beta_6$-bearing CD4$^+$ cells was also demonstrated early after BMT [258]. In a MHC mismatched strain combination, chimerism was shown to disappear with time and clonal deletion was replaced by anergy as a mechanism of tolerance (reviewed in [265]).

Pre-HCT CY has been used in a nonmyeloablative regimen with T-cell depleting antibodies and thymic irradiation in patients to achieve mixed chimerism in HLA-identical and haploidentical combinations [266,267], and organ transplantation tolerance has been achieved with this approach (see below).

Other pharmacologic agents

Recently, combinations of chemotherapeutic agents have been used as nonmyeloablative conditioning in patients with hematologic malignancies who were considered to be at high risk from complications of conventional myeloablative conditioning. High levels of donor reconstitution were achieved in recipients of HLA-matched sibling marrow [268], but more intensive treatment was required to achieve engraftment of matched unrelated donor HCT (reviewed in Chapters 83 and 85). Thus far, these approaches have not been combined with organ transplantation in humans.

Anti-T-cell antibodies

Host cells that mediate alloresistance can be specifically eliminated with the administration of polyclonal sera and MABs against T cells *in vivo*. A fraction of mice pretreated with antilymphocyte serum (ALS) and grafted with donor-type skin several days prior to administration of allogeneic marrow could be rendered specifically tolerant of donor antigens in the presence of certain MHC disparities [269]. Complex mechanisms, including suppressor cells of donor origin, were implicated in this model, and long-term microchimerism was demonstrable (reviewed in [265]). A similar approach has been reported to prolong renal allograft survival in large animals, with the best results being achieved when the donor and recipient share a DR class II MHC allele [270]. In the primate studies, a CD2$^+$CD8$^+$CD16$^+$CD3$^-$DR$^-$ cell population with veto activity has been implicated [271]. Conventional marrow doses are administered in this model without host myelosuppression, so that consistently measurable levels of donor HSC engraftment are not achieved.

Since the development of MAB technology, these reagents have been used more specifically to overcome host resistance to allo- and xeno-engraftment [41,175,272]. *In vivo* depletion of host CD4$^+$ and CD8$^+$ T cells along with TBI (at least 6 Gy) permitted engraftment of allogeneic marrow and induction of skin graft tolerance across complete MHC barriers [41]. Adding a high dose of thymic irradiation (7 Gy) to the regimen permitted engraftment of fully MHC-mismatched allogeneic marrow in animals receiving only 3 Gy TBI [175]. Thymic irradiation is needed because thymocytes become coated with MAB but, unlike T cells in the peripheral lymphoid compartment, are not eliminated [175]. The low dose (3 Gy) of TBI is necessary for the creation of marrow "space" [175]. Permanent mixed chimerism and donor- and host-specific tolerance are reliably induced across complete MHC barriers using this regimen (Fig. 24.1). This approach has been extended to a xenogeneic (rat → mouse) combination by adding anti-NK1.1 and anti-Thy1.2 MABs to the conditioning regimen [272]. These MABs are needed to deplete recipient NK cells and $\gamma\delta$T cells [273], both of which pose a much more significant

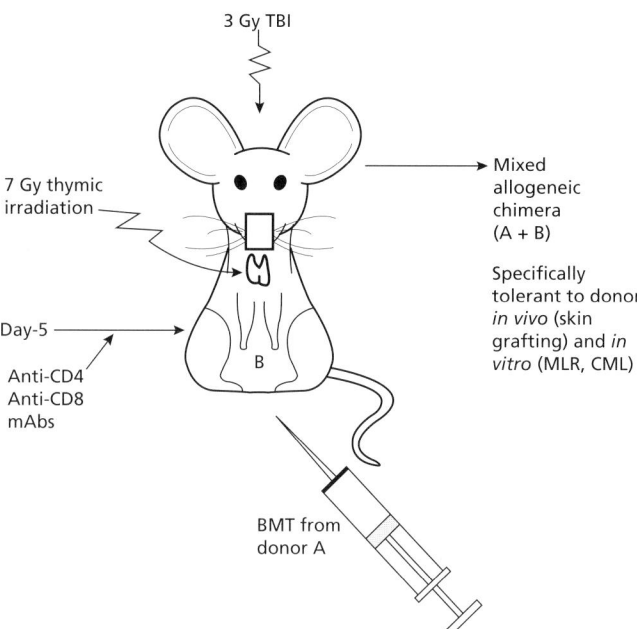

Fig. 24.1 Nonmyeloablative conditioning regimen allowing the induction of mixed allogeneic chimerism and specific transplantation tolerance across complete major histocompatibility complex (MHC) barriers in mice.

barrier to engraftment of xenogeneic than allogeneic HCT. Allogeneic tolerance has been achieved in a nonhuman primate model using this nonmyeloablative approach to inducing mixed chimerism [274]. In both the allogeneic and the xenogeneic rodent systems, intrathymic clonal deletion, rather than peripheral suppression or anergy, is the major mechanism inducing and maintaining long-term donor-specific tolerance [109,176,177,275]. Accordingly, donor class II^{high} cells are present in the thymi of these animals at all times, including 10 days post-BMT, when the first wave of thymopoiesis is underway [109]. Furthermore, tolerance can be broken by depleting donor cells with MABs after stable chimerism has been established [276]. This loss of tolerance correlates with the appearance of T cells bearing donor-reactive $V\beta$ [176]. However, if the host thymus is removed before depletion of donor hematopoietic cells, or if donor-depleted spleen cells are transferred to athymic mice, donor-specific tolerance is maintained and donor-reactive $V\beta$ do not appear [176]. These results demonstrate that intrathymic chimerism is essential to maintain ongoing deletional tolerance in long-term mixed allogeneic chimeras, that peripheral chimerism is not necessary for the maintenance of tolerance and that suppression or anergy do not play significant roles in maintaining long-term tolerance.

The potential toxicity of the regimen shown in Fig. 24.1 can be further minimized by replacing thymic irradiation with a second injection of antidonor MABs on day –1, and deletional tolerance is again attained [277,278]. These thymus-directed host treatments are needed not only to eliminate pre-existing donor-alloreactive thymocytes [279], but also to create "thymic space". Thymic engraftment is regulated independently of marrow engraftment, and specific measures are required to permit donor progenitors to repopulate the recipient thymus at high levels, even in syngeneic mice [180]. For reasons that are not clear, a high donor contribution to early post-transplant thymopoiesis correlates with the development of a state of permanent, stable chimerism and donor-specific tolerance [181,277,278].

In this allogeneic BMT model, TBI can be eliminated from host conditioning by increasing the dose of donor marrow cells administered to mice treated with depleting anti-CD4 and anti-CD8 MAB injections on days –6, –1 and 7, and local thymic irradiation on day 0. Permanent, stable, multilineage mixed chimerism, donor-specific skin graft tolerance, and *in vitro* tolerance were observed in the majority of animals. Abundant donor class II^{high} cells were detected in thymi of long-term chimeras, and their presence was associated with intrathymic deletion of donor-reactive host thymocytes. The treatment was not associated with any clinically significant myelosuppression, toxicity, or GVHD [181]. Thus, high levels of allogeneic hematopoietic repopulation and central deletional tolerance may be achieved with a conditioning regimen that excludes myelosuppressive treatment. In a porcine study based on this model, hematopoietic cell engraftment and donor-specific tolerance have been achieved across a full haplotype barrier using a similar nonmyelosuppressive regimen that includes high stem cell doses [280].

Based on the mouse model in Fig. 24.1, a primate model for tolerance induction has recently been developed. Since effective T-cell-depleting MABs are not available for use in primates, polyclonal ATG and a short (28 day) course of CSP are used in its place. A high percentage of cynomolgus monkeys receiving class I- and II-mismatched marrow with this protocol develop transient mixed chimerism and donor kidney allograft acceptance [274,281].

Several other regimens involving various combinations of anti-T-cell antibodies, irradiation and immunosuppressive drugs have also permitted the achievement of mixed chimerism in mice (reviewed in [282]). Depleting and nondepleting anti-T-cell MABs can also be used to induce tolerance in association with conventional dose BMT without irradiation, though tolerance is then only reliably achieved across minor histocompatibility barriers, and lasting high levels of chimerism are not achieved [41]. $V\beta$ analyses suggest that clonal anergy and not deletion may be the major mechanism of tolerance in this model [41].

The successful induction of tolerance in a primate model using the nonmyeloablative approach to inducing mixed chimerism [274], combined with murine studies demonstrating the utility of mixed chimerism followed by delayed donor lymphocyte infusions (DLI) as an approach to achieving GVLE without GVHD [283–285] has been used as the basis for a clinical trial of mixed chimerism induction followed by DLI for the treatment of patients with hematologic malignancies [266,267]. The experience with this relatively nontoxic protocol provided an opportunity to evaluate the potential of this approach to induce transplantation tolerance in patients with a hematologic malignancy, multiple myeloma, and consequent renal failure. Two patients have received a simultaneous nonmyeloablative BMT and renal allograft from HLA-identical siblings, and have accepted their kidney graft without any immunosuppression for over 2 and 4 years, respectively, while enjoying marked tumor regressions [286,287] (Fig. 24.2 [287]). Similar to the primate model described above, in which BMT has been shown to be essential for tolerance induction [274], chimerism in these patients was only transient [286,287], suggesting that the kidney graft itself may participate in tolerance induction and/or maintenance after chimerism has played its initial role. Because TCD is only partial in these models, it is clear that the pure central, deletional tolerance described above in murine models has not yet been achieved with nonmyeloablative conditioning in large animals or humans. Nevertheless, the promising results obtained in these two patients have provided an important proof of principle, which has led to initiation of a phase I/II trial of tolerance induction with this approach in patients with renal failure due to multiple myeloma.

The mechanisms of T-cell elimination using MABs are not entirely clear. Animals treated with T-cell-depleting MABs after thymectomy show a partial but significant recovery of CD4$^+$ and CD8$^+$ T cells over a period of several weeks [288], suggesting that sequestration rather than destruction may actually account for some of the observed TCD. TCD does not appear to be dependent upon the activity of complement or on antibody-dependent T-cell-mediated cytotoxicity [288]. *In vitro* studies indicate that apoptosis can be induced by signals from crosslinked anti-

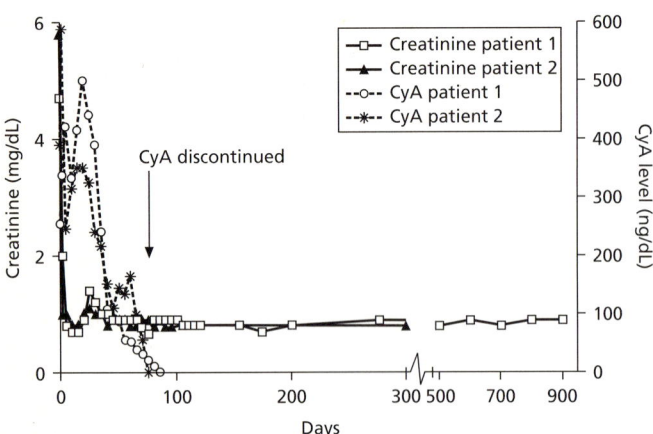

Fig. 24.2 Renal function (measured by serum creatinine) and cyclosporine (CSP) levels (measured by a monoclonal antibody assay) in two patients with multiple myeloma who received combined kidney and bone marrow transplantation (BMT) from human leukocyte antigen (HLA)-identical sibling donors following nonmyeloablative conditioning with cyclophosphamide (CY), pre and post-transplant antithymocyte globulin (ATG) and thymic irradiation. CSP was the only pharmacologic immunosuppressive agent given post-transplant, and it was discontinued in the 3rd month post-transplant. Both patients have sustained normal creatinine levels (now at 2 years and 4 years) following discontinuation of CSP, indicating the presence of tolerance to their kidney allografts. Partial and complete remissions of the multiple myeloma were achieved in the two patients, and no graft-vs.-host disease (GVHD) has occurred. Reprinted with permission from Buhler et al. [287].

CD4 MAB [289]. Memory T cells appear to be more resistant than naive-type T cells to MAB-induced depletion in vivo [290–292].

Costimulatory blockade with HCT

Both thymic irradiation [293] and host T-cell depleting MABs in the conditioning regimen shown in Fig. 24.1 can be replaced by costimulatory blockade [294]. All preconditioning can be eliminated by giving a high dose of fully MHC-mismatched donor marrow followed by a single injection of each of two costimulatory blockers [182] or repeated injections of anti-CD40 ligand [295]. This ability to replace recipient TCD with costimulatory blockade is encouraging for several reasons. First, it has been difficult to achieve TCD with antibodies in large animals and humans that is as exhaustive as that achieved in the above rodent models, perhaps due to the use of inadequate doses or suboptimal reagents. Second, if sufficiently exhaustive TCD could be achieved in humans, T-cell recovery from the thymus might be dangerously slow, especially in older individuals, since thymic function diminishes with age (reviewed in [296]). The ability to minimize the degree and duration of TCD by replacing some [137] or all [182,294,295] of the T-cell depleting antibodies with costimulatory blockers is therefore encouraging.

As in other protocols achieving sustained mixed chimerism, long-term tolerance is maintained by intrathymic deletion in mixed chimeras prepared with costimulatory blockade [137,182,294]. However, since alloreactive T cells are abundant in the peripheral repertoire at the time of BMT with these regimens, these peripheral T cells must be rendered tolerant by BMT under cover of costimulatory blockade. Peripheral deletion of donor-reactive cells occurs through a combination of AICD and "passive cell death", but the latter mechanism seems more important for tolerance induction [182,294,297,298]. However, donor-specific tolerance is complete in mixed lymphocyte reactions by 1 week post-transplant, when deletion of donor-reactive CD4 cells is only partial [299], suggesting that mechanisms in addition to deletion are involved in the early tolerization of peripheral CD4 cells by donor bone marrow in the presence of costimulatory blockade. The mechanisms of CD4 cell tolerance have been studied in isolation in a model involving peripheral CD8 cell depletion with MAB [137]. A single injection of anti-CD40L MAB is sufficient to allow BMT to induce tolerance of CD4 cells in mice receiving depleting anti-CD8 MAB [137]. The anti-CD40L MAB is required only to block the interaction between CD40L and CD40 and not to target activated T cells for depletion or to signal to the CD4 cell [299]. These results indicate that CD4 cell-mediated alloresistance to bone marrow grafts is exquisitely dependent on CD40–CD40L interactions. This is somewhat surprising, since CD40-independent pathways can activate APC to induce antiviral CD4 cell responses. Much remains to be learned about the mechanisms by which CD4 T cells are tolerized to alloantigens when APC activation via CD40 is blocked.

As mentioned above, thymic irradiation was needed in the model shown in Fig. 24.1 to overcome the resistance mediated by mature alloreactive thymocytes that escape depletion with T-cell-depleting MABs [175,279]. However, the use of costimulatory blockade bypasses this need for thymic irradiation [293] in order to achieve lasting chimerism and tolerance. Anti-CD40L rapidly tolerizes alloreactive thymocytes (J. Kurtz and M. Sykes, unpublished data), and the gradual intrathymic engraftment of donor progenitors tolerizes newly developing thymocytes after the costimulatory blocker has been cleared.

GVHD does not occur in the rodent models discussed above, despite the use of unmodified donor bone marrow cells (BMC). This is most readily explained by the continued presence of the T-cell depleting or costimulatory blocking antibodies in the serum of the hosts at the time of BMT [277]. These levels are sufficient to prevent alloreactivity by the relatively small number of mature T cells in the donor marrow.

There are similarities and differences in the mechanisms of tolerance induced by anti-CD40L in combination with BMT vs. DST. Only the BMT model allows engraftment of HSC and intrathymic deletion as a mechanism of long-term tolerance [137,182,293]. Thus, in contrast to BMT, DST and anti-CD40L allows long-term skin graft survival only in thymectomized mice [124]. The inability to maintain tolerance in the presence of a thymus indicates the failure to establish central tolerance in the absence of substantial chimerism. In addition, the inability to resist breaking of tolerance by new thymic emigrants in this model argues that powerful peripheral regulatory mechanisms (suppression) are not operative in these animals, even though regulatory mechanisms may play a role in the initial suppression of CD4-mediated alloresponses [124]. Both CTLA4 and IFN-γ are critical for the induction of tolerance with DST and anti-CD40L [124,300,301]. IFN-γ does not play an important role in the induction of tolerance in recipients in the BMT model, but treatment with anti-CTLA4 MAB blocks the achievement of long-term chimerism and tolerance (J. Kurtz et al., manuscript in preparation). It is unclear whether the inhibition of tolerance by anti-CTLA4 MAB is due to depletion of regulatory cells and/or to blockade of the CTLA4 molecule itself, signaling through which can lead to antiproliferative and anergy-inducing signals, T-cell apoptosis and production of TGF-β (reviewed in [302]).

Studies in mice receiving BMT with anti-CD40L have not shown strong evidence for regulatory mechanisms of tolerance, infectious tolerance or linked suppression (J. Kurtz et al., manuscript in preparation). Since hematopoietic stem cell engraftment ensures complete central deletional tolerance in these long-term chimeras and peripheral deletion is also complete over 1–2 months [137,182,294,303] (J. Kurtz et al., manuscript in preparation), there may be insufficient donor-reactive T cells present to maintain suppressive mechanisms, even if they are involved in the initial peripheral tolerance induction.

It has recently been shown that concurrent viral infections have a deleterious effect on the induction of mixed chimerism under cover of costimulatory blockade [304,305]. Another concern is that successful induction of allogeneic tolerance in the presence of viral infections may also lead to tolerance to the virus and failure to clear it. These results suggest that *de novo* systemic viral infections should be avoided during the period of BMT and tolerance induction, and have considerable implication for the practice of BMT with this approach.

Application of mixed chimerism for the induction of xenogeneic tolerance

For reasons described previously, considerable difficulties have been encountered in achieving high levels of engraftment and hematopoietic function from highly disparate species, such as pig or human hematopoietic cells transferred to immunodeficient mice [306,307]. Xenogeneic hematopoiesis can be enhanced by the administration of donor-specific cytokines [308,309], but much remains to be understood about the physiologic regulation of marrow homing and seeding of the thymus with tolerance-inducing cells from the donor. Previously, HCTs from these species did not result in the migration of donor cells to the recipient thymus [309], as would be needed for the induction of central tolerance. However, this goal has recently been achieved in transgenic mice expressing porcine hematopoietic cytokines, in which the spontaneous migration of porcine class II^{high} cells to the recipient thymus was detected [310]. Recently, an alternative approach, involving removal of the recipient thymus and its replacement with a xenogeneic thymus, has successfully allowed the induction of donor-specific skin graft tolerance across the discordant pig to mouse species barrier [311]. Normal, immunocompetent mice that are thymectomized and treated with T and NK cell-depleting MABs before porcine thymus grafting demonstrate recovery of CD4 T cells in the xenogeneic thymic grafts [312]. These cells repopulate the periphery and are competent to resist infection [236]. Tolerance to both donor and host by intrathymic deletional mechanisms is observed, and this deletion reflects the presence of class II^{high} cells from both species within the graft [311,313]. Since MHC restriction is determined by the MHC of the thymus, and porcine MHC is entirely responsible for positive selection of murine T cells in this model [314,315], it was surprising that T cells that differentiated in xenogeneic thymus grafts were able to respond to peptide antigens presented by host MHC [236]. However, the excellent immune function achieved in humans receiving HLA-mismatched allogeneic thymic transplantation for the treatment of congenital thymic aplasia (DiGeorge syndrome) suggests that this "restriction incompatibility" may not be a major obstacle to the achievement of adequate immune function [316]. Perhaps this high level of crossreactivity, even between species, reflects the fact that MHC reactivity is inherent in unselected TCR sequences [317]. Importantly, it has been demonstrated that human T cells can also develop in porcine thymic grafts (in immunodeficient mice), and that these T cells show specific tolerance toward the MHC of the xenogeneic thymus donor [318].

Induction of B-cell tolerance using HCT

As is mentioned above, mixed chimerism can also induce tolerance across xenograft barriers [232,272]. Pigs are widely believed to be the most suitable xenogeneic donor species for transplantation to humans, but transplantation from this species is impeded by the presence in human sera of NAB that cause hyperacute rejection of porcine vascularized xenografts. In humans, the major specificity recognized by NAB on porcine tissues is a ubiquitous carbohydrate epitope, Galα1-3Galβ1-4GlcNAc-R(αGal). Humans lack a functional α1-3Gal transferase (GalT) enzyme, as do GalT knockout mice, which also make anti-αGal NAB. Both pre-existing and newly developing B cells producing anti-αGal antibodies are tolerized by the induction of mixed chimerism in GalT knockout mice receiving αGal-expressing allogeneic or xenogeneic marrow [206,207]. The induction of mixed xenogeneic chimerism prevents hyperacute rejection, acute vascular rejection and cell-mediated rejection of primarily vascularized cardiac xenografts [208]. Long-term chimeras produced in GalT knockout mice lack anti-Gal surface Ig-bearing cells in the spleen, and show tolerance in Enzyme-Linked Immunosorbent Spot (ELISPOT) assays [207,208], suggesting that clonal deletion and/or receptor editing tolerize B cells developing after BMT. However, tolerance develops by 2 weeks post-BMT, even in mice that are presensitized to Gal antigens, despite the fact that the conditioning regimen does not deplete antibody-producing cells [319]. In $GalT^{-/-}$ mice rendered tolerant by induction of mixed chimerism 2 weeks earlier, cells with anti-Gal receptors are present in the spleen, but do not produce anti-Gal. Anergy may be the nondeletional mechanism responsible for this rapid tolerance of natural antibody-producing cells in mice rendered mixed chimeric with BMT [207,209].

An alternative approach for tolerizing B cells toward the Gal epitope involves retroviral transduction of the *GalT* gene into autologous HSC. Administration of marrow transduced in this manner to lethally irradiated *GalT* knockout mice led to tolerance to the Gal epitope [320]. This strategy using gene therapy has at least one significant advantage over the xenogeneic hematopoietic chimerism approach, because establishing molecular chimerism involves modification of autologous bone marrow stem cells, thereby overcoming difficulties associated with engraftment of pig bone marrow in primates. However, this approach has only been evaluated in lethally irradiated mice, and it is not yet known whether or not a transduced, transplanted bone marrow population could compete sufficiently with host hematopoietic cells to give significant long-term Gal expression in recipients of a more clinically relevant, nonmyeloablative conditioning regimen. Even if this approach were to be successfully applied, non-Gal-reactive xenoreactive NABs and cell-mediated rejection would remain to be overcome. In contrast, all types of rejection can be avoided with a single treatment by induction of mixed xenogeneic hematopoietic chimerism [207–209].

Preventing GVHD by depleting or inducing GvH tolerance among mature donor T cells in the HCT inoculum

It is widely believed that, in order to avoid GVHD, the *de novo* development of host-reactive T cells from progenitors in the marrow must be prevented, and the GVH reactivity of pre-existing mature T cells in the marrow inoculum must be inhibited. While avoidance of GVH alloreactivity is not always desirable (see below), many strategies for preventing GVHD induced by mature T cells in the HCT inoculum involve depletion or tolerization of pre-existing GVH-reactive T cells.

Tolerization of mature T cells in donor marrow could have both beneficial and harmful effects. The beneficial effects of alloreactive T cells include GVLE [321] and promotion of alloengraftment [322]. However, T cells that lack GVH reactivity also have the potential, if given in sufficient numbers, to promote alloengraftment (see Chapter 3), possibly by the veto mechanism described above [256,323]. Additionally, these T cell populations can confer immunity to pathogens [324], thereby avoiding the high risk of opportunistic infection associated with global TCD.

While induction of global GVH tolerance is highly desirable in the use of HCT for the treatment of nonmalignant diseases, such as the induction of transplantation tolerance (discussed above) and the treatment of inborn hematologic, immunologic and metabolic disorders, it could have the deleterious effect of reducing graft-vs.-leukemia/lymphoma (GVL) in the setting of certain malignant diseases. Induction of this type of tolerance could be successful in patients with such diseases if potent leukemia-specific responses could be preserved while responses to normal host antigens were inhibited. Several candidate tumor-specific antigens have recently been identified (see Chapter 28) and CTL activity can be generated against them, resulting in considerable interest in the idea of tolerizing GVH-reactive T cells while maintaining tumor-specific responses. However, the frequency of tumor antigen-specific T cells pre-existing in a given T-cell repertoire is low. These frequencies are even lower than those against multiple minor histocompatibility antigens, and the generation of meaningful tumor-specific responses is likely to necessitate donor presensitization along with *in vitro* expansion of tumor-specific effector cells, a process which can limit the homing capacity of injected cells. Such prolonged cultures may be impractical for use in the setting of BMT, in which leukemia-reactive cells must eliminate exponentially expanding leukemic cells. Immunization of HCT donors with tumor antigens could potentially overcome these limitations. In theory, the less risky strategy of generating tumor-specific responses from autologous T cells could achieve similar outcomes. However, T-cell immunity may be markedly impaired in the tumor-bearing host, and the use of immunologically unimpaired allogeneic donors is therefore attractive.

Minor histocompatibility alloantigens expressed by lymphohematopoietic cells (including leukemias and lymphomas) but not by the epithelial GVHD target tissues may also be targeted using *in vitro* expanded CTL. Several human minor histocompatibility antigens have demonstrated this pattern of expression (see Chapter 29). However, GVH disparities for some of these same minor antigens (e.g. HA-1) have been associated with an increased incidence of GVHD [325,326]. Recently, it was shown that administration of primed T cells specific for a single immunodominant class I-restricted minor histocompatibility antigen could mediate GVL without GVHD. Avoidance of GVHD was dependent on the absence of GVH-reactive T cells with additional specificities in the donor inoculum [327]. Perhaps the response to immunodominant minor antigens induces APC activation and cytokine production which augments responses to additional minor histoincompatibilities that are shared by GVHD target organs.

However, the potency of antitumor effects in BMT is greatest in the setting of MHC disparity [328–330], in which GVH alloresponses are strongest. The potent ability of the anti-MHC GVH alloresponse to mediate GVLE reflects the extraordinarily high frequency of T cells recognizing MHC alloantigens that is present in the unprimed T-cell repertoire. T cells reactive with an allogeneic MHC determinant may represent as many as 2% or more of the total T-cell population, whereas T cells reactive with an exogenous protein generally represent only approximately one in 10 000 of the same T-cell pool [331]. Several reasons for this high frequency of MHC-reactive T cells have been identified. One is the large number of different "nonself" peptide/MHC complexes presented by an allogeneic MHC molecule (i.e. high number of different determinants), resulting in recognition by a large number of different T-cell clones. The second reason is the large number of MHC molecules on an allogeneic cell. This may lead to recognition by large numbers of TCRs that are sufficiently independent of the peptide component for their recognition of the MHC/peptide complex that they bind with relatively low affinity to the MHC molecules regardless of the peptides to which they are complexed. In these instances, the high density of MHC determinants compensates for the low affinity of the TCR recognizing them. In contrast, since minor histocompatibility antigens are peptides, the number of minor antigen/MHC complexes on a given APC will be more limited, perhaps resulting in recognition only by TCR with relatively high affinity. As is discussed later in this section, a number of experimental strategies have been developed that permit exploitation of the GVH alloresponse for GVLE while avoiding GVHD.

Specific depletion or tolerization of mature GVH-reactive T cells present in the donor inoculum at the time of HCT

Several approaches have been developed in efforts to tolerize GVH-reactive mature T cells within donor marrow, including blocking of adhesive and costimulatory interactions of T cells with recipient antigen-presenting cells [332–334]. Additional approaches involve the selective elimination, rather than tolerization, of GVH-reactive T cells. These approaches preserve T-cell populations that may react to tumor-specific antigens and pathogens and perhaps promote engraftment. This goal can be achieved by stimulating donor T cells with host antigens, then depleting the activated cells using antibodies or immunotoxins directed against cell surface markers associated with recent activation, such as CD25 [324] and CD69 [335].

Use of suppressive T-cell populations to induce GVH tolerance

$CD25^+CD4^+$ cells generated by *in vitro* culture with alloantigen and anti-CD40L have been shown to be able to suppress GVHD and to tolerize naive and presensitized T cells via a regulatory cell population [334].

Additional T-cell subsets also have the ability to suppress GVHD. The $\alpha\beta$T-cell subsets that express the $CD4^-CD8^-$ phenotype or that express the NK1.1 marker ordinarily found on NK cells (NK/T cells) make up 30–90% of mouse marrow T cells [336–338]. Marrow NK/T cells are mainly $CD4^-CD8^-$ (double negative) and a smaller population express CD4 [336,338]. $CD4^-CD8^-$ or NK/T cells make up less then 2–5% of all T cells in the peripheral blood or spleen [336,337]. NK/T cells in lymphoid tissues such as the thymus and spleen express a markedly restricted TCR repertoire with an invariant TCR α chain rearrangement of $V\alpha14J\alpha281$ coupled with TCR β chains restricted to the use of $V\beta2$, $V\beta7$ or $V\beta8$ receptors. These restricted TCRs recognize CD1, a nonpolymorphic class I MHC-like molecule associated with $\beta2m$ [339]. The NK/T cells also secrete an unusual pattern of cytokines, including large quantities of both IL-4 and IFN-γ [340]. NK/T cells are the major source of IL-4 detected *in vivo* within 30 min of injection of anti-CD3 MAB [341].

$CD4^-CD8^-$ $\alpha\beta$ T cells in the marrow (the majority of which express NK1.1) have been shown to suppress acute lethal GVHD after coinjection with spleen cells from the same donor into allogeneic irradiated recipients [342] via an IL-4-dependent mechanism [240]. Cloned lines of $CD4^-CD8^-$ T cells derived from the spleen or $CD4^-CD8^-$ NK1.1 T cells derived from the marrow have also been shown to reduce the severity of acute GVHD [93,343]. These cells can suppress MLR *in vitro* [344]. As discussed above, these $CD4^-CD8^-$ T cells showed features of and were originally termed "natural suppressor" cells.

Not all NK/T cells express the invariant chain and recognize CD1, and bone marrow is enriched for the subset that does not recognize CD1 [345]. Furthermore, different subsets of NK/T cells have different cytokine production profiles [346]. Enrichment for IL-4-producing NK/T cells following TLI appears to play an important role in the protection from GVHD [240] and ability to induce HVG tolerance [238,239] in TLI-treated animals. Appropriate mixtures of donor T cells, which are unable to induce GVHD, are still able to retain the capacity to mediate graft-antitumor activity [347]. Recent studies suggest that, in addition to the NK/T cells, T cells lacking NK cell markers that are resident in murine bone marrow have a reduced capacity to produce GVHD, with preserved ability to mediate GVL [348]. The mechanisms of this effect are incompletely understood.

IL-2-activated killer cells for the prevention of GVHD

Studies have demonstrated that LAK cells can inhibit GVHD [81]. These cells, which are derived from the host strain, may inhibit GVHD by eliminating alloreactive donor T cells by the veto mechanism discussed above [80,81].

Approaches to preventing GVHD that do not involve induction of tolerance

TH1 vs. TH2 paradigm in GVHD

Considerable interest has been generated by the notion that GVH-reactive T cells with functional activities that mediate GVL but do not mediate GVHD could separate the two phenomena. Studies involving CD4+ splenic T cells polarized by exposure to alloantigens and cytokines *in vitro* or *in vivo* suggested that the TH1 subset was a potent mediator of acute severe GVHD, but the TH2 subset had little or no GVHD-inducing activity in the same model systems [349,350]. In some experimental systems, TH2 cells ameliorated severe GVHD and associated LPS-induced lethality mediated by TH1 cells [349–351]. Similarly, Tc1 cells mediated severe GVHD in MHC class I mismatched or parent into F1 hybrid combinations, but Tc2 cells were ineffective in the same model systems [350,352]. These observations would suggest that the capacity of mature donor T cells in the allogeneic marrow graft to induce GVHD may be diminished by manipulations which alter the function of TH1 and Tc1 cells, inducing a shift to the TH2 and Tc2 subsets. This is not induction of tolerance *per se*, but instead, represents a selective diminution of the activities of host-reactive T cells that cause tissue injury.

However, the role of TH1 and TH2-associated cytokines in GVHD is complex, as it is in graft rejection. Despite evidence that TH1 and Tc1 T cells appear to play an important role in the induction of acute GVHD and that GVHD may be ameliorated by TH2 or TH2-associated cytokines, systemic administration of TH1-type cytokines such as IL-2 or IFN-γ shortly after BMT in mice ameliorated GVHD [353,354]. Furthermore, T cells from IFN-γ-deficient donors have an increased capacity to cause acute GVHD in lethally irradiated recipients (reviewed in [355]). Early systemic administration of IL-12, a potent inducer of TH1 responses, also ameliorated acute GVHD [356], and this reaction was dependent on the ability to produce IFN-γ (discussed below). The role of IFN-γ in down-modulating graft rejection under certain conditions has already been discussed. While the mechanism by which IFN-γ inhibits graft rejection and GVHD is not fully understood, this cytokine has been shown to have antiproliferative effects on CD4 and CD8 T cells [140,143], to up-regulate the production of nitric oxide [357], which has immunomodulatory properties [358], and to increase T cell apoptosis via the Fas/FasL pathway [359]. Studies in the GVHD model have shown that IFN-γ inhibits both CD4− and CD8 cell-mediated GVHD, and mitigates the expansion of both T-cell subsets (reviewed in [355]). In a viral infection model, IFN-γ plays an important role in the contraction phase of a CD8 CTL response, and that this contraction is impaired in IFN-γ deficient mice, even when virus has been cleared [360].

Further studies have shown that TH2 and TH2-associated cytokines are also capable of contributing significantly to GVHD pathology [361,362], and that this subset is particularly important in causing acute GVHD of the skin and liver in the BALB/c to B6 murine strain combination [361]. The role of TH2 cytokines in mediating graft rejection and autoimmune diseases has already been discussed. Thus, much remains to be learned about the mechanisms by which Th subsets and their secreted cytokines can be either harmful or beneficial.

The potential of exogenously administered immunostimulatory cytokines to separate GVHD and GVL

As is mentioned above, several immunostimulatory cytokines, all of which have been implicated as contributing to GVHD pathophysiology in various models, have the paradoxical capacity to inhibit GVHD. This phenomenon is of considerable interest because these cytokines (IFN-γ, IL-2, IL-12 and IL-18) also have the potential to enhance antitumor effects, and therefore could mediate GVLE while inhibiting GVHD. Indeed, two of these cytokines, IL-2 [363,364] and IL-12 [365], have been shown to preserve antileukemia/lymphoma effects of alloreactive T cells while inhibiting GVHD.

While the mechanisms of GVHD inhibition by IL-2 are not fully understood, they involve a reduction of IFN-γ production in association with GVHD [366,367]. IL-2 inhibits the GVHD-inducing activity of CD4 cells but not of CD4-independent CD8+ T cells [368]. However, the preservation of CD4 cell-mediated GVLE in IL-2-protected mice receiving a myeloid leukemia is unexplained [364].

Early systemic administration of IL-12, a potent immunostimulatory cytokine, inducer of TH1 activity and of CTL function [369], also ameliorates acute GVHD [356]. This effect is dependent on the ability to produce IFN-γ [370,371]. Recent studies showed similar inhibition of GVHD with exogenous administration of IL-18 [372]. Both IL-12 [365,370,373,374] and IL-18 [372] inhibit GVHD in part by promoting Fas-dependent donor T-cell apoptosis and reducing early donor T-cell expansion. IL-12 treatment markedly attenuates all manifestations of the GVH response, including the expansion of host-specific Th. However, IL-12 treatment induces an early surge of IFN-γ production that plays a critical role in its protective effect against GVHD. IFN-γ inhibits the capacity of the CD8 cell subset to mediate GVHD independently of CD4 cells, while playing an important role in CD8 cell-mediated GVL [371] (reviewed in [355,375]). Thus, a single molecule (IFN-γ) both inhibits GVHD and mediates GVLE.

Other approaches

A number of additional approaches to ameliorating GVHD do not involve initial tolerance induction of donor T cells in the HCT graft. One such approach is to transduce donor T cells with suicide genes, such as herpes simplex virus thymidine kinase (TK), so that the alloresponse can be turned off at will, hopefully, after tumor has been eradicated [376]. Initial clinical success with this approach has been somewhat limited, in part due to the fact that ganciclovir, the drug used to kill TK-transduced T cells, is also needed clinically to treat cytomegalovirus reactivation, which is a common and serious complication of HCT. Furthermore, the transduction of GVH-reactive T cells may be incomplete, resulting in escape of some clones from suicide after treatment has been initiated. Finally, the manipulations involved in the transduction process itself might render the donor T cells less effective at eliminating leukemias when transferred back to the patient. The development of new vectors and the use of genes other than TK may lead to further improvements in the utility of this approach. Another approach is to attempt to block the early inflammatory mediators of GVHD, such as IL-1 [377] and TNF-α [378], without blocking the alloresponse *per se*. Recently, keratinocyte growth factor has been shown to ameliorate GVHD without blocking GVL, perhaps by reducing the disruption of the intestinal barrier associated with myeloablative conditioning. However, these factors seem to also affect the immune response, leading to increased TH2 and decreased TH1–type responses in association with GVHD (see Chapter 27).

Delayed donor T-cell administration

In 8- to 10-week established mixed allogeneic chimeras, which are immunologically tolerant of their original marrow donor's antigens, a GVH reaction takes place after administration of DLI, resulting in conversion of the state of mixed hematopoietic chimerism to a state of full donor chimerism. Remarkably, this powerful GVH alloreaction against lymphohematopoietic cells is not associated with any clinically significant GVHD, even though donor T cells are given in numbers that would cause rapidly lethal GVHD in freshly irradiated recipients [283]. Similar results have been obtained in mixed chimeras prepared with non-myeloablative conditioning [284]. This demonstration that GVH reactions could be confined to the lymphohematopoietic system suggested a novel approach to separating GVHD from GVLE. Since hematologic malignancies reside largely in the lymphohematopoietic system, the result suggested that GVH reactions might be confined to this system and would eliminate tumor cells without entering the epithelial GVHD target tissues. DLI have indeed been shown to be capable of mediating powerful GVLE in mouse leukemia models [285,379], in patients with chronic myeloid leukemia who have relapsed late following allogeneic

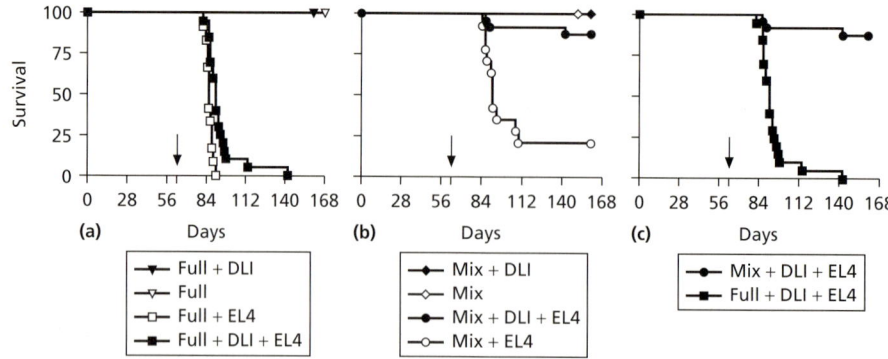

Fig. 24.3 Superior donor lymphocyte infusion (DLI)-mediated graft-vs.-leukemia effect (GVLE) in mixed compared to full allogeneic chimeras. Mixed and full chimeras were prepared by lethally irradiating B6 mice and reconstituting them with either T-cell-depleted allogeneic (B10.A) bone marrow cells (BMC) alone (to produce full chimeras), or a mixture of T-cell-depleted B6 plus B10.A marrow (to produce mixed chimeras). DLI were administered on day 56 post-bone marrow transplantation (BMT) and this step was followed by intravenous (IV) injection of 500 EL4 (a B6 T-cell lymphoma) cells, on day 63 (↓). (a) Full chimeras receiving DLI and EL4 cells (■, $n = 20$) showed a slight, but statistically significant prolongation of survival compared to full chimeras receiving tumor cells only (□, $n = 12$, $p < 0.001$). Full chimeras receiving (▼, $n = 14$) or not receiving DLI (▽, $n = 7$) showed no treatment-related mortality. (b) Mixed chimeras receiving (◆, $n = 11$) or not receiving (◇, $n = 8$) DLI showed no treatment-related mortality. Mixed chimeras receiving DLI and EL4 cells (●, $n = 25$) had a significantly improved survival compared to mixed chimeras receiving EL4 alone (○, $n = 14$, $p < 0.0001$). (c) Mixed chimeras receiving DLI and EL4 cells (●, $n = 25$) had a significantly improved survival compared to full chimeras receiving EL4 + DLI (■, $n = 20$, $p < 0.0001$). Reprinted with permission from Mapara et al. [285].

BMT [380] and in patients with lymphomas and multiple myeloma [266,381,382].

It has been suggested that the recipient's recovery from conditioning-induced tissue injury might reduce the tendency of GVH-reactive donor T cells that recognize host alloantigens to leave the lymphohematopoietic system and cause GVHD [283]. An alternative possibility, that host-type veto or suppressor cells mediate this protection from GVHD in established mixed chimeras, seems less probable, since fully allogeneic chimeras are also resistant to the induction of GVHD by the delayed administration of DLI [283]. Although suppressor cells of donor [383] and host [384] origin have both been implicated in protection from GVHD in mice receiving delayed DLI in various models, studies in the mixed chimera model show that the potent antihost alloresponse occurs despite the absence of GVHD, as alloreactive donor T cells in DLI mediate the destruction of normal host hematopoietic cells and the eradication of host-type leukemias seen in this model [283–285] (Y. Kim, M. Mapara and M. Sykes, manuscript in preparation). Studies in the nonmyeloablative model mentioned above [284] showed no evidence for a role for suppressive host or donor T cells in the resistance to GVHD of mixed chimeras receiving DLI 35 days post-BMT (M. Mapara and M. Sykes, manuscript in preparation).

Based on the murine and nonhuman primate models described above [274,284], a clinical protocol for the induction of mixed chimerism followed by DLI was evaluated for the treatment of hematologic malignancies. Conditioning involved *in vivo* TCD with equine ATG (ATGAM) given pre and post-transplant, CY, thymic irradiation and a short course of CSP as the only post-transplant immunosuppression given in addition to ATG. A remarkably high success rate was achieved with this approach in patients with advanced, refractory lymphoid malignancies [266,267,381,385] in whom other therapies have been uniformly unsuccessful.

In some patients receiving nonmyeloablative HCT and delayed DLI with this approach, powerful antitumor effects against advanced hematological malignancies were observed without or with only mild GVHD [266,381]. The factors predicting the development of GVHD following DLI have not been identified. However, it is this author's opinion that improved TCD of the initial donor stem cell inoculum to avoid even subclinical GVHD, and therefore permit the recovery of a noninflamed environment in the epithelial GVHD target tissues before DLI are given, should allow more reliable avoidance of GVHD with preserved GVLE from DLI. In support of this possibility, recent studies involving *in vivo* TCD of the recipient with a more powerful agent than the ATG used in previous studies, in combination with administration of an increased dose of *ex vivo* T-cell-depleted haploidentical allogeneic HSC, has permitted demonstration in a small number of patients that DLI can convert mixed to full donor T-cell chimerism in this extensively HLA-mismatched setting without causing severe GVHD [386].

The potent antitumor responses seen in patients with advanced lymphoid malignancies who received the transplant protocol described above led to the hypothesis that an initial state of mixed chimerism might permit more powerful graft-vs.-tumor (GVT) effects to be achieved from the GVH alloresponse than is possible in full allogeneic chimeras. To test this hypothesis, the GVLE of DLI were compared in mixed vs. full allogeneic chimeras inoculated with a host-type T-cell lymphoma in a murine model. Remarkably, DLI led to only a slight prolongation of survival in leukemic full allogeneic chimeras, whereas they led to almost complete protection, with 80–100% survival, in mixed chimeras receiving the same tumor inoculum (Fig. 24.3 [285]). This markedly more potent GVT effect of DLI in mixed compared to full chimeras was shown to be dependent on the expression of host class I MHC molecules on recipient-type hematopoietic cells [285]. GVHD was not observed in the mixed chimeras enjoying these potent GVLE from DLI [285]. These data are not inconsistent with an earlier report showing a critical role for recipient hematopoietic APC in initiating GVHD [387]; in that report, the donor T cells were given to freshly lethally irradiated mice, whereas the donor T cells were given as delayed DLI in the studies comparing mixed to full chimeras [285]. The complete absence of GVHD in mixed chimeras enjoying potent GVLE of DLI dramatically illustrates the power to separate GVHD and GVT effects by confining the anti-MHC alloresponse to the lymphohematopoietic system.

GVH tolerance of T cells developing from progenitors in the marrow

As has been discussed above, the mechanism of GVH tolerance in lethally irradiated recipients of T-cell-depleted allogeneic marrow alone (i.e. "full" chimeras) appears mainly to involve T-cell anergy rather than clonal deletion [28]. In contrast, mixed chimeras show excellent clonal deletion of T cells reacting against host antigens [36,109], undoubtedly due to the intrathymic presence of host-type marrow-derived cells in mixed chimeras [109]. However, partial clonal deletion of host-reactive T cells has been described in lethally irradiated mice receiving allogeneic BMT alone [388,389], which may reflect the weaker ability of thymic epithelial cells (compared to hematopoietic cells) to induce intrathymic deletion [390–392]. Perturbations in the thymic environment, such as the destruction of thymic epithelial elements observed in GVHD [393], or thymic injury induced by treatment with CSP [394,395], can impair processes leading to tolerance [396,397]. Defective production of autoregulatory suppressor T cells may contribute to autoimmunity in this setting [397,398].

No *in vitro* evidence for active suppression of GVH reactivity was obtained in long-term recipients of T-cell-depleted allogeneic BMT alone [399], whereas suppression of GVH CTL responses was observed in mixed chimeras prepared with lethal irradiation [245]. These suppressive cell populations show specificities that are consistent with a mixture of veto and NS activity [245]. Cells specifically suppressing GVH reactions have also been described in long-term rat chimeras originally reconstituted with non-T-cell-depleted allogeneic marrow [50] and in human BMT recipients who do not develop GVHD [400].

Summary and future directions

It is clear that BMT has not yet met its full potential to provide a cure for lymphohematopoietic malignancies. There is a need for improved methods of exploiting the immunotherapeutic aspects of GVH alloreactivity without causing GVHD. In view of the new strategies and improved understanding of these phenomena that are developing, it seems likely that this challenge can be met, and that BMT will ultimately be made available to all who could benefit from it, including those lacking an HLA-matched or closely matched donor. In addition, advances in the ability to achieve engraftment of hematopoietic and thymic tissue without ablative treatment of the host, and the demonstration of efficacy in primate models, have brought these approaches closer to clinical application for the treatment of additional nonmalignant diseases, particularly for the induction of solid organ graft tolerance. The recent application of nonmyeloablative conditioning approaches in humans has permitted the demonstration that donor-specific organ allograft tolerance can be achieved clinically using HCT in a manner that avoids excessive toxicity. Improvements in the ability to overcome HVG resistance to HLA-mismatched HSC engraftment without increasing host toxicity should further broaden the applicability of this approach. It will also be desirable to extend this ability to xenogeneic marrow and organ transplantation, which presents additional immunological and physiological hurdles, to overcome the critical organ shortage that currently limits the number of life-saving organ transplants that can be performed. A major goal of transplant immunologists therefore now will be to extend new laboratory findings, first to additional preclinical models in large animals, and then to clinical protocols. In addition, it will be important to continue basic research into the mechanisms by which tolerance is induced and maintained in rodent model systems, so that these mechanisms can be further exploited.

References

1 Allen PM. Peptides in positive and negative selection: a delicate balance. *Cell* 1994; **76**: 593–6.
2 Alam SM, Travers PJ, Wung JL *et al*. T-cell-receptor affinity and thymocyte positive selection. *Nature* 1996; **381**: 616–20.
3 Matzinger P. Why positive selection? *Immunol Rev* 1993; **135**: 81–117.
4 Matzinger P. Tolerance, danger, and the extended family. *Ann Rev Immunol* 1994; **12**: 991–1045.
5 Matzinger P, Guerder S. Does T cell tolerance require a dedicated antigen-presenting cell? *Nature* 1989; **338**: 74–6.
6 Pullen AM, Kappler JW, Marrack P. Tolerance to self antigens shapes the T-cell repertoire. *Immunol Rev* 1989; **107**: 125–39.
7 Marrack P, Kappler J. The staphololococcal enterotoxins and their relatives. *Science* 1990; **248**: 705–11.
8 Sha WC, Nelson CA, Newberry RD, Kranz DM, Russell JH, Loh DY. Positive and negative selection of an antigen receptor on T cells in transgenic mice. *Nature* 1988; **336**: 73–6.
9 Von Boehmer H, Kisielow P. Self–nonself discrimination by T cells. *Science* 1990; **248**: 1369–73.
10 Manilay JO, Pearson DA, Sergio JJ, Swenson KG, Sykes M. Intrathymic deletion of alloreactive T cells in mixed bone marrow chimeras prepared with a non-myeloablative conditioning regimen. *Transplantation* 1998; **66**: 96–102.
11 Ferber I, Schonrich G, Schenkel J, Mellor AL, Hammerling GJ, Arnold B. Levels of peripheral T cell tolerance induced by different doses of tolerogen. *Science* 1994; **263**: 674–6.
12 Webb SR, Hutchinson J, Hayden K, Sprent J. Expansion/deletion of mature T cells exposed to endogenous superantigens *in vivo*. *J Immunol* 1994; **152**: 586–97.

13 Rocha B, Von Boehmer H. Peripheral selection of the T cell repertoire. *Science* 1991; **251**: 1225–8.
14 Renno T, Hahne M, Tschopp J, MacDonald HR. Peripheral T cells undergoing superantigen-induced apoptosis *in vivo* express B220 and upregulate Fas and Fas ligand. *J Exp Med* 1996; **183**: 431–7.
15 Welsh RM, Selin LK, Razvi ES. Role of apoptosis in the regulation of virus-induced T cells responses, immune suppression, and memory. *J Cell Biochem* 1995; **59**: 135–42.
16 Bhandoola A, Cho EA, Yui K, Saragovi HU, Greene MI, Quill H. Reduced CD3-mediated protein tyrosine phosphorylation in anergic CD4$^+$ and CD8$^+$ T cells. *J Immunol* 1993; **151**: 2355–67.
17 Schwartz RH. Costimulation of T lymphocytes: the role of CD28, CTLA-4, and B7/BB1 in interleukin-2 production and immunotherapy. *Cell* 1992; **71**: 1065–8.
18 Jenkins MK, Pardoll DM, Mizuguchi J, Chused TM, Schwartz RH. Molecular events in the induction of a nonresponsive state in interleukin 2-producing helper T-lymphocyte clones. *Proc Natl Acad Sci U S A* 1987; **84**: 5409–13.
19 McKay DB, Irie HY, Hollander G *et al*. Antigen-induced unresponsiveness results in altered T cell signaling. *J Immunol* 1999; **163**: 6455–61.
20 Lafferty KJ. Role of second signals in the induction of T cells and graft rejection. *Immunologist* 1995; **3**: 256–8.
21 Rudd CE. Upstream–downstream. CD28 cosignaling pathways and T cell function. *Immunity* 1996; **4**: 527–34.
22 Grewal IS, Flavell RA. A central role of CD40 ligand in the regulation of CD4$^+$ T-cell responses. *Immunol Today* 1996; **17**: 410–4.
23 Yamada A, Salama AD, Sayegh MH. The role of novel T cell costimulatory pathways in autoimmunity and transplantation. *J Am Soc Nephrol* 2002; **13**: 559–75.
24 Zanders ED, Lamb JR, Feldmann M, Green N, Beverley PCL. Tolerance of T-cell clones is associated with membrane antigen changes. *Nature* 1983; **303**: 625–7.
25 Arnold B, Schonrich G, Hammerling GJ. Multiple levels of peripheral tolerance. *Immunol Today* 1993; **14**: 12–4.
26 Goodnow CC. Transgenic mice and analysis of B-cell tolerance. *Ann Rev Immunol* 1992; **10**: 489–518.
27 Akkaraju S, Ho WY, Leong D, Canaan K, Davis MM, Goodnow CC. A range of CD4 T cell tolerance: Partial inactivation to organ-specific antigen allows nondestructive thyroiditis or insulitis. *Immunity* 1997; **7**: 255–71.
28 Ramsdell F, Fowlkes BJ. Clonal deletion versus clonal anergy: the role of the thymus in inducing self tolerance. *Science* 1990; **248**: 1342–8.
29 van Meerwijk JPM, MacDonald HR. *In vivo* T-lymphocyte tolerance in the absence of thymic clonal deletion mediated by hematopoietic cells. *Blood* 1999; **93**: 3856–62.
30 Vandekerckhove BA, Namikawa R, Bacchetta R, Roncarolo MG. Human hematopoietic cells and thymic epithelial cells induce tolerance via different mechanisms in the SCID-hu mouse thymus. *J Exp Med* 1992; **175**: 1033–43.
31 Rocken M, Urban JF, Shevach EM. Infection breaks T cell tolerance. *Nature* 1992; **359**: 79–82.
32 Morecki S, Leshem B, Eid A, Slavin S. Alloantigen persistence in induction and maintenance of transplantation tolerance. *J Exp Med* 1987; **165**: 1468–80.
33 Rocha B, Tanchot C, Von Boehmer H. Clonal anergy blocks *in vivo* growth of mature T cells and can be reversed in the absence of antigen. *J Exp Med* 1993; **177**: 1517–21.

34 Ramsdell F, Fowlkes BJ. Maintenance of *in vivo* tolerance by persistence of antigen. *Science* 1992; **257**: 1130–4.

35 Pape KA, Merica R, Mondino A, Khoruts A, Jenkins MK. Direct evidence that functionally impaired CD4+ T cells persist *in vivo* following induction of peripheral tolerance. *J Immunol* 1998; **160**: 4719–29.

36 Gao E-K, Lo D, Sprent J. Strong T cell tolerance in parent → F1 bone marrow chimeras prepared with supralethal irradiation. *J Exp Med* 1990; **171**: 1101–21.

37 Salaun J, Bandeira A, Khazaal I *et al*. Thymic epithelium tolerizes for histocompatibility antigens. *Science* 1990; **247**: 1471–4.

38 Burkly LC, Lo D, Flavell RA. Tolerance in transgenic mice expressing major histocompatibility molecules extrathymically on pancreatic cells. *Science* 1990; **248**: 1364–8.

39 Morahan G, Allison J, Miller JFAP. Tolerance of class I histocompatibility antigens expressed extrathymically. *Nature* 1989; **339**: 622–4.

40 Morahan G, Hoffman MW, Miller JFAP. A non-deletional mechanism of peripheral tolerance in T-cell receptor transgenic mice. *Proc Natl Acad Sci U S A* 1991; **88**: 11421–5.

41 Cobbold SP, Qin S, Waldmann H. Reprogramming the immune system for tolerance with monoclonal antibodies. *Sem Immunol* 1990; **2**: 377–87.

42 Ramsdell F, Lantz T, Fowlkes BJ. A nondeletional mechanism of thymic self tolerance. *Science* 1989; **246**: 1038–41.

43 Heath WR, Karamalis F, Donoghue J, Miller JFAP. Autoimmunity caused by ignorant CD8+ T cells is transient and depends on avidity. *J Immunol* 1995; **155**: 2339–49.

44 Hämmerling GJ, Schonrich G, Momburg F *et al*. Non-deletional mechanisms of peripheral and central tolerance: studies with transgenic mice with tissue-specific expression of a foreign MHC class I antigen. *Immunol Rev* 1991; **122**: 47–67.

45 Picarella DE, Kratz A, Li C, Ruddle NH, Flavell RA. Transgenic tumor necrosis factor (TNF)-α production in pancreatic islets leads to insulinitis, not diabetes: distinct patterns of inflammation in TNF-α and TNF-β transgenic mice. *J Immunol* 1993; **150**: 4136–50.

46 Heath WR, Allison J, Hoffman MW *et al*. Autoimmune diabetes as a consequence of locally produced interleukin-2. *Nature* 1992; **359**: 547–9.

47 von Herrath MG, Guerder S, Lewicki H, Flavell RA, Oldstone MBA. Coexpression of B7–1 and viral ("self") transgenes in pancreatic β cells can break peripheral ignorance and lead to spontaneous autoimmune diabetes. *Immunity* 1995; **3**: 727–38.

48 Roser BJ. Cellular mechanisms in neonatal and adult tolerance. *Immunol Rev* 1989; **107**: 179–202.

49 Tomita Y, Mayumi H, Eto M, Nomoto K. Importance of suppressor T cells in cyclophosphamide-induced tolerance to the non-H-2-encoded alloantigens. Is mixed chimerism really required in maintaining a skin allograft tolerance? *J Immunol* 1990; **144**: 463–73.

50 Tutschka PJ, Ki PF, Beschorner WE, Hess AD, Santos GW. Suppressor cells in transplantation tolerance. II. Maturation of suppressor cells in the bone marrow chimera. *Transplantation* 1981; **32**: 321–5.

51 Wilson DB. Idiotypic regulation of T cells in graft-versus-host disease and autoimmunity. *Immunol Rev* 1989; **107**: 159–76.

52 Koide J, Engleman EG. Differences in surface phenotype and mechanism of action between alloantigen-specific CD8+ cytotoxic and suppressor T cell clones. *J Immunol* 1990; **144**: 32–40.

53 Mossman TR, Coffman RL. TH1 and TH2 cells: Different patterns of lymphokine secretion lead to different functional properties. *Ann Rev Immunol* 1989; **7**: 145–73.

54 Salgame P, Abrams JS, Clayberger C, Goldstein H. Differing lymphokine profiles of functional subsets of human CD4 and CD8 T cell clones. *Science* 1991; **254**: 279–82.

55 Sad S, Marcotte R, Mosmann TR. Cytokine-induced differentiation of precursor mouse CD8+ T cells into cytotoxic CD8+ T cells secreting TH1 or TH2 cytokines. *Immunity* 1995; **2**: 271–9.

56 Lowry RP, Takeuchi T. *The TH1, TH2 Paradigm and Transplantation Tolerance*. Austin: R.G. Landes, 1994.

57 Donckier V, Wissing M, Bruyns C *et al*. Critical role of interleukin 4 in the induction of neonatal transplantation tolerance. *Transplantation* 1995; **59**: 1571–6.

58 Onodera K, Hancock WW, Graser E *et al*. Type 2 helper T cell-type cytokines and the development of "infectious" tolerance in rat cardiac allograft recipients. *J Immunol* 1997; **158**: 1572–81.

59 Zheng XX, Steele AW, Nickerson PW, Steurer W, Steiger J, Strom TB. Administration of noncytolytic IL-10/Fc in murine models of lipopolysaccharide-induced septic shock and allogeneic islet transplantation. *J Immunol* 1995; **154**: 5590–600.

60 Piccotti JR, Chan SY, VanBuskirk AM, Eichwald EJ, Bishop DK. Are TH2 helper T lymphocytes beneficial, deleterious, or irrelevant in promoting allograft survival? *Transplantation* 1997; **63**: 619–24.

61 Nickerson P, Steiger J, Zheng XX *et al*. Manipulation of cytokine networks in transplantation. *Transplantation* 1997; **63**: 489–94.

62 Groux H, Powrie F. Regulatory T cells and inflammatory bowel disease. *Immunol Today* 1999; **20**: 442–6.

63 Jonuleit H, Schmitt E, Schuler G, Knop J, Enk AH. Induction of interleukin 10-producing, nonproliferating CD4+ T cells with regulatory properties by repetitive stimulation with allogeneic immature human dendritic cells. *J Exp Med* 2000; **192**: 1213–22.

64 Shevach EM. Certified professionals: CD4+CD25+ suppressor T cells. *J Exp Med* 2001; **193**: F41–F46.

65 Sedon B, Mason D. The third function of the thymus. *Immunol Today* 2000; **21**: 95–9.

66 Piccirillo CA, Shevach EM. Cutting edge: control of CD8+ T cell activation by CD4+CD25+ immunoregulatory cells. *J Immunol* 2001; **167**: 1137–40.

67 Modigliani Y, Pereira P, Thomas-Vaslin V *et al*. Regulatory T cells in thymic epithelium-induced tolerance. I. suppression of mature peripheral non-tolerant T cells. *Eur J Immunol* 1995; **25**: 2563–71.

68 Jordan MS, Boesteanu A, Reed AJ *et al*. Thymic selection of CD4+CD25+ regulatory T cells induced by an agonist self-peptide. *Nat Immunol* 2001; **2**: 301–6.

69 Bensinger SJ, Bandeira A, Jordan MS, Caton AJ, Laufer TM. Major histocompatibility complex class II-positive cortical epithelium mediates the selection of CD4+25+ immunoregulatory T cells. *J Exp Med* 2001; **194**: 427–38.

70 Mars LT, Laloux V, Goude K *et al*. Cutting edge: Vα14-Jα281 NKT cells naturally regulate experimental autoimmune encephalomyelitis in nonobese diabetic mice. *J Immunol* 2002; **168**: 6007–11.

71 Zhang ZX, Yang L, Young KJ, DuTemple B, Zhang L. Identification of a previously unknown antigen-specific regulatory T cell and its mechanism of suppression. *Nat Med* 2000; **6**: 782–9.

72 Liu Z, Tugulea S, Cortesini R, Suciu-Foca N. Specific suppression of T helper alloreactivity by allo-MHC class I-restricted CD8+CD28– T cells. *Int Immunol* 1998; **10**: 775–83.

73 Lombardi G, Sidhu S, Batchelor R, Lechler R. Anergic T cells as suppressor cells *in vitro*. *Science* 1994; **264**: 1587–9.

74 Vendetti S, Chai JG, Dyson J, Simpson E, Lombardi G, Lechler R. Anergic T cells inhibit the antigen-presenting function of dendritic cells. *J Immunol* 2000; **165**: 1175–81.

75 Cobbold SP, Adams E, Marshall SE, Davies JD, Waldmann H. Mechanisms of peripheral tolerance and suppression induced by monoclonal antibodies to CD4 and CD8. *Immunol Rev* 1996; **149**: 5–34.

76 Beschorner WE, Shinn CA, Fischer AC, Santos GW, Hess AD. Cyclosporine-induced pseudograft-versus-host disease in the early post-cyclosporine period. *Transplantation* 1988; **46**: S112–S117.

77 Miller RG. The veto phenomenon and T-cell regulation. *Immunol Today* 1986; **7**: 112–4.

78 Rachamin N, Gan J, Segall H *et al*. Tolerance induction by "megadose" hematopoietic transplants: donor-type human CD34 stem cells induce potent specific reduction of host anti-donor cytotoxic T lymphocyte precursors in mixed lymphocyte culture. *Transplantation* 1998; **65**: 1386–93.

79 Gur H, Krauthgamer R, Berrebi A *et al*. Tolerance induction by megadose hematopoietic progenitor cells: expansion of veto cells by short-term culture of purified human CD34+ cells. *Blood* 2002; **99**: 4174–81.

80 Azuma E, Kaplan J. Role of lymphokine-activated killer cells as mediators of veto and natural suppression. *J Immunol* 1988; **141**: 2601–6.

81 Azuma E, Yamamoto H, Kaplan J. Use of lymphokine-activated killer cells to prevent bone marrow graft rejection and lethal graft-vs-host disease. *J Immunol* 1989; **143**: 1524–9.

82 Nakamura H, Gress RE. Interleukin 2 enhancement of veto suppressor cell function in T-cell-depleted bone marrow *in vitro* and *in vivo*. *Transplantation* 1990; **49**: 931–7.

83 Kast WM, Twuyver WM, Mooijaart RJD *et al*. Mechanism of skin allograft enhancement across an H-2 class I mutant difference. evidence for involvement of veto cells. *Eur J Immunol* 1988; **18**: 2105.

84 Heeg K, Wagner H. Induction of peripheral tolerance to class I major histocompatibility complex (MHC) alloantigens in adult mice: transfused class I MHC-incompatible splenocytes veto clonal response of antigen-reactive Lyt-2+ T cells. *J Exp Med* 1990; **172**: 719–28.

85 Sambhara SR, Miller RG. Programmed cell death of T cells signaled by the T cell receptor and the α-3 domain of class I MHC. *Science* 1991; **252**: 1424–7.

86 Kaplan DR, Hambor JE, Tykocinski ML. An immunoregulatory function for the CD8 molecule. *Proc Natl Acad Sci U S A* 1989; **86**: 8512–5.

87 Verbanac KM, Carver FM, Haisch CE, Thomas JM. A role for transforming growth factor-β in the

88 Maier T, Holda JH, Claman HN. Natural suppressor (NS) cells. Members of the LGL regulatory family. *Immunol Today* 1986; **7**: 312–5.

89 Dorshkind K, Rosse C. Physical, biologic, and phenotypic properties of natural regulatory cells in murine bone marrow. *Am J Anat* 1982; **164**: 1–17.

90 Sykes M, Sharabi Y, Sachs DH. Natural suppressor cells in spleens of irradiated, bone marrow reconstituted mice and normal bone marrow: lack of Sca-1 expression and enrichment by depletion of Mac1-positive cells. *Cell Immunol* 1990; **127**: 260–74.

91 Mortari F, Bains MA, Singhal SK. Immunoregulatory activity of human bone marrow. identification of suppressor cells possessing OKM1, SSEA-1, and HNK-1 antigens. *J Immunol* 1986; **137**: 1133–7.

92 Sugiura K, Ikehara S, Gengozian N et al. Enrichment of natural suppressor activity in a wheat germ agglutinin positive hematopoietic progenitor-enriched fraction of monkey bone marrow. *Blood* 1990; **75**: 1125–31.

93 Sykes M, Hoyles KA, Romick ML, Sachs DH. In vitro and in vivo analysis of bone marrow derived $CD3^+$, $CD4^-$, $CD8^-$, $NK1.1^+$ cell lines. *Cell Immunol* 1990; **129**: 478–93.

94 Hertel-Wulff B, Lindsten T, Schwadron R, Gilbert DM, Davis MM, Strober S. Rearrangement and expression of T cell receptor genes in cloned murine natural suppressor cell lines. *J Exp Med* 1987; **166**: 1168–73.

95 Yamamoto H, Hirayama M, Genyea C, Kaplan J. TGF-β mediates natural suppressor activity of IL-2-activated lymphocytes. *J Immunol* 1994; **152**: 3842–7.

96 Langrehr JM, Hoffman RA, Lancaster JR, JrSimmons RL. Nitric oxide: a new endogenous immunomodulator. *Transplantation* 1993; **55**: 1205–12.

97 Snijdewint FGM, Kalinski P, Wierenga EA, Bos JD, Kapsenberg ML. Prostaglandin E2 differentially modulates cytokine secretion profiles of human T helper lymphocytes. *J Immunol* 1993; **150**: 5321–9.

98 Okada S, Strober S. Spleen cells from adult mice given total lymphoid irradiation or from newborn mice have similar regulatory effects in the mixed leukocyte reaction. I. Generation of antigen-specific cells in the mixed leukocyte reaction after the addition of spleen cells from adult mice given total lymphoid irradiation. *J Exp Med* 1982; **156**: 522–38.

99 Klinman NR. The "clonal selection hypothesis" and current concepts of B cell tolerance. *Immunity* 1996; **5**: 189–95.

100 Nemazee D. Antigen receptor "capacity" and the sensitivity of self-tolerance. *Immunol Today* 1996; **17**: 25–9.

101 Pelanda R, Schwers S, Sonoda E, Torres RM, Nemazee D, Rajewsky K. Receptor editing in a transgenic mouse model. Site, efficiency, and role in B cell tolerance and antibody diversification. *Immunity* 1997; **7**: 765–75.

102 Fang W, Weintraub BC, Dunlap B et al. Self-reactive B lymphocytes overexpressing Bcl-xL escape negative selection and are tolerized by clonal anergy and receptor editing. *Immunity* 1998; **9**: 35–45.

103 Benschop RJ, Aviszus K, Zhang X, Manser T, Cambier JC, Wysocki LJ. Activation and anergy in bone marrow B cells of a novel immunoglobulin transgenic mouse that is both hapten specific and autoreactive. *Immunity* 2001; **14**: 33–43.

104 Cooke MP, Heath AW, Shokat KM et al. Immunoglobulin signal transduction guides the specificity of B cell–T cell interactions and is blocked in tolerant self-reactive B cells. *J Exp Med* 1994; **179**: 425–38.

105 Ohdan H, Swenson KG, Kruger-Gray HW et al. Mac-1-negative B-1b phenotype of natural antibody-producing cells, including those responding to Galα1,3Gal epitopes in α1,3-galactosyltransferase deficient mice. *J Immunol* 2000; **165**: 5518–29.

106 Murakami M, Tsubata T, Okamoto M et al. Antigen-induced apoptotic death of Ly-1 B cells responsible for autoimmune disease in transgenic mice. *Nature* 1992; **357**: 77–80.

107 Alters SE, Shizuru JA, Ackerman J, Grossman D, Seydel KB, Fathman CG. Anti-CD4 mediates clonal anergy during transplantation tolerance induction. *J Exp Med* 1991; **173**: 491–4.

108 Waldmann H, Cobbold S. The use of monoclonal antibodies to achieve immunological tolerance. *Immunol Today* 1993; **14**: 247–51.

109 Tomita Y, Khan A, Sykes M. Role of intrathymic clonal deletion and peripheral anergy in transplantation tolerance induced by bone marrow transplantation in mice conditioned with a nonmyeloablative regimen. *J Immunol* 1994; **153**: 1087–98.

110 Pearson TC, Madsen JC, Larsen CP, Morris PJ, Wood KJ. Induction of transplantation tolerance in adults using donor antigen and anti-CD4 monoclonal antibody. *Transplantation* 1992; **54**: 475–83.

111 Wong W, Morris PJ, Wood KJ. Syngeneic bone marrow expressing a single donor class I MHC molecule permits acceptance of a fully allogeneic cardiac allograft. *Transplantation* 1996; **62**: 1462–8.

112 Eynon EE, Parker DC. Small B cells as antigen-presenting cells in the induction of tolerance to soluble protein antigens. *J Exp Med* 1992; **175**: 131–8.

113 Fuchs EJ, Matzinger P. B cells turn off virgin but not memory T cells. *Science* 1992; **258**: 1156–9.

114 Sonntag KC, Emery DW, Yasumoto A et al. Tolerance to solid organ transplants through transfer of MHC class II genes. *J Clin Invest* 2001; **107**: 65–71.

115 Hara M, Kingsley CI, Niimi M et al. IL-10 is required for regulatory T cells to mediate tolerance to alloantigens in vivo. *J Immunol* 2001; **166**: 3789–96.

116 Bushell A, Niimi M, Morris PJ, Wood KJ. Evidence for immune regulation in the induction of transplantation tolerance: a conditional but limited role for IL-4. *J Immunol* 1999; **162**: 1359–66.

117 Kobata T, Ohnishi Y, Urushibara N, Takahashi TA, Sekiguchi S. UV irradiation can induce in vitro clonal anergy in alloreactive cytotoxic T lymphocytes. *Blood* 1993; **82**: 176–81.

118 Hackstein H, Morelli AE, Thomson AW. Designer dendritic cells for tolerance induction: guided not misguided missiles. *Trends Immunol* 2001; **22**: 437–42.

119 Pearson TC, Alexander DZ, Winn KJ, Linsley PS, Lowry RP, Larsen CP. Transplantation tolerance induced by CTLA4Ig. *Transplantation* 1994; **57**: 1701–6.

120 Lanzavecchia A. Licence to kill. *Nature* 1998; **393**: 413–4.

121 Parker DC, Greiner DL, Phillips NE et al. Survival of mouse pancreatic islet allografts in recipients treated with allogeneic small lymphocytes and antibody to CD40 ligand. *Proc Natl Acad Sci U S A* 1995; **92**: 9560–4.

122 Markees TG, Phillips NE, Noelle RJ et al. Prolonged survival of mouse skin allografts in recipients treated with donor splenocytes and antibody to CD40 ligand. *Transplantation* 1997; **64**: 329–35.

123 Iwakoshi NN, Markees TG, Turgeon N et al. Skin allograft maintenance in a new synchimeric model system of tolerance. *J Immunol* 2001; **167**: 6623–30.

124 Markees TG, Phillips NE, Gordon EJ et al. Long-term survival of skin allografts induced by donor splenocytes and anti-CD154 antibody in thymectomized mice requires $CD4^+$ T cells, interferon-γ, and CTLA4. *J Clin Invest* 1998; **101**: 2446–55.

125 Gordon EJ, Woda BA, Shultz LD, Rossini AA, Greiner DL, Mordes JP. Rat xenograft survival in mice treated with donor-specific transfusion and anti-CD154 antibody is enhanced by elimination of host $CD4^+$ cells. *Transplantation* 2001; **71**: 319–27.

126 Larsen CP, Alexander DZ, Hollenbaugh D et al. CD40–2GP39 interactions play a critical role during allograft rejection: suppression of allograft rejection by blockade of the CD40-gp39 pathway. *Transplantation* 1996; **61**: 4–9.

127 Ensminger SM, Spriewald BM, Witzke O et al. Intragraft interleukin-4 mRNA expression after short-term CD154 blockade may trigger delayed development of transplant arteriosclerosis in the absence of $CD8^+$ T cells. *Transplantation* 2000; **70**: 955–63.

128 Sayegh MH, Akalin E, Hancock WW et al. CD28-B7 blockade after alloantigenic challenge in vivo inhibits TH1 cytokines but spares TH2. *J Exp Med* 1995; **181**: 1869–74.

129 Larsen CP, Elwood ET, Alexander DZ et al. Long-term acceptance of skin and cardiac allografts after blocking CD40 and CD28 pathways. *Nature* 1996; **381**: 434–8.

130 Kirk AD, Harlan DM, Armstrong NN et al. CTLA4-Ig and anti-CD40 ligand prevent renal allograft rejection in primates. *Proc Natl Acad Sci U S A* 1997; **94**: 8789–98.

131 Elwood ET, Larsen CP, Cho HR et al. Prolonged acceptance of concordant and discordant xenografts with combined CD40 and CD28 pathway blockade. *Transplantation* 1998; **65**: 1422–8.

132 Li Y, Zheng XX, Li XC, Zand MS, Strom TB. Combined costimulation blockade plus rapamycin but not cyclosporine produces permanent engraftment. *Transplantation* 1998; **66**: 1387–8.

133 Lehnert AM, Yi S, Burgess JS, O'Connell PJ. Pancreatic islet xenograft tolerance after short-term costimulation blockade is associated with increased $CD4^+$ T cell apoptosis but not immune deviation. *Transplantation* 2000; **69**: 1176–85.

134 Tramblay J, Bingaman AW, Lin A et al. Asialo $GM1^+$ $CD8^+$ T cells play a critical role in costimulation blockade-resistant allograft rejection. *J Clin Invest* 1999; **104**: 1715–22.

135 Kenyon NS, Chatzipetrou M, Masetti M et al. Long-term survival and function of intrahepatic islet allografts in rhesus monkeys treated with humanized anti-CD154. *Proc Natl Acad Sci U S A* 1999; **96**: 8132–7.

136 Kirk AD, Burkly LC, Batty DS *et al*. Treatment with humanized monoclonal antibody against CD154 prevents acute renal allograft rejection in nonhuman primates. *Nature Med* 1999; **5**: 686–93.

137 Ito H, Kurtz J, Shaffer J, Sykes M. CD4 T cell-mediated alloresistance to fully MHC-mismatched allogeneic bone marrow engraftment is dependent on CD40–CD40L interactions, and lasting T cell tolerance is induced by bone marrow transplantation with initial blockade of this pathway. *J Immunol* 2001; **166**: 2970–81.

138 Williams MA, Trambley J, Ha J *et al*. Genetic characterization of strain differences in the ability to mediate CD40/CD28-independent rejection of skin allografts. *J Immunol* 2000; **165**: 6849–57.

139 Li Y, Li XC, Zheng XX, Wells AD, Turka LA, Strom TB. Blocking both signal 1 and signal 2 of T-cell activation prevents apoptosis of alloreactive T cells and induction of peripheral allograft tolerance. *Nature Med* 1999; **5**: 1298–302.

140 Lakkis FG, Dai Z. The role of cytokines, CTLA-4 and costimulation in transplant tolerance and rejection. *Curr Opin Immunol* 1999; **11**: 504–8.

141 Li XC, Li Y, Dodge I *et al*. Induction of allograft tolerance in the absence of Fas-mediated apoptosis. *J Immunol* 1999; **163**: 2500–7.

142 Wagener ME, Konieczny BT, Dai Z, Ring GH, Lakkis FG. Alloantigen-driven T cell death mediated by Fas ligand and tumor necrosis factor-alpha is not essential for the induction of allograft acceptance. *Transplantation* 2000; **69**: 2428–32.

143 Hassan AT, Dai Z, Konieczny BT *et al*. Regulation of alloantigen-mediated T-cell proliferation by endogenous interferon-γ. *Transplantation* 1999; **68**: 124–9.

144 Honey K, Cobbold SP, Waldmann H. CD40 ligand blockade induces CD4+ T cell tolerance and linked suppression. *J Immunol* 1999; **163**: 4805–10.

145 Graca L, Honey K, Adams E, Cobbold SP, Waldmann H. Cutting edge: anti-CD154 therapeutic antibodies induce infectious transplantation tolerance. *J Immunol* 2000; **165**: 4783–6.

146 Tran HM, Nickerson PW, Restifo AC *et al*. Distinct mechanisms for the induction and maintenance of allograft tolerance with CTLA4-Fc treatment. *J Immunol* 1997; **159**: 2232–9.

147 Pescovitz MD, Sachs DH, Lunney JK, Hsu SM. Localization of class II MHC antigens on porcine renal vascular endothelium. *Transplantation* 1984; **37**: 627–30.

148 Choo JK, Seebach JD, Nickeleit V *et al*. Species differences in the expression of major histocompatibility complex class II antigens on coronary artery endothelium: implications for cell-mediated xenoreactivity. *Transplantation* 1997; **64**: 1315–22.

149 Homan WP, Fabre JW, Williams KA, Millard PR, Morris PJ. Studies on immunosuppressive properties of cyclosporin A in rats receiving renal allografts. *Transplantation* 1980; **29**: 361–6.

150 Rosengard BR, Ojikutu CA, Guzzetta PC *et al*. Induction of specific tolerance to class I disparate renal allografts in miniature swine with cyclosporine. *Transplantation* 1992; **54**: 490–7.

151 Gianello PR, Yamada K, Fishbein JM *et al*. Long-term acceptance of primarily vascularized renal allografts in miniature swine. *Transplantation* 1996; **61**: 503–22.

152 Charlton B, Auchincloss H, Jr, Fathman CG. Mechanisms of transplantation tolerance. *Ann Rev Immunol* 1994; **12**: 707–34.

153 Bashuda H, Seino K, Ra C, Yagita H, Okumura K. Lack of cognate help by CD4+ T cells and anergy of CD8+ T cells are the principal mechanisms for anti-leukocyte function-associated antigen-1/intercellular adhesion molecule-1-induced cardiac allograft tolerance. *Transplantation* 1997; **63**: 113–8.

154 Xu XY, Honjo K, Devore-Carter D, Bucy RP. Immunosuppression by inhibition of cellular adhesion mediated by leukocyte function-associated antigen-1/intercellular adhesion molecule-1 in murine cardiac transplantation. *Transplantation* 1997; **63**: 876–85.

155 Bashuda H, Seino K, Ra C, Yagita H, Okumura K. Lack of cognate help by CD4+ T cells and anergy of CD8+ T cells are the principal mechanisms for anti-leukocyte function-associated antigen-1/intercellular adhesion molecule-1-induced cardiac allograft tolerance. *Transplantation* 1997; **63**: 113–8.

156 Sprent J. Stimulating naive T cells. *J Immunol* 1999; **163**: 4629–36.

157 Yang H, Issekutz TB, Wright JR, Jr. Prolongation of rat islet allograft survival by treatment with monoclonal antibodies against VLA-4 and LFA-1. *Transplantation* 1995; **60**: 71–6.

158 Chavin KD, Qin L, Lin J, Yagita H, Bromberg JS. Combined anti-CD2 and anti-CD3 receptor monoclonal antibodies induce donor-specific tolerance in a cardiac transplant model. *J Immunol* 1993; **151**: 7249–59.

159 Krieger NR, Most D, Bromberg JS *et al*. Coexistence of TH1- and TH2-type cytokine profiles in anti-CD2 monoclonal antibody-induced tolerance. *Transplantation* 1996; **62**: 1285–92.

160 Woodward JE, Qin L, Chavin KD *et al*. Blockade of multiple costimulatory receptors induces hyporesponsiveness: inhibition of CD2 plus CD28 pathways. *Transplantation* 1996; **62**: 1011–8.

161 Rothstein DM, Livak MF, Kishimoto K *et al*. Targeting signal 1 through CD45RB synergizes with CD40 ligand blockade and promotes long term engraftment and tolerance in stringent transplant models. *J Immunol* 2001; **166**: 322–9.

162 Myburgh JA, Meyers AM, Thomson PD *et al*. Total lymphoid irradiation: current status. *Transplant Proc* 1989; **21**: 826–8.

163 Najarian JS, Ferguson RM, Sutherland DER *et al*. Fractionated total lymphoid irradiation as preparative immunosuppression in high risk renal transplantation. *Ann Surg* 1982; **196**: 442–51.

164 Myburgh JA, Meyers AM, Margolius L *et al*. Total lymphoid irradiation in clinical renal transplantation: results in 73 patients. *Transplant Proc* 1991; **23**: 2033–4.

165 Strober S, Benike C, Krishnaswamy S, Engleman EG, Grumet FC. Clinical transplantation tolerance twelve years after prospective withdrawal of immunosuppressive drugs: studies of chimerism and anti-donor reactivity. *Transplantation* 2000; **69**: 1549–54.

166 Thomas J, Alqaisi M, Cunningham P *et al*. The development of a posttransplant TLI treatment strategy that promotes organ allograft acceptance without chronic immunosuppression. *Transplantation* 1992; **53**: 247–58.

167 Strober S, Modry DL, Moppe RT *et al*. Induction of specific unresponsiveness to heart allografts in mongrel dogs treated with total lymphoid irradiation and anti-thymocyte globulin. *J Immunol* 1984; **132**: 1013–8.

168 Yamada K, Gianello PR, Ierено FL *et al*. Role of the thymus in transplantation tolerance in miniature swine. I. Requirement of the thymus for rapid and stable induction of tolerance to class I-mismatched renal allografts. *J Exp Med* 1997; **186**: 497–506.

169 Agus DB, Surh CD, Sprent J. Reentry of T cells to the adult thymus is restricted to activated T cells. *J Exp Med* 1991; **173**: 1039–46.

170 Pearce NW, Spinelli A, Gurley KE, Hall BM. Specific unresponsiveness in rats with prolonged cardiac allograft survival after treatment with cyclosporine. V. Dependence of CD4+ suppressor cells on the presence of alloantigen and cytokines, including interleukin-2. *Transplantation* 1993; **55**: 374–9.

171 Oluwole SF, Jin M-X, Chowdhury NC, Ohajewkwe OA. Effectiveness of intrathymic inoculation of soluble antigens in the induction of specific unresponsiveness to rat islet allografts without transient recipient immunosuppression. *Transplantation* 1994; **58**: 1077–81.

172 Sayegh MH, Perico N, Gallon L *et al*. Mechanisms of acquired thymic unresponsiveness to renal allografts. Thymic recognition of immunodominant allo-MHC peptides induces peripheral T cell anergy. *Transplantation* 1994; **58**: 125–32.

173 Ali A, Garrovillo M, Oluwole OO *et al*. Mechanisms of acquired thymic tolerance: induction of transplant tolerance by adoptive transfer of *in vivo* alloMHC peptide activated syngeneic T cells. *Transplantation* 2001; **71**: 1442–8.

174 Odorico JS, O'Connor T, Campos L, Barker CF, Posselt AM, Naji A. Examination of the mechanisms responsible for tolerance induction after intrathymic inoculation of allogeneic bone marrow. *Ann Surg* 1993; **218**: 525–31.

175 Sharabi Y, Sachs DH. Mixed chimerism and permanent specific transplantation tolerance induced by a non-lethal preparative regimen. *J Exp Med* 1989; **169**: 493–502.

176 Khan A, Tomita Y, Sykes M. Thymic dependence of loss of tolerance in mixed allogeneic bone marrow chimeras after depletion of donor antigen. Peripheral mechanisms do not contribute to maintenance of tolerance. *Transplantation* 1996; **62**: 380–7.

177 Lee LA, Sergio JJ, Sykes M. Evidence for non-immune mechanisms in the loss of hematopoietic chimerism in rat-mouse mixed xenogeneic chimeras. *Xenotransplant* 1995; **2**: 57–66.

178 Tomita Y, Sachs DH, Sykes M. Myelosuppressive conditioning is required to achieve engraftment of pluripotent stem cells contained in moderate doses of syngeneic bone marrow. *Blood* 1994; **83**: 939–48.

179 Ramshaw HS, Crittenden RB, Dooner M, Peters SO, Rao SS, Quesenberry PJ. High levels of engraftment with a single infusion of bone marrow cells into normal unprepared mice. *Biol Blood Marrow Transplant* 1995; **1**: 74–80.

180 Sykes M, Szot GL, Swenson K, Pearson DA, Wekerle T. Separate regulation of hematopoietic and thymic engraftment. *Exp Hematol* 1997; **26**: 457–65.

181 Sykes M, Szot GL, Swenson K, Pearson DA. Induction of high levels of allogeneic hematopoietic reconstitution and donor-specific tolerance without myelosuppressive conditioning. *Nature Med* 1997; **3**: 783–7.

182 Wekerle T, Kurtz J, Ito H *et al*. Allogeneic bone marrow transplantation with costimulatory blockade induces macrochimerism and tolerance without cytoreductive host treatment. *Nature Med* 2000; **6**: 464–9.

183 Sharabi Y, Sachs DH, Sykes M. T cell subsets resisting induction of mixed chimerism across various histocompatibility barriers. In: Gergely J, Benczur M, Falus A, Fust Gy, Medgyesi G, Petranyi Gy et al., eds. *Progress in Immunology VIII. Proceedings of the Eighth International Congress of Immunology, Budapest, 1992.* Heidelberg: Springer-Verlag, 1992: 801–5.

184 Hayashi H, LeGuern C, Sachs DH, Sykes M. Alloresistance to K locus mismatched bone marrow engraftment is mediated entirely by CD4[+] and CD8[+] T cells. *Bone Marrow Transplant* 1996; **18**: 285–92.

185 Vallera DA, Taylor PA, Sprent J, Blazar BR. The role of host T cell subsets in bone marrow rejection directed to isolated major histocompatibility complex class I versus class II differences of bm1 and bm12 mutant mice. *Transplantation* 1994; **57**: 249–56.

186 Morita H, Sugiura K, Inaba M et al. A strategy for organ allografts without using immunosuppressants or irradiation. *Proc Natl Acad Sci U S A* 1998; **95**: 6947–52.

187 Fandrich F, Lin X, Chai GX et al. Preimplantation-stage stem cells induce long-term allogeneic graft acceptance without supplementary host conditioning. *Nat Med* 2002; **8**: 171–8.

188 Jin T, Toki J, Inaba M et al. A novel strategy for organ allografts using sublethal (7 Gy) irradiation followed by injection of donor bone marrow cells via portal vein. *Transplantation* 2001; **71**: 1725–31.

189 Moretta L, Ciccone E, Moretta A, Hoglund P, Ohlen C, Karre K. Allorecognition by NK cells: nonself or no self? *Immunol Today* 1992; **13**: 300–6.

190 Kiessling R, Hochman PS, Haller O, Shearer GM, Wigzell H, Cudkowicz G. Evidence for a similar or common mechanism for natural killer activity and resistance to hemopoietic grafts. *Eur J Immunol* 1977; **7**: 655–63.

191 Lee LA, Sergio JJ, Sykes M. Natural killer cells weakly resist engraftment of allogeneic long-term multilineage-repopulating hematopoietic stem cells. *Transplantation* 1996; **61**: 125–32.

192 Aguila HL, Weissman IL. Hematopoietic stem cells are not direct cytotoxic targets of natural killer cells. *Blood* 1996; **87**: 1225–31.

193 Kawai T, Wee SL, Phelan J et al. Association of natural killer cell depletion with induction of mixed chimerism and allograft tolerance in non-human primates. *Transplantation* 2000; **72**: 368–74.

194 Ruggeri L, Capanni M, Urbani E et al. Effectiveness of donor natural killer cell alloreactivity in mismatched hematopoietic transplants. *Science* 2002; **295**: 2097–100.

195 O'Reilly RJ, Brochstein J, Collins N et al. Evaluation of HLA-haplotype disparate parental marrow grafts depleted of T lymphocytes by differential agglutination with a soybean lectin and E-rosette depletion for the treatment of severe combined immunodeficiency. *Vox Sang* 1986; **51**: 81–6.

196 Sykes M, Harty MW, Karlhofer FM, Pearson DA, Szot G, Yokoyama W. Hematopoietic cells and radioresistant host elements influence natural killer cell differentiation. *J Exp Med* 1993; **178**: 223–9.

197 Manilay JO, Waneck GL, Sykes M. Altered expression of Ly-49 receptors on natural killer cells developing in mixed allogeneic bone marrow chimeras. *Int Immunol* 1998; **10**: 1943–55.

198 Manilay JO, Waneck GL, Sykes M. Levels of Ly-49 receptor expression are determined by the frequency of interactions with MHC ligands: evidence against receptor calibration to a "useful" level. *J Immunol* 1999; **163**: 2628–33.

199 Zhao Y, Ohdan H, Manilay JO, Sykes M. NK cell tolerance in mixed allogeneic chimeras. *J Immunol* 2003; **170**: 5398–405.

200 Kung SKP, Miller RG. Mouse natural killer subsets defined by their target specificity and their ability to be separately rendered unresponsive *in vivo*. *J Immunol* 1997; **158**: 2616–26.

201 Johansson MH, Bieberich C, Jay G, Karre K, Hoglund P. Natural killer cell tolerance in mice with mosaic expression of major histocompatibility complex I transgene. *J Exp Med* 1997; **186**: 353–64.

202 Bensinger WI, Dean Buckner C, Donnall Thomas E, Clift RA. ABO-incompatible marrow transplants. *Transplantation* 1982; **33**: 427–9.

203 Barge AJ, Johnson G, Witherspoon R, Torok-Storb B. Antibody-mediated marrow failure after allogeneic bone marrow transplantation. *Blood* 1989; **74**: 1477–80.

204 Galili U. Evolution and pathophysiology of the human natural anti-α-galactosyl IgG (anti-Gal) antibody. *Springer Semin Immunopathol* 1993; **15**: 155–71.

205 Aksentijevich I, Sachs DH, Sykes M. Natural antibodies can inhibit bone marrow engraftment in the rat → mouse species combination. *J Immunol* 1991; **147**: 4140–6.

206 Yang Y-G, deGoma E, Ohdan H et al. Tolerization of anti-Galα1,3Gal natural antibody-forming B cells by induction of mixed chimerism. *J Exp Med* 1998; **187**: 1335–42.

207 Ohdan H, Yang Y-G, Shimizu A, Swenson KG, Sykes M. Mixed bone marrow chimerism induced without lethal conditioning prevents T cell and anti-Galα1,3Gal antibody-mediated heart graft rejection. *J Clin Invest* 1999; **104**: 281–90.

208 Ohdan H, Yang Y-G, Swenson KG, Kitamura H, Sykes M. T cell and B cell tolerance to Galα1,3Gal-expressing heart xenografts is achieved in α1,3-galactosyltransferase-deficient mice by nonmyeloablative induction of mixed chimerism. *Transplantation* 2001; **71**: 1532–42.

209 Ohdan H, Swenson KG, Kitamura H, Yang Y-G, Sykes M. Tolerization of Galα1,3Gal-reactive B cells in presensitized α1,3-Galactosyltransferase-deficient mice by non-myeloablative induction of mixed chimerism. *Xenotransplant* 2002; **8**: 227–38.

210 Anasetti C, Amos D, Beatty PG et al. Effect of HLA compatibility on engraftment of bone marrow transplants in patients with leukemia or lymphoma. *New Engl J Med* 1989; **320**: 197–204.

211 Fulop GM, Phillips RA. Full reconstitution of the immune deficiency in SCID mice with normal stem cells requires low-dose irradiation of the recipients. *J Immunol* 1986; **136**: 4438–43.

212 Owen RD. Immunogenetic consequences of vascular anastomoses between bovine twins. *Science* 1945; **102**: 400–1.

213 Billingham RE, Brent L, Medawar PB. "Actively acquired tolerance" of foreign cells. *Nature* 1953; **172**: 603–6.

214 Flake AW, Roncarolo M-G, Puck JM et al. Treatment of X-linked severe combined immunodeficiency by *in utero* transplantation of paternal bone marrow. *New Engl J Med* 1996; **335**: 1806–10.

215 Carrier E, Lee TH, Busch MP, Cowan MJ. Induction of tolerance in nondefective mice after *in utero* transplantation of major histocompatibility complex-mismatched fetal hematopoietic stem cells. *Blood* 1995; **86**: 4681–90.

216 Mathes DW, Yamada K, Randolph MA et al. In utero induction of transplantation tolerance. *Transplant Proc* 2001; **33**: 98–100.

217 De Villartay J-P, Griscelli C, Fischer A. Self-tolerance to host and donor following HLA-mismatched bone marrow transplantation. *Eur J Immunol* 1986; **16**: 117–22.

218 Lubaroff DM, Silvers WK. The importance of chimerism in maintaining tolerance of skin allografts in mice. *J Immunol* 1973; **111**: 65–71.

219 Streilein JW. Neonatal tolerance of H-2 alloantigens. *Transplantation* 1991; **52**: 1–10.

220 Speiser DE, Schneider R, Hengartner H, MacDonald HR, Zinkernagel RM. Clonal deletion of self-reactive T cells in irradiation bone marrow chimeras and neonatally tolerant mice. Evidence for intercellular transfer of Mlsa. *J Exp Med* 1989; **170**: 595–600.

221 Alard P, Matriano JA, Socarras S, Ortega M-A, Streilein JW. Detection of donor-derived cells by polymerase chain reaction in neonatally tolerant mice. Microchimerism fails to predict tolerance. *Transplantation* 1995; **60**: 1125–30.

222 Smith JP, Kasten-Jolly J, Field LJ, Thomas JM. Assessment of donor bone marrow cell-derived chimerism in transplantation tolerance using transgenic mice. *Transplantation* 1994; **58**: 324–9.

223 Ramseier H. Immunization against abolition of transplantation tolerance. *Eur J Immunol* 1973; **3**: 156–64.

224 Billingham RE, Brent L, Medawar PB. Quantitative studies on tissue transplantation immunity. III. Actively acquired tolerance. *Philos Trans Royal Soc* 1955; **239**: 44.

225 Gruchalla RS, Strome PG, Streilein JW. Analysis of neonatally induced tolerance of H-2 alloantigens. III. Ease of abolition of tolerance of class I, but not class II, antigens with infusions of syngeneic, immunocompetent cells. *Transplantation* 1983; **36**: 318–23.

226 Sykes M, Sheard MA, Sachs DH. Effects of T cell depletion in radiation bone marrow chimeras II. Requirement for allogeneic T cells in the reconstituting bone marrow inoculum for subsequent resistance to breaking of tolerance. *J Exp Med* 1988; **168**: 661–73.

227 Chen N, Field EH. Enhanced type 2 and diminished type 1 cytokines in neonatal tolerance. *Transplantation* 1995; **59**: 933–41.

228 Sarzotti M, Robbins DS, Hoffman PM. Induction of protective CTL responses in newborn mice by a murine retrovirus. *Science* 1996; **271**: 1726–8.

229 Forsthuber T, Yip HC, Lehmann PV. Induction of T$_H$1 and T$_H$2 immunity in neonatal mice. *Science* 1996; **271**: 1728–30.

230 Ridge JP, Fuchs EJ, Matzinger P. Neonatal tolerance revisited. Turning on newborn T cells with dendritic cells. *Science* 1996; **271**: 1723–6.

231 Sykes M, Sheard M, Sachs DH. Effects of T cell depletion in radiation bone marrow chimeras. I. Evidence for a donor cell population which increases allogeneic chimerism but which lacks the potential to produce GVHD. *J Immunol* 1988; **141**: 2282–8.

232 Ildstad ST, Sachs DH. Reconstitution with syngeneic plus allogeneic or xenogeneic bone marrow leads to specific acceptance of allografts or xenografts. *Nature* 1984; **307**: 168–70.

233 Ildstad ST, Wren SM, Bluestone JA, Barbieri SA, Sachs DH. Characterization of mixed allogeneic chimeras. Immunocompetence, *in vitro* reactivity, genetic specificity of tolerance. *J Exp Medical* 1985; **162**: 231–44.

234 Sykes M. Mixed chimerism and transplant tolerance. *Immunity* 2001; **14**: 417–24.

235 Markert ML, Boeck A, Hale LP *et al.* Transplantation of thymus tissue in complete DiGeorge syndrome. *New Engl J Med* 1999; **341**: 1180–9.

236 Zhao Y, Fishman JA, Sergio JJ *et al.* Immune restoration by fetal pig thymus grafts in T cell-depleted, thymectomized mice. *J Immunol* 1997; **158**: 1641–9.

237 Slavin S. Total lymphoid irradiation. *Immunol Today* 1987; **3**: 88–92.

238 Bass H, Mosmann T, Strober S. Evidence for mouse TH1 and TH1 helper T cells *in vivo*: selective reduction of TH1 cells after total lymphoid irradiation. *J Exp Med* 1989; **170**: 1495–511.

239 Zeng D, Ready A, Huie P *et al.* Mechanisms of tolerance to rat heart allografts using posttransplant TLI. *Transplantation* 1996; **62**: 510–7.

240 Lan F, Zeng D, Higuchi M, Huie P, Higgins JP, Strober S. Predominance of NK1.1$^+$TCR$\alpha\beta^+$ or DX5$^+$TCR$\alpha\beta^+$ T cells in mice conditioned with fractionated lymphoid irradiation protects against graft-versus-host disease: "natural suppressor" cells. *J Immunol* 2001; **167**: 2087–96.

241 Raaf J, Monden M, Bray A *et al.* Bone marrow and renal transplantation in canine recipients prepared by total lymphoid irradiation. *Transplant Proc* 1981; **13**: 429–33.

242 Myburgh JA, Smit JA, Browde S. Transplantation tolerance in the primate following total lymphoid irradiation (TLI) and bone marrow (BM) injection. *Transplant Proc* 1981; **13**: 434–8.

243 Gottlieb M, Strober S, Hoppe RT, Grumet FG, Kaplan HS. Engraftment of allogeneic bone marrow without graft-versus-host disease in mongrel dogs using total lymphoid irradiation. *Transplantation* 1980; **29**: 487–91.

244 Millan MT, Shizuru JA, Hoffmann P *et al.* Mixed chimerism and immunosuppressive drug withdrawal after HLA-mismatched kidney and hematopoietic progenitor transplantation. *Transplantation* 2002; **73**: 1386–91.

245 Sachs DH, Sharabi Y, Sykes M. Mixed chimerism and transplantation tolerance. In: Melchers F, Albert ED, Von Boehmer H, eds. *Progress in Immunology*, Vol. VII. Berlin, Heidelberg: Springer-Verlag, 1989; 1171–6.

246 Rapaport FT, Bachvaroff RJ, Akiyama N, Sato T, Ferrebee JW. Specific allogeneic unresponsiveness in irradiated dogs reconstituted with autologous bone marrow. *Transplantation* 1980; **30**: 23–30.

247 Moses RD, Orr KS, Bacher JD, Sachs DH, Clark RE, Gress RE. Cardiac allograft survival across major histocompatibility barriers in the rhesus monkey following T cell-depleted autologous marrow transplantation. II. Prolonged allograft survival with extensive marrow T cell depletion. *Transplantation* 1989; **47**: 435.

248 Norin AJ, Emeson EE. Effects of restoring lethally irradiated mice with anti-Thy1.2-treated bone marrow: graft-vs-host, host-vs-graft, and mitogen reactivity. *J Immunol* 1978; **120**: 754–8.

249 Gao E-K, Kosaka H, Surh CD, Sprent J. T cell contact with Ia antigens on nonhematopoietic cells *in vivo* can lead to immunity rather than tolerance. *J Exp Med* 1991; **174**: 435–46.

250 Bagley J, Tian C, Sachs DH, Iacomini J. Induction of T-cell tolerance to an MHC class I alloantigen by gene therapy. *Blood* 2002; **99**: 4394–9.

251 Clift RA, Storb R. Histoincompatible bone marrow transplants in humans. *Ann Rev Immunol* 1987; **5**: 43–64.

252 Sykes M, Chester CH, Sundt TM, Romick ML, Hoyles KA, Sachs DH. Effects of T cell depletion in radiation bone marrow chimeras. III. Characterization of allogeneic bone marrow cell populations that increase allogeneic chimerism independently of graft-vs.-host disease in mixed marrow recipients. *J Immunol* 1989; **143**: 3503–11.

253 Pierce GE, Watts LM. Effects of Thy-1$^+$ cell depletion on the capacity of donor lymphoid cells to induce tolerance across an entire MHC disparity in sublethally irradiated adult hosts. *Transplantation* 1989; **48**: 289–96.

254 Lapidot T, Lubin I, Terenzi A, Faktorowich Y, Erlich P, Reisner Y. Enhancement of bone marrow allografts from nude mice into mismatched recipients by T cells void of graft-versus-host activity. *Proc Natl Acad Sci U S A* 1990; **87**: 4595–9.

255 de Fazio S, Hartner WC, Monaco AP, Gozzo JJ. Mouse skin graft prolongation with donor strain bone marrow and anti-lymphocyte serum: surface markers of the active bone marrow cells. *J Immunol* 1985; **135**: 3034–8.

256 Martin PJ. Prevention of allogeneic marrow graft rejection by donor T cells that do not recognize recipient alloantigens: potential role of a veto mechanism. *Blood* 1996; **88**: 962–9.

257 Pierce GE. Allogeneic versus semiallogeneic F1 bone marrow transplantation into sublethally irradiated MHC-disparate hosts. effects on mixed lymphoid chimerism, skin graft tolerance, host survival, and alloreactivity. *Transplantation* 1990; **49**: 138–44.

258 Eto M, Mayumi H, Tomita Y, Yoshikai Y, Nomoto K. Intrathymic clonal deletion of Vβ 6$^+$ T cells in cyclophosphamide-induced tolerance to H-2-compatible, Mls-disparate antigens. *J Exp Med* 1990; **171**: 97–113.

259 Mayumi H, Good RA. Long-lasting skin allograft tolerance in adult mice induced across fully allogeneic (multimajor H-2 plus multiminor histocompatibility) antigen barriers by a tolerance-inducing method using cyclophosphamide. *J Exp Med* 1989; **169**: 213–38.

260 Fontes P, Rao AS, Demetris AJ *et al.* Bone marrow augmentation of donor-cell chimerism in kidney, liver, heart and pancreas islet transplantation. *Lancet* 1994; **344**: 151–5.

261 Ciancio G, Miller J, Garcia-Morales RO *et al.* Six-year clinical effect of donor bone marrow infusions in renal transplant patients. *Transplantation* 2001; **71**: 827–35.

262 Kuhr CS, Allen MD, Junghanss C *et al.* Tolerance to vascularized kidney grafts in canine mixed hematopoietic chimeras. *Transplantation* 2002; **73**: 1487–92.

263 Xu H, Exner BG, Cramer DE, Tanner MK, Mueller YM, Ildstad ST. CD8$^+$, $\alpha\beta$-TCR$^+$, and $\gamma\delta$-TCR$^+$ cells in the recipient hematopoietic environment mediate resistance to engraftment of allogeneic donor bone marrow. *J Immunol* 2002; **168**: 1636–43.

264 Luznik L, Jalla S, Engstrom LW, Iannone R, Fuchs EJ. Durable engraftment of major histocompatibility complex-incompatible cells after non-myeloablative conditioning with fludarabine, low-dose total body irradiation, and posttransplantation cyclophosphamide. *Blood* 2001; **98**: 3456–64.

265 Auchincloss H, Jr, Sykes M, Sachs DH. Transplantation immunology. In: Paul WE, ed. *Fundamental Immunology*. Philadelphia: Lippincott-Raven, 1999: 1175–36.

266 Spitzer TR, McAfee S, Sackstein R *et al.* The intentional induction of mixed chimerism and achievement of anti-tumor responses following non-myeloablative conditioning therapy and HLA-matched and mismatched donor bone marrow transplantation for refractory hematologic malignancies. *Biol Blood Marrow Transplant* 2000; **6**: 309–20.

267 Sykes M, Preffer F, McAffee S *et al.* Mixed lymphohematopoietic chimerism and graft-vs.-lymphoma effects are achievable in adult humans following non-myeloablative therapy and HLA-mismatched donor bone marrow transplantation. *Lancet* 1999; **353**: 1755–9.

268 Giralt S, Estey E, Albitar M *et al.* Engraftment of allogeneic hematopoietic progenitor cells with purine analog-containing chemotherapy: harnessing graft-versus-leukemia without myeloablative therapy. *Blood* 1997; **89**: 4531–6.

269 Wood ML, Monaco AP, Gozzo JJ, Liegois A. Use of homozygous allogeneic bone marrow for induction of tolerance with anti-lymphocyte serum: dose and timing. *Transplant Proc* 1970; **3**: 676.

270 Thomas JM, Verbanac KM, Smith JP *et al.* The facilitating effect of one-DR antigen sharing in renal allograft tolerance induced by donor bone marrow in rhesus monkeys. *Transplantation* 1995; **59**: 245–55.

271 Thomas JM, Carver FM, Cunningham PRG, Olson LC, Thomas FT. Kidney allograft tolerance in primates without chronic immunosuppression: the role of veto cells. *Transplantation* 1991; **51**: 198–207.

272 Sharabi Y, Aksentijevich I, Sundt TM, III, Sachs DH, Sykes M. Specific tolerance induction across a xenogeneic barrier. Production of mixed rat/mouse lymphohematopoietic chimeras using a nonlethal preparative regimen. *J Exp Med* 1990; **172**: 195–202.

273 Nikolic B, Cooke DT, Zhao G, Sykes M. Both γ/δ T cells and NK cells inhibit the engraftment of xenogeneic rat bone marrow cells in mice. *J Immunol* 2001; **166**: 1398–404.

274 Kawai T, Cosimi AB, Colvin RB *et al.* Mixed allogeneic chimerism and renal allograft tolerance in cynomologous monkeys. *Transplantation* 1995; **59**: 256–62.

275 Tomita Y, Lee LA, Sykes M. Engraftment of rat bone marrow and its role in negative selection of murine T cells in mice conditioned with a modified non-myeloablative regimen. *Xenotransplant* 1994; **1**: 109–17.

276 Sharabi Y, Abraham VS, Sykes M, Sachs DH. Mixed allogeneic chimeras prepared by a non-myeloablative regimen: requirement for chimerism to maintain tolerance. *Bone Marrow Transplant* 1992; **9**: 191–7.

277 Tomita Y, Khan A, Sykes M. Mechanism by which additional monoclonal antibody injections overcome the requirement for thymic irradiation to achieve mixed chimerism in mice receiving bone marrow transplantation after conditioning with anti-T cell MABs and 3 Gy whole body irradiation. *Transplantation* 1996; **61**: 477–85.

278 Tomita Y, Sachs DH, Khan A, Sykes M. Additional MAB injections can replace thymic irradiation to allow induction of mixed chimerism and tolerance in mice receiving bone marrow transplantation after conditioning with anti-T cell

MABs and 3 Gy whole body irradiation. *Transplantation* 1996; **61**: 469–77.
279 Nikolic B, Khan A, Sykes M. Induction of tolerance by mixed chimerism with non-myeloablative host conditioning: The importance of overcoming intrathymic alloresistance. *Biol Blood Marrow Transplant* 2001; **7**: 144–53.
280 Fuchimoto Y, Huang CA, Yamada K et al. Mixed chimerism and tolerance without whole body irradiation in a large animal model. *J Clin Invest* 2000; **105**: 1779–89.
281 Kimikawa M, Sachs DH, Colvin RB, Bartholemew A, Kawai T, Cosimi AB. Modifications of the conditioning regimen for achieving mixed chimerism and donor-specific tolerance in cynomolgus monkeys. *Transplantation* 1997; **64**: 709–16.
282 Wekerle T, Sykes M. Mixed chimerism and transplantation tolerance. *Annu Rev Med* 2001; **52**: 353–70.
283 Sykes M, Sheard MA, Sachs DH. Graft-versus-host-related immunosuppression is induced in mixed chimeras by alloresponses against either host or donor lymphohematopoietic cells. *J Exp Med* 1988; **168**: 2391–6.
284 Pelot MR, Pearson DA, Swenson K et al. Lymphohematopoietic graft-vs.-host reactions can be induced without graft-vs.-host disease in murine mixed chimeras established with a cyclophosphamide-based non-myeloablative conditioning regimen. *Biol Blood Marrow Transplant* 1999; **5**: 133–43.
285 Mapara MY, Kim Y-M, Wang S-P, Bronson R, Sachs DH, Sykes M. Donor lymphocyte infusions (DLI) mediate superior graft-versus-leukemia (GvL) effects in mixed compared to fully allogeneic. chimeras: a critical role for host antigen-presenting cells. *Blood* 2002; **100**: 1903–9.
286 Spitzer TR, Delmonico F, Tolkoff-Rubin N et al. Combined HLA-matched donor bone marrow and renal transplantation for multiple myeloma with end stage renal disease: The induction of allograft tolerance through mixed lymphohematopoietic chimerism. *Transplantation* 1999; **68**: 480–4.
287 Buhler LH, Spitzer TR, Sykes M et al. Induction of kidney allograft tolerance through mixed lymphohematopoietic chimerism in patients with multiple myeloma and end-stage renal disease. *Transplantation* 2002; **74**: 1405–9.
288 Ghobrial RR, Boublik M, Winn HJ, Auchincloss H Jr. In vivo use of monoclonal antibodies against murine T cell antigens. *Clin Immunol Immunopathol* 1989; **52**: 486–506.
289 Oyaizu N, McCloskey TW, Than S, Hu R, Kalyanaraman VS, Pahwa S. Cross-linking of CD4 molecules upregulates Fas antigen expression in lymphocytes by inducing interferon-γ and tumor necrosis factor-α secretion. *Blood* 1994; **84**: 2622–31.
290 Chace JH, Cowdery JS, Field EH. Effect of anti-CD4 on CD4 subsets. I. Anti-CD4 preferentially deletes resting, naive CD4 cells and spares activated CD4 cells. *J Immunol* 1994; **152**: 405–12.
291 Rice JC, Bucy RP. Differences in the degree of depletion, rate of recovery, and the preferential elimination of naive $CD4^+$ T cells by anti-CD4 monoclonal antibody (GK1.5) in young and aged mice. *J Immunol* 1995; **154**: 6644–54.
292 Zhao Y, Sykes M. Resistance to MAB-induced $CD8^+$ T cell depletion in thymectomized MHC class II deficient mice. *Transplantation* 1997; **64**: 489–94.

293 Wekerle T, Sayegh MH, Ito H et al. Anti-CD154 or CTLA4Ig obviates the need for thymic irradiation in a non-myeloablative conditioning regimen for the induction of mixed hematopoietic chimerism and tolerance. *Transplantation* 1999; **68**: 1348–55.
294 Wekerle T, Sayegh MH, Hill J et al. Extrathymic T cell deletion and allogeneic stem cell engraftment induced with costimulatory blockade is followed by central T cell tolerance. *J Exp Med* 1998; **187**: 2037–44.
295 Durham MM, Bingaman AW, Adams AB et al. Cutting edge: administration of anti-CD40 ligand and donor bone marrow leads to hemopoietic chimerism and donor-specific tolerance without cytoreductive conditioning. *J Immunol* 2000; **165**: 1–4.
296 Haynes BF, Markert ML, Sempowski GD, Patel DD, Hale LP. The role of the thymus in immune reconstitution in aging, bone marrow transplantation, and HIV-1 infection. *Ann Rev Immunol* 2000; **18**: 529–60.
297 Wekerle T, Kurtz J, Sayegh MH et al. Peripheral deletion after bone marrow transplantation with costimulatory blockade has features of both activation-induced cell death and passive cell death. *J Immunol* 2001; **166**: 2311–6.
298 Kurtz J, Sykes M. Activation-induced cell death does not play an essential role in induction of CD4 cell tolerance with costimulatory blockade and allogeneic bone marrow transplantation. *Am J Transplant*, in press.
299 Kurtz J, Ito H, Wekerle T, Shaffer J, Sykes M. Mechanisms involved in the establishment of tolerance through costimulatory blockade and BMT. Lack of requirement for CD40L-mediated signaling for tolerance or deletion of donor-reactive $CD4^+$ cells. *Am J Transplant* 2001; **1**: 339–49.
300 Zheng X-X, Markees TG, Hancock WW et al. CTLA4 signals are required to optimally induce allograft tolerance with combined donor-specific transfusion and anti-CD154 monoclonal antibody treatment. *J Immunol* 1999; **162**: 4983–90.
301 Iwakoshi NN, Mordes JP, Markees TG, Phillips NE, Rossini AA, Greiner DL. Treatment of allograft recipients with donor-specific transfusion and anti-CD154 antibody leads to deletion of alloreactive $CD8^+$ T cells and prolonged graft survival in a CTLA4-dependent manner. *J Immunol* 2000; **164**: 512–21.
302 Wekerle T, Kurtz J, Bigenzahn S, Takeuchi Y, Sykes M. Mechanisms of transplant tolerance induction with costimulatory blockade. *Curr Opin Immunol* 2002; **14**: 592–600.
303 Wekerle T, Sayegh MH, Chandraker A, Swenson KG, Zhao Y, Sykes M. Role of peripheral clonal deletion in tolerance induction with bone marrow transplantation and costimulatory blockade. *Transplant Proc* 1999; **31**: 680.
304 Williams MA, Tan JT, Adams AB et al. Characterization of virus-mediated inhibition of mixed chimerism and allospecific tolerance. *J Immunol* 2001; **167**: 4987–95.
305 Forman D, Welsh RM, Markees TG et al. Viral abrogation of stem cell transplantation tolerance causes graft rejection and host death by different mechanisms. *J Immunol* 2002; **168**: 6047–56.
306 Dick JE, Lapidot T, Pflumio F. Transplantation of normal and leukemic human bone marrow into immune-deficient mice: development of animal models for human hematopoiesis. *Immunol Rev* 1991; **124**: 25–44.

307 Gritsch HA, Glaser RM, Emery DW et al. The importance of non-immune factors in reconstitution by discordant xenogeneic hematopoietic cells. *Transplantation* 1994; **57**: 906–17.
308 Lapidot T, Pflumia F, Doedens M, Murdoch B, Williams DE, Dick JE. Cytokine stimulation of multilineage hematopoiesis from immature human cells engrafted in SCID mice. *Science* 1992; **255**: 1137–43.
309 Yang Y-G, Sergio JJ, Swenson K, Glaser RM, Monroy R, Sykes M. Donor-specific growth factors promote swine hematopoiesis in SCID mice. *Xenotransplant* 1996; **3**: 92–101.
310 Chen AM, Zhou Y, Swenson K, Sachs DH, Sykes M, Yang Y-G. Porcine stem cell engraftment and seeding of murine thymus with class II^+ cells in mice expressing porcine cytokines: toward tolerance induction across discordant xenogeneic barriers. *Transplantation* 2000; **69**: 2484–90.
311 Zhao Y, Swenson K, Sergio JJ, Arn JS, Sachs DH, Sykes M. Skin graft tolerance across a discordant xenogeneic barrier. *Nature Med* 1996; **2**: 1211–6.
312 Lee LA, Gritsch HA, Sergio JJ et al. Specific tolerance across a discordant xenogeneic transplantation barrier. *Proc Natl Acad Sci U S A* 1994; **91**: 10864–7.
313 Zhao Y, Sergio JJ, Swenson KA, Arn JS, Sachs DH, Sykes M. Positive and negative selection of functional mouse CD4 cells by porcine MHC in pig thymus grafts. *J Immunol* 1997; **159**: 2100–7.
314 Zhao Y, Swenson K, Sergio JJ, Sykes M. Pig MHC mediates positive selection of mouse $CD4^+$ T cells with a mouse MHC-restricted TCR in pig thymus grafts. *J Immunol* 1998; **161**: 1320–6.
315 Zhao Y, Rodriguez-Barbosa JI, Zhao G, Shaffer J, Arn JS, Sykes M. Maturation and function of mouse T cells with a transgenic TCR positively selected by highly disparate xenogeneic porcine MHC. *Cell Mol Biol* 2000; **47**: 217–28.
316 Markert ML, Kostyu DD, Ward FE et al. Successful formation of a chimeric human thymus allograft following transplantation of cultured postnatal human thymus. *J Immunol* 1997; **158**: 998–1005.
317 Zerrahn J, Held W, Raulet DH. The MHC reactivity of the T cell repertoire prior to positive and negative selection. *Cell* 1997; **88**: 627–36.
318 Nikolic B, Gardner JP, Scadden DT, Arn JS, Sachs DH, Sykes M. Normal development in porcine thymus grafts and specific tolerance of human T cells to porcine donor MHC. *J Immunol* 1999; **162**: 3402–7.
319 Ohdan H, Yang Y-G, Swenson KG, Thall AD, Sykes M. Vivo T-cell depletion enhances production of anti-Galα1,3Gal natural antibodies in A1,3-galactosyltransferase-deficient mice. *Transplantation* 2000; **69**: 910–13.
320 Bracy JL, Iacomini J. Induction of B-cell tolerance by retroviral gene therapy. *Blood* 2000; **96**: 3008–15.
321 Butturini A, Gale RP. T cell depletion in bone marrow transplantation for leukemia. Current results and future directions. *Bone Marrow Transplant* 1988; **3**: 265–79.
322 Martin PJ, Hansen JA, Torok-Storb B et al. Graft failure in patients receiving T cell-depleted HLA-identical allogeneic marrow transplants. *Bone Marrow Transplant* 1988; **3**: 445–56.
323 Reich-Zeliger S, Zhao Y, Krauthgamer R, Bachar-Lustig E, Reisner Y. Anti-third party $CD8^+$ CTLs as potent veto cells. Coexpression of CD8 and FasL is a prerequisite. *Immunity* 2000; **13**: 507–15.
324 Andre-Schmutz I, Le Deist F, Hacein-Bey-Abina S et al. Immune reconstitution without graft-versus-

host disease after haemopoietic stem-cell transplantation: a phase 1/2 study. *Lancet* 2002; **360**: 130–7.
325 den Haan JMM, Sherman NE, Blokland E et al. Identification of a graft versus host disease-associated human minor histocompatibility antigen. *Science* 1995; **268**: 1476–80.
326 Goulmy E, Schipper R, Pool J et al. Mismatches of minor histocompatibility antigens between HLA-identical donors and recipients and the development of graft-versus-host disease after bone marrow transplantation. *New Engl J Med* 1996; **334**: 281–5.
327 Fontaine P, Roy-Proulx G, Knafo L, Baron C, Roy DC, Perreault C. Adoptive transfer of minor histocompatibility antigen-specific T lymphocytes eradicates leukemia cells without causing graft-versus-host disease. *Nat Med* 2001; **7**: 789–94.
328 Sykes M, Sachs DH. Genetic analysis of the anti-leukemic effect of mixed allogeneic bone marrow transplantation. *Transplant Proc* 1989; **21**: 3022–4.
329 Aizawa S, Sado T. Graft-versus-leukemia effect in MHC-compatible and incompatible allogeneic bone marrow transplantation of radiation-induced, leukemia-bearing mice. *Transplantation* 1991; **52**: 885–9.
330 Beatty PG, Anasetti C, Hansen JA et al. Marrow transplantation from unrelated donors for treatment of hematologic malignancies: effect of mismatching for one HLA locus. *Blood* 1993; **81**: 249–53.
331 Suchin EJ, Langmuir PB, Palmer E, Sayegh MH, Wells AD, Turka LA. Quantifying the frequency of alloreactive T cells *in vivo*: new answers to an old question. *J Immunol* 2001; **166**: 973–81.
332 Blazar BR, Taylor PA, Panoskaltsis-Mortari A et al. Blockade of CD40 ligand–CD40 interactions impairs CD4$^+$ T cell-mediated alloreactivity by inhibiting mature donor T cell expansion and function after bone marrow transplantation. *J Immunol* 1997; **158**: 29–39.
333 Guinan EC, Boussiotis VA, Neuberg D et al. Transplantation of anergic histoincompatible bone marrow allografts. *New Engl J Med* 1999; **340**: 1704–14.
334 Taylor PA, Noelle RJ, Blazar BR. CD4$^+$CD25$^+$ immune regulatory cells are required for induction of tolerance to alloantigen via costimulatory blockade. *J Exp Med* 2001; **193**: 1311–8.
335 Koh MB, Prentice HG, Corbo M, Morgan M, Cotter FE, Lowdell MW. Alloantigen-specific T-cell depletion in a major histocompatibility complex fully mismatched murine model provides effective graft-versus-host disease prophylaxis in the presence of lymphoid engraftment. *Br J Haematol* 2002; **118**: 108–16.
336 Zeng D, Dejbakhsh-Jones S, Strober S. Granulocyte colony-stimulating factor reduces the capacity of mononuclear cells to induce graft-versus-host disease: Impact on blood progenitor cell transplantation. *Blood* 1997; **90**: 453–63.
337 Makino Y, Kanno R, Ito T, Higashino K, Taniguchi M. Predominant expression of invariant Vα14$^+$ TCRα chain in NK1.1$^+$ T cell populations. *Int Immunol* 1995; **7**: 1157–61.
338 Sykes M. Unusual T cell populations in adult murine bone marrow. prevalence of CD3$^+$CD4$^-$CD8$^-$ and αβTCR$^+$NK1.1$^+$ cells. *J Immunol* 1990; **145**: 3209–15.
339 Bendelac A, Lantz O, Quimby ME, Yewdell JW, Bennink JR, Brutkiewicz RR. CD1 recognition by mouse NK1$^+$ T lymphocytes. *Science* 1995; **268**: 863–5.
340 Ballas ZK, Rasmussen WNK. 1.1$^+$ thymocytes: adult murine CD4$^-$, CD8$^-$ thymocytes contain an NK1.1$^+$, CD3$^+$, CD5^{hi}, CD44^{hi}, TCR-Vb8$^+$ subset. *J Immunol* 1990; **145**: 1039–45.
341 Yoshimoto T, Paul WECD, 4$^+$NK. 1.1$^+$ cells promptly produce interleukin 4 in response to *in vivo* challenge with anti-CD3. *J Exp Med* 1994; **179**: 1285–95.
342 Zeng D, Lewis D, Dejbakhsh-Jones S et al. Bone marrow NK1.1$^-$ and NK1.1$^+$ T cells reciprocally regulate acute graft versus host disease. *J Exp Med* 1999; **189**: 1073–81.
343 Strober S, Palathumpat V, Schwadron R, Hertel-Wulff B. Cloned natural suppressor cells prevent lethal graft-vs.-host disease. *J Immunol* 1987; **138**: 699–703.
344 Strober S, Cheng L, Zeng D et al. Double negative (CD4$^-$CD8$^-$αβ$^+$) T cells which promote tolerance induction and regulate autoimmunity. *Immunol Rev* 1996; **149**: 217–30.
345 Eberl G, Lees R, Smiley ST, Taniguchi M, Grusby MJ, MacDonald HR. Tissue-specific segregation of CD1d-dependent and CD1d-independent NK T cells. *J Immunol* 1999; **162**: 6410–9.
346 Hammond KJ, Pelikan SB, Crowe NY et al. NKT cells are phenotypically and functionally diverse. *Eur J Immunol* 1999; **29**: 3768–81.
347 Palathumpat V, Holm B, Dejbakhsh-Jones S, Strober S. Treatment of BCL1 leukemia by transplantation of low-density fractions of allogeneic bone marrow and spleen cells. *J Immunol* 1992; **148**: 3319–26.
348 Zeng D, Hoffmann P, Lan F, Huie P, Higgins J, Strober S. Unique patterns of surface receptors, cytokine secretion, and immune functions distinguish T cells in the bone marrow from those in the periphery: Impact on allogeneic bone marrow transplantation. *Blood* 2002; **99**: 1449–57.
349 Fowler DH, Kurasawa K, Husebekk A, Cohen PA, Gress RE. Cells of the T$_H$2 cytokine phenotype prevent LPS-induced lethality during murine graft-versus-host reaction. regulation of cytokines and CD8$^+$ lymphoid engraftment. *J Immunol* 1994; **152**: 1004–13.
350 Krenger W, Snyder KM, Byon JCH, Falzarano G, Ferrara JLM. Polarized type 2 alloreactive CD4$^+$ and CD8$^+$ donor T cells fail to induce experimental acute graft-versus-host disease. *J Immunol* 1995; **155**: 585–93.
351 Collins BH, Chari RS, Magee JC et al. Mechanisms of injury in porcine livers perfused with blood of patients with fulminant hepatic failure. *Transplantation* 1994; **58**: 1162–71.
352 Fowler DH, Breglio J, Nagel G, Eckhaus MA, Gress RE. Allospecific CD8$^+$ Tc1 and Tc2 populations in graft-versus-leukemia effect and graft-versus-host disease. *J Immunol* 1996; **157**: 4811–21.
353 Sykes M, Romick ML, Hoyles KA, Sachs DH. In vivo administration of interleukin 2 plus T cell-depleted syngeneic marrow prevents graft-versus-host disease mortality and permits alloengraftment. *J Exp Med* 1990; **171**: 645–58.
354 Brok HPM, Heidt PJ, Van der Meide PH, Zurcher C, Vossen JM. Interferon-γ prevents graft-versus-host disease after allogeneic bone marrow transplantation in mice. *J Immunol* 1993; **151**: 6451–9.
355 Yang YG, Sykes M. Graft-versus-host disease and graft-versus-leukemic effect in allogeneic bone marrow transplantation: Role of interferon-γ. *Graft* 2002; **5**: 250–5.
356 Sykes M, Szot GL, Nguyen PL, Pearson DA. Interleukin-12 inhibits murine graft-vs.-host disease. *Blood* 1995; **86**: 2429–38.
357 Willenborg DO et al. IFN-γ is critical to the control of murine autoimmune encephalomyelitis and regulates both in the periphery and in the target tissue: a possible role for nitric oxide. *J Immunol* 1999; **163**: 5278–86.
358 Bogdan C. Nitric oxide and the immune response. *Nat Immunol* 2001; **2**: 907–16.
359 Novelli F, D'Elios MM, Bernabei P et al. Expression and role in apoptosis of the α- and β-chains of the IFN-γ receptor on human T$_H$1 and T$_H$2 clones. *J Immunol* 1997; **159**: 206–13.
360 Badovinac VP, Tvinnereim AR, Harty JT. Regulation of antigen-specific CD8$^+$ T cell homeostasis by perforin and interferon-γ. *Science* 2000; **290**: 1354–8.
361 Nikolic B, Lee S, Bronson RT, Grusby MJ, Sykes M. T$_H$1 and T$_H$2 cells both contribute to acute GVHD, and each subset has distinct end-organ targets. *J Clin Invest* 2000; **105**: 1289–93.
362 Murphy WJ, Welniak LA, Taub DD et al. Differential effects of the absence of interferon-γ and IL-4 in acute graft-versus-host disease after allogeneic bone marrow transplantation in mice. *J Clin Invest* 1998; **102**: 1742–8.
363 Sykes M, Romick ML, Sachs DH. Interleukin 2 prevents graft-vs.-host disease while preserving the graft-vs.-leukemia effect of allogeneic T cells. *Proc Natl Acad Sci U S A* 1990; **87**: 5633–7.
364 Sykes M, Harty MW, Szot GL, Pearson DA. Interleukin-2 inhibits graft-versus-host disease-promoting activity of CD4$^+$ cells while preserving CD4- and CD8-mediated graft-versus-leukemia effects. *Blood* 1994; **83**: 2560–9.
365 Yang Y-G, Sergio JJ, Pearson DA, Szot GL, Shimizu A, Sykes M. Interleukin-12 preserves the graft-versus-leukemia effect of allogeneic CD8 T cells while inhibiting CD4-dependent graft-vs.-host disease in mice. *Blood* 1997; **90**: 4651–60.
366 Szebeni J, Wang M-G, Pearson DA, Szot GL, Sykes M. IL-2 inhibits early increases in serum γ interferon levels associated with graft-vs.-host disease. *Transplantation* 1994; **58**: 1385–93.
367 Wang M-G, Szebeni J, Pearson DA, Szot GL, Sykes M. Inhibition of grafts-vs.-host disease (GVHD) by IL-2 treatment is associated with altered cytokine production by expanded GVH-reactive CD4$^+$ helper cells. *Transplantation* 1995; **60**: 481–90.
368 Sykes M, Abraham VS, Harty MW, Pearson DA. IL-2 reduces graft-vs.-host disease and preserves a graft-vs.-leukemia effect by selectively inhibiting CD4$^+$ T cell activity. *J Immunol* 1993; **150**: 197–205.
369 Trinchieri G. Interleukin-12 and its role in the generation of T$_H$1 cells. *Immunol Today* 1993; **14**: 335–8.
370 Yang Y-G, Dey B, Sergio JJ, Pearson DA, Sykes M. Donor-derived interferon γ is required for inhibition of acute GVHD by interleukin 12. *J Clin Invest* 1998; **102**: 2126–35.
371 Yang Y-G, Qi J, Wang M-G, Sykes M. Donor-derived interferon γ separates graft-versus-leukemia effects and graft-versus-host disease induced by donor CD8 T cells. *Blood* 2002; **99**: 4207–15.
372 Reddy P, Teshima T, Kukuruga M et al. Interleukin-18 regulates acute graft-versus-host disease by

372 enhancing Fas-mediated donor T cell apoptosis. *J Exp Med* 2001; **194**: 1433–40.
373 Dey B, Yang Y-G, Szot GL, Pearson DA, Sykes M. IL-12 inhibits GVHD through a Fas-mediated mechanism associated with alterations in donor T cell activation and expansion. *Blood* 1998; **91**: 3315–22.
374 Yang Y-G, Dey B, Sergio JJ, Sykes M. IL-12 prevents hyperacute GVHD and GVHD-associated immune dysfunction in a full MHC haplotype-mismatched murine bone marrow transplantation model. *Transplantation* 1997; **64**: 1343–52.
375 Yang YG, Sykes M. The role of Interleukin-12 in preserving graft-vs.-leukemia effect of allogeneic CD8 T cells independently of GVHD. *Leuk Lympho* 2002; **33**: 409–20.
376 Bonini C, Ferrari G, Verzeletti S *et al*. HSV-TK gene transfer into donor lymphocytes for control of allogeneic graft-versus-leukemia. *Science* 1997; **276**: 1719–24.
377 Abhyankar S, Gilliland DG, Ferrara JLM. Interleukin-1 is a critical effector molecule during cytokine dysregulation in graft versus host disease to minor histocompatibility antigens. *Transplantation* 1993; **56**: 1518–23.
378 Piguet P-F, Grau GE, Allet B, Vassalli P. Tumor necrosis factor/cachectin is an effector of skin and gut lesions of the acute phase of graft-vs.-host disease. *J Exp Med* 1987; **166**: 1280–9.
379 Johnson BD, Drobyski WR, Truitt RL. Delayed infusion of normal donor cells after MHC-matched bone marrow transplantation provides an anti-leukemia reaction without graft-versus-host disease. *Bone Marrow Transplant* 1993; **11**: 329–36.
380 Kolb HJ, Mittermüller J, Clemm Ch *et al*. Donor leukocyte transfusions for treatment of recurrent chronic myelogenous leukemia in marrow transplant patients. *Blood* 1990; **76**: 2462–5.
381 Spitzer TR, McAfee S, Sackstein R. *et al*. Mixed lymphohematopoietic chimerism and delayed donor leukocyte infusions following non-myeloablative conditioning and HLA-matched and mismatched donor bone marrow transplantation. In: Dicke KA, Keating A., eds. *Autologous Bone Marrow Transplantation. Proceedings of the 10th International Symposium*. Charlottesville, VA: Carden Jennings, 2001: 321–30.
382 Alyea E, Weller E, Schlossman R *et al*. T-cell-depleted allogeneic bone marrow transplantation followed by donor lymphocyte infusion in patients with multiple myeloma: induction of graft-versus-myeloma effect. *Blood* 2001; **98**: 934–9.
383 Johnson BD, Becker EE, LaBelle JL, Truitt RL. Role of immunoregulatory donor T cells in suppression of graft-versus-host disease following donor leukocyte infusion therapy. *J Immunol* 1999; **163**: 6479–87.
384 Blazar BR, Lees CJ, Martin PJ *et al*. Host T cells resist graft-versus-host disease mediated by donor leukocyte infusions. *J Immunol* 2000; **165**: 4901–9.
385 Spitzer TR, McAfee SL, Dey BR *et al*. Durable progression free survival (PFS) following non-myeloablative bone marrow transplantation (BMT) for chemorefractory diffuse large B cell lymphoma (B-LCL). *Blood* 2001; **98**: 672a.
386 Spitzer TRM, Cafee S, Dey BR *et al*. Non-myeloablative haploidentical stem cell transplantation using anti-CD2 monoclonal antibody (MEDI-507) based conditioning for refractory hematologic malignancies. *Transplantation* 2003; **75**: 1748–51.
387 Shlomchik WD, Couzens MS, Tang CB *et al*. Prevention of graft versus host disease by inactivation of host antigen-presenting cells. *Science* 1999; **285**: 412–5.
388 Blackman M, Kappler J, Marrack P. The role of the T cell receptor in positive and negative selection of developing T cells. *Science* 1990; **248**: 1335–41.
389 Sprent J, Gao E-K, Webb SR. T cell reactivity to MHC molecules: immunity versus tolerance. *Science* 1990; **248**: 1357–63.
390 Speiser DE, Pircher H, Ohashi PS, Kyburz D, Hengartner H, Zinkernagel RM. Clonal deletion induced by either radioresistant thymic host cells or lymphohemopoietic donor cells at different stages of class I-restricted T cell ontogeny. *J Exp Med* 1992; **175**: 1277–83.
391 Hoffman MW, Heath WR, Ruschmeyer D, Miller JFAP. Deletion of high-avidity T cells by thymic epithelium. *Proc Natl Acad Sci U S A* 1995; **92**: 9851–5.
392 Laufer TM, DeKoning J, Markowitz JS, Lo D, Glimcher LH. Unopposed positive selection and autoreactivity in mice expressing class II MHC only on thymic cortex. *Nature* 1996; **383**: 81–5.
393 Lapp WS, Ghayur T, Mendes M, Seddik M, Seemayer TA. The functional and histological basis for graft-versus-host-induced immunosuppression. *Immunol Rev* 1985; **88**: 107–31.
394 Cheney RT, Sprent J. Capacity of cyclosporine to induce auto-graft-versus-host disease and impair intrathymic T cell differentiation. *Transplant Proc* 1985; **17**: 528–30.
395 Gao E-K, Lo D, Cheney R, Kanagawa O, Sprent J. Abnormal differentiation of thymocytes in mice treated with cyclosporin A. *Nature* 1988; **336**: 176–9.
396 Parkman R. Graft-versus-host disease: An alternative hypothesis. *Immunol Today* 1989; **10**: 362–4.
397 Rosenkrantz K, Keever C, Kirsch J *et al*. In vitro correlates of graft-host tolerance after HLA-matched and mismatched marrow transplants: Suggestions from limiting dilution analysis. *Transplant Proc* 1987; **19**: 98–103.
398 Hess AD, Fischer AC, Horwitz L, Bright EC, Laulis MK. Characterization of peripheral autoregulatory mechanisms that prevent development of cyclosporin-induced syngeneic graft-versus-host disease. *J Immunol* 1994; **153**: 400–11.
399 Auchincloss H, Jr, Sachs DH. Mechanism of tolerance in murine radiation bone marrow chimeras. *Transplantation* 1983; **36**: 436–41.
400 Tsoi M-S, Storb R, Dobbs S, Thomas ED. Specific suppressor cells in graft-host tolerance of HLA-identical marrow transplantation. *Nature* 1981; **292**: 355–7.

25

Judith A. Shizuru

The Experimental Basis for Hematopoietic Cell Transplantation for Autoimmune Diseases

Introduction

Autoimmune diseases (ADs) are a heterogeneous group of disorders that affect an estimated 3–5% of the population [1,2]. These diseases occur when there is breakdown in the signals that mediate immune tolerance to normal tissues. The result of such breakdown is activation of cellular effector mechanisms and subsequent tissue destruction. Theoretically, all tissue types can be targets of an immune response; however, it is not known why certain organs are involved more commonly than others (Table 25.1). Six of the most common ADs are rheumatoid arthritis, systemic lupus erythematosus (SLE), type 1 diabetes mellitus (T1DM), Graves' disease, multiple sclerosis and pernicious anemia. Collectively these diseases represent ~50% of the ADs [3]. Autoimmune responses are generally sustained, persistent with manifestations of chronic tissue damage, presumably because self-antigens are continually produced on the targeted tissue and, in severe cases, diminution of the response does not occur until the cells expressing the autoantigens are destroyed. More than 30 years ago it was demonstrated that transfer of hematopoietic cells can alter the course of ADs in rodents. Bone marrow transplantations (BMTs) were shown to both transfer disease from autoimmune prone rodents to unaffected ones [4–6] and, conversely, to prevent disease if the hematopoietic cells were transplanted from unaffected rodents to susceptible ones [6–9]. The goals of this chapter are to provide a basis for understanding how and why hematopoietic cell transplantation (HCT) may effectively treat severe ADs and to describe the preclinical studies that have contributed to this understanding. The chapter begins with an over-view of how normal immune responses are regulated followed by a discussion of why autoimmunity develops. Thereafter the studies on preclinical models using HCT for the treatment of autoimmune syndromes are presented.

The immune response

Induction perpetuation of responses

Induction of antigen specific immune responses occurs as a complex cascade of events. The first critical step in turning on a response requires the processing of antigen for presentation to $CD4^+$ T lymphocytes [10]. $CD4^+$ T cells are central to immune response activation because they form the critical link between recognition of foreign antigen and the induction of effector mechanisms that destroy the antigenic source. Most effector cells rely upon ancillary signals provided by activated $CD4^+$ T cells in order to proliferate and differentiate. Because the consequences of nonspecific or inappropriate stimulation of naive $CD4^+$ T cells are potentially disastrous, a number of criteria must be met to activate these cells [11–13]. Only certain specialized cells, designated professional antigen-presenting cells (APCs) fulfill these criteria. The professional APCs include B lymphocytes, macrophages and dendritic cells. As part of their function APCs take up foreign protein antigens by endocytosis. The antigens are then processed via an intracellular pathway into smaller peptide fragments, and the fragments are then bound to class II major histocompatibility complex (MHC) molecules that make their way to the surface of the APC.

The seminal event in the activation of a quiescent and circulating $CD4^+$ T cell is encounter with its cognate antigen, which consists of the appropriate peptide bound to a self-MHC class II molecule. In addition to the binding of a T-cell receptor (TCR) to its cognate antigen, activation cannot be achieved unless this interaction is accompanied by simultaneous delivery of a costimulatory signal(s). In the absence of a costimulatory signal, engagement of the antigen receptor can lead to T-cell anergy—a state of nonresponsiveness to the antigen. Only professional APCs express both high levels of class II MHC molecules on their surface and are capable of delivering the appropriate costimulatory signals.

Table 25.1 Associations of human leukocyte antigen (HLA) serotype with susceptibility to autoimmune disease (AD).

Disease	Affected organ	HLA association	Relative risk
Rheumatoid arthritis	Joints	DR4	4.2
SLE	Systemic	DR3	5.8
T1DM	Pancreatic islets	DR3/DR4	~25.0
Graves' disease	Thyroid	DR3	3.7
Multiple sclerosis	CNS	DR2	4.8
Ankylosing spondylitis	Joints	B27	87.4

CNS, central nervous system; T1DM, type 1 diabetes mellitus; SLE, systemic lupus erythematosus.

Costimulatory molecules expressed by APC include B7-1 (CD80) and B7-2 (CD86)—the ligands for CD28, CD40, inducible costimulator ligand (ICOS-L), and various adhesion molecules [11,12,14]. Following TCR binding plus costimulatory signaling naive T cells respond by rapidly proliferating and differentiating. As part of this process they begin to express new receptor molecules and synthesize and secrete a number of chemokines and cytokines. One of the most important cytokines is interleukin 2 (IL-2) [15–18]. The production of IL-2 determines whether or not a $CD4^+$ T cell will proliferate and continue along its differentiation pathway. IL-2 functions as both a growth hormone and influences the activation state of other T cells, and functions as an autocrine hormone that induces the synthesis and expression of high affinity IL-2 receptor on the $CD4^+$ T cell itself. Signaling through the high affinity IL-2 receptor triggers the cells to progress through the remainder of the cell cycle.

Following CD4 T-cell stimulation and production of IL-2, these cells differentiate into two distinct populations that are distinguishable by the cytokines they produce. One population produces interferon-gamma (IFN-γ), tumor necrosis factor-beta (TNF-β) and IL-2, and the other secretes IL-4 and its congeners. These cell populations have been designated T-helper type 1 subset (TH1) and T-helper type 2 subset (TH2) cells. TH1 cells produce cytokines that drive cell-mediated immunity, while TH2 which elaborate cytokines critical to B-lymphocyte differentiation, provide help for antibody production (humoral immunity) [19,20]. It is clear that these $CD4^+$ T-cell subsets can regulate the growth and effector functions of the opposite T-cell subsets.

Cellular and humoral-based mechanisms mediate the effector phase of an immune response by destroying the pathogenic organisms that bear the target antigens [10]. Effector populations include mature B cells, activated cytotoxic T cells and other inflammatory cells such as natural killer (NK) and phagocytic cells. The humoral components of the effector phase include antibodies and complement protein. Products of activated mononuclear cells include proteolytic enzymes, nitric oxide and oxygen radicals and cytokines such as TNF-α.

Control of immune reactivity

To insure that autoreactivity does not occur during the course of defending host tissues activation of T lymphocytes is highly regulated. In addition, there are at least four ways that self-reactivity is controlled. These mechanisms are termed *clonal deletion*, *immunological ignorance*, *anergy* and *regulation* [21,22] (see also Chapter 24).

Clonal deletion

During development all lymphocytes undergo a rigorous selection process to delete potentially self-reactive cells [23–25]. Hematopoietic stem cells (HSCs) give rise to all lymphoid progenitor cells. For T cells, the progenitors migrate to the thymus, which provides a specialized microenvironment for T-cell maturation and selection. Developing cells that are potentially self-reactive—i.e. those cells with TCRs that bind too strongly to self-peptides plus self-MHC molecules are eliminated, a process termed negative selection or clonal deletion. Only those T cells with receptors that have the potential to recognize self-MHC molecules plus foreign peptides (positive selection) can leave the thymus and enter the bloodstream. Immature B cells that express immunoglobulin receptors that bind too strongly to components of self either die within the bone marrow (BM) or become impaired in their ability to respond to antigen (anergic).

Immunological ignorance

Most self-proteins are expressed at levels that are too low to serve as targets for T-cell recognition, and thus cannot serve as autoantigens. It is likely that only a very few self-proteins contain peptides that are presented by a given MHC molecule at a level that is sufficient for effector T-cell recognition but too low to induce tolerance. T cells able to recognize these rare antigens will be present in the individual but will not normally be activated; they are said to be in a state of immunological ignorance [26,27]. Most autoimmunity likely reflects the activation of such immunologically ignorant cells.

Anergy

A third level of control against nonspecific or self-reactive immune responses occurs if the requirements for lymphocyte activation fail. Quiescent lymphocytes traffic through the blood, lymphatics, and lymphoid organs in search of the cognate antigen that will bind their antigen specific receptors. Engagement of these antigen receptors in the absence of appropriate costimulatory signals (see section above) leads to a state of lymphocyte unresponsiveness called anergy [11,14,21,22]. A lymphocyte that is rendered anergic has an elevated threshold for activation, and thus is more resistant to responsiveness if its cognate antigen is encountered at a later time. Anergy has been observed in both T and B cells.

Regulation or suppression

A fourth way unwanted immune responses can be controlled is through populations that function to actively suppress lymphocyte activity. Experiments from the early 1970s [28] supported the existence of $CD8^+$ cells that down regulated the reactivity of other T cells in an antigen-specific fashion. Although the phenomenon of immune suppression clearly exists the identity of suppressor cells and their mechanism of action was the subject of controversy for many years. More recently lymphocyte subclasses have been identified that demonstrate suppressive activity but have been given the more modern designation of "regulatory" cells [29–32]. Among the most widely studied regulatory cells are $CD4^+CD25^+$ [31,32] and NKT cells [29]. These populations have been identified in both rodents and humans. T cells that coexpress CD4 and CD25 (the IL-2 receptor α chain) are powerful inhibitors of T-cell activation both *in vivo* and *in vitro*. Convincing evidence that $CD4^+CD25^+$ cells suppress AD has been demonstrated in numerous mouse models. Cells that coexpress both NK receptors and TCRs qualify as belonging to a heterogeneous population termed NKT cells. Subclasses of NKT cells have been shown to suppress immune responses, including graft-vs.-host disease (GVHD) responses.

Another form of regulation that has been observed in many autoimmune models involves preferential activation of $CD4^+$ T-cell subsets (TH1 vs. TH2) [19]. There have been several reports showing that ADs are associated with activation of TH1 cells, which drive cellular responses mediated by activated macrophages and inflammatory processes. In certain animal models of AD it has been shown that the relative activation of the T-cell helper subsets can be manipulated to give either a TH1 response, which results in disease, or a TH2 response (humoral), which confers protection from disease. The preferential activation of TH1 and TH2 cells can be achieved by manipulation of the cytokine environment or by administration of antigen by particular routes (such as by feeding). Thus, a hypothesis arose (which predates the revival of regulatory T-cell subsets) designated the "TH1/TH2 paradigm". This hypothesis proposes that skewing of autoimmune responses towards TH2 predominant responses in preference over TH1 responses will be protective. The current consensus is that the TH1/TH2 paradigm is oversimplistic and begs reevaluation [33,34].

Autoimmune pathology

ADs arise when self-antigens become targets for immune destruction. The response may be directed against a single tissue type or a very limited number of tissues. Histologic studies have shown variability in the

Table 25.2 Animal models of autoimmune disease (AD).

Strain or designation	Disease model	Induction/manipulation
NOD mice	T1Dm	Spontaneous
BB rats	T1Dm	Spontaneous
(NZB/NZW)F1 mice	SLE	Spontaneous
MRL-*lpr/lpr* mice	SLE	Spontaneous
BXSB mice	SLE	Spontaneous
NZB/KN mice	Polyarthritis	Spontaneous
C57BL mice	Multiple sclerosis	Induced—peptide of MOG
SJL mice	Multiple sclerosis	Induced—MSCH
DBA1 mice	Rheumatoid arthritis	Induced—Type II collagen
Buffalo rats	Rheumatoid arthritis	Induced—Freund's adjuvant
BDC.2.5 TG mice	T1Dm	Transgenic—TCR
ε-IFN-γ-Tg mice	Myasthenia gravis	Transgenic—IFN-γ on nicotinic acetylcholine receptor
HLA-B27 TG rats	Ankylosing spondylitis	Transgenic—human HLA class II on MHC promoter

HLA, human leukocyte antigen; IFN-γ, interferon-gamma; MHC, major histocompatibility complex; MOG, myelin oligodendrocyte glycoprotein; MSCH, mouse spinal cord homogenate; NOD, nonobese diabetic; NZB, New Zealand black; NZW, New Zealand white; SLE, systemic lupus erythematosus; T1Dm, type 1 diabetes mellitus; TCR, T-cell receptor; TG, transgenic.

apparent causes of tissue destruction since predominance of antibodies, activated T or B lymphocytes, or nonspecific inflammatory cells can be seen in the inflammatory lesions. On the basis of such studies, it was concluded that different diseases are predominantly mediated by either humoral vs. cellular driven immune responses. A traditional categorization of immunologic diseases divides the syndromes into four types, designated as types I–IV hypersensitivity responses. Type I responses are caused by antibodies of the immunoglobulin E (IgE) isotype and are considered to be allergic responses, not classical autoimmune responses. Types II–IV involve tissue damage. Type II responses are mediated by antibodies directed against the targeted tissue, type III responses by antibody-antigen complex deposition and type IV by cellular processes. It should be emphasized, however, that these classifications do not illuminate the more fundamental and important issue of what triggers autoimmune responses since, by the time an autoimmune process becomes clinically evident and classifiable by this scheme, the initiating events are obscured by the downstream effector mechanisms causing the actual tissue damage. At least for the reactions of type II, III and IV, there appears to be a common pathway by which autoreactive lymphocyte clones develop and escape the controls that enforce self-tolerance. From our current understanding of how the immune system functions, and from the cumulative experience in the study of autoimmune syndromes in animals, it is thought that loss of T-cell tolerance is the central pathogenic event.

Genes and environment

Both genetic and environmental factors appear to be required in the development of ADs. Family studies, animal models and human epidemiologic studies all support the role of these factors in AD susceptibility. The importance of genetic predisposition was first identified by analyses of disease incidence in monozygotic twins. The concordance rates in twins ranges from ~15% for rheumatoid arthritis [3,35] to a robust ~57% for SLE [3,36]. Comparisons of these rates with disease incidence in the general population predict that genetic predisposition is a dominant factor. For example, the lifetime risk of developing T1Dm in the general population in the USA is 0.4%, whereas for monozygotic twins the concordance rate is in the range of 30–50% [37,38]. For siblings the rate is still significantly increased above the general population at ~6%, but is lower than for twins. This decrease in the sibling concordance rates as compared with monozygotic twins suggests that multiple genes contribute to genetic predisposition. Thus, while genetic susceptibility is a dominant factor, the pattern of inheritance of ADs is complex [1,3]. The diseases are polygenic, meaning that they arise from several independently segregating genes and, to date, the only clearly defined consistent genetic marker for susceptibility to any AD are certain alleles of the genes located within the MHC (Table 25.1).

Inbred rodent strains exist that reliably develop spontaneous ADs (Table 25.2). These animals are highly inbred, and thus genetically identical. Like human twins, many but not all animals in these inbred colonies develop disease. This lack of 100% concordance in genetically identical humans and rodents gives evidence for the essential role of environmental interactions on AD development. Observations made in rodents where environmental elements can be controlled reveal that some of the factors affecting disease incidence include exposure to infectious pathogens and diet [39–43]. For example, a germ-free environment has been shown to suppress or enhance autoreactivity in mice with spontaneously arising forms of multiple sclerosis [40] and diabetes [41], respectively. Furthermore, it is well known among investigators that raise nonobese diabetic (NOD) mice, a model for T1Dm, that certain common mouse pathogens, such as pinworms, leads to dramatically reduced incidence of diabetes. Oral ingestion of protein antigens has been shown to lead to marked suppression of systemic humoral and cell-mediated immune responses when animals are later immunized with the same antigen. This phenomenon is called oral tolerance [44]. A high-fat, high-protein diet has also been shown to increase the rate and severity of diabetes in NOD mice [45]. Another factor contributing to autoreactivity is sexual dimorphism. Sexual dimorphism refers to a pattern of skewing of disease incidence and/or severity towards one sex. It has been observed in many human ADs, such as SLE and autoimmune thyroid disease, that human females demonstrate a disproportionately higher incidence compared to males [46]. Rodents ADs, including NOD mice, show a similar pattern of sexual dimorphism. In NOD mice castration studies [47] and administration of exogenous male hormones [48,49] have shown that sex-related hormones contribute significantly to the dimorphism.

Data from human epidemiologic studies confirm the contributions of genetic and environmental factors on AD incidence. Such studies show clear associations with race, geography and susceptibility to disease.

Again using T1Dm as an example, the incidence of the disease is ~40 times higher in Finland than in Japan [38].

MHC genes and susceptibility to ADs

The only established genetic association for predisposition to ADs is the genotype of the MHC (reviewed in [50]). This association was noted in the mid-1970s. Initially, correlations were made with the class I MHC type and the spondyloarthropathies. Ankylosing spondylitis, an inflammatory and presumably AD of vertebral joints, was found to be strongly associated with the class I human leukocyte antigen (HLA)-B27 allele. Individuals who are HLA-B27 positive have a ~90–100 times greater chance of developing ankylosing spondylitis than do individuals that lack B27. Later, the emphasis shifted to associations with class II rather than class I MHC molecules since frequent associations were found in subsequent studies with class II gene products and other ADs, such as Graves' disease and T1Dm (Table 25.1).

In the last 20 years, the technology of HLA typing has advanced from serologic assays to the more sensitive molecular based assays that detect variations at the nucleotide level (see Chapter 4). As this technology for HLA genotyping has become more precise, allowing examination of specific regions of the MHC, the associations have become stronger. For example, it has been observed that up to 95% of Caucasians developing T1Dm express the *HLA* alleles *DR3* or *DR4* vs. about 40% of normal individuals, and that individuals heterozygous for both *DR3* and *DR4* have the highest risk of T1Dm development [51]. Subsequent to these observations, it was shown that, in fact, the *DQ*, rather than the *DR*, genotype is a more specific marker for T1Dm susceptibility, and that the previous correlation with *HLA-DR* is due to the fact that *DR* and *DQ* are the products of closely linked genes (linkage disequilibrium) [52]. Thus, for T1Dm the highest risk *DQ* alleles, DQα1*0501/DQβ1*0201 and DQα1*0301/DQβ1*0302, are invariably found in the *DR3* and *DR4* genotype, respectively. Individuals heterozygous for these two *DQ* alleles are at greatest risk of T1Dm development. Such individuals comprise 2% of the US population but 40% of the patients with T1Dm.

A similar evolution in the association of *HLA*-type and disease susceptibility has occurred for Graves' disease. Graves' disease was among the first autoimmune disorders noted to have an association with *HLA* haplotypes and the initial association was with the MHC class I genotype *HLA-B8*. Later, however, it became evident that the stronger association was with *HLA-DR3*, which is tightly linked to *HLA-B8* [53].

Function of MHC in AD pathogenesis

Although genetic associations are firmly established between ADs and defined MHC haplotypes, the way that MHC molecules contribute to autoimmune pathogenesis remains hypothetical. MHC molecules play central roles in both T-cell selection during T-cell ontogeny and in the presentation of antigen to T cells. Thus, it has been hypothesized that certain AD associated MHC haplotypes permit faulty selection of T cells during development and/or allow aberrant presentation of self-peptides to T cells that results in inappropriate T-cell activation [33,54,55]. MHC/peptide-restricted recognition by T cells results from the combined effects of the differences in peptide binding and of direct contact between allotypic portions of the MHC molecule. It is known that certain polymorphic amino acids that form the walls of the peptide-binding groove can result in profound differences in binding affinity of MHC molecules with self-peptides as well as affect the conformation of the MHC/peptide-complexes seen by the antigen specific TCR. Furthermore, other polymorphic residues of the MHC molecules can make direct contact with TCRs and thus affect antigen recognition. Therefore, it is possible that the disease associated MHC haplotypes make certain self-antigens appear foreign and/or the haplotypes generate a strong enough immune response to self-antigens to induce T-cell activation.

Support for this hypothesis of aberrant antigen binding and presentation by disease associated MHC molecules comes from sequence analysis of *DQ* genes from individuals with T1Dm. These analyses suggested that there is a critical single amino acid located in the peptide binding groove at position 57 of the DQβ chain that confers either susceptibility or resistance to T1Dm [56,57]. An aspartic acid, which is present in most persons at that position, appears to decrease the risk of T1Dm, whereas substitution of other amino acids at position 57 is associated with increased risk. Further evidence for the importance of this single amino acid was found in spontaneous diabetic NOD mice. These mice show a similar replacement of serine for aspartic acid at position 57 of the homologous mouse MHC class II molecule (I-Aβ chain) [58]. In humans, amino acid 57 is located at the distal end of the DQβ chain and forms part of the peptide-binding cleft of the DQβ molecule [57]. Aspartic acid, the protective amino acid at this position, forms a salt-bridge with a residue on the opposite side of the binding cleft, and replacement of an uncharged residue at this position disrupts the salt bridge formation.

The above hypothesis presumes that the association of ADs with MHC haplotype derives directly from the function of the MHC gene products. While this hypothesis has been amply supported by data from both humans and rodents, it is not conclusively proved. Disease association clearly maps to the MHC region; however, contained within this region are a number of other genes. Alternative hypotheses include that the MHC-haplotype serves only as a marker and that the true (and as yet undetermined) disease-associated genes are closely linked to the MHC alleles.

Non-MHC genes and susceptibility to ADs

The importance of genetic predisposition in AD susceptibility and the conclusion that several genes contribute to an AD phenotype has motivated the search for predominant non-MHC susceptibility genes [3,59]. It was hoped that genome-wide linkage analysis could aid in the identification of such genes. To achieve this goal international coalitions were formed aimed at collecting large cohorts of families afflicted with specific ADs and employing state-of-the-art technologies to scan their genomes for the location of susceptibility genes. These analyses have confirmed the complex nature of the genetic associations and supported the conclusion that defining the AD susceptibility genes is not easily amenable by such an analysis. The reason for the difficulty is that inheritance of AD susceptibility is multifactorial, arising not only from a combination of multiple contributing susceptibility genes, but that each gene has the possibility to interact with a poorly defined array of environmental and/or stochastic factors. Furthermore, identification of the AD susceptibility loci is complicated by two factors that commonly influence inheritance of multifactorial traits: genetic heterogeneity and epistasis.

Genetic heterogeneity

Genetic heterogeneity means that different combinations of individual genetic abnormalities are capable of causing a similar disease phenotype. Examples of genetic heterogeneity are seen by comparison of the genomic locations of susceptibility genes in separate mouse models of ADs such as T1Dm, SLE and a rodent form of multiple sclerosis (designated experimental autoimmune encephalomyelitis [EAE]) wherein the genomic locations of many susceptibility alleles vary between models. Although emphasis of genetic analyses has been on identification of co-localizing susceptibility genes, it has been determined that most of the genomic segments detected are not shared between the different animal models [3]. Even within the same AD syndrome such as the different rodent models of SLE, susceptibility is mediated by a heterogenous array of genes.

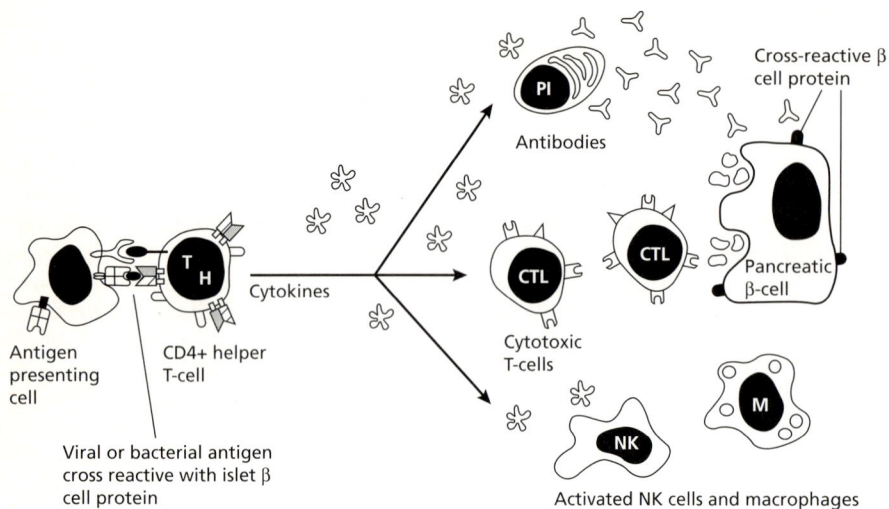

Fig. 25.1 Induction of autoimmunity. Schematic illustration of the events thought to cause an autoimmune response according to the hypothesis of molecular mimicry. A peptide derived from a pathogen is being presented to a CD4+ T cell by a disease-associated class II major histocompatibility complex (MHC) molecule on the surface of a professional antigen-presenting cell (APC). The peptide sequence crossreacts with a component on pancreatic islet β cells. The CD4+ T cell is activated upon receipt of this first signal from its cognate antigen plus MHC molecule, and a second costimulatory signal. Following activation CD4+ T cells secrete a number of cytokines and/or make cell–cell contact with downstream effector cells inducing them to destroy the source of the antigenic stimulus. The pancreatic β cells are also destroyed since they express a protein that contains the same peptide sequence as the inciting antigen.

Epistatic interactions

Epistatic interactions classically refers to interactions in which the genotype at one locus affects the phenotypic expression of the genotype at another locus. A clear example of epistatic interactions in AD pathogenesis comes from a series of studies of congenic mice generated by Wakeland and colleagues [3]. Congenic strains of mice are defined as mice that are genetically identical at all loci except one. The loci may include one or several linked genes. Each strain is generated by repetitive back-crossing of mice carrying the desired trait onto a strain that provides the genetic background. C57BL/6 mice were used as the background strain for different primary susceptibility alleles derived from New Zealand white (NZW) strain mice that spontaneously develop a benign form of SLE. Some of these congenic mice, designated B6.Sle, develop non-pathogenic autoantibodies to nuclear antigens, but do not develop severe autoimmunity. However, when certain of the B6.Sle strains are bred, their bi-congenic F1 offspring develop severe systemic autoimmunity, which is ultimately manifested by fatal glomuerulonephritis [60]. This result is an example of epistasis between two susceptibility alleles leading to a greater increase in disease severity than would be predicted by simply adding together their individual phenotypes. Another type of epistatic interaction exists in which the autoimmune phenotype of the susceptibility alleles are suppressed by epistatic modifiers. Again the clearest example of this concept comes from the B6.Sle congenic mice. When three strains of the B6.Sle mice are crossed which results in triple congenic mice that contain the three susceptibility loci in their genome and are on the C57BL/6 background, nearly 100% of such mice develop fatal lupus nephritis. However, all three of the susceptibility loci were originally derived from NZW mice, a strain in which this genetic combination results in a relatively benign autoimmune syndrome [61].

What triggers autoreactivity?

Several hypotheses exist to explain what triggers and perpetuates AD pathology. Based upon the cumulative data that link autoimmune responses with MHC type, and the central function of T cells in the induction and perpetuation of antigen specific immune responses, these hypotheses have focused primarily on loss of T-cell tolerance, either through inappropriate presentation of antigens to T cells or through the failure to eliminate or silence self-reactive T-cell clones. Although T cells undergo a rigorous selection process during development in the thymus to eliminate self-reactive clones, it is thought that such clonal deletion is imperfect and that circulating self-reactive naive T cells exist which are controlled by the mechanisms of peripheral tolerance.

The predominant view is that one or a few self-peptides can trigger a cascade of cellular events that result in targeted tissue damage [33,62,63]. A typical immune response against a self- or foreign protein is usually focused on one or two peptide sequences (called epitopes) contained within that protein which are termed *dominant epitopes*. Once a response is triggered against the dominant epitope other peptide epitopes from the same protein become targets, thus expanding and perpetuating the immune response. This hierarchical extension of an immune response from dominant epitopes to subdominant ones is termed *epitope spreading* [63]. Most self-peptides cannot serve either as autoantigens simply because they are present at levels that are too low to be detectable by naive T cells. However, a few self-peptides that fail to induce tolerance may be present at high enough levels to be recognized by T cells. These peptides are the breakdown products of tissue specific proteins, and it is likely that only certain proteins can act as autoantigens since there are relatively few distinct autoimmune syndromes, and individuals with a particular AD seem to recognize the same antigenic targets. Thus, autoimmunity can occur if an APC picks up one of these proteins, and presents a dominant epitope of the protein in conjunction with costimulatory molecules resulting in activation of CD4+ T cells. Once autoantigen specific CD4+ T cells are triggered, then barring intervention by suppressive or regulatory subsets, the pathway is set towards elimination of the inciting antigenic stimulus.

Two hypothesis of how spontaneous ADs may be induced are by *molecular mimicry* or *tissue injury*. The hypothesis of *molecular mimicry* (shown in Fig. 25.1) suggests that immune responses directed against infectious agents can crossreact with self-antigens, causing autoimmune destruction. Thus, the inciting antigen could be a bacterium- or virus-derived protein that shares an amino acid sequence with a prevalent tissue-specific protein. Antibodies or cytotoxic T cells directed against the pathogen will also selectively destroy the normal tissue that expresses the crossreactive protein. Relevant examples are from studies in T1DM where correlations exist between congenital rubella and coxsackievirus B4 [42]. For rubella, it has been shown that an immunogenic epitope for the virus capsid protein has structural similarities to an islet β cell protein [64]. In the case of coxsackievirus B4, there is a striking amino acid sequence homology with an enzyme found within β cells called glutamic acid decarboxylase (GAD) [65]. Autoantibodies against GAD may be found in the serum of prediabetic and diabetic patients. The *tissue injury* hypothesis attributes activation of localized inflammatory mechanisms in response to organ injury as an inciting event. During inflammation the release of chemoattractants and cytokines recruits macrophages, lymphocytes and other effector cells. The result may be the release of tissue-specific antigens and uptake by APCs that can result in presentation of self-antigen at high enough levels to act as an immunogen.

Animal models of ADs

Rodent models of ADs have contributed significantly to the understanding of disease pathogenesis. Three major types of animal ADs serve as models for study: (i) ADs that arise spontaneously; (ii) ADs that are induced by immunization or by adoptive transfer of autoreactive mature immune cells; and (iii) ADs that are created by genetic engineering technology. Many of the concepts regarding the causes of autoimmunity have either originated from or have been confirmed by observations made in these animal models. Examples of these models and their homologous human diseases are shown in Table 25.2. The models rely on genetic homogeneity so that recipients and donors are from highly inbred strains.

Spontaneously arising ADs

Animals that spontaneously develop autoimmune syndromes have been instrumental in revealing the complex nature of genetic susceptibility to ADs and in understanding the cellular events that lead to tissue destruction. The observations that even in inbred animals there is reliable but not 100% development of the autoimmune syndromes underscores the importance of the interaction of genetic plus environmental factors in autoimmune pathogenesis [3,66,67]. The essential role of certain MHC alleles as the primary susceptibility genes, the interactions between other minor susceptibility genes, and the role of T lymphocytes in driving autoimmune pathogenesis have all been confirmed by studies in these animals. The most extensively studied models of spontaneously arising ADs are the mice that develop SLE-like syndromes and NOD mice that develop a disease resembling T1DM.

The lupus-prone mice include the F1 hybrid of New Zealand black (NZB) and NZW mice designated (NZBxNZW)F1, MRL-*lpr/lpr* mice and BXSB mice [67,68]. Like human SLE these animals develop autoantibodies to nuclear antigens and progressive severe glomerulonephritis. Extra-renal disease manifestations occur variably in the individual models and include lymphoproliferation with both splenomegaly and lymphadenopathy, hemolytic anaemia, autoimmune thrombocytopenia, vasculitis, thrombosis and arthritis. All of these lupus-prone strains exhibit premature thymic atrophy, the significance of which is unknown. In the (NZBxNZW)F1 model heterozygosity at the MHC (MHC designation $H2^{d/z}$) has shown to directly impact on disease severity. Data on the non-MHC genes linked with murine lupus comes primarily from the New Zealand hybrid model for which genetic crosses have demonstrated confirmed linkage with ~12 loci from the NZB or NZW strains [3,67]. In MRL-strain mice homozygosity for the *lpr* or *gld* mutations results in the acceleration of lupus autoimmunity [69]. *Lpr* is a spontaneous mutation of Fas (CD95) and *gld* is a mutation of Fas ligand. Binding of Fas ligand to Fas results in programmed cell death in the Fas expressing cells. Although the role of these molecules in apoptosis are the subject of intense investigation, the mechanism by which mutations in Fas lead to accelerated autoimmunity is not known. Regardless, the MRL background has been shown to significantly contribute to expression of the lupus-like disease, and neither the genes for Fas or Fas ligand appear to overlap with any of the New Zealand disease loci mapped thus far [69]. BXSB mice carry the *Yaa* (Y chromosome-linked autoimmune acceleration) gene [67,70], which results in more rapid and severe lupus-like disease in male vs. female BXSB mice. This skewing towards higher disease severity in males contrasts the more common pattern of severity seen in female (NZBxNZW)F1 mice, NOD mice and in many human ADs where disease severity is often skewed towards females.

NOD mice develop a syndrome resembling human T1DM and are the most exhaustively studied model of an animal AD [66,71]. The disease pathogenesis begins with the infiltration of mononuclear cells into the insulin producing islets of Langerhans at ~3–4 weeks of age. Infiltration of the islets (termed insulitis) progresses slowly over the course of several months until the islets are destroyed and the mice manifest symptoms of hyperglycemia at ~6–9 months of age. NOD mice express only one MHC class II gene product. As described in detail in the Function of MHC in AD pathogenesis section above, the sequence of this class II molecule, designated I-A^{g7}, is unique to the NOD strain and it binds peptides poorly—a characteristic which has been suggested to explain the association of this genotype with autoreactivity [54,72]. This hypothesis, however, is currently undergoing reevaluation. Progression to overt diabetes can be blocked in these mice by prolonged administration of antibodies directed against CD4$^+$ T cell in the prediabetic phase demonstrating that NOD disease is CD4$^+$ cell mediated [73,74]. Pathogenic T cells capable of transferring the disease have been cloned from these mice and TCRs from such clones have been expressed in non-NOD background transgenic mice thus causing diabetes [75–77]. Once hyperglycemia develops NOD mice can only be cured of their disease with islet or pancreas transplantation.

Immunization and cell transfer models of ADs

Conventional strain rodents may also be induced to develop autoimmune syndromes by immunization with proteins or peptides derived from defined tissues, or by transfer of pathogenic lymphocytes (Table 25.2). Genetic susceptibility plays a major role since certain strains are more prone to mount pathogenic responses than others. One of the best-studied examples of an antigen induced AD is the rodent disease, EAE [62,78,79]. EAE affected mice or rats develop symptoms analogous to the human neurologic disease, multiple sclerosis. The animals show symptoms of paralysis that, like multiple sclerosis, can be either progressive or fluctuating in symptoms. EAE is induced by subcutaneous immunization with components derived from the spinal cord. These components range from the emulsified spinal cord itself, proteins derived from the spinal cord, or defined peptides from spinal cord proteins. The proteins that are known to induce EAE in mice include myelin-basic protein (MBP), proteolipid protein (PLP), or myelin oligodendrocyte glycoprotein (MOG) [80]. Defined peptides derived from these proteins can also induce EAE, and the exact sequence of such peptides depends upon the MHC haplotype of the mouse strain immunized. For any given mouse strain only certain peptide sequences are pathogenic and are termed immunodominant. Figure 25.2 illustrates induction of EAE using a peptide of MOG [35–55]. It was the study of immunodominant peptides in EAE that led to the hypothesis of epitope spreading [62,63] (see What triggers autoreactivity? section above) as a mechanism by which immune responses can be perpetuated and expand to other antigenic specificities. In order to induce pathogenic autoimmune responses by immunization with peptides or proteins it is critical that these antigens be administered as part of a mixture with adjuvants, such as Freund's adjuvant and/or pertussis toxin. Complete Freund's adjuvant is an oil-in-water emulsion containing dead mycobacteria which is thought to enhance immunogenicity in two ways. First, emulsification of antigens in adjuvant serves to convert soluble protein antigens into particulate forms, which are more readily ingested by APCs; and, second, the bacterial products in adjuvant are thought to induce the expression of costimulatory molecules on the surface of APCs so that responding T cells become activated rather than anergized.

Another way to reproducibly induce ADs is by transfer of lymphoid cells from affected to unaffected immunoincompetent recipients.

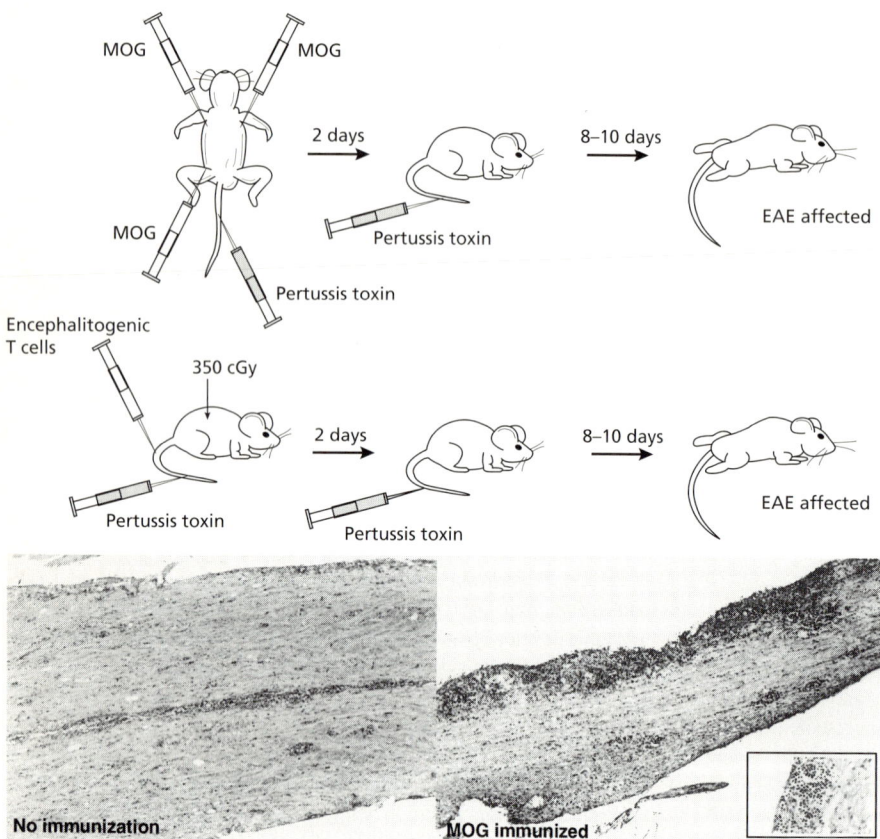

Fig. 25.2 Experimental approach to causing an autoimmune disease (AD). Experimental autoimmune encephalomyelitis (EAE), a rodent disease resembling multiple sclerosis, can be induced by immunization of normal mice with a peptide that crossreacts with components on the spinal cord.

The top panel shows a schematic for EAE induction using a peptide derived from myelin oligodendrocyte glycoprotein (MOG). The peptide is emulsified in Freund's adjuvant. On day 0 the mixture is injected subcutaneoulsy into an inguinal and bilateral axillary regions. Immunized mice receive an additional adjuvant injection (pertusis toxin) by the intravenous route on days 0 and +2. Alternatively, encephalitogenic T-cell lines or clones can be injected into mice prepared with 350 cGy plus pertussis toxin on days 0 and +2. Expected onset of disease is ~8–10 days following immunization or cell transfer. Clinical scoring of EAE is on a scale of 0–5 as follows: 0, no clinical signs; 1, loss of tail tonicity; 2, flaccid tail and hind limb weakness; 3, hind limb paralysis; 4, complete hind limb paralysis; 5, moribund or death.

The bottom panel shows hematoxylin and eosin stained spinal cords from (left) an nonimmunized mouse as compared with (right) a MOG immunized mouse. Note the intense mononuclear cell infiltrate is most prominent in the meningeal areas of the spinal cord of the immunized animal.

Populations capable of transferring disease include cells taken from peripheral lymphoid organs, such as the spleen or lymph nodes [81,82], or cells extracted from autoimmune target tissues, such as infiltrated pancreatic islets in NOD mice. It is also possible to clone pathogenic T cells of a single antigen specificity that can transfer disease [75,76,83]. Cloned T cells are particularly valuable for tracking immune responses *in vivo* since they express a monotonous TCR that can be identified by labeled monoclonal antibodies (MABs) that bind the variable region of the TCR β chain ($V\beta$). Receptors from such clones can also be used to generate transgenic animals. Interestingly, adult T cells from normal mice that are depleted of $CD4^+CD25^+$ T cells can transfer an autoimmune syndrome with a wide spectrum of organ specific manifestations including gastritis, oophoritis, orchitis and thyroiditis. Indeed, this latter observation was one of the ways the existence of regulatory $CD4^+CD25$ T cells was demonstrated [31,32].

Appropriate recipients for adoptive transfer studies are irradiated animals, or genetically immunodeficient strains that cannot produce T and/or B lymphocytes [84]. Two prominent examples of naturally occurring mutations that prevent normal lymphocyte development are a defect in a DNA repair gene resulting in mice with severe combined immunodeficiency syndrome (SCID), and a defect in the Wnt signaling pathway which results in mice that are both hairless and lack a thymus (*nude* mice). Mice with the *nude* defect cannot produce T cells. However, transfer of their BM progenitor cells to recipients with normal thymuses results in normal T development. BM from SCID mice cannot generate functional T or B cells even in a normal recipient. Genetically engineered knockouts of the recombination activating genes (*RAG-1* or *RAG-2*) required for T- and B-cell receptor rearrangement results in defects phenotypically similar to the SCID mutation in that the *RAG-1* or *RAG-2* knockout mice cannot generate functional T or B cells.

Genetic engineering of ADs

Transgenic mice expressing a variety of molecules are now regularly produced in order to model specific aspects of AD pathogenesis. There are four broad categories of the types of transgenic mice that have been studied: (i) MHC transgenic mice; (ii) lymphocyte receptor transgenic mice; (iii) double transgenic mice that express a particular antigen plus the receptor that binds the antigen; and (iv) transgenic mice expressing immunoregulatory molecules.

MHC transgenics

One of the earliest applications of transgenic technology was to ask if ectopic expression of MHC class II molecules on parenchymal tissues that do not normally express these molecules will elicit autoreactivity [85]. For example, chimeric transgenes that contained the insulin promoter fused with an MHC gene resulted in constitutive expression of MHC molecules on islet β cells. An earlier hypothesis had predicted that such ectopic express on nonhematolymphoid tissues would result in presentation of "hidden" tissue specific antigens to potentially autoreactive T-cell clones and induce an immune attack against the islets. The results of a series of independent experiments generating mice that expressed a variety of MHC molecules on the islet β cells were surprising. Although many of the transgenic mice became diabetic, there was no indication that immune reactivity was the cause of the diabetes phenotypes. Rather the data suggested that hyperexpression of the MHC molecules in the islets was detrimental to β cell function, and gave further evidence for the importance of costimulation in T-cell activation. More recently human AD associated MHC alleles have been expressed as xenogeneic proteins in mice [86]. Such mice provide both a surrogate *in vivo* model for studying the development of a TCR repertoire based on human MHC molecules as well as tools to examine aberrant responses as has been shown in *HLA-B27* transgenic rats that develop a syndrome resembling ankylosing spondylitis [87].

Antigen receptor transgenics

Experimental analysis of autoreactivity and immune tolerance has been confounded by difficulty in following the fate of antigen specific cells during development and in the blood and lymphoid tissues where they encounter their cognate antigen. Transgenic technology has permitted a method for generating T and B lymphocytes with defined antigen specificity that dominate an animal's lymphocyte repertoire. MABs specific to the transgenic receptor allow the cells to be tracked throughout the life of an animal and assessed under different conditions, such as challenge with the known antigen. T- or B-cell receptor transgenic mice are generated by using as the transgene the rearranged receptors from antigen specific lymphocyte clones. Because these antigen receptor genes inhibit recombination of the other endogenous antigen receptor gene loci (a phenomenon termed *allelic exclusion*), a large fraction of the T or B cells in these mice express the introduced transgene encoded antigen receptor. Examples in the study of autoimmunity are mice that express a TCR specific for a protein in pancreatic islet β cells (as occurs in T1DM), a TCR specific for myelin basic protein (a target in EAE), and immunoglobulin specific for self-DNA (involved in the pathogenesis of SLE) [88–90]. While BM or lymphoid cells are routinely transferred from these transgenic animals to a variety of types of recipients, the converse experiment has rarely been done. The latter type of experiment wherein transgenic mice serve as recipients rather than donors should be pursued, since the results would allow study of the fate of residual recipient autoreactive cells following autologous or allogeneic HCT.

Double transgenics

A variation for tracking the fate of cells with transgenic antigen receptors is the generation of double transgenic animals that express both the lymphocyte and the cognate antigen (such as a virus) as transgenes [91,92]. The antigen may be expressed in different forms such as secreted, membrane bound or cytoplasmic. Additionally, antigen expression may be constitutive or driven by an inducible promoter. An example of such a system modeled molecular mimicry to show that infectious agents can trigger autoimmunity [93]. The double transgenic mice expressed both a viral nuclear protein driven by the insulin promoter (thus expressed primarily in the islets) and T cells that recognize the viral protein. Virus expression was low in the islet β cells; therefore, T cells that recognized the viral protein remained ignorant, meaning they were neither tolerant to the viral protein nor activated by it. However, when the mice were infected with the live virus, they responded by activating virus specific CD8$^+$ T cells and these CD8$^+$ virus specific T cells could then recognize the viral antigen on the β cells and destroy them causing diabetes.

Immunoregulatory transgenics

A variety of mice have been generated that express transgenes involved in lymphocyte activation or suppression, or that have had specific regulatory genes knocked out [90]. Targeted genes include cytokines, costimulatory molecules, Fas ligand and molecules involved in lymphocyte intracellular signaling pathways. Examples relevant to the study of autoimmunity are transgenic mice that express cytokines, such as IFN-γ in the islets of Langerhans, causing an immune-mediated diabetes [94], enhanced production or knockout in lymphocytes of transforming growth factor beta (TGF-β), which results in progressive glomerulonephritis in the transgenic mice and mononuclear infiltration of multiple organs in the knockout mice, and knockout of the Src tyrosine kinase, *Lyn*, which participates in B-cell receptor signaling results in antinuclear antibody production and glomerulonephritis [67].

HCT and the treatment of ADs

Historical perspective

Preclinical studies and case reports in the human transplantation literature support the use of HCT for the treatment of severe ADs [95–97]. The clinical literature on this topic (reviewed in Chapter 101) contains several case reports demonstrating that patients undergoing allogeneic HCT for conventional indications (i.e. hematologic malignancy) with a coincidental AD experienced long-term improved or even full remission of both disorders. Conversely, there have been case reports of transfer of ADs from AD affected allogeneic HCT donors into previously unaffected recipients. In evaluating the preclinical literature for its relevance to the treatment of human ADs it is important to bear in mind that heterogeneity exists among the experimental systems, and that often the studies were designed to answer basic questions about AD pathogenesis rather than to form a basis for direct translation to human therapy. A goal of the early investigators was to establish what cellular elements transfer or prevent disease. Thus, initial studies were directed towards the creation of allogeneic radiation BM chimeras to determine if transplantation of hematolymphoid elements could alter susceptibility to ADs in rodents.

It was known that certain mouse strains, such as the NZB, develop a syndrome resembling human SLE with manifestations that include production of antinuclear antibodies (ANA), immune complex glomerulonephritis, Coombs-positive hemolytic anemia, and a more general phenomenon of immunological hyperresponsiveness. In 1969, Denman *et al*. [5] demonstrated that transfer of BM or spleen cells from NZB mice to MHC-matched nonautoimmune prone BALB/c mice (both H-2^d) resulted in disease in the recipients. Later, in 1974 Morton and Siegel [4] demonstrated that BM transferred into irradiated recipients could, on the one hand, transfer disease from NZB donors into MHC-matched BALB/c or DBA/2 recipients and, on the other hand, BM from BALB/c or DBA/2 donors could result in transient normalization of ANA titres in NZB recipients. Donor chimerism was not measured in these studies, and one explanation proposed by the authors for the transient rather than persistent nature of ANA depression was that perhaps only short-term chimerism was achieved in the NZB recipients. Other investigators confirmed in different SLE mouse models that BM appeared to be the component capable of transferring disease [8,9]. Cumulatively, these studies were interpreted as demonstrating that the etiology of autoimmunity is determined by the innate properties of the HSC and its differentiated lymphocytic progeny, and independent of the host environment.

ADs as "stem-cell disorders"

These seminal experiments led to the concept that ADs are disorders of HSCs. Indeed, it was later observed by other groups and in different animal systems that the genotypic origins of the BM (i.e. from susceptible or nonsusceptible strains) determined whether or not the animal developed or was protected from disease. However, not all of the studies have been consistent with this concept. For example NOD disease has been transferred by NOD BM into F1 offspring of NOD mice crossed with different strains [82,98]. However, when recipients were genetically disparate such that they did not share one haplotype, radiation chimeras engrafted with NOD BM developed insulitis but most did not progress to overt diabetes [99]. These data show that while anti-islet reactivity can be transferred by BM, the host environment provides additional elements that permit the perpetuation of an immune response, which ultimately results in tissue destruction. That inconsistencies exist in this literature should not be surprising. As discussed in detail in the prior sections, autoreactivity arises from a combination of interacting genetic and stochastic factors that affect hematolymphoid cells as well as other tissues. Furthermore,

BM grafts are complex mixtures of cells with differing functions and the grafts give rise to heterogenous cell populations. Among the populations transferred by BM are those that control antigen specific immune responses—APCs and lymphocytes. APCs express the MHC restricting elements that are instrumental in shaping the T-lymphocyte repertoire. Thus, it is logical that the BM genotype contributes significantly to autoimmune susceptibility. However, the concept that ADs are solely disorders of HSCs is overly simplistic. The other complexities that influence immune reactivity should be considered when interpreting the studies reviewed in the next sections.

Rationale for HCT to treat ADs

Both autologous and allogeneic HCT have been studied in preclinical models of ADs. The rationale for efficacy differs between these two procedures.

The use of *autologous* HCT is based on the idea that near complete ablation of autoreactive cells, primarily T cells, can be achieved by high-dose therapy followed by rescue with a hematopoietic graft that contains few or no pathogenic cells. Such an approach is analogous to the treatment of cancer wherein the conditioning regimen results in cytoreduction of malignant cells and the patient is "rescued" with a hematopoietic graft that contains none or very few passenger cancer cells. It is thought that the aberrant events that induce autoimmunity (such as infection with virus that crossreacts with normal tissues) occur only rarely, and the manifestations of disease in AD patients reflect the perpetuation of effector responses which continue even though the inciting event has passed. Thus, lymphoablation and reconstitution with autologous grafts that lack mature lymphocytes is thought to "reset" the immune system, and the disease will not reoccur assuming that the likelihood a second pathogenic event will trigger autoreactivity is extremely low.

The rationale for *allogeneic* HCT is similarly based on the assumption that replacement of a defective immune system with a normal one will eliminate the autoreactive cells. In addition, donor hematolymphoid cells may express genes that modify immune responses favoring tolerogenic rather than immunogenic responses against autoantigens. The weight of evidence from preclinical animal models favor allogeneic HCT over autologous as the more efficacious approach. However, the current ongoing clinical trials in human disease have been exclusively directed to the use of autologous HCT (see also Chapter 101) [95,96]. The reluctance to perform allogeneic as compared to autologous HCT for ADs is based on concerns of unacceptable procedure-related morbidity and mortality in the former as compared with the latter [9,95].

Definition of terms and experimental approaches

Autologous, syngeneic, congenic

Genuine autologous HCT has only rarely been performed in rodents because of the pragmatic limitations of harvesting autologous hematopoietic cells from small animals. Instead syngeneic donors from the same inbred strain as the recipients, or congenic donors (see Non-MHC genes and susceptibility to ADs section above) that differ from the recipients by one or a limited number of nonhistocompatibility genes, are used. The advantage of using congenic donors is that the gene difference(s) allow determination of the origin of hematopoietic cells (residual host-vs.-graft derived) in the transplanted recipient. For example, mice that are genetically identical except for a congenic difference at the CD45 allele are common laboratory tools. CD45 (previously designated Ly-5) is expressed on all lineages of hematopoietic cells, and in mice there are two alleles, CD45.1 and CD45.2 [100,101]. MABs exist that can distinguish between the two alleles. Thus, staining assays employing labeled MABs, such as fluorescence activated cell sorter (FACS) analysis or immunohistochemistry permit detection of donor-vs.-host hematopoietic cells in transplant recipients. Male into female transplants or vice versa can also be used, in which case the chimerism analysis involves *in situ* hybridization looking for the presence or absence of the Y chromosome. Another type of donor has been termed pseudoautologous. Pseudoautologous means that in models wherein the disease in recipients is induced by antigen immunization [9], the congenic or syngeneic donors undergo similar immunization. Grafts from such donors may contain contaminating autoreactive cells with the potential to cause disease and therefore more accurately reproduce clinical autologous HCT. Grafts from congenic or syngeneic donor strains that develop spontaneous disease are not called pseudoautologous, although there is similar potential to transfer autoreactive cells in unmanipulated hematopoietic grafts. Here, the HCT studies are described as they were originally performed using congenic, syngeneic or pseudoautologous donors with the understanding that all of these graft types serve as models for autologous HCT.

Genetic differences and measurement of chimerism in allogeneic HCT

By definition allogeneic HCT uses donors that are genetically disparate from the recipients. Genetic disparity means that the donor and recipients are mismatched at multiple gene regions and are distinct from congenic pairs wherein the genetic differences are limited. Many of the studies were performed between donors and recipients that were derived from distinct ancestral strains, and thus differ at both MHC and multiple other minor histocompatibility antigen genes. Determination of donor chimerism has been possible using antisera or MABs in cytotoxicity or staining assays. For transplants involving MHC differences (MHC-mismatched and haplo-identical) reagents that recognize MHC determinants have been used. Detection of chimerism between MHC identical strains has been more difficult primarily because the reagents are more limited. In fact, studies that predate the late 1970s when allele specific MABs were developed did not evaluate chimerism. In order to use antibody based assays to measure chimerism allelic differences for defined gene products expressed at the cell surface must exist between donor/recipient strains. Furthermore, antibody reagents that distinguish the allele markers must be available and allelic markers must be expressed on all or on subsets of hematopoietic cells. Examples of antibody reagents used for this purpose are those against Lgp100 [102], a glycoprotein expressed on lymphocytes of certain strains, or CD45 [100,101], an allelic marker expressed on hematopoietic cells. More recently, polymorphisms identified within the mouse genome [103] can be used in polymerase chain reaction assays to differentiate hematopoietic cells between MHC-matched strains.

Preparative regimens

In the vast majority of rodent studies, recipients were prepared for transplantation with lethal radiation. Myeloablative radiation doses are strain specific and require titration studies to determine the dose(s) at which death occurs because of hematopoietic failure, and not from other organ toxicities [9,104]. At such doses mice that would otherwise expire, are rescued by infusion of syngeneic BM cells. For any given strain there is a range of doses that cause myeloablation without other toxicities [104,105], and thus some nonuniformity of radiation dose exists in the literature. Such dose variation can affect both the level of lymphoablation and the degree of resistance to engraftment of allogeneic hematopoietic cells. Therefore, comparisons of outcome between different experiments must take into consideration the potentially relevant effects of radiation dose variability.

Chemotherapy that includes reagents used in human patients such as cyclophosphamide (CY) and busulfan (BU) have been employed in studies wherein the goals were to explicitly model clinical transplantation [106,107]. CY is the best studied of the chemotherapeutic drugs in rodents and reports from the early literature show that this agent alone without hematopoietic cell rescue is highly effective at ameliorating manifestations of Ads, such as EAE in rats [108], and antibody production and immune abnormalities [109,110] in SLE prone mice. Dimethyl myleran is an alkylating agent related to BU with profound marrow suppressive activity and little immunosuppression that has also been used for rodent HCT preparation [111,112]. Fludarabine, an agent that is now widely used in human nonmyeloablative regimens, has also been tested in animals. Unfortunately, mice are highly resistant to the lymphoablative effects of fludarabine and its congeners making it difficult to model homologous nonmyeloablative regimen in mice utilizing this drug. One major advantage of working in rodent systems is the availability of numerous antibody reagents that target specific immune cell subsets. Although there is no study demonstrating that antibodies alone can effectively allow engraftment of allogeneic hematopoietic cells, there are reports demonstrating that antibody treatment can permit engraftment at nonmyeloablative radiation doses in NOD mice [113,114] and other nonautoimmune strains (see also Chapter 24).

Hematopoietic graft types

Unfractionated or T-cell depleted (TCD) BM from wildtype donors or BM from mice with the *nude* defect have been the graft source in most studies. The reason for the use of *nude* mice as donors is that one manifestation of the *nu/nu* gene defect is the absence of a thymus [84]. Thus, BM grafts from *nude* mice do not contain conventional T cells, but when engrafted into recipients with functional thymuses their hematopoietic cells give rise to mature T lymphocytes. Transplantation of purified hematopoietic cell populations have also been studied [115]. Separation techniques to negatively select mature T, B and macrophages in combination with positive selection methods have been used to enrich for progenitor cells. One group of investigators used positive selection by binding to the plant lectin wheat germ agglutinin (WGA) [116]. Their rationale for this approach was the WGA-positive BM cells were enriched for stem and progenitor cells as well as an immunoregulatory "natural suppressor" population [117].

We have used the positively selecting markers Thy1.1, c-Kit and Sca1 in combination with negative selection for mature lineage markers (CD4, CD8, CD3, B220, Mac1, Gr-1 and Terr119) to enrich for an HSC population with a composite phenotype of cKit$^+$Thy1.1^{lo}Lin$^{-/lo}$Sca-1$^+$cKit$^+$ (KTLS) (see also Chapter 8) [115,118,119]. Quantitative assessment of the KTLS population revealed that these cells comprise one in 2000 cells in mouse BM and are, in fact, 2000-fold enriched for HSC activity as measured in *in vivo* radioprotection assays. Further, ~200 KTLS HSC rescues 100% of lethally irradiated mice across CD45 congenic barriers. The T-cell content of KTLS HSC grafts is reduced by >5 logs as compared with BM. Of note, the use of KTLS HSC or other manipulated BM populations in allogeneic transplantation results in profound differences in resistance to engraftment and chimerism outcome as compared to unmanipulated BM [115,120,121]. Thus, graft content can directly affect the outcome of autologous and allogeneic HCT in the treatment of ADs.

Timing of the HCT procedure

Since the progression of ADs in most rodent models is well characterized, it is possible to choose the time of HCT relative to the expected disease course. For example, in antigen induced models, immunized animals have been transplanted either before or following the onset of overt manifestations. In spontaneously arising ADs, the transplantations can be performed during the phase when mice have documented abnormalities in immune function but little clinical signs of impairment or at later disease stages. The studies show that animals are more consistently cured of their ADs if they undergo the HCT procedure at very early stages of disease, even when there is measurable pathology such as insulitis in

NOD mice or evidence of glomerulonephritis in SLE-prone animals, but not at the point when they have suffered endstage organ damage. If a single organ has been destroyed which is itself replaceable by transplantation, then it is possible to perform simultaneous organ plus HCT transplantation (see Chapter 24). The best example of this approach in AD affected animals has been in older NOD mice that have undergone simultaneous allogeneic HCT plus donor matched pancreatic islets in order to cure them of overt diabetes [114,122].

Autologous HCT

There are conflicting reports in the preclinical literature regarding the efficacy of syngeneic or congenic transplantation in curing autoimmune syndromes [9]. Until the late 1980s it was generally believed that syngeneic HCT would have no effect on AD pathogenesis. In fact, mice transplanted from syngeneic donors served as negative controls in allogeneic HCT studies to differentiate the effects of the preparative regimen alone from effect of the allograft—a logical conclusion since syngeneic grafts were thought to merely perpetuate ongoing tissue destruction unless complete elimination of pathogenic cells was achieved. Indeed, in many studies [4,113,123–125] the animals in the syngeneic control groups showed no amelioration of disease whereas allogeneic HCTs were curative. However, a series of reports from a single group of investigators led by van Bekkum emerged beginning in 1989, demonstrating that significant remissions could be achieved with syngeneic transplantation in rats affected with antigen induced ADs [9]. In the original studies of arthritis caused by Freund's adjuvant, the syngeneic BMT "control" group was surprisingly noted to show equal resolution of disease as the allograft recipients [126]. Interestingly, rats that had undergone syngeneic BMT prior to adjuvant exposure developed disease equivalent in frequency and severity as naive rats, whereas reimmunization of rats that were disease affected at the time of syngeneic BMT did not reinduce disease. These data suggest that one element in the effectiveness of HCT may be due to disruption of an ongoing immune response and that antigen exposure at the time of procedure (and not before) is required for shifting the response from an immunogenic to a tolerogenic one. The positive findings were repeated in a genuine autologous transplant study wherein BM was harvested from arthritic rats by surgical removal of a femur, followed by preparation with myeloablative radiation and intravenous return of their own BM cells [127]. In order to reduce the suffering of the affected animals subsequent studies were then performed using pseudoautologous donors with the same stage of disease severity as the recipients at the time of transplantation.

These same investigators confirmed the effect of syngeneic and pseudoautologous BM transplantation in a different AD rat model—EAE. For the EAE studies, rat spinal cord homogenate (RSCH) mixed with Freund's adjuvant was used [107,128,129]. In the initial studies [129] the conditioning regimen of myeloablative radiation (850–1000 cGy) was begun shortly after the appearance of clinical symptoms and a short period of exacerbated disease occurred with the radiation. It was shown that myeloablative radiation followed by transplantation of syngeneic BM from either nonimmunized or disease affected immunized donors lead to complete remission in most rats. However, a certain percentage of these animals spontaneously relapsed. Less intensive conditioning with a nonmyeloablative regimen was also performed using 750 cGy of total body irradiation (TBI) plus CY. Although complete remissions were achieved in many rats, the rate of spontaneous relapse was much higher than what was observed with the myeloablative treatment. Thus, EAE appeared to be more resistant to the curative effects of syngeneic BMT compared with adjuvant induced arthritis.

Success using syngeneic BMT in treating mice with antigen induced EAE or spontaneously arising SLE (MRL-*lpr/lpr*) was also demonstrated by Karussis and colleagues [130–132]. In their studies of EAE [130,131], transplantations were performed at different time intervals following immunization with mouse spinal cord homogenate (MSCH) and recipients received different preparative regimens. Conditioning was begun before to the onset of clinical symptoms on days +6 or +9 following the first immunization, or alternatively on approximately day +17 (2–3 days following the onset of paralysis). Preparative regimens consisted of high-dose radiation (900–1100 cGy) or single dose CY (300 mg/kg). The results were complicated since mice treated at the early (day +6) or later time points (day +17) demonstrated excellent protection from disease, and were resistant to relapse when later rechallenged with the encephalitogenic agent. However, mice treated on day +9 had delayed onset of severe paralysis by 1 week. The reason for this discrepancy is not clear.

One important result of these studies was the use of high-dose CY as a preparative regimen. Given several prior reports demonstrating the efficacy of CY alone in the treatment of rodent ADs [108–110,133] Karussis et al. [130] compared high CY with or without syngeneic BM rescue. Although both treatments were equally effective at ameliorating disease symptoms, survival was superior in the BMT groups. Comparisons of the outcome at the different radiation doses—900 vs. 1100 cGy—showed a superior outcome for the latter group. These investigators extended their studies on syngeneic BMT to the SLE-prone MRL-*lpr/lpr* mice [132]. Mice were prepared with either lethal TBI or high-dose CY followed by rescue with either TCD or unmanipulated syngeneic BM. Improved survival and amelioration of serological and pathological evidence of disease occurred in all treatment groups, unlike untreated controls. However, long-term follow-up at >20 weeks post-transplantation revealed significant incidences of relapse. Under both preparative regimens recipients of TCD BM grafts produced superior results than did unmanipulated BM.

Burt et al. [134] more recently carried out syngeneic BMT studies using a mouse model of EAE that was induced by adoptive transfer of lymphocytes reactive against a PLP peptide. Mice were treated at two time points—in the acute phase or during the chronic phase (day +14 and +74 post-lymphocyte transfer, respectively). Recipients were conditioned with regimens of myeloablative TBI (1100 cGy), TBI plus methylprednisolone, or fractionated TBI (1200 cGy delivered as 200 cGy over 3 days) plus CY (60 mg/kg) and were rescued with unfractionated BM. Histologic analyses of spinal cords were performed on selected mice. Treatment of mice in the acute phase resulted in clinical improvement and prevention of glial scarring in all syngeneic BMT groups as compared to untreated controls. In contrast, mice treated late in the chronic disease phase showed no clinical evidence of disease amelioration and had significant glial scarring. These investigators also measured *in vitro* proliferative responses to the disease associated PLP peptides, production of IFN-γ in splenocytes and an *in vivo* assay of delayed type hypersensitivity responses to peptide challenge. There was no correlation with the *in vitro* studies and clinical outcome, since responses were similar between clinically affected or nonaffected mice. However, the *in vivo* delayed type hypersensitivity assay was more predictive of clinical outcome. The data were interpreted as showing that success with syngeneic BMT in diseases such as multiple sclerosis will likely depend on the stage of disease at treatment—i.e. BMT may be highly effective when there is minimal chronic tissue damage, whereas late intervention initiated after significant tissue damage has occurred will likely not result in clinical improvement.

Autologous grafts

TCD grafts

It can be argued that removal of preformed autoreactive T cells from a hematopoietic graft will reduce the likelihood of relapse following autotransplantation. Indeed, the report of syngeneic BMT by Karussis et al. [132] in the spontaneously arising MRL-*lpr/lpr* model demonstrated improved for the TCD vs. non-TCD groups. The outcomes were different in an antigen-induced rat EAE model wherein comparisons were made between pseudoautologous, syngeneic and TCD BM. No differences were observed in inducing remissions and preventing spontaneous relapses among the various graft types [128]. There were, however, significantly higher incidences of spontaneous relapse in rats that received BM plus peripheral lymphoid cells from pseudoautologous donors. Rodent BM differs from human BM and human mobilized peripheral blood, since rodent BM is extracted directly from bone and has little to no contamination with peripheral T cells. Thus extrapolation from these data leads to the conclusion that T-cell depletion or positive selection of $CD34^+$ cells should be performed for humans undergoing HCT with autologous cells.

Purified HSCs

To test the importance of complete depletion of T cells in autologous HCT we have studied the use of purified syngeneic or congenic HSCs in transplantations into prediabetic NOD mice [113]. KTLS HSCs were isolated from mouse BM as described in the Hematopoietic graft types section above. In our studies doses of ≤1000 HSCs were infused. The T-cell content was, therefore, negligible in these grafts given that HSC purification resulted in a >5 log reduction of T cells from BM, and T cells comprised 2–3% of mouse BM. NOD mice with existing islet infiltrates (8 weeks old) were prepared with myeloablative radiation and transplanted with 200–1000 HSCs from Thy1.1 congenic NOD mice (wildtype NOD are Thy1.2). Donor chimerism was verified in the T-cell lineage by Thy1.1 staining. All HSC recipient mice were partial T-cell chimeras, although the absolute number of NOD Thy1.2 was reduced from ~2000/μL to ~500/μL. Despite this treatment, 80% of mice prepared with radiation and rescued with purified NOD.Thy1.1 HSCs developed hyperglycemia within 6 months post-transplant (Fig. 25.3). The age of diabetes onset was not significantly different from untreated NOD mice ($p > 0.42$). Thus, these studies support the data showing that congenic HCT is ineffective in blocking AD pathogenesis, even if the recipients are rescued with highly purified HSCs.

We next asked if NOD T cells that persist following an irradiation-conditioning regimen are, in the absence of lymphocytes derived from a congenic graft, capable of causing islet destruction. To study this question NOD-SCID mice were used as donors. Because HSCs from NOD-SCID mice cannot give rise to T or B lymphocytes, such grafts are incapable of generating pathogenic T cells. Thus, diabetes could only occur if the residual host cells destroyed the islets. Figure 25.4 demonstrates that NOD-SCID HSC engrafted mice still developed diabetes within 6 months post-transplantation despite very low numbers of endogenous T cells. As compared with unmanipulated NOD mice, the age at which NOD-SCID HSC transplanted mice developed diabetes was delayed, but only by ~2 months. NOD-SCID engrafted mice had persistently reduced absolute counts of $CD3^+$ cells in their peripheral blood as compared to unmanipulated mice (Fig. 25.4). At 2 months post-transplantation, the $CD3^+$ cells remained significantly reduced ($p < 0.001$). Thus, even very low numbers of residual NOD T cells are capable of mediating diabetes pathogenesis.

Translation of autologous HCT to clinical practice

Despite the conflicting results in the preclinical literature using autologous HCT to successfully treat ADs, there are currently a number of patient protocols underway testing if high-dose therapy with or without autologous HCT rescue can effectively treat a variety of human AD syndromes (see also Chapter 101) [95,96]. One hypothesis for the

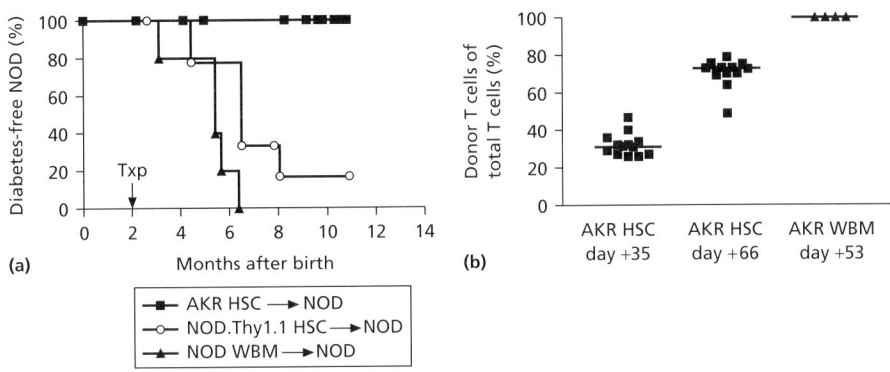

Fig. 25.3 Survival and chimerism in hematopoietic stem cell (HSC) and bone marrow (BM) transplanted mice. Shown in (a) is diabetes onset in nonobese diabetic (NOD) mice that were treated with 950 cGy and 200–1000 NOD.Thy-1.1 congenic HSCs (open circles, $n = 10$), NOD mice treated with 950 cGy plus α-CD4 and α-ASGM1 antibodies and 10^7 NOD syngeneic BM (triangles, $n = 10$), or NOD mice treated with 950 cGy plus α-CD4 and α-ASGM1 antibodies and 10^4 allogeneic AKR HSCs (squares, $n = 15$). Significant differences were noted for AKR HSC transplanted mice vs. mice in all other groups shown (all $p < 0.001$). (b) shows donor T-cell chimerism increased slowly in the blood of NOD mice transplanted with AKR HSC vs. AKR BM. Solid squares represent the percent donor T-cell chimerism as measured in the peripheral blood of individual HSC transplanted mice. The same set of mice were evaluated at 5 and 10 weeks post-HSC transplant, respectively ($n = 13$). These data are compared with AKR BM recipients (triangles; $n = 4$) that were complete T-cell chimeras early post-transplantation.

discrepancies encountered in the animal studies is that antigen induced diseases may be more amenable to treatment with autologous HCT than the spontaneously arising ones. Indeed, all of the reports showing successful treatment with syngeneic HCT have been in animals with antigen induced diseases. Van Bekkum has suggested [9] that antigen induced ADs are the more realistic models of human disease, since their etiology appears to more closely resemble events proposed to induce disease in human counterparts (i.e. exposure to antigens crossreactive to normal tissues). While this latter point is not proved, given the reported successes of autologous HCT in the treatment of rodent ADs, and the more recent results demonstrating positive outcomes in a proportion of patients undergoing the clinical protocols [95,96] (see also Chapter 101), the translation of the autologous HCT approach from the animal studies to clinical practice is not unwarranted.

Allogeneic HCT

In contrast to the conflicting preclinical literature supporting the use of autologous HCT for ADs, several studies have demonstrated that both spontaneous and induced forms of rodent ADs can be successfully treated by allogeneic HCT [7–9]. Indeed, the seminal studies by Morton and Siegel showing success with allogeneic but not syngeneic BMT motivated this area of research [4]. Variability exists among the experiments, including the degree of donor/host genetic disparity, measurements of donor chimerism outcome, the hematopoietic graft type, the preparative regimens and timing of the HCT procedure relative to the onset of disease manifestations. Given these heterogeneities it is, therefore, striking that rodents are consistently cured by an allogeneic HCT approach.

Treatment of advanced stage spontaneous ADs with allogeneic HCT

In 1985, Ikehara and Good began a large series of studies demonstrating that allogeneic BMT could successfully treat AD affected mice with overt clinical symptoms [7,8]. Similar to the prior reports these investigators transplanted mice with spontaneously arising SLE-like syndromes, including MRL-*lpr/lpr* (NZBxNZW)F_1 and BXSB strain mice [135,136]. Resolution of disease was achieved even though treatment was initiated at relatively advanced stages of disease. They further showed protection from progressive insulitis and development of diabetes in young NOD mice [137]. Mice in their series were prepared for transplantation with lethal (myeloablative) radiation and in the initial studies recipients were rescued with either TCD BM from wildtype or BM from mice with the *nu/nu* defect. Thus, mature T cells were not transferred, but the grafts gave rise to functional T cells. Such grafts were incapable of causing GVHD, but were also limited in their ability to eliminate host T cells (see Graft facilitating cells section below). Most of the studies were performed between MHC-mismatched donor/recipient pairs. Donor chimerism was evaluated by H-2 specific antisera plus complement assays, and uniformly revealed that >90% of spleen cells were of donor type. With the exceptions of the MRL-*lpr/lpr* SLE-affected mice [138] and NZB/KN mice that develop a spontaneous inflammatory polyarthritis [139], such allogeneic HCT was uniformly successful at not only blocking disease progression, but also in resolving already established inflammatory lesions [136].

In the case of MRL-*lpr/lpr* and NZB/KN mice it was noted that, while HCT resulted in initial reversal of the clinical manifestations and restoration of other immune aberrations) [7,8], the effects of the transplants were transient and mice regularly relapsed after transplantation [136]. H-2 typing of the relapsed MRL-*lpr/lpr* mice revealed correlation of relapse with the loss of donor chimerism. The major immunologic defect in MRL-*lpr/lpr* is greatly reduced expression of Fas leading to perturbations in lymphocyte apoptosis. These observations by Ikehara and colleagues [138] suggested a high level of engraftment resistance in these mice that the authors attributed to abnormal radioresistant HSCs. In order to enhance engraftment of MHC-mismatched BM, MRL-*lpr/lpr* mice underwent an intensified regimen of increased radiation plus the chemotherapeutic agent CY. In addition, MRL-*lpr/lpr* recipients received both donor BM infusion plus donor bone grafts [138]. The rationale for the added bone grafting was based upon their prior studies that showed colonization and proliferation of donor BM cells could occur in H-2 matched bone grafts [8]. They concluded that such colonization in H-2 compatible BM stroma may enhance hematopoietic cell engraftment. MRL-*lpr/lpr* mice that received this regimen survived long term and were disease free. The principle of simultaneous TCD BM plus bone transplantation from MHC-mismatched donors was also applied to the arthritic NZB/KN mice [139]. The combined transplantations resulted in prevention of joint disease and long-term remissions.

Allogeneic HCT in induced ADs

An important distinction between induced ADs and spontaneous ones is that the latter generally arise in the context of a genetic background with multiple immune system abnormalities, whereas the former are induced in wildtype mice and require purposeful immunizations to break T-cell tolerance. Nonetheless, susceptibility to develop an induced AD also appears to be strain specific, since it has been observed that for any given antigen immunization protocol certain rodent strains are more likely to develop autoimmunity while others are more resistant. Similar to the earlier studies in spontaneously arising ADs, BM transfer experiments were performed from susceptible to resistant rodent strains, and vice versa, in order to identify the cellular elements controlling responsiveness to autoantigens. Therefore, the studies were not designed to examine the curative potential of BMT (i.e. perform BMT after disease induction), rather they focused on disease induction in already established radiation BM chimeras. The majority of investigators reported results similar to those observed for the spontaneously arising ADs, i.e. the BM genotype seemed to determine susceptibility or resistance [9]. Furthermore, there were at least two independent reports from 1981 [140,141] wherein the authors surmised that the mechanism by which the BM genotype exerts its autoreactive or protective effects is at the level of antigen presentation to T cells.

There were, however, notable exceptions to the results demonstrating that BM genotype is the sole determinant of induced AD development. Korngold et al. [125] performed experiments in a model of acute EAE wherein MHC-matched hematopoietic chimeras were generated between SJL strain mice that are highly responsive to MSCH and the low responder B10.S strain. Challenge of chimeras with MSCH derived for SJL led to a high incidence of disease in the B10.S into SJL chimeras, but not in the SJL into B10.S mice. The outcome differed if chimeric mice were immunized with MSCH derived from B10.S mice—both B10.S into SJL and SJL into B10.S chimeras developed severe disease. These data suggested that nonhematopoietic factors, such as elements in the central nervous system, control the development of EAE. This same group published a separate study in a relapsing EAE model [124]. These experiments showed that immunization with MSCH derived from third party MHC-disparate BALB/c or B10.S mice resulted in disease in B10.S into SJL chimeras, but not SJL into B10.S chimeras, indicating once again that restriction in the development of EAE involves elements outside the hematopoietic system.

Treatment of advanced stage induced ADs with allogeneic HCT

Success in curing advanced stage induced ADs with allogeneic HCT was reported beginning in the late 1980s. van Bekkum and coworkers established the adjuvant induced arthritis and EAE models in rats and tested the efficacy of MHC-mismatched transplantations in conjunction with the autologous HCT studies described above (see Autologous HCT section and [9]). It was in the arthritis model that equivalence in the effect of syngeneic as compared with allogeneic BMT was first described [126]. Susceptible strain Buffalo rats (MHC designation RT1A^u) were lethally irradiated and transplanted with BM from nonsusceptible MHC-mismatched WAG/Rij (RT1A^i) or syngeneic BM at either weeks or many months after immunization with the adjuvant (M. tuberculosis). The most effective results were obtained when treatment was initiated shortly after evidence of clinical manifestations 4–7 weeks post-immunization. Animals treated at the later stage had limited recovery with stabilization of disease, but not complete regression. Scarring and permanent joint destruction likely limited the therapeutic effect. Equivalent responses were seen in disease affected recipients of allogeneic or syngeneic BM.

Comparative studies of syngeneic vs. MHC-mismatched allogeneic BMT were then performed in the rat EAE model [107]. RSCH plus adjuvant were used to induce disease and recipients were prepared with lethal radiation or, for some groups of allografted rats, BU plus CY. Syngeneic transplantation was initially effective in inducing complete remissions in all recipients. However, as discussed in an earlier section of this chapter, these results differed from the adjuvant induced arthritis studies, since syngeneic and pseudoautologous recipients demonstrated significantly increased incidences of relapse that occurred spontaneously or following rechallenge with RSCH. In contrast, allografted animals that were given TCD BM or BM from T-cell deficient *nude* rats showed improved outcomes with complete remissions in all animals and markedly reduced spontaneous and induced relapses. The superior outcome of allogeneic HCT was attributed to a subclinical graft-vs.-host reaction, an effect mediated by competent immune cells in the graft against recipient T cells. Turnover of donor CNS cells (perivascular microglial cells) that can potentially function as APCs was measured, and this parameter did not appear to correlate with spontaneous relapse. These EAE studies were extended to the use of largely MHC-matched donor rats using the same preparative regimens [142]. Again allogeneic BMT (unfractionated BM) induced complete remissions and low relapse rates as compared with pseudoautologous recipients. Mixed chimeras were created by using grafts of TCD syngeneic plus TCD allogeneic BM. It was observed that the mixed chimeras relapsed more frequently than the complete chimeras leading the investigators to conclude that clinical protocols for the treatment of multiple sclerosis should be designed for achieving full chimerism. Other studies (see next section), however, do not support the need to convert recipients to full donor type in order to achieve cures of ADs.

Transplantation of purified hematopoietic stem cells

MHC-disparate HSCs

Studies from our laboratory at Stanford University [113] have been directed towards identifying the cells within an allogeneic hematopoietic graft that confer disease protection. To address this question we have examined if grafts composed solely of purified allogeneic KTLS HSCs can block autoimmune pathogenesis in prediabetic NOD mice. Mice were prepared for transplantation with lethal radiation plus antibodies directed against NK and CD4$^+$ cells followed by infusion of MHC-mismatched HSCs. These antibodies were required in the preparative regimen because recipient NOD mice demonstrated high levels of resistance to the allogeneic HSCs, and the antibody treatment reduced this resistance allowing durable engraftment. Figure 25.3 shows that engraftment of purified MHC-mismatched HSCs or BM (not shown) conferred similar protection from diabetes development. Insulitis was also resolved in HSC and BM allografted mice. Of note, although both HSC and BM groups were protected from disease, the pattern of blood chimerism differed (Fig. 25.3). Mice transplanted with purified HSCs remained T-cell chimeras for an extended period of time post-transplantation, whereas BM transplanted animals were complete donor T-cell chimeras only shortly after the time of transplantation. In both groups the other blood cell lineages (B cells, macrophages, granulocytes) were 100% donor derived. The significance of persistent host T cells in animals with spontaneously arising ADs is that these remaining host cells theoretically have the potential for autoreactivity. Evidence that regimen-resistant T cells can, in the absence of an allograft, mediate disease was demonstrated by our studies using NOD-SCID mice as donors (Fig. 25.4). In those studies NOD recipients that underwent myeloablative radiation and rescue with NOD-SCID BM—a congenic graft source that could not contribute lymphocytes to the recovering immune system—developed diabetes. It, therefore, appears that purified allogeneic HSCs alone confer the ability to block autoimmunity and that these grafts have demonstrable effects

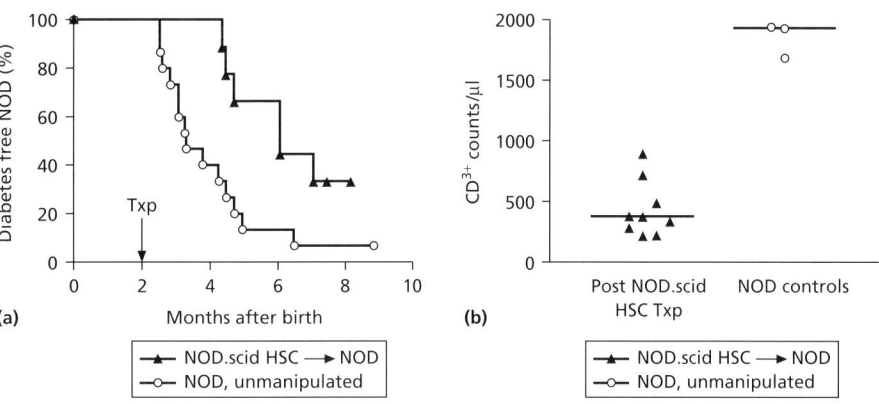

Fig. 25.4 Diabetes-free survival and absolute T-cell levels in nonobese diabetic (NOD) mice following transplantation of non-obese diabetic with severe combined immunodeficiency syndrome (NOD-SCID) hematopoietic stem cells (HSCs). (a) Diabetes onset in NOD mice that were conditioned with 950 cGy and transplanted with 1000 NOD-SCID HSCs (closed triangles, $n = 9$) was compared with untreated NOD control mice (open circles, $n = 15$). Shown in (b) are absolute counts of residual peripheral blood CD3+ cells of NOD mice engrafted with NOD-SCID HSCs that were fourfold reduced even at 2 months post-transplantation (closed triangles, $n = 9$) as compared with unmanipulated NOD mice (open circles, $n = 3$) ($p < 0.001$).

on autoreactive T cells that escape the preparative regimen. This conclusion differs from the one reached by van Gelder et al. [142] since, in our hands, complete replacement of donor T cells does not appear to be required to obtain curative benefit from HSC transplantation.

MHC-matched HSCs

The use of purified allogeneic KTLS HSCs to treat prediabetic NOD mice has been extended in our laboratory to the use of donors that are matched at the MHC. Although the NOD H-2 congenic mice became available in 1992 [143], transplantations of MHC-matched BM into prediabetic NOD mice had not been previously done. The experiments were of particular interest because of the well-studied association of the class II MHC of NOD (IA^{g7}) with susceptibility to diabetes. Thus, it might be predicted that MHC-matched HCT would not confer protective effects comparable to the many prior studies using MHC-mismatched hematopoietic sources [99,113,114,123,144–146]. The donors in our studies were C57BL/6 mice congenic for the entire NOD MHC-region, generated by Wakeland and colleagues [147] and designated B6.H-2^{g7}. The donor were therefore matched at class I and class II loci of NOD mice but differed at multiple minor histocompatibility loci. Prediabetic NOD mice were prepared for transplantation with lethal radiation and infused with BM or KTLS HSCs. Unlike the MHC-mismatched HSC studies (see section above) further antibody treatment was not required in the preparative regimens because the genetic barrier was not as severe. Transplantation of either BM or HSCs from B6.H-2^{g7} donors resulted in 100% protection of prediabetic NOD mice from progression to hyperglycemia. Similar to the chimerism levels observed in the transplants of HSC in MHC-mismatched strains the recipients were partial T-cell chimeras with significant residual host T cells remaining. Thus, the MHC matched allograft also demonstrated the capability to modify the activity of residual host autoreactive cells. The extrapolation of these data to clinical transplantation suggests that inocula of purified HSC from matched related or unrelated donors have the possibility to effectively treat ADs. However, it is possible that not all MHC-matched donor/host combinations will be disease protective unless the critical background genes are homologous between mouse and human. The next important step that requires study in preclinical models is the identification of the background genes expressed in hematopoietic lineages that confer protection.

Graft facilitating cells

The studies demonstrating successful amelioration of NOD disease with purified HSCs show that these grafts are sufficient to protect from development of a spontaneous AD. Moreover, HSCs are the only cells that can permanently engraft in a recipient. Thus HSCs are likely the only population that can confer long-term disease protection. However, non-HSC elements in a hematopoietic graft are known to provide significant beneficial (as well as potentially deleterious) effects. From the studies in nonautoimmune strain mice using TCD BM and our studies with KTLS HSCs, it is evident that unmanipulated grafts contain cells capable of aiding or facilitating engraftment of HSCs. The important contribution of mature immune cells in engraftment is well known in clinical HCT, since it has been observed that TCD leads to higher incidences of graft failure [148,149]. Graft facilitating activity has, therefore, been loosely attributed to T cells. Studies aimed at more precisely identifying allograft-facilitating cells have shown that in MHC-mismatched mice the CD8+ fraction of BM contains the majority of graft facilitating activity [120,150,151]. Studies by Weissman and colleagues [120] examined in detail the phenotypic characteristics of the CD8+ BM cells that can facilitate engraftment of purified KTLS HSC. Those studies showed that the CD8+ population was heterogenous in that there were two morphologically distinct populations that could enhance allogeneic HSC engraftment. One population expressed the α/β TCR, and appeared by microscopy to be conventional lymphocytes, whereas the second did not mark for the TCR and appeared morphologically distinct. This second population was larger than conventional T cells with a granular cytoplasm and low nuclear/cytoplasmic ratio. Cotransfer of the CD8+ facilitating cells with HSCs in lethally irradiated mice enhanced survival and chimerism without GVHD. Chimerism studies comparing mice that received HSCs only vs. HSCs plus facilitating cells [120] or unfractionated BM [121] showed significant decrease in radiation resistant host T cells in the latter groups. Thus, the combined effects of grafts composed of HSC plus facilitating populations provided robust engraftment and significant depletion of residual host immune cells. Such engineered grafts should be considered specifically for treatment in clinical AD wherein engraftment of HSCs from an appropriate donor with depletion of host T cells is likely all that is required to achieve the desired outcome.

Nonmyeloablative allogeneic HCT

One limiting factor in treating human ADs with allogeneic HCT is concern about the morbidity and mortality of the high-dose chemotherapy and radiation used in the preparative regimens. In the last 5 years the field of clinical HCT has markedly changed since allogeneic hematopoietic cell engraftment can now be accomplished with nonmyeloablative conditioning regimens [152,153]. Proof that such an approach is feasible for the treatment of ADs has not been widely tested in different animal models. However, a few reports have been published on nonmyeloablative transplantation (with sublethal radiation) in NOD mice. Ildstad and colleagues [154] prepared 8-week-old NOD mice (H-2^{g7}) with titrated doses of radiation and infusion of MHC-mismatched B10.BR (H-2^k) or

B10 (H-2^b) unmanipulated BM. NOD mice are relatively radioresistant and, consistent with this observation, the investigators found that the nonmyeloablative radiation dose, which permitted engraftment of high quantities of BM cells (6–24 × 10^8 cells/kg), was significantly higher in NOD mice as compared to the nonautoimmune strains that were tested (750 vs. 600 cGy). Control mice that receive these doses of radiation without hematopoietic cell rescue, recover blood-forming capacity without support. Engraftment correlated with high BM dose and despite the nonmyeloablative radiation nearly all engrafted mice exhibited high levels of donor chimerism (>95%). All chimeric animals were protected from disease as compared with the 39% that received radiation conditioning but no cell infusion. Insulitis was also attenuated in the chimeras.

We have also performed nonmyeloablative transplants in NOD mice using low-dose radiation (700 cGy) plus grafts of MHC-matched B6.H-2^{g7} unfractionated BM (1 × 10^7 BM cells). All NOD mice that received this nonmyeloablative treatment engrafted and all were protected from disease development. This regimen resulted in partial chimerism in the T-cell lineage that persisted for an extended period of time (>3 months post-transplantation). In contrast, the other white blood cell lineages converted to near complete donor type within 6 weeks post-transplantation. These studies show that even nonmyeloablative treatment and engraftment of MHC-matched hematopoietic cells can be curative of ADs and that this is a strategy that can be translated directly into clinical practice. Other studies have demonstrated that mixed chimerism, rather than full donor chimerism, is sufficient to protect NOD mice from progression to diabetes [145,155]. However, in those experiments mixed chimerism was achieved by lethal radiation and infusion of grafts that contained both NOD plus donor cells.

Cure of overtly diabetic NOD mice with a combined nonmyeloablative BMT and a donor matched islet graft has been reported [114]. A preparative regimen of sublethal irradiation plus anti-CD40 ligand mAb permitted engraftment with a resultant high level of donor chimerism (>99%) in most mice that received MHC-mismatched (BALB/c) BM. Diabetic chimeric mice were then transplanted with donor matched islets and achieved long-term normoglycemia. The high level of donor chimerism achieved in these studies may be necessary to permit long-term islet allograft acceptance in autoimmune diabetic recipients. We recently showed [113] that the disease outcome was significantly different in diabetic NOD mice that were near full donor chimeras vs. multilineage partial chimeras. NOD mice that received a myeloablative regimen and purified HSCs plus donor type islet allografts were permanently cured of their diabetes, whereas mice that received a nonmyeloablative regimen and developed stable partial chimerism in all white blood cell lineages rejected their donor matched islet grafts after several weeks.

Mechanisms by which allogeneic HCT abrogate autoreactivity

Although many investigators have shown success using allogeneic HCT to block AD pathogenesis, the understanding of the mechanisms that mediate these protective effects is still rudimentary. It is generally thought that allogeneic HCT interrupts AD pathogenesis by a combination of cytoreduction of host immune cells caused by the preparative regimen plus an effect that has been termed graft-vs.-autoimmunity [156]. The latter term refers to the analogous graft-vs.-leukemia effect of allogeneic HCT, wherein the graft mediates elimination of pathogenic cells. This explanation, plus the concept that the allogeneic hematopoietic source replaces a defective HSC leads to a formula that is pervasive in the literature and can be summarized as follows:

$$\text{Elimination of host immune cells} + \text{replacement of defective HSC} = \text{AD cure.}$$

While these two factors clearly play a prominent role in disease protection, the experiments reporting success in treating ADs with transplants of syngeneic, and more recently nonmyeloablative and purified HSC transplants, argue that the formula is overly simplistic. The superior outcomes in allogeneic as compared with autologous models shows that the donor cells, in fact, play a critical role in modifying recipient immune responses. However, the stochastic interactions that occur between a regenerating immune system and the nonhematopoietic factors that drive autoreactivity ultimately determine whether or not immune self-tolerance will be restored. In the broadest of terms it can be surmised that allogeneic HCT demonstrates a higher success rate in curing ADs over autologous HCT because certain hematopoietic specific susceptibility genes have been replaced by donor cells. Furthermore, given the dynamics of immune reactivity, there are likely to be a number of genes or genetic combinations that can favor a protective outcome.

Shifting from the more generalized view to the specific ways allogeneic HCT alters autoreactivity leads to a focus directed towards understanding the effects of the procedure on T cells. T lymphocytes are the primary mediators of pathogenic AD responses. It is therefore logical to conclude that the allogeneic HCT results in changes in the T-cell repertoire and/or T-cell reactivity. The mechanisms of T-cell tolerance described (see Control of immune reactivity section above and Chapter 24) that HCT grafts may affect include: (i) deletion of pathogenic T-cell clones; (ii) alteration in the threshold of reactivity in pathogenic T-cell clones as occurs in the induction of anergy; (iii) skewing of the T-cell response from a T$_H$1 to T$_H$2 type response; and (iv) the emergence of regulatory cells that suppress autoreactive cells.

Depletion of host T cells

Depletion of host T cells is the most extensively studied of the mechanisms by which allogeneic HCT can alter recipient immune function. The advances in antibody based technology has made the measurement of donor-vs.-host T cells accessible to perform. That said, it should be noted that many of the publications on the topic of HCT for the treatment of ADs predates the MAB era and, thus, T-cell chimerism was not directly assessed. There was an apparent assumption in the early reports that if animals survived lethal irradiation with BMT, conversion to donor type must have occurred. In the subsequent studies, particularly by Ikehara and colleagues [123,135–139] wherein chimerism of the blood or spleen was assessed, the data consistently showed chimerism levels of >90%. However, lineage subset analyses were not performed. From more recent studies, including our experiments using purified HSCs [113,121] (Fig. 25.4), clinical studies examining chimerism in patients of TCD grafts [157], and analyses of chimerism following nonmyeloablative transplantation [158], it is evident that the T-cell lineage is the most resistant lineage to conversion to donor type. Furthermore, HSCs and T-cell deficient BM lack graft facilitating populations that mediate elimination of residual host immune cell populations. Transplantation of allogeneic unfractionated BM into lethally irradiated mice results in near complete conversion to donor type shortly after transplantation, whereas HSC transplantation consistently results in partial T-cell chimerism which persists for many months post-transplantation [121,159]. Patients that have received TCD BM also demonstrate long-term mixed chimerism [157,160,161]. Thus, it is reasonable to assume that in the many experiments wherein T chimerism was not assessed, but in which TCD or BM from *nude* mice was used as the graft source, it is highly probably that those autoimmune prone recipients remained partial T-cell chimeras for extended periods of time post-transplantation. Complete deletion of recipient T cells therefore is not a requirement to achieve protection from ADs following allogeneic HCT.

Evidence that even in the absence of a strong graft-vs.-autoimmunity effect (i.e. the graft does not eliminate the host T cells) the donor hematopoietic elements nonetheless modify residual autoreactive cells comes from comparing the results of the experiments in NOD mice using purified allogeneic vs. congenic NOD-SCID HSC grafts (Figs 25.3 & 25.4) [113]. In those experiments the recipients were prepared in an identical manner and following transplantation both groups had similar levels of surviving NOD T cells in the peripheral blood. HSC from NOD-SCID donors cannot contribute T cells to the regenerating immune system, yet recipients engrafted with NOD-SCID HSCs developed diabetes suggesting that the surviving recipient immune cells destroyed the islet tissue. In contrast, mice engrafted with allogeneic HSCs had comparable levels of surviving NOD T cells yet diabetes did not develop and insulitis was reversed.

Although complete depletion of host T cells is not required for disease protection, it is still possible that hematopoietic allografts selectively mediate deletion of autoreactive cells by negative selection. Negative selection is the process that eliminates developing T cells in the thymus whose TCR binds self-antigens too avidly. Although negative selection is thought to apply primarily to the immature T cells in the thymus, this process can also affect peripheral post-thymic cells [162]. BM derived APCs are the most efficient mediators of negative selection. It is virtually impossible to demonstrate directly negative selection of T cells for any particular self-antigen because, generally speaking, antigen specific T cells are too few in number to detect. However, this process can be measured for a class of nonconventional antigens called superantigens (reviewed in [163]). Superantigens are viral or bacterial proteins that bind tightly to both MHC class II molecules and a region of the TCR called the variable region of the β chain ($V\beta$). T cells can be divided into identifiable subsets (by MAB staining) based on this $V\beta$ segment of their receptor. Some superantigens exist as stable endogenous genes in mice of certain strains. The superantigens induce exceptionally strong T-cell responses and T cells bearing the $V\beta$ segment specific for the antigen die by apoptosis resulting in near complete elimination of all cells that are of the responding $V\beta$ subclass. In mice that express endogenous superantigens, the T cells with receptors that have the $V\beta$ segment capable of reacting to these "self-antigens" are deleted by negative selection. Thus, tracking T cells based upon $V\beta$ staining in experimental systems in which exposure to superantigens can be manipulated (such as in BM chimera) serves as a surrogate assay for assessing negative selection.

We followed the fate of superantigen reactive cells in the NOD mice transplanted with purified allogeneic HSCs in order to determine if HSC grafts can mediate negative T-cell selection in these animals [113]. When NOD mice were engrafted with HSCs from a donor mouse strain (AKR/J) which expressed a particular superantigen different from NOD, all of the T cells expressing the $V\beta$ segment ($V\beta_6$) capable of binding the superantigen were absent from the blood of the chimeras [113]. Of particular interest was the $V\beta$ subset analysis of the NOD type cells. Since NOD mice do not normally delete $V\beta_6$ cells, the finding that $V\beta_6$ cells were absent in the blood of chimeras demonstrated that HSC grafts not only mediated the deletion of developing T cells, the grafts also caused the deletion of potentially self-reactive mature post-thymic T cells of NOD origin. Staining of all the different $V\beta$ subsets in the blood of the chimeras revealed that only those $V\beta$ subsets with the potential to bind the discrepant superantigen were deleted in the chimeras. These data, therefore, show that HSC allografts can selectively mediate deletion of potentially autoreactive cells by negative selection.

Replacement of susceptibility genes of the host

The assumption that one fundamental mechanism by which HCT allografts confer protection from autoimmunity is by replacement of susceptibility genes expressed in hematopoietic cells provides the impetus to characterize these genes. The only AD susceptibility genes identified with certainty in mouse and human are specific alleles of MHC molecules [164–166]. Experiments that directly addressed the significance of adding or replacing the MHC susceptibility gene were done by using transgenic technology or genetic approaches in NOD mice. Nishimoto et al. [164] and, later, others [167–169] showed that expression of non-NOD MHC class II transgenes (driven by MHC promoter regions) provided a high degree of protection from insulitis and diabetes. Later, Wicker and colleagues [66,143,170] generated by genetic outcrosses NOD mice that were congenic for non-NOD MHC products and formally showed that replacement of the NOD MHC resulted in failure to develop diabetes. The fact that many of the preclinical studies demonstrating successful treatment of advanced ADs with allogeneic HCT have been done with MHC-mismatched BM raises the very important issue of whether or not similar consistently positive outcomes will be seen when AD affected humans are treated by this approach using HLA-compatible HCT. We [113] and others [4,116,142], have shown that transplantation of MHC-matched HCT can confer similar levels of protection in preclinical models. However, more recent studies from our laboratory in Stanford have revealed that in a model of antigen induced EAE, affected mice prepared in an identical manner were consistently cured of their disease with MHC-mismatched, but not MHC-matched HCT.

There is a vast spectrum of non-MHC genes expressed in hematopoietic cells that can potentially alter the course of autoreactivity. Their identity is not yet known. These genes include those that affect overall immunoreactivity such as cytokines, cell proliferation, lymphocyte or APC cell activation and apoptosis. Another class of candidate genes includes those that affect antigen presentation and recognition. While identification of protective alleles is a formidable challenge, the continued advances in basic sciences such as gene expression profiling by microarrays, sequencing of the mouse and human genome, and other technologies, will aid the determination of these genes. One approach that we have taken is to obtain a series of NOD mice that are congenic at non-MHC gene regions. Although the genetic background in these animals is derived from the NOD (including the MHC) many of these strains do not develop diabetes. We have initiated a series of studies wherein these nondiabetes prone mice serve as HCT donors for prediabetic NOD recipients. We predict that some of the resultant chimeras will demonstrate protection from disease, which will direct us to the genes expressed by donor hematopoietic cells capable of mediating diabetes protective effects to the recipients.

Anergy, subset skewing and regulatory cells

Mechanisms of T-cell tolerance, which include the induction of anergy, skewing of T-cell reactivity to favor nonpathogenic subtypes and/or the emergence of predominant regulatory subsets, have not been studied in the context HCT in the treatment of ADs. Part of the reason for the paucity of data in this area relates to the difficulty in isolating and identifying pathogenic clones that can be followed before and after HCT. The identity of autoantigens has not been achieved with certainty in the spontaneously arising animal ADs, further confounding these types of mechanistic analyses. However, it has been possible to clone autoreactive T cells from animals with spontaneous or antigen induced diseases and adoptively transfer the clones to immune deficient recipients that develop the autoimmune phenotype. The extension of this technology has allowed the generation of transgenic animals that produce a predominant lymphocyte clone with a defined receptor type that develops spontaneous AD. Although these latter two types of animal models are somewhat artificial, they can be used to track the fate and function of autoreactive cells following HCT. Use of these models for this purpose has not been reported to date. Similarly, the emergence of regulatory subsets has not been reported in transplanted AD prone chimeras. In preliminary studies from our laboratory we found no difference in relative numbers of peripheral CD4+CD25+ cells in unmanipulated NOD mice as compared with allogeneic hematopoietic chimeras. Clearly, these are areas of research that will be explored in the near future that are likely to provide further insights to how allogeneic HCT mediate AD protective effects.

Conclusions

The knowledge that autologous and allogeneic HCT results in profound alterations in immune reactivity has been present in the scientific and clinical literature for decades. The animal studies have provided the fundamental basis for understanding both the negative effects as well as the potential beneficial effects that HCT can provide. As summarized in this chapter, there have been numerous studies applying the use of HCT to treat ADs that form the platform for clinical protocols. We believe that these animal models will continue to provide guidelines for translation to clinical practice but, more importantly, they will continue to provide insight into how and why HCT exerts its immune altering effects.

References

1 Vyse TJ, Todd JA. Genetic analysis of autoimmune disease. *Cell* 1996; **85**: 311–8.

2 Jacobson DL, Gange SJ, Rose NR, Graham NM. Epidemiology and estimated population burden of selected autoimmune diseases in the United States. *Clin Immunol Immunopathol* 1997; **84**: 223–43.

3 Wandstrat A, Wakeland E. The genetics of complex autoimmune diseases: non-MHC susceptibility genes. *Nature Immunol* 2001; **2**: 802–9.

4 Morton JI, Siegel BV. Transplantation of autoimmune potential. I. Development of antinuclear antibodies in H-2 histocompatible recipients of bone marrow from New Zealand black mice. *Proc Natl Acad Sci U S A* 1974; **71**: 2162–5.

5 Denman A, Russell A, Denman E. Adoptive transfer of the diseases of New Zealand black mice to normal mouse strains. *Clin Exp Immunol* 1969; **5**: 567–95.

6 Morton JI, Siegel BV. Transplantation of autoimmune potential. IV. Reversal of the NZB autoimmune syndrome by bone marrow transplantation. *Transplantation* 1979; **27**: 133–4.

7 Good RA. Cellular immunology in a historical perspective. *Immunol Rev* 2002; **185**: 136–58.

8 Ikehara S. Treatment of autoimmune diseases by hematopoietic stem cell transplantation. *Exp Hematol* 2001; **29**: 661–9.

9 van Bekkum DW. Experimental basis of hematopoietic stem cell transplantation for treatment of autoimmune diseases. *J Leuk Biol* 2002; **72**: 609–20.

10 Janeway CA, Jr, Travers P, Walport M, eds. *Immunobiology*, 4th edn. London: Elsevier Science Ltd/Garland Publishing, 1999: 262–361.

11 Frauwirth KA, Thompson CB. Activation and inhibition of lymphocytes by costimulation. *J Clin Invest* 2002; **109**: 295–9.

12 Carreno BM, Collins M. The B7 family of ligands and its receptors: new pathways for costimulation and inhibition of immune responses. *Annu Rev Immunol* 2002; **20**: 29–53.

13 Janeway CA Jr. How the immune system protects the host from infection. *Microbes Infect* 2001; **3**: 1167–71.

14 Lenschow DJ, Walunas TL, Bluestone JA. CD28/B7 system of T cell costimulation. *Annu Rev Immunol* 1996; **14**: 233–58.

15 Ullman KS, Northrop JP, Verweij CL, Crabtree GR. Transmission of signals from the T lymphocyte antigen receptor to the genes responsible for cell proliferation and immune function: the missing link. *Annu Rev Immunol* 1990; **8**: 421–52.

16 Minami Y, Kono T, Miyazaki T, Taniguchi T. The IL-2 receptor complex: its structure, function, and target genes. *Annu Rev Immunol* 1993; **11**: 245–68.

17 Paul WE, Seder RA. Lymphocyte responses and cytokines. *Cell* 1994; **76**: 241–51.

18 O'Shea JJ, Ma A, Lipsky P. Cytokines autoimmunity. *Nat Rev Immunol* 2002; **2**: 37–45.

19 Mosmann TR, Coffman RL. TH1 and TH2 cells: different patterns of lymphokine secretion lead to different functional properties. *Annu Rev Immunol* 1989; **7**: 145–73.

20 Constant SL, Bottomly K. Induction of TH1 and TH2 CD4+ T cell responses: the alternative approaches. *Annu Rev Immunol* 1997; **15**: 297–322.

21 van Parijs L, Perez VL, Abbas AK. Mechanisms of peripheral T cell tolerance. *Novartis Found Symp* 1998; **215**: 5–14; discussion: 14–20, 33–40.

22 Ridgway WM, Weiner HL, Fathman CG. Regulation of autoimmune response. *Curr Opin Immunol* 1994; **6**: 946–55.

23 Nossal GJ. Negative selection of lymphocytes. *Cell* 1994; **76**: 229–39.

24 Sant'Angelo DB, Lucas B, Waterbury PG et al. A molecular map of T cell development. *Immunity* 1998; **9**: 179–86.

25 von Boehmer H, Teh HS, Kisielow P. The thymus selects the useful, neglects the useless and destroys the harmful. *Immunol Today* 1989; **10**: 57–61.

26 Strobel S. Oral tolerance, systemic immunoregulation, and autoimmunity. *Ann N Y Acad Sci* 2002; **958**: 47–58.

27 Chen L. Immunological ignorance of silent antigens as an explanation of tumor evasion. *Immunol Today* 1998; **19**: 27–30.

28 Gershon RK. A disquisition on suppressor T cells. *Transplant Rev* 1975; **26**: 170–85.

29 Kronenberg M, Gapin L. The unconventional lifestyle of NKT cells. *Nat Rev Immunol* 2002; **2**: 557–68.

30 Roncarolo MG, Bacchetta R, Bordignon C, Narula S, Levings MK. Type 1 T regulatory cells. *Immunol Rev* 2001; **182**: 68–79.

31 Maloy KJ, Powrie F. Regulatory T cells in the control of immune pathology. *Nat Immunol* 2001; **2**: 816–22.

32 Shevach EM. CD4+ CD25+ suppressor T cells: more questions than answers. *Nat Rev Immunol* 2002; **2**: 389–400.

33 Marrack P, Kappler J, Kotzin BL. Autoimmune disease. Why and where it occurs. *Nat Med* 2001; **7**: 899–905.

34 O'Garra A, Steinman L, Gijbels K. CD4+ T-cell subsets in autoimmunity. *Curr Opin Immunol* 1997; **9**: 872–83.

35 Silman AJ, MacGregor AJ, Thomson W et al. Twin concordance rates for rheumatoid arthritis: results from a nationwide study. *Br J Rheumatol* 1993; **32**: 903–7.

36 Winchester R. Systemic lupus erythematosus. In: Lahita RG, ed. New York: Churchill Livingstone, 1992: 65–85.

37 Barnett AH, Eff C, Leslie RD, Pyke DA. Diabetes in identical twins. A study of 200 pairs. *Diabetologia* 1981; **20**: 87–93.

38 Krolewski AS, Warram JH, Rand LI, Kahn CR. Epidemiologic approach to the etiology of type 1 diabetes mellitus and its complications. *N Engl J Med* 1987; **317**: 1390–8.

39 Maldonado MA, Kakkanaiah V, MacDonald GC et al. The role of environmental antigens in the spontaneous development of autoimmunity in MRL-*lpr* mice. *J Immunol* 1999; **162**: 6322–30.

40 Goverman J, Woods A, Larson L, Weiner LP, Hood L, Zaller DM. Transgenic mice that express a myelin basic protein-specific T cell receptor develop spontaneous autoimmunity. *Cell* 1993; **72**: 551–60.

41 Todd JA. A protective role of the environment in the development of type 1 diabetes? *Diabet Med* 1991; **8**: 906–10.

42 Castano L, Eisenbarth GS. Type 1 diabetes. A chronic autoimmune disease of human, mouse, and rat. *Annu Rev Immunol* 1990; **8**: 647–79.

43 Vaarala O. The gut immune system and type 1 diabetes. *Ann N Y Acad Sci* 2002; **958**: 39–46.

44 Weiner HL. Oral tolerance for the treatment of autoimmune diseases. *Annu Rev Med* 1997; **48**: 341–51.

45 Linn T, Strate C, Schneider K. Diet promotes β-cell loss by apoptosis in prediabetic nonobese diabetic mice. *Endocrinology* 1999; **140**: 3767–73.

46 Lockshin MD. Why do women have rheumatic disease? *Scand J Rheumatol Suppl* 1998; **107**: 5–9.

47 Makino S, Kunimoto K, Muraoka Y, Katagiri K. Effect of castration on the appearance of diabetes in NOD mouse. *Jikken Dobutsu* 1981; **30**: 137–40.

48 Hawkins T, Gala RR, Dunbar JC. The effect of neonatal sex hormone manipulation on the incidence of diabetes in nonobese diabetic mice. *Proc Soc Exp Biol Medical* 1993; **202**: 201–5.

49 Homo-Delarche F, Fitzpatrick F, Christeff N, Nunez EA, Bach JF, Dardenne M. Sex steroids, glucocorticoids, stress and autoimmunity. *J Steroid Biochem Mol Biol* 1991; **40**: 619–37.

50 Rose NR, Mackay IR, eds. *The Autoimmune Diseases*. London: Academic Press, 1999.

51 Wolf E, Spencer KM, Cudworth AG. The genetic susceptibility to type 1 (insulin-dependent) diabetes. analysis of the HLA-DR association. *Diabetologia* 1983; **24**: 224–30.

52 Todd JA, Bell JI, McDevitt HO. HLA-DQ β gene contributes to susceptibility and resistance to insulin-dependent diabetes mellitus. *Nature* 1987; **329**: 599–604.

53 Hunt PJ, Marshall SE, Weetman AP et al. Histocompatibility leucocyte antigens and closely linked immunomodulatory genes in autoimmune thyroid disease. *Clin Endocrinol (Oxf)* 2001; **55**: 491–9.

54 Carrasco-Marin E, Shimizu J, Kanagawa O, Unanue ER. The class II MHC I-Ag7 molecules from non-obese diabetic mice are poor peptide binders. *J Immunol* 1996; **156**: 450–8.

55 McDevitt HO. The role of MHC class II molecules in susceptibility and resistance to autoimmunity. *Curr Opin Immunol* 1998; **10**: 677–81.

56 Bell JI, Todd JA, McDevitt HO. The molecular basis of HLA–disease association. *Adv Hum Genet* 1989; **18**: 1–41.

57 McDevitt H. The role of MHC class II molecules in the pathogenesis and prevention of type 1 diabetes. *Adv Exp Med Biol* 2001; **490**: 59–66.

58 Acha-Orbea H, McDevitt HO. The first external domain of the nonobese diabetic mouse class II, I–A β chain is unique. *Proc Natl Acad Sci U S A* 1987, **84**: 2435–9.

59 Johnson GC, Todd JA. Strategies in complex disease mapping. *Curr Opin Genet Dev* 2000; **10**: 330–4.

60 Morel L, Croker BP, Blenman KR et al. Genetic reconstitution of systemic lupus erythematosus immunopathology with polycongenic murine strains. *Proc Natl Acad Sci U S A* 2000; **97**: 6670–5.

61 Morel L, Tian XH, Croker BP, Wakeland EK. Epistatic modifiers of autoimmunity in a murine model of lupus nephritis. *Immunity* 1999; **11**: 131–9.

62 Kumar V. Determinant spreading during experimental autoimmune encephalomyelitis: is it potentiating, protecting or participating in the disease? *Immunol Rev* 1998; **164**: 73–80.

63 Vanderlugt CL, Miller SD. Epitope spreading in immune-mediated diseases. *Implications for Immunotherapy Nat Rev Immunol* 2002; **2**: 85–95.

64 Karounos DG, Wolinsky JS, Thomas JW. Monoclonal antibody to rubella virus capsid protein recognizes a β-cell antigen. *J Immunol* 1993; **150**: 3080–5.

65 Endl J, Otto H, Jung G et al. Identification of naturally processed T cell epitopes from glutamic acid decarboxylase presented in the context of HLA-DR alleles by T lymphocytes of recent onset IDDM patients. *J Clin Invest* 1997; **99**: 2405–15.

66 Wicker LS, Todd JA, Peterson LB. Genetic control of autoimmune diabetes in the NOD mouse. *Annu Rev Immunol* 1995; **13**: 179–200.

67 Vyse TJ, Kotzin BL. Genetic susceptibility to systemic lupus erythematosus. *Annu Rev Immunol* 1998; **16**: 261–92.

68 Theofilopoulos AN, Dixon FJ. Murine models of systemic lupus erythematosus. *Adv Immunol* 1985; **37**: 269–390.

69 Watson ML, Rao JK, Gilkeson GS et al. Genetic analysis of MRL-*lpr* mice: relationship of the Fas apoptosis gene to disease manifestations and renal disease-modifying loci. *J Exp Med* 1992; **176**: 1645–56.

70 Fossati L, Sobel ES, Iwamoto M, Cohen PL, Eisenberg RA, Izui S. The *Yaa* gene-mediated acceleration of murine lupus: Yaa⁻ T cells from non-autoimmune animals collaborate with Yaa⁺ B cells to produce lupus autoantibodies *in vivo*. *Eur J Immunol* 1995; **25**: 3412–7.

71 Hattori M, Buse JB, Jackson RA et al. The NOD mouse: recessive diabetogenic gene in the major histocompatibility complex. *Science* 1986; **231**: 733–5.

72 Kanagawa O, Shimizu J, Unanue ER. The role of I-Ag7 β chain in peptide binding and antigen recognition by T cells. *Int Immunol* 1997; **9**: 1523–6.

73 Shizuru JA, Taylor-Edwards C, Banks BA, Gregory AK, Fathman CG. Immunotherapy of the nonobese diabetic mouse: treatment with an antibody to T-helper lymphocytes. *Science* 1988; **240**: 659–62.

74 Shizuru JA, Fathman CG. Anti-CD4 antibodies in diabetes. *Immunol Series* 1993; **59**: 237–52.

75 Haskins K, McDuffie M. Acceleration of diabetes in young NOD mice with a CD4⁺ islet-specific T cell clone. *Science* 1990; **249**: 1433–6.

76 Katz JD, Wang B, Haskins K, Benoist C, Mathis D. Following a diabetogenic T cell from genesis through pathogenesis. *Cell* 1993; **74**: 1089–100.

77 Haskins K, Wegmann D. Diabetogenic T-cell clones. *Diabetes* 1996; **45**: 1299–305.

78 Steinman L. Multiple sclerosis and its animal models: the role of the major histocompatibility complex and the T cell receptor repertoire. *Springer Semin Immunopathol* 1992; **14**: 79–93.

79 Raine CS. Biology of disease. Analysis of autoimmune demyelination: its impact upon multiple sclerosis. *Laboratory Invest* 1984; **50**: 608–35.

80 Devaux B, Enderlin F, Wallner B, Smilek DE. Induction of EAE in mice with recombinant human MOG, and treatment of EAE with a MOG peptide. *J Neuroimmunol* 1997; **75**: 169–73.

81 Karussis DM, Vourka-Karussis U, Lehmann D et al. Prevention and reversal of adoptively transferred, chronic relapsing experimental autoimmune encephalomyelitis with a single high dose cytoreductive treatment followed by syngeneic bone marrow transplantation. *J Clin Invest* 1993; **92**: 765–72.

82 Wicker LS, Miller BJ, Mullen Y. Transfer of autoimmune diabetes mellitus with splenocytes from nonobese diabetic (NOD) mice. *Diabetes* 1986; **35**: 855–60.

83 Zamvil S, Nelson P, Trotter J et al. T-cell clones specific for myelin basic protein induce chronic relapsing paralysis and demyelination. *Nature* 1985; **317**: 355–8.

84 Shultz LD, Sidman CL. Genetically determined murine models of immunodeficiency. *Annu Rev Immunol* 1987; **5**: 367–403.

85 Shizuru JA, Sarvetnick N. Transgenic mice for the study of diabetes mellitus. *Trends Endocrin Metab* 1990; **2**: 97–104.

86 Sonderstrup G, Cope AP, Patel S et al. HLA class II transgenic mice: models of the human CD4⁺ T-cell immune response. *Immunol Rev* 1999; **172**: 335–43.

87 Hammer RE, Maika SD, Richardson JA, Tang JP, Taurog JD. Spontaneous inflammatory disease in transgenic rats expressing HLA-B27 and human β2m: an animal model of HLA-B27-associated human disorders. *Cell* 1990; **63**: 1099–112.

88 Boyton RJ, Altmann DM. Transgenic models of autoimmune disease. *Clin Exp Immunol* 2002; **127**: 4–11.

89 Goverman J. Tolerance and autoimmunity in TCR transgenic mice specific for myelin basic protein. *Immunol Rev* 1999; **169**: 147–59.

90 Wong FS, Dittel BN, Janeway CA Jr. Transgenes and knockout mutations in animal models of type 1 diabetes and multiple sclerosis. *Immunol Rev* 1999; **169**: 93–104.

91 Mueller R, Sarvetnick N. Transgenic/knockout mice: tools to study autoimmunity. *Curr Opin Immunol* 1995; **7**: 799–803.

92 Zinkernagel RM, Pircher HP, Ohashi P et al. T and B cell tolerance and responses to viral antigens in transgenic mice: implications for the pathogenesis of autoimmune versus immunopathological disease. *Immunol Rev* 1991; **122**: 133–71.

93 Ohashi PS, Oehen S, Buerki K et al. Ablation of 'tolerance' and induction of diabetes by virus infection in viral antigen transgenic mice. *Cell* 1991; **65**: 305–17.

94 Sarvetnick N, Shizuru J, Liggitt D et al. Loss of pancreatic islet tolerance induced by β-cell expression of interferon-gamma. *Nature* 1990; **346**: 844–7.

95 Burt RK, Slavin S, Burns WH, Marmont AM. Induction of tolerance in autoimmune diseases by hematopoietic stem cell transplantation: Getting closer to a cure? *Blood* 2002; **99**: 768–84.

96 Tyndall A, Koike T. High-dose immunoablative therapy with hematopoietic stem cell support in the treatment of severe autoimmune disease: current status and future direction. *Intern Med* 2002; **41**: 608–12.

97 Tyndall A. Haematological stem cell transplantation in the treatment of severe autoimmune diseases: first experiences from an international project. *Rheumatology* 1999; **38**: 774–6.

98 Serreze DV, Leiter EH, Worthen SM, Shultz LD. NOD marrow stem cells adoptively transfer diabetes to resistant (NODxNON)F1 mice. *Diabetes* 1988; **37**: 252–5.

99 LaFace DM, Peck AB. Reciprocal allogeneic bone marrow transplantation between NOD mice and diabetes-nonsusceptible mice associated with transfer and prevention of autoimmune diabetes. *Diabetes* 1989; **38**: 894–901.

100 Shen FW, Tung JS, Boyse EA. Further definition of the Ly-5 system. *Immunogenetics* 1986; **24**: 146–9.

101 Morse HC 3rd, Shen FW, Hammerling U. Genetic nomenclature for loci controlling mouse lymphocyte antigens. *Immunogenetics* 1987; **25**: 71–8.

102 Ledbetter JA, Goding JW, Tsu TT, Herzenberg LA. A new mouse lymphoid alloantigen (Lgp100) recognized by a monoclonal rat antibody. *Immunogenetics* 1979; **8**: 347–60.

103 Dietrich W, Katz H, Lincoln SE et al. A genetic map of the mouse suitable for typing intraspecific crosses. *Genetics* 1992; **131**: 423–47.

104 Loor F, Jachez B, Montecino-Rodriguez E et al. Radiation therapy of spontaneous autoimmunity: a review of mouse models. *Int J Radiat Biol Relat Stud Phys Chem Med* 1988; **53**: 119–36.

105 Kohn HI, Kallman RF. The influence of strain on acute X-ray lethality in the mouse. I. LD_{50} and death rate studies. *Radiat Res* 1956; **5**: 300–17.

106 Mauch P, Down JD, Warhol M, Hellman S. Recipient preparation for bone marrow transplantation. I. Efficacy of total-body irradiation and busulfan. *Transplantation* 1988; **46**: 205–10.

107 van Gelder M, van Bekkum DW. Treatment of relapsing experimental autoimmune encephalomyelitis in rats with allogeneic bone marrow transplantation from a resistant strain. *Bone Marrow Transplant* 1995; **16**: 343–51.

108 Paterson PY, Drobish DG. Cyclophosphamide. Effect on experimental allergic encephalomyelitis in Lewis rats. *Science* 1969; **165**: 191–2.

109 Russell PJ, Hicks JD. Cyclophosphamide treatment of renal disease in (NZBxNZW)F1 hybrid mice. *Lancet* 1968; **1**: 440–1.

110 Smith HR, Chused TM, Steinberg AD. Cyclophosphamide-induced changes in the MRL-*lpr/lpr* mouse. Effects upon cellular composition, immune function, and disease. *Clin Immunol Immunopathol* 1984; **30**: 51–61.

111 Lapidot T, Faktorowich Y, Lubin I, Reisner Y. Enhancement of T-cell-depleted bone marrow allografts in the absence of graft-versus-host disease is mediated by CD8$^+$CD4$^-$ and not by CD8$^-$CD4$^+$ thymocytes. *Blood* 1992; **80**: 2406–11.

112 Lapidot T, Terenzi A, Singer TS, Salomon O, Reisner Y. Enhancement by dimethyl myleran of donor type chimerism in murine recipients of bone marrow allografts. *Blood* 1989; **73**: 2025–32.

113 Beilhack GF, Scheffold YC, Weissman IL et al. Purified allogeneic hematopoietic stem cell transplantation blocks diabetes pathogenesis in NOD mice. *Diabetes* 2003; **52**: 59–68.

114 Seung E, Iwakoshi N, Woda BA et al. Allogeneic hematopoietic chimerism in mice treated with sublethal myeloablation and anti-CD154 antibody: absence of graft-versus-host disease, induction of skin allograft tolerance, and prevention of recurrent autoimmunity in islet-allografted NOD/Lt mice. *Blood* 2000; **95**: 2175–82.

115 Aguila HL, Akashi K, Domen J et al. From stem cells to lymphocytes: biology and transplantation. *Immunol Rev* 1997; **157**: 13–40.

116 Sardina EE, Sugiura K, Ikehara S, Good RA. Transplantation of wheat germ agglutinin-positive hematopoietic cells to prevent or induce systemic autoimmune disease. *Proc Natl Acad Sci U S A* 1991; **88**: 3218–22.

117 Sugiura K, Ikehara S, Gengozian N et al. Enrichment of natural suppressor activity in a wheat germ agglutinin positive hematopoietic progenitor-enriched fraction of monkey bone marrow. *Blood* 1990; **75**: 1125–31.

118 Spangrude GJ, Heimfeld S, Weissman IL. Purification and characterization of mouse hematopoietic stem cells. *Science* 1988; **241**: 58–62.

119 Uchida N, Weissman IL. Searching for hematopoietic stem cells: Evidence that Thy-1.1^{lo}Lin$^-$ Sca-1$^+$ cells are the only stem cells in C57BL/Ka-Thy-1.1 bone marrow. *J Exp Med* 1992; **175**: 175–84.

120 Gandy KL, Domen J, Aguila H, Weissman IL. CD8$^+$TCR$^+$ and CD8$^+$TCR$^-$ cells in whole bone marrow facilitate the engraftment of hematopoietic stem cells across allogeneic barriers. *Immunity* 1999; **11**: 579–90.

121 Shizuru JA, Jerabek L, Edwards CT, Weissman IL. Transplantation of purified hematopoietic stem cells: requirements for overcoming the barriers of allogeneic engraftment. *Biol Blood Marrow Transplant* 1996; **2**: 3–14.

122 Li H, Kaufman CL, Ildstad ST. Allogeneic chimerism induces donor-specific tolerance to simultaneous islet allografts in nonobese diabetic mice. *Surgery* 1995; **118**: 192–7.

123 Ikehara S, Nakamura T, Sekita K et al. Treatment of systemic and organ-specific autoimmune disease in mice by allogeneic bone marrow transplantation. *Prog Clin Biol Res* 1987; **229**: 131–46.

124 Lublin FD, Knobler RL, Doherty PC, Korngold R. Relapsing experimental allergic encephalomyelitis in radiation bone marrow chimeras between high and low susceptible strains of mice. *Clin Exp Immunol* 1986; **66**: 491–6.

125 Korngold R, Feldman A, Rorke LB, Lublin FD, Doherty PC. Acute experimental allergic encephalomyelitis in radiation bone marrow chimeras between high and low susceptible strains of mice. *Immunogenetics* 1986; **24**: 309–15.

126 van Bekkum DW, Bohre EP, Houben PF, Knaan-Shanzer S. Regression of adjuvant-induced arthritis in rats following bone marrow transplantation. *Proc Natl Acad Sci U S A* 1989; **86**: 10,090–4.

127 Knaan-Shanzer S, Houben P, Kinwel-Bohre EP, van Bekkum DW. Remission induction of adjuvant arthritis in rats by total body irradiation and autologous bone marrow transplantation. *Bone Marrow Transplant* 1991; **8**: 333–8.

128 van Gelder M, van Bekkum DW. Effective treatment of relapsing experimental autoimmune encephalomyelitis with pseudoautologous bone marrow transplantation. *Bone Marrow Transplant* 1996; **18**: 1029–34.

129 van Gelder M, Kinwel-Bohre EP, van Bekkum DW. Treatment of experimental allergic encephalomyelitis in rats with total body irradiation and syngeneic BMT. *Bone Marrow Transplant* 1993; **11**: 233–41.

130 Karussis DM, Slavin S, Lehmann D, Mizrachi-Koll R, Abramsky O, Ben-Nun A. Prevention of experimental autoimmune encephalomyelitis and induction of tolerance with acute immunosuppression followed by syngeneic bone marrow transplantation. *J Immunol* 1992; **148**: 1693–8.

131 Karussis DM, Slavin S, Ben-Nun A et al. Chronic-relapsing experimental autoimmune encephalomyelitis (CR-EAE): treatment and induction of tolerance with high dose cyclophosphamide followed by syngeneic bone marrow transplantation. *J Neuroimmunol* 1992; **39**: 201–10.

132 Karussis DM, Vourka-Karussis U, Lehmann D, Abramsky O, Ben-Nun A, Slavin S. Immunomodulation of autoimmunity in MRL/lpr mice with syngeneic bone marrow transplantation (SBMT). *Clin Exp Immunol* 1995; **100**: 111–7.

133 Russell PJ, Hicks JD, Burnet FM. Cyclophosphamide treatment of kidney disease in (NZBxNZW)F1 mice. *Lancet* 1966; **1**: 1280–4.

134 Burt RK, Padilla J, Begolka WS, Canto MC, Miller SD. Effect of disease stage on clinical outcome after syngeneic bone marrow transplantation for relapsing experimental autoimmune encephalomyelitis. *Blood* 1998; **91**: 2609–16.

135 Ikehara S, Good RA, Nakamura T et al. Rationale for bone marrow transplantation in the treatment of autoimmune diseases. *Proc Natl Acad Sci U S A* 1985; **82**: 2483–7.

136 Ikehara S, Yasumizu R, Inaba M et al. Long-term observations of autoimmune-prone mice treated for autoimmune disease by allogeneic bone marrow transplantation. *Proc Natl Acad Sci U S A* 1989; **86**: 3306–10.

137 Ikehara S, Ohtsuki H, Good RA et al. Prevention of type 1 diabetes in nonobese diabetic mice by allogenic bone marrow transplantation. *Proc Natl Acad Sci U S A* 1985; **82**: 7743–7.

138 Ishida T, Inaba M, Hisha H et al. Requirement of donor-derived stromal cells in the bone marrow for successful allogeneic bone marrow transplantation. Complete prevention of recurrence of autoimmune diseases in MRL/MP-MRL-lpr/lpr mice by transplantation of bone marrow plus bones (stromal cells) from the same donor. *J Immunol* 1994; **152**: 3119–27.

139 Nakagawa T, Nagata N, Hosaka N, Ogawa R, Nakamura K, Ikehara S. Prevention of autoimmune inflammatory polyarthritis in male New Zealand black/KN mice by transplantation of bone marrow cells plus bone (stromal cells). *Arthritis Rheum* 1993; **36**: 263–8.

140 Ben-Nun A, Otmy H, Cohen IR. Genetic control of autoimmune encephalomyelitis and recognition of the critical nonapeptide moiety of myelin basic protein in guinea pigs are exerted through interaction of lymphocytes and macrophages. *Eur J Immunol* 1981; **11**: 311–6.

141 Singer DE, Moore MJ, Williams RM. EAE in rat bone marrow chimeras: analysis of the cellular mechanism of BN resistance. *J Immunol* 1981; **126**: 1553–7.

142 van Gelder M, Mulder AH, van Bekkum DW. Treatment of relapsing experimental autoimmune encephalomyelitis with largely MHC-matched allogeneic bone marrow transplantation. *Transplantation* 1996; **62**: 810–8.

143 Carnaud C, Legrand B, Olivi M, Peterson LB, Wicker LS, Bach JF. Acquired allo-tolerance to major or minor histocompatibility antigens indifferently contributes to preventing diabetes development in non-obese diabetic (NOD) mice. *J Autoimmun* 1992; **5**: 591–601.

144 Yasumizu R, Sugiura K, Iwai H et al. Treatment of type 1 diabetes mellitus in non-obese diabetic mice by transplantation of allogeneic bone marrow and pancreatic tissue. *Proc Natl Acad Sci U S A* 1987; **84**: 6555–7.

145 Mathieu C, Bouillon R, Rutgeerts O, Waer M. Induction of mixed bone marrow chimerism as potential therapy for autoimmune (type 1) diabetes. Experience in the NOD model. *Transplantation Proc* 1995; **27**: 640–1.

146 Georgiou HM, Slattery RM, Charlton B. Bone marrow transplantation prevents autoimmune diabetes in nonobese diabetic mice. *Transplantation Proc* 1993; **25**: 2896–7.

147 Yui MA, Muralidharan K, Moreno-Altamirano B, Perrin G, Chestnut K, Wakeland EK. Production of congenic mouse strains carrying NOD-derived diabetogenic genetic intervals: an approach for the genetic dissection of complex traits. *Mamm Genome* 1996; **7**: 331–4.

148 Ash RC, Casper JT, Chitambar CR et al. Successful allogeneic transplantation of T-cell-depleted bone marrow from closely HLA-matched unrelated donors. *N Engl J Med* 1990; **322**: 485–94.

149 Kernan NA. T-cell depletion for the prevention of graft-versus-host disease. In: Thomas ED, Blume KG, Forman SJ, eds. *Hematopoietic Cell Transplantation*, 2nd edn. Blackwell Science, Inc., Malden, MA: 1999, 186–96.

150 Kaufman CL, Colson YL, Wren SM, Watkins S, Simmons RL, Ildstad ST. Phenotypic characterization of a novel bone marrow-derived cell that facilitates engraftment of allogeneic bone marrow stem cells. *Blood* 1994; **84**: 2436–46.

151 Martin PJ. Donor CD8 cells prevent allogeneic marrow graft rejection in mice: potential implications for marrow transplantation in humans. *J Exp Med* 1993; **178**: 703–12.

152 Maloney DG, Sandmaier BM, Mackinnon S, Shizuru JA. Non-myeloablative transplantation. *Hematology (Am Soc Hematol Educ Program)* 2002: 392–421.

153 Storb R, Yu C, Sandmaier BM et al. Mixed hematopoietic chimerism after marrow allografts. Transplantation in the ambulatory care setting. *Ann N Y Acad Sci* 1999; **872**: 372–5.

154 Li H, Kaufman CL, Boggs SS, Johnson PC, Patrene KD, Ildstad ST. Mixed allogeneic chimerism induced by a sublethal approach prevents autoimmune diabetes and reverses insulitis in nonobese diabetic (NOD) mice. *J Immunol* 1996; **156**: 380–8.

155 Kaufman CL, Li H, Ildstad ST. Patterns of hemopoietic reconstitution in nonobese diabetic mice: dichotomy of allogeneic resistance versus competitive advantage of disease-resistant marrow. *J Immunol* 1997; **158**: 2435–42.

156 Marmont AM. Stem cell transplantation for severe autoimmune disorders, with special reference to rheumatic diseases. *J Rheumatol Suppl* 1997; **48**: 13–8.

157 Mackinnon S, Barnett L, Bourhis JH, Black P, Heller G, O'Reilly RJ. Myeloid and lymphoid chimerism after T-cell-depleted bone marrow transplantation: evaluation of conditioning regimens using the polymerase chain reaction to amplify human minisatellite regions of genomic DNA. *Blood* 1992; **80**: 3235–41.

158 Auffermann-Gretzinger S, Lossos IS, Vayntrub TA *et al*. Rapid establishment of dendritic cell chimerism in allogeneic hematopoietic cell transplant recipients. *Blood* 2002; **99**: 1442–8.

159 Shizuru JA, Weissman IL, Kernoff R, Masek M, Scheffold YC. Purified hematopoietic stem cell grafts induce tolerance to alloantigens and can mediate positive and negative T cell selection. *Proc Natl Acad Sci U S A* 2000; **97**: 9555–60.

160 Bretagne S, Vidaud M, Kuentz M *et al*. Mixed blood chimerism in T cell-depleted bone marrow transplant recipients: evaluation using DNA polymorphisms. *Blood* 1987; **70**: 1692–5.

161 Schouten HC, Sizoo W, van 't Veer MB, Hagenbeek A, Lowenberg B. Incomplete chimerism in erythroid, myeloid and B lymphocyte lineage after T cell-depleted allogeneic bone marrow transplantation. *Bone Marrow Transplant* 1988; **3**: 407–12.

162 Sprent J, Webb SR. Intrathymic and extrathymic clonal deletion of T cells. *Curr Opin Immunol* 1995; **7**: 196–205.

163 Moller G. Superantigens. *Immunol Rev* 1993; **131**: 5–200.

164 Nishimoto H, Kikutani H, Yamamura K, Kishimoto T. Prevention of autoimmune insulitis by expression of I-E molecules in NOD mice. *Nature* 1987; **328**: 432–4.

165 Singer SM, Tisch R, Yang XD, McDevitt HO. An Abd transgene prevents diabetes in nonobese diabetic mice by inducing regulatory T cells. *Proc Natl Acad Sci U S A* 1993; **90**: 9566–70.

166 Reich EP, Sherwin RS, Kanagawa O, Janeway CA Jr. An explanation for the protective effect of the MHC class II, I-E molecule in murine diabetes. *Nature* 1989; **341**: 326–8.

167 Miyazaki T, Uno M, Uehira M *et al*. Direct evidence for the contribution of the unique I-ANOD to the development of insulitis in non-obese diabetic mice. *Nature* 1990; **345**: 722–4.

168 Lund T, O'Reilly L, Hutchings P *et al*. Prevention of insulin-dependent diabetes mellitus in non-obese diabetic mice by transgenes encoding modified I-A β-chain or normal I-E α-chain. *Nature* 1990; **345**: 727–9.

169 Slattery RM, Kjer-Nielsen L, Allison J, Charlton B, Mandel TE, Miller JF. Prevention of diabetes in non-obese diabetic I-Ak transgenic mice. *Nature* 1990; **345**: 724–6.

170 Podolin PL, Pressey A, DeLarato NH, Fischer PA, Peterson LB, Wicker LS. I-E+ nonobese diabetic mice develop insulitis and diabetes. *J Ex Med* 1993; **178**: 793–803.

26

Robert Korngold & Thea M. Friedman

Murine Models for Graft-vs.-Host Disease

Introduction

Graft-vs.-host disease (GVHD) is a major complication of allogeneic hematopoietic cell transplantation (HCT) and is a manifestation of the alloreactive response to host histocompatibility (H) differences mediated by mature donor T cells in the inoculum [1–3] (see also Chapter 3). Before discussing the pathogenesis of GVHD and the cell types involved, it is important to consider the essential features of T-cell specificity and T-effector function.

The specificity of typical T cells expressing αβ T-cell receptor (TCR) molecules is directed to peptide fragments of antigen bound to major histocompatibility complex (MHC) molecules, human leukocyte antigen (HLA) molecules in humans and H-2 molecules in the mouse [4–9]. A more detailed understanding of the MHC molecules can be found in Chapter 4. As the result of a complex process of selection in the thymus, $\alpha\beta^+$ T cells are rendered tolerant to "self" MHC molecules (plus the various endogenous peptides bound to these molecules) but display reactivity to self-MHC molecules complexed to foreign peptides [8,9]. Minor histocompatibility antigens (mHA)—one of the principal targets for GVHD—fall into this category. T-cell specificity also encompasses reactivity to allo (foreign, nonself) MHC molecules [4]. GVHD to MHC alloantigens is intense and reflects that the precursor frequency of T cells for allo-MHC antigens is very high, far higher than for typical foreign peptide antigens complexed to self-MHC molecules. GVHD in the context of MHC differences could also be a reflection of increased antigen concentration on the target tissues where every MHC can elicit T-cell responses. Although the same TCR molecule can recognize both classes of antigens, the biological significance of MHC alloreactivity is poorly understood. In particular, it is still unclear whether alloreactivity is directed to MHC epitopes, MHC-associated peptides or both.

There are two classes of MHC molecules, termed classes I and II [4,7]. Class I molecules are expressed on virtually all nucleated cells and are recognized by the $CD8^+$ subset of T cells. Class II molecules show a more restricted tissue distribution and are recognized by $CD4^+$ T cells. The CD4 and CD8 molecules which define the two major subsets of T cells act as adhesion molecules and bind to nonpolymorphic regions of MHC class II and class I molecules, respectively [6]. Such binding increases the avidity of TCR/MHC interaction and causes each T-cell subset to display MHC class specificity. Thus, the $CD8^+$ subset of T cells reacts much more effectively with class I than class II MHC molecules whereas $CD4^+$ cells show the reverse specificity. As discussed later, this MHC class specificity of $CD4^+$ and $CD8^+$ cells applies to GVHD.

In the case of unprimed cells, T-cell activation depends on contact with MHC-associated peptide (or MHC alloantigens) expressed on specialized antigen-presenting cells (APCs), such as macrophages and dendritic cells [4,8]. These cells reside in the T-dependent areas of the lymphoid tissues, i.e. the periarteriolar lymphocyte sheaths of the splenic white pulp and the paracortical areas of lymph nodes. Recognition of antigen in these sites also applies when T cells are transferred to allogeneic hosts where they encounter host alloantigens expressed constitutively on host APCs in the T-dependent areas of the recipient. After contact with antigen on APCs, T cells proliferate extensively, release various lymphokines and differentiate into T-effector cells; in allogeneic hosts, this chain of events constitutes a GVH reaction (which may or may not progress to overt GVHD). Whereas resting T cells are confined to the recirculating lymphocyte pool (blood, lymphoid tissues and lymph), antigen-activated T cells have the capacity to penetrate the walls of capillary blood vessels and can thus disseminate throughout the body. Activated T cells show a particular propensity for homing to the gut, liver, lung and skin, sites commonly affected by GVHD. When activated T cells reencounter antigen in these sites, the cells express various effector functions.

The effector functions of T cells are complex and difficult to categorize [4]. Direct destruction of target cells by cytotoxic T lymphocytes (CTL) is the simplest type of effector function and is probably a major cause of the protean pathology seen in GVHD. Other T cells have limited CTL activity but, after reencountering antigen on local APCs in the tissue concerned, are able to release large quantities of various lymphokines. By attracting a spectrum of mononuclear cells from the blood and also by causing direct tissue destruction (in the case of toxic lymphokines such as tumor necrosis factor-alpha [TNF-α]), these lymphokines elicit the typical lesions seen in delayed-type hypersensitivity. In many textbooks it is stated that the effector functions of $CD4^+$ and $CD8^+$ cells are quite distinct, with $CD8^+$ cells functioning as CTL and $CD4^+$ cells accounting for delayed-type hypersensitivity. However, this is an oversimplification of effector function because some $CD8^+$ cells can release lymphokines and cause delayed-type hypersensitivity and some $CD4^+$ cells exhibit CTL activity [4].

Target antigens for GVHD

As mentioned earlier, GVHD is directed to two broad categories of alloantigens: major (MHC) antigens and mHA. These antigens also provide the main targets for allograft rejection. Because of the availability of congenic strains, mice are the species of choice for studying GVHD directed to major vs. mHA and for determining the relative contributions of $CD4^+$ and $CD8^+$ cells to GVHD. Before discussing the various models for murine GVHD, it is important to consider the issue of host resistance to GVHD.

Susceptibility to GVHD: the problem of host-vs.-graft (HVG) reactions

GVHD is not an inevitable consequence of transferring T cells across H barriers. Thus, injecting normal adult mice with even large doses of allogeneic lymphoid cells generally causes no pathology; the host mouse mounts a powerful response to the donor alloantigens and the injected T cells are rapidly destroyed. HVG reactions involve three cell types: T cells, B cells and natural killer (NK) cells [10–13]. HVG reactions mediated by T and B cells take several days to develop and cause graft rejection by a combination of CTL activity and production of alloantibody. In adult mice, the simplest approach for inactivating host T and B cells is to expose the host to total body irradiation (TBI), resting T and B cells being highly radiosensitive.

HVG reactions mediated by NK cells are often intense and occur within hours of donor cell transfer [11,12]. The target antigens for NK cells are still poorly defined, but there is accumulating evidence that the specificity of NK cells participating in HVG reactions is directed to cells that lack self-class I molecules [13]. NK-mediated HVG reactions do not apply when hypothetical MHC H-2-heterozygous $(a \times b)F_1$ cells are transferred to their parental homozygous strain a mice because the host strain a class I molecules are fully represented on the donor cells. In this situation, HVG reactions are mediated solely by alloreactive T and B cells, responding to the strain b class I molecules present on the donor cells. A different situation applies in $a \rightarrow b$, $a \rightarrow (a \times b)F_1$ and $(a \times b)F_1 \rightarrow (a \times c)F_1$ strain combinations, where a, b and c each represent a different hypothetical parental MHC H-2 haplotype. In each of these combinations the donor cells do not express the complete set of class I molecules of the host. For example, in the $a \rightarrow (a \times b)F_1$ combination, the host NK cells recognize self-class I^a on the donor cells but do not see self-class I^b: the failure to recognize self-class I^b on the donor cells causes the F_1 hosts to display "hybrid resistance", and their NK cells reject the parental strain cells. Similar lack of self-class I recognition applies in $a \rightarrow b$ and $(a \times b)F_1 \rightarrow (a \times c)F_1$ combinations; here, the GVH reaction by the host NK cells is termed "allogeneic resistance" [14]. In the case of parent $\rightarrow$ F1 combinations, it should be pointed out that the intensity of hybrid resistance varies considerably according to the particular class I disparity involved. In practice, hybrid resistance is only a problem when there is heterozygosity for the $H-2D^b$ class I molecule, e.g. when C57BL (K^bD^b) cells are transferred to [C57BL × CBA (K^{kDak})]F_1 hosts.

NK-mediated HVG reactions are especially strong in MHC H-2 different $a \rightarrow b$ combinations. Inactivating NK cells *in situ* is not easy because these cells are highly radioresistant; injection of anti-NK antibodies can be effective, but this is a cumbersome and expensive procedure. In practice, there are a number of ways to work around the problem of NK-mediated HVG reactions. For example, if it is essential to use fully H-2-different $a \rightarrow b$ combinations, the activity of host NK cells can usually be overcome simply by injecting the donor lymphoid cells in large doses. The easiest solution, however, is to use $a \rightarrow (a \times b)F_1$ combinations; as mentioned above, hybrid resistance in parent $\rightarrow F_1$ combinations is generally insignificant unless $H-2D^b$ heterozygosity is involved. It is worth noting that NK-mediated HVG reactions do not operate in minor H-different combinations since the donor and host are H-2 identical.

In a clinical setting, GVHD seen after HCT is often complicated by concomitant HVG reactions, especially if the host has been presensitized to the donor as the result of blood transfusion. In the case of MHC-incompatible strain combinations, the mouse models outlined below are deliberately designed to avoid the problem of HVG reactions by: (i) using nonimmunized F_1 hybrid mice as hosts for parental strain T cells; (ii) avoiding $H-2D^b$ heterozygosity; and (iii) exposing the host mice to TBI. With this protocol, one can examine "pure" GVHD with little or no interference from host T, B or NK cells. It should be mentioned that all of the models discussed below involve intravenous transfer of cells.

GVHD directed to MHC antigens

Because of the high precursor frequency of T cells for allo-MHC antigens, these antigens elicit a very intense form of GVHD [3,15–20]. Thus, transfer of even small numbers of parental strain T cells ($<10^5$) into irradiated F_1 mice leads to a high incidence of lethal GVHD. GVHD is especially severe when the host expresses combined H-2 class I and class II differences. GVHD directed to whole H-2 differences involves both $CD4^+$ and $CD8^+$ T cells, responding to class II and class I differences, respectively, and either population alone is able to induce lethal GVHD [16–19]. Assessing the relative importance of class I vs. class II antigens as targets for GVHD necessitates using donor/host combinations differing solely at class I or class II loci.

GVHD to H-2 class II antigens

Most mouse strains express two types of class II molecules, I-A and I-E; these molecules are the homologues of HLA-DQ and HLA-DR molecules, respectively. I-E alloantigens are much less immunogenic than I-A antigens, and GVHD directed selectively to I-E antigens tends to be weak and is generally nonlethal. I-A antigens, by contrast, are highly potent inducers of lethal GVHD. In general, the severity and intensity of GVHD varies with the strength of antigenic differences between strain combinations. To study GVHD directed selectively to I-A antigens, the most convenient combination is C57BL/6 (B6) and B6.C-H-2^{bm12} (bm12) [17]. These two strains are identical except for three amino acid differences in the β chain of the I-A molecule. Though seemingly small, this mutation is highly immunogenic for T cells. Indeed, the response of B6 T cells to bm12 and vice versa is as strong as with an allelic (nonmutant) I-A difference [21].

The key feature of GVHD developing in the B6/bm12 combination is that GVHD induction is strictly controlled by $CD4^+$ cells with little or no contribution from $CD8^+$ cells [17,22]. Thus, whereas small numbers of B6 (or bm12) $CD4^+$ cells cause close to 100% mortality in irradiated (B6 × bm12)F_1 hosts under defined conditions (see below), even high doses of B6 (or bm12) $CD8^+$ cells cause no mortality (provided that the $CD8^+$ cells are thoroughly depleted of $CD4^+$ cells). The failure of $CD8^+$ cells to mediate anti-class II GVHD is to be expected because, as mentioned earlier, the specificity of $CD8^+$ cells is strongly skewed to recognition of class I antigens. Proliferative responses of purified B6 $CD8^+$ cells to bm12 APCs are extremely weak, both *in vivo* and *in vitro* [21].

When B6 $CD4^+$ cells are transferred to irradiated (B6 × bm12)F_1 mice, the donor T cells initially home to the T-dependent areas of the spleen and lymph nodes. Here, the T cells respond to host class II antigens expressed on host APCs (typical APCs being highly radioresistant) and then mount a powerful proliferative response [17]. Large numbers of donor-derived blast cells enter the circulation and then percolate throughout the body to reach the skin, gut and liver, among other sites, where the cells mediate their effector functions. The type of GVHD which results from this GVH reaction depends critically on a number of different factors including: (i) the dose of TBI used to condition the host; (ii) the dose of $CD4^+$ cells injected; and (iii) the source of marrow cells (donor or host) used for reconstitution [22].

Donor marrow plus donor $CD4^+$ cells

The simplest model for GVHD is to inject the F_1 host mice with a mixture of donor $CD4^+$ cells and donor marrow cells [22]; under these conditions, the donor CD4+ cells selectively attack the host and do not impair stem cell reconstitution. The severity of GVHD in this situation is quite variable and seems to be a reflection of the general health of the animal colony. If the mice are in excellent health and free from infection, GVHD tends to be quite mild when the conditioning dose of TBI is not above 8 Gy. Mortality rates are low and, except for transient splenomegaly, the mice show minimal pathology. Raising the dose of TBI to 10 Gy, however, leads to acute GVHD and heavy mortality with most deaths occurring within 2 weeks of T-cell injection. This acute pattern of GVHD is characterized by marked weight loss, mild atrophy of the lymphohemopoietic system and a distended small intestine. Exudative enteropathy is apparent, and death is probably largely a reflection of gut damage leading to dehydration and acute infection [20,23,24]. Toxic lymphokines play a key role in gut damage. The key role of toxic lymphokines is apparent from the finding that mice can be protected against gut damage (and death) by injecting anti-TNF-α antibodies [25].

Induction of acute lethal GVHD in heavily irradiated recipients requires surprisingly few CD4+ cells. Doses of 1×10^5 CD4+ cells elicit close to 100% mortality and even 1×10^4 cells cause significant mortality. If the health of the colony is suboptimal, acute lethal GVHD is seen with much lower doses of TBI, e.g. 7 Gy.

Chronic GVHD tends to be sporadic in the above model and is generally seen only when very low numbers of CD4+ cells are transferred. With higher numbers of CD4+ cells, the few mice that survive acute GVHD generally show rapid recovery. When chronic GVHD is seen, the hosts show prolonged weight loss, lymphoid atrophy and evidence of infection, although skin lesions are rare.

Donor marrow plus high doses of donor CD4+ cells

The acute lethal GVHD seen in heavily irradiated recipients applies when the donor CD4+ cells are injected in the range of 3×10^6 cells down to 1×10^4 cells [22]. Injection of higher doses of CD4+ cells paradoxically leads to protection. Thus, whereas doses of 1×10^6 CD4+ cells generally cause close to 100% mortality, increasing the number of CD4+ cells to 2×10^7 reduces the mortality rate to less than 40% [22]. Even lower mortality rates occur when bulk populations of CD4+ cells and B cells are injected. Thus, if 1000 cGy irradiated (B6 × bm12)F_1 mice are injected with a dose of 1×10^8 unseparated B6 spleen cells (a mixture of CD4+ cells, CD8+ cells, B cells and stem cells), mortality rates are less than 10%. In considering the mechanism of this protection, it should be pointed out that mice kept under "germ-free" conditions are relatively resistant to lethal GVHD [26]. It is quite likely therefore that lethal GVHD is largely a consequence of infection, the tissue damage elicited by the GVH reaction making the host susceptible to invasion by pathogens. The capacity of large doses of CD4+ cells and B cells to protect against mortality could thus be attributed to restoration of immunocompetence. Cellular and humoral immunity are restored and the host repels pathogens entering through damaged mucosal surfaces. According to this interpretation, bulk populations of donor lymphoid cells do not limit the intensity of the initial GVH reaction but merely counteract the consequences of this reaction. Here, it is worth mentioning that the bm12 F_1 recipients of bulk populations of donor B6 lymphoid cells do go through a "crisis" at about 2 weeks after transfer (animals show hunched posture and lethargy) but then go on to full recovery.

Host marrow and donor CD4+ cells

A very different pattern of GVHD occurs when donor CD4+ cells are transferred with host rather than donor marrow cells [20,22]. In this situation, the donor CD4+ cells attack the F_1 host stem cells and cause death from hemopoietic failure within 3 weeks; stem cell engraftment is apparent at 1 week post-transfer, but by day 14 the entire lymphohemopoietic system, including the marrow, shows near-total aplasia. Mortality rates approach 100% and are little influenced by either the dose of CD4+ cells injected (1×10^5–2×10^7) or the conditioning dose of TBI used (6–10 Gy). Even with a low dose of 6 Gy, as few as 10^5 CD4+ cells cause close to 100% mortality.

It should be emphasized that the above syndrome of lethal marrow aplasia does not occur when the donor CD4+ cells are transferred with a mixture of donor and host BM. Here, the CD4+ cells attack the host stem cells but do not prevent engraftment of the donor cells. Since semipurified CD4+ cells are often contaminated with stem cells, especially when derived from spleen cells, demonstrating marrow aplasia mediated by CD4+ cells depends critically on using a highly purified population of these cells. Lymph nodes are the best starting population for preparing stem-cell-free CD4+ cells.

GVHD to H-2 class I antigens

As for class II molecules, mice express two class I molecules, H-2K and H-2D. Both types of molecules are potent targets for lethal GVHD. Although a number of class I-different, class II-identical strain combinations are available, the simplest approach for studying anticlass I GVHD is to use class I mutant mice, e.g. the series of "bm" mutant mice [27]. On the basis of skin graft rejection, investigators have isolated more than a dozen different bm mutant strains of mice exhibiting small mutations (1–4 amino acid substitutions) of the H-2K molecules of the B6 (H-2^b) strain. The immunogenicity of these mutant molecules for "wild-type" B6 T cells is quite variable. Some mutants, e.g. bm1, are strongly stimulatory, whereas others, e.g. bm9, elicit only low proliferative and CTL *in vitro* generated responses [21]. Detailed information on the capacity of the various class I mutants to elicit GVHD is not yet available. The data discussed below apply to the B6 (bm1 combination, using (B6 × bm1)F_1 mice as hosts.

Despite the dogma that CD8+ cells function poorly without exogenous help, purified B6 CD8+ cells give spectacularly high proliferative and CTL responses to bm1 stimulators *in vitro* in the absence of CD4+ cells or their products [21]. Helper-independent responses of CD8+ cells also apply *in vivo* [17,21]. Thus, when purified B6 CD8+ cells are transferred to irradiated bm1 F_1 mice, the donor cells proliferate extensively in the lymphoid tissues in the absence of CD4+ cells and then disseminate throughout the body to mediate their effector functions. The end result is GVHD. It should be mentioned that B6 CD4+ cells respond very poorly to bm1, and even large doses of B6 CD4+ cells fail to elicit GVHD in bm1 F_1 hosts [28].

Donor marrow plus donor CD8+ cells

The injection of B6 CD8+ cells into class I-different irradiated (B6 × bm1)F_1 mice, along with B6 marrow cells, causes heavy mortality irrespective of whether the hosts are conditioned with heavy irradiation (10 Gy) or light irradiation (6 Gy) [28]. Mortality rates approaching 100% are observed with a wide range of T-cell numbers, i.e. from 2×10^7 down to 1×10^5 cells. The striking finding is that GVHD tends to be chronic rather than acute. Except for mild weight loss, most of the recipients appear reasonably healthy for the first 3–4 weeks after transfer. Then, often quite suddenly, the mice become obviously ill with hunched posture, diarrhea and marked weight loss. The condition of the mice worsens progressively and deaths occur at around 5–8 weeks after transfer. At autopsy, the mice show the typical signs of chronic GVHD with marked weight loss, lymphohemopoietic atrophy, and lymphocytic infiltrations in various organs. Skin lesions can be severe, although this severity is variable. Gut damage is evident, but is much less severe than in class II-different combinations [23,24].

Effects of adding CD4+ cells

Despite the evidence that CD8+ cells mediate helper-independent responses *in vitro*, one could argue that GVHD elicited to class I antigens *in vivo* reflects help from radioresistant host CD4+ cells. However, the observation that purified CD8+ cells cause lethal GVHD in hosts given multiple injections of anti-CD4 antibody [28] suggests that radioresistant host CD4+ cells do not provide help. Nevertheless, supplementing the injected CD8+ cells with small doses of donor CD4+ cells causes a marked alteration in the pattern of GVHD; instead of developing progressive chronic GVHD, the hosts develop acute GVHD and die at 2–3 weeks after transfer. This finding implies that although CD8+ cells function well in the absence of exogenous help *in vivo*, adding help significantly increases their potency.

Interestingly, the capacity of CD4+ cells to augment GVHD elicited by CD8+ cells only applies when CD4+ cells are injected in small numbers ($\leq 1 \times 10^6$). When high numbers of CD4+ cells are transferred, marked protection occurs [28]. Thus, if an inoculum of 2×10^6 B6 CD8+ cells is supplemented with 2×10^7 B6 CD4+ cells, death rates in irradiated (B6 × bm1)F_1 hosts drop from 100% to 0%. Mortality rates are also very low when a large dose of 1×10^8 unseparated B6 spleen cells is transferred. As for the B6 → bm12 combination, the protective effects of large doses of CD4+ cells in the B6 → bm1 combinations is probably a reflection of restoration of immunocompetence.

GVHD in nonirradiated hosts

All of the patterns of anti-class II and anti-class I GVHD discussed above refer to experiments with irradiated hosts. What happens when nonirradiated hosts are used? The results vary according to the age of the recipients.

If neonatal F_1 hosts are used, the recipients of parental strain T cells develop a lethal form of GVHD characterized by prominent lymphocytic infiltrations in various organs, especially the liver, and enlargement of the spleen [17,29]. Splenomegaly is most pronounced at about 10 days post-injection, and measuring the size of the spleen in neonates has long been a popular model for assessing the severity of GVHD [29]. Induction of splenomegaly is usually attributed to the action of CD4+ cells, but at least in the B6 → bm1 combination, purified CD8+ cells cause prominent spleen enlargement [17]. With large doses of either CD4+ or CD8+ T cells, the host mice usually die after a period of 2–3 weeks.

When nonirradiated adult mice are used as hosts, two distinct patterns of GVHD are seen [30,31]. When GVHD is directed solely to class II MHC antigens, e.g. when purified B6 CD4+ cells are transferred to nonirradiated (B6 × bm12)F_1 mice, the recipients develop a chronic "proliferative" form of sublethal GVHD associated with splenomegaly and prominent autoantibody production. In this situation, the donor CD4+ cells mount a prolonged response against host class II antigens and release large quantities of lymphokines. Autoantibody production is presumed to be a reflection of aberrant T–B interaction: the donor CD4+ cells respond to the alloantigens on the host B cells and drive the B cells to undergo polyclonal activation. This proliferative type of nonlethal GVHD is also seen when purified CD4+ cells are transferred across whole MHC barriers [32].

A quite different type of GVHD occurs when unseparated T cells are transferred to nonirradiated hosts expressing combined class I plus II differences, for example when B6 T cells are transferred to (bm1 × bm12)F_1 mice [30]. Here, the GVH reaction involves both CD4+ and CD8+ cells. In the early stage of this reaction, the host mice exhibit the proliferative form of GVHD discussed above. After a few weeks, however, lymphoproliferation is succeeded by a phase of progressive chronic GVHD associated with lymphoid aplasia; many of the recipients eventually die.

Although this aplastic form of GVHD is known to require the presence of donor CD8+ cells, the chain of events that lead to aplasia is still poorly understood. Some workers argue that the CD8+ cells act as suppressor cells [33,34]. The simplest possibility, however, is that the CD8+ cells act as CTL and cause progressive tissue damage aided by help from the donor CD4+ cells. Such exogenous help seems to be essential because only minimal disease occurs when the donor cells are depleted of CD4+ cells (or unseparated T cells are transferred to hosts expressing only a class I difference rather than a combined class I and II difference). The inability of purified CD8+ cells to cause lethal GVHD applies only to nonirradiated hosts. As discussed earlier, CD8+ cells are highly potent at causing an aplastic form of lethal GVHD in irradiated hosts.

Although transferring unseparated T cells to hosts expressing a combined class I and II difference generally causes an aplastic form of GVHD, this is by no means an invariable finding. For example, when (B6 × DBA/2)F_1 mice ($H-2^b \times H-2^d$) are injected with unseparated DBA/2 T cells, the recipients develop the proliferative type of GVHD rather than aplastic GVHD [34]. By contrast, injecting either B6 or B10.D2 ($H-2^d$) T cells causes aplastic GVHD. Although the disparity in the effect mediated by B10.D2 and DBA/2 (both $H-2^d$) T cells has yet to be resolved, the most likely possibility is that DBA/2 mice have a quantitative and qualitative deficiency of CD8+ cells [35].

GVHD to mHA

Mouse models for GVHD directed to mHA are of obvious clinical relevance because HCT in humans is restricted largely to MHC (HLA)-compatible donor/host combinations. As discussed in Chapter 3, GVHD in HLA-compatible combinations can be very severe. This disease is probably directed largely and perhaps entirely to mHA. In this regard, a few human mHA have been identified and some are ubiquitously expressed by host tissues in the context of appropriate MHC molecules, and others have more tissue-restricted expression, such as HA-1 on hematopoietic cells [36].

The first evidence that mHA provide targets for GVHD in mice came from studies in which untreated marrow cells were transferred to irradiated H-2-compatible hosts expressing a variety of non-H-2 differences [37,38]. A high incidence of lethal GVHD was seen, but only when the donor and host differed at three or more minor H loci. Difference at other loci, e.g. Ly or Mls loci, failed to cause GVHD. Evidence that GVHD was caused by T cells came from the finding that depleting the marrow inoculum of contaminating mature T cells with anti-Thy 1 antibody plus complement abolished GVHD [37]. It should be noted that, in contrast to human marrow, mouse marrow contains only small numbers of mature T cells (1–2%).

mHA target antigens

Although it is clear that lethal GVHD in non-H-2-different combinations requires mHA incompatibility, it is not clear which particular mHA provide the targets for GVHD. Studies with available congenic strains of mice differing selectively at defined mHA have shown that none of these isolated mHA differences elicit lethal GVHD [39,40]. Currently, in only one strain combination, C3H.SW → B6, a single class I-restricted mHA that can cause GVHD has been identified [41]. It would thus appear that only a very limited number of immunodominant mHA may be responsible for GVHD in particular strain combinations that are known to differ at dozens of minor H loci [39,42–45]. Why some mHA are more potent than others in inducing GVHD is obscure. Experiments with B6 → BALB.B and related CXB recombinant inbred strains have indicated that the mHA that act as targets for GVHD do not necessarily correspond with strong *in vitro* CTL responses [46]. In these strain combinations, several strong mHA have now been fully characterized, molecularly and genetically [47–49], but they have proved inadequate when it comes to correlations with GVHD development [39,40,46]. In addition, the curious form of immunodominance, whereby *in vitro* CTL responses to weak antigens are suppressed by responses to stronger antigens [50], does not seem to apply to GVHD (see $V\beta$ analyses below). Instead, it appears that GVHD pathology is caused by a limited number of mHA in each donor/recipient combination that satisfy the criteria of being expressed in appropriate target tissue and are capable of stimulating a large enough T-cell response. Theoretically, all of these mHA may contribute to the development of disease, and given enough responding T cells, each would be capable of inducing GVHD pathology in their own right.

Features of anti-mHA GVHD

Studies with six strain combinations expressing three or more mHA differences have shown that transferring a mixture of purified unprimed donor T cells plus T-depleted donor marrow cells to mice given an intermediate dose of irradiation (7.5–8 Gy) causes heavy mortality in each combination [51]. The most detailed information has come from the CBA → B10.BR combination [37,52,53] in which lethal GVHD approaches 100% and occurs with even very small numbers of T cells ($<1 \times 10^5$). Based on experiments in which donor T cells were negatively selected to class I or class II-restricted mHA by blood to lymph passage through irradiated H-2 recombinant intermediate hosts, the T-cells mediating GVHD in the CBA → B10.BR combination respond to mHA presented by host class I rather than class II molecules [52,53]. These cells comprise a mixture of H-2D- and H-2K-restricted T cells.

The patterns of GVHD elicited by mHA depend on the dose of T cells injected. Large numbers of T cells produce acute GVHD and early deaths whereas smaller numbers of T cells lead to a chronic form of GVHD with late mortality [37] (Fig. 26.1 [37]). Histopathology is most prominent in mice with chronic GVHD and involves lymphoid atrophy, weight loss and lymphocyte infiltration of the skin, liver and lungs [54–58]; involvement of the gut is mild, although some mice develop chronic diarrhea. Symptoms of GVHD tend to be more severe in hosts conditioned with heavy irradiation (8–10 Gy) rather than light irradiation (6–8 Gy) and when the general health of the colony is suboptimal. With regard to the

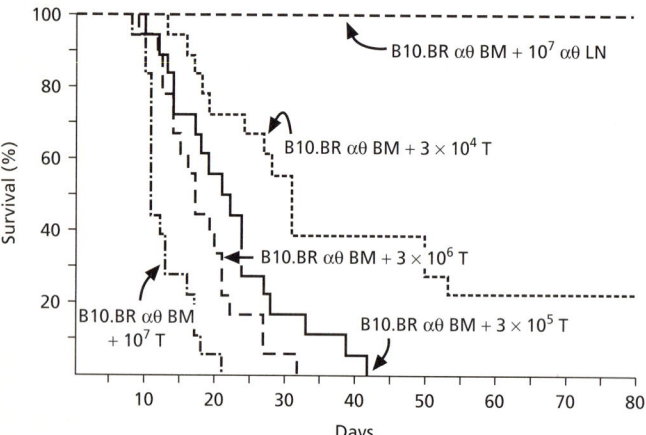

Fig. 26.1 Lethal GVHD in irradiated (750 cGy) CBA/J mice given graded doses of purified B10.BR LN T cells. The data show cumulative mortality after transferring 10^7 anti-Thy 1.2-serum-treated B10.BR marrow cells (B10.BR $\alpha\theta$ BM) supplemented with varying numbers of nylon-wool-purified B10.BR LN T cells or with anti-Thy 1.2 serum-treated B10.BR LN cells ($\alpha\theta$ LN). Data pooled from three experiments involving a total of 18 mice per group. Reproduced with permission from Korngold and Sprent [37].

marrow inoculum, using host rather than donor marrow has little effect in potentiating GVHD [59]. This contrasts with anti-H-2 GVHD where reconstitution with host marrow leads to marked marrow aplasia (see above). It is worth mentioning that the capacity of large doses of $CD4^+$ cells to protect against lethal GVHD does not seem to apply to GVHD directed to mHA [59]. The reason for this difference is unknown.

Role of $CD8^+$ cells

The above finding that the effector cells in the CBA → B10.BR combination were H-2 class I restricted suggested that GVHD to mHA is mediated largely, though not exclusively, by $CD8^+$ cells (Table 26.1 [51]). In this and several other combinations, depleting the injected T cells of $CD4^+$ cells generally has little or no effect in reducing the intensity of GVHD [52], nor does injecting the host mice with anti-CD4 antibody [59]. These findings imply that the capacity of $CD8^+$ cells to mediate GVHD to mHA does not necessarily require help from $CD4^+$ cells. Yet, in some strain combinations like B6 → BALB.B the $CD8^+$ cells will only mediate GVHD in the presence of $CD4^+$ cells [60]. The criteria which dictate $CD8^+$ cell-dependency on exogenous help appears to involve the cytokines available to APCs and their ability to express the 4–1BB ligand molecule which can bind to its counterpart (4–1BB; CD137) on $CD8^+$ T cells and serve as a costimulator for activation and survival [61].

In an effort to investigate the heterogeneity of the T-cell response across a donor-recipient pair disparate at multiple mHA loci, the repertoire of responding $CD8^+$ T cells in the B6 → BALB.B (8.25 Gy) GVHD model was analyzed by TCR $V\beta$ CDR3-size polymerase chain reaction (PCR) spectratyping. This response was found to be oligoclonal in nature, involving T cells from seven $V\beta$ families [62]. With the exception of a single $V\beta$ family, these responses were also found after transplantation of B6 $CD8^+$ T cells into irradiated CXBE mice, a recombinant inbred strain which is derived from a cross between B6 and BALB/c mice and therefore expresses a subset of the mHA found in the BALB.B strain. This overlap in the $CD8^+$ T-cell response repertoire suggested that the phenomenon of competitive immunodominance was not a factor in the recognition of mHA involved in the development of GVHD. In addition, it was demonstrated that lethal GVHD could be induced by the transplantation of T cells from a single purified B6 $CD8^+$ $V\beta$ family into either irradiated BALB.B or CXBE mice, supporting their involvement in disease pathogenesis and suggesting a possible hierarchy of GVHD mediating specificities within the responding T-cell population [62].

Role of $CD4^+$ cells

In the case of the CBA → B10.BR combination and certain other combinations, $CD4^+$ cells play no obvious role in GVHD. The helper function of these cells is not required, and transferring even high doses of purified $CD4^+$ cells generally fails to cause GVHD. Nevertheless in two of six combinations tested from this panel, namely B10.D2 → BALB/c and B10.D2 → DBA/2, purified $CD4^+$ cells do cause a high incidence of lethal GVHD [51,63] (see also Table 26.1). This is also true in the B6 → BALB.B combination, in which $CD4^+$ T cells are required for CD8-mediated GVHD and can cause GVHD on their own account [60]. Why $CD4^+$ cells mediate GVHD in only a limited number of mHA-different strain combinations is obscure. Insight into this problem has been generated from studying the B6 $CD4^+$ mediated GVHD response in BALB.B vs. CXBE recipients, where BALB.B, but not CXBE mice succumb to lethal GVHD despite sharing multiple mHA. A comparison of the responding $CD4^+$ TCR $V\beta$ repertoires from the thoracic duct lymph of irradiated BALB.B and CXBE recipients was made at the early stages of GVHD development (5–6 days) [64]. The spectratype analysis revealed overlapping utilization of nine $V\beta$ families. In addition, the unique skew-

Table 26.1 Lethal graft-vs.-host disease in six minor histocompatibility antigen–different H2-compatible strain combinations: GVHD mediated by purified T cells and T-cell subsets.*

Donor → recipient	H2	Some of the known genetic differences between donor and host	% Mortality (median survival time) after transfer of donor T cells plus donor marrow			
			Whole T	CD4+	CD8+	Marrow alone
C3H.SW → B6	H2^b	H-1, -3, -7, -8, -9, -13, Lyt-1, -2, Mls^b	48 (58)	5 (>80)	77 (45)	0 (>80)
DBA/2 → B10.D2	H2^d	H-1, -3, -4, -8, -13 Lyt-1, -2, Mls^b	26 (>80)	12 (>80)	73 (53)	8 (>80)
B10.BR → CBA/J	H2^k	H-1, -3, -7, -8, -9, -12 Tla, Mls^a, Lyt-1, -2	96 (38)	35 (73)	96 (39)	8 (>80)
B10.S → SJL	H2^s	H-1, -3, -7, -8, -9 H-12, -13, Tla, Mls^c	88 (34)	13 (>80)	88 (35)	0 (>80)
B10.D2 → DBA/2	H2^d	H-1, -3, -4, -8, -13, Mls^a Lyt-1, -2	92 (38)	85 (45)	42 (58)	7 (>80)
B10.D2 → BALB/C	H2^d	H-1, -3, -4, -7, -8, -9, -13 Lyt-1, -2, Mls^c	93 (20)	78 (24)	75 (39)	0 (>80)

*Data were pooled from more than 20 experiments with totals of 15–39 mice for each strain combination. Donor marrow cells (4 × 10^6) were T-cell depleted and injected intravenously along with unseparated (whole) T cells or T-cell subsets (1 × 10^6 cells) into appropriate lethally irradiated (8–10 Gy) recipient mice. Data from Korngold and Sprent [51].

ing of two Vβ families in the B6 → BALB.B response suggested the recognition of BALB.B mHA not expressed in the CXBE recipients. Interestingly, the B6 → CXBE strain combination also exhibited unique skewing of two other Vβ families, which may hint at "immunodominance effects", since one would have expected them to also be present in the B6 → BALB.B response.

Direct evidence that Vβ families found skewed by spectratype analysis were involved in the pathogenesis of GVHD came from immunohistochemical staining of lingual epithelial tissue from BALB.B recipients, which revealed a high correlation between several of the skewed Vβ families and those with increased representation in the epithelial tissue infiltrates [64]. Further proof that the skewed Vβ families were indeed involved with GVHD was provided upon transplantation of those CD4+ Vβ families into irradiated BALB.B recipients, which resulted in a significant level of lethal GVHD. In contrast, mice that received transplants of the unskewed Vβ families survived with minimal symptoms of disease [64].

Applying the above observations concerning differences in responding Vβ repertoires, the capacity of B6 CD4+ T cells to induce lethal GVHD in BALB.B but not CXBE recipients was further examined. Transplantation of highly enriched populations of the two B6 CD4+ Vβ families, that were uniquely skewed in the B6 → BALB.B response, were indeed able to induce lethal GVHD in BALB.B recipients. These data suggested that the BALB.B unique responses contribute in a way that either qualitatively or quantitatively enhances the severity of GVHD. Subsequent data suggested that these cells might preferentially infiltrate the small bowel of BALB.B recipients, thus increasing their importance to the systemic severity of GVHD (unpublished data).

In order to investigate whether the scope of the mHA-driven alloresponse changes during the development of GVHD, the responding B6 T-cell repertoire was examined between days 7 and 40 post-HCT in the B6 → BALB.B strain combination. The results indicated that for the CD8 response, eight Vβ families were consistently skewed throughout the period of observation. It is interesting that skewing in four of those Vβ families had not been detected earlier in the thoracic duct population when examining the single day 5 time point [62]. In addition, skewing of three other Vβ families appeared to develop at later stages post-transplant, which could indicate weaker anti-mHA responses, responses to antigens revealed via tissue destruction, or responses to nonalloantigen, such as to infectious agents. Similar findings were obtained for the CD4 analysis. Eight Vβ families were skewed throughout the course of GVHD development, all of which had been detected earlier in the thoracic duct lymph at day 6 post-transplant [64]. Four additional Vβ families were transiently skewed at later time points. Furthermore, elimination of the eight consistently skewed Vβ families from the CD4+ T-cell donor inoculum delayed the onset in the appearance of most of the remaining four responsive Vβ families. The reason for this delayed appearance is unclear, but would be consistent with them resulting from tissue damage, which would likely be slowed in the absence of dominant GVHD effector cells. These complex relationships in the development of anti-mHA GVHD are in obvious need of further investigation.

One further aspect of the Vβ repertoire studies that remains unclear is the redundant capacity of a single mHA to drive the response of multiple Vβ families via crossreactive TCR binding sites? Insight gained into this issue will provide clues as to the minimum number of mHA required to elicit GVHD in a MHC-matched combination and why some mHA dominate the responses. Overall, the study of Vβ representation in a heterogeneously responding T-cell population in this acute GVHD model has begun to provide valuable insight into the scope of the allogeneic anti-mHA T-cell response.

Approaches for the separation of GVHD and GVL responses

Various strategies have been utilized to minimize GVHD, such as CD4+, CD6+ and CD8+ T-cell-subset depletions; ex vivo tolerization of alloreactive T cells and separation of donor T cells based on functional phenotypes or cytolytic effector mechanisms (discussed in Chapters 3, 28, 29). These approaches all rely on broad differences to activation thresholds and or functional effector mechanisms. However, the alloreactive specificity of the donor T cells, as well as tissue specific expression of the mHA, can also lead to a more targeted immunotherapeutic approach for minimizing GVHD development. The particular goal of any effort in this area is to provide a mechanism for reducing GVHD potential without sacrificing graft-vs.-leukemia (GVL) or the more generalized graft-vs.-tumor (GVT) capability. To this end, *Vβ* spectratype analysis has also recently been used to identify tissue-restricted *Vβ* families in the B6 → BALB.B CD8+ mediated GVHD model. Herein, three *Vβ* families exhibited unique CDR3-size skewing in the gastrointestinal tract of the recipients (unpublished results). Depletion of these *Vβ* families from the donor inoculum could potentially help to reduce the severity of GVHD (and associated gut GVHD) while allowing the remaining T cells to provide a GVL effect.

In conjunction with this analytical approach, *Vβ* spectratyping has also been used to identify antileukemia responses [65]. The GVL activities of both donor B6 CD4+ and CD8+ T cells were studied in the setting of a bone marrow transplant into irradiated (B6xDBA/2)F_1 recipients, challenged one day later with MMB3.19 myeloid leukemia cells, of B6 origin. In comparing B6 CD4+ and CD8+ T-cell responses to either leukemia or host alloantigens, it was apparent that despite several overlapping *Vβ* families, there were a few in each subset that were unique to the antileukemia response. Some of these "leukemia-specific" donor CD4+ *Vβ*+ T cells were selected by monoclonal antibody magnetic separation and were infused into MMB3.19-challenged (B6 × DBA/2)F_1 recipients. These cells were able to provide an effective GVL response without significant development of GVHD [65].

The high inverse correlation between the clinical incidence of GVHD and the rate of leukemic relapse has long suggested that antihost alloreactivity may provide the dominant GVL effect [66]. Therefore, strategies that would involve permitting the initiation of GVHD, presumably with an associated concurrent GVL response that could then be brought under control to avoid full pathological development of disease would be highly desirable. CD4+CD25+ T cells are known to possess potent immunoregulatory properties and are thought to be important for the maintenance of self-tolerance and the prevention of autoimmunity [67–69]. Several studies have demonstrated the capacity of these cells to inhibit alloreactivity [70,71]. Recently, Taylor *et al.* [72] demonstrated that the infusion of *ex vivo* expanded CD4+CD25+ T cells along with donor bone marrow cells were capable of preventing GVHD development. In an effort to separate GVHD from GVL responses, a model to test the potential effects of the delayed infusion of CD4+CD25+ T cells into myeloid leukemia-challenged, HCT-transplanted mice was utilized. To this end, B10.BR CD8+ T cells were transplanted into lethally irradiated mHA-disparate CBA mice, a transplant model in which GVHD is mediated by CD4+ independent CD8+ T cells [51]. One day later the mice received a tumor challenge from a CBA-derived myeloid leukemia and on day 10 they were infused with freshly isolated B10.BR CD4+CD25+ T cells. Transplantation of the immunoregulatory cells ameliorated the development of acute GVHD with significantly prolonged survival. Most importantly, the delayed regulation also allowed for a significant GVL effect in leukemia-challenged recipients (unpublished data). The results of this model may have important potential for future application into the clinical setting.

Immunopathology

As for anti-H-2 GVHD, the effector mechanisms involved in GVHD to mHA are still not fully understood. The histopathology of GVHD mediated by CD4+ cells and CD8+ cells is quite similar in the major target tissues of the skin, liver, and intestinal tract, although gut pathology is more prominent in recipients of CD4+ cells [58]. In the skin, epidermal cytotoxicity is induced by both subsets, albeit by different pathways, but dermal fibrosis seems to be a unique aspect of CD8-mediated GVHD. Mast cell degranulation occurs in the skin early after transplantation of either subset, even before lymphocyte infiltration is detected [73]. In addition, TNF-α (from either mast cells or T cells) does not appear to play a role in initial keratinocyte damage associated with early GVHD stages but is involved in later CD4-mediated pathology, once the cells have infiltrated into the epidermal layers. In the case of CD8+ cells, it would seem that tissue damage, at least in the skin, reflects primarily direct CTL activity, although cytokines other than TNF-α may contribute to pathology. It has also been established that apoptosis has a central role in epithelial injury in acute GVHD [74], and that the primary targets of attack are the follicular stem cells [75,76]. In all, the course and kinetics of pathogenesis in GVHD to mHA may depend on several variables, including the strength of the individual CD4+ and CD8+ cell responses, the levels of expression of antigens in target tissue and the fluctuations of cytokines, both locally and systemically.

Summary

Studies in murine models have provided many important insights into the pathophysiology of GVHD directed across MHC and/or mHA disparities. We now have a workable understanding of the T-cell subsets that can be involved in any given situation of GVHD and clues as to their mechanisms of action. These and future studies in the mouse can help guide us in the development of novel approaches to selectively reduce the risk of GVHD while allowing for the generation of immune responses that can counteract the relapse of leukemia or infectious pathogens.

Acknowledgment

The writing of this chapter was supported by grant HL55593 from the United States Public Health Service.

References

1 Ferrara JL, Levy R, Chao NJ. Pathophysiologic mechanisms of acute graft-vs.-host disease. *Biol Blood Marrow Transplant* 1999; **5**: 347–56.

2 Ferrara J, Deeg JH, Burakoff SJ, eds. *Graft-vs.-Host Disease*. New York: Marcel Dekker, 1997.

3 Korngold R. Biology of graft-vs.-host disease. *Am J Ped Hematol/Oncol* 1993; **15**: 18–27.

4 Sprent J, Webb SR. Function and specificity of T-cell subsets in the mouse. *Adv Immunol* 1987; **41**: 39–133.

5 Hedrick SM, Eidelman FJ. T lymphocyte antigen receptors. In: Paul WE, ed. *Fundamental Immunology*, 3rd edn. New York: Raven Press, 1993: 383–420.

6 Shevach EM. Accessory molecules. In: Paul WE, ed. *Fundamental Immunology*, 3rd edn. New York: Raven Press, 1993: 531–76.

7 Carbone FR, Bevan MJ. Major histocompatibility complex control of T-cell recognition. In: Paul WE, ed. *Fundamental Immunology*, 2nd edn. New York: Raven Press, 1989: 541–70.

8 Sprent J. T lymphocytes and the thymus. In: Paul WE, ed. *Fundamental Immunology*, 3rd edn. New York: Raven Press, 1993: 75–110.

9 von Boehmer H. Developmental biology of T cells in T-cell receptor transgenic mice. *Annu Rev Immunol* 1990; **8**: 531–56.

10 Sprent J, Korngold R. A comparison of lethal graft-versus-host disease to minor-versus-major differences in mice: implications for marrow transplantation in man. *Prog Immunol* 1983; **5**: 1461–75.

11 Bennett M. Biology and genetics of hybrid resistance. *Adv Immunol* 1987; **41**: 333–445.

12 Murphy WJ, Kumar V, Bennett M. Rejection of bone marrow allografts by mice with severe combined immunodeficiency (SCID): evidence that natural killer (NK) cells can mediate the specificity of marrow graft rejection. *J Exp Med* 1987; **165**: 1212–7.

13 Bix M, Liao NS, Zijlstra M, Loring J, Jaenisch R, Raulet D. Rejection of class I MHC-deficient hemopoietic cells by irradiated MHC-matched mice. *Nature* 1991; **349**: 329–31.

14 Moller G, ed. Elimination of allogeneic lymphoid cells. *Immunol Rev* 1983; **73**: 1–126.

15 Vallera DA, Soderling CCB, Kersey JH. Bone marrow transplantation across major histocompatibility barriers in mice. III. Treatment of donor grafts with monoclonal antibodies directed against Lyt determinants. *J Immunol* 1982; **128**: 871–5.

16. Korngold R, Sprent J. Surface markers of T cells causing lethal graft-versus-host disease to class I vs. class II H-2 differences. *J Immunol* 1985; **135**: 3004–10.

17. Sprent J, Schaefer M, Lo D, Korngold R. Properties of purified T-cell subsets. II. *In vivo* responses to class I vs. class II H-2 differences. *J Exp Med* 1986; **163**: 998–1011.

18. Korngold R, Sprent J. Purified T-cell subsets and lethal graft-versus-host disease in mice. In: Gale RP, Champlin R, eds. *Progress in Bone Marrow Transplantation*. New York: Liss, 1987: 213–8.

19. Cobbold S, Martin G, Waldmann H. Monoclonal antibodies for the prevention of graft-versus-host disease and marrow graft rejection. *Transplantation* 1986; **42**: 239–47.

20. Piguet P-F. GVHR elicited by products of class I or class II loci of the MHC: analysis of the response of mouse T lymphocytes to products of class I and class II loci of the MHC in correlation with GVHR-induced mortality, medullary aplasia, and enteropathy. *J Immunol* 1985; **135**: 1637–43.

21. Sprent J, Schaefer M, Lo D, Korngold R. Function of purified L3T4+ and Lyt-2+ cells *in vitro* and *in vivo*. *Immunol Rev* 1986; **91**: 195–218.

22. Sprent J, Schaefer M, Korngold R. Role of T-cell subsets in lethal graft-versus-host disease (GVHD) directed to class I versus class II H-2 differences. II. Protective effects of L3T4+ cells in anti-class II H-2 differences. *J Immunol* 1990; **144**: 2946–54.

23. Guy-Grand D, Vassalli P. Gut injury in mouse graft-versus-host reactions. *J Clin Invest* 1986; **77**: 1584–95.

24. Mowat AM, Sprent J. Induction of intestinal graft-versus-host reactions across mutant major histocompatibility antigens by T lymphocyte subsets in mice. *Transplantation* 1989; **47**: 857–63.

25. Piguet PF, Grau GE, Allet B, Vassalli P. Tumor necrosis factor/cachectin is an effector of skin and gut lesions of the acute phase of graft-vs.-host disease. *J Exp Med* 1987; **166**: 1280–9.

26. Vossen JM, Heidt PJ. Gnotobiotic measures for prevention of acute graft-versus-host disease. In: Burakoff SJ, Deeg HJ, Ferrara JLM, Atkinson K, eds. *Graft-Versus-Host Disease: Immunology, Pathophysiology, and Treatment*. New York: Marcel Dekker Inc, 1990: 403–13.

27. Nathenson SG, Geliebter J, Pfaffenbach GM, Zeff RA. Murine major histocompatibility complex class-I mutants. Molecular analysis and structure-function implications. *Ann Rev Immunol* 1986; **4**: 471–502.

28. Sprent J, Schaefer M, Gao E-K, Korngold R. Role of T-cell subsets in lethal graft-versus-host disease (GVHD) directed to class I versus class II H-2 differences. I. L3T4+ cells can either augment or retard GVHD elicited by Lyt-2+ cells in class I-different hosts. *J Exp Medical* 1988; **167**: 556–9.

29. Simonsen M. Graft-versus-host reactions. Their natural history and applicability as tools of research. *Progr Allergy* 1962; **6**: 349–467.

30. Rolink AG, Pals ST, Gleichmann E. Allosuppressor and allohelper T cells in acute and chronic graft-vs.-host disease. II. F1 recipients carrying mutations at H-2K and/or I-A. *J Exp Medical* 1983; **157**: 755–71.

31. Gleichmann E, Pals ST, Rolink AG, Radaszkiewicz T, Gleichmann H. Graft-versus-host reactions. Clues to the etiopathology of a spectrum of immunological diseases. *Immunol Today* 1984; **5**: 324–32.

32. Rolink AG, Gleichmann E. Allosuppressor and allohelper T cells in acute and chronic graft-vs.-host disease. III. Different Lyt subsets of donor T cells induce different pathological syndromes. *J Exp Med* 1983; **158**: 546–58.

33. Rolink AG, Radaszkiewicz T, Pals ST, van der Meer WGJ, Gleichmann E. Allosuppressor and allohelper T cells in acute and chronic graft-vs.-host disease. I. Alloreactive suppressor cells rather than killer T cells appear to be the decisive cells in lethal graft-vs.-host disease. *J Exp Med* 1982; **155**: 1501–22.

34. van Elven EH, Rolink AG, van der Veen F, Gleichmann E. Capacity of genetically different T lymphocytes to induce lethal graft-versus-host disease correlates with their capacity to generate suppression but not with their capacity to generate anti-F1 killer cells. A non-H-2 locus determines the inability to induce lethal graft-versus-hosts disease. *J Exp Med* 1981; **153**: 1474–88.

35. Via CS, Sharrow SO, Shearer GM. Role of cytotoxic T lymphocytes in the prevention of lupus-like disease occurring in a murine model of graft-vs.-host disease. *J Exp Med* 1987; **139**: 1840–9.

36. Goulmy E. Minor histocompatibility antigens: from T cell recognition to peptide identification. *Hum Immunol* 1997; **54**: 8–14.

37. Korngold R, Sprent J. Lethal graft-versus-host disease after bone-marrow transplantation across minor histocompatibility barriers in mice. Prevention by removing mature T cells from marrow. *J Exp Med* 1978; **148**: 1687–98.

38. Hamilton BL, Bevan MJ, Parkman R. Anti-recipient cytotoxic T lymphocyte precursors are present in the spleens of mice with acute graft-versus-host disease due to minor histocompatibility antigens. *J Immunol* 1981; **126**: 621–5.

39. Korngold R, Leighton C, Mobraaten LE, Berger MA. Inter-strain graft-versus-host disease T cell responses to immunodominant minor histocompatibility antigens. *Biol Blood Marrow Transplant* 1997; **3**: 57–64.

40. Blazar BR, Roopenian DC, Taylor PA, Christianson GJ, Panoskaltsis-Mortari A, Vallera DA. Lack of GVHD across classical, single minor histocompatibility (miH) locus barriers in mice. *Transplantation* 1996; **61**: 619–24.

41. Perreault C, Jutras J, Roy DC, Filep JG, Brochu S. Identification of an immunodominant mouse minor histocompatibility antigen (MiHA). T cell response to a single dominant MiHA causes graft-versus-host disease. *J Clin Invest* 1996; **98**: 622–8.

42. Berger MA, Korngold R. Immunodominant CD4+ T cell receptor Vβ repertoire involved in graft-versus-host disease responses to minor histocompatibility antigens. *J Immunol* 1997; **159**: 77–85.

43. Howell CD, Li J, Roper E, Kotzin BL. Biased liver T cell receptor Vβ repertoire in a murine graft-versus-host disease model. *J Immunol* 1995; **155**: 2350–8.

44. Brochu S, Baron C, Hetu F, Roy DC, Perreault C. Oligoclonal expansion of CTLs directed against a restricted number of dominant minor histocompatibility antigens in hemopoietic chimeras. *J Immunol* 1995; **155**: 5104–14.

45. Perreault C, Roy DC, Fortin C. Immunodominant minor histocompatibility antigens: the major ones. *Immunol Today* 1998; **19**: 69–74.

46. Korngold R, Wettstein PJ. Immunodominance in the graft-vs-host disease T-cell response to minor histocompatibility antigen. *J Immunol* 1990; **145**: 4079–88.

47. Nevala WK, Wettstein PJ. H4 and CTT-2 minor histocompatibility antigens: concordant genetic linkage and migration in two-dimensional peptide separation. *Immunogenetics* 1996; **44**(5): 400–4.

48. Malarkannan S, Shih PP, Eden PA et al. The molecular and functional characterization of a dominant minor H antigen, H60. *J Immunol* 1998; **161**: 3501–9.

49. Malarkannan S, Horng T, Eden PA et al. Differences that matter: major cytotoxic T cell-stimulating minor histocompatibility antigens. *Immunity* 2000; **3**: 333–44.

50. Wettstein PJ. Immunodominance in the T-cell response to multiple non-H-2 histocompatibility antigens. II. Observation of a hierarchy among dominant antigens. *Immunogenetics* 1986; **24**: 24–31.

51. Korngold R, Sprent J. Variable capacity of L3T4+ T cells to cause lethal graft-versus-host disease across minor histocompatibility barriers in mice. *J Exp Med* 1987; **165**: 1522–64.

52. Korngold R, Sprent J. Lethal GVHD across minor histocompatibility barriers: nature of the effector cells and role of the H-2 complex. *Immunol Rev* 1983; **71**: 5–29.

53. Korngold R, Sprent J. Features of T cells causing H-2-restricted lethal graft-versus-host disease across minor histocompatibility barriers. *J Exp Med* 1982; **155**: 872–83.

54. Jaffee BD, Claman HN. Chronic graft-versus-host disease (GVHD) as a model for scleroderma. I. Description of model systems. *Cell Immunol* 1983; **77**: 1–12.

55. Ferrara J, Guillen FJ, Sleckman B, Burakoff SJ, Murphy GF. Cutaneous acute graft-versus-host disease to minor histocompatibility antigens in a murine model. histologic analysis and correlation to clinical disease. *J Invest Dermatol* 1986; **123**: 401–6.

56. Rappaport H, Khalil A, Halle-Pannenko O, Pritchard L, Dantcher D, Mathe G. Histopathologic sequence of events in adult mice undergoing lethal graft-vs-host reaction developed across H-2 and/or non H-2 histocompatibility barriers. *Am J Pathol* 1979; **96**: 121–43.

57. Charley MR, Bangert JL, Hamilton BL, Gilliam JN, Sontheimer RD. Murine graft-versus-host skin disease. A chronologic and quantitative analysis of two histologic patterns. *J Invest Dermatol* 1983; **81**: 412–7.

58. Murphy GF, Whitaker D, Sprent J, Korngold R. Characterization of target injury of murine acute graft-versus-host disease directed to multiple minor histocompatibility antigens elicited by either CD4+ or CD8+ effector cells. *Am J Path* 1991; **138**: 983–90.

59. Korngold R. Lethal graft-versus-host disease in mice directed to multiple minor histocompatibility antigens. Features of CD8+ and CD4+ T-cell responses. *Bone Marrow Transplant* 1992; **9**: 355–64.

60. Berger M, Wettstein PJ, Korngold R. T cell subsets involved in lethal graft-versus-host disease directed to immunodominant minor histocompatibility antigens. *Transplantation* 1994; **57**: 1095–102.

61. Kwon B, Moon CH, Kang S, Seo SK, Kwon BS. 4-1BB: still in the midst of darkness. *Mol Cells* 2000; **10**: 119–26.

62. Friedman TM, Gilbert M, Briggs C, Korngold R. Repertoire analysis of CD8+ T cell responses to minor histocompatibility antigens involved in graft-versus-host disease. *J Immunol* 1998; **161**: 41–8.

63. Hamilton BL. L3T4-positive T cells participate in the induction of graft-vs-host disease in response to minor histocompatibility antigens. *J Immunol* 1987; **139**: 2511–5.

64. Friedman TM, Statton D, Jones SC, Berger MA, Murphy GF, Korngold R. Vβ spectratype analysis reveals heterogeneity of CD4+ T-cell responses to minor histocompatibility antigens involved in graft-versus-host disease: correlations with epithelial

tissue infiltrate. *Biol Blood Marrow Transplant* 2001; **7**: 2–13.
65 Patterson AE, Korngold R. Infusion of select leukemia-reactive TCR *Vβ*+ T cells provides graft-versus-leukemia responses with minimization of graft-versus-host disease following murine hematopoietic stem cell transplantation. *Biol Blood Marrow Transplant* 2001; **7**: 187–96.
66 Kernan NA. T-cell depletion for the prevention of graft-versus-host disease. In: Thomas ED, Blume KG, Forman SJ, eds. *Hematopoietic Cell Transplantation*, 2nd edn. Malden, MA: Blackwell Science, 1999: 186–96.
67 Asano M, Toda M, Sakaguchi N, Sakaguchi S. Autoimmune disease as a consequence of developmental abnormality of a T cell subpopulation. *J Exp Med* 1996; **184**: 387–96.
68 Kuniyasu Y, Takahashi T, Itoh M, Shimizu J, Toda G, Sakaguchi S. Naturally anergic and suppressive CD4+CD25+ T cells as a functionally and phenotypically distinct immunoregulatory T cell subpopulation. *Int Immunol* 2000; **12**: 1145–55.
69 Read S, Powrie, F. CD4+ regulatory T cells. *Current Opinion Immunol* 2001; **13**: 644–9.
70 Johnson BD, Becker EE, LaBelle JL, Truitt RL. Role of immunoregulatory donor T cells in suppression of graft-versus-host disease following donor leukocyte infusion therapy. *J Immunol* 1999; **163**: 6479–87.
71 Taylor PA, Noelle RJ, Blazar BR. CD4+CD25+ immune regulatory cells are required for induction of tolerance to alloantigens via costimulatory blockade. *J Exp Med* 2001; **193**: 1311–7.
72 Taylor PA, Lees CJ, Blazar BR. The infusion of *ex vivo* activated and expanded CD4+CD25+ immune regulatory cells inhibits graft-versus-host disease lethality. *Blood* 2002; **99**: 3493–9.
73 Murphy GF, Sueki H, Teuscher C, Whitaker D, Korngold R. Role of mast cells in early epithelial target cell injury in experimental acute graft-versus-host disease. *J Invest Dermatol* 1994; **102**: 451–61.
74 Gilliam AC, Whitaker-Menezes D, Korngold R, Murphy GF. Apoptosis is the predominant form of epithelial target cell injury in acute experimental graft-versus-host disease. *J Invest Dermatol* 1996; **107**: 377–83.
75 Murphy GF, Lavker RM, Whitaker D, Korngold R. Cytotoxic folliculitis in acute graft-versus-host disease. Evidence of follicular stem cell injury and recovery. *J Cutan Pathol* 1991; **18**: 309–14.
76 Sale GE, Beauchamp M. The parafollicular hair bulge in human GVHD. a stem cell rich primary target. *Bone Marrow Transplant* 1993; **11**: 223–5.

27
James L.M. Ferrara & Joseph Antin

The Pathophysiology of Graft-vs.-Host Disease

Acute GVHD pathophysiology: a three-step model

The pathophysiology of acute graft-vs.-host disease (GVHD) can be considered as a three-step process where the innate and adaptive immune systems interact (Fig. 27.1). The three steps are: (i) tissue damage to the recipient by the radiation/chemotherapy pretransplant conditioning regimen; (ii) donor T-cell activation and clonal expansion; and (iii) cellular and inflammatory factors. This schema underscores the importance of mononuclear phagocytes and other accessory cells to the development of GVHD after complex interactions with cytokines secreted by activated donor T cells.

In *step 1*, the conditioning regimen (irradiation and/or chemotherapy) leads to damage and activation of host tissues throughout the body and the secretion of inflammatory cytokines tumor necrosis factor-alpha (TNF-α) and interleukin 1 (IL-1). These cytokines enhance donor T-cell recognition of host alloantigens by increasing expression of major histocompatibility complex (MHC) antigens and other molecules on host antigen-presenting cells (APCs).

In *step 2*, host APCs present alloantigen in the form of a peptide-human leukocyte antigen (HLA) complex to the resting T cells. Costimulatory signals are required for T-cell activation, and these signals further activate APCs and further enhance T-cell stimulation. Donor T-cell activation is characterized by cellular proliferation and the secretion of cytokines, including IL-2 and interferon-gamma (IFN-γ). IL-2 expands the T-cell clones and induces cytotoxic T-lymphocyte (CTL) responses, whereas IFN-γ primes mononuclear phagocytes to produce TNF-α and IL-1.

In *step 3*, effector functions of mononuclear phagocytes and neutrophils are triggered through a secondary signal provided by mediators, such as lipopolysaccharide (LPS), that leaks through the intestinal mucosa damaged during step 1. Release of inflammatory cytokines stimulates host tissues to produce inflammatory chemokines thus recruiting effector cells into target organs where they adhere due to increased adhesion molecule expression. This mechanism results in the amplification of local tissue injury with and further promotion of a pro-inflammatory response which, together with CTL, leads to target tissue destruction. There is now substantial evidence to implicate the inappropriate production of cytokines as primary effectors of acute GVHD [1,2].

It should be noted from the outset that all these steps do not carry equal weight in the pathogenesis of acute GVHD. The pivotal interaction occurs in step 2, where host APCs activate allogeneic donor T cells. The subsequent cytokine cascade is clearly important, but blockade of individual cytokines may not reverse established GVHD when other cellular effectors such as CTL are present. GVHD can also occur when no conditioning of the host has occurred (e.g. transfusion associated GVHD). This schema is intended to provide perspective on how the innate and adaptive immune systems interact in this complicated, inflammatory disease.

Step 1: effects of HCT conditioning

The first step of acute GVHD starts before donor cells are infused. Prior to hematopoietic cell transplantation (HCT), a patient's tissues have been damaged, sometimes profoundly, by underlying disease and its treatment, infection and transplant conditioning. High intensity chemoradiotherapy characteristic of HCT conditioning regimens activate host APCs that are critical to the stimulation of donor T cells infused in the stem cell inoculum. These important effects help explain a number of unique and seemingly unrelated aspects of GVHD. For example, a number of clinical reports have noted increased risks of GVHD associated with advanced stage leukemia, certain intensive conditioning regimens and histories of viral infections [3–5]. Total body irradiation (TBI) is particularly important in this process because it activates host tissues to secrete inflammatory cytokines, such as TNF-α and IL-1 [6], and it induces endothelial apoptosis that leads to epithelial cell damage in the gastrointestinal (GI) tract [7]. Injury to the gut is transient and self-limited after autologous HCT. However, after allogeneic HCT, further damage by GVHD effectors amplifies GI and systemic GVHD by allowing the translocation of microbial products such as LPS into systemic circulation. This scenario helps to explain the increased risk of GVHD associated with intensive conditioning regimens. The relationship between conditioning intensity, inflammatory cytokines and GVHD severity have been confirmed by animal models [8] and by clinical observations [3,4].

Step 2: donor T-cell activation and cytokine secretion

Donor T-cell activation

Donor T-cell activation occurs during the second step of acute GVHD. Murine studies have demonstrated that host APCs alone are both necessary and sufficient to stimulate donor T cells [2,9] and this process is initiated within secondary lymphoid organs such as lymph nodes and the spleen [10]. In murine models of GVHD to MHC differences between donor and host, robust donor T-cell proliferation is observed in the spleen as early as day 3 after HCT, preceding the engraftment of donor stem cells [2,11,12]. Although the impact of splenectomy prior to HCT on GVHD has yet to be conclusively determined in humans, GVHD can readily develop in mice after splenectomy demonstrating that other secondary lymphoid organs are sufficient to stimulate donor T cells [13].

After allogeneic HCT, both host- and donor-derived APCs are present in secondary lymphoid organs. T-cell receptors (TCRs) of donor T cells can recognize alloantigens either on host APCs (direct presentation) or

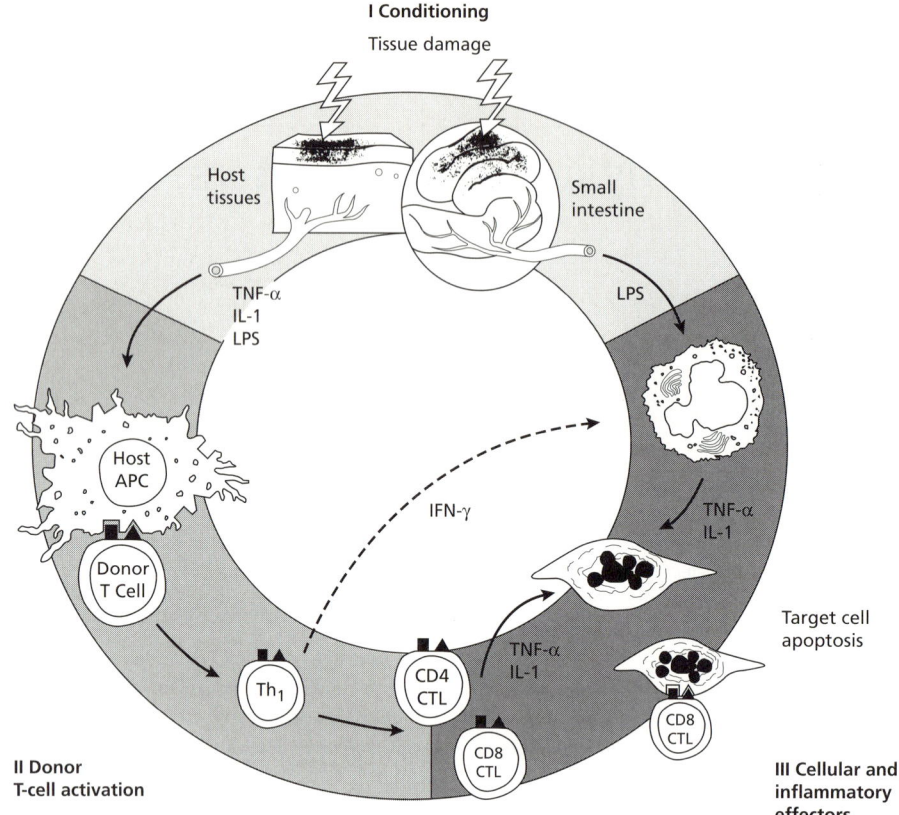

Fig. 27.1 The pathophysiology of acute graft-vs.-host disease (GVHD). GVHD pathophysiology can be summarized in a three-step process. In step 1, the conditioning regimen (irradiation, chemotherapy, or both) leads to the damage and activation of host tissues, especially the intestinal mucosa. This allows the translocation of lipopolysaccharide (LPS) from the intestinal lumen to the circulation, stimulating the secretion of the inflammatory cytokines tumor necrosis factor-alpha (TNF-α) and interleukin 1 (IL-1) from host tissues, particularly macrophages. These cytokines increase the expression of major histocompatibility complex (MHC) antigens and adhesion molecules on host tissues, enhancing the recognition of MHC and minor histocompatibility antigens (mHA) by mature donor T cells.

Donor T-cell activation in step 2 is characterized by the predominance of TH1 cells and the secretion interferon-gamma (IFN-γ), which activates mononuclear phagocytes.

In step 3, effector functions of activated mononuclear phagocytes are triggered by the secondary signal provided by LPS and other stimulatory molecules that leak through the intestinal mucosa damaged during steps 1 and 2. Activated macrophages, along with cytotoxic T lymphocyte (CTL), secrete inflammatory cytokines that cause target cell apoptosis. CD8+ CTL also lyse target cells directly. Damage to the gastrointestinal (GI) tract in this phase, principally by inflammatory cytokines, amplifies LPS release and leads to the "cytokine storm" characteristic of severe acute GVHD. This damage results in the amplification of local tissue injury, and it further promotes an inflammatory response.

donor APCs (indirect presentation). During direct presentation, donor T cells recognize either the peptide bound to allogeneic MHC molecules or the foreign MHC molecules themselves [14]. During indirect presentation, T cells respond to the peptides generated by degradation of the allogeneic MHC molecules that are presented on self-MHC [15]. In GVHD to minor histocompatibility antigens (mHA), direct presentation is dominant because APCs derived from the host rather than from the donor are critical [9].

CD4 and CD8 proteins are coreceptors for constant portions of MHC class II and MHC class I molecules, respectively. MHC class I (HLA-A, B, C) differences stimulate CD8+ T cells and MHC class II (HLA-DR, DP, DQ) differences stimulate CD4+ T cells [16]. In the majority of HLA-identical HCT, GVHD is induced by mHA, which are peptides derived from polymorphic cellular proteins that are presented on the cell surface by MHC molecules [17]. Because the genes for these proteins are located outside of the MHC, two siblings often will have many different peptides in the MHC groove. In this case, different peptides presented by the same MHC are recognized by donor T cells and lead to GVHD. It remains unclear how many of these peptides behave as mHA, although over 50 different mHA genetic loci have been defined among inbred strains of mice [18]. The actual number of so-called "major minor antigens" that can potentially induce GVHD is likely to be limited. Of five previously characterized mHA (HA-1, 2, 3, 4, 5) recognized by T cells in association with HLA-A1 and A2, mismatching of HA-1 alone was significantly correlated with acute grade II–IV GVHD. Theoretical models also predict substantial benefits if multiple minor loci could be typed [19]. Several mHA are encoded on the male-specific Y chromosome. These H-Y antigens are associated with an increased risk of GVHD when male recipients are transplanted from female donors [20,21]. mHA with tissue expression limited to the hematopoietic system are potential target antigens of graft-vs.-leukemia (GVL) reactivity [22], and separation of GVHD and GVL by using CTLs specific for such antigens is an area of intense research [23].

Adhesion molecules mediate the initial binding of T cells to APCs (Table 27.1). TCR signaling after antigen recognition induces a conformational change in adhesion molecules, resulting in higher affinity binding to the APC [24]. Full T-cell activation also requires costimulatory signals provided by APCs in addition to TCR signals. Two primary costimulatory pathways signal through either CD28 or TNF receptors. Currently, there are four known CD28 superfamily members expressed on T cells: CD28, cytotoxic T-lymphocyte antigen 4 (CTLA-4), inducible costimulator (ICOS), and programmed death (PD)-1. In addition,

Table 27.1 T-cell–antigen-presenting cell (APC) interactions.

	T cell	APC
Adhesion	ICAMs	LFA-1
	LFA-1	ICAMs
	CD2 (LFA-2)	LFA-3
Recognition	TCR/CD4	MHC II
	TCR/CD8	MHC I
Costimulation	CD28	CD80/86
	CD152 (CTLA-4)	CD80/86
	ICOS	B7H/B7RP-1
	PD-1	PD-L1, PD-L2
	Unknown	B7-H3
	CD154 (CD40L)	CD40
	CD134 (OX 40)	CD134L (OX40L)
	CD137 (4-1BB)	CD137L (4-1BBL)
	HVEM	LIGHT

HVEM, HSV glycoprotein D for herpesvirus entry mediator; LIGHT, homologous to lymphotoxins, shows inducible expression and competes with herpes simplex virus glycoprotein D for herpesvirus entry mediator (HVEM), a receptor expressed by T lymphocytes.

there are four TNF receptor family members: CD40 ligand (CD154), 4-1BB (CD137), OX40, and herpes simplex virus (HSV) glycoprotein D for herpesvirus entry mediator (HVEM) (Table 27.1). The best-characterized costimulatory molecules, CD80 and CD86, deliver positive signals through CD28 that lower the threshold for T-cell activation and promote T-cell differentiation and survival, while signaling through CTLA-4 is inhibitory [25,26].

The most potent APCs are dendritic cells (DCs); however, the relative contribution of DCs and other semiprofessional APCs, such as monocytes/macrophages and B cells, to the development of GVHD remains to be elucidated. DCs can be matured and activated during HCT by: (i) inflammatory cytokines; (ii) microbial products such as LPS and the dinucleotide CpG entering systemic circulation from intestinal mucosa damaged by conditioning; and (iii) necrotic cells that are damaged by recipient conditioning. All of these stimuli may be considered "danger signals" [27] and may make the difference between an immune response and tolerance [28]. When T cells are exposed to antigens in the presence of adjuvant such as LPS, the migration and survival of T cells are dramatically enhanced *in vivo* [29]. The effect of age in enhancing allostimulatory activity of host APCs may also help explain the increased incidence of acute GVHD in older recipients [30]. The elimination of host APCs by activated natural killer (NK) cells can prevent GVHD [31]. This suppressive effect of NK cells on GVHD has been confirmed in humans: HLA class I differences driving donor NK-mediated alloreactions in the graft-vs.-host (GVH) direction mediate potent GVL effects and produce higher engraftment rates without causing severe acute GVHD [31,32].

Cytokine secretion by donor T cells

T-cell activation involves multiple, rapidly occurring intracellular biochemical changes, including the rise of cytoplasmic free calcium and activation of protein kinase C and tyrosine kinases [33,34]. These pathways in turn activate transcription of genes for cytokines, such as IL-2, IFN-γ, and their receptors. Cytokines secreted by activated T cells are generally classified as T-helper type 1 subset (TH1) (secreting IL-2 and IFN-γ) or T-helper type 2 subset (TH2) (secreting IL-4, IL-5, IL-10 and IL-13) [35]. Several factors influence the ability of DCs to instruct naive CD4$^+$ T cells to secrete TH1 or TH2 cytokines. These factors include the type and duration of DC activation along with the DC/T-cell ratio and the proportions of DC subsets present during T-cell interactions [36,37]. Differential activation of TH1 or TH2 cells has been evoked in the immunopathogenesis of GVHD and the development of infectious and autoimmune diseases. In each setting, activated TH1 cells: (i) amplify T-cell proliferation by secreting IL-2; (ii) lyze target cells by Fas/Fas ligand (FasL) interactions; (iii) induce macrophage differentiation in the bone marrow by secreting IL-3 and granulocyte macrophage colony-stimulating factor (GM-CSF); (iv) activate macrophages by secreting IFN-γ and by their CD40–CD40 ligand interactions; (v) activate endothelium to induce macrophage binding and extravasation; and (vi) recruit macrophages by secreting monocyte chemoattractant protein-1 (MCP-1) [38,39].

During step 2 of acute GVHD pathophysiology, IL-2 has a pivotal role in controlling and amplifying the immune response against alloantigens. IL-2 induces the expression of its own receptor (autocrine effect) and stimulates proliferation of other cells expressing the receptor (paracrine effect). IL-2 is secreted by donor CD4$^+$ T cells in the first several days after GVHD induction [40]. In some studies, the addition of low doses of IL-2 during the 1st week after allogeneic bone marrow transplantation (BMT) enhanced the severity and mortality of GVHD [41,42]. The precursor frequency of host-specific IL-2 producing cells (pHTL) predicts the occurrence of clinical acute GVHD [43–45]. pHTL cells were detectable as early as day 20 after transplant, often preceding the onset of acute GVHD by approximately 2 weeks, and persisted until the GVHD resolved. Monoclonal antibodies (MABs) against IL-2 or its receptor can prevent GVHD when administered shortly after the infusion of T cells [40,46,47], but this strategy was only moderately successful in reducing the incidence of severe GVHD [48,49]. Cyclosporine (CSP) and FK506 dramatically reduce of IL-2 production and effectively prevent GVHD. IL-15 is another critical cytokine in initiating allogeneic T-cell division *in vivo* [50], and elevated serum levels of IL-15 are associated with acute GVHD in humans [51]. IL-15 may, therefore, also be important in the clonal expansion of donor T cells in step 2.

IFN-γ is another crucial cytokine that can be implicated in the second step of the pathophysiology of acute GVHD. Increased levels of IFN-γ are associated with acute GVHD [52–54], and a large proportion of T-cell clones isolated from GVHD patients produce IFN-γ [55]. In animals with GVHD, IFN-γ levels peak between days 4 and 7 after transplantation before clinical manifestations are apparent. CTLs that are specific for mHAs and produce IFN-γ also correlate with the severity of GVH reaction in a skin-explant assay of human disease [56], but serum levels of IFN-γ were not significantly increased in a small series of patients with GVHD [57]. Experimental data demonstrate that IFN-γ modulates several aspects of the pathophysiology of acute GVHD. First, IFN-γ increases the expression of numerous molecules involved in GVHD, including adhesion molecules, chemokines, MHC antigens and Fas, resulting in enhanced antigen presentation and the recruitment of effector cells into target organs [58–60]. Second, IFN-γ alters target cells in the GI tract and skin so that they are more vulnerable to damage during GVHD; the administration of anti-IFN-γ MABs prevents GI GVHD [61] and high levels of both IFN-γ and TNF-α correlate with the most intense cellular damage in the skin [56]. Third, IFN-γ mediates GVHD-associated immunosuppression seen in several experimental HCT systems in part by the induction of nitric oxide (NO) [62–67]. Fourth, IFN-γ primes macrophages to produce pro-inflammatory cytokines and NO in response to LPS [68,69]. At early time points after HCT, IFN-γ may paradoxically reduce GVHD by enhancing Fas-mediated apoptosis of activated donor T cells [11,12,70].

Both cell-mediated and inflammatory cytokine GVHD effector mechanisms can sometimes be inhibited if donor T cells produce less of TH1 cytokines. Transplantation of TH2 cells (generated *in vivo* by treating donor mice with a combination of IL-2 and IL-4) into nonirradiated recipients results in reduced secretion of TNF-α and protection of recipient mice from LPS-induced, TNF-α-mediated lethality [71]. Furthermore, cell mixtures of TH2 donor cells with an otherwise lethal inocula of allogeneic bone marrow and T cells also protects recipient mice from LPS-induced lethality, demonstrating the ability of TH2 cells to modulate TH1 responses after allogeneic transplantation [72]. Similarly, the injection of donor TH2 cells, polarized in a mixed lymphocyte reaction (MLR) with host cells in the presence of IL-4, fails to induce acute GVHD to MHC class I or class II antigens [73]. Polarization of donor T cells toward a TH2 phenotype by pretreating HCT donors with granulocyte colony-stimulating factor (G-CSF) also results in less severe GVHD [74]. Interestingly, GVHD still occurs if donor mice lack the signal transduction and activator of transcription (STAT) 4, which is crucial to a TH1 response, albeit GVHD is less severe than if the donor cells lacked STAT6, a molecule critical for TH2 polarization [75]. These experiments support the concepts that TH1 cells induce GVHD more efficiently than TH2 cells and that the balance of TH1 and TH2 cytokines is critical for the development of a GVH reaction. It should be noted, however, that systemic administration of TH2 cytokines IL-4 or IL-10 as experimental prophylaxis of GVHD was either ineffective or toxic [76–78].

On the other hand, administration of TH1 cytokines can also reduce GVHD. High doses of exogenous IL-2 early after BMT protects animals from GVHD mortality [79]. It has been suggested that IL-2 mediates its protective effect via inhibition of IFN-γ [52]. Furthermore, the injection of IFN-γ itself can prevent experimental GVHD [80], and neutralization of IFN-γ results in accelerated GVHD in lethally irradiated recipients [64]. Interestingly, the use of IFN-γ-deficient donor cells can also accelerate GVHD in lethally irradiated recipients [11,81] but reduces GVHD in sublethally irradiated or unirradiated recipients [82,83]. These paradoxes may be explained by the complex dynamics of donor T-cell activation, expansion, and contraction. Activation-induced cell death (AICD) is a chief mechanism of clonal deletion and is largely responsible for the rapid contraction of activated T cells following an initial massive expansion [84]. IFN-γ contracts the pool of activated CD4$^+$ T cells by inducing AICD, and thus the complete absence of IFN-γ may result in an unrestrained expansion of activated donor T cells, leading to accelerated GVHD. This phenomenon may be of particular importance in recipients of intensified conditioning, which causes greater T-cell activation [8]. Similarly, administration of IFN-γ-inducing cytokines, such as IL-12 or IL-18, early after BMT protects lethally irradiated recipients from GVHD in a Fas dependent fashion [11,12,85,86]. Thus, moderate amounts of TH1 cytokines production after donor T-cell expansion may amplify GVHD; extremes in production (either low or high), particularly during T-cell expansion, may hasten the death of activated donor T cells, aborting T-cell expansion and reducing GVHD.

Subpopulations of regulatory donor T cells can prevent GVHD. Repeated *in vitro* stimulation of donor CD4$^+$ T cells with alloantigens results in the emergence of a population of T-cell clones (Treg cells) that secretes high amounts of IL-10 and TGF-γ [87]. The immunosuppressive properties of these cytokines are explained by their ability to inhibit APC function and to suppress proliferation of responding T cells directly. The addition of IL-10 or TGF-β to MLR cultures induces tolerance [88], with alterations in biochemical signaling similar to costimulatory blockade [89]. Transplantation of HLA mismatched hematopoietic stem cell (HSCs) in patients with severe combined immunodeficiency syndrome (SCID) can result in selective engraftment of donor T cells with complete immunologic reconstitution and tolerance in association with the development of donor derived Treg cells that produce large amounts of IL-10 [90]. Similarly, so called "Th3" cells that produce large amounts of TGF-β can act as regulatory T cells. CD8$^+$ suppressor cells have also been identified in both mice and humans [91–94]. A specific subpopulation of regulatory CD8$^+$ T cells expressing CD57 has been identified in patients with acute and chronic GVHD [94,95]. Natural suppressor (NS) cells reduce GVHD in a variety of experimental BMT models [96]. NK1.1$^+$ T cells (NKT) may possess such NS cell function [97], and both peripheral blood and marrow NKT cells can prevent GVHD by their IL-4 secretion [97–99]. Much recent research has focused on CD4$^+$CD25$^+$ regulatory T cells that can prevent lethal GVHD in several animal models [100].

Step 3: cellular and inflammatory effectors

The pathophysiology of acute GVHD culminates in the generation of multiple cytotoxic effectors that contribute to target tissue injury. At a minimum, step 3 includes: (i) several inflammatory cytokines; (ii) specific antihost CTL activity using Fas and perforin pathways; (iii) large granular lymphocytes (LGLs) or NK cells; and (iv) NO. Significant experimental and clinical data suggest that soluble inflammatory mediators act in conjunction with direct cell-mediated cytolysis by CTL and NK cells to cause the full spectrum of deleterious effects seen during acute GVHD. As such, the effector phase of GVHD involves aspects of both the innate and adaptive immune response and the synergistic interactions of components generated during step 1 and step 2.

Cellular effectors

The Fas/FasL and the perforin/granzyme (or granule exocytosis) pathways are the principal effector mechanisms used by CTLs and NK cells to lyse their target cells [101,102]. Perforin is stored together with granzymes and other proteins in cytotoxic granules of CTLs and NK cells [103]. Following recognition of a target cell through TCR–MHC interaction, perforin is secreted and inserts itself into the target cell membrane forming "perforin pores" that allow granzymes to enter the cell and induce apoptosis through various downstream effector pathways [103]. Ligation of Fas results in the formation of the death-inducing signaling complex and the subsequent activation of caspases [104]. A number of ligands on T cells also possess the capability to trimerize TNF-α receptor (TNFR)-like death receptors (DR) on their targets, such as TNF-related apoptosis inducing ligand (TRAIL : DR4,5 ligand) and TNF-like weak inducer of apoptosis (TWEAK : DR3 ligand) [105–107].

The involvement of these pathways in GVHD has been tested by utilizing donor cells that are genetically deficient in each molecule. Transplantation of perforin deficient T cells results in a marked delay in the onset of acute GVHD in transplants across mHA [108], both MHC and mHA [109], and isolated MHC I or II disparities [110,111]. However, lethal GVHD occurs even in the *absence* of perforin dependent killing demonstrating that the perforin/granzyme pathway plays a significant, but not exclusive, role in target organ damage. Similar findings were noted in experiments employing specific donor T-cell subsets; perforin/granzyme B deficient CD8$^+$ T cells induced significantly less mortality compared to wild type T cells in transplants across a single MHC class I mismatch, whereas this pathway was less important compared to the Fas/FasL pathway in CD4-mediated GVHD [110,112]. Thus CD4$^+$ CTLs preferentially use the Fas/FasL pathway during acute GVHD, while CD8$^+$ CTLs primarily use the perforin/granzyme pathway, consistent with other conditions involving cell mediated cytolysis.

Fas is a TNF-receptor family member that is expressed by many tissues, including GVHD target organs. Inflammatory cytokines such as IFN-γ and TNF-α can increase the expression of Fas during GVHD [113]. FasL expression on donor T cells is also increased during GVHD [114–116]. Elevated serum levels of soluble FasL and Fas have also been observed in some patients with acute GVHD [117–120]. FasL defective donor T cells cause markedly reduced experimental GVHD in liver, skin and lymphoid organs [108,121,122]. The Fas/FasL pathway is particularly important in hepatic GVHD, consistent with the marked sensitivity of hepatocytes to Fas-mediated cytotoxicity in models of murine hepatitis [123]. Fas-deficient recipients are protected from hepatic GVHD, but not from GVHD in other target organs [124]. Administration of anti-FasL (but not anti-TNF) MAB significantly blocked hepatic GVHD damage occurring in one model [125], whereas the use of FasL-deficient donor T cells or the administration of neutralizing FasL MABs had no effect on the development of intestinal GVHD in several studies [108,125,126].

The cytotoxic double deficient (cdd) mouse (absence of both perforin/granzyme and FasL pathways) provides an opportunity to address whether other effector pathways can induce GVHD target organ pathology. An initial study demonstrated that cdd T cells did not induce lethal GVHD across MHC class I and class II disparities after sublethal irradiation [109]. The lack of acute GVHD was probably caused by the rejection of the donor cdd T cells because they lacked cytotoxic effector mechanisms to eliminate host resistance to GVHD [127,128]. When recipients were conditioned with a lethal dose of irradiation, cdd CD4$^+$ T cells produced similar mortality to wild type CD4$^+$ T cells [128]. These results were confirmed by a recent study demonstrating that GVHD target damage can still occur when CTLs cannot interact with target epithelium lacking alloantigen expression (see Fig 27.1) [2].

Inflammatory effectors

In the effector phase of acute GVHD, inflammatory cytokines synergize with CTLs resulting in the amplification of local tissue injury and the development of target organ dysfunction in the transplant recipient. The cytokines TNF-α and IL-1 are produced by an abundance of cell types involved in innate and adoptive immune responses and they have synergistic and redundant during several phases of acute GVHD. A central role for inflammatory cytokines in acute GVHD was confirmed by a recent murine study using bone marrow chimeras in which either MHC class I or MHC class II alloantigens were not expressed on target epithelium but on APCs alone [2]. GVHD target organ injury was induced in these chimeras even in the absence of epithelial alloantigens and mortality and target organ injury was prevented by the neutralization of TNF-α and IL-1. These observations were particularly true for CD4-mediated acute GVHD but also applied, at least in part, for CD8-mediated disease.

A critical role for TNF-α in the pathophysiology of acute GVHD was first suggested almost 15 years ago because mice transplanted with mixtures of allogeneic bone marrow and T cells developed severe skin, gut and lung lesions that were associated with high levels of TNF-α messenger RNA (mRNA) in these tissues [129,130]. Target organ damage could be inhibited by infusion of anti-TNF-α MABs, and mortality could be reduced from 100% to 50% by the administration of the soluble form of the TNF-α receptor (sTNFR) [6]. Extensive experimental data further suggest that TNF-α is involved in the multistep process of GVHD pathophysiology. TNF-α can: (i) cause cachexia, a characteristic feature of GVHD; (ii) induce naturalization of DCs, thus enhancing alloantigen presentation; (iii) recruit effector T cells, neutrophils, and monocytes into target organs through the induction of inflammatory chemokines; and (iv) cause direct tissue damage by inducing apoptosis and necrosis [131]. TNF-α is also involved in donor T-cell activation directly through its signaling via TNFR1 and TNFR2 on T cells; TNF–TNFR1 interactions promote alloreactive T-cell responses [132], whereas TNF–TNFR2 interactions are critical for intestinal GVHD [133]. TNF-α plays a central role in intestinal GVHD in murine and human studies [125,129,134]. TNF-α also seems to be an important effector molecule in GVHD in skin and lymphoid tissue [125,129,135,136] and can contribute to hepatic GVHD, probably by enhancing effector cell migration to the liver via the induction of inflammatory chemokines. Two recent studies in animals demonstrated that neutralization of TNF-α alone or in combination with IL-1 resulted in a significant reduction of hepatic GVHD [2,137].

An important role for TNF-α in clinical acute GVHD has also been suggested by multiple studies. Elevations of TNF-α protein (serum) and mRNA (peripheral blood mononuclear cells) have been measured in patients with acute GVHD and other endothelial complications, such as hepatic veno-occlusive disease (VOD) [138–141]. Furthermore, a phase I/II trial using TNF-α receptor MABs during the conditioning regimen as prophylaxis in patients at high risk for severe acute GVHD showed reduction in lesions of the intestine, skin, and liver. GVHD flared, however, after discontinuation of treatment [134]. Collectively, these data suggest that approaches to limit TNF-α secretion will be a very important avenue of investigation in allogeneic HCT.

IL-1 is the second major pro-inflammatory cytokine that contributes to acute GVHD toxicity. Secretion of IL-1 appears to occur predominantly during the effector phase of GVHD in the spleen and skin, two major GVHD target organs [142]. A similar increase in mononuclear cell IL-1 mRNA has been shown during clinical acute GVHD [140]. Indirect evidence of a role for IL-1 in GVHD was obtained after administration of this cytokine to allogeneic HCT recipients [76]. Mice receiving IL-1 displayed a wasting syndrome with increased mortality that appeared to be an accelerated form of GVHD. Investigations of the role of IL-1 in GVHD intensified after the discovery of IL-1 receptor antagonist (IL-1RA) [143,144]. Intraperitoneal administration of IL-1RA starting on day 10 after stem cell transplantation reversed the development of GVHD in the majority of animals and resulted in a significant survival advantage compared to allogeneic controls [145]. IL-1RA has been used after clinical HCT with mixed results. Although a phase II trial demonstrated that IL-1RA was efficacious in treating GVHD in a subset of patients with steroid refractory disease, an attempt to use IL-1RA to prevent acute GVHD in a randomized trial was not successful [146].

Finally, macrophages can also produce significant amounts of NO as a result of activation during GVHD. Several studies have shown that NO contributes to the deleterious effects of GVHD on target tissues and specifically to GVHD-induced immunosuppression [67,147]. NO also inhibits repair mechanisms of target tissue by inhibiting proliferation of epithelial stem cells in the gut and skin [148]. In humans and rats, development of GVHD is preceded by an increase of NO oxidation products in the serum [149,150].

LPS and innate immunity

As alluded to above, components of the HCT conditioning regimen (in particular TBI) and the secretion of type 1 cytokines (specifically IFN-γ) prime mononuclear phagocytes to produce inflammatory cytokines. However, the actual secretion of soluble cytokines occurs after primed macrophages are triggered or stimulated by a second signal. This stimulus may be provided through Toll-like receptors (TLRs) by LPS and other microbial products that have leaked though an intestinal mucosa damaged initially by HCT conditioning regimens during step 1. Since the GI tract is known to be particularly sensitive to the injurious effects of cytokines [129,151], damage to the GI tract incurred during the effector phase can lead to a positive feed back loop wherein increased translocation of LPS results in further cytokine production and progressive intestinal injury. Thus, the GI tract may be critical to propagating the "cytokine storm" characteristic of acute GVHD; increasing experimental and clinical evidence suggests that damage to the GI tract during acute GVHD plays a major role in the amplification of systemic disease [132].

This conceptual framework underscores the role of LPS in the development of acute GVHD as suggested by several groups [69,151,152]. LPS is a major structural component of gram-negative bacteria and is a potent stimulator of cellular activation and cytokine release [153,154]. LPS shed from bacteria that comprise normal bowel flora can elicit a broad range of inflammatory responses from macrophages, monocytes and neutrophils. In particular, LPS may stimulate gut-associated lymphocytes and macrophages [69]. Following allogeneic HCT, LPS accumulates in both the liver and spleen of animals with GVHD prior to its appearance in the systemic circulation [152]. Elevated serum levels of LPS have been shown to correlate directly with the degree of intestinal histopathology occurring after allogeneic HCT [151,155,156]. The severity of GVHD also appears to be directly related to the level of macrophage priming [69]. Injection of small, normally nonlethal amounts of LPS caused elevated TNF-α serum levels and death in animals with GVHD; this mortality could be prevented with anti-TNF-α antiserum. These experiments strongly support the role of mononuclear phagocytes as major sources of inflammatory cytokines during the effector phase of acute GVHD.

Mice known to be sensitive or resistant to LPS have been used as stem cell donors in order to determine the effect of donor responsiveness to LPS on the development of acute GVHD. C3Heb/Fej animals exhibit normal murine sensitivity to LPS challenge (LPS-s), whereas a genetic mutation in the Toll-like receptor 4 (Tlr4) gene of C3H/Hej mice has made this strain resistant to LPS (LPS-r) [157–160]. These defects are specific to LPS and, importantly, T cells from LPS resistant mice respond normally to mitogen and alloantigen [161,162]. In an irradiated parent (P) → F1 hybrid murine model of GVHD, HCT with LPS-r donor cells resulted in a significant reduction of TNF-α levels, GI tract histopathology and systemic GVHD compared to animals receiving LPS-s SCT [151]. Causality of the association was demonstrated by the systemic neutralization of TNF-α, which further decreased the severity of intestinal and systemic GVHD in LPS-r SCT recipients [151].

These results were complemented by recent experiments using animals deficient in CD14 as HCT donors. CD14 is a cell surface protein that is present on mononuclear cells and macrophages. It is the principal receptor for the complex of LPS and its soluble LPS binding protein (LBP) and is a critical component of the innate immune response [163]. The engagement of CD14 by LPS/LPB results in the association of the CD14 molecules with Toll-like receptors and subsequent intracellular signaling and cytokine synthesis [49]. Mononuclear cells from CD14 deficient (CD14$^{-/-}$) animals are insensitive to LPS stimulation *in vitro*, and such mice are resistant to the lethal effects of LPS challenge *in vivo* [164]. Transplantation of CD14$^{-/-}$ donor cells into irradiated allogeneic recipients resulted in a 60% reduction in serum TNF-α levels by day +7 and a corresponding decrease in gut histopathology compared to mice receiving HCT from normal controls. This reduction in GI toxicity was associated with improved long-term survival and a reduction in systemic GVHD [165].

Data supporting a role for LPS in the GVH response are also provided by both experimental and clinical studies examining the effects of decontamination of the GI tract on the incidence of GVHD. Early animal studies showed that death from GVHD could be prevented if transplanted mice were given antibiotics to decontaminate the gut; normalization of the gut flora at or before day 20 abrogated this effect [166]. After clinical HCT, endotoxemia is associated with biochemical parameters of intestinal injury, hepatic toxicity, acute GVHD and fever in the absence of bacteremia [155,156]. Accordingly, gram-negative gut decontamination during HCT has also been shown to reduce GVHD [167,168], and the intensity of this decontamination can predict GVHD severity [169,170]. Naturally occurring antibody titres to a rough-mutant strain of *Escherichia coli* J5, which protect humans and animals from septic shock, are also associated with a decrease incidence of acute GVHD after allogeneic SCT [171]. Use of a polyclonal antiserum against *E. coli* J5 as prophylaxis for acute GVHD in a prospective, placebo controlled trial found that infusion of the J5 antibody reduced overall GVHD from 63% to 42%. The antiserum was particularly efficacious in a subset of patients with severe GVHD [172].

A more specific approach to the blockade of cellular activation by LPS after allogeneic HCT was recently studied using an irradiated mouse model. B975 is a synthetic analog of *E. coli* lipid A and is one in a family of molecules that are potent antagonists of LPS induced cellular activation [173]. These molecules act as competitive inhibitors to LPS at the cell surface and block NFκB activation and nuclear translocation. They are active both *in vitro* and *in vivo* and are devoid of agonistic activity even at high doses [173]. Treatment of allogeneic BMT recipients with B975 for the first week after transplant blocked the biologic response to LPS and resulted in decreased inflammatory cytokine release and reduced GVHD severity. Importantly, LPS antagonism had no effect on donor T-cell responses to host antigens, and treatment with B975 was associated with preservation of potent GVL effects and improved leukemia-free survival.

Inflammatory chemokines

Regulation of effector cell migration into target tissues during the development of GVHD occurs in a complex milieu of chemotactic signals where several chemokine receptors may be triggered simultaneously or successively. Inflammatory chemokines expressed in inflamed tissues are specialized to recruit effector cells, such as T cells, neutrophils and monocytes [174]. Chemokine receptors are differentially expressed on subsets of activated/effector T cells. Upon stimulation, T cells can rapidly switch chemokine receptor expression, acquiring new migratory capacity [29,175]. The involvement of inflammatory chemokines and their receptors in GVHD has been recently investigated in mouse models of GVHD. MIP-1α recruits CCR5$^+$CD8$^+$ T cells into the liver, lung, and spleen during GVHD [176,177], and levels of several chemokines are elevated in GVHD-associated lung injury [178]. Further studies will determine whether expression of chemokines and their receptors can explain the unusual cluster of GVHD target organs (skin, gut, and liver), and whether these molecules will prove to be potential targets for modulation of GVHD.

GVHD prevention: from animal models to clinical practice

The development of strategies for GVHD prophylaxis and therapy has suffered from a limited understanding of the underlying pathophysiology of acute GVHD. While a good deal more is known about the basis for GVHD, much is left to learn. This conceptual limitation led to approaches that were based on an "oncologic" model of GVHD, i.e. the notion that since GVHD is dangerous and life-threatening, management requires the utilization of high dose immunosuppressant regimens. High doses of multiple immunosuppressive agents have been used much like we use combination chemotherapy to treat malignancies. While there is often reasonable control of the clinical manifestations of GVHD, this "shotgun" approach lacks elegance and is usually associated with opportunistic infections, lymphoproliferative disorders, or relapse of the underlying malignancy. Indeed, it is often infection while GVHD is in remission that results in mortality. The objective should be to reduce the nonspecific tissue damage associated with GVHD, while leaving enough immune function behind to facilitate recognition and control of common organisms. Since it is clear that much of the control of the underlying disorder is related to immunologic targeting of host antigens that have limited expression patterns (e.g. mHA), some degree of functional immunity is critical to the success of transplantation.

In this context, it is important to establish a workable model to explain GVHD. This model should then suggest approaches to control GVHD. The three-phase model described above can be simply summarized. GVHD is an exaggerated and dysregulated response of a normal immune system (that of the donor) to tissue damage that is intrinsic to transplantation. The donor's immune system reacts as if there is a massive and uncontrolled infection, and its efforts to deal with this injury result in the clinical manifestations of GVHD. It is quite possible that the tissue injury intrinsic to the administration of high dose chemoradiotherapy initiates the breakdown of mucosal barriers, allowing endotoxin into the tissues. Toll-like receptors on DCs bind to endotoxin and activate signal transduction pathways that lead to DC maturation and induce inflammation [179]. The up-regulation of costimulatory molecules, MHC molecules, adhesion molecules, cytokines, chemokines, prostanoids and other inflammatory mediators prime and trigger attack on target tissues, fueling the fire. Thus, it is likely that components of cytokine storm [1], the danger hypothesis [27] and more traditional notions of adaptive and innate immunity [180] all apply.

Step 1: reduced intensity conditioning regimens

The three cardinal organs affected by GVHD are the skin, intestinal tract and liver. The common thread would seem to be exposure to the environment. Skin and gut have very obvious barrier functions and a well-developed reticuloendothelial system. Similarly, the liver is the first line of defense downstream of the gut. One would expect the lung to be a similar target; however, its less intense exposure to organisms, particularly gram-negative rods, probably reduces its primacy as a target organ. Nevertheless, recent studies clearly demonstrate pulmonary injury that is likely to reflect GVHD. All of these organs are rich in DCs, a probable prerequisite for generating the injurious cytokines as well as directing the attack of the adaptive immune system. They are all subject to injury from conditioning and breaches of the barrier will allow organisms or endotoxin into the circulation.

One prediction of this model is that less intense conditioning regimens would be associated with less GVHD. This effect was initially observed after donor lymphocyte infusions. The T cells were administered without pharmacologic GVHD prophylaxis, and the resultant GVHD was less frequent and severe than would be expected in the absence of immunosuppressive drugs. It could be inferred that reduced intensity conditioning regimens might similarly be associated with less severe GVHD, both through less cellular injury *per se* and through a reduction in endotoxin exposure by virtue of less mucosal injury. Available data suggest that the rate of GVHD after reduced intensity regimens is similar to the rate seen after conventional dose conditioning [181–184]. Thus, while data on reducing both colonization with bacteria and reducing tissue injury with less intense regimens are suggestive and support the basic concepts described above, the effect is insufficient to control GVHD adequately in human transplantation.

Step 2: modulation of donor T cells

Reduced T-cell numbers

The advent of monoclonal technology in the 1980s led to the logical conclusion that if pharmacologic reduction in T-cell numbers could partially control GVHD, albeit at the risk of drug-induced toxicity, then eliminating the cells with monoclonal antibodies, immunotoxins, lectins, CD34 columns, or physical techniques, might be more effective (reviewed by [185]). Furthermore, the ability to identify and target specific T-cell subsets opened the possibility that the graft could be engineered to control GVHD while allowing immunologic recovery as well as GVL. T-cell depletion (TCD) of marrow is relatively straightforward because the number of T cells in the product is low compared with the total nucleated cell count. This makes marrow relatively easy to manipulate in the laboratory. As the use of peripheral blood hematopoietic cells has become more prevalent, the 10-fold increase in number of T cells represents a technical challenge. A typical unmanipulated marrow transplant entails the infusion of $\sim 10^7$ T cells/kg of recipient weight. Establishment of a clear dose–response relationship is difficult, since the risk of acute GVHD depends on factors beyond simple dosing, e.g. minor histocompatibility disparities, virus exposure, disease and stage, donor age, recipient age, etc. Studies of counterflow elutriation showed that 10^6 T cells/kg plus CSP resulted in a GVHD rate similar to CSP alone, but 5×10^5 T cells/kg plus CSP resulted in an overall rate of 22% and only limited skin involvement was observed [186]. After lectin depletion of T cells in the absence of supplemental immunosuppression, a T-cell dose $\leq 10^5$/kg was associated with complete control of GVHD [187]. More recently the combination of very high stem cell numbers and CD3 T-cell numbers $<3 \times 10^4$/kg allowed haploidentical transplantation without GVHD [188].

Global TCD using a broad panel of monoclonal antibodies has been largely abandoned because of the risk of graft failure [189]. However, it is clear that even depletion of T-cell subsets must be undertaken with caution. Depletion of CD8$^+$ T cells alone can be associated with a high graft failure rate [190,191]. However, depletion of CD5$^+$ or CD6$^+$ T cells seems to be associated with a low graft failure rate [192,193]. The presumption is that radioresistant T cells that survive the initial conditioning are responsible for graft rejection. When the stem cell source is rich in T cells, the GVH reaction will further reduce the residual population capable of alloreactivity, thus decreasing graft rejection. To some degree the higher graft failure rates may be controlled by increasing the intensity of the conditioning regimen [194], adding back T cells [186], or with additional immunosuppressants [190]. Additional problems associated with TCD include a higher incidence of Epstein–Barr virus induced lymphoproliferative disorders, loss of the GVL effect with a consequent increase in relapses and slower immunologic recovery due to reduced passive transfer of donor immunocompetent donor T cells. These concerns also have been approached by increasing the conditioning intensity, delayed T-cell add-back [195], rituximab [196], or infusing specific T-cell lines [197,198]. However, in no case has there been an improvement in survival that can be definitively attributed to TCD. Another interesting and novel approach to restore T-cell function without GVHD is to start by removing T cells from the initial graft using a technique such as CD34 selection. This step is followed by reacting donor and recipient lymphocytes in a MLR in the presence of an anti-IL-2 receptor immunotoxin. This agent removes only activated T cells since it binds to CD25. The remaining resting cells are then infused to enhance immunologic recovery [199]. Alternatively, studies in mice have accomplished a similar effect depleting donor cells activated in a mixed lymphocyte culture with antibodies to the activation antigen CD69 and immunomagnetic bead sorting [200].

Since activated T cells contribute to GVHD and resting T cells presumably have other, potentially useful specificities, selective elimination of activated populations might be of some interest. Treatment of established GVHD with antibodies has produced mixed results. While antithymocyte globulin has definite activity in established GVHD, the nonspecific clearance of T cells may result in increased opportunistic infections and no improvement in survival [201–203]. More specific therapy with humanized anti-IL-2 receptor antibody, daclizumab [204,205], or the humanized anti-CD3 antibody, visilizumab [206], are promising, since they offer the potential of selectively removing the activated T cells. However, an increased risk of infection may still be observed [207].

Reduced T-cell activation

The introduction of CSP in the late 1970s was a significant advance in GVHD prevention. More recently a similar agent, tacrolimus, has been shown to provide similar control of GVHD. Both drugs inhibit T-lymphocyte activation, although the exact mechanism of action is not known. Both drugs bind to immunophilins—CSP binds cyclophilin and tacrolimus binds FKBP12. The complex of drug and binding protein, calcium, calmodulin, and calcineurin is then formed and the phosphatase activity of calcineurin is inhibited. This effect may prevent the dephosphorylation and translocation of nuclear factor of activated T cells, a nuclear component thought to initiate gene transcription for the formation of lymphokines (such as IL-2, interferon-γ). The net result is the inhibition of T-lymphocyte activation (reviewed by [208]).

As a single agent CSP was about as effective as methotrexate (MTX) [209]. However, in combination with MTX, there was a significant reduction in the incidence of GVHD and an improvement in survival [210]. Subsequent trials of tacrolimus and MTX compared with CSP and MTX showed no advantage for either combination [211,212]. The addition of prednisone to the conventional two-drug regimen resulted in similar rates of GVHD and no improvement in survival [213].

DCs appear to be critical to the development of acute GVHD [9]; therefore, interference with DC function would probably prevent GVHD. The goal would be to inhibit function selectively or temporarily until transplanted DC precursors have engrafted and become functional. DC2 seem to foster TH2 responses, which are less likely to result in GVHD. Preliminary data suggest that extracorporeal photopheresis (ECP) may result in attenuation of TH1-mediated cytokine secretion, a shift in the DC1/DC2 ratio favoring plasmacytoid rather than monocytoid DC profiles, and a decrease in antigen responsiveness by dendritic [214,215]. Preliminary results suggest that administering ECP prior to stem cell infusion can accelerate DC turnover and results in a striking reduction in GVHD risk [216]. These provocative results will need to be confirmed. Campath is an anti-CD52 monoclonal antibody that has been extensively used for the prevention of GVHD, primarily in Europe. It is a promiscuous antibody, targeting B cells, T cells, monocytes and other cells. Interestingly, it also appears to target DCs and, when the drug was administered prior to transplantation, host DCs were selectively depleted and the donor DCs repopulated the recipient [217]. These observations are difficult to separate from concomitant TCD, but they may be consistent with the theme that facilitation of DC turnover may ameliorate GVHD. Finally, Flt3 ligand therapy has shown similar effects in mice [2]. Human trials would be very interesting.

Reduced T-cell proliferation

The first generally prescribed GVHD preventive regimen was the administration of intermittent low dose MTX as developed in a dog model by Thomas and colleagues [218]. Another regimen developed by Santos and based on cyclophosphamide [219] was never widely adopted. The principle of this approach is to administer a cell-cycle specific chemotherapeutic agent intermittently immediately after the transplant, when the T cells will have started to divide after exposure to allogeneic antigens. This was an effective approach compared with no prophylaxis [220]; however, GVHD control was incomplete. Subsequently, the addition of antithymocyte globulin or prednisone or both resulted in incremental improvement in the GVHD rate but no improvement in survival [221,222]. Long courses of MTX proved to be associated with a higher risk of interstitial pneumonitis and mucositis, and were abandoned with the advent of CSP. One concern regarding the use of MTX is that the enhanced mucositis might be associated with increased transfer of endotoxin across the mucosa. Ultimately the course of MTX was abbreviated and combined with a T-cell activation inhibitor, such as CSP or tacrolimus.

More recently, mycophenolate mofetil (MMF) has been studied. It is the prodrug of mycophenolic acid (MPA), a selective inhibitor of inosine monophosphate dehydrogenase, and inhibits the *de novo* pathway of guanosine nucleotide synthesis. Since T lymphocytes are dependent on *de novo* synthesis of purines, MPA inhibits proliferative responses of T cells to both mitogenic and allogeneic stimulation. Myeloid and mucosal cells can utilize salvage pathways, so the drug is less toxic to mucosa and myeloid recovery. MPA also prevents the glycosylation of glycoproteins that are involved in adhesion to endothelium and may reduce recruitment of leukocytes into inflammatory sites. MMF does not inhibit the activation of T cells, as such, but blocks the coupling of activation to DNA synthesis and proliferation [223]. Recent limited trials of the combination of MMF with CSP or tacrolimus are promising [184,224–226], but larger definitive trials are necessary to establish the correct dose and schedule, and to compare its effect on GVHD and survival with MTX.

Sirolimus is a macrocyclic lactone immunosuppressant that is similar in structure to tacrolimus and CSP. All three drugs bind to immunophilins; however, sirolimus complexed with FKBP12 inhibits T-cell proliferation by interfering with signal transduction and cell cycle progression. Sirolimus (rapamycin) affects lymphocyte activation at a later stage than either CSP or tacrolimus, and activation stimuli that resist inhibition to the latter agents have been shown to be sensitive to sirolimus. Sirolimus has been shown to inhibit antibody dependent cellular cytotoxicity and the cytolytic effects of NK cells and IL-2 lymphokine-activated killer (LAK) cells. The sirolimus : FKBP12 complex binds to mammalian target of rapamycin (mTOR), which blocks IL-2 mediated signal transduction pathways that prevent G1 → S phase transition. This effect is mediated through a complex pathway involving inhibition of ribosomal protein synthesis at several levels, as well as effects on transcription and translation (reviewed by [227]). The drug has similar effects on proliferation of T cells induced by IL-2, IL-4, IL-7, IL-12 and IL-15. Interestingly, it may also interfere with costimulation [228] by inhibiting CD28-mediated blocking of IκBα and translocation of c-Rel to the nucleus [229]. Sirolimus contributes to massive T-cell apoptosis if signals 1 and 2 of T-cell activation are blocked—an effect that is not seen with CSP [230]. This effect may be related to its ability to inhibit the expression of *bcl-2* and *BAG-1* [231,232]. Sirolimus completely inhibits the kinase activity of the cdk4/cyclin B and cdk2/cyclin E complexes despite normal expression of these proteins and, as a consequence, blocks the hyperphosphorylation of the retinoblastoma gene product (Rb). Interestingly, sirolimus has inhibitory effects on integrin-mediated signal transduction [233], and dermal microvascular injury in a Hu-SCID transplantation model [234]. Sirolimus has excellent antirejection activity in organ transplantation [235], and combination therapy with sirolimus and tacrolimus appears to be extremely effective in human organ allografting [236] and murine models of marrow grafting [111,237]. Since it acts through a separate mechanism from the tacrolimus-FKBP complex (and CSP-cyclophilin complex) which inhibits calcineurin and thus T-cell activation, sirolimus is synergistic with both tacrolimus and CSP. Interestingly, while both tacrolimus and sirolimus bind to FKBP12, there appear to be adequate binding sites for both molecules. Therefore, in contrast to expectations the drugs are not competitive and, in fact, they appear to be synergistic. Since the sirolimus : mTOR complex does not bind to calcineurin, sirolimus also is free of nephrotoxicity and neurotoxicity, making combination therapy appealing. Early clinical trials indicate that sirolimus may be a promising addition to the GVHD armamentarium, but more studies are needed to determine its optimal dosing [238].

Induction of T-cell tolerance or anergy

Engagement of the TCR without appropriate costimulation will result in the inability of T cells to respond to the alloantigen as described earlier. Such an approach was effective in MHC disparate transplantation in animal models, and this success led to a trial of CTLA-4-Ig in MHC mismatched transplantation in humans [239]. In this trial donor cells were treated *ex vivo* with patient stimulator cells and with CTLA-4-Ig. CTLA-4-Ig blocks CD28 : B7 mediated costimulation, and the authors demonstrated a reduction in the frequency of donor T cells capable of recognizing alloantigens of the recipient, while responsiveness to third party alloantigens was unaffected. In 11 evaluable patients the haploidentical bone marrow cells engrafted, and there appeared to be a reduction in acute GVHD. Studies of CD40 : CD40L blockade have demonstrated the development of anergy in mice [240,241], but human trials have not yet been undertaken. Interestingly, administration of anti-CD40 monoclonal antibodies may result in lethal release of inflammatory cytokines, suggesting that attempts to induce tolerization *in vivo* may have unexpected toxicity and must be undertaken with great caution [242,243].

Step 3: blockade of inflammatory stimulation and effectors

Reduced exposure to organisms

Another hypothesis that flows from this model is that reduction of intestinal colonization with bacteria could prevent GVHD. The first indication that elimination of exposure to microorganisms could prevent GVHD was in germ-free experiments in mice, where GVHD was not observed until the mice were colonized with gram-negative organisms [166]. Later, gut decontamination and use of a Laminar air-flow environment was associated with less GVHD and better survival in patients with severe aplastic anaemia [167]. Similarly, studies of intestinal decontamination in patients with malignancies have shown less GVHD in some [169,170] but not all studies [244]. However, despite the power of large number of patients in registry analyses [244], it is possible that the heterogeneity of care in the large number of participating centers obscured an important effect. Viral infections, particularly herpesviruses, may also be associated with GVHD [245].

Blockade of inflammatory effectors

As alluded to above, an important role for TNF-α in clinical acute GVHD was suggested by studies demonstrating elevated levels of TNF-α in the serum of patients with acute GVHD and other endothelial complications such as VOD [138,139,246]. Importantly, the appearance of the increased levels was predictive of the severity of complications and overall survival. Patients with higher serum TNF-α levels during the conditioning regimen (pre-HCT) had a 90% incidence of grade II or greater acute GVHD and an overall mortality of 70%, compared with a mortality of 20% in patients without TNF-α elevations [139]. Murine monoclonal antibodies or F(ab)′$_2$ fragments directed at TNF-α have been studied either as therapy for steroid-resistant GVHD [134] or as prophylaxis [247]. There were no complete responses in the patients with uncontrolled GVHD, but some partial responses were observed. In the majority of patients, GVHD flared after discontinuation of treatment. The prophylactic trial showed a delay in the onset of acute GVHD compared with historical controls but a similar overall incidence of GVHD. Recently, therapy of GVHD with humanized anti-TNF-α (infliximab) [248,249] or a dimeric fusion protein consisting of the extracellular ligand-binding portion of the human TNFR linked to the Fc portion of human IgG1 (etanercept) [250] have shown some promise. More studies are required to understand the pharmacokinetics and proper use of these agents after allogeneic transplantation, since TNF inhibition may increase the risk of opportunistic infections.

The second major proinflammatory cytokine that appears to play an important role in the effector phase of acute GVHD is IL-1. This cytokine is produced mainly by activated mononuclear phagocytes, and it shares with TNF-α a wide variety of biological activities [251]. Secretion of IL-1 appears to occur predominantly during the effector phase of GVHD in the spleen and skin, two major GVHD target organs [142]. IL-1 receptor antagonist (IL-1RA) is a naturally occurring pure competitive inhibitor of IL-1 that is produced by monocytes/macrophages and keratinocytes. Interestingly, the *IL-1RA* gene is polymorphic and the presence in the donor of the allele that is linked to higher secretion of IL-1RA was associated with less acute GVHD [252]. In a murine model of multiple minor MHC incompatibilities, intraperitoneal administration of recombinant IL-1RA starting 10 days after BMT prevented the development of GVHD in the majority of animals [145]. Two phase I/II trials showed promising data that specific inhibition of IL-1 with either the soluble receptor or IL-1RA could result in remissions in 50–60% of patients with steroid-resistant GVHD [253,254]. A subsequent randomized trial of the addition of IL-1RA or placebo to CSP and MTX beginning at the time of conditioning and continuing through day 14 after hematopoietic cell infusion did not show any protective effect of the drug, despite attaining very high plasma levels [146]. Thus, at least as administered in this study, IL-1 inhibition is insufficient to prevent GVHD in humans. IL-11 was able to protect the GI tract in animal models and prevent GVHD [255], but it did not prevent clinical GVHD [215]. Thus not all preclinical data successfully translates to new therapies.

IL-6 might be expected to play a role in the pathophysiology of GVHD, particularly since it is known to have inflammatory properties among its pleiotropic effects, and it is induced in monocytes after stimulation by IFN-γ and TNF-α. Little experimental work has been done in animal models, but there are reports of elevated serum IL-6 levels in patients with acute GVHD and hepatorenal syndrome [256] and with transplant-related toxicities after autologous BMT [257]. In the first study, several patterns of elevated IL-6 levels were observed, but they did not always correlate with active disease among the 22 patients studied. However, IL-6 levels may respond to many stimuli, and the lack of specificity may limit the utility of blood measurements. IL-8, also called neutrophil-activating peptide (NAP-1), may also play a role in GVHD. IL-8 is produced in response to inflammatory mediators such as endotoxin, IL-1, and TNF-α, and its systemic administration inhibits the adhesion of leukocytes to endothelial surfaces. A recent study reported that among patients receiving BMT for β-thalassemia, those with GVHD showed significantly elevated IL-8 blood levels compared to those without GVHD [258]. An interesting implication of this observation is that granulocytes and macrophages may contribute to GVHD pathology. Most GVHD occurs after leukocyte recovery. This observation is typically interpreted to reflect the time necessary for lymphocytes to expand to a critical mass. However, it might equally suggest that the inflammatory cytokine network had similar activation and recruitment effects on neutrophils, and that these newly produced cells follow chemotactic signals to injured epithelium where they contribute to tissue injury by releasing activated oxygen metabolites as well as cytotoxic and proteolytic enzymes.

Chronic GVHD

It is important to recognize that chronic GVHD was originally defined temporally not clinically nor pathophysiologically. The initial clinical reports of chronic GVHD used descriptions of clinical problems occurring at least 150 days after HCT [259]. By convention many transplant clinicians and scientists use day 100 after stem cell infusion as a convenient divider between acute and chronic GVHD. However, it should be recognized that acute manifestations of GVHD may occur after day 100, and problems typically associated with chronic GVHD may occur before day 100. Thus, it is preferable to consider the symptom and signs *per se* rather than the timing of the onset of clinical findings.

Chronic GVHD is often considered an autoimmune disease because of distinctive similarities to various autoimmune disorders, especially collagen-vascular disease. The relationship is difficult to prove clinically, but experimental studies demonstrated an autoimmune aspect of chronic GVHD pathophysiology [260]. Indeed, autoantibody production is commonly observed after transplantation, and some of the clinical manifestations of chronic GVHD are similar to scleroderma, lichen planus, and other autoimmune diseases. T cells from animals with chronic GVHD produce unusual patterns of cytokines, such as IL-4, or IFN-γ in the absence of IL-2. These cytokines can stimulate collagen production by fibroblasts, which can be further amplified by IL-4. Interestingly, there is often an eosinophilia as an early manifestation of chronic GVHD, further supporting the notion that cells with a TH2 phenotype are important mediators of this problem [261]. Donor CD4+ T-cell activation in the absence of appropriate CD8+ T-cell activation can result in abnormalities of Fas/FasL expression autoantibody-mediated response, impaired elimination of autoreactive B cells, and humoral autoimmunity [114]. Another explanation of autoimmunity may be that the massive apoptosis of T cells early in acute GVHD overwhelms the macrophage/DC system resulting in autoantigen presentation [262]. The autoreactive cells of chronic GVHD are associated with a damaged thymus, which may be injured by acute GVHD or the conditioning regimen, or subject to age-related involution and atrophy. Thus, the normal ability of the thymus to delete autoreactive T cells and to induce tolerance may be impaired. Such a relationship has not been demonstrated in human chronic GVHD. However, the anti-CD20 monoclonal antibody (rituximab) has been used clinically to treat severe autoimmune disorders including autoimmune hemolytic anemia, idiopathic thrombocytopenic purpura [263], and a provocative case report suggests that anti-B-cell therapy might be an interesting approach to treating chronic GVHD [264].

Syngeneic GVHD

In experimental models, pathological changes of GVHD were observed in animals receiving marrow transplants from genetically identical donors (or even autologous marrow transplants); findings that substantiate the reports of GVHD occurring in recipients of transplants from their identical twin donors, described over a decade ago (for more details see Chapter 30) [265]. This syngeneic GVHD appears to be mediated by autoreactive lymphocytes directed at MHC class II proteins [266]. Autoreactive T cells are thought to develop in a severely damaged thymic medulla where MHC class II-bearing cells are deficient or absent. T cells thus escape the usual negative selection (clonal deletion) within the thymus and migrate to the periphery where they trigger or mediate target organ damage. Other regulatory lymphocytes, which would normally inactivate or eliminate such autoreactive cells, have themselves been eliminated by TBI (as part of the preparative regimen). The experimental transfer of normal lymphocytes to these irradiated hosts restores the regulatory mechanism and prevents the autoaggressive process. The effects of CSP are important in these models, both in preventing the reestablishment of regulatory cells and in allowing the development of autoreactive cells; these two processes seem related to the damage that CSP inflicts on the thymic medulla [267]. Thus, syngeneic GVHD can be seen as an imbalance between autoreactive and autoregulatory lymphocytes, an imbalance that results from thymic dysfunction. In experimental animals, cutaneous pathological findings of syngeneic and chronic GVHD are similar, and it appears that the efferent arms of syngeneic and chronic GVHD are similar if not identical. In humans the development of chronic GVHD after syngeneic transplantation has not been convincingly demonstrated.

Conclusions

Complications of HCT, particularly GVHD, remain major barriers to the wider application of allogeneic HCT for a variety of diseases. Recent advances in the understanding of cytokine networks, as well as the direct mediators of cellular cytotoxicity, have led to improved understanding of this complex disease process. GVHD can be considered an exaggerated, undesirable manifestation of a normal inflammatory mechanism in which donor lymphocytes encounter foreign antigens in a milieu that fosters inflammation. Tissue injury related to the conditioning regimen or infection is then amplified by direct cytotoxicity via perforin-granzyme and Fas/FasL pathways, through direct cytokine-induced damage, and by recruitment of secondary effectors such as granulocytes and monocytes. Cytokine dysregulation may further result in the production of secondary mediators such as NO. The net effects of this complex system are the severe inflammatory manifestations that we recognize as clinical GVHD.

References

1 Antin JH, Ferrara JLM. Cytokine dysregulation and acute graft-versus-host disease. *Blood* 1992; **80**: 2964–8.

2 Teshima T, Ordemann R, Reddy P et al. Acute graft-versus-host disease does not require alloantigen expression on host epithelium. *Nat Med* 2002; **8**: 575–81.

3 Gale RP, Bortin MM, van Bekkum DW et al. Risk factors for acute graft-versus-host disease. *Br J Haematol* 1987; **67**: 397–406.

4 Clift RA, Buckner CD, Appelbaum FR et al. Allogeneic marrow transplantation in patients with acute myeloid leukemia in first remission: a randomized trial of two irradiation regimens. *Blood* 1990; **76**: 1867–71.

5 Ringden O. Viral infections and graft-vs.-host disease. In: Burakoff S, Deeg H, Ferrara J, Atkinson K, eds. *Graft-vs.-Host Disease*. New York: Marcel Dekker, 1990: 467–86.

6 Xun CQ, Thompson JS, Jennings CD, Brown SA, Widmer MB. Effect of total body irradiation, busulfan-cyclophosphamide, or cyclophosphamide conditioning on inflammatory cytokine release and development of acute and chronic graft-versus-host disease in H-2-incompatible transplanted SCID mice. *Blood* 1994; **83**: 2360–7.

7 Paris F, Fuks Z, Kang A et al. Endothelial apoptosis as the primary lesion initiating intestinal radiation damage in mice. *Science* 2001; **293**: 293–7.

8 Hill G, Crawford J, Cooke K, Brinson Y, Pan L, Ferrara J. Total body irradiation and acute graft-versus-host disease: the role of gastrointestinal damage and inflammatory cytokines. *Blood* 1997; **90**: 3204–13.

9 Shlomchik WD, Couzens MS, Tang CB et al. Prevention of graft versus host disease by inactivation of host antigen-presenting cells. *Science* 1999; **285**: 412–5.

10 Korngold R, Sprent J. Negative selection of T cells causing lethal graft-versus-host disease across minor histocompatibility barriers. Role of the H-2 complex. *J Exp Med* 1980; **151**: 1114–24.

11 Yang YG, Dey BR, Sergio JJ, Pearson DA, Sykes M. Donor-derived interferon gamma is required for inhibition of acute graft-versus-host disease by interleukin 12. *J Clin Invest* 1998; **102**: 2126–35.

12 Reddy P, Teshima T, Kukuruga M et al. Interleukin-18 regulates acute graft-versus-host disease by enhancing Fas-mediated donor T cell apoptosis. *J Exp Med* 2001; **194**: 1433–40.

13 Clouthier SG, Ferrara JL, Teshima T. Graft-versus-host disease in the absence of the spleen after allogeneic bone marrow transplantation. *Transplantation* 2002; **73**: 1679–81.

14 Newton-Nash DK. The molecular basis of allorecognition. Assessment of the involvement of peptide. *Hum Immunol* 1994; **41**: 105–11.

15 Sayegh MH, Perico N, Gallon L et al. Mechanisms of acquired thymic unresponsiveness to renal allografts. Thymic recognition of immunodominant allo-MHC peptides induces peripheral T cell anergy. *Transplantation* 1994; **58**: 125–32.

16 Sprent J, Schaefer M, Gao EK, Korngold R. Role of T cell subsets in lethal graft-versus-host disease (GVHD) directed to class I versus class II H-2 differences. I. L3T4+ cells can either augment or retard GVHD elicited by Lyt–2+ cells in class I different hosts. *J Exp Medical* 1988; **167**: 556–69.

17 Goulmy E, Schipper R, Pool J et al. Mismatches of minor histocompatibility antigens between HLA-identical donors and recipients and the development of graft-versus-host disease after bone marrow transplantation. *N Engl J Med* 1996; **334**: 281–5.

18 Lyon M, Rastan S, Brown S. Catalog of mutant genes and polymorphic loci. In: *Genetic Variants and Strains of Laboratory Mouse*. New York: Oxford University Press, 1996: 17–854.

19 Martin PJ. How much benefit can be expected from matching for minor antigens in allogeneic marrow transplantation? *Bone Marrow Transplant* 1997; **20**: 97–100.

20 Nash RA, Pepe MS, Storb R et al. Acute graft-versus-host disease: analysis of risk factors after allogeneic marrow transplantation and prophylaxis with cyclosporine and methotrexate. *Blood* 1992; **80**: 1838–45.

21 Hansen JA, Gooley TA, Martin PJ *et al*. Bone marrow transplants from unrelated donors for patients with chronic myeloid leukemia. *N Engl J Med* 1998; **338**: 962–8.

22 Goulmy E. Human minor histocompatibility antigens. New concepts for marrow transplantation and adoptive immunotherapy. *Immunol Rev* 1997; **157**: 125–40.

23 Dickinson AM, Wang XN, Sviland L *et al*. In situ dissection of the graft-versus-host activities of cytotoxic T cells specific for minor histocompatibility antigens. *Nat Med* 2002; **8**: 410–4.

24 Dustin ML, Springer TA. T-cell receptor crosslinking transiently stimulates adhesiveness through LFA-1. *Nature* 1989; **341**: 619–24.

25 Alegre ML, Frauwirth KA, Thompson CB. T-cell regulation by CD28 and CTLA-4. *Nat Rev Immunol* 2001; **1**: 220–8.

26 Slavik JM, Hutchcroft JE, Bierer BE. CD28/CTLA-4 and CD80/CD86 families: signaling and function. *Immunol Res* 1999; **19**: 1–24.

27 Matzinger P. The danger model. a renewed sense of self. *Science* 2002; **296**: 301–5.

28 Roncarolo MG, Levings MK, Traversari C. Differentiation of T regulatory cells by immature dendritic cells. *J Exp Med* 2001; **193**: F5–9.

29 Reinhardt RL, Khoruts A, Merica R, Zell T, Jenkins MK. Visualizing the generation of memory CD4 T cells in the whole body. *Nature* 2001; **410**: 101–5.

30 Ordemann R, Hutchinson R, Friedman J *et al*. Enhanced allostimulatory activity of host antigen-presenting cells in old mice intensifies acute graft-versus-host disease. *J Clin Invest* 2002; **109**: 1249–56.

31 Ruggeri L, Capanni M, Urbani E *et al*. Effectiveness of donor natural killer cell alloreactivity in mismatched hematopoietic transplants. *Science* 2002; **295**: 2097–100.

32 Ruggeri L, Capanni M, Martelli MF, Velardi A. Cellular therapy: exploiting NK cell alloreactivity in transplantation. *Curr Opin Hematol* 2001; **8**: 355–9.

33 Nishizuka Y. Studies and perspectives of protein kinase C. *Science* 1986; **233**: 305–12.

34 Samelson LE, Patel MD, Weissman AM, Harford JB, Klausner RD. Antigen activation of murine T cell induces tyrosine phosphorylation of a polypeptide associated with the T cell antigen receptor. *Cell* 1986; **46**: 1083–90.

35 Mosmann TR, Cherwinski H, Bond MW, Giedlin MA, Coffman RL. Two types of murine helper T cell clone. I. Definition according to profiles of lymphokine activities and secreted proteins. *J Immunol* 1986; **136**: 2348–57.

36 Rissoan MC, Soumelis V, Kadowaki N *et al*. Reciprocal control of T helper cell and dendritic cell differentiation. *Science* 1999; **283**: 1183–6.

37 Reid SD, Penna G, Adorini L. The control of T cell responses by dendritic cell subsets. *Curr Opin Immunol* 2000; **12**: 114–21.

38 Carvalho-Pinto CE, Garcia MI, Mellado M *et al*. Autocrine production of IFN-γ by macrophages controls their recruitment to kidney and the development of glomerulonephritis in MRL/*lpr* mice. *J Immunol* 2002; **169**: 1058–67.

39 Lalor PF, Shields P, Grant A, Adams DH. Recruitment of lymphocytes to the human liver. *Immunol Cell Biol* 2002; **80**: 52–64.

40 Via CS, Finkelman FD. Critical role of interleukin-2 in the development of acute graft-versus-host disease. *Int Immunol* 1993; **5**: 565–72.

41 Jadus MR, Peck AB. Lethal murine graft-versus-host disease in the absence of detectable cytotoxic T lymphocytes. *Transplantation* 1983; **36**: 281–9.

42 Malkovsky M, Brenner MK, Hunt R *et al*. T cell-depletion of allogeneic bone marrow prevents acceleration of graft-versus-host disease induced by exogenous interleukin-2. *Cell Immunol* 1986; **103**: 476–80.

43 Theobald M, Nierle T, Bunjes D, Arnold R, Heimpel H. Host-specific interleukin-2-secreting donor T-cell precursors as predictors of acute graft-versus-host disease in bone marrow transplantation between HLA-identical siblings. *N Engl J Med* 1992; **327**: 1613–7.

44 Nierle T, Bunjes D, Arnold R, Heimpel H, Theobald M. Quantitative assessment of posttransplant host-specific interleukin-2-secreting T-helper cell precursors in patients with and without acute graft-versus-host disease after allogeneic HLA-identical sibling bone marrow transplantation. *Blood* 1993; **81**: 841–8.

45 Schwarer AP, Jiang YZ, Brookes PA *et al*. Frequency of anti-recipient alloreactive helper T-cell precursors in donor blood and graft-versus-host disease after HLA-identical sibling bone-marrow transplantation. *Lancet* 1993; **341**: 203–5.

46 Ferrara JLM, Marion A, McIntyre JF, Murphy GF, Burakoff SJ. Amelioration of acute graft-versus-host disease due to minor histocompatibility antigens by *in vivo* administration of anti-interleukin 2 receptor antibody. *J Immunol* 1986; **137**: 1874–7.

47 Herve P, Wijdenes J, Bergerat JP *et al*. Treatment of corticosteroid-resistant acute graft-versus-host disease by *in vivo* administration of anti-interleukin-2 receptor monoclonal antibody (B-B10). *Blood* 1990; **75**: 1017–23.

48 Anasetti C, Martin PM, Hansen JA *et al*. A phase I–II study evaluating the murine anti-IL-2 receptor antibody 2A3 for treatment of acute graft-versus-host disease. *Transplantation* 1990; **50**: 49–54.

49 Belanger C, Esperou-Bourdeau H, Bordigoni P *et al*. Use of an anti-interleukin-2 receptor monoclonal antibody for GVHD prophylaxis in unrelated donor BMT. *Bone Marrow Transplant* 1993; **11**: 293–7.

50 Li XC, Demirci G, Ferrari-Lacraz S *et al*. IL-15 and IL-2: a matter of life and death for T cells *in vivo*. *Nat Med* 2001; **7**: 114–8.

51 Kumaki S, Minegishi M, Fujie H *et al*. Prolonged secretion of IL-15 in patients with severe forms of acute graft-versus-host disease after allogeneic bone marrow transplantation in children. *Int J Hematol* 1998; **67**: 307–12.

52 Szebeni J, Wang MG, Pearson DA, Szot GL, Sykes M. IL-2 inhibits early increases in serum γ-interferon levels associated with graft-versus-host-disease. *Transplantation* 1994; **58**: 1385–93.

53 Wang MG, Szebeni J, Pearson DA, Szot GL, Sykes M. Inhibition of graft-versus-host disease by interleukin-2 treatment is associated with altered cytokine production by expanded graft-versus-host-reactive CD4+ helper cells. *Transplantation* 1995; **60**: 481–90.

54 Troutt AB, Maraskovsky E, Rogers LA, Pech MH, Kelso A. Quantitative analysis of lymphokine expression *in vivo* and *in vitro*. *Immunol Cell Biol* 1992; **70**(1): 51–7.

55 Velardi A, Varese P, Terenzi A *et al*. Lymphokine production by T-cell clones after human bone marrow transplantation. *Blood* 1989; **74**: 1665–72.

56 Dickinson AM, Sviland L, Dunn J, Carey P, Proctor SJ. Demonstration of direct involvement of cytokines in graft-versus-host reactions using an *in vitro* human skin explant model. *Bone Marrow Transplant* 1991; **7**: 209–16.

57 Niederwieser D, Herold M, Woloszczuk W *et al*. Endogenous IFN-γ during human bone marrow transplantation. *Transplantation* 1990; **50**: 620–5.

58 Dufour JH, Dziejman M, Liu MT, Leung JH, Lane TE, Luster AD. IFN-γ-inducible protein 10 (IP-10; CXCL10)-deficient mice reveal a role for IP-10 in effector T cell generation and trafficking. *J Immunol* 2002; **168**: 3195–204.

59 de Veer MJ, Holko M, Frevel M *et al*. Functional classification of interferon-stimulated genes identified using microarrays. *J Leukoc Biol* 2001; **69**: 912–20.

60 Mohan K, Ding Z, Hanly J, Issekutz TB. IFN-γ-inducible T cell α chemoattractant is a potent stimulator of normal human blood T lymphocyte transendothelial migration: differential regulation by IFN-γ and TNF-α. *J Immunol* 2002; **168**: 6420–8.

61 Mowat A. Antibodies to IFN-γ prevent immunological mediated intestinal damage in murine graft-versus-host reactions. *Immunology* 1989; **68**: 18–24.

62 Holda JH, Maier T, Claman HN. Evidence that IFN-γ is responsible for natural suppressor activity in GVHD spleen and normal bone marrow. *Transplantation* 1988; **45**: 772–7.

63 Wall DA, Hamberg SD, Reynolds DS, Burakoff SJ, Abbas AK, Ferrara JL. Immunodeficiency in graft-versus-host disease. I. Mechanism of immune suppression. *J Immunol* 1988; **140**: 2970–6.

64 Wall DA, Sheehan KC. The role of tumor necrosis factor and interferon-γ in graft-versus-host disease and related immunodeficiency. *Transplantation* 1994; **57**: 273–9.

65 Klimpel GR, Annable CR, Cleveland MG, Jerrells TR, Patterson JC. Immunosuppression and lymphoid hypoplasia associated with chronic graft versus host disease is dependent upon IFN-γ production. *J Immunol* 1990; **144**: 84–93.

66 Huchet R, Bruley-Rosset M, Mathiot C, Grandjon D, Halle-Pannenko O. Involvement of IFN-γ and transforming growth factor-β in graft-vs-host reaction-associated immunosuppression. *J Immunol* 1993; **150**: 2517–24.

67 Krenger W, Falzarano G, Delmonte J Jr, Snyder KM, Byon JC, Ferrara JL. Interferon-γ suppresses T-cell proliferation to mitogen via the nitric oxide pathway during experimental acute graft-versus-host disease. *Blood* 1996; **88**: 1113–21.

68 Gifford GE, Lohmann-Matthes M-L. γ-Interferon priming of mouse and human macrophages for induction of tumor necrosis factor production by bacterial lipopolysaccharide. *J Natl Cancer Inst* 1987; **78**: 121–4.

69 Nestel FP, Price KS, Seemayer TA, Lapp WS. Macrophage priming and lipopolysaccharide-triggered release of tumor necrosis factor α during graft-versus-host disease. *J Exp Med* 1992; **175**: 405–13.

70 Liu Y, Janeway CA Jr. Interferon-γ plays a critical role in induced cell death of effector T cell: a possible third mechanism of self-tolerance. *J Exp Med* 1990; **172**: 1735–9.

71 Fowler DH, Kurasawa K, Husebekk A, Cohen PA, Gress RE. Cells of TH2 cytokine phenotype prevent LPS-induced lethality during murine graft-versus-host reaction. Regulation of cytokines and CD8+ lymphoid engraftment. *J Immunol* 1994; **152**: 1004–13.

72 Fowler DH, Kurasawa K, Smith R, Eckhaus MA, Gress RE. Donor CD4-enriched cells of TH2 cytokine phenotype regulate graft-versus-host disease without impairing allogeneic engraftment in sublethally irradiated mice. *Blood* 1994; **84**: 3540–9.

73 Krenger W, Snyder KM, Byon CH, Falzarano G, Ferrara JLM. Polarized type 2 alloreactive CD4+ and CD8+ donor T cells fail to induce experimental acute graft-versus-host disease. *J Immunol* 1995; **155**: 585–93.

74 Pan L, Delmonte J, Jalonen C, Ferrara J. Pretreatment of donor mice with granulocyte colony-stimulating factor polarizes donor T lymphocytes toward type-2 cytokine production and reduces severity of experimental graft-versus-host disease. *Blood* 1995; **86**: 4422–9.

75 Nikolic B, Lee S, Bronson RT, Grusby MJ, Sykes M. TH1 and TH2 mediate acute graft-versus-host disease, each with distinct end-organ targets. *J Clin Invest* 2000; **105**: 1289–98.

76 Atkinson K, Matias C, Guiffre A et al. In vivo administration of granulocyte colony-stimulating factor (G-CSF), granulocyte-macrophage CSF, interleukin-1 (IL-1), and IL-4, alone and in combination, after allogeneic murine hematopoietic stem cell transplantation. *Blood* 1991; **77**: 1376–82.

77 Krenger W, Snyder K, Smith S, Ferrara JLM. Effects of exogenous interleukin-10 in a murine model of graft-versus-host disease to minor histocompatibility antigens. *Transplantation* 1994; **58**: 1251–7.

78 Blazar BR, Taylor PA, Smith S, Vallera DA. Interleukin-10 administration decreases survival in murine recipients of major histocompatibility complex disparate donor bone marrow grafts. *Blood* 1995; **85**: 842–51.

79 Sykes M, Romick ML, Hoyles KA, Sachs DH. In vivo administration of interleukin 2 plus T cell-depleted syngeneic marrow prevents graft-versus-host disease mortality and permits alloengraftment. *J Exp Med* 1990; **171**: 645–58.

80 Brok HPM, Heidt PJ, van der Meide PH, Zurcher C, Vossen JM. Interferon-γ prevents graft-versus-host disease after allogeneic bone marrow transplantation in mice. *J Immunol* 1993; **151**: 6451–9.

81 Murphy WJ, Welniak LA, Taub DD et al. Differential effects of the absence of interferon-γ and IL-4 in acute graft-versus-host disease after allogeneic bone marrow transplantation in mice. *J Clin Invest* 1998; **102**: 1742–8.

82 Ellison CA, Fischer JM, HayGlass KT, Gartner JG. Murine graft-versus-host disease in an F1-hybrid model using IFN-γ gene knockout donors. *J Immunol* 1998; **161**: 631–40.

83 Welniak LA, Blazar BR, Anver MR, Wiltrout RH, Murphy WJ. Opposing roles of interferon-γ on CD4+ T cell-mediated graft-versus-host disease: effects of conditioning. *Biol Blood Marrow Transplant* 2000; **6**: 604–12.

84 Li XC, Strom TB, Turka LA, Wells AD. T cell death and transplantation tolerance. *Immunity* 2001; **14**: 407–16.

85 Sykes M, Szot GL, Nguyen PL, Pearson DA. Interleukin-12 inhibits murine graft-versus-host disease. *Blood* 1995; **86**: 2429–38.

86 Dey BR, Yang YG, Szot GL, Pearson DA, Sykes M. Interleukin-12 inhibits graft-versus-host disease through an Fas-mediated mechanism associated with alterations in donor T-cell activation and expansion. *Blood* 1998; **91**: 3315–22.

87 Jonuleit H, Schmitt E, Schuler G, Knop J, Enk AH. Induction of interleukin 10-producing, nonproliferating CD4+ T cells with regulatory properties by repetitive stimulation with allogeneic immature human dendritic cells. *J Exp Med* 2000; **192**: 1213–22.

88 Zeller JC, Panoskaltsis-Mortari A, Murphy WJ et al. Induction of CD4+ T cell alloantigen-specific hyporesponsiveness by IL-10 and TGF-β. *J Immunol* 1999; **163**: 3684–91.

89 Boussiotis VA, Chen ZM, Zeller JC et al. Altered T-cell receptor + CD28-mediated signaling and blocked cell cycle progression in interleukin 10 and transforming growth factor-β-treated alloreactive T cells that do not induce graft-versus-host disease. *Blood* 2001; **97**: 565–71.

90 Bacchetta R, Bigler M, Touraine JL et al. High levels of interleukin 10 production in vivo are associated with tolerance in SCID patients transplanted with HLA mismatched hematopoietic stem cells. *J Exp Med* 1994; **179**: 493–502.

91 Tsoi MS, Storb R, Dobbs S et al. Nonspecific suppressor cells in patients with chronic graft-vs-host disease after marrow grafting. *J Immunol* 1979; **123**: 1970–6.

92 Rolink AG, Gleichmann E. Allosuppressor- and allohelper-T cells in acute and chronic graft-vs.-host (GVH) disease. III. Different Lyt subsets of donor T cells induce different pathological syndromes. *J Exp Med* 1983; **158**: 546–58.

93 Hurtenbach U, Shearer GM. Analysis of murine T lymphocyte markers during the early phases of GvH-associated suppression of cytotoxic T lymphocyte responses. *J Immunol* 1983; **130**: 1561–6.

94 Autran B, Leblond V, Sadat-Sowti B et al. A soluble factor released by CD8+CD57+ lymphocytes from bone marrow transplanted patients inhibits cell-mediated cytolysis. *Blood* 1991; **77**: 2237–41.

95 Fukuda H, Nakamura H, Tominaga N et al. Marked increase of CD8+S6F1+ and CD8+CD57+ cells in patients with graft-versus-host disease after allogeneic bone marrow transplantation. *Bone Marrow Transplant* 1994; **13**: 181–5.

96 Strober S. Natural suppressor (NS) cells, neonatal tolerance, and total lymphoid irradiation: exploring obscure relationships. *Annu Rev Immunol* 1984; **2**: 219–37.

97 Lan F, Zeng D, Higuchi M, Huie P, Higgins JP, Strober S. Predominance of NK1.1+TCRαβ+ or DX5+TCRαβ+ T cells in mice conditioned with fractionated lymphoid irradiation protects against graft-versus-host disease: "natural suppressor" cells. *J Immunol* 2001; **167**: 2087–96.

98 Zeng D, Lewis D, Dejbakhsh-Jones S et al. Bone marrow NK1.1− and NK1.1+ T cells reciprocally regulate acute graft versus host disease. *J Exp Med* 1999; **189**: 1073–81.

99 Eberl G, MacDonald HR. Rapid death and regeneration of NKT cells in anti-CD3epsilon- or IL-12-treated mice: a major role for bone marrow in NKT cell homeostasis. *Immunity* 1998; **9**: 345–53.

100 Hoffmann P, Ermann J, Edinger M, Fathman CG, Strober S. Donor-type CD4+CD25+ regulatory T cells suppress lethal acute graft-versus-host disease after allogeneic bone marrow transplantation. *J Exp Med* 2002; **196**: 389–99.

101 Kagi D, Vignaux F, Ledermann B et al. Fas and perforin pathways as major mechanisms of T cell-mediated cytotoxicity. *Science* 1994; **265**: 528–30.

102 Lowin B, Hahne M, Mattmann C, Tschopp J. Cytolytic T-cell cytotoxicity is mediated through perforin and Fas lytic pathways. *Nature* 1994; **370**: 650–2.

103 Shresta S, Pham CT, Thomas DA, Graubert TA, Ley TJ. How do cytotoxic lymphocytes kill their targets? *Curr Opin Immunol* 1998; **10**: 581–7.

104 Krammer PH. CD95's deadly mission in the immune system. *Nature* 2000; **407**: 789–95.

105 Chinnaiyan AM, O'Rourke K, Yu GL et al. Signal transduction by DR3, a death domain-containing receptor related to TNFR-1 and CD95. *Science* 1996; **274**: 990–2.

106 Chicheportiche Y, Bourdon PR, Xu H et al. TWEAK, a new secreted ligand in the tumor necrosis factor family that weakly induces apoptosis. *J Biol Chem* 1997; **272**: 32401–10.

107 Pan G, O'Rourke K, Chinnaiyan AM et al. The receptor for the cytotoxic ligand TRAIL. *Science* 1997; **276**: 111–3.

108 Baker M, Altman N, Podack E, Levy R. The role of cell-mediated cytotoxicity in acute GVHD after MHC-matched allogeneic bone marrow transplantation in mice. *J Exp Med* 1996; **183**: 2645–56.

109 Braun M, Lowin B, French L, Aca-Orbea H, Tschopp J. Cytotoxic T cells deficient in both functional Fas ligand and perforin show residual cytolytic activity yet lose their capacity to induce lethal acute graft-versus-host disease. *J Exp Med* 1996; **183**: 657–61.

110 Graubert TA, DiPersio JF, Russell JH, Ley TJ. Perforin/granzyme-dependent and independent mechanisms are both important for the development of graft-versus-host disease after murine bone marrow transplantation. *J Clin Invest* 1997; **100**: 904–11.

111 Blazar BR, Taylor PA, Vallera DA. CD4+ and CD8+ T cells each can utilize a perforin-dependent pathway to mediate lethal graft-versus-host disease in major histocompatibility complex-disparate recipients. *Transplantation* 1997; **64**: 571–6.

112 Graubert TA, Russell JH, Ley TJ. The role of granzyme B in murine models of acute graft-versus-host disease and graft rejection. *Blood* 1996; **87**: 1232–7.

113 Ueno Y, Ishii M, Yahagi K et al. Fas-mediated cholangiopathy in the murine model of graft versus host disease. *Hepatology* 2000; **31**: 966–74.

114 Shustov A, Nguyen P, Finkelman F, Elkon KB, Via CS. Differential expression of Fas and Fas ligand in acute and chronic graft-versus-host disease: up-regulation of Fas and Fas ligand requires CD8+ T cell activation and IFN-γ production. *J Immunol* 1998; **161**: 2848–55.

115 Lee S, Chong SY, Lee JW et al. Difference in the expression of Fas/Fas-ligand and the lymphocyte subset reconstitution according to the occurrence of acute GVHD. *Bone Marrow Transplant* 1997; **20**: 883–8.

116 Wasem C, Frutschi C, Arnold D et al. Accumulation and activation-induced release of preformed Fas (CD95) ligand during the pathogenesis of experimental graft-versus-host disease. *J Immunol* 2001; **167**: 2936–41.

117 Liem LM, van Lopik T, van Nieuwenhuijze AE, van Houwelingen HC, Aarden L, Goulmy E. Soluble Fas levels in sera of bone marrow transplantation recipients are increased during acute graft-versus-host disease but not during infections. *Blood* 1998; **91**: 1464–8.

118 Das H, Imoto S, Murayama T et al. Levels of soluble FasL and FasL gene expression during the development of graft-versus-host disease in DLT-treated patients. *Br J Haematol* 1999; **104**: 795–800.

119 Kanda Y, Tanaka Y, Shirakawa K et al. Increased soluble Fas-ligand in sera of bone marrow trans-

plant recipients with acute graft-versus-host disease. *Bone Marrow Transplant* 1998; **22**: 751–4.
120 Kayaba H, Hirokawa M, Watanabe A et al. Serum markers of graft-versus-host disease after bone marrow transplantation. *J Allergy Clin Immunol* 2000; **106**: S40–4.
121 Baker MB, Riley RL, Podack ER, Levy RB. Graft-versus-host-disease-associated lymphoid hypoplasia and B cell dysfunction is dependent upon donor T cell-mediated Fas-ligand function, but not perforin function. *Proc Natl Acad Sci U S A* 1997; **94**: 1366–71.
122 Via CS, Nguyen P, Shustov A, Drappa J, Elkon KB. A major role for the Fas pathway in acute graft-versus-host disease. *J Immunol* 1996; **157**: 5387–93.
123 Kondo T, Suda T, Fukuyama H, Adachi M, Nagata S. Essential roles of the Fas ligand in the development of hepatitis. *Nat Med* 1997; **3**: 409–13.
124 van Den Brink MR, Moore E, Horndasch KJ et al. Fas-deficient lpr mice are more susceptible to graft-versus-host disease. *J Immunol* 2000; **164**: 469–80.
125 Hattori K, Hirano T, Miyajima H et al. Differential effects of anti-Fas ligand and anti-tumor necrosis factor-α antibodies on acute graft-versus-host disease pathologies. *Blood* 1998; **91**: 4051–5.
126 Stuber E, Buschenfeld A, von Freier A, Arendt T, Folsch UR. Intestinal crypt cell apoptosis in murine acute graft versus host disease is mediated by tumour necrosis factor-α and not by the FasL–Fas interaction: effect of pentoxifylline on the development of mucosal atrophy. *Gut* 1999; **45**: 229–35.
127 Martin PJ, Akatsuka Y, Hahne M, Sale G. Involvement of donor T-cell cytotoxic effector mechanisms in preventing allogeneic marrow graft rejection. *Blood* 1998; **92**: 2177–81.
128 Jiang Z, Podack E, Levy RB. Major histocompatibility complex-mismatched allogeneic bone marrow transplantation using perforin and/or Fas ligand double-defective CD4+ donor T cells. Involvement of cytotoxic function by donor lymphocytes prior to graft-versus-host disease pathogenesis. *Blood* 2001; **98**: 390–7.
129 Piguet PF, Grau GE, Allet B, Vassalli PJ. Tumor necrosis factor/cachectin is an effector of skin and gut lesions of the acute phase of graft-versus-host disease. *J Exp Med* 1987; **166**: 1280–9.
130 Piguet PF, Grau GE, Collart MA, Vassalli P, Kapanci Y. Pneumopathies of the graft-versus-host reaction. Alveolitis associated with an increased level of tumor necrosis factor MRNA and chronic interstitial pneumonitis. *Laboratory Invest* 1989; **61**: 37–45.
131 Laster SM, Wood JG, Gooding LR. Tumor necrosis factor can induce both apoptotic and necrotic forms of cell lysis. *J Immunol* 1988; **141**: 2629–34.
132 Hill GR, Teshima T, Rebel VI et al. The p55 TNF-α receptor plays a critical role in T cell alloreactivity. *J Immunol* 2000; **164**: 656–63.
133 Brown GR, Lee E, Thiele DL. TNF–TNFR2 interactions are critical for the development of intestinal graft-versus-host disease in MHC class II-disparate (C57BL/6J->C57BL/6J,xbm12), F1 mice. *J Immunol* 2002; **168**: 3065–71.
134 Herve P, Flesch M, Tiberghien P et al. Phase I–II trial of a monoclonal anti-tumor necrosis factor-α antibody for the treatment of refractory severe acute graft-versus-host disease. *Blood* 1992; **81**: 1993–9.
135 Murphy GF, Sueki H, Teuscher C, Whitaker D, Korngold R. Role of mast cells in early epithelial target cell injury in experimental acute graft-versus-host disease. *J Invest Dermatol* 1994; **102**: 451–61.
136 Gilliam AC, Whitaker-Menezes D, Korngold R, Murphy GF. Apoptosis is the predominant form of epithelial target cell injury in acute experimental graft-versus-host disease. *J Invest Dermatol* 1996; **107**: 377–83.
137 Cooke KR, Hill GR, Gerbitz A et al. Tumor necrosis factor-α neutralization reduces lung injury after experimental allogeneic bone marrow transplantation. *Transplantation* 2000; **70**: 272–9.
138 Holler E, Kolb HJ, Moller A et al. Increased serum levels of tumor necrosis factor-α precede major complications of bone marrow transplantation. *Blood* 1990; **75**: 1011–6.
139 Holler E, Kolb HJ, Hintermeier-Knabe R et al. Role of tumor necrosis factor-α in acute graft-versus-host disease and complications following allogeneic bone marrow transplantation. *Transplant Proc* 1993; **25**: 1234–6.
140 Tanaka J, Imamura M, Kasai M et al. Cytokine gene expression in peripheral blood mononuclear cells during graft-versus-host disease after allogeneic bone marrow transplantation. *Br J Haematol* 1993; **85**: 558–65.
141 Tanaka J, Imamura M, Kasai M et al. Rapid analysis of tumor necrosis factor-α mRNA expression during venoocclusive disease of the liver after allogeneic bone marrow transplantation. *Transplantation* 1993; **55**: 430–2.
142 Abhyankar S, Gilliland DG, Ferrara JLM. Interleukin 1 is a critical effector molecule during cytokine dysregulation in graft-versus-host disease to minor histocompatibility antigens. *Transplantation* 1993; **56**: 1518–23.
143 Eisenberg SP, Evans RJ, Arend WP et al. Primary structure and functional expression from complementary DNA of a human interleukin-1 receptor antagonist. *Nature* 1990; **343**: 341–6.
144 Hannum CH, Wilcox CJ, Arend WP et al. Interleukin-1 receptor antagonist activity of a human interleukin-1 inhibitor. *Nature* 1990; **343**: 336–40.
145 McCarthy PL, Abhyankar S, Neben S et al. Inhibition of interleukin-1 by an interleukin-1 receptor antagonist prevents graft-versus-host disease. *Blood* 1991; **78**: 1915–8.
146 Antin JH, Weisdorf D, Neuberg D et al. Interleukin-1 blockade does not prevent acute graft versus host disease. Results of a randomized, double blind, placebo-controlled trial of interleukin 1 receptor antagonist in allogeneic bone marrow transplantation. *Blood* 2002; **100**: 3479–82.
147 Falzarano G, Krenger W, Snyder KM, Delmonte J, Karandikar M, Ferrara JLM. Suppression of B cell proliferation to lipopolysaccharide is mediated through induction of the nitric oxide pathway by tumor necrosis factor-a in mice with acute graft-versus-host disease. *Blood* 1996; **87**: 2853–60.
148 Nestel FP, Greene RN, Kichian K, Ponka P, Lapp WS. Activation of macrophage cytostatic effector mechanisms during acute graft-versus-host disease: release of intracellular iron and nitric oxide-mediated cytostasis. *Blood* 2000; **96**: 1836–43.
149 Weiss G, Schwaighofer H, Herold M et al. Nitric oxide formation as predictive parameter for acute graft-versus-host disease after human allogeneic bone marrow transplantation. *Transplantation* 1995; **60**: 1239–44.
150 Langrehr JM, Murase N, Markus PM et al. Nitric oxide production in host-versus-graft and graft-versus-host reactions in the rat. *J Clin Invest* 1992; **90**: 679–83.
151 Cooke KR, Hill GR, Crawford JM et al. Tumor necrosis factor-α production to lipopolysaccharide stimulation by donor cells predicts the severity of experimental acute graft-versus-host disease. *J Clin Invest* 1998; **102**: 1882–91.
152 Price KS, Nestel FP, Lapp WS. Progressive accumulation of bacterial lipopolysaccharide in vivo during murine acute graft-versus-host disease. *Scand J Immunol* 1997; **45**: 294–300.
153 Morrison DC, Ryan JL. Endotoxins and disease mechanisms. *Annu Rev Med* 1987; **38**: 417–32.
154 Raetz CR. Biochemistry of endotoxins. *Annu Rev Biochem* 1990; **59**: 129–70.
155 Fegan C, Poynton CH, Whittaker JA. The gut mucosal barrier in bone marrow transplantation. *Bone Marrow Transplant* 1990; **5**: 373–7.
156 Jackson SK, Parton J, Barnes RA, Poynton CH, Fegan C. Effect of IgM-enriched intravenous immunoglobulin (Pentaglobin) on endotoxaemia and anti-endotoxin antibodies in bone marrow transplantation. *Eur J Clin Invest* 1993; **23**: 540–5.
157 Glode LM, Rosenstreich DL. Genetic control of B cell activation by bacterial lipopolysaccharide is mediated by multiple distinct genes or alleles. *J Immunol* 1976; **117**: 2061–6.
158 Watson J, Kelly K, Largen M, Taylor BA. The genetic mapping of a defective LPS response gene in C3H/HeJ mice. *J Immunol* 1978; **120**: 422–4.
159 Sultzer BM, Castagna R, Bandekar J, Wong P. Lipopolysaccharide nonresponder cells: the C3H/HeJ defect. *Immunobiology* 1993; **187**: 257–71.
160 Poltorak A, He X, Smirnova I et al. Defective LPS signaling in C3H/HeJ and C57BL/10ScCr mice: mutations in Tlr4 gene. *Science* 1998; **282**: 2085–8.
161 Sultzer BM, Goodman GW. Endotoxin protein. A B-cell mitogen and polyclonal activator of C3H/HeJ lymphocytes. *J Exp Med* 1976; **144**: 821–7.
162 Sultzer BM. Lymphocyte activation by endotoxin and endotoxin protein: the role of the C3H/Hej mouse. In: Nowotny A, ed. *Beneficial Effects of Endotoxin*. New York: Plenum Press, 1983: 227–45.
163 Ulevitch RJ, Tobias PS. Receptor-dependent mechanisms of cell stimulation by bacterial endotoxin. *Annu Rev Immunol* 1995; **13**: 437–57.
164 Haziot A, Ferrero E, Kontgen F et al. Resistance to endotoxin shock and reduced dissemination of gram-negative bacteria in CD14-deficient mice. *Immunity* 1996; **4**: 407–14.
165 Cooke KR, Gerbitz A, Crawford JM et al. LPS antagonism reduces graft-versus-host disease and preserves graft-versus-leukemia activity after experimental bone marrow transplantation. *J Clin Invest* 2001; **107**: 1581–9.
166 van Bekkum DW, Roodenburg J, Heidt PJ, van der Waaij D. Mitigation of secondary disease of allogeneic mouse radiation chimeras by modification of the intestinal microflora. *J Natl Cancer Inst* 1974; **52**: 401–4.
167 Storb R, Prentice RL, Buckner CD et al. Graft-versus-host disease and survival in patients with aplastic anemia treated by marrow grafts from HLA-identical siblings. Beneficial effects of a protective environment. *N Engl J Med* 1983; **308**: 302–7.
168 Moller J, Skirhoj P, Hoiby N, Peterson F. Protection against graft versus host disease by gut sterilization? *Exp Haematol* 1982; **10**: 101–2.
169 Beelen DW, Haralambie E, Brandt H et al. Evidence that sustained growth suppression of intestinal anaerobic bacteria reduces the risk of acute graft-versus-host disease after sibling marrow transplantation. *Blood* 1992; **80**: 2668–76.

170 Beelen D, Elmaagacli A, Muller K, Hirche H, Schaefer U. Influence of intestinal bacterial decontamination using metronidazole and ciprofloxacin or ciprofloxacin alone on the development of acute graft-versus-host disease after marrow transplantation in patients with hematologic malignancies: final results and long-term follow-up of an open-label prospective randomized trial. *Blood* 1999; **93**: 3267–75.

171 Cohen JL, Boyer O, Salomon B *et al.* Prevention of graft-versus-host disease in mice using a suicide gene expressed in T lymphocytes. *Blood* 1997; **89**: 4636–45.

172 Bayston K, Baumgartner JD, Clark P, Cohen J. Anti-endotoxin antibody for prevention of acute GVHD. *Bone Marrow Transplant* 1991; **8**: 426–7.

173 Christ WJ, Asano O, Robidoux AL *et al.* E5531, a pure endotoxin antagonist of high potency. *Science* 1995; **268**: 80–3.

174 Moser B, Loetscher P. Lymphocyte traffic control by chemokines. *Nat Immunol* 2001; **2**: 123–8.

175 Sallusto F, Lenig D, Forster R, Lipp M, Lanzavecchia A. Two subsets of memory T lymphocytes with distinct homing potentials and effector functions. *Nature* 1999; **401**: 708–12.

176 Murai M, Yoneyama H, Harada A *et al.* Active participation of CCR5$^+$ CD8$^+$ T lymphocytes in the pathogenesis of liver injury in graft-versus-host disease. *J Clin Invest* 1999; **104**: 49–57.

177 Serody JS, Burkett SE, Panoskaltsis-Mortari A *et al.* T-lymphocyte production of macrophage inflammatory protein-1α is critical to the recruitment of CD8$^+$ T cells to the liver, lung, and spleen during graft-versus-host disease. *Blood* 2000; **96**: 2973–80.

178 Panoskaltsis-Mortari A, Strieter RM *et al.* Induction of monocyte- and T-cell-attracting chemokines in the lung during the generation of idiopathic pneumonia syndrome following allogeneic murine bone marrow transplantation. *Blood* 2000; **96**: 834–9.

179 Schnare M, Barton GM, Holt AC, Takeda K, Akira S, Medzhitov R. Toll-like receptors control activation of adaptive immune responses. *Nat Immunol* 2001; **2**: 947–50.

180 Medzhitov R, Janeway CA Jr. Decoding the patterns of self and nonself by the innate immune system. *Science* 2002; **296**: 298–300.

181 Giralt S, Estey E, Albitar M *et al.* Engraftment of allogeneic hematopoietic progenitor cells with purine analog-containing chemotherapy: harnessing graft-versus-leukemia without myeloablative therapy. *Blood* 1997; **89**: 4531–16.

182 Slavin S, Nagler A, Naparstek E *et al.* Nonmyeloablative stem cell transplantation and cell therapy as an alternative to conventional bone marrow transplantation with lethal cytoreduction for the treatment of malignant and nonmalignant hematologic diseases. *Blood* 1998; **91**: 756–63.

183 Badros A, Barlogie B, Siegel E *et al.* Improved outcome of allogeneic transplantation in high-risk multiple myeloma patients after nonmyeloablative conditioning. *J Clin Oncol* 2002; **20**: 1295–303.

184 McSweeney PA, Niederwieser D, Shizuru JA *et al.* Hematopoietic cell transplantation in older patients with hematologic malignancies: replacing high-dose cytotoxic therapy with graft-versus-tumor effects. *Blood* 2001; **97**: 3390–400.

185 Ho VT, Soiffer RJ. The history and future of T-cell depletion as graft-versus-host disease prophylaxis for allogeneic hematopoietic stem cell transplantation. *Blood* 2001; **98**: 3192–204.

186 Wagner J, Santos G, Noga S *et al.* Bone marrow graft engineering by counterflow centrifugal elutriation: results of a phase I–II clinical trial. *Blood* 1990; **75**: 1370–7.

187 Kernan NA, Collins NH, Juliano L, Cartagena T, Dupont B, O'Reilly RJ. Clonable T lymphocytes in T cell-depleted bone marrow transplants correlate with development of graft-v-host disease. *Blood* 1986; **68**: 770–3.

188 Aversa F, Tabilio A, Velardi A *et al.* Treatment of high-risk acute leukemia with T-cell-depleted stem cells from related donors with one fully mismatched HLA haplotype. *N Engl J Med* 1998; **339**: 1186–93.

189 Martin PJ, Hansen JA, Buckner CD *et al.* Effects of *in vitro* depletion of T cells in HLA-identical allogeneic marrow grafts. *Blood* 1985; **66**: 664–72.

190 Champlin R, Ho W, Gajewski J *et al.* Selective depletion of CD8$^+$ T lymphocytes for prevention of graft-versus-host disease after allogeneic bone marrow transplantation. *Blood* 1990; **76**: 418–23.

191 Martin PJ, Rowley SD, Anasetti C *et al.* A phase I–II clinical trial to evaluate removal of CD4 cells and partial depletion of CD8 cells from donor marrow for HLA-mismatched unrelated recipients. *Blood* 1999; **94**: 2192–9.

192 Antin JH, Bierer BE, Smith BR *et al.* Selective depletion of bone marrow T lymphocytes with anti-CD5 monoclonal antibodies: effective prophylaxis for graft-versus-host disease in patients with hematologic malignancies. *Blood* 1991; **78**: 2139–49.

193 Soiffer RJ, Weller E, Alyea EP *et al.* CD6$^+$ donor marrow T-cell depletion as the sole form of graft-versus-host disease prophylaxis in patients undergoing allogeneic bone marrow transplant from unrelated donors. *J Clin Oncol* 2001; **19**: 1152–9.

194 Papadopoulos EB, Carabasi MH, Castro-Malaspina H *et al.* T-cell-depleted allogeneic bone marrow transplantation as postremission therapy for acute myelogenous leukemia: freedom from relapse in the absence of graft-versus-host disease. *Blood* 1998; **91**: 1083–90.

195 Barrett AJ, Mavroudis D, Tisdale J *et al.* T cell-depleted bone marrow transplantation and delayed T cell add-back to control acute GVHD and conserve a graft-versus-leukemia effect. *Bone Marrow Transplant* 1998; **21**: 543–51.

196 Kuehnle I, Huls MH, Liu Z *et al.* CD20 monoclonal antibody (rituximab) for therapy of Epstein–Barr virus lymphoma after hemopoietic stem-cell transplantation. *Blood* 2000; **95**: 1502–5.

197 Greenberg PD, Riddell SR. Deficient cellular immunity: finding and fixing the defects. *Science* 1999; **285**: 546–51.

198 Walter EA, Greenberg PD, Gilbert MJ *et al.* Reconstitution of cellular immunity against cytomegalovirus in recipients of allogeneic bone marrow by transfer of T-cell clones from the donor. *N Engl J Med* 1995; **333**: 1038–44.

199 Andre-Schmutz I, Le Deist F, Hacein-Bey-Abina S *et al.* Immune reconstitution without graft-versus-host disease after haemopoietic stem-cell transplantation: a phase 1/2 study. *Lancet* 2002; **360**: 130–7.

200 Koh MB, Prentice HG, Corbo M, Morgan M, Cotter FE, Lowdell MW. Alloantigen-specific T-cell depletion in a major histocompatibility complex fully mismatched murine model provides effective graft-versus-host disease prophylaxis in the presence of lymphoid engraftment. *Br J Haematol* 2002; **118**: 108–16.

201 Martin PJ, Schoch G, Fisher L *et al.* A retrospective analysis of therapy for acute graft-versus-host disease: secondary treatment. *Blood* 1991; **77**: 1821–8.

202 Martin PJ, Schoch G, Fisher L *et al.* A retrospective analysis of therapy for acute graft-versus-host disease: initial treatment. *Blood* 1990; **76**: 1464–72.

203 Cragg L, Blazar BR, Defor T *et al.* A randomized trial comparing prednisone with antithymocyte globulin/prednisone as an initial systemic therapy for moderately severe acute graft-versus-host disease. *Biol Blood Marrow Transplant* 2000; **6**: 441–7.

204 Anasetti C, Hansen JA, Waldmann TA *et al.* Treatment of acute graft-versus-host disease with humanized anti-Tac: an antibody that binds to the interleukin-2 receptor. *Blood* 1994; **84**: 1320–7.

205 Przepiorka D, Kernan NA, Ippoliti C *et al.* Daclizumab, a humanized anti-interleukin-2 receptor α chain antibody, for treatment of acute graft-versus-host disease. *Blood* 2000; **95**: 83–99.

206 Carpenter PA, Appelbaum FR, Corey L *et al.* A humanized non-FcR-binding anti-CD3 antibody, visilizumab, for treatment of steroid-refractory acute graft-versus-host disease. *Blood* 2002; **99**: 2712–9.

207 Willenbacher W, Basara N, Blau IW, Fauser AA, Kiehl MG. Treatment of steroid refractory acute and chronic graft-versus-host disease with daclizumab. *Br J Haematol* 2001; **112**: 820–3.

208 Vander Woude AC, Bierer B. Immunosuppression and immunophilin ligands: cyclosporin A, FK506, and rapamycin. In: Ferrara J, Deeg H, Burakoff S, eds. *Graft-vs.-Host Disease*, 2nd edn. New York: Marcel Dekker, Inc., 1997: 111–49.

209 Storb R, Deeg HJ, Thomas ED *et al.* Marrow transplantation for chronic myelocytic leukemia: a controlled trial of cyclosporine versus methotrexate for prophylaxis of graft-versus-host disease. *Blood* 1985; **66**: 698–702.

210 Storb R, Deeg HJ, Pepe M *et al.* Methotrexate and cyclosporine versus cyclosporine alone for prophylaxis of graft versus host disease in patients given HLA-identical marrow grafts for leukemia: long term followup of a controlled trial. *Blood* 1989; **73**: 1729–34.

211 Nash R, Antin J, Karanes C *et al.* A phase III study comparing methotrexate and tacrolimus with methotrexate and cyclosporine for prophylaxis of acute graft-versus-host disease after marrow transplantation from unrelated donors. *Blood* 2000; **96**: 2062–8.

212 Ratanatharathorn V, Nash RA, Przepiorka D *et al.* Phase III study comparing methotrexate and tacrolimus (prograf, FK506) with methotrexate and cyclosporine for graft-versus-host disease prophylaxis after HLA-identical sibling bone marrow transplantation. *Blood* 1998; **92**: 2303–14.

213 Chao NJ, Snyder DS, Jain M *et al.* Equivalence of two effective graft-versus-host disease prophylaxis regimens: results of a prospective double-blind randomized trial. *Biol Blood Marrow Transplant* 2000; **6**: 254–61.

214 Gorgun G, Miller KB, Foss FM. Immunologic mechanisms of extracorporeal photochemotherapy in chronic graft-versus-host disease. *Blood* 2002; **100**: 941–7.

215 Foss FM, Gorgun G, Miller KB. Extracorporeal photopheresis in chronic graft-versus-host disease. *Bone Marrow Transplant* 2002; **29**: 719–25.

216 Chan GW, Gorgun G, Miller KB, Foss FM. Targeting host antigen-presenting cells pre-transplant

217 Klangsinsirikul P, Carter GI, Byrne JL, Hale G, Russell NH. Campath-1G causes rapid depletion of circulating host dendritic cells (DCs) before allogeneic transplantation but does not delay donor DC reconstitution. *Blood* 2002; **99**: 2586–91.

218 Storb R, Epstein R, Graham T, Thomas E. Methotrexate regimens for control of graft-versus-host disease in dogs with allogeneic marrow grafts. *Transplantation* 1970; **9**: 240–6.

219 Santos GW, Sensenbrenner LL, Burke PJ et al. Marrow transplanation in man following cyclophosphamide. *Transplant Proc* 1971; **3**: 400–4.

220 Lazarus HM, Coccia PF, Herzig RH et al. Incidence of acute graft-versus-host disease with and without methotrexate prophylaxis in allogeneic bone marrow transplant patients. *Blood* 1984; **64**: 215–20.

221 Ramsay N, Kersey J, Robison L et al. A randomized study of the prevention of acute graft-versus-host disease. *N Engl J Med* 1982; **306**: 392–7.

222 Blume KG, Beutler E, Bross KJ et al. Bone-marrow ablation and allogeneic marrow transplantation in acute leukemia. *N Engl J Med* 1980; **302**: 1041–6.

223 Allison AC, Eugui EM. Mycophenolate mofetil and its mechanisms of action. *Immunopharmacol* 2000; **47**: 85–118.

224 Bornhauser M, Schuler U, Porksen G et al. Mycophenolate mofetil and cyclosporine as graft-versus-host disease prophylaxis after allogeneic blood stem cell transplantation. *Transplantation* 1999; **67**: 499–504.

225 Busca A, Saroglia EM, Lanino E et al. Mycophenolate mofetil (MMF) as therapy for refractory chronic GVHD (cGVHD) in children receiving bone marrow transplantation. *Bone Marrow Transplant* 2000; **25**: 1067–71.

226 Vogelsang GB, Arai S. Mycophenolate mofetil for the prevention and treatment of graft-versus-host disease following stem cell transplantation: preliminary findings. *Bone Marrow Transplant* 2001; **27**: 1255–62.

227 Sehgal S. Rapamune (RAPA, rapamycin, sirolimus) mechanism of action immunosuppressive effect results from blockade of signal transduction and inhibition of cell cycle progression. *Clin Biochem* 1998; **31**: 335–40.

228 Li Y, Zheng XX, Li XC, Zand MS, Strom TB. Combined costimulation blockade plus rapamycin but not cyclosporine produces permanent engraftment. *Transplantation* 1998; **66**: 1387–8.

229 Lai JH, Tan TH. CD28 signaling causes a sustained down-regulation of IκBα which can be prevented by the immunosuppressant rapamycin. *J Biol Chem* 1994; **269**: 30,077–80.

230 Li Y, Li XC, Zheng XX, Wells AD, Turka LA, Strom TB. Blocking both signal 1 and signal 2 of T-cell activation prevents apoptosis of alloreactive T cells and induction of peripheral allograft tolerance. *Nat Med* 1999; **5**: 1298–302.

231 Shi Y, Frankel A, Radvanyi LG, Penn LZ, Miller RG, Mills GB. Rapamycin enhances apoptosis and increases sensitivity to cisplatin *in vitro*. *Cancer Res* 1995; **55**: 1982–8.

232 Miyazaki T, Liu ZJ, Kawahara A et al. Three distinct IL-2 signaling pathways mediated by *bcl-2*, *c-myc*, and *lck* cooperate in hematopoietic cell proliferation. *Cell* 1995; **81**: 223–31.

233 Malik RK, Parsons JT. Integrin-dependent activation of the p70 ribosomal S6 kinase signaling pathway. *J Biol Chem* 1996; **271**: 29, 785–91.

234 Murray AG, Schechner JS, Epperson DE et al. Dermal microvascular injury in the human peripheral blood lymphocyte reconstituted-severe combined immunodeficient (HuPBL-SCID) mouse/skin allograft model is T cell mediated and inhibited by a combination of cyclosporine and rapamycin. *Am J Pathol* 1998; **153**: 627–38.

235 Groth CG, Backman L, Morales JM et al. Sirolimus (rapamycin)-based therapy in human renal transplantation: similar efficacy and different toxicity compared with cyclosporine. Sirolimus European Renal Transplant Study Group [see comments]. *Transplantation* 1999; **67**: 1036–42.

236 Shapiro AM, Lakey JR, Ryan EA et al. Islet transplantation in seven patients with type 1 diabetes mellitus using a glucocorticoid-free immunosuppressive regimen. *N Engl J Med* 2000; **343**: 230–8.

237 Blazar BR, Taylor PA, Panoskaltsis-Mortari A, Sehgal S, Vallera DA. *In vivo* inhibition of cytokine responsiveness and graft-versus-host disease mortality by rapamycin leads to a clinical–pathological syndrome discrete from that observed with cyclosporin A. *Blood* 1996; **87**: 4001–9.

238 Antin J, Lee S, Harkness S et al. Preliminary results of a phase I/II double-blind placebo-controlled study of recombinant human interleukin-11 (rh-IL11) for mucositis and GVHD prevention in allogeneic transplantation. *Blood* 2000; **96** (Suppl. 1): 786a [Abstract].

239 Guinan EC, Boussiotis VA, Neuberg D et al. Transplantation of anergic histoincompatible bone marrow allografts. *N Engl J Med* 1999; **340**: 1704–14.

240 Taylor PA, Friedman TM, Korngold R, Noelle RJ, Blazar BR. Tolerance induction of alloreactive T cells via *ex vivo* blockade of the CD40: CD40L costimulatory pathway results in the generation of a potent immune regulatory cell. *Blood* 2002; **99**: 4601–9.

241 Tamada K, Tamura H, Flies D et al. Blockade of LIGHT/LTβ and CD40 signaling induces allospecific T cell anergy, preventing graft-versus-host disease. *J Clin Invest* 2002; **109**: 549–57.

242 Hixon J, Anver M, Blazar B, Panoskaltsis-Mort A, Wiltrout R, Murphy W. Administration of either anti-CD40 or interleukin-12 following lethal total body irradiation induces acute lethal toxicity affecting the gut. *Biol Blood Marrow Transplant* 2002; **8**: 316–25.

243 Hixon J, Blazar B, Anver M, Wiltrout R, Murphy W. Antibodies to CD40 induce a lethal cytokine cascade after syngeneic bone marrow transplantation. *Biol Blood Marrow Transplant* 2001; **7**: 136–43.

244 Passweg J, Rowlings P, Atkinson K et al. Influence of protective isolation on outcome of allogeneic bone marrow transplantation for leukemia. *Bone Marrow Transplant* 1998; **21**: 1231–8.

245 Bostrom L, Ringden O, Gratama J et al. A role of herpes virus serology for the development of acute graft-versus-host disease. Leukaemia Working Party of the European Group for Bone Marrow Transplantation. *Bone Marrow Transplant* 1990; **5**: 321–6.

246 Huang XJ, Wan J, Lu DP. Serum TNFα levels in patients with acute graft-versus-host disease after bone marrow transplantation. *Leukemia* 2001; **15**: 1089–91.

247 Holler E, Kolb HJ, Mittermüller J et al. Modulation of acute graft-versus-host disease after allogeneic bone marrow transplantation by tumor necrosis factor α (TNFα) release in the course of pretransplant conditioning: role of conditioning regimens and prophylactic application of a monoclonal antibody neutralizing TNFa (MAK 195F). *Blood* 1995; **86**: 890–9.

248 Kobbe G, Schneider P, Rohr U et al. Treatment of severe steroid refractory acute graft-versus-host disease with infliximab, a chimeric human/mouse antiTNFα antibody. *Bone Marrow Transplant* 2001; **28**: 47–9.

249 Couriel DR, Hicks K, Giralt S, Champlin RE. Role of tumor necrosis factor-α inhibition with inflixiMAB in cancer therapy and hematopoietic stem cell transplantation. *Curr Opin Oncol* 2000; **12**: 582–7.

250 Chiang KY, Abhyankar S, Bridges K, Godder K, Henslee-Downey JP. Recombinant human tumor necrosis factor receptor fusion protein as complementary treatment for chronic graft-versus-host disease. *Transplantation* 2002; **73**: 665–7.

251 Dinarello CA. Interleukin-1 and interleukin-1 antagonism. *Blood* 1991; **77**: 1627–52.

252 Cullup H, Dickinson AM, Jackson GH, Taylor PR, Cavet J, Middleton PG. Donor interleukin 1 receptor antagonist genotype associated with acute graft-versus-host disease in human leucocyte antigen-matched sibling allogeneic transplants. *Br J Haematol* 2001; **113**: 807–13.

253 McCarthy PJ, Williams L, Harris-Bacile M et al. A clinical phase I/II study of recombinant human interleukin-1 receptor in glucocorticoid-resistant graft-versus-host disease. *Transplantation* 1996; **62**: 626–31.

254 Antin JH, Weinstein HJ, Guinan EC et al. Recombinant interleukin-1 receptor antagonist in the treatment of steroid-resistant graft-versus-host disease. *Blood* 1994; **84**: 1342–8.

255 Hill GR, Cooke KR, Teshima T, Crawford JM, Keith JC Jr, Brinson YS et al. Interleukin-11 promotes T cell polarization and prevents acute graft-versus-host disease after allogeneic bone marrow transplantation. *J Clin Invest* 1998; **102**: 115–23.

256 Symington FW, Symington BE, Liu PY, Viguet H, Santhanam U, Sehgal PB. The relationship of serum IL-6 levels to acute graft-versus-host disease and hepatorenal disease after human bone marrow transplantation. *Transplantation* 1992; **54**: 457–62.

257 Rabinowitz J, Petros WP, Stuart AR, Peters WP. Characterization of endogenous cytokine concentrations after high-dose chemotherapy with autologous bone marrow support. *Blood* 1993; **81**: 2452–9.

258 Uguccioni M, Meliconi R, Nesci S et al. Elevated interleukin-8 serum concentrations in β-thalassemia and graft-versus-host disease. *Blood* 1993; **81**: 2252–6.

259 Shulman HM, Sale GE, Lerner KG et al. Chronic cutaneous graft-versus-host disease in man. *Am J Pathol* 1978; **91**: 545–70.

260 Parkman R. Clonal analysis of murine graft-vs.-host disease. I. Phenotypic and functional analysis of T lymphocyte clones. *J Immunol* 1986; **136**: 3543–8.

261 Ellison CA, Bradley DS, Fischer JM, Hayglass KT, Gartner JG. Murine graft-versus-host disease induced using interferon-γ-deficient grafts features antibodies to double-stranded DNA, T helper 2-type cytokines and hypereosinophilia. *Immunology* 2002; **105**: 63–72.

262 Brochu S, Rioux-Masse B, Roy J, Roy DC, Perreault C. Massive activation-induced cell death of alloreactive T cells with apoptosis of bystander

postthymic T cells prevents immune reconstitution in mice with graft-versus-host disease. *Blood* 1999; **94**: 390–400.
263 Saleh MN, Gutheil J, Moore M *et al*. A pilot study of the anti-CD20 monoclonal antibody rituximab in patients with refractory immune thrombocytopenia. *Semin Oncol* 2000; **27**: 99–103.
264 Ratanatharathorn V, Carson E, Reynolds C *et al*. Anti-CD20 chimeric monoclonal antibody treatment of refractory immune-mediated thrombocytopenia in a patient with chronic graft-versus-host disease. *Ann Intern Med* 2000; **133**: 275–9.
265 Einsele H, Ehninger G, Schneider EM *et al*. High frequency of graft-versus-host like syndromes following syngeneic bone marrow transplantation. *Transplantation* 1988; **45**: 579–85.
266 Hess AD, Horowitz L, Beschomer WE, Santos GW. Development of graft-versus-host disease-like syndrome in cyclosporine treated rats after syngeneic bone marrow transplantation. I. Development of cytotoxic T lymphocytes with apparent polyclonal anti-Ia specificity, including autoreactivity. *J Exp Med* 1985; **161**: 718–30.
267 Fischer AC, Beschomer WE, Hess AD. Requirements for the induction and adoptive transfer of cyclosporine-induced syngeneic graft-versus-host disease. *J Exp Med* 1989; **169**: 1031–41.

28 Alexander Fefer

Graft-vs.-Tumor Responses

Introduction

The success of allogeneic hematopoietic cell transplantation (HCT) for advanced hematologic malignancies is limited largely by a high relapse rate. The relapses are thought to reflect both the failure of the conditioning regimens to destroy all residual host tumor cells, and the absence of a sufficiently effective graft-vs.-leukemia effect (GVLE) or, more broadly, graft-vs.-tumor effect (GVTE), mediated by donor lymphocytes. Relapses after autologous HCT may, in addition, reflect the outgrowth of clonogenic tumor cells contaminating the infused cells. Additional chemotherapy as conditioning is limited by cumulative and shared toxicities to organs other than marrow. Consequently, induction and augmentation of GVT responses and the effector cells, targets and mechanisms involved, are being intensively investigated, so as to devise therapies with greater antitumor specificity and less toxicity.

Animal models provide some rationale for studies in humans. Allogeneic marrow infused into lethally irradiated leukemic animals can induce graft-vs.-host disease (GVHD) as well as GVLE. There is now strong evidence for the existence of GVLE and GVTE in humans. Thus, allogeneic HCT often represents a form of adoptive cellular immunotherapy [1]. Efforts to dissociate the lethal effects of GVHD from the desired effects of GVTE continue to dominate both experimental and clinical studies. The possibility of inducing GVTE in the autologous HCT setting is also being explored.

This chapter will briefly review: (a) the cell-mediated GVT response in animal models outside the setting of HCT; (b) GVHD and GVTE in murine models of HCT; (c) the sparse results of adoptive cellular immunotherapy trials without HCT in humans; (d) evidence for the existence of GVTE and its potential effectors and targets in clinical HCT; and (e) approaches to inducing or enhancing GVTE in clinical HCT. Some of the issues are extensively covered in other chapters and will therefore be only briefly summarized here.

Adoptive cellular immunotherapy in murine non-HCT models

A variety of infused syngeneic effector cells can exert antitumor effects. These include T cells specifically reactive to tumor associated antigens (TAA), T cells activated with anti-CD3 monoclonal antibody (MAB), natural killer (NK) cells, interleukin 2 (IL-2)-activated NK cells with lymphokine-activated killer (LAK) activity, and NK-T cells. The different effector cells operate through different mechanisms and probably against different tumor targets.

Syngeneic T lymphocytes specifically reactive to TAA are quite effective when administered 24 h before or after tumor inoculation, but are not usually effective if administered after the transplanted tumors are clinically detectable, even if only 3–5 mm in size [2]. Tumor-specific T cells can, however, be therapeutically effective against established widely disseminated antigenic tumors when used in conjunction with noncurative nonmyeloablative chemotherapy [3,4]. These syngeneic models have served as a prototype of what might be achieved clinically if host T cells reactive to an autologous tumor could be identified, expanded and administered to patients.

The most extensively studied model, which has served as a basis for many similar models, has involved the treatment of a disseminated Friend retrovirus-induced erythroleukemia (FBL-3) in C57Bl/6 mice with a nonmyeloablative but immunosuppressive dose of cyclophosphamide (CY) and syngeneic lymphocytes. Untreated mice die rapidly, as do mice treated only with immune cells; treatment with CY alone, or with CY plus cells immune to antigens not expressed by the tumor, prolongs survival but cures no mice; but treatment with CY plus cells immune to FBL-3 cures the vast majority of leukemic mice [5,6].

Studies in this and other similar models yielded the following observations related to effective syngeneic cellular immunotherapy [3,7–10]: (a) donor T cells had to be specifically reactive to TAA presented in association with major histocompatibility complex (MHC) antigens; (b) the T cells had to proliferate and persist in the recipient for a long time; (c) with rare exceptions [11], IL-2 in vivo augmented the therapeutic efficacy of the transferred T cells; (d) although the prime mediator of tumor eradication was a $CD8^+$ cytotoxic T lymphocyte (CTL) that lysed antigenic tumors with MHC class I-restricted specificity, class II-restricted $CD4^+$ helper T cells could also mediate tumor eradication. Indeed, in some models, the $CD4^+$ T cells did not need to be reactive to TAA to be therapeutically effective. For example, $CD4^+$ T cells activated in vitro with anti-CD3 MAB and administered together with CY plus systemic IL-2 eradicated three types of advanced syngeneic murine tumors [12].

Lymphocytes with non-MHC restricted cytotoxic reactivity can also serve as effector cells in tumor therapy [13]. IL-2 is involved in the generation, activation and/or proliferation of almost all such effector cells in vitro and/or in vivo. IL-2 is a 15-kDa glycoprotein secreted by antigen-stimulated T cells. It promotes the proliferation and differentiation of T, B, and NK cells. Murine lymphocytes cultured in high concentrations of IL-2 acquire the ability to lyse a variety of tumors without MHC restriction, with relative sparing of normal tissue [14,15]. Most cells that mediate LAK activity are activated NK cells, phenotypically $CD3^-CD56^+$, but some arise from T cells. In murine tumor models, exogenous LAK cells alone, without IL-2, have little therapeutic effect, IL-2 alone is often therapeutically effective, and a combination of LAK cells plus IL-2 is therapeutically most effective in inducing regression of established syngeneic tumors and inhibiting metastases [16–18].

NK-T cells express both NK and T-cell markers, i.e. CD3+CD56+. When they are expanded in culture interferon gamma (IFN-γ), IL-2 and anti-CD3 MAB they become predominantly CD8+CD56+ cells which, like LAK cells, exhibit non-MHC-restricted cytotoxicity against many syngeneic and allogeneic NK-sensitive and NK-resistant tumors, with minimal cytotoxicity against normal hematopoietic cells [13,19]. The immunotherapeutic efficacy of NK-T cells against established tumor in mice has not yet been documented.

Murine NK cells express inhibitory and/or activating receptors specific for MHC class I determinants. Binding of the inhibitory receptors by the appropriate MHC class I molecules on target cells leads to inactivation of NK cell function [20]. Accordingly, either MHC class I disparity or blocking of inhibitory NK receptors is required for an antitumor effect. Thus, in one murine model, a blockade of inhibitory NK receptors *in vivo* protected mice from leukemic death, and so did adoptive transfer of IL-2-activated NK cells treated *ex vivo* with a blocker of NK inhibitory receptors [21].

GVL effect of allogeneic BMT in animal models

Historically, syngeneic HCT with lethal total body irradiation (TBI) conditioning was reported to occasionally cure some murine leukemias [22], but most leukemias did not respond [2]. The results probably reflected the variable radiosensitivity and antigenicity of the tumors and a possible syngeneic GVLE. In the most recently reported model, mice bearing established syngeneic *c-myc*-induced leukemia received syngeneic T-cell-depleted bone marrow (BM) plus syngeneic T-cell subsets from mice sensitized to TAA. Both CD4+ T cells, and CD8+ T cells, induced significant GVLE [23].

Barnes *et al.* [22] were the first to postulate that allogeneic marrow infused into a tumor-bearing lethally X-irradiated mouse would "destroy by the action of the immunity these residual leukemia cells . . . and perhaps the host." In their classic studies [22,24], lethally irradiated leukemic mice given syngeneic marrow died of recurrent leukemia, whereas a few of the mice given allogeneic marrow were cured, but almost all ultimately died of what was called "wasting disease" and subsequently renamed "GVHD." The term "GVL" was introduced much later to distinguish it from the GVH reaction [25].

Mathé *et al.* [26] first suggested that one might use the GVH reaction against the tumor, i.e. permit GVHD to occur and exert its GVLE, then treat the GVHD and, thereby, save the cured host. Such exquisite control of GVHD and GVLE is very difficult to achieve even in murine models, but, in practice, now approximates the pragmatic mainstay of current clinical HCT. An alternative approach has been to develop *in vivo* or *in vitro* ways to confer antitumor specificity or preference to the GVH reaction [4]. That approach, which is based on the assumption that the effector(s) and/or targets for GVLE are qualitatively or quantitatively different from those for GVHD, represents a major investigative challenge which, with rare exceptions [27–31], remains largely unmet. For example, some mice bearing a syngeneic advanced antigenic lymphoma could be cured by nonmyeloablative CY plus MHC-compatible spleen cells, without GVHD—but only if the spleen cell donors were preimmunized to TAA; cells from donors preimmunized only to normal host alloantigens were not effective [27]. In the same model, MHC-incompatible cells caused fatal GVHD [32].

The effector cells mediating GVLE and GVHD can vary with the model studied, the degree of donor/host histoincompatibility, the potency of the immunogen and/or the susceptibility of the normal or tumor target to immunologic attack by the different effector cells. The cells mediating GVLE and GVHD have been mainly CD8+ T cells in some models and mainly CD4+ in others [28–31,33–36]. At a clonal level, the relationship between T cells that induce GVLE and those which induce GVHD is unclear. For example, some T cells specifically reactive to host minor histocompatibility antigens (mHA) and cytotoxic to host leukemia cells induce fatal GVHD, while others do not [31].

Moreover, murine allospecific CD8+ T cells can now be subdivided into two phenotypes: the Tc1 subset, which mediates GVLE as well as GVHD, and the Tc2 subset, which mediates GVLE but not GVHD [37]. The differences may reflect the role of cytolysis in GVLE [38] and of type 1 cytokines in the pathogenesis of GVHD [39].

A frequently used approach to identifying effectors of GVLE and GVHD in mice is to study donor lymphocyte infusions (DLIs) after allogeneic HCT. The timing of DLI may be critical for the induction of GVLE. For example, in one model [40], recipients of DLI early after HCT resisted tumor challenge better than did recipients of later DLI; in another model, mixed chimeras resisted tumor better than did full chimeras, suggesting that persistent host antigen-presenting cells (APCs) may present TAA more effectively and, thereby, enhance a mild GVLE [41].

The GVLE-inducing effector in DLI varies among models. For example, in one MHC mismatched murine HCT model, CD8+ T cells in DLI exerted the most potent GVLE, whereas in an MHC-matched model, both CD4+ and CD8+ T cells were required for GVLE [42].

A recently identified T-cell subset, the CD4+CD25+ immune regulatory cell, may also play an important role in GVHD and, possibly, in GVTE. In mice, depletion of CD4+CD25+ cells from DLI or of CD25+ cells in the recipient before HCT increases GVHD. Conversely, infusion of donor CD4+CD25+ cells activated and expanded in culture with anti-CD3 MAB, APCs and IL-2, inhibits the development of lethal GVHD [43]. Their effect on GVTE has not yet been established. Extrapolation of these murine findings to clinical GVTE and GVHD is difficult because these cells are heterogeneous and different methods of activation and expansion may yield different cell populations with potentially different suppressor/effector functions.

Other effector cells have been implicated in GVTE and GVHD. For example, CD8+CD56+ NK-T cells can exert GVTE against an established lymphoma in the setting of syngeneic HCT and GVTE against concurrently inoculated lymphoma cells in the setting of MHC-mismatched HCT—without inducing GVHD [19].

NK cells are now known to play a complex role in GVTE/GVHD [13]. Because of the interaction between NK cell inhibitory receptors and MHC class I molecules, class I similarity between donor and host inhibits NK cell reactivity, whereas disparity promotes it. Therefore, MHC class I-mismatched transplants can trigger NK-cell alloreactivity against host lymphohematopoietic tissue, thereby inducing a strong GVLE. Moreover, since alloreactive NK cells also lyze host APCs, which are responsible for initiating GVHD, but do not lyze nonlymphohematopoietic tissue, no GVHD is induced [44]. In fact, alloreactive NK cells prevented GVHD induction by donor T cells in lethally irradiated mice [45].

IL-2 can potentially influence GVLE/GVHD by its effects on T and NK cell proliferation and function. In several syngeneic HCT models, IL-2 alone [46], or IL-2 plus marrow incubated with IL-2, cured leukemic mice [47]. In allogeneic HCT models, IL-2 can induce or exacerbate GVHD, or protect against it, depending on the model and the timing [48–54]. Thus, IL-2 administered at the time of allogeneic HCT induced GVLE while reducing GVHD, and also enhanced the GVLE of T-cell-depleted HCT [55]. In another, MHC-mismatched, murine HCT model, IL-2 decreased GVHD without diminishing the GVLE [56]. These results all suggest that IL-2 can induce GVLE without inducing or exacerbating GVHD. However, it is not yet clear how/whether these findings will be applicable to clinical HCT.

Adoptive cellular immunotherapy in humans

Murine studies [3,9,57] have identified several advantages of tumor-antigen specific immune T cells over other effector cells for cancer immunotherapy, including: (a) target specificity; (b) ability to "home" to sites of tumor and proliferate there in response to tumor; (c) ability to persist long-term *in vivo*; (d) ability to maintain proliferative and cytolytic function in the presence of low IL-2 concentrations; and (e) acquisition of immunologic memory. Recent advances in cellular and molecular immunology have led to the generation and identification of T cells capable of specifically recognizing and reacting to antigens expressed by a variety of human tumors [58]. The most extensive studies have involved CD8+ CTL reactive to melanoma-associated antigens [58–60].

Most clinical trials of T cells with putative tumor-specificity have been performed in patients with metastatic malignant melanoma. They have involved tumor-infiltrating lymphocytes (TIL) obtained from biopsies of melanoma and expanded in IL-2 [61–64]. In the first TIL trial, nonmyeloablative CY plus autologous TIL plus systemic high dose IL-2, induced a partial response (PR) in 11 of 20 patients [65]. Although response rates in subsequent similar TIL trials for melanoma have been far lower [66,67], the most recent report has yielded particularly encouraging results [68]. Patients with metastatic melanoma refractory to high-dose IL-2 were pretreated with nonmyeloablative CY and fludarabine, and then received billions of autologous polyclonal TIL selected for their cytotoxic reactivity against melanoma-associated antigens and expanded *in vitro*, followed by high-dose systemic IL-2. Objective clinical responses were documented in six of 13 patients. The role and/or necessity of each component of the therapy, especially the particular chemotherapy and the particular IL-2 regimen, has not yet been established. Nevertheless, the clinical use of CTL reactive to TAA is being explored with increasing optimism. This subject is extensively covered in Chapter 29.

Since the usefulness of tumor-specific T cells as therapy may be limited by the need to identify immunodominant tumor-specific peptides and by the highly polymorphic nature of the human MHC complex, cells with non-MHC-restricted cytotoxic activity against tumor but not against normal tissue may have some advantages [19]. Cells with LAK activity have been generated from lymphocytes of healthy people and cancer patients. Most LAK activity is mediated by activated CD3−CD56+ NK cells [69]. LAK cells lyse fresh human leukemia and lymphoma cells without MHC restriction [70–73]. Susceptibility to lysis is noncell-cycle specific and is maintained in cell lines with drug resistance markers [74,75]. LAK cells are particularly lytic to tumors which express few or no MHC class I molecules [76]. Although in many clinical trials infusion of autologous LAK cells accompanied therapy with systemic IL-2 [77], the therapeutic contribution of autologous LAK cells has yet to be documented.

Autologous human NK-T cells expanded in culture (CD8+CD56+) might be more effective than LAK cells. Indeed, NK-T cells inhibited the growth of chronic myeloid leukemia (CML) and Epstein–Barr virus (EBV) lymphoma in severe combined immunodeficiency disease mice more effectively than did LAK cells [13]. In a phase I/II clinical trial of 21 patients with non-Hodgkin's lymphoma (NHL) or Hodgkin's disease (HD) recurring after autologous HCT, treatment with autologous expanded NK-T cells induced objective tumor responses in two patients (see Chapter 102) [19].

All the effector cells being studied can potentially be influenced by IL-2. Thus, IL-2 induces proliferation of T cells reactive to antigenic tumors, promotes expansion and activation of NK cells, induces MHC-unrestricted cytotoxic activity against tumors and induces secretion of cytokines with antitumor activity. IL-2 therefore may, itself, indirectly exert an antitumor effect.

IL-2 has induced some clinical responses of some tumors in some patients [78]. Therapy with IL-2 ± LAK cells induced a PR in 15% and complete remission (CR) in 5–10% of patients with metastatic renal cell carcinoma (RCC) and malignant melanoma [78–82]. Most patients who achieve a CR do not relapse [78,81,82]. In many small trials of various regimens of IL-2 ± autologous LAK cells, about 20% of patients with refractory malignant lymphoma exhibited a PR or CR [83,84]. Although no responses to IL-2 have been reported in the few patients treated for acute lymphoblastic leukemia (ALL), IL-2 induced enduring CR in six of 14 patients with refractory acute myeloid leukemia (AML) or with AML in relapse but with less than 20% blasts in the marrow [84–86]. Another IL-2 regimen [87], demonstrated to be tolerable in children with AML in first CR [88], is being tested in a phase III trial by the Children's Cancer Group (CCG Protocol 2961).

Although the doses of IL-2 which induced clinical responses tended to be the higher ones, the relationship between IL-2 dose, the immunomodulatory effects induced and the clinical outcomes remains unclear, due to the heterogeneity of the patients and of the IL-2 regimens [77,89–91]. Moreover, in contrast to results in murine models, the contribution, if any, of infused LAK cells to the end results is unclear, since the results of a prospectively randomized trial—in RCC—were not definitive [92].

Evidence for a GVL and GVT effect in clinical allogeneic HCT

Temporal association between cessation of immunosuppression and disease remission

Patients have been reported whose disease relapsed after allogeneic bone marrow transplantation (BMT) but disappeared when immunosuppressive therapy for GVHD was stopped. The diseases included ALL, Burkitt's lymphoma, AML, CML, chronic lymphocytic leukemia (CLL), NHL, multiple myeloma, ovarian cancer and small-cell lung cancer [93–103].

The leukemic relapse rate is lower after allogeneic than after syngeneic BMT

This observation (Fig. 28.1 [104]) applies to patients at high risk for relapse, i.e. those transplanted for ALL and AML in second or subsequent CR or in relapse [104], as well as those at low risk for relapse, i.e. AML and ALL in first CR and CML in chronic phase (CML-CP) [105]. The results [106–110], strongly suggest that an antileukemic effect is associated with allogeneic BMT.

The leukemic relapse rate is lower in allogeneic marrow recipients who develop GVHD than in those who do not

Multivariate analyses, including that of 1198 patients transplanted in Seattle for high-risk leukemia, reveal that GVHD is the most significant independent factor associated with a decreased relapse rate [106,107,111–116]. Figure 28.2 [116] presents the probability of leukemic relapse as a function of acute or chronic GVHD. The leukemic relapse rate was

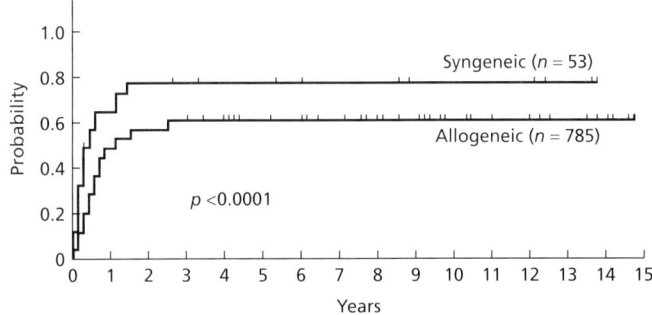

Fig. 28.1 Kaplan–Meier product limit estimates of the probability of relapse of leukemia among recipients of allogeneic and syngeneic marrow. Reproduced with permission from Fefer *et al.* [104], courtesy of Wiley-Liss, Inc., a subsidiary of John Wiley & Sons, Inc.

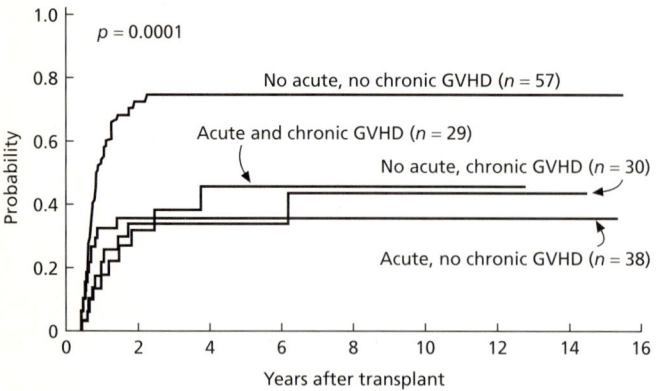

Fig. 28.2 Probability of relapse in 154 patients with acute lymphoblastic leukemia (ALL) or acute myeloid leukemia (AML) transplanted in relapse, grouped by graft-vs.-host disease (GVHD) status. All patients were alive in remission 150 days after bone marrow transplantation (BMT). Reproduced with permission from Sullivan et al. [116].

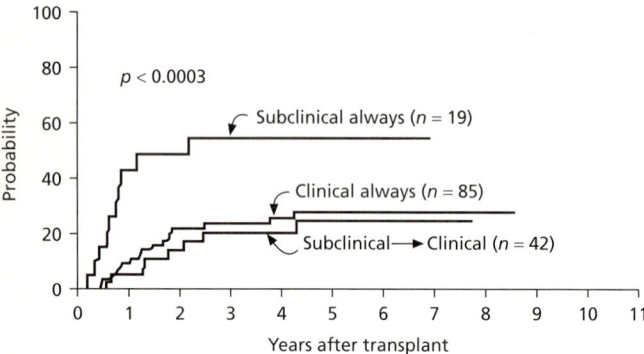

Fig. 28.3 The probability of leukemic relapse after allogeneic bone marrow transplantation (BMT) as a function of the development of clinical chronic graft-vs.-host disease (GVHD). Reproduced with permission from Sullivan et al. [117].

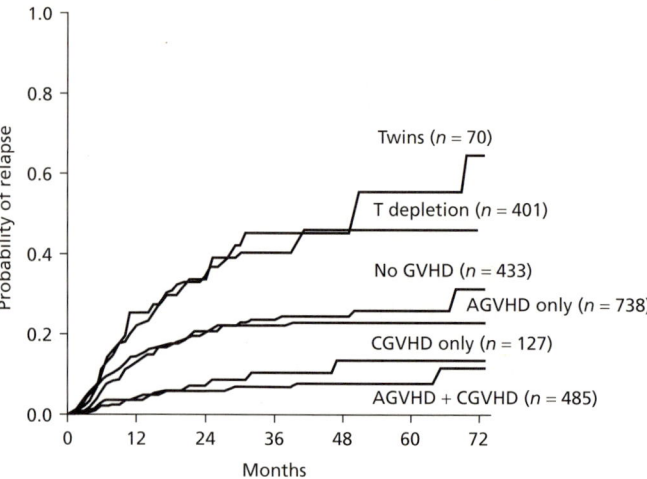

Fig. 28.4 Actuarial probability of leukemic relapse after bone marrow transplantation (BMT) for acute lymphoblastic leukemia (ALL) in first complete remission (CR), acute myeloid leukemia (AML) in first CR and chronic myeloid leukemia (CML) in chronic phase as a function of type of marrow graft and as a function of development of acute or chronic graft-vs.-host disease (GVHD). Reproduced with permission from Horowitz et al. [110].

significantly lower in patients who developed GVHD after BMT for acute leukemia in relapse. Moreover, patients whose chronic GVHD was clinically evident had a significantly lower leukemic relapse rate than did patients whose chronic GVHD remained subclinical (i.e. only histological) (Fig. 28.3) [117]. Thus, clinical acute and/or chronic GVHD is associated with GVLE. Data from the International Bone Marrow Transplant Registry (IBMTR) [110] suggest that although a combination of acute and chronic GVHD was associated with the lowest relapse rate, acute GVHD was most effective in ALL, while chronic GVHD was most effective for AML and CML.

The leukemic relapse rate is lower in recipients of allogeneic marrow *without* GVHD than in recipients of syngeneic marrow

This observation is supported by IBMTR data from patients at low risk for relapse (Fig. 28.4) [110]. Thus, clinical GVHD is not a prerequisite for GVLE. However, recent IBMTR data suggest that without GVHD, GVLE may not occur in patients with NHL or multiple myeloma [103].

The leukemic relapse rate is higher after TCD allogeneic BMT than after unmodified BMT

This observation has been made largely from trials of patients in CML-CP. In one multicenter study [118], the incidence of relapse was 10% in recipients of non-T-cell-depleted BM who had moderate to severe acute GVHD and 50% in recipients of T-cell-depleted BM who had no or mild acute GVHD. Similar observations have been made in patients with CML in the accelerated phase [119].

IBMTR data [110] of allogeneic human leukocyte antigen (HLA)-matched related BMT in patients at low risk for relapse, show that recipients of T-cell-depleted BM who had no GVHD had a far higher relative risk (RR) of relapse than did recipients of unmodified BM who had no GVHD, suggesting that in the absence of clinical GVHD, unmodified allogeneic BM exerted an antileukemic effect, and that this effect depended on the presence of T cells. Moreover, the RR of relapse for recipients of T-cell-depleted BM with GVHD was still significantly higher than that of recipients of unmodified marrow without GVHD. The results support the existence of GVLE independent of clinical GVHD but dependent on the presence of T cells in the infused BM. The higher relapse rates associated with HLA-matched T-cell-depleted BMT have also been documented with BMT from unrelated or HLA-mismatched related donors [103].

Collectively, the clinical observations presented above suggest three antitumor responses after BMT: (i) a GVLE associated with clinically evident acute and/or chronic GVHD; (ii) GVLE that can occur in the absence of clinically evident GVHD; and (iii) GVLE dependent on GVHD, or independent of GVHD but dependent on the presence of T cells.

DLIs induce remissions of leukemias that have recurred after allogeneic BMT

The above observation is the most direct evidence for the existence of a GVLE in allogeneic BMT [120,121]. Remissions after DLI occur in the vast majority of patients who relapse with CML-CP, far less often with AML, in a small number of patients with NHL, HD and multiple myeloma, and very uncommonly in ALL [103,121–123]. Attempts to use chemotherapy before DLI for acute leukemia have yielded disappointing results [124]. Patients with CML-CP treated with DLI exhibit significant GVHD (>50%). Those with morphologic evidence of CML may also develop significant aplasia (>30%). Patients who exhibit GVHD are far more likely to enter a CR than those who do not, suggesting that GVLE and GVHD have effectors and targets in common. However, since the antileukemic response can occur without GVHD, the GVL and GVHD may at times be separable. The subject of DLI is extensively covered in Chapter 84.

Allogeneic HCT after nonmyeloablative conditioning (NM-HCT) induces remissions of hematologic and some nonhematologic malignancies

Given the strong evidence for the existence of GVTE in clinical HCT after conventional myeloablative conditioning regimens, a number of groups have been exploring the possibility that infused allogeneic hematopoietic cells might induce a clinically significant GVTE even when transplanted after NM conditioning regimens which have little, if any, antitumor activity, but which are sufficiently immunosuppressive to permit donor cell engraftment (see Chapter 85) [125]. A variety of NM regimens are being explored to establish mixed or full donor chimerism, and other immunosuppressive regimens are used after HCT in an effort to prevent and/or control GVHD. Successful and sustained engraftment is the rule rather than the exception. CRs have been induced in a variable percentage of patients with a variety of hematologic malignancies by NM-HCT, using HLA-matched related, as well as unrelated donors (see Chapter 85). As with conventional HCT, GVHD after NM-HCT is associated with a significantly lower post-transplant relapse rate of AML and myelodysplastic syndrome [126].

Of particular interest has been the report that a nonhematologic, normally chemo-resistant tumor, namely metastatic RCC, can respond to NM-HCT. Of the first 33 such patients treated at the National Institutes of Health, 11 had a PR and four a CR for up to $3^{1}/_{2}$ years [127]. NM-HCT is extensively covered in Chapters 85 and 86.

Effector cells and targets in clinical GVL effect

Effector cells that could potentially mediate clinical GVLE include mainly: (a) CD8$^+$ CTL that recognize TAA in association with class I MHC antigens; (b) CD4$^+$ T cells that recognize TAA in association with class II MHC and that mediate their effects by direct lysis and/or via secretion of T-helper type 1 subset (TH1) type cytokines, such as IFN-γ, which up-regulates expression of class I MHC molecules on tumors, and IL-2, which promotes expansion and activation, and CD8$^+$ CTL NK cells; and/or (c) NK/LAK and NK-T cells that mediate their antitumor effect via MHC-unrestricted lysis and cytokine secretion, especially against tumors that express few or no MHC class I or II molecules.

GVL effectors may differ with the transplant setting, the degree and nature of donor–host histoincompatibility, and the tumor target involved. The evidence presented above for the existence of a clinical allogeneic GVLE strongly suggests that GVLE is mediated predominantly by CD3$^+$ T cells, especially CD8$^+$ T cells [128]. However, since CD8$^+$ cells may have to persist to exert GVLE, helper CD4$^+$ T cells may also be required.

In allogeneic HCT, potential T-cell targets for GVLE are mHA expressed on tumor cells, normal proteins overexpressed on tumor cells and/or antigens expressed only on tumor cells, i.e. tumor-specific antigens. Some of the mHA are restricted to hematopoietic cells, while others show a broad tissue expression [129–132]. Thus, after allogeneic BMT, leukemia-associated mHA-specific CTL have been generated that can lyse or inhibit the growth of leukemic cells [133,134]. Indeed, mHA-specific CD8$^+$ T-cell clones that lyse host hematopoietic cells—both normal and malignant—but not nonhematopoietic cells can be isolated from most patients after HLA-identical allogeneic HCT [135]. The clinical use of such clones in patients whose leukemia has recurred after HCT is being explored.

Differentiation antigens shared by leukemic and nonleukemic cells may also serve as targets for GVLE. For example, a CD4$^+$ T-cell clone has been generated for which the target antigen is developmentally regulated and expressed only by leukemic cells and CD34$^+$ cells [136].

MHC class II-restricted CD4$^+$ and/or MHC class I-restricted CD8$^+$ T-cell responses have been generated to normal proteins that are overexpressed on tumor cells, such as the Wilms' tumor gene product WT1, proteinase 3 (PR3) [137], and HER-2/*neu* [138], to tumor-specific antigens, such as the immunoglobulin idiotype of B-cell lymphoma and multiple myeloma [139], oncoproteins E6 and E7 expressed by cervical cancer and encoded by human papilloma virus [140], transforming proteins encoded by mutated *ras* [141] and mutated p53 [142], and the joining region of p210 *bcr-abl* [143,144], and PML/RARα [145]. All these antigens can serve as potential targets for a T-cell-mediated GVTE. Some responses have been generated in cells from healthy people and some from cells from patients with malignancies. One patient with CML has been reported to respond clinically to an infusion of leukemia-reactive CTLs [146]. Autologous pre-B leukemia-specific CD8$^+$ CTL lines have been generated from the marrows of 10 out of 15 patients with pre-B-cell leukemia by costimulation via CD28 [147].

The targets for T cells in HCT or DLI in patients with CML may be mHA and/or hematopoietic lineage-related differentiation antigens, as suggested by the finding that the nonmalignant host T cells that persist after HCT disappear after DLI, and that aplasia predicts a CR. However, since T-cell responses have been generated to epitopes of *bcr-abl* [143,144], a leukemia-specific T-cell-mediated GVLE in CML is also a possibility. Moreover, since CD8$^+$ T-cell responses specific for PR3 and WT1 have also been generated, these nonmutated proteins, overexpressed by CML and AML cells, may also be targets of GVLE [137]. This is supported by the report that PR3-reactive T cells were detected in patients with CML who responded clinically to allogeneic HCT or to DLI, but not in patients who did not respond [148].

Activated NK/LAK cells, which lyse autologous or host leukemia cells, are among the earliest cells to be reconstituted after autologous or allogeneic HCT [114,149–153], and therefore might be appropriate candidate GVL effectors, especially early after HCT or after T-cell-depleted HCT. Such cells have not been used after allogeneic HCT and their efficacy after autologous HCT is yet to be determined (see below).

NK cells have now been identified as major GVL effectors against some hematologic malignancies, especially in HLA-mismatched HCT [20]. Human NK cells bear inhibitory receptors, termed killer immunoglobulin-like receptors (KIR), that interact with HLA class I molecules on target cells and inhibit cytotoxicity, thereby protecting normal somatic cells from NK-mediated attack [44]. Thus, interaction between KIR and a class I allele will inhibit the killing of the tumor target by the NK cell. Conversely, when the recipient's class I alleles do not block all donor NK cells, donor alloreactive NK cells are generated which kill lymphohematologic host targets.

In haploidentical HCT, disparity between KIRs expressed by donor NK cells and HLA molecules on recipient leukemic cells favors NK activation. However, since NK cell alloreactivity, in contrast to T-cell alloreactivity, is restricted to host lymphohematopoietic targets—both normal and malignant—but spares other tissues, alloreactive NK cells are likely to exert GVTE against hematologic malignancies without GVHD. Indeed, in high-risk acute leukemia patients who underwent T-cell-depleted HCT from HLA-haplotype-mismatched family donors, transplants from NK cell alloreactive donors protected patients against GVHD and against relapse of AML [45]. Such KIR ligand incompatibility had no effect on ALL [45].

Since NK cell alloreactions, in contrast to T-cell alloreactions, require MHC class I disparity and are restricted to host lymphohematopoietic targets, one would not expect alloreactive NK cells to exert GVLE in the setting of autologous or HLA-matched HCT, or to exert GVTE against nonhematologic malignancies [20]. The role of NK cells in HCT is covered extensively in Chapter 82.

Attempts to induce or enhance the GVL effect

Attempts have been made to induce or enhance GVLE by increasing GVHD or by promoting GVL effectors. In one study, GVHD prophylaxis was not administered to 16 leukemic patients undergoing HLA-identical sibling BMT [154]. Severe and hyper-acute GVHD was observed, without a detectable effect on the leukemic relapse rate. In another trial, leukemic recipients of HLA-identical sibling marrow were randomized to the standard methotrexate (MTX) regimen as GVHD prophylaxis, to a shorter MTX regimen or to standard MTX plus donor buffy-coat cells [155]. Reduction of the MTX or addition of donor buffy-coat cells increased the incidence of acute GVHD, but no effect on the leukemic relapse rate was detectable—partly due to a marked increase in fatal GVHD.

DLIs for relapsed disease have been manipulated in an effort to decrease GVHD but enhance, or, at least, not reduce, the GVLE—largely by controlling the number and subset of T cells infused. Thus, the approximate number of CD3+ T cells or CD8+ T cells which was small enough not to induce significant GVHD and yet large enough to induce a significant GVLE in CML was identified in two trials, but with considerable overlap [156,157].

For HLA-haploidentical T-cell-depleted HCT, donors are already being selected on the basis of KIR mismatching to maximize an NK cell-mediated GVLE without GVHD [13]. The results in patients with AML have been extremely encouraging in one trial [45] but not in another [158].

Since the likely GVL effectors might all be enhanced by IL-2, and since cells with LAK activity against host tumor are detectable soon after allogeneic HCT [73], pharmacologic doses of IL-2 have been administered early after allogeneic BMT, at a time of minimal residual disease, in an effort to induce or augment a GVLE. A 14-week course of low dose IL-2 therapy administered after T-cell-depleted BMT was reported to decrease the leukemic relapse rate without increasing GVHD, as compared with historical controls [159]. IL-2 therapy after unmodified BMT could potentially be more effective but might also induce or exacerbate GVHD. Therefore, a phase I dose escalation trial of IL-2 after unmodified allogeneic matched sibling BMT was performed in children with acute leukemia at high risk for relapse who did not develop GVHD after prophylaxis was stopped [160]. The IL-2 regimen, administered after hematologic recovery, consisted of a 5-day moderate induction dose, a 4-day rest period and a 10-day low maintenance dose. IL-2 induced lymphopenia followed by rebound lymphocytosis, with an increase in CD56+ NK cells and CD8+ T cells, and an increase in LAK activity. No apparent increase in GVHD was noted. The clinical outcomes in this small heterogeneous group of patients were sufficiently encouraging to warrant a phase II trial.

IL-2 has also been used for patients whose leukemia relapsed after allogeneic HCT. Clinical responses were reported in five patients treated with DLI plus IL-2 or donor lymphocytes activated with IL-2 *in vitro*, plus systemic IL-2, plus, in some cases, IFN-α [161]. A trial of DLI plus escalating doses of IL-2 for relapsed acute leukemia is in progress. Since the likelihood of significant GVHD induction by DLI administered late after HCT is low [162], the possibility of using DLI late after allogeneic HCT but before relapse has occurred, i.e. as prophylaxis, is being explored as a way to induce a GVLE and reduce relapses without increasing GVHD [163].

The possibility exists that syngeneic or even autologous HCT might also exert GVLE which, however, hasn't been documented because

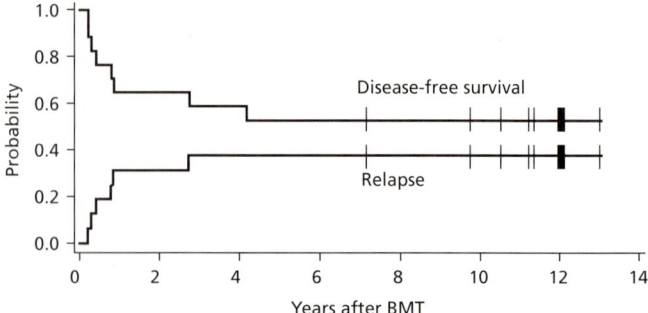

Fig. 28.5 Kaplan–Meier product limit estimates of relapse and of disease-free survival of patients treated with autologous hematopoietic cell transplantation (HCT) plus interleukin 2 (IL-2) for acute myeloid leukemia (AML) = first relapse (*n* = 17).

appropriate controls cannot be identified. Historically, an early attempt to induce a GVLE in leukemic patients after syngeneic BMT consisted of infusion of lymphocytes from the normal twin and injections of killed autologous leukemic cells, in an effort to immunize the infused donor lymphocytes against host leukemic cells [164]. Some patients were cured, but the contribution, if any, of the immunotherapy to the end results, could not be assessed [165].

Based on results in animal models, attempts have been made to induce a GVH reaction for a possible GVTE by administering cyclosporine after autologous HCT [166]. Although self-limited cutaneous acute GVHD can be induced, significant, consistent and reproducible effects on relapse and survival have not yet been observed (see Chapter 30).

The possibility that IL-2 ± LAK cells, as consolidative immunotherapy after autologous HCT, might induce or augment a GVLE, is also being explored [167,168]. If effective, such immunotherapy should destroy not only the residual host disease but also whatever clonogenic malignant cells might be infused with the hematopoietic cells, thereby obviating the need for purging hematopoietic cells of tumor cells. Since relapses after autologous HCT tend to occur early, and since IL-2-responsive lymphocytes have been detected in the circulation within 2–3 weeks [152,169], IL-2 ± LAK cells have been administered after hematologic reconstitution, at a time of minimal residual disease.

Phase I trials have identified the maximum tolerated dose of IL-2 that can be administered in that period after autologous HCT and have documented its immunomodulatory effects [87,170]. The dose-limiting toxicities were hypotension and thrombocytopenia. All toxicities were rapidly reversed by decreasing or stopping IL-2. Neutrophil counts rose during IL-2 treatment. There was transient early lymphopenia followed by a rebound lymphocytosis after stopping the IL-2. This rise reflected increases in the number of CD8+ T cells and CD56+ activated NK cells, and was associated with enhanced ability to lyse tumor lines. The clinical significance of these immunologic changes is unknown. Autologous LAK cells can be generated and infused with IL-2, but with additional toxicity and expense, and without documented benefit [171].

The clinical outcomes for patients with high-risk NHL in phase I/II trials of IL-2 ± LAK cells after autologous HCT were encouraging [172]. A prospectively randomized phase III trial of IL-2 vs. observation after autologous HCT for NHL in relapse is now in progress (SWOG Protocol 9438) to determine whether IL-2 will reduce the relapse rate and improve survival [84].

The results of phase I/II trials of IL-2 after autologous HCT for patients with AML beyond first CR have been inconsistent. In one trial encouraging results were obtained (Fig. 28.5): of the 17 patients treated, one died of infection, six relapsed, one died in CR with a secondary malignancy at 62 months and 10 patients remain in continuous CR for many years [167,171]. In another trial the results with IL-2 were only comparable to historical non-IL-2-treated controls [87]. However, the IL-2 regimen and stem source cell was different, and the patient populations small and heterogeneous. The discrepant results highlight the need for a phase III randomized trial. The same IL-2 regimen [87] is also being tested after autologous HCT for AML in first CR in a pilot trial at The City of Hope National Medical Center, Duarte, California, with encouraging preliminary results [173]. However, phase III trials are essential. The only randomized trial of IL-2 after autologous HCT reported to date involved a different IL-2 regimen in a small number of patients with ALL and was negative [174].

Future directions

With increased knowledge of the effectors and targets of a GVTE and GVHD, approaches will be devised to enhance the former and/or reduce the latter. Such knowledge is most likely to be obtained in the setting of post-transplant DLI and in the setting of NM-HCT. NM-HCT could represent a unique platform for active immunotherapy, i.e. cancer vaccines, and/or adoptive cellular immunotherapy, partly because the new (donor) immune system might bypass whatever factors might have interfered with an effective antitumor response by the host pre-HCT.

Tumor-specific vaccines are likely to be used for immunotherapy in the context of allogeneic or even autologous HCT. Thus, by analogy to murine studies [175–177] in which vaccination of allogeneic BM donors to TAA prior to BMT enhanced GVTE without exacerbating GVHD, a vaccine might be administered to donors whose stem cells or lymphocytes are to be infused, and/or to patients after HCT, in an effort to immunize donor cells in the host.

It is very likely that T cells reactive to antigens associated with or specific for some malignancies will be generated, identified, expanded and infused for tumor therapy in the context of HCT—similar to what has been reported with CMV-specific $CD8^+$ T cells [178,179] or with EBV-specific $CD8^+$ CTL for lymphoproliferative disease [180]. The T cells might be obtained from donors immunized before HCT, or from donors whose T cells are immunized $in\ vitro$, or from recipients who are chimeras and whose donor T cells have acquired reactivity to the relevant antigens. No results of trials with CTLs primed against TAA in the context of HCT are yet available.

NK cells are likely to become clinically more useful in HCT. Since the inhibitory signals delivered by MHC class I molecules expressed on cancer cells will probably limit the usefulness of NK cells in the setting of autologous or even HLA-identical HCT, approaches to blocking the interaction between inhibitory NK cell receptors and MHC class I molecules will be further explored [20], including the possibility of blocking several NK inhibitory receptors simultaneously, so as to promote GVTE [20]. Alternatively, given the limitations of NK cells and of tumor-specific T cells as therapy in the setting of HCT, strategies may be developed to combine both types of cells so as to prevent selection of tumor cell variants attempting to escape destruction by either type of effector cells [181].

Finally, the use of single lymphokines or combinations of lymphokines after HCT will be explored. For example, IL-12 induced cytotoxic antitumor activity in lymphocytes from recipients of autologous and allogeneic hematopoietic cells [182], eradicated some murine tumors [183] and, in one murine BMT model, reduced GVHD without abrogating GVLE [184]. Moreover, exogenous lymphokines, e.g. IL-2, IL-12 and others, might modulate NK receptors and ligand expression on target cells, and might influence the balance between activating and inhibitory receptors on NK cells [20]—possibly in favor of GVTE.

References

1 Appelbaum FR. Haematopoietic cell transplantation as immunotherapy. *Nature* 2001; **411**: 385–9.
2 Fefer A. Tumor immunotherapy. Antineoplastic and immunosuppressive agents. In: Sartorelli A, Johns D, eds. *Handbook of Experimental Pharmacology*. New York: Springer Verlag, 1974: 528–54.
3 Fefer A, Einstein A Jr, Cheever M et al. Models for syngeneic adoptive chemoimmunotherapy of murine leukemias. *Ann NY Acad Sci* 1976; **276**: 573–83.
4 Fefer A, Cheever M, Greenberg P. Overview of prospects and problems of lymphocyte transfer for cancer therapy. In: Fefer A, Goldstein A, eds. *Progress in Cancer Research and Therapy: the Potential Role of T Cells in Cancer Therapy*. New York: Raven Press, 1982: 1–6.
5 Fass L, Fefer A. Studies of adoptive chemoimmunotherapy of a Friend virus-induced lymphoma. *Cancer Res* 1972; **32**: 997–1001.
6 Fass L, Fefer A. Factors related to therapeutic efficacy in adoptive chemoimmunotherapy of a Friend virus-induced lymphoma. *Cancer Res* 1972; **32**: 2427–31.
7 Greenberg PD, Cheever MA, Fefer A. Eradication of disseminated murine leukemia by chemo-immunotherapy with cyclophosphamide and adoptively transferred immune syngeneic Lyt-1^+2^- lymphocytes. *J Exp Med* 1981; **154**: 952–63.
8 Cheever M, Greenberg P, Fefer A et al. Augmentation of the anti-tumor therapeutic efficacy of long-term cultured T lymphocytes by $in\ vivo$ administration of purified interleukin-2. *J Exp Med* 1982; **155**: 968–80.
9 Greenberg PD. Adoptive T cell therapy of tumors: mechanisms operative in the recognition and elimination of tumor cells. *Adv Immunol* 1991; **49**: 281–355.
10 Proietti E, Greco G, Garrone B et al. Importance of cyclophosphamide-induced bystander effect on T cells for a successful tumor eradication in response to adoptive immunotherapy in mice. *J Clin Invest* 1998; **101**: 429–41.
11 Schirrmacher V, Muerkoster S, Umansky V. Antagonistic effects of systemic interleukin 2 on immune T cell-mediated graft-versus-leukemia reactivity. *Clin Cancer Res* 1998; **4**: 2635–45.
12 Saxton ML, Longo DL, Wetzel HE et al. Adoptive transfer of anti-CD3-activated $CD4^+$ T cells plus cyclophosphamide and liposome-encapsulated interleukin-2 cure murine MC-38 and 3LL tumors and establish tumor-specific immunity. *Blood* 1997; **89**: 2529–36.
13 Lowdell MW, Lamb L, Hoyle C et al. Non-MHC-restricted cytotoxic cells: their roles in the control and treatment of leukaemias. *Br J Haematol* 2001; **114**: 11–24.
14 Grimm EA, Mazumder A, Zhang HZ et al. Lymphokine-activated killer cell phenomenon. Lysis of natural killer-resistant fresh solid tumor cells by interleukin 2-activated autologous human peripheral blood lymphocytes. *J Exp Med* 1982; **155**: 1823–41.
15 Ortaldo JR, Mason A, Overton R. Lymphokine-activated killer cells. Analysis of progenitors and effectors. *J Exp Med* 1986; **164**: 1193–205.
16 Mule JJ, Shu S, Rosenberg SA. The anti-tumor efficacy of lymphokine-activated killer cells and recombinant interleukin 2 $in\ vivo$. *J Immunol* 1985; **135**: 646–52.
17 Rosenberg SA, Mule JJ, Spiess PJ et al. Regression of established pulmonary metastases and subcutaneous tumor mediated by the systemic administration of high-dose recombinant interleukin 2. *J Exp Med* 1985; **161**: 1169–88.
18 Lafreniere R, Rosenberg SA. Successful immunotherapy of murine experimental hepatic metastases with lymphokine-activated killer cells and recombinant interleukin 2. *Cancer Res* 1985; **45**: 3735–41.
19 Verneris MR, Baker J, Edinger M et al. Studies of $ex\ vivo$ activated and expanded $CD8^+$ NK-T cells in humans and mice. *J Clin Immunol* 2002; **22**: 131–6.
20 Farag SS, Fehniger TA, Ruggeri L et al. Natural killer cell receptors: new biology and insights into the graft-versus-leukemia effect. *Blood* 2002; **100**: 1935–47.
21 Koh CY, Blazar BR, George T et al. Augmentation of antitumor effects by NK cell inhibitory receptor blockade $in\ vitro$ and $in\ vivo$. *Blood* 2001; **97**: 3132–7.
22 Barnes D, Loutit J, Neal F. Treatment of murine leukemia with X-rays and homologous bone marrow. *Br Med J* 1956; **2**: 626–30.
23 Hsieh MH, Patterson AE, Korngold R. T-cell subsets mediate graft-versus-myeloid leukemia responses via different cytotoxic mechanisms. *Biol Blood Marrow Transplant* 2000; **6**: 231–40.
24 Barnes D, Loutit J. Treatment of murine leukemia with X-rays and homologous bone marrow. *Br J Haematol* 1957; **2**: 241–52.

25 Bortin MM, Rimm AA, Saltzstein EC. Graft versus leukemia. Quantification of adoptive immunotherapy in murine leukemia. *Science* 1973; **179**: 811–3.

26 Mathé G, Amiel J, Niemetz J. Greffe de moelle osseuse apres irradiation totale chez des souris leucémiques suivie de l'administration d'un antimitotique pour réduire la fréquence du syndrome secondaire et ajouter a l'effet antileucémique. *CR Acad Sci (Paris)* 1962; **254**: 3603–5.

27 Fefer A. Adoptive chemoimmunotherapy of a Moloney lymphoma. *Int J Cancer* 1971; **8**: 364–73.

28 Slavin S, Weiss L, Morecki S et al. Eradication of murine leukemia with histoincompatible marrow grafts in mice conditioned with total lymphoid irradiation (TLI). *Cancer Immunol Immunother* 1981; **11**: 155–8.

29 Truitt R, LeFever A, Shih C-Y. Graft-versus leukemia reactions. Experimental models and clinical trials. In: Gale RP, Champlin R, eds. *Progress in Bone Marrow Transplantation*. New York: Alan R Liss, 1987: 219–32.

30 Weiss L, Lubin I, Factorowich I et al. Effective graft-versus-leukemia effects independent of graft-versus-host disease after T cell-depleted allogeneic bone marrow transplantation in a murine model of B cell leukemia/lymphoma. Role of cell therapy and recombinant IL-2. *J Immunol* 1994; **153**: 2562–7.

31 Truitt R, Johnson B, McCabe C et al. Graft versus leukemia. In: Ferrara J, Deeg H, Burakoff S, eds. *Graft Versus Host Disease: Immunology, Pathophysiology, and Treatment*. New York: Dekker, 1996: 385–424.

32 Fefer A. Treatment of a Moloney lymphoma with cyclophosphamide and H-2-incompatible spleen cells. *Cancer Res* 1973; **33**: 641–4.

33 Slavin S, Ackerstein A, Naparstek E et al. The graft-versus-leukemia (GVL) phenomenon: is GVL separable from GVHD? *Bone Marrow Transplant* 1990; **6**: 155–61.

34 Antin JH. Graft-versus-leukemia: no longer an epiphenomenon [editorial]. *Blood* 1993; **82**: 2273–7.

35 Tsukada N, Kobata T, Aizawa Y et al. Graft-versus-leukemia effect and graft-versus-host disease can be differentiated by cytotoxic mechanisms in a murine model of allogeneic bone marrow transplantation. *Blood* 1999; **93**: 2738–47.

36 Pan L, Teshima T, Hill GR et al. Granulocyte colony-stimulating factor-mobilized allogeneic stem cell transplantation maintains graft-versus-leukemia effects through a perforin-dependent pathway while preventing graft-versus-host disease. *Blood* 1999; **93**: 4071–8.

37 Sad S, Marcotte R, Mosmann TR. Cytokine-induced differentiation of precursor mouse $CD8^+$ T cells into cytotoxic $CD8^+$ T cells secreting T_H1 or T_H2 cytokines. *Immunity* 1995; **2**: 271–9.

38 Truitt RL, Johnson BD. Principles of graft-vs.-leukemia reactivity. *Biol Blood Marrow Transplant* 1995; **1**: 61–8.

39 Abhyankar S, Gilliland DG, Ferrara JL. Interleukin-1 is a critical effector molecule during cytokine dysregulation in graft versus host disease to minor histocompatibility antigens. *Transplantation* 1993; **56**: 1518–23.

40 Billiau AD, Fevery S, Rutgeerts O et al. Crucial role of timing of donor lymphocyte infusion in generating dissociated graft-versus-host and graft-versus-leukemia responses in mice receiving allogeneic bone marrow transplants. *Blood* 2002; **100**: 1894–902.

41 Mapara MY, Kim YM, Wang SP et al. Donor lymphocyte infusions mediate superior graft-versus-leukemia effects in mixed compared to fully allogeneic chimeras: a critical role for host antigen-presenting cells. *Blood* 2002; **100**: 1903–9.

42 Johnson BD, Becker EE, Truitt RL. Graft-vs.-host and graft-vs.-leukemia reactions after delayed infusions of donor T-subsets. *Biol Blood Marrow Transplant* 1999; **5**: 123–32.

43 Taylor PA, Lees CJ, Blazar BR. The infusion of *ex vivo* activated and expanded $CD4^+CD25^+$ immune regulatory cells inhibits graft-versus-host disease lethality. *Blood* 2002; **99**: 3493–9.

44 Ruggeri L, Capanni M, Martelli MF et al. Cellular therapy: exploiting NK cell alloreactivity in transplantation. *Curr Opin Hematol* 2001; **8**: 355–9.

45 Ruggeri L, Capanni M, Urbani E et al. Effectiveness of donor natural killer cell alloreactivity in mismatched hematopoietic transplants. *Science* 2002; **295**: 2097–100.

46 Slavin S, Eckerstein A, Weiss L. Adoptive immunotherapy in conjunction with bone marrow transplantation: amplification of natural host defence mechanisms against cancer by recombinant IL-2. *Nat Immun Cell Growth Regul* 1988; **7**: 180–4.

47 Charak BS, Brynes RK, Groshen S et al. Bone marrow transplantation with interleukin-2-activated bone marrow followed by interleukin-2 therapy for acute myeloid leukemia in mice. *Blood* 1990; **76**: 2187–90.

48 Malkovsky M, Brenner MK, Hunt R et al. T-cell depletion of allogeneic bone marrow prevents acceleration of graft-versus-host disease induced by exogenous interleukin 2. *Cell Immunol* 1986; **103**: 476–80.

49 Ghayur T, Seemayer TA, Kongshavn PA et al. Graft-versus-host reactions in the beige mouse. An investigation of the role of host and donor natural killer cells in the pathogenesis of graft-versus-host disease. *Transplantation* 1987; **44**: 261–7.

50 Sprent J, Schaefer M, Gao EK et al. Role of T cell subsets in lethal graft-versus-host disease (GVHD) directed to class I versus class II H-2 differences. I. $L3T4^+$ cells can either augment or retard GVHD elicited by $Lyt-2^+$ cells in class I different hosts. *J Exp Medical* 1988; **167**: 556–69.

51 Toshitani A, Taniguchi K, Himeno K et al. Adoptive transfer of H-2-incompatible lymphokine-activated killer (LAK) cells: an approach for successful cancer immunotherapy free from graft-versus-host disease (GVHD) using murine models. *Cell Immunol* 1988; **115**: 373–82.

52 Clancy J Jr, Goral J, Kovacs EJ et al. Role of recombinant interleukin-2 (rIL-2) and large granular lymphocytes (LGLs) in acute rat graft-versus-host disease (GVHD). *Transplant Proc* 1989; **21**: 88–9.

53 Sykes M, Romick ML, Sachs DH. Interleukin 2 prevents graft-versus-host disease while preserving the graft-versus-leukemia effect of allogeneic T cells. *Proc Natl Acad Sci U S A* 1990; **87**: 5633–7.

54 Sykes M, Romick ML, Hoyles KA et al. In vivo administration of interleukin 2 plus T cell-depleted syngeneic marrow prevents graft-versus-host disease mortality and permits alloengraftment. *J Exp Med* 1990; **171**: 645–58.

55 Sykes M, Abraham VS, Harty MW et al. IL-2 reduces graft-versus-host disease and preserves a graft-versus-leukemia effect by selectively inhibiting $CD4^+$ T cell activity. *J Immunol* 1993; **150**: 197–205.

56 Sykes M, Harty MW, Szot GL et al. Interleukin-2 inhibits graft-versus-host disease-promoting activity of $CD4^+$ cells while preserving $CD4^-$ and CD8-mediated graft-versus-leukemia effects. *Blood* 1994; **83**: 2560–9.

57 Cheever MA, Chen W. Therapy with cultured T cells: principles revisited. *Immunol Rev* 1997; **157**: 177–94.

58 Rosenberg SA. Progress in human tumour immunology and immunotherapy. *Nature* 2001; **411**: 380–4.

59 van der Bruggen P, Traversari C, Chomez P et al. A gene encoding an antigen recognized by cytolytic T lymphocytes on a human melanoma. *Science* 1991; **254**: 1643–7.

60 Yee C, Gilbert MJ, Riddell SR et al. Isolation of tyrosinase-specific $CD8^+$ and $CD4^+$ T cell clones from the peripheral blood of melanoma patients following *in vitro* stimulation with recombinant vaccinia virus. *J Immunol* 1996; **157**: 4079–86.

61 Itoh K, Platsoucas CD, Balch CM. Autologous tumor-specific cytotoxic T lymphocytes in the infiltrate of human metastatic melanomas. Activation by interleukin 2 and autologous tumor cells, and involvement of the T cell receptor. *J Exp Med* 1988; **168**: 1419–41.

62 Topalian SL, Solomon D, Rosenberg SA. Tumor-specific cytolysis by lymphocytes infiltrating human melanomas. *J Immunol* 1989; **142**: 3714–25.

63 Thompson J, Lindgren C, Benz L et al. Tumor-infiltrating lymphocytes (TIL) for the treatment of malignant melanoma (MM): a pilot trial. *Proc Amer Assoc Cancer Res* 1991; **32**: 270a [Abstract].

64 Lindgren C, Thompson J, Higuchi C et al. Growth and autologous tumor lysis by tumor-infiltrating lymphocytes from metastatic melanoma expanded in interleukin-2 or interleukin-2 plus interleukin-4. *J Immunother* 1993; **14**: 322–8.

65 Rosenberg SA, Packard BS, Aebersold PM et al. Use of tumor-infiltrating lymphocytes and interleukin-2 in the immunotherapy of patients with metastatic melanoma. A preliminary report. *N Engl J Med* 1988; **319**: 1676–80.

66 Aebersold P, Hyatt C, Johnson S et al. Lysis of autologous melanoma cells by tumor–infiltrating lymphocytes: association with clinical response. *J Natl Cancer Inst* 1991; **83**: 932–7.

67 Dudley ME, Wunderlich JR, Yang JC et al. A phase I study of nonmyeloablative chemotherapy and adoptive transfer of autologous tumor antigen-specific T lymphocytes in patients with metastatic melanoma. *J Immunother* 2002; **25**: 243–51.

68 Dudley ME, Wunderlich JR, Robbins PF et al. Cancer regression and autoimmunity in patients after clonal repopulation with antitumor lymphocytes. *Science* 2002; **298**: 850–4.

69 Lotzova E, Ades EW. Natural killer cells. Definition, heterogeneity, lytic mechanism, functions and clinical application. Highlights of the Fifth International Workshop on natural killer cells, Hilton Head Island, NC, March 1988. *Nat Immun Cell Growth Regul* 1989; **8**: 1–9.

70 Oshimi K, Oshimi Y, Akutsu M et al. Cytotoxicity of interleukin 2-activated lymphocytes for leukemia and lymphoma cells. *Blood* 1986; **68**: 938–48.

71 Dawson MM, Johnston D, Taylor GM et al. Lymphokine activated killing of fresh human leukaemias. *Leuk Res* 1986; **10**: 683–8.

72 Lotzova E, Savary CA, Herberman RB. Induction of NK cell activity against fresh human leukemia in culture with interleukin 2. *J Immunol* 1987; **138**: 2718–27.

73 Mackinnon S, Hows JM, Goldman JM. Induction of *in vitro* graft-versus-leukemia activity following bone marrow transplantation for chronic myeloid leukemia. *Blood* 1990; **76**: 2037–45.

74 Landay AL, Zarcone D, Grossi CE *et al*. Relationship between target cell cycle and susceptibility to natural killer lysis. *Cancer Res* 1987; **47**: 2767–70.

75 Allavena P, Damia G, Colombo T *et al*. Lymphokine-activated killer (LAK) and monocyte-mediated cytotoxicity on tumor cell lines resistant to antitumor agents. *Cell Immunol* 1989; **120**: 250–8.

76 Andersson ML, Stam NJ, Klein G *et al*. Aberrant expression of HLA class-I antigens in Burkitt lymphoma cells. *Int J Cancer* 1991; **47**: 544–50.

77 Rosenberg SA, Lotze MT, Muul LM *et al*. A progress report on the treatment of 157 patients with advanced cancer using lymphokine-activated killer cells and interleukin-2 or high-dose interleukin-2 alone. *N Engl J Med* 1987; **316**: 889–97.

78 Rosenberg SA. Interleukin-2 and the development of immunotherapy for the treatment of patients with cancer. *Cancer J Sci Am* 2000; **6**: S2–7.

79 West WH, Tauer KW, Yannelli JR *et al*. Constant-infusion recombinant interleukin-2 in adoptive immunotherapy of advanced cancer. *N Engl J Med* 1987; **316**: 898–905.

80 Thompson J, Shulman K, Benyunes M *et al*. Prolonged continuous intravenous infusion interleukin-2 and lymphokine-activated killer cell therapy for metastatic renal cell carcinoma. *J Clin Oncol* 1992; **10**: 960–8.

81 Fyfe G, Fisher RI, Rosenberg SA *et al*. Results of treatment of 255 patients with metastatic renal cell carcinoma who received high-dose recombinant interleukin-2 therapy. *J Clin Oncol* 1995; **13**: 688–96.

82 Gold PJ, Thompson JA, Markowitz DR *et al*. Metastatic renal cell carcinoma: long-term survival after therapy with high-dose continuous-infusion interleukin-2. *Cancer J Sci Am* 1997; **3**: S85–91.

83 Gisselbrecht C, Maraninchi D, Pico JL *et al*. Interleukin-2 treatment in lymphoma: a phase II multicenter study. *Blood* 1994; **83**: 2081–5.

84 Fefer A. Interleukin-2: clinical applications to hematologic malignancies. In: Rosenberg S, ed. *Principles and Practice of the Biologic Therapy of Cancer*, 3rd edn. Philadelphia: Lippincott, Williams & Wilkins, 2000: 83–92.

85 Meloni G, Foa R, Vignetti M *et al*. Interleukin-2 may induce prolonged remissions in advanced acute myelogenous leukemia. *Blood* 1994; **84**: 2158–63.

86 Meloni G, Vignetti M, Andrizzi C *et al*. Interleukin-2 for the treatment of advanced acute myelogenous leukemia patients with limited disease: updated experience with 20 cases. *Leuk Lymphoma* 1996; **21**: 429–35.

87 Robinson N, Benyunes MC, Thompson JA *et al*. Interleukin-2 after autologous stem cell transplantation for hematologic malignancy: a phase I/II study. *Bone Marrow Transplant* 1997; **19**: 435–42.

88 Sievers EL, Lange BJ, Sondel PM *et al*. Feasibility, toxicity, and biologic response of interleukin-2 after consolidation chemotherapy for acute myelogenous leukemia: a report from the Children's Cancer Group. *J Clin Oncol* 1998; **16**: 914–9.

89 Sznol M, Parkinson DR. Clinical applications of IL-2. *Oncology* 1994; **8**: 61–7.

90 Fefer A. Clinical applications of IL-2 reviewed. *Oncology* 1994; **8**: 74–5.

91 Thompson J, Lee D, Lindgren C *et al*. Influence of dose and duration of infusion of interleukin-2 on toxicity and immunomodulation. *J Clin Oncol* 1988; **6**: 669–78.

92 Rosenberg SA, Lotze MT, Yang JC *et al*. Prospective randomized trial of high-dose interleukin-2 alone or in conjunction with lymphokine-activated killer cells for the treatment of patients with advanced cancer. *J Natl Cancer Inst* 1993; **85**: 622–32.

93 Odom L, August C, Githens J *et al*. Remission of relapsed leukaemia during graft-versus-host reaction: a 'graft-versus-leukaemia reaction' in man? *Lancet* 1978; **ii**: 537–40.

94 Odom L, August C, Githens J *et al*. 'Graft-versus-leukemia' reaction following bone marrow transplantation for acute lymphoblastic leukemia. In: O'Kunewick J, Meredith R, eds. *Graft-Versus-Leukemia in Man and Animal Models*. Boca Raton: CRC Press, 1981: 25–43.

95 Sullivan KM, Shulman HM. Chronic graft-versus-host disease, obliterative bronchiolitis, and graft-versus-leukemia effect: case histories. *Transplant Proc* 1989; **21**: 51–62.

96 Higano CS, Brixey M, Bryant EM *et al*. Durable complete remission of acute nonlymphocytic leukemia associated with discontinuation of immunosuppression following relapse after allogeneic bone marrow transplantation. A case report of a probable graft-versus-leukemia effect. *Transplantation* 1990; **50**: 175–7.

97 Collins RH Jr, Rogers ZR, Bennett M *et al*. Hematologic relapse of chronic myelogenous leukemia following allogeneic bone marrow transplantation: Apparent graft-versus-leukemia effect following abrupt discontinuation of immunosuppression. *Bone Marrow Transplant* 1992; **10**: 391–5.

98 Rondon G, Giralt S, Huh Y *et al*. Graft-versus-leukemia effect after allogeneic bone marrow transplantation for chronic lymphocytic leukemia. *Bone Marrow Transplant* 1996; **18**: 669–72.

99 deMagalhaes-Silverman M, Donnenberg A, Hammert L *et al*. Induction of graft-versus-leukemia effect in a patient with chronic lymphocytic leukemia. *Bone Marrow Transplant* 1997; **20**: 175–7.

100 van Besien KW, de Lima M, Giralt SA *et al*. Management of lymphoma recurrence after allogeneic transplantation: the relevance of graft-versus-lymphoma effect. *Bone Marrow Transplant* 1997; **19**: 977–82.

101 Libura J, Hoffmann T, Passweg J *et al*. Graft-versus-myeloma after withdrawal of immunosuppression following allogeneic peripheral stem cell transplantation. *Bone Marrow Transplant* 1999; **24**: 925–7.

102 Moscardo F, Martinez JA, Sanz GF *et al*. Graft-versus-tumour effect in non-small-cell lung cancer after allogeneic peripheral blood stem cell transplantation. *Br J Haematol* 2000; **111**: 708–10.

103 Horowitz MM. Clinical observations of graft-versus-tumor effects after conventional transplantation: what do they teach us? In: Perry MC, ed. *American Society of Clinical Oncology Educational Book, 38th Annual Meeting, Spring 2002*. Alexandria, VA: American Society of Clinical Oncology, 2002: 68–76.

104 Fefer A, Sullivan K, Weiden P *et al*. Graft versus leukemia effect in man. The relapse rate of acute leukemia is lower after allogeneic than after syngeneic marrow transplantation. In: Truitt R, Gale R, Bortin M, eds. *Cellular Immunotherapy of Cancer*. New York: Alan R Liss, 1987: 401–8.

105 Gale R, Champlin R. How does bone-marrow transplantation cure leukaemia? *Lancet* 1984; **ii**: 28–30.

106 Weiden PL, Flournoy N, Thomas ED *et al*. Antileukemic effect of graft-versus-host disease in human recipients of allogeneic-marrow grafts. *N Engl J Med* 1979; **300**: 1068–73.

107 Weiden PL, Sullivan KM, Flournoy N *et al*. Antileukemic effect of chronic graft-versus-host disease: contribution to improved survival after allogeneic marrow transplantation. *N Engl J Med* 1981; **304**: 1529–33.

108 Butturini A, Bortin MM, Gale RP. Graft-versus-leukemia following bone marrow transplantation. *Bone Marrow Transplant* 1987; **2**: 233–42.

109 Ringden O, Horowitz MM. Graft-versus-leukemia reactions in humans. The Advisory Committee of the International Bone Marrow Transplant Registry. *Transplant Proc* 1989; **21**: 2989–92.

110 Horowitz MM, Gale RP, Sondel PM *et al*. Graft-versus-leukemia reactions after bone marrow transplantation. *Blood* 1990; **75**: 555–62.

111 Bacigalupo A, Van-Lint MT, Frassoni F *et al*. Graft-versus-leukemia effect following allogeneic bone marrow transplantation [letter]. *Br J Haematol* 1985; **61**: 749–51.

112 Sanders JE, Flournoy N, Thomas ED *et al*. Marrow transplant experience in children with acute lymphoblastic leukemia: an analysis of factors associated with survival, relapse, and graft vs. host disease. *Med Pediatr Oncol* 1985; **13**: 165–72.

113 Weisdorf DJ, Nesbit ME, Ramsay NK *et al*. Allogeneic bone marrow transplantation for acute lymphoblastic leukemia in remission: prolonged survival associated with acute graft-versus-host disease. *J Clin Oncol* 1987; **5**: 1348–55.

114 Kersey JH, Weisdorf D, Nesbit ME *et al*. Comparison of autologous and allogeneic bone marrow transplantation for treatment of high-risk refractory acute lymphoblastic leukemia. *N Engl J Med* 1987; **317**: 461–7.

115 Sullivan K, Fefer A, Witherspoon R *et al*. Graft-versus-leukemia in man. Relationship of acute and chronic graft-versus-host disease to relapse of acute leukemia following allogeneic bone marrow transplantation. In: Truitt R, Gale R, Bortin M, eds. *Cellular Immunotherapy of Cancer*. New York: Alan R Liss, 1987: 391–9.

116 Sullivan KM, Weiden PL, Storb R *et al*. Influence of acute and chronic graft-versus-host disease on relapse and survival after bone marrow transplantation from HLA-identical siblings as treatment of acute and chronic leukemia. *Blood* 1989; **73**: 1720–8.

117 Sullivan KM, Witherspoon RP, Storb R *et al*. Prednisone and azathioprine compared with prednisone and placebo for treatment of chronic graft-v-host disease: prognostic influence of prolonged thrombocytopenia after allogeneic marrow transplantation. *Blood* 1988; **72**: 546–54.

118 Goldman JM, Gale RP, Horowitz MM *et al*. Bone marrow transplantation for chronic myelogenous leukemia in chronic phase. Increased risk for relapse associated with T-cell depletion. *Ann Intern Med* 1988; **108**: 806–14.

119 Martin PJ, Clift RA, Fisher LD et al. HLA-identical marrow transplantation during accelerated-phase chronic myelogenous leukemia: analysis of survival and remission duration. *Blood* 1988; **72**: 1978–84.

120 Kolb HJ, Mittermuller J, Clemm C et al. Donor leukocyte transfusions for treatment of recurrent chronic myelogenous leukemia in marrow transplant patients. *Blood* 1990; **76**: 2462–5.

121 Kolb HJ, Schattenberg A, Goldman JM et al. Graft-versus-leukemia effect of donor lymphocyte transfusions in marrow grafted patients. European Group for Blood and Marrow Transplantation Working Party Chronic Leukemia. *Blood* 1995; **86**: 2041–50.

122 Collins RH Jr, Shpilberg O, Drobyski WR et al. Donor leukocyte infusions in 140 patients with relapsed malignancy after allogeneic bone marrow transplantation. *J Clin Oncol* 1997; **15**: 433–44.

123 Porter DL, Antin JH. The graft-versus-leukemia effects of allogeneic cell therapy. *Annu Rev Med* 1999; **50**: 369–86.

124 Levine JE, Braun T, Penza SL et al. Prospective trial of chemotherapy and donor leukocyte infusions for relapse of advanced myeloid malignancies after allogeneic stem-cell transplantation. *J Clin Oncol* 2002; **20**: 405–12.

125 Giralt S, Estey E, Albitar M et al. Engraftment of allogeneic hematopoietic progenitor cells with purine analog-containing chemotherapy: Harnessing graft-versus-leukemia without myeloablative therapy. *Blood* 1997; **89**: 4531–6.

126 Martino R, Caballero MD, Simon JA et al. Evidence for a graft-versus-leukemia effect after allogeneic peripheral blood stem cell transplantation with reduced-intensity conditioning in acute myelogenous leukemia and myelodysplastic syndromes. *Blood* 2002; **100**: 2243–5.

127 Childs R, Drachenberg D. Allogeneic stem cell transplantation for renal cell carcinoma. *Curr Opin Urol* 2001; **11**: 495–502.

128 Halverson DC, Schwartz GN, Carter C et al. In vitro generation of allospecific human $CD8^+$ T cells of Tc1 and Tc2 phenotype. *Blood* 1997; **90**: 2089–96.

129 van-Leeuwen A, Schrier PI, Giphart MJ et al. TCA. A polymorphic genetic marker in leukemias and melanoma cell lines. *Blood* 1986; **67**: 1139–42.

130 Voogt PJ, Goulmy E, Veenhof WF et al. Cellularly defined minor histocompatibility antigens are differentially expressed on human hematopoietic progenitor cells. *J Exp Med* 1988; **168**: 2337–47.

131 Falkenburg JH, Goselink HM, van-der-Harst D et al. Growth inhibition of clonogenic leukemic precursor cells by minor histocompatibility antigen-specific cytotoxic T lymphocytes. *J Exp Med* 1991; **174**: 27–33.

132 van-Lochem E, de-Gast B, Goulmy E. In vitro separation of host specific graft-versus-host and graft-versus-leukemia cytotoxic T cell activities. *Bone Marrow Transplant* 1992; **10**: 181–3.

133 Dolstra H, Fredrix H, Preijers F et al. Recognition of a B cell leukemia-associated minor histocompatibility antigen by CTL. *J Immunol* 1997; **158**: 560–5.

134 Faber LM, van-der-Hoeven J, Goulmy E et al. Recognition of clonogenic leukemic cells, remission bone marrow and HLA-identical donor bone marrow by $CD8^+$ or $CD4^+$ minor histocompatibility antigen-specific cytotoxic T lymphocytes. *J Clin Invest* 1995; **96**: 877–83.

135 Warren EH, Greenberg PD, Riddell SR. Cytotoxic T-lymphocyte-defined human minor histocompatibility antigens with a restricted tissue distribution. *Blood* 1998; **91**: 2197–207.

136 Mutis T, Schrama E, van-Luxemburg-Heijs SA et al. HLA class II restricted T-cell reactivity to a developmentally regulated antigen shared by leukemic cells and $CD34^+$ early progenitor cells. *Blood* 1997; **90**: 1083–90.

137 Scheibenbogen C, Letsch A, Thiel E et al. CD8 T-cell responses to Wilms tumor gene product WT1 and proteinase 3 in patients with acute myeloid leukemia. *Blood* 2002; **100**: 2132–7.

138 Disis ML, Cheever MA. Oncogenic proteins as tumor antigens. *Curr Opin Immunol* 1996; **8**: 637–42.

139 Wen YJ, Min R, Tricot G et al. Tumor lysate-specific cytotoxic T lymphocytes in multiple myeloma: promising effector cells for immunotherapy. *Blood* 2002; **99**: 3280–5.

140 Lamikanra A, Pan ZK, Isaacs SN et al. Regression of established human papillomavirus type 16 (HPV-16) immortalized tumors in vivo by vaccinia viruses expressing different forms of HPV-16 E7 correlates with enhanced $CD8^+$ T-cell responses that home to the tumor site. *J Virol* 2001; **75**: 9654–64.

141 Peace DJ, Smith JW, Chen W et al. Lysis of ras oncogene-transformed cells by specific cytotoxic T lymphocytes elicited by primary in vitro immunization with mutated ras peptide. *J Exp Med* 1994; **179**: 473–9.

142 Noguchi Y, Chen YT, Old LJ. A mouse mutant p53 product recognized by $CD4^+$ and $CD8^+$ T cells. *Proc Natl Acad Sci U S A* 1994; **91**: 3171–5.

143 Chen W, Peace DJ, Rovira DK et al. T-cell immunity to the joining region of p210 BCR-ABL protein. *Proc Natl Acad Sci U S A* 1992; **89**: 1468–72.

144 Choudhury A, Gajewski JL, Liang JC et al. Use of leukemic dendritic cells for the generation of antileukemic cellular cytotoxicity against Philadelphia chromosome-positive chronic myelogenous leukemia. *Blood* 1997; **89**: 1133–42.

145 Gambacorti-Passerini C, Grignani F, Arienti F et al. Human CD4 lymphocytes specifically recognize a peptide representing the fusion region of the hybrid protein pml/RARα present in acute promyelocytic leukemia cells. *Blood* 1993; **81**: 1369–75.

146 Falkenburg JH, Wafelman AR, Joosten P et al. Complete remission of accelerated phase chronic myeloid leukemia by treatment with leukemia-reactive cytotoxic T lymphocytes. *Blood* 1999; **94**: 1201–8.

147 Cardoso AA, Seamon MJ, Afonso HM et al. Ex vivo generation of human anti-pre-B leukemia-specific autologous cytolytic T cells. *Blood* 1997; **90**: 549–61.

148 Molldrem JJ, Lee PP, Wang C et al. Evidence that specific T lymphocytes may participate in the elimination of chronic myelogenous leukemia. *Nat Med* 2000; **6**: 1018–23.

149 Hercend T, Takvorian T, Nowill A et al. Characterization of natural killer cells with anti-leukemia activity following allogeneic bone marrow transplantation. *Blood* 1986; **67**: 722–8.

150 Delmon L, Ythier A, Moingeon P et al. Characterization of antileukemia cells' cytotoxic effector function. Implications for monitoring natural killer responses following allogeneic bone marrow transplantation. *Transplantation* 1986; **42**: 252–6.

151 Reittie JE, Gottlieb D, Heslop HE et al. Endogenously generated activated killer cells circulate after autologous and allogeneic marrow transplantation but not after chemotherapy. *Blood* 1989; **73**: 1351–8.

152 Higuchi C, Thompson J, Cox T et al. Lymphokine-activated killer function following autologous bone marrow transplantation for refractory hematologic malignancies. *Cancer Res* 1989; **49**: 5509–13.

153 Rooney CM, Wimperis JZ, Brenner MK et al. Natural killer cell activity following T-cell depleted allogeneic bone marrow transplantation. *Br J Haematol* 1986; **62**: 413–20.

154 Sullivan KM, Deeg HJ, Sanders J et al. Hyperacute graft-v-host disease in patients not given immunosuppression after allogeneic marrow transplantation. *Blood* 1986; **67**: 1172–5.

155 Sullivan KM, Storb R, Buckner CD et al. Graft-versus-host disease as adoptive immunotherapy in patients with advanced hematologic neoplasms. *N Engl J Med* 1989; **320**: 828–34.

156 Mackinnon S, Papadopoulos EB, Carabasi MH et al. Adoptive immunotherapy evaluating escalating doses of donor leukocytes for relapse of chronic myeloid leukemia after bone marrow transplantation: separation of graft-versus-leukemia responses from graft-versus-host disease. *Blood* 1995; **86**: 1261–8.

157 Giralt S, Hester J, Huh Y et al. CD8-depleted donor lymphocyte infusion as treatment for relapsed chronic myelogenous leukemia after allogeneic bone marrow transplantation. *Blood* 1995; **86**: 4337–43.

158 Davies SM, Ruggieri L, DeFor T et al. Evaluation of KIR ligand incompatibility in mismatched unrelated donor hematopoietic transplants. Killer immunoglobulin-like receptor. *Blood* 2002; **100**: 3825–7.

159 Soiffer RJ, Murray C, Gonin R et al. Effect of low-dose interleukin-2 on disease relapse after T-cell-depleted allogeneic bone marrow transplantation. *Blood* 1994; **84**: 964–71.

160 Robinson N, Sanders JE, Benyunes MC et al. Phase I trial of interleukin-2 after unmodified HLA-matched sibling bone marrow transplantation for children with acute leukemia. *Blood* 1996; **87**: 1249–54.

161 Slavin S, Naparstek E, Nagler A et al. Allogeneic cell therapy with donor peripheral blood cells and recombinant human interleukin-2 to treat leukemia relapse after allogeneic bone marrow transplantation. *Blood* 1996; **87**: 2195–204.

162 Johnson BD, Truitt RL. Delayed infusion of immunocompetent donor cells after bone marrow transplantation breaks graft-host tolerance allows for persistent antileukemic reactivity without severe graft-versus-host disease. *Blood* 1995; **85**: 3302–12.

163 Baron F, Beguin Y. Preemptive cellular immunotherapy after T-cell-depleted allogeneic hematopoietic stem cell transplantation. *Biol Blood Marrow Transplant* 2002; **8**: 351–9.

164 Fefer A, Einstein AB, Thomas ED et al. Bone-marrow transplantation for hematologic neoplasia in 16 patients with identical twins. *N Engl J Med* 1974; **290**: 1389–93.

165 Fefer A, Buckner CD, Thomas ED et al. Cure of hematologic neoplasia with transplantation of marrow from identical twins. *N Engl J Med* 1977; **297**: 146–8.

166 Hess AD, Thoburn CJ. Immunobiology and immunotherapeutic implications of syngeneic/autologous graft-versus-host disease. *Immunol Rev* 1997; **157**: 111–23.

167 Fefer A, Robinson N, Benyunes MC *et al*. Interleukin-2 therapy after bone marrow or stem cell transplantation for hematologic malignancies. *Cancer J Sci Am* 1997; **3** (Suppl. 1): S48–53.

168 Fefer A. Interleukin-2 in the treatment of hematologic malignancies. *Cancer J Sci Am* 2000; **6**: S31–2.

169 Neubauer MA, Benyunes MC, Thompson JA *et al*. Lymphokine-activated killer (LAK) precursor cell activity is present in infused peripheral blood stem cells and in the blood after autologous peripheral blood stem cell transplantation. *Bone Marrow Transplant* 1994; **13**: 311–6.

170 Higuchi CM, Thompson JA, Petersen FB *et al*. Toxicity and immunomodulatory effects of interleukin-2 after autologous bone marrow transplantation for hematologic malignancies. *Blood* 1991; **77**: 2561–8.

171 Benyunes MC, Massumoto C, York A *et al*. Interleukin-2 with or without lymphokine-activated killer cells as consolidative immunotherapy after autologous bone marrow transplantation for acute myelogenous leukemia. *Bone Marrow Transplant* 1993; **12**: 159–63.

172 Benyunes MC, Higuchi C, York A *et al*. Immunotherapy with interleukin 2 with or without lymphokine-activated killer cells after autologous bone marrow transplantation for malignant lymphoma: a feasibility trial. *Bone Marrow Transplant* 1995; **16**: 283–8.

173 Stein AS, O'Donnell MR, Slovak ML *et al*. Interleukin-2 following autologous stem cell transplant for adult patients with acute myeloid leukemia in first complete remission. *J Clin Oncol* 2003; 21: 615–23.

174 Attal M, Blaise D, Marit G *et al*. Consolidation treatment of adult acute lymphoblastic leukemia: a prospective, randomized trial comparing allogeneic versus autologous bone marrow transplantation and testing the impact of recombinant interleukin-2 after autologous bone marrow transplantation. BGMT Group. *Blood* 1995; **86**: 1619–28.

175 Kwak LW, Pennington R, Longo DL. Active immunization of murine allogeneic bone marrow transplant donors with B-cell tumor-derived idiotype: a strategy for enhancing the specific antitumor effect of marrow grafts. *Blood* 1996; **87**: 3053–60.

176 Anderson LD Jr, Mori S, Mann S *et al*. Pretransplant tumor antigen-specific immunization of allogeneic bone marrow transplant donors enhances graft-versus-tumor activity without exacerbation of graft-versus-host disease. *Cancer Res* 2000; **60**: 5797–802.

177 Borrello I, Sotomayor EM, Rattis FM *et al*. Sustaining the graft-versus-tumor effect through posttransplant immunization with granulocyte-macrophage colony-stimulating factor (GM-CSF)-producing tumor vaccines. *Blood* 2000; **95**: 3011–9.

178 Riddell SR, Watanabe KS, Goodrich JM *et al*. Restoration of viral immunity in immunodeficient humans by the adoptive transfer of T cell clones. *Science* 1992; **257**: 238–41.

179 Einsele H, Roosnek E, Rufer N *et al*. Infusion of cytomegalovirus (CMV)-specific T cells for the treatment of CMV infection not responding to antiviral chemotherapy. *Blood* 2002; **99**: 3916–22.

180 Heslop HE, Rooney CM. Adoptive cellular immunotherapy for EBV lymphoproliferative disease. *Immunol Rev* 1997; **157**: 217–22.

181 Falk CS, Noessner E, Weiss EH *et al*. Retaliation against tumor cells showing aberrant HLA expression using lymphokine activated killer-derived T cells. *Cancer Res* 2002; **62**: 480–7.

182 Lindgren CG, Thompson JA, Robinson N *et al*. Interleukin-12 induced cytolytic activity in lymphocytes from recipients of autologous and allogeneic stem cell transplants. *Bone Marrow Transplant* 1997; **19**: 867–73.

183 Brunda MJ, Luistro L, Warrier RR *et al*. Antitumor and antimetastatic activity of interleukin 12 against murine tumors. *J Exp Med* 1993; **178**: 1223–30.

184 Sykes M, Szot GL, Nguyen PL *et al*. Interleukin-12 inhibits murine graft-versus-host disease. *Blood* 1995; **86**: 2429–38.

29

Stanley R. Riddell & Philip D. Greenberg

Adoptive Immunotherapy with Antigen-Specific T Cells

Introduction

Adoptive T-cell therapy, in which large numbers of antigen-specific T cells generated *in vitro* are infused into a patient on the premise that establishing a large *in vivo* immune response will provide clinical benefit, offers the potential of overcoming many of the obstacles facing other therapeutic options for cancers, such as the lack of specificity for tumor cells and toxicity associated with chemotherapy, and the difficulties of inducing sufficiently potent *in vivo* immune responses with alternative immunotherapeutic strategies such as vaccination. Studies in rodent models have long suggested that T-cell therapy could be an effective therapeutic strategy [1,2], and there is now ample evidence in humans that transferred T cells can mediate *in vivo* therapeutic effects against human malignancies as well as opportunistic infections. The antileukemic activity of donor T cells which was inferred from the decreased rate of relapse observed in patients who develop graft-vs.-host disease (GVHD) following allogeneic hematopoietic cell transplantation (HCT) has been more formally demonstrated by the achievement of remissions in patients with leukemia that relapsed following HCT by infusion of donor lymphocytes [3–8]. Such donor lymphocytes are now routinely employed as the primary treatment modality for selected solid tumors as well as hematologic malignancies in the context of nonmyeloablative regimens followed by HCT [9–11]. However, in all of these settings, the donor T cells do not necessarily uniquely recognize the tumor but rather potentially broadly expressed antigens, and thus significant and potentially fatal toxicity from GVHD can occur. Such toxicity is not an inherent consequence of the transfer of large numbers of donor T cells with effector functions, since the infusion of billions of T cells preselected for specificity for a virus to prevent and/or treat cytomegalovirus (CMV) or Epstein–Barr virus (EBV) infection following HCT has been shown to be both effective and safe [12–14]. Thus, the potential for routinely employing specific adoptive T-cell therapy in human HCT recipients for opportunistic infections appears well-established, whereas a major obstacle to widespread application for treatment of malignancy remains the necessity to identify target antigens that can be selectively or preferentially recognized on tumor cells rather than normal tissues. Such antigen discovery has consequently become a major area of investigation and, with use of the rapid and precise cellular and molecular technologies now available for screening, several very promising targets have already been uncovered.

Technical issues, such as the optimal *in vitro* methods and conditions that should be employed to generate the large numbers of antigen-specific T cells required for adoptive therapy, still require resolution, but the cell culture process is becoming increasingly efficient and transferable to many laboratories. Studies in malignant melanoma have already demonstrated that it is feasible to generate and expand tumor reactive T-cell clones *in vitro*, and that clones derived with current techniques can traffic to tumor sites and mediate therapeutic antitumor responses *in vivo* [15,16]. Moreover, several biotechnology companies have been formed with the goal of improving the efficiency and reproducibility of the *in vitro* methods for generating and expanding tumor-reactive T cells. Precisely which techniques will be utilized, including variables such as which cytokines should be added during the induction and generation of reactive T cells, how reactive T cells should be isolated from the bulk population, and which and how much growth and survival factors or signals should be provided during the expansion phase, will likely depend on the nature of the responding T cell from which the effector cells are generated and the nature of the effector T cells required for transfer. For example, the addition of interleukin 12 (IL-12) may be important at the initiation of culture if primary responses from a naive T-cell population are being induced, whereas the addition of IL-15 may be helpful for expansion of primed cells [17,18]. Recent studies have also suggested that providing pro-survival signals, as can be delivered by ligation of molecules such as 4–1BB expressed on CD8+ T cells, may greatly enhance the cell yield from culture and shorten the time required to generate a desired cell dose [19].

The *in vivo* conditions established during an HCT may be particularly conducive for studying and establishing effective T-cell responses by adoptive T-cell transfer. Firstly, allogeneic HCT, by virtue of the genetic disparities between host and donor, creates a set of minor histocompatibility antigens (mHAs) that can potentially serve as targets for therapeutic T-cell responses. Secondly, the conditioning regimens administered to patients undergoing either a myeloablative or nonmyeloablative HCT include radiation therapy, chemotherapy and/or fludarabine, all of which deplete the reservoir of host T cells and consequently activate homeostatic mechanisms, such as the production of IL-7 and IL-15, that function to promote *in vivo* expansion of viable T cells [20,21]. A recent study has shown that T cells specific for melanoma antigens administered during a period of severe lymphopenia can expand *in vivo* to extraordinarily high frequencies with retention of function and antitumor activity [16]. At the current time, T-cell transfers after HCT are generally not initiated early post-HCT, but rather are delayed until there is evidence of leukemic relapse or persistence, at which time the size of the T-cell compartment has been largely restored. Thus, after antigens expressed by tumors have been validated as safe and potentially effective to target, administering the reactive T cells at early time points during the period of lymphopenia should both improve efficacy and decrease the technical demands by permitting infusion of smaller numbers of T cells that can subsequently expand *in vivo*. Finally, because of the lymphoablative regimens utilized in the conditioning regimens for HCT, many opportunistic infections develop which might have been controlled if the host had a T-cell response to the pathogen. Studies have already demonstrated that transfer of virus-specific T cells can prevent and/or treat established CMV or EBV infection [12,14]. These viral infections represent not only treatment targets but also provide ideal models for defining the principles for effective T-cell therapy in humans, including the phenotypes and functions of T cells that should be infused, the roles of $CD4^+$ and $CD8^+$ T cells and the requirements to sustain long-term effector and memory $CD8^+$ T-cell responses.

In this chapter we will discuss: (a) the progress that has already been made in specific adoptive T-cell therapy of viral infections post-HCT, in which it has also been possible to extensively investigate the underlying immunobiology; (b) the advances developing in T-cell therapy targeting mHAs expressed predominantly in the lineage from which the malignancy was derived rather than the tissues normally targeted in GVHD; (c) the advances developing in T-cell therapy targeting oncogenic proteins over-expressed in leukemias and lymphomas; and, finally, (d) the potential evolving with new cellular and molecular technologies that will likely influence the future directions, efficacy and applicability of T-cell therapy.

T-cell therapy of CMV infection

Background

Despite advances in antiviral chemotherapy, CMV infection and disease continue to contribute to significant morbidity and mortality after allogeneic HCT. The virology, epidemiology, pathology, diagnosis and standard therapy of CMV in HCT recipients are reviewed in Chapter 53 and the focus here will be on the immunobiology and immunotherapy of CMV. Prior to the use of antiviral chemotherapy, CMV pneumonia or gastrointestinal infection occurred in 40% of CMV-positive (CMV^+) allogeneic HCT recipients [22,23]. Viral load and deficient CMV-specific T-cell immunity were identified as major risk factors for CMV disease leading to optimism that antiviral drugs or T-cell therapy could be employed as therapy [24–27]. The administration of ganciclovir, which has potent activity against CMV, either alone or combined with immunoglobulin (Ig), to patients with established CMV pneumonia failed to reduce the mortality rate below 40% [28–30]. This disappointing result focused efforts on initiating drug therapy at the first sign of CMV reactivation. The administration of ganciclovir as prophylaxis for CMV infection, or as preemptive therapy at the onset of CMV viremia, antigenemia, or rising CMV DNA titres in blood, reduced the incidence of CMV disease to <10% in the first 100 days after HCT [31–36]. However, the use of prophylactic or preemptive ganciclovir was associated with bone marrow suppression, and an improvement in overall survival was difficult to document [33,34,36]. Moreover, although drug therapy reduced the viral load, it did not resolve the underlying T-cell deficiency and the incidence of CMV disease occurring more than 100 days after HCT when antiviral drug therapy was discontinued, increased dramatically to ~18% [37]. Thus, a therapeutic strategy capable of eliminating CMV as a significant problem after allogeneic HCT has not yet been defined.

Rationale for T-cell therapy

Murine models of CMV infection

Studies of the immunobiology and immunotherapy of murine cytomegalovirus (MCMV), which has a similar genomic organization and shares biologic properties with human CMV, have in part provided the rationale for T-cell therapy of human CMV infection. MCMV establishes a persistent latent infection in immunocompetent mice and reactivates and disseminates to visceral organs and bone marrow in mice rendered immunodeficient after treatment with gamma irradiation, corticosteroids, or antilymphocyte serum [38–40]. Studies in BALB/c mice have identified a critical role for adaptive $CD8^+$ T-cell immunity in controlling MCMV infection. The adoptive transfer of MCMV-specific $CD8^+$ cytotoxic T lymphocytes (CTLs) to immunodeficient mice prevented lethal primary infection and reestablished latency after reactivation [38,41,42]. The concurrent administration of $CD8^+$ CTLs and IL-2, normally produced by $CD4^+$ T-cells responding to viral antigens, improved the antiviral efficacy of the transferred $CD8^+$ T cells suggesting an important adjunctive role for virus-specific $CD4^+$ T cells in this model [43].

The specificity of the $CD8^+$ CTL response that provides protective immunity to MCMV in BALB/c mice was examined since it was perceived this would provide insights into the nature of human CMV proteins that might be appropriate targets for T-cell therapy. $CD8^+$ T cells recognize peptides, typically 8–11 amino acids in length, that are derived from the degradation of intracellular proteins by the proteosome, transported into the endoplasmic reticulum (ER) by the transporter-associated with antigen presentation, and delivered to the cell surface as a trimolecular complex with class I major histocompatibility complex (MHC) molecules and β_2-microglobulin [44]. Similar to human CMV, MCMV expresses its genome in three sequential phases termed immediate early (IE), early (E), and late (L). The $CD8^+$ CTL response elicited after MCMV infection of immunocompetent mice was focused on only two peptides—an epitope of the IE-1 protein presented by the L^d class I molecule and an epitope from the m164 E protein presented by D^d [45]. The induction of $CD8^+$ CTL responses specific for either of these epitopes alone is sufficient to protect mice from lethal MCMV challenge [46,47]. The mechanism responsible for the remarkable focus of CTLs on just two epitopes has not been completely elucidated but appears to in part relate to the expression of three MCMV proteins that interfere with the processing and presentation of MCMV antigens by class I MHC, presumably to allow infected cells to evade CTL recognition [48,49]. The IE-1 protein is expressed in infected cells prior to the MCMV immune evasion proteins and m164 is expressed in such abundance in the E phase that it overcomes the inhibitory effects on class I MHC [46,49].

Recovery of CMV-specific T-cell immunity after allogeneic HCT correlates with protection from CMV disease

The role of CMV-specific T cells in controlling human CMV infection has been addressed by examining whether the rate of recovery of functional CMV-specific $CD8^+$ and $CD4^+$ T cells after allogeneic HCT was a determinant in the development of CMV disease. The studies of CMV-specific T-cell reconstitution performed before ganciclovir was available to treat CMV reactivation provided the most informative data. In these studies, the recovery of $CD8^+$ CMV-specific T cells was examined by stimulating peripheral blood mononuclear cells (PBMCs) obtained at various times after HCT with autologous CMV-infected fibroblasts followed by analysis of cytotoxicity against CMV-infected and mock infected target cells. The recovery of $CD4^+$ CMV-specific T cells was examined by stimulating PBMCs with CMV antigen and evaluating ^3H-thymidine incorporation [26,27]. The reconstitution of functional $CD8^+$ and $CD4^+$ CMV-specific T cells was delayed until >60 days in the majority of HCT recipients and CMV disease occurred exclusively in the subset of patients with deficient $CD8^+$ T-cell immunity [26,27].

More recently, novel flow cytometry techniques, that employ fluorochrome labeled monoclonal antibodies specific for intracellular cytokines produced after peptide stimulation or class I MHC/peptide tetramers, have been used to directly quantify T-cells reactive with the CMV pp65 protein, which was identified as a target for the CTL response in CMV^+ donors [50–54]. Similar to the earlier findings using culture techniques, the recovery of $CD8^+$ T cells that produce interferon-gamma (IFN-γ) after stimulation with CMV pp65 peptides was delayed until a median of 90 days after allogeneic HCT [50]. Studies that employed class I MHC tetramers to detect pp65-specific CD8+ T cells demonstrated more rapid recovery than observed with culture methods or IFN-γ staining, and this discrepancy was explained by a lack of effector function in the recovering CD8+ CTLs detected with tetramers [55,56]. Patients in these later studies received preemptive antiviral therapy at the onset of CMV reactivation, and it was not possible to determine if there was a correlation between recovery of CMV-specific T-cell immunity and protection from CMV disease. However, a role for CMV-specific T cells in controlling CMV replication was supported by the observation that an increase in the intensity of immunosuppressive therapy to treat GVHD resulted in a decline in CD8+ CMV-specific T-cell numbers and an increased frequency of subsequent reactivation of CMV [50,55].

The recognition that CMV disease occurring >100 days after HCT is an increasing problem has led to studies evaluating a role for deficient T-cell immunity in the development of late CMV disease. In the largest study, absolute lymphopenia (<100/μL) and a deficiency of CMV-specific CD4+ T-helper (TH) and CD8+ T-cell responses measured by culture methods at day 80 after transplant were predictive of late CMV disease and mortality [37]. Consistent with earlier findings, the need to intensify or reinstitute immunosuppressive drug therapy to treat chronic GVHD resulted in a loss of functional CMV-specific T cells [37]. These findings suggest that stable reconstitution of CMV-specific T cells, particularly CD8+ CTLs, is essential to control persistent CMV infection and provide a rationale for evaluating whether adoptively transferring CMV-specific T cells from the donor to the respective recipient could restore protective responses. However, these studies also provide insight into potential obstacles for T-cell therapy of CMV infection. These include an incomplete understanding of the human CMV antigens recognized by T cells that mediate protective immunity in the immunocompetent host and the potential that immunosuppressive drugs administered to prevent or treat GVHD may inhibit the efficacy of transferred T cells.

Specificity and frequency of CMV-specific T cells in immunocompetent CMV+ donors

CD8+ cytotoxic T cells

The antigens recognized by CD8+ T cells are derived from the processing of intracellular proteins to peptides that are displayed at the cell surface complexed to class I MHC. This mode of presentation suggests that peptides from any of the >160 CMV proteins encoded by the 230 kb viral genome and expressed in infected cells could potentially be recognized by CD8+ CTLs. However, many viruses including CMV, employ mechanisms to evade recognition and elimination by CD8+ CTLs to facilitate their survival in the host [57]. A critical evasion strategy, used by all of the herpesviruses, is to establish latency in a fraction of infected cells since this ensures persistence in each infected host and provides a source of virus for reactivation and subsequent transmission to a new host [58]. The viral genome may be transcriptionally silent in latently infected cells or express a very restricted number of viral proteins, enabling these cells to remain invisible to CD8+ CTLs [59,60]. The situation should be much different for infected cells that are replicating CMV, since these cells express a large number of viral proteins that could provide epitopes for CD8+ CTLs. However, human CMV also interferes with antigen presentation in cells replicating virus by producing four proteins that block various stages in the generation and export of class I MHC/peptide complexes to the cell surface [61]. The US3 protein is expressed rapidly but transiently in the IE phase and acts by binding to and retaining class I molecules in the ER [62,63]. US2 and US11 are expressed in the E phase and cause retrograde translocation of class I molecules from the ER to the cytoplasm where they are subject to proteosomal degradation [64,65]. Finally, US6 is expressed in the E/L phase and binds to the transporter-associated antigen-processing (TAP) molecules on the ER luminal side, blocking the import of cytosolic peptides and limiting the availability of viral peptides for binding to class I MHC [66].

A consequence of the expression of these viral immune evasion proteins is that the expression of class I MHC at the cell surface declines precipitously during the E and L phases of virus replication in infected fibroblasts [61,67,68]. This finding led to the presumption that CMV proteins expressed at E or L times would be poor targets for CD8+ CTLs. Indeed, initial analysis of the specificity of CD8+ CTLs in healthy CMV+ donors with protective immunity appeared to justify this conjecture. Autologous fibroblasts, which express class I but not class II MHC, were infected with the AD 169 isolate of CMV and used as antigen-presenting cells (APCs) to generate CD8+ CMV-specific T cells from CMV+ donors. The CTLs generated in these cultures were examined for recognition of target cells infected with CMV in the presence of metabolic inhibitors that completely prevent viral gene expression, or limit expression to only the IE phase or to the IE and E phase [69,70]. In these experiments, the CD8+ CTLs elicited from CMV+ donors were almost exclusively specific for structural virion proteins that entered the cytosol after viral penetration and were processed and presented to CD8+ CTLs by infected cells without requiring *de novo* synthesis [69].

Vaccinia recombinant viruses encoding individual virion proteins were subsequently used to identify the target antigens recognized by CD8+ CTLs generated by stimulation with CMV-infected fibroblasts. The virion tegument pp65 protein was consistently recognized by CD8+ CTLs from most donors and pp150 was occasionally a target antigen [70–73]. Peptide epitopes of pp65 presented by common class I alleles were identified and class I tetramers were then used to directly quantify the frequency of pp65-specific T cells in the blood of CMV+ donors. These studies, and others using staining of intracellular IFN-γ after stimulation with defined pp65 peptides demonstrated that normal CMV+ donors with latent CMV infection maintained a significant frequency (0.2– >10.0%) of CD8+ T cells specific for pp65 [73–75].

The major IE protein (IE-1) was also considered an attractive antigen for CD8+ CTLs since it is expressed rapidly in infected cells before the decrease in class I MHC, and its homologue in MCMV was an immunodominant target for the CTL response in mice [45,47]. Studies using fibroblasts infected with wild type CMV as APCs suggested there was a low frequency of CD8+ CTLs specific for IE-1 in CMV+ donors [68]. However, subsequent studies that employed stimulation with IE-1 peptides or APCs infected with a recombinant vaccinia virus encoding IE-1 demonstrated a frequency of IE-1-specific CTLs comparable to that of pp65-specific CTLs [75,76]. A surprising characteristic of the IE-1 specific CTLs was that they failed to lyse fibroblasts infected with CMV even if virus gene expression was limited in the target cell to the IE phase with metabolic inhibitors [68,77]. The abrogation of IE-1 presentation in CMV-infected fibroblasts has now been shown to involve sequential evasion mechanisms. Immediately after infection there is a selective interference in the presentation of IE-1, which is thought to be mediated by the virion pp65 protein [77]. However, this interference is limited temporally to the IE phase since fibroblasts infected with a CMV strain (RV798) that contains pp65 but has an engineered deletion of all four *US* genes that block class I presentation, efficiently present IE-1 to CD8+ CTLs in the E and L phase [78]. The inability of IE-1 specific CTLs to recognize fibroblasts infected with wild type CMV *in vitro* has raised questions concerning what role these CTLs might have in containing infection. One possibility is that IE-1 specific CTLs may be uniquely capable of recognizing cells reactivating virus from latency since virion pp65 would not be available in these cells to inhibit processing of IE-1 or as a target for pp65-specific CTLs.

The recognition of pp65 and IE-1 by CD8+ CTLs was consistent with the expectation that the response would be focused on a few viral antigens that were less affected by the viral immune evasion proteins due to their availability, abundance, and/or kinetics of expression. However, recent analysis of the CTL response employing APCs infected with the RV798 CMV strain that is deleted in the immune evasion genes has identified a larger diversity of target antigens and suggested the interplay between viral immune evasion proteins and T-cell immunity *in vivo* is complex [78,79]. The frequency and specificity of CD8+ CTLs in a cohort of healthy CMV+ donors were examined using APCs infected with RV798 to detect responses that might be missed with wild type CMV or with tetramers that detected only pp65 or IE-1 specific T cells. This analysis confirmed earlier work that found a significant frequency of T cells specific for pp65 and IE-1 but identified an even higher frequency of CD8+ T cells specific for other CMV antigens. In all donors studied, a major proportion (29–80%) of the total CD8+ T-cell response to CMV was specific for undefined viral antigens encoded by *IE* or *E* genes that are not presented by fibroblasts infected with common isolates of CMV [79].

The results of studies analyzing the diversity of CMV antigens recognized by CD8+ CTLs suggest that our understanding of the contribution of T cells specific for individual viral antigens in controlling human CMV infection is still incomplete. Cells of several lineages including endothelium, epithelium, smooth muscle, a variety of immature and differentiated hematopoietic cells and neuronal cells are infected with CMV *in vivo*, and it is conceivable that the viral immune evasion proteins may not equivalently impair antigen presentation in all cell types [80]. Moreover, CMV infection induces a cell stress response characterized by the expression of the MHC class I chain-related genes (MICA and MICB), which serve as ligands for the NKG2D receptor that is expressed on CD8+ T cells and natural killer (NK) cells and signals through the DAP 10 or DAP 12 adaptor proteins [81,82]. The engagement of NKG2D by MIC promotes T-cell recognition of CMV-infected cells that display a low level of class I MHC and provides costimulatory signals to T cells [82]. Thus, the MIC/NKG2D interaction may serve as a counter-evasion strategy to facilitate presentation of a large number of CMV antigens, particularly if the class I inhibition mediated by the US proteins is less complete in infected cells *in vivo*. However, even for this host counter-evasion strategy, there is suggestion of an evolutionary battle for supremacy between virus and host since CMV also encodes a protein (UL16) that reduces the expression of one of the MIC molecules (MICB) at the cell surface [83].

CD4+ T helper cells

CD4+ T helper (TH) cells recognize peptides that are derived from lysosomal degradation of phagocytosed exogenous proteins or proteins produced endogenously within the cell, and are loaded onto class II MHC molecules and exported to the cell surface [84]. Many somatic cells that can be infected with CMV *in vivo* lack class II MHC and would not be direct targets for CD4+ TH. However, correlative studies of CD4+ TH recovery after allogeneic HCT suggest CD4+ TH play a crucial role in sustaining CD8+ T cell responses, possibly by producing IL-2 at local sites of infection [26,27,70]. Additionally, CMV can infect a subset of cells with constitutive or inducible expression of class II MHC including monocyte/macrophages, dendritic cells and endothelial cells [80,85]. Thus, CD4+ T cells, which can be cytolytic through both perforin and Fas/Fas ligand pathways may also contribute directly to elimination of some subsets of CMV-infected cells *in vivo* [85].

At present, there is relatively little data concerning the specificity of the CD4+ TH response to CMV. CMV-specific CD4+ TH cells have been quantified in CMV+ donors using crude CMV antigen extracts prepared from infected cells to stimulate PBMCs. A wide range (0.1–44.0%: mean 1.8%) of CD4+ T cells in CMV+ donors were found to be CMV-specific with this approach [86]. Studies using recombinant pp65, IE-1 or gB proteins for stimulation have shown that a subset of the CD4+ TH response is specific for one or more of these antigens [74,85]. Some of the same viral immune evasion proteins that interfere with class I MHC may also subvert direct recognition of infected cells by CD4+ T cells. The selective expression of US2 and US3 in class II+ cells using recombinant adenoviruses reduces class II expression and recognition by CD4+ T cells [87,88].

Clinical trials of adoptive transfer of CMV-specific T cells in allogeneic HCT recipients

Phase I study of adoptive immunotherapy with CD8+ CMV-specific CTL clones

Animal model experiments and studies of the immunobiology of human CMV have provided strong support for pursuing the adoptive transfer of CMV-specific T cells as a strategy for preventing or treating CMV disease in allogeneic HCT recipients that might be more durable and less toxic than antiviral chemotherapy. The first study to address these issues was a phase I trial that examined the safety and immunomodulatory effects of administering CD8+ CMV-specific CTL clones isolated and expanded from the stem cell donor as prophylaxis for CMV disease (Fig. 29.1). The CD8+ CMV-specific CTL clones were generated *in vitro* by stimulation of donor PBMCs with autologous CMV-infected fibroblasts, isolated by limiting dilution, and expanded by repetitive cycles of activation, proliferation and rest [12,13]. An advantage of using CD8+ CMV-specific T-cell clones for therapy was the ability to ensure that all infused cells recognized CMV-infected target cells and not uninfected recipient cells, which should reduce the possibility the transferred T cells would cause GVHD. However, a disadvantage of this approach was the time required for *in vitro* culture, which delayed the initiation of T-cell therapy. Moreover, stimulation of PBMCs with autologous CMV infected fibroblasts would generate T cells that were exclusively specific for virion proteins, such as pp65 or pp150, which was not perceived to be a problem since the available data at the time suggested these antigens were immunodominant targets [69,71–73]. However, in light of recent data that has identified a large CTL response directed against newly synthesized IE and E viral proteins in CMV+ donors, the transfer of CTLs solely specific for virion proteins could limit efficacy, particularly for recognition of cells reactivating CMV from latency [79].

The CD8+ CMV-specific T-cell clones were administered to 14 patients at weekly intervals in four escalating doses of $3.3 \times 10^7/m^2$, $1 \times 10^8/m^2$, $3.3 \times 10^8 m^2$ and $1 \times 10^9/m^2$ beginning 28–42 days after transplant. No serious acute or delayed toxicities were attributed to the T-cell infusions and the only minor side-effects were chills and fever in two of the 14 patients. PBMCs were obtained at multiple time points before and after the T-cell infusions to determine the magnitude and duration of immunologic reconstitution achieved by the T-cell therapy. Prior to receiving T-cell infusions, 11 of the 14 patients were deficient in CD8+ CMV-specific CTLs, and the efficacy of T-cell therapy for restoring immunity could be easily evaluated. In all 11 patients, the infusion of CD8+ CMV-specific CTLs resulted in recovery of CMV-specific T-cell responses after the first infusion and responses equivalent in magnitude to those in healthy CMV+ donors were achieved after the fourth infusion. In a subset of patients, the rearranged Vα and Vβ genes of the T-cell receptor (TCR) were used as unique molecular markers to monitor the long-term persistence of the infused CTLs. These studies documented that the responses detected in patients after completion of the four T-cell infusions were comprised of infused CTLs, and that these CTLs could persist *in vivo* for at least 12 weeks after administration [12,13].

Adoptive transfer of CD8+ CMV-specific CTLs alone was not effective in providing durable reconstitution of CD8+ CTLs responses in all patients. Patients who required therapy with prednisone in addition to cyclosporine to treat GVHD exhibited a gradual decline in the CD8+ CTL

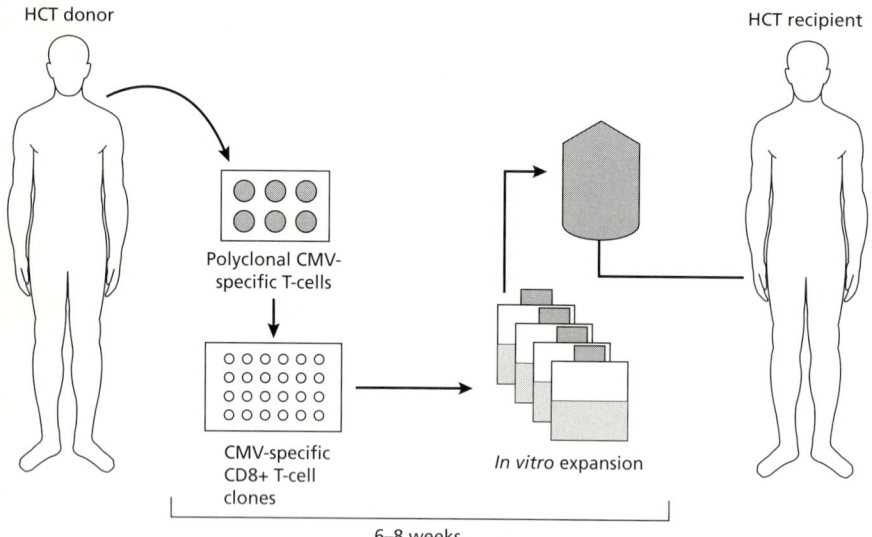

Fig. 29.1 Isolation and expansion of CD8+ cytomegalovirus (CMV)-specific T-cell clones from hematopoietic cell transplantation (HCT) donors for adoptive immunotherapy of HCT recipients. Polyclonal CMV-specific T-cell lines are generated by culturing peripheral blood mononuclear cell (PBMCs) obtained from the donor with autologous CMV-infected fibroblasts. CD8+ T cells are then cloned by limiting dilution and individual T-cell clones are expanded in large scale cultures for adoptive transfer to the HCT recipient.

response to CMV following the discontinuation of T-cell infusions. These patients also differed from patients with sustained CD8+ CTL recovery in that they failed to recover endogenous CD4+ CMV-specific TH responses during the treatment period [12]. This observation was reminiscent of findings in mice rendered deficient in CD4+ T cells by gene knockout technology where transferred virus-specific CTLs failed to persist long-term or became dysfunctional [89,90]. However, in the clinical trial it was not possible to conclude if a deficiency of CD4+ TH, the immunosuppressive drug therapy, or a combination of these factors was responsible for the decline in transferred CTLs.

The patients on the phase I study were followed for virus reactivation by weekly cultures of the blood, urine and throat. A positive culture for CMV from the throat was obtained in one patient before therapy and became negative after the first T-cell infusion. Two patients had a positive urine culture during T-cell therapy. No patient had evidence of CMV viremia and none of the 14 patients developed CMV disease [12]. Thus, the study provided sufficiently encouraging evidence of antiviral activity to proceed with a larger phase II study.

Phase II study of the adoptive transfer of CMV-specific CD8+ and CD4+ CMV-specific T-cell clones as prophylaxis for CMV disease

A phase II study evaluating the immunomodulatory activity and efficacy of the adoptive transfer of CMV-specific T cells as prophylaxis for CMV viremia and disease in allogeneic human leukocyte antigen (HLA)-identical HCT recipients has been performed at the Fred Hutchinson Cancer Research Center in Seattle (unpublished). Based on the findings in the phase I trial suggesting that CD4+ TH responses may be necessary to maintain the CD8+ CTL response, both CMV-specific CD8+ CTL and CD4+ TH clones were administered. Thirty-five patients were treated beginning approximately 1 month after transplant and all were evaluated for 100 days post-transplant. Each patient received two infusions of CD8+ CMV-specific CTL clones (10^9 cells/m^2) 7 days apart and one infusion of CD4+ T-cell clones (10^9 cells/m^2) 2 days following the last CD8+ CTL infusion. As in the phase I trial, all of the CD8+ CTL clones infused were specific for virion proteins, primarily pp65.

The transfer of both CD8+ and CD4+ T-cell clones was safe and associated with immediate recovery or augmentation of CD8+ and CD4+ CMV-specific T-cell responses. However, in contrast to the results of the phase I trial in which none of the 14 patients developed CMV viremia, the virologic outcomes of the phase II trial were less encouraging. All patients had weekly blood samples obtained for quantitative CMV pp65 antigen assays and for viral culture. Patients with antigenemia were not considered treatment failures and did not receive preemptive ganciclovir unless the blood culture also became positive. Twenty-four of the 35 patients (69%) developed CMV antigenemia and 10 of the 35 (28%) developed viremia. Only one of the 35 patients (3%) developed CMV disease, but this patient received treatment with antithymocyte globulin, which would be expected to deplete both endogenous and adoptively transferred T cells. The incidence of antigenemia was similar to historical control data for CMV+ recipients of HCT from a CMV+ donor suggesting the transfer of CTLs specific for virion proteins was not effective in preventing viral reactivation. However, viremia was reduced compared with historical controls, suggesting that T-cell therapy had efficacy, albeit incomplete, for limiting virus dissemination after reactivation.

Additional analysis of the patients on the phase II trial has provided insights into the reasons for the inability of transferred T cells to prevent viremia in a subset of patients. Nine of the 10 patients that developed viremia after T-cell therapy had GVHD and were being treated with prednisone in addition to cyclosporine or FK506. Analysis of the function of transferred CD8+ CTLs and CD4+ TH in these patients suggested that prednisone therapy diminished the ability of these cells to proliferate and produce cytokines. Additionally, studies using polymerase chain reaction (PCR) to detect the unique clone-specific $V\beta$ gene expressed by transferred T cells in PBMCs showed shortened persistence of transferred T cells.

In vitro studies of the effect of glucocorticoids on CMV-specific T-cell clones also showed impaired function and survival of both CD4+ and CD8+ T cells. Dexamethasone did not immediately block cytolytic activity of CD8+ CTLs but inhibited production of IFN-γ by both CD8+ and CD4+ T-cell clones. Dexamethasone also reduced the survival of CMV-specific T-cell clones *in vitro* in a dose and time-dependent fashion. Thus, although the phase II study validated the feasibility and safety of CMV-specific T-cell therapy, it also established intensive post-grafting immunosuppression as the major obstacle to the broad and efficacious application of this approach.

Einsele *et al.* [91] have evaluated the infusion of CMV-specific T cells after HCT as treatment for persistent CMV infection not controlled with antiviral chemotherapy. In this study, CMV reactive T-cell lines containing primarily CD4+ T cells were infused to seven patients. Augmentation of both CD4+ and CD8+ CMV-specific T-cell responses were observed *in vivo* after T-cell therapy and five of the seven patients had a reduction in viral load 1–2 weeks after the T-cell infusions. The two patients that did not respond to therapy received an intensified immune suppressive regimen after the T cells were infused that included prednisolone [91]. These results reaffirm the importance of CD4+ TH and suggest that later administration of CMV-specific T cells may have a therapeutic role if immunosuppression can be safely reduced.

Future directions

The studies of specific T-cell therapy for CMV have identified issues that need to be addressed in future studies to improve efficacy and feasibility. The treatment of GVHD with high doses of steroids appears to be the paramount problem since this interferes with the persistence and function of both adoptively transferred and endogenous CMV-specific T cells. This suggests that CMV-specific T-cell therapy will be most efficacious in HCT recipients in whom T-cell depletion is used for GVHD prophylaxis. In this setting, a post-transplant T-cell deficiency contributes to CMV disease but immunosuppressive drug therapy is rarely required to treat GVHD [92]. For patients who receive unmodified HCT, studies could be designed to determine if patients requiring steroid therapy should temporarily receive ganciclovir or foscarnet to prevent CMV disease, and then receive infusions of CMV-specific T cells when the steroid dose is reduced to reconstitute immunity and protect from late CMV disease.

A second issue to be considered in light of newer data is the specificity of the CMV-specific T cells that are transferred. Although a reduction in the expected incidence of CMV viremia was observed in both the phase I and II trials, more sensitive virologic assays such as measurement of CMV antigenemia or CMV DNA levels in blood provided evidence of reactivation in the majority of patients. In both of these studies, the CD8+ CTLs administered were exclusively specific for virion proteins such as pp65. CTLs of this specificity may be relatively ineffective in eliminating cells reactivating CMV from latency, since structural antigens would not be available in the cell for presentation to CTLs until late stages of the replicative cycle when new virions are being produced. As discussed above, a large fraction of the CTL response in normal CMV+ donors is specific for CMV antigens expressed at IE or E phases of replication and one role for these CTLs may be to eliminate cells reactivating CMV from latency. Thus, it may be essential to transfer T cells with a broader repertoire of antigen specificity to fully restore immunologic control of CMV.

Finally, the initial studies of T-cell therapy for CMV relied on isolating rigorously purified CMV-specific T-cell clones from the stem cell donor and this required substantial time for *in vitro* culture. Novel methods for selection of antigen-specific T cells such as the use of MHC/peptide tetramers or antibodies to capture T cells producing cytokines after antigen stimulation could be employed for the rapid selection of CMV-specific T cells for adoptive therapy [93–95]. These methods should permit the isolation of T cells specific for multiple CMV antigens and eliminate the need for prolonged culture that delays the initiation of therapy and might interfere with homing or survival properties of transferred T cells.

T-cell therapy of EBV-related disease

Background

EBV is a ubiquitous herpesvirus that infects approximately 95% of adults worldwide and is associated with the subsequent development of malignancies including Burkitt lymphoma, Hodgkin's disease (HD), and nasopharyngeal carcinoma in a small subset of infected hosts [96–98]. The virology and pathology of EBV infection are extensively reviewed in Chapter 56, and only issues relevant to T-cell therapy of EBV related disease in the HCT setting will be summarized here. Following primary infection of the immunocompetent host, EBV primarily infects B cells and may either express the full array of viral replication genes and induce cell lysis, a subset of viral genes termed the latency III program that drive cell proliferation, or a more limited subset of viral latency genes [99–105]. The viral latency III proteins expressed in B cells induced to proliferate by EBV *in vivo* are the Epstein–Barr (virus) nuclear antigens (EBNAs) 1, 2, 3A, 3B, 3C, LP and the latent membrane proteins (LMPs) 1, 2A and 2B, which are the same proteins that are expressed in B cells transformed by EBV *in vitro* [104]. Such EBV infected B cells induce a vigorous T-cell response *in vivo* that eradicates a large proportion of the infected cells. However, EBV is never completely eliminated from the host but persists as an episome in a subset of latently infected memory B cells that express only LMP-1, LMP-2A, and EBNA-1 [100,101,103,104,106]. In these cells, EBNA-1 facilitates replication of the viral episome and the LMPs provide survival signals that facilitate cell persistence [100].

Primary infection with EBV or reactivation of latent virus is rarely life-threatening except in the most severely immunocompromised patients who may develop a lymphoproliferative disease (Epstein–Barr virus-associated lymphoproliferative disorder [EBV-LPD]) characterized by proliferation of B cells expressing the EBV latency III proteins [107–110]. Retrospective analysis of >18,000 allogeneic HCT recipients, the majority of whom were HLA-identical siblings, revealed that the risk of EBV-LPD was 1.0% at 10 years [111]. However, the subset of patients who received transplants from partially matched relatives or unrelated donors, which imposes a higher risk of GVHD and results in the use of alternative strategies at some centers to prevent and treat GVHD, resulted in a more severe and prolonged immunodeficiency and an increased incidence of EBV-LPD [109–113]. The major risk factors for EBV-LPD after HCT were transplantation from unrelated or HLA-mismatched (≥2 mismatches) donors, T-cell depletion of the hematopoietic cell inoculum and the use of antithymocyte globulin or anti-T-cell antibodies as prophylaxis or therapy of GVHD [111]. The risk of EBV-LPD with T-cell depletion is much lower if both T and B cells are removed from the graft, presumably because the load of EBV-infected cells introduced with the graft is reduced [114–116].

The clinical presentation of EBV-LPD in HCT recipients is variable and may include pharyngitis, focal or generalized lymphadenopathy, lymphoproliferation in organs including small intestine, liver, spleen, bone marrow, kidney and central nervous system, and constitutional symptoms. After HCT, EBV-LPD almost always originates in donor B cells and commonly exhibits a monomorphic diffuse large cell morphology although plasmacytoid or polymorphic morphology may be seen [117,118]. The majority of EBV-LPD are oligoclonal or monoclonal as shown by analysis of *Ig* gene rearrangements or characterization of repeat sequences at EBV DNA episomal joints [119,120]. Biopsy of involved tissue and demonstration of the presence of EBV in the tumor by Southern blot of tumor DNA using EBV-specific probes or by analysis of *EBV* gene expression in tissue sections establishes the diagnosis [119,120].

Rationale for T-cell therapy

EBV-LPD has historically had a poor prognosis and, with a rising incidence in the context of current transplant regimens, is an increasingly important reason for treatment failure. Chemotherapy, radiation therapy, or immunologic manipulations such as reductions in immunosuppressive therapy or administration of IFN-α, have been used as treatment but rarely result in long-term survival [121]. The administration of anti-B-cell monoclonal antibodies directed at CD21 and CD24 was beneficial in patients with polyclonal EBV-LPD but less effective in patients with oligoclonal or monoclonal disease [122–124]. A similar strategy using a genetically engineered humanized anti-CD20 monoclonal antibody provided more promising results. Anti-CD20 therapy induced remission of EBV-LPD in a majority of HCT recipients and could be used preemptively to treat rising EBV DNA levels [125–129]. However, therapy with anti-CD20 has occasionally resulted in the outgrowth of CD20− tumor variants and caused a prolonged B-cell deficiency that may contribute to other opportunistic infections in these already severely compromised hosts [130].

The association of the development of EBV-LPD with transplant regimens that incorporated T-cell depletion of the stem cell graft or therapy of GVHD with T-cell specific monoclonal antibodies strongly implicated a critical role for T-cell immunity in prevention of EBV-LPD [108,111]. This was supported by studies demonstrating that the growth of EBV-transformed B cells *in vitro* was suppressed by virus-specific T cells [131]. Direct evidence for the activity of EBV-specific CD8+ T cells was provided by studies in a murine model designed for analysis of human EBV-LPD in which the adoptive transfer of EBV-specific CTLs caused tumor regression [132].

Only a few studies have examined the tempo of recovery of EBV-specific T cells after allogeneic HCT and correlated responses with the development of EBV-LPD. The majority of patients transplanted with either unmodified or T-cell-depleted bone marrow exhibited a deficiency of EBV-specific CTLs measured by limiting dilution analysis until 3 months after transplant, and a subset of these patients with the most severe or prolonged deficiency of EBV-specific CTLs developed EBV-LPD [133]. The recovery of EBV-specific CTLs has also been analyzed using class I/EBV peptide tetramers in a small number of recipients who received either matched sibling peripheral blood hematopoietic cell (PBHC) transplant, T-cell-depleted transplant, or cord-blood transplant. EBV-specific T cells recovered rapidly in the matched sibling PBHC transplant recipients despite the administration of post-transplant immunosuppression, but recovery was markedly delayed in the recipients of cord-blood or T-cell-depleted transplants even in response to EBV reactivation [134].

Specificity and frequency of EBV-specific T cells in immunocompetent EBV+ donors

CD8+ cytotoxic T cells

The specificity of the CD8+ CTLs response to EBV in immunocompetent individuals has been studied both in acute infectious mononucleosis and in the subsequent latent state. CD8+ EBV-specific CTLs were found to account for the majority of the activated T cells during the lymphocytosis that develops in individuals with infectious mononucleosis and may comprise up to 44% of the total circulating CD8+ T cells [135]. During this acute phase of EBV infection, the majority of the CTLs are specific for immediate early or early lytic cycle EBV proteins with a smaller component directed against latent proteins, notably EBNA-3A, -3B and -3C [135–137]. In the subsequent latent phase of infection, EBV-specific CTLs may represent 1–5% of the circulating CD8+ T-cell pool [136]. At this stage, CTLs specific for lytic cycle antigens and EBNA-3A, -3B and -3C continue to predominate, CTLs specific for EBNA-2, LP, LMP-1 and LMP-2 represent a minor component of the response, and CTLs specific for EBNA-1 are notably absent [136,138,139].

During chronic infection, the major reservoir of virus is in latently infected B cells, which express only low levels of LMP-1, LMP-2A, and EBNA-1 [100,106]. These cells escape immunologic detection because of a combination of the poor antigen-presenting capability of resting B cells, weak immunogenicity of LMPs, and a unique evasion mechanism utilized by the EBNA-1 protein, which contains Gly/Ala repeats that interfere with its processing and presentation by class I MHC [138,139]. The activation of such B cells can induce expression of the full array of lytic viral genes or expression of the latency III genes that induce B-cell proliferation [140]. Thus, the maintenance of a CTL response to the latency III proteins would appear to be essential for preventing EBV-LPD.

CD4+ T cells

After acute EBV infection, CD4+ T cells do not undergo the same degree of antigen driven expansion as CD8+ T cells suggesting the contribution of EBV-specific CD4+ T cells is primarily mediated by cytokines that promote CD8+ T-cell proliferation [141]. However, studies in latently infected hosts have shown that a significant frequency (~0.5%) of CD4+ T cells specific for EBNA-1 and EBNA-3C are maintained [142,143]. CD4+ T cells specific for EBNA-2 have also been identified in some donors, but responses to LMP-1 and LMP-2 are uniformly present in very low levels [142,144]. In addition to their role in promoting CD8+ T-cell responses, *in vitro* studies suggest CD4+ EBV-specific T cells can exert a direct effect on EBV-infected B cells. CD4+ T cells from EBV+ donors inhibit the initial proliferation of B cells after infection with EBV *in vitro* [145,146], and EBNA-1-specific CD4+ T cells kill EBV transformed lymphoblastoid cell lines (EBV-LCL) by a Fas/Fas ligand interaction [147]. These findings suggest the efficacy of T-cell therapy for EBV may be enhanced by the inclusion of CD4+ EBV-reactive T cells.

Clinical trials of adoptive transfer of EBV-specific T cells for EBV-related LPD in allogeneic HCT recipients

Treatment of EBV-LPD with unselected donor lymphocytes

The evidence that EBV+ LPD may develop as a consequence of an inadequate T-cell response to B cells expressing EBV proteins provided a strong theoretical basis for pursuing EBV-specific T-cell therapy for preventing or treating this disease. Further support for this strategy was provided by a study of five patients who developed EBV-LPD after T-cell-depleted allogeneic HCT and received infusions of unirradiated donor PBMCs containing CD3+ T cells [148]. Regression of the LPD was observed in all five patients and three patients became long-term survivors. Two patients who had pulmonary involvement prior to T-cell therapy developed fatal respiratory failure after the lymphocyte infusions and two of the three patients who survived developed chronic GVHD [148]. In a subsequent report, 16 of the 19 patients with EBV-LPD treated with unselected donor lymphocytes achieved complete resolution of their disease although GVHD developed in 50% of patients [118]. Studies of the frequency of EBV-specific CTLs in the blood before and after therapy demonstrated rapid amplification after T-cell infusion to levels equivalent to normal EBV+ donors. This study provided direct evidence for the benefits of T-cell therapy for EBV-LPD but highlighted the need to isolate EBV-specific T cells for therapy rather than polyclonal donor lymphocytes that also contain T cells capable of causing GVHD, and to treat patients prior to the development of disseminated disease.

Treatment of EBV-LPD by adoptive transfer of EBV-specific T cells

To potentially alleviate the problem of GVHD, donor T-cell lines enriched for reactivity for autologous EBV-transformed B cells and depleted of alloreactivity by *in vitro* culture were evaluated as therapy for EBV-LPD. The adoptive transfer of EBV-specific T-cell lines was effective in two of three HCT recipients with established EBV-LPD without causing GVHD [149]. One patient had progressive disease despite T-cell infusions and analysis of the tumor virus from this patient identified a mutation in the *EBNA-3B* gene that eliminated the region encoding the epitopes which were the predominant targets of the CTL line generated from the donor [150]. In this study, a subset of the transferred T cells were marked with the neomycin phosphotransferase gene to facilitate tracking *in vivo* and the infused T cells could be identified in the regressing tumor and blood for >18 months after infusion [149,151].

Prophylaxis of EBV-LPD by adoptive transfer of EBV-specific T cells

To diminish the toxicity of treating advanced disease and the probability of escape mutants developing, the prophylactic administration of EBV-specific T cells was evaluated for patients at high risk for EBV-LPD. EBV-specific T-cell lines comprised predominantly of $CD3^+$ $CD8^+$ T cells with a smaller subset of $CD3^+$ $CD4^+$ T cells were generated from HCT donors and infused to patients after T-cell-depleted HCT [14]. Most patients received two infusions of T cells at doses of 2×10^7 cells/m^2 and no toxicity was observed. Transfer of EBV-specific CTL immunity was demonstrated by an increase in the frequency of EBV-reactive CTLs in recipient blood after the cell infusions, often to levels equivalent to those in healthy EBV^+ donors. None of the 36 patients who received prophylactic T-cell infusions developed EBV-LPD, while the predicted frequency of LPD in such patients was 14% [14]. Moreover, a small subset of patients had elevated EBV DNA levels measured in the blood prior to treatment and these levels rapidly declined after the EBV-specific T-cell infusions.

EBV-infected B cells accumulate in the blood in immunocompromised patients and monitoring EBV virus DNA after allogeneic HCT can be used to identify patients at high risk for EBV-LPD who would be candidates for EBV-specific T-cell therapy [152–155]. A small study evaluated the administration of EBV-specific CTL lines to recipients of T-cell-depleted HCT after the development of high EBV-DNA levels in the blood. A major reduction of EBV DNA was observed in four of the five recipients while one patient, who received a T-cell line that lacked a major EBV-specific component, progressed to EBV-LPD [156]. Thus, the transfer of EBV-specific T cells to T-cell-depleted HCT recipients at risk of EBV-LPD safely and rapidly reconstituted EBV-specific immunity, mediated antiviral activity and provided protection from EBV-LPD in the majority of patients.

Future directions

The optimal design of prophylaxis and therapy regimens for EBV-LPD with EBV-specific T cells will require better definition of the nature and specificity of the effector T cells mediating the *in vivo* effect. The current trials have employed polyclonal T-cell lines reactive with autologous EBV-transformed B cells and containing variable proportions of $CD4^+$ and $CD8^+$ T cells. Although the precise role of each of these T-cell subsets remains to be defined, $CD8^+$ CTLs are likely to be the essential effector cells and $CD4^+$ T cells are probably responsible for providing helper functions necessary for the *in vivo* persistence and replication of the transferred $CD8^+$ CTLs. Future studies using defined numbers of EBV-reactive $CD4^+$ and $CD8^+$ T cells could provide insights into the relative functions and contributions of each subset, and ultimately lead to a study design that assures all patients receive adequate therapy. Additionally, the specificity of the transferred EBV-reactive T cells for individual viral antigens was not defined in most of the current trials, and it is possible that particular responses may be associated with better protection due to the kinetics and magnitude of protein expression or genetic heterogeneity among EBV isolates. Thus, analysis of the infused T cells to ensure there is sufficient breadth of antigen specificity to minimize the potential for escape variants should facilitate the development of an effective standard therapy that could be directly compared with alternative therapies such as anti-CD20 monoclonal antibodies that are now available.

The promising results of T-cell therapy for EBV-LPD provide the impetus to investigate the potential of this therapy in other EBV-associated malignancies. Approximately 50% of patients with HD have clonal EBV genomes in their malignant Reed–Sternberg cells, consistent with the EBV infection having occurred prior to malignant transformation [157,158]. Moreover, although Reed–Sternberg cells express only EBNA-1, LMP-1 and LMP-2, LMP-1 has transforming potential and likely contributes to the malignant phenotype [158–161]. At the present time, HCT after high-dose cytotoxic therapy is employed for the subset of HD patients who fail primary therapy and have refractory or relapsed disease. Although response rates with most conditioning regimens are high, long-term survival is <30%, primarily due to relapse. Thus, the addition of T-cell therapy targeted to residual EBV^+ tumor cells has the potential to reduce this high relapse rate. One obstacle to this approach is that the EBV proteins expressed in Reed–Sternberg cells are poor immunogens and recognized by a very low frequency of EBV-specific T cells in normal EBV^+ donors [162]. Thus, polyclonal T-cell lines generated by stimulation with EBV-LCL often do not contain CTLs specific for LMP-1 or LMP-2, and their infusion into patients with HD did not exert significant antitumor activity [163]. Several laboratories have now demonstrated that LMP-1 or LMP-2 specific CTLs can be isolated from some EBV^+ donors and HD patients by employing recombinant vectors or RNA transfection to selectively express these proteins in APCs [164–167]. Additional studies are needed to determine how reproducible these strategies will be for eliciting CTLs, but we suggest it may soon be feasible to evaluate adoptive transfer of CTLs specific for EBV antigens expressed in HD.

T-cell therapy of leukemia targeting mHAs

Background

Minor histocompatibility antigens (mHAs) consist of HLA-bound peptides derived from cellular proteins that differ between donor and recipient due to polymorphisms in the genome and are recognized by donor T cells after allogeneic HCT [168,169]. T-cell responses to mHAs are the primary mediators of GVHD after HLA-matched HCT, and both studies in animal models and clinical observations suggest they are critical for the graft-vs.-leukemia effect (GVLE) associated with allogeneic HCT [170–175]. In murine models of HCT, the administration of allogeneic T cells provided a greater antileukemic effect than syngeneic T cells, suggesting that recognition of mHAs on leukemic cells contributed to the GVL response [171,176,177]. Direct evidence for the antileukemic activity of mHA-specific T cells was shown by studies in which the adoptive transfer of donor T cells specific for a single murine mHA that is abundantly expressed on hematopoietic cells eradicated leukemic cells without causing GVHD. These data also suggested that differential tissue expression of individual mHAs might serve as a potential basis for separating GVLE from GVHD [170,178].

Clinical observations also provide strong evidence that mHA-specific T cells contribute to the GVLE. In a large retrospective study, the risk of leukemic relapse was higher for patients treated with allogeneic T-cell-depleted or syngeneic HCT compared with allogeneic unmodified HCT, implying that T cells specific for allogeneic determinants were responsible for the reduction in relapse [175]. The GVLE associated with allogeneic HCT was greatest for patients with acute and/or chronic GVHD, but a reduction in relapse was also observed in chronic myeloid leukemia (CML) and acute myeloid leukemia (AML) patients who did not develop GVHD demonstrating that GVL activity can occur in the absence of GVHD [175,179]. These observations led to the treatment of recurrent leukemia after allogeneic HCT with donor lymphocyte infusions (DLIs) and this has provided additional evidence that allogeneic T cells can eradicate leukemia. The majority of patients with relapse of CML in chronic phase after HCT, and a smaller subset of patients with myeloma, lymphoma, AML, acute lymphoblastic leukemia (ALL) and myelodysplastic syndrome (MDS), achieve a complete remission after DLI [8,180–182]. The ability of alloreactive T cells to eradicate malignancies is also

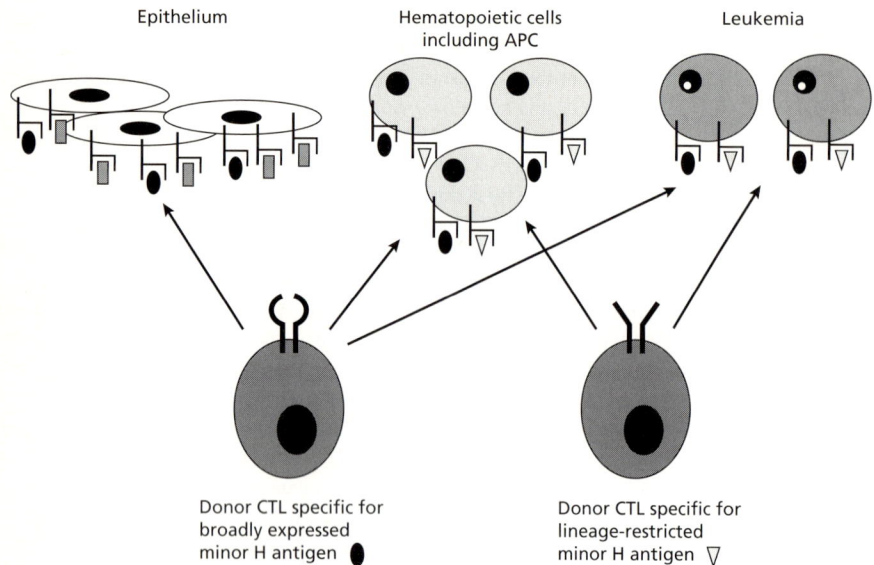

Fig. 29.2 The isolation of donor T cells specific for minor histocompatibility antigens (mHAs) that are selectively expressed on recipient hematopoietic cells may permit separation of the graft-vs.-leukemia (GVL) response from graft-vs.-host disease (GVHD). A subset of mHAs are encoded by genes that are ubiquitously expressed on both hematopoietic and nonhematopoietic cells, while others are encoded by genes that are selectively expressed by hematopoietic cells including leukemic cells. T cells specific for lineage restricted mHAs could selectively mediate GVL activity without GVHD.

illustrated by studies of allogeneic HCT using low intensity, non-myeloablative conditioning regimens, which are not sufficiently cytotoxic to induce tumor regression but suppress host immunity and facilitate engraftment of donor cells [183–185]. This approach has induced complete remission in a subset of patients with CML, chronic lymphocytic leukemia (CLL), multiple myeloma, lymphoma and renal cell carcinoma [9,183,184,186–188]. Unfortunately, DLIs and non-myeloablative HCT are not effective in all patients, particularly those with advanced acute leukemia, and GVHD is a major complication that contributes to morbidity and mortality [8,9,180–184,186–188].

Rationale for developing T-cell therapy targeting mHAs

An attractive strategy for exploiting and potentially increasing the potency of the GVLE is to transfer selected T cells that are specific for defined mHAs expressed on leukemic cells rather than relying on effects mediated by unselected donor lymphocytes. This approach may ultimately require transferring both CD4+ and CD8+ mHA-specific T cells for optimal efficacy. However, murine models have suggested that CD8+ T cells are the primary effector cells responsible for GVL activity, and much of the initial effort in characterizing human mHAs that might be targets for T-cell therapy has also focused on those recognized by CD8+ T cells [189,190]. CD8+ T cells specific for mHAs can be isolated from most allogeneic HCT recipients by in vitro stimulation of PBMCs obtained from the recipient after transplant with γ irradiated cryopreserved pretransplant recipient cells [191]. These mHA-specific T cells efficiently lyse recipient cells including leukemia cells and inhibit leukemia colony formation in vitro [192–194]. Studies in a murine model of human leukemia have analyzed whether the primitive human leukemic stem cell is recognized by mHA-specific CTLs. Transplantation of human AML into nonobese diabetic with severe combined immunodeficiency syndrome (NOD/SCID) mice has identified a rare leukemic progenitor, which has a CD34+CD38− phenotype and is necessary for establishing persistent leukemic hematopoiesis [195,196]. In this model, CD8+ CTLs specific for several human mHAs completely prevented the engraftment of AML by a mechanism that required direct cell/cell contact, demonstrating that leukemic stem cells express mHAs and are susceptible to CTL recognition [197].

These data provide a strong rationale to develop T-cell therapy targeting mHAs to treat leukemia, but this should ideally be accomplished without GVHD. One strategy that could potentially provide this selectivity is to target mHAs that are highly expressed by hematopoietic cells, including leukemia, but have absent or minimal expression in non-hematopoietic tissues (Fig. 29.2). Analysis of CD8+ T-cell clones specific for human mHAs that were isolated from HCT recipients demonstrated that a significant fraction lysed only recipient hematopoietic cells and failed to recognize cells of nonhematopoietic lineages in vitro [169,191,198,199]. These findings encouraged studies to identify the polymorphic genes that encode such mHAs to facilitate the detailed studies of their frequency in the population and expression on various tissues in vivo that are required to define the most appropriate targets for T-cell therapy.

Identification of genes that encode mHAs

Several methods are currently being applied to the discovery of genes encoding human mHAs recognized by CD8+ T cells including peptide elution and mass spectrometry [200–204], complimentary DNA (cDNA) expression cloning [205–207] and genetic linkage analysis [208]. The discovery of genes that encode mHAs has provided insight into the mechanisms operative in generating mHAs, identified mHAs that are preferentially expressed on hematopoietic cells and are attractive candidates as targets for T-cell therapy, and identified mHAs that are ubiquitously expressed and associated with GVHD.

mHAs encoded by autosomal genes and preferentially expressed on hematopoietic cells

The first human gene identified to encode a mHA was the autosomal gene *KIAA0023*, which encodes the HA-1 peptide presented by HLA-A2 [202]. The HA-1 epitope was identified by eluting peptides bound to HLA-A2 molecules, separating fractions that reconstitute recognition by HA-1 specific CTLs when pulsed onto antigen negative cells, and sequencing the active peptides by mass spectrometry. Comparison of the sequence of the HA-1 peptide with protein and DNA databases demonstrated it originated from the *KIAA0023* gene, which has at least 2 alleles that differ by a single amino acid in the epitope region [202]. The peptide for a second mHA (HA-2) presented by HLA-A2 was encoded by the *MYO1G* gene, which has two alleles that differ by one amino acid in the antigenic epitope [201,204]. Both *KIAA0023* and *MYO1G* are selectively expressed in hematopoietic cells, including leukemia cells, and represent potential targets for a GVL response [169,204]. Indeed, one small retrospective study suggested HCT recipients with the antigenic HA-1 allele

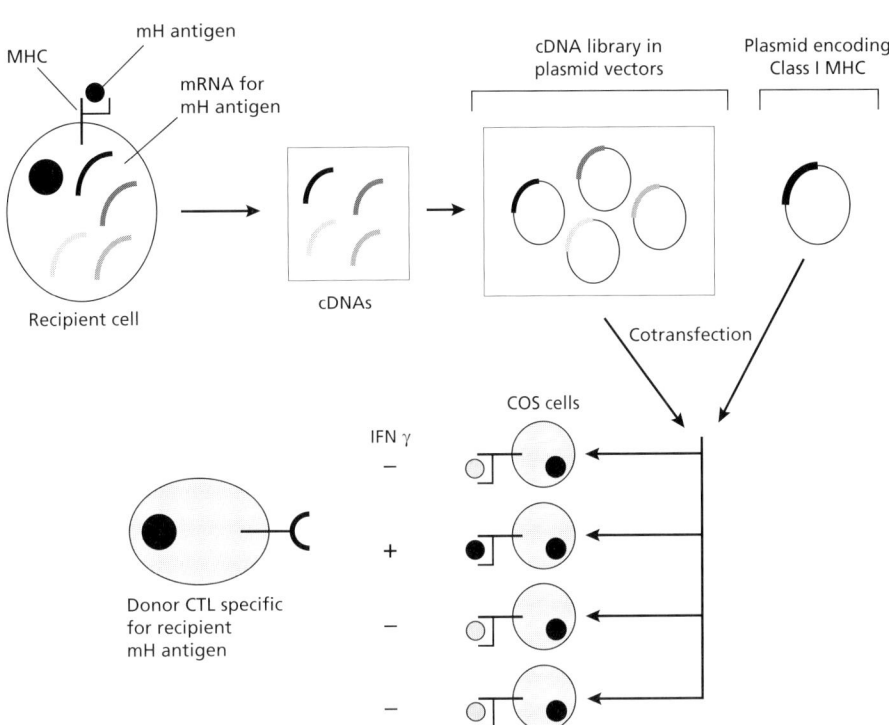

Fig. 29.3 Complimentary DNA (cDNA) expression cloning technique for discovery of genes that encode minor histocompatibility antigens (mHAs). A cDNA library is generated in a mammalian expression plasmid and pools of library cDNA are cotransfected into SV40 transformed monkey kidney (COS) cells with a plasmid encoding the class I major histocompatibility complex (MHC)-restricting allele for the T-cell clone. The transfected COS cells are cocultured with aliquots of the T-cell clone and the supernatant screened for interferon-gamma (IFN-γ) production. Pools of cDNA that are positive in this assay are then subdivided and rescreened to identify a single cDNA that stimulates interferon production by the cytotoxic T lymphocyte (CTL) clone. The plasmid insert is then sequenced and compared to DNA databases to identify the gene encoding the mHA.

and an HA-1-negative donor had a lower rate of leukemic relapse than recipients who were HA-1 compatible with their donors [209]. However, other small studies have implicated HA-1 incompatibility with increased GVHD, although a large retrospective study failed to find a significant association with GVHD [210–212]. The reason for these conflicting results is not immediately clear. One possibility which has been proposed is that local inflammation resulting from T cells responding to the HA-1 on recipient hematopoietic cells at tissue sites may contribute to epitope spreading, that is the activation of T cells reactive with other mHAs that are expressed on epithelium [170,213]. If a careful analysis of the evolution of HA-1 and other mHA-specific T-cell responses in the blood and at tissue sites of GVHD confirms that T-cell responses to HA-1 induce epitope spreading, this result would suggest T-cell therapy targeting lineage restricted mHAs would be best applied after T-cell-depleted HCT to avoid recruiting T-cell responses to other mHAs.

The cDNA expression cloning approach was used to identify an autosomal gene, *HB-1*, which encodes a mHA that is presented by HLA-B44 and expressed only in transformed B cells including B-ALL [206] (Fig. 29.3). The polymorphism in this gene results in a single amino acid difference in the HB-1 peptide presented by donor and recipient cells. The *HB-1* gene is selectively expressed on B-ALL, making it unlikely that T-cell therapy targeted against *HB-1* in HLA-B44+ allogeneic HCT recipients would cause GVHD [206].

These elegant genetic studies have discovered polymorphic genes that encode human mHAs that are attractive targets for T-cell therapy designed to induce a selective GVLE but have so far proven difficult to translate into therapeutic approaches in the clinical setting. The major issue is that to target one of these mHAs, it is essential that the recipient has the appropriate HLA molecule, expresses the mHA and that the donor lacks the mHA. The proportion of individuals who express HA-1, HA-2, and HB-1 are 69%, 95%, and 72%, respectively [193,214]. Thus, even though HLA-A*0201 and HLA-B*4402/03 are relatively common alleles, the actual number of allogeneic transplant recipients who will both express these HLA alleles and be appropriately discordant for one of these three mHAs with their donor is relatively small.

mHAs encoded by Y-chromosome genes and preferentially expressed on hematopoietic cells

Transplantation of hematopoietic stem cells from a female (F) donor into a male (M) recipient (F → M) is a special situation where mHAs encoded by the Y chromosome represent potential targets for a GVLE in all recipients. F → M HCT is associated with both increased GVHD and a reduced risk of leukemic relapse compared with HCT between other donor/recipient gender combinations [215,216]. A recent analysis of transplant outcome depending on donor/recipient gender demonstrated that the GVLE after F → M HCT is evident even after controlling for GVHD [216]. This observation suggested that genes on the Y-chromosome are likely to encode multiple mHAs (H-Y antigens) that make distinct contributions to GVHD and GVL.

A CD8+CTL clone isolated from a male recipient who did not develop GVHD after HCT from his HLA-identical sister recognized a novel H-Y antigen that was presented by HLA-B8 [207]. The B8/HY-specific CTL lysed male hematopoietic cells but not nonhematopoietic cells, and also lysed AML blasts *in vitro* and eliminated leukemic progenitors in NOD/SCID mice [197]. Using a combination of deletion mapping and cDNA expression cloning, the epitope recognized by the B8/HY CTLs was mapped to the *UTY* gene on the Y chromosome. The antigenic UTY peptide differed by two amino acids from the peptide encoded by the homologous sequence of the *UTX* gene, located on the X chromosome [207]. Despite the selective recognition of hematopoietic cells by B8/UTY-specific CTLs *in vitro*, expression of the *UTY* gene is not entirely restricted to hematopoietic cells. Analysis of mRNA in various tissues revealed high levels of *UTY* transcripts in hematopoietic cells and much lower, but still detectable, levels in nonhematopoietic tissues, including those that were not recognized by B8/UTY-specific CTLs *in vitro* [207]. The absence of GVHD in the recipient suggests that this difference in gene expression between hematopoietic and nonhematopoietic tissues was sufficient to prevent recognition of nonhematopoietic cells *in vivo*.

UTY encodes three alternatively spliced transcripts that are predicted to give rise to proteins of 1079, 1240, and 1347 amino acids [217].

Comparison of the sequence of UTY proteins with their UTX homologues revealed only 80–84% identity suggesting that epitopes that could bind to HLA alleles other than HLA-B8 are likely to be present. Computer algorithms that predict peptides likely to bind to common class I MHC molecules were used to analyze polymorphic regions of *UTY*. Several UTY peptides that bind to HLA-A*0201 and elicit T-cell responses in male recipients of HCT from female donors have been identified and candidate peptides that bind to other HLA alleles are now being evaluated [218]. Studies of the ability of CTLs specific for other UTY epitopes to recognize hematopoietic and nonhematopoietic cells are now needed to determine if targeting UTY may be broadly applicable for promoting a GVLE after F → M HCT.

Autosomal and Y-chromosome genes that encode ubiquitously expressed mHAs

Several genes that encode mHAs that are ubiquitously expressed have also been identified and implicated in GVHD, suggesting this class of mHAs will be difficult to exploit for GVL activity unless a strategy to eliminate T cells after leukemia eradication is complete could be employed. The *KIAA0020* gene was found to encode the peptide for an HLA-A2-restricted mHA (HA-8) identified by peptide elution and mass spectrometry [219]. *KIAA0020* encodes at least three alleles and the critical difference in the immunogenic peptide is an arginine substitution for proline at position 1 that facilitates transport of this peptide into the ER. The function of the *KIAA0020* gene is unknown, but it is expressed at high levels in both hematopoietic and nonhematopoietic cells. A retrospective analysis of 577 HLA-A2$^+$ allogeneic HCT recipient–donor pairs showed that HA-8$^+$ recipients with HA-8$^-$ donors had a significantly increased risk of acute GVHD compared with recipients who were HA-8 compatible with their donors (Y. Akatsuka, unpublished data).

Goulmy and Engelhard have identified three broadly expressed H-Y antigens using peptide elution and mass spectrometry [203,220,221]. Comparison of the sequences of these peptides with proteins encoded by the Y chromosome revealed that two of the peptides presented by HLA-A2 and -B7, respectively, were derived from SMCY. The SMCY peptides differ in amino acid sequence from the homologous sequences of SMCX encoded by the X chromosome as a result of nucleotide polymorphism between these two genes [220,221]. The third peptide was presented by HLA-A1 and corresponded to a sequence in DFFRY, which is also polymorphic with its X homologue [203]. SMCY and DFFRY are broadly expressed in both hematopoietic and nonhematopoietic tissues, suggesting that T-cell responses to these antigens may mediate GVHD after allogeneic F → M HCT. Indeed, T cells specific for the SMCY/HLA-A2 mHA induced the histologic features of GVHD in an *in situ* skin explant model and detection of SMCY-reactive T cells by tetramer staining after F → M HCT correlated with the development of acute GVHD [211,213]. The clinical association of GVHD with disparities in mHAs that are ubiquitously expressed supports the hypothesis that sustained T-cell responses to broadly expressed mHAs result in GVHD.

Future strategies for augmenting T-cell responses to mHAs to induce GVL activity

The efforts to identify the molecular basis of mHAs are defining targets that might be exploited for T-cell therapy to induce a selective GVL response and targets that should be avoided due to the risk of inducing GVHD. There are several attributes of hematopoietic-restricted mHAs that make them attractive targets for immunotherapy. First, mHAs are highly immunogenic and donor T cells mediate GVLE after allogeneic HCT despite the administration of immunosuppressive drugs to block alloreactivity. Second, the majority of mHA-specific T-cell clones that have been characterized are of high avidity increasing the likelihood they will recognize malignant cells even if these cells express lower levels of MHC molecules. Third, the T-cell response to mHAs involves both CD8$^+$ and CD4$^+$ T cells. CD4$^+$ Th could directly recognize leukemic cells that express class II MHC molecules and participate in the GVLE by providing help for CD8$^+$ T-cell responses. Finally, T cells may be directed at multiple mHAs expressed on leukemic cells, which may prevent the outgrowth of tumor cells that might evade elimination due to loss or reduced levels of antigen expression.

Specific T-cell therapy targeting mHAs is conceptually attractive but several obstacles have impeded clinical application. The major obstacle is the lack of a sufficiently large number of mHAs that have been molecularly characterized and determined to be suitable candidates for therapy. This primarily reflects the technical complexity of current approaches employed for antigen discovery and it is anticipated that the combination of advances in the human genome project and bioinformatics will facilitate identification of additional candidate antigens that can be evaluated with currently available immunologic tools. A second issue is how to define which of the identified mHAs will be suitable targets for therapy. It would seem most appropriate to attempt to augment T-cell responses to mHAs that are strictly expressed on recipient hematopoietic cells to avoid causing GVHD. However, studies in a murine model have suggested that it may be possible to target mHAs that are not completely limited in their expression to hematopoietic cells [170]. The absence of GVHD in this setting could reflect differential sensitivity of hematopoietic and non-hematopoietic cells to recognition by T cells specific for this mHA *in vivo*, or to the ability of the transferred T cells to survive only long enough to eradicate leukemia but not mount a sustained attack on epithelial tissues. A third issue is to develop culture techniques to rapidly isolate mHA-specific T cells that would be available for therapy of patients who relapse or prophylaxis of patients at high risk for relapse. Current approaches rely on isolating the donor T cells from the recipient post-transplant to allow *in vivo* priming of the response [191]. However, this involves a time delay and may not always be successful. Studies using the HA-1 mHA as a model have shown it is feasible to isolate HA-1 specific T cells from donor blood using dendritic cells that are pulsed with the HA-1 peptide or transfected with the *HA-1* gene as APCs [222,223]. Thus, as additional mHAs are identified, similar approaches for generating T cells for therapy can be evaluated.

A pilot clinical trial has been initiated in which donor CD8$^+$ T-cell clones specific for recipient mHAs that are selectively or preferentially expressed on hematopoietic cells, including leukemia cells, are being adoptively transferred to patients with relapse of AML or ALL after allogeneic HCT [224]. This trial is assisting in identifying mHAs that can be targeted by adoptive transfer without toxicity or GVHD and identifying obstacles that may limit the therapeutic success of T-cell transfer. The elimination of leukemia likely requires migration to the bone marrow and prolonged persistence of the adoptively transferred T cells. Thus, in this study, the T cell receptor (*TCR*) gene is being used as a marker to monitor the presence of transferred CTLs in the blood and bone marrow at intervals after cell transfer. The results of this analysis should aid in determining if CD4$^+$ Th cells or post-infusion IL-2 will be needed to maintain transferred responses. Tumors may also evade T-cell recognition by loss of antigen or MHC expression or by expressing molecules that interfere with T-cell function or survival [225,226]. Thus, if relapse occurs after therapy, the leukemia cells are being evaluated for sensitivity to T-cell recognition *in vitro* and in NOD/SCID mice to determine if antigen loss variants have been selected, which might be overcome by simultaneously targeting multiple antigens. This approach should provide insights into the feasibility, safety, efficacy and limitations of therapy that can then be used to guide the design of subsequent studies.

T-cell therapy targeting normal proteins over-expressed by malignant cells

Background

T cells employed for the therapy of malignancy in association with HCT can potentially be targeted not only to mHAs but also to more "conventional" tumor antigens. Such antigens can be divided into five major categories:
1 Mutational antigens which are tumor-specific, such as p21 *ras* mutations and *BCR-ABL* translocations.
2 Viral antigens which are tumor-specific, such as EBV in HD and HPV in cervical cancer.
3 Tissue-specific differentiation antigens which are not tumor-specific but may be selected as targets if injury to the normal tissue is tolerable, such as MART1 in melanoma and PSA in prostate cancer.
4 Cancer-testes (germ cell) antigens, such as NY-ES0-1 and the MAGE family, which are detected in many tumors, such as myeloma and melanoma, but not in normal adult tissues with the exception of the testes.
5 Over-expressed self-proteins, particularly those associated with the malignant phenotype, such as Her-2/neu in ovarian and breast cancer.

Evaluating tumor antigens as therapeutic targets does not necessarily require the setting of an HCT, but this setting may greatly facilitate such studies, based in part on the advantages of having a normal donor from whom to derive the tumor-reactive T cells rather than a potentially immunosuppressed cancer patient and of performing transfers into recipients with depleted lymphoid compartments. Unique antigens are the obviously preferred targets, and some potentially unique tumor antigens have been predicted in hematological malignancies based on known disease-related translocations that lead to fusion proteins such as BCR-ABL in CML and PML-RARα in acute promyelocytic leukemia (APL) [227,228]. The candidate antigens associated with such translocations would be derived from the region immediately surrounding and containing the fusion site but, as has been observed, only a few epitopes have been shown to bind efficiently to a small subset of class I molecules and to be naturally processed from the protein, making these antigens of limited utility. Thus, most of the tumor antigens identified to date belong in the groups of antigens that are not tumor-specific but rather are also detectable in some normal tissue(s). One limitation with these antigens is that expression of the proteins in peripheral tissues can result in deletion or tolerization of the highest avidity T cells, leaving only a low avidity repertoire. However, the remaining lower avidity T cells may still be capable of recognizing tumor cells, based on the aberrant expression of higher levels of the protein in the tumor as compared to the normal cells which "tolerized" the repertoire. Indeed, it is precisely such significantly higher levels of expression of the protein in tumor cells as revealed by microarray or differential display analyses that have formed the basis by which many of these antigens have been identified. Moreover, following *in vitro* activation of low avidity naive CD8$^+$ T cells, the resulting effector cells generated for adoptive therapy may have less stringent requirements for subsequent activation, with the potential to recognize and kill targets expressing 1–2 logs lower levels of the antigen than the cell required to induce the response [229,230].

Candidate tumor antigens for targeting

The most attractive over-expressed proteins are the subset homogeneously detected in all of the transformed cells of the particular tumor type. These are expressed at levels substantially higher than normal cells (approximately 10-fold or more), associated with the malignant phenotype so that down-regulation results in a survival disadvantage, and endogenously processed efficiently by the tumor cell so that multiple epitopes are presented in association with diverse class I molecules. Several proteins, as described below, which appear to meet these criteria, have already been identified and clinical trials evaluating T-cell therapy targeting these antigens are anticipated in the next few years.

WT1, a zinc finger transcription factor, was first characterized as the gene responsible for cases of childhood Wilm's tumor. It was initially perceived as a tumor suppressor gene, based on the association of Wilm's tumor with loss mutations of *WT1* and on the demonstration that *WT1* can function as a repressor of transcription of growth factor and receptor genes [231–234]. *WT1* has since been shown to exist in many isoforms, interact with many cellular proteins, bind and post-transcriptionally regulate mRNA, and depending on the cellular context transactivate as well as repress expression of a wide range of genes [235–239]. Overexpression of *WT1* has been reported in many malignancies [240–244]. *WT1* is expressed embryonically in the developing kidney and urogenital tract and in supportive structures of mesodermal origin, including the developing pleural sacs, pericardium and splenic capsule, and postnatally can be detected at low levels in adult podocytes of the kidney, sertoli cells of the testes, granulosa cells of the ovary, mesothelial cells of the lung, and the uterus [236,245–248]. Sensitive assays have also revealed low level expression in CD34$^+$ hematopoietic progenitor cells [249,250]. *WT1* is overexpressed in leukemia, including AML, ALL, and CML, with higher levels of expression correlating with worse prognosis [250–256]. A role in oncogenesis has been suggested by inhibition of proliferation and induction of apoptosis of leukemia cells and other tumors following specific down-regulation of *WT1* expression with antisense oligonucleotides [240,257,258]. Additionally, *WT1* increases expression of the antiapoptotic molecule, bcl-2 [259], and constitutive expression of *WT1* in normal hematopoietic progenitor cells increases proliferation and inhibits differentiation of myeloid cells in response to granulocyte colony-stimulating factor (G-CSF) [260,261].

Leukemic cells express approximately 10- to >100-fold the WT1 protein detected in normal CD34$^+$ cells [250,262]. This difference has made it possible to monitor *WT1* expression as a sensitive molecular marker for relapse of leukemia and progression of MDS from refractory anaemia to more malignant forms [252–254,263,264]. Immunologic studies have suggested CD8$^+$ T cells can also distinguish this difference in protein expression. Using peptides representing epitopes predicted by computer algorithms to bind the A2 and A24 human class I molecules or the D^b molecule in mice, CD8$^+$ CTLs have been generated that lyse leukemic CD34$^+$ and not normal CD34$^+$ cells, and inhibit growth of leukemic colonies but not myeloid or erythroid colonies from normal CD34$^+$ cells [262,265–267]. CD8$^+$ CTLs generated in mice eliminated syngeneic *WT1*$^+$ leukemic cells *in vivo* without any evidence of injury to normal tissues, including kidney and bone marrow [262,268,269]. Moreover, CD8$^+$ T cells specific for *WT1* have been detected in the peripheral blood of patients with AML in remission and did not interfere with normal hematopoiesis, suggesting that providing patients with a strong response to this protein may be well tolerated [270].

Another leading candidate protein that has been evaluated is proteinase 3 (PR3), a neutral serine protease with broad proteolytic activity that is detected only in myeloid cells and stored in the azurophilic granules of neutrophils. Gene expression is normally restricted to the promyelocytic stage of granulocytic differentiation [271–274], although the protein is packaged and retained in mature granulocytes [275]. The absence of gene expression with differentiation results from down-regulation of transcription followed by loss of hypersensitivity sites in the regulatory region and ultimately extensive remodeling of this locus in mature granulocytes, implying stringent control mechanisms have evolved to prevent aberrant expression [272]. PR3 is probably best known as the target of autoantibodies diagnostic for Wegener's granulomatosis [276–279], and recent studies have detected a small amount of PR3 on the surface of neutrophils, which upon binding Ab leads to neutrophil degranulation, potentially increasing inflammation and promoting the vascular injury characteristic of the disease [280,281]. PR3 may have roles in normal and abnormal myeloid cell development. Initially identified as a novel serine protease overexpressed in a myeloid leukemia cell line, it was termed myeloblastin (MBN), because expression was found to be downregulated following induced differentiation, and addition of antisense oligonucleotides to leukemic cells led to growth arrest and differentiation [282–284]. Constitutive expression of PR3/MBN with an intact catalytic site also conferred factor-independent growth to a G-CSF dependent hematopoietic cell line [285]. A proform of PR3/MBN secreted by leukemic cells has been shown to selectively interfere with formation of colony forming unit–granulocyte/macrophage (CFU-GM) from normal $CD34^+$ cells but not burst forming unit-erythroid (BFU-E) or leukemic cell growth, potentially providing leukemic progenitors a growth advantage in the confinements of the bone marrow space [286]. Although the mechanisms by which PR3/MBN expression might be prooncogenic still require definition, two proteins which could otherwise promote differentiation of leukemic cells, the transcription factor SP1 and the 28 kDa heat shock protein, are degraded by this enzyme [287,288]. PR3/MBN protein is not detectable in normal hematopoietic stem cells, although very low levels of mRNA are present in normal $CD34^+$ cells [285]. However, the protein is "prematurely" expressed in isolated leukemic blasts, particularly from CML in blast crisis [275] and in the CFU-GM of patients with CML. Leukemic cells express approximately 10- to 25-fold the protein level detected in normal mature granulocytes, which have the highest protein level of normal cells [275,289].

$CD8^+$ T cells specific for PR3/MBN have been generated by repetitive *in vitro* stimulation of PBMCs with a peptide epitope that was initially selected based on the binding motif for the A2 class I allele [289–291], and these CTLs can lyse leukemic cells but not normal bone marrow cells presumably due to the quantitative differences in PR3/MBN expression [290,291]. The CTLs also inhibited the growth of CFU-GM from leukemic precursors but not normal $CD34^+$ cells [289], with leukemic cells from CML in blast crisis appearing particularly sensitive to both lysis and prevention of colony formation [290,291]. The *in vivo* relevance of this response has been assessed with peptide/MHC tetramers containing the epitope and A2 [291]. Although $CD8^+$ CTLs specific for the epitope were not detectable in the PBMCs of normal $A2^+$ individuals or in untreated CML patients, following IFNγ therapy frequencies of up to 1.5% of total $CD8^+$ cells were found in the 11 out of 12 CML patients who responded with reduction of Philadelphia chromosome positive (Ph^+) cells and in none of the seven patients who failed to respond [292]. Additionally, of eight patients analyzed in complete remission at 4–8 months after allogeneic HCT, six had PR3-specific CTLs with frequencies ranging from 0.11% to 12.8%. The CTLs isolated from the blood of patients were functional, directly lysing CML blasts, and progression/recurrence of disease in these patients was associated with loss of the response. The presence of this CTL response, even at high levels, was not associated with any evidence of autoimmune disease or marrow failure, suggesting again that providing patients with a strong response to this antigen should be well tolerated.

Preliminary studies from our laboratory have demonstrated that $CD8^+$ T-cell clones specific for WT1 and PR3/MBN can be generated from the PBMCs of normal individuals, and clinical trials of adoptive therapy using donor-derived clones should be initiated in HCT recipients in the near future. However, there are several additional antigens that may soon be ready to be advanced for clinical testing. Translocations associated with development of leukemia may result not only in potential immunogens from the novel fusion site, but also from increased expression levels or turnover of one or both of the component proteins forming the fusion. The most common translocation in AML, identified in approximately 8% of patients, is t(8;21), which fuses the *AML1(RUNX1)* gene with the *ETO* (also called *MTG8* or *CBFA2T1*) gene, producing a chimeric protein with several proleukemic activities, including functioning as a dominant negative to inhibit the normal transcriptional activity of *AML1/CBF*β [293]. ETO, which is expressed at higher levels in these cells, has very limited expression in normal tissues, and overexpression of ETO in normal $CD34^+$ cells promotes the expansion of hematopoietic stem cells [294]. Additionally, leukemic cells can be induced to differentiate with an antisense molecule to ETO, and mice expressing an *AML1-ETO* knockin gene have a propensity to develop leukemia [295,296]. Preliminary studies suggested that $CD8^+$ T cells specific for target cells expressing increased levels of ETO can be generated [297], and we have recently demonstrated that $CD8^+$ T-cell clones specific for ETO and capable of lysing leukemic cells can be generated *in vitro*.

Survivin, a member of the inhibitor of apoptosis (IAP) family, is a bifunctional protein that suppresses apoptosis and regulates cell division [298,299]. It is a prototypic onco-fetal antigen, which is expressed during early embryonic development, is almost silent in normal adult tissues and is expressed at continuously high levels in most common cancers [300]. Approximately 60% of cases of AML and of large cell lymphomas express survivin, and such expression is associated with a poor prognosis [301,302]. Preliminary studies have suggested that $CD8^+$ CTLs specific for survivin can be generated *in vitro* by stimulation with antigen-pulsed dendritic cells [303], and a low frequency of CTLs specific for survivin has been detected in lymphocytes infiltrating breast cancer and melanoma [304] and in peripheral blood lymphocytes (PBL) from patients with CLL and melanoma [305]. Preliminary studies from the authors' laboratory at the Fred Hutchinson Cancer Research Center have also demonstrated that $CD8^+$ CTL clones specific for surviving and capable of recognizing leukemic cells can be generated from the PBMCs of normal donors.

The human homologue of MDM-2 is another self-protein involved in malignant transformation that is overexpressed in a large fraction of malignancies. MDM-2 both inactivates the p53 tumor suppressor protein and directly promotes cell proliferation by interacting with the Rb protein and stimulating E2F/DP1 transcriptional activity [306,307]. High levels of MDM-2 are frequently detected in hematologic malignancies, particularly in patients with poor prognostic and/or advanced disease [308,309]. MDM-2-specific $CD8^+$ T cells restricted to the class I A2 allele have been generated from normal $A2^+$ donors, but have been reported to generally be of low avidity [310,311]. However, preliminary results from our laboratory have demonstrated that A2-restricted $CD8^+$ CTL clones recognizing several epitopes from MDM-2 with sufficient avidity to lyse leukemic cells can be generated from normal HLA-$A2^+$ donors, suggesting that a more extensive examination of this target protein is warranted.

Future directions

The current technologies being employed to molecularly profile malignancies will undoubtedly suggest many more candidate antigens. Gene expression and, more recently, protein expression are being extensively analyzed in virtually all classes of hematologic malignancies, and characteristic profiles with diagnostic and prognostic implications are being defined [312–314]. Deciding how to utilize the massive amount of data and select individual antigens to pursue will remain a major challenge. Some genes, such as telomerase which functions to prevent senescence and maintain replicative potential, are attractive because they are associated with oncogenesis and over-expressed in most malignancies, and several studies have already suggested that this protein can induce $CD8^+$ CTL responses and might be an appropriate target for T-cell therapy [315,316]. Some genes will be selected because they represent aberrant splice variants that are distinct and characteristic for a particular tumor, and such variants will need to be assessed to determine if the novel protein sequences are immunogenic [317]. Alternatively, some genes may be selected based on evidence that the protein elicits antibody responses in cancer patients, which can be readily detected with serological analysis of recombinant tumor cDNA expression libraries (SEREX), on the assumption that such immunogenicity increases the likelihood that a CD8+ T-cell response could be generated [318]. Regardless of the strategy utilized to select genes for study, an increasing number of immunogenic tumor proteins are certain to be identified, and it will become essential to develop adequate preclinical models and clinical trial designs that can rapidly determine the safety and potential efficacy of a selected protein as a therapeutic target.

Genetic modification as a means to improve efficacy, safety, and applicability of T-cell therapy

Background

Studies in preclinical models and early clinical trials have substantiated the enormous therapeutic potential of adoptive T-cell therapy but have also highlighted the obstacles for success and broad-based application of this approach. One strategy that can be used to potentially overcome many of these obstacles is genetic modification of T cells with the goals of imparting new functions, specificities and/or phenotypes. Such modification can now be readily accomplished in primary T cells with the current generations of viral and nonviral vectors and insights have been obtained into resolution of many of the identified problems.

Transferring T-cell specificity

T-cell therapy in its present format must be individually designed for each patient. However, it is likely that in many donors it will be either difficult or not feasible to isolate in a timely fashion CD8+ T cells with the necessary specificity and avidity for the required tumor antigen or mHA. Although it is not currently possible to create a universal donor T cell as a reagent that could be used for all patients, it is now possible as an alternative to provide the relevant specificity to an autologous or HCT donor T cell. Thus, after a T-cell clone used in adoptive therapy has been demonstrated to be effective with regard to tumor elimination or viral eradication and safe with regard to injury to normal tissues, the rearranged $V\alpha$ and $V\beta$ genes encoding the clonotypic TCR could be cloned, inserted into a retroviral (or alternative shuttle) vector, and transduced into a T cell derived from the HCT donor. Such transduced T cells will express two functional receptors, the endogenous $V\alpha V\beta$ pair and the introduced $V\alpha V\beta$ pair (potentially two alternative receptors from mismatched pairing could additionally be formed, although such pairing may be physically disfavored and would be unlikely to lead to a functionally restricted receptor) (Fig. 29.4). Current retroviral and lentiviral vectors can efficiently introduce genes into the majority of primary CD8+ T cells in a single transduction, and CD8+ cells expressing the two TCR chains can be easily isolated based on surface expression of the TCR without the requirement for any other selectable marker. This approach has already been shown to successfully transfer specificity for a tumor or a virus, and the recipient CD8+ T cells, if selected for expression of wild-type levels of the introduced TCR chains, demonstrate a similar avidity for the target

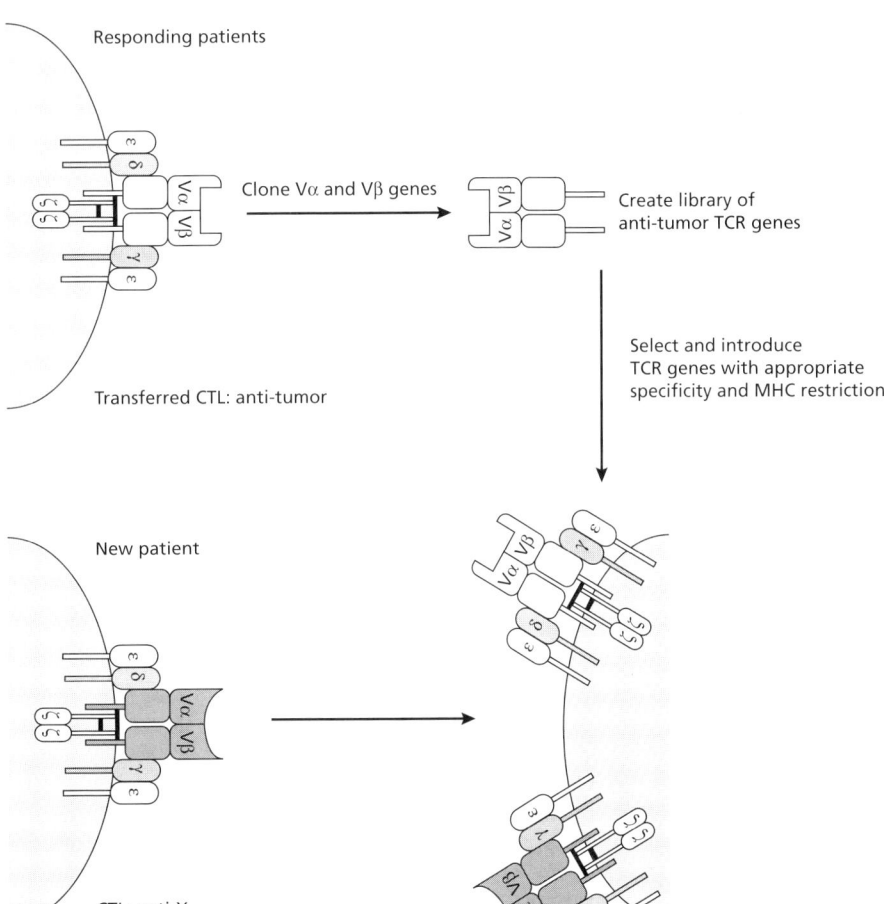

Fig. 29.4 Transferring T-cell specificity. The $V\alpha$ and $V\beta$ TCR genes cloned from CD8+ T cells demonstrated to be effective and safe in adoptive tumor therapy can be collected to form a library of receptors with known specificity and major histocompatibility complex (MHC) restriction. These T-cell receptor (TCR) genes can then be available for immediate expression in CD8+ T cells from patients whose tumor shows the antigen and MHC-restricting allele. Expression of the $V\alpha$ and $V\beta$ genes results in assembly of the complete TCR-signaling molecule, producing a recipient cell with both its natural endogenous specificity and the introduced specificity.

as the clone from which the *TCR* genes were derived [319–323]. Moreover, by introducing the TCR chains into T cells with specificity for a known antigen, such as EBV or an alloantigen, it may be possible to boost the response *in vivo* by triggering the cell through the endogenous TCR [324,325]. Thus, it should be possible to develop and maintain a library of TCRs with known antigen specificity and MHC restriction and, following screening of a patient's tumor for tumor antigen and MHC expression, select the appropriate TCR for use in therapy.

Improving TCR affinity

One problem with pursuing T-cell responses specific for over-expressed tumor antigens that are also expressed in normal tissues is that deletional mechanisms, particularly if the antigen is expressed in the thymus, may eliminate all but the lowest avidity T cells. Such low avidity T cells may prove incapable of recognizing even tumor targets expressing high levels of the protein *in vivo*, particularly if class I expression is down-regulated. However, strategies to manipulate TCR recognition *in vitro* have been developed, in which the $V\alpha$ and $V\beta$ chains are cloned, mutated and compiled into receptor libraries which can be expressed using either a yeast surface single chain TCR display system or retroviral transduction of a TCR-negative T-cell line [326,327]. The expressed TCR library can then be rapidly screened for relative affinity and TCRs with the desired increase in affinity selected. Using this approach, TCRs have been generated with retention of specificity but >100-fold higher affinity than the wild type receptor for the desired peptide/MHC complex. Transfer of such receptors yields T cells with a much improved avidity for the target [327].

As an alternative, naturally occurring high affinity TCRs for candidate antigens can be rescued by generating the peptide/MHC-restricted $CD8^+$ T cells from an allogeneic T-cell population. This approach takes advantage of the facts that tolerance to self-antigens is accomplished by selection against T cells that are restricted to recognition in the context of self-MHC molecules with no negative selection against T cells that happen to recognize a foreign class I molecule with high affinity, and that a proportion of allo-specific $CD8^+$ T-cells reactive with a foreign class I molecule can be as peptide-specific in recognition of the foreign class I/peptide complex as self-restricted $CD8^+$ T cells [328]. Thus, high-affinity $CD8^+$ CTLs from an A2-negative donor but specific for an MDM-2 epitope restricted by the A2 allele were generated *in vitro* by stimulation with a peptide-pulsed $A2^+$ stimulator cell followed by selection of the minor subset of $CD8^+$ T cells from the responding population that only recognized an $A2^+$ target if it expressed the MDM-2 epitope [311]. Such $CD8^+$ CTL clones were of sufficiently high affinity to recognize $A2^+$ leukemia cells that express detectable levels of MDM-2 but not normal $A2^+$ PBMCs. Thus, this rather novel approach could be an alternative means to produce high affinity TCRs specific for a defined epitope in the context of a known class I allele.

Providing alternative specificities for T cells

$CD8^+$ T cells are restricted to recognizing tumor antigens in the context of class I molecules, but one mechanism by which tumors have been shown to evade natural or induced T-cell responses is to down-regulate either expression of class I or the processing machinery that generates the peptide epitopes contained in the class I molecule [329]. Antibodies could provide an alternative and complimentary treatment strategy, since antibodies can recognize an entirely different universe of tumor antigens and, of course, do not require class I expression or an intact processing machinery. However, the effector mechanisms associated with antibodies are usually inadequate to treat established tumors. Thus, one approach to harness both the potential tumor specificity of antibodies generated to surface molecules on tumor cells and the effector activity of $CD8^+$ T cells has been to construct and express in T-cell chimeric receptors with the ectodomains of antibodies and the transmembrane and intracytoplasmic signaling domains of components of the TCR signaling complex. The most extensively investigated of these "T-body" constructs have single chain antibody ectodomains (ScFv) with the V_H and V_L regions attached by a flexible linker and fused in frame to a CD3-ζ or Fc(ϵ)RIγ signaling module [330,331]. Such chimeric receptors retain the specificity of the antibody and deliver an activation signal to the transduced $CD8^+$ T cell that induces cytokine production and cytolytic activity. *In vivo* studies in murine models have demonstrated that adoptive therapy with $CD8^+$ T cells expressing T-bodies can mediate rejection of established tumors [332,333], and preliminary clinical trials have already been initiated targeting antigens on B-cell lymphoma and neuroblastoma.

One problem with the use of the ScFv-based chimeric receptors is that the receptor does not assemble all the signaling components of a normal TCR complex, and the signal induced in the T cell by target recognition, while sufficient to generate tumoricidal activity, may be inadequate to achieve full activation and promote survival. Several strategies, such as changing the signaling module, are being evaluated to address this issue. However, optimal lymphocyte activation usually requires a costimulatory signal in addition to the TCR signal, and one approach has been to create a single receptor that can provide both a TCR and CD28 mediated signal. The most efficient constructs appear to contain the antibody-derived ScFv ectodomain fused in frame to the transmembrane and cytoplasmic tail of CD28 which is then fused to the cytoplasmic signaling domain of CD3ζ. The precise order and relationship of these domains to each other and/or the membrane appears to be important for efficacy [334–336]. Human T cells expressing such multicomponent chimeric receptors have been shown to retain both specificity for the target tumor antigen and cytolytic activity, and also to proliferate and expand in number *in vitro* in response to recognition of the tumor [336]. Murine $CD8^+$ T cells expressing similarly constructed receptors have been shown to secrete increased amounts of IFN-γ, to proliferate following target recognition and to eliminate established tumors and metastases *in vivo* [337]. Further evolution of the chimeric receptor strategy, incorporating either different recognition structures, such as cytokines, to bind molecules expressed preferentially on the surface of tumor cells or different signaling modules to amplify T-cell reactivity can be anticipated and should lead to novel and improved cell-based treatment strategies.

Enhancing T-cell function

Following transfer of T cells that bear a TCR of appropriate specificity and avidity, there may still remain substantial obstacles *in vivo* to achieving the desired therapeutic outcome, including homing to the sites of tumor, receiving an adequate activation signal from recognition of a tumor cell with poor stimulatory capacity and surviving and persisting long enough to provide benefit. Many of these issues might also be addressed by expressing new genes in the T cells prior to infusion. Although enhancing the natural biological activity of T cells still represents an exploratory concept, with all of the studies still in preclinical phases, the potential of this approach suggests that many of these strategies will be advanced to clinical trials in the next few years.

The authors' studies of adoptive T-cell therapy of CMV, human immunodeficiency virus (HIV), metastatic melanoma and leukemia at the Fred Hutchinson Cancer Research Center have all demonstrated that the *in vivo* persistence and therapeutic efficacy of transferred $CD8^+$ T cells is limited in the absence of providing a growth and/or survival factor for the $CD8^+$ cells [12,15,338]. During a normal sustained $CD8^+$ T-cell response to a large persistent antigen burden such as a chronic infection, these factors are provided by concurrently responding $CD4^+$ T helper cells [12,339,340], but in many therapeutic settings it has not been possible to provide both antigen-specific CD4+ and CD8+ T cells. This dependence of effector CD8+ responses on "help" at least in part reflects the fact that most effector CD8+ T cells have lost during differentiation the capacity to produce IL-2 in response to target recognition, and studies in murine models have demonstrated that daily administration of exogenous IL-2 can replace the requirement for CD4+ T cells during the period following CD8+ T-cell transfer [341,342]. This requirement for IL-2 has been confirmed in clinical trials for the treatment of melanoma, in which administration of daily IL-2 in low doses for 14 days was demonstrated to maintain the survival and function and enhance the antitumor activity of CD8+ T-cell clones for at least 14 days [15]. However, this approach is clinically impractical, potentially toxic, may not be effective long-term to maintain a persistent CD8+ response and may be particularly problematic in the context of allogeneic HCT as it could also enhance the GVH response [343]. Thus, we have explored molecular strategies that might provide CD8+ T cells with an autocrine growth signal induced and regulated by target recognition.

The proliferative response of responding T cells is mediated in large part by signals delivered through the IL-2 receptor (IL-2R). The high affinity IL-2R is composed of three chains, which are brought together as a heterotrimer following binding of IL-2. In this complex, the α chain does not contribute to signaling but is essential for maintaining high affinity binding of IL-2, and the activity results from signals that emanate from the β and γc chain. Consequently, strategies that promote dimerization of the cytoplasmic tails of the β and γc chain independent of either the α chain, the ectodomains of the receptor chains, or the IL-2 molecule, can deliver the complete and authentic IL-2 signal [344,345]. Although effector CD8+ T cells do not make IL-2, these cells do continue to make many effector cytokines in a tightly regulated fashion following target recognition, including granulocyte macrophage colony-stimulating factor (GM-CSF) which normally binds to a two chain heterodimeric receptor not expressed by T cells. Therefore, we constructed chimeric receptor chains that have the ectodomains of the α and β chains of the GM-CSF receptor (GMCSFR) fused, respectively, to the cytoplasmic signaling tails of the γ and β chains of the interleukin-2 receptor (IL-2R). These chimeric chains were introduced with retroviral vectors into human effector CD8+ cells, and the cells both retained cytolytic activity and acquired the ability to proliferate in response to target recognition [346]. The activity of this chimeric receptor has been further investigated *in vivo* in preclinical murine models, and CD8+ cells expressing both chains exhibited enhanced responses to tumors and viral infection, established a larger long-lasting memory cell pool, even in the absence of CD4+ T-cell responses, and generated much stronger recall responses following re-exposure to the antigen [347,348]. Thus, expression of these receptors in transferred CD8+ T cells may provide a therapeutic population that upon recognizing a target *in vivo* will not only lyse the cell but also will also receive a regulated signal to survive and replicate to sustain the response.

Trafficking of transferred T cells and accumulation at sites of tumor is also essential for therapeutic activity, but there is evidence that T cells may home poorly or be excluded from some tumor sites [349]. Localization of T cells at particular sites in the body reflects a multistage process requiring rolling and arrest on the vascular endothelium and extravasation and penetration into the tissue, and is based in large part on the differential expression of homing receptors and adhesion molecules on the T cells and the complementary addressins on the relevant vasculature, and on chemokine receptors on T cells responding to chemokines produced in the tissue. By enforcing expression of particular molecules on the surface of T cells it should be possible to facilitate preferential localization at desired sites. For example, expression of the integrin α4β7 should promote localization of infused T cells to mucosal lymphoid tissues that express the complimentary addressin (mucosal addressin cell adhesion molecule [MAdCAM-1]) and might be used for treatment of MALT (mucosa associated lymphoid tissue) lymphomas [350,351]. Alternatively, for treatment of leukemias or tumors metastatic to the bone marrow, constitutive expression of the chemokine receptor CXCR4 might be beneficial—the ligand for this receptor, SDF-1, is produced by marrow stromal cells and normally serves to attract CXCR4+ hematopoietic cells, whereas on T cells this receptor is normally down-regulated following differentiation from naive to effector cells [352–354]. Similarly, expression of CXCR5 or CCR3 on transferred T cells should facilitate localization at sites of follicular lymphoma or HD, respectively [355,356]. Analysis of tumor specimens for chemokine expression could uncover characteristic chemokine production that might be therapeutically exploited. For example, melanomas have been shown to produce CXCL1, whereas T cells do not produce this chemokine and the receptor, CXCR2, is down-regulated in activated T cells. Gene modification of T cells with a retroviral vector to enforce expression of CXCR2 rendered the cells responsive to CXCL1 and attracted to a CXCL1 gradient [357]. Thus, it should be possible using many of these strategies to increase the likelihood that transferred effector cells will find and preferentially accumulate at sites of particular tumors.

An additional strategy to enhance therapeutic activity is to augment the effector functions of the transferred T cells. One approach, which was examined in pilot clinical trials, is to increase secretion of effector cytokines, such as TNF [358]. However, these studies were performed with first generation vectors and promoters that yielded limited expression of the transgene, and this approach will need to be more extensively evaluated. Alternatively, it may be possible to improve effector functions by increasing the sensitivity for TCR signaling. For example, it is now clear that T-cell activation represents the sum of both positive and negative signaling events. Signals delivered through NKG2D decrease the threshold for T-cell activation and increase cytolytic activity, suggesting that up-regulation of expression of this receptor and/or components of the associated signaling complex might be beneficial [82,359]. Conversely, Cbl-b, an adapter protein associated with the TCR, appears to dampen signal strength, presumably by promoting degradation of critical signaling proteins, and disrupting Cbl-b function increases TCR sensitivity and removes the requirement for a costimulatory signal [360–363]. There are obviously many other ways to attempt to modulate T-cell signaling and improve T-cell function, and further studies should provide many potentially useful therapeutic options.

Improving safety of T-cell therapy

The transfer of T cells with specificity for antigens expressed on normal tissues as well as tumor cells, whether these antigens are prooncogenic proteins or mHAs, has the potential to injure normal tissues. Although screening normal tissues for relative expression levels can provide insights into the potential risks and possibly suggest candidate antigens that should not be tested, ultimately safety can only be defined by performing clinical trials in patients. If toxicity is detected after cell transfer, it would be desirable to have a means to rapidly ablate the infused T cells. Therefore, until it has been demonstrated that an antigen is safe to target *in vivo*, it would be helpful to express a conditional "suicide gene" in the transferred T cells. An ideal suicide gene should not interfere with normal T-cell function, and should be capable of being rapidly activated and selectively eliminating the cell expressing it. Initial studies evaluated genes derived from pathogens, such as cytosine deaminase and herpes simplex virus thymidine kinase (HSV-tk), since these genes are capable of converting intracellularly antimicrobial drugs such as 5-fluorocytosine and ganciclovir, respectively, into lethal products [364]. Clinical trials for treatment with DLIs of leukemia that has relapsed post-HCT have been performed with polyclonal donor T cells transduced with a retroviral vector to express HSV-tk. The first study yielded promising results, with the donor T cells mediating an antileukemic effect in some patients, and the GVHD that developed in some patients successfully treated in several cases by ganciclovir administration [365]. However, the study also revealed some of the limitations inherent to this strategy. One patient with chronic GVHD exhibited partial resistance to ganciclovir-mediated elimination of the transduced cells, which presumably reflected the importance of slowly dividing T cells in the pathogenesis of this syndrome coupled with the requirement that cells be synthesizing DNA and actively dividing to succumb to the HSV-tk induced toxicity of ganciclovir. Additionally, several treated patients developed a specific $CD8^+$ T-cell response to HSV-tk that led to selective elimination of the transferred T cells [366]. Similar limitations with the use of HSV-tk modified donor cells have been observed in other post-HCT trials [367]. Indeed, we had previously observed remarkably strong immunogenicity of HSV-tk in a trial in which HIV-infected patients received autologous HIV-specific $CD8^+$ T cells expressing HSV-tk, as evidenced by a strong $CD8^+$ response to HSV-tk and very rapid rejection of the transferred cells [368]. Thus, pathogen-derived genes that encode foreign proteins do not appear ideal for use as suicide genes.

More recent studies have demonstrated the feasibility of harnessing the apoptosis machinery as an inducible suicide switch. Fas is a member of the tumor necrosis factor (TNF) superfamily which upon trimerization assembles intracellularly a death-inducing signaling complex that activates a proteolytic cascade leading to apoptosis. This death signal is effective independent of cell cycle. Therefore, a chimeric chain has been constructed in which the cytoplasmic portion of the Fas sequence is fused at the C-terminus to two copies of FK506-binding protein (FKBP) and anchored to the cell membrane by fusion at the N-terminus to the extracellular and transmembrane portion of the nerve growth factor receptor.

The FKBP binding sites have been modified so that a homodimeric drug AP1903 does not interact with normal cellular FKBP but rather selectively binds and multimerizes the chimeric protein and rapidly induces apoptosis [369]. Since this chimeric protein is derived from human rather than microbial proteins, immunogenicity should be minimal. *In vitro* studies with primary T cells have demonstrated that nanomolar concentrations of AP1903, which can readily and safely be achieved *in vivo*, will rapidly induce death in either proliferating or resting T cells, with 80% of T cells eliminated within 2 h [369,370], and preclinical studies already being performed in macaques suggest this strategy should soon be available to be advanced to clinical trials [370].

Future directions

The use of genetic modification to "build a better T cell" opens up almost limitless possibilities for experimental T-cell therapy. However, clinically evaluating each unique molecular strategy will require substantial effort and resources and, unfortunately, may not be entirely without risks to the patients, both directly as a consequence of the expressed gene and indirectly from unpredicted insertional mutagenesis [371]. Thus, it will be essential to appropriately select both the gene to be evaluated and the clinical setting to be investigated. Precisely how to prioritize such studies should evolve based on the clinical trials being performed with unmodified cells, which undoubtedly will uncover limitations to current approaches and improve understanding of the underlying immunobiology of the disease being targeted. Despite the obstacles and effort that will be required to execute studies with gene-modified T cells, this approach holds the promise of making specific T-cell therapy a more effective and available modality for the treatment of human disease.

References

1 Greenberg PD. Adoptive T cell therapy of tumors: mechanisms operative in the recognition and elimination of tumor cells. *Adv Immunol* 1991; **49**: 281–355.
2 Hanson HL, Donermeyer DL, Ikeda H *et al.* Eradication of established tumors by $CD8^+$ T cell adoptive immunotherapy. *Immunity* 2000; **13**: 265–76.
3 Nash RA, Storb R. Graft-versus-host effect after allogeneic hematopoietic stem cell transplantation. GVHD and GVL. *Curr Opin Immunol* 1996; **8**: 674–80.
4 Porter DL, Antin JH. Graft-versus-leukemia effect of allogeneic bone marrow transplantation and donor mononuclear cell infusions. *Cancer Treat Res* 1997; **77**: 57–85.
5 Giralt SA, Kolb HJ. Donor lymphocyte infusions. *Curr Opin Oncol* 1996; **8**: 96–102.
6 Porter DL, Antin JH. The graft-versus-leukemia effects of allogeneic cell therapy. *Annu Rev Med* 1999; **50**: 369–86.
7 Slavin S, Naparstek E, Nagler A, Kapelushnik Y, Ackerstein A, Or R. Allogeneic cell therapy: the treatment of choice for all hematologic malignancies relapsing post BMT. *Blood* 1996; **87**: 4011–3.
8 Collins RH Jr, Shpilberg O, Drobyski WR *et al.* Donor leukocyte infusions in 140 patients with relapsed malignancy after allogeneic bone marrow transplantation. *J Clin Oncol* 1997; **15**: 433–44.
9 Childs R, Chernoff A, Contentin N *et al.* Regression of metastatic renal-cell carcinoma after nonmyeloablative allogeneic peripheral-blood stem-cell transplantation. *N Engl J Med* 2000; **343**: 750–8.

10 Sandmaier BM, McSweeney PYuC, Storb R. Nonmyeloablative transplants. preclinical and clinical results. *Semin Oncol* 2000; **27**: 78–81.
11 Champlin R, Khouri I, Kornblau S *et al.* Allogeneic hematopoietic transplantation as adoptive immunotherapy. Induction of graft-versus-malignancy as primary therapy. *Hematol Oncol Clin North Am* 1999; **13**: 1041–57.
12 Walter EA, Greenberg PD, Gilbert MJ *et al.* Reconstitution of cellular immunity against cytomegalovirus in recipients of allogeneic bone marrow by transfer of T-cell clones from the donor. *N Engl J Med* 1995; **333**: 1038–44.
13 Riddell SR, Watanabe KS, Goodrich JM, Li CR, Agha ME, Greenberg PD. Restoration of viral immunity in immunodeficient humans by the adoptive transfer of T cell clones. *Science* 1992; **257**: 238–41.
14 Rooney CM, Smith CA, Ng CY *et al.* Infusion of cytotoxic T cells for the prevention and treatment of Epstein–Barr virus-induced lymphoma in allogeneic transplant recipients. *Blood* 1998; **92**: 1549–55.
15 Yee C, Thompson JA, Byrd D *et al.* Adoptive T cell therapy using antigen-specific $CD8^+$ T cell clones for the treatment of patients with metastatic melanoma: *in vivo* persistence, migration, and antitumor effect of transferred T cells. *Proc Natl Acad Sci U S A* 2002; **99**: 16,168–73.
16 Dudley ME, Wunderlich JR, Robbins PF *et al.* Cancer regression and autoimmunity in patients after clonal repopulation with antitumor lymphocytes. *Science* 2002; **298**: 850–4.
17 Schmidt CS, Mescher MF. Peptide antigen priming of naive, but not memory, CD8 T cells requires a third signal that can be provided by IL-12. *J Immunol* 2002; **168**: 5521–9.
18 Liu K, Catalfamo M, Li Y, Henkart PA, Weng NP. IL-15 mimics T cell receptor crosslinking in the induction of cellular proliferation, gene expression, and cytotoxicity in $CD8^+$ memory T cells. *Proc Natl Acad Sci U S A* 2002; **99**: 6192–7.
19 Maus MV, Thomas AK, Leonard DG *et al.* Ex vivo expansion of polyclonal and antigen-specific cytotoxic T lymphocytes by artificial APCs expressing ligands for the T-cell receptor, CD28 and 4-1BB. *Nat Biotechnol* 2002; **20**: 143–8.
20 Prlic M, Lefrancois L, Jameson SC. Multiple choices. regulation of memory CD8 T cell generation and homeostasis by interleukin (IL)-7 and IL-15. *J Exp Med* 2002; **195**: F49–52.
21 Goldrath AW, Sivakumar PV, Glaccum M *et al.* Cytokine requirements for acute and basal homeostatic proliferation of naive and memory $CD8^+$ T cells. *J Exp Med* 2002; **195**: 1515–22.
22 Meyers JD, Flournoy N, Thomas ED. Risk factors for cytomegalovirus infection after human marrow transplantation. *J Infect Dis* 1986; **153**: 478–88.
23 Meyers JD, Ljungman P, Fisher LD. Cytomegalovirus excretion as a predictor of cytomegalovirus disease after marrow transplantation: importance of cytomegalovirus viremia. *J Infect Dis* 1990; **162**: 373–80.
24 Boeckh M, Bowden RA, Goodrich JM, Pettinger M, Meyers JD. Cytomegalovirus antigen detection in peripheral blood leukocytes after allogeneic marrow transplantation. *Blood* 1992; **80**: 1358–64.
25 Gor D, Sabin C, Prentice HG *et al.* Longitudinal fluctuations in cytomegalovirus load in bone

25. marrow transplant patients: relationship between peak virus load, donor/recipient serostatus, acute GVHD and CMV disease. *Bone Marrow Transplant* 1998; **21**: 597–605.
26. Reusser P, Riddell SR, Meyers JD, Greenberg PD. Cytotoxic T-lymphocyte response to cytomegalovirus after human allogeneic bone marrow transplantation. Pattern of recovery and correlation with cytomegalovirus infection and disease. *Blood* 1991; **78**: 1373–80.
27. Li CR, Greenberg PD, Gilbert MJ, Goodrich JM, Riddell SR. Recovery of HLA-restricted cytomegalovirus (CMV)-specific T-cell responses after allogeneic bone marrow transplant: correlation with CMV disease and effect of ganciclovir prophylaxis. *Blood* 1994; **83**: 1971–9.
28. Shepp DH, Dandliker PS, de Miranda P et al. Activity of 9-[2-hydroxy-1-(hydroxymethyl)-ethoxymethyl]guanine in the treatment of cytomegalovirus pneumonia. *Ann Intern Med* 1985; **103**: 368–73.
29. Emanuel D, Cunningham I, Jules-Elysee K et al. Cytomegalovirus pneumonia after bone marrow transplantation successfully treated with the combination of ganciclovir and high-dose intravenous immune globulin. *Ann Intern Med* 1988; **109**: 777–82.
30. Reed EC, Bowden RA, Dandliker PS, Lilleby KE, Meyers JD. Treatment of cytomegalovirus pneumonia with ganciclovir and intravenous cytomegalovirus immunoglobulin in patients with bone marrow transplants. *Ann Intern Med* 1988; **109**: 783–8.
31. Schmidt GM, Horak DA, Niland JC, Duncan SR, Forman SJ, Zaia JA. A randomized, controlled trial of prophylactic ganciclovir for cytomegalovirus pulmonary infection in recipients of allogeneic bone marrow transplants: The City of Hope-Stanford-Syntex CMV Study Group. *N Engl J Med* 1991; **324**: 1005–11.
32. Goodrich JM, Mori M, Gleaves CA et al. Early treatment with ganciclovir to prevent cytomegalovirus disease after allogeneic bone marrow transplantation. *N Engl J Med* 1991; **325**: 1601–7.
33. Goodrich JM, Bowden RA, Fisher L, Keller C, Schoch G, Meyers JD. Ganciclovir prophylaxis to prevent cytomegalovirus disease after allogeneic marrow transplant. *Ann Intern Med* 1993; **118**: 173–8.
34. Winston DJ, Ho WG, Bartoni K et al. Ganciclovir prophylaxis of cytomegalovirus infection and disease in allogeneic bone marrow transplant recipients. Results of a placebo-controlled, double-blind trial. *Ann Intern Med* 1993; **118**: 179–84.
35. Einsele H, Ehninger G, Hebart H et al. Polymerase chain reaction monitoring reduces the incidence of cytomegalovirus disease and the duration and side effects of antiviral therapy after bone marrow transplantation. *Blood* 1995; **86**: 2815–20.
36. Boeckh M, Gooley TA, Myerson D, Cunningham T, Schoch G, Bowden RA. Cytomegalovirus pp65 antigenemia-guided early treatment with ganciclovir versus ganciclovir at engraftment after allogeneic marrow transplantation: a randomized double-blind study. *Blood* 1996; **88**: 4063–71.
37. Boeckh M, Leisenring W, Riddell SR et al. Late cytomegalovirus disease and mortality in recipients of allogeneic hematopoietic stem cell transplants: importance of viral load and T-cell immunity. *Blood* 2003; **101**: 407–14.
38. Reddehase MJ, Weiland F, Munch K, Jonjic S, Luske A, Koszinowski UH. Interstitial murine cytomegalovirus pneumonia after irradiation. Characterization of cells that limit viral replication during established infection of the lungs. *J Virol* 1985; **55**: 264–73.
39. Jordan MC, Shanley JD, Stevens JG. Immunosuppression reactivates and disseminates latent murine cytomegalovirus. *J General Virol* 1977; **37**: 419–23.
40. Steffens HP, Podlech J, Kurz S, Angele P, Dreis D, Reddehase MJ. Cytomegalovirus inhibits the engraftment of donor bone marrow cells by downregulation of hemopoietin gene expression in recipient stroma. *J Virol* 1998; **72**: 5006–15.
41. Polic B, Hengel H, Krmpotic A et al. Hierarchical and redundant lymphocyte subset control precludes cytomegalovirus replication during latent infection. *J Exp Med* 1998; **188**: 1047–54.
42. Steffens HP, Kurz S, Holtappels R, Reddehase MJ. Preemptive CD8 T-cell immunotherapy of acute cytomegalovirus infection prevents lethal disease, limits the burden of latent viral genomes, and reduces the risk of virus recurrence. *J Virol* 1998; **72**: 1797–804.
43. Reddehase MJ, Mutter W, Koszinowski UH. *In vivo* application of recombinant interleukin 2 in the immunotherapy of established cytomegalovirus infection. *J Exp Med* 1987; **165**: 650–6.
44. Solheim JC. Class I MHC molecules. Assembly and antigen presentation. *Immunol Rev* 1999; **172**: 11–9.
45. Holtappels R, Thomas D, Podlech J, Reddehase MJ. Two antigenic peptides from genes *m123* and *m164* of murine cytomegalovirus quantitatively dominate CD8 T-cell memory in the H-2d haplotype. *J Virol* 2002; **76**: 151–64.
46. Holtappels R, Grzimek NK, Simon CO, Thomas D, Dreis D, Reddehase MJ. Processing and presentation of murine cytomegalovirus pORFm164-derived peptide in fibroblasts in the face of all viral immunosubversive early gene functions. *J Virol* 2002; **76**: 6044–53.
47. Del Val M, Schlicht HJ, Volkmer H, Messerle M, Reddehase MJ, Koszinowski UH. Protection against lethal cytomegalovirus infection by a recombinant vaccine containing a single nonameric T-cell epitope. *J Virol* 1991; **65**: 3641–6.
48. Wagner M, Gutermann A, Podlech J, Reddehase MJ, Koszinowski UH. Major histocompatibility complex class I allele-specific cooperative and competitive interactions between immune evasion proteins of cytomegalovirus. *J Exp Med* 2002; **196**: 805–16.
49. Reddehase MJ. Antigens and immunoevasins: opponents in cytomegalovirus immune surveillance. *Nat Rev Immunol* 2002; **2**: 831–44.
50. Hebart H, Daginik S, Stevanovic S et al. Sensitive detection of human cytomegalovirus peptide-specific cytotoxic T-lymphocyte responses by interferon-γ-enzyme-linked immunospot assay and flow cytometry in healthy individuals and in patients after allogeneic stem cell transplantation. *Blood* 2002; **99**: 3830–7.
51. Engstrand M, Tournay C, Peyrat MA et al. Characterization of CMVpp65-specific CD8[+] T lymphocytes using MHC tetramers in kidney transplant patients and healthy participants. *Transplantation* 2000; **69**: 2243–50.
52. Maecker HT, Dunn HS, Suni MA et al. Use of overlapping peptide mixtures as antigens for cytokine flow cytometry. *J Immunol Meth* 2001; **255**: 27–40.
53. Aubert G, Hassan-Walker AF, Madrigal JA et al. Cytomegalovirus-specific cellular immune responses and viremia in recipients of allogeneic stem cell transplants. *J Infect Dis* 2001; **184**: 955–63.
54. Gratama JW, van Esser JW, Lamers CH et al. Tetramer-based quantification of cytomegalovirus (CMV)-specific CD8[+] T lymphocytes in T-cell-depleted stem cell grafts and after transplantation may identify patients at risk for progressive CMV infection. *Blood* 2001; **98**: 1358–64.
55. Cwynarski K, Ainsworth J, Cobbold M et al. Direct visualization of cytomegalovirus-specific T-cell reconstitution after allogeneic stem cell transplantation. *Blood* 2001; **97**: 1232–40.
56. Ozdemir E, St John LS, Gillespie G et al. Cytomegalovirus reactivation following allogeneic stem cell transplantation is associated with the presence of dysfunctional antigen-specific CD8[+] T cells. *Blood* 2002; **100**: 3690–7.
57. Tortorella D, Gewurz BE, Furman MH, Schust DJ, Ploegh HL. Viral subversion of the immune system. *Annu Rev Immunol* 2000; **18**: 861–926.
58. Sissons JG, Bain M, Wills MR. Latency and reactivation of human cytomegalovirus. *J Infect* 2002; **44**: 73–7.
59. Hahn G, Jores R, Mocarski ES. Cytomegalovirus remains latent in a common precursor of dendritic and myeloid cells. *Proc Natl Acad Sci U S A* 1998; **95**: 3937–42.
60. Kondo K, Xu J, Mocarski ES. Human cytomegalovirus latent gene expression in granulocyte-macrophage progenitors in culture and in seropositive individuals. *Proc Natl Acad Sci U S A* 1996; **93**: 11,137–42.
61. Jones TR, Hanson LK, Sun L, Slater JS, Stenberg RM, Campbell AE. Multiple independent loci within the human cytomegalovirus unique short region down-regulate expression of major histocompatibility complex class I heavy chains. *J Virol* 1995; **69**: 4830–41.
62. Jones TR, Wiertz EJ, Sun L, Fish KN, Nelson JA, Ploegh HL. Human cytomegalovirus US3 impairs transport and maturation of major histocompatibility complex class I heavy chains. *Proc Natl Acad Sci U S A* 1996; **93**: 11,327–33.
63. Ahn K, Angulo A, Ghazal P, Peterson PA, Yang Y, Fruh K. Human cytomegalovirus inhibits antigen presentation by a sequential multistep process. *Proc Natl Acad Sci U S A* 1996; **93**: 10990–5.
64. Wiertz EJ, Jones TR, Sun L, Bogyo M, Geuze HJ, Ploegh HL. The human cytomegalovirus *US11* gene product dislocates MHC class I heavy chains from the endoplasmic reticulum to the cytosol. *Cell* 1996; **84**: 769–79.
65. Wiertz EJ, Tortorella D, Bogyo M et al. Sec61-mediated transfer of a membrane protein from the endoplasmic reticulum to the proteasome for destruction. *Nature* 1996; **384**: 432–8.
66. Ahn K, Gruhler A, Galocha B et al. The ER-luminal domain of the HCMV glycoprotein US6 inhibits peptide translocation by TAP. *Immunity* 1997; **6**: 613–21.
67. Beersma MF, Bijlmakers MJ, Ploegh HL. Human cytomegalovirus down-regulates HLA class I expression by reducing the stability of class I H chains. *J Immunol* 1993; **151**: 4455–64.
68. Gilbert MJ, Riddell SR, Li CR, Greenberg PD. Selective interference with class I major histocompatibility complex presentation of the major

immediate-early protein following infection with human cytomegalovirus. *J Virol* 1993; **67**: 3461–9.

69 Riddell SR, Rabin M, Geballe AP, Britt WJ, Greenberg PD. Class I MHC-restricted cytotoxic T lymphocyte recognition of cells infected with human cytomegalovirus does not require endogenous viral gene expression. *J Immunol* 1991; **146**: 2795–804.

70 Riddell SR. Pathogenesis of cytomegalovirus pneumonia in immunocompromised hosts. *Semin Respir Infect* 1995; **10**: 199–208.

71 McLaughlin-Taylor E, Pande H, Forman SJ et al. Identification of the major late human cytomegalovirus matrix protein pp65 as a target antigen for CD8+ virus-specific cytotoxic T lymphocytes. *J Med Virol* 1994; **43**: 103–10.

72 Wills MR, Carmichael AJ, Mynard K et al. The human cytotoxic T-lymphocyte (CTL) response to cytomegalovirus is dominated by structural protein pp65: frequency, specificity, and T-cell receptor usage of pp65-specific CTL. *J Virol* 1996; **70**: 7569–79.

73 Gillespie GM, Wills MR, Appay V et al. Functional heterogeneity and high frequencies of cytomegalovirus-specific CD8+ T lymphocytes in healthy seropositive donors. *J Virol* 2000; **74**: 8140–50.

74 Kern F, Bunde T, Faulhaber N et al. Cytomegalovirus (CMV) phosphoprotein 65 makes a large contribution to shaping the T cell repertoire in CMV-exposed individuals. *J Infect Dis* 2002; **185**: 1709–16.

75 Kern F, Surel IP, Faulhaber N et al. Target structures of the CD8+T-cell response to human cytomegalovirus: the 72-kilodalton major immediate-early protein revisited. *J Virol* 1999; **73**: 8179–84.

76 Gyulai Z, Endresz V, Burian K et al. Cytotoxic T lymphocyte (CTL) responses to human cytomegalovirus pp65, IE1-Exon4, gB.150, and pp28 in healthy individuals: reevaluation of prevalence of IE1-specific CTLs. *J Infect Dis* 2000; **181**: 1537–46.

77 Gilbert MJ, Riddell SR, Plachter B, Greenberg PD. Cytomegalovirus selectively blocks antigen processing and presentation of its immediate-early gene product. *Nature* 1996; **383**: 720–2.

78 Mutimer HP, Akatsuka Y, Manley T et al. Association between immune recovery uveitis and a diverse intraocular cytomegalovirus-specific cytotoxic T cell response. *J Infect Dis* 2002; **186**: 701–5.

79 Manley T, Luy L, Jones T, Riddell SR. Identification of CD8+ CMV-specific cytotoxic T-cell responses to novel viral antigens in normal CMV seropositive individuals. *Blood* 2002; **100**: 3695a [Abstract].

80 Plachter B, Sinzger C, Jahn G. Cell types involved in replication and distribution of human cytomegalovirus. *Adv Virus Res* 1996; **46**: 195–261.

81 Diefenbach A, Tomasello E, Lucas M et al. Selective associations with signaling proteins determine stimulatory versus costimulatory activity of NKG2D. *Nat Immunol* 2002; **3**: 1142–9.

82 Groh V, Rhinehart R, Randolph-Habecker J, Topp MS, Riddell SR, Spies T. Costimulation of CD8αβ T cells by NKG2D via engagement by MIC induced on virus-infected cells. *Nat Immunol* 2001; **2**: 255–60.

83 Sutherland CL, Chalupny NJ, Cosman D. The UL16-binding proteins, a novel family of MHC class I-related ligands for NKG2D, activate natural killer cell functions. *Immunol Rev* 2001; **181**: 185–92.

84 Pieters J. MHC class II-restricted antigen processing and presentation. *Adv Immunol* 2000; **75**: 159–208.

85 Le Roy E, Baron M, Faigle W et al. Infection of APC by human cytomegalovirus controlled through recognition of endogenous nuclear immediate early protein 1 by specific CD4+ T lymphocytes. *J Immunol* 2002; **169**: 1293–301.

86 Sester M, Sester U, Gartner B et al. Sustained high frequencies of specific CD4 T cells restricted to a single persistent virus. *J Virol* 2002; **76**: 3748–55.

87 Hegde NR, Tomazin RA, Wisner TW et al. Inhibition of HLA-DR assembly, transport, and loading by human cytomegalovirus glycoprotein US3: a novel mechanism for evading major histocompatibility complex class II antigen presentation. *J Virol* 2002; **76**: 10929–41.

88 Tomazin R, Boname J, Hegde NR et al. Cytomegalovirus US2 destroys two components of the MHC class II pathway, preventing recognition by CD4+ T cells. *Nat Med* 1999; **5**: 1039–43.

89 Belz GT, Wodarz D, Diaz G, Nowak MA, Doherty PC. Compromised influenza virus-specific CD8+-T-cell memory in CD4+-T-cell-deficient mice. *J Virol* 2002; **76**: 12,388–93.

90 Zajac AJ, Blattman JN, Murali-Krishna K et al. Viral immune evasion due to persistence of activated T cells without effector function. *J Exp Med* 1998; **188**: 2205–13.

91 Einsele H, Roosnek E, Rufer N et al. Infusion of cytomegalovirus (CMV)-specific T cells for the treatment of CMV infection not responding to antiviral chemotherapy. *Blood* 2002; **99**: 3916–22.

92 Ho VT, Soiffer RJ. The history and future of T-cell depletion as graft-versus-host disease prophylaxis for allogeneic hematopoietic stem cell transplantation. *Blood* 2001; **98**: 3192–204.

93 Bissinger AL, Rauser G, Hebart H, Frank F, Jahn G, Einsele H. Isolation and expansion of human cytomegalovirus-specific cytotoxic T lymphocytes using interferon-γ secretion assay. *Exp Hematol* 2002; **30**: 1178–84.

94 Szmania S, Galloway A, Bruorton M et al. Isolation and expansion of cytomegalovirus-specific cytotoxic T lymphocytes to clinical scale from a single blood draw using dendritic cells and HLA-tetramers. *Blood* 2001; **98**: 505–12.

95 Keenan RD, Ainsworth J, Khan N et al. Purification of cytomegalovirus-specific CD8 T cells from peripheral blood using HLA-peptide tetramers. *Br J Haematol* 2001; **115**: 428–34.

96 Takada K. Role of Epstein–Barr virus in Burkitt's lymphoma. *Curr Top Microbiol Immunol* 2001; **258**: 141–51.

97 Dolcetti R, Boiocchi M, Gloghini A, Carbone A. Pathogenetic and histogenetic features of HIV-associated Hodgkin's disease. *Eur J Cancer* 2001; **37**: 1276–87.

98 Sam CK, Brooks LA, Niedobitek G, Young LS, Prasad U, Rickinson AB. Analysis of Epstein–Barr virus infection in nasopharyngeal biopsies from a group at high risk of nasopharyngeal carcinoma. *Int J Cancer* 1993; **53**: 957–62.

99 Qu L, Rowe DT. Epstein–Barr virus latent gene expression in uncultured peripheral blood lymphocytes. *J Virol* 1992; **66**: 3715–24.

100 Babcock GJ, Thorley-Lawson DA. Tonsillar memory B cells, latently infected with Epstein–Barr virus, express the restricted pattern of latent genes previously found only in Epstein–Barr virus-associated tumors. *Proc Natl Acad Sci U S A* 2000; **97**: 12,250–5.

101 Thorley-Lawson DA. Epstein–Barr virus: exploiting the immune system. *Nat Rev Immunol* 2001; **1**: 75–82.

102 Babcock GJ, Hochberg D, Thorley-Lawson AD. The expression pattern of Epstein–Barr virus latent genes *in vivo* is dependent upon the differentiation stage of the infected B cell. *Immunity* 2000; **13**: 497–506.

103 Tierney RJ, Steven N, Young LS, Rickinson AB. Epstein–Barr virus latency in blood mononuclear cells. Analysis of viral gene transcription during primary infection and in the carrier state. *J Virol* 1994; **68**: 7374–85.

104 Laytragoon-Lewin N, Chen F, Avila-Carino J, Klein G, Mellstedt H. Epstein–Barr virus (EBV) gene expression in lymphoid B cells during acute infectious mononucleosis (IM) and clonality of the directly growing cell lines. *Int J Cancer* 1997; **71**: 345–9.

105 Schaefer BC, Strominger JL, Speck SH. Host-cell-determined methylation of specific Epstein–Barr virus promoters regulates the choice between distinct viral latency programs. *Mol Cell Biol* 1997; **17**: 364–77.

106 Joseph AM, Babcock GJ, Thorley-Lawson DA. EBV persistence involves strict selection of latently infected B cells. *J Immunol* 2000; **165**: 2975–81.

107 Wagner HJ, Rooney CM, Heslop HE. Diagnosis and treatment of posttransplantation lymphoproliferative disease after hematopoietic stem cell transplantation. *Biol Blood Marrow Transplant* 2002; **8**: 1–8.

108 Gross TG, Steinbuch M, DeFor T et al. B cell lymphoproliferative disorders following hematopoietic stem cell transplantation: risk factors, treatment and outcome. *Bone Marrow Transplant* 1999; **23**: 251–8.

109 Shapiro RS, McClain K, Frizzera G et al. Epstein–Barr virus associated B cell lymphoproliferative disorders following bone marrow transplantation. *Blood* 1988; **71**: 1234–43.

110 Zutter MM, Martin PJ, Sale GE et al. Epstein–Barr virus lymphoproliferation after bone marrow transplantation. *Blood* 1988; **72**: 520–9.

111 Curtis RE, Travis LB, Rowlings PA et al. Risk of lymphoproliferative disorders after bone marrow transplantation: a multi-institutional study. *Blood* 1999; **94**: 2208–16.

112 Gerritsen EJ, Stam ED, Hermans J et al. Risk factors for developing EBV-related B cell lymphoproliferative disorders (BLPD) after non-HLA-identical BMT in children. *Bone Marrow Transplant* 1996; **18**: 377–82.

113 Chiang KY, Hazlett LJ, Godder KT et al. Epstein–Barr virus-associated B cell lymphoproliferative disorder following mismatched related T cell-depleted bone marrow transplantation. *Bone Marrow Transplant* 2001; **28**: 1117–23.

114 Cavazzana-Calvo M, Bensoussan D, Jabado N et al. Prevention of EBV-induced B-lymphoproliferative disorder by *ex vivo* marrow B-cell depletion in HLA-phenoidentical or non-identical T-depleted bone marrow transplantation. *Br J Haematol* 1998; **103**: 543–51.

115 Hale G, Waldmann H. Risks of developing Epstein–Barr virus-related lymphoproliferative disorders after T-cell-depleted marrow transplants. CAMPATH users. *Blood* 1998; **91**: 3079–83.

116 Meijer E, Slaper-Cortenbach IC, Thijsen SF, Dekker AW, Verdonck LF. Increased incidence of EBV-associated lymphoproliferative disorders after allogeneic stem cell transplantation from matched unrelated donors due to a change of T cell depletion technique. *Bone Marrow Transplant* 2002; **29**: 335–9.

117 Knowles DM, Cesarman E, Chadburn A et al. Correlative morphologic and molecular genetic analysis demonstrates three distinct categories of posttransplantation lymphoproliferative disorders. *Blood* 1995; **85**: 552–65.

118 O'Reilly RJ, Small TN, Papadopoulos E, Lucas K, Lacerda J, Koulova L. Biology and adoptive cell therapy of Epstein–Barr virus-associated lymphoproliferative disorders in recipients of marrow allografts. *Immunol Rev* 1997; **157**: 195–216.

119 Cleary ML, Nalesnik MA, Shearer WT, Sklar J. Clonal analysis of transplant-associated lymphoproliferations based on the structure of the genomic termini of the Epstein–Barr virus. *Blood* 1988; **72**: 349–52.

120 Ambinder RF, Mann RB. Detection and characterization of Epstein–Barr virus in clinical specimens. *Am J Pathol* 1994; **145**: 239–52.

121 Benkerrou M, Durandy A, Fischer A. Therapy for transplant-related lymphoproliferative diseases. *Hematol Oncol Clin North Am* 1993; **7**: 467–75.

122 Fischer A, Blanche S, Le Bidois J et al. Anti-B-cell monoclonal antibodies in the treatment of severe B-cell lymphoproliferative syndrome following bone marrow and organ transplantation. *N Engl J Med* 1991; **324**: 1451–6.

123 Blanche S, Le Deist F, Veber F et al. Treatment of severe Epstein–Barr virus-induced polyclonal B-lymphocyte proliferation by anti-B-cell monoclonal antibodies. Two cases after HLA-mismatched bone marrow transplantation. *Ann Intern Med* 1988; **108**: 199–203.

124 Benkerrou M, Jais JP, Leblond V et al. Anti-B-cell monoclonal antibody treatment of severe post-transplant B-lymphoproliferative disorder: prognostic factors and long-term outcome. *Blood* 1998; **92**: 3137–47.

125 Faye A, Quartier P, Reguerre Y et al. Chimaeric anti-CD20 monoclonal antibody (rituximab) in post-transplant B-lymphoproliferative disorder following stem cell transplantation in children. *Br J Haematol* 2001; **115**: 112–8.

126 McGuirk JP, Seropian S, Howe G, Smith B, Stoddart L, Cooper DL. Use of rituximab and irradiated donor-derived lymphocytes to control Epstein–Barr virus-associated lymphoproliferation in patients undergoing related haplo-identical stem cell transplantation. *Bone Marrow Transplant* 1999; **24**: 1253–8.

127 Kuehnle I, Huls MH, Liu Z et al. CD20 monoclonal antibody (rituximab) for therapy of Epstein–Barr virus lymphoma after hemopoietic stem-cell transplantation. *Blood* 2000; **95**: 1502–5.

128 Milpied N, Vasseur B, Parquet N et al. Humanized anti-CD20 monoclonal antibody (rituximab) in post transplant B-lymphoproliferative disorder: a retrospective analysis on 32 patients. *Ann Oncol* 2000; **11**: 113–6.

129 Carpenter PA, Appelbaum FR, Corey L et al. A humanized non-FcR-binding anti-CD3 antibody, visilizumab, for treatment of steroid-refractory acute graft-versus-host disease. *Blood* 2002; **99**: 2712–9.

130 Verschuuren EA, Stevens SJ, van Imhoff GW et al. Treatment of posttransplant lymphoproliferative disease with rituximab: the remission, the relapse, and the complication. *Transplantation* 2002; **73**: 100–4.

131 Moss DJ, Rickinson AB, Pope JH. Long-term T-cell-mediated immunity to Epstein–Barr virus in man. I. Complete regression of virus-induced transformation in cultures of seropositive donor leukocytes. *Int J Cancer* 1978; **22**: 662–8.

132 Lacerda JF, Ladanyi M, Louie DC, Fernandez JM, Papadopoulos EB, O'Reilly RJ. Human Epstein–Barr virus (EBV)-specific cytotoxic T lymphocytes home preferentially to and induce selective regressions of autologous EBV-induced B cell lymphoproliferations in xenografted C.B-17 scid/scid mice. *J Exp Med* 1996; **183**: 1215–28.

133 Lucas KG, Small TN, Heller G, Dupont B, O'Reilly RJ. The development of cellular immunity to Epstein–Barr virus after allogeneic bone marrow transplantation. *Blood* 1996; **87**: 2594–603.

134 Marshall NA, Howe JG, Formica R et al. Rapid reconstitution of Epstein–Barr virus-specific T lymphocytes following allogeneic stem cell transplantation. *Blood* 2000; **96**: 2814–21.

135 Callan MF, Tan L, Annels N et al. Direct visualization of antigen-specific CD8+ T cells during the primary immune response to Epstein–Barr virus in vivo. *J Exp Med* 1998; **187**: 1395–402.

136 Tan LC, Gudgeon N, Annels NE et al. A re-evaluation of the frequency of CD8+ T cells specific for EBV in healthy virus carriers. *J Immunol* 1999; **162**: 1827–35.

137 Catalina MD, Sullivan JL, Brody RM, Luzuriaga K. Phenotypic and functional heterogeneity of EBV epitope-specific CD8+ T cells. *J Immunol* 2002; **168**: 4184–91.

138 Khanna R, Burrows SR, Kurilla MG et al. Localization of Epstein–Barr virus cytotoxic T cell epitopes using recombinant vaccinia: implications for vaccine development. *J Exp Med* 1992; **176**: 169–76.

139 Dantuma NP, Sharipo A, Masucci MG. Avoiding proteasomal processing. The case of EBNA1. *Curr Top Microbiol Immunol* 2002; **269**: 23–36.

140 Rowe M, Lear AL, Croom-Carter D, Davies AH, Rickinson AB. Three pathways of Epstein–Barr virus gene activation from EBNA1-positive latency in B lymphocytes. *J Virol* 1992; **66**: 122–31.

141 Maini MK, Gudgeon N, Wedderburn LR, Rickinson AB, Beverley PC. Clonal expansions in acute EBV infection are detectable in the CD8 and not the CD4 subset and persist with a variable CD45 phenotype. *J Immunol* 2000; **165**: 5729–37.

142 Leen A, Meij P, Redchenko I et al. Differential immunogenicity of Epstein–Barr virus latent-cycle proteins for human CD4+ T-helper 1 responses. *J Virol* 2001; **75**: 8649–59.

143 Rajnavolgyi E, Nagy N, Thuresson B et al. A repetitive sequence of Epstein–Barr virus nuclear antigen 6 comprises overlapping T cell epitopes which induce HLA-DR-restricted CD4+ T lymphocytes. *Int Immunol* 2000; **12**: 281–93.

144 Munz C, Bickham KL, Subklewe M et al. Human CD4+ T lymphocytes consistently respond to the latent Epstein–Barr virus nuclear antigen EBNA1. *J Exp Med* 2000; **191**: 1649–60.

145 Nikiforow S, Bottomly K, Miller G. CD4+ T-cell effectors inhibit Epstein–Barr virus-induced B-cell proliferation. *J Virol* 2001; **75**: 3740–52.

146 Wilson AD, Hopkins JC, Morgan AJ. In vitro cytokine production and growth inhibition of lymphoblastoid cell lines by CD4+ T cells from Epstein–Barr virus (EBV) seropositive donors. *Clin Exp Immunol* 2001; **126**: 101–10.

147 Paludan C, Bickham K, Nikiforow S et al. Epstein–Barr nuclear antigen 1-specific CD4+ TH1 cells kill Burkitt's lymphoma cells. *J Immunol* 2002; **169**: 1593–603.

148 Papadopoulos EB, Ladanyi M, Emanuel D et al. Infusions of donor leukocytes to treat Epstein–Barr virus-associated lymphoproliferative disorders after allogeneic bone marrow transplantation. *N Engl J Med* 1994; **330**: 1185–91.

149 Rooney CM, Smith CA, Ng CY et al. Use of gene-modified virus-specific T lymphocytes to control Epstein–Barr-virus-related lymphoproliferation. *Lancet* 1995; **345**: 9–13.

150 Gottschalk S, Ng CY, Perez M et al. An Epstein–Barr virus deletion mutant associated with fatal lymphoproliferative disease unresponsive to therapy with virus-specific CTLs. *Blood* 2001; **97**: 835–43.

151 Heslop HE, Ng CY, Li C et al. Long-term restoration of immunity against Epstein–Barr virus infection by adoptive transfer of gene-modified virus-specific T lymphocytes. *Nat Med* 1996; **2**: 551–5.

152 Qu L, Green M, Webber S, Reyes J, Ellis D, Rowe D. Epstein–Barr virus gene expression in the peripheral blood of transplant recipients with persistent circulating virus loads. *J Infect Dis* 2000; **182**: 1013–21.

153 Babcock GJ, Decker LL, Freeman RB, Thorley-Lawson DA. Epstein–Barr virus-infected resting memory B cells, not proliferating lymphoblasts, accumulate in the peripheral blood of immunosuppressed patients. *J Exp Med* 1999; **190**: 567–76.

154 Hoshino Y, Kimura H, Tanaka N et al. Prospective monitoring of the Epstein–Barr virus DNA by a real-time quantitative polymerase chain reaction after allogenic stem cell transplantation. *Br J Haematol* 2001; **115**: 105–11.

155 van Esser JW, van der Holt B, Meijer E et al. Epstein–Barr virus (EBV) reactivation is a frequent event after allogeneic stem cell trans-plantation (SCT) and quantitatively predicts EBV-lymphoproliferative disease following T-cell-depleted SCT. *Blood* 2001; **98**: 972–8.

156 Gustafsson A, Levitsky V, Zou JZ et al. Epstein–Barr virus (EBV) load in bone marrow transplant recipients at risk to develop posttransplant lymphoproliferative disease: prophylactic infusion of EBV-specific cytotoxic T cells. *Blood* 2000; **95**: 807–14.

157 Wu TC, Mann RB, Charache P et al. Detection of EBV gene expression in Reed–Sternberg cells of Hodgkin's disease. *Int J Cancer* 1990; **46**: 801–4.

158 Weiss LM. Epstein–Barr virus and Hodgkin's disease. *Curr Oncol Rep* 2000; **2**: 199–204.

159 Deacon EM, Pallesen G, Niedobitek G et al. Epstein–Barr virus and Hodgkin's disease: transcriptional analysis of virus latency in the malignant cells. *J Exp Med* 1993; **177**: 339–49.

160 Wang D, Liebowitz D, Kieff E. An EBV membrane protein expressed in immortalized lymphocytes transforms established rodent cells. *Cell* 1985; **43**: 831–40.

161 Kulwichit W, Edwards RH, Davenport EM, Baskar JF, Godfrey V, Raab-Traub N. Expression of the Epstein–Barr virus latent membrane protein 1 induces B cell lymphoma in transgenic mice. *Proc Natl Acad Sci U S A* 1998; **95**: 11,963–8.

162 Meij P, Leen A, Rickinson AB et al. Identification and prevalence of CD8+ T-cell responses directed against Epstein–Barr virus-encoded latent membrane protein 1 and latent membrane protein 2. *Int J Cancer* 2002; **99**: 93–9.

163 Roskrow MA, Suzuki N, Gan Y et al. Epstein–Barr virus (EBV)-specific cytotoxic T lymphocytes for the treatment of patients with EBV-positive relapsed Hodgkin's disease. *Blood* 1998; **91**: 2925–34.

164 Sing AP, Ambinder RF, Hong DJ et al. Isolation of Epstein–Barr virus (EBV)-specific cytotoxic T lymphocytes that lyse Reed–Sternberg cells: implications for immune-mediated therapy of EBV+ Hodgkin's disease. *Blood* 1997; **89**: 1978–86.

165 Gahn B, Siller-Lopez F, Pirooz AD et al. Adenoviral gene transfer into dendritic cells efficiently amplifies the immune response to LMP2A antigen: a potential treatment strategy for Epstein–Barr virus-positive Hodgkin's lymphoma. *Int J Cancer* 2001; **93**: 706–13.

166 Su Z, Peluso MV, Raffegerst SH, Schendel DJ, Roskrow MA. The generation of LMP2a-specific cytotoxic T lymphocytes for the treatment of patients with Epstein–Barr virus-positive Hodgkin disease. *Eur J Immunol* 2001; **31**: 947–58.

167 Gottschalk S, Edwards OL, Huls MH et al. Generating CTL against the subdominant Epstein–Barr virus LMP1 antigen for the adoptive immunotherapy of EBV-associated malignancies. *Blood* 2003; **101**: 1905–12.

168 Warren EH, Gavin M, Greenberg PD, Riddell SR. Minor histocompatibility antigens as targets for T-cell therapy after bone marrow transplantation. *Curr Opin Hematol* 1998; **5**: 429–33.

169 Goulmy E. Human minor histocompatibility antigens. New concepts for marrow transplantation and adoptive immunotherapy. *Immunol Rev* 1997; **157**: 125–40.

170 Fontaine P, Roy-Proulx G, Knafo L, Baron C, Roy DC, Perreault C. Adoptive transfer of minor histocompatibility antigen-specific T lymphocytes eradicates leukemia cells without causing graft-versus-host disease. *Nat Med* 2001; **7**: 789–94.

171 Bortin MM, Truitt RL, Rimm AA, Bach FH. Graft-versus-leukaemia reactivity induced by alloimmunisation without augmentation of graft-versus-host reactivity. *Nature* 1979; **281**: 490–1.

172 Friedman TM, Gilbert M, Briggs C, Korngold R. Repertoire analysis of CD8+ T cell responses to minor histocompatibility antigens involved in graft-versus-host disease. *J Immunol* 1998; **161**: 41–8.

173 Weiden PL, Flournoy N, Thomas ED et al. Antileukemic effect of graft-versus-host disease in human recipients of allogeneic-marrow grafts. *N Engl J Med* 1979; **300**: 1068–73.

174 Weiden PL, Sullivan KM, Flournoy N, Storb R, Thomas ED. Antileukemic effect of chronic graft-versus-host disease: contribution to improved survival after allogeneic marrow transplantation. *N Engl J Med* 1981; **304**: 1529–33.

175 Horowitz MM, Gale RP, Sondel PM et al. Graft-versus-leukemia reactions after bone marrow transplantation. *Blood* 1990; **75**: 555–62.

176 Bortin MM, Truitt RL, Shih CY, Tempelis LD, LeFever AV, Rimm AA. Alloimmunization for induction of graft-versus-leukemia reactivity in H-2-compatible donors: critical role for incompatibility of donor and alloimmunizing strains at non-H-2 loci. *Transplant Proc* 1983; **15**: 2114–7.

177 Korngold R, Leighton C, Manser T. Graft-versus-myeloid leukemia responses following syngeneic and allogeneic bone marrow transplantation. *Transplantation* 1994; **58**: 278–87.

178 Meunier MC, Roy-Proulx G, Labrecque N, Perreault C. Tissue distribution of target antigen has a decisive influence on the outcome of adoptive cancer immunotherapy. *Blood* 2003; **101**: 766–70.

179 Ringden O, Labopin M, Gorin NC et al. Is there a graft-versus-leukaemia effect in the absence of graft-versus-host disease in patients undergoing bone marrow transplantation for acute leukaemia? *Br J Haematol* 2000; **111**: 1130–7.

180 Kolb HJ, Mittermuller J, Clemm C et al. Donor leukocyte transfusions for treatment of recurrent chronic myelogenous leukemia in marrow transplant patients. *Blood* 1990; **76**: 2462–5.

181 Porter DL, Collins RH Jr, Hardy C et al. Treatment of relapsed leukemia after unrelated donor marrow transplantation with unrelated donor leukocyte infusions. *Blood* 2000; **95**: 1214–21.

182 Levine JE, Braun T, Penza SL et al. Prospective trial of chemotherapy and donor leukocyte infusions for relapse of advanced myeloid malignancies after allogeneic stem-cell transplantation. *J Clin Oncol* 2002; **20**: 405–12.

183 Champlin R, Khouri I, Shimoni A et al. Harnessing graft-versus-malignancy: non-myeloablative preparative regimens for allogeneic haematopoietic transplantation, an evolving strategy for adoptive immunotherapy. *Br J Haematol* 2000; **111**: 18–29.

184 McSweeney PA, Niederwieser D, Shizuru JA et al. Hematopoietic cell transplantation in older patients with hematologic malignancies: replacing high-dose cytotoxic therapy with graft-versus-tumor effects. *Blood* 2001; **97**: 3390–400.

185 Appelbaum FR. The current status of hematopoietic cell transplantation. *Ann Rev Med* 2003; **54**: 494–512.

186 Khouri IF, Saliba RM, Giralt SA et al. Nonablative allogeneic hematopoietic transplantation as adoptive immunotherapy for indolent lymphoma: low incidence of toxicity, acute graft-versus-host disease, and treatment-related mortality. *Blood* 2001; **98**: 3595–9.

187 Corradini P, Tarella C, Olivieri A et al. Reduced-intensity conditioning followed by allografting of hematopoietic cells can produce clinical and molecular remissions in patients with poor-risk hematologic malignancies. *Blood* 2002; **99**: 75–82.

188 Rini BI, Zimmerman T, Stadler WM, Gajewski TF, Vogelzang NJ. Allogeneic stem-cell transplantation of renal cell cancer after nonmyeloablative chemotherapy: feasibility, engraftment, and clinical results. *J Clin Oncol* 2002; **20**: 2017–24.

189 O'Kunewick JP, Kociban DL, Machen LL, Buffo MJ. The role of CD4 and CD8 T cells in the graft-versus-leukemia response in Rauscher murine leukemia. *Bone Marrow Transplant* 1991; **8**: 445–52.

190 Palathumpat V, Dejbakhsh-Jones S, Strober S. The role of purified CD8+ T cells in graft-versus-leukemia activity and engraftment after allogeneic bone marrow transplantation. *Transplantation* 1995; **60**: 355–61.

191 Warren EH, Greenberg PD, Riddell SR. Cytotoxic T-lymphocyte-defined human minor histocompatibility antigens with a restricted tissue distribution. *Blood* 1998; **91**: 2197–207.

192 Faber LM, van der Hoeven J, Goulmy E et al. Recognition of clonogenic leukemic cells, remission bone marrow and HLA-identical donor bone marrow by CD8+ or CD4+ minor histocompatibility antigen-specific cytotoxic T lymphocytes. *J Clin Invest* 1995; **96**: 877–83.

193 Dolstra H, Fredrix H, Preijers F et al. Recognition of a B cell leukemia-associated minor histocompatibility antigen by CTL. *J Immunol* 1997; **158**: 560–5.

194 van der Harst D, Goulmy E, Falkenburg JH et al. Recognition of minor histocompatibility antigens on lymphocytic and myeloid leukemic cells by cytotoxic T-cell clones. *Blood* 1994; **83**: 1060–6.

195 Bonnet D, Dick JE. Human acute myeloid leukemia is organized as a hierarchy that originates from a primitive hematopoietic cell. *Nat Med* 1997; **3**: 730–7.

196 Lapidot T, Sirard C, Vormoor J et al. A cell initiating human acute myeloid leukaemia after transplantation into SCID mice. *Nature* 1994; **367**: 645–8.

197 Bonnet D, Warren EH, Greenberg PD, Dick JE, Riddell SR. CD8+ minor histocompatibility antigen-specific cytotoxic T lymphocyte clones eliminate human acute myeloid leukemia stem cells. *Proc Natl Acad Sci U S A* 1999; **96**: 8639–44.

198 de Bueger M, Bakker A, Van Rood JJ, Van der Woude F, Goulmy E. Tissue distribution of human minor histocompatibility antigens. Ubiquitous versus restricted tissue distribution indicates heterogeneity among human cytotoxic T lymphocyte-defined non-MHC antigens. *J Immunol* 1992; **149**: 1788–94.

199 Voogt PJ, Goulmy E, Veenhof WF et al. Cellularly defined minor histocompatibility antigens are differentially expressed on human hematopoietic progenitor cells. *J Exp Med* 1988; **168**: 2337–47.

200 Hunt DF, Henderson RA, Shabanowitz J et al. Characterization of peptides bound to the class I MHC molecule HLA-A2.1 by mass spectrometry. *Science* 1992; **255**: 1261–3.

201 den Haan JM, Sherman NE, Blokland E et al. Identification of a graft versus host disease-associated human minor histocompatibility antigen. *Science* 1995; **268**: 1476–80.

202 den Haan JM, Meadows LM, Wang W et al. The minor histocompatibility antigen HA-1: a diallelic gene with a single amino acid polymorphism. *Science* 1998; **279**: 1054–7.

203 Pierce RA, Field ED, den Haan JM et al. Cutting edge: the HLA-A*0101-restricted HY minor histocompatibility antigen originates from DFFRY and contains a cysteinylated cysteine residue as identified by a novel mass spectrometric technique. *J Immunol* 1999; **163**: 6360–4.

204 Pierce RA, Field ED, Mutis T et al. The HA-2 minor histocompatibility antigen is derived from a diallelic gene encoding a novel human class I myosin protein. *J Immunol* 2001; **167**: 3223–30.

205 Van Pel A, van der Bruggen P, Coulie PG et al. Genes coding for tumor antigens recognized by cytolytic T lymphocytes. *Immunol Rev* 1995; **145**: 229–50.

206 Dolstra H, Fredrix H, Maas F et al. A human minor histocompatibility antigen specific for B cell acute lymphoblastic leukemia. *J Exp Med* 1999; **189**: 301–8.

207 Warren EH, Gavin MA, Simpson E et al. The human *UTY* gene encodes a novel HLA-B8-restricted H-Y antigen. *J Immunol* 2000; **164**: 2807–14.

208 Warren EH, Otterud BE, Linterman RW et al. Feasibility of using genetic linkage analysis to identify the genes encoding T cell-defined minor histocompatibility antigens. *Tissue Antigens* 2002; **59**: 293–303.

209 Murata M, Emi N, Hirabayashi N et al. No significant association between HA-1 incompatibility and

209 incidence of acute graft-versus-host disease after HLA-identical sibling bone marrow transplantation in Japanese patients. *Int J Hematol* 2000; **72**: 371–5.
210 Goulmy E, Schipper R, Pool J et al. Mismatches of minor histocompatibility antigens between HLA-identical donors and recipients and the development of graft-versus-host disease after bone marrow transplantation. *N Engl J Med* 1996; **334**: 281–5.
211 Mutis T, Gillespie G, Schrama E, Falkenburg JH, Moss P, Goulmy E. Tetrameric HLA class I-minor histocompatibility antigen peptide complexes demonstrate minor histocompatibility antigen-specific cytotoxic T lymphocytes in patients with graft-versus-host disease. *Nat Med* 1999; **5**: 839–42.
212 Lin MT, Gooley T, Hansen JA et al. Absence of statistically significant correlation between disparity for the minor histocompatibility antigen-HA-1 and outcome after allogeneic hematopoietic cell transplantation. *Blood* 2001; **98**: 3172–3.
213 Dickinson AM, Wang XN, Sviland L et al. In vitro dissection of the graft-versus-host activities of cytotoxic T cells specific for minor histocompatibility antigens. *Nat Med* 2002; **8**: 410–4.
214 van Els CA, D'Amaro J, Pool J et al. Immunogenetics of human minor histocompatibility antigens: their polymorphism and immunodominance. *Immunogenetics* 1992; **35**: 161–5.
215 Gratwohl A, Hermans J, Niederwieser D, van Biezen A, van Houwelingen HC, Apperley J. Female donors influence transplant-related mortality and relapse incidence in male recipients of sibling blood and marrow transplants. *Hematol J* 2001; **2**: 363–70.
216 Randolph SB, Gooley TA, Warren EH, Riddell SR. Impact of donor/patient gender on relapse and graft versus host disease in matched related hematopoietic stem cell transplant. *Blood* 2002; **100**: 546a [Abstract].
217 Lahn BT, Page DC. Functional coherence of the human Y chromosome. *Science* 1997; **278**: 675–80.
218 Randolph SB, Warren EH, Riddell SR. Identification of novel minor histocompatibility antigen encoded by the Y chromosome gene, *UTY*. *Blood* 2002; **100**: 2421a [Abstract].
219 Brickner AG, Warren EH, Caldwell JA et al. The immunogenicity of a new human minor histocompatibility antigen results from differential antigen processing. *J Exp Med* 2001; **193**: 195–206.
220 Meadows L, Wang W, den Haan JM et al. The HLA-A*0201-restricted H-Y antigen contains a posttranslationally modified cysteine that significantly affects T cell recognition. *Immunity* 1997; **6**: 273–81.
221 Wang W, Meadows LR, den Haan JM et al. Human H-Y: a male-specific histocompatibility antigen derived from the SMCY protein. *Science* 1995; **269**: 1588–90.
222 Mutis T, Ghoreschi K, Schrama E et al. Efficient induction of minor histocompatibility antigen HA-1-specific cytotoxic T-cells using dendritic cells retrovirally transduced with HA-1-coding cDNA. *Biol Blood Marrow Transplant* 2002; **8**: 412–9.
223 Mutis T, Verdijk R, Schrama E, Esendam B, Brand A, Goulmy E. Feasibility of immunotherapy of relapsed leukemia with ex vivo-generated cytotoxic T lymphocytes specific for hematopoietic system-restricted minor histocompatibility antigens. *Blood* 1999; **93**: 2336–41.
224 Warren EH, Kelly DM, Brown ML, Koo KK, Xuereb SM, Riddell SR. Adoptive GVL therapy targeting minor histocompatibility for the treatment of post-transplant leukemic relapse. *Blood* 2002; **100**: 2493a [Abstract].
225 Seliger B, Cabrera T, Garrido F, Ferrone S. HLA class I antigen abnormalities and immune escape by malignant cells. *Semin Cancer Biol* 2002; **12**: 3–13.
226 Lee PP, Yee C, Savage PA et al. Characterization of circulating T cells specific for tumor-associated antigens in melanoma patients. *Nat Med* 1999; **5**: 677–85.
227 Yotnda P, Firat H, Garcia-Pons F et al. Cytotoxic T cell response against the chimeric p210 BCR-ABL protein in patients with chronic myelogenous leukemia. *J Clin Invest* 1998; **101**: 2290–6.
228 Gambacorti-Passerini C, Grignani F, Arienti F, Pandolfi PP, Pelicci PG, Parmiani G. Human CD4 lymphocytes specifically recognize a peptide representing the fusion region of the hybrid protein pml/RARα present in acute promyelocytic leukemia cells. *Blood* 1993; **81**: 1369–75.
229 Viola A, Schroeder S, Sakakibara Y, Lanzavecchia A. T lymphocyte costimulation mediated by reorganization of membrane microdomains. *Science* 1999; **283**: 680–2.
230 Sykulev Y, Joo M, Vturina I, Tsomides TJ, Eisen HN. Evidence that a single peptide-MHC complex on a target cell can elicit a cytolytic T cell response. *Immunity* 1996; **4**: 565–71.
231 Drummond IA, Madden SL, Rohwer-Nutter P, Bell GI, Sukhatme VP, Rauscher FJ, 3rd. Repression of the insulin-like growth factor II gene by the Wilms tumor suppressor *WT1*. *Science* 1992; **257**: 674–8.
232 Gashler AL, Bonthron DT, Madden SL, Rauscher FJ, 3rd, Collins T, Sukhatme VP. Human platelet-derived growth factor A chain is transcriptionally repressed by the Wilms tumor suppressor *WT1*. *Proc Natl Acad Sci U S A* 1992; **89**: 10,984–8.
233 Harrington MA, Konicek B, Song A, Xia XL, Fredericks WJ, Rauscher FJ, 3rd. Inhibition of colony-stimulating factor-1 promoter activity by the product of the Wilms' tumor locus. *J Biol Chem* 1993; **268**: 21,271–5.
234 Werner H, Re GG, Drummond IA et al. Increased expression of the insulin-like growth factor I receptor gene, *IGF1R*, in Wilms tumor is correlated with modulation of *IGF1R* promoter activity by the *WT1* Wilms tumor gene product. *Proc Natl Acad Sci U S A* 1993; **90**: 5828–32.
235 Little M, Holmes G, Walsh P. *WT1*: what has the last decade told us? *Bioessays* 1999; **21**: 191–202.
236 Menke AL, van der Eb AJ, Jochemsen AG. The Wilms' tumor 1 gene: oncogene or tumor suppressor gene? *Int Rev Cytol* 1998; **181**: 151–212.
237 Scharnhorst V, Menke AL, Attema J et al. EGR-1 enhances tumor growth and modulates the effect of the Wilms' tumor 1 gene products on tumorigenicity. *Oncogene* 2000; **19**: 791–800.
238 Laity JH, Dyson HJ, Wright PE. Molecular basis for modulation of biological function by alternate splicing of the Wilms' tumor suppressor protein. *Proc Natl Acad Sci U S A* 2000; **97**: 11,932–5.
239 Scharnhorst V, Dekker P, van der Eb AJ, Jochemsen AG. Internal translation initiation generates novel WT1 protein isoforms with distinct biological properties. *J Biol Chem* 1999; **274**: 23456–62.
240 Oji Y, Ogawa H, Tamaki H et al. Expression of the Wilms' tumor gene *WT1* in solid tumors and its involvement in tumor cell growth. *Jpn J Cancer Res* 1999; **90**: 194–204.
241 Campbell CE, Kuriyan NP, Rackley RR et al. Constitutive expression of the Wilms tumor suppressor gene (*WT1*) in renal cell carcinoma. *Int J Cancer* 1998; **78**: 182–8.
242 Viel A, Giannini F, Capozzi E et al. Molecular mechanisms possibly affecting *WT1* function in human ovarian tumors. *Int J Cancer* 1994; **57**: 515–21.
243 Silberstein GB, Van Horn K, Strickland P, Roberts CT Jr, Daniel CW. Altered expression of the *WT1* Wilms tumor suppressor gene in human breast cancer. *Proc Natl Acad Sci U S A* 1997; **94**: 8132–7.
244 Rodeck U, Bossler A, Kari C et al. Expression of the *WT1* Wilms' tumor gene by normal and malignant human melanocytes. *Int J Cancer* 1994; **59**: 78–82.
245 Pritchard-Jones K, Fleming S, Davidson D et al. The candidate Wilms' tumour gene is involved in genitourinary development. *Nature* 1990; **346**: 194–7.
246 Armstrong JF, Pritchard-Jones K, Bickmore WA, Hastie ND, Bard JB. The expression of the Wilms' tumour gene, *WT1*, in the developing mammalian embryo. *Mech Dev* 1993; **40**: 85–97.
247 Kreidberg JA, Sariola H, Loring JM et al. WT-1 is required for early kidney development. *Cell* 1993; **74**: 679–91.
248 Mundlos S, Pelletier J, Darveau A, Bachmann M, Winterpacht A, Zabel B. Nuclear localization of the protein encoded by the Wilms' tumor gene *WT1* in embryonic and adult tissues. *Development* 1993; **119**: 1329–41.
249 Baird PN, Simmons PJ. Expression of the Wilms' tumor gene (*WT1*) in normal hemopoiesis. *Exp Hematol* 1997; **25**: 312–20.
250 Inoue K, Ogawa H, Sonoda Y et al. Aberrant overexpression of the Wilms tumor gene (*WT1*) in human leukemia. *Blood* 1997; **89**: 1405–12.
251 Menssen HD, Renkl HJ, Rodeck U et al. Presence of Wilms' tumor gene (*WT1*) transcripts and the WT1 nuclear protein in the majority of human acute leukemias. *Leukemia* 1995; **9**: 1060–7.
252 Inoue K, Ogawa H, Yamagami T et al. Long-term follow-up of minimal residual disease in leukemia patients by monitoring *WT1* (Wilms tumor gene) expression levels. *Blood* 1996; **88**: 2267–78.
253 Bergmann L, Miething C, Maurer U et al. High levels of Wilms' tumor gene (*WT1*) mRNA in acute myeloid leukemias are associated with a worse long-term outcome. *Blood* 1997; **90**: 1217–25.
254 Sugiyama H. Wilms tumor gene (*WT1*) as a new marker for the detection of minimal residual disease in leukemia. *Leuk Lymphoma* 1998; **30**: 55–61.
255 Im HJ, Kong G, Lee H. Expression of Wilms tumor gene (*WT1*) in children with acute leukemia. *Pediatr Hematol Oncol* 1999; **16**: 109–18.
256 Niegemann E, Wehner S, Kornhuber B, Schwabe D, Ebener U. *WT1* gene expression in childhood leukemias. *Acta Haematol* 1999; **102**: 72–6.
257 Algar EM, Khromykh T, Smith SI, Blackburn DM, Bryson GJ, Smith PJ. A WT1 antisense oligonucleotide inhibits proliferation and induces apoptosis in myeloid leukaemia cell lines. *Oncogene* 1996; **12**: 1005–14.
258 Yamagami T, Sugiyama H, Inoue K et al. Growth inhibition of human leukemic cells by *WT1* (Wilms tumor gene) antisense oligodeoxynucleotides: implications for the involvement of *WT1* in leukemogenesis. *Blood* 1996; **87**: 2878–84.
259 Mayo MW, Wang CY, Drouin SS et al. *WT1* modulates apoptosis by transcriptionally upregulating

the bcl-2 proto-oncogene. *Embo J* 1999; **18**: 3990–4003.

260 Tsuboi A, Oka Y, Ogawa H *et al.* Constitutive expression of the Wilms' tumor gene *WT1* inhibits the differentiation of myeloid progenitor cells but promotes their proliferation in response to granulocyte-colony stimulating factor (G-CSF). *Leuk Res* 1999; **23**: 499–505.

261 Inoue K, Tamaki H, Ogawa H *et al.* Wilms' tumor gene (*WT1*) competes with differentiation-inducing signal in hematopoietic progenitor cells. *Blood* 1998; **91**: 2969–76.

262 Gaiger A, Reese V, Disis ML, Cheever MA. Immunity to *WT1* in the animal model and in patients with acute myeloid leukemia. *Blood* 2000; **96**: 1480–9.

263 Tamaki H, Ogawa H, Ohyashiki K *et al.* The Wilms' tumor gene *WT1* is a good marker for diagnosis of disease progression of myelodysplastic syndromes. *Leukemia* 1999; **13**: 393–9.

264 Patmasiriwat P, Fraizer G, Kantarjian H, Saunders GF. *WT1* and *GATA1* expression in myelodysplastic syndrome and acute leukemia. *Leukemia* 1999; **13**: 891–900.

265 Ohminami H, Yasukawa M, Fujita S. HLA class I-restricted lysis of leukemia cells by a CD8+ cytotoxic T-lymphocyte clone specific for WT1 peptide. *Blood* 2000; **95**: 286–93.

266 Oka Y, Elisseeva OA, Tsuboi A *et al.* Human cytotoxic T-lymphocyte responses specific for peptides of the wild-type Wilms' tumor gene (*WT1*) product. *Immunogenetics* 2000; **51**: 99–107.

267 Gao L, Bellantuono I, Elsasser A *et al.* Selective elimination of leukemic CD34+ progenitor cells by cytotoxic T lymphocytes specific for *WT1*. *Blood* 2000; **95**: 2198–203.

268 Oka Y, Udaka K, Tsuboi A *et al.* Cancer immunotherapy targeting Wilms' tumor gene *WT1* product. *J Immunol* 2000; **164**: 1873–80.

269 Tsuboi A, Oka Y, Ogawa H *et al.* Cytotoxic T-lymphocyte responses elicited to Wilms' tumor gene *WT1* product by DNA vaccination. *J Clin Immunol* 2000; **20**: 195–202.

270 Scheibenbogen C, Letsch A, Thiel E *et al.* CD8 T-cell responses to Wilms tumor gene product *WT1* and proteinase 3 in patients with acute myeloid leukemia. *Blood* 2002; **100**: 2132–7.

271 Sturrock A, Franklin KF, Hoidal JR. Human proteinase-3 expression is regulated by PU.1 in conjunction with a cytidine-rich element. *J Biol Chem* 1996; **271**: 32392–402.

272 Wong ET, Jenne DE, Zimmer M, Porter SD, Gilks CB. Changes in chromatin organization at the neutrophil elastase locus associated with myeloid cell differentiation. *Blood* 1999; **94**: 3730–6.

273 Sturrock AB, Franklin KF, Rao G *et al.* Structure, chromosomal assignment, and expression of the gene for proteinase-3. The Wegener's granulomatosis autoantigen. *J Biol Chem* 1992; **267**: 21,193–9.

274 Zimmer M, Medcalf RL, Fink TM, Mattmann C, Lichter P, Jenne DE. Three human elastase-like genes coordinately expressed in the myelomonocyte lineage are organized as a single genetic locus on 19pter. *Proc Natl Acad Sci U S A* 1992; **89**: 8215–9.

275 Dengler R, Munstermann U, al-Batran S *et al.* Immunocytochemical and flow cytometric detection of proteinase 3 (myeloblastin) in normal and leukaemic myeloid cells. *Br J Haematol* 1995; **89**: 250–7.

276 Jenne DE, Tschopp J, Ludemann J, Utecht B, Gross WL. Wegener's autoantigen decoded. *Nature* 1990; **346**: 520.

277 Jennette JC, Hoidal JR, Falk RJ. Specificity of anti-neutrophil cytoplasmic autoantibodies for proteinase 3. *Blood* 1990; **75**: 2263–4.

278 Gross WL, Csernok E, Flesch BK. 'Classic' anti-neutrophil cytoplasmic autoantibodies (cANCA), 'Wegener's autoantigen' and their immunopathogenic role in Wegener's granulomatosis. *J Autoimmun* 1993; **6**: 171–84.

279 Wiik A. What you should know about PR3-ANCA. An introduction. *Arthritis Res* 2000; **2**: 252–4.

280 Campbell EJ, Campbell MA, Owen CA. Bioactive proteinase 3 on the cell surface of human neutrophils: quantification, catalytic activity, and susceptibility to inhibition. *J Immunol* 2000; **165**: 3366–74.

281 Kurosawa S, Esmon CT, Stearns-Kurosawa DJ. The soluble endothelial protein C receptor binds to activated neutrophils: involvement of proteinase-3 and CD11b/CD18. *J Immunol* 2000; **165**: 4697–703.

282 Bories D, Raynal MC, Solomon DH, Darzynkiewicz Z, Cayre YE. Down-regulation of a serine protease, myeloblastin, causes growth arrest and differentiation of promyelocytic leukemia cells. *Cell* 1989; **59**: 959–68.

283 Labbaye C, Zhang J, Casanova JL *et al.* Regulation of myeloblastin messenger RNA expression in myeloid leukemia cells treated with all-trans retinoic acid. *Blood* 1993; **81**: 475–81.

284 Zimber A, Chedeville A, Abita JP, Barbu V, Gespach C. Functional interactions between bile acids, all-trans retinoic acid, and 1,25-dihydroxyvitamin D3 on monocytic differentiation and myeloblastin gene down-regulation in HL60 and THP-1 human leukemia cells. *Cancer Res* 2000; **60**: 672–8.

285 Lutz PG, Moog-Lutz C, Coumau-Gatbois E, Kobari L, Di Gioia Y, Cayre YE. Myeloblastin is a granulocyte colony-stimulating factor-responsive gene conferring factor-independent growth to hematopoietic cells. *Proc Natl Acad Sci U S A* 2000; **97**: 1601–6.

286 Skold S, Rosberg B, Gullberg U, Olofsson T. A secreted proform of neutrophil proteinase 3 regulates the proliferation of granulopoietic progenitor cells. *Blood* 1999; **93**: 849–56.

287 Spector NL, Hardy L, Ryan C *et al.* 28-kDa mammalian heat shock protein, a novel substrate of a growth regulatory protease involved in differentiation of human leukemia cells. *J Biol Chem* 1995; **270**: 1003–6.

288 Rao J, Zhang F, Donnelly RJ, Spector NL, Studzinski GP. Truncation of Sp1 transcription factor by myeloblastin in undifferentiated HL60 cells. *J Cell Physiol* 1998; **175**: 121–8.

289 Molldrem JJ, Clave E, Jiang YZ *et al.* Cytotoxic T lymphocytes specific for a nonpolymorphic proteinase 3 peptide preferentially inhibit chronic myeloid leukemia colony-forming units. *Blood* 1997; **90**: 2529–34.

290 Molldrem J, Dermime S, Parker K *et al.* Targeted T-cell therapy for human leukemia: cytotoxic T lymphocytes specific for a peptide derived from proteinase 3 preferentially lyse human myeloid leukemia cells. *Blood* 1996; **88**: 2450–7.

291 Molldrem JJ, Lee PP, Wang C, Champlin RE, Davis MM. A PR1-human leukocyte antigen-A2 tetramer can be used to isolate low-frequency cytotoxic T lymphocytes from healthy donors that selectively lyse chronic myelogenous leukemia. *Cancer Res* 1999; **59**: 2675–81.

292 Molldrem JJ, Lee PP, Wang C *et al.* Evidence that specific T lymphocytes may participate in the elimination of chronic myelogenous leukemia. *Nat Med* 2000; **6**: 1018–23.

293 Downing JR, Higuchi M, Lenny N, Yeoh AE. Alterations of the AML1 transcription factor in human leukemia. *Semin Cell Dev Biol* 2000; **11**: 347–60.

294 Mulloy JC, Cammenga J, MacKenzie KL, Berguido FJ, Moore MA, Nimer SD. The AML1-ETO fusion protein promotes the expansion of human hematopoietic stem cells. *Blood* 2002; **99**: 15–23.

295 Sakakura C, Yamaguchi-Iwai Y, Satake M *et al.* Growth inhibition and induction of differentiation of t(8;21) acute myeloid leukemia cells by the DNA-binding domain of PEBP2 and the *AML1/MTG8* (ETO)–specific antisense oligonucleotide. *Proc Natl Acad Sci U S A* 1994; **91**: 11,723–7.

296 Higuchi M, O'Brien D, Kumaravelu P, Lenny N, Yeoh EJ, Downing JR. Expression of a conditional *AML1-ETO* oncogene bypasses embryonic lethality and establishes a murine model of human t(8;21) acute myeloid leukemia. *Cancer Cell* 2002, 1bv: 63–74.

297 Maeda M, Otsuka T, Kimura N *et al.* Induction of MTG8-specific cytotoxic T-cell lines: MTG8 is probably a tumour antigen that is recognized by cytotoxic T cells in *AML1-MTG8*-fused gene-positive acute myelogenous leukaemia. *Br J Haematol* 2000; **111**: 570–9.

298 Reed JC. The Survivin saga goes *in vivo*. *J Clin Invest* 2001; **108**: 965–9.

299 Li F, Ambrosini G, Chu EY *et al.* Control of apoptosis and mitotic spindle checkpoint by survivin. *Nature* 1998; **396**: 580–4.

300 Altieri DC. The molecular basis and potential role of survivin in cancer diagnosis and therapy. *Trends Mol Med* 2001; **7**: 542–7.

301 Adida C, Recher C, Raffoux E *et al.* Expression and prognostic significance of survivin in *de novo* acute myeloid leukaemia. *Br J Haematol* 2000; **111**: 196–203.

302 Ambrosini G, Adida C, Altieri DC. A novel anti-apoptosis gene, survivin, expressed in cancer and lymphoma. *Nat Med* 1997; **3**: 917–21.

303 Schmitz M, Diestelkoetter P, Weigle B *et al.* Generation of survivin-specific CD8+ T effector cells by dendritic cells pulsed with protein or selected peptides. *Cancer Res* 2000; **60**: 4845–9.

304 Andersen MH, Pedersen LO, Capeller B, Brocker EB, Becker JC, thor Straten P. Spontaneous cytotoxic T-cell responses against survivin-derived MHC class I-restricted T-cell epitopes *in vitro* as well as *ex vivo* in cancer patients. *Cancer Res* 2001; **61**: 5964–8.

305 Andersen MH, Pedersen LO, Becker JC, Straten PT. Identification of a cytotoxic T lymphocyte response to the apoptosis inhibitor protein survivin in cancer patients. *Cancer Res* 2001; **61**: 869–72.

306 Momand J, Zambetti GP, Olson DC, George D, Levine AJ. The *mdm-2* oncogene product forms a complex with the p53 protein and inhibits p53-mediated transactivation. *Cell* 1992; **69**: 1237–45.

307 Xiao ZX, Chen J, Levine AJ *et al.* Interaction between the retinoblastoma protein and the oncoprotein MDM2. *Nature* 1995; **375**: 694–8.

308 Bueso-Ramos CE, Manshouri T, Haidar MA, Huh YO, Keating MJ, Albitar M. Multiple patterns of

308 *MDM-2* deregulation in human leukemias: implications in leukemogenesis and prognosis. *Leuk Lymphoma* 1995; **17**: 13–8.

309 Watanabe T, Ichikawa A, Saito H, Hotta T. Overexpression of the *MDM2* oncogene in leukemia and lymphoma. *Leuk Lymphoma* 1996; **21**: 391–7.

310 Dahl AM, Beverley PC, Stauss HJ. A synthetic peptide derived from the tumor-associated protein mdm2 can stimulate autoreactive, high avidity cytotoxic T lymphocytes that recognize naturally processed protein. *J Immunol* 1996; **157**: 239–46.

311 Stanislawski T, Voss RH, Lotz C et al. Circumventing tolerance to a human *MDM2*-derived tumor antigen by TCR gene transfer. *Nat Immunol* 2001; **2**: 962–70.

312 Radich JP. The promise of gene expression analysis in hematopoetic malignancies. *Biochim Biophys Acta* 2002; **1602**: 88–95.

313 Staudt LM. Gene expression profiling of lymphoid malignancies. *Annu Rev Med* 2002; **53**: 303–18.

314 Claudio JO, Masih-Khan E, Tang H et al. A molecular compendium of genes expressed in multiple myeloma. *Blood* 2002; **100**: 2175–86.

315 Vonderheide RH, Hahn WC, Schultze JL, Nadler LM. The telomerase catalytic subunit is a widely expressed tumor-associated antigen recognized by cytotoxic T lymphocytes. *Immunity* 1999; **10**: 673–9.

316 Arai J, Yasukawa M, Ohminami H, Kakimoto M, Hasegawa A, Fujita S. Identification of human telomerase reverse transcriptase-derived peptides that induce HLA-A24-restricted antileukemia cytotoxic T lymphocytes. *Blood* 2001; **97**: 2903–7.

317 Mercatante DR, Sazani P, Kole R. Modification of alternative splicing by antisense oligonucleotides as a potential chemotherapy for cancer and other diseases. *Curr Cancer Drug Targets* 2001; **1**: 211–30.

318 Chen YT. Cancer vaccine. Identification of human tumor antigens by SEREX. *Cancer J* 2000; **6**: S208–17.

319 Clay TM, Custer MC, Sachs J, Hwu P, Rosenberg SA, Nishimura MI. Efficient transfer of a tumor antigen-reactive TCR to human peripheral blood lymphocytes confers anti-tumor reactivity. *J Immunol* 1999; **163**: 507–13.

320 Cooper LJ, Kalos M, Lewinsohn DA, Riddell SR, Greenberg PD. Transfer of specificity for human immunodeficiency virus type 1 into primary human T lymphocytes by introduction of T-cell receptor genes. *J Virol* 2000; **74**: 8207–12.

321 Willemsen RA, Weijtens ME, Ronteltap C et al. Grafting primary human T lymphocytes with cancer-specific chimeric single chain and two chain TCR. *Gene Ther* 2000; **7**: 1369–77.

322 Orentas RJ, Roskopf SJ, Nolan GP, Nishimura MI. Retroviral transduction of a T cell receptor specific for an Epstein–Barr virus-encoded peptide. *Clin Immunol* 2001; **98**: 220–8.

323 Kessels HW, Wolkers MC, van den Boom MD, van der Valk MA, Schumacher TN. Immunotherapy through TCR gene transfer. *Nat Immunol* 2001; **2**: 957–61.

324 Rossig C, Bollard CM, Nuchtern JG, Rooney CM, Brenner MK. Epstein–Barr virus-specific human T lymphocytes expressing antitumor chimeric T-cell receptors: potential for improved immunotherapy. *Blood* 2002; **99**: 2009–16.

325 Kershaw MH, Westwood JA, Hwu P. Dual-specific T cells combine proliferation and anti-tumor activity. *Nat Biotechnol* 2002; **20**: 1221–7.

326 Holler PD, Holman PO, Shusta EV, O'Herrin S, Wittrup KD, Kranz DM. *In vitro* evolution of a T cell receptor with high affinity for peptide/MHC. *Proc Natl Acad Sci U S A* 2000; **97**: 5387–92.

327 Kessels HW, van Den Boom MD, Spits H, Hooijberg E, Schumacher TN. Changing T cell specificity by retroviral T cell receptor display. *Proc Natl Acad Sci U S A* 2000; **97**: 14,578–83.

328 Rotzschke O, Falk K, Faath S, Rammensee HG. On the nature of peptides involved in T cell alloreactivity. *J Exp Med* 1991; **174**: 1059–71.

329 Marincola FM, Jaffee EM, Hicklin DJ, Ferrone S. Escape of human solid tumors from T-cell recognition: molecular mechanisms and functional significance. *Adv Immunol* 2000; **74**: 181–273.

330 Eshhar Z. Tumor-specific T-bodies: towards clinical application. *Cancer Immunol Immunother* 1997; **45**: 131–6.

331 Eshhar Z, Waks T, Bendavid A, Schindler DG. Functional expression of chimeric receptor genes in human T cells. *J Immunol Meth* 2001; **248**: 67–76.

332 Altenschmidt U, Klundt E, Groner B. Adoptive transfer of *in vitro*-targeted, activated T lymphocytes results in total tumor regression. *J Immunol* 1997; **159**: 5509–15.

333 Hwu P, Yang JC, Cowherd R et al. In vivo antitumor activity of T cells redirected with chimeric antibody/T-cell receptor genes. *Cancer Res* 1995; **55**: 3369–73.

334 Alvarez-Vallina L, Hawkins RE. Antigen-specific targeting of CD28-mediated T cell co-stimulation using chimeric single-chain antibody variable fragment-CD28 receptors. *Eur J Immunol* 1996; **26**: 2304–9.

335 Haynes NM, Trapani JA, Teng MW et al. Rejection of syngeneic colon carcinoma by CTLs expressing single-chain antibody receptors co-delivering CD28 costimulation. *J Immunol* 2002; **169**: 5780–6.

336 Maher J, Brentjens RJ, Gunset G, Riviere I, Sadelain M. Human T-lymphocyte cytotoxicity and proliferation directed by a single chimeric TCRzeta/CD28 receptor. *Nat Biotechnol* 2002; **20**: 70–5.

337 Haynes NM, Trapani JA, Teng MW et al. Single-chain antigen recognition receptors that costimulate potent rejection of established experimental tumors. *Blood* 2002; **100**: 3155–63.

338 Brodie SJ, Lewinsohn DA, Patterson BK et al. In vivo migration and function of transferred HIV-1-specific cytotoxic T cells. *Nat Med* 1999; **5**: 34–41.

339 Matloubian M, Concepcion RJ, Ahmed R. $CD4^+$ T cells are required to sustain $CD8^+$ cytotoxic T-cell responses during chronic viral infection. *J Virol* 1994; **68**: 8056–63.

340 Rosenberg ES, Billingsley JM, Caliendo AM et al. Vigorous HIV-1-specific $CD4^+$ T cell responses associated with control of viremia. *Science* 1997; **278**: 1447–50.

341 Greenberg PD. Therapy of murine leukemia with cyclophosphamide and immune $Lyt-2^+$ cells: cytolytic T cells can mediate eradication of disseminated leukemia. *J Immunol* 1986; **136**: 1917–22.

342 Kast WM, Offringa R, Peters PJ et al. Eradication of adenovirus E1-induced tumors by E1A-specific cytotoxic T lymphocytes. *Cell* 1989; **59**: 603–14.

343 Robinson N, Sanders JE, Benyunes MC et al. Phase I trial of interleukin-2 after unmodified HLA-matched sibling bone marrow transplantation for children with acute leukemia. *Blood* 1996; **87**: 1249–54.

344 Nelson BH, Lord JD, Greenberg PD. Cytoplasmic domains of the interleukin-2 receptor β and γ chains mediate the signal for T-cell proliferation. *Nature* 1994; **369**: 333–6.

345 Nakamura Y, Russell SM, Mess SA et al. Heterodimerization of the IL-2 receptor β- and γ-chain cytoplasmic domains is required for signalling. *Nature* 1994; **369**: 330–3.

346 Evans LS, Witte PR, Feldhaus AL et al. Expression of chimeric granulocyte-macrophage colony-stimulating factor/interleukin 2 receptors in human cytotoxic T lymphocyte clones results in granulocyte-macrophage colony-stimulating factor-dependent growth. *Hum Gene Ther* 1999; **10**: 1941–51.

347 Cheng LE, Ohlen C, Nelson BH, Greenberg PD. Enhanced signaling through the IL-2 receptor in $CD8^+$ T cells regulated by antigen recognition results in preferential proliferation and expansion of responding $CD8^+$ T cells rather than promotion of cell death. *Proc Natl Acad Sci U S A* 2002; **99**: 3001–6.

348 Cheng LE, Greenberg PD. Selective delivery of augmented IL-2 receptor signals to responding $CD8^+$ T cells increases the size of the acute antiviral response and of the resulting memory T cell pool. *J Immunol* 2002; **169**: 4990–7.

349 Ganss R, Hanahan D. Tumor microenvironment can restrict the effectiveness of activated antitumor lymphocytes. *Cancer Res* 1998; **58**: 4673–81.

350 Briskin MJ, Rott L, Butcher EC. Structural requirements for mucosal vascular addressin binding to its lymphocyte receptor alpha 4 beta 7. Common themes among integrin–Ig family interactions. *J Immunol* 1996; **156**: 719–26.

351 Dogan AM, Koulis A, Briskin MJ, Isaacson PG. Expression of lymphocyte homing receptors and vascular addressins in low-grade gastric B-cell lymphomas of mucosa-associated lymphoid tissue. *Am J Pathol* 1997; **151**: 1361–9.

352 Peled A, Petit I, Kollet O et al. Dependence of human stem cell engraftment and repopulation of NOD/SCID mice on CXCR4. *Science* 1999; **283**: 845–8.

353 Peled A, Grabovsky V, Habler L et al. The chemokine SDF-1 stimulates integrin-mediated arrest of $CD34^+$ cells on vascular endothelium under shear flow. *J Clin Invest* 1999; **104**: 1199–211.

354 Sallusto F, Kremmer E, Palermo B et al. Switch in chemokine receptor expression upon TCR stimulation reveals novel homing potential for recently activated T cells. *Eur J Immunol* 1999; **29**: 2037–45.

355 Husson H, Freedman AS, Cardoso AA et al. CXCL13 (BCA-1) is produced by follicular lymphoma cells: role in the accumulation of malignant B cells. *Br J Haematol* 2002; **119**: 492–5.

356 Jundt F, Anagnostopoulos I, Bommert K et al. Hodgkin/Reed–Sternberg cells induce fibroblasts to secrete eotaxin, a potent chemoattractant for T cells and eosinophils. *Blood* 1999; **94**: 2065–71.

357 Kershaw MH, Wang G, Westwood JA et al. Redirecting migration of T cells to chemokine secreted from tumors by genetic modification with CXCR2. *Hum Gene Ther* 2002; **13**: 1971–80.

358 Treisman J, Hwu P, Yannelli JR et al. Upregulation of tumor necrosis factor-α production by retrovirally transduced human tumor-infiltrating lymphocytes using trans-retinoic acid. *Cell Immunol* 1994; **156**: 448–57.

359 Groh V, Wu J, Yee C, Spies T. Tumour-derived soluble MIC ligands impair expression of NKG2D and T-cell activation. *Nature* 2002; **419**: 734–8.

360 Fang D, Wang HY, Fang N, Altman Y, Elly C, Liu YC. Cbl-b, a RING-type E3 ubiquitin ligase, targets phosphatidylinositol 3-kinase for ubiquitination in T cells. *J Biol Chem* 2001; **276**: 4872–8.

361 Krawczyk C, Bachmaier K, Sasaki T *et al.* Cbl-b is a negative regulator of receptor clustering and raft aggregation in T cells. *Immunity* 2000; **13**: 463–73.

362 Bachmaier K, Krawczyk C, Kozieradzki I *et al.* Negative regulation of lymphocyte activation and autoimmunity by the molecular adaptor Cbl-b. *Nature* 2000; **403**: 211–6.

363 Chiang YJ, Kole HK, Brown K *et al.* Cbl-b regulates the CD28 dependence of T-cell activation. *Nature* 2000; **403**: 216–20.

364 Springer CJ, Niculescu-Duvaz I. Prodrug-activating systems in suicide gene therapy. *J Clin Invest* 2000; **105**: 1161–7.

365 Bonini C, Ferrari G, Verzeletti S *et al.* HSV-TK gene transfer into donor lymphocytes for control of allogeneic graft-versus-leukemia. *Science* 1997; **276**: 1719–24.

366 Verzeletti S, Bonini C, Marktel S *et al.* Herpes simplex virus thymidine kinase gene transfer for controlled graft-versus-host disease and graft-versus-leukemia: clinical follow-up and improved new vectors. *Hum Gene Ther* 1998; **9**: 2243–51.

367 Tiberghien P. Use of suicide gene-expressing donor T-cells to control alloreactivity after haematopoietic stem cell transplantation. *J Intern Med* 2001; **249**: 369–77.

368 Riddell SR, Elliott M, Lewinsohn DA *et al.* T-cell mediated rejection of gene-modified HIV-specific cytotoxic T lymphocytes in HIV-infected patients. *Nat Med* 1996; **2**: 216–23.

369 Thomis DC, Marktel S, Bonini C *et al.* A Fas-based suicide switch in human T cells for the treatment of graft-versus-host disease. *Blood* 2001; **97**: 1249–57.

370 Berger C, Blau CA, Clackson T, Riddell SR, Heimfeld S. CD28 costimulation and immuno-affinity-based selection efficiently generate primary gene-modified T cells for adoptive immunotherapy. *Blood* 2003; **101**: 476–84.

371 Baum C, Duellmann J, Li Z *et al.* Side effects of retroviral gene transfer into hematopoietic stem cells. *Blood* 2003; **101**: 2099–114.

30

Allan D. Hess & Richard J. Jones

Autologous Graft-vs.-Host Disease

Introduction

Graft-vs.-host disease (GVHD) is a major life-threatening complication of allogeneic hematopoietic cell transplantation (HCT) due primarily to the response of donor lymphocytes contained in the bone marrow graft to the foreign histocompatibility antigens on the cells of the recipient [1,2]. In addition to the direct lymphocyte-mediated destruction of cells, the release of cytokines indirectly potentiates the clinical complexity of GVHD [3]. Although histocompatibility differences are thought to initiate the antihost response of the graft, a GVHD-like syndrome can occur after marrow transplants performed between identical twins (syngeneic) and even after autologous HCT [4–7]. The occurrence of GVHD after autologous or syngeneic HCT was initially met with great skepticism since it directly challenged the dogma that histo'in'compatibility between donor and host is an absolute requirement for the induction of GVHD [8]. Current understanding, however, suggests that GVHD can include the aberrant recognition of self-major histocompatibility (MHC) antigens when there is a failure in reconstituting the immunobiological mechanisms that govern self-tolerance.

Tolerance to self-MHC antigens is, in fact, one of the fundamental tenets of immunology. To account for tolerance to self-antigens, Burnet put forth the concept of clonal selection whereby self-reactive clones are deleted centrally in the thymus during the ontogeny of the neonatal immune system while maintaining the capacity to respond to environmental antigens [9]. This concept has received strong experimental support [10,11]. Moreover, self-tolerance in the peripheral compartment is also safeguarded by regulatory T cells that control autoreactive T lymphocytes, which escape clonal deletion [12]. Recent studies suggest that $CD4^+CD25^+$ T cells play a critical role in self-immunoregulation [13]. Failure of this peripheral regulatory system leads to autoimmune disease.

Acquisition of tolerance to self-MHC antigens is not limited to the developing immune system in the neonate but also occurs after autologous or syngeneic HCT. Perturbation of the developing immune system by disrupting the reconstitution of the mechanisms governing self-tolerance can lead to autoaggression. Administration of drugs that alter T-cell differentiation in the thymus such as cyclosporine (CSP) or FK 506 during immunologic reconstitution induces an autoimmune syndrome with pathology identical to allogeneic GVHD [14–16]. This syndrome termed autologous or syngeneic GVHD is due to the dysregulation of the central and peripheral mechanisms that control self-reactivity [17]. The failure to reconstitute and maintain tolerance to self-antigens leads to the autoimmune destruction of "host" tissue realizing the *horror autotoxicus* postulated by Ehrlich over a century ago [18]. Despite this realization, the ability to induce autoaggression by manipulating central and peripheral control mechanisms provides a unique model to dissect further autoimmune self-recognition and self-tolerance. Principles established in this model also underlie the mechanisms required for the reconstitution of self-tolerance and donor to host tolerance in allogeneic HCT. In addition, elucidating mechanisms of self/nonself-recognition in the syngeneic GVHD model may also facilitate the development of novel antitumor immunotherapeutic strategies since this autoimmune syndrome can mobilize effector T cells that effectively target and eliminate tumor cells.

Autologous/syngeneic GVHD—basic mechanisms

Preclinical studies

The experimental induction of syngeneic GVHD after autologous or syngeneic HCT with CSP was first reported in the mid-1980s [14,15]. In this model, lethally irradiated rats are reconstituted with either syngeneic or autologous bone marrow and treated with a limited course of CSP. Upon discontinuation of CSP treatment, the recipients develop a severe autoimmune syndrome (see Plate 30.1, *facing p. 296*). The initial onset of this syndrome is characterized by erythroderma and dermatitis, classical clinical signs of acute GVHD. The histologic changes (dyskeratosis, epidermal lymphocyte infiltration) are virtually identical with the pathology observed during acute allogeneic GVHD. The majority of the infiltrating lymphocytes are $CD8^+$ T cells, findings consistent with the epithelial destruction observed histologically. After the onset of syngeneic GVHD, there can be a rapid progression to a chronic form of GVHD (alopecia, scleroderma and fibrosis) along with its relevant histologic features. During this phase, there is an accumulation of $CD4^+$ T cells (although $CD8^+$ T cells are still present) mirroring the infiltrates observed in chronic allogeneic GVHD [17,19–21].

The mechanisms accounting for the production of the autoreactive cells and the subsequent development of syngeneic GVHD are not yet fully understood. In addition to CSP treatment, an intact thymus and lymphoablative treatment are also critical requirements.

A number of studies clearly demonstrate that an intact thymus and the effect of CSP on the thymus are major components required for the induction of syngeneic GVHD [22,23]. The definitive finding implicating the thymus is that thymectomy prior to HCT and CSP therapy prevents the development of syngeneic GVHD. Moreover, CSP treatment also directly affects thymic function. Pharmacologic doses of CSP induce architectural changes in the thymus characterized by a rapid involution of the thymic medulla with a remarkable loss of epithelial cells, interdigitating cells, dendritic cells and macrophages [24,25]. As a consequence, total MHC class II antigen expression in the medulla is reduced [26,27]. In contrast, cortical areas show little change after CSP treatment. These structural changes in the medulla alter the microenvironment that governs

T-cell differentiation [28,29]. CSP treatment also directly alters thymocyte development and T-cell differentiation, a process directly related to the ability of this drug to inhibit the calcineurin/calmodulin pathway [30]. Treatment with CSP induces a maturational arrest of thymocyte development and stops the usual progression of CD4$^+$CD8$^+$ thymocytes to mature CD4 or CD8 single positive cells [30]. In addition, CSP also inhibits the clonal deletion of autoreactive T cells in the thymus (including antiself-MHC class II reactive T lymphocytes). Interestingly, both the thymic architecture and T-cell maturation quickly return to normal once CSP treatment is discontinued. Nevertheless, during CSP treatment, the autoreactive T cells emigrate to the peripheral lymphoid compartment and peripheral tissues where they can manifest autoaggression [31–33].

Despite the attractive hypothesis that the induction of syngeneic GVHD is primarily due to the inhibition of clonal deletion by CSP, this hypothesis, by itself, is insufficient. A permissive environment is required for the autoreactive T cells to manifest autoaggression. The permissive environment is provided by the second factor critically important for the successful induction of syngeneic GVHD, irradiation or other lymphoablative therapy [34–36]. The principal effect of irradiation or other cytotoxic therapy is the elimination of a peripheral T-lymphocyte-dependent regulatory system [34,36]. In the presence of this peripheral regulatory mechanism, the autoreactive T cells fail to initiate active autoaggression.

Further support for the importance of an autoregulatory system is provided by the findings that normal splenic T lymphocytes, when cotransferred with autoimmune effector cells, prevent the development of syngeneic GVHD in secondary recipients [37,38]. The regulatory effect of normal splenic T lymphocytes is dose-dependent and sensitive to irradiation and cyclophosphamide [34]. Additional studies reveal that there is a CD4$^+$ subset of autoregulatory T cells in normal animals that specifically recognizes and responds to the autoreactive lymphocytes [34,37]. In this setting, recognition requires the specific interaction between the α/β T-cell receptor (TCR) on the regulatory cells and MHC class II determinants on the autoreactive T lymphocytes. In accord are recent studies demonstrating that the regulation of CSP-induced syngeneic GVHD is mediated by a CD4$^+$CD25$^+$ subset of T cells that are recent thymic emigrants [39,40]. Although CSP treatment directly retards the development of CD4$^+$CD25$^+$ regulatory T cells in the thymus, the reconstitution of this subset after syngeneic HCT and CSP treatment occurs quite rapidly [39,40]. The regulatory T cells can be detected in the peripheral lymphoid compartment just 4 days after discontinuation of CSP treatment and may, ultimately, limit the progression of autoimmune disease [39,40]. The specificity of the regulatory system and the mechanism by which it controls the autoreactive effector T cells remain unknown. Recent studies suggest that the regulatory T-cell subset can induce apoptotic death of the effector T cells via a Fas/Fas ligand interaction leading to a peripheral clonal deletion of the autoreactive effector T cells [41]. On the other hand, the regulatory T cells can also down regulate type 1 cytokine production by the effector T-cell subset thus limiting their ability to manifest autoaggression [21]. Furthermore, the initiation and progression of autoaggressive disease (i.e. acute to chronic) also may be subject to distinct immunoregulatory mechanisms [21].

The absence of immunoregulatory mechanisms allows both the initiation and the progression of syngeneic GVHD. The initiation of acute syngeneic GVHD and progression to the chronic phase requires the collaboration between autoreactive CD8$^+$ and CD4$^+$ T-lymphocyte subsets with distinct cytokine profiles as defined in the adoptive transfer studies (see Fig. 30.1) [20]. CD8$^+$ T cells from animals with syngeneic GVHD introduced into secondary recipients transfer a self-limited acute disease that resolves within 2 weeks. The CD4$^+$ subset by itself is ineffective. Progression of CD8$^+$ mediated disease to the chronic phase, however, requires the addition of the CD4$^+$ T helper cell subset. These data suggest that CD4$^+$ autoreactive T helper cells play an essential role in syngeneic

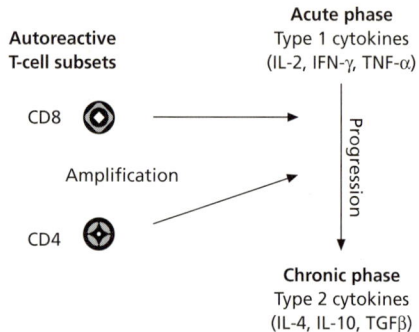

Fig. 30.1 Autoreactive T-cell subsets and the role of cytokines in acute and chronic syngeneic graft-vs.-host disease (GVHD). CD8$^+$ autoreactive T cells mediate acute syngeneic GVHD. Progression and development of chronic syngeneic GVHD requires the CD4$^+$ autoreactive T-cell subset. Furthermore, the transition from acute to chronic also correlates with the cytokine profile of the infiltrating lymphocytes.

GVHD, possibly amplifying the activity of the autoreactive CD8$^+$ cytolytic T cells. The autoreactive T helper subset may provide a cytokine amplification signal for CD8$^+$ autocytotoxic T cells allowing subsequent clonal expansion and development of disease. The CD4$^+$ (and other CD8$^+$) T cells may also act directly by releasing cytokines that induce the tissue response characteristic of chronic GVHD [21].

Interestingly, recent studies indicate that the transition from acute to chronic autoaggressive disease correlates with a change in the cytokine profile of the infiltrating autoreactive T cells [21]. Analysis of the target tissue during acute syngeneic GVHD reveals that mRNA for type 1 cytokines (interleukin 2 [IL-2], interferon-gamma [IFN-γ], tumor necrosis factor-alpha [TNF-α]) is preferentially detected whereas mRNA for type 2 cytokines (IL-4, IL-10 and transforming growth factor-beta [TGF-β]) is predominantly found in the target tissues of animals with chronic syngeneic GVHD [21]. Recent studies also confirm that type 1 cytokines, including IL-2, IL-12 and TNF-α, play a critical role in the initial induction of syngeneic GVHD [42,43]. Interestingly, subsets of autoreactive T-cell clones with polarized type 1 or type 2 cytokine profiles can also be isolated from animals with acute and chronic syngeneic GVHD, respectively [21,43]. These autoreactive T-cell subsets can induce similar pathologies as assessed in a local graft-vs.-host reaction (GVHR) assay and confirm their participation in the development of acute and chronic syngeneic GVHD [21,44,45]. In addition to the direct killing of the target cells, the cytokines produced by these autoreactive T-lymphocyte subsets may further accentuate their pathogenic potential. For instance, secretion of TNF-α can trigger apoptotic death of epithelial cells, a hallmark of acute GVHD [46]. On the other hand, local production of type 2 cytokines particularly IL-4 and TGF-β in the target tissue can lead to fibrosis, pathologic changes consistent with chronic GVHD [47,48].

Recent studies indicate that the repertoire of the CSP-induced autoreactive T lymphocytes in the acute phase of syngeneic GVHD is highly conserved and predominantly restricted to cells expressing the Vβ 8.5 TCR gene element [20]. Moreover, expression of Vα TCR genes may also be restricted. Clonal analysis reveals the preferential expression of the Vα 10 and Vα 11 TCR elements. During the chronic phase of syngeneic GVHD, however, the repertoire broadens with respect to Vβ TCR gene utilization but appears to maintain the Vα restriction as assessed by analysis of clones established from animals with acute and chronic syngeneic GVHD [45]. Moreover, lymphocytes expressing these specific TCR determinants can also be detected infiltrating the target tissues in syngeneic GVHD [21].

The highly restricted expression of Vα/Vβ TCR determinants utilized by the syngeneic GVHD effector T lymphocytes indicates that there is limited oligoclonality of the autoreactive T-cell population. In sharp contrast to the limited diversity of the effector T-cell population, there is promiscuous recognition of MHC class II determinants across histocompatibility barriers. The onset of acute syngeneic GVHD is associated with the development of autoreactive CD8$^+$Vβ8.5$^+$ cytotoxic T cells (and CD4$^+$ T helper cells) that recognize MHC class II (I-A) determinants *in vitro* and *in vivo* [44,49,50]. The CSP-induced autoreactive T cells not only recognize self-MHC class II antigens but can also recognize these determinants on several different MHC-disparate strains of rats. Moreover, recognition of the MHC class II antigens *in vivo* and *in vitro* by the syngeneic GVHD effector T lymphocytes can be effectively blocked with anti-MHC class II monoclonal antibodies. On the other hand, anti-MHC class I monoclonal antibodies are ineffective, confirming restriction of the autoreactivity to MHC class II antigens.

The novel specificity of the CD8$^+$Vβ8.5$^+$ CSP-induced autoreactive T cells even in the absence of the appropriate cell-surface-restricting element (i.e. CD4) for MHC class II recognition suggest that there is nontraditional recognition of this antigen. Either a highly conserved structural element or an endogenous superantigen governs the recognition of MHC class II target antigens. Recent studies provide insight into the molecular mechanisms that may account for the promiscuous recognition of MHC class II determinants by the syngeneic GVHD effector T cells and their restriction to common *V-region TCR* genes. Analysis of the fine specificity of the effector mechanisms in syngeneic GVHD reveals that the pathogenic T lymphocytes recognize a highly conserved peptide from the MHC class II invariant chain, termed the class II invariant chain peptide (CLIP), and presented by MHC class II molecules [44,51–54]. In support are the findings that pretreatment of the target cells with antibody to CLIP completely blocks lysis mediated by the CD8$^+$Vβ8.5$^+$ CSP-induced autoreactive T lymphocytes, while loading of CLIP onto the target cells markedly enhances their susceptibility to recognition and lysis [44].

The highly conserved nature and ubiquitous expression of CLIP with MHC class II molecules may explain, in part, the observed promiscuity of the syngeneic GVHD effector T cells. An additional requirement, however, is the apparent functional interaction between the TCR and the flanking regions of CLIP (peptide sequences that extend beyond the peptide binding domain of the MHC class II molecule) that also contributes to the novel specificity of the effector T cells (see Fig. 30.2). The flanking regions of CLIP appear to interact directly with the V-regions of the autoreactive TCR outside of complementarity determining region 3 (CDR3), a domain of the TCR that governs peptide specificity [44,45]. Particularly important is the interaction between the *N*-terminal flanking region of CLIP and the Vβ chain of the TCR, an interaction that may also explain the restriction of the autoreactive T-cell repertoire [44]. In support are the findings from the TCR CDR3 region analysis of the clones [45,48,55]. Although *TCR J-region* gene utilization was limited, sequences in the nucleotide-diversity-nucleotide (*N-D-N*) region were quite diverse. These results suggest that the specificity of the peptide-binding domain of the autoreactive TCR may be less important compared to the interaction between the flanking region of CLIP and the TCR Vβ chain. This interaction may override any "looseness of fit" between the MHC class II-peptide complex and the TCR [45]. Interestingly, recent studies demonstrate that CLIP can modify the T-cell response to the superantigen *Staphylococcal enterotoxin* B (SEB) by disrupting the ligation of the TCR with MHC class II molecules [56]. Based on the finding that the autoreactive T cells primarily express a Vβ TCR element that confers responsiveness to SEB (i.e. Vβ 8.5) and that SEB pretreatment of the autoreactive T lymphocytes inhibits their activity, the *N*-terminal flanking region of CLIP may interact with the TCR at or near the SEB-binding site [44]. The requirement for a TCR β chain sequence that can bind the *N*-terminal flanking region of CLIP appears to account for the restricted repertoire of autoreactive T cells [44,45,48,49]. The additional

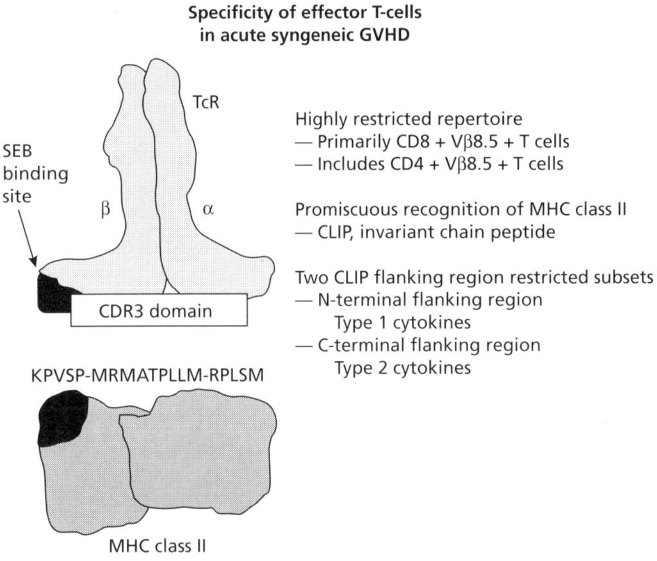

Specificity of effector T-cells in acute syngeneic GVHD

Highly restricted repertoire
— Primarily CD8 + Vβ8.5 + T cells
— Includes CD4 + Vβ8.5 + T cells

Promiscuous recognition of MHC class II
— CLIP, invariant chain peptide

Two CLIP flanking region restricted subsets
— *N*-terminal flanking region Type 1 cytokines
— *C*-terminal flanking region Type 2 cytokines

KPVSP-MRMATPLLM-RPLSM

Fig. 30.2 Schematic model of the interaction between the autoreactive T-cell receptor (TCR) and the major histocompatibility complex (MHC) class II invariant chain peptide (CLIP) complex. The *N*-terminal flanking region of CLIP appears to directly interact with the Vβ chain of the TCR at or near the *Staphylococcal enterotoxin* B (SEB) super antigen-binding site. This interaction increases the avidity of the TCR-MHC class II-CLIP complex overriding any "looseness of fit" between the MHC-peptide complex and the complementarity determining region 3 (CDR3) domain of the TCR.

interaction between the flanking regions of CLIP and the TCR may strengthen the avidity of the TCR-peptide-MHC class II complex bypassing the requirement for classical cell surface restriction elements and facilitating promiscuous recognition of MHC class II determinants.

Interestingly, clonal analysis reveals two populations of CLIP restricted autoreactive T-cell subsets that are functionally distinct and may play discrete roles in syngeneic GVHD. These two subsets can be separated based on their requirement for the *N*-terminal or *C*-terminal flanking region of CLIP, their cytokine profile and their pathogenic potential [21,44,45]. The autoreactive T-cell clones that recognize the MHC class II-CLIP complex and restricted by the *N*-terminal flanking region of CLIP produce type 1 (IL-2, IFN-γ, TNF-α) cytokines and mediate histologic changes consistent with acute GVHD (marked epithelial cell destruction, dyskeratosis) as assessed in a local GVHR assay. In contrast, clones requiring the *C*-terminal flanking region of CLIP produce type 2 (IL-4, IL-10, TGF-β) cytokines and do not mediate epithelial cell destruction. Rather, in the local GVHR assay, these clones can induce pathologic damage in the deep dermis including dermal and glandular destruction, swelling and myositis. These changes are similar to the early stages of chronic GVHD [21,57]. However, the *C*-terminal restricted clones can only mediate pathology if the target antigen (MHC class II-CLIP) is up regulated after local IFN-γ administration. Taken together, these two subsets of CLIP autoreactive T cells may differentially participate in the acute and chronic phases of syngeneic GVHD.

Clinical studies

A number of clinical studies over the past decade provide substantial evidence that an autoimmune GVHD can be induced in humans by CSP treatment after autologous HCT [58–60]. Moreover, these early studies revealed some interesting insights into the complexity of this novel autoaggression syndrome. Initially, patients with a variety of chemotherapy resistant hematologic malignancies or with metastatic breast cancer

Table 30.1 Clinical cyclosporine (CSP)-induced autologous graft-vs.-host disease (GVHD).

Can be induced in the majority of patients
    Factors influencing the incidence of autologous GVHD:
        ↓Delayed engraftment—"purged" marrow grafts
        ↓Transfer of mature T cells—mobilized peripheral blood stem cells
        ↑ Extent of previous chemotherapy—elimination of immunoregulation
        ↑ IL-10 promoter polymorphism associated with high IL-10 production
        ↑ Dose of CSP: 1–2 mg/kg/day IV

Confined primarily to skin; rare involvement of internal organs:
    Rare progression to the chronic phase

Onset coincides with initial phases of engraftment:
    Can occur 1–2 weeks after CSP treatment
    Lasts 1–3 weeks
    Usually resolves spontaneously
    Low-dose steroid therapy may be required in some patients

Treatment with IFN-γ or IL-2 increases severity:
    No effect on incidence

Can occur spontaneously:
    Dysregulation of autoreactivity and autoregulation

IFN-γ, interferon-gamma; IL, interleukin; IV, intravenous.

underwent autologous HCT and CSP treatment for 28 days starting on the day of transplantation. Histologically confirmed grade II GVHD of the skin developed in a large number of patients usually at the time of initial hematologic recovery. The disease was confined to the skin (erythematous maculopapular rash affecting the face, ears, trunk, hands, and feet) with no evidence of extra cutaneous involvement (see Plate 30.2, *facing p. 296*). The autologous GVHD resolved within 1–3 weeks either spontaneously or after a short course of corticosteroids. Since these initial reports, the results from several subsequent studies have established important characteristics and factors that influence the induction of clinical autologous GVHD as summarized in Table 30.1 [60–66].

Autologous GVHD can be induced in the majority of patients after autologous HCT with the onset primarily occurring during the initial phases of engraftment while CSP treatment is ongoing. A number of factors, however, can influence the ability to induce this autoaggression syndrome. For instance, the incidence of autologous GVHD is reduced in recipients receiving modified hematopoietic stem cell grafts. Chemical tumor-cell purging of the bone marrow delays engraftment and reduces the incidence of autologous GVHD [61]. In addition, recent studies also suggest that the ability to induce autologous GVHD is significantly reduced in patients receiving mobilized peripheral blood progenitor cells [67,68]. Rigorous T-cell depletion or CD34 enrichment of the stem cell product, however, restores the ability to induce this syndrome [68]. Interestingly, autologous GVHD can occur in a small number of patients after CD34$^+$ peripheral blood stem cell transplantation *without* CSP treatment, suggesting that reconstitution of autoreactivity and autoregulation is precariously balanced [69]. Recent studies indicate that IL-2 therapy after HCT can induce effects that histologically and clinically mimic cutaneous autologous GVHD in the absence of any CSP treatment [70]. The immunobiological mechanisms responsible for this response after IL-2 administration remain unclear. In a permissive environment, administration of IL-2 may lead to the amplification of other autoreactive T cells that are released prematurely from the thymus that was damaged due to the HCT preparative regimen. Certainly, the evidence suggests that CSP treatment accentuates the development of autoreactive cells. These results also support the hypothesis that unpurified peripheral blood progenitor stem cell grafts contain mature regulatory T lymphocytes that prevent the induction of autologous GVHD [34,64,68]. The ability to induce autologous GVHD is also greatest in patients (particularly in patients with lymphoma) who have received multiple cycles of chemotherapy [71]. Previous chemotherapy may compromise or reduce peripheral regulatory T-cell activity facilitating the induction of this autoaggression syndrome.

Recent studies evaluating the cytokine and chemokine profiles in autologous GVHD reveal that the induction of autologous GVHD correlates with the level of IL-10 mRNA detected in peripheral blood mononuclear cells from patients with this autoaggression syndrome [72]. Moreover, the susceptibility to autologous GVHD is associated with inheritance of an allelic variant in the IL-10 promoter region [72]. The ability to induce autologous GVHD correlated primarily with patients who inherit the IL-10^{-1082} G/G single nucleotide polymorphism locus, an allelic variant associated with high IL-10 production. These findings suggest that the immunoregulatory cytokine IL-10 plays an unexpected role in the induction of autologous GVHD. Although IL-10 has a wide variety of biologic activities, recent studies suggest that this cytokine not only enhances IFN-γ production by CD8$^+$ T cells, but can also provide a proliferative signal for autoreactive T cells prematurely released from the thymus [73,74]. Both of these properties certainly could potentiate the induction of autologous GVHD.

The results from several clinical trials also reveal that the autoaggression syndrome is, in most cases, confined to the skin without any clinical evidence of internal organ disease and spontaneously resolves within a few weeks. Progressive disease and development of chronic autologous GVHD occurs rarely [65,66]. Of further importance is the finding that administration of IFN-γ significantly increases the severity (greater incidence of grade II disease) of the autologous GVHD [59]. The up regulation of class II MHC antigens in the target tissue from IFN-γ treatment probably accounts for the increased severity of the skin lesions [59].

The immune mechanisms associated with human autologous GVHD are remarkably similar to the effector mechanisms defined in the animal model system. For instance, the CSP-induced autoaggression syndrome in humans is also associated with the development of autocytotoxic T cells that promiscuously recognize the MHC class II-CLIP complex [54,58,67]. The appearance of these autoreactive T cells coincides with the onset of autologous GVHD, persists through CSP treatment and subsides upon resolution of autoaggression [54,67]. It is noteworthy, however, that this population of autocytolytic T cells can be detected in a subset of patients who do not develop clinical evidence of GVHD after an autologous peripheral blood stem cell graft; only a subclinical GVHD develops. The activity of these cells, however, wanes very quickly [67]. There may be a failure to amplify the autocytolytic T cells or the immunoregulatory T-cell system rapidly reconstitutes in these patients limiting the activity of the autoaggressive T cells. The autoreactive cells associated with autologous GVHD are also primarily CD8$^+$CD4$^-$ α/β TCR$^+$ T lymphocytes; however, in some patients, the lytic T cells appear to express both the CD8 and CD4 cell surface accessory molecules [54,75]. Interestingly, recent findings suggest that the autoreactive T cells do not express CD28, the conventional costimulatory receptor [76]. The requirements for classic costimulation of the autoreactive T cells may be limited.

Similar to the findings in the animal model, the T-cell repertoire in human autologous GVHD appears to be highly conserved. CDR3 domain and clonotype analysis of the peripheral blood T-cell compartment in patients with autologous GVHD reveal a clonal expansion of T lymphocytes that preferentially express either the *V*β15, *V*β16 or *V*β22 *TCR* gene elements [76]. Importantly, in a limited number of patients evaluated, lymphocytes that express these *TCR V*-region gene elements can be detected infiltrating into the skin of patients with autologous GVHD

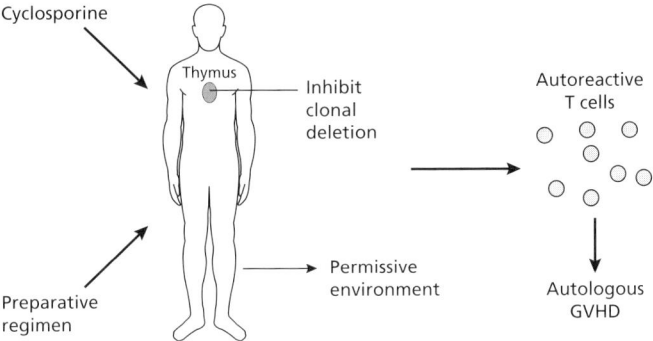

Fig. 30.3 Induction of autologous graft-vs.-host disease (GVHD). The induction of clinical autologous GVHD is two-tiered. Administration of cyclosporine (CSP) inhibits the clonal deletion of autoreactive T cells that emigrate to the periphery. The autologous hematopoietic cell transplantation (HCT) preparative regimen eliminates a peripheral regulatory or resistance mechanism providing a permissive environment for the autoreactive T cells.

[77,78]. Additional studies indicate that the clonal expansion of T cells with a given *V*-region determinant, however, is dependent on the *HLA-DRB1* genotype of the patient. Further analysis sequencing the CDR3 domain reveals that *TCR J*-region gene utilization is limited [77]. Additionally, although common sequences can be detected in the *N-D-N* region, there appears to be remarkable diversity within this domain.

Despite remarkable similarities, there are a few differences between autologous/syngeneic GVHD in humans compared to the rat model. One major difference is that autologous GVHD develops in the patients while they are being treated with CSP. In the rat model, CSP usually must be discontinued prior to the onset of disease. This difference may be related to the higher doses of CSP administered to the animals, whereas lower doses in humans allow for the activation of the autoreactive T cells. The activation of the autoreactive T cells may be functionally resistant to CSP or they utilize alternative activation pathways. The second major difference is that a chronic phase of the disease develops in a large proportion of the animals while the development of a chronic phase in humans is rare. Since the development of the chronic phase appears principally due to type 2 cytokine producing autoreactive T cells, it seems likely that a similar population of autoreactive T cells may develop infrequently in humans or may develop discordantly with the CD8$^+$ autoreactive T cells. Alternatively, a regulatory mechanism may be reconstituted more quickly in humans, thus limiting the activity of the autoreactive T-cell subset. Nevertheless, the immune mechanisms in humans and in rats are remarkably similar.

Based on the results from both the preclinical and initial clinical studies, a simplified working model of CSP-induced autologous GVHD can be constructed (see Fig. 30.3). Treatment with CSP leads to the production of MHC class II-CLIP autoreactive T cells. This occurs either by inhibiting clonal deletion in the thymus (through inhibition of the TCR signaling apoptotic process) or by altering normal selection mechanisms. These autoreactive T cells are then exported into the periphery. Upon discontinuation of CSP treatment and in a permissive environment (elimination of regulatory T cells by the preparative regimens), the autoreactive T cells can mediate autoaggression.

Antitumor activity of autologous GVHD

Several recent studies in animal model systems indicate that this "autoimmune" GVHD syndrome can be mobilized to mediate a significant antitumor effect [79–84]. This finding is particularly important since one of the major limitations of autologous therapy for malignancy is the unacceptably high rate of tumor recurrence compared to the rate of tumor

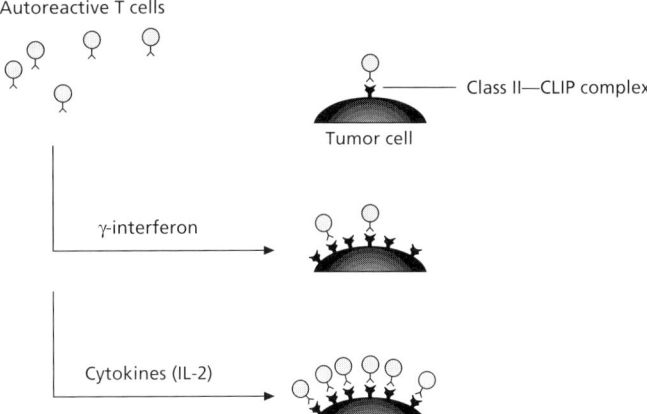

Fig. 30.4 Antitumor effect of cyclosporine (CSP) induced autologous/syngeneic graft-vs.-host disease (GVHD). The autoreactive T cells can target and lyse tumor cells that express the major histocompatibility complex (MHC) class II invariant chain peptide (CLIP) target antigen complex. Inducing up regulation of the target antigen on the tumor cells and clonally expanding the effector T-cell population can amplify the antitumor response. Moreover, natural killer (NK) cell activity reconstitutes quickly and may work in concert with the autoreactive T cells.

recurrence after allogeneic HCT, regardless of the preparative regimen employed [85–90]. The enhanced antitumor effect of allogeneic HCT is currently thought to be due to the occurrence of GVHD and implies that tumor cells can be eliminated by immune mechanisms [84–89]. Furthermore, adoptive transfer of donor T cells (donor lymphocyte infusion) can also induce remissions in patients who relapse after allogeneic HCT indicating that effective targeting of the tumor cells by the immune system does occur [91,92]. Although autologous HCT avoids the morbidity and mortality associated with GVHD after allogeneic HCT, the graft-vs.-tumor effect is absent. Immunologic approaches to eradicate tumor cells in this setting may be particularly effective because it would occur at a time of minimal residual disease, thus limiting the number of tumor cells that have to be eliminated by the immune system. Moreover, immune targeting appears to be noncross-resistant with high-dose chemotherapy since cytolytic T cells can recognize and destroy tumor cells that are resistant to conventional cytotoxic drugs [93].

The induction of syngeneic/autologous GVHD as antitumor therapy after autologous bone marrow transplantation (BMT) is attractive for several reasons. Immune recognition of tumor cells by the autoreactive T lymphocytes appears to be dependent on expression of the MHC class II-CLIP target antigen complex (see Fig. 30.4). This target antigen of the autologous/syngeneic GVHD effector T cells is commonly expressed on many human malignancies, particularly malignancies of the lymphohematopoietic system [94]. In addition, several strategies can be utilized to potentiate tumor targeting. For instance, the up regulation of the target antigen on the tumor cells and the expansion of the autoreactive T-cell population can be readily accomplished by administration of recombinant cytokines such as IFN-γ and IL-2, respectively [95,96]. Furthermore, the reconstitution of natural killer (NK) cell activity occurs quite rapidly after autologous HCT even with CSP treatment [42,54,67]. This population of cells provides another potential antitumor immune mechanism that can work in concert with the CSP-induced autoreactive T cells.

Preclinical studies

Initial preclinical studies clearly established that syngeneic GVHD had significant antitumor activity *in vitro* and *in vivo*. *In vitro*, CD8$^+$ splenic T cells from rats that develop syngeneic GVHD were able to lyse myeloma cells [79]. Lysis was blocked by pretreatment of the tumor cells with antibody to MHC class II determinants but not with antibody to MHC class I antigens. Furthermore tumor cell susceptibility to immune recognition and killing by the effector T cells was enhanced by IFN-γ. These studies demonstrated that syngeneic GVHD can manifest significant antitumor activity *in vitro* and confirmed that the effector T cells recognize MHC class II antigens on the tumor cell. Additional studies *in vivo* indicated that syngeneic GVHD mediated a modest but significant antitumor effect achieving a 1–2 log tumor cell kill [80–82]. Importantly, the antitumor effect of syngeneic GVHD could be potentiated by administration of either IFN-γ or low dose IL-2 [80,81]. Moreover, combining the administration of IFN-γ maximized the antitumor activity of syngeneic GVHD and IL-2 achieving a 4 log tumor cell kill.

It is of interest that other antitumor immune mechanisms may also play a significant role in the autologous/syngeneic GVHD setting. Recent studies indicate that MHC class II negative tumor cells can be effectively targeted and eliminated *in vivo* following syngeneic HCT and CSP treatment [84]. The principal effector population that mediates the antitumor effect includes NK cells amplified by type 1 cytokines that are produced during the period of active syngeneic GVHD. Similarly, studies by Charak *et al.* [83] suggest that IL-2 administration after syngeneic HCT and CSP therapy induces a very potent antitumor mechanism mediated by an activated NK cell population.

Clinical studies

Based on the results in animal model systems and encouraged by the fact that autologous GVHD can be induced in humans, several phase I/II clinical trials were initiated to evaluate the antitumor activity of this experimental autoaggression syndrome. A number of phase I studies conducted in a wide variety of hematological malignancies, including chemotherapy-resistant lymphoma, chemotherapy-resistant Hodgkin's disease and acute lymphoblastic leukemia, suggested that there is significant antitumor activity of autologous GVHD [71,97–100]. Both overall survival and disease-free survival were improved in patients undergoing autologous GVHD induction with CSP compared to historical controls. A phase II trial in intermediate or high-grade non-Hodgkin's lymphoma in sensitive relapse (still responsive to conventional salvage therapy prior to HCT) revealed that the patients on the autologous GVHD induction protocol had a decreased relapse rate and an event-free survival benefit compared to historical controls [100]. Moreover, the antitumor effect of autologous GVHD was potentiated by the administration of IFN-γ [100]. In patients with high-risk chemotherapy-resistant malignancies, immune modulation with CSP and IFN-γ after autologous HCT resulted in an improvement in disease-free survival (44%) compared to historical controls (disease-free survival, <10%). In accord are the results of a small-randomized trial in patients with resistant hematological malignancies. Overall survival was significantly improved in patients who developed autologous GVHD compared to those who did not (81% vs. 58%) [101]. Certainly, the antitumor activity of autologous GVHD needs to be confirmed in larger randomized clinical trials.

Recent studies have also described a novel approach to potentiate the induction of antitumor activity after HCT combining the induction of autologous GVHD with CSP plus IFN-α followed by additional cycles of IFN-α and chemotherapy in children with high-risk acute lymphoblastic leukemia (immnunochemotherapy). At 2 years, disease-free survival and overall survival of the patients on this treatment protocol were significantly greater compared to patients receiving CSP plus IFN-α alone after autologous HCT (69% vs. 13%; 85% vs. 25%, respectively) [102]. Unfortunately, the effect of the additional cycles of chemotherapy on the antitumor response in this study was not determined. Nevertheless, therapeutic strategies combining immunotherapy and chemotherapy after HCT may be necessary to induce a more effective autologous graft-vs.-tumor effect.

This autoaggression syndrome can also be induced in patients undergoing autologous HCT for metastatic breast cancer although higher doses of CSP are required to induce the syndrome [59,60]. The higher doses may stem from residual host immunoregulatory mechanisms that were not eliminated by the preparative regimen. Nevertheless, there does not appear to be significant antitumor activity in the breast cancer patients developing autologous GVHD [67,103,104]. This observation is not surprising as, in contrast to most hematological malignancies, breast cancer cells usually do not constitutively express MHC class II antigen and are more resistant to immune targeting [105,106]. Even the use of IFN-γ to induce up regulation of MHC class II-expression on the breast cancer tumor cells was largely unsuccessful [67,103]. Although the severity of autologous GVHD was markedly increased, no significant effect on tumor progression was observed. The tumor load in patients with metastatic breast cancer may have exceeded the capacity of the autologous GVHD effector mechanisms to inhibit or alter tumor progression. The induction of autologous GVHD as adjuvant therapy for patients with limited disease may have greater success. Certainly, other strategies are required for patients with metastatic breast cancer.

Conclusion

The full antitumor potential of autologous GVHD has not yet been fully realized. New approaches are still being developed. At present, the combination of IFN-γ and low-dose IL-2 appears to be the most effective strategy for enhancing the efficacy of CSP-induced autologous GVHD. This approach, amplifying the effector T-cell arm and inducing the up-regulation of the target antigen in autologous GVHD, yields a greater degree of antitumor activity as demonstrated in the animal model. Surprisingly, current studies suggest that the immunoregulatory cytokine, IL-10 may play a critical role in enhancing the antitumor activity of autologous GVHD. Furthermore, combining the induction of autologous GVHD with post-transplant immunochemotherapy may enhance antitumor activity. Underlying the success or failure of this or any approach, however, are regulatory T cells. Transfer of these cells contained in the stem cell inoculum not only compromises the ability to induce autologous GVHD, but may also compromise other immunotherapeutic approaches after autologous HCT [106].

References

1 Santos GW, Cole LJ. Effect of donor and host lymphoid and myeloid tissue injections in lethally X-irradiated mice treated with rat bone marrow. *J Natl Cancer Inst* 1958; **21**: 279–93.

2 Billingham RE, Brent L. Quantitative studies on tissue transplantation immunity IV. Induction of tolerance in newborn mice and studies on the phenomenon of runt disease. *Phil Transact Roy Soc London, B* 1959; **242**: 439–77.

3 Holler E, Ferrara JLM. Antagonists of inflammatory cytokines: prophylactic and therapeutic applications. In: Ferrara JLM, Deeg HJ, Burakoff SJ, eds. *Graft-vs.-Host Disease*. New York: Marcel Dekker Inc, 1996: 667–92.

4 Gluckman E, Devergie A, Sohier J, Sauret JH. Graft-versus-host disease in recipients of syngeneic bone marrow. *Lancet* 1980; **1**: 253–5.

5 Rappeport J, Reinhertz E, Mihm M, Lopanski S, Parkman R. Acute graft-versus-host disease in recipients of bone marrow transplantation from identical twin donors. *Lancet* 1979; **2**: 717–8.

6 Thien SW, Goldman JM, Galton DG. Acute graft-versus-host disease after autografting for chronic granulocytic leukemia in transplantation. *Ann Intern Med* 1981; **94**: 210–4.

7 Hood AF, Vogelsang GB, Black LP, Farmer ER, Santos GW. Acute graft-versus-host disease.

Development following autologous and syngeneic bone marrow transplantation. *Arch Dermatol* 1987; **123**: 745–50.
8. Billingham RE. The biology of graft-versus-host reactions. *Harvey Lect* 1966–67; **62**: 21–78.
9. Burnet F. *The Clonal Selection Theory of Acquired Immunity*. Cambridge: Cambridge University Press, 1959.
10. Kappler J, Staerz U, White J *et al*. Self-tolerance eliminates T cells specific for Mls-modified products of the major histocompatibility complex. *Nature* 1988; **332**: 35–8.
11. Kappler JW, Staerz U, White J *et al*. T cell tolerance by clonal elimination in the thymus. *Cell* 1987; **49**: 273–80.
12. Fowell D, Mason D. Evidence that the T cell repertoire of normal rats contains cells with potential to cause diabetes. Characterization of the CD4+ T cell subset that inhibits this autoimmune potential. *J Exp Med* 1993; **177**: 627–36.
13. Shevach E. Regulatory T cells in autoimmunity. *Ann Rev Immunol* 2000; **18**: 423–49.
14. Glazier A, Tutschka PJ, Farmer ER *et al*. Graft-versus-host disease in cyclosporin A treated rats after syngeneic and autologous bone marrow reconstitution. *J Exp Med* 1983; **158**: 1–8.
15. Glazier A, Tutschka PJ, Farmer ER. Studies on the immunobiology of syngeneic and autologous graft-versus-host disease in cyclosporine treated rats. *Trans Proc* 1983; **15**: 3035–41.
16. Cooper MH, Hartman GG, Starzl TE, Fung JJ. The induction of pseudo-graft-host disease following syngeneic bone marrow transplantation using FK506. *Trans Proc* 1991; **23**: 3234–5.
17. Hess AD, Thoburn CJ. Immunobiology and immunotherapeutic implications of syngeneic/autologous graft-vs.-host disease. *Immunol Rev* 1997; **157**: 111–23.
18. Ehrlich P. The Croonian lecture: on immunity. *Proc Roy Soc London (Biol)* 1900; **66**: 424–79.
19. Beschorner WE, Shinn CA, Fischer A *et al*. Cyclosporine (CsA) induced pseudo-graft-vs.-host disease (CIPGvHD) in the early post CsA period. *Transplantation* 1988; **46** (Suppl.): 112–7.
20. Hess AD, Fischer AC, Beschorner WE. Effector mechanisms in cyclosporine A induced syngeneic graft-vs.-host disease: role of CD4+ and CD8+ T lymphocyte subsets. *J Immunol* 1990; **140**: 526–33.
21. Hess AD, Thoburn CJ, Chen W, Horwitz LR. Complexity of effector mechanisms in cyclospoine-induced syngeneic graft-vs.-host disease. *Biol Blood Marrow Trans* 2000; **6**: 13–24.
22. Sorokin R, Kimura H, Schroder K, Wilson D. Cyclosporine-induced autoimmunity. Conditions for expressing disease: requirement for intact thymus, and potency estimates of autoimmune lymphocytes in drug-treated rats. *J Exp Med* 1986; **164**: 1615–6.
23. Babock S, Niswender K, Wilson DB, Bellgrau D. Cyclosporine-induced autoimmunization in rats carrying thymus allografts. *Transplantation* 1990; **50**: 1278–81.
24. Beijleveld LJ, Damoiseaux JG, Van Breda Vreiesman PJ. Differential effects of X-irradiation and cyclosporin-A administration on the thymus with respect to the generation of cyclosporin-A-induced autoimmunity. *Dev Immunol* 1995; **4**: 127–38.
25. De Waal EJ, Rademakers LH, Schuurman HJ, Vos JG, Van Loveren H. Alterations of dendritic cells in the rat thymus without epithelial cell loss during cyclosporine treatment and recovery. *Toxicology* 1996; **110**: 1333–151.
26. Ryffel B, Deysseroth R, Borel JF. Cyclosporin A. effects on the mouse thymus. *Agents Actions Suppl* 1981; **11**: 373–81.
27. Beschorner WE, Namnoun JD, Hess AD, Shinn C, Santos GW. Cyclosporin A and the thymus. *Immunopathol Am J Pathol* 1987; **126**: 487–96.
28. Urdahl KB, Pardoll DM, Jenkins MK. Cyclosporin A inhibits positive selection and delays negative selection in α/β TCR transgenic mice. *J Immunol* 1994; **152**: 2853–9.
29. von Boehmer H. The developmental biology of T lymphocytes. *Annu Rev Immunol* 1988; **6**: 309–76.
30. Hollander GA, Fruman DA, Bierer BE, Burakoff SJ. Disruption of T cell development and repertoire selection by calcineurin inhibition *in vivo*. *Transplantation* 1994; **58**: 1037–43.
31. Jenkins MK, Schwartz RH, Pardoll DM. Effects of cyclosporine A on T cell development and clonal deletion. *Science* 1988; **241**: 1655–7.
32. Gao EK, Lo D, Cheney R, Kanagawa O, Sprent J. Abnormal differentiation of thymocytes in mice treated with cyclosporin A. *Nature* 1988; **336**: 176–9.
33. Urdahl KB, Pardoll DM, Jenkins MK. Self-reactive T cells are present in the peripheral lymphoid tissues of cyclosporin A-treated mice. *Int Immunol* 1992; **4**: 1341–9.
34. Fischer AC, Beschorner WE, Hess AD. Requirements for the induction and adoptive transfer of cyclosporine-induced syngeneic graft-vs.-host disease. *J Exp Med* 1989; **169**: 1031–104.
35. Hess AD, Fischer AC. Immune mechanisms in cyclosporine-induced syngeneic graft-vs.-host disease. *Transplantation* 1989; **48**: 895–900.
36. Fischer AC, Hess AD. Age related factors in cyclosporine-induced syngeneic graft-vs.-host disease. Regulatory role of marrow derived T lymphocytes. *J Exp Med* 1990; **172**: 85–94.
37. Fischer AC, Laulis MK, Horwitz L, Beschorner WE, Hess AD. Host-resistance to cyclosporine induced syngeneic graft-vs.-host disease. *J Immunol* 1989; **143**: 827–32.
38. Hess AD, Fischer AC, Horwitz L, Bright EC, Laulis MK. Characterization of peripheral autoregulatory mechanisms that prevent devleopment of cyclosporin-induced syngeneic graft-vs.-host disease. *J Immunol* 1994; **153**: 400–11.
39. Wu DY, Goldschneider I. Tolerance to cyclosporin A-induced autologous graft-versus-host disease is mediated by a CD4+CD25+ subset of recent thymic emigrants. *J Immunol* 2001; **166**: 7158–64.
40. Wu DY, Goldschneider I. Cyclosporin A-induced autologous graft-versus-host disease. A prototypical model of autoimmunity and active (dominant) tolerance coordinately induced by recent thymic emigrants. *J Immunol* 1999; **162**: 6926–33.
41. Hess AD, Horwitz LR, Thoburn CJ. Immune tolerance to self MHC class II antigens after bone marrow transplantation. *Trans Proc* 1999; **31**: 688–9.
42. Flanagan DL, Jennings CD, Bryson JS. Th1 cytokines and NK cells participate in the development of murine syngeneic graft-versus-host disease. *J Immunol* 1999; **163**: 1170–7.
43. Beijleveld LJ, Groen H, Broeren CP *et al*. Susceptibility to clinically manifest cyclosporine A (CsA)-induced autoimmune disease is associated with interferon-gamma (IFN-gamma)-producing CD45RC+RT6− T helper cells. *Clin Exp Immunol* 1996; **105**: 486–96.
44. Hess AD, Thoburn CJ, Horwitz L. Promiscuous recognition of major histocompatiblity class II determinants in cyclosporine-induced syngeneic graft-versus-host disease. *Transplantation* 1998; **65**: 785–92.
45. Chen W, Thoburn CJ, Hess AD. Characterization of the pathogenic autoreactive T cells in cyclosporine-induced syngeneic graft-versus-host disease. *J Immunol* 1998; **161**: 7040–6.
46. Ashkenazi A, Dixit VM. Death receptors, signaling and modulation. *Science* 1998; **281**: 1305–10.
47. Ferrara JLM, Antin JH. The pathophysiology of graft-versus-host disease. In: Thomas ED, Blume KG, Forman SJ, eds. *Hematopoietic Cell Transplantation*, 2nd edn. Malden, MA: Blackwell Science, 1999: 305–25.
48. Fischer AC, Ruvolo P, Burt R *et al*. Characterization of autoreactive T cell repertoire in cyclosporine-induced syngeneic graft-versus-host disease: a highly conserved repertoire mediates autoaggression. *J Immunol* 1995; **154**: 3713–25.
49. Hess AD, Horwitz L, Beschorner WE, Santos GW. Development of graft-vs.-host disease-like syndrome in cyclosporine-treated rats after syngeneic bone marrow transplantation. I. Development of cytotoxic-T lymphocytes with apparent polyclonal anti-Ia specificity including autoreactivity. *J Exp Med* 1985; **161**: 718–30.
50. Hess AD, Horwitz LR, Laulis MK. Cyclosporine induced syngeneic graft-vs.-host disease. Prevention of autoaggression by treatment with monoclonal antibodies to T lymphocyte cell surface determinants and to MHC class II antigens. *Clin Immunol Immunopathol* 1993; **69**: 341–50.
51. Malcherek G, Gnau V, Jung G, Rammensee HG, Melms A. Supermotifs enable natural invariant chain-derived peptides to interact with many major histocompatibility complex class II molecules. *J Exp Med* 1995; **181**: 527–30.
52. Freisewinkel IM, Schench K, Koch N. The segment of the invariant chain that is critical for association with major histocompatibility complex class II molecules contains the sequence of a peptide eluted from class II polypeptides. *Proc Natl Acad Sci U S A* 1993; **90**: 9703–7.
53. Chicz RM, Urban RG, Gorga JC, Vignali DA, Lane WS, Strominger JL. Specificity and promiscuity among naturally processed peptides bound to HLA-DR alleles. *J Exp Med* 1993; **178**: 27–38.
54. Hess AD, Bright EC, Thoburn C, Vogelsang GB, Jones RJ, Kennedy MJ. Specificity and antitumor activity of effector T lymphocytes in autologous graft-vs.-host disease: Role of the MHC class II invariant chain peptide. *Blood* 1997; **89**: 2203–9.
55. Pannetier CM, Cochet S, Darche A, Casrouge M, Zoller M, Kourilsky P. The sizes of the CDR3 hypervariable regions of the murine T cell receptor β chain vary as a function of the recombined germline segments. *Proc Natl Acad Sci U S A* 1993; **90**: 4319–23.
56. Ericson ML, Sundstrom M, Sansom DM, Charron DJ. Mutually exclusive binding of peptide and invariant chain to major histocompatibility complex class II antigens. *J Biol Chem* 1994; **269**: 26531–8.
57. Sale GE, Shulman HM, Hackman RC. Pathology of hematopoietic cell transplantation. In: Thomas ED, Blume KG, Forman SJ, eds. *Hematopoietic Cell Transplantation*, 2nd edn. Malden, MA: Blackwell Science, 1999: 24–49.
58. Jones RJ, Vogelsang GB, Hess AD *et al*. Induction of graft-versus-host disease after autologous bone marrow transplantaion. *Lancet* 1989; **i**: 754–7.

59 Kennedy MJ, Vogelsang GB, Beveridge RA et al. Phase I trial of intravenous cyclosporine to induce graft-versus-host disease in women undergoing autologous bone marrow transplantation for breast cancer. *J Clin Oncol* 1993; **11**: 478–84.

60 Kennedy MJ, Vogelsang GB, Jones RJ et al. Phase I trial of interferon-gamma to potentiate cyclosporine A-induced graft-versus host disease in women undergoing autologous bone marrow transplantation for breast cancer. *J Clin Oncol* 1994; **12**: 249–57.

61 Yeager AM, Vogelsang GB, Jones RJ et al. Induction of cutaneous graft-versus-host disease by administration of cyclosporine to patients undergoing autologous bone marrow transplantation for acute myeloid leukemia. *Blood* 1992; **79**: 3031–5.

62 Carella AM, Gaozza E, Congiu A et al. Cyclosporine-induced graft-versus-host disease after autologous bone marrow transplantation in hematological malignancies. *Ann Hematol* 1991; **62**: 156–9.

63 Giralt S, Weber D, Colome M et al. Phase I trial of cyclosporine-induced autologous graft-versus-host disease in patients with multiple myeloma undergoing high-dose chemotherapy with autologous stem-cell rescue. *J Clin Oncol* 1997; **15**: 667–73.

64 Pati AR, Godder KT, Abhyankar SH et al. Cyclosporine-induced autologous graft-versus-host disease following autologous blood stem cell transplantation for lymphoma. *Bone Marrow Transplant* 1996; **17**: 1081–3.

65 Barredo JC, Yusuf U, Hahn A et al. Progressive autologous graft-versus-host disease induced by cyclosporine A. *Bone Marrow Transplant* 1996; **18**: 659–62.

66 Martin RW, Farmer ER, Altomonte VL et al. Lichenoid graft-vs.-host disease in an autologous bone marrow transplant recipient. *Arch Dermatol* 1995; **131**: 333–5.

67 van der Wall E, Horn T, Bright E et al. Autologous graft-versus-host disease induction in advanced breast cancer: role of peripheral blood progenitor cells. *Br J Cancer* 2000; **83**: 1405–11.

68 Miura Y, Ueda M, Zeng W et al. Induction of autologous graft-versus-host disease with cyclosporine A after peripheral blood stem cell transplantation: analysis of the factors affecting induction. *J Allergy Clin Immunol* 2000; **106**: 51–7.

69 Sica S, Chiusolo P, Salutari P et al. Autologous graft-versus-host disease after CD34+-purified autologous peripheral blood progenitor cell transplanation. *J Hematotherapy Stem Cell Res* 2000; **9**: 375–9.

70 Massumoto C, Benyunes MC, Sale G et al. Close simulation of acute graft-versus-host-disease by interleukin-2 administered after autologous bone marrow transplantation for hematologic malignancy. 1996; **17**: 351–6.

71 Gothot BF, Salmon JP, Hermanne JP, Pierard GE, Fillet G, Beguin Y. Clinical course and predictive factors for cyclosporine-induced autologous graft-versus-host disease after autlogous haematopoietic stem cell transplantation. *Br J Haematol* 2000; **111**: 745–53.

72 Miura Y, Thoburn CJ, Bright EC, Chen W, Nakao S, Hess AD. Cytokine and chemokine profiles in autologous graft-versus-host disease (GVHD): interleukin 10 and interferon-γ may be critical mediators for the development of autologous GVHD. *Blood* 2002; **100**: 2650–8.

73 Blazar B, Taylor PA, Smith S. Vallera DA. Interleukin 10 administration decreases survival in murine recipients of major histocompatibility complex disparate bone marrow grafts. *Blood* 1995; **85**: 842–51.

74 MacNeil IA, Suda T, Moore KW, Mosmann TR, Zlotnik A. IL-10, a novel growth cofactor for mature and immature T cells. *J Immunol* 1990; **145**: 4167–73.

75 Ruvolo PP, Bright EC, Kennedy MJ et al. Cyclosporine-induced autologous graft-versus-host disease: assessment of cytolytic effector mechanisms and the Vβ T cell receptor repertoire. *Transplant Proc* 1995; **27**: 1363–5.

76 Garin L, Rigal D, Souillet G et al. Strong increase in the percentage of the CD8 bright+ CD28− T cells and delayed engraftment associated with cyclosporine-induced autologous GVHD. *Eur J Haematol* 1996; **56**: 119–23.

77 Miura Y, Thoburn CJ, Bright EC et al. Characterization of the T-cell repertoire in autologous graft-versus-host disease (GVHD): evidence for the involvement of antigen-driven T-cell response in the development of autologous GVHD. *Blood* 2001; **98**: 868–76.

78 Ruvolo PP, Fischer AC, Vogelsang GB et al. Analysis of the Vβ T-cell receptor repertoire in autologous graft-versus-host disease. *Ann NY Acad Sci* 1995; **756**: 432–4.

79 Geller RB, Esa AH, Beschorner WE, Frondoza CG, Santos GW, Hess AD. Successful in vitro graft-versus-tumor effect against an Ia-bearing tumor using cyclosporine-induced syngeneic graft-versus-host disease in the rat. *Blood* 1989; **74**: 1165–71.

80 Noga SJ, Horwitz L, Kim H, Laulis MK, Hess AD. Interferon-γ potentiates the antitumor effect of cyclosporine-induced autoimmunity. *J Hematotherapy* 1992; **1**: 75–84.

81 Hess AD, Kennedy MJ, Ruvolo PP, Vogelsang GB, Jones RJ. Antitumor activity of syngeneic/autologous graft-vs.-host disease. *N Y Acad Sci* 1995; **770**: 189–202.

82 Hess AD, Noga SJ. Cyclosporine-induced syngeneic graft-versus-host disease: An immunotherapeutic approach after autologous bone marrow transplantation. *Int J Cell Cloning* 1992; **10** (Suppl. 1): 179–80.

83 Charak BS, Agah R, Mazumder A. Synergism of interleukin-2 and cyclosporine A in induction of a graft-versus-tumor effect without graft-versus-host disease after syngeneic bone marrow transplantation. *Blood* 1992; **80**: 179–84.

84 Bryson JS, Jennings CD, Lowery DM et al. Rejection of an MHC class II negative tumor following induction of murine syngeneic graft-versus-host disease. *Bone Marrow Transplant* 1999; **23**: 363–72.

85 Weiden PL, Flournoy N, Thomas ED et al. Anti-leukemic effect of graft-versus-host disease in human recipients of allogeneic marrow grafts. *N Engl J Med* 1979; **300**: 1068–73.

86 Weiden PL, Sullivan KM, Flournoy N, Storb R, Thomas ED. Anti-leukemic effect of chronic graft-versus-host disease. *N Engl J Med* 1981; **304**: 1529–33.

87 Kersey JH, Weisdorf D, Nesbit M et al. Comparison of autologous and allogeneic bone marrow transplantation for treatment of high-risk refractory acute lymphoblastic leukemia. *N Engl J Med* 1987; **317**: 461–7.

88 Butturini A, Bortin MM, Gale RP. Graft-versus-leukemia following bone marrow transplantation. *Bone Marrow Transplant* 1987; **2**: 233–42.

89 Horowitz MM, Gale RP, Sondel PM et al. Graft-versus-leukemia ractions after bone marrow transplantation. *Blood* 1990; **75**: 555–62.

90 Jones RJ, Ambinder RF, Piantadosi S, Santos GW. Evidence of a graft-versus-lymphoma effect associated with allogeneic bone marrow transplantation. *Blood* 1991; **77**: 649–53.

91 Mackinnon S, Papadopoulos EB, Carabasi MH et al. Adoptive immunotherapy evaluating escalating doses of donor leukocytes for relapse of chronic myeloid leukemia after bone marrow transplantation: separation of graft-versus-leukemia responses from graft-versus-host disease. *Blood* 1995; **86**: 1261–8.

92 Kolb HJ, Schattenberg A, Goldman JM et al. Graft-versus-leukemia effect of donor lymphocyte transfusions in marrow grafted patients. European Group for Blood and Marrow Transplantation Working Party for Chronic Leukemia. *Blood* 1995; **86**: 2041–50.

93 Fuchs EJ, Bedi A, Jones RJ, Hess AD. Cytotoxic T cells overcome *BCR-ABL*-mediated resistance to apoptosis. *Cancer Res* 1995; **55**: 463–6.

94 Foon KA, Todd RF III. Immunologic classification of leukemia and lymphoma. *Blood* 1986; **68**: 1–31.

95 Baldini L, Cortelezzi A, Polli N et al. Human recombinant interferon α-2C enhances the expression of class II HLA antigens on hairy cells. 1986; **67**: 458–64.

96 Gressier VH, Weinkauff RE, Franklin WA, Golomb HM. Modulation of the expression of major histocompatibility antigens on splenic hairy cells: differential effect upon *in vitro* treatment with α-2β-interferon, γ-interferon, and interleukin-2. *Blood* 1988; **72**: 1048–53.

97 Vogelsang GB, Bitton R, Piantadosi S et al. Immune modulation in autologous bone marrow transplantation: cyclosporine and gamma-interferon trial. *Bone Marrow Transplant* 1999; **24**: 637–40.

98 Gruhn B, Hafer R, Kosmehl H, Fuchs D, Zintl F. Cyclosporin A-induced graft-versus-host disease following autologous bone marrow and stem cell transplantation in hematological malignancies of childhood. *Bone Marrow Transplant* 1998; **21**: 901–7.

99 Gryn J, Johnson E, Goldman N et al. The treatment of relapsed or refractory intermediate grade non-Hodgkin's lymphoma with autologous bone marrow transplantation followed by cyclosporine and interferon. *Bone Marrow Transplant* 1997; **19**: 221–6.

100 Jones RJ, Vogelsang GB, Ambinder RF et al. Autologous marrow transplantation (ABMT) with cyclosporine (CsA)-induced autologous graft-versus-host disease (GVHD) for relapsed aggressive non-Hodgkin's lymphoma (NHL). *Blood* 1991; **78**: 287 [Abstract].

101 Marin GH, Prates PA, Etchegogen NJ et al. Graft-versus-host disease in autologous stem cell transplantation. *J Exp Clin Cancer Res* 1999; **18**: 201–8.

102 Houtenbos I, Bracho F, Davenport V et al. Autologous bone marrow transplantataion for childhood acute lymphoblastic leukemia: a novel combined approach consisting of *ex vivo* marrow purging, modulation of multi-drug resistance, induction of autograft vs. leukemia effect and post-

transplant immuno- and chemotherapy (PITC). *Bone Marrow Transplant* 2001; **27**: 145–53.
103 Kennedy MJ, Vogelsang GB, Jones RJ, Hess AD. Post-transplant immunotherapy by induction of autologous GVHD. *Autologous Marrow Blood Transplantation* 1997; **8**: 601–8.
104 Zuk JA, Walker RA. HLA class II sublocus expression in benign and malignant breast epithelium. *J Pathol* 1988; **155**: 301–9.
105 Gastl G, Marth C, Leiter E *et al*. Effects of human recombinant α_2 arg-interferon and γ-interferon on human breast cancer cell lines: dissociation of anti-proliferative activity and induction of HLA-DR antigen expression. *Cancer Res* 1985; **45**: 2957–61.
106 Hess AD. Autologous graft-versus-host disease [editorial]. *J Hematotherapy Stem Cell Res* 2000; **9**: 397–8.

31 Biostatistical Methods in Hematopoietic Cell Transplantation

Joyce C. Niland

With the tremendous strides and newly emerging science within the field of hematopoietic cell transplantation (HCT), advances in study design, biostatistical methodology and biomedical informatics are required to keep pace. Clinical trial design and analysis methodology has been evolving over the past decade [1], providing the tools needed to obtain valid results and advances in evidence-based medicine based on HCT studies. This chapter provides an overview of the study cycle for new treatment discoveries, from observational studies through the phases of clinical trials as applied to HCT. The principles for designing such studies and the fundamentals regarding study conduct and monitoring are described. Subtleties and potential pitfalls of various study designs and analytic approaches are given, along with the requirements for full and complete reporting of study results. Special issues that must be considered during the conduct of human clinical trials are discussed, including appropriate monitoring through independent data and safety boards, along with international standards for the conduct and reporting of human research.

The future availability of high-resolution maps of the human genome and the ability to determine rapidly the allelic variation in individuals will change the nature of clinical trials research. With the postgenome era of biologic research underway, the clinical trial database, design, conduct and analytic tools required to manage the huge amounts of genomic data must by considered. Our greatest challenge will be understanding the meaning of these data, and applying this new understanding to develop targeted interventions and approaches to treatment. Because of the far-reaching future impact of genomics data on clinical research, for each section of this chapter the potential influence of human genome data on the study cycle is forecasted. The need for evolving advanced biomedical informatics tools to support study design, data management and analysis of these data also is addressed.

Throughout Chapter 31 formulas and calculations are avoided in favor of emphasizing the underlying concepts and theories of biostatistical methodology. It is hoped that this approach will provide physicians, fellows, medical students and health care professionals involved in HCT research with a basic understanding of and guide to appropriate approaches in study design, conduct, statistical analysis and data computerization. Frequent references to related biostatistical/clinical trials articles and textbooks are included to promote better understanding. For those seeking a more detailed treatment of the history, rationale and methodology underlying clinical trials, the texts by Meinert and Tonascia [2], Pocock [3] and Friedmen *et al*. [4] provide these underpinnings. For a comprehensive overview of clinical trial informatics applied to the field of oncology the reader is referred to the text by Silva *et al*. [5].

The study cycle

Figure 31.1 provides an overview of the study cycle for new treatment discoveries. Often initial insights into the potential value of certain therapeutic approaches are gleaned through observational studies. These observations must be substantiated by the development of a sound biologic hypothesis that holds promise of explaining the underlying mechanism of action for the new therapy. Animal studies are then conducted to assess dosing, toxicities and possible efficacy in humans. Only at this critical juncture can an investigator engage in experimentation via clinical trials, i.e. planned interventional studies to assess the efficacy of treatments in humans.

The final phase of the study cycle is to observe the use of successful treatments stemming from the clinical trial results, now offered to the entire patient population. The application of evidence-based medical approaches to the general population may lead to observations that cycle back into the next phase of research to advance medical discoveries. Often disparate or diminished results are observed when new treatments are first applied as the standard of care, as the careful selection process applied during clinical trial conduct is no longer in effect, and the patients being treated post clinical trials represent the gamut of stages, phases and demographics. This field of study, known as outcomes research, is not covered in this chapter, as this topic is discussed in detail in Chapter 32.

The following sections focus on two of the key designs for observational studies, a frequent starting point of the study cycle.

Observational study designs

Table 31.1 suggests that there is a hierarchy of study designs, from the least convincing (anecdotal case reports), to the most convincing (the confirmed randomized controlled clinical trial) [6]. The key differential between observational studies and clinical trials is that the former does not involve any type of intervention with the subjects under study, while clinical trials by definition are experimental in nature and involve an investigator controlled intervention. Much can be learned from conducting well-designed observational studies, and they may serve as a valuable precursor to the next novel treatment approach to be tested in clinical trials, particularly at the point when a randomized trial in HCT is not ethical or practical. While true experiments (i.e. clinical trials) allow an investigator to establish causal associations more conclusively, observational studies can provide major contributions to the understanding of disease processes.

In an observational study, the association between the outcome of interest and membership in study groups formed by the patient's experience, exposure or health-related behavior (the antecedent or "independent"

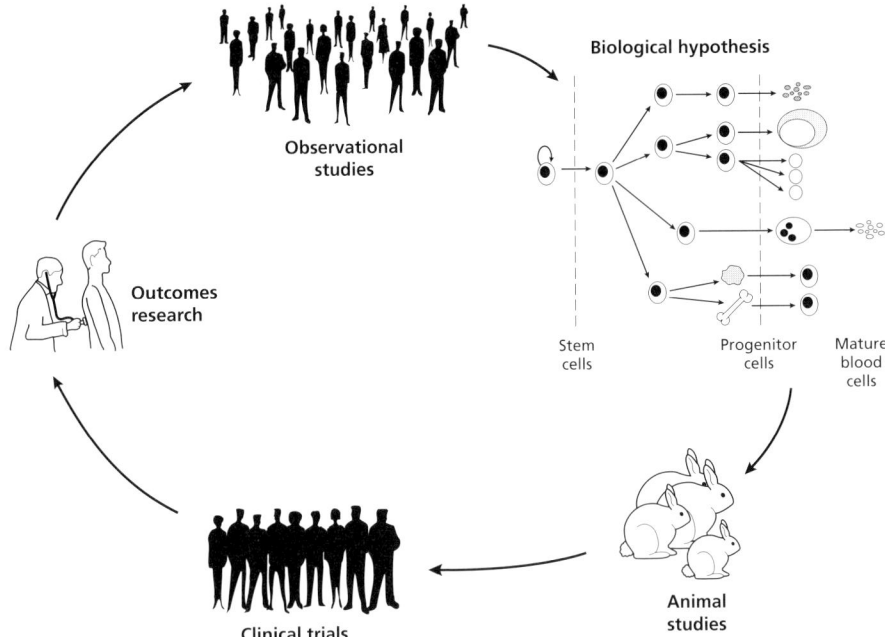

Fig. 31.1 The study cycle of new treatment discoveries.

Table 31.1 Hierarchy of strength of evidence concerning efficacy of treatment. (Adapted from [6].)

1 Confirmed randomized controlled clinical trial
2 Single randomized controlled clinical trial
3 Case series with historical controls
4 Retrospective case–control study
5 Analyses of existing databases
6 Series with literature controls
7 Case series without controls
8 Anecdotal case reports

variable) are observed and analyzed relative to the disease outcome of interest (the "dependent" variable). A difficulty with observational studies is that the observed groups under comparison usually differ naturally with respect to other characteristics beyond the specific factor under study. For example, people in various occupations differ not only with respect to their exposures to occupational hazards, but also with respect to their prior and current lifestyles. Such differences may come about by one or more mechanism such as self-selection, education level, fitness for a particular occupation or hiring practices. These potential influences on the outcome under study are known as "confounding factors". While a good study design will anticipate and measure confounding factors, many such factors are difficult, costly or impossible to measure fully. In this instance the role of the primary factor under investigation is more difficult to demonstrate, and the statistical analyses are more challenging.

When observational studies are designed carefully, one may be able to control some of the biases that are inherent in patient selection or outcome assessment. Two major types of design approaches for observational studies—prospective and retrospective—can be applied in the area of HCT research. Each design has attendant features, analytical methods and advantages or disadvantages, as described in the subsequent sections.

Prospective cohort studies

In a prospective cohort design, groups or "cohorts" of subjects are selected based on an observed common exposure to some naturally occurring factor. For example, patients who have a matched sibling donor and receive an allogeneic bone marrow transplant (BMT) may be compared to patients with a similar disease status for whom no donor is available. Even through such a natural group assignment process there could be inherent selection bias between the two groups. As an example, donor availability is likely to correlate with family size, which in turn may correlate with the educational and economic levels of the study subjects. Furthermore, the decision to take a patient to transplant is not dictated solely by the availability of the donor, e.g. a physician could withhold BMT because of the worsened clinical condition of a patient. Matching on as many potentially confounding factors as possible helps to reduce some of the bias. (However, then care must be taken to take the matching into account via the appropriate statistical techniques when analyzing the data.)

There also is potential bias related to the length of time that a patient waits for an allogeneic HCT procedure. Transplant recipients may be at lower risk than all patients intended to receive a BMT, as the recipients not only responded to induction chemotherapy but also survived relapse-free long enough to identify an appropriate donor. This "waiting time" to transplant causes bias as the transplant group excludes those who would have undergone a BMT had they survived long enough. To analyze data of this nature properly, time-varying covariates need to be incorporated into the model, via techniques such as the one described by Mantel and Byar [7].

An advantage of the prospective cohort design is that it permits the calculation of incidence rates among those "exposed" and those "not exposed" to the antecedent factor of interest, providing a direct estimate of the true relative risk (RR). With this study design one also can calculate the difference in incidence rates between groups, known as the attributable risk. A primary disadvantage of prospective cohort studies is that they usually are quite expensive and require a long follow-up period to observe a sufficient number of outcome events. Just as with a controlled clinical trial, hypotheses for the observed difference of clinical importance between the groups, the alpha (type I) error that is allowable, and the desired power must be clearly established at the outset of the study, so that the requisite sample size can be calculated.

Retrospective case–control studies

When the outcome of interest is relatively rare, a retrospective case–control study may be the best design for evaluating potential factors associated with an outcome of interest [8]. In a case–control study, the cases are defined as subjects with a particular type and stage of disease. Controls who are free from the disease under study are chosen, matched to the cases based on certain known confounding factors such as age and gender. Care must be taken not to overmatch cases and controls on more than a few key factors, because of the increased difficulty of identifying appropriate matched controls, the increased complexity of the analyses and the resultant inability to study any of the matching factors with respect to association with the outcome.

A drawback of the retrospective case–control design is that incidence rates cannot be directly estimated, as no appropriate denominators are available (populations at risk). Instead an odds ratio (OR) is calculated to estimate the RR between cases and controls, quantifying the odds of having the disease when the factor of interest is present versus when it is absent. The OR is an accurate estimate of the true RR if, and only if, three assumptions hold true:
1 the controls are representative of the general population;
2 the assembled cases are representative of all cases; and
3 the frequency of the disease in the population is rare.

Like the prospective cohort study design, case–control studies are subject to uncontrolled variation and potential biases. If a case–control study yields a modest difference in outcome between treatments this must be interpreted cautiously, as it is difficult to conclude whether a true treatment effect actually exists, or the results are confounded by other factors. Case–control studies can be strengthened through several means, including larger sample sizes, adjustment or matching for potential confounding factors, careful testing of model assumptions, and adjustment for multiple comparisons.

Quality of life and cost-effectiveness studies

Two burgeoning areas of observational study over the past several years include the study of quality of life (QOL) and of cost-effectiveness. Many clinical trials now incorporate these endpoints in the protocol to corroborate the success of new interventions, particularly as the margin for improvement decreases as more successful treatment options become routinely available [9]. Literature review has shown that citations for QOL studies grew from less than 30 in 1977 to more than 1000 some 20 years later [10].

Analysis of QOL associated with clinical trials may involve multiple scales assessed repeatedly over time, raising the challenge of appropriate statistical handling of multiple measurements and comparisons [11]. To reduce the number of hypotheses and facilitate the interpretation of trial results for the primary question, "Does the overall QOL differ between treatment arms?", summary measures collapsing over the multiple QOL items and scales often are used. With multiple QOL assessments over time, missing data can strongly influence the choice of methodology and analytic strategy.

Methods have been developed to incorporate QOL into survival analysis, such as the "Q-TWiST" method for quality-adjusted survival analysis using the Cox proportional hazards model [12]. The Q-TWiST model assumes that following HCT, patients progress through a series of health states that differ in QOL. The Kaplan–Meier product limit estimate is used to calculate the mean duration of each state, and quality-adjusted survival is estimated given a set of covariate values (Kaplan–Meier/Cox models are described in more detail in the "Analysis" section of this chapter). The results can be useful for investigating how prognostic factors might affect treatment benefits in terms of QOL. Further discussion of QOL and cost-effectiveness studies is provided in Chapter 32.

Impact of genetic data on observational studies

Through the mapping and sequencing of the human genome it has become possible to explore how genotypic differences lead to phenotypic variation, and to begin to understand the genetically influenced mechanisms that underlie human disease [13]. Initial exploratory studies will involve "data mining" of existing genetic databanks to look for correlations and begin to generate hypotheses. This initial data mining should be "unsupervised" in nature, employing methods that will allow nonmathematical biologists to browse and manipulate the vast data already available in genetic databases such as GenBank and the Online Mendelian Inheritance in Man (OMIM) database. Investigators are beginning to use automated sequencing and analysis of DNA as an inexpensive screening of multiple loci for polymorphisms. Sharing of data across all research groups worldwide will be required to expedite discoveries of critical genetic patterns.

As we move into the next phase of attempting to relate genetic information to clinical phenotypic data, DNA databanks oriented toward future hypotheses not framed at the outset will need to be created. Such databanks will consist of repositories of identified specimens, and will be able to serve many different "parent" clinical studies in future. To examine genotype–phenotype correlations it will be critical that the genetic data are linked to repositories of detailed biologic, medical history and treatment data on the same individuals. The standard endpoints used in clinical trials (e.g. efficacy, safety) will give way to less clear outcomes such as "classification" and "correlation". Epidemiologic trials will be increasingly important to tease out environmental versus genetic contributions to disease, and familial history data will become critical. This collection and exploration of complex phenotypic, intervention and environmental data may prove to be a more daunting information management feat than the amassing of the genetic information, comprised of data elements with a very simple structure by comparison. Guidelines for the use of genomics in clinical research (and in clinical practice) will be required, using an interdisciplinary approach involving clinical investigators, geneticists, biostatisticians and bioinformaticists.

Clinical trial design in HCT research

A clinical trial involves a true experimental design in which the investigator controls the intervention. The National Institutes of Health (NIH) define a clinical trial as a prospective biomedical or behavioral research study of human subjects that is designed to answer specific questions about new interventions (drugs, treatments, devices or new ways of using known interventions). Clinical trials are used to determine whether the new interventions are safe, efficacious and effective. Such trials in humans can be conducted only in a very narrow window of select circumstances.

The field of oncology is well-suited to the application of clinical trials [14]. Outcomes generally are well-defined and measurable, and the participation, compliance and follow-up rates tend to be better in the face of such serious illness than they would be for less life-threatening diseases.

Precursors of modern clinical trials date as far back as informal human experiments conducted in the 1700s, and modern trial methods began to appear in the medical literature in the 1930s. It is generally agreed that the earliest trial using today's formal methods such as patient selection and treatment assignment was the Medical Research Council (MRC) trial of streptomycin for the treatment of tuberculosis, designed by Austin Bradford Hill [15]. In this trial two measures of success (endpoints) were defined as survival and improvement on chest X-rays, as interpreted by a radiologist who was unaware of (i.e. masked to) the type of treatment that the patients had received.

There are four possible phases of clinical trial in the development of a new therapeutic intervention:

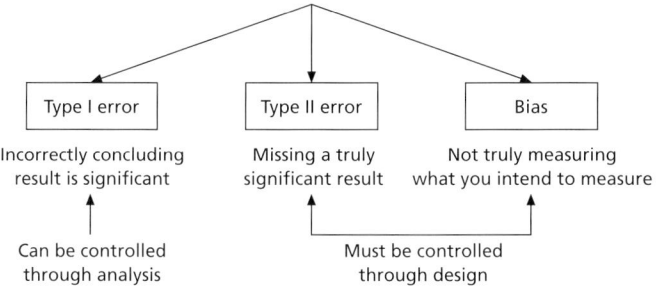

Fig. 31.2 Possible errors in clinical trials.

- Phase 1 Determine the appropriate dose ("How much therapy can be given safely?")
- Phase 2 Demonstrate effectiveness ("Does it work in a group of target patients?")
- Phase 3 Compare against the standard ("Is it better than what we can offer now?")
- Phase 4 Evaluate effects postmarketing ("Will the effect hold in the general population?")

A number of legal requirements must be in place before conducting a clinical trial, including outside review of the protocol by an independent body, determination that the participant's risk/benefit ratio is reasonable, and a procedure for obtaining the participant's informed consent prior to enrollment on the trial. (Note that "participant" often is the favored term for individuals enrolled on a clinical trial, rather than patients or subjects, emphasizing consideration of the enrollee's human rights and expectation of an acceptable quality of life, as well as acknowledging that some trials enroll healthy individuals, e.g. vaccine development trials.) An in-depth treatment on human subject protections and regulatory requirements is beyond the scope of the current chapter; however, a comprehensive overview can be found in the recent text edited by Amdur and Bankert [16].

The fundamental core of a clinical trial must be based on the scientific question to be answered. However, the design also must incorporate an ethical concern for the participants, and a wise use of available financial, therapeutic and human resources. The trial must be designed such that the results will be persuasive to the intended audience(s), including the health care and patient populations, and the regulatory bodies responsible for approval of new drugs/devices. The study design also must provide appropriate statistical control against potentially erroneous conclusions.

By their nature, clinical trials tend to include lower risk patients within a certain age group and with particular clinical characteristics. In the real world, patients are less well-defined and do not fit the inclusion and exclusion criteria of the trial, such that the trial results will apply only to a proportion of all the patients with the same disease. Ideally, a registry of all *potential* trial patients should be an essential part of any clinical trial; however, maintenance of such a registry often is overlooked.

As can be seen from Fig. 31.2, at least three major errors can occur within a clinical trial, leading to potentially spurious or misleading results. Type I error involves an incorrect conclusion of a statistically significant result when none is actually present. Type II error reflects an inability to detect a significant result when it truly is present. Bias is the third type of error, occurring when the data do not actually measure the intended results, but rather are influenced systematically by other existing factors. While type I errors can be diminished through the correct analytic approaches, avoidance of type II errors and bias must occur up front through the appropriate study design, sample size and robust definition and collection of endpoints.

Readers of published studies may wonder why several trials conducted to examine the same therapeutic regimen and endpoints in similar patients with a given disease entity often draw differing conclusions. Variation in clinical trial results can be explained by several factors which must be considered to ensure valid intertrial comparisons. These include, but are not limited to:

- specific participant selection criteria;
- exact response definitions;
- interobserver variability in assessing response;
- dosage modifications proscribed by the protocol;
- participant compliance with dosing rules;
- completeness of the reporting of results; and
- overall sample size of the trial.

Prior to contrasting results across clinical trials, the astute reader should assess the comparability of the studies with respect to these critical points (provided that the report is complete enough to allow such an assessment, another frequent downfall in published studies).

The primary tool to help control variability of these components *within* a clinical trial is strict specification of a detailed protocol, and measurement of protocol adherence during the conduct of the trial. The typical components to be specified when authoring a clinical trial protocol are shown in Table 31.2. Some items apply more in certain phases of clinical trials (e.g. randomization typically occurs in phase 3 trials, although randomized phase 1 and 2 designs also are possible). All of these protocol sections should at least be considered for inclusion when authoring a clinical trial protocol, and most are mandatory to create a valid protocol document.

Table 31.3 provides a synopsis of the core elements of the first three phases of clinical trials typically conducted at research institutions. The table summarizes the primary aim, sample to be studied, general procedure and pertinent notes relevant to each phase of study, as discussed in more detail in the following sections.

Phase 1 clinical trials

A phase 1 clinical trial is conducted to test a new intervention in a small group of people (e.g. less than 80) for the first time, to evaluate the

Table 31.2 Key components of a clinical trial protocol.

- Objectives
- Background
- Hypotheses
- Drug information
- Staging criteria
- Patient eligibility
- Descriptive/stratification factors
- Randomization scheme
- Treatment plan
- Dosage modifications
- Toxicities monitored
- Study parameters
- Endpoint definitions
- Criteria for evaluation
- Pathology review
- Special instructions
- Statistical considerations
- Registration guidelines
- Data submission schedule
- Inclusion of women, minorities and children
- Ethical and regulatory considerations
- References

Table 31.3 Core elements of phase 1–3 clinical trials.

Phase 1 trials
Primary aim	Identify the safe range and maximum tolerated dose (MTD) for a new drug (or a new combination of drugs)
Sample	Volunteers with advanced cancer no longer responding to standard therapy, or homogeneous subsets of high-risk patients
Procedure	Gradually increase dose in successive groups of patients until "significant" toxicity occurs
Notes	Response is rarely seen and is not a primary aim of a phase 1 trial

Phase 2 trials
Primary aim	Determine whether new drug has sufficient biologic activity to warrant further investigation
Sample	Patients with a given type of cancer who have measurable disease
Procedure	Stop after first stage of accrual if insufficient response; otherwise continue to full accrual
Notes	Biologic activity does not necessarily imply therapeutic benefit, e.g. if drug has serious side-effects

Phase 3 trials
Primary aim	Evaluate in a randomized trial the therapeutic role of a new drug with known biologic activity vs. standard
Sample	Patients with a given type of cancer randomized to new vs. standard
Procedure	Test for differences between groups in major endpoints reflecting benefit
Notes	Usually expensive and requires large number of patients

toxicity profile, determine a safe dosage range and begin to look at possible efficacy. This phase of trial is used to confirm which organ systems are affected (with initial information stemming from animal studies); to evaluate the extent, duration and reversibility of toxicities; and to observe any possible antitumor activity. Because of this emphasis on determining toxicities, some investigators see an ethical dilemma in enrolling patients in a phase 1 trial, as response is not necessarily the primary objective. While the probability of therapeutic benefit of a phase 1 intervention is unknown, the possibility of a response does exist, such that a phase 1 trial often is a means of continuing active therapy with the hope that the treatment will benefit some of the individual patients, even during this early testing.

Standard phase 1 trial design

For the typical phase 1 trial in solid tumors, the study sample consists of a heterogeneous group of volunteers with any type of advanced cancer that is no longer responsive to standard therapy. In contrast, phase 1 trials in HCT often are performed on a homogeneous subset of high-risk patients who share the same disease type. Phase 1 trials for acute leukemia often are more aggressive with respect to hematologic toxicities, as it is generally accepted that antileukemic activity will be accompanied by myelosuppression. If the mortality in a subset of patients is quite high using an existing therapy then the potential gain may be great, even with accompanying high levels of toxicity.

While less complex in terms of statistical analysis when compared to randomized phase 3 studies, phase 1 trials still require rigorous "statistical thinking" in terms of design and decision-making. Requirements for entry into a phase 1 study typically include:
1 minimum estimated life expectancy of 8–12 weeks;
2 reasonably good performance status (e.g. minimum Karnofsky Performance Status score of 80);
3 cessation of all prior experimental therapy for the last 2–6 weeks; and
4 adequate major organ function to allow normal metabolism of the new agent.

In addition, with molecular or immunologic targeted therapies, phase 1 trials usually are restricted to patients with the specific target. Many new HCT therapies under investigation for the first time have specific molecular targets, such that a primary endpoint is the ability to shut down a specific enzyme or pathway. This is the case in the testing of new biologics, where once a dose that saturates a target is reached, what happens at higher doses is not of interest.

Although response rates are examined within a phase 1 trial, because these trials generally consist of very small pilot studies, lack of response should not necessarily deter the investigator from proceeding to a phase 2 trial for estimation of therapeutic effect. Conversely, responses observed during the phase 1 trial should not be used as a substitute for performing a full phase 2 or 3 study.

Dose-escalating phase 1 designs

For traditional interventions with no specific molecular target, the phase 1 trial involves a dose-escalation scheme to determine the maximum tolerated dose (MTD) as a primary endpoint. This primary aim is carried out under the assumption that a larger dose or more aggressive regimen is more likely to provide therapeutic benefit to the patient, but will also increase the risk of adverse events. Because adverse events occurring at high doses may be irreversible and life-threatening, the MTD is a relative concept that weighs an acceptable level of toxicity against potential clinical gain. Establishment of the MTD is required not only for a new individual drug, but also for any new drug combination, as the cumulative effect of combining therapeutics with known toxicities becomes a critical unknown that must be established.

The study plan must avoid overaccruing patients to subtherapeutic doses that are unlikely to be beneficial, while avoiding overexposure of patients to unacceptably high toxicity levels [17]. A dose-escalating study design should specify the starting dose, steps in the dose escalation, number of patients to be tested at each dose level, and the criteria for moving to the next level and for specifying the estimated MTD. A dose range must be selected that is considered to be relatively safe yet likely to encompass the MTD (i.e. based on the predefined level of toxicity considered to be unacceptable). A safe starting dose is selected based on preclinical pharmacology, animal toxicity or use in other types of patients [18]. Typically, one-tenth of the mouse equivalent dose that is lethal to 10% of nontumor-bearing animals (MELD 10) is used, although arriving at a precise starting dose estimate can be difficult [19].

The usual study procedure in a dose-escalating phase 1 trial is to increase the dose gradually in successive groups of three patients, until the predetermined level of unacceptable toxicity is observed. The most common dose escalation method is the "modified Fibonacci scheme", a

Table 31.4 Examples of phase 1 dose-escalation schema.*

Modified Fibonacci scheme (mg)†	Unit step-size scheme (mg)‡	Constant step-size scheme (mg)§
30	30	30
60	60	40
100	90	50
150	120	60
200	150	70

* For comparison, all three dose-escalation schema examples were set at a starting dose of 30 mg.
†Escalation factors are: 100%, 67%, 50%, 33%, 33% . . .
‡Escalation factors are set equal to the starting dose, e.g. 30 mg in this example.
§Escalation factors are set equal to an arbitrary constant, e.g. 10 mg in this example.

gradually diminishing escalation series adapted from the mathematician Leonardo Pisano Fibonacci, who lived from 1170 to 1240. The second dose is incremented by 100% over the first dose, then successive doses are incremented by 67, 50 and 33% above each prior dose. Escalation then proceeds at 33% increments until the MTD is reached. Alternative dose-escalation schema include the unit step-size scheme in which a constant step-size equal to the initial dose is applied, and the constant step-size scheme in which each dose is increased by a constant fixed increment over the previous dose (Table 31.4).

While the sample size necessary to progress to the MTD cannot be anticipated within a phase 1 plan, in our experience the typical number of dose levels ranges from 5 to 8, and the total number of patients accrued ranges from 6 to 30. In HCT trials, the study regimen often will have been used in other types of patients, so that the types of toxicities and a crude estimate of the MTD are available for planning purposes. However, patterns of toxicity can change markedly from one type of patient to another, such that caution is still required.

A dose-escalation procedure commonly in use is shown in Fig. 31.3. Three patients are accrued to the first dose level. If no grade III or IV toxicity is observed in those three patients (after one complete course *plus* any predesignated waiting period to observe drug-related toxicity), the dose is escalated to the next level specified by the protocol. If a single patient experiences grade III toxicity, three additional patients are treated at the same dose level; the dose may continue to be escalated only if no additional grade III or IV toxicity is observed in the additional patients treated at that level. If a second grade III or any grade IV toxicity is detected, the MTD is estimated to be the preceding dose level. Six patients are accrued at the estimated MTD dose level, with the occurrence of no grade IV and at most one grade III toxicity, before the trial is considered complete.

A recent criticism of phase 1 trials is that "the recommended dose has no interpretation as an estimate of the dose that yields a specified rate of severe side-effects" [20]. With the usual schema only 3–6 patients are observed at the estimated MTD, and no measure of statistical precision (standard error [SE] or confidence interval [CI]) can be calculated. This is particularly troubling when the target is a dose with a specified amount of severe toxicity, in an attempt to achieve a favorable risk/benefit ratio. Statisticians have examined the operating characteristics of phase 1 designs to try to improve upon the rather *ad hoc* design described above. Storer [21] provides an introduction to work in this area, showing how poorly the usual designs perform with respect to providing a reliable estimate of the MTD. He proposes some simple variations in the designs that may perform better, and methods for obtaining confidence limits for the MTD. The article by Korn *et al.* [22] provides a discussion of Storer's approach along with other alternatives, and evaluates their performance via computer simulations. Ivanova *et al.* [23] have described an up-and-down design for the sequential allocation of subjects to dose levels, yielding a local estimate of the toxicity probability calculated from all previous responses.

Most new phase 1 designs have met with hesitancy in practice, because of concerns such as length of time to complete the trial, potential for excessive toxicity and the complexity of updating the models for dose escalation throughout the trial, without an automated system in the clinic. (As more institutions adopt electronic medical records, the capability and access to computers at the point of care may change this last situation.) Before implementation in the clinic, computer simulation studies must be carried out to compare the performance of the proposed designs. Such comparisons traditionally use the following performance criteria: proportion of patients treated at the recommended MTD; average number of patients required to complete the trial; and the probability of toxicity. In future simulation studies it will be important to incorporate the actual time to trial completion as a performance measure, as it is unethical to spend excessive time examining an unpromising regimen before moving on to the next therapeutic approach. Clarke *et al.* [24] have investigated a new phase 1 approach intended to minimize the time to trial completion by

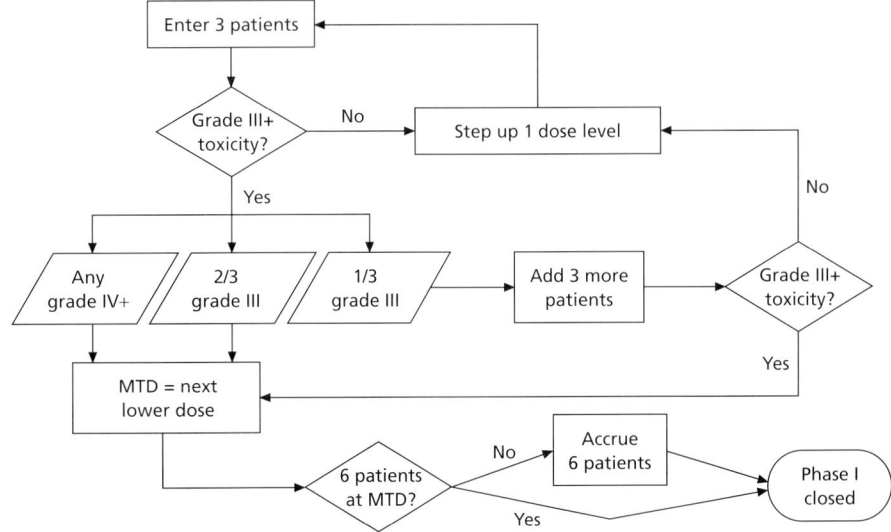

Fig. 31.3 Traditional Phase I trial schema.

allowing new patients to enter the trial without waiting for toxicity evaluation on the full prior cohort of patients, yet conditioned on all available toxicity information to that point.

Regardless of the particular study design, uncertainty in estimating the MTD requires investigators to be cautious and monitor toxicities in a phase 2 trial very carefully, and to be prepared to adjust the phase 2 treatment dose as additional information accumulates.

Phase 2 clinical trials

Following establishment of the safety and toxicity profiles of a new intervention, a phase 2 clinical trial is conducted to determine whether the new therapy has sufficient evidence of biologic activity to warrant further investigation. Phase 2 trials are performed not only for antitumor activity, but also to prevent relapse, for prophylaxis and treatment of graft-vs.-host disease (GVHD), for treatment of symptoms of other therapies (e.g. pain) and for prophylaxis against and treatment of specific infections. The primary components of a phase 2 trial are summarized in Table 31.3.

Standard phase 2 trial design

Phase 2 trials typically are conducted in those patients who are most likely to respond favorably to a new regimen, so that potential activity of the new treatment is not missed. Therefore, participants with maximum performance status and a minimum amount of prior therapy should be selected whenever ethically possible. In addition, all patients in a phase 2 trial should demonstrate measurable disease, so that the regimen's activity can be assessed objectively. Subjective methods of assessing treatment effect make the outcome of the phase 2 study more problematical, but may be necessary in certain studies.

A frequent approach to phase 2 trials is the single group design, with no control group. Like the phase 1 study, the single group phase 2 trial is subject to the problems of any uncontrolled clinical trial. However, these studies are intended as low-cost screens for choosing safe doses and for eliminating treatments that do not have sufficient promise for further study. Similar to the phase 1 study, the uncontrolled phase 2 group study design depends on careful definition of the eligibility criteria, and uniform application of these criteria in admitting patients to the study throughout the accrual period. It also is extremely important to define clearly within the study protocol the response endpoint and its method of measurement.

The number of patients to be studied in a phase 2 trial depends on the specified degree of disease activity required for the new treatment to be of therapeutic value, typically specified as the percentage of patients expected to respond to the treatment. The study should be large enough to furnish information that will rule out with high probability (e.g. 95%) a treatment that does not have this desired degree of activity, taking into account possible random variation in the limited sequence of patients studied. An upper 95% confidence limit can be computed, and if this limit is less than the desired activity level, the treatment would be rejected as of little interest. If the upper limit is greater than the desired level, investigation would proceed to determine just how active the regimen might be, via a phase 3 trial. (Other factors might preclude further study, such as additional evidence of unacceptable toxicities or a higher MTD than indicated by the phase 1 study results.) Statistical methods for computing the upper (one-sided) confidence limit are found in most elementary statistical texts, such as in chapter 5 of Glantz [25] or chapter 14 of Pagano and Gauvreau [26].

Commonly, a single sample two-stage design is employed in phase 2 trials, thereby allowing early termination of the study after the first accrual stage if the new regimen does not appear to be promising with some level of specified confidence. Table 31.5 shows the number of patients required in the first stage of accrual if one desires either 95%

Table 31.5 Number of patients required for phase 2 trial of an agent for given levels of therapeutic effectiveness and type II error. (From [27].)

Rejection error (β)	Therapeutic effectiveness (%)								
	5	10	15	20	25	30	35	40	45	50
5%	59	29	19	14	11	9	7	6	6	5
10%	45	22	15	11	9	7	6	5	4	4

confidence (rejection error or β = 5%) or 90% confidence (β = 10%) for efficacy levels ranging from 5 to 50% [27]. The new treatment is rejected as not sufficiently active if no responses are seen among n patients treated. For example, if the study produced no responses among the first 11 patients, one would have 95% confidence in rejecting the new treatment as being active in less than 25% of patients.

If one or more responses are seen among the first set of patients, accrual is continued into the second stage, until a large enough study group is reached to estimate the response rate with a prespecified level of precision based on the final sample size. As an example, with 35 subjects entered after concluding both stages of accrual, the response rate could be estimated with a maximum standard error of approximately 8% (95% CI width of approximately 16%).

The typical phase 2 study uses a binary endpoint of response or no response. Response could be defined to include only complete response (CR), or to include both complete and partial responses (CR plus PR), as the outcome of interest. However, the counts themselves usually are based on quantitative measurements (e.g. estimates of the amount of reduction in tumor volume, or counts of cutaneous lesions in herpes zoster). Using quantitative information for the response decision, rather than a binary endpoint, provides a more precise measure of disease and requires fewer patients for the same degree of statistical discrimination between regimens, with as much as a 50% decrease in the required study size.

Variants of the phase 2 trial design

Important work has been done on designs that control both risks of error (α and β) and achieve significant savings in numbers of patients required. Simon [28] provides a thorough review of different approaches to phase 2 trials. He has developed an optimized two-stage design with a smaller sample size in situations where the efficacy becomes clear early in the accumulation of the data, allowing the possibility of earlier stopping at the end of the first stage of accrual [29]. Simon concludes that two-stage designs with a target sample size of 35–50 and a substantial probability of early termination are generally appropriate, and that two to three such studies usually are needed to estimate the response rate with reasonable precision. Fleming [30] offers other commonly used procedures for two-stage designs.

Storer [31] has proposed that designs for control of both alpha and beta risks be expanded to consider three possible decision outcomes: response rate unacceptable; response rate acceptable; and an intermediate region in which further study is required before a decision can be made. Several statisticians have carried out work on combining decision-making risks with estimation, where the precision of the estimates is based on confidence limits. Chang and O'Brien [32] have created a method and offer a computer program for obtaining confidence limits for the response rates from the results of multistage phase 2 studies. Another area of interest is Bayesian methods, the quantitative expression of prior beliefs about the treatment to be tested, using this quantitative information and a measure of its precision in the study design and final analysis. Phase 2 trials are a likely arena for using this approach, and Thall and Simon [33] provide a useful introduction to this topic.

In a two-stage phase 2 trial, participant accrual typically must be suspended while the results of the first stage accrual are examined to determine whether or not to continue into the second stage accrual. This temporary suspension has drawbacks in that the momentum for patient accrual is lost, and the overall time to completion of the study is lengthened. In addition there may be logistical problems in reactivating the trial if the data show that it is warranted to proceed to the second stage, particularly in a multicentered study setting. Herndon [34] has proposed an alternative "hybrid" design that allows accrual to continue while the results from the first stage of accrual are being examined to determine whether the study should continue to the next stage.

Other variations on the standard phase 2 design include adding a phase 2 treatment arm to a phase 3 clinical trial [35], randomized phase 2 trials (or "active control phase 3 trials") to select the most promising of several new agents [36] and "calibrated" phase 3 trials, in which a subgroup of patients are randomized to a standard treatment to verify that the population under study is capable of responding to an active treatment [37]. In these designs one does not enroll typical phase 3 sample sizes or make direct statistical comparisons of the groups; rather, the conventional sample sizes and early stopping rules of nonrandomized phase 2 trials are used.

Phase 3 clinical trials

After the efficacy of a new HCT drug or regimen has been established in a single group of participants through phase 1/2 trials, the new therapy is tested against a standard (or a placebo in the case where no standard exists) within a phase 3 trial. As shown in Table 31.3, in this phase of trial participants are assigned to therapeutic strategies by random or probabilistic assignment, to determine which therapy is superior. The phase 3 clinical trial requires an extremely detailed protocol to serve as a guide to the organization and conduct of the study, and provide a plan for analysis of the results, allowing replication and confirmation of the study results. The protocol must specify the eligibility criteria for deciding whether the patient qualifies for the clinical trial, based on the scientific question being asked. Hypothesis testing is used to determine whether any differences observed are significantly greater than would be expected by chance alone.

Often, historical controls are suggested in lieu of random concurrent controls, i.e. comparing patients treated earlier at the same institution(s) using a therapy that is different from the new therapy under consideration, or using historical control results from the literature. While it has been argued that historical controls are convincing in certain situations [38,39], many scientists consider such comparisons to be suggestive of benefit only, rather than providing a valid reliable basis for evaluation of a new therapy. A few medical advances have been so clear-cut that historical controls would suffice (e.g. the penicillin discovery); however, such quantum leaps in clinical discovery are rare. The more typical, modest advances in oncology need more careful scientific evaluation through clinical experiments, and the phase 3 clinical trial is the accepted "gold standard" for separating fact from random noise.

International guidelines have been established that generally require randomized comparisons as proof of the efficacy and safety of new drugs and therapeutic devices as the final step in approval for marketing. The International Conference on Harmonization (ICH) Technical Requirements for Registration of Pharmaceuticals for Human Use were developed by the US Food and Drug Administration (FDA) and the comparable regulatory bodies in Japan and the European Union, resulting in publication of the *ICH Tripartite Guideline for General Considerations for Clinical Trials* [40]. The ICH E9 guideline *Statistical Principles for Clinical Trials* [41] was adopted by the Committee for Proprietary Medicinal Products in 1998. The principles within this document are scientifically sound, and are being followed by the three ICH regions, although at the current time some regions may be applying these guidelines more stringently than others. To prevent delays in receiving marketing authorizations for new drugs, it is strongly recommended that the statistical guidelines provided in ICH E9 are consulted, and that planned statistical analysis strategies are modified to reflect these principles when designing drug development studies [42].

Standard phase 3 trial design

The primary rationale for randomization within a phase 3 trial is to ensure that the study arms can be compared in an unbiased fashion. Although the need to evaluate competing therapeutic strategies on comparable groups has been acknowledged for many years [43], the difficulty of ensuring that groups of patients treated in different manners are truly comparable often has been underappreciated. The randomized trial balances treatment groups statistically, not only with respect to known and recorded factors, but also with respect to unknown patient factors. While the randomized groups will not be identical, any observed differences in therapeutic outcomes between them can be evaluated relative to differences expected through random chance alone. The group comparison is based on probability theory, and provides a measure of the statistical precision of the treatment difference estimate, accounting for random variation. This precision is measured by the SE of the estimate, the CI and/or the p-value, as described in introductory statistical texts [25,26].

In addition to utilizing randomization to minimize patient variability that might confound the evaluation of treatment effects, HCT protocols also often attempt to minimize the variability in supportive treatments. However, strict requirements to a protocol-specified supportive care regimen may greatly impair participation among centers and accrual within centers, such that allowing for a more general supportive care regimen within wider guidelines may be necessary in HCT studies.

The phase 3 study plan is based on information stemming from the preceding phase 1/2 studies, and calls for accrual and follow-up of participants over a specified period of time. All participants are observed until the occurrence of a specified endpoint has occurred, such as death, progression of target disease or relapse, or to the administratively defined time for analysis at the end of the predefined observation period.

HCT studies that include courses of nontransplant treatment as an integral part of the strategy must enroll and follow patients from the time that nontransplant treatment is begun. If the pretransplant treatment strategy differs between the two arms, care must be taken to ensure that patients are enrolled and followed from a similar time point for both arms. Randomization should occur immediately after ascertaining eligibility, as undue delay between randomization and transplantation could lead to high patient drop-out, complicating valid interpretation of the trial results.

Randomization process

The randomization procedures in a phase 3 clinical trial should be clearly described and justified in the protocol. To obtain valid trial results, it is crucial that the research team has no knowledge of the treatment assignment at the time of decision for study entry for any given study participant; otherwise the advantage of the random assignment may be lost as a result of selection bias.

The usual procedure is to screen the patient for eligibility, and if the participant is deemed fully eligible and gives his or her consent, contact the data center to obtain a random assignment to one of the treatment groups. This assignment is made according to a series of random numbers, with the sequence being computer-generated in advance or as the patients are entered into the study.

It is desirable to minimize heterogeneity in the participant group to avoid imbalances in patient characteristics. However, the benefits of a homogeneous study population must be balanced against the need to accrue sufficient numbers of patients in a timely manner, and the need to have the study sample reflect the population in which the treatment eventually will be used, to be able to generalize the study results. If accrual at each site is expected to be modest, the randomization schedule often is balanced at successive points during accrual, by ensuring that the patients within a "block" (e.g. every six patients) are evenly assigned to the randomization groups as accrual progresses at each site. To protect the research team from being able to anticipate treatment group assignment, the block sizes can be varied, and block size information should not be specified in the protocol.

If considerable variation in prognosis among the study patients is anticipated, more of the higher risk patients may be assigned randomly to one treatment group and more lower risk patients to the other group, making it difficult to detect a true treatment difference as a result of the unfair comparison. Heterogeneity among patients can be addressed in the design phase by using "stratified randomization", in which patients are divided into risk groups (strata) based on a small number of known prognostic variables, such as age (younger/older) and remission status at transplant (first complete remission/beyond first remission). Randomization is carried out within each age/transplant status group to remove the "noise" associated with different prognoses.

Because the number of strata grows rapidly with each new characteristic, stratification should be confined to only a few proven prognostic variables. For example, if there are four stratification factors, each of which takes on one of two possible values (e.g. male or female, disease stage III or IV, age young or old, and previous radiation therapy received or not received) this results in 16 possible randomization strata. Therefore designs that stratify on more than three factors generally are unnecessary and unwise. Furthermore, stratified trials often are more complicated to carry out logistically. The number of patients in some groups will be small and unequal across strata, making it difficult to account for heterogeneity through the analysis. An alternative to stratified randomization is to conduct covariate adjustment to adjust for any imbalance in treatment arms. In this case the covariates must be specified a priori as part of the protocol.

If the study is to be carried out at several sites (clinics, hospitals, study centers), the variability among centers in transplant trials may be quite considerable, even for tightly written protocols. In the case of such multi-centered HCT trials, stratified randomization should be used to generate separate randomization assignments for each site, to ensure that the treatment arms are statistically balanced within each center. In their seminal 1976 paper on clinical trials design, Peto *et al*. [44] recommended that, unless the trial size is quite small, there generally is little need for prerandomization stratification, other than for treatment center in the case of a multicenter trial.

Another approach to obtaining balance on participant covariates is to use Efron's "biased coin" design, or recent variations on this idea [45,46]. An example would be to balance a study adaptively on gender and age as new patients are accrued to the study, instead of randomizing within each of four gender/age strata. With this method, as each new participant is enrolled in the study, the degree of balance between the two treatment arms is examined separately for gender and by age. Randomization proceeds with a skewed probability favoring assignment to the treatment group that reduces any existing imbalance in prognostic factors between the two arms. One caution is that applying correct analytic methods within adaptive randomization can be complex, as discussed by Lachin *et al*. [47] and Simon [48].

Study sample size

Planning the size of the study is crucial to determine the number of participants required to acquire sufficient information for comparing the treatment groups. While controlled trials tend to reduce the inherent bias in the data through the study design, extremely small sample sizes may limit the ability to avoid bias fully. Most treatments have relatively minor effects on disease, and it has become appreciated that trials can be heavily influenced by chance [49]. Establishing the reality of small differences between treatments often requires a very large sample size, making such studies expensive. Recruitment may have to occur from many hospitals, or even across several countries, making control of data quality difficult. Attaining a sufficient sample size for a phase 3 BMT trial requiring a human leukocyte antigen (HLA) identical sibling donor can be particularly problematic, as only about one-third of otherwise eligible transplant candidates have such a donor. For trials studying interventions designed to prevent later complications, e.g. trials to prevent chronic GVHD, relapse or late organ failure, early attrition from transplant-related mortality decreases the effective sample size available (and could bias the analysis of the longer term endpoint if not handled appropriately).

In calculating the desired sample size, several parameters must be specified by the investigator, based on prior data, past experience and clinical relevance. The investigator must specify whether the statistical evaluation of the hypothesis is to test for no difference between the two arms, or prespecify a desired direction of the test, e.g. that the new treatment is better than the standard treatment. These are known as two- and one-sided alternative hypotheses, respectively, with the two-sided approach being the more conservative method preferred by most peer-reviewed journals (unless strong biologic evidence or the use of a placebo comparison arm dictates that the direction of the test should be one-sided). The investigator also must determine the difference between treatment arms that would be clinically important, generally based on his or her clinical experience and the historical success rate in similar patients. The alpha error rate for the null hypothesis of no difference must be specified in advance, i.e. the probability of declaring that the two treatments differ when they are really equivalent, with the apparent difference being caused by random variation. (A traditional alpha error level is 5%, but may be set smaller when critical to further avoid this type of error.) The beta error rate also must be declared in calculating the study sample size, representing the probability of missing the specified clinical important treatment difference (often set at 20% or below, such that the power of the test $[1 - \beta]$ is 80% or higher).

While this overview of the phases of clinical trials may make it seem relatively straightforward to move from phase 1 to 2, and from phase 2 to 3, often this is not the case. Evidence for safety and dosing may be based on an accumulation of results from several trials, and when appropriate or necessary because of few available patients for study, phases 1 and 2 may be combined in a single trial. There is much to be learned in the field of HCT, particularly with the advent of the human genome. At times it may become necessary to study more than one intervention in the same patient, such as enrolling the same individual in both an experimental transplant trial and the follow-on trial of a new GVHD prophylaxis. In such instances, very careful planning of entry criteria, measurement of potential confounding factors, and adjustment for primary treatment arm must be considered in the conduct and analysis of these companion trials.

Impact of genetic data on clinical trials design

Since the beginning of the "genomic revolution", specific genetic events involving oncogenes, tumor suppressor genes and DNA repair enzymes have been characterized for many tumor types [50]. Knowledge of these molecular markers of malignancy now can be exploited within clinical trials being conducted for the detection and treatment of cancer.

Four avenues of expanding genomic research that impact future clinical trials design are made possible through the availability of the human genome mapping. First, genetic testing will provide earlier detection of the genetic risk of disease, and improved sensitivity and specificity in the diagnosis of disease. With the growing availability of genetic markers for presymptomatic conditions in hematologic malignancies, early intervention and prevention protocols will become more feasible and prevalent. Eligibility will be developed to include disease specificity as determined by genetic testing. In addition, genetic testing may be used to refine detection of disease as the primary endpoint of a clinical trial [51]. Detection of minimal residual disease (MRD) can be approached through the detection of the unusual expression of a gene in leukemia cells, such as the aberrant expression of the *WT1* gene in acute myeloid leukemia (AML) or the presence of very subtle genetic lesions, such as the detection of *ras* point mutations in AML [52,53]. However, it can be technically difficult to discriminate the rare aberrant expression or mutated allele from normal background expression or wild-type alleles, such that using genetic targets as a marker of MRD generally suffers from less sensitivity and specificity compared to the detection of translocations or gene rearrangements. Because of this concern, qualitative polymerase chain reaction (PCR) assays require controls to detect false-positive results from contamination or a suboptimal assay, or false-negative results because of reaction failure and/or contamination of the assay.

The second new scientific area of pharmacogenomics is advancing greatly our knowledge of the human ability to metabolize, tolerate or respond to drugs based on the individual's genetic makeup [13]. In this field, large-scale genomic technologies such as gene sequencing, statistical genetics and gene expression analysis are systematically applied to speed discovery of drug response markers, whether they act at the level of the drug target, drug metabolisms or disease pathways. Pharmacogenomics offers the prospect of predicting an individual's susceptibility to side-effects when undergoing a new therapy, and to individualize treatment selection based on his or her genetic profile [54; for further information also see Chapter 12].

Future clinical trials will involve genetic prescreening and treatment "run-in" periods as part of the study eligibility, to ensure that the participants can metabolize and tolerate the drug, to individually calibrate the most potentially efficacious dose, and/or to stratify subjects by their genetic ability to respond to the study drug. Defining patient populations genetically could greatly improve the outcomes, safety and efficacy profiles achieved within therapeutic oncology research. As an example, an ongoing phase 2 study being conducted at City of Hope National Medical Center has as its specific aim the determination of the frequency of genetic polymorphism of UGT1A1 in Hispanics with colorectal cancer, and to determine whether the pharmacokinetics of CPT11 are associated with the genotype of UGT1A1.

The third emerging scientific area, pharmacogenetics, involves the development of new drugs based on information about genes and gene targets. Knowledge of molecular characteristics of certain cancers has made it possible to identify patients who could benefit from therapies that target those features [50]. For example, in the majority of patients with chronic myeloid leukemia (CML), leukemic cells have a "telltale" chromosomal abnormality involving "swapping" of genetic material between chromosome 9 and 22, resulting in development and proliferation of leukemic cells. Effective pharmacologic intervention may be designed to target and specifically inhibit this faulty enzyme. Based on a randomized phase 3 trial of 1106 patients, in December 2002 the FDA granted accelerated approval of a drug involving a genetic target, imatinib mesylate (Gleevec®, Novartis), for the initial treatment of newly diagnosed Philadelphia chromosome (Ph) positive CML patients. The approval was granted in a record time of just under 6 months from receipt of the application, and was based on a statistically significant decrease in the risk of disease progression detected at the first interim analysis.

In the fourth new scientific avenue, clinical trials exploring novel gene therapies that provide exciting possibilities of repairing or replacing defective genes will impact study design and conduct. Gene therapy is predicated on the ability to clone and manipulate genes responsible for human disease, and to reintroduce functional copies of normal genes into living cells and tissues [50; see also Chapters 10 and 11]. For some diseases, introducing a functional homolog of the defective gene that produces even small amounts of the missing gene product can have beneficial effects, making these diseases strong candidates for gene therapy. An example of a pilot study in gene therapy is underway at City of Hope National Medical Center, in a limited series of five patients with advanced glioma. The goal is to assess the feasibility and safety of cellular immunotherapy utilizing *ex vivo* expanded autologous $CD8^+$ T-cell clones, genetically modified to express the interleukin 13 (IL-13) zetakine chimeric immunoreceptor.

With the availability of genomic data, more exploratory and "data mining" studies will be needed prior to designing the subsequent clinical trials, to find correlations and identify the constellation of genes that may determine the toxicity and efficacy of new therapies to be tested within a trial. Both randomized clinical trials and prospective observational studies that include storage of genetic tissue will provide opportunities to gain insights into the genetic basis of variation in response to treatments [55]. Ideally, all future clinical trials will include the banking of genetic samples, to continue to build extensive databases linking clinical and genetic data for future exploratory "data mining" and the discovery of new patterns and predictors. Future clinical practice may require that all trial results be coupled with genetic information to determine treatment choices by genotype.

Based on the availability of results from the initial "data mining" involving huge genetic databases, subsequent phase 1 and 2 trials are likely to be smaller, as probabilities of toxicity and response will be more predictable and genetic information can make the samples under study more homogeneous, obviating the need for larger sample sizes. By identifying those patients most likely to respond to novel drugs, it will be easier to demonstrate efficacy and safety, leading to smaller, faster, more effective clinical trials with corresponding cost savings. In addition, this focused approach will be more ethical as it is more likely that a suitable efficacious drug will be administered to the appropriate patients in a safe manner.

While these new trials will be faster to complete, they will be more complex to analyze, as genetic information will be collected and correlated with clinical results within the trial plan. Novel trial designs will arise involving not only gene-based eligibility criteria and stratification by genetic risk/response data, but also multifaceted designs combining observational with experimental arms to maximize our understanding of the genetic impact on disease and response. For gene therapy trials, data monitoring and early stopping rules will become even more crucial as a core component of the study protocol. The rapid pace of development of new therapies for experimentation will put rising pressure on standardization within the entire clinical trials arena, to support the requirement for even more efficient flexible study design tools.

At the end of 2002, a review of the NIH-sponsored website, clinicaltrials.gov identified 249 active breast cancer trials and 111 CML trials. Among these 360 trials, 61 (17%) included a genetic component. Of the 249 breast cancer trials, 26 were using *HER2* to characterize disease, four included testing for *BRCA1/BRCA2* for eligibility and stratification purposes, and three included microarray expression data for exploratory analyses. Among the 111 CML trials, 35 were utilizing the presence of the Ph chromosome as either an eligibility or stratification factor.

Clinical trial conduct

Single vs. multicenter studies

While phase 1 and 2 HCT trials usually can be completed within a single institution, randomized phase 3 clinical trials frequently require collaboration among several or many sites to achieve the targeted sample size.

National cooperative groups such as the South-West Oncology Group (SWOG) and the BMT Clinical Trials Network have been established to conduct randomized trials that may require thousands of patients to attain sufficient power. Alternatively, several transplant centers may join forces to achieve sufficient sample sizes to conduct trials within a smaller consortium setting, such as the City of Hope National Medical Center–Fred Hutchinson Cancer Research Center–Stanford University Medical Center consortium for the conduct of regional HCT trials. National and international registries such as the International Bone Marrow Transplant Registry (IBMTR) are conducting large-scale observational studies based on the results that are routinely reported to them from hundreds of HCT centers.

Each of these multicenter approaches creates new challenges and obstacles that must be conquered to conduct a valid study. One central location must be established as the data coordinating center (DCC) responsible for final protocol documentation and dissemination, case report form development, data quality assurance, protocol adherence monitoring, database programming and statistical analysis. Central registration of patients, review of eligibility and incoming data records by trained staff, centralized audit procedures for review of data records against the original source data, and ensuring appropriate reporting of Institutional Review Board (IRB) approvals, amendments and severe adverse events at all sites are responsibilities of the DCC in a multicenter model.

In both single and multicenter studies, an effective, convenient and accurate mechanism for data capture and transmission needs to be developed and distributed to all participating sites. Implementation of a system for data collection ranges from paper-based data collection forms to online data entry systems. Mailing of paper forms for central data entry at the DCC has been the more traditional mode to date. However, electronic data transfer from distributed sites of data entry has been available since the 1980s, and is becoming more commonplace [56]. In this case, a secure mode of data transfer with redundancy checking and audit trails must be established. At City of Hope National Medical Center we have over 6 years' experience with directing a national DCC for cancer research that has established online data capture via the Internet using web-based forms [57]. Numerous additional considerations arise when transmitting data via the Internet, such as ensuring security of the data via encryption, and fault tolerance of the online system.

Data and Safety Monitoring Boards

The Data and Safety Monitoring Board (DSMB) plays an essential part in protecting the safety of cancer clinical trial participants and in assuring the integrity of the research being conducted [58]. DSMBs serve a data-monitoring function above and beyond that traditionally served by IRBs, and as such are particularly important for studies that involve blinded or masked data, and cooperative clinical trials involving several centers. Generally, the DSMB monitors ongoing phase 3 trials; however, their purview also may include phase 1 trials with specified dose-escalation rules and adverse drug reaction reporting to ensure that the toxicity profiles of these studies are within acceptable limits.

DSMB members are charged with monitoring the accumulating trial data at regular intervals and making recommendations regarding appropriate protocol and operational changes based on the data. The DSMB must ensure that trials do not continue beyond the point when the objective(s) have been met and a clinically meaningful answer of importance to the scientific community and the public has been obtained. However, the decision to continue or to stop a trial, or to modify the protocol in a major way is rarely straightforward. Such deliberations require considerable judgement and attention to numerous factors, to protect the safety of the research participants while ensuring the highest quality scientific research.

The size and composition of a DSMB panel are driven by the nature of the study involved, but generally the panel consists of 5–8 members whose expertise encompasses the scientific area under study, ethics, clinical trials methodology, regulatory affairs, and biostatistics. The committee should be multidisciplinary in nature, and made up of individuals who are free of any significant conflict of interest [59]. Once the DSMB membership has been established and charged with its responsibilities, the DSMB chair, coordinator and biostatistician typically agree to a basic format and schedule for the presentation of ongoing data, so that DSMB members will receive adequate reports within a sufficient time frame for the decision-making process. The study principal investigator (PI) may participate as an *ex officio* member of the DSMB; however, for phase 3 trials the data should remain "blinded" to the PI during all discussions of the interim results. Although exceptions can be considered by the DSMB chair on a case-by-case basis, this principle is particularly important if the PI is involved with patient care during the course of the study.

The DCC will provide interim results to the DSMB on the study progress, safety and relative efficacy of treatment arms, subject to restrictions of the protocol design. Methods such as group sequential designs satisfy the valid objectives of interim monitoring, while avoiding undesirable consequences such as increased alpha error [58]. After each meeting, the DSMB members will make a recommendation regarding the continuation of the trial(s) under review. Critical issues that should be incorporated in this assessment include:

- increased morbidity/mortality related to the study intervention;
- severe or increased adverse reactions;
- unsatisfactory performance of the DCC or study sites;
- suspicion of fraud;
- inability to complete the study in a timely manner because of lack of patient enrollment;
- failure to comply satisfactorily to recruitment criteria; and
- any other issues concerning possible important protocol deviations or suggested protocol changes.

Depending on the findings and circumstances, actions to be taken by the DSMB include expanding the number of trial centers involved, extending the period of recruitment, stopping recruitment because of inadequate rate of accrual, modifying the protocol because of safety or accrual issues, discontinuing the protocol because of poor protocol compliance, or terminating the study early following a planned interim analysis with highly significant results. An interim analysis that strongly suggests that the protocol cannot be successfully completed, e.g. if the initial study design estimates are found to be invalid or seriously inaccurate, also can lead to the recommendation for early study termination. However, such a decision must be carefully balanced with the potential for useful findings resulting from the trial. Other issues of concern in monitoring trial conduct include the problems of premature publication and exaggerated estimation in trials that are stopped early [60].

Impact of genetic data on clinical trials conduct

The introduction of genomics into clinical trials will influence future organizational structures to provide the optimal infrastructure for management and analysis of the complex merging of genetic and clinical data. The application of industrial processing and quality improvement techniques may emerge more prominently to help decrease the attendant possibility for errors with such complex data [61]. Clearly, the addition of genomic data to clinical trials raises new ethical questions regarding confidentiality, particularly in light of the recent enactment of the Health Insurance Portability and Accountability Act (HIPAA). In the past there was relatively unrestricted access by third parties for secondary uses of data, and inadequate data anonymization, neither of which will be

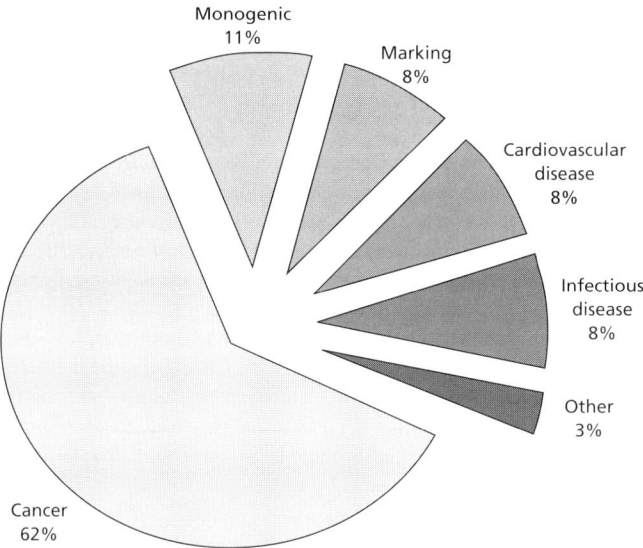

Fig. 31.4 Gene transfer trials by type of application.

tolerated in the future under the HIPAA regulations which came into effect as of April 2003.

There are significant technologic and policy issues that must be addressed in protecting participant confidentiality and security of their data. Concerns about subjects' rights, informed consent, privacy, and ownership of genetic material require strict attention in the development of DNA banks [13]. The biggest challenges to data access likely will stem from the complex organizational, social, political and ethical issues that must be resolved to allow linkage of clinical and DNA information.

Genetic data are more reliable, persistent and specific than ordinary identifiers such as name, social security number, etc. As genetic research proceeds such data may come to be highly predictive of current and future health status, making it extremely sensitive in nature. It is likely that a separate consent process and/or wording for genetic tissue analysis will be required in the future. It may be necessary to move the consenting process to earlier in the participant recruitment activities whenever genetic testing is a key component of eligibility screening for a clinical trial. Within the clinical trial setting, some test results may be noninterpretable with respect to the impact on health or treatment decisions, and should remain within the realm of the research team and database, at least until such interpretation becomes available.

Safeguards will be critical when genetic data are incorporated into routine clinical practice. Privacy policies and procedures will be required to minimize the risk of inappropriate disclosure of private information for linked samples. HIPAA mandates both high standards of data privacy, as well as the extent of patient access to their own data, and extends to clinical data generated by researchers who also are clinicians providing patient care.

The use of genetic manipulations to create novel interventions dictates the need for greatly increased monitoring of protocol conduct, decision support for patient treatment, identification of adverse events in real time, and strict regulatory reporting of severe adverse events (SAEs). Figure 31.4 shows the number and type of gene transfer trials ongoing in 2002, with cancer being the predominant focal area, encompassing two-thirds of all such trials. As the number of gene transfer trials has grown, so has the number of SAE reports, from 285 reported from 1988–99, to 3263 reported in the period 1999–2002. In an attempt to enhance the safety of such highly experimental trials, the NIH has recently developed a system for the automated reporting of SAEs stemming from gene transfer trials, called the Genetic Modification Clinical Research Information System (GeMCRIS). This system is intended to facilitate the evaluation and analysis of safety information across all gene transfer clinical trials, and to provide database reports that will inform diverse user groups of this safety data, including IRBs, bioethics committees, DSMBs, investigators and research participants. Security features are in place within GeMCRIS to protect trade secrets and confidential commercial information contained in the database. GeMCRIS is web-based and could provide the basis for continuous review of studies involving humans, even being suggested for extension to nongene transfer trials in the future. It is hoped that the use of such systems will optimize patient safety, while providing useful data to inform the design and conduct of both ongoing and future trials.

The critical nature of such SAE reporting recently was highlighted by the closure of a French trial studying human gene transfer as a possible treatment for X-linked severe combined immunodeficiency (X-SCID), after enrolling 11 patients. The strategy of the experiment was to correct the early block in T-cell and natural killer lymphocyte differentiation by transducing the subjects' $CD34^+$ cells *ex vivo* with a defective Moloney murine leukemia retroviral vector. This vector contains the common gamma chain gene for the cytokine receptors responsible for the delivery of growth, survival and differentiation signals to the early lymphoid progenitors. While nine of the 11 subjects experienced significant restoration of their immune systems following the gene transfer intervention, two of the nine also experienced SAEs that appear to be directly related to the experimental therapy. Both children developed a T-cell leukemia that appeared to be caused by insertional mutagenesis after receiving the gene transfer product.

Calls for tightening of government oversight of gene therapy research in humans also were heard following the death of an 18-year-old participant in a gene therapy experiment at the University of Pennsylvania, involving transferring DNA to treat a genetic defect that reduces liver function. However, as of the time of writing, this single death is the only one directly attributable to gene therapy research. It is hoped that future government oversight will not restrict genetic research unreasonably, as it holds such great promise for the eradication of life-threatening disease.

Database management for clinical research

The choice of software tools for research data management depends on the complexity of the study design, and the volume and types of data to be collected. Options range from simple spreadsheets such as Excel for a very small straightforward study, to an Access database for a study of intermediate size and complexity, to MS SQL Server, SAS or Oracle databases for larger, more complex data collection efforts. For any approach chosen, however, some basic principles of database design hold true. Each entity (e.g. person) in the database requires a unique identifying code. More than one type of datum should not be mixed within the same data field, e.g. entering both the value for weight and the code for kilograms as one data point within the field. Continuous values should always follow the same format and convention for data entry (e.g. white blood cells [WBC] $\times 10^3$) and categorical data should be entered using invariant coding schemes (e.g. M for male, F for female). Deviations from these basic rules make the ultimate data analysis and interpretation of the database difficult if not impossible without a major reworking of the entire dataset.

Options for statistical analysis software also range widely, depending on the complexity of the required analyses and the expertise of the individual doing the programming. Data entered into an Excel spreadsheet can be manipulated directly within this system for simple statistics such as frequencies and means. Anything more complex than this is best run in an actual statistical analysis package, with the simplest being menu-driven systems such as Systat, and the more complex but powerful choice for biomedical research often being the SAS statistical package. Typically, few physicians have the time or inclination to learn to program such a system adequately, and would be better off consulting a biostatistician for analyses at this level of sophistication.

In the future, the health care institution within which clinical trials are being conducted is likely to be fully networked, facilitating the deployment of electronic data capture and decision support tools, and allowing health care providers and biomedical researchers ready access to electronic information for health care that could be used for biomedical research activities [61]. However, there are many challenges in integrating data from electronic clinical care systems into a clinical trials data system, including information access, data flow, coding schemas (or lack of coded data in the case of free text information), compatibility of the rules and timing for data collection, comparability of field definitions, political and organizational boundaries, and data security and confidentiality.

In large part because of all these challenges, the current clinical trials process is coordinated and monitored offline rather than dynamically, requiring duplicate data entry and resulting in inconsistencies, increased errors, and delays in reporting and analysis. Documentation of protocols is nonstandard, and there is no consistent means of locating them or determining eligibility for them. Future health care data networks will need to be able to translate to and from any electronic medical record system to allow data to be collected at the point of use in a structured form, to facilitate clinical trials and outcomes analysis. Furthermore, a unifying information "architecture" needs to be developed for cancer clinical trials, so that data can be exchanged across systems and institutions in a seamless fashion, based on protocols written in a standard format and structure.

At City of Hope National Medical Center we have received funding to develop *Fully Integrated Research Standards and Technology (FIRST)*, an electronic clinical research database model and prototype system, which will be extended nationwide if successful. We also have developed a web-based system that delivers protocol information dynamically from our clinical trials database [62], and are working with the Association of American Cancer Institutes to achieve virtual exchange of protocol information nationwide from any existing database structure. The National Cancer Institute's Center for Biomedical Informatics should strive to further harmonize the informatics approaches to cancer center clinical trials information management across the nation's cancer centers.

Impact of genetic data on clinical trial information systems

The rapid pace of future genetic discoveries and trials will result in extremely demanding data integration requirements. Much more flexible and responsive clinical trial data management systems will be needed to incorporate the high throughput of genomic data, while establishing the correct IDs and appropriate key structure to be able to merge these data with incoming correlative clinical information. In addition to data from DNA or other genetic tissue from the participants in the dataset, a high-quality large-sample clinical dataset with well-characterized participant and longitudinal follow-up for effects of treatments will be needed, both to store analyzable data for the clinical trials and to provide the databanks for exploratory mining for future discoveries and new hypothesis generation [13]. A new generation of professionals with both biomedical and computer science skills will be required to provide advanced biomedical informatics and biostatistical expertise to build and use the critical tools for data retrieval, storage, classification, retrieval, and correlative analysis capabilities for complex clinical and genetic data.

With the advent of clinical trials that incorporate genomic components, the need for electronic data integration standards across systems and institutions becomes even greater. To facilitate sharing and pooling of genetic results worldwide, standards must be adopted for the coding and exchange of such data, and genetic protocol results will need to be published in a sharable electronic form, for merging into existing resources such as GenBank and OMIM.

Analysis of clinical research data

Increasingly more sophisticated statistical techniques are required for HCT research, along with the application of sound biostatistics principles. The protocol needs to define clearly the primary and secondary endpoints to be analysed, and the statistical plan for conducting the analyses. Certain biologic measurements may have more than one usage, and our understanding of the meaning of these endpoints may be evolving over time with new discoveries, such that definitions need to address how the information will be applied within the specific protocol. For example, the study of MRD generally aims to understand the biology and clinical significance of leukemia that persists in patients who are in complete pathologic remission [49]. Following marrow transplantation, the detection of MRD usually has been associated with subsequent relapse in childhood acute lymphoblastic leukemia (ALL), t(15;17)-positive AML and in CML. However, MRD also has been detected in patients enjoying long-term remission. Therefore, the study of MRD has evolved from the objective of identifying patients at high risk for relapse, to explaining how leukemia can persist for years in an otherwise "cured" patient.

This section on statistical analysis first covers some of the general principles and guidelines to be observed in the analysis of clinical research data, and then discusses more specific forms of analysis that frequently are applicable to HCT data.

The intent-to-treat principle

Biases and misinterpretations can be caused by careless use of the definitions of censoring in the statistical analysis, such as assuming that losses to follow-up due to withdrawal from the study are not related to differential risk of the endpoint. More obvious risks of bias can arise through the common practice of eliminating patients from the analysis after entry into the study by declaring them to be "inevaluable". The argument is that if the purpose is to determine whether a new treatment is effective in forestalling or preventing disease, then a patient who fails to go through the assigned cycle of treatment (e.g. because of failure to take the full course of drugs) should not be regarded as contributing valid information on the question. While the concept itself is valid, it is clear that deleting patients who are unwilling or unable to take the assigned regimen provides only one picture of the difference between treatment efficacies. Including in the comparison all patients thought to be candidates for the treatments at the time of randomization can provide quite a different view, and answer quite a different question.

The inclusion of all patients in the analysis is called the "intent-to-treat" approach. Both approaches are reasonable, however the plans and logic should appear in the protocol. Generally, the FDA will want an intent-to-treat analysis because the treatment difference expected in practice, taking account of drop-outs, is most relevant in approving a new drug for the market.

Subgroup analyses

Another common pathway to faulty conclusions lies in searching for possible treatment differences by analyzing multiple subgroups of the patients, with the idea that although the new treatment may not be efficacious for all patients who are believed to be reasonable candidates for the study, it may be efficacious for certain subgroups (e.g. women vs. men, younger persons vs. more frail older persons, less seriously diseased vs. more advanced diseased patients). Planning such searches and the specific analyses at the writing of the protocol is important. Unplanned searches at the end of the study will increase the possibility of uncovering differences that are caused by random variation alone, and hence the risk of erroneously concluding that the treatment is effective in some subgroup. If such searches are planned beforehand, the size of the study can be enlarged to minimize the chance of such errors when examining subgroups. In reporting the results of clinical trials investigators should clearly point out the degree to which conclusions may have arisen through unplanned searches for subgroup treatment differences, and readers should be aware of the possible dangers of undisclosed subgroup analysis.

Interim analyses

The protocol should clearly state the plan for accruing patients to the trial, the target time and number of patients to be accrued, and the plan for stopping the trial and carrying out the target analysis. However, it is common to analyze the data at some preliminary points in the accrual and follow-up of the patients. Interim evaluations are conducted to protect patients against unexpected excessive or severe toxicities and to allow earlier termination of the trial if needed, either for unforeseen difficulties in execution of the trial or for data suggesting a large and persuasive efficacy for the experimental treatment. It is important to protect both the patient and the study against overinterpretation of what may be chance variations in early data (see the section on Data and Safety Monitoring Boards, and also a comment in the next section on statistical guidelines for early stopping of clinical trials).

Group sequential methods call for analyzing accumulating responses in groups as they become available. The strategy is to identify a priori stopping boundaries at each interim analysis time point that preserve the desired type I and II statistical errors. An adaptive design is one in which the data accumulating in a trial are examined periodically or even continually, with the goal of modifying the trial's design depending on what the data show about the unknown hypotheses. Among the possible modifications are stopping early, extending the trial beyond its original sample size if the conclusion of the trial is still unclear, or dropping or adding arms or doses. Although adaptive designs can be conducted using the frequentist approach, in classical models flexibility is penalized and adaptation is difficult to effect, while the Bayesian approach is more flexible. Berry [63,64] gives a general introduction of the Bayesian approach and describes its role in clinical trials.

Returning to the example of the recent accelerated FDA approval of Gleevec®, the protocol-specified analysis was to have occurred at 5 years. However, an interim analysis conducted after a median follow-up time of 14 months revealed a statistically significantly lower time to treatment failure (i.e. disease progression) in the Gleevec arm over the arm receiving interferon and cytarabine. It is important to note that while Gleevec has received FDA approval for use in CML patients, because this decision was based on an early interim analysis the long-term effects of treatment with Gleevec currently are unknown. Further extension of the follow-up time is needed for the initial study that led to approval, and additional studies with sufficient sample size and power to study long-term survival as the primary endpoint should be conducted.

Equivalency testing

While the majority of HCT trials are interested in demonstrating a significant difference in efficacy, equivalency studies also are being reported more often in HCT, to demonstrate that there is a nonsignificant difference in efficacy. Often, the classical test of significance is applied inappropriately, with the danger of incorrectly accepting the null hypothesis of no difference solely because of inadequate sample size. If one wishes to use significance testing, the appropriate "null" hypothesis is that the standard therapy is more effective than the experimental therapy by at least some specified amount [65,66]. Because correct interpretation of significance tests relies heavily on sample size, and statistical significance often is used inappropriately as a binary decision rule [67], some investigators evaluate equivalency trials using confidence intervals [68]. This approach is more intuitively appealing and allows for sequential monitoring using repeat confidence intervals.

It is impossible to demonstrate that a new treatment is exactly equivalent to a standard treatment. Therefore, to examine therapeutic equivalence, a maximum "acceptable" difference (delta) in the effectiveness of two treatments must be specified in advance. With a fatal outcome, the new treatment can only be considered equivalent to the standard if no more than a very small decline in efficacy is allowed; with less toxic outcomes, larger differences may be clinically acceptable. Other parameters that must be specified are the confidence level (alpha) for the upper limit of the true difference between the new and the standard treatment, and the probability $(1 - \beta)$ that the confidence limit for the true difference will not exceed the specified value of delta [67].

Because the acceptable difference between two equivalent treatments usually is small (particularly in contrast to the larger differences desired when demonstrating superior therapeutic efficacy), the required sample sizes tend to be large. Estimated sample sizes for equivalency testing are given in Table 31.6, assuming a true common response rate between the two treatments (ranging from 70% to 90%), and values of the acceptable difference in these response rates between 5% and 15%. Typical values for alpha and $(1 - \beta)$ in this setting (0.10 and 0.80, respectively) are assumed.

Table 31.6 shows that whenever the common response rate is greater than the quantity $(1 + \delta)/2$, sample sizes for equivalency testing are lower than those required if the same trial were to be (inappropriately) conducted using the traditional significance testing approach [42]. This equation frequently holds true in HCT studies, because if the response rate is too low (e.g. less than 50%) investigators are more likely to conduct efficacy trials in an attempt to identify better treatments. It is only when response rates are satisfactorily high that equivalence tests become of paramount importance. It also should be noted that if the assumption of a true common response rate does not hold (e.g. one therapy is actually slightly better), the required sample size might be increased greatly over those shown.

Analysis of recurrent states

The statistical discussions so far apply to events that occur once during follow-up, e.g. the risk of first progression after HCT, death, or first occurrence of GVHD. However, often there is interest not only in the occurrence of a state (e.g. GVHD, pulmonary infection or hospitalization for any reason) but also how long it persists and how often it recurs. Describing such data for a group of transplant patients followed over time with censoring, and comparing groups of patients present statistical challenges.

One measure of the importance of the state of interest (e.g. GVHD) is the proportion of surviving patients, uncensored as defined in the protocol, who are presently in that state at each time post-transplant. This can be estimated by the prevalence curve [68], taken from Storb *et al.* [69] and shown in Fig. 31.5, which suggests that chronic GVHD is more prevalent among disease-free surviving patients who received prednisone than among those who did not. The figure also indicates that chronic GVHD is higher among the patients who had developed acute GVHD earlier. However as the investigators point out, one must be cautious in drawing causal conclusions, as the groups compared are defined by events that could be linked causally to the occurrence of chronic GVHD in ways that might obscure or complicate the interpretation. Examples

True response rate*	Acceptable δ (%)	Required sample size per group†	
		Efficacy testing‡	Equivalency testing
70%	5	790	756
	10	204	189
	15	93	84
80%	5	628	576
	10	168	144
	15	79	64
90%	5	394	324
	10	114	81
	15	57	36

Table 31.6 Sample sizes required for efficacy testing vs. equivalency testing for differences in the range of 5–15%.

*Assuming true response rates are equal in the two groups.
†Assuming $\alpha = 0.10$ and $(1 - \beta) = 0.80$.
‡Using the χ-square test of proportions, without Yates continuity correction.

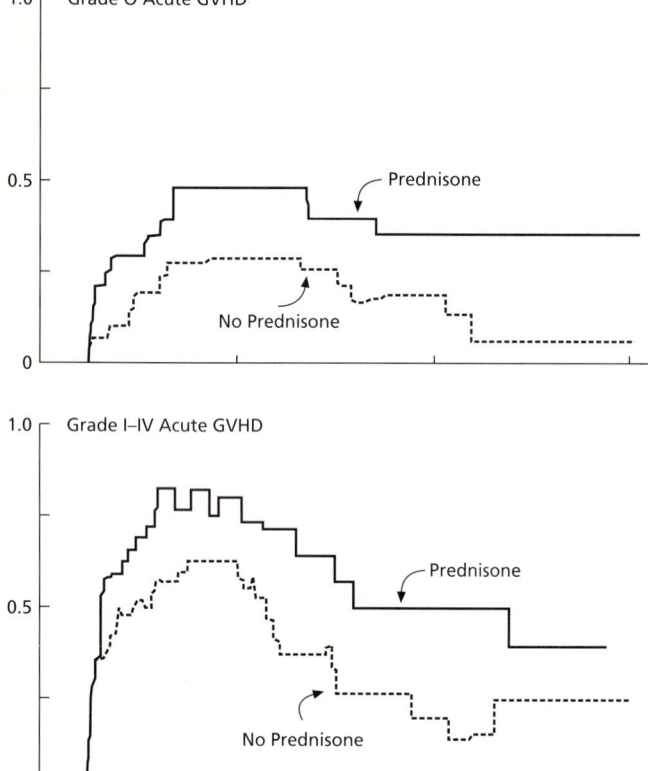

Fig. 31.5 Prevalence curves for active chronic GVHD, stratified by grade of acute GVHD.

would be the relationship between survival and the use of prednisone, or the preceding occurrence of acute GVHD and its concomitant implications for prednisone treatment and survival.

As another technique for states that may recur and are sequential in nature, the probability that a patient is in a given state can be modelled by Markov or semi-Markov multistate models. These models have been used by Klein *et al.* [70] and Keiding *et al.* [71] to study the antileukemic effect of GVHD on relapse and death following transplantation.

Surrogate endpoints

Cancer clinical trials often experience difficulties in recruiting patients to studies, and/or sustaining the length of follow-up necessary to accumulate sufficient endpoint events (e.g. disease progression or death) to obtain meaningful statistically reliable results. Studies of acquired immune deficiency syndrome (AIDS), having the same problems and pressing urgency of impending fatality as cancer, prompted the statistical considerations of earlier endpoints as substitute or "surrogate" markers of later fatality, with the idea of drawing reliable conclusions about comparative risks of death from earlier results. Disease progression in cancer and in HCT also has been used as a surrogate marker for length of life, however, with some reservations about the reliability of translating progression comparisons to valid prediction of differences in mortality and RR. As more is learned about early markers in HCT, the interest in time-efficacy in research becomes more acute, and interest in the use of early markers as surrogates to guide research grows. Two papers in this area, one by Prentice [72], dealing with statistical aspects of the definition and operational use of surrogate markers, and another by Ellenberg and Hamilton [73] on surrogate markers in cancer, provide useful introductions to these concepts and their related applications.

Analysis of time to an event

While most phase 1 and 2 studies focus on a binary endpoint, such as toxicity or response to therapy, phase 3 studies generally concentrate on longer term events, such as time to progression of disease or survival time after transplant. The data for a given patient will include the time from HCT to occurrence of the event or to the time of data analysis, if the patient is treated successfully. Because the times of transplant vary over the study accrual period, each patient will have his or her own data point consisting of the time from HCT to event or end of the study at time of analysis. There also will be information regarding whether or not the patient experienced the event of interest (e.g. relapse, death). The patient who avoids the event by the time of analysis is said to have a "censored" data point, as all that is known for that patient is that the event has not happened thus far. This form of censoring is called "administrative" censoring, because the incomplete information on the patient is a result of the administration of the study, rather than any irregularities in the data collection. More information will not be known about the censored data unless the study is extended by further follow-up of all surviving patients and then is reanalyzed.

In comparing the results for two groups of censored data points, standard methods for comparing means, such as the two-sample *t*-test, should not be used, as they do not take into account the censored aspect of the data. Methods for handling censored data are covered in several recent statistical texts [25,26], and several texts that describe methods that are more advanced yet intended for the clinical scientist rather than the statistician also are available [74–76].

An extended period of follow-up often is required to observe sufficient endpoints to allow a statistically precise determination of the relative superiority of one or the other treatment. Long periods of study will necessarily mean that some patients will be lost to follow-up other than because of "administrative" censoring, e.g. moving away from the study site or decision of the patient to leave the study for personal reasons. These losses to follow-up will result in censored data points also, and can be treated in the same way as administratively censored data points in the analysis. However, losses to follow-up for reasons other than administrative censoring can be brought about by reasons that build biases into the study and the analysis. If the patients tend to drop-out of one of the treatment arms for reasons that might be associated with the treatment itself and/or with the risks of the endpoint of interest (e.g. because of excessive toxicity), then an analysis that treats this as administrative censoring has this bias built into it. The analysis may then be seriously misleading, particularly if such biased losses to follow-up occur relatively frequently. On the other hand, administrative censoring should not create a similar possibility of bias, as the patients are blindly and randomly assigned to the treatments over time. This form of censoring is considered to be "uninformative", meaning that the reasons for censoring should not be expected to be related to the risk of event if the patient were to stay in the study.

Kaplan–Meier survival analysis

The Kaplan–Meier graph is used for describing the typical censored clinical trial dataset, plotting estimates of the probability of "surviving" to time *t* post-transplant (i.e. the probability of not experiencing the endpoint, such as progression, from transplant to time *t*). The graph indicates the times of death by dropping down a fraction of its value at each time of death (the event of interest). The surviving (censored) data points typically are denoted by hash marks on the survival function graph.

In HCT studies, the survival pattern often differs from more common survival distributions, with a high early mortality rate followed by a marked decrease or plateau in mortality after transplantation. Unfortunately, interest is highest exactly where the data are least informative—at the end of the curve where few patients are still at risk. This uncertainty should be quantified by reporting either point-wise confidence intervals or confidence bands. Standard errors can be computed for the Kaplan–Meier curve at any time point, and the estimated survival curve graphed with a *plus* and *minus* distance (confidence limits) around the curve.

Analysis of multivariate interval-censored survival data

Multivariate failure time data are observed in biomedical studies when subjects are followed for the occurrence of multiple events, such as recurrent infections or GVHD. In some studies the multivariate events can be interval-censored [77]. Interval-censored survival times occur when the outcomes are not directly observable, but are detected from periodic clinical examinations or laboratory tests, such as periodic PCR testing for positivity for the Ph chromosome, or cytogenetic testing for signs of disease relapse. The exact times of events are not known because the events could have happened at any time during the interval between the last visit when the subject was determined to be negative for the outcome and the first positive visit. Also, the timing and width of the interval often differ across subjects. Another example of multivariate interval-censored data involve the time to multiple tumor recurrences, usually diagnosed from periodic clinical examinations. If all study subjects were monitored according to the same examination schedule and no appointments were missed, then this type of data could be treated as multivariate grouped survival data and analyzed using the approach of Guo and Lin [78], a grouped data version of Wei *et al.* [79]. However, the approach is not applicable to the more common situation when there are missed visits. In the proposed approach in this latter situation, the marginal distributions are based on a proportional hazards model for discrete survival data that has been utilized by Finkelstein [80] for singly interval-censored data and Kim *et al.* [81] for doubly censored data.

Weighted Kaplan–Meier estimator for matched data

Studies on the comparison of transplantation with respect to standard therapy present a number of statistical challenges: they usually are not randomized, often are based on retrospective registry data, and the treatment assignment is time dependent (waiting time to transplant). These challenges motivate the use of matching a set of known prognostic factors and the waiting time to transplant, to identify a set of "controls" from the group of nontransplanted patients. Usually the latter is a larger group than the transplanted one, and thus is likely to have more than one control for many of the cases. When a variable number of patients treated with conventional therapy matches each transplanted patient, the standard estimating and testing procedures need to be modified to account for the fact that matched data are highly stratified, with strata containing a few—possibly censored—observations.

A weighted version of the Kaplan–Meier estimator that accounts for a variable proportion of matching, recently has been proposed and its statistical properties studied [82]. The problem of comparing the survival experience between two treatment groups was addressed and two tests were examined through simulations, with the aim of obtaining an unbiased estimate of the effect of BMT. The procedures proposed then were applied to data collected from an Italian study whose aim was the evaluation of BMT compared to intensive chemotherapy for pediatric patients with ALL. Although the focus was on a retrospective observational study, the methods proposed also would be applicable to prospective studies.

Log–rank test

The analysis for comparing two curves that represent two treatment groups in a phase 3 study is carried out by a log–rank test of statistical significance (sometimes called the Cox actuarial or proportional rank analysis). In the log–rank analysis, the Kaplan–Meier probabilities of death are estimated for each group at each time *t* where one or more deaths occur. The relative risk (RR) of death is estimated, along with an average of the RR (or "proportional hazards", as the log–rank method is developed under the assumption that the RR of the event for the two treatments is a constant proportion over time). Several texts describe these calculations in detail [25,26,74–76].

If the average RR is greater than 1, then the data favor the control group; if it is less than 1, then the experimental group is favored. The 95% confidence interval (CI) for the RR can be obtained, along with a *p*-value, giving the probability of obtaining an RR as far from unity or further, under the null hypothesis of no difference in average risk of death between the two treatments.

In the accelerated FDA approval of Gleevec® mentioned earlier, the risk of progression was compared by the log–rank test. The RR was calculated to be 0.183, with a 95%CI of 0.117–0.285, and a *p*-value much less than 0.001. The results from such a log–rank analysis might be represented by the layout found in Table 31.7. The line of information refers to the experimental group receiving Gleevec in the phase 3 randomized study, with the RR of disease progression, relative to the risk

Table 31.7 Results of log–rank analysis.

Treatment group	Relative risk	95%CI	p-value
Gleevec	0.183	(0.117–0.285)	<0.001

in the standard treatment group receiving interferon and cytarabine. The last three columns show the estimated risk of progression for the experimental treatment relative to the risk for the control treatment (0.183) suggesting that the Gleevec treatment group treatment will have only 18% the risk of the control group, thereby reducing the risk by 82% over the interferon-treated group. The confidence limits indicate a statistical precision of the RR estimate, ranging from approximately 12% to 28%. The p-value of <0.001 indicates that in a study of this size, an estimate as far from the null value of equal risk (RR = 1.00) as the observed RR of 0.183 would occur by chance alone less than once in 1000 repetitions.

Most log–rank analyses adjust the estimate of the treatment effect, the interval estimate and the p-value for baseline differences in the treatment groups. However, sometimes it is of interest to ask whether the RR of the experimental treatment compared with the standard treatment seems to change throughout the time of follow-up, when a change occurs in some covariate. For example, some marker of tumor burden might be monitored at specified time points, and the RR estimated as a function of the measured marker. Such an analysis is an extension of the log–rank approach and can be carried out with current readily accessible statistical software. However, as both the marker and the endpoint (e.g. clinical disease progression and mortality) are now allowed and even expected to differ in the two treatment groups, interpretation of the results with regard to causal linkage must be handled carefully.

Because of the high early mortality in HCT followed by a relative plateau, inferences based on the log–rank statistic are not well-suited to studying long-term survival, as this statistic may report a difference between study arms even though no long-term survival benefit exists. An alternative approach is to conduct a separate analysis of long-term survival, modeling the population as a mix of long-term survivors and patients undergoing an earlier failure process [83]. The failure distribution used involves a mixed model, where a probability of long-term survival is postulated. Such techniques have been implemented in S-*plus* [84]. This parametric approach has its own set of limitations however; in particular, model misspecification can inflate the type I error [85].

Cox proportional hazards model

The Cox proportional hazards model can be used to detect and estimate effects in both a univariate and multivariate setting. The validity of the estimate is dependent on the proportionality assumption, and a variety of techniques exist for testing this assumption (for discussion see [74]). If the violation is detected, time-dependent covariates can be used, although this approach makes interpretation more difficult.

If the phase 3 study design was stratified by a factor such as gender, then the analysis could be performed for each gender separately, as above. However, the results also could be averaged over the two gender strata to obtain one overall estimate of the RR, on the assumption that the RR is approximately the same across all characteristics and times within each gender and across the two gender strata. The analysis is simply an extension of the proportional hazards model, using the log–rank or Cox approach. If a baseline variable was used as a stratifying factor in the randomization, it is prudent to include it in the analysis, as presumably it was believed to be predictive of the endpoint, and care in balancing the groups within strata would provide more statistical precision in estimating the RR. Inclusion of this additional variable in the log–rank analysis reaps that benefit and also provides information on the degree to which the variable (e.g. gender) is indeed predictive of the endpoint. Other prognostic or predictive variables not even used in the randomization but measured at baseline (e.g. stage of disease before transplant or age of the patient at transplant) also can be used in the Cox proportional hazards analysis. It is important to test for the presence of center effects in case of either survival outcomes [86] or the Cox model [87].

Competing risks

Transplant recipients face multiple competing risks of adverse events especially in the early post-transplant period. While many HCT clinical trials target a single outcome such as transplant complication, e.g. GVHD or hepatic veno-occlusive disease, often there is interest in several types of endpoints. One interest is in the risk of treatment failure as a result of the transplant itself, such as severe toxicities associated with the transplant and possible engraftment failure. On the other hand, there is interest in the failure of the transplantation process in preventing progression of the target disease and enhanced survival of the patient. The protocol should provide clear-cut methods for defining and distinguishing the two types of failure as two types of endpoints, along with their times of occurrence.

In the case of two types of endpoints, two different analyses can be carried out, using the same log–rank analysis. One can regard one of the events (e.g. death as a result of disease progression) as the event of interest, and regard the other event (e.g. death resulting from the transplant procedures) as a censoring of the data relative to knowledge of the risk of the treated target disease. The data also will have administratively censored data points, and perhaps a few other censored points as a result of other losses to follow-up (e.g. patients moving out of the range of observation). A second analysis can then be performed for the other endpoint, this time considering death caused by the target disease as a censoring event that prevents observation of an event attributable to the transplant itself. Here the attribution of risk to the types of failure is subject to questions of informative censoring, and definitions and procedures need careful consideration. Interpretation of the results can be problematic, even though the log–rank analyses themselves are well-defined.

Ignoring the presence of competing risks in the calculation of the sample size could lead to strongly underpowered studies: the larger the competing risks the more underpowered the study. In addition, it is universally agreed that the Kaplan–Meier analysis overestimates the probability of the event of interest in the presence of competing risks [88]. Kalbfleisch and Prentice [89] recommend using the cumulative incidence as an estimate of the probability of an event of interest. However, there is no consensus on how to test the effect of a covariate in the presence of competing risks. Using simulations, their paper illustrates that the Cox proportional hazards model gives valid results when employed in testing the effect of a covariate on the hazard rate and when estimating the hazard ratio. A method to calculate the sample size for testing the effect of a covariate on outcome in the presence of competing risks also is provided. The main aim of the paper is to show that the Cox proportional hazards model can be used to test the significance of the effect of a covariate on the hazard rate of the event of interest in the presence of competing risks. The Wald test, as well as the score test and the log–likelihood test, give the correct type I and II error. The hazard ratio obtained from the model is centered on the theoretical hazard ratio.

Impact of genetic data on clinical trials analyses

The eventual goal of connecting the billions of genomic sequences to disease occurrences in the clinic requires the disciplines of bioinformatics, clinical research informatics and biostatistics. It will be possible to begin to answer the question regarding why some people fail and some succeed within the same clinical trial, possibly explained by a specific genotype. In the past, successful drugs have been withdrawn because of a few severe adverse reactions. With the advent of genetic information we may be able to predict in advance who will be able to tolerate a new drug to more fairly assess the probability of a successful impact on the disease. Clinical trials incorporating genomic data will lead to the capability of "personalizing" medicine.

New biostatistical methods and novel applications of standard biostatistical techniques will be required for genetic trials. These new methods will involve "supervised analyses" including hierarchical clustering of tumors to look for differences in risks, drug uptake, or outcomes. Future approaches will include stratification and testing of genetic subtypes related to survival, correlation between microarray quantitative and PCR data, and novel approaches to applying traditional principles to massive quantities of data. The amount of "noise" in microarray data often is ignored. Small changes in expression that are indistinguishable from such random noise easily can lead to false-positives. Several such false-positive findings were inadvertently published in leading journals in 1999. Calculation of specificity rates in gene expression can be achieved via applying the log–normal distribution.

In future semiautomated discovery of patterns, associations and statistically significant genetic structures will be accomplished via "data mining". This area borrows from the fields of artificial intelligence and neural networks, and allows the discovery of information hidden within huge datasets. Algorithms for analyzing genetic determinants of cancer susceptibility will need to be developed, sample size programs will need to be extended to determining the necessary power to detect genetic disease associations, interaction tests will be needed to detect genes involved in multilocus models, and association tests of observed vs. predicted allele sharing probabilities will be required.

Reporting of clinical trials results

Increasingly more sophisticated statistical techniques are being utilized for HCT research, requiring more advanced expertise to apply them correctly. The omission of key elements from the design and conduct of such research studies limits their usefulness, as well as the ability of readers to interpret the results and draw informed conclusions. Accurate complete reporting is critical to be persuasive to the audience at hand, and to allow the critical reader to assess the validity, comparability and generalizability of the study conclusions.

A survey article reviewed the transplantation literature to determine the quality and variety of analytical techniques being employed for 255 HCT articles included in several leading journals [90]. It was found that 20% of studies lacked some key elements within the analysis, 10% employed statistical methods that were inappropriate, and an additional 10% provided insufficient information to allow an assessment of the statistical methods. There were 63 articles that reported nonsignificant results based on small sample sizes; however, 86% of these failed to provide an estimation of the study power, essential to interpreting the true meaning of these results. It is imperative to include sufficient detail to allow the reader to evaluate the appropriateness of the statistical techniques employed and the validity of the results.

Although room for improvement remains, the past decade has seen substantial efforts to establish meaningful guidelines for the reporting of clinical trials in the medical literature. Detailed publication guidelines have been given by George *et al.* [91], Bailar and Mosteller [92], Zelen [93], Simon and Wittes [94], Mosteller *et al.* [95] and Simon and Altman [96]. Table 31.8 provides a suggested publication checklist for prospective authors of HCT studies, synthesized from several of the articles listed above.

Table 31.8 Publications checklist.

1 All important study-related dates should be given, such as the date the study opened, the closing date and the approximate date of analysis (which could differ substantially from the date of publication)
2 The population under study should be fully specified, including the eligibility requirements, exclusion criteria, and selection methods
3 The type of study design should be specified, including whether it is a phase of clinical trial, prospective cohort study, retrospective case–control study, prognostic study, etc.
4 The objectives and hypotheses should be clearly elucidated
5 Details of the clinical trial or study design should be given based on the type of study, such as dose-escalation rules for a phase 1 trial, stages of accrual in a phase 2 trial, blinding techniques for a randomized phase 3 trial, matching criteria for an observational study, etc.
6 In all cases some justification of sample size and power considerations must be included
7 Any intervention involved should be described with sufficient detail so that it could be reproduced
8 The choice of controls should be well justified, including potential biases for nonrandomized studies, patient or physician self-selection, and any known differences among patients, such as diagnosis, staging supportive care, evaluation, follow-up or prognostic factors
9 All registered patients must be accounted for, including withdrawals or exclusions
10 Mechanisms for ensuring data quality should be described, including quality control checks, review of response and toxicity assessments, etc.
11 The follow-up for each patient should be summarized, including the distribution of time between the data analysis and the last patient accrual, and the last dates of contact for all patients who remain at risk of failure
12 Sufficient detail should be provided to allow the reader to reproduce the analyses if the data were available. There should be a statement regarding adjustments made for multiple comparisons or multiple endpoints. Estimates of precision (CI or SE) should be provided. Modeling, step-wise procedures and the creation of cutpoints need to be fully described

The Consolidated Standards of Reporting Trials (CONSORT) was developed to alleviate the suboptimal reporting of randomized controlled trials [97]. A recent article recorded the reporting of 11 key methodologic factors within 105 randomized clinical trials from 29 medical journals published subsequent to the CONSORT statement. The quality of reporting was examined in relationship to whether a journal was a "CONSORT promoter", as defined by inclusion of the CONSORT checklist in a journal's "information to authors" section or a requirement that authors, manuscript reviewers or copyeditors complete the CONSORT checklist. It was found that the number of methodologic factors reported was greater in CONSORT promoters than in journals not promoting CONSORT (6.4 vs. 4.8 of 11 methodologic factors, respectively, p-value = 0.0001) analyses.

While journals that promote CONSORT demonstrated superior reporting of randomized clinical trials (RCTs), persistent inadequacies in reporting remain. The items that fell below the 50% reporting level were concealment of randomization (46%); data collector blinding status (37%); health care provider blinding status (34%); cointerventions for each group during the study (30%); and data analyst blinding status (4%).

Other recommendations to help investigators improve their ability to interpret and apply medical statistics appropriately include additional medical school and postgraduate courses in statistics for physicians, increased recognition of the importance of medical statistics by the research community and more attention to the statistical aspect of papers in medical journals. Furthermore, an effective collaborating relationship between investigators and biostatisticians can be the key to the successful conduct of medical research. Central to such a successful collaboration is two-way communication regarding both the scientific area of interest and the study design and analytical issues. Early interaction with the biostatistician during the study concept and design stage can help to avoid intractable problems with the study conduct and data collection. Engaging the biostatistician solely to program analyses in isolation from the other stages of the study creation and conduct is suboptimal, and can lead to inappropriate models or misinterpretation of the data. It also is important to involve the biostatistician in writing the statistical methods and results of the final manuscript, and to give him or her an opportunity to review the manuscript in its entirety, to ensure that these sections have not been misinterpreted by the medical authors inadvertently. The biostatistician should take responsibility for verifying the consistency of results in the text and tables, and guarding that the conclusions drawn in the discussion section are supported by the analyses.

If the recommended guidelines and principles included in this chapter are adhered to by investigators and biostatisticians, the quality of HCT research and literature should continually be further improved and enhanced, resulting in more rapid advancement in this critical scientific area, and more effective dissemination of high-quality HCT research findings.

References

1 Simon R. A decade of progress in statistical methodology for clinical trials. *Stat Med* 1991; **10**: 1789–817.
2 Meinert CL, Tonascia S. Clinical trials design, conduct and analysis. *Monographs in Epidemiology and Biostatistics*, Vol. 8. New York: Oxford University Press, 1986.
3 Pocock SJ. *Clinical Trials: a Practical Approach*. New York: John Wiley and Sons, 1983.
4 Friedman L, Furberg C, Demets I. *Fundamentals of Clinical Trials*, 2nd edn. Boston: PSG Publishing, 1985.
5 Silva J, Ball M, Chute C *et al*. *Cancer Informatics: Essential Technologies for Clinical Trials*. New York: Springer-Verlag, 2002.
6 Green S, Byar DE. Using observational data from registries to compare treatments: the fallacy of omnimetrics. *Stat Med* 1984; **3**: 361–70.
7 Mantel N, Byar DP. Evaluation of response-time data involving transient states: an illustration using heart-transplant data. *J Am Stat Soc* 1974; **69**: 81–6.
8 Breslow NE, Day NE. *Statistical Methods in Cancer Research*. Vol. 1. *The Analysis of Case-Control Studies*. Oxford: Oxford University Press, 1980.
9 Schumacher M, Olschewski M, Schulgen G. Assessment of quality of life in clinical trials. *Stat Med* 1991; **101**: 1915–30.
10 Grant M, Padilla CV, Ferrell BR, Rhiner M. Assessment of quality of life with a single instrument. *Semin Oncol Nurs* 1990; **6**: 260–70.
11 Fairclough DL. Summary measures and statistics for comparison of quality of life in a clinical trial of cancer therapy. *Stat Med* 1997; **16**: 1197–209.
12 Cole BE, Gelber RD, Goldhirsch A. Cox regression niodels for quality adjusted survival analysis. *Stat Med* 1993; **12**: 975–87.
13 Lavori PW, Krause-Steinrauf H, Brophy M *et al*. Principles, organization, and operation of a DNA bank for clinical trials: a Department of Veterans Affairs cooperative study. *Controlled Clin Trials* 2002; **23**: 222–39.
14 Green S, Benedetti J, Crowley J. *Clinical Trials in Oncology*. London, New York: Chapman & Hall, 1997.
15 Medical Research Council Investigation. Streptomycin treatment of pulmonary tuberculosis. *Br Med J* 1948; **2**: 669–782.
16 Amdur R, Bankert E. *Institutional Review Board: Management and Function*. Sudbury, MA: Jones & Bartlett Publishers, 2002.
17 Collins JM, Zaharko DS, Dedrick RL, Chabner BA. Potential roles for preclinical pharmacology in phase I clinical trials. *Cancer Treat Rep* 1986; **70**: 73–80.
18 Woolley PV, Schein PS. Clinical pharmacology and phase 1 trial design. In: DeVita VT Jr, Busch H, eds. *Methods in Cancer Research*, Vol. 17. New York: Academic Press, 1979: 177–98.
19 Guarino AM, Rozencweig M, Kline I *et al*. Adequacies and inadequacies in assessing murine toxicity data with antineoplastic agents. *Cancer Res* 1979; **39**: 2204–10.
20 O'Quigley J, Pepe M, Fisher L. Continual reassessment method: a practical design for phase 1 clinical trials in cancer. *Biometrics* 1990; **46**: 33–48.
21 Storer BE. Design and analysis of phase 1 clinical trials. *Biometrics* 1989; **45**: 925–37.
22 Korn EL, Midthune D, Chen TT, Rubinstein LV, Christian MC, Simon RM. A comparison of two phase 1 trial designs. *Stat Med* 1994; **13**: 1799–806.
23 Ivanova A, Montazer-Haghighi A, Mohanty SG, Durham SD. Improved up-and-down designs for phase 1 trials. *Stat Med* 2003; **22**: 69–82.
24 Clarke KG, Odom-Maryon T, Niland JC. *Comparison of Novel Phase 1 Designs Incorporating Time to Trial Completion*. Anaheim, CA: American Statistical Association Annual Meeting, 1997.
25 Glantz SA. *Primer of Biostatistics*, 4th edn. New York: McGraw-Hill, 1997.
26 Pagano M, Gauvreau K. *Principles of Biostatistics*. Belmont, CA: Wadsworth, 1993.
27 Gehan EA, Schneiderman MA. Experimental design of clinical trials. In: Holland JF, Frei E III, eds. *Cancer Medicine*, 2nd edn. Philadelphia: Lea & Febiger, 1982: 531–53.
28 Simon R. How large should a phase 2 trial of a new drug be? *Cancer Treat Rep* 1987; **71**: 1079–985.
29 Simon R. Optimal two-stage designs for phase 2 clinical trials. *Control Clin Trials* 1989; **10**: 1–10.
30 Fleming TR. One-sample multiple testing procedures for phase 2 clinical trials. In: Holland JF, Frei E III, eds. *Cancer Medicine*, 2nd edn. Philadelphia: Lea & Febiger, 1982: 521–33.
31 Storer BE. A class of phase 2 designs with three possible outcomes. *Biometrics* 1992; **48**: 55–60.
32 Chang MN, O'Brien PC. Confidence intervals following group sequential tests. *Control Clin Trials* 1986; **7**: 18–26.
33 Thall PF, Simon R. A Bayesian approach to establishing sample size and monitoring criteria for phase 2 clinical trials. *Control Clin Trials* 1994; **15**: 463–81.
34 Herndon JE. A design alternative for two-stage, phase 2, multicenter cancer clinical trials. *Control Clin Trials* 1998; **19** (5): 440–50.
35 Schaid DJ, Ingle JN, Wieand S, Ahmann DL. A design for phase 2 testing of anticancer agents within a phase 3 clinical trial. *Control Clin Trials* 1988; **9**: 107–18.
36 Simon R, Wittes RE, Ellenberg SS. Randomized phase 2 clinical trials. *Cancer Treat Rep* 1985; **69**: 1375–81.
37 Herson J, Carter SK. Calibrated phase 2 clinical trials in oncology. *Stat Med* 1986; **5**: 441–7.
38 Gehan EA, Freireich EJ. Nonrandomized controls in cancer clinical trials. *N Engl J Med* 1974; **290**: 198–203.
39 Gehan EA. Design of controlled clinical trials: use of historical controls. *Cancer Treat Rep* 1982; **66**: 1089–93.
40 http://www.ich.org/ich5e.html.
41 Phillips A, Haudiquet V. ICH E9 guideline. Statistical principles for clinical trials: a case study. *Stat Med* 2003; **22**: 1–11.
42 Brown DJ. ICH E9 guideline. Statistical principles for clinical trials: a case study. Response to A. Phillips and V. Haudiquet. *Stat Med* 2003; **22**: 13–17.
43 Gehan BA. Progress of therapy in acute leukemia 1948–81: randomized versus nonrandomized clinical trials. *Control Clin Trials* 1982; **3**: 199–207.
44 Peto R, Pike MC, Armitage P, Breslow NE *et al*. Design and analysis of randomized clinical trials requiring prolonged observation of each patient. I. Introduction and design. *Br J Cancer* 1976; **34**: 585–612.
45 Efron B. Forcing a sequential experiment to be balanced. *Biometrika* 1971; **58**: 403–17.
46 Efron B. Randomizing and balancing a complicated sequential experiment. In: Miller R Jr, Efron B, Brown BW Jr, Moses L, eds. *Biostatistics Casebook*. New York: John Wiley and Sons, 1980.
47 Lachin JM, Matts JR, Wei LJ. Randomization in clinical trials: conclusions and recommendations. *Control Clin Trials* 1988; **9**: 365–74.
48 Simon R. Restricted randomization designs in clinical trials. *Biometrics* 1979; **35**: 503–12.
49 Hampton JR. Size isn't everything. *Stat Med* 2002; **21**: 2807–14.
50 Emilien G, Ponchon M, Caldas C, Isacson O, Maloteaux JM. Impact of genomics on drug discovery and clinical medicine. *Q J Med* 2000; **93**: 391–423.
51 Radich JP. The use of PCR technology for detecting minimal residual disease in patients with leukemia. *Rev Immunogenet* 1999; **1**: 265–78.
52 Inoue K, Sugiyama H, Ogawa H *et al*. WT1 as a new prognostic factor and a new marker for the detection of minimal residual disease in acute leukemia. *Blood* 1994; **84**: 3071–9.
53 Radich JP, Kopecky KJ, Willmann CL *et al*. N-ras mutations in adult *de novo* acute myelogenous leukemia: prevalence and significance. *Blood* 1990; **76**: 801–6.
54 Evans WE, Relling MV. Pharmacogenomics: translating functional genomics into rational therapeutics. *Science* 1999; **286**: 487–91.

55 *Report of the Special Emphasis Panel (SEP) on Opportunities and Obstacles to Genetic Research in BHLBI Clinical Studies*. Bethesda, MD: National Heart, Lung and Blood Institute, 1997.
56 Niland-Weiss J, Azen SP, Odom-Maryon T, Lui F, Hagerty C. Transfusion Safety Study Group. A microcomputer based distributed data management system for a large cooperative study of transfusion associated acquired immune deficiency syndrome (AIDS). *Comput Biomed Res* 1987; **20**: 225–43.
57 Niland JC. Internet-based data system for outcomes research. In: Silva J, Ball MJ, Chute C *et al.* eds. *Cancer Informatics: Essential Technologies for Clinical Trials*. New York: Springer-Verlag, 2002.
58 Siebert C, Clark C. Operational and policy considerations of data monitoring in clinical trials: the diabetes control and complications trial experience. *Control Clin Trials* 1993; **14**: 30–44.
59 Fleming T, DeMets D. Monitoring of clinical trials: issues and recommendations. *Control Clin Trials* 1993; **14**: 183–97.
60 Pocock S. Statistical and ethical issues in monitoring clinical trials. *Stat Med* 1993; **12**: 1459–69.
61 Greenes RA, Lorenzi NM. Audacious goals for health and biomedical informatics in the new millennium. *J Am Med Inform Assoc* 1998; **5**: 395–400.
62 Niland JC, Stahl DC. Increasing clinical trial awareness and accrual via the web. In: Silva J, Ball MJ, Chute C *et al.* eds. *Cancer Informatics: Essential Technologies for Clinical Trials*. New York: Springer-Verlag, 2002.
63 Berry DA. *Statistics: A Bayesian Perspective*. Belmont, CA: Duxbury Press, 1996.
64 Berry DA. A case for Bayesianism in clinical trials [with discussion]. *Stat Med* 1993; **12**: 1377–404.
65 Dunnett CW, Gent M. Significance testing to establish equivalence between treatments, with special reference to data in the form of 2 × 2 tables. *Biometrics* 1977; **33**: 593–602.
66 Blackwelder WC. "Proving the null hypothesis" in clinical trials. *Control Clin Trials* 1982; **3**: 345–53.
67 Makuch R, Simon R. Sample size requirements for evaluating a conservative therapy. *Cancer Treat Rep* 1978; **62**: 1037–411.
68 Pepe MS, Longton C, Thornquist M. A qualifier Q for the survival function to describe the prevalence of a transient condition. *Stat Med* 1991; **10**: 413–21.
69 Storb R, Pepe MS, Appelbaum FR *et al*. What role for prednisone in prevention of acute graft-versus-host disease in patients undergoing marrow transplants? *Blood* 1990; **76**: 1037–45.
70 Klein JP, Szydlo RM, Craddock C, Goldman JM. Estimation of current leukemia-free survival following donor lymphocyte infusion therapy for patients with leukemia who relapse after allografting: application of a multistate model. *Stat Med* 2000; **19**: 3005–16.
71 Keiding N, Klein JP, Horowitz MM. Multistate models and outcome prediction in bone marrow transplantation. *Stat Med* 2001; **20** (12): 1871–85.
72 Prentice RL. Surrogate endpoints in clinical trials: definition and operational criteria. *Star Med* 1989; **8**: 431–40.
73 Ellenberg SS, Hamilton JM. Surrogate endpoints in clinical trials. *Cancer Star Med* 1989; **8**: 405–14.
74 Marubini E, Valsecchi MG. *Analysing Survival Data Front Clinical Trials and Observational Studies*. Chichester, England: John Wiley and Sons, 1995.
75 Parmar MKB, Machin D. *Survival Analysis, a Practical Approach*. Chichester, England: John Wiley and Sons, 1995.
76 Armitage P, Berry G. *Statistical Methods in Medical Research*, 2nd edn. Boston, MA: Blackwell Scientific Publications, 1987.
77 Kim MY, Xue X. The analysis of multivariate interval-censored survival data. *Stat Med* 2002; **21**: 3715–26.
78 Guo SW, Lin Dy. Regression analysis of multivariate grouped survival data. *Biometrics* 1994; **50**: 632–9.
79 Wei LJ, Lin DY, Weissfeld L. Regression analysis of multivariate incomplete failure time data by modeling marginal distributions. *J Am Statist Assoc* 1989; **84**: 1065–73.
80 Finkelstein DM. A proportional hazards model for interval-censored failure time data. *Biometrics* 1986; **42**: 845–54.
81 Kim MY, DeGruttola VG, Lagakos SW. Analyzing doubly censored data with covariates, with application to AIDS. *Biometrics* 1993; **49**: 13–22.
82 Galimberti S, Sasieni P, Valsecchi MG. A weighted Kaplan–Meier estimator for matched data with application to the comparison of chemotherapy and bone marrow transplant in leukemia. *Stat Med* 2002; **21**: 3847–64.
83 Gamel JW, Vogel RL. A model of long-term survival following adjuvant therapy for stage 2 breast cancer. *Br J Cancer* 1993; **68**: 1167–70.
84 Frankel P, Longmate J. Parametric models for accelerated and long-term survival: a comment on proportional hazards. *Stat Med* 2002; **21**: 3279–89.
85 Li Y, Klein JP, Moeschberger ML. Effects of model misspecification in estimating covariate effects in survival analysis for small sample sizes. *Comput Stat Data Anal* 1996; **22**: 177–92.
86 Anderson PK, Klein JP, Zhang MJ. Testing for center effects in multicenter survival studies: a Monte Carlo comparison of fixed and random effects. *Stat Med* 1995; **18**: 1489–500.
87 Commenges D, Andersen PK. Score test of homogeneity for survival data. *Lifetime Data Anal* 1995; **1** (2): 145–60.
88 Pintilie Melania. Dealing with competing risks: testing covariates and calculating sample size. *Stat Med* 2002; **21**: 3317–24.
89 Kalbfleisch JD, Prentice RL. *The Statistical Analysis of Failure Time Data*. New York: Wiley, 1980: 163–71.
90 Niland JC, Gebhardt JA, Lee J, Forman SJ. Study design, statistical analyses, and results reporting in the bone marrow transplantation literature. *Biol Blood Marrow Transplant* 1995; **1**: 47–53.
91 George SL. Statistics in medical journals: a survey of current policies and proposals for editors. *Med Pediatr Oncol* 1985; **13**: 109–12.
92 Bailar JC, Mosteller F. Guidelines for statistical reporting in articles for medical journals. *Ann Intern Med* 1988; **108**: 266–73.
93 Zelen M. Guidelines for publishing cancer clinical trials: responsibilities of editor and authors. *J Clin Oncol* 1983; **1**: 164–9.
94 Simon R, Wittes RE. Methodologic guidelines for reports of clinical trials. *Cancer Treat Rep* 1985; **69**: 1–3.
95 Mosteller F, Gilbert JP, McPeek B. Reporting standards and research strategies for controlled trials. *Control Clin Trials* 1980; **1**: 37–58.
96 Simor R, Altman DG. Statistical aspects of prognostic factor studies in oncology. *Br J Cancer* 1994; **69**: 979–85.
97 Devereaux PJ, Manns B, Ghali WA, Quan H, Guyatt GH. The reporting of methodologic factors in randomized controlled trials and the association with a journal policy to promote adherence to the Consolidated Standards of Reporting Trials (CONSORT) checklist. *Control Clin Trials* 2002; **23**: 380–8.

32

Stephanie J. Lee

Outcomes Research in Hematopoietic Cell Transplantation

Introduction

The field of hematopoietic cell transplantation (HCT) has grown dramatically since the first successful allogeneic transplant procedure was performed in 1968. However, as the subspecialty has matured, questions about costs and cost-effectiveness, quality of life (QOL), patient preferences, medical decision making and aggregation of different data sources to guide treatment decisions have become relevant. These questions are best addressed by "outcomes" research, a field of study focused on obtaining the best results, broadly defined, given the available medical knowledge and limited healthcare resources. A closely related discipline, health services research, is concerned with social and political determinants of outcome such as access to health care and quality of care. A chapter on outcomes research is new to the third edition of this book, and the research methods employed to study these issues may be new to many readers.

There are several features of HCT that make outcomes studies especially relevant: (i) HCT involves high treatment-related risks compared to other medical interventions; (ii) significant practice variation exists; (iii) costs are high; and (iv) the long-term results, considering both disease-free survival (DFS) and QOL, have much room for improvement. Issues of medical decision making, quality of care, resource allocation and QOL are material to HCT, and all fall under the rubric of outcomes and health services research.

On the other hand, several characteristics of HCT make outcomes studies challenging. For example, HCT patients are often not represented in large, administrative databases that collect standardized clinical, outcome and resource utilization data. The most active transplant centers still perform only several hundred procedures per year, and smaller centers may do fewer than 10. Thus, the overall impact of HCT on the health of the general population and health care finances is relatively small. Also, the field is changing rapidly, and adequate information on long-term results is available for few diseases and procedures.

This chapter will present a brief history of outcomes research in American medicine to help frame the research topics and methods. The remainder of the chapter is organized around several specific questions in HCT that outcomes research is well-suited to answer. Representative HCT studies are used whenever possible to illustrate the principles discussed. Readers are referred to Chapter 31 (Biostatistical Methods in Hematopoietic Cell Transplantation), Chapter 39 (Assessment of Quality of Life in Hematopoietic Cell Transplantation Recipients) and Chapter 49 (Hematopoietic Cell Donor Registries) for detailed information on related research methods and data sources.

Definition

It is difficult to state a precise definition of "outcomes research." At some level, all results can be considered outcomes; thus, most scientific investigation is concerned with measurement and interpretation of outcomes. However, generally excluded from the definition of "outcomes research" are phase I, II and III clinical studies addressing efficacy questions when the primary endpoints are toxicity, disease control and survival. Similarly excluded are clinical epidemiology studies that describe an institutional experience with a disease or treatment. However, when the research question begins to consider how well a treatment works outside of a clinical trial or institutional setting ("effectiveness"), subjective endpoints (e.g. QOL, patient preferences), nonbiologic influences on outcomes (e.g. access, quality of care, physician–patient communication, medical decision making), health care policy (e.g. economic evaluation), or aggregation of data from multiple sources (e.g. decision analysis, meta-analysis), then the title of "outcomes research" may be legitimately applied. A conceptual framework that distinguishes outcomes research from other types of clinical research is presented in Fig. 32.1 [1].

Major questions for outcomes research in HCT:
- What are the costs of HCT and how can they be reduced? (Resource utilization, cost minimization.)
- Are the clinical benefits of HCT worth the monetary cost? (Cost-benefit, cost-effectiveness, cost-utility analysis.)
- How can one combine knowledge available from several different data sources to reach broader conclusions about HCT than are possible from any one study? (Registry studies, decision analysis, quality time without symptoms of toxicity [Q-TWiST], meta-analysis, evidence-based medicine.)
- What is the patient's experience with HCT? (Qualitative research, QOL.)
- How are new tools to measure subjective or clinical endpoints developed? (Instrument development, scale development.)
- How can the practice of HCT be improved through health services research? (Access, quality of care.)

History

The ultimate goal of outcomes research is to improve the practice of medicine through the provision of data about the effectiveness, costs, risks and benefits of treatment options, incorporating both individual and societal level considerations [2,3]. Approaches to achieve this goal in the USA have varied over the decades. Initially, it seemed that funding large-scale research projects would help establish which clinical practices worked and which did not, so that effective practices could be promulgated.

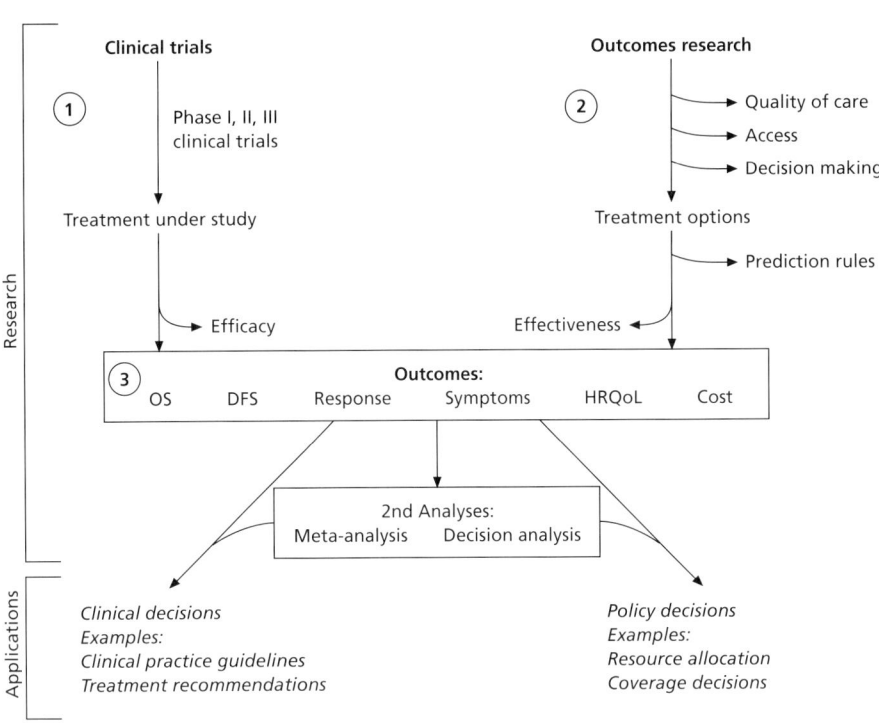

Fig. 32.1 Conceptual framework. Interaction is shown between research topics, end points, analytic techniques, and applications in defining outcomes research. In **1** are depicted the classic clinical trials and analytic techniques that are not outcomes research. **2** shows the study topics, end points and analytic techniques that are considered to be outcomes research. Outcomes depicted in **3** may or may not constitute outcomes research, depending on the context. For example, overall survival as measured in a phase III trial is not an outcomes study (efficacy), whereas it is if observed in a large community cohort (effectiveness). Symptoms have both efficacy and outcomes influences. Applications are indicated in *italic* and may emanate from either clinical trials or outcomes research. DFS, disease-free survival; HRQOL, health-related quality of life; OS, overall survival. Reproduced with permission from Lee *et al.* [1].

However, this attempt was soon followed by a realization that definitive conclusions about the most effective therapies were elusive because there were so many diverse factors (patient characteristics, patient preferences and societal priorities) to consider. More recently, outcomes researchers recognized that, while it is important to know what works at a population level and to establish treatment guidelines, scientific methods to incorporate patient values and individualize treatment are also important. This more encompassing view of the situation recognizes the complexity of medical decisions and the often contradictory influences affecting patient outcomes.

The "father" of the American outcomes movement was a surgeon named Ernst Codman who, as early as 1914, argued that the quality of hospitals could be judged only if procedure success rates were made available on a routine basis [4]. He advocated standardized measures of outcomes so that different institutions could be compared on a level playing field. In 1966, Avides Donabedian reintroduced the term "outcomes" when he developed his concept of quality assessment and its three components: *structure*, *process* and *outcome*. He broadened the endpoints of interest: "Although some outcomes are generally unmistakable and easy to measure (death, for example), other outcomes, not so clearly defined, can be difficult to measure. These include patient attitudes and satisfactions, social restoration, and physical disability, and rehabilitation." He echoed Codman in stating "Outcomes, by and large, remain the ultimate validators of the effectiveness and quality of medical care" [5].

In the 1970s and 1980s the need to understand medical outcomes reached political prominence because of its association with health care costs. Archie Cochrane, after whom the Cochrane evidence-based database is named, warned that the medical system would become bankrupt if expensive technologies were routinely applied without evidence of benefit [6]. In 1973, Wennberg and Gittelsohn documented surprising geographic variation in resource utilization, expenditures and rates of hospitalization and procedures [7]. For example, rates of tonsillectomy varied dramatically within the state of Vermont without seeming to influence health outcomes. This observation focused attention on practice variation and the possible savings that could be realized by eliminating unnecessary procedures.

Several national databases were established to study practice variation in the USA. These included the Patterns of Care Study (focusing on radiation therapy practices) [8,9], the National Cancer Data Base (focusing on surgical practice) [10] and the linkage of Medicare billing and Surveillance, Epidemiology and End Results (SEER) data (providing resource utilization and cancer-specific information on patients common to these databases) [11]. In addition, the Federal government entered the fray directly by establishing the Agency for Health Care Research and Quality (AHRQ). Although this organization has been renamed and refocused several times, it is probably most famous for developing the Patient Outcomes Assessment Research Teams (PORTs). The goal of this funding mechanism was to support large teams investigating the effectiveness of treatments for common diseases.

Discourse in the medical journals throughout this period reflected the outcomes movement. In 1988, Arnold Relman labeled "assessment and accountability" the "third revolution in medical care," following the earlier revolutions of health care expansion and the backlash of cost containment [12]. In 1990, Arnold Epstein further defined the "outcomes movement" as research efforts to address "the effectiveness of different interventions, the use of this information to make possible better decision making by physicians and patients, and the development of standards to guide physicians and aid third-party payers in optimizing the use of resources" [13].

The 1990s were a period of national economic growth in the USA, and concerns about health care financing for specific procedures faded into the background behind debate about the overall structure of health care coverage. Managed care and health maintenance organizations thrived, and physicians practiced in a more constrained setting with new concerns about financial risk. The incentive to save money may have replaced the original goal of outcomes research, which is to spend money wisely to improve overall health. Treatment guidelines proliferated in the late 1990s but these efforts grew out of a desire to standardize physician practice to improve patient outcomes rather than to contain costs.

It is difficult to tell what the future holds for outcomes research, especially in HCT. HCT is a highly specialized practice that for many will fall outside of health care policy and economic considerations. Nevertheless, there are many aspects of HCT that may make outcomes research more relevant. Attention to long-term outcomes, patient decision making and guidance based on what is known about short-term outcomes is especially critical for the field.

Specific questions for the field of HCT

What are the costs of HCT, and how can they be reduced?

On a per patient basis, the costs of HCT are high relative to other available medical interventions, ranging from approximately $30,000 for an uncomplicated autologous procedure to $200,000 for an allogeneic, myeloablative procedure using an unrelated donor [14–16]. (For information regarding charges for the different HCT procedures, see Table 34.1 in Chapter 34.) The investment in infrastructure is immense, requiring support of the transplant centers and national resources such as the National Marrow Donor Program. In the USA, insurance companies have tried to limit access to some HCT procedures by designating them "experimental," but are often forced by state law or by threat of patient lawsuits to acquiesce and finance the procedures. When it comes to HCT, society has shown itself to be quite willing to follow "the rule of rescue," defined as the human imperative to help those facing an otherwise tragic death without regard for the resources consumed or the ultimate likelihood of success.

Well-established research methods are available for quantifying monetary costs [17–19]. "Direct medical" cost refers to the monetary value of goods and services provided. These costs are usually captured through administrative billing systems or other itemized methods of determining resource utilization. Units of goods and services are then converted to charges or costs. The distinction between "charges" and "costs" is important in the USA. Charges are the amount billed to the patient or insurance company, and are almost always higher than costs. In contrast, costs should reflect the actual resources needed to provide a service and are usually lower than charges. Because health care organizations offset one expense against another, and usually include some amount of profit, charges are not directly linked to the resources needed to provide a service.

Outcomes studies favor the use of costs since they reflect the actual resources expended. When costs are not available directly, conversion between charges and costs is determined by "ratios of costs to charges" (RCCs), a fraction recalculated on an annual basis. Institutions often aggregate logical groups such as clinical departments when setting their RCCs. Fixed costs (such as physical space, personnel) and variable costs (supplies) are totaled and divided by the amount billed by the department during the same period of time.

Direct *nonmedical* costs are expenditures related to health care, but not directly used for goods and services (e.g. transportation to the hospital, hotel charges for family members accompanying patients). These costs have proven much more difficult to quantify since they must be captured directly from patients through cost diaries or receipts. *Indirect* nonmedical costs are even harder to quantify and include time off work and the loss of future earnings. Which costs to include depends on the perspective of the analysis. The "societal" perspective includes all costs to the system regardless of who pays. Other perspectives can be imagined, such as the hospital, insurance company or patient, and would include costs borne by that payer.

One important feature of costs is that they vary by year because of inflation. Thus, it is important to consider the year in which the study was performed and the specific items that are included in the analysis. For example, health care inflation is calculated from a "basket" of goods similar to the methodology used for the Consumer Price Index, and at 3–9% has outpaced general inflation. These conversion factors, published by the Bureau of Labor Statistics by month and year, help to "inflation-adjust" costs and allow comparability of studies performed at different times (http://stats.bls.gov). "Discounting" is distinct from inflation-adjustment, and is normally set at 3% per annum. Discounting reflects the fact that costs and benefits in the future are valued less than those that are immediately available, and allows conversion of future dollars or future improvements in health to their current value.

Once the relevant costs are captured, they can be analyzed in a variety of ways. Some studies simply report the costs of an intervention. Others look for patterns of costs, predictors of costs or ways to decrease costs. Totals, breakdowns by specific categories, trends over time and association with clinical characteristics or treatments have all been reported in HCT. For example, several studies have evaluated the costs or lengths of stay associated with specific complications or patient characteristics [20–22].

Cost-minimization studies compare the costs of treatment approaches that result in similar clinical patient outcomes. In these cases, adoption of the least costly approach does not compromise patient outcomes. Table 32.1 shows some examples of cost-minimization studies in HCT [15,23–32].

Are the clinical benefits of HCT worth the monetary costs?

Deciding whether the clinical benefits of HCT are worth the monetary costs may seem to conflict with a physician's duty as a patient's advocate. However, in a society where health care dollars are constrained, spending money for one person's procedure ultimately means that another person may not receive some necessary treatment. As discussed below, the various forms of economic analysis (cost-benefit, cost-effectiveness and cost-utility) differ primarily in how they quantify clinical benefits.

Table 32.1 Examples of cost-minimization studies.

Ref.	Less costly approach	More costly approach
[15,23,24]	Peripheral blood progenitor cells for autologous HCT	Bone marrow
[25]	Delayed growth factor support in autologous HCT	Early growth factor support
[26]	Growth factor support in T-cell-depleted BMT	No growth factor support
[27]	Acute GVHD prophylaxis with T-cell depletion in unrelated donor BMT	Methotrexate, cyclosporine
[28–31]	Outpatient transplantation	Inpatient transplantation
[32]	Hyperhydration to prevent hemorrhagic cystitis after cyclophosphamide conditioning	Mesna

BMT, bone marrow transplantation; GVHD, graft-vs.-host disease; HCT, hematopoietic cell transplantation.

Table 32.2 Economic analyses.

Type	Equation	Illustration	Conclusion
Cost–benefit	Cost of providing treatment ($) minus benefits of treatment ($)	For treatment X: $100,000 – 0.50*$1,000,000 = –$400,000 For treatment Y: $50,000 – 0.30*$1,000,000 = –$250,000	Treatment X is the preferred approach, although society should support both treatments because they "save" money
Cost-effectiveness	(Cost of X minus cost of Y)/ (benefit of X minus benefit of Y)	($100,000–$50,000)/ (0.5 lives–0.3 lives)*20 years = $12,500/LY	Treatment X is cost-effective relative to other well-accepted medical procedures
Cost-utility	Same numerator as cost-effectiveness but denominator is (quality-adjusted benefit of X effectiveness quality-adjusted benefit of Y)	($100,000–$50,000)/(0.5 lives*0.85 – 0.3 lives*1.0)*20 yrs = $20,000/QALY	Quality-adjustment raises the cost/effectiveness ratio of treatment X but it is still very favorable

For illustration purposes, consider treatment X and treatment Y. Treatment X costs on average $100,000 per patient but cures 50% of patients, while Treatment Y costs $50,000 and cures 30%. Survivors live for another 20 years. However, patients undergoing treatment X suffer from long-term complications, so that their utility is 0.85 compared to patients undergoing treatment Y who have a utility of 1.0. Separate studies suggest that for the purposes of cost–benefit analysis, a life saved through medical intervention is worth $500,000–$1,000,000 [33–35]. See text for details.
LY, life year; QALY, quality-adjusted life year.

However, all are designed to provide information that may be used by policy makers to allocate resources and maximize the health and welfare of the entire population. Table 32.2 contrasts the types of economic analyses [33–35].

Cost–benefit analysis requires that clinical benefits be converted into monetary values to determine the net financial impact of an intervention. This is sometimes straightforward (inexpensive prophylactic antibiotics may prevent costly infections later) but is often quite complicated and fraught with unpalatable value judgements. For example, what is the economic value of a life extended or saved? Attempts to use income as a surrogate lead to the uncomfortable conclusion that the lives of high-wage earners are more valuable than homemakers or retired people [17]. Placing monetary values on goods that are not normally for sale (such as medical procedures or health) can be performed by creating a hypothetical market for that good ("contingent valuation"), but the amounts derived from such market exercises have been questioned because they seem too high [36]. As a consequence, cost–benefit analysis is rarely performed in health care; it is much more common in business and environmental applications.

Cost-effectiveness analysis avoids such value judgements by calculating a "cost/effectiveness ratio" expressed as dollars per unit of clinical benefit [18]. To facilitate comparison across interventions, clinical benefit is usually measured in years of life gained (life-years, or LYs), but may be any clinically recognized unit of benefit (e.g. cases of acute graft-vs.-host disease [GVHD] prevented, days of hospitalization, lives saved). Cost/effectiveness ratios are by definition comparisons of one treatment approach vs. another (which may be "no treatment") since they are calculated as:

(cost of treatment X minus cost of treatment Y)/(benefit of X minus benefit of Y).

When several possible treatment options are available, one or more may be "dominated" (found to be both more costly and less effective than another option) and eliminated from further consideration. Because cost-effectiveness analysis are intended for policy makers, it is important to specify the perspective (e.g. government program, hospital, health plan, etc.) and time horizon (e.g. 1 year, 100 years, etc.) of the analysis in order to reflect which costs and benefits were included. The strategy most cost-effective for a health maintenance organization may not be the one that is best for a hospital, patient or society.

Many people use the term "cost-effectiveness analysis" and "cost-utility analysis" interchangeably. However, a *cost-utility analysis* specifically incorporates QOL considerations and usually has a denominator of quality-adjusted life years (QALYs). In these analyses, survival time is adjusted for the QOL associated with that survival. For example, for some people, a year of life in good health may be worth several years in poor health. These adjustment factors are called "patient utilities" and usually range from 0 (equivalent to being dead) to 1.0 (the year of life is fully valued). A utility less than 0 represents a health state worse than death. Utilities fulfill the mathematical condition of linearity so that one year of perfect health is considered equal in value to two years of life with a utility of 0.5. For example, some quoted patient utilities for health states are 0.98 for suffering the side-effects of beta-blockers [37], 0.8 when 1 year after autologous transplantation for non-Hodgkin's lymphoma (NHL) [38] and 0.5 following a stroke [39–41].

Patient utilities may be assessed using several techniques: standard gamble, time trade-off and multiattribute utility theory. *Standard gambles* ask people what risk of death they would accept to reach perfect health, with one minus risk of death equal to patient utility. For example, if a patient is willing to assume a 15% chance of death to reach perfect health, then the utility of their current, compromised health state is 0.85 (1.0 minus 15%). Assessment of patient utilities by standard gamble is limited by people's ability to consider life and death risks hypothetically and rationally. However, the decision to undergo HCT is very much like a standard gamble. Patients may either opt for best supportive care or standard chemotherapy, or they accept some chance of treatment-related mortality from the transplant procedure in order to cure their diseases. *Time trade-off* questions ask people how much life expectancy they would trade for perfect health in their remaining time, with utility equal to time in perfect health divided by time in current compromised state of health. For example, let's assume that a patient has a life expectancy of 10 years, but has a painful, debilitating disease. If that patient was willing to trade-off (i.e. give up) 1.5 years of life so that the remaining 8.5 years would be in perfect health, his utility would be 8.5/10 or 0.85. Similar to utility assessment, time trade-off questions require people to consider hypothetical scenarios in which perfect health is guaranteed, but at a cost of some decrease in life expectancy. *Multiattribute utility theory* calculates utilities from QOL or functional status data. The conversion equations are derived from studies in which subjects complete validated surveys and have their utilities assessed by standard gamble or time

Table 32.3 Examples of cost-effectiveness and cost-utility studies in hematopoietic cell transplantation (HCT) and medicine.

Ref.	Year of pub.	Treatment	Alternative	Cost/effectiveness ratio
[42]	1989	Allogeneic BMT for AML	Conventional chemotherapy	$10,000/LY
[43]	1992	Autologous BMT for HD in 2nd CR	Conventional chemotherapy	$26,000/LY
[44]	1997	Autologous BMT for relapsed NHL	Conventional chemotherapy	$9,200/LY
[16]	1998	Unrelated donor BMT for stable phase CML	IFN-α	$51,800/QALY
[45]	1999	Second allogeneic transplantation after relapse of acute leukemia	Conventional chemotherapy	$52,000/LY
[46]	2001	Autologous PBSCT for MM	Conventional chemotherapy	$23,300/LY*
[47]	1989	Smoking cessation program	No intervention	$1,300/LY
[48]	1987	Hemodialysis	No dialysis	$50,000/LY
[49]	1990	Captopril for hypertension	No therapy	$72,000/LY

*£0.64 = $1.00

AML, acute myeloid leukemia; BMT, bone marrow transplantation; CML, chronic myeloid leukemia; CR, complete remission; HD, Hodgkin's disease; IFN, interferon; LY, life year; MM, multiple myeloma; NHL, non-Hodgkin's lymphoma; PBSCT, peripheral blood stem cell transplantation; QALY, quality-adjusted life year.

trade-off at the same time. Use of the equations allows utility estimates to be based on patient self-reported data without the need for interviewers to administer standard gamble and time trade-off questions.

What makes cost-effectiveness and cost-utility analyses powerful is that diverse interventions may be compared and selected for their ability to provide maximal health benefit for money spent. For example, if health care dollars are limited, these methods allow some rational basis for recommending whether society should routinely provide coverage for a patient with acute myeloid leukemia (AML) in third complete remission scheduled for an unrelated donor HCT, or instead cover patients with congestive heart failure and severe diabetes who need heart transplants. Similarly, one can compare the health care gain of one high-cost treatment procedure, such as an autologous HCT for relapsed NHL, vs. the preventive strategy of providing statin therapy to several middle-age men. Based on the cost/effectiveness ratio for hemodialysis, a procedure covered separately by the federally funded Medicare program and thus available to all people, an acceptable cost/effectiveness ratio of <$50,000 per QALY has been proposed. A ratio >$100,000 is questionable because that money applied elsewhere may buy better health for the population. A ratio between $50,000 and $100,000 per QALY is in the gray zone, as we found for unrelated donor transplantation for stable phase chronic myeloid leukemia (CML) compared to interferon-alpha (IFN-α) therapy [16]. Some countries, such as Australia and Canada, require information on cost-effectiveness prior to drug approval. Table 32.3 shows examples of published cost-effectiveness and cost-utility studies in HCT and some comparisons in other fields [42–49]. League tables have been published to help put cost-effectiveness [50,51] and cost-utility ratios [52,53] into perspective. Online resources such as http://www.hsph.harvard.edu/organizations/hcra/cuadatabase contain comprehensive lists of cost analyses and patient utilities that may be downloaded [54].

How can one combine knowledge available from several different data sources to reach broader conclusions about HCT than are possible from any one study?

Registry studies

Several large transplant registries were established to provide national and international information on the outcomes of HCT. These include the International Bone Marrow Transplant Registry (IBMTR, http://www.ibmtr.org), the National Marrow Donor Program (NMDP, http://www.nmdp.org), the European Group for Blood and Marrow Transplantation Registry (EBMT Registry, http://www.ebmt.org) and Eurocord. These registries collect, computerize and make available data for analyses. While they suffer from limitations common to registries, including incomplete capture of all procedures, problems with data standardization, validation issues and difficulty obtaining detailed clinical information, they also provide the only means for determining the effectiveness of HCT as practiced outside of clinical trials and single institutions. Many important research questions can only be answered by registry studies because large patient numbers are required. Rarer diseases and clinical situations for which no single institution has adequate experience are also best approached by registry studies.

Decision analysis

There is rarely a definitive clinical trial or report that provides all the data necessary to settle a clinical question. People believe they can weigh complicated decisions fairly, but research shows that this *ad hoc* approach is subject to serious cognitive biases and frequently results in suboptimal decisions. Decision analysis uses computer modeling to determine the optimal treatment choice based on what is known about the probabilities and consequences of different treatment options [55]. In order to construct a computer model, an explicit description of the decision to be made and the likelihood of different outcomes emanating from each possible treatment choice are necessary. The analyst also decides which health states are relevant (e.g. dead, alive with disease, alive without disease, alive with chronic GVHD). Health states need to be broad enough to allow accurate estimation of the percentage of the population within them at any time but narrow enough to discriminate different clinical circumstances. The analyst also decides how often people can transition between different health states (cycle length) based on data available from clinical trials or observational studies.

Decision-analysis models are often depicted as "trees." A square represents the decision to be made (choice node), while branches off of circles (chance node) represent possible clinical consequences. A prudent analyst only includes clinical consequences material to the decision or else a decision tree can quickly become "too leafy" with small, perhaps inconsequential branches for which solid clinical data may be unavailable. Advanced programming capabilities allow the probabilities of

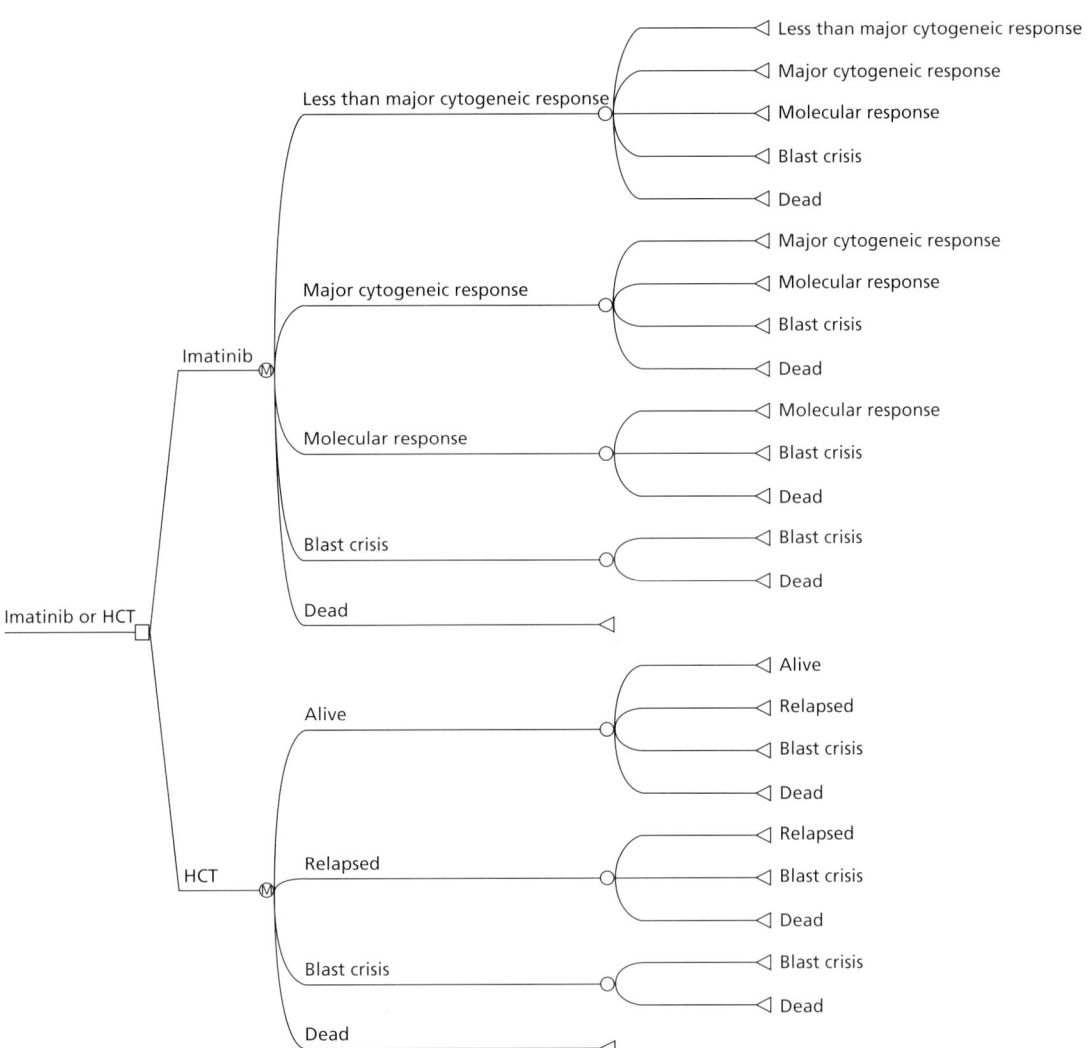

Fig. 32.2 Simplified structure of a decision analysis of imatinib mesylate (STI571, Gleevec®) vs. hematopoietic cell transplantation (HCT) for treatment of chronic myeloid leukemia (CML) in first chronic phase.

different outcomes to vary depending upon a patient's characteristics, time from diagnosis or prior clinical course, assuming such data are available. Figure 32.2 shows the structure of a simplified decision tree using the example of imatinib mesylate (STI571, Gleevec®) vs. allogeneic HCT for CML in the first chronic phase. Note that this simplified model does not account for combination therapy, crossover between imatinib mesylate and HCT, prognostic information based on response to imatinib mesylate or complications of HCT such as chronic GVHD.

The results of decision analysis provide a population-based approach to determine the optimal treatment choice. Treatment options are compared based on the area-under-the-survival-curve (life years-LYs) or the quality-adjusted area under the survival curve (QALY). In practical terms, a decision analysis may not distinguish between one individual surviving an extra 10 years and five individuals surviving an extra 2 years, although patients may view these outcomes differently. Such value judgements are incorporated into the model using discounting functions that value early survival greater than distant years of life. While a decision analysis obviously can not predict what will happen to any particular individual, if the information put into the model is correct, results should accurately reflect what happens to the population on which it is based [56].

Comparison of LYs or QALYs obtained from a decision analysis are not amenable to statistical testing in the classic sense, since p-values and confidence intervals (CIs) reflect the uncertainty in measurements and likelihood of chance findings. In decision analysis, it is up to the reader to compare the gains in LYs or QALYs and determine if one treatment is optimal. Obviously such comparison is easier when the survival benefit associated with one option is several years and the other offers several weeks. Published league tables can help put gains in life expectancy into perspective [57]. Sometimes decision analysis can identify key pieces of information that should influence treatment decisions and, conversely, point out which considerations should *not* affect a rational decision. When assumptions and estimates have to be made because sufficient clinical data are not available, sensitivity analysis helps determine whether results hinge on those estimates. If conclusions are the same despite drastically changing an assumption, then the analysis is "robust" and not dependent on that variable. Several assumptions may be tested at the same time to see if any combination of values would change conclusions.

Several decision analyses have been performed in HCT. For example, an analysis of autologous HCT vs. conventional combination therapy for a 50-year-old woman with progressively erosive, active rheumatoid arthritis after initial therapy suggests equivalent QALYs with either approach [58]. Similarly, a decision analysis of allogeneic bone marrow transplantation (BMT) vs. periodic blood transfusion for patients with sickle cell anaemia and elevated cerebral blood velocities suggested that

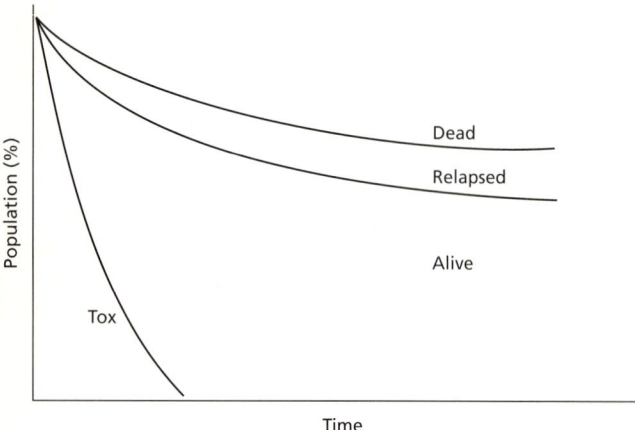

Fig. 32.3 Schematic of a Q-TWiST analysis. The population is divided into Dead, Relapsed, Alive (without disease or toxicity) and Tox (alive with toxicity from treatment).

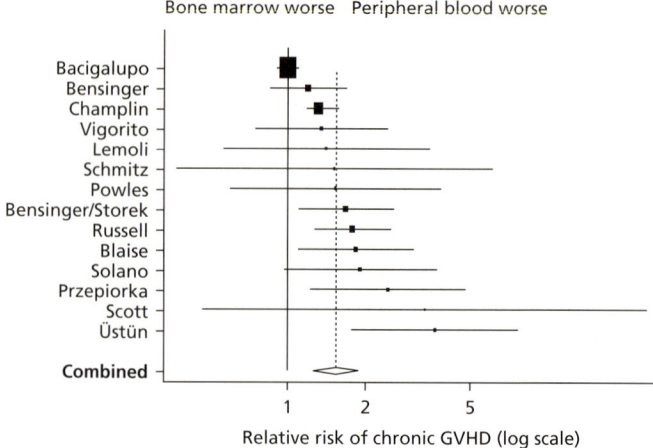

Fig. 32.4 Results of a meta-analysis of the risk of chronic graft-vs.-host disease (GVHD) associated with peripheral blood or bone marrow transplantation (BMT). Reproduced with permission of the American Society of Clinical Oncology from Cutler et al. [66].

either treatment approach was reasonable [59]. A decision analysis of unrelated donor BMT for chronic phase CML vs. IFN-α (prior to the approval of imatinib mesylate) suggested that early transplantation maximized quality-adjusted survival [60,61]. The widespread use of imatinib mesylate illustrates how decision analyses need to be updated as new treatments and data become available.

Q-TWiST

Q-TWiST stands for "*q*uality *t*ime *wi*thout *s*ymptoms of *t*oxicity." It is another method of integrating QOL and survival data [62,63]. Although concurrent data on QOL, survival and DFS may be obtained in a single clinical trial, information on symptoms and QOL are often derived independently. Figure 32.3 shows a schematic of a Q-TWiST analysis in which patients are divided up into four mutually exclusive categories: alive without disease or treatment toxicity, alive with symptoms of toxicity, alive in relapse and dead. Quality-adjustment is applied to the different health states, and the area-under-the-curves are aggregated. If there are two available treatments, the option that provides the greatest quality-adjusted survival is judged superior. This type of analysis has been used to suggest that autologous HCT is better than chemotherapy for aggressive NHL in first complete remission [64] and that allogeneic transplantation is better than chemotherapy or autologous transplantation for pediatric AML in first complete remission [65].

Meta-analysis

Meta-analysis is another technique that allows the results of several studies to be aggregated, increasing the power of the analysis and enhancing confidence in the results. This statistical technique is particularly useful in detecting treatment differences if negative studies are due to small sample size and lack of power. Study-level meta-analyses use individual studies as the unit of analysis. Patient-level meta-analyses actually retrieve and analyze data on individual patients, although each patient's participation in a particular study is incorporated into the analysis. Analyses can either use "fixed-effect" or "random-effect" models. In fixed-effect models, one true effect of the treatment is assumed and any differences in studies from that effect are considered part of variability. In random-effect models, each study estimate may be true because of differences in studies and the analysis allows for a range of "true" values. Tests for homogeneity/heterogeneity can address whether the reported effect sizes from different studies could vary due to chance, although these tests lack power and should only be minimally reassuring. Both randomized, controlled trials and observational studies are often included in meta-analyses, although effect sizes are usually smaller in randomized trials. Sensitivity analyses that exclude lower quality studies can be performed to increase confidence in the conclusions. The results of meta-analyses are displayed as point estimates and confidence intervals for each study with the width of the box reflecting relative study size. A diamond is used to depict the aggregate estimate.

All meta-analyses depend upon data available in the literature or otherwise attainable. Thus, publication bias may significantly affect results. A funnel plot is a graphic that can help determine if a meta-analysis is likely to suffer from publication bias. Effect size is plotted vs. study size. If all studies are published and available regardless of their conclusions, then the plot should result in a funnel shape with the apex centered on the true value. This pattern occurs because the ranges of effect sizes are wider for the smaller studies due to statistical factors, while larger studies should provide results closer to the actual truth. For example, Cutler and colleagues published a meta-analysis of acute and chronic GVHD and hematopoietic stem cell source ($n = 16$ studies) [66]. They found that rates of both acute and chronic GVHD were elevated when peripheral blood served as the source of the graft instead of marrow. Figure 32.4 shows the study results.

Evidence-based medicine

Critical reviews of the literature summarize the available evidence for or against certain practices, and they are often translated into practice guidelines. The methodology is very well established and several organizations, such as the Cochrane Collaboration, the Agency for Healthcare Research and Quality, Cancer Care of Ontario, the American Society of Clinical Oncology and the American Society of Hematology, have performed critical reviews. The American Society for Blood and Marrow Transplantation has produced evidence-based reviews of HCT for NHL and multiple myeloma (http://www.absmt.org). A typical grading system for critical reviews is shown in Table 32.4, and is based on the type, frequency and consistency of evidence [67]. One practical limitation of evidence-based reviews compared to consensus statements or clinical reviews is that the published evidence is strictly interpreted [68]. For example the American Society of Hematology guidelines on the management of CML deferred comment on the relative value of transplantation vs. nontransplantation strategies because randomized studies have not been conducted [69]. In contrast, editorials, book chapters and clinical reviews are not held to the same high standard of evidence, and thus some reasonable triage strategies have been suggested [61,70–73]. However, these algorithms predate the widespread availability of imatinib mesylate.

Table 32.4 Levels of evidence and grade of recommendations. Reproduced with permission from the American Society of Hematology [67].

Level	Types of evidence
I	Evidence obtained from meta-analysis of multiple, well-designed, controlled studies. Randomized trials with low false-positive and low false-negative errors (high power)
II	Evidence from at least one well-designed experimental study. Randomized trials with high false-positive and/or high false-negative errors (low power)
III	Evidence obtained from well-designed, quasi-experimental studies such as nonrandomized, controlled, single-group, prepost, cohort, time, or matched case–control series
IV	Evidence from well-designed, nonexperimental studies such as comparative and correlational descriptive and case studies
V	Evidence from case reports and clinical examples
Grade	Grade of recommendation
A	There is evidence of type I or consistent findings from multiple studies of types II, III or IV
B	There is evidence of types II, III, or IV, and findings are generally consistent
C	There is evidence of types II, III, or IV, but findings are inconsistent
D	There is little or no systematic empiric evidence

Many organizations have produced practice guidelines. A nonexhaustive list relevant to transplantable diseases includes the American Society of Clinical Oncology, American Society for Blood and Marrow Transplantation, National Comprehensive Cancer Network (NCCN, http://www.nccn.org), and the Physician Data Query (PDQ, http://www.nci.nhi.gov/cancer_information/pdq). However, relatively little research has evaluated the influence of practice guidelines on clinical practice and patient outcomes, and what has been published suggests less improvement than hoped [74–76].

What is the patient's experience with HCT?

Beyond the traditional biological endpoints of survival and relapse reported in HCT studies, outcomes research tries to measure and put into perspective other factors that determine whether an intervention is ultimately judged a success or failure. Many of these factors are subjective (not directly observable) and are referred to as "constructs." For example, measurement of health-related quality of life (HRQOL, the QOL related to health, disease and medical treatment), satisfaction and patient utilities are considered part of outcomes research. Measuring these endpoints relies heavily on survey research, the collection of data directly from patients.

Qualitative methods

The goal of qualitative studies is to capture the breadth of possible patient attitudes or experiences. One forum is a focus group, in which 8–10 people are lead by a moderator and discuss particular topics. Focus groups usually last about 2 h, and participants may be paid a nominal amount for participation. They are often audio- or videotaped, with an additional researcher taking notes. The interactive nature of the communication process allows topics to be probed and ideas developed under the influence of group dynamics, which may lead to unexpected insights about the topic under discussion. Focus groups are often used for formative research to explore patient attitudes and opinions prior to launching a formal study.

Qualitative information is also collected through interviews or open-ended survey questions. In contrast to quantitative studies in which generalizability is critical, the goal in qualitative studies is not to obtain a representative sample. In fact, "purposive" or targeted sampling can be performed in order to ensure the spectrum of possible patient experiences is represented. For example, if 80% of the population has a typical experience, 5% has a less typical experience and the remaining 15% all have unique experiences, the goal would be to interview 17 people, one from the majority, one from the minority and all 15 who had unique experiences. Usually, transcriptions are made of the interviews, and qualitative coding software is used to mark the transcripts for easier analysis. Transcripts are reviewed by a limited number of individuals who code them for themes, aggregate the concepts into broader groups if possible, and report on the range of patient experiences.

Qualitative methods have been used in several studies to evaluate aspects of recovery following HCT [77–80]. These studies revealed several themes that are not particularly well covered in standardized instruments; for example, strategies that patients use to compensate for limitations, multiple losses in all aspects of their lives and the greater appreciation for life brought about by the HCT experience.

Quality of life

Quality of life (QOL) is composed of diverse determinants including physical abilities, symptoms, social well-being, psychoemotional status and spiritual/existential experiences. It reflects how well people feel, what they can accomplish, how satisfied they are with their lives and whether their lives have meaning and purpose (for details regarding QOL after HCT see Chapter 39). Capturing these domains requires multidimensional instruments. QOL studies in HCT have generally sought to: (i) describe the long-term QOL, adaptation, and recuperation of patients; (ii) find predictors of better or worse QOL; and (iii) compare populations treated with different procedures. With the availability of numerous validated instruments, QOL is generally measured quantitatively with questionnaires. One commonly used instrument is the Medical Outcomes Study Short Form 36 (SF-36) a generic multidimensional 36 item instrument that has been used on thousands of patients and healthy people to measure physical and mental health status [81,82]. Other cancer-specific instruments, such as the European Organization for Research and Treatment of Cancer (EORTC) Quality of Life Questionnaire (QLQ) C30 (30 items) [83] and the Functional Assessment of Chronic Illness Therapies (27 items) [84], are designed for use in cancer populations. Both of these instruments also offer HCT-specific modules that can be added to the core form to capture issues specific to HCT. When scored according to psychometrically tested methods, they provide standardized QOL information that may be compared with other populations, and that describe the QOL and functioning of patients. Figure 32.5 shows an example of the physical functioning scales from these instruments. Of note, comparative studies have shown that despite similarly named subscales, instruments are actually measuring different constructs and it is difficult to compare studies unless they use identical instruments [85,86].

Many QOL surveys have been translated into other languages, an arduous process that first requires translation, then back-translation to see if

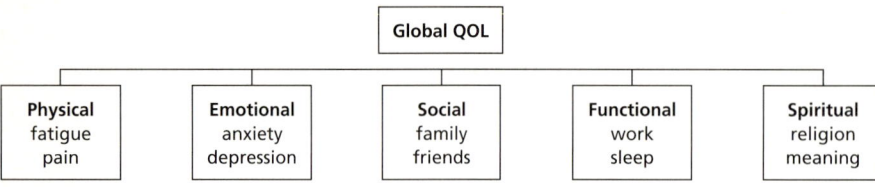

SF-36 (physical)
Does your health now limit you in:
- Vigorous activities, such as running, lifting heavy objects, participating in strenuous sports
- Moderate activities, such as moving a table, pushing a vacuum cleaner, bowling or playing golf
- Lifting or carrying groceries
- Climbing several flights of stairs
- Climbing one flight of stairs
- Bending, kneeling, or stooping
- Walking more than a mile
- Walking several blocks
- Walking one block
- Bathing or dressing yourself

EORTC (physical)
- Do you have any trouble with strenuous activities, like carrying a heavy shopping bag or a suitcase?
- Do you have any trouble taking a long walk?
- Do you have any trouble taking a short walk outside of the house?
- Do you have to stay in bed or in a chair for most of the day?
- Do you need help with eating, dressing, washing yourself or using the toilet?

FACT (physical)
- I have a lack of energy
- I have nausea
- Because of my physical condition, I have trouble meeting the needs of my family
- I have pain
- I am bothered by side effects of treatment
- I feel ill
- I am forced to spend time in bed

Fig. 32.5 Dimensions of quality of life and examples of the physical domain from validated questionnaires.

meaning is preserved. It is a common mistake to assume that interpreters can administer English instruments to a non-English speaker. Instead, the validated version in the subject's native language should be used since interpreters may unintentionally change the meanings of items and responses.

Ideally, any QOL report should include information about the instruments used, reasons for missing data, a comparison of respondents and those who choose not to participate, and response rates at each assessment point to assist in interpretation of study quality. Missing data are a great problem in QOL and survey research for several reasons. First, 10–50% of data may be missing due to logistical problems and patient refusal to complete questionnaires. One barrier may be literacy, since studies have shown that approximately 25% of the US population is functionally illiterate [87]. Second, data are often not missing at random, but rather reflect poor health or other characteristics that could influence QOL. Many validated scales are long, and ill HCT patients are more likely to refuse to complete them. This consideration is called "respondent burden" and is an important part of planning any survey-based study.

Biostatistical methods for analyzing QOL data can be complicated because they must address issues of longitudinal data analysis, informatively missing data and other problems exacerbated by the nature of QOL data [88,89]. Repeated measures analysis and mixed models allow differences between populations and over time to be studied, but methods of reporting results might not be intuitive to physicians. Also, it is important to remember that QOL studies are often cross-sectional and represent only those patients surviving the procedure at a particular point [90,91].

Developing methods to place QOL differences into their clinical context is an active area of research. Although validated scales are psychometrically sound and allow comparison of treatment groups by statistical testing, the results of QOL studies are not intuitive to patients and physicians. For example, a survival difference of 10% is easily interpretable. But many find it harder to interpret a QOL difference of 50 vs. 35 on a given scale and place such an observation in its clinical context. There is no intuitive feeling for what a person with a score of 50 feels like compared to someone with a score of 35.

A group of QOL researchers began meeting in 2000 to address the issue of clinical significance for QOL measures. A "clinically meaningful difference" is defined as the difference in QOL that would prompt adoption of the intervention or a change in practice. Two approaches have been suggested: anchor-based and distribution-based. Anchor-based methods rely on patient-reported differences to determine clinically meaningful differences. For example, patients are asked a global change question such as, "Overall, is your QOL a lot better, a little better, somewhat better, somewhat worse, a little worse or a lot worse." This overall category is then compared to their QOL scores [92–94]. However, this method uses patient-perceived differences in QOL as the gold standard, raising the question of why we cannot just ask patients directly about changes in their QOL. The second approach is based on the statistical distribution of QOL scores. Generally, a difference of 0.5 standard deviation is considered to be clinically meaningful.

Results and conclusions of specific QOL studies are discussed in more depth in Chapter 39.

Patient satisfaction

Patient satisfaction has proven an elusive construct to measure in medicine. Although patient satisfaction with care and the results of treatments are undoubtedly important, most validated scales have shown a ceiling effect, defined as an inability to distinguish variations in satisfaction because most people are highly satisfied with their personal care. Patient satisfaction as a primary outcome of HCT studies awaits more responsive instruments that can distinguish gradations of satisfaction.

How are new tools to measure subjective or clinical endpoints developed?

Instrument development

Instrument (or survey) development is considered a facet of outcomes research because it establishes the validity of clinical tools to measure subjective endpoints. In order for an instrument to be useful, it needs to reflect what it purports to measure (validity), be an accurate measure (reliability), separate people into clinically meaningful groups (discrimination) and detect important changes (sensitivity). Instrument development from scratch is a demanding process. First, a list of relevant concepts should be created from prior literature, focus groups or other means of formative research. Then, a draft scale is created. Attention should be given to the wording of specific questions and response items to allow sufficient variability to capture the range of clinical conditions. Then, a pilot study is conducted with cognitive interviewing to ensure that patients understand the questions and are selecting response options consistent with their intent. Finally, a larger study is performed to document validity, reliability and sensitivity. Many survey developers neglect the final step of confirming sensitivity to change. This is an important feature since many instruments are intended to describe the experiences of population subgroups, compare one population to another, or show changes over time.

Reliability refers to whether a measure is consistently reflecting the true status of a subject. Internal reliability is usually reported as a Cronbach's *alpha* with acceptable values greater than 0.7. Cronbach's *alpha* measures whether items are correlated with each other and measure the same underlying construct. Stability of measurements is reported as "test–retest reliability," the correlation between two measurements separated in time when an individual's status has not changed. The range is from 0 to 1.0, with higher values reflecting greater stability and values >0.5 generally considered acceptable. If test–retest reliability is <0.5 and the subject's clinical situation has not changed, the scale is probably susceptible to influences unrelated to the clinical status of the person.

Validity refers to whether an instrument is truly reflecting what it is supposed to measure, and is usually expressed as correlation coefficients or effect sizes. Content validity refers to how well the scale measures the different aspects of the construct. Convergent validity is demonstrated when the scale correlates highly with other scales measuring similar constructs, while discriminant validity means there is little correlation with scales measuring unrelated concepts. Discrimination refers to the ability of the scale to separate people into clinically meaningful groups, while sensitivity to change means that as a person's clinical situation changes, they should score differently on the instrument.

Several surveys have been developed specifically for HCT. For example, McQuellon and colleagues developed and validated a HCT module for the Functional Assessment of Chronic Illness Therapies (FACT) that assesses additional transplant-specific symptoms [84]. A leukemia module for the EORTC QLQ C30 has been used in a study comparing chemotherapy to autologous and allogeneic transplantation for AML [83,95]. Lee and colleagues have developed a chronic GVHD symptom scale [96]. This scale was designed to be self-administered and brief (5 min) and to follow patients with chronic GVHD over time to detect improvement or worsening in their symptoms. It includes questions about bothersome eye, mouth, lung, skin, nutrition, emotional and energy symptoms. Comparison with the SF-36 and FACT-BMT showed adequate convergent and discriminant validity, discrimination between patients with self-assessed mild, moderate or severe chronic GVHD, and sensitivity to change using an anchor-based method of assessment.

Scale development

Clinical syndromes such as acute and chronic GVHD have been notoriously difficult to measure, yet they are important endpoints in almost every allogeneic HCT report (for details see Chapter 50). The greatest challenge arises from the heterogeneous clinical manifestations complicating standardization of severity grading. Martin *et al.* [97] showed that interobserver differences in acute GVHD grading from medical records were substantial, and suggested a more objective way of coding this complication. However, his approach has not been widely adopted. A second barrier to scale development is the need to validate the scale against a gold standard. Since a gold standard does not exist for GVHD severity, developers have used survival or chronic GVHD mortality as objective endpoints.

In acute GVHD, several grading systems have been proposed including the Glucksberg scale [98], the modified Glucksberg scale [99], the Consensus Conference grading system [100] and the IBMTR index [101]. Application of these grading systems first requires ascertainment of performance status and staging of skin, liver and gastrointestinal involvement, followed by aggregation into five grades (0–IV or 0, A, B, C, D). With the exception of the IBMTR index, all the grading systems were developed by observation and consensus. The IBMTR used one large set of patients undergoing human leukocyte antigen (HLA)-matched sibling BMT for acute or chronic leukemia ("training set," $n = 2129$ given cyclosporine and methotrexate) to develop the index, then validated it in an independent dataset ("testing set," $n = 752$ receiving T-cell depletion) using survival as the primary endpoint [101]. Additional validation studies in separate cohorts have yielded conflicting results [102,103].

Several scales have also been proposed for grading the severity of chronic GVHD. Akpek and colleagues identified three dichotomous variables (extensive skin involvement, thrombocytopenia and progressive onset) that could be combined to distinguish three groups at different risks of chronic GVHD-specific mortality [104]. A multicenter validation study has been performed to show that the scale successfully predicts survival in four independent cohorts (G. Akpek, manuscript submitted). Lee and colleagues took a similar approach to devising a chronic GVHD severity score using IBMTR and NMDP data [105]. The resulting grading scheme is complicated and difficult to use in clinical practice, but does predict survival and treatment-related mortality.

How can the practice of HCT be improved through health services research?

Access

Studies seeking to understand the nonmedical barriers to appropriate health care are termed "access" studies. They generally focus on socioeconomic, political, cultural and other nonbiological factors. For example, ethnic and racial minorities have long been under-represented in HCT statistics for unclear reasons. In addition, survival varies by racial group even after controlling for disease and transplant characteristics (F.R. Loberiza, manuscript submitted). While similar observations have been made in other areas of medicine, issues of access and social determinants of outcome are only starting to be evaluated in HCT. Kollman and colleagues at the NMDP studied reasons why only a third of promising initial searches proceed to transplantation [106]. They identified death of the patient, worsening of the patient's health and length of the search process as major barriers accounting for up to a quarter of failures to proceed to transplantation. The importance of financial issues could not be adequately evaluated in this study, but 41% of coordinators listed insurance coverage as a potential barrier at the time of initial search. Importantly, 34% of white- compared to 13% of African-Americans went on to transplantation. In another study, a survey of 589 African-Americans was conducted to examine barriers to participation in an unrelated donor program. The cost of donation, limited opportunities to donate and lack of knowledge about the life-saving potential of HCT from an unrelated donor were found to be important barriers to donation. Importantly, with introduction of an educational program, the African-American donor pool at the Medical College of Virginia increased substantially [107].

Unfortunately, one of the best data sources for access studies is not relevant for HCT. The linked SEER-Medicare database provides cancer-specific information and inpatient and outpatient billing data on approximately 14% of the US population, but is limited to patients aged 65 or older [11]. Oncology studies using this and other databases suggest that African-Americans are less likely than white Americans to receive screening exams for cancer, to be diagnosed with cancer in its early stages and to receive adjuvant therapy and aggressive care [108–114]. African-Americans are also less likely to undergo some procedures than white Americans, such as renal transplantation, even after correcting for clinical characteristics [115] and patient preferences [116]. However, once access to treatment is controlled, survival and DFS is similar between African-American and white American patients, suggesting that the biological response to treatment is comparable [117,118].

Quality of care

HCT has been relatively spared from scrutiny about quality of care. Significant practice variation has been tolerated and, in fact, encouraged, as a means of testing different approaches that could eventually improve the field of transplantation. The relatively low volume of procedures per center and the inevitable case mix differences have made it nearly impossible to provide standardized center statistics, although the NMDP is required to report center-specific disease activity and risk-adjusted survival information. Nevertheless, a volume-outcome and experience-outcome relationship is probably operating in HCT similar to what has been observed in other technologically sophisticated procedures such as solid organ transplantation and complicated surgical procedures [119–122]. A time-series study of costs during autologous HCT for NHL suggested that technological advances and learning curve effects (institutional familiarity with a procedure tends to improve outcomes) probably both contribute to falling costs, although the study was not designed to compare clinical outcomes [123]. There is every reason to believe that greater attention to institutional and programmatic factors contributing to patient outcome may identify ways to improve care and decrease costs [122]. For example, a study documented significant variation in vaccination practices following HCT [124], and recommendations for infectious disease prophylaxis have subsequently been published [125].

Summary

Outcomes and health services research seeks to answer questions that are relevant as a procedure matures beyond the experimental phase: What are the costs of providing these services? Is society getting its money's worth? How do you pull together disparate sources of data (now that they are available)? What do patients experience with the procedure? Can we develop new or better tools to measure results of treatments? Is the procedure equally available to all people and of the highest possible quality? Answers to these questions are moving targets as HCT evolves. Nevertheless, for people afflicted with diseases treated by HCT and societies trying to control health care spending, decisions have to be made today. Outcomes research tries to provide the necessary data so that personal and societal decisions can be based on the best information available.

References

1 Lee SJ, Earle CC, Weeks JC. Outcomes research in oncology. History, conceptual framework, and trends in the literature. *J Natl Cancer Inst* 2000; **92**: 195–204.

2 Weeks JC. Outcomes assessment. In: Holland JF, Frei EJ, eds. *Cancer Medicine*. Baltimore: Williams & Wilkins, 1996: 1451–8.

3 Weeks J. Overview of outcomes research and management and its role in oncology practice. *Oncology (Huntingt)* 1998; **12**: 11–3.

4 Codman EA. The product of a hospital. *Surgery, Gynecology and Obstetrics* 1914; **18**: 491–6.

5 Donabedian A. Evaluating the quality of medical care. *Milbank Memorial Fund Q* 1966; **44** (Suppl.): 166–206.

6 Cochrane AL. *Effectiveness and Efficiency: Random Reflections on Health Services*. London: Nuffield Provincial Hospitals Trust, 1972.

7 Wennberg J, Gittelsohn A. Small area variations in health care delivery. *Science* 1973; **182**: 1102–8.

8 Hanks GE, Kramer S, Diamond JJ, Herring DF. Patterns of Care Outcome Survey: national outcome data for six disease sites. *Am J Clin Oncol* 1982; **5**: 349–53.

9 Kramer S, Hanks GE, Diamond JJ, MacLean CJ. The study of the patterns of clinical care in radiation therapy in the United States. *CA Cancer J Clin* 1984; **34**: 75–85.

10 Steele GD Jr, Winchester DP, Menck HR, Murphy GP. Clinical highlights from the National Cancer Data Base: 1993. *CA Cancer J Clin* 1993; **43**: 71–82.

11 Potosky AL, Riley GF, Lubitz JD, Mentnech RM, Kessler LG. Potential for cancer related health services research using a linked Medicare-tumor registry database. *Med Care* 1993; **31**: 732–48.

12 Relman AS. Assessment and accountability: the third revolution in medical care [editorial]. *N Engl J Med* 1988; **319**: 1220–2.

13 Epstein AM. The outcomes movement: will it get us where we want to go? *N Engl J Med* 1990; **323**: 266–70.

14 Bennett CL, Armitage JL, Armitage GO *et al.* Costs of care and outcomes for high-dose therapy and autologous transplantation for lymphoid malignancies. Results from the University of Nebraska 1987 through 1991. *J Clin Oncol* 1995; **13**: 969–73.

15 Hartmann O, Le Corroller AG, Blaise D *et al.* Peripheral blood stem cell and bone marrow transplantation for solid tumors and lymphomas: hematologic recovery and costs. A randomized, controlled trial. *Ann Intern Med* 1997; **126**: 600–7.

16 Lee SJ, Anasetti C, Kuntz KM, Patten J, Antin JH, Weeks JC. The costs and cost-effectiveness of unrelated donor bone marrow transplantation for chronic phase chronic myelogenous leukemia. *Blood* 1998; **92**: 4047–52.

17 Drummond MF, Stoddart GL, Torrance GW. *Methods for the Economic Evaluation of Health Care Programmes*. Oxford: Oxford University Press, 1987.

18 Gold MR, Siegel JE, Russell LB, Weinstein MC. *Cost-Effectiveness in Health and Medicine*. New York: Oxford University Press, Inc., 1996.

19 Waters TM, Bennett CL, Pajeau TS *et al.* Economic analyses of bone marrow and blood stem cell transplantation for leukemias and lymphoma: what do we know? *Bone Marrow Transplant* 1998; **21**: 641–50.

20 Griffiths RI, Bass EB, Powe NR, Anderson GF, Goodman S, Wingard JR. Factors influencing third party payer costs for allogeneic BMT. *Bone Marrow Transplant* 1993; **12**: 43–8.

21 Lee SJ, Klar N, Antin JH, Weeks JC. Predicting costs of stem cell transplantation. *J Clin Oncol* 1999; **18**: 64–71.

22 Prieto JM, Blanch J, Atala J *et al.* Psychiatric morbidity and impact on hospital length of stay among hematologic cancer patients receiving stem-cell transplantation. *J Clin Oncol* 2002; **20**: 1907–17.

23 Smith TJ, Hillner BE, Schmitz N *et al.* Economic analysis of a randomized clinical trial to compare filgrastim-mobilized peripheral-blood progenitor-cell transplantation and autologous bone marrow transplantation in patients with Hodgkin's and non-Hodgkin's lymphoma. *J Clin Oncol* 1997; **15**: 5–10.

24 Vellenga E, van Agthoven M, Croockewit AJ *et al.* Autologous peripheral blood stem cell transplantation in patients with relapsed lymphoma results in accelerated haematopoietic reconstitution, improved quality of life and cost reduction compared with bone marrow transplantation. The Hovon 22 Study. *Br J Haematol* 2001; **114**: 319–26.

25 Colby C, McAfee SL, Finkelstein DM, Spitzer TR. Early vs. delayed administration of G-CSF following autologous peripheral blood stem cell transplantation. *Bone Marrow Transplant* 1998; **21**: 1005–10.

26 Lee SJ, Weller E, Alyea EP, Ritz J, Soiffer RJ. Efficacy and costs of granulocyte colony-stimulating factor in allogeneic T-cell depleted bone marrow transplantation. *Blood* 1998; **92**: 2725–9.

27 Lee SJ, Zahrieh D, Alyea EA *et al.* Comparison of T-cell depleted and non-T-cell depleted unrelated donor transplantation for hematologic diseases: clinical outcomes, quality of life and costs. *Blood* 2002; **100**: 2697–702.

28 Jagannath S, Vesole DH, Zhang M *et al.* Feasibility and cost-effectiveness of outpatient autotransplants in multiple myeloma. *Bone Marrow Transplant* 1997; **20**: 445–50.

29 Meisenberg BR, Ferran K, Hollenbach K, Brehm T, Jollon J, Piro LD. Reduced charges and costs associated with outpatient autologous stem cell transplantation. *Bone Marrow Transplant* 1998; **21**: 927–32.

30 Rizzo JD, Vogelsang GB, Krumm S, Frink B, Mock V, Bass EB. Outpatient-based bone marrow transplantation for hematologic malignancies. Cost saving or cost shifting? *J Clin Oncol* 1999; **17**: 2811–8.

31 Ener RA, Meglathery SB, Cuhaci B *et al.* Use of granulocyte colony-stimulating factor after high-dose chemotherapy and autologous peripheral blood stem cell transplantation: what is the optimal timing? *Am J Clin Oncol* 2001; **24**: 19–25.

32 Ballen KK, Becker P, Levebvre K *et al.* Safety and cost of hyperhydration for the prevention of hemorrhagic cystitis in bone marrow transplant recipients. *Oncology* 1999; **57**: 287–92.

33 Zeckhauser R. Procedures for valuing lives. *Public Policy* 1975; **23**: 419–64.

34 Schelling TC. The life you save may be your own. *Choice and Consequence*. Cambridge: Harvard University Press, 1984.

35 Hirth RA, Chernew ME, Miller E, Fendrick AM, Weissert WG. Willingness to pay for a quality-adjusted life year. In search of a standard. *Med Decis Making* 2000; **20**: 332–42.

36 Mitchell RC, Carson RT. *Using Surveys to Value Public Good: the Contingent Valuation Method*. Washington, D.C.: Resources for the Future, 1989.

37 Nease RF Jr, Owens DK. A method for estimating the cost-effectiveness of incorporating patient preferences into practice guidelines. *Med Decis Making* 1994; **14**: 382–92.

38 Uyl-de Groot CA, Okhuijsen SY, Hagenbeek A et al. Costs of introducing autologous BMT in the treatment of lymphoma and acute leukaemia in The Netherlands. *Bone Marrow Transplant* 1995; **15**: 605–10.

39 Eckman MH, Beshansky JR, Durand-Zaleski I, Levine HJ, Pauker SG. Anticoagulation for non-cardiac procedures in patients with prosthetic heart valves. Does low risk mean high cost? *JAMA* 1990; **263**: 1513–21.

40 Derdeyn CP, Powers WJ. Cost-effectiveness of screening for asymptomatic carotid atherosclerotic disease. *Stroke* 1996; **27**: 1944–50.

41 Post PN, Stiggelbout AM, Wakker PP. The utility of health states after stroke: a systematic review of the literature. *Stroke* 2001; **32**: 1425–9.

42 Welch HG, Larson EB. Cost effectiveness of bone marrow transplantation in acute nonlymphocytic leukemia. *N Engl J Med* 1989; **321**: 807–12.

43 Desch CE, Lasala MR, Smith TJ, Hillner BE. The optimal timing of autologous bone marrow transplantation in Hodgkin's disease patients after a chemotherapy relapse. *J Clin Oncol* 1992; **10**: 200–9.

44 Messori A, Bonistalli L, Costantini M, Alterini R. Cost-effectiveness of autologous bone marrow transplantation in patients with relapsed non-Hodgkin's lymphoma. *Bone Marrow Transplant* 1997; **19**: 275–81.

45 Messori A, Bosi A, Bacci S et al. Retrospective survival analysis and cost-effectiveness evaluation of second allogeneic bone marrow transplantation in patients with acute leukemia. Gruppo Italiano Trapianto Midollo Osseo. *Bone Marrow Transplant* 1999; **23**: 489–95.

46 Sampson FC, Beard SM, Scott F, Vandenberghe E. Cost-effectiveness of high-dose chemotherapy in first-line treatment of advanced multiple myeloma. *Br J Haematol* 2001; **113**: 1015–9.

47 Cummings SR, Rubin SM, Oster G. The cost-effectiveness of counseling smokers to quit. *JAMA* 1989; **261**: 75–9.

48 Garner TI, Dardis R. Cost-effectiveness analysis of end-stage renal disease treatments. *Med Care* 1987; **25**: 25–34.

49 Edelson JT, Weinstein MC, Tosteson AN, Williams L, Lee TH, Goldman L. Long-term cost-effectiveness of various initial monotherapies for mild to moderate hypertension. *JAMA* 1990; **263**: 407–13.

50 Smith TJ, Hillner BE, Desch CE. Efficacy and cost-effectiveness of cancer treatment: rational allocation of resources based on decision analysis. *J Natl Cancer Inst* 1993; **85**: 1460–74.

51 Tengs TO, Adams ME, Pliskin JS et al. Five-hundred life-saving interventions and their cost-effectiveness. *Risk Anal* 1995; **15**: 369–90.

52 Chapman RH, Stone PW, Sandberg EA, Bell C, Neumann PJ. A comprehensive league table of cost-utility ratios and a sub-table of 'panel-worthy' studies. *Med Decis Making* 2000; **20**: 451–67.

53 Stone PW, Teutsch S, Chapman RH, Bell C, Goldie SJ, Neumann PJ. Cost-utility analyzes of clinical preventive services: published ratios, 1976–97. *Am J Prev Med* 2000; **19**: 15–23.

54 Bell CM, Chapman RH, Stone PW, Sandberg EA, Neumann PJ. An off-the-shelf help list. A comprehensive catalog of preference scores from published cost-utility analyses. *Med Decis Making* 2001; **21**: 288–94.

55 Weinstein MC, Fineberg HV, Elstein AS et al. *Clinical Decision Analysis*. Philadelphia: W.B. Saunders & Co., 1980.

56 Sonnenberg FA, Beck JR. Markov models in medical decision making: a practical guide. *Med Decis Making* 1993; **13**: 322–38.

57 Wright JC, Weinstein MC. Gains in life expectancy from medical interventions: standardizing data on outcomes. *N Engl J Med* 1998; **339**: 380–6.

58 Verburg RJ, Sont JK, Vliet Vlieland TP et al. High dose chemotherapy followed by autologous peripheral blood stem cell transplantation or conventional pharmacological treatment for refractory rheumatoid arthritis? A Markov decision analysis. *J Rheum* 2001; **28**: 719–27.

59 Nietert PJ, Abboud MR, Silverstein MD, Jackson SM. Bone marrow transplantation versus periodic prophylactic blood transfusion in sickle cell patients at high risk of ischemic stroke: a decision analysis. *Blood* 2000; **95**: 3057–64.

60 Lee SJ, Kuntz KM, Horowitz MM et al. Unrelated donor bone marrow transplantation for chronic myelogenous leukemia: a decision analysis. *Ann Intern Med* 1997; **127**: 1080–8.

61 Lee SJ, Anasetti C, Horowitz MM, Antin JH. Initial therapy for chronic myelogenous leukemia: playing the odds [editorial]. *J Clin Oncol* 1998; **16**: 2897–903.

62 Gelber RD, Goldhirsch A. A new endpoint for the assessment of adjuvant therapy in postmenopausal women with operable breast cancer. *J Clin Oncol* 1986; **4**: 1772–9.

63 Glasziou PP, Simes RJ, Gelber RD. Quality adjusted survival analysis. *Stat Med* 1990; **9**: 1259–76.

64 Mounier N, Haioun C, Cole BF et al. Quality of life-adjusted survival analysis of high-dose therapy with autologous bone marrow transplantation versus sequential chemotherapy for patients with aggressive lymphoma in first complete remission. Groupe d'Etude les Lymphomes de l'Adulte (GELA). *Blood* 2000; **95**: 3687–92.

65 Parsons SK, Gelber S, Cole BF et al. Quality-adjusted survival after treatment for acute myeloid leukemia in childhood: a Q-TWiST analysis of the Pediatric Oncology Group Study 8821. *J Clin Oncol* 1999; **17**: 2144–52.

66 Cutler C, Giri S, Jeyapalan S, Paniagua D, Viswanathan A, Antin JH. Acute and chronic graft-versus-host disease after allogeneic peripheral-blood stem-cell and bone marrow transplantation: a meta-analysis. *J Clin Oncol* 2001; **19**: 3685–91.

67 Rizzo JD, Lichtin AE, Woolf SH et al. Use of epoetin in patients with cancer: evidence-based clinical practice guidelines of the American Society of Clinical Oncology and the American Society of Hematology. *Blood* 2000; **100**: 4083–107.

68 Pater JL, Browman GP, Brouwers MC, Nefsky MF, Evans WK, Cowan DH. Funding new cancer drugs in Ontario: closing the loop in the practice guidelines development cycle. *J Clin Oncol* 2001; **19**: 3392–6.

69 Silver RT, Woolf SH, Hehlmann R et al. An evidence-based analysis of the effect of busulfan, hydroxyurea, interferon, and allogeneic bone marrow transplantation in treating the chronic phase of chronic myeloid leukemia. Developed for the American Society of Hematology. *Blood* 1999; **94**: 1517–36.

70 Hughes TP, Goldman JM. Chronic myeloid leukemia. In: Hoffman R, Benz EJ, Shattil SJ, Furie B, Cohen HJ, eds. *Hematology: Basic Principles and Practice*. New York: Churchill Livingstone Inc., 1991: 854–69.

71 Deisseroth AB, Kantarjian H, Andreeff M et al. Chronic leukemias. In: DeVita VT, Hellman S, Rosenberg SA, eds. *Cancer Principles and Practice of Oncology*, Vol. 2. Philadelphia: Lippincott-Raven, 1997: 2321–43.

72 Sawyers CL. Chronic myeloid leukemia. *N Engl J Med* 1999; **340**: 1330–40.

73 Faderl S, Talpaz M, Estrov Z, Kantarjian HM. Chronic myelogenous leukemia. Biology and therapy. *Ann Intern Med* 1999; **131**: 207–19.

74 Kosecoff J, Kanouse DE, Rogers WH, McCloskey L, Winslow CM, Brook RH. Effects of the National Institutes of Health Consensus Development Program on physician practice. *JAMA* 1987; **258**: 2708–13.

75 Fineberg HV. Clinical evaluation. How does it influence medical practice? *Bull Cancer* 1987; **74**: 333–46.

76 Smith TJ, Hillner BE. Ensuring quality cancer care by the use of clinical practice guidelines and critical pathways. *J Clin Oncol* 2001; **19**: 2886–97.

77 Ferrell B, Grant M, Schmidt GM et al. The meaning of quality of life for bone marrow transplant survivors. Part 1. The impact of bone marrow transplant on quality of life. *Cancer Nurs* 1992; **15**: 153–60.

78 Ferrell B, Grant M, Schmidt GM et al. The meaning of quality of life for bone marrow transplant survivors. Part 2. Improving quality of life for bone marrow transplant survivors. *Cancer Nurs* 1992; **15**: 247–53.

79 Haberman M, Bush N, Young K, Sullivan KM. Quality of life of adult long-term survivors of bone marrow transplantation: a qualitative analysis of narrative data. *Oncol Nurs Forum* 1993; **20**: 1545–53.

80 Baker F, Zabora J, Polland A, Wingard J. Reintegration after bone marrow transplantation. *Cancer Pract* 1999; **7**: 190–7.

81 Ware JE, Snow KK, Kosinski M, Gandek B. *SF-36 Health Survey. A Manual and Interpretation Guide*. Boston: The Health Institute, New England Medical Center, 1993.

82 Ware JE, Kosinski M, Keller SD. *SF-36 Physical and Mental Health Summary Scales: a User's Manual*. Boston: The Health Institute, New England Medical Center, 1994.

83 Watson M, Zittoun R, Hall E, Solbu G, Wheatley K. A modular questionnaire for the assessment of long-term quality of life in leukaemia patients. The MRC/EORTC QLQ-LEU. *Qual Life Res* 1996; **5**: 15–9.

84 McQuellon RP, Russell GB, Cella DF et al. Quality of life measurement in bone marrow transplantation. Development of the Functional Assessment of Cancer Therapy-Bone Marrow Transplant (FACT-BMT) scale. *Bone Marrow Transplant* 1997; **19**: 357–68.

85 Kopp M, Schweigkofler H, Holzner B et al. EORTC QLQ-C30 and FACT-BMT for the measurement of quality of life in bone marrow transplant recipients: a comparison. *Eur J Haematol* 2000; **65**: 97–103.

86 Holzner B, Kemmler G, Sperner-Unterweger B et al. Quality of life measurement in oncology: a matter of the assessment instrument? *Eur J Cancer* 2001; **37**: 2349–56.

87 Kirsch I, Jungeblut A, Jenkins L, Kolstad A. *Adult Literacy in America. A First Look at the Results of the National Adult Literacy Survey*. Washington, D.C.: National Center for Education Statistics, U.S. Department of Education, 1993.

88 Littell RC, Milliken GA, Stroup WW, Wolfinger RD. *SAS System for Mixed Models*. Cary, NC: SAS Institute Inc., 1996: 1–633.

89 Fairclough DL. *Design and Analysis of Quality of Life Studies in Clinical Trials*. Boca Raton, FL: CRC Press LLC, 2002: 1–307.

90 Bush NE, Donaldson GW, Haberman MH, Dacanay R, Sullivan KM. Conditional and unconditional estimation of multidimensional quality of life after hematopoietic stem cell transplantation: a longitudinal follow-up of 415 patients. *Biol Blood Marrow Transplant* 2000; **6**: 576–91.

91 Lee SJ, Fairclough D, Parsons SK et al. Recovery after stem-cell transplantation for hematologic diseases. *J Clin Oncol* 2001; **19**: 242–52.

92 Jaeschke R, Singer J, Guyatt GH. Measurement of health status. Ascertaining the minimal clinically important difference. *Control Clin Trials* 1989; **10**: 407–15.

93 Lydick E, Epstein RS. Interpretation of quality of life changes. *Qual Life Res* 1993; **2**: 221–6.

94 Juniper EF, Guyatt GH, Willan A, Griffith LE. Determining a minimal important change in a disease-specific quality-of-life questionnaire. *J Clin Epidemiol* 1994; **47**: 81–7.

95 Zittoun R, Suciu S, Watson M et al. Quality of life in patients with acute myelogenous leukemia in prolonged first complete remission after bone marrow transplantation (allogeneic or autologous) or chemotherapy: a cross-sectional study of the EORTC-GIMEMA AML 8A trial. *Bone Marrow Transplant* 1997; **20**: 307–15.

96 Lee SJ, Cook EF, Soiffer RJ, Antin JH. Development and validation of a scale to measure symptoms of chronic graft-versus-host disease. *Biol Blood Marrow Transplant* 2002; **8**: 444–52.

97 Martin P, Nash R, Sanders J et al. Reproducibility in retrospective grading of acute graft-versus-host disease after allogeneic marrow transplantation. *Bone Marrow Transplant* 1998; **21**: 273–9.

98 Glucksberg H, Storb R, Fefer A et al. Clinical manifestations of graft-versus-host disease in human recipients of marrow from HL-A-matched sibling donors. *Transplantation* 1974; **18**: 295–304.

99 Sullivan KM. Acute and chronic graft-versus-host disease in man. *Int J Cell Cloning* 1986; **4**: 42–93.

100 Przepiorka D, Weisdorf D, Martin P et al. 1994 consensus conference on acute GVHD grading. *Bone Marrow Transplant* 1995; **15**: 825–8.

101 Rowlings PA, Przepiorka D, Klein JP et al. IBMTR Severity Index for grading acute graft-versus-host disease: retrospective comparison with Glucksberg grade. *Br J Haematol* 1997; **97**: 855–64.

102 Martin PJ, Schoch G, Gooley T et al. Methods for assessment of graft-versus-host disease [letter]. *Blood* 1998; **92**: 3479–81.

103 Martino R, Romero P, Subira M et al. Comparison of the classic Glucksberg criteria and the IBMTR Severity Index for grading acute graft-versus-host disease following HLA-identical sibling stem cell transplantation. The International Bone Marrow Transplant Registry. *Bone Marrow Transplant* 1999; **24**: 283–7.

104 Akpek G, Zahurak ML, Piantadosi S et al. Development of a prognostic model for grading chronic graft-versus-host disease. *Blood* 2001; **97**: 1219–26.

105 Lee SJ, Klein JP, Barrett AJ et al. Severity of chronic graft-versus-host disease: association with treatment-related mortality and relapse. *Blood* 2002; **100**: 406–14.

106 Kollman C, Weis T, Switzer GE et al. Non-HLA barriers to unrelated donor stem cell transplantation. *Bone Marrow Transplant* 2001; **27**: 581–7.

107 Laver JH, Hulsey TC, Jones JP, Gautreaux M, Barredo JC, Abboud MR. Assessment of barriers to bone marrow donation by unrelated African-American potential donors. *Biol Blood Marrow Transplant* 2001; **7**: 45–8.

108 Ayanian JZ, Udvarhelyi IS, Gatsonis CA, Pashos CL, Epstein AM. Racial differences in the use of revascularization procedures after coronary angiography. *JAMA* 1993; **269**: 2642–6.

109 Ball JK, Elixhauser A. Treatment differences between blacks and whites with colorectal cancer. *Med Care* 1996; **34**: 970–84.

110 Burns RB, McCarthy EP, Freund KM et al. Black women receive less mammography even with similar use of primary care. *Ann Intern Med* 1996; **125**: 173–82.

111 Klabunde CN, Potosky AL, Harlan LC, Kramer BS. Trends and black/white differences in treatment for nonmetastatic prostate cancer. *Med Care* 1998; **36**: 1337–48.

112 Bach PB, Cramer LD, Warren JL, Begg CB. Racial differences in the treatment of early-stage lung cancer. *N Engl J Med* 1999; **341**: 1198–205.

113 Potosky AL, Harlan LC, Kaplan RS, Johnson KA, Lynch CF. Age, sex, and racial differences in the use of standard adjuvant therapy for colorectal cancer. *J Clin Oncol* 2002; **20**: 1192–202.

114 Shavers VL, Brown ML. Racial and ethnic disparities in the receipt of cancer treatment. *J Natl Cancer Inst* 2002; **94**: 334–57.

115 Epstein AM, Ayanian JZ, Keogh JH et al. Racial disparities in access to renal transplantation: clinically appropriate or due to underuse or overuse? *N Engl J Med* 2000; **343**: 1537–44.

116 Ayanian JZ, Cleary PD, Weissman JS, Epstein AM. The effect of patients' preferences on racial differences in access to renal transplantation. *N Engl J Med* 1999; **341**: 1661–9.

117 McCollum AD, Catalano PJ, Haller DG et al. Outcomes and toxicity in African-American and Caucasian patients in a randomized adjuvant chemotherapy trial for colon cancer. *J Natl Cancer Inst* 2002; **94**: 1160–7.

118 Bach PB, Schrag D, Brawley OW, Galaznik A, Yakren S, Begg CB. Survival of blacks and whites after a cancer diagnosis. *JAMA* 2002; **287**: 2106–13.

119 Hosenpud JD, Breen TJ, Edwards EB, Daily OP, Hunsicker LG. The effect of transplant center volume on cardiac transplant outcome. A report of the United Network for Organ Sharing Scientific Registry. *JAMA* 1994; **271**: 1844–9.

120 Begg CB, Cramer LD, Hoskins WJ, Brennan MF. Impact of hospital volume on operative mortality for major cancer surgery. *JAMA* 1998; **280**: 1747–51.

121 Edwards EB, Roberts JP, McBride MA, Schulak JA, Hunsicker LG. The effect of the volume of procedures at transplantation centers on mortality after liver transplantation. *N Engl J Med* 1999; **341**: 2049–53.

122 Showstack J, Katz PP, Lake JR et al. Resource utilization in liver transplantation: effects of patient characteristics and clinical practice. NIDDK Liver Transplantation Database Group. *JAMA* 1999; **281**: 1381–6.

123 Freeman M, Vose J, Bennett C et al. Costs of care associated with high-dose therapy and autologous transplantation for non-Hodgkin's lymphoma: results from the University of Nebraska Medical Center 1989–95. *Bone Marrow Transplant* 1999; **24**: 679–84.

124 Henning KJ, White MH, Sepkowitz KA, Armstrong D. A national survey of immunization practices following allogeneic bone marrow transplantation. *JAMA* 1997; **277**: 1148–51.

125 The American Society for Blood and Marrow Transplantation. Guidelines for preventing opportunistic infections among hematopoietic stem cell transplant recipients. *Biol Blood Marrow Transplant* 2000; **6**: 659–713; 715; 717–27.

Section 2

Patient-Related Issues in Hematopoietic Cell Transplantation

33

Karl G. Blume & Michael D. Amylon

The Evaluation and Counseling of Candidates for Hematopoietic Cell Transplantation

Aegroti salus suprema lex

Introduction

Most chapters of this book rely on scientific information that has been derived from laboratory studies or from controlled clinical trials. Not so this chapter. It refers mostly to the experiences and opinions of the two authors who have spent the better part of the past quarter-of-a-century as physicians taking care of transplant recipients and carrying out clinical research studies. The recommendations the reader finds in this chapter are—at least on occasion—based on personal observations and preferences. We ask for your understanding as we know there are "many ways to Rome" and other physicians in other programs may choose approaches different from ours.

Patients who are under consideration for high-dose chemotherapy (with or without total body irradiation [TBI]) or treatment with an intensity-reduced regimen followed by hematopoietic cell transplantation (HCT) require a careful clinical evaluation and in-depth counseling by experienced physicians, nurses and a knowledgeable social worker at the respective transplant center. Most transplant candidates are referred by practicing hematologists or oncologists to the tertiary center where the transplant procedure will be performed. Information regarding the prior course, including initial diagnostic studies, previous drug and radiation treatments and responses to these interventions, as well as psychosocial aspects of the transplant candidate are of utmost importance.

Written information for patients

Prior to the time of the initial meeting with the medical and paramedical staff at the transplant center, patients should have received at least some written educational material regarding the rationale, principle, potential complications and the projected treatment results of HCT. An increasing number of patients are obtaining information from the Internet and may be quite knowledgeable and informed (or misinformed) based on the quality of the knowledge that they are able to acquire.

Many transplant centers have developed their own center-specific written information, as well as educational videotapes which are mailed to future patients and their families in advance of their first clinic visit. Another excellent source of general information is the Blood and Marrow Transplant Information Network. This organization was founded 12 years ago by a former HCT patient (the author of Chapter 36) who provides well-written handbooks to patients and publishes updated information concerning new aspects of HCT in regularly appearing newsletters. The Network also maintains a website (for further details, see Chapter 36).

It may be extremely helpful for transplant candidates to communicate with former transplant recipients who can share their experience with the future patient. Such contacts are much more valuable than the visit to so-called Internet "chat rooms" which the authors of this chapter consider "goldmines for misinformation" (this statement about the "chat rooms" may reflect a generational prejudice).

The patient's first visit to the transplant center

The first meeting with the candidate and relevant family members is intended mainly for information gathering and not for decision-making, i.e. the physician should form an impression as to whether the examination and the medical data identify the patient as a suitable transplant candidate. Conversely, the patient should be provided with well-organized general and also individualized information about the intended treatment course, potential complications, expected transplant outcome and alternative procedures. The communication with the patient should occur in lay language. Technical terms should be explained and abbreviations be avoided whenever possible. Simple illustrations can be particularly valuable and a glossary may prove to be very helpful.

Until they become ill, most patients have never heard words like: allogeneic, autologous, haplo-type, graft-vs.-host disease (GVHD), etc. The concept that a small number of donor stem cells can restore the entire bone marrow with all its production of blood cells needs to be explained. If one would ask 100 random people in Cleveland in Ohio, Dortmund in Germany or Adelaide in Australia what they know about the vital functions of their bone marrow, one would most likely get very few correct answers. It is therefore most important to take ample time to explain the rationale behind HCT. A well-informed patient is much more likely to participate actively in his or her future care.

Finally, we need to be most careful with the terminology we introduce to our patients. A word like "mini-transplant" implies to most listeners that this must be a minor procedure and nothing can go wrong. "Transplant-lite" is an equally misleading term. Consider that even at the most experienced centers, the day 100 non-relapse mortality after dose-intensity-reduced therapy and allogeneic HCT is at least 5%.

Advice on counseling new patients

Each physician and clinical investigator should develop his or her own approach to the education of patients and the counseling process. Over the years, I (Karl G. Blume) have developed, for my own use, a simple four question–answer system (*why*, *how*, *when* and *what*) for my counseling meetings:

1 *Why* is transplantation being done, i.e. the rationale for the procedure and discussion of alternative therapies.

Table 33.1 Issues and topics which should be addressed during counseling meetings of transplant candidates and their families.

I *Rationale* (Why is HCT offered to you?)
II *Principle* (How is HCT performed?)
  A Autologous vs. allogeneic transplantation
  B Preparatory regimen
    1 Choice of a high-dose or intensity-reduced regimen (with or without irradiation)
    2 Risks associated with high-dose therapy
      (a) Nausea, emesis, diarrhea
      (b) Fluid retention
      (c) VOD
      (d) Pancytopenia, immunosuppression and associated infectious complications
      (e) Mucositis and pain in oral cavity and throat
      (f) Hemorrhagic cystitis after cyclophosphamide
      (g) Cardiomyopathy after cyclophosphamide
      (h) Dermatitis after etoposide
      (i) Pneumonitis after nitrosoureas
      (j) Need for transfusional support
      (k) Temporary or permanent alopecia, especially after busulfan
      (l) Infertility
      (m) Cataracts
      (n) Second or secondary malignancies
  C Hematopoietic cell grafting
    1 Marrow vs. peripheral blood cell graft
    2 Risks associated with infusion of hemopoietic cell graft
      (a) Allergic reactions
      (b) Discomfort from cryoprotectant
      (c) Graft failure and graft rejection
  D Risks for GVHD
    1 Symptoms and prognosis of acute GVHD
    2 Need for drugs to prevent/treat acute GVHD
    3 Side-effects of immunosuppressive drugs
    4 Symptoms and prognosis of chronic GVHD
    5 Drugs to prevent/treat chronic GVHD
    6 Immunodeficiency resulting from GVHD including bacterial, fungal, viral and other infections
  E Risk of relapse after HCT
  F Risk of mortality after HCT
    1 Financial affairs, Will
    2 Durable Power of Attorney for Health Care
    3 Use of life support
III *Timing of transplant* (When should the procedure be performed?)
    1 Very soon, e.g. acute leukemia
    2 Within weeks or a few years, e.g. CML
    3 Elective HCT, e.g. follicular small cleaved lymphoma in first remission
IV *Projected result* (What can the candidate expect from HCT?)
    1 Underlying disease and remission status
    2 Compatibility of donor/recipient pair
    3 Performance status of candidate
    4 Comorbid conditions
    5 Prior therapies
    6 Nutrititional status
    7 Age of HCT candidate
    8 Previous infections
    9 Transfusion history
    10 Other individual aspects
V *Other important issues*
    1 Banking of sperm, *in vitro* fertilized eggs
    2 Habits such as nicotine, alcohol or drug addiction
    3 Need for active participation by patient and caregiver during entire course
    4 Rationale and need for clinical trials including randomization
    5 Duration of stay in the area of the transplant center
    6 Return to home and work
    7 Sexual activities
    8 Time to full recovery
    9 Quality-of-life issues

CML, chronic myeloid leukemia; GVHD, graft-vs.-host disease; HCT, hematopoietic cell transplantation; VOD, veno-occlusive disease.

2 *How* is the procedure performed including the explanation of side-effects from the preparatory regimen, the transplant process itself (including the impact on an allogeneic donor), the description of the reason for and clinical presentation of GVHD, the efforts for the prevention of GVHD as well as the potential risks for other early or late side-effects and relapse.

3 *When* should the procedure be performed, e.g. very soon, in case of relapsed acute leukemia or electively, for patients with chronic myeloid leukemia (CML) who may have several weeks or a few years until the preparation for transplantation is begun.

4 *What* is the projected treatment outcome for the individual patient who is being evaluated. It is advisable to quote a range of percentages for disease-free survival (DFS) and not a precise figure which would be arbitrary at best.

Patients may elect to tape the conversations in order to review the information presented at their leisure. The physician should also encourage the patient to take notes and to write down questions which may come up between meetings or at a later time. An atmosphere of trust between patients and their families and the transplant team is of greatest importance for the long weeks before, during and after the transplant procedure. The more carefully a patient is prepared for the difficult phases of transplantation and the more he or she understands the rationale for diagnostic and therapeutic procedures, the significance of expected (and sometimes unexpected) events and the risk of the entire medical approach, the easier will be the task for the health team to guide the often (or maybe always) frightened individual through one of the physically and emotionally most challenging times of their life. Issues such as the potential use of life support and the Durable Power of Attorney for Health Care need to be addressed before the preparation for transplantation is begun. Between 5% and 10% of HCT recipients require invasive life support, most often during the first 2 months after transplantation, and only very few of such unfortunate patients recover [1,2]. Patients should also be advised to make sure their financial affairs are in order and that they have a will.

It may take years for the physician to gain the necessary experience, medical knowledge and sound clinical judgement to "perfectly" counsel his or her patients. It obviously requires a high level of comfort to present a medical procedure which is offered with curative intent but which is also associated with a significant risk to life, i.e. with procedure-related morbidity and mortality. Even under optimal conditions, autologous HCT is associated with a 2–5% early fatality rate and still 10–25% of recipients of allogeneic HCT succumb sooner or later to GVHD or GVHD-associated complications such as overwhelming infections, veno-occlusive disease (VOD), prolonged immunodeficiency or secondary malignancies.

The patient and the family members need to hear from the counseling physician that the intended treatment planned to provide a cure of the life-threatening disease may—in the case of one of the potentially severe complications—lead to the patient's early demise. Still, much of what is explained during the pretransplant meetings is frequently forgotten when devastating complications occur later on. The special situations of desperate patients and their families explain why often little information from the counseling meeting is retained.

To avoid miscommunications or misinterpretation of information early after the first meeting or at a later time, it may be useful to provide the patient with a copy of the consultation letter directed to the referring physician.

Table 33.1 lists issues and topics that should be addressed during the counseling meetings with transplant candidates. This list is only a guideline and should be reduced or expanded as appropriate by each transplant physician and for each patient under evaluation.

The problem of permanent infertility

For many young transplant candidates, the high probability of permanent infertility after high-dose therapy and HCT represents a major problem. Modern technologies, such as cryopreservation of sperm and fertilized eggs, can be used to overcome this serious issue in only a limited number of patients. Unfortunately, the ejaculates of many younger men are aspermic or hypospermic due to the effects of prior combination chemotherapy used for remission–induction treatment. In the case of many younger women, the procedures to harvest eggs for *in vitro* fertilization fail. Despite successful fertilization, the number of those in whom a viable post-transplant pregnancy occurs is still extremely low.

A small number of patients, men and women, have spontaneously recovered reproductive function with healthy children being born during the years after transplantation. These patients were usually children or adolescents at the time of transplantation. It cannot be predicted at the time of transplantation which patient will be able to regain fertility. However, it should be noted that patients conditioned with high-dose cyclophosphamide as therapy for aplastic anaemia often are able to have children during the years following transplantation (see Chapter 71).

Regarding the psychologic and physiologic aspects of infertility, sexuality, quality of life and delayed long-term effects after HCT, the reader is referred to Chapters 36–40, 68 and 69.

The recent introduction of intensity-reduced regimens into the field of HCT may result in a higher number of patients from both genders who retain or recover fertility. Since such regimens have so far included mainly older individuals, the information regarding this important issue is still lacking; however, cautious optimism seems to be justified.

The choice of the transplant procedure

Most patients arriving at a transplant center have been told by their referring physician that they are in need of a transplant procedure. Many of them are surprised when they hear that there are many different types of transplantation: autologous HCT (hematopoietic cells from the patient's own marrow or blood), allogeneic HCT (grafts from a donor's marrow, blood or cord blood) and, occasionally, syngeneic HCT (using marrow or blood hematopoietic cells from an identical twin donor). The counseling physician has to use his or her best judgement and knowledge, as well as the experience at the respective transplant center to advise the patient concerning the type of procedure which most likely will be successful for the candidate's particular condition.

Not all centers can or should offer all the different procedures mentioned above. For example, HCT using cord blood cells for an adult recipient should be limited to clinical research centers with pertinent expertise and specific research protocols. Likewise, HCT from haplotype matched donors requires a transplant team with a commitment to clinical research including a trained group of specialists in the graft engineering laboratory.

Which outcomes data should one quote?

The single most important issue for the patient is the expected survival. Information described below indicates that the remission status and the patient's age are the most predictive factors—with age losing some of its prognostic power in the days of dose-intensity-reduced regimens. Ideally, each transplant center would have a rich database from which one could generate information pertaining to each disease, remission status, age, etc. In the absence of such a powerful tool, which data should be quoted by the counseling physician? For example, a 40-year-old-patient with CML transplanted during first chronic phase from an human leukocyte antigen (HLA)-identical sibling donor at the Fred Hutchinson Cancer Research Center has a >80% chance for long-term DFS [3] (see Fig. 73.4 in Chapter 73). The data at a less experienced center are likely to be less favorable. The patient counseled at that center should either be quoted center-specific results (if available) or the relatively representative

Table 33.2 Discrepancies between patient and physician estimates for the success of hematopoietic cell transplantation (HCT). From: Lee et al. [4] with permission of the authors and the American Medical Association.

Type of transplant	No. of patients*	Estimate				Actual % with DFS (95% CI)†
		Cure without stem cell transplantation %		Cure with stem cell transplantation %		
		Patient	Physician	Patient	Physician	
Autologous‡	94	20	7	70	32	44 (30–58)
Allogeneic disease status	169					
Early	78	20	8	80	62	52 (40–64)
Intermediate	71	13	7	73	42	32 (21–44)
Advanced	20	19	7	80	31	10 (0–23)

*Five patients did not provide an estimate of cure without stem cell transplantation and three did not provide an estimate of cure with stem cell transplantation.
†At 2 years.
‡Ninety patients with intermediate and four patients with advanced disease.
CI, clearance interval; DFS, disease-free survival.

data from the large national and international bone marrow transplant registries.

What does the patient hear and remember?

The patient comes to the transplant center with the expectation of being cured. Much of the information provided during the counseling meetings is viewed and interpreted by the patient in a more favorable light than is actually realistic. An important analysis has recently been reported from the Dana Farber Cancer Institute indicating significant discrepancies between patient and physician estimates for the success of HCT [4]. In this prospective study, 313 autologous or allogeneic HCT recipients and their physicians responded to baseline and follow-up questionnaires concerning their expectations for cure with or without HCT and for treatment-related mortality. Information of actual treatment-related mortality and disease-free 1-year survival was subsequently available for 263 patients. The data are shown in Table 33.2 [4]. Patients and their physicians had the most concordant and accurate expectations when the outcome of HCT was likely to be favorable. However, patients with more advanced diseases failed to recognize the higher risk associated with their situations. This important study illustrates the urgent need to improve further the communication with transplant candidates.

The second counseling meeting

After the first visit to the transplant center, the patient should be allowed adequate time (several days) to consider the often-overwhelming information. In a second meeting, the transplant physician should assure him or herself that the patient understands the whole impact of the proposed treatment, both in general and in its details. An adequate amount of time should be set aside to address all issues and questions concerning the planned treatment and its potential complications.

When to advise against transplantation

No firm rules for a minimal success rate can be established that would be generally applicable. The patient and the entire healthcare team need to keep in mind that a long-term 10% DFS rate implies that nine of 10 patients sooner or later succumb to either relapse or non-relapse mortality. For example, most patients with active central nervous system (CNS) leukemia have already received CNS therapy including irradiation prior to arrival at the transplant center. They will require further CNS treatment (irradiation and intrathecal drug instillations) which put them at a high risk for leukoencephalopathy, a devastating, debilitating complication. Although not all such patients end up with extensive intellectual deficits, such long-term complications need to be considered carefully, especially because even less extensive manifestations can severely affect the future quality of life of the transplant recipient.

Patients whose disease has recurred several times represent a similar dilemma. The chances that their underlying disease will persist or recur after HCT are exceedingly high, especially after autologous HCT. Unless innovative treatment concepts to overcome resistance are pursued in the form of exploratory research trials, these patients should be advised against HCT. Miracles are rare!

Finally, subjecting a volunteer unrelated donor to the physical and emotional stress of marrow donation for a patient with refractory disease and a very poor prognosis requires serious consideration. How often in our decision-making process before HCT do we think about the donor, and how often do we think about this volunteer once the graft is infused? Honestly, the answer would be rarely. A negative outcome of a transplant effort affects many donors for months or even years. They may suffer feelings of loss, failure and, quite often, guilt, especially if the patient dies of GVHD. Needless to say, the same issues apply to all related donors; for details concerning HCT donors (see Chapter 42).

How to counsel patients seeking multiple opinions

Receiving the diagnosis of cancer is one of the most devastating events in the life of any human being. It is certainly understandable that patients are very concerned about their future health and wish to obtain the best treatment which could restore their natural life expectancy. Therefore, many patients seek second or even more opinions, especially when it comes to risky procedures such as HCT. We all have met these traveling patients who arrive at the transplant center with stacks of computer printouts to obtain another opinion. They are clearly in need of very careful guidance. These consultations often take several hours.

We need to explain that the HCT procedures performed at most centers differ only in one or the other detail. In principle, we employ the same concepts, be it high-dose or intensity-reduced regimens followed by infusion of hematopoietic cells. It is the experience and the care provided at the transplant center that make the difference. Moreover, many academic centers may offer innovative approaches which are tested in the setting of clinical research trials and are not available at other institutions.

It is the task of the counseling physician to guide the concerned and often confused patient to a most important decision while objectively explaining the pros and cons of one vs. the other method; for example, T cell depletion of the graft at the Memorial Sloan Kettering Cancer Center in New York vs. post-transplant immunosuppression of the host at the Fred Hutchinson Cancer Research Center or at the Stanford University Medical Center. In this situation, the patient–physician relationship returns to its basic meaning. There is no room for dogma! Ultimately, most patients will decide in favor of the center at which they feel most comfortable and where they understand the rationale for one or the other approach.

The new foreign patient

The number of foreign transplant patients may vary considerably from center to center. Approximately 7% of transplant recipients treated at Fred Hutchinson Cancer Research Center come from another country compared to <1% at Stanford University Medical Center.

Many patients from other countries are unused to the American insistence of discussing all pertinent issues openly with them and their families. They may be more accustomed to having unpleasant facts glossed over. Also, there may be many different dietary preferences and regulations making it advisable to involve a dietitian early on. Rules on body invasion (endoscopy, biopsy, autopsy) are important considerations requiring particular explanations and greatest sensitivity. No detailed rules can be provided in this chapter as the expectations and needs will vary with patients from different countries of origin.

The issue of clinical trials

All progress made during the past 50 years in the field of HCT is based on well-designed preclinical experiments and carefully conducted prospective clinical trials. Almost every transplant center is engaged in one or, more commonly, several clinical trials. Without patient participation, such important investigations are never possible. Therefore, all patients should be informed about clinical research trials as early as possible and be encouraged to consider enrollment in studies as part of their HCT procedure. The concept that a patient simultaneously serves as a research subject and the physician accepts also the role and responsibility of a clinical investigator should be explained during the first and subsequent counseling meetings.

Most patients and some referring physicians do not have a clear understanding for the rationale and need for randomized trials. These clinical research efforts are made to define how a new treatment compares to a previously utilized approach. It should be explained to the patient that the "new arm" might be better, the same or worse than the "old arm". If the answer were known, the trial would be superfluous.

Either during the first or second meeting, the patient should receive a copy of the written informed consent for his or her perusal. The consenting process itself should be completed only after all questions have been satisfactorily answered and should meet both institutional and federal standards. Investigators with a conflict of interest need to provide pertinent information to their patients.

Conditions affecting treatment outcomes

A number of pretransplant factors and conditions strongly influence the treatment outcome and thus impact the advice to patients regarding their candidacy for transplantation. These factors are described below.

Disease and remission status

This book will provide the most up-to-date information on the treatment outcome of autologous or allogeneic HCT for the many different diseases during the various remission stages. The extent of the underlying disease and its sensitivity to chemotherapy strongly influence the treatment result for recipients of autologous and allogeneic hematopoietic transplants. Figure 33.1 demonstrates the statistically significant effect of the remission status at the time of HCT on post-transplant overall survival, event-free survival, relapse and non-relapse mortality in a sample of 2597 consecutive patients transplanted between 1986 and 2001 at Stanford University Medical Center. Throughout this book, the reader will find multiple examples of the effect of the pretransplant remission status on long-term DFS, e.g. acute leukemia, non-Hodgkin's lymphoma, breast cancer and most other conditions.

In order to evaluate a patient's candidacy for HCT the most recent clinical information regarding the extent of the underlying disorder must be reviewed or must be obtained newly if the previous information is no longer considered to be accurate. For example, a patient with acute leukemia referred during first complete remission should undergo another bone marrow examination if the previous study was performed more than one month earlier. Patients with extramedullary leukemia with involvement of the CNS or other manifestation (chloromas of skin, skeletal system or testicular involvement) have a considerably reduced chance for a successful transplant procedure as compared to patients whose leukemia is limited to the bone marrow–blood system [5–7]. Appropriate diagnostic procedures (biopsies, cytogenetic and molecular methods) must be selected to assess the extent of current disease activity.

Patients with acute bone marrow injury following exposure to toxic agents may require a new assessment of their marrow cellularity and function to detect if there are signs of spontaneous recovery obviating the need for the transplant procedure.

Candidates referred for autologous transplantation who have received extensive and prolonged therapy with drugs (especially alkylating agents) and irradiation require detailed cytologic, cytogenetic and molecular analyses of their bone marrow to rule out any clonal abnormalities that would predispose them for later myelodysplastic or leukemic conditions [8,9].

Patients with breast cancer—regardless of their assumed stage—should be restaged to rule out new metastatic disease to the brain, liver or elsewhere, conditions which are considered strong prognostic indicators for early relapse.

Compatibility of the donor-recipient pair

Virtually all patients referred to a transplant center for allogeneic transplantation have been previously tissue-typed and an intended donor has been identified at that time. The transplant center should, however, repeat the histocompatibility testing at their own laboratory to confirm the accuracy of the typing data. After all, the transplant team assumes responsibility for the future care of the transplant candidate and thus the expense of renewed laboratory procedures is fully justified.

Tissue-typing information influences the candidacy for allogeneic transplantation and therefore the discussion with future patients during the counseling meeting. Marrow grafting from a genotypically matched sibling donor is still the most widely used allogeneic transplant approach for patients with hematologic malignancies, bone marrow failure conditions and certain inherited disorders. Highly reproducible clinical data from the matched sibling donor-recipient pair combination have become available during the past three decades.

It is generally accepted that transplantation from related donors who are either phenotypically identical or matched at five of six loci results

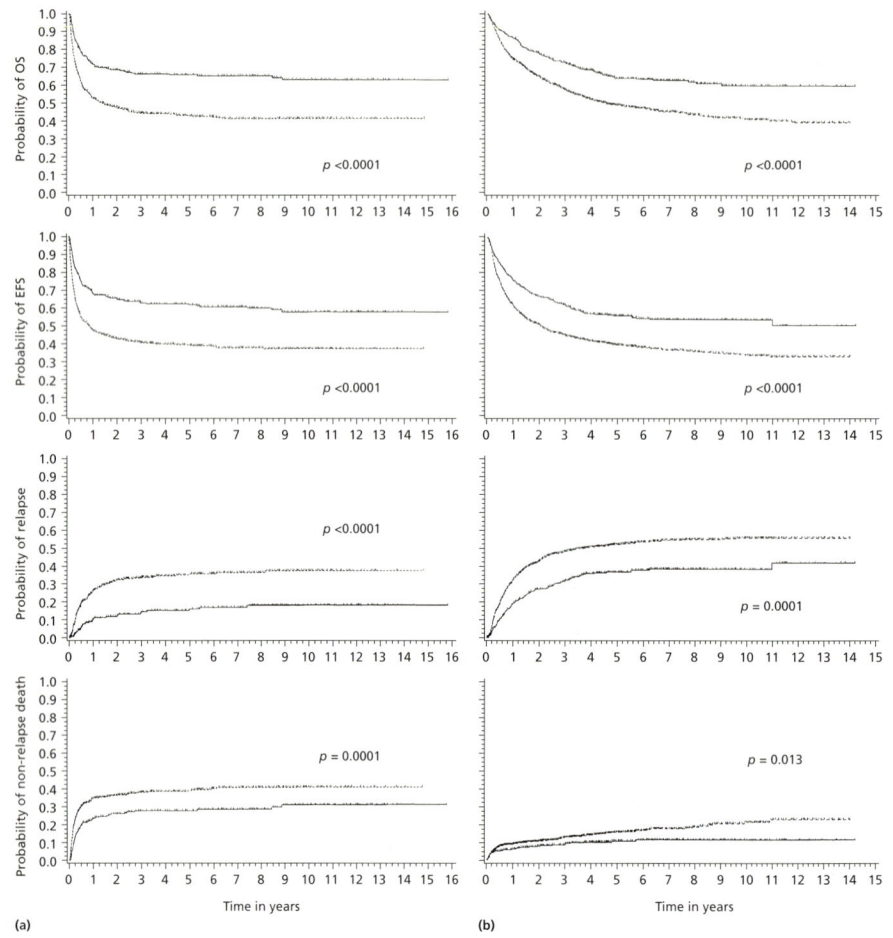

Fig. 33.1 Effect of remission status on treatment outcome (overall survival, OS; event-free survival, EFS) and causes for failure (relapse and non-relapse mortality) as demonstrated in 2597 consecutive recipients of hematopoietic cell transplants (HCT) treated between 1986 and 2001 at Stanford University Medical Center. In all eight analyses, the difference between the two groups of candidates for allogeneic or autologous transplantation with respect to outcomes and events was statistically significant, favoring HCT at the time of minimal tumor burden. (a) 882 patients (369 female, 513 male; median 31 years; range: <1–71 years) received *allogeneic* grafts from related ($n = 683$) or unrelated donors ($n = 199$). The underlying diseases included acute myeloid leukemia (AML; $n = 208$), acute lymphoblastic leukemia (ALL; $n = 213$), biphenotypic acute leukemia ($n = 10$), chronic lymphocytic leukemia (CLL; $n = 15$), chronic myelogenous leukemia (CML; $n = 185$), myelodysplastic syndromes (MDS; $n = 68$), myelofibrosis (MF; $n = 12$), lymphoma (NHL; $n = 50$), Hodgkin's disease (HD; $n = 2$), multiple myeloma (MM; $n = 29$) or other less frequent bone marrow disorders ($n = 90$). The group considered to be at minimal residual disease (———) consisted of 252 patients in either first complete remission (CR) of acute leukemia or in first chronic phase (CP) of CML. The other 630 patients had more advanced hematologic malignancies ($n = 560$) or other hematologic conditions ($n = 70$) not responding to conventional management (– – –). (b) 1719 patients (886 female, 823 male; median age 41 years; range 1–75 years) received *autologous* ($n = 1698$) or *syngeneic* grafts ($n = 11$). The diseases treated included AML ($n = 132$), ALL ($n = 23$), CLL ($n = 6$), CML ($n = 5$), NHL ($n = 598$), HD ($n = 247$), MM ($n = 223$), breast cancer (BC; $n = 348$), ovarian cancer ($n = 14$), germ cell tumors (GCT; $n = 28$), neuroblastoma (NB; $n = 31$) or other less frequent malignancies ($n = 54$). The group of HCT recipients in first CR, first CP or with minimal disease (———) consisted of 369 patients. The underlying diseases included hematologic malignancies ($n = 184$) or BC ($n = 185$) in stages II (with 10 or more positive lymph nodes) or stages IIIA or IIIB. A group of 1340 patients (– – –) had failed standard dose therapies at least once or had persistent or recurrent hematologic malignancies ($n = 1050$) or had stage IV BC ($n = 163$), ovarian cancer ($n = 14$), GCT ($n = 28$), NB ($n = 31$) or other solid tumors ($n = 54$).

in outcomes similar to those from HLA identical siblings [10] (see also Chapter 82).

Through successful preclinical and clinical efforts, HCT from HLA haplotype matched donors has now become possible and has opened up an entirely new and exciting area of transplantation [11–15]. The majority of potential transplant candidates have a haplo-identical family member and could proceed to HCT. However, this approach requires an experienced graft-engineering laboratory and is as yet limited to very few clinical research centers. Moreover, alloreactivity of donor natural killer cells derived from such mismatched grafts against the leukemic blasts seems to be most potent in transplant recipients with acute myeloid leukemia (AML) whereas there is little reactivity—and thus a high relapse rate—in patients with acute lymphoblastic leukemia (ALL) [14,15].

The field of HCT from unrelated donors has made remarkable strides during the past decade, in particular, through the improved understanding of the major histocompatibility complex (see Chapter 4) and the introduction of molecular HLA typing methods for donor selection [16–20]. It is the transplant center that should assume the primary direction and the responsibility in the search for the unrelated donor. The success rate of HCT from unrelated donors is improving continuously as demonstrated by large clinical trials [21,22]. Both types of grafts—from marrow harvests or from apheresis—have yielded similar outcomes [23] (more details are provided in Chapters 49 and 83).

Table 33.3 Karnofsky score [24], modified for hematopoietic cell transplantation (HCT) [25].

General	Score (%)	Description
Able to carry on normal activity, no special care needed	100	Normal, no complaints, no evidence of disease
	90	Able to carry on normal activity, minor signs or symptoms of disease
	80	Normal activity with effort, some signs or symptoms of disease
Unable to work, able to live at home and to care for most personal needs. Varying amount of assistance needed	70	Cares for self, unable to carry on normal activity or to do work
	60	Requires occasional assistance from others but able to care for most needs
	50	Requires considerable assistance from others and frequent medical care
Unable to care for self; requires institutional or hospital care or equivalent. Disease may be progressing rapidly	40	Disabled, requires special care and assistance
	30	Severely disabled, hospitalization indicated, death not imminent
	20	Very sick, hospitalization necessary, active support treatment necessary
	10	Moribund
	0	Dead

Performance status

The invasive nature of high-dose cancer therapy, with or without irradiation, always causes some extent of regimen-related toxicity (RRT), sometimes resulting in little and at other times in extensive morbidity. Therefore, the transplant candidate must be in good to excellent condition when preparation for HCT is begun. The performance score system introduced more than 50 years ago by Karnofsky and colleagues is still a most useful tool for the clinician in the assessment of patients [24]. It has been generally accepted that a patient's performance score should be 70% or above to qualify for transplantation. Most cooperative groups follow this requirement for patient enrollment although some groups have introduced their own scoring system, for example, the Eastern Cooperative Oncology Group uses a 0–3 score with 0 being asymptomatic and without any evidence of disease.

The Karnofsky scoring system has been adapted for bone marrow transplantation patients by Sullivan and Siadak [25] (see Table 33.3 [24,25]). This grading system can also be used to describe the performance status following transplantation. By definition, the best score early after transplantation is 70% (on day +100 following allogeneic HCT).

The previous need to be a young, vigorous patient even to be considered for HCT has changed considerably over the past 5 years. Dose intensity-reduced conditioning regimens have been introduced and explored in rapidly growing clinical trials [26–33]. This novel approach relies heavily on the graft-vs.-malignancy effect derived from donor T cells. Because of the less toxic side-effects of the low-dose preparatory regimen as compared to the previously used high-dose combinations, the extensive morbidity of the first few weeks following HCT is not encountered in this setting, and it is possible to perform these kinds of procedures on an outpatient basis. With intensity-reduced regimens, it is possible to treat older patients (up to the age of 75 years) and others who would have been excluded previously because of serious comorbid conditions. This approach has been greeted with a great deal of enthusiasm, partially explaining the poorly chosen term "mini-transplant". However, we should realize that these HCT recipients still face all the serious clinical transplant-related problems of allografting for malignancy, namely GVHD, infections and relapse. The only major aspect that has changed is the lack of toxicity previously observed during the first post-transplant month. Long-term survival data (beyond 5 years) are not yet available.

We should also keep in mind that the comorbid conditions may continue to affect the patient's life and life expectancy after a non-myeloablative regimen and HCT procedure. For example, a 52-year-old patient of ours with CML underwent such a transplant from her histocompatible brother in spite of having serious coronary artery disease, type II diabetes mellitus and morbid obesity. She is now, 2 years later, in hematologic, cytogenetic and molecular remission of her disease but recently suffered another myocardial infarct and her future is much more compromised by her heart disease, diabetes, obesity and some chronic GVHD rather than by CML.

At the time of arrival at the transplant center, most patients with malignancies have undergone combination chemotherapy for remission induction. Others have received multiple courses of treatment for cytoreduction following a relapse of their tumors. It is the combination of "standard" dose therapy and the nature of the underlying disorders that greatly affect the general condition of the transplant candidate. The transplant physician should try to assess the expected cumulative toxicity from prior treatments and the planned high-dose or dose intensity-reduced preparatory regimen to determine whether the patient will be able to tolerate the intended therapy. Every component of therapy administered from the date of the original diagnosis adds in a cumulative fashion to the ultimate toxicity, including the development of secondary cancers after transplantation. The circumstances of prior "conventional" cancer therapy are often not sufficiently considered when the risks for malignancies after HCT are discussed [34]. In addition, one should remember that there are not only *secondary* but also *second* malignancies, i.e. patients who survive one type of cancer are at risk to develop another malignancy regardless of the type of their prior therapy.

Comorbid conditions

Although—or maybe even because—the number of patients treated with intensity-reduced regimens and HCT is growing rapidly, the need for a careful history and a physical examination, as well as objective tests which allow for a determination of the patient's organ functions, must be stressed. In addition, RRT remains an important issue for all candidates for autologous HCT who will be exposed to maximum tolerated doses of chemotherapeutic agents (with or without radiotherapy). Ideal eligibility criteria for adult candidates for high-dose therapy followed by allogeneic or autologous HCT are described in Table 33.4. In the following paragraphs, some of the most important aspects of compromised organ function are discussed.

Cardiac evaluation

Patients over the age of 50 years or those with a history of extensive exposure to anthracycline drugs may be at risk for future cardiac complications, especially if high doses of cyclophosphamide are part of the planned conditioning regimen [35–37]. In our experience and that of other centers, life-threatening cardiotoxicity after HCT is rare, occurring

Table 33.4 Ideal eligibility criteria for adult candidates for high-dose therapy followed by allogeneic or autologous hematopoietic cell transplantation (HCT).

	Allogeneic HCT	Autologous HCT
Age (years)	0–60	0–75
Karnofsky performance score	70–100	70–100
Left ventricular ejection fraction	≥45%	≥45%
PFT; FVC	≥60%	≥60%
DLCO	≥60%	≥60%
Serum creatinine	≤1.5 mg/%	≤1.5 mg
Serum bilirubin	≤2 mg/%	≤2 mg
ALT	1–2 × normal	1–2 × normal
AST	1–2 × normal	1–2 × normal
Body weight	95–145% of IBW	95–145% of IBW

ALT, alanine aminotransferase; AST, aspartate aminotransferase; DLCO, diffusion capacity; FVC, force volume capacity; IBW, ideal body weight; PFT, pulmonary function test.

in less than 2% of all transplant recipients [38]. An ejection fraction of less than 50% as measured by two-dimensional echocardiography and a prior history of congestive heart failure are significant independent correlates of clinical cardiotoxicity [39]. Many cooperative cancer research groups and also insurance companies have made the use of radionuclide tests of ventricular function a requirement for enrollment of patients to clinical transplant trials or for authorization of financial coverage, respectively. There is little reason to insist that all transplant candidates be evaluated with multigated acquisition (MUGA) scans [40]. Considerable financial resources can be saved by relying on two-dimensional echocardiography if a test is needed at all for a given patient.

Respiratory evaluation

Pulmonary function tests such as diffusion capacity (DLCO), forced expiratory volume (FEV) and forced vital capacity (FVC) have gained a firm place in the pretransplant evaluation of HCT candidates [41–44]. A decrease in these parameters before transplantation predicts for post-transplant respiratory impairment, especially if chronic GVHD occurs, both in children and adults [45–47]. The data are not as clear in recipients of autologous grafts. Exercise tolerance with pulmonary function tests did not predict for later respiratory compromise in 191 patients who underwent autologous HCT for non-Hodgkin's lymphoma [46].

Hepatic evaluation

Liver function tests are routinely obtained before and after marrow transplantation in an attempt to predict or detect hepatic compromise (for details, see Chapter 58). An elevation of transaminases at the time of admission for HCT was significantly associated with post-transplant hepatic VOD. Other risk factors associated with this complication included vancomycin therapy during cytoreductive therapy, acyclovir therapy before transplantation and radiation therapy to the abdomen at any time before transplantation [48]. The occurrence of VOD after transplantation varies greatly between transplant centers ranging from less than 2% to over 50% of patients [48,49]. Possibly patient selection, donor–recipient matching, the use of prophylactic anticoagulation with heparin at the time of the administration of the preparatory regimen and during the 1st week after HCT, as well as a tight control of the patient's fluid status, may play an important role in the occurrence or prevention of VOD.

Renal evaluation

Testing of renal function is a standard requirement at all HCT centers. Serum creatinine of under 1.5 mg percentage (for adult patients) and a creatinine clearance over 60 mL/min are considered adequate as eligibility criteria for transplant candidates. Considering the potential nephrotoxicity of several drugs that are used frequently after transplantation, such as cyclosporine, vancomycin, aminoglycosides, amphotericin, acyclovir and other agents, adequate kidney function seems to be mandatory. However, in patients with multiple myeloma who are treated with high-dose melphalan and autologous HCT, even highly abnormal kidney function still permits a successful transplant outcome [50].

Nutritional status

A nutritional assessment by an experienced dietitian, including an exploration of the patient's dietary habits, should be part of the evaluation process of each transplant candidate (for details, see Chapter 65). It appears that for the assessment of most patients the clinical impression of the nutritional status suffices and that sophisticated laboratory tests and anthropometric measurements are not contributory [51]. However, a baseline albumin value (or better prealbumin) should be part of the evaluation.

Extreme nutritional conditions, such as cachexia or morbid obesity, require special considerations and counseling. Malnourished patients may require pretransplant enteral or parenteral nutrition to improve their general condition, and patients suffering from excessive obesity may be advised to reduce their body weight under the guidance of a dietitian—provided the underlying disease permits the delay of the transplant procedure.

The dosing of drugs in the preparatory regimen is frequently adjusted to ideal body weight (IBW) which may be considerably different from the patient's actual body weight (ABW). In the case of very obese patients this dosing policy would result in serious underdosing with all its inherent consequences, i.e. insufficient immunosuppression and decrease in tumor cell kill. To overcome this problem some transplant centers have made provisions in their clinical protocols by using a formula to calculate an adjusted ideal body weight (AIBW), i.e. IBW plus 50% of the difference between ABW and IBW. For example, if a patient's IBW is 80 kg and ABW is 130 kg then AIBW would be 105 kg. Similar calculations apply if the patient's body surface is used to determine drug doses.

It has been demonstrated in a large clinical study of 2238 patients at Fred Hutchinson Cancer Research Center that body weight impacts on non-relapse mortality after allogeneic transplantation [52]. This analysis indicated that in those patients whose ABW ranged between 95% and 145% of ideal experienced comparable non-relapse mortality whereas patients whose weight was less than 95% or above 145% had decreased survival. The treatment outcome was poorest in those patients whose body weight was less than 85% of IBW.

We have performed a similar analysis at Stanford University Medical Center in 473 consecutive adult patients with hematologic malignancies who received high-dose combination therapy followed by autologous HCT. Again, those patients who were malnourished or those who were extremely obese fared the worst [53].

Age of the transplant candidate

Age of allogeneic HCT candidates

During the early years of allogeneic transplantation successful outcome was limited mostly to children, adolescents and younger adults. Even 15 years ago, many transplant centers would not have accepted patients above the age of 50 years because of concerns regarding early mortality and the high incidence of chronic GVHD in older patients. In 1986, two groups reported encouraging results after high-dose therapy and allogeneic marrow transplantation in older adults, ages 32–54 years and 45–68 years, respectively [54,55]. Data now available for patients with

CML in the age group of 50–60 years indicate excellent survival outcomes [56]. Likewise, the results of older patients with acute leukemia are improved compared to 15 or 20 years ago [57].

The arrival of less toxic, intensity-reduced regimens has allowed the extension of allogeneic HCT to patients in the age group of 60–75 years. In this—as in all other settings—the advice to proceed to HCT should be individualized and based upon physiological rather than chronological age. After all, the 70-year-old patient with CML can be cured by HCT but the comorbid conditions still persist.

Age of autologous HCT candidates

Several transplant centers have analyzed the effect of age on the outcome of autologous transplantation [58–62]. Although there appears to be an increased risk of non-relapse mortality during the early phase after transplantation in those patients over the age of 50 years, it does not seem to be warranted to exclude older patients from autologous HCT. Over the past 15 years, we have autografted 146 patients between the ages of 60 and 75 years with various forms of hematologic malignancies or selected solid tumors at Stanford Medical Center; seven patients (4.8%) in this group died within the first 100 days from RRT. DFS for the 146 older patients was not statistically different from that of the 1578 patients who were under the age of 60 years and were treated with identical protocols during the same period.

Ethnic background

One study has dealt with the effect of race on the outcome of allogeneic transplantation [63]. The only significant difference in this study was found for patients of African-American background with AML who fared worse than patients of Caucasian, Hispanic or Asian-American origin. No such difference was detected for ALL or aplastic anaemia. To our knowledge, there are currently no data available regarding ethnic background and the result of autologous HCT.

Previous infections

Beginning with the time of their initial presentation of a malignant disorder or a bone marrow failure condition, patients enter a phase in their lives when they become more susceptible to infections than healthy individuals. Their conditions are even more compromised by antineoplastic treatments with chemotherapy and/or irradiation or in the case of marrow failure exposure to immunosuppressive drugs such as cyclosporine, antithymocyte globulin or glucocorticosteroids. Many of the patients referred to transplant centers have a history of prior infections with bacteria, fungi or viruses. Modern medicine has provided us with powerful antibacterial drugs and also with agents that are effective against viral infections. However, the currently available drugs to treat fungal infections, especially infections with the *Aspergillus* species, are less potent.

The evaluation process of transplant candidates, in particular those who are scheduled to undergo allogeneic HCT, should include a meticulous search for any signs of subclinical infectious sources. Such studies include standard X-rays as well as computerized tomography (CT) scans and magnetic resonance imaging (MRI) scans if clinically indicated. In addition, a dental examination is recommended.

Clearly, patients with any significant infectious history acquired during prior therapy are at risk for reactivation of the infectious process and need to be counseled accordingly. Issues related to prior or current infections of the hemopoietic cell donor are discussed in detail in Chapters 42 and 58.

Fortunately, much is changing to the better in the field of HCT through basic and clinical research. Five years ago, when the previous edition of this book was published, it was stated in this very chapter that "patients infected with the human immunodeficiency virus (HIV) cannot be considered for HCT". With combined use of powerful antiviral agents, patients with HIV-associated lymphoid malignancies can now be transplanted successfully as demonstrated by a recent clinical trial reported from the City of Hope National Medical Center [64].

Concerning specific infections, the reader is referred to Chapters 51–57. The issue of hepatitis of donors and recipients is specifically dealt with in Chapter 58.

This is probably the right place in this chapter to mention that the incidence of certain infectious complications in patients treated with intensity-reduced regimens followed by allografting is by no means different compared to the infectious complication rate of patients treated with myeloablative regimens (e.g. infections with the cytomegalovirus) [65,66] (for further details, see Chapter 85).

Transfusion history

Most patients with acute leukemia receive multiple transfusions during their remission induction therapy and some patients are refractory to platelet transfusions at the time of referral for HCT. Other patients may have never been transfused, namely those with CML in first chronic phase, breast cancer, non-Hodgkin's lymphoma or multiple myeloma.

Twenty-five years ago, patients with aplastic anaemia used to be referred for transplantation after extensive transfusional support, sometimes even with blood products from their relatives, a circumstance which is associated with an increased risk for marrow graft rejection [67]. Consistent educational efforts have been successful, and it is now quite rare that aplastic anaemia patients are sensitized in this manner [68,69]. Conversely, it seems that transfusions from blood relatives and even from the future hematopoietic cell donor do not interfere with the subsequent engraftment process in patients transplanted for hematologic malignancies—probably because of the strong immunosuppressive effect of high doses of TBI [70].

It is not yet entirely clear how far the prior exposure to blood products influences the outcome of those transplant procedures that involve the use of intensity-reduced regimens. It could be that the rejection rate is increased in polytransfused patients.

For those patients who have been transfused, a detailed transfusion history should be obtained, i.e. number and response to red blood cell and platelet transfusions. It is also important to monitor the number of transfusions in order to assess cumulative iron load [71]. Recent studies indicate that many long-term transplant survivors have secondary hemosiderosis and may need iron mobilization therapy [72], especially patients with thalassemia [73].

Psychosocial assessment

It is the goal of the psychosocial assessment to get to know the candidates' personalities and related issues in order to maximize patients' participation in their own care and to lay the foundation for the successful return to their personal and professional life after HCT. It is furthermore the goal to minimize problem areas that would interfere in any way with the transplant procedure and the recovery phase. Pretransplant family conflicts are among other factors associated with impaired medical and psychosocial recovery [74]. The patient's psychosocial history and condition has the potential to enhance or detract from the transplant procedure. The assessment including evaluation of previous response to pain control should be made by a qualified professional at the time the patient's medical candidacy is being evaluated. In addition, appropriate insurance funding for HCT is part of the evaluation process. The purpose of the psychosocial assessment is summarized in Table 33.5.

Substance abuse is associated with a poor outcome of HCT [75] and drug, nicotine and alcohol dependence are exclusion criteria. The State

Table 33.5 Goals of the psychosocial assessment of adult hematopoietic cell transplantation (HCT) candidates.

Purpose of psychosocial assessment
1 Documentation of psychosocial stability
2 Identification of patient and family strengths and weaknesses in coping mechanisms
3 Assistance with preplanning for the HCT procedure, e.g. arrangement for child care, transportation, state and federal program linkages, etc
4 Coordination of any corrective action if necessary for the success of the transplant procedure, e.g. referral for psychiatric evaluation, compliance contract, drug testing, etc

Individual areas of patient assessment should include
1 Previous methods of dealing with treatment issues and crises
2 Past and present drug, alcohol and tobacco usage
3 Past and present psychiatric history
4 Understanding of diagnosis, treatment plan and prognosis
5 Compliance with previous therapy needs
6 Motivation
7 Unique cultural, religious, literacy and language needs
8 The ability to use information given
9 Previous activity and interest levels

Other important areas for assessment are
1 Emotional support for patient during all phases of transplantation
2 Caregiver availability, i.e. family members or friends
3 Employment issues
4 Advanced directives, e.g. durable Power of Attorney for health care
5 Stability of the environment to which the patient is expected to return
6 Family adjustment to diagnosis, therapy and prognosis
7 Ability to relocate geographically for transplantation
8 Other stressors, i.e. parents, children, insurance, transportation, etc

Insurance System in California (Medi-Cal) does not provide coverage unless the transplant candidate has proven abstinence for an adequate length of time. A history of any substance dependence indicates the need for a formal psychiatric evaluation prior to acceptance for HCT. Non-compliance in the context of HCT is a major issue in the case of many adult patients [76].

Often adult transplant candidates do not initially understand why a caregiver would be needed. A recently reported observation indicates that the presence of a reliable person throughout the entire transplant course is a very powerful prognostic factor for survival following allogeneic HCT [77].

Several of the issues mentioned on psychosocial assessment overlap with what has been stated in earlier paragraphs describing the patient/physician interaction. It is actually desirable that some of the psychosocial issues be assessed by more than one person, i.e. the attending physician and the medical social worker. The impression by both examiners should be presented in a formal meeting in order to create an impression of the patient's candidacy for HCT. During such a meeting all medical and social issues should be presented to an institutional group of transplant physicians, social workers, research nurses, dietitians, etc., and the candidacy for HCT of the referred patient including enrollment to institutional or national clinical trials be determined.

Special considerations for pediatric transplant candidates

Most of the considerations involved with the evaluation of the pediatric HCT candidate are quite similar to those described for adult transplant candidates. The physician must explore thoroughly with the patient and family the rationale for the procedure and the alternative treatment approaches that are available (*why*); the specific protocol being recommended including the risks and side-effects of the procedure and the implications of the source of stem cells (*how*); time considerations based upon the patient's disease status and the availability of a donor (*when*); and the possible outcomes including a projection of the expected odds for survival and the quality of life for the patient under consideration (*what*).

Issues of informed consent

There are, however, some considerations which are unique to the evaluation of the pediatric transplant candidate which may present unusual challenges to the transplant team. The most obvious difference in the conduct of the initial consultation visits is that the person for whom the procedure is intended is not the one who will give consent. The parents or other legal guardians of the minor child have responsibility for decision-making, and must therefore have access to all of the necessary information to evaluate the risks and benefits of the transplant procedure. The child nonetheless is still the patient, and the one upon whom the transplant will be performed. The physician must make every effort to meet the needs of both child and parents or other caregivers [78–82].

I (Michael D. Amylon) make a point to direct the discussion to the child who is old enough and mature enough to understand the implications (usually aged 11 years or older). This means establishing a relationship and engaging the child in the discussion, maintaining eye contact, and encouraging questions from the child before asking the parents for questions. On the other hand, an infant or young toddler will not be able to understand most of this very complex discussion, and the child's presence may, in fact, be a distraction to the parents. In this situation, one of the care team members can bring some quiet toys or coloring materials to engage the child during the meeting, or even take the child back to the playroom. This allows the parents to focus more easily on the discussion and decreases their stress level considerably. There is a wide range of "in between" situations, where the child is present for parts of the discussion. This conversation must be conducted at a level appropriate to the child's ability to understand the rationale and outlines of the transplant procedure without causing undue fear or anxiety. Specific details of possible outcomes and toxicities are then discussed with the parents alone to allow them to ask about issues they do not wish to bring up in front of the child. This is often the appropriate time to discuss potentially fatal side-effects and the issues of intensive care unit (ICU) transfer and intensive life support.

Disease status and the decision not to proceed to HCT

The specific disease and remission status of the patient is one of the most important indicators of the likelihood of a successful outcome following HCT. Weighing the potential risks against this potential benefit and making the decision not to proceed with the procedure is sometimes appropriate for children with advanced malignancies and little chance for a successful outcome. This decision is very difficult even for medically sophisticated adults to make for themselves, and can be extraordinarily stressful for parents making the decision on behalf of a child. In such situations, it is important for the physician to give the parents permission to make such a choice. The likely failure of the procedure and the high risk for severe side-effects should be pointed out gently but clearly. The parents should be able to articulate their understanding of the pain and discomfort that the child will need to endure if the procedure is undertaken and of the odds for a good outcome.

A decision to forgo a potentially helpful therapy (albeit with little likelihood of success) is very difficult for a parent to make on behalf of a

Table 33.6 The Lansky Play–Performance Scale [83] (for patients aged 1–14 years).

Score (%)	Description
100	Fully active, normal
90	Minor restrictions in physically strenuous activity
80	Active but tires more quickly
70	Both greater restriction of, and less time spent in, play activities
60	Up and around but minimal active play; keeps busy with quieter activities
50	Gets dressed but lies around much of the day. No active play; able to participate in all quiet play and activities
40	Mostly in bed; participates in quiet activities
30	In bed; needs assistance even for quiet play
20	Often sleeping; play entirely limited to very passive activities
10	Unresponsive
0	Dead

child. On the other hand, however, physicians also need to take into consideration that the potential benefit to a young child may also be greater than for an adult. It may be worthwhile to accept greater risks for a smaller chance of cure in a young child with a whole life ahead than would be appropriate for an adult. In terms of potential years of life saved, the benefit is objectively greater in a child. To measure the value of a chance at life for a child who has not yet had the opportunity to reach adulthood is difficult. When the parents' hopes and dreams for their child's future are added to the mix, it can be extremely difficult to sort out what is in the best interest of the child and what aspects reflect the hopes of the parents. It is important to help the parents as much as possible to separate their own needs and wants from the child's as they come to a decision.

Pretransplant evaluation

The pretransplant performance status and potential comorbid conditions are equally important in children and adults. The methods by which they are evaluated, however, are sometimes different. The Lansky Play–Performance Scale (see Table 33.6 [83]) is more appropriate for evaluation of transplant candidates less than 16 years of age [83]. In general, a performance status of less than 60% may disqualify a patient for transplantation. Children are remarkably resilient, however, and can sometimes improve their performance status dramatically within a few weeks. Specific suggestions can be provided to parents (with consultation from the pediatric physical therapist, occupational therapist, recreation therapist and nutritionist) for interventions that will enhance the recuperative potential of their child.

The issue of obesity in a pediatric transplant candidate can also present unique challenges. The interactions between parents and children involving food can be quite complex. Mothers in particular (although fathers potentially also) often see feeding the child as one of the most basic ways they can nurture and protect. It is very difficult to convince such a parent that limiting food intake is in their child's best interest. Childhood obesity is also often a reflection of family patterns of food choices and exercise. To be successful in helping a child lose weight the entire family food environment may have to be altered. More healthy and less fattening foods need to be available in the household, and a pattern of family walks or some other kind of family exercise regimen may be necessary to encourage success for the child.

Specific organ function evaluations are performed in all pediatric transplant candidates as for adults. The creatinine value of 1.5 mg/% may reflect significant renal dysfunction in a young child with a baseline creatinine value of 0.3 mg/%, however. A more accurate predictor in any child with an increase in the serum creatinine over the pretreatment baseline would be a nuclear medicine renal scan or creatinine clearance. Because of the need for patient cooperation for pulmonary function testing, many young children will be unable to perform these tests successfully. In the absence of symptoms, a history of pulmonary dysfunction, or a risk factor such as prior bleomycin exposure, no specific testing is indicated. When the degree of suspicion is moderate, a chest X-ray and percutaneous oxygen saturation should be performed to rule out significant pulmonary dysfunction. If there is a high degree of suspicion, then a set of arterial blood gases should be obtained.

The age of the transplant candidate is a consideration in pediatrics as it relates to the potential for long-term complications of treatment, especially failure of normal growth and development. Younger and smaller patients are at greater risk of growth abnormalities, which may also have a greater impact on their eventual quality of survival. This is a particularly vexing problem when considering the risk/benefit ratio for transplantation options in infants with leukemia. Infants with recurrent ALL or AML are at very high risk for treatment failure. Careful consideration needs to be given to the choice of the preparative regimen in these very young patients. The potential for significant toxicity exists with TBI-based regimens that may be most effective in eradicating the leukemia and in facilitating engraftment of inocula from alternative donors.

Intensity-reduced conditioning regimens for children

Many pediatric diseases such as hemoglobinopathies and other genetic diseases may be well suited to intensity-reduced conditioning regimens (non-myeloablative regimens) with establishment of mixed donor chimerism. Since there is no necessity to ablate a malignant clone, high intensity conditioning is not required if the survival of the hematopoietic cell graft can be assured. The improved risk/benefit ratio (if the acute procedure related toxicities are reduced) might make HCT available to a broader patient population.

It must be stressed that these "intensity-reduced" regimens followed by allogeneic HCT still carry considerable potential for morbidity and mortality. The risks of infections and GVHD are similar to a "conventional" transplant procedure. For this reason, the use of such terms as "mini-transplant", which might tend to give a false sense of assurance of success, should be avoided.

Psychosocial and family issues

Even under the best of circumstances, a family facing HCT will be significantly stressed. The emotional cost to parents of having a child undergo a potentially life-threatening procedure is obvious. Many families currently are dependent upon two incomes to maintain their lifestyle and meet their financial obligations. HCT requires extended in-patient time, during which one parent must take considerable time away from work to be with the ill child. Additionally, there are often costs associated with the procedure (such as travel, meals away from home, even some of the medical costs) which are not covered by third-party payers. These and other factors can cause very real financial difficulties.

The transplant center is often at a great distance from the family home. This leads to the necessity to maintain two households during the transplant hospitalization and period of post-discharge outpatient follow-up care. It forces prolonged separation for many families, and raises child care issues for siblings. Parents' relationships as a couple are strained by the separation and difficulties in communication. Siblings may be sent to a friend or relative to live during some or all of this time, and they lack the usual attention that they need from their parents. They may feel

Table 33.7 Factors to be explored in the evaluation of a child referred for hematopoietic cell transplantation (HCT).

Factors to be explored in the initial evaluation of the child
1. History of developmental delay
2. Behavior problems
3. School difficulties
4. Problems with peer relationships
5. History of sexual or physical abuse or neglect
6. Past psychiatric history or treatment
7. History of suicide attempts
8. Substance abuse history
9. Past exposure to trauma
10. Medical compliance issues
11. Problems with prior hospitalization experiences

Factors to be explored in the evaluation of the family structure
1. Financial resources
2. Social supports
3. Past psychiatric history of treatment
4. Family history of substance abuse
5. Child protective services involvement
6. Marital/family conflict
7. Cultural/ethnic/religious issues

neglected, rejected, unloved; they often are jealous of the attention that the ill child receives, but then feel guilty because they know that their brother or sister is going through something very difficult and dangerous. This is a time when all of the resources which a family can mobilize are needed, including other family members, neighbors and friends, support groups, church groups and other community agencies.

It is often in the area of psychosocial assessment that the most unique challenges arise in considering pediatric candidates for HCT. Some of the practical issues involved in the conduct of the consultation visit and the medical decision-making process have already been discussed. There are very real issues, however, in decisions regarding suitability of a candidate for transplant, which are complicated by the fact that the patient is a minor child. An adult candidate who has an immediate history of drug or alcohol abuse may legitimately be turned down because of the implications of this behavior on medical compliance and follow-up care. A child whose parents are substance abusers, however, still has the right to undergo the procedure even though adult caregivers will necessarily be responsible for the same complex follow-up care. Behavioral problems may make it very difficult to care for a child during the intense phases of transplant. Some of these perceived "problems" may be developmentally appropriate reactions to the stress of a difficult and perhaps poorly understood medical procedure. However, such problems should be anticipated and dealt with proactively.

The psychosocial assessment of a pediatric transplant candidate must include a thorough evaluation of the minor child and the family structure, particularly as it relates to the safety of the home environment for post-transplant follow-up care. Factors to be explored in the initial psycho-social evaluation of the child are listed in Table 33.7.

Significant findings that in the judgement of the transplant team might put the patient at risk for complications may demand unusual interventions. Such findings might include a history of parental substance abuse, compliance problems, inadequacies of the home environment, inadequate support to deal with the patients' medical needs as well as other family demands (other children in particular) or other issues. A variety of support systems may be present in the community to help mitigate these issues, and the social worker can be invaluable to the family in helping them to access these services. In some cases a more radical intervention is required, including a change of custody to another family member or even emergency medical foster care placement during the most critical parts of the procedure and recovery period. Such a placement ideally would be voluntary and be perceived by the parents as helpful in a difficult situation. In some cases, however, when the parents cannot appreciate the need for alternative placement, child protective services intervention is necessary.

Child development and compliance

Children at different developmental stages can be predicted to react in certain ways to the loss of control necessarily experienced during HCT. In particular, adolescent patients are likely to become oppositional and uncooperative when their independence and control are taken from them. Every attempt should be made to reserve some areas of control for the adolescent patient where possible, and to maximize the patient's understanding of the need for the various medical interventions. I (Michael D. Amylon) always tell preteen and adolescent patients that we need them to be members of the care team; a transplant is not a procedure that can be done to someone without their cooperation and involvement. These young patients must be sufficiently involved in the consultation and decision-making process that they can choose to proceed based on their knowledge and understanding of the risk/benefit ratio.

I (Michael D. Amylon) have found that adolescents generally do well with an explicit behavioral contract which is signed in advance of the transplant hospitalization. This contract states our expectations for co-operation by the adolescent patient in the plan of care, but also explicitly states what the patient may expect from the care team in terms of respect, information, availability, resources, support, etc. Adolescent patients wish to be treated as mature and responsible individuals, while at the same time they often need support and protection. An open and honest relationship with the medical team with clearly stated expectations up front can go a long way to prevent some very difficult interactions during the transplant procedure.

The entire counseling process can take on another level of complexity when the parents of the patient are themselves still adolescents. In these situations another generation becomes involved in the decision process. Whether or not the young parents are married, the grandparents often compete for influence and control, which makes an already stressful situation that much worse. The transplant physician, with the help of the psychosocial support staff, must keep the discussion and the decision-making process focused clearly on the needs of the patient. The lines of communication throughout the evaluation and the transplant process must be clear. The parents should be positioned as the primary decision-makers, and communication should be channeled through them at all times. Appropriate support and guidance must be provided to these young and frightened parents, and the grandparents should be given appropriate guidelines to allow them to be supportive of their children (who are trying hard to parent a critically ill child) while not interfering with the delivery of care. In these situations a pretransplant contract is often useful to the parents, as it is with adolescent patients, to state clearly expectations and define appropriate parameters of behavior to help them in their interactions with their child, with the members of the health care team, and with other family members.

Some final considerations

HCT requires a cooperative, educated and insightful patient. Through the educational efforts of the transplant team and the informed consent process the patient should have acquired the high level of understanding and knowledge which is a prerequisite for participation throughout the long

HCT process both at the transplant center and subsequently in the domestic environment. It is sometimes forgotten or ignored that the transplant process is not completed with the return of the white blood cell count to the normal range. Deficiencies of the immune system persist for many months and sometimes years.

Allogeneic marrow graft recipients especially are at risk for late infectious complications even if all *in vitro* tests are showing a return of normal immune function. The transplant patient should be instructed to seek medical advice for even relatively harmless-appearing symptoms. A well functioning communication system between the transplant center, the patient and his or her local physician has to be a permanent part of the post-transplant course.

During our more than 25 years in the field of HCT, we can remember several sad circumstances which led to the demise of patients where a timely telephone call either from the patient to his or her local physician or from the local physician to the transplant center might have saved the patient's life. It is our responsibility to educate and to educate again!

This chapter can never be complete. There are simply too many medical or social circumstances that cannot be described in detail or even be anticipated. There are no rules for common sense and no substitute for professional judgement or rapid communication. Regarding many of the patient care issues before and after transplantation, we refer the reader to Chapters 34–39 of this book.

References

1 Rubenfeld GD, Crawford SW. Withdrawing life support from mechanically ventilated recipients of bone marrow transplants: a case for evidence-based guidelines. *Ann Intern Med* 1996; **125**: 625–33.

2 Bach PS, Schrag D, Nierman DM *et al.* Identification of poor prognostic features among patients requiring mechanical ventilation after hematopoietic stem cell transplantation. *Blood* 2001; **98**: 3234–40.

3 Radich JP, Gooley T, Clift R *et al.* Allogeneic-related transplantation for chronic phase chronic myeloid leukemia (CML) using a targeted busulfan and cytocan preparative regimen. *Blood* 2001; **98**: 778a [Abstract].

4 Lee SJ, Fairclough D, Antin JH *et al.* Discrepancies between patient and physician estimates for the success of stem cell transplantation. *J Am Med Assoc* 2001; **285**: 1034–8.

5 Harrison DT, Flournoy N, Ramberg R *et al.* Relapse following marrow transplantation for acute leukemia. *Am J Hematol* 1978; **5**: 191–202.

6 Spruce WE, Forman SJ, Krance RA *et al.* Outcome of bone marrow transplantation in patients with extramedullary involvement of acute leukemia. *Blut* 1983; **48**: 75–9.

7 Thompson CB, Sanders JE, Flournoy N *et al.* The risks of central nervous system relapse and leukoencephalopathy in patients receiving marrow transplants for acute leukemia. *Blood* 1986; **67**: 195–9.

8 Chao NJ, Nademanee AP, Long GD *et al.* Importance of bone marrow cytogenetic evaluation before autologous bone marrow transplantation for Hodgkin's disease. *J Clin Oncol* 1991; **9**: 1575–9.

9 Gilliland G, Gribben JG. Therapy-related MDS/AML after stem cell transplantation. *Biol Blood Marrow Transplant* 2002; **8**: 9–16.

10 Beatty PG, Clift RA, Mickelson EM *et al.* Marrow transplantation from related donors other than HLA-identical siblings. *N Engl J Med* 1985; **313**: 765–71.

11 Aversa F, Tabilio A, Terenzi A *et al.* Successful engraftment of T-cell-depleted haploidentical "three-loci" incompatible transplants in leukemia patients by addition of factor-mobilized peripheral blood progenitor cells to bone marrow inoculum. *Blood* 1994; **84**: 3948–55.

12 Henslee-Downey PJ, Abhyankar SH, Parrish RS *et al.* Use of partially mismatched related donors extends access to allogeneic marrow transplant. *Blood* 1997; **89**: 3864–72.

13 Soiffer RJ, Mauch P, Fairclough D *et al.* CD6+ T cell depleted allogeneic bone marrow transplantation from genotypically HLA nonidentical related donors. *Biol Blood Marrow Transplant* 1997; **3**: 11–7.

14 Aversa F, Tabilio A, Velardi A *et al.* Treatment of high-risk acute leukemia with T-cell-depleted stem cells from related donors with one fully mismatched HLA haplotype. *N Engl J Med* 1998; **339**: 1186–93.

15 Ruggeri L, Capanni M, Urbani E *et al.* Effectiveness of donor natural killer cell alloreactivity in mismatched hematopoietic transplants. *Science* 2002; **295**: 2097–100.

16 Petersdorf EW, Longton GM, Anasetti C *et al.* The significance of HLA-DRB1 matching on clinical outcome after HLA-A, B, DR identical unrelated donor marrow transplantation. *Blood* 1995; **86**: 1606–13.

17 Speiser DE, Tiercy J-M, Rufer N *et al.* High resolution HLA matching associated with decreased mortality after unrelated bone marrow transplantation. *Blood* 1996; **87**: 4455–62.

18 Petersdorf EW, Kollman C, Hurley CK *et al.* Effect of HLA class II gene disparity on clinical outcome in unrelated donor hematopoietic cell transplantation for chronic leukemia: the US National Marrow Donor Program Experience. *Blood* 2001; **98**: 2922–9.

19 Petersdorf EW, Hansen JA, Martin PJ *et al.* Major-histocompatibility-complex class I alleles and antigens in hematopoietic-cell transplantation. *N Engl J Med* 2001; **345**: 1794–800.

20 Drobyski WR, Klein J, Flomenberg N *et al.* Superior survival associated with transplantation of matched unrelated versus one-antigen-mismatched unrelated or highly human leukocyte antigen-disparate haploidentical family donor marrow grafts for the treatment of hematologic malignancies: establishing a treatment algorithm for recipients of alternative donor grafts. *Blood* 2002; **99**: 806–14.

21 Hansen JA, Gooley TA, Martin PJ *et al.* Bone marrow transplants from unrelated donors for patients with chronic myeloid leukemia. *N Engl J Med* 1998; **338**: 962–8.

22 Weisdorf DJ, Anasetti C, Antin JH *et al.* Allogeneic bone marrow transplantation for chronic myelogenous leukemia: comparative analysis of unrelated versus matched sibling donor transplantation. *Blood* 2002; **99**: 1971–7.

23 Remberger M, Ringen O, Blau I-W *et al.* No difference in graft-versus-host disease, relapse, and survival comparing peripheral stem cells to bone marrow using unrelated donors. *Blood* 2001; **98**: 1739–45.

24 Karnofsky DA, Abelmann WH, Craver LF *et al.* The use of the nitrogen mustards in the palliative treatment of carcinoma. *Cancer* 1948; **1**: 634–56.

25 Sullivan KM, Siadak MF. Stem cell transplantation. In: Johnson FE, Virgo KS, eds. *Cancer Patient Follow-up*. St. Louis: Mosby Inc, 1997: 490–501.

26 Slavin S, Nagler A, Naparstek E *et al.* Non-myeloablative stem cell transplantation and cell therapy as an alternative to conventional bone marrow transplantation with lethal cytoreduction for the treatment of malignant and nonmalignant hematologic diseases. *Blood* 1998; **91**: 756–63.

27 Khouri IF, Keating M, Körbling M *et al.* Transplant-lite: induction of graft-versus-malignancy using fludarabine-based nonablative chemotherapy and allogeneic blood progenitor-cell transplantation as treatment for lymphoid malignancies. *J Clin Oncol* 1998; **16**: 2817–24.

28 Sykes M, Preffer F, McAfee S *et al.* Mixed lymphohaemopoietic chimerism and graft-versus-lymphoma effects after non-myeloablative therapy and HLA-mismatched bone-marrow transplantation. *Lancet* 1999; **353**: 1755–9.

29 Childs R, Chernoff A, Contentin N *et al.* Regression of metastatic renal-cell carcinoma after non-myeloablative allogeneic peripheral-blood stem-cell transplantation. *N Engl J Med* 2000; **343**: 750–8.

30 McSweeney PA, Niederwieser D, Shizuru JA *et al.* Hematopoietic cell transplantation in older patients with hematologic malignancies: replacing high-dose cytotoxic therapy with graft-versus-tumor effects. *Blood* 2001; **97**: 3390–400.

31 Khouri IF, Saliba RM, Girald SA *et al.* Nonablative allogeneic hematopoietic transplantation as adoptive immunotherapy for indolent lymphoma: low incidence of toxicity, acute graft-versus-host disease, and treatment-related mortality. *Blood* 2001; **98**: 3595–9.

32 Devine SM, Hoffman R, Verman A *et al.* Allogeneic blood cell transplantation following reduced-intensity conditioning is effective therapy for older patients with myelofibrosis with myeloid metaplasia. *Blood* 2002; **99**: 2255–8.

33 Chakraverty R, Peggs K, Chopra R *et al.* Limiting transplantation-related mortality following unrelated donor stem cell transplantation by using a non-myeloablative conditioning regimen. *Blood* 2002; **99**: 1071–8.

34 Curtis RE, Rowlings PA, Deeg HJ *et al.* Solid cancers after bone marrow transplantation. *N Engl J Med* 1997; **336**: 897–904.

35 Appelbaum FR, Strauchen JA, Graw RG. Acute lethal carditis caused by high-dose combination chemotherapy. *Lancet* 1976; i: 58–62.

36 Cazin B, Gorin NC, Laportee JP. Cardiac complications after bone marrow transplantation. *Cancer* 1986; **57**: 2061–9.

37 Trigg ME, Finlay JL, Bozdech M *et al.* Fatal cardiac toxicity in bone marrow transplant patients

receiving cytosine arabinoside, cyclophosphamide, and total body irradiation. *Cancer* 1987; **59**: 38–42.
38 Hertenstein M, Stefanic T, Schmeiser T *et al.* Cardiac toxicity of bone marrow transplantation: predictive value of cardiologic evaluation before transplant. *J Clin Oncol* 1994; **12**: 998–1004.
39 Braverman AC, Antin JH, Plapper MT *et al.* Cyclophosphamide cardiotoxicity in bone marrow transplantation: a prospective evaluation of new dosing regimens. *J Clin Oncol* 1991; **9**: 1215–23.
40 Bearman SI, Petersen FB, Schor RA *et al.* Radionuclide ejection fractions in the evaluation of patients being considered for bone marrow transplantation: risk for cardiac toxicity. *Bone Marrow Transplant* 1990; **5**: 173–7.
41 Depledge MH, Barrett A, Powles RL. Lung function after bone marrow grafting. *Int J Rad Onc Biol Phys* 1983; **9**: 145–51.
42 Clark JG, Schwartz DA, Flournoy N *et al.* Risk factors for airflow obstruction in recipients of bone marrow transplants. *Ann Intern Med* 1987; **107**: 648–56.
43 Prince DS, Wingard JR, Saral R *et al.* Longitudinal changes in pulmonary function following bone marrow transplantation. *Chest* 1989; **96**: 301–6.
44 Crawford SW, Fisher L. Predictive value of pulmonary function tests before marrow transplantation. *Chest* 1992; **101**: 1257–64.
45 Clark JG, Crawford SW, Madtes DK *et al.* Obstructive lung disease after allogeneic marrow transplantation. *Ann Intern Med* 1989; **111**: 368–76.
46 Nichols DG, Walker LK, Wingard JR *et al.* Predictors of acute respiratory failure after bone marrow transplantation in children. *Crit Care Med* 1994; **22**: 1485–91.
47 Jain B, Floreani AA, Anderson JR *et al.* Cardiopulmonary function and autologous bone marrow transplantation: results and predictive value for respiratory failure and mortality. *Bone Marrow Transplant* 1996; **17**: 561–8.
48 McDonald GB, Hinds MS, Fisher LD *et al.* Veno-occlusive disease of the liver and multiorgan failure after bone marrow transplantation: a cohort study of 355 patients. *Ann Intern Med* 1993; **118**: 255–67.
49 Locasciulli A, Bagigalupo A, Alberti A *et al.* Predictability before transplant of hepatic complications following allogeneic bone marrow transplantation. *Transplantation* 1989; **48**: 68–72.
50 Badros A, Barlogie B, Siegel E *et al.* Results of autologous stem cell transplant in multiple myeloma patients with renal failure. *Br J Haematol* 2001; **114**: 822–9.
51 Baker JP, Detsky AS, Wesson DE *et al.* Nutritional assessment: a comparison of clinical judgement and objective measurements. *N Engl J Med* 1982; **306**: 969–72.
52 Deeg JJ, Siegel K, Bruemmer B *et al.* Impact of patient weight on non-relapse mortality after marrow transplantation. *Bone Marrow Transplant* 1995; **15**: 461–8.

53 Coghlin Dickson TM, Kusnierz-Glaz CR, Blume KG *et al.* Impact of body weight and dose adjustment on ABMT. *Biol Blood Marrow Transplant* 1999; **5**: 299–305.
54 Blume KG, Forman SJ, Nademanee AP *et al.* Bone marrow transplantation for hematologic malignancies in patients aged 30 years or older. *J Clin Oncol* 1986; **4**: 1489–92.
55 Klingemann JG, Storb R, Fefer A *et al.* Bone marrow transplantation in patients aged 45 years and older. *Blood* 1986; **67**: 770–6.
56 Clift RA, Appelbaum FR, Thomas ED. Treatment of chronic myeloid leukemia by marrow transplantation. *Blood* 1993; **82**: 1954–6.
57 Soiffer RJ, Fairclough D, Robertson M *et al.* CD6-depleted allogeneic bone marrow transplantation for acute leukemia in first complete remission. *Blood* 1997; **89**: 3039–47.
58 Sweetenham JW, Pearce R, Philip T *et al.* High-dose therapy and autologous bone marrow transplantation for intermediate and high grade non-Hodgkin's lymphoma in patients aged 55 years and over: results from the European Group for Bone Marrow Transplantation. *Bone Marrow Transplant* 1994; **14**: 981–7.
59 Cahn JY, Labopin M, Mandelli F. Autologous bone marrow transplantation for first remission acute myeloblastic leukemia in patients older than 50 years. a retrospective analysis of the European bone marrow transplant group. *Blood* 1995; **85**: 575–9.
60 Miller CB, Piantadosi S, Vogelsang GB *et al.* Impact of age on outcome of patients with cancer undergoing autologous bone marrow transplant. *J Clin Oncol* 1996; **14**: 1327–32.
61 Kusnierz-Glaz CR, Schlegel PG, Wong RM *et al.* Influence of age on the outcome of 500 autologous bone marrow transplant procedures for hematologic malignancies. *J Clin Oncol* 1997; **15**: 18–25.
62 Siegel DS, Desikan KR, Mehta J *et al.* Age is not a prognostic variable with autotransplants for multiple myeloma. *Blood* 1999; **93**: 51–4.
63 Klingemann HG, Deeg HJ, Self S *et al.* Is race a risk factor for allogeneic marrow transplantation? *Bone Marrow Transplant* 1986; **1**: 87–94.
64 Krishnan A, Molina A, Zaia J *et al.* Autologous stem cell transplantation for HIV-associated lymphoma. *Blood* 2001; **98**: 3857–9.
65 Junghanss C, Boeckh M, Carter RA *et al.* Incidence and outcome of cytomeg-alovirus following non-myeloablative compared with myeloablative allogeneic stem cell transplantation, a matched control study. *Blood* 2002; **99**: 1978–85.
66 Chakrabarti S, Mackinnon S, Chopra R *et al.* High incidence of cytomegalovirus infection after non-myeloablative stem cell transplantation: potential role of Campath-1H in delaying immune reconstitution. *Blood* 2002; **99**: 4357–63.
67 Storb R, Prentice RL, Thomas ED. Marrow transplantation for treatment of aplastic anemia. *N Engl J Med* 1977; **296**: 61–6.

68 Anasetti C, Doney KC, Storb R *et al.* Marrow transplantation for severe aplastic anemia. *Ann Intern Med* 1986; **104**: 461–6.
69 Deeg HJ, Self S, Storb RL *et al.* Decreased incidence of marrow graft rejection in patients with severe aplastic anemia: changing impact of risk factors. *Blood* 1986; **68**: 1363–8.
70 Ho WG, Champlin RW, Winston DJ *et al.* Bone marrow transplantation in patients with leukaemia previously transfused with blood products from family members. *Br J Haematol* 1987; **67**: 67–70.
71 Brittenham GM. Iron and the pathophysiology of bone marrow transplantation. *Bone Marrow Transplant* 1997; **19**: 116–8.
72 McKay PJ, Murphy JA, Cameron S *et al.* Iron overload and liver dysfunction after allogeneic or autologous bone marrow transplantation. *Bone Marrow Transplant* 1996; **17**: 63–6.
73 Angelucci E, Muretto P, Lucarelli G *et al.* Phlebotomy to reduce iron overload in patients cured of thalassemia by bone marrow transplantation. *Blood* 1997; **90**: 994–8.
74 Syrjala KL, Chapko MK, Vitaliano PP *et al.* Recovery after allogeneic marrow transplantation: prospective study of predictors of long-term physical and psychosocial functioning. *Bone Marrow Transplant* 1993; **11**: 319–27.
75 Chang G, Antin JH, Orav EJ *et al.* Substance abuse and bone marrow transplant. *Am J Drug Alcohol Abuse* 1997; **23**: 301–8.
76 Bishop MM, Rodrigue JR, Wingard JR. Mismanaging the gift of life: noncompliance in the context of adult stem cell transplantation. *Bone Marrow Transplant* 2002; **29**: 875–80.
77 Bolwell BJ, Foster L, McLellan L *et al.* The presence of a caregiver is a powerful prognostic variable of survival following allogeneic bone marrow transplantation. *Blood* 2001; **98**: 202a [Abstract].
78 American Academy of Pediatrics Committee on Drugs. Guidelines for the ethical conduct of studies to evaluate drugs in pediatric populations. *Pediatrics* 1995; **95**: 286–94.
79 Susman EJ, Dorn LD, Fletcher JC. Participation in biomedical research. The consent process as viewed by children, adolescents, young adults, and physicians. *J Pediatrics* 1992; **121**: 547–52.
80 Weithorn I, Campbell SB. The competency of children and adolescents to make informed treatment decisions. *Child Dev* 1982; **53**: 1589–98.
81 Mammel KA, Kaplan DW. Research consent by adolescent minors and institutional review boards. *J Adolescent Health* 1995; **17**: 328–30.
82 Sullivan KM, Walters MC, Ohene-Frempong K. Bone marrow transplantation for sickle cell disease. *N Engl J Med* 1996; **355**: 1845–6 [letter].
83 Lansky SB, List MA, Lansky LL *et al.* The measurement of performance in childhood cancer patients. *Cancer* 1987; **60**: 1651–6.

34

Laura L. Adams & Angela A. Johns

Clinical and Administrative Support for Hematopoietic Cell Transplant Programs

Introduction

Patient care, clinical outcomes and research are the cornerstones upon which a hematopoietic cell transplantation (HCT) program is built. But there are many other contributing factors that must be present in order to establish a program that is administratively as well as clinically successful. These factors, which are sometimes overlooked and often misunderstood, create the foundation upon which the program can grow and prosper within the parent hospital or health care system.

The roles of physicians and nurses within a HCT program are generally well understood. But a HCT program is comprised of a variety of clinical and administrative functions that create the framework upon which the program relies. In this chapter we will discuss key clinical and administrative functions, and staff which might perform these functions including nurse program manager, nurse case manager, clinical nurse specialist, administrative director/business manager, financial coordinator and search coordinator (for unrelated donor transplants). While there are certainly other key roles and functions within a program—HCT laboratory, pharmacy, social work, data management, dietary, physical therapy and support staff, such as transcriptionists and secretaries, a discussion of these roles is beyond the scope of this chapter.

Successful HCT programs have structures that support excellence in patient care and incorporate good business practices. An ideal scenario is one in which the clinical and administrative leadership of the HCT program routinely collaborate on practice changes considering the clinical as well as the financial impact on the individual patient and the entire program. This goal can be accomplished through many different structures or organizational models, but the key remains the melding of clinical and administrative aspects of the program. In addition to the complement of attending HCT physicians, a program needs staff which can provide clinical expertise in patient care management, resource utilization, development of clinical pathways to optimize patient outcomes, and staff with administrative expertise in business and financial management, contracting with third-party payers, marketing and outreach.

In this chapter we will explore key responsibilities assigned to designated personnel within our respective organizations, which are academic medical centers (Stanford University and Duke University) with HCT programs that perform in excess of 200 adult transplants annually at the time of this writing. We present this chapter as one model for successful management of a HCT program. There are a myriad of factors that will affect the organization and structure of a HCT program. These factors include but are in no way limited to: academic medical center or community-based HCT program; annual program volume (program volumes across the country range from fewer than 20 transplants annually to over 500 transplants annually); type of transplants performed—autologous only, autologous and allogeneic from related donors, autologous and allogeneic from related and unrelated donors, adult and/or pediatric patients, etc. However, regardless of academic or community status, program volume, type of transplants performed or organizational structure, for optimal success it is important that the functions described are performed by individuals within the HCT program or individuals who work with the HCT program.

To most health care professionals the importance of the clinical functions within a HCT program are self-evident, but some may wonder about the necessity of administrative or business functions within a HCT program. In addition to serving as a curative therapy for patients, HCT also has business and economic components which, in today's health care environment, at least in the USA, cannot be ignored. A HCT program represents both significant expense and revenue in any US hospital or health care system. In 1999, there were an estimated 16,700 HCT procedures performed in the USA and the proportion of transplants at that time was projected at 25% from related donors, 10% from unrelated donors and 65% autologous HCT [1].

Table 34.1 illustrates the estimated charges for HCTs in the USA in 1999, using volumes derived from Hauboldt's estimated proportion of transplants, and their estimated average 1st-year charges for HCT (which include charges for evaluation, candidacy/pretransplant, procurement of marrow/stem cells, hospital, physician, follow-up and, for allogeneic transplant recipients, immunosuppressants) [1].

HCT programs in the USA were estimated to generate over $3 billion in charges in 1999, as reflected in Table 34.1. These significant dollars illustrate why hospitals and health care systems are committed to successfully managing HCT programs, why third-party payers are concerned about the expenditures for this procedure, and why HCT program leadership (physician, clinical and administrative) must do everything possible to assure that the HCT program is fiscally responsible and financially viable.

A HCT program may not have sufficient volume to support, or its organization or structure may not support a dedicated administrative director/business manager. In those situations it remains important for the program's long-term success that key people within the organization be identified to perform the responsibilities of such a role, and that these individuals work in close collaboration with the HCT program.

Clinical roles

Nurse program manager (NPM)

The NPM is a registered nurse with advanced education in nursing and administration. The traditional head nurse role can be expanded to that of

Table 34.1 Estimated Charges for US transplants, 1999. Adapted from Hauboldt [1].

	No. of transplants	Estimated average charge	Estimated total charge
Autologous transplants	10,855	$144,400	$1,567,462,000
Allogeneic related transplants	4175	$232,600	$971,105,000
Allogeneic unrelated transplants	1670	$293,100	$489,477,000
Total	16,700		$3,028,044,000

Table 34.2 Quality indicators for hematopoietic cell transplantation (HCT) programs.

Clinical indicators

Transplant-related complications	Patient satisfaction
Infectious complications	Quality of life
Intensive care utilization	Disease-free survival
Transplant-related mortality	

Administrative indicators

Length of stay	Patient satisfaction
Unplanned readmissions	Referring physician satisfaction
Resource utilization	

NPM if the position includes the oversight of patient care throughout the continuum. Through the course of a HCT procedure the patient will be cared for in the clinic, in the outpatient treatment center and in the inpatient unit. The NPM can oversee the nursing practice in all three settings so that continuity of care and a consistent standard of nursing practice can be assured.

The NPM is responsible for keeping abreast of the changes in medical practice and interpreting the impact on patients and the HCT program. New approaches to HCT may require changes in the care delivery system. Movement of protocols to the outpatient setting requires an integrated professional team to assure 24-h a day coverage for acute patient needs. Patients undergoing reduced intensity, nonmyeloablative HCT may never need an inpatient admission but still require 7-days a week access to experienced HCT physicians and nurses. The NPM organizes the nursing structure to meet the patient care requirements and monitors the outcomes.

An important aspect of the NPM role is to carefully review patient care on a regular basis to assure that changes in medical or nursing practice do not adversely impact patient outcomes. Third-party payers are also interested in basic clinical and administrative quality indicators. Table 34.2 outlines key clinical and administrative indicators requested by payers, including the number and type of transplants performed, complication rates, transplant-related mortality, disease-free survival, length of stay and readmission rates.

For HCT programs that do not have a single nursing leader with the responsibility for coordination of clinical care, one nurse may be responsible for case management, providing direct patient care and providing the nursing leadership for the program. In programs that transplant fewer than 20 patients per year the key team members may only consist of a physician and nurse(s), and be supported by a larger oncology division. In contrast, some centers that transplant over 200 patients per year have divided their teams to better manage the large number of patients. Several HCT programs have outpatient and inpatient teams with physician, nursing and administrative leadership in both settings.

Regardless of the program size and organizational structure, the nursing leader is accountable to the hospital or health care system leadership for the quality of care provided to HCT patients. The nursing leadership must be able to collaborate closely with the medical director of the HCT program in order to assure that program goals are in compliance with the overall health care system objectives, and also work closely with the administrative director/business manager and other key members of the HCT team.

Nurse case manager (NCM)

Case management is a term used to define the process whereby patients have one individual who helps to coordinate medical care. Social workers and nurses have traditionally filled these roles. Case management models differ significantly based on the patient population served, the country's health care system and the existing regional and/or national economic conditions. NCMs can work for the government, an insurance company, a hospital or a clinic. In each setting the NCM's role may have unique features, although the overall goal is to provide comprehensive patient care services within economic constraints [2]. The NCM working for the insurance company serves as an economic "gatekeeper" and frequently is the person who will authorize treatment. Government employed NCMs usually are assisting patients with chronic diseases who need help coordinating complex therapies. Hospital or clinic based NCMs represent the interests of the patient, the physicians and the health care system. NCMs have been credited with reducing costs of care while maintaining quality and satisfaction with managed care [3–6]. The title used for nurses responsible for the coordination of patients throughout the course of transplantation varies among HCT programs but is usually one of the following: nurse clinicians, nurse coordinators or NCMs.

Because there are no representative data on the optimal number of active HCT patients that each NCM full-time equivalent (FTE) can and should manage, an informal survey on staffing ratios was conducted by the administrative director's Special Interest Group from the American Society for Blood and Marrow Transplantation (ASBMT) in December 2001. The survey results for NCM ratios are summarized in Table 34.3.

There is no consistent ratio of NCM FTEs to number of transplants performed due to the wide variation in the scope and responsibilities of the position. Some HCT programs have the financial coordinator (see later in this chapter) assume a great deal of the approval process and in other centers the NCM assumes most of that responsibility. NCMs may also assume responsibility for ongoing monitoring of patients after their return to the referring physician, while in other HCT programs administrative staff perform the follow-up. The number of NCM FTEs may also be dependent upon on the complexity of the care required by each patient or protocol. As the number of recipients of nonmyeloablative transplants increases, managing the patients through a longer continuum of care becomes more challenging and requires more NCM time.

NCMs in most HCT programs serve as the main communication link between the HCT physician, the referring physician, the patient, and the third-party payer representative(s). A NCM can be a major asset to the HCT physicians and to the program. The roles and responsibilities of the NCM generally include patient and family teaching prior to

Table 34.3 Number of hematopoietic cell transplantation (HCT) patients per nurse case manager (NCM).

Transplant center	No. of adult transplant patients	No. of NCM (FTEs)
A	240	8
B	175–200	4
C	150	6.5
D	160–180	2
E	135	2
F	120	2
G	100	3
H	70	4
I–K	Under 30	1

FTE, full-time equivalent.

transplantation, coordinating the pretransplant testing, assuring compliance with protocol criteria, communicating with the third-party payer NCM and facilitating the patient's return to the referring physician practice. The NCM can also be responsible for obtaining informed consent after the HCT physician has thoroughly explained the risks and benefits associated with HCT. The role of the research nurse clinician is also included in the NCM role in some HCT programs. The research nurse clinician, in addition to fulfilling the case manager responsibilities, also facilitates the clinical research process. The research nurse clinician/case manager assures compliance with protocol eligibility requirements, collection of data elements and adverse event reporting.

Patient teaching

Patient and family teaching has always been an important responsibility for nurses. NCMs are the first and most consistent educators for patients considering the option of HCT. As more transplantation procedures are performed on an outpatient basis, the education of patients and families is of critical importance in order to provide safe and effective care [7]. There are a number of published books and webpages dedicated to educating HCT recipients. The material in print ranges from accurate and well written to biased and poorly presented. Susan Stewart, a former HCT patient and author of Chapter 36, has developed a number of excellent resources for patients and families. Experienced transplant physicians and nurses review the content. The website, www.bmtinfonet.org, contains current information including several books for patients and families. The most recent publications include *Bone Marrow and Blood Stem Cell Transplants a Guide for Patients* (2002), *Autologous Stem Cell Transplants: a Handbook for Patients* (2001) and *Across the Chasm, a Caregiver's Story* (2002), all published by Blood and Marrow Transplant Information Network, Highland Park, Illinois.

Even the best information available needs to be individualized for each patient and discussed at a time when the patient is ready to hear the information or read the material. Tailoring the education to the individual patient, timing the amount and content of information and assessing comprehension are included among the responsibilities of the NCM. If the patient or caregiver is unable to process information the lack of knowledge can result in poor outcomes [7]. NCMs need to have the skill to identify the learning styles of patients and families and be able to present information in a useful and timely fashion. Many patients are overwhelmed at the first visit to the HCT program and do not hear or comprehend much of the information presented (see Chapter 33). The NCM assigned to the individual should be able to assess the patient's ability to comprehend new information and to structure the teaching times and modify the materials necessary to assure understanding of the material.

It is helpful for patients, families and the NCM if the HCT physician includes the NCM in the discussion about the treatment plan. As new approaches and more treatment options become available it is not always clear what the most appropriate plan is for the individual patient. If the NCM hears the physician's discussion with the patient and family, it is then easier for the NCM to provide clear and accurate follow-up communication with the patient and family. The NCM can also use this opportunity to evaluate the patient's understanding of the discussion by observing the patient's verbal and nonverbal interactions.

Many HCT programs have handbooks for patients and families which are intended to guide them through the complex transplant process. Some patients are sophisticated, educated and compulsive about reading and carrying their handbook with them throughout the course of their treatment. Other patients do not have the intellectual capacity or, in some cases, the desire to know all of the details contained in the written material. NCMs can help the patient to understand the important information necessary to safely proceed with the transplant process and develop a plan to meet the needs of each patient. Individualized teaching by the NCM is essential for patient compliance with the treatment plan and contributes to successful outcomes [7].

Psychosocial assessment

Most HCT programs have a licensed clinical social worker assess patients prior to transplantation. These initial assessments are helpful to screen patients for obvious psychosocial issues and to help patients develop a plan for handling the stress associated with HCT. During the work-up phase for transplantation the NCM has many interactions with the patient and family. During these meetings or phone conversations the NCM assesses the patient's ability to comprehend information and comply with instructions. In addition, the NCM can assess the patient's ability to handle stress and help to identify coping strategies. Assessing psychological status prior to starting the transplant process can help the team plan for emotional difficulties during the transplant course [8]. The NCM can bring key members of the HCT team together to discuss appropriate interventions to help the patient handle the stress of transplantation.

Communication

In our model the NCM coordinates the testing and evaluation prior to HCT with the referring physician's office. There may be several weeks or months of preparation prior to starting the transplant process. The NCM can be the major link to the referring physician's office to obtain new information regarding the patient's status and to assist with scheduling return visits to the HCT program. Written and verbal communication from the transplant physician and NCM to the referring physician helps to facilitate a smooth transition from one health care provider to another. It is also reassuring to the patient to know that both medical teams are in communication regarding the treatment plan.

Authorization process

Obtaining authorization for testing or treatments is usually either the responsibility of the NCM or the financial coordinator. When the NCM has the role of obtaining authorization he or she can describe to the third-party payer the patient's clinical course and articulate the need for the requested procedure. The NCM can frequently reduce the need for the HCT physician to become involved in the more routine requests from the third-party payer. If the patient's HCT treatment plan is not an accepted standard of care or is a more novel approach to transplantation, the NCM can supply the protocol or the published data that are required in order for the third-party payer to consider the treatment for coverage. If the HCT program has a financial coordinator, this position works closely with the NCM.

Clinical nurse specialist (CNS)

A CNS is an advanced practice nurse with a master's degree in oncology nursing and additional experience or education in HCT. CNSs collaborate with all of the HCT team members to provide expert consultation regarding patient care. The traditional CNS role includes education, research and patient care. The CNS facilitates the ongoing professional development of nursing staff by providing orientation, bedside consultation with staff nurses, clinical updates and ongoing education regarding new protocols. The CNS develops and coordinates clinical research, collects data and assists with the analysis of the research. The CNS is a clinical expert who consults with members of the HCT team when planning new protocols and can assist in the development of systems to maximize positive outcomes [9]. Some HCT programs have incorporated the NCM role into the CNS role. In a smaller program the CNS may have additional responsibilities for the education of the general oncology nurses or assume some case management responsibilities. The transition from CNS to CNS/NCM involves a shift in emphasis from education and research to patient care management. This shift can result in a positive impact on the HCT program but will reduce the resources necessary for staff education and development [9].

There is certainly debate regarding the role of an advanced practice nurse within health care systems [10,11]. The continuing shortage of experienced nurses in oncology supports the role of educator and clinical expert in the CNS role. When the CNS is also responsible for case management, the education and training of HCT nurses may be adversely impacted. HCT programs that conduct clinical research studies may also be adversely affected by the shift in emphasis from research to case management. It is the opinion of the authors of this chapter that expanding the role of CNS to include case management is a decision that will ultimately undermine the strength of the nursing care in the HCT program.

Administrative roles

Administrative director/business manager

The administrative director/business manager is a position that is dedicated to the HCT program and one that has responsibility for the business and administrative components of the program, including strategic planning, financial performance, marketing, outreach, operating and capital budgets, fund-raising, and supervision of nonclinical staff. As stated previously, if a HCT program does not have someone dedicated to this role it is important that the members of the program understand which individuals within their organization perform these functions on the program's behalf, and that the program develops a strong working relationship with those administrators. Additionally, we suggest that the role should have direct involvement in contracting with third-party payers and other financial arrangements that directly affect reimbursement of services provided by the program; monitoring hospital and physician charges, costs, billings, collections, revenue and profit/loss; and physician and hospital billing of services provided by the program. The administrative director/business manager serves as the liaison between the HCT program and hospital/health care system administration. An individual in this position might possess a graduate degree or a bachelor's degree with extensive work experience in health care administration or a similar field.

An example of a key responsibility of an administrative director/business manager is the creation of a strategic business plan for the HCT program. A strategic plan for the HCT program serves many purposes including defining the program's goals and objectives for the upcoming 3–5 years, projecting growth and revenue, assuring that resources are committed to the program in order to meet the stated growth and resulting revenue, and identifying any current or future issues that could affect the program's ability to grow.

Key components of a HCT strategic plan might include:
- Executive summary.
- Program overview (combined, as well as separate adult and pediatric HCT program overviews if both services exist within the organization).
- Mission and vision of the program.
- SWOT analysis, i.e. **s**trengths of the program, **w**eaknesses of the program, **o**pportunities for growth and expansion, **t**hreats to growth and expansion.
- Strategic objectives for the stated time period (usually 3 years but no more than 5 years).
- Reimbursement issues and strategies.
- Cost reduction initiatives.
- Staffing.
- Finances.
- Program development resource plan.
- Marketing and outreach plan.
- Contingency scenarios.

The creation of the strategic plan brings together the key clinical and administrative team members from within the HCT program and from within the health care system, and enables them to mutually agree to the goals and objectives of the HCT program and the resources necessary to achieve these goals. Furthermore, the strategic plan serves as a document that can be used to educate others, including hospital/health care system senior leadership and boards of directors as well as potential financial donors, about the current state and future vision of the HCT program.

Once the strategic plan is presented (usually to the hospital or health care system chief executive officer and other senior leaders) and endorsed, it is the responsibility of the administrative director/business manager to assure that the key components are in place to implement the strategic plan and to proactively monitor the progress of the implementation. Ideally, the administrative director/business manager should meet with the key clinical and administrative HCT program team members on an annual basis so that the program can reassess all of the major areas, the strategic plan can be updated and modifications can be made as needed to implementing strategies.

A dedicated administrative director/business manager is accountable to the hospital or health care system leadership for the overall financial health of the HCT program. The administrative director works closely with the medical director of the HCT program, the NPM and other key members of the HCT team.

Financial coordinator

According to a recent report from the American Hospital Association, many of the hospitals in the USA are "sitting on the edge of financial viability" [12]. In fact, it is stated that in 2000, 32% of hospitals have negative total margins; that is, overall they are paid less than the cost of delivering care [12]. As noted earlier in this chapter the life-saving treatment that HCT programs offer comes at significant expense. While the estimated average charge for an unrelated allogeneic HCT procedure was stated as $293,100, a patient with serious complications can have charges in excess of $1 million or even $2 million. As payments to hospitals from third-party payers have continued to decrease, more pressure is placed on programs, particularly programs with high charges such as HCT, to assure that adequate reimbursement will be received from the patient or his or her third-party payer.

A role that serves the needs of both the patient and the health care system is that of a dedicated financial coordinator. A financial coordinator can ensure patient access as well as maximum financial reimbursement for patients undergoing treatment in the HCT program. This goal is accomplished by coordination of financial clearances and treatment authorizations required for meeting patient, third-party payer, health care system and HCT program needs. Treatment authorizations from third-party payers assure that the hospital and physicians are paid for the technical and professional services that are provided to the patient, and that the patient is only liable for the monies that his or her third-party payer does not cover. Without appropriate approval from the third-party payer the patient and/or the health care system could be responsible for literally hundreds of thousands of dollars, or more, for care provided.

The financial coordinator performs a complete financial assessment for the patient at the time of initial consultation in the HCT program. This assessment includes researching and verifying the patient's third-party payer coverage and its limitations (including transplant benefit maximum, lifetime maximum, outpatient pharmacy benefits, home infusion benefits), discussing with the patient and family the out-of-pocket expenses for which the patient will be responsible during the course of care, and providing financial counseling related to the cost of the HCT treatment. Another role of the financial coordinator is to pursue every avenue in order to obtain the optimal level of coverage from the patient's third-party payer. Related activities include appealing denials, benefit maximum and other limiting events and managing these appeals until they are resolved.

There are patients who do not have health care coverage through a third-party payer or may not have adequate coverage to pay for their HCT. In the USA alone the number of people without health insurance was 38.7 million in 2000 [13]. In those unfortunate situations the financial coordinator works with the patient and his/her family to explore all available options, including government-funded programs and self-funding by the patient/family.

The financial coordinator interfaces with representatives from the third-party payers to discuss protocol appropriateness and to educate regarding the necessity for various types of HCT, working closely with the HCT program physicians and NCMs in presenting this information. This role is that of an integral member of the HCT team and one that must establish credibility with the team in matters that deal with patient health care coverage and reimbursement. He or she presents patient financial profiles at meetings and succinctly summarizes financial issues with a recommended course of action for resolution.

Search coordinator

The National Marrow Donor Program (NMDP) facilitates unrelated donor transplants through a worldwide network with over 130 NMDP transplant centers in the USA and many foreign countries [14]. Programs that participate in the NMDP as a transplant center for matched unrelated donor transplants are obligated via their contract with the NMDP to have a designated marrow coordinator position [15]. In addition to this individual's various responsibilities within the HCT program, the NMDP states that his or her responsibilities with the NMDP include, but are not limited to, coordination with NMDP protocols and procedures and arranging for hematopoietic cell collection and transportation [15].

Depending on the size of the HCT program this function may be incorporated into an existing position (including a NCM or financial coordinator) or it may be a separate and distinct position(s) such as a search coordinator. This role is typically responsible for managing the search process for unrelated donors beginning with the HCT physician's request to search unrelated donor registries and continuing until a match is found or until the search process is terminated. Throughout this process the search coordinator engages in regular communication with the NMDP and other registries, the HCT team (including physicians, NCMs, HCT laboratory, human leukocyte antigen (HLA) laboratory, data management, financial coordinators and others), the patient's referring physician, and the patient.

If a donor is located the search coordinator works in close and constant contact with the NMDP, the donor collection center, the transplant center HCT laboratory and the transplant center HCT team as the plans are developed to harvest bone marrow or to collect blood hematopoietic cells, to transport the graft and, ultimately, to administer the graft.

The NMDP recently estimated that there is an average of 3000 patients searching the NMDP registry at any given time; as of March 31, 2002, the total number of potential volunteer donors was 4,646,701 [16]. As treatment options utilizing unrelated donor hematopoietic cells continue to increase, so will the work of the search coordinators.

Conclusion

Clinical and administrative leadership is essential for successful HCT programs. The physician leadership sets the clinical and research goals and the nonphysician leadership operationalizes these goals within the health care system. Hospital and nursing administrative structures do not always support the model of designated clinical and administrative leaders for the HCT program. Many hospitals employ "silo management"—the HCT outpatient clinic reports to clinic administration, the HCT inpatient unit reports to nursing administration, the nonclinical staff may report to the cancer service line and the physicians may be a separate entity from all of these other components. For optimum success, a HCT program should consider having key leadership roles managing or responsible for all of the clinical and administrative components that represent the HCT continuum of care. The model of a dedicated NPM and administrative director is one way to assure that the needs of the entire HCT program are represented.

A HCT program is a marvelously unique and dynamic enterprise: it combines patient care, technology and research; it offers a potentially curative treatment for patients who otherwise face an uncertain future; it employs a multidisciplinary team that encompasses many clinical disciplines and includes administrative functions; it often represents a source of significant cost, staff, resources and income to its parent health care system. The success of a HCT program today is measured by more than its treatment results alone—it is measured by success in every facet of its operation, including patient care, clinical outcomes, research and administration.

As in all clinical programs and businesses, one of the keys to success is having a motivated and educated staff collaborating with one another for a common goal. HCT programs with dedicated physician leadership and involved and committed individuals with clinical and administrative responsibilities have the greatest opportunity to provide high-quality patient care and to also sustain financial viability. The HCT programs that employ an encompassing view of success will be best positioned to treat patients for many years to come.

References

1. Hauboldt R. Research report. Cost implications of human organ and tissue transplantation, an update. Milliman and Roberston, Inc. Available at http://www.milliman.com, accessed June 14, 2002.
2. Sherman JJ, Johnson PK. Nursing care management. *Qual Assur Util Rev* 1991; **6**: 142–5.
3. Barry TL, Davis DJ, Meara JG et al. Case management: an evaluation at children's hospital of Los Angeles, CA, USA. *Nurs Econ* 2002; **20**: 22–7.
4. Aliotta SL. Case management programs: investment in the future. *HMO Prac* 1995; **9**: 174–8.
5. Yarmo D. Research directions for case management. *Care Manag J* 1998; **7**: 84–91.
6. Schroeder C, Trehearne B, Ward D. Expanded role of nursing in ambulatory care. Part II. Impact on outcomes of cost, quality and patient satisfaction. *Nurs Econ* 2000; **18**: 71–8.

7 Sagehorn KK, Russell CL, Ganong LH. Implementation of a patient-family pathway: effects on patients and families. *Clin Nurse Spec* 1996; **13**: 119–22.
8 Molassiotis A. Further evaluation of a scale to screen for risk of emotional difficulties in bone marrow transplant recipients. *J Advan Nurs* 1999; **29**: 922–7.
9 Wells N, Erickson S, Spinella J. Role transition from clinical nurse specialist to clinical nurse specialist/case manager. *J Nurs Admin* 1996; **26**: 23–8.
10 Alvarez CA. When is the case manager role best filled by an advanced practice nurse? *Clin Nurse Spec* 1996; **10**(2): 106.
11 Sohl-Kreiger R, Lagaard MW, Scherrer J. Nursing case management: relationships as a strategy to improve care. *Clin Nurse Spec* 1996; **10**: 107–13.
12 American Hospital Association. AHA White Paper. The state of hospitals' financial health. Available at: http://www.aha.org/ar/Advocacy/Content/Wp2002HospFinances.doc, accessed June 14, 2002.
13 US Census Bureau. US Department of Commerce News, September 28, 2001 [press release, CB01-162]. Available at: *http://www.census.gov/Press-Relase/www/2001/cb01–162html*, accessed June 14, 2002.
14 National Marrow Donor Program. NMDP US transplant centers. Available at: *http://www.marrow.org/NMDP/transplant_centers.html*, accessed June 14, 2002.
15 National Marrow Donor Program. Transplant center participation agreement, revised. 11598; Section 2(f),(i), 1999, p. 6.
16 National Marrow Donor Program. General facts and figures. Available at: *http://www.marrow.org/NMDP/general_facts_figures.html*, accessed June 14, 2002.

35
Rosemary C. Ford, Judy Campbell & Juanita Madison

Nursing Issues in Hematopoietic Cell Transplantation

Introduction

Caring for patients undergoing hematopoietic cell transplantation (HCT) is one of the most challenging and rewarding of all the subspecialties of nursing. These patients require nurses with expertise in assessing the acute, subtle and unique clinical changes of HCT. In addition to the knowledge base of oncology nursing, the specialty of HCT nursing requires expertise in addressing diseases unique to HCT patients such as veno-occlusive disease (VOD) and graft-vs.-host disease (GVHD). Most of the nursing effort is focused on the post-transplant phase with managing side-effects, toxicities and preventing complications caused by the high-dose chemo-radiotherapy given to prepare for HCT and the consequences of GVHD [1]. Nurses are the members of the HCT multidisciplinary team that spend the most time with the patients, and often are the first to identify the need for specific interventions. Nurses must have expert psychosocial skills as they support the patients and their significant others through decisions and acute clinical changes encountered during the process.

Supporting medical research, the foundation of HCT care, is another factor that attracts nurses to this subspecialty. Integrating new research initiatives into clinical care and being on the front line as new therapies evolve to change standard practice is very exciting. Nurses feel they are working in a medical arena offering the best possible therapy to their patients. Those nurses who stay with this specialty over a number of years have witnessed therapies used in phase I research studies become the standards upon which current clinical research is based. These nurses can readily identify the improvements in patient outcomes that have occurred in the field of HCT over the past three decades in curing specific diseases, as well as prophylaxis and treatment of GVHD, VOD, infectious diseases and symptom management. In addition, expanding HCT to treat additional diseases, such as autoimmune diseases and solid tumors, has required nurses to become familiar with disease processes beyond hematologic malignancies. The recent efforts to treat patients using non-myeloablative-conditioning regimens have presented new challenges to HCT nurses. Not only are these patients often older than those eligible for myeloablative regimens, but patterns in their clinical courses in areas such as acute GVHD presentation do not match those of myeloablative transplants.

There has been a major change in the site of HCT care from inpatient units to outpatient clinics with the goal of containing costs while maintaining quality care [2]. This change was made possible by major improvements in antiemetics, antibiotics with less frequent dosing and improved ambulatory infusion devices [3]. Patients often receive all of their conditioning and hematopoietic stem cell (HSC) infusion in a clinic setting, and are admitted for clinical reasons usually fever or mucositis pain. Patients are also discharged from the hospital based on more liberal criteria than in the past. This change has resulted in increasingly complex ambulatory clinics where the focus of nursing-care shifts from first-hand assessment and care to teaching the caregivers to provide some of these services [4]. In addition, the average acuity of the HCT patient populations on inpatient units has markedly increased with patients acutely ill with complicated multisystem issues. It has also led to most patients having multiple admissions and discharges in the months after transplant. Nurses are responsible for ensuring continuity of care and safety as the responsibility for care passes from one site to another [5].

The intensity of therapy requires further specialization of HCT nurses to meet the care needs of these patients. Transplant centers organize nursing support in a variety of ways depending on their operational structure. At most centers, specific nurses have a role in the initial intake of patients into the program. Most outpatient clinics have a case manager structure, which allows for continuity of care coordination throughout the transplant process. HCT patients often spend large amounts of time in outpatient infusion areas. These patients require nursing expertise different from that of other oncology outpatients. Inpatient units either have a transplant unit or designate a portion of an oncology unit for HCT care with specific nurses assigned to this area. Each center needs to give serious consideration as to whether to keep HCT patients requiring intensive care on the HCT unit or to transfer them to an intensive care unit (ICU). In either case, nurses with expertise in both HCT and intensive care are required. Discharging HCT patients from an inpatient unit to the outpatient setting is often complicated, and many centers have specific nurses with expertise in managing these transitions.

Complex research protocols often require the coordination of a specific nurse who works closely with the principal medical investigator. These nurses are responsible for ensuring protocol data documentation and the reporting of adverse advents. They are key in ensuring that protocol coordination is seamless when patients transfer to and from the inpatient and outpatient settings. They are the primary resource for medical and nursing staff regarding protocol implementation. In addition, HCT patient care provides ideal opportunities for nursing research. Nursing studies have been conducted in a number of areas including quality of life and symptom management.

Achieving and maintaining an expert nursing staff is a constant challenge for institutions with HCT programs. Initial orientation of a nurse with oncology experience generally takes 6–8 weeks. After this time the nurse can be counted in staffing patterns, but is not considered fully competent until they have completed their 1st year. The nurse/patient ratio is also an issue that must be considered when planning a HCT unit. Most inpatient units staff on a one nurse to two–three patient ratio. This is usually a much lower ratio than on other oncology units and may need to be justified to hospital administrators. Patients develop strong feelings of trust and confidence in specific nurses, and facilitating work schedules to maximize these relationships can be a challenge for nurse managers.

The purpose of this chapter is to describe the nurse's role at the various phases of the HCT process. Tables detail the key nursing responsibilities of assessment, teaching and care coordination at each phase. They do not list basics such as vital signs and weighing the patient.

Assessment includes not only the basics of physical assessment, but also the ability of the patient and caregivers to cope with this intense experience.

Teaching must be individualized to each specific patient and caregiver situation. There is no substitution for one-on-one assessment and teaching by the patient's primary nurse [6]. One-on-one encounters allow for assessment of the patient's assimilation of the required information and a time for the patient to ask whatever questions are of foremost concern. Teaching can be accomplished in a variety of methods, including written materials with photographs or illustrations and videotapes. Classes are also an effective method for centers that perform a large number of transplants.

Coordination of care for these patients is extremely complex. Nurses assess the patient's and family's strengths and weaknesses and plan interventions to assist them to integrate this intense process into their lives. Nurses must include clinical issues, operational resources, research requirements and the patient's needs and desires when planning care.

Prework-up/prior to arrival at transplant center
(Table 35.1)

The first interface many patients have with an HCT transplant program occurs at the time when they come for a second opinion. Other patients make a consultation appointment to compare a particular program with other centers they are considering. These patients meet with a transplant physician to review their options, a financial counselor and a nurse. The nurse's role is to assist the patient with this decision by explaining the logistics of the program including the usual length of stay on the inpatient unit and how much of the transplant process will be managed on an outpatient basis [7]. Many patients are interested in the nursing services at the program they are considering and ask questions about the nurse/patient ratio. The responsibilities of the patient's caregiver are reviewed as well. At that time many families are concerned with the logistics of relocating and incorporating this intense therapy into their lives. These patients present with a myriad of questions and the nurse must be versatile in meeting the patients' and families' informational needs. Nurses often are also responsible for giving information regarding the transplant program to physicians and nurses from the referring center as well as third-party payers.

Table 35.1 Prework-up/prior to patient's arrival at transplant center.

Assessment
Understanding of overall transplant process and time commitment
Current symptoms from previous therapies or disease
Current coping ability
Current pain
Current blood product requirements
Sedation preference for procedures

Teaching
Length of time for work-up, mobilization and transplant process
Role of caregiver

Care coordination
Contact referring physician's office to obtain report
Confirm financial clearance
Confirm housing plan

Table 35.2 Work-up.

Assessment
Patient's current fears and concerns
Barriers to learning
Current pain
Knowledge of disease status
Knowledge of transplant process
Knowledge of patient's rights and responsibilities when participating in medical research
Usual coping strategies
Level of fatigue and usual sleep patterns
Patient's experience in other health care environments
Identified caregiver(s)' commitment
Identified caregiver(s)' barriers to learning
Allergies
Current medications and knowledge of purpose
Compliance in taking medications
Current central venous access
History of central venous access

Teaching
Clinic logistics including how to access care after-hours
Importance of having a caregiver during various phases of transplant process
Purpose of procedures, laboratory tests and scans required for work-up
Overall transplant process
Usual complications of transplant
Central venous catheter preop teaching

Care coordination
Assess ability to adhere to work-up schedule
Confirm financial clearance for transplant
Social work assessment
Nutrition assessment

Work-up (Table 35.2)

Once a patient has met initial screening and has decided to undergo HCT at a specific center, the nurse's primary responsibility becomes education. The patient must understand the specifics of the rigorous evaluation. The coordination of care during this phase is especially critical if the patient has an unrelated donor. The completion of work-up and the initiation of conditioning must start on an exact date to allow HSC infusion on the planned date of HSC procurement. The generosity of the volunteer donors must be respected and accommodated.

Preconditioning (Table 35.3)

The nurse plays an important role in the informed consent process, supporting the medical staff's explanations and plans to ensure, as much as possible, that the patient is making an informed decision regarding HCT.

Donor preparation (Table 35.4)

Donors have been called the "forgotten patients" of transplant. The HCT recipient, appropriately, is the center of focus for the transplant team.

Table 35.3 Preconditioning.

Assessment
Knowledge of need for compliance during conditioning regimen
Knowledge of side-effects to report during conditioning
Caregiver's ability to report symptoms
Caregiver's ability to utilize ambulatory infusion pump if required
History of antiemetics
Assure appropriate patient central venous access
Purpose of viral and/or fungal prophylaxis
Purpose of GVHD prophylaxis if appropriate

Teaching
Treatment plan and schedule for chemotherapy and TBI
Antiemetic schedule and importance of compliance
Care of central venous access
Caregiver education for ambulatory infusion pump if hydration given in ambulatory setting
Importance of laboratory monitoring
Purpose of hydration
Symptoms to report
Differences between previous chemotherapy and conditioning chemotherapy
Purpose of allopurinol if ordered
Importance of compliance with pneumocystis prophylaxis compliance

Care coordination
Research consents
Chemotherapy and TBI order verification with protocol
Dosimetry and simulation appointment with radiation oncology if applicable
Plasma exchange if required
Pager/cell phone for patient if conditioning to start in the clinic

GVHD, graft-vs.-host disease; TBI, total body irradiation.

Table 35.4 Donor work-up.

Assessment
Current fears and concerns
Barriers to learning
Donor screening per American Association of Blood Bank requirements
Knowledge of donation process
Knowledge of patient's rights and responsibilities when participating in medical research
Allergies

Teaching
Donation plan and schedule
Importance of laboratory monitoring
Preop teaching if applicable
Symptom management

Care coordination
Assess ability to adhere to work-up schedule
Research consents
Storage of autologous red cells if marrow donation planned

However, donors also have concerns about their own health and the procedures they will undergo. It is ideal for donors to have a primary nurse with whom they can establish a relationship who can prepare them for the hematopoietic cell collection and monitor them throughout the procedure.

Table 35.5 Mobilization and collection (autologous patients and allogenic donors). From [8].

Assessment
Adequacy of veins for apheresis if applicable
Knowledge of care of central venous access (if applicable)

Teaching
Purpose of monitoring CBC, $CD34^+$ cells, electrolytes
Purpose and care of central venous catheter if applicable
Specific medications used to mobilize and usual side-effects if applicable
Subcutaneous injections if applicable
Temperature monitoring
Importance of increasing calcium intake
Medications to avoid (i.e. aspirin)

Care coordination
Subcutaneous injections—in clinic or self-administered

Mobilization and collection (autologous patients and allogeneic donors) (Table 35.5 [8])

Nursing care during mobilization must be individualized to the specific medical protocols being utilized as well as the response of the donor or autologous patient [9]. The nurse must stay in daily contact with the patient during this time as collection schedules can change based on cell yield. The nurse needs to assist in determining whether it is necessary to have a long-term central venous access catheter inserted before mobilization, if a short-term central venous access catheter is sufficient or if vein-to-vein access may be possible.

Conditioning (Table 35.6)

Conditioning regimens may be administered in the outpatient or inpatient setting, based upon the type of preparatory regimen chosen, the availability of 24-h triage and supportive services, and the available level of caregiver support. Chemotherapy used for traditional myeloablative transplants is administered at higher doses than conventional chemotherapy. Acute toxicities may manifest more rapidly and intensely than with standard-dose therapy [9]. The nurse's role is key in supporting the patient and caregiver in the management of acute needs [3]. Toxicities associated with high-dose chemotherapy and/or irradiation therapy require vigilant monitoring with special emphasis on assessment of fluid, gastrointestinal tract and renal status.

Care must be available to outpatients 24 h a day, 7 days a week in order to safely provide for patients whose conditions may rapidly deteriorate. In general, successful management in the outpatient setting during the conditioning phase of transplant requires a high level of continuous caregiver support. Outpatient teaching places special emphasis on use of ambulatory infusion pumps, patient and caregiver ability to assess, report and manage the side-effects of high-dose therapy (Table 35.7), and access to 24 h emergency care and support telephone numbers [6]. Printed patient and caregiver teaching reference materials containing outpatient guidelines and how to access emergency care are useful tools for the reinforcement of patient and caregiver teaching [3].

Bone marrow harvest (Table 35.8 on p. 475)

The technique of harvesting marrow is essentially the same for allogeneic related donors, unrelated donors and autologous patients Patient education will prepare donors for anticipated side-effects, emphasizing those to

Table 35.6 Conditioning.

Assessment

Knowledge of potential side-effects of high-dose chemotherapy or radiation therapy

Response to high-dose chemotherapy and/or TBI

Ability to perform self-care and infection control preventative measures (hand washing, personal hygiene, oral care, etc.)

Renal and fluid status: intake and output; postural vital signs; daily or BID weights; breath sounds, heart sounds, skin turgor; laboratory tests: serum electrolytes, blood urea nitrogen, creatinine

Nutritional status: weight, skin turgor, amount, content and patterns of nutritional intake

Outpatients:
- Patient/caregiver ability to assess, report, and manage side-effects of high-dose chemotherapy and/or TBI
- Knowledge of phone numbers to access emergency care and support 24 h a day

Teaching

Treatment plan and schedule, including administration of IV hydration, antiemetics, uroprotectants and/or other medications

Potential side-effects of high-dose chemotherapy and/or irradiation therapy (nausea, vomiting, mucositis, diarrhea, fever, etc.)

Prevention and management of side-effects

Level of caregiver support required

Guidelines for preventing infection:
- Handwashing
- Personal hygiene
- Nutrition/diet guidelines for immunosuppressed patients
- Avoiding activities with high risk for infection

Outpatients:
- Signs/symptoms requiring inpatient hospitalization
- Access to 24 h triage and emergency care phone numbers

Care coordination

Clinic appointment schedules or admission to inpatient unit

Pre and post-conditioning therapy IV hydration and medications (antiemetics, uroprotectants, etc.)

Chemotherapy administration

TBI schedules

Patient and caregiver education: one-on-one instruction or attendance at caregiver classes

BID, twice daily; IV, intravenous; TBI, total body irradiation.

---

report to health care providers. Nurses educating donors should emphasize the expectations for the marrow harvest, including pain at sites of marrow aspirations, admission to hospital day-surgery settings, anticipated discharge from day-surgery to home, site care post-harvest and follow-up visits.

Patients receiving unrelated donor marrow will need instruction regarding when and how the donor marrow will arrive for infusion. Donor marrow is harvested at the medical center closest to the donor's resident state or country and the marrow flown to the patient's location accompanied by an Unrelated Donor Program courier.

Autologous patients will have their marrow harvested and cryopreserved (frozen) prior to receiving conditioning therapy.

Transplant phase (Table 35.9 on p. 476)

The actual stem-cell product infusion is very similar to a blood transfusion. The rate of infusion and potential side-effects depend on whether the product is cryopreserved or noncryopreserved. Dimethylsulfoxide (DMSO) is generally used as a preservative for cryopreserving autologous marrow, periperal blood stem cells or umbilical cord blood. Infusion of products cryopreserved with DMSO tends to cause a significant number of transient, self-limited side-effects amenable to premedication [10]. Complications from infusion of noncryopreserved products may include volume overload and pulmonary abnormalities from fat or cellular debris emboli. In addition, patients may experience symptoms similar to blood transfusion reactions (chills, urticaria, fever, etc.) [6]. Patients and caregivers benefit from nursing descriptions of the steps in the infusion procedure, potential side-effects, premedications and treatments to minimize side-effects. Important care coordination considerations for nursing staff include ensuring initiation of GVHD prophylaxis pretransplant for allogeneic patients per institution-specific protocols and timing stem-cell product prehydration and premedications with the arrival of the products on the unit or the patient care area.

Pre-engraftment (Table 35.10 on p. 477)

The majority of complications that occur prior to engraftment are the result of high-dose conditioning regimen associated toxicities and/or administration of immunosuppressive medications [6]. Nursing care is directed at strategies to prevent potential complications, early detection and prompt implementation of appropriate interventions if complications develop. Systematic and astute assessment skills are required to identify subtle clues indicative of multiple potential complications [1].

Coordination of care can be very complex during this phase. Patients often require administration of multiple red blood cell and platelet transfusions, intravenous fluids and parenteral nutrition, and multiple intravenous medications. Whether in the inpatient or ambulatory clinic setting, infusing all required intravenous medications and fluids presents

Table 35.7 Quick reference for symptoms. Reproduced with permission from the Seattle Cancer Care Alliance Patient Education Program.

Areas of concern	Critical emergency **DIAL 911** Tell medics to take patient to University of Washington Medical Center Hospital	Call clinic now 8:00 am—12:00 am call clinic 12:00 am—8:00 am after hours
Alertness, consciousness, activity	• Unconscious • Unable to arouse • Seizure	• New or increased confusion • Change in level of alertness • Mood changes: irritable, tearful, agitated • Change in vision • Sleeplessness • Falling down • Numbness, tingling or loss of movement in limbs • Dizziness • Lethargic • Change in energy level • Tremors/shakiness • Unable to get around • Difficulty swallowing
Bleeding	• Uncontrollable, consistent bleeding • Patient is unconscious	• New or increased bleeding • Bloody urine • New bruising • Unable to stop nosebleed • Bloody diarrhea • Vomiting of blood • Patient falls or is injured • One or more feminine pad per hour is used • Little red or purple spots on the skin
Breathing	• Not breathing • Choking—not moving air into chest	• Trouble breathing • Gets "winded" more easily with minimal activity • Feeling as if cannot get enough air • Trouble breathing when laying flat • Wheezing with breaths • New or recurrent cough • Persistent continuous cough • Coughing blood or green/yellow material
Central venous catheter (Hickman line)	• Line open to air and patient short of breath • Clamp line immediately	• Line broken or leaking • Face, neck, exit site swelling • Inability to flush • Line fell out • Headache related to infusions • Redness, swelling or tenderness at exit site • Drainage from exit site • Constant or uncontrolled diarrhea
Diarrhea		• New onset diarrhea • Diarrhea with fever and abdominal cramping • Whole pills passed in stool • Greater than five times each day • Stool which is bloody, burgundy or black • Mild abdominal cramping
Fatigue	• Unable to wake up	• Dizziness • Fatigue is getting worse • Too tired to get out of bed or walk to the bathroom • Staying in bed all day
Fever/chills		• Fever >1°C (1.8°F) above usual • Cold symptoms (runny nose, watery eyes, sneezing, coughing) • Shaking chills, temperature may be normal • Temperature >38.3°C (100.9°F) by mouth

Table 35.7 (cont'd)

Areas of concern	Critical emergency **DIAL 911** Tell medics to take patient to University of Washington Medical Center Hospital	Call clinic now 8:00 am—12:00 am call clinic 12:00 am—8:00 am after hours
Mouth pain/mucositis	• Not breathing	• Having difficulty breathing • Cannot swallow • Choking • Bright red blood in mouth • Pain not controlled by medication • White patches or sores appear on gums or mouth • Difficulty swallowing food or fluid
Nausea/vomiting		• Nausea persists without control from antinausea medications • Vomit shoots out for a distance (projectile vomiting) • Uncontrolled, constant nausea and vomiting • Blood or "coffee ground" appearing material in the vomit • Medicine not kept down because of vomiting • Weakness or dizziness along with nausea/vomiting • Severe stomach pain while vomiting
Pain	• Severe chest/arm pain • Severe squeezing or pressure in chest	• New or uncontrolled pain in body • New headache • Chest discomfort • Pounding heart • Heart "flip-flop" feeling • Painful central line site or area of "tunnel" • Burning in chest or stomach • Pain or burning while urinating • Strong stomach pain • Pain with infusion of medications or fluids into central line • New abdominal or back pain
Rash		• Sudden onset body rash • Rash with severe pain
Swelling		• Sudden swelling with or without pain • Swollen legs, hands
Urination		• Unable to urinate for more than 8 h • Bloody urine • Painful urination

a major challenge. Many transplant centers place double lumen central venous catheters for use throughout the transplant. Patients may require additional intravenous access during the pre-engraftment phase in order to administer all of the required intravenous medications and fluids. Additionally, patients usually require frequent collections of blood specimens, diagnostic procedures, examinations or appointments with various members of the health care team, coupled with ongoing needs for education, completing activities of daily living and psychosocial support. The nurse is responsible for collaborating with the patient, caregiver(s) and other health care professionals to develop plans that incorporate all patient care needs into manageable schedules.

Early post-engraftment (Table 35.11 on p. 478)

GVHD in the allogeneic transplant recipient may be difficult to distinguish from symptoms caused by infections or residual side-effects of high-dose conditioning regimens. Nurses, often the first to assess patients' signs and symptoms, must have a thorough understanding of the pathophysiology, clinical manifestations and management of GVHD [6,8].

The nurse plays a key role in preparing the patient and family for discharge from the hospital.

Criteria for transition from inpatient to outpatient settings will differ based on institutional policies, the patient's condition, the availability of skilled outpatient teams and family caregiver support. Caregivers must be knowledgeable in recognizing, managing and appropriately reporting complications, and be competent in performing aspects of the patient's care. Detailed and structured discharge teaching is necessary to ensure adequate understanding of critical information by patients and caregivers [11].

Table 35.8 Bone marrow harvest.

Assessment

Results of preharvest donor work-up
Preharvest physical reassessment
Verification of informed consent
Understanding of bone marrow harvest process and potential complications
Understanding of signs/symptoms to report to health care team post-harvest
Ability to access 24-h triage and emergency care phone numbers

Teaching

Bone marrow harvest process and procedures:
- Hospital admission—location, schedule
- Marrow aspiration sites
- Autologous blood transfusions
- Hospital discharge criteria
- Site care post-bone marrow harvest
- Post-harvest iron supplements

Potential complications:
- Pain
- Infection
- Anemia related to blood loss
- Nausea and vomiting (if general anesthesia used)
- Dehydration

Signs/symptoms to report to health care team
Access to 24-h triage and emergency care phone numbers
Patients receiving unrelated donor marrow:
- Marrow harvested at donor residence state/country
- Marrow arrives via courier
- Anticipated time of unrelated donor marrow arrival (often late evening)

Care coordination

Operating room scheduling
Type and cross-match for autologous stored unit, if stored
Day surgery hospital admission time and location
Discharge teaching
Discharge medications
Post-harvest outpatient appointment and lab draws (generally, CBC with differential and platelets)

CBC, complete blood count.

Hospital readmissions after initial hospital discharge to the ambulatory care setting frequently occur during the early engraftment phase. Coordination and communication of patient care issues between the nursing staff of the inpatient unit and the ambulatory care setting allows for smooth transition and continuity of care. Particular attention needs to be given to caregivers' ability to continuously cope with their multiple demands and roles [8].

Intensive care management of the transplant patient

Most transplant patients require complex, high acuity levels of care throughout their inpatient stay [12]. It is estimated that up to 40% of patients undergoing HCT will require nursing skills typical of most ICUs, including hemodynamic monitoring, noninvasive cardiac monitoring, administration of inotropic and vasoactive medications to support blood pressure, and mechanical ventilatory support [13,14]. The need for ICU support varies from center to center, especially in relation to the type of HCT performed (autologous, allogenic and, especially, unrelated).

Management of critically ill transplant patients combines the complexity of oncology and critical care nursing skills, presenting significant challenges to the provision of expert nursing care. Oncology nurses generally are not trained or skilled in the management of critically ill patients. Conversely, critical care nurses generally do not have an oncology background. Patients with critical care complications may be transferred to a critical care unit. However, many institutions have worked towards merging the two specialties of oncology nursing and critical care nursing to meet the needs of these patients by training transplant nurses to provide intensive care on the transplant unit or by cross-training ICU staff to specialized transplant procedures [12]. Challenges to each approach include the maintenance of nurses' competency. Transplant nurses may find it difficult to keep critical care skills up-to-date if the volume of transplant patients requiring critical care is low. Critical care nurses may face similar issues in maintaining transplant competencies and skills. Each institution must evaluate the available resources, outcomes of care and the cost-effectiveness of cross-training staff and maintaining clinical competencies when determining models for providing critical care to transplant patients [12,15]. Despite substantial progress in treating the complications of HCT, the mortality rate in ICUs remains high, especially in those patients requiring mechanical ventilation [14].

Relapse post-transplant

Some patients may fail to respond to treatment or, after initial response, relapse of underlying disease may occur [16]. For patients with disease recurrence, options for care may include standard chemotherapy, a second HCT or palliative care. Nurses play a significant role in clarifying the treatment options presented by the medical staff. Nurses also serve as advocates for the patient and family, helping to communicate the patient's individual goals clearly to the health care team.

Discharge (Table 35.12 on p. 479)

Preparation for long-term recovery begins during the treatment phase and is part of the ongoing nursing-care process. Discharge education is provided by nurses to review possible late effects of transplantation, such as chronic GVHD and infectious risks, and make recommendations related to activities of daily living for the 1st year after HCT (Table 35.13 on p. 480). It is also a good opportunity to discuss possible cognitive, sexual and emotional concerns. Some large centers accomplish this educational goal through individual classes. This effort facilitates the transition from the transplant center to the care of the referring physician. Patients often express feelings of anxiety when leaving the security of the transplant program that they have relied on so heavily. If the patient is being discharged from the transplant center to their referring physician, identifying a designated contact person or group at the transplant center for both the patient and the referring physician for consultation on transplant-related problems is essential. This contact person can decrease the anxiety of the patient and caregiver and provide the referring physician access to transplant expertise and continuity of the medical plan. General guidelines should be provided by the transplant center for the referring physician that details the important aspects of long-term care of the transplant recipient [17].

Long-term recovery (Table 35.14 on p. 481)

Nurses, under the guidance of the transplant center medical team, can successfully act as liaison between the referring physician and the transplant physicians. They can collect important and pertinent information to triage transplant-related problems and, after discussion with the

Table 35.9 Transplant.

Assessment

Preinfusion:
- Knowledge of stem cell infusion process
- Renal and fluid status: intake and output; postural vital signs; weight; breath sounds; skin turgor; laboratory tests: serum electrolytes, blood urea nitrogen, creatinine
- Response to prior red blood cell transfusions
- Adequacy of venous access for infusion of stem cells (central venous access required for infusion of cryopreserved stem cell products due to hyperosmolar infusate; central venous access preferred for noncryopreserved nonmanipulated products)
- Availability emergency medications

During infusion:
- Frequent assessment to detect the early onset of potential infusion-related complications

Post-infusion:
- Tolerance of cell infusion
- Renal function and fluid status: intake and output (general goal—maintain urine output 2–3 mL/kg/h); presence of hematuria)

Teaching

Location for stem cell infusion (inpatient vs. outpatient setting)
Anticipated timing of stem cell product arrival on unit or in outpatient department
Stem cell infusion procedure:

Cryopreserved
- Prehydration
- Premedications (e.g. antiemetics, diphenhydramine, hydrocortisone, acetaminophen, etc.)
- Transport of cryopreserved cells
- Thawing of cells at bedside
- Infusion of cells via central venous catheter

Noncryopreserved
- Premedication (if patient previously experienced transfusion reactions to red blood cell transfusions)
- Transport of cells to patient care area

Infusion (generally, via central venous catheter)
Potential complications:

Cryopreserved
- Reactions to cryoprotectant (DMSO) including nausea/vomiting, facial flushing, hypertension, hypotension, bradycardia, tachycardia, cardiac arrhythmia, chest tightness, cough, chills, fever, abdominal cramping, diarrhea, headache, transient taste and smell of DMSO, appearance of red urine post-infusion
- Prevention/treatment of nausea secondary to DMSO by sucking on or inhaling smell of fresh cut up oranges
- Transfusion reactions (if allogeneic)
- Volume overload (although volume generally <10 mL/kg)
- Allergic reaction
- Pulmonary microembolism (clumps of cell debris may occur after thawing): shortness of breath, dyspnea, cough

Non-cryopreserved
- Fluid overload
- Pulmonary microembolism secondary to fat emboli (may occur with infusions of bone marrow): shortness of breath, dyspnea, cough
- Transfusion reactions (allogeneic cell sources)
- Allergic reactions
- Excessive anticoagulation: may occur with rapid or large volume infusions (marrow and blood cells anticoagulated with heparin and/or citrate solutions).

Care coordination

Initiation of GVHD prophylaxis pretransplant
Arrival of stem cell product coordinated with department or service handling and/or processing cells:
- Apheresis unit—allogeneic peripheral blood cells
- Cryopreservation laboratory—cryopreserved cell products (bone marrow, umbilical cord blood, peripheral blood cells)
- Operating room—allogeneic bone marrow
- Unrelated donor program—unrelated donor peripheral blood cells or bone marrow

Administration of prehydration and premedications appropriately timed with arrival of stem cell product

DMSO, dimethylsulfoxide; GVHD, graft-vs.-host disease.

Table 35.10 Pre-engraftment.

Assessment

Assessments for potential conditioning-related toxicities:
- **Mucositis**: color/integrity of oral mucosa; volume and consistency of oral mucous; airway patency; general level of consciousness; subjective complaints of pain and/or difficulty swallowing; ability to perform oral care
- **Nausea/vomiting**: subjective reports of nausea; frequency and appearance of emesis, including gastroccult for presence of blood; abdominal assessment; fluid status, including intake and output, postural vital signs; effectiveness of antiemetic therapy
- **Diarrhea**: amount, frequency, appearance of stool, presence of blood; abdominal assessment; fluid status, including intake and output; subjective complaints of fullness, cramping, pain
- **Infection**: fever and/or chills unrelated to blood products or other medications; skin integrity, including oral, rectal and vaginal mucosa; presence adventitious breath sounds or cough; subjective reports of pain, weakness, fatigue; microbiology culture reports; hematologic laboratory values; chest X-ray report
- **Bleeding**: appearance and integrity of skin, sclera, mucous membranes; appearance of oral secretions; presence of frank of occult blood in urine, stool and emesis; mentation and level of consciousness, vital signs—noting hypotension or tachycardia; laboratory values (hematocrit, platelet count, coagulation studies, hepatic and renal function tests)
- **VOD**: weight gain; increased abdominal girth; abdominal distention; right upper quadrant pain; hepatomegaly; mentation and level of consciousness; jaundice (skin and/or sclera); laboratory values (liver function tests including serum bilirubin, SGOT, alkaline phosphatase)
- **Pain**: onset, location, description, intensity (using rating scale), aggravating and relieving factors; effectiveness of interventions; psychosocial assessment
- **Renal insufficiency**: strict intake and output; daily or BID weight; postural blood pressure and heart rate; pulmonary assessment including respiratory rate, quality and presence of adventitious breath sounds; cardiac assessment, neck vein distention; presence of edema or ascites; administration of nephrotoxic drugs; laboratory values (serum blood urea nitrogen, creatinine, electrolytes; urine specific gravity)
- **Pulmonary**: respiratory rate, rhythm, depth, quality; breath sounds; existence and quality of cough; sputum production; mentation and level of consciousness; presence of cyanosis or skin mottling; subjective complaints of shortness of breath, dyspnea, or pain; oxygen saturation

Knowledge of patient/caregiver of potential complications
Ability to participate in self-care measures to treat and/or prevent complications
Ability of caregiver to participate in patient support

Teaching

Recognition, reporting and management of post-transplant complications:
- Mucositis
- Nausea/vomiting
- Diarrhea
- Infection
- Bleeding
- VOD
- Pain
- Renal insufficiency
- Pulmonary complications

Reinforcement of guidelines for preventing infections:
- Handwashing
- Personal hygiene
- Nutrition/diet guidelines for immunosuppressed patients
- Avoiding activities with high risk for infection

Rationale and procedures for administration of blood products, parenteral fluids and nutrition, medications
Anticipated time to engraftment:
- Peripheral blood stem cell transplant: 7–11 days
- Bone marrow transplant: 14–21 days
- Umbilical cord blood transplant: 21–28$^+$ days

Signs and symptoms of engraftment (consistent rise in WBCC)

Care coordination

Blood product administration:
- Platelet transfusions (often daily or multiple times per day)
- RBC or whole blood transfusions

Intravenous fluids:
- Total parenteral nutrition/lipids
- Hydration fluids
- Patient-controlled analgesia (inpatients)

Medication administration:
- GVHD prophylaxis (allogeneic patients)
- Antibiotics, antivirals, antifungals
- Antiemetics
- Opioid/nonopioid analgesia
- Investigational drugs

Multiple health-care provider appointments (outpatient) or health-care provider examinations (inpatient)
Multiple laboratory draws
Frequent physical assessments and vital signs (inpatient: every 4-h—inpatient and as needed; outpatient—weekly clinic visit and as needed)
Physical care and ADL:
- Bath—skin care
- Oral care
- Dressing/central venous catheter changes
- Exercise/ambulation

Patient and caregiver education: one-on-one instruction or attendance at caregiver classes

ADL, activities of daily living; BID, twice daily; GVHD, graft-vs.-host disease; RBC, red blood cell; SGOT, serum glutamic-oxaloacetic transaminase; VOD, veno-occlusive disease; WBCC, white blood cell count.

Table 35.11 Early post-engraftment.

Assessment

On-going assessment for conditioning-related toxicities (see Table 35.10)

Signs and symptoms of GVHD:

- **Skin**: itching; redness or maculopapular rash on palms of hands, soles of feet, ears, trunk, extremities; erythroderma
- **Liver**: right upper quadrant pain; hepatomegaly; jaundice; laboratory values (elevated serum bilirubin, SGOT, alkaline phosphatase)
- **GI tract**: nausea; vomiting; anorexia; diarrhea; abdominal cramping and pain; diarrhea

Readiness for discharge from hospital:

- Availability of caregiver on discharge
- Competency of patient and caregiver to: (i) recognize, report and manage post-transplant complications; (ii) manage outpatient schedules and treatments; and (iii) administer outpatient IV fluids and medications
- Knowledge of phone numbers to access emergency care and support 24 h a day on discharge

Caregiver ability to provide support

Teaching

Acute GVHD

Signs and symptoms

Rationale and procedures for GVHD diagnostic testing if signs and symptoms develop (e.g. skin biopsy, liver biopsy and/or endoscopy)

Management of GVHD (adding immunosuppressive medications to current GVHD prophylaxis), dietary restrictions

Hospital discharge planning:

- Criteria for discharge from inpatient to outpatient setting (e.g. nausea/vomiting/pain controlled; blood counts supportable; number and type of IV infusions or medications)
- Level of caregiver support required on discharge (generally constant support required first 2–3 weeks post-discharge)
- Outpatient administration of IV fluids and medications
- Discharge medication schedule: GVHD prophylaxis and/or treatment immunosuppressant medications (allogeneic patients), PCP prophylaxis, antivirals, antibacterials, antifungals, electrolyte replacements, antiemetics (etc.)
- Importance of reporting inability to take medications prescribed
- Outpatient appointment schedules on discharge

Recognition and management of post-transplant complications

Likelihood of readmission to hospital post-initial discharge

Care coordination

Blood product administration:

- Platelet transfusions (often daily or multiple times per day)
- RBC or whole blood transfusions

Intravenous fluids:

- Total parenteral nutrition/lipids
- Hydration fluids
- Patient controlled analgesia (inpatients)

Medication administration:

- GVHD prophylaxis
- Antibiotics, antivirals, antifungals
- Opioid/nonopioid analgesics
- Electrolyte replacements
- Investigational drugs
- Antiemetics

Multiple health-care provider appointments (outpatient) or health-care provider examinations (inpatient)

Multiple laboratory draws

Frequent physical assessments and vital signs (inpatient: every 4-h—inpatient and as needed; outpatient—each clinic visit and as needed)

Physical care and ADL:

- Bath—skin care
- Oral care
- Dressing/central venous catheter changes
- Exercise/ambulation

Scheduling procedures (marrow aspirations, chest-X-rays, etc.)

Transitioning care from inpatient to outpatient setting

ADL, activities of daily living; GI, gastrointestinal; GVHD, graft-vs.-host disease; IV, intravenous; PCP, peumocystis carinii pneumonia; RBC, red blood cell; SGOT, serum glutamic-oxaloacetic transaminase.

Table 35.12 Discharge from transplant program.

Assessment
Knowledge of infectious risks
Knowledge of expected follow-up office visits and laboratory testing
Nutritional needs
Need for continuance or removal of central venous catheter
Allogeneic patients:
- Current symptoms of GVHD
- Visual exam of skin
- Skin biopsy
- Schirmer's test
- Knowledge of chronic GVHD

Teaching
Symptoms of chronic GVHD
Recovery of immunity
Recommendations for minimizing daily infectious risks (see Table 35.13)
Recommendations for returning to work or school
Management of fatigue
Management of possible problems related to sexual function
Management of cognitive and emotional issues
When to report fever
Necessity for consistent medical follow-up for life

Care coordination
Medication list
Nursing-care plan for local nursing-care provider
Home health care agency if needed
Special transfusion requirements and preparation of products (irradiation and CMV screening if CMV negative)
Interface with health insurance carriers as needed
Assist with research coordination
Time after transplant

CMV, cytomegalovirus; GVHD, graft-vs.-host disease.

transplant physicians, relay possible solutions to the team providing care at home. One organized approach is to conduct long-term follow-up rounds on a regular basis to discuss nonurgent problems. Issues most frequently requiring the expertise of the transplant team are the diagnosis and treatment of chronic GVHD, pulmonary complications, gastrointestinal symptoms, engraftment issues, treatment of serious and life threatening infections, booster immunization, recurrent disease and the development of secondary malignancies [18]. The need for the transplant team to act as a resource may persist from a few months to several years. While patients who live at a distance from the transplant center benefit from periodic follow-up visits to the transplant center, the general oncologist or hematologist at home can provide the routine follow-up care.

Transplant nurses can also provide ongoing support in the outlying communities by offering educational programs and by sending out educational material when the need is recognized. Facilitation of support groups is another way for transplant nurses to provide ongoing education and support for local patients in the long-term recovery phase.

If the transplant center is involved in ongoing research, the research nurse plays an integral role in continuing with the collection of data and following research protocols. In some research centers, patient health questionnaires are regularly mailed to post-transplant patients to update demographics, quality-of-life information and survival documentation. Research nurses can triage problem issues that are identified from the questionnaires.

The role of the nurses working with the HCT patients during long-term recovery requires patience and perseverance when considering the recurring nature of chronic GVHD and other long-term issues. As in other phases of HCT nursing, the work is rewarding and challenging and it allows for establishment of long-term and trusting relationships. While nurses working in the office setting may find the problems of this population to be daunting at times, the eventual recovery and return of patients to a satisfying and full life is a reward experienced by those who are fortunate enough to work with these patients.

Summary

Expert nursing care is essential to the success of a HCT program. Dr E. Donnall Thomas, founding Medical Director of the Fred Hutchinson Cancer Research Center's Transplant Program, and recipient of the 1990 Nobel Prize in Physiology and Medicine, called transplant nurses "his secret weapons" [19]. Nurses who are drawn to this subspecialty within oncology, and are successful in mastering the required skills, are rewarded by intense and intimate relationships with the patients during this time of crisis in their lives. There is great satisfaction knowing that they have made a positive difference in the lives of these patients.

References

1 Ford R, McDonald J, Mitchell-Supplee K, Jagels B. Marrow transplant and peripheral blood stem cell transplantation. In: McCorkle R, Grant M, Frank-Stromborg M, Baird S, eds. *Cancer Nursing: a Comprehensive Textbook*. Philadelphia: W.B. Saunders & Co., 1996: 504–30.
2 Herrmann RP, Leather M, Leather HL, Leen K. Clinical care for patients receiving autologous hematopoietic stem cell transplantation in the home setting. *Oncol Nurs Forum* 1998; **25**(8): 1427–32.
3 Kelley CH, Randolph S. The role of the homecare nurse throughout the continuum of blood cell transplantation. *J Intraven Nurs* 1998; **21**(6): 361–6.
4 Holmes W, Kapustay PM, Walker F, Williams L, Ezzone S, eds. *Peripheral Blood Stem Cell Transplantation: Recommendations for Nursing Education and Practice*. Pittsburgh, PA: Oncology Nursing Press, Inc., 1997: 1–44.
5 Nelson JP. The blood cell transplant program. *Semin Oncol Nurs* 1997; **13**(3): 208–15.
6 Buchsel PC, Leum E, Randolph SR. Nursing care of the blood cell transplant recipient. *Semin Oncol Nurs* 1997; **13**(3): 172–83.
7 Johns A. Overview of bone marrow and stem cell transplantation. *J Intraven Nurs* 1998; **21**(6): 356–60.
8 Gorlin JB. Transfusion reactions associated with hematopoietic progenitor cell reinfusion. In: Popovsky MA, ed. *Transfusion Reactions*, 2nd edn. Bethesda, MD: AABB Press, 2001: 235–54.
9 Wagner ND, Quinones VW. Allogeneic peripheral blood stem cell transplantation: clinical overview and nursing implications. *Oncol Nurs Forum* 1998; **25**(6): 1049–57.
10 Kapustay PM, Buchsel PC. Process, complications, and management of peripheral stem cell transplantation. In: Buchsel PC, Kapustay PM, eds. *Stem Cell Transplantation: a Clinical Textbook*. Pittsburgh, PA: Oncology Nursing Press, Inc., 2000: 5.1–28.
11 Kapustay PM. Blood cell transplantation: concepts and concerns. *Semin Oncol Nurs* 1997; **13**: 151–63.
12 Shapiro TW. Intensive care management of the BMT patient: administrative and clinical issues. In: Buchsel P, Wheedon MP, eds. *Bone Marrow Transplantation: Administrative Strategies and Clinical Concerns*. Boston, MA: Jones & Bartlett Publishers, 1995: 69–96.
13 Crawford SW. Critical care and respiratory failure. In: Thomas ED, Blume KG, Forman SJ, eds. *Hematopoietic Cell Transplantation*, 2nd edn. Malden, MA: Blackwell Science, 1999: 712–22.
14 Horak DA, Forman SJ. Critical care of the hematopoietic stem cell patient. *Crit Care Clin* 2001; **17**: 671–95.
15 Plunkett P. Ethical issues in transplantation. In: Whedon MB, Wujcik D, eds. *Marrow and Blood Stem Cell Transplantation: Principles, Practice, and Nursing Insights*, 2nd edn. Boston, MA: Jones & Bartlett Publishers, 1997: 506–23.

Table 35.13 Common questions asked by hematopoietic stem cell transplantation and long-term follow-up (LTFU) patients. Reproduced with permission from the Fred Hutchinson Cancer Research Center Long-term Follow-up Program.

Questions often asked	Time after transplant			
The general guidelines below may not apply to your case. You must discuss with your physician to assess if these rules apply to you	All patients <6 months	Not receiving immunosupression 6–12 months	Receiving immunosupression 6–12 months	Receiving immunosupression >1 year
School	No	No	No	OK
Hot tubs*	No	OK*	No	No
Swimming (avoid head submersion and diving, use sun screen)*	No	OK*	No	No
Gardening (digging in soil); mowing the lawn; raking leaves	No	No	No	OK
Having plants in the home (not handling)§	No	No	No	No
Making/kneading yeast breads	OK	OK	OK	OK
Carpenter work	OK	OK	OK	OK
Occasional woodworking (sawdust)	No	No	No	No
	No	OK	OK	OK
Animals, birds, reptiles, fish, other (not handling feces, litter boxes, cleaning utensils or cages/tanks, etc.)				
New pets in patient's household	No	No	No	No
Cats/dogs (not sleeping with pets)	OK	OK	OK	OK
Domestic birds (parakeets, parrots, etc.) (not with respiratory problems)	No	OK	OK	OK
Poultry and wild birds (pigeons, chickens, ducks, geese, other wild birds, etc.)	No	No	No	No
Small cage rodents (gerbils, rabbits, hamsters, guinea pigs, hedge hogs, prairie dogs, etc.) (do not handle)	No	OK	OK	OK
Reptiles (snakes, turtles, lizards, iguanas, etc.); ferrets	No	No	No	No
Farm animals (pigs, horses, cows, llamas, etc.) (do not handle; stay out of barns full of hay)	No	OK	OK	OK
Wild and game animals (deer, elk, squirrels, bear, etc.); exotic animals (i.e. monkeys, etc.) (do not handle)	No	No	No	No
Zoos and petting zoos	No	No	No	No
Public aquariums (do not touch marine life in handling tanks)‡	OK‡	OK‡	OK‡	OK‡
Animal trophy mounts in the house	OK	OK	OK	OK
Fishing (fresh and salt water) (OK to handle fish if wearing gloves; do not bait hooks)	OK	OK	OK	OK
Hunting (wild game and birds) and sport shooting (wear latex gloves when handling game; do not clean game; without venous catheter device)†	No	OK†	OK†	OK†
Horseback riding (stay out of barns full of hay)	No	OK	OK	OK
Golfing (sun protection required; without venous catheter device)†	No	OK	OK	OK
Spectator events and crowds (no hand shaking)‡	No	OK‡	OK‡	OK‡
Sexual activity	OK	OK	OK	OK
Working with mechanical equipment (oil changes, working on cars and engines, etc.)	OK	OK	OK	OK
Camping and hiking	OK	OK	OK	OK
Down comforters (with cover)	OK	OK	OK	OK

Other reminders:
- **Minimize**: exposure to dirt and aerosolized material
- **Minimize**: sun exposure and use of sunscreen (SPF >15)
- **Use**: hat, long sleeve shirts and pants if outside for long period of time
- **Avoid**: contact with people with respiratory illness or other transmissible diseases

*No swimming if venous access device still in place (i.e. catheter). No patient history of sinusitis. Chlorinated and well-maintained pools preferable over uncertain water conditions of lakes, rivers and sea for swimming. Do not recommend swimming in pools used by nontoilet-trained babies and children. Water aerobics OK.
†Shooting of rifles and shotguns and golfing is not recommended if venous access device still in place (i.e. catheter).
‡Recommend caution and an understanding of the risk involved when participating in public events or going to locations with large crowds.
§Real Christmas trees: in the water reservoir of the tree stand, use water solution of 1 part chlorine solution (Clorox™) in 10 parts water.

Table 35.14 Long-term recovery.

Assessment

Fatigue
Pain
Functional status
Complete blood count
Kidney function
Liver function
Magnesium level
Drug levels
Chronic GVHD symptoms (allogeneic patients):
- **Skin**: erythema, dryness, macular or urticarial rash and pruritis, hyperpigmentation, vitiligo, mottling, lichenoid plaques, hyperkeratosis, exfoliation scleroderma or morphia
- **Mouth**: dryness, mucositis, erythema, lichenoid changes, striae, tightness around the mouth, sensitivity to hot, cold or spicy foods and gingivitis
- **Eyes**: dryness, grittiness, blurring, excessive tearing, photophobia and pain
- **Liver**: elevated liver function tests not attributable to other causes and sometimes jaundice
- **GI**: anorexia, nausea, vomiting, diarrhea, dysphagio, malabsorption, weight loss
- **Lungs**: cough, wheezing, dyspnea on exertion, history of recurrent brochiolitis or sinusitis, bronchiolitis obliterans
- **Nails**: ridging, onychodystrophy, onycholysis
- **Hair**: premature graying of scalp hair, eyelashes, eyebrows, thinning of scalp hair, allopecia and decreased body hair
- **Vagina**: dryness, dyspareunia, stricture or stenosis, erythema, atrophy or lichenoid changes not induced by ovarian failure or other causes
- **Myofascia**: stiffness and tightness with restriction of movement, sometimes with swelling, pain, cramping, erythema and induration, most commonly affecting the forearms, wrists and hands, ankles, legs and feet, contractures
- **Muscles**: proximal muscle weakness, cramping
- **Skeletal**: arthralgia of large proximal girdle joints and, sometimes, smaller joints
- **Serosal**: unexplained effusions involving the pleural, pericardial or peritoneal cavities
- Thrombocytopenia, eosinophilia and hypogammaglobulinemia
- **Energy level**: unusual fatigue

Medication compliance
Nutritional needs
Symptoms of infection
Hormonal issues
Neurological symptoms
Sexual dysfunction

Teaching

Symptoms to be reported: skin changes, nausea, anorexia, weight loss, diarrhea, dysphagia, dry or sensitive mouth, dry, gritty eyes or excessive tearing, coughing, wheezing or shortness of breath, thinning of scalp hair, ridged nails, loss of range of motion or stiffness, vaginal symptoms)
When to report fever
How to access medical help after hours
Review of infection prevention
Importance of medication compliance
Importance of reporting abnormal lesions or lumps, bowel changes or abnormal vaginal bleeding
Importance of regular exercise

Care coordination

Health-care provider appointments
Medication administration
Laboratory draws
Return visit to transplant center at 1-year anniversary of transplant and thereafter as needed
Vaccinations after the 1st year
Allogeneic patients:
- Plans for work-up of chronic GVHD symptoms based on assessment
- Plans for treatment of chronic GVHD

GI, gastrointestinal; GVHD, graft-vs.-host disease.

References (continued from p. 479)

16 Whedon MB, Fliedner MC. Nursing issues in hematopoietic cell transplantation. In: Thomas ED, Blume KG, Forman SJ, eds. *Hematopoietic Cell Transplantation*, 2nd edn. Malden, MA: Blackwell Science, 1999: 381–5.

17 Flowers MED, McDonald GB, Boeckh M et al. *Long-Term Follow-Up after Hematopoietic Stem Cell Transplant: General Guidelines for Referring Physicians*. Seattle, WA: Fred Hutchinson Cancer Research Center/Seattle Cancer Care Alliance, 2002.

18 Deeg HJ. Delayed complications after hematopoietic cell transplantation. In: Thomas ED, Blume KG, Forman SJ, eds. *Hematopoietic Cell Transplantation*, 2nd edn. Malden, MA: Blackwell Science, 1999: 776–88.

19 Lilleby K. A nursing history of bone marrow and peripheral stem cell transplantation: recollections. In: Buchsel PC, Kapustay PM, eds. *Stem Cell Transplantation: a Clinical Textbook*. Pittsburgh, PA: Oncology Nursing Press, Inc., 2000: 15.1–8.

36

Susan K. Stewart

The Patient's Perspective

Patients arrive at the door of the transplant center from a variety of cultural backgrounds and experiences. One thing they all share is tremendous fear: fear of pain, fear of death and fear of leaving dependent loved ones behind.

In addition, many, if not most, arrive at the transplant center angry or depressed, or both. They are angry that a disease has stripped them of control over their own bodies. They are angry that they must depend on others whom they barely know to cure them of their illnesses. They are depressed because no matter what treatment option they pursue, there is no guarantee that it will be successful.

Transplant centers must be completely honest with patients about the risks involved in undergoing hematopoietic cell transplant (HCT). Sometimes, however, the educational process unnecessarily increases the patient's emotional trauma. While discussions about the risks associated with HCT are difficult for patients under the best of circumstances, it is possible to minimize their emotional distress by keeping a few key principles in mind.

Assess patient's informational needs

Preparing patients for the rigors of an HCT against this backdrop of fear, anger and depression is challenging. It helps both the patient and physician if the patient's style of coping with troubling medical information is first assessed.

Some patients want complete, detailed information about the treatment, risks and side-effects up front so that there are no surprises during treatment. They want to be engaged as partners in their care and obtaining detailed information gives them a sense of control in a situation that, otherwise, seems largely out of control. Others are unable to process a large volume of technical information, particularly during initial consultations with the medical team, and need simpler explanations delivered incrementally. Asking patients what level of detail they need to hear helps physicians present the information in an appropriate manner and may help avert feelings by some patients that important details are being withheld or that their intelligence is not being respected.

A patient's cultural background may influence the amount and type of information that the patient is ready to hear. For example, in some cultures it is believed that discussing illness or death promotes both events. When dealing with a patient whose cultural background is different from the physician's, consulting with a neutral party about accepted practices and taboos in that culture can help to overcome communication barriers that may arise during pretreatment and treatment.

Put the risks in perspective

When a patient meets with the transplant team, a long list of potential treatment-related complications is recited and described in graphic detail. Often, however, little or no mention is made of how likely it is that each complication will arise. The prospect of developing all the various complications is frightening and overwhelming and, as a consequence, many patients leave the transplant center more depressed than when they arrived.

Patients need help putting the possible risks associated with HCT into proper perspective. They should not leave the interview under the impression that they are just as likely to develop serious liver damage as mucositis. Assigning a probability of occurrence to each complication or discussing complications in groups, according to their likelihood of occurrence, will help the patient feel less overwhelmed. For example, complications might be grouped as: (i) those that nearly all patients experience; (ii) those that many, but not all, patients experience; and (iii) those that are possible, but that most patients do *not* experience. The prospect of undergoing HCT is far less daunting if the patient understands that there is a *chance* that the most serious complications will occur but not high *likelihood*.

It also helps the patient's emotional well-being if he or she is explicitly told what will be done to treat various complications. When no mention is made of how complications are treated, patients sometimes incorrectly assume that no treatment is available. Some are so overwhelmed that it does not occur to them to ask if and how the problems will be addressed. Knowing that the most common complications are treatable, and that the more serious are often treatable and reversible, will help ease a patient's anxiety.

Communicate in lay language

Although many patients are well educated, most are unfamiliar with the medical jargon routinely used by medical professionals. Terms such as CBC, aspirate, Hickman, bilirubin, lymphocyte, TPN, or stem cells are foreign to most persons without medical training. Even more commonly used words such as prognosis or remission are meaningless to many patients.

It is important to describe HCT in language that patients can understand. Today's print media is written in language that can be understood by a person with a sixth grade education. Given that all HCT patients are under a great deal of emotional stress and may not be able to process information as easily as the average person, medical procedures and terms should be described as simply as possible. Words that are not understood or that are misunderstood can cause additional, and unnecessary, emotional stress.

Repeat information

It is important to check that patients understand what has been said, not only at the initial interview but throughout the course of treatment. Most patients are overwhelmed by the volume of information presented to them at their initial meeting with the transplant team and may forget much of it after they leave. Some will only partially hear what was said or block out the information altogether. Repeating the information at critical junctures and encouraging patients to ask questions will help to ensure that they actually process the information that they have been given.

Encouraging patients to ask questions consists of more than telling them that it is all right to do so. Patients often feel that they should not ask questions because they are afraid of embarrassing themselves, because their upbringing taught them not to question doctors, or because they feel they have little entitlement to the quality of medical care that they are receiving, let alone the right to understand treatment. If patients sense that a physician or nurse is busy or hassled, they may be reluctant to articulate their concerns and have them addressed.

Creating an atmosphere that encourages questions is important. I recall that when I was a patient undergoing an autologous bone marrow transplant (BMT) procedure in 1989, one of the attending physicians would come in each morning, examine me and then sit down in a relaxed manner to write a few notes. He would then talk with me and encourage me to ask questions. He never seemed rushed (although I am sure he was very busy) and always gave me sufficient time to recall questions and understand the answers. During my 2nd month of hospitalization a different attending physician took over. He arrived each morning and talked mostly to the bevy of students who accompanied him on rounds. He examined me thoroughly and told me what he needed to say, finishing the last sentence as he stepped over the threshold of the door and out into the hall. I could barely muster the strength to call him back in, let alone recall my questions. Needless to say, many questions were left unanswered.

Suggesting that patients write down their questions so that they are not forgotten, sitting down with patients in a relaxed manner, giving them plenty of time to recall and formulate their questions, and assuring them that it is normal to need answers repeated or explained differently will help patients feel more comfortable. Providing patients with a phone number where physicians can be contacted if questions arise is also helpful, particularly if the patient's spouse or caregiver cannot be present during rounds.

Providing patients with written, illustrated information about the transplant process is also very helpful. While many patients more easily process audio/visual information, others find it helpful to have printed information to which they can refer when they are ready to focus on a particular question. Being able to read about a subject before discussing it with a physician makes some patients feel more comfortable during the discussion. They have at least a rudimentary understanding of the topic and may be able to ask more meaningful questions as a consequence of this preparation.

Some patients find that tape-recording or videotaping discussions with their physicians enables them to double-check their understanding later on. Some patients may be reluctant to record conversations, however. Suggesting that they do so will not only assure them that it is all right but also will assure them that their physician truly wants them to understand and participate in their treatment.

Discuss pain management

Many patients fear pain even more than death. Yet while all transplant teams inform patients about potential painful complications, some neglect to explain what steps will be taken to relieve the pain. They assume the patient knows that pain medications are available and will be administered as needed. Many patients, however, have had little experience with hospitalization or medical treatment and so do not make such assumptions about pain control. Others may have already undergone painful procedures, such as a bone marrow aspiration, without the benefit of adequate pain medication and have little reason to assume that their pain will be properly managed at the transplant center. Thus, the already distraught patient hears a litany of painful scenarios that may develop during treatment and is unable to relieve his or her anxiety about pain by reflecting on what will be done to control it.

It is important to emphasize to the patient that pain medications are available to control pain and will be administered as needed. If patient-administered pain medication devices are used at the center, it helps to tell patients that they will have some control over when pain medication is administered. Some patients may have had experience with under-medication or delays in delivery of pain medication in the past. Knowing that they will have some control over pain medication will help ease their anxiety.

Many patients, and the family members who stay with them during hospitalization, are unprepared for changes in mental status that can occur while patients are on certain pain and antidepressant medications. Lack of warning about these temporary changes can result in unnecessary anxiety for patients and family members alike. Observing a loved one hallucinating or talking nonsense is extremely upsetting if the family member is not advised in advance that a medication may temporarily produce this result. It can be even more frightening for the patient who slips in and out of coherence and realizes at some point that his or her mental abilities are impaired. Talking about the possible side-effects of pain and antidepressant medications before they are given, and emphasizing that the effects are temporary, can eliminate one source of anxiety. It is important that the medical personnel "legitimize" the use of pain medications. Most patients have never before undergone a procedure that involved as much pain as an HCT. Many will come to the experience with a bias against pain medications—either a fear that they will become addicted or a sense that they will be perceived as cowards if they request pain relief too often. Patients should be advised that not only is it all right to request pain medication but that it is recommended. Treating pain after it becomes severe is more difficult than controlling it at the outset. Patients need to know that pain medications are a routine part of the treatment and that they will not become dependent on them long-term.

Discuss psychological difficulties

While potential physical complications are usually thoroughly discussed with patients at the initial interview with the HCT team, possible psychological complications are not. In some cases, nothing is said about the emotional difficulty involved in undergoing HCT. In other cases, patients may simply be told that this will be a "difficult" or "stressful" experience, words that convey little specificity about the type and depth of emotions that the patient is likely to experience.

Thus, when patients become angry, belligerent or deeply depressed during treatment and recovery, they assume that there is something wrong with themselves and that they are weaklings who are not coping with the stress as well as other patients. After all, they reason, if these emotional difficulties were common among HCT patients, the medical team would have warned them in advance. Their anger with themselves for coping poorly exacerbates their emotional distress.

It is important that the HCT team be as explicit with patients about the psychological distress that may be experienced during treatment and recovery as they are about the physical complications that the patient may face. Patients need to know that it is normal to feel angry about their lack of control over their disease and treatment, to resent their dependence on medical personnel for routine bodily care, to be fearful about medical procedures and to become depressed when recovery is slow or a new complication arises. Family members should be advised that some patients lash out at those closest to them during these times of distress or at the medical personnel caring for them. They need not be embarrassed if this occurs; the medical team has seen it all before and understands why it is happening.

Patients need to understand that an HCT is an extraordinary experience. They should not expect to deal with it as calmly and rationally as they deal with most of life's mishaps. They need assurance that no one will think badly of them if they cry or ask for psychological help. Extraordinary circumstances require extraordinary interventions. Patients need to know that even persons who have never before sought psychiatric help may need it during this stressful period. Helping patients set reasonable expectations for themselves and legitimizing the use of psychiatric help and antidepressant medications will help patients better cope with the psychological stress during transplant.

For some patients, the period of greatest psychological stress is during hospitalization. Others weather the hospitalization in high spirits but fall apart emotionally upon their return home. Suddenly, they have lost the safety net of the medical personnel who attended to their every need. They are back in a familiar setting but unable to function normally. As Jim King [1], who survived a BMT for myelofibrosis in 1994, put it:

> When I left the hospital, I thought the tough part was over. I've never been so wrong. The inpatient part was the easiest part of the bone marrow transplant process. I was focused and fired up.... All the worldly things, such as my role as a husband and father, were secondary to winning the in-patient battle. Other routine things such as house payments, medical bills, career and church weren't even on my mind. Nurses and doctors took care of me. It wasn't easy, but I felt I was making significant progress toward beating my disease.
>
> The clarity of purpose and sense of progress were lost when I came home. Instead of feeling like a successful patient, I felt like a failed person. All those worldly things, such as my role as husband and father that I had ignored in the hospital came roaring back. They were once again important, and I felt woefully inadequate in those roles.
>
> The steroids and cyclosporine made me extremely emotional and irrational. I would cry because I had too much milk on my cereal. I couldn't sleep (steroids), couldn't shower (Hickman), couldn't read (no concentration), couldn't drink coffee in the morning (nausea), couldn't exercise (no strength) and couldn't get close to my children (might get infection). Even taking my medicine was confusing and overwhelming. I spent time worrying about things I couldn't control. I was convinced I was going to run out of money, lose my house, my dog, etc. There was no measured progress anymore. I felt I was regressing. I was in an emotional rut.

Patients should be advised at discharge that psychological stress can develop or continue after they leave the transplant facility. Medications they take may leave them feeling depressed. Rehospitalization for infections or the host of other problems that can develop following a patient's release takes its emotional toll on the patient and his or her family. Many patients begin to wonder if they will ever again be able to wake up and enjoy a day without thinking about their disease and treatment.

Some patients experience something akin to post-traumatic stress syndrome following their discharge. They have difficulty sleeping. A sight or smell will cause them to recall some unpleasant experience they had during hospitalization and they will be stunned and upset. Some will start crying in the middle of a conversation, an embarrassing situation at best. Just knowing that these emotions are common and temporary goes a long way toward helping patients overcome their anger and depression when it occurs.

Encouraging patients to talk about their emotional difficulties and providing them with sources of help are also important. For patients who live near the transplant facility, professional counselors or support groups, or both, may be available. Those who live out of town may benefit from local support groups, local therapists or phone conversations with survivors who have experienced similar emotions and can provide patients with peer emotional support. Some organizations such as the Blood and Marrow Transplant Information Network (BMT InfoNet) (888-597-7674) and the National BMT-Link (800-546-5268) link patients with supportive survivors.

HCT patients with access to the Internet may find the following websites helpful:

- *Blood and Marrow Transplant Information Network* (BMT InfoNet) at www.bmtinfonet.org. Provides electronic access to books and newsletters about HCT. Also offers a patient–survivor link service, an attorney referral service for patients who have insurance reimbursement difficulties, a directory of transplant centers in the USA and Canada, and news of interest to HCT patients.
- *National Marrow Donor Program* at http://www.marrow.org. Information about becoming or searching for an unrelated bone marrow donor; a directory of transplant centers in the USA that perform unrelated HCT transplants with donors supplied by the program, including outcome data; medical information for patients and health care professionals about HCT for specific diseases and other patient resources.
- *BMT-Talk* at http://listserv.acor.org/archives/bmt-talk.html. Home page for the mailing list BMT-Talk that hosts communications between more than 400 HCT patients, survivors and caregivers.
- *BMT Support Online* at www.bmtsupport.org. Provides two online support groups—one for patients and another for caregivers—that chat weekly.
- *National BMT Link* www.bmtlink.org. Links HCT patients with survivors who can provide emotional support.
- *International Bone Marrow Transplant Registry* at www.ibmtr.org. Offers reports on autologous and allogeneic BMTs, based on data collected from 300 transplant centers, and can respond to some patient inquiries.

Discussing clinical trials

Patients considering an HCT have a life-threatening disease. For them, the top priority is finding a therapy that will cure them of their diseases and/or prolong their lives. The patient is sick *now* and needs to decide *today* which treatment will enable him or her to achieve these objectives.

Thus, when offered the opportunity to participate in a clinical trial, patients often view the trial from a much different perspective than the physician does. Physicians see clinical trials for what they are: research that may provide answers tomorrow about the optimal way to treat patients with a particular disease or disorder. The patient, on the other hand, is evaluating a clinical trial to determine if it is the optimal therapy for him or her today.

This difference in the way physicians and patients view clinical trials frequently result in patient confusion and misunderstanding. Patients want outcome data about the therapy offered as part of a clinical trial so that they can compare it to data about other available therapies. When a physician is unable to provide detailed data, patients may suspect that the doctor is not being completely candid with them. While it may be obvious to a physician that reliable outcome data cannot be provided until a substantial number of patients undergo a particular therapy and are followed for many years, this is not intuitively obvious to the patient who must make a critical treatment decision today.

Language used to describe a clinical trial sometimes contributes to a patient's confusion. Although a physician may not explicitly say that one therapy is superior to another, explanations about why, theoretically, a new therapy may work and references to preliminary data about the efficacy of the treatment can be highly suggestive. Most patients are not familiar enough with clinical research to understand that therapies which look promising in the laboratory or in early clinical trials often prove to be no better, and sometimes worse, than existing therapies when tested on a larger number of patients. This misunderstanding often underlies a patient's reluctance to be randomized to a particular therapy.

Patients need help understanding that, by definition, a clinical trial is research, and that the physicians conducting the trial are asking exactly the same question that the patient is asking: is this therapy superior to other therapies? They need *examples* of why it is dangerous to presume that a newer therapy is more effective than another therapy, based on preliminary trial results. They need assurance that a physician is not promoting a particular clinical trial because he or she has a vested interest, either monetary or professionally, in the outcome.

Acknowledging the difficulty of deciding whether or not to undergo a particular treatment based on incomplete data, and empathizing with a patient who must do so, may stop some patients from attempting the impossible: predicting the outcome of a clinical trial before mature data are available.

The National Cancer Institute (NCI) publishes an excellent series of booklets and videos that are designed to be used with patients. Some are accompanied with guides for health care professionals who will be discussing trials with patients. The publications/videos clearly explain what a clinical trial is, how it is conducted and suggest questions patients should ask before agreeing to participate in a clinical trial. These publications, some of which are also available in Spanish, can be ordered online from the Cancer Information Service at http://cis.nci.gov. Additional patient-friendly online resources about clinical trials can be found at the NCI's website at www.clinicaltrials.gov. Providing a patient with these resources can help them better understand the clinical trial process and enhance their trust in the physician who is providing them the opportunity to participate in a trial.

Quality of life post-treatment

From the patient's perspective, a successful HCT does not mean only that the patient survives. Patients also want a good quality of life after transplant. Certain issues that affect quality of life are sometimes not discussed with patients in the same depth as those that affect survival, although they are just as important to the patient. Patients need preparation for permanent changes that may occur in their lifestyle long-term and should be referred to persons who can help them deal with some of the more troubling chronic problems that are beyond the expertise of the HCT team.

One example is the issue of infertility. For some patients, the prospect of infertility post-transplant is as upsetting as the diagnosis itself. Disappointment over the prospect of infertility is not limited to patients who have never had children but extends to some individuals who already have children and would like to expand their family.

Patients' emotional distress can be lessened if they are advised that it is sometimes possible to conceive a child post-transplant. Men may be able to bank a sufficient quantity of viable sperm before treatment to enable attempts at pregnancy post-transplant. Some women may be able to conceive a child with assisted reproduction techniques and a donor oocyte. While these steps are not guaranteed to result in a successful pregnancy, it comforts many patients to know that at least a chance exists.

Women are usually advised that they will be infertile post-transplant but many are not warned that they may be prematurely menopausal as well. For some women, this is a serious quality-of-life issue. When menopause occurs, it can shock and anger the unprepared patient. It is important to advise patients that they may become menopausal and to assure them that steps can be taken to overcome some of the consequences of premature menopause, such as osteoporosis. Women who hope to become pregnant after transplant, with help of assisted reproduction techniques, should be assured that premature menopause will not eliminate this option.

Many transplant survivors experience significant, long-term changes in sexuality following treatment. Problems include lack of libido, inability to perform and pain, and are reported both by persons with normal and abnormal hormone levels post-transplant. As one man stated at a conference of transplant survivors, "It seems like my brain has been cut off from the rest of my body. I can conjure up all sorts of juicy sexual images in my brain, but can't get the rest of my body to perform." Little research has been done on the issue of sexuality post-transplant. That which has been done suggests that women experience difficulty with sexuality post-HCT more frequently than men [2]. It also appears that women who begin hormone replacement therapy within a year after their HCT experience fewer difficulties with sexuality than those who do not [2].

Changes in sexuality can seriously stress a relationship, particularly if the survivor's partner believes that the problem is purely psychological rather than physical. While fatigue and psychological trauma do, indeed, affect sexuality, it is important that patients and their partners know that physical changes occur following transplant that may affect the survivor's sexuality as well. Patients should be advised that they may need to develop new approaches to intimacy after transplant to enable both partners to have a satisfying sexual relationship. Patients should be encouraged to report sexual difficulties and be provided with referrals to experts who may be able to help resolve some of the problems.

A final issue that is often overlooked in discussions with patients is changes in cognitive abilities that they may experience, both short-term and long-term. Much has been written about learning difficulties observed in children following HCT but little note has been taken of the cognitive changes experienced by some adult HCT survivors. Problems reported by survivors include poor concentration, memory problems, stuttering, difficulty in spelling, inability to perform jobs that were previously mastered and difficulty in learning new tasks. Many survivors have been able to overcome these problems by changing the way that they manage information; for example, making lists, writing down all appointments, keeping notes and so forth. For others, the solution is not so simple and the problems may interfere with their ability to perform a job or learn a new skill. For example, one survivor who was a sculptor, said, "Before my BMT, conceptualizing the design and drawing it was the most difficult part of my work. When it came to the actual sculpting, I could do it without even thinking. However, after my BMT, I could barely concentrate on the sculpting. Conceptualizing and drawing the design became impossible. No one has been able to explain why this happened or to suggest what I can do to relieve the problem."

One woman who underwent high-dose chemotherapy and an autologous BMT for breast cancer was delighted that her company held her computer operator job for her while she underwent treatment. However, when she returned to work 4 months later she found that the nature of the job had changed. She needed extensive training to perform the new tasks. After 2 weeks of training, she feared she would be fired. As she explained, "When I'm at work and in training, all the explanations make perfect sense. But then I come home, fix dinner and clean up. When I sit down to review the day's lesson I'm totally confused. By the following morning, I've completely forgotten everything I learned the previous day." Although most patients do not develop cognitive problems as severe as those experienced by the two persons described above, patients should be advised that changes in cognitive abilities sometimes occur. If cognitive problems do develop, survivors will be less frustrated if they know that their problem is not unique. Advance warning about this potential problem can also relieve tension in the home. Tired and distraught family members will understand that the survivor's new forgetfulness is not simply laziness but a consequence of the treatment.

While it is impossible to predict what any individual's quality of life will be post-transplant, it is encouraging for patients to hear about survivors or to speak with them directly. Sharing the results of one quality-of-life study performed in 1990 at the Fred Hutchinson Cancer Research Center, in which 74% of the 125 long-term survivors said that their quality of life was as good or better than it was pre-HCT, can buoy a frightened patient's spirits [3,4]. Offering patients the opportunity to talk with an HCT survivor can, for some, be very encouraging. Sometimes just hearing a live voice of someone who has undergone similar treatment energizes a patient and gives him or her hope.

Conclusion

Undergoing HCT is a very difficult experience both physically and emotionally. Working with a compassionate medical team that is attuned not only to the patient's physical needs but also to his or her emotional needs is a blessing that all patients will deeply appreciate. Being fully armed with information about long-term quality-of-life issues will help make the HCT patient's transition from being a successful patient to a successful survivor much easier.

References

1 King J. It's not a 10 K, it's a marathon. *BMT Newsletter* 1996; **7**: 4–7.

2 Syrjala K, Abrams J. Ask the Doctor *Blood & Marrow Transplant Newsletter* 1977; **8**: 1–11.

3 Haberman M, Bush N, Young K, Sullivan K. Quality of life of adult long-term survivors of bone marrow transplantation: a qualitative analysis of narrative data. *Oncol Nurs Forum* 1993; **20**: 1545–53.

4 Bush N, Haberman M, Donaldson G, Sullivan K. Quality of life of adult long-term survivors of bone marrow transplantation. *Soc Sci Med* 1995; **40**: 479–90.

37

David S. Snyder

Ethical Issues in Hematopoietic Cell Transplantation

Introduction

Many of the ethical issues raised in hematopoietic cell transplantation (HCT) are common to those involved in other forms of medical therapy utilizing advanced technologies. These issues revolve around the traditional principles of patient autonomy and the importance of informed consent and confidentiality; justice, that is, the fair allocation of limited resources; beneficence and nonmaleficence; and fidelity or nonabandonment when the goals of treatment shift from cure to supportive care. However, certain unique features of HCT compound the complexity of these ethical issues, including: the young age of most patients; the fact that most of the diseases are life-threatening and often fatal within a short time in the absence of an HCT, yet are potentially curable with this treatment; the fact that a living donor is required who is often a minor; the great financial expense of the procedure and controversies about reimbursement; and the fact that survivors of HCT may be cured of their primary malignant disease but may face other serious complications, such as sterility, chronic graft-vs.-host disease (GVHD), psychological distress, sexual dysfunction, cognitive impairments and occupational disability. In this chapter, some of the ethical issues in HCT are reviewed under the following general headings: Who receives an HCT?, Informed consent for the patient, Informed consent for the donor, Alternative sources of stem cells, HCT for nonmalignant diseases and End-of-life issues.

Who receives an HCT?

Case scenario 1

A 49-year-old-man with stage II multiple myeloma has a human leukocyte antigen (HLA)-identical sibling. He is eligible for a protocol utilizing tandem autologous HCT followed by a nonmyeloablative allogeneic HCT. His physicians feel this approach represents his best chance for long-term, disease-free survival, and possible cure of his myeloma. His insurance plan considers this treatment plan experimental and will only authorize a single autologous HCT.

Case scenario 2

A 32-year-old man with chronic myeloid leukemia (CML) has no sibling donors available for allogeneic HCT. Though his company's insurance plan covers the costs of procurement and the actual transplant for a matched-unrelated donor HCT, it will not pay for the search costs, which the patient cannot afford. Although the company sponsors a donor drive in the name of this patient, he cannot access any of the donors who might be identified.

These two scenarios, which are based on actual cases, help to highlight some of the difficult issues involved in determining who undergoes an HCT procedure. This process involves both medical decision making based on clinical and protocol-determined criteria and third-party payer decision making. Each of these processes is ethically complex. First, the medical decision making. In the interest of justice, it is imperative that transplant teams develop standardized sets of criteria by which patients are selected for HCT. Some of these criteria are straightforward, such as the patient's diagnosis and stage of disease, age and adequacy of major organ function. Other criteria are more subjective and often relate to psychosocial issues that may influence the patient's ability either to tolerate the HCT procedure or to comply with the long-term follow-up regimen. Multidisciplinary teams are needed that include not only physicians, but also nurses, psychologists, and social workers.

It is important to avoid arbitrary and inconsistent decision making in deciding when not to offer HCT to a patient. For example, an HCT center may decide that a young patient with acute leukemia who has Down syndrome is not an acceptable candidate because of expected psychosocial management problems that might compromise the outcome. In one survey of 58 pediatric HCT centers, 16 leukemic children with Down syndrome had been transplanted at 10 centers. This was only about 20–25% of the predicted number based on incidence data. In fact, the outcomes were not different than those expected from a similar cohort of patients with acute leukemia who did not have Down syndrome. The author cautioned against physician bias toward these patients [1]. In an accompanying editorial, physicians were advised to use a utilitarian approach; that is, to recommend against HCT for children with Down syndrome only if data show poorer outcomes for them.

Many HCT teams are concerned that patients with a history of active substance abuse may be poor candidates because of expectations of higher complication rates and poor compliance in their long-term care. A retrospective study from one transplant center identified 17 of 468 HCT patients as lifetime substance abusers (alcohol in 71%, marijuana in 30% and opiates in 30%). When these 17 patients were paired with matched control subjects, a significant difference in survival probability was seen, 60% vs. 10% ($p = 0.0022$) [2]. More data may be needed to substantiate these findings, but they do support the current practice at many HCT centers of excluding such patients.

Decision making regarding third-party payer reimbursement is seen as a conflict over fairness and justice. Physicians as patient advocates are often in conflict with the insurers who argue that HCT for certain diagnoses and disease stages is experimental and unproven. Physicians often believe that it is unfair to have patients accepted or denied access based on geography, their position in society, or their ability to pay when a therapy is investigational, or high-cost, or both. In analyzing patterns of utilization in four states, Mitchell *et al*. [3] found that African-American patients, those enrolled in health maintenance organizations, those covered by Medicaid and self-pay patients were less likely to receive an HCT when admitted for either leukemia or lymphoma. Insurers believe that it is unfair, and uneconomical, to be pressured by physicians and patients to pay for care that is not standard therapy [4].

Uniform and fair methodologies are needed to bridge these two views, rather than relying on costly litigation [5]. One approach is taxonomic, with a treatment modality labeled as experimental or standard. Third-party payers would cover experimental therapy if it meets certain criteria, such as a phase III trial approved by the appropriate government agency, for example, the Food and Drug Administration (FDA), and if the treatment is likely to benefit the patient. The treatment should be medically necessary, safe and effective. The therapy must be as beneficial as any established alternative, and the improvement must be attainable outside of the investigational setting [6].

It is necessary to balance the premature dissemination of poorly studied, toxic and expensive therapies to desperate patients by accepting limitations to HCT on the one hand, and by accepting that the patients' best interests may be served by an experimental therapy on the other. Legal authorities caution that although insurers may deny autologous transplant for a patient with cancer because the treatment is experimental, the more relevant question may be, "Is it the best option available for that particular patient with that particular disease?" The controversy over the last 10 years related to autologous HCT for breast cancer exemplifies these dilemmas. Welch and Mogielnicki [7] recently highlighted some of the lessons that could be gleaned from this experience, including: (i) it is premature to discuss cost effectiveness of an intervention when its clinical effectiveness is unknown; (ii) the National Institutes of Health should have an important role in determining what is experimental therapy; (iii) public officials should not mandate coverage in the absence of clear data; and (iv) the news media watchdog role should be extended to health care.

An alternative approach is to reach a consensus based on available data of efficacy, duration of expected benefit and the quality of well-being after the treatment [8]. Panels of expert physicians and insurers could review available data on a regular basis and develop grids that designate which diagnoses and disease stages will be covered, based on outcome analyses. Different categories could be considered, such as: (i) diseases for which HCT is curative and may be the only curative therapy available, for example, CML; (ii) diseases for which HCT may not be curative, but definitely prolongs survival; for example, autologous transplant for CML, and possibly breast cancer and multiple myeloma; and (iii) diseases for which the benefits of HCT are not yet known; for example, autologous transplant for autoimmune diseases such as multiple sclerosis. One model is the Oregon Medicaid system, which adopted such an approach and covered HCT for all major hematological malignancies including chronic lymphocytic leukemia, but did not cover chemotherapy for metastatic renal cell carcinoma. Such an approach is followed in California for Medi-Cal patients and by Blue Cross/Blue Shield. Another component of this approach is to restrict payments to "centers of excellence" that have demonstrated track records in their field.

One of the most difficult challenges that the medical profession and the public at large face is how to assure that progress in developing new therapies will continue in a managed care system designed to minimize health care expenses and to reimburse only for medically necessary and proven treatments. Who is going to pay for ongoing research that will lead to the breakthroughs of the future? One could argue that third-party payers have an ethical obligation to participate in this process by helping to underwrite the expenses involved in clinical research, and thereby to help establish which new treatment modalities are in fact effective and superior to established methods. Such new therapies may in fact be cheaper in the long run if they lead to definitive cures for patients and obviate the need for years of expensive, supportive chronic care.

Informed consent for patients undergoing HCT

Case scenario 3

An 18-year-old woman with relapsed acute myeloid leukemia (AML) has an HLA-matched brother available for allogeneic HCT. She has expressed an interest and willingness to undergo a transplant. However, during the informed consent process, she refuses to listen to any discussion about possible risks and complications from HCT. Can her doctors assume that she has given her consent and proceed to HCT?

Respect for patient autonomy is reflected most critically in the informed consent process, in which patients are informed of their diagnosis, prognosis, potential benefits and risks of the proposed therapy, and alternative treatments available. Although this statement is true for any type of medical intervention, in the setting of HCT there are extra complexities, including the facts that many patients are minors, that almost all patients being considered for HCT have diseases that will likely be fatal without a transplant and are potentially curable with the procedure, and that patients who survive their original disease and the early transplant mortality are at risk for development of a wide variety of chronic complications that may impair their quality of life in many ways. After a patient has been told that he or she has a fatal disease and that a potentially curative procedure is available, how much does the patient really hear and/or retain about the potential risks and complications? How accurate are the available data about details of mortality and morbidity—including the risk of veno-occlusive disease (VOD), acute and chronic GVHD, cytomegalovirus (CMV) and other infections, chronic radiation effects, avascular necrosis, sterility, the risk of second malignancies and quality of life after transplant—and how many of these data are revealed to prospective HCT patients? If patients choose not to hear all of these specifics and make choices solely on the options of life and death, is this really informed consent? Must we insist on inflicting them with these truths? Can patients exercise their autonomy by choosing not to be fully informed?

One study in 1987 compared the process of informed consent as viewed by physicians or nurses in comparison to the view of patients [9]. For the HCT nurses, it was most important that patients know about the side-effects and complications of the procedure. The physicians wanted the patients to know about the diagnosis, therapeutic options and outcomes of treatment. The physicians' views matched the patients' most closely, as they made decisions based mainly on outcome and life or death. In another study of adult and pediatric patients and their physicians published in 1989, the three main reasons that patients, and where applicable, their parents chose HCT were: (i) trust in their physician; (ii) fear that their illness would get worse without the transplant; and (iii) belief that the HCT would be a cure. Most of the adult patients remembered that complications could occur, but they could recall fewer than half of those mentioned. Most of the patients believed they had been given adequate information and that it was not too technical, although the physicians thought the information conveyed was in fact too technical and excessive. Most of the patients believed that their physician wanted them to undergo the bone marrow transplantation, and the patients made their decision based on that advice. One HCT nursing director suggested that the role of the HCT nurse in this process may be to ensure that patients have been completely informed, although the nurse must realize that patients may not be able to comprehend the complex details of treatment, and that the intensity of the choice between life and death may overshadow the risks of potentially life-threatening complications. The nurse can function as a patient advocate, which may create conflicts with the physician at times, and the nurse must not take away hope from the patient [9].

Andrykowski *et al.* [10] focused on the question of whether patients had "returned to normal" following HCT, and examined differences between their expectations and actual outcomes, and the impact these differences might have on their sense of well-being. They studied 172 disease-free survivors from five HCT centers and found that only a minority felt they were back to normal. Pre-HCT, only 19% of patients had not expected to return to normal, and 47% anticipated they would. Following HCT, 32% (possibly up to 52%) stated they had not returned to normal. The discordance between pre-HCT expectations and their current functional status was associated with greater current psychological stress. Despite this discrepancy, the survivors' evaluation of their decision to pursue HCT was generally quite positive.

The investigators asked why would there be such differences between pre-HCT expectations and actual outcomes? Some patients may hear the word "cure" pre-HCT and therefore expect that they will be "as good as new" after the transplant. Patients may not have been adequately informed of potential sequelae at the time of the HCT. Some patients may underestimate the risk of bad things happening to them, the so-called optimistic bias. This may be an adaptive mechanism to deny threats and to be unrealistically optimistic in the face of stress or adversity. In the short term, this adaptive mechanism may be beneficial but, in the long run, it may promote psychological distress because of unrealistic expectations. These findings suggest that providing details of risks and benefits during the informed consent process may have little impact on the patients' decision making. Only a minuscule number of patients actually turn down HCT if it is offered, mainly because they view HCT as their sole chance of disease cure and survival. These studies suggest, however, that following HCT, periodic discussions of possible complications and outcomes should continue to take place between patients and their physicians to help optimize the patients' psychological well-being.

Other investigators have studied the quality of life for HCT survivors, focusing on physical, psychological, social, sexual, spiritual and vocational issues [11]. Up to 25% of survivors report moderate to severe problems after HCT [12]. More work is needed to generate useful data using prospective, well-designed methodologies with appropriate control groups and baseline data. Identification of some of the factors that predict poor outcomes after HCT might provide a basis for targeted support programs [12]. Baker [13] reviewed the psychological sequelae for HCT survivors, including concerns about loss of control, physical complications, sexual dysfunction, cognitive dysfunction, difficulties in social relationships, occupational disability and financial troubles. He stressed the importance of individualizing and optimizing patient education pre-HCT to help patients have more realistic expectations of their condition after HCT. The physician needs to assess the needs and abilities of each patient and tailor the education process accordingly. Family members or close friends, or both, should be present at initial meetings to help patients recall what was covered. Audio- or videotaping of information sessions may be helpful, along with written materials. Referring physicians may be in a position to help by providing basic information to their patients and by balancing realism and optimism.

The issue of involving children in medical decision making is important since many candidates for HCT are minors. Most investigators recognize that children's capacity for decision making and autonomy develops over time. The parents or guardians must give consent for their minor child, but the wishes and concerns of the child should be taken into account [14]. The American Academy of Pediatricians states that one "should not exclude children and adolescents from decision making without persuasive reasons" [15]. It is generally accepted that children aged 7 or 8 are capable of giving assent to any proposed intervention, and that their assent should be required to proceed. The assumption is made that the parents will act as surrogate decision-makers for their children and make choices based on the best interests of the child. The courts may need to become involved if parents do not seem to be following this approach; for example, if a parent is a Jehovah's Witness and refuses blood transfusion for the child.

Informed consent for donors of hematopoietic cells

Case scenario 4

A mother leaves the country with her 16-year-old son who is HLA-matched with his 22-year-old brother who has acute leukemia because she fears her younger son will die or get leukemia too. She feels she is going to lose one son and does not want to lose the other. The older son dies from refractory leukemia without HCT.

Case scenario 5

In performing HLA typing on members of a large family because a relative has leukemia, it becomes evident that one of the siblings has a different father from the rest of the children.

The source of cells for an allogeneic transplant is usually a living donor who may be closely related to the patient, who may be a minor, or who may be an unrelated volunteer. In each of these situations, the autonomy of the donor must be respected, as reflected in an appropriate informed consent process. Donors must be informed of the specifics of the procedure that they may undergo, especially the potential risks involved. The process must be free of coercion and must respect the confidentiality of the donor and the family when it is a family donor in question. Cultural diversity issues may complicate the search for a potential donor if unusual or irrational beliefs are brought to bear. Special and important considerations are raised when the donor is a minor.

It is generally accepted that the risks involved in being a marrow donor are very small. Buckner *et al.* [16] found an overall complication rate of 27% in reviewing 1549 marrow donations performed at the Fred Hutchinson Cancer Research Center between 1983 and 1990. These events included hypotension, bleeding that required transfusions, pain and fevers. Life-threatening complications occurred in 0.4% of all donors, but only in 0.1% of "normal" donors between the ages of 18 and 55. A potential benefit of the donation process is that pre-existing medical problems that require intervention may be detected in the donor. In this study from Seattle, 206 medical problems were observed in the 1549 donor evaluations, with hypertension, obesity and cardiac problems the most common (see also Chapter 42) [16].

Currently most centers are using granulocyte colony-stimulating factor (G-CSF) mobilized peripheral blood cells (PBCs) from matched siblings as their preferred source of cells [17–19]. Hematopoietic cells collected in this manner seem to promote rapid engraftment and do not appear to carry increased risks of GVHD. Many of the risks associated with marrow harvests are minimized or prevented, such as complications from general anesthesia, the pain from multiple iliac crest punctures, local hematomas and/or infection at the aspiration sites. In a recently reported randomized study comparing PBC to bone marrow donations, the donors found the PBC collections to be the less burdensome and the preferred method [20].

In reviewing the experiences and attitudes of the first 20 volunteer unrelated donors at the University of Minnesota, Stroncek *et al.* [21] found no serious physical or emotional after effects. Nine of the 20 donors reported that a friend or family member had discouraged them. Nineteen said they would donate again and 17 would advise others to donate. One donor had orthostatic hypotension for 1 day, and all donors received 1 or 2 U of autologous blood.

The benefits of being a marrow donor for a family member or an unrelated recipient are a matter of debate. At one extreme it is argued that there are no benefits to the donor and, therefore, even the small risk of complications becomes more significant. Others state strongly that there are remarkable benefits to the donor of a psychological nature, especially when donating to a family member, such as the satisfaction of helping to saved a loved one's life [22]. On balance, the very low risks associated with marrow donation and the fact that marrow is a renewable resource, like blood, and that significant benefits are derived by the donor, make it ethically appropriate to encourage PBC and marrow donation.

Of course, it is imperative that any coercion of potential donors be avoided. To that end, the HCT center should keep results of HLA typing confidential (or not even initiate testing) until all family members have had the opportunity to discuss privately their desire to proceed [9]. Another argument for strict confidentiality related to HLA typing results is that previously hidden facts about paternity may be brought to light to an unsuspecting family. Revelation of such information could have devastating effects on the entire family unit.

The psychological state of the donor must be respected. If the outcome is poor, especially if the patient fails because of GVHD, there will be a natural tendency for donors to blame themselves for the patient's death. Appropriate counseling before and after the HCT can help lessen this burden for the donor. In light of these concerns, it has become the legal standard that no court can force anyone to undergo medical testing or a procedure that is intended only to benefit another individual.

Confidentiality and noncoercion are especially important issues in relation to unrelated donors. The National Marrow Donor Program (NMDP) has very explicit policies and procedures designed to respect potential donors' autonomy by requiring informed consent at every step of the process, including the time at which a donor is first listed in the registry; before collection of blood for confirmatory typing, infectious disease markers and research samples; prior to notification of the transplant center that a donor is willing to proceed to donation; and before general anesthesia [23]. The donor's privacy is of utmost importance to avoid any extraneous influences or pressures as the donor decides whether or not to donate. The identity of the donor is known only to the individual donor center, and many precautions are put in place to ensure this. The recipient and donor are allowed to contact each other directly only by mutual consent 1 year after the HCT. The NMDP considers these measures to be critical in promoting increased participation in the program by altruistic individuals.

The process by which decisions are made to use minors as marrow donors is somewhat controversial [24–26]. Some authors have questioned the manner in which informed consent is obtained to collect marrow from minors and have asked whether parents can truly give informed consent. The need to involve the minor in the consent process by seeking his or her assent is a widely accepted concept, especially for children over the age of 7 or 8 years.

Delany has questioned whether it is really legal to harvest marrow from a minor and has labeled the process "altruism by proxy" [26]. One legal concept permits a medical procedure only if it serves the best interests of the child who undergoes it. If there is disagreement between caregivers, then it may be necessary to go to court. A second concept argues that parents can give valid consent to treatments that are "not against the interests of the child." This approach was developed to allow blood drawing from children whose legitimacy or parentage was at issue. Some have argued that this principle is relevant to any medical intervention carried out on children purely for other people's benefit. Delany argues that marrow donation is not in the best interest of the donor, and that it may be against the child's interests, especially if the potential donor is too young to have established an emotional bond with the intended recipient. She also contends that the parents are not well-suited to give informed consent for the donor due to conflict of interests related to the sick child and that an informal tribunal or other forum independent of the parents and medical advisors should be responsible for approving each proposed donation. This procedure would be analogous to the strategy developed by the Law Commission in England to safeguard mentally incapacitated adults from being inappropriately volunteered for marrow extraction.

Month disagreed strongly with this interpretation of the issues [26]. She believed that the positive aspects for the child donor are considerable, and include the saving of a sibling's life and the benefit of many years of a whole family not burdened by the psychological trauma of the death of a child. Furthermore, since HCT is an accepted therapeutic option that can be life saving and often offers the best cure rate, is there really any reason a morally competent sibling would not want to donate? The risks of donation are minimal, especially when compared to the risks of not donating marrow, that is, the death of a sibling.

Savulescu argued that though the bone marrow donation is not in the donor's medical interests, it may be in his or her overall interest [26]. To save the life of a loved one is one of the most important things one can do. Even for donors who are too young to understand at the time, the potential for a future sense of achievement and the love and gratitude of the saved sibling is important. There are benefits to the family unit as well. Parents should be the ones to give informed consent after they are educated about the risks and benefits of the donation, just as parents often make decisions with conflicting interests of their children, but with a commitment to the overall good of the family.

The formal process for approving the use of a minor for marrow donation varies between countries and between centers within the same country. A survey of 52 HCT centers in Europe and the USA found that some centers have an ethics committee decide the validity of the therapeutic proposal [25]. In France, there is a law that requires a committee of three experts to assess the psychological and medical consequences of donation of the organ by a minor and notes that "the refusal of the minor donor to accept the removal shall always be respected." In the USA, a Washington State court ruling stated that the advantages to the donor are undoubtedly greater than the risks, and defers to the parents to give informed consent. Some institutions require an authority outside the family and hospital, for example, a "tutelary judge," or commission of experts to make the decision.

A questionnaire was sent to 70 HCT centers in North America by pediatricians at the M.D. Anderson Cancer Center to poll the HCT teams on their approaches to marrow donations by minors [27]. The impetus for sending the questionnaire was a case brought to the M.D. Anderson pediatricians in which they were asked to collect marrow from a young child which was to be donated to the child's parent. There was a significant difference in size between the child and the parent and three HLA mismatches. The parent had relapsed AML. Ethical concerns were raised by hospital staff members. As a result, M.D. Anderson developed a process in which the minor donor and surrogate are interviewed by a social worker, pediatrician and anesthesiologist, none of whom are involved in the care of the recipient. If any concerns are raised, the case is referred to the ethics committee for consultation.

Fifty-six (80%) of the centers responded to the questionnaire. There was consensus in endorsing the validity of parental consent. Most centers would use donors as young as 6 months old—and would use them more than once if needed. The centers were willing to use minor donors for patients on experimental protocols, and the projected outcome of the HCT did not affect the decision to use the minor as a donor. Issues raised included the nontherapeutic nature of the donation, the vulnerability of the minor and the potential conflict of interest when a parent acts as a surrogate for both the donor and a sick family member. Even greater conflict was seen if a parent is the intended recipient of the marrow, and most agreed that the other parent or both should be involved in the informed consent procedure. The majority of the centers and physicians had policies or practices of using the parents as the surrogate; a minority preferred to use a parent plus a child advocate or child protection agency. If there were disagreements between the parents, eight centers would cancel the HCT and the rest would either seek consultation with the ethics committee, use an unrelated donor, refer the parents for another opinion or refer the decision to a child protection agency. When asked if the use of a child intentionally conceived as a marrow donor were ethical, most of the physicians answered that they would be willing to use such a donor. They would consider using umbilical cord blood in that case as being safer for the donor.

Alternative sources of hematopoietic cells

Case scenario 6

A couple decides to reverse a vasectomy to create a new baby to be a possible donor for their teenage daughter with CML who has no family or unrelated donors.

HLA-matched siblings are usually considered the primary source of cells for HCT. For the 70% of patients who lack such a donor, alternative sources of stem cells include matched related donors other than siblings, unrelated volunteer donors and, possibly, autologous stem cells in the appropriate clinical setting. Allogeneic PBCs are becoming a preferred source of cells at many centers. In this section, the ethical issues raised by three additional potential sources of stem cells are discussed, namely, umbilical cord blood [14,28–30], "children conceived to give life" [31] and xenografts from baboons or other primates.

Kurtzberg *et al.* [32] reported on the results of unrelated cord blood stem cell transplants in 25 patients. In previous reports of sibling donors of cord blood stem cells, there was successful engraftment and a lower incidence of GVHD. For these 25 patients who received unrelated cord blood grafts, all engrafted, successfully reconstituted their immune systems and developed treatable GVHD. The advantages of cord blood over adult marrow include the lower risk of carrying viruses; a reduction in procurement time from the 4–6 months needed for an unrelated marrow donor, to 1–2 weeks; and the fact that cord blood cells are potentially usable across greater HLA disparities. The major disadvantages are the limited number of cells available, the fact that one cannot go back to the donor for more cells if needed and the risk of transmitting a genetic disease not previously diagnosed in the donor's family.

Marshall [33] raised several ethical issues related to cord blood cell collections and cord blood banks, starting with consent and privacy. Is informed consent required for a product that is otherwise discarded as waste? Is the mother (or parents) the appropriate one(s) to give consent? Is consent required to conduct a battery of tests to detect possible infectious or genetic diseases, or both? Should donors, that is, the parents, be informed of the results of such tests? Who owns the cord blood? Obviously the donor him or herself cannot give informed consent, yet an extensive medical profile about the donor may be generated, raising concerns about invasion of privacy. Should consent be obtained for follow-up tests that are not directly consented to? What should be done with abnormal results from such tests? Should banks maintain medical files and genetic data but in such a way that names and identifiers are delinked from the donated sample [34]? What are the obligations to inform the family if evidence of human immunodeficiency virus (HIV) or an abnormal gene is found?

Some authors argue that the infant donors should be the first to benefit from use of their own cord blood cells [35]. Records should be kept of diseases detected and parents informed. Therapy should be offered for treatable diseases. Commercialization of cord blood cells for therapy should include a financial benefit for infants; for example, royalties from each donation should be placed in a national trust fund for research and treatment of children with serious diseases. Kurtzberg *et al.* argued that cord blood that was previously discarded material should be a public resource with no financial gain to any party [32]. Regulation of donor banks by an agency such as the FDA is needed. For example, there are companies that try to persuade parents that they should store the cells as insurance against future needs, when in fact the chances are remote that the donor would ever need or want to use the cord blood cells. There is a pressing need to protect the confidentiality of the information collected, to notify parents and children of the test results and to assure equitable access to cord blood samples. For the health of the mother and baby, the collection process should be restricted to full-term, uncomplicated pregnancies and should not interfere with good obstetrical practice at delivery.

Considerable attention and debate were generated in response to the actual case outlined above as Case scenario 6. The practice of "conceiving a child to give life" is not a rare event [36]. Some question whether a good outcome for the recipient lessens the ethical dilemmas posed. It was argued that such a practice does not impose harm on persons or relationships within the family, and does not show lack of respect for the child conceived [9]. Others raised their concerns about performing prenatal testing to diagnose the genetic disease affecting the intended recipient and for HLA typing, and the potential for aborting in the case of a mismatch.

One hematologist's view of the concept is that such a child is conceived not to replace the sick sibling but to give life to the sibling who would not survive without a transplant [36]. The benefits of this approach include the fact that the cord blood is disposable material and that no anesthesia or blood transfusions are needed for the donor. From the recipient's perspective, the transplant can be performed earlier since a marrow transplant could require a delay of 6 months or more.

Alby [31] described three characteristics of pregnancies conceived for HCT: (i) families in that situation face the trauma of the impending death of the sick child; (ii) the pregnancy outcome with respect to HLA matching and the HCT results are both uncertain; and (iii) biology has intruded into the family dynamics. A family may attempt a cure at any cost, especially in an emergent situation such as acute leukemia. A child may be viewed subconsciously as a replacement child but should never be reduced to the role of a therapeutic tool. In terms of family dynamics, a child may be viewed as bad or good based on HLA matching. Many are concerned that such a child is being conceived only for transplantation. Yet a child is always born for something: to maintain the integrity of a couple, to gratify the parents' need for a family, to repair their vulnerability. All parents must go beyond the idealized view of their child and accept that he or she has an identity of her own, and all children have some symbolic role in the family fantasy. In that light, is there really anything wrong with conceiving a child to donate cells for the purpose of saving the life of a sibling?

There are risks for children born for HCT, of both a physical and a psychological nature. The physical risks are less from cord blood collection than from marrow harvesting. Such a child would be born into a psychologically stressed family dealing with the emotional and financial trauma of caring for a sick child. In case of the death of the recipient, the new child is exposed to parental depression, identification with the deceased sibling, loss of identity if the parents cannot accept the death and shared guilt with the parents. When the procedure is successful, the donor is seen as the savior, and both the child and the family must find a normal way of life again.

Advances in *in vitro* fertilization techniques have opened the door to preimplantation genetic diagnosis (PGD). Candidate embryos can be screened *in vitro* for various genetic traits as the basis for selecting which embryos to implant. HLA typing of embryos to select a potential stem cell donor for an afflicted relative has been proposed as a legitimate means of securing a donor for a patient that is in need of a life-saving transplant. The ethics of this approach were reviewed recently, and the conclusions were that using PGD to choose a stem cell donor is unlikely to cause harm to anyone, is likely to be beneficial to some, is a reasonable use of limited health resources and should be permitted in countries where PGD is already allowed [37]. As a recent case in point, in the United Kingdom the Human Fertilization and Embryology Authority gave permission for PGD to be utilized to select an unaffected embryo to serve as a future hematopoietic cell donor for a sibling with thalassemia. The technique has been used in the USA since 2000 [38]. Pennings *et al.* [39] argued that PGD-guided selection of embryos for this purpose is morally defensible on the condition that the procedure to be performed on the future child is acceptable for an existing child and that the "instrumentalization" of the donor child does not demonstrate disrespect for the child's autonomy and intrinsic worth.

The ability to create multipotential stem cells *in vitro* from pluripotential embryonic stem cells is a subject of wide public debate. Legal and ethical distinctions have been drawn between human reproductive cloning and nuclear transplantation for the production of stem cells for therapeutic applications. Only the latter will be discussed here as a potential source of hematopoietic cells for use in HCT in the future. Many scientists, ethicists, government bodies and medical organizations in the USA, Canada and Europe have advocated for the legalization of research for the purpose of therapeutic cloning [40–45]. The potential to utilize such cells to treat a variety of medical conditions appears to be great, though significant technical hurdles are yet to be overcome before there can be clinical applications. Many serious ethical issues must be considered including the protection of human dignity, the source of unfertilized eggs and/or embryos to be used for research, informed consent from potential donors, the privacy of donors and financial incentives to donate eggs and/or embryos.

The utilization of an unusual source of stem cells generated considerable media attention when investigators attempted to reconstitute the immune system of a patient with acquired immune deficiency syndrome (AIDS) using stem cells collected from a baboon [46]. A number of scientific and safety issues are raised including: the risks of the baboon cells attacking the human host; the unknown ability of the baboon cells to mount an immune response against pathogens to which the AIDS patient is exposed; the concern that the patient will be made sicker by the conditioning regimen; and the question of whether the patient will have to fight off baboon viruses. Ethically, there are concerns about how to protect the rights of the first patients treated this way. How does one select the first patients for procedures that are not likely to benefit them, that is, the so-called "patient-pioneer" or "human guinea pig?" It is critical that the patient understands how unlikely it is that he or she will benefit, and that the experiments are done in a rigorous way so that the specialists in the field can learn from the experience. There are fears of transmission of animal pathogens to humans, perhaps necessitating germ-free colonies of donor animals. Pigs are being used for solid organ transplants to humans, perhaps as a bridge to tide the patient over until a human organ becomes available. Barker and Polcrack proposed caution in xenotransplantation and a postponement of solid organ xenotransplants until the issue of informed consent to the infectious disease risks is adequately addressed in an open public policy process [47].

Transplantation for nonmalignant diseases

Most HCT procedures are performed to treat malignant diseases for which HCT often represents the only curative option. Many nonmalignant diseases are also treated by HCT, especially in the pediatric patient population, and include primary marrow failure such as severe aplastic anaemia and a variety of congenital immune deficiency syndromes. The balance of risk and benefit for patients with these diseases is clearly in favor of HCT since the diseases are often rapidly fatal and curative alternative options are generally not available. The balance may not be so clearly defined for a variety of diseases that affect marrow-derived cells, which may be a source of significant morbidity for affected patients and possibly shortened life span, but are not considered to be rapidly fatal. Furthermore, the data that demonstrate the long-term benefit from HCT for these conditions may be inconclusive or even nonexistent. Examples of this category of diseases would include hemoglobinopathies, such as sickle cell disease, certain metabolic storage diseases, autoimmune diseases, such as multiple sclerosis or rheumatoid arthritis, and acquired immune deficiency diseases, specifically AIDS. How does one select the right patient to be treated by a procedure that carries significant risk of morbidity and possibly early mortality? How can one demonstrate the efficacy of HCT in diseases that usually progress over years rather than weeks or months? How does a parent decide to consent to an HCT for a child with such a disease?

This discussion focuses on hemoglobinopathies as a paradigm for these issues since there has already been a broad experience in performing transplants for thalassemia [48], and a body of literature about the ethical dilemmas involved is available. These issues were discussed at an international meeting on HCT in children held in March 1994 [28]. In regard to hemoglobinopathies, the difficult questions are whom to treat and when, and whether to offer HCT as a curative procedure to all affected children as early as possible. Some participants favored HCT for all patients with sickle cell disease who have an HLA-matched sibling in early childhood, given the high risk of morbidity in adult life. Others argued that it should be reserved for those who show clinical indicators of poor prognosis, as adopted by the ongoing national trial to recruit 30–60 children over a 5-year period. For thalassemia, the clinical course is more variable. Some proposed that HCT should be offered before any morbidity has occurred, while others would reserve it for children whose iron overload was well-controlled and were without liver disease.

Giardini discussed the ethical issues of HCT for thalassemia in an editorial in 1995 [49]. He argued in favor of HCT since the risk of mortality from disease-related complications remains high even with desferrioxamine chelation. The success of standard therapy depends on compliance of the patient and a health care system that is able to carry it out. The cost of this effort is about $32,000 per patient per year in developing countries and about $60,000 per year for adults in the USA. These patients require the input of specialists, including cardiologists, hepatologists, psychologists and endocrinologists. In comparison, an HCT for hemoglobinopathies in 1991 cost about $173,250 in the USA and about half that in Europe. Giardini argued that it is ethically and economically appropriate to recommend HCT for thalassemia, especially given the progress in dealing with GVHD and CMV, the availability of newer antibiotics, and so forth. Estimated outcomes for patients with class of risk I are 3% probability of death, 4% rejection and 93% disease-free survival. For patients in class of risk II and III with organ damage from iron overload, the mortality from HCT is higher, but their expected survival with standard therapy is much lower. Although other experimental approaches show promise, such as artificial hemoglobin, new oral iron chelators, gene therapy and agents to stimulate fetal hemoglobin, the fact is that currently HCT offers the only chance of cure of the disease.

Kodish and associates examined the issue of parents' decision making concerning HCT for children who are affected with sickle cell disease [50]. A questionnaire was presented to parents with hypothetical chances of cure vs. mortality to see how they balanced these two outcomes. In the study of 67 parents, 54% were willing to accept some risk of short-term mortality. Thirty-seven percent would accept at least a 15% mortality risk in the short term and 12% were willing to accept a 50% or more risk. Sixteen (24%) of the 67 parents would not accept HCT even if there was a 0% mortality risk.

Differences were found between the group of parents who would accept some risk vs. those who would not. Parents who were high school graduates, who were employed outside of the home or who had more than one child with sickle cell disease were more willing to take the risks. Of note, parents were more willing to take risks for girls than for boys. The parents' decisions were not related to the clinical severity of their children's illness, unlike the way the doctors might make such a decision. For parents with more than one child, their willingness may reflect their knowledge of the disease or the burden of caring for children with sickle cell disease. Clearly the concerns and values of the parents must be considered along with weighing the medical issues of risks and benefits. The difficult issue is what criteria to use to select patients to undergo HCT for sickle cell disease. As one model, the Institutional Review Board at the University of Chicago in 1988 allowed two groups of children to be treated with HCT: children who already had had a stroke and therefore were receiving monthly transfusions to prevent the next stroke and those with recurrent painful crises who had required hospitalization for at least 60% of the preceding year [50].

Recent advances in HCT, such as the use of peripheral blood hematopoietic cells from allogeneic donors and reduced intensity conditioning regimens, have been utilized in the treatment of hemoglobinopathies [51,52]. These advances help reduce the risks of short- and long-term toxicities for either the donor or the recipient, and thus create a more favorable risk—benefit ratio. Parents of minors with hemoglobinopathies will need to be informed about these innovations to help them make an appropriate decision for their children who may be candidates for HCT.

End-of-life issues

Case scenario 7

A 50-year-old physician with CML is dying from VOD and GVHD with liver and respiratory failure early after HCT. He has no written advanced directive. He made his second wife promise that she would not let him stay on life support for more than a week if he had no hope of recovery. She is devoutly Catholic but feels she made a commitment to her husband to withdraw life support. His adult children from his first marriage, who are atheists, say their father would never agree to withdrawal of life support, that he is ardently opposed to euthanasia and that to him withdrawal of life support is no different from euthanasia.

Respect for patient autonomy requires caregivers to determine the wishes of their patient with respect to resuscitation and life support. Advanced directives, such as a Power of Attorney for Health Care, are extremely effective vehicles to facilitate discussions between patients and their doctors, for patients to convey their wishes and to name a surrogate to speak for them when they become incapacitated. Yet very few patients execute such documents or discuss these matters with their doctor. Such discussions about end-of-life issues are difficult for most physicians, nurses and patients. They are even more difficult in the context of HCT where the patients are generally young and, though they have potentially fatal diseases, often have a significant chance for cure with this treatment. During the informed consent process that leads up to the HCT, physicians are obligated to discuss the risks and complications of the planned therapy, including the chance of early mortality. As discussed above in the section on informed consent for patients, when faced with life and death choices, patients often block out the details of possible complications in the decision-making process. Physicians have trouble raising end-of-life issues in the context of proposing a potentially life-saving therapy, in part for fear that patients will take away a negative message about their prognosis [53].

The fact remains that up to 15–20% of patients may succumb to early allogeneic transplant-related mortality. HCT patients often decompensate rapidly and unpredictably; for example, from severe VOD or GVHD. There may not be an opportunity to discuss end-of-life issues when the patient is in respiratory failure on the way to the intensive care unit. The quality of patient care would be much enhanced if such discussions and appropriate documentation of patients' wishes were carried out well before this point and were then acted upon as dictated by the patient or the surrogate. Many of these patients will be maintained by intensive life support for extended periods of time, despite generally poor chances of recovery. At some point in the course of the HCT procedure, the goals of therapy must shift from cure and aggressive interventions to palliation and supportive care for a dying patient. Rigorous attention to pain control is essential throughout the HCT process and certainly during the period of dying.

The principles of fidelity and nonabandonment require caregivers to make it clear to patients and their families that they will not be abandoned as the goals of treatment shift from cure to caring for the dying patient. Though it may be appropriate to withhold interventions that are medically futile, how is this to be determined? How much of our limited health care resources should be expended providing what is ultimately futile medical care? How great an emotional cost do families have to pay? These are difficult questions that need to be addressed at both the macro level of society and the micro level of individual patients and families. It is the patient (or surrogate) who is best able to understand and decide on the issues of his or her ability to pay for a treatment and the possibility of financial destitution of a family by continuing futile care. The surrogate must utilize substituted judgement to relay the decisions that the patient would have made if he or she had the capacity. In cases in which no surrogate is legally designated, an ethics committee may need to be involved to consider quality of life issues and death with dignity.

To explore the variables involved in instituting do-not-resuscitate (DNR) orders for HCT patients, a retrospective review of 40 patients who died on the Seattle Veterans Administration Medical Center HCT unit was carried out [54]. This center has a DNR policy that requires physicians to document the discussion held with the patient or surrogate and for the patient or surrogate to sign a DNR consent. Patients with fatal diseases often suspend their feelings about terminal illness in hopes of a cure through HCT. The dying trajectory of these patients is often sudden and unpredictable. The health care providers often focus on aggressive medical management when these situations arise and, as a result, the topic of death is avoided. The process of executing DNR orders was believed to facilitate the transition from aggressive care to supportive care in critically ill HCT patients.

Of the 42 deaths that occurred on the HCT unit during a 5-year period, six patients had a resuscitation attempt and 36 had DNR orders (two records were not available for review). The DNR consent was signed 26% of the time by the patients themselves, 32% by spouses, 24% by mothers and 18% by other family members. The two groups of patients did not vary in terms of age, diagnosis or type of HCT. The non-DNR group developed life-threatening complications earlier in their course, whereas multisystem organ failure was the common factor among the DNR patients. The death of non-DNR patients may not have been anticipated because the complications that developed were emergent and were considered reversible. These conditions may have precluded discussions regarding DNR status. For the DNR patients, this designation occurred close to the time of death: 32% on the same day as death, 82% <5 days before death and 18% 5–14 days prior to death.

In 11 studies of HCT patients who required mechanical ventilation, the rates of survival to discharge from the hospital ranged from 0% to 11.1%

with a mean of 4.7% [55]. It would be clinically useful to define a subgroup of patients whose chance of survival is so low that both patients/surrogates and physicians can agree that intensive care can no longer fulfill the original goals of the HCT. Criteria to identify patients who are destined to die after HCT are needed to help reduce emotional and financial expenditures of families and institutions. At the Fred Hutchinson Cancer Research Center, 25% of all HCT patients were ventilated from 1980 to 1992. Patients who were more than 20 years old, had disease in relapse and had grafts that were not HLA-identical had a 50% chance of needing ventilation. Only 6.1% survived. To identify predictors of death in mechanically ventilated HCT patients, Rubenfeld and Crawford conducted a nested case-control study comparing all 53 survivors of ventilatory support to 106 matched control subjects who did not survive [55]. These patients were selected from the 865 individuals who were mechanically ventilated for at least 24 h during that 12-year period. Survivors were defined as those who were alive for 30 days after extubation and who were discharged from the hospital.

Survival was statistically associated with younger age, lower score on the Acute Physiology, Age, Chronic Health Evaluation (APACHE) III scale, and shorter time from HCT to intubation. Of the 106 control subjects who died, 82% died while on the ventilator and the remaining 18% died in the hospital a median of 18 days after extubation. Of the 53 survivors, median survival after extubation was 634 days (range from 54 days to 12 years). Eighteen (34%) survived for <6 months and five (9%) for <1 year; 30 (57%) lived for more than 1 year. No patient who was intubated for more than 149 days survived. The survival rates changed from 5% to 16% over the most recent 5 years, which was not explained by changes in the age of patients, the rate or timing of intubation, or the percentage of allogeneic transplants that *were* not HLA-identical. The improved survival may be due to better antimicrobials and the use of cytokines.

There were no survivors among the 398 patients who had lung injury and either required more than 4 h of vasopressors or had sustained hepatic and renal failure. Using these three criteria, an accurate prediction of death could be made in the first 4 days for more than half of the patients who did not survive. Of the 60% of patients who developed any two of these three risk factors, half had done so by day 2 and 90% by day 4. On average, these risk factors developed 6 ventilator days and 9 hospital days before death. If life support had been withdrawn on the 1st day that two out of three risk factors were met, and if death had followed swiftly, then more than 7300 hospital days and 4800 ventilator days could have been avoided for the 812 patients who died.

A recent multiinstitutional study has confirmed these observations in adult HCT patients, for whom the combination of mechanical ventilation, hepatic and renal dysfunction was associated with a probability of death of 98–100% [56]. A scoring system for pediatric patients undergoing allogeneic HCT called the oncologic pediatric risk of mortality (O-PRISM) may be useful in predicting fatal events and thus help parents decide to establish a supportive care strategy for their children [57].

Though most physicians and ethicists may agree that futile, inappropriate or unreasonable medical care should not be provided even if requested, how are these terms to be defined and by whom? In cases in which the patient or surrogate continues to request treatments that the caregivers consider futile, the physician is not ethically required to provide that care but is obligated based on the principle of nonabandonment to facilitate the transfer of the patient to another physician who will. Consultation with the institutional ethics committee may be helpful in these most difficult situations.

Closing remarks

The indications for HCT have expanded over the years to encompass a wide range of diagnoses and disease stages, including patients with early stages of hematologic malignancies considered to be at high risk of relapse, solid tumors, congenital disorders and autoimmune diseases. Potential sources of stem cells have also expanded to include autologous or allogeneic cells from bone marrow, peripheral blood or cord blood from related or unrelated HLA-matched donors. It is imperative that the rights of both patients and donors are respected in step with these technologic advances. The ethical principle of justice requires caregivers and insurers to provide potentially life-saving, yet high-risk, procedures to HCT candidates in an open and equitable manner. Patient autonomy, nonmaleficence and nonabandonment are guiding principles in making decisions about end-of-life care.

References

1 Arenson EB Jr, Forbe MD. Bone marrow transplantation for acute leukemia and Down syndrome: report of a successful case and results of a national survey. *J Pediatr* 1989; **114**(1): 69–72.

2 Chang G, Antin JH, Orav EJ, Randall U, McGarigle C, Behr HM. Substance abuse and bone marrow transplant. *Am J Drug Alcohol Abuse* 1997; **23**(2): 301–8.

3 Mitchell JM, Meehan KR, Kong J, Schulman K. Access to bone marrow transplantation for leukemia and lymphoma: the role of sociodemographic factors. *J Clin Oncol* 1997; **15**(7): 2644–51.

4 Vaughan WP, Purtilo RB, Butler CD, Armitage JO. Symposium: ethical and financial issues in autologous marrow transplantation: a symposium sponsored by the University of Nebraska Medical Center. *Ann Intern Med* 1986; **105**: 134–5.

5 Faber-Langendoen K. Ethical issues in the allocation and reimbursement of bone marrow transplantation. *Leukemia* 1993; **7**(7): 1117–21.

6 Beatty PG. Bone marrow transplantation for the treatment of hematologic disease: status in 1994. *Exp Hematol* 1995; **23**: 277–88.

7 Welch GH, Mogielnicki J. Presumed benefit: lessons from the American experience with marrow transplantation for breast cancer. *Br Med J* 2002; **324**: 1008–92.

8 Vaughan WP, Purtilo RB, Butler CD, Armitage JO. Symposium: ethical and financial issues in autologous marrow transplantation. *Ann Intern Med* 1986; **105**: 134–5.

9 Downs S. Ethical issues in bone marrow transplantation. *Semin Oncol Nurs* 1994; **10**(1): 58–63.

10 Andrykowski MA, Brady MJ, Greiner CB *et al.* "Returning to normal" following bone marrow transplantation: outcomes, expectations and informed consent. *Bone Marrow Transplant* 1995; **15**: 573–81.

11 Winer EP, Sutton LM. Quality of life after bone marrow transplantation. *Oncology* 1994; **8**(1): 19–31.

12 Hjermstad MJ, Kaasa S. Quality of life in adult cancer patients treated with bone marrow transplantation: a review of the literature. *Eur J Cancer* 1995; **31**(2): 163–73.

13 Baker F. Psychosocial sequelae of bone marrow transplantation. *Oncology* 1994; **8**(10): 87–101.

14 Massimo L. Ethical problems in bone marrow transplantation in children. *Bone Marrow Transplant* 1996; **18** (Suppl. 2): 8–12.

15 Harrison C, Kenny NP, Sidarous M, Rowell M. Bioethics for clinicians. 9. Involving children in medical decisions. *Can Med Assoc J* 1997; **156**: 825–8.

16 Buckner CD, Petersen FB, Bolonesi BA. Bone marrow donors. In: Forman SJ, Blume KG, Thomas ED, eds. *Bone Marrow Transplantation*. Boston: Blackwell Scientific Publications, 1994: 259–69.

17 Anderlini P, Przepiorka D, Lauppe J *et al.* Collection of peripheral blood stem cells from normal donors 60 years of age or older. *Br J Haematol* 1997; **97**: 485–7.

18 Bishop MR, Tarantolo SR, Jackson JD *et al.* Allogeneic-blood stem-cell collection following mobilization with low-dose granulocyte colony-stimulating factor. *J Clin Oncol* 1997; **15**: 1601–7.

19 Pavletic ZS, Bishop MR, Tarantolo SR *et al.* Hematopoietic recovery after allogeneic blood stem-cell transplantation compared with bone marrow transplantation in patients with hematologic malignancies. *J Clin Oncol* 1997; **15**: 1608–16.

20 Heldal D, Brinch L, Tjonnfjord G *et al.* Donation of stem cells from blood or bone marrow: results of a randomised study of safety and complaints. *Bone Marrow Transplant* 2002; **29**(6): 479–86.

21 Stroncek D, Strand R, Scott E *et al.* Attitudes and physical condition of unrelated bone marrow donors immediately after donation. *Transfusion* 1989; **29**(4): 317–22.

22 Anonymous. Ethics of organ transplantation from living donors. *Transplant Proc* 1992; **24**(5): 2236–7.

23 National Marrow Donor Program (NMDP) Transplant Center. *Policy Matters. National Marrow Donor Program Transplant Center Manual of Operations.* Minneapolis, MN: NMDP center, 1996: 3–1–3–25.

24 Curran WJ. Beyond the best interests of a child: bone marrow transplantation among half-siblings. *N Engl J Med* 1991; **324**(25): 1818–9.

25 Burgio GR, Nespoli L, Varrasi G, Buzzi F. Bone marrow transplantation in children: between therapeutic and medico-legal problems. *Bone Marrow Transplant* 1989; **4** (Suppl. 4): 34–7.

26 Delany L, Month S, Savulescu J, Browert P, Palmer S. Altruism by proxy: volunteering children for bone marrow donation. *BMJ* 1996; **312**: 240–3.

27 Chan K-W, Gajewski JL, Supkis D, Pentz R, Champlin R, Bleyer WA. Use of minors as bone marrow donors: current attitude and management. *J Pediatr* 1996; **128**(5): 644–8.

28 Roberts I. Bone marrow transplantation in children: current results and controversies. *Bone Marrow Transplant* 1994; **14**: 197–9.

29 Gluckman E. Eurocord Network Organisation. Ethical and legal aspects of placental/cord blood banking and transplant. *Hematol J* 2000; **1**(1): 67–9.

30 Dame L, Sugarman J. Blood money: ethical and legal implications of treating cord blood as property. *J Pediatr Hematol Oncol* 2001; **23**: 409–10.

31 Alby N. The child conceived to give life. *Bone Marrow Transplant* 1992; **9** (Suppl. 1): 95–6.

32 Kurtzberg J, Laughlin M, Graham ML *et al.* Placental blood as a source of hematopoietic stem cells for transplantation into unrelated recipients. *N Engl J Med* 1996; **335**: 157–66.

33 Marshall E. Clinical promise, ethical quandary. *Science* 1996; **271**: 586–8.

34 Rubinstein P, Stevens CE, Adamson JW, Migliaccio G. Umbilical cord blood cells: informed consent. *Bone Marrow Transplant* 1995; **15**: 160.

35 Ammann AJ. Placental-blood transplantation. *N Engl J Med* 1997; **336**(1): 68.

36 Schaison GS. The child conceived to give life. The point of view of the hematologist. *Bone Marrow Transplant* 1992; **9** (Suppl. 1): 93–4.

37 Boyle RJ, Savulescu J. Ethics of using preimplantation genetic diagnosis to select a stem cell donor for an existing person. *Br Med J* 2001; **323**(7323): 1240–3.

38 Watchdog approves embryo selection to treat 3-year-old child. *Br Med J* 2002; **324**: 503–5.

39 Pennings G, Schots R, Liebaers I. Ethical considerations on preimplantation genetic diagnosis for HLA typing to match a future child as a donor of haematopoietic stem cells to a sibling. *Hum Reprod* 2002; **17**(3): 534–8.

40 Weissman IL. Stem cells: scientific, medical, and political issues. *N Engl J Med* 2002; **346**(20): 1576–9.

41 Anonymous. The environments of stem cells: biology, ethics, and policy. *Can Med Assoc J* 2002; **166**(8): 1005.

42 American Academy of Pediatrics: Committee on Pediatric Research, Committee on Bioethics. Human embryo research. *Pediatrics* 2001; **108**(3): 813–6.

43 McLaren A. Ethical and social considerations of stem cell research. *Nature* 2001; **414**: 129–31.

44 Evers K. European perspectives on therapeutic cloning. *N Engl J Med* 2002; **346**(20): 1579–82.

45 Bruce DM. Stem cells, embryos and cloning: unravelling the ethics of a knotty debate. *J Mol Biol* 2002; **319**(4): 917–25.

46 Nowak R. Xenotransplants set to resume. *Science* 1994; **266**: 1148–51.

47 Barker JH, Polcrack L. Respect for persons, informed consent and the assessment of infectious disease risks in xenotransplantation. *Med Health Care Philos* 2001; **4**(1): 53–70.

48 Lucarelli G, Andreani M, Angelucci E. The cure of thalassemia by bone marrow transplantation. *Blood Rev* 2002; **16**(2): 81–5.

49 Giardini C. Ethical issues of bone marrow transplantation for thalassemia [editorial]. *Bone Marrow Transplant* 1995; **15**: 657–8.

50 Kodish E, Lantos J, Stocking C, Singer PA, Siegler M, Johnson FL. Bone marrow transplantation for sickle cell disease: a study of parents' decisions. *N Engl J Med* 1991; **325**: 1349–53.

51 Yesilipek MA, Hazar V, Küpesiz A, Kizilörs A, Uguz A, Yegin O. Peripheral blood stem cell transplantation in children with beta-thalassemia. *Bone Marrow Transplant* 2001; **28**: 1037–40.

52 Schleuning M, Stoetzer O, Waterhouse C, Schlemmer M, Ledderose G, Kolb H-J. Hematopoietic stem cell transplantation after reduced-intensity conditioning as treatment of sickle cell disease. *Exp Hematol* 2002; **30**: 7–10.

53 Crawford SW. Decision making in critically ill patients with hematologic malignancy. *West J Med* 1991; **155**: 488–93.

54 Kern D, Kettner P, Albrizio M. An exploration of the variables involved when instituting a do-not-resuscitate order for patients undergoing bone marrow transplantation. *Oncol Nurs Forum* 1992; **19**(4): 635–40.

55 Rubenfeld GD, Crawford SW. Withdrawing life support from mechanically ventilated recipients of bone marrow transplants: a case for evidence-based guidelines. *Ann Intern Med* 1996; **125**: 625–33.

56 Bach PB, Schrag D, Nierman DM *et al.* Identification of poor prognostic features among patients requiring mechanical ventilation after hematopoietic stem cell transplantation. *Blood* 2002; **98**(12): 3234–40.

57 Schneider DT, Cho J, Laws HJ, Dilloo D, Göbel U, Nürnberger W. Serial evaluation of the oncological pediatric risk of mortality (O-PRISM) score following allogeneic bone marrow transplantation in children. *Bone Marrow Transplant* 2002; **29**(5): 383–9.

38

Michael A. Andrykowski & Richard P. McQuellon

Psychosocial Issues in Hematopoietic Cell Transplantation

Hematopoietic cell transplantation (HCT) is a class of complex medical procedures used in the treatment of a variety of life-threatening diseases. Common diseases for which HCT is indicated, morbidity and mortality risks associated with these procedures, and the nuances of medical management have all been discussed in great detail in other chapters in this volume. We focus on identification and discussion of the complex psychological and social issues associated with HCT. Recognition and management of these issues is a significant challenge to the health care team. In some respects, management of these psychological and social issues can be more difficult and frustrating than management of the medical issues posed by HCT.

Throughout this chapter, we use the term "psychosocial" to collectively refer to issues which are psychological or social (or both) in nature. Similarly, we use the term HCT to refer to a class of medical procedures that involve the transplantation of hematopoietic stem cells (HSCs) derived from peripheral blood, cord blood, or bone marrow. Technically, bone marrow transplantation (BMT) refers only to the latter. For the most part, however, the scientific literature examining psychosocial issues in HCT does not make this distinction. Regardless of the source of HSCs, HCT is associated with a common set of psychosocial issues. Similarly, HCT is used to treat a variety of diseases and a set of generic psychosocial issues are germane regardless of the underlying disease. Again, we focus on these generic psychosocial issues while indicating issues unique to a specific disease, when appropriate. Finally, we focus our discussion upon psychosocial issues pertinent to adult HCT recipients, while providing some additional discussion of psychosocial issues pertinent to HCT donors, family caregivers and medical staff.

Psychosocial issues in HCT: recipients

HCT recipients confront a variety of physical and psychosocial stressors during the course of treatment and recovery. Two general sources of stress can be identified. First, HCT typically occurs in a life-threatening context. The diseases for which this procedure is indicated are virtually always life threatening and HCT is often used after other treatment options have been exhausted. Furthermore, HCT itself is associated with significant mortality risk, with the possibility that HCT may actually hasten a patient's death relative to what might have been expected had conventional treatment, or no treatment, been employed. Additionally, HCT carries no guarantee of success in eradicating a recipient's underlying disease. This context of uncertain, yet ever present, life-threat serves as a significant source of stress for all individuals involved in the HCT setting: patients, family caregivers, HSC donors and medical staff. Second, HCT is an aggressive form of treatment. Marrow-ablative therapy, consisting of high-dose chemotherapy with or without localized and/or total body irradiation (TBI), is usually employed prior to HCT. The acute (e.g. nausea, mucositis, hair loss, fatigue) and long-term (e.g. chronic GVHD, secondary malignancies, etc.) side-effects associated with high-dose chemotherapy and radiation can be significant sources of distress. Furthermore, medical management of HCT recipients typically requires administration of many drugs and therapies; each associated with its own profile of acute and chronic side-effects ranging from mildly discomforting to painful and debilitating. In short, HCT recipients experience an array of taxing physical stressors within the context of the psychological and social stressors associated with medical uncertainty and life-threat.

Stages of HCT

As HCT unfolds, patients are confronted with a fairly predictable sequence of treatment-related events. Each of these "stages" of HCT treatment is associated with a fairly predictable set of physical and psychosocial stressors. The number and nature of stages of HCT that have been identified have varied [1–3]. We will organize our discussion of psychosocial issues confronting the HCT recipient around five stages: (i) the decision to undergo HCT; (ii) pre-HCT preparation; (iii) post-HCT hospitalization; (iv) hospital discharge and early recovery; and (v) long-term recovery. We will identify and discuss the psychosocial issues germane to each of these five stages. Table 38.1 provides a short summary of the psychosocial issues relevant to each stage.

Stage one: the decision to undergo HCT

The decision to undergo HCT is very stressful for most potential recipients. At best, recipients can expect a host of toxic short and long-term side-effects, typically exceeding those associated with conventional therapeutic options. At worst, the recipient may die during the course of HCT, experiencing an earlier death relative to that which might have occurred had other conventional or palliative therapeutic options been selected. Despite the critical nature of the decision to opt for HCT, little research has examined this decision-making process. Most of the extant research has focused upon recipients' provision of informed consent for HCT. The formal consent process, however, is only the final step in an often protracted decision-making process. Earlier steps in the decision sequence include the decision to even consider HCT as a treatment option and to undergo formal evaluation for HCT suitability (i.e. medical referral for HCT). Finally, the medical team must decide that an individual is a suitable candidate for HCT.

Medical referral for treatment

The decision to undergo HCT begins with its initial consideration as a treatment option. In most cases, the possibility of HCT is raised initially

Table 38.1 Psychological and social issues germane to each stage of hematopoietic cell transplantation (HCT).

Stage	Issues
I. The decision to undergo HCT	*Theme: active decision making* Confronting the possibility of death Managing the uncertainty of treatment outcome Considering alternative treatments Financial considerations/insurance limitations Psychosocial evaluation Informed consent process Symptoms of anxiety, depression, and distress
II. Pre-HCT preparation	*Theme: aggressive treatment* Managing acute treatment side-effects Adapting to isolation and hospital routine Maintaining morale and hope Confronting unfamiliar procedures and treatment (e.g. TBI) Separation from family and friends Altered body image with Hickman catheter
III. Post-HCT hospitalization	*Theme: watchful waiting* Waiting for engraftment Heightened physical and emotional vulnerability Contending with the boredom of isolation Dealing with life-threatening complications Encountering acute psychological distress Managing discouragement
IV. Hospital discharge and early recovery	*Theme: transition from intense medical surveillance* Managing the loss of daily psychosocial support of medical team and allied health care professionals (e.g. pastoral care) Contending with the stress of frequent medical appointments, readmissions, and set-backs Reintegration into valued social roles (e.g. parent, spouse, or social companions) Managing unexpected sequelae (e.g. profound fatigue) Adapting to potential frustration, depressive symptoms, and anger Complying with self-care guidelines and daily medicine regimen
V. Long-term recovery	*Theme: readaptation to a normal life* Full recovery of valued roles Adjust to losses associated with transplantation, e.g. fertility Return to employment Accepting the possibility and reality of long-term effects (e.g. cataracts, second malignancies) Adoption of nonpatient identity

TBI, total body irradiation.

by the medical oncologist managing the patient's care. However, in other instances, the patient may initially raise the possibility of HCT on their own and press for consideration of this option. Regardless of the source of referral, up-to-date knowledge regarding HCT is critical at this juncture. This is particularly true when HCT is viewed as the only viable hope for disease cure. In these instances, patients are likely to quickly embrace HCT as their only alternative, disregarding the alternative of no further curative treatment. In effect, a psychological commitment to HCT may be made at the time this option is first considered [4,5], perhaps before the patient possesses any substantial knowledge of the risks and benefits associated with HCT. This commitment may be immutable by the time the patient arrives at the transplant center for initial evaluation. The referring physician therefore plays a critical role in ensuring that the decision to undergo HCT is truly an "informed" decision [6].

Selection of candidates

Some form of psychiatric or psychosocial assessment is recommended during the medical evaluation of HCT candidates [7]. The intent of this assessment is to obtain information about current psychological distress, past or present psychiatric disorder, current support systems, coping style, history of medical noncompliance and past or current problems with alcohol or substance abuse. How this psychosocial information is used can vary considerably. While psychosocial considerations, such as a history of alcohol abuse or medical noncompliance, may be used to screen candidates for solid organ transplantation [8], rejection of an HCT candidate strictly on the basis of psychosocial considerations is uncommon. Psychosocial information obtained during the pre-HCT evaluation is most likely used to anticipate problems in caring for the patient and to develop an individualized plan for the patient's care over the course of HCT. For example, to facilitate care planning, Molassiotis [9] developed a brief scale to prospectively identify patients prone to emotional difficulties during post-HCT hospitalization.

Standardized approaches to the pre-HCT psychosocial evaluation have been described, including the Psychosocial Levels System (PLS) [10], the Transplant Evaluation Rating Scale (TERS) [11] and the Psychosocial Assessment of Candidates for Transplantation Scale (PACT) [12].

All three approaches focus, for the most part, upon the content areas indicated above. The PACT and the TERS yield comparable information [13], while the TERS appears to possess somewhat better psychometric properties than its precursor, the PLS [14]. The clinical utility of these standardized approaches to the pre-HCT psychosocial evaluation for selecting appropriate candidates for HCT remains to be empirically established. As a result, reliance upon pre-HCT psychosocial data for making HCT treatment decisions is likely unwarranted at this time.

There is a critical need for more research in this area. In addition to the considerable monetary costs associated with HCT, HCT can involve the allocation of scarce, often finite resources. This is particularly true when unrelated individuals serve as the source of hematatopoietic stem cells. Thus, similar to solid organ transplantation, there is strong justification for ensuring that HCT be offered to suitable candidates (i.e. those most likely to evince a successful outcome), based upon the relevant information available, both medical and psychosocial. Critical to the use of psychosocial information in the selection of candidates or development of care plans for individual patients are sound data linking critical post-HCT outcomes (e.g. noncompliance, physical and psychological morbidity, survival) to information obtained in the psychosocial evaluation. While it might be anticipated that inadequate social support, a history of medical noncompliance or substance abuse problems, would be associated with poorer post-HCT outcomes, this linkage has not been demonstrated. However, several recent studies suggest a link between psychosocial status at the time of HCT and important post-HCT outcomes such as survival [15–18] and risk for medical complications [17,19]. For example, Loberiza et al. [15] reported recipients evidencing a depressive syndrome at the time of HCT were three times more likely to die between 6 and 12 months post-HCT, even after adjustment for other prognostic factors. While research has found no link between pre-HCT psychosocial variables and post-HCT survival [20], this is a provocative research area and merits further investigation. In particular, identification of biopsychosocial mechanisms linking psychosocial variables to poorer post-HCT clinical outcomes should be a research priority.

Provision of informed consent

The decision to undergo HCT is formalized by the provision of informed consent. In theory, the consent process allows patients to make an informed and voluntary decision regarding whether to proceed with HCT [21]. In practice, however, this ideal is unlikely to be realized in the HCT setting [4,22]. As noted above, the decision to undergo HCT is difficult. Significant elevations in psychological distress have been observed in adult HCT recipients [23] and parents of pediatric HCT recipients [24] within the 48 h after provision of informed consent. Such elevations in distress are not surprising. Most consent forms contain exhaustive descriptions and listings of the medical risks associated with HCT—enough to frighten even the most psychologically stable adult. Furthermore, research has documented that many recipients are considerably distressed in the days prior to HCT [25–29]. For example, Grassi et al. [27] found that 30–50% of their sample evidenced moderate to severe symptoms of anxiety and depression at the time of hospital admission for autologous HCT. Similarly, Baker et al. [25] found that 31% of their sample of 437 HCT candidates (both autologous and allogeneic) evidenced clinically significant levels of depressive symptoms. In a longitudinal study, Fife et al. [26] found that emotional distress was highest after hospital admission but prior to HCT. While these data do not necessarily implicate the consent process as the *cause* of distress in potential HCT recipients, these data do suggest that the consent process occurs within a context of considerable distress. The presence of distress can compromise the consent process by inhibiting communication with health care providers, limiting rational consideration of risks and benefits of HCT and inhibiting comprehension or memory for information communicated during the important consent discussions. Indeed, research suggests that distressed individuals might be more likely to agree to undergo experimental therapies [30]. In addition, the presence of mild to moderate cognitive impairment may further compromise the pre-HCT decision-making and consent processes. Such impairment may be common in HCT candidates, likely due to the candidate's underlying disease and treatment [31,32].

Historically, HCT began as a treatment of "last resort" that was offered only to patients with otherwise fatal diseases and only when all other potentially curative or life-prolonging treatment options had been exhausted. Under these conditions, the decision to undergo HCT is simpler (though still stressful) since potential HCT recipients are likely to believe they have no other choice [22,33]. Increasingly, however, HCT is used as a "first-line" therapy for some medical conditions, making the treatment decision even more complex and distressing for patients. While HCT may increase the likelihood of cure or prolonged remission relative to other therapeutic options, these other options (e.g. conventional oral or intravenous chemotherapy) may be associated with less morbidity and virtually no short-term mortality risk. A good example of this dilemma lies in the treatment of chronic myeloid leukemia (CML). Conventional therapy for CML, while fairly benign, is not curative and the disease will ultimately accelerate and result in death. Patients with a suitable donor may be advised to consider undergoing HCT before their disease accelerates. Given the increased morbidity and mortality associated with HCT, an optimal strategy might be to postpone HCT as long as possible. However, if CML enters an accelerated phase, risks for HCT-related morbidity and mortality increase relative to what the risks would have been if HCT had been implemented during the chronic, stable phase of the disease. This decision is now even more complicated with the success of the oral chemotherapeutic agent, imatinib mesylate (STI571, Gleevec®), as this agent has produced prolonged remissions in some CML patients and may even produce cure.

The scenario described above illustrates that the decision of whether and when to undergo HCT fundamentally involves a trade-off between the increased toxicity associated with HCT and the increased potential for disease cure or at least long-term disease-free survival. In other words, quality of life (QOL) considerations must be balanced against quantity of life considerations. There is evidence that patients are willing to risk substantial toxicity and increased risk of mortality for increased survival even if the outcome of treatment is uncertain [34,35]. Given the significance and psychological complexity of this type of treatment decision, information about how patients (or parents) make decisions regarding HCT would be useful. Only two studies have explored the decisional process employed in making a decision to accept or reject HCT [36,37]. Using a standard reference-gamble paradigm, parents of children with sickle cell disease were asked to indicate the level of risk they would accept in exchange for a possible disease cure [36]. Despite the fact that the natural course of sickle cell disease is one of chronic debilitation, over one-third of parents were willing to accept a 15% risk of death within 30 days of HCT in exchange for a possible cure. Based on the premise that the HCT decision is based upon patients' knowledge of HCT and their preferences for certain mortality and morbidity (e.g. QOL) outcomes, Sebban et al. [37] developed a bedside decision board to assist CML patients and their physicians in deciding between HCT and other more conservative management options for CML. They tested the decision board with 42 healthy hospital personnel, not patients. Satisfaction with treatment preference was higher for those exposed to the decision board compared to those presented with an abbreviated version of the decision board.

In addition to the decision whether and when to undergo HCT, patients and their families are also confronted with decisions regarding participation in a variety of clinical trials associated with the treatment process.

Again, these decisions can be very difficult. The number of potential clinical trials that a patient might be eligible for might be substantial, and comprehension and consideration of the risks and benefits associated with each potential clinical trial can be daunting. Finally, the stress associated with the HCT setting makes informed decision making regarding clinical trial participation challenging. Because clinical trial participation is critical to treatment innovation and improvement, decision making regarding clinical trial participation merits exploration in the HCT setting.

Discussion of risks and benefits associated with HCT, as well as alternative courses of action, is fundamental to the informed consent process. Nevertheless, patients may be reticent to engage in this type of discussion [38]. Such reticence may occur because the patient's (or parents') decision to undergo HCT has been made well before the formal consent discussion occurs. Disclosure and discussion of information regarding mortality and morbidity risks in these instances may be quite threatening, triggering attempts to avoid or minimize important information [39]. While it may seem maladaptive for patients to deny, distort or avoid information provided in the consent discussion, such avoidance may be critical to the mobilization of the psychological strength necessary to embark upon the arduous, uncertain and life-threatening course of HCT [4]. Recognition that avoidance of critical information might be adaptive from the patient's perspective does not suggest, however, that critical information should be withheld from patients during the consent process. Rather, this recognition suggests that provision of informed consent in the HCT setting might best be considered a process rather than a discrete event. Complete and accurate information should be presented prior to HCT, with additional supplementary discussions throughout the course of HCT to review critical information presented earlier. While threatening information might be avoided prior to HCT, this same information might be accepted later in the course of post-HCT recovery. Accurate expectations for post-HCT outcomes are important since poorer post-HCT psychological adjustment is associated with violated expectations for post-HCT outcomes [4].

Stage two: pre-HCT preparation

The second stage begins when the patient begins pre-HCT preparative therapy. This therapy consists of high-dose chemotherapy, often in combination with TBI. In most instances, preparative therapy is administered over a 3–10-day period immediately prior to HCT. Typically, the recipient is hospitalized while undergoing preparative therapy. More recently, it has become more common for preparative therapy to be administered on an outpatient basis over a more extended period of time, perhaps several weeks. The acute side-effects of this preparative, "conditioning" therapy include nausea and vomiting, hair loss, diarrhea, fatigue and mucositis. Side-effects are often severe, even with appropriate supportive care, and may continue after preparative therapy has been completed. Pain from mucositis, in particular, is likely to peak from 4 to 14 days after conclusion of preparative therapy.

Critical psychosocial issues at this stage center on adaptation to the hospital routine and infection control procedures and maintenance of the recipient's psychological strength and coping capacity. Effective management of the demoralizing and painful side-effects of pre-HCT preparative therapy is critical. Pain and nausea are typically controlled through liberal use of antiemetic and analgesic medications. Cognitive-behavioral therapies can also be used as adjunctive therapy for symptom control, especially with patients who are averse to antiemetic and analgesic medications. In a pair of well-designed studies, Syrjala *et al.* [40,41] examined the utility of several cognitive-behavioral interventions (e.g. hypnosis, relaxation and imagery, cognitive behavioral coping skills training), for controlling pain and nausea associated with pre-HCT preparative therapy. While hypnosis and coping skills training appeared to have little impact upon nausea and vomiting [40], all three interventions reduced oral pain associated with mucositis. As all study participants received routine pharmacologic therapy for their symptoms, results suggest that hypnosis can significantly *add* to effects obtained with standard analgesic medications. While these results are promising, incorporation of cognitive-behavioral therapies into the management of HCT recipients may be limited since implementation of these therapies is typically time-consuming and costly, even when patients are trained to implement them on their own. However, more abbreviated cognitive-behavioral interventions could be developed and could be effective. For example, a recent study found a single session psychoeducational intervention designed to enhance coping with treatment side-effects was effective in reducing nausea, fatigue and anxiety in a group of autologous HCT recipients [42].

The pre-HCT preparative period should also be devoted to planning for management of recipients' psychosocial needs as they will inevitably emerge during post-HCT recovery [43]. If not completed earlier, a detailed psychosocial evaluation should be performed at this time. As indicated earlier, several structured approaches to the psychosocial evaluation are available [10–12]. All share a focus on identification of potential risk factors for poor coping with the stressors posed by HCT. These risk factors include inadequate social support, past or current depression or substance abuse and an inflexible coping style, among others. Recognition of these potential risk factors for psychosocial difficulties post-HCT is key to prevention or management of these difficulties. Regardless of whether risk factor information is obtained using a structured or unstructured interview, a proactive approach is critical. Elements of this approach include identification of coping resources and deficits, discussion of psychosocial difficulties that might be anticipated and training in behavioral skills to improve symptom management and facilitate coping. A proactive approach is beneficial as it establishes a relationship between the HCT recipient and a health care professional, usually a social worker, psychologist or psychiatrist, who might later help manage any emerging psychosocial difficulties.

Stage three: post-HCT hospitalization

Upon conclusion of preparative therapy, the actual transplantation ushers in a period of vulnerability and watchful waiting. The recipient is left without a functioning immune system and is susceptible to a spectrum of life-threatening infectious complications. During the weeks after HCT, recipients are monitored for evidence of engraftment and immune system reconstitution. Once the side-effects of preparative therapy have resolved, and if no serious infectious complications have arisen, the recipient enters a period of relative quiescence. While weakness and fatigue are common at this time, the recipient may actually feel relatively good. Should serious medical complications develop, however, this state of quiescence quickly ends. Given the life-threatening nature of many medical complications during this early post-HCT period, recipients often react to medical setbacks with anxiety and/or depression. Furthermore, the number and extent of post-HCT medical complications is a good barometer of the length of post-HCT hospitalization required. A prolonged hospitalization can be profoundly demoralizing, especially if a tentative discharge date had been set only later to be postponed. Some recipients respond to a prolonged hospitalization with depression and lethargy. Others respond with anger and agitation, stating they can tolerate no further hospitalization and demanding to be discharged. In extreme cases, a recipient may leave the hospital against medical advice. At these times, the psychosocial team can play a critical, if not life-saving, role by helping the recipient to better cope with the stresses, disappointments and lack of control endemic to the HCT setting.

The primary psychosocial issues during this early period of post-HCT recovery center on promotion of continued effective coping with the physical and psychological stresses associated with HCT and management of any emergent psychological or psychiatric symptoms. In addition to anxiety and depressive reactions [44], recipients may experience neurocognitive symptoms or neurological complications [45–47]. Episodes of delirium may occur and may last several hours to several days. Symptoms can include: alterations in level of consciousness; altered sensory or perceptual function (e.g. hallucinations); impairments in memory, concentration and higher cognitive processes; mood swings; impaired judgement; and sleep disturbance [48]. Management of these symptoms is challenging due to their multifactorial etiology. The HCT setting is replete with potential neuropathological mechanisms including central nervous system disease, infection, metabolic imbalance due to graft-vs.-host-disease (GVHD) induced liver or renal dysfunction, immunosuppressive medications, respiratory compromise due to interstitial pneumonia or withdrawal or intoxication associated with psychoactive substances [48,49], and this is only a partial list of potential etiological factors! Resolution of the underlying pathology often results in symptom resolution. However, it is often difficult to pinpoint the underlying pathology given the sheer number of neuropathological mechanisms that might be involved.

HCT recipients can differ in the amount of time they are required to spend in a dedicated hospital unit before and after HCT. Some recipients experience HCT strictly as an inpatient procedure while others are treated on an outpatient basis. The point along this inpatient–outpatient continuum that characterizes a recipient's experience is critical to understanding the particular psychosocial difficulties they may encounter. The more HCT is experienced as an inpatient procedure, the more likely recipients are to evidence psychosocial difficulties associated with prolonged confinement in an institutional setting (e.g. boredom, loss of control, loss of identity, social and physical isolation, interrupted sleep, etc.). As an outpatient procedure, psychosocial difficulties associated with isolation and prolonged confinement are mitigated to a degree. However, other difficulties may be substituted. For example, while hospitalization and strict infection control procedures can be stressful, the immediate availability of supportive care from the medical team can be enormously reassuring to the recipient. While assistance with an emergency medical crisis is immediately available for inpatients, it may not be as available in the outpatient setting. This seeming small difference can have a profoundly discomforting effect on some recipients. Some recipients might even prefer the psychological security afforded by hospitalization on a specialized unit in lieu of the freedoms associated with more outpatient-based HCT procedures. There is a need for research examining the different psychosocial challenges posed by HCT in the outpatient and inpatient settings, since understanding of these differences is critical to provision of appropriate support to recipients and their families [50].

The transplant process is extremely difficult even under the best of circumstances. The stressors associated with HCT can bring out both the best and the worst in both patients and their families. The so-called "difficult" patient or family member can pose many challenges. Generally, when HCT staff refer to a "difficult" patient or family member, they mean someone who is angry, demanding and often uncooperative with the HCT team. Unfortunately, there is no one recipe for successfully managing the difficult patient or family member. However, certain principles that can underlie the management of such individuals should be borne in mind. These include frequent communication among medical team members, formulation of a reasonable treatment care plan and consistent implementation of this treatment plan by all members of the HCT team. Of course, continued effective communication with the difficult patient or family member is critical along with continued attempts to identify, convey understanding of, and address the fears and anxieties likely underlying their difficult behavior.

Stage four: hospital discharge and early post-HCT recovery

When engraftment has occurred, blood counts are near normal and recipients are medically stable, they are ready to leave the HCT unit. Patients are often moved to a less restrictive setting such as a "step down" unit in the hospital or a hotel close to the HCT center. This move allows those who live distant from the medical center to continue to be monitored carefully. Frequent medical follow-up on an outpatient basis is the norm during the first several weeks or months post-HCT. Frequent follow-up is especially important for older recipients, those with allogeneic, partially mismatched or unrelated transplants and those with pre-existing health problems.

Hospital discharge and a return home marks the beginning of an often long process of convalescence, recovery and life reintegration. Critical psychosocial issues associated with this early recovery period include coping with anxiety generated by the progressive weaning from intensive medical care and frequent clinic follow-up, as well as coping with the physical debilitation typically experienced at this time. Promotion of appropriate self-care behaviors to reduce risk of infection is also a significant issue at this time.

While hospital discharge and a return home is an eagerly anticipated milestone, it can be highly distressing. Many recipients report anxiety at the realization they will no longer be under the constant surveillance and care of medical staff. Fears that life-threatening difficulties might emerge when appropriate medical assistance is not easily available can temper any excitement surrounding the release from the hospital and a return home.

Upon returning home, recipients may discover they remain physically compromised and easily fatigued. It is not uncommon for recipients to report generalized, often profound, weakness and fatigue during the 6–12 months after HCT [51–53]. These symptoms can drastically interfere with resumption of routine activities characteristic of the recipient's premorbid lifestyle. How recipients react to these symptoms and their functional limitations can be influenced by expectations for post-HCT recovery. While most recipients anticipate some limitations, the anticipated time line for post-HCT recovery varies considerably. Recipients and family members are often overly optimistic in their expectations. Many anticipate a quick return to a healthy, fully functioning, "normal" life. Frustration, depression and anger can result when these expectations are not met. Family and friends can exacerbate these reactions by suggesting the failure to achieve a rapid and full recovery is due to a lack of motivation or malingering.

Practice of a regimen of self-care behaviors is critical to successful recovery. This regimen is intended to reduce risk of infection and includes both behavioral restrictions and prescriptions. Failure to adhere to this regimen can result in death or serious medical complications. Despite the importance of appropriate self-care after HCT, little research has examined this issue. One study reviewed nursing records of 54 pediatric HCT recipients and found reports of significant noncompliance during hospitalization in 52% [54]. Our own experience suggests that adherence to self-care guidelines can be a significant problem after HCT in both adult and pediatric settings. Skill or knowledge deficits underlie some instances of nonadherence. If detected, these deficits are usually easily corrected. More difficult to remedy are instances when nonadherence is due to a motivational deficit. Recipients may not automatically adhere to self-care guidelines simply because it is the "rational" thing to do. Given the long history of illness of many HCT recipients, it is not surprising they are often highly motivated to feel that they are no longer "sick" and are essentially a "normal" person. The need to practice a daily regimen of self-care behaviors or to observe certain behavioral restrictions suggests otherwise, however. As a result, recipients may decide to abandon portions of their self-care regimen to "test" whether these behaviors or restrictions are necessary [55]. This testing can have disastrous consequences. Management of nonadherence in the HCT setting requires education of both recipients and family members as well as attention to recipients' perceptions of the costs and benefits of adherence to self-care guidelines. These perceptions may differ from those held by medical staff. While recipients' health and safety should never be compromised, some flexibility on the part of medical staff is helpful. It may be necessary to condone less than optimal adherence to less critical aspects of the self-care regimen in exchange for more rigorous adherence to more critical behaviors.

Stage five: long-term recovery

Successful recovery after HCT is characterized by waning of physical side-effects of treatment, decreased symptoms of disease, a return to pre-morbid levels of psychosocial and physical functioning and resumption of valued life roles. This process usually begins 3–6 months after HCT and may continue for up to 2 years or more. It is critical to recognize, however, the wide variability in the "the trajectory of recovery" following HCT. Unfortunately, some recipients never fully recover, both physically and psychosocially, from their HCT experience, while for others recovery requires a lengthy journey.

One of the benchmarks of long-term recovery consists of recipients' perception they have "returned to normal" [4]. What is "normal" is generally dependent upon each recipient's perspective. However, even with the return of what they consider a "normal" lifestyle, few recipients are left unchanged by their HCT experience. Recipients may evidence a variety of late physical effects, such as pulmonary problems, cataracts, sterility, endocrine dysfunction, chronic GVHD and weakness and fatigue [56–58]. Even without late physical effects, most recipients experience some interruption in normal developmental tasks; for example, attending school and developing peer group relationships in the case of pediatric recipients, and maintaining a career and establishing satisfactory marital and family relationships in the case of adult recipients. Psychosocial sequelae of HCT, such as anxiety, depression, strained interpersonal relationships, or even post-traumatic stress disorder [59], may persist for months or years after HCT [25]. It is perhaps a testimony to the resilience of the human spirit that many HCT recipients consider themselves to have "returned to normal" despite the acknowledged presence of one or more of the aforementioned physical or psychosocial "late effects" [4].

It is useful to recognize that long-term recovery from HCT is a process and not a discrete event. Research has suggested that recovery may be characterized by gradual passage through a series of psychosocial transitions [60]. These transitions are characterized by the changing physical and psychosocial concerns of primary importance to the HCT recipient [53,61]. Early in the course of post-HCT recovery, recipients are most concerned about surviving the transplant and achieving a measure of medical stability. Psychosocial concerns are few at this time. As months and years pass, however, recipients focus more upon psychosocial concerns revolving around sexuality, occupational adjustment, social relationships, fears of recurrence and coping with chronic physical limitations. Ultimately, most recipients achieve a level of psychosocial equilibrium and "move on with their life" [60]. This view of recovery as a process has clear clinical implications. Specifically, staff should be aware that psychosocial concerns emerge over time as recipients' gradually come to grips with what has changed in their life. A recipient might evince no interest in addressing issues of sexual or occupational functioning, for example, early in the course of recovery. Later, however, they may show great concern regarding deficits in these areas. As a result, clinical efforts to assist recipients' recovery must focus on appropriate areas of concern at the appropriate time in the course of recovery [61].

It is important to note the long-term impact of HCT is not uniformly negative. Positive psychosocial sequelae can stem from the HCT experience. These include improved self-esteem, perception of a new meaning in life, redirected and reestablished life priorities, enhanced capacity for compassion, improved family and social relationships and renewed spiritual faith [62,63]. Hence, post-HCT recovery can involve more than adjustment to the potential negative sequelae of HCT and reestablishment of the premorbid status quo. Rather, recovery can involve establishment of a fundamentally altered life equilibrium, one that incorporates both the negative as well as positive impact of the experience.

Clinical experience and empiric research both suggest the sense that one has "returned to normal" is often present within the first 1–2 years following HCT for most disease-free recipients [4,53,64]. However, it is not uncommon for even disease-free recipients to acknowledge that their life "will never be the same." Indeed, even though the majority of surviving HCT recipients report relatively satisfactory QOL, a small, but not inconsequential, proportion of recipients report some continuing difficulties in physical and psychosocial functioning [65]. For example, Broers *et al.* [66] reported 90% of their sample of HCT recipients reported good to excellent QOL 3 years post-HCT. However, about 25% of this sample continued to experience significant functional limitations 3 years after HCT. Thus, while recipients might acknowledge having quite good QOL, they might still be experiencing significant functional difficulties. While complacency might be an understandable response to widespread reports of satisfactory QOL in HCT recipients, continued effort must be devoted to improving both medical and psychosocial management of the long-term sequelae of HCT.

There is a need for additional research focusing upon the long-term recovery of HCT recipients. While we know a fair amount about the types of psychosocial difficulties confronted by HCT recipients during the course of recovery, we know less about psychosocial and medical factors that either increase or minimize risk for psychosocial difficulties. Some recent research has suggested that better long-term psychosocial adjustment in HCT survivors may be linked to more aggressive conditioning regimens [67], enhanced social support, fewer social constraints, a more cohesive and flexible family environment [59,68] and greater global meaning [69]. Identification of such risk and protective factors is critical for targeting HCT survivors at greatest risk for long-term psychosocial difficulties, thus enabling clinical management efforts to be focused upon these individuals.

Psychosocial issues in HCT: stem cell donors

Both allogeneic and syngeneic HCT use hematopoietic grafts from a healthy donor for subsequent transplantation into a diseased recipient. While the HCT donor is "matched" to the recipient with regard to human leukocyte antigen (HLA)-typing, the donor may be either related or unrelated to the recipient. While other registries are available both in the USA and worldwide, most unrelated donors in the USA are identified from a registry maintained by the National Marrow Donor Program [70]. The nature of HCT donation has evolved over the years. Until the mid-1980s, donors were almost exclusively drawn from the ranks of HLA-matched relatives and donation of bone marrow was the norm. The growth of the National Marrow Donor Program, as well as other registries, has resulted in increased numbers of unrelated donors. Most recently, collection of HSCs from peripheral blood has become increasingly common among both related and unrelated donors.

Critical psychosocial issues surrounding the act of HSC donation revolve around understanding the physical and psychosocial outcomes associated with donation and understanding the motivation underlying donation. Some parallels can be drawn between HSC donation and both blood and solid organ donation [71]. However, significant differences exist among these types of donation regarding the risks associated with donation, the prior relationship between the donor and recipient and the donor's knowledge and direct experience of the medical outcomes experienced by the recipient of their donation. These differences are critical and preclude simple translation of what is known about blood and solid organ donation to the HSC donation context. For example, HSC donation requires a higher level of commitment and health risk than that associated with blood donation but less commitment and risk than that associated with solid organ donation. Thus, while parallels can be drawn among these types of donation, the uniqueness of HSC donation needs to be considered.

A number of studies have examined physical outcomes, primarily pain and physical disability, following donation of bone marrow or peripheral stem cells [72–75]. While serious physical complications after donation are uncommon, the degree and extent of pain and disability experienced following donation of HSCs may be slightly underestimated, and thus likely to be undertreated [74]. While the procedures associated with bone marrow and peripheral stem cell donation suggest that the former might be associated with less favorable physical outcomes, the data provide inconsistent support for this expectation [72,75].

In addition to the acute physical impact of HSC donation, research has examined the long-term psychosocial outcomes associated with HSC donation [71,76–81]. Several studies have examined post-donation outcomes in related bone marrow donors [82–84]. In general, related marrow donors tend to report little emotional distress associated with marrow donation and little change in their relationship with the recipient. Typically, few if any regrets regarding donation are expressed. As might be expected, reports of increased self-esteem, happiness and life satisfaction are common among donors. While the experience of related marrow donation is generally positive, the minority of donors who report negative experiences (e.g. estrangement from the recipient) should not be overlooked. More research in this area is merited. In particular, it might be expected that outcomes associated with related marrow donation might differ as a function of whether or not the recipient dies or otherwise experiences difficulties associated with the marrow graft. The available data suggest the negative impact of a recipient's death on donor adjustment and attitudes may be less than what might be expected [83].

Most of what is known about long-term psychosocial outcomes associated with HSC donation comes from a comprehensive study of several hundred adult unrelated marrow donors recruited through the National Marrow Donor Program [71,76,77,79,81]. Donors were assessed at several points including after provision of informed consent for donation as well as 1–2 weeks and 1 year post-donation. Results of the 1–2 week post-donation assessment indicated a sizable minority of donors experienced donation as stressful and inconvenient with 12% admitting to a degree of worry about their health [77]. Nevertheless, donors ultimately were generally quite positive about their donation. One year post-donation, 87% of donors stated they believed their donation experience was "very worthwhile" while 91% indicated they would be willing to donate again. Some evidence suggested donors with longer marrow collection times and those experiencing lower back pain or difficulty walking following donation viewed their experience as more stressful and experienced less positive psychosocial outcomes.

Unrelated HCT relies upon recruitment and maintenance of a large pool of volunteer hematopoietic cell donors. As a result, it is important to understand the motivations that underlie unrelated donors' actions. Simmons et al. [79] reported that unrelated donors believed the act of donation actualized certain central traits in their identity—most notably that of being a helpful and generous person. Switzer et al. [81] identified six types of donor motives: exchange-related, idealized helping, normative, positive feeling, empathy-related and past experience-based. Female donors were more likely to cite anticipated positive feelings following donation, empathy and a desire to help someone as critical factors in their donation. Additionally, donor motives predicted donor reactions to donation. Donors characterized by exchange motives or simple-helping motives reported greater predonation ambivalence and more negative post-donation reactions. Donors who reported empathy and positive feeling motives evidenced less predonation ambivalence and more positive post-donation reactions.

A critical issue relevant to marrow donation is the extent to which long-term donor outcomes vary as a function of HCT outcome. Suggestions that donors may experience "survivor guilt" following death of the HCT recipient can be found in the literature [84–86]. It has also been suggested that donors may experience guilt and self-blame should their marrow fail to engraft or should GVHD contribute to the recipient's death. While these are plausible reactions to these medical events, the virtual absence of research on this topic makes drawing conclusions in this area impossible. In the large study of unrelated donors described above, Butterworth et al. [77] found that death of the recipient rarely produced feelings of guilt and responsibility. In contrast, grief was an almost universal response to the recipient's death and was often surprisingly intense given the recipient was a stranger. Of course, these data describe the experience of unrelated donors. Given the existence of a prior donor-recipient relationship and the likelihood the donor may be attendant to the recipient's death, more negative reactions, perhaps involving guilt and anger in addition to profound grief, might be expected among related donors. However, the single study which has compared bereaved and nonbereaved related donors did not discover major differences in adjustment and attitudes as a function of recipient outcome [83].

In summary, the assumption that HSC donation is a completely benign experience is likely a faulty one. While serious physical and psychosocial complications are uncommon among both related and unrelated donors, such reactions at least occasionally occur. Long-term monitoring of donor reactions is thus justified. Current research priorities include early identification of donors at greatest risk for negative responses to donation as well as development of brief, supportive psychosocial interventions to minimize any negative post-donation reactions.

Finally, this section has focused upon the adult HCT donor. It is not uncommon for children to be called upon to serve as an HSC donor for a seriously ill sibling or even parent. Pediatric HSC donation raises important ethical and legal issues and the psychosocial consequences of such remain to be adequately identified [87–89]. Clearly, this is an area in need of more research and informed ethical and legal deliberation.

Psychosocial issues in HCT: family caregivers

Family caregivers that stay with their loved one during hospitalization for HCT are exposed to many of the same psychological stressors as HSC recipients themselves. These include geographic dislocation, radical change of normal daily activities, interrupted sleep, isolation from other family members, financial stressors and helplessness or a sense of inadequacy in the midst of the patient's suffering. While the caregiver does not experience the physical demands of transplantation, they also do not benefit from the care of medical staff. In addition, caregivers are not permitted to assume the patient role, a role that is acceptable for the recipient. In large part, assumption of this patient role gives the recipient implicit permission to depend on caregivers for help with even the most basic of functional activities and to temporarily suspend regular responsibilities. Caregivers, however, are not afforded the luxury of such reduced expectations. In fact, caregivers are often subjected to the increased expectations associated with the role of caregiver, expectations which typically involve serving as a primary source of physical care and emotional support for the HCT recipient. Both the recipient as well as the medical staff can hold these expectations. It is remarkable how well most caregivers respond to the demands of their role during the course of HCT and surprising that so little research has examined the experience of the HCT caregiver. However, there are some representative studies that shed light on this experience [90–93]. Perhaps the reason so few studies exist is the complexity of studying the caregiver. For example, while many patients may have a spouse who is the primary caregiver, a sibling or child may supplement the work of the primary caregiver, resulting in two and sometimes three or four "primary" caregivers. Which should be the focus of study? On the other hand, some recipients may have no caregiver readily available during hospitalization due to work or family demands (e.g. young children in the home). The "caregivers" in this example would likely experience quite different stressors than those who stay with the patient during hospitalization. This heterogeneity in the caregiving experience can frustrate research efforts.

Two general issues have been the focus of caregiver research in the HCT setting. First, researchers have tried to document the nature, extent, trajectory and consequences of distress and caregiver burden experienced by HCT caregivers. Relative to HCT recipients, caregivers have been found to report more impairment in family relationships and similar levels of distress [91]. In a prospective study of 28 recipients and their close relative caregivers, 88% of caregivers reported considerable psychological distress both prior to and 3 months after HCT [94]. Fortunately, distress generally diminished by 12 months post-HCT. Finally, Foxall and Gaston-Johansson [95] interviewed 24 family caregivers regarding the burden of care and health outcomes (anxiety, depression, symptom distress and fatigue) experienced prior to and during HCT hospitalization. Not surprisingly, they found higher care burden was linked to more negative health outcomes.

The second issue which has been the focus of caregiver research in the HCT setting involves comparison of caregiver burden and distress associated with HCT in the inpatient setting *vis a vis* HCT in the outpatient setting. In general, few differences have been found in caregiver distress between HCT in the inpatient vs. outpatient setting [90,92]. In fact, some evidence suggests that caregivers associated with HCT administered in a combined inpatient/outpatient setting reported less mood disturbance than caregivers associated with HCT in an inpatient setting. This is a bit of a surprise as caregiver burden has been assumed to increase in the outpatient setting due to increased responsibility upon the caregiver to provide for the recipient's needs. While this research is limited due to a lack of random assignment to inpatient or outpatient HCT, it raises important questions for researchers attempting to understand variations in caregiver burden in different HCT settings.

It is likely that caregiver well-being is influenced by a host of factors including the support they are able to gather from relatives and/or medical staff, the relative difficulty and the physical demands of the HCT procedure itself, their own pre-HCT functional health status and their capacity for coping with the demands of the hospital setting. Clearly, their presence on the hospital unit and their availability to the patient during post-HCT recovery are crucial to the well-being of the recipient in terms of helping with instrumental tasks (e.g. preparing food, helping the recipient dress, arranging for daily medications) and providing emotional support and companionship. Interestingly, some data suggest the presence of a caregiver during the hospitalization stage of HCT is linked to better survival during the 1st year post-HCT [96].

Psychosocial issues in HCT: medical staff

The medical and psychological care of HCT recipients requires highly trained nursing, medical and allied health care professionals to work under conditions of high stress. Most HCT units are equipped as intensive care facilities to account for a range of patient needs, including life support, during treatment. Due to side-effects of medications or life-threatening infections, a patient who undergoes HCT in relatively good health could quickly require intubation and hover in a life-threatening situation for many days. This potential for rapid and profound shifts in patient status requires professionals vigilant enough to manage an array of machines and medications as well as respond appropriately to worried family caregivers who are in the same room, closely observing their every action. Several studies have surveyed nurses and physicians in the HCT setting regarding the stressful nature of this work. Molassiotis *et al.* [97] surveyed 129 nurses and 26 doctors from 16 HCT centers. One half reported emotional exhaustion and 80% reported feelings of low personal accomplishment. While overt depression was lower than would be expected in the normal population, signs of clinically significant anxiety were seen in more than 10% of respondents. Reported specific sources of distress included regularly working with dying patients, excessive responsibility, rapid advances in HCT technology and excessive demands of patients and family members. A second study of burnout and job satisfaction in HCT nurses found burnout was low and job satisfaction was high [98]. While most respondents reported a sense of personal accomplishment in their work setting, about 25% of respondents presented with manifestations of anxiety.

The work of health care providers on HCT units is demanding and stressful, particularly when patients are critically ill and nurses are short-staffed. The HCT unit requires highly flexible personnel who can respond quickly to medical emergencies while at the same time sustaining motivation when the pace of the unit moves more slowly. Remarkably, these units often serve as models of cohesion even under the extraordinary pressures of day-to-day care.

Finally, the psychological impact of the transplant outcome on medical staff should not be understated. In the HCT setting, the stakes are very high and often amount to an "all or nothing" wager. The patient either engrafts and has a chance at extended life or does not engraft and faces a very poor prognosis. These high stakes, coupled with frequent, lengthy and often intense interactions with the HCT medical team, create a fertile environment for distress. It is not unusual for members of the HCT team to become deeply attached to patients and family members. The consequences of this deep attachment can range across the spectrum of human emotional experience, from deep feelings of sadness and distress when a patient dies to joy and celebration when a patient "beats the odds" and is rewarded with extended life. While psychosocial support programs for HCT staff have been described [99,100], more effort needs to be devoted to the development, implementation and maintenance of staff support programs.

Conclusion

HCT is not a monolithic procedure and broad and sweeping generalizations about the experience of recipients, donors, caregivers and medical staff are necessarily limited. However, the core of the HCT experience is similar for nearly all recipients. Fundamentally, HCT is a life-threatening treatment for a life-threatening disease and can produce a range of physical and psychosocial morbidities. We have summarized issues for each stage of the HCT process in Table 38.1 (see p. 498). While not all issues will be germane to all HCT recipients, this listing can alert those concerned with the psychosocial adjustment of HCT recipients to areas of potential difficulty.

There is a growing literature addressing psychosocial issues associated with HCT. However, most research in this area has focused upon the adult HCT recipient. There is a need for more psychosocial research germane to the pediatric HCT setting. Finally, while the literature is replete with studies describing the physical and psychosocial difficulties encountered by HCT recipients, there is a critical need for research addressing the design, implementation and evaluation of interventions to prevent or minimize these difficulties. Intervention studies examining the use of cognitive-behavioral or hypnotic techniques [40,41], aerobic exercise [101], massage therapy [102], or a coping strategy training program [42] to enhance physical performance and reduce distress and physical symptoms in HCT recipients can serve as useful models in this regard.

References

1 Brown HN, Kelly MJ. Stages of bone marrow transplantation: a psychiatric perspective. *Psychosom Med* 1976; **38**: 439–46.

2 Pfefferbaum B, Lindamood M, Wiley FM. Stages in pediatric bone marrow transplantation. *Pediatrics* 1978; **61**: 625–8.

3 McQuellon RP, Andrykowski MA. Psychosocial complications of bone marrow transplantation. In: Atkinson K, ed. *Clinical Bone Marrow and Blood Stem Cell Transplantation*, 2nd edn. Oxford: Oxford University Press, 2000: 1045–52.

4 Andrykowski MA, Brady MJ, Greiner CB et al. "Returning to normal" following bone marrow transplantation: outcomes, expectations and informed consent. *Bone Marrow Transplant* 1995; **15**: 573–81.

5 Patenaude AF, Rappeport JM, Smith BR. The physician's influence on informed consent for bone marrow transplantation. *Theor Med* 1986; **7**: 165–79.

6 Chauvenet AR, Smith NM. Referral of pediatric oncology patients for marrow transplantation and the process of informed consent. *Med Pediatr Oncol* 1988; **16**: 40–4.

7 Phipps S, Brenner M, Heslop H, Krance R, Jayawardene D, Mulhern R. Psychological effects of bone marrow transplantation on children and adolescents: preliminary report of a longitudinal study. *Bone Marrow Transplant* 1995; **15**: 829–35.

8 Frierson RL, Lippmann SB. Heart transplant candidates rejected on psychiatric indications. *Psychosomatics* 1987; **28**: 347–55.

9 Molassiotis A. Further evaluation of a screen for risk of emotional difficulties in bone marrow transplant recipients. *J Advanced Nurs* 1999; **29**: 922–7.

10 Futterman AD, Wellisch DK, Bond G, Carr CR. The Psychosocial Levels System. A new rating scale to identify and assess emotional difficulties during bone marrow transplantation. *Psychosomatics* 1991; **32**: 177–86.

11 Twillman RK, Manetto C, Wellisch DK, Wolcott DL. The Transplant Evaluation Rating Scale. A revision of the psychosocial levels system for evaluating organ transplant candidates. *Psychosomatics* 1993; **34**: 144–53.

12 Olbrisch ME, Levenson JL, Hamer R. The PACT. A rating scale for the study of clinical decision-making in psychological screening of organ transplant candidates. *Clin Transplant* 1989; **3**: 164–9.

13 Presberg BA, Levenson JL, Olbrisch ME, Best AM. Rating scales for the psychosocial evaluation of organ transplant candidates: comparison of the PACT and TERS with bone marrow transplant patients. *Psychosomatics* 1995; **36**: 458–61.

14 Hoodin F, Kalbfleisch KR. How psychometrically sound is the transplant evaluation rating scale for bone marrow transplant recipients? *Psychosomatics* 2000; **42**: 490–6.

15 Loberiza FR Jr, Rizzo JD, Bredeson CN et al. Association of depressive syndrome and early deaths among patients after stem-cell transplantation for malignant diseases. *J Clin Oncol* 2002; **20**: 2118–26.

16 Molassiotis A, van den Akker OB, Milligan DW, Goldman JM. Symptom distress, coping style, and biological variables as predictors of survival after bone marrow transplantation. *J Psychosom Res* 1997; **42**: 275–85.

17 Sullivan AK, Szkrumelak N, Hoffman LH. Psychological risk factors and early complications after bone marrow transplantation in adults. *Bone Marrow Transplant* 1999; **24**: 1109–20.

18 Tschuschke V, Hertenstein B, Arnold R, Bunjes D, Denzinger R, Kaechele H. Associations between coping and survival time of adult leukemia patients receiving allogeneic bone marrow transplantation: Results of a prospective study. *J Psychosom Res* 2001; **50**: 277–85.

19 Gregurek R, Labar B, Mrsic M et al. Anxiety as a possible predictor of GVHD. *Bone Marrow Transplant* 1996; **18**: 585–9.

20 Broers S, Hengeveld MW, Kaptein AA, Le Cessie S, van de Loo F, de Vries T. Are pretransplant psychological variables related to survival after bone marrow transplantation? A prospective study of 123 consecutive patients. *J Psychosom Res* 1998; **45**: 341–51.

21 Annas GJ. Informed consent. *Ann Rev Med* 1978; **29**: 9–14.

22 Andrykowski MA. Psychosocial factors in bone marrow transplantation. A review and recommendations for research. *Bone Marrow Transplant* 1994; **13**: 357–75.

23 Dermatis H, Lesko LM. Psychosocial correlates of physician–patient communication at time of informed consent for bone marrow transplantation. *Cancer Invest* 1991; **9**: 621–8.

24 Dermatis H, Lesko LM. Psychological distress in parents consenting to child's bone marrow transplantation. *Bone Marrow Transplant* 1990; **6**: 411–7.

25 Baker F, Marcellus D, Zabora J et al. Psychological distress among adult patients being evaluated for bone marrow transplantation. *Psychosomatics* 1997; **38**: 10–9.

26 Fife BL, Huster GA, Cornetta KG, Kennedy UN, Akard LP, Broun ER. Longitudinal study of adaptation to the stress of bone marrow transplantation. *J Clin Oncol* 2000; **18**: 1539–49.

27 Grassi L, Rosti G, Albertazzi L, Marangolo M. Psychological stress symptoms before and after autologous bone marrow transplantation in patients with solid tumors. *Bone Marrow Transplant* 1996; **17**: 843–7.

28 Leigh S, Wilson KC, Burns R, Clark RE. Psychosocial morbidity in bone marrow transplant recipients: a prospective study. *Bone Marrow Transplant* 1995; **16**: 635–40.

29 Trask PC, Paterson A, Riba M et al. Assessment of psychological distress in prospective bone marrow transplant patients. *Bone Marrow Transplant* 2002; **29**: 917–25.

30 Mehta P, Rodrigue J, Nejame C, Gaa R, Wingard JR. Acquiescence to adjunctive experimental therapies may relate to psychological distress: pilot data from a bone marrow transplant center. *Bone Marrow Transplant* 2000; **25**: 673–6.

31 Andrykowski MA, Schmitt FA, Gregg ME et al. Neuropsychologic impairment in adult bone marrow transplant candidates. *Cancer* 1992; **70**: 2288–97.

32 Meyers CA, Weitzner M, Byrne K, Valentine A, Champlin RE, Przepiorka D. Evaluation of the neurobehavioral functioning of patients before, during and after bone marrow transplantation. *J Clin Oncol* 1994; **12**: 820–6.

33 Prows CA, McCain GC. Parental consent for bone marrow transplantation in the case of genetic disorders. *J Soc Pediatr Nurs* 1997; **2**: 9–18.

34 McQuellon RP, Muss HB, Hoffman SL et al. Patient preferences for treatment of metastatic breast cancer: a study of women with early-stage breast cancer. *J Clin Oncol* 1995; **13**: 858–68.

35 Yellen SB, Cella DF. Someone to live for. Social well-being, parenthood status, and decision-making in oncology. *J Clin Oncol* 1995; **13**: 1255–64.

36 Kodish E, Lantos J, Siegler M et al. Bone marrow transplantation in sickle cell disease: the trade-off between early mortality and quality of life. *Clin Res* 1990; **38**: 694–700.

37 Sebban C, Browman G, Gafni A et al. Design and validation of a bedside decision instrument to elicit a patient's preference concerning allogenic bone marrow transplantation in chronic myeloid leukemia. *Am J Hematol* 1995; **48**: 221–7.

38 Lesko LM, Dermatis H, Penman D, Holland JC. Patients', parents', and oncologists' perceptions of informed consent for bone marrow transplantation. *Med Pediatr Oncol* 1989; **17**: 181–7.

39 Shatz D. Autonomy, beneficence, and informed consent: rethinking the connections. *Cancer Invest* 1986; **4**: 353–61.

40 Syrjala KL, Cummings C, Donaldson GW. Hypnosis or cognitive behavioral training for the reduction of pain and nausea during cancer treatment: a controlled clinical trial. *Pain* 1992; **48**: 137–46.

41 Syrjala KL, Donaldson GW, Davis MW, Kippes ME, Carr JE. Relaxation and imagery and congitive-behavioral training reduce pain during cancer treatment: a controlled clinical trial. *Pain* 1995; **63**: 189–98.

42 Gaston-Johansson F, Fall-Dickson JM, Nanda J et al. The effectiveness of the comprehensive coping strategy program on clinical outcomes in breast cancer autologous bone marrow transplantation. *Cancer Nur* 2000; **23**: 277–85.

43 Bryant LH, Heiney SP, Henslee-Downey PJ, Cornwell P. Proactive psychosocial care of blood or marrow transplant patients. *Cancer Pract* 1997; **5**: 234–40.

44 Sasaki T, Akaho R, Sakamaki H et al. Mental disturbances during isolation in bone marrow transplant patients with leukemia. *Bone Marrow Transplant* 2000; **25**: 315–8.

45 Ahles TA, Tope DM, Furstenberg C et al. Psychologic and neuropsychologic impact of autologous bone marrow transplantation. *J Clin Oncol* 1996; **14**: 1457–62.

46 Antonini G, Ceschin U, Morino S et al. Early neurologic complications following allogeneic bone marrow transplant for leukemia: a prospective study. *Neurology* 1998; **50**: 1441–5.

47 Snider S, Bashir R, Bierman P. Neurologic complications after high-dose chemotherapy and autologous bone marrow transplantation for Hodgkin's disease. *Neurology* 1994; **44**: 681–4.

48 Wellisch DK, Wolcott DL. Psychological issues in bone marrow transplantation. In: Forman SJ, Blume KB, Thomas ED, eds. *Bone Marrow Transplantation*. Boston: Blackwell Scientific Publications, 1994: 554–71.

49 Gallardo D, Ferra C, Berlanga JJ et al. Neurologic complications after allogeneic bone marrow transplantation. *Bone Marrow Transplant* 1996; **18**: 1135–9.

50 Amato JJ, Williams M, Greenberg C, Bar M, Lo S, Tepler I. Psychological support to an autologous bone marrow transplant unit in a community hospital: a pilot experience. *Psychooncology* 1998; **7**: 121–5.

51 Andrykowski MA, Bruehl S, Brady MJ, Henslee-Downey PJ. Physical and psychosocial status of adults one-year after bone marrow transplantation: a prospective study. *Bone Marrow Transplant* 1995; **15**: 837–44.

52 Andrykowski MA, Carpenter JS, Greiner CB et al. Energy level and sleep quality following bone marrow transplantation. *Bone Marrow Transplant* 1997; **20**: 669–79.

53 McQuellon RP, Russell GR, Rambo TD et al. Quality of life and psychological distress of bone marrow transplantation recipients: the "time trajectory" to recovery over the first year. *Bone Marrow Transplant* 1998; **21**: 477–86.

54 Phipps S, DeCuir-Whalley S. Adherence issues in pediatric bone marrow transplantation. *J Pediatr Psychol* 1990; **15**: 459–75.

55 Conrad P. The meaning of medications: another look at compliance. *Soc Sci Med* 1985; **20**: 29–37.

56 Kolb HJ, Portscher C. Late effects after allogeneic bone marrow transplantation. *Curr Opin Hematol* 1997; **4**: 401–7.

57 Niethammer D, Mayer E. Long-term survivors. An overview of late effects, sequelae and second neoplasias. *Bone Marrow Transplant* 1998; **21** (Suppl. 2): S61–3.

58 Vose JM, Kennedy BC, Bierman PJ et al. Long-term sequelae of autologous bone marrow or peripheral stem cell transplantation for lymphoid malignancies. *Cancer* 1992; **69**: 784–9.

59 Widows MR, Jacobsen PB, Fields KK. Relation of psychological vulnerability factors to posttraumatic stress disorder symptomatology in bone marrow transplant recipients. *Psychosom Med* 2000; **62**: 873–82.

60 Molassiotis A. Psychosocial transitions in the long-term survivors of bone marrow transplantation. *Eur J Cancer Care* 1997; **6**: 100–7.

61 Andrykowski MA, Cordova MJ, Hann DM, Jacobson PB, Fields KM, Phillips G. Patients' psychosocial concerns following stem cell transplantation: Findings from two transplant centers. *Bone Marrow Transplant* 1999; **24**: 1121–9.

62 Curbow B, Somerfield MR, Baker F et al. Personal changes, dispositional optimism, and psychological adjustment to bone marrow transplantation. *J Behav Med* 1993; **16**: 423–43.

63 Fromm K, Andrykowski MA, Hunt J. Positive and negative psychosocial sequelae of bone marrow transplantation: implications for quality of life assessment. *J Behav Med* 1996; **19**: 221–40.

64 Syrjala KL, Chapko MK, Vitaliano PP et al. Recovery after allogeneic marrow transplantation: prospective study of predictors of long-term physical and psychosocial functioning. *Bone Marrow Transplant* 1993; **11**: 319–27.

65 Hjermstad MJ, Kaasa S. Quality of life in adult cancer patients treated with bone marrow transplantation: a review of the literature. *Eur J Cancer* 1995; **31**(A): 163–73.

66 Broers S, Kaptein AA, Le Cessie S, Fibbe W, Hengeveld MW. Psychological functioning and quality of life following bone marrow transplantation: a 3-year follow-up study. *J Psychosom Res* 2000; **48**: 11–21.

67 Molassiotis A. Late psychosocial effects of conditioning for BMT. *Br J Nursing* 1996; **5**: 1296–302.

68 Molassiotis A, van den Akker OB, Boughton BJ. Perceived social support, family environment, and psychosocial recovery in bone marrow transplant long-term survivors. *Soc Sci Med* 1997; **44**: 317–25.

69 Johnson Vickberg SM, Duhmel KW, Smith MM et al. Global meaning and psychological adjustment among survivors of bone marrow transplant. *Psychooncology* 2001; **10**: 29–39.

70 McCullough J, Hansen J, Perkins H et al. The National Marrow Donor Program: how it works, accomplishments to date. *Oncology* 1989; **3**: 63–74.

71 Switzer GE, Dew MA, Butterworth VA et al. Understanding donors' motivations: a study of unrelated bone marrow donors. *Soc Sci Med* 1997; **45**: 137–47.

72 Auquier P, Macquart-Moulin G, Moatti JP et al. Comparison of anxiety, pain and discomfort in two procedures of hematopoietic stem cell collection: leukacytapheresis and bone marrow harvest. *Bone Marrow Transplant* 1995; **16**: 541–7.

73 Chang G, McGarigle C, Spitzer TR et al. A comparison of related and unrelated donors. *Psychosom Med* 1998; **60**: 163–7.

74 Hill HF, Chapman CR, Jackson TL, Sullivan KM. Assessment and management of donor pain following marrow harvest for allogeneic bone marrow transplantation. *Bone Marrow Transplant* 1989; **4**: 57–161.

75 Rowley SD, Donaldson G, Lilleby K, Bensinger WI, Appelbaum FR. Experiences of donors enrolled in a randomized study of allogeneic marrow or peripheral blood stem cell transplantation. *Blood* 2001; **97**: 2541–8.

76 Butterworth VA. When altruism fails. Reactions of unrelated bone marrow donors when the recipient dies. *Omega* 1992; **26**: 161–73.

77 Butterworth VA, Simmons RG, Bartsch G et al. Psychosocial effects of unrelated bone marrow donation: Experiences of the National Marrow Donor Program. *Blood* 1993; **81**: 1947–59.

78 Molassiotis A, Holroyd E. Assessment of psychosocial adjustment in Chinese unrelated bone marrow donors. *Bone Marrow Transplant* 1999; **24**: 903–10.

79 Simmons RG, Schimmel M, Butterworth VA. The self-image of unrelated bone marrow donors. *J Health Soc Behav* 1993; **34**: 285–301.

80 Stroncek D, Strand R, Scott E et al. Attitudes and physical condition of unrelated bone marrow donors immediately after donation. *Transfusion* 1989; **29**: 317–22.

81 Switzer GE, Simmons RG, Dew MA. Helping unrelated strangers. Physical and psychological reactions to the bone marrow donation process among anonymous donors. *J Appl Soc Psychol* 1996; **26**: 469–90.

82 Christopher KA. The experience of donating bone marrow to a relative. *Oncol Nurs Forum* 2000; **27**: 693–700.

83 Switzer GE, Dew MA, Magistro CA et al. The effects of bereavement on adult sibling bone marrow donors' psychological well-being and reactions to donation. *Bone Marrow Transplant* 1998; **21**: 181–8.

84 Wolcott DL, Wellisch DK, Fawzy FI, Landsverk J. Psychological adjustment of adult bone marrow transplant donors whose recipient survives. *Transplantation* 1986; **41**: 484–8.

85 Gardner GG, August CS, Githens J. Psychological issues in bone marrow transplantation. *Pediatrics* 1977; **60**: 625–31.

86 Wolcott DL, Fawzy FI, Wellisch DK. Psychiatric aspects of bone marrow transplantation: a review and current issues. *Psychiatr Med* 1986; **4**: 299–317.

87 Shama WI. The experience and preparation of pediatric sibling bone marrow donors. *Soc Work Health Care* 1998; **27**: 89–99.

88 Weisz V. Psycholegal issues in sibling bone marrow donation. *Ethics Behav* 1992; **2**: 185–201.

89 Weisz V, Robbennolt JK. Risks and benefits of pediatric bone marrow donation: a critical need for research. *Behav Sci Law* 1996; **14**: 375–91.

90 Grimm PM, Zawacki KL, Mock V, Krumm S, Frink BB. Caregiver responses and needs. An ambulatory bone marrow transplant model. *Cancer Pract* 2000; **8**: 120–8.

91 Siston AK, List MA, Daugherty CK et al. Psychosocial adjustment of patients and caregivers prior to allogeneic bone marrow transplantation. *Bone Marrow Transplant* 2001; **27**: 1181–8.

92 Summers N, Dawe U, Stewart DAA. Comparison of inpatient and outpatient ASCT. *Bone Marrow Transplant* 2000; **26**: 389–95.

93 Stetz KM, McDonald JC, Compton K. Needs and experiences of family caregivers during marrow transplantation. *Oncol Nurs Forum* 1996; **23**: 1422–7.

94 Keogh F, O'Riordan J, McNamara C, Duggan C, McCann SR. Psychosocial adaptation of patients and families following bone marrow transplantation: a prospective longitudinal study. *Bone Marrow Transplant* 1998; **22**: 905–11.

95 Foxall MJ, Gaston-Johansson F. Burden and health outcomes of family caregivers of hospitalized bone marrow transplant patients. *J Adv Nurs* 1996; **24**: 915–23.

96 Bolwell BJ, Foster L, McLellan L et al. The presence of a caregiver is a powerful prognostic variable of survival following allogeneic bone marrow transplantation. *Proc Am Soc Hematol* 2001; **98**: 845.

97 Molassiotis A, van den Akker OB, Boughton BJ. Psychological stress in nursing and medical staff on bone marrow transplant units. *Bone Marrow Transplant* 1995; **15**: 449–54.

98 Molassiotis A, Haberman M. Evaluation of burn-out and job satisfaction in marrow transplant nurses. *Cancer Nurs* 1996; **19**: 360–7.

99 Kiss A. Support of the transplant team. *Suppor Care Cancer* 1994; **2**: 56–60.

100 Sarantos S. Innovations in psychosocial staff support. A model program for the marrow transplant nurse. *Semin Oncol Nurs* 1988; **4**: 69–73.

101 Dimeo F, Bertz H, Finke J, Fetscher S, Mertelsmann R, Keul J. An aerobic exercise program for patients with haemotological malignancies after bone marrow transplantation. *Bone Marrow Transplant* 1996; **18**: 1157–60.

102 Ahles TA, Tope DM, Pinkson B et al. Massage therapy for patients undergoing autologous bone marrow transplantation. *J Pain Symptom Manage* 1999; **18**: 157–63.

39

Karen Syrjala

Assessment of Quality of Life in Hematopoietic Cell Transplantation Recipients

Cross-sectional surveys have tracked health-related quality of life (QOL) for hematopoietic cell transplant (HCT) patients from pretransplant through approximately 10 years post-transplant [1–9]. As a result, much is known about QOL outcomes of transplant over time for autologous and allogeneic myeloablative transplant recipients within and across diagnoses. The central consistent findings of these studies are that:

1 physical function returns to pretransplant level for approximately 75% of survivors by 1 year;
2 by 3 years 80–90% of survivors are back to full-time work;
3 the majority of patients navigate the challenges of HCT with good psychologic health; and
4 a minority of patients will have major residual problems with a variety of QOL functions.

Excellent measures for evaluating QOL have been tested with HCT patients in the past decade. Additional measures have been tested with cancer patients and are appropriate for use with HCT patients. With increasing emphasis on population-based screening and evidence-based care, measures are being tested with a variety of technologies to facilitate routine, rapid assessment and immediately usable results.

Even with the many descriptive studies of QOL in HCT, there are gaps in knowledge resulting from the wide array of transplant types as well as people receiving them. For instance, we have only clinical observation to inform us of QOL outcomes after nonmyeloablative HCT. Clinical reports and early toxicity data suggest that these patients' course of morbidity and function will differ from patients receiving myeloablative HCT [10,11]. Chapters 85 and 86 discuss the differences in eligibility as well as treatment for nonmyeloablative HCT recipients. There also remain gaps in our knowledge of long-term pediatric QOL outcomes. Caregivers and families of patients who die have been minimally examined. In addition, clinical trials to improve identified QOL deficits are few.

This chapter reviews what is known about QOL during and after HCT and considers the measurement issues to understand when interpreting or carrying out research that includes QOL outcomes. Other chapters discuss the applications of QOL within outcomes research, in the psychosocial domain and with sexual problems (see Chapters 32, 38 and 40).

Definition of health-related quality of life

Most QOL researchers would concur that: "Health-related QOL refers to the extent to which one's usual or expected physical, emotional and social well-being are affected by a medical condition or its treatment" [12]. Elements essential to any definition of QOL are multidimensionality and the patient's perspective. With time, QOL has grown to encompass not only subjective evaluation, but also those behaviors that may be reported by patients but go beyond subjective experience to include function and activity reports. QOL is often described as change over time rather than comparing peak toxicity grade or time to an event such as relapse or death. A central tenet is that QOL is *relative* to the current situation and the *expectations* of patients within the circumstances they find themselves. As an example, patients with major toxicities during transplant can report good psychosocial QOL and satisfaction with QOL because they believe they are doing as well as possible in a difficult situation, and they have the support they need from people important to them [1]. Despite this subjectivity, QOL correlates with medical, functional and observational outcomes [13–15].

Dimensions

Concepts of QOL continue to adhere to a three-level "pyramid" first described by Spilker [16]. He topped the pyramid with global assessment of well-being. The middle level included multidimensional assessment of physical, psychologic, economic, spiritual and social domains. The base detailed subcomponents of each domain, e.g. work and symptoms are aspects of the physical domain. Other subcomponents include social and recreational activities; sexual function; relationship with the medical team; religion; perspective on life; personal control; and components of health and treatment that add stress or worry for the patient. Ferrell *et al.* [17] interviewed 119 adult bone marrow transplant survivors at least 100 days post-transplant to determine what QOL meant to these patients. They categorized the many positives and negatives noted by survivors into themes and then into four domains matching Spilker: physical; psychologic; social; and spiritual/existential well-being. All broad QOL measures used with HCT patients include physical, psychologic and social function questions. Each measure then develops specific areas of interest more fully. Thus, selection of measures depends on which dimensions are judged to be of greatest relevance in the situation being measured. Table 39.1 lists a selection of measures used to assess QOL components in HCT.

Smith *et al.* [18] found that patients perceived health status and QOL as distinct from each other. Physical function weighed more heavily in assessments of health status while emotional health weighed more heavily in judgements of QOL. Social function was not prominently considered in either global rating.

Researchers are attending more to understanding resilience as they document that most patients with cancer and HCT do very well. Four concepts being examined in detail are spirituality; optimism; benefit-finding; and "post-traumatic growth" [19–22]. In essence, the ability to find purpose beyond the disease, and to perceive gains as well as losses in the disease and transplant process, predict better long-term adaptation.

Table 39.1 Selected quality of life (QOL) measures used in hematopoietic cell transplantation (HCT).

Relevant measures tested in HCT*	Minutes to complete	Number of items	Scores
Multidimensional QOL			
EORTC-QLQ-C30 (European Organization for Research and Treatment of Cancer–Quality of Life–C30) (BMT module not yet published)	12	30	9 subscales No total score
FACT-BMT (Functional Assessment of Cancer Therapy–General + BMT module)	10	34 + 24	5 subscales plus BMT module and overall score
PedsQL (Pediatric Quality of Life Inventory) plus PCQL (Pediatric Cancer Quality of Life)	4	23	4 subscales, physical and psychological summary score and total score
	5	32	5 subscales, and total score
SF36 (Short Form 36 Health Survey)	5	36	8 subscales plus physical and mental components No total score
SIP (Sickness Impact Profile)	20	136 (check items that apply)	12 subscales plus physical and psychosocial dimensions and overall score
Symptoms			
MDASI (M.D. Anderson Symptom Inventory)	3	13	Total score
RSCL (Rotterdam Symptom Checklist)	8	38	3 subscales and global score
Mental health, emotional well-being			
BDI (Beck Depression Inventory)	5	21	Total score
BSI (Brief Symptom Inventory–Short Form)	4	18	3 dimensions and global severity
CESD (Center for Epidemiologic Studies–Depression)	5	20	Total score
HADS (Hospital Anxiety and Depression Scale)	4	14	2 scores
HCT Distress	3	18	5 subscales and mean total score
MAC (Mental Adjustment to Cancer Scale)	10	40	5 subscales
POMS-SF (Profile of Mood States–Short Form)	5	30	6 subscales and total score
Coping style			
COPE (Coping Orientations to Problems Experienced Scale)	10–15	60 at most	13 subscales in 3 groups; can select from subscales
MAC (Mental Adjustment to Cancer Scale)	10	40	5 subscales
WCCL (Ways of Coping Checklist)	10	50	8 subscales
Social function			
MOS Social Support (Medical Outcomes Study)	4	19	4 subscales and overall index
Spiritual, existential well-being			
FACIT-SP (Functional Assessment of Chronic Illness Therapy–Spirituality and Well-Being Scale)	3	12	Total score
Sexuality			
SFQ (Sexual Function Questionnaire)	10	40	9 subscales, overall score and medical impact score
Caregiver and family impact			
Caregiver QOL–Cancer	10	35	4 subscales and total score

*Updated measure information is available from websites for many of the measures listed.

Those noted below can be located with a web search of the name or with the web address listed. If not listed no website was found and the author needs to be contacted.

- Beck Depression Inventory (http://www.psychcorp.com/)
- BSI (Brief Symptom Inventory)
- CESD (Center for Epidemiologic Studies–Depression)
- CQOLC (Caregiver Quality of Life–Cancer)
- EORTC-QLQ-C30 (European Organization for Research and Treatment of Cancer–Quality of Life Questionnaire)
- FACIT-SP (under Functional Assessment of Chronic Illness Therapy)
- FACT (Functional Assessment of Cancer Therapy)
- HCT Distress (ksyrjala@fhcrc.org for form and manual)
- MAC (Mental Adjustment to Cancer Scale)
- MDASI (M.D. Anderson Symptoms Inventory)
- MOS Social Support Survey
- PCQOL (Pediatric Quality of Life–Cancer: check website for PedsQL below)
- PedsQL (Pediatric Quality of Life Inventory)
- POMS (Profile of Mood States)
- SF36 (Health Survey Short Form 36)
- SFQ (Sexual Function Questionnaire: ksyrjala@fhcrc.org for form and manual)
- SIP (Sickness Impact Profile)

Most often gains are reported as greater appreciation for life, closer relationships, reprioritizing "what really matters", feeling closer to God, inner strength and a sense of peace and thankfulness [17,23,24]. While these concepts might not appear in most health-related QOL measurement, they are usually noted as important outcomes by patients, clinicians and researchers examining qualitative outcomes of HCT [22,25]. Benefit-finding, optimism and growth are all associated with improved outcomes in studies that have solid methodology [19–21].

As measured by most scales, spirituality includes finding connection and meaning in life as well as practising organized religion [23,26]. A challenge for QOL experts has been to determine a definition of spirituality distinct from religion and still specific enough to be measured rather than being all-inclusive of peaceful positive feelings. Although research has reported relationships between spirituality and mortality, as well as numerous other health outcomes, recent reviews conclude that most studies finding relationships between spirituality and health outcomes are methodologically flawed [23,24]. A survey of 1422 individuals from the general population in the USA reports that those who describe themselves as both spiritual and religious have less psychologic distress than those who are religious and not spiritual [26]. However, associations to health status have not been adequately tested because significant sociodemographic differences cannot be controlled between these groups [26].

The relevance of specific QOL dimensions within the population and treatment being examined merit consideration when designing an assessment plan. For instance, a study assessing African-American elderly and the health-related QOL relevancy of items found that spirituality was more relevant for these males and females than many of the usual QOL content items [27]. As another example, examining the QOL impacts of an antiviral prophylaxis will require careful thought about side-effects to assess, but may not need evaluation of social function.

In summary, QOL is always evaluated from the patient's perspective. It is rated in part by internal comparisons with how much worse things could be. Thus, patients with poor physical health may report good psychologic or overall QOL. Many different dimensions of QOL can be considered for evaluation, but physical health and psychologic health are always included. The ability to see positive elements of disease and treatment relates to improved psychologic outcomes.

Phases of HCT

Transplantation is both an individual and dynamic process [25]. While fairly consistent patterns can be described, a patient will have his or her own trajectory of illness and recovery depending on both medical and psychosocial factors [28]. There are two methodologic concerns in past research that contribute some instability to results across studies. One is that much of the research is cross-sectional, clustering patients with widely varying times since transplant and diverse diseases or treatments. Another is the range of assessment instruments used to evaluate QOL outcomes. This prevents ready comparison across studies. None the less, outcomes are more similar than different, lending confidence to the robustness of these results. The psychosocial components of these phases are only summarized here (see Chapter 38 for detailed review).

Pretransplant

Patients arrive at transplant with differing diseases, histories of treatment, levels of physical function, and psychologic, social and financial resources. Psychosocial predictors of outcome have received the most attention, although data indicate that physical QOL also predicts transplant outcomes [1,8,29]. Distress, in particular, predicts acute transplant symptom course, especially for pain and distress [2,29–31]. Psychosocial needs are greatest just prior to transplant if judged by the percentage of patients with clinically significant anxiety or depression at different phases of treatment and recovery [1,29]. The conclusion from review of numerous studies is that pretransplant physical condition and psychologic status predict later physical and psychologic adaptation in addition to survival [1,4,5,32–36]. These replicated findings support recent guidelines calling for routine assessments of psychosocial function [37].

Acute treatment

During the immediate post-transplant weeks, assessments find that survival is the axis around which other aspects of QOL are evaluated. In consequence, patients attribute their experiences to physical rather than psychologic cause during this phase [1,29,32]. Mouth pain, nausea, hair loss, fevers, adhering to treatment requirements, managing acute graft-vs.-host disease (GVHD) and efforts to maintain self-care dominate patient focus.

The first year

Multiple studies report that the same factors predict slower or poorer return of function: physical health pretransplant; medical complications during recovery in particular chronic GVHD; depression; lack of social support; lower education level; and female sex [1,2,4,5]. While most investigators find that older age at HCT is a risk factor for poorer QOL, others have reported the opposite [28]. For patients with chronic GVHD, osteoporosis and asceptic necrosis from steroid use can impair QOL [2,38]. As one of the most consistent long-term deficits found across studies and time points after treatment, both men and women have lower rates of sexual activity and satisfaction after HCT than the general population, with women's sexual dysfunction one of the most frequent and persistent long-term QOL problems [9,35,39–43]. Chapter 40 details these sexual function issues following HCT.

Long-term function

Survivors have more difficulty in the years following transplant if they struggle with chronic GVHD, pulmonary disease, infection or other medical complications [2,44,45]. However, in looking at survivors post-resolution of extensive chronic GVHD, function matches levels with those patients who do not have chronic GVHD [7]. Similarly, patients receiving allogeneic transplants may have more physical difficulties in the first year, but by 12 months physical and psychologic difficulties do not differ between types of transplant [7]. After the first year post-transplant, QOL issues arise that may have received minimal attention during transplant, such as work, family relations, infertility and sexual function [28,46]. All studies, whether longitudinal or cross-sectional, find that a large majority of adult survivors of HCT function well in their return to "normal" life in the domains of physical, psychologic, social, existential and overall subjective QOL [8,9,47–50].

Return to work justifiably receives a good deal of attention in recovery and long-term function reports. While 30–60% of survivors begin to return to work by the end of their first year post-transplant, return to full-time work continues to occur for patients into the third year [8,51,52]. Fortunately, by 3 years post-transplant studies agree that at least 80–90% of patients have returned to productive full-time work or school [2,8,53]. It appears that rates of return to work may differ to some extent according to the country a patient is in, perhaps as a result of differing financial and social or rehabilitation aids available [35,54,55].

Fatigue

Fatigue is the most persistent symptom beyond the first year of recovery [56,57]. It should be noted that fatigue is not a symptom specific to oncology. It is listed among common symptoms or side-effects for a large proportion of medical, pharmacologic, behavioral and psychologic diseases and treatments. Many biologic mechanisms have been postulated to explain fatigue following HCT or other cancer treatments. Considered among potential causes are effects of interleukins and interferons, anemia, systemic medications such as steroids, metabolic abnormalities, infection, treatment-related hormone and immunosuppression, total body irradiation (TBI), sleep disruption, lack of physical activity, depression and many medications [58].

Knobel et al. [59] examined fatigue in autologous survivors 3 years or longer post-transplant. While men did not differ from the general population, women differed significantly. Neither disease factors nor time since treatment predicted level of fatigue. For women, those treated in first remission reported more fatigue than women transplanted at more advanced stages of disease. Because biologic explanations were not detectable, this finding may reflect the relativity of subjective report. Women with less prior treatment may have noticed a greater contrast in their energy than women who came to transplant fatigued from prior treatment. Gonadal dysfunction also was not associated with post-transplant fatigue. Follicle-stimulating hormone and luteinizing hormone levels did not predict fatigue level, nor did estradiol or testosterone levels in male or female survivors. Likewise, hemoglobin and thyroid levels were unrelated to fatigue in HCT survivors. Immune markers tested, including interleukin 6 and soluble tumor necrosis factor receptors p55 and p75 did not predict fatigue either. On the other hand, interleukins, interferons, depression and numerous medications have been associated with fatigue in other non-HCT cancer studies [60].

Although common pathways continue to be investigated, successful treatments have included psychostimulants, antidepressants, erythropoietin and exercise [60,61]. Regardless of etiology, the behavioral component of this problem merits consideration in treating HCT patients. More than one researcher has demonstrated improvement of fatigue with exercise interventions [62,63].

In summary, the etiology of fatigue is almost certainly multifactorial. Varying sets of cause and effect components likely operate. However, there may be common pathways that respond to the same interventions such as exercise, psychostimulants or erythropoietin.

Cognitive function

Cognitive performance is an area of great individual variability pretransplant. Studies indicate that 20–56% of patients enter transplant with cognitive deficits that could interfere with function [64–66]. Andrykowski et al. [64] first noted that transplant candidates frequently had deficits in neuropsychologic function before starting HCT conditioning.

In children, cognitive effects of cranial irradiation are well-recognized [67]. Less consistent are findings on the stability or change in children's cognitive abilities as a result of HCT treatment. In a prospective study of 102 patients, Phipps et al. [68] report that no decline is evident in 1- or 3-year follow-up testing in patients over the age of 5 years at transplant. However, younger patients, particularly those under 3 years, do have some risk of IQ decline over time post-transplant [67,68]. Long-term outcomes do not differ based on TBI vs. chemotherapy-only conditioning regimens [68–70]. For adults, to date there is no indication that cognitive abilities decline more rapidly after HCT than with nontransplanted adults [71].

By 2 years post-transplant, 60% of allogeneic HCT survivors have some evidence of cognitive impairment on objective tests [72]. Harder et al. [72] report the central neuropsychologic difficulty for adult transplant recipients is found in information processing speed. Memory deficits occur if the speed at which information is presented outpaces patient ability to encode the information received. As a result, patients may be aware of memory problems, but not their source. In this study, no specific treatments could be identified as predictors of deficits; rather, accumulated difficulties in overall health, fatigue, mood and physical function were significant predictors.

As an indication of the variability in findings, van Dam et al. [73] reported on objective neuropsychologic function in 34 women who had autologous transplant plus ongoing tamoxifen for at least 2 years prior to testing. They found that 32% of their sample were impaired vs. 17% of women in a comparison group who received standard dose chemotherapy. Disparity in findings, with researchers reporting cognitive deficits in one-third to two-thirds of survivors, may be attributable to inclusion requirements of the samples (e.g. autologous vs. allogeneic, age range, history of prior treatment). Alternatively, some disparity may result from differences in tests selected, from time points at which testing was done or from differences in HCT treatment at the sites where patients were examined.

Padovan et al. [74] reported on 66 patients given neurologic examination, magnetic resonance imaging and neuropsychologic examinations from 8 months to 5 years after transplant. While 37% had neuropsychologic deficits, the deficits seen on one type of examination did not correlate with those seen on other forms of testing. Pathology in neurologic and magnetic resonance imaging was greater for patients with chronic GVHD, corticosteroid or cyclosporine use. Meanwhile, long-term cyclosporine use and age increased the risk for neuropsychologic impairment. Disease, donor status and conditioning regimen were unrelated to neuropsychologic results.

Several investigators have described neuropsychologic disorders in patients taking cyclosporine, tacrolimus or prednisone. For the most part, these have been case reports. A number of mechanisms have been postulated as the cause, and unless stroke or other permanent brain events occur, reports have indicated that these effects resolve with discontinuation of the drug [75–77].

In considering neuropsychologic function before and after transplant, it is important to recognize that performance is susceptible to disruption from virtually any source. Similar to fatigue, cognitive dysfunction is a common endpoint of many physiologic and mental strains. A large proportion of patients have cognitive deficits at any time point that has been tested thus far. As etiologies are further examined, causes will likely be numerous and will differ between patients, treatments and time points. Chapter 59 reviews neurologic toxicities of HCT.

In summary, a large proportion of patients test as cognitively impaired prior to transplant. The number grows somewhat at 1 year post-transplant, but long-term outcomes are not yet known. It remains uncertain whether etiologies differ at pretransplant vs. post-transplant and which factors, if any, during HCT cause permanent cognitive deficits. Longer prospective follow-up is required to answer these questions.

Late effects

As late effects are more closely studied, medical risks continue at a higher level for long-term survivors than for nontransplanted adults and children [6,35,44,78]. Chronic GVHD continues for some patients [6]. Bone mineral density declines measurably by 12 months post-transplant in both males and females receiving allogeneic HCT, particularly if treated for chronic GVHD [38]. Investigators report nontraumatic fractures in 11% of patients and avascular necrosis in 10% by 3 years post-transplant. In a different sample of survivors 10 years post-transplant, osteoporosis rate was 18% and restricted to women [6]. Second cancers and relapse of primary disease remain risks [52,78]. Consistent with earlier results, limited available QOL data indicate that survivors 5–10 plus years after HCT continue to be psychosocially very healthy, but vulnerable to late complications that might impact physical QOL if not overall life satisfaction [6,25,44,78].

We recently completed a survey of 135 10-year survivors compared with matched nontransplant controls. Results of similarities and differ-

Table 39.2 Rates of common problems in adult survivors of hematopoietic cell transplantation (HCT) and matched nontransplant comparisons.*

Common symptoms	10 years' survivors (%)	Matched comparisons (%)
Fatigue/stamina	13	6
Muscle weakness	15	7
Sleep difficulty	7	8
Eye problems	28	21
Cataract surgery	39	1
Mouth and throat problems	12	15
Breathing difficulties	12	6
On psychotherapeutic medications	28	13
Divorced or separated	41	41

*$n = 135$ allogeneic and autologous survivors 10 years post-transplant; $n = 135$ nontransplanted siblings or friends of the survivors, known prior to transplant, within 5 years of the 10 year survivors' age, same gender and ethnicity.

ences can be seen in Table 39.2. Fundamentally, HCT survivors look much like other adults their age, with the exception of highly specific areas of difficulty. Chapter 69 presents a complete review of late medical risks.

Relapse

A lacuna exists in QOL research on patients who relapse. Issues of family, social connection and spiritual needs become vital to patient evaluations of their QOL as their physical health is jeopardized. The symptoms and course of QOL whether proceeding to death or returning to remission remain unexplored, in part because patients are usually censored from studies when they relapse and so are no longer followed. This needs to change as more patients live with active disease or move between relapse and remission status several times following HCT.

In summary, the physiologic, psychological and existential phases of HCT have been well-defined. Common problems post-transplant include fatigue, cognitive difficulties, sexual dysfunction for men and women, and efforts to manage continuing uncertainty and fear. Thus far, social interactions have been examined primarily in regard to patient needs. Pretransplant QOL predictors of outcomes have been identified along with long-term strengths and difficulties. Late effects have not been well-defined for psychologic and functional dimensions of QOL, nor has the interaction between medical and QOL domains been well-examined. Finally, a number of interventions have improved outcomes, particularly in the areas of acute symptoms and management of fatigue. However, interventions to improve QOL are few in number and isolated to those problems just mentioned.

Diversity of HCT

Clearly, all transplants are not the same. Differences in medical course and outcome have been documented for autologous and allogeneic stem cell recipients, for patients with different diseases or risk factors, and for patients who receive TBI vs. those who receive chemotherapy-only regimens. Another area of diversity is the wide range of patients and others affected by transplant who respond within their own developmental phase of life or within their roles: adult or child patients; caregivers who are parents of children or spouses of adults; donors both related and unrelated; and males or females whether as patients or as caregivers. As with treatment, toxicities and medical outcomes, QOL varies with these diverse patient factors.

Conditioning regimen

Few sustained QOL differences have been confirmed relative to the use of TBI or chemotherapy-only as conditioning regimens. Early differences indicate that TBI is the best predictor of neuropsychologic deficits at 80 days post-transplant, but differences are no longer measurable after 1 year [66]. This remains true 5–10 years post-transplant [44]. Two medical differences that could influence QOL are greater incidence of cataracts in patients receiving TBI and greater likelihood of alopecia in patients receiving busulfan/cyclophosphamide [52]. Few studies document other differences predicted by conditioning regimen except for the increased risk of second cancers with higher doses of TBI [44,78].

Autologous, allogeneic related or unrelated HCT

Type of donor has been compared directly in numerous studies, and is considered a confounding factor in most regressions predicting QOL outcomes. Few studies have found measurable differences in psychologic QOL over time between autologous, allogeneic and unrelated transplant recipients, despite their medical and treatment differences [79,80]. One study reported that autologous HCT survivors had better QOL in all domains than allogeneic transplant recipients [80]. Another found autologous advantages only in psychologic function at 3 years post-transplant [1]. Other results are more consistent with the findings reported by Lee et al. [7]; autologous patients had fewer physician visits, fewer hospital admissions, fewer symptoms, were more likely to be off medication and had a higher rate of return to work or school at 6 months. However, most of these advantages disappeared by 1 year and all of them disappeared by 2 years. Another study found that allogeneic HCT recipients had better QOL in all domains pretransplant, but at 1 year only cognitive function differed [81]. The change that occurred between pretransplant and 1 year post-transplant could be accounted for by improvement in QOL in the autologous patients by 1 year. In other words, allogeneic patients were back to pretransplant baseline by 1 year, while autologous patient QOL had improved from their pretransplant levels by 1 year.

Several conclusions are evident. One is that these transplant recoveries are more similar than different, particularly in the psychologic domains. Another is that, between related and unrelated allogeneic HCT recipients, no differences in outcomes have been identified.

Age effects among adults

Older adults have more difficulties with medical recovery from high-dose treatment and are less likely to return to work or social activities [2,7,44,57,79]. In QOL domains, the direction of greater effect depends on several factors. Risk of chronic GVHD or other medical sequelae increase with age. On the other hand, younger age at time of transplant and higher doses of TBI put survivors at greater risk for second cancers [78]. Andrykowski et al. [28] found that younger women had poorer performance status and more psychosocial concerns. In all, while medical risks vary significantly with age, QOL is more noteworthy for lack of differences based on age to 50 years than for any remarkable distinctions based on age. A caveat in this conclusion is the open question of long-term outcomes in pediatric HCT recipients who survive to adulthood. Also, inadequate data prevent any conclusions on QOL for patients over age 50.

Pediatric QOL

Long-term and late medical outcomes of HCT in children have been defined to some extent. In contrast, research on both physical and psychosocial function is limited and cross-sectional to date. Nevertheless, what has been reported testifies to the resilience of children not unlike the resilience in the adults who have been studied. We assessed 120 adult survivors who had HCT as children and compared them with 114 adult survivors of childhood leukemia who had received chemotherapy without transplant and an age- and gender-matched group of non-transplanted comparison subjects [82]. Time since treatment was set at 5 or more years for eligibility; average time was more than 10 years post-transplant, average age was 27 years for the HCT and healthy comparison groups and 24 years for the chemotherapy without transplant group. The pediatric HCT survivors reported more major illness, physician visits, diabetes and second malignancies than either of the other two groups. HCT survivors reported mental health equivalent to the comparison subjects, but were lower in physical health scales of the SF36 than the other groups. Both survivor groups reported more health or life insurance refusals (25% and 33% vs. 3% for comparison subjects). Marital status did not differ between groups and other psychosocial factors measured did not differentiate the groups.

Other researchers have found generally similar results. In examining adolescents and young adults 2–13 years post-transplant, Felder-Puig et al. [3] compared an HCT sample with bone cancer survivors. The groups did not differ in most areas of adjustment or in perceived overall QOL, with the exception that HCT survivors reported higher anxiety, feelings of sensitivity and vulnerability. Other researchers have reported that pediatric survivors do better than their peers in psychosocial domains [83]. The rate of successful return to school (85–95%) is quite similar to rates of return to work in adult survivors [84].

The restriction to these overall positive outcomes is that it has not been possible yet to track many survivors past the age of 27 years. Survivor samples of mature adults are not yet large enough to adequately evaluate their adult QOL as indicated by physical limits, psychologic stability, marital relationships, work history, sexual function or management of infertility.

Male or female

Unlike survival and toxicities, little attention has focused explicitly on gender effects in QOL outcomes. None the less, nearly all research documents some gender effects within QOL surveys or interventions. In reviewing these outcomes, it becomes rapidly apparent that female recovery is more complex than male recovery, at least based on self-reports [2,5,44,50,57,79]. Norms for males and females on psychologic tests are always separated because of the well-established fact that women endorse more symptoms than men given the same levels of health. These inherent differences emphasize the value of norm-based standardized scores when interpreting self-report forms. Women report more fatigue and they generally report higher levels of distress, even when using standardized scores within gender normed measures [85]. Two additional consistent findings across studies are that women have more sexual problems and are slower to return to work [39,44].

Donors

Related and unrelated donors are critical to HCT success. Their needs and research examining their QOL are fully reviewed in Chapter 38. In short, the large majority of donors find the experience rewarding and are not permanently traumatized or injured by their donation. For the smaller group of patients (perhaps 9–13%) who find the process stressful or otherwise problematic, little is known about predictors or long-term outcomes [86].

Caregivers

It is questionable whether medical staff and patients could manage HCT and recovery without the presence of a family caregiver or multiple caregivers. As central a role as families have, research on family caregivers is only now making headway in recognizing QOL needs and in comparing patients, caregivers and norms. A small number of studies have defined the course of caregiver fatigue, burden and emotions over time. These studies report that fatigue peaks at 3 months [87], but that emotional distress in caregivers peaks during the first 2 weeks of treatment [88].

Langer et al. [89] find that caregivers report both more anxiety and depression than patients consistently over the first year. Female spousal caregivers report less marital satisfaction than male spousal caregivers [89]. Despite this decreased marital satisfaction, rates of divorce among long-term HCT survivors and spouses do not differ from that reported by matched controls (see Table 39.2).

Although one might hypothesize that inpatient care would be less stressful for caregivers given the greater availability of professional support, this hypothesis is rejected by surveys [90]. From pretransplant to discharge to the patient's primary physician, ambulatory-patient caregivers not only report more positive mood during acute treatment, but also report greater satisfaction with the extent to which their needs were met. Similar results have been found for patient outcomes; autologous HCT recipients do as well or better in all QOL domains when treated during the first month in ambulatory care rather than inpatient care [91].

Mothers of pediatric HCT patients seem to suffer the greatest trauma in the course of their child's treatment [92]. Other caregivers manage remarkably well from early evidence, despite their levels of acute distress.

Interventions to improve QOL outcomes

Randomized controlled trials (RCTs) to improve predictable QOL problems have been regrettably infrequent in HCT populations. During acute treatment several studies have demonstrated that pain is improved with hypnosis or other psychologic care [93,94]. For a sample of autologous breast cancer patients, Gaston-Johansson et al. [95] found that a "coping strategies program", including preparatory information, cognitive restructuring and relaxation with imagery, reduced nausea along with fatigue at 7 days into transplant. Sustained effects were not reported. In another RCT, massage had immediate effects on distress, fatigue and nausea in an RCT [96]. However, these results were not maintained into future days.

Several RCTs and nonrandomized trials by two independent groups of investigators demonstrate that fatigue is reduced in HCT patients who participate in exercise programs [62,63,97,98]. Given that these are the rare nonpharmacologic clinical trials indicating both subjective and objective improvement in fatigue, results justify including exercise programs as standard care. A phase 2 trial indicates that fatigue is reduced for allogeneic HCT patients infused with recombinant human erythropoietin after day 35 [61]. Another nonrandomized controlled trial comparison found that post-transplant patients who received a 3–4-week inpatient rehabilitation program demonstrated no difference in employment when compared with a group of patients who did not receive this rehabilitation [54].

Several issues stand out after a review of this limited RCT research. The RCTs in this population have had modest effects, while the cost-effectiveness can be questioned: more is not necessarily better. Few attempts have been made to implement clinical trials designed to improve QOL using nonpharmacologic methods for patients or others affected by HCT. Instead, most QOL interventions are provided as clinical care without demonstration of efficacy. More RCT are needed to examine which

QOL deficits respond to what interventions, in which high-risk patients, at what points in time.

Interventions to address the needs of caregivers are provided clinically (e.g. family support groups, activities, classes in managing the caregiving role), but minimal research has tested interventions in RCTs. In one non-randomized study, caregivers who were provided with two 30-min massages twice a week for 3 weeks reported declines in anxiety, depression and fatigue [99]. Little can be concluded without randomized trials that include an active control. As it stands, placebo effect and motivation to please in nonrandomized and nonblinded studies restrict confidence in the results.

Measurement

In QOL measurement a "response shift" is expected as patient medical conditions change. Patients naturally reprioritize concerns, and self-report is relative to expectation rather than being tied to medical status. In this process, health may decline, but many patients still report good psychologic function [1]. Another factor that can shift response is the changing relevance of assessment dimensions. While physical symptoms may be the central focus during acute treatment, focus shifts in long-term follow-up to functional abilities and emotional adaptation [28,46]. This is a major reason why excellent measures in one circumstance may be of less value at a different time. For instance, if no patients work in the 3 months after HCT, there is no gain from asking about work and to do so would seem out of touch with patient experiences. However, after the first year, not asking about work would be a major oversight.

Generic assessments

There are three QOL measures routinely selected when providing a "generic" assessment of HCT outcomes: the Short Form 36 Health Survey (SF36), the Functional Assessment of Cancer Therapy–Bone Marrow Transplant (FACT-BMT) and the European Organization for Research and Treatment of Cancer Quality of Life Questionnaire-C30 (EORTC QLQ-C30). One of these is used in most cancer QOL studies. Each of these well-standardized, reliable and valid measures has some questions in common with the others and asks some questions that are not represented in the others. Yet each of them has been used effectively in HCT research. The FACT-BMT asks questions specific to treatment of cancer and the HCT process and focuses its emotional well-being content on concerns specific to the disease and treatment. It does not evaluate physical ability. As such it is quite disease and treatment oriented. The "BMT module" of added questions contains items that elaborate the more common HCT symptoms and concerns [100]. The EORTC QLQ-C30, in contrast, has a more explicit focus on function, what a patient is able to do physically, specific symptoms and rather brief psychologic review. While an HCT-specific module is in development and some have been tested, one is not yet available from the instrument developers [9,101]. The SF36, meanwhile, is a health-related QOL measure not specific to disease [102]. Its evaluation of physical ability corresponds most closely to the EORTC QLQ-C30 [103]; it provides a full although brief assessment of psychologic function, and it has minimal emphasis on physical symptoms. Given its general health orientation across populations, the SF36 is appropriate for use multiple years post-transplant as issues become less transplant-specific.

Numerous studies have documented that these QOL measures are correlated but do not share enough variance to be considered equivalent [103]. Investigators find that the instruments have analogous global health items (correlation: $r = 0.82$; 67% of the variance is shared). However, physical and psychologic dimensions of the EORTC QLQ-C30 and FACT share only limited variance. Virtually no variance is shared between the EORTC QLQ-C30 and FACT on scales of social well-being, relationship with the doctor or cognitive function [103]. With its focus on treatment related issues, the FACT covers the areas of greatest influence on patients during acute treatment, whereas the EORTC QLQ-C30 provides assessments that may be relevant beyond the acute transplant period and through recovery.

Selection of which instrument to use depends on the goals and time frame of assessment. Giving multiple generic measures is not recommended because of patient burden and tolerance for responding to similar questions. As the most extensively studied comparison, data are clear that results of the FACT cannot be directly compared with the EORTC QLQ-C30 [104].

Each of these measures has normative information on use with HCT. Each has translations in multiple languages, and all are appropriate to capture issues faced by HCT patients. These scales have particular value for their abilities to provide a normative reference for a sample or an individual patient. The SF36 offers the most extensive norms, grouped by gender, age and illness, and also normed on general population samples. For comparison, Table 39.3 lists the subscales for these three QOL measures.

Numerous other measures exist that are relevant to HCT, but are not as widely used. Hence, comparative data are not as readily available. The Sickness Impact Profile (SIP) [105], with 12 subscales, effectively tracks decline and recovery in health-related QOL before and after HCT [8]. Other scales have relevance in specific circumstances, but do not have the extent of testing in HCT to provide normative information. Still, these multidimensional measures of QOL might be of greater relevance depending on the target of assessment. The Cancer Rehabilitation Evaluation System–Short Form (CARES) and the Functional Living Index–Cancer (FLIC) are two notable examples [106,107]. For a detailed consideration of measures, the reader is referred to books on this topic or articles comparing measures [108].

Assessment of specific dimensions

Because generic measures are unlikely to have the sensitivity to capture details of main interest in a clinical trial, measures specific to anticipated outcomes may need to be added to a generic tool. Considering physical adaptation helps to clarify this point. Patients can be assessed for general physical function with a measure such as the EORTC QLQ-C30 or SF36, but if an intervention is targeted explicitly to reducing fatigue, these scales may not have the sensitivity to capture outcome changes [59]. A specific fatigue measure will provide more sensitivity to differences in outcomes. These focused forms will also inform investigators of where changes are occurring: is sleep improved, is stamina better or does the patient feel more alert?

An element central to HCT QOL is the concept of transplant-specific distress: what are the worries, stresses or distress unique to a patient having a transplant that contribute to how he or she is doing? To address this concern, we have developed an HCT distress measure composed of 18 items which fit into five categories. The measure has been tested in 732 patients prior to HCT. Survivors have been reassessed through 5 years post-transplant. Figure 39.1 shows the mean level of transplant-specific distress in patients over time in comparison to their general depression scores. The difference in these two measures visually demonstrates why a generic measure may not always be specific or sensitive enough to capture selective information. HCT distress is a better predictor of pain, nausea and stress responses during acute treatment than is depression or other general mood indicators [30,31], while depression is a better predictor of long-term outcomes [Syrjala, unpublished data].

Table 39.3 Subscales of the three most widely used global health-related quality of life (QOL) measures.

EORTC-QLQ-C30	FACT-G	SF36
Subscales		
Physical function	Physical well-being	Physical function
Role function	Social/family well-being	Role: physical
Emotional function	Relationship with the doctor	Body pain
Cognitive function	Emotional well-being	Vitality (fatigue)
Social function	Functional well-being	Social function
Plus 9 symptom scales	BMT module (includes work; side-effects; appearance; fatigue; memory; finances; family burden)	Role: emotional
Global health status		Mental health
		General health perception
Summary scores		
No, only subscales	Total score	Physical composite T score
		Mental health composite T score
Number of items		
30 in core	34 in core	36
BMT module in development	24 added in BMT module	

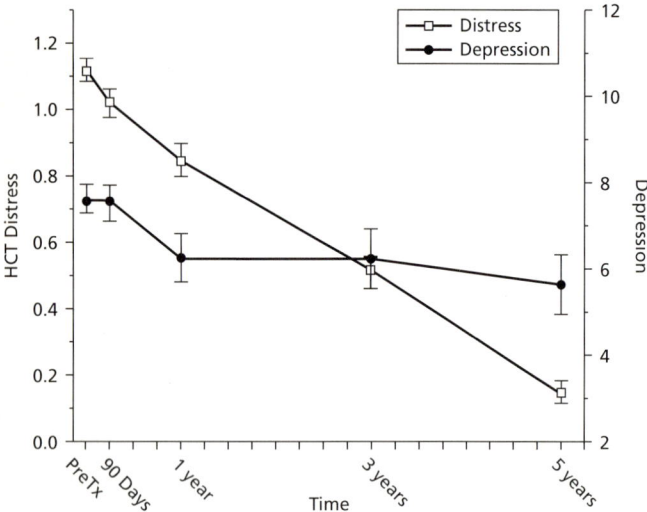

Fig. 39.1 Comparison of mean depression and hematopoietic cell transplantation (HCT)-specific distress scores from prior to transplant to 5 years. Depression and distress differed from each other in repeated measures analysis of variance for time course ($p < 0.001$). In this case, measuring depression would not provide the same information gained by measuring distress. At each time point distress and depression correlated significantly ($r = 0.44–0.65$) demonstrating some share variance, but not redundancy. Mean depression scores changed only from 90 days to 1 year ($p < 0.01$), remaining unchanged between other time points. Distress changed significantly between each successive time point ($p < 0.05$). Patients were 319 adult male and female recipients of allogeneic or autologous HCT who had been treated with myeloablative therapy, with survivors followed to 5 years.

Alternative QOL measurement strategies

The gold standard for QOL assessment is a patient face to face with a staff person who is available to answer questions and to assure that the patient is competent and responding in the proper format. However, there are times when the choice is between no information and either someone responding for the patient or the patient responding through mailed forms or telephone interviews.

Parent or proxy assessment

When a patient is unable to provide self-report of QOL, a proxy responder may be the only option. This proxy is often a nurse who is providing care for the patient, a parent of a young child or the family member of a patient unable to communicate. Research on the validity of proxy responses indicates that, on average, parents and other proxies differ equally in responses when compared with patient reports [109]. Proxies, including parents, tend to underestimate patients' symptoms. In contrast, they tend to rate global QOL and mental health lower than patient self-reports [109]. Fortunately, proxies are more accurate when they are rating concrete observable events. Another finding from this research is that clinicians and parents underestimate the QOL information a child or patient with limited communication ability can still transmit. Of interest, children's self-reports of their own health status significantly match physician ratings but not parent ratings [13].

When choosing to have a parent respond for a child over 5 years, there are several pediatric assessments to consider [13]. The Pediatric Quality of Life Inventory includes both a patient report and a parent report evaluating health-related QOL for pediatric cancer patients on dimensions parallel to the FACT or EORTC QLQ-C30 [110]. Multiple versions suited to the developmental ages of children are comparable. A companion measure, the Pediatric Cancer QOL Inventory, provides treatment specific assessment of symptoms [111]. Both of these measures have well-established reliability and validity, although it is unclear whether they have been used with HCT patients.

Given the large number of measures translated for age, language and culture, it should be possible for the majority of patients to complete a general QOL measure appropriate to their needs.

Written, mailed, phone interview, computer-based assessment

The shortening of QOL measures, the increased attention to symptoms and the unremitting brevity of physician time have led researchers to explore the use of automated assessment systems with some success. Testing of QOL assessment across modalities with HCT or other cancer patients substantiates the transferability of written measures to touch-screen or other bedside computer [112–115]. Measures confirmed to be

Table 39.4 Correlations between objective and subjective measures of neuropsychologic performance. Fred Hutchinson Cancer Research Center data: 150 allogeneic and autologous adults tested pretransplant.

	Subjective report	
	Memory	Thinking/concentration
Objective tests		
Verbal learning (HVLT)	0.02	0.04
Word finding (COWAT)	0.25	0.32
Cognitive flexibility (Trails B)	0.20	0.05

NOTE: These correlations indicate that patients who self-report memory or concentration complaints are not consistently the same people who test as impaired. The correlations do not indicate that patients do not have objectively measurable deficits.
HVLT, Hopkin's verbal learning test; COWAT, controlled oral word association test.

equally reliable and valid with written, mailed and computer formats include the EORTC QLQ-C30, SF36 and the Memorial Symptom Assessment Scale [112–115]. If any trend exists, it is for patients to rate needs or difficulties slightly lower using a touch-screen [114]. On the other hand, Ryan *et al.* [113] note that the quality of data was better with a computerized version of the SF36. The software corrected skipped items or double responses, yielding a dataset with no missing data or errors. In contrast, one error or another occurred in 44% of paper response forms. Further, patients preferred the electronic response version, and the touch-screen took slightly less time to complete. One investigator tested several different QOL measures using touch-screen technology and found the method reliable as long as the format and content of the written form is precisely replicated [112].

Automated telephone symptom monitoring for HCT recipients has been successfully tested and compared with written report [116]. A computerized system (Interactive Voice Response) can be set to contact patients at home at any designated day or time selected by the patient. If the patient does not respond, the system will call after set periods as often as programmed to do so. Responses are easily given using the telephone keypad or they can be spoken. The technology can be programmed to download information to a physician or nurse if critical set points are reached. In a comparison of the Interactive Voice Response vs. paper and pen, HCT patients responded at the same rate as on paper and reported the same symptom severity. In addition, 98% found the system easy to use [116].

Clinically meaningful differences

The topic of what constitutes a clinically meaningful difference on QOL measures is still under discussion. Even so, general consensus is building that one-half a standard deviation on most tests will be meaningful, or alternatively, one standard error of measurement [117,118].

There are situations when self-reporting is not dependable as a sole source for outcomes. One example is the relationship between subjective experience of cognitive deficits and objective tests of deficits. As seen in Table 39.4, the greatest overlap in variance between objective neuropsychologic tests and self-report of cognitive difficulties is 11% in our sample at 1 year. While this says nothing about the *validity* of patient complaints of impairment, it indicates that self-report is not a *reliable* indicator of who has which problems. Lack of correlation on neuropsychologic tests between self-report and objective test results is the norm across samples of medical patients.

Psychometrics: evaluating reliability, validity, sensitivity and specificity

Analyses that tell us whether a measure is capturing what we want it to and how well the measure is assessing the concept targeted are generally grouped together as "psychometric" qualities of a test [60]. Psychometric properties are used to examine the strength, generalizability and value of a self-report or observation measure.

As with laboratory values, normal individual variation is often large and any one person or single response may fall outside the group norm or the patient's own norm on related questions. The subjective nature of QOL requires the use of psychometric analyses to establish the reliability, validity, sensitivity and specificity of these tests. Recent studies indicate that cancer patient self-report is generally consistent with medical record reports, with the exception that symptoms are less often noted in records and when noted are rated less severely than the patient's self-report [14,15].

In brief, *reliability* is most often used to answer the questions:
1 am I asking questions that fit together as a construct? and
2 am I measuring something that is stable to the extent I want it to be stable?
The aim to establish reliability and reduce measurement error is a major reason why we ask more than one question when assessing QOL.

Internal consistency is a form of reliability that asks, "how strongly are these questions related to each other?" If people who are depressed endorse the same symptoms of depression, then we find that these items have high internal consistency. There is no single standard for what is considered acceptable internal consistency. As in a correlation, a score of 1 would mean the items are all answered exactly the same way. As a general rule of thumb, internal reliability between 0.80 and 0.90 is ideal. If internal reliability for a scale or subscale goes below 0.80, one might think of looking at whether items can be deleted because they are not measuring the same construct. If this reliability rises above 0.90, then one might consider that there are more items than needed, adding unnecessarily to patient burden.

Test–retest reliability addresses the stability of responses. In medical treatment, where change is expected, the correlation between scores at two time points needs to be tested within a time frame when change is not expected. This may be 2 days in a row for mucositis pain or an interval of 7 days for long-term follow-up questions, such as ability to climb stairs.

When a scale has multiple subscales, *factor analytic* strategies, such as principal components analysis, are used to determine which items cluster together to form a subscale. As an example, the SF36 has subscales of physical function and body pain. To be separate scales, it is necessary for physical function items to load on a different factor than body pain items in a principal components analysis. The internal reliability of each subscale should be held to the same standards as the internal reliability requirements of the overall scale score.

Validity is usually assessed after reliability for the obvious reason that a scale cannot be valid if it is not reliable. While reliability speaks to the internal qualities of a measure, validity speaks to how well a measure is assessing what it is purporting to assess. Tests of validity are done with two primary methods. The first looks at the measure content, considering the way it was developed and making a judgement of its adequacy in capturing the content it is designed to score. The second, criterion validity and its subtypes, are tested with correlations between the test instrument and other established instruments to demonstrate that the new measure correlates as hypothesized. An example is subjective report of cognitive difficulty and neuropsychologic testing as demonstrated in Table 39.4. The validity of self-report in this case is called into question because the well-established standard for evaluating cognitive function is objective testing. Because asking about cognitive difficulties is more highly correlated with distress than with the objective test results, we would conclude that self-report in this case is invalid. This does not mean that patients do not have cognitive deficits, because formal neuropsychologic testing clearly defines that they do. Rather, the lack of relationship indicates that patients are not a best source of knowledge about who has how much difficulty within specific cognitive functions.

Conclusions

QOL before, during and after HCT has been well-described. All studies agree that most patients regain high levels of physical and psychologic QOL by 3 years following transplant. At the same time, a subset of 5–20% of patients will have medical problems, such as chronic GVHD or pulmonary disease, that impinge on QOL for 5 or even 10 years after transplant. Even for the patients who return to full-time work and normal social activities, who have good psychologic and physical function, specific areas of common difficulty have been identified. Recognized long-term problems include fatigue, cognitive deficits and sexual dysfunction for both males and females. The QOL impact of medical late effects is beginning to be defined, but is still an area of limited investigation. Understanding of QOL in relapsed patients, caregivers, adult survivors of pediatric transplant and in nonmyeloablative transplant recipients remain largely unknown. To date, few clinical trials have been published that improve QOL during either acute treatment or long-term recovery. For those that have been successful, cost-effectiveness and effect size can both be improved by targeting high-risk patients with specific problems for which effective treatments exist or can be developed.

By nature, QOL shifts with the situation a patient is in, reflecting not only observable abilities but also experiences relative to expectations for the immediate circumstance. As a result, very ill patients can report good QOL in some areas. In assessing QOL, many options have been tested with HCT patients and work well. A generic QOL measure provides valuable normative information that permits comparison of scores with patients of comparable age, gender and/or disease. At the same time, a specific, more focused measure such as a fatigue or sexual function scale may be needed to provide adequate sensitivity when defining the scope and nature of a targeted problem or intervention. Fortunately, there are many effective examples of QOL evaluation with HCT patients, at all stages of treatment and survivorship.

References

1 Broers S, Kartein AA, Le Cessie S *et al.* Psychological functioning and quality of life following bone marrow transplantation: a 3 year follow-up study. *J Psychosom Res* 2000; **48**: 11–21.

2 Duell T, van Lint MT, Ljungmann P *et al.* Health and functional status of long-term survivors of bone marrow transplantation. *Ann Intern Med* 1997; **126**: 184–92.

3 Felder-Puig R, Peters C, Matthes-Martin S *et al.* Psychosocial adjustment of pediatric patients after allogeneic stem cell transplantation. *Bone Marrow Transplant* 1999; **24**: 75–80.

4 Hjermstad MJ, Evensen SA, Kvaloy SO *et al.* Health-related quality of life 1 year after allogeneic or autologous stem-cell transplantation: a prospective study. *J Clin Oncol* 1999; **17**: 706–18.

5 Heinonen H, Volin L, Uutela A *et al.* Quality of life and factors related to perceived satisfaction with quality of life after allogeneic bone marrow transplantation. *Ann Hematol* 2001; **80**: 137–43.

6 Kiss TL, Abdolell M, Jamal N *et al.* Long-term medical outcomes and quality-of-life assessment of patients with chronic myeloid leukemia followed at least 10 years after allogeneic bone marrow transplantation. *J Clin Oncol* 2002; **20**: 2334–43.

7 Lee SJ, Fairclough D, Parsons SK *et al.* Recovery after stem-cell transplantation for hematologic diseases. *J Clin Oncol* 2001; **19**: 242–52.

8 Syrjala KL, Chapko MK, Vitaliano PP *et al.* Recovery after allogeneic marrow transplantation: prospective study of predictors of long-term physical and psychosocial functioning. *Bone Marrow Transplant* 1993; 11: 319–27.

9 Bush NE, Donaldson GW, Haberman MH *et al.* Conditional and unconditional estimation of multidimensional quality of life after hematopoietic stem cell transplantation: a longitudinal follow-up of 415 patients. *Biol Blood Marrow Transplant* 2000; **6**: 576–91.

10 Marks DI, Lush R, Cavenagh J *et al.* The toxicity and efficacy of donor lymphocyte infusions given after reduced-intensity conditioning allogeneic stem cell transplantation. *Blood* 2002; **100**: 3108–14.

11 Mielcarek M, Sandmaier BM, Maloney DG *et al.* Nonmyeloablative hematopoietic cell transplantation: status quo and future perspectives. *J Clin Immunol* 2002; **22**: 70–4.

12 Cella D. Quality of life. In: Holland J, ed. *Psycho-oncology*. Oxford: Oxford University Press, 1998: 1135–46.

13 Parsons SK, Barlow SE, Levy SL *et al.* Health-related quality of life in pediatric bone marrow transplant survivors: according to whom? *Int J Cancer* 1999; **12**: 46–51.

14 Velikova G, Wright P, Smith AB *et al.* Self-reported quality of life of individual cancer patients: concordance of results with disease course and medical records. *J Clin Oncol* 2001; **19**: 2064–73.

15 Stromgren AS, Groenvold L, Pedersen AK *et al.* Symptomatology of cancer patients in palliative care: content validation of self-assessment questionnaires against medical records. *Eur J Cancer* 2002; **38**: 788–94.

16 Spilker B, ed. *Quality of Life and Pharmacoeconomics in Clinical Trials*, 2nd edn. Philadelphia: Lippincott-Raven Press, 1996: 1–10.

17 Ferrell B, Grant M, Schmidt G *et al.* The meaning of quality of life for bone marrow transplant survivors. I. The impact of bone marrow transplant on quality of life. *Cancer Nurs* 1992; **15**: 153–60.

18 Smith KW, Avis NE, Assmann SF. Distinguishing between quality of life and health status in quality of life research: a meta analysis. *Qual Life Res* 1999; **8**: 447–59.

19 Anderson BL. Biobehavioral outcomes following psychological interventions for cancer patients. *J Consult Clin Psychol* 2002; **70**: 590–610.

20 Antoni MH, Lehman JM, Kilbourn KM *et al.* Congitive–behavioral stress management intervention decreases the prevalence of depression and enhances benefit finding among women under treatment for early-stage breast cancer. *Health Psychol* 2001; **20**: 20–32.

21 Folkman S, Greer S. Promoting psychological well-being in the face of serious illness: when theory, research and practice inform each other. *Psychooncology* 2000; **9**: 11–19.

22 Matthews DA, McCullough ME, Larson DB *et al.* Religious commitment and health status: a review of the research and implications for family medicine. *Arch Fam Med* 1998; **7**: 118–24.

23 Thoreson CE, Harris AH. Spirituality and health: what's the evidence and what's needed? *Ann Behav Med* 2002; **24**: 3–13.

24 Sloan RP, Bagiella E. Claims about religious involvement and health outcomes. *Ann Behav Med* 2002; **24**: 14–21.

25 Haberman M, Bush N, Young K *et al.* Quality of life of adult long-term survivors of bone marrow transplantation: a qualitative analysis of narrative data. *Oncol Nurs Forum* 1993; **20**: 1545–53.

26 Shahabi L, Powell L, Musick M. Correlates of self-perceptions of spirituality in American adults. *Ann Behav Med* 2002; **24**: 59–68.

27 Cunningham WE, Burton TM, Hawes-Dawson J *et al.* Use of relevancy ratings by target respondents to develop health-related quality of life measures: an example with African-American elderly. *Qual Life Res* 1999; **8**: 749–68.

28 Andrykowski MA, Cordova MJ, Hann DM *et al.* Patients' psychosocial concerns following stem cell transplantation. *Bone Marrow Transplant* 1999; **24**: 1121–9.

29 Fife B, Huster GA, Cornetta KG *et al.* Longitudinal study of adaptation to the stress of bone marrow transplantation. *J Clin Oncol* 2000; **18**: 1539–49.

30 Syrjala KL, Chapko ME. Evidence for a biopsychosocial model of cancer treatment-related pain. *Pain* 1995; **61**: 69–79.

31 Schulz-Kindermann F, Hennings U, Ramm G *et al.* The role of biomedical and psychosocial factors for the prediction of pain and distress in patients undergoing high-dose therapy and BMT/PBST. *Bone Marrow Transplant* 2002; **29**: 341–51.

32 Andrykowski MA, Brady MJ, Henslee-Downey PJ. Psychosocial factors predictive of survival after allogeneic bone marrow transplantation for leukemia. *Psychosom Med* 1994; **56**: 432–9.

33 Loberiza FR, Rizzo JD, Bredeson CN *et al.* Association of depressive syndrome and early deaths among patients after stem-cell transplantation for malignant diseases. *J Clin Oncol* 2002; **20**: 2118–26.

34 Tschuschke V, Hertenstein B, Arnold R et al. Associations between coping and survival time of adult leukemia patients receiving allogeneic bone marrow transplantation: results of a prospective study. *J Psychosom Res* 2001; **50**: 277–85.

35 Molassiotis A, van den Akker OB, Milligan DW et al. Quality of life in long-term survivors of marrow transplantation: comparison with a matched group receiving maintenance chemotherapy. *Bone Marrow Transplant* 1996; **17**: 249–58.

36 Hjermstad MJ, Loge JH, Evensen SA et al. The course of anxiety and depression during the first year after allogeneic or autologous stem cell transplantation. *Bone Marrow Transplant* 1999; **24**: 1219–28.

37 Holland JC. Preliminary guidelines for treatment of distress. *Oncology* 1997; **11**: 109–14.

38 Stern JM, Sullivan KM, Ott SM et al. Bone density loss after allogeneic hematopoietic stem cell transplantation: a prospective study. *Biol Blood Marrow Transplant* 2001; **7**: 257–64.

39 Syrjala KL, Roth SL, Abrams JR et al. Prevalence and predictors of sexual dysfunction in long-term survivors of bone marrow transplantation. *J Clin Oncol* 1998; **16**: 3148–57.

40 Syrjala KL, Schroeder TC, Abrams JR et al. Sexual function measurement and outcomes in cancer survivors and matched controls. *J Sex Res* 2000; **37**: 213–25.

41 Howell SJ, Radford JA, Smets EM et al. Fatigue, sexual function and mood following treatment for haematological malignancy: the impact of mild Leydig cell dysfunction. *Br J Cancer* 2000; **82**: 789–93.

42 Schimmer AD, Ali V, Stewart AK et al. Male sexual function after autologous blood or marrow transplantation. *Biol Blood Marrow Transplant* 2001; **7**: 279–83.

43 Wingard JR, Curbow B, Baker F et al. Sexual satisfaction in survivors of bone marrow transplantation. *Bone Marrow Transplant* 1992; **9**: 185–90.

44 Socie G, Clift RA, Blaise D et al. Busulfan plus cyclophosphamide compared with total-body irradiation plus cyclophosphamide before marrow transplantation for myeloid leukemia: long-term follow-up of four randomized studies. *Blood* 2001; **98**: 3569–74.

45 Chiodi S, Spinelli S, Ravera G et al. Quality of life in 244 recipients of allogeneic bone marrow transplantation. *Br J Haematol* 2000; **110**: 614–9.

46 McQuellon RP, Russell GB, Rambo TD et al. Quality of life and psychological distress of bone marrow transplant recipients: the "time trajectory" to recover over the first year. *Bone Marrow Transplant* 1998; **21**: 477–86.

47 Andrykowski MA. Psychosocial factors in bone marrow transplantation: a review and recommendations for research. *Bone Marrow Transplant* 1994; **13**: 357–75.

48 Bush NE, Haberman M, Donaldson G et al. Quality of life of 125 adults surviving 6–18 years after bone marrow transplantation. *Soc Sci Med* 1995; **40**: 479–90.

49 Fife B, Baker F, Zabora J et al. Reintegration after bone marrow transplantation. *Cancer Pract* 1999; **7**: 190–7.

50 Baker F, Wingard JR, Curbow B et al. Quality of life of bone marrow transplant long-term survivors. *Bone Marrow Transplant* 1994; **13**: 589–96.

51 Deeg HJ, Leisenring W, Storb R et al. Long-term outcome after marrow transplantation for severe aplastic anemia. *Blood* 1998; **91**: 3637–45.

52 Socie G, Mary JY, Esperou H et al. Health and functional status of adult recipients 1 year after allogeneic haematopoietic stem cell transplantation. *Br J Haematol* 2001; **113**: 194–201.

53 Edman L, Larsen J, Hagglund H et al. Health-related quality of life, symptom distress and sense of coherence in adult survivors of allogeneic stem-cell transplantation. *Eur J Cancer Care* 2001; **10**: 124–30.

54 Hensel M, Egerer G, Schneeweiss A et al. Quality of life and rehabilitation in social and professional life after autologous stem cell transplantation. *Ann Oncol* 2002; **13**: 209–17.

55 Molassiotis A, Boughton BJ, Burgoyne T, van den Akker OB. Comparison of the overall quality of life in 50 long-term survivors of autologous and allogeneic bone marrow transplantation. *J Adv Nurs* 1995; **22**: 509–16.

56 Andrykowski MA, Carpenter JS, Greiner CB et al. Energy level and sleep quality following bone marrow transplantation. *Bone Marrow Transplant* 1997; **20**: 669–79.

57 Molassiotis A, Morris PJ. The meaning of quality of life and the effects of unrelated donor bone marrow transplants for chronic myeloid leukemia in adult long-term survivors. *Cancer Nurs* 1998; **21**: 205–11.

58 Cella D, Peterman A, Passik S et al. Progress toward guidelines for the management of fatigue. *Oncology* 1998; **12**: 369–77.

59 Knobel H, Loge JH, Nordoy T et al. High level of fatigue on lymphoma patients treated with high dose therapy. *J Pain Symptom Manage* 2000; **19**: 446–55.

60 Cella D. Quality of life. In: Holland J, ed. *Psychooncology*. Oxford: Oxford University Press, 1998; 1135–46.

61 Baron F, Sautois B, Baudoux E et al. Optimization of recombinant human erythropoietin therapy after allogeneic hematopoietic stem cell transplantation. *Exp Hematol* 2002; **30**: 546–54.

62 Dimeo FC, Tilmann MH, Bertz H et al. Aerobic exercise in the rehabilitation of cancer patients after high dose chemotherapy and autologous peripheral stem cell transplantation. *Cancer* 1997; **79**: 1717–22.

63 Courneya KS, Keats MR, Turner AR. Physical exercise and quality of life in cancer patients following high dose chemotherapy and autologous bone marrow transplantation. *Psychooncology* 2000; **9**: 127–36.

64 Andrykowski MA, Schmitt FA, Gregg ME et al. Neuropsychologic impairment in adult bone marrow transplant candidates. *Cancer* 1992; **70**: 2288–97.

65 Meyers CA, Weitzner M, Byrne K et al. Evaluation of the neurobehavioral functioning of patients before, during and after bone marrow transplantation. *J Clin Oncol* 1994; **12**: 820–6.

66 Syrjala KL, Dikmen S, Roth-Roemer S et al. Neuropsychological function after marrow or stem cell transplantation: prospective longitudinal results. *Psychooncology* 1998; **7**: 4.

67 Cool VA. Long-term neuropsychological risks in pediatric bone marrow transplant: what do we know? *Bone Marrow Transplant* 1996; **18** (Suppl. 3): S45–9.

68 Phipps S, Dunavant M, Srivastava DK et al. Cognitive and academic functioning in survivors of pediatric bone marrow transplantation. *J Clin Oncol* 2000; **18**: 1004–11.

69 Kramer JH, Crittenden MR, DeSantes K et al. Cognitive and adaptive behavior 1 and 3 years following bone marrow transplantation. *Bone Marrow Transplant* 1997; **19**: 607–13.

70 Simms S, Kazak AE, Gannon T et al. Neuropsychological outcome of children undergoing bone marrow transplantation. *Bone Marrow Transplant* 1998; **22**: 181–4.

71 Wenz F, Steinvorth S, Lohr F et al. Prospective evaluation of delayed central nervous system (CNS) toxicity of hyperfractionated total body irradiation (TBI). *Int J Radiat Oncol Biol Phys* 2000; **48**: 1497–501.

72 Harder H, Cornelissen JJ, Van Gool AR et al. Cognitive functioning and quality of life in long-term adult survivors of bone marrow transplantation. *Cancer* 2002; **95**: 183–92.

73 van Dam FS, Schagen SB, Muller MJ et al. Impairment of cognitive function in women receiving adjuvant treatment for high-risk breast cancer: high-dose versus standard-dose chemotherapy. *J Natl Cancer Inst* 1998; **90**: 210–8.

74 Padovan CS, Yousry TA, Schleuning M et al. Neurological and neuroradiological findings in long-term survivors of allogeneic bone marrow transplantation. *Ann Neurol* 1998; **43**: 627–33.

75 Provenzale JM, Graham ML. Reversible leukoencephalopathy associated with graft-versus-host disease: MR findings. *Am J Neuroradiol* 1996; **17**: 1290–4.

76 Openshaw H, Slatkin NE, Smith E. Eye movement disorders in bone marrow transplant patients on cyclosporin and ganciclovir. *Bone Marrow Transplant* 1997; **19**: 503–5.

77 Shah AK. Cyclosporine A neurotoxicity among bone marrow transplant recipients. *Clin Neuropharmacol* 1999; **22**: 67–73.

78 Curtis RE, Rowlings PA, Deeg HJ et al. Solid cancers after bone marrow transplantation. *N Engl J Med* 1997; **336**: 897–904.

79 Prieto JM, Saez R, Carreras E et al. Physical and psychosocial functioning of 117 survivors of bone marrow transplantation. *Bone Marrow Transplant* 1996; **17**: 1133–42.

80 Zittoun R, Suciu S, Watson M et al. Quality of life in patients with acute myelogenous leukemia in prolonged first complete remission after bone marrow transplantation (allogeneic or autologous) or chemotherapy: a cross-sectional study of the EORTC-GIMEMA AML 8A trial. *Bone Marrow Transplant* 1997; **20**: 307–15.

81 Hjermstad M, Holte H, Evensen S et al. Do patients who are treated with stem cell transplantation have a health-related quality of life comparable to the general population after 1 year? *Bone Marrow Transplant* 1999; **24**: 911–18.

82 Sanders JE, Syrjala KL, Hoffmeister PA et al. Quality of life (QOL) of adult survivors of childhood leukemia treated with chemotherapy (CT) or bone marrow transplant (BMT). *Blood* 2001; **98**: 741a–742a.

83 Badell I, Igual L, Gomez P et al. Quality of life in young adults having received a BMT during childhood: a GETMON study. *Bone Marrow Transplant* 1998; **21** (Suppl. 2): S68–71.

84 Schmidt GM, Niland JC, Forman SJ et al. Extended follow-up in 212 long-term allogeneic bone marrow transplant survivors. *Transplantation* 1990; **50**: 399–406.

85 Heinonen H, Volin L, Uutela A et al. Gender-associated differences in the quality of life after allogeneic BMT. *Bone Marrow Transplant* 2001; **28**: 503–9.

86 Butterworth VA, Simmons RG, Bartsch G et al. Psychosocial effects of unrelated bone marrow

donation: experiences of the National Marrow Donor Program. *Blood* 1993; **81**: 1947–59.

87 Zabora JR, Smith ED, Baker F *et al*. The family: the other side of bone marrow transplantation. *J Psychosoc Oncol* 1992; **10**: 35–46.

88 Foxall MJ, Gaston-Johansson F. Burden and health outcomes of family caregivers of hospitalized bone marrow transplant patients. *J Adv Nurs* 1996; **24**: 915–23.

89 Langer S, Abrams J, Syrjala K. Caregiver and patient marital satisfaction and affect following hematopoietic stem cell transplantation: a prospective, longitudinal investigation. *Psychooncology* 2003; **12**: 239–53.

90 Grimm PM, Zawacki KL, Mock V *et al*. Caregiver responses and needs: an ambulatory bone marrow transplant model. *Cancer Prac* 2000; **8**: 120–8.

91 Summers N, Dawe U, Stewart DA. A comparison of inpatient and outpatient ASCT. *Bone Marrow Transplant* 2000; **26**: 389–95.

92 Manne S, DuHamel K, Nereo N *et al*. Predictors of PTSD in mothers of children undergoing bone marrow transplantation: the role of cognitive and social processes. *J Pediatr Psychol* 2002; **27**: 607–17.

93 Syrjala KL, Cummings C, Donaldson G. Hypnosis or cognitive–behavioral training for the reduction of pain and nausea during cancer treatment: a controlled clinical trial. *Pain* 1992; **48**: 137–46.

94 Syrjala KL, Donaldson GW, Davis MW *et al*. Relaxation and imagery and cognitive–behavioral training reduce pain during cancer treatment: a controlled clinical trial. *Pain* 1995; **63**: 189–98.

95 Gaston-Johansson F, Fall-Dickson J, Nanda J *et al*. The effectiveness of the comprehensive coping strategy program on clinical outcomes in breast cancer autologous bone marrow transplantation. *Cancer Nurs* 2000; **23**: 277–85.

96 Ahles TA, Tope DM, Pinkson B *et al*. Massage therapy for patients undergoing autologous bone marrow transplantation. *J Pain Symptom Manage* 1999; **18**: 157–63.

97 Dimeo F, Fetscher S, Lange W *et al*. Effects of aerobic exercise on the physical performance and incidence of treatment-related complications after high-dose chemotherapy. *Blood* 1997; **90** (9): 3390–4.

98 Dimeo FC, Stieglitz RD, Novelli-Fischer U *et al*. Effects of physical activity on the fatigue and psychologic status of cancer patients during chemotherapy. *Cancer* 1999; **85**: 2273–7.

99 Rexilius SJ, Mundt C, Erickson MM *et al*. Therapeutic effects of massage therapy and handling touch on caregivers of patients undergoing autologous hematopoietic stem cell transplant. *Oncol Nurs Forum* 2002; **29**: E35–44.

100 McQuellon RP, Russell GB, Cella DF *et al*. Quality of life measurement in bone marrow transplantation: development of the Functional Assessment of Cancer Therapy–Bone Marrow Transplant (FACT-BMT). *Bone Marrow Transplant* 1997; **19**: 357–68.

101 Velikova G, Wies J, Sezer O *et al*. Development of an EORTC questionnaire module to be used in health-related QOL assessment for oncology patients receiving myeloablative therapy with blood or marrow transplantation. *Bone Marrow Transplant* 2000; **25**: 78 [Abstract].

102 Ware JE, Snow KK, Kosinski M *et al*. SF-36 Health Survey: Manual and Interpretation Guide. Boston: Health Institute, New England Medical Center, 1997.

103 Holzner B, Kemmler G, Sperner-Unterweger B *et al*. Quality of life measurement in oncology: a matter of the assessment instrument? *Eur J Cancer* 2001; **37**: 2349–56.

104 Kemmler G, Holzner B, Kopp M *et al*. Comparison of two quality-of-life instruments for cancer patients: the functional assessment of cancer therapy-general and the European Organization for Research and Treatment of Cancer Quality of Life Questionnaire–C30. *J Clin Oncol* 1999; **17**: 2932–40.

105 Bergner M, Bobbitt RA, Carter WB *et al*. The Sickness Impact Profile: development and final revision of health status measure. *Med Care* 1981; **19**: 787–805.

106 Schag CA, Ganz PA, Heinrich RL. Cancer Rehabilitation Evaluation System–Short Form (CARES-SF). a cancer specific rehabilitation and quality of life instrument. *Cancer* 1991; **68**: 1406–13.

107 Schipper H, Clinch J, McMurrary A *et al*. Measuring the quality of life in cancer patients. the Functional Living Index–Cancer: development and validation. *J Clin Oncol* 1984; **2**: 472–83.

108 Kemmler G, Holzner B, Kopp M *et al*. Comparison of two quality-of-life instruments for cancer patients: the functional assessment of cancer therapy-general and the European Organization for Research and Treatment of Cancer Quality of Life Questionnaire–C30. *J Clin Oncol* 1999; **17**: 2932–40.

109 Sprangers, MA, Aaronson, NK. The role of health care providers and significant others in evaluating the quality of life of patients with chronic disease: a review. *J Clin Epidemiol* 1992; **45**: 743–60.

110 Varni JW, Seid M, Kurtin PS. PedsQL 4.0: reliability and validity of the pediatric quality of life inventory version 4.0 generic core scales in healthy and patient populations. *Med Care* 2001: **39** (8): 800–12.

111 Seid M, Varni JW, Rode CA *et al*. The Pediatric Cancer Quality of Life Inventory: a modular approach to measuring health-related quality of life in children with cancer. *Int J Cancer Suppl* 1999; **12**: 71–6.

112 Boyes A, Newell S, Girgis A. Rapid assessment of psychosocial well-being: are computers the way forward in a clinical setting? *Qual Life Res* 2002; **11**: 27–35.

113 Ryan JM, Corry JR, Attewell R *et al*. A comparison of an electronic version of the SF-36 General Health Questionnaire to the standard paper version. *Qual Life Res* 2002; **11**: 19–26.

114 Velikova G, Wright EP, Smith AB *et al*. Automated collection of quality-of-life data: a comparison of paper and computer touchscreen questionnaires. *J Clin Oncol* 1999; **17**: 998–1007.

115 Wilkie DJ, Huang HY, Berry DL *et al*. Cancer symptom control: feasibility of a tailored, interactive computerized program for patients. *Fam Community Health* 2001; **24**: 48–62.

116 Cleeland CS, Mendoza TR, Wang XS *et al*. Assessing symptom distress in cancer patients: the M.D. Anderson Symptom Inventory. *Cancer* 2000; **89**: 1634–46.

117 Cella D, Hahn EA, Dineen K. Meaningful change in cancer-specific quality of life scores: differences between improvement and worsening. *Qual Life Res* 2002; **11**: 207–21.

118 Wyrwich KW, Tierney WM, Wolinsky FD. Further evidence supporting a SEM-based criterion for identifying meaningful intra-individual changes in health-related quality of life. *J Clin Epidemiol* 1999; **52**: 861–73.

40

D. Kathryn Tierney

Sexuality after Hematopoietic Cell Transplantation

Introduction

Exciting advances have occurred in the field of hematopoietic cell transplantation (HCT) and the brisk pace of change continues with the acquisition of new knowledge in the fields of hematopoiesis, immunology, cancer cell biology, pharmacology and other related areas. HCT is a curative approach for a variety of malignant and nonmalignant disorders. Recipients of this aggressive treatment modality are susceptible to numerous short-term and long-term toxicities that insult the physical, psychological and social well-being of survivors. In order to appraise the overall value of HCT it is important to measure not only the traditional outcome variables such as overall survival, disease-free survival, morbidity, mortality and cost, but also quality of life (QOL).

While QOL research is hampered by a number of issues such as lack of a consensual definition, measurement difficulties and methodological challenges, many investigators have begun to explore dimensions of QOL in HCT recipients. During the 1990s many studies were conducted that identified variables that both positively and negatively impact recovery and QOL following HCT. One aspect of QOL profoundly affected by HCT is sexuality.

This chapter will begin by defining sexuality and QOL and by providing a conceptual model clarifying the relationship between sexuality and QOL. A review of the physiologic, psychological and social variables impacting the sexual response cycle will be provided. The incidence of identified problems of sexuality for HCT recipients will be reviewed and finally, assessment and intervention strategies for addressing disorders of the sexual response cycle will be addressed.

Sexuality and the sexual response cycle

The integration of somatic, emotional, intellectual and social aspects of sexual beings in ways that enrich and enhance personality, communication and love is the definition of sexual health provided by the World Health Organization [1]. Sexuality includes the feelings one has about oneself as a sexual being and the way these feelings are expressed. The developmental stage of the individual and cultural norms will influence the expression of sexuality [2]. Cultural norms define what is considered normal sexual expression. Spiritually, sexuality is an integration of mind and body and is a vehicle for experiencing and expressing emotions. An individual's sexuality is often expressed in the context of a bond formed with another individual. Sexuality includes various aspects of intimacy such as fantasy and masturbation as well as hugging, touching, kissing and the various expressions of sexual intercourse.

Issues of sexuality and sexual functioning following treatment for a life-threatening malignancy are complex. Sexual dysfunction in transplant recipients results from physiologic, psychological and social variables, and the complex interactions among these variables.

The sexual response cycle is divided into four phases: desire, arousal, orgasm and resolution [3]. Desire includes sexual fantasy and thoughts and is strongly linked to arousal [4]. Desire is a complex and poorly understood phenomenon encompassing biologic, behavioral and cognitive components [2,4]. Arousal includes the subjective experience of excitement and pleasure and associated physiologic changes. In men, the arousal phase involves a complex integration of neurovascular and cellular physiologic changes leading to an erection [5,6]. Vaginal lubrication and swelling secondary to vasocongestion occur during the arousal phase in women [4]. Orgasm is a period of intense sexual pleasure and is accompanied by the release of sexual tension and rhythmic muscular contractions of the perineal tissues and reproductive organs. Emission and ejaculation are the two phases of orgasm in men. Relaxation is noted in the final phase of the sexual response cycle, resolution.

Quality of life (QOL)

QOL has been defined in many ways. There is no consensual definition of QOL, but it is generally agreed that QOL is a multidimensional construct that defines an individual's assessment of well-being. A number of domains are included when defining and evaluating this abstract construct. These dimensions include physical health, morbidity associated with illness or treatment, functional status, role functioning, life satisfaction, treatment satisfaction, social well-being, spirituality and psychological well-being [7–10]. QOL is a construct that encompasses the individual's physical, psychological and social response to illness and treatment and the extent to which changes in these areas affect the individual's level of satisfaction and sense of self-worth [11]. A modification of the definition of health by the World Health Organization provides a working definition of QOL, which would read: QOL is a state of complete physical, mental and social well-being in the absence of or successful adaptation to health problems [12]. Broadly speaking, health problems would refer to physical, psychological or social morbidity following illness or treatment. QOL is a subjective phenomenon with differences from individual to individual and even within the same individual over time.

Figure 40.1a is a model that includes the physical, psychological, social and spiritual domains of QOL and highlights the dynamic interplay between these dimensions [13]. This same figure can be modified (Fig. 40.1b [13]) to show the interactions between physical, psychological, social and spiritual aspects of sexuality. The inclusion of both subjective

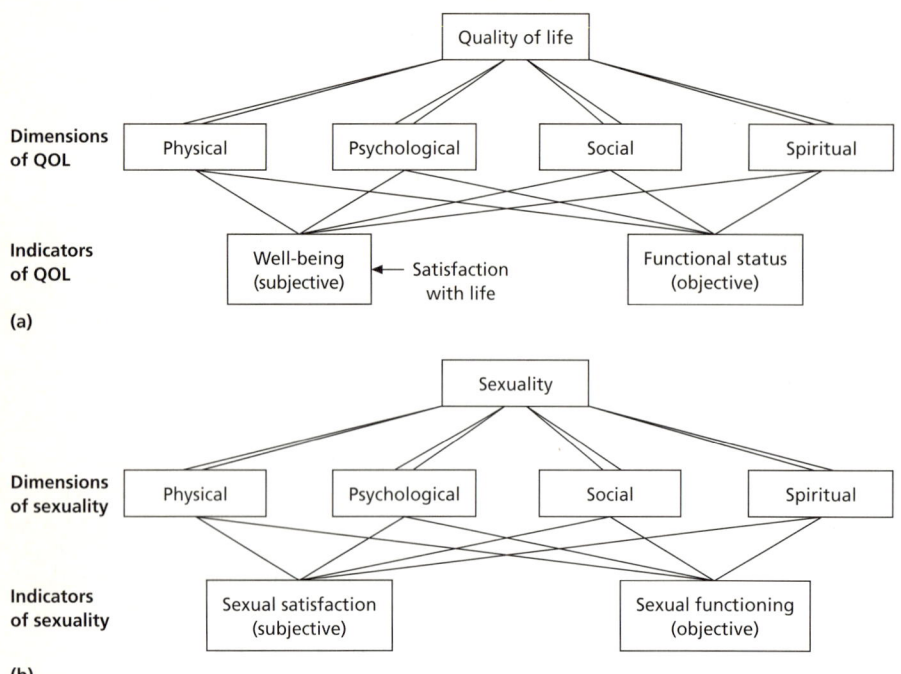

Fig. 40.1 (a) Well-being and functional status as subjective and objective components of quality of life (QOL). (b) Dimensions of sexuality with objective and subjective indicators. Modified and reproduced with permission from Haas [13] with permission of the author and Sigma Theta Tau, publisher.

and objective indicators of QOL and sexuality and the emphasis on the dynamic interplay between these dimensions are strengths of the models. The model in Fig. 40.1b will be used later in the chapter as a framework for assessing sexual dysfunction and satisfaction.

Significance of changes in sexuality and the impact on QOL in HCT recipients

The diagnosis of cancer, the underlying malignancy, therapy antecedent to transplantation, the preparatory regimen used, the complications of HCT and the treatment of complications may lead to disruption in feelings of sexuality and the sexual response cycle leading to sexual dissatisfaction or dysfunction. One QOL study of long-term cancer patients found that two variables, family distress and sexuality, exerted the most negative effect on measures of social well-being [14]. In a recent study asking cancer patients to rank the severity of side-effects from chemotherapy treatment, loss of sexual feeling ranked sixth in severity following affects on my family or partner, loss of hair, feeling constantly tired, affects on my work/home duties and affects on my social activities, respectively [15]. Sexual dysfunction and dissatisfaction are regularly cited as negatively impacting QOL in HCT recipients [16–19]. Decreased libido, infertility, erectile and ejaculatory dysfunction and premature menopause can all contribute to sexual difficulties [20–22]. Additionally, body image, psychological well-being and social relationships are impacted by transplant and may contribute to sexual dissatisfaction or dysfunction after HCT.

The incidence of sexual dissatisfaction or dysfunction following transplantation is pervasive. Anderson reports the incidence of sexual dysfunction in cancer patients is estimated to be as high as 90% [23] and sexual dysfunction following HCT ranges from 22% to 70% [24,25]. Fifty-five percent of allogeneic patients and 42% of autologous patients reported that their sex life was worse following treatment [26]. Table 40.1 [16–19, 27–32] is a review of QOL studies that have identified one or more aspects of sexuality as a variable adversely influencing QOL. For some transplant recipients sexual dissatisfaction may be pervasive for years [17,33,34].

Physical, psychological and social variables impacting the sexual health of HCT recipients

Physiologic and biologic changes in males

A number of biologic and physiologic changes affecting the gonads and hypothalamic–pituitary–gonad axis occur in men following HCT. Physiologic alterations include neurovascular damage, erectile dysfunction, dry ejaculation and infertility. These alterations may disrupt one or more phases of the sexual response cycle and adversely affect sexual functioning and satisfaction.

Figure 40.2 [35] demonstrates the relationships within the hypothalamic–pituitary–gonad axis. Control of this axis begins with the secretion of gonadotropin-releasing hormone (GnRH) from the hypothalamus into circulation. The GnRH in turn stimulates the pituitary to release the gonadotropins, follicle-stimulating hormone (FSH) and lutenizing hormone (LH). FSH and LH control gonadal function resulting in production of gametes and the synthesis of sex steroids. The Leydig cells in the testicles start androgen synthesis and secretion under the influence of LH. Spermatogenesis is maintained by testosterone but initiated by FSH [36]. Negative feedback to the hypothalamus and pituitary occurs when testosterone and inhibin levels rise inhibiting the secretion of GnRH and the gonadotropins [35]. Damage to the gonads from the preparatory regimen leads to a loss or reduction in the secretion of sex steroids leading to an absence of negative feedback to the hypothalamus and pituitary. Thus levels of FSH and LH rise, which is the hallmark of gonadal failure [36].

Damage to the gonads and disruption of endocrine function in men results in infertility and the potential for changes in sexual functioning. The degree of damage will depend on age, the dose of radiation and chemotherapy and the type of chemotherapy administered [36,37]. Alkylating chemotherapeutic agents are often utilized in transplantation and are strongly linked to infertility [38]. With both radiation and chemotherapy, there is a dose-dependent depletion of the germinal epithelium lining the seminiferous tubule of the testes and this depletion results in azoospermia, testicular atrophy and infertility [37,39]. Features of germinal cell depletion consist of small testicular size, 3.7 cm long × 2.3 cm wide (normal being 5.0 cm × 3.0 cm) and reduced testicular volume

Table 40.1 Quality-of-life (QOL) studies identifying negative impact on sexuality.

Article [ref.]	Factors negatively impacting recovery and QOL	Factors positively impacting recovery and QOL	Findings related to sexual activity
2-year adjustment of BMT survivors [27]			14 subjects representing over half of the sample noted changes for the worse in sexual functioning
Physical and psychosocial status of adults 1-year after BMT: a prospective study [28]	Older age at the time of transplant was a consistent predicator of declines in both physical and psychological status. Males had a greater decline in functional status and an increase in illness related dysfunction compared to women		Sexual relationships were significantly worse 1-year post-transplant compared to pretransplant assessment
QOL of BMT long-term survivors [16]	Older age was associated with less life satisfaction	Higher self-esteem and family support associated with improved QOL indicators	Overall relatively dissatisfied with sex life
QOL of 125 adults surviving 6–18 years after BMT [17]	Decreasing support over time was noted as a distressing hardship of long-term survival Greater age at the time of transplant was associated with decreased QOL measures post-transplant		27% report dissatisfaction with appearance. Dissatisfaction with sexual appeal, ability to share warmth and intimacy or interest in sexual thoughts or feelings was reported by 26–36% 32% of females indicated physical problems that led to decreased sexual satisfaction and intimacy
Dynamic assessment of QOL after autologous BMT [7]		Individuals working reported better QOL than those not working or working part time	36% reported less satisfying sexual activity compared to pretransplant
QOL and psychological distress of BMT recipients: the "time trajectory" to recovery over the 1st year [29]	Patients with depressive symptoms reported lower QOL scores	Patients with higher performance scores at 1 year had higher QOL scores	Over the course of the 1st year, 35% of patients reported increasing concern over intimate relations
QOL in breast cancer patients before and after autologous BMT [30]	Study showed general improvement in mood and physical functioning post-transplant compared to pretransplant, but did not correlate any variables that specifically impacted recovery or QOL		33% reported concerns with personal or intimate physical relations
Comparison of the overall QOL in 50 long-term survivors of autologous and allogeneic BMT [21]	Predictors of lower QOL scores included the presence of physical symptoms, vocational adjustment and depression		35% of autologous recipients and 20% of allogeneic recipients reported decreased sexual interest
QOL in long-term survivors of marrow transplantation Comparison with a matched group receiving maintenance chemotherapy [31]	Depression negatively impacted overall QOL	Social support positively impacted QOL	45% of men and 33% of women reported a deterioration in their sexual life post-transplant
Physical and psychosocial functioning of 117 survivors of BMT [18]	Women reported worse QOL, higher psychiatric morbidity and a higher percentage of medical problems than men	Patients transplanted at a younger age have a better QOL and decreased psychosocial distress Employed individuals had increased QOL and less psychosocial distress compared to those not working	25% of women reported menopausal symptoms and 20% of men reported impotence 23% of men and 41% of females reported health problems related to sex life
Extended follow-up in 212 long-term allogeneic BMT survivors [19]	Poorer QOL ratings were associated with regular medication use and sexual dissatisfaction		31% reported decreased sexual satisfaction from pretransplant
QOL following BMT: a comparison of patient reports with population norms [32]	Factors that negatively impacted health-related QOL included <3 years from transplant, older age, presence of acute GVHD and greater disparity in donor match	Individuals >3-years post-transplant reported better QOL	68% satisfied, 12% neutral and 20% not satisfied with ability to attain sexual satisfaction

BMT, bone marrow transplantation; GVHD, graft-vs.-host disease.

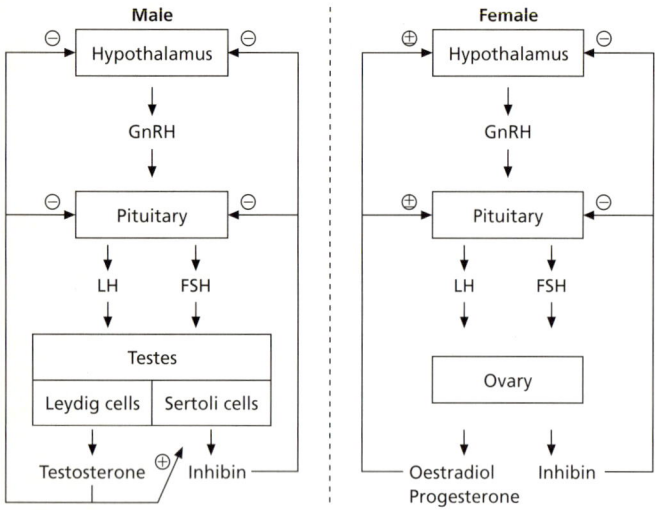

Fig. 40.2 Hypothalamic–pituitary–gonadal axis. Reproduced with permission from Brook and Marshall [35].

8–15 cc (normal is 16–30 cc) [37]. Endocrine values in men with germinal cell depletion follow (with normal values given in parentheses): FSH 25–90 mIU/mL (4–25 mIU/mL), LH 8–25 mIU/mL (4–20 mIU/mL), testosterone 200–700 ng/100 mL (250–1200 ng/mL), testosterone production rate 3.5 mg/day (7.5 mg/day) and free testosterone 8.6 ng/100 mL (15.3 ng/100 mL) [37].

Leydig cells are relatively resistant to the effects of chemotherapy and radiation and as a result testosterone levels generally remain within the normal range [40]. However, more extensive hormonal testing indicates that there may be subtle damage to the Leydig cells evidenced by a reduction in the amount of testosterone produced and a decrease in the levels of circulating free testosterone [41]. Additionally, an increased incidence of testosterone insufficiency in men over the age of 45 has been reported [42]. A low response to GnRH has been seen in some patients indicating potential damage at the hypothalamic-pituitary level [39]. Elevated prolactin levels have been observed in some men following HCT and suggest damage to the hypothalamus [39,40]. The exact role of prolactin is not entirely clear but hyperprolactinemia has been associated with infertility, erectile dysfunction and decreased libido [4,43]. Some studies indicate subclinical hypothyroidism secondary to radiation damage to the thyroid [39,40].

In men, the arousal phase may be disrupted due to neurovascular damage secondary to the preparatory regimen. Chemotherapeutic agents that cause peripheral neuropathies may also cause erectile problems and diminish the intensity of orgasm [44]. Radiation results in neurovascular damage leading to difficulty with erections in some men [45]. Radiation can potentiate hardening or narrowing of the pelvic arteries contributing further to the potential for erectile dysfunction. Vascular problems secondary to smoking, hyperlipidemia, diabetes and the use of cyclosporine are additional risk factors for erectile dysfunction. In some men, radiation may result in an inability to achieve orgasm or decrease the intensity of orgasm. Fatigue and decreased physical stamina are common following HCT and may further contribute to erectile dysfunction and difficulty achieving orgasm [2,45].

Physiologic and biologic changes in females

A number of biologic and physiologic changes affecting the gonads, the hypothalamic–pituitary–gonad axis and estrogen-dependent tissues occur in women following HCT. Alterations include amenorrhea, vaginal alterations secondary to radiation and chemotherapy and chronic graft-vs.-host disease (GVHD) of the vagina. These alterations may disrupt one or more phases of the sexual response cycle and adversely influence sexual functioning, satisfaction and QOL.

Again the reader is referred to Fig. 40.2 demonstrating the function of the hypothalamic–pituitary–gonad axis. As in men, control of this axis is initiated with the release of GnRH from the hypothalamus leading to the secretion of FSH and LH from the pituitary. In women, FSH initiates growth and maturation of the ovarian follicles and LH controls ovulation and corpus luteum formation [36]. The negative feedback from the rise in estrogen causes a decrease in the release of GnRH from the hypothalamus and decrease in the secretion of FSH and LH from the pituitary. Both radiation and high-dose chemotherapy damage ovarian tissue leading to decreased secretion of sex steroids and thus a loss of the negative feedback inhibition at the level of the hypothalamus and pituitary. The result is the characteristic finding of elevated levels of FSH and LH indicative of infertility and menopause [36].

Alkylating agents and radiation therapy have cytotoxic effects on both dividing and resting ovarian cells. The sensitivity of the ovary to radiation and chemotherapy is dependent upon the dose administered, the site of radiation, the type of chemotherapy agent and the age of the female, with women over the age of 25 being more susceptible to ovarian failure [37,46]. A single high dose of total body irradiation produces ovarian failure in all women [36]. Alkylating agents such as cyclophosphamide, nitrosoureas or melphan are particularly toxic to ovarian tissue, especially in the doses employed in HCT. Decreased levels of estradiol and elevated levels of FSH and LH are indicative of infertility and premature menopause [40,46]. The majority of female HCT recipients will have elevated FSH and LH and low levels of estradiol. A small number of women tested had evidence of abnormal androgen function [39].

Fatigue has been noted as a common problem following HCT and can negatively influence the desire, arousal and orgasm phase of the sexual response cycle.

In physiologic (natural) menopause the symptoms of estrogen deficiency develop gradually over the peri-menopausal and post-menopausal years. In contrast, in HCT recipients these changes occur within 6 months of ovarian failure and are more severe due to the abrupt withdrawal of estrogen [25,47]. Premature menopause leads to symptoms of estrogen deficiency resulting in hot flashes, night sweats, insomnia, mood swings, irritability, depression, vaginal dryness, vaginal atrophy and fibrosis, pruritus, urogenital symptoms, changes in cognitive function and changes in appearance [48–50].

Several studies describe the incidence of menopausal symptoms in females post-transplant. One study of 15 women following transplant found that 53% developed hot flashes, 40% noted decreased libido, 53% experienced painful intercourse, 33% described mood changes, 40% suffered from insomnia, 25% described urogenital symptoms and 73% of participates in this study reported depression [51]. Of note, only 10% of patients had resumed sexual activity during the first 3 months post-transplant. A valuable contribution of this study is that the 15 women evaluated were menopausal before transplant and findings revealed that the ovaries suffered additional insults as measured by hormone levels and ultrasound studies following the preparative regimen.

Menopausal symptoms were assessed in a sample of 37 women who were a minimum of 1-year post-transplant [25]. Specifically, hot flashes were reported by 83% and dyspareunia, vaginal dryness and dysuria were described by 76%. Dyspareunia was the most distressing symptom reported and associated with sexual difficulties in 70% of these women.

A third study on the incidence of menopausal symptoms in post-transplant females indicates that, of the 44 women evaluated, 67% of those receiving total body irradiation and chemotherapy and 38% of those receiving chemotherapy without radiation experienced vasomotor symptoms (hot flashes, night sweats, insomnia and irritability) [22]. Of the 30 women in this group who had resumed sexual activity 77% noted vaginal dryness, 53% described decreased libido and 60% experienced dyspareunia. Eighty percent of this sample of 44 women had gynecologic abnormalities following allogeneic HCT, which included tissue atrophy, loss of pubic hair, pale mucous membranes, small uterus and cervical size, introital stenosis and atrophic vulvovaginitis. Finally, a study of 79 female recipients of allogeneic transplant found that 78% experienced hot flashes and 94% of the sexually active women reported difficulties with intercourse [47].

Infrequent and mild hot flashes were reported within the first few months following transplant, but 6 months later 78% of women complained of hot flashes, which were often severe [47]. The pathophysiology of hot flashes is not entirely understood, but believed to be secondary to vasomotor instability. Hot flashes begin with a decrease in estrogen output from the ovaries, the more gradual the drop the less severe the symptoms. Hot flashes are uncomfortable feelings of extreme heat that come on unexpectedly. The face, chest or entire body becomes warm and flushed. Hot flashes may last up to 5 min and skin temperature may rise measurably (2–3°C).

Premature menopause may affect the desire, arousal or orgasm phase of the sexual response cycle. Loss of or decreased desire is often cited as a consequence of menopause and as stated earlier is a complex and poorly understood phenomenon. The role of hormones in regulating sex drive in females is debated [4,52]. Libido may or may not be significantly influenced by the loss of hormone production from the ovary [53]. Loss of desire may occur as a secondary reaction to dyspareunia.

Vaginal alterations occur earlier and are more severe in HCT recipients than during physiologic menopause due to a combination of insults that include the preparative regimen, the abruptness of the estrogen loss and vaginal chronic GVHD [22,47,54]. Vaginal changes include dryness, narrowing, fibrosis and atrophy as well as an increased susceptibility to infection [47]. After menopause when estrogen levels are low, swelling and lubrication of the vagina take place slowly. Even when aroused the vagina may remain narrow and dry leading to dyspareunia. Radiation may contribute to vaginal stenosis and narrowing [45]. The majority of women have vaginal atrophy post-transplant and nearly all will experience dyspareunia [47].

The incidence of vaginal GVHD is not known. Biopsy of tissue is helpful in the evaluation of GVHD, but generally the diagnosis of GVHD is based on physical findings and subjective symptoms. Epithelial cell damage, mononuclear cell inflammatory infiltration, fibrosis and atrophy are histological features of chronic GVHD [55]. Additional features of chronic vaginal GVHD include inflammation, stricture formation and narrowing [56]. Arousal and orgasm dysfunction has been reported in women with extensive chronic GVHD [34]. These vaginal alterations may interfere with gynecologic examinations and the ability of the woman to monitor her long-term health care needs appropriately.

Urogenital changes associated with menopause include atrophy of the urethra and bladder with the associated symptoms of dysuria, urinary frequency, incontinence and cystitis [53,54]. Additionally, chronic GVHD of the bladder has been reported and presents as severe cystitis [57].

Women who undergo HCT are generally young (<50 years) and will spend a significantly longer period of time in menopause. A 30-year-old female who undergoes transplantation for a diagnosis of acute leukemia will spend an additional 20 years in menopause (with the average age of menopause being 50 years) and thus have an additional 20 years of risk of menopause-related health problems. The increased period of time spent in an estrogen deficient state may increase the risks of osteoporosis and heart disease.

Psychosocial variables affecting sexuality in both genders

Psychological factors that may disrupt the sexual response cycle in HCT recipients include changes in body image, depression, decreased self-confidence, anxiety, concurrent life stresses, somatization, fear of recurrence, anger, despair and infertility [2,26,33]. Body image scores were significantly lower in HCT recipients of both genders compared to a healthy sample [33]. Infertility in women may negatively impact their sense of femininity and self-esteem and in men infertility may be associated with decreased feelings of masculinity and lead to decreased self-confidence [44]. Findings of one study demonstrated that higher global psychological distress was correlated with less sexual satisfaction, poorer body image and increased disruption in sexual relationships [32]. In men, higher levels of psychological distress pretransplant were significantly predictive for sexual dissatisfaction at 3-years post-transplant [34].

Infertility may lead to discordance in existing relationships, difficulty establishing intimate relationships, and decreased self-esteem and confidence [33,42,58]. Younger age in one study accounted for most of the concern related to infertility [26] and a second study showed that infertility was a common concern among younger, unmarried and nulliparous women [58]. Psychological distress, especially depression and anxiety, can alter the desire, arousal and orgasm phase of the sexual response cycle [2,59]. Additionally, individuals with rigid views of sexuality, a narrow range of sexual behavior and those with pessimistic attitudes towards the future are at higher risk for sexual problems [23,24].

Social variables impacting sexual health in both genders

Social variables also contribute to sexual dissatisfaction in transplant recipients. In regards to sexuality, the most important social relationship is that of the intimate partner. Factors influencing this relationship include partner uncertainty and anxiety, role shifting within the couple during treatment and difficulty communicating [59–61]. The transplant course is often complicated, uncertain and lengthy. A caregiver is required and assumes a large burden of care for the recovering transplant recipient. Often this caregiver is the sexual partner. Role changes and the impact they have on sexual relationships are not yet understood. The forced absence of sexual intimacy due to lengthy treatments and hospitalization may leave some couples uncertain as to how to reestablish sexual relations [59]. If upon resuming sexual activity the couple encounters problems both may withdraw from further contact and silence envelops these sensitive issues [2]. Furthermore, the partner may develop sexual dysfunction secondary to anxiety and depression.

Social support has been cited by several investigators as an important variable in the psychosocial adjustment of patients following HCT [16,17,62]. Social support has been found to facilitate healthy adjustment following HCT, with strong family relationships predictive of better psychosocial adjustment [63]. Other investigators have noted that social support for HCT recipients dwindled over time and decreased social support adversely influenced psychosocial coping [17]. Younger patients and single individuals are at high risk for sexual dysfunction because cancer and its treatment can complicate the development of new relationships and subsequent intimacy [2,61,64].

Assessment and interventions for improving sexual health in HCT recipients

While sexuality is a much broader concept than the sexual response cycle, the sexual response cycle remains a standardized means of assessing and diagnosing sexual dysfunction. The *Diagnostic and Statistical Manual of Mental Disorders* collectively describes sexual dysfunction as a group of disorders that may affect one or more phases of the sexual response cycle [65]. These disorders are characterized by physiologic or psychological changes that adversely influence sexual functioning leading to psychological distress or stress within relationships. Diagnoses for disorders of the sexual response cycle include hypoactive sexual desire disorder, female sexual arousal disorder, male erectile disorder, orgasmic disorders and sexual pain disorders including dyspareunia and vaginismus [65]. In making the diagnosis of a sexual disorder, considerations include the onset of the symptoms, the situational context, the frequency of occurrence and the psychological and physiologic conditions that may be contributory.

One barrier to assessing sexuality is reluctance on the part of many health care professionals to discuss sensitive issues. Reasons cited for this reluctance include health care providers feeling embarrassed, concerns about embarrassing the patient, lack of education regarding sexuality, feeling inadequately trained to address issues of sexuality and believing it is not relevant to their practice [66]. Increasing one's awareness of the types of sexual problems experienced in the population served, gaining experience in assessing sexual dysfunction and acquiring knowledge of interventions that can be utilized to address issues of sexuality are strategies that health care providers can utilize to overcome this reluctance [67]. Additionally, clinicians can identify available resources and make referrals as needed.

A number of health care professionals have an opportunity in the pretransplant period to address issues of sexuality. An essential element of informed consent for HCT recipients is revealing the risk of infertility. At this point in time potential changes in sexual functioning can be disclosed. Simply informing patients that decreased libido in the first 3–6 months post-transplant is common will pave the way to discussing issues of sexuality in the post-transplant setting. The health care providers who have identified sexual concerns with HCT candidates in the pretransplant period have identified themselves as a resource for patients during recovery and have validated that sexuality is a legitimate area of concern. Additionally, data have shown that the greater the disparity between expectations and outcomes the higher the degree of psychological distress [68]. This discrepancy between expectations and outcomes suggests that one intervention for improving post-transplant sexual functioning and QOL is preparing individuals for changes that will occur in sexual functioning, thereby closing the gap between expectations and realities. Ideally, this discussion of sexuality prior to transplantation includes the sexual partner. Inclusion of the sexual partner facilitates a discussion between the couple, may identify the partner's anxieties and enlists the partner's support for coping with changes. It has been shown that individuals have a remarkable capacity to adapt to changes and reestablish norms [69]. Enabling individuals and their partners to establish realistic expectations of changes in sexual functioning following transplantation will allow them to maximize their ability to adapt to these changes.

Perhaps the simplest way of beginning an assessment of sexuality is asking patients if they have resumed sexual activity. One report demonstrated that by asking two specific questions during an office visit; "Are you sexually active?" and "Are you having any sexual difficulties or problems at this time?" the number of sexual concerns revealed increased from 3% who spontaneously disclosed concerns to 16% [70]. Findings from one study indicated that discussions with a health care provider immediately after transplant would have been helpful as a means of dealing with changes in sexual functioning [58].

Isolating the various biologic, physiologic, psychological and social factors is a useful way to improve the understanding of sexual dissatisfaction and dysfunction, however, these variables are interrelated in very complex ways and it is unlikely that sexual problems will be isolated to one of these domains exclusively. Consequently, an assessment of sexuality will require an assessment of each of these dimensions. Figure 40.1b is a schematic representation of the complex and interactive relationships between physical, psychological, social and spiritual aspects of sexuality and its expression.

In using the model in Fig. 40.1b, assessment of the physical dimensions of sexuality could include hormonal testing, pelvic exams, tests of erectile function, fatigue, medications and other health problems, such as hyperlipidemia, hypertension, anemia and chronic GVHD. In assessing the psychological dimensions of sexuality depression, anxiety, self-esteem, body image changes and emotional response to infertility need to be considered. Interpersonal relationships, particularly intimate relationships, need to be examined for stress and discordance of expectations as well as adequacy of communication regarding issues of sexuality. Partner anxiety, depression and uncertainty must also be assessed. As an assessment guide Fig. 40.1b is useful in that both objective indicators of sexual functioning and the subjective experience of sexual satisfaction are included in the overall assessment of sexuality. Figure 40.1b may also guide the clinician in selecting intervention strategies. If the problem lies principally in the physical dimension, the interventions will be different than if the problem lies within the dynamics of the relationship.

Addressing infertility and its emotional impact for those who have not yet completed their childbearing requires a sensitive health care provider knowledgeable of currently available reproductive techniques for assisting couples to maintain fertility. A discussion of reproductive technologies is beyond the scope of this chapter; however, keeping abreast of recent advances in order to counsel individuals in the pretransplant period is essential. A lack of disclosure of options to maintain fertility constitutes a breech of the informed consent process, although it is recognized that much of this burden rests with the referring oncologist as most patients have already received therapy that may have affected fertility prior to arriving at the transplant center.

Hypoactive sexual desire disorder

Of all phases of the sexual response cycle, desire is the least well understood and the most difficult aspect to treat. Desire is strongly linked to sexual arousal, the second phase of the sexual response cycle. Many studies have demonstrated that decreased desire and arousal are common problems in the post-transplant setting. Decreased libido in female HCT recipients has been reported to be 40–53% [22,51]. Twenty percent of male HCT recipients report depressed libido and arousal problems in one report [34] and a second study reported decreased libido in 38% of male HCT recipients [43]. Pretransplant assessment of a group of men and women indicated that 56% indicated overall sexual dissatisfaction and this finding was not statistically different in post-transplant assessments suggesting that many problems of sexuality predate HCT [71]. Significant negative correlations were found for both genders between sexual interest and arousal difficulty and between arousal difficulties and sexual satisfaction [34].

The dynamic relationships between the phases of the sexual response cycle cannot be over emphasized. For example, decreased libido in men may be a reaction to erectile dysfunction. Similarly, if a woman experiences dyspareunia, she may rapidly loose desire. If decreased libido is a result of other disruptions of the sexual response cycle, specific interventions aimed at those disruptions must be initiated.

In many cases, the discussion of sexual difficulties with the HCT recipient and partner can be therapeutic. The information, reassurance and opportunity to explore sexual issues with the health care provider can often effectively address many areas of concern [72].

Key variables to assess in relationship to hypoactive sexual desire are depression and anxiety. Depression and anxiety will decrease sexual desire in both men and women. Referral to a mental health professional may be needed. Additionally, antidepressant therapy can be useful. Support groups can be a valuable resource for couples during recovery and in the process of reintegrating into "normal" life. A visit to any HCT Internet chat room will reveal that issues of sexuality are frequently discussed.

The American Cancer Society also provides two well-written books for cancer survivors on sexuality entitled *Sexuality and Cancer* [73]. There is one version for women and one for men.

Much of the current literature on the treatment of sexual dysfunction is not directed to the assessment and treatment of sexual difficulties that arise following the diagnosis and treatment of cancer and therefore there are few, if any, resources specific to the treatment of sexual dysfunction following HCT. The reader should keep this in mind when exploring interventions for sexual dysfunction in HCT recipients.

Treatment of sexual dysfunction in women

Female sexual arousal disorder and sexual pain disorder—dyspareunia

Hormone replacement therapy (HRT) can decrease or improve many of the common symptoms associated with menopause. HRT is effective in relieving hot flashes, improving sleep if sleep is disturbed due to hot flashes, maintaining vaginal elasticity and lubrication and decreasing changes in the appearance of the skin and changes in breast size. One study found that symptoms of estrogen deficiency were eliminated in 22 of 27 women [58]. HRT alone, however, may not improve sexual satisfaction [24].

There are many gaps in knowledge relating to the use HRT in the treatment of premature menopause. There are several studies that suggest that currently prescribed HRT may not be adequate for HCT recipients [24,39,58]. The evidence for questioning the adequacy of currently prescribed HRT is the findings of low estradiol levels despite HRT, the large number of women receiving HRT not having menstrual cycles and the degree of vaginal dryness found despite HRT. Data from one study revealed that at 3-years post-transplant, 76% of the women were taking HRT yet 52% cited lubrication and arousal problems, 33% had pain with sexual intercourse and 46% experienced difficulties with orgasm [34].

The appropriate time to begin HRT is unclear. Closer evaluation and monitoring of the efficacy of HRT therapy in women with treatment induced premature menopause is required. There are currently no data available on how well HRT protects these women from the long-term problems of osteoporosis and cardiovascular disease given the longer period of risk. Although HRT has long been a subject of debate and controversy, recent findings have seriously questioned the risk/benefit balance of HRT in women who have transitioned through physiologic "natural" menopause. There remain many unanswered questions regarding the role of HRT in those women who are prematurely menopausal as a result of cancer therapies. After all, these women would still be exposed to endogenous estrogen had they not been treated for a malignancy and prematurely suffered ovarian failure. Given the fact that there are currently more questions than answers regarding the use of HRT, the prudent course of action is to refer female HCT recipients to a gynecologist for a thorough evaluation and individualized approach to HRT. This individualized approach must encompass a broad assessment of factors that may increase the risks or benefits associated with HRT. These factors include family history of cardiovascular disease, family history of cancer, genetic markers, hypertension, and hyperlipidemia and well as life style issues such as the amount of daily exercise, obesity, diet and smoking history.

Demographic, medical and psychological factors will influence the choices a woman makes post-transplant regarding the use of HRT. Those women who receive transplants for a hormonally dependent tumor (such as breast cancer) and are currently advised to avoid HRT will need to explore other interventions to relieve menopausal symptoms. Alternative strategies are available but the efficacy of alternative approaches in ameliorating the problems impacting sexuality and the long-term health risks of osteoporosis and heart disease is not clear.

The use of herbs, vitamins, yoga, acupressure, acupuncture, exercise and diet modifications are interventions that have been suggested, but few of these interventions have been rigorously tested. Nevertheless, resources are available to women for the management of menopausal symptoms. Several that have been well received by female HCT recipients include *The Estrogen Decision* [74] and *Natural Menopause* [75]. These books provide information of the role of HRT and alternative strategies in alleviating symptoms of menopause. Nonhormonal strategies for managing menopausal symptoms will require a consistent commitment by the woman to maximize potential benefits.

Another nonhormonal strategy that may alleviate some symptoms of menopause is the use of antidepressants. Hot flashes were reduced by 60% with the use of venlafaxine (Wyeth-Ayerst Laboratories, Philadelphia, PA) [76].

Specific interventions for women with vaginal dryness and dyspareunia include the use of lubricants and dilators. A number of vaginal lubricants are available. The lubricant should be water soluble to avoid the risk of infections. Vaseline is not water soluble and should not be used as a lubricant. Vitamin E, Replens® (LDS Consumer Products, Cedar Rapids, IA) and Astroglide® (Biofilm Inc., Vista, CA) can be used as a lubricant prior to sexual intercourse. Replens® (LDS Consumer Products, Cedar Rapids, IA) can be used as a vaginal moisturizer as well as a lubricant. As a vaginal moisturizer, one applicator of Replens® (LDS Consumer Products, Cedar Rapids, IA) can be inserted into the vagina three to four times per week at bedtime. Astroglide® (Biofilm Inc., Vista, CA) has been reported by some users to last longer during sexual activity. These products are often found at the local drug store or can be obtained over the Internet. One Internet source is www.drugstore.com.

Dilators can be obtained from a gynecologist or often through the radiation therapy department. Women should lubricate the dilator and then insert the dilator into the vagina until it is slightly uncomfortable and then lay with the dilator in place for 10–15 minutes three to four times per week. As the vaginal tissues begin to stretch, she can increase the depth of penetration and gradually increase the size of the dilator. A high level of commitment for pursuing these measures in a consistent manner will optimize results.

Women experiencing dyspareunia should assume a position during coitus that allows her to control both the rate and depth of penetration. This will allow her to stop penetration if she becomes uncomfortable. A relationship with open communication will enable the couple to slowly work through these problems. Strain and stress within the relationship will make it difficult to overcome sexual dysfunction.

A number of medications may affect sexual functioning in women including antiandrogens, sedatives, antidepressants and stimulants [77]. Evaluation of the medication profile and adjustment of medications may improve sexual functioning.

Additionally, if GVHD of the vagina is contributing to dyspareunia, systemic and local therapy for GVHD should be instituted.

Treatment of sexual dysfunction in men

Male erectile disorder

A number of studies of HCT recipients report erectile dysfunction: 38% in one study [43] and in another study the incidence was 24%, with 13% reporting problems with ejaculation [24]. Similarly, 3-years post-transplant 38% of men reported erectile problems, 20% reported arousal problems and 6% noted difficulty with orgasm [34].

For an excellent and thorough article of the evaluation and treatment of sexual disorders in men, the reader is referred to Kandeel *et al*. [78]. Evaluation of erectile dysfunction should include a medical history and physical exam, a review of the medication profile and an endocrine evaluation including total testosterone, serum hormone binding globulin, free androgen index (FAI), FSH, LH and prolactin. Extensive evaluation of the functional and structural capacity of the penis can be accomplished with the following: penile imaging, penile biopsy, cavernosal electrical activity, nocturnal or daytime penile tumescence monitoring, pharmaco-penile duplex ultrasound, dynamic infusion cavernosometry and cavernosography, penile angiography, radionuclear scintigraphy, cavernous oxygen tension and neurological testing of somatic and autonomic innervation [78].

For the majority of men studied testosterone levels remain normal and this hormone is strongly associated with libido and sexual functioning. However, a subset of men have low levels of testosterone production and a low FAI and may benefit from hormone replacement with an improvement in libido or erectile functioning. Testosterone replacement therapy is available as an intramuscular injection, transdermal patches and in oral forms. Testosterone enanthate (BTG Pharmaceuticals, Iselin, NJ) and testosterone cypionate (Pharmacia Corp, Peapack, NJ) are two testosterone replacement products available [78]. These agents are administered intramuscularly every 2–4 weeks at doses of 100–200 mg [78]. Testosterone replacement is contraindicated in men with a history of prostate carcinoma and routine monitoring of levels of prostate specific antigen should be performed at 6-month intervals [79]. Testosterone replacement therapy can contribute to coronary artery disease by its effect of lowering high-density lipoproteins [78].

Hyperprolactinemia has been observed in some male HCT recipients suggesting damage at the level of the hypothalamus. High prolactin levels have been associated with low sexual desire, erectile difficulties and infertility. The use of bromocriptine mesylate (Medisca, Plattsburgh, NY) can be effective in treating lowering prolactin levels [80].

Performance anxiety can lead to erectile dysfunction and subsequently decreased libido. Suggesting that the male patient masturbate may increase his confidence in his erectile capabilities and decrease performance anxiety. Suggesting that the couple prolong foreplay will help to ensure that the male is aroused and improve his erection. Advising the male to adapt a very self-centered focus on sensations during sexual foreplay and intercourse will distract him from negative thoughts and performance concerns.

There are many medications that can interfer with sexual functioning in men including antihypertensives, anticholinergics, antihistamines, cardiac medications, antidepressants as well as alcohol and other recreational drugs. Reviewing the medication profile and trying alternative medications may result in improved sexual functioning.

Sildenafil (Pfizer Inc., New York, NY) has made an important contribution to the effective treatment of men with erectile dysfunction. Sildenafil inhibits cyclic guanosine monophosphate and thereby increases the penile response to sexual stimulation [5]. Sildenafil does not increase sexual desire. The dose of sildenafil ranges from 20 mg to 100 mg orally and is taken approximately 1 hour prior to sexual activity. Side-effects were generally mild and well tolerated and include disturbed color vision, headache, flushing and dyspepsia [5]. Sildenafil is contraindicated in men taking nitrates for angina or hypertenstion.

A number of medications are available as intracavernosal injections for the treatment of erectile dysfunction. These medications include prostaglandin E_1, papaverin, phentolamine. Prostaglandin E_1 is also available as an intraurethral pellet. Vacuum devices and surgical interventions are other strategies for the management of erectile dysfunction.

Conclusion

The picture emerging regarding sexuality following HCT is far from complete. It is clear that biologic and physiologic factors influence the severity and type of sexual dysfunction that may occur. It is also apparent that social and psychological variables will influence the degree of sexual satisfaction. There are complex interactions between these dimensions.

Sexuality and its expression are an important aspect of being human. This sensitive but essential aspect of the human experience is profoundly altered by the diagnosis and treatment of cancer. The physical and psychosocial impact of HCT on a recipient's sexuality and sexual functioning is an area of interest to health care providers seeking to improve the QOL of transplant recipients. While the current understanding of issues related to sexuality is incomplete, enough knowledge exists to allow health care professionals to begin to address this critical aspect of QOL. By addressing issues of sexuality in the pretransplant period a pathway is paved to helping couples adjust and cope with changes that occur as a result of high-dose cancer therapy and HCT. While the focus of this chapter has been on sexual dysfunction it must be remembered that many HCT recipients enjoy satisfying sexual relationships and that sometimes just the opportunity to discuss sexual concerns is the only intervention required. As knowledge grows researchers will be in a position to develop and test additional interventions with the goal of improving the QOL of HCT recipients.

References

1 World Health Organization. *Education and Treatment in Human Sexuality*. Technical Report. Geneva: World Health Organization, 1975.
2 Auchincloss S. Sexual dysfunction after cancer treatment. *J Psychosocial Oncol* 1991; **9**: 23–42.
3 Masters WH, Masters VJ. Human sexual response. In: Masters WH, Johnson VE, eds. 1st edn. Boston: Little Brown, 1966: 3–9.
4 Schiavi RC, Segraves RT. The biology of sexual function. *Psychiatr Clin North Am* 1995; **18**: 7–23.
5 Goldstein I, Lue TF, Padma-Nathan H, Rosen RC, Steers WD, Wicker PA. Oral sildenafil in the treatment of erectile dysfunction. Sildenafil Study Group. *N Engl J Med* 1998; **338**: 1397–404.
6 Lue TF. Erectile dysfunction. *N Engl J Med* 2000; **342**: 1802–13.
7 Chao NJ, Tierney DK, Bloom JR *et al*. Dynamic assessment of quality of life after autologous bone marrow transplantation. *Blood* 1992; **80**: 825–30.
8 Mast ME. Definition and measurement of quality of life in oncology nursing research: review and theoretical implications. *Oncol Nurs Forum* 1995; **22**: 957–64.
9 Osoba D. Lessons learned from measuring health-related quality of life in oncology. *J Clin Oncol* 1994; **12**: 608–16.
10 Skeel RT. Quality of life dimensions that are most important to cancer patients. *Oncology* 1993; **7**: 55–61.
11 Bowling A. *Measuring Health*. Buckingham: Open University Press, 1997.
12 World Health Organization. *Constitution of the World Health Organization*. Geneva: World Health Organization, 1946: 1–19.
13 Haas BK. Clarification and integration of similar quality of life concepts. *J Nursing Scholarship* 1999; **31**: 215–20.
14 Ferrell BR, Dow KI. Quality of life among long-term cancer survivors. *Oncology* 1997; **11**: 565–76.
15 Carelle N, Piotto E, Ballanger A, Germanaud J, Thuillier A, Khayat D. Changing patient perceptions of the side effects of cancer chemotherapy. *Cancer* 2002; **95**: 155–63.
16 Baker F, Wingard JR, Curbow B *et al*. Quality of life of bone marrow transplant long-term survivors. *Bone Marrow Transplant* 1994; **13**: 589–96.
17 Bush NE, Haberman M, Donaldson G, Sullivan KM. Quality of life of 125 adults surviving 6–18 years after bone marrow transplantation. *Soc Sci Med* 1995; **40**: 479–90.
18 Prieto JM, Saez R, Carreras E *et al*. Physical and psychosocial functioning of 117 survivors of bone marrow transplantation. *Bone Marrow Transplant* 1996; **17**: 1133–42.
19 Schmidt GM, Niland JC, Forman SJ *et al*. Extended follow-up in 212 long-term allogeneic bone marrow transplant survivors. Issues of quality of life. *Transplantation* 1993; **55**: 551–7.
20 Marks D, Friedman SH, Delli Carpini L, Neuz CM,

Neuz AM. A prospective study of the effects of high-dose chemotherapy and bone marrow transplantation on sexual function in the first year after transplant. *Bone Marrow Transplant* 1997: **19**: 819–22.

21 Molassiotis A, Boughton BJ, Burgoyne T, van den Akker OB. Comparison of the overall quality of life in 50 long-term survivors of autologous and allogeneic bone marrow transplantation. *J Adv Nurs* 1995; **22**: 509–16.

22 Schubert MA, Sullivan KM, Schubert MM et al. Gynecological abnormalities following allogeneic bone marrow transplantation. *Bone Marrow Transplant* 1990; **5**: 425–30.

23 Andersen BL. Sexual functioning morbidity among cancer survivors. Current status and future research directions. *Cancer* 1985; **55**: 1835–42.

24 Wingard JR, Curbow B, Baker F, Zabora J, Piantadosi S. Sexual satisfaction in survivors of bone marrow transplantation. *Bone Marrow Transplant* 1992; **9**: 185–90.

25 Chiodi S, Spinelli S, Cohen A et al. Cyclic sex hormone replacement therapy in women undergoing allogeneic bone marrow transplantation: aims and results. *Bone Marrow Transplant* 1991; **8** (Suppl. 1): 47–9.

26 Watson M, Wheatley K, Harrison GA et al. Severe adverse impact on sexual functioning and fertility of bone marrow transplantation, either allogeneic or autologous, compared with consolidation chemotherapy alone: analysis of the MRC AML 10 trial. *Cancer* 1999; **86**: 1231–9.

27 Altmaier EM, Gingrich RD, Fyfe MA. Two-year adjustment of bone marrow transplant survivors. *Bone Marrow Transplant* 1991; **7**: 311–6.

28 Andrykowski MA, Bruehl S, Brady MJ, Henslee-Downey PJ. Physical and psychosocial status of adults one-year after bone marrow transplantation: a prospective study. *Bone Marrow Transplant* 1995; **15**: 837–44.

29 McQuellon RP, Russell GB, Rambo TD et al. Quality of life and psychological distress of bone marrow transplant recipients: the 'time trajectory' to recovery over the first year. *Bone Marrow Transplant* 1998; **21**: 477–86.

30 McQuellon RP, Craven B, Russell GB et al. Quality of life in breast cancer patients before and after autologous bone marrow transplantation. *Bone Marrow Transplant* 1996; **18**: 579–84.

31 Molassiotis A, van den Akker OB, Milligan DW et al. Quality of life in long-term survivors of marrow transplantation: comparison with a matched group receiving maintenance chemotherapy. *Bone Marrow Transplant* 1996; **17**: 249–58.

32 Sutherland HJ, Fyles GM, Adams G et al. Quality of life following bone marrow transplantation: a comparison of patient reports with population norms. *Bone Marrow Transplant* 1997; **19**: 1129–36.

33 Mumma GH, Mashberg D, Lesko LM. Long-term psychosexual adjustment of acute leukemia survivors: impact of marrow transplantation versus conventional chemotherapy. *General Hosp Psychiatry* 1992; **14**: 43–55.

34 Syrjala KL, Roth-Roemer SL, Abrams JR et al. Prevalence and predictors of sexual dysfunction in long-term survivors of marrow transplantation. *J Clin Oncol* 1998; **16**: 3148–57.

35 Brook CGD, Marshall NJ (eds). *Essential Endocrinology*, 4th edn. London: Blackwell Science, 2001.

36 Klein CE, Glode LM. Gonadal complications. In: Armitage JO, Antman KH, eds. *High-Dose Cancer Therapy. Pharmacology, Hematopoietins, Stem Cells.* Baltimore: Williams & Wilkins, 1992: 555–66.

37 Sherins RJ. Gonadal dysfunction. In: Devita VT, Hellman S, Rosenberg SA, eds. *Cancer, Principles and Practice of Oncology*, 4th edn. Philadelphia: Lippincott; 1993: 2395–406.

38 Averette HE, Boike GM, Jarrell MA. Effects of cancer chemotherapy on gonadal function and reproductive capacity. *CA Cancer J Clin* 1990; **40**: 199–209.

39 Kauppila M, Koskinen P, Irjala K, Remes K, Viikari J. Long-term effects of allogeneic bone marrow transplantation (BMT) on pituitary, gonad, thyroid and adrenal function in adults. *Bone Marrow Transplant* 1998; **22**: 331–7.

40 Littley MD, Shalet SM, Morgenstern GR, Deakin DP. Endocrine and reproductive dysfunction following fractionated total body irradiation in adults. *Q J Med* 1991; **78**: 265–74.

41 Kauppila M, Viikari J, Irjala K, Koskinen P, Remes K. The hypothalamus–pituitary–gonad axis and testicular function in male patients after treatment for haematological malignancies. *J Intern Med* 1998; **244**: 411–6.

42 Chatterjee R, Goldstone AH. Gonadal damage and effects on fertility in adult patients with haematological malignancy undergoing stem cell transplantation. *Bone Marrow Transplant* 1996; **17**: 5–11.

43 Molassiotis A, van den Akker OB, Milligan DW, Boughton BJ. Gonadal function and psychosexual adjustment in male long-term survivors of bone marrow transplantation. *Bone Marrow Transplant* 1995; **16**: 253–9.

44 Thaler-DeMers D. Intimacy issues: sexuality, fertility and relationships. *Seminars Oncol Nursing* 2001; **17**: 255–62.

45 Krebs LU. Sexual and reproductive dysfunction. In: Groenwald SL, ed. *Cancer Nursing: Principles and Practice*, 3rd edn. Boston: Jones and Bartlett, 1993: 696–718.

46 Gradishar WJ, Schilsky RL. Ovarian function following radiation and chemotherapy for cancer. *Semin Oncol* 1989; **16**: 425–36.

47 Spinelli S, Chiodi S, Bacigalupo A et al. Ovarian recovery after total body irradiation and allogeneic bone marrow transplantation: long-term follow up of 79 females. *Bone Marrow Transplant* 1994; **14**: 373–80.

48 Albertazzi P, Natale V, Barbolini C, Teglio L, Di Micco R. The effect of tibolone versus continuous combined norethisterone acetate and oestradiol on memory, libido and mood of postmenopausal women: a pilot study. *Maturitas* 2000; **36**: 223–9.

49 Dennerstein L, Dudley EC, Hopper JL, Guthrie JR, Burger HG. A prospective population-based study of menopausal symptoms. *Obstetrics Gynecol* 2000; **96**: 351–8.

50 Zichella L. Clinical management of the menopausal woman. *Int J Fertil Menopausal Stud* 1993; **38** (Suppl. 1): 15–22.

51 Chatterjee R, Mills W, Katz M, McGarrigle HH, Goldstone AH. Prospective study of pituitary-gonadal function to evaluate short-term effects of ablative chemotherapy or total body irradiation with autologous or allogenic marrow transplantation in post-menarcheal female patients. *Bone Marrow Transplant* 1994; **13**: 511–7.

52 Myers LS. Methodological review and meta-analysis of sexuality and menopause research. *Neuroscience Biobehavioral Rev* 1995; **19**: 331–41.

53 Lichtman R. Perimenopausal and postmenopausal hormone replacement therapy. Part 1. An update of the literature on benefits and risks. *J Nurse Midwifery* 1996; **41**: 3–28.

54 Soltes BA. Therapeutic options for menopause in cancer survivors. *Oncol Nursing Updates* 1997; **4**: 1–12.

55 Atkinson K. Chronic graft versus host disease. *Bone Marrow Transplant* 1990; **5**: 69–82.

56 Corson SL, Sullivan K, Batzer F, August C, Storb R, Thomas ED. Gynecologic manifestations of chronic graft-versus-host disease. *Obstetrics Gynecol* 1982; **60**: 488–92.

57 Atkinson K. Chronic graft versus host disease following marrow transplantation. *Marrow Transplant Rev* 1992; **2**: 1–7.

58 Cust MP, Whitehead MI, Powles R, Hunter M, Milliken S. Consequences and treatment of ovarian failure after total body irradiation for leukaemia. *BMJ* 1989; **299**: 1494–7.

59 Moadel AB, Ostroff JS, Lesko LM. Fertility and sexuality. In: Whedon BM, ed. *Bone Marrow Transplantation: Principles, Practice, and Nursing Insights.* Boston: Jones and Bartlett, 1991: 377–99.

60 Anderson BJ, Wolf FM. Chronic physical illness and sexual behavior: psychological issues. *J Consult Clin Psychol* 1986; **54**: 168–75.

61 Dobkin PL, Bradley I. Assessment of sexual dysfunction in oncology patients: review, critique, and suggestions. *J Psychosocial Oncol* 1991; **9**: 43–74.

62 Syrjala KL, Chapko MK, Vitaliano PP, Cummings C, Sullivan KM. Recovery after allogeneic marrow transplantation. Prospective study of predictors of long-term physical and psychosocial functioning. *Bone Marrow Transplant* 1993; **11**: 319–27.

63 Molassiotis A, van den Akker OB, Boughton BJ. Perceived social support, family environment and psychosocial recovery in bone marrow transplant long-term survivors. *Soc Sci Med* 1997; **44**: 317–25.

64 Puukko LR, Hirvonen E, Aalberg V, Hovi L, Rautonen J, Siimes MA. Sexuality of young women surviving leukaemia. *Arch Dis Child* 1997; **76**: 197–202.

65 American Psychiatric Association. *Diagnostic and Statistical Manual of Mental Disorders*, 4th edition, revised (DSM-IV-R). Washington, DC: American Psychiatric Association, 2000.

66 Warner PH, Rowe T, Whipple B. Shedding light on the sexual history. *Am J Nursing* 1999; **99**: 34–40.

67 Hughs MK. Sexuality issues: keeping your cool. *Oncol Nurs Forum* 1996; **23**: 1597–600.

68 Andrykowski MA, Brady MJ, Greiner CB et al. 'Returning to normal' following bone marrow transplantation: outcomes, expectations and informed consent. *Bone Marrow Transplant* 1995; **15**: 573–81.

69 Ferrell B, Grant M, Schmidt GM et al. The meaning of quality of life for bone marrow transplant survivors. Part 2. Improving quality of life for bone marrow transplant survivors. *Cancer Nurs* 1992; **15**: 247–53.

70 Bachmann GA, Leiblum SR, Grill J. Brief sexual inquiry in gynecologic practice. *Obstet Gynecol* 1989; **73**: 425–7.

71 Marks DI, Friedman SH, Delli Carpini L, Nezu CM, Nezu AM. A prospective study of the effects of high-dose chemotherapy and bone marrow transplantation on sexual function in the first year after transplant. *Bone Marrow Transplant* 1997; **19**: 819–22.

72 Gregoire A. ABC of sexual health: assessing and

managing male sexual problems. *BMJ* 1999; **318**: 315–7.

73 Schover LR. *Sexuality and Cancer*. Atlanta, Ga: American Cancer Society, 2001.

74 Lark S. *The Estrogen Decision*. Berkeley, CA: Celestial Arts, 1999.

75 Perry S, O'Hanlan K. *Natural Menopause*. Reading, MA: Persus Books, 1997.

76 Barton D, LaVasseur B, Loprinzi C, Novotny P, Wilwerding B, Sloan J. Venlafaxine for the control of hot flashes: results of a longitudinal continuation study. *Oncol Nurs Forum* 2002; **29**: 33–40.

77 Butcher J. ABC of sexual health: female sexual problems I. Loss of desire: what about fun? *BMJ* 1999; **318**: 41–3.

78 Kandeel FR, Koussa VKT, Swerdloff RS. Male sexual function and its disorders: physiology, pathyophysiology, clinical investigation, and treatment. *Endocrine Rev* 2001; **22**: 342–88.

79 Dinsmore W, Evans C. ABC of sexual health: erectile dysfunction. *BMJ* 1999; **318**: 387–90.

80 Buvat J, Lemaire A. Endocrine screening in 1022 men with erectile dysfunction. Clinical significance and cost-effective strategy. *J Urol* 1997; **158**: 1764–7.

Section 3

Sources of Hematopoietic Cells for Human Transplant

41

Phyllis I. Warkentin, Lewis Nick & Elizabeth J. Shpall

Hematopoietic Cell Procurement, Processing and Transplantation: Regulation and Accreditation

Introduction

Hematopoietic cell transplantation (HCT) is now established therapy for many serious congenital and acquired diseases of hematopoietic origin, as well as many high-risk malignancies [1]. Significant improvements in supportive care, histocompatibility matching, chemoradiotherapy and hematopoietic graft manipulation have contributed to improvements in the clinical outcome of patients. Because of the curative potential of such transplants, the number of centers now performing these procedures throughout the world has increased dramatically over the past several years. Combined with the emergence of other novel therapeutic strategies, the indications for transplantation are continually changing. Hematopoietic cells are also being used in novel ways, such as post-transplant donor lymphocyte infusions, to improve patient survival [2]. Cellular therapies have now expanded beyond hematopoietic and immunologic reconstitution to exciting new therapies using mesenchymal stem cells, dendritic cells, targeted lymphocytes, gene-modified and other cells.

The source of hematopoietic cells has also expanded from the traditional bone marrow graft employed in the earliest transplants to peripheral blood hematopoietic cells (PBHCs) now commonly used as the major source of hematopoietic support for both autologous [3] and allogeneic [4,5] transplantation. In addition, unrelated marrow and PBHC donors are now increasingly available. Since the number of potential unrelated volunteers in the National Marrow Donor Registry exceeds four million, unrelated donors can be identified and grafts obtained more rapidly; and high-resolution histocompatibility typing has improved HCT outcome [6,7]. Cell selection and selective T-cell-depletion techniques have become common, making haplo-identical donors a viable alternative [8]. There is also increasing use of umbilical cord blood cells, known to be a rich source of hematopoietic cells (HCs), for transplantation. Umbilical cord blood cells have been shown to reconstitute pediatric patients, as well as small cohorts of adult patients, who have received high-dose therapy [9,10]. The use of umbilical cord blood is likely to produce substantial benefits in the treatment of malignant and nonmalignant disease in the next several years, given the rapid advances in purification and expansion of umbilical cord blood that are currently under investigation.

Proliferation of HC technology has also stimulated the involvement of corporations whose research, in many cases, has contributed to the rapid advances made in this field. Recently, new businesses have begun promoting the elective storage of autologous umbilical cord blood for use as part of cancer treatment at some later date.

The rapid advances in many aspects of HC procurement, processing and transplantation have resulted in substantial variability in procedures and standards within the field, even in seemingly fundamental issues. What constitutes an adequate HC product continues to be the subject of extensive debate and little consensus. A number of parameters have been used to determine an adequate graft, including the number of total nucleated or mononuclear cells [11], the presence or number of colony forming unit–granulocyte/macrophage (CFU-GM) [12] and the $CD34^+$ cell content [13]. While this latter assay appears to be the most consistent and clinically relevant measure of graft quality available, the number of $CD34^+$ cells required for a satisfactory transplant varies widely, depending on the clinical situation, size of the patient and type of transplant. There also remains substantial variability in the performance of the CD34 flow cytometric assay [3]. A variety of graft manipulations are now relatively common, including removal or enrichment of various cell populations, expansion of HC populations and cryopreservation.

The proliferation of new transplant facilities, donor and graft sources, and processing and matching technologies, in conjunction with the risks associated with the transplant procedure, has raised legitimate concerns about the safety and quality of HCs obtained for clinical use.

HC therapies are being subjected to increasing and rapidly evolving regulation. Serious issues about the safety of human tissue used for transplantation have been raised since at least the early 1990s, when the primary concern was the potential for transmission of human immunodeficiency virus (HIV) and/or one of the hepatitis viruses through transplantation from an infected donor. Interim regulations from the Food and Drug Administration (FDA) regarding donor infectious disease screening were implemented in 1993 and finalized in 1997, with the intent to add more extensive requirements in the future [14,15]. At the same time, there is considerable debate concerning the appropriateness and necessity of governmental regulation, as well as the effectiveness, benefit and burden of voluntary accreditation.

Governmental regulation

Governmental regulation occurs at the federal and state levels. At the federal level, the FDA regulates human cells, tissues and cellular and tissue-based products (HCT/Ps) under the authority of the Public Health Services (PHS) Act and the Federal Food, Drug and Cosmetic Act (FDCA). Within FDA, the Center for Biologic Evaluation and Research (CBER) and the Center for Devices and Radiological Health (CDRH) have oversight of various activities. CBER regulates human tissues intended for transplantation that are recovered, processed, stored or distributed by methods that do not change tissue function or characteristics and that are not currently regulated as a human drug, biological product or medical device. Regulations require registration of the facility with the FDA, compliance with all applicable regulations, and cooperation with periodic on-site inspections.

In the past, FDA oversight of HCT/Ps has been fragmented, inconsistent and sometimes confusing. In 1997, FDA proposed a unified and tiered approach to the regulation of traditional and new products, including HCs, which would provide a more uniform review of applications within the FDA and the amount of regulation necessary to protect the public health [16]. Products that are expected to be at a higher risk for disease transmission or at risk for contamination, such as allogeneic cells or cells highly manipulated *ex vivo*, would be subject to more regulation than those products with less risk, such as autologous or minimally manipulated products. A Tissue Reference Group, comprising of representatives of both the CBER and the CDRH, was formed in 1998 to provide a single reference point within the FDA for all regulatory questions about HCT/Ps and for the development and implementation of regulations. The FDA-proposed regulations are based on five public health and regulatory concerns:

1 Prevention of the transmission of communicable disease.
2 Assurance that necessary processing controls exist to prevent the contamination of cells and tissues, and to preserve their integrity and function.
3 Assurance of clinical safety and effectiveness.
4 Assurance of necessary product labeling, including permissible promotion for proper product use.
5 Establishment of a mechanism for FDA to communicate with the cell and tissue industry [16].

The proposed regulations have been published in the Federal Register for public comment and will create a new section of the Code of Federal Regulations, Title 21, Part 1271 that will contain cell and tissue regulations [17–19]. The three proposed rules are the Registration rule, the Donor Suitability rule and the current Good Tissue Practices (cGTP) rule. The final FDA registration rule, published in January 2001, became effective April 4, 2001 [17]. This rule requires that any establishment that manufactures HCT/Ps regulated under Section 361 of the PHS Act must register with the FDA, update registration annually and update product listings every 6 months.

Under the proposed Donor Suitability rule [18], the FDA considers communicable disease screening and testing to be part of manufacturing and, therefore, subject to regulation. Donor screening is the review of relevant medical records for indications of past or present infection and for risk factors for a relevant communicable disease. Donor testing is performing laboratory tests on a specimen, generally a blood specimen, collected from the donor to determine if he or she has been exposed to or infected with a relevant communicable disease or its agent. Under this proposed rule, infectious disease screening and testing requirements will be based on risk. The allogeneic donor will have a long list of requirements because of the higher risk of infectious disease transmission. The autologous donor screening and testing will likely be a shorter list of recommendations. The final Donor Suitability rule has not yet been published.

The proposed cGTP rule is a set of regulations intended to prevent the introduction, transmission, and spread of communicable disease by helping to ensure that products do not contain relevant communicable disease agents, that products are not contaminated during manufacturing, and that the function and integrity of products are not impaired through improper processing [19]. Good Tissue Practice regulations include requirements for adequate organizational structure; sufficient personnel; adequate facilities; environmental control and monitoring; adequate equipment, supplies and reagents for the processes carried out in the facility; proper processing, including process change and process validation; proper labeling, claims and labeling controls; storage, receipt, distribution and other records; maintenance of complaint files; reporting adverse reactions and product deviations; and the establishment of a quality plan.

Governmental regulation of HC therapy at the state level is fragmented, often voluntary and, in the opinion of the FDA, inadequate to prevent the transmission of disease [15]. Many states have little specific regulation. Some states have adopted mechanisms of qualifying HCT programs and facilities, such as the Certificate of Need process. Other states have developed a licensure process, often heavily dependent on the standards established by professional societies. Some states, such as New York, have identified the public health concerns in cellular transplantation, and have adopted direct and specific regulations for HCT/Ps processing and storage facilities [20,21]. A number of states have adopted, or are considering, a mechanism of approval for transplantation that requires accreditation by a professional organization. At the time of writing (2003), both Massachusetts and Maryland require accreditation by the Foundation for the Accreditation of Cellular Therapy (FACT) to perform HCT within those states.

Voluntary accreditation

In contrast to governmental regulation, accreditation by professional organizations is voluntary. Accredited programs are required to follow the standards of the accrediting organization; those who choose not to participate are not required to follow the standards. This is one of the limitations of voluntary self-monitoring within an industry. There is no certainty that all who will participate in an activity will choose to participate in the accreditation process and, hence, follow the professional standards. In the field of HCT, there are three professional organizations that set standards and accredit various aspects. These three are the Foundation for the Accreditation of Cellular Therapy (FACT), the American Association of Blood Banks (AABB), and the National Marrow Donor Program (NMDP).

The Foundation for the Accreditation of Cellular Therapy (FACT)

Historical background

FACT was founded in 1995 by investigators active in the field of HCT who determined that both standards and voluntary professional accreditation for the procurement, manipulation and transplantation of HC products were necessary to promote quality patient care, quality laboratory practices, and to preserve the flexibility required to nurture continued rapid scientific evolution of the field. FACT was originally founded as the Foundation for the Accreditation of Hematopoietic Cell Therapy (FAHCT), but the name was changed in December 2001 to reflect the dramatic expansion of cellular therapies, beyond HC therapeutics, to exciting new therapies using mesenchymal stem cells, dendritic cells, targeted lymphocytes, genetically modified cells, pancreatic islets, and others. This change followed the lead of one of FACT's parent organizations, the International Society for Hematotherapy and Graft Engineering (ISHAGE), that also changed its name in 2001 to the International Society for Cellular Therapy (ISCT).

FACT is a partnership between two organizations, one clinically based and the other laboratory based. Both are dedicated to the improvement of the practice of cellular therapy. In 1992, ISHAGE (now ISCT) was formed as a professional society representing scientists and physicians working in the area of HC manipulation. Its membership represents most of the major HCT centers in the world. The ISHAGE Regulatory Affairs Committee, under the Chairperson, Dr Scott D. Rowley, developed the first draft of the Standards for Hematopoietic Cell Collection and Processing in 1994.

In 1993, the American Society for Blood and Marrow Transplantation (ASBMT) was formed as a professional organization representing physicians and investigators involved in the clinical conduct of HCT. The membership of this society represents transplant centers located predominantly in the USA and Canada. A subcommittee of the ASBMT Clinical

Affairs Committee, under the Chairperson, Dr Gordon Phillips, developed the first draft of the Clinical Standards for Hematopoietic Cell Transplantation in 1994. Believing that quality care could only be achieved if both clinical and laboratory issues were addressed, the ISHAGE laboratory standards and the ASBMT clinical standards were merged into a single document in December 1994. FACT was established to develop and implement a voluntary accreditation program based on these standards, the major objective of which is to promote high quality medical and laboratory practice in HC therapy.

The merged laboratory and clinical standards of the ISHAGE and the ASBMT underwent considerable debate and revision over a 2-year period, including the input from individual members of the ISHAGE (now ISCT) and the ASBMT. After each comment had been reviewed and incorporated as appropriate, the first edition of FAHCT *Standards for Hematopoietic Progenitor Cell Collection, Processing & Transplantation* for North America was published in September 1996 [22].

A companion *Accreditation Manual* was subsequently published to provide guidance to applicant facilities and personnel, and to FAHCT (now FACT) inspectors [23]. The *Accreditation Manual* lists each Standard, the checklist items related to that Standard that will be evaluated at the time of the on-site inspection and additional guidance information, including the rationale for Standards, explanations and definitions, and examples of alternative methods, approaches and organizations that would be considered to be in compliance with the Standards. The manual also contains specific information that addresses questions and concerns that were submitted in writing during the period of member comment.

FACT is now an established nonprofit organization with a national office and staff in Omaha, Nebraska. An infrastructure has been developed that includes technical staff, a Standards Committee and a Quality Improvement Committee. The core of FACT is its active Board of Directors, comprised of an equal number of representatives from ISCT and ASBMT, the Presidents of these two parent organizations during their terms of office and the Chairpersons of the Accreditation Program and the Standards Committee, who represent ASBMT, ISCT, or both. The FACT Board of Directors approves all publications, determines the accreditation status of all applicant programs and sets the future agenda for the Foundation.

In 1997, it became apparent that the field of placental and umbilical cord blood banking is more complex than addressed in the first edition of FAHCT's (now FACT's) *Standards for Hematopoietic Progenitor Cell Collection, Processing & Transplantation* [22]. Representatives of FACT, ISCT and ASBMT collaborated with members of NETCORD, an international organization of independent cord blood banks, to draft additional standards and establish a parallel accreditation program. The first edition of NETCORD/FACT *International Standards for Cord Blood Processing, Testing, Banking, Selection and Release* was developed by consensus, circulated for member and public comment, adopted by the Boards of NETCORD and FACT, and published in June, 2000 [24]. These Standards were revised in December 2000 and a second edition published in July 2001 [25]. These Standards supersede all relevant sections relating to cord blood in the first edition of the FAHCT *Standards for Hematopoietic Progenitor Cell Collection, Processing & Transplantation* [22] excepting those clinical standards related to the transplantation of cord blood cells.

Recently, cooperation in Europe between the European Group for Blood and Marrow Transplantation (EBMT) and ISHAGE-Europe (now ISCT-Europe), in collaboration with North American colleagues, established a structure similar to FACT in Europe known as the Joint Accreditation Committee of ISHAGE-Europe and EBMT (JACIE) [26]. Based on the first edition of the FAHCT (now FACT) *Standards for Hematopoietic Progenitor Cell Collection, Processing & Transplantation* [22], JACIE created a Standards document that was approved by the EBMT and the ISHAGE-Europe to be the basis for accreditation programs throughout Europe [27]. Three collaborative training workshops have been held in Barcelona, Spain (January 2000, March 2001 and May 2002) to share accreditation tools and experience, and to implement the European accreditation programs. Two different general strategies are used in the European community. In countries with national cooperative blood and marrow transplant groups and national regulatory agencies, training of inspectors and inspections are organized by the national group under the auspices and in cooperation with JACIE. JACIE ascertains that the Standards remain the same and are updated as appropriate. In contrast, in countries with no national groups or in small countries with only one or two blood and marrow transplantation programs, JACIE will organize the inspection process similar to the FACT program.

FACT Standards

The first edition of FAHCT's (now FACT's) *Standards for Hematopoietic Progenitor Cell Collection, Processing & Transplantation* was unique in the breadth and depth of activities covered [22]. FACT Standards are applied to all sources of HCs, and to all phases of collection, processing and administration of these cells. HCs include primitive pluripotent HCs capable of self-renewal as well as maturation into any of the hematopoietic lineages, including committed and lineage restricted progenitor cells and therapeutic cells. This includes, but is not limited to, cells isolated from marrow, peripheral blood or placental and umbilical cord blood, and any of a variety of manipulations including removal or enrichment of various cell populations, expansion of HC populations, cryopreservation, infusion, expansion or activation of lymphocyte populations for immunological therapy and genetic modification of lymphoid or HCs, when these cells are intended to permanently or transiently engraft in the recipient or to be used in the treatment of disease. FACT Standards do not address the collection, processing or administration of erythrocytes, mature granulocytes, platelets, plasma or plasma-derived components, or products intended for transfusion support.

FACT Standards define an infrastructure required for the safe and efficacious collection, processing, storage and use of HCs. They define the minimum education and experience necessary for staff participating in these activities and require an ongoing assessment of activities. There is a minimum requirement that patient outcome be monitored by at least the tracking of neutrophil and platelet engraftment. FACT Standards do not define a required structure or form for the transplant program, nor do they prescribe the clinical use of HCs.

Every effort was made to incorporate sound recommendations fostering quality medical and laboratory practice in HCT. However, no standards can guarantee the successful outcome of such therapies. FACT Standards are minimal guidelines for facilities and individuals performing HCT and therapy or providing support services for such procedures. FACT Standards may be exceeded as deemed appropriate by responsible personnel in individual facilities. FACT Standards are not intended to include all procedures and practices that a facility or individual should implement if the standard of practice in the community or governmental laws or regulations establish additional requirements, nor are they intended to be an exclusive means of complying with the standard of care in the industry or community. Attempts have been made to conform these Standards to existing US federal regulations; however, regulations are changed often and compliance with Standards does not guarantee compliance with all regulations. In all cases, personnel are expected to follow all applicable laws and regulations.

Hematopoietic cell (HC) collection

The intent of the HC collection standards is to provide a framework for donor evaluation and HC collection that will foster good, safe care for both patient and donor. These collection standards are divided into bone marrow and PBHC sections. Each section addresses collection from autologous and allogeneic donors separately. Informed consent must be obtained and documented for each collection procedure. Each facility is required to have written criteria for the donation of HCs that take into account the safety of the donor as well as the safety and efficacy of the product. Critical factors include lack of microbial contamination, adequacy of progenitor cell number, and accurate matching of donor and recipient HLA type.

Histocompatibility testing (HLA-A, -B, and -DR) must be performed by a laboratory accredited by the American Society for Histocompatibility and Immunogenetics (ASHI). All other laboratory testing must be performed by laboratories accredited by the College of American Pathologists (CAP), the Joint Commission on Accreditation of Health Care Organizations (JCAHO) or the Health Care Financing Administration (HCFA).

Hematopoietic cell (HC) processing

The intent of FACT Standards is to establish that the laboratory is run in a responsible and responsive manner, that aberrations in results are noted and that the recipient's physician is aware of any adverse event that could compromise the graft. The production of a safe HC product for clinical use depends on good biosafety procedures in a secure, adequately designed laboratory space using appropriate equipment. HC products should not be exposed to radioactive materials during processing.

Assurance of patient safety and maintenance of the ability to conduct responsible research are equally important goals central to the mission of FACT. These goals can be accomplished by adequately defining the conditions under which the manipulation of HCs may take place. The investigators must either use reagents or devices previously approved for the specific procedure or demonstrate that they have complied with applicable governmental regulations (Investigational New Drug, Investigational Device Exemption, etc.). Institutional Review Board (IRB) approval demonstrates compliance for procedures not covered by governmental regulations. The IRB review ensures that there will be independent third-party evaluation of the proposed HC manipulations. It is understood that early clinical studies may involve partial treatment of grafts by investigational protocols. However, when the manipulation is entirely experimental, IRB approval should be obtained. Detailed written procedures for these investigational manipulations should always be available for review.

Hematopoietic cell (HC) transplantation

The clinical transplantation program facility consists of an integrated medical team housed in a geographically contiguous or proximate space with a program director, common staff training programs, protocols and quality assessment systems. The program must use HC collection and processing facilities that meet FACT Standards with respect to their interactions with that clinical program.

Standards in the clinical section define the training and experience necessary for physicians, nurses and other members of the transplant team to ensure optimal care and safety of HCT patients and ensure that the transplant outcomes are generally compatible with expected norms. FACT Standards require that clinical research is carried out using IRB-approved protocols in an appropriate clinical environment with adequate support staff. Clinical records must be complete and accurate, obviously an important element of good clinical care as well as clinical investigation. Prior to FACT accreditation, consecutive allogeneic and autologous transplant patient records are reviewed during the on-site inspection. Records are assessed for completeness by documenting the presence of key pieces of transplant-related data, and for accuracy by comparing the patient record provided with a primary hospital record. Data points are verified against a primary pathology report, a laboratory report or record, or similar data from another source.

The second edition of *Standards for Hematopoietic Progenitor Cell Collection, Processing & Transplantation* [28] was developed after a detailed review of the first edition by the FACT Standards Committee. Draft standards were submitted for comment from the public and from the memberships of ISCT and ASBMT. Following review of comments, revision, and legal review, the second edition was adopted by the FACT Board of Directors and published in March 2002, and became effective June 1, 2002 [28]. Concepts retained in the second edition include the requirement that all programs have a quality management program, which includes at least the following components: a system for detecting, evaluating and reporting errors, accidents and suspected adverse reactions; quality audits; corrective actions; the documentation, review and reporting of quality program initiatives; and a safety program. In addition all clinical, collection and laboratory processing facilities must evaluate and report clinical outcomes.

The second edition of *Standards for Hematopoietic Progenitor Cell Collection, Processing & Transplantation* [28] differs from the first edition [22] in several ways. Section A now contains only terminology, definitions and abbreviations; and individual items in each section have been reorganized as applicable in a parallel fashion. Product names have been changed to be consistent with the International Council for Commonality in Blood Banking Automation nomenclature, to facilitate international cooperation and bar coding in the future.

In the Clinical Section B, data management standards now include the specific items required on the Transplant Essential Data (TED) forms of the International Bone Marrow Transplant Registry (IBMTR) and the Autologous Blood and Marrow Transplant Registry (ABMTR). Specific standards have been added for pediatric transplantation. Standards for HC donor evaluation and selection have been moved from the Collection Section to the Clinical section; and the therapy administration standards have been expanded.

In the Collection Section C, responsibilities for donor evaluation have been clarified, and the relevant labeling standards have been added. In the Laboratory Section D, labeling standards have been consolidated into a single table; and packaging and transportation standards have been clarified.

FACT process for accreditation

FACT accreditation is a voluntary process based on documented compliance with the published Standards as judged by an evaluation of submitted written information and an on-site inspection of the applicant program or facility. The evaluation of submitted materials is completed by the Accreditation Program Chairperson, a designee or the appropriate member of the inspection team. One of the strengths of the program is that all inspectors are active in the field of HC therapy and meet the minimum qualifications for all inspectors for the FACT Accreditation Program. All inspectors are unpaid volunteers who meet minimum FACT inspector qualifications as listed in Table 41.1. To promote uniformity and consistency in the process and fairness to applicant facilities, it is important that inspectors have a common, up-to-date understanding of the principles of FACT Standards and the approach it takes to inspection and accreditation.

The formal process for initial FACT accreditation is illustrated in Fig. 41.1, and is as follows:

1 *Registration.* A program or facility director will notify the FACT Accreditation Office in Omaha, Nebraska, of its interest in becoming accredited by FACT for one or more of the transplant-related services. FACT staff will send an inspection registration form to the applicant program or facility. Alternatively, a director may register electronically by accessing the registration form on the Internet (http://www.factwebsite.org).

Table 41.1 Foundation for the Accreditation of Cellular Therapy (FACT) Accreditation Program: inspector qualifications.

1 Each inspector shall be an individual member of ISCT, ASBMT, or both
2 Each inspector shall be affiliated with a FACT-accredited or applicant program
3 Each inspector shall document that she or he is qualified by training and experience to perform the FACT on-site inspection
4 An inspector of a clinical transplant program shall hold a medical degree and license to practice medicine in the USA or Canada, and have a minimum of 5 years of clinical marrow transplant experience
5 An inspector of a hematopoietic cell collection facility shall hold a relevant doctoral degree (MD or PhD) and have 5 years of experience in hematopoietic cell collection procedures, including apheresis; or shall have 5 years of experience as the nurse or technician supervising the collection of PBHCs by apheresis
6 An inspector of a cell processing laboratory shall hold a relevant doctoral degree (MD or PhD) or a professional degree in biological sciences or medical technology, and have 5 years of experience as a laboratory director, medical director, or supervisor of a hematopoietic cell processing laboratory
7 Each inspector shall have completed at least one training course for new inspectors, participated in at least one inspection as an inspector-trainee with an experienced inspector, and successfully completed the inspector's written examination
8 Each inspector shall complete the required inspections and reports in a timely manner and receive satisfactory evaluations as submitted by the inspected applicant facilities and the FACT technical staff

ASBMT, American Society of Blood and Marrow Transplantation; ISCT, International Society for Cellular Therapy; PBHCs, peripheral blood hematopoietic cells.

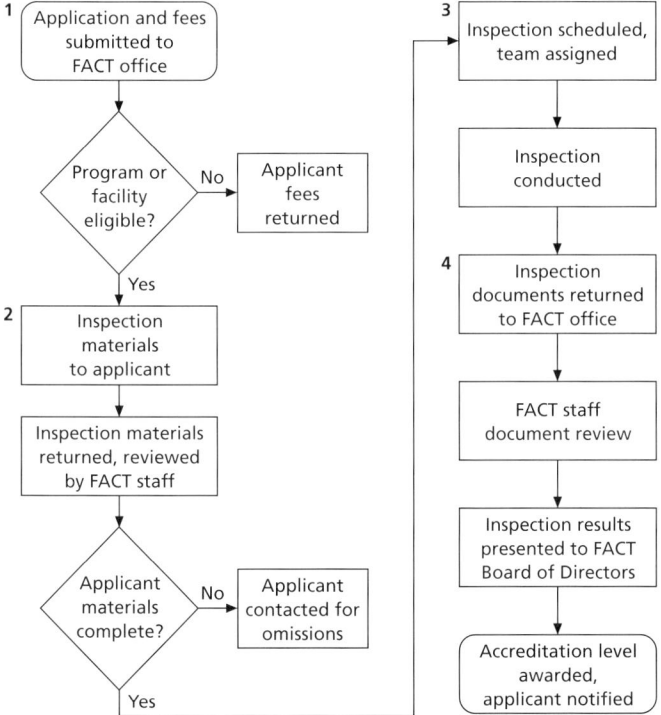

Fig. 41.1 Foundation for the Accreditation of Cellular Therapy (FACT) Accreditation Program: accreditation process. Time allotted to each step is limited to a maximum total time of 12–17 months (if reinspection is required) from application to accreditation.

The inspection registration form contains basic demographic information about the program or facility, its scope and its personnel. The FACT Accreditation Office staff will review the registration information and determine if the program or facility is eligible for accreditation.

2 *Application.* Eligible applicants are sent an inspection packet that details the accreditation requirements and process. Included in these materials are (i) instructions to the applicant for completion of the formal application process; (ii) a list of documents that must accompany the formal application; and (iii) the inspection checklist that lists all of the items to be inspected during the on-site inspection. The applicant facility personnel answer each item on the checklist pertaining to their program, and submit the checklist to the FACT office. The inspector will verify each of these items at the on-site inspection, using the checklist as part of the formal report. Completion of the checklist is expected within 12 months of receipt by the applicant.

3 *On-site Inspection.* The submitted materials are reviewed by the FACT technical staff upon receipt from the applicant, and an inspection team and date are selected. The date is chosen by the applicant at a time when all key personnel will be available to participate in the process. The inspection team selection is based on the size and complexity of the applicant program; so that members of the team have the training and experience necessary to assess the transplant-related services and activities performed by the applicant. The on-site inspection is coordinated by the FACT office staff. At the conclusion of the on-site inspection, the inspection team members summarize the findings for the program director and other facility personnel, emphasizing that the final accreditation decision will be made by the FACT Board of Directors. A written report of the observations by the inspection team is submitted to the FACT office as soon as possible after the on-site inspection, including any documents collected on-site, the completed checklist and a report of all citations observed.

4 *Review.* The FACT technical staff will review the inspectors' report and all submitted documents, prepare a summary report, and present this report to the FACT Board of Directors. The Board will review and discuss the inspection report at its next meeting, and assign an accreditation level based upon its determination of the program's compliance with FACT Standards. The possible accreditation levels are listed in Table 41.2. FACT staff will assist those programs that were not fully in compliance with FACT Standards after initial inspection to correct any deficiencies cited, to document these corrections and to achieve full accreditation. Programs in compliance with FACT Standards will be accredited for 3 years.

5 *Annual report.* All accredited programs and facilities report annually on the changes made within their program, the number of transplants performed in the previous 12 months and any significant changes in personnel, location or complexity of service.

6 *Accreditation renewal.* Between 6 and 9 months prior to the expiration of accreditation, each accredited program will receive information and documents from the FACT Accreditation Office to begin the application for accreditation renewal. The renewal process is essentially identical to initial accreditation. The applicable Standards will be the edition that is current at the time of the on-site inspection.

The goal of the accreditation process is to raise the bar of performance for all HCT programs and the support services that contribute to the activities, in the expectation that these improvements will lead to better patient outcomes. It is not the goal to be punitive, but rather to be educational and helpful to enable capable and committed personnel to achieve accreditation. Assessments by peers and experts in the field contribute to the ability of FACT to accomplish this goal.

The first FACT on-site inspection occurred in September 1997 and the first accreditation was awarded in March 1998. Since that time, over 200 programs have submitted initial applications for accreditation and over

Table 41.2 Foundation for the Accreditation of Cellular Therapy (FACT) Accreditation Program: potential inspection outcomes. Copyright (2003), FACT.

Level	Description
1	No deficiencies or variances from recommendation observed at the on-site inspection or documented on submitted materials. Full accreditation for 3 years awarded effective on the date of the Board decision
2	Few minor deficiencies and/or variances from recommendation noted at the on site inspection and/or documented on the submitted materials. Full accreditation can be awarded upon written documentation by the Program Director of correction of all deficiencies and a satisfactory response to all variances from recommendation. The Chairperson of the Accreditation Program may determine the adequacy of the facility's response and award full accreditation without further Board deliberation. Incomplete or unsatisfactory responses may be referred back to the Board
3	Significant deficiency or deficiencies with or without variances from recommendations documented at the site inspection. Full accreditation requires the Program Director's documentation of correction of all deficiencies and satisfactory response to recommendations. The Board of Directors will review the facility's documentation and responses prior to making the decision regarding accreditation. The Board may require reinspection of all or part of a program or facility based upon the responses submitted
4	Significant deficiency or deficiencies observed at the on site inspection, primarily involving one or two areas in the Hematopoietic Progenitor Cell (HPC) Program (clinical, collection, laboratory) or one area (collection or laboratory) of the applicant Cord Blood Bank (CBB). Full accreditation requires correction of all deficiencies, written documentation of these corrections, a satisfactory response to all variances and recommendations, and satisfactory completion of a focused reinspection of the one or two areas where excessive deficiencies were noted. Unless specifically requested, the same inspector(s) will be responsible to conduct the focused reinspection. The results of the focused reinspection will be reviewed by the Board of Directors, who will determine the accreditation status of the program
5	Significant deficiencies observed during the on site inspection involving all three areas of an applicant HPC Program or both areas of an applicant CBB. Full accreditation requires correction of all deficiencies, written documentation of these corrections, a satisfactory response to all variances and recommendations, and satisfactory completion of a focused reinspection of all areas of the applicant program or facility. Full Board review of the reinspection results and the submitted documentation is required prior to accreditation
6	Non-accreditation. Reapplication and submission of *all* documents required

100 programs have been accredited. Over 300 inspectors have been trained at one or more of 11 North American Training Workshops. Additionally, cord blood bank inspectors have been trained at three International Training Workshops and several cord blood bank on-site inspections have been completed.

In the FACT accreditation process, observations made at the on-site inspection are recorded on the checklist and are determined to be in compliance with Standards or not in compliance. A deficiency is the failure to comply with a mandatory requirement, stated in FACT Standards as "shall". A variance from recommendation is the failure to follow a recommended practice, stated in FACT Standards as "should."

The inspection summaries of the 145 programs or facilities inspected under the first edition of FAHCT (now FACT) *Standards for Hematopoietic Progenitor Cell Collection, Processing & Transplantation* [22] were reviewed by the FACT Accreditation Office to determine the most frequently cited deficiencies and variances from recommendation. This review included only the initial inspection results for these programs, although several accreditation renewal inspections were also performed under this first edition. The results from the first 76 programs have been published [29].

The most common deficiencies cited across all areas of the HCT programs were deficiencies related to standard operating procedures (SOPs), both in format and content. In many cases, the SOPs for entire processes were absent. In addition, clinical programs frequently had deficiencies in data management, in defining and performing quality management activities and in documentation of personnel qualifications. Cell-collection facilities often had not validated processes in use, and often had elements missing in both the informed consent process and on the product collection label. Cell-processing laboratories also frequently omitted required label information. SOPs most often missing or incomplete were those for assessment of staff training and competency, microbial monitoring of products, resolution of ABO/Rh discrepancies and processes for return and reissue of previously released HC products.

The American Association of Blood Banks (AABB)

The AABB is the professional society of 8500 individuals involved in blood banking and transfusion medicine. It also represents over 2200 institutional members, including community and American Red Cross blood collection centers, hospital-based blood banks, transfusion services and cell processing laboratories that collect, process, distribute and transfuse blood components and HC products [30]. The AABB has a long history of standard-setting activity, having published its first edition of *Standards for a Transfusion Service* in 1958, the same year when it began its program of on-site inspections and accreditation. Approximately 160 programs involved in HC collection or processing worldwide have been accredited by the AABB.

The AABB has current standards for hematopoietic progenitor cells and a separate volume dedicated to cord blood services [31,32]. AABB Standards documents are based upon a quality management framework. All Standards within the documents are of equal importance. Each Standard is stated once; then it applies throughout. The quality management Standards, combined with the technical requirements, form the total requirements of AABB. Although very different in structure, the content of AABB Standards for HC services parallels the FACT Standards as published in the first edition of FAHCT (now FACT) *Standards for Hematopoietic Progenitor Cell Collection, Processing & Transplantation* [22].

The National Marrow Donor Program (NMDP)

The NMDP was founded in 1987 as a cooperative effort of the AABB, the American Red Cross, the Council of Community Blood Centers and the US Navy to facilitate volunteer, unrelated donor marrow transplantation. It is comprised of a network of cooperating facilities, including transplant centers, donor centers, marrow collection centers, apheresis centers, cord blood banks, recruitment groups, cooperative donor registries, contract laboratories and cell and serum repositories. The Health Resources and Services Administration (HRSA) has regulatory authority over the NMDP. Since its inception, NMDP has established Standards for membership participation. A Standards Committee composed of experts in various aspects of transplantation is in place to provide continuous review and revision of these Standards. NMDP Standards cover cells obtained from marrow, peripheral blood and umbilical cord blood. The Standards include Standards for participating centers and groups, personnel qualifications, required support services, policy and procedure requirements, confidentiality, recruitment of the unrelated donor, donor medical and laboratory screening and testing, informed consent, donation and transplant process, a few collection, packaging, labeling and processing Standards, and records requirements. NMDP Standards also cover the informed consent process, standards for progenitor cell packaging, labeling and transportation, quality control and patient rights. Standards for laboratory processing are not as detailed as those of FACT or AABB, since most of the processing laboratories and the procedures performed are an integral part of the recipient's transplant program. Oversight of investigational procedures is from the Institutional Review Board, the FDA, if applicable, and FACT or AABB if the program participates. NMDP Standards are intended to serve the discrete function of qualifying groups, centers and banks for participation in the registry. NMDP Standards include standards for quality assessment and improvement, and are generously supplemented by operational policies and procedures of the registry.

Conclusions

In this era of rapid advances in cellular therapies, both regulations and voluntary standards will coexist and, hopefully, improve the safety and efficacy of such therapies. Historically, HC standards were limited to laboratory practices and the reporting of transfusion-related toxicities. Hematopoietic engraftment, the duration of cytopenias, the frequency of concomitant infections, and the incidence and severity of GVHD and similar outcomes are now considered essential components of the hematopoietic graft performance. In this new era, appropriate standards in this field are critical to ensure quality patient care. Inappropriate practice of HC therapies will limit their future application in the treatment of life-threatening illnesses and slow scientific advancement in HCT.

References

1 Gratwohl A, Baldomero H, Horisberger B, Schmid C, Passweg J, Urbano-Ispizua A. Current trends in hematopoietic stem cell transplantation in Europe. *Blood* 2002; **100**: 2374–86.

2 Marks DI, Lush R, Cavenagh J *et al.* The toxicity and efficacy of donor lymphocyte infusions given after reduced-intensity conditioning allogeneic stem cell transplantation. *Blood* 2002; **100**: 3108–14.

3 Shpall EJ, Cagnoni PJ, Bearman SI *et al.* Peripheral blood stem cells for autografting. *Annu Rev Med* 1997; **48**: 241–51.

4 Couban S, Simpson DR, Barnett MJ *et al.* A randomized multicenter comparison of bone marrow and peripheral blood in recipients of matched sibling allogeneic transplants for myeloid malignancies. *Blood* 2002; **100**: 1525–31.

5 Flowers MED, Parker PM, Johnston LJ *et al.* Comparison of chronic graft-versus-host disease after transplantation of peripheral blood stem cells versus bone marrow in allogeneic recipients: long-term follow-up of a randomized trial. *Blood* 2002; **100**: 415–9.

6 McGlave PB, Shu XO, Wen W *et al.* Unrelated donor marrow transplantation for chronic myelogenous leukemia: 9 years' experience of the National Marrow Donor Program. *Blood* 2000; **95**: 2219–25.

7 Petersdorf EW, Hansen JA, Martin PJ *et al.* Major-histocompatibility-complex class I alleles and antigens in hematopoietic-cell transplantation. *N Engl J Med* 2001; **345**: 1794–800.

8 Henslee-Downey PJ, Abhyankar SH, Parrish RS *et al.* Use of partially mismatched related donors extends access to allogeneic marrow transplant. *Blood* 1997; **89**: 3864–72.

9 Kurtzberg J, Laughlin M, Graham ML *et al.* Placental blood as a source of hematopoietic stem cells for transplantation into unrelated recipients. *N Engl J Med* 1996; **335**: 157–66.

10 Wagner JE, Barker JN, DeFor TE *et al.* Transplantation of unrelated donor umbilical cord blood in 102 patients with malignant and nonmalignant diseases: influence of CD34 cell dose and HLA disparity on treatment-related mortality and survival. *Blood* 2002; **100**: 1611–8.

11 Kessinger A, Armitage JO, Landmark JD *et al.* Autologous peripheral hematopoietic stem cell transplantation restores hematopoietic function following marrow ablative therapy. *Blood* 1988; **71**: 723–7.

12 Juttner C, To LB. Peripheral blood stem cells: mobilization by myelosuppressive chemotherapy. In: Dicke KA, Armitage JO, Dicke-Evinger MJ, eds. *Proceedings of the 5th International Symposium on Autologous Bone Marrow Transplant*. Omaha, NE: University of Nebraska Press, 1991: 783–8.

13 Siena S, Bregni M, Brando B *et al.* Flow cytometry for clinical estimation of circulating hematopoietic progenitors for autologous transplantation in cancer patients. *Blood* 1991; **77**: 400–6.

14 Food and Drug Administration Health and Human Services. Interim rule for human tissue intended for transplantation. *Federal Register* December 14, 1993; **58**: 65,514–21.

15 Food and Drug Administration Health and Human Services. Human tissue for transplantation. Final rule. *Federal Register* July 29, 1997; **62**: 40,429–47.

16 Food and Drug Administration Health and Human Services. A proposed approach to the regulation of cellular and tissue-based products. *Federal Register* March 4, 1997; **62**: 9721–2.

17 Food and Drug Administration Health and Human Services. Human cells, tissues, and cellular and tissue-based products; establishment registration and listing. Final rule. *Federal Register* January 19, 2001; **66**: 5447–69.

18 Food and Drug Administration Health and Human Services. Suitability determination for donors of human cellular and tissue-based products. *Federal Register* September 30, 1999; **64**: 52,696–723.

19 Food and Drug Administration Health and Human Services. Current good tissue practice for manufacturers of human cellular and tissue-based products; inspection and enforcement. *Federal Register* January 8, 2001; **66**: 1508–59.

20 Ciavarella D, Linden JV. The regulation of hematopoietic stem cell collection and storage: the New York State approach. *J Hemather* 1992; **1**: 201–14.

21 Linden JV, Preti RA, Dracker R. New York State Guidelines for cord blood banking. *J Hemather* 1997; **6**: 535–41.

22 Foundation for the Accreditation of Hematopoietic Cell Therapy. *Standards for Hematopoietic Progenitor Cell Collection, Processing & Transplantation*, 1st edn. Omaha, NE: Foundation for the Accreditation of Hematopoietic Cell Therapy, 1996.

23 Foundation for the Accreditation of Hematopoietic Cell Therapy. *Accreditation Manual*. Omaha, NE: Foundation for the Accreditation of Hematopoietic Cell Therapy, 1996.

24 NETCORD/Foundation for the Accreditation of Hematopoietic Cell Therapy. *International Standards for Cord Blood Processing, Testing, Banking, Selection and Release*, 1st edn. Omaha, NE: NETCORD and the Foundation for the Accreditation of Cellular Therapy, 2000.

25 NETCORD/Foundation for the Accreditation of Cellular Therapy. *International Standards for Cord Blood Processing, Testing, Banking, Selection and Release*, 2nd edn. Omaha, NE: NETCORD and the Foundation for the Accreditation of Cellular Therapy, 2002.

26 Kvalheim G, Urbano-Ispizua A, Gratwohl A. FAHCT-JACIE workshop on accreditation for blood and marrow progenitor cell processing, collection and transplantation. Barcelona, Spain. *Cytotherapy* 2000; **2**: 223–4.

27 Joint Accreditation Committee of ISHAGE-Europe, EBMT. Standards for blood and marrow progenitor cell processing, collection and transplantation. *Cytotherapy* 2000; **2**: 225–46.

28 Foundation for the Accreditation of Cellular Therapy. *Standards for Hematopoietic Progenitor Cell Collection, Processing & Transplantation*, 2nd edn. Omaha, NE: Foundation for the Accreditation of Cellular Therapy, 2002.

29 Warkentin PI, Nick L, Shpall EJ. FAHCT accreditation: common deficiencies during on-site inspections. *Cytotherapy* 2000; **2**: 213–20.

30 Warkentin PI. Regulations and standards for hematopoietic progenitor cell facilities. In: Snyder EL, Haley NR, eds. *Hematopoietic Progenitor Cells: a Primer for Medical Professionals*. Bethesda, MD: AABB Press, 2000: 210–20.

31 American Association of Blood Banks. *Standards for Hematopoietic Progenitor Cell and Cellular Product Services*, 3rd edn. Bethesda, MD: American Association of Blood Banks, 2002.

32 American Association of Blood Banks. *Standards for Cord Blood Services*, 1st edn. Bethesda, MD: American Association of Blood Banks, 2001.

42

Dennis L. Confer

Hematopoietic Cell Donors

Introduction

Hematopoietic cell (HC) donors provide bone marrow or peripheral blood hematopoietic cells (PBHCs) for more than 15,000 allogeneic hematopoietic cell transplantation (HCT) recipients annually [1]. Donations from related allogeneic HC donors continue to outnumber those from unrelated donors by 3 : 1, even though at least 70% of HCT candidates lack HLA-matched sibling donors. The less frequent application of unrelated donor HCT is not from lack of suitable donors or available cord blood units. There are currently more than 8 million registered volunteer unrelated HC donors and 110,000 cord blood units available worldwide [2]. The less frequent use on unrelated donor HCs in part reflects differing opinions about the indications for allogeneic transplantation using HLA-matched sibling donors, unrelated donors and cord blood units.

Bone marrow was until recently the most common source for allogeneic HCT [3,4], but in recent years use of PBHCs has increased dramatically. Data from the International Bone Marrow Transplant Registry (IBMTR) show that between 1998 and 2000 PBHCs comprised 40% of related donor HCT grafts [1]. In July of 1999, the National Marrow Donor Program (NMDP) launched an investigational protocol for PBHC products from unrelated HC donors. As of September 2002, more than 1600 PBHC transplants had been facilitated by the NMDP. As of the end of 2002, 40% of NMDP-facilitated transplants used PBHC products.

This chapter discusses the evaluation of HC donors, the risks and side-effects of donation, and the logistics of HC collections. Cord blood, which represents an important evolving source of HCs for transplantation, and cord blood donors are discussed in Chapter 43.

Evaluation of HC donors

Prior to HC donation, donors must be evaluated to ensure that: (i) their HCs will be safe for the recipient; (ii) they can safely donate; and (iii) they fully understand what they are being asked to do [5–7].

Assessing the risks for transmitting disease to the recipient

There are numerous infectious diseases that if present in the HC donor would pose definite or theoretical risk to the transplant recipient. It is clear that HCs can transmit many of the same infections that are transmissible by blood transfusion including hepatitis B virus (HBV), hepatitis C virus (HCV) and human immunodeficiency virus (HIV). In addition, some congenital or acquired conditions in the donor, such as genetic defects and immune system abnormalities, may be potentially transmissible to the recipient.

Minimizing the risk of disease transmission requires combining the information obtained from a targeted behavioral/medical history, a search for the physical signs of disease and the results of laboratory testing for specific pathogens [8].

HC donors, similar to blood donors, should complete a written questionnaire which has been specifically designed to elicit medical history and identify behaviors or activities that may increase the risk of infectious disease transmission [5–8]. Questions regarding sexual behaviors, nonprescription drug use and skin-breaching procedures, such as tattooing and piercing, are included, as well as questions to assess residence in regions where exposure to malaria or the agent of bovine spongiform encephalopathy (BSE) may occur. The donor-screening questionnaire is intended to detect information that may place the transplant recipient at increased risk for transplantation-transmissible diseases. Testing of the donor's blood cannot substitute for direct questioning because blood tests may be falsely negative and, more importantly, testing does not include all potentially transmissible diseases. Indeed, suitable screening blood tests for some disorders, such as the West Nile Virus, Creutzfeldt–Jakob disease and variant Creutzfeldt–Jakob disease, do not currently exist. Positive responses on a proper donor-screening questionnaire may lead to donor disqualification or, at a minimum, careful donor evaluations and a thorough assessment of risk vs. benefit. Decisions to proceed with donors who may present increased risk to their recipients are discussed later in this section.

The donor physical examination, also discussed in greater detail below (see History and physical section), should detect behavioral and experiential stigmata, such as recent tattoos, piercings, illicit drug use, etc., as well as signs of significant illnesses. In addition, a sample of the donor's blood must be tested for at least the following infectious diseases: HIV 1 and 2, HBV, HCV, *Treponema pallidum*, human T-cell lymphotropic virus 1 and 2 (HTLV 1 & 2) and cytomegalovirus (CMV). The results of this testing must be available and reviewed prior to the initiation of preparative conditioning therapy for the recipient [6,7]. Repeat testing may be necessary closer to donation or at the time of donation to minimize the window period between a new exposure and seroconversion [8]. It is also desirable to perform testing for prior infections with varicella-zoster virus, Epstein–Barr virus and possibly others, such as toxoplasmosis.

Donors with a confirmed positive test for HIV must not donate. Donors with prior exposure to HBV and HCV may be used when there are no suitable alternatives and the potential gain outweighs the risk. Strategies for managing hepatitis exposure in donors and recipients have been reviewed [9]. When antibodies to HCV are detected, polymerase chain reaction (PCR) testing may be performed to detect circulating HCV RNA [10]. Failure to detect RNA, however, does not ensure absence of HCV transmission to the marrow recipient. In one instance, interferon-alpha pretreatment of a marrow donor apparently prevented transmission of HCV to the recipient [11]. These issues are fully discussed in Chapter 58.

Donors who have recovered from HBV infection may safely donate marrow [12]. HCT recipients with active HBV infections may, in fact, benefit from transplantation with a donor who shows evidence of hepatitis B immunity [13–18]. Further, it may be that natural immunity, reflecting recovery from HBV infection, is more likely to benefit the transplant recipient than vaccination-related immunity [18]. Transplant recipients whose donors are positive for hepatitis BsAg, however, are at high risk for post-transplant hepatic complications and transplant-related mortality [19,20].

CMV seronegative recipients may benefit from having CMV seronegative donors, but this is a controversial issue. An analysis of data from the NMDP recently showed that, although recipients who are CMV seropositive have poorer outcomes, donor CMV status has no impact on transplant outcome [21]. It has been suggested that CMV seropositive patients may benefit from CMV seropositive donors [22]. A study of chronic myeloid leukemia (CML) recipients showed that those with seropositive donors experienced a more rapid rise of high avidity anti-CMV antibodies following transplant [23]. CMV seropositive recipients with seronegative donors had a slower rise of anti-CMV antibodies, which were initially of low avidity. CMV-related issues are further discussed in Chapter 53.

Assessing the risks to the donor

HC donation is not without risk. As described below, adverse events are uniformly encountered, but these are generally minor and short-lived (see The risks and adverse events associated with HC donation section below). Serious adverse events, including death, may, however, occur. It is essential that prior to donation each donor is assessed to ensure the absence of conditions that might increase donor risk to unacceptable levels.

History and physical

The donor receives a medical history and physical examination appropriate for the anticipated donation procedure. The history, which addresses risk to the donor, as opposed to the screening history described above, should focus on matters relevant for the anticipated donation, including the psychological issues addressed below. For all donors, these would include a review of known health problems, a listing of medication and allergies, and review of the family history. Marrow donors should be questioned about prior surgical procedures and types of anesthesia received. Marrow donors should also have a careful review of systems directed toward neurological, respiratory, cardiovascular and musculoskeletal problems. PBHC donors should be questioned about prior whole blood or apheresis donations. The review of systems for PBHC donors should include a careful cardiovascular and neurological review as well as specific questions about a history of venous access problems, autoimmune diseases and splenic disorders.

The donor's physical examination should focus upon the neurological, respiratory and cardiovascular systems. In addition, marrow donors need an assessment of the oral airways and an evaluation of access to the iliac crests. Among obese donors, the ease of palpating the posterior, superior iliac spine varies widely. Donors with a history of musculoskeletal symptoms need a careful examination of the spine and lower extremities. The examination of PBHC donors should additionally include evaluation of venous access and an abdominal examination for splenomegaly.

It is important to recognize that the history and physical examination of HC donors is not a comprehensive evaluation. Routine health care screening, e.g. fecal blood testing, PAP smears, mammograms, etc., is irrelevant for HC donations. Donors who are delinquent with their general health care should be advised to visit their personal physician or clinic.

Psychological aspects of marrow donation

The psychological condition of the donor should be assessed. In particular, what are the donor's motivations for considering the HC donation? Is the donor acting out of a genuine desire to help, or are there other motives involved—perhaps an unrealistic expectation of reward or personal gain?

Switzer et al. [24] interviewed 343 unrelated marrow donors predonation, then immediately and one year post-donation. They determined that donor motives could be classified into six categories and that an individual donor might express motives in more than one category. The most common motives were "exchange-related," that is, where the donor is conducting an analysis of risk vs. benefit. "Idealized-helping" motives describes motives based on a more or less spontaneous response to help, not unlike the Good Samaritan. Idealized-helping motives are relatively superficial and much less deep-seated than "normative motives," which create the conviction that there is no doubt about the decision to donate. Normative motives may be founded on religious beliefs or personal values. "Positive-feeling" motives are those that directly benefit the donor because the donor believes their personal self-worth is enhanced by the donation. In contrast, "empathy-related" motives are based upon the donor's concern about the recipient. Finally, "past-experience motives" arise from the donor's personal experiences. Switzer et al. [24] determined that positive-feeling and empathy-based motives were more common among women. Positive-feeling motives also predicted low levels of predonation ambivalence, while higher ambivalence resulted from exchange-related (cost/benefit) motives. Idealized-helping motives, which are simplistic, were associated with both psychological and physical difficulties post-donation.

Related donors may have different motivations and may be subject to increased emotional and physical stress associated with donation [25,26]. Discussions of the psychological issues affecting donors post-donation are presented in Chapter 38.

Occasionally donors may be subjected to coercion [27,28]. In the United Kingdom, a potential donor's unwillingness to donate for her sister attracted media attention forcing the donor to reconsider her decision [27]. Switzer et al. [24] have reported that unrelated donors who feel they were pressured, either encouraged or discouraged about donation, are less likely to have a positive donation experience. In an early report of unrelated donors, nine of 20 reported being discouraged from donation by a relative or a friend [29].

Children who are being evaluated as potential marrow donors deserve special attention. Their fears and concerns may be complex and accompanied by significant ambivalence [30,31].

Laboratory and procedural evaluations of donors

The laboratory evaluation of all HC donors should include the following: complete blood count with white blood cell differential, serum electrolytes, alanine aminotransferase (ALT), bilirubin, creatinine or blood urea nitrogen (BUN), total serum protein and albumin [7]. PBHC donors should also have determinations of alkaline phosphatase (AP) and lactate dehydrogenase (LDH). Some physicians will also recommend evaluations of immunoglobulin levels and a screen for monoclonal proteins in the blood [32]. Additional evaluations of donors may include urinalysis, chest X-ray and electrocardiogram (ECG).

HC donors whose intended recipients suffer from inherited conditions, such as hemoglobinopathies or inborn errors of metabolism, may require specific testing to rule out carrier states that could affect transplant outcome. Donors with sickle cell trait and thalassemia minor can serve as donors in successful bone marrow transplants [33]. As discussed below, however, donors with S-β thalassemia, SC or other complex sickle hemoglobinopathies should not receive recombinant human granulocyte colony-stimulating factor (RHuG-CSF). Successful transplantation from a donor with hemoglobin H disease has also been reported [34]. Barquinero et al. [35] suggested that marrow donors with trisomy 21 and Fanconi syndrome heterozygotes may be less suitable. Case reports describe successful transplants from donors with severe rheumatoid arthritis, systemic lupus erythematosis and classical hemophilia [36–38].

A pregnancy assessment must be performed for female donors with childbearing potential [6,7]. Pregnancy is usually considered a contraindication to marrow donation; however, successful marrow collection from a pregnant donor at 26 weeks gestation has been reported [39]. Pregnant women cannot be PBHC donors as hematopoietic growth-factor administration is contraindicated. One PBHC donor has been reported, however, who inadvertently received filgrastim while 2 weeks pregnant without any adverse impact on the pregnancy or delivery [40].

Ethical and legal aspects of donation

Donor consent for HC donation

HC donors must provide written consent prior to donation [6,7]. The model of informed consent for research, as detailed in multiple documents [41–43], is appropriate for the HC donor. Like the research subject, the HC donor is a volunteer who must be provided full and complete information about their donation. This means that donors must receive a clear description of the proposed procedure, its risks and the alternatives to the procedure. They must also have the opportunity to raise questions and to have these satisfactorily addressed. Materials and programs have been developed to assist with providing donor education and information [30,44–47].

Consent for children presents special concerns. In general, children are only considered for related-donor HC donation. In most instances, parents are expected to consent for their children, which may create conflict of interest situations. A survey of pediatric transplant physicians in the USA confirmed that most felt the role of consent appropriately rested with the parents [48]. Outside the USA, "altruism by proxy" has stirred debate in the medical literature [31,49–54]. In some countries, it remains the standard practice to appoint legal guardians to determine whether HC donation is in the child's best interest. When governing law allows parents to render consent, it is incumbent on the physician, at a minimum, to recognize the potential for conflict of interest, to seek expert ethical guidance when needed, and to ensure to the extent possible that the child donor is a willing and informed participant. Children who are able should provide assent for donation [55].

Whether children can serve as unrelated HC donors is a matter of debate. The Washington State Legislature recently passed a law intended to pave the way for minors to become unrelated HC donors [56]. The law states simply, "A person's status as a minor may not disqualify him or her from bone marrow donation." This legislation was the direct result of a campaign by a 15-year-old-male who wanted to be tested as a potential donor for a young Hawaiian man with leukemia [57]. Legislation was also introduced in the 2002 Massachusetts State Legislature that would allow minors 15 years of age and older to serve as unrelated HC donors with parental consent.

HC donors as research subjects

It is important to determine the circumstances that make the HC donor a bona fide research subject. Several tests may be applied to help determine whether a particular activity constitutes research involving the HC donor. These include the following: (i) Is there collection of information for the purpose of peer-reviewed publication? (ii) Is there collection of information in support of a Food and Drug Administration (FDA) investigational new drug (IND) application or an FDA investigational device exemption (IDE)? (iii) Is there any interaction with a donor that would not be occurring in the absence of the research? Affirmative responses to any of these questions serve to define research. Examples of research wherein the HC donor becomes a research subject include the following: *ex vivo* culture or "expansion" of donor cells, insertion of new genes into donor cells, establishment of immortal donor cell lines and nonstandard genetic analysis of donor DNA. Standard genetic analysis includes, for example, DNA-based HLA typing or the identification of polymorphisms in long-terminal repeats for the purpose of assessing donor/recipient chimerism. An example of genetic research would be the identification of single nucleotide polymorphisms within particular donor genes for the purpose of assessing impact upon transplant outcomes. The complex risks and consent issues created by genetic analysis of DNA have been reviewed [58].

Finally, it is worth emphasizing that donors are research subjects when they are asked to provide HCs for patients on experimental transplant protocols where the patient could not otherwise receive a transplant were it not for the protocol. This would include allogeneic transplantation for totally new indications, e.g. lung cancer or breast cancer, and allogeneic transplantation with a new preparative regimen wherein patients are only eligible for the new regimen if they are ineligible for standard regimens. In both of these situations, the HC donation, even if it is a standard donation, is occurring because of the research protocol.

The risks and adverse events associated with HC donation

An adverse event is any untoward medical occurrence [59]. Serious adverse events are those adverse events that pose a threat to the individual's life or functioning. Serious adverse events include, at a minimum, those adverse events that are (i) fatal; (ii) immediately life threatening; (iii) require or prolong hospitalization; (iv) result in a significant or persistent disability; (v) represent a new cancer; or (vi) represent a congenital anomaly [59]. Both marrow and PBHC donations are associated with adverse events. Fortunately, serious adverse events are not common.

Adverse events associated with marrow donation

Marrow donors routinely experience minor adverse events [60–63]. In a review of 1270 related-donor marrow collections in Seattle, it was reported that all donors experienced some component of pain [61]. Stroncek et al. [63] reviewed the experiences of the first 493 unrelated marrow donors in the NMDP. When surveyed 2 days after donation, 75% reported fatigue, 68% had pain at the collection site and 52% were reporting lower back pain. In a 2001 analysis of 9601 NMDP marrow collections, reported by donor sex, are shown in Table 42.1. Women report more adverse events in general. Only bandage pain is reported more often in men. Older donors report significantly fewer adverse events related to pain, nausea, lightheadedness and vomiting. Fever is more likely to be reported by older donors.

Not surprisingly, in the NMDP experience some adverse events are dependent upon how the collection procedure is performed. For example, regarding the type of anesthesia, general anesthesia was administered in 78% of cases, epidural anesthesia in 15% and spinal anesthesia in 7%. Nausea, vomiting and sore throat are all significantly more common following general anesthesia than following regional anesthesia; whereas fever and fainting are less likely to occur. Similar results were seen in a small controlled study [64].

Observations among unrelated donors may not apply to related marrow donors. In a Seattle study of post-donation pain, male donors tended to report more pain and used more codeine-containing analgesics than did

Table 42.1 Symptoms reported by National Marrow Donor Program (NMDP) bone marrow donors, 1987–2000 (n = 9601).

Symptom	Women (4106) (%)	Men (5495) (%)
Tired*	85	76
Collection site pain*	78	75
Back pain	67	68
Nausea*	63	40
Sore throat*	62	57
Pain sitting*	62	57
Lightheadedness*	53	42
Headache*	40	32
Vomiting*	39	17
Intravenous site pain*	37	23
Fever	22	22
Bandage pain*	19	26
Bleeding at site*	10	8
Fainting*	7	5

*$p < 0.05$ between men and women.

Table 42.2 Major bone marrow donor complications reported to the International Bone Marrow Transplant Registry (IBMTR), 1980–89 (n = 8296). Source: IBMTR, M.M. Horowitz.

Complication	No. of reports
Myocardial infarction	3
Severe anemia	3
Anaphylaxis during anesthesia	2
Prolonged paralysis after anesthesia	2
Pulmonary embolism	2
Severe back pain	2
Acute renal failure from incompatible blood transfusion	1
Anaphylaxis from incompatible blood transfusion	1
Hepatitis B virus infection	1
Intervertebral disk prolapse	1
Malignant hyperthermia	1
Paroxysmal tachycardia	1
Pulmonary edema	1
Retroperitoneal hematoma	1
Severe hypotension during anesthesia	1
Severe vasovagal reaction	1

female donors [62]. This study also concluded that pain relief was incomplete with acetaminophen plus codeine, and that donors might benefit from more potent narcotic analgesics.

Stroncek et al. [63] examined how side-effects and recovery varied with respect to marrow volume collected, duration of the marrow collection and duration of anesthesia. The total marrow volume removed, measured as milliliter per kilogram of donor weight, was only modestly correlated with most symptoms. The duration of the marrow collection procedure, which reflects not only the volume collected but also the ease of the collection, was the single factor most strongly correlated with increased frequencies of immediate and delayed symptoms, and with longer time to complete recovery. Longer collections increased the frequency of symptoms and prolonged recovery. Sixty-three percent of the 493 NMDP donors reported complete recovery, as defined by the donor, within 14 days. An additional 24% recovered between 2 weeks and 1 month, but 13% of donors took more than a month until they felt fully recovered.

Minor complications occur in 6–20% of marrow donations [61,63,65]. These include such events as hypotension, syncope, severe post-spinal headache, excess pain, unexpected hospitalization and minor infections. By definition, these complications resolve within a few to several days of onset.

Laboratory and radiological abnormalities also accompany marrow donation. Anemia is the most significant laboratory finding. The severity of anaemia is determined entirely by the donor's preoperative hemoglobin level and the net blood loss, which is calculated by subtracting the red cell volume transfused from that removed. Marrow harvesting also causes significant, but transient, elevations in serum AP and ostoecalcin [66]. X-rays, computerized tomography (CT) scans and radionuclide scans disclose abnormalities in the pelvis and sacrum that may persist for weeks or months [67].

Serious adverse events following marrow donation

The frequency of serious adverse events following marrow donation is estimated at 0.1–0.3%. A review of data collected between 1969 and 1983 on 2248 allogeneic marrow donations reported to the IBMTR and 1160 additional donations occurring in Seattle revealed nine total incidents (0.27%) [68]. These included one case of aspiration pneumonia, two cases of deep vein thrombosis (including one occurrence of pulmonary embolism), three serious bacterial infections (including two with bacteremia), two instances of serious cardiac arrhythmia and one case of cerebral infarction.

The IBMTR data were updated in 1991 in an examination of 8296 allogeneic donations occurring between 1980 and 1989 (M.M. Horowitz, personal communication). Twenty-four instances of life-threatening or incapacitating complications were identified for an incidence of 0.29% (Table 42.2). In a review of the first 493 NMDP marrow donors, only one case was identified with a potential life-threatening complication (apnea and bradycardia) (0.2%) [63].

The NMDP has classified major and/or life-threatening complications into five risk categories: (i) anesthesia, (ii) infection, (iii) mechanical injury, (iv) transfusion and (v) others.

Anesthesia risks

These are related to procedures employed and the agents administered. Rarely do significant complications accompany procedures such as intravenous line insertion, endotracheal intubation and lumbar puncture. Reactions to the anesthetic agents administered may be adverse reactions, hypersensitivity reactions or idiosyncratic reactions. One NMDP donor experienced laryngospasm following extubation that required urgent treatment and several hours of mechanical ventilation. Recovery was prompt and complete. Additionally, several NMDP donors have experienced profound bradycardia during anesthesia, including regional anesthesia (spinal or epidural), that required emergency treatment. In each case recovery was prompt and complete. In no case was the marrow collection aborted.

Five serious cases of potential anesthetic complications, including hypotension, hypoxia or cardiac arrest, were identified among 1549 marrow donors at Seattle [65], who were not included in earlier reports [61,68]. A marrow donor who developed life-threatening malignant hyperthermia has also been reported [69].

Infection risks

Infections may occur at the sites of marrow collection or line insertions. Infections at distant sites, for example pneumonia, have also been reported [68]. Infections frequently require prompt therapy with antibiotics, which may themselves produce adverse reactions, hypersensitivity reactions or idiosyncratic reactions. Serious infections have been rare in the NMDP experience. One donor developed bacterial sepsis shortly after marrow donation. The medical literature also contains additional reports of serious infections following marrow collection [61,68]. Two cases of osteomyelitis have been reported following marrow collection [65,70].

Mechanical injury risks

The procedure of marrow collection (described below) may lead to local tissue injuries. These may include bone damage, nerve damage or entry of a collection needle into a blood vessel, an organ or the spinal canal. Hemorrhage, which may be delayed, can create severe pain from compression of soft tissues [71]. NMDP donors have experienced significant injuries to bone and nerve tissues, which have required medical and physical therapy lasting weeks or months. Sciatic pain lasting up to 18 months has been reported in a related marrow donor [61]. One NMDP donor has had an operation intended to correct an injury to the sacroiliac joint. Prolonged and significant pain may occur following marrow collection, leading to permanent disabilities.

Fractures of the iliac crests have also been reported among non-NMDP donors [61,72]. Visceral injuries are apparently very rare, although a case of retroperitoneal hematoma has been reported to the IBMTR (Table 42.2).

Transfusion risks

Neither autologous nor allogeneic blood transfusion is free of serious risks. Allogeneic transfusions may cause transfusion reactions, transmit viral infections and, rarely, transmit bacterial infections. The IBMTR analysis (Table 42.2) included a case of HBV transmission and two cases of incompatible blood transfusion.

Autologous blood has largely replaced allogeneic blood for transfusion of both related and unrelated marrow donors. Buckner et al. [61], describing the Seattle experience through 1983, reported allogeneic blood transfusions in 21% of 1135 related marrow donors. Allogeneic blood was more often used in women (35%) and in children under the age of 10 years (38%). Among 23 infants under the age of 2 years whose marrow was harvested between 1975 and 1986, 22 received allogeneic blood transfusions [73]. In an update of the Seattle experience, only 10% of 1126 adult donors with autologous blood stored required allogeneic blood transfusions [65].

Most NMDP donors receive autologous blood transfusions [63]. NMDP Standards prohibit the administration of allogeneic blood except in emergencies [7]. Units of autologous blood are collected from NMDP donors according to the planned nucleated cell dose for the recipient. More than 85% of NMDP donors receive autologous blood transfusions. Among 6277 NMDP marrow collections, allogeneic blood was administered in only 16 instances (0.25%). In seven of these, transfusion of allogeneic blood was probably avoidable.

Another strategy for avoiding allogeneic transfusion is to recover autologous red cells from the collected bone marrow. This process has been successfully applied in children donors without compromising the quality of the marrow product [74].

Administration of epoetin alfa (recombinant human erythropoietin [RHuEPO]) may also diminish the likelihood of allogeneic blood transfusion following marrow donation [75,76]. Among 10 donors in Seattle, including two children under 6 years of age, who were treated preoperatively with epoetin alfa at 100 U/kg daily for 9–22 days, post-donation hematocrits declined an average of 3% (predonation hematocrit normalized to 100%, range: −6.9 to +6.7) [75]. No donor required an allogeneic blood transfusion. A theoretical concern about pretreatment of donors with epoetin alfa is diminished quality of the collected marrow. In this study, all nine evaluable recipients engrafted without apparent problems. Similar results were reported in a smaller study from Japan [76].

Other risks

Fat embolism has been documented following marrow donation [77]. An unusual case of small bowel mechanical obstruction, which necessitated an exploratory laparotomy, has also been reported [78]. The donor had a distant history of prior intestinal obstruction following appendectomy. It was postulated that perhaps the prone positioning of the donor during the marrow collection had allowed an intestinal volvulus to develop. In another report, a donor with unsuspected Addison's disease experienced grand mal seizures and acute adrenal insufficiency following marrow collection [79]. A flare of systemic lupus erythematosis following marrow donation has also been reported [37].

Marrow donation and the risk of death

Death has occurred among normal marrow donors. A recent review of 7857 marrow collections reported to the IBMTR revealed two deaths [80]. Table 42.3 lists nine documented deaths occurring within a few days of HC donation [81–84]. The aforementioned cases from the IBMTR are not included in Table 42.3 because it cannot be determined whether they may represent duplicate reports. As is evident in Table 42.3, two deaths actually occurred prior to scheduled marrow donations. Whether the stress of impending donation somehow contributed to these

Table 42.3 Death occurring in association with hematopoietic cell (HC) donation.

Reference	Age (years)	Sex	HSC source	Proximity to donation	Cause of death
Blazar et al. 1986 [81]	40	M	Marrow	Prior	Cardiac arrest
D.L. Confer, pers. comm. 1994	46	M	Marrow	Prior	Cardiac arrest
U.W. Scheafer, pers. comm. 1997	57	F	Marrow	Immediate	Ventricular fibrillation
Y. Onozawa, pers. comm. 1997	35	M	Marrow	Immediate	Respiratory arrest
Martin 1988 [82]	35	F	Marrow	Immediate	Myocardial infarction
Boogaerts, pers. comm. 1997	35	M	Marrow	After	Pulmonary embolism
Adler et al. 2001 [83]	47	F	PBHCs	Immediate	Sickle crisis
Anderlini et al. 1997 [84]; J. Gajewski, pers. comm. 1997	57	F	PBHCs	After	Stroke
C. Aul & A. Heyll, pers. comm. 1997	62	F	PBHCs	After	Cardiac arrest

HSC, hematopoietic stem cell; PBHCs, peripheral blood hematopoietic cells; pers. comm, personal communication.

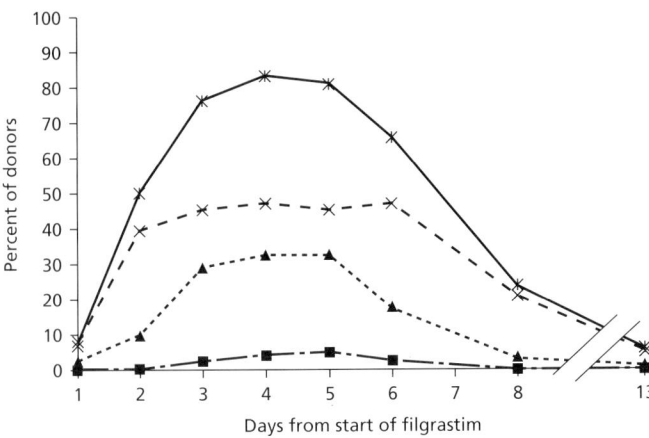

Fig. 42.1 Percentage of National Marrow Donor Program (NMDP) peripheral blood hematopoietic cell (PBHC) donors reporting bone pain during mobilization, collection and follow-up. Filgrastim was administered starting on day 1 and continuing through day 4 or 5. Bone pain was assessed prior to the filgrastim injection on each day. Filgrastim was not administered during follow-up, days 6–13. Apheresis was performed on day 5 for all donors ($n = 1084$) and on day 6 for the majority ($n = 787$). ———, Total reports; – – – –, mild pain; ----------, moderate pain; —·—·—, severe pain.

Table 42.4 Symptoms reported by National Marrow Donor Program (NMDP) peripheral blood hematopoietic cell (PBHC) donors, excluding reports of bone pain, 1997–2002.

Symptom	All donors (1080) (%)
Myalgia	54
Headache	52
Malaise	49
Insomnia	28
Nausea	15
Sweats	14
Other flu-like symptoms	12
Anorexia	11
Fever	6
Chills	6
Vomiting	2

events is unknown. Similarly, it is difficult to know whether death in the days immediately following HC donation is causally related. Overall, with an estimated 100,000 allogeneic HC donations worldwide, it appears the risk of death in proximity to the procedure is approximately 1 : 10,000.

Adverse events associated with PBHC donation

Like marrow donors, most PBHC donors will also experience adverse events. Most of these are related to the administration of hematopoietic growth factors, most commonly filgrastim (RHuG-CSF, r-metHUG-CSF), lenograstim (a glycosylated RHuG-CSF formulation, not marketed in the USA) or sargramostim (recombinant human granulocyte macrophage colony-stimulating factor [RHuGM-CSF]), that are intended to increase the concentration of HCs in the donor's blood. Rowley et al. [85] reported the experiences of 69 sibling donors who participated in a randomized comparison of bone marrow and PBHC transplantation. The frequency and intensity of symptoms between the two groups of donors was no different.

Bone pain is the most prominent adverse event among PBHC donors occurring in 25–86% of donors receiving filgrastim [86–94]. Bone pain most likely results from altered bone metabolism, which is reflected by increased bone-derived AP and decreased serum osteocalcin [95]. The pain is typically diffuse but most prominent in the spine, hips or pelvis and ribs [91]. Headache is also common, occurring in 38–70% [90,91]. The discomfort from bone pain improves with mild analgesic therapy, such as acetaminophen or a nonsteroidal anti-inflammatory drug (NSAID). Other symptoms seen with filgrastim include nausea and vomiting (~10%), myalgia (~20%), fatigue (~15%), insomnia (~10%) and injection site reactions (rare). Symptoms are probably less frequent at filgrastim doses below 10 μg/kg daily. Pain symptoms resolve promptly with discontinuation of filgrastim, and are rarely sufficient to cause premature cessation, or even dose reduction [90,91,93,94,96,97].

The NMDP has evaluated data on more than 1000 adult unrelated PBHC donors, all receiving filgrastim at 10 μg/kg/day for 4 or 5 days. Bone pain is reported by 85% of these donors and is the single most common adverse event. The pain begins after a single filgrastim injection and plateaus after two to three injections (Fig. 42.1). Bone pain resolves promptly after discontinuation of filgrastim. Additional side-effects among NMDP donors are summarized in Table 42.4.

HC mobilization with filgrastim also causes numerous alterations in serum chemistries and blood cell counts. LDH, AP and ALT increase two- to four-fold after five daily doses of filgrastim [90,91,93,94]. Anderlini et al. [90] reported that isoenzymes LDH-4 and LDH-5 comprise most of the LDH increase. Gamma glutamyl transferase levels are unaffected by filgrastim, suggesting that increased AP is not hepatic in origin. The serum levels of potassium, BUN and magnesium may show minimal declines during filgrastim treatment [91].

The white blood cell count (WBC) and, in particular, the absolute neutrophil count (ANC) increase dramatically during filgrastim therapy [90,91,93,94]. These increases are dose-dependent. At daily filgrastim doses of ≥ 10 μg/kg, the total WBC may reach $70-80 \times 10^9$/L by day 5. Eighty to ninety percent of the WBC will be neutrophils or band forms. Although leukostasis has never been reported in a PBHC donor, it is generally recommended that the filgrastim dose be reduced if the WBC exceeds $70-75 \times 10^9$/L [84,98]. In the NMDP experience, only five of 1084 donors (0.5%) receiving filgrastim at 10 μg/kg/day demonstrated WBC $>75 \times 10^9$/L in the preapheresis blood sample on day 5. The median WBC among NMDP donors preapheresis was 36.8×10^9/L with the 25th and 75th percentiles at 29.9 and 45.2×10^9/L, respectively.

A decline in platelet counts accompanies daily filgrastim administration [91,99]. Among NMDP donors the median decline from the baseline to day 5 preapheresis is modest, only 16×10^9/L. However, the range in platelet count change is large, from a decline of 156×10^9/L to an increase of 103×10^9/L. Frank thrombocytopenia (platelets $<140 \times 10^9$/L) was present in 17 of 1084 (1.6%) of NMDP donors by day 5 preapheresis. The platelet decline appears to be dose-independent and occurs even at filgrastim doses of 2 μg/kg daily [91].

The apheresis procedure (described below) used in PBHC collection is also a source of adverse events. Securing peripheral venous access at the antecubital veins may produce bruising, hematoma or minor bleeding. Anticoagulation with acid-citrate-dextrose (ACD) solution may elicit symptoms of hypocalcemia—perioral numbness, paresthesias and carpo-pedal spasms [98,100]. These symptoms may be ameliorated with oral calcium supplementation, but are more effectively managed with an intravenous infusion of calcium during apheresis. Reducing the blood flow rate may also improve symptoms of hypocalcemia, but at the expense of prolonging the collection procedure. Another approach that has been used is to supplement the anticoagulation with heparin to diminish the amount of ACD required [101].

Peripheral WBC will fall after the collection of mobilized PBHCs. Mild neutropenia is usual for a few weeks [102]. Decreases in the hemoglobin and hematocrit are minimal, although in one report hemoglobin levels decreased an average of 1.2 g/dL (range 0.3–2.2 g/dL) with each apheresis procedure [103]. Thrombocytopenia is the most consistent and significant finding with PBHC apheresis [90–92,97,99,100,103–106]. The preapheresis platelet count reproducibly declines between 20% and 30% with each collection, and does not begin to recover until 3–4 days after the last collection. Following two procedures, it is common to encounter total platelet counts below $100 \times 10^9/L$ [90,92,97,99,100,103–105]. In the NMDP experience, the incidence of thrombocytopenia $<75 \times 10^9/L$ is 1% (11 out of 1084 patients) after a single apheresis procedure (median blood volume processed of 12 L) but rises to 11% (90 out of 787 patients) after two procedures. No instances of hemorrhage secondary to thrombocytopenia have been reported. Nevertheless, avoidance of aspirin during mobilization and collection, and NSAID therapy during collection is prudent. Some authors have recommended discontinuing PBHC leukapheresis if the platelet count falls below $70–80 \times 10^9/L$ [84,98]. An alternative to discontinuation of PBHC collection is the recovery and reinfusion of platelet-rich plasma from the leukapheresis product. Each product obtained by standard technique may contain $3–5 \times 10^{11}$ total platelets, which is approximately equal to a platelet apheresis product.

Mild lymphocytopenia is routine following PBHC donation and persists for 8–10 weeks [105,107]. The cause of this lymphocytopenia has not been determined, but clinical sequelae have not been reported.

The most significant immediate problem of PBHC apheresis is inadequate venous access. Central lines to perform apheresis are required in 0–8% of collections [84,88,91,103,105]. The NMDP has tried to minimize the use of central venous lines. In spite of this, 41 of the first 395 NMDP PBHC donors required a central line. Central lines were 10 times more common among women than men (37 out of 179 women [21%] vs. four out of 216 men [2%]).

Central line complications are uncommon but include pneumothorax, hemorrhage and infection. To eliminate the risk of pneumothorax, some authors have recommended the femoral approach to central venous access for PBHC collections [98]. A disadvantage of femoral catheterization is the requirement for immobility, which, if more than one apheresis procedure is necessary, will force overnight hospitalization of the donor. Large volume leukapheresis, which involves the processing of more than three total donor blood volumes, allows the collection of large numbers of HCs in a single procedure and may be appropriate when femoral catheterization is required [100].

Serious adverse events following PBHC donation

Filgrastim administration may precipitate severe sickle crisis in persons with sickle cell anaemia or complex sickle cell hemoglobinopathies [83,108]. Indeed, a 47-year-old-woman with Hb SC disease, who had never had any symptoms from her condition, suffered a fatal sickle crisis during filgrastim mobilization of PBHCs intended for her sister with CML [83]. It remains to be clarified whether persons with sickle trait (Hb AS) are at any increased risk from filgrastim. Kang et al. [109] safely mobilized and collected PBHCs from nine donors with sickle trait. These donors did experience higher symptom scores during mobilization than did eight simultaneous control donors, but there were no symptoms suggestive of painful sickle crisis.

Spontaneous splenic rupture has been reported in two normal PBHC donors [110,111]. In both cases the spleen was surgically removed and disclosed extensive extramedullary hematopoiesis. Platzbecker et al. [112] performed ultrasound evaluations of spleen size before and after granulocyte colony-stimulating factor (G-CSF) mobilization in 91 healthy PBHC donors. Although no adverse splenic events occurred in this group, significant increases in spleen length and width were routinely documented. No donor factors or clinical findings (change in WBC, increase in AP, etc.) correlated with the degree of splenic enlargement.

Growth factor should not be given to donors with a history of autoimmune disorders [113–117]. Flares of rheumatoid arthritis and ankylosing spondylitis have been reported in non-PBHC donors following therapy with filgrastim or sargramostim [113,114]. In patients with normal thyroid function, but pre-existing antithyroid antibodies, therapy with sargramostim caused thyroid dysfunction and one case of goiter [115]. A variety of eye inflammatory responses have been reported among allogeneic PBHC donors. These have included marginal keratitis, episcleritis and iritis occurring during therapy with filgrastim [116–118].

Chest pain in association with PBHC donation is occasionally encountered and is noncardiac in origin [91,104]. However, an instance of myocardial infarction following PBHC leukapheresis has been reported [97]. The donor in this instance had a history of coronary artery disease and had previously suffered myocardial infarction. The donor recovered uneventfully, but a planned second leukapheresis procedure had to be cancelled.

The long-term safety profile of growth-factor therapy in normal individuals has not been established. There have been several reports providing 1–5 years follow-up on limited numbers of PBHC donors [92,103,119–121]. In no instance have serious adverse events attributable to filgrasim been identified. Cavallaro et al. [40] evaluated 101 PBHC or granulocyte donors who had received filgrastim between 3 and 6 years previously. Ninety-four donors were interviewed; one of the remaining had died 15 months after donation from a drug overdose and the six others could not be interviewed. Among the 94 donors, 11 had experienced adverse medical events during the follow-up period, but none of these related to the hematopoietic system. Two donors had developed cancer during the follow-up period: one breast cancer and the other prostate cancer. Anderlini et al. [122] recently reported on the follow-up of 343 PBHC donors, of whom 281 (82%) they were able to interview. With a median follow-up of 39 months (range: 7–80), there were no instances of leukemia or other hematopoietic adverse events.

PBHC donation and the risk of death

As with bone marrow donation, death at the time of, or in close proximity to, PBHC donation has been reported [83,84]. Table 42.3 lists three deaths among PBHC donors. Only one of these, the 47-year-old woman with Hb SC disease was clearly related to the PBHC donation [83]. Given the relatively limited experience with allogeneic PBHC donations, the risk of death cannot currently be estimated.

Marrow collection procedure (technique)

Marrow is typically collected from the posterior iliac crest of the donor under general or regional anesthesia [60]. The posterior superior iliac spine is the primary landmark for initiating the marrow collection. Marrow is aspirated through large bore needles into glass or plastic syringes that have been rinsed with a heparin-containing solution.

Typically the iliac crest is entered through a skin puncture or a small skin incision. Once the cortical bone has been penetrated, a small amount of marrow (5–10 mL) is aspirated by applying vigorous suction. The syringe is removed and its contents are immediately transferred to an anticoagulant solution. Commonly, the aspiration needle is then advanced several millimeters and the process repeated. Several aspirations may be obtained from a single bone puncture as the needle is repeatedly advanced. Through a single skin entry site, the bone may be entered multiple times. A typical collection may involve 200–300 marrow aspirations obtained through a few or several skin punctures/incisions. Occasionally, marrow is also collected from the anterior iliac crests or the sternum. In a report from Seattle, prior to 1983, the anterior crests were aspirated in 69% of collections and the sternum in 9% [61]. Current practice employs these supplemental sites only when the target cell dose cannot be reached by aspiration from the posterior iliac crests. This may occur if the marrow space of the crest has been compromised by trauma, radiation or some other insult.

The aspiration of marrow produces an admixture of marrow cells from the bone cavity and capillary blood. The ratio of marrow to blood depends upon the technique employed. Short, vigorous aspirations are generally thought to produce a higher concentration of marrow cells relative to peripheral blood. Because the dilution of marrow cells with peripheral blood is variable, the adequacy of the collection is determined by the nucleated cell count of the marrow collection. Sierra *et al.* [123] evaluated the effect of marrow cell dose in 174 unrelated-donor bone marrow transplant patients with high-risk acute leukemia. Their analysis showed a beneficial effect of marrow cell doses above the study group median (3.65×10^8 nucleated cells/kg recipient body weight).

Overnight hospitalization of donors was once routine but is now uncommon at many centers. When the marrow collection is completed in the morning, most donors will be ready for discharge by late afternoon. Donors are given instructions about care for their dressings, and precautions about fever or signs of infection. Some centers will routinely provide codeine- or oxycodone-containing analgesics upon discharge. Women are often treated with several weeks of oral iron, but this measure is probably unnecessary for male donors.

Decisions regarding transfusions of blood vary between collection physicians. When autologous blood units are available, some physicians will routinely transfuse these either intraoperatively or following completion of the collection. Other physicians will not transfuse even autologous blood unless there is an indication upon completion of the collection.

PBHC collection procedure

Requirements for establishment of a PBHC collection program have been reviewed [98]. The PBHC collection site is usually a blood center or the apheresis unit of a hospital. Donors typically remain as outpatients throughout the mobilization and collection process. Filgrastim is currently the most commonly used mobilizing agent. It is usually administered at a daily dose of 10–16 µg/kg donor weight, which may be given as a single subcutaneous injection or divided into twice-daily injections. Daily doses of less than 10 µg/kg donor weight yield smaller numbers of HCs.

PBHCs are collected using a continuous-flow cell separation device. Collections begin after the fourth or fifth dose of filgrastim. Success with shorter courses of G-CSF has been described [124]. Usually cannulae are placed in the antecubital veins. From one line, blood is withdrawn into the apheresis machine at a rate of 30–70 mL/min. The continuous-flow centrifuge is set to separate a fraction composed predominantly of mononuclear cells and platelets from the other blood elements. The mononuclear cell/platelet fraction, which is rich in HCs, is retained while the remainder is reinfused to the donor via the return line.

During a single 3 h procedure, it is possible to process between 9 and 12 L of whole blood. The resulting yield of $CD34^+$ cells is correlated with the precollection concentration of $CD34^+$ cells in the donor's blood. In an effort to reduce donor inconvenience, expedite PBHC collection and reduce overall cost, there has been increasing interest in large volume (16–25 L) leukapheresis. Following large volume leukapheresis, the total yield of $CD34^+$ cells may exceed the calculated maxima based upon the donor's peripheral blood $CD34^+$ content [100]. This observation suggests that during the leukapheresis procedure, $CD34^+$ cells are continually released into the blood stream.

Several effective apheresis devices are available. Stroncek *et al.* [106] compared two different cell separators commonly employed for PBHC collection. Although the two machines differed in the proportion of mononuclear cells and granulocytes in the final product, they were very similar in $CD34^+$ collection efficiency.

There is wide variability between donors in the number of $CD34^+$ cells that will be mobilized and collected following stimulation with filgrastim [125]. The exact dose of $CD34^+$ cells appropriate for allogeneic transplantation has also not been established, but the usual target is $4-6 \times 10^6$ $CD34^+$ cells/kg recipient weight [92,100,103,120,126,127]. For the majority of adult recipients, it appears that one or two 12 L aphereses, or a single large volume procedure, will provide sufficient HCs for successful engraftment [90,125].

Special considerations

Growth-factor-mobilized bone marrow

One attraction of PBHCs over bone marrow is more rapid engraftment of neutrophils and platelets [128–130]. Rather than reflecting intrinsic properties of the circulating peripheral blood HCs, this beneficial effect may result from pretreatment with hematopoietic growth factors. Several groups have explored filgrastim administration prior to bone marrow collection [131–134]. These reports, a combination of single arm trials and comparison studies, suggest indeed that G-CSF pretreatment of the marrow donor may accelerate recovery of neutrophils and platelets. When G-CSF was administered in one report at relatively low-dose (2 µg/kg/day), accelerated engraftment was not observed [135]. Morton *et al.* [136] reported a randomized comparison between PBHCs and filgrastim-primed bone marrow. Engraftment of neutrophils and platelets was not different between the two groups, but patients receiving filgrastim-primed bone marrow had significantly less steroid-refractory acute graft-vs.-host disease (GVHD), less chronic GVHD and fewer days of immunosuppressive therapy. Taken together, these preliminary observations suggest that it may be possible to achieve the rapid engraftment of PBHCs without the added risk for increased acute and chronic GVHD [136,137].

These studies, however, have important implications for HC donors because many of the most significant and nonoverlapping adverse events of PBHC and marrow donation are combined in a single procedure. While reduced volumes of marrow collection may be possible [94,131], this is unlikely to fully offset the added risks of filgrastim administration. This would seem to be an area where carefully designed, prospective clinical trials are essential.

Second donations of HCs

Second donations of marrow have occurred weeks to months after the first donation. In most instances the donor is donating for the same recipient, although several unrelated marrow donors have provided marrow for more than one recipient. Buckner *et al.* [61] reporting on 1160 marrow donors identified 99 who donated marrow twice, usually within a 2-month period. There was a modest decline in the average total nucleated cells collected with the second donation. Stroncek *et al.* [138] reported on 16 second-donation donors in Minnesota. There was a trend toward lower total cells and lower cell concentrations in the second collections. When fewer than 90 days separated the collections, the decrement in cell concentration was statistically significant [138]. Importantly, donors whose second donation occurred within 60 days of the first were frequently transfused with allogeneic blood (five of eight donors within 60 days vs. none of eight donors later than 60 days).

Through early 1997, with more than 5500 transplants, the NMDP had received 265 requests (5%) for donors to provide additional HC support for their original marrow recipients. Among these 265 requests, 117 second donations ultimately occurred. Seventy-six donors provided a second marrow donation, 40 provided PBHCs and one provided both. No major donor complications have been encountered during second marrow or PBHC collections. Switzer et al. [139] compared the reactions of second-time donors to PBHC and to marrow. All of these donors had initially provided marrow as their HC product. Although the donors asked to provide PBHCs as a second-time product expressed more initial reluctance, they ultimately reported fewer donation-related side-effects than did second-marrow donors. The donors who had provided bone marrow followed by PBHCs expressed strong preferences for the latter procedure [139].

The feasibility of consecutive PBHC donations has also been reported. Stroncek et al. [121] collected PBHC products 1 year apart in 19 healthy volunteers. There were no differences in premobilization blood counts, the response to filgrastim stimulation or the $CD34^+$ cell yield between the first and second collections. Similar results were reported by Anderlini et al. [120] who described 13 allogeneic PBHC donors providing a second donation at a median of 5 months (range: 1–13 months). No differences were identified in preapheresis WBC counts of the donors or in the yield of $CD34^+$ HCs.

It is anticipated that increasingly allogeneic HC donors will be asked to provide lymphocyte donations as immunomodulatory and graft-vs.-tumor support for their recipients [140]. As strategies for post-transplant cellular support evolve, it will be necessary to include this information in the initial donor education materials and to ensure that donors are made aware of the potential for subsequent requests at the time of initial consent.

Infants and children as HC donors

Children may safely donate marrow [48,61,73,141,142]. They are probably more likely than are adults to receive allogeneic blood transfusion, but serious complications among children donors have been rare [61,73,142]. The use of children as HC donors must include consideration of the ethical and legal issues that were addressed above (see Ethical and legal aspects of donation section).

Sanders et al. [73] reported on 23 marrow donors under 2 years of age. Harvested volumes were between 11.5 and 19.3 mL/kg donor weight. One 14-month-old donor was discovered during predonation evaluation to have a stage 1 neuroblastoma. The tumor was resected at the time of marrow donation. Aside from this case, no serious complications were encountered, but 22 of the 23 infants required allogeneic blood [73]. For children especially, recovery of autologous red blood cells from the collected bone marrow product may by a useful strategy [74].

Successful marrow collection from a 3.95-kg donor has also been reported [142]. The collection volume represented two-thirds of the donor's total blood volume, essentially necessitating exchange transfusion. Another case reported collecting 335 mL of marrow from a 9.4-kg infant (total blood volume 750 mL) [141]. In this instance, recovery of autologous red cells from the collected marrow enabled avoidance of allogeneic blood transfusion.

In a survey of pediatric marrow transplant physicians, only seven of 56 responders were unwilling to collect marrow from infant donors 0–6 months old [48]. There was little agreement, however, on the management of large volume collections. Of 52 respondents, six would limit collections to 25% or less of the donor's blood volume, whereas 24 placed the limit at 50% or higher. Twenty-two respondents preferred to manage large volume collections in two stages [48].

Children appear similar to adults with respect to their response to filgrastim and PBHC collection [143]. They tolerate filgrastim similarly and provide high yields of $CD34^+$ cells. Central venous access may be required more often for successful collection from children [143]. A report described PBHC collections in five children 4–13 years old [101]. The children each received filgrastim at a dose of 6 μg/kg every 12 h for 3 or 4 days. One or two leukapheresis procedures were performed. Three children were donating for siblings and two were donating for a parent. No child required a central venous line and no immediate complications were encountered.

Cryopreservation of allogeneic HCs

Allogeneic marrow and PBHCs can be safely cryopreserved (see Chapter 47) [81,101,144]. Concerns about potential damage to primitive stem cells during the freezing process have been largely dispelled. In a study of 10 recipients of cryopreserved related donor marrow, successful engraftment occurred in all cases [144].

Cryopreservation and storage of cadaver marrow is also feasible [81,145]. Large-scale banking of cadaver marrow for unrelated HC transplantation is impractical because of the huge inventory that would be required (see Chapter 49). Because of less stringent HLA-matching requirements, the banking of cord blood is more likely to be cost-effective [146–150]. Further, marrow from cadaver solid organ donors is currently being evaluated for induction of solid organ graft tolerance. Cadaver marrow may ultimately prove most useful in this setting.

Summary

Allogeneic HC donation is safe. Serious adverse events are uncommon and death is exceedingly rare. Nevertheless, all donors must be carefully evaluated and fully informed prior to HC donation. Donors need to understand that newer transplantation strategies increase the likelihood that they may be asked for second-donation or even third-donation products for their recipients. Additional special considerations apply to children.

Requests for PBHC donations have increased dramatically and may ultimately prove better for both donors and their recipients, but long-term safety data about growth-factor therapy in the normal population remain incomplete. Strategies that combine growth-factor mobilization with marrow collection deserve careful prospective evaluations.

References

1 International Bone Marrow Transplant Registry/Autologous Blood and Marrow Transplant Registry. IBMTR/ABMTR slide set. In: Horowitz MM, ed. *State of the Art in Transplantation*. Milwaukee, 2002.

2 http://www.bmdw.org.

3 Bortin MM, Horowitz MM, Rimm AA. Increasing utilization of allogeneic bone marrow transplantation. *Ann Int Med* 1992; **116**: 505–12.

4 Armitage J. Bone marrow transplantation. *N Engl J Med* 1994; **330**: 827–38.

5 American Association of Blood Banks. *Standards for Hematopoietic Progenitor Cell Services*. Bethesda: American Association of Blood Banks, 2000.

6 Foundation for the Accreditation of Cellular Therapy. *Standards for Hematopoietic Progenitor Cell Collection, Processing & Transplantation*, 2nd edn. Omaha, NE: Foundation for the Accreditation of Cellular Therapy, 2002.

7 National Marrow Donor Program. *National Marrow Donor Program Standards*, 18th edn. Minneapolis: National Marrow Donor Program, 2002.

8 Food and Drug Administration. Suitability determination for donors of human cellular and tissue-based products: proposed rule. *Federal Register* 1999; **64**: 52,696–723.

9 Strasser SI, McDonald GB. Hepatitis viruses and hematopoietic cell transplantation: a guide to patient and donor management. *Blood* 1999; **93**: 1127–36.

10 Shuhart MC, Myerson D, Childs BH *et al.* Marrow transplantation from hepatitis C virus positive donors: transmission rate and clinical course. *Blood* 1994; **84**: 3229–35.

11 Vance EA, Soiffer RJ, McDonald GB, Myerson D, Fingeroth J, Ritz J. Prevention of transmission of hepatitis C virus in bone marrow transplantation by treating the donor with α-interferon. *Transplantation* 1996; **62**: 1358–60.

12 Chen P-M, Fan S, Liu C-J *et al.* Changing of hepatitis B virus markers in patients with bone marrow transplantation. *Transplantation* 1990; **49**: 708–13.

13 Ilan Y, Nagler A, Adler R *et al.* Adoptive transfer of immunity to hepatitis B virus after T cell-depleted allogeneic bone marrow transplantation. *Hepatology* 1993; **18**: 246–52.

14 Ilan Y, Nagler A, Adler R, Tur-Kaspa R, Slavin S, Shouval D. Ablation of persistent hepatitis B by bone marrow transplantation from a hepatitis B-immune donor. *Gastroenterology* 1993; **104**: 1818–21.

15 Ilan Y, Nagler A, Shouval D *et al.* Development of antibodies to hepatitis B virus surface antigen in bone marrow transplant recipient following treatment with peripheral blood lymphocytes from immunized donors. *Clin Exp Immunol* 1994; **97**: 299–302.

16 Brugger SA, Oesterreicher C, Hofmann H, Kalhs P, Greinix HT, Muller C. Hepatitis B virus clearance by transplantation of bone marrow from hepatitis B immunised donor [letter]. *Lancet* 1997; **349**: 996–7.

17 Lau GK, Liang R, Lee CK, Lim WL. Is vaccination of donor adequate for clearance of hepatitis B virus after bone-marrow transplantation [Letter]? *Lancet* 1997; **349**: 1626–7.

18 Lau GKK, Liang R, Lee CK *et al.* Clearance of persistent hepatitis B virus infection in Chinese bone marrow transplant recipients whose donors were anti-hepatitis B core- and anti-hepatitis B surface antibody-positive. *J Infect Dis* 1998; **178**: 1585–91.

19 Locasciulli A, Alberti A, Bandini G *et al.* Allogeneic bone marrow transplantation from HBsAg+ donors: a multicenter study from the Gruppo Italiano Trapianti di Midolio Osseo (GITMO). *Blood* 1995; **86**: 3236–40.

20 Lau GKK, Lie AKW, Kwong YL *et al.* A case-controlled study on the use of HBsAg-positive donors for allogeneic hematopoietic cell transplantation. *Blood* 2000; **96**: 452–8.

21 Kollman C, Howe CWS, Anasetti C *et al.* Donor characteristics as risk factors in recipients after transplantation of bone marrow from unrelated donors: the effect of donor age. *Blood* 2001; **98**: 2043–51.

22 Grob JP, Grundy JE, Prentice HG *et al.* Immune donors can protect marrow-transplant recipients from severe cytomegalovirus infections. *Lancet* 1987; **1**: 774–6.

23 Lutz E, Ward KN, Szydlo R, Goldman JM. Cytomegalovirus antibody avidity in allogeneic bone marrow recipients. Evidence for primary or secondary humoral responses depending on donor immune status. *J Med Virol* 1996; **49**: 61–5.

24 Switzer GE, Dew MA, Butterworth VA, Simmons RG, Schimmel M. Understanding donors' motivations. A study of unrelated bone marrow donors. *Soc Sci Med* 1997; **45**: 137–47.

25 Chang G, McGarigle C, Spitzer TR *et al.* A comparison of related and unrelated marrow donors. *Psychosomatic Med* 1998; **60**: 163–7.

26 Christopher KA. The experience of donating bone marrow to a relative. *Oncol Nursing Forum* 2000; **27**: 693–9.

27 Davies S. Bone marrow transplant raises issues of privacy. *Br Med J* 1997; **314**: 1356.

28 Warwick R. Anonymity for unrelated bone marrow donors should remain [letter]. *Br Med J* 1997; **315**: 548–9.

29 Stroncek D, Strand R, Scott E *et al.* Attitudes and physical condition of unrelated bone marrow donors immediately after donation. *Transfusion* 1989; **29**: 317–22.

30 Kinrade LC. Preparation of sibling donor for bone marrow transplant harvest procedure. *Cancer Nursing* 1987; **10**: 77–81.

31 Kent G. Volunteering children for bone marrow donation. Studies show large discrepancies between views of surrogate decision makers and patients [letter]. *Br Med J* 1996; **313**: 49–50.

32 Peters SO, Stockschlader M, Zeller W *et al.* Monoclonal gammopathy of unknown significance in a bone marrow donor. *Ann Hematol* 1993; **66**: 93–5.

33 Centis F, Delfini C, Agostinelli F *et al.* Soluble transferrin receptor following bone marrow transplantation from donors heterozygous for beta thalassemia. *Haematologica* 1994; **79**: 448–51.

34 Peltier JY, Girault D, Debre M, Galacteros F, Fischer A, Girot R. Donor for BMT with haemoglobin H disease. *Bone Marrow Transplant* 1993; **12**: 81–4.

35 Barquinero J, Witherspoon R, Sanders J *et al.* Allogeneic marrow grafts from donors with congenital chromosomal abnormalities in marrow cells. *Br J Haematol* 1995; **90**: 595–601.

36 D'Amico EA, Villaca PR, Prado SS *et al.* Bone marrow harvesting from haemophilia A donor [letter]. *Lancet* 1993; **341**: 254.

37 Sturfelt G, Lenhoff S, Sallerfors B, Nived O, Truedsson L, Sjoholm AG. Transplantation with allogenic bone marrow from a donor with systemic lupus erythematosus (SLE). Successful outcome in the recipient and induction of an SLE flare in the donor. *Ann Rheum Dis* 1996; **55**: 638–41.

38 Snowden JA, Atkinson K, Kearney P, Brooks P, Biggs JC. Allogeneic bone marrow transplantation from a donor with severe active rheumatoid arthritis not resulting in adoptive transfer of disease to recipient. *Bone Marrow Transplant* 1997; **20**: 71–3.

39 DeFour Jones M, Petrikovsky BM, Sahdev I, Prisco M. Continuous fetal heart rate monitoring during bone marrow harvesting in pregnancy. *Am J Perinatol* 1995; **12**: 243–4.

40 Cavallaro AM, Lilleby K, Majolino I *et al.* Three to six year follow-up of normal donors who receive recombinant human granulocyte colony-stimulating factor. *Bone Marrow Transplant* 2000; **25**: 85–9.

41 US National Archives and Records Administration. *Code of Federal Regulations*, 21 CFR, Part 50. Washington, DC: GPO, 1998.

42 US National Commission for the Protection of Human Subjects of Biomedical and Behavioral Research. *The Belmont Report: Ethical Principles and Guidelines for the Protection of Human Subjects of Research*. Washington, DC: GPO, 1978.

43 World Medical Association. *Declaration of Helsinki (2000). Ethical Principles for Medical Research Involving Human Subjects. Bull Med Ethics* 2000; **162**: 8–11.

44 Holcombe A. Patient education. Bone marrow harvest. *Oncol Nursing Forum* 1987; **14**: 63–5.

45 Ruggiero MR. The donor in bone marrow transplantation. *Sem Oncol Nursing* 1988; **4**: 9–14.

46 National Marrow Donor Program. *Questions and Answers: You Could Be the Missing Piece*. Minneapolis, 2001.

47 National Marrow Donor Program. *Now That You Are a Match*. Minneapolis: 2001.

48 Chan KW, Gajewski JL, Supkis D, Jr, Pentz R, Champlin R, Bleyer WA. Use of minors as bone marrow donors: current attitude and management. A survey of 56 pediatric transplantation centers. *J Pediatrics* 1996; **128**: 644–8.

49 Delaney L. Altruism by proxy: volunteering children for bone marrow donation. Protecting children from forced altruism: the legal approach. *Br Med J* 1996; **312**: 240.

50 Month S. Altruism by proxy: volunteering children for bone marrow donation. Preventing children from donation may not be in their interests. *Br Med J* 1996; **312**: 240–1.

51 Savulescu J. Altruism by proxy: volunteering children for bone marrow donation. Substantial harm but substantial benefit. *Br Med J* 1996; **312**: 241–2.

52 Browett P, Palmer S. Altruism by proxy: volunteering children for bone marrow donation. Legal barriers might have catastrophic effects. *Br Med J* 1996; **312**: 242–3.

53 Osmun WE. Volunteering children for bone marrow donation. Children's views should have been represented in discussion [letter]. *Br Med J* 1996; **313**: 50.

54 Alderson P, Montgomery J. Volunteering children for bone marrow donation. Children may be able to make their own decisions [letter]. *Br Med J* 1996; **313**: 50.

55 US National Archives and Records Administration. *Code of Federal Regulations*, 45 CFR, 48.408. Washington, DC: GPO, 1991.

56 Revised Code of Washington: Bone Marrow Donation, sec. 70.54.305. Washington State Legislature, 2000.

57 The Associated Press. "Young Would-be Marrow Donor to Be Tested After All." *The Seattle Times*, August 11, 1999.

58 Clayton EW, Steinberg KK, Khoury MJ *et al.* Consensus statement. Informed consent for genetic research on stored tissue samples. *JAMA* 1995; **274**: 1786–92.

59 Food and Drug Administration. International Conference on Harmonization; Guideline on clinical safety data management: definitions and standards for expedited reporting. *Federal Register* 1995; **60**: 11,284–7.

60 Thomas ED, Storb R. Technique for human marrow grafting. *Blood* 1970; **36**: 507–15.

61 Buckner CD, Clift RA, Sanders JE *et al.* Marrow harvesting from normal donors. *Blood* 1984; **64**: 630–4.

62 Hill HF, Chapman CR, Jackson TL, Sullivan KM. Assessment and management of donor pain following marrow harvest for allogeneic bone marrow transplantation. *Bone Marrow Transplant* 1989; **4**: 157–61.

63 Stroncek DF, Holland PV, Bartch G *et al.* Experiences of the first 493 unrelated marrow donors in the National Marrow Donor Program. *Blood* 1993; **81**: 1940–6.

64 Burmeister MA, Standl T, Brauer P et al. Safety and efficacy of spinal vs. general anaesthesia in bone marrow harvesting. *Bone Marrow Transplant* 1998; **21**: 1145–8.

65 Buckner CD, Petersen FB, Bolonski BA. Bone marrow donors. In: Forman SJ, Blume KG, Thomas ED, eds. *Bone Marrow Transplantation*. Malden, MA: Blackwell Scientific Publications, 1994: 259–69.

66 Foldes J, Naparstek E, Statter M, Menczel J, Bab I. Osteogenic response to marrow aspiration. Increased serum osteocalcin and alkaline phosphatase in human bone marrow donors. *J Bone Mineral Res* 1989; **4**: 643–6.

67 Fondriest JE, Pitt MJ, Williams WH, Dalton WS. Radiologic abnormalities at the harvest site in patients undergoing bone marrow transplantation. *Am J Roentgenol* 1992; **159**: 226–7.

68 Bortin MM, Buckner CD. Major complications of marrow harvesting for transplantation. *Exp Hematol* 1983; **11**: 916–21.

69 Hosoya N, Miyagawa K, Mimura T et al. Malignant hyperthermia induced by general anesthesia for bone marrow harvesting. *Bone Marrow Transplant* 1996; **19**: 509–11.

70 Riley D, Evans TG. Osteomyelitis complicating bone marrow harvest [letter]. *Clin Infect Dis* 1992; **14**: 980–1.

71 Drake P. Hemorrhage after bone marrow harvest: a case presentation. *Clin J Oncol Nursing* 2000; **4**: 29–31.

72 Klumpp TR, Mangan KF, MacDonald JS, Mesgarzadeh M. Fracture of the ilium: an unusual complication of bone marrow harvesting. *Bone Marrow Transplant* 1992; **9**: 503–4.

73 Sanders J, Buckner CD, Bensinger WI, Levy W, Chard R, Thomas ED. Experience with marrow harvesting from donors less than 2 years of age. *Bone Marrow Transplant* 1987; **2**: 45–50.

74 Kletzel M, Olezewski M, Danner-Koptik K, Coyne K, Haut PR. Red cell salvage and reinfusion in pediatric bone marrow donors. *Bone Marrow Transplant* 1999; **24**: 385–8.

75 York A, Clift RA, Sanders JE, Buckner CD. Recombinant human erythropoietin (rh-Epo) administration to normal marrow donors. *Bone Marrow Transplant* 1992; **10**: 415–7.

76 Akiyama H, Tanikawa S, Takamoto S, Sakamaki H, Sasaki T, Onozawa Y. Recombinant human erythropoietin (rhEPO) administration to marrow donors. Bone Marrow Transplantation (BMT) Team. *Int J Hematol* 1995; **62**: 145–9.

77 Baselga J, Reich L, Doherty M, Gulati S. Fat embolism syndrome following bone marrow harvesting. *Bone Marrow Transplant* 1991; **7**: 485–6.

78 Wolf HH, Heyll A, Hesterberg R et al. Mechanical ileus following bone marrow harvesting: an unusual complication [letter]. *Bone Marrow Transplant* 1994; **14**: 179–80.

79 Agura ED. Seizure in a normal marrow donor: Addison's disease unmasked. *Bone Marrow Transplant* 1994; **13**: 215–6.

80 Anderlini P, Rizzo JD, Nugent ML, Schmitz N, Champlin RE, Horowitz MM. Peripheral blood stem cell donation. An analysis from the International Bone Marrow Transplant Registry (IBMTR) and European Group for Blood and Marrow Transplant (EBMT) databases. *Bone Marrow Transplant* 2001; **27**: 689–92.

81 Blazar BR, Lasky LC, Perentesis JP et al. Successful donor cell engraftment in a recipient of bone marrow from a cadaveric donor. *Blood* 1986; **67**: 1655–60.

82 Martin J. "Offer to Give All a Chilling Prophecy before Surgery." *South Bend Tribune*, September 1, 1998.

83 Adler BK, Salzman DE, Carabasi MH, Vaughan WP, Reddy VVB, Prchal JT. Fatal sickle cell crisis after granulocyte colony-stimulating factor administration. *Blood* 2001; **97**: 3313–4.

84 Anderlini P, Körbling M, Dale D et al. Allogeneic blood stem cell transplantation. Considerations for donors [Editorial]. *Blood* 1997; **90**: 903–8.

85 Rowley SD, Donaldson G, Lilleby K, Bensinger WI, Appelbaum FR. Experiences of donors enrolled in a randomized study of allogeneic bone marrow or peripheral blood stem cell transplantation. *Blood* 2001; **97**: 2541–8.

86 Dreger P, Haferlach T, Eckstein V et al. G-CSF-mobilized peripheral blood progenitor cells for allogeneic transplantation: safety, kinetics of mobilization, and composition of the graft. *Br J Haematol* 1994; **87**: 609–13.

87 Bensinger WI, Weaver CH, Appelbaum FR et al. Transplantation of allogeneic peripheral blood stem cells mobilized by recombinant human granulocyte colony-stimulating factor. *Blood* 1995; **85**: 1655–8.

88 Schmitz N, Dreger P, Suttorp M et al. Primary transplantation of allogeneic peripheral blood progenitor cells mobilized by filgrastim (granulocyte colony-stimulating factor). *Blood* 1995; **85**: 1666–72.

89 Grigg AP, Roberts AW, Raunow H et al. Optimizing dose and scheduling of filgrastim (granulocyte colony-stimulating factor) for mobilization and collection of peripheral blood progenitor cells in normal volunteers. *Blood* 1995; **86**: 4437–45.

90 Anderlini P, Przepiorka D, Seong D et al. Clinical toxicity and laboratory effects of granulocyte-colony-stimulating factor (filgrastim) mobilization and blood stem cell apheresis from normal donors, and analysis of charges for the procedures. *Transfusion* 1996; **36**: 590–5.

91 Stroncek DF, Clay ME, Petzoldt ML et al. Treatment of normal individuals with granulocyte-colony-stimulating factor: donor experiences and the effects on peripheral blood CD34+ cell counts and on the collection of peripheral blood stem cells. *Transfusion* 1996; **36**: 601–10.

92 Majolino I, Cavallaro AM, Bacigalupo A et al. Mobilization and collection of PBSC in healthy donors: a retrospective analysis of the Italian Bone Marrow Transplantation Group (GITMO). *Haematologica* 1997; **82**: 47–52.

93 Anderlini P, Donato M, Chan K-W et al. Allogeneic blood progenitor cell collection in normal donors after mobilization with filgrastim. The M.D. Anderson Cancer Center experience. *Transfusion* 1999; **39**: 555–60.

94 Murata M, Harada M, Kato S et al. Peripheral blood stem cell mobilization and apheresis: analysis of adverse events in 94 normal donors. *Bone Marrow Transplant* 1999; **24**: 1065–71.

95 Froberg MK, Garg UC, Stroncek DF, Geis M, McCullough J, Brown DM. Changes in serum osteocalcin and bone-specific alkaline phosphatase are associated with bone pain in donors receiving granulocyte-colony-stimulating factor for peripheral blood stem and progenitor cell collection. *Transfusion* 1999; **39**: 410–4.

96 Lane TA, Law P, Maruyama M et al. Harvesting and enrichment of hematopoietic progenitor cells mobilized into the peripheral blood of normal donors by granulocyte-macrophage colony-stimulating factor (GM-CSF) or G-CSF. Potential role in allogeneic marrow transplantation. *Blood* 1995; **85**: 275–82.

97 Bensinger WI, Buckner CD, Rowley S, Storb R, Appelbaum FR. Treatment of normal donors with recombinant growth factors for transplantation of allogeneic blood stem cells. *Bone Marrow Transplant* 1996; **17**: S19–21.

98 Stroncek D, McCullough J. Policies and procedures for the establishment of an allogeneic blood stem cell collection programme. *Transfus Med* 1997; **7**: 77–87.

99 Murata M, Kanie T, Hamaguchi M et al. Unrelated bone marrow transplantation from the National Marrow Donor Program. *Int J Hematol* 1997; **66**: 239–43.

100 Kobbe G, Soehngen D, Heyll A et al. Large volume leukapheresis maximizes the progenitor cell yield for allogeneic peripheral blood progenitor donation. *J Hematother* 1997; **6**: 125–31.

101 Körbling M, Chan KW, Anderlini P et al. Allogeneic peripheral blood stem cell transplantation using normal patient-related pediatric donors. *Bone Marrow Transplant* 1996; **18**: 885–90.

102 Anderlini P, Prezpiorka D, Seong D, Champlin R, Körbling M. Transient neutropenia in normal donors after G-CSF mobilization and stem cell apheresis. *Br J Haematol* 1996; **94**: 155–8.

103 Miflin G, Charley C, Stainer C, Anderson S, Hunter A, Russell N. Stem cell mobilization in normal donors for allogeneic transplantation. Analysis of safety and factors affecting efficacy. *Br J Haematol* 1996; **95**: 345–8.

104 Majolino I, Buscemi F, Scime R et al. Treatment of normal donors with rhG-CSF 16 μg/kg for mobilization of peripheral blood stem cells and their apheretic collection for allogeneic transplantation. *Haematologica* 1995; **80**: 219–26.

105 Martinez C, Urbano-Ispizua A, Rozman C et al. Effects of G-CSF administration and peripheral blood progenitor cell collection in 20 healthy donors. *Ann Hematol* 1996; **72**: 269–72.

106 Stroncek DF, Clay ME, Smith J, Jaszcz WB, Herr G, McCullough J. Comparison of two blood cell separators in collecting peripheral blood stem cell components. *Transfus Med* 1997; **7**: 95–9.

107 Körbling M, Anderlini P, Durett A et al. Delayed effects of rhG-CSF mobilization treatment and apheresis on circulating CD34+ and CD34+Thy-1dim CD38– progenitor cells and lymphoid subsets in normal stem cell donors for allogeneic transplantation. *Bone Marrow Transplant* 1996; **18**: 1073–9.

108 Wei A, Grigg A. Granulocyte colony-stimulating factor-induced sickle cell crisis and multiorgan dysfunction in a patient with compound heterozygous sickle cell/B+ thalassemia. *Blood* 2001; **97**: 3998–9.

109 Kang E, Areman E, David-Ocampo V et al. Mobilization, collection, and processing of peripheral blood stem cells in individuals with sickle cell trait. *Blood* 2002; **99**: 850–5.

110 Becker PS, Wagle M, Matous S et al. Spontaneous splenic rupture following administration of granulocyte colony-stimulating factor (G-CSF): occurrence in an allogeneic donor of peripheral blood stem cells. *Biol Blood Marrow Transplant* 1997; **3**: 45–9.

111 Falzetti F, Aversa F, Minelli O, Tabilio A. Spontaneous rupture of spleen during peripheral blood stem-cell mobilisation in a healthy donor. *Lancet* 1999; **353**: 555.

112 Platzbecker U, Prange-Krex G, Bornhäuser M *et al.* Spleen enlargement in healthy donors during G-CSF mobilization of PBPCs. *Transfusion* 2001; **41**: 184–9.

113 De Vries EGE, Willemse PHB, Biesma B, Stern AC, Limburg PC, Vellenga E. Flare-up of rheumatoid arthritis during GM-CSF treatment after chemotherapy [letter]. *Lancet* 1991; **338**: 517–8.

114 Storek J, Glaspy JA, Grody WW, Susi E, Slater ED. Adult-onset cyclic neutropenia responsive to cyclosporine therapy in a patient with ankylosing spondylitis. *Am J Hematol* 1993; **43**: 139–43.

115 Hoekman K, von Blomberg-van der Flier BME, Wagstaff J, Drexhage HA, Pinedo HM. Reversible thyroid dysfunction during treatment with GM-CSF. *Lancet* 1991; **338**: 541–2.

116 Huhn RD, Yurkow EJ, Tushinski R *et al.* Recombinant human interleukin-3 (rhIL-3) enhances the mobilization of peripheral blood progenitor cells by recombinant human granulocyte colony-stimulating factor (rhG-CSF) in normal volunteers. *Exp Hematol* 1996; **24**: 839–47.

117 Parkkali T, Volin L, Siren MK, Ruutu T. Acute iritis induced by granulocyte colony-stimulating factor used for mobilization in a volunteer unrelated peripheral blood progenitor cell donor. *Bone Marrow Transplant* 1996; **17**: 433–4.

118 Esmaeli B, Ahmadi A, Kim S, Onan H, Korbling M, Anderlini P. Marginal keratitis associated with administration of filgrastim and sargramostim in a healthy peripheral blood progenitor cell donor. *Cornea* 2002; **21**: 621–2.

119 Sakamaki S, Matsunaga T, Hirayama Y, Kuya T, Niitsu Y. Haematological study of healthy volunteers 5 years after G-CSF. *Lancet* 1995; **346**: 1432–3.

120 Anderlini P, Lauppe J, Przepiorka D, Seong D, Champlin R, Korbling M. Peripheral blood stem cell apheresis in normal donors. Feasibility and yield of second collections. *Br J Haematol* 1997; **96**: 415–7.

121 Stroncek D, Clay ME, Herr G, Smith J, Ilstrup S, McCullough J. Blood counts in healthy donors 1 year after the collection of granulocyte-colony-stimulating factor-mobilized progenitor cells and the results of a second mobilization and collection. *Transfusion* 1997; **37**: 304–8.

122 Anderlini P, Chan FA, Champlin RE, Korbling M, Strom SS. Long-term follow-up of normal peripheral blood progenitor cell donors treated with filgrastim: no evidence of increased risk of leukemia development. *Bone Marrow Transplant* 2002; **30**: 661–3.

123 Sierra J, Storer B, Hansen JA *et al.* Transplantation of marrow cells from unrelated donors for treatment of high-risk acute leukemia: the effect of leukemia burden, donor HLA-matching, and marrow cell dose. *Blood* 1997; **89**: 4226–35.

124 de Fabritiis P, Paola Iori A, Mengarelli A *et al.* $CD34^+$ cell mobilization for allogeneic progenitor cell transplantation: efficacy of a short course of G-CSF. *Transfusion* 2001; **41**: 190–5.

125 Stroncek DF, Clay ME, Smith J *et al.* Composition of peripheral blood progenitor cell components collected from healthy donors. *Transfusion* 1997; **37**: 411–7.

126 Körbling M, Przepiorka D, Huh YO *et al.* Allogeneic blood stem cell transplantation for refractory leukemia and lymphoma: potential advantage of blood over marrow allografts. *Blood* 1995; **85**: 1659–65.

127 Körbling M, Huh YO, Durett A *et al.* Allogeneic blood stem cell transplantation: peripheralization and yield of donor-derived primitive hematopoietic progenitor cells ($CD34^+Thy-1^{dim}$) and lymphoid subsets, and possible predictors of engraftment and graft-versus-host disease. *Blood* 1995; **86**: 2842–8.

128 Couban S, Simpson DR, Barnett MJ *et al.* A randomized multicenter comparison of bone marrow and peripheral blood in recipients of matched sibling allogeneic transplants for myeloid malignancies. *Blood* 2002; **100**: 1525–31.

129 Champlin R, Schmitz N, Horowitz M *et al.* Blood stem cells compared with bone marrow as a source of hematopoietic cells for allogeneic transplantation. *Blood* 2000; **95**: 3702–9.

130 Bensinger WI, Martin PJ, Storer B *et al.* Transplantation of bone marrow as compared with peripheral-blood cells from HLA-identical relatives in patients with hematologic cancers. *N Engl J Med* 2001; **344**: 175–81.

131 Couban S, Messner HA, Andreou P *et al.* Bone marrow mobilized with granulocyte colony-stimulating factor in related allogeneic transplant recipients: a study of 29 patients. *Biol Blood Marrow Transplant* 2000; **6**: 422–7.

132 Isola L, Scigliano E, Fruchtman S. Long-term follow-up after allogeneic granulocyte colony-stimulating factor-primed bone marrow transplantation. *Biol Blood Marrow Transplant* 2000; **6**: 428–33.

133 Ji S-Q, Chen H-R, Wang H-X, Yan H-M, Pan S-P, Xun C-Q. Comparison of outcome of allogeneic bone marrow transplantation with and without granulocyte colony-stimulating factor (lenograstim) donor-marrow priming in patients with chronic myelogenous leukemia. *Biol Blood Marrow Transplant* 2002; **8**: 261–7.

134 Serody JS, Sparks SD, Lin Y *et al.* Comparison of granulocyte colony-stimulating factor (G-CSF)-mobilized peripheral blood progenitor cells and G-CSF-stimulated bone marrow as a source of stem cells in HLA-matched sibling transplantation. *Biol Blood Marrow Transplant* 2000; **6**: 434–40.

135 Machida U, Tojo A, Takahashi S *et al.* The effect of granulocyte colony-stimulating factor administration in healthy donors bone marrow harvesting. *Br J Haematol* 2000; **108**: 747–53.

136 Morton J, Hutchins C, Durrant S. Granulocyte-colony stimulating factor (G-CSF)-primed allogeneic bone marrow. Significantly less graft-versus-host disease and comparable engraftment to G-CSF-mobilized peripheral blood stem cells. *Blood* 2001; **98**: 3186–91.

137 Donato M, Champlin R. Granulocyte colony-stimulating factor-primed allogeneic bone marrow transplants. Capturing the advantages of blood stem cell transplants without increased risk of chronic graft-versus-host disease. *Biol Blood Marrow Transplant* 2000; **6**: 419–21.

138 Stroncek DF, McGlave P, Ramsay N, McCullough J. Effects on donors of second bone marrow collections. *Transfusion* 1991; **31**: 819–22.

139 Switzer GE, Goycoolea JM, Dew MA, Graeff EC, Hegland J. Donating stimulated peripheral blood stem cells vs. bone marrow: do donors experience the procedures differently? *Bone Marrow Transplant* 2001; **27**: 917–23.

140 Porter D, Collins R, Hardy C *et al.* Treatment of relapsed leukemia after unrelated donor marrow transplantation with unrelated donor leukocyte infusions. *Blood* 2000; **95**: 1214–21.

141 Chan KW, Stanley CE, Wadsworth LD. Bone marrow collection from a 9.4-kg donor avoiding allogeneic blood transfusion [letter]. *Transfusion* 1987; **27**: 441–2.

142 Urban C, Weber G, Slavc I, Kerbl R. Anesthetic management of marrow harvesting from a 7-week-old premature baby. *Bone Marrow Transplant* 1990; **6**: 443–4.

143 de la Rubia J, Diaz M, Verdeguer A *et al.* Donor age-related differences in PBPC mobilization with rHuG-CSF. *Transfusion* 2001; **41**: 201–5.

144 Eckardt JR, Roodman GD, Boldt DH *et al.* Comparison of engraftment and acute GVHD in patients undergoing cryopreserved or fresh allogeneic BMT. *Bone Marrow Transplant* 1993; **11**: 125–31.

145 Ferebee JW, Atkins L, Gochte HL, Thomas ED. The collection, storage and preparation of viable cadaver bone marrow for intravenous use. *Blood* 1959; **14**: 140–7.

146 Rubinstein P, Rosenfield RE, Adamson JW, Stevens CE. Stored placental blood for unrelated bone marrow reconstitution. *Blood* 1993; **81**: 1679–90.

147 Rubinstein P, Dobrila L, Rosenfield R *et al.* Processing and cryopreservation of placental/umbilical cord blood for unrelated bone marrow reconstitution. *Proc Natl Acad Sci U S A* 1995; **92**: 10,119–22.

148 Kurtzberg J, Laughlin M, Graham M *et al.* Placental blood as a source of hematopoietic stem cells for transplantation into unrelated recipients. *N Engl J Med* 1996; **335**: 157–66.

149 Wagner J, Rosenthal J, Sweetman R *et al.* Successful transplantation of HLA-matched and HLA-mismatched umbilical cord blood from unrelated donors: analysis of engraftment and acute graft-versus-host disease. *Blood* 1996; **88**: 795–802.

150 Gluckman E, Rocha V, Boyer-Chammard A *et al.* Outcome of cord blood transplantation from unrelated and related donors. *N Engl J Med* 1997; **337**: 373–81.

Hal E. Broxmeyer & Franklin O. Smith

Cord Blood Hematopoietic Cell Transplantation

Introduction

Bone marrow transplantation (BMT) from human leukocyte antigen (HLA)-matched related donors has been successfully used for the treatment of children and adults with a high risk of recurrent hematological malignancies, genetic immunodeficiencies, metabolic disorders, or marrow failure syndromes. Unfortunately, the majority of patients who could potentially benefit from allogeneic BMT do not have suitably matched related donors. To address this problem, the National Marrow Donor Program (NMDP) was established in 1986 [1,2]. Despite the success of this program, suitable HLA-compatible bone marrow and peripheral blood (PB) donors cannot be identified for all patients in need of allogeneic transplantation [3]. Therefore, clinical investigators have, over the past decade, explored the suitability of umbilical cord blood (CB) hematopoietic cells as an alternative source of hematopoietic stem cells (HSCs). While prospective clinical trials are still in progress, the world's experience now suggest that CB is an acceptable alternative to bone marrow (BM).

History of CB transplantation

The potential use of umbilical CB as a source of HSCs was proposed in 1982 in private discussions held by Edward A. Boyse, Hal E. Broxmeyer and Judith Bard [4,5]. Subsequent to these discussions, a number of *in vitro* studies with human CB [6,7] and *in vivo* studies with mouse blood [7] were performed to document the feasibility of this proposal. Initial studies used hematopoietic progenitor cell (HPC) assays, which served as surrogate assays for HSCs, to compare numbers of primitive cells in CB as compared to BM [6–8]. Specifically, these early studies assessed whether previously untrained obstetrical health care professionals were able to collect CB that was free of bacterial and fungal contamination, determine the range and average volume of CB collected, and assay samples for the total number of nucleated cells and HPCs using *in vitro* culture methods following overnight shipment of CB units. During the course of these experiments, a number of CB units were cryopreserved and stored in liquid nitrogen freezers at the Indiana University School of Medicine for potential clinical use. These studies were followed by experiments in which lethally irradiated mice received transplantations of blood from near-term or term donors. Since it is not possible to get CB cells from mice because of the small size of the placenta and CB, the closest one can get to study of CB cells in mice is to use the blood of near-term and term mice which would be equivalent to the blood found in the cord. It was demonstrated that the blood of near-term and term mice contained sufficient numbers of HSCs capable of reconstituting hematopoiesis [7].

The first CB hematopoietic cell transplantation (HCT) was performed for a 5-year-old child with Fanconi anemia by Gluckman and colleagues in October 1988 [9]. CB from the patient's HLA-identical sibling was collected in Durham, NC, by Gordon Douglas, then at the New York University Medical Center in New York; it was then shipped to Indiana University where it was cryopreserved by Broxmeyer's laboratory and then hand-delivered to Paris where the patient underwent his preparative regimen and CB-HCT [4,5,9]. Events leading up to this first CB-HCT transplantation are given in more detail elsewhere [4–6,10]. The patient had durable engraftment of donor hematopoiesis and survived without hematological manifestations of the treated disease. The next four CB transplantations, for three children with Fanconi anemia and one with juvenile myelomonocytic leukemia, were performed using CB also collected at a distant obstetrical unit by Douglas and banked at Indiana University [4–7,9–12]. Four of the first five CB recipients had engraftment of donor cells, with only one patient with Fanconi anemia having graft failure. In 1991, two children with leukemia received myeloablative preparative regimens for CB-HCT from related donors [11,13].

Following these first, largely successful transplant procedures, CB as an alternative source of HSCs was utilized by others and these transplantations were initially reported by an International Cord Blood Transplant Registry (ICBTR) [14]. It is now estimated that more than 70,000 CB units have been banked with at least 2000 CB transplantations performed worldwide [15–19]. CB has now been utilized as a stem cell source for numerous malignant and nonmalignant diseases.

Collection of CB

CB can be collected for several purposes [20]. Public (not-for-profit) CB banks collect CB for the allogeneic transplantation of any recipient for whom the CB unit is a suitable HLA-match. CB can be collected and stored by expectant parents for potential use by the newborn infant (e.g. autologous transplantation) or a family member in need of a stem cell transplantation procedure (e.g. directed allogeneic donor transplantation). While autologous and directed allogeneic collections and storage have typically been performed by private (for-profit) banks, the National Heart, Lung and Blood Institute (NHLBI) of the National Institutes of Health (NIH) now supports a public CB bank at the Children's Hospital Oakland in California for this purpose. This federally funded CB bank stores CB from children with hemoglobinopathies, genetic diseases and from the normal siblings of children with malignant and nonmalignant disease who are in need of a transplant procedure [21]. Finally, CB can be collected from anonymous donors, on local Institutional Review Board approved studies, for laboratory-based research.

A number of techniques have been proposed for the optimal collection of CB. An optimal collection is generally considered to be a CB unit with sufficient volume of blood, total nucleated cells, and CD34$^+$ cells. In addition, the unit would contain a low number of maternal T cells [22] and would be free of transmissible infectious agents.

As engraftment is closely correlated with the number of infused cells [18], numerous variables in the CB collection process have been examined in attempts to maximize the cell dose. Factors that may increase these numbers include volume of CB collected, number of nucleated cells or number of CD34$^+$ cells, larger birth weight, fewer prior live births and birth order with a larger number of cells in first-born children [23]. Other factors that appear to increase cell dose include prolonged stress during delivery, placing the infant on the mother's abdomen after delivery [24], collection prior to delivery of the placenta, cesarean section [25–27], early clamping of the umbilical cord [24,28] and normal saline flush of the umbilical vessels [27,29]. In addition, there is a direct correlation of gestational age with nucleated cell count, but an inverse relation to CD34$^+$ cell count [23,30]. Factors that do not appear to effect the number of collected cells include maternal age, race and sex [28,31,32]. Despite this information, there remains considerable debate about the optimal collection method, with no consensus about the most appropriate process. While there appears to be little clinical impact on the newborn infant or the mother with these different techniques, the American College of Obstetrics and Gynecology [33] and the American Academy of Pediatrics [34] have strongly recommended that standard obstetric procedures not be altered to facilitate CB collections.

CB for public allogeneic use is generally collected at a limited number of sites in a single geographic location, with dedicated, trained personnel performing the collections according to standard operating procedures established by the CB bank [19,35]. These collection sites generally perform collections on only term infants. For directed allogeneic or autologous use, CB is generally collected at the birth location by local obstetrical care providers. The CB unit is then shipped to the CB bank for cryopreservation.

Despite these variable methodologies, the cellular characteristics of CB units are reasonably constant and distinct from BM and mobilized PB. Single CB units generally contain a 10-fold smaller dose of nucleated cells and CD34$^+$ cells than that typically transplanted with BM or mobilized PB [23]. However, these units are enriched in HPCs [6,8].

Despite efforts to bank as many CB units as possible, it has been shown that a very large percentage of potential CB donors are ineligible for donations to public CB banks [36–38]. Chief reasons for not using potential CB donors is the presence of sexually transmitted diseases in the mother, maternal fever during delivery, medications administered to the mother, maternal diseases, complications of delivery, presence of infections and complications and problems with the placenta or umbilical cord. This high deferral rate of donors must be taken into account as the costs associated with CB collection and banking are considerable.

Given the uncertainty about the optimal method of CB collection that results in the best quality CB product, but also preserves the health of the newborn infant and maternal donor, some CB collection programs and banks have instituted outcomes programs to evaluate the mother and baby after CB donation [38]. While diseases in the baby have on rare occasions been identified, resulting in the discarding of their CB units from public bank, the overall experience suggests that CB donation is a safe procedure for both mother and newborn.

CB banking

The first CB bank was created at the Indiana University School of Medicine, with the first CB-HCT performed using units cryopreserved and stored in this bank [4–7]. As a result of the interest in CB transplantation generated from this preliminary transplant experience, CB banks were established in 1993 in New York City, USA, in Düsseldorf, Germany, and in Milan, Spain. Subsequently, CB banks have been created worldwide in Austria, Belgium, Canada, China, United Kingdom, Finland, France, Germany, Ireland, Italy, Japan, Korea, the Netherlands, Poland, Singapore, Spain, Switzerland, Thailand and throughout the USA [16,21,35,39–45]. It is estimated that more than 70,000 CB units have been collected, tested and cryopreserved by these banks [16]. CB banking is a very complex and expensive process. The establishment of a quality CB bank requires attention to a number of specific issues including donor recruitment, donor consent, donor evaluation, labeling, CB collection, CB processing (e.g. red-cell depletion, volume reduction and stem cell selection) cryopreservation, histocompatibility testing, infectious disease testing, genetic disease testing, confirmation of recipient histocompatibility testing, tracking and allocation methods, transportation of CB from the collection site to the bank, transportation from the CB bank to the transplant center, thawing methods and protection of confidentiality of donors and recipients [16,46,47]. Therefore, a number of organizations have created standards to ensure the quality of CB banks and CB units, including the American Association of Blood Banks (AABB), the American Red Cross (ARC), the NHLBI Cord Blood Transplantation Study (COBLT), the European Group for Blood and Marrow Transplantation (EBMT), EUROCORD/NETCORD, the Foundation for the Accreditation of Cellular Therapy (FACT), the Group for the Collection and Expansion of Hematopoietic Cells (GRACE), the International Society for Cellular Therapy (ISCT), the Joint Accreditation Committee of ISHAGE-Europe and EBMT (JACIE) and the NMDP [16]. While minor differences exist in these standards, they are generally consistent, with few areas of conflict.

Over the past 35 years, techniques for the cryopreservation of human HSCs have developed empirically with little information about the cryobiology of these cells (see Chapter 47). With these techniques, survival rates for purified HSCs can be variable, with loss of cells due to clumping and the toxic effects of the cryoprotectants. While these techniques of cryopreservation have been generally acceptable for BM and PB sources of HSCs, where the number of cells preserved is usually in large excess of what is needed for successful engraftment and can compensate for higher degrees of cell loss due to the technical aspects of the process, these techniques may be inadequate for CB given the lower and limited number of nucleated cells.

Because of concerns about the loss of nucleated cells, CB that was initially collected for transplantation was cryopreserved without removal of red blood cells or further separation [6]. With this method of cryopreservation, large volumes of unseparated CB required a large freezer for storage. Subsequently, numerous investigators explored different methods of CB separation including the use of Ficoll, Percoll, methylcellulose, gelatin, starch and lysis to remove red blood cells and recover nucleated cells [28,48–51]. These methods have allowed for more efficient storage of CB units, although it is not yet clear what the best separation procedure is in terms of efficient recovery of stem and progenitor cells.

In clinical practice, many CB investigators and transplant physicians currently utilize the method of Rubinstein and colleagues for cryopreservation, thawing and infusion of separated and unseparated CB units [48]. However, investigators are now examining the cryobiologic properties of CB to determine how these differ from BM and mobilized PB and how best to optimize the cryopreservation and thawing of CB [52]. The cryobiologic properties may identify modifications of the Rubinstein method that will improve the recovery of viable HSCs from CB units.

CB units that are banked for allogeneic transplantation undergo histocompatibility typing using conventional serological and molecular, DNA-based techniques for class I antigens and molecular HLA typing for class II alleles. Because the amount of CB that is available for HLA typing and infectious disease testing is limited, molecular methods, including the polymerase chain reaction (PCR) and sequence-specific

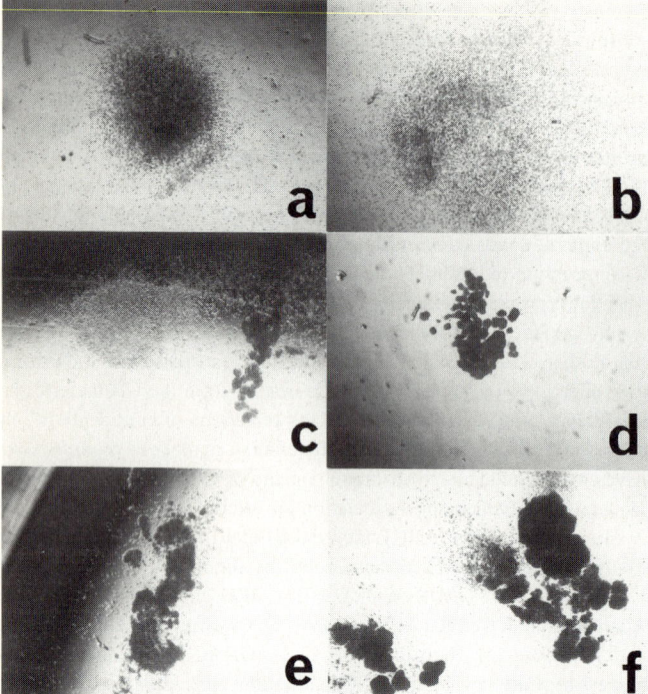

Fig. 43.1 Colony formation by granulocyte-macrophage (CFU-GM), erythroid (BFU-E) and multipotential (CFU-GEMM) progenitor cells from cord blood defrosted and plated in semisolid culture medium after being stored frozen for 15 years.

oligonucleotide probe (SSOP) methods, are used to better define class I and class II alleles while using very small amounts of CB cells (see Chapter 4) [53,54]. While these molecular techniques better define specific alleles, the optimal level of HLA typing for CB and the clinical impact of higher degrees of resolution are not currently known.

In addition to ABO, rhesus and HLA typing, CB banked for transplantation is tested for infectious agents in accordance with the requirements and recommendations of regulatory bodies as listed above. Specifically, CB units and the mother's blood are routinely tested for hepatitis B and C, human immunodeficiency virus (HIV), human T-cell lymphotropic virus (HTLV), cytomegalovirus (CMV) and syphilis [39,40,55].

Since some infectious agents can be transferred in liquid nitrogen, newly collected CB units are typically kept in quarantine until infectious disease testing is complete. If newly collected CB units are found to be free of potentially transmissible infectious agents, the units are placed into long-term liquid nitrogen storage. In addition to this testing, CB banks also elicit a history of genetic diseases in the family, travel of donors to places that have a high frequency of transmissible infections and other high-risk behavior, including intravenous drug use and high risk sexual behavior, upon which CB units may be excluded from the bank. These screening questions are similar to these used for blood donor screening by the AABB.

It is currently unclear how long CB can be viably cryopreserved, although theoretically this should be for at least the lifetime of an individual, assuming no practical mishaps. It has been shown that upon thawing, units of CB that were cryopreserved for up to 15 years contained $83 \pm 12\%$ of nucleated cells, with $95 \pm 16\%$, $84 \pm 25\%$ and $85 \pm 25\%$ recovery of granulocyte macrophage, erythroid and multipotential progenitor cell [56] values essentially equal to 10 years defrosts [57]. Moreover, the proliferative capacity of these early progenitor cells were intact (Fig. 43.1) for colonies formed from the cryopreserved cells and self-renewal potential of multipotential progenitors was high, as assessed by replating of colonies into secondary dishes *in vitro* and extensive *ex vivo* expansion was possible. Most importantly, CD34[+] cells separated from the 15 years defrosts were able to multilineage engraft sublethally irradiated nonobese diabetic with severe combined immunodeficiency syndrome (NOD/SCID) mice, suggesting high-quality recovery of HSCs [56]. Laboratory studies demonstrated that CB cells frozen for several years can be thawed, gene transduced and *ex vivo* expanded [56,58–60].

The unique paradigm created by CB banking has raised a number of ethical, regulatory and legal issues, including questions about recruitment, confidentiality, ownership, informed consent and fairness in the allocation of this valuable resource. Considerable efforts have been made to define these issues to ensure the appropriate operation of CB banks [46,47,61–65].

Searching for a CB donor

Several potential advantages of unrelated donor CB transplantation over unrelated donor BM or mobilized PB is the ready availability of banked CB units, a shorter time to acquisition of CB with a more rapid time to transplantation and the ability to tolerate greater degrees of HLA disparity. A recent analysis of the NMDP suggest that if 4 out of 6 and 3 out of 6 antigen matches are clinically acceptable, donors would be identified 99% of the time for patients of all races [66]. The clinical experience with CB suggest that HLA mismatches of up to 3 antigens result in acceptable clinical outcome. Thus, the availability of a suitable number of CB units would allow for the transplantation of the majority of patients. Further, the theoretical ability to target minority populations for inclusion in CB banks would further reduce the need to extend HLA mismatches to 2–3 antigens. However, it is not yet clear that CB banks have achieved success in diversifying the necessary HLA types by targeting minority populations [24].

Based upon traditional search methods and strategies, several groups have demonstrated that the time required for identification of a suitable stem cell source and the time to transplantation is more rapid for unrelated donor CB than for unrelated donor BM [67,68]. This shortened time interval may be as long as 4 weeks. However, it is not yet clear that CB transplantation will maintain this advantage with the recent initiation of the NMDP's urgent search process.

Finally, the ability to safely and effectively perform preimplantation genetic diagnosis, histocompatibility testing and *in vitro* fertilization allows parents with children with diseases in need of transplantation the option of creating a suitable CB donor [69]. While the ethical issues involved in this process continue to be debated [69], the advent of this technology will undoubtedly have a tremendous impact upon the practice of clinical transplantation.

Clinical results

While there is now extensive clinical experience for the transplantation of related and unrelated donor CB, to date, there are no prospective, randomized clinical trials comparing CB to BM or mobilized PB. Further, until recently, there were no retrospective cohort controlled studies to compare these different stem cell sources. The vast majority of clinical reports to date represent descriptive, retrospective case series of patients. While prospective, randomized studies involving CB, BM and PB are unlikely to occur, ongoing prospective trials of CB as the single stem cell source are in progress [35].

Related donor CB transplantation

Two large case series of related donor CB transplants have been reported by the International Bone Marrow Transplant Registry (IBMTR) [71] and EUROCORD [72]. These retrospective series have shown survival rates of approximately 60% at 1 year. However, of greater importance are results of the IBMTR and EUROCORD report in a retrospective cohort controlled analysis of children <15 years of age transplanted for malignant and nonmalignant diseases with HLA-identical CB or BM [72]. In this study, 2052 unmanipulated BM recipients were compared to 113 CB recipients. Transplants were performed between 1990 and 1997 at 207 transplant centers worldwide. The median period of follow-up was 27 months (range: 3–85). Significant differences in these two patient groups were identified, with CB recipients being younger (5 years vs. 8 years, $p <0.001$), of lower weight (median weight 17 kg vs. 26 kg, $p <0.001$) and less likely to receive methotrexate (MTX) for graft-vs.-host disease (GVHD) prophylaxis (28% vs. 65%, $p <0.001$). The median CB cell dose was 4.7×10^7 nucleated cells/kg (range: $<1.0 \times 10^8$–36×10^7/kg). The cumulative incidence of neutrophil engraftment by day 60 was 0.89 (95%CI: 0.82–0.94) for CB vs. 0.98 (95%CI: 0.97–0.99) for BM ($p <0.001$). The cumulative incidence of platelet recovery to 20,000/mm^3 was 44 days after CB and 24 days after BM, with a cumulative incidence of platelet engraftment by day 180 of 0.86 (95%CI: 0.78–0.92) for CB vs. 0.96 (95%CI: 0.94–0.97) after BM ($p <0.001$).

The cumulative incidence of grades II–IV acute GVHD was 0.14 (95%CI: 0.08–0.22) for CB vs. 0.24 (95%CI: 0.22–0.26) for BM ($p = 0.02$). The 3-year cumulative incidence of chronic GVHD was 0.06 (95%CI: 0.02–0.13) for CB vs. 0.15 (95%CI: 0.13–0.17) for BM ($p = 0.02$). However, there was no difference in the probability of overall survival at 3 years (0.64 (95%CI: 0.53–0.74) for CB vs. 0.66 (95%CI: 0.64–0.68) for BM with no difference in relapse-related deaths. Taken together, this study demonstrated a lower risk of acute and chronic GVHD with CB, a slower rate of neutrophil and platelet recovery in the 1st month post-transplant with CB, but similar survival in both CB and BM recipients. These findings support the use of HLA-matched related donor CB as an acceptable alternate to BM for children with HLA-identical siblings.

Unrelated donor CB transplantation

As with related donor CB transplantation, the vast majority of the experience with unrelated donor CB transplantation is the result of retrospective case reports of patients [18,70–74], rather than the result of prospective clinical trials [75]. The largest of these retrospective series [74] has been recently updated [19]. The large series of 861 patients reports the outcome of unrelated donor CB transplantation as facilitated by the New York Cord Blood Program.

The majority of CB recipients in this series were children (age 0–11 years) (67%) and patients with hematologic malignancies (67%) [19]. The majority of patients received CB grafts that were HLA mismatched at HLA-A, -B or -DRB1 with 87% of grafts mismatched for 1 or 2 antigens. The Kaplan–Meier estimate for neutrophil engraftment (absolute neutrophil count [ANC] ≥500/mm^3) was 0.93. As in other reports [73,75,76], the most powerful factor predictive of neutrophil engraftment was the cell dose of the CB unit. However, the analysis also found that the time to neutrophil recovery was associated with HLA disparity, with a median neutrophil engraftment on day 23 for recipients of HLA matched CB vs. day 28 for recipients of HLA mismatched CB ($p = 0.0027$). Acute GVHD was also associated with increasing HLA disparity. The incidence of grade III–IV acute GVHD was 0.08 for recipients of HLA-A, -B, -DRB1 matched CB and 0.28 in mismatched CB recipients ($p = 0.006$). Multivariate analysis demonstrated GVHD and stage of disease as the best predictors of disease relapse. In this series, the Kaplan–Meier estimate at 3 years for overall survival was 0.27 (95%CI: 0.40–0.55) for patients with hematologic malignancies and 0.48 (95%CI: 0.40–0.55) for patients with genetic diseases.

Among the largest single institution unrelated donor CB studies is that reported by investigators at the University of Minnesota [18]. In the retrospective study, 102 patients (median age 7.4 years; range: 0.2–56.9) received CB grafts between 1994 and 2001. Patients had malignant ($n = 65$, 63%) and nonmalignant ($n = 37$, 37%) disorders. Fourteen percent of CB grafts were fully matched with 86% of grafts mismatched for 1–3 antigens. The incidence of neutrophil and platelet engraftment was 0.88 (95%CI: 0.81–0.95) and 0.65 (95%CI: 0.53–0.77) at a median of 23 days and 86 days, respectively.

The probability of severe acute GVHD and chronic GVHD were 0.11 (95%CI: 0.05–0.17) and 0.10 (95%CI: 0.04–0.16), respectively. The probability of survival at 1 year was 0.58 (95%CI: 0.48–0.68). Cell dose as measured by transplanted CD34$^+$ was significantly associated with the rate of engraftment, transplant related mortality and survival.

Two recent reports have compared the results of unrelated donor CB transplantation with that of unrelated donor BMT [77,78]. In the first of these case controlled retrospective reports, recipients of 0–3 HLA antigen mismatched CB were compared with recipients of HLA-A, -B, -DRB1-matched unrelated donor BM [77]. Analyses were based upon the type of GVHD prophylaxis administered. All CB recipients received cyclosporine (CSP) and methylprednisone. BM recipients received either CSP and MTX (26 pairs) or CSP and methylprednisone and T-cell depletion (31 pairs). This analysis demonstrated a probability of neutrophil engraftment at day 45 of 0.88 (95%CI: 0.75–1.00) for CB vs. 0.96 (95%CI: 0.89–1.00) for BM (CSP plus MTX) ($p = 0.41$) and 0.85 (95%CI: 0.72–0.98) for CB vs. 0.90 (95%CI: 0.80–1.0) for BM (T-cell depletion) ($p = 0.32$). The probability of platelet engraftment by day 180 was 0.72 (95%CI: 0.50–0.94) for CB vs. 0.76 (95%CI: 0.54–0.98) for BM (CSP plus MTX), and 0.84 (95%CI: 0.64–1.00) for CB compared to 0.84 (95%CI: 0.64–1.00) for T-cell-depleted BM. Analyses were performed using matched-pair analysis based on the type of GVHD prophylaxis administered. The incidences of acute and chronic GVHD were similar for both stem cell sources.

The Kaplan–Meier estimate of overall survival at 2 years was 0.53 (95%CI: 0.31–0.75) for CB recipients vs. 0.41 (95%CI: 0.22–0.60) for BM (CSP plus MTX) ($p = 0.40$) and 0.52 (95%CI: 0.30–0.73) for CB vs. 0.56 (95%CI: 0.30–0.70) for BM (T-cell depletion) ($p >0.80$). The single institution, case controlled analysis suggested that despite significantly greater HLA disparity among CB recipients, the probabilities of neutrophil and platelet engraftment, acute and chronic GVHD and survival were similar between recipients of 0–3 antigen-mismatched unrelated donor CB and HLA-matched unrelated donor BM.

Similar results were demonstrated in an analysis performed by EUROCORD [68]. In this analysis, 541 children with acute leukemia who received either 0–4 HLA antigen mismatched CB ($n = 99$) were compared with recipients of 0–3 HLA antigen mismatched T-cell-depleted unrelated donor BM ($n = 180$) or recipients of 0–2 HLA antigen mismatched T-replete BM ($n = 262$). While comparisons were made after adjustments to these three groups, distinct differences were noted among the three groups. Most notably, CB recipients received a higher number of HLA mismatched grafts (92%) vs. recipients of T-cell-depleted BM (43%) vs. T-replete BM recipients (18%) ($p <0.001$). The probability of neutrophil engraftment by day 60 was 0.80 (95%CI: 0.70–0.90) for CB, 0.90 (95%CI: 0.84–0.96) for T-cell-depleted BM and 0.96 (95%CI: 0.95–0.97) for T-replete BM at a median of 32 days (range: 11–56), 16 days (9–40) and 18 days (range: 10–40) ($p <0.001$), respectively. Platelet recovery occurred at a median of 81 days (range: 16–159) for CB, 29 days (range: 8–165) for T-cell-depleted BM and 28 days for T-replete BM ($p <0.001$). The probability of grades III–IV acute GVHD was less in recipients of CB (0.22) and T-cell-depleted BM (0.08) vs. T-replete BM ($p = 0.30$). Further, the probability of chronic GVHD was lower in CB and T-cell-depleted marrow recipients as compared to T-replete BM

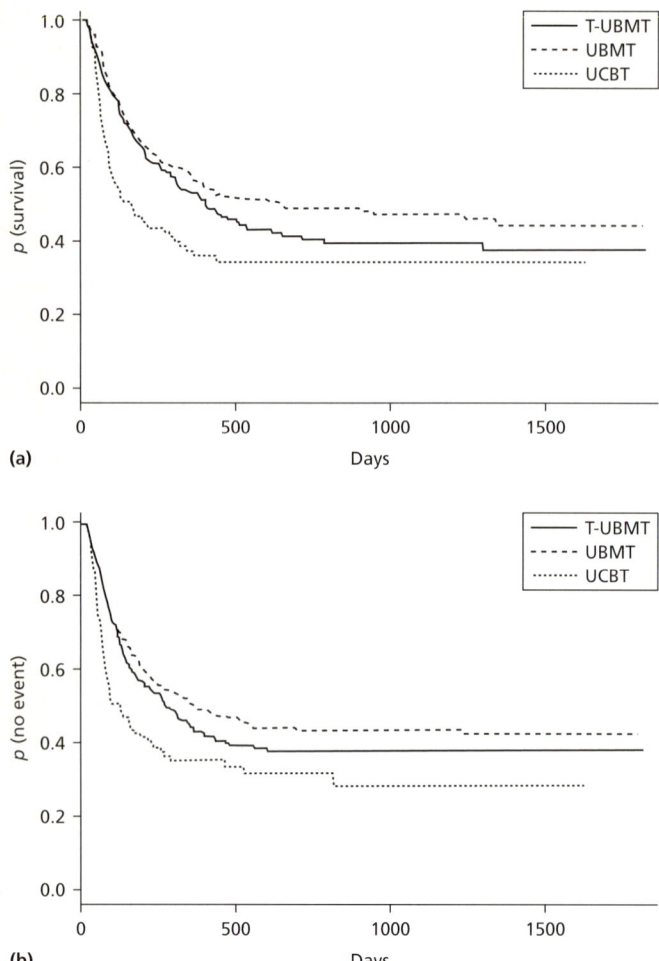

Fig. 43.2 Kaplan–Meier estimate of overall survival (a) and event-free survival (b) of all children with acute leukemia receiving unrelated stem cell transplants (UBMT, T-UBMT and UCBT) nonadjusted for patient, disease and transplant differences. Reproduced with permission from Rocha et al. [68], courtesy of the American Society of Hematology.

($p = 0.02$). While early transplant-related mortality was highest among CB recipients ($p < 0.01$), nonadjusted estimates of survival (for patient, disease and transplant differences) at 2 years were similar: 0.35 (95%CI: 0.25–0.45) for CB, 0.41 (95%CI: 0.33–0.49) for T-cell-depleted BM and 0.49 (95%CI: 0.43–0.55) for T-replete BM (Fig. 43.2 [68]). Overall mortality was greatest in recipients of T-cell-depleted BM ($p < 0.07$).

Taken together, the retrospective analyses suggest that unrelated donor CB, T-cell-depleted unrelated donor BM CB and T-replete BM have different risks and potential advantages, with similar overall survival. The data support the overall findings suggesting that unrelated donor CB is a reasonable stem cell source for children without a matched related donor, giving comparable survival results to unrelated donor BM.

CB transplantation in adults

As a result of the limited number of cells available in the finite volume of collected CB, there was initial concern that CB may not contain a sufficient number of cells to reliably engraft larger children, adolescents and adults. However, with the growth of CB banks and improvements in CB collection techniques, CB units with a large number of nucleated cells are becoming increasingly available. As a result, while there are still no prospective clinical trials in adults, there is an emerging experience for CB transplantation in adults [15,16,79–83].

The first large series of CB transplantation in adults reported 68 adults (median age 31.4 years; range: 17.6–58.1) with hematologic malignancies, marrow failure syndromes and a single patient with an inborn error of metabolism [79]. The median weight of patients was 69.2 kg (range: 40.9–115.5). Seventy-one percent of patients received CB grafts that were mismatched for 2 or more HLA antigens with patients receiving a median cell dose of 1.6×10^7 nucleated cells/kg (range: 0.6×10^7–4×10^7) and a median of 1.2×10^5 CD34$^+$/kg (range: 0.2×10^5–16.7×10^5). The probability of neutrophil engraftment was 0.90 (95%CI: 0.85–1.0) at a median of 27 days (range: 13–59). Similar to other reports, this study also demonstrated an association between a higher number of cells in the cryopreserved CB unit and the rate of neutrophil recovery. Platelet recovery (>50,000/mm^3) occurred at a median of 99 days (range: 42–228).

The probability of acute GVHD of grades III–IV by day 100 was 0.20 (95%CI: 0.11–0.29) without a significant association between the grade of acute GVHD and the degree of HLA mismatching ($p = 0.70$). The probability of chronic GVHD was 0.38 (95%CI: 0.23–0.52). At a median follow-up of 22 months (range: 11–51), 19 of 68 patients were alive (28%) with 18 of them disease-free. Thirty-two of 68 (47%) patients died of transplant-related complications. Patients receiving CB grafts containing more than 1.2×10^5 CD34$^+$ cells/kg had longer survival than patients receiving less than this number of CD34$^+$ cells ($p = 0.05$). However, event-free survival was not associated with HLA disparity ($p = 0.07$), patient age ($p = 0.42$), or the type of malignancy. The results are similar to those reported by EUROCORD for 107 adults [78].

Taken together, the experience in adults suggests that the probability of engraftment and incidence of acute and chronic GVHD are tolerable, but nonrelapse mortality is high. While this may be the result of performing CB transplantation in only high-risk patients, prospective studies and case controlled comparisons of CB to BM in adults are required to better define the use of CB in adults.

Immune reconstitution after CB transplantation

As a result of the low number of transplanted cells and the "naive" pattern of immune cells in CB, it was initially thought that immune reconstitution following CB transplantation was delayed in comparison to BM and mobilized PB. It was reported that CB transplant recipients had a high incidence of infectious complications, although it was not apparent if these infections were the result of delayed immune recovery, delayed neutrophil engraftment, or the general use of high-dose steroids for GVHD prophylaxis in CB recipients.

The pattern of immune recovery following CB transplantation has now been well described for children and adults [75,76,84–90]. The reports demonstrate a remarkably similar pattern, with prompt recovery of natural killer (NK) cells by 2–3 months post-transplant, recovery of B cells by 6–9 months post-transplant, CD8$^+$ T cells by 8–9 months, but delayed recovery of CD4$^+$ T cells with a return to normal numbers at approximately 1 year. In studies involving both children and adults, the recovery of CD4$^+$ T cells is slower in adults, consistent with the pattern of recovery for BM and PB [90]. Mitogen stimulation responses are noted in the normal range by 6–9 months post-transplant. More recent studies of the T-cell receptor diversity [88] and T-cell receptor excision circles [86–88] further suggest efficient thymic regeneration mechanisms following CB transplantation that are similar, if not superior, to that of BM.

Future directions for clinical CB transplantation

Slower neutrophil and platelet engraftments, as well as a lower probability of engraftment compared to other graft sources, has been consistently reported in children and adults following CB transplantation. Several strategies have been explored to address this problem. The expansion of CB banks with an increasingly large number of CB units with a larger cell dose is making larger CB units more available for transplantation. The use of hematopoietic growth factors (e.g. granulocyte colony-stimulating factor [G-CSF]) has been routinely used after CB transplantation. More limited is the use of other growth factors (e.g. interleukin 11 [IL-11]). However, to date, there are no reliable data to suggest the benefit of growth factors following CB transplantation.

Another approach for facilitation of neutrophil and platelet engraftment is the *ex vivo* expansion of CB prior to transplantation [91,92]. In the largest series to date [91] 25 adults and 12 children with hematologic malignancies ($n = 34$) or breast cancer ($n = 3$) received the infusion of CB expanded in G-CSF, megakaryocyte growth and development factor and stem cell factor (also called steel factor). Patients received a median of 0.99×10^7 nucleated cells/kg (expanded plus unexpanded CB). The median time to neutrophil and platelet engraftment was 28 days (range: 15–49) and 106 days (range: 38–345) with engraftment in all patients who survived 28 days. Grade III–IV acute GVHD occurred in 40% of patients, with extensive chronic GVHD in 63% of patients. This information notes a greatly increased rate of acute and chronic GVHD compared to noncultured cells. With a median follow-up of 30 months, 35% of patients survive. Future studies will continue to explore the safety and efficacy of *ex vivo* expansion, different expansion conditions and the use of gene-marking to better understand the contribution of expanded CB cells to short and long-term hematopoiesis.

Finally, the pooling of two or more CB units from different donors is now being explored. However, the safety and efficacy of this approach is currently unknown. The initial report of this approach [93] involved the transplantation of two units of CB into an 84-kg adult recipient. Neutrophil engraftment occurred on day 25 with both units contributing to blood production. Whether engraftment by both, one or none of the units is maintained remains to be determined. The prospective use of multiple CB units is currently ongoing.

Characteristics of primitive hematopoietic stem and progenitor cells in CB

The numbers of nucleated cells available for CB transplantation are greatly limited compared to that available and used for BMT. How has CB served as a source of transplantable cells when the numbers of nucleated cells used are generally less than or equal to one-tenth that used for BMT? It is clear that the frequency of primitive cells in CB, as assessed by progenitor cell numbers as determined by assays of colony-forming cells [6,8], is greater than that of BM. The numbers of granulocyte-macrophage, erythroid, and multipotential progenitor cells, respectively, assessed as colony-forming unit–granulocyte/macrophage (CFU-GM), burst forming units-erythroid (BFU-E) and colony-forming unit–granulocyte/erythrocyte/macrophage/megakaryocyte (CFU-GEMM) present in the first 65 CB collections performed in the Broxmeyer laboratory have been published [57]. The numbers included those used for the first five and two of the next five transplantations. While the wide range of values within a category demonstrates the variability of CB content, most of these values fell within the limits of the corresponding numbers present in BM used for successful BMT [8]. For example, there were $12.5 \pm 23.6\%$ (mean ± 1 SD; range: 0.3–47.1) CFU-GM and $11.3 \pm 12.8\%$ (range: 0.9–70.7) CFU-GEMM colonies, which responded to stimulation *in vitro* by the combination of erythropoietin (EPO), IL-3 and stem cell factor, and $9.5 \pm 9.9\%$ (range: 0.9–44.8) BFU-E colonies, which formed from cells stimulated by EPO plus IL-3. In one report, it was noted that the progenitor cell content of CB units was more rigorously associated with major covariants of post-transplantation survival than was the nucleated cell count, and that progenitor cell content was a better indication of

CB grafts [94]. Numbers of progenitor cells alone, however, do not tell the whole story. As important, or more important, than absolute numbers are the quality of these cells in CB compared to BM. Functional characterization of primitive cells in CB includes cells with extensive proliferative capacity and replating ability (the latter being a measure used to estimate self-renewal capacity) *in vitro* [6,8,95–118]. While CB progenitors are usually in a slow or noncycling state compared to those in BM, they respond very rapidly to stimulation by combinations of cytokines including EPO, granulocyte macrophage colony-stimulating factor (GM-CSF), IL-3, stem cell factor and Flt3 ligand (Flt3L). Moreover, primitive human CB cells appear to have great capacity to engraft/repopulate the hematopoietic system of mice with SCID.

Transplantation of human cells into mice with SCID, especially those with the NOD genotype, has been used to evaluate the engrafting capability of primitive human cells in the hopes of providing an assay for the earliest subset of human HSCs that has long-term marrow repopulating capacity. Studies suggest that CB cells repopulate in SCID mice more effectively than do BM cells [109–118]. Both CB and BM are mainly in a quiescent state, with these cells in the G_0 and G_1 phases of the cell cycle. CB CD34$^+$ cells in G_0 and G_1 phases of the cell cycle have similar ability to repopulate the hematopoietic system of NOD/SCID mice [119]. The G_0 and G_1 values are of interest in light of a report that demonstrated that G_0 CD34$^+$ cells from CB have a 1000-fold greater capacity than G_1 CD34$^+$ cells for generating progenitors *in vitro* [120]. Whether the differences in these two studies reflect homing characteristics (discussed below) or other characteristics of cells at different stages of the cell cycle remains to be determined.

The proliferative characteristics of primitive CB cells noted above are extensive and are no doubt an important measure responsible for the engrafting capability of CB in patients. However, investigations have not yet clearly defined why engraftment of neutrophils and, especially, platelets is slower with CB than BM cells. This difference may in part reflect the more immature nature of CB vs. BM primitive cells. While there is as yet no evidence that CB contains a primitive population unique to CB, the more immature status of CB primitive cells as a total population is suggested by studies evaluating the loss of telomeric DNA with age [121] and a higher ratio of more immature to the mature colony-forming cells in CB than in BM [8]. A recent review on the capacity for functional activity of HSCs during aging has suggested that HSCs do show signs of aging and may have a limited functional lifespan that may limit longevity in mammals [122]. If there is less loss of telomeric DNA in CB cells then it is likely that HSCs from CB would be more functionally competitive than HSCs from BM and perhaps a more appropriate source for long-term repopulation. The information is consistent with the observation of more telomeric DNA in CB than BM CD34$^+$ cells [121] and recent studies in mice demonstrating that BM cells from mice deficient in telomerase, which have critically short telomeres, have reduced *in vitro* proliferative, *in vitro* replating and *in vivo* long-term repopulating capacities [123].

Efforts to accelerate neutrophil recovery in recipients of CB transplantation have not been very rewarding. There is no clear evidence that administration of G-CSF to patients receiving a CB transplant have decreased the time to neutrophil engraftment. It has been suggested, but not yet proven, that perhaps engraftment of *ex vivo* treated CB cells, which are known to enhance numbers of progenitors and more mature cells, would have faster mature cell engraftment as an end product [124]. Low numbers of megakaryocyte progenitors in CB grafts have been implicated in the delay in platelet recovery after CB transplantation [125], but the problem may also be in the maturation capacity of the megakaryocytes from CB. It has been noted that CB megakaryocytes derived from megakaryocyte progenitors do not complete maturation as well as cells from BM or PB in an *in vitro* situation where CB megakaryocytes were associated with impaired endomitosis after stimulation with thrombopoietin (TPO) [126]. TPO is currently being evaluated for clinical efficacy in accelerating platelet production [127], but whether or not TPO will have benefits for CB, or other forms of HSC transplantation, is not clear. More intricate knowledge of cytokine regulation of blood cell production in the context of stromal cell interactions may be necessary for development of better intervention methodologies to accelerate engraftment of CB cells.

There are a number of cell surface phenotypic markers of primitive cells that help to define these populations. For the most part, these markers, which include CD34 [128], CD38, Thy1, c-kit, Flt3, and rhodamine-123, are the same for primitive cells found in CB and BM [99,103,129–136]. These primitive cells express CD34 antigens and low levels of CD38, thy1, c-kit and rhodamine-123, and are positive for Flt3. Only expression of HLA-DR seems to be different in that primitive populations of CB cells express HLA-DR, but these populations in BM either do not express it or do so at a very low level [135,137]. CD34 is a glycophosphoprotein [128] and the earliest cells contain a higher density distribution of CD34 than do the later, more mature cells [138]. However, human $CD34^+$ cells contain HSCs and HPCs, and since CD34 is also found on other cells (e.g. endothelial cells) this marker alone is not a perfect indicator of the actual number of HSCs or the composition of HSCs and HPCs of a graft. The possibility that HSCs were in a $CD34^-$ population was suggested by studies demonstrating long-term lymphohematopoietic reconstitution in mice with a single CD34 low or negative cell [139] and then by human studies highlighted by a report demonstrating $CD34^-lin^-$ human SCID-repopulating cells (SRCs) [140]. The problem of whether HSCs resided in a lineage negative population of $CD34^+$ or $CD34^-$ cells became even more complicated when it became clear that the CD34 cell surface component was inducible and variable, and its detection in human cells clearly depended on the sensitivity of the technology and background settings used to determine its expression on the cell surface. Presently, it is not clear if the intense discussions of $CD34^+/CD34^-$ lineage negative cells, which have decreased to the point where few or no publications even continue to report on the issue, have changed the thinking or processing of cells for transplantation. Most clinicians still consider CD34 a reasonable marker for an engraftable population of primitive cells. In the human system, $CD34^+$ cells can be subtyped into a $CD38^-$ population, considered to contain the earliest cells including HSCs, and a $CD38^+$ population in which HPCs are highly enriched and HSCs are few or absent. The complexity and heterogeneity of the $CD34^+CD38^-$ population is highlighted by the demonstration that in the human SRC assay, fewer than 1 : 600 $CD34^+CD38^-$ cells appear to be a human SRC [115], and the SCID assay is currently our best assay for evaluating human HSCs. At present it is possible to more rigorously define a murine, than a human, HSCs phenotypically. Mouse HSCs functional assays depend on repopulation of lethally irradiated mice in either a competitive or noncompetitive situation. In the human SRC assay, only sublethal irradiation dosages are given to recipient mice, and human cells have not been proven to rescue lethally irradiated SCID mice. Murine HSCs [141,142] are phenotypically characterized into long (Sca-1^{hi} Thy1^{lo}, Lin$^-$Mac-1^-, c-kit$^+$) and short-term (Sca-1^{hi} Thy-1^{lo}, Lin$^-$, Mac-1^{lo}, c-kit$^+$) repopulating cells [143]. More rigorous phenotyping of murine, than human, HPCs is also available [144,145]. More definitive phenotypic categorizing of human HSCs and HPCs is needed. In this regard, a clonogenic subpopulation of $CD34^+CD38^-$ cells were identified that expressed high levels of CD7 and possessed only potential for lymphoid cell development [146]. These cells also expressed CD45RA and HLA-DP, but were low or absent in expression of c-kit and Thy-1. While phenotyping of cells has been of some use in a clinical setting in that the read-out of cell types is quick compared to that of functional assays, and primitive populations can be enriched using these markers, phenotypes do not offer definitive information on the self-renewal, proliferation and differentiation capacity of these cells.

The next step in HSC biology is likely to be a comprehensive molecular profile of HSC and HPC populations. This molecular profile, which has already begun in terms of phenotypically defined populations of murine adult BM, murine embryonic stem cells, murine fetal liver cells and human fetal liver cells [147–149] will no doubt be accelerated for human cells by advances in technology, but may be hindered by lack of more precise phenotypic-markers of human HSCs and HPCs that better recapitulate subset functional heterogeneity.

The possibility of adult stem cell plasticity/transdifferentiation evolved recently. The intrigue in this area centered on the supposition that HSCs might have a previously unrecognized capacity to give rise to cells of other tissues. This potential for plasticity would greatly expand the uses of HSCs, including those found in CB, and hence the excitement. During embryonic development, the germ layer gives rise to endoderm (internal organs, gastrointestinal epithelium), mesoderm (blood, bone, muscle, connective tissue) and ectoderm (nervous system, skin). The question being asked was whether or not HSCs from adult BM and CB had this enhanced developmental capacity inherent in them. Most recently, caution with regards to the plasticity concept has surfaced [150,151]. None of the original reports definitively provided complete and rigorous proof that HSCs had this pluripotenciality. If plasticity of adult cells truly exists, it may be a rare event that may not readily lend itself to clinical utility in the near future. A rigorous definition of plasticity/transdifferentiation is that a single cell of one type (e.g. HSCs) can give rise to functional cells of another lineage (e.g. bone, muscle, nervous system, skin, etc.). Because this involves one cell becoming another, only the most rigorous experimental proof will satisfy the question as to whether this cell truly exists in the adult. This requires proof of the single cell origin of the donor cell and the identification of functional activity of the cell(s) of another lineage that the donor cell gave rise to. If rigorous proof for this concept is attained, efforts will be needed to study the regulation of growth of these multitissue stem cells and their production of lineage specific cells. Questions here include the following: Will there be a hierarchy of these multitissue stem cells? Do HSCs have this potentiality? Will HSCs have the capability of giving rise to all three germ cell lines or will they be more lineage restricted to one or more germ cell lines? And, finally, since these cells may be extremely rare, can they be expanded without loss of their multipotentialities?

Ex vivo expansion of CB stem cells

Since the numbers of HSCs and HPCs that can be obtained from single collections of CB is limited [6,8,57,95] and that these numbers appear to be dose-limiting, especially in the context of higher-weight individuals and adults [9,79], a number of different options to deal with this problem have been evaluated (see Chapter 9). These include attempts at *ex vivo* expansion of HSCs and HPCs, the use of combined collections of CB, and enhancement in the homing capacity of HSCs and HPCs. Investigators have placed extensive laboratory efforts into expanding CB HSCs *ex vivo*. Such expansion could also potentially allow a single CB collection to be used for multiple transplant recipients, thus enhancing the efficacy of CB banking. It is clear that primitive CB cells can be greatly expanded *ex vivo* [8,97–99,101,102,104,105]. However, these studies point to a far greater expansion of the more mature cells than the most immature cells in this primitive population. Also a dissociation of SRC phenotype and function was noted during expansion of CB $CD34^+CD38^-$ cells [152], and the fate of functional SRCs has varied greatly amongst groups studying their expansion *ex vivo*. These studies leave the question of whether the long-term marrow repopulating HSCs are truly being expanded under these conditions and, if so, by how much?

Clearly, loss of these most primitive cells is undesirable, although, for *ex vivo* expansion procedures to be clinically useful, it may be sufficient to use a collection that has been expanded for HPCs and at least maintained for HSCs. While CB cells that have been subjected to *ex vivo* expansion culture maneuvers have been transplanted into recipients [91], clinical benefit of these cells has not yet been convincingly demonstrated.

The capacity to *ex vivo* expand HSCs is most likely limited by our knowledge of the process of self-renewal, and what it actually takes in terms of known or unknown cytokines and stromal cell interactions to accomplish this process. Without doubt, a clearer understanding of self-renewal and the mechanisms mediating these effects will accelerate our ability to expand HSCs *ex vivo* and also *in vivo*. In this context, *HOXB4*, a member of the HOX family of transcriptional factors, has been implicated in the expansion of adult, embryonic, and yolk sac murine HSCs [153–155]. Future efforts to enhance expression of *HOXB4*, and other to be identified genes, that may be involved in self-renewal, through the use of cytokine, stromal and/or gene transfer methods may prove useful in *ex vivo* expansion procedures as long as it is proven that such maneuvers do not inadvertently confer abnormal growth characteristics on these treated cells that result in leukemia, proliferative or aplastic conditions.

Gene therapy of CB stem cells

Gene therapy has been considered a potential treatment possibility for at least 20 years [156] and there are over 600 such clinical trials completed, ongoing or pending worldwide (see Chapter 11) [157]. Efforts in this regard have used gene therapy in order to try to myeloprotect HSCs from cytotoxic chemotherapeutics [158,159] as well as to replace defective genes. In this continued effort, CB HSCs are logical cellular vehicles for the dissemination of the products of newly introduced genes, since transferring a gene into the earliest subsets of HSCs, those with long-term marrow repopulating capacity, offers the opportunity for lifetime expression of the new gene. There is *in vitro* evidence that primitive CB cells may be more efficiently transduced than equivalent cells in BM using retroviral vectors [138,160]. Primitive CB cells, including subsets within the CB HSC pool, are efficiently transduced by retroviral vectors [58,138,159–161], although the rate of successful gene transfer into the cell that repopulates the hematopoietic system of SCID mice, and which might be a long-term marrow repopulating human cell, is relatively low [114]. In laboratory studies, retroviral vectors have been used to replace genetically defective genes, and to place genes for growth factor receptors and growth factors into primitive cells, with resultant enhanced functional activities for these cells [58,160,162–167]. Additional viral vectors have been evaluated [168] and include lentiviruses [169,170] and adeno-associated viral vectors [171–173].

A limited number of attempts at gene therapy have been performed utilizing CB in a clinical setting [174]. Three children with adenosine deaminase (ADA)-deficient SCID received transplants of noncryopreserved autologous CB CD34+ *ADA* gene-transduced cells in a nonmyeloablated setting. Engraftment of the retrovirally *ADA* gene-transduced cells was successful, but the level of engraftment was low [175,176]. Enhanced effectiveness of this procedure as a clinical effort will most likely have to await the elucidation of better viral or other types of vectors and improved methodology to transduce the earliest noncycling HSCs, with maintenance of the self-renewal capacity of the transduced cells and high, but controlled, expression of the introduced genes. It is hoped that technical advances will accelerate the use of gene transfer for gene therapy using CB HSCs as vehicles for the transduced genes. In this context, it is of interest that the messenger RNA expression of receptors for certain retroviral vectors is significantly increased after, compared to before, cryopreservation of CB cells [177].

Homing of CB stem cells

While *ex vivo* expansion of HSCs from CB is potentially a viable possibility for enhancing the utility of CB transplantation for higher weight individuals (including adults), enhanced homing of the small numbers of HSCs found in single collections of CB is another potential option to increase the applicability of CB transplantation. Little is known regarding the migration and homing of CB HSCs and HPCs, or even why CB is so highly enriched in these primitive cells compared to nonmobilized adult PB. As in studies in which mouse cells are infused into mice, it is likely that only a minority of the population of HSCs that are infused into human recipients actually home to an appropriate microenvironment that is conducive for the self-renewal, proliferation and differentiation of the HSCs and HPCs. A future scenario can be envisioned in which it is possible to successfully induce or activate the cell surface of CB HSCs, or any HSCs, or modify the microenvironment, such that the percentage of cells homing to the appropriate microenvironment is greatly enhanced. This ability of enhanced homing could result in a reduction in the number of cells necessary for engraftment and might even shorten the time to engraftment. A clearer understanding of adhesion molecules, such as the integrins [178–185], and the agents that enhance expression and activation of these adhesion molecules will no doubt be of use. Whether there are specific homing receptors on HSCs remains to be determined, but it is possible that the cytokine family of chemokine molecules, along with other cytokines, may be intimately involved in the migration and homing of HSCs. Chemokines were so-named because they were chemoattractant chemokines involved in chemotaxis (directed cell movement, as contrasted to chemokinesis, random cell movement) of leukocytes [186]. Amongst the more than 50 known chemokines within the CC, CXC, C and CX_3C family, few have actually shown chemotaxis activity for HSCs or HPCs. For example, the chemokines stromal cell-derived factor (SDF)-1/CXCL12 [187,188], CKβ-11/CXCL19 [189] and SLC/CCL21 [190] have been implicated in the *in vitro* chemotactic migration of primitive cells from CB and BM, and these chemokines act in concert with stem cell factor [188,189], CXβ-11/CCL19 and SLC/CCL21 and are relatively specific for chemotaxis of macrophage progenitor cells [189,190], while SDF-1/CXCL12 is chemotactic for a wide range of progenitor cells (CFU-E, BFU-E, CFU-GEMM, etc.) [187,188]. Further, amongst all chemokines selective for chemotaxis of phenotypically defined populations of murine HSCs [191]. SDF-1/CXCL12 and its receptor CXCR4 have been implicated in homing of human stem cells into SCID mice [192–194]. While there is information on intracellular signaling in cell lines associated with SDF-1/CXCL12 actions [reviewed in 195], the only intracellular signals thus far definitely linked mechanistically to SDF-1/CXCL12 chemotaxis of primary HPCs are the phosphatases SHIP [196] and SHP-1 [195] in which HPCs from mice functionally deleted in SHIP and SHP-1 were enhanced in sensitivity to SDF-1/CXCL12 chemotaxis, suggesting that they act to negatively regulate SDF-1/CXCL12 induced chemotaxis. Since SDF-1/CXCL12 also acts as a survival factor for HPCs and HSCs [reviewed in 197–199] this chemokine may play a dual role in homing to, as well as survival within, the marrow microenvironment.

In addition, mice that are null for chemokine receptors, such as CXCR4 (the receptor for SDF-1/CXCL12) [200], CXCR2 (a receptor for IL-8) [201] and CCR1 (a receptor for MIP-1α) [202], have been used to suggest that these chemokine receptors may also be involved in trafficking of murine HPCs. $CXCR4^{-/-}$ mice die perinatally with little or no hematopoiesis in the marrow. $CXCR2^{-/-}$ mice demonstrate a hyperplasia of hematopoietic cells, especially in the spleen, and $CCR1^{-/-}$ mice have abnormal tissue distribution of progenitor cells.

Treating CB HSCs or HPCs *ex vivo* with cytokines, or transducing these cells with genes for receptors or cytokines involved in homing, may permit the use of fewer HSCs for optimal engraftment. In this context, decreasing the amount or activity of CD26/DPPIV (dipeptidylpeptidase IV), a membrane bound extracellular peptidase that cleaves dipeptides from the N-terminus of polypeptide chains, may result in enhanced homing [203]. CD26/DPPIV can cleave the chemokine CXCL12/SDF-1α at its position two proline and inactivate CXCL12/SDF-1. CD26/DPPIV is expressed by a subpopulation of $CD34^+$ cells isolated from CB and these cells have DPPIV activity. It was found that N-terminal truncated CXCL12/SDF-1α lacked the ability to induce migration of $CD34^+$ CB cells, but acted to inhibit normal CXCL12/SDF-1α induced migration. Inhibition of endogenous CD26/DPPIV activity on $CD34^+$ CB cells enhanced the migratory response of these cells to CXCL12/SDF-1α. CD26/DPPIV is only expressed on 8–10% of $CD34^+$ CB cells, and this process of CXCL12/SDF-1α cleavage by CD26/DPPIV on a subpopulation of $CD34^+$ cells may represent a mechanism in HSCs and HPCs for migration, homing and mobilization of these cells. Thus, inhibition of the CD26/DPPIV peptidase activity may represent a means to increase homing and engraftment during CB transplantation.

Immune cells

An original concern with CB transplantation was that CB collections might contain maternal cell contamination and, thus, elicit a severe and life-threatening GVHD reaction [7,9,10,204]. However, the original studies using relatively insensitive methods did not find any maternal T-cell contamination [7,9–11]. Further studies using much more sensitive technology found that maternal T cells do contaminate CB collections in many cases [22,205–209], but the frequency of contaminating T cells was extremely low. This low frequency of contaminating T cells, in the absence of clinical data suggesting an enhanced incidence of GVHD in CB transplantation [7,9,14,70–74,76,210,211], brings into question the clinical meaning of such a low frequency of T-cell contamination. This observation does not imply that it is not a worthwhile venture to continue to monitor for such contamination. Although the incidence of GVHD is apparently low in CB transplant recipients, even in an unrelated, HLA-disparate setting [70–74,76], GVHD is noted in some recipients, although the extent of GVHD has thus far not correlated well with the disparity of HLA between donor and recipient [71,76]. Of interest, the *ex vivo* expansion of CB cells did not lead to coexpansion of contaminating maternal mononuclear cells [209].

The apparently low incidence of GVHD noted in most CB transplant recipients may reflect the biological activities of CB T lymphocytes [212,213]. CB T lymphocytes generate less cytotoxic T-cell activity than do adult T cells, even after repeated allogeneic stimulation *in vitro* [213,214].

Whereas CB T lymphocytes respond as well as adult BM or blood T lymphocytes to the proliferation-inducing activity of a primary allogeneic stimulation, CB T cells become unresponsive to secondary allogeneic stimulation, whereas adult T cells proliferate to an even greater extent in response to secondary allogeneic stimulation compared to their response to the primary allogeneic stimulation [215]. Investigation into the possible mechanisms mediating this CB T lymphocyte unresponsiveness to secondary allogeneic stimulation has implicated the *ras* intracellular signal transduction pathway [216]. Responsiveness to allogeneic stimulation is associated with activation of *ras* to the guanosine triphosphate (GTP)-bound form from the inactive guanosine diphosphate (GDP)-bound form, whereas the nonresponsive cells maintain *ras* in the inactive GDP-bound form.

Stimulated lymphocytes from CB have reduced production of cytokines, such as interferon-γ (IFN-γ) and tumor necrosis factor-alpha (TNF-α), which may be involved in the pathophysiology of GVHD. As transcription factors of the nuclear factor of activated T cell (NF-AT) family play a role in transcription of *IL-4*, *IFN-γ*, *GM-CSF*, *IL-13*, *TNF-α*, *CD69*, *FasL*, and *CD40L* genes [217], it is possible that NF-AT-1, found to be low or not expressed in CB T cells [218], might be involved in the lowered amplification of donor CB T-cell alloresponsiveness against recipient antigens and in the reduced GVHD noted in CB transplantation. CB T cells have also been shown to manifest distinct chemokine responsiveness by different chemokine receptor repertoires than T cells from adult blood [219], which may also be involved in differences noted in the extent of GVHD after CB compared to BMT.

Further analysis of CB T cells focused on $CD8^+$ T cells [220]. CD28 is a costimulatory molecule. It is the $CD28^-CD8^+$ T-cell subset that has been associated with cytotoxic T lymphocyte (CTL) effector function. CB is composed of $CD8^+$ T cells with few or no $CD28^-$ CTLs. However, a combination of cytokine stimulation and activation of another costimulatory molecule (41BB) leads to CTL effector function in the following sequence. IL-15 and IL-12 preferentially induced 41BB on $CD28^-CD8^+$ CB T cells. Costimulation of these cells with anti-41BB restored expression of CD28 on these cells as well as memory markers such as CD45RO and CCR6. The memory-type $CD28^+$ T cells so generated acquired greatly enhanced CTL activity in association with increased content of granzyme B, a cytolytic mediator. Interestingly, the CTL activity could be almost completely abrogated by a soluble form of 41BB. This observation implicated 41BB in the developmental production of CTLs, effects that probably occur in the child over time following birth.

It has been suggested that *ex vivo* expanded, matured and activated CB T cells with IL-2, IL-12, anti-CD3 and IL-7 may be of value for adoptive cellular immunotherapy post-umbilical CB transplantation [221]. It is possible that 41BB activation is also of importance and useful in this type of adaptive immunotherapy.

It was originally thought that a lower GVHD incidence inherent in CB transplantation, might manifest in a lowered graft-vs.-leukemia effect (GVLE) with CB cells. While increased relapse rates have not been obvious so far in CB transplantation for malignant disease, more experience in this area is needed before any firm conclusions can be drawn. NK cells have been implicated in mediating GVLE [222,223]. While CB generally manifests low NK activity compared to that found in adult BM and blood, NK cell activity of CB and adult cells is readily activated *in vitro* by cytokines, such as IL-2 and IL-12 [222–224], suggesting that CB NK cells should be as capable as adult BM or blood NK cells to mediate GVLE. Interestingly, a subset of NK cells with the surface phenotype $CD16^+56^-$, which has not yet been identified in adult blood of normal individuals, has low lytic activity and might represent a precursor of mature NK cells [220]. The lytic activity of $CD16^+56^-$ cells can be enhanced by cytokine stimulation [225].

In addition to the immune cell activities of CB cells noted above, the functional quantitative activities of other CB immune cells are also distinct from their counterparts found in the adult [212,222]. For example, selected cytokine production by T cells and dendritic cell (DC) antigen presentation are reported to be lower in CB than adult blood cells.

DCs are active antigen presenting cells that initiate and maintain adaptive immune responses. Both lymphoid ($HLA-DR^+$, $CD123^{3+}$, $CD11c^-$, $CD33^-$) and myeloid ($HLA-DR^{2+}$, $CD123^+$, $CD11c^+$, $CD33^+$) DCs have been identified in CB, although the majority of these cells had a lymphoid morphology [226]. The 41BB ligand was found to mediate maturation of $CD11c^+$ myeloid DCs derived from $CD34^+$ CB [227]. In addition to enhanced expression of CD11c, other antigens, such as MHC class II, CD86 and 41BB ligand, were increased after stimulation of CB $CD34^+$ cells with GM-CSF, TNF-α, Flt3L and stem cell factor. Stimulation of the 41BB ligand on these DCs resulted in the capacity of these cells to produce IL-12, results that may be of use in the design of DC-based vaccines with enhanced activity.

Freshly isolated CB lymphoid DCs did not induce a potent allo-stimulation for naive CB T cells. $CD34^+$ CB cells can generate DCs. A $CD7^+CD45RA^+$ subpopulation of $CD34^+$ CB cells was found to have the dual capacity to generate NK cells and DCs [228]. This result is in contrast to the $CD7^-CD45RA^+$, and $CD7^+CD45RA^-$ subsets of $CD34^+$ CB cells.

Differences between the immune cells in CB and adult BM and blood heighten the need to more fully analyze the immune system of recipients of CB transplantation. It is also important that studies of CB immune cell activity and the mechanisms involved in these activities continue, as this information will probably be of use in designing appropriate clinical trials to best utilize CB for HCT.

Conclusions

The experience with CB-HCT is extremely encouraging. However, the worldwide experience with CB transplantation is still limited. Controlled clinical trials are lacking. CB offers a number of potential advantages as an alternative source of HSC. Specifically, CB is readily available and appears to present no risk to the donor. It offers the potential of targeting collections in minority populations, groups that are currently underrepresented in the NMDP registry, although this possibility has not yet reached practicality [24]. If the incidence and severity of acute and chronic GVHD are found in controlled trials to reflect the information already available and to be less than that proved with comparably matched or mismatched BM, greater degrees of HLA disparity may be tolerated, further increasing the donor pool. As allogeneic CB banks reach sufficient size, the time required to acquire a donor unit may decrease further, allowing transplantation to occur at an earlier time. Finally, due to the vast amount of CB continually available for banking, it may be possible to bank only CB units negative for all the viruses for which screening tests are currently available, thereby providing a safer HSC product to the recipient.

Despite these potential advantages, there are several disadvantages. Since the volume of each CB available for collection is limited, means to enhance the number or quality of HSCs in CB is needed. Manipulation of CB through *ex vivo* expansion is still a sought after endpoint, but enhancing the capacity of the CB HSCs to home to an appropriate microenvironment in the marrow may serve a similar purpose. In fact, a problem with *ex vivo* expanded cells may be their loss of effective homing capacity. In the unrelated CB setting, it is not possible to reacquire CB from the donor when the recipient experiences graft failure or relapse. *Ex vivo* expanded cells stored for future use or the use of another stored CB unit may circumvent these possible problems. Despite proposals to require long-term tracking of unrelated CB donors, there is currently little clinical information available on unrelated CB donors, such that the possibility exists that genetic diseases may be inadvertently transferred to CB recipients. Enhanced genetic testing in the future will be of use here, and time will tell if this is a significant problem with current collections. Neutrophil and, especially, platelet engraftment in CB recipients is prolonged. *In vivo* or *ex vivo* use of cytokines or expanded mature cells may be of help, but the appropriate cytokines to enhance these endpoints do not appear to have been identified.

CB HSC transplantation has many potential advantages. However, it is clear that CB collection, banking and transplantation presents the transplant community with a number of medical, scientific, technical, ethical and regulatory challenges. True potential advantages and disadvantages of CB HSCs should emerge as experience in this still relatively new field continues.

References

1. McCullough J, Hansen J, Perkins H, Stroncek D, Bartsch G. The National Marrow Donor Program: how it works, accomplishments to date. *Oncology* 1989; **3**: 63–8; discussion 72–4.
2. Perkins HA, Hansen JA. The US National Marrow Donor Program. *Am J Pediatr Hematol Oncol* 1994; **16**(1): 30–4.
3. Kernan NA, Bartsch G, Ash RC *et al*. Analysis of 462 transplantations from unrelated donors facilitated by the National Marrow Donor Program. *N Engl J Med* 1993; **328**: 593–602.
4. Broxmeyer HE. Introduction. The past, present, and future of cord blood transplantation. In: Broxmeyer HE, ed. *Cellular Characteristics of Cord Blood and Cord Blood Transplantation*. Bethesda, MD: AABB Press, 1998: 1–9.
5. Broxmeyer HE. Introduction. Cord blood transplantation: looking back and to the future. In: Cohen SBA, Gluckman E, Rubinstein P, Madrigal JA, eds. *Cord Blood Characteristics: Role in Stem Cell Transplantation*. London: Dunitz, 2000: 1–12.
6. Broxmeyer HE, Douglas GW, Hangoc G *et al*. Human umbilical cord blood as a potential source of transplantable hematopoietic stem/progenitor cells. *Proc Natl Acad Sci U S A* 1989; **86**: 3828–32.
7. Broxmeyer HE, Kurtzberg J, Gluckman E *et al*. Umbilical cord blood hematopoietic stem and repopulating cells in human clinical transplantation. *Blood Cells* 1991; **17**: 313–29.
8. Broxmeyer HE, Hangoc G, Cooper S *et al*. Growth characteristics and expansion of human umbilical cord blood and estimation of its potential for transplantation in adults. *Proc Natl Acad Sci U S A* 1992; **89**: 4109–13.
9. Gluckman E, Broxmeyer HA, Auerbach AD *et al*. Hematopoietic reconstitution in a patient with Fanconi's anemia by means of umbilical-cord blood from an HLA-identical sibling. *N Engl J Med* 1989; **321**: 1174–8.
10. Broxmeyer HE, Gluckman E, Auerbach A *et al*. Human umbilical cord blood: a clinically useful source of transplantable hematopoietic stem/progenitor cells. *Int J Cell Cloning* 1990; **8** (Suppl. 1): 76–89; discussion 89–91.
11. Wagner JE, Broxmeyer HE, Byrd RL *et al*. Transplantation of umbilical cord blood after myeloablative therapy: analysis of engraftment. *Blood* 1992; **79**: 1874–81.
12. Kohli-Kumar M, Shahidi NT, Broxmeyer HE *et al*. Haemopoietic stem/progenitor cell transplant in Fanconi anaemia using HLA-matched sibling umbilical cord blood cells. *Br J Haematol* 1993; **85**: 419–22.
13. Vilmer E, Sterkers G, Rahimy C *et al*. HLA-mismatched cord-blood transplantation in a patient with advanced leukemia. *Transplantation* 1992; **53**: 1155–7.
14. Wagner JE, Kernan NA, Steinbuch M, Broxmeyer HE, Gluckman E. Allogeneic sibling umbilical-cord-blood transplantation in children with malignant and non-malignant disease. *Lancet* 1995; **346**: 214–9.
15. Gluckman E. Hematopoietic stem-cell transplants using umbilical-cord blood. *N Engl J Med* 2001; **344**: 1860–1.
16. Ballen K, Broxmeyer HE, McCullough J *et al*. Current status of cord blood banking and transplantation in the United States and Europe. *Biol Blood Marrow Transplant* 2001; **7**: 635–45.
17. Gluckman E. Current status of umbilical cord blood hematopoietic stem cell transplantation. *Exp Hematol* 2000; **28**: 1197–205.
18. Wagner JE, Barker JN, DeFor TE *et al*. Transplantation of unrelated donor umbilical cord blood in 102 patients with malignant and non-malignant diseases: influence of CD34 cell dose and HLA disparity on treatment-related mortality and survival. *Blood* 2002; **100**: 1611–8.
19. Rubinstein P, Stevens CE. Placental blood for bone marrow replacement. The New York Blood Center's program and clinical results. *Baillieres Best Pract Res Clin Haematol* 2000; **13**: 565–84.
20. Smith FO, Thomson BG. Umbilical cord blood collection, banking, and transplantation: current status and issues relevant to perinatal caregivers. *Birth* 2000; **27**: 127–35.
21. Reed W, Walters M, Lubin BH. Collection of sibling donor cord blood for children with thalassemia. *J Pediatr Hematol Oncol* 2000; **22**: 602–4.
22. Scaradavou A, Carrier C, Mollen N, Stevens C, Rubinstein P. Detection of maternal DNA in placental/umbilical cord blood by locus-specific amplification of the noninherited maternal *HLA* gene. *Blood* 1996; **88**: 1494–500.
23. Ballen KK, Wilson M, Wuu J *et al*. Bigger is better: maternal and neonatal predictors of hematopoietic potential of umbilical cord blood units. *Bone Marrow Transplant* 2001; **27**: 7–14.
24. Pafumi C, Zizza G, Russo A *et al*. Placing the newborn on the maternal abdomen increases the volume of umbilical cord blood collected. *Clin Laboratory Haematol* 2001; **23**: 397–9.
25. Yamada T, Okamoto Y, Kasamatsu H, Horie Y, Yamashita N, Matsumoto K. Factors affecting the

26 Surbek DV, Visca E, Steinmann C et al. Umbilical cord blood collection before placental delivery during cesarean delivery increases cord blood volume and nucleated cell number available for transplantation. *Am J Obstet Gynecol* 2000; **183**: 218–21.

27 Surbek DV, Aufderhaar U, Holzgreve W. Umbilical cord blood collection for transplantation: which technique should be preferred? *Am J Obstet Gynecol* 2000; **183**: 1587–8.

28 Ballen KK, Hicks J, Dharan B et al. Racial and ethnic composition of volunteer cord blood donors: comparison with volunteer unrelated marrow donors. *Transfusion* 2002; **42**: 1279–84.

29 Elchalal U, Fasouliotis SJ, Shtockheim D et al. Postpartum umbilical cord blood collection for transplantation: a comparison of three methods. *Am J Obstet Gynecol* 2000; **182**: 227–32.

30 Hiett AK, Britton KA, Hague NL, Brown HL, Stehman FB, Broxmeyer HE. Comparison of hematopoietic progenitor cells in human umbilical cord blood collected from neonatal infants who are small and appropriate for gestational age. *Transfusion* 1995; **35**: 587–91.

31 Bertolini F, Lazzari L, Lauri E et al. Comparative study of different procedures for the collection and banking of umbilical cord blood. *J Hematother* 1995; **4**: 29–36.

32 Lasky L, Lane TA, Miller JP et al. In utero or ex utero cord blood collection: which is better? *Transfusion* 2002; **42**: 1261–7.

33 American College of Obstetricians and Gynecologists committee opinion. Routine storage of umbilical cord blood for potential future transplantation. *Int J Gynaecol Obstet* 1997; **58**(2): 257–9.

34 American Academy of Pediatrics Work Group on Cord Blood Banking. Cord blood banking for potential future transplantation: subject review. *Pediatrics* 1999; **104**: 116–8.

35 Fraser JK, Cairo MS, Wagner EL et al. Cord blood transplantation study (COBLT): cord blood bank standard operating procedures. *J Hematother* 1998; **7**: 521–61.

36 McCullough J, Clay M. Reasons for deferral of potential umbilical cord blood donors. *Transfusion* 2000; **40**: 124–5.

37 Jeffries LC, Alberto M, Morgan MA, Muolten D. High deferral rate for maternal–neonatal donor pairs for an allogeneic umbilical cord blood bank. *Transfusion* 1999; **39**: 415–9.

38 Lecchi L, Rebulla P, Ratti I et al. Outcomes of a program to evaluate mother and baby 6 months after umbilical cord blood donation. *Transfusion* 2001; **41**: 606–10.

39 Gluckman E. Cord blood banking and transplantation in Europe. In: Broxmeyer HE, ed. *Cellular Characteristics of Cord Blood and Cord Blood Transplantation*. Bethesda, MD: AABB Press, 1998: 147–64.

40 Peterson RK, Clay M, McCullough J. Unrelated cord blood baking. In: Broxmeyer HE, ed. *Cellular Characteristics of Cord Blood and Cord Blood Transplantation*. Bethesda, MD: AABB Press, 1998: 165–97.

41 Rubinstein P, Rosenfield RE, Adamson JW, Stevens CE. Stored placental blood for unrelated bone marrow reconstitution. *Blood* 1993; **81**: 1679–90.

42 Rubinstein P, Taylor PE, Scaradavou A et al. Unrelated placental blood for bone marrow reconstitution: organization of the placental blood program [see comments]. *Blood Cells* 1994; **20**: 587–600.

43 Pafumi C, Bosco P, Cavallaro A et al. Two CD34+ stem cells from umbilical cord blood enrichment methods. *Pediatr Hematol Oncol* 2002; **19**: 239–45.

44 Kato S, Nishihira H, Hara H et al. Cord blood transplantation and cord blood bank in Japan. *Bone Marrow Transplant* 2000; **25** (Suppl. 2): S68–70.

45 Donaldson C, Buchanan R, Webster J et al. Development of a district Cord Blood Bank: a model for cord blood banking in the National Health Service. *Bone Marrow Transplant* 2000; **25**: 899–905.

46 Vawter DE, Rogers-Chrysler G, Clay M et al. A phased consent policy for cord blood donation. *Transfusion* 2002; **42**: 1268–74.

47 Askari S, Miller J, Clay M, Moran S, Chrysler G, McCullough J. The role of the paternal health history in cord blood banking. *Transfusion* 2002; **42**: 1275–8.

48 Rubinstein P, Dobrila L, Rosenfield RE et al. Processing and cryopreservation of placental/umbilical cord blood for unrelated bone marrow reconstitution. *Proc Natl Acad Sci U S A* 1995; **92**: 10,119–22.

49 Denning-Kendall P, Donaldson C, Nicol A, Bradley B, Hows J. Optimal processing of human umbilical cord blood for clinical banking. *Exp Hematol* 1996; **24**: 1394–401.

50 Nagler A, Peacock M, Tantoco M, Lamons D, Okarma TB, Okrongly DA. Separation of hematopoietic progenitor cells from human umbilical cord blood. *J Hematother* 1993; **2**: 243–5.

51 Newton I, Charbord P, Schaal JP, Herve P. Toward cord blood banking. density-separation and cryopreservation of cord blood progenitors. *Exp Hematol* 1993; **21**: 671–4.

52 Woods EJ, Liu J, Derrow CW, Smith FO, Williams DA, Critser JK. Osmometric and permeability characteristics of human placental/umbilical cord blood CD34+ cells and their application to cryopreservation. *J Hematother Stem Cell Res* 2000; **9**: 161–73.

53 Pollack MS, Auerbach AD, Broxmeyer HE, Zaafran A, Griffith RL, Erlich HA. DNA amplification for DQ typing as an adjunct to serological prenatal HLA typing for the identification of potential donors for umbilical cord blood transplantation. *Hum Immunol* 1991; **30**: 45–9.

54 Trachtenberg EA, Erlich HA. DNA-based HLA typing for cord blood stem cell transplantation. *J Hematother* 1996; **5**: 295–300.

55 Fisher CA, McGrath MB, Cannon ME. Related and autologous cord blood banking. In: Broxmeyer HE, ed. *Cellular Characteristics of Cord Blood and Cord Blood Transplantation*. Bethesda, MD: AABB Press, 1998: 199–216.

56 Broxmeyer HE, Srour EF, Hangoc G, Cooper S, Anderson JA, Bodine D. High efficiency recovery of hematopoietic progenitor cells with extensive proliferative and *ex-vivo* expansion activity and of hematopoietic stem cells with NOD/SCID mouse repopulation ability from human cord blood stored frozen for 15 years. *Proc Natl Acad Sci U S A* 2003; **100**: 645–50.

57 Broxmeyer HE, Cooper S. High-efficiency recovery of immature haematopoietic progenitor cells with extensive proliferative capacity from human cord blood cryopreserved for 10 years. *Clin Exp Immunol* 1997; **107** (Suppl. 1): 45–53.

58 Lu L, Ge Y, Li ZH, Freie B, Clapp DW, Broxmeyer HE. CD34 stem/progenitor cells purified from cryopreserved normal cord blood can be transduced with high efficiency by a retroviral vector and expanded *ex vivo* with stable integration and expression of Fanconi anemia complementation C gene. *Cell Transplant* 1995; **4**: 493–503.

59 DiGiusto DL, Lee R, Moon J et al. Hematopoietic potential of cryopreserved and *ex vivo* manipulated umbilical cord blood progenitor cells evaluated *in vitro* and *in vivo*. *Blood* 1996; **87**: 1261–71.

60 Li ZH, Broxmeyer HE, Lu L. Cryopreserved cord blood myeloid progenitor cells can serve as targets for retroviral-mediated gene transduction and gene-transduced progenitors can be cryopreserved and recovered. *Leukemia* 1995; **9** (Suppl. 1): S12–6.

61 Sugarman J, Kaalund V, Kodish E et al. Ethical issues in umbilical cord blood banking. Working Group on Ethical Issues in Umbilical Cord Blood Banking. *JAMA* 1997; **278**: 938–43.

62 Wils JP. Umbilical cord blood stem cell transplantation: ethical problems. *Biomed Ethics* 1999; **4**: 92–101.

63 Cohen SB. Blood money. *Biologist (London)* 2000; **47**: 280.

64 Munzer SR, Smith FO. Limited property rights in umbilical cord blood for transplantation and research. *Am J Pediatr Hematol Oncol* 2001; **23**: 203–7.

65 Munzer SR. The special case of property rights in umbilical cord blood for transplantation. *Rutgers Law Rev* 1999; **51**: 493–568.

66 Beatty PG, Boucher KM, Mori M, Milford EL. Probability of finding HLA-mismatched related or unrelated marrow or cord blood donors. *Hum Immunol* 2000; **61**: 834–40.

67 Barker JN, Krepski TP, DeFor TE, Davies SM, Wagner JE, Weisdorf DJ. Searching for unrelated donor hematopoietic stem cells. Availability and speed of umbilical cord blood versus bone marrow. *Biol Blood Marrow Transplant* 2002; **8**: 257–60.

68 Rocha V, Cornish J, Sievers EL et al. Comparison of outcomes of unrelated bone marrow and umbilical cord blood transplants in children with acute leukemia. *Blood* 2001; **97**: 2962–71.

69 Robertson JA, Kahn JP, Wagner JE. Conception to obtain hematopoietic stem cells. *Hastings Cent Rep* 2002; **32**: 34–40.

70 Wagner JE, Kurtzberg J. Allogeneic umbilical cord blood transplantation. In: Broxmeyer HE, ed. *Cellular Characteristics of Cord Blood and Cord Blood Transplantation*. Bethesda, MD: AABB Press, 1998: 113–46.

71 Gluckman E, Rocha V, Boyer-Chammard A et al. Outcome of cord-blood transplantation from related and unrelated donors. EUROCORD Transplant Group and the European Blood and Marrow Transplantation Group. *N Engl J Med* 1997; **337**: 373–81.

72 Rocha V, Wagner JE, Sobocinski KA et al. Graft-versus-host disease in children who received a cord-blood or bone marrow transplant from an HLA-identical sibling. *New Engl J Med* 2000; **342**: 1846–54.

73 Wagner JE, Rosenthal J, Sweetman R et al. Successful transplantation of HLA-matched and HLA-mismatched umbilical cord blood from unrelated donors: analysis of engraftment and acute graft-versus-host disease. *Blood* 1996; **88**: 795–802.

74 Rubinstein P, Carrier C, Scaradavou A et al. Outcomes among 562 recipients of placental-blood

transplants from unrelated donors. *N Engl J Med* 1998; **339**: 1565–77.

75 Thomson BG, Robertson KA, Gowan D *et al*. Analysis of engraftment, graft-versus-host disease, and immune recovery following unrelated donor cord blood transplantation. *Blood* 2000; **96**: 2703–11.

76 Kurtzberg J, Laughlin M, Graham ML *et al*. Placental blood as a source of hematopoietic stem cells for transplantation into unrelated donors [see comments]. *N Engl J Med* 1996; **335**: 157–66.

77 Barker JN, Davies SM, DeFor T, Ramsay NK, Weisdorf DJ, Wagner JE. Survival after transplantation of unrelated donor umbilical cord blood is comparable to that of human leukocyte antigen-matched unrelated donor bone marrow: results of a matched-pair analysis. *Blood* 2001; **97**(10): 2957–61.

78 Gluckman E, Rocha V, Chevret S. Results of unrelated umbilical cord blood hematopoietic stem cell transplant. *Transfus Clin Biol* 2001; **8**(3): 146–54.

79 Laughlin MJ, Barker J, Bambach B *et al*. Hematopoietic engraftment and survival in adult recipients of umbilical-cord blood from unrelated donors. *N Engl J Med* 2001; **344**: 1815–22.

80 Sanz GF, Saavedra S, Jimenez C *et al*. Unrelated donor cord blood transplantation in adults with chronic myelogenous leukemia: results in nine patients from a single institution. *Bone Marrow Transplant* 2001; **27**: 693–701.

81 Ooi J, Iseki T, Takahashi S *et al*. A clinical comparison of unrelated cord blood transplantation and unrelated bone marrow transplantation for adult patients with acute leukaemia in complete remission. *Br J Haematol* 2002; **118**: 140–3.

82 Sanz GF, Saavedra S, Planelles D *et al*. Standardized, unrelated donor cord blood transplantation in adults with hematologic malignancies. *Blood* 2001; **98**: 2332–8.

83 Abu-Ghosh A, Goldman S, Slone V *et al*. Immunological reconstitution and correlation of circulating serum inflammatory mediators/cytokines with the incidence of acute graft-versus-host disease during the first 100 days following unrelated umbilical cord blood transplantation. *Bone Marrow Transplant* 1999; **24**: 535–44.

84 Niehues T, Rocha V, Filipovich AH *et al*. Factors affecting lymphocyte subset reconstitution after either related or unrelated cord blood transplantation in children: a EUROCORD analysis. *Br J Haematol* 2001; **114**: 42–8.

85 Giraud P, Thuret I, Reviron D *et al*. Immune reconstitution and outcome after unrelated cord blood transplantation: a single paediatric institution experience. *Bone Marrow Transplant* 2000; **25**: 53–7.

86 Klein AK, Patel DD, Gooding ME *et al*. T-cell recovery in adults and children following umbilical cord blood transplantation. *Biol Blood Marrow Transplant* 2001; **7**: 454–66.

87 Weinberg K, Blazar BR, Wagner JE *et al*. Factors affecting thymic function after allogeneic hematopoietic stem cell transplantation. *Blood* 2001; **97**: 1458–66.

88 Talvensaari K, Clave E, Douay C *et al*. A broad T-cell repertoire diversity and an efficient thymic function indicate a favorable long-term immune reconstitution after cord blood stem cell transplantation. *Blood* 2002; **99**: 1458–64.

89 Moretta A, Maccario R, Fagioli F *et al*. Analysis of immune reconstitution in children undergoing cord blood transplantation. *Exp Hematol* 2001; **29**: 371–9.

90 Smith F, Thomson B. Immune reconstitution and stem cell sources. *Pediatric Pathol Mol Med* 2000; **19**: 187–203.

91 Shpall EJ, Quinones R, Giller R *et al*. Transplantation of *ex vivo* expanded cord blood. *Biol Blood Marrow Transplant* 2002; **8**: 368–76.

92 Fernandez MN, Regidor C, Cabrera R *et al*. Cord blood transplants: early recovery of neutrophils from co-transplanted sibling haploidentical progenitor cells and lack of engraftment of cultured cord blood cells, as ascertained by analysis of DNA polymorphisms. *Bone Marrow Transplant* 2001; **28**: 355–63.

93 Barker JN, Weisdorf DJ, Wagner JE. Creation of a double chimera after the transplantation of umbilical-cord blood from two partially matched unrelated donors. *N Engl J Med* 2001; **344**: 1870–1.

94 Migliaccio AR, Adamson JW, Stevens CE, Dobrila NL, Carrier CM, Rubinstein P. Cell dose and speed of engraftment in placental/umbilical cord blood transplantation: Graft progenitor cell content is a better predictor than nucleated cell quantity. *Blood* 2000; **96**: 2717–22.

95 Broxmeyer HE. Phenotypic and proliferative characteristics of cord blood hematopoietic stem and progenitor cells and gene transfer. In: Broxmeyer HE, ed. *Cellular Characteristics of Cord Blood and Cord Blood Transplantation*. Bethesda, MD: AABB Press, 1998: 11–43.

96 Nakahata T, Ogawa M. Hemopoietic colony-forming cells in umbilical cord blood with extensive capability to generate mono- and multipotential hemopoietic progenitors. *J Clin Invest* 1982; **70**: 1324–8.

97 Ruggieri L, Heimfeld S, Broxmeyer HE. Cytokine-dependent *ex vivo* expansion of early subsets of CD34$^+$ cord blood myeloid progenitors is enhanced by cord blood plasma, but expansion of the more mature subsets of progenitors is favored. *Blood Cells* 1994; **20**: 436–54.

98 Lansdorp PM, Dragowska W, Mayani H. Ontogeny-related changes in proliferative potential of human hematopoietic cells. *J Exp Med* 1993; **178**: 787–91.

99 Cardoso AA, Li ML, Batard P *et al*. Release from quiescence of CD34$^+$CD38$^-$ human umbilical cord blood cells reveals their potentiality to engraft adults. *Proc Natl Acad Sci U S A* 1993; **90**: 8707–11.

100 Lu L, Xiao M, Grigsby S *et al*. Comparative effects of suppressive cytokines on isolated single CD34^{3+} stem/progenitor cells from human bone marrow and umbilical cord blood plated with and without serum. *Exp Hematol* 1993; **21**: 1442–6.

101 Traycoff CM, Abboud MR, Laver J, Clapp DW, Srour EF. Rapid exit from G_0/G_1 phases of cell cycle in response to stem cell factor confers on umbilical cord blood CD34$^+$ cells an enhanced *ex vivo* expansion potential. *Exp Hematol* 1994; **22**: 1264–72.

102 Moore MA, Hoskins I. *Ex vivo* expansion of cord blood-derived stem cells and progenitors. *Blood Cells* 1994; **20**: 468–79.

103 Lu L, Xiao M, Shen RN, Grigsby S, Broxmeyer HE. Enrichment, characterization, and responsiveness of single primitive CD34 human umbilical cord blood hematopoietic progenitors with high proliferating and replating potential. *Blood* 1993; **81**: 41–8.

104 Hows JM, Bradley BA, Marsh JC *et al*. Growth of human umbilical cord blood in long-term haemopoietic cultures [see comments]. *Lancet* 1992; **340**: 73–6.

105 Xiao M, Broxmeyer HE, Horie M, Grigsby S, Lu L. Extensive proliferative capacity of single isolated CD34 human cord blood cells in suspension culture. *Blood Cells* 1994; **20**: 455–66.

106 Carow CE, Hangoc G, Cooper SH, Williams DE, Broxmeyer HE. Mast cell growth factor (c-kit ligand) supports the growth of human multipotential progenitor cells with a high replating potential. *Blood* 1991; **78**: 2216–21.

107 Carow CE, Hangoc G, Broxmeyer HE. Human multipotential progenitor cells (CFU-GEMM) have extensive replating capacity for secondary CFU-GEMM. An effect enhanced by cord blood plasma. *Blood* 1993; **81**: 942–9.

108 Broxmeyer HE, Cooper S, Hague N *et al*. Human chemokines: enhancement of specific activity and effects *in vitro* on normal and leukemic progenitors and a factor-dependent cell line and *in vivo* in mice. *Ann Hematol* 1995; **71**: 235–46.

109 Bodine D. Animal models for the engraftment of human hematopoietic stem and progenitor cells. In: Broxmeyer HE, ed. *Cellular Characteristics of Cord Blood and Cord Blood Transplantation*. Bethesda, MD: AABB Press, 1998: 45–65.

110 Vormoor J, Lapidot T, Pflumio F *et al*. Immature human cord blood progenitors engraft and proliferate to high levels in severe combined immunodeficient mice. *Blood* 1994; **83**: 2489–97.

111 Orazi A, Braun SE, Broxmeyer HE. Commentary: immunohistochemistry represents a useful tool to study human cell engraftment in SCID mice transplantation models. *Blood Cells* 1994; **20**: 323–30.

112 Bock TA, Orlic D, Dunbar CE, Broxmeyer HE, Bodine DM. Improved engraftment of human hematopoietic cells in severe combined immunodeficient (SCID) mice carrying human cytokine transgenes. *J Exp Med* 1995; **182**: 2037–43.

113 Lowry PA, Shultz LD, Greiner DL *et al*. Improved engraftment of human cord blood stem cells in NOD/LtSz$^-$SCID/SCID mice after irradiation or multiple-day injections into unirradiated recipients. *Biol Blood Marrow Transplant* 1996; **2**: 15–23.

114 Larochelle A, Vormoor J, Hanenberg H *et al*. Identification of primitive human hematopoietic cells capable of repopulating NOD/SCID mouse bone marrow: implications for gene therapy. *Nat Med* 1996; **2**: 1329–37.

115 Bhatia M, Wang JC, Kapp U, Bonnet D, Dick JE. Purification of primitive human hematopoietic cells capable of repopulating immune-deficient mice. *Proc Natl Acad Sci U S A* 1997; **94**: 5320–5.

116 Hogan CJ, Shpall EJ, McNulty O *et al*. Engraftment and development of human CD34$^+$-enriched cells from umbilical cord blood in NOD/LtSz$^-$SCID/SCID mice. *Blood* 1997; **90**: 85–96.

117 Wang JC, Doedens M, Dick JE. Primitive human hematopoietic cells are enriched in cord blood compared with adult bone marrow or mobilized peripheral blood as measured by the quantitative *in vivo* SCID-repopulating cell assay. *Blood* 1997; **89**: 3919–24.

118 Tanavde VM, Malehorn MT, Lumkul R *et al*. Human stem-progenitor cells from neonatal cord blood have greater hematopoietic expansion capacity than those from mobilized adult blood. *Exp Hematol* 2002; **30**: 816–23.

119 Wilpshaar J, Falkenburg JHF, Tong X et al. Similar repopulating capacity of mitotically active and resting umbilical cord blood CD34+ cells in NOD/SCID mice. *Blood* 2000; **96**: 2100–7.

120 Summers YJ, Heyworth CM, de Wynter EA, Chang J, Testa NG. Cord blood G_0 CD34+ cells have a thousand-fold higher capacity for generating progenitors *in vitro* than G_1 CD34+ cells. *Stem Cells* 2001; **19**: 505–13.

121 Vaziri H, Dragowska W, Allsopp RC, Thomas TE, Harley CB, Lansdorp PM. Evidence for a mitotic clock in human hematopoietic stem cells. Loss of telomeric DNA with age. *Proc Natl Acad Sci U S A* 1994; **91**: 9857–60.

122 Geiger H, Van Zant G. The aging of lympho-hematopoietic stem cells. *Nature Immunol* 2002; **3**: 329–33.

123 Samper E, Fernandez P, Eguia R et al. Long-term repopulating ability of telomerase-deficient murine hematopoietic stem cells. *Blood* 2002; **99**: 2767–75.

124 McNiece I, Briddell R. Ex vivo expansion of hematopoietic progenitor cells and mature cells. *Exp Hematol* 2001; **29**: 3–11.

125 Kanamaru S, Kawano Y, Watanabe T et al. Low numbers of megakaryocyte progenitors in grafts of cord blood cells may result in delayed platelet recovery after cord blood cell transplant. *Stem Cells* 2000; **18**: 190–5.

126 Bornstein R, Garcia-Vela J, Gilsanz F, Auray C, Cales C. Cord blood megakaryocytes do not complete maturation, as indicated by impaired establishment of endomitosis and low expression of G_1/S cyclins upon thrombopoietin-induced differentiation. *Br J Haematol* 2001; **114**: 458–65.

127 Kuter DJ, Begley CG. Recombinant human thrombopoietin. Basic biology and evaluation of clinical studies. *Blood* 2002; **100**: 3457–69.

128 Krause DS, Fackler MJ, Civin CI, May WSC. D34. Structure, biology, and clinical utility. *Blood* 1996; **87**: 1–13.

129 Hao QL, Shah AJ, Thiemann FT, Smogorzewska EM, Crooks GM. A functional comparison of CD34+CD38− cells in cord blood and bone marrow. *Blood* 1995; **86**: 3745–53.

130 Mayani H, Lansdorp PM. Thy-1 expression is linked to functional properties of primitive hematopoietic progenitor cells from human umbilical cord blood. *Blood* 1994; **83**: 2410–7.

131 Broxmeyer HE, Maze R, Miyazawa K et al. The kit receptor and its ligand, steel factor, as regulators of hemopoiesis. *Cancer Cells* 1991; **3**: 480–7.

132 Laver JH, Abboud MR, Kawashima I, Leary AG, Ashman LK, Ogawa M. Characterization of c-kit expression by primitive hematopoietic progenitors in umbilical cord blood. *Exp Hematol* 1995; **23**: 1515–9.

133 Rappold I, Ziegler BL, Kohler I et al. Functional and phenotypic characterization of cord blood and bone marrow subsets expressing FLT3 (CD135) receptor tyrosine kinase. *Blood* 1997; **90**: 111–25.

134 Broxmeyer HE, Lu L, Cooper S, Ruggieri L, Li ZH, Lyman SD. Flt3 ligand stimulates/costimulates the growth of myeloid stem/progenitor cells. *Exp Hematol* 1995; **23**: 1121–9.

135 Traycoff CM, Abboud MR, Laver J et al. Evaluation of the *in vitro* behavior of phenotypically defined populations of umbilical cord blood hematopoietic progenitor cells. *Exp Hematol* 1994; **22**: 215–22.

136 Cicuttini FM, Welch KL, Boyd AW. The effect of cytokines on CD34+ Rh^{123} high and low progenitor cells from human umbilical cord blood. *Exp Hematol* 1994; **22**: 1244–51.

137 Traycoff CM, Abboud MR, Laver J et al. Human umbilical cord blood hematopoietic progenitor cells: are they the same as their adult bone marrow counterparts? *Blood Cells* 1994; **20**: 382–90.

138 Lu L, Xiao M, Clapp DW, Li ZH, Broxmeyer HE. High efficiency retroviral mediated gene transduction into single isolated immature and replatable CD34[3+] hematopoietic stem/progenitor cells from human umbilical cord blood. *J Exp Med* 1993; **178**: 2089–96.

139 Osawa M, Hanada K, Hamada H, Nakauchi H. Long-term lymphohematopoietic reconstitution by a single CD34− low/negative hematopoietic stem cell. *Science* 1996; **273**: 242–5.

140 Bhatia M, Bonnet D, Murdoch B, Gan OI, Dick JE. A newly discovered class of human hematopoietic cells with SCID-repopulating activity. *Nat Med* 1998; **4**: 1038–45.

141 Spangrude GJ, Heimfeld S, Weissman IL. Purification and characterization of mouse hematopoietic stem cells. *Science* 1988; **241**: 58–62. Erratum: *Science* 1989; **244**: 1030.

142 Uchida N, Weissman IL. Searching for hematopoietic stem cells: evidence that Thy-1.1[lo]Lin−Sca-1+ cells are the only stem cells in C57BL/Ka-Thy-1.1 bone marrow. *J Exp Med* 1992; **175**: 175–84.

143 Morrison SJ, Wandycz AM, Hemmati HD, Wright DE, Weissman IL. Identification of a lineage of multipotent hematopoietic progenitors. *Development* 1997; **124**: 1929–39.

144 Akashi K, Traver D, Miyamoto T, Weissman IL. A clonogenic common myeloid progenitor that gives rise to all myeloid lineages. *Nature* 2000; **404**: 193–7.

145 Kondo M, Weissman IL, Akashi K. Identification of clonogenic common lymphoid progenitors in mouse bone marrow. *Cell* 1997; **91**: 661–72.

146 Hao QL, Zhu J, Price MA, Payne KJ, Barsky LW, Crooks GM. Identification of a novel, human multilymphoid progenitor in cord blood. *Blood* 2001; **97**: 3683–90.

147 Phillips RL, Ernst RE, Brunk B et al. The genetic program of hematopoietic stem cells. *Science* 2000; **288**: 1635–40.

148 Ramalho-Santos M, Yoon S, Matsuzaki Y, Mulligan RC, Melton DA. 'Stemness': transcriptional profiling of embryonic and adult stem cells. *Science* 2002; **298**: 597–600.

149 Ivanova NB, Dimos JT, Schaniel C, Hackney JA, Moore KA, Lemischka IR. A stem cell molecular signature. *Science* 2002; **298**: 601–4.

150 Hawley RG, Sobieski D. Somatic stem cell plasticity: To be or not to be.... *Stem Cells* 2002; **20**: 195–7.

151 Wagers AJ, Sherwood RI, Christensen JL, Weissman IL. Little evidence for developmental plasticity of adult hematopoietic stem cells. *Science* 2002; **297**: 2256–9.

152 Dorrell C, Gan OI, Pereira DS, Hawley RG, Dick JE. Expansion of human cord blood CD34+CD38− cells in *ex vivo* culture during retroviral transduction without a corresponding increase in SCID repopulating cell (SRC) frequency: dissociation of SRC phenotype and function. *Blood* 2000; **95**: 102–10.

153 Antonchuk J, Sauvageau G, Humphries RK. HOXB4-induced expansion of adult hematopoietic stem cells ex vivo. *Cell* 2002; **109**: 39–45.

154 Antonchuk J, Sauvageau G, Humphries RK. HOXB4 overexpression mediates very rapid stem cell regeneration and competitive hematopoietic repopulation. *Exp Hematol* 2001; **29**: 1125–34.

155 Kyba M, Perlingeiro RC, Daley GQ. HoxB4 confers definitive lymphoid-myeloid engraftment potential on embryonic stem cell and yolk sac hematopoietic progenitors. *Cell* 2002; **109**: 29–37.

156 Bordignon C, Roncarolo MG. Therapeutic applications for hematopoietic stem cell gene transfer. *Nat Immunol* 2002; **3**(4): 318–21.

157 Bonetta L. Leukemia case triggers tighter gene-therapy controls. *Nat Med* 2002; **8**: 1189.

158 Sorrentino BP. Gene therapy to protect haematopoietic cells from cytotoxic cancer drugs. *Nat Rev Cancer* 2002; **2**: 431–41.

159 Abonour R, Williams DA, Einhorn L et al. Efficient retrovirus-mediated transfer of the multidrug resistance 1 gene into autologous human long-term repopulating hematopoietic stem cells. *Nat Med* 2000; **6**: 652–8.

160 Moritz T, Keller DC, Williams DA. Human cord blood cells as targets for gene transfer: potential use in genetic therapies of severe combined immunodeficiency disease. *J Exp Med* 1993; **178**: 529–36.

161 Clapp DW, Williams DA. The use of umbilical cord blood as a cellular source for correction of genetic diseases affecting the hematopoietic system. *Stem Cells* 1996; **13**: 613–21.

162 Lu L, Xiao M, Clapp DW, Li ZH, Broxmeyer HE. Stable integration of retrovirally transduced genes into human umbilical cord blood high-proliferative potential colony-forming cells (HPP-CFC) as assessed after multiple HPP-CFC colony replatings *in vitro*. *Blood Cells* 1994; **20**: 525–30.

163 Lu L, Ge Y, Li ZH et al. Retroviral transfer of the recombinant human erythropoietin receptor gene into single hematopoietic stem/progenitor cells from human cord blood increases the number of erythropoietin-dependent erythroid colonies. *Blood* 1996; **87**: 525–34.

164 Xiao M, Yang YC, Yang L et al. Transduction of human interleukin-9 receptor gene into human cord blood erythroid progenitors increases the number of erythropoietin-dependent erythroid colonies. *Bone Marrow Transplant* 1996; **18**: 1103–9.

165 Lu L, Ge Y, Li ZH, Xiao M, Broxmeyer HE. Influence of retroviral-mediated gene transduction of both the recombinant human erythropoietin receptor and interleukin-9 receptor genes into single CD34+CD33− or low cord blood cells on cytokine-stimulated erythroid colony formation. *Exp Hematol* 1996; **24**: 347–51.

166 Braun SE, Aronica SM, Ge Y et al. Retroviral mediated gene transfer of Flt3 ligand enhances proliferation and MAP kinase activity of AML5 cells. *Exp Hematol* 1997; **25**: 51–6.

167 Balduini A, Braun SE, Cornetta K, Lyman S, Broxmeyer HE. Comparative effects of retroviral-mediated gene transfer into primary human stromal cells of Flt3-ligand, interleukin 3 and GM-CSF on production of cord blood progenitor cells in long-term culture. *Stem Cells* 1998; **16** (Suppl. 1): 37–49.

168 Emery DW, Nishino T, Murata K, Fragkos M, Stamatoyannopoulos G. Hematopoietic stem cell gene therapy. *Int J Hematol* 2002; **75**: 228–36.

169 Miyoshi H, Smith KA, Mosier DE, Verma IM, Torbett BE. Transduction of human CD34+ cells that mediate long-term engraftment of NOD/SCID mice by HIV vectors. *Science* 1999; **283**: 682–6.

170 Guenechea G, Gan OI, Inamitsu T et al. Transduction of human CD34+CD38− bone marrow and cord blood-derived SCID-repopulating cells with third-generation lentiviral vectors. *Mol Ther* 2000; **1**: 566–73.

171 Russell DW, Kay MA. Adeno-associated virus vectors and hematology. *Blood* 1999; **94**: 864–74.

172 Hanazono Y, Brown KE, Handa A et al. In vivo marking of rhesus monkey lymphocytes by adeno-associated viral vectors: direct comparison with retroviral vectors. *Blood* 1999; **94**: 2263–70.

173 Srivastava A. Obstacles to human hematopoietic stem cell transduction by recombinant adeno-associated virus 2 vectors. *J Cell Biochem* 2002; **38** (Suppl.): 39–45.

174 Kohn DB, Weinberg KI, Nolta JA et al. Engraftment of gene-modified umbilical cord blood cells in neonates with adenosine deaminase deficiency. *Nat Med* 1995; **1**: 1017–23.

175 Kohn DB, Hershfield MS, Carbonaro D et al. T lymphocytes with a normal ADA gene accumulate after transplantation of transduced autologous umbilical cord blood CD34+ cells in ADA-deficient SCID neonates. *Nat Med* 1998; **4**: 775–80.

176 Kohn DB. Adenosine deaminase gene therapy protocol revisited. *Mol Ther* 2002; **5**: 96–7.

177 Orlic D, Girard LJ, Anderson SM et al. Identification of human and mouse hematopoietic stem cell populations expressing high levels of mRNA encoding retrovirus receptors. *Blood* 1998; **91**: 3247–54.

178 Hynes RO. Integrins. Versatility, modulation, and signaling in cell adhesion. *Cell* 1992; **69**: 11–25.

179 Williams DA, Rios M, Stephens C, Patel VP. Fibronectin and VLA-4 in haematopoietic stem cell–microenvironment interactions. *Nature* 1991; **352**: 438–41.

180 Verfaillie CM, McCarthy JB, McGlave PB. Differentiation of primitive human multipotent hematopoietic progenitors into single lineage clonogenic progenitors is accompanied by alterations in their interaction with fibronectin. *J Exp Med* 1991; **174**: 693–703.

181 Simmons PJ, Zannettino A, Gronthos S, Leavesley D. Potential adhesion mechanisms for localisation of haemopoietic progenitors to bone marrow stroma. *Leuk Lymphoma* 1994; **12**: 353–63.

182 Levesque JP, Leavesley DI, Niutta S, Vadas M, Simmons PJ. Cytokines increase human hemopoietic cell adhesiveness by activation of very late antigen (VLA)-4 and VLA-5 integrins. *J Exp Med* 1995; **181**: 1805–15.

183 Takahira H, Gotoh A, Ritchie A, Broxmeyer HE. Steel factor enhances integrin-mediated tyrosine phosphorylation of focal adhesion kinase (pp125FAK) and paxillin. *Blood* 1997; **89**: 1574–84.

184 Gotoh A, Takahira H, Geahlen RL, Broxmeyer HE. Cross-linking of integrins induces tyrosine phosphorylation of proto-oncogene product vav and protein tyrosine kinase Syk in a human factor-dependent myeloid cell line. *Cell Growth Differ* 1997; **8**: 721–9.

185 Gotoh A, Ritchie A, Takahira H, Broxmeyer HE. Thrombopoietin and erythropoietin activate inside-out signal of integrin and enhance adhesion to immobilized fibronectin in human growth-factor-dependent hematopoietic cells. *Ann Hematol* 1997; **75**: 207–13.

186 Kim CH, Broxmeyer HE. Chemokines. Signal lamps for trafficking of T and B cells for development and effector function. *J Leukoc Biol* 1999; **65**: 6–15.

187 Aiuti A, Webb IJ, Bleul C, Springer T, Guttierrez-Ramas JC. The chemokine SDF-1 is a chemoattractant for human CD34+ progenitors to peripheral blood. *J Exp Med* 1997; **185**: 111–20.

188 Kim CH, Broxmeyer HE. In vitro behavior of hematopoietic progenitor cells under the influence of chemoattractants: stromal cell-derived factor-1, steel factor, and the bone marrow environment. *Blood* 1998; **91**: 100–10.

189 Kim CH, Pelus LM, White JR, Broxmeyer HE. CKb-11/MIP-3b/ELC, a CC chemokine, is a chemoattractant with a specificity for macrophage progenitors amongst myeloid progenitor cells. *J Immunology* 1998; **25**: 80–5.

190 Kim CH, Broxmeyer HE. SLC/exodus2/6Ckine/TCA4 induces chemotaxis of hematopoietic progenitor cells: differential activity of ligands of CCR7, CXCR3, or CXCR4 in chemotaxis versus suppression of progenitor proliferation. *J Leukoc Biol* 1999; **66**: 455–61.

191 Wright DE, Bowman EP, Wagers AJ, Butcher EC, Weissman IL. Hematopoietic stem cells are uniquely selective in their migratory response to chemokines. *J Exp Med* 2002; **195**: 1145–54.

192 Peled A, Petit I, Kollet O et al. Dependence of human stem cell engraftment and repopulation of NOD/SCID mice on CXCR4. *Science* 1999; **283**: 845–8.

193 Kollet O, Petit I, Kahn J et al. Human CD34+CXCR4− sorted cells harbor intracellular CXCR4, which can be functionally expressed and provide NOD/SCID repopulation. *Blood* 2002; **100**: 2778–86.

194 Lapidot T, Kollet O. The essential roles of the chemokine SDF-1 and its receptor CXCR4 in human stem cell homing and repopulation of transplanted immune-deficient NOD/SCID and NOD/SCID/B2m(null) mice. *Leukemia* 2002; **16**: 1992–2003.

195 Kim CH, Qu CK, Hangoc G et al. Abnormal chemokine-induced responses of immature and mature hematopoietic cells from motheaten mice implicate the protein tyrosine phosphatase SHP-1 in chemokine responses. *J Exp Med* 1999; **190**: 681–90.

196 Kim CH, Hangoc G, Cooper S et al. Altered responsiveness to chemokines due to targeted disruption of SHIP. *J Clin Invest* 1999; **104**: 1751–9.

197 Lee Y, Gotoh A, Kwon HJ et al. Enhancement of intracellular signaling associated with hematopoietic progenitor cell survival in response to SDF-1/CXCL12 in synergy with other cytokines. *Blood* 2002; **99**: 4307–17.

198 Broxmeyer HE, Cooper S, Kohli L et al. Transgenic expression of stromal cell derived factor-1/CXCL12 enhances myeloid progenitor cell survival/anti-apoptosis in vitro. Response to growth factor withdrawal and enhances myelopoiesis in vivo. *J Immunol* 2003; **170**: 421–9.

199 Broxmeyer HE, Kohli L, Kim CH et al. Stromal cell derived factor-1/CXCL12 enhances survival/anti-apoptosis of hematopoietic stem and myeloid progenitor cells: Direct effects mediated through CXCR4 and Gαi proteins. *J Leuk Biol* 2003; **73**: 630–8.

200 Nagasawa T, Hirota S, Tachibana K et al. Defects of B-cell lymphopoiesis and bone-marrow myelopoiesis in mice lacking the CXC chemokine PBSF/SDF-1. *Nature* 1996; **382**: 635–8.

201 Broxmeyer HE, Cooper S, Cacalano G, Hague N, Bailish E, Moore MW. Interleukin-8 receptor is involved in negative regulation of myeloid progenitor cells in vivo: evidence from mice lacking the murine IL-8 receptor homolog. *J Exp Med* 1996; **184**: 1825–32.

202 Gao JL, Wynn TA, Chang Y et al. Impaired host defense, hematopoiesis, granulomatous inflammation and type 1/type 2 cytokine balance in mice lacking cc chemokine receptor 1. *J Exp Med* 1997; **185**: 1959–68.

203 Christopherson KW, II, Hangoc G, Broxmeyer HE. Cell surface petidose CD26/DPPIV regulates CXCL12/SDF-1α mediated chemotaxis of human CD34+ progenitor cells. *J Immunol* 2002; **169**: 7000–8.

204 Broxmeyer HE. Questions to be answered regarding umbilical cord blood hematopoietic stem and progenitor cells and their use in-transplantation. *Transfusion* 1995; **35**: 694–702.

205 Socie G, Gluckman E, Carosella E, Brossard Y, Lafon C, Brison O. Search for maternal cells in human umbilical cord blood by polymerase chain reaction amplification of two minisatellite sequences. *Blood* 1994; **83**: 340–4.

206 Hall JM, Lingenfelter P, Adams SL, Lasser D, Hansen JA, Bean MA. Detection of maternal cells in human umbilical cord blood using fluorescence in situ hybridization. *Blood* 1995; **86**: 2829–32.

207 Petit T, Gluckman E, Carosella E, Brossard Y, Brison O, Socie G. A highly sensitive polymerase chain reaction method reveals the ubiquitous presence of maternal cells in human umbilical cord blood. *Exp Hematol* 1995; **23**: 1601–5.

208 Poli F, Crespiatico L, Lecchi L et al. Highly sensitive chemiluminescent method for the detection of maternal cell contamination in human cord blood stored for allotransplantation: The experience of the Milano cord blood bank [letter]. *Blood* 1997; **89**: 3061–2.

209 Fietz T, Hilgenfeld E, Berdel WE et al. Ex vivo expansion of human umbilical cord blood does not lead to co-expansion of contaminating maternal mononuclear cells. *Bone Marrow Transplant* 1997; **20**: 1019–26.

210 Brichard B, Vermylen C, Ninane J, Cornu G. Persistence of fetal hemoglobin production after successful transplantation of cord blood stem cells in a patient with sickle cell anemia. *J Pediatr* 1996; **128**: 241–3.

211 Laporte JP, Gorin NC, Rubinstein P et al. Cord-blood transplantation from an unrelated donor in an adult with chronic myelogenous leukemia. *N Engl J Med* 1996; **335**: 167–70.

212 Roncarolo MG, Vaccarinom E, Saracco P, Miniero R, Madon E, Yssel H. Immunologic properties of cord blood. In: Broxmeyer HE, ed. *Cellular Characteristics of Cord Blood and Cord Blood Transplantation.* Bethesda, MD: AABB Press, 1998: 67–81.

213 Risdon G, Gaddy J, Stehman FB, Broxmeyer HE. Proliferative and cytotoxic responses of human cord blood T-lymphocytes following allogeneic stimulation. *Cell Immunol* 1994; **154**: 14–24.

214 Risdon G, Gaddy J, Broxmeyer HE. Allogeneic responses of human umbilical cord blood. *Blood Cells* 1994; **20**: 566–70.

215 Risdon G, Gaddy J, Horie M, Broxmeyer HE. Alloantigen priming induces a state of unresponsiveness in human umbilical cord blood T cells. *Proc Natl Acad Sci U S A* 1995; **92**: 2413–7.

216 Porcu P, Gaddy J, Broxmeyer HE. Alloantigen-induced unresponsiveness in cord blood T lymphocytes is associated with defective activation of Ras. *Proc Natl Acad Sci U S A* 1998; **95**: 4538–43.

217 Hodge MR, Ranger AM, Charles de la Brousse F, Hoey T, Grusby MJ, Glimcher LH. Hyperproliferation and dysregulation of IL-4 expression in NF-ATp-deficient mice. *Immunity* 1996; **4**: 397–405.

218 Kadereit S, Mohammad SF, Miller RE *et al.* Reduced NFAT1 protein expression in human umbilical cord blood T lymphocytes. *Blood* 1999; **94**: 3101–7.

219 Sato K, Kawasaki H, Nagayama H *et al.* Chemokine receptor expressions and responsiveness of cord blood T cells. *J Immunol* 2001; **166**: 1659–66.

220 Kim Y-J, Brutkiewicz R, Broxmeyer HE. Role of 4-1BB (CD137) in the functional activation of cord blood CD28$^-$CD8$^+$ T cells. *Blood* 2002; **100**: 3253–60.

221 Robinson KL, Ayello J, Hughes R *et al. Ex vivo* expansion, maturation, and activation of umbilical cord blood-derived T lymphocytes with IL-2, IL-12, anti-CD3, and IL-7. Potential for adoptive cellular immunotherapy post-umbilical cord blood transplantation. *Exp Hematol* 2002; **30**: 245–51.

222 Gaddy J, Porcu P, Broxmeyer HE. Clinical and basic science studies of human umbilical cord blood: implications for the GVL effect following cord blood transplantation. In: Barrett J, Jiang YZ, eds. *Allogeneic Immunotherapy for Malignant Disease*. New York: Marcel Dekker, 2000: 267–84.

223 Gaddy J, Broxmeyer HE. Cord blood natural killer cells. Implication for cord blood transplantation and insights into natural killer cell differentiation. In: Broxmeyer HE, ed. *Cellular Characteristics of Cord Blood and Cord Blood Transplantation*. Bethesda, MD: AABB Press, 1998: 83–111.

224 Gaddy J, Risdon G, Broxmeyer HE. Cord blood natural killer cells are functionally and phenotypically immature but readily respond to interleukin-2 and interleukin-12. *J Interferon Cytokine Res* 1995; **15**: 527–36.

225 Gaddy J, Broxmeyer HE. Cord blood CD16$^+$56$^-$ cells with low lytic activity are possible precursors of mature natural killer cells. *Cell Immunol* 1997; **180**: 132–42.

226 Borras FE, Matthews NC, Lowdell MW, Navarrete CV. Identification of both myeloid CD11c$^+$ and lymphoid CD11c$^-$ dendritic cell subsets in cord blood. *Br J Haematol* 2001; **113**: 925–31.

227 Kim Y-J, Li G, Broxmeyer HE. 4-1BB ligand stimulation enhances myeloid dendritic cell maturation from hman umbilical cord blood CD34$^+$ progenitor cells. *J Hematother Stem Cell Res* 2002; **11**: 895–904.

228 Canque B, Camus S, Dalloul A *et al.* Characterization of dendritic cell differentiation pathways from cord blood CD34$^+$CD7$^+$CD45RA$^+$ hemato-poietic progenitor cells. *Blood* 2000; **96**: 3748–56.

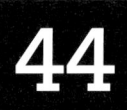

Alan W. Flake & Esmail D. Zanjani

In Utero Transplantation

Introduction

For most of human history, the fetus has been shrouded in mystery, obscured by multiple layers of maternal tissue and protected from the scrutiny and intervention of well meaning physicians. In the past 3 decades, this private world of the fetus has been invaded by a vast array of imaging techniques and methods for fetal tissue sampling, allowing the early gestational diagnosis of selected congenital hematologic disorders. Over the past 5 years, progress has accelerated in a number of technologies that are destined to revolutionize the field of prenatal diagnosis. The convergence of knowledge from the human genome project, molecular genetic diagnosis, isolation of fetal cells or DNA from the maternal circulation and techniques of high through-put gene analysis will in all likelihood allow population screening and diagnosis of every genetically based hematologic disorder early in gestation. In many instances the early prenatal diagnosis of a disease provides a rationale for prenatal treatment [1]. This rationale is particularly compelling for diseases that cause death or irreversible organ damage before birth. In this circumstance, by the time of birth, the damage has already been done. Examples of successful treatment of lethal fetal disease are now numerous and include fetal transfusion for *erythroblastosis fetalis* [2] and prenatal correction of selected anatomical malformations [3]. Another compelling rationale for fetal therapy exists when there are biological advantages to prenatal therapy relative to postnatal therapy. In this circumstance, unique aspects of fetal development may allow treatment of a disease with reduced morbidity, mortality, and cost compared to treatment after birth. This is the rationale for *in utero* hematopoietic stem cell (HSC) transplantation. It is the purpose of this chapter to review the theoretical, experimental and, at the present time, limited clinical support for this approach.

An experiment of nature

Perhaps the most compelling argument for the potential of *in utero* hematopoietic cell transplantation (IU-HCT) comes from an experiment of nature. Owen [4], in 1945, observed that dizygotic cattle twins that shared placental circulation were chimeric for their sibling's blood cells after birth. Subsequent investigators confirmed that chimeric animals were specifically tolerant for skin grafts [5] and organ grafts [6] from their sibling donor. Natural chimerism arising from shared placental circulation has also been observed in a number of other species, most notably primates [7] and humans [8]. The cotton-top tamarin, a New World primate species, has a high incidence of natural chimerism, with documentation of stable donor cell chimerism of >80% in some animals. The incidence of human chimerism in monochorionic dizygotic pregnancies is around 8% when sensitive detection methodology is utilized, and natural human chimeras with all levels of donor cell chimerism, including marked donor cell predominance [9], have been observed. These observations are proof in principal for IU-HCT. They confirm that circulating allogeneic stem cells can effectively compete and stably engraft an early gestational recipient and that, at least under specific circumstances, normal host hematopoiesis is not prohibitive to the engraftment of donor cells. The primary question is: what are the ideal circumstances to permit experimental and clinical recapitulation of this experiment of nature?

Fetal immunologic tolerance

Owen's observations of natural chimerism [4] were followed by Burnet's [10] theory of immunity, which subsequently led to the experimental work of Billingham and colleagues [11] promoting the concept of "acquired" immunologic tolerance. These studies suggested that the early presentation of cellular antigen resulted in specific immunologic tolerance. Their studies documented that tolerance could only be achieved during a period of immunologic immaturity and was best accomplished by the transplantation of living cells.

More recent studies have documented the role of the fetal thymus in self-recognition and tolerance induction [12,13]. The human thymus becomes populated by prethymocytes at 8–9 weeks' gestation [14]. Thymocytes undergo a series of differentiation and selection events in the thymus before becoming mature functional lymphocytes. The details of thymic processing are still being investigated, but the critical events have now been defined. Thymocytes are positively selected for recognition of self-class I or class II major histocompatability complex (MHC) antigens, which are presented by thymic epithelial cells of thymic stromal origin. Lack of MHC recognition results in programmed cell death. Thymocytes that recognize self-MHC are then negatively selected by high-affinity recognition of "self"-antigen in association with self-MHC. Self-antigen presentation is directed by thymic dendritic cells that are derived from HSCs. The end result is a repertoire of single positive ($CD4^+$ or $CD8^+$) functionally competent lymphocytes that recognize foreign antigen in association with self-MHC. Single positive (post-thymic) lymphocytes are first seen in the peripheral blood circulation at around 12–14 weeks' gestation [15]. Theoretically, the introduction of foreign cells prior to completion of this process would result in thymic processing of foreign cells as "self" with secondary specific tolerance on the basis of clonal deletion. It is important to emphasize, however, that the presence of phenotypically mature lymphocytes does not necessarily equate to their immunological function and the capacity for rejection, and that the gestational limit of tolerance induction in the human fetus has not been defined. It is also important to emphasize that the mechanism of

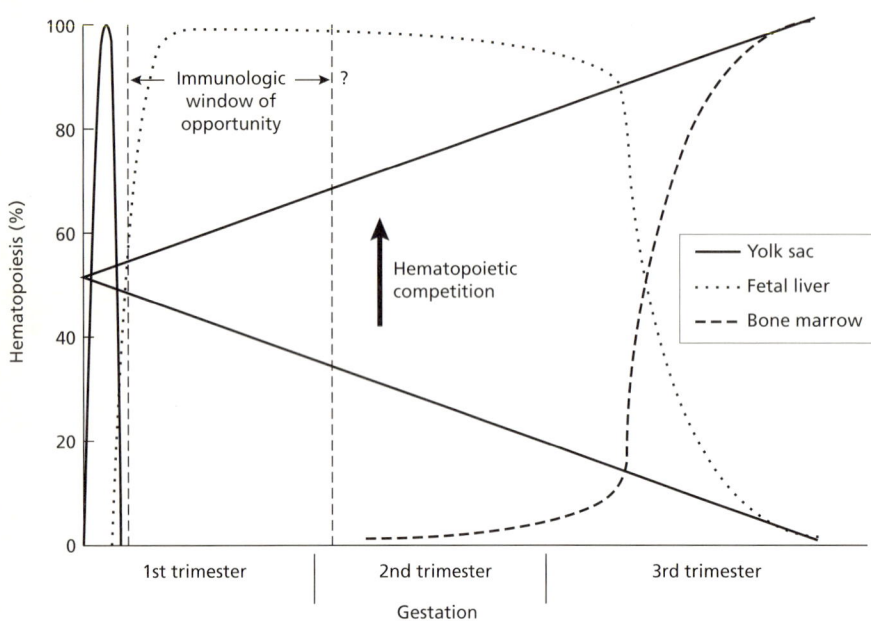

Fig. 44.1 A schematic of normal hematopoietic ontogeny depicting the concepts of an early immunologic "window of opportunity" and increasing host hematopoietic competition. The late limit of immunologic tolerance in humans has not been defined and may extend into later gestation in immunodeficiency disorders such as severe combined immunodeficiency syndrome (SCID).

central thymic tolerance has been defined primarily in T-cell receptor (TCR) transgenic mice. In these mice, thymic maturation of lymphocytes occurs in an environment of unregulated high level expression of TCR with high affinity for a specific self-antigen, which is expressed from the earliest to the latest stages of thymic development [16–18]. This is distinct from the clinical situation following IU-HCT in which there are a large number of circulating antigens interacting with recipient TCR's of varying affinity for donor antigen. Differences in thymic maturation of lymphocytes in normal mice from the defined mechanisms in TCR transgenic mice have been recognized [19,20]. In addition, there are other mechanisms of rejection including natural killer (NK)-cell or B-cell mediated response that are relatively poorly understood.

The fetal hematopoietic environment

A biologically unique aspect of IU-HCT is the fetal receptive environment. Whereas, postnatal bone marrow transplantation (BMT) generally requires myeloablative or at least minimally myeloablative conditioning to achieve engraftment, such conditioning would be prohibitively toxic to the fetus. Thus, engraftment following in utero HSC, by necessity, must depend upon competitive population of available receptive sites with the goal of achieving an adequate level of mixed chimerism to have therapeutic effect for a given target disorder. The receptive sites in the early gestational environment are undoubtedly dynamic and are dependent upon the gestational age of the fetus. Fetal hematopoiesis is characterized by an orderly series of migrational events that proceed from the yolk sac or peri-aortic splanchnopleura, or both, to the fetal liver and, finally, to the bone marrow (BM) [21,22]. Thus the migration of fetal hematopoiesis is probably best viewed as a sequential development of organ-specific microenvironmental niches of increasing HSC affinity. At the developmental stage that corresponds to fetal immunologic immaturity in multiple species, the primary receptive site is the fetal liver. Studies in which tracking of transplanted cells have been performed in the sheep [23] and mouse [24] models suggest that the pattern of engraftment after IU-HCT recapitulates ontogeny, i.e. prior to BM formation cells home to the fetal liver but once the BM forms, even fetal liver derived cells will preferentially home to the fetal BM.

The early dogma of this field predicted that the rapid expansion of the fetal hematopoietic compartment would favor the availability of open niches for engraftment of donor cells, and that there would be a "window of opportunity" prior to immune competence. While "space" is available prior to population of the BM, this has proven to be only partially true (Fig. 44.1). While it is certainly true that the immunologic opportunity exists, the efficiency of engraftment of BM cells after in utero transplantation is no better than that after postnatal myeloablative BMT with only approximately 5% of cells homing to and engrafting receptive sites in the fetal liver [24]. This suggests that the fetal receptive environment, with a few disease-specific exceptions, is highly competitive and that strategies will need to be developed to improve the competitive capacity of donor cells to achieve significant engraftment.

Animal studies that support in utero transplantation

The first experimental studies that supported engraftment of donor cells after in utero transplantation were the classic studies of Billingham and colleagues [11], who documented donor-specific tolerance for skin grafts after fetal or neonatal transplantation in mice. Although chimerism was not analyzed, it can now be assumed that tolerant animals were chimeric for donor cells. The next important study was the correction of genetic anaemia by Fleischman and Mintz [25] in W/W^v mice by transplacental injection of normal HSC. The W/W^v mouse strain is genetically deficient in the c-*kit* receptor resulting in a selective advantage for normal stem cells [26]. In this model a single normal stem cell can engraft and reconstitute normal hematopoiesis [27]. Blazer et al. [28] demonstrated in a murine severe combined immunodeficiency syndrome (SCID) model that in utero transplantation of congenic or fully allogeneic adult BM could result in full T-cell and partial B-cell reconstitution and a functionally intact immune system. Thus, in experimental circumstances of a selective donor stem cell or lineage advantage, IU-HCT can result in functional reconstitution and disease correction.

In order to determine whether engraftment of allogeneic HSC could be achieved in a large animal model, the authors developed an in utero HSC transplant approach in sheep that results in multilineage allogeneic engraftment without the need for myeloablation [29] and, under appropriate conditions, without graft-vs.-host-disease (GVHD) [30]. Although limited by the lack of characterized differentiation markers, the sheep model has provided a number of basic observations that define some of the parameters that allow long-term engraftment of donor HSC in the fetus.

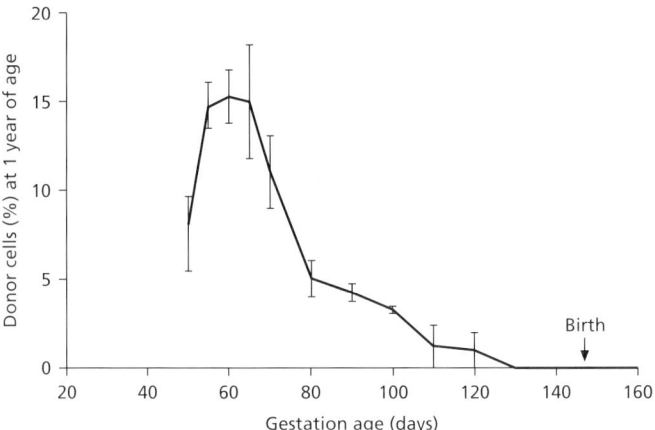

Fig. 44.2 Maximal donor cell engraftment occurs during the mid- to latter stages of the preimmune period. This period is associated with the development of bone marrow (BM) in sheep, which is populated by donor stem cells in competition with endogenous hematopoietic cells. The failure of donor cells to engraft in very young fetuses may be explained by the absence of suitable receptive sites.

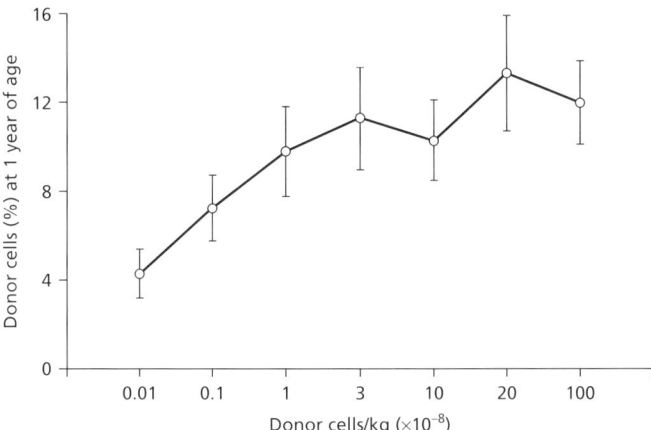

Fig. 44.3 Levels of engraftment plateau with transplantation of log-fold increases in donor cells. This is most consistent with a model of saturation kinetics with engraftment limited by available receptive sites. An identical curve is seen in the xenogeneic human-sheep model.

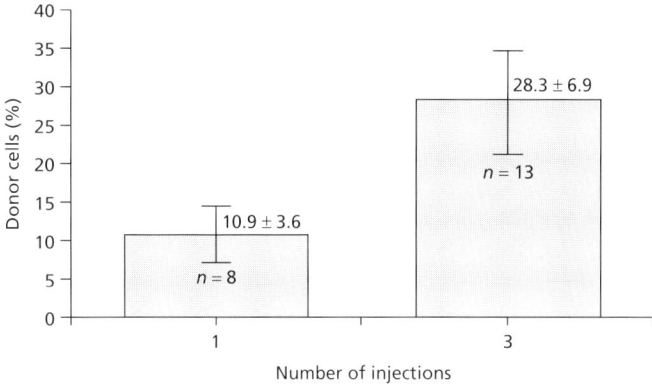

Fig. 44.4 The effect of dividing cell dose on engraftment. Transplantation of the same total number of cells as a single injection vs. a series of three injections given 1 week apart is shown. The engraftment with divided doses is significantly higher supporting the concept that engraftment is limited at any particular time by the number of available receptive sites.

The relationship of gestational age at transplantation and engraftment has been examined with confirmation of the concept of a presumed immunologic "window of opportunity." Late gestational transplantation results in failure of engraftment, with loss of the ability to engraft roughly corresponding to the gestational age at which fetal lambs reject allogeneic skin grafts (75 days gestation) (Fig. 44.2). In another study in the sheep model, the relationship between dose of donor cells and engraftment was examined. Log-fold increases in doses of transplanted cells initially increased engraftment but this rise rapidly plateaued, suggesting saturation of available receptive sites (Fig. 44.3) [31]. If this theory were true, then transplantation of cells in divided doses should allow the development of new receptive sites between transplants and should improve engraftment. Indeed, in the allogeneic sheep model, transplantation of the same total number of cells in three divided doses increases engraftment by a considerable margin (Fig. 44.4). The importance of route of administration of donor cells has also been examined in sheep. Higher levels of donor cell engraftment have been obtained when cells are administered by intraperitoneal (IP) injection than by intravenous injection. Although the authors are unable to provide an explanation for this finding, this difference has been observed on many occasions and for that reason we have utilized the IP approach for most studies.

Among the many potentially important variables for *in utero* transplantation is the source of donor cells. This, by necessity, is influenced by the important clinical issues of susceptibility of the early gestational fetus to GVHD and the risk to the maternal–fetal unit of transmissible viral, bacterial and fungal infection. It makes intuitive sense that HSC from preimmune fetal sources may offer immunologic and functional advantages over adult-derived HSC with respect to engraftment and the risk for GVHD. In fact, in the sheep, baboon and murine models, fetal liver derived cells provide significantly better engraftment than adult BM without the risk of GVHD [29–34]. However, the use of fetal liver for human *in utero* transplantion presents practical problems that may severely limit its use. The authors found that more than 85% of human fetal livers obtained from abortus specimens over a 3-year period were contaminated with bacterial and fungal pathogens, and only three of 18 ectopic/spontaneous abortus tissues were genetically normal. Rice *et al.*, using the US Pharmacopoeia Assay, reported a 79% rate of bacterial and fungal contamination, making the specimens unsuitable for clinical use [35]. Even when the tissues were sterile, quality control evaluations required that the tissue be frozen until used.

In contrast to fetal sources, newborns (cord blood) and adults are readily available sources of donor HSC that do not present any significant quality control or ethical issues. However, the presence of mature T cells in both sources raises concern for GVHD. The concern is justified by experimental data. BM mononuclear cells from adult sheep were transplanted into unrelated normal fetuses of different gestational ages and pregnancy was allowed to go to term. The results demonstrated significant donor-cell engraftment in a number of recipients, but all chimeric lambs developed severe GVHD and died. GVHD occurred at different times after transplant and was not accompanied by significant graft loss. Severe GVHD occurred regardless of the gestational age of the recipient at the time of the transplant, suggesting that GVHD is related to the immune status of the donor rather than the recipient [36]. Two lines of evidence confirm that GVHD is secondary to the innoculum of mature donor T cells given at the time of transplantation rather than from *de novo* generation of T cells from donor progenitors. The first is that removal of T cells before transplantation prevents GVHD and incremental readdition of T cells results in GVHD in a dose-dependent fashion [37]. Second, in the murine model, the presence of significant levels of chimerism with secondary donor specific tolerance is associated with high-level deletion of donor host reactive $V\beta$-TCR bearing lymphocytes. This deletion is present early, and in the murine model is ongoing throughout the lifetime of the animal, even with subsequent retransplantation of donor HSCs

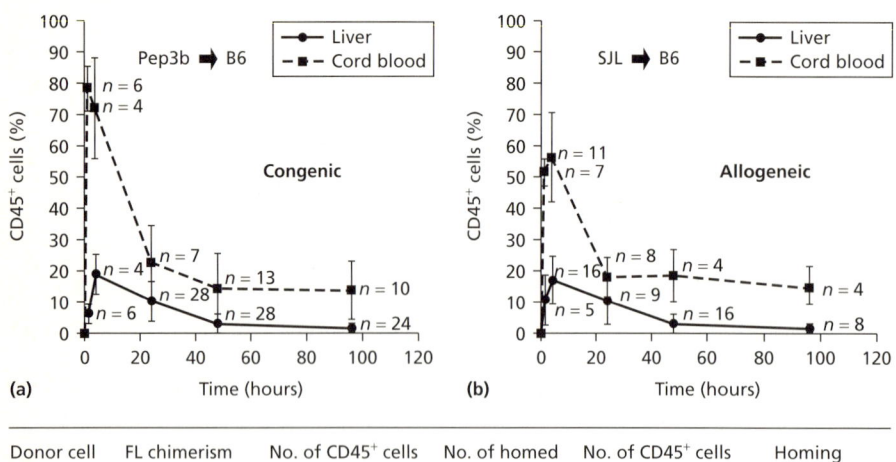

Fig. 44.5 These graphs depict the triphasic kinetic profiles for the frequency of donor cells circulating within the recipient fetal peripheral blood (cord blood) or lodged within the fetal liver at various time points (1.5–96.0 h) after *in utero* transplantation in the murine model. The nearly identical profiles for both the congenic (a) and the fully allogeneic (b) strain combinations are shown. The donor cell frequency is calculated as the percentage of cells expressing the donor CD45.1 isoform among all CD45.1 cells within the host cord blood or fetal liver. (c) Represents the efficiency calculations for homing of donor hematopoietic cells to fetal liver in this model. Only approximately 5% of transplanted cells home and engraft. Adapted with permission from Shaaban *et al.* [24].

Donor cell type	FL chimerism at 4 hours (%)	No. of CD45+ cells per recipient FL	No. of homed CD45+ cells	No. of CD45+ cells in donor innoculum	Homing efficiency (%)
Pep 3b BM	19 ± 6.3	2.6 ± 0.8 × 10^5	4.8 ± 1.6 × 10^4	9.9 × 10^5	4.9 ± 1.6
SJL BM	16.9 ± 7.7	2.6 ± 0.8 × 10^5	4.3 ± 1.9 × 10^4	9.9 × 10^5	4.4 ± 2.0

or following donor lymphocyte infusion (DLI) [38,39]. The potential of cord blood to cause GVHD in the fetus has not been fully evaluated. We have observed GVHD after allogeneic cord blood transplantation but not after xenogeneic cord blood transplantation (E.D. Zanjani, unpublished results). As there are significant engraftment benefits of cord blood, the use of cord blood as a donor source needs further evaluation in animal models. One approach to decreasing the risk of GVHD is to simultaneously T-cell deplete and enrich for HSC. In general, the use of highly enriched HSC populations for *in utero* transplantation has been disappointing. We have had no success in the murine model transplanting even very large numbers of Sca1+lin− BM cells (A.W. Flake, unpublished data) and clinical experience under optimal circumstances has likewise shown no engraftment [40]. This suggests the need for an as yet undefined cell population to facilitate engraftment of HSC in the prenatal recipient, analogous to the situation in postnatal allogeneic BMT.

A remarkable feature of fetal tolerance is that it extends across even widely disparate species barriers. Xenogeneic hematopoietic chimerism after IU-HCT has now been documented in the human–sheep [32,41], human–baboon [33], human–mouse [42], pig–sheep [43] and rat–mouse [44] species combinations. The human–sheep model has been the most studied and the most informative with respect to clinical transplantation. The human–sheep model allows the engraftment of long-term repopulating human HSC and is uniquely suited for the *in vivo* study of engraftment and differentiation potential of human HSC [45–51]. In addition, it appears that in some aspects, at least, human HSC in this model display similar biology in their homing and engraftment patterns to those established in other models [52].

Despite the success of the sheep model, engraftment in other models has been difficult to achieve. Until recently, the sheep was the only model in which engraftment greater than "microchimerism" was possible. The likely barriers to engraftment in most species, including humans, were recently reviewed and can be categorized as: a lack of available space; host cell competition; and undefined immunologic barriers [53]. In order to systematically examine the relative importance of these barriers and to develop strategies to overcome them, the development of the murine model was critical. The available inbred and transgenic strains, defined immunology, large litter size, minimal cost and short gestation period of the mouse, allows studies to be performed that simply cannot be considered in other species. In addition, the mouse is stage-for-stage very similar to the human with respect to hematopoietic and immunologic ontogeny. *In utero* HSC transplants can be performed early in gestation (11–15 days) during a time when hematopoiesis is confined to the fetal liver, and prior to completion of thymic processing and the appearance of mature lymphocytes in the peripheral circulation. Finally, the normal mouse proved very difficult to engraft, making it a legitimate model for investigation of barriers to engraftment. The authors, and other researchers, were only able to achieve microchimerism for several years in hematopoietically competitive strains [42,54–58]. To assess the reason for failure we performed a kinetic study of homing and engraftment after *in utero* transplantation [24]. The study clearly demonstrated that engraftment efficiency was no better in the fetal recipient than in the adult and that one reason for inability to achieve measurable levels of chimerism was the inability to engraft an adequate number of stem cells (Fig. 44.5). In response to this study, we improved our cell preparations and performed a dose escalation study to investigate the effect of increasing cell doses. With improved delivery of higher numbers of HSC we were able to achieve macrochimerism in multiple allogeneic strain combinations. The level of chimerism was dependent upon cell dose, cell source, with fetal liver being far superior to adult BM at equivalent doses, and on strain combination (Fig. 44.6). The second barrier of host cell competition may be the most important. It is clear from studies of *in utero* transplantation utilizing mouse strains that have a genetic deficiency in HSC [25] or a specific lineage deficiency [28,59,60], that hematopoietic repopulation or lineage replacement can be achieved with very low levels of HSC engraftment and, in the case of c-*kit* deficient mice, engraftment of a single HSC [27]. Similarly, as described below, the conferment of a competitive advantage after birth to donor cells after establishment of low-level chimerism by *in utero* transplantation results in conversion to high-level or complete chimerism [38,39]. Thus, after initial engraftment, the size of the donor-derived hematopoietic compartment will depend upon the ability of donor cells to compete with host hematopoiesis. Finally, the immunologic barriers to engraftment remain to be defined. The fact that clinical success has only been achieved in the setting of SCID [61,62] has been used by some to argue that the primary barrier to *in utero* transplantation is the immune response. However, SCID also confers a defect in proliferation and survival of the T-cell lineage, providing a selective advantage to donor cells. The absence of significant donor representation in other lineages supports the argument that it is primarily competition rather than immune rejection that limits chimerism. In the murine model Flake and colleagues have confirmed the ability to achieve donor specific

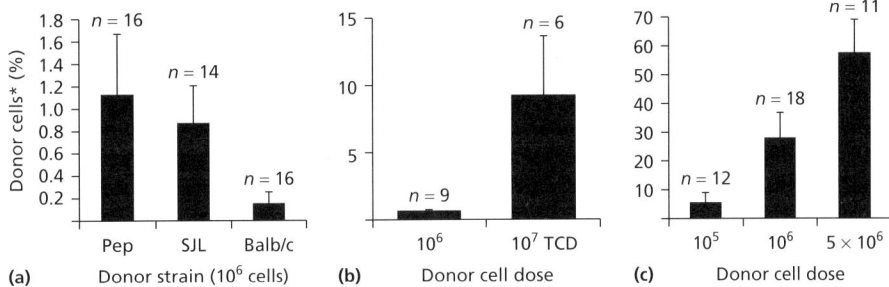

Fig. 44.6 The effect of strain combination, dose, and cell source on donor cell engraftment after *in utero* hematopoietic cell transplantation (IU-HCT). (a) Peripheral blood chimerism in B6 recipients of adult bone marrow (BM) from three different strain donors. (b) Peripheral blood chimerism of Balb/c recipients of B6 BM at low and high doses. (c) Peripheral blood chimerism in B6 recipients of various doses of SJL fetal liver demonstrating the dramatically higher levels of dose-dependent engraftment achieved with fetal liver derived donor cells. (All levels measured at 6 months of age.) *Note the difference in scale of the Y axis for the three figures. B6, C57BL6; FL, fetal liver; PB, peripheral blood; Pep, C57BL/6; Ly5.1:Pep3B; TCD, T-cell depleted.

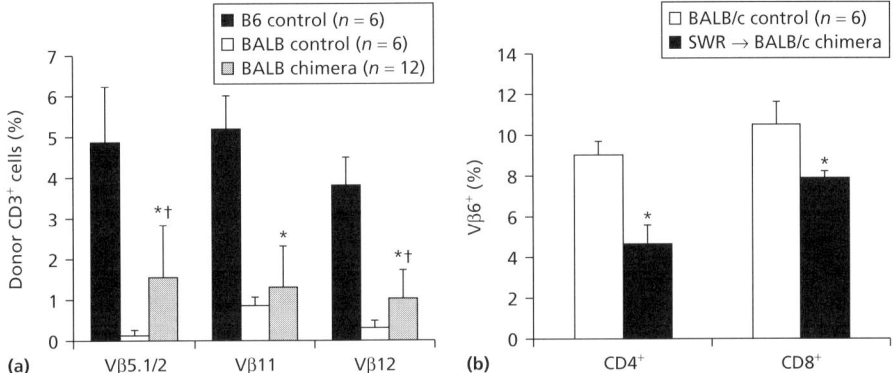

Fig. 44.7 Evidence of bidirectional clonal deletion as a mechanism of tolerance in macrochimeric animals created by *in utero* hematopoietic cell transplantation (IU-HCT). Donor and host strains are chosen based on the presence or absence of Class II I–E, which is required for presentation of mammary tumor virus (mtv) antigens. Mtv antigens are superantigens encoded by Mtv oncogenes in the host genome that are normally deleted in the host strain but not the donor strain. Thus donor antigen presentation in the thymus can be limited to donor derived antigen-presenting cells (APCs), i.e. direct antigen presentation, or to host derived APC, i.e. indirect antigen presentation. (a) Efficient deletion of donor host specific $V\beta TCR$ in chimeric mice by direct antigen presentation after IU-HCT. $*p <0.001$ Chimeric mice vs. B6 control; $†p <0.05$ chimeric mice vs. Balb/c control. (b) Partial deletion of host donor specific $V\beta TCR$ by indirect antigen presentation in SWR >Balb/c chimeras after IU-HCT $*p <0.001$. Adapted with permission from Hayashi *et al.* [38].

tolerance with transplantation at, or prior to, 15 days gestation. Tolerance is consistently present in animals with levels of peripheral blood chimerism of >1% (macrochimerism) [38] but inconsistent in microchimeric animals [58]. We have documented a predominant mechanism of high-level clonal deletion in macrochimeric animals by analysis of relevant $V\beta$-TCR consistent with thymic processing of donor antigen (Fig. 44.7). This and other evidence suggests that there is not a T-cell mediated barrier to engraftment if the transplant is performed early enough in gestation to allow thymic processing. Whether NK or other nonspecific immune barriers may exist that limit initial engraftment, particularly of highly enriched HSC, remains to be determined.

In summary, experimental results from animal models support the rationale and feasibility of IU-HCT. Although engraftment can be achieved clinically in circumstances of a donor cell selective advantage, the primary limitation to clinical application for most target disorders is the relatively low level of donor cell expression achieved. The future of IU-HCT depends upon developing successful strategies to overcome the barriers to engraftment, particularly host cell competition. There are a number of strategies being tested in animal models that show considerable promise and will be discussed below.

Strategies for successful *in utero* HSC transplantation

The potential clinical applications of IU-HCT fall into two general categories. The first is reconstitution or replacement of a stem cell or lineage defect or deficit. The second is prenatal tolerance induction for facilitation of postnatal cellular transplantation. In order for either strategy to be successful, an adequate number of donor HSCs must initially engraft to provide ongoing hematopoiesis at a therapeutic level or to provide adequate thymic presentation of antigen for stable tolerance induction. One of the major problems clinically is the inability to achieve greater than polymerase chain reaction-detectable engraftment using enriched cell populations. The achievement of "microchimerism" is probably inadequate for either purpose as it appears to be associated with the engraftment of very few, if any, HSC and does not reliably induce tolerance by a mechanism of clonal deletion. Therefore, one of the major clinical challenges is to achieve higher initial levels of HSC engraftment. As myeloablation is not an attractive option in the fetus, an alternative approach has been to attempt to increase available "space" by stromal cotransplantation [63,64]. Although the mechanism remains unclear, it has now been documented in both the allogeneic and xenogeneic sheep models that stromal cotransplantation leads to increased short and long-term levels of donor cell engraftment in the BM and donor cell expression in peripheral blood. In the allogeneic model the cotransplantation of adult stroma resulted in greater enhancement of early donor peripheral blood expression (60 days after transplantation) than fetal-derived stroma and the enhancement of expression was sustained for at least 30 months (Fig. 44.8). This observation, in combination with previous findings of delayed contribution of BM engrafted donor cells to peripheral expression in the sheep model [23], suggests that fetal stroma may be

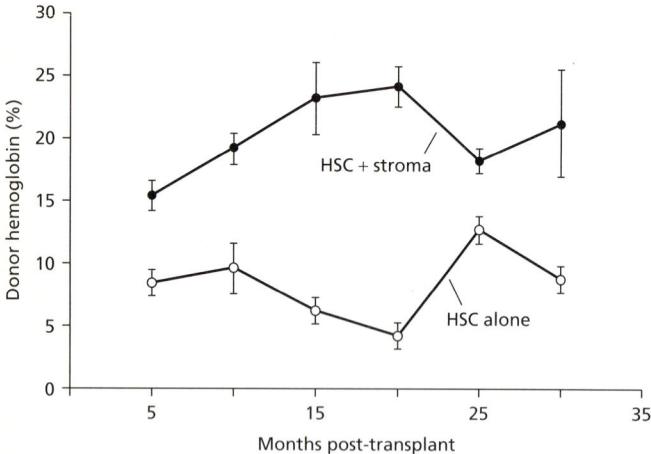

Fig. 44.8 Cotransplantation of adult sheep stromal cells results in a sustained increase in donor-derived hematopoiesis. Sustained long-term engraftment that has persisted for more that 30 months after transplantation is shown, where the donor hemoglobin levels in peripheral blood in animals receiving adult bone marrow (BM) stroma ($n = 4$) are significantly higher ($p < 0.01$) than those receiving adult T-depleted BM mononuclear cells alone ($n = 3$). Reproduced with permission from Almeida-Porada et al. [63]

deficient or immature in its capacity to support definitive hematopoiesis, adding an additional rationale for the cotransplantation of stroma, particularly in circumstances where high levels of donor cells are required early after *in utero* transplantation. There are a variety of other potential approaches to improvement of initial engraftment but these await experimental support. At the present time, attempts at *in utero* reconstitution or replacement have only been successful under circumstances where a competitive advantage exists for donor cells. It would therefore follow that, in order to achieve replacement of host cells in a competitive environment, one would need to either increase the competitive capacity of donor cells or reduce the competitive capacity of host cells, or both.

A particularly promising approach is to increase the competitive capacity of donor cells postnatally after establishing low level chimerism and tolerance by IU-HCT. This approach is based on the observation that engraftment can be achieved without cytoreduction in syngeneic models, arguing that in the presence of tolerance or effective immunosuppression, cytoreduction may not be required [65,66]. This observation has been validated in allogeneic systems by the success of a variety of nonmyeloablative strategies for postnatal BMT in circumstances of host immune deficiency or tolerance [67,68]. Flake and colleagues have applied two nonmyeloablative strategies in the mouse model to alter the competitive balance of the donor and host cell compartments in tolerant mixed chimeric animals after IU-HCT. In the first strategy, DLI was utilized to induce a graft-vs.-host hematopoietic effect. This resulted in a donor lymphocyte dose-dependent conversion of mixed chimerism to complete donor chimerism across a fully MHC mismatched strain combination (Fig. 44.9). Surprisingly, only one out of 56 animals receiving the high dose of donor lymphocytes with conversion to complete donor chimerism developed evidence of GVHD, suggesting that the mixed chimeric recipient created by IU-HCT may be a favorable candidate for DLI-induced enhancement of engraftment relative to the postnatal irradiation-induced chimera. Potential reasons for reduced GVHD in our study include the lack of irradiation with its accompanying proinflammatory cytokine milieu which may lower the threshold for GVHD in nonhematopoietic tissues, or the presence of a highly active, nonirradiated thymus for the production of regulatory T-cell populations. These animals maintain donor specific tolerance with bi-directional deletion of alloreactive lymphocytes and normal immune response to third party or novel T-cell dependent antigens. This study is indicative of the potential for this approach as it is, to our knowledge, the first time that complete allogeneic chimerism has been achieved across full MHC barriers in the complete absence of cyto-reductive or immunosuppressive therapy [38]. The second minimally ablative approach that we have investigated was suggested by results of marked enhancement of engraftment in the syngeneic nonmyeloablative model when low dose total body irradiation (TBI) was administered prior to transplantation [69]. When we administered graded doses of minimal TBI to our tolerant mixed chimeric animals following IU-HCT and then retransplanted the animals with 30 million T-cell-depleted donor BM cells, we observed a TBI dose-dependent enhancement of engraftment to levels of >90% donor peri-pheral blood expression with the highest TBI dose of 276 cGy [39] (Fig. 44.10). These studies confirm the predominant importance of competitive capacity for maintenance and expansion of the donor cell compartment in circumstances of mixed chimerism and suggest that similar strategies could be clinically successful once adequate chimerism is established by IU-HCT for induction and maintenance of donor specific tolerance.

Considerations for clinical application

Consideration of the above supports the rationale for prenatal HSC transplantation in selected circumstances. The potential clinical advantages of the prenatal approach over postnatal BMT are summarized in Table 44.1. These potential advantages must be weighed against the associated maternal and fetal risk. It should be emphasized that prenatal transplantation does not preclude conventional postnatal therapy. From an ethical perspective, it would be inappropriate to withhold beneficial postnatal therapy if prenatal transplantation fails or is only partially effective [70].

Maternal and fetal risk

Maternal and fetal risk can be divided into procedural and nonprocedural risk. The risk of fetal loss with chorionic villous sampling (CVS) has been well documented and is <1% [71]. The risk of procedure-related fetal loss with intraperitoneal or intravascular transplantation of HSC in the first to second trimester is unknown, but extrapolation from the extensive experience with intraperitoneal transfusion for fetal rhesus (Rh) disease is reasonable. There are differences, however, which need elaboration. A number of factors increase the risk of fetal loss in treatment of Rh disease that are not present with IU-HCT. Intraperitoneal transfusion when used for Rh disease involves placement of a catheter into the fetal peritoneal cavity via the lumen of a 16-gauge needle with infusion of a relatively large volume of cells. In contrast, IU-HCT is usually carried out using no larger than a 22-gauge needle and involves less than 1 mL of injectate. The early gestational age and small size of the fetal recipient of IU-HCT, on the other hand, may increase the relative risk of *in utero* stem cell transplantation. On balance, the increased risk of fetal loss following a single *in utero* transplant procedure is probably on the lower end of the range of risk for intraperitoneal transfusion, which has been estimated to be between 0.8% and 3.5% in various series [72], and the authors currently estimate a risk of around 1% per transplant when counseling patients. It goes without saying that these risk estimates apply only to centers with extensive experience with these techniques.

Nonprocedural risk to the mother and fetus include transmissible infectious disease and GVHD. The risk of transmissible infectious disease is dependent upon the donor cell source and the donor cell screening process. This represents the primary obstacle to the use of fetal tissue, as there currently exists no quality controls on procurement, processing and donor screening. With adult-derived tissues, standard protocols and procedures used to screen donors for BMT can be utilized. Clinical BM or

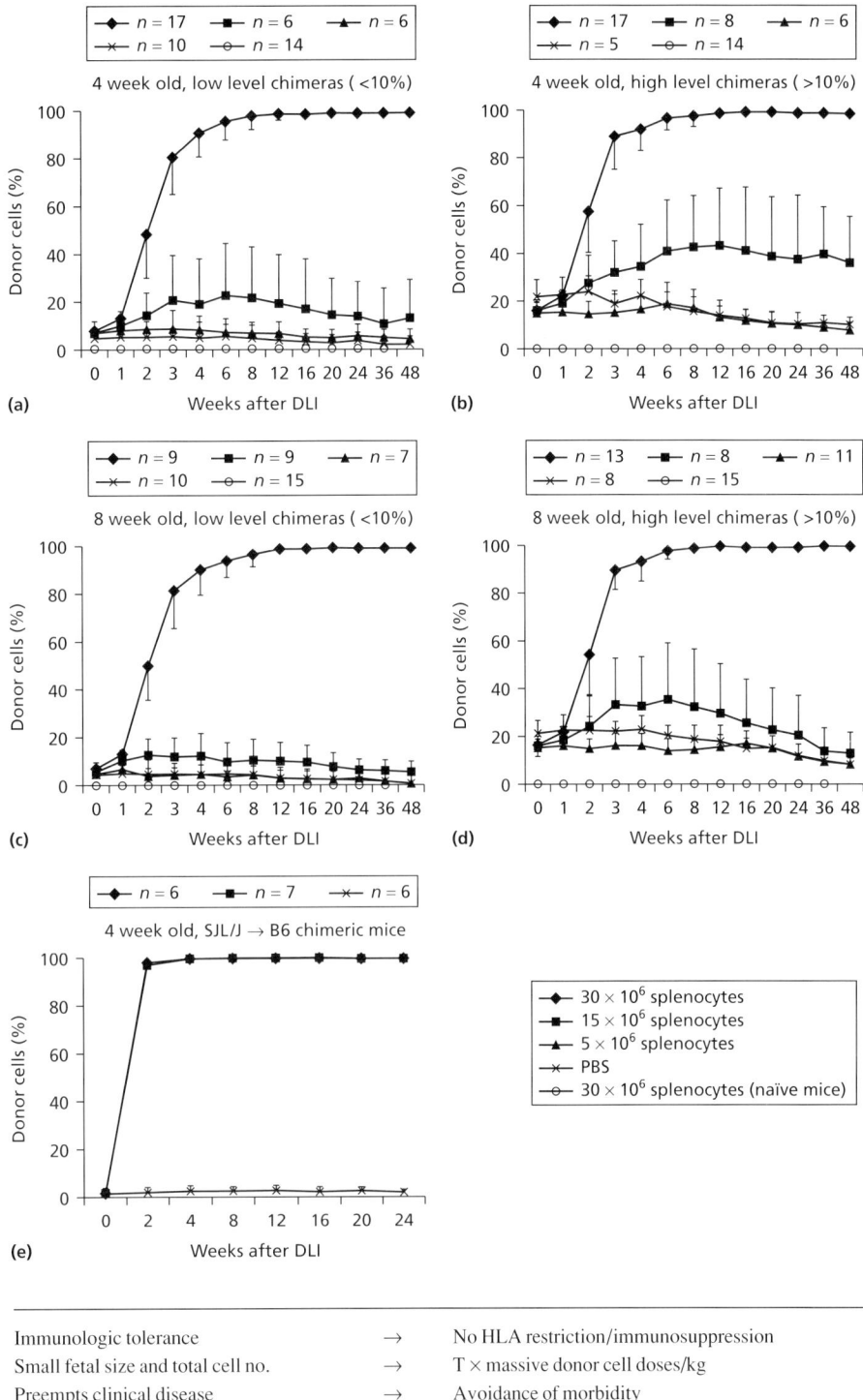

Fig. 44.9 Engraftment profiles following postnatal donor lymphocyte infusion (DLI) in chimeric animals created by *in utero* hematopoietic cell transplantation (IU-HCT). DLI was performed in 4- (a, b) or 8- (c, d) week-old chimeras with either low-level (a, c) or high-level (b, d) chimerism using three doses of donor splenocytes. (e) Results of DLI performed at 4 weeks of age in a second allogeneic strain combination. Reproduced with permission from Hayashi *et al.* [38].

Table 44.1 Potential advantages of *in utero* hematopoietic stem cell transplantation.

Immunologic tolerance	→	No HLA restriction/immunosuppression
Small fetal size and total cell no.	→	T × massive donor cell doses/kg
Preempts clinical disease	→	Avoidance of morbidity
Stem cell biology: expansion, migration	→	Expansion and distribution of engrafted donor cells*

*Assumes equal or superior competitive capacity of donor cells.
HLA, human leukocyte antigen.

stem cell laboratories can be utilized and the high level of quality control established for cell processing for BMT can be maintained. The risk of fetal GVHD is also dependent on the donor tissue used. Postnatal experience in immunocompromised BMT recipients suggests that transplantation of more than 1×10^5 mature T cells/kg introduces the risk of GVHD [73]. Undoubtedly, fetuses with immune deficiency disorders are at greater risk than other disease groups for this complication. It is well docu-

mented that newborns with SCID have a significant incidence of maternal vs. fetal GVHD related to transplacental passage of maternal T cells [74,75]. The two reported recipients of CD34-enriched paternal marrow with X-linked severe combined immunodeficiency syndrome (XSCID) received doses of 1.1×10^5 T cells/kg fetal weight, or less, per injection and neither had clinical evidence of GVHD [61,62]. Thus, based on available evidence, this appears to be a relatively safe minimal dose of T cells

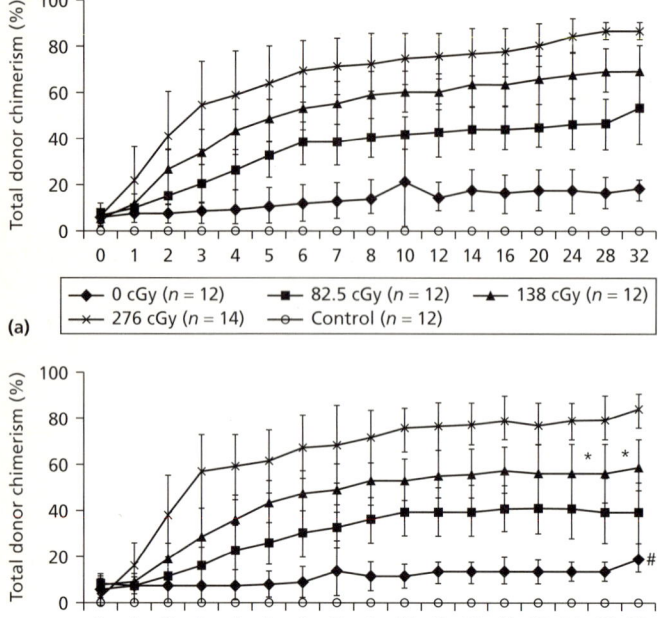

Fig. 44.10 *In utero* hematopoietic cell transplantation (IU-HCT) followed by a postnatal low-dose total body irradiation/bone marrow transplantation (TBI/BMT) regimen results in high levels of allochimerism. Chimeric mice after IU-HCT received one of four doses of TBI followed by a postnatal T-cell-depleted BMT with cells congenic (B6Pep3b) to the allogeneic prenatal donor at 4 (a) or 8 (b) weeks of age. Control mice were 4-week-old-naive Balb/c males that received 276 cGy TBI followed by tail vein infusion of 30×10^6 T-cell-depleted B6 BM cells. At all time points there is no difference between chimerism levels in mice boosted at 8 and 4 weeks of age ($p < 0.05$) with the exception of the two marked points [*]. Levels of chimerism were statistically different between each irradiation dose ($p < 0.05$) with the exception of the # marked point. Reproduced with permission from Peranteau et al. [39].

Table 44.2 Diseases potentially amenable to *in utero* hematopoietic stem cell transplantation.

Rationale = selective advantage for donor cells
SCID:
    X-linked*
    ZAP 70
    Jak 3
    ADA deficency
Wiskott–Aldrich syndrome
Chromosal breakage syndromes:
    Fanconi anemia
    Bloom syndrome

Rationale = minimal engraftment requirement
Hyper IgM syndrome
Chronic granulomatous disease

*Has been successfully treated by *in utero* hematopoietic stem cell transplantation.
ADA, adenosine deaminase; IgM, immunoglobulin M; SCID, severe combined immunodeficiency syndrome.

for clinical *in utero* transplantation. An important area in the future will be definition of facilitating populations required to achieve higher levels of engraftment after IU-HCT in hematopoietically competitive recipients. These populations will need to be carefully assessed in experimental models for their propensity to induce GVHD prior to clinical application.

Diseases that are potentially amenable to IU-HCT

Theoretically, in the future, any disease that can be diagnosed early in gestation and can be cured by postnatal BMT could potentially be treated by IU-HCT. In reality, each disease is biologically unique, and with the limitations of current knowledge regarding the requirements for engraftment, only a few are reasonable candidate diseases to consider (Table 44.2).

Diseases with a selective advantage for normal cells

By far the most favorable biology for IU-HCT are circumstances in which there is a survival or proliferative advantage for normal cells. This is clearly the case in the majority of SCID disorders. The most common type of SCID is X-linked (XSCID) and is due to a mutation in the gene encoding the common gamma chain (γc), a member of the cytokine receptor superfamily, and an essential component for normal function of the interleukin 2 (IL-2) and multiple other cytokine receptors [76]. The resultant cytokine unresponsiveness causes a block in T-cell development, and a severe deficiency of mature T cells. B cells, although present in normal or even increased numbers, are also dysfunctional. Other characterized mutations in cytokine receptor signaling pathways (i.e. Jak 3 or ZAP-70), or adenosine deaminase (ADA) deficiency, resulting in SCID, should also be favorable candidate diseases for IU-HCT. Based on the available clinical and experimental evidence, it is likely that any member of this group of disorders can be effectively treated by IU-HCT, using established protocols, with results comparable to the reported results for XSCID. Ideally, clinical trials of IU-HCT for SCID would be established, and the results compared to early postnatal transplantation protocols, to determine whether there is a biologic advantage favoring IU-HCT. Unfortunately, such trials may not be possible due to the rarity of these diseases and the perception that postnatal therapy is adequate [77]. In addition, the recent impressive results of postnatal gene therapy for XSCID may make prenatal treatment unnecessary [78], although recent concerns regarding insertional mutagenesis may require reexamination of the gene therapy approach.

Another immunodeficiency disorder where a selective advantage for normal cells exists is the Wiskott–Aldrich syndrome (WAS). WAS is a severe immunodeficiency and platelet deficiency disease arising from mutation(s) in the *WASP* gene, which in normal cells encodes an intracellular protein able to interact with other proteins relevant to the control of cytoskeletal organization [79]. Immunodeficiency is mainly due to progressive T-cell malfunction. Salient defects of WAS T cells are a CD3-restricted impairment in proliferative responses and cytoskeletal abnormalities, including the frequent appearance of T cells with atypical morphology [80]. Direct evidence of a selective advantage for normal cells is documentation of nonrandom inactivation of the X chromosome in multiple lineages of peripheral blood cells and early lineage hematopoietic cells in carriers of WAS, similar to that seen in the T-cell lineage in carriers of XSCID [81,82]. The combination of a selective advantage for normal hematopoietic progenitors and a proliferative defect in host T cells should provide favorable biology for successful IU-HCT. This disease has been successfully treated with matched sibling BMT, but the results of mismatched marrow transplants have been poor [83,84], adding to the justification for attempting IU-HCT. However, IU-HCT has not yet been appropriately tested in a fetus with WAS.

Another group of diseases that could benefit from IU-HCT are those in which somatic mosaicism and *in vivo* selection have been documented to occur. In these diseases there is presumably a survival advantage for the spontaneously corrected cells [85]. Such correction has been noted in ADA-SCID [86], Fanconi anemia [87] and Bloom syndrome [88]; the latter two of which are chromosomal breakage syndromes. In both Fanconi anemia and Bloom syndrome, mitotic recombination was documented as the molecular mechanism of somatic reversion. This represents an experiment of nature documenting the improvement in a disease by clonal expansion of a single spontaneously corrected HSC and suggests that low level engraftment achieved *in utero* could eventually replace host hematopoiesis as progressive BM failure occurred. True clinical cure of either disease is unlikely as they are associated with other pleiotropic manifestations, such as an increased rate of malignancy, that are unlikely to be reversed by hematopoietic reconstitution alone.

Although the target disorders remain limited, it is not unreasonable to consider further attempts at IU-HCT using current methodology in the context of the discussion and disease entities described above. Having said that, it is clear that this remains an experimental approach and should be limited to institutions with active research programs, IU-HCT, appropriate clinical protocols in place and the clinical expertise to optimally test the approach for this limited subset of disorders. It should be emphasized that at the present time, because of the extremely limited clinical experience at individual centers, the optimal approach to IU-HCT remains debatable.

Clinical experience with IU-HCT

The clinical experience with IU-HCT thus far supports the existence of the barriers discussed above, and the inadequacy of current approaches to overcome them. There have now been well over 40 attempts to transplant fetuses for a variety of congenital disorders. Most of these cases have been adequately presented in recent reviews [89,90] and will not be revisited here. The majority of these efforts have been performed in a suboptimal fashion with respect to the gestational age of the fetus, the disease entity chosen for treatment or the donor cells utilized, and with current knowledge would be predicted to fail. However, more recently, there have been a number of optimally performed transplants with high doses of appropriate donor cells delivered at early gestational time points [40,61,62,91–93]. The only clear successes have been in XSCID, with results reported thus far in a few patients that are comparable to results with nonmyeloablated postnatal transplantation. As discussed above, XSCID offers a selective advantage for donor T-cell development, proliferation and function because of the common γc deficiency present in host cells. Fetuses that have been successfully transplanted have stable split chimerism with the T-cell lineage of donor origin, and all other lineages of host origin. They maintain a partial B-cell functional deficit; however, a detailed comparison of B-cell function and T-cell/B-cell cooperation between pre and postnatal nonmyeloablated recipients has not been performed [94]. All other target diseases, i.e. other immune deficiency disorders, hemoglobinopathies and inborn errors of metabolism have either failed to engraft or have had inadequate engraftment for therapeutic effect.

Conclusions

IU-HCT is currently in its early stages of development but holds considerable promise as a therapeutic approach for the treatment of a large number of congenital hematological diseases. Despite only recent limited evidence of clinical efficacy, interest in the field continues to gain momentum. Parallel advances in prenatal screening, molecular diagnosis and the human genome project make it highly likely that opportunities for application of this approach will increase. However, at this point in the evolution of IU-HCT there are more questions than answers. Widespread clinical application is premature based on the extremely limited clinical success that has been achieved. The biology of each disease is unique and expectations of success or failure can only be based on sound clinical investigation guided by experimental work in relevant animal models. The barriers to prenatal engraftment need to be investigated and understood prior to further clinical efforts in diseases where host cell competition is prohibitive. Clinical centers should be associated with an active research effort to solve the remaining problems with this potentially promising clinical approach. In the near future, advances in our understanding of stem cell biology in the context of the prenatal microenvironment may allow IU-HCT to achieve its full potential.

References

1. Harrison M. The fetus as a patient: historical perspective. In: Harrison M, Golbus M, Filly R, eds. *The Unborn Patient. Prenatal Diagnosis and Treatment*, 2nd edn. Philadelphia: W.B. Saunders Co., 1990: 1–7.
2. Moise K. Intrauterine transfusion with red cells and platelets. *West J Med* 1993; **159**: 318–24.
3. Kitano Y, Flake AW, Crombleholme TM, Johnson MP, Adzick NS. Open fetal surgery for life-threatening fetal malformations. *Semin Perinatol* 1999; **23**: 448–61.
4. Owen RD. Immunogenetic consequences of vascular anastomoses between bovine cattle twins. *Science* 1945; **102**: 400–1.
5. Anderson D, Billingham R, Lampkin G, Medawar P. The use of skin grafting to distinguish between monozygotic and dizygotic twins in cattle. *Heredity* 1951; **5**: 379–97.
6. Simonsen M. The acquired immunity concept in kidney homotransplantation. *Ann NY Acad Sci* 1955; **59**: 448–52.
7. Picus J, Aldrich W, Letvin N. A naturally occurring bone-marrow chimeric primate. *Transplantation* 1985; **39**: 297–303.
8. van Dijk B, Bommsma D, de Man A. Blood group chimerism in human multiple births is not rare. *Am J Med Genet* 1996; **61**: 264–8.
9. Gill T. Chimerism in humans. *Transplant Proc* 1977; **9**: 1423–31.
10. Burnet M. *The Clonal Selection Theory of Acquired Immunity*. London: Cambridge University Press, 1959.
11. Billingham R, Brent L, Medawar PB. Actively acquired tolerance of foreign cells. *Nature* 1953; **172**: 603–7.
12. Sprent J. Central tolerance of T cells. *Int Rev Immunol* 1995; **13**: 95–105.
13. Anderson G, Moore N, Owen J, Jenkinson E. Cellular interactions in thymocyte development. *Ann Rev Immunol* 1996; **14**: 73–99.
14. Haynes BF, Martin ME, Kay HH, Kurtzberg J. Early events in human T-cell ontogeny. Phenotypic characterization and immunohistologic localization of T-cell precursors in early human fetal tissues. *J Exp Med* 1988; **168**: 1061–80.
15. Strominger JL. Developmental biology of T cell receptors. *Science* 1989; **244**: 943–9.
16. Sha WC, Nelson CA, Newberry RD, Kranz DM, Russell JH, Loh DY. Positive and negative selection of an antigen receptor on T-cells in transgenic mice. *Nature* 1988; **336**: 73–6.
17. Schwartz R. Acquisition of immunologic self tolerance. *Cell* 1989; **57**: 1073–81.
18. Blackman M, Kappler J, Marrack P. The role of the T-cell receptor in positive and negative selection of developing T-cells. *Science* 1990; **248**: 1335–42.
19. Guidos CJ, Danska JS, Fathman CG, Weissman IL. T cell receptor-mediated negative selection of autoreactive T lymphocyte precursors occurs after commitment to the CD4 or CD8 lineages. *J Exp Med* 1990; **172**: 835–45.
20. Weissman IL. Developmental switches in the immune system. *Cell* 1994; **76**: 207–18.
21. Metcalf D, Moore MAS. Embryonic aspects of haemopoiesis. In: Neuberger A, Tatum EL, eds. *Haemopoietic Cells*. Amsterdam: North-Holland Publishing Co., 1971: 4–38.
22. Tavian M, Coulombel L, Luton D, San Clemente H, Dieterlen-Lievre F, Peault B. Aorta-associated CD34+ hematopoietic cells in the early human embryo. *Blood* 1996; **87**: 67–72.
23. Zanjani ED, Ascensao JL, Tavassoli M. Liver-derived fetal hematopoietic stem cells selectively and preferentially home to the fetal bone marrow. *Blood* 1993; **81**: 399–404.
24. Shaaban AF, Kim HB, Milner R, Flake AW. A

24 kinetic model for homing and migration of prenatally transplanted marrow. *Blood* 1999; **94**: 3251–7.
25 Fleischman R, Mintz B. Prevention of genetic anemias in mice by microinjection of normal hematopoietic cells into the fetal placenta. *Proc Natl Acad Sci U S A* 1979; **76**: 5736–40.
26 Geissler E, Ryan M, Housman D. The dominant-white spotting (W) locus of the mouse encodes the c-kit proto-oncogene. *Cell* 1988; **55**: 185–91.
27 Mintz B, Anthony K, Litwin S. Monoclonal derivation of mouse myeloid and lymphoid lineages from totipotent hematopoietic stem cells experimentally engrafted in fetal hosts. *Proc Natl Acad Sci U S A* 1984; **81**: 7835–9.
28 Blazer B, Taylor P, Vallera D. *In utero* transfer of adult bone marrow cells into recipients with severe combined immunodeficiency disorder yields lymphoid progeny with T- and B-cell functional capabilities. *Blood* 1995; **86**: 4353–66.
29 Flake AW, Harrison MR, Adzick NS, Zanjani ED. Transplantation of fetal hematopoietic stem cells *in utero*: the creation of hematopoietic chimeras. *Science* 1986; **233**: 776–8.
30 Zanjani ED, Ascensao JL, Flake AW, Harrison MR, Tavassoli M. The fetus as an optimal donor and recipient of hemopoietic stem cells. *Bone Marrow Transplant* 1992; **10**: 107–14.
31 Flake A, Zanjani E. Cellular therapy. New trends and controversies in fetal diagnosis and therapy. *Obstet Gynecol Clin North Am* 1997; **24**: 159–77.
32 Zanjani ED, Pallavicini MG, Ascensao JL *et al.* Engraftment and long-term expression of human fetal hemopoietic stem cells in sheep following transplantation *in utero*. *J Clin Invest* 1992; **89**: 1178–88.
33 Shields L, Bryant E, Easterling T, Andrews R. Fetal liver cell transplantation for the creation of lymph-hematopoietic chimerism in the fetal baboon. *Am J Obstet Gynecol* 1995; **173**: 1157–60.
34 Shaaban AF, Milner R, Kim HB, Flake AW. Fetal liver is a superior donor source for the engraftment of prenatally transplanted allogeneic hematopoietic stem cells. *Exp Hematol* 1999; **121**: 320 [Abstract].
35 Rice HE, Hedrick MH, Flake AW, Donegan E, Harrison MR. Bacterial and fungal contamination of human fetal liver collected transvaginally for hematopoietic stem cell transplantation. *Fetal Diagn Ther* 1993; **8**: 74–8.
36 Zanjani ED, Mackintosh FR, Harrison MR. Hematopoietic chimerism in sheep and nonhuman primates by *in utero* transplantation of fetal hematopoietic stem cells. *Blood Cells* 1991; **17**: 349–63.
37 Crombleholme TM, Harrison MR, Zanjani ED. *In utero* transplantation of hematopoietic stem cells in sheep: the role of T cells in engraftment and graft-versus-host disease. *J Pediatr Surg* 1990; **25**: 885–92.
38 Hayashi S, Peranteau WH, Shaaban AF, Flake AW. Complete allogeneic hematopoietic chimerism achieved by a combined strategy of *in utero* hematopoietic stem cell transplantation and postnatal donor lymphocyte infusion. *Blood* 2002; **100**: 804–12.
39 Peranteau WF, Hayashi S, Hsieh M, Shaaban AF, Flake AW. High level allogeneic chimerism achieved by prenatal tolerance induction and postnatal non-myeloablative bone marrow transplantation. *Blood* 2002; **100**: 2225–34.
40 Muench MO, Rae J, Barcena A *et al.* Transplantation of a fetus with paternal Thy-1^+CD34^+ cells for chronic granulomatous disease. *Bone Marrow Transplant* 2001; **27**: 355–64.

41 Zanjani ED, Flake AW, Rice H, Hedrick M, Tavassoli M. Long-term repopulating ability of xenogeneic transplanted human fetal liver hematopoietic stem cells in sheep. *J Clin Invest* 1994; **93**: 1051–5.
42 Pallavicini MG, Flake AW, Madden D *et al.* Hemopoietic chimerism in rodents transplanted *in utero* with fetal human hemopoietic cells. *Transplant Proc* 1992; **24**: 542–3.
43 Hedrick MH, Rice HE, Sachs DH, Zanjani ED, Flake AW. Creation of pig–sheep xenogeneic hematopoietic chimerism by the *in utero* transplantation of hematopoietic stem cells. *Transplant Sci* 1993; **3**: 23–6.
44 Rice HE, Hedrick MH, Flake AW. *In utero* transplantation of rat hematopoietic stem cells induces xenogeneic chimerism in mice. *Transplant Proc* 1994; **26**: 126–8.
45 Zanjani ED, Srour EF, Hoffman R. Retention of long-term repopulating ability of xenogeneic transplanted purified adult human bone marrow hematopoietic stem cells in sheep. *J Laboratory Clin Med* 1995; **126**: 24–8.
46 Zanjani ED, Almeida-Porada G, Livingston AG, Flake AW, Ogawa M. Human bone marrow CD34$^-$ cells engraft *in vivo* and undergo multilineage expression that includes giving rise to CD34$^+$ cells. *Exp Hematol* 1998; **26**: 353–60.
47 Zanjani ED, Almeida-Porada G, Livingston AG, Porada CD, Ogawa M. Engraftment and multilineage expression of human bone marrow CD34$^-$ cells *in vivo*. *Ann N Y Acad Sci* 1999; **872**: 220–31.
48 Verfaillie CM, Almeida-Porada G, Wissink S, Zanjani ED. Kinetics of engraftment of CD34$^-$ and CD34$^+$ cells from mobilized blood differs from that of CD34$^-$ and CD34$^+$ cells from bone marrow. *Exp Hematol* 2000; **28**: 1071–9.
49 Lewis ID, Almeida-Porada GJ, Du J *et al.* Umbilical cord blood cells capable of engrafting in primary, secondary, and tertiary xenogeneic hosts are preserved after *ex vivo* culture in a noncontact system. *Blood* 2001; **97**: 3441–9.
50 Civin C, Almeida-Porada G, Lee M-J, Olweus J, Terstappen L, Zanjani E. Sustained, retransplantable, multilineage engraftment of highly purified adult human bone marrow stem cells *in vivo*. *Blood* 1996; **88**: 4102–9.
51 Tsai EJ, Malech HL, Kirby MR *et al.* Retroviral transduction of IL2RG into CD34$^+$ cells from X-linked severe combined immunodeficiency patients permits human T- and B-cell development in sheep chimeras. *Blood* 2002; **100**: 72–9.
52 Zanjani ED, Flake AW, Almeida-Porada G, Tran N, Papayannopoulou T. Homing of human cells in the fetal sheep model: modulation by antibodies activating or inhibiting very late activation antigen-4-dependent function. *Blood* 1999; **94**: 2515–22.
53 Flake AW, Zanjani ED. *In utero* hematopoietic stem cell transplantation. Ontogenic opportunities and biologic barriers. *Blood* 1999; **94**: 2179–91.
54 Carrier E, Lee TH, Busch MP, Cowan MJ. Induction of tolerance in nondefective mice after *in utero* transplantation of major histocompatibility complex-mismatched fetal hematopoietic stem cells. *Blood* 1995; **86**: 4681–90.
55 Carrier E, Gilpin E, Lee TH, Busch MP, Zanetti M. Microchimerism does not induce tolerance after *in utero* transplantation and may lead to the development of alloreactivity. *J Laboratory Clin Med* 2000; **136**: 224–35.
56 Blazar BR, Taylor PA, Vallera DA. Adult bone marrow-derived pluripotent hematopoietic stem

cells are engraftable when transferred *in utero* into moderately anemic fetal recipients. *Blood* 1995; **85**: 833–41.
57 Kim HB, Shaaban AF, Yang EY, Liechty KW, Flake AW. Microchimerism and tolerance after *in utero* bone marrow transplantation in mice. *J Surg Res* 1998; **77**: 1–5.
58 Kim HB, Shaaban AF, Milner R, Fichter C, Flake AW. *In utero* bone marrow transplantation induces tolerance by a combination of clonal deletion and anergy. *J Pediatr Surg* 1999; **34**: 726–30.
59 Blazer BR, Taylor PA, McElmurry R *et al.* Engraftment of severe combined immune deficient mice receiving allogeneic bone marrow via *in utero* or postnatal transfer. *Blood* 1998; **92**: 3949–59.
60 Archer DR, Turner CW, Yeager AM, Fleming WH. Sustained multilineage engraftment of allogeneic hematopoietic stem cells in NOD/SCID mice after *in utero* transplantation. *Blood* 1997; **90**: 3222–9.
61 Flake A, Roncarolo M-G, Puck J *et al.* Treatment of X-linked severe combined immunodeficiency by *in utero* transplantation of paternal bone marrow. *N Engl J Med* 1996; **335**: 1806–10.
62 Wengler G, Lanfranchi A, Frusca T *et al.* In-utero transplantation of parental CD34 haematopoietic progenitor cells in a patient with X-linked severe combined immunodeficiency (SCIDX1). *Lancet* 1996; **348**: 1484–7.
63 Almeida-Porada G, Flake AW, Glimp HA, Zanjani ED. Cotransplantation of stroma results in enhancement of engraftment and early expression of donor hematopoietic stem cells *in utero*. *Exp Hematol* 1999; **27**: 1569–75.
64 Almeida-Porada G, Porada CD, Tran N, Zanjani ED. Cotransplantation of human stromal cell progenitors into preimmune fetal sheep results in early appearance of human donor cells in circulation and boosts cell levels in bone marrow at later time points after transplantation. *Blood* 2000; **95**: 3620–7.
65 Brecher G, Tjio JH, Haley JE, Narla J, Beal SL. Transplantation of murine bone marrow without prior host irradiation. *Blood Cells* 1979; **5**: 237–46.
66 Stewart FM, Crittenden RB, Lowry PA, Pearson-White S, Quesenberry PJ. Long-term engraftment of normal and post-5-fluorouracil murine marrow into normal nonmyeloablated mice. *Blood* 1993; **81**: 2566–71.
67 Slavin S, Nagler A, Shapira M, Panigrahi S, Samuel S, Or A. Non-myeloablative allogeneic stem cell transplantation focusing on immunotherapy of life-threatening malignant and non-malignant diseases. *Crit Rev Oncol Hematol* 2001; **39**: 25–9.
68 Sykes M, Preffer F, McAfee S *et al.* Mixed lymphohaemopoietic chimerism and graft-versus-lymphoma effects after non-myeloablative therapy and HLA-mismatched bone-marrow transplantation. *Lancet* 1999; **353**: 1755–9.
69 Stewart FM, Zhong S, Wuu J, Hsieh C-C, Nilsson SK, Quesenberry PJ. Lymphohematopoietic engraftment minimally myeloablated hosts. *Blood* 1998; **91**: 3681–7.
70 Flake AW. Prenatal intervention. Ethical considerations for life-threatening and non-life-threatening anomalies. *Semin Pediatr Surg* 2001; **10**: 212–21.
71 Rhoads G, Jackson L, Schlesselman S *et al.* The safety and efficacy of chorionic villus sampling for early prenatal diagnosis of cytogenetic abnormalities. *N Engl J Med* 1989; **320**: 609–17.
72 Bowman J. Hemolytic disease (*erythroblastosis fetalis*). In: Creasy R, Resnick R, eds. *Maternal-Fetal Medicine. Principles and Practice*, 3rd edn. Philadelphia: W.B. Saunders Co., 1994: 730–3.

73 McKinnon S, Papadopoulos E, Carabasi M *et al*. Adoptive immunotherapy. Evaluating escalating doses of donor leukocytes for relapse of CML after BMT. Separation of GvL responses from GvHD. *Blood* 1995; **86**: 1261–8.

74 Alain G, Carrier C, Beaumier L, Bernard J, Lemay M, Lavoie A. *In utero* acute graft-versus-host disease in a neonate with severe combined immunodeficiency. *J Am Acad Dermatol* 1993; **29**: 862–5.

75 Sottini A, Quiros-Roldan E, Notarangelo LD, Malagoli A, Primi D, Imberti L. Engrafted maternal T cells in a severe combined immunodeficiency patient express T-cell receptor variable beta segments characterized by a restricted *V-D-J* junctional diversity. *Blood* 1995; **85**: 2105–13.

76 Puck JM, Deschenes SM, Porter JC *et al*. The interleukin-2 receptor γ chain maps to Xq13.1 and is mutated in X-linked severe combined immunodeficiency, SCIDX1. *Hum Mol Genet* 1993; **2**: 1099–104.

77 Buckley RH, Schiff SE, Schiff RI *et al*. Hematopoietic stem-cell transplantation for the treatment of severe combined immunodeficiency. *N Engl J Med* 1999; **340**: 508–16.

78 Cavazzana-Calvo M, Hacein-Bey S, de Saint Basile G *et al*. Gene therapy of human severe combined immunodeficiency (SCID)-X1 disease. *Science* 2000; **288**: 669–72.

79 Gallego MD, Santamaría M, Peña J, Molina IJ. Defective actin reorganization and polymerization of Wiskott–Aldrich T cells in response to CD3-mediated stimulation. *Blood* 1997; **90**: 3089–97.

80 Prchal JT, Carroll AJ, Prchal JF *et al*. Wiskott–Aldrich syndrome: cellular impairments and their implication for carrier detection. *Blood* 1980; **56**: 1048–54.

81 Puck JM, Siminovitch KA, Poncz M, Greenberg CR, Rottem M, Conley ME. Atypical presentation of Wiskott–Aldrich syndrome: diagnosis in two unrelated males based on studies of maternal T cell X chromosome inactivation. *Blood* 1990; **75**: 2369–74.

82 Wengler G, Gorlin JB, Williamson JM, Rosen FS, Bing DH. Nonrandom inactivation of the X chromosome in early lineage hematopoietic cells in carriers of Wiskott–Aldrich syndrome. *Blood* 1995; **85**: 2471–7.

83 Mullen CA, Anderson KD, Blaese RM. Splenectomy and/or bone marrow transplantation in the management of the Wiskott–Aldrich syndrome: long-term follow-up of 62 cases. *Blood* 1993; **82**: 2961–6.

84 Filipovich AH, Shapiro RS, Ramsay NK *et al*. Unrelated donor bone marrow transplantation for correction of lethal congenital immunodeficiencies. *Blood* 1992; **80**: 270–6.

85 Kvittengen EA, Rootwelt H, Brandtzaeg P, Bergan A, Bergan R. Hereditary tyrosinemia type I. Self induced correction of the fumarylacetoacetase defect. *J Clin Invest* 1993; **91**: 1816–23.

86 Hirschhorn R, Yang DR, Puck JM, Huie ML, Jiang CK, Kurlandsky LE. Spontaneous *in vivo* reversion to normal of an inherited mutation in a patient with adenosine deaminase deficiency. *Nat Genet* 1996; **13**: 290–6.

87 D'Andrea AD, Grompe M. Molecular biology of Fanconi anemia: implications for diagnosis and therapy. *Blood* 1997; **90**: 1725–36.

88 Ellis NA, Lennon DJ, Proytcheva M, Aldadeff B, Henderson EE, German J. Somatic intragenic recombination within the mutated locus BLM can correct the high sister-chromatid exchange phenotype of Bloom syndrome cells. *Am J Hum Genet* 1995; **57**: 1019–27.

89 Flake AW, Zanjani ED. *In utero* hematopoietic stem cell transplantation. A status report. *JAMA* 1997; **278**: 932–7.

90 Jones DR, Bui TH, Anderson EM *et al*. In utero haematopoietic stem cell transplantation: current perspectives and future potential. *Bone Marrow Transplant* 1996; **18**: 831–7.

91 Hayward A, Ambruso D, Battaglia F *et al*. Microchimerism and tolerance following intrauterine transplantation and transfusion for α-thalassemia-1. *Fetal Diagn Ther* 1998; **13**: 8–14.

92 Westgren M, Ringden O, Sturla E-N *et al*. Lack of evidence of permanent engraftment after *in utero* fetal stem cell transplantation in congenital hemoglobinopathies. *Transplantation* 1996; **61**: 1176–9.

93 Westgren M, Ringden O, Bartmann P *et al*. Prenatal T-cell reconstitution after *in utero* transplantation with fetal liver cells in a patient with X-linked severe combined immunodeficiency. *Am J Obstet Gynecol* 2002; **187**: 475–82.

94 Flake AW, Zanjani ED. Treatment of severe combined immunodeficiency [Letter]. *N Engl J Med* 1999; **341**: 291.

45

Judith Ng-Cashin & Thomas Shea

Mobilization of Autologous Peripheral Blood Hematopoietic Cells for Support of High-Dose Cancer Therapy

Introduction

High-dose chemotherapy has become an important therapeutic strategy for many malignancies. These regimens are often severely myelosuppressive or myeloablative, and autologous peripheral blood progenitor cells (PBPCs) have been used to provide rapid and sustained hematopoietic recovery to support such treatment. In the past, autologous bone marrow transplantation was used in this setting but, because of the less invasive collection methods and more rapid resolution of neutropenia and thrombocytopenia, PBPC transplantation has largely replaced bone marrow transplantation for the support of high-dose chemotherapy [1–3].

Both hematopoietic stem cells and progenitor cells populate the resting bone marrow. Stem cells are single cells that are clonal precursors capable of giving rise to both identical stem cells (self-renewal) and a defined set of differentiated progenitors. Progenitor cells are multipotent precursor cells that lack the ability to self-renew but, like stem cells, maintain the capacity to differentiate and proliferate. Despite this important difference, these terms often are used interchangeably in the literature [4].

The ability of PBPC to reconstitute hematopoiesis was first described in 1980 and followed by additional reports in 1985 and 1986 [5–9]. Under steady-state conditions, hematopoietic progenitor cells circulate in the peripheral blood compartment at a frequency of approximately 100 cells/mL of whole blood. This low frequency of PBPC in the circulation made collecting adequate numbers of these cells a cumbersome process. As a result, methods to mobilize these cells from the marrow compartment and increase their numbers in the peripheral circulation have been developed to foster collection of sufficient cells for clinical use. The work by Abrams and Richman in animal models demonstrating an increase in PBPC following subablative chemotherapy administration and by Socinski and Gianni in patients following cytokine administration have led to the widespread application of this approach for supporting high-dose therapy [10–13].

Identification and enumeration

Human hematopoietic stem cells express CD34 and Thy-1 at a high level and c-kit at a low level and do not express Lin and CD38 [4]. The ability of a mobilized pheresis product to engraft and permanently repopulate the bone marrow depends on its content of both stem cells and progenitor cells. In the transplant setting, this can be evaluated using several assays. Long-term culture-initiating cells (LTC-IC) have been used to assess the ability of mobilized cells to repopulate the bone marrow but this assay is time consuming and subject to inconsistency between laboratories. Functional assays measuring the quantity of cells committed to a particular lineage include colony-forming unit (CFU) and burst-forming unit (BFU) assays. Colony-forming unit-granulocyte/macrophage (CFU-GM), colony-forming unit-granulocyte/erythrocyte/macrophage/megakaryocyte (CFU-GEMM), and burst-forming unit-erythroid (BFU-E) have been correlated with time to engraftment [14]. Because these assays require significant laboratory manipulation, results often reflect technical variability and are difficult to compare.

More recently, quantification of CD34 expressing cells has been used to assess the quality of the pheresis product and its adequacy for repopulating the bone marrow. $CD34^+$ cell content correlates closely with CFU-GM, BFU-E and CFU-GEMM, as well as time to engraftment of both neutrophils and platelets [15–20]. $CD34^+$ cell quantification also is subject to intralaboratory variation, but standardization of procedures can reduce this variation [21–23]. Efforts also have been undertaken to identify subsets of the CD34 cell population that are critical to bone marrow reconstitution, such as $CD34^+CD33^-$, $CD34^+CD33^+$ or $CD34^+CD38^-$ cells [19,20,24–26]. One study found $CD34^+CD33^-$ cells more reliably predictive of hematopoietic recovery rates than $CD34^+$ cells [24], but others have not.

Mechanisms of progenitor cell mobilization

Although the indications for the clinical use of mobilized PBPC are well established and expanding, the mechanisms by which these cells are mobilized into the peripheral blood are poorly understood. Several steps seem to be involved, including enhanced proliferation of early progenitor cells and subsequent migration out of the bone marrow. Stem cell expansion alone may lead to egress of stem cells to the peripheral blood [27]. The hematopoietic cells are surrounded by stromal cells that include endothelial cells, macrophages, fibroblasts, adipocytes and barrier cells. These stromal cells provide signals through direct cell–cell interactions and through the extracellular matrix (ECM) that they produce [28]. The ECM primarily is composed of collagens, glycoproteins and glycosaminoglycans, and interacts with progenitor cells through specific cell surface receptors and growth factors [28]. Adhesive interactions between $CD34^+$ cells and their progenitors with cellular and matrix components of the bone marrow environment also are involved in mobilization and homing.

Adhesion molecules

The interactions between hematopoietic stem cells and components of the bone marrow play a central role in migration, circulation, and proliferation of progenitor cells. β_1- and β_2-integrins and selectins are involved in these adhesive interactions [29]. The β_1-integrins, very-late antigen-4 (VLA-4 [CD29CD49d]) and VLA-5 (CD29CD49e), are important in the adhesion of hematopoietic progenitor cells to the bone marrow stroma [30]. VLA-4 is expressed on progenitor cells and binds to vascular cell adhesion molecule-1 (VCAM-1) and fibronectin, both of which are found on bone marrow stromal cells [31]. In mouse and primate animal models, when this adhesion interaction was disrupted by monoclonal antibodies binding to VLA-4, a significant increase in PBPCs was seen [32,33]. Anti-VLA-4 antibodies also inhibit the adhesions of purified CD34$^+$ cells to bone marrow stromal cells [34]. The β_2-integrins, leukocyte function-associated antigen-1 (LFA-1 [CD18CD11a]) and macrophage antigen-1 (Mac-1 [CD11b]) are expressed by CD34$^+$ bone marrow cells. LFA-1 and Mac-1 bind to the intracellular adhesion molecules (ICAMs), ICAM-1 and ICAM-2, both expressed in the bone marrow stroma. The fact that both VLA-4 and LFA-1 are expressed at lower levels in mobilized CD34$^+$ cells compared to bone marrow CD34$^+$ cells [35], implies a down-regulation of these adhesion molecules that may be important for the release of these progenitor cells into the peripheral blood. In a mouse model, granulocyte colony-stimulating factor (G-CSF) induced stem cell mobilization was enhanced by the administration of antibodies to LFA-1 and Mac-1, implying that attenuation of these adhesive interactions potentiates mobilization [31]. However, this effect was not reproduced when antibodies to ICAM-1 were administered with G-CSF, suggesting that the mechanism through which β_2-integrins augmented mobilization is independent of ICAM binding. In addition, there was no enhancement of G-CSF induced mobilization in LFA-1$^{-/-}$ knockout mice. One hypothesis for these data is that LFA-1 exerts its effect on mobilization through a rapidly recruited or expanded cell such as the neutrophil as opposed to a more long-lived stromal cell [31]. Recent studies suggest that neutrophil proteases may be induced in G-CSF mobilization and may cleave VCAM-1, as its cleavage products are increased in the plasma after G-CSF administration [36].

Cytokines

Cytokines are secreted cellular proteins that act as intercellular mediators. Because hematopoietic cytokines have been found to effectively mobilize PBPCs, cytokines are thought to play a critical role in mobilization, but the exact mechanism through which they act remains largely undefined. The hematopoietic cytokine, G-CSF is the most commonly used agent to mobilize PBPCs. G-CSF is involved in the differentiation of myeloid progenitors into mature granulocytes, but this property may not be essential for its ability to mobilize hematopoietic progenitors. The expression of receptors for G-CSF is very low on primitive progenitor cells and increases with myeloid differentiation [37]. In a mouse model, the absence of the G-CSF receptor on CD34$^+$ cells did not impair their mobilization by exogenous G-CSF, demonstrating that the stimulation of growth and differentiation of hematopoietic progenitors is not the mechanism through which G-CSF induces mobilization [38]. The direct mechanism by which progenitor cells are mobilized by G-CSF may not be through the CD34$^+$ cells themselves, but through receptors present on the bone marrow stromal cells. Other cytokines that have been investigated as mobilization agents include granulocyte macrophage colony-stimulating factor (GM-CSF), interleukin-3 (IL-3), IL-8, IL-11, stem cell factor (SCF), and Flt3 ligand [27,39–46]. As single agents, these compounds are inferior to G-CSF for mobilization of PBPCs and the pathways through which they induce PBPC mobilization remain poorly understood. However, SCF, GM-CSF or IL-3 have been shown to increase the activation of VLA-4 and VLA-5 [47,48], demonstrating an interaction between cytokines and cell adhesion.

Chemokines

Chemokines are chemoattractant cytokines that usually act on differentiated cells, but they also play a role in hematopoietic cell homing and migration. Chemokines are classified based on the position and spacing of the first two conserved cysteines. Most chemokines fall into two subfamilies: the C–X–C and the C–C chemokines. Stromal derived factor-1 (SDF-1) is a CXC chemokine. SDF-1 binds CXC chemokine receptor 4 (CXCR4), which is found on many cells including CD34$^+$ cells [49]. The expression of SDF-1 in mobilized CD34$^+$ cells is decreased compared to bone marrow CD34$^+$ cells, suggesting that SDF-1 may be involved in hematopoietic cell migration and hematopoiesis. IL-8 is a CXC chemokine that is chemotactic for neutrophils and T cells, binding receptors CXCR1 and CXCR2. In mouse and primate models, IL-8 is a potent and rapid inducer of PBPCs. It is thought that IL-8 attracts and activates neutrophils to release proteases, such as matrix metalloproteinase 9 (MMP9), which are able to degrade ECM components and may participate in mobilization [50,51]. In fact, in a mouse model, neutrophils were found to be essential for IL-8 induced PBPC mobilization [52]. MMP9 levels in mobilized peripheral blood also have been found to be increased compared to that found in steady state [53]. GROβ is another CXC chemokine that, like IL-8, binds to CXCR2 and is a chemoattractant and activator of neutrophils. A recombinant, truncated form of the N-terminal of GROβ, SB-251353, has been used successfully in mice and monkeys to mobilize PBPCs. Single agent SB-251353-mobilized CFU-GM were capable of reconstituting lethally irradiated animals. When given in combination with G-CSF, the progenitor cell mobilization was increased fivefold [54]. GROβ also is thought to stimulate the release of MMP9, which may be partly responsible for its mobilization capacities.

Clinical applications

PBPCs have become the preferred source of autologous stem cells to support the use of high-dose, myeloablative chemotherapy in a variety of hematologic malignancies and solid tumors [1,3] and are being evaluated widely for use in allogeneic transplants [55–62]. Current mobilization regimens include single agent and cytokine combinations as well as combinations of chemotherapy and cytokines. Following mobilization, PBPCs are collected using a variety of leukapheresis techniques.

Collection techniques

Once PBPC mobilization is initiated, the timing and volume of leukapheresis is critical to maximizing yield. For steady-state mobilization with recombinant growth factors (in the absence of chemotherapy), the peak values of mobilized progenitor cells are observed after 4–6 days of treatment in most series [11,12,25,63–74]. Chemotherapy based mobilization results in an increase in the time required to initiate collection, as maximal mobilization occurs following resolution of the hematologic nadirs produced with chemotherapy induced myelosuppression. Collections are usually initiated when the white blood cell count (WBC) recovers to >1–>3 × 10^9/L WBC/L [75,76]. Monitoring daily CD34$^+$ cell content in the peripheral blood has also been studied as a predictor of PBPC yield. In one study, a CD34$^+$ cell count of ≥50 cell/mL peripheral blood predicted a CD34$^+$ cell yield of ≥2.5 × 10^6 CD34$^+$ cells/kg body weight in a single leukapheresis [77]. Other studies have found that a percentage of peripheral blood CD34$^+$ cells ≥0.5% predicted a high mobilization yield and early engraftment [78,79].

In harvesting PBPCs, the goal is to minimize the number of pheresis procedures required to achieve the target progenitor cell dose. To date, the optimal pheresis volume that achieves this goal has not been defined. Large volume leukapheresis (>15 L) has been investigated as a way to decrease the number of apheresis. Initially, there was concern that the large volumes would impair CD34$^+$ cell quantity harvested over collection time. In one study evaluating large volume leukapheresis in myeloma patients being mobilized for autologous transplant, the quantity

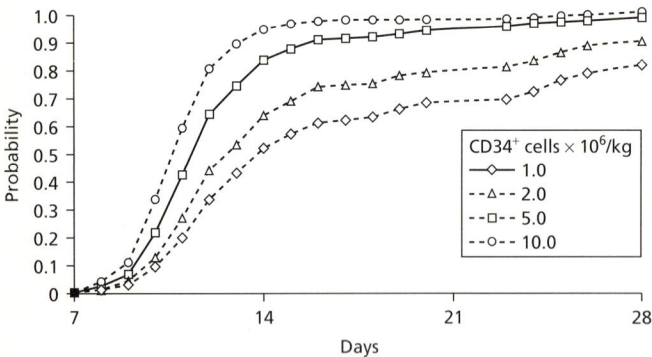

Fig. 45.1 This figure demonstrates the achievement of platelet recovery to >50,000/μL post-transplant on the Y axis and days post-transplant on the X axis as a function of the number of CD34+ cells infused. Note that the median days to platelet recovery does not change but that the frequency of patients with prolonged time to recovery decreases markedly as doses exceed 5×10^6 CD34 cells/kg infused. Adapted with permission from Glaspy et al. [92].

of CD34+ cells harvested during the 1st h of collection was similar to that collected during the last 2 h while the CD34+ cell content collected during subsequent days was not affected [80]. This demonstrates that large volume leukapheresis can allow collection of more CD34 cells per session than smaller volumes. Another study examining the kinetics of large volume leukapheresis showed that CD34+ cell recruitment from the bone marrow to the peripheral blood starts in the second half hour of the collection and remains steady during the next 4 h [81]. However, other groups have not shown an advantage for using larger pheresis volumes to collect PBPCs. In one randomized trial comparing 7-L and 10-L pheresis volumes, the use of a 10-L volume did not decrease the number of leukapheresis required to collect $\geq 2 \times 10^6$ CD34+ cells/kg [82]. Another group compared an 8-L to a 12-L volume after cyclophosphamide (CY) and etoposide mobilization followed by G-CSF. The median number of CD34+ cells collected per leukapheresis did not differ between the two volumes and the larger volume increased the time on the pheresis machine by 1 h [83]. Most reports have demonstrated a correlation between total CD34+ cell yield and the blood volume processed, resulting in varied approaches among institutions that are frequently based on practical issues such as scheduling and cost.

Identifying the optimal cell yield

Several groups have attempted to determine a minimum threshold CD34+ cell dose necessary for rapid and sustained engraftment [78,84–86]. These groups have identified thresholds ranging from 1×10^6 to 3×10^6 CD34+ cells/kg body weight. Other investigators have suggested an optimal CD34+ cell dose of ≥5 to ≥8 × 10^6 CD34+ cells/kg, with which neutrophil and platelet recovery is accelerated, the demand for other supportive measures (antibiotics, transfusion) is decreased and therapy schedule is more likely to be preserved [16,87–91]. One report highlighted the fact that although a higher dose of CD34+ cells is unlikely to shorten the median duration of neutropenia or thrombocytopenia in a broad patient population, it will reduce the number of "outlier" patients with prolonged times to engraftment requiring prolonged transfusion support (Fig. 45.1) [92]. While some investigators suggest that more primitive CD34+ cell subsets such as CD34+CD33− or CD34+CD38− cells are better predictors of durable engraftment, most centers continue to rely on total CD34+ cell numbers as the most reliable indicator of an adequate PBPC population [19,24,89].

Cytokine-induced mobilization

G-CSF and GM-CSF have been used alone to mobilize PBPCs from cancer patients at doses from 3 to 24 μg/kg/day by subcutaneous injection. Most studies evaluating single agent cytokines report increases in circulating CD34+ cells or in peak levels of CD34+ cells or CFU-GMs compared to that found in the unmobilized, steady state [11,12,63–74]. A number of studies have compared the use of G-CSF and GM-CSF for mobilization both alone and in conjunction with chemotherapy [25,74,93–95]. While most have found that G-CSF provides a higher yield of PBPC, both growth factors reliably mobilize cells into the circulation with minimal toxicity (Table 45.1 [25,74,93,95]). A dose–response to G-CSF, with higher doses resulting in increased CD34+ peripheral cells, has been demonstrated. One group compared G-CSF doses of 5 and 10 μg/kg/day [68] while other groups compared G-CSF doses of 10 or 24 μg/kg/day [96]. In these studies, the higher dose resulted in superior collections of CD34+ cells (Table 45.2 [68,73,95–103]). Higher doses of GM-CSF also have been shown to improve yield of CD34+ cells [73]. When given after myelosuppressive chemotherapy, G-CSF dose escalation has produced inconsistent results (Table 45.2). One group compared G-CSF doses of 8 and 16 μg/kg following chemotherapy, with the higher dose resulting in a 1.7-fold increase in CD34+ cell yield [97]. Another group compared G-CSF doses of 5 and 10 μg/kg after chemotherapy and found no difference in CD34+ cell numbers [98]. Dosing schedule of G-CSF has been evaluated comparing once a day to twice a day doses of G-CSF in normal donors. Administering G-CSF 5 μg/kg twice daily rather than 10 μg/kg once daily resulted in higher CD34+ cell yield and a fewer number of pheresis procedures [104]. Similar findings have been reported by Ponisch et al. [105] and Quittet et al. [106]. Pegylated G-CSF (Ro 25–8315) has been evaluated for mobilization when administered in conjunction with chemotherapy. This compound is a long-acting

Table 45.1 Comparison of mobilization with granulocyte colony-stimulating factor (G-CSF) vs. granulocyte macrophage colony-stimulating factor (GM-CSF).

No. of patients	Comparison	Observation	Ref.
262	G-CSF + chemo vs. GM-CSF + chemo	G-CSF group: 1.7-fold increase in CD34+ cell yield	93
29	G-CSF at 6 μg/kg vs. GM-CSF at 8 or 16 μg/kg	G-CSF group: 5.4-fold higher CD34+ cell yield	25
44		No difference in G-CSF vs. GM-CSF induced CD34+ cell yield	74
156	G-CSF + chemo vs. GM-CSF + chemo	G-CSF group: 3.5-fold increase in CD34+ cell yield	95

chemo, chemotherapy.

Table 45.2 Comparisons of cytokine doses and combinations for mobilization.

No. of patients	Comparison	Observation	Ref.
Cytokine doses			
95	G-CSF: 5 µg/kg/day vs. 10 µg/kg/day	G-CSF 10 µg/kg qd group: fourfold increase in CD34$^+$ cell yield	68
75	G-CSF: 10 µg/kg/day vs. 6 µg/kg bid	G-CSF 6 µg/kg bid group: 1.8-fold increase in CD34$^+$ cell yield	96
50	Chemo + G-CSF: 8 µg/kg vs. 16 µg/kg	G-CSF 16 µg/kg group: 1.7-fold increase in CD34$^+$ cell yield	97
144	No growth factor vs. GM-CSF: 125 µg/m^2/day vs. 250 µg/m^2/day	GM-CSF 125 µg/m^2/day and 250 µg/m^2/day groups: five and 12-fold increase in PBSCs compared to no growth factor	73
128	Chemo + G-CSF: 5 µg/kg vs. 10 µg/kg G-CSF	No benefit from higher dose G-CSF	98
Cytokine combinations			
30	Chemo + G-CSF vs. chemo + GM-CSF followed by G-CSF	No difference in CD34$^+$ cell yield	99
35	Chemo + G-CSF vs. chemo + GM-CSF vs. GM-CSF followed by G-CSF	No difference in CD34$^+$ cell yield	100
156	Chemo + G-CSF vs. chemo + GM-CSF followed by G-CSF	No difference in CD34$^+$ cell yield (but both regimens yielded 3.5-fold more CD34$^+$ cells than chemo + GM-CSF)	95
40	G-CSF or GM-CSF vs. GM-CSF followed by G-CSF	GM-CSF f/b G-CSF group: 2.3-fold increased yield of CD34$^+$ cells	101
48	GM-CSF vs. GM-CSF + G-CSF vs. GM-CSF followed by G-CSF	GM-CSF f/b G-CSF group: increased yield of CD34$^+$ cells compared to GM-CSF alone or concurrent GM-CSF + G-CSF	102
174	G-CSF vs. GM-CSF followed by G-CSF (in allogeneic donors)	GM-CSF f/b G-CSF group: 1.4-fold increase in CD34$^+$ cell yield no difference in OS, DFS, relapse or GVHD	103

bid, twice daily; chemo, chemotherapy; DFS, disease-free survival; f/b, followed by; G-CSF, granulocyte colony-stimulating factor; GM-CSF, granulocyte macrophage colony-stimulating factor; OS, overall survival; PBSCs, peripheral blood stem cells; qd, every day.

polyethylene glycol conjugate of recombinant human G-CSF that is cleared more slowly and has a much longer half-life. A single dose of 100 µg/kg/week of pegylated G-CSF seems equivalent to conventional G-CSF 10 µg/kg/day for 7 days [107]. Other cytokines capable of PBPC mobilization as a single agent include IL-12, IL-3 and SCF [108–110], but none to date offers a compelling advantage over G-CSF or GM-CSF.

The timing of leukapheresis initiation also has been examined. One study of normal donors receiving G-CSF at 10 µg/kg/day showed that CD34$^+$ cell yield was threefold higher when pheresis was started at day 5 vs. day 6 [25,68,111]. On the day of pheresis, the optimal time at which CD34$^+$ cell yield was maximized was found to be 3–7 h after G-CSF administration [111].

Combination cytokine-induced mobilization

Cytokine combination regimens continue to be investigated as avenues through which mobilization of PBPCs might be improved. These cytokine combinations have been used both with and without antecedent chemotherapy. Concurrent and sequential use of G-CSF and GM-CSF has been investigated (Table 45.2). While some trials have found no significant difference in progenitor cell yields following G-CSF alone compared to sequential GM-CSF and G-CSF [95,99,100], others have found a significant increase in yields in both the autologous [101,102] and the allogeneic setting [103]. However, the additional yield of PBPCs resulting from such approaches does not seem warranted, given the added expense and fairly small improvement in PBPC yield compared to the yield from G-CSF alone.

SCF is a cytokine that acts on primitive multilineage hematopoietic progenitor cells. In a randomized controlled phase III trial of patients with high-risk breast cancer, steady-state mobilization with G-CSF alone was compared to G-CSF plus SCF. The administration of G-CSF plus SCF resulted in a significant reduction in the number of leukapheresis required to achieve the desired CD34$^+$ cell yield [112]. In a phase II study in heavily pretreated lymphoma patients, patients receiving G-CSF plus SCF had a higher median CD34$^+$ cell collection than patients receiving G-CSF alone [113]. Because the improvement in PBSC yield following the addition of SCF to G-CSF was relatively modest, and the use of SCF increased the risk of histamine related side-effects, it is unlikely that this drug will become widely available for use in the USA despite its potential utility in hard-to-mobilize patients.

IL-3 has been used alone and in combination with G-CSF or GM-CSF with or without mobilization chemotherapy [114–116]. In these studies, both cytokines acted synergistically with IL-3 to mobilize PBPCs. When given sequentially after mobilization chemotherapy in heavily pretreated patients, the G-CSF/IL-3 combination resulted in an adequate CD34$^+$ cell yield for autologous stem cell support [117], but the additional IL-3-associated toxicity including headache, fever and malaise, has prevented its widespread availability for this purpose. A synthetic fusion molecule combining IL-3 and G-CSF has been developed but was found inferior when compared to G-CSF alone for mobilization [118]. IL-11, a cytokine used to stimulate platelet generation, has been studied as a mobilization agent in conjunction with chemotherapy and G-CSF. The pheresis products mobilized with this regimen contained adequate numbers of CD34$^+$ cells and reconstituted the bone marrow following myeloablative therapy [119], but the value of this combination over G-CSF alone has not been demonstrated clearly.

Because IL-2 stimulates cellular immunity and T-cell progenitors, it has the potential to promote antitumor immunity within an autograft.

Table 45.3 Comparison of cytokine alone vs. cytokine + chemotherapy.

No. of patients	Comparison	Observation	Ref.
85	G-CSF alone vs. chemo + G-CSF	Chemo + G-CSF group: decreased no. of phereses to achieve targeted CD34$^+$ cell yield	125
47	G-CSF alone vs. chemo + G-CSF	Chemo + G-CSF group: 2.9-fold increase in CD34$^+$ cell yield	126
96	GM-CSF followed by G-CSF vs. chemo + G-CSF	Chemo + G-CSF: 2.7-fold increase in CD34$^+$ cell yield	127
21	CSF alone vs. chemo alone vs. chemo + GM-CSF	G-CSF alone and chemo + GM-CSF groups: fourfold increase in CD34$^+$ cell yield compared to chemo alone group	94
152	G-CSF alone vs. standard chemo + G-CSF vs. intensive chemo (di-CEP) + G-CSF	Standard chemo + G-CSF group: 2.1-fold increase in CD34$^+$ cell yield. Intensive chemo + G-CSF group: 5.5-fold increase in CD34$^+$ cell yield	128

chemo, chemotherapy; di-CEP, di-cyclophosphamide, etoposide and cisplatin; G-CSF, granulocyte colony-stimulating factor; GM-CSF, granulocyte macrophage colony-stimulating factor.

These characteristics make IL-2 an attractive candidate for costimulation of immunologic effector cells in concert with other cytokines, such as G-CSF, that are more effective for progenitor cell mobilization. Although IL-2 may enhance the number and function of antitumor effector cells, it impairs the mobilization of the CD34$^+$ cells [120,121]. Even so, as long as the CD34$^+$ dose was adequate, IL-2 mobilized progenitor cells were able to repopulate the bone marrow after myeloablative chemotherapy [122].

Combination chemotherapy and cytokine-induced mobilization

Myelosuppressive therapy stimulates stem cell and progenitor cell proliferation. This results in a larger pool of progenitors than exists at baseline steady state. Some of these progenitors will egress into the peripheral blood. Early mouse studies demonstrated that combination therapy with CY plus G-CSF resulted in an increased egress of stem cells and progenitor cells from the bone marrow compared to G-CSF alone and CY alone [123]. Human studies have shown that patients mobilized with CY plus G-CSF had more rapid platelet engraftment following their autograft than patients mobilized with CY alone, suggesting that the combination regimen resulted in increased numbers of mobilized PBPCs (Table 45.3) [94,125–129]. In a randomized trial comparing mobilization with G-CSF alone with CY plus G-CSF in patients with refractory lymphoma, the addition of CY resulted in a threefold increase in CD34$^+$ cell yield, but this did not translate into a shorter time to engraftment [126]. Another study comparing CD34$^+$ cell yield within the same patient found that 21 out of 22 patients who did not mobilize an adequate CD34$^+$ cell dose following G-CSF alone were successfully mobilized with high-dose CY plus G-CSF [130]. A randomized, cross-over trial compared CY plus G-CSF with GM-CSF plus G-CSF within the same patients. The CY-containing regimen resulted in a 2.7-fold increase in CD34$^+$ PBPCs over that resulting from the cytokines alone [127]. Another randomized, phase III trial compared regimens of (i) G-CSF, (ii) GM-CSF and (iii) sequential GM-CSF then G-CSF following myelosuppressive chemotherapy. Compared to patients receiving GM-CSF alone, patients receiving G-CSF alone yielded more CD34$^+$ cells/kg, had fewer aphereses and had a faster time to neutrophil recovery. There were no significant differences between groups receiving G-CSF alone and sequential GM-CSF followed by G-CSF [95]. These studies illustrate the improved potency of regimens containing both myelosuppressive chemotherapy and hematopoietic growth factors. At the same time, these increased PBPC yields have been accompanied by greater toxicity as a result of the concurrent administration of chemotherapy compared to the use of cytokines alone.

The optimal doses of G-CSF have been investigated in a number of studies. In a randomized controlled trial, patients received either 8 or 16 mg/kg/day G-CSF following standard mobilization chemotherapy. With the higher dose of G-CSF, the CD34$^+$ PBPC yield was significantly increased over threefold and the time to WBC engraftment was significantly decreased [97]. While these results demonstrate a dose–response to G-CSF following mobilization chemotherapy, other trials have failed to demonstrate a difference between 5 and 10 mg/kg when used in conjunction with moderately intensive doses of CY [98]. Efforts have been made to determine an optimal CY mobilization dose as well. Intermediate dose CY, 4 g/m^2, has been used with G-CSF to collect PBPCs. Several studies have shown that a higher dose, 7 g/m^2, results in higher PBPC yield but also leads to increased toxicity without a significant reduction in time to engraftment [94]. However, in a more recent historical cohort study, multiple myeloma patients received either 4 or 7 g/m^2 CY and the higher dose did not result in a higher yield of CD34$^+$ PBPCs but increased the patients' risk of febrile neutropenia [131]. Even with higher doses, some patients will not mobilize an adequate CD34$^+$ cell product with CY. Often these patients are quite heavily pretreated. In patients who failed mobilization with CY, etoposide [132,133] and high-dose cytarabine [134] have been used with good results.

Because no single mobilization chemotherapy regimen is clearly superior to the others, another mobilization approach is to incorporate PBPC mobilization into a cycle of disease specific chemotherapy. In patients with hematologic malignancies, regimens containing ifosfamide, carboplatin and etoposide (ICE, mini-ICE) and the etoposide, cytosine arabinoside, cisplatin and prednisone regimen have been used successfully for concurrent tumor cytoreduction and mobilization chemotherapy [135–141]. Taxane-based regimens have been used similarly in patients with breast cancer with good mobilization results [142–148]. In choosing a mobilization chemotherapy regimen that is disease specific and cytoreductive, it is important to avoid stem cell toxic agents, such as melphalan and carmustine, as both the quantity and quality of the progenitor cells will be impaired [149,150].

Factors affecting yield of PBPC mobilization

It is important to note that most patients mobilize adequate numbers of CD34$^+$ cells using a regimen of G-CSF alone. Although the addition of chemotherapy improves CD34$^+$ yield, this comes at the expense of increased short-term toxicity and, possibly, the increased risk of secondary myelodysplastic syndrome [151]. Even with chemotherapy–growth factor combination regimens, it may be difficult to achieve an adequate CD34$^+$ cell yield in some patients. Often, cancer patients undergoing

Table 45.4 Guidelines for the "hard to mobilize" patient.

1 Increase chemotherapy dose: 4–7 g/m² CY appears more effective than 2–4 g/m²
2 Increase growth factor dose (up to 24 μg/kg G-CSF) and use bid schedule
3 Consider bone marrow harvest
4 Prolong duration between last chemotherapy and planned collection
5 Use investigational agents such as SCF, IL-11, GRO-β, Flt3 ligand

bid, twice daily; CY, cyclophosphamide; G-CSF, granulocyte colony-stimulating factor; IL, interleukin; SCF, stem cell factor.

mobilization therapy for PBPC harvest to support high-dose chemotherapy have been treated extensively with chemotherapeutic agents and may have malignancy involving their bone marrow. These factors impair the ability to mobilize PBPCs. Even in normal, previously untreated donors, mobilization with G-CSF results in a wide variability of CD34+ cell doses with 5–15% of donors mobilizing a suboptimal yield of less than $2.5–5 \times 10^6$ CD34+ cells/kg [152]. This variability makes predicting how well any one patient will mobilize quite difficult. However, several studies have identified predictors of poor PBPC yield. The amount of myelosuppressive therapy (both chemotherapy and radiation therapy) received prior to mobilization is the most important factor affecting CD34+ yield [16,153–155]. In particular, stem cell toxic agents including nitrogen mustard, procarbazine, melphalan, carmustine and >7.5 g CY, were strongly associated with poor mobilization [8,150,155]. The number of chemotherapeutic regimens, >6 [156] and ≥11 [155], and duration of exposure to chemotherapy (>12 months) [153] also predict poor mobilization. Timing of most recent cytotoxic drug administration relative to mobilization and stem cell collection may also influence mobilization. Short time interval since last chemotherapy, <6 months [157] and <65 days [158], was found to be predictive of poor mobilization. Finally, previous radiation, hypocellular marrow and refractory disease have been associated with poor mobilization [159].

Strategies to manage patients who do not mobilize well include dose escalation of cytokines, bone marrow harvesting and remobilization with a more intensive or novel regimen (Table 45.4) [160]. One center has found that infusing a suboptimal PBPC product in combination with harvested bone marrow can achieve short and long-term engraftment [161]. In some patients with inadequate CD34+ cell yield following G-CSF mobilization, a second mobilization using G-CSF plus SCF can mobilize enough additional CD34+ cells to allow myeloablative therapy and autologous transplant [162,163]. Others have used high-dose G-CSF at 16 and 32 μg/kg/day to successfully mobilize patients previously failing standard myelosuppressive chemotherapy plus G-CSF mobilization [164–166]. In fact, one study found G-CSF alone superior to chemotherapy plus G-CSF for second mobilization in patients failing their first mobilization regimen [167].

Techniques to prospectively identify poor mobilizers have been investigated. One group found the peripheral blood CD34+ and CFU-GM response to a single dose of 12 μg/kg G-CSF predictive of PBPC mobilization [168]. Other groups have found that steady-state peripheral blood CD34+ cells predicted response to G-CSF mobilization [91,169,170]. Identifying these poor mobilizers prospectively would assist clinicians in choosing an appropriate mobilization regimen.

Tumor contamination

Although PBPC products are less frequently contaminated with tumor cells than bone marrow, tumor cells have been detected in patients with breast cancer, small-cell lung cancer, lymphoma, multiple myeloma and leukemia [126,171–174]. In fact, it has been shown that PBPC mobilization can also cause breast cancer and small-cell lung cancer cell recruitment into the peripheral blood [171]. In one study, all of the 16 multiple myeloma patients mobilized tumor cells with CD34+ cells at the time of PBPC harvest [130]. In one study that compared outcomes of patients with non-Hodgkin's lymphoma receiving high-dose therapy followed by autologous transplantation, patients receiving tumor-free autografts had a significantly improved survival over those receiving minimally contaminated autografts, demonstrating the importance of decontaminating the PBPC product [173]. One group attempted to predict tumor cell contamination in the mobilized product by examining preharvest peripheral blood and bone marrow. There was no association between the presence of tumor cells in the preharvest samples and the harvested PBPC product [175]. Comparing cytokine mobilization with G-CSF vs. SCF plus G-CSF did not impact on the incidence of tumor contamination in one series of breast cancer patients [176].

One strategy to reduce tumor contamination in mobilized PBPCs is to perform a positive CD34+ cell selection. This approach resulted in a 2–5 log decrease in malignant cells [171,177], but it can only be applied to CD34− malignancies. In patients with CML receiving autologous PBPCs, positive selection of CD34+ human leukocyte antigen (HLA)-DR− cells was associated with a superior cytogenetic response, suggesting successful purging of *BCR/ABL* expressing cells [178]. In multiple myeloma patients, both positively selected CD34+Thy-1+Lin− progenitor cells and B-cell lineage depleted PBPCs have been transplanted to support high-dose chemotherapy with elimination of detectable tumor contamination and good engraftment [174,179]. Although these techniques are promising, they require a larger mobilized PBPC product, as PBPCs are depleted in the selection process. In addition, the impact of these strategies on survival is still being evaluated.

Future directions

While the majority of patients receiving conventional mobilization regimens do produce adequate PBPC products, a significant, and not always predictable, portion of the population does not. Patients at risk for poor mobilization yields represent a challenging clinical scenario requiring improved mobilization strategies. Higher cytokine and marrow suppressive chemotherapy doses can produce improved CD34+ cell yields [64,68,97,126]; however, these higher yields do not always translate into a shorter time to engraftment. Cytokine combinations have also been used in heavily pretreated patients resulting in modestly increased CD34+ PBPC yield [113]. Clearly, innovative approaches are needed to address these patients.

Novel means of mobilizing PBPCs continue to be investigated (Tables 45.5 & 45.6 [3,31,45,46,54,107,112,118,119,180–2]). Manipulation of the adhesive interactions between hematopoietic progenitor cells and the bone marrow stroma has much promise. The expression of adhesion molecules on mobilized CD34+ cells by different growth factors is being investigated [183]. Pharmacological modification of the expression or functional state of adhesion receptors could improve PBPC collection. These interactions could be blocked using monoclonal antibodies or competitive inhibitors of receptor-ligand binding. Anti-integrin monoclonal antibodies already have been shown to increase circulating hematopoietic progenitor cells in nonhuman primates [33,180] and in mice [31]. In a mouse model, the addition of an anti-VCAM immunoglobulin to both G-CSF and CY plus G-CSF has been shown to increase the cumulative number of CFUs mobilized into the peripheral blood [181]. Manipulation of the chemokine environment also represents an opportunity for improving mobilization. A truncated GROβ chemokine agonist has been shown to induce a rapid mobilization of hematopoietic stem cells in mice

Table 45.5 Preclinical mobilization studies.

Preclinical compound	System	Observation	Ref.
GRO-β (SB-251353)	Mice/primates	Fivefold increase in CFU and CD34$^+$ cells relative to G-CSF alone	54
Flt3 ligand	Mice/primates	Marked increase in CFU or CD34$^+$ cells and synergy with G-CSF	45,46
Antibodies to LFA-1/Mac integrins	Mice	2.7-fold increase in cobblestone and CFU/mL	31
Antibodies to VLA-4	Mice	2–4-fold increase in CFU/mL	3,181,182
IL-8	Mice/primates	Increase in CFU/mL	42,43
IL-17	Mice	Increase in CFU/mL	183

CFU, colony-forming unit; G-CSF, granulocyte colony-stimulating factor; IL, interleukin.

Table 45.6 Clinical mobilization studies with investigational compounds.

Compound	No. of patients	Observation	Ref.
Pegylated G-CSF (Ro 25–8315)	36	Pegylated G-CSF 100 µg/kg × 1 dose: equivalent to G-CSF 10 µg/kg qd × 7 doses	107
G-CSF vs. G-CSF + IL-3 fusion protein (leridistim)	267	G-CSF + IL-3 fusion protein: increased toxicity but no increase in PBPC yield	118
IL-11 + G-CSF + ICE chemo	8 children	Good yield with combination but no comparison available	119
G-CSF + SCF vs. G-CSF alone	203	G-CSF + SCF group: 63% achieved target of 5 × 10^6 CD34$^+$ cells/kg G-CSF alone group: 47% achieved target of 5 × 10^6 CD34$^+$ cells/kg	112

G-CSF, granulocyte colony-stimulating factor; ICE; ifosfamide, carboplatin and etoposide regimen; IL, interleukin; PBPC, peripheral blood progenitor cell; SCF, stem cell factor; qd, every day.

Table 45.7 Recommendations for "standard" mobilization regimens

Regimen	Advantages	Disadvantages
G-CSF: 10–24 µg/kg/day by bid schedule	Adequate yield in most patients Low toxicity Reliable scheduling Low risk of MDS Appropriate for use in allogeneic patients	Lower yield than G-CSF + chemo
GM-CSF followed by G-CSF	Higher CD34$^+$ cell yield than G-CSF alone Appropriate to consider for use in allogeneic patients	More expensive than G-CSF alone No proven benefit over G-CSF alone in allogeneic or autologous patients
Chemotherapy + G-CSF: CY 2–4 g/m^2 CY ± VP16 Paclitaxel Standard chemotherapy regimen	Higher CD34$^+$ cell yield than cytokine alone Enhanced cytoreduction pretransplant	Greater toxicity Increased risk of MDS/AML post transplant Uncertain scheduling Inappropriate for allogeneic patients

AML, acute myeloid leukemia; bid, twice daily; chemo, chemotherapy; CY, cyclophosphamide; G-CSF, granulocyte colony-stimulating factor; GM-CSF, granulocyte macrophage colony-stimulating factor; MDS, myelodysplastic syndrome; VP16, etoposide.

and primates [54], as has IL-8 [42]. Preclinical studies with compounds, such as Flt3 ligand and IL-8, also hold promise but require additional study prior to clinical use [42–46], as do investigational compounds such as pegylated G-CSF, SCF, leridistim (an IL-3 fusion protein), IL-8 and IL-17 [107,112,118,119,182]. Whether these newer cytokines or efforts to manipulate the progenitor cell–bone marrow stroma interactions can provide a synergistic approach to PBPC mobilization remains to be determined.

Summary

The use of high-dose therapy and autologous PBPC-supported transplantation has become an essential component of contemporary therapy for hematologic malignancies. The majority of patients will undergo successful mobilization and collection of sufficient PBPC with standard approaches to permit safe and effective autologous transplant procedures (Table 45.7). Despite these advances in PBPC acquisition, a significant minority of patients will have inadequate yields of PBPC and will continue to be the focus of research efforts designed to understand better the mechanisms of PBPC mobilization and to identify improved methods for their collection and administration.

References

1 Hartmann O, Le Corroller AG, Blaise D et al. Peripheral blood stem cell and bone marrow transplantation for solid tumors and lymphomas; hematologic recovery and costs. A randomized, controlled trial. *Ann Intern Med* 1997; **126**: 600–7.

2 Siena S, Schiavo R, Pedrazzoli P, Carlo-Stella C. Therapeutic relevance of CD34+ cell dose in blood cell transplantation for cancer therapy. *J Clin Oncol* 2000; **18**: 1360–77.

3 To LB, Haylock DN, Simmons PJ, Juttner CA. The biology and clinical uses of blood stem cells. *Blood* 1997; **89**: 2233–58.

4 Weissman IL, Anderson DJ, Gage F. Stem and progenitor cells: origins, phenotypes, lineage commitments, and transdifferentiations. *Ann Rev Cell Dev Biol* 2001; **17**: 387–403.

5 Abrams RA, Glaubiger D, Appelbaum FR et al. Result of attempted hematopoietic reconstitution using isologous, peripheral blood mononuclear cells: a case report. *Blood* 1980; **56**: 516–20.

6 Kessigner A, Armitage JO, Landmark JD et al. Reconstitution of human hematopoietic function with autologous cryopreserved circulating stem cells. *Exp Hematol* 1986; **14**: 192–6.

7 Körbling M, Dörken B, Ho AD et al. Autologous transplantation of blood-derived hemopoietic stem cells after myeloablative therapy in a patient with Burkitt's lymphoma. *Blood* 1986; **67**: 529–32.

8 Juttner CA, To LB, Haylock DN et al. Circulating autologous stem cells collected in very early remission from acute non-lymphoblastic leukaemia produce prompt but incomplete haemopoietic reconstitution after high dose melphalan or supralethal chemoradiotherapy. *Br J Haematol* 1985; **61**: 739–45.

9 To LB, Dyson PG, Juttner CA. Cell-dose effect in circulating stem-cell autografting. *Lancet* 1986; **2**: 404–5.

10 Abrams RA, McCormack K, Bowles C, Deisseroth AB. Cyclophosphamide treatment expands the circulating hematopoietic stem cell pool in dogs. *J Clin Invest* 1981; **67**: 1392–9.

11 Richman CM, Weiner RS, Yankee RA. Increase in circulating stem cells following chemotherapy in man. *Blood* 1976; **47**: 1031–9.

12 Socinski MA, Cannistra SA, Elias A, Antman KH, Schnipper L, Griffin JD. Granulocyte-macrophage colony stimulating factor expands the circulating haemapoietic progenitor cells compartment in man. *Lancet* 1988; **1**(28): 1194–8.

13 Gianni AM, Siena S, Bregni M et al. Granulocyte-macrophage colony-stimulating factor to harvest circulating haemopoietic stem cells for autotransplantation. *Lancet* 1989; **2**: 580–5.

14 Bender JG, Williams SF, Myers S et al. Characterization of chemotherapy mobilized peripheral blood progenitor cells for use in autologous stem cell transplantation. *Bone Marrow Transplant* 1992; **10**: 281–5.

15 Vogel W, Kunert C, Blumenstengel K, Fricke HG, Kath R, Sayer HG. Correlation between granuloycte/macrophage-colony-forming units and CD34+ cells in apheresis products from patients treated with different chemotherapy regimens and granuloycte-colony-stimulating factor to mobilize peripheral blood progenitor cells. *J Cancer Res Clin Oncol* 1998; **124**: 341–5.

16 Bensinger WI, Appelbaum FR, Rowley S et al. Factors that influence collection and engraftment of autologous peripheral blood stem cells. *J Clin Oncol* 1995; **13**: 2547–55.

17 Roscoe RA, Rybka WB, Winkelstein A, Houston AM, Kiss JE. Enumeration of CD34+ hematopoietic stem cells for reconstitution following myeloablative therapy. *Cytometry* 1994; **16**: 74–9.

18 Bender JG, Lum L, Unverzagt KL et al. Correlation of colony-forming cells, long-term culture initiating cells and CD34+ cells in apheresis products from patients mobilized for peripheral blood progenitors with different regimens. *Bone Marrow Transplant* 1994; **13**: 479–85.

19 Siena S, Bregni M, Brando B et al. Flow cytometry for clinical estimation of circulating hematopoietic progenitors for autologous transplantation in cancer patients. *Blood* 1991; **77**: 400–9.

20 To LB, Haylock DN, Dowse T et al. A comparative study of the phenotype and proliferative capacity of peripheral blood (PB) CD34+ cells mobilized by four different protocols and those of steady-phase PB and bone marrow CD34+ cells. *Blood* 1994; **84**: 2930–9.

21 Sutherland DR, Anderson L, Keeney M et al. The ISHAGE guidelines for CD34+ cell determination by flow cytometry. *J Hematother* 1996; **5**: 213–26.

22 Brecher ME, Sims L, Schmitz J, Shea T, Bentley SA. North American multicenter study on flow cytometric enumeration of CD34+ hematopoietic stem cells. *J Hematother* 1996; **5**: 277–36.

23 Ross A, Ruud E, Sharp JG. Report of the Tumor Evaluation Committee workshops at ISHAGE 2001. *Cytotherapy* 2002; **4**: 79–81.

24 Pecora AL, Preti RA, Gleim GW et al. CD34+CD33− cells influence days to engraftment and transfusion requirements in autologous blood stem-cell recipients. *J Clin Oncol* 1998; **16**: 2093–104.

25 Peters WP, Rosner G, Ross M et al. Comparative effects of granuloycte-macrophage colony-stimulating factor (GM-CSF) and granuloycte colony-stimulating factor (G-CSF) on priming peripheral blood progenitor cells for use with autologous bone marrow after high-dose chemotherapy. *Blood* 1993; **81**: 1709–19.

26 deBoer F, Drager AM, Van Haperen MJ et al. The phenotypic profile of CD34-positive peripheral blood stem cells in different mobilization regimens. *Br J Haematol* 2000; **111**: 1138–44.

27 Brasel K, McKenna HJ, Morrissey PJ et al. Hematologic effects of Flt3 ligand *in vivo* in mice. *Blood* 1996; **88**: 2004–12.

28 Link DC. Mechanisms of granuloycte colony-stimulating factor-induced hematopoietic progenitor-cell mobilization. *Semin Hematol* 2000; **37**: 25–32.

29 Teixido J, Hemler ME, Greenberger JS, Anklesaria P. Role of β_1 and β_2 integrins in the adhesion of human CD34^{hi} stem cells to bone marrow stroma. *J Clin Invest* 1992; **90**: 358–67.

30 Mohle R, Murea S, Kirsch M, Haas R. Differential expression of L-selectin, VLA-4, and LFA-1 on CD34+ progenitor cells from bone marrow and peripheral blood during G-CSF-enhanced recovery. *Exp Hematol* 1995; **23**: 1535–42.

31 Velders GA, Pruijt JF, Verzaal P et al. Enhancement of G-CSF-induced stem cell mobilization by antibodies against the β_2 integrins LFA-1 and Mac-1. *Blood* 2002; **100**: 327–33.

32 Papayannopoulou T, Craddock C, Nakamoto B, Priestley GV, Wolf NS. The VLA4/VCAM-1 adhesion pathway defines contrasting mechanisms of lodgement of transplanted murine hemopoietic progenitors between bone marrow and spleen. *Proc Natl Acad Sci U S A* 1995; **92**: 9647–51.

33 Papayannopoulou T, Nakamoto B. Peripheralization of hemopoietic progenitors in primates treated with anti-VLA4 integrin. *Proc Natl Acad Sci U S A* 1993; **90**: 9374–8.

34 Simmons PJ, Masinovsky B, Longenecker BM et al. Vascular cell adhesion molecule-1 expressed by bone marrow stromal cells mediates the binding of hematopoietic progenitor cells. *Blood* 1992; **80**: 388–95.

35 Gazitt Y. Recent developments in the regulation of peripheral blood stem cell mobilization and engraftment by cytokines, chemokines, and adhesion molecules. *J Hematother Stem Cell Res* 2001; **10**: 229–36.

36 Levesque JP, Takamatsu Y, Nilsson SK, Haylock DN, Simmons PJ. Vascular cell adhesion molecule-1 (CD106) is cleaved by neutrophil proteases in the bone marrow following hematopoietic progenitor cell mobilization by granulocyte colony-stimulating factor. *Blood* 2001; **98**: 1289–97.

37 Wognum AW, de Jong MO, Wagemaker G. Differential expression of receptors for hemapoietic growth factors on subsets of CD34+ hemapoietic cells. *Leuk Lymphoma* 1996; **24**: 11–25.

38 Liu F, Poursine-Laurent J, Link DC. Expression of the G-CSF receptor on hematopoietic progenitor cells is not required for their mobilization by G-CSF. *Blood* 2000; **95**: 3025–31.

39 Brugger W, Bross K, Frisch J et al. Mobilization of peripheral blood progenitor cells by sequential administration of interleukin-3 and granuloycte-macrophage colony-stimulating factor following polychemotherapy with etoposide, ifosfamide, and cisplatin. *Blood* 1992; **79**: 1193–200.

40 Haas R, Ehrhardt R, Witt B et al. Autografting with peripheral blood stem cells mobilized by sequential interleukin-3/granuloycte-macrophage colony-stimulation factor following high-dose chemotherapy in non-Hodgkin's lymphoma. *Bone Marrow Transplant* 1993; **12**: 643–9.

41 Jacobsen SE, Okkenhaug C, Myklebust J et al. The FLT3 ligand potently and directly stimulates the

41 growth and expansion of primitive murine bone marrow progenitor cells in vitro: synergistic interactions with interleukin (IL) 11, IL-12, and other hematopoietic growth factors. *J Exp Med* 1995; **181**: 1357–63.

42 Laterveer L, Lindley IJ, Heemskerk DP et al. Rapid mobilization of hematopoietic progenitor cells in rhesus monkeys by a single intravenous injection of interleukin-8. *Blood* 1996; **897**: 781–8.

43 Laterveer L, Lindley IJ, Hamilton MS, Willemze R, Fibbe WE. Interleukin-8 induces rapid mobilization of hematopoietic stem cells with radioprotective capacity and long-term myelolymphoid repopulating ability. *Blood* 1995; **85**: 2269–75.

44 De Revel T, Appelbaum FR, Storb R et al. Effects of granulocyte colony-stimulating factor and stem cell factor, alone and in combination, on the mobilization of peripheral blood cells that engraft lethally irradiated dogs. *Blood* 1994; **83**: 3795–801.

45 Molineux G, McCrea C, Yan XQ et al. Flt-3 ligand synergizes with granuloycte colony-stimulating factor to increase neutrophil numbers and to mobilize peripheral blood stem cells with long-term repopulating potential. *Blood* 1997; **89**: 3998–4004.

46 Brasel K, McKenna HJ, Charrier K, Morrissey PJ, Williams DE, Lyman SD. Flt3 ligand synergizes with granuloycte-macrophage colony-stimulating factor or granuloycte colony-stimulating factor to mobilize hematopoietic progenitor cells into the peripheral blood of mice. *Blood* 1997; **90**: 3781–8.

47 Kovach NL, Lin N, Yednock T et al. Stem cell factor modulates avidity of ∝4β1 and ∝5β1 integrins expressed on hematopoietic cell lines. *Blood* 1995; **85**: 159–67.

48 Levesque J-P, Leavesley DI, Niutta S et al. Cytokines increase human hemopoietic cell adhesiveness by activation of very late antigen (VLA)-4 and VLA-5 integrins. *J Exp Med* 1995; **181**: 1805–15.

49 Möhle R, Bautz F, Rafii S et al. The chemokine receptor CXCR-4 is expressed on CD34+ hematopoietic progenitors and leukemia cells and mediates transendothelial migration induced by Stromal cell-derived factor-1. *Blood* 1998; **91**: 4523–30.

50 Fibbe WE, Pruijt JFY, van Kooyk Figdor CG, Opdenakker G, Willemze R. The role of metalloproteinase and adhesion molecules in interleukin-8-induced stem cell mobilization. *Semin Hematol* 2000; **37** (Suppl. 2): 19–24.

51 Pruijt JF, Fibbe WE, Laterveer L et al. Prevention of interleukin-8-induced mobilization of hematopoietic progenitor cells in rhesus monkeys by inhibitory antibodies against the metalloproteinase gelatinase B (MMP-9). *Proc Natl Acad Sci U S A* 1999; **96**: 10,893–68.

52 Pruijt JF, Verzaal P, van Os R et al. Neutrophils are indispensable for hematopoietic stem cell mobilization induced by interleukin-8 in mice. *Proc Natl Acad Sci U S A* 2002; **99**: 6228–33.

53 Carion A, Benboubker L, Herault O et al. Evaluation of marrow and blood levels of SDF-1 and MMP-9 during progenitor cell mobilization: correlation with mobilizing capacity. *Blood* 2001; **98**: 175a [Abstract].

54 King AG, Horowitz D, Dillon SB et al. Rapid mobilization of murine hematopoietic stem cells with enhanced engraftment properties and evaluation of hematopoietic progenitor cell mobilization in rhesus monkeys by a single injection of SB-251353, a specific truncated form of the human CXC chemokine GROβ. *Blood* 2001; **97**: 1534–42.

55 Brown RA, Adkins D, Khoury H et al. Long term follow-up of high-risk allogenic peripheral-blood stem-cell transplant recipients: graft-vs.-host disease and transplant-related mortality. *J Clin Oncol* 1999; **17**(3): 806–12.

56 Schmitz N, Beksac M, Hasenclever D et al. Transplantation of mobilized peripheral blood cells to HLA-identical siblings with standard-risk leukemia. *Blood* 2002; **100**: 761–7.

57 Guardiola P, Runde V, Bacigalupo A et al. Subcommittee for Myelodysplastic Syndromes of the Chronic Leukaemia Working Group of the European Blood and Marrow Transplantation Group. Retrospective comparison of bone marrow and granulocyte colony-stimulating factor-mobilized peripheral blood progenitor cells for allogeneic stem cell transplantation using HLA identical sibling donors in myelodysplastic syndromes. *Blood* 2002; **99**: 4370–8.

58 Bensinger WI, Martin PJ, Storer B et al. Transplantation of bone marrow as compared with peripheral-blood cells from HLA-identical relatives in patients with hematologic cancers. *N Engl J Med* 2001; **344**: 175–81.

59 Flowers ME, Parker PM, Johnston LJ et al. Comparison of chronic graft-versus-host disease after transplantation of peripheral blood stem cells versus bone marrow in allogeneic recipients: long-term follow-up of a randomized trial. *Blood* 2002; **100**: 415–9.

60 Korbling M, Huh YO, Durett A et al. Allogeneic blood stem cell transplantation: peripheralization and yield of donor-derived primitive hematopoietic progenitor cells (CD34+Thy-1^{dim}) and lymphoid subsets, and possible predictors of engraftment and graft-versus-host disease. *Blood* 1995; **86**: 2842–8.

61 Schmitz N, Dreger P, Suttorp M et al. Primary transplantation of allogeneic peripheral blood progenitor cells mobilized by filgrastim (granulocyte colony-stimulating factor). *Blood* 1995; **85**: 1666–72.

62 Korbling M, Anderlini P. Peripheral blood stem cell versus bone marrow allotransplantation: does the source of hematopoietic stem cells matter? *Blood* 2001; **98**: 2900–8.

63 Duhrsen U, Villeval JL, Boyd J, Kannourakis G, Morstyn G, Metcalf D. Effects of recombinant human G-CSF on hematopoietic progenitor cells in cancer patients. *Blood* 1998; **72**: 2074–81.

64 Sheridan WP, Begley CG, To LB et al. Phase II study of autologous filgrastim (G-CSF)-mobilized peripheral blood progenitor cells to restore haemopoiesis after high-dose chemotherapy for lymphoid malignancies. *Bone Marrow Transplant* 1994; **14**: 105–11.

65 Bensinger WI, Longin K, Appelbaum F et al. Peripheral blood stem cells collected after recombinant granuloycte colony stimulating factor (rhG-CSF): an analysis of factors correlating with the tempo of engraftment after transplantation. *Br J Haematol* 1994; **87**: 825–31.

66 Chao NJ, Schriber JR, Grimes K et al. Granulocyte colony-stimulating factor 'mobilized' peripheral blood progenitor cells accelerate granuloycte and platelet recovery after high-dose chemotherapy. *Blood* 1993; **81**: 2031–5.

67 Basser RL, To LB, Begley CG et al. Adjuvant treatment of women with high-risk breast cancer using multiple cycles of high-dose chemotherapy supported by filgrastim-mobilized peripheral blood progenitor cells. *Clin Cancer Res* 1995; **1**: 715–20.

68 Nademanee A, Sniecinski I, Schmidt GM et al. High dose therapy followed by autologous peripheral-blood stem cell transplantation for patients with Hodgkin's disease and non-Hodgkin's lymphoma using unprimed and granulocyte colony-stimulating factor-mobilized peripheral-blood stem cells. *J Clin Oncol* 1994; **12**: 2176–86.

69 Mahe B, Milpied N, Hermouet S et al. G-CSF alone mobilizes sufficient peripheral blood CD34+ cells for positive selection in newly diagnosed patients with myeloma and lymphoma. *Br J Haematol* 1996; **92**: 263–8.

70 Aglietta M, Piacibello W, Savavio F et al. Kinetics of human hemapoietic cells after in vivo administration of granulocyte-macrophage colony-stimulating factor. *J Clin Invest* 1989; **83**: 551–7.

71 Haas R, Ho AD, Bredthauer U et al. Successful autologous transplantation of blood stem cells mobilized with recombinant human granuloycte-macrophage colony-stimulating factor. *Ex Hematol* 1990; **18**: 94–8.

72 Villeval J, Dührsen U, Morstyn G, Metcalf D. Effect of recombinant human granuloycte-macrophage colony stimulating factor on progenitor cells in patients with advanced malignancies. *Br J Haematol* 1990; **74**: 36–44.

73 Bishop MR, Anderson JR, Jackson JD et al. High-dose therapy and peripheral blood progenitor cell transplantation: effects of recombinant human granuloycte-macrophage colony-stimulating factor on the autograft. *Blood* 1994; **83**: 610–6.

74 Bolwell BJ, Goormastic M, Yanssens T, Dannley R, Baucco P, Fishleder A. Comparison of G-CSF with GM-CSF for mobilizing peripheral blood progenitor cells and for enhancing marrow recovery after autologous bone marrow transplant. *Bone Marrow Transplant* 1994; **14**: 913–8.

75 Pettengell R, Morgenstern GR, Woll PJ et al. Peripheral blood progenitor cell transplantation in lymphoma and leukemia using a single apheresis. *Blood* 1993; **82**: 3770–7.

76 Ho AD, Gluck S, Germond C et al. Optimal timing for collections of blood progenitor cells following induction chemotherapy and granuloyctemacrophage colony-stimulating factor for autologous transplantation in advanced breast cancer. *Leukemia* 1993; **7**: 1738–44.

77 Haas R, Moos M, Karcher A et al. Sequential high-dose therapy with peripheral blood progenitor cell support in low-grade non-Hodgkin's lymphoma. *J Clin Oncol* 1994; **12**: 1685–92.

78 Passos-Coelho JL, Braine HG, David JM et al. Predictive factors for peripheral-blood progenitor-cell collection using a single large-volume leukapheresis after cyclophosphamide and granulocyte-macrophage colony-stimulating factor mobilization. *J Clin Oncol* 1995; **13**: 705–14.

79 Bandarenko N, Sims LC, Brecher ME. Circulating CD34+ cell counts are predictive of CD34+ peripheral blood progenitor cell yields [letter]. *Transfusion* 1997; **37**: 1218–20.

80 Desikan KR, Jagannath S, Siegel D et al. Collection of more hematopoietic progenitor cells with large volume leukapheresis in patients with multiple myeloma. *Leuk Lymphoma* 1998; **28**: 501–8.

81 Moller AKH, Dickmeiss E, Geisler CH, Christensen LD. Recruitment of CD34+ cells during large-volume leukapheresis. A research report. *J Hemather Stem Cell Res* 2001; **10**: 837–53.

82 Schwarer AP, Messino NM, Gibson M, Akers C, Taouk Y. A randomized trial of leukapheresis volumes, 7 L versus 10 L. An assessment of efficacy

and patient tolerance. *J Hematother Stem Cell Res* 2000; **9**: 269–74.

83. Demirer T, Dagli M, Ilhan O et al. A randomized trial of assessment of efficacy of leukapheresis volumes, 8 liters vs. 12 liters. *Bone Marrow Transplant* 2002; **29**: 893–7.

84. Reiffers J, Faberes C, Boiron JM et al. Peripheral blood progenitor cell transplantation of 118 patients with hematological malignancies: analysis of factors affecting the rate of engraftment. *J Hematother* 1994; **3**: 185–91.

85. Vescio RA, Hong CH, Cao J et al. The hematopoietic stem cell antigen, CD34, is not expressed on the malignant cells in multiple myeloma. *Blood* 1994; **84**: 3283–90.

86. Haas R, Möühle R, Frühauf S et al. Patient characteristics associated with successful mobilizing and autografting of peripheral blood progenitor cells in malignant lymphoma. *Blood* 1994; **83**: 3787–94.

87. Van der Wall E, Richel DJ, Holtkamp MJ et al. Bone marrow reconstitution after high-dose chemotherapy and autologous peripheral blood progenitor cell transplantation: effect of graft size. *Ann Oncol* 1994; **5**: 795–802.

88. Beguin Y, Baudoux E, Sautois B et al. Hematopoietic recovery in cancer patients after transplantation of autologous peripheral blood CD34+ cells or unmanipulated peripheral blood stem and progenitor cells. *Transfusion* 1998; **38**: 199–208.

89. Dercksen MW, Rodenhuis S, Dirkson MKA et al. Subsets of CD34+ cells and rapid hematopoietic recovery after peripheral-blood stem-cell transplantation. *J Clin Oncol* 1995; **13**: 1922–32.

90. Klumpp TR, Goldberg SL, Magdalinski AJ et al. Phase II study of high-dose cyclophosphamide, etoposide and carboplatin (CED) followed by autologous hematopoietic stem cell rescue in women with metastatic or high-risk non-metastatic breast cancer: multivariate analysis of factors affecting survival and engraftment. *Bone Marrow Transplant* 1997; **20**: 273–81.

91. Brown RA, Adkins D, Goodnough LT et al. Factors that influence the collection and engraftment of allogeneic peripheral-blood stem cells in patients with hematologic malignancies. *J Clin Oncol* 1997; **15**: 3067–74.

92. Glaspy JA, Shpall EJ, LeMaistre CF et al. Peripheral blood progenitor cell mobilization using stem cell factor in combination with filgrastim in breast cancer patients. *Blood* 1997; **90**: 2939–51.

93. Bojko P, Waschek S, Seeber S, Nowrousian MR. Comparison of G-CSF and GM-CSF in combination with chemotherapy for peripheral blood stem cell (PBSC) mobilization. *Blood* 2001; **98**: 177a [Abstract].

94. Sutherland HJ, Eaves CJ, Lansdorp PM et al. Kinetics of committed and primitive blood progenitor mobilization after chemotherapy and growth factor treatment and their use in autotransplants. *Blood* 1994; **83**: 3808–14.

95. Weaver CH, Schulman KA, Wilson-Relyea B, Birch R, West W, Buckner CD. Randomized trial of filgrastim, sargramostim, or sequential sargramostim and filgrastim after myelosuppressive chemotherapy for the harvesting of peripheral-blood stem cells. *J Clin Oncol* 2000; **18**: 43–53.

96. Englehardt M, Bertz H, Afting M, Waller CF, Finke J. High-versus standard-dose filgrastim (rhG-CSF) for mobilization of peripheral-blood progenitor cells from allogeneic donors and CD34+ immunoselection. *J Clin Oncol* 1999; **17**: 2160–72.

97. Demirer T, Ayli M, Ozcan M et al. Mobilization of peripheral blood stem cells with chemotherapy and recombinant human granulouycte colony-stimulating factor (rhG-CSF): a randomized evaluation of different doses of rhG-CSF. *Br J Haematol* 2002; **116**: 468–74.

98. Beguin Y, Andre M, Baudoux E et al. An open, randomized, phase III study of transplantation with PBPC mobilized with chemotherapy and 5 vs. 10 µg/kg/d filgrastim in patients with non-myeloid malignancies. *Blood* 2000; **96**: 518a [Abstract].

99. Comenzo RL, Sanchorawala V, Fisher C et al. Intermediate-dose intravenous melphalan and blood stem cells mobilized with sequential GM + G-CSF or G-CSF alone to treat AL (amyloid light chain) amyloidosis. *Br J Haematol* 1999; **104**: 553–9.

100. Gazitt Y, Callander N, Freytes CO, Shaughnessy P, Tsai TW, Devore P. Peripheral blood stem cell mobilization with cyclophosphamide in combination with G-CSF, GM-CSF, or sequential GM-CSF followed by G-CSF in non-Hodgkin's lymphoma patients: a randomized prospective study. *J Hematother Stem Cell Res* 2000; **9**: 737–48.

101. Winter JN, Lazarus H, Rademaker A et al. Phase I/II study of combined granulouycte colony-stimulating factor and granulouycte-macrophage colony-stimulating factor administration for the mobilization of hematopoietic progenitor cells. *J Clin Oncol* 1996; **14**: 277–86.

102. Sohn SK, Kim JG, Seo KW et al. GM-CSF-based mobilization effect in normal healthy donors for allogeneic peripheral blood stem cell transplantation. *Bone Marrow Transplant* 2002; **30**: 81–6.

103. Brown RA, Adkins D, Haug J et al. Mobilization of allogeneic peripheral blood stem cell donors with both G- and GM-CSF increases progenitor yield without impacting graft-vs.-host disease (GVHD), relapse risk or progression-free survival (PFS). *Blood* 2000; **96**: 181a [Abstract].

104. Kroger N, Renges H, Kruger W et al. A randomized comparison of once versus twice daily recombinant human granulouycte colony-stimulating factor (filgrastim) for stem cell mobilization in healthy donors for allogeneic transplantation. *Bri J Haematol* 2000; **111**: 761–5.

105. Ponisch W, Leiblein S, Edel E et al. Mobilization of peripheral blood progenitor cells (PBPC) in normal donors for allogeneic PBPC transplantation: comparison between once a day vs. twice a day G-CSF administration. *Blood* 1999; **94**: 137a [Abstract].

106. Quittet PJM, Becht C, Legouffe E et al. Mobilization of CD34 peripheral stem cells (PSC) by lenograstim (Gly-G-CSF) given in a single dose compared to same split dose after cyclophosphamide (CPM): results of a randomized study in 60 patients. *Blood* 2001; **98**: 178a [Abstract].

107. Viens P, Chabannon C, Pouillard P et al. Randomized, controlled, dose-range study of Ro 25–8315 given before and after a high-dose combination chemotherapy regimen in patients with metastatic or recurrent breast cancer patients. *J Clin Oncol* 2002; **20**: 24–36.

108. Jackson JD, Yan Y, Brunda MJ, Kelsey LS, Talmadge JE. Interleukin-12 enhances peripheral hematopoiesis *in vivo*. *Blood* 1995; **85**: 2371–6.

109. Rosenfeld CS, Blowell M, LeVevre A, Taylor R, List A, Collins R. Comparison of four cytokine regimens for mobilization of peripheral blood stem cells: IL-3 alone and in combination with GM-CSF for G-CSF. *Bone Marrow Transplant* 1997; **17**: 179–83.

110. Bodine DM, Seidel NE, Zsebo KM, Orlic D. *In vivo* administration of stem cell factor to mice increases the absolute number of pluripotent hematopoietic stem cells. *Blood* 1993; **82**: 445–55.

111. Fischer J, Kiesel U, Herda A, Wernet P. Factors influencing yield of G-CSF mobilized PBPC from unrelated donors: interim results from an ongoing phase III study. *Blood* 2001; **98**: 173a [Abstract].

112. Shpall EJ, Wheeler CA, Turner SA et al. A randomized phase 3 study of peripheral blood progenitor cell mobilization with stem cell factor and filgrastim in high-risk breast cancer patients. *Blood* 1999; **93**: 2491–501.

113. Stiff P, Gingrich R, Luger S et al. A randomized phase 2 study of PBPC mobilization by stem cell factor and filgrastim in heavily pretreated patients with Hodgkin's disease or non-Hodgkin's lymphoma. *Bone Marrow Transplant* 2000; **26**: 471–81.

114. D'Hondt V, Guillaume T, Humblet Y et al. Tolerance of sequential or simultaneous administration of IL-3 and G-CSF in improving peripheral blood stem cells harvesting following multi-agent chemotherapy: a pilot study. *Bone Marrow Transplant* 1994; **13**: 261–4.

115. Geissler K, Peschell C, Niederwieser D et al. Effect of interleukin-3 pretreatment on granulocyte/macrophage colony-stimulating factor induced mobilization of circulating haemopoietic progenitor cells. *Br J Haematol* 1995; **91**: 299–305.

116. Brugger W, Frisch J, Schulz G, Pressler K, Mertelsmann R, Kanz L. Sequential administration of interleukin-3 and granulocyte-macrophage colony-stimulating factor following standard-dose combination chemotherapy with etoposide, ifosfamide, and cisplatin. *J Clin Oncol* 1992; **10**: 1452–9.

117. Kolbe K, Peschel C, Rupilius B et al. Peripheral blood stem cell (PBSC) mobilization with chemotherapy followed by sequential IL-3 and G-CSF administration in extensively pretreated patients. *Bone Marrow Transplant* 1997; **20**: 1027–32.

118. Mayer J, Indrak K, Koza V et al. Leridistim vs. G-CSF mobilization of peripheral blood stem cells when used with cyclophosphamide and etoposide in patients with lymphoma. *Blood* 2000; **96**: 518a [Abstract].

119. Goldman SC, Bracho F, Davenport V et al. Feasibility study of IL-11 and granulocyte colony-stimulating factor after myelosuppressive chemotherapy to mobilize peripheral blood stem cells from heavily pretreated patients. *J Pediatr Hematol Oncol* 2001; **23**: 300–5.

120. Burns LJ, Weisdorf DJ, DeFor TE, Repka TL, Ogle KM, Hummer C. Enhancement of the anti-tumor activity of a peripheral blood progenitor cell graft by mobilization with interleukin 2 plus granulocyte colony-stimulating factor in patients with advanced breast cancer. *Exp Hematol* 2000; **28**: 96–103.

121. Sosman JA, Stiff P, Moss SM et al. Pilot trial of interleukin-2 with granulouycte colony-stimulating factor for the mobilization of progenitor cells in advanced breast cancer patients undergoing high-dose chemotherapy: expansion of immune effectors within the stem-cell graft and post-stem-cell infusion. *J Clin Oncol* 2001; **19**: 634–44.

122. Schiller G, Wong S, Lowe T et al. Transplantation of IL-2-mobilized autologous peripheral blood progenitor cells for adults with acute myelogenous leukemia in first remission. *Leukemia* 2001; **15**: 757–63.

123 Neben S, Marcus K, Mauch P. Mobilization of hematopoietic stem and progenitor cell subpopulations from the marrow to the blood of mice following cyclophosphamide and/or granulocyte colony-stimulating factor. *Blood* 1993; **81**: 1960–7.

124 Siena S, Bregni M, Brando B, Ravagnani F, Bonadonna G, Gianni AM. Circulation of CD34+ hematopoietic stem cells in the peripheral blood of high-dose cyclophosphamide-treated patients: enhancement by intravenous recombinant human granulocyte-macrophage colony-stimulating factor. *Blood* 1989; **11**: 1905–14.

125 Gajewski J, Ron don G, Mehra R et al. Preliminary results of a randomized trial comparing intensive chemotherapy with growth factor (GF) for peripheral blood progenitor cell (PBPC) mobilization to growth factor alone for hematopoietic rescue after high dose chemotherapy (HDC). *Blood* 1998; **92**: 270a [Abstract].

126 Narayanasami U, Kanteti R, Morelli J et al. Randomized trial of filgrastim versus chemotherapy and filgrastim mobilization of hematopoietic progenitor cells for rescue in autologous transplantation. *Blood* 2001; **98**: 2059–64.

127 Koc ON, Gerson SL, Cooper BW et al. Randomized cross-over trial of progenitor-cell mobilization: high-dose cyclophosphamide plus granulocyte colony-stimulating factor (G-CSF) versus granulocyte-macrophage colony-stimulating factor plus G-CSF. *J Clin Oncol* 2000; **18**: 1824–30.

128 Stewart DA, Guo D, Morris D et al. Superior autologous blood stem cell mobilization from dose-intensive cyclophosphamide, etoposide, cisplatin plus G-CSF than from less intensive chemotherapy regimens. *Bone Marrow Transplant* 1999; **23**: 111–7.

129 Sheridan WP, Begley CG, Juttner CA et al. Effect of peripheral-blood progenitor cells mobilized by filgrastim (G-CSF) on platelet recovery after high-dose chemotherapy. *Lancet* 1992; **339**: 640–4.

130 Knudsen LM, Rasmussen T, Nikolaisen K, Johnsen HE. Mobilisation of tumour cells along with CD34+ cells to peripheral blood in multiple myeloma. *Eur J Haematol* 2001; **67**: 289–95.

131 Fitoussi O, Perreau V, Boiron JM et al. A comparison of toxicity following two different doses of cyclophosphamide for mobilization of peripheral blood progenitor cells in 116 multiple myeloma patients. *Bone Marrow Transplant* 2001; **27**: 837–42.

132 Reiser M, Josting A, Draube A et al. Successful peripheral blood stem cell mobilization with etoposide (VP-16) in patients with relapsed or resistant lymphoma who failed cyclophosphamide mobilization. *Bone Marrow Transplant* 1999; **23**: 1223–8.

133 Ashihara E, Shimazaki C, Okano A, Hatsuse M, Inaba T, Nakagawa M. Feasibility and efficacy of high-dose etoposide followed by low-dose G-CSF as a mobilization regimen in patients with non-Hodgkin's lymphoma. *Haematologica* 2000; **85**: 1112–4.

134 Tarella C, Di Nicola M, Caracciolo D et al. High-dose ara-C with autologous peripheral blood progenitor cell support induces a marked progenitor cell mobilization: an indication for patients at risk for low mobilization. *Bone Marrow Transplant* 2002; **30**: 725–32.

135 Holowiecki J, Wojciechowska M, Giebel S, Krawczyk-Kulis M, Wojnar J, Kachel L. Ifosfamide, etoposide, epirubicine, and G-CSF. An effective mobilization regimen for PBSCT in heavily pretreated patients. *Transplant Proc* 2000; **32**: 1412–5.

136 Arland M, Leuner S, Lange S et al. Ifosamide, epirubicin and granuloycte colony-stimulating factor: a regimen for successful mobilization of peripheral blood progenitor cells in patients with multiple myeloma. *Hematol Oncol* 2001; **19**: 59–66.

137 Carella AM, Lerma E, Celesti L et al. Effective mobilization of Philadelphia-chromosome-negative cells in chronic myelogenous leukaemia patients using a less intensive regimen. *Br J Haematol* 1998; **100**: 445–8.

138 Moskowitz CH, Bertino JR, Glassman JR et al. Ifosfamide, carboplatin, and etoposide: a highly effective cytoreduction and peripheral-blood progenitor-cell mobilization regimen for transplant-eligible patients with non-Hodgkin's lymphoma. *J Clin Oncol* 1999; **17**: 3776–85.

139 Sureda A, Petit J, Brunet S et al. Mini-ICE regimen as mobilization therapy for chronic myelogenous leukaemia patients at diagnosis. *Bone Marrow Transplant* 1999; **24**: 1285–90.

140 Petit J, Boque C, Cancelas JA et al. Feasibility of ESHAP+ G-CSF as peripheral blood hematopoietic progenitor cell mobilization regimen in resistant and relapsed lymphoma: a single-center study of 22 patients. *Leukemia Lymph* 1999; **34**: 119–27.

141 Berdeja JG, Ambinder RF, Jones RJ et al. Stem cell mobilization with G-CSF following standard ESHAP chemotherapy in patients with lymphoma. *Blood* 2001; **98**: 179a [Abstract].

142 Fleming DR, Goldsmith J, Goldsmith GH, Stevens DA, Herzig RH. Mobilization of peripheral blood stem cells in high-risk breast cancer patients using G-CSF after standard dose docetaxel. *J Hemather Stem Cell Res* 2000; **9**: 855–60.

143 Zibera C, Pedrazzoli P, Ponchio L et al. Efficacy of epirubicin/paclitaxel combination in mobilizing large amounts of hematopoietic progenitor cells in patients with metastatic breast cancer showing optimal response to the same chemotherapy regimen. *Haematologica* 1999; **84**: 924–9.

144 Shea TC. Mobilization of peripheral blood progenitor cells with paclitaxel-based chemotherapy. *Semin Oncol* 1997; **24**(1) (Suppl. 2): S105–7.

145 Gomez-Espuch J, Moraleda JM, Ortuno F et al. Mobilization of hematopoietic progenitor cells with paclitaxel (Taxol) as a single chemotherapeutic agent, associated with rhG-CSF. *Bone Marrow Transplant* 2000; **25**: 231–5.

146 Demirer T, Buckner CD, Storer B et al. Effect of different chemotherapy regimens on peripheral-blood stem-cell collections in patients with breast cancer receiving granuloycte colony-stimulating factor. *J Clin Oncol* 1997; **15**: 684–90.

147 Shea TC, Mason JR, Breslin M, Bissent E, Mullen M, Taetle R. Reinfusion and serial measurements of carboplatin-mobilized peripheral-blood progenitor cells in patients receiving multiple cycles of high-dose chemotherapy. *J Clin Oncol* 1994; **12**: 101–21.

148 Weaver CH, Schwartzberg LS, Zhen B et al. Mobilization of peripheral blood stem cells with docetaxel and cyclophosphamide (CY) in patients with metastatic breast cancer: a randomized trial of 3 vs. 4 g/m² of CY. *Bone Marrow Transplant* 1999; **23**: 421–5.

149 To LB, Shepperd DM, Haylock DN et al. Single high doses of cyclophosphamide enable the collection of high numbers of hemopoietic stem cells from the peripheral blood. *Exp Hematol* 1990; **18**: 442–7.

150 Weaver Ch, Zhen B, Buckner CD. Treatment of patients with malignant lymphoma with mini-BEAM reduces the yield of CD34+ peripheral blood stem cells. *Bone Marrow Transplant* 1998; **21**: 1169–70.

151 Krishnan A, Bhatia S, Slovak M et al. Predictors for therapy-related leukemia and myelodysplasia following autologous transplantation for lymphoma: an assessment of risk factors. *Blood* 2000; **95**: 1588–93.

152 Bensinger WI, Weaver CH, Appelbaum FR et al. Transplantation of allogeneic peripheral blood stem cells mobilized by recombinant human granulocyte colony-stimulating factor. *Blood* 1995; **85**: 1655–8.

153 Tricot G, Jagannath S, Vesole D et al. Peripheral blood stem cell transplants for multiple myeloma: identification of favorable variables for rapid engraftment in 225 patients. *Blood* 1995; **85**: 588–96.

154 Dreger P, Kloss M, Petersen B et al. Autologous progenitor cell transplantation: prior exposure to stem cell-toxic drugs determines yield and engraftment of peripheral blood progenitor cell but not of bone marrow grafts. *Blood* 1995; **86**: 3970–8.

155 Moskowitz CH, Glassman JR, West D et al. Factors affecting mobilization of peripheral blood progenitor cells in patients with lymphoma. *Clin Cancer Res* 1998; **4**: 311–6.

156 Kobbe G, Sohngen D, Bauser U et al. Factors influencing G-CSF-mediated mobilization of hematopoietic progenitor cells during steady-state hematopoiesis in patients with malignant lymphoma and multiple myeloma. *Ann Hematol* 1999; **78**: 456–62.

157 Perry AR, Watts MJ, Peniket AM, Goldstone AH, Linch DC. Progenitor cell yields are frequently poor in patients with histologically indolent lymphomas especially when mobilized within 6 months of previous chemotherapy. *Bone Marrow Transplant* 1998; **21**: 1201–5.

158 Tarella C, Zallio F, Caracciolo D, Cherasco C, Bondesan P, Gavarotti P. Hemopoietic progenitor cell mobilization and harvest following an intensive chemotherapy debulking in indolent lymphoma patients. *Stem Cells* 1999; **17**: 55–61.

159 Seong D, Anderson B, Korbling M et al. Predicting parameters of successful peripheral blood stem cell (PBSC) collection after chemo/cytokine primed mobilization in relapsed Hodgkin's disease. *Proc ASCO* 1995; **14**: 943 [Abstract].

160 Stiff PJ. Management strategies for the hard-to-mobilize patient. *Bone Marrow Transplant* 1999; **23** (Suppl. 2): 29–33.

161 Bentley SA, Brecher ME, Powell E, Serody JS, Wiley JM, Shea TC. Long-term engraftment failure after marrow ablation and autologous hematopoietic reconstitution: differences between peripheral blood stem cell and bone marrow recipients. *Bone Marrow Transplant* 1997; **19**: 557–63.

162 Bashford J, Durrant S, Schwarer A et al. Ancestim (r-metHsSCF) plus filgrastim (r-metHuG-CSF) allows mobilization of peripheral blood stem cells (PBSC) for transplantation in patients filing mobilization with filgrastim alone. *Blood* 2000; **96**: 178a [Abstract].

163 Azar N, Vantelon JM, Hashmati P et al. Ancestim (r-metHuSCF): mobilization of peripheral blood stem cells (PBSC) in patients with prior unsuccessful mobilization with G-CSF. Experience of 67

cases of compassionate use in France. *Blood* 2000; **96**: 178a [Abstract].

164 Lie AKW, Hui CH, Rawling T *et al*. Granulocyte colony-stimulating factor (G-CSF) dose-dependent efficacy in peripheral blood stem cell mobilization in patients who had failed initial mobilization with chemotherapy and G-CSF. *Bone Marrow Transplant* 1998; **22**: 853–7.

165 Gazitt Y, Freytes C, Callander N *et al*. Successful PBSC mobilization with high-dose G-CSF for patients failing a first round of mobilization. *J Hematother* 1999; **8**: 173–83.

166 Voralia M, Nagy T, Trip K, Chen C, Keating A, Crump M. Effectiveness of high-dose G-CSF (32 µg/kg) for stem cell mobilization after failure of chemotherapy + standard dose G-CSF (10 µg/kg) for autologous stem cell transplantation. *Blood* 2000; **96**: 178a [Abstract].

167 Fraipont V, Sautois B, Baudoux E *et al*. Successful mobilization of peripheral blood HPCs with G-CSF alone in patients failing to achieve sufficient numbers of CD34[+] cells and/or CFU-GM with chemotherapy and G-CSF. *Transfusion* 2000; **40**: 339–47.

168 Mijovic A, Pagliuca A, Mufti GJ. The 'G-CSF test.' The response to a single dose of granulocyte colony-stimulating factor predicts mobilization of hemopoietic progenitors in patients with hematologic malignancies. *Exp Hematol* 1999; **27**: 1204–9.

169 Fruehauf S, Schmitt K, Veldwijk MR *et al*. Peripheral blood progenitor cell (PBPC) counts during steady-state haemopoiesis enable the estimation of the yield of mobilized PBPC after granulocyte colony-stimulating factor supported cytotoxic chemotherapy: an update on 100 patients. *Br J Haematol* 1999; **105**: 786–94.

170 Fernandez-Jimenez MC, Arrieta R, Quevedo E, Hernandez-Navarro F. Blood CD34[+] cell count in the steady state as a predictor factor for PBSC mobilization in patients with hematologic malignancies. *Blood* 2001; **98**: 176a [Abstract].

171 Brugger W, Bross KJ, Glatt M, Weber F, Mertelsmann R, Kanz L. Mobilization of tumor cells and hematopoietic progenitor cells into peripheral blood of patients with solid tumors. *Blood* 1994; **83**: 636–40.

172 Passos Coelho JL, Ross AA, Kahn DJ *et al*. Similar breast cancer cell contamination of single-day peripheral-blood progenitor-cell collections obtained after priming with hematopoietic growth factor alone or after cyclophosphamide followed by growth factor. *J Clin Oncol* 1996; **14**: 2569–75.

173 Sharp JG, Kessinger A, Mann S *et al*. Outcome of high-dose therapy and autologous transplantation in non-Hodgkin's lymphoma based on the presence of tumor in the marrow or infused hematopoietic harvest. *J Clin Oncol* 1996; **14**: 214–9.

174 Tricot G, Gazitt Y, Leemhuis T *et al*. Collection, tumor contamination, and engraftment kinetics of highly purified hematopoietic progenitor cells to support high dose therapy in multiple myeloma. *Blood* 1998; **91**: 4489–95.

175 Kruger W, Kroger N, Togel F *et al*. Influence of preharvest tumor cell contamination in bone marrow or blood does not predict resultant tumor cell contamination of granuloycte colony-stimulating factor mobilized stem cells. *J Hematother Stem Cell Res* 2001; **10**: 303–7.

176 Franklin WA, Glaspy J, Pflaumer SM *et al*. Incidence of tumor-cell contamination in leukapheresis products of breast cancer patients mobilized with stem cell factor and granuloycte colony-stimulating factor (G-CSF) or with G-CSF alone. *Blood* 1999; **94**: 340–7.

177 Shpall EJ, Jones RB, Bearman SI *et al*. Transplantation of enriched CD34-positive autologous marrow into breast cancer patients following high-dose chemotherapy: influence of CD34-positive peripheral-blood progenitors and growth factors on engraftment. *J Clin Oncol* 1994; **12**: 28–36.

178 Verfaillie CM, Bhatia R, Steinbuch M *et al*. Comparative analysis of autografting in chronic myelogenous leukemia: effects of priming regimen and marrow or blood origin of stem cells. *Blood* 1998; **92**: 1820–31.

179 Lemoli RM, Martinelli G, Olivieri A *et al*. Selection and transplantation of autologous CD34[+] B-lineage negative cells in advanced-phase multiple myeloma patients: a pilot study. *Br J Haematol* 1999; **107**: 419–28.

180 Craddock CF, Nakamoto B, Andrews RG *et al*. Antibodies of VLA4 integrin mobilize long-term repopulating cells and augment cytokin-induced mobilization in primates and mice. *Blood* 1997; **90**: 4779–88.

181 Tsuruta T, Ohno N, Tojo A *et al*. Enhancement by VCAM-Ig of granuloycte colony stimulating factor-induced progenitor cell mobilization in mice. *Blood* 2001; **98**: 177a [Abstract].

182 Schwarzenberger P, Huang W, Oliver P *et al*. Il-17 mobilizes peripheral blood stem cells with short- and long-term repopulating ability in mice. *J Immunol* 2001; **167**: 2081–6.

183 Gazitt Y, Shaughnessy P, Liu Q. Expression of adhesion molecules on CD34[+] cells in peripheral blood of non-Hodgkin's lymphoma patients mobilized with different growth factors. *Stem Cells* 2001; **19**: 134–43.

46

Norbert Schmitz

Peripheral Blood Hematopoietic Cells for Allogeneic Transplantation

Introduction

The existence of hematopoietic cells (HCs) in the peripheral blood (PB) was postulated in 1909 by Alexander Maximow [1]. In 1962, Goodman and Hodgson were first to prove that circulating HCs were capable of restoring irradiation-induced marrow aplasia in mice [2]. The first clinical transplantation was published in 1980 by Abrams *et al.* [3] who transfused large numbers of syngeneic blood leukocytes to a patient with Ewing's sarcoma. In 1985 and 1986 four different teams of investigators reported successful hematopoietic reconstitution by autologous blood-derived HCs in cancer patients [4–7].

Although these latter case reports provided the long-sought proof of principle, the low concentration of HCs in unmanipulated PB remained a major obstacle to the wider use of clinical transplants from PB, especially in the allogeneic setting where the exposure of healthy individuals to cytotoxic drugs was not possible.

Only with the advent of granulocyte colony-stimulating factor (G-CSF) and the discovery that this and related cytokines were able to substantially increase the concentration of CD34$^+$ cells in PB [8,9] did autologous and—5–6 years later—allogeneic peripheral blood hematopoietic cell transplantation (PBHCT) begin to enter the clinic. With regard to PBHCT, in 1989 Kessinger *et al.* [10] showed that T-cell-depleted blood HCs were able to restore hematopoiesis after myeloablative therapy. Because of fears that the high numbers of T lymphocytes contained in PBHC harvests would induce graft-vs.-host disease (GVHD) in most recipients, allogeneic PBHCT replete of T cells was first used in emergency situations such as the failure of a previous marrow graft [11] or the inability of the donor to undergo general anesthesia for marrow collection [12].

After the first successful pilot studies using unmanipulated PB from human leukocyte antigen (HLA)-identical sibling donors were published in 1995 [13–15] a surge of allogeneic PBHCTs ensued. Currently, close to 60% of all allogeneic transplants in Europe are performed with PB instead of marrow [16], and there is no reason to believe that further development will not duplicate the situation in autologous transplantation where, within few years, PB had largely replaced bone marrow (BM) as the source of HCs.

The donors

When allogeneic HCT using PB entered the clinical arena the experience with healthy individuals donating HCs mobilized into the blood was also limited. The major issues that had to be addressed were the following:
1 How could HCs be harvested most effectively?
2 Did harvest products from the PB contain stem cells in the quantity and quality which would allow for timely, complete and durable engraftment of allogeneic lymphohematopoiesis?
3 What were the acute side-effects and long-term sequelae of the mobilization and collection procedure?

For further information regarding donors for HCT see also Chapter 42.

Mobilization and collection of HCs from PB

The first attempts to "mobilize" HCs into the PB of normal donors followed the experience gained with granulocyte transfusions [17] and the mobilization of autologous HCs in patients with lymphoma and other diseases where the stem cell pool was not compromised by marrow infiltration or extensive cytotoxic therapy [18,19]. Accordingly, G-CSF at doses between 5 and 16 µg/kg/day was administered to the potential donor for 5–7 days. Such treatment allowed the collection of CD34$^+$ cell numbers ranging from around two to more than 20×10^6/kg body weight when 1–4 leukaphereses were performed 4–7 days after initiation of G-CSF administration. Infusion of the harvest products into recipients with leukemia or lymphoma after myeloablative therapy resulted in reliable and surprisingly fast engraftment [13–15].

Thousands of healthy individuals have now undergone mobilization and collection of PBHCs using a large variety of harvest protocols [20–34]. A recent analysis from International Bone Marrow Transplant Registry (IBMTR) and European Group for Blood and Marrow Transplantation (EBMT) [35] summarized the experience with 1488 donations of PBHCs from HLA-identical siblings ($n = 1322$), other relatives ($n = 149$) or unrelated donors ($n = 15$). Nearly all donors had received G-CSF (filgrastim, lenograstim) for mobilization. Approximately 40% of the donors had undergone a single apheresis only, 45% underwent two, 11% underwent three and 5% underwent four or more leukaphereses to collect the number of HCs deemed necessary for engraftment by the investigator. An activity report from the Spanish National Donor Registry specified that G-CSF was administered to 466 donors at a median dose of 10 µg/kg/day (range: 4–20 µg/kg) for a median of 5 days (range: 4–8 days). The mean CD34$^+$ cell dose collected was 6.9×10^6/kg (range: $1.3–36 \times 10^6$/kg) with only 14 donors (2.9%) not achieving the minimum target number of 2×10^6 CD34$^+$ cells/kg [36]. Because of the short half-life of G-CSF (3–4 h), some physicians prefer a twice-daily schedule over a single injection of G-CSF per day although the data supporting this practice are somewhat controversial [31–33,37,38].

Based on these and similar data, G-CSF at doses between 5 and 16 µg/kg given for 4 or 5 consecutive days may be considered the standard for mobilization of allogeneic HCs [39,40]. Commencing leukapheresis on day 4 or 5 with any commercially available continuous flow blood cell separator will allow the collection of adequate numbers of HCs in the vast majority of healthy individuals with one to three daily collections if two to four times the donor's blood volume is processed.

G-CSF doses as low as 2 µg/kg [22] or as high as 40 µg/kg (in the autologous setting [41]) have been used with a clear trend towards higher CD34$^+$ cell numbers being collected after administration of higher doses of growth factor. Systematic studies investigating the relationship between G-CSF administration and HC yield over a wider dose range have not been published. However, CD34$^+$ concentrations in PB decrease when G-CSF is continued for 7 days and beyond. Therefore, adequate timing of aphereses and effective collection procedures are the key to achieve optimum harvest products. Other variables like age, sex, body weight or baseline CD34$^+$ cell concentration in the blood of the donor have also been described to correlate with the stem cell yield, but these findings have not always been confirmed [42,43] and none of these parameters will allow to individually predict the stem cell yield.

Growth factors other than G-CSF, mostly granulocyte macrophage colony-stimulating factor (GM-CSF) in conjunction with G-CSF, have occasionally been used for mobilization in healthy individuals without obvious advantages over the administration of G-CSF alone [44,45]. Interleukin 3 (IL-3) [46], stem cell factor [47] and other experimental cytokines, such as Flt3 ligand [48], have been shown to increase the CD34$^+$ cell concentration in the PB of rodents, primates or humans, but were not broadly used clinically because of their side-effects, which would put healthy volunteers at unnecessary and potentially severe risks.

Specific clinical situations, i.e. T-cell depletion of the graft, non-myeloablative preparatory regimens or unrelated, mismatched and haplo-identical transplants [49] will need much higher CD34$^+$ cell numbers to safeguard against the increased risk of graft failure associated with any of these procedures. It is for these reasons that the search for the optimum mobilization and collection procedure is ongoing.

Characteristics and dose of HC from PB or marrow

As the human hematopoietic stem cell has not yet been fully described, the precise answer to the question if true hematopoietic stem cells are contained in sufficient numbers in a typical PB collection product awaits further study. It is, however, possible to describe the quality and quantity of committed and more immature HCs as they appear in mobilized PB and compare the findings to marrow-derived HCs. This comparison would indicate that primitive and committed HCs are present in mobilized PB at least as frequently as in a typical BM harvest.

Using the CD34$^+$ antigen, which can easily be detected by flow cytometry as a surrogate marker for the human stem cell, pilot studies found that mobilized PB would contain 2–5 times more HCs than BM. This has been confirmed by the results of the large randomized trials [114–116, 120].

What is the minimum CD34$^+$ cell number to guarantee quick and durable engraftment? Should a certain number of CD34$^+$ cells not be exceeded? A definite answer to both questions is not really possible. However, it seems reasonable to recommend the collection of at least $1-2 \times 10^6$ CD34$^+$ cells/kg because clinical experience indicates that the risk of graft failure is increased if less than this threshold number is transplanted. It is also difficult to tell if there should be an upper limit for CD34$^+$ cell numbers and if higher numbers would be harmful if transferred to the recipient. Animal experiments [50] and clinical data [151] indicate that the desirable number of HCs needed to ensure engraftment will depend on a number of interdependent parameters, the most important of which are the immunosuppressive potential of the conditioning regimen, the HLA-disparity between donor and recipient, the number of T cells infused and the regimen used for GVHD prophylaxis. For a "standard" transplant from an HLA-identical sibling donor after myeloablative conditioning, doses between 3 and 5×10^6 CD34$^+$ cells/kg may be optimal while haplo-identical recipients will need much higher numbers of

Table 46.1 Characteristics of CD34$^+$ hematopoietic cells (HCs) from bone marrow (BM) or mobilized peripheral blood (PB).

Characteristics	BM	Mobilized PB
Phenotype		
CD13$^+$, CD33$^+$	Standard	Higher
CD38$^-$	Standard	Higher
HLA-DR$^-$	Standard	Higher
CD10$^+$, CD19$^+$	Standard	Less
CD7$^+$	Standard	Less
c-kit	Standard	Less
VLA-4	Standard	Less
Metabolic activity		
CD71$^+$	High	Low
Rhodamine	High	Low retention
Clonogenicity		
Colony formation	Normal	Increased
LTC-IC	Normal	Increased
Cycling status	Active	Nonactive
Genotype cell cycle progression	Standard	Less
DNA synthesis	Standard	Less
GATA 2		Increased
N-*myc*		Increased
Apoptotic activity		Increased

CD34$^+$ cells, perhaps 10×10^6 CD34$^+$ cells/kg, to secure engraftment [49]. Recently, high CD34$^+$ cell numbers have generally been recommended because several investigators were able to demonstrate a significant correlation with improved survival [51,52]. It probably is not important if high CD34$^+$ cell numbers come from BM or PB [53] but only mobilized blood will allow collection of higher numbers regularly. On the other hand, because PBHC collection products containing high CD34$^+$ cell numbers also contain more T cells it has been postulated that transplants from PB with very high CD34$^+$ cell numbers should not be used. Przepiorka *et al.* [54] evaluated risk factors for acute GVHD after allogeneic PBHCT and found a sharp increase of GVHD if more than of $6.3-10.0 \times 10^6$ CD34$^+$ cells/kg were transplanted. However, it will be difficult to confirm this finding with prospective data because such high numbers of PBHCs are harvested from a small fraction of donors only.

A number of investigators have looked at immunophenotypically, genotypically or functionally characterized subtypes of HCs in more detail. Körbling *et al.* [55,56] reported that G-CSF at a dose of 12 µg/kg/day increased the concentrations of PB CD34$^+$ cells and more primitive subsets such as CD34$^+$Thy-1^{dim} and CD34$^+$Thy-1^{dim}CD38 cells by 16.3-, 24.2- and 23.2-fold, respectively. The mean apheresis yield of CD34$^+$Thy-1^{dim} and CD34$^+$Thy-1^{dim}CD38 cells/kg of recipient body weight and per liter of donor blood processed was 48.9×10^4 and 27.2×10^4, respectively, indicating an additional "peripheralization" effect of G-CSF on primitive CD34$^+$ cell subsets [55,56]. Other reports [57] confirmed these findings but also showed that the immunophenotypic profiles of HCs from blood or marrow differ in several respects (Table 46.1) (for review see [58]). The low expression of CD71 and the decreased retention of rhodamine-123 in CD34$^+$ cells from mobilized PB suggest that these cells are not actively proliferating or metabolically active [59]. Kinetic data corroborate the phenotypic findings, further demonstrating that relatively more CD34$^+$ cells from PB exhibit characteristics of quiescent cells [60].

Recently, Steidl *et al.* [61] reported on the molecular phenotype of BM-derived and circulating CD34$^+$ cells from mobilized PB. Gene expression profiling confirmed that CD34$^+$ cells from BM cycle more rapidly whereas CD34$^+$ cells from PB include more quiescent stem and progenitor cells.

Prosper et al. [62] investigated the number of long-term culture initiating cells (LTC-IC) in the PB of normal donors treated with G-CSF (7.5–10.0 µg/kg/day) and found that CD34$^+$ CD38$^+$ cells and CD34$^+$ HLA-DR$^+$ cells sorted from mobilized PB contained 0.5–5.0% of cells capable of sustaining hematopoiesis in long-term culture for up to 5 weeks. This is at least five times more than the number of LTC-IC found in steady-state BM or nonmobilized PBHC. However, 90–95% of the LTC-IC present in CD34$^+$ CD38$^+$ or CD34$^+$ HLA-DR$^+$ fractions of mobilized PB were not able to sustain hematopoiesis for 8 weeks, as was the case with almost one-third of CD34$^+$ CD38$^+$ and CD34$^+$ HLA-DR$^+$ cells from nonmobilized PB [62]. Taken together, phenotypic, genotypic and functional analyses of HCs from BM or PB demonstrate that stem and progenitor cells are contained in both compartments. While HCs from PB may be enriched in LTC-IC and other clonogenic cells, they are metabolically less active, they cycle less intensely and they show increased apoptotic activity. Stem cell biology including the differences of CD34$^+$ cells from mobilized PB or BM remains an area of active research because better understanding of basic phenotypes and function is paramount to optimize peripheralization, harvesting and clinical use of HCs.

T lymphocytes and other immune cells in mobilized blood

There are many differences in the composition of PBHC harvests and marrow grafts if cells other than the HCs are considered. Most importantly, PB harvests contain approximately 10 times more T cells than BM; however, the ratio of CD4$^+$/CD8$^+$ lymphocytes remains unaffected. This had already been noticed with autologous PBHC harvests [63] and was the most important reason why allogeneic transplants with PB were accepted as an alternative to BM only after pilot studies had demonstrated that the infusion of such high T cell numbers was not regularly followed by the occurrence of severe GVHD [13–15]. To some extent, the numbers of T cells contained in PBHC harvests relative to the number of CD34$^+$ positive cells seem to depend on the mobilization protocol and the day of apheresis. Leukapheresis on day 5 after administration of G-CSF should give the highest stem cell yield with relatively low numbers of T cells contained in the final product [26,63].

The observation that the high number of T cells in PB harvests did not lead to a dramatic increase in the incidence and severity of GVHD in patients allografted with mobilized PB prompted researchers to investigate the effects of G-CSF administration on the number and function of immune cells in more detail. With regard to T cells, Pan et al. [64] were first to show that pretreatment of healthy individuals with G-CSF polarizes T cells towards the production of type-2 cytokines (IL-4, IL-10) while type-1 cytokine production (interferon-γ, IL-2) is reduced. These observations were confirmed by others [65]. Other effects capable of explaining the surprisingly low incidence of severe GVHD after transplantation of allogeneic PBHCs are down-regulation of allogeneic immune responses by post-transcriptional inhibition of tumor necrosis factor-alpha (TNF-α) production [66] or the comobilization of CD4$^+$ and CD8$^+$ T cells. Kusnierz-Glaz et al. [67] demonstrated that CD4$^+$CD8$^+$αβ T cells are markedly enriched in leukapheresis products of G-CSF treated normal donors and that these cells further enriched in low-density fractions of mobilized PB significantly suppress the mixed-lymphocyte reaction.

Mielcarek et al. [68,69] calculated that the number of CD14$^+$ cells in mobilized PB was 50-fold greater than in marrow. These large numbers of monocytes then suppress T-cell proliferative responses to alloantigen [68,69]. Recently, Arpinati et al. [70] demonstrated that the numbers of T helper type 2 subset (TH2)-inducing dendritic cells (pre-DC2s) are increased in mobilized PB. As pre-DC2s lead to polarization of naive CD4$^+$ T cells toward a TH2 phenotype, this finding also may explain why transplantation of allogeneic PBHC does not lead to more severe GVHD in a larger fraction of patients [70].

Natural killer (NK) cells are fivefold to 10-fold more frequent in mobilized PB than in BM. Joshi and colleagues analyzed peripheral blood mononuclear cells (PBMC) from G-CSF-mobilized blood cell harvests for their immunological function and compared them with PBMC from steady-state nonmobilized donors [71]. They found a significant decrease in NK- and lymphokine-activated killer cell-mediated cytotoxicity for G-CSF-mobilized effector cells. They also reported a significant decrease in both T-cell and B-cell mitogen responses with G-CSF mobilized vs. nonmobilized cells.

Neutrophils not only increase in numbers after administration of G-CSF but their function is also enhanced immediately after G-CSF administration as shown by up-regulation of Fcγ RIII receptors, cell surface CD11b and CD66 molecules and elevated levels of plasma elastase [72].

It is currently not clear if any of the mechanisms described above can fully explain the striking clinical phenomenon that the infusion of 1–2 log more T cells into the recipient does not result in the development of severe GVHD in more patients grafted with PB.

There are certainly other, yet undetected, effects of G-CSF on the number and function of cells from mobilized PB. Among others, the question how G-CSF mobilizes HCs into the blood needs further study. Although recent work has demonstrated that G-CSF administration causes a reduced expression of very-late antigen-4 (VLA-4) integrin [73] and c-kit on HCs, and induces proteolytic cleavage of vascular cell adhesion molecule-1 (VCAM-1) on CD34$^+$ cells [74], this may not be the full explanation and research is ongoing.

Side-effects and long-term sequelae of mobilization and collection of HCs

The short- and long-term effects of G-CSF have recently been reviewed [75]. The acute toxicities of G-CSF experienced by normal donors are now described reasonably well and generally parallel those observed earlier in cancer patients. Bone pain, headache and fatigue are the most frequent side-effects of G-CSF administration, but myalgias, chest pain, anxiety, insomnia, night sweats, fever, anorexia, weight gain, nausea and/or vomiting and local reactions at the injection site have also been described [31,36,75,76]. Side-effects have been mild to moderate in the vast majority of donors and usually resolve within 48 h of discontinuation of G-CSF. They can be treated successfully by the administration of minor analgesics (acetaminophen or ibuprofen) in most instances and these side-effects have not been reported to require cessation of G-CSF administration or cancellation of the PBHC harvest. There is some indication that the frequency and severity of side-effects of G-CSF is dose-dependent [77,78]. Therefore, the use of doses as low as possible has been recommended.

A number of side-effects of G-CSF administration and the harvest procedure on blood chemistry, the coagulation system and baseline hematologic parameters, already described in patients with hematological malignancies, also occur in normal individuals. Laboratory abnormalities caused by G-CSF include transient increases of lactate dehydrogenase and alkaline phosphatase, uric acid, alanine aminotransferase and/or-glutamyl transpeptidase and a decrease in serum potassium and/or magnesium [21,39,79].

Several authors have shown that G-CSF can induce a mild hypercoagulable state as indicated by in vitro testing. Increases in fibrinogen and factor VIII levels, a reduction in protein C and S levels [80], increases in prothrombin fragments, thrombin–antithrombin complexes, D-dimers and platelet aggregation have all been reported [81–83]. Mild to moderate decrements in platelet, lymphocyte and granulocyte levels have been described following the collection of PBHCs [17,84]. Thrombocytopenia may partly be due to the administration of G-CSF itself [85] or due to the leukapheresis procedure. Cytopenias are usually mild and self-limited, although more profound thrombocytopenia following repeated large volume leukaphereses has been reported [86].

Serious or lethal complications of G-CSF administration and leukapheresis are rare. Two cases of splenic rupture associated with the harvest procedure have been reported [87,88]. Also, single cases of cardiovascular events have been described. However, the reports by Cavallaro et al. [89] on a case of myocardial infarction, Anderlini et al. [39] on a case of stroke and others on less serious cardiovascular complications [152] should engender caution when donors with a history of vascular disease are considered. Other serious side-effects reported to date are acute iritis [90], pyogenic infections [91], gouty arthritis [92] and anaphylactoid reactions [93]. These phenomena have mainly been reported in patients suffering from autoimmune and inflammatory disease. Therefore, potential donors with any of these disorders should be given special attention and G-CSF administration should be avoided whenever possible.

The leukapheresis itself is generally well tolerated but side-effects caused by the anticoagulant and placement of central venous access have been reported. Although every effort should be made to avoid a central venous access, 2–7% of donors ultimately will need it because peripheral veins cannot be used or the necessary blood flow cannot be established [116,120]. Rarely, donors have experienced tetany or severe symptoms of hypocalcemia caused by the anticoagulant used throughout the leukapheresis procedure [94].

Recently, a number of studies have been presented which compare the experience of donors who participated in one of the randomized trials comparing BMT with PBHCT [94–97]. Most importantly, it was reassuring to read that none of these reports described life-threatening complications or long-lasting discomfort in any of the donors. The study reports generally confirm that the side-effects of PBHC harvesting are related mainly to G-CSF administration while the side-effects of BM harvesting are caused by the harvest procedure itself. The incidence of adverse events occurring in ≥5% of donors of PB or BM who participated in the large European trial are presented in Table 46.2 [94].

Some of these studies also measured the emotional status and pain of donors prior to the harvest procedure and at defined time points after the collection of BM or PB. In general, the symptom burden, the levels of maximal and average pain, and anxiety were similar although symptom peaks occurred at different time points during G-CSF administration (in PB donors) or shortly after BM harvesting. A quicker resolution of symptoms in PBHC donors was also described [95,96]. Only the Scandinavian trial reported a significant difference in the total burden of complaints in the two groups of donors favoring the PB donors [97]. This study also found that donors would prefer to donate PB rather then BM if asked to donate again [97]. This observation is in line with a report from unrelated donors [98] and a previous report in cancer patients who also preferred to donate autologous PB rather than BM [99].

No long-term effects of G-CSF administration and PBHC collection have been reported so far. However, the maximum observation period of healthy donors is limited and rare events may have escaped detection so far. Because of concerns that G-CSF might perturbate normal hematopoiesis and increase the risk to develop malignant disorders of the blood including myelodysplastic syndrome (MDS) and leukemia it was proposed to establish an international donor registry for PBHC donors [39]. These requests have only partly been met so far because of statistical considerations questioning this approach [100] and the lack of financial resources necessary to capture all PBHC donors worldwide. The cases of leukemic transformation seen after G-CSF treatment in patients with severe chronic neutropenia (SCN) [101] likely reflect the inherent

Table 46.2 Subject incidence of adverse events occurring in >5% of donors. Data from the EBMT study comparing bone marrow transplantation (BMT) with peripheral blood progenitor cell transplantation (PBPCT) [94].

	BM donors (n = 166)	PBHC donors (n = 164)
Any adverse event	95 (57%)	107 (65%)
Harvesting procedure-related adverse events		
Any harvest-related	91 (55%)	61 (37%)
Access pain	39 (23%)	2 (1%)
Anemia	17 (10%)	0 (0%)
Back pain	16 (10%)	4 (2%)
Nausea	10 (6%)	1 (1%)
Arthralgia	8 (5%)	1 (1%)
Vomiting	8 (5%)	0 (0%)
Skeletal pain	3 (2%)	10 (6%)
Filgrastim-related adverse events		
Any filgrastim-related		96 (59%)
Musculoskeletal		71 (43%)
Headache		19 (12%)
LDH increased		14 (9%)
Alkaline phosphatase increased		8 (5%)

BM, bone marrow; LDH, lactate dehydrogenase; PBHC, peripheral blood hematopoietic cell.

propensity of SCN patients to develop leukemia rather than being a consequence of G-CSF administration.

Overall, there is no compelling evidence to date suggesting the superiority of BM or PB if only donor aspects are taken into account. The advantages of PBHC collection include avoidance of general anesthesia, blood transfusions and local discomfort. For most donors, PBHC collection will be an outpatient procedure, and return to normal daily activity is usually quicker than after BM harvesting. BM harvesting is not without risk, and significant to life-threatening complications have occasionally been reported [102]. There have also been unreported deaths after general anesthesia and BM harvesting in at least two elderly donors. Thus, the decision of the donor to undergo BM or PB harvesting will depend on his or her personal choice after the advantages and disadvantages of both procedures have been thoroughly explained. Donor information should include that knowledge of the long-term effects of G-CSF administration and PBHC harvesting may be incomplete at this time.

The recipients

Small pilot studies performed in Houston, TX, Seattle, WA, and Kiel, Germany, all published in 1995 [13–15], indicated that transplantation of allogeneic PBHCs resulted in fast and stable engraftment, and GVHD did not seem to occur more frequently than after marrow grafting. Larger series from other transplant centers or cooperative groups [103–108], as well as retrospective comparisons with BMT [109–112], were reported during subsequent years and confirmed that transplantation of allogeneic HCs from PB without devastating GVHD was feasible. The largest retrospective analysis was presented by IBMTR and EBMT and compared results of 288 PBHCTs with 536 BMT procedures from HLA-identical sibling donors [113]. The major conclusion from this paper was that recipients of PBHCs attained more rapid recovery of neutrophils and platelets; significant differences in relapse rates and the incidence of grades II–IV acute GVHD were not observed. However, the incidence of chronic GVHD at 1 year after transplantation was significantly higher after PBHCT (65%) than after BMT (53%). Treatment-related mortality was lower and leukemia-free survival rates were higher with PBHCT in patients with advanced leukemias but were comparable in standard-risk leukemias.

The randomized trials

Between 1998 and 2002, the results of eight prospective randomized trials comparing transplantation of allogeneic PBHCs with BM were published [114–121]. These studies were almost exclusively done in patients with leukemia; patients with other hematological malignancies were only rarely included, and patients with nonmalignant disorders were not included at all. The donors were HLA-identical siblings and BM or PBHCs were infused without any manipulation. It is important to realize that the design of these trials differed substantially with respect to the numbers of patients included, the status of the diseases, the conditioning regimes used, the doses of HCs and T cells infused, the GVHD-prophylaxis administered and a number of other variables that may have influenced outcome. Keeping in mind that these differences exist, the results available from these trials allow a number of important conclusions that are summarized below.

Engraftment

Transplantation of allogeneic PBHCs results in faster engraftment of HCs of all lineages as compared to BMT. Neutrophils exceed a threshold of 0.5×10^9 cells/L between 2 and 6 days earlier with PBHC than after BMT. In the US trial the neutrophils surpassed 0.5×10^9/L on day 16 (range: 11–29 days) with PB and on day 21 (range: 13–36 days) with BM ($p < 0.001$) [114]. The Canadian study reported neutrophil recovery on day 19 (range: 12–35 days) with PB and on day 23 (range: 13–68 days) with BM [116]. Patients in the EBMT study had the shortest time interval from transplantation to an absolute neutrophil count (ANC) $>0.5 \times 10^9$/L: 12 days for PB and 15 days for BM [120]. However, this trial was the only one of the randomized studies which used G-CSF (5 µg/kg/day) after transplantation as well and day 11 methotrexate (MTX) was not included. Two other randomized trials proved that the administration of G-CSF at a dose of 10 µg/kg/day after PBHCT can accelerate neutrophil recovery by 3–4 days [122,123]. Platelet recovery after allogeneic PBHCT is also faster by approximately 6 days. A platelet count of 20×10^9/L was reached on day 13 (range: 5–41 days) with PB and on day 19 (range: 7–74 days) with BM in the US study ($p < 0.001$) [114]. The Canadian study reported platelet recovery after 16 days (range: 0–100 days) for patients grafted with PB and 22 days (0–100 days) for patients grafted with BM ($p < 0.0001$) [116]. The EBMT study had a median time to platelet recovery $>20 \times 10^9$/L of 15 days for patients transplanted with PB and 20 days for patients transplanted with BM ($p > 0.0001$) [120]. This difference translated into a median of 8 days (range: 1–68 days) of platelet transfusions in the PBHCT group and a median of 10 days (range: 2–71 days) in the BMT group ($p = 0.0029$).

It is well recognized that factors other than the source of HCs influence the pace of hematological recovery. While G-CSF accelerates neutrophil recovery, MTX given for prophylaxis of GVHD retards hematopoietic reconstitution [124]. Occurrence of GVHD, infection, the grade of genetic disparity between recipient and donor and splenomegaly have all been reported to affect the speed of hematopoietic recovery and could explain the slight variations in times to neutrophil and platelet recovery seen in the randomized trials. Graft failures after PBHCT are not more frequent than after BMT. Comparative studies of hematopoietic chimerism developing after PBHCT and BMT support the notion that transplantation of PB results in fast, complete and durable chimerism [125].

Table 46.3 Acute graft-vs.-host disease (GVHD) grades II–IV.

Reference	PB (%)	BM (%)	p-value
Bensinger et al. [114]	64	57	$p = 0.35$
Blaise et al. [115]	44	42	Not given
Couban et al. [116]	44	44	$p > 0.9$
Heldal et al. [117]	21	10	Not given
Powles et al. [119]	50	47	Not given
Schmitz et al. [120]	52	39	$p = 0.013$
Vigorito et al. [121]	27	19	$p = 0.53$

All percentages represent cumulative incidences at day +100 post-transplant except for the studies by Blaise et al. [115], Heldal et al. [117] and Powles et al. [119] where the actual percentage of patients with acute GVHD at day +100 is given.

Immune recovery

Recovery of immunity after allogeneic PBHCT is at least as quick as after BMT but may be faster with respect to some subgroups of cells with immune functions. Circulating naive (CD4$^+$CD45RA$^+$) and memory (CD4$^+$CD45RO$^+$) helper T cells, B cells and monocytes are found in higher numbers after PBHCT as compared to BMT between 1 and 11 months post-transplant [126]. NK cell numbers did not significantly differ between patients grafted with PB or marrow over the same time period. Proliferative responses to T- and B-cell mitogens (phytohemagglutinine A [PHA], pokeweed mitogen [PWM], tetanus toxoid, Candida) were significantly increased in recipients of PB from HLA-identical donors [126]. Storek et al. [127] studied 115 patients who had been randomly assigned to receive allogeneic marrow or mobilized PB from HLA-identical donors. Between 1 month and 1 year after transplantation the counts of CD4$^+$CD45RA^{high} and CD4$^+$CD45RA$^{low/-}$ T cells were significantly higher after PBHCT. T cells appeared equally functional when challenged by PHA or herpesvirus antigen. Median serum immunoglobulin G levels were similar in both groups of patients. Of note, these authors also reported that infections and severe infections in particular were significantly reduced after PBHCT. The reduced risk was most prominent for fungal infections, intermediate for bacterial infections and least important for viral infections. It remains to be explored to what extent the earlier neutrophil, monocyte and lymphocyte recovery or other, as yet undetected, mechanisms contribute to the reduced risk of infections seen after PBHCT.

Another interesting observation recently published by Lapierre et al. [128] was that 30 days after PBHCT anti-A and/or anti-B titres were significantly increased as compared to BMT. Overall, their data strongly suggest that immunohematological reconstitution after PBHCT is also quicker than after BMT. This observation could explain the cases of acute hemolysis described after ABO-incompatible PBHCT [129,130].

Acute GVHD

The incidences of acute GVHD grades II–IV were similar for both groups of patients in all larger studies except for the largest one by EBMT [120]. The EBMT study noted a 13% increase of acute GVHD grades II–IV ($p = 0.013$) with BM and a 12% increase of acute GVHD grades III–IV with PB ($p = 0.0088$) (Table 46.3 [114–117,119–121]). The EBMT study was also the only study where the maximum grade of acute GVHD was the primary endpoint and randomization was stratified for some of the known risk factors of GVHD. Other differences in the design of the EBMT study and the other trials were the inclusion of good-risk patients only, the omission of MTX on day 11 and the use of G-CSF post-transplant. Omission of day 11 MTX has been reported to predispose

Table 46.4 Chronic graft-vs.-host disease (GVHD).

Reference	First report			Reference	Follow-up report at 3 years		
	PB	BM	p-value		PB	BM	p-value
Bensinger et al. [114]	(46%)	(35%)	0.54	Flowers et al. [131]	(63%)	(52%)	0.33
Blaise et al. [115]	(50%)	(28%)	<0.03	Mohty et al. [132]	65%	36%	0.004
Couban et al. [116]	85% (40%)	69% (30%)	0.62 (0.37)				
Schmitz et al. [120]	(67%)	(54%)	0.0066	Schmitz, unpublished data	73% (36%)	55% (19%)	0.003

%, overall chronic GVHD; (% in brackets), extensive chronic GVHD.
BM, bone marrow; PB, peripheral blood.

recipients to develop GVHD, but other causes for the higher frequency of GVHD observed in that study cannot be excluded [124]. It also remains in question if the high numbers of T cells transferred with a typical PBHC graft are responsible for the higher incidence of acute GVHD. Although a correlation between GVHD and T-cell numbers was detected in the EBMT study [120], lower numbers of NK cells in the graft and the source of stem cells—independent from the number of T and NK cells—also significantly correlated with the occurrence of acute GVHD.

Chronic GVHD

The large randomized studies all showed a trend towards more chronic GVHD with PBHCs (Table 46.4 [114–116,131,132]), and two studies reported statistically significantly more chronic GVHD after PBHCT [115,120]. There was also more extensive chronic GVHD in patients who had received PBHCs compared with BM cells. This difference was significant in the EBMT trial [120] and in the studies chaired by Blaise et al. [115] and Vigorito et al. [121]. Because the median follow-up of patients in the randomized trials was between 24 and 33 months only further follow-up was necessary to confirm these findings. Recently, follow-up reports from the US [131] and French [132] trials have been published with a median follow-up of 41 months. Flowers et al. [131] still did not observe more chronic GVHD after PBHCT and the clinical characteristics of chronic GVHD were similar after PBHCT or BMT. However, the updated study showed that chronic GVHD was more difficult to control when it occurred after PBHCT as compared to BMT. The number of successive treatments needed to control chronic GVHD was higher after PBHCT and the duration of glucocorticoid treatment was also longer ($p = 0.03$ for both endpoints). In contrast, Mohty et al. [132] found a highly significant difference in the 3-year cumulative incidence of chronic GVHD in the PBHC group compared with the BM group (65% vs. 36%, $p = 0.004$). They also observed significantly more extensive chronic GVHD. Chronic GVHD needed further immunosuppression and led to longer periods of hospitalization. No survival difference was observed so far. Three-year follow-up of the prospective EBMT trial showed more chronic GVHD in patients transplanted with PB as compared to BM (Table 46.4). More detailed analyses are ongoing. The 5-year follow-up of the retrospective IBMTR and EBMT study also revealed more chronic GVHD in patients after PBHCT [133]. Overall, the massive fears created by early reports of frequent and severe chronic GVHD [134–136] were not confirmed by the randomized studies. However, there is evidence that PBHCT causes more chronic GVHD or at least chronic GVHD that is more difficult to treat. The picture is not yet complete, however, and further updates from the large randomized trials are eagerly awaited.

Relapse rates

Knowing that the graft-vs.-leukemia effect (GVLE) is exerted mainly by donor T cells and that around 10 times more T cells are transferred with a typical PB collection product, it was anticipated that transplantation of PB cells would result in a reduction of relapse rates after PBHCT. Animal studies [137] and results of nonrandomized studies [138] also pointed in that direction. The randomized studies have not generally confirmed these expectations so far, although the US study [114] and the small British study [119] indeed reported significantly less patients with relapse after PBHCT than after BMT. Again, follow-up, particularly for good-risk patients treated within the randomized trials, is short and only time will tell if relapse rates after PBHCT and BMT are different.

Transplant-related mortality

Retrospective analyses had suggested a trend in favor of lower transplant-related mortality (TRM) after PBHCT. Specifically, the EBMT and IBMTR study showed a significant advantage in 1-year TRM for patients transplanted with PB for advanced leukemias [113]. The randomized US study reported a cumulative incidence of transplantation-related deaths of 21% in the PB group and 30% in the BM group; however, this difference was not significant [114]. The Canadian study also found a reduction in nonrelapse deaths after PBHCT as opposed to BMT. At day +100 the actuarial probabilities of death were 7.4% for the PB group and 16.1% for the BM group, respectively ($p = 0.07$) [116]. Until now, significant differences have not been reported from any of the randomized studies and it remains to be determined if subgroups of patients with specific diseases or disease status benefit from the transplantation of PB because TRM is reduced.

Survival

Survival is the most relevant endpoint of studies comparing BMT with PBHCT. It is of particular interest in this setting because different sources of HCs may have different effects on secondary endpoints like TRM, relapse rate or GVHD, and the interplay of these may give different results for overall survival if different clinical situations are considered. The three largest randomized studies came to different conclusions with respect to survival. The EBMT study had overlapping survival curves for patients grafted with PB or BM [120]. The US study reported a difference in overall survival of 12% at 2 years between both groups of patients favoring PBHCT: this difference was borderline significant ($p = 0.06$) [114]. The subgroup of patients with more advanced disease had a statistically significantly better survival (57%) with PB than with BM (33%) ($p = 0.04$). The Canadian study reported better overall survival for the whole group of patients transplanted with PB (68%) compared with the BMT group (60%) at 30 months ($p = 0.04$) [112]. As in the US study, the survival benefit mainly rested with the advanced disease patients while patients with early disease did not show significant differences. In a subgroup analysis survival was significantly better for patients with chronic myeloid leukemia (CML) and a trend in this direction was observed for patients with MDS, while patients with acute myeloid leukemia (AML) had comparable survival with either source of HCs. Taking these data and the experience of the other randomized or retrospective analyses into account, one may conclude that transplantation of allogeneic PBHCs will result in survival rates at least as good as those seen after BMT. Patients with advanced leukemias may have better outcomes after PBHCT than after BMT. For many patients and clinical situations, however, further studies will be necessary before definite conclusions can be drawn.

Mobilized BM for allogeneic transplantation

Several investigators have used G-CSF stimulated BM for hematopoietic reconstitution after myeloablative therapy and compared engraftment and development of GVHD to patients who were rescued with G-CSF-mobilized PB [139]. A small prospective study (57 patients were randomized) comparing G-CSF primed BM with G-CSF mobilized PBHCs concluded that engraftment after transplantation of either source of HCs was comparable; however, more steroid refractory acute GVHD, chronic GVHD and prolonged requirement for immunosupppressive therapy was found after PBHCT [140]. Survival did not significantly differ. Larger randomized studies are needed to clearly define the role of G-CSF stimulated BM as compared to G-CSF mobilized blood.

Allogeneic peripheral blood progenitor cell transplantation (PBPCT) in diseases other than leukemia

The prospective studies comparing BMT with PBHCT, as well as most retrospective analyses, include patients with leukemia and a few cases with lymphoma or myeloma. It is therefore largely unknown how patients with diseases other than leukemia would fare after either procedure. Recently, EBMT published their experience with BMT or PBHCT in patients with MDS [141]. The results of this retrospective study were similar to the results of the large retrospective analysis of patients with acute leukemias and CML published by IBMTR and EBMT: earlier hematopoietic recovery, similar incidences of acute but more chronic GVHD with PB [113]. The 2-year TRM was significantly reduced with PB except for patients who had refractory anemia or high-risk cytogenetics. Treatment failure incidence was significantly decreased with PB. Estimates of the 2-year event-free survival were 50% with PBHC vs. 39% with BM. Gahrton et al. [142] compared PBHCT with BMT in patients with multiple myeloma. They did not find significant differences between BMT and PBHCT for TRM, acute and chronic GVHD, progression-free survival or relapse rates: overall survival tended to be better in the BMT group (53% vs. 44% at 3 years, $p = 0.05$). No comparisons of BMT with PBHCT are available so far for patients with lymphoma or nonmalignant diseases. In these and other entities, prospective studies are needed to help clinicians decide whether patients should receive HCs from PB or from BM.

T-cell-depleted mobilized blood

From the beginning the interest in T-cell-depletion strategies was high because of concerns that the large numbers of T cells contained in mobilized PB would cause more frequent and severe GVHD. Soon after the first transplants with mobilized PB were reported, a number of studies using T-cell-depleted mobilized PB were initiated [143,144]. Early results, however, were disappointing because—among other causes—depletion methods were far from optimal. With residual T-cell numbers in excess of 1×10^5 T cells/kg recipient body weight in the graft it was not too surprising to see that acute and severe GVHD still occurred with incidences comparable to those observed after transplantation of unmanipulated PBHCs.

With further experience technical problems were solved and it became possible to routinely purge PB collection products to a residual T-cell content of below 1×10^4 T cells/kg. Such minimal T-cell load is not sufficient to elicit clinical GVHD even in the haplo-identical setting [49]. When BM was exclusively used as the source of HCs, one of the major problems of T-cell depletion was the increase in graft failures occurring after transplantation. Because CD34$^+$ cell numbers are much higher in mobilized PB, and the eventual loss of HCs caused by the depletion process can be compensated for by further leukaphereses, graft failure is less of a problem after transplantation of T-depleted mobilized PB. Urbano-Ispizua et al. [145] reported that the graft failure rate was still 18% after T-cell-depleted PBHCT if $<2 \times 10^5$ CD3$^+$ T cells remained in the graft while the incidence was very low (1%) if $>2 \times 10^5$ T cells were infused. It should be noted, however, that in this study relatively low numbers of CD34$^+$ cells (3.4×10^6/kg) had been infused into patients who subsequently suffered graft failure. Other studies suggest that transplantation of very high numbers of CD34$^+$ cells can overcome the graft failure risk in the HLA-identical [146] and the mismatched setting [49] regardless of the residual number of T cells in the graft.

Transplantation of CD34$^+$ selected cells from mobilized PB to patients with early myeloid malignancies may result in less GVHD, less TRM and better disease-free survival if compared to unmanipulated PBHCT [147]. Although moderate T-cell depletion achieved by CD34$^+$ selection may be one strategy to improve outcome in early disease patients, there is little hope that T-cell depletion will be of much help in more advanced disease. Previous experience with BM [148] and experimental data in mice [149] clearly indicate that T-cell depletion abrogates the GVL-activity and thus leads to increased relapse rates.

In summary, the availability of HCs from PB is important in the context of T-cell-depletion strategies because GVHD can virtually be eliminated without a dramatic increase of graft failure rates when high to very high numbers of HCs are transferred. T cells, however, are mediators of the GVLE and contribute to quick immune reconstitution after transplantation. For these reasons transplantation of T-depleted mobilized blood will have a limited role in allogeneic transplantation of patients with advanced or chemoresistant disease. Rather, T-depleted mobilized PB should be seen as a versatile source of practically unlimited numbers of HCs. These can then be used for various types of manipulation to the benefit of the patient.

Unrelated donor transplants

In contrast to the HLA-identical setting no randomized trials comparing allogeneic PBHCT with BMT in unrelated donors have been published. Concerns regarding the side-effects of G-CSF administration to healthy volunteers, and the big logistical problems with such an inevitably worldwide effort, have so far prevented the scientific community from performing such a trial. However, most donor registries have become more open to the idea of having their donors donate mobilized PB instead of BM and activities in this direction continue (see Chapter 42). For the time being, the available information on the outcome of transplants with mobilized PB in unrelated donors is limited. The largest study so far was published in 1999 by Ringdén et al. [150]. In a retrospective comparison with BMT they reported faster engraftment with PB: acute GVHD, 1-year TRM and overall survival did not significantly differ after PBHCT or BMT. The study had only 45 patients in each arm, 18 more patients had received CD34-selected PB. Therefore, observations must be rated as preliminary and no definite conclusions can yet be drawn.

Conclusions and future developments

A clear-cut picture of the advantages and disadvantages of G-CSF administration and the collection of HCs from PB has evolved over recent years. Unexpected long-term effects of PBHC harvesting, however, cannot be totally excluded at this time. Because the demand for HCs will steadily increase and older individuals as well as donors with comorbidities will increasingly be involved, continued observation of PBHC donors is mandatory. Many potential donors and medical community members currently prefer to work with HCs from PB. This is a consequence of the results of the clinical trials available so far, but it is also dictated by recent developments in other areas of blood and marrow transplantation including nonmyeloablative conditioning, exhaustive T-cell depletion and transplantation across major HLA barriers, all of which require high to extremely high numbers of HCs, which usually cannot be harvested from BM. In the near future patients will likely receive cocktails of HCs plus an array of other cells with distinct immune functions tailored to each patient's needs. Probably, all of these cells can be harvested or grown from the PB. One of the most exciting questions today is if, with our increased understanding of basic immunology, it will be possible to dissect GVHD from the GVLE, both exerted by donor T cells. Future work will also show if blood can act as a source of truly pluripotent stem cells that can be used in the treatment of nonhematopoietic diseases, including cardiac failure or Parkinson's disease.

References

1 Maximow A. Der Lymphozyt als gemeinsame Stammzelle der verschiedenen Blutelemente in der embryonalen Entwicklung und im postfetalen Leben der Säugetiere. *Folia Haemat (Lpz)* 1909; **8**: 125–41.

2 Goodman JW, Hodgson GS. Evidence for stem cells in the peripheral blood of mice. *Blood* 1962; **19**: 702–14.

3 Abrams RA, Glaubiger D, Appelbaum FR et al. Result of attempted hematopoietic reconstitution using isologous, peripheral blood mononuclear cells: a case report. *Blood* 1980; **56**: 516–20.

4 Juttner CA, To LB, Haylock DN et al. Circulating autologous stem cells collected in very early remission from acute non-lymphoblastic leukemia produce prompt but incomplete haemopoietic reconstitution after high dose melphalan or supralethal chemoradiotherapy. *Br J Haematol* 1985; **61**: 739–45.

5 Körbling M, Dörken B, Ho AD et al. Autologous transplantation of blood-derived hemopoietic stem cells after myeloablative therapy in a patient with Burkitt's lymphoma. *Blood* 1986; **67**: 529–32.

6 Kessinger A, Armitage JO, Landmark JD et al. Reconstitution of human hematopoietic function with autologous cryopreserved circulating stem cells. *Exp Hematol* 1986; **14**: 192–6.

7 Reiffers J, Bernard P, David B et al. Successful autologous transplantation with peripheral blood hemopoietic cells in a patient with acute leukemia. *Exp Hematol* 1986; **14**: 312–5.

8 Socinski MA, Elias A, Schnipper L et al. Granulocyte-macrophage colony stimulating factor expands the circulating haemopoietic progenitor cell compartment in man. *Lancet* 1988; **1**: 1194–8.

9 Dührsen U, Villeval JL, Boyd J et al. Effects of recombinant human granulocyte colony-stimulating factor on hematopoietic cells in cancer patients. *Blood* 1988; **72**: 2074–81.

10 Kessinger A, Smith DM, Strandjord SE et al. Allogeneic transplantation of blood-derived, T cell-depleted hemopoietic stem cells after myeloablative treatment in a patient with acute lymphoblastic leukemia. *Bone Marrow Transplant* 1989; **4**: 643–6.

11 Dreger P, Suttorp M, Haferlach T et al. Allogeneic granulocyte colony-stimulating factor-mobilized peripheral blood progenitor cells for treatment of engraftment failure after bone marrow transplantation. *Blood* 1993; **81**: 1404–7.

12 Russell NH, Hunter A, Rogers S et al. Peripheral blood stem cells as an alternative to marrow for allogeneic transplantation. *Lancet* 1993; **341**: 1482.

13 Bensinger WI, Weaver CH, Appelbaum FR et al. Transplantation of allogeneic peripheral blood stem cells mobilized by recombinant human granulocyte colony-stimulating factor. *Blood* 1995; **85**: 1655–8.

14 Körbling M, Przepiorka D, Huh YO et al. Allogeneic blood stem cell transplantation for refractory leukemia and lymphoma: potential advantage of blood over marrow allografts. *Blood* 1995; **85**: 1659–65.

15 Schmitz N, Dreger P, Suttorp M et al. Primary transplantation of allogeneic peripheral blood progenitor cells mobilized by filgrastim (granulocyte colony-stimulating factor). *Blood* 1995; **85**: 1666–72.

16 Gratwohl A, Baldomero H, Passweg J. et al. Increasing use of reduced intensity conditioning transplants: report of the EBMT activity survey. *Bone Marrow Transplant* 2002; **30**: 813–31.

17 Bensinger WI, Price TH, Dale DC et al. The effects of daily recombinant human granulocyte colony-stimulating factor administration on normal granulocyte donors undergoing leukapheresis. *Blood* 1993; **81**: 1883–8.

18 Chao NJ, Schriber JR, Grimes K et al. Granulocyte colony-stimulating factor 'mobilized' peripheral blood progenitor cells accelerate granulocyte and platelet recovery after high-dose chemotherapy. *Blood* 1993; **81**: 2031–5.

19 Schmitz N, Linch DC, Dreger P et al. Randomised trial of filgrastim-mobilized peripheral progenitor cell transplantation versus autologous bone-marrow transplantation in lymphoma patients. *Lancet* 1996; **347**: 353–7.

20 Matsunaga T, Sakamaki S, Kohgo Y et al. Recombinant human granulocyte colony-stimulating factor can mobilize sufficient amounts of peripheral blood stem cells in healthy volunteers for allogeneic transplantation. *Bone Marrow Transplant* 1993; **11**: 103–8.

21 Dreger P, Haferlach T, Eckstein V et al. G-CSF-mobilized peripheral blood progenitor cells for allogeneic transplantation: safety, kinetics of mobilization, and composition of the graft. *Br J Haematol* 1994; **87**: 609–13.

22 Sato N, Sawada K, Takahashi TA et al. A time course study for optimal harvest of peripheral blood progenitor cells by granulocyte-stimulating factor in healthy volunteers. *Exp Hematol* 1994; **22**: 973–8.

23 Grigg AP, Roberts AW, Raunow H et al. Optimizing dose and scheduling of filgrastim (granulocyte colony-stimulating factor) for mobilization and collection of peripheral blood progenitor cells in normal volunteers. *Blood* 1995; **86**: 4437–45.

24 Miflin G, Charley C, Stainer C et al. Stem cell mobilization in normal donors for allogeneic transplantation: analysis of safety and factors affecting efficacy. *Br J Haematol* 1996; **95**: 345–8.

25 Tanaka R, Matsudaira T, Aizawa J et al. Characterization of peripheral blood progenitor cells (PBPC) mobilized by filgrastim (rHuG-CSF) in normal volunteers: dose–effect relationship for filgrastim with the character of mobilized PBPC. *Br J Haematol* 1996; **92**: 795–03.

26 Anderlini P, Prezpiorka D, Huh Y et al. Duration of filgrastim mobilization and apheresis yield of CD34$^+$ progenitor cells and lymphoid subsets in normal donors for allogeneic transplantation. *Br J Haematol* 1996; **93**: 940–2.

27 Höglund M, Smedmyr B, Simonsson B et al. Dose-dependent mobilization of haematopoietic progenitor cells in healthy volunteers receiving glycosylated rHuG-CSF. *Bone Marrow Transplant* 1996; **18**: 19–27.

28 Bishop MR, Tarantolo SR, Jackson JD et al. Allogeneic-blood stem-cell collection following mobilization with low-dose granulocyte colony-stimulating factor. *J Clin Oncol* 1997; **15**: 1601–7.

29 Arbona C, Prosper F, Benet I et al. Comparison between once a day vs. twice a day G-CSF for mobilization of peripheral blood progenitor cells (PBPC) in normal donors for allogeneic PBPC transplantation. *Bone Marrow Transplant* 1998; **22**: 39–45.

30 Engelhardt M, Bertz H, Afting M et al. High- versus standard-dose filgrastim (rhG-CSF) for mobilization of peripheral-blood progenitor cells from allogeneic donors and CD34$^+$ immunoselection. *J Clin Oncol* 1999; **17**: 2160–72.

31 Martinez C, Urbano-Ispizua A, Marin P et al. Efficacy and toxicity of a high-dose G-CSF schedule for peripheral blood progenitor cell mobilization in healthy donors. *Bone Marrow Transplant* 1999; **24**: 1273–8.

32 Kröger N, Renges H, Krüger W et al. A randomized comparison of once versus twice daily recombinant human granulocyte colony-stimulating factor (filgrastim) for stem cell mobilization in healthy donors for allogeneic transplantation. *Br J Haematol* 2000; **111**: 761–5.

33 Anderlini P, Donato M, Lauppe MJ et al. A comparative study of once-daily versus twice-daily filgrastim administration for the mobilization and collection of CD34$^+$ peripheral blood progenitor cells in normal donors. *Br J Haematol* 2000; **109**: 770–2.

34 Basara N, Schmetzer B, Blau IW et al. Lenograstim-mobilized peripheral blood progenitor cells in volunteer donors: an open label randomized split

dose escalating study. *Bone Marrow Transplant* 2000; **25**: 371–6.

35 Anderlini P, Rizzo JD, Nugent ML *et al.* Peripheral blood stem cell donation: an analysis from the International Bone Marrow Transplant Registry (IBMTR) and European Group for Blood and Marrow Transplant (EBMT). *Bone Marrow Transplant* 2001; **27**: 689–92.

36 de la Rubia J, Martínez C, Solano C *et al.* Administration of recombinant human granulocyte colony-stimulating factor to normal donors: results of the Spanish National Donor Registry. *Bone Marrow Transplant* 1999; **24**: 723–8.

37 Carlo-Stella C, Cesana C, Regazzi E *et al.* Peripheral blood progenitor cell mobilization in healthy donors receiving recombinant human granulocyte colony-stimulating factor. *Exp Hematol* 2000; **28**: 216–24.

38 Lee V, Li CK, Shing MM *et al.* Single vs. twice daily G-CSF dose for peripheral blood stem cells harvest in normal donors and children with non-malignant diseases. *Bone Marrow Transplant* 2000; **25**: 931–5.

39 Anderlini P, Körbling M, Dale D *et al.* Allogeneic stem cell transplantation: considerations for donors. *Blood* 1997; **90**: 903–8.

40 Russell NH, Gratwohl A, Schmitz N. The place of blood stem cells in allogeneic transplantation. *Br J Haematol* 1996; **93**: 747–53.

41 Weaver CH, Birch R, Greco FA *et al.* Mobilization and harvesting of peripheral blood stem cells: randomized evaluations of different doses of filgrastim. *Br J Haematol* 1998; **100**: 338–47.

42 Anderlini P, Przepiorka D, Seong D *et al.* Factors affecting mobilization of CD34$^+$ cells in normal donors treated with filgrastim. *Transfusion* 1997; **37**: 507–12.

43 Brown RA, Adkins D, Goodnough LT *et al.* Factors that influence the collection and engraftment of allogeneic peripheral-blood stem cells in patients with hematologic malignancies. *J Clin Oncol* 1997; **15**: 3067–74.

44 Lane TA, Law P, Maruyama M *et al.* Harvesting and enrichment of hematopoietic progenitor cells mobilized into the peripheral blood of normal donors by granulocyte-macrophage colony-stimulating factor (GM-CSF) or G-CSF. Potential role in allogeneic marrow transplantation. *Blood* 1995; **85**: 275–82.

45 Sohn SK, Kim JG, Seo KW *et al.* GM-CSF-based mobilization effect in normal healthy donors for allogeneic peripheral blood stem cell transplantation. *Bone Marrow Transplant* 2002; **30**: 81–6.

46 Huhn RD, Yurkow EJ, Tushinski R *et al.* Recombinant human interleukin-3 (rhIL-3) enhances the mobilization of peripheral blood progenitor cells by recombinant human granulocyte colony-stimulating factor (rhG-CSF) in normal volunteers. *Exp Hematol* 1996; **24**: 839–47.

47 Andrews RG, Briddell RA, Knitter GH *et al. In vivo* synergy between recombinant human stem cell factor and recombinant human granulocyte colony-stimulating factor in baboons: enhanced circulation of progenitor cells. *Blood* 1994; **84**: 800–10.

48 Papayannopoulou T, Nakamoto B, Andrews RG *et al. In vivo* effects for Flt3/Flk2 ligand on mobilization of hematopoietic progenitors in primates and potent synergistic enhancement with granulocyte colony-stimulating factor. *Blood* 1997; **90**: 620–9.

49 Martelli MF, Aversa F, Bachar-Lustig E *et al.* Transplants across human leukocyte antigen barriers. *Semin Hematol* 2002; **39**: 48–56.

50 Uharek L, Gassmann W, Glass B *et al.* Influence of cell dose and graft-versus-host reactivity on rejection rates after allogeneic bone marrow transplantation. *Blood* 1992; **79**: 1612–21.

51 Singhal S, Powles R, Treleaven J *et al.* A low CD34$^+$ cell dose results in higher mortality and poorer survival after blood or marrow stem cell transplantation from HLA-identical siblings: should 2×10^6 CD34$^+$ cells/kg be considered the minimum threshold? *Bone Marrow Transplant* 2000; **26**: 489–96.

52 Mavroudis D, Read E, Cottler-Fox M *et al.* CD34$^+$ cell dose predicts survival, posttransplant morbidity, and rate of hematologic recovery after allogeneic marrow transplants for hematologic malignancies. *Blood* 1996; **88**: 3223–9.

53 Bittencourt H, Rocha V, Chevret S *et al.* Association of CD34 cell dose with hematopoietic recovery, infections, and other outcomes after HLA-identical sibling bone marrow transplantation. *Blood* 2002; **99**: 2726–33.

54 Przepiorka D, Smith TL, Folloder J *et al.* Risk factors for acute graft-versus-host disease after allogeneic blood stem cell transplantation. *Blood* 1999; **94**: 1465–70.

55 Körbling M, Huh YO, Durett A *et al.* Allogeneic blood stem cell transplantation: peripheralization and yield of donor-derived primitive hematopoietic progenitor cells (CD34$^+$Thy-1^{dim}) and lymphoid subsets, and possible predictors of engraftment and graft-versus-host disease. *Blood* 1995; **86**: 2842–8.

56 Körbling M, Anderlini P, Durett A *et al.* Delayed effects of rhG-CSF mobilization treatment and apheresis on circulating CD34$^+$ and CD34$^+$Thy-1^{dim}CD38$^-$ progenitor cells, and lymphoid subsets in normal stem cell donors for allogeneic transplantation. *Bone Marrow Transplant* 1996; **18**: 1073–9.

57 To LB, Haylock DN, Dowse T *et al.* A comparative study of the phenotype and proliferative capacity of peripheral blood (PB) CD34$^+$ cells mobilized by four different protocols and those of steady-phase PB and bone marrow CD34$^+$ cells. *Blood* 1994; **84**: 2930–9.

58 Gyger M, Stuart RK, Perreault C. Immunobiology of allogeneic peripheral blood mononuclear cells mobilized with granulocyte-colony stimulating factor. *Bone Marrow Transplant* 2000; **26**: 1–16.

59 Tjonnford GE, Stein R, Evensen AS *et al.* Characterization of CD34$^+$ peripheral blood cells from healthy adults mobilized by recombinant human granulocyte colony-stimulating factor. *Blood* 1994; **84**: 2795–801.

60 Uchida N, He D, Friera AM *et al.* The unexpected G_0/G_1 cell cycle status of mobilized hematopoietic stem cells from peripheral blood. *Blood* 1997; **89**: 1189–96.

61 Steidl U, Kronenwett R, Rohr UP *et al.* Gene expression profiling identifies significant differences between the molecular phenotypes of bone marrow-derived and circulating human CD34$^+$ hematopoietic stem cells. *Blood* 2002; **99**: 2037–44.

62 Prosper F, Stroncek D, Verfaillie M. Phenotypic and functional characterization of long-term culture-initiating cells present in peripheral blood progenitor collections of normal donors treated with granulocyte colony-stimulating factor. *Blood* 1996; **88**: 2033–42.

63 Weaver CH, Longin K, Buckner CD *et al.* Lymphocyte content in peripheral blood mononuclear cells collected after the administration of recombinant human granulocyte colony-stimulating factor. *Bone Marrow Transplant* 1994; **13**: 411–5.

64 Pan L, Delmonte J, Jalonen CK *et al.* Pretreatment of donor mice with granulocyte colony-stimulating factor polarizes donor T lymphocytes toward type-2 cytokine production and reduces severity of experimental graft-versus-host disease. *Blood* 1995; **86**: 4422–9.

65 Sloand EM, Kim S, Maciejewski JP *et al.* Pharmacologic doses of granulocyte colony-stimulating factor affect cytokine production by lymphocytes *in vitro* and *in vivo*. *Blood* 2000; **95**: 2269–74.

66 Kitabayashi A, Hirokawa M, Hatano Y *et al.* Granulocyte colony-stimulating factor downregulates allogeneic immune responses by posttranscriptional inhibition of tumor necrosis factor-α production. *Blood* 1995; **86**: 2220–7.

67 Kusnierz-Glaz CR, Still BJ, Amano M *et al.* Granulocyte colony-stimulating factor-induced comobilization of CD4$^-$CD8$^-$ T cells and hematopoietic progenitor cells (CD34$^+$) in the blood of normal donors. *Blood* 1997; **89**: 2586–95.

68 Mielcarek M, Roecklein BA, Torok-Storb B. CD14$^+$ cells in granulocyte colony-stimulating factor (G-CSF)-mobilized peripheral blood mononuclear cells induce secretion of interleukin-6 and G-CSF by marrow stroma. *Blood* 1996; **87**: 574–80.

69 Mielcarek M, Martin PJ, Torok-Storb B. Suppression of alloantigen-induced T-cell proliferation by CD14$^+$ cells derived from granulocyte colony-stimulating factor-mobilized peripheral blood mononuclear cells. *Blood* 1997; **89**: 1629–34.

70 Arpinati M, Green CL, Heimfeld S *et al.* Granulocyte-colony stimulating factor mobilizes T helper 2-inducing dendritic cells. *Blood* 2000; **95**: 2484–70.

71 Joshi SS, Lynch JC, Pavletic SZ *et al.* Decreased immune functions of blood cells following mobilization with granulocyte colony-stimulating factor: association with donor characteristics. *Blood* 2001; **98**: 1963–70.

72 de Haas M, Kerst JM, van der Schoot E *et al.* Granulocyte colony-stimulating factor administration to healthy volunteers: analysis of the immediate activating effects on circulating neutrophils. *Blood* 1994; **84**: 3885–94.

73 Papayannopoulon T, Nakamoto B. Peripheralization of hemopoietic progenitor in primates treated with anti-VLA-4 integrin. *Proc Natl Acad Sci U S A* 1993; **90**: 9374–8.

74 Levesque JP, Takamatsu I, Nilsson SK *et al.* Mobilization of hemopoietic progenitor cells into peripheral blood is associated with VCAM-1 proteolytic cleavage in the bone marrow. *Blood* 2000; **96**: 221a [Abstract].

75 Anderlini P, Przepiorka D, Champlin R *et al.* Biologic and clinical effects of granulocyte colony-stimulating factor in normal individuals. *Blood* 1996; **88**: 2819–25.

76 Anderlini P, Lauppe J, Przepiorka D *et al.* Peripheral blood stem cell apheresis in normal donors: feasibility and yield of second collections. *Br J Haematol* 1997; **96**: 415–7.

77 Murata M, Harada M, Kato S *et al.* Peripheral blood stem cell mobilization and apheresis: analysis of adverse events in 94 normal donors. *Bone Marrow Transplant* 1999; **24**: 1065–71.

78 Stroncek DF, Clay ME, Petzoldt ML *et al.* Treatment of normal individuals with granulocyte-colony-stimulating factor: donor experiences and the effects on peripheral blood CD34$^+$ cell counts

and on the collection of peripheral blood stem cells. *Transfusion* 1996; **36**: 601–10.
79 Fossa SD, Poulsen JP, Aaserud A. Alkaline phosphatase and lactate dehydrogenase changes during leucocytosis induced by G-CSF in testicular cancer. *Lancet* 1992; **340**: 1544.
80 Söhngen D, Wienen S, Siebler M et al. Analysis of rhG-CSF-effects on platelets by *in vitro* bleeding test and transcranial Doppler ultrasound examination. *Bone Marrow Transplant* 1998; **22**: 1087–90.
81 LeBlanc R, Roy J, Demers C et al. A prospective study of G-CSF effects on hemostasis in allogeneic blood stem cell donors. *Bone Marrow Transplant* 1999; **23**: 991–6.
82 Falanga A, Marchetti M, Evangelista V et al. Neutrophil activation and hemostatic changes in healthy donors receiving granulocyte colony-stimulating factor. *Blood* 1999; **93**: 2506–14.
83 Shimoda K, Okamura S, Inaba S et al. Granulocyte colony-stimulating factor and platelet aggregation. *Lancet* 1993; **341**: 633.
84 Anderlini P, Przepiorka D, Seong D et al. Transient neutropenia in normal donors after G-CSF mobilization and stem cell apheresis. *Br J Haematol* 1996; **94**: 155–8.
85 Lindemann A, Herrmann F, Oster W et al. Hematologic effects of recombinant human granulocyte colony-stimulating factor in patients with malignancy. *Blood* 1989; **74**: 2644–51.
86 Wiesneth M, Schreiner T, Friedrich W et al. Mobilization and collection of allogeneic peripheral blood progenitor cells for transplantation. *Bone Marrow Transplant* 1998; **21**: 21–4.
87 Becker PS, Wagle M, Matous S et al. Spontaneous splenic rupture following administration of granulocyte colony-stimulating factor (G-CSF): occurrence in an allogeneic donor of peripheral blood stem cells. *Biol Blood Marrow Transplant* 1997; **3**: 345–9.
88 Falzetti F, Aversa F, Minelli O et al. Spontaneous rupture of spleen during peripheral blood stem-cell mobilization in a healthy donor. *Lancet* 1999; **353**: 555.
89 Cavallaro AM, Lilleby K, Majolino I et al. Three to six year follow-up of normal donors who received recombinant human granulocyte colony stimulating factor. *Bone Marrow Transplant* 2000; **25**: 85–9.
90 Parkkali T, Volin L, Sirèn MK et al. Acute iritis induced by granulocyte colony-stimulating factor used for mobilization in a volunteer unrelated peripheral blood progenitor cell donor. *Bone Marrow Transplant* 1996; **17**: 433–4.
91 Hilbe W, Nussbaumer W, Bonatti H et al. Unusual adverse events following peripheral blood stem cell (PBSC) mobilization using granulocyte colony stimulating factor (G-CSF) in healthy donors (Case Report). *Bone Marrow Transplant* 2000; **26**: 811–3.
92 Spitzer T, McAfee S, Poliquin C et al. Acute gouty arthritis following recombinant human granulocyte colony-stimulating factor therapy in an allogeneic blood stem cell donor (Correspondence). *Bone Marrow Transplant* 1998; **21**: 966–7.
93 Adkins DR. Anaphylactoid reaction in a normal donor given granulocyte colony-stimulating factor. *J Clin Oncol* 1998; **16**: 812–3.
94 Favre G, Beksac M, Bacigalupo A et al. Blood or bone marrow? Graft product and donor aspects. *Bone Marrow Transplant*, in press.
95 Rowley SC, Donaldson G, Lilleby K et al. Experiences of donors enrolled in a randomized study of allogeneic bone marrow or peripheral blood stem cell transplantation. *Blood* 2001; **97**: 2541–8.

96 Fortanier C, Kuentz M, Sutton L et al. Healthy sibling donor anxiety and pain during bone marrow or peripheral blood stem cell harvesting for allogeneic transplantation: results of a randomised study. *Bone Marrow Transplant* 2002; **29**: 145–9.
97 Heldal D, Brinch L, Tjonnfjord G et al. Donation of stem cells from blood or bone marrow: results of a randomised study of safety and complaints. *Bone Marrow Transplant* 2002; **29**: 479–86.
98 Switzer GE, Goycoolea JM, Dew MA et al. Donating stimulated peripheral blood stem cells vs. bone marrow: do donors experience the procedures differently? *Bone Marrow Transplant* 2001; **27**: 917–23.
99 Auquier P, Macquart-Moulin G, Moatti JP et al. Comparison of anxiety, pain and discomfort in two procedures of hematopoietic stem cell collection: leukacytapheresis and bone marrow harvest. *Bone Marrow Transplant* 1995; **16**: 541–7.
100 Hasenclever D, Sextro M. Safety of allo PBPCT donors: biometrical considerations on monitoring long-term risks. *Bone Marrow Transplant* 1996 (Suppl.); **17**: S28–30.
101 Cottle TE, Fier CJ, Donadieu J et al. Risk and benefit of treatment of severe chronic neutropenia with granulocyte colony-stimulating factor. *Sem Hematol* 2002; **39**: 134–40.
102 Buckner CD, Petersen FB, Bolonesi BA. Bone marrow donors. In: Forman SJ, Blume KG, Thomas ED, eds. *Bone Marrow Transplantation*. Malden, MA: Blackwell Scientific Publications, 1994: 259–70.
103 Schmitz N, Bacigalupo A, Labopin M et al. Transplantation of peripheral blood progenitor cells from HLA-identical sibling donors. *Br J Haematol* 1996; **836**: 1–9.
104 Azevedo WM, Aranha FJP, Gouvea JV et al. Allogeneic transplantation with blood stem cells mobilized by rhG-CSF for hematological malignancies. *Bone Marrow Transplant* 1995; **16**: 647–53.
105 Bacigalupo A, van Lint MT, Valbonesi M et al. Thiotepa cyclophosphamide followed by granulocyte colony-stimulating factor mobilized allogeneic peripheral blood cells in adults with advanced leukemia. *Blood* 1996; **88**: 353–7.
106 Urbano-Ispizua A, Solano C, Brunet S et al. Allogeneic peripheral blood progenitor cell transplantation: analysis of short-term engraftment and acute GVHD incidence in 33 cases. *Bone Marrow Transplant* 1996; **18**: 35–40.
107 Przepiorka D, Anderlini P, Ippoliti C et al. Allogeneic blood stem cell transplantation in advanced hematologic cancers. *Bone Marrow Transplant* 1997; **19**: 455–60.
108 Miflin G, Russell NH, Hutchinson RM et al. Allogeneic peripheral blood stem cell transplantation for haematological malignancies: an analysis of kinetics of engraftment and GVHD risk. *Bone Marrow Transplant* 1997; **19**: 9–13.
109 Lickliter JD, McGlave PB, DeFor TE et al. Matched-pair analysis of peripheral blood stem cells compared to marrow for allogeneic transplantation. *Bone Marrow Transplant* 2000; **26**: 723–8.
110 Bensinger WI, Clift R, Martin P et al. Allogeneic peripheral blood stem cell transplantation in patients with advanced hematologic malignancies: a retrospective comparison with marrow transplantation. *Blood* 1996; **88**: 2794–800.
111 Russell JA, Brown C, Bowen T et al. Allogeneic blood cell transplants for haematological malignancy: preliminary comparison of outcomes with bone marrow transplantation. *Bone Marrow Transplant* 1996; **17**: 703–8.
112 Pavletic ZS, Bishop MR, Tarantolo ST et al. Hematopoietic recovery after allogeneic blood stem-cell transplantation compared with bone marrow transplantation in patients with hematologic malignancies. *J Clin Oncol* 1997; **15**: 1608–16.
113 Champlin RE, Schmitz N, Horowitz MM et al. Blood stem cells compared with bone marrow as a source of hematopoietic cells for allogeneic transplantation. *Blood* 2000; **95**: 3702–9.
114 Bensinger WI, Martin PJ, Storer B et al. Transplantation of bone marrow as compared with peripheral-blood cells from HLA-identical relatives in patients with hematologic cancers. *N Engl J Med* 2001; **344**: 175–81.
115 Blaise D, Kuentz M, Fortanier C et al. Randomized trial of bone marrow versus lenograstim-primed blood cell allogeneic transplantation in patients with early-stage leukemia: a report from the Société Francaise de Greffe de Moelle. *J Clin Oncol* 2000; **18**: 537–46.
116 Couban S, Simpson DR, Barnett MJ et al. A randomized multicenter comparison of bone marrow and peripheral blood in recipients of matched sibling allogeneic transplants for myeloid malignancies. *Blood* 2002; **100**: 1525–31.
117 Heldal D, Tjonnfjord G, Brinch L et al. A randomised study of allogeneic transplantation with stem cells from blood or bone marrow. *Bone Marrow Transplant* 2000; **25**: 1129–36.
118 Mahmoud HK, Fahmy OA, Kamel A et al. Peripheral blood vs. bone marrow as a source for allogeneic hematopoietic stem cell transplantation. *Bone Marrow Transplant* 1999; **24**: 355–8.
119 Powles R, Mehta J, Kulkarni S et al. Allogeneic blood and bone-marrow stem-cell transplantation in haematological malignant diseases: a randomised trial. *Lancet* 2000; **355**: 1231–7.
120 Schmitz N, Beksac M, Hasenclever D et al. Transplantation of mobilized peripheral blood cells to HLA-identical sibling with standard-risk leukemia. *Blood* 2002; **100**: 761–71.
121 Vigorito AC, Azevedo WM, Marques JFC et al. A randomised, prospective comparison of allogeneic bone marrow and peripheral blood progenitor cell transplantation in the treatment of hematological malignancies. *Bone Marrow Transplant* 1998; **22**: 1145–51.
122 Bishop MR, Tarantolo SR, Geller RB et al. A randomized, double-blind trial of filgrastim (granulocyte colony-stimulating factor) versus placebo following allogeneic blood stem cell transplantation. *Blood* 2000; **96**: 80–5.
123 Przepiorka D, Smith TL, Folloder J et al. Controlled trial of filgrastim for acceleration of neutrophil recovery after allogeneic blood stem cell transplantation from human leukocyte antigen-matched related donors. *Blood* 2001; **97**: 3405–10.
124 Nash RA, Pepe MS, Storb R et al. Acute graft-versus-host disease: analysis of risk factors after allogeneic marrow transplantation and prophylaxis with cyclosporine and methotrexate. *Blood* 1992; **80**: 1838–45.
125 Beelen DW, Ottinger HD, Elmaagacli A et al. Transplantation of filgrastim-mobilized peripheral blood stem cells from HLA-identical sibling or alternative family donors in patients with hematologic malignancies: a prospective comparison on clinical outcome, immune reconstitution, and hematopoietic chimerism. *Blood* 1997; **90**: 4725–35.

126 Ottinger HD, Beelen DW, Scheulen B et al. Improved immune reconstitution after allotransplantation of peripheral blood stem cells instead of bone marrow. *Blood* 1996; **88**: 2775–9.

127 Storek J, Dawson MA, Storer B et al. Immune reconstitution after allogeneic marrow transplantation compared with blood stem cell transplantation. *Blood* 2001; **97**: 3380–9.

128 Lapierre V, Oubouzar N, Aupéring A et al. Influence of the hematopoietic stem cell source on early immunohematologic reconstitution after allogeneic transplantation. *Blood* 2001; **97**: 2580–6.

129 Oziel-Taieb S, Faucher-Barbey C, Chabannon C et al. Early and fatal immune haemolysis after so-called 'minor' ABO-incompatible peripheral blood stem cell allotransplantation. *Bone Marrow Transplant* 1997; **19**: 1155–6.

130 Salmon JP, Michaux S, Hermanne JP et al. Delayed massive immune hemolysis mediated by minor ABO incompatibility after allogeneic peripheral blood progenitor cell transplantation. *Transfusion* 1999; **39**: 824–7.

131 Flowers ME, Parker PM, Johnston LJ et al. Comparison of chronic graft-versus-host disease after transplantation of peripheral blood stem cells versus bone marrow in allogeneic recipients: long-term follow-up of a randomized trial. *Blood* 2002; **100**: 415–9.

132 Mohty M, Kuentz M, Michallet M et al. Chronic graft-versus-host disease after allogeneic blood stem cell transplantation: long-term results of a randomized study. *Blood* 2002; **100**: 3128–34.

133 Schmitz N, Champlin RE, Loberiza FR et al. Long term follow-up of allogeneic blood stem cell and bone marrow transplantation: a collaborative study of EBMT and IBMTR. *Blood* 2001; **1**: 744a [Abstract].

134 Majolino I, Saglio G, Scime R et al. High incidence of chronic GVHD after primary allogeneic peripheral blood stem cell transplantation in patients with hematologic malignancies. *Bone Marrow Transplant* 1996; **17**: 555–60.

135 Storek J, Gooley T, Siadak M et al. Allogeneic peripheral blood stem cell transplantation may be associated with a high risk of chronic graft-versus-host disease. *Blood* 1997; **90**: 4705–9.

136 Solano C, Martinez C, Brunet S et al. Chronic graft-versus-host disease after allogeneic peripheral blood progenitor cell or bone marrow transplantation from matched related donors. A case-control study. *Bone Marrow Transplant* 1998; **22**: 1129–35.

137 Glass B, Uharek L, Zeis M et al. Allogeneic peripheral blood progenitor cell transplantation in an murine model: evidence for an improved graft-versus-leukemia effect. *Blood* 1997; **90**: 1694–700.

138 Elmaagacli AH, Beelen DW, Opalka B et al. The risk of residual molecular and cytogenetic disease in patients with Philadelphia-chromosome positive first chronic phase chronic myelogenous leukemia is reduced after transplantation of allogeneic peripheral blood stem cells compared with bone marrow. *Blood* 1999; **94**: 384–9.

139 Serody JS, Sparks SD, Lin Y et al. Comparison of granulocyte colony-stimulating factor (G-CSF)-mobilized peripheral blood progenitor cells and G-CSF stimulated bone marrow as a source of stem cells in HLA-matched sibling transplantation. *Biol Blood Marrow Transplant* 2000; **6**: 434–40.

140 Morton J, Hutchins C, Durrant S. Granulocyte-colony stimulating factor (G-CSF)-primed allogeneic bone marrow. Significantly less graft-versus-host disease and comparable engraftment to G-CSF-mobilized peripheral blood stem cells. *Blood* 2001; **98**: 3186–90.

141 Guardiola P, Runde V, Bacigalupo A et al. Retrospective comparison of bone marrow and granulocyte colony-stimulating factor-mobilized peripheral blood progenitor cells or allogeneic stem cell transplantation using HLA identical sibling donors in myelodysplastic syndromes. *Blood* 2002; **99**: 4370–8.

142 Gahrton G, Apperley J, Bacigalupo A et al. An update of allogeneic transplantation with peripheral blood stem cells (PBSCT) as compared to bone marrow (BMT) in multiple myeloma. *Bone Marrow Transplant* S13: [Abstract 0124].

143 Bensinger WI, Buckner CD, Shannon-Dorcy K et al. Transplantation of allogeneic CD34$^+$ peripheral blood stem cells in patients with advanced hematologic malignancy. *Blood* 1996; **88**: 4132–8.

144 Link H, Arseniev L, Bähre O et al. Transplantation of allogeneic CD34$^+$ blood cells. *Blood* 1996; **87**: 4903–9.

145 Urbano-Ispizua A, Rozman C, Pimentel P et al. The number of donor CD3$^+$ cells is the most important factor for graft failure after allogeneic transplantation of CD34$^+$ selected cells from peripheral blood from HLA-identical siblings. *Blood* 2001; **97**: 383–7.

146 Beelen DW, Peceny R, Elmaagacli A et al. Transplantation of highly purified HLA-identical sibling donor peripheral blood CD34$^+$ cells without prophylactic post-transplant immunosuppression in adult patients with first chronic phase chronic myeloid leukemia: results of a phase II study. *Bone Marrow Transplant* 2000; **26**: 823–9.

147 Urbano-Ispizua A, Brunet S, Solano C et al. Allogeneic transplantation of CD34$^+$-selected cells from peripheral blood in patients with myeloid malignancies in early phase: a case control comparison with unmodified peripheral blood transplantation. *Bone Marrow Transplant* 2001; **28**: 349–54.

148 Marmont AM, Horowitz MM, Gale RP et al. T-cell depletion of HLA-identical transplants in leukemia. *Blood* 1991; **78**: 2120–30.

149 Uharek L, Glass B, Zeis M et al. Abrogation of graft-vs.-leukemia activity after depletion of CD3$^+$ T cells in a murine model of MHC-matched peripheral blood progenitor cell transplantation (PBPCT). *Exp Hematol* 1998; **26**: 93–9.

150 Ringdén O, Remberger M, Runde V et al. Peripheral blood stem cell transplantation from unrelated donors: a comparison with marrow transplantation. *Blood* 1999; **94**: 455–64.

151 Niederwieser D, Maris M, Shizuru JA. Low dose total body irradiation (TBI) and fludarabine followed by hematopoietic cell transplantation (HCT) from HLA-matched or mismatched unrelated donors and postgrafting immunosuppression with cyclosporine and mycophenolate Mofetil (MMF) can induce durable complete chimerism and sustained remissions in patients with hematological diseases. *Blood* 2003; **101**: 1620–9.

152 Russell JA, Luider J, Weaver M. Collection of progenitor cells for allogeneic transplantation from peripheral blood of normal donors. *Bone Marrow Transplant* 1995; **15**: 111–5.

47

Scott D. Rowley

Cryopreservation of Hematopoietic Cells

Introduction

Storage of hematopoietic cells (HCs) is required for transplantation, whether for the brief period required to deliver a freshly harvested bone marrow (BM) or peripheral blood hematopoietic cell (PBHC) product to an allogeneic recipient, or the long-term (potentially decades) banking of cord blood hematopoietic cells (CBHCs) intended for unrelated-donor transplantation. Room temperature or refrigerated (4°C) storage may be appropriate for products stored for a few hours to a few days. Cryopreservation allows longer-term storage and is the storage technique for virtually all products intended for autologous hematopoietic cell transplantation (HCT). Although cryopreservation of HCs is not a requirement for treatment with myeloablative, dose-intensive conditioning regimens, and patients have recovered marrow function after reinfusion of HCs stored for several days at 4°C, a progressive loss of HCs occurs during nonfrozen storage. Definition of ideal conditions (e.g. temperature of storage, initial processing of the cells, cell concentration, additives) for nonfrozen storage of cells may slow this loss. In contrast, although some unavoidable loss of HCs occurs with marrow or PBHC processing and cryopreservation, progressive loss over months to years of proper storage is not obvious and may not occur if optimal storage conditions are maintained. Cryopreservation allows the administration of multiple-day transplant conditioning regimens as well as elective storage of cells for patients to be transplanted at a subsequent point in a course of treatment.

That HCs can be successfully cryopreserved is evident from the successes of autologous and allogeneic HCT in regenerating marrow function after marrow-lethal conditioning regimens. Engraftment failure is generally not attributed to HC cryopreservation. Although some investigators correlated poor HC cryopreservation with delayed engraftment after transplantation [1,2], this deleterious effect is most likely to be observed, however, with products containing borderline quantities of HCs. Most cryopreservation laboratories use a variation of the technique outlined in Table 47.1, including differences in cryoprotectant concentration, product volume and storage temperature [3,4]. Cryopreservation research, however, has been a focus of few transplantation teams, and the biological consequences of HC cryopreservation is one of the least understood aspects of HC processing. This lack of understanding of the effects of cell freezing on the cellular structure and the function of the cell populations required for hematological and immunological reconstitution of the patient hinders the ability to adapt techniques to handle modified cell collections, such as cells expanded *in vitro*, or to assess the consequences of accidental or intentional deviations from laboratory protocol. Although easily performed, HC cryopreservation and reinfusion are not

Table 47.1 Hematopoietic cell (HC) cryopreservation: basic technical considerations.

Item	Principle	Example
Prefreeze processing	Reduction of mature blood cells that are poorly cryopreserved	Separation of buffy-coat cells or light-density cells
Cryoprotectant	Protection of the cells from ice formation and dehydration. May be "colligative" or "polymeric" or combination of both	Colligative: DMSO, glycerol Polymeric: HES
Plasma protein	Reduces cryopreservation injury	Autologous plasma or plasma protein concentrates
Solvent	Provides suspension of cells and diluent for cryoprotectants	Saline solutions, tissue-culture media
Cooling	Cooling rates are dependent on the cell being frozen and the cryoprotectant used	HCs in DMSO are cooled at 1–3°C/min
Storage	Storage temperature must protect from ice recrystallization and progressive cell damage	Nitrogen liquid or vapor-phase. Addition of polymeric cryoprotectant may allow storage at warmer temperatures

DMSO, dimethylsulfoxide; HCs, hematopoietic cells; HES, hydroxyethyl starch.

without risk of toxicity to both the HC inoculum and the recipient. There are multiple aspects to successful cryopreservation of HCs. Each of these variables affects the survival of the cells and, as with any manufacturing process, must be rigidly controlled for reproducible results.

Nonfrozen storage of HC products

Cryopreservation is not required for short-term storage of HCs. Nonfrozen storage is a less-costly alternative, especially for immediate transportation of products and for transplantation of patients conditioned with brief courses of chemotherapeutic agents with short *in vivo* half-lives. Although most products are infused or processed within a few hours of collection, products collected for unrelated donor HCT may be shipped over long distances, requiring, sometimes, over 24 h of transit time. Similarly, products intended for autologous HCT may be transported to regional processing centers, again requiring 24–48 h of transit time before processing [5,6]. The major advantages of cryopreservation are the lack of progressive loss of HCs over time and the greater flexibility in timing of HCT relative to collection of HCs, including the ability to modify or postpone a transplant conditioning regimen already started.

A progressive loss of HCs occurs during nonfrozen storage. One author reported a 61% loss of myeloid colony-forming progenitor cells (colony-forming unit–granulocyte/macrophage [CFU-GM]) from marrow after 72 h of storage at 4°C [7]. Yet, another found only a 3% loss of CFU-GM from marrow stored for 96 h, but a 95% loss if the source of the cells was peripheral blood [8]. As part of a clinical trial described below, Preti *et al.* [9] compared the survival of mature hematopoietic progenitor cells isolated from marrow during frozen or nonfrozen storage, and reported an immediate loss of myeloid (CFU-GM) progenitors of 33% during cryopreservation and thawing. In contrast, cells stored at 4°C showed a progressive, linear loss of total nucleated cells, cell viability and HCs cloned *in vitro*. The quantity of erythroid colony-forming progenitor cells (burst-forming units-erythroid [BFU-E]) in these nonfrozen samples became significantly less than cryopreserved samples only after 5 days of storage. The difference for myeloid progenitor cells (CFU-GM) was not yet significant even after 9 days of storage. These differing reports demonstrate that storage conditions, such as concentration of cells, chemicals added, product volume, storage bag and temperature of storage, will affect the survival of cells kept in nonfrozen storage [10].

Most published reports of noncryopreserved storage describe storage at 4°C. This condition provides a stable temperature compared to storage at ambient temperatures, which can be quite variable (and which must be considered during the shipping of products). What temperature is optimal is not known and will probably depend upon such concerns as the prestorage processing, the quantity and concentration of mature blood cells, the buffering capacity of the solution and the gas-diffusion capacity of the storage container. Beaujean *et al.* [6], for example, reported a much lower pH for PBHC products stored overnight at room temperature compared to storage at 4°C. Although they did not find a difference in the recovery of progenitor cells in their experiments, this effect may be damaging to HCs under other circumstances. Yet another report describes better survival of HCs stored at 37°C and at 25°C compared to cells stored at 4°C [11]. These warmer storage temperatures are comparable to techniques being developed for the *in vitro* expansion of HCs (see Chapter 9). None of these studies entailed marrow reconstitution as the experimental endpoint. The conflicting reports about optimal storage temperatures are therefore difficult to interpret. Storage conditions for nonfrozen storage have not been tested in an engraftment model, so proper storage conditions are not adequately defined. For laboratories intending to store HCs for prolonged periods without freezing, rigorous validation of the storage conditions must be pursued.

There is limited experience with the autologous transplantation of noncryopreserved HCs. Used primarily in conjunction with high-dose melphalan or cyclophosphamide (CY) conditioning [7,9,12–14], refrigerated storage was supplanted by cryopreservation as most transplant centers developed multiday conditioning regimens. HCs appear to maintain viability for several days after collection if carefully stored. Preti *et al.* [9] compared, in a nonrandomized retrospective analysis, the engraftment kinetics of 54 patients who received cryopreserved marrow cells to 45 patients who received refrigerated cells. The refrigerated cells were stored for a median of 4 days (range: 3–9). The cryopreserved cells were stored a median of 69 days (range: 5–981) at –80°C using a cryoprotectant mixture of dimethylsulfoxide (DMSO) and hydroxyethyl starch (HES). Almost all patients were conditioned with a regimen consisting of carmustine (1,3-*bis*(2-chloroethyl)-1-nitrosourea[BCNU]), etoposide and CY. This group found no significant difference in engraftment kinetics for these two groups, although a small, few days difference would not have been detected with the limited numbers of patients in this study.

Cryopreservation theory

The chemistry and biology of mammalian cell cryopreservation

The recovery of viable mammalian cells after cryopreservation and thawing became possible with the discovery that glycerol could be used for the freezing of bovine sperm [15]. Subsequent experiments demonstrated that marrow cells frozen with glycerol could be used to reconstitute the marrow function of irradiated mice [16,17]. Considerable exploration of the cryobiology of various mammalian and nonmammalian cells ensued. Those studies defined the mechanism of cell damage incurred during cryopreservation and techniques to moderate that damage. The current understanding of cryobiology contends that ice crystal formation during cooling is the primary cause of cell damage [18]. This damage can be classified into two categories: at rapid rates of cooling, intracellular ice crystals may form, resulting in *mechanical* disruption of the cell and immediate cell death. At slower rates of cooling ice crystal formation preferentially occurs in the extracellular space, resulting in increasing osmolality as free water is incorporated into the growing ice crystals. This loss of free water results in the concentration of extracellular solutes, such as sodium, that do not freely penetrate the cell membrane, extreme hyperosmolality and *dehydration* injury. For example, the molality of NaCl in a saline solution at –10°C is about 5.3 m and at –20°C about 10.5 m.

Intracellular ice formation may be limited by cooling cells slowly. At slow rates, it is probable that ice nucleation will occur first in the larger volume outside the cell. Progressive dehydration of the cell will result if the rate of cooling is slow enough to allow water to shift to the extracellular space and be incorporated into the growing ice crystals. The optimal cooling rate differs for different cell types and appears to be defined by the permeability of water through the cell membrane [19]. Progressive dehydration with concentration of intracellular solutes prevents supercooling of intracellular water and protects the cells from the formation of intracellular ice crystals. Ice that happens by chance to nucleate first within a cell will result in the death of that cell but will also serve to promote the freezing of extracellular water as the ice crystal penetrates the cell membrane. The corollary is not true in that extracellular ice does not penetrate into the cell and promote intracellular ice formation, presumably because of some feature of the cell membrane.

Glycerol and DMSO are colligative cryoprotectants that prevent dehydration injury by moderating the increased concentration of nonpenetrating extracellular solutes during ice formation, and by decreasing the amount of water absorbed by (in equilibrium with) the ice crystals at a defined temperature. Colligative refers to properties dependant upon the number of particles (solute), not the composition of the particles. Freezing is the crystallization of water and the freezing point is the temperature at which ice crystals can be sustained in equilibrium with water. The freezing point of water is depressed by the addition of solute. For any particular mixture of solute(s) and water, there will be a defined temperature at which ice crystals can initially form. Unlike pure water, ice crystal formation and growth in aqueous solutions occurs over a temperature range. Growing ice crystals absorb free water and exclude solute particles. The incorporation of water into ice results in concentration of the solute and further depression of the freezing temperature of the remaining water, thereby preventing additional ice formation unless further cooling occurs. Thus, temperature (and pressure) defines the equilibrium between ice and the nonfrozen solution. With further cooling a temperature is eventually reached at which the solute itself crystallizes (eutectic point). The molality of a solution in equilibrium with ice therefore is determined by the temperature of the solution, not the initial concentration of the solute, as depicted by the equation in which m represents the osmolal concentration of the solute and T is the temperature in degrees Kelvin [20].

$$m \approx \frac{273 - T}{1.9} \qquad (47.1)$$

Similarly, the fraction of water not frozen (q) is defined by the equation:

$$q \approx \frac{1.9\, Mo}{273 - T} \qquad (47.2)$$

where Mo is the osmolal concentration of the solution before freezing.

In our example above, a saline solution at –20°C has a NaCl molality of about 10.5 M. For a three component system, such as DMSO and NaCl in water, both solutes will contribute to the molality of the unfrozen solution in the same relative proportion found in the initial solution. The molality (before freezing) of 10% DMSO (v/v) in normal saline (140 mM) solution is about 1.6 M, with DMSO contributing about 10-times the molality contributed by NaCl to the medium. At –20°C, this molal ratio between DMSO and NaCl will be maintained. The molality contributed by NaCl will be about 1.05 M, or about 7-times the molality of NaCl in a solution without ice. DMSO freely penetrates the HC cell membrane so that the intracellular concentration of DMSO will equal the extracellular concentration throughout the temperature range, assuming adequate movement of water from the cell as the extracellular ice crystals form and grow. The addition of a penetrating cryoprotectant to an aqueous saline solution therefore reduces the osmotic stress across the cell membrane at –20°C from about 75-times to about seven-times that of an ice-free solution. According to this theory, colligative cryoprotectants must be capable of penetrating the cell to avoid merely contributing to the molality of the extracellular medium and must be nontoxic to the cells at the concentration required for this effect.

The tolerance of cells to freezing at slow cooling rates depends on the ability of the cells to withstand osmotic stress, and initial studies of the osmotic behavior of HCs have been reported [21]. The osmotic tolerance of granulocytes is much less than that for lymphocytes or CFU-GM, probably accounting at least in part for the difference in survival after cryopreservation [22,23]. With DMSO concentrations <10%, the degree of dehydration caused by concentration of the nonpenetrating solutes during freezing will be greater because nonpenetrating solutes will contribute proportionately more to the molality of the nonfrozen solution in the extracellular medium. With higher concentrations of DMSO, the osmotic stress will be less. The optimal concentration for a colligative cryoprotectant depends upon the osmotic tolerance of the cell to be frozen, the toxicity to the cell of high concentrations of the cryoprotectant [24–26], and the presence of other cryoprotectants. The ability of a cryoprotectant to penetrate the cell and its subcellular organelles explains, at least in part, the relative efficacy of different colligative cryoprotectants for different cell species.

Table 47.2 Recoveries of nucleated cells and hematopoietic cells (HCs) after cryopreservation with ethylene glycol or dimethylsulfoxide (DMSO).

Cryoprotectant solution	Cell recovery	CFU-GM recovery
8 M ethylene glycol	89.5 ± 8.5	66.6 ± 20.8
4 M ethylene glycol	83.6 ± 9.4	36.4 ± 23.6
2 M ethylene glycol	75.0 ± 17.4	14.7 ± 24.6
10% (v/v) DMSO	88.5 ± 12.4	69.1 ± 9.7

CFU-GM, colony-forming unit–granulocyte/macrophage; DMSO, dimethylsulfoxide.
Adapted from Kurata et al. [30].

Colligative properties do not explain the cryoprotection achieved by freezing cells in solutions of macromolecules such as HES. Solutions of high-molecular weight, polymeric cryoprotectants, contain relatively few particles and, moreover, do not freely penetrate the cell. These cryoprotectants may protect the cell by forming a viscous, glassy shell that retards the movement of water thereby preventing progressive dehydration as water is incorporated into the extracellular ice crystals [27]. Solutions of some compounds, when present in sufficiently high concentrations, will solidify to an amorphous glass without first forming ice crystals, a process termed vitrification [28]. The "glass-transition temperature" (Tg) depends upon both the structure and concentration of the solute. At very high concentrations of cryoprotectants (6.3 M for DMSO [28]) the Tg is higher (warmer) than the temperature at which ice crystals can form, thereby preventing crystallization during cooling and its resulting mechanical and osmotic stresses. The practical difficulty with achieving vitrification arises from the necessity to use these very high concentrations of cryoprotectants. Vitrification has been used for the cryopreservation of murine embryos, for example, with a solution of 20% DMSO, 15.5% acetamide, 10% propylene glycol and 6% polyethylene glycol [29]. Prolonged exposure to this solution was toxic, however, with complete loss of viability after 30 min at 4°C. Kurata et al. [30] plunged cord blood HCs protected by high concentrations of ethylene glycol directly into liquid nitrogen. The recovery of HCs in samples preserved with the highest concentrations of ethylene glycol were similar to that for samples more conventionally cryopreserved with 10% DMSO (Table 47.2 [30]). The toxicity of the cryoprotectant solution was not addressed by these authors. Also, the rapid cooling and warming rates required are easier to achieve with the small cell aliquots (0.5 mL) tested than with the large volumes characteristic of HC products.

With lower concentrations of cryoprotectants, including extracellular macromolecular compounds and many sugars, crystallization occurs at warmer temperatures than the vitrification temperature and ice crystals will form during cooling. Yet, glass transition may occur even in the presence of ice crystallization. With the formation of ice crystals and resulting loss in free water, the concentration of the cryoprotectant in the nonfrozen water will increase. With decreasing temperature causing increasing cryoprotectant concentration, a point will be reached at which the solution forms a glass. At this Tg the solution suddenly becomes viscous, retarding if not stopping the flow of water through the extracellular matrix. This has been proposed as the mechanism for cryoprotection afforded by the extracellular cryoprotectants [27]. In one study of peripheral blood monocyte cryopreservation using extracellular cryoprotectants, a limiting glass-transition temperature of –20°C was optimal, which was achieved using a 20% solution of HES [27]. Substances forming glasses at higher or lower temperatures were less effective. Pure water forms a glass at about –139°C [31]. The addition of cryoprotectants such as DMSO, glycerol or HES raises the Tg [32]. This model of cryopreservation requires adequate dehydration to occur to concentrate intracellular solutes and decrease the probability of intracellular ice formation, but glass formation at an appropriate temperature (please recall that temperature defines the osmolality of the unfrozen aqueous solution) to prevent excessive dehydration of the cell.

Cells are not frozen in simple two- or three-component solutions but rather in complex solutions containing salts, sugars, penetrating cryoprotectants, with or without extracellular cryoprotectants, and plasma proteins. Phase transition temperatures (such as Tg) for these solutions have not been published. The improved survival observed with increasing protein concentration [33] and, possibly, by combined penetrating and extracellular cryoprotectants [34,35], may be explained at least in part by these theories on ice and glass formation and their effects on the cell. Moreover, the existence of glass formation may explain the relationship between storage temperature and survival of HCs over time. Below the Tg temperature, enlargement of previously formed ice crystals by recrystallization of unfrozen water cannot occur, and the cells are protected from progressive mechanical disruption. (The growth of an existing ice crystal through the process of recrystallization is thermodynamically more favorable than the nucleation of a new ice crystal.) The optimal storage temperature is below the Tg for the cryoprotectant solution used. Warmer temperatures may be used, but at risk of cell damage, a risk that is dependent upon the temperature of storage and the stability (viscosity) of the solution at that temperature.

This simplified review of the effects of freezing and the cryoprotectant properties of penetrating and polymeric cryoprotectants does not completely explain the processes involved during freezing, and more detailed reviews of the freezing of aqueous solutions and mammalian cells have been published [36,37]. This discussion ignores the specific damaging effects of dehydration on cell function. In addition to mechanical and dehydration injuries, cooling itself may be damaging to the cell [38]. Finally, colligative effects alone are not sufficient to explain the cryoprotectant properties of DMSO or glycerol. Other freely penetrating chemicals, such as urea and dimethylsulfone ($DMSO_2$), do not function as cryoprotectants for mammalian cells [39,40] and some chemicals, such as ethanol and guanidine, may actually function as cryosensitizers [41]. Obviously, the chemical structure of the cryoprotectant is important in the survival of mammalian cells, and a molecular interaction between the cryoprotectant and protein or lipid molecules appears necessary for optimal cryopreservation [42–45]. Examples of selective damage to cell membrane proteins or structure from freezing is illustrated by the loss of response to giant cell tumor (GCT)-conditioned medium of myeloid progenitor cells after cryopreservation [46], the decrease in L-selectin expression by $CD34^+$ cells after cryopreservation and thawing [47], and the lineage-specific effects on granulocyte recovery for patients receiving cells frozen with HES and DMSO in combination [48].

The physics of cooling and warming of cell products

The rationale for slow rates of cooling and rapid rates of warming are explained by the mechanical and dehydration injuries resulting from the formation and growth of ice crystals. Heat transfer is a physical process, not a biological or chemical process. Cooling is a physical process dependent on properties of the object being cooled such as the difference in temperature between the object and its environment, and the size and thermal conductivity of the object. The rate of heat transfer is described by the equation:

$$q(r,t) = -k\nabla T(r,t) \qquad (47.3)$$

in which $q(r,t)$ represents the heat-flux vector at a particular point on the object and a particular time, $-k$ represents the thermal conductivity of the material, and $T(r,t)$ represents the temperature gradient vector at that particular time and place. Objects with a greater thermal conductivity

Table 47.3 Effect of product volume on cooling rate after immersion into a –70°C freezer.

Volume (mL)	Cooling velocity (°C/min)		Duration of transition phase (min)
	Pretransition	Post-transition	
30	6.1	2.0	0.5
60	3.1	1.6	3.0
90	1.6	1.0	8.6
120	1.8	1.0	12.8

Shown are the rates of cooling before and after the transition phase, and the duration of transition phase for samples of the stated volumes immersed into a –70°C refrigerator.
Adapted from Clark *et al*. [52].

because of composition or smaller size will gain or lose heat more rapidly, as will objects placed in an environment with a much larger difference in temperature between the object and its environment. Most centers use electronic-rate controllers to achieve an optimal cooling rate, but satisfactory rates of cooling can be achieved by immersing an appropriate volume of marrow or PBHCs into a –80°C mechanical freezer [49–52]. Rowley [49] cooled 50 mL aliquots in storage bags and found reproducible cooling rates of about 3°C/min when placed in a –80°C freezer, but rates between 10°C/min and 16°C/min when placed in a –135°C freezer. Clark *et al*. [52] studied the effects of marrow volume on the cooling rates before and after the transition phase, and the duration of the transition phase for cells placed either in freezing bags or vials. As would be predicted by the equation describing heat transfer, bags containing larger volumes cooled much more slowly and required longer duration of the transition phase (Table 47.3 [52]). Before immersion techniques are adopted by individual laboratories, the rate of cooling and reproducibility for the type of bag and volume of cells must be determined and documented. The advantages of immersion cooling techniques are the avoidance of a rate-controlled apparatus and the decrease in personnel time required. The disadvantages are the lack of a recording documenting the rate of cooling, the limited adaptability to different volumes and containers, and possible detrimental effects related to the duration of transition phase, which may be critical if borderline quantities of cells are harvested.

Cryoprotectant solutions

Dimethylsulfoxide (DMSO)

DMSO, glycerol and a variety of other chemicals may serve as colligative cryoprotectants that protect the cell from excessive dehydration as extracellular water is drawn into growing ice crystals. The cryoprotectant properties of glycerol were described in 1949 [15], and those of DMSO 10 years later [53]. Both have been used for the cryopreservation of marrow. The rapid diffusion of DMSO through the cell membrane and the difficulty in removing glycerol before reinfusion (infusion of DMSO-containing products is generally tolerated) have made DMSO the favored agent for HC cryopreservation.

DMSO, a byproduct of paper manufacturing, is a hygroscopic polar compound developed originally as a solvent for chemicals such as insecticides, fungicides, and herbicides [54]. Pure DMSO is a colorless, virtually odourless liquid (sp.gr. 1.108, m.w. 78.13 g/mol) although industrial grades may have a strong sulfur odour [55]. The serum half-life of DMSO is about 20 h, although that of $DMSO_2$, a renal-excreted metabolite, is 72 h [55]. A small proportion of DMSO is reduced to dimethylsulfide (DMS), which is expired through the lungs for about 24 h after administration,

Table 47.4 Engraftment kinetics for patients receiving peripheral blood hematopoietic cells (PBHCs) frozen in dimethylsulfoxide (DMSO) or DMSO and hydroxyethyl starch (HES).

Outcome	Patients below the median*			Patients above the median*		
	DMSO	DMSO/HES	p-value	DMSO	DMSO/HES	p-value[†]
Granulocyte engraftment						
WBC $\geq 1.0 \times 10^9$/L	11	11	0.71	11	10	0.02
ANC $\geq 0.1 \times 10^9$/L	10	10	0.86	10	9	0.03
ANC $\geq 0.5 \times 10^9$/L	11	11	0.87	11	10	0.01
ANC $\geq 1.0 \times 10^9$/L	13	12	0.87	12	11	0.02
Platelet engraftment						
Platelet $\geq 20 \times 10^9$/L	11	12	0.25	9	9	0.36
Platelet $\geq 50 \times 10^9$/L	14	15	0.10	12	12	0.28
Last transfusion	9	9	0.67	8	8	0.75

*Shown are the median times to achieve the designated outcome for patients classified by cryoprotectant used and stratified by quartile of $CD34^+$ cell dose/kg (1st and 2nd quartiles combined vs. 3rd and 4th quartiles combined). The median cell doses for patients receiving products frozen with DMSO alone was 6.4×10^6/kg and for those receiving cells frozen with DMSO/HES was 6.5×10^6/kg.
†p-values are based on weighted log-rank test, which compares the two estimated recovery curves.
ANC, absolute neutrophil count; WBC, white blood cell count.
Reproduced with permission from Rowley et al. [48].

and which accounts for the characteristic odour resulting from DMSO infusion.

The optimal concentration of either DMSO or glycerol for the cryoprotection of HCs appears to be about 10%, although concentrations as low as 5% have been used successfully for HCT [56]. In their original report, Lovelock and Bishop [53] demonstrated a dose–response with improving red cell survival as the concentration of DMSO was increased to 15%. The effect of yet higher concentrations was not reported. Subsequently, Ragab et al. [33] studied the survival of HCs from human donors after freezing with various concentrations of DMSO. They found a significant increase in progenitor cell recovery when the concentration of DMSO was increased from 7.5% to 10.0%. No further improvement was found with an increase to 12.5%. This improvement resulted from an increase in nucleated cell recovery from 17.2% to 35.6% and 32.1%, respectively, after washing. Cell recovery before the post-thaw wash did not differ, nor were the numbers of colonies per 10^5 cells plated. The loss of cells during the wash steps that was found in this study may or may not reflect events occurring during direct intravenous infusion commonly used clinically. Donaldson et al. [57] studied the recovery of $CD34^+$ cells cryopreserved in varying concentrations of DMSO and HES and reported an increase in $CD34^+$ cell recovery from $12.2 \pm 10.0\%$ (mean ± SD) to $85.4 \pm 28.4\%$ as the concentration of DMSO was increased from 2.5% to 5.0%, but no further improvement with further increase in concentration to 10% (HES concentration was kept constant at 4% [w/v]). Varying the concentration of HES in the presence of 5% (v/v) DMSO had no effect on $CD34^+$ cell recovery.

Hydroxyethyl starch (HES)

HES is a polymeric substance containing chains of different molecular weights. Initially explored as a cryoprotectant for red blood cells, it was found also to be an effective cryoprotectant for a variety of other cells [27,58]. Macromolecular cryoprotectants may be used as single agents, but the major focus in the study of HC cryopreservation using extracellular cryoprotectants has been their use in combination with penetrating cryoprotectants. In one early study, the addition of polyvinylpyrrolidone (PVP), another macromolecular cryoprotectant, to glycerol or DMSO improved the cryopreservation of murine cells compared to the use of a penetrating agent alone [59]. Stiff et al. [34] froze human cells in a combination of 5% DMSO, 6% HES and 4% human serum albumin, and reported improved progenitor cell survival as determined using *in vitro* cultures. They subsequently successfully used this mixture of cryoprotectants to cryopreserve the marrow of 60 patients [50]. No engraftment failure was attributed to this technique, or after the cryopreservation of peripheral blood-derived HCs [51].

Only two clinical studies comparing engraftment outcomes for patients receiving products stored in DMSO/HES or DMSO alone have been reported. The first trial, limited to 12 patients in each arm, did not detect any difference in the kinetics of engraftment, although the small numbers of patients treated limited the power of the study to detect the small differences in engraftment speed that might be expected from small differences in cryoprotectant efficacy [60]. The other trial, a single-blind phase III study of 294 patients found 1-day differences in the times to achieve a white blood cell count (WBC) $\geq 1 \times 10^9$/L and absolute neutrophil count (ANC) $\geq 0.5 \times 10^9$/L and time to discontinuation of antibiotics for recipients of cells frozen with the combination cryoprotectant solution [48]. No differences were found for times to achieve endpoints of platelet engraftment (either 20×10^9/L or 50×10^9/L), indicating that this effect was probably lineage-specific. Furthermore, the effect was more pronounced for recipients who received more than the median number of $CD34^+$ cells suggesting a specific effect on a limited cell population (Table 47.4 [48]). No adverse effects from the use of the combination cryoprotectant were noted by these authors.

Protein

Plasma proteins exert cryoprotectant effects, possibly by modifying the viscosity or the glass-transition temperature of the cryoprotectant solution. Lymphocytes can be cryopreserved using serum alone [39,61]. The addition of serum proteins to the cryoprotectant solution appears to improve HC survival. In one study using human marrow cells, myeloid progenitor cell survival, which was $41.1 \pm 8.0\%$ in the absence of serum, increased significantly to $64.8 \pm 14.2\%$ with 15% serum and $75.4 \pm 14.8\%$ with 50% serum [33]. Similarly, murine spleen colony-forming cells (colony-forming unit–spleen [CFU-S]) recovery increased from 18.2% to 100.5% when frozen in 10% DMSO with 10% serum added

[62]. In this second study, cryopreservation with 10% fetal bovine serum was less effective (25.4% recovery) than homologous serum, which may reflect the low protein content that is a characteristic of fetal sources of serum. The effect of protein content or source on engraftment speed has not been defined but anecdotal experience would suggest that the presence of protein is important. Engraftment will occur for CD34+ cells frozen without the addition of protein [63]. The 33 days (median) to achieve an ANC >500/µL and 46 days to achieve a platelet count >20,000/µL in that study, which did not use protein in the cryoprotectant solution, however, were much slower than the 23 days and 22 days for ANC and platelet engraftment reported by Shpall et al. [64] using a similar marrow processing technique but different cryoprotectant solution containing protein.

Virtually all cryopreservation solutions currently in use contain plasma proteins added as either part of the cryopreservation solution or during cell processing. The range in concentration and source of protein varies among the various transplant groups, with some groups using up to 90% plasma [65]. The source of protein is similarly diverse, although fetal bovine serum (used in some early trials of marrow transplantation [66,67]) is no longer used. The use of albumin solutions is appealing because of the ability to achieve high, uniform concentrations of protein while avoiding the marrow fat, cellular debris, anticoagulants and risk of cryoglobulins associated with the use of autologous plasma collected during initial processing of the HC product.

A unique group of proteins are the antifreeze glycoproteins found in some species adapted to survival in cold environments. Some of these proteins are extremely efficient at preventing the recrystallization of ice and have been shown to enhance the cryopreservation of pig and murine embryos [68]. In studies of red cell cryopreservation, this effect was limited to a narrow concentration range with higher concentrations actually increasing the growth of extracellular ice with concomitant cell damage [69]. It can not be assumed that the addition of these proteins will improve HC cryopreservation survival.

Salt and sugar content

Metabolically inactive cryopreserved cells do not require the complex media preparations used for *ex vivo* growth of HCs. Successful cryopreservation has been achieved using commercially available pharmacological salt solutions. However, the solution in which the cells are suspended should not be viewed as inert. For example, many tissue culture media contain compounds that may increase the sensitivity of cells to freezing (cryosensitizers) [41]. Also, as noted in Equation 47.1, the fraction of unfrozen water is determined by the initial osmolarity of the solution. At least for red cells, cryopreservation in hypotonic solutions increases post-thaw hemolysis [70].

Various sugars may function as cryoprotectants. Leibo et al. [71] found 50% survival of CFU-S after cryopreservation of murine marrow cells in 0.35 M sucrose without protein or other cryoprotectants. Optimal rates of cooling, as with other extracellular cryoprotectants, were between 16 and 70°C/min. Cooling at slower rates (<10°C/min) was associated with much poorer cryosurvival. Using a cell line derived from human kidney, Vos and Kaalen [39] showed cryoprotectant properties for a number of sugars, including glucose, mannitol and sorbitol, at concentrations >0.1 M. The amount of glucose in tissue culture media is in the millimolar range, which is negligible compared to the concentration shown by Vos and Kaalen [39] to be an effective cryoprotectant in their system. These sugars do not freely penetrate the cell membrane and function as extracellular cryoprotectants. Sugars may serve to stabilize the cell membrane during freezing or dehydration [43,44]. It has also been suggested that glucose may protect against the cytotoxicity observed with high concentrations of DMSO [72].

Table 47.5 Protective effect of various additives for murine marrow cryopreservation.

Cryoprotectant	Viability by vital stain (%)	Animal survival (%)
DMSO (15%)	91	70
Glycerol (15%)	75	70
Serum (30%)	90	0
BSA (15%)	100	19
Dextran (15%)	62	24
Saline	3	0

Shown is the viability of bone marrow cells cryopreserved with various additives as shown by vital dye stains and the ability of these cells to rescue an animal from irradiation.
BSA, bovine serum albumin; DMSO, dimethylsulfoxide.
Adapted from Rowe [77].

Cryopreservation technique

Evaluation of cryopreservation efficacy

A major impediment to the study of HC cryobiology is the inability to culture primitive HCs *in vitro*. The only "assay" for the cryosurvival of these cells is engraftment after transplantation, the rate of which depends more on patient diagnosis and marrow function, quantity of cells harvested and any *ex vivo* treatment performed than on the cryosurvival of HCs as reflected by *in vitro* cultures [2,73,74]. Experimental models include engraftment of human cells in immunodeficient nonobese diabetic with severe combined immunodeficiency syndrome (NOD/SCID) mice [75]. Initial studies of blood and HC cryobiology used either metabolic assays or dye-exclusion assays [76]. These assays are irrelevant, if only because the rarity of HCs in the harvested cells precludes a correlation between cell metabolism or dye uptake and HC cryosurvival. Techniques that measure the viability of the whole population of cells are of no use in determining HC viability. Complete kill of HCs would change the proportion of cells with dye uptake by <1%. HCs cannot be identified morphologically and, moreover, metabolic and dye-exclusion tests do not measure the proliferative capacity of these cells (Table 47.5) [77].

Progenitor cell assays such as culture for CFU-GM after thawing can be predictive of engraftment [1,2], but the validity of these assays must be determined for each group of patients and the assay used. DMSO must not be present in concentrations >0.1% in *in vitro* cultures [78,79], so some technique of dilution must be undertaken before cell culture. Rapid dilution of DMSO after thawing exposes the cells to osmotic shock. Some authors have reported satisfactory recovery of HCs after rapid dilution of thawed cells [1,80]. Others, however, have demonstrated a distinct advantage to serial dilution [33,79,81]. Deoxyribonuclease (DNAse) can be added to lyse clumps that form. The addition of sorbitol or other macromolecular substances after thawing may be of value to help prevent osmotic shock [82,83]. These techniques, of course, differ from direct intravenous infusion.

Some centers routinely freeze "test vials" containing small aliquots of cells alongside the greater quantity of cells contained in freezing bags. The different cooling properties of vials compared to bags diminishes the reliability of these small aliquots for determining cryosurvival [52,84]. If an attempt is made to use small aliquots for clinical decisions, a system of cooling, thawing, washing and culture that correlates with engraftment kinetics must first be developed.

Processing of HC products for cryopreservation

One of the basic concepts of clinical HC cryopreservation is the heterogeneity of marrow and blood cell populations. HC cryopreservation involves not only the cryobiology of HCs, but also of the mature blood cells contained in the harvested product. HCs comprise a very small portion (generally, <1%) of the marrow, PBHC or CBSC product. Furthermore, HC products consist of HCs heterogeneous over a range of cell maturation; accessory cells are also important to engraftment. Marrow consists of HCs, mature blood cells and noncellular material such as fat. Cryopreservation techniques that are optimal for HCs will not preserve mature blood cells. The standard technique for red cell cryopreservation uses glycerol; granulocytes cannot be cryopreserved successfully; platelets are frozen with lower concentrations of DMSO, which must be added at a controlled rate to avoid osmotic shock to the cell [85]. The presence of mature blood cells affects HC cryopreservation in at least three ways. First, the large proportion of mature blood cells collected may hinder the laboratory processing if clumping before freezing or after thawing is induced by damaged granulocytes or platelets. Second, damaged cells may cause infusion-related toxicity. The infusion of marrow that was frozen without depletion of mature blood cells was associated with acute renal failure in three of 33 patients in one study [86]. This problem presumably resulted from massive hemolysis of the poorly preserved red blood cells. Third, if the cells are frozen at a set concentration, the presence of large numbers of mature blood cells requires that the cells be frozen in large volumes. Patients receiving such products are at considerable risk for serious infusion-related toxicity from the large quantities of cryoprotectant used. In addition, concentration of HCs before storage reduces the space required, which is a logistical consideration for the management of large banks of cells. CBHCs intended for unrelated donor transplantation are routinely concentrated to minimize the space required for the large numbers of products necessary in the banks providing products for patients lacking other sources of HCs.

Therefore, cryopreservation of HCs can be facilitated by the prefreeze depletion of mature blood elements. A number of apheresis or cell washing devices are capable of processing the large quantities of cells harvested. Some apheresis devices provide enrichment of mononuclear cells relative to granulocytes, providing a "cleaner" preparation for processing and cryopreservation. Density-gradient separation of light-density cells further enriches for HCs, although at the expense of additional cell losses and cost of processing. At the extreme of prefreeze processing is the extensive purification of HCs by isolation of CD34$^+$ cells, which reduces the quantity of mature blood cells, the amount of cryoprotectant infused and the DMSO-related toxicity [87]. Collection of buffy-coat cells with depletion of red blood cells is the minimum processing required for cryopreservation of marrow. PBHCs collected by apheresis contain small proportions of red cells and generally do not require further separation, although volume reduction will decrease the amount of cryoprotectant used. Cord blood cells are processed to reduce the storage volume required for the large banks of cells intended for allogeneic transplantation [83].

Cell concentration

The cell concentrations used in most protocols are often driven by practical considerations, such as the desire to freeze more than one bag or to minimize the total volume and number of bags of product stored. PBHCs differ from marrow products because of their much larger nucleated cell quantity that must be processed by the laboratory. Although many protocols set limits for the concentration of nucleated cells, few also define the maximum or minimum concentrations or quantities of red cells, granulocytes, or platelets. The effect of these cells on HC cryopreservation is

Table 47.6 Effect of cryoprotectant on optimal cooling rate for murine colony-forming unit–spleen (CFU-S).

Cryoprotectant	Optimal cooling rate	CFU-S survival (%)
0.4 M glycerol	100°C/min	18
0.8 M glycerol	18°C/min	40
1.25 M glycerol	1.8°C/min	65
0.35 M sucrose	16–70°C/min	54

Adapted from Leibo et al. [71].

not defined, but a potential effect is illustrated by a report of poor post-thaw recovery of red blood cells frozen at high cell concentrations, which may relate to the limited space in channels of nonfrozen water between the growing ice crystals during cooling and increased packing of cells [88]. Most studies involving cryopreservation of HCs at high cell concentrations were not designed to detect subtle damage from this practice. The cryopreservation of PBHCs at an average 3.7×10^8 nucleated cells/mL (range: $0.4-8.0 \times 10^8$/mL) with no obvious correlation between cell concentration and engraftment kinetics has been reported [89]. Although there also was no correlation between cell concentration during freezing and the post-thaw recovery of CD34$^+$ cells, the recovery of CFU-GM appeared to decrease at higher cell concentrations. This observation has been confirmed by others [90]. Although cell cryopreservation at high concentrations of nucleated cells is feasible, Rowley et al. [91] suggested that infusion of PBHCs frozen at high concentrations resulted in increased risk for neurological events during or shortly after cell infusion.

The development of techniques that enrich for CD34$^+$ cells presents a different challenge to the cryopreservation laboratory. These techniques typically recover about 1% of the nucleated cells initially present. Cryopreservation of these cells in the same volume used for unselected cells would result in very low cell concentrations. Dicke et al. [81] cites one study of murine marrow cryopreservation that showed stable CFU-S cryosurvival at cell concentrations between 5×10^6 and 2×10^8 cells/mL. At cell concentrations of 1×10^6 cells/mL and below, however, CFU-S cryosurvival dropped precipitously. This decline may be related to nonspecific losses such as adhesion to surfaces and post-thaw wash steps. Similar studies of the effect of cell concentration have not been reported for human HCs. CD34$^+$ cell-enriched products may be frozen in small vials or bags with adjustment of the cooling technique for the smaller volume.

Rates of cooling and warming

Different cells have different optimal cooling rates, and the optimal cooling rate is also dependent on the type and concentration of cryoprotectant used. In general, the higher the concentration of a colligative cryoprotectant, the slower the optimal cooling rate (Table 47.6 [71]). The optimal cooling rate when using a colligative cryoprotectant also falls within a narrow range. In contrast, optimal rates for cooling when using extracellular cryoprotectants are generally more rapid, and the cells tolerate a broader range (Table 47.6). Ma et al. [92] used in vitro cultures of human BM to show optimal cooling at 1°C/min for human hematopoietic progenitor cells suspended in 10% DMSO. The recovery of colony-forming cells fell at rates slower than 1°C, or faster than 3°C/min. Lewis et al. [93] studied the impact of cooling rates before and after the plateau phase (immediately after the "heat of fusion"), and of the duration of the plateau phase on the recovery of murine CFU-S frozen in 12% glycerol. No difference was found for preplateau cooling rates ranging from 0.8 to 4°C/min. Increasing the duration of the plateau phase from 0 to 16 min resulted in a drop in spleen colonies from 16.7 to 12.0. Increasing the rate of the postplateau cooling similarly decreased CFU-S recovery. Clinically, Gorin et al. [94] associated a rapid cooling rate with delayed engraftment for eight recipients of autologous marrow.

Virtually all the reports regarding the optimal rate of cooling for HCs do not discuss the temperature at which time rate becomes irrelevant. This author (S.D. Rowley) routinely increased the rate to 10°C/min when the product has reached −40°C and transferred the bags to the storage refrigerators when a temperature of −80°C was reached [48]. At −40°C, water will spontaneously nucleate so supercooled water cannot exist below this temperature [95]. Leibo et al. [71] reported that most cell damage in their murine model occurred at temperatures between −10°C and −45°C. Therefore, HCs may be tolerant of higher cooling rates after initial freezing of water.

The warming rate is more critical when rapid rates of cooling are used because of the intracellular ice nucleation that occurs with rapid cooling. If warming is slow during the thawing process, growth of these ice crystals by recrystallization can occur. Cooling at slow rates limits intracellular ice nucleation and mechanical disruption of the cell from ice recrystallization during warming is less likely. Leibo et al. [71] found no difference in CFU-S recovery for cells in 1.25 M glycerol cooled at 1.7°C/min and warmed at either 1.8 or 910°C/min. Therefore, rapid warming is appropriate.

Storage of cryopreserved cells

Most laboratories store HCs below −120°C in mechanical (electric) freezers or in either the vapor or liquid phase of nitrogen. The rationale for this method is the possible progressive growth of ice crystals at warmer temperatures as water migrates from smaller to larger crystals (recrystallization), a process that does not occur in pure water at temperatures below about −130 to −139°C [31,32] or in cryopreservation solutions cooled below the phase transition temperatures of the mixture [32]. Critical phase-transition temperatures for HC cryoprotectant solutions containing DMSO or DMSO/HES have not been fully explored. Nor has the effect of storage or intermittent warming above these phase-transition temperatures on HC viability been determined. Initial attempts of autologous transplantation infused cells stored at −80°C, although the mild, probably marrow-sparing, pretransplant conditioning regimens used in those initial trials hinder interpretation of the results [96,97]. In other, preclinical studies, however, progressive loss of HCs was demonstrated for cryopreserved cells stored at relatively warm temperatures. Marrow cells stored for 25 weeks in 10% DMSO at −30°C failed to rescue mice from marrow-lethal irradiation, compared to 80% survival after 22 weeks storage at −70°C and 72% survival after 26 weeks storage in liquid nitrogen [98]. The need to maintain stable storage temperatures for long-term HC cryopreservation is illustrated by Appelbaum et al.'s [99] report, using a dog model of autologous transplantation, of the failure of engraftment in 30%, 66% and 100% of recipients of 0.5×10^8 marrow cells/kg stored in the vapor phase of nitrogen for 9, 12 and 18 months, respectively. Storage at ultra-low temperatures is not a requirement for successful engraftment if adequate numbers of HCs are harvested and if the duration of storage is limited. Under such conditions, moderate losses of HCs may occur without obvious delay in engraftment kinetics. The engraftment failure observed by Appelbaum et al. [99] can be explained by their intentional cryopreservation and transplantation of borderline quantities of marrow cells and the probable instability of the storage temperature of their cells. Nitrogen vapor-phase refrigerators are noted for the temperature gradient formed. Temperatures as warm as −100°C may exist at the top of the refrigerator. Cells stored at this location will be exposed to additional warming upon opening of the refrigerator or lifting of the rack to gain access to the storage cassettes. Over prolonged storage time, cells may be repetitively exposed to warming during normal operation of the refrigerator, and this warming may be progressively damaging to HCs. This temperature gradient in the vapor phase can be minimized by constructing frames from metals with better heat conductivity such as aluminum. Rowley and Byrne [100] found a gradient of only 5.9°C at 55.88 cm (22″) above the liquid when using an aluminum racking system compared to a gradient of 86°C for a similar refrigerator containing a racking system constructed of steel. This design achieved stable low-temperature storage throughout the refrigerator.

In addition to the issue of temperature gradients in vapor-phase refrigerators, many laboratories perceive storage in the liquid phase to be safer because of the larger quantity of nitrogen present. However, liquid nitrogen can serve as a reservoir for viruses, which may be of clinical importance for high-potency pathogens that require only a few organisms contaminating the bag port for transmission of disease [101]. This problem was dramatically illustrated by the transmission of hepatitis B infection to at least three patients whose cells were immersed in the same liquid nitrogen refrigerator as those of the index case [102]. Molecular typing of the virus and its isolation from the detritus of the refrigerator on subsequent investigation confirmed this mode of transmission.

It is possible that different cryoprotectant solutions may permit storage at warmer temperatures although this has not been prospectively tested using appropriate models of engraftment. Many centers have adopted storage at −80°C because of its simplicity for short-term storage for patients expected to undergo transplantation within a few weeks or months of cell harvest. Mostly, this storage is used in conjunction with DMSO/HES cryoprotection. Stiff [103] reported successful transplantation of products stored for up to 22 months at this temperature. Whether this accomplishment results from the addition of HES to the cryoprotectant solution, thereby affecting the stability of the solution at this relatively warm temperature, or because enough HCs were harvested to allow progressive loss was not analyzed. Galmes et al. [104] reported a progressive loss of CFU-GM and BFU-E from PBHC products stored at −80°C in either 5% or 10% DMSO (without HES) and recommended that time of storage at this temperature be limited.

The duration of storage may be indefinite if adequate temperatures are maintained and appropriate cryopreservation techniques are used. Evidence supporting this premise is found in both laboratory and clinical experience. Parker et al. [105] found no loss of colony-forming unit-culture (CFU-C) after storage of human marrow in vapor-phase nitrogen for a median of 42 months. Furthermore, limited numbers of patients have received HC products stored for prolonged periods of time. One report of experience from multiple centers reported transplantation of cells stored for up to 11 years [106]. In that study of 33 patients, however, the median duration of storage was only 2.8 years, the authors did not correlate duration of storage with engraftment kinetics or other markers of HC survival, and some products were treated ex vivo with mafosfamide, which is known to delay engraftment. Some patients experienced markedly prolonged post-transplant aplasia (up to 119 days), and two patients failed to engraft. Another study reported the outcome of transplantation for 36 patients who received marrow stored for 2.0–7.8 years and found, in retrospective comparison to a control group who received cells stored for less than 2 years, no differences in success or speed of engraftment [107]. The products in that report were stored either in nitrogen vapor-phase refrigerators or mechanical freezers at −135°C.

The temperature of storage should be maintained during transportation of marrow. The availability of "dry shippers" in which the nitrogen is absorbed into the wall of the container simplifies the transportation of frozen cells. These "shippers" can maintain nitrogen vapor-phase temperatures of about −180°C for periods of 7–10 days (if stored upright).

The amount of residual nitrogen at any time after filling is determined by weighing the container.

Cells may be stored either in bags or vials constructed of plastics tolerant to cryogenic temperatures. The advantage of vials relates to the ease with which samples may be thawed for analysis. The large numbers of vials required for storage, the risk of explosion on warming from nitrogen seepage into poorly sealed vials and the higher risk of microbial contamination during handling are reasons that favor bags.

Post-thaw manipulation

DMSO and HES need not be removed before infusion if consideration is given to the potential toxicities of these agents. Most products may be frozen at sufficiently high cell concentrations that the total cryoprotectant dose is held within tolerable limits. Clumping of damaged cells may occur after thawing, especially if the cells are manipulated [108]. For these reasons, most centers infuse cells within a few minutes after thawing and without any post-thaw processing other than filtration.

Most DMSO-associated toxicities are related to the quantity of DMSO infused, which can be reduced by washing of the cells after thawing. The techniques described generally involve serial dilution to avoid osmotic shock and resuspension in a protein-containing medium [109–111]. Beaujean et al. [110] reported an average 73.9 ± 6.4% CFU-GM recovery (±SE; range: 20.5–158.2%) for 50 density-gradient separated marrows after thawing and washing. The recovery for 12 peripheral blood products was 93.9 ± 7.0% (range: 67.4–135.6%). Twelve of the marrow bags were stored at room temperature for 4 h after washing with an additional 20–25% loss of cells and CFU-GM. These authors did not describe the speed of engraftment, compare engraftment kinetics to similar patients receiving unmanipulated cells, or correlate engraftment speed with either total cell or CFU-GM recoveries. However, there is no unequivocal evidence published to date that dilution of DMSO from HC products significantly affects engraftment kinetics.

The risk of post-thaw clumping can be diminished by removing granulocytes and platelets from the cell product before freezing, or by the addition of acid-citrate-dextrose (ACD [112]) or DNAse [65]. Symptomatic hypocalcemia occurs with the infusion of citrate anticoagulants, which may predispose the patient to adverse neurological events during the infusion [91]. DNAse is effective at lysing clumps but poses the risk of allergic or febrile reactions if a pharmaceutical-grade reagent is not used. Unlike DNAse, ACD will not lyse clumps that have already formed. Thawed cells should be infused through a standard blood administration set with an in-line filter of 170 μm pore size. It is possible to process HC products extensively after thawing, including the separation of CD34+ cells from cryopreserved PBHC products [113,114]. Cell clumping during the processing is, as stated, a complication that appears related to the quantity of mature blood cells contained in the product.

Cryoprotectant toxicity

Toxicity to HCs

High concentrations of cryoprotectants may incur direct toxicity to the cells being cryopreserved (cf. effects of vitrification solutions on murine embryos previously discussed: Cryopreservation therapy, p. 600). In general, cells are more tolerant to cryoprotectants at reduced temperatures. For example, DMSO is also concentrated during the formation of ice. Optimal cryopreservation requires a balance between protection from freeze damage and the occurrence of cryoprotectant-induced toxicity. The toxicity of DMSO to the HC has been described and most laboratories minimize the time of exposure to DMSO of cells before and after cryopreservation. Using in vitro cultures, Douay et al. [115] described a 23.5% recovery of CFU-C after 60 min exposure (at 4°C, without cryopreservation) and a 15% recovery after 120 min. However, Rowley and Anderson [78] were unable to confirm their findings of DMSO-induced progenitor cell loss in similar studies and surmised the difference between these reports may relate to the purity of the DMSO used. DMSO is a potent solvent, easily contaminated. In the latter study, which used pharmaceutical grade DMSO, recoveries of nucleated cells, CFU-GM and BFU-E were virtually 100% after exposure to 10% DMSO at either 4°C or 37°C. Only at 20% concentration of DMSO did cell clumping cause a decrease in cell recovery to 21.7% (and total CFU-GM quantity to 27.1%). The numbers of myeloid and erythroid progenitors per 5×10^4 cells plated dropped only after exposure to 40% DMSO (3.3% of control after 60 min incubation). Similarly, they found no loss of progenitor cells after thawing if the removal of DMSO was delayed even up to 60 min Others have also reported no toxicity to HCs with short exposure to DMSO [92], although direct addition of DMSO at 1% or greater concentration is toxic to cell culture [78,79].

Toxicity to the HCT recipient

In contrast, a high incidence of generally mild, infusion-related morbidity with the reinfusion of either marrow or PBHCs has been reported by several centers [116–118]. DMSO itself has a variety of pharmacological effects [54], which may be compounded by the presence of lysed blood cells, foreign proteins from tumor-cell purging procedures, or contaminants from nonpharmaceutical grades of reagents used in the processing. The LD50 values (amount of DMSO required to kill 50% of test animals) reported for intravenous infusion of DMSO are 3.1–9.2 g/kg for mice, and 2.5 g/kg for dogs [55]. The acute toxic dose of DMSO for humans has not been determined. If a large amount of cryopreserved material is to be infused, the infusion can be separated over 2 days to avoid complications from infusion of excessive amounts of DMSO.

The most dramatic toxicity is the rare anaphylactic reaction occurring during the initial administration of thawed cells. This appears to be an allergic reaction to DMSO or products of tissue culture medium used for cryopreservation. Treatment of this complication is the same as for anaphylactic reactions to other medications and, after resuscitation of the recipient, the remainder of the cells may be administered cautiously. Nonallergic, profound hypotension may result from the intravenous infusion of DMSO, presumably from histamine-induced vasodilatation [54]. Skin flushing, dyspnea, abdominal cramping, nausea and diarrhea, reported to varying degrees after HC infusion, can also all be attributed to DMSO-induced histamine release. These complaints resolve over a few hours and are treated symptomatically.

DMSO has a variety of cardiovascular effects. In a series of 82 patients who were premedicated with diphenhydramine, Davis et al. [116] observed increased blood pressure and decreased heart rate, which were maximal about 1 h after the completion of the marrow infusion. A number of authors have noted cardiac arrest or high-degree heart block occurring during or immediately after the infusion of cryopreserved marrow or PBHCs [119–122]. In two series, the incidence of bradycardia (heart rate <60 bpm) was 48.8% and 65%, second-degree heart block was 9.7% and 24%, and complete (third-degree) heart block was 4.8% and 5.9% [121,122]. In both reports, the median time of onset was about 3 h after the completion of the infusion. In one series, the authors noted that the heart block was often episodic, occurring with episodes of emesis [121]. In both series, the cardiac rhythm abnormalities resolved spontaneously within 24 h of infusion. In contrast, Lopez-Jimenez et al. [123] found no cardiac rhythm changes in a prospective series of 29 patients. A break of 20 min was allowed between bags of thawed cells in this last series, and it may be the slower overall infusion rate that accounted for the lack of rhythm changes.

Although headache in up to 70% of recipients of cryopreserved cells has been reported [118], other central nervous system complications are rare and generally related to the amount of DMSO infused. Two recipients who received HC products containing a total of 225 mL and 120 mL, respectively, of DMSO developed reversible encephalopathy [124]. The first patient underwent plasmapheresis with prompt improvement in mental status; the second patient recovered over 5 days without specific treatment. The weights of the patients were not cited in this report, but both patients probably received over 2 g of DMSO/kg of body weight. The use of DMSO to reduce cerebral edema has been associated with severe hyperosmolality in a patient who received the equivalent of about 10 g of DMSO/kg of body weight [125]. In an attempt to reduce the volume of DMSO used during the cryopreservation of PBHCs, Rowley et al. [89] concentrated cells to very high concentrations, averaging over 3.7×10^8 nucleated cells/mL. They subsequently reported several patients who experienced seizures during the administration of these cells [91]. The average cell concentration for these patients was 6.9×10^8 nucleated cells/mL (range: $0.8–12.9 \times 10^8$ cells/mL) but the maximum amount of DMSO administered was only 0.6 g/kg of body weight. Administration of similar quantities of DMSO during the infusion of marrow frozen at much lower cell concentrations has not been associated with seizures, so it is likely that these events are related to the cell concentration, cell quantity or types of cells cryopreserved in a PBHC product. This laboratory previously added ACD (formula A) after thawing to prevent clumping. This practice was stopped after a high incidence of citrate toxicity was observed. The incidence of seizures has also decreased with the removal of ACD from the infusate. Marrows frozen in 10% DMSO (which itself is 1.4 M) have an average osmolality of 1794 mOsm/kg H_2O after thawing [52], and infusion through a central venous catheter is preferred. Painful irritation may occur if thawed cells are infused through a peripheral vein. Despite the hyperosmolality of the products, serum osmolality is not greatly affected for patients receiving less than about 1 g of DMSO/kg of body weight. Although intravascular hemolysis has been reported after DMSO administration to cats [126] and possibly humans [127], Davis et al. [116] did not detect significant hemolysis in their clinical study as reflected by a major change in hematocrit. Hemoglobinuria occurs frequently [118], presumably resulting from cryopreservation-induced hemolysis of red cells within the HC inoculum. In anticipation of the infusion of hemolysed red blood cells, many centers manage patients with urinary alkylinization and mannitol diuresis using a strategy recommended for the treatment of acute hemolytic reaction to red cell infusion. This author (S.D. Rowley) discontinued this practice (but maintained prophylactic mediation with an antihistaminic agent and a corticosteroid) without an increase in postinfusion renal failure [48]. The infusion of large quantities of red blood cells in marrow products that were not red cell depleted before cryopreservation was associated with the development of acute renal failure in three of 33 patients at one transplant center [86].

In contrast to the extensive studies of DMSO-induced toxicities, little attention has been given to the toxicity of nonpenetrating cryoprotectants. HES toxicity to HCs has not been reported. HES is widely used as a blood volume expander during surgery and to enhance the collection of granulocytes from healthy donors by apheresis methodology, and significant systemic toxicity from the infusion of HES is rare.

Special considerations

Cryopreservation of HCs intended for allogeneic transplantation

Cryopreserved HC products are not commonly used in allogeneic transplantation. The availability of a volunteer donor obviates the cost and risks inherent with cryopreservation of cells. However, when concerns about the availability of the donor arise (e.g. foreign nationals, prisoners, substance abusers, overly apprehensive donors), collection and cryopreservation of cells before initiation of a myeloablative conditioning regimen may be justified. There is growing interest in the use of CBHCs for the use in related or unrelated donor transplantation. Obviously, the only practical method of storage of CBHCs involves cryopreservation, potentially for decades. HC products harvested from cadavers similarly may be frozen.

Limited experience in the allogeneic transplantation of cryopreserved marrow from related or unrelated donors has been published [128–132]. The probability and rate of engraftment were similar for recipients of cryopreserved cells and retrospective control groups of patients in the two studies that performed this analysis (Table 47.7 [129,130,132]). Long-term survival of these patients also appeared similar. Eckardt et al. [129], however, described a significantly lower incidence of acute graft-vs.-host disease (GVHD) for the recipients of cryopreserved cells. Stockschlader et al. [130,131] reported a similar study that found no difference in incidence of either acute or chronic GVHD. Both studies used total body irradiation or busulfan-based conditioning regimens and cyclosporine and methotrexate for prophylaxis against GVHD for most patients. Stockschlader et al. [132] subsequently published their experience with cryopreserved cells from unrelated donors (Table 47.7). The incidence of severe acute GVHD for recipients of cryopreserved marrow was 75%, which is similar to the reported experience of transplantation of noncryopreserved cells from unrelated donors transplanted at a number of centers.

Recipients of CBHC experience slower engraftment compared to recipients of either marrow or PBHCs [133–135]. It is likely that these observations result from the limited cell dose available in this source of HCs and not from the cryopreservation process. The observation that granulocyte engraftment kinetics could be hastened by the post-thaw removal of DMSO for recipients of CBHC products could also be attributed to changes in the post-transplant immunosuppressive regimen or other modifications of the transplant regimen for the small number of patients reported [136].

These data indicate that HCs intended for allogeneic transplantation may be cryopreserved, but with the increased costs of the additional processing and the increased risks inherent with the use of cryopreserved cells. A potential benefit from the reduced risk of GVHD proposed by one center has not been confirmed by another [129,130]. For these reasons, it

Table 47.7 Engraftment and outcome for transplantation of cryopreserved marrow from allogeneic donors.

	Study 1		Study 2		Study 3
	Fresh	Frozen	Fresh	Frozen	Frozen
No. of patients	33	10	19	18	10
Days to ANC >500/µL	16	19	17	18	21
Days to platelet >50,000/µL	28	23	ND	ND	ND
aGVHD 3 grade II	57.5%	20%*	64%	78%	75%
cGVHD	ND	ND	38%	55%	20%
Day 100 mortality	39.4%	30%	32%	26%	44.4%

*Difference between fresh and frozen is significant ($p = 0.037$).
ANC, absolute neutrophil count; aGVHD, acute graft-vs.-host disease; cGVHD, chronic graft-vs.-host disease; ND, no data provided.
Study 1 adapted from Eckardt et al. [129]. Study 2 adapted from Stockschlader et al. [130]. Study 3 adapted from Stockschlader et al. [132].

is likely that cryopreservation of cells from allogeneic donors will be limited to specific situations in which the practicality of having cryopreserved cells outweighs these risks.

Tumor cell purging

Some investigators have suggested that cryopreservation provides a purging mechanism that will reduce the risk of relapse after autologous HCT [137,138]. In one study, which used a rat model of acute myeloid leukemia (AML), Hagenbeek and Martens [137] demonstrated a 30.% recovery of normal CFU-S but only a 1.4% survival of splenic colonies derived from the leukemic cell line. Allieri et al. [138] cloned leukemia progenitor cells (AML-CFU) from the peripheral blood of five patients with AML before and after cryopreservation and compared the recovery of these cells to the recovery of CFU-GM and BFU-E from marrow specimens from healthy donors. The percent recovery of AML-CFU was always <50% of the percent recovery of the normal cells in a series of cryopreservation experiments. Questions about the relevance of the models studied by these investigators can be raised and whether cryopreservation of cells reduces the risk of relapse after autologous transplantation is not answered by these two studies. The demonstration using genetically marked cells that cryopreserved marrow products can be a source of relapse in patients treated for AML, neuroblastoma and chronic myeloid leukemia suggest that cryopreservation is not a highly efficient purging technique [139–141].

Summary

The cryopreservation of HCs was explored during the earliest attempts to understand HCT [142–144]. It should be obvious from this discussion that current cryopreservation techniques are satisfactory for the treatment of many patients, but there has been no comprehensive study of HC cryobiology to quantify the cell losses resulting from cell freezing. Virtually all centers freeze cells with DMSO alone or in combination with HES. The similarities between the techniques used by different transplant centers are much greater than the differences. Current cryopreservation techniques may reduce the HC content of the product with a potential delay in engraftment if inadequate quantities of HCs are harvested and stored. Moreover, there is considerable, but generally minor, toxicity from the currently used cryoprotectants, and the equipment and processing techniques are expensive. The ideal cryopreservation solution is one that will achieve reproducible high cell recoveries, allow rapid cooling to minimize laboratory processing times and is free of the toxicities associated with DMSO.

References

1 Gorin NC. Collection, manipulation and freezing of haemopoietic stem cells. In: Goldstone AH, ed. *Clinics in Haematology*. London: Saunders & Co., 1986: 19–48.

2 Rowley SD, Piantadosi S, Santos GW. Correlation of hematologic recovery with CFU-GM content of autologous bone marrow grafts treated with 4-hydroperoxycyclophosphamide. Culture after cryopreservation. *Bone Marrow Transplant* 1989; **4**: 553–8.

3 Areman EM, Sacher RA, Deeg HJ. Processing and storage of human bone marrow: a survey of current practices in North America. *Bone Marrow Transplant* 1990; **6**: 203–9.

4 Elliot C, McCarthy D. A survey of methods of processing and storage of bone marrow and blood stem cells in the EBMT. *Bone Marrow Transplant* 1994; **14**: 419–23.

5 Lazarus HM, Pecora AL, Shea TC et al. CD34+ selection of hematopoietic blood cell collections and autotransplantation in lymphoma: overnight storage of cells at 4°C dose not affect outcome. *Bone Marrow Transplant* 2000; **25**: 559–66.

6 Beaujean F, Pico J, Norol F et al. Characteristics of peripheral blood progenitor cells frozen after 24 hours of storage. *J Hematother* 1996; **5**: 681–6.

7 Burnett AK, Tansey P, Hills C et al. Haematological reconstitution following high dose and supralethal chemo-radiotherapy using stored, noncryopreserved autologous bone marrow. *Br J Haematol* 1983; **54**: 309–16.

8 Delforge A, Ronge-Collard E, Stryckmans P, Spiro T, Malarme MA. Granulocyte-macrophage progenitor cell preservation at 4°C. *Br J Haematol* 1983; **53**: 49–54.

9 Preti RA, Razis E, Ciavarella D et al. Clinical and laboratory comparison study of refrigerated and cryopreserved bone marrow for transplantation. *Bone Marrow Transplant* 1994; **13**: 253–60.

10 Kohsake M, Yanes B, Ungerleider JS, Murphy MJ. Nonfrozen preservation of committed hematopoietic stem cells from normal human bone marrow. *Stem Cells* 1981; **1**: 111–23.

11 Niskanen E. Preservation of human granulopoietic precursors following storage in the nonfrozen state. *Transplantation* 1983; **36**: 341–3.

12 Sierra J, Conde E, Iriondo A et al. Frozen vs. nonfrozen bone marrow for autologous transplantation in lymphomas: a report from the Spanish GEL/TAMO Cooperative Group. *Ann Hematol* 1993; **67**: 111–4.

13 Ruiz-Arguelles GJ, Ruiz-Arguelles A, Perez-Romano B, Marin-Lopez A, Larregina-Diez A, Apreza-Molina MG. Filgrastim-mobilized peripheral blood stem cells can be stored at 4°C and used in autografts to rescue high-dose chemotherapy. *Am J Hematol* 1995; **48**: 100–3.

14 Seymour LK, Dansey RD, Bezwoda WR. Single high-dose etoposide and melphalan with noncryopreserved autologous marrow rescue as primary therapy for relapsed, refractory and poor-prognosis Hodgkin's disease. *Br J Cancer* 1994; **70**: 526–30.

15 Polge C, Smith AU, Parkes AS. Revival of spermatozoa after vitrification and dehydration at low temperatures. *Nature* 1949; **164**: 666.

16 Barnes DWH, Loutit JF. The radiation recovery factor: preservation by the Polge–Smith–Parkes technique. *J Natl Cancer Inst* 1955; **15**: 901–5.

17 Ferrebee JW, Billen D, Urso IM, Lu WC, Thomas ED, Congdon CC. Preservation of radiation recovery factor in frozen marrow. *Blood* 1957; **12**: 1096–100.

18 Karow AM, Webb WR. Tissue freezing. A theory for injury and survival. *Cryobiology* 1965; **2**: 99–108.

19 Mazor P. Theoretical and experimental effects of cooling and warming velocity on the survival of frozen and thawed cells. *Cryobiology* 1966; **2**: 181–92.

20 Mazur P. Cryobiology. The freezing of biological systems. *Science* 1970; **168**: 939–49.

21 Gao DY, Chang Q, Liu C et al. Fundamental cryobiology of human hematopoietic progenitor cells. I. Osmotic characteristics and volume distribution. *Cryobiology* 1998; **36**: 40–8.

22 Dooley DC, Takahashi T. The effect of osmotic stress on the function of the human granulocyte. *Exp Hematol* 1981; **9**: 731–41.

23 Law P, Alsop P, Dooley DC, Meryman HT. Studies of cell separation: a comparison of the osmotic response of human lymphocytes and granulocyte-monocyte progenitor cells. *Cryobiology* 1983; **20**: 644–51.

24 Karow AM, Webb WR. Toxicity of various solute moderators used in hypothermia. *Cryobiology* 1965; **1**: 270–3.

25 Fahy GM. The relevance of cryoprotectant "toxicity" to cryobiology. *Cryobiology* 1986; **23**: 1–13.

26 Arakawa T, Carpenter JF, Kita YA, Crowe JH. The basis for toxicity of certain cryoprotectants: a hypothesis. *Cryobiology* 1990; **27**: 401–15.

27 Takahashi T, Hirsh A, Erbe E, Williams RJ. Mechanism of cryoprotection by extracellular polymeric solutes. *Biophys J* 1988; **54**: 509–18.

28 Fahy GM, MacFarlane DR, Angell CA, Meryman HT. Vitrification as an approach to cryopreservation. *Cryobiology* 1984; **21**: 407–26.

29 Rall WF, Fahy GM. Ice-free cryopreservation of mouse embryos at −196°C by vitrification. *Nature* 1985; **313**: 573–5.

30 Kurata H, Takakuwa K, Tanaka K. Vitrification of hematopoietic progenitor cells obtained from human cord blood. *Bone Marrow Transplant* 1994; **14**: 261–3.

31 Grout BWW. The effects of ice formation during cryopreservation of clinical systems. In: Fuller BJ, Grout BWW, eds. *Clinical Application of Cryobiology*. Boca Raton, FL: CRC Press, 1991: 81–94.

32 Luyet B. On various phase transitions occurring in aqueous solutions at low temperatures. *Ann N Y Acad Sci* 1960; **85**: 549–69.

33 Ragab AH, Gilkerson E, Myers M. Factors in the cryopreservation of bone marrow cells from children with acute lymphocytic leukemia. *Cryobiology* 1977; **14**: 125–34.

34 Stiff PJ, Murgo AJ, Zaroulis CG et al. Unfractionated human marrow cell cryopreservation using dimethylsulfoxide and hydroxyethyl starch. *Cryobiology* 1983; **20**: 17–24.

35 Conscience J-F, Fischer F. An improved preservation technique for cells of hemopoietic origin. *Cryobiology* 1985; **22**: 495–8.
36 Karow AM, Pegg DE, eds. *Organ Preservation for Transplantation*. New York: Marcel Dekker, 1981.
37 Fuller BJ, Grout BWW, eds. *Clinical Application of Cryobiology*. Boca Raton, FL: CRC Press, 1991.
38 Fuller BJ. The effects of cooling on mammalian cells. In: Fuller BJ, Grout BWW, eds. *Clinical Application of Cryobiology*. Boca Raton, FL: CRC Press, 1991: 1–21.
39 Vos O, Kaalen MCAC. Prevention of freezing damage to proliferating cells in tissue culture. A quantitative study of a number of agents. *Cryobiology* 1965; **2**: 249–60.
40 McGann LE, Walterson ML. Cryoprotection by dimethyl sulfoxide and dimethyl sulfone. *Cryobiology* 1987; **24**: 11–6.
41 Kruuv J, Glofcheski DJ, Lepock JR. Interactions between cryoprotectors and cryosensitizers. *Cryobiology* 1990; **27**: 232–46.
42 Anchordoguy TJ, Cecchini CA, Crowe JH, Crowe LM. Insights into the cryoprotective mechanism of dimethyl sulfoxide for phospholipid bilayers. *Cryobiology* 1991; **28**: 467–73.
43 Carpenter JF, Crowe JH. The mechanism of cryoprotection of proteins by solutes. *Cryobiology* 1988; **25**: 244–55.
44 Crowe JH, Crowe LM, Carpenter JF, Aurell-Wistrom C. Stabilization of dry phospholipid bilayers and proteins by sugars. *Biochem J* 1987; **242**: 1–10.
45 Crowe JH, Carpenter JF, Crowe LM, Anchordoguy TJ. Are freezing and dehydration similar stress vectors? A comparison of modes of interaction of stabilizing solutes with biomolecules. *Cryobiology* 1990; **27**: 219–31.
46 Gilmore MJML. GCT-conditioned medium: an unsuitable stimulus for monitoring granulocyte-macrophage colony-forming cells in cryopreserved bone marrow. *Cryobiology* 1983; **20**: 106–10.
47 De Boer F, Drager AM, Van der Wall E, Pinedo HM, Schuurhuis GJ. Changes in L-selectin expression on CD34-positive cells upon cryopreservation of peripheral blood stem cell transplants. *Bone Marrow Transplant* 1998; **22**: 1103–10.
48 Rowley SD, Feng Z, Chen L et al. A randomized phase III clinical trial of autologous blood stem cell transplantation comparing cryopreservation using dimethylsulfoxide versus dimethylsulfoxide with hydroxyethylstarch. *Bone Marrow Transplant* 2003; **31**: 1043–51.
49 Rowley SD. Techniques of bone marrow and stem cell cryopreservation and storage. In: Sacher R, AuBuchon J, eds. *Marrow Transplantation: Practical and Technical Aspects of Stem Cell Reconstitution*. Bethesda, MD: American Association of Blood Banks, 1992: 105–27.
50 Stiff PJ, Koester AR, Weidner MK et al. Autologous bone marrow transplantation using unfractionated cells cryopreserved in dimethylsulfoxide and hydroxyethyl starch without controlled-rate freezing. *Blood* 1987; **70**: 974–8.
51 Makino S, Harada M, Akashi K et al. A simplified method for cryopreservation of peripheral blood stem cells at −80°C without rate-controlled freezing. *Bone Marrow Transplant* 1991; **8**: 239–44.
52 Clark J, Pati A, McCarthy D. Successful cryopreservation of human bone marrow does not require a controlled-rate freezer. *Bone Marrow Transplant* 1991; **7**: 121–5.
53 Lovelock JE, Bishop MWH. Prevention of freezing damage to living cells by dimethylsulphoxide. *Nature* 1959; **183**: 1394–5.
54 David NA. The pharmacology of dimethyl sulfoxide 6544. *Ann Rev Pharmacol* 1972; **12**: 353–74.
55 Willhite CC, Katz PI. Dimethyl sulfoxide. *J Appl Toxicol* 1984; **4**: 155–60.
56 Galmes A, Besalduch J, Bargay J et al. Cryopreservation of hematopoietic progenitor cells with 5% dimethyl sulfoxide at −80°C without rate-controlled freezing. *Transfusion* 1996; **36**: 794–7.
57 Donaldson C, Armitage WJ, Denning-Kendall PA, Nicol AJ, Bradley BA, Howes JM. Optimal cryopreservation of human umbilical cord blood. *Bone Marrow Transplant* 1996; **18**: 725–31.
58 Ashwood-Smith MJ, Warby C, Connor KW, Becker G. Low-temperature preservation of mammalian cells in tissue culture with polyvinylpyrrolidone (PVP), dextrans, and hydroxyethyl starch (HES). *Cryobiology* 1972; **9**: 441–9.
59 van Putten LM. Monkey and mouse bone marrow preservation and the choice of technique for human application. *Proceedings of the 11th Congress of the International Society for Blood Transfusion*, Sydney, Australia. Basel/New York: Karger, 1968: 797–801.
60 Takaue Y, Abe T, Kawano Y et al. Comparative analysis of engraftment after cryopreservation of peripheral blood stem cell autografts by controlled-versus uncontrolled-rate methods. *Bone Marrow Transplant* 1994; **13**: 801–4.
61 Knight SC, Farrant J, McGann LE. Storage of human lymphocytes by freezing in serum alone. *Cryobiology* 1977; **14**: 112–5.
62 Grilli G, Porcellini A, Lucarelli G. Role of serum on cryopreservation and subsequent viability of mouse bone marrow hemopoietic stem cells. *Cryobiology* 1980; **17**: 516–20.
63 Berenson RJ, Bensinger WI, Hill RS et al. Engraftment after infusion of CD34+ marrow cells in patients with breast cancer or neuroblastoma. *Blood* 1991; **77**: 1717–22.
64 Shpall EJ, Jones RB, Bearman SI et al. Transplantation of enriched CD34-positive autologous marrow into breast cancer patients following high-dose chemotherapy: influence of CD34-positive peripheral-blood progenitors and growth factors on engraftment. *J Clin Oncol* 1994; **12**: 28–36.
65 Sallan SE, Niemeyer CM, Billett AL. Autologous bone marrow transplantation for acute lymphoblastic leukemia. *J Clin Oncol* 1989; **7**: 1594–601.
66 Dicke KA, McCredie KB, Spitzer G et al. Autologous bone marrow transplantation in patients with adult acute leukemia in relapse. *Transplantation* 1978; **26**: 169–73.
67 Lowenberg B, Abels J, van Bekkum DW et al. Transplantation of nonpurified autologous bone marrow in patients with AML in first remission. *Cancer* 1984; **54**: 2840–3.
68 Rubinsky B, Arav A, Devries AL. The cryoprotective effect of antifreeze glycopeptides from Antarctic fishes. *Cryobiology* 1992; **29**: 69–79.
69 Carpenter JF, Hansen TN. Antifreeze protein modulates cell survival during cryopreservation. Mediation through influence on ice crystal growth. *Proc Natl Acad Sci USA* 1992; **89**: 8953–7.
70 Mazur P, Cole KW. Roles of unfrozen fraction, salt concentration, and changes in cell volume in the survival of frozen human erythrocytes. *Cryobiology* 1989; **26**: 1–29.
71 Leibo SP, Farrant J, Mazur P et al. Effects of freezing on marrow stem cells suspensions: interactions of cooling and warming rates in the presence of PVP, sucrose or glycerol. *Cryobiology* 1970; **6**: 315–32.
72 Clark P, Fahy GM, Karow AM. Factors influencing renal cryopreservation. II. Toxic effects of three cryoprotectants in combination with three vehicle solutions in nonfrozen rabbit cortical slices. *Cryobiology* 1984; **21**: 274–84.
73 Visani G, Dinota A, Tosi P et al. Cryopreserved autologous bone marrow transplantation in patients with acute nonlymphoid leukemia: chemotherapy before harvesting is the main factor in delaying hematological recovery. *Cryobiology* 1990; **27**: 103–6.
74 Rowley SD, Piantadosi S, Marcellus DC et al. Analysis of factors predicting speed of hematologic recovery after transplantation with 4-hydroperoxycyclophosphamide-purged autologous bone marrow grafts. *Bone Marrow Transplant* 1991; **7**: 183–91.
75 Tokushima Y, Sasayama N, Takahashi TA. Repopulating activities of human cord blood cells separated by a stem cell collection filter in NOD/SCID mice: a comparison study of filter method and HES method. *Transfusion* 2001; **41**: 1014–9.
76 Pegg DE. *In vitro* assessment of cell viability in human bone marrow preserved at −79°C. *J Appl Physiol* 1964; **19**: 123–6.
77 Rowe AW. Biochemical aspects of cryoprotective agents in freezing and thawing. *Cryobiology* 1966; **3**: 12–8.
78 Rowley SD, Anderson GL. Effect of DMSO exposure without cryopreservation on hematopoietic progenitor cells. *Bone Marrow Transplant* 1993; **11**: 389–93.
79 Goldman JM, Th'ng KH, Park DS et al. Collection, cryopreservation and subsequent viability of haemopoietic stem cells intended for treatment of chronic granulocytic leukaemia in blast-cell transformation. *Br J Haematol* 1987; **40**: 185–95.
80 Visani G, Ricci P, Motta MR et al. Recovery of CFU-GM after freezing of normal human bone marrow: effect of three dilution techniques after thawing. *Cryobiology* 1983; **20**: 587–90.
81 Dicke KA, Vellekoop L, Spitzer G et al. The role of autologous bone marrow transplantation in neoplasia. In: Okunewick JP, Meredith RE, eds. *Graft-Versus-Leukemia in Man and Animal Models*. Boca Raton, FL: CRC Press, 1981: 68–96.
82 de Loecker R, Goossens W, Bruneel P et al. The prevention of erythrocyte swelling upon dilution after freezing and thawing. *Cryobiology* 1991; **28**: 237–45.
83 Rubinstein P, Dobrila L, Rosenfield RE et al. Processing and cryopreservation of placental/umbilical cord blood for unrelated bone marrow reconstitution. *Proc Natl Acad Sci USA* 1995; **92**: 10,119–22.
84 Douay L, Lopez M, Gorin NC. A technical bias. Differences in cooling rates prevent ampoules from being a reliable index of stem cell cryopreservation in large volumes. *Cryobiology* 1986; **23**: 296–301.
85 Sputtek A, Korber C. Cryopreservation of red blood cells, platelets, lymphocytes, and stem cells. In: Fuller BJ, Grout BWW, eds. *Clinical Application of Cryobiology*. Boca Raton, FL: CRC Press, 1991: 95–147.
86 Smith DM, Weisenberger DD, Bierman P, Kessinger A, Vaughn WP, Armitage JO. Acute renal failure associated with autologous bone

marrow transplantation. *Bone Marrow Transplant* 1987; **2**: 195–201.

87 Berenson RJ, Shpall EJ, Auditore-Hargreaves K, Heimfeld S, Jacobs C, Krieger MS. Transplantation of CD34+ hematopoietic progenitor cells. *Cancer Invest* 1996; **14**: 589–96.

88 Mazur P, Cole KW. Influence of cell concentration on the contribution of unfrozen fraction and salt concentration to the survival of slowly frozen human erythrocytes. *Cryobiology* 1985; **22**: 509–36.

89 Rowley SD, Bensinger WI, Gooley TA, Buckner CD. Effect of cell concentration on bone marrow and peripheral blood stem cell cryopreservation. *Blood* 1994; **83**: 2731–6.

90 Keung Y-K, Cobos E, Morgan D et al. High cellular concentration of peripheral blood progenitor cells during cryopreservation adversely affects CFU-GM but not hematopoietic recovery. *J Hematother* 1996; **5**: 73–7.

91 Rowley SD, MacLeod B, Heimfeld S, Holmberg L, Bensinger WI. Severe central nervous system toxicity associated with the infusion of cryopreserved PBSC components. *Cytotherapy* 1999; **1**: 311–7.

92 Ma DDF, Johnson LA, Chan PM, Biggs JC. Factors influencing myeloid stem cell (CFU-C) survival after cryopreservation of human marrow and chronic granulocytic leukemia cells. *Cryobiology* 1982; **19**: 1–9.

93 Lewis JP, Passovoy M, Trobaugh RE. Studies on the effect of controlled rate cooling on marrow viability. *Proceedings of the 10th Congress of the International Society for Blood Transfusion*, Stockholm, Sweden. Basel/New York: Karger, 1964: 656–61.

94 Gorin NC, Douay L, David R et al. Delayed kinetics of recovery of haemopoiesis following autologous bone marrow transplantation. The role of excessively rapid marrow freezing rates after the release of fusion heat. *Eur J Cancer Clin Oncol* 1983; **19**: 485–91.

95 Karow AM. Biophysical and chemical considerations in cryopreservation. In: Karow AM, Pegg DE, eds. *Organ Preservation for Transplantation.* New York: Marcel Dekker, 1981: 113–41.

96 Kurnick NB, Feder BH, Montano A et al. Some observations on the treatment of postirradiation hematopoietic depression in man by the infusion of stored autogenous bone marrow. *Ann Intern Med* 1959; **51**: 1204–19.

97 Pegg DE, Humble JG, Newton KA. The clinical application of bone marrow grafting. *Br J Cancer* 1962; **16**: 417–35.

98 Bender MA, Tran PT, Smith LH. Preservation of viable bone marrow cells by freezing. *J Appl Physiol* 1960; **15**: 520–4.

99 Appelbaum FR, Herzig GP, Graw RG et al. Study of cell dose and storage time on engraftment of cryopreserved autologous bone marrow in a canine model. *Transplantation* 1976; **26**: 245–8.

100 Rowley SD, Byrne DV. Low-temperature storage of bone marrow in nitrogen vapor-phase refrigerators: decreased temperature gradients using aluminum racking systems. *Transfusion* 1992; **32**: 750–4.

101 Schafer TW, Everett J, Silver GH, Came PE. Biohazard-virus contaminated liquid nitrogen [letter]. *Science* 1976; **191**: 24.

102 Tedder RS, Zuckerman MA, Goldstone AH et al. Hepatitis B transmission from contaminated cryopreservation tank. *Lancet* 1995; **346**: 137–40.

103 Stiff PJ. Simplified bone marrow cryopreservation using dimethyl sulfoxide and hydroxyethyl starch as cryoprotectants. In: Gee AP, ed. *Bone Marrow Processing and Purging. A Practical Guide.* Boca Raton, FL: CRC Press, 1991: 341–9.

104 Galmes A, Besalduch J, Bargay J et al. Long-term storage at –80°C of hematopoietic progenitor cells with 5-percent dimethyl sulfoxide as the sole cryoprotectant. *Transfusion* 1999; **39**: 70–3.

105 Parker LM, Binder N, Gelman R et al. Prolonged cryopreservation of human bone marrow. *Transplantation* 1981; **31**: 454–7.

106 Aird W, Labopin M, Gorin NC, Antin JH. Long-term cryopreservation of human stem cells. *Bone Marrow Transplant* 1992; **9**: 487–90.

107 Attarian H, Feng Z, Buckner CD, MacLeod B, Rowley SD. Long-term cryopreservation of bone marrow for autologous transplantation. *Bone Marrow Transplant* 1996; **17**: 425–30.

108 Beaujean F, Hartmann O, Le Forestier C, Bayet S, Duedari N, Parmentier C. Successful infusion of 40 cryopreserved autologous bone-marrows. *In vitro* studies of the freezing procedure. *Biomed Pharmacother* 1984; **38**: 348–52.

109 Abrams RA, Polacek L, Buck P. Postcryopreservation growth of human CFU-GM. Sequential examination of methodologic factors. *Exp Hematol* 1985; **13**: 1089–93.

110 Beaujean F, Hartmann O, Kuentz M et al. A simple, efficient washing procedure for cryopreserved human hematopoietic stem cells prior to reinfusion. *Bone Marrow Transplant* 1991; **8**: 291–4.

111 Rubinstein P, Dobrila L, Rosenfield RE et al. Processing and cryopreservation of placental/umbilical cord blood for unrelated bone marrow reconstitution. *Proc Nat Acad Sci U S A* 1995; **92**: 10,119–22.

112 Weiner RS, Tobias JS, Yankee RA. The processing of human bone marrow for cryopreservation and reinfusion. *Biomedicine* 1976; **24**: 226–31.

113 Alcorn MJ, Holyoake TL, Richmond L et al. CD34-positive cells isolated from cryopreserved peripheral-blood progenitor cells can be expanded *ex vivo* and used for transplantation with little or no toxicity. *J Clin Oncol* 1996; **14**: 1839–47.

114 Bohbot A, Lioure B, Faradji A et al. Positive selection of CD34+ cells from cryopreserved peripheral blood stem cells after thawing: technical aspects and clinical use. *Bone Marrow Transplant* 1996; **17**: 259–64.

115 Douay L, Gorin NC, David R et al. Study of granulocyte-macrophage progenitor (CFU$_c$) preservation after slow freezing of bone marrow in the gas phase of liquid nitrogen. *Exp Hematol* 1982; **10**: 360–6.

116 Davis JM, Rowley SD, Braine HG, Piantadosi S, Santos GW. Clinical toxicity of cryopreserved bone marrow graft infusion. *Blood* 1990; **75**: 781–6.

117 Stroncek DF, Fautsch SK, Lasky LC, Hurd DD, Ramsay NKC, McCullough J. Adverse reactions in patients transfused with cryopreserved marrow. *Transfusion* 1991; **31**: 521–6.

118 Okamoto Y, Takaue Y, Saito S et al. Toxicities associated with cryopreserved and thawed peripheral blood stem cell autografts in children with active cancer. *Transfusion* 1993; **33**: 578–81.

119 Vriesendorp R, Aalders JG, Sleijfer DT et al. Effective high-dose chemotherapy with autologous bone marrow infusion in resistant ovarian cancer. *Gynecol Oncol* 1984; **17**: 271–6.

120 Rapoport AP, Rowe JM, Packman CH, Ginsberg SJ. Cardiac arrest after autologous marrow infusion. *Bone Marrow Transplant* 1991; **7**: 401–3.

121 Styler MJ, Topolsky DL, Crilley PA et al. Transient high grade heart block following autologous bone marrow infusion. *Bone Marrow Transplant* 1992; **10**: 435–8.

122 Keung Y-K, Lau S, Elkayam U, Chen S-C, Douer D. Cardiac arrhythmia after infusion of cryopreserved stem cells. *Bone Marrow Transplant* 1994; **14**: 363–7.

123 Lopez-Jimenez J, Cervero C, Munoz A et al. Cardiovascular toxicities related to the infusion of cryopreserved grafts: results of a controlled study. *Bone Marrow Transplant* 1994; **13**: 789–93.

124 Dhodapkar M, Goldberg SL, Tefferi A, Gertz MA. Reversible encephalopathy after cryopreserved peripheral blood stem cell infusion. *Am J Hematol* 1994; **45**: 187–8.

125 Runckel DN, Swanson JR. Effect of dimethyl sulfoxide on serum osmolality. *Clin Chem* 1980; **26**: 1745–7.

126 DiStefano V, Klahn JJ. Observations on the pharmacology and hemolytic activity of dimethyl sulfoxide. *Toxicol Appl Pharmacol* 1965; **7**: 660–6.

127 Samoszuk M, Reid ME, Toy PTCY. Intravenous dimethylsulfoxide therapy causes severe hemolysis mimicking a hemolytic transfusion reaction [letter]. *Transfusion* 1983; **23**: 405.

128 Lasky LC, Van Buren N, Weisdorf DJ et al. Successful allogeneic cryopreserved marrow transplantation. *Transfusion* 1989; **29**: 182–4.

129 Eckardt JR, Roodman GD, Boldt DH et al. Comparison of engraftment and acute GVHD in patients undergoing cryopreserved or fresh allogeneic BMT. *Bone Marrow Transplant* 1993; **11**: 125–31.

130 Stockschlader M, Kruger W, Kroschke G et al. Use of cryopreserved bone marrow in allogeneic bone marrow transplantation. *Bone Marrow Transplant* 1995; **15**: 569–72.

131 Stockschlader M, Hassan HT, Krog C et al. Long-term follow-up of leukaemia patients after related cryopreserved allogeneic bone marrow transplantation. *Br J Haematol* 1997; **96**: 382–6.

132 Stockschlader M, Kruger W, tom Dieck A et al. Use of cryopreserved bone marrow in unrelated allogeneic transplantation. *Bone Marrow Transplant* 1996; **17**: 197–9.

133 Laughlin MJ, Barker J, Bamback B et al. Hematopoietic engraftment and survival in adult recipients of umbilical-cord blood from unrelated donors. *N Engl J Med* 2001; **344**: 1815–22.

134 Barker JN, Davies SM, DeFor T et al. Survival after transplantation of unrelated donor umbilical cord blood is comparable to that of human leukocyte antigen-matched unrelated donor bone marrow: results of a matched-pair analysis. *Blood* 2001; **97**: 2957–61.

135 Rocha V, Cornish J, Sievers EL et al. Comparison of outcomes of unrelated bone marrow and umbilical cord blood transplants in children with acute leukemia. *Blood* 2001; **97**: 2962–71.

136 Kurtzberg J, Laughlin M, Graham ML et al. Placental blood as a source of hematopoietic stem cells for transplantation into unrelated recipients. *N Engl J Med* 1996; **335**: 157–66.

137 Hagenbeek A, Martens ACM. Cryopreservation of autologous marrow grafts in acute leukemia: Survival of *in vivo* clonogenic leukemic cells and normal hemopoietic stem cells. *Leukemia* 1989; **3**: 535–7.

138 Allieri MA, Lopez M, Douay L, Mary JYN, Guyen L, Gorin NC. Clonogenic leukemic progenitor cells in acute myelocytic leukemia are highly

sensitive to cryopreservation: possible purging effect for autologous bone marrow transplantation. *Bone Marrow Transplant* 1991; **7**: 101–5.
139 Brenner MK, Rill DR, Holladay MS *et al.* Gene marking to determine whether autologous marrow infusion restores long-term haemopoiesis in cancer patients. *Lancet* 1993; **342**: 1134–7.
140 Rill DR, Santana VM, Roberts WM *et al.* Direct demonstration that autologous bone marrow transplantation for solid tumors can return a multiplicity of tumorigenic cells. *Blood* 1994; **84**: 380–3.
141 Deisseroth AB, Zu Z, Claxton D *et al.* Genetic marking shows that Ph+ cells present in autologous transplants of chronic myelogenous leukemia (CML) contribute to relapse after autologous bone marrow in CML. *Blood* 1994; **83**: 3068–76.
142 Ferrebee JW, Lochte HL, Swanberg H, Thomas ED. The collection and storage of viable human fetal hematopoietic tissue for intravenous use. *Blood* 1959; **14**: 1173–9.
143 Ferrebee JS, Atkins L, Lochte HL *et al.* The collection, storage and preparation of viable cadaver marrow for intravenous use. *Blood* 1959; **14**: 140–7.
144 Cavins JA, Scheer SC, Thomas ED, Ferrebee JW. The recovery of lethally irradiated dogs given infusion of autologous leukocytes preserved at −80°C. *Blood* 1964; **23**: 38–43.

48

Jürgen Finke & Roland Mertelsmann

Recombinant Growth Factors after Hematopoietic Cell Transplantation

The field of autologous and allogeneic hematopoietic cell transplantation (HCT) has changed considerably during the last decade due to the availability of cytokine mobilized peripheral blood hematopoietic cells as a graft source. Despite the more rapid hematopoietic reconstitution compared to the use of marrow-derived grafts, high-dose chemotherapy preceding HCT still induces a period of severe marrow aplasia with the risk of infections and bleeding, requiring prophylactic and therapeutic interventions. Sepsis during the time of neutropenia represents a major problem and may result in transplant-related death.

Hematopoietic growth factors and other cytokines contribute to the regulation of cellular growth and differentiation of the lympho-hematopoietic system. Early acting growth factors contribute to the differentiation of pluripotent stem cells, capable of self-renewal, into multipotent and committed progenitor cells, and late-acting growth factors lead to further differentiation, eventually giving rise to mature cell elements with distinct function (Fig. 48.1). However, almost all growth factors have multiple biologic activities, partly overlapping or synergistic with other hematopoietic growth factors, and can act on more than one cell type (Table 48.1). It has been demonstrated in murine models that, in addition to very primitive long-term hematopoietic cells, other progenitor cells with a lower proliferative potential and restricted differentiation capabilities contribute to the hematopoietic reconstitution after HCT [1–3]. Xenotransplantation of human hematopoietic cells into severely immunodeficient mice revealed heterogeneity in the human transplantable stem cell compartment [4,5]. Kinetic as well as cell purification studies suggested that hematopoietic reconstitution in humans is dominated by different types of short-term repopulating cells during the first months after HCT [6,7]. Myeloid-restricted short-term repopulating cells play a major role during the 1st month after transplantation and are followed by a second type of short-term repopulating cells able to regenerate myeloid as well as lymphoid lineages for a still undefined period of time [4].

Engraftment kinetics after HCT can be influenced by the use of recombinant hematopoietic growths factors and numerous studies, including randomized trials, have demonstrated the effects and established the role of specific growth factors after HCT.

Erythropoietin (EPO)

EPO was the first growth factor to be identified experimentally and to be made available as a recombinant protein. EPO is widely used for the successful treatment of anemia associated with renal failure. The anemia encountered in HCT recipients is partly due to a relative EPO deficiency. Frequently, patients are already anaemic prior to transplantation and present with elevated serum EPO levels [8]. Inappropriately low EPO levels in relation to the severity of anemia during the period following HCT is attributed to several causes such as toxic effects of high-dose therapy and drugs like cyclosporine on EPO-producing cells of the kidney, as well as inhibitory effects of inflammatory cytokines like tumor necrosis factor alpha (TNF-α) on hypoxia-induced EPO production.

Recombinant human EPO (rHuEPO) after autologous HCT

Several trials have addressed the value of rHuEPO after transplantation to accelerate red cell regeneration and to decrease the need for red blood cell (RBC) transfusions. After autologous bone marrow transplantation (BMT), rHuEPO has been used in phase 2 as well randomized phase 3 trials alone or in combination with granulocyte colony-stimulating factor (G-CSF) or granulocyte macrophage colony-stimulating factor (GM-CSF) [9–13]. Although EPO was tolerated without side-effects and an increase in reticulocyte counts was attained, no obvious benefit regarding transfusional requirements, engraftment or treatment outcome was observed.

RHuEPO after allogeneic HCT

After allogeneic marrow transplantation rHuEPO did enhance reticulocytosis, increased hemoglobin (Hb) levels and reduced time to transfusion independence, resulting in the need for fewer RBC transfusions. In a large multicenter, placebo controlled, randomized trial 106 patients were treated with rHuEPO after allogeneic BMT and 109 patients with placebo [11]. Patients received either 150 IU/kg/day C127 mouse-cell-derived rHuEPO or placebo as continuous intravenous infusion. Therapy started after the bone-graft infusion and was continued until independence from RBC transfusions for 7 consecutive days with stable Hb levels ≥90 g/L or until day 41 after BMT. The reticulocyte counts were significantly higher with rHuEPO from day 21 to day 42 after BMT. The median time to RBC transfusion independence was 19 days (range, 16.3–21.6) with rHuEPO and 27 days (range, 22.3 to >42) with placebo ($p < 0.003$). The mean (± SD) numbers of RBC transfusions until day 20 after BMT were 6.6 ± 4.8 with rHuEPO and 6.0 ± 3.8 with placebo. However, from day 21 to day 41, the rHuEPO-treated patients received 1.4 ± 2.5 (median: 0) transfusions and the control group received 2.7 ± 4.0 (median: 2) transfusions ($p = 0.004$). In the follow-up period from day 42 to day 100, 2.4 ± 5.6 transfusions were required with rHuEPO and 4.5 ± 9.6 were required with placebo ($p = 0.075$). A multivariate analysis showed that acute graft-vs.-host disease (GVHD), major ABO blood group incompatibility, age above 35 years and hemorrhage significantly increased the need for transfusions. However, after day 20, rHuEPO significantly reduced the number of RBC transfusions in these patient groups. For the whole study period, rHuEPO reduced the transfusion requirements in patients with

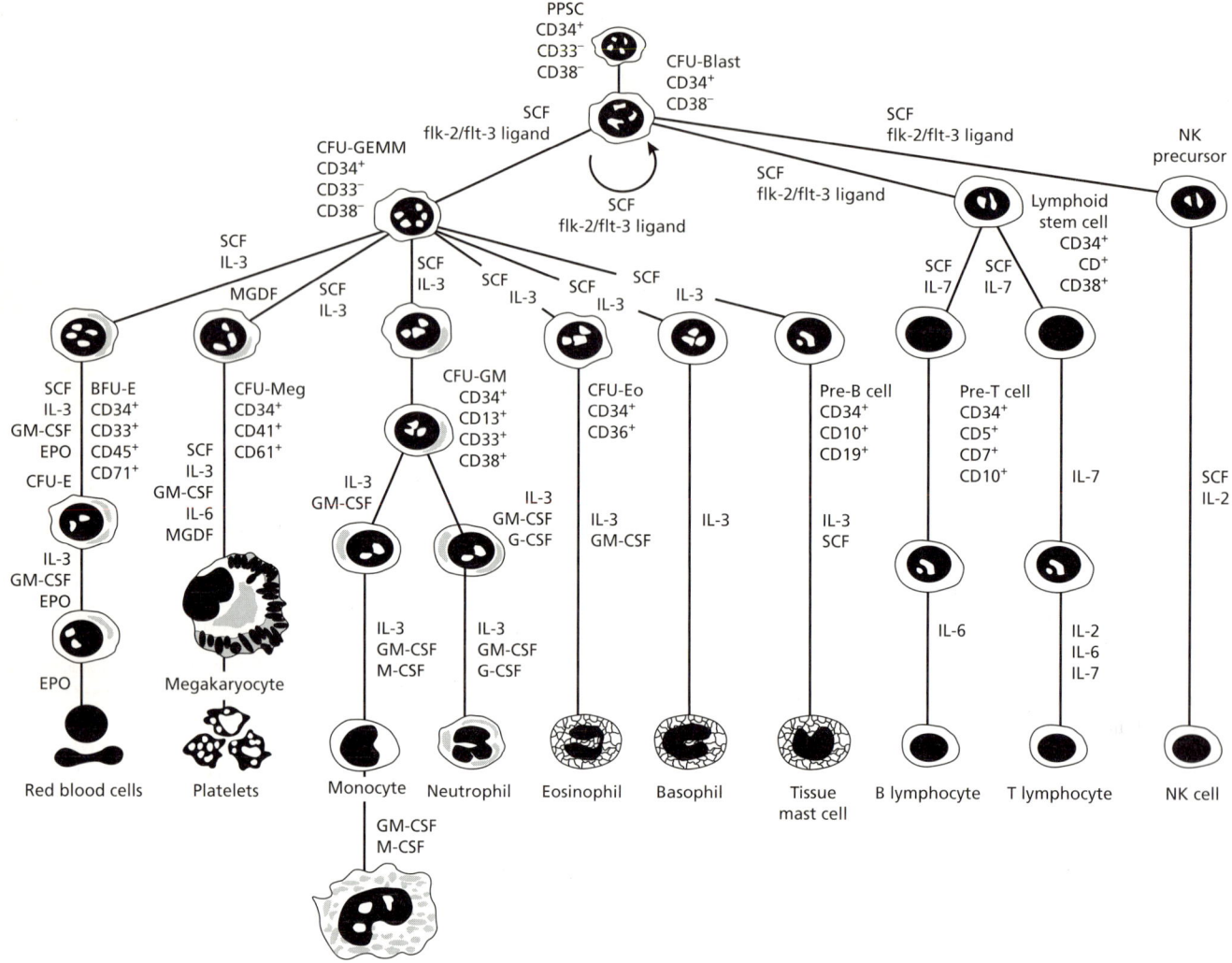

Fig. 48.1 Schematic illustration of the hematopoeitic lineages and the respective growth factors that promote proliferation and differenteition of stem cells into mature effector cells. BFU, burst forming unit; CFU, colony forming unit; IL, interleukin; EPO, erythropietin; G-CSF, granulocyte colony-stimulating factor; GM-CSF, granulocyte macrophage colony-stimulating factor; PPSC, pluripotent progenitor stem cell; SCF, stem-cell factor.

Table 48.1 Growth factors available for clinical use.

Growth factor	Gene localization	Naturally induced by	Main effector lineage	Generic name
EPO	7q21	Hypoxia	Erythroid	Epoetin alpa, beta
G-CSF	17q11.2-q12	IL-1, TNF-α, endotoxin	Myeloid	Filgrastim, lenograstim
GM-CSF	5q31.1	TNF-α, lipopolysaccharide	Myeloid/macrophage	Molgramostin, sargramostim
IL-3	5q31.1	Activation	Progenitor/myeloid/lymphoid	n.a.
SCF	12q22-24	Constitutive	Myeloid/lymphoid	Ancestim
MGDF/TPO	3q2-28	Constitutive (thrombocytopenia)	Megakaryocytic/progenitor	n.a.
IL-11	19q13.3-13.4	IL-1	Lymphoid/myeloid/megakaryocytic	Oprelvekin

EPO, erythropoietin; G-CSF, granulocyte colony-stimulating factor; GM-CSF, granulocyte macrophage colony-stimulating factor; IL, interleukin; MGDF, megakaryocyte growth and differentiation factor; n.a., not applicable; SCF, stem-cell factor; TNF-α, tumor necrosis factor alpha; TPO, thrombopoietin.

GVHD grade III and grade IV from 18.4 ± 8.6–8.5 ± 6.8 U ($p = 0.05$) [11].

In another phase 3 trial in allogeneic BMT, 50 patients were randomized to treatment with rHuEPO ($n = 25$) or placebo ($n = 25$) [8]. RHuEPO was given at 200 U/kg daily for 4 weeks and 200 U/kg twice weekly for a further 4 weeks. There were no differences between the two groups regarding time to engraftment, fever, hospitalization, GVHD, infections, hemorrhages, transplant-related mortality, relapse and survival. However, more patients in the control group had an elevated serum creatinine (43% vs. 14%; $p = 0.04$). RBC transfusion requirements for the first 2 months after BMT were significantly lower in the rHuEPO group compared with the control group (5 U vs. 10 U; $p = 0.04$). Time to unsupported

Hb >70 g/L was less in patients treated with rHuEPO (14 days vs. 24 days; $p = 0.03$). No effect was seen on platelet engraftment or the number of transfused platelet units. According to the protocol, the study drug was reduced (Hb >100 g/L) or discontinued (Hb >120 g/L) for a mean of 3.6 weeks among 11 rHuEPO patients compared with 1.9 weeks among seven controls ($p = 0.02$) [8].

Ninety-one patients between the ages of 17 and 58 years undergoing allogeneic transplants from sibling donors were entered into a double-blind randomized trial to evaluate the effect of rHuEPO at a dose of 300 U/kg/day given thrice weekly by intravenous injection. Treatment ended when the Hb exceeded 120 g/L and recommenced if the Hb fell below 120 g/L, at 150 U/kg/day. If the Hb exceeded 120 g/L on a further occasion, the dose of rHuEPO was not given. Patients received 2 U of erythrocytes when the Hb dropped below 85 g/L. Univariate analysis revealed a significantly higher reticulocyte count, Hb concentration and bone marrow erythropoiesis after day 14 in the group receiving rHuEPO, but this was not reflected in decreased RBC transfusions (7 ± 5 transfusions in controls vs. 6 ± 5 transfusions in rHuEPO group). However, in the multivariate analysis, the administration of rHuEPO was associated with an 18% reduction in RBC transfusion requirement when other variables were taken into account [14].

Allogeneic HCT with major ABO blood group incompatibility may be associated with markedly prolonged time to RBC engraftment, immune hemolysis or pure red cell aplasia. Several reports suggested a curative effect of rHuEPO for these patients [15,16]. In a patient with normal neutrophil and platelet engraftment and pure red cell aplasia despite documentation of an elevated endogenous EPO level (360 mU/mL; normal value, <19 mU/mL) during the 230-day period of absent erythropoiesis, erythroid engraftment was observed soon after the initiation of human recombinant EPO at a dose of 50 U/kg daily [15]. A 32-year-old AML patient developed pure red cell aplasia after major ABO incompatible BMT. After receiving rHuEPO and methylprednisolone she developed reticulocytosis and hemolysis. She promptly recovered from hemolysis and pure red cell aplasia after plasmapheresis [16]. In the era of reduced intensity conditioning using fludarabine based conditioning regimens, a higher incidence of pure red cell aplasia may be expected in patients with high antidonor isoagglutinins in comparison to myeloablative regimens [17]. No randomized trial has addressed the role of rHuEPO late after HCT for slow RBC engraftment. However, in individual patients with inappropriate reticulocyte counts and relatively low serum EPO levels the application of rHuEPO may be of benefit.

In summary, rHuEPO stimulates erythroid engraftment after BMT resulting in a small but significant reduction of RBC transfusion requirements. Whereas trials after autologous transplantation showed negative results the beneficial effect after allogeneic BMT was more prominent. Later after allogeneic HCT individual patients with delayed erythropoiesis benefit from the application of rHuEPO.

Granulocyte colony-stimulating factor (G-CSF)

G-CSF is produced by many cell types and is rapidly induced by inflammatory stimuli. In vivo studies demonstrated that G-CSF is a potent myeloid growth and differentiation factor. The dose dependent increase of peripheral blood neutrophils is caused by expansion of the myeloid compartment in the marrow, an accelerated production of mature neutrophils and a rapid shift of mature neutrophils from the marrow sinusoids into the peripheral blood [18].

Side-effects of rHuG-CSF administration are usually mild and include bone pain, occasionally low grade fever and weight gain. After high-dose therapy and HCT transient pulmonary infiltrates that cause dyspnea, especially during the early phase of hematopoietic engraftment, can occasionally be observed radiologically and clinically. High-dose corticosteroids and diuretics are the treatment of choice. The entity of the clinical findings of fever, capillary leak and pulmonary infiltrates, also including skin rash, observed during engraftment after HCT, has been termed "engraftment syndrome" and post-transplant G-CSF increased the incidence of this syndrome [19].

Two recombinant preparations of G-CSF are commonly in use, filgrastim produced in *Escherichia coli* and the glycosylated form lenograstim produced in a Chinese hamster ovary cell line.

RHuG-CSF after autologous HCT

Early data suggested that, after autologous BMT, neutrophil recovery was accelerated in G-CSF treated patients, compared with historical controls, exceeding 0.5×10^9/L at a mean of 11 days after marrow infusion, compared with 20 days for controls; a significant difference. This reduction led to significantly fewer days of parenteral antibiotic therapy, 11 days vs. 18 days in controls, and less isolation in reverse barrier nursing, 10 days vs. 18 days [20]. Similar data were obtained after autologous BMT in lymphoma patients [21].

Several large randomized trials have confirmed the significantly accelerated neutrophil engraftment after autologous BMT or peripheral blood stem cell transplantation (PBSCT) compared to placebo (Table 48.2 [22–30]). Lenograstim was given to 315 patients after autologous or allogeneic BMT in a prospective randomized placebo controlled multicenter trial [22]. One day after bone marrow infusion, 163 patients received lenograstim 5 µg/kg/day by 30-min infusion and 152 patients received placebo daily for 28 days or until neutrophil recovery. Patients were stratified by age and by type of BMT. Neutrophil recovery to above 10^9/L for 3 consecutive days was seen earlier in lenograstim-treated patients (16 days vs. 27 days, $p < 0.001$). Time to neutrophil recovery above 0.5×10^9/L was reduced (14 days vs. 20 days, $p < 0.001$). The difference was significant both in autograft (20 days vs. 14 days, $p < 0.001$) and allograft (20 days vs. 14 days, $p < 0.01$) patients, in children (20 days vs. 13 days, $p < 0.001$), and adults. Lenograstim-treated patients had fewer days of infection, of antibiotic administration and also spent less time in hospital. However, clinical and microbiological sepsis was similar in both groups. There was no significant toxicity ascribed to lenograstim. Survival was similar between groups at both days 100 and 365 after transplantation [22].

Patients with lymphoma were treated in a randomized, open-label trial to study the use of filgrastim as an adjunct to high-dose chemotherapy and autologous BMT [23]. Of 43 assessable patients, 19 were randomized to receive filgrastim by continuous subcutaneous infusion at a dose of 10 µg/kg/day, 10 to filgrastim 20 µg/kg/day and 14 to a parallel control group that received no filgrastim after autologous BMT. The median time to neutrophil recovery, $\geq 0.5 \times 10^9$/L after the day of autologous BMT, was significantly accelerated to 10 days in the combined G-CSF groups compared with 18 days in control patients ($p = 0.0001$). The median number of platelet transfusions was identical in both groups. Clinical parameters, including the median number of days with fever (1 days vs. 4 days, $p = 0.0418$) and neutropenic fever (5 days vs. 13.5 days, $p = 0.0001$) were significantly improved in the filgrastim compared to the control group. For patients treated with the two different dose levels of filgrastim, the neutrophil recovery and clinical results were similar [23].

Forty-one patients undergoing high-dose therapy followed by infusion of autologous peripheral blood stem cells (PBSC) with or without bone marrow were randomized to receive G-CSF 5 µg/kg/day beginning on day +1 following transplant or standard post-transplant supportive care without G-CSF [24]. The median time to a neutrophil count $\geq 500/\mu L$ was 10.5 days in the G-CSF group vs. 16 days in the control group ($p = 0.0001$). G-CSF was associated with statistically significant reductions in the time to neutrophil engraftment among patients who received

Table 48.2 Randomized placebo controlled trials of G-CSF following HCT.

No. of patients enrolled	Type of transplant	G-CSF given from day	ANC >500/µL (day after transplantation)		p value	Reference
			G-CSF	Placebo		
315	Auto/allo BMT	+1	14	20	0.001	[22]
43	Auto BMT	+1	10	18	0.0001	[23]
41	Auto PBSCT +/−BMT	+1	10	18	0.0001	[24]
54	Auto BMT	+1	12 (14)	20	0.0004	[25]
38	Auto PBSCT	+1	10	14	0.0001	[26]
62	Auto PBSCT	+1	9	12.5	0.0001	[27]
62	Auto PBSCT	+5	10	12	0.0008	[28]
54	Allo PBSCT	±0	11	15	0.0082	[29]
42	Allo PBSCT	+1	12	15	0.002	[30]

allo, allogeneic; ANC, absolute neutrophil count; auto, autologous; BMT, bone marrow transplantation; G-CSF, granulocyte colony-stimulating factor; PBSCT, peripheral blood stem cell transplantation.

PBSC alone (11 days vs. 17 days, $p = 0.0003$) and in those patients who received PBSC in conjunction with bone marrow (10 days vs. 14 days, $p = 0.02$) [24].

In 54 patients with malignant lymphoma, hematopoietic recovery after high-dose chemotherapy and autologous BMT was compared between patients randomized to receive 10 or 30 µg/kg/day of rHuG-CSF (filgrastim) or no growth factor [25]. After standard high-dose chemotherapy with cyclophosphamide, etoposide (VP16), BCNU (CVB) or BCNU, VP16, cytosine arabinoside, melphalan (BEAM) regimen followed by autologous BMT, rHuG-CSF was administered by continuous intravenous infusion from the 1st day after autologous BMT until neutrophil recovery. When the rHuG-CSF groups were compared with the control group the major findings were: the median time to reach an absolute neutrophil count (ANC) $\geq 0.5 \times 10^9$/L was 20 days in the control group and 12 and 14 days, respectively, in the rHuG-CSF groups ($p = 0.0004$). The duration of neutropenia (ANC $<0.5 \times 10^9$/L) was reduced from 27 days in the control group to 11 and 13 days in the rHuG-CSF groups ($p = 0.0001$). In addition, fewer days of febrile neutropenia were observed in the rHuG-CSF groups (5 and 6 days) than in the control group (10 days; $p = 0.036$). No significant effects on the total number of days with fever was observed [25].

An accelerated neutrophil engraftment was observed in 41 consecutive children undergoing autologous BMT for hematologic malignancies in comparison with a similar historical control group of 38 children who did not receive rHuG-CSF after autologous BMT. Their ages ranged from 2 to 16 years (mean 7.2 years). RHuG-CSF was given at a dose of 10 µg/kg/day IV in a 2-h infusion from day +1 until day +28 or until the ANC was $>1 \times 10^9$/L [31].

The results obtained after autologous BMT were essentially confirmed in several phase 2 and 3 trials (Table 48.2) addressing the role of G-CSF after myeloablative chemotherapy and autologous cytokine mobilized PBSCT [26–28, 32].

Thirty-eight patients with lymphoproliferative disorders were randomized to receive low-dose filgrastim (19 patients) or placebo (19 patients) beginning on the 1st day after HCT [26]. All patients received more than 2.5×10^6 CD34$^+$ cells/kg, which had been mobilized with chemotherapy and filgrastim 300 µg from day 5. Neutrophil engraftment was significantly more rapid in patients who received filgrastim with a median number of days until ANC was $>0.5 \times 10^9$/L of 10 days [9–13] vs. 14 days (9–19 days; $p <0.0001$). The time to reach an ANC $>1 \times 10^9$/L was 12 days [9–14] vs. 16 days (10–25 days; $p <0.0001$). The total number of patients who required intravenous antibiotic therapy was lower in the filgrastim-treated group (68%) compared with the placebo group (89%); also, the median number of days with fever and the duration of antibiotic therapy were shorter, although these differences did not reach statistical significance. However, although only three of the 19 (16%) patients who received filgrastim required amphotericin, 11 of the 19 (58%) who received placebo did require it, and amphotericin usage was significantly less in the filgrastim group ($p = 0.029$). Finally, in-patient stay was significantly shortened in those who received filgrastim from 16 days (13 to 23 days) to 13 days (11–18 days; $p = 0.0003$) [27].

In another prospective study 34 patients had been randomized to receive lenograstim 263 µg/day subcutaneously and 28 to no growth factor [27]. The median time to ANC $>0.5 \times 10^9$/L was 9 days in the lenograstim arm vs. 12.5 days in the no-lenograstim arm ($p = 0.0001$). This was associated with a median duration of time in hospital after PBSCT of 13 days in the lenograstim arm vs. 15.5 days in the no-lenograstim arm ($p = 0.0002$). Median days to platelet independence, platelet transfusions, incidence of infection and RBC transfusion were the same in both arms [27].

Factors influencing hematopoietic engraftment were analyzed within the French multicenter LNH93-3 trial treating patients with aggressive high-grade non-Hodgkin's lymphoma with intensive chemotherapy including BEAM and autologous PBSCT [32]. In the patient population treated with the same first-line regimen, bone marrow involvement and infusion of fewer CD34$^+$ cells delayed platelet recovery. Administration of G-CSF after peripheral blood progenitor cell significantly reduced neutropenia [32].

The effect on accelerated neutrophil engraftment by G-CSF appears to be preserved when the start of application is delayed to day +5 after HCT. Sixty-two adult patients were randomized to receive filgrastim after PBSC infusion ($n = 30$) and 32, the control group, received no cytokines [28]. G-CSF was administered subcutaneously from day +5 in the treated group at a dose of 5 µg/kg body weight/day. The numbers of CD34$^+$ and mononuclear cell (MNC) infused were similar in each group. Faster granulocyte engraftment was evident in the treated group (mean of 10 days vs. 12 days to achieve $>0.5 \times 10^9$/L granulocytes, $p = 0.0008$), without differences in incidence and severity of infections, days of fever or duration of antibiotic treatment between groups. Considering the economic costs, the median expenditure per inpatient stay was €5961 (range €4386–€17,186) in the G-CSF group compared with €5751 (range €3676–€15,640) in the control group ($p = 0.47$) [28].

Several randomized trials show no delayed neutrophil engraftment when G-CSF is not given before days +3, +5, +6, or +7 after PBSCT [33–35]. Early (day +1) or delayed (day +7) G-CSF after immunoselected CD34$^+$ autologous PBSCT significantly accelerated ANC recovery but did not reduce the amount of supportive treatment or the duration of hospitalization in 21 consecutive patients with hematological malignancies [36].

RHuG-CSF after allogeneic HCT

Initial concerns over potential aggravation of GVHD or an increase of relapse in patients with myeloid leukemias tempered the use of growth factors after allogeneic BMT. Essentially, after allogeneic BMT the same effects as after autologous transplantation can be observed. Schriber et al. [37] reported the experience with 50 patients treated at a single institution using G-CSF after allogeneic sibling ($n = 30$) and matched-unrelated ($n = 20$) BMT. The time to an ANC $\geq 500/\mu L$ was significantly faster in patients who received G-CSF and cyclosporine and prednisone for GVHD prophylaxis when compared to historical control patients receiving the same GVHD prophylaxis (10 days vs. 13 days, $p <0.01$). A similar accelerated myeloid engraftment was observed for patients who received additional methotrexate for GVHD prophylaxis when compared to historical control patients receiving the same GVHD prophylaxis regimen (16 days vs. 19 days, $p <0.05$). The median time to engraftment for patients receiving a matched-unrelated BMT and G-CSF was 17 days (range 13–26 days) [37]. Similar results were obtained in children [38]. Effects of rHuG-CSF, filgrastim, in patients undergoing allogeneic BMT from volunteer unrelated donors were analyzed retrospectively [39]. Cohorts of patients received rHuG-CSF ($n = 22$) or no rHuG-CSF ($n = 25$) in a nonrandomized manner. Median time to ANC >500/μL was 14 days with rHuG-CSF vs. 16 days without rHuG-CSF ($p = 0.048$). Neutrophil recovery was accelerated in patients receiving more than the median mononuclear cell dose of 2.54×10^8/kg with a median time to ANC >1000/μL of 13 days vs. 19 days ($p = 0.017$). RHuG-CSF did not influence platelet recovery nor the incidence of infectious complications [39].

Delayed treatment with G-CSF resulted in a reduction of G-CSF treatment from 19 days to 14 days ($p = 0.0017$) in 38 patients randomly assigned to receive G-CSF starting day +1 or day +6 after allogeneic BMT [40]. Reducing the length of treatment by 5 days lowered G-CSF treatment costs by 26.3% and postponing treatment with G-CSF had no influence on the hematologic recovery after allogeneic BMT. The authors detected an economical benefit of postponing G-CSF use without any clinical disadvantages [40]. Similar results were obtained in 69 patients after unrelated donor BMT randomly assigned to rHuG-CSF starting days 0, +5, or +10 resulting in equivalent rapid neutrophil engraftment [41].

A randomized, double-blind, placebo controlled study was performed by Bishop et al. [29] to determine the effects of filgrastim on hematopoietic recovery after allogeneic PBSCT. Fifty-four patients with hematologic malignancies undergoing a related, human leukocyte antigen (HLA)-matched allogeneic HCT were randomly assigned to receive daily filgrastim at 10 µg/kg or placebo starting on the day of transplantation. The median time to achieve an ANC >0.5×10^9/L was 11 days (range, 9–20 days) for patients who received filgrastim compared with 15 days (range, 10–22 days) for patients who received placebo ($p = 0.0082$). The median time to achieve a platelet count >20×10^9/L was 13 days (range, 8–35 days) for patients who received filgrastim compared with 15.5 days (range, 8–42 days) for patients who received placebo ($p = 0.79$). There were no significant differences for RBC transfusion independence, in the incidence of acute GVHD, or 100-day mortality between the groups. The authors concluded that the administration of filgrastim appears to be a safe and effective supportive care measure following allogeneic peripheral blood HCT [29].

Forty-two adult recipients of allogeneic PBSCT from HLA-matched related donors were randomized to receive filgrastim 10 µg/kg/day subcutaneously from day 1 through neutrophil recovery or no growth factor support after transplantation [30]. There was no significant difference between the two groups in the number of CD34$^+$ cells infused (median, 4.8 vs. 4.3×10^6/kg). GVHD prophylaxis consisted of tacrolimus and steroids for nine patients and tacrolimus and mini-methotrexate for 33 patients. The group receiving filgrastim had a shorter time to neutrophil levels above 0.5×10^9/L (day 12 vs. day 15, $p = 0.002$) and to neutrophil levels over 1.0×10^9/L (day 12 vs. day 16, $p = 0.01$) [30].

G-CSF in murine allogeneic transplant models

Apart from these clinical findings, data obtained in murine animal models of allogeneic HCT point towards possible clinically relevant effects of G-CSF on the immune system. G-CSF polarized donor T cells towards a T$_H$2 cell type resulting in decreased alloreactivity [42] and, furthermore, decreased the allostimulatory capacity of antigen-presenting cells [43].

Administration of recombinant G-CSF to C57BL/Ka mice markedly increased the capacity of peripheral blood mononuclear cells (PBMC) to reconstitute lethally irradiated syngeneic hosts. T- and B-lineage lymphocytes were depleted about 10-fold in the bone marrow of the treated mice, and the T-cell yield in the blood was increased about fourfold. The ability of PBMC or purified CD4$^+$ and CD8$^+$ T cells to induce acute lethal GVHD in irradiated BALB/c mice was reduced after the administration of G-CSF. This effect was associated with decreased secretion of interferon-gamma (IFN-γ), interleukin 2 (IL-2) and an increased secretion of IL-4. The donor cell inoculum, which was most successful in the rescue of irradiated allogeneic hosts, was the low-density fraction of PBMC from G-CSF treated mice. These low-density cells were enriched for CD4$^-$CD8$^-$NK1.1$^+$ T cells and secreted about 10-fold more IL-4 than the unfractionated cells from the G-CSF-treated donors [42]. In another study it was investigated whether G-CSF administration to peripheral blood HCT recipients, both with and without donor G-CSF pretreatment, further modulated acute GVHD in a murine model of peripheral blood HCT [43]. Recipients of G-CSF mobilized splenocytes showed a significantly improved survival ($p <0.001$) and a reduction in GVHD score and serum lipopolysaccharide levels compared with control recipients. G-CSF treatment of donors, rather than recipients, had the most significant effect on reducing levels of TNF-α 7 days after transplantation. As a potential mechanism of the reduction in TNF-α, G-CSF was shown to decrease dendritic cell TNF-α and IL-12 production to lipopolysaccharide. G-CSF modulated GVHD predominantly by its effects on donor cells, reducing the production of TNF-α. The authors concluded that G-CSF treatment of BMT recipients, without pretreatment of the donor, does not have an impact on acute GVHD [43].

After full haplotype-mismatched HCT in humans, the application of G-CSF after transplantation markedly delayed T-lymphocyte reconstitution and omitting G-CSF led to a more rapid increase of T cells and improved anti-infectious defense in this specific situation [44].

In summary, G-CSF application after allogeneic or autologous bone marrow or peripheral blood HCT is safe and significantly accelerates the time to neutrophil engraftment without negatively influencing other parameters like platelet engraftment or GVHD. This effect is more prominent after BMT and is preserved when the start of G-CSF application is delayed from day +1 to day +5 or to day +7 after HCT. Apart from this, present randomized trials fail to show a clear beneficial effect on other factors like outcome of patients after HCT. However, the present data do not allow definite conclusions regarding specific patient situations, especially after allogeneic HCT. The positive effect of G-CSF on acute GVHD in murine allogenic HCT models is not clearly seen in humans. This is likely to be due to a more complex situation in clinical transplantation of patients with different malignant diseases, state of remission and other influencing factors. The potential immune modulating effects of G-CSF on mobilized stem cell grafts, as well as G-CSF application to the recipient and a possible aggravation of an "engraftment syndrome", should be kept in mind when treating patients with G-CSF after allogeneic HCT.

Granulocyte macrophage colony-stimulating factor (GM-CSF)

GM-CSF can be produced by many different cell types, particularly activated T cells. *In vitro*, GM-CSF promotes the growth and expansion of granulocytic and monocytic and, in combination with EPO, also multilineage colony forming units. Multiple functions of mature neutrophils and macrophages, such as tumoricidal activity, superoxide production, antibody-dependent cell-mediated cytotoxicity, phagocytic activity, microbial killing, and secretion of other cytokines are stimulated [45,46]. Furthermore, GM-CSF, when used *in vitro*, induces the differentiation of malignant antigen-presenting cells with potent T-cell stimulatory capacity [47].

In humans, GM-CSF causes a dose-dependent increase, mainly in blood neutrophils and eosinophils but also macrophages and lymphocytes. There is no effect on the erythroid or megakaryocytic lineage. After application, patients may suffer from low-grade fever, fatigue, myalgias and dyspnea. After higher doses, significant fluid retention, pericarditis, pleuritis and a capillary leak syndrome may develop [48,49].

Commercially available recombinant preparations of GM-CSF (molgramostin and sargramostim) differ in their state of glycosylation. However, this difference does not appear to be clinically relevant.

RHuGM-CSF after autologous HCT

One-hundred and twenty-eight patients undergoing autologous BMT for lymphoid malignancies were enrolled in a randomized, double-blind, placebo controlled trial [50]. Sixty-five patients received rHuGM-CSF in a 2-h intravenous infusion daily for 21 days, starting within 4 h of the marrow infusion, and 63 patients received placebo. The patients given rHuGM-CSF had a recovery of the neutrophil count to 500×10^6/L 7 days earlier than the patients who received placebo (19 days vs. 26 days, $p < 0.001$), had fewer infections, required 3 fewer days of antibiotic administration (24 days vs. 27 days, $p = 0.009$), and required 6 fewer days of initial hospitalization (median, 27 days vs. 33 days; $p = 0.01$). There was no difference in the survival rate at day +100 after HCT. The authors concluded that in patients undergoing autologous BMT for lymphoid neoplasia, rHuGM-CSF significantly lessens morbidity [50]. The data were essentially confirmed by other large randomized trials in autologous BMT [51] and peripheral blood HCT [52] (Table 48.3 [50–56]), and in a trial where GM-CSF and G-CSF were used sequentially after autologous transplantation [57]. In contrast, no statistical difference with regard to hematopoietic engraftment of any lineage or clinical parameters was seen in 50 patients of a randomized trial comparing GM-CSF with placebo after autologous PBSCT with GM-CSF mobilized grafts [53].

GM-CSF was compared with G-CSF post-autologous transplantation in a randomized trial with 42 patients with breast cancer randomized to receive filgrastim vs. molgramostim subcutaneously at a dose of 5 µg/kg starting on day 6 after peripheral blood HCT. PBMC were collected in all patients after stimulation with filgrastim and infused following high-dose chemotherapy. The median days to reach $>0.5 \times 10^9$/L granulocytes was similar for patients receiving filgrastim (10.5 ± 0.8 days) and molgramostim (10.2 ± 0.9 days). No significant differences were observed in platelet engraftment or in the number of platelets transfused. Time of discharge was 2 days earlier in the filgrastim arm (15 ± 4.2 days vs. 17.4 ± 4.7 days, $p = 0.04$). Finally, the incidence of adverse side-effects attributable to the cytokines (filgrastim or molgramostim) was equivalent and only present in 19% of the patients [58].

Another study compared the use of G-CSF (5 µg/kg/day) with sargramostim (GM-CSF) 500 µg/day from day 0 until neutrophil recovery (ANC >1500/µL) in patients with breast cancer or myeloma who had PBSC mobilized with the combination of cyclophosphamide, VP16, and G-CSF [59]. Twenty patients (13 breast cancer and 7 myeloma) received GM-CSF and 26 patients (14 breast cancer and 12 myeloma) received G-CSF. The patients were comparable for age and stage of disease, and received grafts that were not significantly different. Platelet recovery, transfusion requirements, fever days and use of antibiotics were similar in both groups. The recovery of neutrophils, however, was faster using G-CSF. ANC >500/µL and >1000/µL were reached in the GM-CSF group at 10.5 ± 1.5 and 11.0 ± 1.7 days, respectively, whereas with G-CSF only 8.8 ± 1.2 and 8.9 ± 2.2 days were required ($p < 0.001$). As a result, patients given G-CSF received fewer injections than the GM-CSF patients (10.9 vs. 12.3). This study suggests that neutrophil recovery occurs more quickly when using G-CSF in comparison to GM-CSF at the specific doses used following autologous peripheral blood HCT, but the

Table 48.3 Randomized placebo controlled trials of GM-CSF following stem cell transplantation.

| No. of patients enrolled | Type of transplant | GM-CSF given from day | ANC >500/µL (day after transplantation) | | p value | Reference |
			GM-CSF	Placebo		
128	auto BMT	±0	19	26	0.001	[50]
81	auto BMT	±0	15	28	0.001	[51]
343	auto BMT	+1	19	27	0.001	[52]
44	auto PBSCT	+1	14	21	0.001	[52]
50	auto PBSCT	+1	12	14	0.22 (n.s.)	[53]
40	allo BMT (sib)	+1	13	16	n.s.	[54]
57	allo BMT (sib, T-deplet)	±0	16	20	n.s.	[55]
109	allo BMT (sib; CyA, Pred)	±0	13	17	0.0001	[56]

allo, allogeneic; ANC, absolute neutrophil count; auto, autologous; BMT, bone marrow transplantation; CyA, Pred, GVHD prophylaxis with cyclosporine A and prednisone; GM-CSF, granulocyte macrophage colony-stimulating factor; n.s., not significant; PBSCT, peripheral blood stem cell transplantation; sib, matched sibling donor; T-deplet, T-cell depleted graft.

difference is not large enough to result in lower total cost [59]. In a randomized trial, San Miguel *et al.* [60] studied the *in vivo* effect of GM-CSF and G-CSF administration on the immune recovery of patients who underwent autologous BMT. For that purpose, 14 different T, B and NK lymphoid cell subsets using appropriate dual staining were sequentially analyzed during the 1st year following HCT. Twenty-four patients with lymphoproliferative disorders who had undergone autologous BMT were included in the study. G-CSF contributed to a significantly faster recovery of $CD8^+$ cells ($p = 0.03$). The $CD8^+$ cell regeneration consisted mainly of activated cells ($CD38^+/HLA-DR^+$) which lacked the CD11b antigen. In contrast, GM-CSF favored the regeneration of $CD4^+$ cells (through both the $CD45RO^+$ and $CD45RA^+$ subset), leading to a higher $CD4^+/CD8^+$ ratio ($p = 0.007$). Furthermore, the use of hematopoietic growth factors did not seem to exert a significant influence on the recovery of NK cells and B lymphocytes [60].

RHuGM-CSF after allogeneic HCT

GM-CSF was also tested in randomized trials after allogeneic transplantation. In a randomized double-blind trial in patients undergoing HCT for leukemia, 20 received GM-CSF and 20 received placebo, for 14 days after allogeneic, matched sibling BMT [54]. The neutrophil count recovered to $0.5 \times 10^9/L$ 3 days earlier in the GM-CSF group than in the placebo group (not significant). No difference in GVHD or relapse was reported.

In a prospective randomized placebo controlled trial involving 57 patients receiving T-cell depleted marrow transplants, rHuGM-CSF led to higher neutrophil and monocyte counts for 6–10 days during the time period of 2–3 weeks after transplantation resulting in less pneumonias [55].

In a prospective, multicenter, randomized, double-blind, placebo controlled trial, yeast-derived rHuGM-CSF or placebo was administered by 4-h intravenous infusion starting on the day of marrow infusion (day 0) to day 20 [56]. All patients received marrow grafts from HLA-identical siblings and cyclosporine and prednisone for GVHD prophylaxis. Fifty-three patients received rHuGM-CSF and 56 received placebo. The time to achieve an ANC of $>0.5 \times 10^9$ cells/L was shortened in rHuGM-CSF treated patients (day 13 vs. day 17, $p = 0.0001$). The incidence of grade III–IV mucositis and infection were significantly reduced ($p = 0.005$, $p = 0.001$, respectively). Duration of hospitalization was modestly shortened by 1 day ($p = 0.02$) in rHuGM-CSF treated patients. No differences in platelet recovery, erythrocyte recovery, incidence of veno-occlusive disease, GVHD severity, relapse or survival were observed [56].

Long delay in hematologic recovery after BMT, especially graft failure, can extend and amplify the risks of infection and hemorrhage, compromise patients' survival and increase the duration and cost of hospitalization. RHuGM-CSF was evaluated in 37 patients with marrow graft failure after allogeneic ($n = 15$), autologous ($n = 21$), or syngeneic ($n = 1$) BMT [61]. RHuGM-CSF was administered by 2-h infusion at doses between 60 and 1000 $\mu g/m^2$/day for 14 or 21 days. At doses of $<500 \mu g/m^2$, rHuGM-CSF was well tolerated and did not exacerbate GVHD in allogeneic transplant recipients. No patient with myelogenous leukemia relapsed while receiving rHuGM-CSF. Twenty-one patients reached an ANC greater equal or above $0.5 \times 10^9/L$ within 2 weeks of starting therapy while 16 did not. None of the seven patients who received chemically purged autologous marrow grafts responded to rHuGM-CSF. The survival rates of GM-CSF treated patients were significantly better than those of a historical control group [61].

A prospective, randomized trial compared GM-CSF (250 $\mu g/m^2$/day $\times$ 14 days) vs. sequential GM-CSF $\times$ 7 days followed by G-CSF (5 $\mu g/m^2$/day $\times$ 7 days) as treatment for primary or secondary graft failure after BMT [62]. Eligibility criteria included failure to achieve a white blood cell (WBC) count $\geq 100/\mu L$ by day +21 or $\geq 300/\mu L$ by day +28, no ANC $\geq 200/\mu L$ by day +28, or secondary sustained neutropenia after initial engraftment. Forty-seven patients were enrolled: 23 received GM-CSF (10 unrelated, eight related allogeneic and five autologous), and 24 received GM-CSF followed by G-CSF (12 unrelated, seven related allogeneic and five autologous). For patients receiving GM-CSF alone, neutrophil recovery (ANC $\geq 500/\mu L$) occurred between 2 and 61 days (median, 8 days) after therapy, while those receiving GM-CSF + G-CSF recovered at a similar rate of 1–36 days (median, 6 days; $p = 0.39$). Recovery to RBC transfusion independence was slow, occurring 6–250 days (median, 35 days) after enrollment with no significant difference between the two treatment groups (GM-CSF: median, 30 days; GM-CSF + G-CSF: median, 42 days; $p = 0.24$). Similarly, platelet transfusion independence was delayed until 4–249 days (median, 32 days) after enrollment, with no difference between the two treatment groups (GM-CSF: median, 28 days; GM-CSF + G-CSF: median, 42 days; $p = 0.38$). Recovery times were not different between patients with unrelated donors and those with related donors or autologous transplant recipients. Survival at 100 days after enrollment was superior after treatment with GM-CSF alone, yielding Kaplan–Meier 100-day survival estimates of $96\% \pm 8\%$ for GM-CSF vs. $71\% \pm 18\%$ for GM-CSF + G-CSF ($p = 0.026$). Sequential growth factor therapy with GM-CSF followed by G-CSF offered no advantage over GM-CSF alone in accelerating trilineage hematopoiesis or preventing lethal complications in patients with poor graft function after BMT [62].

In summary, GM-CSF accelerates neutrophil engraftment after autologous and allogeneic transplantation. GM-CSF has been used effectively in bone marrow failure states. The immunostimulating effects of GM-CSF with its capacity to differentiate antigen-presenting cells are currently employed and tested with or without concomitant donor lymphocyte infusions for relapse after allogeneic transplantation. Furthermore GM-CSF may have a place as an adjunct in post-transplant vaccination trials as well as in anti-infectious strategies.

Interleukin 3 (IL-3) and derivatives

IL-3, also known as multi-CSF, is a multilineage hematopoietic growth factor produced by T lymphocytes and mast cells that acts on early and committed cell populations of all lineages. *In vivo*, IL-3 administration is often accompanied by severe side-effects, with fever, malaise, chills, headache, arthralgias and urticaria [63]. Because of these side-effects, a dose escalating study using IL-3 alone had to be stopped at 2 $\mu g/kg/day$ [63]. Used alone, IL-3 did not enhance neutrophil engraftment compared to the use of GM-CSF [64].

IL-3 was used in combination with G-CSF in 54 consecutive patients with refractory or relapsed lymphoma [65]. Patients were assigned sequentially to one of three treatment groups: group 1, G-CSF 5 $\mu g/kg/$day subcutaneously from day +1 after reinfusion of autologous marrow ($n = 23$); group 2, G-CSF from day +1 combined with IL-3 10 $\mu g/kg/day$ subcutaneously from day +6 ($n = 22$, overlapping schedule); and group 3, G-CSF treatment discontinued at day +6 before start of IL-3 administration ($n = 9$, sequential schedule). No side-effects were observed when G-CSF was given alone. Four of 31 patients (12.9%) who received IL-3 subcutaneously experienced one severe adverse event defined as World Health Organization grade 3–4 toxicity (fever, $n = 2$; pulmonary toxicity, $n = 2$) and were withdrawn from the study. Groups 2 and 3 did not differ as for the ability to tolerate treatment, whereas a trend toward faster hematopoietic recovery when IL-3 was administered concomitantly with G-CSF from day 6 (i.e. group 2) was observed. Grouped together, patients who received IL-3 showed a median time to a granulocyte count >0.1 and $>0.5 \times 10^9/L$ of 8 and 11 days, respectively. When the hematologic reconstitution of patients in groups 2 and 3 was compared with that of patients in group 1, the addition of IL-3 resulted in a significant improvement of multilineage hematopoietic recovery, lower transfusion requirements, fewer documented infections and shorter stays in the hospital [65].

In vivo the complementary biological effects of IL-3 and GM-CSF and cross competition for receptor binding prompted the development of PIXY321, a synthetic hybrid protein of GM-CSF and IL-3. PIXY321 binds to cell lines expressing specific receptors for either ligand, and it exhibits enhanced biological activity in human hematopoietic progenitor cell assays [66]. A large randomized trial compared PIXY321 with GM-CSF alone. One-hundred and seventy-seven patients with NHL receiving autologous blood and marrow transplant (ABMTR) were randomized to receive either PIXY321, 750 µg/m^2/day divided into two subcutaneous doses or GM-CSF 250 µg/m^2/day as a 2-h intravenous infusion starting on day 0 post-ABMTR for a maximum of 28 days. The median time to reach an ANC ≥500/µL in the PIXY321 group was 17 days vs. 19 days in the GM-CSF group ($p = 0.07$) and the median time to reach platelet transfusion independence in the PIXY321 group was 25 days vs. 23 days in the GM-CSF group ($p = 0.30$). The toxicity profiles of the two agents appeared to be equivalent with the exception that more patients in the PIXY321 group developed a rash (64%) compared to the GM-CSF group (48%; $p = 0.028$). A logistic regression model identified the use of a regimen without total body irradiation (TBI) and/or the use of an unpurged marrow graft and a body-surface area >2.0 m^2 as predictive of faster neutrophil engraftment. Those three factors, as well as the receipt of two or less prior chemotherapy regimens were predictive for rapid platelet engraftment. No differences could be identified between the two agents with respect to the time to platelet transfusion independence [67].

Another development within the IL-3 system is a synthetic IL-3 receptor agonist, Synthokine-SC55494, which was tested alone or in combination with rHuG-CSF on platelet and neutrophil recovery in non-human primates exposed to total body ^{60}Co gamma radiation of 700 cGy. The combination of Synthokine and rHuG-CSF further decreased the cytopenic periods and nadirs for both platelets and neutrophils relative to Synthokine and rHuG-CSF monotherapy [68].

In summary, due to the side-effects and only modest positive impact on hematopoiesis, IL-3 or its modifications have not been licensed for clinical use after HCT.

Stem cell factor (SCF)

Stem cell factor, also known as steel factor, kit ligand, or mast cell growth factor promotes the proliferation and differentiation of the most primitive hematopoietic progenitor cells into committed progenitor cells. Recombinant SCF (rHuSCF, ancestim) has been developed and licensed for clinical use in combination with rHuG-CSF to optimize stem cell mobilization from the marrow into the peripheral blood for apheresis and to provide a sustained increase in the number of hematopoietic stem cell (HSC) capable of engraftment [69]. When used for hematopoietic cell mobilization, a considerable number of patients reacted with delayed type hypersensitivity such as skin rash, dyspnea, angiedema and cardiovascular symptoms.

No trials with the use of SCF after HCT have been published. In a single case report an unexpectedly rapid rise in platelet counts was observed with complete hematological recovery after the BEAM regimen, in a patient who could not be rescued by autologous transplant but who received filgrastim, epoetin alfa, and ancestim (rHuSCF) [70]. The authors attributed these findings to this specific growth factor combination, including ancestim [70].

Presently, there is no proven indication for rHuSCF after transplantation. It remains to be shown whether rHuSCF in combination with other growth factors has a potential in marrow failure after transplantation.

Thrombopoietin (TPO)/megakaryocyte growth factor

TPO stimulates the growth and differentiation of megakaryocytes and proplatelets via the receptor c-mpl. It is predominantly produced by hepatocytes and serum levels are inversely correlated with platelet counts.

Two ligands for the mpl receptor with broad *in vitro* megakaryocytic proliferative, maturational, and differentiation capacity have been developed and tested in clinical trials. One is a modified (PEGylated) form of a recombinant truncated mpl ligand, called the megakaryocyte growth and development factor (MGDF) [71]. The other is the recombinant glycosylated version of the naturally occurring TPO molecule [72].

In a randomized trial, 47 patients with stage II, III, or IV breast cancer undergoing autologous HCT were allocated to placebo ($n = 13$) or to one of five sequential dose cohorts of PEG-rHuMGDF (1.0, 2.5, 5.0, 7.5, or 10.0 µg/kg/day; $n = 34$). Blinded study drug was started on the day of transplantation and was continued until the platelet count was ≥100 × 10^9/L or a maximum of 21 days. HSC were mobilized with filgrastim and all patients received filgrastim starting on day +2 after transplantation. The nadir platelet count was not affected by treatment. The median time to platelet recovery was 11 and 12 days for the placebo and combined PEG-rHuMGDF groups, respectively [73].

In an open label phase 1 study rHuTPO was administered intravenously by bolus injection at doses ranging from 0.3 to 4.8 µg/kg/day every 3 days to 30 patients and 0.6 µg/kg daily to three patients. RHuTPO was begun the day after marrow infusion and continued until platelet recovery to >20,000/µL. G-CSF was concomitantly administered to promote myeloid recovery. Median platelet recovery after autologous BMT was 19 days (range, 11–41). Neither the dose nor the schedule of rHuTPO appeared to have any impact upon the time course of platelet recovery. In this phase 1 study, rHuTPO was found to be well tolerated without the development of neutralizing antibodies [72].

A case of pancytopenia associated with the development of neutralizing antibodies to TPO occurred in a patient who had undergone chemotherapy repeatedly with multiple cycles of subcutaneous administration of pegylated recombinant human MGDF [74]. Samples of the patient's bone marrow showed trilineage hypoplasia with absence of myeloid, erythroid, and megakaryocyte progenitor cells but with elevated endogenous levels of EPO, G-CSF, and SCF. The subcutaneous route of application of TPO in this trial may have been of importance for the development of anti-TPO antibodies.

The role of recombinant megakaryocyte growth factors after HCT has not been thoroughly tested and remains unclear. Furthermore, due to reports on the development of neutralizing antibodies and thrombophilia *in vivo*, the above mentioned recombinant products have not been licensed for clinical use and are presently being reevaluated.

Interleukin 11 (IL-11)

IL-11 is a naturally occurring cytokine produced by fibroblasts and bone marrow stromal cells and is a growth factor with pleiotropic effects overlapping with other growth factors. *In vivo*, IL-11 administration stimulates megakaryopoiesis and increases peripheral platelet and neutrophil counts [75], an effect that can be enhanced by the combination with IL-3. A recombinant preparation of IL-11, oprelvekin, produced in *Escherichia coli*, is licensed for clinical use for the prevention of severe thrombocytopenia and the reduction of the need for platelet transfusions following myelosuppressive chemotherapy. Major side-effects include fluid retention and edema.

A placebo controlled randomized trial with 80 breast cancer patients tested the effects of recombinant IL-11 on platelet recovery after high-dose chemotherapy and autologous transplantation with peripheral blood hematopoietic cell support. The results did not demonstrate that rHuIL-11 treatment significantly decreased platelet transfusion [76].

In a murine allogeneic BMT model of GVHD directed against major histocompatibility complex (MHC) and minor antigens, an immunomodulating effect of IL-11 with prevention of lethal GVHD while preserving the graft-vs.-leukemia effect (GVLE) was demonstrated [77]. IL-11 decreases cytokine release and increases survival in murine BMT models. In these systems, it reduces gut permeability, partially polarizes T cells to a TH2 phenotype, down-regulates IL-12, prevents mucositis, and accelerates recovery of oral and bowel mucosa.

In a randomized double-blind pilot study, rHuIL-11 was administered with cyclosporine/methotrexate (MTX) prophylaxis after cyclophosphamide/TBI conditioning and allogeneic stem cell transplantation for hematologic malignancies [78]. Patients received rHuIL-11, 50 μg/kg subcutaneously daily or placebo in a 3 : 1 ratio. Treatment was administered prior to the start of conditioning and continued up to 21 days. The study was designed to assess safety with stopping rules for cardiac arrhythmias and mortality. Although projected to accrue 20 patients, only 13 patients (10 IL-11, three placebo) were enrolled because the early stopping rule for mortality was enforced. Of 10 evaluable patients who received IL-11, four died by day 40 and one died on day 85. Deaths were attributable to transplant-related toxicity. One of three placebo recipients died by suicide, the other two are still alive. Patients receiving IL-11 had severe fluid retention and early mortality, making it impossible to determine whether IL-11 given in this schedule can reduce the rate of GVHD. Grade II–IV acute GVHD occurred in two of eight evaluable patients on IL-11 and one of three patients on placebo. The primary adverse events of the study were severe fluid retention resistant to diuresis (average weight gain 9% ± 4%) and multiorgan failure in five of 10 evaluable patients. The authors concluded that IL-11 as administered in this trial for GVHD prophylaxis in allogeneic transplantation cannot be recommended [78].

Keratinocyte growth factor (KGF)

KGF, also called fibroblast growth factor 7 (FGF-7), is a mediator of epithelial cell proliferation and a growth factor for hepatocytes and pneumocytes. KGF has been shown to be protective in radiation or chemotherapy induced organ damage. In murine models of allogeneic transplantation it protected the gut from lethal GVHD [79]. Interestingly, in murine transplantation models KGF protected thymic epithelial cells from cytotoxic damage when given prior to conditioning [80]. Furthermore, pharmacological doses of KGF allow regeneration of GVHD induced thymic damage and therefore KGF appears to exert a potent effect on thymic epithelial cell function, which in turn allows for normal T lymphopoiesis to occur during acute GVHD [81].

A phase 1 multicenter dose escalating trial was performed with rHuKGF for mucositis prevention in lymphoma patients conditioned with the BEAM protocol prior to autologous HCT [82]. A dose of 60 μg/kg/day × 3 prior to BEAM high-dose chemotherapy was chosen based on safety and preliminary efficacy. With this dose, a reduction in duration of severe ulcerative mucositis from 4.6 days (placebo) to 0.8 days was observed [82].

Definitive data from the field of clinical autologous or allogeneic HCT are presently lacking. However, the drug is under development and due to the promising data obtained in animal models it may be of special interest for the field of allogeneic transplantation.

Conclusion

In several situations hematopoietic growth factors have a defined role after HCT. In particular, randomized trials documented faster erythroid engraftment with EPO after allogeneic BMT, and G-CSF resulted in accelerated neutrophil engraftment after allogeneic and autologous marrow as well as peripheral blood HCT. Regarding other endpoints the results are equivocal. The value of these growth factors given after HCT has to be seen in the light of pros and cons of the individual patient and the specific transplant situation. Beyond faster engraftment, days in hospital or in isolation, transfusion requirements, possible cytokine-induced engraftment syndromes, or influence on the immune system, especially after allogeneic HCT, as well as costs only highlight some of the aspects to be taken into consideration. Of special interest will be growth factors preventing or repairing tissue damage, modulating the immune system post-transplantation and optimizing platelet engraftment. Preclinical and early clinical data suggest that some of these objectives could possibly be achieved in the near future.

References

1 Morrison SJ, Weissman IL. The long-term repopulating subset of hematopoietic stem cells is deterministic and isolatable by phenotype. *Immunity* 1994; **1**: 661–73.

2 Weissman IL. Stem cells: units of development, units of regeneration, and units in evolution. *Cell* 2000; **100**: 157–68.

3 Akashi K, Traver D, Miyamoto T, Weissman IL. A clonogenic common myeloid progenitor that gives rise to all myeloid lineages. *Nature* 2000; **404**: 193–7.

4 Glimm H, Eisterer W, Lee K et al. Previously undetected human hematopoietic cell populations with short-term repopulating activity selectively engraft NOD/SCID-beta2 microglobulin-null mice. *J Clin Invest* 2001; **107**: 199–206.

5 Guenechea G, Gan OI, Dorrell C, Dick JE. Distinct classes of human stem cells that differ in proliferative and self-renewal potential. *Nat Immunol* 2001; **2**: 75–82.

6 Hao QL, Smogorzewska EM, Barsky LW, Crooks GM. In vitro identification of single CD34+. *Blood* 1998; **91**: 4145–51.

7 Kim HJ, Tisdale JF, Wu T et al. Many multipotential gene-marked progenitor or stem cell clones contribute to hematopoiesis in nonhuman primates. *Blood* 2000; **96**: 1–8.

8 Klaesson S, Ringden O, Ljungman P, Lonnqvist B, Wennberg L. Reduced blood transfusion requirements after allogeneic bone marrow transplantation: results of a randomised, double-blind study with high-dose erythropoietin. *Bone Marrow Transplant* 1994; **13**: 397–402.

9 Pene R, Appelbaum FR, Fisher L et al. Use of granulocyte-macrophage colony-stimulating factor and erythropoietin in combination after autologous marrow transplantation. *Bone Marrow Transplant* 1993; **11**: 219–22.

10 Ayash LJ, Elias A, Hunt M et al. Recombinant human erythropoietin for the treatment of the anemia associated with autologous bone marrow transplantation. *Br J Haematol* 1994; **87**: 153–61.

11 Link H, Boogaerts MA, Fauser AA et al. A controlled trial of recombinant human erythropoietin after bone marrow transplantation. *Blood* 1994; **84**: 3327–35.

12 Vannucchi AM, Bosi A, Ieri A et al. Combination therapy with G-CSF and erythropoietin after autologous bone marrow transplantation for lymphoid malignancies: a randomized trial. *Bone Marrow Transplant* 1996; **17**: 527–31.

13 Chao NJ, Schriber JR, Long GD et al. A randomized study of erythropoietin and granulocyte colony-stimulating factor (G-CSF) versus placebo and G-CSF for patients with Hodgkin's and non-Hodgkin's lymphoma undergoing autologous bone marrow transplantation. *Blood* 1994; **83**: 2823–8.

14 Biggs JC, Atkinson KA, Booker V et al. Prospective randomised double-blind trial of the in vivo use of recombinant human erythropoietin in bone marrow transplantation from HLA-identical sibling donors. The Australian Bone Marrow Transplant Study Group. *Bone Marrow Transplant* 1995; **15**: 129–34.

15 Paltiel O, Cournoyer D, Rybka W. Pure red cell aplasia following ABO-incompatible bone marrow transplantation: response to erythropoietin. *Transfusion* 1993; **33**: 418–21.

16 Fujisawa S, Maruta A, Sakai R et al. Pure red cell aplasia after major ABO-incompatible bone marrow transplantation: two case reports of treatment with recombinant human erythropoietin. *Transpl Int* 1996; **9**: 506–8.

17 Veelken H, Wäsch R, Behringer D, Bertz H, Finke. J. Pure red cell aplasia after allogeneic stem cell transplantation with reduced conditioning. *Bone Marrow Transplant* 2000; **26**: 911–5.

18 Welte K, Gabrilove J, Bronchud MH, Platzer E, Morstyn G. Filgrastim (r-metHuG-CSF): the first 10 years. *Blood* 1996; **88**: 1907–29.

19 Lee CK, Gingrich RD, Hohl RJ, Ajram KA. Engraftment syndrome in autologous bone marrow and peripheral stem cell transplantation. *Bone Marrow Transplant* 1995; **16**: 175–82.

20 Sheridan WP, Morstyn G, Wolf M et al. Granulocyte colony-stimulating factor and neutrophil recovery after high-dose chemotherapy and autologous bone marrow transplantation. *Lancet* 1989; **2**: 891–5.

21 Schriber JR, Negrin RS, Chao NJ, Long GD, Horning SJ, Blume KG. The efficacy of granulocyte colony-stimulating factor following autologous bone marrow transplantation for non-Hodgkin's lymphoma with monoclonal antibody purged bone marrow. *Leukemia* 1993; **7**: 1491–5.

22 Gisselbrecht C, Prentice HG, Bacigalupo A et al. Placebo-controlled phase III trial of lenograstim in bone-marrow transplantation. *Lancet* 1994; **343**: 696–700.

23 Stahel RA, Jost LM, Cerny T et al. Randomized study of recombinant human granulocyte colony-stimulating factor after high-dose chemotherapy and autologous bone marrow transplantation for high-risk lymphoid malignancies. *J Clin Oncol* 1994; **12**: 1931–8.

24 Klumpp TR, Mangan KF, Goldberg SL, Pearlman ES, Macdonald JS. Granulocyte colony-stimulating factor accelerates neutrophil engraftment following peripheral-blood stem-cell transplantation: a prospective, randomized trial. *J Clin Oncol* 1995; **13**: 1323–7.

25 Schmitz N, Dreger P, Zander AR et al. Results of a randomized, controlled, multicentre study of recombinant human granulocyte colony-stimulating factor (filgrastim) in patients with Hodgkin's disease and non-Hodgkin's lymphoma undergoing autologous bone marrow transplantation. *Bone Marrow Transplant* 1995; **15**: 261–6.

26 McQuaker IG, Hunter AE, Pacey S, Haynes AP, Iqbal A, Russell NH. Low-dose filgrastim significantly enhances neutrophil recovery following autologous peripheral-blood stem-cell transplantation in patients with lymphoproliferative disorders: evidence for clinical and economic benefit. *J Clin Oncol* 1997; **15**: 451–7.

27 Linch DC, Milligan DW, Winfield DA et al. G-CSF after peripheral blood stem cell transplantation in lymphoma patients significantly accelerated neutrophil recovery and shortened time in hospital: results of a randomized BNLI trial. *Br J Haematol* 1997; **99**: 933–8.

28 Ojeda E, Garcia-Bustos J, Aguado M et al. A prospective randomized trial of granulocyte colony-stimulating factor therapy after autologous blood stem cell transplantation in adults. *Bone Marrow Transplant* 1999; **24**: 601–7.

29 Bishop MR, Tarantolo SR, Geller RB et al. A randomized, double-blind trial of filgrastim (granulocyte colony-stimulating factor) versus placebo following allogeneic blood stem cell transplantation. *Blood* 2000; **96**: 80–5.

30 Przepiorka D, Smith TL, Folloder J et al. Controlled trial of filgrastim for acceleration of neutrophil recovery after allogeneic blood stem cell transplantation from human leukocyte antigen-matched related donors. *Blood* 2001; **97**: 3405–10.

31 Madero L, Muonz A, Diaz DH et al. G-CSF after autologous bone marrow transplantation for malignant diseases in children. Spanish Working Party for Bone Marrow Transplantation in Children. *Bone Marrow Transplant* 1995; **15**: 349–51.

32 Langouet AM, Brice P, Simon D et al. Factors affecting hematopoietic recovery after autologous peripheral blood progenitor-cell transplantation in aggressive non-Hodgkin's lymphoma: a prospective study of 123 patients. *The Hematol J* 2001; **2**: 81–6.

33 Bolwell BJ, Pohlman B, Andresen S et al. Delayed G-CSF after autologous progenitor cell transplantation: a prospective randomized trial. *Bone Marrow Transplant* 1998; **21**: 369–73.

34 Faucher C, Le Corroller AG, Chabannon C et al. Administration of G-CSF can be delayed after transplantation of autologous G-CSF-primed blood stem cells: a randomized study. *Bone Marrow Transplant* 1996; **17**: 533–6.

35 Bence-Bruckler I, Bredeson C, Atkins H et al. A randomized trial of granulocyte colony-stimulating factor (Neupogen) starting day 1 vs day 7 post-autologous stem cell transplantation. *Bone Marrow Transplant* 1998; **22**: 965–9.

36 Piccirillo N, Sica S, Laurenti L et al. Optimal timing of G-CSF administration after CD34+ immunoselected peripheral blood progenitor cell transplantation. *Bone Marrow Transplant* 1999; **23**: 1245–50.

37 Schriber JR, Chao NJ, Long GD et al. Granulocyte colony-stimulating factor after allogeneic bone marrow transplantation. *Blood* 1994; **84**: 1680–4.

38 Locatelli F, Pession A, Zecca M et al. Use of recombinant human granulocyte colony-stimulating factor in children given allogeneic bone marrow transplantation for acute or chronic leukemia. *Bone Marrow Transplant* 1996; **17**: 31–7.

39 Berger C, Bertz H, Schmoor C et al. Influence of recombinant human granulocyte colony-stimulating factor (filgrastim) on hematopoietic recovery and outcome following allogeneic bone marrow transplantation (BMT) from volunteer unrelated donors. *Bone Marrow Transplant* 1999; **23**: 983–90.

40 Ciernik IF, Schanz U, Gmur. J. Delaying treatment with granulocyte colony-stimulating factor after allogeneic bone marrow transplantation for hematological malignancies: a prospective randomized trial. *Bone Marrow Transplant* 1999; **24**: 147–51.

41 Hagglund H, Ringden O, Oman S, Remberger M, Carlens S, Mattsson. J. A prospective randomized trial of Filgrastim (r-metHuG-CSF) given at different times after unrelated bone marrow transplantation. *Bone Marrow Transplant* 1999; **24**: 831–6.

42 Zeng D, Dejbakhsh-Jones S, Strober S. Granulocyte colony-stimulating factor reduces the capacity of blood mononuclear cells to induce graft-versus-host disease: impact on blood progenitor cell transplantation. *Blood* 1997; **90**: 453–63.

43 Reddy V, Hill GR, Pan L et al. G-CSF modulates cytokine profile of dendritic cells and decreases acute graft-versus-host disease through effects on the donor rather than the recipient. *Transplantation* 2000; **69**: 691–3.

44 Martelli MF, Aversa F, Bachar-Lustig E et al. Transplants across human leukocyte antigen barriers. *Semin Hematol* 2002; **39**: 48–56.

45 Gasson JC, Weisbart RH, Kaufman SE et al. Purified human granulocyte-macrophage colony-stimulating factor: direct action on neutrophils. *Science* 1984; **226**: 1339–42.

46 Nemunaitis J, Cox J, Meyer W et al. Comparison of neutrophil and monocyte function by microbicidal cell-kill assay in patients with cancer receiving granulocyte colony-stimulating factor, granulocyte-macrophage colony-stimulating factor, or no cytokine after cytotoxic chemotherapy: a phase II trial. *Am J Clin Oncol* 1998; **21**: 308–12.

47 Chen X, Regn S, Raffegerst S, Kolb HJ, Roskrow M. Interferon-alpha in combination with GM-CSF induces the differentiation of leukaemic antigen-presenting cells that have the capacity to stimulate a specific anti-leukaemic cytotoxic T-cell response from patients with chronic myeloid leukaemia. *Br J Haematol* 2000; **111**: 596–607.

48 Antman KS, Griffin JD, Elias A et al. Effect of recombinant human granulocyte-macrophage colony-stimulating factor on chemotherapy-induced myelosuppression. *N Engl J Med* 1988; **319**: 593–8.

49 Brandt SJ, Peters WP, Atwater SK et al. Effect of recombinant human granulocyte-macrophage colony-stimulating factor on hematopoietic reconstitution after high-dose chemotherapy and autologous bone marrow transplantation. *N Engl J Med* 1988; **318**: 869–76.

50 Nemunaitis J, Rabinowe SN, Singer JW et al. Recombinant granulocyte-macrophage colony-stimulating factor after autologous bone marrow transplantation for lymphoid cancer. *N Engl J Med* 1991; **324**: 1773–8.

51 Link H, Boogaerts MA, Carella AM et al. A controlled trial of recombinant human granulocyte-macrophage colony-stimulating factor after total body irradiation, high-dose chemotherapy, and autologous bone marrow transplantation for acute lymphoblastic leukemia or malignant lymphoma. *Blood* 1992; **80**: 2188–95.

52 Greenberg P, Advani R, Keating A et al. GM-CSF accelerates neutrophil recovery after autologous hematopoietic stem cell transplantation. *Bone Marrow Transplant* 1996; **18**: 1057–64.

53 Legros M, Fleury J, Bay JO et al. rhGM-CSF vs. placebo following rhGM-CSF-mobilized PBPC transplantation: a phase III double-blind randomized trial. *Bone Marrow Transplant* 1997; **19**: 209–13.

54 Powles R, Smith C, Milan S et al. Human recombinant GM-CSF in allogeneic bone-marrow transplantation for leukaemia: double-blind, placebo-controlled trial. *Lancet* 1990; **336**: 1417–20.

55 de Witte T, Gratwohl A, Van Der LN et al. Recombinant human granulocyte-macrophage colony-stimulating factor accelerates neutrophil and monocyte recovery after allogeneic T-cell-depleted bone marrow transplantation. *Blood* 1992; **79**: 1359–65.

56 Nemunaitis J, Rosenfeld CS, Ash R et al. Phase III randomized, double-blind placebo-controlled trial of rhGM-CSF following allogeneic bone marrow transplantation. *Bone Marrow Transplant* 1995; **15**: 949–54.

57 Spitzer G, Adkins DR, Spencer V et al. Randomized study of growth factors post-peripheral-blood stem-cell transplant: neutrophil recovery is improved with modest clinical benefit. *J Clin Oncol* 1994; **12**: 661–70.

58 Caballero MD, Vazquez L, Barragan JM et al. Randomized study of filgrastim versus molgramostim after peripheral stem cell transplant in breast cancer. *Haematologica* 1998; **83**: 514–8.

59 Jansen J, Thompson EM, Hanks S et al. Hematopoietic growth factor after autologous peripheral blood transplantation: comparison of G-CSF and GM-CSF. *Bone Marrow Transplant* 1999; **23**: 1251–6.

60 San Miguel JF, Hernandez MD, Gonzalez M et al. A randomized study comparing the effect of GM-CSF

and G-CSF on immune reconstitution after autologous bone marrow transplantation. *Br J Haematol* 1996; **94**: 140–7.
61 Nemunaitis J, Singer JW, Buckner CD *et al*. Use of recombinant human granulocyte-macrophage colony-stimulating factor in graft failure after bone marrow transplantation. *Blood* 1990; **76**: 245–53.
62 Weisdorf DJ, Verfaillie CM, Davies SM *et al*. Hematopoietic growth factors for graft failure after bone marrow transplantation: a randomized trial of granulocyte-macrophage colony-stimulating factor (GM-CSF) versus sequential GM-CSF plus granulocyte-CSF. *Blood* 1995; **85**: 3452–6.
63 Nemunaitis J, Appelbaum FR, Singer JW *et al*. Phase I trial with recombinant human interleukin-3 in patients with lymphoma undergoing autologous bone marrow transplantation. *Blood* 1993; **82**: 3273–8.
64 Albin N, Douay L, Fouillard L *et al*. In vivo effects of GM-CSF and IL-3 on hematopoietic cell recovery in bone marrow and blood after autologous transplantation with mafosfamide-purged marrow in lymphoid malignancies. *Bone Marrow Transplant* 1994; **14**: 253–9.
65 Lemoli RM, Rosti G, Visani G *et al*. Concomitant and sequential administration of recombinant human granulocyte colony-stimulating factor and recombinant human interleukin-3 to accelerate hematopoietic recovery after autologous bone marrow transplantation for malignant lymphoma. *J Clin Oncol* 1996; **14**: 3018–25.
66 Vadhan-Raj S. PIXY321 (GM-CSF/IL-3 fusion protein): biology and early clinical development. *Stem Cells* 1994; **12**: 253–61.
67 Vose JM, Pandite AN, Beveridge RA *et al*. Granulocyte-macrophage colony-stimulating factor/interleukin-3 fusion protein versus granulocyte-macrophage colony-stimulating factor after autologous bone marrow transplantation for non-Hodgkin's lymphoma: results of a randomized double-blind trial. *J Clin Oncol* 1997; **15**: 1617–23.
68 MacVittie TJ, Farese AM, Herodin F, Grab LB, Baum CM, McKearn JP. Combination therapy for radiation-induced bone marrow aplasia in non-human primates using synthokine SC-55494 and recombinant human granulocyte colony-stimulating factor. *Blood* 1996; **87**: 4129–35.
69 Basser RL, To LB, Begley CG *et al*. Rapid hematopoietic recovery after multicycle high-dose chemotherapy: enhancement of filgrastim-induced progenitor-cell mobilization by recombinant human stem-cell factor. *J Clin Oncol* 1998; **16**: 1899–908.
70 Blaise D, Faucher C, Vey N, Caraux J, Maraninchi D, Chabannon C. Rescue of haemopoiesis by a combination of growth factors including stem-cell factor. *Lancet* 2000; **356**: 1325–6.
71 Basser RL, Rasko JE, Clarke K *et al*. Randomized, blinded, placebo-controlled phase I trial of pegylated recombinant human megakaryocyte growth and development factor with filgrastim after dose-intensive chemotherapy in patients with advanced cancer. *Blood* 1997; **89**: 3118–28.
72 Wolff SN, Herzig R, Lynch J *et al*. Recombinant human thrombopoietin (rhTPO) after autologous bone marrow transplantation: a phase I pharmacokinetic and pharmacodynamic study. *Bone Marrow Transplant* 2001; **27**: 261–8.
73 Bolwell B, Vredenburgh J, Overmoyer B *et al*. Phas1 study of pegylated recombinant human megakaryocyte growth and development factor (PEG-rHuMGDF) in breast cancer patients after autologous peripheral blood progenitor cell (PBPC) transplantation. *Bone Marrow Transplant* 2000; **26**: 141–5.
74 Basser RL, O'Flaherty E, Green M *et al*. Development of pancytopenia with neutralizing antibodies to thrombopoietin after multicycle chemotherapy supported by megakaryocyte growth and development factor. *Blood* 2002; **99**: 2599–602.
75 Nash RA, Seidel K, Storb R *et al*. Effects of rhIL-11 on normal dogs and after sublethal radiation. *Exp Hematol* 1995; **23**: 389–96.
76 Vredenburgh JJ, Hussein A, Fisher D *et al*. A randomized trial of recombinant human interleukin-11 following autologous bone marrow transplantation with peripheral blood progenitor cell support in patients with breast cancer. *Biol Blood Marrow Transplant* 1998; **4**: 134–41.
77 Teshima T, Hill GR, Pan L *et al*. IL-11 separates graft-versus-leukemia effects from graft-versus-host disease after bone marrow transplantation. *J Clin Invest* 1999; **104**: 317–25.
78 Antin JH, Lee SJ, Neuberg D *et al*. A phase I/II double-blind, placebo-controlled study of recombinant human interleukin-11 for mucositis and acute GVHD prevention in allogeneic stem cell transplantation. *Bone Marrow Transplant* 2002; **29**: 373–7.
79 Hill GR, Ferrara JL. The primacy of the gastrointestinal tract as a target organ of acute graft-versus-host disease: rationale for the use of cytokine shields in allogeneic bone marrow transplantation. *Blood* 2000; **95**: 2754–9.
80 Min D, Taylor PA, Panoskaltsis-Mortari A *et al*. Protection from thymic epithelial cell injury by keratinocyte growth factor: a new approach to improve thymic and peripheral T-cell reconstitution after bone marrow transplantation. *Blood* 2002; **99**: 4592–600.
81 Rossi S, Blazar BR, Farrell CL *et al*. Keratinocyte growth factor preserves normal thymopoiesis and thymic microenvironment during experimental graft-versus-host disease. *Blood* 2002; **100**: 682–91.
82 Durrant S, Picot JL, Schmitz N *et al*. A phase 1 study of recombinant human keratinocyte growth factor (rHuKGF) in lymphoma patients receiving high-dose chemotherapy (HDC) with autologous peripheral blood progenitor cell transplantation (autoPBSCT). *Blood* 1999; **94** (Suppl. 1): 708a [Abstract].

49

Jeffrey W. Chell

Hematopoietic Cell Donor Registries

Introduction

The growth and development of registries of unrelated potential donors of adult hematopoetic cells (HCs) and umbilical cord blood (UCB) have been successful because of two basic human needs. The first is the need for a source of hematopoietic stem cells for the 70% of the population that does not have an available identical human leukocyte antigen (HLA) match within their immediate family. The second need is that of the voluntary unrelated donor. The need to help, to be of service to another human, to have a hand in saving another life is strong [1] and an integral part of what makes a registry of unrelated potential HC donors a reality.

This chapter will examine the history of unrelated HC donor registries, methods of recruiting and retaining donors, evolution of HLA-matching techniques and technologies, emergence of UCB as a source of HCs and ethical considerations of the unrelated donation process.

History

In the early 1970s case reports first appeared documenting the use of unrelated HCs for the treatment of a variety of hematologic disorders [1–4]. Early on, unrelated donors were identified and recruited from platelet donors who had been HLA typed [5]. If a compatible platelet donor was not available, then the patient and family made a general appeal to the community. The response by platelet donors and the general community was quite positive and stimulated interest in the potential of unrelated registries. As the outcomes of these early case reports documented engraftment, graft-vs.-tumor effect, prolonged survival and cure, patients, families and their physicians considered unrelated hematopoietic cell transplantation (HCT) as a potentially viable option in the face of a life-threatening hematologic disorder when an acceptably matched related donor was not available.

Early development of registries in Great Britain and the USA were inspired or led by families searching for a potential match [5,6]. As families encouraged members of their communities to be tested, awareness built and those touched by the message joined these early registry efforts and/or donated time and money to make these general appeals more successful. By 1983, the Anthony Nolan Registry in Great Britain had recruited and HLA typed over 50,000 volunteers. Anthony Nolan was a child with Wiscott–Aldrich syndrome, after whom the recruiting efforts and registry were eventually named.

In the USA, a 10-year-old girl's struggle with acute lymphoblastic leukemia was one of the forces that led to a national registry [4]. Laura was transplanted with marrow from an unrelated donor in 1979. The marrow engrafted, but Laura died of recurrent leukemia 2 years later. Laura's father, Robert Graves, established the Laura Graves Foundation in 1981 and worked tirelessly to bring the issue of unrelated transplantation to national attention. The National Marrow Donor Program (NMDP) of the US was established in 1986 as a consequence of these efforts [7].

As a result of those early efforts and other similar stories worldwide, there are currently 7.9 million donors represented by 51 HC registries in 37 countries and 28 cord blood banks in 18 countries [8]. This donor base supports approximately 5000 unrelated HCTs per year.

Donor registries

A registry of potential volunteer donors of HC consists of several common elements. The first are contact data that enable the registry to contact the donor in the event that a potential match for a searching patient has occurred. The contact data are also important to periodically update the donors on their participation in the registry and to solicit any changes in their address, health or interest in the program. The second is the results of HLA testing. HLA typing has undergone a number of iterations over the past 20 years. Many donors have been typed by serologic methods. Over time, many registries have adopted DNA-based typing methods as the standard typing method for new donors entering the registry. Most registries provide at a minimum HLA-A and -B results using serologic methods. Currently the standard for unrelated donor registries is HLA-A, -B and -DR by DNA-based methods. Most registries have a number of donors who are typed only at the HLA-A and -B loci. These tend to be donors who were recruited early in the history of the registry. Some registries continue to collect only these loci, often to reduce the overall typing expense, allowing the registry to add more potential donors. However, the more complete the initial typing, the more likely the donor will be chosen [9]. The experience of the NMDP is that 98% of the HC product requests are from the 67% of the registry that is HLA-A, -B and -DR typed. The third most common element is demographic information regarding the potential donor. This information serves as a tool for the requesting transplant center. If the searching patient is large, the transplant center may choose a male donor if there are two or more donors who would serve as a match for the searching patient. Race and ethnicity data are also often included. Fourth is screening healthcare information on the potential donor. This baseline information assists in determining eligibility of donors. It is also a helpful reminder to potential donors of the types of medical conditions that may make them ineligible to donate in the future.

The NMDP of the US partners with a group of organizations to recruit donors to its registry. There are 91 Donor Centers in the NMDP network. The Donor Centers may be freestanding, associated with a blood center or a healthcare institution that performs unrelated HCTs. Each of these Donor Centers works within their communities to recruit donors from the general population and educate them about the process of donation. The Donor Center may work with a local civic group, a college fraternity/sorority or any other of a number of organizations to promote HC donation and encourage participation in the registry. The NMDP also contracts with 10 Recruitment Groups that aid Donor Centers in recruiting donors from minority populations. Donor Centers may be independent or are part of another organization. They may be commonly affiliated with a blood center or an academic healthcare institution.

In addition to recruiting donors, the Donor Center contacts the potential donor if they have been chosen as a potential match for a patient. The Donor Center then arranges for collection of a blood sample for further testing of the donor's HLA type (confirmatory typing). That testing is usually performed at the potential recipient's transplant center. If the donor is chosen to continue to donation of HCs, the Donor Center conducts or arranges for the donor's preprocedure physical exam and then the donation itself, either marrow or peripheral blood hematopoietic cells (PBHCs). The role of the Donor Center is critical in ensuring that the process of donation assures safety and confidentiality for the donor.

Table 49.1 outlines the international registries that currently submit data to Bone Marrow Donors Worldwide (BMDW). BMDW is a continuing effort to collect the HLA phenotypes on volunteer HC and cord blood units from member registries around the world. This allows searching transplant centers to identify the registry where potential donors that are likely to match the patient are listed [8]. It began in 1988 as an initiative of the Immunobiology Working Party of the European Group for Blood and Marrow Transplantation (EBMT). The goals of BMDW are to:

1 Maximize the chance of finding a donor by providing access to all donors and cord blood units available in the world.
2 Minimize the effort put into donor searches—only registries with potential donors need to be contacted.
3 Provide an estimate of the chance of finding a donor for a given patient.
4 Provide advanced search programs to identify partially matched donors.
5 Facilitate improvements in family search strategy.
6 Provide relevant general information for the benefit of the patient.
7 Facilitate search request advice via the internet [10].

The BMDW is a valuable tool in a worldwide quest for matched unrelated donors and for research. A transplanter who queries the BMDW database will identify those registries that potentially have a match for their patient. This allows the physician to limit their subsequent search to only those registries that are likely to yield a potential match. The BMDW can also provide information regarding the number of unique phenotypes (defined as HLA-A, -B, -DR split) that are likely to exist. The approximately 400,000 unique phenotypes that were listed in the BMDW in 1999 represent <1% of the theoretical number that could exist. As new donors are added to the BMDW, the number that represents new phenotypes is <15%. This is down from 25% in 1994. This implies that the genes that encode the HLA antigens are closely linked and are inherited as a cluster, a haplotype. For example, in North American Caucasians the frequency of HLA-A1 is 13.8% and the frequency of HLA-B8 is 9%. Therefore, one would expect the HLA-A1, B8 haplotype to naturally occur 1.3% of the time in North American Caucasians. Instead, the actual haplotype frequency is 6% [11]. The implication of this close linkage for transplantation is significant. Less close linkage would profoundly increase the variation in *HLA* gene inheritance and make the likelihood of finding an acceptable match among potential donors more difficult. Also, as these common haplotypes are common in one race and rarely seen in others, the value of racial diversity in a registry becomes important.

The presence of a phenotypic match in BMDW doesn't necessarily mean that the potential donor will be an adequate match or that the donor is available. But it is a valuable tool to efficiently screen for potential donors worldwide and focus the search for the best match available. As can be surmised from Table 49.1, there is a great deal of variation in the size of the registries and the percentage HLA-A, -B, and -DR typed. This is related to the age of the registry and the resources available to it to recruit and type donors. It is unclear what impact cultural differences may play in a national registry's ability to recruit its citizens to participate in a registry of unrelated HC donors.

Each registry has developed its own standards, policies and procedures to facilitate its function. These govern all of the aspects of managing an unrelated donor registry. Donor recruitment and management are critical aspects usually covered in these standards and procedures. Less evident is the need to develop standards, policies and procedures for handling blood specimens, level of typing of the specimens, a means of capturing the information in a database and making it readily accessible to searching patients without compromising donor confidentiality. For a discussion regarding donor confidentiality see the Ethical considerations section below. Other responsibilities of the registry that are documented in their standards, policies and procedures include assessment of a potential donor's fitness to donate, HC collection procedures, quality and quantity standards of the product and the handling and transportation of the product [12].

Although most donors donate to a patient in their own country, there is a significant amount of international exchange. The experience of the NMDP reflects this well. Approximately 20% of the collections performed in the USA, facilitated by the NMDP, are for international recipients. Interestingly, the percentage of NMDP-facilitated transplants that utilize an international donor is also 20%. Given this robust level of international exchange [13], there has arisen a need to create an international body of physicians, scientists and administrators to develop guidelines to aid in the exchange [14].

The World Marrow Donor Association (WMDA) performs such a role. The WMDA serves as a forum to develop consensus on and make recommendations for standards for international exchange of HCs. The WMDA has developed a statement of purpose to "promote the exchange of information and development of standards in order to facilitate the exchange of hematopoietic stem cells across international borders" [14]. The WMDA has broad international participation and the opportunity to build consensus among the leaders in transplantation. It communicates its recommendations through semiannual meetings and consensus papers submitted to peer-reviewed journals.

Donor recruitment

As noted previously, nearly eight million potential donors have been recruited to become unrelated HC donors. Early recruitment initiatives focused on whole blood and platelet apheresis donors. They were an obvious choice as many donor centers were begun by blood centers. Blood and platelet donors had already shown their altruism by their donation history. The blood centers had contact information and were able to recruit a number of blood and platelet donors to also register as potential stem cell donors. Since then, some registries continue to focus their recruitment efforts on blood and platelet donors. Other registries have used a variety of techniques and populations within which to recruit potential donors [15].

As families held recruitment drives to find a match, those recruited were soon asked to donate to anyone in need as they were likely not a match for the patient for whom the donor drives was organized. Patient-focused drives can be very successful as potential donors can better see and understand the issues through the eyes of a patient and family. Patient-focused drives can also attract local and media attention as well as community financial support. The challenge of patient-focused drives is to retain the interest of the potential donors if they do not match the index patient. Often a potential donor may be prepared at that point in time to help that unique patient. At a later time, when they may match

Table 49.1 Registries listed with Bone Marrow Donors Worldwide (BMDW), 2002, reproduced with permission.

Registry	Registry country	Registry size	HLA-A % -B, -DR typed	Last updated
Argentina MDP & New Zealand	Argentina	158,214	55	June 2002
Austria BMD	Austria	49,241	32	June 2002
MDP Belgium	Belgium	51,389	76	April 2002
Canadian Blood Services UBMDR	Canada	219,431	35	June 2002
Croatian BMDR	Croatia	94	69	December 2001
Cyprus Paraskevaidio BMDR	Cyprus	2410	21	June 2002
Cyprus BMDR	Cyprus	73,193	16	April 2002
Czech National BMDR	Czech Republic	20,763	61	June 2002
Czech BMDR	Czech Republic	14,638	13	June 2002
Danish BMDR	Denmark	6641	81	June 2002
BMD Copenhagen	Denmark	1574	53	June 2002
Finnish BMDR	Finland	18,224	97	June 2002
France Greffe de Moelle	France	108,734	74	June 2002
German National BMDR	Germany	1,786,814	38	June 2002
Athens BMDR	Greece	8089	13	April 2002
Macedonian BMDR	Greece	1806	71	April 2002
Hong Kong Marrow Match Foundation	Hong Kong	39,114	32	April 2002
Hungarian BMDR	Hungary	3316	18	April 2002
Asian Indian DMR	India	1205	0	October 2001
Irish UBM Panel	Ireland	14,270	98	June 2002
Ezer Mizion BMDR	Israel	119,189	7	June 2002
Hadassah BMDR.	Israel	17,956	24	June 2002
Sheba Med. Center DR	Israel	884	11	June 2002
Italian BMDR	Italy	286,648	45	June 2002
Japan MDP	Japan	154,811	99	June 2002
Mexican BMDR	Mexico	2555	100	June 2002
EuropDonor Foundation	The Netherlands	31,950	95	June 2002
Norwegian BMDR	Norway	20,244	89	June 2002
Polish NBMDR	Poland	1462	82	April 2002
Against Leukaemia MDR	Poland	1098	53	June 2002
UBMD—Warsaw	Poland	3568	11	June 2002
Portuguese BMDR	Portugal	1116	54	June 2002
Russian BMDR	Russia	13,517	8	March 2002
San Marino BMDR	San Marino	620	100	April 2002
Slovak NBMDR	Slovakia	215	3	March 1999
Slovenia BMDR	Slovenia	343	90	June 2002
South African BMR	South Africa	22,689	7	June 2002
REDMO	Spain	40,910	55	June 2002
Tobias Registry	Sweden	39,991	46	June 2002
Swiss BMDR	Switzerland	18,110	99	June 2002
Tzu Chi Taiwan MDR	Taiwan	219,674	73	June 2002
Ankara University	Turkey	492	34	May 2001
BM Bank of Istanbul	Turkey	25,436	1	April 2002
Anthony Nolan Trust	Great Britain	323,418	69	June 2002
British BMR	Great Britain	140,191	81	June 2002
Welsh BMDR	Wales	32,596	100	June 2002
American BMDR	USA	31,394	9	January 2002
Caitlin Raymond IR	USA	46,256	10	June 2002
Gift of Life	USA	69,702	58	June 2002
National MDP	USA	3,546,200	72	June 2002
Total		7,914,773		

B, Bone; D, Donor; I, International; M, Marrow; N, National; R, Registry.

Table 49.2 Change in National Marrow Donor Program (NMDP) Registry size by race/ethnicity following focused minority recruitment, reproduced with permission.

Race/ethnic group	June 1993	February 2002
Black & African-American	13,217	390,893
American Indian & Alaskan Native	3281	61,489
Asian & Pacific Islander	10,425	320,475
Caucasian	143,193	2,577,987*
Hispanic	10,687	413,411
Multi-race	1507	109,952
Total	182,301	3,874,207*

*Excludes 1,035,459 potential donors recruited in Europe that are listed on the NMDP Registry. These donors are predominately Caucasian.

Table 49.3 Percent likelihood that a patient will find at least one HLA-A, -B or -DR match in the National Marrow Donor Program (NMDP) Registry by year, reproduced with permission.

Race/ethnic group	1988	1995	2002
Black & African-American	5	35	60
Asian & Pacific Islander	5	50	75
Hispanic	15	60	78
Multi-race	18	70	80
American Indian & Alaskan Native	18	72	82
Caucasian	25	75	85

Table 49.4 Effect of donor recruitment on the likelihood of patient finding a match on the National Marrow Donor Program (NMDP) Registry, reproduced with permission.

Race	No. with at least one matching donor (%)	Incremental effect of adding 10,000 donors of same race (%)
White	87	0.17
African-American	60	0.85
Asian/Pacific Islander	75	0.85
Hispanic	85	Not applicable

another patient, their connection to the need of an anonymous patient may not be as strong. This is covered in more detail in the Donor retention section below.

Since the early 1990s the NMDP has been proactive in increasing the diversity of the registry. In addition to asking each donor center to recruit from each racial and ethnic minority, the NMDP supported Recruitment Groups that focus on specific minority populations. The Recruitment Groups have been able to make connections within minority communities to aid in improving the diversity of the registry managed by the NMDP. Table 49.2 shows the impact of a proactive approach to the increased focus on minority recruitment.

Initially a goal of the NMDP was to ensure that minorities were represented in the registry in the same proportion as they are represented in the population of the USA. Although this has been a laudable goal, it is clear that the likelihood of finding a matched and available donor in the US is more difficult for a minority than for a Caucasian. This discrepancy is due to more genetic diversity among some minority groups compared to Caucasians and a higher incidence of deferral from donation for medical or other reasons among minorities. Table 49.3 shows the likelihood of at least one HLA-A, -B, -DR match within the registry for patients searching the NMDP database. The likelihood of minorities finding at least one matching donor has increased significantly over the past 10 years. Therefore, the NMDP has focused on achieving comparable access to HCT among all racial groups. Working with community leaders, minority press, social and professional organizations and NMDP Donor Centers and Recruitment Groups, the NMDP is working toward "over representation" of minorities in the registry in order to improve progress toward comparable access. In 2003, the Office of Management and Budget (OMB) of the US Federal Government will implement new race codes [16]. These include "White," "Native Hawaiian and Other Pacific Islander," "Black or African-American," "Asian" and "American Indian or Alaska Native." Hispanic or Latino has been designated as an ethnicity. Ethnicity is defined as the nationality group, lineage or country of birth of the person, the person's parents or ancestors before their arrival in the USA. People who identify their origin as Hispanic or Latino may be of any race: most likely "White," "Central or South American Indian" and "African or Caribbean Black."

All of the registries listed by BMDW and noted in Table 49.1 have identified age limits for participation in the registry as a potential donor. The NMDP uses 18–60 years of age. The lower age limit was chosen as it represents the most commonly used age of consent. The upper age limit was chosen as a means of limiting the potential for medical complications of the donation process. The procedures associated with HC donation serve no medical benefit to the donor and the tenet of "do no harm" to donors is an important part of a registry's policies and procedures. An argument could be made that the upper and lower age limits are arbitrary. There is a great deal of variation among young adults in their level of maturity and ability to make informed decisions about the donation process, free of parental or peer influence. The upper age limit could also be challenged as most otherwise healthy 60 years olds could tolerate an HC collection without complication. However, most transplant physicians, when given a choice of two donors, will choose the younger one. An important point to make is whether adding potential donors outside the ages of the current guidelines would significantly add to the diversity of the registry. Table 49.4 shows the likelihood of a searching patient finding a match as donors are added to the NMDP registry. The first column shows the likelihood of finding at least one HLA-A, -B, -DR matched donor in the NMDP registry as of 2002. The second column shows the incremental increase in the likelihood of finding a donor after 10,000 donors of the same race are added. As noted, there are only incremental improvements in the likelihood of finding a match for every 10,000 people added to the NMDP registry. The goal of the registry is to add as much diversity of HLA types as possible given the financial limitations of recruiting, retaining and HLA typing the donors. Expanding the age range alone does not accomplish that goal. Table 49.4 also reveals a common issue as a registry matures. As new donors are added, a progressively smaller percentage of the new donors recruited represent the addition of new HLA types to the registry. Instead, duplication of common HLA types is added. Some duplication is of great value as some donors aren't available at the time their HLA type is needed. Also, as donors pass the age of 60, new, younger recruits should replace them in the registry.

Donor retention

One of the most significant issues in managing a registry of unrelated volunteer donors of HCs is donor availability. At the time a person is recruited to join the registry, they declare their interest in joining the registry and making themselves available for a patient in need. They declare that their health is such that they are able to undergo a marrow collection or apheresis procedure. They also commit to keeping the registry aware

Table 49.5 Donor deferral in the National Marrow Donor Program (NMDP) Registry, reproduced with permission.

Reason for donor "not available"	Percent of registry
Unable to contact	8
Temporarily unavailable	6
Medically deferred	7
Not interested	4
Total	25

of any change in their health, contact information and continuing interest in participation in the registry. However, at the time of the formal search when donors are requested for further testing to determine if they are the best match for a patient, 25% of the donors listed on the NMDP registry are not available to continue on as a potential donor. The most common reasons are listed in Table 49.5. These include "Unable to contact," "Temporarily unavailable," "Medically deferred" and "Not interested." "Unable to contact" usually means that the donor has not provided updated information to find them if they move. "Temporarily unavailable" means that they are still interested in participating but cannot donate at present. Examples include pregnancy, recent surgery, certain types of military service (i.e. submarine duty), family crisis, etc. "Medical deferral" is usually permanent and the donor is removed from the registry. This includes diagnosis of a malignancy or a medical condition that increases the donor's risk of complications of the HC collection process. "Not interested" is also a reason to remove someone from the registry. This is often related to a change in a person's living situation or relationships.

Donor deferrals have a significant impact on the integrity and performance of unrelated donor registries. Physicians, patients and families are dismayed to find that potentially compatible donors are no longer available. Staff at donor centers attempt to locate donors they are initially unable to contact but this can be time-consuming and unproductive. Delays in contact and further evaluation of the donor can cause delays in the care of the patient with the potential for a poorer outcome [17]. A number of strategies have been employed to reduce the rate of donor deferral. First is to properly educate donors at the time of recruitment. The education session should stress the importance of keeping contact information updated. Newsletters or other means to regularly communicate with donors is also important. These communications can keep donors apprised of the need to update contact information, give donors the chance to hear stories about patients and donors involved with successful transplants and remind them of their previous commitment to become a donor. The circumstances under which a donor is recruited can also have an impact on availability [18]. Recruitment drives should encourage but not coerce participation.

Unrelated donor selection

The medical indications for unrelated HCT are similar to related HCT. Once a physician makes the decision to consider allogeneic HCT for their patient, the search for a compatible donor usually begins among first-degree relatives [19]. This will yield an acceptable donor 30% of the time. If there is no close family match, the physician may consider expanding the family search or performing a transplant using a family member with the closest compatible match as the source of HCs. The next step would be to access and search the registries most likely to yield an acceptable match for the patient. This goal can be accomplished by starting with the registry in the country in which the transplant will be performed or with BMDW. The physician typically submits the patient's HLA typing information to the registry and receives back a list of potential donors' HLA data. The list is generated through application of the registry's search algorithm against the database of donors. The list may contain a few possible matched donors or hundreds. This step is often called a "preliminary search." Most algorithms have the ability to prioritize the potential donors based on the degree of the match. Identical matches would be given first consideration, with single mismatches given next consideration. More than a single mismatch would also be listed but at a lower priority. The matching and prioritization process the algorithm uses is complicated by the methodology employed by the registry to type its donors. As mentioned previously, many donors are typed only at the HLA-A and -B level using serological methods. As more sophisticated and accurate means of typing are employed and more loci are utilized (e.g. HLA-C, -DP and -DQ), the complexity of the algorithm and its ranking of potential donors increases.

At the preliminary search point in the search process, the physician has available the HLA data, age, sex and race of the donors. The next step is to identify the donor or donors that represent the most likely matches for the index patient and request further testing of the donors. The physician will identify the specific donors based on HLA typing and demographic data. This process often includes a higher resolution of HLA typing of the donor. Infectious disease marker (IDM) testing is also performed at that time to assess whether the donor has been exposed to human immunodeficiency virus (HIV), hepatitis, cytomegalovirus (CMV) or other diseases that may make the donor ineligible or would have an impact on post-transplant outcomes for the patient. The sample is used to confirm the original typing (confirmatory typing) and expand the detail of the typing if the existing level of typing is inadequate for decision-making.

Once a donor has been identified as the best choice, the donor work-up begins. The donor center conducts an information session to ensure that the donor understands the collections procedures and the risks associated with donation. The information session allows the donor to provide informed consent for the donation. The work-up includes a physical exam to assess the donor's status to undergo a marrow collection or apheresis procedure. The collection is then scheduled and the process of preparing the patient for transplantation begins. The HCs are collected and transported to the patient's bedside. Ideally, the collection arrives within 24 h of collection. Marrow HC is transported at 20–25°C although some transplant centers request that it be transported at a cooler temperature. Peripheral blood HC is transported at 2–6°C [12].

Characteristics that affect post-transplant outcome, other than degree of match have also been studied [20]. The age of the donor can be significant with younger donors preferred. CMV status compared to the patient is significant with a CMV-negative donor preferred. Sex of donor is also significant with male donors preferred. Males are preferred as the HC harvest may yield larger volumes. Female donors who have had one or more pregnancies may also have developed antibodies during pregnancy, which may increase the risk of post-transplant graft-vs.-host disease (GVHD).

Umbilical cord blood (UCB) registries

UCB was initially used for transplantation in the related setting in 1988 [21]. The first unrelated donor UCB was performed in 1993 [22]. From 1993 to 2001 over 1500 UCB transplants have been performed worldwide and reported to the WMDA [14]. There are some potential advantages of UCB and UCB registries over adult volunteer donation. The supply of UCB is nearly limitless and there is great potential to develop a large HLA-diverse pool of UCB units internationally. UCB, once processed, tested and stored, is nearly immediately available for HCT. Adult volunteer donors move and lose contact, may develop medical conditions that preclude donating HCs or may no longer be interested in being a

Table 49.6 Cord blood registries listed with the Bone Marrow Donors Worldwide (BMDW), reproduced with permission.

Cord blood registry	Country	No. of units	Last updated
Bancel—Argentina CBB	Argentina	70	December 2001
Australian CBR	Australia	6449	June 2002
Austrian CBR	Austria	3	June 1999
Belgium CBR	Belgium	3881	April 2002
Leuven CBB	Belgium	2814	June 2002
China—Sinocord	China	5238	June 2002
Czech CBR	Czech Republic	714	June 2002
Finnish CBR	Finland	1389	June 2002
French CBR	France	3134	June 2002
ZKRD—German CBB	Germany	2605	June 2002
German Branch of European CBB	Germany	4820	June 2002
Hadassah CBB	Israel	425	June 2002
Emilia Romagna CBB	Italy	176	February 2002
Milan CBR	Italy	6521	June 2002
Eurocord Netherlands	Netherlands	944	June 2002
Warsaw CBR	Poland	42	September 2001
Bratislava Placental Stem Cells Registry	Slovak Republic	37	October 2001
Spanish CBR	Spain	11,890	June 2002
Swiss CBR	Switzerland	378	June 2002
British Bone Marrow Registry—Cord Blood	United Kingdom	4920	June 2002
American Red Cross CBP	USA	5565	June 2002
Elie Katz Umbilical CBP	USA	1390	June 2002
Caitlin Raymond International Registry	USA	2122	June 2002
Michigan Community Blood Centers CBB	USA	741	June 2002
National Marrow Donor Program	USA	16,279	June 2002
New York CBR	USA	14,200	June 2002
StemCyte, Inc.	USA	8555	June 2002
University of Colorado CBB	USA	6708	June 2002
Total		112,010	

CBB, Cord Blood Bank; CBP, Cord Blood Program; CBR, Cord Blood Registry.

donor. GVHD represents a major complication and cause of mortality and morbidity for patients undergoing allogeneic HCT. The risk of GVHD increases as the rate of HLA mismatch between donor and recipient increases. The incidence of GVHD appears less in UCB transplant, even in circumstances when the degree of mismatch is as much as two HLA antigens [23].

There are disadvantages to using UCB as a source of HC for transplantation [24]. The total nucleated cell dose is critical for engraftment and for ultimate survival. The progenitor cells available in UCB may not be enough to reconstitute the recipient's hematopoetic system [25]. Associated with the lower cell counts is delayed engraftment and poor immune reconstitution. There also remains uncertainty about the degree of graft-vs.-leukemia effect associated with UCB transplants. Lastly, if the recipient needs further HC from the donor, there would be no opportunity with a UCB unit.

Chapter 43 describes the process of transplantation using UCB. UCB registries have developed in response to the need for this source of HCs and to the promise of UCB as an effective therapy [26]. The recruitment of donors usually begins during pregnancy and often through an obstetrician's office. At that time, the mother can be informed of the procedure and consent obtained. At the time of delivery, trained staff is available to collect and process the cord blood, collect a sample for HLA, infectious disease testing, volume and cell count assessment and then packaging for cryopreservation. The units of cord blood can then be stored. Table 49.6 lists the current cord blood banks listed with BMDW.

Ethical considerations

The foundation of an unrelated registry is the good will of its volunteer donors. They are willing to sign up and offer a sample of blood for tissue typing. They give the registry contact information and confidential health information. Subsequently, if chosen, they must suspend their usual activities to undergo a reassessment of their capacity and eligibility as a donor, eventually undergoing some discomfort and post-donation inconvenience for which they receive no direct benefit or remuneration. Yet, over eight million people worldwide have registered to become donors. More would do so if the resources were available to develop and maintain a registry in countries where one does not exist, if transplantation were a priority health care issue in the country or community, and the funds were available to recruit and register potential donors.

As there is no direct benefit to the individual undergoing the donation procedure, it is a unique health care situation. One in which it is incumbent that the health care system takes extraordinary precautions that no avoidable harm occurs to the donor. The policies and procedures developed by a registry can mitigate, to some extent, that potential harm. Age restrictions are a good example. Most registries consider a donor eligible between the ages of 18 and 60. Certainly donation usually is safe as evidenced by thousands of related transplants occurring with donors above and below the age restrictions imposed by unrelated registries. Yet, there is a clear benefit to a donor providing HCs to a relative. In the case of related donation, the potential loss of a loved one outweighs the potential harm of the donation procedure. As unrelated HC donation is anonymous, there is no prior relationship between the donor and the recipient. There would be no loss of companionship or relationship if the donation does not occur. Therefore, although the setting of age restrictions may seem arbitrary and represent as much art as science, the goal is laudable. That is, to reduce as much as possible the risk to the donor.

The same holds true for the medical contraindications for donation. These also are more restrictive for unrelated donors than they would be for related donors or for an individual undergoing a medical procedure for their own benefit. Again the first tenet is "Do no harm." Therefore, a history of back problems, difficulty with general anaesthesia, heart problems, etc., even though relatively mild, may make a donor candidate ineligible. Even if the planned procedure is a PBHC collection by apheresis, the donor may not be eligible to donate if they have difficulties with general anesthesia. If the donor does not mobilize well with granulocyte colony-stimulating factor (G-CSF) and a peripheral collection will not yield adequate numbers of stem cells, then a marrow collection would be necessary. As the recipient will have already begun the preparative regimen, a delay at this late juncture would put the recipient at great risk. Once a donor is chosen and the recipient begins myeloablative chemotherapy and radiation, the need for that donor to complete the process of donation is critical and there may not be time to prepare a second unrelated donor.

What then of the potential donor who backs out at the final stages, after the potential recipient has already begun preparation? This is one of the most difficult dilemmas and ethical issues for a registry to face. Ultimately, one must respect the wishes of the donor and not subject the donor to coercion of any kind. The natural tendency might be to shame the donor or blame them for any poor outcome the recipient may face. The time to prevent a potential donor from backing out at the "11th hour" is well before the recipient's myeloablative regimen has begun. It starts at recruitment and continues with regular communication while on the registry and when the donor is initially contacted as a potential donor for a specific patient. The staff that work with the donor and guide him or her through the process should be attuned to any concerns or fears that the donor might express. They should elicit from the donor any concerns he or she may have and, if it appears they may have difficulty assuaging the fears and concerns, the registry should develop a backup plan with the transplanter. This may include a backup donor from the registry or a related transplant with the best-matched relative. The incidence of donors backing out after the recipient has begun myeloablative preparation is not reported by the registries, but anecdotally appears to be very rare.

There are ethical issues beyond the health of the donor and the potential for coercion that are worthy of consideration. Donors entrust the registry with a significant amount of information. This information includes HLA typing, contact information, government identification number (Social Security Number in the US) and contact information for friends and family members who can help locate the donor, if necessary, and preliminary health information. In addition, the registry may have a sample of blood in a repository. If the individual is chosen as a potential donor, the registry will have more comprehensive health information and more blood samples for tests that will include infectious disease testing. All of this information on an individual or a group of volunteer donors represents a potential for less than ethical use. The names and contact information could be given or sold to other organizations for their purposes (e.g. fund raising, credit card applications). The information may be stolen if care is not taken in developing security measures to reduce that likelihood. The donors could be entered into research studies using their information and blood samples, the purpose of which was not given to the donors at the time the information and samples were collected and without their consent, then or in the future. These issues need to be carefully considered when a registry is developed and safeguards implemented.

Systems, processes and procedures should be developed that ensure a donor's safety, security and confidentiality. Equally important to the system approach is the attitude and culture of the registry, a culture of protecting the registry's greatest asset, the altruism of the volunteer unrelated donor.

Conclusion

The development, evolution and maturation of an international system of cooperating registries of volunteer unrelated donors represent an achievement that is remarkable given their humble beginnings. As outcomes for allogeneic transplant improve, the demand for unrelated donors will significantly increase. Changes in HLA testing, non-HLA match criteria, search algorithms, diseases for which HCT represents appropriate therapy, and a myriad of other changes and innovations will challenge the world's registries to adapt. It will also allow the world's registries of unrelated donors to contribute to the health and well-being of thousands more for whom there is no other viable alternative therapy.

References

1 Speck B, Zwan FE, Rood JJV, Eernisse JG. Allogeneic bone marrow transplantation in a patient with aplastic anemia using a phenotypically HLA-identical unrelated donor. *Transplantation* 1973; **16**: 24–8.

2 Horowitz SD, Bach FH, Groshong T, Hong R, Yunis EJ. Treatment of severe combined immunodeficiency with bone marrow from an unrelated, mixed leukocyte culture non-reactive donor. *Lancet* 1975; **2**: 432–3.

3 Foroozonfar N. Bone marrow transplant from an unrelated donor for chronic granulomatous disease. *Lancet* 1977; **1**: 210–3.

4 Hansen JA, Clift RA, Thomas ED, Buckner CD, Storb R, Giblett ER. Transplantation of marrow from an unrelated donor to a patient with acute leukemia. *N Engl J Med* 1980; **303**: 565–7.

5 James DCV. Organization of a hospital bone marrow panel. In: Smit-Sibinga CTH, Das PC, Opelz G, eds. *Transplantation and Blood Transfusion*. Boston: Martinus Nijoff, 1984: 131–9.

6 Dupont B. Immunology of hematopoietic stem cell transplantation: a brief review of its history. *Immunol Rev* 1997; **157**: 5–12.

7 McCullough J, Hansen J, Perkins H, Stroncek D, Bartsch G. The National Marrow Donor Program: how it works, accomplishments to date. *Oncology* 1989; **3**: 63–72.

8 Bone Marrow Donors Worldwide. *Annual Report 2001–2002*. Leiden, NE: Bone Marrow Donors Worldwide, 2002.

9 Confer DL. Unrelated marrow donor registries. *Curr Opin Hematol* 1997; **4**: 408–12.

10 Oudshoorn M, Leeuwen AV, Zanden HGMV, Rood JJV. Bone Marrow Donors Worldwide: a successful exercise in international cooperation. *Bone Marrow Transplant* 1994; **14**: 3–8

11 Lee G et al. *Wintrobe's Clinical Hematology*, 10th edn. Baltimore: Williams & Wilkins, 1999: 774–816.

12 National Marrow Donor Program. *National Marrow Donor Program Standards*, 16th edn. Minneapolis: National Marrow Donor Program, 1997.

13 Buskard N, Stroncek D. Bone marrow donor registries and international cooperation. *Transfus Med Rev* 1993; **7**: 11–6.

14 World Marrow Donor Association. *Annual Report*. Leiden, NE: World Marrow Donor Association, 2001.

15 Coppo PA. Unrelated bone marrow donor registries. In: Chapman JR, Deierhoi M, Wight C, eds. *Organ and Tissue Donation for Transplantation*. London: Arnold, 1997: 430–45.

16 US Federal Government, Office of Management and Budget. *No. 00–02, Guidance on Associations and Allocation of Data on Race for Use in Civil Rights Monitoring and Enforcement*, 2000. www.whitehouse.gov/omb/bulletins/b00-02.html

17 Barker J, Krepski T, DeFor T, Davies S, Wagner J, Weisdorf D. Searching for unrelated donor hematopoietic stem cells. Availability and speed of umbilical cord blood vs. bone marrow. *Biol Blood Marrow Transplant* 2002; **8**: 257–60.

18 National Marrow Donor Program. *Effectiveness in Retaining Donors*. Washington, DC: Office of

Inspector General, US Department of Health and Human Services, 2002.
19 Schipper RF, D'Amaro J, Oudshoorn M. The probability of finding a suitable related donor for bone marrow transplantation in extended families. *Blood* 1996; **87**(2): 800–4.
20 Hansen JA, Gooley TA, Martin PJ *et al*. Bone Marrow transplants from unrelated donors for patients with chronic myeloid leukemia. *N Engl J Med* 1998; **338**: 962–8.
21 Gluckman E, Broxmeyer HA, Auerbach AD *et al*. Hematopoietic reconstitution in a patient with Fanconi's anemia by means of umbilical cord blood from an HLA-identical sibling. *N Engl J Med* 1989; **321**: 1174–8.
22 Barker JN, Wagner JE. Umbilical cord blood transplantation: current state of the art. *Curr Opin Oncol* 2002; **14**: 160–4.
23 Grewal SS, Barker JN, Davies SM, Wagner JE. Unrelated donor hematopoietic cell transplantation. Marrow or umbilical cord blood? *Blood* 2003; **101**: 4233–43.
24 Wadlow RC, Porter DL. Umbilical cord blood transplantation: where do we stand? *Biol Blood Marrow Transplant* 2002; **8**: 637–47.
25 Paulin T. Importance of bone marrow cell dose in bone marrow transplantation. *Clin Transplant* 1992; **6**: 48–54.
26 Rubinstein P, Carrier C, Scaradavou A *et al*. Outcomes among 562 recipients of placental-blood transplants from unrelated donors. *N Eng J Med* 1998; **339**: 1565–77.

Section 4

Complications and Their Management

50

Keith M. Sullivan

Graft-vs.-Host Disease

Background

Historical development

In 1955 a description of graft-vs.-host disease (GVHD) in animals, then known as secondary disease, was reported by Barnes and Loutit [1]. Named to differentiate it from the primary disease of radiation sickness, fatal secondary disease was observed in irradiated mice given allogeneic spleen cells but not in recipients of syngeneic cells. By the late 1950s, it was apparent that the skin abnormalities and diarrhea of secondary disease and runt disease (a wasting syndrome in unirradiated newborn mice given allogeneic spleen cells) were the result of immunologically competent cells introduced into an immunoincompetent host. The term graft-vs.-host was introduced to describe the vector of this immunologic assault [2,3].

Human graft-vs.-host disease

Early human transplants of allogeneic marrow were often complicated by GVHD [4–8]. Features were remarkably similar to those seen in animal studies of GVHD [9] and to reports of GVHD developing in immunodeficient children who received blood transfusions [10]. Because it has been difficult to separate the illness caused by immunologic attack from the consequences of this assault (including immunodeficiency, organ dysfunction and infection), both aspects have been considered a part of human GVHD. The term *acute* GVHD describes a distinctive syndrome of dermatitis, hepatitis and enteritis developing within 100 days of allogeneic hematopoietic cell transplantation (HCT). The term *chronic* GVHD describes a more pleiotropic syndrome that develops after day 100.

Pathogenesis

In a remarkably perceptive summary in 1966, Billingham [11] defined the criteria for the development of GVHD as follows.

1 The graft must contain immunologically competent cells.
2 The host must possess important transplantation alloantigens that are lacking in the donor graft, so that the host appears foreign to the graft, and is, therefore, capable of stimulating it antigenically.
3 The host itself must be incapable of mounting an effective immunological reaction against the graft, at least for sufficient time for the latter to manifest its immunological capabilities; that is, it must have the security of tenure.

These criteria now require some modification to incorporate current understanding of the biology of GVHD (see Chapters 27 and 30). The occurrence of autologous GVHD suggests that inappropriate recognition

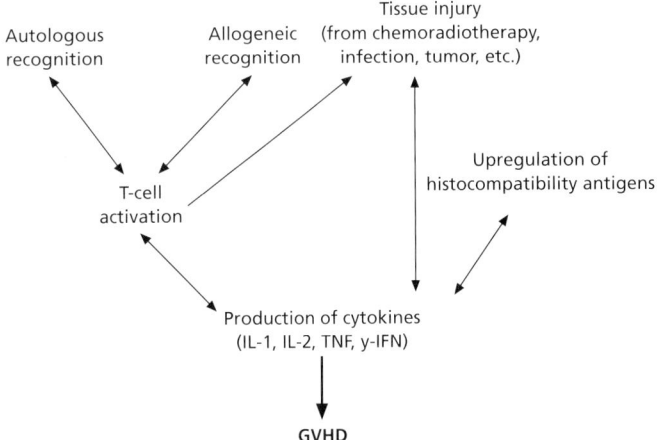

Fig. 50.1 Interactive events that lead to graft-vs.-host disease (GVHD). T-cell activation and tissue injury release cytokines that produce the clinical manifestations of GVHD. IL, interleukin; IFN, interferon; TNF, tumor necrosis factor. (Adapted from [12].)

of host self-antigens may occur, and transfusion-associated GVHD (T-GVHD) may develop in certain immunocompetent individuals. A multi-step model of antigen expression, cytokine production, T-cell activation and tissue injury has been described and Fig. 50.1 depicts this interactive construct [12,13].

Alloreactivity

Abundant animal data demonstrate that T lymphocytes contained in the donor inoculum proliferate and differentiate *in vivo* in response to disparate histocompatibility antigens on host tissues and directly, or through secondary mechanisms, attack recipient cells, thus producing the signs and symptoms of acute GVHD (see Chapter 26) [9,11,14]. The afferent arm of acute GVHD consists of antigen presentation, activation of individual T cells, clonal proliferation and differentiation [15,16]. Cell death of host targets results from alloreactivity of donor-derived T cells. In the efferent phase, release of cytokines from activated lymphocytes contributes to cell death, either directly or through recruitment of secondary effectors, such as natural killer (NK) cells [17]. Based on mechanistic roles postulated for interleukin-1 (IL-1), IL-2, lipopolysaccharide (LPS), and proinflammatory cytokines such as IL-6, interferon-γ (IFN-γ) and tumor necrosis factor (TNF), immunomodulatory agents have been administered *in vivo* to control GVHD.

Microbial environment

The microbial mileu of the host may also influence the development of GVHD. Compared with conventionally housed irradiated mice, enteric GVHD was significantly reduced in germ-free mice given incompatible marrow [18]. Human studies confirm this gnotobiotic effect [19,20]. Microorganisms could act as triggers of GVHD, perhaps by sharing antigenic epitopes with gut epithelial cells or by activating latent virus-inducing antigens on cell surfaces to become targets of alloreactivity [21]. Gut damage could also lead to leakage of LPS into the circulation, thereby releasing cytokine effectors of GVHD [22].

Tolerance

Chapter 24 reviews the mechanisms of graft–host tolerance after allogeneic HCT. Tolerance can be achieved by elimination (clonal deletion) in the thymus of host reactive cells; accordingly, thymic damage could abrogate self-tolerance [23,24]. Alternatively, functional suppressor T cells may be important in transplantation tolerance [25]. Alterations in this regulatory immune balance could explain the development of GVHD-like syndromes following autologous HCT.

Autologous graft-vs.-host disease

Histocompatibility differences between donor and recipient may not always be needed to produce GVHD; instead, inappropriate recognition of self-antigens may produce a GVHD-like syndrome [26–28]. A syndrome similar to GVHD develops upon withdrawal of cyclosporine (CSP) in lethally irradiated animals administered CSP after syngeneic HCT. Autoreactive T cells can be found in a damaged thymus in which class II-bearing cells are absent and clonal deletion of antiself autoreactive cells does not occur. Administration of CSP in the context of thymic damage appears to be key to preventing development of immune regulatory cells and permitting development of autoreactive CD8$^+$ T cells which recognize class II determinants (see Chapter 30 for further details of these instructive experiments).

Mild and usually self-limited episodes of dermal GVHD occasionally are seen in patients who are undergoing syngeneic or autologous bone marrow transplantation (BMT) [29,30]. One clinical series reported these findings in seven of 96 autologous and two of 19 syngeneic marrow transplants [31]. Hepatic and gastrointestinal abnormalities consistent with acute GVHD have also been described [32] (see Plate 23.28, *facing p. 296*). Findings of GVHD-like lesions have also been noted after administration of CSP and IL-2 to autologous marrow recipients [33,34]. Recent reports of gene expression analysis reveal a marked increase in IL-10 messenger ribonucleic acid (mRNA) levels in peripheral blood mononuclear cells (PBMCs) of individuals given CSP after autologous HCT who subsequently develop autologous GVHD [35]. Although controversy surrounds the interpretation of such clinical reports, the biology of this syndrome holds considerable importance, especially if clinical protocols could be developed to successfully augment any associated graft-vs.-leukemia (GVL) effect (see Chapter 28).

Transfusion-associated graft-vs.-host disease

Etiology and incidence

The pathobiology of T-GVHD appears similar to the sequence of events following allogeneic HCT [36]. For example, cytotoxic clones of CD8$^+$ and CD4$^+$ T cells from a transfusion donor (the son) reacting against parental antigens not shared by the son were isolated from the peripheral blood of a postoperative patient (the father) suffering from T-GVHD. Other isolated CD4$^+$ clones were found to secrete TNF. T-GVHD was initially recognized in children with immunodeficiencies [10,37]. Since these original descriptions almost 40 years ago, over 100 patients have been reported [38]. A Medline search of articles on T-GVHD published in English since 1960 indicates that most were published between 1985 and 1996, reflecting perhaps more effective current prevention [39]. In most reported cases, patients with congenital or acquired immunodeficiencies (including HCT) had received whole blood, packed red cells, platelet or granulocyte transfusions, or fresh plasma [40,41]. No cases have been observed in patients with acquired immune deficiency syndrome (AIDS), and no cases have resulted from transfusion of cryoprecipitate or fresh frozen plasma [38,39].

This syndrome has also been reported in immunocompetent individuals [42,43]. In Japan, the incidence is estimated to be approximately 1/500 open heart operations [42]. In inbred populations sharing common human leukocyte antigen (HLA) haplotypes, it is likely that blood from a donor homozygous for an extended HLA haplotype could be transfused into a recipient who is heterozygous for the same haplotype [44,45]. In this setting, donor cells would not be rejected as foreign by the recipient and could precipitate GVHD. Accordingly, transfusion guidelines in Japan call for irradiated blood support during surgery and severe trauma [46].

Diagnosis and clinical features

Histocompatibility typing demonstrates marrow and peripheral blood cells to be of donor origin and skin biopsy confirms characteristic lesions of acute GVHD. In neonates, the diagnosis may be more difficult to establish because the onset after transfusion is often more delayed than in adults (28 days vs. 10 days, respectively) [47]. Rapid methods to detect donor-derived DNA polymorphisms and diagnose GVHD have been described [48]. In general, this syndrome develops 4–30 days after transfusion and resembles hyperacute GVHD following allogeneic HCT; unfortunately, fever, erythroderma, diarrhea and liver abnormalities progress despite therapy with corticosteroids, CSP or antithymocyte globulin (ATG). In immunocompetent hosts, the rash often resembles epidermal necrolysis or severe erythema multiforme. Lichenoid histology, a common feature of GVHD following HCT, is a less frequent finding [49]. Marrow aplasia is not usual following allogeneic HCT (marrow being of donor origin), but in the case of transfusion-associated disease the marrow is of host origin and can serve as a target for GVHD. Thus, marrow aplasia is frequently observed with T-GVHD and contributes to the 90% case fatality [38]. Treatment with CSP and OKT3 has rarely been successful and, because the immediate mortality is so high, few patients with chronic GVHD have been reported [50].

Prevention

The efficacy of blood product irradiation has long been recognized, and initial BMT practice routinely employed irradiation of blood products with 1500 cGy [51]. This dose of gamma irradiation from cobalt-60 (^{60}Co) or cesium-137 (^{137}Cs) sources effectively prevents lymphocyte proliferation without adverse effect on blood cell morphology or function [52]. Although there has been variation across individual centers, 97% of institutions surveyed by the American Association of Blood Banks employ doses of 1500–3500 cGy [53]. This practice appeared to be highly effective and only a single case of T-GVHD has been reported in a patient given blood components irradiated with 2000 cGy from a ^{137}Cs source [54]. Based upon more sensitive limiting dilution assays of T-cell inactivation, more recent studies have called for higher doses of blood production irradiation and since July 1993, the Food and Drug Administration (FDA) has required a dose of 2500 cGy to the internal midplane of the canister with well-defined procedures for quality assurance, dose mapping and storage times (see Chapter 61) [55,56]. Currently, methods are in development to use photoactive dyes or psoralen and ultraviolet A (PUVA) light to inactivate infectious organisms in blood components. In preclinical models this approach appears to be an effective means to inhibit lymphocyte proliferation and prevent T-GVHD [57]. At present, however, gamma irradiation remains the standard. Although debate continues as to which patients should receive irradiated blood products, it is universally recommended for HCT recipients. This practice continues for at least 6 months post-HCT, but may be needed for longer periods in patients with active chronic GVHD and severe immunodeficiency.

Acute graft-vs.-host disease

Incidence and predictive factors

Donor–host factors

HLA disparity between the hematopoietic cell donor and recipient is the most powerful factor governing the severity and kinetics of GVHD. The incidence of acute GVHD is much increased with HLA-nonidentical related marrow donors (Fig. 50.2) [58]. Among haploidentical sibling transplants, mismatches for noninherited paternal antigens appear associated with higher rates of GVHD, suggesting that exposure to maternal HLA antigens *in utero* could have a lifelong effect on immune response [59]. A high incidence of acute GVHD has also been observed with HLA-matched unrelated donors (reviewed in Chapter 83) [60]. Although some studies have identified certain HLA antigens associated with increased rates of GVHD [61,62], these correlations have not been observed consistently [63,64]. Chapter 4 details the evolving precision of molecular HLA typing. The importance of class I and II allele matching in reducing the risk for GVHD has been widely demonstrated in unrelated donor HCT cohorts [65–68]. In a recent National Marrow Donor Program (NMDP) analysis of individuals undergoing HCT from HLA-A and -B matched unrelated donors, HLA-DRB1 allele disparity was independently associated with an increased risk of severe acute GVHD [69]. Minor HLA peptides have been identified and sequenced, and minor histocompatibility antigen (mHA) disparities appear correlated with the risk for GVHD in adults given HLA-identical donor grafts [70–72]. The importance of mHA matching is further supported by the observed low rate of GVHD in populations that feature genetic homogeneity [73]. In more genetically heterogeneous racial groups, data are less consistent as to increased rates of GVHD [74–76]. Both class I and class II disparities have been associated with GVHD [77,78]. Altered peptide ligands may have profound effects on alloreactivity and tolerance (see Chapter 24).

Sex mismatching and donor parity have been associated with an increased risk of acute GVHD [62–64]. Female donor T cells could recognize H-Y minor antigens on host Y chromosome-containing cells. Moreover, previously parous donors could have experienced maternal alloimmunization as a result of unshared minor antigens of the fetus [79]. These presensitized cells would then mount a vigorous secondary type response when transplanted.

Age is another key factor associated with the development of acute GVHD [62,63,80]. Among patients under 20 years of age given a 102-day course of intermittent methotrexate (MTX) as GVHD prophylaxis, the incidence of significant (grade II–IV) acute GVHD was approximately 20% [81]. In contrast, the incidence of acute GVHD was 30% in patients 45–50 years old, and 79% in those 51–62 years old [82]. In a recursive partition model of factors which influence GVHD development among HLA-identical marrow recipients, the risk of GVHD varied from 19% to 66%, depending on recipient age, donor–recipient sex matching and donor parity [62]. Because sibling ages are often closely linked covariates, an effect of donor age has been difficult to detect in this setting. Among unrelated transplant recipients, increasing donor age is associated with an increased risk of developing GVHD [67,83]. In a recent report from the NMDP describing donor risk factors for development of GVHD in unrelated transplants, donor age (but not race, cytomegalovirus [CMV] serostatus or ABO incompatibility) was associated with increasing incidence of severe acute GVHD [84]. Perhaps the relative paucity of naive T-cells and an abundance of mature T-cells in older donors could account for these increased rates of GVHD. However, difficulty in establishing the diagnosis and grade of GVHD, as discussed below, may influence center or registry studies of incidence and risk factors.

Source of hematopoietic cells

The source of allogeneic hematopoietic cells may also influence the development of GVHD. For more than two decades, experience was derived from marrow transplant cohorts describing rates and risk factors for GVHD [8,62–64]. Virtually all marrow grafts were infused as fresh products, although one group reported apparent reduction in rates of GVHD with cryopreserved marrow [85].

Of considerable interest to stem cell biologists, umbilical cord blood cells appear less immunologically reactive than bone marrow cells [86]. When applied in human HCT, there is an apparent reduction in rates of GVHD in recipients who are usually of younger age [87–89]. With a relative abundance of immature stem cells and naive T cells in the inoculum, crossing HLA barriers is met with relatively little acute and chronic GVHD. In a study of unrelated donor transplants, the incidence of acute GVHD was 37% with cord blood, compared with an expected 83% rate in comparable pediatric recipients of unrelated marrow [90]. Ongoing research focuses on methods to expand the number of cord blood cells *ex vivo* to yield sufficient cells to transplant into adults (see Chapter 43).

Allogeneic peripheral blood hematopoietic cells (PBHCs) have also received considerable recent attention as a source for HCT. Initial reports suggested no significant increase in the rates of acute and chronic GVHD when compared to the historical BMT experience [91,92]. However, with longer follow-up, the increased risk for chronic GVHD appears established [93], and a number of controlled trials comparing outcomes in related marrow or PBHC transplantations (PBHCTs) have been reported.

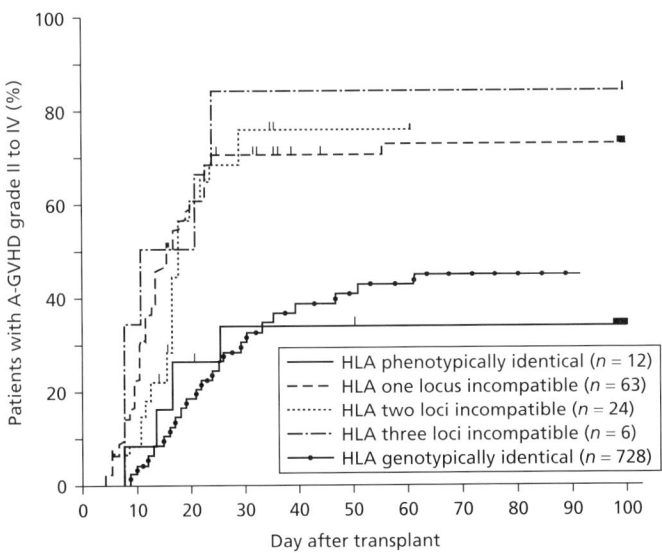

Fig. 50.2 Cumulative probability of grade II–IV acute graft-vs.-host disease (GVHD) after allogeneic bone marrow transplantation (BMT) from a genotypically human leukocyte antigen (HLA) identical sibling or other family members mismatched for 0–3 loci on the nonshared haplotype. (Adapted from [58].)

Faster engraftment, fewer hospitalizations, less donor morbidity and economic advantages are noted with PBHCTs. A meta-analysis conducted in June 2000 of 16 studies (five randomized and 11 cohort) found that the relative risk (RR) for acute GVHD after PBHCT was 1.16-fold greater ($p = 0.006$) when compared to BMT [94]. There was also a trend toward lessened rates of relapse with PBHCT. In a cohort study of PBHCT compared with BMT from unrelated donors, GVHD rates were similar but nonrelapse mortality (NRM) was lower and survival was higher after PBHCT (see Chapter 46) [95].

Hematopoietic cell dose

Studies of CD34+ cell dose have shown advantages in resource utilization and cost in autologous PBHCT. In allogeneic PBHCT, a higher (6.3–10.0×10^6 CD34+ cells/kg) hematopoietic cell dose was associated with a sharp increase in GVHD risk among CSP recipients [96]. In contrast, CD34+ cell dose did not appear to influence the occurrence or severity of acute or chronic GVHD in allogeneic BMT [97]. Of interest, a low PBHC dose ($<3 \times 10^6$ CD34+ cells/kg) was associated with slower hematologic recovery, increased rates of fungal infections and NRM, and decreased overall survival.

Immunomodulation

The incidence of acute GVHD after matched sibling BMT varies inversely with the efficacy of post-transplant immunosuppressive prophylaxis. Multivariate analysis revealed that an increased dose of pretransplant total body irradiation (TBI) was associated with an increased risk of GVHD. Among HLA-identical HCT recipients who received GVHD prophylaxis with MTX and CSP, acute GVHD developed in 48% of patients given 1575 cGy TBI, compared with 21% of patients given 1200 cGy TBI ($p = 0.02$) [98]. One hypothesis is that more intensive myeloablative conditioning might eliminate persisting host cells and restrict the development of mixed donor–host chimerism, which has been associated with a decreased probability of GVHD [99,100]. Alternatively, more intensive conditioning could increase gastrointestinal damage, modify microbial environment, release cytokine mediators and/or attenuate the dose of administered GVHD prophylaxis. Some studies indicate that donor or host infection (as denoted by seropositivity for the herpesviruses) predicts the subsequent development of GVHD [101], whereas others find no predictive association [64,102].

Cytokine levels and gene polymorphisms

As shown in Fig. 50.1, activated donor T cells release proinflammatory cytokines which upregulate HLA expression (see Chapter 27). Compared with IFN-γ or IL-12, serum levels of IL-18 appear to have an even greater sensitivity and specificity for GVHD [103]. Accordingly, investigators have asked if cytokine gene polymorphisms which alter function and regulation might be predictive of GVHD. An initial study in blood and tissue samples failed to show a clear correlation or prediction of GVHD [104]. Another report found that the genotype in the donor of IL-1 receptor antagonist (allele 2) was protective against severe GVHD developing in the recipient [105]. Single nucleotide polymorphisms were determined in sibling transplants and recipient genotypes for IFN-γ intron 1, IL-10^{-1064} and TNF d3 were found to be associated with acute GVHD, whereas IL-6^{174} genotype was associated with chronic GVHD [106]. In a similar study of genetic and clinical factors, polymorphisms of IL-10 (an inhibitor of TNF-α) in both donor (RR 3.5) and recipient (RR 7.9) predicted for acute GVHD along with donor CMV seropositivity and mHA mismatching [107].

Predictive assays

The frequencies of alloreactive cytotoxic T-lymphocyte precursors and helper T-lymphocyte precursors may have pretransplant predictive value in selecting donor–recipient pairs with a reduced risk of GVHD (see Chapters 4 and 5) [108,109]. Skin-explant models have been developed in which donor lymphocytes sensitized *in vitro* against recipient cells are cultured with recipient skin [110,111]. In other models, a mixed epidermal cell lymphocyte reaction is used to detect incompatibility [112]. Although correlations with GVHD appear to be statistically significant, individual variations have been observed [113]. More recent reports suggest a tighter correlation by combining cytokine gene polymorphisms and explant results [114].

Clinical features

Dermal

The initial manifestation of acute GVHD is often a maculopapular exanthem [115]. Among the first 43 patients given MTX prophylaxis and transplanted in Seattle from HLA-identical donors, the median time of onset of skin rash was 19 days (range 5–47 days) post-transplant [116]. Lesions may be pruritic or painful and red to violaceous in color, and may initially involve the palms and soles (see Plate 23.16, *facing p. 296*). The characteristic predilection for these sites appears related to concentration of stem cells in the rete ridges (see Plate 23.18, *facing p. 296*) [117]. As the rash intensifies, confluent involvement of the cheeks, ears, neck and trunk is noted, often associated with papule formation (see Plate 23.22, *facing p. 296*). A hyperacute form of GVHD has been described, which includes fever, generalized erythroderma and desquamation developing 7–14 days after transplantation [118]. Epidermal necrosis is the most severe form of cutaneous GVHD, and bullae formation and epidermal separation may resemble toxic epidermal necrolysis (see Plate 23.17, *facing p. 296*). Rarely, a necrolytic rash may be caused by a staphylococcal scalded skin syndrome, which can respond to appropriate antibiotics [119]. The differential diagnosis of post-transplant skin rash includes chemoradiotherapy effects, drug allergy and viral exanthem. Topography and review of serial skin biopsies help establish the diagnosis. Chapter 23 presents the histopathologic features of GVHD.

Hepatic

The liver is the next most frequently involved target of acute GVHD [120]. Cholestatic jaundice commonly occurs; however, hepatic failure with encephalopathy caused solely by hepatic GVHD is unusual. Hypoalbuminemia is not usually a result of liver failure, but rather of GVHD-associated intestinal protein leak and negative nitrogen balance [121]. The differential diagnosis includes hepatic veno-occlusive disease (VOD), infection and drug toxicity. Hepatotoxicity caused by CSP can cause isolated hyperbilirubinemia, which improves within several days as the dosage of drug is modified. Although not usually required in patients with typical manifestations of dermal and intestinal GVHD, liver biopsy may be useful in some patients because bile duct damage from GVHD is often characteristic (see Chapter 58; Plates 23.32 and 23.33, *facing p. 296*).

Gastrointestinal

Symptoms of acute GVHD of the distal small bowel and colon include profuse diarrhea, intestinal bleeding, crampy abdominal pain and ileus. The diarrhea is often green, mucoid, watery and mixed with exfoliated cells, forming fecal casts. Even with cessation of oral intake, voluminous secretory diarrhea may persist, and stool volumes should be recorded to quantify the severity of involvement and response to treatment. Bloody diarrhea often requires frequent transfusion support. In general, signs of enteric GVHD develop as the chemoradiotherapy effects resolve following the first several weeks after transplantation. A variant of enteric GVHD has been described in 13% of patients who received HLA-identical

Table 50.1 Clinical staging of acute graft-vs.-host disease (GVHD): Seattle criteria. (Adapted from [116].)

Stage	Skin*	Liver bilirubin	Gut†‡
+	Maculopapular rash <25% body surface	2–3 mg/dL	Diarrhea, 500–1000 mL/day or persistent nausea
++	Maculopapular rash 25–50% body surface	3–6 mg/dL	Diarrhea, 1000–1500 mL/day
+++	Generalized erythroderma	6–15 mg/dL	Diarrhea, >1500 mL/day
++++	Desquamation and bullae	>15 mg/dL	Pain ± ileus

*Use "rule of nines" or burn chart to determine extent of rash.
†Diarrhea volumes apply to adults.
‡Persistent nausea requires endoscopic biopsy evidence of GVHD histology in the stomach or duodenum.

Table 50.2 Clinical grading of acute graft-vs.-host disease (GVHD): Seattle criteria. (Adapted from [116].)

Overall grade	Skin	Liver	Gut	Functional impairment
0 (none)	0	0	0	0
I (mild)	+ to ++	0	0	0
II (moderate)	+ to +++	+	+	+
III (severe)	++ to +++	++ to +++	++ to +++	++
IV (life-threatening)	+ to ++++	++ to ++++	++ to ++++	+++

transplants [122]. Presenting symptoms include anorexia and dyspepsia, and patients with upper gastrointestinal disease may not manifest lower tract involvement. Apparently more common in older patients, upper tract disease responds well to immunosuppressive therapy, although a high proportion (74%) of patients progress to chronic GVHD.

The differential diagnosis includes residual effects of chemoradiotherapy and intestinal infection including *Clostridium difficile* and CMV enteritis. Endoscopic findings of enteric GVHD range from normal to extensive edema (see Plates 23.24, 23.26 & 23.27, *facing p. 296*) and mucosal sloughing (see Plate 23.30, *facing p. 296*). Lesions may be most prominent in the cecum, ileum and ascending colon, but may also involve the stomach, duodenum and rectum. Histology reveals crypt-cell necrosis and drop-out (see Plates 23.25, 23.26 and 23.27, *facing p. 296*). Gastrointestinal endoscopy and biopsy are mandatory for the diagnosis of upper tract disease [122,123]. Routine endoscopic biopsy of patients with unexplained nausea and vomiting can reveal herpesvirus infection with or without associated acute GVHD (reviewed in Chapter 58) [124]. However, the great majority of patients with nausea and vomiting persisting after day 20 post-transplant will have enteric acute GVHD [125].

Other findings

Ocular symptoms have been described in patients with acute GVHD [126]. Photophobia, hemorrhagic conjunctivitis, pseudomembrane formation and lagophthalmos can be observed within 50 days of BMT. Individuals with acute GVHD and conjunctival involvement are reported to have a poorer survival than patients with GVHD without ocular disease [127]. Acute GVHD has been associated with an increased risk for infectious and noninfectious pneumonia and sterile effusions [128–131]. Severe hypogammaglobulinemia may also be noted. Hemorrhagic cystitis with infective agents recovered from urine has been reported in patients with acute GVHD [132]. Thrombocytopenia and anemia have been reported in patients with GVHD and failure of platelet recovery was shown to be 3.5-fold more common in patients with acute GVHD [133,134]. A hemolytic–uremic syndrome of microangiopathy, hemolysis and thrombocytopenia has also been observed in CSP recipients developing severe GVHD [135].

Diagnosis and grading

Staging

Acute GVHD is a clinicopathologic syndrome involving the skin, liver and gut [116]. Characteristic findings in biopsies of skin (eosinophilic bodies), liver (bile duct damage) and gut (crypt-cell degeneration) early after BMT may be difficult to distinguish from the effects of chemoradiotherapy conditioning (see Chapter 23) [136,137]. Serial biopsies and observations help establish the diagnosis and severity of GVHD [138].

Grading

Tables 50.1 and 50.2 present the commonly used Glucksberg *et al.* [116] Seattle criteria for the staging and grading of acute GVHD. In general, grade I acute GVHD has a favorable prognosis and does not require treatment. Grade II GVHD is a moderately severe disease, which requires therapy and usually consists of multiorgan involvement. Occasionally, patients with a 3+ skin rash and impaired performance will qualify for grade II severity in the absence of liver or gut involvement. A more recent modification of grade II disease includes symptoms of nausea, anorexia, food intolerance or vomiting confirmed to be enteric GVHD on upper intestinal biopsy [122,139]. Grade III disease is severe multiorgan GVHD, and grade IV disease is life-threatening or fatal acute GVHD. The overall grade of acute GVHD usually predicts the clinical course [19,116]. Figure 50.3 illustrates outcome in 325 recipients of HLA-identical BMT given GVHD prophylaxis with a combination of MTX and CSP [64].

Differential diagnosis and severity scores

Within 96 h of neutrophil engraftment, GVHD may be difficult to distinguish from a constellation of findings (fever without infection, erythroderma and noncardiogenic pulmonary edema) known as the engraftment syndrome [140]. Dermal biopsies help establish a diagnosis of GVHD when clinical features are consistent with the syndrome, but they are of limited value in the early post-transplant period or in predicting visceral disease [141]. Upper gastrointestinal endoscopy and biopsy in patients with anorexia and vomiting may yield a variety of diagnoses, including GVHD, peptic ulceration, or mycotic or viral infections [123,124]. Liver

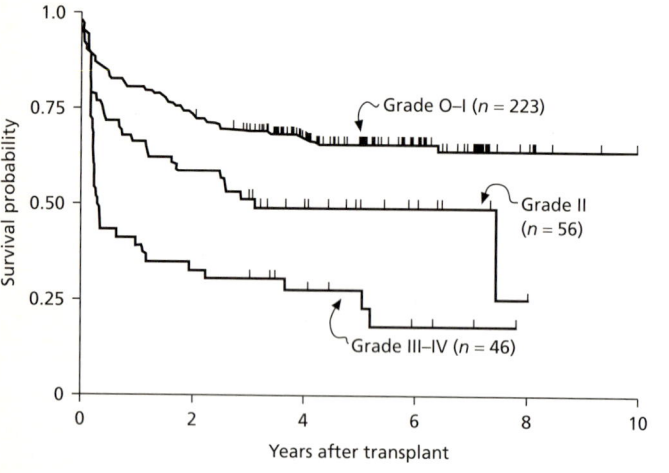

Fig. 50.3 Kaplan–Meier estimates of survival based on the clinical grade of acute graft-vs.-host disease (GVHD). For this analysis, 325 patients without advanced malignancy were studied. (Adapted from [64].)

function abnormalities may cause diagnostic dilemmas even on review of hepatic histology.

Given differing approaches for diagnostic testing, procedures and interpretations, it is not surprising that there is inconsistency in the grading of acute GVHD [142]. As shown in Table 50.3, revised criteria have been proposed to reflect disease progression and amount of immunosuppressive therapy required to control GVHD [143]. Another system shown in Table 50.4 is based on the extent of organ involvement exclusive of subjective evaluation of functional performance of the patient and corresponding rates of NRM are shown in Fig. 50.4 [144]. Whether this revision of the Seattle grading system is more sensitive and specific for predicting outcome remains unclear given inherent difficulties in distinguishing morbidity resulting from GVHD and other causes [83,145]. Along with GVHD response, future trials should always report survival and NRM when evaluating GVHD prevention and treatment [146].

Prevention

Donor and host factors

Because histocompatability is a key determinant of the kinetics of GVHD [147], molecular characterization of class I and II antigens can be a powerful asset in selection of the best available family member or unrelated donor (see Chapters 4 and 83). For CMV-seronegative BMT recipients, matching with seronegative donors also appears to reduce the risk of both CMV infection and GVHD [62]. Laminar airflow (LAF) protective isolation with gut decontamination has been shown to decrease the incidence of acute GVHD and improve survival in patients with aplastic anemia prepared with cyclophosphamide (CY) alone [19]. Findings in patients with leukemia are more inconsistent, perhaps because of poorer compliance with nonabsorbable oral antibiotics in patients prepared with TBI [148,149]. However, more recent reports further our understanding of gnotobiosis and BMT. Preclinical models demonstrate that administration of an LPS antagonist reduces TNF levels and intestinal GVHD histopathology after HCT [22]. Updated analyses of two previously reported randomized clinical trials of antimicrobial prophylaxis show significant lessening of enteric GVHD after administration of either antifungal prophylaxis with fluconazole compared with placebo [150], or anerobic intestinal decontamination with metronidazole plus ciprofloxacin, compared with ciprofloxacin alone [20]. Newer approaches aimed at preservation of enteric epithelial integrity are currently under study. Keratinocyte growth factor has a specificity for gut epithelial cells and can prevent epithelal injury from chemoradiotherapy, reduce levels of LPS and TNF and decrease enteric GVHD in animal models [151]. Administration of recombinant human IL-11 protects gastrointestinal

Table 50.3 Revised Seattle criteria for grading acute graft-vs.-host disease (GVHD). (Based upon [116], adapted from [143].)

Grade	Criteria*
0	No convincing evidence of GVHD at any time *before day 100*; all abnormalities in skin, liver and gut fully accountable by processes other than GVHD; no immunosuppressive treatment *for acute GVHD* given except for the originally planned prophylaxis
II	Rash characteristic of *acute* GVHD in clinical presentation and time of onset (with or without visceral GVHD) or biopsy *or autopsy-proven visceral GVHD without rash*; improvement without need for treatment or progressive improvement *in at least one organ without deterioration in others* within 2–3 weeks after starting treatment *for acute GVHD*; no need for secondary treatment *during an appropriately paced taper of primary systemic treatment*
III	Clinical presentation as described for grade II but without progressive improvement *in any organ* after starting treatment, or requiring multiple cycles of treatment or extended hospitalization *before day 100 because of failure* to achieve control *after an adequate trial of initial systemic treatment, or requiring reversal during taper of primary systemic treatment because of recurrent manifestations before day 100*, but without GVHD as a clinically significant contributing cause of death
IV	Clinical presentation as described for grade II but with GVHD *or GVHD-related complication* as a clinically significant contributing cause of death

*Expanded criteria are given in italics.

Table 50.4 International Bone Marrow Transplant Registry (IBMTR) Severity Index for acute GVHD. (Adapted from [144]).

Index*	Skin involvement		Liver involvement		Gastrointestinal involvement	
	Stage (max)	Extent of rash	Stage (max)	Total bilirubin (nmol/L)	Stage (max)	Volume of diarrhea (mL/day)
A	1	<25%	0	<34	0	<500
B	2	25–50% or	1–2	34–102 or	1–2	550–1500
C	3	>50% or	3	103–255 or	3	>1500
D	4	Bullae or	4	>255 or	4	Severe pain and ileus

*Assign Index based on maximum involvement in an individual organ.

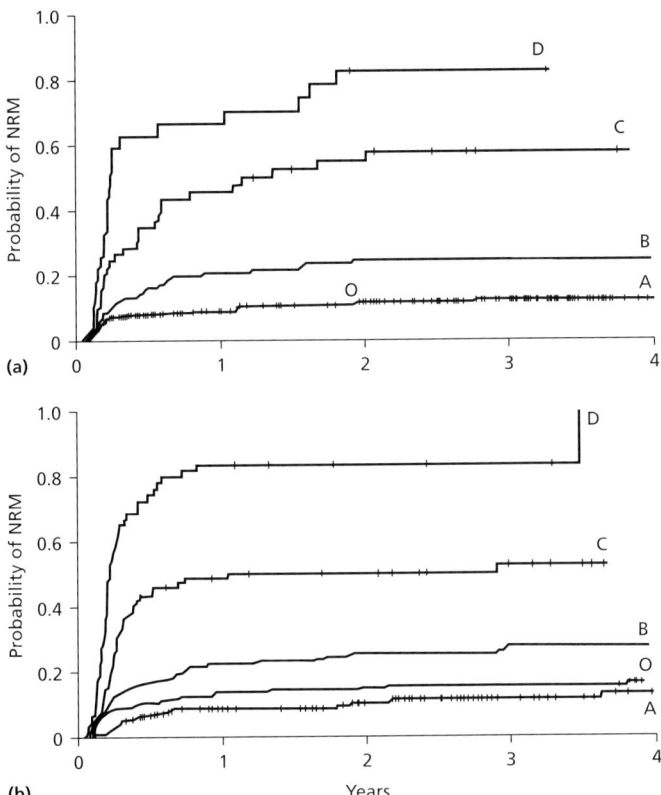

Fig. 50.4 Probability of nonrelapse mortality (NRM) for patients with early leukemia: (a) aged 16–30 years; or (b) >30 years by the International Bone Marrow Transplant Registry (IBMTR) Severity Index (see Table 50.4 for individual index criteria). (Adapted from [144].)

cells from cytotoxic damage with resulting reduction in the frequency and load of bacteremia in leukemia patients given conventional chemotherapy [152]. Trials of these approaches in HCT recipients are eagerly awaited.

Single-agent immunosuppression

On the basis of animal studies outlined in Chapter 1, post-transplant immunosuppression to prevent GVHD was incorporated into initial clinical practice [8,153]. Procarbazine, CY and MTX were found to be effective prophylaxis in murine and canine models [154,155]. Standard MTX prophylaxis was given at a dose of 15 mg/m^2 on day 1 and 10 mg/m^2 on days 3, 6, 11 and weekly thereafter to day 102. One study reported no apparent differences in the incidence or severity of acute GVHD in young patients who did or did not receive MTX [156]. However, in a subsequent report of young patients not given immunosuppression following unmodified HLA-identical BMT, hyperacute GVHD developed in all 15 patients who engrafted [118]. In comparison, age-matched historical control subjects who received standard (102 day) MTX had a 25% incidence of grade II–IV acute GVHD ($p < 0.0001$). Attempts have been made to shorten the duration of immunoprophylaxis. A prospective randomized trial comparing standard 102-day MTX prophylaxis with an abbreviated course of MTX found a significant increase in the incidence of grade II–IV acute GVHD when immunosuppression was discontinued at day 11 (25% vs. 59%; $p < 0.002$) [81].

Initial pilot studies demonstrated effective prevention of GVHD with CSP prophylaxis. Cyclosporine was given intravenously at a dosage of 1.5 mg/kg every 12 h starting the day before BMT and was continued until oral dosing (6.25 mg/kg every 12 h) was tolerated [157]. Starting at day 50, oral CSP was tapered 5% each week and discontinued on day 180. While subsequent studies have not shown direct correlation of blood levels of CSP metabolites with clinical outcome, CSP doses are commonly adjusted to maintain steady state trough concentrations within therapeutic ranges [158]. Chapter 16 details the toxicities of CSP, interactions with other drugs that can increase or decrease CSP levels and adjustments of CSP and MTX dosing for impaired renal and hepatic function. Controlled trials comparing standard MTX with a 6-month course of CSP monotherapy showed no significant difference in the rates of acute and chronic GVHD, leukemic relapse, interstitial pneumonia or event-free survival [157,159].

More recently, monotherapy with tacrolimus (FK-506) has been administered to prevent GVHD. Initial studies were aimed at determining dose schedules, pharmacokinetics and toxicity profiles [160,161]. The therapeutic window of this drug appears narrow: blood levels >20 ng/mL doubled renal toxicity without further modifying GVHD [162]. Tacrolimus is administered as a continuous intravenous (IV) infusion at 0.03–0.04 mg/kg/day and is switched to oral dosing (0.15 mg/kg/day given in two divided oral doses with monitoring of trough levels) when oral intake recovers. Administered as single-agent prophylaxis in a randomized trial of 136 Japanese patients, acute GVHD was significantly reduced in tacrolimus recipients compared with CSP recipients in both matched (13% vs. 41%) and mismatched (21% vs. 54%) BMT [163]. However, neither chronic GVHD nor survival differed between the two prophylaxis groups.

Combination immunosuppression

As outlined in Chapter 16, the mechanisms of action of immunosuppressive drugs differ widely and provide a rationale for effective use in combination (Table 50.5, [164–77]). A randomized trial from the Minnesota group compared standard MTX with a combination of MTX, ATG and prednisone (PSE; 40 mg/m^2 on days 8–20) and found that acute GVHD developed in 48% and 21% of patients, respectively [164]. Overall survival and chronic GVHD did not differ. The City of Hope team combined standard MTX with PSE (0.5–1.0 mg/kg/day) starting at day 15 and tapering throughout the first year. In a follow-up randomized study, these investigators compared MTX/PSE with CSP/PSE [168]. The incidence of acute GVHD in the two groups was 47% and 28%, respectively ($p = 0.05$). Others have compared steroids combined with CSP or CY [169].

A combined regimen of MTX, given on days 1, 3, 6 and 11, and a 180-day course of CSP given twice a day was compared to either drug used alone and was shown to reduce GVHD and improve survival [165–167]. Attempts to further enhance the efficacy of MTX/CSP prophylaxis have been reported. The addition of PSE given from day 0 through day 21 at 1 mg/kg/day and reduced from day 22 to day 35 to 0.5 mg/kg/day was not of benefit [170]. In another randomized trial, PSE given from day 7 to day 180, combined with MTX on days 1, 3 and 6, and CSP given to day 180 resulted in a 9% incidence of acute GVHD, compared with a 23% incidence in patients randomized to CSP/PSE [171]. In another trial comparing methylprednisolone (MP; given from days 7 to 72 post-transplant) combined with CSP compared with CSP alone, acute GVHD was less frequent but chronic GVHD was more common in the steroid recipients [172]. This unexpected finding that MP was not effective in preventing chronic GVHD and promoting tolerance was similar to that found in another controlled study [170].

Two controlled trials have compared MTX/CSP with MTX/CSP/PSE. In one there was a significant reduction in acute GVHD with the triple regimen [175], but in neither was there a significant difference in chronic GVHD or overall survival [174,175]. In one of the few randomized studies showing a survival advantage, MTX/CSP was associated with improved survival compared to CSP alone in patients with aplastic anemia [176]. In another study, survival was better in the group given MTX/CSP compared to MTX/tacrolimus, despite the latter group's lower rate of acute

Table 50.5 Randomized trials of combination immunosuppression for prevention of acute GVHD.

Investigator (year, reference)	Disease groups	Patients (n)	Regimens compared	Median age (year)	Acute GVHD (%)	Chronic GVHD (%)	Overall survival (%)
HLA-identical sibling donors							
Ramsay et al. (1982 [164])	Nonmalignant and malignant diseases	32	MTX + ATG + PSE vs.	16	21 ($p = 0.01$)	6 (n.s.)	52 (n.s.)
		35	MTX	16	48	9	44
Storb et al. (1989 [165])	Severe aplastic anemia	22	MTX + CSP vs.	23	18 ($p = 0.01$)	58 (n.s.)	73 (n.s.)
		24	MTX	23	53	36	58
Storb et al. (1986, 1989 [166,167])	AML in CR1 and CML in CP	43	MTX + CSP vs.	30	33 ($p = 0.01$)	26 (n.s.)	65 (n.s.)
		50	CSP	30	54	24	54
Forman et al. (1987 [168])	Acute leukemia and CML	53	MTX + PSE vs.	26	47 ($p = 0.05$)	?	53 (n.s.)
		54	CSP + PSE	26	28	?	57
Santos et al. (1987 [169])	Nonmalignant and malignant diseases	42	CSP + MP vs.	23	32 ($p = 0.05$)	40 (n.s.)	38 ($p = 0.03$)
		40	CY + MP	24	68	18	20
Sullivan et al. (1989 [81])	Advance-stage malignant diseases	25	Long MTX + BC vs.	19	82 ($p = 0.016$)	44 (n.s.)	24 (n.s.)
		40	Short MTX vs.	18	59 ($p = 0.0016$)	51 (n.s.)	30 (n.s.)
		44	Long MTX	19	25	33	41
Storb et al. (1990 [170])	Nonmalignant and malignant diseases	59	MTX + CSP + PSE vs.	32	46 ($p = 0.02$)	62 ($p = 0.01$)	52 (n.s.)
		63	MTX + CP	28	25	40	46
Chao et al. (1993 [171])	Malignant diseases	74	CSP + PSE vs.	32	23 ($p = 0.02$)	60 (n.s.)	59 (n.s.)
		75	MTX + CSP + PSE	28	9	57	46
Deeg et al. (1997 [172])	Hematologic malignant diseases	60	CSP vs.	36	73 ($p = 0.01$)	21 (n.s.)	26 (n.s.)
		62	CSP + MP	39	60	44	23
Ratanatharathorn et al. (1998 [173])	Hematologic malignant diseases	164	MTX + CSP vs.	40	44 ($p = 0.01$)	49 (n.s.)	57 ($p = 0.02$)
		165	MTX + TACR	40	32	56	47
Chao et al. (2000 [174])	Hematologic malignant diseases	96	MTX + CSP vs.	34	20 (n.s.)	52 (n.s.)	51 (n.s.)
		90	MTX + CSP + PSE	34	18	46	60
Ruutu et al. (2000 [175])	Hematologic malignant diseases Severe aplastic anemia	55	MTX + CSP vs.	41	56 ($p = 0.001$)	48 ($p = 0.06$)	72 (n.s.)
		53	MTX + CSP + PSE	42	19	36	65
Locatelli et al. (2000 [176])	Severe aplastic anemia	37	MTX + CSP vs.	20	30 (n.s.)	44 (n.s.)	94 ($p = 0.05$)
		34	CSP	18	38	30	78
HLA-nonidentical donors							
Nash et al. (2000 [177])	Nonmalignant and malignant diseases	90	MTX + CSP vs.	35	74 ($p = 0.001$)	70 (n.s.)	50 (n.s.)
		90	MTX + TACR	34	56	76	54

AML, acute myeloid leukemia; ATG, antithymocyte globulin; BC, donor buffy coat cells; CML, chronic myeloid leukemia; CP, chronic phase; CR, complete remission; CSP, cyclosporine; CY, cyclophosphamide; GVHD, graft-vs.-host disease; MP, methylprednisolone; MTX, methotrexate; n.s., not significant; PSE, prednisone, TACR, tacrolimus.

GVHD [173]. When studied in relation to International Bone Marrow Transplantation (IBMTR) control cohorts, these results were shown to be a result of imbalance in the underlying risk factor for death within two prophylaxis groups [178].

In over a dozen randomized controlled trials of combination immunosuppression to prevent acute GVHD in HLA-identical sibling HCT, no regimen to date has been found to be superior to the widely used MTX/CSP regimen developed by the Seattle team. As new combinations and approaches become available, this regimen should be designated the standard control arm. Using such a design, MTX/tacrolimus was recently studied in recipients of unrelated donor BMT [177]. While the tacrolimus-based regimen led to significantly lower rates of acute GVHD in this multicenter trial, chronic GVHD and survival did not differ. Investigations of novel regimens remain of key importance in preventing GVHD, especially in HLA mismatched and unrelated donor transplants.

Many of these regimens have side-effects that limit full dosing. Hepatic and renal toxicity are well-recognized side-effects of CSP and tacrolimus, whereas infection or microangiopathy may be more difficult to ascribe to treatment [179,180]. Several pilot studies have adopted regimen revisions with reduced drug dose or regimen [181,182]. Modifications could attenuate the effectiveness of immunosuppressive prophylaxis. A retrospective analysis found that a reduction of MTX to <80% of the scheduled dose was an independent risk factor for the development of grade II–IV acute GVHD [64]. Moreover, even if centers report the same regimen of GVHD prophylaxis, there appears to be wide variations in their standard practice. A survey of European BMT centers found significant variations in CSP infusion practices, target blood levels and duration of prophylaxis [183]. Moreover, nearly one-half of the 87 responding centers reported that folinic acid rescue was given after MTX administration. Such variations in clinical practice contribute to the potential heterogeneity of outcome assessments and registry reports.

Antibody prophylaxis

Two prospective studies assigned patients receiving standard MTX to receive or not receive additional ATG prophylaxis [184,185]. Neither study showed a change in the incidence or severity of GVHD. In a recent trial, 109 patients undergoing BMT from unrelated donors participated in two consecutive trials of rabbit ATG (at two dose levels) compared with no ATG in the pretransplant conditioning regimen [186]. Grade III–IV acute GVHD was less frequent in the second trial employing 15 mg/kg ATG, but lethal infections were also more common. In an uncontrolled trial, Campath-1H (a humanized antibody against the CD52 antigen) was added to the conditioning regimen and resulted in a low rate of acute GVHD and a low (11%) rate of NRM following nonmyeloablative HCT [187].

Monoclonal antibodies (MAB) against the IL-2 receptor were infused to deplete activated T cells and prevent acute GVHD [188,189]. Some benefit was seen during antibody administration but this effect was not sustained. Murine models showed a reduction of GVHD mortality after antibody inhibition of IL-1 and TNF [17,190]. However, human trials failed to show a reduction in the incidence of acute GVHD with anticytokine prophylaxis [191,192]. Similarly, an anti-CD5-immunotoxin conjugate did not appear to be of benefit in preventing GVHD [193,194]. Polyvalent intravenous immunoglobulin (IVIg) has been beneficial in several autoimmune disorders with immunopathologic features [195]. Initial studies of IVIg use in BMT focused on infection prophylaxis [196], but subsequent studies found that IVIg reduced the frequency of acute GVHD [197]. This benefit was most apparent in patients ≥20 years and was associated with a reduction in related donor BMT mortality [198]. Meta-analysis of published controlled trials confirmed a reduction in transplant-related complications [199]. However, more recent trials with lower doses of IVIg did not show benefit in reducing acute GVHD [200,201].

Marrow T-cell depletion

Several techniques have been developed for *in vitro* treatment of donor marrow to remove T cells and prevent GVHD (see Chapter 17) [202–208]. Almost all studies show a significant reduction in the incidence and severity of acute GVHD, but most results to date have been offset by an increase in the rate of graft failure, prolonged immunodeficiency and recurrent leukemia [83,209,210]. It may be that newer approaches at depleting only antihost alloreactive T cells may obviate problems with prolonged immune recovery [211].

Other approaches

A trial attracting considerable interest reported a nontoxic and inexpensive agent that was originally studied to prevent hepatic complications after allogeneic HCT [212]. Ursodeoxycholic acid (UDCA) is a hydrophilic bile acid that when administered by mouth reduces the concentration of hydrophobic (hepatotoxic) bile acids. It also reduces release of proinflammatory cytokines, reduces rates of heptic VOD after HCT and decreases expression of class I antigens on hepatocytes in cholestatic liver diseases [213]. In a study of the Nordic BMT Group, related and unrelated HCT recipients were randomized to receive ($n = 123$) or not receive ($n = 119$) 12 mg/kg/day UDCA orally, starting before conditioning and continuing to day 90 post-transplant. Severe hyperbilirubinemia was lessened in the UDCA group, as was the incidence of grade III–IV acute GVHD (five of 123 vs. 17 of 119; $p = 0.01$) and NRM (19% vs. 34%; $p = 0.01$). Importantly, survival was improved (71% vs. 55%; $p = 0.02$) and CSP blood levels were similar in the two groups, making altered pharmacokinetics an unlikely explanation of results [212]. Given the few side-effects (5% had diarrhea), this approach is an attractive adjunct to GVHD prophylaxis.

New immunosuppressive agents are being placed into clinical trials as single agents or in combinations to prevent GVHD. Trimetrexate, fludarabine, rapamycin (sirolimus) and UV irradiation are of interest [214–219]. Mycophenolate mofetil (MMF) is an inhibitor of *de novo* purine synthesis during cell division. Unlike other cells, activated lymphocytes depend primarily on the *de novo* rather than the salvage pathway; hence, MMF selectively impairs lymphocyte proliferation. Unfortunately, the number, size and follow-up of clinical trials of this novel agent in HCT are still too limited to draw firm conclusions [220,221]. Agents to prevent T-cell activation or proliferation, to prevent expansion of alloreactive T cells or to promote donor-specific anergy via blockage of B7 family costimulation are moving toward clinical trials [222–227]. Chapter 16 describes the mechanisms of actions, toxicities and preliminary clinical experience with these and other new agents.

Treatment

Primary therapy

Glucocorticoids have been the most effective initial treatment of established acute GVHD [8,154,155,228,229]. The mechanism of action of MP is thought a result of lympholysis and suppression of proinflammatory cytokines. Although clinical responses have been observed at dosages of MP varying from 1 to 60 mg/kg/day, fatal infections have been observed with ultra high-dose regimens, and most clinicians employ a tapering schedule starting with 2 mg/kg/day MP given in divided doses [229–233]. In a prospective trial comparing MP at 2 mg/kg/day vs. 10 mg/kg/day, response rates and progression to grade III–IV disease were similar in the two groups as were rates of NRM and overall survival [234]. Importantly, patients could be identified at day 5 of treatment with the 2 mg/kg MP regimen who required prompt alternate therapy to

Table 50.6 Randomized trials of primary treatment of acute GVHD.

Investigator (year, reference)	Patients (n)	Regimens compared	Median age (year)	Response (flare) (%)	Chronic GVHD (%)	Overall survival (%)
Doney et al. (1981 [236])	20	MP	24	65	56 (n.s.)	40 (n.s.)
	17	vs. ATG	24	35	45	24
Kennedy et al. (1985 [237])	39	MP	27	41 ($p = 0.039$)	?	28 (n.s.)
	38	vs. CSP	26	61	?	24
Deeg et al. (1985 [238])	27	ATG + CSP*	25	48	89	67
	18	vs. ATG + CSP + MP*	20	33	83	25
Hings et al. (1993 [235])	16	MP long taper	33	(13) (n.s.)	67 (n.s.)	81 (n.s.)
	14	vs. MP short taper	29	(29)	57	66
Cahn et al. (1995 [239])	34	MP + CSP + placebo	29	63 (n.s.)	?	59 (n.s.)
	35	vs. MP + CSP + CD25mAb	25	70	?	66
Martin et al. (1996 [240])	114	MP + placebo	30	25 ($p = 0.019$)	72 (n.s.)	(45) (n.s.)
	129	vs. MP + CD5-IT	29	40	65	49
Van Lint et al. (1996 [234])	47	MP 2 mg/kg	26	68 (n.s.)	35 (n.s.)	63 (n.s.)
	48	vs. MP 10 mg/kg	28	71	38	62
McDonald et al. (1998 [241]) (Enteric GVHD)	29	MP + placebo	39	41 ($p = 0.02$)	45 (n.s.)	?
	31	vs. MP + Beclo	34	71	35	?
Cragg et al. (2000 [242])	46	MP	28	55 ($p = 0.02$)	50 (n.s.)	50 (n.s.)
	50	vs. MP + ATG	23	27	64	40

ATG, antithymocyte globulin; Beclo, beclomethasone; CSP, cyclosporine; GVHD, graft-vs.-host disease; IT, immunotoxin; MAB, monoclonal antibody; MP, methylprednisolone; n.s., not significant; PSE, prednisone.
*Alternating concurrent pilot trials.

control GVHD. Plates 50.20 and 50.21 (facing p. 296) illustrate the clinical response to MP treatment. Treatment is mandated for grade II–IV acute GVHD and consists of continuing the original immunosuppressive prophylaxis (CSP or tacrolimus) and adding MP [183]. Most centers employ a steroid taper schedule based on patient response rather than a fixed dose regimen. In a prospective trial, the Minneapolis team randomized patients with acute GVHD who were responding by day 14 of corticosteroid treatment to a fast taper of PSE (2275 mg/m^2) over 86 days ($n = 14$) or a slow taper (6300 mg/m^2) over 147 days ($n = 16$) [235]. The median time to acute GVHD resolution was 42 days (range 12–74 days) in the short treatment group, compared with 30 days (range 6–30 days) for the long taper schedule ($p = 0.01$). The groups did not significantly differ in the number of patients with flare of acute GVHD, chronic GVHD, median dose of PSE administered, infection or death. Although the size of the trial was small, the authors concluded that in patients who responded to initial therapy, short-term treatment to a cumulative PSE dosage of 2000 mg/m^2 appeared effective and might be expected to minimize steroid-related complications.

Although initial pilot studies demonstrated benefit of ATG in controlling human acute GVHD, subsequent randomized comparisons of intravenous ATG (15 mg/kg every other day for 6 doses) and MP (2 mg/kg/day) showed no difference in efficacy or survival between the two treatments [236]. As shown in Table 50.6 [234–42], a number of controlled trials have tested other agents combined with standard MP as primary treatment of acute GVHD. The addition of ATG has not shown overall benefit [242]. Of note, MP and MP/CSP have not been compared in randomized trials. Administration of enteric beclomethasone capsules appears of benefit in patients with intestinal GVHD receiving systemic MP [241]. While initial reports of therapy with CSP appeared encouraging [243], subsequent randomized trials found a similar 25% survival in patients treated with either intravenous CSP (3–5 mg/kg/day) or standard MP [237]. Sequential administration of ATG/CSP (with or without MP) was evaluated as primary treatment of acute GVHD: long-term survival was 49% in the ATG/CSP group but only 11% in the triple-therapy group [238].

In the past decade, several pilot studies have reported potentially useful new agents for treatment of acute GVHD. MMF exerts a cytostatic effect on activated lymphocytes and has demonstrated efficacy in preventing solid organ allograft rejection [244,245]. Initial clinical studies for treatment of acute GVHD appear encouraging [221,246]. Satisfactory response rates were also observed with anti-IL-2 receptor, or an anti-CD5-specific immunotoxin [247–250]. A controlled study of anti-IL-2 receptor antibody in 69 patients treated in 13 centers showed no overall benefit in survival or response in patients who received the antibody and CSP/MP compared with CSP/MP alone [239]. In another phase 3 trial, MP and placebo ($n = 114$) were found to yield similar overall outcome as MP and Xoma-Zyme® (a pan T-cell ricin-A-chain immunotoxin; $n = 129$) [240]. Manifestations of acute GVHD responded more quickly to the immunoconjugate, but benefits were not durable.

The critical importance of response of acute GVHD to primary therapy was analyzed in 740 patients [251]. Treatment failure (defined as initiation of secondary treatment or NRM) was increased with ATG therapy compared with either CSP or MP. Patients given MTX and CSP prophylaxis were less likely to experience treatment failure than those who were given other prophylaxis regimens. Consequently, MP is the best initial therapy for individuals given MTX and CSP prophylaxis. However, considerable room for improvement is apparent because of the 70–80% NRM observed in the one-half of patients in whom initial treatment failed [251,252].

Secondary therapy

Patients in whom initial therapy fails (commonly defined as progression after 3 days, no change after 7 days or incomplete response after 14 days of MP treatment) have been given a variety of salvage regimens. To date, there is no clear standard for salvage treatment. Administration of ATG at the first sign of MP failure has been reported to lead to a durable 20% complete response rate and 32% overall survival [253]. Other groups, however, have noted much poorer outcome with salvage ATG, reporting only 5% long-term survival [254]. Treatment with OKT3 MAB has shown some benefit [255] but is counterbalanced by toxicity and TNF release [256]. Secondary therapy with a mitogenic anti-CD3 antibody was complicated by a 24% incidence of Epstein–Barr virus-associated lymphoproliferative syndrome [257–259]. A nonmitogenic anti-CD3 antibody appears to modulate T-cell function safely and to lessen GVHD [260]. Pilot studies of anti-CD3/anti-CD7 immunotoxins and humanized anti-CD3 MAB have recently been reported [261,262].

In an attempt to target activated T cells, antibody therapy specific for the IL-2 receptor has been analyzed [263]. In individuals with steroid-resistant acute GVHD, 65% had a complete response and 19% a partial response to secondary treatment [249]. However, another study demonstrated that only one of 10 patients achieved a complete response [248]. A humanized anti-Tac antibody to the IL-2 receptor has been developed [264], but clinical trials in BMT patients with acute GVHD refractory to corticosteroids showed only a 40% response rate to salvage treatment [265]. This result was similar to response rates of ATG, CSP or multiple pulses of MP given for salvage treatment [266]. More recent trials with daclizumab (a humanized anti-IL-2 receptor antibody) have been more encouraging [267,268]. Daclizumab is a competitive inhibitor of IL-2 on activated lymphocytes. Another novel approach to secondary treatment employed ABX-CBL, an anti-CD147 MAB. This antibody targets activated but not resting lymphocytes for a more specific lympholysis [269]. Of 27 patients with refractory acute GVHD, 51% responded and 44% survived 6 months. Therapies to downregulate IL-1 yielded response rates of 57–63% in pilot trials [270,271]. Salvage therapy with an antibody directed against activated T and B lymphocytes and NK cells produces better results, with response seen in nine of 10 patients with steroid-resistant acute GVHD [272]. Other MABs have also been targeted against the efferent arm of GVHD. A murine IgG1 antibody specific for TNF-α was evaluated in 19 patients with acute GVHD refractory to MP and anti-IL-2 receptor treatment [273]. Five patients had no improvement, and 14 had a partial response to anti-TNF therapy. However, all responders had a return of GVHD after discontinuing treatment.

The results of secondary treatment of GVHD with tacrolimus and sirolimus were recently published. When combined with ATG, 14 of 20 patients had a response to tacrolimus salvage therapy with a median survival of 86 days [274]. In a study of conversion of CSP to tacrolimus, several important observations were made: (a) only rarely did patients resistant to GVHD treatment with CSP respond to tacrolimus; (b) CSP-associated hemolytic uremic syndrome did not improve with conversion; and (c) eight of 11 patients with CSP-associated neurotoxicity improved with conversion to tacrolimus [275]. Secondary treatment with sirolimus showed that 12 of 21 patients responded and seven survived [276]. However, hematologic toxicity was observed and dose optimization studies are still required.

An alternative approach employs use of UV irradiation to control refractory cutaneous GVHD [219]. Psoralan and ultraviolet A irradiation (PUVA) appears of benefit for cutaneous lesions of GVHD [277–279] (see Plates 23.22 & 23.23, *facing p. 296*). High response rates have been reported, although many patients go on to develop chronic GVHD [280,281]. Considerable recent interest has focused on extracorporeal photopheresis (ECP) in management of refractory acute GVHD [282,283]. In this approach, white cells of the patient are exposed *ex vivo* to 8-methoxypsoralen and UVA irradiation. Between 60 and 83% of patients manifest response in cutaneous GVHD, 67% in hepatic but none in enteric GVHD. Mechanisms of action include apoptosis and phagocytosis of ECP-treated lymphocytes [284]. In patients with chronic GVHD, ECP modulates NK and antigen-presenting cells and allo-targeted effector T cells [285,286]. Ongoing studies examine the value of ECP as adjunctive therapy of GVHD.

Response and outcome of secondary therapy of acute GVHD have been described in 427 patients [251]. Highest rates of response were observed in patients in whom GVHD recurred during a steroid taper and for whom the dose of PSE was subsequently increased. Overall, less than half the patients had sustained improvement. Administration of additional agents most often included addition of ATG or MABs [183].

Supportive care

Gut rest, hyperalimentation, pain control and antibiotic prophylaxis are routine elements of supportive care of patients with GVHD [287]. Oral beclometasone appears to be free of systemic or local toxicity and improves oral intake, nausea and diarrhea [241,288]. Octreotide (a somatostatin analog) controls secretory diarrhea in many patients with enteric GVHD [289,290]. Antiviral prophylaxis may be especially important in preventing interstitial pneumonia in patients with refractory GVHD [291]. Similarly, new antifungal agents, such as the triazols and echinocandins, may be useful in preventing and treating mycotic infections [292]. Not unexpectedly, development of GVHD substantially contributes to the morbidity and cost of HCT [293].

Prognosis

Clinical severity

Outcome is predicted by the overall grade of acute GVHD [116]. Response to treatment is another key determinant as shown in Fig. 50.5, [294]; mortality in patients with grade II–IV acute GVHD is lowest in those who achieve a complete response to initial treatment [251]. Consistently across studies, dermal disease responds promptly but lower gastro-intestinal involvement responds poorly to therapy [295].

Prognostic factors

Factors associated with impaired survival include HLA-nonidentical marrow donors, liver abnormalities in addition to GVHD, and early time to onset and treatment of GVHD. Similar times to treatment failure and similar determinants of outcome were observed in patients who received

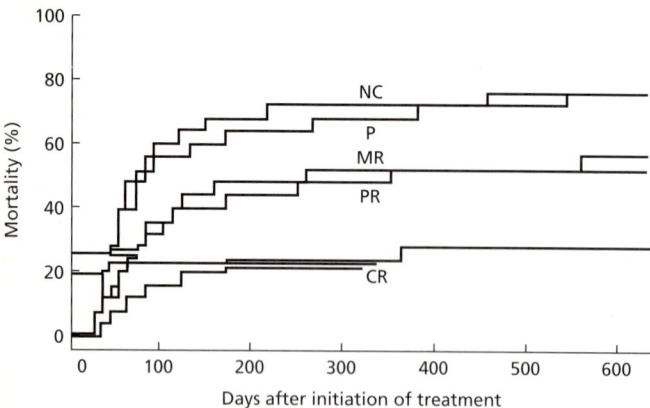

Fig. 50.5 Non-relapse mortality of patients displayed by outcome to primary treatment of acute GVHD. CR, complete response; MR, mixed response; NC, no change; P, progression; PR, partial response. (Adapted from [251].)

primary and secondary therapy [251,266]. Taken together, these findings support the validity of testing new modalities in patients with inadequate response to primary treatment of GVHD.

Chronic graft-vs.-host disease

Pathogenesis

Alloreactivity contributes to the pathogenesis of chronic GVHD, and some investigators consider chronic GVHD to be a later phase of acute GVHD caused by minor antigen recognition. Others believe it incorporates features of an autoimmune-like process. In both experimental and clinical studies of chronic GVHD, thymic atrophy (see Plate 23.61, facing p. 296), lymphocyte depletion and loss of thymic epithelial secretory function are noted [296–299]. Absence of thymic function either by age or injury may contribute to immune dysregulation, similar to the pathogenesis of autologous GVHD [26]. This hypothesis is supported by experiments in which T cells from animals with chronic GVHD specifically react to host class II determinants [300]. Similarities of clinical features of chronic GVHD and several autoimmune diseases have been commonly observed. Autoantibody formation has been noted in experimental models of chronic GVHD [301,302] and clinical studies also report these findings [303–305]. Occurrence of antinuclear, anti-double-stranded DNA and antismooth muscle autoantibodies ranges in frequency from 11% to 62% of patients with chronic GVHD, while anticytoskeletal and antinucleolar antibodies have also been detected [306,307]. Although specific nucleolar phosphoproteins have been identified as targets of GVHD [308], the pathogenetic role for antibodies in chronic GVHD is still poorly defined [309].

Incidence and predictive factors

Donor–host factors

Among patients who survived 150 days after allogeneic BMT, chronic GVHD was observed in 33% of HLA-identical sibling transplants, in 49% of HLA-nonidentical related transplants and in 64% of matched unrelated donor transplants [310]. Data from single institution and registry studies indicate that the incidence of chronic GVHD may be as high as 80% in one-antigen HLA-nonidentical unrelated transplants. Among more homogeneous ethnic populations sharing mHA, rates of chronic GVHD are lower [311]. In addition to HLA disparity, prior acute GVHD and increasing patient age are independent factors associated with an increased risk of developing chronic GVHD [61,312–317]. As shown in Fig. 50.6, for recipients of HLA-identical marrow who survived beyond day 150, the probability of developing chronic GVHD was 13% in children <10 years, 28% in adolescents 10–19 years old, and 42–46% in adults >20 years [310]. In contrast, there appeared to be little reduction in GVHD rates in young patients given HLA-nonidentical and unrelated marrow. However, among recipients of unrelated marrow, increasing donor age is associated with an increased incidence of chronic GVHD [67,84]. Chronic GVHD has been reported in one randomized trial of conditioning regimens to be more common in recipients of busulfan than TBI (59% vs. 47%; $p = 0.05$) [318]. This was not confirmed on a larger analysis of four studies [319]. Pretransplant IFN was reported to increase mortality from chronic GVHD in one study [320], but was subsequently reported to have no influence on the incidence or outcome of chronic GVHD [321]. Similarly, hormone replacement therapy did not appear to influence the development of chronic GVHD [322].

Source and dose of hematopoietic cells

Cord blood HCT is associated with low to absent rates of chronic GVHD [90]. Among allogeneic PBHCT recipients, higher $CD34^+$ cell doses ($>8.0 \times 10^5$/kg) were associated with significantly increased risk (RR 2.3) of clinical extensive chronic GVHD [323]. Initial reports suggested no increased incidence of chronic GVHD after allogeneic PBHCT

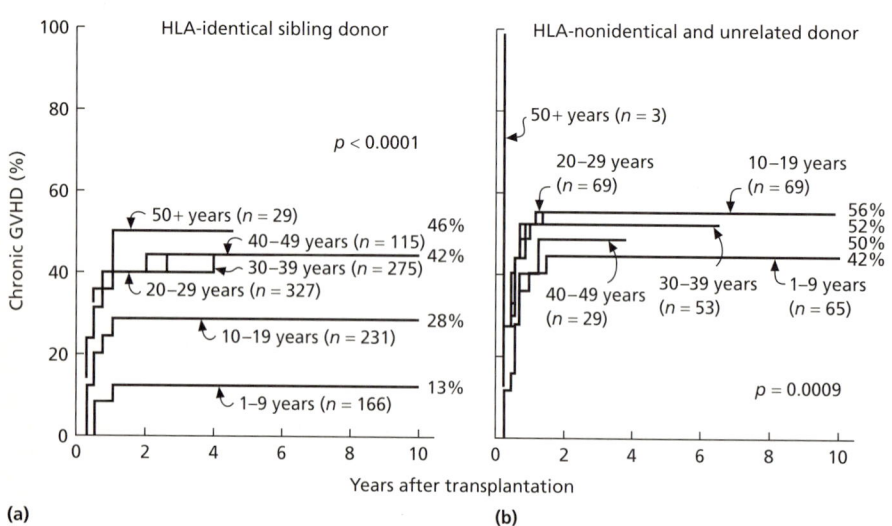

Fig. 50.6 Probability of developing clinical extensive chronic GVHD in patients with hematologic malignancies who survived at least 150 days after BMT from HLA-identical siblings (a) or HLA-nonidentical family members or unrelated donors (b). (Adapted from [310].)

[91,92], but subsequent studies revealed more frequent chronic GVHD following allogeneic PBHCT than with BMT [93,324–328]. Meta-analysis indicates the magnitude to be RR 1.66 ($p = 0.001$) of developing chronic GVHD with PBHCT [94]. Although some studies indicate a threshold dose of T-lymphocytes that is sufficient to dissociate GVHD and GVL during donor lymphocyte infusions (DLI) [329], a report of 140 patients in North America given donor cell infusions found that chronic GVHD developed in 60% and was highly predictive of leukemia remission [330]. Because of this high risk of GVHD with DLI, clinical protocols for suicide gene modification of donor lymphocytes have been proposed [331,332].

Immunomodulation

In contrast to the experience with acute GVHD, abbreviation or deletion of MTX prophylaxis did not appear to influence the development of chronic GVHD [333]. Random red cell transfusions given shortly before HCT have been associated with a decreased risk of chronic GVHD, whereas unirradiated donor buffy coat or second marrow reinfusions are linked to an increased risk for GVHD development [334,335]. In one publication, splenectomy appeared to increase the risk for development of chronic GVHD, possibly resulting from increased rates of infection in splenectomized patients [336], but another report could not confirm this finding [337]. The relationship between infection and subsequent chronic GVHD remains rather unclear. European investigators report that seropositivity for latent herpesvirus in the marrow donor or recipient may be an important predictor for the development of acute and chronic GVHD [101,338]. In other reports, no association of CMV infection with subsequent onset of chronic GVHD was observed [339].

Cytokine levels and gene polymorphisms

The development of chronic GVHD has been shown to be independently associated with older patient age (RR 2.5), prior acute GVHD (RR 9.7) and recipient IL-6 gene polymorphism (RR 4.2; $p = 0.02$) [107]. Expression of OX40 (a member of the TNF receptor family) on T cells was signficantly higher in patients who subsequently manifest chronic GVHD [340]. Levels increased shortly before the onset of clinical disease; moreover, higher levels were associated with poorer response to treatment.

Clinical features

Dermal

Two types of cutaneous involvement have been described [115,341]. An early phase resembles lichen planus. Lesions may be scanty or evanescent, ranging from polygonal papules to more typical lesions (see Plates 23.46 and 23.54, *facing p. 296*). Inspection with side-angle lighting more clearly defines these raised flat-topped lesions. During later phases, poikiloderma is observed (see Plates 23.48 and 23.49, *facing p. 296*). In patients with the localized type of histology, epidermal atrophy and dense focal dermal fibrosis are noted in the absence of significant inflammation. As shown in Plate 23.50, clinical features may resemble morphea. In other patients, a generalized type of histology is noted, with inflammation in eccrine coils and pilar units resulting in fibrosis throughout the dermis and the adnexal structures (see Plate 23.47, *facing p. 296*). Generalized scleroderma may lead to joint contractures and severe debility (see Plates 23.51 and 23.52, *facing p. 296*) [342,343].

The tempo of dermal abnormalities may show wide variation. In some patients erythema, hyperkeratosis and desquamation develop rapidly, sometimes after solar exposure. Erythema may begin in the malar area and resembles lupus erythematosus but soon spreads to sun-exposed and sun-shielded areas. In others the onset is insidious, with patchy hypo- and hyperpigmentation, reticular mottling, perifollicular papules and papulosquamous plaques. Total leukoderma has also been observed [344]. Guttate lesions appear on the trunk as shiny indurated areas or can be localized to areas of pressure-point trauma, prior irritation, injury, zoster or irradiation [345–347]. Rarely, vesicles, bullae or bullous pemphigoid lesions have been reported [348]. Alopecia and nail loss are not uncommon (see Plate 23.53, *facing p. 296*), and regrowth of body hair and return of sweat gland function usually herald disease improvement. Skin lesions are sometimes incorrectly attributed to reactions to drugs such as trimethoprim-sulfamethoxazole (TMP-SMX) and skin biopsies can be very useful in establishing the correct diagnosis. The differential diagnosis from dyskeratosis congenita may be difficult and should be considered in patients with aplastic anemia who are undergoing allogeneic HCT [349,350].

Hepatic

Liver function tests manifest predominantly cholestatic abnormalities. The degree of hyperbilirubinemia correlates less closely with clinical outcome than in patients with acute GVHD [343]. Although reported, development of portal hypertension, cirrhosis and death from hepatic failure are surprisingly rare despite years of hepatic abnormalities [351]. The differential diagnosis of late hepatic abnormalities is broad and includes viral infection, hepatotoxic drug reactions, gallstones and infiltrative hepatic abnormalities, including fungal infection and neoplastic disease. Liver biopsies are helpful in establishing a diagnosis. Naturally occurring primary biliary cirrhosis and chronic GVHD show similarities in bile duct damage as well as ocular and oral sicca syndrome [352].

Ocular

Ophthalmic symptoms of keratoconjunctivitis sicca include burning, irritation, photophobia and pain [353,354]. Tear function is evaluated by Schirmer's testing and fluorescein biomicroscopy of the cornea. Punctate keratopathy can range from minimal stippling to massive erosions. Even in the absence of symptoms, patients should be screened for ocular sicca and started on artificial tear replacement if indicated. Ligation of the lacrimal puncti may be of benefit to conserve corneal wetting in the severely dry eye. A more common cause of impaired vision acuity is the development of cataracts following BMT [355,356]. Analyses found that use of PSE after day 100 to treat chronic GVHD and use of TBI in conditioning promote cataract formation. Fortunately, cataract repair can be performed safely even in the presence of ocular sicca syndrome.

Oral

Oral dryness, sensitivity to acidic or spicy foods and increasing pain after day 100 strongly suggest the development of chronic GVHD [353,357,358]. In a prospective study of 60 long-term survivors after allogeneic BMT, oral atrophy, erythema and lichenoid lesions of the buccal and labial mucosa were significantly correlated with development of chronic GVHD [357]. A common clinical error is to confuse lichen planus-like lesions of chronic GVHD with oral candidiasis. Lichenoid reactions range from fine white reticular striae on buccal surfaces to large plaques on the buccal surface or the lateral tongue (see Plate 23.56, *facing p. 296*). Oral herpes simplex can exacerbate the pain associated with chronic GVHD and serial viral cultures may be required to establish the diagnosis and direct appropriate antiviral therapy.

Pulmonary

Several noninfectious pulmonary complications can be associated with chronic GVHD [359,360]. Bronchodilator-resistant obstructive lung disease can be a clinical feature of chronic GVHD [361,362] and histopathology reveals characteristic lesions of obliterative bronchiolitis (see Plate 23.60, *facing p. 296*). The frequency of this complication was increased in patients with chronic GVHD who received a 102-day course of MTX for GVHD prophylaxis as compared to chronic GVHD patients given CSP prophylaxis without long MTX [361]. In addition, patients with chronic GVHD and hypogammaglobulinemia or IgG subclass deficiencies appear to be at increased risk for late obstructive airway disease [363,364]. The 3-year mortality in patients with chronic GVHD was significantly increased in individuals developing obstructive lung disease compared with chronic GVHD patients who have normal pulmonary function [365]. In patients with obstructive airway disease otherwise refractory to systemic immunosuppression, lung transplants have been successfully conducted [366,367].

Gastrointestinal

Intestinal involvement is uncommon in chronic GVHD. Dysphagia, pain and insidious weight loss may be presenting symptoms of chronic GVHD of the esophagus [368]. Manometric studies demonstrate poor acid clearance, and motor abnormalities range from aperistalsis to high-amplitude contractions. Radiographic findings feature web formation, ring-like narrowings and tapering of structures in the mid and upper esophagus [369]. It was possible to distinguish esophageal involvement of chronic GVHD from that of naturally occurring progressive systemic sclerosis in a coded review of autopsy material [368]. Nerve fibers and silver stains of the myenteric plexus were of normal appearance in all patients with chronic GVHD, in contrast to findings in patients with scleroderma.

Neuromuscular

There is no compelling evidence for a central nervous system component of chronic GVHD [370]. Metabolic and infectious etiologies are common causes of post-transplant neurologic impairment, although one case report suggested cerebral involvement in a patient with chronic GVHD [371]. Results of sural nerve biopsy and response of neuropathy to immunosuppressive therapy demonstrate that the peripheral nervous system may be a target of chronic GVHD [372]. Myasthenia gravis has been reported in several patients with chronic GVHD [373,374]. Clinical and laboratory features mirror those of classic autoimmune myasthenia gravis, including the development of acetylcholine receptor antibodies; moreover, all patients responded to cholinesterase inhibitors and immunosuppressive drugs. Polymyositis has also been reported in a number of patients with chronic GVHD (see Plate 23.58, *facing p. 296*) [343,375,376]. Muscle strength commonly improves following corticosteroid treatment.

Other findings

Vaginitis and vaginal strictures have been noted in women with chronic GVHD [377]. In a study of women examined 1 year after allogeneic BMT, the gynecologic effects of chronic GVHD could be distinguished from those of primary ovarian failure as a result of TBI [378]. Recurrent sterile effusions have also been reported in patients with chronic GVHD [131,343]. Less easy to attribute to chronic GVHD were the effects on renal and marrow function in long-term survivors [379–381]. In one study, chronic GVHD was associated with poor growth of hematopoietic progenitor cells [382]. In other reports, autoimmune-like thrombocytopenia and anemia have been described [133,383,384]. Hypogammaglobulinemia and factor VIII deficiency have also been noted in patients developing GVHD [385,386]. The treatment of chronic GVHD with long-term corticosteroids in turn increases the risk of cataract formation, avascular necrosis and osteoporosis [356,387–390]. In children, weight loss and growth arrest (runting) are observed during active GVHD, and growth and development abnormalities improve when the disease resolves and corticosteroid therapy is withdrawn [391]. In adults, weight loss appears to be caused by increased resting energy expenditures, often resulting from increased actions of glucagon and norepinephrine [392].

Changing features

The protean manifestations of chronic GVHD have been likened to those of progressive systemic sclerosis, systemic lupus erythematosus, lichen planus, Sjögren syndrome, eosinophilic fasciitis, rheumatoid arthritis and primary biliary cirrhosis [303,343,352,393,394]. However, correlations are not exact, as evidenced by the rarity of characteristic esophageal or renal involvement, which is common to several autoimmune diseases [368,380,394]. The spectrum of abnormalities in chronic GVHD appears to be changing as a result of earlier diagnosis and institution of immunosuppressive therapy. Figure 50.7 presents a comparison of clinical features in patients in an initial cohort [343], compared with those transplanted later when earlier diagnosis and treatment were standard [395]. Ocular, esophageal, pulmonary and serosal involvement have occurred less commonly in recent years.

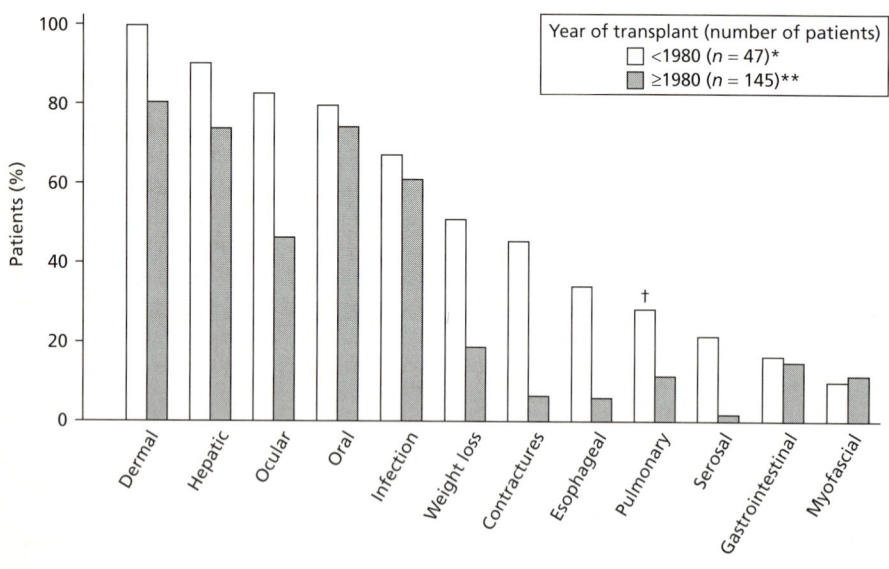

Fig. 50.7 Features of clinical extensive chronic GVHD in patients transplanted before 1980 (open columns) and since 1980 (shaded columns) in Seattle.

Blood **57**:267, 1981.
Blood* **72:546, 1988.
†*Ann Intern Med* **107**:648, 1987 (Methotrexate only).

Table 50.7 Seattle classification of chronic GVHD.

Limited chronic GVHD
Either or both
1 Localized skin involvement
2 Hepatic dysfunction as a result of chronic GVHD

Extensive chronic GVHD
Either
1 Generalized skin involvement
or
2 Localized skin involvement and/or hepatic dysfunction as a result of chronic GVHD
plus
3 (a) Liver histology showing chronic aggressive hepatitis, bridging necrosis, or cirrhosis; or
  (b) Involvement of eye (Schirmer test with <5 mm wetting); or
  (c) Involvement of minor salivary glands or oral mucosa demonstrated on labial biopsy; or
  (d) Involvement of any other target organ

Diagnosis and grading

Staging

Clinicians rely on histologic review of oral and skin biopsies to diagnose disease and gauge response to therapy [396]. Table 50.7 presents a summary of the clinicopathologic classification of chronic GVHD [394]. Patients with *limited* disease involving the skin or liver have a favorable course, even if untreated [343]. In contrast, patients with *extensive* disease involving multiple organs have an adverse natural course. This staging system is easily derived and highly reproducible when tested in an international survey [397].

Grading

Morbidity and mortality are highest in patients with *progressive* onset of chronic GVHD directly following acute GVHD, intermediate in those with a *quiescent* onset following resolution of acute GVHD and lowest in patients with a *de novo* onset [343]. Approximately 20% of patients with chronic GVHD have a *de novo* onset without prior acute GVHD. Because the classification in Table 50.7 does not capture prognostic outcome based on organ involvement or type of chronic GVHD onset, investigators have proposed additional classifications. The Baltimore group found that NRM after the diagnosis of chronic GVHD was independently associated with extensive skin involvement (>50% body surface area), thrombocytopenia and progressive-type of onset [398]. In another study, which was validated with IBMTR and NMDP datasets, Karnofsky performance score (KPS), weight loss, chronic diarrhea and skin or oral involvement were found to be key prognostic variables [399]. This classification system is presented in Table 50.8.

Diagnosis

The median time to diagnosis in HLA-identical sibling recipients is 201 days after transplant; in contrast, HLA-nonidentical related and unrelated donor marrow recipients have an earlier diagnosis and onset (159 and 133 days, respectively) [310]. Few patients develop chronic GVHD beyond day 500. Screening studies to detect early clinical chronic GVHD are routinely conducted on all allogeneic HCT recipients 100 days after transplantation [400]. Even in the absence of active signs or symptoms of chronic GVHD, a positive random skin biopsy or a history of prior acute GVHD independently predicts a threefold increase in the relative risk of subsequent chronic GVHD. Analysis of day 100 screening studies in patients who received MTX/CSP prophylaxis showed that corticosteroid-dependent acute GVHD (i.e. patients unable to taper successfully and discontinue PSE by day 100) was the most significant factor for development of subsequent chronic GVHD [401]. To establish an early diagnosis of chronic GVHD, real-time monitoring of patients leaving the transplant center is of critical importance for preventing late complications and disability. Long-term follow-up contact by telephone, fax and letter to patients and primary care physicians combined with regular on-site evaluations at the transplant center are of central importance [402]. Similarly, establishing an early and correct diagnosis is essential. In a referral cohort of 123 patients thought to have chronic GVHD, 7% had other disorders and 20% were found to have inactive chronic GVHD [403].

Prevention

Thymic factors

Based on the hypothesis that impaired thymic regulation of autoreactive T cells contributes to the immunopathogenesis of chronic GVHD, attempts have been made to prevent chronic GVHD by modification of thymic function. Transplantation of thymic tissue grafts or administration of thymic factors did not reduce the incidence or severity of chronic GVHD [404,405].

T-cell depletion

The risk of chronic GVHD was found to be reduced by >50% after T-cell depletion of HLA-identical marrow [83]. However, overall survival was not improved. Moreover, chronic GVHD was still noted in 85% of long-term survivors who received T-cell-depleted marrow from unrelated donors [204].

Antibody prophylaxis

Weekly administration of IVIg through day 90 post-transplant reduced the incidence and mortality of acute GVHD [198]. When the same dose of 500 mg/kg IVIg was given on a monthly schedule from day 90 to day 360 post-transplant, median serum IgG levels decreased from 1600 to 900 mg/dL, and the cumulative incidence of chronic GVHD was not different from that of patients randomized not to receive IVIg [406]. A controlled trial performed in 109 unrelated donor BMT recipients found

Table 50.8 International Bone Marrow Transplant Registry (IBMTR) severity scoring of chronic GVHD. (Adapted from [399].)

KPS at diagnosis	Mild (low risk)	Moderate (intermediate risk)	Severe (high risk)
≥80	No weight loss, no diarrhea	Either weight loss or diarrhea	Both weight loss and diarrhea
<80	No weight loss, no skin involvement (or) one or two of above with oral involvement	Diarrhea, weight loss and/or skin involvement (one or two of above)	Weight loss, diarrhea and skin involvement (or) one or two of above without oral involvement

KPS; Karnofsky performance score.

that individuals randomized to receive ATG in the preparative regimen had a significant reduction in grades III–IV acute GVHD [186]. This study also showed a reduction in chronic GVHD in those who received ATG conditioning compared with those not who did not (39% vs. 62%, respectively). However, overall survival and NRM did not improve. In contrast, an uncontrolled trial of 44 patients conditioned with a Campath-1H regimen reported only one case of chronic GVHD and a low 11% NRM following nonmyeloablative stem cell transplantation [187].

Immunosuppressive drugs

In a retrospective registry review of the effect of GVHD prophylaxis on transplant outcome in patients with aplastic anemia, 5-year survivals were shown to be improved in recipients of CSP or CSP/MTX prophylaxis ($n = 341$), compared with those given MTX alone ($n = 254$) [407]. In this nonrandomized study, patients who received a CSP-containing regimen had a decreased risk of developing chronic GVHD. However, prospective controlled trials did not confirm this observation. As shown in Table 50.5, several trials demonstrate a significant reduction of acute GVHD in CSP recipients but no alteration in the rate of chronic GVHD [166,168], a finding consistent with that of other publications of combination immunosuppression showing reduction in acute but not in chronic GVHD [81,164,171–173,177,408].

Prolonged immunosuppression

Several pilot studies suggest that the incidence of chronic GVHD may be reduced with an extended course of CSP prophylaxis [409–411]. These findings are further supported by the observation that chronic GVHD usually develops during or shortly after the routine 6-month taper of CSP. Additional insights were provided by a trial of 103 patients given CSP/MTX prophylaxis. Those who had no active acute GVHD at day 60 were randomized to stop CSP at day 60 ($n = 52$) or continue to day 180 ($n = 51$) post-transplant [412]. In the former group, the onset of chronic GVHD was significantly more rapid in onset, but not significantly greater in incidence than that of the day 180 control group. Among those with no prior acute GVHD, NRM was similar in the two groups; however, among those with prior acute GVHD, mortality was 38% in the day 60 cohort and 17% in the day 180 group. These findings suggest that for patients at high risk to develop chronic GVHD, extended prophylaxis or additional immunosuppressive agents may be required.

Prophylaxis that extended beyond day 180 was studied by the Stanford University and City of Hope teams [413]. Starting at day 80, patients received long-term prophylaxis with thalidomide (200 mg twice a day; $n = 28$) or placebo ($n = 26$) in a double blind randomized trial. At the interim analysis, the study was discontinued by the Data and Safety Monitoring Board when the thalidomide group was found to have increased rates of chronic GVHD and mortality. While thalidomide is effective in treating GVHD, the reason for this paradoxical effect on preventing chronic GVHD was unclear. In another controlled study to test whether prolonged administration was of value in preventing chronic GVHD, individuals without clinical manifestations of GVHD on day 80 post-transplant were randomized to receive 24 months (89 patients) or to complete 6 months (73 patients) of CSP prophylaxis [414]. Clinical extensive chronic GVHD developed in 39% and 51% of the patients, respectively (RR 0.76; $p = 0.25$). Moreover, there were no significant differences in NRM or survival. Thus, the need for an effective regimen to prevent chronic GVHD remains an unmet challenge to the field.

Treatment

Natural history

An initial report established the clinicopathologic criteria for diagnosis and grading [394]. Thirteen patients with clinical extensive chronic

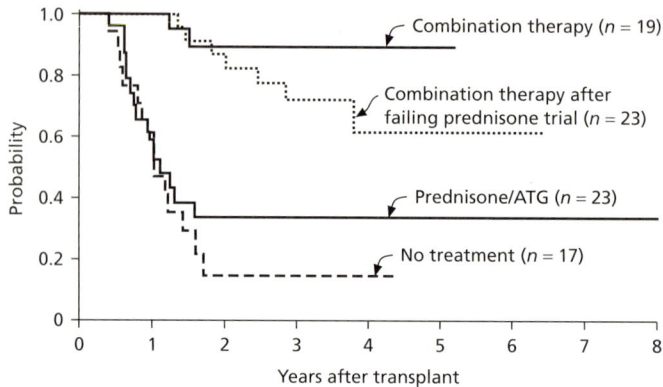

Fig. 50.8 Kaplan–Meier estimates of survival without disability (i.e. Karnofsky performance) in patients with clinical extensive chronic GVHD transplanted in Seattle before 1980. (Adapted from [415].)

GVHD were not treated and only two survived (KPS >70%) [343]. There appeared to be no spontaneous improvement in disabled survivors despite years of observation.

Primary treatment

Another 13 patients received a brief course of ATG or a prolonged course of corticosteroids given late in the course of disease, and only three survived without disability [343]. Similar experience with other immunosuppressive drugs or plasmapheresis given late in the disease had little apparent benefit [303]. In 21 patients with extensive chronic GVHD, PSE (1.0 mg/kg every other day) was given with either CY, procarbazine or azathioprine (all 1.5 mg/kg/day) early in the course of disease before clinical deterioration [343]. Procarbazine appeared to be less effective, and CY was associated with hemorrhagic cystitis. Chronic GVHD responded to a median of 13 months of combination therapy with PSE and azathioprine (see Plates 23.54 & 23.55, *facing p. 296*). Figure 50.8 presents these and additional patients treated before 1980 [415]. Results after administration of late PSE or ATG appeared little different than if no treatment were given. Combination therapy given as either primary or secondary treatment was associated with improved disability-free survival. However, results could not be compared directly because patients given combination therapy were treated in later years when treatment was given earlier in their disease.

To determine the benefit of early combination therapy, a double-blind randomized trial was conducted comparing PSE and azathioprine with PSE and placebo [395]. Patients with persisting thrombocytopenia were not randomized as a result of concern about using cytotoxic drugs in cytopenic patients; instead, these patients were placed into treatment with an equivalent dose of alternate-day PSE. All three groups received prophylaxis with TMP-SMX. NRM was significantly higher (40% vs. 21%) in standard-risk patients randomized to PSE and azathioprine ($p = 0.003$; Table 50.9 [395,414,416–419]). This mortality was caused by an increase in fatal infections in patients who received cytotoxic treatment. Survival was 61% in patients randomized to PSE and placebo. This survival rate was significantly higher than the 26% survival observed in high-risk patients with thrombocytopenia treated with an identical PSE regimen. The reason for the increased infectious mortality in high-risk patients was unclear because granulocyte counts were normal. It appeared that the hypomegakaryocytic thrombocytopenia was a marker for more severe chronic GVHD, often of progressive-type onset in patients with prior acute GVHD.

The addition of oral CSP (6 mg every 12 h every other day) in patients at high risk for GVHD with thrombocytopenia was next studied [418]. Renal toxicity was modest [420]. As shown in Table 50.9, survival appeared improved with this regimen [421]. Functional performance of

Table 50.9 Trials of combination immunosuppression after marrow transplantation: chronic GVHD studies.

Investigator (year, reference)	Patients (n)	Regimens compared	Chronic GVHD (%)	GVHD response (%)	Non-relapse mortality (%)	Overall survival (%)
Prevention						
Kansu et al. (2001 [414])	73	6 month CSP	51			84
		vs.	(n.s.)			(n.s.)
	89	24 month CSP	39			88
Initial treatment						
Sullivan et al. (1988 [395])	63	PSE + placebo	62		21	61
(Standard risk)		vs.	(n.s.)		($p = 0.003$)	($p = 0.03$)
	63	PSE + AZ	64		40	47
Koc et al. (2002 [416])	145	PSE	53		13	54
(Standard risk)		vs.	(n.s.)		(n.s.)	(n.s.)
	142	PSE + CSP	54		17	66
Arora et al. (2001 [417])	27	PSE + CSP	73			72
(Standard and high risk)		vs.	(n.s.)			(n.s.)
	27	PSE + CSP + Thal	88			67
Sullivan et al. (1988 [395])	38	PSE (placebo) (thrombocytopenia)	32		58	26
(High risk)						
Sullivan et al. (1988 [418])	40	PSE + CSP	56		40	52
(High risk)						
Koc et al. (2000 [419])	26	PSE + [CSP or TACR] + placebo	23			47
(High risk)	26	vs.	(n.s.)			(n.s.)
		PSE + [CSP or TACR] + Thal	39			49

AZ, azathioprine; CSP, cyclosporine; GVHD, graft-vs.-host disease; n.s., not significant; PSE, prednisone; TACR, tacrolimus; Thal, thalidomide.

the long-term survivors was maintained near normal, and the incidence of disabling scleroderma was decreased from 43% to 6% (see Fig. 50.7). As shown in Fig. 50.9, the average duration of treatment was 1–2 years [422]. However, infections remained a frequent cause of morbidity and contributed to transplant-related mortality in patients with high-risk chronic GVHD. The value of initial treatment with CSP + PSE in standard-risk (platelets >100,000/μL) chronic GVHD was prospectively compared to PSE alone [416]. Although the combination may reduce steroid-related toxicity, there was no beneficial effect on NRM or survival (Table 50.9).

A report from the Baltimore team described the use of thalidomide in high-risk patients [423]. The 3-year survival was 48% in 21 patients who received primary treatment, and infections seemed to be diminished in the long-term survivors. Part of the benefit of this therapy may be a result of modulation of TNF production [424]. The value of thalidomide has been studied in two controlled trials of initial treatment of chronic GVHD. In one trial of standard and high-risk patients, PSE + CSP was compared with PSE + CSP + thalidomide and no clinical benefit for the addition of thalidomide was found [417]. Poorer outcome was seen in individuals with thrombocytopenia, progressive-type onset of chronic GVHD, unrelated and sex mismatched donors. In a placebo-controlled study enrolling high-risk patients with thrombocytopenia or progressive-type onset of chronic GVHD, administration of thalidomide (200 mg/day increasing to 800 mg/day) was associated with neutropenia and neurologic toxicity [419]. In that study, 92% of thalidomide and 65% of placebo patients had study drug stopped before resolution of GVHD ($p = 0.02$).

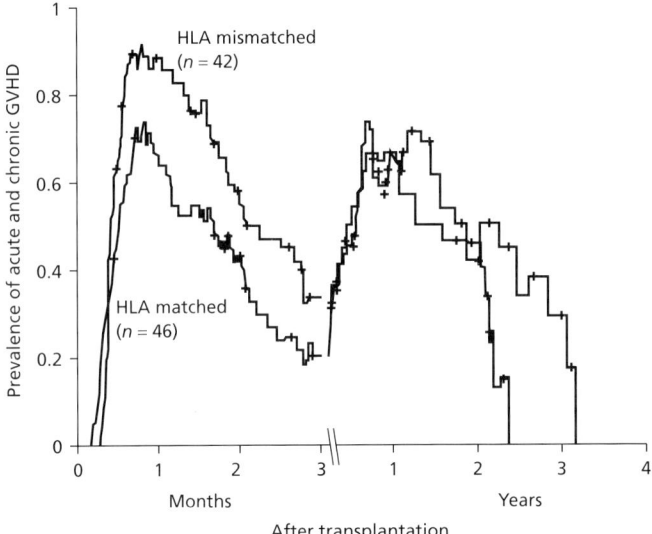

Fig. 50.9 Prevalence of acute GVHD of grades II–IV and clinical extensive chronic GVHD according to HLA compatibility. Resolution of clinical acute GVHD was scored despite continued immunosuppression. Conversely, resolution of chronic GVHD was scored only when patients discontinued immunosuppression indefinitely. (Adapted from [422].)

Secondary treatment

As with acute GVHD, to date there is no clear standard salvage regimen for chronic GVHD treatment [425,426]. Evaluation of therapy is sometimes difficult, as shown by investigator responses to six clinical vignettes sent to transplant programs [427]. While there was agreement as to diagnosis (limited/extensive), need for treatment and supportive care, there was less agreement in cases with atypical presentation or management of less severe or stable disease.

Azathioprine, alternating CSP/PSE, high-dose pulse MP, tacrolimus and thalidomide give surprisingly similar 2–3 year survival rates (approximately 75%) for patients failing initial steroid therapy [423,428–432]. As with the primary treatment studies, significant side-effects were noted with thalidomide [433]. For several of these regimens, approximately 30% of patients can successfully discontinue treatment after 2–3 years of salvage therapy without return of active GVHD [430,432]. Similar to thalidomide, clofazimine is used in treating leprosy and immunomediated skin disorders. It also has activity in the cutaneous and oral lesions of chronic GVHD [434]. Side-effects and infectious complications appear minimal and this agent may be useful as adjunctive steroid-sparing therapy.

Other investigations have explored the use of PUVA in treating patients with refractory cutaneous chronic GVHD [277–279]. Dermal responses were observed in 31 of 40 patients, and some improvement was noted at extracutaneous sites [278,435] (see Plates 23.22 & 23.23, *facing p. 296*). ECP has demonstrated benefit in reversing cardiac allograft rejection [436] and has been reported to improve oral manifestations, sclerodermatous involvement and joint contractures in patients with refractory chronic GVHD [283,437–441]. Response to ECP does not appear to correlate with psoralen levels or number of treated lymphocytes [440]. Low-dose total lymphoid irradiation was also reported to lead to partial or complete improvement in nine patients who received 100 cGy thoracoabdominal irradiation [442]. Secondary treatment of cutaneous chronic GVHD has shown some benefit with halofuginone (an inhibitor of collagen) and etretinate (a synthetic retinoid) [443–445]. Apparent activity in steroid-refractory chronic GVHD has also been reported with daclizumab (an anti-IL-2 receptor MAB) and etanercept (anti-TNF antibody) [268,446]. Other clinical trials found responses with MMF and hydroxychloroquine [246,447,448]. In other reports, three or more agents have been given in combination, but with a high rate of infectious complications and NRM [449]. As shown in Fig. 50.10, tolerance can be achieved and many patients can have immunosuppression discontinued [450]. Over the past two decades there appear to be fewer skin contractures and serious infections, but NRM remains a challenge and better means to prevent chronic GVHD and infections are still required.

Supportive care

Severe dermal involvement of chronic GVHD may benefit from burn care management to speed reepithelialization and closure of portals of infection. Skin allografting from the marrow donor without further immunosuppression has been performed successfully [451]. Ocular sicca may respond to retinoic acid and oral sicca to pilocarpine [452,453]. Neuromuscular manifestations of chronic GVHD (muscular aches, cramping and carpal spasm) have improved with clonazepam treatment [454]. Liver function abnormalities in patients with refractory hepatic chronic GVHD have improved by approximately 30% following bile acid displacement therapy with UDCA [455]. For patients who are receiving long-term corticosteroid therapy, estrogen replacement in women, calcium supplements and antiosteoporosis agents should be considered for individuals at risk for bone loss and fracture [388,389]. Antimicrobial prophylaxis is another important aspect of the treatment of patients with

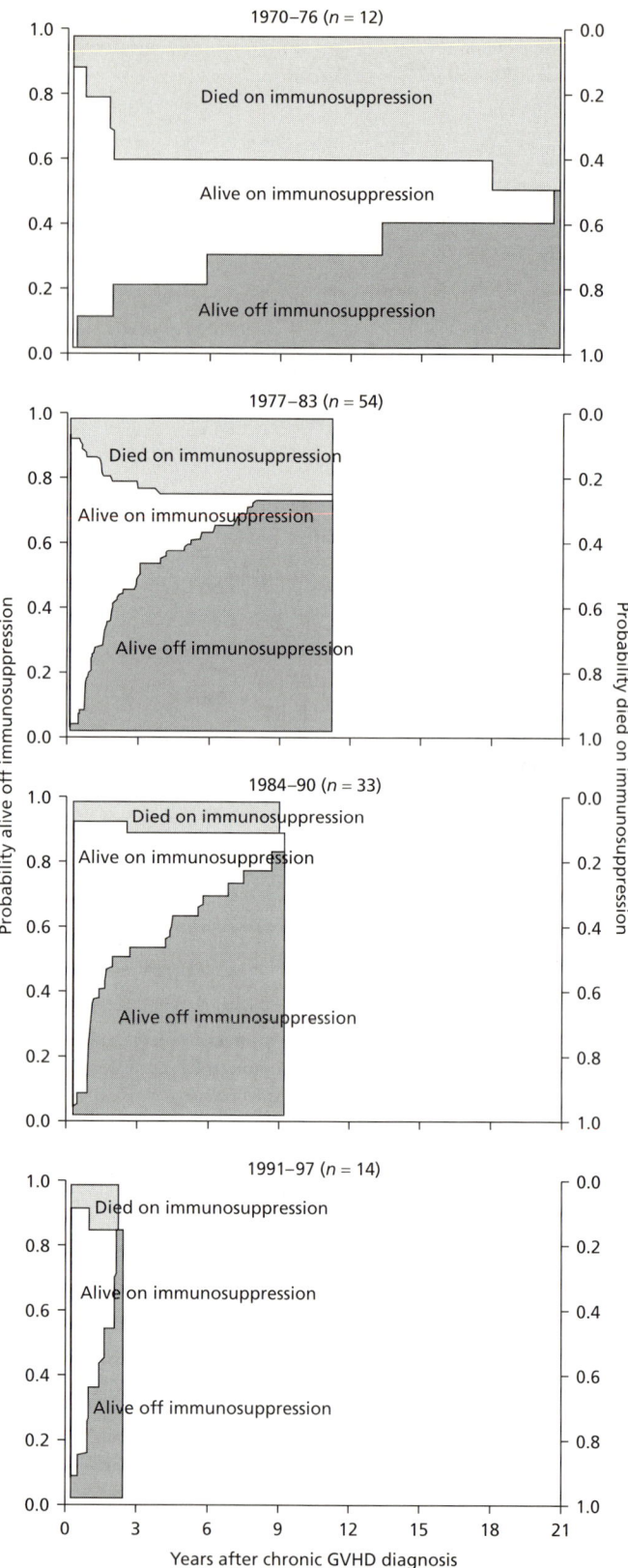

Fig. 50.10 Probabilities of death during continued immunosuppressive therapy and probabilities to discontinue immunosuppression among 113 patients with extensive chronic GVHD. The arc between the two curves represents patients alive but still receiving immunosuppressive therapy for chronic GVHD. (Adapted from [450].)

chronic GVHD. The relationships between immunodeficiency, GVHD-associated immunosuppression and infection are complex interactions that are of critical importance in the management of patients with GVHD.

Late infections

Immunodeficiency

Multiple immune defects are observed in patients with chronic GVHD (see Chapter 62). Thymic injury, impaired mucosal defense, chemotactic defects, functional asplenia, T-cell alloreactivity and qualitative and quantitative B-cell abnormalities contribute to the susceptibility to late infection. Chronic GVHD and its treatment retard thymopoiesis as well as B-cell lymphopoiesis [299,456,457].

Spectrum of infection

Bacteremia and sinopulmonary infections resulting from *Streptococcus pneumoniae* and *Haemophilus influenzae* frequently develop in patients with chronic GVHD [395,458–460]. The probability of developing pneumococcal sepsis by 10 years post-transplant in patients with chronic GVHD is estimated at 14% [461]. Of note, none of the patients with fatal infections were taking prophylaxis for *Pneumococcus*. Pulmonary infection after day 100 post-transplant developed in 50% of those recipients with chronic GVHD, 21% of those free of chronic GVHD and 2% of autograft recipients [428]. Late infections appear to be particularly increased in mismatched and unrelated marrow recipients. The probability of bacteremia or septicemia after day 100 was 22% in 364 HLA-identical sibling transplant recipients and 38% in 38 unrelated transplant recipients ($p = 0.008$) [310]. Chronic GVHD and HLA nonidentity contribute to this increased rate of infection in unrelated marrow recipients, as does the frequent presence of hypogammaglobulinemia [428]. Figure 50.11 depicts the time to first late infection by type of allogeneic marrow donor and GVHD status [462]. Among patients with chronic GVHD, first infection and first septicemia/bacteremia were more common and had an earlier onset in individuals with progressive-type onset of chronic GVHD (Fig. 50.12) [428].

Antimicrobial prophylaxis

Most BMT patients receive *Pneumocystis carinii* prophylaxis through day 120 post-transplant or for as long as they continue on chronic GVHD therapy with corticosteroids. Prophylaxis with TMP-SMX significantly reduced the incidence of late interstitial pneumonia from 28% to 8% in patients with chronic GVHD [463]. Given the risk for infection with encapsulated organisms, penicillin prophylaxis is recommended for at

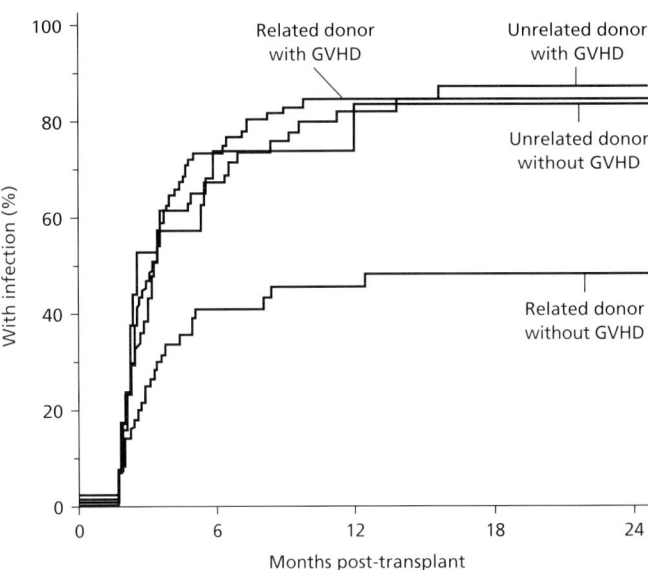

Fig. 50.11 Incidence of late infections. The effect of donor source and GVHD on the incidence of late infection in related donor (RD) and unrelated donor (URD) BMT recipients with advance GVHD is considered as a time-dependent covariate. Recipients of RD BMT had a statistically significant increase of infection among those in whom advanced GVHD developed ($p < 0.00001$). The incidence of infection was different in URD recipients with or without advanced GVHD and was similar to that seen in RD recipients with advances GVHD. (Adapted from [462].)

least 6 months after all immunosuppressive therapy for chronic GVHD has been discontinued [402,426,464].

Immunizations

After the first year, healthy patients free of chronic GVHD are likely to respond to influenza, pneumococcal polysaccharide, inactivated poliovirus, diphtheria, pertussis, tetanus toxoid, and *H. influenzae* type b conjugate vaccines (see Chapter 63). Patients being treated for chronic GVHD who are receiving immunosuppressive therapy may or may not form an adequate antibody response [457,465]. Live virus vaccines such as measles–mumps–rubella (MMR), oral poliovirus, oral typhoid and bacillus Calmette–Guérin carry risk in the immunocompromised host [464]. Clinical studies suggest that MMR can be given safely after the second year after transplantation in individuals who are free of chronic GVHD [466].

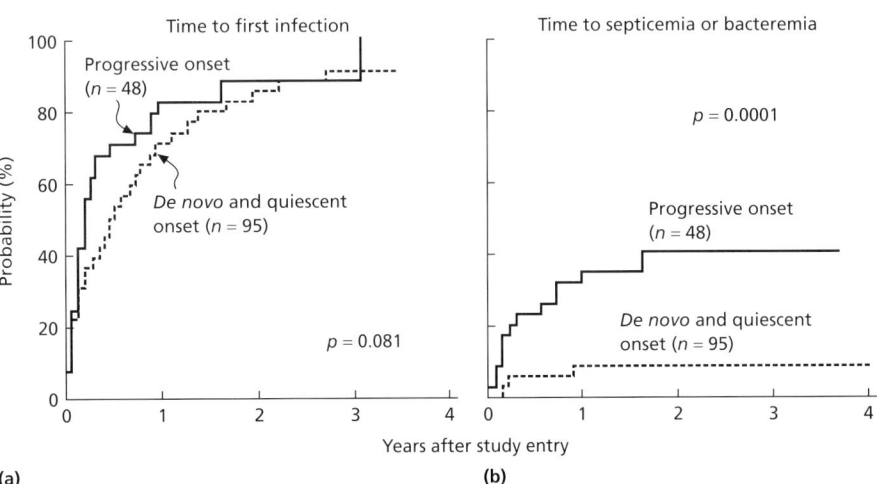

Fig. 50.12 Probability of developing infection in 143 standard-risk and high-risk patients with extensive chronic GVHD treated with cyclosporine/prednisone. (a) represents time to any infection (excluding upper respiratory illnesses) and (b) represents septicemia or bacteremia. (Adapted from [428].)

Table 50.10 Baltimore prognostic model for chronic graft-vs.-host disease (GVHD). (Adapted from [398].)

Prognostic factors*	10-year survival after diagnosis of chronic GVHD (%)
None	82
1 or 2 ± 3	68
1 + 2 or 3	34
1 + 2 + 3	3

* Factor 1: Extensive skin involvement (>50% body surface area).
Factor 2: Thrombocytopenia (<100,000/μL).
Factor 3: Progressive-type onset of chronic GVHD.

Prognosis

Transplant-related mortality

Mortality is increased in patients with extensive disease, progressive-type onset, thrombocytopenia, impaired KPS, weight loss and HLA-non-identical marrow donors [343,395,399,467]. A severity model has been developed by the IBMTR (Table 50.8). The Baltimore team reviewed 151 patients with chronic GVHD, outcome and relation to 23 variables at diagnosis of chronic GVHD [398]. Survival 10 years after diagnosis is listed in Table 50.10. Future studies of chronic GVHD should include the prognostic factors listed in Tables 50.8 and 50.10 when reporting results of clinical trials.

Malignancy-related mortality

Chronic GVHD appears to be associated with a GVL effect, which contributes to improved survival in patients transplanted in advanced stages of leukemia (see Chapter 28) [468]. The effect appears less beneficial in patients transplanted in remission [469]. Table 50.11 illustrates the prognostic influence of acute or chronic GVHD on treatment failure (relapse or death from any cause) following HLA-identical sibling transplantation [470].

Although immunodeficiency and chronic antigenic stimulation have been associated with lymphomagenesis in animal models, no clear evidence has been shown of an association of chronic GVHD with secondary malignancies in an initial analysis of 2246 patients undergoing marrow transplantation [259]. However, of five patients in whom secondary neoplasms developed among 320 individuals transplanted for aplastic anemia, all five had chronic GVHD and were treated for extended periods with azathioprine and PSE [471]. In more recent studies, azathioprine treatment of chronic GVHD was found to be associated with an increased risk for secondary neoplasms among non-Fanconi patients with aplastic anemia [472]. Among patients in whom solid cancers developed after BMT, chronic GVHD was significantly associated with development of squamous cell neoplasms of the skin and buccal mucosa [473]. Chapter 70 details more fully these factors related to development of secondary cancers.

Quality of life

Chronic GVHD remains the prime determinant of late transplant-related morbidity, including abnormalities of growth and development in children [391], sexual satisfaction and employment in adults [378,474] and functional performance status [475–482]. Symptoms resulting from chronic GVHD have been studied in relation to self-assessed severity and recently reported as a 30-item measure of GVHD manifestations [483]. Issues of quality of life are further detailed in Chapters 39 and 40.

Conclusions

Of fundamental interest to cell biologists and immunologists, the control of GVHD is of critical importance to transplant patients and physicians. The past four decades have witnessed considerable progress in the understanding and control of GVHD. During the 1950s and 1960s, animal

Table 50.11 Multivariate analysis of relapse and treatment failure according to GVHD factors.*

Disease status of transplantation	Relapse of leukemia			Treatment failure (relapse or death)		
	GVHD factor	Relative risk	p value	GVHD factor	Relative risk	p value
AML in 1st remission ($n = 251$)	MTX/CSP	2.34	0.017	A-GVHD	2.33	<0.001
AML in 2nd remission ($n = 55$)	A-GVHD	0.21	0.42	None	—	—
AML in relapse ($n = 020$)	A- or C-GVHD	0.42	0.003	None	—	—
	MTX	0.58	0.038	—	—	—
ALL in 1st remission ($n = 56$)	A-GVHD	0.11	0.006	CSP	13.85	0.024
ALL ≥2nd remission ($n = 147$)	A-GVHD	0.48	0.045	None	—	—
ALL in relapse ($n = 202$)	A- or C-GVHD	0.33	<0.001	A- or C-GVHD	0.70	0.033
	MTX/CSP	2.78	<0.001	MTX/CSP	1.69	0.016
CML in chronic phase ($n = 174$)	None	—	—	A- and C-GVHD	3.29	<0.001
				MTX	1.85	0.013
CML in accelerated phase ($n = 61$)	None	—	—	MTX	0.45	0.024
				MTX/SCP	0.24	0.003
CML in blast crisis ($n = 50$)	MTX/CSP	6.03	0.012	A- or C-GVHD	0.37	0.009

* Proportional hazards regression analysis using four time-dependent GVHD covariates (acute no chronic, $n = 337$; chronic no acute, $n = 145$; either acute or chronic, $n = 482$; both acute and chronic, $n = 21$) and four GVHD prophylaxis regimens (CSP alone, $n = 178$; MTX alone, $n = 754$; MTX + CSP, $n = 249$; other regimens, $n = 21$). Patient age, donor/patient gender, and pretransplant preoperative regimens were also included in the models but are not displayed in this table.

A, acute; ALL, acute lymphoblastic leukemia; AML, acute myeloid leukemia; C, chronic; CML, chronic myeloid leukemia; CSP, cyclosporine prophylaxis; GVHD, graft-vs.-host disease; MTX, methotrexate prophylaxis. (Adapted from [470]).

models defined the biology of GVHD. In the 1970s, initial clinical descriptions, grading systems for acute and chronic GVHD and treatment results were reported. During the 1980s, prognostic factors for the development and severity of GVHD were described by several groups. The first randomized trials of immunosuppressive agents, used alone or in combination, provided a basis for more effective prevention and treatment. The successful experience with HLA-identical siblings led to wider application of HCT from more HLA-disparate donors.

In the 1990s, improved control of GVHD prompted studies of HCT to improve the quality of life for patients with hematologic and immunologic diseases featuring considerable immediate morbidity but little early mortality. It is likely that results of allogeneic HCT will continue to improve during the current decade with improved techniques of molecular HLA typing and new approaches to enhance graft–host tolerance. Refinements in current immunosuppressive regimens are being studied and compared with other new approaches, and this continuing research in GVHD is reflected in more than 2900 scientific reports published during the past 5 years. This chapter highlights the clinical features, diagnosis, prevention and treatment of acute and chronic GVHD and outlines areas of future investigation in this singularly important aspect of allogeneic HCT.

References

1 Barnes D, Loutit J. Spleen protection: the cellular hypothesis. In: Bacq ZM, ed. *Radiobiology Symposium*. London: Butterworth, 1955.
2 Billingham R. A simple method of inducing tolerance of skin homografts in mice. *Transplant* 1957; **4**: 67–71.
3 Simonsen M. Graft-versus-host-reactions: the history that never was, and the way things happened to happen. *Immunol Rev* 1985; **88**: 5–23.
4 Mathe G, Amiel J, Schwarzenberg L *et al.* Haematopoietic chimera in man after allogeneic (homologous) bone-marrow transplantation (Control of the secondary syndrome. Specific tolerance due to the chimerism). *Br Med J* 1963; **5373**: 1633–5.
5 Graw RG Jr, Rogentine GN Jr, Leventhal BG *et al.* Graft-versus-host reaction complicating HLA-matched bone-marrow transplantation. *Lancet* 1970; **2**: 1053–5.
6 Kersey JH, Meuwissen HJ, Good RA. Graft versus host reactions following transplantation of allogeneic hematopoietic cells. *Hum Pathol* 1971; **2**: 389–402.
7 Gatti RA, Kersey JH, Yunis EJ *et al.* Graft-versus-host disease. *Prog Clin Pathol* 1973; **5**: 1–18.
8 Thomas D, Storb R, Clift R. Bone-marrow transplantation. *N Engl J Med* 1975; **2292**: 823–843; 895–902.
9 Grebe SC, Streilein JW. Graft-versus-host reactions: a review. *Adv Immunol* 1976; **22**: 119–221.
10 Hathaway WE, Githens JH, Blackburn WR *et al.* Aplastic anemia, histiocytosis and erythrodermia in immunologically deficient children: probable human runt disease. *N Engl J Med* 1965; **273**: 953–8.
11 Billingham R. The biology of graft-versus-host reactions. *The Harvey Lectures*, Vol. 62. Academic Press, 1966: 21–78.
12 Vogelsang GB, Hess AD. Graft-versus-host disease: new directions for a persistent problem. *Blood* 1994; **84**: 2061–7.
13 Antin JH, Ferrara JL. Cytokine dysregulation and acute graft-versus-host disease. *Blood* 1992; **80**: 2964–8.
14 Korngold R, Sprent J. T cell subsets and graft-versus-host disease. *Transplantation* 1987; **44**: 335–9.
15 Ferrara JL, Deeg HJ. Graft-versus-host disease. *N Engl J Med* 1991; **324**: 667–74.
16 Ferrara JL, Levy R, Chao NJ. Pathophysiologic mechanisms of acute graft-vs.-host disease. *Biol Blood Marrow Transplant* 1999; **5**: 347–56.
17 Piguet PF, Grau GE, Allet B *et al.* Tumor necrosis factor/cachectin is an effector of skin and gut lesions of the acute phase of graft-vs.-host disease. *J Exp Med* 1987; **166**: 1280–9.
18 van Bekkum DW, Roodenburg J, Heidt PJ *et al.* Mitigation of secondary disease of allogeneic mouse radiation chimeras by modification of the intestinal microflora. *J Natl Cancer Inst* 1974; **52**: 401–4.
19 Storb R, Prentice RL, Buckner CD *et al.* Graft-versus-host disease and survival in patients with aplastic anemia treated by marrow grafts from HLA-identical siblings: beneficial effect of a protective environment. *N Engl J Med* 1983; **308**: 302–7.
20 Beelen DW, Elmaagacli A, Muller KD *et al.* Influence of intestinal bacterial decontamination using metronidazole and ciprofloxacin or ciprofloxacin alone on the development of acute graft-versus-host disease after marrow transplantation in patients with hematologic malignancies: final results and long-term follow-up of an open-label prospective randomized trial. *Blood* 1999; **93**: 3267–75.
21 Grundy JE, Shanley JD, Shearer GM. Augmentation of graft-versus-host reaction by cytomegalovirus infection resulting in interstitial pneumonitis. *Transplantation* 1985; **39**: 548–53.
22 Cooke KR, Gerbitz A, Crawford JM *et al.* LPS antagonism reduces graft-versus-host disease and preserves graft-versus-leukemia activity after experimental bone marrow transplantation. *J Clin Invest* 2001; **107**: 1581–9.
23 Atkinson K, Storb R, Weiden PL *et al. In vitro* tests correlating with presence or absence of graft-vs.-host disease in DLA nonidentical canine radiation chimeras: evidence that clonal abortion maintains stable graft-host tolerance. *J Immunol* 1980; **124**: 1808–14.
24 Fukushi N, Arase H, Wang B *et al.* Thymus: a direct target tissue in graft-versus-host reaction after allogeneic bone marrow transplantation that results in abrogation of induction of self-tolerance. *Proc Natl Acad Sci U S A* 1990; **87**: 6301–5.
25 Rosenkrantz K, Keever C, Bhimani K *et al.* Both ongoing suppression and clonal elimination contribute to graft–host tolerance after transplantation of HLA mismatched T-cell-depleted marrow for severe combined immunodeficiency. *J Immunol* 1990; **144**: 1721–8.
26 Hess AD, Horwitz L, Beschorner WE *et al.* Development of graft-vs.-host disease-like syndrome in cyclosporine-treated rats after syngeneic bone marrow transplantation. I. Development of cytotoxic T lymphocytes with apparent polyclonal anti-Ia specificity, including autoreactivity. *J Exp Med* 1985; **161**: 718–30.
27 Hess AD, Fischer AC, Beschorner WE. Effector mechanisms in cyclosporine A-induced syngeneic graft-versus-host disease: role of CD4$^+$ and CD8$^+$ T lymphocyte subsets. *J Immunol* 1990; **145**: 526–33.
28 Fischer AC, Hess AD. Age-related factors in cyclosporine-induced syngeneic graft-versus-host disease: regulatory role of marrow-derived T lymphocytes. *J Exp Med* 1990; **172**: 85–94.
29 Gluckman E, Devergie A, Sohier J *et al.* Graft-versus-host disease in recipients of syngeneic bone marrow. *Lancet* 1980; **1**: 253–4.
30 Thein SL, Goldman JM, Galton DA. Acute 'graft-versus-host disease' after autografting for chronic granulocytic leukemia in transformation. *Ann Intern Med* 1981; **94**: 210–1.
31 Hood AF, Vogelsang GB, Black LP *et al.* Acute graft-vs-host disease: development following autologous and syngeneic bone marrow transplantation. *Arch Dermatol* 1987; **123**: 745–50.
32 Einsele H, Ehninger G, Schneider EM *et al.* High frequency of graft-versus-host-like syndromes following syngeneic bone marrow transplantation. *Transplantation* 1988; **45**: 579–85.
33 Yeager AM, Vogelsang GB, Jones RJ *et al.* Induction of cutaneous graft-versus-host disease by administration of cyclosporine to patients undergoing autologous bone marrow transplantation for acute myeloid leukemia. *Blood* 1992; **79**: 3031–5.
34 Massumoto C, Benyunes MC, Sale G *et al.* Close simulation of acute graft-versus-host disease by interleukin-2 administered after autologous bone marrow transplantation for hematologic malignancy. *Bone Marrow Transplant* 1996; **17**: 351–6.
35 Miura Y, Thoburn CJ, Bright EC *et al.* Cytokine and chemokine profiles in autologous graft-versus-host disease (GVHD): interleukin 10 and interferon gamma may be critical mediators for the development of autologous GVHD. *Blood* 2002; **100**: 2650–8.
36 Nishimura M, Uchida S, Mitsunaga S *et al.* Characterization of T-cell clones derived from peripheral blood lymphocytes of a patient with transfusion-associated graft-versus-host disease: *Fas*-mediated killing by CD4$^+$ and CD8$^+$ cytotoxic T-cell clones and tumor necrosis factor beta production by CD4$^+$ T-cell clones. *Blood* 1997; **89**: 1440–5.
37 Hathaway WE, Fulginiti VA, Pierce CW *et al.* Graft-vs-host reaction following a single blood transfusion. *J Am Med Assoc* 1967; **201**: 1015–20.
38 Greenbaum BH. Transfusion-associated graft-versus-host disease: historical perspectives, incidence, and current use of irradiated blood products. *J Clin Oncol* 1991; **9**: 1889–902.
39 Schroeder ML. Transfusion-associated graft-versus-host disease. *Br J Haematol* 2002; **117**: 275–87.
40 Parkman R, Mosier D, Umansky I *et al.* Graft-versus-host disease after intrauterine and exchange transfusions for hemolytic disease of the newborn. *N Engl J Med* 1974; **290**: 359–63.
41 Weiden PL, Zuckerman N, Hansen JA *et al.* Fatal graft-versus-host disease in a patient with lymphoblastic leukemia following normal granulocyte transfusion. *Blood* 1981; **57**: 328–32.
42 Juji T, Takahashi K, Shibata Y *et al.* Post-transfusion graft-versus-host disease in immunocompetent

43 Capon SM, DePond WD, Tyan DB et al. Transfusion-associated graft-versus-host disease in an immunocompetent patient. Ann Intern Med 1991; 114: 1025–6.

44 Kruskall M, Alpher C, Awdeh Z et al. HLA-homozygous donors and transfusion-associated graft-versus-host disease. N Engl J Med 1990; 322: 1005–6.

45 Shivdasani RA, Haluska FG, Dock NL et al. Brief report: graft-versus-host disease associated with transfusion of blood from unrelated HLA-homozygous donors. N Engl J Med 1993; 328: 766–70.

46 Asai T, Inaba S, Ohto H et al. Guidelines for irradiation of blood and blood components to prevent post-transfusion graft-vs.-host disease in Japan. Transfus Med 2000; 10: 315–20.

47 Ohto H, Anderson KC. Post-transfusion graft-versus-host disease in Japanese newborns. Transfusion 1996; 36: 117–23.

48 Wang L, Juji T, Tokunaga K et al. Brief report: polymorphic microsatellite markers for the diagnosis of graft-versus-host disease. N Engl J Med 1994; 330: 398–401.

49 Tanaka K, Aki T, Shulman HM et al. Two cases of transfusion-associated graft-vs.-host disease after open heart surgery. Arch Dermatol 1992; 128: 1503–6.

50 Siimes MA, Koskimies S. Chronic graft-versus-host disease after blood transfusions confirmed by incompatible HLA antigens in bone marrow. Lancet 1982; 1: 42–3.

51 Thomas D, Herman E Jr, Greenough WI. Irradiation and marrow infusion in leukemia. Arch Intern Med 1961; 107: 829–45.

52 Button LN, DeWolf WC, Newburger PE et al. The effects of irradiation on blood components. Transfusion 1981; 21: 419–26.

53 Anderson KC, Goodnough LT, Sayers M et al. Variation in blood component irradiation practice: implications for prevention of transfusion-associated graft-versus-host disease. Blood 1991; 77: 2096–102.

54 Drobyski W, Thibodeau S, Truitt RL et al. Third-party-mediated graft rejection and graft-versus-host disease after T-cell-depleted bone marrow transplantation, as demonstrated by hypervariable DNA probes and HLA-DR polymorphism. Blood 1989; 74: 2285–94.

55 Pelszynski MM, Moroff G, Luban NL et al. Effect of gamma irradiation of red blood cell units on T-cell inactivation as assessed by limiting dilution analysis: implications for preventing transfusion-associated graft-versus-host disease. Blood 1994; 83: 1683–9.

56 Moroff G, Luban NL. The irradiation of blood and blood components to prevent graft-versus-host disease: technical issues and guidelines. Transfus Med Rev 1997; 11: 15–26.

57 Grass JA, Wafa T, Reames A et al. Prevention of transfusion-associated graft-versus-host disease by photochemical treatment. Blood 1999; 93: 3140–7.

58 Beatty PG, Clift RA, Mickelson EM et al. Marrow transplantation from related donors other than HLA-identical siblings. N Engl J Med 1985; 313: 765–71.

59 van Rood JJ, Loberiza FR Jr, Zhang MJ et al. Effect of tolerance to noninherited maternal antigens on the occurrence of graft-versus-host disease after bone marrow transplantation from a parent or an HLA-haploidentical sibling. Blood 2002; 99: 1572–7.

60 Kernan NA, Bartsch G, Ash RC et al. Analysis of 462 transplantations from unrelated donors facilitated by the National Marrow Donor Program. N Engl J Med 1993; 328: 593–602.

61 Storb R, Prentice RL, Sullivan KM et al. Predictive factors in chronic graft-versus-host disease in patients with aplastic anemia treated by marrow transplantation from HLA-identical siblings. Ann Intern Med 1983; 98: 461–6.

62 Weisdorf D, Hakke R, Blazar B et al. Risk factors for acute graft-versus-host disease in histocompatible donor bone marrow transplantation. Transplantation 1991; 51: 1197–203.

63 Bross DS, Tutschka PJ, Farmer ER et al. Predictive factors for acute graft-versus-host disease in patients transplanted with HLA-identical bone marrow. Blood 1984; 63: 1265–70.

64 Nash R, Pepe M, Storb R. Acute graft-versus-host disease: analysis of risk factors after allogeneic marrow transplantation and prophylaxis with cyclosporine and methotrexate. Blood 1992; 80: 1838–45.

65 Beatty PG, Anasetti C, Hansen JA et al. Marrow transplantation from unrelated donors for treatment of hematologic malignancies: effect of mismatching for one HLA locus. Blood 1993; 81: 249–53.

66 Petersdorf EW, Longton GM, Anasetti C et al. The significance of HLA-DRB1 matching on clinical outcome after HLA-A, B, DR identical unrelated donor marrow transplantation. Blood 1995; 86: 1606–13.

67 Nademanee A, Schmidt GM, Parker P et al. The outcome of matched unrelated donor bone marrow transplantation in patients with hematologic malignancies using molecular typing for donor selection and graft-versus-host disease prophylaxis regimen of cyclosporine, methotrexate, and prednisone. Blood 1995; 86: 1228–34.

68 Gajewski J, Gjertson D, Cecka M et al. The impact of T-cell depletion on the effects of HLA DR beta 1 and DQ beta allele matching in HLA serologically identical unrelated donor bone marrow transplantation. Biol Blood Marrow Transplant 1997; 3: 76–82.

69 Petersdorf EW, Kollman C, Hurley CK et al. Effect of HLA class II gene disparity on clinical outcome in unrelated donor hematopoietic cell transplantation for chronic myeloid leukemia: the US National Marrow Donor Program Experience. Blood 2001; 98: 2922–9.

70 den Haan JM, Sherman NE, Blokland E et al. Identification of a graft versus host disease-associated human minor histocompatibility antigen. Science 1995; 268: 1476–80.

71 Goulmy E, Schipper R, Pool J et al. Mismatches of minor histocompatibility antigens between HLA-identical donors and recipients and the development of graft-versus-host disease after bone marrow transplantation. N Engl J Med 1996; 334: 281–5.

72 Martin PJ. How much benefit can be expected from matching for minor antigens in allogeneic marrow transplantation? Bone Marrow Transplant 1997; 20: 97–100.

73 Morishima Y, Kodera Y, Hirabayashi N et al. Low incidence of acute GVHD in patients transplanted with marrow from HLA-A, B, DR-compatible unrelated donors among Japanese. Bone Marrow Transplant 1995; 15: 235–9.

74 Klingemann HG, Deeg HJ, Self S et al. Is race a risk factor for allogeneic marrow transplantation? Bone Marrow Transplant 1986; 1: 87–94.

75 Easaw SJ, Lake DE, Beer M et al. Graft-versus-host disease: possible higher risk for African American patients. Cancer 1996; 78: 1492–7.

76 Walters MC, Patience M, Leisenring W et al. Bone marrow transplantation for sickle cell disease. N Engl J Med 1996; 335: 369–76.

77 Balduini CL, Noris P, Giorgiani G et al. Incompatibility for CD31 and human platelet antigens and acute graft-versus-host disease after bone marrow transplantation. Br J Haematol 1999; 106: 723–9.

78 Vogt MH, van den Muijsenberg JW, Goulmy E et al. The DBY gene codes for an HLA-DQ5-restricted human male-specific minor histocompatibility antigen involved in graft-versus-host disease. Blood 2002; 99: 3027–32.

79 Flowers M, Pepe M, Longton G. Previous donor pregnancy as a risk factor for acute graft-versus-host disease in patients with aplastic anemia treated by allogenic marrow transplantation. Br Haematol 1990; 74: 492–6.

80 Popplewell LL, Forman SJ. Is there an upper age limit for bone marrow transplantation? Bone Marrow Transplant 2002; 29: 277–84.

81 Sullivan KM, Storb R, Buckner CD et al. Graft-versus-host disease as adoptive immunotherapy in patients with advanced hematologic neoplasms. N Engl J Med 1989; 320: 828–34.

82 Klingemann HG, Storb R, Fefer A et al. Bone marrow transplantation in patients aged 45 years and older. Blood 1986; 67: 770–6.

83 Marmont AM, Horowitz MM, Gale RP et al. T-cell depletion of HLA-identical transplants in leukemia. Blood 1991; 78: 2120–30.

84 Kollman C, Howe CW, Anasetti C et al. Donor characteristics as risk factors in recipients after transplantation of bone marrow from unrelated donors: the effect of donor age. Blood 2001; 98: 2043–51.

85 Eckardt JR, Roodman GD, Boldt DH et al. Comparison of engraftment and acute GVHD in patients undergoing cryopreserved or fresh allogeneic BMT. Bone Marrow Transplant 1993; 11: 125–31.

86 Broxmeyer HE, Hangoc G, Cooper S et al. Growth characteristics and expansion of human umbilical cord blood and estimation of its potential for transplantation in adults. Proc Natl Acad Sci U S A 1992; 89: 4109–13.

87 Wagner JE, Kernan NA, Steinbuch M et al. Allogeneic sibling umbilical-cord-blood transplantation in children with malignant and non-malignant disease. Lancet 1995; 346: 214–19.

88 Kurtzberg J, Laughlin M, Graham ML et al. Placental blood as a source of hematopoietic stem cells for transplantation into unrelated recipients. N Engl J Med 1996; 335: 157–66.

89 Gluckman E, Rocha V, Boyer-Chammard A et al. Outcome of cord-blood transplantation from related and unrelated donors. Eurocord Transplant Group and the European Blood and Marrow Transplantation Group. N Engl J Med 1997; 337: 373–81.

90 Thomson BG, Robertson KA, Gowan D et al. Analysis of engraftment, graft-versus-host disease, and immune recovery following unrelated donor cord blood transplantation. Blood 2000; 96: 2703–11.

91 Bensinger WI, Clift R, Martin P et al. Allogeneic peripheral blood stem cell transplantation in patients with advanced hematologic malignancies: a retrospective comparison with marrow transplantation. Blood 1996; 88: 2794–800.

92 Schmitz N, Bacigalupo A, Labopin M. Transplantation of peripheral blood progenitor cells from HLA-identical sibling donors. Br J Haematol 1996; 95: 715–23.

93 Storek J, Gooley T, Siadak M et al. Allogeneic peripheral blood stem cell transplantation may be associated with a high risk of chronic graft-versus-host disease. *Blood* 1997; **90**: 4705–9.

94 Cutler C, Giri S, Jeyapalan S et al. Acute and chronic graft-versus-host disease after allogeneic peripheral blood stem cell and bone marrow transplantation: a meta-analysis. *J Clin Oncol* 2001; **19**: 3685–91.

95 Elmaagacli AH, Basoglu S, Peceny R et al. Improved disease-free-survival after transplantation of peripheral blood stem cells as compared with bone marrow from HLA-identical unrelated donors in patients with first chronic phase chronic myeloid leukemia. *Blood* 2002; **99**: 1130–5.

96 Przepiorka D, Smith TL, Folloder J et al. Risk factors for acute graft-versus-host disease after allogeneic blood stem cell transplantation. *Blood* 1999; **94**: 1465–70.

97 Bittencourt H, Rocha V, Chevret S et al. Association of CD34 cell dose with hematopoietic recovery, infections, and other outcomes after HLA-identical sibling bone marrow transplantation. *Blood* 2002; **99**: 2726–33.

98 Clift RA, Buckner CD, Appelbaum FR et al. Allogeneic marrow transplantation in patients with acute myeloid leukemia in first remission: a randomized trial of two irradiation regimens. *Blood* 1990; **76**: 1867–71.

99 Hill RS, Petersen FB, Storb R et al. Mixed hematologic chimerism after allogeneic marrow transplantation for severe aplastic anemia is associated with a higher risk of graft rejection and a lessened incidence of acute graft-versus-host disease. *Blood* 1986; **67**: 811–6.

100 Petz LD, Yam P, Wallace RB et al. Mixed hematopoietic chimerism following bone marrow transplantation for hematologic malignancies. *Blood* 1987; **70**: 1331–7.

101 Gratama JW, Zwaan FE, Stijnen T et al. Herpesvirus immunity and acute graft-versus-host disease. *Lancet* 1987; **1**: 471–4.

102 Miller W, Flynn P, McCullough J et al. Cytomegalovirus infection after bone marrow transplantation: an association with acute graft-vs.-host disease. *Blood* 1986; **67**: 1162–7.

103 Fujimori Y, Takatsuka H, Takemoto Y et al. Elevated interleukin (IL) 18 levels during acute graft-versus-host disease after allogeneic bone marrow transplantation. *Br J Haematol* 2000; **109**: 652–7.

104 Carayol G, Bourhis JH, Guillard M et al. Quantitative analysis of T helper 1, T helper 2, and inflammatory cytokine expression in patients after allogeneic bone marrow transplantation: relationship with the occurrence of acute graft-versus-host disease. *Transplantation* 1997; **63**: 1307–13.

105 Cullup H, Dickinson AM, Jackson GH et al. Donor interleukin 1 receptor antagonist genotype associated with acute graft-versus-host disease in human leucocyte antigen-matched sibling allogeneic transplants. *Br J Haematol* 2001; **113**: 807–13.

106 Cavet J, Dickinson AM, Norden J et al. Interferon-gamma and interleukin-6 gene polymorphisms associate with graft-versus-host disease in HLA-matched sibling bone marrow transplantation. *Blood* 2001; **98**: 1594–600.

107 Socie G, Loiseau P, Tamouza R et al. Both genetic and clinical factors predict the development of graft-versus-host disease after allogeneic hematopoietic stem cell transplantation. *Transplantation* 2001; **72**: 699–706.

108 Schwarer AP, Jiang YZ, Brookes PA et al. Frequency of anti-recipient alloreactive helper T-cell precursors in donor blood and graft-versus-host disease after HLA-identical sibling bone-marrow transplantation. *Lancet* 1993; **341**: 203–5.

109 Weston LE, Geczy AF, Farrell C. Donor helper T-cell frequencies as predictors of acute graft-versus-host disease in bone marrow transplantation between HLA-identical siblings. *Transplantation* 1997; **64**: 836–41.

110 Vogelsang GB, Hess AD, Berkman AW et al. An *in vitro* predictive test for graft versus host disease in patients with genotypic HLA-identical bone marrow transplants. *N Engl J Med* 1985; **313**: 645–50.

111 Sviland L, Dickinson AM, Carey PJ et al. An *in vitro* predictive test for clinical graft-versus-host disease in allogeneic bone marrow transplant recipients. *Bone Marrow Transplant* 1990; **5**: 105–9.

112 Bagot M, Mary JY, Heslan M et al. The mixed epidermal cell lymphocyte-reaction is the most predictive factor of acute graft-versus-host disease in bone marrow graft recipients. *Br J Haematol* 1988; **70**: 403–9.

113 Sahin S, Akoglu TF, Gurbuz O et al. Reevaluation of skin-explant model in graft-versus-host disease prediction. *Clin Transplant* 1995; **9**: 370–4.

114 Dickinson AM, Cavet J, Cullup H et al. GvHD risk assessment in hematopoietic stem cell transplantation: role of cytokine gene polymorphisms and an *in vitro* human skin explant model. *Hum Immunol* 2001; **62**: 1266–76.

115 Saurat JH. Cutaneous manifestations of graft-versus-host disease. *Int J Dermatol* 1981; **20**: 249–56.

116 Glucksberg H, Storb R, Fefer A et al. Clinical manifestations of graft-versus-host disease in human recipients of marrow from HL-A-matched sibling donors. *Transplantation* 1974; **18**: 295–304.

117 Sale GE, Shulman HM, Gallucci BB et al. Young rete ridge keratinocytes are preferred targets in cutaneous graft-versus-host disease. *Am J Pathol* 1985; **118**: 278–87.

118 Sullivan KM, Deeg HJ, Sanders J et al. Hyperacute graft-vs.-host disease in patients not given immunosuppression after allogeneic marrow transplantation. *Blood* 1986; **67**: 1172–5.

119 Goldberg NS, Ahmed T, Robinson B et al. Staphylococcal scalded skin syndrome mimicking acute graft-vs-host disease in a bone marrow transplant recipient. *Arch Dermatol* 1989; **125**: 85–7.

120 McDonald GB, Shulman HM, Sullivan KM et al. Intestinal and hepatic complications of human bone marrow transplantation. *Gastroenterology* 1986; **90**: 460–77; 770–84.

121 Weisdorf SA, Salati LM, Longsdorf JA et al. Graft-versus-host disease of the intestine: a protein losing enteropathy characterized by fecal alpha 1-antitrypsin. *Gastroenterology* 1983; **85**: 1076–81.

122 Weisdorf DJ, Snover DC, Haake R et al. Acute upper gastrointestinal graft-versus-host disease: clinical significance and response to immunosuppressive therapy. *Blood* 1990; **76**: 624–9.

123 Roy J, Snover D, Weisdorf S et al. Simultaneous upper and lower endoscopic biopsy in the diagnosis of intestinal graft-versus-host disease. *Transplantation* 1991; **51**: 642–6.

124 Spencer GD, Hackman RC, McDonald GB et al. A prospective study of unexplained nausea and vomiting after marrow transplantation. *Transplantation* 1986; **42**: 602–7.

125 Wu D, Hockenberry DM, Brentnall TA et al. Persistent nausea and anorexia after marrow transplantation: a prospective study of 78 patients. *Transplantation* 1998; **66**: 1319–24.

126 Jack MK, Jack GM, Sale GE et al. Ocular manifestations of graft-v-host disease. *Arch Ophthalmol* 1983; **101**: 1080–4.

127 Jabs DA, Wingard J, Green WR et al. The eye in bone marrow transplantation. III. Conjunctival graft-vs.-host disease. *Arch Ophthalmol* 1989; **107**: 1343–8.

128 Weiner RS, Bortin MM, Gale RP et al. Interstitial pneumonitis after bone marrow transplantation: assessment of risk factors. *Ann Intern Med* 1986; **104**: 168–75.

129 Piguet P, Garu GE, Collar MA, Vassalli P, Kapanci Y. Pneumopathies of the graft-versus-host disease reaction: alveolitis associated with an increased level of tumor necrosis factor mRNA and chronic pheumonia. *Lab Invest* 1989; **61**: 37–45.

130 Crawford SW, Longton G, Storb R. Acute graft-versus-host disease and the risks for idiopathic pneumonia after marrow transplantation for severe aplastic anemia. *Bone Marrow Transplant* 1993; **12**: 225–31.

131 Seber A, Khan SP, Kersey JH. Unexplained effusions: association with allogeneic bone marrow transplantation and acute or chronic graft-versus-host disease. *Bone Marrow Transplant* 1996; **17**: 207–11.

132 Russell SJ, Vowels MR, Vale T. Haemorrhagic cystitis in paediatric bone marrow transplant patients: an association with infective agents, GVHD and prior cyclophosphamide. *Bone Marrow Transplant* 1994; **13**: 533–9.

133 Anasetti C, Rybka W, Sullivan KM et al. Graft-vs.-host disease is associated with autoimmune-like thrombocytopenia. *Blood* 1989; **73**: 1054–8.

134 Bruno B, Gooley T, Sullivan KM et al. Secondary failure of platelet recovery after hematopoietic stem cell transplantation. *Biol Blood Marrow Transplant* 2001; **7**: 154–62.

135 Holler E, Kolb HJ, Hiller E et al. Microangiopathy in patients on cyclosporine prophylaxis who developed acute graft-versus-host disease after HLA-identical bone marrow transplantation. *Blood* 1989; **73**: 2018–24.

136 Sale GE, Lerner KG, Barker EA et al. The skin biopsy in the diagnosis of acute graft-versus-host disease in man. *Am J Pathol* 1977; **89**: 621–35.

137 Snover DC, Weisdorf SA, Ramsay NK et al. Hepatic graft versus host disease: a study of the predictive value of liver biopsy in diagnosis. *Hepatology* 1984; **4**: 123–30.

138 Vogelsang GB, Hess AD, Santos GW. Acute graft-versus-host disease: clinical characteristics in the cyclosporine era. *Medicine (Baltimore)* 1988; **67**: 163–74.

139 Przepiorka D, Weisdorf D, Martin P et al. 1994 Consensus conference on acute GVHD grading. *Bone Marrow Transplant* 1995; **15**: 825–8.

140 Spitzer TR. Engraftment syndrome following hematopoietic stem cell transplantation. *Bone Marrow Transplant* 2001; **27**: 893–8.

141 Kohler S, Hendrickson M, Chao N et al. Value of skin biosies in assessing prognosis and progression of acute graft-versus-host disease. *Am J Surg Path* 1997; **214**: 988–96.

142 Atkinson K, Horowitz MM, Biggs JC et al. The clinical diagnosis of acute graft-versus-host disease: a diversity of views amongst marrow transplant centers. *Bone Marrow Transplant* 1988; **3**: 5–10.

143 Martin P, Nash R, Sanders J et al. Reproducibility in retrospective grading of acute graft-versus-host

144 Rowlings PA, Przepiorka D, Klein JP et al. IBMTR Severity Index for grading acute graft-versus-host disease: retrospective comparison with Glucksberg grade. Br J Haematol 1997; **97**: 855–64.

145 Al-Ghamdi H, Leisenring W, Bensinger WI et al. A proposed objective way to assess results of randomized prospective clinical trials with acute graft-versus-host disease as an outcome of interest. Br J Haematol 2001; **113** (2): 461–9.

146 Clift R, Goldman J, Gratwohl A et al. Proposals for standardized reporting of results of bone marrow transplantation for leukaemia. Bone Marrow Transplant 1989; **4**: 445–8.

147 Storb R, Prentice RL, Hansen JA et al. Association between HLA-B antigens and acute graft-versus-host disease. Lancet 1983; **2**: 816–9.

148 Peterson FB, Bucker CD, Clift R. Laminar air flow isolation and decontamination: a prospective randomized study of the effects of prophylactic systemic antibiotics in bone marrow transplant patients. Infection 1986; **14**: 115–21.

149 Beelen DW, Haralambie E, Brandt H et al. Evidence that sustained growth suppression of intestinal anaerobic bacteria reduces the risk of acute graft-versus-host disease after sibling marrow transplantation. Blood 1992; **80**: 2668–76.

150 Marr KA, Seidel K, Slavin MA et al. Prolonged fluconazole prophylaxis is associated with persistent protection against candidiasis-related death in allogeneic marrow transplant recipients: long-term follow-up of a randomized, placebo-controlled trial. Blood 2000; **96**: 2055–61.

151 Krijanovski OI, Hill GR, Cooke KR et al. Keratinocyte growth factor separates graft-versus-leukemia effects from graft-versus-host disease. Blood 1999; **94**: 825–31.

152 Ellis M, Zwaan F, Hedstrom U et al. Recombinant human interleukin 11 and bacterial infection in patients with haemological malignant disease undergoing chemotherapy: a double-blind placebo-controlled randomised trial. Lancet 2003; **361**: 275–80.

153 Uphoff D. Alteration of homograft reaction by A-methopterin in lethally irradiated mice treated with homologous marrow. Proc Soc Exp Biol Med 1958; **99**: 651–3.

154 Santos GW, Owens AH. Production of graft-versus-host disease in the rat and its treatment with cytotoxic agents. Nature 1966; **210**: 139–40.

155 Storb R, Epstein RB, Graham TC et al. Methotrexate regimens for control of graft-versus-host disease in dogs with allogeneic marrow grafts. Transplantation 1970; **9**: 240–6.

156 Lazarus HM, Coccia PF, Herzig RH et al. Incidence of acute graft-versus-host disease with and without methotrexate prophylaxis in allogeneic bone marrow transplant patients. Blood 1984; **64**: 215–20.

157 Deegs HJ, Storb R, Thomas ED et al. Cyclosporine as prophylaxis for graft-versus-host disease in man after allogeneic bone marrow transplantation. Lancet 1980; **1**: 327–9.

158 Atkinson K, Downs K, Ashby M et al. Clinical correlations with cyclosporine blood levels after allogeneic bone marrow transplantation: an analysis of four different assays. Transplant Proc 1990; **22**: 1331–4.

159 Storb R, Deeg HJ, Fisher L et al. Cyclosporine vs. methotrexate for graft-vs.-host disease prevention in patients given marrow grafts for leukemia: long-term follow-up of three controlled trials. Blood 1988; **71**: 293–8.

160 Nash RA, Etzioni R, Storb R et al. Tacrolimus (FK506) alone or in combination with methotrexate or methylprednisolone for the prevention of acute graft-versus-host disease after marrow transplantation from HLA-matched siblings: a single-center study. Blood 1995; **85**: 3746–53.

161 Fay JW, Wingard JR, Antin JH et al. FK506 (tacrolimus) monotherapy for prevention of graft-versus-host disease after histocompatible sibling allogenic bone marrow transplantation. Blood 1996; **87**: 3514–19.

162 Przepiorka D, Nash RA, Wingard JR et al. Relationship of tacrolimus whole blood levels to efficacy and safety outcomes after unrelated donor marrow transplantation. Biol Blood Marrow Transplant 1999; **5**: 94–7.

163 Hiraoka A, Ohashi Y, Okamoto S et al. Phase III study comparing tacrolimus (FK506) with cyclosporine for graft-versus-host disease prophylaxis after allogeneic bone marrow transplantation. Bone Marrow Transplant 2001; **28**: 181–5.

164 Ramsay NK, Kersey JH, Robison LL et al. A randomized study of the prevention of acute graft-versus-host disease. N Engl J Med 1982; **306**: 392–7.

165 Storb R, Deeg HJ, Pepe M et al. Graft-versus-host disease prevention by methotrexate combined with cyclosporin compared to methotrexate alone in patients given marrow grafts for severe aplastic anaemia: long-term follow-up of a controlled trial. Br J Haematol 1989; **72**: 567–72.

166 Storb R, Deeg HJ, Whitehead J et al. Methotrexate and cyclosporine compared with cyclosporine alone for prophylaxis of acute graft versus host disease after marrow transplantation for leukemia. N Engl J Med 1986; **314**: 729–35.

167 Storb R, Deeg HJ, Pepe M et al. Methotrexate and cyclosporine versus cyclosporine alone for prophylaxis of graft-versus-host disease in patients given HLA-identical marrow grafts for leukemia: long-term follow-up of a controlled trial. Blood 1989; **73**: 1729–34.

168 Forman SJ, Blume KG, Krance RA et al. A prospective randomized study of acute graft-vs.-host disease in 107 patients with leukemia: methotrexate/prednisone vs. cyclosporine A/prednisone. Transplant Proc 1987; **19**: 2605–7.

169 Santos GW, Tutschka PJ, Brookmeyer R. Cyclosporine plus methylprednisolone vs. cyclophosphamide plus methylprednisolone as prophylaxis for graft-versus-host disease: a randomized doubleblind study in patients undergoing allogeneic marrow transplantation. Clin Transplant 1987; **1**: 21–8.

170 Storb R, Pepe M, Anasetti C et al. What role for prednisone in prevention of acute graft-versus-host disease in patients undergoing marrow transplants? Blood 1990; **76**: 1037–45.

171 Chao NJ, Schmidt GM, Niland JC et al. Cyclosporine, methotrexate, and prednisone compared with cyclosporine and prednisone for prophylaxis of acute graft-versus-host disease. N Engl J Med 1993; **329**: 1225–30.

172 Deeg HJ, Lin D, Leisenring W et al. Cyclosporine or cyclosporine plus methylprednisolone for prophylaxis of graft-versus-host disease: a prospective, randomized trial. Blood 1997; **89**: 3880–7.

173 Ratanatharathorn V, Nash RA, Przepiorka D et al. Phase III study comparing methotrexate and tacrolimus (prograf, FK506) with methotrexate and cyclosporine for graft-versus-host disease prophylaxis after HLA-identical sibling bone marrow transplantation. Blood 1998; **92**: 2303–14.

174 Chao NJ, Snyder DS, Jain M et al. Equivalence of two effective graft-versus-host disease prophylaxis regimens: results of a prospective double-blind randomized trial. Biol Blood Marrow Transplant 2000; **6**: 254–61.

175 Ruutu T, Volin L, Parkkali T et al. Cyclosporine, methotrexate, and methylprednisolone compared with cyclosporine and methotrexate for the prevention of graft-versus-host disease in bone marrow transplantation from HLA-identical sibling donor: a prospective randomized study. Blood 2000; **96**: 2391–8.

176 Locatelli F, Bruno B, Zecca M et al. Cyclosporin A and short-term methotrexate vs. cyclosporin A as graft versus host disease prophylaxis in patients with severe aplastic anemia given allogeneic bone marrow transplantation from an HLA-identical sibling: results of a GITMO/EBMT randomized trial. Blood 2000; **96**: 1690–7.

177 Nash RA, Antin JH, Karanes C et al. Phase 3 study comparing methotrexate and tacrolimus with methotrexate and cyclosporine for prophylaxis of acute graft-versus-host disease after marrow transplantation from unrelated donors. Blood 2000; **96**: 2062–8.

178 Horowitz MM, Przepiorka D, Bartels P et al. Tacrolimus vs. cyclosporine immunosuppression: results in advanced-stage disease compared with historical controls treated exclusively with cyclosporine. Biol Blood Marrow Transplant 1999; **5**: 180–6.

179 Sayer HG, Longton G, Bowden R et al. Increased risk of infection in marrow transplant patients receiving methylprednisolone for graft-versus-host disease prevention. Blood 1994; **84**: 1328–32.

180 Kalhs P, Brugger S, Schwarzinger I et al. Microangiopathy following allogeneic marrow transplantation: association with cyclosporine and methylprednisolone for graft-versus-host disease prophylaxis. Transplantation 1995; **60**: 949–57.

181 Stockschlaeder M, Storb R, Pepe M et al. A pilot study of low-dose cyclosporin for graft-versus-host prophylaxis in marrow transplantation. Br J Haematol 1992; **80**: 49–54.

182 Atkinson K, Downs K. Omission of day 11 methotrexate does not appear to influence the incidence of moderate to severe acute graft-versus-host disease, chronic graft-versus-host disease, relapse rate or survival after HLA-identical sibling bone marrow transplantation. Bone Marrow Transplant 1995; **16**: 755–8.

183 Ruutu T, Niederwieser D, Gratwohl A et al. A survey of the prophylaxis and treatment of acute GVHD in Europe: a report of the European Group for Blood and Marrow Transplantation (EBMT). Chronic Leukaemia Working Party EBMT. Bone Marrow Transplant 1997; **19**: 759–64.

184 Weiden PL, Doney K, Storb R et al. Antihuman thymocyte globulin for prophylaxis of graft-versus-host disease: a randomized trial in patients with leukemia treated with HLA-identical sibling marrow grafts. Transplantation 1979; **27**: 227–30.

185 Doney KC, Weiden PL, Storb R et al. Failure of early administration of antithymocyte globulin to lessen graft-versus-host disease in human allogeneic marrow transplant recipients. Transplantation 1981; **31**: 141–3.

186 Bacigalupo A, Lamparelli T, Bruzzi P et al. Antithymocyte globulin for graft-versus-host disease prophylaxis in transplants from unrelated donors:

two randomized studies from Gruppo Italiano Trapianti Midollo Osseo (GITMO). *Blood* 2001; **98**: 2942–7.
187 Kottaridis PD, Milligan DW, Chopra R *et al. In vivo* Campath-1H prevents graft-versus-host disease following nonmyeloablative stem cell transplantation. *Blood* 2000; **96**: 2419–25.
188 Anasetti C, Martin PJ, Storb R *et al.* Prophylaxis of graft-versus-host disease by administration of the murine anti-IL-2 receptor antibody 2A3. *Bone Marrow Transplant* 1991; **7**: 375–81.
189 Blaise D, Olive D, Hirn M *et al.* Prevention of acute GVHD by *in vivo* use of anti-interleukin-2 receptor monoclonal antibody (33B3.1): a feasibility trial in 15 patients. *Bone Marrow Transplant* 1991; **8**: 105–11.
190 McCarthy PL Jr, Abhyankar S, Neben S *et al.* Inhibition of interleukin-1 by an interleukin-1 receptor antagonist prevents graft-versus-host disease. *Blood* 1991; **78**: 1915–8.
191 Clift RA, Bianco JA, Appelbaum FR *et al.* A randomized controlled trial of pentoxifylline for the prevention of regimen-related toxicities in patients undergoing allogeneic marrow transplantation. *Blood* 1993; **82**: 2025–30.
192 Holler E, Kolb HJ, Mittermuller J *et al.* Modulation of acute graft-versus-host-disease after allogeneic bone marrow transplantation by tumor necrosis factor alpha (TNF alpha) release in the course of pretransplant conditioning: role of conditioning regimens and prophylactic application of a monoclonal antibody neutralizing human TNF alpha (MAK 195F). *Blood* 1995; **86**: 890–9.
193 Weisdorf D, Filipovich A, McGlave P *et al.* Combination graft-versus-host disease prophylaxis using immunotoxin (anti-CD5-RTA [Xomazyme-CD5]) plus methotrexate and cyclosporine or prednisone after unrelated donor marrow transplantation. *Bone Marrow Transplant* 1993; **12**: 531–6.
194 Przepiorka D, LeMaistre CF, Huh YO *et al.* Evaluation of anti-CD5 ricin A chain immunoconjugate for prevention of acute graft-vs.-host disease after HLA-identical marrow transplantation. *Ther Immunol* 1994; **1**: 77–82.
195 Dwyer JM. Manipulating the immune system with immune globulin. *N Engl J Med* 1992; **326**: 107–16.
196 Sullivan KM. Immunoglobulin therapy in bone marrow transplantation. *Am J Med* 1987; **83**: 34–45.
197 Winston DJ, Ho WG, Lin CH *et al.* Intravenous immune globulin for prevention of cytomegalovirus infection and interstitial pneumonia after bone marrow transplantation. *Ann Intern Med* 1987; **106**: 12–8.
198 Sullivan KM, Kopecky KJ, Jocom J *et al.* Immunomodulatory and antimicrobial efficacy of intravenous immunoglobulin in bone marrow transplantation. *N Engl J Med* 1990; **323**: 705–12.
199 Bass EB, Powe NR, Goodman SN *et al.* Efficacy of immune globulin in preventing complications of bone marrow transplantation: a meta-analysis. *Bone Marrow Transplant* 1993; **12**: 273–82.
200 Feinstein LC, Seidel K, Jocum J *et al.* Reduced dose intravenous immunoglobulin does not decrease transplant-related complications in adults given related donor marrow allografts. *Biol Blood Marrow Transplant* 1999; **5**: 369–78.
201 Winston DJ, Antin JH, Wolff SN *et al.* A multicenter, randomized, double-blind comparison of different doses of intravenous immunoglobulin for prevention of graft-versus-host disease and infection after allogeneic bone marrow transplantation. *Bone Marrow Transplant* 2001; **28**: 187–96.

202 Reisner Y, Kapoor N, Kirkpatrick D *et al.* Transplantation for acute leukaemia with HLA-A and B nonidentical parental marrow cells fractionated with soybean agglutinin and sheep red blood cells. *Lancet* 1981; **2**: 327–31.
203 Hale G, Cobbold S, Waldmann H. T cell depletion with Campath-1 in allogeneic bone marrow transplantation. *Transplantation* 1988; **45**: 753–9.
204 Ash RC, Casper JT, Chitambar CR *et al.* Successful allogeneic transplantation of T-cell-depleted bone marrow from closely HLA-matched unrelated donors. *N Engl J Med* 1990; **322**: 485–94.
205 Wagner JE, Santos GW, Noga SJ *et al.* Bone marrow graft engineering by counterflow centrifugal elutriation: results of a phase I–II clinical trial. *Blood* 1990; **75**: 1370–7.
206 Champlin R, Ho W, Gajewski J *et al.* Selective depletion of $CD8^+$ T lymphocytes for prevention of graft-versus-host disease after allogeneic bone marrow transplantation. *Blood* 1990; **76**: 418–23.
207 Antin JH, Bierer BE, Smith BR *et al.* Selective depletion of bone marrow T lymphocytes with anti-CD5 monoclonal antibodies: effective prophylaxis for graft-versus-host disease in patients with hematologic malignancies. *Blood* 1991; **78**: 2139–49.
208 Ho VT, Soiffer RJ. The history and future of T-cell depletion as graft-versus-host disease prophylaxis for allogeneic hematopoietic stem cell transplantation. *Blood* 2001; **98**: 3192–204.
209 Martin PJ, Hansen JA, Buckner CD *et al.* Effects of *in vitro* depletion of T cells in HLA-identical allogeneic marrow grafts. *Blood* 1985; **66**: 664–72.
210 Goldman JM, Gale RP, Horowitz MM *et al.* Bone marrow transplantation for chronic myelogenous leukemia in chronic phase: increased risk for relapse associated with T-cell depletion. *Ann Intern Med* 1988; **108**: 806–14.
211 Andre-Schmutz I, Le Deist F, Hacein-Bey-Abina S *et al.* Immune reconstitution without graft-versus-host disease after haemopoietic stem-cell transplantation: a phase 1–2 study. *Lancet* 2002; **360**: 130–7.
212 Ruutu T, Eriksson B, Remes K *et al.* Ursodeoxycholic acid for the prevention of hepatic complications in allogeneic stem cell transplantation. *Blood* 2002; **100**: 1977–83.
213 Calmus Y, Gane P, Rouger P *et al.* Hepatic expression of class I and class II major histocompatibility complex molecules in primary biliary cirrhosis: effect of ursodeoxycholic acid. *Hepatology* 1990; **11**: 12–15.
214 Doney KC, Storb R, Beach K *et al.* A toxicity study of trimetrexate used in combination with cyclosporine as acute graft-versus-host disease prophylaxis in HLA-mismatched, related donor bone marrow transplants. *Transplantation* 1995; **60**: 55–8.
215 Khouri IF, Przepiorka D, van Besien K *et al.* Allogeneic blood or marrow transplantation for chronic lymphocytic leukaemia: timing of transplantation and potential effect of fludarabine on acute graft-versus-host disease. *Br J Haematol* 1997; **97**: 466–73.
216 Dumont FJ, Staruch MJ, Koprak SL *et al.* Distinct mechanisms of suppression of murine T cell activation by the related macrolides FK506 and rapamycin. *J Immunol* 1990; **144**: 251–8.
217 Morris RE, Meiser BM, Wu J *et al.* Use of rapamycin for the suppression of alloimmune reactions *in vivo*: schedule dependence, tolerance induction, synergy with cyclosporine and FK506, and effect on host-versus-graft and graft-versus-host reactions. *Transplant Proc* 1991; **23**: 521–4.

218 Blazar BR, Taylor PA, Panoskaltsis-Mortari A *et al. In vivo* inhibition of cytokine responsiveness and graft-versus-host disease mortality by rapamycin leads to a clinical–pathological syndrome discrete from that observed with cyclosporin A. *Blood* 1996; **87**: 4001–9.
219 Deeg HJ. Ultraviolet irradiation in transplantation biology: manipulation of immunity and immunogenicity. *Transplantation* 1988; **45**: 845–51.
220 Bornhauser M, Schuler U, Porksen G *et al.* Mycophenolate mofetil and cyclosporine as graft-versus-host disease prophylaxis after allogeneic blood stem cell transplantation. *Transplantation* 1999; **67**: 499–504.
221 Vogelsang GB, Arai S. Mycophenolate mofetil for the prevention and treatment of graft-versus-host disease following stem cell transplantation: preliminary findings. *Bone Marrow Transplant* 2001; **27**: 1255–62.
222 Wallace PM, Johnson JS, MacMaster JF *et al.* CTLA4Ig treatment ameliorates the lethality of murine graft-versus-host disease across major histocompatibility complex barriers. *Transplantation* 1994; **58**: 602–10.
223 Schlegel PG, Chao NJ. Immunomodulatory peptides with high binding affinity for class II MHC molecules for the prevention of graft-versus-host disease. *Leuk Lymphoma* 1996; **23**: 11–6.
224 Townsend RM, Briggs C, Marini JC *et al.* Inhibitory effect of a CD4-CDR3 peptide analog on graft-versus-host disease across a major histocompatibility complex–haploidentical barrier. *Blood* 1996; **88**: 3038–47.
225 Blazar BR, Taylor PA, Linsley PS *et al. In vivo* blockade of CD28/CTLA4: B7/BB1 interaction with CTLA4-Ig reduces lethal murine graft-versus-host disease across the major histocompatibility complex barrier in mice. *Blood* 1994; **83**: 3815–25.
226 Gribben JG, Guinan EC, Boussiotis VA *et al.* Complete blockade of B7 family-mediated costimulation is necessary to induce human alloantigen-specific anergy: a method to ameliorate graft-versus-host disease and extend the donor pool. *Blood* 1996; **87**: 4887–93.
227 Chen B, Liu C, Cui X *et al.* Prevention of graft-versus-host disease by a novel immunosuppressant, PG490-88, through inhibition of alloreactive T cell expansion. *Transplantation* 2000; **70**: 1442.
228 Glucksberg H, Fefer A. Combination chemotherapy for clinically established graft-versus-host disease in mice. *Cancer Res* 1973; **33**: 859–61.
229 Goker H, Haznedaroglu IC, Chao NJ. Acute graft-vs-host disease: pathobiology and management. *Exp Hematol* 2001; **29**: 259–77.
230 Kendra J, Barrett AJ, Lucas C *et al.* Response of graft versus host disease to high doses of methyl prednisolone. *Clin Lab Haematol* 1981; **3**: 19–26.
231 Bacigalupo A, van Lint MT, Frassoni F *et al.* High-dose bolus methylprednisolone for the treatment of acute graft versus host disease. *Blut* 1983; **46**: 125–32.
232 Kanojia MD, Anagnostou AA, Zander AR *et al.* High-dose methylprednisolone treatment for acute graft-versus-host disease after bone marrow transplantation in adults. *Transplantation* 1984; **37**: 246–9.
233 Deeg HJ, Henslee-Downey PJ. Management of acute graft-versus-host disease. *Bone Marrow Transplant* 1990; **6**: 1–8.
234 Van Lint MT, Uderzo C, Locasciulli A *et al.* Early treatment of acute graft-versus-host disease with high- or low-dose 6-methylprednisolone: a

235 Hings IM, Filipovich AH, Miller WJ et al. Prednisone therapy for acute graft-versus-host disease: short- versus long-term treatment: a prospective randomized trial. *Transplantation* 1993; **56**: 577–80.

236 Doney KC, Weiden PL, Storb R et al. Treatment of graft-versus-host disease in human allogeneic marrow graft recipients: a randomized trial comparing antithymocyte globulin and corticosteroids. *Am J Hematol* 1981; **11**: 1–8.

237 Kennedy MS, Deeg HJ, Storb R et al. Treatment of acute graft-versus-host disease after allogeneic marrow transplantation: randomized study comparing corticosteroids and cyclosporine. *Am J Med* 1985; **78**: 978–83.

238 Deeg HJ, Loughran TP Jr, Storb R et al. Treatment of human acute graft-versus-host disease with antithymocyte globulin and cyclosporine with or without methylprednisolone. *Transplantation* 1985; **40**: 162–6.

239 Cahn JY, Bordigoni P, Tiberghien P et al. Treatment of acute graft-versus-host disease with methylprednisolone and cyclosporine with or without an anti-interleukin-2 receptor monoclonal antibody: a multicenter phase III study. *Transplantation* 1995; **60**: 939–42.

240 Martin PJ, Nelson BJ, Appelbaum FR et al. Evaluation of a CD5-specific immunotoxin for treatment of acute graft-versus-host disease after allogeneic marrow transplantation. *Blood* 1996; **88**: 824–30.

241 McDonald GB, Bouvier M, Hockenbery DM et al. Oral beclomethasone dipropionate for treatment of intestinal graft-versus-host disease: a randomized controlled trial. *Gastroenterology* 1998; **115**: 28–35.

242 Cragg L, Blazar BR, Defor T et al. A randomized trial comparing prednisone with antithymocyte globulin/prednisone as an initial systemic therapy for moderately severe acute graft-versus-host disease. *Biol Blood Marrow Transplant* 2000; **6**: 441–7.

243 Powles RL, Barrett AJ, Clink H et al. Cyclosporin A for the treatment of graft-versus-host disease in man. *Lancet* 1978; **2**: 1327–31.

244 Allison AC, Eugui EM. Purine metabolism and immunosuppressive effects of mycophenolate mofetil (MMF). *Clin Transplant* 1996; **10**: 77–84.

245 European Mycophenolate Mofetil Cooperative Study Group. Placebo-controlled study of mycophenolate mofetil combined with cyclosporin and corticosteroids for prevention of acute rejection. *Lancet* 1995; **345**: 1321–5.

246 Basara N, Blau WI, Romer E et al. Mycophenolate mofetil for the treatment of acute and chronic GVHD in bone marrow transplant patients. *Bone Marrow Transplant* 1998; **22**: 61–5.

247 Byers VS, Henslee PJ, Kernan NA et al. Use of an anti-pan T-lymphocyte ricin A chain immunotoxin in steroid-resistant acute graft-versus-host disease. *Blood* 1990; **75**: 1426–32.

248 Anasetti C, Martin PJ, Hansen JA et al. A phase I–II study evaluating the murine anti-IL-2 receptor antibody 2A3 for treatment of acute graft-versus-host disease. *Transplantation* 1990; **50**: 49–54.

249 Herve P, Wijdenes J, Bergerat JP et al. Treatment of corticosteroid resistant acute graft-versus-host disease by *in vivo* administration of anti-interleukin-2 receptor monoclonal antibody (B-B10). *Blood* 1990; **75**: 1017–23.

250 Belanger C, Esperou-Bourdeau H, Bordigoni P et al. Use of an anti-interleukin-2 receptor monoclonal antibody for GVHD prophylaxis in unrelated donor BMT. *Bone Marrow Transplant* 1993; **11**: 293–7.

251 Martin P, Schoch G, Fisher L et al. A retrospective analysis of therapy for acute graft-versus host disease after allogeneic marrow transplantation. *Blood* 1990; **76**: 1464–72.

252 Hings IM, Severson R, Filipovich AH et al. Treatment of moderate and severe acute GVHD after allogeneic bone marrow transplantation. *Transplantation* 1994; **58**: 437–42.

253 MacMillan ML, Weisdorf DJ, Davies SM et al. Early antithymocyte globulin therapy improves survival in patients with steroid-resistant acute graft-versus-host disease. *Biol Blood Marrow Transplant* 2002; **8**: 40–6.

254 Arai S, Margolis J, Zahurak M et al. Poor outcome in steroid-refractory graft-versus-host disease with antithymocyte globulin treatment. *Biol Blood Marrow Transplant* 2002; **8**: 155–60.

255 Gratama JW, Jansen J, Lipovich RA et al. Treatment of acute graft-versus-host disease with monoclonal antibody OKT3: clinical results and effect on circulating T lymphocytes. *Transplantation* 1984; **38**: 469–74.

256 Gleixner B, Kolb HJ, Holler E et al. Treatment of aGVHD with OKT3: clinical outcome and side-effects associated with release of TNF alpha. *Bone Marrow Transplant* 1991; **8**: 93–8.

257 Martin PJ, Shulman HM, Schubach WH et al. Fatal Epstein–Barr-virus-associated proliferation of donor B cells after treatment of acute graft-versus-host disease with a murine anti-T-cell antibody. *Ann Intern Med* 1984; **101**: 310–5.

258 Martin PJ, Hansen JA, Anasetti C et al. Treatment of acute graft-versus-host disease with anti-CD3 monoclonal antibodies. *Am J Kidney Dis* 1988; **11**: 149–52.

259 Witherspoon RP, Fisher LD, Schoch G et al. Secondary cancers after bone marrow transplantation for leukemia or aplastic anemia. *N Engl J Med* 1989; **321**: 784–9.

260 Anasetti C, Martin PJ, Storb R et al. Treatment of acute graft-versus-host disease with a nonmitogenic anti-CD3 monoclonal antibody. *Transplantation* 1992; **54**: 844–51.

261 van Oosterhout YV, van Emst L, Schattenberg AV et al. A combination of anti-CD3 and anti-CD7 ricin A-immunotoxins for the *in vivo* treatment of acute graft versus host disease. *Blood* 2000; **95**: 3693–701.

262 Carpenter PA, Appelbaum FR, Corey L et al. A humanized non-FcR-binding anti-CD3 antibody, visilizumab, for treatment of steroid-refractory graft-versus-host disease. *Blood* 2002; **99**: 2712–9.

263 Ferrara JL, Marion A, McIntyre JF et al. Amelioration of acute graft vs. host disease due to minor histocompatibility antigens by *in vivo* administration of anti-interleukin 2 receptor antibody. *J Immunol* 1986; **137**: 1874–7.

264 Brown PS Jr, Parenteau GL, Dirbas FM et al. Anti-Tac-H, a humanized antibody to the interleukin 2 receptor, prolongs primate cardiac allograft survival. *Proc Natl Acad Sci U S A* 1991; **88**: 2663–7.

265 Anasetti C, Hansen JA, Waldmann TA et al. Treatment of acute graft-versus-host disease with humanized anti-Tac: an antibody that binds to the interleukin-2 receptor. *Blood* 1994; **84**: 1320–7.

266 Martin PJ, Schoch G, Fisher L et al. A retrospective analysis of therapy for acute graft-versus-host disease: secondary treatment. *Blood* 1991; **77**: 1821–8.

267 Przepiorka D, Kernan NA, Ippoliti C et al. Daclizumab, a humanized anti-interleukin-2 receptor alpha chain antibody, for treatment of acute graft-versus-host disease. *Blood* 2000; **95**: 83–9.

268 Willenbacher W, Basara N, Blau IW et al. Treatment of steroid refractory acute and chronic graft-versus-host disease with daclizumab. *Br J Haematol* 2001; **112**: 820–3.

269 Deeg HJ, Blazar BR, Bolwell BJ et al. Treatment of steroid-refractory acute graft-versus-host disease with anti-CD147 monoclonal antibody ABX-CBL. *Blood* 2001; **98**: 2052–8.

270 Antin JH, Weinstein HJ, Guinan EC et al. Recombinant human interleukin-1 receptor antagonist in the treatment of steroid-resistant graft-versus-host disease. *Blood* 1994; **84**: 1342–8.

271 McCarthy PL Jr, Williams L, Harris-Bacile M et al. A clinical phase I–II study of recombinant human interleukin-1 receptor in glucocorticoid-resistant graft-versus-host disease. *Transplantation* 1996; **62**: 626–31.

272 Heslop HE, Benaim E, Brenner MK et al. Response of steroid-resistant graft-versus-host disease to lymphoblast antibody CBL1. *Lancet* 1995; **346**: 805–6.

273 Herve P, Flesch M, Tiberghien P et al. Phase I–II trial of a monoclonal anti-tumor necrosis factor alpha antibody for the treatment of refractory severe acute graft-versus-host disease. *Blood* 1992; **79**: 3362–8.

274 Durrant S, Mollee P, Morton AJ et al. Combination therapy with tacrolimus and anti-thymocyte globulin for the treatment of steroid-resistant graft-versus-host disease developing during cyclosporine prophylaxis. *Br J Haematol* 2001; **113**: 217–23.

275 Furlong T, Storb R, Anasetti C et al. Clinical outcome after conversion to FK506 (tacrolimus) therapy for acute graft-versus-host disease resistant to cyclosporine or for cyclosporine-associated toxicities. *Bone Marrow Transplant* 2000; **26**: 985–91.

276 Benito AI, Furlong T, Martin PJ et al. Sirolimus (rapamycin) for the treatment of steroid-refractory acute graft-versus-host disease. *Transplantation* 2001; **72**: 1924–9.

277 Eppinger T, Ehninger G, Steinert M et al. 8-Methoxypsoralen and ultraviolet A therapy for cutaneous manifestations of graft-versus-host disease. *Transplantation* 1990; **50**: 807–11.

278 Deeg HJ, Erickson K, Storb R et al. Photoinactivation of lymphohemopoietic cells: studies in transfusion medicine and bone marrow transplantation. *Blood Cells* 1992; **18**: 151–61; discussion 161–2.

279 Aubin F, Brion A, Deconinck E et al. Phototherapy in the treatment of cutaneous graft-versus-host disease: our preliminary experience in resistant patients. *Transplantation* 1995; **59**: 151–5.

280 Wiesmann A, Weller A, Lischka G et al. Treatment of acute graft-versus-host disease with PUVA (psoralen and ultraviolet irradiation): results of a pilot study. *Bone Marrow Transplant* 1999; **23**: 151–5.

281 Furlong T, Leisenring W, Storb R et al. Psoralen and ultraviolet A irradiation (PUVA) as therapy for steroid-resistant cutaneous acute graft-versus-host disease. *Biol Blood Marrow Transplant* 2002; **8**: 206–12.

282 Greinix HT, Volc-Platzer B, Kalhs P et al. Extracorporeal photochemotherapy in the treatment of severe steroid-refractory acute graft-versus-host disease: a pilot study. *Blood* 2000; **96**: 2426–31.

283 Dall'Amico R, Messina C. Extracorporeal photochemotherapy for the treatment of graft-versus-host disease. *Ther Apher* 2002; **6**: 296–304.

284 Bladon J, Taylor PC. Extracorporeal photopheresis in cutaneous T-cell lymphoma and graft-versus-host disease induces both immediate and progressive apoptotic processes. *Br J Dermatol* 2002; **146**: 59–68.

285 Alcindor T, Gorgun G, Miller KB *et al*. Immunomodulatory effects of extracorporeal photochemotherapy in patients with extensive chronic graft-versus-host disease. *Blood* 2001; **98**: 1622–5.

286 Gorgun G, Miller KB, Foss FM. Immunologic mechanisms of extracorporeal photochemotherapy in chronic graft-versus-host disease. *Blood* 2002; **100**: 941–7.

287 Gauvreau JM, Lenssen P, Cheney CL *et al*. Nutritional management of patients with intestinal graft-versus-host disease. *J Am Diet Assoc* 1981; **79**: 673–7.

288 Baehr PH, Levine DS, Bouvier ME *et al*. Oral beclomethasone dipropionate for treatment of human intestinal graft-versus-host disease. *Transplantation* 1995; **60**: 1231–8.

289 Bianco JA, Higano C, Singer J *et al*. The somatostatin analog octreotide in the management of the secretory diarrhea of the acute intestinal graft-versus-host disease in a patient after bone marrow transplantation. *Transplantation* 1990; **49**: 1194–5.

290 Ippoliti C, Champlin R, Bugazia N *et al*. Use of octreotide in the symptomatic management of diarrhea induced by graft-versus-host disease in patients with hematologic malignancies. *J Clin Oncol* 1997; **15**: 3350–4.

291 Goodrich JM, Mori M, Gleaves CA *et al*. Early treatment with ganciclovir to prevent cytomegalovirus disease after allogeneic bone marrow transplantation. *N Engl J Med* 1991; **325**: 1601–7.

292 Goodman JL, Winston DJ, Greenfield RA *et al*. A controlled trial of fluconazole to prevent fungal infections in patients undergoing bone marrow transplantation. *N Engl J Med* 1992; **326**: 845–51.

293 Lee SJ, Klar N, Weeks JC *et al*. Predicting costs of stem-cell transplantation. *J Clin Oncol* 2000; **18**: 64–71.

294 Weisdorf D, Haake R, Blazar B *et al*. Treatment of moderate–severe acute graft-versus-host disease after allogeneic bone marrow transplantation: an analysis of clinical risk features and outcome. *Blood* 1990; **75**: 1024–30.

295 MacMillan ML, Weisdorf DJ, Wagner JE *et al*. Response of 443 patients to steroids as primary therapy for acute graft-versus-host disease: comparison of grading systems. *Biol Blood Marrow Transplant* 2002; **8**: 387–94.

296 Beschorner WE, Tutschka PJ, Santos GW. Chronic graft-versus-host disease in the rat radiation chimera. I. Clinical features, hematology, histology, and immunopathology in long-term chimeras. *Transplantation* 1982; **33**: 393–9.

297 Tutschka P, Teasdall R, Beschorner WE, Santos GW. Chronic graft-versus-host disease in the rat radiation chimera. II. Immunological evaluation in long-term chimera. *Transplantation* 1982; **34**: 289–94.

298 Atkinson K, Incefy GS, Storb R *et al*. Low serum thymic hormone levels in patients with chronic graft-versus-host disease. *Blood* 1982; **59**: 1073–7.

299 Weinberg K, Blazar BR, Wagner JE *et al*. Factors affecting thymic function after allogeneic hematopoietic stem cell transplantation. *Blood* 2001; **97**: 1458–66.

300 Parkman R. Clonal analysis of murine graft-vs.-host disease. I. Phenotypic and functional analysis of T lymphocyte clones. *J Immunol* 1986; **136**: 3543–8.

301 Fialkow P, Gilchrist C, Allison AC. Autoimmunity in chronic graft-versus-host disease. *Clin Exp Immunol* 1973; **13**: 479–86.

302 Beschorner W, Tutschka PJ, Santos GW. Chronic graft-versus-disease in the rat radiation chimera. III. Immunology and immunopathology in rapidly induced models. *Transplantation* 1983; **35**: 224–30.

303 Graze PR, Gale RP. Chronic graft versus host disease: a syndrome of disordered immunity. *Am J Med* 1979; **66**: 611–20.

304 Lister J, Messner H, Keysteon E *et al*. Autoantibody analysis of patients with graft-versus-host disease. *J Clin Lab Immunol* 1987; **24**: 19–23.

305 Rouquette-Gally AM, Boyeldieu D, Prost AC *et al*. Autoimmunity after allogeneic bone marrow transplantation: a study of 53 long-term-surviving patients. *Transplantation* 1988; **46**: 238–40.

306 Dighiero G, Intrator L, Cordonnier C *et al*. High levels of anti-cytoskeleton autoantibodies are frequently associated with chronic GVHD. *Br J Haematol* 1987; **67**: 301–5.

307 Kier P, Penner E, Bakos S *et al*. Autoantibodies in chronic GVHD: high prevalence of antinucleolar antibodies. *Bone Marrow Transplant* 1990; **6**: 93–6.

308 Wesierska-Gadek J, Penner E, Hitchman E *et al*. Nucleolar proteins B23 and C23 as target antigens in chronic graft-versus-host disease. *Blood* 1992; **79**: 1081–6.

309 Bell SA, Faust H, Mittermuller J *et al*. Specificity of antinuclear antibodies in scleroderma-like chronic graft-versus-host disease: clinical correlation and histocompatibility locus antigen association. *Br J Dermatol* 1996; **134**: 848–54.

310 Sullivan KM, Agura E, Anasetti C *et al*. Chronic graft-versus-host disease and other late complications of bone marrow transplantation. *Semin Hematol* 1991; **28**: 250–9.

311 Remberger M, Aschan J, Lonnqvist B *et al*. An ethnic role for chronic, but not acute, graft-versus-host disease after HLA-identical sibling stem cell transplantation. *Eur J Haematol* 2001; **66**: 50–6.

312 Niederwieser D, Pepe M, Storb R *et al*. Factors predicting chronic graft-versus-host disease and survival after marrow transplantation for aplastic anemia. *Bone Marrow Transplant* 1989; **4**: 151–6.

313 Atkinson K, Horowitz MM, Gale RP *et al*. Risk factors for chronic graft-versus-host disease after HLA-identical sibling bone marrow transplantation. *Blood* 1990; **75**: 2459–64.

314 Ochs LA, Miller WJ, Filipovich AH *et al*. Predictive factors for chronic graft-versus-host disease after histocompatible sibling donor bone marrow transplantation. *Bone Marrow Transplant* 1994; **13**: 455–60.

315 Carlens S, Ringden O, Remberger M *et al*. Risk factors for chronic graft-versus-host disease after bone marrow transplantation: a retrospective single centre analysis. *Bone Marrow Transplant* 1998; **22**: 755–61.

316 Wagner JL, Seidel K, Boeckh M *et al*. De novo chronic graft-versus-host disease in marrow graft recipients given methotrexate and cyclosporine: risk factors and survival. *Biol Blood Marrow Transplant* 2000; **6**: 633–9.

317 Remberger M, Kumlien G, Aschan J *et al*. Risk factors for moderate-to-severe chronic graft-versus-host disease after allogeneic hematopoietic stem cell transplantation. *Biol Blood Marrow Transplant* 2002; **8**: 674–82.

318 Ringden O, Remberger M, Ruutu T *et al*. Increased risk of chronic graft-versus-host disease, obstructive bronchiolitis, and alopecia with busulfan vs. total body irradiation: long-term results of a randomized trial in allogeneic marrow recipients with leukemia. Nordic Bone Marrow Transplantation Group. *Blood* 1999; **93**: 2196–201.

319 Socie G, Clift RA, Blaise D *et al*. Busulfan plus cyclophosphamide compared with total-body irradiation plus cyclophosphamide before marrow transplantation for myeloid leukemia: long-term follow-up of four randomized studies. *Blood* 2001; **98**: 3569–74.

320 Morton A, Gooley T, Hansen JA *et al*. Association between pretransplant interferon-alpha and outcome after unrelated donor marrow transplantation for chronic myelogenous leukemia in chronic phase. *Blood* 1998; **92**: 394–401.

321 Lee SJ, Klein JP, Anasetti C *et al*. The effect of pretransplant interferon therapy on the outcome of unrelated donor hematopoietic stem cell transplantation for patients with chronic myelogenous leukemia in first chronic phase. *Blood* 2001; **98**: 3205–11.

322 Balleari E, Garre S, Van Lint MT *et al*. Hormone replacement therapy and chronic graft-versus-host disease activity in women treated with bone marrow transplantation for hematologic malignancies. *Ann N Y Acad Sci* 2002; **966**: 187–92.

323 Zaucha JM, Gooley T, Bensinger WI *et al*. CD34 cell dose in granulocyte colony-stimulating factor-mobilized peripheral blood mononuclear cell grafts affects engraftment kinetics and development of extensive chronic graft-versus-host disease after human leukocyte antigen-identical sibling transplantation. *Blood* 2001; **98**: 3221–7.

324 Majolino I, Saglio G, Scime R *et al*. High incidence of chronic GVHD after primary allogeneic peripheral blood stem cell transplantation in patients with hematologic malignancies. *Bone Marrow Transplant* 1996; **17**: 555–60.

325 Champlin RE, Schmitz N, Horowitz MM *et al*. Blood stem cells compared with bone marrow as a source of hematopoietic cells for allogeneic transplantation. IBMTR Histocompatibility and Stem Cell Sources Working Committee and the European Group for Blood and Marrow Transplantation (EBMT). *Blood* 2000; **95**: 3702–9.

326 Przepiorka D, Anderlini P, Saliba R *et al*. Chronic graft-versus-host disease after allogeneic blood stem cell transplantation. *Blood* 2001; **98**: 1695–700.

327 Korbling M, Anderlini P. Peripheral blood stem cell versus bone marrow allotransplantation: does the source of hematopoietic stem cells matter? *Blood* 2001; **98**: 2900–8.

328 Mohty M, Kuentz M, Michallet M *et al*. Chronic graft-versus-host disease after allogeneic blood stem cell transplantation: long-term results of a randomized study. *Blood* 2002; **100**: 3128–34.

329 Mackinnon S, Papadopoulos EB, Carabasi MH *et al*. Adoptive immunotherapy evaluating escalating doses of donor leukocytes for relapse of chronic myeloid leukemia after bone marrow transplantation: separation of graft-versus-leukemia responses from graft-versus-host disease. *Blood* 1995; **86**: 1261–8.

330 Collins RH Jr, Shpilberg O, Drobyski WR *et al*. Donor leukocyte infusions in 140 patients with

relapsed malignancy after allogeneic bone marrow transplantation. *J Clin Oncol* 1997; **15**: 433–44.
331 Bonini C, Ferrari G, Verzeletti S *et al.* HSV-TK gene transfer into donor lymphocytes for control of allogeneic graft-versus-leukemia. *Science* 1997; **276**: 1719–24.
332 Cohen JL, Boyer O, Klatzmann D. Suicide gene therapy of graft-versus-host disease: immune reconstitution with transplanted mature T cells. *Blood* 2001; **98**: 2071–6.
333 Sullivan K, Storb R, Witherspoon RP *et al.* Deletion of immunosuppressive prophylaxis after marrow transplantation increases hyperacute graft-versus-host disease but does not influence chronic graft-versus-host disease or relapse in patients with advanced leukemia. *Clin Transplant* 1989; **3**: 5–11.
334 Bolger GB, Sullivan KM, Storb R *et al.* Second marrow infusion for poor graft function after allogeneic marrow transplantation. *Bone Marrow Transplant* 1986; **1**: 21–30.
335 deGast GC, Beatty PG, Amos D *et al.* Transfusions shortly before HLA-matched marrow transplantation for leukemia are associated with a decrease in chronic graft-versus-host disease. *Bone Marrow Transplant* 1991; **7**: 293–5.
336 Bostrom L, Ringden O, Jacobsen N *et al.* A European multicenter study of chronic graft-versus-host disease. The role of cytomegalovirus serology in recipients and donors: acute graft-versus-host disease, and splenectomy. *Transplantation* 1990; **49**: 1100–5.
337 Kalhs P, Schwarzinger I, Anderson G *et al.* A retrospective analysis of the long-term effect of splenectomy on late infections, graft-versus-host disease, relapse, and survival after allogeneic marrow transplantation for chronic myelogenous leukemia. *Blood* 1995; **86**: 2028–32.
338 Bostrom L, Ringden O, Sundberg B *et al.* Pretransplant herpes virus serology and chronic graft-versus-host disease. *Bone Marrow Transplant* 1989; **4**: 547–52.
339 Ljungman P, Niederwieser D, Pepe MS *et al.* Cytomegalovirus infection after marrow transplantation for aplastic anemia. *Bone Marrow Transplant* 1990; **6**: 295–300.
340 Kotani A, Ishikawa T, Matsumura Y *et al.* Correlation of peripheral blood OX40+ (CD134+) T cells with chronic graft-versus-host disease in patients who underwent allogeneic hematopoietic stem cell transplantation. *Blood* 2001; **98**: 3162–4.
341 Shulman HM, Sale GE, Lerner KG *et al.* Chronic cutaneous graft-versus-host disease in man. *Am J Pathol* 1978; **91**: 545–70.
342 Lawley TJ, Peck GL, Moutsopoulos HM *et al.* Scleroderma, Sjögren-like syndrome, and chronic graft-versus-host disease. *Ann Intern Med* 1977; **87**: 707–9.
343 Sullivan KM, Shulman HM, Storb R *et al.* Chronic graft-versus-host disease in 52 patients: adverse natural course and successful treatment with combination immunosuppression. *Blood* 1981; **57**: 267–76.
344 Nagler A, Goldenhersh MA, Levi-Schaffer F *et al.* Total leucoderma: a rare manifestation of cutaneous chronic graft-versus-host disease. *Br J Dermatol* 1996; **134**: 780–3.
345 Fenyk JR Jr, Smith CM, Warkentin PI *et al.* Sclerodermatous graft-versus-host disease limited to an area of measles exanthem. *Lancet* 1978; **1**: 472–3.
346 Socie G, Gluckman E, Cosset JM *et al.* Unusual localization of cutaneous chronic graft-versus-host disease in the radiation fields in four cases. *Bone Marrow Transplant* 1989; **4**: 133–5.
347 Freemer CS, Farmer ER, Corio RL *et al.* Lichenoid chronic graft-vs-host disease occurring in a dermatomal distribution. *Arch Dermatol* 1994; **130**: 70–2.
348 Ueda M, Mori T, Shiobara S *et al.* Development of bullous pemphigoid after allogeneic bone marrow transplantation: report of a case. *Transplantation* 1986; **42**: 320–2.
349 Ling NS, Fenske NA, Julius RL *et al.* Dyskeratosis congenita in a girl simulating chronic graft-vs.-host disease. *Arch Dermatol* 1985; **121**: 1424–8.
350 Ivker R, Woosley J, Resnick S. Dyskeratosis congenita or chronic graft-versus-host disease? A diagnostic dilemma in a child 8 years after bone marrow transplantation for aplastic anemia. *Pediatr Dermatol* 1993; **10**: 362–5.
351 Yau JC, Zander AR, Srigley JR *et al.* Chronic graft-versus-host disease complicated by micronodular cirrhosis and esophageal varices. *Transplantation* 1986; **41**: 129–30.
352 Epstein O, Thomas HC, Sherlock S. Primary biliary cirrhosis is a dry gland syndrome with features of chronic graft-versus-host disease. *Lancet* 1980; **1**: 1166–8.
353 Gratwhol AA, Moutsopoulos HM, Chused TM *et al.* Sjögren-type syndrome after allogeneic bone-marrow transplantation. *Ann Intern Med* 1977; **87**: 703–6.
354 Tichelli A, Duell T, Weiss M *et al.* Late-onset keratoconjunctivitis sicca syndrome after bone marrow transplantation: incidence and risk factors. European Group or Blood and Marrow Transplantation (EBMT) Working Party on Late Effects. *Bone Marrow Transplant* 1996; **17**: 1105–11.
355 Deeg HJ, Flournoy N, Sullivan KM *et al.* Cataracts after total body irradiation and marrow transplantation: a sparing effect of dose fractionation. *Int J Radiat Oncol Biol Phys* 1984; **10**: 957–64.
356 Benyunes MC, Sullivan K, Deeg HJ. Cataracts after bone marrow transplantation: long-term follow-up of adults treated with fractionated total body irradiation. *Int J Radiat Oncol Biol Phys* 1995; **32**: 661–70.
357 Schubert MM, Sullivan KM, Morton TH *et al.* Oral manifestations of chronic graft-vs.-host disease. *Arch Intern Med* 1984; **144**: 1591–5.
358 Schubert MM, Sullivan KM. Recognition, incidence, and management of oral graft-versus-host disease. *NCI Monogr* 1990; **9**: 135–43.
359 Schwarer AP, Hughes JM, Trotman-Dickenson B *et al.* A chronic pulmonary syndrome associated with graft-versus-host disease after allogeneic marrow transplantation. *Transplantation* 1992; **54**: 1002–8.
360 Duncker C, Dohr D, Harsdorf S *et al.* Non-infectious lung complications are closely associated with chronic graft-versus-host disease: a single center study of incidence, risk factors and outcome. *Bone Marrow Transplant* 2000; **25**: 1263–8.
361 Clark JG, Schwartz DA, Flournoy N *et al.* Risk factors for airflow obstruction in recipients of bone marrow transplants. *Ann Intern Med* 1987; **107**: 648–56.
362 Sullivan KM, Shulman HM. Chronic graft-versus-host disease, obliterative bronchiolitis, and graft-versus-leukemia effect: case histories. *Transplant Proc* 1989; **21**: 51–62.
363 Holland HK, Wingard JR, Beschorner WE *et al.* Bronchiolitis obliterans in bone marrow transplantation and its relationship to chronic graft-vs.-host disease and low serum IgG. *Blood* 1988; **72**: 621–7.
364 Sullivan KM. Intravenous immune globulin prophylaxis in recipients of a marrow transplant. *J Allergy Clin Immunol* 1989; **84**: 632–8; discussion 638–9.
365 Clark JG, Crawford SW, Madtes DK *et al.* Obstructive lung disease after allogeneic marrow transplantation: clinical presentation and course. *Ann Intern Med* 1989; **111**: 368–76.
366 Boas SR, Noyes BE, Kurland G *et al.* Pediatric lung transplantation for graft-versus-host disease following bone marrow transplantation. *Chest* 1994; **105**: 1584–6.
367 Rabitsch W, Deviatko E, Keil F *et al.* Successful lung transplantation for bronchiolitis obliterans after allogeneic marrow transplantation. *Transplantation* 2001; **71**: 1341–3.
368 McDonald GB, Sullivan KM, Schuffler MD *et al.* Esophageal abnormalities in chronic graft-versus-host disease in humans. *Gastroenterology* 1981; **80**: 914–21.
369 McDonald G, Sullivan KM, Plumley TF. Radiographic features of esophageal involvement in chronic graft-versus-host disease. *Am J Roentgenol* 1984; **142**: 501–6.
370 Nelson KR, McQuillen MP. Neurologic complications of graft-versus-host disease. *Neurol Clin* 1988; **6**: 389–403.
371 Marosi C, Budka H, Grimm G *et al.* Fatal encephalitis in a patient with chronic graft-versus-host disease. *Bone Marrow Transplant* 1990; **6**: 53–7.
372 Greenspan A, Deeg HJ, Cottler-Fox M *et al.* Incapacitating peripheral neuropathy as a manifestation of chronic graft-versus-host disease. *Bone Marrow Transplant* 1990; **5**: 349–52.
373 Smith C, Aarli J, Biberfeld P. Myasthenia gravis after bone marrow transplantation. *N Engl J Med* 1983; **309**: 1565–8.
374 Bolger GB, Sullivan KM, Spence AM *et al.* Myasthenia gravis after allogeneic bone marrow transplantation: relationship to chronic graft-versus-host disease. *Neurology* 1986; **36**: 1087–91.
375 Parker P, Chao NJ, Ben-Ezra J *et al.* Polymyositis as a manifestation of chronic graft-versus-host disease. *Medicine (Baltimore)* 1996; **75**: 279–85.
376 Stevens AM, Sullivan KM, Nelson JL. Polymyositis as a manifestation of chronic graft-versus-host disease. *Rheumatology (Oxford)* 2003; **42**: 34–9.
377 Corson SL, Sullivan K, Batzer F *et al.* Gynecologic manifestations of chronic graft-versus-host disease. *Obstet Gynecol* 1982; **60**: 488–92.
378 Schubert MA, Sullivan KM, Schubert MM *et al.* Gynecological abnormalities following allogeneic bone marrow transplantation. *Bone Marrow Transplant* 1990; **5**: 425–30.
379 Peralvo J, Bacigalupo A, Pittaluga PA *et al.* Poor graft function associated with graft-versus-host disease after allogeneic marrow transplantation. *Bone Marrow Transplant* 1987; **2**: 279–85.
380 Gomez-Garcia P, Herrera-Arroyo C, Torres-Gomez A *et al.* Renal involvement in chronic graft-versus-host disease: a report of two cases. *Bone Marrow Transplant* 1988; **3**: 357–62.
381 Miralbell R, Bieri S, Mermillod B *et al.* Renal toxicity after allogeneic bone marrow transplantation: the combined effects of total-body irradiation and graft-versus-host disease. *J Clin Oncol* 1996; **14**: 579–85.

382 Atkinson K, Norrie S, Chan P et al. Hematopoietic progenitor cell function after HLA-identical sibling bone marrow transplantation: influence of chronic graft-versus-host disease. *Int J Cell Cloning* 1986; **4**: 203–20.

383 Godder K, Pati AR, Abhyankar SH et al. De novo chronic graft-versus-host disease presenting as hemolytic anemia following partially mismatched related donor bone marrow transplant. *Bone Marrow Transplant* 1997; **19**: 813–7.

384 Ratanatharathorn V, Carson E, Reynolds C et al. Anti-CD20 chimeric monoclonal antibody treatment of refractory immune-mediated thrombocytopenia in a patient with chronic graft-versus-host disease. *Ann Intern Med* 2000; **133**: 275–9.

385 Siadak MF, Kopecky K, Sullivan KM. Reduction in transplant-related complications in patients given intravenous immunoglobulin after allogeneic marrow transplantation. *Clin Exp Immunol* 1994; **97** (Suppl. 1): 53–7.

386 Seidler C, Mills L, Flowers M et al. Spontaneous factor VIII inhibitor occurring in association with chronic graft-versus-host disease. *Am J Hematol* 1994; **45**: 240–3.

387 Socie G, Selimi F, Sedel L et al. Avascular necrosis of bone after allogeneic bone marrow transplantation: clinical findings, incidence and risk factors. *Br J Haematol* 1994; **86**: 624–8.

388 Stern JM, Chesnut CH III, Bruemmer B et al. Bone density loss during treatment of chronic GVHD. *Bone Marrow Transplant* 1996; **17**: 395–400.

389 Fink JC, Leisenring WM, Sullivan KM et al. Avascular necrosis following bone marrow transplantation: a case–control study. *Bone* 1998; **22**: 67–71.

390 Stern JM, Sullivan KM, Ott SM et al. Bone density loss after allogeneic hematopoietic stem cell transplantation: a prospective study. *Biol Blood Marrow Transplant* 2001; **7**: 257–64.

391 Sanders J. Effects of chronic graft-versus-host disease on growth and development. In: Burakoff SJ, Deeg HJ, Ferrara J, Atkinson K, eds. *Graft-versus-Host Disease: Immunology, Pathophysiology and Treatment*. New York: Marcel Dekker, 1990: 37; 665–80.

392 Zauner C, Rabitsch W, Schneeweiss B et al. Energy and substrate metabolism in patients with chronic extensive graft-versus-host disease. *Transplantation* 2001; **71**: 524–8.

393 Furst DE, Clements PJ, Graze P et al. A syndrome resembling progressive systemic sclerosis after bone marrow transplantation: a model for scleroderma? *Arthritis Rheum* 1979; **22**: 904–10.

394 Shulman HM, Sullivan KM, Weiden PL et al. Chronic graft-versus-host syndrome in man: a long-term clinicopathologic study of 20 Seattle patients. *Am J Med* 1980; **69**: 204–17.

395 Sullivan KM, Witherspoon RP, Storb R et al. Prednisone and azathioprine compared with prednisone and placebo for treatment of chronic graft-vs.-host disease: prognostic influence of prolonged thrombocytopenia after allogeneic marrow transplantation. *Blood* 1988; **72**: 546–54.

396 Loughran T, Sullivan K. Early detection and monitoring of chronic graft-versus-host disease. In: Burakoff SJ, Deeg HJ, Ferrara J, Atkinson K, eds. *Graft-versus-Host Disease: Immunology, Pathophysiology and Treatment*. New York: Marcel Dekker, 1990: 631–6.

397 Atkinson K, Horowitz MM, Gale RP et al. Consensus among bone marrow transplanters for diagnosis, grading and treatment of chronic graft-versus-host disease. Committee of the International Bone Marrow Transplant Registry. *Bone Marrow Transplant* 1989; **4**: 247–54.

398 Akpek G, Zahurak ML, Piantadosi S et al. Development of a prognostic model for grading chronic graft-versus-host disease. *Blood* 2001; **97**: 1219–26.

399 Lee SJ, Klein JP, Barrett AJ et al. Severity of chronic graft-versus-host disease: association with treatment-related mortality and relapse. *Blood* 2002; **100**: 406–14.

400 Loughran TP Jr, Sullivan K, Morton T et al. Value of day 100 screening studies for predicting the development of chronic graft-versus-host disease after allogeneic bone marrow transplantation. *Blood* 1990; **76**: 228–34.

401 Wagner JL, Flowers ME, Longton G et al. The development of chronic graft-versus-host disease: an analysis of screening studies and the impact of corticosteroid use at 100 days after transplantation. *Bone Marrow Transplant* 1998; **22**: 139–46.

402 Sullivan K, Siadak M. Stem cell transplantation. In: Johnson FL, Virgo KS, eds. *Cancer Patient Follow-Up*. St. Louis: Mosby, 1997: 490–518.

403 Jacobsohn DA, Montross S, Anders V et al. Clinical importance of confirming or excluding the diagnosis of chronic graft-versus-host disease. *Bone Marrow Transplant* 2001; **28**: 1047–51.

404 Atkinson K, Storb R, Ochs HD et al. Thymus transplantation after allogeneic bone marrow graft to prevent chronic graft-versus-host disease in humans. *Transplantation* 1982; **33**: 168–73.

405 Witherspoon RP, Sullivan KM, Lum LG et al. Use of thymic grafts or thymic factors to augment immunologic recovery after bone marrow transplantation: brief report with 2–12 years' follow-up. *Bone Marrow Transplant* 1988; **3**: 425–35.

406 Sullivan KM, Storek J, Kopecky KJ et al. A controlled trial of long-term administration of intravenous immunoglobulin to prevent late infection and chronic graft-vs.-host disease after marrow transplantation: clinical outcome and effect on subsequent immune recovery. *Biol Blood Marrow Transplant* 1996; **2**: 44–53.

407 Gluckman E, Horowitz MM, Champlin RE et al. Bone marrow transplantation for severe aplastic anemia: influence of conditioning and graft-versus-host disease prophylaxis regimens on outcome. *Blood* 1992; **79**: 269–75.

408 Ross M, Schmidt GM, Niland JC et al. Cyclosporine, methotrexate, and prednisone compared with cyclosporine and prednisone for prevention of acute graft-vs.-host disease: effect on chronic graft-vs.-host disease and long-term survival. *Biol Blood Marrow Transplant* 1999; **5**: 285–91.

409 Ruutu T, Volin L, Elonen E. Low incidence of severe acute and chronic graft-versus-host disease as a result of prolonged cyclosporine prophylaxis and early aggressive treatment with corticosteroids. *Tranplant Proc* 1988; **20**: 491–3.

410 Lonnquist B, Aschan J, Ljungman P et al. Long-term cyclosporin therapy may decrease the risk of chronic graft-versus-host disease. *Br J Haematol* 1990; **74**: 547–8.

411 Bacigalupo A, Maiolino A, Van Lint MT et al. Cyclosporin A and chronic graft versus host disease. *Bone Marrow Transplant* 1990; **6**: 341–4.

412 Storb R, Leisenring W, Anasetti C et al. Methotrexate and cyclosporine for graft-vs.-host disease prevention: what length of therapy with cyclosporine? *Biol Blood Marrow Transplant* 1997; **3**: 194–201.

413 Chao NJ, Parker PM, Niland JC et al. Paradoxical effect of thalidomide prophylaxis on chronic graft-vs.-host disease. *Biol Blood Marrow Transplant* 1996; **2**: 86–92.

414 Kansu E, Gooley T, Flowers ME et al. Administration of cyclosporine for 24 months compared with 6 months for prevention of chronic graft-versus-host disease: a prospective randomized clinical trial. *Blood* 2001; **98**: 3868–70.

415 Sullivan KM, Deeg HJ, Sanders JE et al. Late complications after marrow transplantation. *Semin Hematol* 1984; **21**: 53–63.

416 Koc S, Leisenring W, Flowers ME et al. Therapy for chronic graft-versus-host disease: a randomized trial comparing cyclosporine plus prednisone vs. prednisone alone. *Blood* 2002; **100**: 48–51.

417 Arora M, Wagner JE, Davies SM et al. Randomized clinical trial of thalidomide, cyclosporine, and prednisone vs. cyclosporine and prednisone as initial therapy for chronic graft-versus-host disease. *Biol Blood Marrow Transplant* 2001; **7**: 265–73.

418 Sullivan KM, Witherspoon RP, Storb R et al. Alternating-day cyclosporine and prednisone for treatment of high-risk chronic graft-vs.-host disease. *Blood* 1988; **72**: 555–61.

419 Koc S, Leisenring W, Flowers ME et al. Thalidomide for treatment of patients with chronic graft-versus-host disease. *Blood* 2000; **96**: 3995–6.

420 Sullivan KM, Siadak MF, Witherspoon RP. Cyclosporine treatment of chronic graft-versus-host disease following allogeneic bone marrow transplantation. *Transplant Proc* 1990; **22**: 1336–8.

421 Siadak M, Sullivan KM. The management of chronic graft-versus-host disease. *Blood Rev* 1994; **8**: 154–60.

422 Balduzzi A, Gooley T, Anasetti C et al. Unrelated donor marrow transplantation in children. *Blood* 1995; **86**: 3247–56.

423 Vogelsang GB, Farmer ER, Hess AD et al. Thalidomide for the treatment of chronic graft-versus-host disease. *N Engl J Med* 1992; **326**: 1055–8.

424 Sampaio EP, Sarno EN, Galilly R et al. Thalidomide selectively inhibits tumor necrosis factor alpha production by stimulated human monocytes. *J Exp Med* 1991; **173**: 699–703.

425 Gaziev D, Galimberti M, Lucarelli G et al. Chronic graft-versus-host disease: is there an alternative to the conventional treatment? *Bone Marrow Transplant* 2000; **25**: 689–96.

426 Vogelsang GB. How I treat chronic graft-versus-host disease. *Blood* 2001; **97**: 1196–201.

427 Lee SJ, Vogelsang G, Gilman A et al. A survey of diagnosis, management, and grading of chronic GVHD. *Biol Blood Marrow Transplant* 2002; **8**: 32–9.

428 Sullivan KM, Mori M, Sanders J et al. Late complications of allogeneic and autologous marrow transplantation. *Bone Marrow Transplant* 1992; **10** (Suppl. 1): 127–34.

429 Mookerjee B, Altomonte V, Vogelsang G. Salvage therapy for refractory chronic graft-versus-host disease with mycophenolate mofetil and tacrolimus. *Bone Marrow Transplant* 1999; **24**: 517–20.

430 Carnevale-Schianca F, Martin P, Sullivan K et al. Changing from cyclosporine to tacrolimus as salvage therapy for chronic graft-versus-host disease. *Biol Blood Marrow Transplant* 2000; **6**: 613–20.

431 Browne PV, Weisdorf DJ, DeFor T et al. Response to thalidomide therapy in refractory chronic graft-versus-host disease. *Bone Marrow Transplant* 2000; **26**: 865–9.

432 Akpek G, Lee SM, Anders V et al. A high-dose pulse steroid regimen for controlling active chronic graft-versus-host disease. Biol Blood Marrow Transplant 2001; 7: 495–502.

433 Parker PM, Chao N, Nademanee A et al. Thalidomide as salvage therapy for chronic graft-versus-host disease. Blood 1995; 86: 3604–9.

434 Lee SJ, Wegner SA, McGarigle CJ et al. Treatment of chronic graft-versus-host disease with clofazimine. Blood 1997; 89: 2298–302.

435 Vogelsang GB, Wolff D, Altomonte V et al. Treatment of chronic graft-versus-host disease with ultraviolet irradiation and psoralen (PUVA). Bone Marrow Transplant 1996; 17: 1061–7.

436 Barr M, Meiser BM, Kur F. Immunomodulation with photopheresis: clinical results of the multi-center cardiac transplantation study—reduction of the incidence of rejection by adjunct immunosuppression with photochemotherapy after heart transplantation. Transplantation 1994; 57: 563–8.

437 Owsianowski M, Gollnick H, Siegert W et al. Successful treatment of chronic graft-versus-host disease with extracorporeal photopheresis. Bone Marrow Transplant 1994; 14: 845–8.

438 Rossetti F, Zulian F, Dall'Amico R et al. Extracorporeal photochemotherapy as single therapy for extensive, cutaneous, chronic graft-versus-host disease. Transplantation 1995; 59: 149–51.

439 Rabitsch W, Reiter E, Keil F et al. Extracorporeal photopheresis (ECP) in extensive chronic graft-versus-host disease (GVHD). Blood 1997; 90 (Suppl.): 376a.

440 Smith EP, Sniecinski I, Dagis AC et al. Extracorporeal photochemotherapy for treatment of drug-resistant graft-vs.-host disease. Biol Blood Marrow Transplant 1998; 4: 27–37.

441 Greinix HT, Volc-Platzer B, Rabitsch W et al. Successful use of extracorporeal photochemotherapy in the treatment of severe acute and chronic graft-versus-host disease. Blood 1998; 92: 3098–104.

442 Socie G, Devergie A, Cosset JM et al. Low-dose (1 Gy) total-lymphoid irradiation for extensive, drug-resistant chronic graft-versus-host disease. Transplantation 1990; 49: 657–8.

443 Halevy O, Nagler A, Levi-Schaffer F et al. Inhibition of collagen type I synthesis by skin fibroblasts of graft versus host disease and scleroderma patients: effect of halofuginone. Biochem Pharmacol 1996; 52: 1057–63.

444 Nagler A, Pines M. Topical treatment of cutaneous chronic graft versus host disease with halofuginone: a novel inhibitor of collagen type I synthesis. Transplantation 1999; 68: 1806–9.

445 Marcellus DC, Altomonte VL, Farmer ER et al. Etretinate therapy for refractory sclerodermatous chronic graft-versus-host disease. Blood 1999; 93: 66–70.

446 Chiang KY, Abhyankar S, Bridges K et al. Recombinant human tumor necrosis factor receptor fusion protein as complementary treatment for chronic graft-versus-host disease. Transplantation 2002; 73: 665–7.

447 Lopez F, Parker P, Rodriquez D et al. Efficacy of mycophenolate mofetil (MMF) in the treatment of chronic graft-versus-host disease. Blood 2001; 98 (Suppl.): 398a [Abstract].

448 Gilman AL, Chan KW, Mogul A et al. Hydroxychloroquine for the treatment of chronic graft-versus-host disease. Biol Blood Marrow Transplant 2000; 6: 327–34.

449 Gaziev D, Lucarelli G, Polchi P et al. A three or more drug combination as effective therapy for moderate or severe chronic graft-versus-host disease. Bone Marrow Transplant 2001; 27: 45–51.

450 Goerner M, Gooley T, Flowers ME et al. Morbidity and mortality of chronic GVHD after hematopoietic stem cell transplantation from HLA-identical siblings for patients with aplastic or refractory anemias. Biol Blood Marrow Transplant 2002; 8: 47–56.

451 Knobler HY, Sagher U, Peled IJ et al. Tolerance to donor-type skin in the recipient of a bone marrow allograft: treatment of skin ulcers in chronic graft-versus-host disease with skin grafts from the bone marrow donor. Transplantation 1985; 40: 223–5.

452 Murphy PT, Sivakumaran M, Fahy G et al. Successful use of topical retinoic acid in severe dry eye due to chronic graft-versus-host disease. Bone Marrow Transplant 1996; 18: 641–2.

453 Singhal S, Powles R, Treleaven J et al. Pilocarpine hydrochloride for symptomatic relief of xerostomia due to chronic graft-versus-host disease or total-body irradiation after bone-marrow transplantation for hematologic malignancies. Leuk Lymphoma 1997; 24: 539–43.

454 Adams F, Messner H. Neuropharamacologic therapy of the neuromuscular manifestations of graft-versus-host disease. Proc Am Soc Clin Oncol 1987; 6: 145.

455 Fried R, Murakami CS, Fisher LD et al. Ursodeoxycholic acid treatment of refractory chronic graft-versus-host disease of the liver. Ann Intern Med 1992; 116: 624–9.

456 Storek J, Wells D, Dawson MA et al. Factors influencing B lymphopoiesis after allogeneic hematopoietic cell transplantation. Blood 2001; 98: 489–91.

457 Maury S, Mary JY, Rabian C et al. Prolonged immune deficiency following allogeneic stem cell transplantation: risk factors and complications in adult patients. Br J Haematol 2001; 115: 630–41.

458 Winston DJ, Schiffman G, Wang DC et al. Pneumococcal infections after human bone marrow transplantation. Ann Intern Med 1979; 91: 835–41.

459 Atkinson K, Farewell V, Storb R et al. Analysis of late infections after human bone marrow transplantation: role of genotypic nonidentity between marrow donor and recipient and of nonspecific suppressor cells in patients with chronic graft-versus-host disease. Blood 1982; 60: 714–20.

460 Engelhard D, Cordonnier C, Shaw PJ et al. Early and late invasive pneumococcal infection following stem cell transplantation: a European Bone Marrow Transplantation survey. Br J Haematol 2002; 117: 444–50.

461 Kulkarni S, Powles R, Treleaven J et al. Chronic graft versus host disease is associated with long-term risk for pneumococcal infections in recipients of bone marrow transplants. Blood 2000; 95: 3683–6.

462 Ochs L, Shu XO, Miller J et al. Late infections after allogeneic bone marrow transplantations: comparison of incidence in related and unrelated donor transplant recipients. Blood 1995; 86: 3979–86.

463 Sullivan KM, Meyers JD, Flournoy N et al. Early and late interstitial pneumonia following human bone marrow transplantation. Int J Cell Cloning 1986; 4 (Suppl. 1): 107–21.

464 Guidelines for preventing opportunistic infections among hematopoietic stem cell transplant recipients. Biol Blood Marrow Transplant 2000; 6: 659–713.

465 Winston DJ, Ho WG, Schiffman G et al. Pneumococcal vaccination of recipients of bone marrow transplants. Arch Intern Med 1983; 143: 1735–7.

466 Ljungman P, Fridell E, Lonnqvist B et al. Efficacy and safety of vaccination of marrow transplant recipients with a live attenuated measles, mumps, and rubella vaccine. J Infect Dis 1989; 159: 610–5.

467 Wingard JR, Piantadosi S, Vogelsang GB et al. Predictors of death from chronic graft-versus-host disease after bone marrow transplantation. Blood 1989; 74: 1428–35.

468 Weiden PL, Sullivan KM, Flournoy N et al. Antileukemic effect of chronic graft-versus-host disease: contribution to improved survival after allogeneic marrow transplantation. N Engl J Med 1981; 304: 1529–33.

469 Horowitz MM, Gale RP, Sondel PM et al. Graft-versus-leukemia reactions after bone marrow transplantation. Blood 1990; 75: 555–62.

470 Sullivan KM, Weiden PL, Storb R et al. Influence of acute and chronic graft-versus-host disease on relapse and survival after bone marrow transplantation from HLA-identical siblings as treatment of acute and chronic leukemia. Blood 1989; 73: 1720–8.

471 Witherspoon RP, Storb R, Pepe M et al. Cumulative incidence of secondary solid malignant tumors in aplastic anemia patients given marrow grafts after conditioning with chemotherapy alone. Blood 1992; 79: 289–91.

472 Deeg HJ, Socie G, Schoch G et al. Malignancies after marrow transplantation for aplastic anemia and Fanconi anemia: a joint Seattle and Paris analysis of results in 700 patients. Blood 1996; 87: 386–92.

473 Curtis RE, Rowlings PA, Deeg HJ et al. Solid cancers after bone marrow transplantation. N Engl J Med 1997; 336: 897–904.

474 Wingard JR, Curbow B, Baker F et al. Sexual satisfaction in survivors of bone marrow transplantation. Bone Marrow Transplant 1992; 9: 185–90.

475 Andrykowski MA, Altmaier EM, Barnett RL et al. The quality of life in adult survivors of allogeneic bone marrow transplantation: correlates and comparison with matched renal transplant recipients. Transplantation 1990; 50: 399–406.

476 Wingard JR, Curbow B, Baker F et al. Health, functional status, and employment of adult survivors of bone marrow transplantation. Ann Intern Med 1991; 114: 113–8.

477 Syrjala KL, Chapko MK, Vitaliano PP et al. Recovery after allogeneic marrow transplantation: prospective study of predictors of long-term physical and psychosocial functioning. Bone Marrow Transplant 1993; 11: 319–27.

478 Bush NE, Haberman M, Donaldson G et al. Quality of life of 125 adults surviving 6–18 years after bone marrow transplantation. Soc Sci Med 1995; 40: 479–90.

479 Duell T, van Lint M, Ljungman P. Health and functional status of long-term survivors of bone marrow transplantation. EBMT Working Party on Late Effects and EULEP Study Group on Late Effects. European Group for Blood Marrow Transplantation. Ann Intern Med 1997; 126: 184–92.

480 Deeg HJ, Leisenring W, Storb R et al. Long-term outcome after marrow transplantation for severe aplastic anemia. Blood 1998; 91: 3637–45.

481 Chiodi S, Spinelli S, Ravera G et al. Quality of life in 244 recipients of allogeneic bone marrow transplantation. Br J Haematol 2000; 110: 614–9.

482 Bush NE, Donaldson GW, Haberman MH et al. Conditional and unconditional estimation of multidimensional quality of life after hematopoietic stem cell transplantation: a longitudinal follow-up of 415 patients. Biol Blood Marrow Transplant 2000; 6: 576–91.

483 Lee S, Cook EF, Soiffer R et al. Development and validation of a scale to measure symptoms of chronic graft-versus-host disease. Biol Blood Marrow Transplant 2002; 8: 444–52.

51

John R. Wingard & Helen L. Leather

Bacterial Infections

Introduction

Susceptibility to infection has posed one of the most formidable challenges in the clinical management of patients undergoing hematopoietic cell transplantation (HCT) from the earliest days of this treatment. A variety of advances in infection control have permitted major strides in the supportive care of transplant recipients and these have translated into improved outcomes. Increased understanding of the pathogenesis of infectious syndromes, introduction of new antimicrobial agents, adoption of empirical antibiotics during aplasia before engraftment, development of novel strategies to prevent and treat infections, and recognition of the contributory role of infectious pathogens to the morbidity of other transplant complications, especially graft-vs.-host disease (GVHD), have all been responsible for improved survival rates. Advances including peripheral blood hematopoietic cells as alternative sources of bone marrow cells have resulted in faster engraftment of both platelets and neutrophils, leading to shorter length of stay, fewer days of fever and less antibiotic use. The increasing use of nonmyeloablative transplants, which are associated with less gastrointestinal (GI) and overall chemotherapy-induced toxicity, are also associated with reduced infectious complications. However, shifts in the patterns of opportunistic pathogens, changing antimicrobial susceptibility, differences in host immunodeficiency with implementation of new immunosuppressive regimens for GVHD, introduction of new conditioning regimens for use in the treatment of solid tumors and the increasing use of alternate donors continue to pose new and different challenges and opportunities for the management of infectious complications.

Biology of bacterial pathogens

Bacteria are found in a great variety of environments. They are classified as prokaryotic microorganisms distinguished by absence of a membrane enclosing their DNA and absence of other membrane-bound organelles. More than 2500 species of bacteria are known. Classification consists of the broad grouping of medically significant bacteria based on their staining properties using the Gram stain (positive or negative), morphology (cocci, bacilli) and oxygen tolerance (aerobic, anaerobic). Other properties, including DNA and RNA homology, ribosomal RNA homology, biochemical properties, specialized growth requirements and antigenic attributes, have also been used for further characterization.

In general, bacteria have cell walls made of peptidoglycan, a molecule unique to bacteria and thus a target for many antimicrobial agents. The cell wall provides the basic shape of the organism and confers rigidity. The Gram stain detects differences in the cell wall structure of bacteria. These differences are useful in distinguishing both antibiotic susceptibility and the potential for interacting with host defenses. Gram-positive bacteria have walls that consist of thick layers of peptidoglycan, teichoic acids, teichuronic acids and other polysaccharides. Inhibition of peptidoglycan synthesis is the mechanism of action of a variety of antibiotics, including penicillins, cephalosporins and glycopeptides. The cell wall of gram-negative organisms consists of an outer membrane composed of protein, lipopolysaccharide (LPS) and phospholipid and a thin inner layer of peptidoglycan. Protein components of the membrane, known as porins, serve as permeability conduits for hydrophilic molecules. The size and number of porins determine permeability to various molecules, including antibiotics.

Several properties are important in the ability of a given bacterial species to colonize or invade the human host (Table 51.1). These include adherence to host cells, the capacity to acquire iron from the host, elaboration of toxins and successful competition with other microbial colonizers for nutrients. Adhesins on the surface of bacteria interact with specific receptors on host tissue targets. Differences in either the adhesin molecules or host cell receptor binding determine tissue tropism. Various structures exist on the surface of medically important bacterial pathogens, which are important virulence factors. A capsule of polysaccharide can afford protection against phagocytosis. Immunological diversity of such capsules within species is common (the basis for serotyping) and can permit evasion of the normal host defenses since opsonizing antibodies directed against the specific antigens of the capsule are important for phagocytosis. In gram-negative bacteria, pili are important means by which bacteria adhere to epithelial cells. Gram-positive bacteria may have surface proteins (e.g. the M protein of group A streptococci or staphylococcal protein A) that serve as virulence factors. Bacterial products such as superantigens may provoke host responses that are deleterious to maintenance of host physiology. Exotoxins produced during exponential growth and released by both gram-positive and gram-negative bacteria interfere with normal host cell metabolism and contribute to host toxicity. Certain toxins, known as bacteriocins, are elaborated to enhance an organism's competition with other microorganisms within the normal flora to establish an ecological niche. The production of certain extracellular enzymes, such as hyaluronidase, neuraminidase, elastase and collagenase, facilitates overcoming anatomical barriers and promotes spread past tissue barriers. Proteins may be produced that facilitate entry into host cells. Disruption of host humoral responses by proteases permits traversing of mucosal barriers and survival in extracellular tissue as well as serum.

Avoidance of phagocytosis or killing of microorganisms once ingested is the role of a variety of virulence factors. The polysaccharide capsule of many organisms is designed both to resist humoral immunity and impede phagocytosis. Bacterial LPS (endotoxin) serves as an important barrier

Table 51.1 Bacterial virulence factors.

Molecule	Effects on host
Adhesins	Adhere to mucus or mucosal cells
Exotoxins	Interfere with cellular physiology
Endotoxins	Elicit sepsis syndrome
Bacteriocins	Establish ecological niche in host flora
Exoenzymes	Disrupt anatomical barriers, facilitate tissue invasion
Proteases	Degrade humoral immune responses and complement
Polysaccharide capsules	Resist humoral immunity and phagocytosis
Plasmids, phages, transposons	Confer antibiotic resistance, multiple virulence properties, rapid adaptation to environment
Regulatory factors	Allow rapid adaptation to environmental changes
Biofilms	Form barrier to exclude antibiotics

Table 51.2 Targets for various antibiotics.

Bacterial targets	Antibiotics
Peptidoglycan synthesis	Penicillins, cephalosporins, glycopeptides
Lipopolysaccharide	Antibodies to endotoxins or cytokines mediating sepsis syndrome
Penicillin-binding proteins	Penicillins, cephalosporins, carbapenems
Beta-lactamases	Clavulanic acid, sulbactam, tazobactam
Ribosomes	Aminoglycosides, macrolides, tetracyclines, chloramphenicol
RNA polymerases	Rifamycins
Folic acid synthesis	Sulfonamides, trimethoprim
DNA gyrase	Fluoroquinolones

against bile salts, lytic enzymes, DNA and heavy metals. LPS also contains a carbohydrate moiety (the O antigen) that resists complement binding and differs antigenically from strain to strain. The generation of such antigenic diversity is a mechanism that bacteria use to evade host humoral immune responses. LPS induces the sepsis syndrome by causing the release of a variety of proinflammatory cytokines, such as tumor necrosis factor-alpha (TNF-α), interleukin 1 (IL-1), interferon-gamma (IFN-γ) and various colony-stimulating factors by monocytes and macrophages and triggering a variety of host enzymatic mechanisms, including complement, clotting, fibrinolytic and kinin pathways.

A number of gene products on extrachromosomal elements, such as plasmids, phages, insertion elements and transposons, provide bacteria with mechanisms to rapidly adapt to a competitive environment, conferring antibiotic resistance and multiple virulence properties, which can be shared between a wide variety of unrelated microbes. A variety of regulatory proteins provide bacteria with the capacity to respond favorably to rapid shifts in the environment, such as temperature, iron and pH. These proteins facilitate adherence and invasiveness and modify expression of other proteins on the cell surface to optimize the organism's competitive stance. Antigenic variation of these proteins are the mechanisms used by bacteria to evade host immune responses. These characteristics of bacteria offer a range of bacterial targets for antimicrobial agents (Table 51.2).

The host microbial flora itself may act as a barrier against opportunistic pathogens. Ordinarily, complex bacterial communities reside on the body's surfaces and within the GI tract without deleterious effects. However, when the interactions are altered by the use of antimicrobial agents or other infection control measures, this natural barrier may be compromised and overgrowth of pathogens that might otherwise not be capable of establishing a niche can occur. The normal commensal flora prevent the establishment of opportunistic pathogens by competition for the same nutrients or receptors on host cells through the production of toxic products, fatty acids or other metabolites that inhibit growth of potential competitors and stimulation of the host immune system.

Some bacteria routinely cause disease in susceptible hosts who have normal defenses and these certainly can cause morbidity in the HCT recipient. However, more commonly infectious morbidity in the HCT recipient is caused by bacterial organisms (such as many gram-negative bacteria, α-streptococci and *Staphylococcus epidermidis*) that ordinarily are not pathogens. These organisms, known as opportunistic pathogens, exploit deficits in host defenses that occur as a result of the transplant procedure or nosocomial procedures, or they exploit microbial shifts caused by infection control measures. Whether or not an opportunistic pathogen causes disease is a reflection of an interplay between its own inherent virulence, whether it has access to the host in sufficient numbers and the state of the host defenses. Thus, effective infection control measures must address issues related to minimizing exposure to potential pathogens, the strategic use of antimicrobial agents to suppress microbial burden and, where possible, bolstering host defenses.

Antibiotic resistance

One of the most successful attributes bacteria have to enhance survival is the capacity for genetic variability. This capacity is frequently used by bacterial organisms to foil clinicians' attempts to control infection by antibiotics. Through point mutations, rearrangement of entire sequences of DNA to different locations within the bacterial genome (e.g. transposons), or the transfer of DNA from one bacterial organism to another (e.g. via plasmids), development of antibiotic resistance can occur in a variety of ways (Table 51.3).

A common mechanism is inactivation of antibiotics by enzymes. For example, staphylococci and many gram-negative bacteria produce a class of enzymes known as beta-lactamases that render inactive beta-lactam antibiotics, the group of molecules that includes the penicillins, multiple cephalosporins (e.g. cephalothin, cefuroxime, ceftazidime, moxalactam, cefoxitin, cefaclor, etc.), carbapenems (e.g. imipenem, meropenem) and monobactams (e.g. aztreonam). Beta-lactamase genes found on

Table 51.3 Mechanisms of antibiotic resistance.

Mechanism	Examples	Genetic basis	Types of bacteria	Antibiotic affected
Inhibition of antibiotic by enzymes	Beta-lactamases	Chromosomal, plasmids, transporons	Staphylococci, many gram-negative bacteria	Penicillins, cephalosporins
	Acetyl transferases	Plasmids	Many gram-negative bacteria	Aminoglycosides, chloramphenicol
	Phosphotransferases	Plasmids	Many gram-negative bacteria	Chloramphenicol, aminoglycosides
	Nucleotidyltransferases	Plasmids	Many gram-negative bacteria	Aminoglycosides
Reduced membrane permeability of antibiotic	Mutations involving porins	Chromosomal	Many gram-negative bacteria	Beta-lactams, aminoglycosides, carbapenems, nalidixic acid, fluoroquinolones
Increased efflux of antibiotics	New proteins	Chromosomal, plasmids, transporons	Many gram-negative bacteria and staphylococci	Tetracyclines, macrolides, flouroquinolones
Altered targets	Changes in ribosomal binding sites	Chromosomal, plasmids	Gram-positive and -negative bacteria	Tetracyclines, macrolides, aminoglycosides, lincosamides
	Changes in cell wall	Chromosomal, plasmids	Gram-positive bacteria	Vancomycin, other glycopeptides
	Changes in penicillin-binding proteins	Chromosomal, plasmids	Gram-positive and some gram-negative bacteria	Penicillins, cephalosporins
	Changes in dihydropteroate synthetase	Plasmids	Many gram-negative	Sulfonamides
	Changes in dihydrofolate reductase	Chromosomal, plasmids	Gram-negative bacteria	Trimethoprim
	Changes in DNA gyrases	Chromosomal, plasmids	Gram-negative bacteria	Nalidixic acid, fluoroquinolones
Exclusion barrier	Biofilm formation	Chromosomal	*Staphylococcus epidermidis*, *Pseudomonas aeruginosa*	Multiple

transposons or plasmids permit spread of resistance widely. Unfortunately, prevalent use of the beta-lactam class of antibiotics, particularly third-generation cephalosporins, has resulted in selection pressure to give advantage to resistant organisms and further encourage spread.

Reduced entry of the antibiotic into bacterial organisms by alteration of permeability can be caused by mutations involving different porins. Such changes are potential mechanisms for resistance to nalidixic acid, fluoroquinolones (such as norfloxacin, ciprofloxacin, gatifloxacin, levofloxacin, ofloxacin), aminoglycosides and beta-lactams, among others. Alternatively, resistance to some antibiotics may occur by an increase in efflux of antibiotics from the bacterial organism. This can take place by mutations in chromosomal genes or acquisition of new genes from plasmids that lead to new membrane proteins which reduce the retention of certain antibiotics, such as tetracyclines in gram-negative bacteria and macrolides (such as erythromycin, azithromycin, clarithromycin) in gram-positive bacteria.

Alteration of the target of the antibiotic is another strategy. Multiple examples are notable. Changes in ribosomal binding sites may lead to resistance to tetracyclines, aminoglycosides or macrolides, while changes in the constituents of the cell wall or their building blocks may confer resistance to antibiotics such as vancomycin. Mutations in the genes that encode for penicillin-binding proteins (PBPs) alter susceptibility to beta-lactams, such as the penicillins and cephalosporins. A variety of target enzymes (as shown in Table 51.3) that can be changed by mutations can potentially lead to resistance to sulfonamides, trimethoprim, nalidixic acid and fluoroquinolones, among other antibiotics.

The emergence of widespread antibiotic resistance can impede the best efforts of clinicians to control infections by various bacterial pathogens. Clearly, a cornerstone of any infection control program is the wise use of antibiotics. Repeated pleas by the Centers for Disease Control and Prevention (CDC) and other authoritative bodies [1–3] for clinicians to practice antimicrobial stewardship have regrettably failed to slow the continuing emergence of drug resistance. However, several strategies have been offered [1–4]. Patients colonized or infected with resistant organisms should be isolated [2]. Each institution should maintain a program of surveillance for resistance to detect shifts in susceptibility and trends of problem organisms. Certain antimicrobial agents may need to be restricted to reduce the prevalence of specific resistant organisms [4,5]. Certain antibiotics initiated empirically for suspected organisms (e.g. vancomycin) should be discontinued once it has been determined that they are not needed. Such efforts will reduce selection pressures and spread of antibiotic resistance among microbial populations.

Compromised host defenses

Host defenses are compromised by a variety of factors following HCT. The degree and type of compromise of host defenses change over time [6]. Three periods have been described: (i) early recovery, corresponding to the first several weeks after transplantation, the pre-engraftment phase; (ii) mid-recovery, corresponding to the 2nd and 3rd months after transplant, the early post-engraftment phase; and (iii) late recovery, corresponding to the interval beyond 3 months. Table 51.4 lists the predominant deficits that are present at various intervals.

Early recovery (phase I)

The cytoreductive agents used in conventional conditioning regimens damage rapidly dividing cell populations, particularly bone marrow progenitors and mucosal epithelial cells. For several weeks after HCT, pancytopenia and damage to the mucosal barriers are predominant deficits in the host defenses against infectious pathogens.

The duration of neutropenia varies according to the number of stem

Table 51.4 Host defenses compromised by hematopoietic cell transplantation (HCT) that make patients vulnerable to bacterial infections.

Early recovery
Neutropenia
Oral and gastrointestinal mucosal damage due to cytoreductive therapy
Skin barrier compromised by CVCs

Mid-recovery
Skin and gastrointestinal mucosal damage due to GVHD
Decreased cellular immunity due to GVHD and immunosuppressive therapy
Skin barrier compromised by CVCs
Decreased cellular immunity due to viral infections, especially CMV

Late recovery
Decreased cellular immunity; persistent with chronic GVHD
Nonspecific suppressor cells with chronic GVHD
Reduced opsonization
Decreased reticuloendothelial function
IgG subclass deficiencies

CMV, cytomegalovirus; CVCs, central venous catheters; GVHD, graft-vs.-host disease; IgG, immunoglobulin G.

cells used to effect reconstitution, the occurrence of certain viral infections, especially cytomegalovirus (CMV), the use of immunosuppressive agents after transplantation as part of the GVHD prophylaxis, the use of agents to purge the marrow stem cells *ex vivo* from contaminating tumor cells and the use of cytokines to stimulate recovery. In the autologous transplant setting, the number of prior treatment regimens, the prior use of radiotherapy and the use of certain chemotherapeutic agents that are known to damage hematopoietic cells, such as nitrosoureas and melphalan, negatively influence the ability to obtain stem cells, leading to delays in engraftment. In the allogeneic transplant setting, human leukocyte antigen (HLA) disparity between donor and recipient, T-lymphocyte depletion of the graft and inadequate conditioning of the recipient to eliminate host immune cells can impede robust engraftment as well.

The duration and the depth of neutropenia independently influence the risk for infection [7,8]. Although the risk for bacterial infection increases incrementally as the circulating neutrophil count falls below 1000/μL, the risk becomes substantial below 500/μL. Bacteremia and life-threatening bacterial infection occur mostly at neutrophil counts below 100/μL. Indeed, in HCT recipients, 90% of the bacterial infections occur at neutrophil counts below 100/μL [9–11].

The degree of mucosal damage varies according to the preparative regimen. Busulfan, etoposide (VP16), melphalan, cytarabine, cyclophosphamide and total body irradiation (TBI) are associated with varying degrees of mucositis. Although stomatitis is readily observable, damage to the mucosa of the entire GI tract occurs. Attempts to reliably quantify the degree of mucosal damage are primitive and have hampered efforts to correlate the degree of mucosal damage with infection risk along the same lines that the neutrophil count and the risk for infection have been quantified. However, the use of the D-xylose absorption test, a measure of mucosal functional integrity, has been evaluated in leukemic patients. An association between the degree of D-xylose absorption and the risk for infection has been noted [12,13]. Reactivation of herpes simplex virus (HSV) type 1 (which occurs in approximately 70% of seropositive patients, usually during the 1st or 2nd week after HCT unless acyclovir prophylaxis is given) can lead to diffuse or localized ulceration of the mucosa of the oral cavity and the lower oesophagus. This change has been associated with bacteremia from organisms that reside on the buccal mucosa. Reactivation of HSV type II occurs in seropositive patients and can result in urethral, labial, perineal and perianal skin and mucosal breakdown. The use of cytotoxic agents after HCT, such as methotrexate (MTX) or cyclophosphamide (CY) to prevent GVHD, can also result in exacerbation of mucositis and delays in healing, as can the corticosteroids.

The nearly universal use of indwelling central venous catheters (CVCs) today poses a risk for infection, both early and late after HCT. Such catheters compromise the integrity of the integument as a physical barrier to potential pathogens residing on the skin. Marrow puncture sites and peripheral venous catheters can also compromise the skin barrier.

The use of nonmyeloablative HCT is increasing, utilizing the immune system rather than chemotherapy to achieve disease control. The lower intensity conditioning regimens that are used limit the development of neutropenia and mucositis is also significantly diminished. As a consequence, this new type of HCT has demonstrated differences in infection patterns compared with conventional allogeneic HCT [14,15]. The incidence of early bacteremias (day 0–30) is low and this accounts for a low rate of bacteremia during the first 100 days.

Mid-recovery (phase II)

Following engraftment, patients enter a period of profound deficiency of cellular and humoral immunity. The degree and duration of immunodeficiency are influenced by the type of HCT, the degree of donor and recipient histocompatibility, whether T lymphocytes have been eliminated from the allogeneic marrow graft, the use of immunological or pharmacological purging of autologous marrow, the post-transplant immunosuppressive treatment given as GVHD prophylaxis, the occurrence of certain viral infections (especially CMV) and the occurrence and severity of GVHD. The integrity of mucosal barriers may continue to be compromised by recurrent HSV infections, the use of cytotoxic agents and intestinal involvement by GVHD. Indwelling venous catheters typically remain in place during this period, adding to the patient's vulnerability for infection from skin bacterial flora.

Late recovery (phase III)

With time, there is gradual recovery of both cellular and humoral immunity (discussed in Chapter 62). Generally, immune recovery is more rapid after autologous than allogeneic HCT. Among autograft recipients, those given myeloablative preparative regimens (as typically used for acute leukemia) are more immunodeficient, and are more immunodeficient for longer intervals, than those given less intensive, nonablative regimens, such as those used for solid tumor therapy. Immune recovery following peripheral blood autotransplantation may be more rapid than after autologous marrow transplantation. Recipients of CD34 selected grafts have slower T-cell immune reconstitution [16]. Immune recovery after matched-related HLA-identical transplantation appears to be more rapid than after HLA-disparate or HLA-matched unrelated donor transplantation.

The occurrence of GVHD also influences the tempo of immune recovery and is associated with dysregulated immune responses (see Chapter 50). If chronic GVHD occurs, cellular and humoral immunodeficiency may persist for months and even years [17,18]. Reticuloendothelial function can also be severely impaired, especially in patients with chronic GVHD. Immunoglobulin (Ig) deficiencies can occur. Even in the face of normal levels of the isotypes, IgG subclass deficiencies, especially of subclass II, can be present.

By 1 year, immune recovery is nearly complete in recipients of matched-related transplants. However, in matched-unrelated donor and mismatched family-related donor transplants, immune recovery may lag substantially. Even in the absence of overt GVHD, vulnerability for recurrent sinopulmonary infections can persist for much longer periods than for those seen after HLA-matched sibling transplants [19,20]. Responses to immunizations may be impaired up to 1 year or longer.

Spectrum of bacterial infections

Just as the defects in host immunity vary over time, so does the spectrum of infections. In Fig. 51.1, the various infectious syndromes that occur at different times after HCT are portrayed [6]. As noted previously, relative to viral and fungal infections, bacterial infections predominate during the early recovery phase whereas viral and fungal infections predominate during the mid- and late recovery phases. However, there are important differences that vary over time, as noted in Tables 51.5 and 51.6.

Early recovery (phase I)

Between 48% and 60% or more of neutropenic patients with fever have infection, either established or occult. Because signs and symptoms of infection are attenuated during neutropenia [21], and untreated bacterial infections during neutropenia may be rapidly life threatening, neutropenic fevers should operationally be regarded as infectious until proven otherwise.

Bacterial pathogens account for more than 90% of the first infections during neutropenia. Gram-negative bacteria are the most virulent bacterial pathogens during neutropenia and historically have been major causes of morbidity and mortality. Over the past 20 years the percentage of infections caused by gram-negative organisms has steadily decreased from 70% to 30%. However, several centers have again started to notice an increase in the incidence of gram-negative bacterial infections [22].

The most common gram-negative bacteria have been *Escherichia coli*, *Klebsiella* spp. and *Pseudomonas aeruginosa*. In recent years several other organisms such as *Acinetobacter* spp., *Stenotrophomonas* spp. [23,24], *Alcaligenes xylosoxidans* [25], *Serratia* spp. [26], *Legionella* [25] and *Burkholderia cepacia* [25] have increased. The portal of entry for these organisms generally is the damaged mucosa of the GI tract. Perianal fissures or skin breakdown are other potential sources, especially for *P. aeruginosa*. Occasionally, venous catheters can also serve as an entry site for gram-negative bacteria.

Gram-positive bacteria have emerged as major pathogens and bacteremia rates for gram-positive organisms now exceed those for gram-negative bacteria [22,27–29]. Gram-positive bacteria now account for 70% of bacterial infections, compared with 30% 25 years ago. This increase is in large part attributable to the nearly universal use of indwelling CVCs. The widespread use of antibiotics with gram-negative coverage to decontaminate the gut and reduce gram-negative infections has also contributed to the proliferation of gram-positive infections. Occasionally, gram-positive organisms may invade the host via the GI tract as well. *Staphylococcus epidermidis*, *Staphylococcus aureus*, α-hemolytic streptococci and *Corynebacterium* spp. [30] are the most common organisms.

The portal of entry for α-hemolytic streptococci is frequently the oral mucosa [31]. Thus, patients with stomatitis due to chemotherapy, radiotherapy, or HSV-induced mucosal ulcerations are particularly at risk. Several large series have reported bacteremia rates of 15–25% in HCT populations [32–36]. Where speciated, *Streptococcus mitis*, an organism that normally resides on the buccal mucosa, is the most common α-hemolytic streptococcus. Although gram-positive bacteria are less virulent than gram-negative bacteria, approximately 10% of α-hemolytic streptococcal bacteremias are associated with a toxic shock-like syndrome that can be fatal even with prompt antimicrobial therapy [32,33,37]. The use of fluoroquinolones in several series has been associated with an increased risk for streptococcal infection [36,38,39]. *Corynebacterium jeikeium* infections are associated with infected marrow

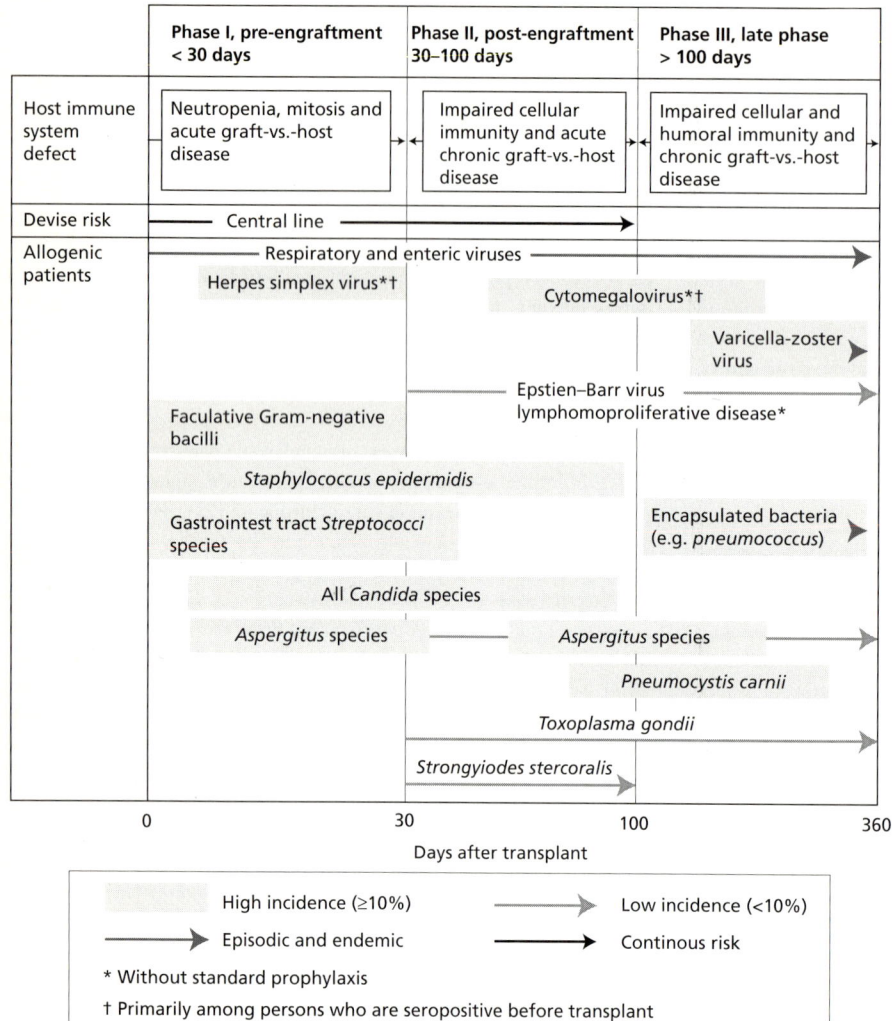

Fig. 51.1 Phases of opportunistic infections among allogenic hematopoietic stem cell (HSC) transplantation recipients.

Table 51.5 Bacterial and fungal infectious syndromes encountered early after hematopoietic cell transplantation (HCT) and during the pre-engraftment phase (early recovery or phase I).

Syndrome	Relative frequency*	Relative life-threatening potential
First fever		
Staphylococci	+++	+
α-Hemolytic streptococci	+	++
Gram-negative bacilli	+	+++
Subsequent fevers		
Antibiotic-resistant gram-negative bacilli	+	+++
Staphylococci	+++	+
Fungi	++	+++

*Increasing frequency and life-threatening potential depicted by increased number of "+" signs.

Table 51.6 Bacterial infections encountered after engraftment (mid- and late recovery).

	Relative frequency*		
Infection	Allogeneic HCT with no GVHD	Allogeneic HCT with GVHD	Autologous HCT
Mid-recovery (phase II)			
Staphylococci	++	++	++
Fungi	++	+++	+
Gram-negative bacilli	–	+	–
Late recovery (phase III)			
Encapsulated bacteria	–	++	–
Fungi	–	+	–

*Increasing frequency depicted by increased number of "+" signs; "–" indicates uncommon infections.
HCT, hematopoietic cell transplantation; GVHD, graft-vs.-host disease.

needle puncture sites or infected peripheral venous catheters, often with associated thrombophlebitis. Typically they are resistant to multiple antibiotics and frequently require catheter removal [30].

After institution of antibiotics during first fever, the microbial flora changes. Superinfections, as manifest by recurrent or persistent fever during the 2nd or subsequent week of neutropenia, are more heterogeneous in etiology (see Table 51.5). Gram-negative bacteria, especially those that are resistant to the antibiotic regimen used to treat the first febrile episode, are of paramount concern [40]. These bacteria account for only roughly 10% of superinfections but are the most virulent and have rapid

Table 51.7 Causes of fevers of obscure origin after engraftment.

Cytomegalovirus
Central venous catheter infections
Occult sinusitis
Hepatosplenic candidiasis
Pulmonary or disseminated *Aspergillus* infection

life-threatening potential if appropriate antibiotic modification is not made.

The most common etiologic agent is *Staphylococcus epidermidis*, which accounts for roughly half of superinfections. These organisms are less virulent than gram-negative bacteria and are quickly isolated from blood cultures of bacteremic patients. Thus, clinicians can wait until multiple blood cultures are positive to ensure that the isolate is a true pathogen rather than a harmless contaminant. Other potential causes of superinfection include fungal pathogens.

Mid-recovery (phase II)

With recovery of the neutrophil count, most bacterial infections resolve and antimicrobial agents can be discontinued. Fever of obscure etiology is occasionally noted in the mid-recovery period (Table 51.7). Sinusitis is a common cause of fever of uncertain etiology during this period [41]. Frequently it is without specific focal signs or symptoms but can readily be detected by either radiographs or computed tomographic scans of the sinuses [42]. Another cause of a fever could be an occult infection of the CVC. Blood cultures are helpful but may be unrevealing initially. Removal of the catheter is occasionally required to exclude this possibility in a patient with persistent obscure fever and is discussed under Treatment of intravascular catheter-related infections (p. 676).

Patients who have undergone allogeneic HCT are more susceptible to infections during the mid-recovery period than are autograft recipients [43], particularly if acute GVHD occurs and more intensive immunosuppression is necessary (see Table 51.6). Although viral and fungal infections predominate during this period, occasionally gram-negative bacteremias can occur as a result of GI mucosa barrier disruption from acute GVHD. Also, gram-positive bacteremia frequently occurs related to infections associated with the CVCs [44–47].

Late recovery (phase III)

Over time, with gradual immune recovery, the risk for infection progressively declines. Autograft recipients have a very low risk for bacterial infection late after the procedure. If the indwelling CVC remains in place, however, infections related to the catheter can continue to occur, especially if the catheter continues to be used or if fibrin sheaths develop. In the absence of chronic GVHD, allogeneic transplant recipients have a progressively declining risk for bacterial infection. However, patients with chronic GVHD are highly susceptible to recurrent bacterial infections, especially from encapsulated bacteria, including *Streptococcus pneumoniae*, *Hemophilus influenzae* and *Neisseria meningitidis*, due to low CD4-lymphocyte counts, poor reticuloendothelial function and low levels of opsonizing antibodies [17,19,20,48–50]. The continuing use of immunosuppressive therapy, especially corticosteroids with their deleterious effects on phagocytosis, renders the patient susceptible for recurrent infection. As noted earlier, patients who are the recipients of mismatched or matched-unrelated donor transplants, even in the absence of chronic GVHD, are vulnerable to recurrent infections [19,20], especially sinopulmonary infections.

Treatment strategies

First fever during neutropenia

With the recognition that most febrile episodes during neutropenia are infectious in origin, awareness of their life-threatening potential and knowledge that most first infections are due to bacteria, evaluation should be prompt and thorough. Special attention should be directed to the oral cavity, catheter sites and perianal area. Cultures of suspected sites of infection should be obtained and in all patients at least two sets of blood samples should be submitted for bacterial and fungal cultures. Patients with respiratory signs or symptoms should have a chest X-ray, in addition to physical examination and routine blood cultures.

Two or three blood cultures should be obtained either simultaneously or separated by 30–60 min [51]. According to the Infectious Disease Society of America (IDSA) guidelines for the management of febrile neutropenia, at least one of these cultures should be from a peripheral venous puncture and the other can be from an intravenous (IV) line [47]. Many centers do not draw peripheral blood cultures, preferring to draw two sets of cultures from the indwelling catheter. There appears to be no value in obtaining more than a single set of cultures per 24-h period. Preferably 20–30 mL per culture set for an adult is recommended [52], with proportionately smaller volumes for children: 1–2 mL blood per culture for neonates; 2–3 mL for infants aged 1 month to 2 years; 3–5 mL for older children; and 10–20 mL for adolescents are recommended. Numerous satisfactory manual or instrumental culture systems are commercially available (reviewed in [51]). Most systems perform well but no one medium or system is capable of detecting all microorganisms. Several systems are suitable for special considerations. There are products to minimize the inhibitory influence of antibiotics for patients who are already receiving antibiotics and systems that are useful for detecting filamentous fungi or mycobacteria (such as the lysis centrifugation system). Each has its strengths and shortcomings (reviewed in [51]). Because of declining rates of isolation of anaerobes, some authorities have questioned the common practice of routinely using a combination of aerobic and anaerobic bottles except in patients who are at high risk for anaerobic bacteremia. In general, it is advisable that each transplant team meets periodically with the director of the hospital microbiology laboratory to review the blood culture system in place at that institution and the infections encountered in the HCT patients to accommodate specific situations where special media would be advisable.

After evaluation, antibacterial agents should be instituted promptly on an empirical basis. This strategy has reduced the morbidity and mortality associated with infection from more than 50% to less than 10% in the last 25 years [53], and has become universally adopted as the standard of care for management of the initial fever during neutropenia. A variety of antibiotic regimens have been evaluated in controlled clinical trials. It remains debatable as to whether one regimen is superior to another. What is generally agreed upon, however, is that antibiotics should be begun promptly at the first sign of fever, without waiting for isolation of an organism in blood or other cultures, even in the absence of signs or symptoms of infection, since the host is unable to mount an effective inflammatory response [21].

When choosing an antibiotic, a number of factors must be considered, such as local susceptibility patterns, as well as the susceptibility of organisms to available antibiotics. Other important considerations include toxicity of the individual agents (particularly in individuals with impaired organ function), allergic history, the likelihood of the emergence of drug resistance, the risk for superinfection (both frequency and the type of superinfection) and cost. A consensus committee of the IDSA first provided guidelines for the management of fever during neutropenia in 1990, and these were updated in 1997 and 2002 [54]. Although developed

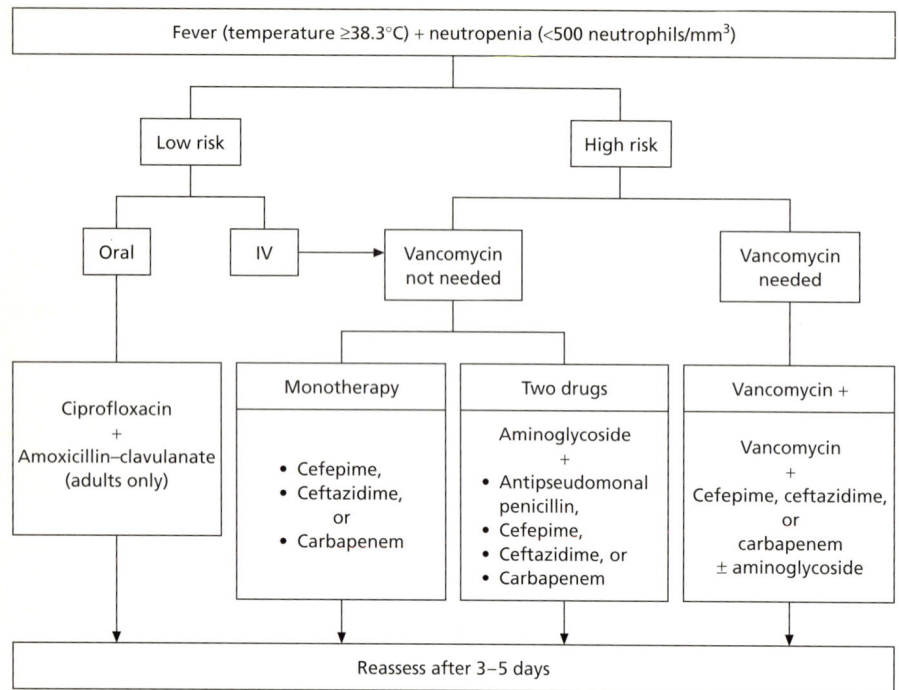

Fig. 51.2 Algorithm for initial management of febrile neutropenic patients. Reproduced with permission from Hughes et al. [54], courtesy of The University of Chicago Press.

primarily for hospitalized patients with neutropenia following conventional chemotherapy, they have been updated to include outpatient management of febrile neutropenia and are suitable for HCT patients as well. These guidelines are evidence based, ranking both the strength and the quality of evidence of each recommendation.

The IDSA's suggested strategies for first fever are indicated in Fig. 51.2 [54]. The first decision to be made concerns where the patient will be managed, inpatient or outpatient. With the increasing role of non-myeloablative regimens followed by HCT and rapid recovery seen with autologous peripheral blood cell autologous transplants, many patients are managed exclusively as outpatients. Management of neutropenic fever should be no exception provided the patient is stable. Indications and candidates for outpatient management of febrile neutropenia will be discussed under Outpatient management of neutropenia (p. 674).

In hospitalized individuals with bacteremia, there are three potential management options. The first strategy is treatment with a single agent, or monotherapy [54,55]. Successfully studied agents include the third-generation cephalosporin ceftazidime [56–59], the fourth-generation cephalosporin cefepime [58–62] and carbapenems including imipenem [57,60] and meropenem [63,64]. Several studies have demonstrated no difference in outcomes between monotherapy and combinations of two or three drugs in the empirical treatment of uncomplicated febrile neutropenia, including two recent meta-analyzes [65,66]. Disadvantages of the monotherapy approach include limited gram-positive activity, particularly with ceftazidime and lack of efficacy against viridans streptococci. Cefepime and the carbapenems have excellent activity against viridans streptococci and pneumococci. None, however, have activity against methicillin-resistant *Staphylococcus aureus* (MRSA) which must be considered in hospitals with high MRSA rates. Other organisms that are poorly covered by monotherapy include vancomycin resistant enterococci (VRE), penicillin resistant *Streptococcus pneumoniae* and coagulase negative *Staphylococcus aureus*.

In the era of increasing bacterial resistance to antimicrobial agents, particularly VRE, clinicians need to implement strategies to reduce unnecessary antibiotic consumption. Cefepime in particular has reduced the need for the addition of vancomycin to the empirical regimen when compared to ceftazidime [67]. In a recent study vancomycin was added to the empirical regimen in 51% and 80% of cases, respectively [68]. When appropriateness of vancomycin use was evaluated against IDSA guidelines, patients receiving cefepime had less inappropriate use compared to ceftazidime patients (28% vs. 58%, $p < 0.001$) [68]. Concerns with monotherapy include emergence of resistant strains. Extended spectrum beta-lactamases have been shown to reduce the utility of ceftazidime monotherapy [69,70]. Fourth-generation cephalosporins have not been subject to the same problem and in fact ceftazidime resistant strains of *Enterobacter cloacae* remain susceptible to cefepime [70]. Institutions that have adopted an "antibiotic cycling" program, or have changed their preference of cephalosporin from ceftazidime to cefepime, have seen a reversal in the resistance patterns of ceftazidime to inducible Enterobacteriaceae [71].

Imipenem and meropenem have also been extensively evaluated in the management of febrile neutropenia [60,63,64]. In trials comparing carbapenems to third- and fourth-generation cephalosporins, there were no appreciable differences in time to recrudescence of fever, days of therapy or breakthrough infections. One potential concern with the routine use of carbapenems is the lack of coverage against *Stenotrophomonas maltophilia*, an organism that is increasingly isolated in HCT patients. Depending upon individual institutions' susceptibility patterns, carbapenems are a suitable choice for monotherapy.

Other agents that have been evaluated less extensively include fluoroquinolones such as ciprofloxacin [72,73] and levofloxacin and the beta-lactam/beta-lactamase combination piperacillin–tazobactam [74,75]. Ciprofloxacin has been studied with varying results. One potential concern is development of resistance, based on widespread prophylactic use as part of "gut decontamination." If a patient develops a fever while on oral ciprofloxacin, changing to intravenous ciprofloxacin is probably a poor choice since the cause of fever may be an organism not susceptible to fluoroquinolones.

A second option for high-risk febrile neutropenia patients is a combination of two agents, such as an aminoglycoside in combination with either an antipseudomonal penicillin, cefepime, ceftazidime, or a carbapenem. In general, the two-drug combinations have similar response rates to monotherapy regimens. An advantage of combination therapy is

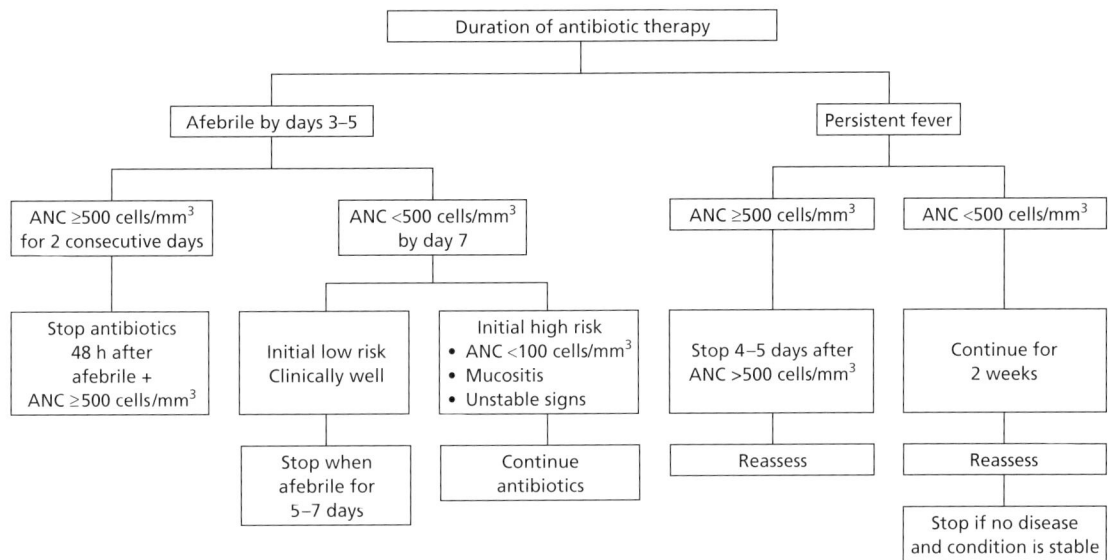

Fig. 51.3 Suggested scheme for estimating the duration of antibiotic administration under various conditions. See Table 51.8 for rating system for patients at low risk. ANC, absolute neutrophil count. Reproduced with permission from Hughes *et al.* [54], courtesy of The University of Chicago Press.

a broad coverage of pathogens, including organisms that might be resistant to individual agents. A second advantage is potential synergy against gram-negative bacteria and coverage against anaerobes. A third advantage is potential reduction in the emergence of antimicrobial resistance. Combination regimens are attractive for patients at high risk for *P. aeruoginosa* infections, although the role of combination therapy for such infections has recently been challenged [76]. Disadvantages include nephrotoxicity, ototoxicity, hypokalemia, the need for monitoring of aminoglycoside levels to assure therapeutic levels and to minimize toxicity, and a lack of coverage against most gram-positive bacteria. A regimen of two beta-lactams, such as a cephalosporin plus an ureidopenicillin, for example, piperacillin or mezlocillin, has been evaluated at some centers and appears effective. Such combinations offer broad-spectrum activity with little toxicity and good anaerobic coverage, but there is little coverage against gram-positive organisms, it is more costly and antagonism is possible in certain bacterial infections [77].

The final option is to combine the glycopeptide vancomycin with either option one or two [78]. This combination offers the advantage of excellent coverage against gram-positive bacteria in addition to the advantages and disadvantages noted in the first option. Opinion is divided as to the need for empirical vancomycin because many gram-positive infections are easily controlled once they are identified, and because of concerns as to the emergence of resistance if the agent is overused [79]. Certainly, the emergence of VRE in many centers has led to calls for restricted use of this drug from the CDC as well as multiple infectious disease committees [80]. Vancomycin resistant enterococcal infections will be discussed under Vancomycin resistant enterococci (VRE) (p. 74). However, inclusion of vancomycin in first-line therapy could be considered in seriously ill patients with suspected staphylococcal infections or with infected catheters, or in centers where fulminant gram-positive bacterial infections are common. If cultures prove negative, its use should be curtailed.

Subsequent fever during neutropenia

The response to the initial antibiotic regimen dictates subsequent management decisions. If the patient defervesces, then the initial regimen can be continued without modification until resolution of neutropenia (absolute neutrophil count [ANC] $\geq 500/mm^3$ for 2 consecutive days), regardless of whether an infection was documented. Occasionally, if the

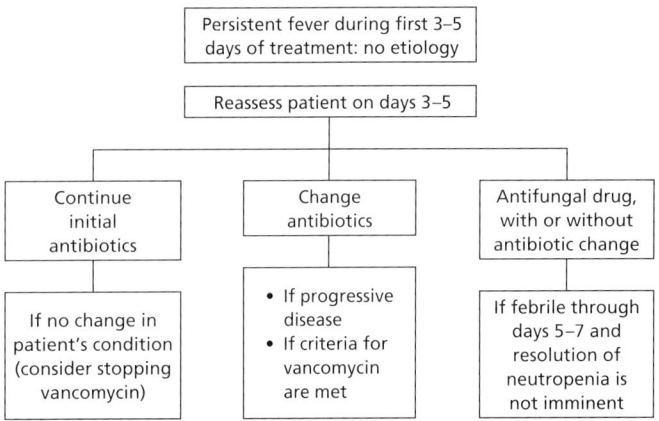

Fig. 51.4 Guide to treatment of patients who have persistent fever after 3–5 days of treatment and for whom the cause of fever is not found. Reproduced with permission from Hughes *et al.* [54], courtesy of The University of Chicago Press.

patient has defervesced and no infection has been documented, antibiotics can be stopped before resolution of neutropenia. However, this step should be taken only with caution, preferably in patients who have been afebrile for 5–7 days. The patient should be monitored closely and therapy resumed if fever should recur (Fig. 51.3 [54]). Generally, it is advisable to avoid stopping antibiotics if ongoing active oral or GI mucositis is present. In the past, it was customary to operationally define neutropenic resolution at $500/mm^3$. However, studies in children undergoing cancer chemotherapy have suggested that stopping antibiotics at lower levels, such as $250/mm^3$, is also satisfactory as long as the counts are rising.

If fever persists, patients require continued careful monitoring. If no infection has been documented and no signs of progressive infection are seen, then the initial regimen can be continued without modification. If an infection has been documented, then therapy targeted against the pathogens should be instituted. If signs of progressive infection occur, modification of the initial regimen should be instituted to cover suspected pathogens that were not covered by the initial regimen (Fig. 51.4 [54]).

If fever persists or recurs 5 or more days after initiation of antibiotics and the patient is likely to remain profoundly neutropenic, the patient is at

Table 51.8 Scoring index for identification of low-risk febrile neutropenic patients at time of presentation with fever. Reproduced with permission from Klastersky et al. [85], courtesy of The University of Chicago Press.

Characteristic	Score
Extent of illness*	
No symptoms	5
Mild symptoms	5
Moderate symptoms	3
No hypertension	5
No chronic obstructive pulmonary disease	4
Solid tumor or no fungal infection	4
No dehydration	3
Outpatient at onset fever	3
Age <60 years[†]	2

Note: highest theoretical score is 26. A risk index score of ≥21 indicates that the patient is likely to be at low risk for complications and morbidity. The scoring system is derived from MASCC [85].
*Choose one item only.
[†]Does not apply to patients ≤16 years of age.

high risk for fungal infection. Consideration should be made to initiation of antifungal therapy, as discussed in Chapter 52, and the patient worked up clinically and radiologically. Antibiotics may be continued without modification, depending upon patient status.

Fever following resolution of neutropenia

In the HCT population, patients occasionally remain febrile following neutrophil recovery. In this febrile, nonneutropenic population, where reassessment for undiagnosed infection is negative, antibiotics can be stopped after 4–5 days of an ANC >500/mm^3 [54] (see Fig. 51.3).

Outpatient management of neutropenia

In recent years, a variety of considerations have led to the development of outpatient antibiotic regimens including the development of programmable infusion pumps, the widespread availability of home-care services, the desire for patients to receive more of their care in the outpatient setting, the introduction of highly effective and nontoxic antibiotic regimens and an emphasis on cost containment. A variety of studies have identified factors that distinguish patients who are at low risk for serious morbidity from those who are at risk for septic shock and other complications of neutropenic fever [81–85]. Factors such as the presence of comorbid diseases, the development of fever as an inpatient, underlying hematological malignancy, prolonged neutropenia (>10 days) and recipients of allogeneic HCT identify those at high-risk. Low-risk patients include those with underlying solid tumors receiving conventional chemotherapy, those with a short anticipated duration of neutropenia (<7 days) and those with no comorbid conditions.

Following the stratification of the different clinical risk groups, further research has been centered on developing an internationally validated scoring system to identify low-risk patients at the onset of a febrile illness [85]. In a multivariate model several characteristics have been identified that are considered independent predictive factors of favorable outcome. Integer weights were applied to these characteristics to develop a risk-index score, which was subsequently validated (Table 51.8 [85]). A risk-index score of ≥21 identified low-risk patients with a positive predictive value of 91%, specificity of 68% and a sensitivity of 71% [85]. This scoring system demonstrated lower misclassification rates and better sensitivity compared to earlier models. One of the limitations of the model is the applicability to the HCT setting. A small percentage of the patients studied were HCT recipients, but this model requires further validation in a larger cohort of transplant recipients. If applicable to this population, it could be possible to select low-risk patients for early IV-to-oral switch programs while remaining neutropenic.

Outpatient antibiotic therapy or early discharge of patients at low risk for serious sequelae has been evaluated in non-HCT patient groups [81,82,86]. Outpatient antibiotic regimens have also been evaluated in autologous HCT patients [87,88] and appear to be quite promising for some HCT patients at low risk for serious sequelae. Stable febrile and neutropenic patients who received a nonmyeloablative regimen are also candidates for outpatient therapy.

Vancomycin resistant enterococci (VRE)

Enterococcal infections are the third most common cause of hospital-acquired bacteremia in hospitalized patients [89]. *Enterococcus faecalis* and *E. faecium* are the most frequently identified species, although *E. faecium* is overtaking *E. faecalis* as the predominant organism. Of great concern is the development of resistance of *Enterococcus* to multiple antimicrobial agents. Enterococci are intrinsically resistant to beta-lactams (particularly cephalosporins and penicillinase resistant penicillin), low concentration aminoglycosides, clindamycin, fluoroquinolones and trimethoprim–sulfamethoxazole. Acquired resistance to high concentration of beta-lactams and aminoglycosides, glycopeptides (vancomycin, teicoplanin), tetracycline, erythromycin, fluoroquinolones, rifampin, chloramphenicol, fusidic acid and nitrofurantoin, is also well documented [90].

Colonization and infection with VRE is the greatest concern in high-risk neutropenic patients, particularly as several outbreaks have been reported in oncology and HCT units over the last decade [91,92]. There are five vancomycin-resistant enterococcal phenotypes, namely VanA, VanB, VanC, VanD and VanE [90,93], of which VanA and VanB are the most common. VanA resistance, characterized by resistance to high concentrations of vancomycin (minimum inhibitory concentration [MIC] ≥64 µg/mL) and teicoplanin (MIC ≥16 µg/mL), can be induced by the presence of either drug. VanB-resistant enterococci are resistant to low to high concentration of vancomycin (MIC 4–>1064), but sensitive to teicoplanin. Both VanA and VanB VRE phenotypes are most common amongst *E. faecium* and *E. faecalis* and less common among other *Enterococcus* spp. such as *E. gallinarum* and *E. casseliflavus*, which are typically associated with the VanC phenotype [90,93].

Several risk factors have been identified that are associated with colonization or infection with VRE [90,94–96]. Antibiotic exposure, particularly to vancomycin, cephalosporins and antianaerobic agents such as metronidazole and imipenem are widely reported to increase risk [97]. Other variables that increase risk are a longer duration of hospitalization, greater severity of underlying illness, presence of feeding tubes and a close proximity to colonized or infected patients. Enterococci are resilient organisms and are able to be easily transmitted via health care workers, contaminated medical equipment, as well as inadequately cleaned rooms following occupation with a VRE positive patient.

It is essential that standard infection control measures, as suggested by the CDC guidelines for preventing opportunistic infections in HCT recipients [6], be strictly adhered to. These measures include handwashing with antibacterial soap before and after entering HCT recipients' rooms and disinfecting patients' rooms and equipment, including structural surfaces (e.g. walls, floors, bed-frames) with an approved Food and Drug Administration (FDA) or Environmental Protection Authority-registered disinfectant [6]. Patients must also be placed under contact precautions until all antibiotics are discontinued and repeat cultures are negative.

Initial treatment of VRE infected patients includes draining any collections if present, which is less likely in severely neutropenic patients with an absence of neutrophils. All indwelling vascular access devices should be removed immediately. There are a number of drugs that have been used in the management of VRE infection, with traditional approaches including ampicillin, gentamicin, chloramphenicol [98], tetracycline [99] and nitrofurantoin [90]. More recently the availability of quinupristin–dalfopristin, a combination of streptogrammins, as well as linezolid, an oxazolidinone have shown better response rates. Choice of agent should be guided by species of *Enterococcus*, particularly as quinupristin–dalfopristin has limited activity against *E. faecalis*. Due to the severity of VRE infections in the immunocompromised patients, as well as high mortality rates, combination therapy with quinupristin–dalfopristin and minocycline has been evaluated with impressive success rates [100].

A more rational approach is to attempt to reduce colonization, or at least prevent colonization from developing into a subsequent bacteremia. Ramoplanin, a glycolipodepsipeptide with bactericidal activity against all enterococci is in clinical trials to evaluate its ability to reduce GI carriage of VRE. Phase II results demonstrate effective suppression of VRE in asymptomatic GI carriers while receiving ramoplanin [101]. Seven days following discontinuation of active drug, 81% and 90% of the ramoplanin 100 mg and 400 mg recipients, respectively, were VRE free, compared to none in the placebo-treated group. Similarly at 14 days following discontinuation of ramoplanin 100 mg, 400 mg, or placebo, 28%, 41% and 10% of patients, respectively, were VRE free. At day 21 following discontinuation, there was no difference between the three arms. The observations would suggest that ramoplanin could be an effective agent to be administered to high-risk VRE colonized HCT recipients during periods of severe neutropenia to prevent development of VRE bacteremia. Phase III trials evaluating the efficacy of ramoplanin in preventing VRE bacteremias are ongoing.

Clostridium difficile associated diarrhea (CDAD)

Clostridium difficile is thought to be the cause of a quarter of all cases of antibiotic-associated diarrhea and a higher percentage of colitis associated with antibiotic treatment [102,103]. In a large series of neutropenic patients receiving myelosuppressive chemotherapy, *C. difficile* infection occurred in 7% of all chemotherapy cycles [104]. In 8.2% of these, severe enterocolitis developed. Among HCT recipients, CDAD is reported to occur in five to 15% of patients with diarrhea [105–109]. Antibiotics most frequently associated with antibiotic associated diarrhea are clindamycin, penicillins and cephalosporins.

Clostridium difficile, a gram-negative, aerobic bacillus, from endogenous or exogenous origin, can establish itself in the colon and proliferate. *Clostridium difficile* usually produces two toxins, namely toxin A and toxin B. Patients are classified as *C. difficile* positive when either toxin A or B is detected in the stool. There are several methods of detecting *C. difficile*, of which the enzyme immunoassay (ELISA) method is the most common. The ELISA test can detect both toxin A and B, or only toxin A depending on the reagent used. Reagents that detect both toxin A and toxin B are prefered as a small number of cases of *C. difficile* (i.e. 1–2%) involve strains of *C. difficile* that only produce toxin B. The enzyme immunoassay is capable of detecting 100–1000 pg of toxin, which results in a relatively high false negative rate [102]. As a consequence, between 5% and 20% of patients need greater than one stool sample to detect toxin. Good clinical practice involves sending multiple stool specimens (up to three), to increase the diagnostic yield by 5–10% [102,103]. The ELISA test is sensitive (71–94%) and has a high specificity (92–98%) [102] and also has the advantage of a quick turnaround for results. Other tests that have been used include cytotoxic tissue culture, polymerase chain reaction, latex agglutination and counter immunoelectrophoresis. Many of these tests are less sensitive and take considerably longer to generate a result, delaying implementation of treatment. In HCT patients with diarrhea, symptomatic remedies, including loperamide and other antimotility agents should be withheld until the results of *C. difficile* testing is known.

Where possible, treatment of CDAD involves discontinuation or streamlining of antibiotic therapy. Among HCT recipients, this is often not feasible due to underlying infection. Substituting a quinolone and an aminoglycoside for penicillins or cephalosporins may be considered. First-line treatment options for CDAD include metronidazole and vancomycin. Two comparative trials have shown similar response rates with these agents [110,111]. Metronidazole 250 mg orally four times a day, or 500 mg orally three times a day, is the preferred treatment. It is significantly cheaper and is not associated with the VRE resistance issues that plague vancomycin therapy. If alternative treatment is necessary due to intolerance or failure to respond to initial therapy, vancomycin 125 mg orally four times daily should be initiated. Treatment failure in immunocompetent patients is often defined as failure to stop diarrhea after 4–5 days of therapy. This definition may not be applicable in immunocompromised patients, with recent data in neutropenic patients demonstrating a longer time to response [104]. If clinical symptoms progress, alternative treatment options should be considered. Vancomycin must be administered orally, not IV. Oral therapy results in high concentrations in the stool, whereas intravenous therapy does not achieve therapeutic concentrations in the stool. If intravenous therapy is indicated due to mucositis, metronidazole can be administered IV, as bactericidal concentrations are achieved in the colon when administered via this route [102]. Other treatment options that have been investigated for CDAD incude bacitracin and rifampin. More recently an *in vitro* study demonstrated that linezolid has activity against *C. difficile* isolates with decreased susceptibility to vancomycin and metronidazole [112]. The *in vivo* implications of this *in vitro* study are unknown. Patients with CDAD should be treated with appropriate therapy for 10–14 days.

Relapses are reported to occur following successful treatment in up to 25% of cases [103], although relapse rates among neutropenic patients are reported to be lower, i.e. 3.3% [104]. Relapses can be treated with another 10–14 days of therapy. Relapses are primarily due to reinfection with a new strain and are not associated with bacterial resistance [102]; therefore, the drug used for the initial infection can be used for the relapse. In patients who have multiple relapses, addition of cholestyramine, a nonabsorbable anion exchange resin which acts to bind the toxin can be considered. Other treatment options that have been investigated include a slow tapering schedule of oral vancomycin over a period of 6 weeks, or in appropriate candidates, intracolonic vancomycin. The use of probiotic therapy to restore normal colonic fecal flora has also been investigated. Administration of *Lactobacillus* or *Saccharomyces boulardii* are reported to protect agains *C. difficile* incudes colitis. These approaches should be avoided in neutropenic patients. Finally intravenous immunoglobulin (IVIg) therapy has been used with some success. The basis of decreasing transmission of *C. difficile* is good infection control. This is discussed later under preventive strategies (p. 676).

Treatment of late bacterial infections

Recurrent sinopulmonary infections are frequently associated with chronic GVHD or Ig deficiency [17,19,20,48–50]. They can be treated successfully by a variety of antibiotics, including penicillin, trimethoprim–sulfamethoxazole, cefaclor, cefuroxime and the new-generation macrolide antibiotics. If Ig deficiency is present (i.e. IgG <400 mg/dL), IVIg can be helpful [6] but is very costly.

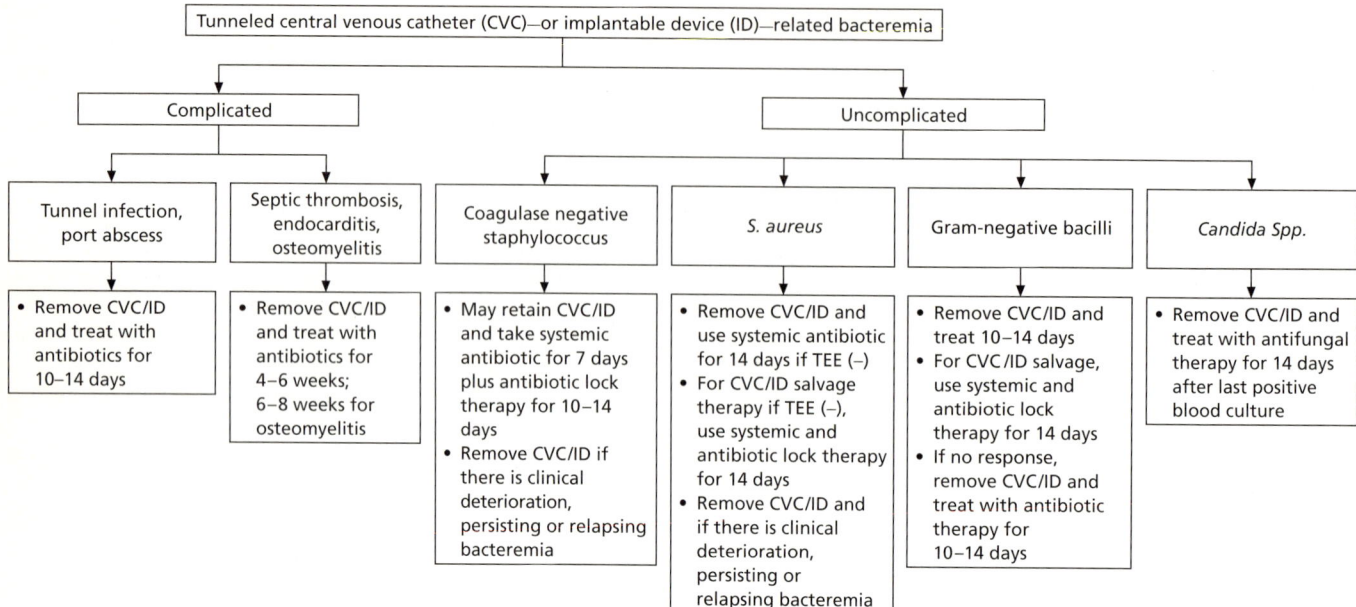

Fig. 51.5 Approach to the management of a patient with a tunneled central venous catheter (CVC) or a surgically implanted device-related bloodstream infection. Reproduced with permission from Mermel et al. [47], courtesy of The University of Chicago Press.

Treatment of intravascular catheter-related infections

Intravascular catheters are used almost universally in HCT recipients. Tunneled CVCs such as Hickman, Broviac and Groshong catheters, as well as implantable devices such as the PortACath are most commonly used. The majority of infections are caused by gram-positive organisms, particularly *Staph. aureus*, coagulase-negative *Staph. aureus* and *Corynebacterium* speices, although gram-negative infections with *Pseudomonas* spp., *Acinetobacter baumanni* and *Stenotrophomonas* spp. are increasingly documented.

The IDSA has, as previously mentioned, developed guidelines for the management of intravascular catheter-related infections [47] and these are useful in therapeutic decision-making processes. For those patients with a suspected CVC-related infection, the guidelines recommend that two sets of blood cultures should be drawn, with one set drawn percutaneously. This approach is most helpful if the blood sample drawn through the CVC is negative, as it excludes CVC-related infection. Once results are available identifying the organism, choice of antibiotic therapy must be based on susceptibilities. Guidelines for managing tunneled CVC infections are outlined in Fig. 51.5 [47] and specifically address when to remove the catheter and duration of antibiotic therapy. Patients should be educated on how to best access their lines if they are performing catheter care at home to minimize the risk of catheter-associated infection.

Preventive strategies

General measures

The foremost principle of infection prophylaxis is minimization of the possibility that encounters with the health care team and exposure to the hospital environment place patients at greater risk for acquiring infection. Accordingly, clinical procedures, especially the placement of venous and urinary catheters, should be avoided when possible. General consensus guidelines for prevention of infection in HCT patients have been published [6]. Hand washing by care providers is of utmost importance to avoid transmission of infectious agents from one patient to another or from staff to patients. Opinion is divided as to the need for decontaminating regimens to reduce the endogenous flora and the use of pathogen-free diets. However, abstinence from fresh fruits and vegetables is frequently advised.

Particular attention has been placed on the need for minimizing exposure to airborne organisms. Opinion again is divided as to the value of various isolation strategies. The consensus guidelines for the prevention of opportunistic infections in HCT recipients has recommended that all allogeneic HCT patients be placed in rooms with greater than 12 air exchanges per hour and point-of-use high-efficiency particulate air (HEPA) filters capable of removing particles ≥0.3 μm in diameter be used [6]. The relative merits of laminar air flow vs. HEPA filtered rooms have not been clarified.

Knowledge that most infectious pathogens originate from the endogenous flora, as well as the observations that in many instances these organisms are acquired after entry to the hospital environment, have led to investigation of the utility of bacterial and fungal surveillance cultures. Bacterial surveillance cultures have been found to be useful in detecting antibiotic-resistant bacteria [113]. Such surveillance culture programs have been useful primarily in the setting of prolonged neutropenia for detecting causes of superinfection. The disadvantage of routine use of surveillance cultures is its high cost, the enormous workload for the microbiology laboratories and frequent low predictive value [114]. Accordingly, routine surveillance of individual patients has not been used widely. Nevertheless, there is consensus that ongoing hospital-wide and unit-specific infection surveillance programs need to be in place to detect shifts in infectious pathogens as well as patterns of antibiotic resistance [113,115].

Clostridium difficile is a major cause of diarrhea in HCT patients, most often in those who are receiving antibiotics [116]. Nosocomial transmission of the organism occurs frequently [117]. Contaminated environmental surfaces and the hands of health care personnel are major sources of organism transmission to susceptible patients. Minimization of antibiotic exposure and attention to infection control measures to reduce person-to-person contact are of paramount importance in preventing outbreaks [118,119].

A variety of factors influence the risk for infection associated with CVCs: the type of catheter, the site of insertion, catheter size, the duration of use, the degree of host immunodeficiency, the type of precautions used during catheter insertion and the skill with which the catheter is inserted. The Hospital Infection Control Practices Advisory Committee has published guidelines for prevention of infections related to intravascular devices [120] and they include: training of the health care team that will place and maintain the lines, monitoring infection rates with different kinds of catheters over time, hand washing before and after handling catheters or their dressings, the use of barrier precautions during catheter insertion and care, the use of skin antiseptics before catheter insertion, the use of either sterile gauze or transparent dressings for covering the catheter site, change of dressings when they are soiled or wet, avoiding touching of the catheter exit site when the dressing is changed, the use of a single-lumen rather than a multilumen catheter when possible, the use of a tunneled catheter if long-term use is anticipated and the use of a subclavian rather than a jugular or femoral site unless necessary. Several controlled trials have evaluated the use of silver and antibiotic-impregnated catheters to reduce the risks for infection in non-HCT recipients [121–123]. This promising strategy was successful in the context of these clinical trials; however, the long-term effects in terms of antibiotic resistance are not known. Further, since the studies were not conducted with tunneled catheters, how applicable the results are to the HCT setting is yet to be tested.

Antibiotic prophylaxis during neutropenia

The frequency and severity of gram-negative bacterial infections during neutropenia and concomitant GI mucosal damage led to an early emphasis on suppressing the intestinal flora to prevent invasive infection. Early efforts to prevent bacterial infections employed the use of oral non-absorbable agents. Agents such as vancomycin, gentamicin, neomycin, colistin and polymyxin B have been advocated in various combinations. A variety of controlled trials have been conducted, and some have shown a beneficial effect. Unfortunately, difficulties with patient compliance, concerns about the emergence of resistance and the high cost of several of these regimens have led to poor acceptance.

Trimethoprim–sulfamethoxazole has also been found to reduce both gram-positive and gram-negative bacterial infections. These studies have been conducted mainly in patients undergoing treatment for a variety of hematological malignancies, but not HCT. Its broad-spectrum activity against a number of gram-negative organisms is offset by its lack of activity against *P. aeruginosa*, a major pathogen in HCT patients. Moreover, concerns about delays in engraftment, patient tolerance and selection of resistant organisms have limited its use [124,125]. Because of these concerns and the paucity of data in HCT patients, this regimen has not been adopted widely.

The fluoroquinolones have been shown in controlled trials to significantly reduce gram-negative bacterial infections, appear to be as or more effective than other oral antibiotic regimens and have been evaluated in HCT patients [126,127]. Norfloxacin, ciprofloxacin, ofloxacin, levofloxacin and gatifloxacin have been used most widely. Ciprofloxacin has an advantage over norfloxacin in that it achieves systemic blood levels, however, it is not active against most methicillin-resistant staphylococci (the majority of staphylococcal isolates). The availability of gatifloxacin and levofloxacin offer greater activity against gram-positive organisms, including *Staphylococcus* and *Streptococcus* spp.

Concerns about the emergence of fluoroquinolone resistance have also been raised. The risk for streptococcal infection may also be greater [36,38,39]. The addition of penicillin or rifampin to the fluoroquinolone can reduce the risk for streptococcal infection [128–131]. However, resistance to penicillin is also high in the community and may not confer additional protection [132]. Historically, preservation of the anaerobic flora has generally been believed to offer protection against more virulent pathogens. Little activity against anaerobes is a feature of many quinolones and this may be desirable in protecting against the more virulent pathogens.

Two meta-analyses have examined the value of the fluoroquinolones as prophylaxis. The first meta-analysis published in 1996 evaluated more than 2000 patients in 19 eligible studies [133]. Fluoroquinolones, while effective in preventing gram-negative bacteremia, had no effect on days of fever or on infection related-mortality. Surprisingly, in addition, there was no increase in the number of cases with gram-positive bacteremia as initially feared. A subsequent analysis published in 1998 [134], also found fluoroquinolones to significantly reduce the incidence of gram-negative bacterial infections, microbiologically documented infections and total infectious episodes and fever. However there was no difference in the incidence of gram-positive bacterial infection, clinically documented infection or infection-related deaths. Based on such considerations, the CDC/IDSA/ASBMT consensus panel does not recommend the routine use of gut decontamination in HCT recipients [6].

Bacterial prophylaxis after engraftment

Morbidity and mortality from chronic GVHD are frequently due to infection. Antibiotic prophylaxis while not providing universal protection against encapsulated organisms, significantly reduces the mortality from chronic GVHD [135,136]. Accordingly, all patients with chronic GVHD should be placed on daily antibiotic prophylaxis with either penicillin, trimethoprim–sulfamethoxazole or a suitable alternative guided by local susceptibility patterns for as long as active GVHD therapy is prescribed [6]. If penicillin is used, additional prophylaxis for *Pneumocystis carinii* should also be administered. Even in the absence of chronic GVHD, patients with recurrent sinopulmonary infections and autograft recipients undergoing HCT with TBI-containing regimens [136] should be considered for prophylaxis to prevent infection from encapsulated organisms. Agents such as penicillin, cefaclor, cefuroxime, trimethoprim–sulfamethoxazole and the new-generation macrolides are particularly useful. Moreover, patients who have previously undergone splenectomy should be considered for antibiotic prophylaxis against encapsulated bacteria.

Adjunctive measures

Growth factors

Growth factors such as granulocyte colony-stimulating factor (G-CSF) or granulocyte macrophage colony-stimulating factor (GM-CSF) to stimulate more rapid hematopoietic recovery, as well as to obtain an enriched hematopoietic cell product, have become widespread in the field of HCT, and are especially useful in autologous HCT. Unfortunately, although neutrophil recovery is hastened in most prospective randomized trials, the effects on preventing bacterial infections have either been nonexistent [137–148] or marginal [149–152]. In some studies, the impact on bacterial infections was not addressed [153–155]. Of interest is the use of hematopoietic growth factors as an adjunct for antibiotic therapy for established infection or for patients with persistent fever. However, controlled trials have failed to show improved outcomes in either HCT [156] or non-HCT neutropenic patients [157–162] other than shortening of neutropenia duration and antibiotic utilization. The advantages, disadvantages and indications for the use of these cytokines are discussed in more detail elsewhere in the book (see Chapter 48).

Several cytokines, including transforming growth factor-beta (TGF-β) [163] and keratinocyte growth factor (KGF) [164–166], have been shown in preclinical studies to enhance mucosal stem cell regrowth. Early clinical trials have shown that both recombinant human KGF and repifermin are able to reduce the severity of mucositis [167,168]. Since mucositis is associated with infection [12,13,31], whether or not these molecules reduce the risk for infection will be an important consideration. GM-CSF mouthwash has been suggested as a potential agent to decrease mucosal toxicity and subsequent infections in cancer patients. A recent randomized, placebo-controlled, double-blind trial demonstrated a lack of efficacy by GM-CSF, with mucositis rates similar to the placebo arm [169].

Granulocyte transfusions

During the 1970s, granulocyte transfusions were frequently used to treat or prevent infections in severely neutropenic patients [170–172]. Unfortunately, they were found to have only marginal benefit in most individuals, perhaps in part due to low number of granulocytes mobilized. Moreover, they often transmitted CMV from donors and morbidity frequently developed from the acquired CMV infection. Today, with modern antibiotic regimens, the need for granulocyte transfusions has diminished. However, they can be useful where bacterial infection from an organism resistant to multiple antibiotics is present or the infection progresses despite the administration of optimal antimicrobial agents [173,174]. The use of granulocyte donors who are serologically negative for CMV eliminates the risk of transmitting CMV.

The use of growth factors such as G-CSF or GM-CSF, alone or in combination with dexamethasone, to stimulate granulocyte production and mobilization into the peripheral blood has led to the potential for collecting large numbers of granulocytes from normal donors [173–177], and the use of these "enhanced" granulocyte transfusion products for the treatment of severe infection [178–180]. It has yet to be demonstrated whether this approach offers significant clinical benefit.

Immunobiological agents

Several studies have shown that the use of IVIg reduces bacterial, fungal and viral infections after allogeneic HCT [181–184], but others have not [185–187], including a controlled trial in autologous HCT patients [187]. The relative merits of IVIg as a general antimicrobial measure vs. the specific antimicrobial agents mentioned above remain unclear. Generally speaking, IVIg is well tolerated. Its disadvantages include its high cost, large fluid volumes, need for parenteral administration and occasional side-effects. Beyond day 90, IVIg given as a monthly infusion was of no benefit in reducing bacterial infections and routine use is not recommended in the CDC guidelines [6,182]. Moreover, there was no reduction in the incidence of bronchiolitis obliterans, overall survival, or survival from chronic GVHD and serum IgG and IgA levels in patients who received IVIg were lower than those of control subjects, suggesting that the use of IVIg might retard humoral immune recovery. Although there may be other reasons to consider the use of immune globulin (e.g. to reduce GVHD or interstitial pneumonia), its high cost and cheaper antibiotic alternatives do not make this approach attractive for prevention of bacterial infections.

Monoclonal antibodies against endotoxin appeared promising as adjunctive treatment of gram-negative sepsis when there is a risk for septic shock [188,189]. Unfortunately, even though well tolerated, randomized controlled trials in gram-negative sepsis demonstrated no survival advantage for the monoclonal antibody compared to placebo [188]. More recently activated protein C has been shown to be effective in the treatment of sepsis syndrome, which frequently complicates HCT and is associated with significant morbidity and mortality. This syndrome is the end result of the activation of inflammatory and coagulation cascades in response to infection [190]. Activated protein C is an endogenous protein that is important in maintaining circulatory homeostasis. In sepsis, concentrations are depleted, a factor that has been associated with poor outcomes in septic patients.

Activated protein C has several actions, those of most importance in sepsis are the anti-inflammatory, pro-fibrinolytic and anticoagulant activities. Drotecogin alfa, a recombinant human activated protein C has been shown to reduce the relative and absolute risks of death in septic individuals [190]. In the pivotal FDA licensing trial HCT recipients were excluded due to increased risk from bleeding complications in an already thrombocytopenic population. Since FDA approval, several centers have used this agent in the high-risk thrombocytopenic HCT recipients with success [191], although the benefits of administration should be weighed against the potential risks of treatment.

Conclusion

The morbidity and mortality from infection have dramatically improved in recent years as insights into the deficits in host defenses, bacterial pathogenesis and epidemiology of infections, the introduction of more effective and less toxic antimicrobial regimens and improved strategies of using various antimicrobial agents have translated into effective therapeutic approaches. Such advances have facilitated enormous strides in reducing transplant-associated mortality, thereby improving the acceptability of HCT as a treatment option for an ever-widening array of malignant and nonmalignant diseases.

Variations in the epidemiology of opportunistic pathogens, the ever-continuing emergence of antimicrobial resistance among microorganisms, changes in host characteristics due to new preparative and immunosuppressive regimens, the application of HCT to new patient populations (older ages, different hematopoietic stem cell sources, different underlying diseases) and the adoption of post-transplant immunoadjuvant therapies to reduce the risk for relapse in the autologous transplant setting require continuing vigilance, and will pose new challenges for the control of bacterial infections. Better diagnostic tools to detect pathogens more accurately and rapidly and to detect them earlier in the course of infection are needed. Newer antimicrobial agents that are safer and more effective, with a broader spectrum of activity must be sought. The expanding array of biological agents to modify pathogen virulence and host responses to infection offer the opportunity to reduce host susceptibility to infection and will likely prove important adjuncts to antimicrobial agents directed against the growing repertoire of opportunistic pathogens.

References

1 Goldmann DA, Weinstein RA, Wenzel RP et al. Strategies to prevent and control the emergence and spread of antimicrobial-resistant microorganisms in hospitals: a challenge to hospital leadership. *JAMA* 1996; **275**: 234–40.

2 Garner JS. Guideline for isolation precautions in hospitals. The hospital infection control practices advisory committee. *Infect Control Hosp Epidemiol* 1996; **17**: 53–80.

3 Shlaes DM, Gerding DN, John JF et al. Society for Healthcare Epidemiology of America and Infectious Diseases Society of America Joint Committee on the prevention of antimicrobial resistance: guidelines for the prevention of antimicrobial resistance in hospitals. *Clin Infect Dis* 1997; **25**: 584–99.

4 McGowan JE Jr. Do intensive hospital antibiotic control programs prevent the spread of antibiotic resistance? *Infect Control Hosp Epidemiol* 1994; **15**: 478–83.

5 Shaikh ZHA, Osting CA, Hanna HA et al. Effectiveness of a multifaceted infection control policy in reducing vancomycin usage and vancomycin-resistant enterococci at a tertiary care cancer centre. *J Hosp Infect* 2002; **51**: 52–8.

6 Dykewicz CA, Jaffe HW, Kaplan JE in collaboration with The Guidelines Working Group Members

from the CDC, the Infectious Diseases Society of America and the American Society of Blood and Marrow Transplantation. Guidelines for preventing opportunistic infections among hematopoietic stem cell transplant recipients. *Biol Blood Marrow Transplant* 2000; **6**: 659–737.

7 Bodey GP, Buckley M, Sathe YS *et al*. Quantitative relationships between circulating leukocytes and infection in patients with acute leukemia. *Ann Intern Med* 1966; **64**: 328–40.

8 Winston DJ, Gale RP, Meyer DV *et al*. Infectious complications of human bone marrow transplantation. *Medicine* 1979; **58**: 1–31.

9 Tsakona CP, Khwaja A, Goldstone AH. Does treatment with haematopoietic growth factors affect the incidence of bacteraemia in adult lymphoma transplant recipients? *Bone Marrow Transplant* 1993; **11**: 433–6.

10 Linch DC, Scarffe H, Proctor S *et al*. Randomized vehicle-controlled dose-finding study of glycosylated recombinant human granulocyte colony stimulating factor after bone marrow transplantation. *Bone Marrow Transplant* 1993; **11**: 307–11.

11 Khaja A, Linch DC, Goldstone AH *et al*. Recombinant human granulocyte-macrophage colony-stimulating factor after bone marrow transplantation for malignant lymphoma: a British National Lymphoma Investigation double-blind, placebo-controlled trial. *Br J Haematol* 1992; **82**: 317–23.

12 Bow EJ, Loewen R, Cheang MS *et al*. Invasive fungal disease in adults undergoing remission-induction therapy for acute myeloid leukemia: the pathogenetic role of the antileukemia regimen. *Clin Infect Dis* 1995; **21**: 361–9.

13 Bow EJ, Loewen R, Cheang MS *et al*. Cytotoxic therapy—induced D-xylose malabsorption and invasive infection during remission-induction therapy for acute myeloid leukemia in adults. *J Clin Oncol* 1997; **15**: 2254–61.

14 Junghanss C, Marr KA, Carter RA *et al*. Incidence and outcome of bacterial and fungal infections after nonmyeloablative compared with myeloablative allogeneic hematopoietic stem cell transplantation: a matched control study. *Biol Blood Marrow Transplant* 2002; **8**: 515–20.

15 Mohty M, Faucher C, Vey N *et al*. High rate of secondary viral and bacterial infections in patients undergoing allogeneic bone marrow mini-transplantation. *Bone Marrow Transplant* 2000; **26**: 251–5.

16 Crippa F, Holmberg L, Carter RA *et al*. Infectious complications after autologous CD34-selected peripheral blood stem cell transplantation. *Biol Blood Marrow Transplant* 2002; **8**: 281–9.

17 Atkinson K, Storb R, Prentice RL *et al*. Analysis of late infections in 89 long-term survivors of bone marrow transplantation. *Blood* 1979; **53**: 720–31.

18 Aucouturier P, Barra A, Intrator L *et al*. Long lasting IgG subclass and antibacterial polysaccharide antibody deficiency after allogeneic bone marrow transplantation. *Blood* 1987; **70**: 779–85.

19 Atkinson K, Farewell V, Storb R *et al*. Analysis of late infections after human bone marrow transplantation: role of genotypic nonidentity between marrow donor and recipient and of nonspecific suppressor cells in patients with chronic graft-versus-host disease. *Blood* 1982; **60**: 714–20.

20 Ochs L, Shu XO, Miller J *et al*. Late infections after allogeneic bone marrow transplantation: comparison of incidence in related and unrelated donor transplant recipients. *Blood* 1995; **86**: 3979–86.

21 Sickles EA, Green WH, Wiernick PH. Clinical presentation of infection in granulocytopenic patients. *Arch Intern Med* 1975; **135**: 715–9.

22 Collin BA, Leather HL, Wingard JR *et al*. Evolution, incidence and susceptibility of bacterial bloodstream isolates from 519 bone marrow transplant patients. *Clin Infect Dis* 2001; **33**: 947–53.

23 Labarca JA, Leber AL, Kern VL *et al*. Outbreak of *Stenotrophomonas maltophilia* bacteremia in allogeneic bone marrow transplant patients: role of severe neutropenia and mucositis. *Clin Infect Dis* 2000; **30**: 195–7.

24 Micozzi A, Venditti M, Monaco M *et al*. Bacteremia due to *Stenotrophomonas maltophilia* in patients with hematologic malignancies. *Clin Infect Dis* 2000; **31**: 705–11.

25 Zinner SH. Changing epidemiology of infections in patients with neutropenia and cancer: emphasis on gram-positive and resistant bacteria. *Clin Infect Dis* 1999; **29**: 490–4.

26 Knowles S, Herra C, Devitt E *et al*. An outbreak of multiply resistant *Serratia marcescens*: the importance of persistent carriage. *Bone Marrow Transplant* 2000; **25**: 873–7.

27 Rubin M, Hathorn JW, Marshall D *et al*. Gram-positive infections and the use of vancomycin in 550 episodes of fever and neutropenia. *Ann Intern Med* 1988; **108**: 30–5.

28 Lowder JN, Lazarus HM, Herzig RH. Bacteremias and fungemias in oncologic patients with central venous catheters: changing spectrum of infection. *Arch Intern Med* 1982; **142**: 1456–9.

29 Karp JE, Dick JD, Angelopulos C *et al*. Empiric use of vancomycin during prolonged treatment-induced granulocytopenia. Randomized, double-blind, placebo-controlled clinical trial in patients with acute leukemia. *Am J Med* 1986; **81**: 237–42.

30 Wang CC, Mattson D, Wald A. *Corynebacterium jeikeium* bacteremia in bone marrow transplant patients with Hickman catheters. *Bone Marrow Transplant* 2001; **27**: 445–9.

31 Wingard JR. Infectious and noninfectious systemic consequences. Oral complications of cancer therapies. *Diagnosis, Prevention, Treatment NCI Monogr* 1990; **9**: 21–6.

32 Villablanca JG, Steiner M, Kersey J *et al*. The clinical spectrum of infections with viridans streptococci in bone marrow transplant patients. *Bone Marrow Transplant* 1990; **5**: 387–93.

33 Steiner M, Villablanca J, Kersey J *et al*. Viridans streptococcal shock in bone marrow transplantation patients. *Am J Hematol* 1993; **42**: 354–8.

34 Valteau D, Hartmann O, Brugieres L *et al*. Streptococcal septicemia following autologous bone marrow transplantation in children treated with high-dose chemotherapy. *Bone Marrow Transplant* 1991; **7**: 415–9.

35 Classen DC, Burke JP, Ford CD *et al*. *Streptococcus mitis* sepsis in bone marrow transplant patients receiving oral antimicrobial prophylaxis. *Am J Med* 1990; **89**: 441–6.

36 Bochud PY, Calandra T, Francioli P. Bacteremia due to viridans streptococci in neutropenic patients: a review. *Am J Med* 1994; **97**: 256–64.

37 Marron A, Carratala J, Gonzalez-Barca E *et al*. Serious complications of bacteremia caused by viridans streptococci in neutropenic patients with cancer. *Clin Infect Dis* 2000; **31**: 1126–30.

38 Kern W, Kurrle E, Schmeiser T. Streptococcal bacteremia in adult patients with leukemia undergoing aggressive chemotherapy. A review of 55 cases. *Infection* 1990; **18**: 138–45.

39 de Pauw BE, Donnelly JP, de Witte T *et al*. Options and limitations of long-term oral ciprofloxacin as antibacterial prophylaxis in allogeneic bone marrow transplant recipients. *Bone Marrow Transplant* 1991; **5**: 179–82.

40 Wingard JR, Santos GW, Saral R. Differences between first and subsequent fevers during prolonged neutropenia. *Cancer* 1987; **59**: 844–9.

41 Gussack GS, Burson JG, Hudgins P *et al*. Sinusitis in the bone marrow transplant patient. *Diagnosis Manage Am J Rhinol* 1995; **9**: 1–5.

42 Deutsch JH, Hudgins PA, Siegel JL *et al*. The paranasal sinuses of patients with acute graft-versus-host disease. *Am J Neuroradiol* 1995; **16**: 1287–91.

43 Yuen KY, Woo PC, Hui CH *et al*. Unique risk factors for bacteremia in allogeneic bone marrow transplant recipients before and after engraftment. *Bone Marrow Transplant* 1998; **21**: 1137–43.

44 Sanders JE, Hickman RO, Aker S *et al*. Experience with double lumen right atrial catheters. *J Parenter Enteral Nutr* 1982; **6**: 95–9.

45 Ulz L, Petersen FB, Ford R *et al*. A prospective study of complications in Hickman right-atrial catheters in marrow transplant patients. *J Parenter Enteral Nutr* 1990; **14**: 27–30.

46 Petersen FB, Clift RA, Hickman RO *et al*. Hickman catheter complications in marrow transplant recipients. *J Parenter Enteral Nutr* 1986; **10**: 58–62.

47 Mermel LA, Farr BM, Sherertz RJ *et al*. Guidelines for the management of intravascular catheter-related infections. *Clin Infect Dis* 2001; **32**: 1249–72.

48 Sullivan KM, Nims J, Leisenring W *et al*. Determinants of late infection following marrow transplantation for aplastic anemia and myelodysplastic syndrome. *Blood* 1995; **86** (Suppl. 1): 213a [Abstract 841].

49 Hoyle C, Goldman JM. Life-threatening infections occurring more than 3 months after BMT. *Bone Marrow Transplant* 1994; **14**: 247–52.

50 Winston DJ, Schiffman G, Wang DC *et al*. Pneumococcal infections after human bone-marrow transplantation. *Ann Intern Med* 1979; **91**: 835–41.

51 Weinstein MP. Current blood culture methods and systems: Clinical concepts, technology and interpretation of results. *Clin Infect Dis* 1996; **23**: 40–6.

52 Reller LB, Murray PR, MacLowry JD. Blood cultures II. In: Washington JA II, ed. Cumitech 1A. Washington, DC: American Society for Microbiology, 1982.

53 Dranitsaris G. Clinical and economic considerations of empirical antibacterial therapy of febrile neutropenia in cancer. *Pharmacoeconomics* 1999; **16**: 343–53.

54 Hughes WT, Armstrong D, Bodey GP *et al*. Guidelines for the use of antimicrobial agents in neutropenic patients with cancer. *Clin Infect Dis* 2002; **34**: 730–51.

55 Rubin M, Pizzo PA. Monotherapy for empirical management of febrile neutropenic patients. *NCI Monogr* 1990; **9**: 111–6.

56 Pizzo PA, Hathorn JW, Hiemenz J *et al*. A randomized trial comparing ceftazidime alone with combination antibiotic therapy in cancer patients with fever and neutropenia. *N Engl J Med* 1986; **315**: 552–8.

57 Freifeld AG, Walsh T, Marshall D *et al*. Monotherapy for fever and neutropenia in cancer patients: a randomized comparison of ceftazidime versus imipenem. *J Clin Oncol* 1995; **13**: 165–76.

58 Mustafa MM, Carlson L, Tkaczerwki I et al. Comparative study of cefepime verus ceftazidime in the empiric treatment of pediatric cancer patients with fever and neutropenia. Pediatr Infect Dis J 2001; **20**: 362–9.

59 Chuang YY, Hung IJ, Yang CP et al. Cefepime versus ceftazidime as empiric monotherapy for fever and neutropenia in children with cancer. Pediatr Infect Dis J 2002; **21**: 203–9.

60 Biron P, Fuhrmann C, Cure H et al. Cefepime versus imipenem–cilastatin as empirical monotherapy in 400 febrile patients with short duration neutropenia. J Antimicrob Chemother 1998; **42**: 511–8.

61 Engervall P, Kalin M, Dornbusch K et al. Cefepime as empirical monotherapy in febrile patients with hematological malignancies and neutropenia: a randomized, single-center phase II trial. J Chemother 1999; **11**: 278–86.

62 Chandrasekar PH, Arnow PM. Cefepime versus ceftazidime as empiric therapy for fever in neutropenic patients with cancer. Ann Pharmacother 2000; **34**: 989–95.

63 Feld R, DePauw B, Berman S et al. Meropenem versus ceftazidime in the treatment of cancer patients with febrile neutropenia: a randomized, double-blind trial. J Clin Oncol 2000; **18**: 3690–8.

64 Vandercam B, Gerain J, Humblet Y et al. Meropenem versus ceftazidime as empirical monotherapy for febrile neutropenic cancer patients. Ann Hematol 2000; **79**: 152–7.

65 Furno P, Bucaneve G, Del Favero A. Monotherapy or aminoglycoside-containing combinations for empirical antibiotic treatment of febrile neutropenic patients: a meta-analysis. Lancet Infect Dis 2002; **2**: 231–42.

66 Paul M, Soares-Weiser K, Grozinsky S et al. Beta-lactam versus beta-lactam-aminoglycoside combination therapy in cancer patients with neutropaenia. Cochrane Database Syst Rev 2002; **2**: CD003038.

67 Breen J, Ramphal R, Cometta A et al. Cefepime versus ceftazidime as empiric therapy of febrile episodes in neutropenic patients. In: Klastersky JA, ed. Febrile Neutropenia. New York: Springer Verlag, 1997: 63–75.

68 Owens RC, Owens CA, Holloway WJ. Reduction in vancomcyin (VANC) consumption in patients with fever and neutropenia. Infectious Disease Society of America Abstracts New Orleans, Abstract 458.

69 Johnson MP, Ramphal R. Beta-lactam-resistant Enterobacter bacteremia in febrile neutropenic patients receiving monotherpy. J Infect Dis 1990; **162**: 981–3.

70 Mimoz O, Leotard S, Jacolot A et al. Efficacies of imipenem, meropenem, cefepime and ceftazidime in rats with experimental pneumonia due to a carbapenem-hydrolyzing beta-lactamase-producing strain of Enterobacter cloacae. Antimicrob Agents Chemother 2000; **44**: 885–90.

71 Mebis J, Goossens H, Bruyneel P et al. Decreasing antibiotic resistance of Enterobacteriaceae by introducing a new antibiotic combination therapy for neutropenic fever patients. Leukemia 1998; **12**: 1627–9.

72 Winston DJ, Lazarus HM, Beveridge RA et al. Randomized double-blind multicenter trial comparing clinafloxacin with imipenem as empirical monotherapy for febrile granulocytopenic patients. Clin Infect Dis 2001; **32**: 381–90.

73 Giamarellou H, Bassaris HP, Petrikkos G et al. Monotherapy with intravenous followed by high-dose ciprofloxacin versus combination therapy with ceftazidime plus amikacin as initial empiric therapy for granulocytopenic patients with fever. Antimicrob Agents Chemother 2000; **44**: 3264–71.

74 Del Favero A, Menichetti F, Martino P et al. A multicenter, double-blind, placebo-controlled trial comparing piperacillin-tazobactam with and without amikacin as empiric therapy for febrile neutropenia. Clin Infect Dis 2001; **33**: 1295–301.

75 Hess U, Bohme C, Rey K et al. Monotherapy with piperacillin/tazobactam versus combination therapy with ceftazidime plus amikacin as an empiric therapy for fever in neutropenic cancer patients. Support Care Cancer 1998; **6**: 402–9.

76 Chatzinikolaou I, Abi-Said D, Bodey GP et al. Recent experience with Pseudomonas aeruginosa bacteremia in patients with cancer: retrospective analysis of 245 episodes. Arch Intern Med 2000; **160**: 501–9.

77 Gutman L, Williamson R, Kitzic MD, Acar JF. Synergism and antagonism in double β-lactam antibiotic combinations. Am J Med 1986; **80**: 21–9.

78 Attal M, Schlaifer D, Rubie H et al. Prevention of gram-positive infections after bone marrow transplantation by systemic vancomycin: a prospective, randomized trial. J Clin Oncol 1991; **9**: 865–70.

79 Schwalbe RS, Stapleton JT, Gilligan PH. Emergence of vancomycin resistance in coagulase-negative staphylococci. N Engl J Med 1989; **316**: 927–31.

80 Centers for Disease Control and Prevention. Recommendations for preventing the spread of vancomycin resistance recommendations of the Hospital Infection Control Practices Advisory Committee (HICPAC). Morbid Mortal Weekly Rep 1995; **44**: 1–13.

81 Talcott JA, Finberg R, Mayer RJ, Goldman L. The medical course of cancer patients with fever and neutropenia: clinical identification of a low-risk subgroup at presentation. Arch Intern Med 1988; **148**: 2561–8.

82 Talcott JA, Siegel RD, Finberg R, Goldman L. Risk assessment in cancer patients with fever and neutropenia: a prospective, two-center validation of a prediction rule. J Clin Oncol 1992; **10**: 316–22.

83 Rolston KV. New trends in patient management: risk-based therapy for febrile patients with neutropenia. Clin Infect Dis 1999; **29**: 515–21.

84 Freifeld A, Marchigiani D, Walsh T et al. A double-blind comparison of empirical oral and intravenous antibiotic therapy for low risk febrile patients with neutropenia during cancer chemotherapy. New Engl J Med 1999; **341**: 305–11.

85 Klastersky J, Paesmans M, Rubenstein EB et al. The multinational association for supportive care in cancer risk index: a multinational scoring system for identifiying low-risk febrile neutropenic cancer patients. J Clin Oncol 2000; **18**: 3038–51.

86 Shenep JL, Flynn PM, Baker DK et al. Oral cefixime is similar to continued intravenous antibiotics in the empirical treatment of febrile neutropenic children with cancer. Clin Infect Dis 2001; **32**: 36–43.

87 Gilbert C, Meisenberg B, Vrendenburgh J et al. Sequential prophylactic oral and empiric once-daily parenteral antibiotics for neutropenia and fever after high-dose chemotherapy and autologous bone marrow support. J Clin Oncol 1994; **12**: 1005–11.

88 Meisenberg B, Gollard R, Brehm T, McMillan R, Miller W. Prophylactic antibiotics eliminate bacteremia and allow safe outpatient management following high-dose chemotherapy and autologous stem cell rescue. Support Care Cancer 1996; **4**: 364–9.

89 Edmond MB, Wallace SE, McClish DK et al. Noscomial bloodstream infections in United States hospitals: a three-year analysis. Clin Infect Dis 1999; **29**: 239–44.

90 Gold HS. Vancomycin-resistant enterococci: mechanisms and clinical observations. Clin Infect Dis 2001; **33**: 210–9.

91 Montecalvo MA, Horowitz H, Gedris C et al. Outbreak of vancomycin-, ampicillin- and aminoglycoside-resistant Enterococcus faecium bacteremia in an adult oncology unit. Antimicrob Agents Chemother 1994; **38**: 1363–7.

92 Kirkpatrick BD, Harrington SM, Smith D et al. An outbreak of vancomycin-dependent Enterococcus faecium in a bone marrow transplant unit. Clin Infect Dis 1999; **29**: 1268–73.

93 Levison ME, Mallela S. Increasing antimicrobial resistance: therapeutic implications for enterococcal infections. Curr Infect Dis Rep 2000; **2**: 417–23.

94 Edmond MB, Ober JF, Weinbaum DL et al. Vancomycin-resistant Enterococcus faecium bacteremia: risk factors for infection. Clin Infect Dis 1995; **20**: 1126–33.

95 Vergis EN, Hayden MK, Chow JW et al. Determinants of vancomycin resistance and mortality rates in enterococcal bacteremia. A prospective multicenter study. Ann Intern Med 2001; **135**: 484–92.

96 Husni R, Hachem R, Hanna H et al. Risk factors for vancomycin-resistant Enterococcus (VRE) infection in colonized patients with cancer. Infect Control Hosp Epidemiol 2002; **23**: 102–3.

97 Fridkin SK, Edwards JR, Courval JM et al. The effect of vancomycin and third-generation cephalosporins on prevalence of vancomycin-resistant-enterococci in 126 US adult intensive care units. Ann Intern Med 2001; **135**: 175–83.

98 Norris AH, Reilly JP, Edelstein PH et al. Chloramphenicol for the treatment of vancomycin-resistant enterococcal infections. Clin Infect Dis 1995; **20**: 1137–44.

99 Moreno F, Jorgensen JH, Weiner MH. An old antibiotic for a new multiple-resistant Enterococcus faecium? Diagn Microbiol Infect Dis 1994; **20**: 41–3.

100 Raad I, Hachem R, Hanna H et al. Treatment of vancomycin-resistant enterococcal infections in the immunocompromised host: quinupristin-dalfopristin in combination with minocycline. Antimicrob Agents Chemother 2001; **45**: 3202–4.

101 Wong MT, Kauffman CA, Standiford HC et al. Effective suppression of vancomycin-resistant Enterococcus species in asymptomatic gastrointestinal carriers by a novel glycolipodepsipeptide, ramoplanin. Clin Infect Dis 2001; **33**: 1476–82.

102 Malnick S, Zimhony O. Treatment of Clostridium difficile-associated diarrhea. Ann Pharmacother 2002; **36**: 1767–75.

103 Bartlett SG. Antibiotic-associated diarrhea. N Engl J Med 2001; **346**: 334–9.

104 Gorschluter M, Glasmacher A, Hahn C et al. Clostridium difficile infection in patients with neutropenia. Clin Infect Dis 2001; **33**: 786–91.

105 Bilgrami S, Feingold JM, Dorsky D et al. Incidence and outcome of Clostridium difficile infection following autologous peripheral blood stem cell transplantation. Bone Marrow Transplant 1999; **23**: 1039–42.

106 Avery R, Pohlman B, Adal K et al. High prevalence of diarrhea but infrequency of documented Clostridium difficile in autologous peripheral blood progenitor cell transplant recipients. Bone Marrow Transplant 2000; 25: 67–9.

107 Tomblyn M, Fordon L, Singhal S et al. Rarity of toxigenic Clostridium difficile infections after hematopoietic stem cell transplantation: implications for symptomatic management of diarrhea. Bone Marrow Transplant 2002; 30: 517–9.

108 Yolken RH, Bishop CA, Townsend TR et al. Infectious gastroenteritis after marrow transplantation: a prospective study. Gastroenterology 1994; 107: 1398–407.

109 Blakey JL, Barnes GL, Bishop RF et al. Infectious diarrhea in children undergoing bone-marrow transplantation. Aust NZ J Med 1989; 19: 31–6.

110 Teasley DG, Gerding DN, Olson MM et al. Prospective randomized trial of metronidazole versus vancomycin for Clostridium difficile associated diarrhea and colitis. Lancet 1982; 2: 1043–6.

111 Wenisch C, Parschalk B, Hasenhundl M et al. Comparison of vancomycin, metronidazole and fusidic acid for the treatment of Clostridium difficile-associated diarrhea. Clin Infect Dis 1996; 72: 813–8.

112 Pelaez T, Alonso R, Perez C et al. In vitro activity of linezolid against Clostridium difficile. Antimicrob Agents Chemother 2002; 46: 1617–8.

113 Wingard JR, Dick JD, Charache P, Saral R. Antibiotic-resistant bacteria in surveillance stool cultures of patients with prolonged neutropenia. Antimicrob Agents Chemother 1986; 30: 435–9.

114 Riley DK, Pavia AT, Beatty PG, Denton D, Carroll KC. Surveillance cultures in bone marrow transplant recipients: worthwhile or wasteful? Bone Marrow Transplant 1995; 15: 469–73.

115 Schimpff SC. Oral complications of cancer therapies: surveillance cultures. NCI Monogr 1990; 9: 37–42.

116 Yolken RH, Bishop CA, Townsend TR et al. Infectious gastroenteritis after marrow transplant recipients. N Engl J Med 1982; 306: 1010–2.

117 Gerding DN, Johnson S, Peterson LR, Mulligan ME, Silva J. Clostridium difficile-associated diarrhea and colitis. Infect Control Hosp Epidemiol 1995; 16: 459–77.

118 Lai KK, Melvin ZS, Menard MJ et al. Clostridium difficile-associated diarrhea: epidemiology, risk factors and infection control. Infect Control Hosp Epidemiol 1997; 18: 628–32.

119 Mayfield JL, Leet T, Miller J et al. Environmental control to reduce transmission of Clostridium difficile. Clin Infect Dis 2000; 31: 995–1000.

120 Pearson ML. Guideline for prevention of intravascular device-related infections. Hospital Infection Control Practices Advisory Committee. Infect Control Hosp Epidemiol 1996; 17: 438–73.

121 Maki DG, Stolz SM, Wheeler S, Mermel LA. Prevention of central venous catheter-related bloodstream infection by use of an antiseptic-impregnated catheter. Ann Intern Med 1997; 124: 257–66.

122 Raad I, Darouiche R, Dupuis J et al. Central venous catheters coated with minocycline and rifampin for the prevention of catheter-related colonization and bloodstream infections: a randomized, double-blind trial. The Texas Medical Center Catheter Study Group. Ann Intern Med 1997; 127: 267–74.

123 Pearson ML, Abrutyn E. Reducing the risk for catheter-related infections: a new strategy. Ann Intern Med 1997; 127: 304–6.

124 Murray BE, Rensimer ER, DuPont HL. Emergence of high-level trimethoprim resistance in fecal Escherichia coli during oral administration of trimethoprim or trimethoprim–sulfamethoxazole. N Engl J Med 1982; 306: 130–5.

125 Wilson JM, Guiney DG. Failure of oral trimethoprim–sulfamethoxazole prophylaxis in acute leukemia: isolation of resistant plasmids from strains of Enterobacteriaceae causing bacteremia. N Engl J Med 1982; 306: 16–20.

126 Lew MA, Kehoe K, Ritz J et al. Ciprofloxacin versus trimethoprim/sulfamethoxazole for prophylaxis of bacterial infections in bone marrow transplant recipients: a randomized, controlled trial. J Clin Oncol 1995; 13: 239–50.

127 Jansen J, Cromer M, Akard L, Black JR, Wheat LJ, Allen SD. Infection prevention in severely myelosuppressed patients. A comparison between ciprofloxacin and a regimen of selective antibiotic modulation of the intestinal flora. Am J Med 1994; 96: 335–41.

128 Broun ER, Wheat JL, Kneebone PH, Sundblad K, Hromas RA, Tricot G. Randomized trial of the addition of gram-positive prophylaxis to standard antimicrobial prophylaxis for patients undergoing autologous bone marrow transplantation. Antimicrob Agents Chemother 1994; 38: 576–9.

129 Kern WV, Hay B, Kern P, Marre R, Arnold R. A randomized trial of roxithromycin in patients with acute leukemia and bone marrow transplant recipients receiving fluoroquinolone prophylaxis. Antimicrob Agents Chemother 1994; 38: 465–72.

130 International Antimicrobial Therapy Group of the European Organization for Research and Treatment of Cancer. Reduction of fever and streptococcal bacteremia in granulocytopenic patients with cancer. JAMA 1994; 272: 1183–9.

131 Gomez-Martin C, Sola C, Hornedo J et al. Rifampin does not improve the efficacy of quinolone antibacterial prophylaxis in neutropenic cancer patients: results of a randomized clinical trial. J Clin Oncol 2000; 18: 2126–34.

132 Guiot HFL, Corel LJ, Bossen JMHJ. Prevalence of penicillin-resistant viridans streptococci in healthy children and in patients with malignant haematological disorders. Eur J Clin Microbiol Infect Dis 1994; 13: 645–50.

133 Cruciani M, Rampazzo R, Malena M et al. Prophylaxis with fluoroquinolones for bacterial infections in neutropenic patients: a meta-analysis. Clin Infect Dis 1996; 23: 795–805.

134 Engels EA, Lau J, Barza M. Efficacy of quinolone prophylaxis in neutropenic cancer patients: a meta-analysis. J Clin Oncol 1998; 16: 1179–87.

135 Sullivan KM, Dahlberg S, Storb R et al. Infection prophylaxis with chronic graft-versus-host disease. Exp Hematol 1993; 1: 193.

136 Kulkarni S, Powers R, Treleaven J et al. Chronic graft versus host disease is associated with long-term risk for pneumococcal infections in recipients of bone marrow transplants. Blood 2000; 95: 3683–6.

137 Gorin NC, Coiffier B, Hayat M et al. Recombinant human granulocyte-macrophage colony-stimulating factor after high-dose chemotherapy and autologous bone marrow transplantation with unpurged and purged marrow in non-Hodgkin's lymphoma: a double-blind placebo-controlled trial. Blood 1992; 80: 1149–57.

138 Gulati SC, Bennett CL. Granulocyte-macrophage colony-stimulating factor (GM-CSF) as adjunct therapy in relapsed Hodgkin disease. Ann Intern Med 1992; 116: 177–82.

139 Nemunaitis J, Rabinowe SN, Singer JW et al. Recombinant granuclocyte-macrophage colony-stimulating factor after autologous bone marrow transplantation for lymphoid cancer. N Engl J Med 1991; 324: 1773–8.

140 Schmitz N, Dreger P, Zander AR et al. Results of a randomized controlled multicenter study of recombinant human granulocyte colony-stimulating factor (filgrastim) in patients with Hodgkin's disease and non-Hodgkin's lymphoma undergoing autologous bone marrow transplantation. Bone Marrow Transplant 1995; 15: 261–6.

141 Stahel RA, Jost LM, Cerny T et al. Randomized study of recombinant human granulocyte colony-stimulating factor after high-dose chemotherapy and autologous bone marrow transplantation for high-risk lymphoid malignancies. J Clin Oncol 1994; 12: 1931–8.

142 Legros M, Fleury J, Cure H et al. rhGM-CSF after high dose chemotherapy and PBPC. A unicenter randomized study of 50 patients. Blood 1994; 84 (Suppl. 1): 90a [Abstract 348].

143 Spitzer G, Adkins DR, Spencer V et al. Randomized study of growth factors post-peripheral-blood stem-cell transplant: neutrophil recovery is improved with modest clinical benefit. J Clin Oncol 1994; 12: 661–70.

144 De Witte T, Gratwohl A, Van Der Lely N et al. Recombinant human granulocyte-macrophage colony-stimulating factor accelerates neutrophil and monocyte recovery after allogeneic T-cell-depleted bone marrow transplantation. Blood 1992; 79: 1359–65.

145 Powles R, Smith C, Milan S et al. Human recombinant GM-CSF in allogeneic bone-marrow transplantation for leukaemia: double-blind, placebo-controlled trial. Lancet 1990; 336: 1417–20.

146 Anasetti C anderson G, Appelbaum FR et al. Phase III study of rh-GM-CSF in allogeneic bone marrow transplantation from unrelated donors. Blood 1993; 82 (Suppl. 1): 454a [Abstract 1799].

147 Larsson K, Bjorkstrand B, Ljungman P. Faster engraftment but no reduction in infectious complications after peripheral blood stem cell transplantation compared to autologous bone marrow transplantation. Support Care Cancer 1998; 6: 378–83.

148 Przepiorka D, Smith TL, Folloder J et al. Controlled trial of filgrastim for acceleration of neutrophil recovery after allogeneic blood stem cell transplantation from human leukocyte antigen-matched related donors. Blood 2001; 97: 3405–10.

149 Link H, Boogaerts MA, Carella AM. A controlled trial of recombinant human granulocyte-macrophage colony-stimulating factor after total body irradiation, high-dose chemotherapy and autologous bone marrow transplantation for acute lymphoblastic leukemia or malignant lymphoma. Blood 1992; 80: 2188–95.

150 Advani R, Chao NJ, Horning SJ et al. Granulocyte-macrophage colony-stimulating factor as an adjunct to autologous hematopoietic stem cell transplantation for lymphoma. Ann Intern Med 1992; 116: 183–9.

151 Gisselbrecht C, Prentice HG, Bacigalupo A et al. Placebo-controlled phase III trial of lenograstim in

152 Nemunaitis J, Rosenfeld CS, Ash R et al. Phase III randomized, double-blind placebo-controlled trial of rhGM-CSF following allogeneic bone marrow transplantation. *Bone Marrow Transplant* 1995; **15**: 949–54.

153 Klumpp TR, Mangan KF, Goldberg SL et al. G-CSF accelerates neutrophil engraftment following PBSC transplantation: a prospective, randomized trial. *J Clin Oncol* 1995; **13**: 1323–7.

154 Linch DC, Milligan DW, Winfield DA et al. G-CSF significantly accelerates neutrophil recovery after PBSC transplantation in lymphoma patients and shortens the time in hospital: preliminary results of a randomized BNLI trial. *Blood* 1995; **86** (Suppl. 1): 221a [Abstract 873].

155 Blaise D, Vernant JP, Fiere D et al. A randomized, controlled, multicenter trial of recombinant human granulocyte colony stimulating factor (filgrastim) in patients treated by bone marrow transplantation (BMT) with total body irradiation (TBI) for acute lymphoblastic leukemia (ALL) or lymphoblastic leukemia (LL). *Blood* 1992; **80**(Suppl.): 248a [Abstract 982].

156 Mitchell PLR, Morland B, Stevens MCG et al. Granulocyte colony-stimulating factor in established febrile neutropenia: a randomized study of pediatric patients. *J Clin Oncol* 1997; **15**: 1163–70.

157 Maher DW, Lieschke GJ, Green M et al. Filgrastim in patients with chemotherapy-induced febrile neutropenia. A double-blind, placebo-controlled trial. *Ann Intern Med* 1994; **121**: 538–40.

158 Mayordomo JI, Rivera F, Diaz-Puente MT et al. Improving treatment of chemotherapy-induced neutropenic fever by administration of colony-stimulating factors. *J Natl Cancer Inst* 1995; **87**: 803–8.

159 Anaissie EJ, Vartivarian S, Bodey GP et al. Randomized comparison between antibiotics alone and antibiotics plus granulocyte–macrophage colony-stimulating factor (*E. coli*-derived) in cancer patients with neutropenia and fever. *Am J Med* 1996; **100**: 17–23.

160 Biesma B, de Vries EG, Willemse PH et al. Efficacy and tolerability of recombinant human granulocyte–macrophage colony-stimulating factor in patients with chemotherapy-related leukopenia and fever. *Eur J Cancer* 1990; **26**: 932–6.

161 Riikonen P, Saarinen UM, Makipernaa A et al. Recombinant human granulocyte-macrophage colony-stimulating factor in the treatment of febrile neutropenia: a double blind placebo-controlled study in children. *Pediatr Infect Dis J* 1994; **13**: 197–202.

162 Vellenga E, Uyl-de Groot CA, de Wit R et al. Randomized placebo controlled trial of granulocyte-macrophage colony-stimulating factor in patients with chemotherapy-related febrile neutropenia. *J Clin Oncol* 1996; **14**: 619–27.

163 Sonis ST, Lindquist L, Van Vugt A et al. Prevention of chemotherapy-induced ulcerative mucositis by transforming growth factor beta 3. *Cancer Res* 1994; **54**: 1135–8.

164 Housley RM, Morris CF, Boyle W et al. Keratinocyte growth factor induced proliferation of hepatocytes and epithelial cells throughout the rat gastrointestinal tract. *J Clin Invest* 1994; **94**: 1764–77.

165 Yi ES, Shabaik AS, Lacey DL et al. Keratinocyte growth factor causes proliferation of urothelium *in vivo*. *J Urol* 1995; **154**: 1566–70.

166 Yi ES, Yin S, Harclerode DL et al. Keratinocyte growth factor induces pancreatic ductal epithelial proliferation. *Am J Pathol* 1994; **145**: 80–5.

167 Spielberger RT, Stiff P, Emmanouilides C et al. Efficacy of recombinant human keratinocyte growth factor (rHuKGF) in reducing mucositis in patients with hematologic malignancies undergoing autologous peripheral blood progenitor cell transplantation (auto-PBPCT) after radiation-based conditioning. Results of a phase 2 trial. *Proc Am Soc Clin Oncol* 2001; **20**: 7a [Abstract 25].

168 Freytes C, LeVeque F, Meisenberg B et al. Safety and efficacy of repifermin (KGF-2) in reducing mucositis in patients undergoing autologous hematopoietic stem cell transplantation (auto-HCT): results of a phase 2a trial. *Blood* 2001; **98** (Suppl. 11): 346b [Abstract 5154].

169 Valcarcel D, Sanz MA, Sureda A et al. Mouth-washings with recombinant human granulocyte-macrophage colony stimulating factor (rhGM-CSF) do not improve grade III–IV oropharyngeal mucositis (OM) in patients with hematological malignancies undergoing stem cell transplantation. Results of a randomized double-blind placebo-controlled study. *Bone Marrow Transplant* 2002; **29**: 783–7.

170 Clift RA, Sanders JE, Thomas ED et al. Granulocyte transfusions for the prevention of infection in patients receiving bone marrow transplants. *N Engl J Med* 1978; **298**: 1052–7.

171 Ruthe RC, Andersen BR, Cunningham BL et al. Efficacy of granulocyte transfusions in the control of systemic candidiasis in the leukopenic host. *Blood* 1981; **52**: 493–8.

172 Winston DJ, Ho WG, Young LS et al. Prophylactic granulocyte transfusions during human bone marrow transplantation. *Am J Med* 1980; **68**: 893–7.

173 Price TH, Bowden RA, Boeckh M et al. Phase I/II trial of neutrophil transfusions from donors stimulated with G-CSF and dexamethasone for treatment of patients with infections in hematopoietic stem cell transplantation. *Blood* 2000; **95**: 3302–9.

174 Illerhaus G, Wirth K, Dwenger A et al. Treatment and prophylaxis of severe infections in neutropenic patients by granulocyte transfusions. *Ann Hematol* 2002; **81**: 273–81.

175 Bensinger WI, Price TH, Dale DC et al. The effects of daily recombinant human granulocyte colony-stimulating factor administration on normal granulocyte donors undergoing leukapheresis. *Blood* 1993; **81**: 1883–8.

176 Caspar CB, Seger RA, Burger J et al. Effective stimulation of donors for granulocyte transfusions with recombinant methionyl granulocyte colony-stimulating factor. *Blood* 1993; **81**: 2866–71.

177 Dale DC, Liles WC, Llewellyn C et al. Neutrophil transfusions: kinetics and functions of neutrophils mobilized with granulocyte-colony-stimulating factor and dexamethasone. *Transfusion* 1988; **38**: 713–21.

178 Dignani MC, Anaissie EJ, Hester JP et al. Treatment of neutropenia-related fungal infections with granulocyte colony-stimulating factor-elicited white blood cell transfusions: a pilot study. *Leukemia* 1997; **11**: 1621–30.

179 Leitman SF, Obiltas JM, Emmons R et al. Clinical efficacy of daily G-CSF-recruited granulocyte transfusions in patients with severe neutropenia and life threatening infections. *Blood* 1996; **88** (Suppl. 1): 331a [Abstract 1313].

180 Taylor K, Moore D, Kelly C et al. Safety and logistical use of filgrastim (FG) mobilized granulocytes (FMG) in early management of severe neutropenic sepsis (SNS) in acute leukemia (AL)/autograft. *Blood* 1996; **88** (Suppl. 1): 349a [Abstract 1384].

181 Sullivan KM, Kopecky J, Jocom J et al. Immunomodulatory and antimicrobial efficacy of intravenous immunoglobulin in bone marrow transplantation. *N Engl J Med* 1990; **323**: 705–12.

182 Sullivan KM, Storek J, Kopecky J et al. A controlled trial of long-term administration of intravenous immunoglobulin to prevent late infection and chronic graft-vs.-host disease after marrow transplantation: Clinical outcome and effect on subsequent immune recovery. *Biol Blood Marrow Transplant* 1996; **2**: 44–53.

183 Graham-Pole J, Camitta B, Casper CJ et al. Intravenous immunoglobulin may lessen all forms of infection in patients receiving allogeneic bone marrow transplantation for acute lymphoblastic leukemia: a pediatric oncology group study. *Bone Marrow Transplant* 1988; **3**: 559–66.

184 Petersen FB, Bowden RA, Thornquist M et al. The effect of prophylactic intravenous immune globulin on the incidence of septicemia in marrow transplant recipients. *Bone Marrow Transplant* 1987; **2**: 141–7.

185 Emanuel DJ, Taylor J, Brochstein J et al. The use of intravenous immune globulin as prophylaxis for the infectious complications of allogeneic marrow transplantation. *Blood* 1992; **80** (Suppl. 1): 271a [Abstract 1075].

186 Winston D, Antin JH, Wolff SN et al. Multi-center, randomized, double-blind doses of intravenous immunoglobulin for the prevention of graft versus host disease and infection after allogeneic bone marrow transplantation. *Bone Marrow Transplant* 2001; **28**: 187–91.

187 Wolff SN, Fay JW, Herzig RH et al. High-dose weekly intravenous immunoglobulin to prevent infections in patients undergoing autologous bone marrow transplantation or severe myelosuppressive therapy. A study of the American Bone Marrow Transplant Group. *Ann Intern Med* 1993; **118**: 937–42.

188 Angus DC, Birmingham MC, Balk RA et al. E5 murine monoclonal antiendotoxin antibody in gram-negative sepsis: a randomized controlled trial E5 Study Investigation. *JAMA* 2000; **283**: 1723–30.

189 Ziegler EJ, Fisher CJ, Sprung CL et al. Treatment of gram-negative bacteremia and septic shock with HA-1A human monoclonal antibody against endotoxin—a randomized, double-blind, placebo-controlled trial. The HA-1A Sepsis Study Group. *N Engl J Med* 1991; **324**: 429–36.

190 Bernard GR, Vincent JL, Laterre PF et al. Efficacy and safety of recombinant human activated protein C for severe sepsis. *N Engl J Med* 2001; **344**: 699–709.

191 Pastores SM, Papadopoulos E, Van Den Brink M et al. Septic shock and multiple organ failure after hematopoietic stem cell transplantation: treatment with recombinant human activated protein C. *Bone Marrow Transplant* 2000; **30**: 131–4.

52
Janice (Wes) M.Y. Brown

Fungal Infections after Hematopoietic Cell Transplantation

Introduction

Invasive fungal infections (IFIs) are increasingly recognized as the leading infectious causes of mortality following allogeneic hematopoietic cell transplantation (HCT) in adults and children [1–4]. The rising incidence of these infections, the emergence of noncandidal, nonaspergillus infections, the refinement of new diagnostic modalities and the introduction of the broadest array of antifungal drugs in the history of medicine have resulted in a renaissance in the study of IFIs. Although the incidence of these infections following HCT is significant, the substantially higher mortality rate in patients with IFIs reflects the unique degree and nature of immunosuppression resulting from allogeneic HCT.

There are three major classes of clinically important fungi—yeasts, molds and dimorphic fungi. One genus of yeast, *Candida* spp., and one genus of molds, *Aspergillus* spp., cause more than 80% of all IFIs following HCT. *Candida* spp. are distinguished by their lack of true hyphae or branching forms and exist primarily as unicellular forms known as blastoconidia or blastospores. Molds, such as *Aspergillus* spp., are most commonly transmitted via inhalation of the conidial (spore) forms and have true hyphae. The dimorphic fungi, such as *Coccioidomycosis imitis* or *Histoplasma capsulatum*, have both yeast forms and true hyphae and are still relatively uncommon in nonendemic areas following transplantation.

This chapter will focus on infections due to *Aspergillus* and *Candida* spp., the two clinically most important fungi following HCT. Since the epidemiology and pathophysiology of *Candida* spp. and *Aspergillus* spp. are unique they will be discussed separately.

The European Organization for Research and Treatment of Cancer (EORTC) and the Mycoses Study Group (USA) have devised classifications of IFIs based on the degree of certainty of the diagnosis. Infections are classified as *definite*, *probable*, or *possible* based on the underlying clinical condition and the results of histopathology, culture and radiologic studies. The classifications differ slightly with respect to HCT recipients as the likelihood that invasion has occurred is great, specific radiologic findings may not be present and invasive diagnostic procedures are not always feasible. *Definite* infection requires evidence of infection on histopathologic specimens or the isolation of fungus from typically sterile sites. Although the culture of fungus from nonsterile specimens, e.g. sputum, and radiographic findings consistent with IFIs define *probable* infection in other populations, following HCT an X-ray consistent with IFIs is generally considered sufficient even in the absence of supporting microbiological data. Therefore, the classification of *possible* fungal infections, formally defined as an X-ray consistent with IFIs but without positive cultures, has little clinical significance following HCT.

While these classifications are of importance for clinical studies of antifungal therapy, there is no difference in the outcome/survival of patients classified as having *definite* vs. *probable* IFIs, especially aspergillosis. Following HCT, even patients who meet the formal criteria for *probable* and *possible* IFIs should be treated aggressively with appropriate antifungal medications. Every reasonable attempt should be made to obtain samples necessary to properly identify the pathogen to ensure appropriate treatment. This principle takes on renewed significance in light of the increasing number of reports of a variety of infections due to fungi other than *Aspergillus* spp. or *Candida* spp.

Epidemiology of IFIs

In several retrospective analyses, the overall incidence of IFIs was between 8% and 15% of all patients undergoing HCT [3–6]. IFIs due to *Candida* or *Aspergillus* spp. occur following autologous or allogeneic HCT, although the incidence and outcome differ in these two groups. Practices and demographics at individual centers will influence the rate and type IFIs; however, many centers report that the incidence of infection due to *Aspergillus* spp. is between 2% and 6% and 5% and 9% following autologous and allogeneic transplantation, respectively [7]. Although the incidence of invasive candidal infections has generally decreased at institutions where prophylactic fluconazole therapy is used an increase in invasive aspergillus infections has been described [8]. In a systematic review of the literature, the case fatality rate in patients with invasive aspergillosis following allogeneic HCT was 86.7% compared to a case fatality rate of 8–60% in hematology and solid organ transplant patients despite prompt institution of aggressive antifungal therapy [9–11].

There is a bimodal pattern to the occurrence of IFIs. This pattern was recognized early in the history of HCT and the specific associated risk factors were identified [5]. Interestingly, the pattern persists, although a shift in the pathogens associated with early and late infections has occurred, reflecting changes that include the shortening of time to neutrophil engraftment, the use of prophylactic antifungal agents, and issues associated with graft-vs.-host disease (GVHD). Currently, although the incidence of infections due to candidal species is lower than was reported in the earlier years of HCT, the mean time to diagnosis of candidal infections remains at 2 weeks post-transplantation, during or immediately following the period of neutropenia and disruption of the mucocutaneous barriers. Invasive aspergillus infections also occur during this period and are generally associated with either colonization of the airways or protracted neutropenia peri-transplantation. Thus, although neutropenia remains a risk for invasive aspergillosis, the majority (58–100%) of patients currently are diagnosed following the resolution of neutropenia. In most large studies, the first peak of invasive aspergillus infection occurs at approximately day +15 and the second, larger peak occurs at

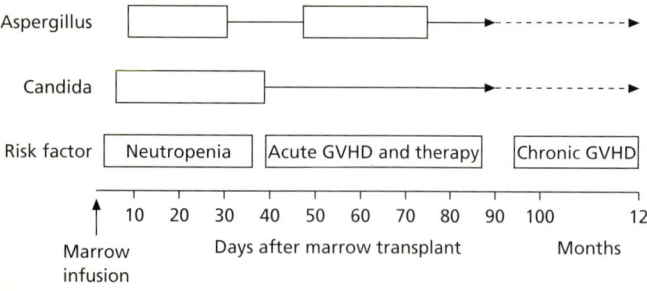

Fig. 52.1 Risk for fungal infection after HCT.

between day +60 and day +136 post-transplant in association with GVHD and systemic corticosteroid use [1,6,12–15]. The timing of IFIs in relation to specific risks is represented schematically in Fig. 52.1.

Specific risk factors for the development of invasive aspergillus infection differ based on when patients are diagnosed in temporal relation to their transplant. For patients diagnosed prior to day +40, risk factors include increases in genetic disparities between donor and recipient, certain conditioning and GVHD prophylactic regimens, and undergoing HCT in a room lacking laminar air-flow. Mortality was higher if IFIs was associated with bacteremia or viral infections [5,16]. For patients diagnosed after day +40, risk factors included systemic steroid administration, late-onset cytomegalovirus (CMV), certain underlying malignancies and hematopoietic disorders, genetic disparities between donor and recipient, prolonged neutropenia, acute grades III–IV GVHD, or extensive chronic GVHD [1,5,13,15,17]. One study reported that ≥21 days of steroid of ≥1 mg/kg/day was specifically associated with increased risk [1]. Recipients of BMT from matched-unrelated donors have been reported to be at a high risk, especially for late fungal disease [16]. Other risk factors include the history of IFIs prior to transplantation and the underlying disease that serves as the indication for transplantation. Examples of underlying conditions that increase the risk for fungal infection, particularly due to *Aspergillus* spp., include chronic granulomatous disease, aplastic anemia and myelodysplastic syndrome.

IFIs are not limited to adult HCT recipients. A recent retrospective analysis reports a 16% incidence of IFIs, including invasive candida and aspergillus, after allogeneic HCT and 8% after autologous HCT in children with a mortality rate comparable to that of adults. There was an association with severe GVHD and with steroid administration. Children who received a total of 0.25–1.00 g/day methylprednisolone for 5 days had a significantly higher incidence of invasive aspergillosis (77%) than patients receiving 2 mg/kg/day prednisone (5%, $p < 0.001$) [3]. IFIs have also been described as one of the most common causes of pneumonia death in pediatric HCT recipients [18].

There are increasing numbers of reports of serious invasive infections caused by less commonly encountered fungi—as a group, these are often referred to as "emerging fungal infections" and include *Pseudoallescheria boydii*, *Blastoschizomyces capitatus*, *Fusarium* spp. (see Plate 23.45, facing p. 296), *Malassezia furfur*, *Scedosporium* spp., *Mucormycosis* and *Trichosporon* spp. [12,19,20–30]. Although the increase may in part be due to improving fungal identification and speciation, concern remains that this trend may in part be due to the growing use of antifungal agents. Little is known about the epidemiology and treatment of infections due to these fungi following HCT. As these fungi often exhibit intrinsic resistance to many antifungal agents, this trend underscores the need for a detailed history of prior antifungal therapy, definitive identification of the pathogen and appropriate use of antifungal susceptibility testing.

The most important principle in understanding the pathophysiology of IFIs is to understand the nature of the immunodeficiencies that render HCT recipients so susceptible to lethal infection. Armed with this knowledge, rational immunologic strategies may be formulated to improve antifungal immune reconstitution. In the case of candidal infections, animal models demonstrate that the crucial determinant of fungal clearance is specific host immune reactivity and not the administration of antifungal agents [31].

Biology and pathophysiology

Candida

Candidal organisms are commensurals, residing on the skin, airways and gastrointestinal (GI) tract. HCT results in numerous conditions and risk factors that have been demonstrated to predispose individuals to candidal invasion, including mucositis, neutropenia, GVHD, coinfections of the urogenital tract (such as herpes simplex virus), administration of broad-spectrum antibiotics, total parenteral nutrition and central venous catheters. Antibiotics including penicillins, quinolones and cephalosporins alter GI colonization [32–34]. Sulfonamides, aminoglycosides and doxycycline may also increase the risk of invasive candidal infection via decreased antifungal neutrophil activity. Ample evidence exists to demonstrate the important roles of both GI and skin disruption in the development of invasive candidal infection [35–37]. It is generally believed that the GI tract is the most common source of the introduction [38]. Thus, while invasive infections must be distinguished from colonization, identification of the colonizing organism may be helpful in the selection of the appropriate antifungal agent in the setting of presumed or proven invasive disease.

Of the numerous species of *Candida*, only *C. albicans*, *C. glabrata*, *C. guillermondi*, *C. krusei*, *C. lusitaniae*, *C. dublineniensis*, *C. tropicalis*, *C. pseudotropicalis*, *C. parapsilosis* and *C. inconspicua* are associated with fungal disease [39,40]. Certain species exhibit intrinsic resistance to specific antifungals. *Candida krusei* is intrinsically resistant to fluconazole and *C. lusitaniae* is resistant to amphotericin. *Candida glabrata* exhibits variable resistance to fluconazole and amphotericin [37,41]. Prior to the widespread use of fluconazole prophylaxis, candidal organisms represented 10–20% of all bloodstream isolates and 5–50% of nosocomial sepsis [42]. While many reports confirm a decrease in invasive candidal infections following HCT, since the administration of prophylactic fluconazole became a more widely used practice an increase in the relative incidence of nonalbicans *Candida* spp. has been inconsistently reported [35,43,44]. Currently, following HCT for adult patients, *C. albicans* is the most common isolated species (52–64%), followed by *C. tropicalis* (11–25%), *C. parapsilosis* (7–24%), *C. glabrata* (8–20%) and *C. krusei* (1–5%). Pediatric programs often report a relatively increased incidence of *C. parapsilosis* [35,45,46].

There is a great deal of ongoing investigation into the factors that are associated with candidal invasion and/or virulence. The nature of the germ tube, pseudohyphal formation, production of proteases, adherence factors, integrin-like substances and specific antigen expression are some of the areas of active investigation; however, the clinical significance of these factors remains unknown.

Syndromes of candidal infection

Although distinguishing colonization from infection is frequently difficult, multiple clinical syndromes associated with *Candida* spp. have been described. The unifying feature of these syndromes is that a high degree of clinical suspicion is required in order to make a premortem diagnosis.

Mucocutaneous infection

Involvement of the skin or GI tract in HCT recipients should be treated, as colonization in these locations pose greater risks for invasion in this setting. Esophagitis or involvement of other areas of the GI tract is a well-recognized entity and may occur in the absence of thrush. Symptoms of candidal esophagitis may be indistinguishable from esophagitis due to other etiologies and include dysphagia, substernal chest pain, nausea, vomiting, or upper GI bleeding. The stomach is the second most common site GI of candidal infection, followed by the large and small bowel. Definitive diagnosis of GI candidiasis is made by endoscopic examination. Findings at endoscopy include white plaques, single or multiple ulcers, erosions, or pseudomembrane formation. Rarely, patients may present with perforation.

Candidemia

Methods used to culture blood are insensitive in the isolation of *Candida* spp. and, as a result, fewer than 50% of patients with proven dissemination have positive blood cultures. Despite the insensitivity of this test, *Candida* spp. are some of the most common organisms isolated from blood cultures at large medical centers. Techniques such as the lysis-centrifugation system (Isolator system) have not significantly improved the sensitivity of blood cultures. Following HCT there is a higher incidence of dissemination associated with candidemia; therefore, clinical suspicion should be high that dissemination has occurred.

Candidal species are capable of producing glycocalyx, potentially contributing to a biofilm on intravenous catheters. Thus, candidemia is highly associated with infection of a central venous catheter and most data support the recommendation to remove any catheters present at the time of diagnosis of candidemia. Removal of catheters, particularly if accomplished very early during the infection, significantly shortens the period of candidemia and reduces the risk for recurrent candidemia. Changing catheters over a wire does not appear to reduce the risk. It would be ideal to delay replacement of central venous catheter until blood cultures are negative. Some patients were described as having a spontaneous resolution of symptoms (primarily fever) following the removal of the central venous catheter; however, given the high risk for dissemination and the difficulty confirming that dissemination has occurred, it is ill-advised to presume that removal of the intravenous catheter is sufficient treatment. Parenteral administration of antifungal agents should be administered [47–50].

Dissemination with deep-tissue infection

Following HCT the risk for visceral dissemination is high especially in patients with a history of documented candidemia; however, dissemination is frequently not diagnosed until post-mortem examination. Although the liver, spleen and lungs are most frequently affected, virtually all other organs are at risk for seeding including the kidneys, brain, heart (myocarditis or endocarditis), central nervous system (CNS), vascular endothelium, bone, endocrine glands and eye (endophthalmitis). Microabscesses are the hallmark of candidal tissue invasion and are not necessarily accompanied by a marked inflammatory response especially following HCT [51]. Histologic examination may reveal a granulomatous response with epithelioid or histiocyte response. Special stains (periodic acid Schiff or methenamine silver stains) may increase the identification of fungal organisms present in the microabscesses.

Hepatosplenic candidiasis is probably the most common syndrome of disseminated infection and is believed to require candidal entry via the portal system. Patients do not usually have signs and symptoms associated with organ involvement; therefore, radiologic imaging is recommended in high-risk patients such as patients with candidemia. With a reported >90% sensitivity, computerized tomography (CT) scans of the abdomen following the administration of intravenous contrast are more sensitive than ultrasound examinations. However, in one retrospective analysis of autopsy-proven cases of hepatic candidiasis, CT scans or ultrasound exams revealed evidence of tissue infection in only 18% of patients prior to their death. Other imaging modalities may be more useful. One prospective study examined the role of magnetic resonance imaging (MRI) scans in patients with suspected hepatosplenic candidiasis. Patients were divided into groups based on whether they received acute (<2 weeks), subacute (>2 weeks but <3 months), or chronic (>3 months or completed) antifungal treatment. MRI scanning offers high positive and negative predictive values (85% and 100%, respectively, with a sensitivity of 100%) and a specificity of 96% in the diagnosis of hepatosplenic candidiasis in the acute setting. In 11 of 13 patients with hepatoplenic abnormalities, the lesions were <1 cm in diameter and were described as well-defined high signal intensity foci on T1-weighted images. Additionally, the MRI may be able to distinguish active from chronic lesions that are presumed to be healed and which tend to be larger (1–3 cm) with irregular, more angular margins [52].

The lungs are often involved in disseminated candidiasis representing delivery of organisms by nonportal perfusion. As with hepatosplenic candidiasis, patients may have fever but infrequently complain of symptoms referable to the respiratory tract. Unfortunately, cultures of sputum or bronchoalveolar lavage fluid have limited sensitivity and specificity and are therefore of limited diagnostic value. CT scans of the chest are recommended in the setting of candidemia following HCT [4,53]. The early institution of antimycotic therapy improves survival. In one series, therapy started within 10 days of the diagnosis of pulmonary candidiasis resulted in 41% mortality compared to >90% mortality if therapy was started after 10 days of symptoms [54]. An endovascular source of infection should be considered in patients believed to have disseminated candidiasis who persistently exhibit symptoms or develop new lesions despite appropriate antifungal therapy [55].

Cardiovascular system

Candida spp. are capable of attaching to the endothelium and to catheters which may explain the presence of endovascular infections, such as endocarditis and thrombophlebitis, with or without concomitant deep venous thrombosis. Thrombophlebitis is most commonly a post-mortem diagnosis; however, the classic presentation includes a patient with localizing extremity edema and a history of protracted broad spectrum antibiotic and/or total parenteral nutrition administration via a central venous catheter [56]. Although rare, *Candida* spp. are the most common cause of fungal endocarditis. Most of the symptoms are indistinguishable from bacterial endocarditis and it is notable that patients may have minimal symptoms. One clue that a patient may have fungal endocarditis may be the occurrence of large peripheral embolic lesions as fungal vegetations tend to be large and friable. Blood cultures are frequently positive and endophthalmitis is a common finding. Formal ophthalmologic evaluation is recommended in HCT recipients with visual complaints and is mandatory in the setting of disseminated candidal infection. Vitreous biopsy may be necessary to diagnose candidal endophthalmitis. Endovascular candidal infections have high mortality rates, but significantly improved outcomes have been consistently reported if surgical intervention is part of the therapy of thrombophlebitis or endocarditis [56–62].

CNS disease

In retrospective analyses, candida was identified as one of the most common causes of CNS infection following HCT. In two large retrospective analyses performed prior to the widespread use of fluconazole prophylaxis in allogeneic HCT, *Candida* spp. were identified as the responsible pathogen in 18% and 33% of CNS lesions. Candida meningitis or brain abscess often occurred in association with fungemia (63% of cases) or neutropenia (63%) and widespread dissemination [27,29,63]. The high incidence of CNS involvement following HCT mandates that the treatment or prevention of IFIs should take into account the CNS compartment.

Skin lesions

Skin lesions may be overlooked or obscured by other presentations of dermatitis including drug eruptions or GVHD. The early post-transplant period is the time of highest risk for disseminated candidal infection, a time period that overlaps with the period of broad-spectrum antibiotic administration (febrile neutropenia) and acute GVHD, which most commonly affects the skin. The cutaneous lesions of disseminated candidiasis may be subtle or dramatic and include macronodular lesions (0.5–1.0 cm diameter, pink or red), lesions resembling ecthyma gangrenosum, or purpura fulminans. Diagnosis requires biopsy and culture of the lesions [64].

Aspergillus

Aspergillus spores are thermotolerant and resistant to dessication. Although molds are not commensurals, exposure to spores likely occurs frequently as they are found throughout nature, particularly associated with decaying vegetation and soil. High spore concentrations have been associated with barns and compost piles, but significant exposure have also been ascribed to indoor potted plants, peppers, spices and smoking marijuana [65]. Filamentous fungi, including *Aspergillus*, have also been isolated from water in a pediatric bone marrow transplantation (BMT) unit; however, the clinical significance of this finding is not clear as there have not yet been large studies confirming nosocomial transmission via the water supply, even in high risk populations [66].

There are numerous species of *Aspergillus*, but virtually all clinical illness described has been caused by five species, probably due to the fact that these pathogenic species can grow at 37°C in contrast to nonpathogenic species that lack this trait. The five species most commonly associated with disease are *A. fumigatus*, *A. flavus*, *A. niger*, *A. terreus* and *A. nidulans*. The marked predominance of *A. fumigatus* may be explained in part by its ubiquity in nature and its very rapid growth rate, with hyphal extension occurring at a rate as high as 1–2 cm/h.

The small size and hydrophobic coating of the spores result in a reduction in electrostatic forces and ensure efficient aerosolization and possibly facilitate immune escape. Inhalation by immunocompetent hosts in the absence of corticosteroid therapy very rarely results in invasive infections. The association between inoculum size and disease is unknown but is suspected to be minimal in severely immunocompromised individuals. This hypothesis is supported by (i) the occurrence of nosocomial outbreaks of *Aspergillus* spp. infections with highest incidence in the most immunocompromised patients, even in the absence of documentation of high ambient spore counts; and (ii) the lower frequency of positive cultures of the respiratory tracts of HCT recipients when compared to patients with other risk factors. Additionally, patients may have been colonized for an extended period and develop disease after subsequent immunocompromise.

The inhaled conidia that escape mucociliary defenses are rapidly ingested by the alveolar macrophages. Soon after tissue infection by this angioinvasive organism, the hyphae are damaged and destroyed by neutrophils and, to some degree, by platelets and monocytes. A variety of different antigens are expressed during the morphologic changes as soon as the conidia begins germination as the initial stages of hyphal formation.

The hallmark of aspergillus disease is angioinvasion and it is by this method that the fungus disseminates. Due to the angioinvasive tendencies of this pathogen hemorrhage and infarction are hallmarks of infection. Similarly, cavitation may appear as a consequence of vascular compromise. As *Aspergillus* spp. can thrive in an acidic environment with low oxygen tension, vascular disruption establishes these growth conditions and impairs the delivery of antifungal agents and immune effectors. These findings may help explain the observation that complete eradication is very difficult with medical therapy alone and that the patient remains at risk following further immunotherapy.

Hydrocortisone *in vitro* causes a 30–40% acceleration in the growth rate of some species of *Aspergillus* [67]. Steroids have also been shown to inhibit the control of fungal infection by a variety of mechanisms. Steroids impair the ingestion and/or killing of aspergillus conidia and hyphae by alveolar macrophage, monocyte and neutrophil killing. Delayed cytokine production and cell recruitment in response to aspergillus challenge has also been documented [68,69]. Impaired anticandidal response in the setting of pharmacologic doses of dexamethasone included the marked reduction of tumor necrosis factor (TNF) production and therefore an attenuation of monocyte activation [70].

Pathogen-specific virulence determinants have not yet been defined for *Aspergillus* spp. In addition to the ability to grow at body temperature, pathogenic species of *Aspergillus* demonstrate efficient binding to laminin and fibrinogen, and they produce elastases, phospholipases, several superoxide dismutases and catalases; however, the specific role of each of these biochemical characteristics in the pathogenesis of invasive infection has yet to elucidated [71–73].

Aspergillosis: clinical syndromes

The term "aspergillosis" is currently used in reference to invasive disease in contrast to "aspergilloma" which refers to a focal lesion, typically in the lung. In settings other than following HCT, each of these terms has a distinct histopathologic and clinical significance. Following HCT, however, even the patient with, for example, a single lesion identified on chest CT, must be considered to have microscopic invasion or to be at imminent risk for invasion even at the time of first diagnosis. This risk for and likelihood of invasive disease has important therapeutic ramifications.

As the biology of aspergillus would predict, the most common sites of inoculation are the bronchial tree and the paranasal sinuses. Therefore, concomitant pneumonia and sinusitis should suggest fungal disease [74]. Pulmonary aspergillosis following HCT is most commonly accompanied only by fever but many patients may be completely asymptomatic. Symptoms of infection, if present, may be organ-specific but are not specific to fungal infection. The paucity and nonspecific nature of the symptoms likely accounts for the fact that as many as two-thirds of cases are diagnosed at autopsy [75–77]. Necrotic skin or mucosal lesions, invasive sinusitis, hemoptysis and pneumonia with pain are findings that should raise suspicion of an invasive infection due to *Aspergillus* spp.

As the risk factors for invasive aspergillosis have changed over time, the spectrum of radiologic findings have changed. Likely as a result of a limited immune response, parenchymal lesions due to *Aspergillosis* spp. may appear in a multitude of forms including nodules, with or without a circumferential hemorrhage (often described as a "halo") or central cavitation, infiltrates, or a combination of both. Radiographic findings may be highly variable following HCT and requiring the presence of "classic" lesions, such as halos, or crescents will ensure missing the diagnosis in some cases.

Sinusitis is usually symptomatic and is usually not distinguishable from inflammation resulting from a variety of etiologies. Due to the pigments produced by *Aspergillus* and the invasive nature of the fungus, drainage may be green, black, or bloody. Other ominous signs or symptoms suggestive of an invasive process include erosive lesions of the nasal septum, cavernous sinus thrombosis, pain with eye movement, extraocular muscle plegias, diplopia, or periorbital swelling [78].

Infections limited to the lower airways are the next step in the spectrum from colonization to parenchymal invasion. These infections include laryngitis, tracheitis and tracheobronchitis [79]. The invasive potential for tracheobronchitis is documented by the detection of aspergillus antigen in the blood prior to initial clinical presentation and subsequent development of parenchymal lesions [80]. A high degree of clinical suspicion must exist in order to diagnose tracheobronchitis as airway thickening may be absent or not appreciated. Sputum samples may persistently yield colonies of mold—often more than a few colonies—but negative cultures do not rule out this diagnosis. Bronchoscopy should be considered in patients with unexplained or chronic cough which may be productive and refractory to antibacterial therapy. A variety of bronchoscopic and post-mortem findings have been described including pseudomembranes, plaques, and balls of fungus.

Sites of skin trauma including catheter insertion sites are also portals of fungal entry; however, these infections are relatively uncommon. Cutaneous aspergillosis may invade and become fatal [81,82]. Skin lesions typically start as focal lesions and necrosis is characteristic. If the lesion is not at a site of known trauma or there is more than one lesion, the possibility of hematogenous spread from an intravascular focus of infection including endocarditis should be considered [75]. Histopathologic examination and culture of biopsies of the lesion should be performed to confirm the diagnosis.

Although not studied prospectively, a high incidence of CNS involvement has frequently been noted and this has potential significance with respect to the pharmacokinetics and tissue distribution of the antifungal agent selected. In a retrospective study, CNS involvement was reported in 10 of 18 HCT patients diagnosed with invasive aspergillosis [11]. Manifestations of CNS disease include microabscesses, macroabscesses, meningitis and extension from sinus disease. In retrospective analyses of brain abscesses following BMT, fungal organisms were isolated in almost all cases (60–92%) and *Aspergillus* spp. was the most common organism isolated [27,29,63]. It is important to note that although pulmonary disease was present in the vast majority (87%) of cases of aspergillus brain abscess, this finding was not invariably present [27].

Dissemination to virtually every tissue has been described including the myocardium, thyroid, kidneys, eyes and GI tract. Although there is no clear pattern of *Aspergilllus* spp. dissemination, there are a number of published reports of renal, GI and eye involvement. With the exception of fungal endophthalmitis, tissue biopsy is necessary in order to establish the diagnosis. In contrast to candidal endophthalmitis, biopsy of vitreal tissue often fails to identify the organism in aspergillus infection. Thus, empiric broad-spectrum antifungal therapy is mandated in this infection. Treatment may include vitrectomy and/or intravitreal instillation of amphotericin B even in the absence of a confirmed diagnosis. Although still investigational, molecular diagnostic tests may be helpful in the future evaluation of this infection.

GI involvement may result from direct invasion or angioinvasive spread and should be a diagnostic consideration for persistent symptomatology in the setting of protracted therapy for GI GVHD. Any region of the GI tract may be involved and a variety of findings, including diffuse infiltration, necrotizing lesions and pseudomembrane formation, have been described [83]. To further complicate matters, there is a particularly high association with CMV in this setting. Thus, the diagnosis of GVHD should heighten suspicion of both concomitant viral and fungal infections and the risk of infection increases with protracted GVHD therapy.

Diagnostic testing for IFIs not based on cultures

Blood cultures are rarely positive, even in invasive aspergillosis, and they have an unacceptably low sensitivity in candidemia. Decades of investigation have led to the development of nonculture based diagnostic tests. Currently, the most promising for clinical use include tests to detect fungal components and tests based on molecular techniques to detect fungal nucleic acids.

Galactomannans (GMs) are cell wall components of fungi and measurement of this antigen in the blood and urine has been studied for over two decades as a potential diagnostic test for IFIs. The two most studied GM antigenemia tests are the latex agglutination (LA) test and enzyme-linked immunosorbent assay (ELISA). A number of recent studies reported that the LA test failed to distinguish between infection and exposure to noninfectious *Aspergillus* spp. antigens [84], and was less sensitive and persistently less positive than ELISA [85,86]. ELISA has a sensitivity of 60–90% and a specificity of 82–98%, but repeated/serial sampling is necessary. Nonaspergillus molds were not detected [87]. Although use of ELISA did not result in the detection of invasive aspergillosis prior to the development of signs or symptoms [88], it may be useful as a confirmatory test in probable or possible aspergillosis. In one study of 37 patients being treated for invasive aspergillosis following HCT the temporal changes in quantitative serum GM as measured by ELISA was found to have some utility in the determination of response of aspergillosis to therapy despite a sensitivity of 44% [89].

A variety of polymerase chain reaction (PCR)-based assays have been developed and appear to hold more promise in the early diagnosis of both invasive candidiasis and aspergillosis. In some assays, specific primers have been paired with species-specific probes permitting the identification of the pathogenic fungus. Retrospective and prospective PCR assays of the blood have been reported. While no direct comparative trial of the different PCR assays has been reported, results are consistent following HCT. Assays are capable of identifying genus and species of pathogenic fungi with a reported 100% sensitivity, 98% specificity. In one large study, colonization was infrequently associated with a positive PCR signal in the blood. However, the signal was positive only 4–7 days prior to a radiologic diagnosis and 5.7 days prior (range 0–14 days) to the institution of antifungal therapy. Additionally, the sensitivity decreases and the specificity increases depending if two rather than one test is considered to be the threshold for a diagnosis [90–92]. The utility of a PCR assay has also been studied in the clinical evaluation of 197 bronchoalveolar lavage samples from 102 immunocompromised patients. A variety of patients were included in the study and the sensitivity, specificity and a negative predictive value were 94.0%, 94.0% and 98.1%, respectively, when a combination of culture, radiographic and histologic studies were used to confirm the diagnosis [93].

One advantage to molecular-based assays in the diagnosis of IFIs is that the test may be completed rapidly. A multiplex PCR, designed to amplify unique sequences of *C. albicans*, was run in parallel with standard blood cultures. The sensitivity of the assay was 96.9% and the test was completed within 8 h. The identification of nonalbicans species was less optimal [94]. Despite the encouraging data, one prospective study of three serum assays including PCR-based detection of *Candida* spp., concentration of $(1,3)$-β-D-glucan, a key component of the fungal cell wall, and two commercial candidal GM antigens assays in 40 allogeneic BMT and solid-organ transplant recipients demonstrated that no single test was sufficient for the diagnosis [95]. In addition to aiding in the diagnosis of IFIs, nonculture based diagnostic modalities offer great potential in the development of strategies to stratify risk and/or pre-emptively treat patients both pre and post-transplantation.

Immune response to *Candida* spp. and *Aspergillus* spp.

The association between neutropenia and IFIs has long been recognized; however, the significant increase in IFIs in immunocompromised hosts has brought into focus the role of other immune effectors in defense against infection. The morphologic changes the fungi undergo in the course of invasion with the attendant changes in surface molecule expression adds to the complexity of host–pathogen interaction. The high incidence of invasive candidal infection associated with human immunodeficiency virus (HIV)-infection first highlighted the clinically significant role of the $CD4^+$ cell in anticandidal defense. Studies demonstrate that invasive candidal infection follows adhesion of the organism to cell surfaces, which induces pro-inflammatory cytokine production [96]. Various immune effectors are involved in response to candidal infections. Neutrophils damage candidal pseudohyphae and phagocytose the blastospores [97,98]. Both dendritic cells (DCs) and macrophages attach to mannose-fucose receptors and ingest candidal blastospores, presenting fungal antigens to T cells. Unlike macrophages, DCs do not require opsonization of the candida and serum does not enhance ingestion. DCs that ingest heat-killed candida induced lymphocyte proliferation [99]. *In vitro* and mouse studies demonstrate that following DC or macrophage presentation of candidal antigens recovery from infection is dependent on CD4$^+$TH1-type cytokine enhancement of monocyte and neutrophil function. In adoptive transfer studies, naive CD4$^+$ but not CD8$^+$ cells were demonstrated to protect against death due to candida [100]. Studies using antibodies and/or knockout mice have demonstrated that interferon-gamma (IFN-γ), TNF and interleukin 18 (IL-18) are important in the defense against invasive candidal disease. Additionally, neutralization of IL-18, IL-1, or IL-12 results in a decrease in candida-induced IFN production. Therefore, the production and secretion of epithelial cytokines of the TH1-type appear to recruit activated lymphocytes in response to infection with *Candida* spp. [101].

The cellular immune response to *Candida* spp. is complex and evidence suggests that specific effector populations may be linked to the route of invasion. Gamma/delta and alpha/beta T-cell knockout mice were more resistant than wild-type mice to disseminated candidiasis following intravenous injection. However, these mice are highly susceptible to candidal dissemination following high-dose oral challenge [102]. In contrast, transgenic mice with combined natural killer and T-cell defects are highly susceptible to oral challenge [103].

The immune response against *Candida* spp. is not purely beneficial to the host. The role of antibodies in infection with *Candida* spp. is complex. Patients with disseminated disease may have high titers of immunoglobulin G (IgG); however, serum is not protective against infection. Studies in mice reveal that administration of subsets of antibodies may actually potentiate disease progression whereas others agglutinate blastospores, assisting with clearance of fungus. However, antibody-mediated agglutination of candidal organisms is not sufficiently protective. To complicate matters, *Candida* spp. produce proteases that digest IgG and IgA.

The role of alveolar macrophages is equally complex. The ability of alveolar macrophages to ingest and destroy candidal organisms has been well established *in vitro*. Alveolar macrophage-deficient mice demonstrated reduced candidal clearing and fewer recruited neutrophils due to a reduction in the level of the neutrophil chemoattractant macrophage inflammatory protein-2 and decreased myeloperoxidase activities. However, this attenuated immune response was associated with an improved survival.

Fungal determinants of pathogenicity are not well understood but are, in part, due to varying degrees of immunogenicity. Species of *Candida* differ in their association with invasive disease. These differences may be explained by fungal determinants of virulence as well as variations in the intricacies of immunomodulation induced by the organism. Illustrative of these principles is the fact that *C. glabrata* is considered to be intrinsically less virulent. However, studies in mice demonstrate that the improved survival following *C. glabrata* infection may in part be due to an associated vigorous IFN-γ, TNF and IL-12 response and a minimal production of the anti-inflammatory cytokine, IL-10. In contrast, death due to infection with *Candida albicans* is associated with a delayed and severely reduced IFN-γ, TNF and IL-12 response [104,105]. The immune response to different candidal forms is also specific. DCs appear to differentiate yeast from hyphae as ingestion of early hyphal forms inhibit IL-12 production to a degree far greater than the quiescent yeast cells [106].

A few studies have begun to elucidate the dysregulation of TH-type cytokine production in mice following T-cell-depleted allogeneic BMT. Early post-transplant, production of the TH2 type cytokines, IL-4 and IL-10, was substantial in contrast to a significantly impaired production of TH1-type cytokines IL-12, IFN-γ and TNF. TH1-type antifungal resistance could be restored following treatment with TH2 cytokine antagonists. In the haploidentical model, this shift to a TH2-type immunoreactivity was seen despite the establishment of full, donor-type chimerism by the 2nd week post-transplantation and the mice were profoundly susceptible to lethal fungal infections. By 5 weeks post-transplantation, the susceptibility to infection had resolved and was temporally correlated with an improved TH1-type response [107].

The significantly higher mortality due to IFIs following HCT compared to patients in other risk groups is further evidence that the recovery of an effective immune response is crucial to effective clearance of fungus. Studies in immunosuppressed mice confirm that antifungal therapy did not result in optimal antifungal clearance unless a favorable cytokine response was restored. In this model, the concomitant administration of soluble IL-4 receptor, IL-12, or antibodies against IL-10 was synergistic with the administration of antifungal agents.

A growing body of work is beginning to elucidate the immune response to *Aspergillus* spp. As observed with *Candida* spp., different morphologic forms of the fungus elicit different immune responses. The current understanding of the immune response to the conidia and hyphal forms of *Aspergillus* spp. is represented schematically in Fig. 52.2. Following inhalation of conidia, the alveolar macrophages and DCs are the first line of defense. Any conidial forms that escape are subject to clearance by tissue macrophages. Invasive aspergillosis is associated with hyphal germination and subsequent tissue destruction. Neutrophils are crucial in the clearance of the earliest hyphal (germlings) as well as the full hyphal forms [68].

A limited number of early animal studies demonstrated the importance of the acquired immune response. These reports demonstrated the prevention of aspergillosis following vaccination of turkey poults and the adoptive transfer of immune splenic macrophages in immunoincompetent mice [108,109]. DCs have been shown to have pivotal role in the defense against aspergillosis both in mice and human cells [110]. In addition to phagocytosing both conidia and hyphae, DCs migrate to lymph nodes and spleen, influencing T-cell reactivity [111]. Multiple recent animal and clinical studies have consistently demonstrated that the specific nature of the resultant T-cell reactivity influences the host's ability to resist invasive aspergillosis. As documented in the immune response to *Candida* spp., a TH1-type immunoreactivity, as indicated by production of TNF-α, IL-12, IFN-γ and IL-2, is protective against intravenous or inhaled challenge with *A. fumigatus*. In contrast, TH2-type immunoreactivity is deleterious and high production of IL-4 and IL-10 correlates with an increased susceptibility to infection. These observations have been confirmed using appropriate knockout mice and cytokine neutralization [112,113]. Immunocompetent or immunized mice produce significant quantities of IFN-γ and IL-12 in the lungs and spleen in contrast to susceptible cortisone-treated mice that had an increase in IL-10 production in these organs [114].

Increased levels of IFN-γ, granulocyte macrophage colony-stimulating factor (GM-CSF), TNF-α and IL-2, but not IL-10 or IL-4, were detected in supernatants of cocultured *A. fumigatus* and human peripheral blood mononuclear cells [115]. The role of natural killer (NK) cells has not been extensively studied, although in one study activated lymphocytes but not NK cells were capable of interfering *in vitro* with adherence of *Aspergillus* to a surface [116].

Effect of immunosuppressive agents

Virtually all clinical studies have identified systemic corticosteroid use as a key risk factor for the development of IFIs. Other immunosuppressive agents commonly used post-transplantation have not yet been shown to

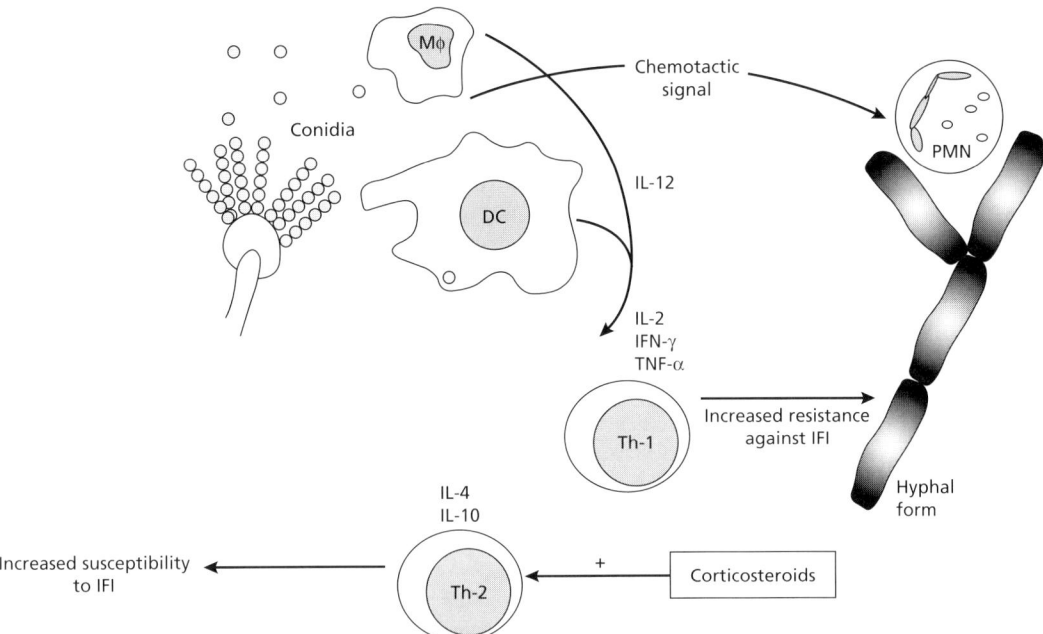

Fig. 52.2 Immune response to conidia and hyphal forms of *Aspergillus* spp.

be similarly associated with increased risk. Hydrocortisone *in vitro* causes a 30–40% acceleration in the growth rate of some species of *Aspergillus* [67]. Steroids have also been shown to impair alveolar macrophages, monocytes and the neutrophil killing of fungi [70,117,118]. Steroid-treated mice had a delayed initial clearance of the conidia, increased splenic production of IL-10, poorly regulated IL-6 and IL-2β production, and an inflammatory response with few lymphocytes [68,114]. The immunologic sequelae of GVHD, however, further confounds the clear understanding of the precise additional risk of IFIs resulting from the administration of corticosteroids.

Preparative regimen, graft manipulation, progenitor cells

The preparative regimen for HCT may influence the incidence of IFIs. Protocols that result in significant mucositis were associated with an increase in invasive candidal infections. Protracted neutropenia increased the risk for invasive infections with both *Candida* and *Aspergillus* spp. Insufficient data are available at this time regarding the precise risks for and ability to clear opportunistic infections following nonmyeloablative preparative regimens. It is notable that patients with a history of IFIs, including bilateral pulmonary infiltrates due to invasive aspergillosis, have survived and even cleared infection following nonmyeloablative preparative regimens, which suggests the potential benefit for rapid immune reconstitution with a minimal period of neutropenia. In studies with a limited number of patients, the incidence of CMV reactivations and disease was comparable following nonmyeloablative vs. myeloablative preparative regimens; however, there were insufficient numbers of patients to determine risk for IFIs. The incidence of late invasive aspergillosis following nonmyeloablative transplant would be predicted to be dependent on the incidence of grade III or IV GVHD and the dose of steroid administration as with all other HCT [119–121].

Prevention and treatment

It is very difficult to sterilize tissue that has been invaded with fungus; thus, relapse can occur in the event of subsequent immunosuppression. Given the morbidity and mortality associated with IFIs, preventative measures as well as therapeutic maneuvers are essential.

Prevention of infection

Given the seriousness of the infection, the difficulty of early diagnosis and the high mortality rate despite early institution of antifungal therapy, prevention of IFIs would be predicted to be the ideal way of reducing deaths due to these infections after HCT.

Transplantation strategies that reduce the duration and degree of mucosal injury, the duration of myeloid, macrophage, and TH1-type immunodeficiency, the severity of GVHD, and the need for corticosteroids, parenteral nutrition, or intravenous catheters would all contribute to a decrease in IFIs. *Candida* spp. is a mucocutaneous commensural organism and violating the integrity of these surfaces is directly related to the risk for infection. Outbreaks of candidal infections have also been associated with transmission via the skin and nails of healthcare workers. In contrast, the incidence of aspergillus has been shown to be related to environmental exposures, which may have occurred prior to the diagnosed infection.

Environmental considerations

Although not a common occurrence, transmission of candidal species has been documented from infections or colonization of the skin and nails of healthcare workers. Simple maneuvers, such as strict hand-washing protocols, prohibition of direct patient contact by healthcare personnel who have fungal skin or nail infections, and staff education are successful. Interestingly, false or acrylic nails and dermatitis are associated with increased risk for superficial fungal infection and, therefore, nosocomial transmission.

Central to the prevention of aspergillosis is the avoidance of inhalation of spores. In the outpatient setting, there are no proven methods to decrease risk of colonization. Given published associations, avoidance of contact with soil and plants including marijuana smoking, gardening, or maintenance of compost piles would be prudent. The optimal duration of this prohibition is not clear [122]. The efficacy of wearing high-efficiency particulate air (HEPA)-filtered air masks has also not been proven. Behavioral modifications that result from wearing the mask may theoretically decrease the transmission of other infections such as those due to respiratory viruses, especially as an outpatient.

In the inpatient setting, although some inconsistent observations have been reported, a number of studies have demonstrated the benefit of laminar airflow rooms and HEPA-filtered air. These structural considerations have been incorporated into most large transplant centers for high-risk patients who are neutropenic [123]. Although it is noteworthy that aspergillus has been isolated from water, a post-transplantation prohibition of showers or bathing has not been demonstrated to reduce infection. The Centers for Disease Control publishes recommendations regarding the reduction of environmental risks for reducing IFIs [122,124].

Administration of antifungal agents

In addition to attempts to decrease exposures or risk for IFIs, prevention of invasive disease typically includes the administration of antifungal agents. The efficacy of antifungals in the prevention of IFIs is an area of active investigation. Strategies include (i) *primary prophylaxis*, defined as the administration of antifungal drugs in the absence of any evidence or history of infection; (ii) *secondary prophylaxis*, defined as the administration of agents to patients with a history of prior IFIs; and (iii) *empiric treatment*, defined as the administration of agents based on a defined but nondiagnostic clinical indication, but without proven IFIs. The prototypic empiric therapy is the use of antifungals in patients with fever during neutropenia.

Primary prophylaxis

The concept of primary chemoprophylaxis of IFIs has been supported by *in vitro* data and by clinical studies with respect to candidiasis. Studies in animal models of HCT demonstrated that administration of antifungal prior to infection was successful in improving mortality even when compared to therapy given early post-infection [125]. Numerous clinical studies have been reported and are included in Table 52.1; however, few had a study design that would provide statistically significant results [126]. Administration of fluconazole during the early post-transplant period through engraftment [127] or day +75 post-transplantation [128] has been shown to reduce the incidence of all invasive candidal infections (27% vs. 8%) and, in particular, hepatic candidal infection (16% vs. 3%) [8]. Additionally, after 8 years of follow-up, 68 of 152 patients who received fluconazole at a dose of 400 mg/day, survived following allogeneic HCT compared to 41 of 148 patients who received placebo from day +0 through day +75 ($p = 0.001$). In this same study, the incidence and mortality rate of severe GVHD was significantly higher in the placebo group; however, these observations could not be attributed specifically to a decrease in IFIs [129].

Despite the efficacy of fluconazole prophylaxis in allogeneic HCT, questions remain. The optimal dose and duration of prophylactic administration of fluconazole has not yet been determined. Studies have yielded conflicting results regarding the efficacy of lower dosages of fluconazole. In one randomized study of 253 pediatric and adult HCT patients comparing 400 mg/day vs. 200 mg/day of fluconazole during the neutropenic period, no significant difference was observed in IFIs by day +50. However, other studies have failed to demonstrate any protective benefit of 100 mg/day [130]. Similarly, the role of fluconazole prophylaxis following autologous transplantation has not been thoroughly studied; however, it would be prudent to consider fluconazole prophylaxis if significant mucositis or prolonged neutropenia is expected to result.

One major concern is that widespread implementation of fluconazole prophylaxis may result in the emergence of resistance in previously susceptible species of candida or an increase in the incidence of infection with species intrinsically resistant to fluconazole. Although some centers have reported the emergence of such species, this shift in pathogens has not been consistently reported; however, the development of azole resistance is a well-documented occurrence in the setting of therapy. In fact, candidal species have been shown to develop a relative resistance to fluconazole during treatment and require significant dose escalation to inhibit growth. Administration of antifungal agents may have unexpected effects on the spectrum of fungal diseases. An interesting observation in one large retrospective analysis of patient outcomes and autopsy data is that, although there was no increase in infections due to resistant candidal species, there was an increase in the incidence of invasive aspergillosis following the institution of routine fluconazole prophylaxis [8]. The investigators postulated that the reduction in death due to invasive candidal infections prolonged survival so patients eventually succumbed to mold infection. Finally, the administration of fluconazole may decrease the sensitivity of blood cultures especially with respect to *C. albicans* [131].

Prior to the introduction of lipid formulations of amphotericin and itraconazole, the only licensed, broad-spectrum antifungal agent was amphotericin B deoxycholate (D-Amb, Fungizone®). The high incidence of nephrotoxicity associated with D-Amb limited the tolerated dose in high-risk patients (e.g. myeloablative allogeneic HCT recipients) as the majority of these patients were receiving at least one other nephrotoxic agent. Of the numerous reports of equivalence or intolerance of drug, one group reported a decrease in mortality due to fungal infections after changing their clinical practice and administering low dose (5–10 mg/day) D-Amb from day +0 through engraftment following allogeneic HCT [132]. However, this is a report of a retrospective analysis using historical controls. Even in the absence of significant changes in practice that may have changed steroid use, incidence of GVHD, or graft composition, the marked and rapidly varying incidence of invasive aspergillosis makes all retrospective analyses flawed.

Due to the documented intolerability of higher doses of parenteral D-Amb, the efficacy of aerosolized D-Amb was also studied; however, all studies published to date lack a design that would provide statistically significant results [133,134]. Lipid-associated forms of amphotericin accumulate in alveolar macrophages and the enhanced killing of aspergillus spores when ingested by macrophages preloaded with liposomal amphotericin has been reported in mouse studies and inhalation of these agents as prophylaxis are being studied. Randomized trials to date have included investigations of prophylactic administration of lipid-associated amphotericin and itraconazole. Two randomized trials of lower dose lipid-associated amphotericin have been published. Although underpowered to demonstrate a significance difference, a trend toward a decrease in IFIs was noted in which patient received 1–2 mg/kg three times per week of lipid-associated amphotericin during neutropenia. No difference in mortality was observed during a short follow-up period between the groups.

One center described a successful strategy for prophylaxis against IFIs in high-risk post-transplant patients utilizing oral itraconazole or intravenous AmBisome® (for those intolerant) until the resolution of neutropenia, prednisone dose below 10 mg/day, or the disappearance of aspergillus colonization [135]. Although this is a descriptive trial, prophylactic strategies such as these are ongoing. The demonstration of tolerability of newer antifungals, including lipid-associated formulations of amphotericin, new formulations of azoles and echinocandins, has made the prophylaxis of IFIs a possibility. The results of one such large, multicenter, randomized trial compared micafungin, an investigational agent of the echinocandin class, with fluconazole in the neutropenic HCT recipient was recently presented and demonstrated that micafungin was as well-tolerated and efficacious as fluconazole in the prophylaxis of candidal infections and superior with respect to the reduction in the incidence of mold infections [136]. However, this study only addressed prophylaxis during the early post-transplant period when a minority of mold infections following HCT are diagnosed. Although universal prophylaxis is not ideal, the multicenter trials in progress should help identify the highest risk patients.

Table 52.1 Studies of antifungal prophylaxis.

Study	n =	Drug	Dose	Duration of treatment	Effect of treatment on fungal-related conditions	Comments
Alangaden (1994) [170]	112	Fluconazole	100–200 mg/day	Until PMN engraftment	↓ IFIs and *Candida albicans* colonization ↑ *Candida glabrata* colonization ↓ Ampho B use	Historical controls
Winston (2003) [171]	140	Itraconazole or fluconazole	200–400 mg/day (Itra) vs. 400 mg/day (Flu)	Day +100	IFIs in Itra group	Included 10 pediatric patients (100 mg/day)
Ehninger (1996) [172]	53	Fluconazole	200 mg/day	≤Day +393	No infections in either group	
Slavin (1995) [128] and Marr (2000) [129]	300	Fluconazole	400 mg/day	Day +75	↓ Early candidal death ↓ GI GVHD ↑ Survival	8-year follow-up
van Burik (1988) [8]	355	Fluconazole	400 mg/day	At least 5 days	↓ Hepatic candidiasis ↑ Mold infections	Autopsy
MacMillan (2002) [130]	253	Fluconazole	400 mg/day vs. 200 mg/day	Until PMN engraftment then 100 mg/day through D+100	No significant difference in IFIs	Randomized, HCT Pediatric and adult patients
Nucci (2000) [173]	210	Itraconazole vs. placebo	100 mg b.i.d.	Until PMN engraftment	↓ IFIs	Included chemotherapy ↓ Ampho B use if protracted neutropenia
Foot (1999) [174]	103	Itraconazole solution	5 mg/kg/day	Until PMN engraftment	26 received ampho for persistent fever during neutropenia	Pediatric, majority (90%) HCT
Wolff (2000) [175]	355	Fluconazole vs. ampho B	400 mg/day vs. 0.2 mg/kg/day	Until PMN engraftment	Trend toward decrease in IFIs in fluconazole group	Amphotericin associated with greater toxicity
O'Donnell (1994) [132]	331	Ampho B	5–10 mg/day	2–3 months	↓ IFIs	All allogeneic, retrospective
Riley (1994) [176]	35	Ampho B vs. placebo	0.1 mg/kg/day	Until PMN engraftment	↓ IFIs ↓ High-dose ampho	Fewer days of antibiotic therapy Trend toward decreased hospitalization and improved survival
Tollemar (1993) [177]	76	AmBisome® vs. placebo	1 mg/kg/day	Until PMN engraftment	↓ Colonization	
Kelsey (1999) [178]	161	AmBisome® vs. placebo	2 mg/kg/day t.i.w.	Until PMN engraftment	No significant difference in IFIs ↓ Rate of colonization	Included chemotherapy

ampho B, amphotericin B; b.i.d., twice daily; GI, gastrointestinal; GVHD, graft-vs.-host disease; HCT, hematopoietic cell transplantation; IFIs, invasive fungal infections; PMN, polymorphonuclear leukocyte; t.i.w., thrice weekly.

An ideal strategy would parallel the pre-emptive strategies used for CMV infection and involve repetitive screening patients with a sensitive test, such as the molecular diagnostics currently being studied, and the results of which would be used to further refine the risk for IFIs.

Secondary prophylaxis

It is difficult to determine the precise degree to which risk of mortality is increased by a pretransplant history of IFIs. Outcome depends on a variety of factors, most notably the pathogenic organism, whether or not the infection has been cleared or, at least, stabilized, and the preparative regimen. Representative of several case reports is a series of 15 patients with a history of stable hepatosplenic candidiasis who underwent transplantation while receiving 0.5 mg/kg/day of amphotericin B. In 11 of the 15 patients, the abnormalities seen on CT scans were either improved or resolved and, in one patient, the lesions were stable. The remaining three patients died with evidence of fungal disease; however, the pathogen identified was not the same as that identified prior to transplantation [137].

A history of aspergillus likely represents greater risk than one of invasive candidiasis and adds to the mortality risk of HCT, particularly following the transplantation of grafts from matched-unrelated donors. Most reports confirmed a higher mortality rate following HCT after a myeloablative preparative regimen in patients with a history of invasive aspergillosis; however, the cause of death may not be directly attributable to the fungus [138]. Successful transplantation has been demonstrated following the stabilization of disease and the administration of at least 0.5–1.0 mg/kg/day amphotericin B during the peri-transplant period. Additionally, common themes of these successful cases were the aggressive primary therapy of the initial infections including surgical debridement, attempts at immunotherapy including IFN-γ and the transfusion of granulocyte colony-stimulating factor (G-CSF) mobilized white blood cells prior to engraftment [134,137,139,140]. However, other studies report a significantly worse outcome despite a similar approach [138]. A history of invasive aspergillosis is clearly associated with increased mortality following transplantation of grafts from a mismatched or matched-unrelated donor following a myeloablative preparative regimen. Although there are reports of successful transplantation in patients with a history of aspergillosis treated prior to matched-unrelated donor transplantation for chronic granulomatous disease, most would consider aspergillosis to be a contraindication to matched-unrelated donor transplantation following a myeloablative preparative regimen [141].

Nonmyeloablative preparative regimens may offer an option to patients with a history of aspergillosis. Successful allogeneic transplantation following a nonmyeloablative preparative regimen has been reported in patients with a either a history of or evidence of refractory invasive aspergillosis. In one report, three of four patients with active aspergillus demonstrated regression of fungal lesions and one with slight progression on chest CT. Antifungal treatments peritransplant included administration of an antifungal agent (amphotericin B or lipid-associated amphotericin) and G-CSF-mobilized white blood cell transfusions with or without additional G-CSF [142,143].

Although published reports represent a set of moderate sized but nonrandomized series, the surgical excision of solitary or large fungal lesions prior to planned immunosuppression is reasonable to consider in carefully selected patients. It would also be prudent to perform imaging of the brain to confirm absence of CNS lesions in the case of a history of IFIs prior to transplantation. All patients with a history of IFIs should receive ongoing antifungal therapy at therapeutic or near-therapeutic doses throughout the preparative regimen and until resolution of the pertinent lesions. It is notable that transfusions of G-CSF-mobilized neutrophils prior to engraftment were a component of the therapy of many of the successful cases reported; however, there are no randomized studies to confirm the efficacy of these treatments.

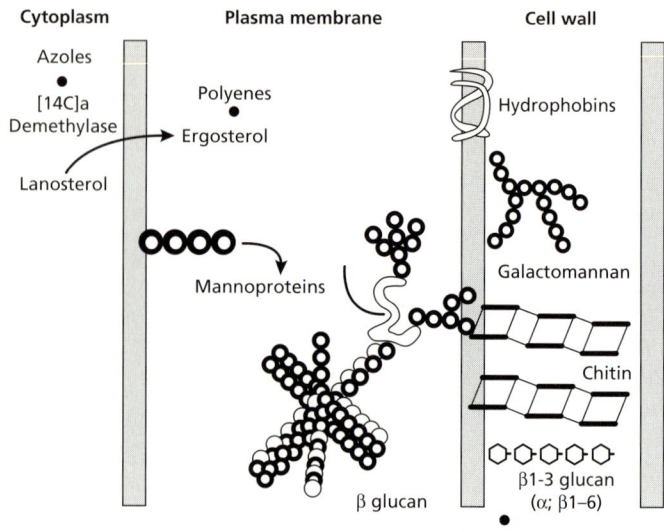

Fig. 52.3 Site of action of licensed antifungal drugs.

Fever during neutropenia

The empiric administration of antifungal agents following a period of fever during neutropenia unresponsive to antibacterial agents is a widely accepted practice. A variety of multicenter studies using amphotericin B, lipid-preparations of amphotericin, fluconazole, itraconazole and voriconazole have not identified a superior drug or regimen. Recently published studies of voriconazole are discussed. The use of weekly screening chest X-rays is recommended although CT scans of the chest are more likely to detect lesions earlier and may be associated with an improved outcome in neutropenic patients, even in the absence of fever [144].

Antifungal agents

The armamentarium of available antifungal agents with a variety of mechanisms of action and routes of administration continues to grow. All licensed agents offer improved tolerability when compared to amphotericin B following HCT. The mechanism of action of the currently licensed agents is represented schematically in Fig. 52.3. Available formulations of licensed agents, dosing schedules, commonly encountered toxicities and drug interactions are summarized in Table 52.2.

Polyenes

Amphotericins: amphotericin B deoxycholate (Fungizone®) and lipid-associated amphotericin preparations

The binding of these drugs to ergosterol, a key element of the fungal cell membrane, results in the physical disruption of that membrane. The efficacy of amphotericin B, the first drug in this class, is limited by significant toxicities. Most common adverse effects include potentially severe infusion-related symptoms (fevers, rigors, cardiovascular instability, hypoxemia), nephrotoxicity, hypokalemia and anemia. The risk of nephrotoxicity increases with concomitant administration of other nephrotoxic agents. Thus, it is no surprise that extensive clinical experience and studies demonstrate that full dose amphotericin B is frequently not tolerated following HCT. Three lipid-associated preparations of amphotericin—amphotericin B colloidal dispersion, amphotericin B lipid complex (ABLC) and liposomal amphotericin—were formulated to decrease the toxicities associated with amphotericin B. These preparations differ in many respects due to the lipid with which they are complexed. Although none of these formulations have been shown to provide

Table 52.2 Currently licensed antifungal agents.

	Trade name	Spectrum	Route	Dose	Dose adjustment	Most common toxicities	Drug interactions
Polyenes							
Amphotericin B	Fungizone®	Broad	IV	0.5–1.0 mg/kg	Renal	Infusion-related, nephrotoxicity, hypokalemia, hemolysis	Concomitant administration of other nephrotoxic agents increases risk for ampho-induced renal failure
			Oral topical		Renal	GI	
ABCD	Amphotec®	Broad	IV	2.5–5.0 mg/kg	Renal	Infusion-related, nephrotoxicity	Less potential for nephrotoxicity than ampho B
ABLC	Abelcet®	Broad	IV	2.5–7.5 mg/kg	Renal	Nephrotoxicity	Less potential for nephrotoxicity than ampho B
Liposomal amphotericin	AmBisome®	Broad	IV	2.5–15.0 mg/kg	Renal	Neprotoxicity	Less potential for nephrotoxicity than ampho B
Azoles							
Fluconazole	Diflucan®	*Candida* spp.	IV	200–400 mg	Renal	Hepatic	Decreases fluconazole levels: rifampin Flu increases levels of: CSA, phenytoin, glipizide, glyburide, warfarin
			PO	200–800 mg	Renal		
Itraconazole	Sporonox®	Broad	IV	100–400 mg	Renal, hepatic	Hepatic, hypokalemia, edema	Decreases itraconazole levels: increased gastric pH, rifampin, INH, phenytoin, carbamazepine, cisapride
			PO capsules	200–600 mg	Renal, hepatic	GI, hypokalemia, edema (hepatic)	Itraconazole increases levels of: CSA, tacrolimus, steroids, digoxin, astemizole, cisapride, warfarin, vinca alkaloids, busulfan
			PO solution	200–600 mg	Renal, hepatic	GI, hypokalemia, edema (hepatic)	
Voriconazole	Vfend®	Broad	IV	6 mg/kg × 2 4 mg/kg b.i.d.	Renal, hepatic	Visual disturbances, hepatic, mental status, rash, neutropenia	As above for itraconazole except potentially more pronounced and more numerous
			PO	200–300 mg b.i.d.	Hepatic		
Candins							
Caspofungin		Broad	IV	70 mg × 1 50 mg	Hepatic	Hepatic	Increases caspofungin levels: CSA

ABCD, amphotericin B colloidal dispersion; ABLC, amphotericin B lipid complex; b.i.d. twice daily; CSA, cyclosporin; GI, gastrointestinal; INH, isoniazid; IV, intravenous; PO, *per os* (oral administration).

superior efficacy when compared to the other formulations in the treatment of IFIs, all are tolerated better than amphotericin B. In separate comparative studies with amphotericin B, infusion-related toxicities were significantly lower with ABLC and liposomal amphotericin, and all three lipid-associated preparations were significantly less nephrotoxic. Additionally, the majority of patients switched to a lipid preparation due to amphotericin B-induced nephrotoxicity, serum creatinine either remained stable or improved.

The precise treatment dose of lipid preparations is still not clear. There are no randomized dose–response studies, although there are a growing number of published reports of clinical response following dose escalation to as high as 15 mg/kg/day of liposomal amphotericin for infections involving the CNS.

Echinocandins

Caspofungin

Caspofungin is an echinocandin lipopeptide that interferes with the synthesis of the major component of the cell wall of many clinically important fungi including *Candida* and *Aspergillus* spp. Sites of *Aspergillus* hyphal growth appear to be particularly affected. Echinocandins inhibit the synthesis of (1,3)-β-D-glucan and do not demonstrate cross-resistance with other licensed antifungal agents in *in vitro* susceptibility studies.

The response efficacy of caspofungin treatment is equivalent to amphotericin B and fluconazole in the treatment of candidal esophagitis [145,146]. However, a significantly improved tolerability of caspofungin resulted in the discontinuation of the drug is only 4–7% of patients vs. 24% of patients on amphotericin B. It is important to note that, due to the effect of cyclosporine on serum levels of caspofungin, limited data are available regarding concomitant administration of these agents [146]. Tacrolimus does not appear to affect levels of caspofungin. Although licensed for the treatment of the treatment of invasive aspergillus infections refractory to other licensed therapy, a very limited number of patients with invasive aspergillosis were reported and further study is required to determine the true safety and efficacy of caspofungin in the treatment of this IFI following HCT. Hope remains for the use of this agent in combination therapy of IFIs.

Other echinocandins currently under study include anidulfungin (LY303366) and micafungin (FK463). Findings of a multicenter randomized trial of micafungin as prophylaxis during the early post-transplant period is discussed above.

Azoles

Azoles inhibit production of ergosterol, an essential component of the fungal cytoplasmic membrane. Early drugs of this class include ketoconazole, which exhibited a unique toxicity associated with the inhibition of cortisol and testosterone production. This mechanism results from binding of cytochrome P450 enzymes and, in fungus, results in the inhibition of C-14-α demethylation of lanosterol. Resistance may result from increased drug efflux, or altered C-14-α demethylase. Currently, the four most important drugs of this class for use in HCT recipients include fluconazole, itraconazole, voriconazole and posaconazole. Unlike earlier drugs in this class, the newer triazoles do not significantly affect hormone production. Cross-resistance between the triazoles is variable and may become a clinically more important issue following widespread use of these agents.

Fluconazole (Diflucan®)

After well-designed multicenter trials demonstrated that fluconazole, 400 mg daily, was efficacious in preventing invasive candidiasis and in reducing mortality due to fungal infection following allogeneic HCT [127–129], its prophylactic use in this setting has become widespread.

The most important principle regarding the use of this drug in immunocompromised hosts is that, while it has excellent activity against most *Candida* spp., it is not useful in the treatment of infections due to *Aspergillus* spp. As mentioned previously, certain species of *Candida*, including *C. glabrata* and *C. krusei*, demonstrate innate resistance to fluconazole.

Fluconazole is available for parenteral and oral administration. Oral fluconazole is well absorbed, even in the setting of some GI disruption. The distribution of drug includes blood, tissue, bladder and the cerebral spinal fluid. Dose reduction in renal failure is recommended. Blood levels of cyclosporine, warfarin, phenytoin and oral hypoglycemic agents may increase when administered with fluconazole. Adverse effects are distinctly uncommon, the most important of which is that elevations in aminotransferase levels may occur in as many of 10% of patients.

Itraconazole (Sporonox®)

Itraconazole is a broad-spectrum agent available in two oral formulations and one intravenous formulation. The absorption of the original capsular formulation is so erratic that it is generally considered to be inadequate following HCT. The solubilization of itraconazole in cyclodextrin solution results in excellent oral bioavailability; however, the most common toxicity of both oral formulations is dose-related nausea and GI distress. The intravenous form increases the potential utility of this drug. Unlike the oral formulations, however, dose reduction is recommended in significant renal insufficiency (creatinine clearance <50 mL/min) due to potential accumulation of the intravenous carrier, hydroxypropyl-β-cyclodextrin. Dose adjustment of both the oral and intravenous forms should also be considered in significant hepatic insufficiency. Great inter- and intrapatient variability of plasma levels has been observed and monitoring of levels, although not readily available at all centers, is ideal. Other toxicities include hypokalemia and edema, also primarily associated with higher doses. Rash is infrequent but a variety of dermatologic eruptions have been described, including pustular lesions. Itraconazole has been demonstrated to increase the blood levels of several drugs including cyclosporine, tacrolimus, methylprednisolone, vinca alkaloids, benzodiazepines and busulfan [147]. Therefore, the potential for toxicity associated with itraconazole administration may result from its effect on other agents.

Perhaps of greatest concern is the potential for antagonism between itraconazole and amphotericin. Although published results are conflicting, some *in vitro* and animal studies have demonstrated an antagonistic interaction between the drugs, particularly if amphotericin is started subsequent to treatment with itraconazole [148–150].

Voriconazole (Vfend®)

Voriconazole is a recently licensed triazole that is structurally related to fluconazole but has activity against both *Candida* and *Aspergillus* spp. Like itraconazole, it also has activity against *Histoplasma* spp., *Blastomyces* spp. and *Cryptococcus neoformans*. It is unique in its activity against scedosporiosis and fusariosis.

A great deal of attention has been paid to two recent randomized, multicenter trials involving voriconazole [151,152]. The first trial compared voriconazole with liposomal amphotericin B for empiric antifungal therapy in patients with fever and neutropenia [151]. Of the 837 patients included in the analysis, 415 had undergone HCT, including 76 (18.3%) and 79 (18.7%) recipients of allogeneic HCT who were assigned to the voriconazole and liposomal amphotericin arms, respectively. Voriconazole was administered intravenously at a dose of 4 mg/kg twice daily after two doses of 6 mg/kg. Oral administration of voriconazole (200 mg twice daily) was permitted after 2 days of intravenous administration. The target dose of intravenous liposomal amphotericin was 3 mg/kg/day; however, dose reduction to 1.5 mg/kg/day was permitted. The voriconazole group (median duration of therapy 7 days, range 1–113 days) had fewer cases of severe infusion-related reactions ($p<0.01$) and of nephrotoxicity ($p<0.001$). However, a significantly higher incidence of visual disturbances (22% vs. 1%, $p<0.001$) and hallucinations (4.3% vs. 0.5%, $p<0.001$) than those receiving liposomal amphotericin B (median duration of 7 days, range 1–81 days) was also reported. It is also notable that there were fewer documented breakthrough fungal infections in patients treated with voriconazole than in those treated with liposomal amphotericin B (1.9% vs. 5.0%, $p = 0.02$). The significantly higher 30-day mortality in patients with break-through fungal infections demonstrated the limitations of empiric therapy. Thus, although voriconazole did not fulfill the protocol-defined criteria for noninferiority to liposomal amphotericin B with respect to overall response to empiric therapy, these results suggest a role in the empiric treatment of patients with persistent fever during neutropenia although breakthrough infections still occurred [151].

In a separate multicenter, randomized trial, voriconazole was compared to amphotericin B for the treatment of invasive aspergillosis [152]. A total of 144 patients in the voriconazole group and 133 patients in the amphotericin B group with definite or probable aspergillosis received at least one dose of treatment. Thirty-seven (25.7%) and 30 (22.6%) recipients of allogeneic HCT were assigned to the voriconazole and amphotericin B arms, respectively. A detailed discussion of this study is beyond the scope of this chapter; however, a few key points are worth discussing. First, a total of 102 patients were excluded from the modified intention-to-treat population. The most common reason for the lack of confirmation was the inability of the data-review committee to confirm the presence of a halo or air-crescent sign in patients without supporting mycologic or pathological evidence (35 in the voriconazole group and 25 in the amphotericin B group). Following HCT, halo and air-crescent signs are frequently not visualized and, as described previously, these findings may represent an immune response. One of the most important observations of the study was that the mean duration of therapy was significantly different between the groups. The median duration of voriconazole treatment was 77 days and other licensed antifungal therapy was given to 52 patients in the voriconazole group. The median duration of amphotericin B treatment was 10 days and, during the first 14 days of therapy, administration of amphotericin B was suspended for more than 1 day in 13 patients. Other licensed antifungal therapy was given to 107 patients in the amphotericin B group. The survival rate at 12 weeks was 70.8% in the voriconazole group and 57.9% in the amphotericin B group, although the percentage of patients with a complete response was similar. Adverse effects of voriconazole included visual disturbances (44%) and hallucinations or confusion (10.4%), skin reactions including rash, pruritus, or photosensitivity (8.2%) and hepatic inflammation (3.6%). In contrast, a significant percentage of patients receiving amphotericin B therapy experienced infusion-related (24.9%) and renal toxicity. Thus, the inability to administer full-dose amphotericin B, especially early after the identification of aspergillus infection, may explain the difference in outcome between the two groups. Perhaps the most notable observation of the study was that 24% of patients with CNS aspergillosis survived, which may be due to the measurable brain tissue levels achieved during voriconazole treatment [152].

Voriconazole is available in an intravenous form and a highly bioavailable oral form. As noted, adverse effects include visual symptoms, hepatotoxicity, rash, fever, GI distress, headache and peripheral edema. In healthy subjects, anaphylactoid type reactions have been described. The visual disturbances require some mention as they occur in as many of 44% of patients and are often infusion related. A variety of disturbances have been described including altered or enhanced visual perception, blurred vision, changes in color vision, or photophobia. They may persist throughout the course of therapy; however, no long-term visual sequelae have been noted in animals or in clinical trials. Rashes, with or without photosensitivity, occurred in 6% of patients. Hepatotoxicity may occur more frequently following HCT due to drug interactions with other potentially hepatotoxic medications. The list of known drug interactions is lengthy and concomitant administration may result in increased levels of cyclosporine, tacrolimus, benzodiazepines, vinca alkaloids, ergot alkaloids and omeprazole. Like itraconazole, the metabolism of the drug has been shown to be highly variable, although further study is necessary to demonstrate correlation between plasma or tissue levels and clinical outcome. Because of potential accumulation of the intravenous vehicle, patients with moderate to severe renal insufficiency (creatinine clearance <50 mL/min) should receive the drug orally, or be closely monitored if parenteral therapy is more appropriate. In the case of significant hepatic insufficiency the maintenance dose should be halved.

Other agents

In addition to the investigational echinocandins and triazoles referred to above, other agents being evaluated include liposomal formulations of nystatin, inhibitors of fungal elongation factor-2 or chitin synthesis and immunomodulators [153].

Immunotherapy

Although the availability of more antifungal agents offers the possibility of improved survival from IFIs, all clinical and laboratory data support the need to improve reconstitution of an effective immune response to ensure fungal clearance. Adjunctive immunotherapy may take the form of administration of antibodies against well-defined antigens, transfer of adoptive immune effects, modification of graft composition, active immunization, or the administration of immunomodulators.

Hematopoietic cell growth factors

The role of hematopoietic cell growth factors in the prevention or adjunctive treatment of IFIs is not clear. A number of *in vitro* studies confirm the salutatory effect of macrophage-colony stimulating factor (M-CSF), G-CSF and GM-CSF on cellular response to fungus and the shortening of the neutropenic period following chemotherapy and transplantation of bone marrow cells. GM-CSF has been shown to enhance the killing of *Aspergillus* hyphae and *Candida* spp. as well as prevent the suppression of neutrophil killing of *A. fumigatus* hyphae resulting from steroid administration [117,154,155]. M-CSF has also been demonstrated to enhance the ingestion and killing of fungi but this agent is no longer being developed [156]. Despite these findings, there has yet to be a definitive study documenting the reduction in the incidence of or mortality due to IFIs. Changes in the graft composition have shortened the time to neutrophil engraftment, which has resulted in a significant reduction in the incidence of IFIs during the early post-transplant period. Therefore, it may be difficult to statistically appreciate any further reduction in the risk of IFIs resulting from the shortening of the median duration neutropenia from 14 days to 10.5 days due to G-CSF following myeloablative HCT.

In fact, post-transplantation administration of hematopoietic growth factors may have deleterious effects. Recent studies demonstrate that G-CSF treatment influences post-transplantation lymphocyte recovery resulting in a potentially detrimental shift towards a lymphocyte profile associated with increased susceptibility to fungal infection. In a study of patients following T-cell-depleted haploidentical HCT, G-CSF administration post-transplant impaired T-cell reconstitution without influencing the rate of engraftment or the incidence of GVHD. The most important observation with respect to intracellular pathogens and fungi was that the administration of G-CSF resulted in a profound TH2-type immunoreactivity as measured by increased production of IL-4 and IL-10, concomitant decreased IL-12 production and the absence of IL-12 receptor β_2 chain expression by CD4[+] cells. The appearance of IL-12 producing cells took >12 months following G-CSF administration in contrast to 1–3 months post-transplant in patients who did not receive G-CSF. CD4+ and antifungal reactivity *in vitro* recovered more rapidly in the absence of G-CSF. Thus, in recipients of T-cell-depleted grafts, functional lymphoid immune response to IFIs may be negatively influenced by the administration of hematopoietic growth factors [157].

Adjunctive therapy with IFN-γ is actively being studied with a particular focus on the treatment of invasive aspergillosis and the influence on the incidence of GVHD.

Antifungal vaccine strategies

The antibody response to invasive candidal infection is complex and has been demonstrated to be both protective as well as deleterious. The role of antibodies in aspergillosis is not well understood. Therefore, a passive antibody approach for either fungus is not yet near development. A natural offshoot of the demonstration of the potentially significant non-myeloid response to aspergillosis and the ability to adoptively transfer some degree of resistance to disease in mouse models is the study of the efficacy of vaccination. In fact, killed vaccines against aspergillosis were reported decades ago when such fungal infections were clinical rarities. Potential advantages to a successful vaccine strategy against IFIs would be to obviate the need for antifungal prophylactic administration and therefore avoid the potential issues of toxicity and resistance. Differences in fungal strain tropism and virulence may influence the specific nature of the immunoreactivity; therefore, further study is needed in the development of this strategy. Vaccination prior to challenge appears more effective in fungal clearance than vaccination or antibody administration following infection. The primary question would be whether strategies should include vaccination of the donor and/or recipient and whether the immunodeficient patient could generate an adequate response post-transplantation. Vaccines against invasive candidal infections are being studied and include heat-killed candida or various, well-characterized candidate antigens.

The study of possible vaccine strategies for aspergillosis is in its infancy. Vaccination of mice with a crude extract induces a TH1-type response comparable to that resulting from nasal instillation of conidia. Protection against invasive pulmonary aspergillosis was documented following adoptive transfer of antigen-specific CD4+ lymphocytes from these vaccinated mice. In contrast, vaccination with a recombinant antigen, Asp f 2, led to an increase in IL-4 production without an increase in IL-12, consistent with a TH2-type response, which would be predicted to increase susceptibility to fungus [158]. These complexities must be further understood prior to the development of an effective vaccine.

Other investigational immunotherapy: pulsed dendritic cells and graft modification

In mouse models, splenic or bone marrow derived DCs pulsed with candidal yeasts, or yeast RNA, enhanced reconstitution of IFN-producing CD4+ candidal-specific cells and protect against IFIs following allogeneic HCT. These cells also expressed fungal mannoproteins, upregulate major histocompatibility complex (MHC) class II antigens and costimulatory molecules and produce IL-12 [159]. Similar findings were reported using *ex-vivo* generated human DCs derived from CD34+ progenitors or monocytes harvested prior to autologous or allogeneic HCT. Following exposure of these DCs to *Aspergillus* antigens, these cells partially restored the fungal immunoreactivity of lymphocytes collected from patients 1 month post-transplantation. These findings suggest that antigen-pulsed DCs, including those generated *ex vivo*, have the potential to effectively enhance immunity after HCT when antibody response may be inadequate [110].

Enhancement of immune reconstitution may also be achieved via modification of graft composition. In studies of murine hematopoietic stem cell transplantation, cotransplantation of lineage-restricted progenitors known as common myeloid progenitors (CMPs) and granulocyte macrophage progenitors (GMPs) resulted in a significant increase in the absolute number of myeloid cells, the majority of which were CMP/GMP-derived. Cotransplantation of GMP/GMP with hematopoietic stem cells protected against death following lethal challenge with either of two lethal pathogens associated with neutropenia: *A. fumigatus* and *Pseudomonas aeruginosa*. Survival correlated with the measurable appearance of progenitor-derived myeloid cells in the spleen despite persistent peripheral neutropenia [160].

Surgical approaches to IFIs

The role of surgery in invasive candidal infections is limited to intravascular lesions such as endocarditis and thrombophlebitis. However, there is a growing body of data to support combination medical and surgical therapy for invasive mold infections in patients with hematologic malignancies, most of whom were neutropenic at the time of surgery [144,161,162]. Given the comorbid conditions and the likelihood of dissemination with aspergillosis, determining the potential risks vs. benefits is typically more difficult following HCT. Small series have been published describing survival following both open and thoracoscopic approaches in the excision following HCT, even in the setting of GVHD, but this success was not universally observed [163,164]. All series include patients with single lesions (aspergillomas) or multiple lesions. Therefore, resection should be considered in patients who are deemed acceptable surgical candidates with (i) a single lesion; (ii) one predominant, large lesion; or (iii) lesions abutting vascular structures given the high risk for hemorrhage. Even in the setting of disseminated or CNS disease, there may be a role for surgical intervention, which may include drainage, excision and/or instillation of antifungal agents [165,166]. Successful surgical approaches often include the intraoperative frozen section demonstration that the margins of the excision are free of disease. This approach is perhaps of greatest importance in surgery involving the sinus or periorbital regions. Intralesional administration of antifungal agents (typically amphotericin B) has also been described in cavitary pulmonary and CNS lesions, with and without an attempt at excision, but the data are limited to individual case reports. Surgical debridement is almost invariably necessary for the successful treatment of fungal sinusitis, skin lesions and intravascular lesions following HCT [167,168]; however, survival benefit has not been definitively demonstrated.

Fungal eye infections deserve special mention given their high risk for dissemination and the diagnostic and therapeutic challenges. These infections should not be treated without the active participation of an experienced ophthalmologist to determine the accurate diagnosis and response to treatment. Fluid and/or tissue sampling or intravitreal instillation of antifungal agents is frequently necessary. Conflicting data exist regarding the optimal antifungal agent.

Approach to the patient with suspected invasive fungal disease following HCT

Outcomes are better for patients who are diagnosed and treated as early and as aggressively as can be tolerated. Patients with persistent, unexplained fever should be treated empirically while being evaluated for IFIs. Although diagnostic blood tests have not been validated, if they are available, they may provide adjunctive data; however, further evaluation should proceed immediately including appropriate radiologic tests and biopsies (see Plate 23.45, *facing p. 296*).

In the setting of documented candidemia, immediate central venous catheter removal is strongly recommended. A CT scan with intravenous contrast or MRI of the chest and abdomen should be performed to determine the extent of disease in order to select the appropriate antifungal agent as well as the necessary duration of therapy. There are no randomized trials to guide the duration of therapy in either disseminated candidal infections or invasive aspergillosis. However, symptomatic and/or radiologic exaccerbations are not uncommon if therapy is stopped while patients remain on immunosuppressive agents or have persistent radiologic abnormalities. Two to six months of therapy are the rule, rather than the exception, during which time serial CT scans should be performed. The variety of antifungals now offers options when protracted therapy is indicated.

In vitro susceptibility testing should be performed on any nonalbicans *Candida* spp. or *C. albicans* isolates obtained in the setting of fluconazole therapy. Amphotericin B, lipid-associated amphotericin preparations, azoles and caspofungin have all been demonstrated to have efficacy against candidal infections. The vast majority of *C. albicans* remains susceptible to all agents; however, the intrinsic resistance patterns of certain species, including *C. krusei* (intrinsically resistant to fluconazole), *C. glabrata* (variably resistant to fluconazole and amphotericin) and *C. lusitanea* (resistant to amphotericin), should be considered and appropriate agents chosen pending the results of *in vitro* susceptibility testing [169].

As patients with invasive aspergillosis may not develop fever, especially in the setting of corticosteroid administration, the clinician should remain vigilant, especially in patients at high risk such as allogeneic HCT recipients with GVHD on higher doses of steroids. Abnormal findings on CT scans should prompt attempts to isolate the organism, including induction of sputum, bronchoalveolar lavage and/or biopsy for accessible lesions. Culture of the specimens is crucial to confirm identification of fungus and determination of *in vitro* antifungal susceptibility. Given the potential of CNS involvement in invasive aspergillosis following HCT, it would be prudent to consider a magnetic resonance scan of the head in invasive disease. Symptoms of sinus involvement should prompt a CT scan of the sinuses. Prompt surgical evaluation is warranted if invasive sinusitis is documented on a CT scan. In the case of invasion, aggressive surgical debridement should be considered as an important part of therapy.

For all IFIs, empiric therapy should not be delayed during clinical evaluation. The choice of agent—or combination of agents—should be determined by balancing any existing or potential for organ dysfunction with known toxicities of the drug. Antifungal CNS penetration should also be considered if CNS disease is documented. First choice should be given to drugs that can be safely administered at full dose. Even with agents with excellent oral bioavailablity, it is prudent to administer agents parenterally until stabilization or improvement of infection can be demonstrated, especially in the setting of GI pathology such as GVHD. Trends toward isolating noncandidal, nonaspergillus, or fungi resistant to various antimicrobials with increasing frequency underscores the importance of aggressive attempts to isolate the organism. Although the correlation between *in vitro* fungal susceptibility testing and clinical outcome has not yet been proven, it is prudent to avoid agents against which the fungus demonstrates *in vitro* resistance. *In vitro* fungal susceptibility testing will likely be of increasing importance [169]. As discussed, there is potentially a role for surgical excision or debridement in selected patients. Reducing steroid dosage as rapidly as possible is also crucial to clearance of fungus.

Conclusion

IFIs remain the leading cause of infectious death following allogeneic HCT at most large centers. Strategies to reduce the incidence of GVHD, to lower the dose of corticosteroids and to enhance the immune response to fungi following HCT, coupled with a growing armamentarium of better tolerated antifungal agents, offer hope for a reduction in the morbidity and mortality of these infections. Surgery in selected cases may also result in improved survival. Prophylactic and empiric strategies based on improved diagnostic assays are currently under study. Modification of the graft composition designed to accelerate the recapitulation of fungal immune response without increasing GHVD would be ideal. The specter of emergent fungal infections cannot be overlooked, especially following protracted administration of broad-spectrum antifungal drugs and as the use of these drugs becomes more widespread.

References

1 Grow WB, Moreb JS, Roque D *et al*. Late onset of invasive aspergillus infection in bone marrow transplant patients at a university hospital. *Bone Marrow Transplant* 2002; **29**: 15–9.

2 Kruger W, Russmann B, Kroger N *et al*. Early infections in patients undergoing bone marrow or blood stem cell transplantation: a 7 year single centre investigation of 409 cases. *Bone Marrow Transplant* 1999; **23**: 589–97.

3 Hovi L, Saarinen-Pihkala UM, Vettenranta K *et al*. Invasive fungal infections in pediatric bone marrow transplant recipients: single center experience of 10 years. *Bone Marrow Transplant* 2000; **26**: 999–1004.

4 Allan BT, Patton D, Ramsey NK *et al*. Pulmonary fungal infections after bone marrow transplantation. *Pediatr Radiol* 1988; **18**: 118–22.

5 Meyers JD. Fungal infections in bone marrow transplant patients. *Semin Oncol* 1990; **17**: 10–3.

6 Martino R, Subira M, Rovira M *et al*. Invasive fungal infections after allogeneic peripheral blood stem cell transplantation: incidence and risk factors in 395 patients. *Br J Haematol* 2002; **116**: 475–82.

7 Iwen PC, Reed EC, Armitage JO *et al*. Nosocomial invasive aspergillosis in lymphoma patients treated with bone marrow or peripheral stem cell transplants. *Infect Control Hosp Epidemiol* 1993; **14**: 131–9.

8 van Burik JH, Leisenring W, Myerson D *et al*. The effect of prophylactic fluconazole on the clinical spectrum of fungal diseases in bone marrow transplant recipients with special attention to hepatic candidiasis. An autopsy study of 355 patients. *Medicine (Baltimore)* 1998; **77**: 246–54.

9 Lin SJ, Schranz J, Teutsch SM. Aspergillosis case fatality rate. A systematic review of the literature. *Clin Infect Dis* 2001; **32**: 358–66.

10 Nosari A, Oreste P, Cairoli R *et al*. Invasive *Aspergillosis* in hematological malignancies: clinical findings and management for intensive chemotherapy completion. *Am J Hematol* 2001; **68**: 231–6.

11 Saugier-Veber P, Devergie A, Sulahian A *et al*. Epidemiology and diagnosis of invasive pulmonary aspergillosis in bone marrow transplant patients: results of a 5 year retrospective study. *Bone Marrow Transplant* 1993; **12**: 121–4.

12 De Bock R. Epidemiology of invasive fungal infections in bone marrow transplantation. EORTC Invasive Fungal Infections Cooperative Group. *Bone Marrow Transplant* 1994; **14** (Suppl. 5): S1–2.

13 Jantunen E, Ruutu P, Niskanen L *et al*. Incidence and risk factors for invasive fungal infections in allogeneic BMT recipients. *Bone Marrow Transplant* 1997; **19**: 801–8.

14 McWhinney PH, Kibbler CC, Hamon MD *et al*. Progress in the diagnosis and management of aspergillosis in bone marrow transplantation: 13 years' experience. *Clin Infect Dis* 1993; **17**: 397–404.

15 Wald A, Leisenring W, van Burik JA *et al*. Epidemiology of *Aspergillus* infections in a large cohort of patients undergoing bone marrow transplantation. *J Infect Dis* 1997; **175**: 1459–66.

16 Williamson EC, Millar MR, Steward CG *et al*. Infections in adults undergoing unrelated donor bone marrow transplantation. *Br J Haematol* 1999; **104**: 560–8.

17 Baddley JW, Stroud TP, Salzman D *et al*. Invasive mold infections in allogeneic bone marrow transplant recipients. *Clin Infect Dis* 2001; **32**: 1319–24.

18 Heurlin N, Bergstrom SE, Winiarski J *et al*. Fungal pneumonia: the predominant lung infection causing death in children undergoing bone marrow transplantation. *Acta Paediatr* 1996; **85**: 168–72.

19 Morrison VA, McGlave PB. Mucormycosis in the BMT population. *Bone Marrow Transplant* 1993; **11**: 383–8.

20 Arrese JE, Pierard-Franchimont C, Pierard GE. Fatal hyalohyphomycosis following *Fusarium onychomycosis* in an immunocompromised patient. *Am J Dermatopathol* 1996; **18**: 196–8.

21 Gaziev D, Baronciani D, Galimberti M *et al*. Mucormycosis after bone marrow transplantation: report of four cases in thalassemia and review of the literature. *Bone Marrow Transplant* 1996; **17**: 409–14.

22 Jantunen E, Kolho E, Ruutu P *et al*. Invasive cutaneous mucormycosis caused by *Absidia corymbifera*

23 Leleu X, Sendid B, Fruit J et al. Combined antifungal therapy and surgical resection as treatment of pulmonary zygomycosis in allogeneic bone marrow transplantation. *Bone Marrow Transplant* 1999; **24**: 417–20.

24 Groll AH, Walsh TJ. Uncommon opportunistic fungi: new nosocomial threats. *Clin Microbiol Infect* 2001; **7** (Suppl. 2): 8–24.

25 Jahagirdar BN, Morrison VA. Emerging fungal pathogens in patients with hematologic malignancies and marrow/stem-cell transplant recipients. *Semin Respir Infect* 2002; **17**: 113–20.

26 Berenguer J, Rodriguez-Tudela JL, Richard C et al. Deep infections caused by *Scedosporium prolificans*. A report on 16 cases in Spain and a review of the literature. *Scedosporium prolificans* Spanish Study Group. *Medicine (Baltimore)* 1997; **76**: 256–65.

27 Hagensee ME, Bauwens JE, Kjos B et al. Brain abscess following marrow transplantation: experience at the Fred Hutchinson Cancer Research Center, 1984–92. *Clin Infect Dis* 1994; **19**: 402–8.

28 de Medeiros CR, Bleggi-Torres LF, Faoro LN et al. Cavernous sinus thrombosis caused by zygomycosis after unrelated bone marrow transplantation. *Transpl Infect Dis* 2001; **3**: 231–4.

29 de Medeiros BC, de Medeiros CR, Werner B et al. Central nervous system infections following bone marrow transplantation: an autopsy report of 27 cases. *J Hematother Stem Cell Res* 2000; **9**: 535–40.

30 Walsh TJ, Groll AH. Emerging fungal pathogens. Evolving challenges to immunocompromised patients for the twenty-first century. *Transpl Infect Dis* 1999; **1**: 247–61.

31 Mencacci A, Cenci E, Bacci A et al. Host immune reactivity determines the efficacy of combination immunotherapy and antifungal chemotherapy in candidiasis. *J Infect Dis* 2000; **181**: 686–94.

32 Maraki S, Hajiioannou I, Anatoliotakis N et al. Ceftriaxone and dexamethasone affecting yeast gut flora in experimental mice. *J Chemother* 1999; **11**: 363–6.

33 Maraki S, Mouzas IA, Kontoyiannis DP et al. Prospective evaluation of the impact of amoxicillin, clarithromycin and their combination on human gastrointestinal colonization by *Candida* species. *Chemotherapy* 2001; **47**: 215–8.

34 Mavromanolakis E, Maraki S, Cranidis A et al. The impact of norfloxacin, ciprofloxacin and ofloxacin on human gut colonization by *Candida albicans*. *Scand J Infect Dis* 2001; **33**: 477–8.

35 Berrouane YF, Herwaldt LA, Pfaller MA. Trends in antifungal use and epidemiology of nosocomial yeast infections in a university hospital. *J Clin Microbiol* 1999; **37**: 531–7.

36 Ferretti GA, Ash RC, Brown AT et al. Control of oral mucositis and candidiasis in marrow transplantation: a prospective, double-blind trial of chlorhexidine digluconate oral rinse. *Bone Marrow Transplant* 1988; **3**: 483–93.

37 Verfaillie C, Weisdorf D, Haake R et al. Candida infections in bone marrow transplant recipients. *Bone Marrow Transplant* 1991; **8**: 177–84.

38 Cole GT, Halawa AA, Anaissie EJ. The role of the gastrointestinal tract in hematogenous candidiasis: from the laboratory to the bedside. *Clin Infect Dis* 1996; **22** (Suppl. 2): S73–88.

39 Krcmery V, Barnes AJ. Non-albicans *Candida* spp. causing fungaemia. pathogenicity and antifungal resistance. *J Hosp Infect* 2002; **50**: 243–60.

40 Pfaller MA. Nosocomial candidiasis. Emerging species, reservoirs, and modes of transmission. *Clin Infect Dis* 1996; **22** (Suppl. 2): S89–94.

41 Klepser ME. Antifungal resistance among *Candida* species. *Pharmacotherapy* 2001; **21**: S124–32.

42 Jarvis WR. Epidemiology of nosocomial fungal infections, with emphasis on *Candida* species. *Clin Infect Dis* 1995; **20**: 1526–30.

43 Marr KA, Seidel K, White TC et al. Candidemia in allogeneic blood and marrow transplant recipients: evolution of risk factors after the adoption of prophylactic fluconazole. *J Infect Dis* 2000; **181**: 309–16.

44 Singh N. Changing spectrum of invasive candidiasis and its therapeutic implications. *Clin Microbiol Infect* 2001; **7** (Suppl. 2): 1–7.

45 Baran J Jr, Muckatira B, Khatib R. Candidemia before and during the fluconazole era: prevalence, type of species and approach to treatment in a tertiary care community hospital. *Scand J Infect Dis* 2001; **33**: 137–9.

46 Fraser VJ, Jones M, Dunkel J et al. Candidemia in a tertiary care hospital: epidemiology, risk factors, and predictors of mortality. *Clin Infect Dis* 1992; **15**: 414–21.

47 Rex JH, Walsh TJ, Sobel JD et al. Practice guidelines for the treatment of candidiasis. *Infect Dis Clin North Am* 2000; **30**: 662–78.

48 Edwards JE Jr, Bodey GP, Bowden RA et al. International conference for the development of a consensus on the management and prevention of severe candidal infections. *Clin Infect Dis* 1997; **25**: 43–59.

49 Eppes SC, Troutman JL, Gutman LT. Outcome of treatment of candidemia in children whose central catheters were removed or retained. *Pediatr Infect Dis J* 1989; **8**: 99–104.

50 Dato VM, Dajani AS. Candidemia in children with central venous catheters. Role of catheter removal and amphotericin B therapy. *Pediatr Infect Dis J* 1990; **9**: 309–14.

51 Rossetti F, Brawner DL, Bowden R et al. Fungal liver infection in marrow transplant recipients: prevalence at autopsy, predisposing factors, and clinical features. *Clin Infect Dis* 1995; **20**: 801–11.

52 Semelka RC, Kelekis NL, Sallah S et al. Hepatosplenic fungal disease: diagnostic accuracy and spectrum of appearances on MR imaging. *AJR Am J Roentgenol* 1997; **169**: 1311–6.

53 Kontoyiannis DP, Reddy BT, Torres HA et al. Pulmonary candidiasis in patients with cancer: an autopsy study. *Clin Infect Dis* 2002; **34**: 400–3.

54 von Eiff M, Roos N, Schulten R et al. Pulmonary aspergillosis: early diagnosis improves survival. *Respiration* 1995; **62**: 341–7.

55 Rose HD, Sheth NK. Pulmonary candidiasis. A clinical and pathological correlation. *Arch Intern Med* 1978; **138**: 964–5.

56 Strinden WD, Helgerson RB, Maki DG. Candida septic thrombosis of the great central veins associated with central catheters. Clinical features and management. *Ann Surg* 1985; **202**: 653–8.

57 Jarrett F, Maki DG, Chan CK. Management of septic thrombosis of the inferior vena cava caused by *Candida*. *Arch Surg* 1978; **113**: 637–9.

58 Kelly RF, Yellin AE, Weaver FA. Candida thrombosis of the innominate vein with septic pulmonary emboli. *Ann Vasc Surg* 1993; **7**: 343–6.

59 Roush K, Scala-Barnett DM, Donabedian H et al. Rupture of a pulmonary artery mycotic aneurysm associated with candidal endocarditis. *Am J Med* 1988; **84**: 142–4.

60 Johnston PG, Lee J, Domanski M et al. Late recurrent *Candida endocarditis*. *Chest* 1991; **99**: 1531–3.

61 Leung WH, Lau CP, Tai YT et al. Candida right ventricular mural endocarditis complicating indwelling right atrial catheter. *Chest* 1990; **97**: 1492–3.

62 Martino P, Micozzi A, Venditti M et al. Catheter-related right-sided endocarditis in bone marrow transplant recipients. *Rev Infect Dis* 1990; **12**: 250–7.

63 Mohrmann RL, Mah V, Vinters HV. Neuropathologic findings after bone marrow transplantation: an autopsy study. *Hum Pathol* 1990; **21**: 630–9.

64 Edwards JE Jr, Lehrer RI, Stiehm ER et al. Severe candidal infections: clinical perspective, immune defense mechanisms, and current concepts of therapy. *Ann Intern Med* 1978; **89**: 91–106.

65 Hamadeh R, Ardehali A, Locksley RM et al. Fatal aspergillosis associated with smoking contaminated marijuana, in a marrow transplant recipient. *Chest* 1988; **94**: 432–3.

66 Warris A, Gaustad P, Meis JF et al. Recovery of filamentous fungi from water in a paediatric bone marrow transplantation unit. *J Hosp Infect* 2001; **47**: 143–8.

67 Ng TT, Robson GD, Denning DW. Hydrocortisone-enhanced growth of *Aspergillus* spp. implications for pathogenesis. *Microbiology* 1994; **140**(9): 2475–9.

68 Duong M, Ouellet N, Simard M et al. Kinetic study of host defense and inflammatory response to *Aspergillus fumigatus* in steroid-induced immunosuppressed mice. *J Infect Dis* 1998; **178**: 1472–82.

69 Waldorf AR, Levitz SM, Diamond RD. In vivo bronchoalveolar macrophage defense against *Rhizopus oryzae* and *Aspergillus fumigatus*. *J Infect Dis* 1984; **150**: 752–60.

70 Heidenreich S, Kubis T, Schmidt M et al. Glucocorticoid-induced alterations of monocyte defense mechanisms against *Candida albicans*. *Cell Immunol* 1994; **157**: 320–7.

71 Neth O, Jack DL, Dodds AW et al. Mannose-binding lectin binds to a range of clinically relevant microorganisms and promotes complement deposition. *Infect Immun* 2000; **68**: 688–93.

72 Bromley IM, Donaldson K. Binding of *Aspergillus fumigatus* spores to lung epithelial cells and basement membrane proteins: relevance to the asthmatic lung. *Thorax* 1996; **51**: 1203–9.

73 Haido RM, Silva MH, Ejzemberg R et al. Analysis of peptidogalactomannans from the mycelial surface of *Aspergillus fumigatus*. *Med Mycol* 1998; **36**: 313–21.

74 Savage DG, Taylor P, Blackwell J et al. Paranasal sinusitis following allogeneic bone marrow transplant. *Bone Marrow Transplant* 1997; **19**: 55–9.

75 Chim CS, Ho PL, Yuen ST et al. Fungal endocarditis in bone marrow transplantation: case report and review of literature. *J Infect* 1998; **37**: 287–91.

76 Chandrasekar PH. Empirical antifungal therapy for persistent fever in patients with neutropenia. *Clin Infect Dis* 2001; **32**: 320–1.

77 Jantunen E, Piilonen A, Volin L et al. Diagnostic aspects of invasive *Aspergillus* infections in allogeneic BMT recipients. *Bone Marrow Transplant* 2000; **25**: 867–71.

78 Siberry GK, Costarangos C, Cohen BA. Destruction of the nasal septum by *Aspergillus* infection after autologous bone marrow transplantation. *N Engl J Med* 1997; **337**: 275–6.

79 van Assen S, Bootsma GP, Verweij PE et al. Aspergillus tracheobronchitis after allogeneic bone marrow transplantation. *Bone Marrow Transplant* 2000; **26**: 1131–2.

80 Machida U, Kami M, Kanda Y et al. Aspergillus tracheobronchitis after allogeneic bone marrow transplantation. Bone Marrow Transplant 1999; 24: 1145–9.

81 van Burik JA, Colven R, Spach DH. Cutaneous aspergillosis. J Clin Microbiol 1998; 36: 3115–21.

82 Bretagne S, Bart-Delabesse E, Wechsler J et al. Fatal primary cutaneous aspergillosis in a bone marrow transplant recipient: nosocomial acquisition in a laminar-air flow room. J Hosp Infect 1997; 36: 235–9.

83 Choi JH, Yoo JH, Chung IJ et al. Esophageal aspergillosis after bone marrow transplant. Bone Marrow Transplant 1997; 19: 293–4.

84 Ansorg R, Heintschel von Heinegg E, Rath PM. Aspergillus antigenuria compared to antigenemia in bone marrow transplant recipients. Eur J Clin Microbiol Infect Dis 1994; 13: 582–9.

85 Machetti M, Feasi M, Mordini N et al. Comparison of an enzyme immunoassay and a latex agglutination system for the diagnosis of invasive aspergillosis in bone marrow transplant recipients. Bone Marrow Transplant 1998; 21: 917–21.

86 Sulahian A, Tabouret M, Ribaud P et al. Comparison of an enzyme immunoassay and latex agglutination test for detection of galactomannan in the diagnosis of invasive aspergillosis. Eur J Clin Microbiol Infect Dis 1996; 15: 139–45.

87 Maertens J, Verhaegen J, Lagrou K et al. Screening for circulating galactomannan as a noninvasive diagnostic tool for invasive aspergillosis in prolonged neutropenic patients and stem cell transplantation recipients: a prospective validation. Blood 2001; 97: 1604–10.

88 Williamson EC, Oliver DA, Johnson EM et al. Aspergillus antigen testing in bone marrow transplant recipients. J Clin Pathol 2000; 53: 362–6.

89 Boutboul F, Alberti C, Leblanc T et al. Invasive aspergillosis in allogeneic stem cell transplant recipients: increasing antigenemia is associated with progressive disease. Clin Infect Dis 2002; 34: 939–43.

90 Einsele H, Hebart H, Roller G et al. Detection and identification of fungal pathogens in blood by using molecular probes. J Clin Microbiol 1997; 35: 1353–60.

91 Hebart H, Loffler J, Reitze H et al. Prospective screening by a panfungal polymerase chain reaction assay in patients at risk for fungal infections: implications for the management of febrile neutropenia. Br J Haematol 2000; 111: 635–40.

92 Williamson EC, Leeming JP, Palmer HM et al. Diagnosis of invasive aspergillosis in bone marrow transplant recipients by polymerase chain reaction. Br J Haematol 2000; 108: 132–9.

93 Buchheidt D, Baust C, Skladny H et al. Clinical evaluation of a polymerase chain reaction assay to detect Aspergillus species in bronchoalveolar lavage samples of neutropenic patients. Br J Haematol 2002; 116: 803–11.

94 Chang HC, Leaw SN, Huang AH et al. Rapid identification of yeasts in positive blood cultures by a multiplex PCR method. J Clin Microbiol 2001; 39: 3466–71.

95 Chryssanthou E, Klingspor L, Tollemar J et al. PCR and other non-culture methods for diagnosis of invasive Candida infections in allogeneic bone marrow and solid organ transplant recipients. Mycoses 1999; 42: 239–47.

96 Clemons KV, Calich VL, Burger E et al. Pathogenesis I. Interactions of host cells and fungi. Med Mycol 2000; 38 (Suppl. 1): 99–111.

97 Lal S, Mitsuyama M, Miyata M et al. Pulmonary defence mechanism in mice. A comparative role of alveolar macrophages and polymorphonuclear cells against infection with Candida albicans. J Clin Lab Immunol 1986; 19: 127–33.

98 Kullberg BJ, Netea MG, Vonk AG et al. Modulation of neutrophil function in host defense against disseminated Candida albicans infection in mice. FEMS Immunol Med Microbiol 1999; 26: 299–307.

99 Newman SL, Holly A. Candida albicans is phagocytosed, killed, and processed for antigen presentation by human dendritic cells. Infect Immun 2001; 69: 6813–22.

100 Farah CS, Elahi S, Drysdale K et al. Primary role for $CD4^+$ T lymphocytes in recovery from oropharyngeal candidiasis. Infect Immun 2002; 70: 724–31.

101 Farah CS, Elahi S, Pang G et al. T cells augment monocyte and neutrophil function in host resistance against oropharyngeal candidiasis. Infect Immun 2001; 69: 6110–8.

102 Jones-Carson J, Vazquez-Torres A, Warner T et al. Disparate requirement for T cells in resistance to mucosal and acute systemic candidiasis. Infect Immun 2000; 68: 2363–5.

103 Balish E, Warner T, Pierson CJ et al. Oroesophageal candidiasis is lethal for transgenic mice with combined natural killer and T-cell defects. Med Mycol 2001; 39: 261–8.

104 Brieland J, Essig D, Jackson C et al. Comparison of pathogenesis and host immune responses to Candida glabrata and Candida albicans in systemically infected immunocompetent mice. Infect Immun 2001; 69: 5046–55.

105 Brieland JK, Jackson C, Menzel F et al. Cytokine networking in lungs of immunocompetent mice in response to inhaled Aspergillus fumigatus. Infect Immun 2001; 69: 1554–60.

106 Liu L, Kang K, Takahara M et al. Hyphae and yeasts of Candida albicans differentially regulate interleukin-12 production by human blood monocytes: inhibitory role of C. albicans germination. Infect Immun 2001; 69: 4695–1.

107 Mencacci A, Perruccio K, Bacci A et al. Defective antifungal T-helper 1 (TH1) immunity in a murine model of allogeneic T-cell-depleted bone marrow transplantation and its restoration by treatment with TH2 cytokine antagonists. Blood 2001; 97: 1483–90.

108 de Repentigny L, Petitbois S, Boushira M et al. Acquired immunity in experimental murine aspergillosis is mediated by macrophages. Infect Immun 1993; 61: 3791–802.

109 Richard JL, Thurston JR, Cutlip RC et al. Vaccination studies of aspergillosis in turkeys: subcutaneous inoculation with several vaccine preparations followed by aerosol challenge exposure. Am J Vet Res 1982; 43: 488–92.

110 Grazziutti M, Przepiorka D, Rex JH et al. Dendritic cell-mediated stimulation of the in vitro lymphocyte response to Aspergillus. Bone Marrow Transplant 2001; 27: 647–52.

111 Bozza S, Gaziano R, Spreca A et al. Dendritic cells transport conidia and hyphae of Aspergillus fumigatus from the airways to the draining lymph nodes and initiate disparate TH responses to the fungus. J Immunol 2002; 168: 1362–71.

112 Cenci E, Mencacci A, Fe d'Ostiani C et al. Cytokine- and T helper-dependent lung mucosal immunity in mice with invasive pulmonary aspergillosis. J Infect Dis 1998; 178: 1750–60.

113 Cenci E, Mencacci A, Del Sero G et al. Interleukin-4 causes susceptibility to invasive pulmonary aspergillosis through suppression of protective type I responses. J Infect Dis 1999; 180: 1957–68.

114 Centeno-Lima S, Silveira H, Casimiro C et al. Kinetics of cytokine expression in mice with invasive aspergillosis: lethal infection and protection. FEMS Immunol Med Microbiol 2002; 32: 167–73.

115 Grazziutti ML, Rex JH, Cowart RE et al. Aspergillus fumigatus conidia induce a TH1-type cytokine response. J Infect Dis 1997; 176: 1579–83.

116 Martins MD, Rodriguez LJ, Savary CA et al. Activated lymphocytes reduce adherence of Aspergillus fumigatus. Med Mycol 1998; 36: 281–9.

117 Roilides E, Uhlig K, Venzon D et al. Prevention of corticosteroid-induced suppression of human polymorphonuclear leukocyte-induced damage of Aspergillus fumigatus hyphae by granulocyte colony-stimulating factor and γ-interferon. Infect Immun 1993; 61: 4870–7.

118 Roilides E, Blake C, Holmes A et al. Granulocyte-macrophage colony-stimulating factor and interferon-γ prevent dexamethasone-induced immunosuppression of antifungal monocyte activity against Aspergillus fumigatus hyphae. J Med Vet Mycol 1996; 34: 63–9.

119 Chakrabarti S, Mackinnon S, Chopra R et al. High incidence of cytomegalovirus infection after nonmyeloablative stem cell transplantation: potential role of Campath-1H in delaying immune reconstitution. Blood 2002; 99: 4357–63.

120 Mossad SB, Avery RK, Longworth DL et al. Infectious complications within the first year after nonmyeloablative allogeneic peripheral blood stem cell transplantation. Bone Marrow Transplant 2001; 28: 491–5.

121 Junghanss C, Marr KA. Infectious risks and outcomes after stem cell transplantation: are nonmyeloablative transplants changing the picture? Curr Opin Infect Dis 2002; 15: 347–53.

122 Oren I, Haddad N, Finkelstein R et al. Invasive pulmonary aspergillosis in neutropenic patients during hospital construction: before and after chemoprophylaxis and institution of HEPA filters. Am J Hematol 2001; 66: 257–62.

123 Alberti C, Bouakline A, Ribaud P et al. Relationship between environmental fungal contamination and the incidence of invasive aspergillosis in haematology patients. J Hosp Infect 2001; 48: 198–206.

124 Munoz P, Burillo A, Bouza E. Environmental surveillance and other control measures in the prevention of nosocomial fungal infections. Clin Microbiol Infect 2001; 7 (Suppl. 2): 38–45.

125 BitMansour A, Brown JM. Prophylactic administration of liposomal amphotericin B is superior to treatment in a murine model of invasive aspergillosis after hematopoietic cell transplantation. J Infect Dis 2002; 186: 134–7.

126 Wingard JR. Antifungal chemoprophylaxis after blood and marrow transplantation. Clin Infect Dis 2002; 34: 1386–90.

127 Goodman JL, Winston DJ, Greenfield RA et al. A controlled trial of fluconazole to prevent fungal infections in patients undergoing bone marrow transplantation. N Engl J Med 1992; 326: 845–51.

128 Slavin MA, Osborne B, Adams R et al. Efficacy and safety of fluconazole prophylaxis for fungal infections after marrow transplantation: a prospective, randomized, double-blind study. J Infect Dis 1995; 171: 1545–52.

129 Marr KA, Seidel K, Slavin MA et al. Prolonged fluconazole prophylaxis is associated with persistent protection against candidiasis-related death in allogeneic marrow transplant recipients: long-term follow-up of a randomized, placebo-controlled trial. Blood 2000; 96: 2055–61.

130 MacMillan ML, Goodman JL, DeFor TE et al. Fluconazole to prevent yeast infections in bone marrow transplantation patients: a randomized trial of high versus reduced dose, and determination of the value of maintenance therapy. *Am J Med* 2002; **112**: 369–79.

131 Kami M, Machida U, Okuzumi K et al. Effect of fluconazole prophylaxis on fungal blood cultures: an autopsy-based study involving 720 patients with haematological malignancy. *Br J Haematol* 2002; **117**: 40–6.

132 O'Donnell MR, Schmidt GM, Tegtmeier BR et al. Prediction of systemic fungal infection in allogeneic marrow recipients: impact of amphotericin prophylaxis in high-risk patients. *J Clin Oncol* 1994; **12**: 827–34.

133 Conneally E, Cafferkey MT, Daly PA et al. Nebulized amphotericin B as prophylaxis against invasive aspergillosis in granulocytopenic patients. *Bone Marrow Transplant* 1990; **5**: 403–6.

134 Trigg ME, Morgan D, Burns TL et al. Successful program to prevent aspergillus infections in children undergoing marrow transplantation: use of nasal amphotericin. *Bone Marrow Transplant* 1997; **19**: 43–7.

135 Grigg A. Prophylaxis and treatment of patients with aspergillosis: an overview, including the Royal Melbourne Hospital experience. *J Antimicrob Chemother* 2002; **49** (Suppl. 1): 75–80.

136 van Burik JH, Ratanatharathorn V, Lipton J et al. Randomized, double-blind trial of micafungin versus fluconazole for prophylaxis of invasive fungal infections in patients undergoing hematopoietic cell transplant, NIAID/BAMSG Protocol 46. 42nd ICAAC (Abstracts). San Diego, CA: American Society for Microbiology, 2002: 401.

137 Bjerke JW, Meyers JD, Bowden RA. Hepatosplenic candidiasis: a contraindication to marrow transplantation? *Blood* 1994; **84**: 2811–4.

138 Offner F, Cordonnier C, Ljungman P et al. Impact of previous aspergillosis on the outcome of bone marrow transplantation. *Clin Infect Dis* 1998; **26**: 1098–103.

139 Verschraegen CF, van Besien KW, Dignani C et al. Invasive *Aspergillus* sinusitis during bone marrow transplantation. *Scand J Infect Dis* 1997; **29**: 436–8.

140 Ozsahin H, von Planta M, Muller I et al. Successful treatment of invasive aspergillosis in chronic granulomatous disease by bone marrow transplantation, granulocyte colony-stimulating factor-mobilized granulocytes, and liposomal amphotericin-B. *Blood* 1998; **92**: 2719–24.

141 Watanabe C, Yajima S, Taguchi T et al. Successful unrelated bone marrow transplantation for a patient with chronic granulomatous disease and associated resistant pneumonitis and *Aspergillus* osteomyelitis. *Bone Marrow Transplant* 2001; **28**: 83–7.

142 Singhal S, Safdar A, Chiang KY et al. Nonmyeloablative allogeneic transplantation ("microallograft") for refractory myeloma after two preceding autografts: feasibility and efficacy in a patient with active aspergillosis. *Bone Marrow Transplant* 2000; **26**: 1231–3.

143 Hermann S, Klein SA, Jacobi V et al. Older patients with high-risk fungal infections can be successfully allografted using non-myeloablative conditioning in combination with intensified supportive care regimens. *Br J Haematol* 2001; **113**: 446–54.

144 Caillot D, Casasnovas O, Bernard A et al. Improved management of invasive pulmonary aspergillosis in neutropenic patients using early thoracic computed tomographic scan and surgery. *J Clin Oncol* 1997; **15**: 139–47.

145 Arathoon EG, Gotuzzo E, Noriega LM et al. Randomized, double-blind, multicenter study of caspofungin versus amphotericin B for treatment of oropharyngeal and esophageal candidiases. *Antimicrob Agents Chemother* 2002; **46**: 451–7.

146 Villanueva A, Arathoon EG, Gotuzzo E et al. A randomized double-blind study of caspofungin versus amphotericin for the treatment of candidal esophagitis. *Clin Infect Dis* 2001; **33**: 1529–35.

147 Buggia I, Zecca M, Alessandrino EP et al. Itraconazole can increase systemic exposure to busulfan in patients given bone marrow transplantation. GITMO (Gruppo Italiano Trapianto Midollo Osseo). *Anticancer Res* 1996; **16**: 2083–8.

148 Kontoyiannis DP, Lewis RE, Sagar N et al. Itraconazole-amphotericin B antagonism in *Aspergillus fumigatus*: an E-test-based strategy. *Antimicrob Agents Chemother* 2000; **44**: 2915–8.

149 Schaffner A, Bohler A. Amphotericin B refractory aspergillosis after itraconazole: evidence for significant antagonism. *Mycoses* 1993; **36**: 421–4.

150 Sugar AM, Liu XP. Interactions of itraconazole with amphotericin B in the treatment of murine invasive candidiasis. *J Infect Dis* 1998; **177**: 1660–3.

151 Walsh TJ, Pappas P, Winston DJ et al. Voriconazole compared with liposomal amphotericin B for empirical antifungal therapy in patients with neutropenia and persistent fever. *N Engl J Med* 2002; **346**: 225–34.

152 Herbrecht R, Denning DW, Patterson TF et al. Voriconazole versus amphotericin B for primary therapy of invasive aspergillosis. *N Engl J Med* 2002; **347**: 408–15.

153 Walsh TJ, Viviani MA, Arathoon E et al. New targets and delivery systems for antifungal therapy. *Med Mycol* 2000; **38** (Suppl. 1): 335–47.

154 Roilides E, Uhlig K, Venzon D et al. Enhancement of oxidative response and damage caused by human neutrophils to *Aspergillus fumigatus* hyphae by granulocyte colony-stimulating factor and γ-interferon. *Infect Immun* 1993; **61**: 1185–93.

155 Roilides E, Holmes A, Blake C et al. Effects of granulocyte colony-stimulating factor and interferon-γ on antifungal activity of human polymorphonuclear neutrophils against pseudohyphae of different medically important *Candida* species. *J Leukoc Biol* 1995; **57**: 651–6.

156 Roilides E, Lyman CA, Sein T et al. Antifungal activity of splenic, liver and pulmonary macrophages against *Candida albicans* and effects of macrophage colony-stimulating factor. *Med Mycol* 2000; **38**: 161–8.

157 Volpi I, Perruccio K, Tosti A et al. Postgrafting administration of granulocyte colony-stimulating factor impairs functional immune recovery in recipients of human leukocyte antigen haplotype-mismatched hematopoietic transplants. *Blood* 2001; **97**: 2514–21.

158 Cenci E, Mencacci A, Bacci A et al. T cell vaccination in mice with invasive pulmonary aspergillosis. *J Immunol* 2000; **165**: 381–8.

159 Bacci A, Montagnoli C, Perruccio K et al. Dendritic cells pulsed with fungal RNA induce protective immunity to *Candida albicans* in hematopoietic transplantation. *J Immunol* 2002; **168**: 2904–13.

160 BiMansour A, Burns SM, Traver D et al. Myeloid progenitors protect against invasive aspergillosis and *Pseudomonas aeruginosa* infection following hematopoietic stem cell transplantation. *Blood* 2002; **100**: 4660–7.

161 Caillot D, Mannone L, Cuisenier B et al. Role of early diagnosis and aggressive surgery in the management of invasive pulmonary aspergillosis in neutropenic patients. *Clin Microbiol Infect* 2001; **7** (Suppl. 2): 54–61.

162 Pidhorecky I, Urschel J, Anderson T. Resection of invasive pulmonary aspergillosis in immunocompromised patients. *Ann Surg Oncol* 2000; **7**: 312–7.

163 Gossot D, Validire P, Vaillancourt R et al. Full thoracoscopic approach for surgical management of invasive pulmonary aspergillosis. *Ann Thorac Surg* 2002; **73**: 240–4.

164 Salerno CT, Ouyang DW, Pederson TS et al. Surgical therapy for pulmonary aspergillosis in immunocompromised patients. *Ann Thorac Surg* 1998; **65**: 1415–9.

165 Erdogan E, Beyzadeoglu M, Arpaci F et al. Cerebellar aspergillosis: case report and literature review. *Neurosurgery* 2002; **50**: 874–6; discussion 876–7.

166 Imai T, Yamamoto T, Tanaka S et al. Successful treatment of cerebral aspergillosis with a high oral dose of itraconazole after excisional surgery. *Intern Med* 1999; **38**: 829–32.

167 Choi SS, Milmoe GJ, Dinndorf PA et al. Invasive *Aspergillus* sinusitis in pediatric bone marrow transplant patients: evaluation and management. *Arch Otolaryngol Head Neck Surg* 1995; **121**: 1188–92.

168 Iwen PC, Rupp ME, Hinrichs SH. Invasive mold sinusitis: 17 cases in immunocompromised patients and review of the literature. *Clin Infect Dis* 1997; **24**: 1178–84.

169 Pfaller MA, Rex JH, Rinaldi MG. Antifungal susceptibility testing. Technical advances and potential clinical applications. *Clin Infect Dis* 1997; **24**: 776–84.

170 Alangaden G, Chandrasekar PH, Bailey E et al. Antifungal prophylaxis with low-dose fluconazole during bone marrow transplantation. The Bone Marrow Transplantation Team. *Bone Marrow Transplant* 1994; **6**: 919–24.

171 Winston DJ, Maziarz RT, Chandrasekar PH et al. Intravenous and oral itraconazole versus intravenous fluconazole for long-term antifungal prophylaxis in allogeneic hematopoietic stem-cell transplant recipients. A multi-center, randomized trial. *Ann Intern Med* 2003; **9**: 705–13.

172 Ehninger G, Schuler HK, Sarnow E. Fluconazole in the prophylaxis of fungal infection after bone marrow transplantation. *Mycoses* 1996; **7–8**: 259–63.

173 Nucci M, Biasoli I, Akiti T et al. A double-blind, randomized, placebo-controlled trial of itraconazole capsules as antifungal prophylaxis for neutropenic patients. *Clin Infect Dis* 2000; **2**: 300–5.

174 Foot AB, Veys PA, Gibson BE. Itraconazole oral solution as antifungal prophylaxis in children undergoing stem cell transplantation or intensive chemotherapy for haematological disorders. *Bone Marrow Transplant* 1999; **10**: 1089–93.

175 Wolff SN, Fay J, Stevens D, Herzig RH et al. Fluconazole vs. low-dose amphotericin B for the prevention of fungal infections in patients undergoing bone marrow transplantation: a study of the North American Marrow Transplant Group. *Bone Marrow Transplant* 2000; **8**: 853–9.

176 Riley DK, Pavia AT, Beatty PG et al. The prophylactic use of low-dose amphotericin B in bone marrow transplant patients. *Am J Med* 1994; **6**: 509–14.

177 Tollemar J, Ringden O, Andersson S et al. Randomized double-blind study of liposomal amphotericin B (Ambisome) prophylaxis of invasive fungal infections in bone marrow transplant recipients. *Bone Marrow Transplant* 1993; **6**: 577–82.

178 Kelsey SM, Goldman JM, McCann S et al. Liposomal amphotericin (AmBisome) in the prophylaxis of fungal infections in neutropenic patients: a randomised, double-blind, placebo-controlled study. *Bone Marrow Transplant* 1999; **2**: 163–8.

53

John A. Zaia

Cytomegalovirus Infection

Introduction

The sequential occurrence of different specific infections after hematopoietic cell transplantation (HCT) has historically formed the basis for certain management decisions post-transplantation [1,2]. Foremost among these infectious complications have been those associated with human cytomegalovirus (CMV) [3–9]. In the past decade, however, the introduction of improved methods for detection of CMV has enhanced the early or pre-emptive use of antiviral agents that had been poorly effective during the 1980s. As a result, although approximately 50–70% of persons who have had a prior CMV infection continue to develop a reactivation of this infection after allogeneic HCT, the occurrence of CMV-associated disease and mortality in the first 3 months after HCT has been significantly reduced. This iatrogenic manipulation of the natural course of CMV infection has not eliminated the problem of CMV after HCT and, in fact, it has introduced new problems, such as later onset of disease and the occurrence of side-effects of antiviral therapy. In addition, the increasing use of nonmyeloablative HCT procedures, which have lessened the procedure-related morbidity of HCT, has not lessened the incidence of CMV infection. Also, the increased use of HCT as a mode of therapy for nonhematopoietic diseases indicates that there will be expanding areas in which the natural course of CMV infection needs to be defined.

The pathogenesis of CMV disease has become better understood in the past decade. In the past few years, several mechanisms by which this virus escapes immune surveillance have been demonstrated. In addition, with the understanding of the specific cellular immunodeficiency that places HCT recipients at risk for CMV disease, potential methods of passive immunotherapy have been introduced. An immunologic understanding of the peptide structures of the virus and of host responses to CMV have introduced quantitative methods for characterizing this immune response and suggest methods for antiviral drug management of the HCT recipient.

This chapter brings to the student, the transplant physician and other interested medical care-providers an awareness of the extensive background regarding the natural history of CMV after HCT, derived from the carefully designed studies performed when there were few adequate methods for treatment of CMV infection. The chapter focuses on the current methods for detection, prevention and treatment of CMV. Finally, a description of the pathophysiology of CMV infection and of host response to this infection is intended to provide the setting for understanding how future improvements in the management of CMV infection should occur.

Virology and epidemiology

Structure of human CMV

CMV is classified as a beta herpesvirus, which groups it with those herpesviruses that have a restricted host range [10], a relatively dynamic reproductive cycle [11], and repeated reactivation of virus infection with or without the eventual occurrence of disease [2]. CMV is a DNA virus that has the typical herpes virion structure consisting of (i) a core containing linear, double-stranded DNA; (ii) an icosahedral capsid of approximately 150 nm diameter containing 162 capsomeres; (iii) an amorphic, asymmetric material surrounding the capsid and designated the tegument or matrix; and (iv) an envelope containing viral glycoproteins on its surface. As shown in Fig. 53.1, CMV infection *in vitro* is associated with intact herpesvirus particles, defective virions and CMV-dense bodies. Only the intact virions are thought to be infectious; the defective particles and viral dense bodies contain nucleocapsid and matrix viral proteins. The clinical significance of defective virions in the CMV-associated syndromes is unknown. The genomic size of the DNA is approximately 240-kb pairs, which is the largest of the known herpesviruses [12]. This large genome encodes nearly 200 proteins based on an analysis of open

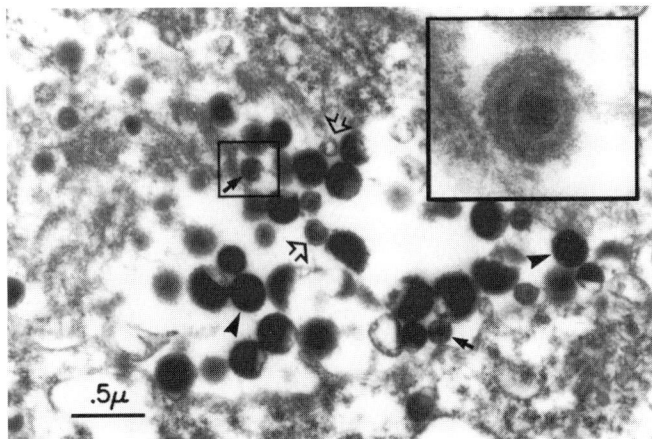

Fig. 53.1 Electron micrograph of cytomegalovirus (CMV) virions and defective particles. CMV-infected human foreskin fibroblasts were subjected to glutaraldehyde and osmium tetroxide fixation and electron microscopy, revealing intact virions (solid arrows), defective virions (open arrows) and dense bodies (arrowheads). (×38,750; inset: magnification ×182,500). Photomicrograph prepared by John Hardy, City of Hope National Medical Center.

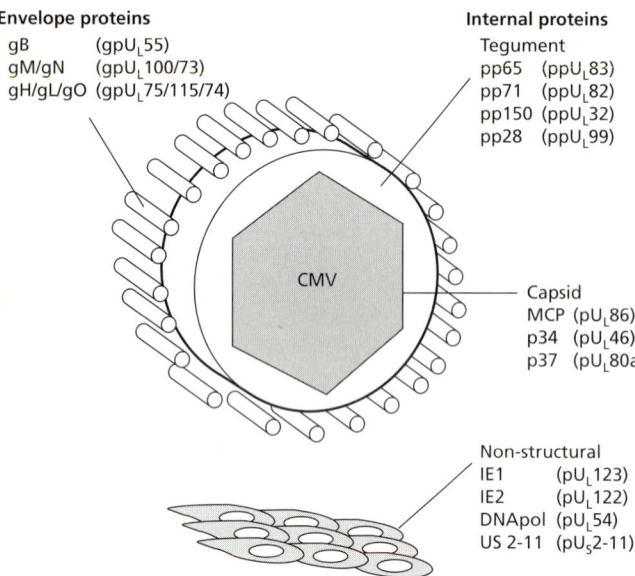

Fig. 53.2 Significant proteins of human cytomegalovirus (CMV). A schematic cross-sectional representation of the CMV virion and infected cells is shown indicating the components of the viral envelope, the internal proteins, and the nonstructural proteins. The alpha-numeric labels refer to the usual names of these proteins with the official nomenclature in parenthesis.

reading frames [13], but only a few of these proteins have been characterized (see below). A more detailed virologic description of CMV is beyond the scope of this chapter, and the interested reader is referred to reviews of this subject [10,14].

Characteristics of virus growth

From a clinical standpoint, a significant aspect of viral replication is the ability of the CMV genome to exist in cells in either an active or in a quiescent state of transcription. In the active state of transcription, there is a sequential expression of three categories of genomic elements termed immediate early (IE), early, or late viral proteins [15]. The major IE transcripts are transactivated by an in-coming virion protein, the 71 kDa tegument protein [16], in the absence of virion DNA replication, and these *IE* gene products then regulate the synthesis of the "early" proteins which facilitate viral DNA replication and can also affect host cell transcription (Fig. 53.2). By 12–18 h post-infection, viral DNA replication occurs and "late" proteins, derived from transcription of the newly synthesized DNA, are generated and assembled into the structural elements of the virion. The importance of this phenomenon to the clinician is that the inhibition of viral DNA replication does not stop *IE* gene transcription and, although it can restrict new virus production, it would not affect potentially pathological processes mediated by IE proteins. Interestingly, virus-induced cytopathology is present *in vitro* at times when only *IE* gene expression has occurred. For example, immediately after infection, basic housekeeper proteins are down-regulated [17], and a family of proteins encoded in the unique short (U_s) region of the genome interferes with peptide processing in the cytosol and endoplasmic reticulum (ER) [10,18]. Although the actual role of these IE-early virus proteins in the pathogenesis of CMV disease is only beginning to be understood, it is possible that a component of CMV pathology is contributed by these gene products. The ineffectiveness of the CMV inhibitors, which act by blocking viral DNA replication, to effectively treat advanced CMV infection suggests that this concept might have some clinical relevance.

CMV latency

The term latency refers to the presence of viral genome in the absence of immediate and active production of infectious virus. Certain diagnostic assays for CMV infection can establish whether the infection is active; i.e. a positive tissue culture assay indicates infectious CMV, rising titer of CMV in blood using a PCR-based assay, or an antigen-based assay indicates active infection. If the person under study is seronegative for CMV-specific antibody and has no detectable infectious virus, then it is likely that there is no latent infection present. It should be noted that with newer assays for CMV, virus has been detected in CMV seronegative blood donors [19,20]; however, seronegative marrow donors virtually never transmit CMV to seronegative recipients. The person who is seropositive for CMV antibody and has no detectable evidence for infectious virus is assumed to have latent CMV infection, and the blood products from this person are infectious for the marrow recipient.

The evidence for latency of CMV is based on such circumstantial evidence in humans in which virus infection follows tissue or cellular transfer, but latency is more solidly established in the murine model of CMV infection [21]. Here, lymphoid cells from previously infected mice, which show no active viral infection, undergo activation of infection when cocultivated with allogeneic fibroblasts. It is likely, although not proven conclusively, that latency is nothing more than the functional absence of sufficient cellular transcription factors for permissive replication. Looked at from this standpoint, virus (re)activation to the permissive state involves induction of these transcription factors [22]. In this regard, Söderberg-Nauclér *et al.* [19] have demonstrated the ability to isolate infectious virus from peripheral blood mononuclear cells that were placed in long-term culture with allogeneic stimulation. Thus, it appears that a site of latency of CMV is the blood monocyte and, following certain signal transduction events, the virus can be activated from latency.

One of the frustrating aspects of understanding CMV latency has been the attempt to localize the tissue source from which virus reactivates. In humans, virus transmission is well-documented in blood transfusions, solid organ transplantation and HCT [23]. However, in transplant settings, short-term cultures from specimen aliquots have been negative for virus, but the specimen nevertheless transferred infection to the recipient. Clinical observations have indicated that transmission of virus by blood is relatively inefficient compared to transmission by solid organs such as kidney and heart [23]. The actual activation of the virus within these cells appears to be dependent on cellular activation signals [19,24]. It is possible that other cells of the blood can serve as a vehicle for transmission of CMV with transfusions, and Salzberger *et al.* [25] have demonstrated CMV in circulating endothelial cells after HCT.

Epidemiology of CMV infection in marrow transplantation

The changing pattern of CMV epidemiology

The epidemiological description of CMV infection in the HCT population is among the best described and has established that CMV infection can originate from both endogenous and exogenous sources [26]. Yet, because of differences in the incidence of infection and/or disease at different HCT centers, there is some confusion regarding the risks for infection and for disease. Contributing to this confusion is the fact that the incidence of CMV disease in this population has changed over the past two decades because of the major changes in patient management. The first important change was the curtailment of CMV exposure via granulocyte transfusion therapy and decreased use of CMV-seropositive blood product support in the susceptible recipient. The second was the use of antiviral therapy to limit CMV reactivation.

The incidence of unmodified CMV infection and disease is best described by the control groups from the blinded studies that attempted to

Table 53.1 Changing epidemiology of cytomegalovirus (CMV) disease after allogeneic hematopoietic cell transplantation (HCT).*

Reference	Pre-emptive Rx	CMV disease (%)	Median day disease onset
Winston et al. 1987 [29]	No	17/37 (46)	52
Bowden et al. 1991 [30]	No	12/60 (20)	60
Schmidt et al. 1991 [31]	No	30/84 (36)	51
Zaia et al. 1995 [46]	Yes—BAL	11/103 (1)[†]	60[†]
		4/60 (7)[‡]	125[‡]
Einsele et al. 1995 [32]	Yes—BC	13/34 (38)[§]	<100[§]
	Yes—PCR	5/37 (14)[¶]	>100[¶]
Boeckh et al. 1996 [33]	Yes—AG	23/114 (20)**	160**
Zaia et al. 1997 [34]	Yes—BAL/BC	10/117 (8.5)[††]	176[††]
Boeckh et al. 2002 [70]	Yes—AG	26/146 (18)**	169**

*Results include only control groups from clinical studies in which there was no pre-emptive treatment strategy, except for Schmidt et al. [31] in which the pre-emptive treatment control group is used.
†Data are from subjects undergoing routine BAL who received early ganciclovir treatment for positive CMV culture in BAL specimens.
‡Data are from subjects undergoing routine BAL who did not receive ganciclovir because of negative CMV culture in BAL specimen.
§Data are from subjects undergoing routine CMV BC surveillance who received early ganciclovir treatment for positive CMV culture.
¶Data are from subjects undergoing routine CMV leukocyte PCR assay and received early ganciclovir treatment for positive CMV PCR.
**Data are from subjects undergoing routine CMV leukocyte AG and received early ganciclovir treatment for positive CMV AG.
††Data are from subjects undergoing routine CMV culture of BAL and blood and received early ganciclovir treatment for positive CMV BAL or BC.
AG, antigenemia assay; BAL, bronchoalveolar lavage; BC, blood culture; PCR, polymerase chain reaction; Rx, therapy.

Table 53.2 Incidence of cytomegalovirus (CMV) infection in marrow allograft recipients by donor/recipient CMV serology.*

Reference	CMV antibody In donor	CMV antibody in recipient R+ (%[†])	R− (%[†])
Meyers et al. 1986 [37]	D−	81/118 (69)	58/208 (28)
	D+	97/140 (69)	44/77 (57)
Miller et al. 1986 [6]	D−	15/21 (71)	20/107 (19)
	D+	13/23 (57)	6/30 (20)
Nichols et al. 2002 [38]	D−	220/393 (56)	13/628 (2)
	D+	268/467 (57)	31/262 (12)

*CMV antibody determination prior to HCT.
†Percent with CMV infection documented post-HCT.
D, donor; R, recipient.

alter the occurrence of CMV complications after HCT. Thus, the incidence of CMV infection in CMV-seronegative recipients of seronegative donor marrow dropped from 60–70% to nearly 0% with the introduction of CMV-seronegative blood support [27,28]. In the CMV-seropositive recipients, the course of CMV disease was fairly stable until the introduction of preventive antiviral chemotherapy. Pre-emptive antiviral treatment strategies dramatically reduced the early occurrence of CMV disease but moved disease occurrence to later times after HCT. As shown in Table 53.1, in the 1980s the disease occurred at a median time of 50–60 days post-HCT [29–31], but with the introduction of pre-emptive ganciclovir therapy, the median time of onset has shifted to a median time of 160–176 days HCT [32–34]. The therapeutic maneuvers used to prevent early CMV disease altered the natural history of infection and resulted in late-onset disease. Thus, an understanding of the natural history of CMV disease must be divided into that of the preantiviral era and the antiviral era.

Infection rate in marrow allograft recipients

Preantiviral era

The first descriptions of CMV-associated disease in marrow allograft recipients appeared in the 1970s and described a relatively new disease, CMV-associated interstitial pneumonia (CMV-IP) (see Plate 23.41, facing p. 296) [35,36]. CMV infection, defined as virus-positive culture from a clinical specimen or seroconversion of CMV antibody, occurred in 42–69% if the HCT recipient was CMV seropositive and in 13–36% if the recipient was CMV seronegative. The rate of CMV disease, defined as evidence of virus in association with organ-specific pathology (see Plates 23.34 and 23.35, facing p. 296), usually in lungs, gastrointestinal tract, or liver, also followed this pattern and, in the CMV seropositive population, occurred in 15–25%. The most detailed early analysis of CMV infection in marrow allograft recipients was performed by Meyers et al. [37] in a prospective assessment of infection in 545 patients studied between 1979 and 1982. Because this study so accurately reflects the epidemiology of CMV in the period prior to effective intervention, the details of this study are worth reviewing. Evidence of CMV infection was present in 51% of patients and infectious virus was cultured from 43%. CMV seroconversion was noted in 31% of patients. Among the infected patients, approximately 40% had virus recovered without undergoing antibody seroconversion, indicating the poor reliability of antibody determinations in this population, and an additional 16% underwent seroconversion without isolation of virus. The median time to infection in the throat and urine was 54 and 59 days, respectively, after HCT. The excretion of virus and seroconversion was significantly associated with the serological status of the recipient and donor prior to HCT. The incidence of CMV infection among sero-negative patients was significantly increased by the use of a seropositive marrow donor (26% vs. 53%, $p < 0.001$). This risk factor for CMV infection persisted even when other seropositive blood support was used in the seronegative HCT recipient. This observation underlines the importance of the donor marrow in contributing to an exogenous source of CMV infection. In the seropositive HCT recipients, CMV infection was significantly more common (69% vs. 28%) and was not affected by the serology of the marrow donor nor by the use of CMV seropositive blood support. Excretion of virus, but not seroconversion, increased significantly with increasing age. When age and serological status were considered, the age effect was observed only for CMV excretion among seronegative patients. The excretion of CMV was highest among recipients transplanted for acute myeloid leukemia (AML), and again this was related to the increased proportion of CMV seropositives among the group with AML.

The most striking aspect of CMV epidemiology in the pretreatment era becomes apparent when the attack rates are analyzed according to donor and recipient pre-HCT CMV antibody (Table 53.2). Here, the CMV seronegative recipient group had an infection rate as high as or even higher than those with prior CMV infection [27,28]. Today, this group would be expected to have minimum risk for CMV infection because of protection from exogenous CMV exposure [38]. Thus, prior to 1985, CMV disease occurred at a higher rate in the seronegative recipients, in marked contrast to subsequent observations [38,39].

The incidence of CMV infection and disease during this pretreatment era is recorded in the control arms of clinical trials of the various

Table 53.3 Historic incidence of cytomegalovirus (CMV) infection and disease.*

Reference	CMV antibody in recipient Pretransplantation	Infection (%)	Time	Disease (%)	Time
Bowden et al. 1986 [40]	No	8/20 (40)	Day 56	3/20 (15)	Day 58
Winston et al. 1987 [29]	No	21/37 (57)	Day 53	17/37 (46)	Day 52
Sullivan et al. 1990 [39]†	No	1/58 (2)	NA	0/61 (0)	NA
De Witte et al. 1990 [41]‡	No	0/28 (0)	NA	0/28 (0)	NA
Bowden et al. 1991 [30]	No	26/60 (43)	Day 54	12/60 (20)	Day 60
Bowden et al. 1991 [27]	No	7/30 (23)	Day 59	2/30 (7)	NP
Miller et al. 1991 [28]	No	21/61 (34)	NP	3/55 (5)	NP
Nichols et al. 2002 [38]	No	44/890 (5)	NP	21/890 (2)	NP
Meyers et al. 1988 [44]	Yes	49/65 (75)	Day 40	20/65 (31)	NP
Sullivan et al. 1990 [39]	Yes	NP (50)	NP	67/308 (22)	NP
De Witte et al. 1990 [41]	Yes	42/48 (86)	NP	10/48 (21)	NP
Schmidt et al. 1991 [31]	Yes	56/104 (54)§	Day 35	84 (36)	Day 51
Goodrich et al. 1991 [42]	Yes	107/194 (55)	Day 40	15/35 (43)	NP
Goodrich et al. 1993 [43]	Yes	14/31 (45)	NP	9/31 (29)	NP
Nichols et al. 2002 [38]	Yes	488/860 (57)	NP	164/860 (19)	NP

*Results include only control groups from these clinical trials, except for De Witte et al. [41], which was a prospective but uncontrolled study, and Schmidt et al. [31] and Goodrich et al. [42] in which CMV infection data were collected prior to therapy and hence include all patients.
†Data from the subgroup of subjects who were CMV-seronegative recipients of a CMV-seronegative donor marrow and who received CMV-seronegative blood support.
‡Study includes only CMV-seronegative recipients receiving leukocyte-poor blood support.
§Study includes only CMV-infection rate for bronchoalveolar lavage (BAL) specimens.
Abbreviations: NA, does not apply; NP, data not provided in source document.

candidate agents evaluated for anti-CMV effect in allograft populations (Table 53.3). These data from five HCT centers are shown separately for marrow recipients with and without pretransplant CMV antibody and compared to results obtained when more current pre-emptive anti-CMV strategies were in place. Again, the high rates of infection and disease [29,40] fell dramatically with the introduction of CMV-negative blood support [39,41]. Note that even in the latter part of the 1980s, the control groups that did not receive selected blood support had high infection rates, suggesting that other anticancer or antigraft-vs.-host-disease (GVHD) management regimen changes did not account for the decrease in CMV attack rates [27,28,42,43]. In the current era, approximately 10–15% of CMV seronegative recipients will develop CMV blood infection and up to one-half of these will get CMV disease [38]. The vast majority of CMV seronegative recipients who develop CMV-related adverse events have a seropositive donor [38].

For CMV-seropositive recipients, infection rates have remained as high as first described, ranging from 45% to 86%, and prevalence rates for CMV disease ranged from 21% to 43% [31,39,41–44]. Of note, CMV reactivation in recent times continues to occur in up to two-thirds of all CMV seropositive recipients [38,45]. It was thought that if this reactivation of CMV could be controlled by anti-CMV chemotherapy, the problem of CMV infection should be mitigated. The historical data in Table 53.3 indicate that CMV disease has been decreased, but antiviral agents have not entirely solved the problem.

Antiviral era

As indicated in the studies of pre-emptive ganciclovir therapy over the past decade, the incidence of CMV reactivation has remained 60–70% despite the fact that the diagnostic methods that confirm this infection rate have improved considerably in sensitivity [45,46]. For example, compare the prevalence of CMV infection from past observations using blood culture or antigenemia as a virus detection method [31–33,42] with the observations made using polymerase chain reaction (PCR) methods [32,47]. On the other hand, the use of antiviral agents at the time of engraftment or when CMV infection first occurs reduces the incidence of CMV disease in the first 100 days post-HCT to 1–2%. However, when treatment ends, the eventual incidence of CMV disease can be expected to be as high as 16% [33,43]. In the largest analysis of outcomes since the onset of pre-emptive anti-CMV treatment of HCT recipients, Nichols et al. [38] have reported that in 1750 HCT recipients treated between 1992 and 1998, CMV disease occurred in 10.6% overall and in 15.8% of those transplants in which either the recipient or donor or both were CMV seropositive. A recent report from Einsele et al. [45] confirms the continued high rate of CMV blood infection after HCT. Importantly, the advent of nonmyeloablative HCT has not changed the incidence of CMV reactivation [48].

Infection rates in autologous/syngeneic recipients

Wingard et al. [49] have reported that the incidence of CMV infection in a cohort of 143 autologous marrow recipients was 45%. This observation is not very different from the infection rate (~50%) in the allogeneic setting [37]. However, in the autologous HCT recipients, there was only a 2% rate of CMV disease, suggesting that pathogenesis is a function of alloreactivity. In that study, the incidence of CMV-IP was not different than that of the allograft recipients having no acute GVHD. Reusser et al. [50] have also studied the epidemiology of CMV in autologous marrow recipients and noted a rate of approximately 10% CMV disease in this same population. Boeckh et al. [51] reported that in a group of 67 autologous marrow or blood hematopoietic cell recipients, CMV reactivated in 39%, as determined by antigenemia assay, and CMV disease occurred in 4 (6%) of the 67. In a comparable group analyzed by leukocyte PCR, Hebart et al. [52] described a similar rate of CMV reactivation, with a

7.5% incidence of disease. Recent studies of autologous HCT, including those in which selected CD34+ stem cells were used, indicate the variable incidence of associated CMV disease [53–55]. The risk for CMV disease in this population has been linked to heavy pre-HCT chemotherapy, concomitant anti-T-cell therapy and use of CD34-selected peripheral blood stem cells. In syngeneic transplants, on the other hand, Appelbaum *et al.* [4] reported that, despite a similar occurrence of CMV infection, there was no CMV disease in 100 recipients of syngeneic marrow. Rare occurrence of CMV disease among this group would likely be due to the same risk factors as noted for autologous HCT recipients.

Clinical significance of virus strain differences

An epidemiological question frequently raised concerns the strain of CMV that occurs in the HCT recipient—does this CMV originate from the patient, from the donor, or from the blood products used in patient management? It is recognized that there is great variability among CMV isolates based on genetic polymorphism analyses [56]. These genetic polymorphisms occur throughout the entire CMV genome and, as a result, although the restriction endonuclease profiles of various CMV strains show many similarities, no two strains are identical unless they are related by epidemiology, e.g. mother-to-infant or blood donor-to-patient transmissions [57,58]. The human CMV genomes are colinear and have at least 80% sequence homology [13,22]. However, when specific coding regions are compared, certain strains have as little as 40% sequence identity. CMV strains have been typed based on variation in surface glycoproteins gB and gH [59]. Because of this diversity, questions exist regarding potential biological differences among the human CMV strains. It is of clinical importance that repeated infection may occur with different strains of CMV in one person and, for immunodeficient persons, it has been shown that multiple strains of CMV can be present at the same time [60,61]. In the marrow allograft setting, recipients can have multiple strains present in urine and blood simultaneously, and a strain can be present in lung tissue that is different from that in the urine [62]. The study of Winston *et al.* [63] demonstrated in four marrow allograft recipients, from whom isolates were obtained prior to HCT, that the CMV isolated subsequently was similar to the original CMV type in two and was different in two. It is recognized that CMV can infect and cause serious disease from either an endogenous or an exogenous source. The experience of Miller *et al.* [28] in CMV-seronegative recipients of seropositive donor marrow, in which those who received no CMV seropositive blood support had a similar CMV infection rate as those receiving CMV-seropositive blood support, indicates that the marrow itself is a significant source of CMV. Whether certain strains have virulence factors is currently being investigated and, in this regard, Torok-Storb *et al.* [64] and Boeckh *et al.* [65] have reported that CMV isolates from marrow of HCT recipients dying with graft failure have a significant prevalence of CMVgB types 3 and 4. This finding suggests that strain-specific virulence factors might exist which influence the occurrence of CMV disease after HCT.

Clinical approaches to management

Natural course of infection in the HCT recipient

General considerations

Since the discovery of CMV in animals and humans more than 35 years ago, two issues are apparent in considering the management of infection. The first is that these viruses are frequently found in many different tissues, and the second is that they are not always clearly associated with disease at times of active infection. CMV isolates frequently can be obtained from urine, blood and even the lung in asymptomatic individuals. In addition, these viruses are ubiquitous, with different species-specific strains occurring in virtually all vertebrate animals. Yet, despite this, in the natural setting, they cause few, if any, serious veterinary or human diseases. It has taken the iatrogenic alteration of normal immune function or the chronic immunodeficiency induced by human immunodeficiency virus-1 (HIV-1) to produce life-threatening infection by this virus. In addition, the mononucleosis syndromes of malaise, fatigue, thrombocytopenia and neutropenia, and even the more organ-specific syndromes, such as hepatitis and pneumonitis, can represent a broad differential diagnosis. In most situations, the diagnostic evaluation must exclude other explanations for the symptomatology before the diagnosis of CMV disease is made. In addition, in HCT recipients, contrary to the general rule that primary CMV infection is more severe than reactivation-associated disease, the clinician is more likely to be confronted with severe CMV-associated disease in persons with reactivation of their prior infection [1]. This situation occurs because primary infection can be prevented at present by the use of selected blood product support and because the CMV-seropositive population forms the majority of HCT recipients in most centers. The general approach to the CMV-specific management of the HCT recipient requires an understanding of the definition of CMV disease and of the risks of severe disease, and the use of this information for preventive intervention strategies in an effort to minimize disease.

Definitions of CMV disease

CMV infection *per se* in HCT recipients is usually defined as the isolation of CMV in tissue culture; the identification of CMV in tissue specimens by histological and histochemical means, or by specific antigen staining; direct CMV DNA/RNA or CMV antigen detection; or by a fourfold or higher rise in CMV antibody titer [66]. *CMV pneumonia* is defined as a progressive interstitial pulmonary process, as evidenced by chest X-ray, with concomitant evidence of CMV infection in the lung and without evidence for other causes of pneumonitis. *CMV enteritis* is defined as a gastrointestinal disease with pain, nausea and vomiting, or diarrhea and evidence of CMV infection at the site of an erythematous or ulcerative mucosal lesion. In general, other CMV-associated organ-related syndromes, such as hepatitis and encephalitis, are defined as syndromes with specific organ dysfunction and concomitant presence of active CMV infection. With the exception of CMV retinitis, the diagnosis of CMV disease cannot be made with confidence without histologic evidence of CMV infection in the involved organ.

Analysis of risk for disease

Although it would appear to be obvious, the most significant risk factor for the occurrence of CMV-associated disease after allogeneic HCT is the development of CMV infection. This is important to note because it is a strong confirmation that the heterogeneous syndromes that can present during CMV disease are, in fact, due to this infection and that this ubiquitous agent is not merely present and masking another pathologic process. In addition, it allows us to focus on management of patients by recognizing the factors that predict for CMV infection and disease. In the preganciclovir era, the analyses of risk for CMV disease after HCT demonstrated the following risk factors: (i) host factors, such as previous CMV infection, age, and diagnosis/remission disease status and delayed immune reconstitution post-HCT; (ii) treatment factors such as total body irradiation, preparative chemotherapy and GVHD prophylaxis; and (iii) the degree of allogeneic mismatch of the recipient and donor [5–9,37,67–69]. These risk factors continue to be important, but the ability to intervene with pre-emptive anti-CMV treatment has focused attention on the importance and understanding of these risk factors. Boeckh *et al.* [70] have evaluated the risk for late occurrence of CMV disease at 3 months after HCT and found that CMV virus load, any GVHD, post-engraftment lymphocytopenia <100/mm^3, CD4 counts <50/mm^3 and CMV-specific

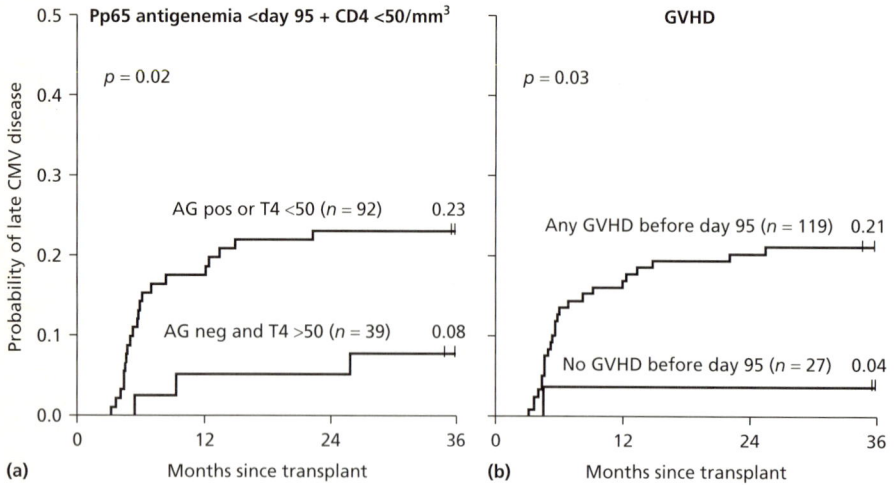

Fig. 53.3 Cumulative incidence of late cytomegalovirus (CMV) disease in patients with presence and absence of risk factors present at 3 months. Panel (a) compares patients with any pp65 antigenemia before day 95 or CD4 count <50/mm^3 with patients having no CMV antigenemia or CD4 count <50/mm^3. Panel (b) compares patients with any graft-vs.-host disease (GVHD) (grade 2–4 or clinical chronic) with patients having no GVHD before day 95. Reproduced with permission from Boeckh et al. [70].

T-cell immunodeficiency are the important predictors. Any CMV antigenemia before day 95 post-HCT or a CD4 count <50/mm^3 or any GVHD before day 95 post-HCT significantly increase the probability of late CMV disease (Fig. 53.3). Ljungman et al. [71] and Krause et al. [72] have demonstrated that T-lymphocyte immunity post-HCT signals diminished risk for CMV complications. Thus, from a practical standpoint, the central risks that define how the patient should be managed relative to probability of CMV disease are defined by the chances that the individual will develop CMV infection and the likelihood that inadequate immune function exists for resolution of the infection. When considered in this way, the important risk factors for development of severe CMV disease are patient age, pretransplantation seropositivity of donor or recipient for CMV antibody, human leukocyte antigen (HLA)-mismatch, recipient-donor status, occurrence of acute GVHD and ongoing immunologic function post-HCT.

Once the risk for CMV infection is present, several other significant risk factors deserve attention. The use of corticosteroids for management of GVHD is the single most important risk factor. Nichols et al. [38] have shown that 1–2 mg/kg corticosteroid was associated with significant rise in CMV DNA in blood during ganciclovir therapy. At doses of 2 mg/kg or higher, there was a 10-fold likelihood of a rising CMV DNA load while on therapy. Einsele et al. [45] have reported that risk factors for late-onset CMV disease are chronic GVHD and the need to treat with anti-CMV therapy for 4 weeks or more prior to day 100 when treatment is based on clearance of blood infection. The importance of donor (D) and recipient (R) CMV seropositive (+) and seronegative (−) status as risk factors for outcome in the current era has recently been evaluated [38]. CMV disease prevalence and overall mortality was higher in CMV seropositive recipients than in seronegative recipients (viz. CMV disease was seen in 17.6% D$^+$/R$^+$, in 20.9% D$^-$/R$^+$, in 5.3% D$^+$/R$^-$ and in 1.1% D$^-$/R$^-$). The D$^+$/R$^+$ and D$^+$/R$^-$ groups had the highest risk for mortality, and CMV-associated morbidity, including ganciclovir-related neutropenia, explained the increase in the D$^+$/R$^+$ group. However, the increased mortality in the D$^+$/R$^-$ group was explained not by overt CMV infection but by an increased occurrence of bacterial and fungal infections, which was mitigated in those receiving ganciclovir therapy. The implication of this observation is that it is likely that even subclinical CMV infection in CMV D$^+$/R$^-$ settings appears to contribute to poor outcome, presumably by the influence of occult CMV infection on immune reconstitution. Thus, marrow allograft recipients must be managed based on their various risks for CMV disease. Yet, even those in the lowest-risk groups face some chance of CMV-related disease after HCT and, therefore, it is important for the transplant team to consider all HCT recipients when considering anti-CMV strategies and to base treatment on relative risks of CMV disease.

CMV-associated interstitial pneumonia (CMV-IP)

Description of disease after HCT

As described in the epidemiology section, prior to the development of methods for prevention of CMV infection, CMV-IP (see Plate 23.41, facing p. 296) occurred in 15–30% of marrow allograft recipients [1,5,8,73]. The prevalence rates for infection, noted in Table 53.3, are the most accurate that are available, but institutional rates of late CMV-IP vary based on risk status of the referral population. No matter whether CMV-IP occurs before or after day 100 after HCT, hypoxia is the major physiological abnormality observed, and radiological abnormalities suggestive of interstitial pneumonitis are the frequent pattern on X-ray films (Fig. 53.4). Although infiltrates usually become diffuse and are basilar, there is considerable variation in the X-ray pattern, which can reveal segmental, lobar, or diffuse interstitial or nodular infiltrates [73,74]. The differential diagnosis includes radiation-induced pulmonary disease, cytotoxic chemotherapy-induced pulmonary damage, pulmonary hemorrhage, pulmonary edema, metastatic neoplasia and other infections of fungal, viral, or bacterial etiology. As illustrated in Fig. 53.5, the histopathology of CMV-IP involves thickening of the interalveolar membranes with cellular infiltrates and edema [35,36,74]. Of interest, CMV infections occur in an erratic distribution and are not clearly related to sites of typical CMV pathology [75,76]. Zaia [77] analyzed clinical and virologic aspects of 32 consecutive autopsied cases of CMV-IP. The amount of CMV/g lung, as measured by infectious titer or by amount of CMV DNA, did not significantly correlate with the duration of disease. Similarly, Slavin et al. [78] reported that quantitative assessment of infectious CMV in the bronchoalveolar lavage (BAL) specimens from allograft recipients could not distinguish patients in terms of disease severity, and virus burden was not predictive of individual outcome. However, as noted earlier, it is recognized that CMV level in blood is predictive of risk for late onset CMV disease [70].

Although the diagnostic procedure of choice in the past was lung biopsy, since the mid-1980s BAL has become the preferred method of diagnosis of CMV-IP [79,80]. The specimen should be analyzed for infectious virus and for cytological evidence of CMV. As shown in Fig. 53.5, inclusion bodies typical for CMV can often be seen in the CMV-positive BAL samples.

The historical use of antiviral agents for treatment of CMV-IP

Although pre-emptive ganciclovir use has improved in the past decade

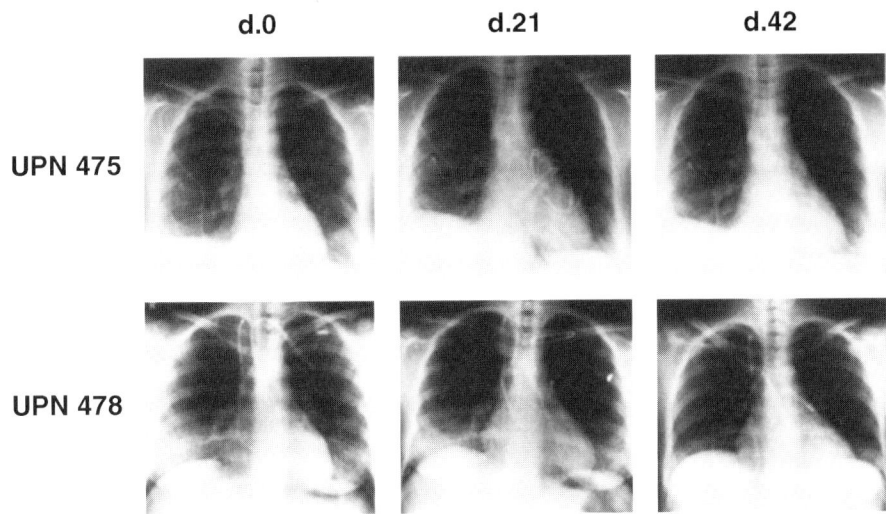

Fig. 53.4 Clinical course of treated cytomegalovirus-associated interstitial pneumonia (CMV-IP). This series of X-ray films from two patients (UPN475 and UPN478) treated with ganciclovir as described in Table 53.5. X-rays are from days 0, 21 and 42 of treatment. Note the resolution of the right lower lobe pneumonitis in both patients.

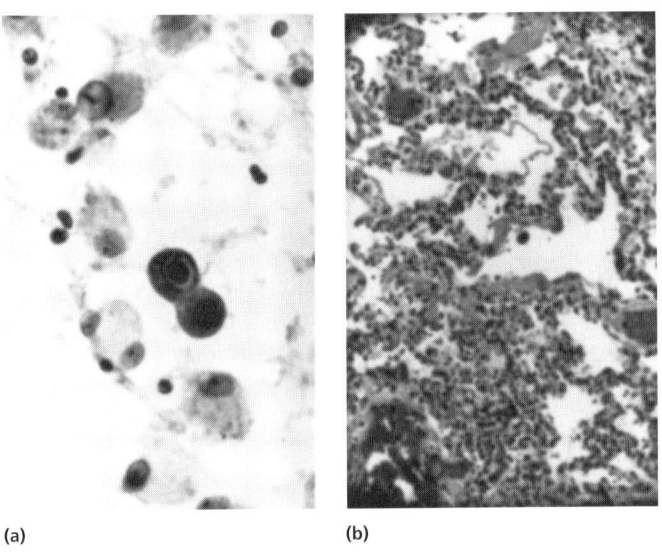

Fig. 53.5 Histopathology of cytomegalovirus-associated interstitial pneumonia (CMV-IP). (a) Photomicrograph of thin section of lung from a patient with CMV-IP stained with hematoxylin and eosin. Note the cell in alveolar space containing Cowdry type A intranuclear inclusion typical of CMV (×640). (b) Photomicrograph of Papanicolaou-stained bronchoalveolar lavage specimen from a patient with CMV-IP. Note similar CMV-induced "owl's eye" intranuclear inclusions (×1000) (see also Plate 23.41, facing p. 296).

Table 53.4 Historic treatment of cytomegalovirus-associated interstitial pneumonia (CMV-IP) with antiviral agents.

Reference	Agent	Survival rate at 3 months (%)
Kraemer et al. 1978 [82]	Vidarabine	16.6
Meyers et al. 1980 [83]	Leukocyte IFN	0.0
Meyers et al. 1982 [84]	IFN & vidarabine	14.2
Wade et al. 1982 [85]	Acyclovir	12.5
Wade et al. 1983 [86]	IFN & acyclovir	23.0
Meyers et al. 1983 [87]	rDNA IFN	0.0
Winston et al. 1983 [88]	rDNA IFN	60.0
Shepp et al. 1984 [89]	IFN & acyclovir	12.5
Shepp et al. 1985 [81]	Ganciclovir	10.0
Winston et al. 1988 [90]	Ganciclovir	22.2
Erice et al. 1987 [91]	Ganciclovir	45.0
Reed et al. 1986 [92]	Ganciclovir & steroid	16.6
Blacklock et al. 1985 [93]	CMVIg	50.0
Reed et al. 1987 [94]	CMVIg	21.4
Ringden et al. 1985 [95]	Foscarnet	0.0
Reed et al. 1988 [101]	Ganciclovir/IVIg	48.0
Emmanuel et al. 1988 [102]	Ganciclovir/IVIg	65.0
Schmidt et al. 1988 [103]	Ganciclovir/IVIg	85.0
Ljungman et al. 1992 [104]	Ganciclovir/IVIg	31.0
Aschan et al. 1992 [150]	Foscarnet	0.0

CMVIg, cytomegalovirus immunoglobulin; IFN, interferon; IVIg, intravenous immunoglobulin; rDNA IFN, recombinant interferon.

and changed the epidemiology of CMV-IP [32–34,46], the treatment of overt disease has not changed significantly. The treatment of CMV-IP has had mixed success in immunocompromised persons, probably due to variations in patient groups, that is, different diagnoses, different levels of immunosuppression, and varying contribution from host factors, known and unknown, that modify CMV infection. Overall, the outcome for the untreated disease has historically been very poor, with a mortality in the initial reports in the 1970s of 65% [36] and in the 1980s of approximately 85% (Table 53.4). Attempts to treat CMV disease with antiviral agents were uniformly unsuccessful despite the fact that many of these agents had produced a dramatic *in vitro* antiviral effect [81–95]. Thus, for example, the use of vidarabine [82], leukocyte interferon [83], vidarabine plus interferon [84], acyclovir [85], interferon plus acyclovir [86,89], recombinant DNA-derived interferon [87,88], ganciclovir [81,90,91], ganciclovir plus corticosteroids [92], CMV immunoglobulin (CMVIg) [93,94] and foscarnet [95] did not produce a significant improvement in the outcome of CMV-IP. In the first report of ganciclovir therapy for CMV-IP in this population by Shepp et al. [81], ganciclovir was used at a total dose ranging from 7.5 to 15.0 mg/kg/day in 10 persons, with only one surviving patient. In a study reported by Winston et al. [90], ganciclovir used at a dose of 10 mg/kg/day resulted in a survival rate of 22% in nine marrow recipients with CMV-IP. Erice et al. [91] reported that ganciclovir used at 7.5 mg/kg/day was associated with a 45% survival rate, in a study that included nonmarrow transplant patients. Thus, unlike the initial experience in the use of ganciclovir for treatment of CMV diseases in acquired immune deficiency syndrome (AIDS) patients, in which prompt clinical response was the rule [96], ganciclovir alone did not improve the outcome of CMV-IP in the HCT recipient.

Combination of antiviral agent and corticosteroids: the inability of agents that act only to suppress virus replication to treat CMV-IP successfully has suggested that there are additional factors contributing to pathogenesis besides virus cytopathology. Because CMV-IP could be caused by both CMV infection and the host response to infection, it was suggested that antiviral therapy be combined with immune response modification [76]. The initial use of combined treatment, reported by Reed *et al.* [92] involved ganciclovir (7.5 mg/kg/day) plus methyl prednisolone (16 mg/kg/day) in 6 marrow recipients. Only one patient survived and severe marrow and renal toxicities were observed in five patients. Clearly, this regimen produced no improvement.

The use of a CMVIg was evaluated for the treatment of CMV-IP, with mixed results. In the initial study of Blacklock *et al.* [93], nine of 18 marrow recipients survived CMV-IP, but the only other reported use of CMVIg for treatment of CMV-IP by Reed *et al.* [94] did not confirm this result.

Combination of antiviral agent and CMVIg: animal studies provided observations relevant to the combination of ganciclovir and Ig. In a mouse model of CMV-IP, Shanley and Pesanti [97] found that ganciclovir, while decreasing the amount of murine CMV infection in mouse lung, failed to prevent interstitial pneumonia. However, Wilson *et al.* [98] demonstrated that the combination of ganciclovir and mouse immune serum would protect from a lethal challenge with murine CMV. In this study neither ganciclovir nor immune serum alone provided protection.

These studies set the stage for regimens that combined ganciclovir and intravenous Ig (IVIg) for the treatment of CMV-IP. Reed *et al.* [99] and Bratanow *et al.* [100] provided the initial reports of this combination with improved outcome of CMV-IP. Subsequently, several centers published results using this regimen. The results are included in Table 53.4 [101–104]. In the study reported by Reed *et al.* [101], two IVIg products were used in conjunction with ganciclovir. One product contained high-titer CMV-specific antibody and was given at a dose of 400 mg/kg on days 1, 2 and 7, and then at half this dose on days 14 and 21. Of 50 patients in this group, 25 (50%) had at least a 6-week survival time and 16 patients (32%) were alive at 6 months, at a median follow-up time of 9 months. In an additional trial, patients were treated with a standard, commercially available Ig containing a lower-titer CMV-specific antibody given at 500 mg/kg every other day for nine doses. Thirteen patients were entered into this group; (38%) were alive at 6 weeks and at 6 months, with a median follow-up time of 5 months.

In the study reported by Emmanuel *et al.* [102], 20 patients received a regimen of IVIg consisting of 500 mg/kg every other day for 10 doses and then every 2 weeks for 8 doses. Fourteen (70%) of the 20 patients were alive at 6 weeks and 10 (30%) were alive at 6 months, with a median follow-up time of 24 months. In the study of Schmidt *et al.* [103], 40 patients were treated with therapy which included antiviral induction treatment lasting 3 weeks, or until there was documented clearing of pulmonary CMV infection, followed by a maintenance treatment lasting until immunosuppressive medications were stopped. In this regimen, ganciclovir was given at 10 mg/kg daily and Ig at 500 mg/kg every other day for 21 days, followed by ganciclovir at 5 mg/kg daily 5 days/week and IVIg at 500 mg/kg weekly until day 180 after HCT. With this treatment, 32 (80%) marrow recipients were alive at 6 weeks after treatment was started and 16 (40%) were alive at a median follow-up time of 18 months. Ganciclovir Ig treatment of CMV-IP has met with varying success in some HCT centers, probably due to variations in patient populations. For example, Ljungman *et al.* [104] noted that patients who did not receive total body irradiation compared to those who did benefited more from ganciclovir Ig treatment of CMV-IP (75% vs. 27% survival rates at 30 days, respectively, $p = 0.009$) and, in general, the patient with multiple organ dysfunction or respiratory failure was less likely to respond to antiviral therapy [105].

Thus, ganciclovir combined with IVIg has produced improvement in the outcome of this disease. Although these results were derived from uncontrolled studies, ganciclovir plus Ig has become the recommended

Table 53.5 Treatment of cytomegalovirus-associated interstitial pneumonia (CMV-IP).*

Induction phase—21 days
GCV	5 mg/kg IV q.12 h
IVIg*	500 mg/kg IV q.o.d. **or**
CMVIg*	125 mg/kg IV q.o.d.

Maintenance phase—during continued immunosuppression
GCV	5 mg/kg IV q.d. 5days/week
IVIg*	500 mg/kg IV q. week **or**
CMVIg*	125 mg/kg IV q. week

*IVIg or CMVIg used only for CMV-IP and not for other organ-specific syndromes.
†If the absolute neutrophil count (ANC) <1000/mL for 2 consecutive days, then stop GCV until count recovers; consider use of granulocyte (G-) or granulocyte macrophage colony-stimulating factor (GM-CSF).
CMVIg, cytomegalovirus immunoglobulin; GCV, ganciclovir; IV, intravenous; IVIg, intravenous immunoglobulin; q, every; q.d., every day; q.o.d., every other day.

treatment for CMV-IP in the HCT recipient; a method of treatment is outlined in Table 53.5. Repeat BAL is suggested after the initial 21 days of treatment if there is any question regarding response to the initial antiviral therapy. Reactivation of CMV is the usual course when ganciclovir is stopped and, therefore, it is recommended that maintenance therapy be continued for the duration of major immunosuppressive treatment. The expected course of resolution of CMV-IP on treatment is shown in Fig. 53.4. Fever and hypoxia usually resolve within the 1st week of treatment, but X-ray changes persist for many weeks. The patient with a slow response to treatment prompts the consideration of ganciclovir-resistant CMV or raises questions of the accuracy of the original diagnosis (Fig. 53.6). Both of these concerns can be addressed by repeat BAL. CMV infection is usually eliminated from the lavage specimen by 21 days after the start of treatment, and deterioration of pulmonary function with continued CMV lung infection at this time suggests ganciclovir resistance [106], although this event is rare in the setting of HCT.

If ganciclovir resistance occurs, or if ganciclovir cannot be used because of marrow toxicity, then foscarnet is indicated [105]. As derived from experience with treatment of retinitis in persons with AIDS, foscarnet is given at a dose of either 90 mg/kg twice daily or 60 mg/kg three times daily with saline infusion over 2 h during an initial 7-day induction period. Maintenance therapy follows this at a dose of 90 mg/kg/day for an extended period of time, determined by the immunosuppression of the patient. Foscarnet is nephrotoxic and it is recommended that the calculation of the dosage be determined by creatinine clearance. There has been no systematic evaluation of the efficacy of foscarnet plus Ig for the treatment of CMV-IP.

CMV-associated enteritis

Gastrointestinal syndromes associated with CMV are an increasingly important problem in allogeneic HCT recipients. Ulcerations associated with CMV infection can be identified in the esophagus (see Plates 23.34 and 23.35, *facing p. 296*), the stomach, the small bowel and the large intestine [107,108]. The diagnosis is made by the association of CMV infection with mucosal pathology and appropriate symptoms. Although the optimal method for treatment of this disease is not known, based on experiences with CMV retinitis, it is common practice to use ganciclovir alone for CMV-enteritis according to the dosing schedule shown for CMV-IP (Table 53.5). One controlled study using ganciclovir showed

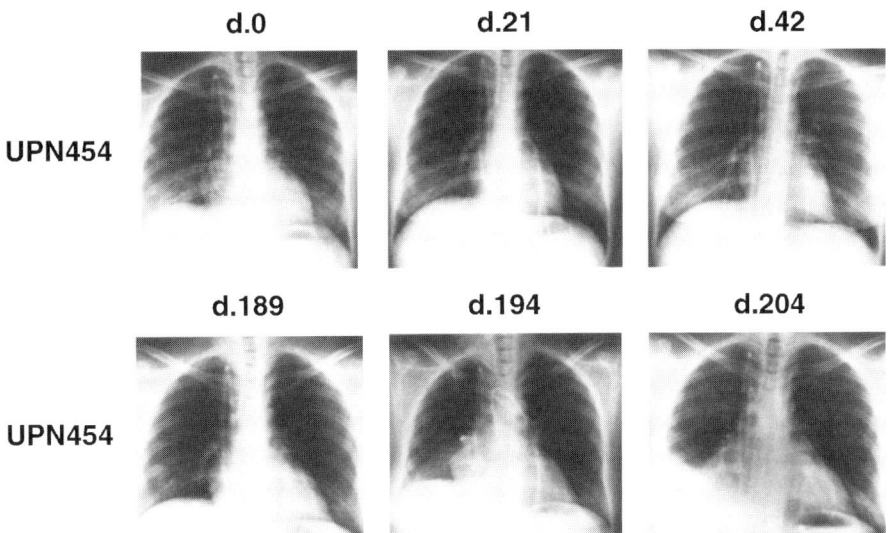

Fig. 53.6 Late complication of treated cytomegalovirus-associated interstitial pneumonia (CMV-IP). Patient (UPN454) was treated on day 0 (d.0) with ganciclovir according to the regimen in Table 53.5, with resolution of pneumonitis (d.21 and d.42). Subsequently, the patient developed a right-lower-lobe nodule (d.189), progressing to right-lower-lobe pneumonia (d.194 and d.204) and then death from Aspergillus infection and chronic graft-vs.-host disease (GVHD).

that despite antiviral effect, there was no significant improvement in the clinical course [109]. van Burik *et al.* [110] has recently reported a median onset of CMV enteritis at day 91 post-HCT (range 17–527 days) and a 2-year overall survival rate in this population of 35%.

Other CMV-associated syndromes

Since approximately two-thirds of all at-risk transplant recipients develop CMV infection, the accurate association of other syndromes with this infection can be difficult. Nevertheless, in addition to mononucleosis-like syndrome with fever, arthralgia and malaise, both hepatitis and suppressed marrow function, including neutropenia and thrombocytopenia, have been associated with acute CMV infection [65]. The course of asymptomatic CMV infection is not well described in the allogeneic marrow graft recipient, but it appears that febrile episodes are a significant part of this infection. In order to understand the clinical effects of asymptomatic CMV infection, Zaia [77] evaluated consecutive patients with CMV infection during HCT and found a significant association of fever between days 42 and 56 in those with otherwise asymptomatic infection. There was no increased rate of neutropenia in this group. However, neutropenia is associated with CMV infection during this same time period; for example, in 66 patients examined by Meyers and Thomas [1], there was a fall in leukocyte and platelet count compared to the control group (59% vs. 36%, *p*-value nonsignificant). Boeckh *et al.* [65] documented a case of CMV-associated marrow suppression with response to therapy using a growth factor and an antiviral agent. In addition, pre-emptive ganciclovir has been used for treatment of marrow failure after marrow transplantation [111].

Complications of CMV therapy

The major complications associated with ganciclovir treatment are neutropenia and renal dysfunction. Neutropenia occurs in approximately 30% of patients and, based on the experience of Goodrich *et al.* [43], it lasts for a median of 12 days with an upper range of 74 days. Salzberger *et al.* [112] analyzed ganciclovir-associated neutropenia in 278 HCT recipients and noted that neutropenia occurred significantly more frequently when there was an elevated bilirubin level (≥ 6 mg/dL) during the first 20 days after HCT, or a serum creatinine level of 2 mg/dL or higher after day 21 of transplantation, or low marrow cellularity between days 21 and 28. Persons with one risk factor had a 21% incidence of neutropenia, but those with more factors had a 57% occurrence of neutropenia.

Of importance, this treatment-related neutropenia was an independent risk factor for overall survival (relative risk [RR] 3.8, $p = 0.001$), for event-free survival (RR 2.1, $p < 0.0001$) and for relapse (RR 1.7, $p = 0.03$) [112]. Therefore, in the event of ganciclovir-induced neutropenia, in addition to cessation of therapy or switching to foscarnet treatment, the use of granulocyte colony-stimulating factor (G-CSF) or granulocyte macrophage colony-stimulating factor (GM-CSF) is recommended. To minimize this problem, a stopping rule for ganciclovir use must be employed such as cessation of drug when the absolute neutrophil count (ANC) is lower than 1000/µL on 2 consecutive days.

Prevention of CMV infection after HCT

There are two general approaches to the prevention of CMV disease using either ganciclovir or foscarnet: (i) treatment of early blood-borne CMV infection prior to onset of disease and (ii) treatment of all at-risk patients for the defined period of risk. The first approach is a "pre-emptive" strategy and was first shown to be effective in the setting of HCT where the period of risk is well-defined [31,42]. With this method the requirement for accurate detection of CMV infection is the limiting feature, but the benefit is that fewer patients are exposed to the antiviral chemotherapy. The second approach, termed "general prophylaxis" is used when select patients can be defined as at particularly high risk for CMV infection, and all patients are treated for the period of risk. For both strategies, the risk of CMV disease governs the management, and this risk is determined by analysis for host-specific factors as discussed above.

Pre-emptive treatment strategy for prevention of CMV after HCT

Implementation of pre-emptive anti-CMV treatment

Patients should be monitored for CMV infection using one of several methods for detection of CMV [113]. Surveillance is started based on medical history, such that patients with a history of CMV infection in the past 6 months should have a preconditioning test and all others should begin at approximately 21 days post-HCT. Monitoring can be done using a variety of methods including CMV blood culture, CMV antigenemia assay, DNA-based assays, such as PCR and hybrid capture, and RNA-based assays (see the Diagnosis section, below) [32,34,46,51,114–120]. When less sensitive assays such as blood cultures are used, twice-weekly monitoring can be effective [46] but, in general, once weekly surveillance

Table 53.6 Cytomegalovirus (CMV) prophylaxis in hematopoietic cell transplantation (HCT) recipients.

I. Pre-emptive treatment
Treat all recipients with documented CMV infection in blood or lung; for PCR assays, require two positive results within a 3–7-day period, unless a highly sensitive assay is used (e.g. quantitative PCR) in which case, treatment might be based on a slight positive result

Induction therapy:
  Ganciclovir, 5 mg/kg IV b.i.d. for 7–14 days*†
  Foscarnet, 60 mg/kg IV b.i.d. for 7–14 days†‡

Maintenance therapy:
  Ganciclovir, 5 mg/kg IV q.d. 5–6 days/week, or 1 g p.o. t.i.d. (adults) or 30 mg/kg p.o. t.i.d. (children)
  Foscarnet, 60 mg/kg b.i.d. or 90 mg/kg q.d.*
  Duration of 2–5 weeks, on the basis of (a) time to significant reduction in immunosuppression (long course) or (b) time to return of CMV infection indicator to negative (short course)

II. General prophylaxis
Treat all HCT recipients at highest risk for CMV on the basis of immunosuppressive regimen using ganciclovir or foscarnet§

Dosage:
  Ganciclovir, 5 mg/kg b.i.d. for 7 days, then q.d. 5–6 days/week†
  Foscarnet 60 mg/kg b.i.d. for period of prophylaxis‡

Doses must be adjusted for renal insufficiency.
*If no maintenance therapy is used, the induction period continues until the CMV detection assay result becomes negative. Note that the CMV load can initially increase and treatment should continue until the CMV load is negative.
†When ganciclovir is not available, valganciclovir can be substituted.
‡Patients should be prehydrated with normal saline before foscarnet is provided and the Mg^{2+} and Ca^{2+} levels in serum should be maintained with appropriate supplements.
§Start therapy when the absolute neutrophil count is 750×10^9 neutrophils/L and stop therapy when the immunosuppression is significantly reduced or the absolute neutrophil count is $<1000 \times 10^9$ neutrophils/L for 2 consecutive days.
b.i.d., twice daily intradermal; PCR, polymerase chain reaction; p.o., *per os* (oral administration); t.i.d., three times daily intradermal; q.d., four times daily. Modified with permission from Zaia, CID 2002.

---

is preferred using the more sensitive antigenemia assay and the DNA-based assays [121]. Documented CMV blood infection should be pre-emptively treated starting with ganciclovir for at least 2–3 weeks [32,114] [115,116], and at most for 10 weeks [33,46,122]. With the availability of methods to measure CMV blood levels, the antiviral treatment is monitored to document the effect of treatment [47,123].

Routine dosing schedule

As shown in Table 53.6, ganciclovir is the drug of choice for pre-emptive treatment and is administered at an "induction" dose of 5 mg/kg twice daily for at least 7 days or until evidence of falling CMV load. CMV infection will clear in most patients within 2 weeks [32,33,124] but for those with stable or increasing CMV levels, the induction period should continue. Maintenance therapy consists of ganciclovir 5 mg/kg/day for 5–7 days/week for an additional period of time based on the patient's risk factors. For example, if the CMV levels are negative on two occasions, and the subject is not receiving corticosteroids or *in vivo* T-lymphocyte depletion, then maintenance can stop after 3–6 weeks. For patients on steroid or other secondary therapy for GVHD, treatment should continue for up to day 100 post-HCT. Monitoring should continue after treatment stops to observe for relapsed infection, which then requires additional treatment using the induction/maintenance regimen as before. Sporadic CMV positive surveillance can occur during maintenance and does not require additional treatment unless consecutive positive results are seen (see below; concern for antiviral T drug resistance).

After day 100 post-HCT, patients in the high-risk category are defined as those who just had a treated CMV blood infection, those receiving steroid therapy or other secondary therapy for GVHD and those with lymphopenia [70]. Although controlled experience with pre-emptive management does not exist with these patients, careful monitoring of CMV blood infection should continue with treatment as necessary.

Rules for stopping pre-emptive treatment and surveillance

Since the risk for ganciclovir toxicity is proportional to total drug exposure, it is important to treat pre-emptively only during the period of significant risk [125]. For patients for whom immunosuppressive therapy of GVHD is lessening and in whom there are at least 2 weeks of negative surveillance points for CMV in blood, pre-emptive ganciclovir can be stopped. The reconstitution of CMV-specific T-lymphocyte function has been shown to serve as a sign that the period of risk has ended [71,72]. Similarly, the risk for late CMV pneumonia has been linked to T-lymphocyte function [70]. For patients in the 2nd and 3rd months after HCT, for whom there are no major risk factors relating to GVHD and immunosuppressive therapy, pre-emptive management can be tentatively stopped. However, if secondary treatment for GVHD is required, and corticosteriod use is ≥1 mg/kg/day, the pre-emptive surveillance program should be reactivated.

Should a pre-emptive strategy be used for receipients of autologous HCT?

All CMV-seropositive recipients of HCT are at risk for CMV reactivation and, in the autologous HCT population, the rate of reactivation ranges from 25% to 45% with CMV disease occurring in 2–10% [49–52]. The risk of disease in this group appears to be related to immune reconstitution post-HCT [126]. Nevertheless, CMV disease occurs in some recipients of autologous HCT, and the risk factors in this population include prior amount of pre-HCT chemotherapy, treatment with corticosteroids after HCT and the use of $CD34^+$-selected peripheral blood progenitor cells [53,55]. Autologous HCT recipients with these risk factors should be managed with pre-emptive monitoring and early treatment with ganciclovir.

Should a pre-emptive strategy be used for recipients of nonmyeloablative regimens?

Although there are several methods for nonmyeloablative conditioning of allogeneic HCT, the risk for CMV-associated disease in these patients does not appear to be any less than for more routine allogeneic recipients [48]. In addition, if the graph is manipulated, there may be an increased risk for CMV infections [53,118]. Hence, recipients of nonmyeloablative regimens should receive pre-emptive monitoring of and early treatment for CMV infection [113].

Concern for antiviral drug resistance

Breakthrough CMV infection while on seemingly adequate therapy can be a difficult clinical problem. Boeckh *et al.* [124] documented that ganciclovir therapy used at engraftment results in breakthrough CMV-positive blood in 50% of patients monitored by antigenemia and in 66% of those followed by PCR. For this reason, two positive assays should be documented before treating relapsed infection and, using this rule, studies have shown that approximately 15–25% of patients treated pre-emptively with ganciclovir or foscarnet will require retreatment

[32,114,116]. Rising CMV DNA levels are probably the best laboratory criteria for assessing potential antiviral drug resistance. In patients already receiving ganciclovir, therapy should be switched to foscarnet in the following situations: (i) whenever there is marrow toxicity and the CMV assays remain persistently positive or show rising CMV blood load; (ii) when persistent infection is present at the time of increased treatment of GVHD with corticosteroids or other secondary anti-GVHD drugs; and (iii) when there are changing clinical symptoms suggestive of CMV disease.

General prophylactic anti-CMV treatment

Implementation of general prophylaxis

Not all HCT recipients will do well with pre-emptive anti-CMV management, especially those at the highest risk for CMV infection [127]. The alternative approach to prevention of CMV in high-risk patients is to treat all patients with ganciclovir, usually at the time of engraftment [33,43,128,129]. Atkinson et al. [128] assessed the early routine use of ganciclovir in a nonrandomized study in which ganciclovir was given at a dose of 5 mg/kg IV twice daily from day −8 to −1 pre-HCT and resumed when the ANC equaled 1,000/μL at 5 mg/kg IV three times/week until day 84 post-HCT. This regimen was found to eliminate the early occurrence of CMV-IP. Subsequently, in a randomized, placebo-controlled trial, Goodrich et al. [43] studied the effect of ganciclovir given at a dose of 5 mg/kg IV twice daily for 5 days and then every day until day 100 after HCT in patients who were CMV seropositive at the time of engraftment. This method significantly reduced CMV excretion (3% vs. 45%, $p = 0.0001$) and CMV-associated disease (10% vs. 29%, $p = 0.0008$). CMV-IP and CMV gastroenteritis occurred only in those receiving placebo or in those no longer receiving ganciclovir. Subsequent CMV disease occurred in 10% of the treated group after cessation of therapy at day 100. There was no difference between control and treated groups in terms of mortality, either during treatment (19% vs. 12%, respectively, $p = 0.4$) or at day 180 (26% vs. 30%, respectively, = n.s.). This lack of effect of ganciclovir treatment on mortality is different from the effect observed with pre-emptive use of ganciclovir [32,42]. The prophylactic treatment was marrow toxic and resulted in some neutropenia-associated complications. Finally, in a study by Winston et al. [129], in which ganciclovir was given at a dose of 2.5 mg/kg IV every 8 h from day −8 to −1 before HCT and was resumed when the ANC was above 1×10^9/L at 6 mg/kg given 5 days/week until day 120 after HCT, the group receiving ganciclovir had a significant reduction in the rate of CMV infection (20% vs. 56%, $p = 0.009$) but no significant reduction of CMV disease (10% vs. 24%, $p = 0.09$).

Problem of universal therapy with ganciclovir

Prophylactic ganciclovir used in all at-risk HCT recipients has effectively reduced CMV infection but has not been unequivocally associated with a beneficial outcome [33,43]. Not all CMV-seropositive HCT recipients will develop progressive CMV infection during the course of transplantation, but all recipients receiving ganciclovir are at risk for the toxic side-effects of the drug. The exposure to marrow suppression in the more-than 70% of patients who do not develop CMV disease defeats the purpose of the therapy, and this problem is unavoidable with the universal-use strategy. Ganciclovir-associated neutropenia has been reported in 30–60% of HCT recipients [42,112], creating a new risk for infection to substitute for the risk of CMV infection. Drug-related neutropenia occurs at a significant rate compared to a nontreated group (30% vs. 0%, $p = 0.0014$), and the median duration of neutropenia is 12 days (range: 4–20 days) [112]. Patients on ganciclovir who became neutropenic had a significantly increased risk of bacterial infection, and there was one septic death in this group. Furthermore, the cost of treating all allogeneic marrow transplant recipients in this way is not inconsiderable. Therefore, because of the toxicity of these agents and their expense, general use of ganciclovir in all CMV-seropositive persons is currently not recommended [125].

Risk-adapted prophylaxis

Verdonck et al. [130] were the first to recognize that certain HCT recipients were at such high risk for CMV that a short course of prophylactic ganciclovir would probably be safer than pre-emptive therapy. They have used a risk-adapted strategy in which patients with GVHD requiring increased steroid therapy were given a 2-week course of ganciclovir. Other patients in this study were followed with antigenemia assays and treated pre-emptively. This approach was used in 41 patients; half of the patients never received ganciclovir and, of those treated, 26% required a second 2-week course. Using this approach, there was no CMV disease and no neutropenia [130]. In general, HCT recipients of grafts from matched-unrelated donors fare well with pre-emptive anti-CMV management. But if T-cell depletion plus antithymocyte globulin is used for matched-unrelated or haploidentical HCT, then anti-CMV chemotherapy should be initiated early after HCT. Similarly, if the risk for CMV disease increases in the course of any allogeneic HCT, the method of risk-adapted general prophylaxis can be adopted. In such patients, subsequent routine surveillance for CMV is not necessary and CMV diagnostic assays should be based on clinical issues [125].

Other considerations in prevention of CMV infection and disease after HCT

Which clinical specimen should be used for CMV monitoring?

CMV detection in blood is considered the preferred specimen for detection of CMV because the predictive value of a positive result is high [37]. BAL is a site of early reactivation of CMV, and was used in the initial demonstration of the effectiveness of pre-emptive therapy [31]. But it has been demonstrated that the positive predictive value of results from BAL are no better than from blood specimens [131–133] and that monitoring of blood for CMV is better that using BAL [134,135].

The initial studies of pre-emptive management are informative in regards to understanding the importance of choice of clinical specimen. When Schmidt et al. [31] used asymptomatic pulmonary CMV infection as the determinant for use of ganciclovir, the purpose of this study was to determine if ganciclovir could prevent the development of CMV-IP after virus reactivation had already occurred in the lung [31]. Allogeneic HCT recipients were randomly assigned to receive ganciclovir after routine CMV-positive BAL day 35 after HCT, and study subjects were free of pulmonary symptoms and had normal chest X-ray findings at the time of BAL. Of the 104 patients enrolled in this study, 40 (39%) were found to have asymptomatic pulmonary CMV infection as judged by CMV culture from BAL specimens, and 20 patients were randomized to receive ganciclovir therapy and 20 were randomized to receive no treatment. The occurrence of either CMV-IP or death was significantly reduced in the ganciclovir-treated group (25% vs. 70%, $p = 0.01$) (Fig. 53.7a). No patients who completed the full course of induction and maintenance therapy with ganciclovir developed CMV-IP, yet among those patients who had negative BAL findings on day 35, 12 (21%) out of 55 subsequently developed CMV pneumonia. The antiviral effects of this regimen are shown in Fig. 53.7b. Among the 40 BAL positive specimens obtained on day 35, 38 were positive as determined by the rapid centrifugal culture method and two were positive by the cytological method and subsequently confirmed by conventional culture. Among the treated subjects, 33% remained CMV positive at repeat BAL 14 days after ganciclovir was started. All untreated CMV-positive individuals remained positive at repeat BAL on day 49. Interestingly, 52% of those who were CMV

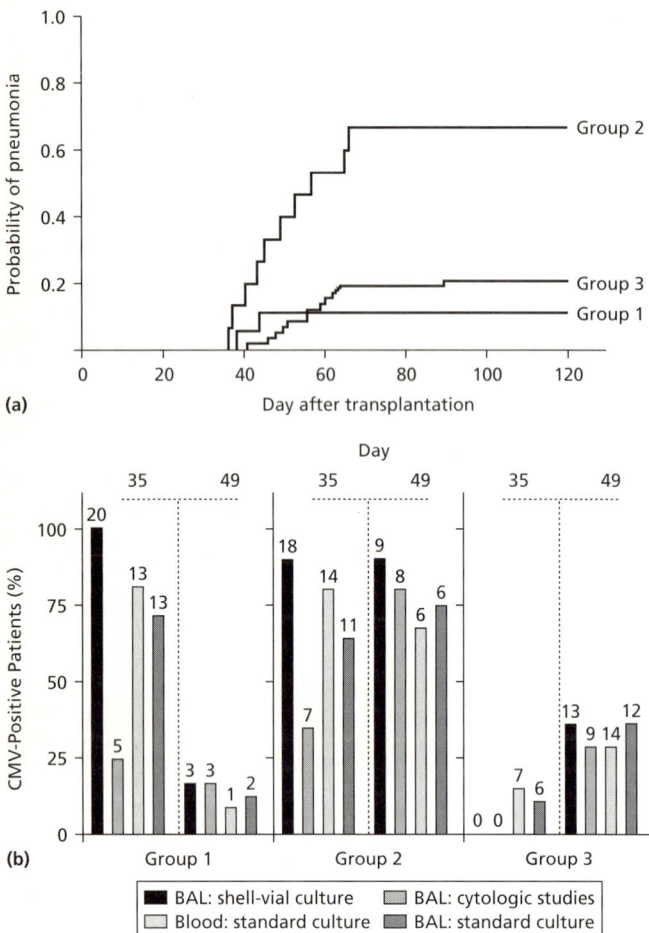

Fig. 53.7 Effects of pre-emptive therapy for prevention of cytomegalovirus (CMV) disease. (a) Kaplan–Meier product-limit estimates of the probability of cytomegalovirus-associated interstitial pneumonia (CMV-IP) in subjects with asymptomatic CMV lung infection on day 35 after HCT, treated with ganciclovir (group 1) or no ganciclovir (group 2), or with no detectable CMV lung infection on day 35 after hematopoietic cell transplantation (HCT) (group 3). (b) Results of CMV cultures and cytological studies of specimens obtained on days 35 and 49 according to study group. Inset legend refers to methods used to detect CMV in blood or bronchoalveolar lavage (BAL) specimens. Reproduced with permission from Schmidt et al. [31].

negative at BAL on day 35 were positive at BAL on day 49, suggesting that infection, when it occurred in this group, was progressing at a different time course than in the other group.

In an early method for pre-emptive therapy, Goodrich et al. [42] treated allogeneic HCT recipients with ganciclovir at the time of first CMV infection as monitored in weekly cultures of throat, urine and blood. Based on positive cultures, patients were randomly assigned to treatment with placebo or ganciclovir. Ganciclovir treatment significantly reduced the occurrence of CMV-associated disease (3% vs. 43%, $p < 0.00001$) and had a profound effect on mortality (2.7% vs. 17%, $p = 0.041$). As with the BAL-based study, 12% of subjects developed CMV-associated disease because detection of CMV culture occurred either prior to or simultaneously with the development of clinical signs and symptoms. In this study, throat infection was less reliable than blood, and urine was nonpredictive of subsequent disease [42].

What is the optimal assay for detecting CMV?

Pre-emptive management strategy places a burden on the transplant team to detect CMV infection before progression to overt disease, and clearly the window of opportunity for such early treatment varies with the sensitivity of the assay. There are two general types of assays for detection of CMV: replication/antigen assays and DNA/RNA assays (see the Diagnosis section, below). The tissue culture assay for CMV, called the "shell vial" assay [136], and the detection of a CMV antigen called "CMVpp65," rely on CMV replication and become positive at a median time of 42 days after HCT [124]. Since CMV-IP occurs at a median time of 50–60 days post-HCT, the use of these assays present a small margin of safety for negative assays. Nevertheless, these assays are easy to perform, are relatively inexpensive and have been associated with successful patient management [46,122]. With the development of DNA/RNA-based methods of CMV detection, detection in blood can be made at approximately 35 days post-HCT [32,120,137]. Thus, the DNA/RNA-based assays widen the opportunity for early treatment by 1 week. Although this seems small, Einsele et al. [32] demonstrated that this was sufficient to significantly reduce CMV disease and overall mortality. As important, the quantitative aspects of these tests allow them to be useful for monitoring the response to treatment [47,123,138].

What is the role of acyclovir and related agents in pre-emptive strategies?

Acyclovir is not a first-line agent for prevention of CMV infection, but it does have an important role in the management of the HCT patient. Initial attempts to suppress the reactivation of CMV infection in transplant recipients used either oral or intravenous acyclovir [44,139,140]. Both an oral regimen in renal transplant recipients, using a dose of 800 mg given four times daily, and an intravenous regimen in HCT recipients, using a dose of 500 mg/m^2 given three times daily, significantly reduced CMV reactivation and disease. Since the mean 50% inhibitory dose of acyclovir for CMV strains is 63.1 ± 30.2 μM [141] and, since peak acyclovir levels in the plasma with these regimens can be expected to range from 25 to 100 μM, it is not surprising that acyclovir had some ability to modify CMV infection. However, of interest, the prophylactic administration of acyclovir in allogeneic HCT recipients and in renal allograft recipients significantly lowered patient mortality [44,139,140]. In the study from Meyers et al. [44], although the incidence of active CMV infection in HCT recipients dropped from 75% in the control patients to 59% in the acyclovir-treated group, the overall probability of CMV reactivation remained high in both groups (0.70 in the acyclovir-treated group vs. 0.87 in the control group). Nevertheless, there was a reduction in the infection-associated clinical syndromes, such as CMV-IP and CMV enteritis, and a significant reduction in mortality in the treated group (54% vs. 29%, respectively, $p < 0.01$). In addition, there were fewer deaths associated with any infectious cause in the acyclovir group (45% vs. 22%, respectively, $p < 0.01$). Of note, when acyclovir was used in the same dose and at the same institution but in autologous marrow recipients, there was no significant effect on CMV infection or disease compared to a control group [142].

A most interesting result of acyclovir prophylaxis was reported by the European Group for Blood and Marrow Transplantation (EBMT) [143,144]. Recipients of matched-related or unrelated HCT were randomly assigned to receive: (i) acyclovir (500 mg/m^2 IV three times daily) from day –5 to day 30 post-HCT and then oral acyclovir (800 mg four times daily) for 6 months; (ii) the same intravenous dose of acyclovir followed by an oral placebo for 6 months; or (iii) a standard herpes simplex prevention regimen (400 mg orally four times a day) for 30 days followed by an oral placebo for 6 months. The use of high-dose acyclovir (groups 1 and 2) was associated with reduced CMV infection compared with group 3. The occurrence of procedure-related morbidity, including CMV disease, was the same for all groups, but there was a 19% survival advantage at 3 months and at 1 year in the group with long-term acyclovir use [143,144]. This result suggests that either CMV infection or some other virus or viruses influence fatal complications without recognizable overt viral disease. The use of short-term high-dose acyclovir as a supplement to ganciclovir preventive treatment had no such outcome advantage [145].

Valacyclovir has been used for primary CMV prophylaxis or for suppressive anti-CMV therapy after ganciclovir induction therapy in recent studies [146,147]. In the randomized, double-blinded study of Ljungman et al. [147], in which 748 patients received acyclovir 500 mg/m^2 IV three times daily for the initial 28 days post-HCT and then either oral valacyclovir 2 g four times daily or acyclovir 800 mg four times daily until 18 weeks post-HCT, valacyclovir was significantly more effective in suppressing CMV reactivation (28% vs. 40%, respectively, $p <0.0001$). In this study, pre-emptive ganciclovir or foscarnet was used for CMV blood infection, and there were fewer patients with infections that initiated anti-CMV treatment in the valacyclovir group compared with the acyclovir group (23% vs. 37%, respectively) and significantly more time to onset of indicator infection in the valacyclovir group. If cost-effectiveness studies and other studies of outcome can confirm the benefit of supplementing pre-emptive strategies with valacyclovir, it is possible that valacyclovir will eventually have a role in the prevention of CMV infection in the HCT recipient.

How is foscarnet used in the HCT patient?

Foscarnet is a phosphonate that requires no metabolism for activity and, because of its excellent antiviral profile, has become an important agent in the treatment of CMV infection in the immunosuppressed population [114–117,148–150]. Initial experiences with this agent indicated that nephrotoxicity, hypocalcemia and hypophosphatemia were significant problems [149,150]. The importance of hydration has been emphasized [148], and safe use of foscarnet has been demonstrated in the HCT population [114,115–117]. Bacigalupo et al. [114] first showed that foscarnet could be used in place of ganciclovir for pre-emptive management of CMV after marrow transplantation. In this study, if the white blood count was <2500/μL, foscarnet was used at a dose of 90 mg/kg IV twice daily. This group further showed that for recipients at high risk for CMV disease, foscarnet and ganciclovir could be used in combination [115], at the same doses as before [114], and with maintenance therapy for an additional 2 weeks if needed, by alternating each drug every other day. The transplant-related mortality was significantly reduced compared to a historical control group treated with only one agent (0.13 vs. 0.47, $p = 0.02$).

Ljungman et al. [116] showed that for PCR-based pre-emptive therapy, foscarnet effectively prevents CMV disease when used at 60 mg/kg twice daily for 14 days. Thus, foscarnet appears to have a role in the pre-emptive management of the transplant recipient. However, the choice of foscarnet is often difficult in patients receiving other nephrotoxic agents after HCT and, for this reason, ganciclovir is usually started when CMV infection occurs. Ippoliti et al. [117] reported that for persons unable to continue on ganciclovir, foscarnet can be successfully substituted for continued pre-emptive therapy.

What is the role of oral formulations of ganciclovir?

Orally administered ganciclovir (1000 mg three times daily; pediatric dosage, 30 mg/kg three times daily) is poorly absorbed but achieves levels that are sufficient to suppress CMV infection [151,152]. Use of oral ganciclovir during the maintenance phase of pre-emptive treatment has been successful, with no change in the marrow-suppressive toxicity of the drug. Valganciclovir has more bioavailability and, based on the experience in liver transplant recipients, an oral dose of 900 mg can result in a blood level of drug exposure (area-under-the-curve) similar to an intravenous dose of 5 mg/kg ganciclovir. Neither oral ganciclovir nor valganciclovir have an approved indication in HCT recipients, but studies are actively exploring the role of these agents in the treatment and prevention of CMV.

When should cidofovir be used in the HCT recipient?

Cidofovir has been used for the pre-emptive management of the HCT patient [153]. The dosage for cidofovir is 5 mg/kg per dose in two doses given 1 week apart, followed by maintenance therapy provided every other week. The drug is given with probenecid and adequate preinfusion hydration. Cidofovir is not approved for the prevention of CMV infection in the HCT recipient. It is nephrotoxic, and its use in this setting is as a second-line agent when pre-emptive use of ganciclovir or foscarnet has failed.

Prevention of CMV using selected blood products

As described, CMV infection arises either from exogenous introduction of virus via blood elements and transplanted tissue or from reactivation of endogenous virus. Persons who have had CMV infection prior to HCT form the group at risk for most problems relating to CMV after HCT (Table 53.3). The seronegative transplant recipient is at much lower risk for serious infection so long as exposure to exogenous sources of infection can be minimized. Meyers et al. [154] and Bowden et al. [40], have provided convincing evidence that granulocytes are a major source of exogenous CMV after HCT. Several other studies [9,155] suggest that exposure to CMV after HCT arises by contact with random blood products.

For this reason, CMV-seronegative HCT recipients of stem cells from seronegative donors need to be protected from potentially infectious blood products. The controlled comparisons of selected blood support for prevention of CMV infection in CMV-seronegative marrow allograft recipients is summarized in Table 53.7. Bowden et al. [40] initially studied this issue and the use of Ig to prevent CMV infection. Passive immunization did not reduce infection, but the use of CMV-seronegative blood donor support significantly reduced both CMV infection and CMV disease. Subsequently, Bowden et al. [27] performed a randomized controlled trial comparing the use of leukocyte-depleted platelets plus CMV seronegative red blood cells with standard unscreened blood products for the prevention of primary CMV infection during the first 100 days after autologous HCT. In this study, platelets were depleted of leukocytes by centrifugation, and blood products were screened for CMV seronegativity

Table 53.7 Prevention of cytomegalovirus (CMV) using CMV-seronegative blood support.*

Reference	Selected blood (%)	Standard blood (%)	p-value
Bowden et al. 1986 [40]†	1/32 (3)	8/25 (32)	<0.007
Bowden et al. 1991 [27]‡	0/35 (0)	7/30 (23)	0.0013
Miller et al. 1991 [28]§,¶	8/64 (13)	21/61 (34)	0.002
HCT donor –	(6)	(37)	0.0006
HCT donor +	(62)	(42)	0.8

*Unless noted, marrow allograft recipients were CMV-seronegative and had a CMV-seronegative marrow donor.
†Combines groups receiving selected seronegative blood or no screened blood with groups receiving or not receiving CMV immunoglobulin.
‡Blood product selection used CMV-seronegative donors of red blood cells (RBCs) and leukocyte-depleted RBCs and platelets.
§Blood product selection used CMV-seronegative donors of blood products; marrow donor CMV-serologic status is indicated as negative (–) or positive (+).
¶Number of CMV-seronegative and -seropositive HCT donors was not provided in source material.
HCT, hematopoietic cell transplantation.

by latex agglutination assay and enzyme immunoassay. The probability of developing CMV infection was significantly greater in patients receiving standard unscreened blood products (0% vs. 23%, $p = 0.0013$), with no infection occurring in the 35 patients who received the leukocyte-poor platelets and the screened CMV-seronegative red blood cells. Miller et al. [28] confirmed the effectiveness of screened CMV seronegative blood products in a randomized trial in 125 patients. Among the subjects receiving marrow grafts from CMV-seronegative donors, CMV infections were significantly reduced in those receiving screened blood products (6% vs. 37%, $p = 0.0006$).

Use of filtered blood products has been shown to reduce the risk of CMV transmission and is now in general use for support of the HCT recipient [156–158]. In a study of Bowden et al. [156], a comparison of CMV-seronegative screened vs. filtered blood products showed no significant differences between the probability of CMV infection (1.3% vs. 2.4%, respectively, $p = 1.00$), disease (0% vs. 2.4%, respectively, $p = 1.00$), or survival. The rate of CMV infection after blood product filtration was approximately 2.5% in both the study of Bowden et al. [156] and of Narvios et al. [158], and explains the persistently low risk of CMV infection even in the D−/R− HCT recipient. Of note, in the study of Miller et al. [28], blood product screening did not effectively reduce the CMV infection rates in the groups receiving unscreened vs. screened products if the marrow donor was seropositive (62% vs. 42%, respectively, $p = 0.8$), and exposure to CMV infection from any blood source, either seropositive donor or unscreened blood products, resulted in statistically similar infection rates (62% vs. 38%, $p = 0.5$). Thus, the use of screened seronegative donor blood support is usually limited to those who are seronegative at the time of transplantation and are receiving grafts from seronegative donors.

Immune response to CMV infection

Cellular immunity to CMV

Cytotoxic T lymphocyte (CTL) function is most critical for protection from severe disease and mortality in the setting of HCT. Meyers et al. [159] recognized that CMV-specific cellular immunity was suppressed in marrow recipients with CMV infection. Quinnan and colleagues initially demonstrated that CMV-specific, HLA-restricted CTL function was associated with survival from CMV-IP in this patient population [160,161]. Subsequently, Reusser et al. [162] confirmed the role of virus-specific CTLs in an analysis of allograft recipients with and without CMV-IP. Ljungman et al. [163] and Krause et al. [72] demonstrated that patients lacking CD4-specific CMV recognition were at higher risk for CMV complications.

Borysiewicz et al. [164] first described the role of specific CMV proteins in the induction of CTL function in humans. They demonstrated that nonvirion, IE proteins of CMV as well as the virion envelope glycoprotein, CMVgB, could induce CTL immunity [164]. The most important targets of the cellular immune responses are the internal matrix proteins, especially CMVpp65 [165–170] and the 72 kDa IE protein (IE72) [171–175]. More recent studies suggest that 75% of all CMV-specific CTL clones recognize either CMVpp65 or CMV-IE72 [173,175,176]. Importantly, both of these proteins can be present early in virus infection and in the absence of active virus replication [167]. Thus, the persistence of viral antigens, in the absence of continued viral replication, could serve as a stimulus for cellular-mediated immunity in the human host. In fact, oligoclonal expansion of these CMV-specific CTLs occurs to remarkably high proportions of total CD8+ lymphocytes [177–179], and this oligoclonal expansion over a life-time has been suggested to have potential negative effects, presumably on immune function, late in life, possibly with an effect on longevity [180–182].

A major advance in the understanding of the response to CMV by CD8+ lymphocytes has been the elucidation of HLA allele-specific peptide epitopes of CMVpp65 and CMV-IE72 [169,170,172,175,176,183]. The specific CMVpp65 peptide recognized by some HLA allele-specific CTL clones has been defined [169,170]. Analysis of T-cell receptor (TCR) usage among such peptide-responsive clones indicates that the CTL function is focused in a very narrow range of $V\beta$ TCR-bearing cells, suggesting that it should be possible to elucidate a limited number of peptide epitopes to cover the HLA-specificities in humans [183].

By linking these peptide epitopes to recombinant fluorescence-labeled human HLA molecules, the fine specificity of the immune response can be measured by fluorescence activated cell sorter (FACS) [178]. Cwynarski et al. [184] first applied this technology to HCT recipients and demonstrated that expansion of CD8+ lymphocytes occurs and suggested that those with at least 10^7 CMV specific CD8+ cells/L appeared to be protected from CMV disease. Gratama et al. [185] have reported that after T-cell-depleted HCT, CMV disease occurred only in those with no FACS-detectable CMV-specific CD8+ lymphocytes. Lacey et al. [186] have demonstrated that the CMV-specific CD8+ cell expansions can occur prior to day 40 post-HCT and reach levels as high as 25% of total CD8+ cells. Based on analysis of two donor–recipient pairs, these cells represented clonal expansions and were derived from the donor [186]. It appears that such responses are induced in HCT recipients only after CMV reactivation, and it remains to be shown how an epitope-based FACS assay would assist in management decisions. Nevertheless, this immunologic analysis of the cellular immune response to CMV after HCT should help to define the population that has reconstituted its immune response and is protected from further CMV complications.

CMV-mediated escape from immune surveillance

Down-regulation of HLA class I expression

HLA class I consists of a membrane-anchored heavy chain that is non-covalently associated with a secretory protein called β_2-microglobulin [187]. The HLA class I molecule binds short peptides derived from host proteins or from pathogens and presents these to CD8+ T cells (reviewed in [188]). These peptides usually derive from proteolytic processes in the cytosol, and formation of stable class I complexes with these peptides occurs in the ER [189]. From the ER, these complexes are transported to the Golgi membranes and then to the cell surface [190]. Thus, there is a series of interactive mechanisms involving chaperone proteins and the transporter associated with antigen processing (TAP) that facilitates the process by which peptide antigen is displayed to the immune system in the context of specific HLA alleles.

Viruses have evolved strategies that reduce class I expression in an effort to escape the immune system. Several groups [191–193] have showed an increased turnover of major histocompatibility complex (MHC) class I heavy-chain complexes after CMV infection. In these infected cells, class I HLA heavy chains undergo rapid turnover within the ER and do not become expressed on the surface of the cell. Jones et al. [18,194], using deletion mutants of CMV, identified three early viral genes (U_S2, U_S3, and U_S11), whose gene products were associated with increased turnover of class I HLA heavy chains. Wiertz et al. [195] showed that this is due to a dislocation of the HLA molecule from the ER into the proteosome. The gene products of U_S2 can also influence class II HLA processing [196]. Thus, there are at least three *CMV* genes that are active after infection that appear to protect the infected cell from immune recognition and cytotoxic attack [197,198].

Inhibition of HLA-dependent mechanisms

The essential transport of antigen from the cytosol to the ER via the TAP system and from there to the cell surface is critical to MHC-restricted cellular events [188]. CMV inhibits this TAP system, thus blocking the translocation of peptides into the ER lumen [199]. Lehner et al. [200] showed that this inhibition is associated with the protein product of CMV US6, a 22-kDa glycoprotein that binds the TAP complex and inhibits peptide translocation from the cytosol to the ER. US6 closely resembles the herpes simplex virus-encoded ICP47 protein, which also binds TAP and inhibits peptide transport [201]. US6 contains an ER retention signal in its C-terminal cytoplasmic domain, which is thought to account for this inhibitory function [200].

In the 1980s, it was noted that the CMV genome encodes polypeptide sequences with molecular mimicry to HLA class I and class II peptides [202,203]. Grundy et al. [204] reported that CMV infection *in vitro* could be neutralized using β_2-microglobulin, a protein component of class I HLA antigens. It was conjectured that CMV could influence immune function either by binding to HLA molecules or by inducing differences in HLA and preventing cell-to-cell interactions necessary for either CTL induction or for natural killer (NK) cell binding. CMVgpU_L18 has homology to HLA class I and is expressed late in infection, presumably at a time when NK killing could be important [205]. CMVgpU_L18 binds to a subclass of NK cells that have a leukocyte Ig-like receptor [206]. Nevertheless, at present there is mixed evidence regarding the role played by CMVgpU_L18 in protection from NK cell killing [207,208]. CMV also encodes a surface glycoprotein, CMVgpU_L40, which serves as a negative signal for NK recognition. CMVgpU_L40 inhibits NK cells by mimicking class I HLA-E [209–211]. HLA-E inhibits NK cell killing by interaction of its signal peptide with the NK cell receptor. CMVgpU_L40 encodes a peptide that is identical to this ligand, thereby serving as a negative signal for NK cells [210].

Thus, CMV encodes intriguing mechanisms of immune escape [212]. One strategy down-regulates the class I HLA process required for functional CD8$^+$ cell response, leaving NK killing as a significant concern. The other strategy alters the ability of NK cells to recognize and kill. It has been suggested that the multiplicity of HLA-based immune escape mechanisms developed by CMV may have been necessary because of the heterogeneity of the HLA system [213]. In turn, this heterogeneity might be necessary in order to prevent any single virus mechanism from shutting off the antigen presentation by class I alleles.

Humoral immunity to CMV

Despite the many potential polypeptides encoded in the CMV genome, only a small number of proteins and glycoproteins are known to be recognized by the immune system. Neutralizing antibody is directed towards the surface glycoproteins, principally the gB and gH herpesvirus homologues (Fig. 53.2). In nature, the discrete glycoproteins noted in Fig. 53.2 exist as molecular complexes, gcI, consisting of gB, gcII, consisting of gM and gN, and gcIII, consisting of gH, gL and gO [214,215]. Using synthetic peptides, investigators have defined the humoral response to CMV [216]. In marrow recipients, the humoral immune response to CMV has been described and is the same as that observed in normal persons with predominant antibody responses to gB, gH, CMVpp65 and the capsid proteins [217]. In the HCT allograft recipient with prior CMV infection, there is no clear evidence that CMV-specific antibody protects from severe disease, although specific antibody production might well serve as a marker for overall immune responsiveness to this infection.

In the earliest experience with CMV-IP in HCT, the most serious occurrence of disease was seen in those having minimal antibody response to CMV [35]. Subsequent studies of pretransplantation CMV antibody levels did not substantiate a protective effect [9,37]. In the analysis of polypeptide-specific CMV antibody responses in marrow allograft recipients with and without CMV-IP, Zaia et al. [217] reported a variable response in patients and no clear correlation between range of protein-specific antibody response and outcome. Thus, although CMV antibody might play some role in the control of CMV infection, it has not been found to be essential for recovery.

The use of Ig in HCT

Overview

One of the most controversial areas in the management of the transplant patient in regards to CMV infection is the use of passive immunization with IVIg [218,219]. In solid organ transplantation, in which CMVIg is an approved product, there is convincing evidence for a protective effect but without improved survival [220]. In the HCT recipient, because early experience [35] showed that favorable outcome was associated with elevated CMV antibody, the use of standard IVIg was evaluated in many centers. These passive immunization studies utilized either conventional IVIg or CMVIg [221]. In general, this method decreased the incidence of CMV infection compared to control, but the effect on CMV-associated disease was variable, with no effect seen in some studies. Recently, a controlled use of passive immunization with a monoclonal antibody (MSL-109) to CMVgH failed to protect CMV seropositive recipients from CMV reactivation, ganciclovir exposure, GVHD, or bacterial and fungal infections [222]. Of interest, the D$^+$/R$^-$ patients, a group known to be at higher risk for poor survival due to bacterial and fungal infections compared to D$^-$/R$^-$ recipients [38], had improved survival at 100 days post-HCT if treated with the MSL-109 antibody. This improved survival effect was lost at 1-year post-HCT [222]. In summary, at present there is no general recommendation to use Igs to protect HCT recipients from CMV [223]. If there were a group that might benefit from passive immunization with such antibody, it would be the D$^+$/R$^-$ patient.

Adoptive cellular immunotherapy and/or active vaccination for CMV

Adoptive cellular immunotherapy (for details see Chapter 29), utilizing CTLs that are reactive to specific CMV proteins, is feasible for protection of marrow allograft recipients [224,225]. In this approach, donor CD8$^+$ class I MHC-restricted CMV-specific CTLs are cloned, expanded in the presence of CMV antigens plus interleukin 2 (IL-2) and administered to the HCT recipient. The safety of this form of passive immunization has been demonstrated [225] and phase 2 efficacy studies are currently under investigation. Lucas et al. [226] and Kondo et al. [227] have reported on the production of antigen-presenting autologous B cells using retroviral vectors as a means of deriving polyclonal T cells. Einsele et al. [228] have reported on the use of polyclonal T-lymphocyte infusions late after HCT to treat recipients that have failed antiviral therapy. Recently it has been shown that by FACS CMV-specific T lymphocytes can be efficiently isolated and expanded *in vitro* [229] and that artificial surfaces can be used to support efficient T cell growth *in vitro* [230], illustrating that improved technology promises to make cellular therapy more practical. Thus, adoptive cellular immunotherapy offers an exciting new potential preventive approach to CMV management.

This method suggests an alternative approach, namely, the stimulation of CMV immunity in the donor and transfer of precursor CTLs to the recipient. Boland et al. [231] reported that some component of donor immunity to CMV is transferred to the recipient. In this study, among CMV seropositive allograft recipients, those receiving marrow from CMV-seropositive donors had an earlier lymphocyte proliferative response to CMV than did those with seronegative marrow donors. Lacey et al. [186] have shown that the CMV-specific CTLs, that respond early after HCT, derive from the donor. In this regard, several types of CMV vaccines have been suggested [170,232–235], including subunit peptide vaccines [170,233], nucleotide-based vaccines [236] and live recombinant viral vaccines [235]. Purified CMV glycoproteins, CMVgA and gB, have even been used in human volunteers to induce humoral and cellular immune responses [233]. As noted, there is evidence that peptide epitopes can be elucidated and used to induce CMV-specific CTLs [170]. Also, naked DNA encoding CMVpp65 can induce immunity in mice after direct injection [236]. Thus, although the method for optimal induction of protective CMV immunity is not yet known, it is currently recognized that the principal risk for CMV disease after HCT is the absence of virus-specific CTL function. Passive or active immunization is likely to provide the essential method that could further improve the management of the HCT recipient in regard to CMV disease prevention.

Diagnosis

Overview of the methods of detection of CMV

The methods for surveillance of CMV in the setting of HCV have been recently reviewed [121]. There are two general categories of CMV diagnostic assays: (i) those that depend on virus infection in tissue culture for a positive endpoint and (ii) the molecular methods that require virus protein, RNA, or DNA without a need for *in vitro* infection. The detection of infectious CMV involves observation of the cytopathogenic effects in tissue culture or in tissue specimens, and the interested reader is referred to technological references that describe the methodology for culturing CMV from clinical specimens [237]. Briefly, the CMV-IE72 protein is used as a marker for infection, since it is present within hours of culture and even in the absence of permissive virus replication. With this approach, as shown in Fig. 53.8, the rapid centrifugal culture method, originally using "shell vials," remains a simple and valuable diagnostic test for CMV infection [136,238,239]. As applied in many laboratories today, assays are performed in microtiter plates, permitting efficient processing of multiple specimens. Conventional long-term (2–4-week) culture in human fibroblast monolayer tissue culture is used as a "backup" for this test, and of these two assays, the shell vial test is usually preferred because of rapid result [240]. However, the molecular detection assays are more sensitive and, since the purpose of surveillance is the early detection and treatment of CMV reactivation, these tests have generally replaced the tissue culture assays. These tests include the antigenemia assay, the CMV DNA-based assays, and a CMV RNA-based assay [241].

Molecular methods of detection

The antigenemia assay

As indicated, virus isolation takes considerable time and can produce significant delay in diagnosis. Therefore, supplemental assays are now used to directly detect viral antigens or DNA in clinical specimens and provide more rapid methods for detection of CMV. It is recognized from *in vitro* studies that within 2 h after CMV infection, an early/late matrix protein CMVpp65 is present in the nuclei of infected cells [22]. CMVpp65 is nucleotropic and enters the cell as part of the infecting virion. Detection of this antigen in granulocytic nuclei is used to document early CMV dissemination in immunocompromised patients (Fig. 53.9). This CMV antigenemia method, first described by van der Bij *et al.* [242], utilizes monoclonal antibody staining of peripheral blood leukocytes. The initial reports of this method referred to this antigen as an IE protein, implying that it detected infection prior to the onset of permissive virus infection. However, it was later recognized that the monoclonal antisera used in this assay recognized CMVpp65 [243]. The presence of this antigen in leukocytes means that the phagocytes either ingested viral particles or were actually infected by the virus. Gerna *et al.* [244] studied the presence of both CMVpp65 and CMV-IE72 in both polymorphonuclear leukocytes and monocyte/macrophages in an immunocompromised population, composed mainly of heart transplant recipients, and noted that 73% of CMVpp65-positive leukocytes expressed CMV-IE with evidence of CMV-IE72-specific RNA in most cells. This observation suggests that the granulocytes are actually infected by CMV in the process of virus dissemination.

In the 1990s, considerable clinical experience using the antigenemia

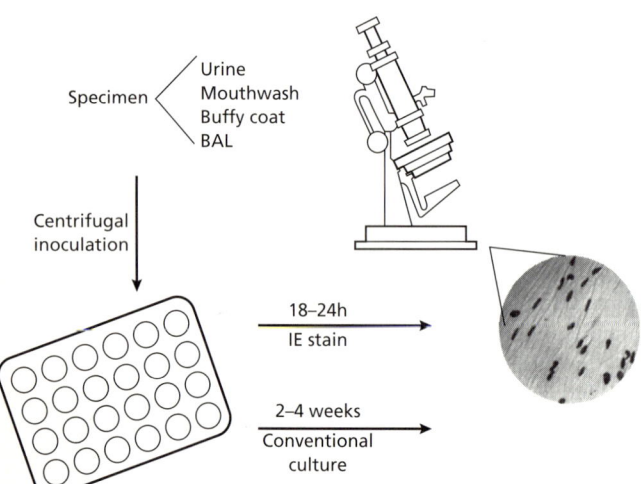

Fig. 53.8 Laboratory detection of infectious cytomegalovirus (CMV). This is a schematic description of the rapid centrifugal and conventional tissue culture methods for detection of infectious CMV in clinical specimens. The photomicrograph shows MRC5 human lung fibroblasts stained with immunoperoxidase and monoclonal antibody to the major immediate early protein (mIE p72) (×640).

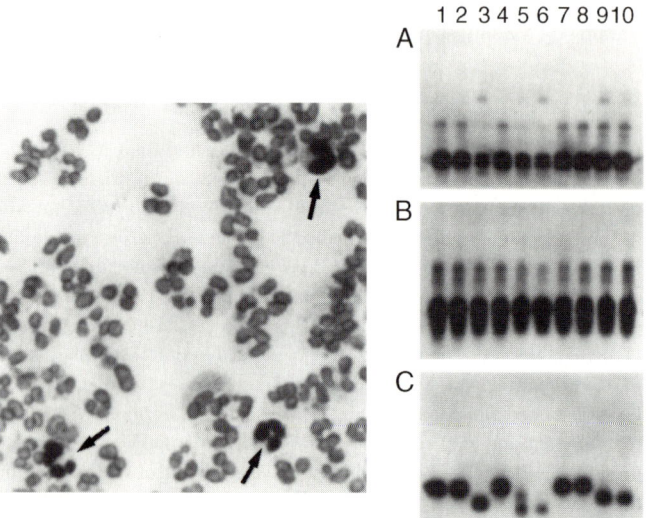

Fig. 53.9 Antigenemia and polymerase chain reaction (PCR) assays for cytomegalovirus (CMV). (Left) Photomicrograph showing three CMV antigen-positive polymorphonuclear leukocytes as detected with the CMV antigenemia assay (×640) Reproduced with permission from Grefte *et al.* [243]. (Right) Southern blot hybridization of polymerase chain reaction-amplified DNA from 10 wild isolates of CMV with amplification of genomic DNA encoding an immediate early protein (A), an early/late protein pp65 (B), or the hypervariable a sequence of CMV (C). Reproduced with permission from Zaia *et al.* [62].

assay showed that this assay correlates with CMV blood infection [33,122,245–249]. CMV antigenemia detection in organ transplantation indicates that the onset of antigenemia precedes the detection of "infectious" CMV, using the culture-based assays. Boeckh et al. [248] first applied this method in a systematic way to marrow transplantation, comparing the antigenemia assay to the rapid centrifugal culture method in 59 CMV-seropositive marrow allograft recipients. The antigenemia assay was positive in 21 of 22 CMV culture-positive individuals (sensitivity, 95%; specificity, 91%). As important, however, the median time to onset of antigenemia was significantly shorter for the antigenemia assay (day 47 vs. day 55, $p = 0.0006$), as had been described in other transplant populations [245–247]. In addition, of the nine patients who developed CMV disease without preceding positive viral cultures, CMV was detected by antigenemia in eight cases. Levels of antigenemia were also significantly higher in patients who subsequently developed disease. Thus, the antigenemia assay is a surrogate marker for CMV blood infection and, as such, has become a valuable tool for determining pre-emptive use of antiviral agents [33,122,248–251].

PCR detection methods

Methods that utilize the detection of CMV DNA directly or indirectly are now used regularly for diagnosis of CMV infection [62,75,252–265]. *In situ* cytohybridization has been available for nearly a decade and is currently able to detect single infected cells [75,252–254]. Nevertheless, *in situ* cytohybridization technology remains labor-intensive, which limits its use except in the research setting. The PCR assay is more versatile and can be used for quantitative characterization of CMV infection. It was first developed as a sensitive method for CMV detection [255–257] but, because of its ability to distinguish small DNA sequence differences, it can be used to differentiate strains of CMV by selective amplification of hypervariable regions of the viral genome (see example in Fig. 53.9) [62,258,259]. With this method, strain differentiation or other CMV genomic characterizations are possible without the necessity of virus isolation [258].

Einsele et al. [260] applied PCR detection of CMV to marrow transplant recipients. In 28 patients followed at weekly intervals, the PCR assay detected CMV blood infection more frequently than did the conventional culture method (83% vs. 67%) and the results were positive for all patients with CMV-IP diagnosed by conventional means. In addition, the detection of CMV infection by PCR was possible at very early times (weeks 1 and 2) compared to conventional detection methods (weeks 5 and 6). Einsele et al. [261] reported that PCR is useful for evaluating the recipient with CMV disease who is receiving ganciclovir therapy. In a pilot study, the PCR assay was more accurate for evaluation of virus clearance than blood cultures [261]. Subsequently, Einsele et al. [32] compared the use of a leukocyte PCR assay with blood culture as a basis for pre-emptive ganciclovir use after HCT. In this study, patients were randomly followed to day 100 after allogeneic HCT with either blood cultures or PCR and received ganciclovir, 5 mg/kg of body weight twice daily for 14 days and then continued at 5 mg/kg daily only if the CMV PCR test result remained positive. The group followed with PCR was treated earlier, required less treatment and had improved survival compared to the group followed with blood cultures. Clearly, PCR is a valuable tool for CMV management and will become even more helpful when commercial test kits are available for general use.

The detection of CMV by PCR can be applied to both serum [262] and to plasma [263]. CMV DNA in plasma correlates with presence of CMV infection in BAL samples [264], and the risk of late CMV disease has been shown to correlate with high CMV plasma DNA [34,70]. More recently, the quantitative plasma assays performed by real-time PCR methods have been described and are becoming essential in the management of bone marrow transplantation recipients by defining the population at high risk for CMV disease that requires pre-emptive antiviral treatment [47,123,138].

Regarding the relative diagnostic performance of the PCR assay and the CMV antigenemia assay, several studies compared these tests in prospective analyses in transplant populations [124,266–268]. In 16 subjects with CMV blood infection, Jiwa et al. [266] found that the antigenemia assay was positive for a mean of 2.5 weeks, and the PCR assay remained positive for a mean of 4.4 weeks. Boeckh et al. [124] compared shell vial culture, antigenemia assay, leukocyte PCR result and plasma PCR, and confirmed that the leukocyte PCR remains positive for a median time of 23 days after ganciclovir treatment, compared to 12 days for antigenemia and a 13-day median for plasma PCR. Woo et al. [268] confirmed that the leukocyte PCR result becomes positive prior to the plasma CMV DNA assay. Nevertheless, because the plasma-based assay can detect virus during neutropenia and is predictive of late CMV disease, it appears to be a useful method for evaluating patients [34,47,123].

DNA hybrid capture assay

Hybrid capture systems use a synthetic strand of RNA to "find" a strand of homologous DNA from a clinical specimen and then this "hybrid" RNA/DNA is captured in a tube coated with antibody to RNA/DNA complexes [121]. At least two such systems are available for diagnostic testing (Digene Corporation, USA, and Murex Diagnostica GmbH, Germany,). The amount of captured material is then detected using an antibody-based assay, and the clinical DNA is measured without a requirement for PCR-based amplification. Mazzulli et al. [269] have reported that the specificity of the CMV hybrid capture assay is similar to the antigenemia assay (95% and 94%, respectively). Hebart et al. [119] compared this assay with PCR in the management of HCT patients and found good concordance between the hybrid capture test and the PCR results. Both the hybrid capture and PCR detected CMV reactivation at approximately the same times post-HCT (median day 35 and day 34, respectively) and, importantly, none of the hybrid capture negative patients develop CMV disease. In addition, the capture assay performed well in the documentation of response to antiviral therapy. Because of its relative simplicity and ease of implementation, the CMV hybrid capture is useful in the management of the HCT patient.

Nucleic acid sequence-based amplification

The nucleic acid sequence-based amplification (NASBA) assay detects CMV using an RNA amplification technique. The principle of the NASBA assay is that a specific RNA molecule can be made into DNA and will then serve as a template for amplification of RNA copies, which can then be detected [121]. A potential advantage of the RNA amplification system is that a positive result indicates the presence of actively replicating virus. The NASBA assay also features an internal system control using CMV RNA control having specific internal sequences for confirmation that the clinical specimens do not contain inhibitors of the assay. Blok et al. [270] have reported that, in solid organ transplant recipients, the NASBA assay was more sensitive than the antigenemia assay. However, this observation was not confirmed in a later experience in liver transplant recipients in which the antigenemia assay was superior to the NASBA assay [271]. Hebart et al. [120] have compared the NASBA with PCR and blood culture in 33 HCT recipients. The PCR and NASBA were similar in documenting infection (88% concordance of positive patients), no NASBA negative patients developed CMV disease, and approximately 10% of patients treated with ganciclovir based on PCR were NASBA negative. Of note, there was more rapid return to negative NASBA blood tests while on anti-CMV therapy [120]. At present, the experience with NASBA for HCT patient management is limited, and its utility must await controlled evaluation in this population.

Table 53.8 Comparison of cytomegalovirus (CMV) diagnostic methods used in pre-emptive ganciclovir therapy.

Assay	Median days to first positive* (range)	Median days until clearance* (range)
Antigenemia	42 (27–75)†	13 (7–41)†
PCR$_{PL}$	45 (18–56)†	12 (7–41)†
PCR$_{PBL}$	32 (18–46)†	23 (14–53)†
	35 (2–90)‡	12 (7–49)‡
	28 (8–82)§	19 (6–43)§
Hybrid capture	34 (16–84)‡	10 (7–49)‡
NASBA	21 (4–82)§	19 (2–32)§
Blood culture	51 (37–93)†	0 (0–7)†
	59 (48–81)‡	NA‡

*Median day to initial positive based on weekly testing and days to negative test after start of pre-emptive antiviral therapy.
†Adapted from Boeckh et al. [124].
‡Adapted from Hebart et al. [119].
§Adapted from Hebart et al. [120].
Antigenemia, CMV antigenemia assay; NASBA, nucleic acid sequence based assay; PCR$_{PL}$, plasma polymerase chain reaction; PCR$_{PBL}$, leukocyte polymerase chain reaction.

Summary: which diagnostic test to choose for the HCT patient?

There is probably no "best" assay for CMV surveillance in management of the HCT recipient [121]. In a recent survey of tests used in the USA, 25% used tissue culture methods, 25% used an antigenemia assay and ~50% used PCR or DNA/RNA assays [272]. The choice of assay should be based on clinical need, and the most important needs are detection of CMV infection early enough to prevent disease and confirmation of treatment response or failure. Table 53.8 compares the various assays in terms of time to CMV detection and time to clearance of infection after start of antiviral treatment. Using the data of Boeckh et al. [124] and the experiences of Hebart et al. [119,120,137], it is clear that the PCR, hybrid capture and NASBA assays report the earliest times of CMV reactivation. For example, the median first day showing positivity has been reported as day 32 (range: 18–46) for leukocyte PCR, day 35 for hybrid capture, day 42 (range: 27–75) for antigenemia assay, day 45 (range: 18–56) for plasma PCR, and day 51 (range: 37–93) for blood culture. Antigenemia and plasma PCR results can be expected to become negative on therapy at approximately 12–13 days, and leukocyte PCR results become negative at 23 days. But the choice of assay must be made based on the resources at each medical center, and the type of HCT patients treated [121].

Pathogenesis

Overview

The usual course of CMV infection in most persons is not associated with specific signs or symptoms of disease, and this is true, too, with CMV infection after marrow or solid organ transplantation [67,273]. Furthermore, when renal, heart/lung and marrow transplant recipient populations are compared, the rates of infection with CMV and the incubation periods are nearly identical, yet the types of disease vary, with CMV-IP being a more frequent problem for the allogeneic HCT recipients [23,274–276]. It is important to appreciate this heterogeneity for what it tells us about the mechanism of disease. In AIDS patients and in fetuses, CMV infection is progressive and unchecked and, in these settings, the virus demonstrates its neurotropism with direct tissue damage in the central nervous system (CNS). The neurotropic aspect of CMV infection is rarely ever seen in the HCT recipient [5]. The principal difference in presentation of CMV disease between the transplantation population and the groups in which CNS complications of CMV infection are more common is the predominance of mononucleosis-like symptoms in the transplantation patients (compare findings [67,273–279]). The cardinal features of CMV infection in such patients are fever, neutropenia, thrombocytopenia and malaise, symptoms that are more frequently observed without other organ-specific involvement. This observation has suggested an aspect of disease pathogenesis that is separate from the organ-tropic features of viral disease. Furthermore, because these symptoms have been associated with immunological abnormalities specific for transplant populations, such as host-vs.-graft reaction or GVHD, and increase in bacterial and fungal infections, the symptom complex associated with CMV could be due not so much to the virus as to effect on the host responses to infection [77,280]. Thus, the pathogenesis of CMV disease in HCT involves (i) the role of progressive virus infection; (ii) the effect of CMV infection on cellular functions including immune response; and (iii) the interaction of CMV with selective hematopoietic cell lineages.

Role of progressive or recurrent infection

In the simplest terms, certain disease syndromes occur because of persistent virus infection, which leads to organ dysfunction, and others occur because the host is reacting to the infection, causing functional abnormalities based on immunopathology. The fact that inhibition of CMV infection with therapeutic effect occurs with use of appropriate antiviral agents, such as ganciclovir or foscarnet for retinitis and enteritis in AIDS patients, means that the virus infection *per se*, with resultant specific tissue cytopathology, causes the disease. It is recognized that CMV infection is very active in the retina during CMV retinitis based on electron microscopic analysis [281], and inhibition of virus replication is associated with restoration of organ function [282]. On the other hand, antiviral agents when used alone can produce an anti-CMV effect but often fail to affect clinical improvement of disease in the HCT recipient. For example, both CMV-IP and CMV-associated enteritis in marrow allograft recipients often fail to respond to ganciclovir treatment even though the treatment effectively inhibits CMV excretion [81,283].

In the HCT population, the occurrence of CMV infection at sites such as the kidney or throat does not correlate with incidence of subsequent CMV disease [31,44,67]. However, CMV blood and asymptomatic pulmonary infections strongly correlate with disease [31,43,67]. Thus, it appears that the progression of CMV from regional infection to disseminated infection is necessary prior to the onset of serious CMV disease in this setting. Schmidt et al. [31] observed that asymptomatic pulmonary CMV infection and CMV blood infection both strongly correlated with rates of subsequent CMV-IP (Fig. 53.7a). In this study, a subgroup of patients with CMV-negative BAL on day 35 after HCT remained at risk for CMV-IP. As shown in Fig. 53.7b, these individuals developed late-onset CMV blood infection in association with the later-onset CMV-IP. Thus, the progression of CMV infection to the peripheral blood, whether in the 4–7-week period or in the 8–10-week period after transplantation, occurs in association with the development of CMV-IP and is a major risk for CMV-IP. An obvious implication of this observation is that CMV infection, despite temporary interruption, is the central factor for disease pathogenesis. Any secondary factors that promote continued CMV replication are risk factors for CMV disease.

Effect of infection on cellular functions including immune response

As noted, CMV enters the host cell and expresses a cascade of proteins leading to the production of infectious viral particles [15]. Two events happen during this time which alter cellular function. The first is the activation of the signal transduction system at the time of virus binding to the cell surface, and the second is the introduction to the cytoplasm of proteins that have influence on cellular metabolism and function. Boldogh et al. [284] first showed that CMV infection alters the second messenger systems of the cell with changes in diacylglycerol, inositol triphosphate, intracellular calcium and protein kinase C. The effect of this activation is to up-regulate protein and DNA synthetic cellular pathways resulting in oncogene expression and heightened cellular metabolic activity. When the relatively large and complex CMV virion (see Figs 53.1 & 53.2) enters the infected cell, structural proteins of the virus having biologic function enter and contribute to the regulation of IE viral protein synthesis, which subsequently affects transcription of selective cell proteins. The exact function of these IE proteins is only generally understood, these proteins are necessary for further viral protein expression and for permissive virus replication [22,285].

Another function of *IE* viral gene expression is to repress other cellular transcriptional events [286]. In this regard, selected cellular proteins are either down-regulated or up-regulated during CMV infection; for example, fibronectin and fibronectin-specific RNA is down-regulated immediately after infection without concomitant alteration in β-actin-specific RNA [17]. The effect on housekeeper gene down-regulation might well begin the process of cell enlargement that is recognized as characteristic of CMV pathology. As important, it is also recognized that the *IE* gene products are transcriptionally activated by DNA response elements nearly identical to those required for host genes, such as IL-2 [287–290]. For example, Hunninghake et al. [289] reported that the promoter/enhancer region of the *IE* gene contains cyclic adenosine monophosphate response elements and Sambucetti et al. [290] described within this region consensus binding sites for the cellular transcription factors CREB/ATF, NF-kB and AP-1. The biologic significance of these observations is not fully appreciated, but it suggests that CMV replication is facilitated by events which activate these cellular systems [24].

Interaction of CMV with selective hematopoietic cell lineages

It has been recognized for nearly 2 decades that the function of certain hematopoietic cell lineages, especially neutrophils, platelets and monocyte/macrophages, are altered during CMV infection, and the mechanisms involved in this process are gradually being understood. The cells in which CMV is latent are thought to be those of myeloid elements from which macrophages and dendritic cells are derived [19]. Thus, the monocyte has been postulated to be the central site for CMV-induced interference with immune function [291–296]. Human monocytes, for example, exhibit an inhibited response to concanavalin A-induced proliferation after CMV infection [292]. It has been reported that CMV infection of these cells results in diminished production of IL-1 and 2, and it has been suggested that CMV influences these cells by impairing their ability to produce and to respond to cytokines or growth factors [294–296]. These responses are mediated at the cellular level via protein kinase C-dependent and inositol triphosphate-dependent signal-transduction pathways and, as noted, both of these pathways are altered by CMV infection [284]. Thus, it is possible that CMV infection results in a metabolic derangement that impairs the ability of cells of the immune system to produce or to react to mediators of the immune response. Fas-ligand mediated apoptosis of blood cells has been linked to murine CMV infection [297], and human CMV appears to influence Fas-mediated cell loss in CMV retinitis in humans [298].

These interactions of CMV and host cell, and the potential influences of CMV for escape from the immune surveillance noted above suggest that there are unrecognized effects of CMV on the infected patient that contributes to disease. The question that remains unanswered is how do these *in vitro* observations translate to relevant aspects of transplantation medicine. Despite the observation that neutropenia, thrombocytopenia and graft failure can be part of CMV-associated pathology after HCT, there is only circumstantial evidence that CMV induces these changes. The recent observation of Nichols et al. [38] that the D^+/R^- HCT recipient is at higher risk for early death from bacterial and fungal infection than the D^-/R^- patient suggests again that there are indirect effects of primary CMV infection that deserve further study. However, until there is evidence that inhibition of CMV using antiviral drugs can alter these events, these aspects of CMV disease pathogenesis will remain unknown.

Conclusions

Despite the fact that antiviral agents are available, the management of the allogeneic HCT recipient remains less than optimal—because the available antiviral drugs are toxic and, even when used successfully to prevent early disease, the patient often remains at risk for late-onset disease. An immune deficiency underlies prolonged susceptibility to CMV in this population, and this continued inability of the host to develop protective immunity suggests that antiviral agents alone will not solve the problem. In the future, CMV-specific immunological reconstitution, using either adoptive cellular immunotherapy or active vaccination, or both, will be developed, and this approach, in combination with less-toxic antiviral agents, will provide a more effective method for preventing CMV disease in this population.

References

1 Meyers JD, Thomas ED. Infection complicating bone marrow transplantation. In: Rubin RH, Young LS, eds. *Clinical Approach to Infection in the Compromised Host.* New York: Plenum, 1981: 525–56.

2 Zaia JA. Infections in organ transplant recipients. In: Richman DD, Whitley RJ, Hayden FG, eds. *Clinical Virology.* Washington, DC: ASM Press, 2002: 79–100.

3 Winston DJ, Gale RP, Meyers DV, Young LS. Infectious complications of human bone marrow transplantation. *Medicine* 1979; **58**: 1–31.

4 Appelbaum FR, Meyers JD, Fefer A et al. Nonbacterial nonfungal pneumonia following marrow transplantation in 100 identical twins. *Transplantation* 1982; **33**: 265–8.

5 Meyers JD, Flournoy N, Thomas ED. Nonbacterial pneumonia after allogeneic marrow transplantation. A review of ten years' experience. *Rev Infect Dis* 1982; **4**: 1119–32.

6 Miller WJ, Flynn P, McCullough J. Cytomegalovirus infection after bone marrow transplantation: an association with acute graft-versus-host disease. *Blood* 1986; **69**: 1162–7.

7 Wingard JR, Mellits ED, Sostrin MB. Interstitial pneumonitis after allogeneic bone marrow transplantation. Nine-year experience at a single institution. *Medicine* 1988; **71**: 175–86.

8 Winston DJ, Ho WG, Champlin RE. Cytomegalovirus infections after allogeneic bone marrow transplantation. *Rev Infect Dis* 1990; **12**: S776–92.

9 Wingard JR, Piantadosi S, Burns WH, Zahurak ML, Santos GW, Saral R. Cytomegalovirus infections in bone marrow transplant recipients given intensive cytoreductive therapy. *Rev Infect Dis* 1990; **12** (Suppl. 7): S793–804.

10 Griffiths PD, Emery VC. Cytomegalovirus. In: Richman DD, Whitley RJ, Hayden FG, eds. *Clinical Virology.* Washington, DC: ASM Press, 2002: 433–61.

11 Emery VC, Cope AV, Bowen EF, Gor D, Griffiths PD. The dynamics of human cytomegalovirus replication *in vivo*. *J Exp Med* 1999; **190**: 177–82.

12 DeMarchi JM, Blankship ML, Brown GD, Kaplan AS. Size and complexity of human cytomegalovirus DNA. *Virology* 1978; **89**: 643–6.

13 Chee MA, Bankier AT, Beck S. An analysis of the protein coding content of the sequence of human

cytomegalovirus strain AD169. *Curr Top Microbiol Immunol* 1990: 125–69.
14 Mocarski ES Jr. Cytomegalovirus biology and replication. In: Roizman B, Whitley RJ, Lopez C, eds. *The Human Herpesviruses*. New York: Raven Press, 1993: 173–226.
15 Walthen M, Stinski MF. Temporal patterns of human cytomegalovirus transcription: mapping the viral RNAs synthesized at immediate early, and late times after injection. *J Virol* 1982; **41**: 462–77.
16 Liu B, Stinski MF. Human cytomegalovirus contains a tegument protein that enhances transcription from promoters with upstream ATF and AP-1 cis-acting elements. *J Virol* 1992; **66**: 4434–44.
17 Pande H, Terramani T, Churchill MA, Hawkins GG, Zaia JA. Regulation of fibronectin gene expression by human cytomegalovirus. *J Virol* 1990; **64**: 1366–9.
18 Jones TR, Wiertz EJ, Sun L, Fish KN, Nelson JA, Ploegh HL. Human cytomegalovirus US3 impairs transport and maturation of major histocompatibility complex class I heavy chains. *Proc Natl Acad Sci U S A* 1996; **93**: 11,327–33.
19 Söderberg-Nauclér C, Fish KN, Nelson JA. Reactivation of latent human cytomegalovirus by allogeneic stimulation of blood cells from healthy donors. *Cell* 1997; **91**: 119–26.
20 Zhang L, Hanff P, Rutherford C, Churchill WH, Crumpacker CS. Detection of human cytomegalovirus DNA, RNA, and antibody in normal donor blood. *J Infect Dis* 1995; **171**: 1002–6.
21 Dutko FJ, Oldstone MBA. Cytomegalovirus causes a latent infection in undifferentiated cells and is activated by induction of cell differentiation. *J Exp Med* 1981; **154**: 1636–51.
22 Stinski MF. Cytomegalovirus and its replication. In: Fields BN, Knipe DM, eds. *Virology*. New York: Raven Press, 1990: 1959–80.
23 Ho M. *Cytomegalovirus. Biology and Infection*. New York: Plenum Publishing, 1991.
24 Söderberg-Nauclér C, Fish KN, Nelson JA. Interferon-γ and tumor necrosis factor-α specifically induce formation of cytomegalovirus-permissive monocyte-derived macrophages that are refractory to the antiviral activity of these cytokines. *J Clin Invest* 1997; **100**: 3154–63.
25 Salzberger B, Boeckh M, Myerson D. Circulating cytomegalovirus (CMV)-infected endothelial cells in marrow transplant patients with CMV disease and CMV infection. *J Infect Dis* 1997; **176**: 778–81.
26 Meyers JD. Prevention of cytomegalovirus infection after marrow transplantation. *Rev Infect Dis* 1989; **11** (Suppl. 7): S1691–705.
27 Bowden RA, Slichter SJ, Sayers MH, Mori M, Cays MJ, Meyers JD. Use of leukocyte-depleted platelets and cytomegalovirus-seronegative red blood cells for prevention of primary cytomegalovirus infection after marrow transplant. *Blood* 1991; **78**: 246–509.
28 Miller WJ, McCullough J, Balfour HH Jr et al. Prevention of cytomegalovirus infection following bone marrow transplantation: a randomized trial of blood product screening. *Bone Marrow Transplant* 1991; **7**: 227–34.
29 Winston DJ, Ho WG, Lin CH et al. Intravenous immune globulin for prevention of cytomegalovirus infection and interstitial pneumonia after bone marrow transplantation. *Ann Intern Med* 1987; **106**: 12–8.
30 Bowden RA, Fisher LK, Rogers K, Cays M, Meyers JD. Cytomegalovirus (CMV)-specific intravenous immunoglobulin for the prevention of primary CMV infection and disease after marrow transplant. *J Infect Dis* 1991; **164**: 483–7.
31 Schmidt GM, Horak DA, Niland JC, Duncan SR, Forman SJ, Zaia JA. A randomized controlled trial of prophylactic ganciclovir for cytomegalovirus pulmonary infection in recipients of allogeneic bone marrow transplants. *N Engl J Med* 1991; **324**: 1005–11.
32 Einsele H, Ehninger G, Hebart H et al. Polymerase chain reaction monitoring reduces the incidence of cytomegalovirus disease and the duration and side effects of antiviral therapy after bone marrow transplantation. *Blood* 1995; **86**: 2815–20.
33 Boeckh M, Gooley TA, Myerson D, Cunningham T, Schoch G, Bowden RA. Cytomegalovirus pp65 antigenemia-guided early treatment with ganciclovir at engraftment after allogeneic marrow transplantation: a randomized double-blind study. *Blood* 1996; **10**: 4063–71.
34 Zaia JA, Gallez-Hawkins GM, Tegtmeier BR et al. Late cytomegalovirus disease in marrow transplantation is predicted by virus load in plasma. *J Infect Dis* 1997; **176**: 782–5.
35 Neiman PE, Wasserman PB, Wentworth B. Interstitial pneumonia and cytomegalovirus infection as complications of human marrow transplantation. *Transplantation* 1973; **15**: 478–85.
36 Neiman PE, Reeves W, Ray G et al. A prospective analysis interstitial pneumonia and opportunistic viral infection among recipients of allogeneic bone marrow grafts. *J Infect Dis* 1977; **136**: 754–67.
37 Meyers JD, Flournoy N, Thomas ED. Risk factors for cytomegalovirus infection after human marrow transplantation. *J Infect Dis* 1986; **153**: 478–88.
38 Nichols WG, Corey L, Gooley T, Davis C, Boeckh M. High risk of death due to bacterial and fungal infection among cytomegalovirus (CMV)-seronegative recipients of stem cell transplants from seropositive donors: evidence for indirect effects of primary CMV infection. *J Infect Dis* 2003; **101**: 407–14.
39 Sullivan KM, Kopecky KJ, Jocom J et al. Immunomodulatory and antimicrobial efficacy of intravenous immunoglobulin in bone marrow transplantation. *N Engl J Med* 1990; **323**: 705–12.
40 Bowden RA, Sayers M, Flournoy N et al. Cytomegalovirus immune globulin and seronegative blood products to prevent primary cytomegalovirus infection after marrow transplantation. *N Engl J Med* 1986; **314**: 1006–10.
41 DeWitte T, Schattenberg A, Dijk V et al. Prevention of primary cytomegalovirus infection after allogeneic bone marrow transplantation by using leukocyte-poor random blood products from cytomegalovirus-unscreened blood-bank donors. *Transplantation* 1990; **50**: 964–8.
42 Goodrich JM, Mori M, Gleaves CA et al. Early treatment with ganciclovir to prevent cytomegalovirus disease after allogeneic bone marrow transplantation. *N Engl J Med* 1991; **325**: 1601–7.
43 Goodrich JM, Bowden RA, Fisher L, Keller C, Schoch BA, Meyers JD. Ganciclovir prophylaxis to prevent cytomegalovirus disease after allogeneic marrow transplant. *Ann Intern Med* 1993; **118**: 173–8.
44 Meyers JD, Reed EC, Shepp DH. Acyclovir for prevention of cytomegalovirus infection and disease after allogeneic marrow transplantation. *N Engl J Med* 1988; **318**: 70–5.
45 Einsele H, Hebart H, Kauffmann-Schneider C et al. Risk factors for treatment failures in patients receiving PCR-based preemptive therapy for CMV infection. *Bone Marrow Transplant* 2000; **25**: 757–63.
46 Zaia JA, Schmidt GM, Chao NJ et al. Preemptive ganciclovir administration based solely on asymptomatic pulmonary cytomegalovirus infection in allogeneic bone marrow transplant recipients: long-term follow-up. *Biol Blood Marrow Transplant* 1995; **1**: 88–93.
47 Yun Z, Lewensohn-Fuchs I, Ljungman P, Vahlne A. Real-time monitoring of cytomegalovirus infections after stem cell transplantation using the TaqMan polymerase chain reaction assays. *Transplantation* 2000; **69**: 1733–6.
48 Junghans C, Boeckh M, Carter RA et al. Incidence and outcome of cytomegalovirus infections following nonmyeloablative compared with myeloablative allogeneic stem cell transplantation, a matched control study. *Blood* 2002; **99**: 1978–85.
49 Wingard JR, Chen DY, Burns WH et al. Cytomegalovirus infection after autologous bone marrow transplantation with comparison to infection after allogeneic bone marrow transplantation. *Blood* 1988; **71**: 1432–7.
50 Reusser P, Fisher LD, Buckner CD, Thomas ED, Meyers JD. Cytomegalovirus infection after autologous bone marrow transplantation. Occurrence of cytomegalovirus disease and effect on engraftment. *Blood* 1990; **75**: 1888–94.
51 Boeckh M, Stevens-Ayers T, Bowden RA. Cytomegalovirus pp65 antigenemia after autologous marrow and peripheral blood stem cell transplantation. *J Infect Dis* 1996; **174**: 907–12.
52 Hebart H, Schroder A, Loffler J et al. Cytomegalovirus monitoring by polymerase chain reaction of whole blood samples from patients undergoing autologous bone marrow or peripheral blood progenitor cell transplantation. *J Infect Dis* 1997; **175**: 1490–3.
53 Holmberg LA, Boeckh M, Hooper H et al. Increased incidence of cytomegalovirus disease after autologous CD34-selected peripheral blood stem cell transplantation. *Blood* 1999; **94**: 4029–35.
54 Mohty M, Faucher C, Vey N et al. High rate of secondary viral and bacterial infections in patients undergoing allogeneic bone marrow minitransplantation. *Bone Marrow Transplant* 2000; **26**: 251–5.
55 Peggs KS, Mackinnon S. Cytomegalovirus infection and disease after autologous peripheral blood stem cell transplantation. *Br J Haematol* 2001; **115**: 1032–3.
56 Huang E-S, Alford CA, Reynolds DW, Stagno S, Pass RF. Molecular epidemiology of cytomegalovirus infection in women and their infants. *N Engl J Med* 1980; **303**: 958–62.
57 Spector SA, Spector DH. Molecular epidemiology of cytomegalovirus infection in premature twin infants and their mother. *Pediatr Infect Dis* 1982; **1**: 405–9.
58 Yow MD, Lakeman AD, Stagno S, Reynolds RB, Plavidal FJ. Use of restriction enzymes to investigate the source of a primary cytomegalovirus infection in a pediatric nurse. *Pediatrics* 1982; **70**: 713–6.
59 Chou SW. Differentiation of cytomegalovirus strains by restriction analysis of DNA sequences amplified from clinical specimens. *J Infect Dis* 1990; **162**: 738–42.
60 Collier AC, Chandler SH, Handsfield HH, Corey L, McDougall JK. Identification of multiple strains of cytomegalovirus in homosexual men. *J Infect Dis* 1989; **159**: 123–6.

61 Drew WL, Sweet ES, Miner RC, Mocarski ES. Multiple infections by cytomegalovirus in patients with acquired immunodeficiency syndrome: documentation by Southern blot hybridization. *J Infect Dis* 1984; **150**: 952–3.

62 Zaia JA, Gallez-Hawkins G, Churchill MA *et al*. Comparative analysis of human cytomegalovirus: a sequence in multiple clinical isolates using polymerase chain reaction and restriction fragment length polymorphism assays. *J Clin Microbiol* 1990; **38**: 2602–7.

63 Winston DJ, Huang ES, Miller MJ *et al*. Molecular epidemiology of cytomegalovirus infections associated with bone marrow transplantation. *Ann Intern Med* 1985; **102**: 16–20.

64 Torok-Storb B, Boeckh M, Hoy C, Leisenring W, Myerson D, Gooley T. Association of specific cytomegalovirus genotypes with death from myelosuppression after marrow transplantation. *Blood* 1997; **90**: 2097–102.

65 Boeckh M, Hoy C, Torok-Storb B. Occult cytomegalovirus infection of marrow stroma. *Clin Infect Dis* 1998; **26**: 209–10.

66 Ljungman P, Griffiths P, Paya C. Definitions of cytomegalovirus infection and disease in transplant recipients. *Clin Infect Dis* 2002; **34**: 1094–7.

67 Meyers JD, Ljungman P, Fisher LD. Cytomegalovirus excretion as a predictor of cytomegalovirus disease after marrow transplantation: importance of cytomegalovirus viremia. *J Infect Dis* 1990; **162**: 373–80.

68 Weiner RS, Bortin MM, Gale RP. Interstitial pneumonitis after bone marrow transplantation. Assessment of risk factors. *Ann Intern Med* 1986; **104**: 168–75.

69 Humar A, Wood S, Lipton J *et al*. Effect of cytomegalovirus infection on 1-year mortality rates among recipients of allogeneic bone marrow transplants. *Clin Infect Dis* 2003; **101**: 407–14.

70 Boeckh M, Leisenring W, Riddell SR *et al*. Late cytomegalovirus disease and mortality in allogeneic hematopoietic stem cell transplant recipients: importance of viral load and T cell immunity. *Blood* 2003; **101**: 407–14.

71 Ljungman P, Aschan J, Azinge JN *et al*. Cytomegalovirus viraemia and specific T-helper cell responses as predictors of disease after allogeneic marrow transplantation. *Br J Haematol* 1993; **83**: 118–24.

72 Krause H, Hebart H, Jahn G, Muller CA, Einsele H. Screening for CMV-specific T cell proliferation to identify patients at risk of developing late onset CMV disease. *Bone Marrow Transplant* 1997; **19**: 1111–6.

73 Khouri NF, Saral R, Armstrong EM. Pulmonary interstitial changes following bone marrow transplantation: a complex, multifactor disorder. *Radiology* 1979; **133**: 587–92.

74 Beschorner WE, Hutchins GM, Burns WH, Saral R, Tutschka PJ, Santos GW. Cytomegalovirus pneumonia in bone marrow transplant recipients. Miliary and diffuse patterns. *Am Rev Respir Dis* 1980; **122**: 107–14.

75 Myerson D, Hackman RD, Nelson JA, Ward DC, McDougall JK. Widespread presence of histologically occult cytomegalovirus. *Hum Pathol* 1984; **15**: 430–9.

76 Zaia JA. The biology of human cytomegalovirus infection after bone marrow transplantation. *Int J Cell Cloning* 1986; **4** (Suppl. 1): 135–54.

77 Zaia JA. Understanding human cytomegalovirus infection. In: Champlin RE, Gale RP, eds. *New Strategies: Bone Marrow Transplantation*. UCLA Symposia on Molecular and Cellular Biology New Series. New York: Wiley-Liss, Inc., 1990: 319–34.

78 Slavin MA, Gleaves CA, Schoch HG, Bowden RA. Quantification of cytomegalovirus in bronchoalveolar lavage fluid after allogeneic marrow transplantation by centrifugation culture. *J Clin Microbiol* 1992; **30**: 2776–9.

79 Stover DE, Zaman MB, Jajdu SI, Lange M, Gold J, Armstrong D. Bronchoalveolar lavage in the diagnosis of diffuse pulmonary infiltrates in the immunosuppressed host. *Ann Intern Med* 1984; **101**: 1–7.

80 Springmeyer SC, Hackman RC, Holle R. Use of bronchoalveolar lavage to diagnose acute diffuse pneumonia in the immunocompromised host. *J Infect Dis* 1986; **154**: 604–10.

81 Shepp DH, Dandliker PS, de Miranda P *et al*. Activity of 9-[2-hydroxy-1-(hydroxymethyl) ethoxymethyl]guanine in the treatment of cytomegalovirus pneumonia. *Ann Intern Med* 1985; **103**: 368–73.

82 Kraemer KG, Neiman PE, Reeves WC, Thomas ED. Prophylactic adenine arabinoside following marrow transplantation. *Transplant Proc* 1978; **10**: 237–40.

83 Meyers JD, McGuffin RW, Neiman PE, Singer JW, Thomas ED. Toxicity and efficacy of human leukocyte interferon for treatment of cytomegalovirus pneumonia after marrow transplantation. *J Infect Dis* 1980; **141**: 555–62.

84 Meyers JD, McGuffin RW, Bryson YJ, Cantell K, Thomas ED. Treatment of cytomegalovirus pneumonia after marrow transplant with combined vidarabine and human leukocyte interferon. *J Infect Dis* 1982; **146**: 80–4.

85 Wade JC, Hintz M, McGuffin RW, Springmeyer SC, Connor JD, Meyers JD. Treatment of cytomegalovirus pneumonia with high dose acyclovir. *Am J Med* 1982; **73**: 249–56.

86 Wade JC, McGuffin RW, Springmeyer SC, Newton B, Singer JW, Meyers JD. Treatment of cytomegaloviral pneumonia with high-dose acyclovir and human leukocyte interferon. *J Infect Dis* 1983; **148**: 557–62.

87 Meyers JD, Day LM, Lum LG, Sullivan KM. Recombinant leukocyte α interferon for the treatment of serious viral infection after marrow transplant: a phase I study. *J Infect Dis* 1983; **148**: 551–6.

88 Winston DJ, Ho WG, Schroff RW, Champlin RE, Gale RP. Safety and tolerance of recombinant leukocyte α interferon in bone marrow transplant recipients. *Antimicrob Agents Chemother* 1983; **23**: 846–51.

89 Shepp DH, Newton BA, Meyers JD. Intravenous lymphoblastoid interferon and acyclovir for treatment of cytomegaloviral pneumonia. *J Infect Dis* 1984; **150**: 776–7.

90 Winston DJ, Ho WG, Bartoni K. Ganciclovir therapy for cytomegalovirus infections in recipients of bone marrow transplants and other immunosuppressed patients. *Rev Infect Dis* 1988; **10**: S547–53.

91 Erice A, Jordan MC, Chace BA, Fletcher C, Chinnock BJ, Balfour HHJ. Ganciclovir treatment of cytomegalovirus disease in transplant recipients and other immunocompromised hosts. *J Am Med Assoc* 1987; **257**: 3082–7.

92 Reed EC, Dandliker PS, Meyers JD. Treatment of cytomegalovirus pneumonia with 9-[2-hydroxy-1-(hydroxymethyl)ethoxymethyl]guanine and high dose corticosteroids. *Ann Intern Med* 1986; **105**: 214–6.

93 Blacklock HA, Griffiths P, Stirk P, Prentice HG. Specific hyperimmune globulin for cytomegalovirus pneumonitis. 1985; **2**: 152–3.

94 Reed EC, Bowden RA, Dandliker PS, Gleaves CA, Meyers JD. Efficacy of cytomegalovirus immunoglobulin in marrow transplant recipients with cytomegalovirus pneumonia. *J Infect Dis* 1987; **156**: 641–5.

95 Ringden O, Wilczek H, Lonnqvist Gahrton G, Wahren AB, Lernestedt J-O. Foscarnet for cytomegalovirus infections. *Lancet* 1985; **1**: 1503–4.

96 Masur H, Lane HC, Palestine A. Effect of 9-(1,3-dihydroxy-2-propoxymethyl)guanine on serious cytomegalovirus disease in eight immunosuppressed homosexual men. *Ann Intern Med* 1986; **104**: 41–4.

97 Shanley JD, Pesanti EL. The relation of viral replication to interstitial pneumonitis in murine cytomegalovirus lung infection. *J Infect Dis* 1985; **151**: 454–8.

98 Wilson EJ, Medearis DN Jr, Hansen LA, Rubin RH. 9-(1–3-dihydroxy-2-propoxymethyl)guanine prevents death but not immunity in murine cytomegalovirus-infected normal and immunosuppressed BALB/c mice. *Antimicrob Agents Chemother* 1987; **31**: 1017–20.

99 Reed EC, Bowden RA, Dandliker PS, Meyers JD. Treatment of cytomegalovirus (CMV) pneumonia in bone marrow transplant (BMT) patients (PTS) with ganciclovir (GCV) and CMV immunoglobulin (CMV-IG). *Blood* 1987; **70**: 313 [Abstract].

100 Bratanow N, Ash RC, Turner P. The use of 9(1,3-dihydroxy-2-propoxymethyl)guanine (ganciclovir, DHPG) and intravenous immunoglobulin (IVIG) in the treatment of serious cytomegalovirus (CMV) infections in thirty-one allogeneic bone marrow transplant (BMT) patients. *Blood* 1987; **70**: 302 [Abstract].

101 Reed EC, Bowden RA, Dandliker PS, Lilleby KE, Meyers JD. Treatment of cytomegalovirus pneumonia with ganciclovir and intravenous cytomegalovirus immunoglobulin in patients with bone marrow transplants. *Ann Intern Med* 1988; **109**: 783–8.

102 Emmanuel D, Cunningham I, Jule-Elysee K. Cytomegalovirus pneumonia after bone marrow transplantation successfully treated with the combination of ganciclovir and high-dose intravenous immune globulin. *Ann Intern Med* 1988; **109**: 777–82.

103 Schmidt GM, Kovacs A, Zaia JA *et al*. Ganciclovir/immunoglobulin combination therapy for the treatment of human cytomegalovirus-associated interstitial pneumonia in bone marrow allograft recipients. *Transplantation* 1988; **46**: 905–7.

104 Ljungman P, Englehard D, Link H. Treatment of interstitial pneumonitis due to cytomegalovirus with ganciclovir and intravenous immune globulin: experience of European Bone Marrow Transplant Group. *Clin Infect Dis* 1992; **14**: 831–5.

105 Ljungman P. Cytomegalovirus infections in transplant patients. *Scand J Infect Dis* 1996; **100**: 59–63.

106 Drew WL, Miner RC, Busch DF. Prevalence of resistance in patients receiving ganciclovir for serious cytomegalovirus infection. *J Infect Dis* 1990; **163**: 716–9.

107 McDonald GB, Sharma P, Hackman RC, Meyers JD, Thomas ED. Esophageal infections in immunosuppressed patients after marrow transplantation. *Gastroenterology* 1985; **88**: 1111–7.

108 Page MJ, Dreese JC, Poritz LS, Koltun WA. Cytomegalovirus enteritis. A highly lethal condition requiring early detection and intervention. *Dis Colon Rectum* 1998; **41**: 619–23.

109 Reed EC, Wolford JL, Kopecky KJ et al. Ganciclovir for the treatment of cytomegalovirus gastroenteritis in bone marrow transplant patients. A randomized, placebo-controlled trial. Ann Intern Med 1990; 112: 505–10.

110 van Burik JA, Lawatsch EJ, DeFor TE, Weisdorf DJ. Cytomegalovirus enteritis among hematopoietic stem cell transplant recipients. Biol Blood Marrow Transplant 2001; 7: 674–9.

111 Choi JH, Kim KJ, Kim CC. Pre-emptive ganciclovir treatment can play a role in restoration of hematopoiesis after allogeneic bone marrow transplantation. Bone Marrow Transplant 1997; 19: 187–90.

112 Salzberger B, Bowden RA, Hackman RC, Davis C, Boeckh M. Neutropenia in allogeneic marrow transplant recipients receiving ganciclovir for prevention of cytomegalovirus disease: risk factors and outcome. Blood 1997; 90: 2502–8.

113 Zaia JA. Prevention and management of CMV-related problems after hematopoietic stem cell transplantation. Bone Marrow Transplant 2002; 29: 633–8.

114 Bacigalupo A, Van Lint E, Tedone F et al. Early treatment of CMV infections in allogeneic bone marrow transplant recipients with foscarnet or ganciclovir. Bone Marrow Transplant 1994; 13: 753–4.

115 Bacigalupo A, Bregante S, Tedone E et al. Combined foscarnet-ganciclovir treatment for cytomegalovirus infections after allogeneic hemopoietic stem cell transplantation. Bone Marrow Transplant 1996; 2 (Suppl.): 110–4.

116 Ljungman P, Oberg G, Aschan J et al. Foscarnet for pre-emptive therapy of CMV infection detected by a leukocyte-based nested PCR in allogeneic bone marrow transplant patients. Bone Marrow Transplant 1996; 18: 565–8.

117 Ippoliti C, Morgan A, Warkentin D. Foscarnet for prevention of cytomegalovirus infection in allogeneic marrow transplant recipients unable to receive ganciclovir. Bone Marrow Transplant 1997; 20: 491–5.

118 Hebart H, Brugger W, Grigoleit U et al. Risk for cytomegalovirus disease in patients receiving polymerase chain reaction-based preemptive antiviral therapy after allogeneic stem cell transplantation depends on transplantation modality. Blood 2001; 97: 2183–5.

119 Hebart H, Wuchter P, Loeffler J et al. Evaluation of the Murex CMV DNA hybrid capture assay version 2.0 for early diagnosis of cytomegalovirus infection in recipients of an allogeneic stem cell transplant. Bone Marrow Transplant 2001; 28: 213–8.

120 Hebart H, Rudolph T, Loeffler J et al. Evaluation of the NucliSens CMV pp67 assay for detection and monitoring of human cytomegalovirus infection after allogeneic stem cell transplantation. Bone Marrow Transplant 2002; 30: 181–7.

121 Zaia JA, Molinder KM. Advances in CMV diagnostic testing and their implications for the management of CMV infection in transplant recipients. In: Singh N, Aguado JM, eds. Infectious Complications in Transplant Patients. Boston: Kluwer Academic Publishers, 2000: 75–92.

122 Boeckh M, Bowden RA, Gooley T, Myerson D, Corey L. Successful modification of a pp65 antigenemia-based early treatment strategy for prevention of cytomegalovirus disease in allogeneic marrow transplant recipients. Blood 1999; 93: 1781–2.

123 Limaye AP, Huang ML, Leisenring W, Stensland L, Corey L, Boeckh M. Cytomegalovirus (CMV) DNA load in plasma for the diagnosis of CMV disease before engraftment in hematopoietic stem-cell transplant recipients. J Infect Dis 2001; 183: 377–82.

124 Boeckh M, Gallez-Hawkins GM, Myerson D, Zaia JA, Bowden RA. Plasma polymerase chain reaction for cytomegalovirus DNA after allogeneic marrow transplantation. Comparison with polymerase chain reaction using peripheral blood leukocytes, 65 antigenemia, and viral culture. Transplantation 1997; 64: 108–13.

125 Zaia JA. Prevention of cytomegalovirus disease in hematopoietic stem cell transplantation. Clin Infect Dis 2002; 35: 999–1004.

126 Reusser P, Attenhofer R, Hebart H, Helg C, Chapuis B, Einsele H. Cytomegalovirus-specific T-cell immunity in recipients of autologous peripheral blood stem cell or bone marrow transplants. Blood 1997; 89: 3873–9.

127 Kroger N, Zabelina T, Kruger W et al. Patient cytomegalovirus seropositivity with or without reactivation is the most important prognostic factor for survival and treatment-related mortality in stem cell transplantation from unrelated donors using pretransplant in vivo T-cell depletion with antithymocyte globulin. Br J Haematol 2001; 113: 1060–71.

128 Atkinson K, Downs K, Golenia M et al. Prophylactic use of ganciclovir in allogeneic bone marrow transplantation: absence of clinical cytomegalovirus infection. Br J Haematol 1991; 79: 57–62.

129 Winston DJ, Ho WG, Bartoni K. Ganciclovir prophylaxis of cytomegalovirus infection and disease in allogeneic bone marrow transplant recipients. Ann Intern Med 1993; 118: 179–84.

130 Verdonck LF, Van den Hoek MR, Rozenberg-Arska M, Dekker AW. A risk-adapted approach with a short course of ganciclovir to prevent cytomegalovirus (CMV) pneumonia in CMV-seropositive recipients of allogeneic bone marrow transplants. Clin Infect Dis 1997; 24: 901–7.

131 Slavin MA, Gooley TA, Bowden RA. Prediction of cytomegalovirus pneumonia after marrow transplantation from cellular characteristics and cytomegalovirus culture of bronchoalveolar lavage fluid. Transplantation 1994; 58: 915–9.

132 Sakamaki H, Yuasa K, Goto H et al. Comparison of cytomegalovirus (CMV) antigenemia and CMV in bronchoalveolar lavage fluid for diagnosis of CMV pulmonary infection after bone marrow transplantation. Bone Marrow Transplant 1997; 20: 143–7.

133 Machida U, Kami M, Kanda Y et al. Comparison of the antigenemia assay and screening bronchoscopy for detection of cytomegalovirus infection after bone marrow transplantation. Bone Marrow Transplant 1999; 24: 1153–7.

134 Reddy V, Hao Y, Lipton J et al. Management of allogeneic bone marrow transplant recipients at risk for cytomegalovirus disease using a surveillance bronchoscopy and prolonged pre-emptive ganciclovir therapy. J Clin Virol 1999; 13: 149–59.

135 Humar A, Lipton J, Welsh S, Moussa G, Messner H, Mazzulli T. A randomised trial comparing cytomegalovirus antigenemia assay vs screening bronchoscopy for the early detection and prevention of disease in allogeneic bone marrow and peripheral blood stem cell transplant recipients. Bone Marrow Transplant 2001; 28: 485–90.

136 Gleaves CA, Smith TF, Shuster EA, Pearson GR. Rapid detection of cytomegalovirus in MRC-5 cells inoculated with urine specimens by using low-speed centrifugation and monoclonal antibody to an early antigen. J Clin Microbiol 1984; 19: 917–9.

137 Hebart H, Gamer D, Loeffler J et al. Evaluation of Murex CMV DNA hybrid capture assay for detection and quantitation of cytomegalovirus infection in patients following allogeneic stem cell transplantation. J Clin Microbiol 1998; 36: 1333–7.

138 Emery VC, Sabin CA, Cope AV, Gor D, Hassan-Walker AF, Griffiths PD. Application of viral-load kinetics to identify patients who develop cytomegalovirus disease after transplantation. Lancet 2000; 355: 2032–6.

139 Balfour HH Jr, Chace BA, Stapleton JT, Simmons RL, Fryd DS. A randomized, placebo-controlled trial of oral acyclovir for the prevention of cytomegalovirus disease in recipients of renal allografts. N Engl J Med 1989; 320: 1381–7.

140 Fletcher CV, Englund JA, Edelman CK. Pharmacologic basis for high-dose oral acyclovir prophylaxis of cytomegalovirus disease in renal allograft recipients. Antimicrob Agents Chemother 1991; 35: 938–43.

141 Cole NL, Balfour HH Jr In vitro susceptibility of cytomegalovirus isolates from immunocompromised patients to acyclovir and ganciclovir. Diagn Microbiol Infect Dis 1987; 6: 255–61.

142 Boeckh M, Gooley TA, Reusser P, Buckner CD, Bowden RA. Failure of high-dose acyclovir to prevent cytomegalovirus disease after autologous marrow transplantation. J Infect Dis 1995; 172: 939–43.

143 Prentice HG, Gluckman E, Powles RL et al. Impact of long-term acyclovir on cytomegalovirus infection and survival after allogeneic bone marrow transplantation. European Acyclovir for CMV Prophylaxis Study Group. Lancet 1994; 343: 749–53.

144 Prentice HG, Gluckman E, Powles RL et al. Long-term survival in allogeneic bone marrow transplant recipients following acyclovir prophylaxis for CMV infection. The European Acyclovir for CMV Prophylaxis Study Group. Bone Marrow Transplant 1997; 19: 129–33.

145 Boeckh M, Gooley TA, Bowden RA. Effect of high-dose acyclovir on survival in allogeneic marrow transplant recipients who received ganciclovir at engraftment or for cytomegalovirus pp65 antigenemia. J Infect Dis 1998; 178: 1153–7.

146 Vusirikala M, Wolff SN, Stein RS et al. Valacyclovir for the prevention of cytomegalovirus infection after allogeneic stem cell transplantation: a single institution retrospective cohort analysis. Bone Marrow Transplant 2001; 28: 265–70.

147 Ljungman P, de La Camara R, Milpied N et al. Randomized study of valacyclovir as prophylaxis against cytomegalovirus reactivation in recipients of allogeneic bone marrow transplants. Blood 2002; 99: 3050–6.

148 Deray G, Martinez F, Katlama C. Foscarnet nephrotoxicity. Mechanism, incidence and prevention. Am J Nephrol 1989; 9: 316–21.

149 Reusser P, Gambertoglio JG, Lilleby K, Meyers JD. Phase I–II trial of foscarnet for prevention of cytomegalovirus infection in autologous and allogeneic marrow transplant recipients. J Infect Dis 1992; 166: 473–9.

150 Aschan J, Ringdén O, Ljungman P. Foscarnet for treatment of cytomegalovirus infections in bone

marrow transplant recipients. *Scan J Inf Dis* 1992; **24**: 143–50.
151 Boeckh M, Zaia JA, Jung D, Skettino S, Chauncey TR, Bowden RA. A study of the pharmacokinetics, antiviral activity, and tolerability of oral ganciclovir for CMV prophylaxis in marrow transplantation. *Biol Blood Marrow Transplant* 1998; **4**: 13–9.
152 Frenkel LM, Capparelli EV, Dankner WM *et al*. Oral ganciclovir in children: pharmacokinetics, safety, tolerance, and antiviral effects. The Pediatric AIDS Clinical Trials Group. *J Infect Dis* 2000; **182**: 1616–24.
153 Ljungman P, Deliliers GL, Platzbecker U *et al*. Cidofovir for cytomegalovirus infection and disease in allogeneic stem cell transplant recipients. The Infectious Diseases Working Party of the European Group for Blood and Marrow Transplantation. *Blood* 2001; **97**: 388–92.
154 Meyers JD, Leszcynski J, Zaia JA. Prevention of cytomegalovirus infection by cytomegalovirus immune globulin after marrow transplantation. *Ann Intern Med* 1983; **98**: 442–6.
155 Winston DJ, Ho WG, Howell CL. Cytomegalovirus infections associated with leukocyte transfusions. *Ann Intern Med* 1980; **93**: 671–5.
156 Bowden RA, Slichter SJ, Sayers M *et al*. A comparison of filtered leukocyte-reduced and cytomegalovirus (CMV) seronegative blood products for the prevention of transfusion-associated CMV infection after marrow transplant. *Blood* 1995; **86**: 3598–603.
157 Landaw EM, Kanter M, Petz LD. Safety of filtered leukocyte-reduced blood products for prevention of transfusion-associated cytomegalovirus infection. *Blood* 1996; **87**: 4910.
158 Narvios AB, Przepiorka D, Tarrand J, Chan KW, Champlin R, Lichtiger B. Transfusion support using filtered unscreened blood products for cytomegalovirus-negative allogeneic marrow transplant recipients. *Bone Marrow Transplant* 1998; **22**: 575–7.
159 Meyers JD, Flournoy N, Thomas ED. Cytomegalovirus infection and specific cell-mediated immunity after marrow transplantation. *J Infect Dis* 1980; **142**: 816–24.
160 Quinnan GV Jr, Kirmani N, Rook AH *et al*. Cytotoxic T cells in cytomegalovirus infection: HLA-restricted T-lymphocyte and non-T-lymphocyte cytotoxic responses correlate with recovery from cytomegalovirus infection in bone-marrow-transplant recipients. *N Engl J Med* 1982; **307**: 7–13.
161 Rook AH, Quinnan GV, Frederick WJR. Importance of cytotoxic lymphocytes during cytomegalovirus infection in renal transplant recipients. 1984; **76**: 385–92.
162 Reusser P, Riddell SR, Meyers JD, Greenberg PD. Cytotoxic T-lymphocyte response to cytomegalovirus after human allogeneic bone marrow transplantation. Pattern of recovery and correlation with cytomegalovirus infection and disease. *Blood* 1991; **78**: 1373–80.
163 Ljungman P, Lonnqvist B, Gahrton G, Ringden O, Wahren B. Cytomegalovirus-specific lymphocyte proliferation and *in vitro* cytomegalovirus IgG synthesis for diagnosis of cytomegalovirus infections after bone marrow transplantation. *Blood* 1986; **68**: 108–12.
164 Borysiewicz LK, Graham S, Hickling JK, Mason PD, Sissions JGP. Human cytomegalovirus-specific cytotoxic T cells. Their precursor frequency and stage specificity. *Eur J Immunol* 1988; **18**: 269–75.

165 Forman SJ, Zaia JA, Clark BR. *In vitro* cellular response to the late 64K glycoprotein of cytomegalovirus: evidence for T-cell activation. *Transplant Proc* 1985; **1**: 507–9.
166 McLaughlin-Taylor E, Pande H, Forman SJ *et al*. Identification of the major late human cytomegalovirus matrix protein pp65 as a target antigen for CD8+ virus-specific cytotoxic T lymphocytes. *J Med Virol* 1994; **43**: 103–10.
167 Riddell SR, Rabin M, Geballe AP, Britt WJ, Greenberg PD. Class I MHC-restricted cytotoxic T-lymphocyte recognition of cells infected with human cytomegalovirus does not require endogenous viral gene expression. *J Immunol* 1991; **146**: 2795–804.
168 Boppana SV, Britt WJ. Recognition of human cytomegalovirus gene products by HCMV-specific cytotoxic T-cells. *Virology* 1996; **222**: 293–6.
169 Wills MR, Carmichael AJ, Mynard K *et al*. The human cytotoxic T-lymphocyte (CTL) response to cytomegalovirus is dominated by structural protein pp65: frequency, specificity, and T-cell receptor usage of pp65-specific CTL. *J Virol* 1996; **70**: 7569–79.
170 Diamond DJ, York J, Sun JY, Wright CL, Forman SJ. Development of a candidate HLA A*0201 restricted peptide-based vaccine against human cytomegalovirus infection. *Blood* 1997; **90**: 1751–67.
171 Alp NJ, Allport TD, Van Zanten J, Rodgers B, Sissons JG, Borysiewicz LK. Fine specificity of cellular immune responses in humans to human cytomegalovirus immediate-early 1 protein. *J Virol* 1991; **65**: 4812–20.
172 Kern F, Surel IP, Faulhaber N *et al*. Target structures of the CD8+ T-cell response to human cytomegalovirus: the 72-kDa major immediate-early protein revisited. *J Virol* 1999; **73**: 8179–84.
173 Gyulai Z, Endresz V, Burian K *et al*. Cytotoxic T lymphocyte (CTL) responses to human cytomegalovirus pp65, IE1-Exon4, gB.150, and pp28 in healthy individuals: reevaluation of prevalence of IE1-specific CTLs. *J Infect Dis* 2000; **181**: 1537–46.
174 Peggs K, Verfuerth S, Pizzey A, Ainsworth J, Moss P, Mackinnon S. Characterization of human cytomegalovirus peptide-specific CD8+ T-cell repertoire diversity following *in vitro* restimulation by antigen-pulsed dendritic cells. *Blood* 2002; **99**: 213–23.
175 Khan N, Cobbold M, Keenan R, Moss PA. Comparative analysis of CD8+ T cell responses against human cytomegalovirus proteins pp65 and immediate early 1 shows similarities in precursor frequency, oligoclonality, and phenotype. *J Infect Dis* 2002; **185**: 1025–34.
176 Kern F, Bunde T, Faulhaber N *et al*. Cytomegalovirus (CMV) phosphoprotein 65 makes a large contribution to shaping the T cell repertoire in CMV-exposed individuals. *J Infect Dis* 2002; **185**: 1709–16.
177 Wang EC, Moss PA, Frodsham P, Lehner PJ, Bell JI, Borysiewicz LK. CD8highCD57+ T lymphocytes in normal, healthy individuals are oligoclonal and respond to human cytomegalovirus. *J Immunol* 1995; **155**: 5046–56.
178 Gillespie GM, Wills MR, Appay V *et al*. Functional heterogeneity and high frequencies of cytomegalovirus-specific CD8+ T lymphocytes in healthy seropositive donors. *J Virol* 2000; **74**: 8140–50.
179 Jin X, Demoitie MA, Donahoe SM *et al*. High frequency of cytomegalovirus-specific cytotoxic T-effector cells in HLA-A*0201-positive subjects during multiple viral coinfections. *J Infect Dis* 2000; **181**: 165–75.
180 Olsson J, Wikby A, Johansson B, Lofgren S, Nilsson BO, Ferguson FG. Age-related change in peripheral blood T-lymphocyte subpopulations and cytomegalovirus infection in the very old: the Swedish longitudinal OCTO immune study. *Mech Ageing Dev* 2000; **121**: 187–201.
181 Khan N, Shariff N, Cobbold M *et al*. Cytomegalovirus seropositivity drives the CD8 T cell repertoire toward greater clonality in healthy elderly individuals. *J Immunol* 2002; **169**: 1984–92.
182 Wikby A, Johansson B, Olsson J, Lofgren S, Nilsson BO, Ferguson F. Expansions of peripheral blood CD8 T-lymphocyte subpopulations and an association with cytomegalovirus seropositivity in the elderly: the Swedish NONA immune study. *Exp Gerontol* 2002; **37**: 445–53.
183 Longmate J, York J, La Rosa C *et al*. Population coverage by HLA class-I restricted cytotoxic T-lymphocyte epitopes. *Immunogenetics* 2001; **52**: 165–73.
184 Cwynarski K, Ainsworth J, Cobbold M *et al*. Direct visualization of cytomegalovirus-specific T-cell reconstitution after allogeneic stem cell transplantation. *Blood* 2001; **97**: 1232–40.
185 Gratama JW, van Esser JW, Lamers CH *et al*. Tetramer-based quantification of cytomegalovirus (CMV)-specific CD8+ T lymphocytes in T-cell-depleted stem cell grafts and after transplantation may identify patients at risk for progressive CMV infection. *Blood* 2001; **98**: 1358–64.
186 Lacey SF, Gallez-Hawkins G, Crooks M *et al*. Characterization of cytotoxic function of CMV-pp65-specific CD8+ T-lymphocytes identified by HLA tetramers in recipients and donors of stem-cell transplants. *Transplantation* 2002; **74**: 722–32.
187 Hsu VW, Yuan JG, Nuchtern K. A recycling pathway between the endoplasmic reticulum and the golgi apparatus for retention of unassembled MHC class I molecules. *Nature* 1991; **352**: 352–441.
188 Townsend A, Bodmer H. Antigen recognition by class I restricted T-lymphocytes. *Ann Rev Immunol* 1989; **7**: 601–24.
189 Benham A, Tulp A, Neefjes J. Synthesis and assembly of MHC-peptide complexes. *Immunol Today* 1995; **16**: 359–62.
190 Elliot T. How does TAP associate with MHC class I molecules? *Immunol Today* 1997; Aug.
191 Beersma MFC, Bijlmakers MJE, Ploegh HL. Human cytomegalovirus down-regulates HLA class I expression by reducing the stability of class I H chains. *J Immunol* 1993; **151**: 4455–64.
192 Warren ADD, Pj L, LKB. Human cytomegalovirus-infected cells have unstable assembly of major histocompatibility complex class I complexes and are resistant to lysis by cytotoxic T lymphocytes. *J Virol* 1994; **68**: 2822–9.
193 Yamashita Y, Shimokata K, Saga S. Rapid degradation of the heavy chain of class I major histocompatibility complex antigens in the endoplasmic reticulum of human cytomegalovirus-infected cells. *J Virol* 1994; **68**: 7933–43.
194 Jones TR, Hanson LK, Sun L. Multiple independent loci within the human cytomegalovirus unique sort region down-regulate expression of major. *J Virol* 1995; **69**: 4930–841.
195 Wiertz EJ, Tortorella D, Bogyo M *et al*. Sec61-mediated transfer of a membrane protein from the endoplasmic reticulum to the proteasome for destruction. *Nature* 1996; **384**: 432–8.

196 Tomazin R, Boname J, Hegde NR et al. Cytomegalovirus US2 destroys two components of the MHC class II pathway, preventing recognition by CD4+ T cells. Nat Med 1999; **5**: 1039–43.

197 Jones TR, Sun L. Human cytomegalovirus US2 destabilizes major histocompatibility complex class I heavy chains. J Virol 1997; **71**: 2970–9.

198 Gewurz BE, Gaudet R, Tortorella D, Wang EW, Ploegh HL. Virus subversion of immunity: a structural perspective. Curr Opin Immunol 2001; **13**: 442–50.

199 Hengle H, Flohr T, Hämmerline G, Koszinowski UH. Human cytomegalovirus inhibits peptide translocation into the endoplasmic reticulum for MHC class I assembly. J Gen Virol 1996; **77**: 2287–96.

200 Lehner PJ, Karttunen JT, Wilkinson GWG, Cresswell P. The human cytomegalovirus US6 glycoprotein inhibits transporter associated with antigen processing-dependent peptide translocation. Proc Natl Acad Sci U S A 1997; **94**: 6904–9.

201 York IA, Roop C, Andrews DW. A cytosolic herpes simplex virus protein inhibits antigen presentation to CD8+ T lymphocytes. Cell 1994; **77**: 525–35.

202 Beck S, Barrell GB. Human cytomegalovirus encodes a glycoprotein homologous to MHC class-I antigens. Nature 1988; **331**: 269–72.

203 Fujinami RS, Nelson JA, Walker L, Oldstone MA. Sequence homology and immunologic cross-reactivity of human cytomegalovirus with HLA-DR β chain: a means for graft rejection and immunosuppression. J Virol 1988; **62**: 100–5.

204 Grundy JE, McKeating JA, Ward PJ, Sanderson AR, Griffiths PD. β$_2$ microglobulin enhances the infectivity of cytomegalovirus and when bound to the virus enables class 1 HLA molecules to be used as a virus receptor. J Gen Virol 1987; **68**: 793–803.

205 Hassan-Walker AF, Cope AV, Griffiths PD, Emery VC. Transcription of the human cytomegalovirus natural killer decoy gene, UL18, in vitro and in vivo. J Gen Virol 1998; **79**(9): 2113–6.

206 Vitale M, Castriconi R, Parolini S et al. The leukocyte Ig-like receptor (LIR)-1 for the cytomegalovirus UL18 protein displays a broad specificity for different HLA class I alleles: analysis of LIR-1 + NK cell clones. Int Immunol 1999; **11**: 29–35.

207 Leong CC, Chapman TL, Bjorkman PJ et al. Modulation of natural killer cell cytotoxicity in human cytomegalovirus infection: the role of endogenous class I major histocompatibility complex and a viral class I homolog. J Exp Med 1998; **187**: 1681–7.

208 Odeberg J, Cerboni C, Browne H et al. Human cytomegalovirus (HCMV)-infected endothelial cells and macrophages are less susceptible to natural killer lysis independent of the downregulation of classical HLA class I molecules or expression of the HCMV class I homologue, UL18. Scand J Immunol 2002; **55**: 149–61.

209 Ulbrecht M, Martinozzi S, Grzeschik M et al. Cutting edge: the human cytomegalovirus UL40 gene product contains a ligand for HLA-E and prevents NK cell-mediated lysis. J Immunol 2000; **164**: 5019–22.

210 Tomasec P, Braud VM, Rickards C et al. Surface expression of HLA-E, an inhibitor of natural killer cells, enhanced by human cytomegalovirus gpUL40. Science 2000; **287**: 1031.

211 Wang EC, McSharry B, Retiere C et al. UL40-mediated NK evasion during productive infection with human cytomegalovirus. Proc Natl Acad Sci U S A 2002; **99**: 7570–5.

212 Vink C, Beisser PS, Bruggeman CA. Molecular mimicry by cytomegaloviruses. Function of cytomegalovirus-encoded homologues of G protein-coupled receptors, MHC class I heavy chains and chemokines. Intervirology 1999; **42**: 342–9.

213 Machold RP, Wiertz EJHJ, Jones TR, Ploegh HL. The HCMV gene products US11 and US2 differ in their ability to attack allelic forms of murine major histocompatibility complex (MHC) class I heavy chains. J Exp Med 1997; **185**: 363–6.

214 Gretch DR, Kari B, Rasmussen L, Gehrz RC, Stinski MF. Identification and characterization of three distinct families of glycoprotein complexes in the envelopes of human cytomegalovirus. J Virol 1988; **62**: 875–81.

215 Simpson JA, Chow JC, Baker J et al. Neutralizing monoclonal antibodies that distinguish three antigenic sites on human cytomegalovirus glycoprotein H have conformationally distinct binding sites. J Virol 1993; **67**: 489–96.

216 Van Zanten J, Lazzarotto T, Campisi B et al. Comparative immunoblot analysis with ten different, partially overlapping recombinant fusion proteins derived from five different cytomegalovirus proteins. New Microbiol 1995; **18**: 223–8.

217 Zaia JA, Forman SJ, Ting YP, Vanderwal-Urbina E, Blume KG. Polypeptide-specific antibody response to human cytomegalovirus after infection in bone marrow transplant recipients. J Infect Dis 1986; **153**: 780–7.

218 Snydman DR. Historical overview of the use of cytomegalovirus hyperimmune globulin in organ transplantation. Transpl Infect Dis 2001; **3** (Suppl. 2): 6–13.

219 Zaia JA. Cytomegalovirus infections. In: Thomas ED, Blume KG, Forman SF, eds. Hematopoietic Cell Transplantation. Malden, MA: Blackwell Scientific Publications, 1998: 560–83.

220 Couchoud C, Cucherat M, Haugh M, Pouteil-Noble C. Cytomegalovirus prophylaxis with antiviral agents in solid organ transplantation: a meta-analysis. Transplantation 1998, **65**. 641–7.

221 Zaia JA, Levin MJ, Leszczynski J, Wright GG, Grady GF. Cytomegalovirus immune globulin: production from selected normal donor blood. Transplantation 1979; **27**: 66–7.

222 Boeckh M, Bowden RA, Storer B et al. Randomized, placebo-controlled, double-blind study of a cytomegalovirus-specific monoclonal antibody (MSL-109) for prevention of cytomegalovirus infection after allogeneic hematopoietic stem cell transplantation. Biol Blood Marrow Transplant 2001; **7**: 343–51.

223 Dykewicz CA. Summary of the guidelines for preventing opportunistic infections among hematopoietic stem cell transplant recipients. Clin Infect Dis 2001; **33**: 139–44.

224 Riddell SR, Watanabe KS, Goodrich JM, Li CR, Agha ME, Greenberg PD. Restoration of viral immunity in immunodeficient humans by the adoptive transfer of T-cell clones. Science 1992; **257**: 238–41.

225 Walter EA, Greenberg PD, Gilbert MJ et al. Reconstitution of cellular immunity against cytomegalovirus in recipients of allogeneic bone marrow by transfer of T-cell clones from the donor. N Engl J Med 1995; **333**: 1038–44.

226 Lucas KG, Sun Q, Burton RL et al. A phase I–II trial to examine the toxicity of CMV- and EBV-specific cytotoxic T lymphocytes when used for prophylaxis against EBV and CMV disease in recipients of CD34-selected/T cell-depleted stem cell transplants. Hum Gene Ther 2000; **11**: 1453–63.

227 Kondo E, Topp MS, Kiem HP et al. Efficient generation of antigen-specific cytotoxic T cells using retrovirally transduced CD40-activated B cells. J Immunol 2002; **169**: 2164–71.

228 Einsele H, Roosnek E, Rufer N et al. Infusion of cytomegalovirus (CMV)-specific T cells for the treatment of CMV infection not responding to antiviral chemotherapy. Blood 2002; **99**: 3916–22.

229 Keenan RD, Ainsworth J, Khan N et al. Purification of cytomegalovirus-specific CD8 T cells from peripheral blood using HLA-peptide tetramers. Br J Haematol 2001; **115**: 428–34.

230 Maus MV, Thomas AK, Leonard DG et al. Ex vivo expansion of polyclonal and antigen-specific cytotoxic T lymphocytes by artificial APCs expressing ligands for the T-cell receptor, CD28 and 4-1BB. Nat Biotechnol 2002; **20**: 143–8.

231 Boland GJ, Vlieger AM, Ververs C, De Gast GC. Evidence for transfer of cellular and humoral immunity to cytomegalovirus from donor to recipient in allogeneic bone marrow transplantation. Clin Exp Immunol 1992; **88**: 506–11.

232 Plotkin SA. Cytomegalovirus vaccine development: past and present. In: Zaia JA, Hooper JA, eds. Pathogenesis of cytomegalovirus-associated diseases. Transplant Proc 1991; **23**: S85–9.

233 Gönczöl E, Ianacone J, Ho W, Starr S, Meignier B, Plotkin S. The isolated gA/gB glycoprotein complex of human cytomegalovirus envelope induces humoral and cellular immune-responses in human volunteers. Vaccine 1990; **8**: 130–6.

234 Pande H, Campo K, Tanamachi B, Forman SJ, Zaia JA. Direct DNA immunization of mice with plasmid DNA encoding the tegument protein pp65 of human cytomegalovirus induces high levels of circulating antibody to the encoded protein. Scan J Inf Dis 1995; **99**: 117–20.

235 Berencsi K, Rando RF, Plotkin SA et al. The N-terminal 303 amino acids of the human cytomegalovirus envelope glycoprotein B (UL55) and the exon 4 region of the major immediate early protein 1 (UL123) induce cytotoxic T-cell response. Vaccine 1996; **14**: 369–74.

236 Gallez-Hawkins G, Lomeli NA, Li X et al. Kinase-deficient CMVpp65 triggers a CMVpp65 specific T-cell immune response in HLA-A*0201.Kb transgenic mice after DNA immunization. Scand J Immunol 2002; **55**: 592–8.

237 Gregory WW, Menegus MA. Practical protocol for cytomegalovirus isolation. Use of MRC-5 cell monolayers incubated for 2 weeks. J Clin Microbiol 1983; **17**: 605–9.

238 Swenson PD, Kaplan MH. Rapid detection of cytomegalovirus in cell culture by indirect immunoperoxidase staining with monoclonal antibody to an early nuclear antigen. J Clin Microbiol 1985; **21**: 669–73.

239 Stirk PR, Griffiths PD. Use of monoclonal antibodies for the diagnosis of cytomegalovirus infection by the detection of early antigen fluorescent foci (DEAFF) in cell culture. J Med Virol 1987; **21**: 329–37.

240 Gleaves CA, Smith TF, Shuster EA, Pearson GR. Comparison of standard tube and shell vial cell culture techniques for the detection of cytomegalovirus in clinical specimens. J Clin Microbiol 1985; **21**: 217–21.

241 Zaia JA, Sissons JG, Riddell S et al. Status of cytomegalovirus prevention and treatment in 2000. *Hematology (Am Soc Hematol Educ Program)* 2000; pp. 339–55.

242 van der Bij W, Torensma R, van Son WJ. Rapid immunodiagnosis of active cytomegalovirus infection by monoclonal antibody staining of blood leukocytes. *J Med Virol* 1988; **25**: 179–88.

243 Grefte JMM, van der Gun BTF, Schmolke S. Cytomegalovirus antigenemia assay: identification of the viral antigen as the lower matrix protein pp65. *J Infect Dis* 1992; **166**: 683–4.

244 Gerna G, Zipeto D, Percivalle E. Human cytomegalovirus infection of the major leukocyte subpopulations and evidence for initial viral replication in polymorphonuclear leukocytes from viremic patients. *J Infect Dis* 1992; **166**: 1236–44.

245 van den Berg AP, van der Bij W, van Son WJ. Cytomegalovirus antigenemia as a useful marker of symptomatic cytomegalovirus infection after renal transplantation: a report of 130 consecutive patients. *Transplantation* 1989; **48**: 991–5.

246 Revello MG, Percivalle E, Zavattoni M, Parea M, Grossi P, Gerna G. Detection of human cytomegalovirus immediate early antigen in leukocytes as a marker of viremia in immunocompromised patients. *J Med Virol* 1989; **29**: 88–93.

247 Boland GJ, de Gast GC, Hene RJ. Early detection of active cytomegalovirus (CMV) infection after heart and kidney transplantation by testing for immediate early antigenemia and influence of cellular immunity of the occurrence of CMV infection. *J Clin Microbiol* 1990; **28**: 2069–75.

248 Boeckh M, Bowden RA, Goodrich JM, Pettinger M, Meyers JD. Cytomegalovirus antigen detection in peripheral blood leukocytes after allogeneic marrow transplantation. *Blood* 1992; **80**: 1358–64.

249 Boeckh M, Woogerd PM, Stevens-Ayers T. Factors influencing detection of quantitative cytomegalovirus antigenemia. *J Clin Microbiol* 1994; **32**: 832–4.

250 Koehler M, Rinaldo C, Neudorf SM. Prevention of CMV disease in allogeneic BMT recipients by cytomegalovirus antigenemia-guided preemptive ganciclovir therapy. *J Pediatr Hematol Oncol* 1997; **19**: 43–7.

251 Nicholson VA, Whimbey E, Champlin R et al. Comparison of cytomegalovirus antigenemia and shell vial culture in allogeneic marrow transplantation recipients receiving ganciclovir prophylaxis. *Bone Marrow Transplant* 1997; **19**: 37–41.

252 Myerson D, Hackman RC, Meyers JD. Diagnosis of cytomegalovirus pneumonia in *in situ* hybridization. *J Infect Dis* 1984; **150**: 272–7.

253 Dankner WM, McCutchan JA, Richman DD, Hirata K, Spector SA. Localization of human cytomegalovirus in peripheral blood leukocytes by *in situ* hybridization. *J Infect Dis* 1990; **161**: 31–6.

254 Stockl E, Popow-Kraupp T, Heinz FX, Hulbacher F, Balcke P, Kunz C. Potential of *in situ* hybridization for early diagnosis of productive cytomegalovirus infection. *J Clin Microbiol* 1988; **26**: 2536–40.

255 Demmler GJ, Buffone GJ, Schimbor CM, May RA. Detection of cytomegalovirus in urine from newborns by using polymerase chain reaction DNA amplification. *J Infect Dis* 1988; **158**: 1177–84.

256 Cassol SA, Poon M-C, Pal R. Primer-mediated enzymatic amplification of cytomegalovirus (CMV) DNA. *J Clin Invest* 1989; **83**: 1109–15.

257 Hsia K, Spector DH, Lawrie J, Spector SA. Enzymatic amplification of human cytomegalovirus sequences by polymerase chain reaction. *J Clin Microbiol* 1989; **27**: 1802–9.

258 Chow SN, Ouyang PC, Chu CT, Lee CY. Rapid and simple immunoassays for measurement of human chorionic gonadotropin using monoclonal antibodies. *J Formos Med Assoc* 1990; **89**: 792–8.

259 Chou S, Dennison KM. Analysis of interstrain variation in cytomegalovirus glycoprotein B sequences encoding neutralization-related epitopes. *J Infect Dis* 1991; **163**: 1229–34.

260 Einsele H, Steidle M, Vallbracht A, Saal JG, Ehninger G, Muller CA. Early occurrence of human cytomegalovirus infection after bone marrow transplantation as demonstrated by the polymerase chain reaction technique. *Blood* 1991; **77**: 1104–10.

261 Einsele H, Ehninger G, Steidle M. Polymerase chain reaction to evaluate antiviral therapy for cytomegalovirus disease. *Lancet* 1991; **2**: 1170–2.

262 Ishigaki S, Takeda M, Kura T, Ban N, Saitoh T. Cytomegalovirus DNA in the sera of patients with cytomegalovirus pneumonia. *Br J Haematol* 1991; **79**: 198–204.

263 Spector SA, Merrill R, Wolf D, Dankner WM. Detection of human cytomegalovirus in plasma of AIDS patients during acute visceral disease by DNA amplification. *J Clin Microbiol* 1992; **30**: 2359–65.

264 Aspin MM, Gallez-Hawkins GM, Giugni TD et al. Comparison of plasma PCR and bronchoalveolar lavage fluid culture for detection of cytomegalovirus infection in adult bone marrow transplant recipients. *J Clin Microbiol* 1994; **32**: 2266–9.

265 Gallez-Hawkins GM, Tegtmeier BR, Ter Veer A. Evaluation of a quantitative plasma PCR plate assay for detecting CMV infection in marrow transplant recipients. *J Clin Microbiol* 1997; **35**: 788–90.

266 Jiwa NM, Van Gemert GW, Raap AK. Rapid detection of human cytomegalovirus DNA in peripheral blood leukocytes of viremic transplant recipients by the polymerase chain reaction. *Transplantation* 1989; **48**: 72–6.

267 Boland GJ, de Weger RA, Tilanus MGJ, Ververs C, Bosboom-Kalsbeek K, de Gast GC. Detection of cytomegalovirus (CMV) in granulocytes by polymerase chain reaction compared with the CMV antigen test. *J Clin Microbiol* 1992; **30**: 1763–7.

268 Woo PC, Chan TK, Liang RH. Detection of CMV DNA in bone marrow transplant recipients: plasma versus leukocyte polymerase chain reaction. *J Clin Pathol* 1997; **50**: 231–5.

269 Mazzulli T, Drew LW, Yen-Lieberman B et al. Multicenter comparison of the digene hybrid capture CMV DNA assay version 2.0, the pp65 antigenemia assay, and cell culture for detection of cytomegalovirus viremia. *J Clin Microbiol* 1999; **37**: 958–63.

270 Blok MJ, Goossens VJ, Vanherle SJ et al. Diagnostic value of monitoring human cytomegalovirus late pp67 mRNA expression in renal-allograft recipients by nucleic acid sequence-based amplification. *J Clin Microbiol* 1998; **36**: 1341–6.

271 Blok MJ, Lautenschlager I, Goossens VJ et al. Diagnostic implications of human cytomegalovirus immediate early-1 and pp67 mRNA detection in whole-blood samples from liver transplant patients using nucleic acid sequence-based amplification. *J Clin Microbiol* 2000; **38**: 4485–91.

272 Avery RK, Adal KA, Longworth DL, Bolwell BJ. A survey of allogeneic bone marrow transplant programs in the United States regarding cytomegalovirus prophylaxis and preemptive therapy. *Bone Marrow Transplant* 2000; **26**: 763–7.

273 Betts RF, Freeman RB, Douglas RG Jr. Clinical manifestations of renal allograft derived primary cytomegalovirus infection. *Am J Dis Child* 1977; **131**: 759–63.

274 Zaia JA. Ganciclovir treatment of bone marrow transplant recipients with cytomegalovirus disease. In: SA Spector, ed. *Ganciclovir Therapy for Cytomegalovirus Infection*. New York: Marcel Dekker, Inc., 1991: 155–83.

275 Dummer JS, White LT, Ho M. The morbidity of cytomegalovirus infection in heart and heart-lung treatment recipients on cyclosporine. *J Infect Dis* 1985; **152**: 1182–91.

276 Rubin RB, Cosimi AB, Tolkoff-Rubin NE et al. Infectious disease syndromes attributable to cytomegalovirus and their significance among renal transplant recipients. *Transplantation* 1977; **24**: 458–64.

277 Jacobson MA, Mills J. Serious cytomegalovirus disease in the acquired immunodeficiency syndrome (AIDS). *Ann Intern Med* 1988; **108**: 585–94.

278 Zaia JA, Lang DJ. Cytomegalovirus infection of the fetus and neonate. *Neurol Clin* 1984; **2**: 387–410.

279 Klemola E. Cytomegalovirus infection in previously healthy adults. *Ann Intern Med* 1973; **79**: 267–8.

280 Grundy JE, Shanely JD, Griffith PD. Is cytomegalovirus interstitial pneumonitis in transplant recipients an immunopathological condition? *Lancet* 1987; **2**: 996–9.

281 D'Amico DJ, Talamo JH, Felsenstein D, Hirsch MS, Albert DM, Schooley RT. Ophthalmoscopic and histologic findings in cytomegalovirus retinitis treated with BW-B759U. *Arch Ophthalmol* 1986; **104**: 1788–93.

282 Group AR. Mortality in patients with the acquired immunodeficiency syndrome treated with either foscarnet or ganciclovir for cytomegalovirus retinitis. *N Eng J Med* 1992; **326**: 213–20.

283 Reed EC, Wolford JL, Kopecky KJ. Ganciclovir for the treatment of cytomegalovirus pneumonia. *Ann Intern Med* 1990; **112**: 505–10.

284 Boldogh I, AbuBakar S, Albrecht T. Activation of proto-oncogenes: an immediate early event in human cytomegalovirus infection. *Science* 1990; **247**: 561–4.

285 Mocarski ES Jr. Initial events involved in cytomegalovirus–cell interactions. In: JA Zaia, JA Hooper, eds. Pathogenesis of cytomegalovirus-associated diseases. *Transplant Proc* 1991; **23** (Suppl. 3): 43–7.

286 Sternberg RM, Stinski MF. Autoregulation of the human cytomegalovirus major immediate-early gene. *J Virol* 1985; **56**: 676–82.

287 Pizzorno M, O'Hara P, Sha L, LaFemina RL, Hayward GS. Transactivation and autoregulation of gene expression by the immediate-early region 2 gene products of human cytomegalovirus. *J Virol* 1988; **62**: 1167–79.

288 Hennighausen L, Fleckenstein B. Nuclear factor 1 interacts with five DNA elements in the promoter region of the human cytomegalovirus major immediate early gene. *EMBO J* 1986; **5**: 1367–71.

289 Hunninghake GW, Monick MM, Liu B, Stinski MF. The promoter-regulatory region of the major immediate-early gene of human cytomegalovirus responds to T-lymphocyte stimulation and contains

functional cyclic AMP-response elements. *J Virol* 1989; **63**: 3026–33.
290 Sambucetti LC, Cherrington JM, Wilkinson GWG, Mocarski ES. NF-kB activation of the cytomegalovirus enhancer is mediated by a viral transactivator and by T cell stimulation. *EMBO J* 1989; **8**: 4251–8.
291 Carney WP, Hirsch MS. Mechanisms of immunosuppressive in CMV mononucleosis. II. Virus–monocyte interactions. *J Infect Dis* 1981; **144**: 47–54.
292 Dudding LR, Garnett HM. Interaction of strain AD169 and a clinical isolates of cytomegalovirus with peripheral monocytes: the effect of lipopolysaccharide stimulation. *J Infect Dis* 1987; **155**: 891–6.
293 Ibanez E, Schrier R, Ghazal P. Human cytomegalovirus productively infects primary differentiated macrophages. *J Virol* 1991; **65**: 6581–8.
294 Rodgers BC, Scott DM, Mundin J, Sissons JGP. Monocyte-derived inhibitor of interleukin 1 induced by human cytomegalovirus. *J Virol* 1985; **55**: 527–32.
295 Kapasi K, Rice GPA. Cytomegalovirus infection of peripheral blood mononuclear cells: effects on interleukin-1 and -2 production and responsiveness. *J Virol* 1988; **62**: 3603–7.
296 Movassagh M, Gozlan J, Senechal B. Direct infection of CD34+ progenitor cells by human cytomegalovirus: evidence for inhibition of hematopoiesis and viral replication. *Blood* 1996; **88**: 1277–83.
297 Mori T, Ando K, Tanaka K, Ikeda Y, Koga Y. Fas-mediated apoptosis of the hematopoietic progenitor cells in mice infected with murine cytomegalovirus. *Blood* 1997; **89**: 3565–73.
298 Chiou SH, Liu JH, Hsu WM *et al*. Up-regulation of Fas ligand expression by human cytomegalovirus immediate-early gene product 2: a novel mechanism in cytomegalovirus-induced apoptosis in human retina. *J Immunol* 2001; **167**: 4098–103.

54

James I. Ito

Herpes Simplex Virus Infections

Introduction

Members of the herpesvirus family are the cause of significant morbidity and mortality in the post-hematopoietic cell transplantation (HCT) setting. They all possess the unique characteristics of latency and reactivation, and each virus emerges during a specific time period after transplantation. Herpes simplex virus (HSV) infections occur during the early, neutropenic or pre-engraftment period soon after the initiation of immunosuppressive therapy [1,2]. In the days prior to the use of antiviral prophylaxis, approximately 70% of HSV seropositive HCT recipients would shed the virus and, of these, 70% would develop HSV disease [3]. With the advent of acyclovir prophylaxis, the incidence of HSV disease has dropped below 5% [3–5]. But while the problem of HSV infection after HCT has substantially diminished in the early post-transplant period, HSV infection has shifted to the period after prophylaxis has ended, and the occurrence of acyclovir-resistant HSV strains has emerged.

Virology

HSVs, HSV-1 and HSV-2, belong to the group of human herpesviruses designated alphaherpesviruses. Varicella-zoster virus (VZV) rounds out this group. All herpesviruses are morphologically similar and consist of four components: (i) an electron-dense core containing viral DNA; (ii) an icosadeltahedral capsid consisting of 162 capsomeres; (iii) an amorphous layer of proteins surrounding the capsid called tegument; and (iv) a lipid envelope [6]. The HSV genome is a linear, double-stranded DNA molecule containing at least 152-kb pairs encoding at least 84 different polypeptides.

For viral replication to occur, infection of the human host cell must take place. HSV attaches to cell surface receptors, fuses its envelope to the plasma membrane, the capsid is de-enveloped and the DNA is transported to the nucleus. Viral replication then proceeds in the nucleus with transcription, DNA synthesis, capsid assembly, DNA packaging and envelopment. Synthesis of viral proteins takes place in three sequential periods designated α (immediate-early), β (early) and γ (late). The α proteins shut off host protein synthesis and initiate synthesis of β proteins. The β proteins are responsible for viral nucleic acid metabolism and are the main target of current antiviral therapy. These include viral DNA polymerase and viral thymidine kinase. The antiviral drug acyclovir, for example, is a nucleoside analog that is a substrate for the HSV thymidine kinase. Acyclovir is selectively phosphorylated by HSV-infected cells to acyclovir-monophosphate. It is then phosphorylated by host cellular enzymes to acyclovir-triphosphate, a competitive inhibitor of the viral DNA polymerase. Acyclovir-triphosphate is incorporated into the growing viral DNA chain causing chain termination. Resistance to acyclovir occurs because of spontaneously arising mutations (at a frequency of 10^{-4}) in the viral thymidine kinase or DNA polymerase genes. The γ proteins are the structural components of the virion. A more detailed description of the virology of HSV can be found in recent reviews [6].

Pathogenesis and immunology

HSV possesses two unique properties that it shares with the other alphaherpesvirus, VZV: neurotropism and latency. These two related characteristics explain a great deal of the pathogenesis and pathology of HSV infection and disease.

HSV infection begins after close contact of a susceptible individual with someone excreting virus. This usually involves exposure to HSV at mucosal surfaces or abraded skin. For HSV-1, it is usually the oral mucosa, and for HSV-2, it is usually the genital mucosa. However, either virus type can infect at the other site. Viral replication takes place at these mucosal sites and progresses to the sensory or autonomic nerve endings [7]. Virus is then transported intra-axonally to the nerve cell bodies in the dorsal root ganglia [8]. For oral HSV-1 infection, this usually results in trigeminal ganglion infection, and for HSV-2 genital infection, this usually produces sacral nerve root ganglia (S2–S5) infection. Virus continues to replicate in these ganglia and in contiguous neural tissues, and then can spread to other mucosal or skin surfaces through centrifugal migration via peripheral sensory nerves.

After primary infection resolves, a state of latency is established. During latency, infectious HSV can no longer be recovered from the ganglia, but viral DNA can be recovered from some ganglion cells. The viral genome remains in an episomal state for the life of the infected human host. The mechanism(s) whereby latency is established and maintained is not understood. Latency allows the virus to survive in a sequestered state not vulnerable to the inhibitory effects of antiviral agents or the host's immune system.

What the property of latency allows is subsequent reactivation of virus. Again, the mechanism whereby reactivation occurs is not known. But a number of stimuli have been closely associated with reactivation: physical or emotional stress, fever, exposure to ultraviolet (UV) light, tissue damage and immune suppression. These are all (if one substitutes radiation therapy for UV light) present during the early phase of HCT. It is likely that tissue damage and the repair process may have a greater influence on reactivation than immune suppression.

The immunologic response to primary and reactivation infection involves both humoral and cell-mediated immune responses. It is assumed that the more crucial immune response is the cell-mediated response since agammaglobulinemic patients handle HSV infection well, and the presence of neutralizing antibody does not prevent reactivation. Also, patients with T-cell immune deficiencies (transplant recipients, human immunodeficiency virus (HIV)-infected persons, congenital T-cell-deficient patients) tend to have more widespread, invasive and disseminated disease. In animal models, it appears that T cells play the major role in preventing dissemination of HSV [9], although antibodies can reduce the viral titers. Monoclonal antibodies have been shown to protect animals against HSV challenge and reduced subsequent disease and latency [10,11]. Other cell populations (CD4 and CD8 T lymphocytes, natural killer (NK) cells, macrophages) and various cytokines also play a role in limiting and terminating infection [12].

HSV is capable of modulating and subverting the host immune response. Programmed death (apoptosis) of a virus-infected cell is one host response intended to prevent spread of virus to uninfected cells. HSV has been shown to prevent apoptosis in differentiated cells. HSV can also prevent the immune activation of $CD8^+$ cytotoxic T lymphocytes. It does this via the $\alpha 47$-gene product (ICP-47), which induces retention of the major histocompatibility complex (MHC) class 1 molecules in the cytoplasm, resulting in a lack of peptide presentation on the cell surface [13].

HSV immunology in the HCT recipient

Almost all of the components of both the innate immune system and the adaptive immune system are deficient after the conditioning regimen for HCT is administered [14]. It is probably the combination of the stimuli of mucosal damage, induced by the cytotoxic agents of the conditioning regimen and global, but primarily T-cell-mediated immune deficiency, that is responsible for the high reactivation rate seen after HCT. Certainly the more severe and invasive HSV infections that occur in the early transplantation period are related to a cellular immunodeficiency. Virtually all HSV infection in HCT is due to reactivation and not primary infection. In one early study, 62 (82%) of 76 seropositive patients but only one (1.5%) of 65 seronegative patients developed HSV infection [1]. Approximately 80% of seropositive immunocompetent persons have a positive lymphocyte proliferation response to HSV antigens with a mean lymphocyte stimulation index of 10.4. This compares to only 7% of seronegative persons with a mean stimulation index of $1.5 \times$ control. Of note, patients pre-HCT have similar lymphocyte stimulation index profiles, although the mean lymphocyte stimulation index of seropositive patients is lower, i.e. 4.5. Immediately after HCT, the lymphocyte response to HSV drops in these seropositive recipients. However, after day 40, the lymphocyte response returns to pretransplant levels. This return of response occurred in those who developed HSV reactivation and it was not related to the immune status of the donor. Seronegative recipients continued to show no HSV specific lymphocyte response. Thus, it appears that the return of specific lymphocyte-mediated immunity to HSV requires exposure to antigen in the form of reactivation infection, and that passively transferred donor immune lymphocytes are insufficient to establish immune reactivity in the recipient.

It was also observed that acyclovir treatment of HSV infection after HCT was associated with a delay in restoration of the lymphocyte response [15], and that this delay in HSV-specific immune reconstitution was manifested clinically as more frequent HSV recurrences as well as a shorter interval between recurrences in those treated with acyclovir. In this regard, in an oral acyclovir prophylaxis study, seropositive patients on acyclovir had a significantly lower lymphocyte response than those on placebo within the first 7 weeks of HCT [5]. This response slowly improved until it matched the placebo group at 3 months after transplantation. This was reflected in a 68% incidence of HSV reactivation in the placebo group compared to a 21% incidence in the acyclovir prophylaxis group during the 4-week prophylaxis period. Ultimately, however, after acyclovir was stopped, 58% of the prophylaxis group had HSV infection. Thus, in recipients undergoing prophylaxis, there may be a delay in HSV-specific immune reconstitution.

Epidemiology

As virtually all HSV disease occurring in the HCT setting is due to reactivation, the serologic status of the recipient determines risk for disease and, therefore, the requirement for prophylaxis. The likelihood of any one patient being HSV-1 or -2 seropositive is proportionate to a number of factors including age, geographic origin, socioeconomic status, race and, in the case of HSV-2, past sexual activity. However, once the transplantation process is initiated, these factors have no bearing on the risk of reactivation, although other factors do, such as the type and severity of the cytotoxic conditioning regimen.

HSVs have a worldwide distribution and there are no animal vectors or reservoirs. HSV-1 infection is more prevalent and acquired earlier in life than HSV-2.

HSV-1

Primary HSV-1 infections usually occur in young children under the age of 5 years and are usually asymptomatic. The seroprevalence of HSV-1 slowly increases with age until a 90% rate is achieved by the 5th decade of life [16]. Prevalence of HSV-1 antibody correlates with socioeconomic status and with higher prevalence in the lower socioeconomic groups [17]. In the USA, African-Americans appear to acquire HSV-1 earlier in life, but the prevalence rates in the white population becomes similar to the African-American rates (90%) by the 5th decade of life [16].

HSV-2

Antibodies to HSV-2 appear later in life than HSV-1 antibodies. They begin to appear in puberty and correlate with past sexual activity. The HSV-2 seroprevalence of adults in the USA is approximately 22% [18] and represents a significant increase over the previous two decades. In the USA, there is an ethnic difference in seroprevalence of HSV-2 antibody with 25% in white women, 20% in white men, 80% in African-American women and 60% in African-American men [18]. Thus, it is highly likely that an adult candidate for HCT will be seropositive for HSV-1 and fairly likely to be seropositive for HSV-2.

Epidemiology of HSV infection in the HCT recipient

Prior to the use of antiviral prophylaxis, 82% of seropositive patients reactivated infection after HCT [1]. The median time to infection was during the 3rd week post-HCT. Only 1.5% of seronegative patients had HSV infection. Approximately 90% of infections involved the oral mucous membranes, while 6% involved the genital area.

Since the advent of antiviral prophylaxis, the incidence of HSV infection has diminished and shifted to a later time period. While on prophylaxis, few patients, 0% and 21%, respectively, in two separate studies, reactivated HSV infection compared to those on placebo (70% and 68%, respectively) [3,5]. However, in one study, when prophylaxis was discontinued after 4 weeks, 38% of treated seropositive patients reactivated at a median time of 8 weeks after stopping drug [5]. In another study, where prophylaxis was administered for 18 days, 70% (7 out of 10) of seropositive patients on prophylaxis reactivated at a median time of 25 days after cessation of the drug [3]. Five (71%) of these patients developed symptomatic skin lesions while two (29%) had asymptomatic shedding.

Clinical manifestations

Prior to the antiviral prophylaxis era, the majority (92%) of HSV reactivations presented as oropharyngeal or orofacial lesions, and only 6% presented as genital eruption [1]. Two (3%) had esophageal involvement and two (3%) had lung involvement following oropharyngeal infection. In the prophylaxis era it appears that the distribution is 85% oropharyngeal and 15% genital presentation [19], possibly reflecting the relatively higher acyclovir resistance of HSV-2 compared to HSV-1. However, HSV infection now occurs predominantly after prophylaxis cessation. In addition, the infections are probably less severe [3,5].

Oropharyngeal HSV infection can be confused with the mucositis that frequently occurs after conditioning therapy for HCT (see Plates 23.2 and 23.3, *facing p. 296*). The painful mucosal ulcerations appear similar. The pain suffered by the patient can become a major management problem, but the damage done to the oral mucosa can lead to portals of entry and sites of infection for bacteria (*Viridans streptococci*) and fungi (*Candida*). It can also lead to extension of infection into the esophagus and lung. But, again, with prophylaxis, the severity of oropharyngeal reactivation is much less. Oral labial and facial reactivation is less likely to be confused with regimen-induced mucositis. Also, although the cutaneous lesions are usually classically appearing herpetic lesions, presenting as clusters of vesicular lesions, they can be quite severe and extensive, especially in someone who is not receiving or has not received antiviral prophylaxis. Genital HSV infection usually presents as patches of vesicular lesions in or around the genital area. It can appear in the rectum, perianal area and the buttocks and hips. If it occurs unilaterally it can be confused with VZV infection. This differentiation becomes important as these two infections are treated differently. HSV-2 can also present as a cystitis or urethritis.

Oropharyngeal HSV infection can spread contiguously to the esophagus and the lungs. HSV esophagitis can be severe and, clinically, it cannot be distinguished from cytomegalovirus (CMV) (see Plates 23.34 and 23.35, *facing p. 296*) or *Candida* esophagitis. Morphologically, HSV infection can be distinguished from *Candida* esophagitis upon endoscopic inspection, but it requires a biopsy to distinguish it from CMV infection. HSV can also cause disease further down the gastrointestinal tract, including the small intestine [20] (see Plate 23.36, *facing p. 296*) and colon [21]. It is not clear, however, whether lower gastrointestinal tract involvement is due to the extension of higher tract infection or blood-borne dissemination, or whether it is even the primary etiology of disease at these sites as other etiologies (CMV, *Clostridium difficile*, graft-vs.-host disease) are often coexistent.

HSV pneumonia probably results as an extension of oropharyngeal infection and usually presents as an interstitial pneumonitis. HSV interstitial pneumonitis has a high fatality rate [22] and does not appear to have changed in the era of prophylaxis [23]. Also, it does not appear that the acyclovir-resistant strains of HSV are any less virulent in the lung. One also has to be careful with regard to attributing pneumonia to HSV when the patient may have an ongoing oropharyngeal reactivation and the bronchoscopically obtained specimen is contaminated by virus in the upper airway or aspirated virus in the lung (see the Diagnosis section, below).

HSV hepatitis is fairly rare. In one series, eight cases were found over a 14-year period in a transplantation population base of 3000 [24]. HSV hepatitis probably represents true HSV dissemination as multiple organ involvement was found in the majority of cases. Also, HSV-2 has been reported to cause fulminant hepatitis in early HCT despite antiviral prophylaxis [25]. The mortality rate was 100% in this small series [24]. Cases from the preprophylaxis era occurred before day 20, while those who received prophylaxis did not develop disease until after day 40. Common presenting signs and symptoms included fever, abdominal pain, and elevated serum transaminase levels. Fulminant hepatitis was also seen.

HSV encephalitis is a rare complication after HCT. It occurs in the general population with a frequency of 1 : 250,000–1 : 500,000 persons per year, and does not appear to be more common in HCT [26]. The clinical presentation consists of acute onset of fevers and focal, primarily temporal lobe, neurologic signs and symptoms.

Diagnosis

Diagnosis of HSV infection relies upon both clinical and laboratory criteria. A clinical diagnosis of cutaneous HSV infection can be made when clumps of vesicular lesions on an erythematous base near or around the perioral or genital areas are present. However, there may be difficulty in differentiating HSV infection from VZV infection if these lesions appear to be unilateral and in a limited dermatomal distribution, e.g. a cluster of lesions on the hip or on one side of the face. In the past, rapid diagnosis of cutaneous lesions was made with adequate scrapings of fresh, early lesions examined microscopically after Giemsa (Tzanck preparation), Wright or Papanicolaou staining. The demonstration of intranuclear inclusions and/or giant cells confirmed a diagnosis of herpesvirus infection. But these staining techniques do not differentiate between HSV or VZV and, therefore, the preferred test is for HSV (and VZV) antigens or DNA. These scrapings can be submitted for antigen detection by direct fluorescent antibody (DFA), peroxidase or enzyme-linked (EIA) methods. These are highly specific and sensitive tests if the specimens are obtained early in newly erupted lesions. Polymerase chain reaction (PCR) can be used to detect HSV DNA in swabs or scrapings from mucocutaneous lesions.

The standard of diagnosis of HSV infection is virus isolation. The positive culture will also provide the laboratory with an isolate that can subsequently be tested for antiviral resistance. Culture for HSV is recommended when acyclovir resistance is suspected, e.g. emergence of infection during acyclovir prophylaxis. Clinical specimens submitted for culture should be transported on ice and immediately inoculated into a cell culture system. Cytopathic effect may develop within 24–48 h, but definitive identification may take from 48 to 96 h. A more rapid cultural technique is the spin-amplified culture, or shell vial, technique with subsequent staining for specific HSV antigen. The turnaround time for this method can be less than 24 h.

A tissue biopsy is usually required to make a diagnosis of visceral HSV infection (see Plate 23.36, *facing p. 296*). The tissue should be submitted for culture and histologic examination. The demonstration of tissue pathology is important in differentiating between HSV disease and HSV excretion and contamination.

A positive culture from bronchioalveolar lavage fluid can result from contamination of the fluid from oropharyngeal excretion rather from the pneumonia. Likewise a positive culture from tissue or fluid obtained from the esophagus or stomach during an endoscopic procedure might also have come from oropharyngeal excretion of HSV.

The standard of diagnosis for HSV encephalitis is isolation of the virus from brain tissue. However, the current method of choice is the much less invasive test of HSV DNA determination by PCR of cerebrospinal fluid [27].

In the post-HCT setting, serologic testing for HSV specific antibody is of very little use. What defines reactivation and infection is detection of HSV in specimens from mucous membranes and tissue. Antibody testing in the HCT candidate is useful in determining past-HSV exposure. It is only the seropositive patient who is likely to reactivate HSV infection after HCT, defining those at risk for reactivation during HCT and, therefore, the optimal candidate for anti-HSV prophylaxis (see below). Moreover, it has been reported that the risk of HSV reactivation is proportional to the pretransplant HSV immunoglobulin G titer [28].

Table 54.1 Prophylaxis and treatment guidelines for herpes simplex virus (HSV) infections in hematopoietic cell transplantation (HCT).

Drug	Route	Dose	Interval
Prophylaxis:			
Acyclovir	IV	250 mg/m^2 or 5 mg/kg	q. 12 h
Acyclovir	p.o.	200 mg	t.i.d.
Valacyclovir	p.o.	500 mg	q.d.
Treatment:			
Acyclovir	IV	250 mg/m^2 or 5 mg/kg	q. 8 h
Acyclovir	p.o.	400 mg	5×/day
Valacyclovir	p.o.	500–1000 mg	b.i.d.
Famciclovir	p.o.	500 mg	b.i.d.
For visceral or disseminated disease:			
Acyclovir	IV	500 mg/m^2 or 10 mg/kg	q. 8 h
For acyclovir-resistant HSV:			
Foscarnet	IV	40–60 mg/kg	q. 8 h
For acyclovir/foscarnet-resistant HSV:			
Cidofovir	IV	5 mg/kg	weekly × 2, then q. 2 weeks

b.i.d., twice daily; IV, intravenous; p.o., *per os* (oral administration); t.i.d., three times daily; q.d., four times daily.

Treatment

The drug of choice for the treatment of HSV mucocutaneous infection in the HCT recipient is acyclovir (Table 54.1). It is usually given intravenously but can be given orally if the patient is capable of taking and absorbing the oral formulation. An early study demonstrated that intravenous acyclovir shortened the time to resolution of pain, crusting of lesions, total healing and excretion of virus [29]. Unfortunately, recurrent infection was more common in the acyclovir-treated group. This study is the basis for the current standard of therapy: 250 mg/m^2 acyclovir (or 5 mg/kg) intravenously (IV) every 8 h for at least 7 days. A study of oral acyclovir therapy for mucocutaneous HSV infections in HCT recipients demonstrated similar benefits [30]. Acyclovir was given as 400 mg orally five times a day for 10 days. The choice of oral vs. intravenous therapy is based on the ability to take oral medications and on the severity of disease. Newer oral drugs that result in higher serum levels can probably also be used although they have not been studied extensively in HCT patients. These include valacyclovir, a prodrug of acyclovir, and famciclovir, a prodrug of penciclovir. Valacyclovir is administered at 500–1000 mg orally three times a day for 7 days while famciclovir is administered at 500 mg orally three times a day for 7 days. If the patient has more severe, visceral, disseminated, or central nervous system disease, acyclovir at 10 mg/kg (or 500 mg/m^2) IV every 8 h is recommended.

If infection with acyclovir-resistant HSV is suspected or proven, the drug of choice is foscarnet, a nonthymidine kinase-dependent agent. It is given at 40 mg/kg IV every 8 h. For more severe or visceral involvement, 60 mg/kg every 8 h is recommended. The major and limiting toxicity of foscarnet is nephrotoxicity, making it very difficult to use in the HCT setting. Recently, there have been reports of HSV strains resistant to both acyclovir and foscarnet [31–33]. In such cases, cidofovir has shown some benefit and is recommended at 5 mg/kg IV once weekly times two doses, then once every 2 weeks. But this drug is also nephrotoxic.

Prophylaxis

Acyclovir prophylaxis should be offered to all HSV-seropositive allogeneic recipients to prevent HSV reactivation during the early post-transplant period. This is the recommendation of the Centers for Disease Control and Prevention, the Infectious Disease Society of America and the American Society for Blood and Marrow Transplantation [34]. The recommended regimen is either acyclovir 200 mg orally three times a day or acyclovir 250 mg/m^2 IV every 12 h. It is also recommended that acyclovir be started at the beginning of conditioning therapy and continue until engraftment or until mucositis resolves, i.e. approximately 30 days after HCT for allogeneic HCT recipients. The duration of acyclovir prophylaxis can be extended beyond 30 days for persons with "frequent recurrent HSV." A recommended alternative to acyclovir is valacyclovir. If a patient is already receiving ganciclovir, acyclovir is not necessary. If a patient is placed on long-term (i.e. 1 year) prophylaxis for VZV reactivation prophylaxis, there should be no break between the end of HSV and the end of VZV prophylaxis.

Despite this strong recommendation and the fact that most HCT centers use HSV prophylaxis, the decision to use universal prophylaxis is not without controversy. Furthermore, the duration of prophylaxis varies among centers. Although antiviral prophylaxis has clearly been shown to dramatically reduce the incidence of viral shedding and disease during the period of prophylaxis, reactivation and disease still occurs after prophylaxis has ended [3–5]. If the duration of prophylaxis is extended much beyond the recommended 30 days to either 75 days or 6 months, there appears to be fewer reactivations and less severe disease [28,35,36]. Also, prophylaxis not only delays reactivation but also delays immunologic reactivity to HSV antigens and specific immune reconstitution to this virus [5]. Whether this delay is detrimental or beneficial to the HCT recipient is unknown. Another argument for prophylaxis is the observation that resistant virus often emerges in the treatment setting but rarely in the prophylactic setting [5,37]. There may be other benefits of using HSV prophylaxis in the HCT setting. Meyers *et al.* [38] demonstrated a significant decrease in CMV infection and disease and significantly improved survival in those HCT recipients given high doses (500 mg/m^2 every 8 h) of intravenous acyclovir prophylaxis until 30 days after HCT. However, others using lower doses (250 mg/m^2) of acyclovir could demonstrate no effect on the frequency of CMV infections [36]. A more recent study demonstrated that valacyclovir was even more effective as a CMV-prophylactic agent when given after the initial intravenous/high-dose acyclovir prophylaxis [39]. There were also fewer HSV infections in the valacyclovir group vs. the acyclovir group (7% and 10%, respectively), but the difference was not significant. There have also been reports of earlier engraftment in patients receiving acyclovir prophylaxis [5], but this has not been confirmed by others [40,41].

The ultimate preventive measure is the development of a vaccine that will prevent primary HSV infection in the general population. Preferably it would be a killed, subunit, replication-defective viral or naked DNA vaccine, as a live vaccine would have the unknown potential of reactivating during HCT. Work is in progress [42], but there will be no effective vaccine in the near future, and it will not be of help to those who are already seropositive. It is unlikely that a vaccine could ever prevent HSV reactivation in the profoundly immunocompromised seropositive population of HCT recipients.

Conclusions

Since the inception of acyclovir prophylaxis, the incidence of HSV reactivation and disease has dramatically decreased during the early period of HCT. However, prophylaxis has resulted in a delay of HSV-specific immune reconstitution, and reactivation now occurs during a later period in HCT. However, severe, visceral and disseminated HSV infection still occurs and demands rapid and specific diagnosis in order to initiate effective therapy, and, although resistant virus is less likely to occur under prophylactic conditions, it still remains a significant problem in treating patients with HSV infection after HCT.

References

1 Meyers JD, Flournoy N, Thomas ED. Infection with herpes simplex virus and cell-mediated immunity after marrow transplantation. *J Infect Dis* 1980; **142**: 338–46.
2 Meyers JD. Infections in marrow recipients. In: Mandell GL, Douglas RG, Bennett JE, eds. *Principles and Practice of Infectious Diseases*, 2nd edn. New York: John Wiley & Sons, 1984: 1674–6.
3 Saral R, Burns WH, Laskin OL, Santos GW, Lietman PS. Acyclovir prophylaxis of herpes simplex virus infections: a randomized, double-blind controlled trial in bone marrow transplant recipients. *N Engl J Med* 1981; **305**: 63–7.
4 Gluckman E, Lotsberg J, Devergie A et al. Prophylaxis of herpes infections after bone marrow transplantation by oral acyclovir. *Lancet* 1983; **2**(8352): 706–8.
5 Wade JC, Newton B, Flournoy N, Meyers JD. Oral acyclovir for prevention of herpes simplex reactivation after marrow transplantation. *Ann Intern Med* 1984; **100**: 823–8.
6 Whitley RJ. Herpes simplex viruses. In: Fields BN, Knipe DM, Howley PM, Griffin DE, eds. *Fields Virology*, 4th edn. Philadelphia: Lippincott, Williams & Wilkins, 2001: 2461–509.
7 Stanberry LR, Kern ER, Richards JT et al. Genital herpes in guinea pigs: pathogenesis of primary infection and description of recurrent disease. *J Infect Dis* 1983; **146**: 397–404.
8 Bastian FO, Rabson AS, Yee CL, Tralka TS. Herpesvirus hominis: isolation from human trigeminal ganglion. *Science* 1972; **178**: 306–7.
9 Kapoor AK, Nash AA, Wildy P et al. Pathogenesis of herpes simplex virus in congenitally athymic mice: the relative roles of cell-mediated and humoral immunity. *J General Virol* 1982; **60**: 225–33.
10 Balachandran N, Bacchetti S, Rawls WE. Protection against lethal challenge of BALB/c mice by passive transfer of monoclonal antibodies to five glycoproteins of herpes simplex virus type-2. *Infect Immun* 1982; **37**: 1132–7.
11 Eisenberg R, Cerini CP, Heilman CJ et al. Synthetic glycoprotein D-related peptides protect mice against herpes simplex virus challenge. *J Virol* 1985; **55**: 1014–7.
12 Manickan E, Rouse BT. Role of different T-cell subsets in control of herpes simplex virus infection determined by using T-cell-deficient mouse models. *J Virol* 1995; **69**: 8178–9.
13 York IA, Roop C, Andrews DW et al. A cytosolic herpes simplex virus protein inhibits antigen presentation to CD8+ T lymphocytes. *Cell* 1994; **77**: 525–35.
14 Storek J, Witherspoon RP. Immunologic reconstitution after hematopoietic stem cell transplantation. In: Atkinson K, ed. *Clinical Bone Marrow and Blood Stem Cell Transplantation*. Cambridge, UK: Cambridge University Press, 2000: 111–46.
15 Wade JC, Day LM, Crowley JJ, Meyers JD. Recurrent infection with herpes simplex virus after marrow transplantation. Role of the specific immune response and acyclovir treatment. *J Infect Dis* 1984; **149**: 750–6.
16 Nahmias AJ, Lee FK, Bechman-Nahmias S. Sero-epidemiological and sociological patterns of herpes simplex virus infection in the world. *Scand J Infect Dis* 1990; **69**: 19–36.
17 Rawls WE, Iwamoto K, Adam E, Melnick JL. Measurement of antibodies to herpesvirus type 1 and 2 in human sera. *J Immunol* 1970; **104**: 599–606.
18 Fleming DT, McQuillan GM, Johnson RE et al. Herpes simplex virus type 2 in the United States, 1976–94. *N Engl J Med* 1997; **337**: 1105–11.
19 Sable CA, Donowitz GR. Infections in bone marrow transplant recipients. *Clin Infect Dis* 1994; **18**: 273–84.
20 Kingreen D, Nitsche A, Beyer J, Siegert W. Herpes simplex infection of the jejunum occurring in the early post-transplantation period. *Bone Marrow Transplant* 1997; **20**: 989–91.
21 Naik HR, Chandrasekar PH. Herpes simplex virus (HSV) colitis in a bone marrow transplant recipient. *Bone Marrow Transplant* 1996; **17**: 285–6.
22 Ramsey PG, Fife KH, Hackman RC, Meyers JD, Corey L. Herpes simplex virus pneumonia. *Ann Intern Med* 1982; **97**: 813–20.
23 Ljungman P, Ellis MN, Hackman RC, Shepp DH, Meyers JD. Acyclovir-resistant herpes simplex virus causing pneumonia after marrow transplantation. *J Infect Dis* 1990; **162**: 244–8.
24 Johnson JR, Egaas S, Gleaves CA, Hackman R, Bowden RA. Hepatitis due to herpes simplex virus in marrow-transplant recipients. *Clin Infect Dis* 1992; **14**: 38–45.
25 Gruson D, Hilbert G, Le Bail B, Portel L, Boiron JM, Reiffers J, Gbikpi-Benissan G. Fulminant hepatitis due to herpes simplex virus-type 2 in early phase of bone marrow transplantation. *Hematol Cell Ther* 1998; **40**: 41–4.
26 Whitley RJ. Viral encephalitis. *N Engl J Med* 1990; **323**: 242–50.
27 Lakerman FD, Whitley RJ, the National Institute of Allergy and Infectious Diseases Collaborative Antiviral Study Group. Diagnosis of herpes simplex encephalitis: application of polymerase chain reaction 50 cerebrospinal fluid from brain biopsied patients and correlation with disease. *J Infect Dis* 1995; **171**: 857–63.
28 Lundgren G, Wilczek H, Lonnqvist B, Lindholm A, Wahren B, Ringden O. Acyclovir prophylaxis in bone marrow transplant recipients. *Scand J Infect Dis* 1985; **47** (Suppl.): 137–44.
29 Wade JC, Newton B, McLaren C, Flournoy N, Keeney RE, Meyers JD. Intravenous acyclovir to treat mucocutaneous herpes simplex virus infection after marrow transplantation: a double-blind trial. *Ann Intern Med* 1982; **96**: 265–9.
30 Shepp DH, Newton BA, Dandliker PS, Flournoy N, Meyers JO. Oral acyclovir mucocutaneous herpes simplex virus infections in immunocompromised marrow transplant recipients. *Ann Intern Med* 1985; **102**: 783–5.
31 Bryant P, Sasadeusz J, Carapetis J, Waters K, Curtis N. Successful treatment of foscarnet-resistant herpes simplex stomatitis with intravenous cidofovir in a child. *Pediatr Infect Dis J* 2001; **20**: 1083–6.
32 Blot N, Schneider P, Young P, Janvresse C, Dehesdin D, Tron P, Vannier JP. Treatment of an acyclovir and foscarnet-resistant herpes simplex virus infection with cidofovir in a child after an unrelated bone marrow transplant. *Bone Marrow Transplant* 2000; **26**: 903–5.
33 Darville JM, Ley BE, Roome AP, Foot AB. Acyclovir-resistant herpes simplex virus infections in a bone marrow transplant population. *Bone Marrow Transplant* 1998; **22**: 587–9.
34 Center for Disease Control and Prevention. Guidelines for preventing opportunistic infections among hematopoietic stem cell transplant recipients: recommendations of the CDC, the Infectious Disease Society of America, and the American Society of Blood and Marrow Transplantation. *MMWR* 2000; **49** (RR-10): 15–16.
35 Shepp DH, Dandliker PS, Fournoy N, Meyers JD. Sequential intravenous and twice-daily oral acyclovir for extended prophylaxis of herpes simplex virus infection in marrow transplant patients. *Transplantation* 1987; **43**: 654–8.
36 Ljungman P, Wilczek H, Gahrton G et al. Long-term acyclovir prophylaxis in bone marrow transplant recipients and lymphocyte proliferation responses to herpesvirus antigens *in vitro*. *Bone Marrow Transplant* 1986; **1**: 185–92.
37 Wade JC, McLaren C, Meyers JD. Frequency and significance of acyclovir-resistant herpes simplex virus isolated from marrow transplant patients receiving multiple courses of treatment with acyclovir. *J Infect Dis* 1983; **48**: 1077–82.
38 Meyers JD, Reed EC, Shepp DH et al. Acyclovir for prevention of cytomegalovirus infection and disease after allogeneic marrow transplantation. *N Engl J Med* 1988; **318**: 70–5.
39 Ljungman P, de la Camara R, Milpied N et al. Randomized study of valacyclovir as prophylaxis against cytomegalovirus reactivation in recipients of allogeneic bone marrow transplants. *Transplantation* 2002; **99**: 3050–6.
40 Perren TJ, Powles RL, Easton D, Stolle K, Selby PS. Prevention of herpes zoster in patients by longer-term oral acyclovir after allogenic bone marrow transplantation. *Am J Medical* 1988; **85** (*Suppl. 2A*): 99–101.
41 Lundgren G, Wilczek H, Lonnqvist B, Lindholm A, Wahren B, Ringden O. Acyclovir prophylaxis in bone marrow transplant recipients. *Scan J Infect Dis* 1985; **47**: 137–44.
42 Whitley RJ, Roizman B. Herpes simplex viruses: is a vaccine tenable? *J Clin Invest* 2002; **109**: 145–51.

55

Ann M. Arvin

Varicella-Zoster Virus Infections

Introduction

Varicella-zoster virus (VZV), like other pathogens of the herpesvirus family, can cause severe infections in hematopoietic cell transplantation (HCT) recipients [1,2]. As in other immunodeficient patients, serious VZV disease after transplantation is related to the compromise of T-lymphocyte function [3,4]. VZV infections are encountered in HCT patients who are experiencing their initial contact with the virus or who have recurrent disease due to the reactivation of latent virus. Primary VZV infection is manifest clinically as varicella or "chicken pox", in which the exposure of a susceptible individual, who has not had previous VZV infection, to the virus results in systemic symptoms of fever and malaise, and a characteristic vesicular rash. After primary infection, VZV establishes latency in cells of the dorsal root ganglia. Serum immunoglobulin G (IgG) antibodies to VZV provide evidence of a past primary infection and indicate that the individual is latently infected with the virus. The reactivation of endogenous latent VZV usually causes herpes zoster, in which the vesicular eruption appears in a localized, dermatomal distribution. Recurrent VZV infection also presents as atypical, nonlocalized herpes zoster in HCT recipients that cannot be distinguished from varicella by its clinical manifestations.

In addition to describing the clinical patterns of VZV infection after HCT, significant progress has been made towards understanding viral pathogenesis and the host response to VZV among HCT recipients. Fortunately, most disease caused by either primary or recurrent VZV infection, when recognized promptly, can now be treated effectively with antiviral therapy.

The virus

VZV is a member of the alphaherpesvirus subgroup of the herpesvirus genus. It is an enveloped virus that has a double-stranded DNA genome that is surrounded by an icosahedral capsid [5,6]. VZV DNA contains approximately 125,000 base pairs, arranged as long unique and short unique segments, each of which contains terminal repeat sequences. The VZV genome has coding regions for at least 70 distinct genes. Information about most of the *VZV* gene products is limited, but VZV proteins regulate viral gene transcription during replication and form the viral capsid, tegument and virion envelope structures. Probable functions for some VZV proteins have been deduced from homologies with herpes simplex virus, type 1 (HSV-1), which is the prototype of the alphaherpesvirus subgroup. Like HSV, replication of VZV usually involves synthesis and activation of a viral thymidine kinase which makes the virus susceptible to inhibition by the antiviral agent, acyclovir. Since the thymidine kinase is not required for VZV replication, mutant strains that do not express this antiviral target can be selected by exposure to the drug. The viral glycoproteins, gB, gC, gE, gH and gI, as well as viral proteins with structural and regulatory functions, including the IE4, IE62 and IE63 proteins, are known to be targets of the host response following VZV infection.

Epidemiology

Primary VZV infection

Primary VZV infection, or varicella, is much less common than disease caused by VZV reactivation during the 1st year after HCT, accounting for only about 5% of VZV infections in this population. The lower incidence of varicella is due to the fact that more than 85% of individuals in the USA have had primary VZV infection by 8 years of age as a result of the annual varicella epidemics that occur in this and other temperate regions of the world. Nevertheless, if an HCT recipient has never had VZV infection before, the attack rate for varicella after close exposure to an index case will reflect the risk of transmission to any susceptible individual, defined as an individual who has not been infected previously. Attack rates range from about 30% with classroom exposure to 90% with household contact. Direct contact with lesions is not required since, in contrast to other herpesviruses, VZV is transmissible by the respiratory route. The incidence of primary VZV infection is higher in pediatric HCT recipients and, as expected, the risk correlates inversely with the age of the child. In one series, 10 of 54 children (18%) with VZV infections after HCT had primary VZV infection demonstrated serologically [6]. Although 25 adult patients presented with a disseminated cutaneous VZV exanthem, only two patients had serologic evidence of primary VZV infection [1]. While the possibility of reinfection cannot be eliminated in some cases, the epidemiologic evidence suggests that patients who have been infected previously are usually protected against infection following a new VZV exposure, presumably because VZV IgG titres are maintained despite immunosuppressive disease or therapies. The addition of the varicella vaccine to the routine childhood immunization schedule has reduced the extent of the annual epidemics, making it less likely that HCT recipients who have no pre-existing immunity to VZV will be exposed to varicella and making it more likely that pediatric HCT recipients will have vaccine-induced immunity to VZV.

Recurrent VZV infection

The reported incidence of recurrent VZV infection after HCT ranges from 23% to 59% [1,6–22] (Table 55.1 [1,7,8,10–13, 18–20, 23]). This incidence is higher than that observed among organ transplant recipients,

Table 55.1 Incidence of varicella-zoster virus (VZV) infections following hematopoietic cell transplantation (HCT).

Year [ref.]	Underlying disease	Transplant type	n	VZV infection (%)	Localized zoster (%)	Atypical zoster (%)	Varicella (%)
1980 [8]	Leukemia	Allogeneic/syngeneic	33	21			
1982 [10]	Leukemia/aplastic anemia	Allogeneic/syngeneic	98	52			
1985 [1]	Leukemia/aplastic anemia	Allogeneic	1394	17	85	15	0
1986 [11]	Hematological malignancy	Allogeneic	73	36	91	7	2
1989 [7]	Leukemia/solid tumors	Autologous	236	23	75	13	18*
1989 [12]	Leukemia/lymphoma	Autologous	153	28	77	20	2
1991 [13]	Hodgkin's diseaese	Autologous	28	32	100	0	0
1992 [23]	Leukemia/lymphoma/other	Autologous/allogeneic	51	31	100	0	0
2000 [18]	Leukemia/other	Allogeneic	100	41	100	0	
2000 [19]	Leukemia/other	Allogeneic	151	38	100	0	
2001 [20]	Leukemia/lymphoma/other	Autologous	164	15.8	92	4	4

*This study evaluated pediatric patients only.

which is about 7%, but it is comparable to rates of VZV reactivation in patients with Hodgkin's disease receiving combined modality therapy. For purposes of comparison, the estimated annual incidence of herpes zoster in adults without underlying disease is 0.5% [18].

The reactivation of herpesviruses follows a predictable temporal pattern after HCT [2,24,25]. HSV-1 causes clinically apparent disease at about 2–3 weeks and cytomegalovirus (CMV) disease usually occurs during the 2nd to 3rd month after transplantation. Epstein–Barr virus (EBV) may also reactivate in the 3rd month whereas VZV recurrences present at a median of 5 months after HCT. In general, the risk of recurrent VZV infection is highest between 2 and 10 months after transplantation, although cases have been reported within the 1st week and continue to occur after the 1st year (Fig. 55.1 [1]). Locksley et al. [1] found that 80% of patients who developed VZV infection following HCT had disease within 9 months. When options for antiviral therapy were limited, 21% of these patients had visceral dissemination of the virus and 12% died from complications of recurrent VZV. In a review of 100 consecutive patients who received allogeneic HCT between 1992 and 1997, 41% developed VZV reactivation at a median of 227 days (range 45–346 days) [18]. Of these episodes, 12% occurred in the first 100 days; the attack rate was 59% among patients who survived for at least 2 years.

Factors that are associated with higher rates of VZV reactivation following HCT include genotypic nonidentity for human leukocyte antigen (HLA) between donor and recipient, and acute or chronic graft-vs.-host disease (GVHD), which are linked variables [10,19]. In one series, 64% of patients whose donor was HLA nonidentical had herpes zoster compared to 44% of HCT recipients with matched donors and no GVHD. The risk of late VZV infection was increased fourfold (Table 55.2 [9]). In a second series, patients with a limited chronic GHVD had a lower incidence of VZV reactivation compared with those with extensive chronic GVHD [18]. The presence of nonspecific suppressor cells associated with chronic GVHD correlated with a higher risk of recurrent VZV (Table 55.2) [10]. A CD4 T-cell count <200 cells/μL and a CD8 T-cell count <800 cells/μL at 30 days after transplantation correlated with an increased risk of zoster within the 1st year [20]. The cumulative evidence indicates that patients undergoing allogeneic or autologous HCT have about the same overall risk of recurrent VZV disease (Table 55.1). In one study, 28% of autologous transplant patients developed recurrent VZV infection [12]. The initial manifestation of recurrence was localized dis-

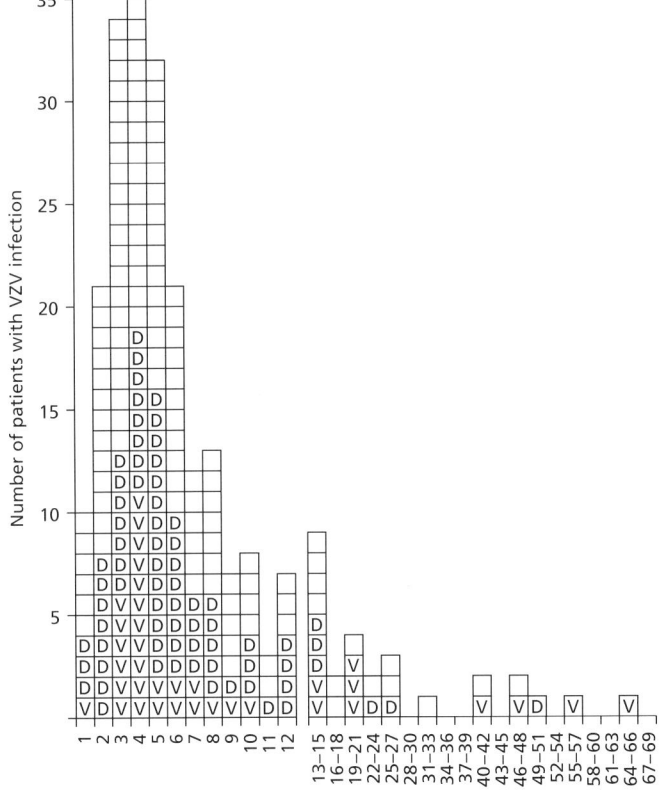

Fig. 55.1 Varicella-zoster virus (VZV) infections by month after marrow transplantation. (□) uncomplicated herpes zoster; (V) varicella; (D) herpes zoster with subsequent dissemination. Reproduced with permission of the Chicago University Press from Locksley et al. [1].

ease in 77% of these patients while 23% had atypical nonlocalized zoster, which is comparable to the distribution of these clinical syndromes among allogeneic HCT recipients. In a pediatric HCT population, 23% of children given an autologous HCT had VZV disease at a median interval of 3 months after transplant but this series also included patients with

Table 55.2 Risk of recurrent varicella-zoster virus (VZV) infection after hematopoietic cell transplantation (HCT) in relation to human leukocyte antigen (HLA) matching of recipient and donor and the occurrence of graft-versus-host disease (GVHD) in the recipient. Adapted from Atkinson et al. [9].

	HLA Identical				
		With GHVD			
	No GHVD	No Suppressor Cells	With Suppressor Cells	HLA Nonidentical	Syngeneic
No. of patients	25	21	19	14	19
Late VZV infections	24%	38%	47%	36%	11%
VZV at any time	44%	57%	79%	64%	21%

Nonspecific suppressor cells were detected in cocultures with donor lymphocytes, assessing their effect on the proliferation responses to alloantigens or concanavalin-A.

primary VZV infection [7]. Thirty-two percent of patients who received an autologous HCT for Hodgkin's lymphoma had VZV infection [13], which is consistent with experience in Hodgkin's and non-Hodgkin's lymphoma patients [26]. The somewhat higher incidence of zoster in lymphoma patients may account for the fact that patients who receive autologous HCT have rates of VZV reactivation that are similar to those in allogeneic HCT recipients even though GVHD is less common. Morbidity and mortality caused by VZV infection after autologous HCT cannot be compared with the original analyses of VZV-related disease after allogeneic HCT because antiviral therapy was available when the studies of autologous HCT patients were done. In the series by Schuchter et al. [12], 15% of autologous HCT recipients had cutaneous dissemination, 5% had visceral dissemination and 25% had morbidity, including post-herpetic neuralgia and neurologic dysfunction.

The underlying disease that provides the indication for HCT probably does not influence VZV reactivation. However, a history of symptomatic herpes zoster before marrow transplantation was associated with a higher risk of early post-transplant VZV disease among Hodgkin's disease patients undergoing autologous HCT [13]. VZV reactivation has not been found to predict relapse of the underlying disease in HCT recipients [7].

Reinfection with VZV

Although symptomatic reinfection with VZV is extremely rare among immunocompetent individuals [27], it probably occurs occasionally among severely immunocompromised patients who had primary VZV infection previously. However, this hypothesis is difficult to confirm because the distinction between atypical nonlocalized herpes zoster and reinfection requires a comparison of the VZV isolates causing the initial infection and the new episode by DNA sequence analysis. Based on clinical criteria only, children with leukemia have been reported to have second episodes of varicella following close contact despite a past history of varicella and serologic evidence of pre-existing immunity. Nevertheless, anecdotal experience suggests that exposure of HCT patients who have had past primary VZV infection rarely causes any clinically apparent signs of reinfection [2].

Mechanisms of pathogenesis and viral immune evasion

Primary VZV infection

While several phases of viral replication are likely to occur during the 10–21 day incubation period, events during primary VZV infection have been difficult to document with laboratory methods. The epidemiologic evidence suggests that infection is initiated by the inoculation of respiratory mucosal sites [5,28]. Infectious virus is then presumed to be transported to regional lymphoid tissue, possibly undergoing a phase of local replication at these sites. VZV causes a cell-associated viremia, which appears to target T lymphocytes, although the possibility that other mononuclear cells become infected has not been definitively eliminated. Recent studies demonstrate that tonsillar T cells are highly permissive for VZV infection, suggesting that VZV could be transferred efficiently from respiratory epithelial cells into these local T-cell-rich tissues as a first stage of spread within the naive host [29]. Cell-associated viremia has been demonstrated late in the incubation period, just before and after the appearance of varicella skin lesions. VZV was isolated by viral culture from 24% of samples of peripheral blood mononuclear cells (PBMCs) taken within 24 h after the onset of rash [30]. Cell-associated VZV viremia was detected by in situ hybridization with a probe for VZV DNA, which showed viral DNA in lymphocytic cells, and by polymerase chain reaction (PCR) testing for viral DNA in PBMC specimens from 67% of otherwise healthy subjects tested immediately after the appearance of skin lesions [31,32]. VZV infection of tonsillar T lymphocytes was enhanced in activated, memory CD4 T lymphocytes that expressed skin homing markers, which suggests that cell-associated viremia may be particularly associated with T-lymphocyte infection [29]. When the cutaneous exanthem develops, VZV replication in epithelial cells may amplify viremia by transfer of infectious virus into migrating T-lymphocyte populations, leading to secondary "crops" of skin lesions. These observations about the pathogenesis of primary VZV infection suggest that the efficiency with which cell-associated viremia and replication at skin sites is terminated, either by the host response or by antiviral therapy, is likely to influence the extent of the cutaneous exanthem and the risk of visceral dissemination.

The study of VZV pathogenesis in animal models has been hampered by the restricted replication of the virus in nonhuman species. Mice that have inherited severe combined immunodeficiency syndrome (SCID) can be used to support grafts of human tissues that differentiate to contain the usual human cell populations. These animals, which are referred to as SCID-hu mice, provide an unique opportunity to examine VZV–cell interactions in intact human tissues independently of the effects of the host immune response on viral replication [33,34]. Conditions in the model are similar to those in the period immediately after bone marrow transplantation, since VZV-specific immunity is absent. Experiments in the SCID-hu mouse model demonstrate that VZV infects CD4+ and CD8+ human T lymphocytes, proving that VZV shares pathogenic mechanisms that are characteristic of the lymphotropic as well as the neurotropic herpesviruses (Figs 55.2 & 55.3 [33,34]). The tropism of VZV for human T cells and its infectivity for skin are both essential elements of its pathogenicity in human disease but comparative analyses of VZV strains demonstrate that these tropisms are mediated by different virulence determinants. For example, the VZV strain used to make the live attenuated varicella vaccine, the vaccine Oka

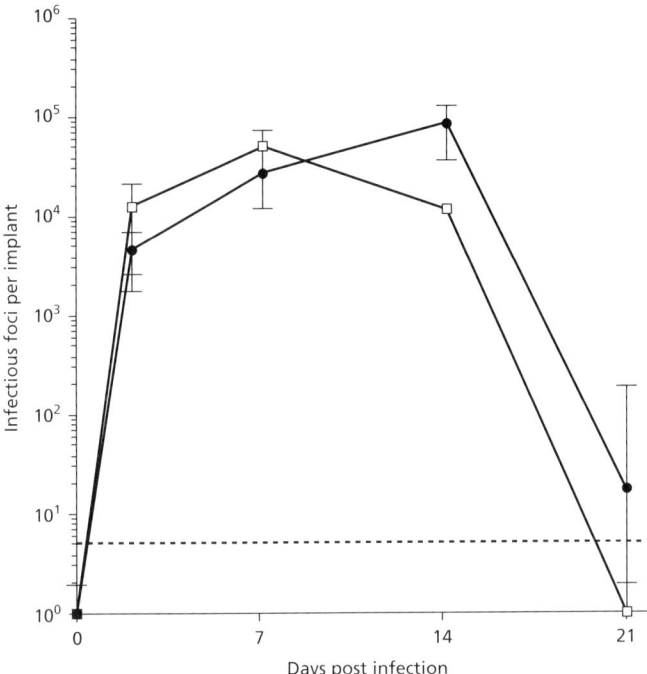

Fig. 55.2 Replication of varicella-zoster virus (VZV) in thy/liv implants. The number of infectious foci per implant was determined by titration of infected lymphocytes on Vero cell monolayers. The titre of the inoculum of infected MRC-5 cells from four experiments is shown at day 0. The scattergraph (panel A) shows the total number of infectious foci for each thy/liv implant infected with wildtype (□) and Oka (●) strains of VZV. Panel B shows the geometric means of the scatter data; the bars represent the SE of the mean. Only positive samples were used to calculate the data shown for day 14. Dotted lines represent the level of detection of the assay. Reproduced with permission from Moffat et al. [33].

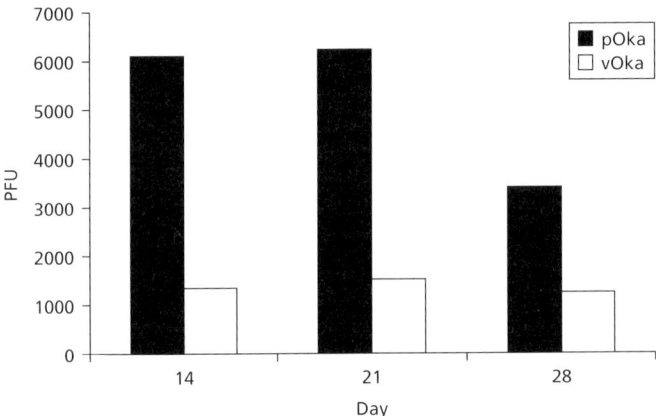

Fig. 55.3 Infectious virus in varicella-zoster virus (VZV)-infected skin implants. Implants were inoculated with P-Oka (■) or V-Oka (□) and harvested 14, 21 or 28 days after infection. Cell-associated virus was measured in an infectious focus assay and plaque-forming units per implant was calculated. Error bars indicate the SE of the mean. On day 21, all differences between strains were statistically significant ($p = 0.02$, student's t-test). Reproduced with permission from Moffat et al. [33].

strain, was indistinguishable from low passage VZV in its infectivity for CD4+ and CD8+ T cells (Fig. 55.2), whereas its pathogenic potential in human skin was reduced substantially compared to the parent Oka strain, as assessed by the extent of the cutaneous lesions, viral protein synthesis, infectious virus yields and release of infectious virus (Fig. 55.3). Investigations of VZV and HSV-1 replication in the SCID-hu model also revealed significant differences in cell tropisms that correlate with clinical observations about their pathologic effects in intact and immunocompromised individuals. In SCID-hu mice, VZV caused extensive necrosis in deeper dermal layers of skin implants, but HSV-1 was confined to the epidermis. In contrast to VZV, HSV-1 was not infectious for human CD4+ or CD8+ T cells, which is consistent with the clinical differences, since primary HSV infection is not associated with viremia in the intact host. HCT recipients and other immunocompromised patients are also susceptible to cell-associated viremia when VZV reactivates, whereas HSV viremia is a rare occurrence during recurrent HSV infection even with intensive immunosuppression.

Recurrent VZV infection

The hypothesis that VZV becomes latent in sensory ganglia following primary infection and that herpes zoster is caused by its reactivation from latency was proved by using restriction enzyme analysis to demonstrate that a single VZV strain caused both varicella and a subsequent episode of herpes zoster in a child with Wiskott–Aldrich syndrome [35]. During the primary attack, VZV is postulated to pass centripetally from the skin to the corresponding ganglia; hematologic seeding of the ganglia secondary to cell-associated viremia is also possible. Once in the ganglia, VZV establishes latency, apparently without viral replication and without causing cell damage. In contrast to HSV, infectious VZV has not been recovered from ganglion tissue by explant culture or cocultivation techniques. However, the presence of VZV nucleic acid sequences has been documented in human ganglia taken at autopsy from individuals with no evidence of recent VZV infection [6,36–40]. Multiple VZV RNA sequences have been detected by *in situ* hybridization and PCR, in contrast to HSV in which only limited gene transcription has been identified in latently infected neurons. Latent infection appears to be more common in the trigeminal ganglion than in any of the thoracic ganglia [38]. Investigations using molecular probes for VZV DNA sequences and methods to detect viral proteins indicate that the virus persists in both neuronal and satellite cells, although neuronal infection appears to predominate [6,37]. The protein encoded by the immediate early gene, *IE63*, appears to be made in latently infected human ganglia, confirming observations made in the rat model of VZV neurotropism [37,41,42]. The maintenance of VZV latency, as defined by the absence of symptomatic VZV reactivation, is also influenced directly by the host response to VZV, as is evident from the high incidence of VZV reactivation after HCT when VZV immunity is impaired. Although HSV reactivation causes little or no damage to ganglion cells, VZV reactivation is associated with extensive viral replication in the affected ganglia, producing pathologic changes including necrosis, inflammation and destruction of neural cell bodies.

In contrast to HSV, CMV and EBV, which can be recovered from asymptomatic patients by viral culture methods, technical problems have interfered with the detection of subclinical VZV reactivation. Episodes of subclinical VZV reactivation, consisting of cell-associated viremia in HCT recipients detected by VZV PCR, were documented in 19% of patients tested at a mean of 94 days after transplantation [43]. Disseminated VZV infection has been diagnosed at autopsy in HCT patients who had no cutaneous lesions [1,44,45]. However, testing PBMCs with the VZV PCR assay provided the first virologic evidence that these severely immunocompromised patients can experience VZV reactivation in the absence of clinically apparent cutaneous infection and resolve the infection without developing signs of visceral dissemination. Herpes zoster, like recurrent HSV, has been attributed to the spread of the reactivated virus along neural pathways from the site of latency in dorsal root ganglia. Some immunodeficient patients with localized herpes zoster develop VZV viremia, presumably because PBMCs become infected at the site of local cutaneous replication [46]. Subclinical, cell-associated viremia in HCT patients without cutaneous disease suggests that the virus also may be taken up directly by circulating lymphocytes at the neuronal site of viral reactivation. This mechanism for causing viremia could account for the clinical observation of atypical, generalized herpes zoster in some HCT recipients. Since the activation of T lymphocytes makes this cell population more permissive for VZV infection *in vitro* [29], cell-associated VZV viremia in HCT patients may be potentiated by the characteristic persistence of activated T lymphocytes in circulation for a prolonged period after transplant [47].

Viral immune evasion

Like many viruses, VZV has mechanisms to inhibit recognition by the host immune system. Abendroth and colleagues have found that VZV causes a significant reduction of the cell surface expression of major histocompatibility complex (MHC) class I protein on infected fibroblasts and on infected T cells, as demonstrated in the SCID-hu model [48]. Although their synthesis was not affected, MHC class I molecules were retained in the Golgi in VZV-infected cells. This effect may enable the virus to evade CD8+ T-cell immune recognition during VZV pathogenesis, including the critical phase of T-lymphocyte-associated viremia. In related experiments, Abendroth and colleagues showed that VZV has the capacity to block the up-regulation of MHC class II protein that is usually induced when cells are exposed to interferon-gamma (IFN-γ) [49]. Induction of MHC class I expression is required for recognition of virus-infected cells by antiviral CD4 T cells. When skin biopsies of varicella lesions were analyzed by *in situ* hybridization, MHC class II RNA transcripts were detected in cells near the lesion but not in cells that were infected with VZV. VZV infection inhibited transcription of interferon regulatory factor 1 (IRF-1) in the IFN-γ signaling pathway and expression of Stat1a and Jak2 proteins. The inhibition of MHC class II expression on VZV-infected cells *in vivo*, may transiently protect cells from CD4 T-cell immune surveillance, facilitating local virus replication during the first few days of cutaneous lesion formation during primary or recurrent VZV infection, and could allow a period of viral replication in skin cells even when the host has VZV-specific CD4 T cells.

The host response

Primary VZV infection is associated with the development of virus-specific IgG and IgM antibodies and the acquisition of cellular immunity, which can be demonstrated by proliferation of PBMCs that are stimulated with VZV antigens *in vitro*. Although VZV IgG antibodies can neutralize virus infectivity and function in antibody-mediated cellular cytotoxicity, humoral immunity seems to be less important in the host response to VZV than cell-mediated immunity. Progressive varicella occurs in immunocompromised children despite the production of VZV IgG and IgM antibodies whereas these children fail to develop VZV-specific T-lymphocyte proliferation [50]. Immunocompromised patients, including HCT recipients, develop VZV reactivation in spite of high concentrations of circulating antibodies to VZV. No quantitative relationship between VZV antibody titres in the donor or the recipient and the subsequent development of herpes zoster has been established in HCT patients [51]. However, periods of diminished VZV-specific T-lymphocyte proliferation have been correlated with an increase in susceptibility to herpes zoster among immunocompromised patient populations, including HCT recipients. In the individual patient, the loss of T-cell proliferation to VZV is a necessary, but not a sufficient condition for symptomatic reactivation [52]. Conversely, VZV-specific T-lymphocyte proliferation has been correlated with a decreased risk of herpes zoster.

Analyses of VZV-specific cell-mediated immunity have demonstrated a gradual recovery of T-cell proliferation to VZV antigens, with a larger

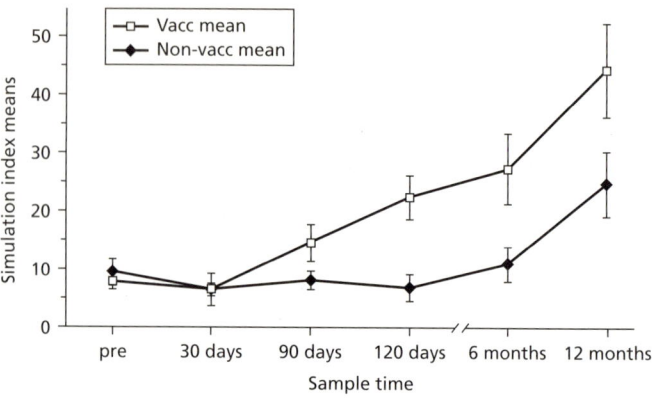

Fig. 55.4 CD4 T-cell proliferation in response to varicella-zoster virus (VZV) antigen. T-cell proliferation in response to VZV antigen, measured as the stimulation index (SI) is shown as the mean SI (*y* axis) for vaccinated (□) and unvaccinated (♦) participants; the time of immunologic evaluation is shown on the *x*-axis in relation to time of hematopoietic cell transplantation (HCT). Inactivated varicella vaccine was given pretransplant, and at 30, 60 and 90 days; the SI for vaccinees at 30 days represents responses after the pretransplant dose; at 90 days, three doses had been given, and at 120 days, 6 months and 12 months, vaccinees had received four doses. The error bars represent SEs. The number of patients tested at each time point were: pretransplantation, 58 unvaccinated/53 vaccinated; 30 days, 50 unvaccinated/49 vaccinated; 90 days, 43 unvaccinated/42 vaccinated; 120 days, 34 unvaccinated/39 vaccinated; 6 months, 30 unvaccinated/34 vaccinated; 12 months, 27 unvaccinated/33 vaccinated. Reproduced with permission from Hata *et al.* [26].

percentage of HCT patients having detectable responses as the interval following transplant increases [3,11,43,53,54]. The interval to recovery may be somewhat shorter in autologous HCT recipients [55]. This reconstitution of cell-mediated immunity to VZV antigens is generally observed by 9–12 months after HCT, which correlates with the time when VZV reactivation and susceptibility to severe VZV disease become less common. In HCT patients, IFN-γ production was associated with the recovery of T-cell proliferation to VZV antigen and increased with time following transplantation. Interleukin 10 (IL-10) production by PBMCs stimulated with VZV antigen was also observed consistently after HCT and was highest in patients who recovered T-cell proliferation to VZV antigen [53].

When VZV T-cell proliferation responses were followed prospectively in unvaccinated patients in a study of inactivated varicella vaccine, autologous transplant patients had a mean VZV stimulation index (SI) of 9.9 ± 2.32 within 30 days before transplantation, responses were undetectable at 30 days, and then increased to 8.0 ± 1.63 by 90 days; mean responses continued to increase over the 1st year (Figs 55.4 & 55.5 [26]). Evaluation of VZV immunity at 6 months after transplantation, using a quantitative flow cytometry method, showed that the frequencies of CD4 T cells that made tumor necrosis factor-alpha (TNF-α) in response to VZV stimulation was 0.19%, compared to 0.30% in VZV immune adults without underlying disease; the mean percentage of CD4 T cells that made IFN-γ was 0.11%, which was equivalent to frequencies in healthy adults [26,56] (Fig. 55.5). These analyses excluded patients who developed herpes zoster, indicating that VZV-specific T-cell responses can recover either as a result of subclinical VZV reactivation, as documented by VZV PCR testing of HCT recipients who had no signs of infection, or through reexpansion of memory T-cell populations that persisted through the preparative regimen for transplantation [43]. In this prospective study, the risk of zoster was reduced by 19% per unit increase in SI >1.6; a SI >5.0 correlated with >93% protection [26]. Pretransplant immunity in both the donor and the recipient may facilitate the reconstitution of VZV specific cell mediated immunity [57].

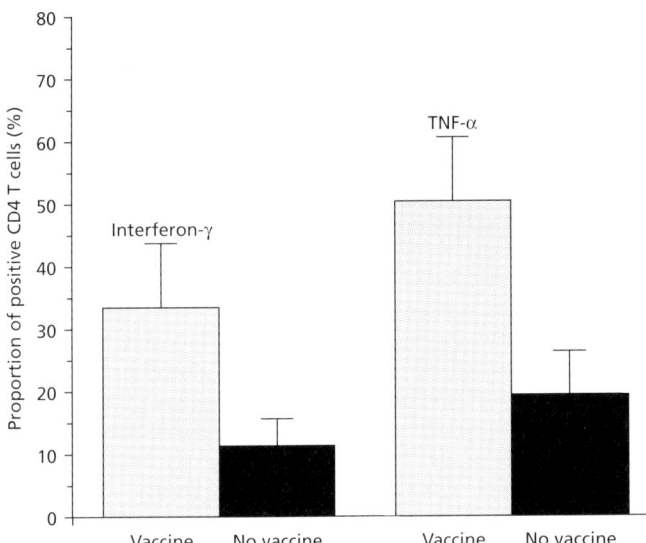

Fig. 55.5 Intracellular production of interferon-gamma (IFN-γ) or tumor necrosis factor-alpha (TNF-α) in T cells incubated with varicella-zoster virus (VZV). The percentage of CD4+ T cells that expressed CD69 and intracellular cytokine, IFN-γ (■) or TNF-α (□), was determined at 6 months after hematopoietic cell transplantation (HCT) in 19 vaccinated and 19 unvaccinated patients. Results are shown as mean percent responder cells ± SE. Differences in VZV-specific responder cell frequencies in vaccinated and unvaccinated subjects were analyzed by unpaired t-test; for CD4+ CD69+ and IFN-γ, $p = 0.07$, and for TNF-α, $p = 0.03$. Reproduced with permission from Hata et al. [26].

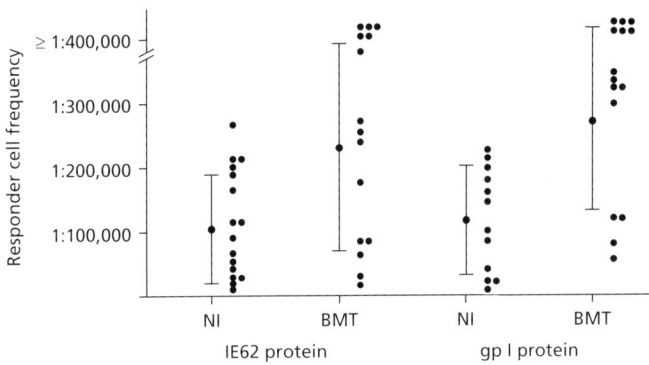

Fig. 55.6 Precursor frequencies of cytotoxic T lymphocytes (CTLs) specific for the immediate early protein (IE62) and glycoprotein I (gp I) of varicella-zoster virus (VZV) in bone marrow transplant recipients and healthy subjects. The mean + SD for precursor frequency estimates are indicated next to the individual data points (●) generated by testing individual HCT recipients and healthy immune subjects. Reproduced with permission from Wilson et al. [43].

Nevertheless, it is apparent that the recovery of virus-specific cellular immunity is delayed for months and recovery of VZV-specific T-cell immunity often does not occur until after the patient has had an episode of herpes zoster, which provides *in vivo* reexposure to VZV antigens. Meyers et al. [3] detected T-lymphocyte proliferation to VZV in 16 of 18 patients (89%) following symptomatic recurrences of VZV compared to 15 of 29 patients (51%) who did not develop herpes zoster. When herpes zoster occurs, HCT recipients show an increase in VZV-specific CD4 T-cell proliferation. Hata and colleagues found that the mean SI response before onset of herpes zoster was 2.2 ± 0.4 compared to 28.1 ± 6.68 when the episode of VZV reactivation had resolved [26], which is likely to explain why HCT recipients are usually not susceptible to repeated episodes of herpes zoster.

During the 1st year, HCT patients recover cytotoxic T cells that recognize and lyse autologous target cells expressing VZV proteins [43]. Fifty percent of HCT patients showed recovery of VZV-specific cytotoxic T-lymphocyte (CTL) function when tested at a mean of 155 days after transplant (Fig. 55.6 [43]). However, the mean precursor frequency of T lymphocytes that recognized the VZV IE62 protein or glycoprotein E (formerly designated gp I) was more than twofold lower among HCT recipients than the frequency of CTL that recognized these viral proteins in PBMCs from healthy immune subjects. In these experiments, cultures from HCT recipients showed a significant reduction in the proliferation of CD4+ T cells when compared to the pattern of cell phenotypes in cultures from healthy subjects. CD8+ T cells predominated in VZV-stimulated cultures, reflecting the relative increase in circulating CD8+ T cells that is common after HCT [58]. Although CD8+ T lymphocytes have been defined as the "classic" cytotoxic effecter cell, human CD4+ cells also function effectively as antiviral CTL against many viruses, including VZV [59]. The diminished CD4+ T-cell response to VZV antigen may explain why the overall frequencies of CTL precursors specific for the IE62 or gE (gp I) proteins remained significantly lower after HCT than in healthy, VZV immune individuals. Helper and cytotoxic T-cell responses specific for the IE63 protein as well as proteins encoded by open reading frames 4 and 10 are maintained for decades after primary VZV infection in the intact host [60,61], and their absence could be related to the high risk of VZV reactivation causing herpes zoster.

In contrast to virus-specific T-cell immunity, natural killer (NK) cell activity comparable to that of healthy subjects is recovered during the first few months after HCT [62]. Some HCT recipients had a predominance of NK cells, expressing CD16 surface antigen, in assays for cytotoxicity against VZV-infected targets [43]. The capacity of lymphocytes from some HCT patients to lyse targets expressing VZV proteins by a mechanism that is not antigen-specific may help to limit VZV replication prior to the recovery of virus-specific T cells.

Clinical manifestations

Primary VZV infection

The diagnosis of varicella is usually suspected clinically in high-risk as well as healthy children when the characteristic vesicular exanthem appears [4,21,63,64]. The interval from exposure of the nonimmune child to the appearance of the rash is about 14 days, with a range of 10–21 days; the incubation period may be somewhat shorter in immunocompromised children.

Because of its low incidence, specific descriptions of the clinical course of varicella after HCT are limited, but it is reasonable to generalize from the literature about varicella in other high-risk populations [63–65]. The initial manifestations of varicella in immunocompromised children are similar to those observed in healthy children. Prodromal symptoms may precede the rash by 24–48 h, usually consisting of headache, irritability, malaise and fever. Cutaneous lesions most often appear first on the scalp, face or trunk, and are usually pruritic. Each lesion begins as a small erythematous macule which evolves into a vesicle of 1–4 mm diameter, on an irregular erythematous base, the classic "dewdrop on a rose petal." In high-risk children, including HCT recipients, the vesicles may be unusually large and can involve deeper skin layers. Vesicles on mucous membranes, including the conjunctiva, the oropharynx, the rectum or the vagina are common even among otherwise healthy children. Varicella is typically accompanied by low-grade fever but temperature elevations may be as high as 40.5°C in high-risk patients, and fever often persists beyond the usual 3–4 days.

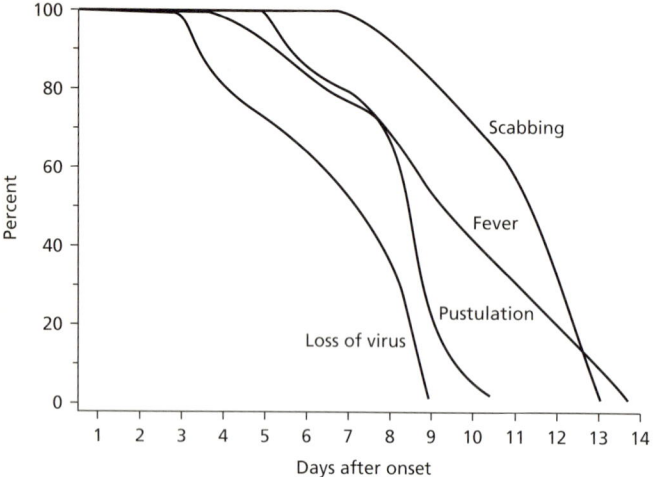

Fig. 55.7 The clinical course of varicella among immunocompromised children. Reproduced with permission from Whitley [65].

New vesicle formation typically continues for about 3 days, with a range of 1–7 days, among healthy children. This phase is often prolonged in immunocompromised children, with more than half of patients developing new lesions for more than 7 days (Fig. 55.7 [65]). Although the majority of immunocompetent children with varicella have fewer than 500 lesions, it is not unusual for patients on immunosuppressive therapy to develop more than 1500 lesions. Successive crops of varicella vesicles develop in a centrifugal pattern, appearing last on the extremities. These later crops of lesions tend to be more extensive in immunocompromised patients, and may involve the palms and soles as well as arms and legs. In lesions that are resolving normally, the vesicle fluid rapidly becomes cloudy and the lesion may develop an umbilicated appearance as it becomes crusted. Among healthy children, the lesions that erupt later in the disease sometimes resolve after a maculopapular phase, but many of the late lesions also progress through the vesicular stage in immunocompromised patients. In general, the time to complete crusting of lesions is prolonged. Extensive hypopigmentation and scarring may be seen as the crusts resolve, presumably because of the involvement of deeper layers of the dermis in immunocompromised patients.

Patients who acquire the infection during the first 9–12 months after transplantation appear to be at highest risk of developing severe varicella [1]. The potential complications of varicella after HCT can be anticipated from the clinical experience with primary VZV infection in other immunocompromised patient populations. HCT recipients can be compared with patients whose immunosuppression is due to treatment of lymphoproliferative malignancies or solid tumors. In one large series, 32% of these patients developed visceral dissemination in the course of varicella, with VZV infection of the lungs, liver, and central nervous system (CNS) [64]. The mortality rate was 7% overall, with an increase to 25% in patients who developed varicella pneumonia. The risk for visceral involvement was significantly higher among patients whose absolute lymphocyte counts were <500/μL, and the rate of visceral dissemination increased to 71% when the lymphocyte count declined to <100 cells/μL. Visceral dissemination was associated with new lesion formation for a median of 10 days in more than half of patients who were evaluated before effective antiviral therapy for VZV was available. Based on the analysis of placebo recipients in the original studies of antiviral treatment of varicella in high-risk children, the mortality rate was 17%; 27% of the patients developed varicella pneumonia, 19% had hepatitis (see Plate 23.44, *facing p. 296*) and 6% had CNS disease [65].

Among the complications of primary VZV infection, varicella pneumonia is the most common cause of life-threatening illness. Respiratory symptoms, except for mild rhinitis and cough, are unusual in uncomplicated varicella and require urgent evaluation in the immunocompromised patient. Pneumonia most often develops within 3–7 days after the appearance of the rash and progresses rapidly to respiratory failure. Clinical signs of pneumonia may be limited to tachypnea, cough, and dyspnea with no accompanying abnormal findings by auscultation. The degree of hypoxemia may be marked even when abnormalities on the chest X-ray are minimal.

Varicella can be associated with abnormal liver function tests in the immunocompetent host but hepatic involvement is usually subclinical. In contrast, immunocompromsied children are at risk of fulminant varicella hepatitis (see Plate 23.44, *facing p. 296*), with progression to hepatic failure. Severe varicella is usually accompanied by signs of disseminated intravascular coagulopathy (DIC), including epistaxis, hematuria, and gastrointestinal bleeding. Hemorrhage into the cutaneous lesions is recognized as a poor prognostic sign in high-risk patients. Bleeding is most often due to DIC and hepatic failure, but isolated thombocytopenia can occur. Vomiting and abdominal pain are uncommon in children with uncomplicated varicella. Severe abdominal or back pain should be considered a sign of life-threatening infection, and may be associated with inappropriate antidiuretic hormone secretion in the absence of any obvious CNS disease. This atypical presentation of VZV infection has been reported after HCT [66,67]. While the pathogenic mechanism is not understood, disseminated VZV infection can cause pancreatitis and disease of the gastrointestinal tract, such as esophagitis, which may account for these symptoms, or pre-eruptive infection of sensory ganglia may occur.

Varicella meningoencephalitis is unusual in immunocompromised children but, when it occurs, it is usually associated with other signs of visceral involvement. Some patients develop a rapidly deteriorating course progressing to death. Symptoms of CNS disease most often occur between 2 and 6 days after the eruption of the rash and can progress rapidly to coma. Encephalitis may precede the appearance of the rash [68] The clinical signs include vomiting, headache, altered sensorium and seizures. The cerebrospinal fluid usually shows a mild to moderate pleocytosis and elevated protein. Inappropriate antidiuretic hormone secretion may occur in patients who have meningoencephalitis [69].

Severe hypertension is a poor prognostic sign in immunocompromised patients with varicella. The mechanism is uncertain except in cases that are associated with nephritis. Adrenal cortical necrosis is noted at autopsy in patients with disseminated VZV infection.

In addition to complications directly related to viral replication, secondary bacterial infections are a risk in immunocompromised patients with primary VZV infection, as they are in otherwise healthy children. *Staphylococcous aureus* and *Streptococcus pyogenes* (group A streptococcus) are the most common pathogens, causing cellulitis, subcutaneous abscesses, and lymphadenitis. Varicella gangrenosa, a very rare syndrome of necrotizing fasciitis caused by *Streptococcus pyogenes*, is life threatening even in the intact host. Secondary bacterial infection of sites other than the skin, including bacterial pneumonia, septic arthritis and osteomyelitis, may follow varicella. Staphylococcal sepsis can occur, and children with indwelling catheters can develop line-related infections.

Although information is limited, varicella occurring late after HCT is usually not associated with complications. Four children who had varicella 2 years after transplantation had clinical disease that resembled primary VZV infection in children with no immunodeficiency and four children who developed varicella from 105 to 350 days after HCT had no complications [1,57]. However, progressive varicella with severe pneumonia was reported in one child who acquired varicella 6 years after successful HCT [70].

Table 55.3 Distribution of dermatomal involvement with herpes zoster in bone marrow transplant recipients and healthy individuals with reucrrent varicella-zoster virus (VZV) infections.

	HCT recipients*	Healthy individuals†
No. of patients	195	116
Dermatomes involved (%)		
Cranial	16	15
Cervical	17	22
Thoracic	47	53
Lumbar	20	18
Sacral	12	8
Dissemination (%)		
Cutaneous	23	0
Visceral	13	0
Mortality (%)	7	0

*Adapted from Locksley et al. [1].
†Adapted from Brunell [73].

Recurrent VZV infection

Localized herpes zoster

Localized herpes zoster is the most common clinical presentation of VZV infection in HCT recipients who are seropositive at the time of transplantation, accounting for 85% of cases in 231 HCT recipients in the study by Locksley et al. [1]. The rash of localized herpes zoster is usually preceded by pain and parasthesias in the involved dermatome [5,16,63]. These symptoms may begin as long as 5 days before the eruption and vary from mild discomfort to very severe debilitating pain. The etiology of the initial pain is sometimes misdiagnosed as pleurisy, myocardial infarct, cholecystitis or renal colic. In some instances the prodrome is not followed by any skin eruption, but a typical antibody response is observed; this syndrome is referred to as "zoster sine herpete" [71,72].

In healthy subjects, herpes zoster involves the thoracic dermatomes in about half of the cases, and cranial nerve disease occurs in 13–20% of cases [63]. Recurrent VZV affects similar dermatomes in HCT patients, with thoracic dermatomal disease in 41–47% of cases and cranial nerve involvement in 16% [18,52] (Table 55.3 [1,73]).

The cutaneous lesions of localized herpes zoster appear as clusters of varicella-like vesicles in one or several sites anteriorly and posteriorly along the dermatome; typically, the lesions do not cross the midline, but some cases of bilateral dermatomal involvement have been described. Discrete vesicles often enlarge to form confluent lesions. In immunocompromized patients, including HCT recipients, the local vesicular eruption may be very extensive, evolving to occupy the whole dermatome, the lesions may become hemorrhagic, and the duration of cutaneous disease is prolonged [63]. In the normal host, new lesion formation usually continues for 3–7 days followed by a phase of pustulation and crust formation; complete healing is expected by 2–3 weeks. In high-risk patients, the average time for cessation of new lesion formation was 8 days, and crusting was not complete until an average of 18 days. Immunosuppressed patients may occasionally develop a chronic cutaneous reactivation of VZV that persists for months [16,74]. As clinical experience with severely immunocompromised patients due to human immunodeficiency virus (HIV) infection increases, knowledge about the spectrum of disease caused by VZV continues to expand [75]. Many of these complications are now recognized in HCT recipients with VZV reactivation.

When VZV reactivation involves cranial nerves, complications are more likely in both immunocompromised and immunocompetent patients [4]. In one series, corneal damage, facial scarring, cranial nerve VII palsy or hearing loss occurred in 35% of patients [1]. The distribution of the ophthalmic branch of the trigeminal nerve is a common site of herpes zoster. The development of vesicular lesions on the nose is a sign of involvement of the ophthalmic branch and indicates a risk for ocular complications. The clinical findings of ocular herpes zoster include conjunctivitis, keratitis, anterior uveitis or, rarely, panophthalmitis. Although corneal lesions are common, blindness is an unusual complication of herpes zoster ophthalmicus [76]. Loss of vision associated with herpes zoster is usually secondary to retrobulbar neuritis. VZV reactivation may produce facial palsy when it involves cranial nerve VII. Although it is less common than CMV retinitis, chorioretinopathy caused by VZV is observed after HCT [77]. Herpes zoster oticus is associated with VZV reactivation from the geniculate ganglion, producing the Ramsay–Hunt syndrome with unilateral deafness and vestibular symptoms. Oral lesions of the palate may develop without any cutaneous lesions when the second branch of cranial nerve V is affected.

Cerebral angiitis is a syndrome of cerebral vascular inflammation with thrombosis and microinfarcts associated with VZV reactivation in cranial nerve ganglia. In severe cases, massive thrombosis with contralateral hemiparesis may result [78]. Infarct in the distribution of the middle cerebral artery can be demonstrated by computerized tomography (CT) scan. Pathologic findings include a granulomatous inflammatory process in the arterial wall, mononuclear cell infiltrates, vascular necrosis and viral particles within the smooth muscle cells of the affected arteries. The syndrome is rare and there is no evidence that HCT or other immunocompromised patients are at increased risk for cerebral angiitis. However, it is important to recognize this complication in patients who develop hemiparesis about 6–8 weeks after the symptoms of herpes zoster.

When the anterior horn cells are involved in VZV reactivation, inflammation and necrosis may follow with resulting motor deficits [72]. In otherwise healthy individuals, motor paralysis was present in 11.5% of patients with cervical herpes zoster, 7% with lumbosacral disease and 0.3% of those with thoracic zoster [79]. Full recovery of the motor deficit is expected in 85–90% of the cases. Transverse myelitis and ascending paralysis are rare neurologic syndromes caused by recurrent VZV infection with or without immunosuppression.

Immunocompromised patients are at increased risk of post-herpetic neuralgia, which is the most common complication of herpes zoster in all patient populations. The definition of post-herpetic pain varies from any pain lasting after the crusts of the cutaneous lesions have disappeared to pain that persists more than 2 months. Estimates of the incidence of post-herpetic neuralgia vary depending upon the definition used. In one study of healthy individuals, 9% of patients with herpes zoster developed post-herpetic neuralgia, whereas Locksley et al. [1] observed post-herpetic neuralgia in 25% of patients with herpes zoster after HCT and Offidani et al. [20] reported an incidence of 32%. Koc et al. [18] found that post-herpetic neuralgia and peripheral neuropathy were the most common complications of VZV reactivation after HCT, occurring in 68 of 100 consecutively identified cases. Post-herpetic neuralgia is uncommon in children, even in those who are immunocompromised [15–17]; only 2–3% pediatric HCT recipients who developed herpes zoster have persistent pain [7,21].

Secondary bacterial infection of skin lesions and local scarring are common in HCT recipients with herpes zoster, occurring with an incidence of 17% and 19%, respectively.

Cutaneous and visceral dissemination

In contrast to otherwise healthy subjects, HCT patients often develop cutaneous dissemination, defined as more than five vesicular lesions beyond the primary dermatome. Cutaneous dissemination has been reported in 17–24% of HCT recipients and was equally common among those who had recurrent VZV during the early or late period after transplant [1,18]. HCT recipients are also at risk of visceral dissemination during episodes of VZV reactivation (Fig. 55.1). Since it is a sign of VZV infection of circulating lymphocytes, cutaneous dissemination provides a marker for the risk for visceral dissemination. However, visceral dissemination also occurs in patients whose cutaneous lesions are localized to the primary dermatome. Without antiviral therapy, visceral dissemination was observed in 13% of HCT patients with herpes zoster [18]. The potential sites of visceral dissemination with recurrent VZV are the same as those with disseminated primary VZV infection. The clinical complications that result include pneumonia, hepatitis, DIC and encephalitis. The mortality that accompanies VZV reactivation is almost always due to viral pneumonia, but fatal fulminant hepatitis and DIC without VZV pneumonia have been reported [80]. Acute GVHD is the only risk factor associated significantly with VZV dissemination. VZV has also been identified as the causative agent of late interstitial pneumonia in HCT patients with chronic GVHD [81].

Occasionally HCT recipients present with signs of visceral dissemination 24–96 h before the localized cutaneous eruption of recurrent VZV becomes evident, resulting in misdiagnosis as GVHD or other complications. Among these patients, the clinical presentation is characterized by abdominal pain, often mid-epigastric or peri-umbilical, with or without associated nausea, vomiting or fever. Pancreatitis, hepatitis (see Plate 23.44, *facing p. 296*), gastrointestinal hemorrhage, intestinal necrosis, DIC and inappropriate secretion of antidiuretic hormone have been described in patients with abdominal symptoms preceding the rash [44,45,82–86]. In a recent description of 10 cases, patients had abdominal pain and elevated aminotransferases and pancreatic enzymes, associated with nausea (60%), fever >38°C (60%), and vomiting (50%) [87]. Four patients had a skin rash, which appeared at an interval of 4–14 days after the onset of abdominal pain, five patients had pneumonitis, and VZV infection was fatal in five cases. Visceral dissemination can also occur without any signs of cutaneous disease. Three HCT patients had fatal VZV infection and no skin lesions during the course of their illness despite evidence of widespread organ infection at autopsy [1].

Immunosuppression also predisposes to CNS infection with recurrent VZV, although symptomatic neurologic complications of herpes zoster are rare [88,89]. Two of 100 consecutively identified patients with recurrent VZV after HCT developed VZV encephalitis [18]. In evaluating these patients, it is important to note that abnormal cerebrospinal fluid findings are common even in immunocompetent patients with herpes zoster. Lymphocytic pleocytosis and elevated protein were observed in about 40% of healthy individuals who had no abnormalities by neurologic examination whereas the incidence of herpes zoster-associated encephalitis is estimated to be only 0.2–0.5% in this population [13,90–92]. The clinical symptoms and signs of CNS disease are headache, photophobia, meningismus and altered state of consciousness [91,92]. The neurologic symptoms usually appear within a few days after the exanthem. The temperature is usually normal or mildly elevated. Seizures are rare but the electroencephalogram may show diffuse slowing or epileptiform activity.

As would be expected, the occurrence of visceral dissemination increases the mortality of recurrent VZV infection substantially from an overall death rate of 7% to 55%. The mortality rate is higher in patients who develop both pneumonia and encephalitis than in those patients who have encephalitis only.

Atypical nonlocalized herpes zoster

Atypical nonlocalized herpes zoster after HCT is sometimes categorized as varicella because the HCT recipient is presumed to lack VZV immunity, regardless of prior immune status. However, identifying the syndrome as a distinct clinical presentation is useful because the pathogenesis of infection and the timing of the host response may be affected by differences between the endogenous and exogenous routes of infection and residual immunity may modify the clinical course. The incidence of atypical nonlocalized herpes zoster is variable, with reports of its occurrence ranging from none to as many as 25% of episodes of VZV reactivation after HCT. Clinically, patients with atypical nonlocalized herpes zoster have cutaneous vesicles that are identical to those of varicella. The number of lesions is quite variable but the eruption is often extensive, involving face, trunk, extremities, palms and soles. This syndrome occurs in autologous as well as allogeneic HCT recipients, accounting for 21% of episodes of recurrent VZV in one series [13]. The morbidity of untreated infection is high, with 45% of patients developing visceral dissemination, resulting in a mortality rate of 28% during the period before antiviral therapy was available [1].

Second episodes of recurrent VZV

Second episodes of VZV reactivation after HCT are uncommon. About 2% of patients had two episodes of herpes zoster, occurring at an average of 25 months after transplantation, with a range of 4–41 months. Most of the reported second episodes after HCT have involved the same dermatome but reactivation from another ganglia may occur [1].

Subclinical reactivation of latent VZV

The occurrence of subclinical VZV reactivation in HCT recipients has been shown by using a PCR method to demonstrate cell-associated VZV viremia [43]. Subclinical VZV reactivation was detected in 19% of 37 HCT patients who were screened randomly and had no signs of infection. Two of the seven patients who had subclinical VZV viremia developed clinical signs of herpes zoster subsequently, at intervals of 60 days and 130 days later. Three patients who had subclinical VZV viremia between 17 and 85 days after HCT had cleared the cell-associated viremia when they were retested by VZV PCR; two patients were not reevaluated by VZV PCR but did not develop herpes zoster. Thus, five of seven patients (71%) who had subclinical viremia did not progress to clinical infection.

Laboratory diagnosis

Direct detection of VZV-infected cells by immunofluorescence

The optimal method for the rapid diagnosis of cutaneous VZV infection is to obtain epithelial cells from a fresh lesion and to stain the specimen using fluorescein-conjugated monoclonal antibodies to VZV antigens [93–95]. The VZV-specific monoclonal antibodies bind to viral proteins that are synthesized within infected cells; fixing the cells prior to staining makes the cell membrane permeable, allowing the detection of VZV proteins in the cytoplasm and the nucleus as well as on the cell surface. This method is referred to as the direct fluorescence antigen (DFA) test or DFA technique. The most important step in obtaining the specimen is to disrupt the roof of the vesicle in order to collect intact cells from the base of the lesion. Cells can be recovered efficiently by rotating the blunt end of a wooden applicator stick in the unroofed lesion or by scraping with a scapel and transferring the material to a glass slide. Unless at least five intact cells are visible on the slide, the specimen should not be considered adequate for processing by the DFA method. It is important to include parallel staining of a portion of the specimen with reagents to detect HSV since VZV and HSV lesions are often indistinguishable clinically, and to provide a control for the specificity of the assay. The proper interpretation of DFA slides requires experience; the most common error is to identify false positive results because of lack of expertise at distinguishing background nonspecific fluorescence. If the clinical course of the patient is not consistent with a diagnosis of VZV infection that was based on the DFA method, the laboratory result should be questioned. DFA and indirect immunofluorescence or immunoperoxidase methods can also be used to demonstrate the presence of VZV in properly prepared tissue sections of lung, liver and other organs from patients with disseminated VZV infections.

Enzyme immunoassay methods are also useful for detecting VZV antigens in specimens from skin lesions [93]. When laboratory facilities for DFA testing are not available, the Tzanck stain and other cytologic methods can be used to detect multinucleated giant cells in a lesion scraping; however, it is essential to realize that false negatives are common and that these methods do not differentiate VZV from HSV infection. Herpes viral particles can be detected by electron microscopy but few diagnostic laboratories are equipped to perform this procedure, the method is not rapid and the morphology of herpesviruses is too similar to distinguish these viruses by electron microscopy.

Viral isolation in tissue culture cells

VZV can be detected in clinical samples using standard tissue culture methods for viral isolation [93,96,97]. The highest yield for viral culture depends upon obtaining vesicular fluid along with infected cells from the base of the cutaneous lesion. Vesicular fluid can be collected in a tuberculin syringe or by using a cotton or a dacron swab. Swabs should be put in viral transport medium immediately, agitated and pressed against the side of the vial to remove absorbed fluid; the swab should be taken out of the vial before it is sent to the laboratory. If storage for more than a few hours is required, the specimen should be kept on dry ice or frozen at −70°C; storing the specimen at −20°C in a standard refrigerator freezer for 24 h usually inactivates the virus.

The optimal recovery of infectious virus in tissue culture requires the use of diploid cell lines or human embryonic lung fibroblasts [96,97]. The cytopathic effect appears within 2–4 days after inoculation. Since the average time to detection of the virus in tissue culture is 7 days, diagnosis by viral culture is not rapid enough to influence clinical decisions in most circumstances. The sensitivity of tissue culture for detection of VZV is also substantially less than for identification of HSV and CMV. Procedures such as centrifugation enhancement may shorten the time required to detect cytopathic effect [97,98]. There are some differences in the morphology of plaques produced by VZV compared to these other herpesviruses but the identity of the virus isolate must be proved by immunofluorescence staining with virus-specific antisera. As in the case of CMV, the shell vial culture method improves the sensitivity of VZV isolation and permits earlier identification of positive specimens. This method combines centrifugation and staining with fluorescein-conjugated monoclonal antibodies to VZV; positive results may be available within 1–3 days after inoculation. In a recent study, VZV was detected in 79% of specimens by shell vial culture compared to a 64% rate of detection by standard tissue culture methods, but viral diagnosis by either tissue culture method was less sensitive than DFA, which was positive in 92% of clinically diagnosed cases [95].

The likelihood of recovery of VZV from cutaneous lesions is directly related to the stage of the lesion, with clear vesicles being much more likely to be positive than specimens from lesions that have become pustular or crusted. Varicella lesions are usually positive for 3 days, while virus can be recovered for a week or longer in herpes zoster. VZV can be isolated from PBMCs by tissue culture inoculation of specimens from immunocompromised patients with recurrent as well as primary VZV infections [46]. In contrast to meningoencephalitis associated with primary VZV infection, the virus has been isolated from the cerebrospinal fluid of patients with herpes zoster [90]. Bronchial washings may yield VZV in patients with pneumonia. The lungs are the most common autopsy organ from which VZV has been isolated, but the virus has been recovered from many sites, including heart, liver, pancreas, gastrointestinal tract, brain and eyes.

Viral DNA detection

VZV DNA sequences can be detected using radiolabeled or biotinylated nucleic acid probes for *in situ* hybridization or Southern blot procedures [31,99,100]. *In situ* hybridization was more sensitive than viral culture for demonstrating viremia in patients with varicella [31]. The presence of VZV gene sequences in human ganglion tissue has been demonstrated using probe methods [38–40,100]. PCR is a sensitive method for detecting VZV in clinical samples from patients with varicella and herpes zoster but it may not be available for routine diagnosis [32,101,102].

Serologic diagnosis

Serologic screening of prospective HCT recipients for VZV antibodies is a valuable tool to establish immune status before transplantation. Many serological methods are available for measuring IgG antibodies to VZV [4,93]. The most sensitive serologic assays for detection of VZV antibodies are fluorescent-antibody staining of membrane antigen (FAMA) and radioimmunoassay (RIA). Other methods that are relatively reliable for establishing immune status include enzyme immunoassay (ELISA) and anticomplement immunofluorescence (ACIF). While the commercially available ELISA kits for detecting VZV antibodies have a high degree of specificity, these methods are not as sensitive as research laboratory procedures such as FAMA. While these methods do not usually yield false positive results, from 10% to 15% of immune individuals may be wrongly identified as not having had previous VZV infection. Complement fixation methods are not satisfactory for determining immune status. Latex agglutination is a sensitive and specific method for establishing VZV immune status [103–105].

Although seroconversion can be documented with primary VZV infection and boosts in antibody titres accompany recurrent VZV, the serologic diagnosis of acute infection requires paired sera and is rarely helpful for clinical purposes. There are no reliable commercial methods to test for VZV IgM antibodies but they can be detected in patients with varicella using research methods. The majority of patients with recurrent infection also produce VZV IgM [106]. Testing for VZV IgM antibodies is not useful in clinical practice.

Antiviral therapy for VZV infection

Acyclovir

At the present time, acyclovir is the drug of choice for the treatment of primary and recurrent VZV infections. The antiviral activity of acyclovir (9,2 hydroxy-ethoxy-methylguanine) against VZV follows the same pathway that mediates its interference with the replication of HSV. The metabolism of the drug to the triphosphate form by the viral thymidine kinase produces a compound that functions as a competitive inhibitor and chain terminator of viral DNA polymerase. However, while HSV-1 and HSV-2 isolates are usually inhibited *in vitro* by 0.125 µg/mL and 0.215 µg/mL of acyclovir, respectively, the mean concentrations required to inhibit VZV isolates are often 0.82–4.64 µg/mL, with ranges as low as 0.3 and as high as 10.8 µg/mL [107,108].

The plasma concentrations achieved by the intravenous administration of acyclovir at doses of 10 mg/kg or 250–500 mg/m^2 range from 15 to 25 µg/mL [109]. These concentrations are several-fold above the *in vitro* inhibitory concentrations for most VZV isolates. In contrast, only about 20% of the oral dose of acyclovir is absorbed. Oral administration to pediatric patients at doses of 600 mg/m^2 given four times produced peak plasma concentrations of approximately 1.0–1.5 µg/mL [110]. The oral dose of 200 mg of acyclovir given five times a day to adults (approximately 115 mg/m^2 for an adult male) produces plasma concentrations of approximately 0.5 µg/mL; increasing the unit dose to 600 mg resulted in plasma concentrations of 1.3 µg/mL [111]. Thus, acyclovir concentrations required to inhibit some VZV isolates can be expected to be significantly above the mean peak plasma concentration achieved by oral dosing.

Antiviral treatment of varicella

The administration of intravenous acyclovir to immunocompromised children with varicella has the potential to terminate the cell-associated viremia that produces malignant progressive varicella in these patients and to prevent the onset of varicella pneumonitis, each of which is correlated with a high risk of fatal infection [4,5,64,112]. The dosage of intravenous acyclovir for varicella in high-risk patients is 500 mg/m^2/dose every 8 h, with administration continuing for 7 days. When this dosage was tested in placebo-controlled trials, the effect of the drug on the number of days to defervescence and resolution of cutaneous lesions was not signficant, but varicella pneumonitis was prevented in the acyclovir recipients [113,114]. The efficacy of acyclovir and its superiority to vidarabine in preventing the visceral dissemination of VZV was confirmed by Feldman and Lott who found that none of 16 children with cancer given acyclvoir developed varicella pneumonitis while six of 21 (29%) patients treated with vidarabine progressed to pneumonia [64]. The clinical impact of specific antiviral therapy was illustrated by the fact that none of 37 children with varicella who received vidarabine or acyclovir had fatal infection [64].

Primary VZV infection in HCT recipients occurring within the 1st year after transplant should be considered to require intravenous acylovir therapy. The goal of antiviral therapy for varicella in high-risk patients is to initiate drug treatment within 72 h after the appearance of the cutaneous rash. Parents and patients need to be educated about the typical appearance of varicella lesions because many cases occur without any known exposure, and prompt diagnosis during the early phase of infection is important to the success of antiviral therapy. Since there are other causes of vesicular rashes in childhood and in immunocompromised patients, the clinical diagnosis should be confirmed by the laboratory using the DFA technique. While most children do not have clinical signs of dissemination immediately, the interval during which preventive therapy can be initiated is very short. The decision to initiate antiviral therapy must be made before progression of the rash becomes obvious because visceral dissemination takes place at the same time. The average period to onset of varicella pneumonitis is 6 days, with most cases occurring within 4–8 days among untreated high-risk patients. In addition to preventing life-threatening dissemination, acyclovir therapy can also be expected to minimize the extent of the cutaneous disease and shorten the time to complete healing significantly [64]. More rapid resolution of the cutaneous lesions may reduce the risk of secondary bacterial infections as well.

Immunocompromised children or adults who present with signs of disseminated VZV infection should receive immediate treatment with intravenous acyclovir. The efficacy of acyclovir for the treatment of established varicella pneumonia or other visceral sites of infection has not been determined in a controlled trial. Five recipients of placebo in the original acyclovir trial who developed pneumonitis were placed on the drug approximately 6–8 days after the appearance of the varicella rash, and all of these patients improved after initiation of the drug [113]. However, in another series, three of four high-risk patients who were not treated until at least 5 days after the onset of the cutaneous lesions had evidence of visceral dissemination at the initiation of treatment; all three patients had progressive varicella and two patients died [115].

Varicella zoster immunoglobulin (VZIG) administration is indicated for high-risk children and adults who have never had VZV infection, whose exposure to VZV is identified within 96 h. Nevertheless, clinicians must be aware that severe varicella develops in some immunocompromised patients despite the timely administration of VZIG. The incidence of varicella despite VZIG prophylaxis is significantly higher for children with household exposures than for those who have less prolonged contact with the index case, and the attack rate is affected by the VZV IgG titre of the preparation [116]. In the placebo controlled trial of intravenous acyclovir, one of six (17%) placebo recipients who had recieved ZIG (zoster immunoglobulin) or ZIP (zoster immunoplasma) before entry required reassignment to open drug because of progressive varicella [113]. In the St Jude experience, the risk of varicella pneumonitis was reduced significantly by passive antibody prophylaxis but 11% of children developed pneumonia despite receiving ZIG, ZIP or VZIG [64]. Because of these risks, HCT recipients who develop varicella should be treated with intravenous acyclovir even if passive antibody prophylaxis was given at the time of exposure.

Beyond 9–12 months after HCT, it may be acceptable to monitor the clinical course of varicella without giving acyclovir, assuming that the patient has no evidence of GVHD and is not receiving immunosusppressive therapy. However, given the predictable benefits of a short course of acyclovir for varicella, even in healthy children, its administration is justified.

Antiviral treatment of herpes zoster

Acyclovir has been shown to be effective for the treatment of recurrent VZV infection in immunocompromised patients in placebo-controlled trials and through extensive clinical experience with the drug. The dose of acyclovir is 500 mg/m^2 or 10 mg/kg intravenously (IV) given every 8 h. Therapy should be continued for 7 days or for 2 days after cessation of new lesion formation, whichever provides the longer treatment course.

In an early study of the efficacy of acyclovir, all immunocompromised patients with herpes zoster experienced improvement of symptoms within 24 h, no new skin lesions were noted after 24 h and none had visceral dissemination [117]. In a subsequent placebo-controlled trial, local progression and progression of cutaneous dissemination was terminated with acyclovir therapy [118]. One of 52 treated patients had progressive VZV disease compared to 11 of 42 placebo recipients. Meyers *et al.* [119] showed that intravenous acyclovir had clinical benefit in a study enrolling only HCT patients with herpes zoster. Treatment resulted in a shorter time to cessation of new lesion formation, more rapid crusting and healing and prevention of cutaneous and visceral dissemination in patients who presented with localized herpes zoster (Fig. 55.8 [118]). When acyclovir was compared to vidarabine for the treatment of herpes zoster, none of 12 acyclovir recipients developed cutaneous dissemination compared with five of 10 patients given vidarabine [120]. Acyclovir decreased the duration of local viral replication, with viral cultures remaining positive for VZV for only 4 days after the initiation of treatment. Based on this experience, acyclovir therapy initiated within 72 h after the onset of VZV reactivation can be expected to reduce the duration of new lesion formation in HCT patients to approximately 3 days. On average, early antiviral treatment should cause the cessation of acute pain within 4 days, crusting of lesions by 7 days and complete healing by 2–3 weeks (Fig. 55.8).

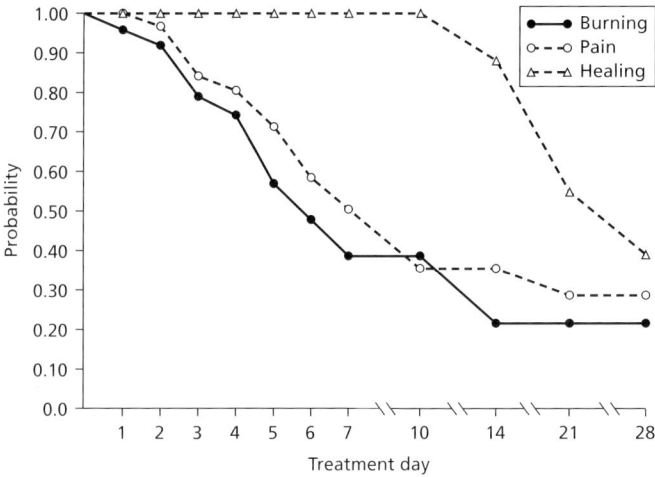

Fig. 55.8 Probability of lesion burning (23 patients [●—●]), of lesion pain (31 patients [○- - -○]), and of not having total healing (31 patients [△- - -△]) by treatment day. Reproduced with permission from Balfour et al. [118].

Although early acyclovir treatment is likely to produce the best results, clinical benefit can still occur when therapy is delayed for more than 3 days [118]. None of 29 immunocompromised patients whose therapy was initiated more than 3 days after the onset of the rash had progressive herpes zoster compared to three of 17 patients in the placebo group.

Although the drug eliminates the life-threatening complications of VZV reactivation in most patients, relapse of herpes zoster is a clinical problem in some HCT patients who are treated with acyclovir. In one series, five of 40 patients (12%) developed new lesions, with relapse occurring less than 4 days after treatment was stopped in three of the five patients [120]. Early acyclovir therapy may delay the recovery of VZV specific immunity in some patients. Nevertheless, most patients respond to treatment with a second course of acyclovir.

Although acyclovir is clearly beneficial for the treatment of acute herpes zoster, its effect on the incidence of post-herpetic neuraliga has been more difficult to establish. Varying definitions of post-herpetic neuralgia have complicated assessments of antiviral and adjunctive therapies. A meta-analysis of several placebo-controlled trials of oral acyclovir therapy for herpes zoster in otherwise healthy individuals indicates that long-term pain is diminished [121,122]. However, among HCT recipients, 21% of 40 patients had recurrence of pain after cessation of therapy [119]. Based upon experience in immunocompetent patients, extending the duration of acyclovir therapy from 7 to 21 days does not improve outcome [123]. Recent evaluations of the administration of steroids as adjunctive therapy in patients without malignancy have yielded conflicting results about clinical benefit [123,124]. Whether the use of steroids along with antiviral therapy reduces the severity of zoster-associated pain in HCT recipients has not been assessed. The fact that acyclovir ameliorates the acute pain associated with herpes zoster more effectively than long-term pain suggests that a different mechanism is responsible for post-herpetic neuralgia. Continued VZV replication is not likely to account for post-herpetic pain. Instead, it has been suggested that the initial neuronal infection and associated inflammation, which can persist for months, results in deafferentation, ectopic activity of damaged afferents nerves and enhanced excitability of neurons relaying central pain signals. Current approaches to the management of post-herpetic neuralgia include tricyclic antidepressants, topical lidocaine patches and gabapentin as well as opioids; nerve blocks have little benefit for post-herpetic neuralgia [125]. Medical interventions are often used in combination, or sequentially, because no single approach is beneficial in most patients.

The efficacy of oral acyclovir for herpes zoster in HCT patients has not been firmly established in prospective studies but this route of administration is appropriate for selected patients who have localized herpes zoster occurring in the late period after HCT. Since the bioavailability of oral acyclovir is low, this route of administration requires giving 800 mg/dose, five times a day. Patients receiving oral acyclovir should be monitored for signs of progressive VZV infection and should be treated with the intravenous drug if complications arise. When patients are treated with the standard intravenous regimen, there is no need to provide further treatment with oral acyclovir after discharge. However, in some cases, the full course of therapy may be achieved by a combination of intravenous and oral acyclovir.

Acyclovir toxicity

The safety of acyclovir has been established in numerous clinical trials. While HCT patients also tolerate the drug well, the incidence of side-effects is higher. In one series, gastrointestinal symptoms of nausea and vomiting occurred in 40% of treated patients [120]. Nephrotoxicity, defined as a 50% rise in serum creatinine, was also more common than in other patient populations treated with acyclovir; 10–25% of HCT patients receiving acyclovir are reported to have an abnormal serum creatinine but these elevations may be caused by other medications given concurrently [120]. In any case, since acyclovir is excreted by glomerular filtration, other drugs that affect renal function, such as cyclosporin, can interact to cause elevated plasma concentrations of the drug.

The dosage and dose interval for acyclovir administration should be adjusted based on the relative impairment of creatinine clearance. The dosage interval should be lengthened to every 12 h for clearances of 25–50 mL/min and to 24 h for clearances of 10–25 mL/min; if the clearance is 0–10 mL/min, the dosage should be reduced to 250 mg/m^2, given every 24–48 h. It is also important to maintain adequate hydration in patients receiving acyclovir to avoid precipitation of the drug in renal tubules. A few cases of acute neurotoxicity have been reported in patients with deficient renal clearance who were receiving acyclovir. Abnormal liver function tests should be considered possible evidence of VZV hepatitis rather than drug toxicity. Acyclovir does not have hematologic toxicity and does not interfere with engraftment in HCT recipients.

Other antiviral compounds

Famciclovir and valaciclovir are nucleoside analog drugs that have been licensed for treatment of herpes zoster in the immunocompetent host [126–128]. Like acyclovir, these drugs inhibit VZV primarily by the thymidine kinase pathway. Their advantage is a much better absorption after oral administration than acyclovir, coupled with a safety profile that resembles that of acyclovir. Although controlled trials to establish the clinical efficacy of these antiviral agents in HCT patients have not been done, valaciclovir or famciclovir may be useful in selected patients who are considered to be at low risk of visceral dissemination during recurrent VZV reactivation. Attention to the dosage to these very efficiently absorbed drugs is essential, since toxicity of valaciclovir, manifest as thrombocytopenic purpura and hemolytic uremic syndrome, has been reported in HCT recipients [129]. Plasma concentrations approach those achieved by intravenous administration of acyclovir unless the patient has altered gastrointestinal function, which may be an obstacle to their use in some HCT recipients. Famciclovir and valaciclovir require less frequent administration and are more convenient for patients but these drugs are more expensive than oral acyclovir.

Although VZV resistance to acyclovir has not been common in HCT recipients, it has been reported in these patients and patients with the acquired immunodeficiency syndrome [130–132]. Among HCT recipients, the failure of VZV infections to resolve or their recurrence shortly after antiviral therapy is discontinued, is usually a function of the limited host response and should not be attributed to acyclovir resistance in most cases. When it occurs, antiviral resistance is usually mediated by thymidine kinase mutations. As a result, valaciclovir and famciclovir are not useful for treating VZV infections caused by acyclovir-resistant strains [130–132].

Foscarnet, a pyrophosphate analog, has antiviral activity against VZV through inhibition of the viral DNA polymerase and has activity against isolates that are not inhibited by acyclovir or famciclovir [75,131]. Its clinical use is complicated by potential liver toxicity and the emergence of resistance [133,134].

Cidofovir is a nucleotide agent that may be useful for resistant strains but clinical experience is limited [135]. There is no evidence that combinations of these antiviral drugs improve the treatment of VZV infection and adverse drug interactions may occur.

Vidarabine, the first antiviral agent shown to have clinical benefit for the treatment of VZV infections in immunocompromised patients, inhibits VZV by a different pathway, but was less effective than acyclovir and is no longer available [120]. Although it might have been useful for managing resistant VZV, the development of sorivudine (BVaraU) has been terminated in the USA because of its lethal interactions with 5-fluoro-uracil and concern that it might be administered inadvertently to patients who were receiving this drug [136,137]. Alternative nucleoside analog drugs with activity against VZV are being developed [138]. Human and recombinant leukocyte interferon were shown to have significant clinical efficacy in immunocompromized patients with herpes zoster in early studies and provide an alternative to the nucleoside analog drugs for the treatment of resistant VZV infection [139,140]. Although VZV strains resistant to acyclovir may emerge during therapy, particularly when the drug is given for prolonged courses and at low doses, VZV strains isolated from later recurrences in patients whose resistant infections have resolved are usually again susceptible to acyclovir.

Dihydroxy-propoxy-methylguanine (Ganciclovir, DHPG) has *in vitro* activity against VZV that is equivalent to acyclovir but clinical studies of its efficacy for the treatment of VZV infections have not been done because of its greater toxicity. However, it is possible that the administration of ganciclovir to HCT recipients who have CMV infection could alter the course of concurrent VZV infection.

Prophylaxis for VZV infection

Varicella-zoster immunoglobulin (VZIG)

VZIG is a passive antibody preparation containing VZV IgG antibodies which is prepared from high titer immune human serum. VZIG is distributed by the American Red Cross Blood Service and can be obtained by calling the local Red Cross Blood Center. The dosage is 1 vial/10 kg body weight given intramuscularly.

VZIG is indicated for the prophylaxis of primary VZV infection in VZV seronegative, immunocompromised children or adults who have not had previous VZV infection, including HCT recipients [128]. Its effect depends upon administration within 96 h, and preferably within 48 h after exposure. Varicella exposure is defined as household contact, shared hospital room, or indoor play for at least 1 h with a child who is in the contagious phase of varicella, which is the interval from 2 days before to 5 days after the onset of the rash. If a patient has received any of the commercial preparations of high-dose intravenous immunoglobulin (100–400 mg/kg) for other indications within 3 weeks before the exposure, it is not necessary to administer VZIG [121]. A second dose of VZIG should be given if a new exposure occurs more than 2 weeks after a dose of VZIG has been given; protective titers may persist longer, but data

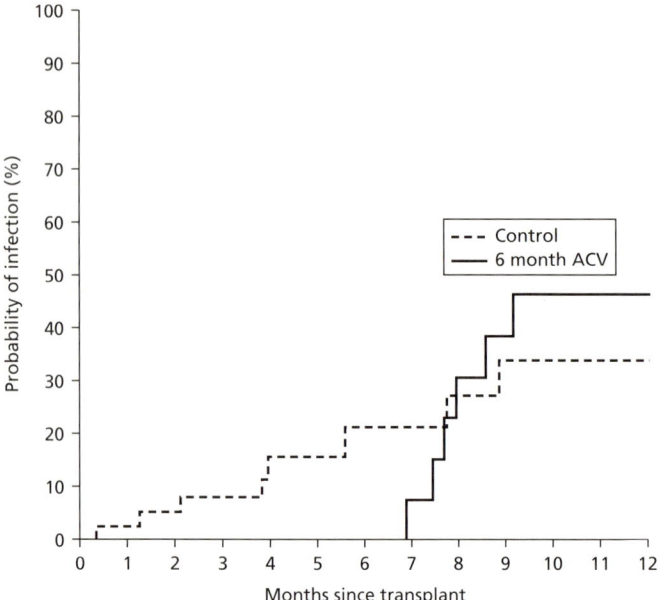

Fig. 55.9 Cumulative probability of varicella-zoster virus (VZV) infection in patients receiving acyclovir (——) or placebo (- - - -). Reproduced with permission from Ljungman *et al.* [143].

about VZV IgG titers at later time points is not available. While the risk of VZV transmission from an individual with herpes zoster is low, close contact between an HCT patient who has never been infected with VZV, and a patient with recurrent VZV lesions also justifies the administration of VZIG.

Since the live attenuated varicella vaccine is now recommended for universal administration to children in the USA at age 12–15 months, some children will have had vaccine-induced immunity before HCT [141,142]. These children should be given VZIG prophylaxis for exposure to wild type varicella because the protective efficacy of varicella vaccine is not defined in these circumstances. High-risk children may also have close exposure to an immunized child or adult who has breakthrough varicella caused by the wild type virus or, rarely, to a healthy contact with a varicella vaccine-related rash. Immunocompromised children who have such an exposure should receive VZIG.

There is no indication that passive antibody prophylaxis will reduce the risk of VZV reactivation after HCT in patients who have serologic evidence of prior VZV infection. Passive antibody administration is not effective for the treatment of herpes zoster.

Acyclovir prophylaxis

The efficacy of acyclovir prophylaxis for preventing recurrent VZV infection in HCT recipients was shown in three placebo-controlled trials, involving a total of 202 patients [143–146]. The prophylactic doses of acyclovir that have been tested were 250 mg/m^2 given IV twice a day for a period of 5 weeks after transplant followed by 400 mg orally every 8 h for 6 months and 5 mg/kg IV every 8 h for 3 weeks followed by 800 mg orally every 6 h for 6 months. None of the acyclovir recipients developed herpes zoster during the period of therapy compared to a 15% incidence in the placebo group. The lower dose was as effective as the higher dose regimen. However, VZV reactivation occurred when acyclovir was discontinued, so that there was no overall reduction in the number of episodes at 1 year (Fig. 55.9 [144]). The infections in the acyclovir group were concentrated in the second half of the year. The suppressive effect of antiviral drugs was confirmed in clinical experience in allogeneic HCT patients who received acyclovir and/or ganciclovir, but rapid occurrence of herpes zoster was observed when the drugs were discontinued [18,19].

While it may reduce episodes of VZV reactivation, giving acyclovir as prophylaxis to prevent herpes zoster in HCT recipients is not recommended as routine practice, as stated in the CDC guidelines for preventing opportunistic infections after transplantation [129]. Although herpes zoster early after HCT has a risk of causing disseminated disease, prompt initiation of acyclovir for the treatment of recurrent VZV infections has proved to be very effective. None of the placebo recipients in the acyclovir prophylaxis studies had fatal dissemination when given intravenous acyclovir at the onset of recurrent VZV infection [126,127]. Nevertheless, clinical practice varies, and some institutions elect to use acyclovir or related antiviral drugs for suppression of recurrent VZV infections after transplantation. Antiviral prophylaxis may be indicated for selected patients at high risk, such as those with GVHD who remain severely immunodeficient [19]. The rationale for avoiding routine use is that prolonged administration of antiviral prophylaxis enhances the emergence of VZV strains that are resistant to the drug.

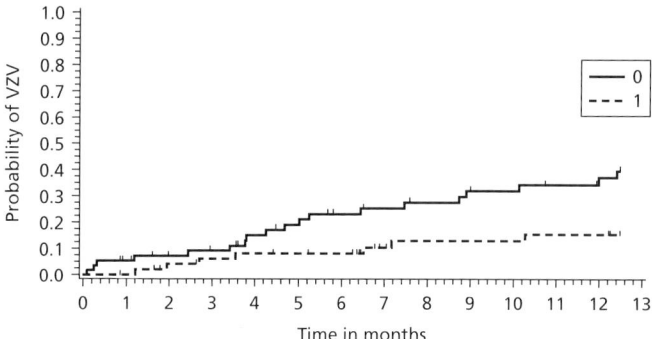

Fig. 55.10 The occurrence of zoster in autologous hematopoietic cell transplantation (HCT) recipients randomized to receive inactivated varicella vaccine or no vaccine. The Kaplan–Meier plot shows the probability of zoster in study participants who were randomized to receive inactivated vaccine (- - - -) and those who were unvaccinated (——), from enrollment until 12.5 months after HCT. The incidence of zoster was significantly higher in the unvaccinated group ($p = 0.01$). When the two cases of zoster that occurred before transplant were excluded, the difference remained significant ($p = 0.02$). Reproduced with permission from Hata et al. [26].

Varicella vaccine

The investigational live attenuated varicella vaccine (Oka–Merck strain) has been given to children with leukemia in remission [136,142]. However, it is not appropriate for administration to HCT recipients for prevention of varicella because it contains infectious virus. Immunizing healthy household contacts who are not immune to varicella with this vaccine may be useful for some families in order to reduce the risk of household exposure of the HCT recipient to varicella in siblings [147]. Health care workers in contact with HCT patients should be evaluated for susceptibility to VZV and immunized, with provisions to avoid patient contact if a vaccine-related rash occurs [129]. Since some vaccine recipients become candidates for HCT, post-transplant reactivation of vaccine virus has been demonstrated in a few instances. However, the vaccine virus appears to reactivate less commonly than wild type VZV [148]. If symptomatic reactivation occurs, the vaccine virus is susceptible to inhibition by acyclovir and episodes of vaccine-related herpes zoster can be treated with this drug [149].

Whether immunization with an inactivated preparation of the live attenuated varicella vaccine could substitute for the "natural" resensitization caused by VZV reactivation after HCT and whether the early restoration of immunity modified the clinical course of recurrent VZV disease has been evaluated in two prospective studies [26,150]. The administration of the live attenuated varicella vaccine to elderly individuals without underlying disease boosts VZV-specific immunity and immunization is being evaluated as a strategy to reverse the decline of T-cell responses which is associated with the increased risk of herpes zoster in this population [151]. Although live attenuated varicella vaccine cannot be given to immunocompromised patients, the vaccine can be heat-inactivated without loss of immunogenicity [152]. HCT recipients recover VZV immunity but reconstitution is delayed for months and often does not occur until after the patient has experienced herpes zoster [3,26,43,54]. A single dose regimen of inactivated varicella vaccine induced short-term immunologic enhancement but did not result in clinical benefit. A three dose regimen in which vaccine was given to allogeneic or autologus transplant recipients at 30, 60 and 90 days after HCT boosted cell-mediated immunity and modified the clinical severity of herpes zoster, but did not reduce the overall incidence of herpes zoster after HCT [150].

When inactivated varicella vaccine was given to autologous HCT recipients in a regimen that included a pretransplantation dose, as well as doses given at 30, 60 and 90 days after HCT, the risk of herpes zoster was reduced and protection correlated with reconstitution of VZV CD4 T-cell immunity [26]. In this study, 19 of 58 unvaccinated patients (33%) developed herpes zoster compared to seven of 53 (13%) of vaccine recipients ($p = 0.01$) (Fig. 55.10 [26]). The difference was 30% compared to 13% ($p = 0.02$) when two patients who developed zoster before transplant were excluded. VZV-specific CD4 T-cell proliferation was significantly higher in vaccinees by 90 days, following three doses of vaccine ($p = 0.04$), and the differences remained significant at 120 days, after four doses ($p = 0.0001$), at 6 months ($p = 0.004$) and at 12 months ($p = 0.02$) (Fig. 55.4).

As noted in the section on host response, this prospective study demonstrated that VZV-specific CD4 T-cell proliferation was a correlate of protection against VZV reactivation [26]. The risk of zoster was reduced by 19% per unit increase in SI >1.6 and a SI >5.0 correlated with >93% protection. The relationship between a high SI and reduced risk of herpes zoster could reflect the direct contribution of VZV-specific CD4 T cells to controlling VZV replication, since these cells make IFN-γ and other cytokines, and have cytotoxic function. Reconstitution of VZV-specific CD4 T cells by vaccination may also provide helper functions necessary to expand VZV-specific CD8 T-cell populations that are essential for preserving VZV latency.

In terms of basic immunobiology, the reduced frequency of VZV reactivation observed after active immunization of HCT recipients establishes the critical role of virus-specific T-cell responses in preserving the balance between VZV and the host. Sustaining these host responses by repeated doses is likely to be necessary to preserve clinical efficacy against herpesvirus reactivation while immunosuppressive therapy continues. Immunization of HCT patients against herpesviruses represents a particular challenge because disease is usually due to the reactivation of endogenous viruses during the first several months after transplantation. However, this experience with inactivated varicella vaccine indicates that immunotherapy with vaccines against herpesviruses has the potential to reduce the morbidity caused by these common pathogens after HCT.

Conclusion

Primary and recurrent VZV infections remain a serious threat to HCT recipients. Nevertheless, early recognition of the clinical signs of varicella and herpes zoster permits effective intervention with antiviral drugs. Immunization with inactivated varicella vaccine has the potential to reduce the morbidity of VZV reactivation after HCT.

References

1 Locksley RM, Flournoy N, Sullivan KM, Meyers JD. Infection with varicella-zoster virus after marrow transplantation. *J Infect Dis* 1985; **152**: 1172–8.

2 Zaia J. Viral infections with bone marrow transplantation. *Hematology/Oncol Clin North Am* 1990; **4**: 603–23.

3 Meyers JD, Flournoy N, Thomas ED. Cell-mediated immunity to varicella-zoster virus after allogeneic marrow transplant. *J Infect Dis* 1980; **141**: 479–87.

4 Arvin AM. Varicella-zoster virus. *Clin Microbiol Rev* 1996; **9**: 361–81.

5 Arvin AM. Varicella-zoster virus. In: Knipe DM, Howley P, eds. *Fields' Virology*, 4th edn. Philadelphia: Lippincott-Williams & Wilkins, 2001: 2731–68.

6 Cohen JI, Straus SE. Varicella-zoster virus and its replication. In: Knipe DM, Howley P, eds. *Fields' Virology*, 4th edn. Philadelphia: Lippincott-Williams & Wilkins, 2001: 2702–30.

7 Wacker P, Hartmann O, Salloum E, Lemerle J. VZV infections after bone marrow transplantation in children. *Bone Marrow Transplant* 1989; **4**: 191–4.

8 Blume K, Beutler E, Bross K *et al.* Bone marrow ablation and allogeneic bone marrow transplantation in acute leukemias. *N Engl J Med* 1980; **302**: 1041–6.

9 Atkinson K, Meyers J, Storb R *et al.* VZV infection after marrow transplantation for aplastic anemia or leukemia. *Transplantation* 1980; **29**: 47–50.

10 Atkinson K, Farwell V, Storb R *et al.* Analysis of late infections after human bone marrow transplantation: role of genotypic nonidentity between marrow donor and recipient and of nonspecific suppressor cells in patients with chronic graft-versus-host disease. *Blood* 1982; **60**: 714–20.

11 Ljungman P, Lonnqvist B, Gahrton G *et al.* Clinical and subclinical reactivation of VZV in immunocompromised patients. *J Infect Dis* 1986; **153**: 840–7.

12 Schuchter L, Wingard J, Piantadosi S *et al.* Herpes zoster infection after autologous bone marrow transplantation. *Blood* 1989; **74**: 1424–7.

13 Christiansen N, Haake R, Hurd D. Early herpes zoster in adult patients with Hodgkin's disease undergoing bone marrow transplant. *Bone Marrow Transplant* 1991; **7**: 435–7.

14 Han CS, Miller W, Haake R, Weisdorf D. Varicella zoster infection after bone marrow transplantation. Incidence, risk factors and complications. *Bone Marrow Transplant* 1994; **13**: 277–83.

15 Kawasaki H, Takayama J, Ohira M. Herpes zoster infection after bone marrow transplantation in children. *J Pediatr* 1996; **128**: 355–6.

16 Feldman S. Varicella zoster infections in bone marrow transplants. *Recent Results Cancer Res* 1993; **132**: 175–84.

17 Nakayama H, Okamura J, Ohga S *et al.* Herpes zoster in children with bone marrow transplantation: report from a single institution. *Acta Paediatr Jpn* 1995; **37**: 302–7.

18 Koc Y, Miller KB, Schenkein DP *et al.* Varicella zoster virus infections following allogeneic bone marrow transplantation: frequency, risk factors, and clinical outcome. *Biol Blood Marrow Transplant* 2000; **6**: 44–9.

19 Steer CB, Szer J, Sasadeusz J, Matthews JP, Beresford JA, Grigg A. Varicella-zoster infection after allogeneic bone marrow transplantation. Incidence, risk factors and prevention with low-dose aciclovir and ganciclovir. *Bone Marrow Transplant* 2000; **25**: 657–64.

20 Offidani M, Corvatta L, Olivieri A *et al.* A predictive model of varicella-zoster virus infection after autologous peripheral blood progenitor cell transplantation. *Clin Infect Dis* 2001; **32**: 1414–22.

21 Leung TF, Chik KW, Li CK *et al.* Incidence, risk factors and outcome of varicella-zoster virus infection in children after haematopoietic stem cell transplantation. *Bone Marrow Transplant* 2000; **25**: 167–72.

22 Ragozzino M, Melton L, Kurland L *et al.* Population based study of herpes zoster and its sequelae. *Medicine* 1982; **61**: 310–6.

23 Cohrs RJ, Barbour M, Gilden DH. Varicella-zoster virus (VZV) transcription during latency in human ganglia. Detection of transcripts mapping to genes 21, 29, 62, and 63 in a cDNA library enriched for VZV RNA. *J Virol* 1996; **70**: 2789–96.

24 Saral R, Burns WH, Prentice HG. Herpes virus infections. Clinical manifestations and therapeutic strategies in immunocompromised patients. *Clin Haematol* 1984; **13**: 645–60.

25 Wingard JR. Viral infections in leukemia and bone marrow transplant patients. *Leuk Lymphoma* 1993; **2**: 115–25.

26 Hata A, Asanuma H, Rinki M. *et al.* Use of an inactivated varicella vaccine in recipients of hematopoietic-cell transplants. *N Engl J Med* 2002; **347**: 26–34.

27 Wallace MR, Chamberlin CJ, Zerboni L *et al.* Lack of evidence for recurrent varicella in immunocompetent adults. *J Am Med Assoc* 1997; **278**: 1520–2.

28 Grose C. Varicella zoster virus. Pathogenesis of the human diseases, the virus and viral replication. In: Hyman R, ed. *The Natural History of Varicella Zoster Virus*. Boca Raton: CRC Press, 1987: 1–66.

29 Ku CC, Padilla J, Grose C, Butcher EC, Arvin AM. Tropism of varicella-zoster virus for human tonsillar $CD4^+$ T lymphocytes that express activation, memory and skin homing markers. *J Virol* 2002; **76**: 11425–33.

30 Asano Y, Itakura N, Hiroishi Y *et al.* Viral replication and immunologic responses in children naturally infected with varicella-zoster virus and in varicella vaccine recipients. *J Infect Dis* 1985; **152**: 863–8.

31 Koropchak CM, Solem S, Diaz PS, Arvin AM. Investigation of varicella-zoster virus infection of lymphocytes by *in situ* hybridization. *J Virol* 1989; **63**: 2392–5.

32 Koropchak CM, Graham G, Palmer J *et al.* Investigation of varicella-zoster virus infection by polymerase chain reaction in the immunocompetent host with acute varicella. *J Infectdis* 1991; **163**: 1016–22.

33 Moffat JF, Stein MD, Kaneshima H, Arvin AM. Tropism of varicella-zoster virus for human $CD4^+$ and $CD8^+$ T lymphocytes and epidermal cells in SCID-hu mice. *J Virol* 1995; **69**: 5236–42.

34 Moffat J, Zerboni L, Stein M, Grose C, Kaneshima H, Arvin A. The attenuation of the vaccine Oka strain of varicella-zoster virus and the role of glycoprotein C in alphaherpesvirus virulence demonstrated in the SCID-hu mouse. *J Virol* 2002; **76**: 8468–71.

35 Straus S, Reinhold W, Smith H *et al.* Endonuclease analysis of viral DNA from varicella and subsequent zoster in the same patient. *N Engl J Med* 1984; **311**: 1326–8.

36 Gilden D, Mahlingham R, Dueland N, Cohrs R. Herpes zoster. Pathogenesis and latency. *Prog Med Virol* 1992; **39**: 19–75.

37 Lungu O, Annunziato PW, Gershon A *et al.* Reactivated and latent varicella-zoster virus in human dorsal root ganglia. *Proc Natl Acad Sci U S A* 1995; **92**: 10,980–4.

38 Mahalingam R, Wellish M, Wolf W *et al.* Latent VZV DNA in human trigeminal and thoracic ganglia. *N Engl J Med* 1990; **323**: 627–31.

39 Silverstein S, Straus SE. Varicella-zoster virus. Pathogenesis of latency and reactivation. In: Arvin AM, Gershon AA, eds. *Varicella-Zoster Virus: Virology and Clinical Practice*. Cambridge: Cambridge Press, 2000: 123–41.

40 Kennedy PG, Grinfeld E, Bell JE. Varicella-zoster gene expression in latently infected and explanted human ganglia. *J Virol* 2000; **74**: 11,893–8.

41 Mahalingam R, Wellish M, Cohrs R *et al.* Expression of protein encoded by varicella-zoster virus open reading frame 63 in latently infected human ganglionic neurons. *Proc Natl Acad Sci U S A* 1996; **93**: 2122–4.

42 Debrus S, Sadzot DC, Nikkels AF, Piette J, Rentier B. Varicella-zoster virus gene 63 encodes an immediate-early protein that is abundantly expressed during latency. *J Virol* 1995; **69**: 3240–1.

43 Wilson A, Sharp M, Koropchak CM, Ting SF, Arvin AM. Subclinical varicella-zoster virus viremia, herpes zoster and recovery of T-lymphocyte responses to varicella-zoster viral antigens after allogeneic and autologous bone marrow transplantation. *J Infect Dis* 1992; **165**: 119–26.

44 Rogers SY, Irving W, Harris A, Russell NH. Visceral varicella zoster infection after bone marrow transplantation without skin involvement and the use of PCR for diagnosis. *Bone Marrow Transplant* 1995; **15**: 805–7.

45 Stemmer SM, Kinsman K, Tellschow S, Jones RB. Fatal noncutaneous visceral infection with varicella-zoster virus in a patient with lymphoma after autologous bone marrow transplantation. *Clin Infect Dis* 1993; **16**: 497–9.

46 Feldman S, Epp E. Isolation of varicella-zoster virus from blood. *J Pediatr* 1976; **88**: 265–8.

47 Atkinson K, Hansen JA, Strob R, Goehle S, Goldstein G, Thomas ED. T cell subpopulations identified by monoclonal antibodies after human bone marrow transplantation. Helper-inducer and cytotoxic-suppressor subsets. *Blood* 1982; **59**: 1292–8.

48 Abendroth A, Slobedman B, Lee E, Mellins E, Wallace M, Arvin AM. Modulation of major histocompatibility class II expression by varicella zoster virus. *J Virol* 2000; **74**: 1900–7.

49 Abendroth A, Lin I, Slobedman B, Ploegh H, Arvin AM. Varicella zoster virus retains major histocompatibility complex class I proteins in the Golgi of infected cells. *J Virol* 2001; **75**: 4878–88.

50 Arvin M, Koropchak CM, Williams BR, Grumet FC, Foung SK. Early immune response in healthy and immunocompromised subjects with primary varicella-zoster virus infection. *J Infect Dis* 1986; **154**: 422–9.

51 Webster A, Grint P, Brenner MK, Prentice HG, Griffiths PD. Titration of IgG antibodies against varicella zoster virus before bone marrow trans-

plantation is not predictive of future zoster. *J Med Virol* 1989; **27**: 117–9.
52 Arvin AM, Pollard RB, Rasmussen LE, Merigan TC. Cellular and humoral immunity in the pathogenesis of recurrent herpes viral infections in patients with lymphoma. *J Clin Invest* 1980; **65**: 869–78.
53 Arvin AM. Varicella-zoster virus. In: Ahmed R, Irvin S, Chen Y, eds. *Persistent Viral Infections*. West Sussex, England: John Wiley & Sons Ltd, 1999: 183–208.
54 Takaue Y, Okamoto Y, Kawano Y et al. Regeneration of immunity and varicella-zoster virus infection after high-dose chemotherapy and peripheral blood stem cell autografts in children. *Bone Marrow Transplant* 1994; **14**: 219–23.
55 Gratama JW, Verdonck LF, Van der Linden JA et al. Cellular immunity to vaccinations and herpes virus infections after bone marrow transplantation. *Transplantation* 1986; **41**: 719–24.
56 Asanuma H, Sharp M, Maecker HT, Maino VC, Arvin AM. Frequencies of memory T cells specific for varicella-zoster virus, herpes simplex virus and cytomegalovirus determined by intracellular detection of cytokine expression. *J Infect Dis* 2000; **181**: 859–66.
57 Kato S, Yabe MY, Kimura M et al. Studies on transfer of varicella-zoster-virus specific T-cell immunity from bone marrow donor to recepient. *Blood* 1990; **75**: 806–9.
58 Ault KA, Antin JH, Ginsburg D et al. Phenotype of recovery lymphoid cell populations after marrow transplantation. *J Exp Med* 1985; **161**: 1483–501.
59 Arvin AM, Sharp MS, Smith S et al. Equivalent recognition of a varicella-zoster virus immediate early protein (IE62) and glycoprotein I by cytotoxic T-lymphocytes of either CD4+ or CD8+ phenotype. *J Immunol* 1991; **146**: 257–64.
60 Sadzot-Delvaux C, Kinchington P, Arvin AM. Humoral and cell-mediated immune responses to the ORF63 protein of varicella-zoster virus. *J Immunol* 1997; **159**: 2802–6.
61 Arvin AM, Sharp M, Moir M et al. Memory cytotoxic T cell responses to viral tegument and regulatory proteins encoded by open reading frames 4, 10, 29 and 62 of varicella-zoster virus. *Viral Immunol* 2002; **15**: 1–10.
62 Neiderwieser D, Gastl G, Rumpold H, Kraft MD, Huber C. Rapid reappearance of large granular lymphocytes (LGL) with concomitant reconstitution of natural killer (NK) activity after human bone marrow transplantation. *Br J Haematol* 1987; **65**: 301–5.
63 Whitley RJ. Varicella zoster virus infections. In: Galasso G, Whitley R, Merigan T, eds. *Antiviral Agents and Viral Diseases of Man*. New York: Lippincott-Raven Press, 1997: 279–304.
64 Feldman S, Lott L. Varicella in children with cancer. Impact of antiviral therapy and prophylaxis. *Pediat* 1987; **80**: 465–71.
65 Whitley RJ. Chickenpox in the immunocompromised host. In: Balfour HH, ed. *Advances in Therapy Against Herpes Virus Infections in Immunocompromised Hosts*. New York: Park Row Publications, 1985: 25–39.
66 Szabo F, Horvath N, Seimon S, Hughes T. Inappropriate antidiuretic hormone secretion, abdominal pain and disseminated varicella-zoster virus infection: an unusual triad in a patient 6 months post mini-allogeneic peripheral stem cell transplant for chronic myeloid leukemia. *Clin Laboratory Haematol* 2001; **23**: 255–4.
67 Yagi T, Karasuno T, Hasegawa T et al. Acute abdomen without cutaneous signs of varicella zoster virus infection as a late complication of allogeneic bone marrow transplantation: importance of empiric therapy with acyclovir. *Bone Marrow Transplant* 2000; **25**: 1003–5.
68 Tenenbaum T, Kramm CM, Laws HJ, Nurnberger W, Lenard HG, Gobel U. Pre-eruptive varicella zoster virus encephalitis in two children after haematopoietic stem cell transplantation. *Med Pediatr Oncol* 2002; **38**: 288–9.
69 Ingraham J, Estes N, Bern M, De Girolami P. Disseminated varicella zoster virus infection and the syndrome of inappropriate ADH. *Arch Intern Med* 1983; **143**: 1270–3.
70 Ballow M, Hirschhorn R. Varicella pneumonia in a bone marrow transplanted immune-reconstituted adenosine deaminase deficient patient with severe combined immunodeficiency disease. *J Clin Immunol* 1985; **5**: 180–6.
71 Gilden DH, Beinlich BR, Rubinstien EM et al. Varicella-zoster virus myelitis: an expanding spectrum. *Neurol* 1994; **44** (10): 1818–23.
72 Meylan PR, Miklossy J, Iten A et al. Myelitis due to varicella-zoster virus in an immunocompromised patient without a cutaneous rash. *Clin Infect Dis* 1995; **20**: 206–8.
73 Brunell PA. Varicella-zoster virus. In: Mandell GL, Douglas RG, Bennett JE, eds. *Principles and Practice of Infectious Diseases*. New York: Wiley, 1985: 952–60.
74 Gallagher J, Merigan T. Prolonged herpes zoster infection associated with immunosuppressive therapy. *Ann Intern Med* 1979; **91**: 842–4.
75 Whitley RJ, Gnann JW. Herpes zoster in patients with human immunodeficiency virus infection: an ever-expanding spectrum of disease. *Clin Infect Dis* 1995; **21**: 989–90.
76 Womack L, Liesegang T. Complications of herpes zoster ophthalmicus. *Arch Ophthalm* 1983; **101**: 42–51.
77 Roberts TV, Francis IC, Kappagoda MB, Dick AD. Herpes zoster chorioretinopathy. *Eye* 1995; 594–8.
78 Linneman C, Alvira M. Pathogenesis of varicella-zoster angiitis in the central nervous system. *Arch Neurol* 1980; **37**: 239–43.
79 Jamsek J, Greenberg S, Taber L. Herpes zoster associated encephalitis. Clinicopathologic report of 12 cases and review of the literature. *Medicine* 1983; **62**: 81–8.
80 Morishita K, Kodo H, Asano S et al. Fulminant varicella hepatitis following bone marrow transplantation. *JAMA* 1985; **253**: 511.
81 Sullivan K, Meyers J, Flournoy N et al. Early and late interstitial pneumonia following human bone marrow transplantation. *Int J Cell Cloning* 1986; **4** (Suppl.): 107–24.
82 Schiller G, Nimer S, Gajewski J et al. Abdominal presentation of VZV infection in recipients of allogeneic bone marrow transplantation. *Bone Marrow Transplant* 1991; **7**: 489–91.
83 Nomdedeu JF, Nomdedeu J, Martino R et al. Ogilvie's syndrome from disseminated varicella-zoster infection and infarcted celiac ganglia. *J Clin Gastroenterol* 1995; **20**: 157–9.
84 Sanz Moreno J, Lopez-Rubio M, Calero-Garcia MA, Ratia-Jimenez T, Arranz-Caso A, Martinez-Martinez J. Acute abdomen and intestinal necrosis produced by varicella-zoster virus in an immunocompromised host. *Clin Infect Dis* 1996; **22**: 857–8.
85 Perez-Oteyza J, Pascual C, Garcia-Larana J, Odriozola J, Rocamora A, Navarro JL. Abdominal presentation of varicella zoster infection in recipients of allogeneic bone marrow transplantation. *Bone Marrow Transplant* 1992; **9**: 21–3.
86 Drakos P, Weinberger M, Delukina M et al. Inappropriate antidiuretic hormone secretion (SIADH) preceding skin manifestations of disseminated varicella zoster virus infection post-HCT. *Bone Marrow Transplant* 1993; **11**: 407–8.
87 David DS, Tegtmeier BR, O'Donnell MR, Paz IB, McCarty TM. Visceral varicella-zoster after bone marrow transplantation. Report of a case series and review of the literature. *Am J Gastroenterol* 1998; **93**: 810–3.
88 Flamholc L. Neurological complications in herpes zoster. *Scand J Infect Dis Suppl* 1996; **100**: 35–40.
89 Kleinschmidt-DeMasters BK, Amlie-Lefond C, Gilden DH. The patterns of varicella zoster virus encephalitis. *Hum Pathol* 1996; **27**: 927–38.
90 Gold E, Robin F. Isolation of herpes zoster from the spinal fluid of a patient. *Virol* 1958; **6**: 293–5.
91 McKendall R, Klawns H. Nervous system complications of varicella zoster. In: Vinken P, Bruyn G, eds. *Handbook of Clinical Neurology. Infection of the Nervous System*. Amsterdam: North Holland Press, 1978: 161–7.
92 Reichman R. Neurologic complications of varicella zoster infections. *Ann Intern Med* 1978; **375**: 89–96.
93 Gershon AA, LaRussa P, Steinberg S. Varicella-zoster virus. In: Murray P, ed. *Manual of Clinical Microbiology*. Washington, DC: American Society for Microbiology, 1999: 900–11.
94 Schmidt NJ, Gallo D, Devlin V, Woodie JD, Emmons RW. Direct immunofluorescence staining for detection of herpes simplex and varicella-zoster virus antigens in vesicular lesion and certain tissue specimens. *J Clin Microbiol* 1980; **12**: 651–5.
95 Gleaves CA, Lee CF, Bustamante CI, Meyers JD. Use of murine monoclonal antibodies for laboratory diagnosis of varicella-zoster virus infection. *J Clin Microbiol* 1988; **26**: 1623–5.
96 Levin M, Leventhal S, Masters H. Factors influencing quantitative isolation of varicella zoster virus. *J Clin Microbiol* 1984; **19**: 880–3.
97 Brinker JP, Doern GV. Comparison of MRC-5 and A-549 cells in conventional culture tubes and shell vial assays for the detection of varicella-zoster virus. *Diagn Microbiol Infect Dis* 1993; **17**: 75–7.
98 West PG, Aldrich A, Hartwig A, Haller G. Increased detection rate for varicella-zoster virus with combination of two techniques. *J Clin Microbiol* 1988; **26**: 2680–1.
99 Forghani BYuG, Hurst J. Comparison of biotinylated DNA and RNA probes for rapid detection of varicella-zoster virus genome by *in situ* hybridization. *J Clin Microbiol* 1991; **29**: 583–91.
100 Annunziato P, Lungu O, Gershon A, Silvers DN, LaRussa P, Silverstein SJ. *In situ* hybridization detection of varicella zoster virus in paraffin-embedded skin biopsy samples. *Clin Diagn Virol* 1996; **7**: 69–76.
101 Bergstrom T. Polymerase chain reaction for diagnosis of varicella zoster virus central nervous system infections without skin manifestations. *Scand J Infect Dis Suppl* 1996; **100**: 41–5.
102 LaRussa P, Steinberg S, Shapiro E et al. Viral strain identification in varicella vaccines with disseminated rashes. *Pediatr Infect Dis J* 2000; **19**: 1037–9.
103 Steinberg S, Gershon A. Measurement of antibodies to VZV by using a latex agglutination test. *J Clin Microbiol* 1991; **29**: 1527–30.

104 Gleaves CA, Schwarz KA, Campbell MB. Determination of varicella-zoster virus (VZV) immune status with the VIDAS VZV immunoglobulin G automated immunoassay and the VZVScan latex agglutination assay. *Clin Diagn Laboratory Immunol* 1996; **3**: 365–7.

105 Klevjer AP, Anderson LW. Comparison of a new latex agglutination assay with indirect immunofluorescence to detect varicella-zoster antibodies. *Diagn Microbiol Infect Dis* 1993; **17**: 247–9.

106 Schmidt N, Arvin AM. Sensitivity of different assay systems for immunoglobulin M, responses to varicella zoster virus in reactivated infection. *J Clin Microbiol* 1986; **23**: 978–9.

107 Biron KK, Elion GB. *In vitro* susceptibility of varicella-zoster to acyclvoir. *Antimicrob Ag Chemother* 1980; **18**: 443–7.

108 Crumpacker CS, Schnipper LE, Zaia JA, Levin MJ. Growth inhibition by acycloguanosine of herpes viruses isolated from human infections. *Antimicrob Ag Chemother* 1979; **15**: 642–5.

109 Bryson YJ. The use of acyclovir in children. *Ped Infect Dis* 1984; **3**: 345–51.

110 Sullender W, Arvin AM, Diaz P et al. Acyclovir pharmacokinetics following suspension administration to children. *Antimicrob Ag Chemo* 1987; **31**: 1722–6.

111 de Miranda P, Blum MR. Pharmacokinetics of oral acyclovir after intravenous and oral administration. *J Antimicrob Chemother* 1983; **12** (Suppl. B): 29–33.

112 Myers M. Viremia caused by varicella–zoster virus: association with malignant progressive varicella. *J Infect Dis* 1979; **140**: 229–34.

113 Prober C, Kirk E, Keeney R. Acyclovir therapy of chickenpox in immunosuppressed children, a collaborative study. *J Pediatr* 1984; **101**: 622–5.

114 Balfour HJ Jr, McMonigal K, Bean B. Acyclovir therapy of VZV infections in immunocompromised patients. *J Antimicrob Chemother* 1983; **12** (Suppl. B): 169–79.

115 Balfour HH Jr. Intravenous acyclvoir therapy for varicella in immunocompromised children. *J Pediatr* 1984; **104**: 134–6.

116 Zaia JA, Levin MJ, Preblud SR et al. Evaluation of varicella-zoster immune globulin: protection of immunosuppressed children after household exposure to varicella. *J Infect Dis* 1983; **147**: 737–43.

117 Selby P, Jameson B, Watson J et al. Parenteral acyclovir for herpes virus infections of man. *Lancet* 1979; **1**: 1267–70.

118 Balfour H, Dean B, Laskin O et al. Acyclovir halts the progression of herpes zoster in immunocompromised patients. *N Engl J Med* 1983; **308**: 1448–53.

119 Meyers J, Wade J, Shepp D et al. Acyclovir treatment of VZV infection in the compromised host. *Transplantation* 1984; **37**: 571–4.

120 Shepp D, Dandliker P, Meyers J. Treatment of varicella zoster infections in severely immunocompromized patients. *N Engl J Med* 1986; **314**: 208–12.

121 Wood MJ, Kay R, Dworkin RH, Soong SJ, Whitley RJ. Oral acyclovir therapy accelerates pain resolution in patients with herpes zoster. A meta-analysis of placebo-controlled trials. *Clin Infect Dis* 1996; **22**: 341–7.

122 Jackson JL, Gibbons R, Meyer G, Inouye L. The effect of treating herpes zoster with oral acyclovir in preventing post-herpetic neuralgia. A meta-analysis. *Arch Intern Med* 1997; **157**: 909–12.

123 Wood MF, Johnson RW, McKendrick MW, Taylor J, Mandal B, Crooks J. A randomized trial of acyclovir for 7 days or 21 days with and without prednisolone for treatment of acute herpes zoster. *N Engl J Med* 1994; **330**: 896–900.

124 Whitley RJ, Weiss H, Gnann JW Jr et al. Acyclovir with and without prednisone for the treatment of herpes zoster. A randomized, placebo-controlled trial. The National Institute of Allergy and Infectious Diseases Collaborative Antiviral Study Group. *Ann Intern Med* 1996; **125**: 376–83.

125 Rowbotham MC, Petersen KL. Zoster-associated pain and neural dysfunction. *Pain* 2001; **93**: 1–5.

126 Beutner KR, Friedman DJ, Forszpaniak C, Andersen PL, Wood MJ. Valaciclovir compared with acyclovir for improved therapy for herpes zoster in immunocompetent adults. *Antimicrob Agents Chemother* 1995; **39**: 1546–53.

127 Saltzman R, Boon R. The safety of famciclovir in patients with herpes zoster. *Curr Therapeu Res* 1995; **56**: 219–25.

128 Tyring S, Barbarash RA, Nahlik JE et al. Famciclovir for the treatment of acute herpes zoster: effects on acute disease and post-herpetic neuralgia. A randomized, double-blind, placebo-controlled trial. Collaborative Famciclovir Herpes Zoster Study Group. *Ann Intern Med* 1995; **123**: 89–96.

129 Centers for Disease Control. Guidelines for preventing opportunistic infections among hematopoietic-cell transplant recipients. *Morbidity and Mortality Weekly Report* October 20, 2000; **49**.

130 Reusser P, Cordonnier C, Einsele H et al. European survey of herpes virus resistance to antiviral drugs in bone marrow transplant recipients. Infectious Diseases Working Party of the European Group for Blood and Marrow Transplantation (EHCT). *Bone Marrow Transplant* 1996; **17**: 813–7.

131 Balfour HH, Benson C, Braun J et al. Management of acyclovir-resistant herpes simplex and varicella-zoster infections. *J Acquir Imm Def Synd* 1994; **7**: 254–60.

132 Boivin G, Edelman CK, Pedneault L, Talarico CL, Biron K, Balfour H. Phenotypic and genotypic characterization of acyclovir-resistant varicella-zoster viruses isolated from persons with AIDS. *J Infect Dis* 1994; **170**: 68–75.

133 Fillet AM, Visse B, Caumes E, Dumont B, Gentilini M, Huraux JM. Foscarnet-resistant multidermatomal zoster in a patient with AIDS. *Clin Infect Dis* 1995; **21**: 1348–9.

134 Lietman PS. Clinical pharmacology: foscarnet. *Am J Med* 1992; **92** (Suppl. 2A): S8–11.

135 De Clercq E. Therapeutic potential of HPMPC as an antiviral drug. *Rev Med Virol* 1993; **3**: 85–96.

136 Wallace MR, Chamberlin CJ, Sawyer MH et al. Treatment of adult varicella with sorivudine: a randomized, placebo-controlled trial. *J Infect Dis* 1996; **174**: 249–55.

137 Okuda H, Nishiyama T, Ogura Y et al. Lethal drug interactions of sorivudine, a new antiviral drug, with oral 5-fluorouracil prodrugs. *Drug Metab Dispos* 1997; **25**: 270–3.

138 Fiddian AP. Antiviral drugs in development for herpes zoster. *Scand J Infect Dis Suppl* 1996; **100**: 51–4.

139 Merigan T, Rand K, Pollard R et al. Human leukocyte interferon for the treatment of herpes zoster in patients with cancer. *N Engl J Med* 1987; **298**: 981–7.

140 Paryani SG, Arvin AM, Koropchak CM et al. A comparison of varicella-zoster antibody titers in patients given intravenous immune serum globulin or varicella zoster immune globulin. *J Pediatr* 1984; **105**: 201–5.

141 Krause PR, Klinman DM. Efficacy, immunogenicity, safety, and use of live attenuated chickenpox vaccine. *J Pediatr* 1995; **127**: 518–25.

142 Arvin AM, Gershon AA. Live attenuated varicella vaccine. *Annu Rev Microbiol* 1996; **50**: 59–100.

143 Ljungman P, Wilczek H, Gahrton G et al. Long-term acyclovir prophylaxis in bone marrow transplant recipients and lymphocyte proliferation responses to herpes virus *in vitro*. *Transplantation* 1986; **1**: 185–92.

144 Selby P, Powles R, Easton D et al. The prophylactic role of intravenous and long-term oral acyclovir after allogeneic bone marrow transplantation. *Br J Cancer* 1989; **59**: 434–8.

145 Perren T, Powels R, Easton D et al. Prevention of herpes zoster in patients by long term acyclovir after bone marrow transplantation. *Am J Med* 1988; **85**: S99–101.

146 Gershon AA, LaRussa P, Steinberg S. The varicella vaccine. Clinical trials in immunocompromised individuals. *Infect Dis Clin North Am* 1996; **10**: 583–94.

147 Diaz PS, Smith S, Hunter E, Au D, Arvin AM. Lack of transmission of the live attenuated varicella vaccine to immmunocompromised children following immunization of their siblings. *Pediatrics* 1991; **87**: 166–70.

148 Hardy I, Chu B, Gershon AA, Steinberg SP, LaRussa P. The incidence of zoster after immunization with live attenuated varicella vaccine. *N Engl J Med* 1991; **325**: 1545–50.

149 Shiraki K, Matsui S, Aiba N. Susceptibility of Oka varicella vaccine strain to antiviral drugs. *Vaccine* 1993; **11**: 1380–2.

150 Redman RL, Nader S, Zerboni L et al. Early reconstitution of immunity and decreased severity of herpes zoster in bone marrow transplant recipients immunized with inactivated varicella vaccine. *J Infect Dis* 1997; **176**: 578–85.

151 Levin MJ, Hayward AR. The varicella vaccine. Prevention of herpes zoster. *Infect Dis Clin North Am* 1996; **10**: 657–75.

152 Sperber SJ, Smith BV, Hayden FG. Serologic response and reactogenicity to booster immunization of healthy seropositive adults with live or inactivated varicella vaccine. *Antiviral Res* 1992; **17**: 213–22.

56

Richard F. Ambinder

Epstein–Barr Virus Infection

Introduction

Herpesvirus-associated complications after hematopoietic cell transplantation (HCT) include mucositis associated with herpes simplex virus (HSV), pneumonitis and enteritis associated with cytomegalovirus (CMV), zoster associated with varicella-zoster virus (VZV) and encephalitis associated with human herpesvirus-6 (HHV-6). These diseases are either prevented or treated with antiviral agents that inhibit lytic infection and the tissue damage that accompanies it. In contrast, Epstein–Barr virus-associated lymphoproliferative disorder (EBV-LPD) is a fundamentally different process in that it is associated with latent rather than lytic viral infection. Although EBV-LPD is not reliably prevented or treated with conventional antiviral agents, this once usually fatal complication of HCT can nonetheless be prevented or treated in most instances. EBV is also associated with other diseases, such as Hodgkin's disease (HD) and nasopharyngeal carcinoma, which lead patients to treatment with HCT or adoptive cellular immunotherapy. This chapter reviews the biology of the virus, EBV-LPD in HCT patients, aspects of its detection and characterization in clinical specimens, and other EBV tumor associations with an emphasis on the possible application of HCT strategies to their treatment.

EBV biology

EBV infection is ubiquitous in all adult human populations [1,2]. EBV is a gammaherpesvirus. Like other herpesviruses, EBV infection may be either latent or lytic (productive of new virions). In contrast to most other human herpesviruses, the latent states of EBV predominate *in vitro* and, in most infected tissues, *in vivo*. The virus is most commonly transmitted in the saliva. Usually asymptomatic in childhood, when primary infection is delayed to adolescence or young adulthood it is often associated with the syndrome of infectious mononucleosis characterized by fever, pharyngitis, lymphadenopathy and splenomegaly. Infected B cells proliferate and thus expand the pool of latently infected cells throughout the B-cell compartment. Early on in the infection several percent of the lymphocytes may be infected by virus.

Early in infection the full range of latency viral transcripts, including the immunodominant Epstein–Barr nuclear antigens (EBNAs), are expressed. These latency proteins "drive" proliferation of the infected lymphocytes. However, with time, as the cellular immune response is established, expression of these antigens serves to target these proliferating B cells for destruction by virus-specific cytotoxic T lymphocytes (CTLs). Ultimately, viral DNA persists in resting B lymphocytes as episomes with very limited viral gene expression [3–6].

In seropositive individuals virus is periodically shed in the saliva. The source of virion shedding, B cells in the mucosa vs. epithelial cells, is unknown. However, observations of patients treated with acyclovir suggest that maintenance of the infected B-cell reservoir does not require lytic infection. Treatment with acyclovir eliminates lytic viral replication as evidenced by the inability to detect EBV in throat washings, but does not affect the number of latently infected B cells in the blood [7].

The EBV virion is enveloped and carries a double stranded linear viral genome approximately 172,000 bp in length. The genome encodes more than 80 open reading frames. Most of these are expressed in lytic infection, some are expressed in latent infection and some are expressed in both. EBV has a predominant tropism for B lymphocytes, although it can also infect a variety of other cell types including monocytes and epithelial cells [8,9]. In the nucleus, the left and right termini of the linear viral genomes fuse to form episomes. In cells that proceed to lytic infection these episomes give rise to linear multigenome length concatemers that are then cleaved to generate genome length linear molecules. Generation of concatemers requires the viral DNA polymerase and other virus encoded lytic cycle enzymes. In cells that maintain the genome in a latent state, viral episomes persist. Viral episomes replicate once per cell division cycle and maintain stable copy numbers over many generations. The only viral protein required for this process is EBNA-1, a sequence-specific DNA binding protein expressed in all forms of EBV latency [10]. Although in some circumstances the viral DNA may integrate such as when proliferating cells are infected, integration is not site specific nor is it a regular feature of EBV infection [11].

Several key aspects of the biology of the virus are illuminated by considering the infection of B lymphocytes *in vitro* and resultant growth transformation [1,12]. *In vitro* infection drives lymphocytes from G_0 into G_1 and S phase and continuous proliferation. The resulting EBV-immortalized lines are referred to as lymphoblastoid cell lines (LCLs). These LCLs will grow indefinitely in tissue culture and form human B-cell tumors in severe combined immunodeficiency syndrome (SCID) mice. They produce few progeny virions and are predominantly latently infected. As such they are not sensitive to inhibitors of the viral DNA polymerase. These inhibitors do not inhibit immortalization or the passage of LCLs in culture.

Latency does not imply transcriptional silence. On the contrary, viral genes profoundly alter the growth properties of the latently infected cells [13]. Among the viral proteins expressed are the six EBNAs, three latent membrane proteins (LMPs) and poorly characterized proteins encoded by the Bam HI A rightward transcripts. In addition, two small polymerase III transcripts, EB encoded RNAs (EBER-1 and -2), which do not code for protein, are expressed.

The use of recombinant virus lacking individual latency genes has demonstrated that immortalization is the result of the coordinated expression of several viral genes [12]. EBNA-1 functions to initiate viral DNA replication, to enhance the expression of other viral latency proteins and to partition the viral episomes during cell division [14]. The protein appears not to directly alter expression of cellular genes except insofar as it maintains the viral episome [15]. EBNA-2 is a transcriptional transactivator that regulates the pattern of EBV latency gene expression in B cells and modifies cellular gene expression by mimicry of activated Notch signaling [16,17]. Among the genes up-regulated are viral genes *LMP-1* and *LMP-2*, and cellular genes *CD21*, *CD23* and *c-myc*. EBNA-2 also interacts directly with Nur77 and blocks cell death. EBNA-3A and -3B are also required for immortalization and also modulate transcription of viral and cellular genes. LMP-1 is an integral membrane protein that functionally resembles a constitutively activated member of the tumor necrosis factor receptor superfamily, particularly CD40 [13]. In contrast to CD40 and other members of the superfamily, LMP-1 in the cell membrane constitutively aggregates forming patches and caps in the absence of ligand. *In vitro* expression is associated with transformation of immortalized rodent fibroblast cell lines as marked by loss of contact inhibition, anchorage independent growth and tumorigenesis in nude mice. In transgenic mice, expression under the control of an immunoglobulin heavy chain regulatory locus leads to B-cell lymphomagenesis. Many of the effects of the protein are mediated by the carboxyl terminal domain of the protein engaging cellular signaling pathways, including NFKB, AP-1 and Stats 1 and 3.

The immune response to EBV infection

Neutralizing antibodies may play a role in interrupting the spread of infection and blocking superinfection with other strains in seropositive individuals, but the humoral response is thought to have little impact on established latent infection as the target antigens are either not expressed in latently infected cells or are nuclear antigens. Early on, after primary infection, CD8$^+$ T-cell responses to lytic antigens predominate [18–20]. Ultimately, responses to latency antigens emerge. Across many human leukocyte antigen (HLA) types, EBNA-3A, EBNA-3B and EBNA-3C dominate the CD8$^+$ T-cell response and cells expressing these latency antigens are killed. The B cells that chronically harbor the virus show limited antigen expression. LMP-2 a subdominant antigen and, perhaps, EBNA-1, which blocks its own presentation in the class I major histocompatibility complex (MHC) pathway are expressed. Absence of target antigens and the resting state of the infected B cells may combine to make these cells relatively "invisible" to cytotoxic T cells. Nonetheless, CD8$^+$ T-cell responses to latency viral are chronically maintained at high levels (Fig. 56.1 [20]).

Epstein–Barr virus-associated lymphoproliferative disorder (EBV-LPD)

Incidence and risk factors

The disease manifestations associated with EBV in the setting of HCT are EBV-LPD or EBV-HD. The incidence of EBV-LPD in marrow and blood hematopoietic cell recipients varies widely according to the source of hematopoietic cells, the associated cell manipulations, and the details of immunosuppressive regimens used [21–28]. In many series, a substantial fraction of cases were diagnosed only at autopsy and, as many deceased patients were never autopsied, it seems likely that published estimates are too low [29]. Unmanipulated allogeneic bone marrow transplantations (BMTs) have a risk of approximately 1%, while, at the other extreme, T-cell depletion (TCD) using antibodies specific for CD2 and CD3 was associated with EBV-LPD in five out of seven patients (71%) [30]. Risk factors have been most completely assessed in an International Bone Marrow Transplant Registry (IBMTR) study of more than

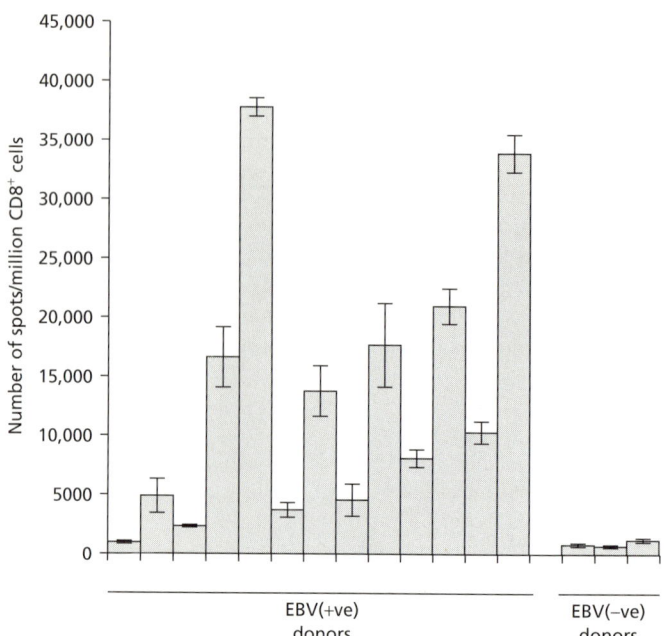

Fig. 56.1 Numbers of CD8$^+$ T cells responding to Epstein–Barr virus (EBV) lymphoblastoid cell lines (LCLs) from EBV-seropositive and EBV-seronegative healthy individuals. Adapted from Yang *et al.* [20].

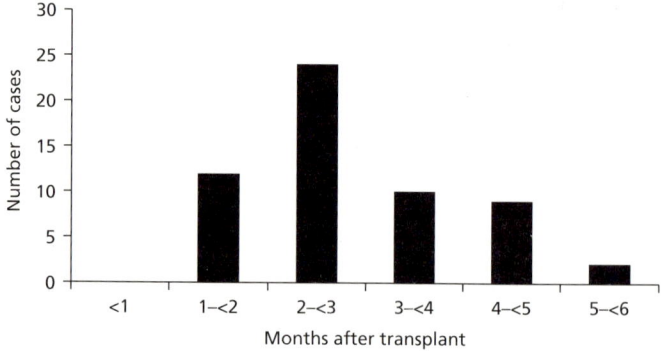

Fig. 56.2 Numbers of cases of lymphoproliferative disorder (LPD) after allogeneic bone marrow transplantation (BMT). Adapted from Curtis *et al.* [31].

18,000 allogeneic BMT recipients who showed the cumulative incidence of LPD to be 1% at 10 years [31]. More than 80% of cases occurred in the 1st year after transplant, with the incidence of LPD highest at 2–3 months (Fig. 56.2 [31]). A multivariate analysis identified the risk factors for early disease as shown in Table 56.1 [31]. The risk factor that conferred the greatest relative risk was the use of a monoclonal anti-CD3 antibody to treat graft-vs.-host disease (GVHD). TCD was also a risk factor, but the risk associated with various approaches to depletion varied substantially. The use of sheep red blood cell (SRBC) rosetting, anti-T or anti-T and natural killer (NK) monoclonal antibodies was associated with relative risks of LPD of 15 and 12, respectively. The use of lectins, Campath-1 monoclonal antibody or elutriation were not associated with a statistically significant increased relative risk.

High risk of LPD was associated with selective TCD whether in the context of systemic therapy to prevent or treat GVHD or marrow product manipulations to prevent GVHD. In contrast, the use of methods that resulted in balanced loss of B cells and T cells were not associated with significantly increased risk. Smaller studies reinforce these conclusions [30,32–35]. Whether the protective effects of B-cell depletion mainly

Table 56.1 Risk factors for lymphoproliferative disorder (LPD).

EBV-LPD <1 year	Relative risk
Anti-CD3 monoclonal antibody	43.2
T-cell depletion	12.7
Antithymocyte globulin	6.4
Unrelated donor or ≥2 HLA-mismatched related donor	4.1
Acute GVHD: grade II–IV	1.9

EBV-LPD, Epstein–Barr virus-associated lymphoproliferative disorder; GVHD, graft-vs.-host disease; HLA, human leukocyte antigen.
Adapted from Curtis et al. [31].

reflects decreased numbers of virus carrying donor lymphocytes or the elimination of the target cell for transformation is not clear. Other risk factors identified include the use of unrelated and mismatched donors, although HCT from related donors with mismatch at a single HLA locus did not differ from HCT using matched donors. The reasons for this observation are not well understood, but the suggestion has been made that chronic antigenic stimulation may play a role [26]. Chronic antigenic stimulation similarly seems likely to play a role in the development of LPD in organ transplant recipients where tumors are commonly found in association with the transplanted organ.

In contrast to EBV-LPD in the solid-organ transplant setting, neither the age of the recipient, EBV seronegativity nor underlying disease were risk factors for allogeneic BMT recipients [31]. Chemotherapy used in the preparative regimen also had not been identified as a risk factor. T-cell depleted haploidentical transplantation seems to be associated with a marked increase in risk [29,36].

Cases that occur late after HCT differ in their risk factors, pathology and their EBV association. The only statistically significant risk factor in the IBMTR study was extensive chronic GVHD [31]. These tumors are sometimes of T-cell rather than of B-cell origin and sometimes not EBV-associated [37,38]. Late cases of LPD not associated with EBV have also been described in solid-organ transplant recipients [39].

HD was also identified as occurring at increased frequency following allogeneic BMT. In an IBMTR study of more than 18,000 allogeneic BMT recipients, eight developed HD in contrast to 78 who developed LPD. Although the frequency is an order of magnitude less than other LPDs after transplantation this nonetheless indicates a sixfold-increased risk of HD in BMT recipients in comparison with the general population —similar to the increase in risk in human immunodeficiency virus (HIV) positive patients [40]. In contrast to other LPD, HD is almost always a late event. The median time to developing a tumor is 4.2 years, and it is always more than 2.5 years. It is also always EBV-associated, just as it is when it occurs in association with congenital immunodeficiency or HIV infection. Histologically, the mixed cellularity subtype predominates. As with other late LPDs, TCD and HLA disparity are not risk factors for HD. The occurrence of severe acute or chronic GVHD was a risk factor. In contrast to other LPDs in BMT recipients the outcome was strikingly better. Most patients were alive and well after therapy.

Recipients of allogeneic peripheral blood hematopoietic cell (PBHC) transplants also are at risk for LPD [29]. The median time to the diagnosis of LPD is similar to that of bone marrow recipients. TCD of the PBHC product and underlying diagnosis of immune deficiency in the recipient are both identified as risk factors in multivariate analysis.

Since EBV generally does not cross the blood–placenta barrier, cord blood hematopoietic cell (CBHC) transplantation might be anticipated to be associated with a lower incidence of EBV-LPD than transplantation from other donor sources. Alternatively, CBHC transplant recipients might be anticipated to have a higher incidence of lymphoma because they resemble T-depleted bone marrow and blood hematopoietic cell products insofar as they lack EBV-specific cytotoxic T cells. These factors appear to approximately balance one another and CBHC recipients do not appear to have an incidence of EBV-LPD different from recipients of unmanipulated bone marrow grafts [41,42].

Autologous BMT or PBHC transplantation has also occasionally been associated with EBV-LPD, although much less frequently than with allogeneic transplantation. TCD appears to be the major risk factor, but EBV-LPD has also occurred in association with CD34 selection [43–45]. Reduced intensity transplants have also been associated with EBV-LPD [46,47]. Fludarabine alone may be associated with the development of EBV-LPD [48,49], and so the contribution of transplantation to the problem is not yet clear.

The major determinants of the risk period for LPD are presumed to be immunologic and several investigators have presented evidence that reconstitution of $CD8^+$ T-cell immunity to EBV generally occurs during the 6-month period following allogeneic BMT [33]. It may occur even more rapidly following autologous PBHC transplantation [50,51]. Hierarchies of cellular responses to classes of EBV antigens (latent vs. lytic) and to particular antigens are well recognized [18,19,52]. Thus different peptide epitopes elicit different magnitudes of T-cell response. Magnitude and patterns of response differ between individuals. In allogeneic PBHC, recipients' evidence has been presented that suggests similarities in pattern between patients and their respective donors, suggesting that homeostatic mechanisms in the donor have been recapitulated in the matched sibling recipient [53]. Evidence has been presented suggesting a relationship between EBV $CD8^+$ T-cell frequencies and viral load in peripheral blood mononuclear cells (PBMCs). However, the relative importance of $CD8^+$ and $CD4^+$ responses, responses to latent vs. lytic viral antigens expressed on tumor cells, or responses to specific individual viral antigens remains to be determined. Several but not all investigators have presented evidence that $CD4^+$ T cells targeting EBV antigens may be lytic or may suppress outgrowth of EBV transformed B-cell lines [54–58].

Clinical features

LPD most commonly presents early after transplantation and as disseminated disease [21,29,31,37,59]. Fever, generalized lymphadenopathy, respiratory compromise and rising liver transaminases are typical and have usually been associated with a rapidly progressive course with multiorgan failure and death, often within several days. Lesions are nodal and extranodal, frequently involving Waldeyer's ring, the gastrointestinal tract, the liver and the central nervous system. In some instances circulating clonally restricted B cells have been detected by flow cytometry. Approximately one third of cases are diagnosed only at autopsy, but LPD is fairly consistently the primary or a contributing cause of death. Later after transplantation (>1 year), tumors are more commonly localized and have a more indolent course. Late, localized LPD is occasionally recognized at autopsy as an incidental finding.

A variety of morphologic classifications have been suggested [60–63]. These have been studied mainly in solid-organ transplant recipients. There is the suggestion in the literature that in BMT recipients, LPD lesions tend to be more aggressive and with higher proliferative activity than in solid-organ transplant recipients [64]. Monoclonal and polyclonal lesions are recognized with determination by immunoglobulin gene rearrangements standard. It has been argued that monoclonal disease is more aggressive and less likely to respond to immune interventions, but it remains unclear as to whether either morphology or clonality generally correlates with clinical course or prognosis [21,24,26,59,64]. However, it is clear that on occasion patients with monoclonal disease will have spontaneous remissions and that patients with polyclonal disease will progress despite aggressive therapy including donor lymphocyte infusion (DLI) as discussed below [29]. In most instances, EBV-LPD developing in allogeneic HCT recipients arises in donor B lymphocytes although occasionally it arises in host lymphocytes when there is autologous recovery [65–70]. In contrast, in solid-organ transplant recipients EBV-LPD most commonly arises in host B cells.

Virologic aspects

Myeloablative therapy destroys the viral B-cell reservoir and, at least in some cases, seems to eliminate the host virus [71]. EBV-seropositive BMT recipients receiving allografts from seronegative donors may become seronegative and, in EBV-seropositive BMT recipients receiving allografts from seropositive donors, the host strain of virus may be replaced by the donor strain. These observations are consistent with the observation that B cells are required for long-term maintenance of infection as exemplified by the absence of viral infection in patients with X-linked agammaglobulinemia [72].

Viral strain or "biotype" has been studied. The A strain, which is also known as the type 1 virus, is most common in LPD in the transplant setting [73,74]. This strain is the most prevalent in the general population and so its predominance in LPD may not reflect increased pathogenicity—although *in vitro* and in murine studies it is more efficient in immortalization and transformation than the less common B strain [75]. Many variations in viral genes have been described, including variants in EBNA-1 and LMP-1 [76–78]. However, there is little evidence for a high-risk donor strain.

Expression of the full spectrum of latency viral antigens is often detected in LPD following BMT [79] as it is following organ transplantation [80,81]. The antigens expressed parallel those expressed in LCLs and the antigens targeted by T-cell products expanded using LCL stimulators (as described in HCT for EBV-associated tumors, p. 753) are generally expected to target LPD. Antigen escape by mutation in EBV-LPD following transplantation would appear to be a rare event, although in one instance a deletion mutation has been documented [74,82].

Diagnosis

Definitive diagnosis of EBV-LPD requires biopsy and immunohistochemistry or flow cytometry. Lesions are typically CD19+ and CD20+, and often show restricted light chain expression [62,83]. EBV detection requires *in situ* hybridization for the EBER transcripts or the detection of viral antigens. Because of variability of antigen expression in EBV-LPD, the inability to detect particular viral antigens, such as LMP-1 or EBNA-2, should not be regarded as evidence that the lesion is not virus associated [65,84]. Some EBV-associated tumors, such as Burkitt's lymphoma, and a subset of EBV-LPD will not express any viral antigens other than EBNA-1, and reagents to detect EBNA-1 are not widely used because of lack of commercial availability and issues related to crossreactivity.

With the availability of effective interventions for the prevention or treatment of LPD in BMT recipients, diagnosis and early diagnosis have become clinically more important. Whereas serology is useful in the diagnosis of primary EBV infection in the general population, in the post-transplant setting it is difficult to interpret because blood products passively transfer antibodies to the viral capsid antigen (VCA) and EBNA. Thus, most patients who are seronegative prior to transplant and have seronegative marrow or stem cell donors show antibodies to VCA and EBNA within a few days after transplant if they have been transfused (since most blood products are from EBV-seropositive donors). In addition the typical serologic changes of infectious mononucleosis, i.e. a rise

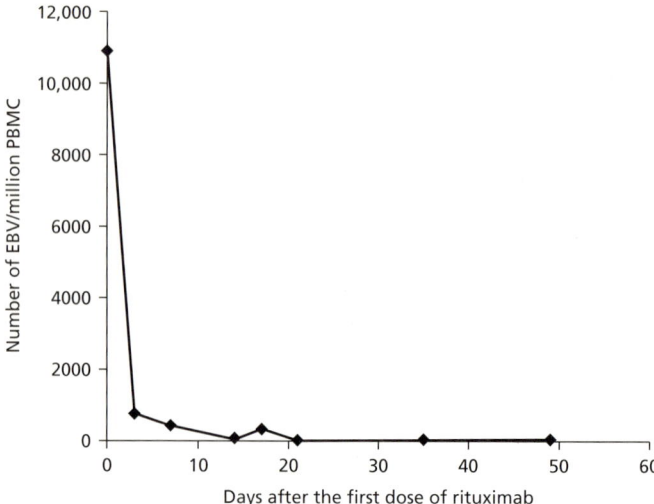

Fig. 56.3 Fall in Epstein–Barr virus (EBV) genome copy number per million peripheral blood mononuclear cells (PBMCs) following treatment with rituximab in a patient with Epstein–Barr virus-associated lymphoproliferative disorder (EBV-LPD).

in the immunoglobulin M anti-VCA antibody or the appearance of heterophile antibodies, do not generally occur in the BMT setting.

In contrast to serology, PCR amplification of viral DNA shows promise in facilitating diagnosis and guiding early interventions to prevent or treat EBV-LPD. There is general agreement that the number of EBV genomes in PBMCs is increased in association with EBV-LPD, although there is striking variability in the absolute values in healthy seropositives across the studies [5,66–68,85,86]. Monitoring viral genome copy number has also been thought to be useful in monitoring response to therapy [68,69]. However, for rituximab therapy at least (Fig. 56.3), there is a very consistent fall in viral copy number in PBMCs, even in those patients whose tumors are progressing [5]. Mainly resting B cells harbor virus in PBMCs—and thus, although the cellular viral load may mirror LPD, LPD cells and circulating virus-infected lymphocytes constitute distinct compartments.

Some investigators have measured virus load in whole blood, while others have measured virus load in serum or plasma [70,87–94]. Whether cell-free DNA (plasma or serum) reflects the presence of infectious virus or the presence of DNA released by dying cells in these patients is unclear. However, it is clear that tumor cell DNA can often be detected in plasma or serum, and that the presence of EBV DNA in serum can be used to monitor therapy in another EBV-associated tumor, nasopharyngeal carcinoma [95,96].

Treatment

A variety of treatments have been explored [88]. Discontinuation of immunosuppression is sometimes associated with regression of LPD in solid-organ transplant recipients, but it is very rarely effective in BMT recipients. The use of antivirals, such as acyclovir, ganciclovir or their congeners, has been advocated, but there is little evidence to suggest therapeutic efficacy against EBV in any setting [7,97–99]. These drugs do not inhibit the proliferation of lymphocytes latently infected by EBV either *in vitro* or *in vivo*. Furthermore, high rates of EBV-LPD have been noted in recipients of T-cell-depleted grafts despite the use of these drugs [21,27,29]. Interferon-alpha (IFN-α) has also been used with some success [29]. Cytotoxic chemotherapy has been curative in organ transplant recipients with LPD, but there was no similar track record of success in a series of BMT recipients [100].

Immune therapies with antibodies, DLI, or adoptive T-cell transfer of EBV-specific cytotoxic T cells have all met with impressive successes. Experience with DLI to treat EBV-LPD was first reported from the Memorial Sloan Kettering Cancer Center where patients with EBV-LPD following TCD allogeneic marrow transplantation were treated with a relatively low dose of donor leukocytes (1×10^6 CD3$^+$ cells/kg) [101]. Durable remissions were rapidly achieved (14–30 days after infusion) with only modest GVHD. Since donor origins of the EBV-LPD were demonstrated, the effectiveness of the therapy is presumed to reflect EBV-specific reactivity rather than alloreactivity. DLI has also been used in other settings, but not always successfully. In recipients of mismatched-related transplants, DLI given to prevent primary disease did not prevent late LPD (>15 months) [102]. Similarly, in the allogeneic peripheral blood HCT setting, DLI has been used with mixed results [29].

This use of DLI in the treatment of EBV-LPD after BMT was followed by the demonstration that infusion of EBV-specific T cells can also induce tumor regression or prevent the development of tumors [69]. Expanded EBV-specific donor T-cell lines were prepared by stimulating donor lymphocytes with irradiated donor-derived LCLs. The resultant cell lines were mixes of CD8$^+$ and CD4$^+$ T cells as well as NK cells. Patients responded to four weekly T-cell infusions with cell doses ranging from 1×10^7 to $5 \times 10^7/m^2$ with return of viral load to normal values and resolution of fever, lymphadenopathy and pulmonary infiltrates. High-risk patients were treated prophylactically. These infusions prevented the development of EBV-LPD, restored EBV cellular immune responses and established populations of cytotoxic T-cell precursors that could respond to *in vivo* or *ex vivo* challenge with the virus for as long as 18 months [69,103,104].

Anti-B-cell antibodies have also been used to treat EBV-LPD [5,105–108]. These include antibodies with specificity for CD21, CD24 and CD20 (rituximab). Each of the monoclonals have met with substantial success and been associated with very modest or no toxicity. They are effective in many instances, particularly when used early. However, the complete response rate in established LPD is likely to be <50%.

The ready availability of rituximab and its lack of toxicity suggest that it should be considered appropriate as first-line therapy, or as a part of first-line therapy, in most instances. It may be most effective when used preemptively in high-risk patients receiving TCD peripheral blood stem cell transplantation in whom rising viral loads suggest early disease [89]. EBV-specific T cells, when available, are an attractive alternative or adjunct. Similarly, DLI from allogeneic HCT donors is often effective, even at lymphocyte doses not usually associated with GVHD.

The different incidences of EBV-LPD associated with various methods of TCD, the response to anti-B-cell monoclonal antibody therapy in some patients with EBV-LPD, and the response to adoptive cellular immunotherapy all suggest that, with attention to maintaining a balance between T cells and the EBV B-cell reservoir, this potentially fatal disease may be prevented or successfully treated in the marrow transplant setting in most instances.

HCT for EBV-associated tumors

The successes in the treatment of EBV-LPD in BMT recipients has stimulated interest in the treatment of other EBV-associated lymphoid tumors. Two issues need to be considered in regard to such immunotherapeutic approaches. The first relates to the ability of tumor cells to present antigens and to be killed by cognate T cells. The second relates to the pattern of viral antigen expression associated with the tumor.

Defects in antigen processing, down-regulation of MHC class I molecules and down-regulation of adhesion molecules are well recognized in Burkitt's lymphoma [109,110]. At least some HD tumors are not likely to be susceptible to CD8$^+$-mediated killing because Reed–Sternberg cells often fail to express MHC class I antigens [111]. However, down-regulation of MHC class I antigens is almost exclusively a phenomenon of HD not associated with EBV [112,113]. EBV-associated HD very consistently expresses MHC class I and high levels of transporter associated proteins (TAP-1 and -2), irrespective of the presence of latent EBV infection. Studies of the HD cell lines support susceptibility to lysis by antigen-specific CTLs in a class I-restricted manner [114]. In HD there is also the possibility that there may be suppression of the CTL response in tumor tissue, perhaps related to production of cytokines that perturb the cellular immune response.

The spectrum of viral antigen expression may also be an obstacle. Tumor types have characteristic patterns of viral gene expression. Three such patterns of expression are recognized. Burkitt's lymphoma expresses only a single viral antigen in most tumor cells [115,116]. HD expresses EBNA-1 and the latency membrane antigens (LMP-1 and -2) [113,117]. Nasopharyngeal carcinoma has a similar pattern of antigen expression, although membrane antigens are less consistently expressed [118,119]. EBV-LPD in organ transplant recipients often expresses the complete spectrum of latency antigens [80,81]. The patterns of expression are of key importance because the viral latency antigens (EBNA-3A, -3B and -3C) most commonly targeted by EBV-specific T cells expanded *in vitro* with LCLs are not expressed in HD, nasopharyngeal carcinoma and many other EBV-associated malignancies.

Thus, adoptive T-cell therapy using LCL stimulators for T-cell expansion has been explored in small studies of patients with LPD following organ transplantation, nasopharyngeal carcinoma and HD [120–125]. In LPD, the tumors are generally sensitive to T-cell killing and there is likely to be a match between antigens expressed by tumor cells and antigens targeted by expanded T cells. Thus there have been some promising results [120]. However, the approach is limited by the time required (several weeks) to expand autologous EBV-specific T-cell products. An alternative approach has been to use partially matched products expanded from allogeneic donors [121]. Early results with this approach have been encouraging. In other tumors, such as HD and nasopharyngeal carcinoma, the results with LCL expanded T-cell products have been less certain [122,123]. Promising new approaches to expanding antigen-specific T cells, which will more specifically target viral antigens expressed in a given tumor type, are emerging [124,125].

Summary

EBV infection is ubiquitous. Following primary infection, latency is established in B cells and infection is spread throughout the B-cell compartment by virus-"driven" proliferation of infected B cells. An EBV-specific cytotoxic T-cell response helps to limit the proliferation. A reservoir of resting infected B cells with very limited viral antigen expression escapes immune surveillance. With myeloablative regimens and marrow transplantation, the host reservoir of latently infected B cells may be replaced by infected donor B cells. In the 6-month period following HCT, patients are at risk for developing EBV-LPD. This tumor usually arises in the donor B cells. The major risk factors are TCD and HCT from unrelated or mismatched donors. Treatment with adoptive cellular immunotherapy, either DLI or EBV-specific T-cell infusion, has been associated with impressive clinical results in a small number of patients, as has treatment with monoclonal antibodies. Adoptive immunotherapy in the setting of HCT may also have a role to play in the management of EBV-associated malignancies such as HD.

References

1 Rickinson ABKE. Epstein–Barr virus. In: Fields BN, Knipe DM, Howley PM, Griffin DE, eds. *Fields Virology*, 4th edn. Philadelphia: Lippincott, Williams & Wilkins, 2001: 2575–627.

2 Cohen JI. Epstein–Barr virus infection. *N Engl J Med* 2000; **343**: 481–92.

3 Miyashita EM, Yang B, Babcock GJ, Thorley-Lawson DA. Identification of the site of Epstein–Barr virus persistence *in vivo* as a resting B cell. *J Virol* 1997; **71**: 4882–91.

4 Tierney RJ, Steven N, Young LS, Rickinson AB. Epstein–Barr virus latency in blood mononuclear cells: analysis of viral gene transcription during primary infection and in the carrier state. *J Virol* 1994; **68**: 7374–85.

5 Yang J, Tao Q, Flinn IW *et al.* Characterization of Epstein–Barr virus-infected B cells in patients with posttransplantation lymphoproliferative disease: disappearance after rituximab therapy does not predict clinical response. *Blood* 2000; **96**: 4055–63.

6 Thorley-Lawson DA. Epstein–Barr virus: exploiting the immune system. *Nat Rev Immunol* 2001; **1**: 75–82.

7 Yao QY, Ogan P, Rowe M, Wood M, Rickinson AB. Epstein–Barr virus-infected B cells persist in the circulation of acyclovir-treated virus carriers. *Int J Cancer* 1989; **43**: 67–71.

8 Li L, Liu D, Hutt-Fletcher L, Morgan A, Masucci MG, Levitsky V. Epstein–Barr virus inhibits the development of dendritic cells by promoting apoptosis of their monocyte precursors in the presence of granulocyte macrophage-colony-stimulating factor and interleukin-4. *Blood* 2002; **99**: 3725–34.

9 Borza CM, Hutt-Fletcher LM. Alternate replication in B cells and epithelial cells switches tropism of Epstein–Barr virus. *Nat Med* 2002; **8**: 594–9.

10 Lee MA, Diamond ME, Yates JL. Genetic evidence that EBNA-1 is needed for efficient, stable, latent infection by Epstein–Barr virus. *J Virol* 1999; **73**: 2974–82.

11 Hurley EA, Agger S, McNeil JA *et al.* When Epstein–Barr virus persistently infects B-cell lines, it frequently integrates. *J Virol* 1991; **65**: 1245–54.

12 Kieff ERAB. Epstein–Barr virus and its replication. In: Fields BN, Knipe DM, Howley PM, Griffin DE, eds. *Fields Virology*, 4th edn. Philadelphia: Lippincott, Williams & Wilkins, 2001: 2511–73.

13 Raab-Traub N. Epstein–Barr virus in the pathogenesis of NPC. *Semin Cancer Biol* 2002; **12**: 431–41.

14 Wu H, Kapoor P, Frappier L. Separation of the DNA replication, segregation, and transcriptional activation functions of Epstein–Barr nuclear antigen 1. *J Virol* 2002; **76**: 2480–90.

15 Kang MS, Hung SC, Kieff E. Epstein–Barr virus nuclear antigen 1 activates transcription from episomal but not integrated DNA and does not alter lymphocyte growth. *Proc Natl Acad Sci U S A* 2001; **98**: 15,233–8.

16 Lee JM, Lee KH, Weidner M, Osborne BA, Hayward SD. Epstein–Barr virus EBNA2 blocks Nur77-mediated apoptosis. *Proc Natl Acad Sci U S A* 2002; **99**: 11,878–83.

17 Hsieh JJ, Henkel T, Salmon P, Robey E, Peterson MG, Hayward SD. Truncated mammalian Notch1 activates *CBF1/RBPJk*-repressed genes by a mechanism resembling that of Epstein–Barr virus EBNA2. *Mol Cell Biol* 1996; **16**: 952–9.

18 Hislop AD, Annels NE, Gudgeon NH, Leese AM, Rickinson AB. Epitope-specific evolution of human CD8+ T cell responses from primary to persistent phases of Epstein–Barr virus infection. *J Exp Med* 2002; **195**: 893–905.

19 Redchenko IV, Rickinson AB. Accessing Epstein–Barr virus-specific T-cell memory with peptide-loaded dendritic cells. *J Virol* 1999; **73**: 334–42.

20 Yang J, Lemas VM, Flinn IW, Krone C, Ambinder RF. Application of the ELISPOT assay to the characterization of CD8+ responses to Epstein–Barr virus antigens. *Blood* 2000; **95**: 241–8.

21 Zutter MM, Martin PJ, Sale GE *et al.* Epstein–Barr virus lymphoproliferation after bone marrow transplantation. *Blood* 1988; **72**: 520–9.

22 Martin PJ, Shulman HM, Schubach WH *et al.* Fatal Epstein–Barr-virus-associated proliferation of donor B cells after treatment of acute graft-versus-host disease with a murine anti-T-cell antibody. *Ann Intern Med* 1984; **101**: 310–5.

23 Antin JH, Bierer BE, Smith BR *et al.* Selective depletion of bone marrow T lymphocytes with anti-CD5 monoclonal antibodies: effective prophylaxis for graft-versus-host disease in patients with hematologic malignancies. *Blood* 1991; **78**: 2139–49.

24 Gerritsen EJ, Stam ED, Hermans J *et al.* Risk factors for developing EBV-related B cell lymphoproliferative disorders (BLPD) after non-HLA-identical BMT in children. *Bone Marrow Transplant* 1996; **18**: 377–82.

25 Jabado N, Le Deist F, Cant A *et al.* Bone marrow transplantation from genetically HLA-nonidentical donors in children with fatal inherited disorders excluding severe combined immunodeficiencies: use of two monoclonal antibodies to prevent graft rejection. *Pediatrics* 1996; **98**: 420–8.

26 Shapiro RS, McClain K, Frizzera G *et al.* Epstein–Barr virus associated B cell lymphoproliferative disorders following bone marrow transplantation. *Blood* 1988; **71**: 1234–43.

27 Witherspoon RP, Fisher LD, Schoch G *et al.* Secondary cancers after bone marrow transplantation for leukemia or aplastic anemia. *N Engl J Med* 1989; **321**: 784–9.

28 Bhatia S, Ramsay NK, Steinbuch M *et al.* Malignant neoplasms following bone marrow transplantation. *Blood* 1996; **87**: 3633–9.

29 Gross TG, Steinbuch M, DeFor T *et al.* B cell lymphoproliferative disorders following hematopoietic stem cell transplantation: risk factors, treatment and outcome. *Bone Marrow Transplant* 1999; **23**: 251–8.

30 Meijer E, Slaper-Cortenbach IC, Thijsen SF, Dekker AW, Verdonck LF. Increased incidence of EBV-associated lymphoproliferative disorders after allogeneic stem cell transplantation from matched unrelated donors due to a change of T cell depletion technique. *Bone Marrow Transplant* 2002; **29**: 335–9.

31 Curtis RE, Travis LB, Rowlings PA *et al.* Risk of lymphoproliferative disorders after bone marrow transplantation: a multi-institutional study. *Blood* 1999; **94**: 2208–16.

32 Gross TG, Hinrichs SH, Davis JR, Mitchell D, Bishop MR, Wagner JE. Depletion of EBV-infected cells in donor marrow by counterflow elutriation. *Exp Hematol* 1998; **26**: 395–9.

33 Lucas KG, Small TN, Heller G, Dupont B, O'Reilly RJ. The development of cellular immunity to Epstein–Barr virus after allogeneic bone marrow transplantation. *Blood* 1996; **87**: 2594–603.

34 O'Donnell PV, Jones RJ, Vogelsang GB *et al.* CD34+ stem cell augmentation of elutriated allogeneic bone marrow grafts: results of a phase II clinical trial of engraftment and graft-versus-host disease prophylaxis in high-risk hematologic malignancies. *Bone Marrow Transplant* 1998; **22**: 947–55.

35 Hale G, Waldmann H. Risks of developing Epstein–Barr virus-related lymphoproliferative disorders after T-cell-depleted marrow transplants: Campath users. *Blood* 1998; **91**: 3079–83.

36 Smogorzewska EM, Brooks J, Annett G *et al.* T cell depleted haploidentical bone marrow transplantation for the treatment of children with severe combined immunodeficiency. *Arch Immunol Ther Exp (Warsz)* 2000; **48**: 111–8.

37 Zutter MM, Durnam DM, Hackman RC *et al.* Secondary T-cell lymphoproliferation after marrow transplantation. *Am J Clin Pathol* 1990; **94**: 714–21.

38 Trimble MS, Waye JS, Walker IR, Brain MC, Leber BF. B-cell lymphoma of recipient origin 9 years after allogeneic bone marrow transplantation for T-cell acute lymphoblastic leukaemia. *Br J Haematol* 1993; **85**: 99–102.

39 Leblond V, Davi F, Charlotte F *et al.* Posttransplant lymphoproliferative disorders not associated with Epstein–Barr virus: a distinct entity? *J Clin Oncol* 1998; **16**: 2052–9.

40 Goedert JJ, Cote TR, Virgo P *et al.* Spectrum of AIDS-associated malignant disorders. *Lancet* 1998; **351**: 1833–9.

41 Barker JN, Martin PL, Coad JE *et al.* Low incidence of Epstein–Barr virus-associated posttransplantation lymphoproliferative disorders in 272 unrelated-donor umbilical cord blood transplant recipients. *Biol Blood Marrow Transplant* 2001; **7**: 395–9.

42 Ohga S, Kanaya Y, Maki H *et al.* Epstein–Barr virus-associated lymphoproliferative disease after a cord blood transplant for Diamond–Blackfan anemia. *Bone Marrow Transplant* 2000; **25**: 209–12.

43 Anderson KC, Soiffer R, DeLage R *et al.* T-cell-depleted autologous bone marrow transplantation therapy: analysis of immune deficiency and late complications. *Blood* 1990; **76**: 235–44.

44 Peniket AJ, Perry AR, Williams CD *et al.* A case of EBV-associated lymphoproliferative disease following high-dose therapy and CD34-purified autologous peripheral blood progenitor cell transplantation. *Bone Marrow Transplant* 1998; **22**: 307–9.

45 Lones MA, Kirov I, Said JW, Shintaku IP, Neudorf S. Post-transplant lymphoproliferative disorder after autologous peripheral stem cell transplantation in a pediatric patient. *Bone Marrow Transplant* 2000; **26**: 1021–4.

46 Ho AY, Adams S, Shaikh H, Pagliuca A, Devereux S, Mufti GJ. Fatal donor-derived Epstein–Barr virus-associated post-transplant lymphoproliferative disorder following reduced intensity volunteer-unrelated bone marrow transplant for myelodysplastic syndrome. *Bone Marrow Transplant* 2002; **29**: 867–9.

47 Milpied N, Coste-Burel M, Accard F *et al.* Epstein–Barr virus-associated B cell lymphoproliferative disease after non-myeloablative

47 allogeneic stem cell transplantation. *Bone Marrow Transplant* 1999; **23**: 629–30.
48 Shields DJ, Byrd JC, Abbondanzo SL, Lichy JH, Diehl LF, Aguilera NI. Detection of Epstein–Barr virus in transformations of low-grade B-cell lymphomas after fludarabine treatment. *Mod Pathol* 1997; **10**: 1151–9.
49 Abruzzo LV, Rosales CM, Medeiros LJ *et al*. Epstein–Barr virus-positive B-cell lymphoproliferative disorders arising in immunodeficient patients previously treated with fludarabine for low-grade B-cell neoplasms. *Am J Surg Pathol* 2002; **26**: 630–6.
50 Nolte A, Buhmann R, Straka C, Emmerich B, Hallek M. Assessment and characterization of the cytolytic T lymphocyte response against Epstein–Barr virus in patients with non-Hodgkin's lymphoma after autologous peripheral blood stem cell transplantation. *Bone Marrow Transplant* 1998; **21**: 909–16.
51 Nolte A, Buhmann R, Emmerich B, Schendel D, Hallek M. Reconstitution of the cellular immune response after autologous peripheral blood stem cell transplantation in patients with non-Hodgkin's lymphoma. *Br J Haematol* 2000; **108**: 415–23.
52 Annels NE, Callan MF, Tan L, Rickinson AB. Changing patterns of dominant TCR usage with maturation of an EBV-specific cytotoxic T cell response. *J Immunol* 2000; **165**: 4831–41.
53 Marshall NA, Howe JG, Formica R *et al*. Rapid reconstitution of Epstein–Barr virus-specific T lymphocytes following allogeneic stem cell transplantation. *Blood* 2000; **96**: 2814–21.
54 Nikiforow S, Bottomly K, Miller G. CD4+ T-cell effectors inhibit Epstein–Barr virus-induced B-cell proliferation. *J Virol* 2001; **75**: 3740–52.
55 Bickham K, Munz C, Tsang ML *et al*. EBNA1-specific CD4+ T cells in healthy carriers of Epstein–Barr virus are primarily TH1 in function. *J Clin Invest* 2001; **107**: 121–30.
56 Munz C, Bickham KL, Subklewe M *et al*. Human CD4+ T lymphocytes consistently respond to the latent Epstein–Barr virus nuclear antigen EBNA1. *J Exp Med* 2000; **191**: 1649–60.
57 Khanolkar A, Yagita H, Cannon MJ. Preferential utilization of the perforin/granzyme pathway for lysis of Epstein–Barr virus-transformed lymphoblastoid cells by virus-specific CD4+ T cells. *Virology* 2001; **287**: 79–88.
58 Koehne G, Smith KM, Ferguson TL *et al*. Quantitation, selection, and functional characterization of Epstein–Barr virus-specific and alloreactive T cells detected by intracellular interferon-γ production and growth of cytotoxic precursors. *Blood* 2002; **99**: 1730–40.
59 Micallef IN, Chhanabhai M, Gascoyne RD *et al*. Lymphoproliferative disorders following allogeneic bone marrow transplantation: the Vancouver experience. *Bone Marrow Transplant* 1998; **22**: 981–7.
60 Chadburn A, Chen JM, Hsu DT *et al*. The morphologic and molecular genetic categories of posttransplantation lymphoproliferative disorders are clinically relevant. *Cancer* 1998; **82**: 1978–87.
61 Knowles DM, Cesarman E, Chadburn A *et al*. Correlative morphologic and molecular genetic analysis demonstrates three distinct categories of posttransplantation lymphoproliferative disorders. *Blood* 1995; **85**: 552–65.
62 Harris NL, Ferry JA, Swerdlow SH. Posttransplant lymphoproliferative disorders: summary of the Society for Hematopathology Workshop. *Semin Diagn Pathol* 1997; **14**: 8–14.
63 Swerdlow SH. Classification of the posttransplant lymphoproliferative disorders: from the past to the present. *Semin Diagn Pathol* 1997; **14**: 2–7.
64 Orazi A, Hromas RA, Neiman RS *et al*. Posttransplantation lymphoproliferative disorders in bone marrow transplant recipients are aggressive diseases with a high incidence of adverse histologic and immunobiologic features. *Am J Clin Pathol* 1997; **107**: 419–29.
65 Ambinder RF, Mann RB. Epstein–Barr-encoded RNA *in situ* hybridization: diagnostic applications. *Hum Pathol* 1994; **25**: 602–5.
66 Rose C, Green M, Webber S *et al*. Detection of Epstein–Barr virus genomes in peripheral blood B cells from solid-organ transplant recipients by fluorescence *in situ* hybridization. *J Clin Microbiol* 2002; **40**: 2533–44.
67 Johannessen I, Haque T, N'Jie-Jobe J, Crawford DH. Non-correlation of *in vivo* and *in vitro* parameters of Epstein–Barr virus persistence suggests heterogeneity of B cell infection. *J General Virol* 1998; **79**(7): 1631–6.
68 Orii T, Ohkohchi N, Satomi S, Hoshino Y, Kimura H. Decreasing the Epstein–Barr virus load by adjusting the FK506 blood level. *Transpl Int* 2002; **15**: 529–34.
69 Rooney CM, Smith CA, Ng CY *et al*. Infusion of cytotoxic T cells for the prevention and treatment of Epstein–Barr virus-induced lymphoma in allogeneic transplant recipients. *Blood* 1998; **92**: 1549–55.
70 Gartner BC, Schafer H, Marggraff K *et al*. Evaluation of use of Epstein–Barr viral load in patients after allogeneic stem cell transplantation to diagnose and monitor posttransplant lymphoproliferative disease. *J Clin Microbiol* 2002; **40**: 351–8.
71 Gratama JW, Oosterveer MA, Zwaan FE, Lepoutre J, Klein G, Ernberg I. Eradication of Epstein–Barr virus by allogeneic bone marrow transplantation: implications for sites of viral latency. *Proc Natl Acad Sci U S A* 1988; **85**: 8693–6.
72 Faulkner GC, Burrows SR, Khanna R, Moss DJ, Bird AG, Crawford DH. X-Linked agammaglobulinemia patients are not infected with Epstein–Barr virus. Implications for the biology of the virus. *J Virol* 1999; **73**: 1555–64.
73 Frank D, Cesarman E, Liu YF, Michler RE, Knowles DM. Posttransplantation lymphoproliferative disorders frequently contain type A and not type B Epstein–Barr virus. *Blood* 1995; **85**: 1396–403.
74 Tao Q, Yang J, Huang H, Swinnen LJ, Ambinder RF. Conservation of Epstein–Barr virus cytotoxic T-cell epitopes in posttransplant lymphomas: implications for immune therapy. *Am J Pathol* 2002; **160**: 1839–45.
75 Cohen JI, Picchio GR, Mosier DE. Epstein–Barr virus nuclear protein 2 is a critical determinant for tumor growth in SCID mice and for transformation *in vitro*. *J Virol* 1992; **66**: 7555–9.
76 Fassone L, Cingolani A, Martini M *et al*. Characterization of Epstein–Barr virus genotype in AIDS-related non-Hodgkin's lymphoma. *AIDS Res Hum Retroviruses* 2002; **18**: 19–26.
77 Schafer H, Berger C, Aepinus C *et al*. Molecular pathogenesis of Epstein–Barr virus associated posttransplant lymphomas: new insights through latent membrane protein 1 fingerprinting. *Transplantation* 2001; **72**: 492–6.
78 Gutierrez MI, Kingma DW, Sorbara L *et al*. Association of EBV strains, defined by multiple loci analyses, in non-Hodgkin lymphomas and reactive tissues from HIV positive and HIV negative patients. *Leuk Lymphoma* 2000; **37**: 425–9.
79 Gratama JW, Zutter MM, Minarovits J *et al*. Expression of Epstein–Barr virus-encoded growth-transformation-associated proteins in lymphoproliferations of bone-marrow transplant recipients. *Int J Cancer* 1991; **47**: 188–92.
80 Young L, Alfieri C, Hennessy K *et al*. Expression of Epstein–Barr virus transformation-associated genes in tissues of patients with EBV lymphoproliferative disease. *N Engl J Med* 1989; **321**: 1080–5.
81 Murray PG, Swinnen LJ, Constandinou CM *et al*. BCL-2, but not its Epstein–Barr virus-encoded homologue, BHRF1, is commonly expressed in posttransplantation lymphoproliferative disorders. *Blood* 1996; **87**: 706–11.
82 Gottschalk S, Ng CY, Perez M *et al*. An Epstein–Barr virus deletion mutant associated with fatal lymphoproliferative disease unresponsive to therapy with virus-specific CTLs. *Blood* 2001; **97**: 835–43.
83 Knowles DM. Immunodeficiency-associated lymphoproliferative disorders. *Mod Pathol* 1999; **12**: 200–17.
84 Ambinder RF, Mann RB. Detection and characterization of Epstein–Barr virus in clinical specimens. *Am J Pathol* 1994; **145**: 239–52.
85 Holmes RD, Orban-Eller K, Karrer FR, Rowe DT, Narkewicz MR, Sokol RJ. Response of elevated Epstein–Barr virus DNA levels to therapeutic changes in pediatric liver transplant patients: 56-month follow up and outcome. *Transplantation* 2002; **74**: 367–72.
86 Green M. Management of Epstein–Barr virus-induced post-transplant lymphoproliferative disease in recipients of solid organ transplantation. *Am J Transplant* 2001; **1**: 103–8.
87 Stevens SJ, Verschuuren EA, Pronk I *et al*. Frequent monitoring of Epstein–Barr virus DNA load in unfractionated whole blood is essential for early detection of posttransplant lymphoproliferative disease in high-risk patients. *Blood* 2001; **97**: 1165–71.
88 Wagner HJ, Rooney CM, Heslop HE. Diagnosis and treatment of posttransplantation lymphoproliferative disease after hematopoietic stem cell transplantation. *Biol Blood Marrow Transplant* 2002; **8**: 1–8.
89 van Esser JW, Niesters HG, van der Holt B *et al*. Prevention of Epstein–Barr virus-lymphoproliferative disease by molecular monitoring and preemptive rituximab in high-risk patients after allogeneic stem cell transplantation. *Blood* 2002; **99**: 4364–9.
90 Stevens SJ, Verschuuren EA, Verkuijlen SA, Van Den Brule AJ, Meijer CJ, Middeldorp JM. Role of Epstein–Barr virus DNA load monitoring in prevention and early detection of post-transplant lymphoproliferative disease. *Leuk Lymphoma* 2002; **43**: 831–40.
91 Lankester AC, van Tol MJ, Vossen JM, Kroes AC, Claas E. Epstein–Barr virus (EBV)-DNA quantification in pediatric allogenic stem cell recipients: prediction of EBV-associated lymphoproliferative disease. *Blood* 2002; **99**: 2630–1.
92 van Esser JW, van der Holt B, Meijer E *et al*. Epstein–Barr virus (EBV) reactivation is a frequent event after allogeneic stem cell transplantation (SCT) and quantitatively predicts EBV-lymphoproliferative disease following T-cell-depleted SCT. *Blood* 2001; **98**: 972–8.

93 van Esser JW, Niesters HG, Thijsen SF et al. Molecular quantification of viral load in plasma allows for fast and accurate prediction of response to therapy of Epstein–Barr virus-associated lymphoproliferative disease after allogeneic stem cell transplantation. Br J Haematol 2001; 113: 814–21.

94 Hoshino Y, Kimura H, Tanaka N et al. Prospective monitoring of the Epstein–Barr virus DNA by a real-time quantitative polymerase chain reaction after allogenic stem cell transplantation. Br J Haematol 2001; 115: 105–11.

95 Chan AT, Lo YM, Zee B et al. Plasma Epstein–Barr virus DNA and residual disease after radiotherapy for undifferentiated nasopharyngeal carcinoma. J Natl Cancer Inst 2002; 94: 1614–9.

96 Johnson PJ, Lo YM. Plasma nucleic acids in the diagnosis and management of malignant disease. Clin Chem 2002; 48: 1186–93.

97 Hanto DW, Frizzera G, Gajl-Peczalska KJ et al. Epstein–Barr virus-induced B-cell lymphoma after renal transplantation: acyclovir therapy and transition from polyclonal to monoclonal B-cell proliferation. N Engl J Med 1982; 306: 913–8.

98 Davis CL, Harrison KL, McVicar JP, Forg PJ, Bronner MP, Marsh CL. Antiviral prophylaxis and the Epstein Barr virus-related post-transplant lymphoproliferative disorder. Clin Transplant 1995; 9: 53–9.

99 Yao QY, Ogan P, Rowe M, Wood M, Rickinson AB. The Epstein–Barr virus: host balance in acute infectious mononucleosis patients receiving acyclovir anti-viral therapy. Int J Cancer 1989; 43: 61–6.

100 Swinnen LJ, Mullen GM, Carr TJ, Costanzo MR, Fisher RI. Aggressive treatment for postcardiac transplant lymphoproliferation. Blood 1995; 86: 3333–40.

101 Papadopoulos EB, Ladanyi M, Emanuel D et al. Infusions of donor leukocytes to treat Epstein–Barr virus-associated lymphoproliferative disorders after allogeneic bone marrow transplantation. N Engl J Med 1994; 330: 1185–91.

102 Chiang KY, Hazlett LJ, Godder KT et al. Epstein–Barr virus-associated B cell lymphoproliferative disorder following mismatched related T cell-depleted bone marrow transplantation. Bone Marrow Transplant 2001; 28: 1117–23.

103 Heslop HE, Ng CY, Li C et al. Long-term restoration of immunity against Epstein–Barr virus infection by adoptive transfer of gene-modified virus-specific T lymphocytes. Nat Med 1996; 2: 551–5.

104 Liu Z, Savoldo B, Huls H et al. Epstein–Barr virus (EBV)-specific cytotoxic T lymphocytes for the prevention and treatment of EBV-associated post-transplant lymphomas: recent results. Cancer Res 2002; 159: 123–33.

105 Fischer A, Blanche S, Le Bidois J et al. Anti-B-cell monoclonal antibodies in the treatment of severe B-cell lymphoproliferative syndrome following bone marrow and organ transplantation. N Engl J Med 1991; 324: 1451–6.

106 Zilz ND, Olson LJ, McGregor CG. Treatment of post-transplant lymphoproliferative disorder with monoclonal CD20 antibody (rituximab) after heart transplantation. J Heart Lung Transplant 2001; 20: 770–2.

107 Serinet MO, Jacquemin E, Habes D, Debray D, Fabre M, Bernard O. Anti-CD20 monoclonal antibody (rituximab) treatment for Epstein–Barr virus-associated, B-cell lymphoproliferative disease in pediatric liver transplant recipients. J Pediatr Gastroenterol Nutr 2002; 34: 389–93.

108 Kuehnle I, Huls MH, Liu Z et al. CD20 monoclonal antibody (rituximab) for therapy of Epstein–Barr virus lymphoma after hemopoietic stem-cell transplantation. Blood 2000; 95: 1502–5.

109 Frisan T, Sjoberg J, Dolcetti R et al. Local suppression of Epstein–Barr virus (EBV)-specific cytotoxicity in biopsies of EBV-positive Hodgkin's disease. Blood 1995; 86: 1493–501.

110 Frisan T, Zhang QJ, Levitskaya J, Coram M, Kurilla MG, Masucci MG. Defective presentation of MHC class I-restricted cytotoxic T-cell epitopes in Burkitt's lymphoma cells. Int J Cancer 1996; 68: 251–8.

111 Poppema S, Visser L. Absence of HLA class I expression by Reed–Sternberg cells. Am J Pathol 1994; 145: 37–41.

112 Oudejans JJ, Jiwa NM, Kummer JA et al. Analysis of major histocompatibility complex class I expression on Reed–Sternberg cells in relation to the cytotoxic T-cell response in Epstein–Barr virus-positive and -negative Hodgkin's disease. Blood 1996; 87: 3844–51.

113 Murray PG, Constandinou CM, Crocker J, Young LS, Ambinder RF. Analysis of major histocompatibility complex class I, TAP expression, and LMP2 epitope sequence in Epstein–Barr virus-positive Hodgkin's disease. Blood 1998; 92: 2477–83.

114 Sing AP, Ambinder RF, Hong DJ et al. Isolation of Epstein–Barr virus (EBV)-specific cytotoxic T lymphocytes that lyse Reed–Sternberg cells: implications for immune-mediated therapy of EBV+ Hodgkin's disease. Blood 1997; 89: 1978–86.

115 Tao Q, Robertson KD, Manns A, Hildesheim A, Ambinder RF. Epstein–Barr virus (EBV) in endemic Burkitt's lymphoma. Molecular analysis of primary tumor tissue. Blood 1998; 91: 1373–81.

116 Niedobitek G, Agathanggelou A, Rowe M et al. Heterogeneous expression of Epstein–Barr virus latent proteins in endemic Burkitt's lymphoma. Blood 1995; 86: 659–65.

117 Deacon EM, Pallesen G, Niedobitek G et al. Epstein–Barr virus and Hodgkin's disease: transcriptional analysis of virus latency in the malignant cells. J Exp Med 1993; 177: 339–49.

118 Pathmanathan R, Prasad U, Chandrika G, Sadler R, Flynn K, Raab-Traub N. Undifferentiated, nonkeratinizing, and squamous cell carcinoma of the nasopharynx. Variants of Epstein–Barr virus-infected neoplasia. Am J Pathol 1995; 146: 1355–67.

119 Brooks L, Yao QY, Rickinson AB, Young LS. Epstein–Barr virus latent gene transcription in nasopharyngeal carcinoma cells: coexpression of EBNA1, LMP1, and LMP2 transcripts. J Virol 1992; 66: 2689–97.

120 Khanna R, Bell S, Sherritt M et al. Activation and adoptive transfer of Epstein–Barr virus-specific cytotoxic T cells in solid organ transplant patients with posttransplant lymphoproliferative disease. Proc Natl Acad Sci U S A 1999; 96: 10391–6.

121 Haque T, Wilkie GM, Taylor C et al. Treatment of Epstein–Barr-virus-positive post-transplantation lymphoproliferative disease with partly HLA-matched allogeneic cytotoxic T cells. Lancet 2002; 360: 436–42.

122 Roskrow MA, Suzuki N, Gan Y et al. Epstein–Barr virus (EBV)-specific cytotoxic T lymphocytes for the treatment of patients with EBV-positive relapsed Hodgkin's disease. Blood 1998; 91: 2925–34.

123 Chua D, Huang J, Zheng B et al. Adoptive transfer of autologous Epstein–Barr virus-specific cytotoxic T cells for nasopharyngeal carcinoma. Int J Cancer 2001; 94: 73–80.

124 Savoldo B, Goss J, Liu Z et al. Generation of autologous Epstein–Barr virus-specific cytotoxic T cells for adoptive immunotherapy in solid organ transplant recipients. Transplantation 2001; 72: 1078–86.

125 Gottschalk S, Edwards OL, Huls MH et al. Generating CTL against the subdominant Epstein–Barr virus LMP1 antigen for the adoptive immunotherapy of EBV-associated malignancies. Blood 2003; 101: 1905–12.

Michael Boeckh

Other Viral Infections after Hematopoietic Cell Transplantation

Viral infections have been a major cause of morbidity and mortality after hematopoietic cell transplantation (HCT). There has been significant progress in the management of herpes simplex virus, varicella-zoster virus (VZV) and cytomegalovirus (CMV) after HCT but, at the same time, other viruses have gained importance. Herpesviruses 1–5 (HSV 1 and 2, VZV, CMV and Epstein–Barr virus [EBV]) are reviewed in Chapters 53–56. This chapter reviews the significance of adenovirus, herpesviruses 6–8, community respiratory viruses, papovaviruses (papillomavirus, polyomaviruses), parvovirus B19, enteroviruses, rotavirus and Norwalk virus in the HCT setting.

Adenovirus

Virology

Adenovirus is a nonenveloped DNA virus that replicates and assembles in the nucleus. Virions are released when the cell is lysed. Adenovirus causes both lytic and latent infection [1]. Infection may persist from days to years and may occur in host tissue (e.g. adenoidal) without causing apparent symptoms in immunocompetent hosts.

All adenoviruses share a common group-specific complement-fixing antigen. Adenoviruses are categorized in subgroups A–F, and there are presently 51 human serotypes known, although only approximately half have been implicated in human disease. Serotypes from all five subgroups can cause disease in both immunocompetent and immunocompromised subjects, although the disease spectrum associated with strains may differ [2,3]. After primary infection, adenovirus establishes latency in adenoidal tissues with lifelong persistence of specific antibodies [2].

Pathogenesis and immunity

Transmission of adenovirus is by either respiratory droplet or the oral–fecal route. Adenovirus enters the mucosa and infects epithelial cells, resulting in inflammation and necrosis. Subsequent viremia may lead to infection of kidney, bladder, liver and lungs in HCT recipients; central nervous system (CNS) disease is rare. After HCT, reactivation from latency is probably more important than exogenous infection [4]. It has been reported that immunosuppressed children have a higher rate of adenovirus infections compared to adults. The reasons for this phenomenon are poorly understood.

Epidemiology and clinical manifestations

Primary infection is usually established in early life with either asymptomatic or symptomatic infection. By age 5 years, most people have been infected by one or more serotypes of adenovirus.

Adenovirus infections are common after HCT [3–6], and some recent reports suggest that they may be increasing, possibly related to transplantation practices (e.g. T-cell depletion) [7]. However, the incidence of adenovirus disease is dependent on the degree of immunosuppression and seems to be increasing only in recipients of T-cell-depleted grafts [7]. Clinical manifestations include pneumonia, hepatitis, gastrointestinal disease, nephritis, cystitis and eye infection [4,6–8].

Risk factor analyses have been performed for adenovirus infection at any site and for adenovirus disease. Risk factors for adenovirus infection include graft-vs.-host disease (GVHD), unrelated donor graft, use of total body irradiation, T-cell depletion and lower age [4,5,7,9]. The degree of T-cell depletion and post-transplant immunosuppression directed at T-cell function seems to be important. For example, transplant protocols utilized for haploidentical grafts are associated with a particularly high incidence of adenovirus infection and invasive disease [10]. Almost all studies report a higher incidence in children [4,11,12].

Adenovirus invasive disease is rare in non-T-cell-depleted transplant recipients and seems to be restricted to allogeneic transplant recipients [4,9]. However, cases of disease in reduced-toxicity regimens that include T-cell depletion have been reported [13]. Disease is more common in T-cell-depleted transplant recipients. Risk factors for adenovirus disease include younger age [12], viremia and shedding from more than two sites [9,12,14], total body irradiation [5], GVHD [7] and transplantation from an unrelated donor [9].

Adenovirus disease is associated with a fatality rate of 30–50% [4,7,15]. Response to treatment seems to be particularly poor in patients with pneumonia or disseminated disease [15]. A recent multivariable analysis in non-T-cell-depleted HCT recipients indicated that adenovirus infection is independently associated with mortality [4].

Diagnostic techniques

Direct detection methods are necessary to establish the diagnosis of adenovirus infection and disease in HCT. As with other viral infections in HCT recipients, serology is not recommended. Adenovirus can be grown in cell culture. Shell vial assays and direct antigen detection methods are used routinely in clinical practice. For detection of adenovirus in stool, enzyme immunoassays or polymerase chain reaction (PCR) are required because enteropathogenic serotypes (40, 41) usually do not grow in culture. Quantitative PCR assays have been developed to diagnose adenovirus. These assays are especially promising for detection of adenovirus DNA in blood [10,14,16,17]. For diagnosis of adenovirus disease, detection of the virus in bronchoalveolar lavage (BAL) or tissue samples is required using rapid culture techniques or direct fluorescent antibody (DFA) tests on BAL and immunohistochemistry or *in situ* hybridization techniques for tissue samples. The role of quantitative PCR in BAL and tissue is currently not defined.

Prevention and treatment

There are no controlled treatment studies for adenovirus infection in the immunocompromised host. Intravenous ribavirin has been used but results are conflicting [18–21]. Recently, cidofovir has been shown to have *in vitro* activity and initial small case series show promising results [15,16,20,22–24], although no randomized comparison with ribavirin has been performed. Ganciclovir has *in vitro* activity against adenovirus and has a moderate effect in prevention of adenovirus infection in non-T-cell-depleted patients [4]. Ganciclovir is not recommended for treatment of adenovirus disease. Specific and nonspecific T-cell therapy have been reported in some cases [13,25].

In high-risk settings such as HCT from haploidentical donors or cord blood transplantation [10,26], prevention strategies are needed because of the high risk of fatal adenovirus disease. Because viremia seems to be predictive for disease [10,13], one approach would be to use PCR surveillance for viremia and pre-emptive treatment with cidofovir [10]. It has also been suggested that adenovirus DNA in stool may be predictive for disease in highest risk patients [10], which might represent an earlier opportunity to intervene. Randomized trials are needed to evaluate prevention strategies because all available agents are associated with significant toxicity.

Respiratory viruses

Community acquired respiratory virus infections are an important cause of morbidity and mortality after HCT. The best studied viruses include respiratory syncytial virus (RSV), parainfluenza viruses and influenza viruses. Less information is available on rhinoviruses and coronavirus and the recently described metapneumovirus. The infection epidemiology in HCT recipients usually parallels that observed in the community, as these viruses circulate in immunocompetent individuals (including health care personnel and family members). RSV, influenza viruses, rhinovirus and metapneumovirus have a seasonal distribution, while parainfluenza virus infections often occur year around. The biggest impact on morbidity and mortality after HCT has been from RSV, parainfluenza viruses and influenza viruses [27–30]. Whether rhinovirus can cause lower tract disease remains controversial [31,32].

Several methods exist for the diagnosis of respiratory viruses [33]. Because viral load in immunocompromised adults may be very low, appropriate specimen handling is important for recovery of the virus. Nasal wash specimens should be placed on ice or in the refrigerator immediately and transported to the laboratory without delay [33]. Specimen set-up in the laboratory should occur within 2–4 h. Methods available for testing include standard viral cultures (results available in several days), shell vial centrifugation cultures using RSV-specific monoclonal antibodies (results after 1–3 days), DFA tests (2 h), enzyme immunoassays (2 h) and, more recently, reverse transcription-polymerase chain reaction (RT-PCR). A problem with the rapid test methods is a relatively low sensitivity in immunocompromised hosts where viral load may be low [33]. This problem can be overcome in part by combining two rapid tests. On tissue sections from lung biopsy or autopsy specimens, virus-specific monoclonal antibody staining can be used. Isolation of rhinovirus requires lower incubation temperatures. Molecular detection techniques are rapidly replacing traditional methods [17,34,35].

Respiratory syncytial virus

Clinical significance

RSV is an RNA virus (paramyxovirus) that causes a wide spectrum of respiratory diseases ranging from life-threatening bronchiolitis in infants and potentially fatal pneumonia in transplant recipients to a mild upper

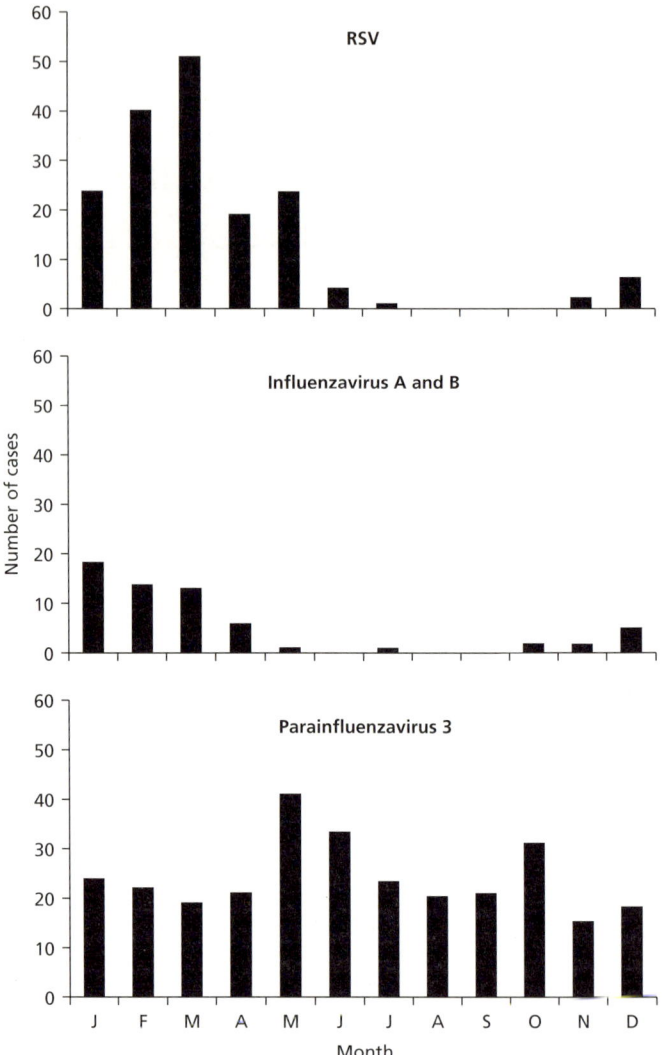

Fig. 57.1 Monthly distribution of respiratory syncytial virus (RSV), parainfluenza virus 3 and influenza infections after hematopoietic cell transplantation (HCT) between 1990 and 1999 at Fred Hutchinson Cancer Research Center [38–40].

respiratory infection (URI) in immunocompetent adults and older children. The virus is implicated increasingly in a number of respiratory illnesses in immunocompetent or mildly immunosuppressed individuals, such as exacerbation of chronic obstructive lung disease and community acquired pneumonia. RSV has also been described as a cause of otitis media. After HCT and also in severely immunosuppressed nontransplant patients with hematologic malignancies [36], RSV causes URI, which may progress to fatal pneumonia [37]. During the respiratory virus season (Fig. 57.1 [38–40]) the incidence may be as high as 10%, and both allogeneic and autologous HCT recipients may be infected (Table 57.1 [38–48]) [27,41]. Most of the infections occur during the first 2 months after HCT; however, late cases have been reported (Fig. 57.2) [49].

Risk factors

In a large study, winter season, male gender and use of bone marrow as stem cell source were identified for the acquisition of RSV in HCT recipients [27]. URI precedes pneumonia in 80% of patients and approximately 40–50% of patients with RSV URI progress to pneumonia after a median of 7 days; however, in 20% of patients with RSV pneumonia, URI is not present or very mild, or occurs only concurrently with the

Table 57.1 Respiratory virus infections after hematopoietic cell transplantation (HCT): comparison of respiratory syncytial virus (RSV), parainfluenza virus 3 and influenza viruses [38–47].

Virus	Incidence of infection (%)	Progression from URI to pneumonia (%)	Time from URI to pneumonia (median)	Proportion of pneumonia without URI (%)	Pulmonary copathogens in cases with pneumonia (%)	Overall mortality at 1 month after diagnosis of pneumonia (%)
RSV	1.8–6*	40	7 days	20–50	2.5–33	45
Parainfluenza virus 3	4–7	18–44	7 days	31	53	35–37
Influenza viruses A and B	1.3–2.6†	18	11 days	18	50	25–28

RSV, respiratory syncytial virus; URI, upper respiratory infection.
*During the winter season, the incidence may be as high as 10%.
†May be significantly higher during outbreaks [48].

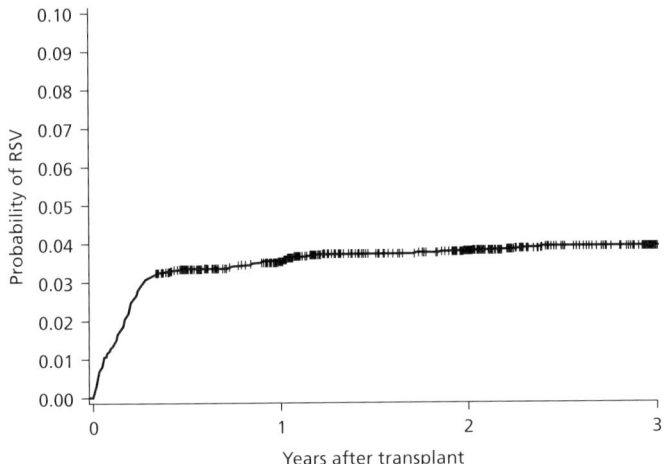

Fig. 57.2 Time to first respiratory syncytial virus (RSV) infection after hematopoietic cell transplantation (HCT).

onset of pneumonia. Strongest risk factors for progression to pneumonia are older age and lymphopenia [27]. One study in pediatric HCT recipients indicates that asymptomatic shedding of RSV can occur [50]. An earlier study in adult HCT recipients using monthly surveillance by culture did not detect asymptomatic shedding [51]. A prospective surveillance study using molecular detection methods is ongoing.

Treatment and prevention

Without treatment, RSV pneumonia is almost uniformly fatal in hematopoietic cell transplantation (HCT) recipients [37]. Pulmonary copathogens are detected in one-third of the patients with RSV pneumonia and require aggressive treatment. No controlled trials exist for the treatment of RSV infection and pneumonia in the hematopoietic transplantation setting. Available evidence comes from small uncontrolled cohort studies. The data suggest that treatment of early pneumonia (i.e. prior to mechanical ventilation) is associated with improved outcome (Table 57.2 [27,30,37,41,52–56]). Intermittent short duration (2 g over 2 h three times daily) or continuous aerosolized ribavirin (16–18 h) is considered the treatment of choice for RSV pneumonia. With this regimen, the 30-day all-cause mortality is approximately 40% (Table 57.2). In a large multivariable analysis, RSV pneumonia (but not URI) was independently associated with mortality (M. Boeckh, unpublished observation, 2003). Systemic ribavirin alone does not seem to be effective [56,57]. Whether combined oral and aerosolized ribavirin is more effective than aerosolized ribavirin alone has not been studied. The role of concomitant intravenous immunoglobulin (IVIg) or RSV-specific immunoglobulin or palivizumab, an RSV-specific monoclonal antibody directed at the F protein of RSV, remains unclear. Uncontrolled data suggest that high-titer antibody preparations or palivizumab may be required if such adjunctive therapy is given [41,54,55]; however, this issue has not been studied in a controlled fashion. Outcome results of recent series are depicted in Table 57.2. There are several factors that may account for differences in outcome in the available cohort studies. Perhaps the most important factor seems to be the timing of initiation of therapy. Several studies suggest that treatment that is started after respiratory failure has occurred is almost uniformly unsuccessful (Table 57.2). Other factors that may be important and that may explain the differences in outcome between studies include the presence of lymphopenia at the time of diagnosis, presence of copathogens (e.g. invasive molds, CMV) and the use of immunosuppressive agents. Recent data suggest that lymphocyte rather than neutrophil engraftment is an important risk factor for progression and outcome [30]. Available studies are too small to control for these parameters, making the interpretation of results of pharmacologic interventions difficult. Most centers now agree that aerosolized ribavirin should be given to HCT patients with lower respiratory tract RSV disease. There is no consensus on the role of antibody preparations.

Because of the high mortality rate of RSV pneumonia, much interest has focused on prevention. Possible strategies are similar to those employed for prevention of CMV. While it is well-established that RSV URI precedes pneumonia in the majority of cases [38], limited information is available on the extent of asymptomatic shedding of respiratory viruses in HCT recipients [50,51]. Currently, controlled studies are underway to evaluate the efficacy and toxicity of pre-emptive antiviral therapy based on RSV shedding [50] or based on RSV URI [38].

Prophylactic measures recommended throughout the respiratory virus season included isolation of infected patients, hand washing prior to every patient contact, educational efforts targeted at health care personnel and family members, avoiding patient contact of health care personnel and family members with uncontrolled secretions, as well as influenza vaccination of health care personnel and family members [58,59]. Whether pharmacologic prophylaxis (e.g. palivizumab, RSV-Ig) throughout the respiratory virus season is effective in preventing infection and disease in HSCT recipients has not been studied.

For pretransplant infections with RSV, parainfluenza virus or influenza virus, most transplant centers postpone the transplantion until resolution and cessation of viral shedding, especially when an allogeneic HCT procedure is planned. Indeed, Centers for Disease Control and Prevention (CDC) guidelines suggest postponing transplantation in all patients with URI symptoms [60]. This approach is supported by a recent study of pretransplant RSV infection, which showed rapid progression to RSV pneumonia in patients in whom the transplant procedure was not postponed [61].

Table 57.2 Outcome of radiographic and virologic documented respiratory syncytial virus (RSV) pneumonia with antiviral therapy (only series of ≥5 patients considered).

Author/year	Reference	Number of patients	Survival (%)	Respiratory failure at start of treatment
Aerosolized ribavirin alone				
Harrington et al. 1992	[37]	13	22	NR
Ljungman 2001	[30]	9	66	NR
Nichols et al. 2002	[27]	5	60	NR
Aerosolized ribavirin + pooled IVIG				
Whimbey et al. 1995	[52]	12	58	Survival 78% if therapy was started before respiratory failure; 0% after respiratory failure
Ghosh et al. 2000	[53]	6	66	Survival 80% if therapy was started before respiratory failure; 0% after respiratory failure
Ljungman 2001	[30]	5	60	NR
Nichols et al. 2002	[27]	19	68	NR
Aerosolized ribavirin + palivizumab				
Boeckh et al. 2001	[54]	12	83	None of the patients had respiratory failure at start of treatment
Aerosolized ribavrin + RSV-specific Ig				
DeVincenco et al. 2000	[55]	7*	86%	None of the patients had respiratory failure at start of treatment
Small et al. 2002	[41]	11	91	Including two patients with respiratory failure at start of treatment; both survived†
IV ribavirin alone				
Lewinsohn et al. 1996	[56]	10	20	Survival 40% if therapy was started before respiratory failure; 0% after respiratory failure
IV ribavirin + aerosolized ribavirin				
Ljungman 2001	[30]	5	40	NR

Ig, immunoglobulin; IV, intravenous; NR, not reported.
*Only patients with radiologic signs of lower tract involvement considered.
†T. Small, personal communication, 2003.

However, there is some evidence that low-risk autologous transplant patients may be transplanted without adverse outcome [62]. Also, outcome of respiratory virus infections may be less severe with nonmyeloablative or reduced-toxicity conditioning regimens [42]. Thus, more studies are needed to define which patients require postponing the transplantation procedure. Until these data are available delaying the transplant procedures based on URI symptoms is recommended. Use of prophylaxis (e.g. RSV-Ig, palivizumab) during transplantation in patients with pretransplant respiratory virus infections has not been studied.

Parainfluenza viruses

Clinical significance

Parainfluenza, an enveloped paramyxovirus containing single-stranded RNA, is classified into four serotypes. Of the four types of parainfluenza viruses, parainfluenza virus serotype 3 is most common (approximately 90%), followed by serotypes 1 and 2. The incubation time is 1–4 days. Parainfluenza virus infection usually does not follow a seasonal pattern (Fig. 57.1). The incidence of 7% in two studies is higher than that reported for RSV (4%) [39,63].

Risk factors

Only HCT from an unrelated donor has been identified as a risk factor for acquisition of the parainfluenza virus [39]. In recipients of T-cell-depleted grafts, the degree of CD4 lymphopenia has been reported to increase the risk of all respiratory virus infections, including parainfluenza virus [42].

Similar to RSV, URI is the predominant presentation. Progression to pneumonia seems to be less common than with RSV (Table 57.1) [39]. The most important risk factors for the progression from URI to pneumonia is use of systemic corticosteroids and lymphopenia [39,42]. Although the overall progression rate to pneumonia is only 18%, in allograft recipients with >1 mg/kg prednisone, the risk is 40%, and 65% with 2 mg/kg [39]. Parainfluenza 3 pneumonia may also occur after autologous transplantation but mainly in the setting of CD34 selection or after use of high-dose steroids [39]. Parainfluenza 3 pneumonia is often associated with serious pulmonary copathogens (53%) such as *Aspergillus fumigatus*. Factors associated with poor outcome after pneumonia include presence of copathogens and mechanical ventilation [39]. Thus, aggressive diagnostic intervention (i.e. BAL) and therapy are indicated in patients with suspected parainfluenza pneumonia. In a large retrospective analysis, both URI and pneumonia caused by parainfluenza virus 3 were associated with overall mortality in multivariable models [39].

Treatment and prevention

Mortality of pneumonia is approximately 35% in patients who are treated with myeloablative regimens [28,39,43]. Outcome may be improved in reduced toxicity conditioning regimens [42]. In a retrospective analysis, neither aerosolized ribavirin nor IVIg led to improved outcome of pneumonia or a reduction in viral shedding following pneumonia [39].

Systemic ribavirin has only been reported in case observations [44]. Randomized treatment studies have not been performed. Whether earlier antiviral treatment (i.e. pre-emptive treatment for URI) is effective in the prevention of pneumonia is unknown [44]. The association of high-dose steroid treatment with progression to disease might suggest that reduction of immunosuppression may be useful [39]; however, such an approach has not been tested. The role of immunoglobulin in treatment is also poorly defined. One retrospective analysis did not find a benefit of pooled immunoglobulin given for parainfluenza pneumonia [39]. However, antibody content in pooled preparations is highly variable. The highest titers can be found in RSV-specific immunoglobulin, which also contains high titer of antibodies directed against parainfluenza [64].

Infection control is the mainstay of prevention strategies. Unfortunately, current infection control practices seem to be far from perfect in keeping parainfluenza away from HCT units, as indicated by the high incidence figures (Table 57.2). Parainfluenza virus has been prone to persistent outbreaks in HCT units [39,65,66]. Possible explanations for the difficulty in preventing parainfluenza from entering HCT units include lack of a vaccine for health care workers and close contacts, very mild or absence of symptoms in immunocompetent individuals in combination with prolonged shedding, prolonged asymptomatic shedding in infected patients and persistence of the virus on environmental surfaces [67].

Influenza viruses

Clinical significance

Influenza viruses belong to the family of orthomyxoviruses and are enveloped, single-stranded pleomorphic RNA viruses. Influenza is classified into three major types, of which type A is most common, followed by type B [29,68,69]. Influenza type C is very uncommon, even in the immunocompetent patient population; there are no reports of influenza C in HCT recipients. Influenza virus infections seem to be less common than RSV and parainfluenza virus infections. Both subtypes can cause infection, although type A appears to be more common. Clinical characteristics are listed in Table 57.1.

Risk factors

Acquisition of influenza is increased in patients with high-risk underlying disease [40]. Progression to severe pneumonia can occur similar to RSV and parainfluenza virus [69]; however, progression appears to be less common and risk factors for progression differ (Table 57.1). In contrast to parainfluenza virus infection where corticosteroids are an important risk factor for the development of pneumonia, lower tract infection with influenza virus appears to be less common in patients treated with corticosteroids [40]. Interestingly, the clinical presentation in HCT often lacks myalgia and high fever, which is commonly seen in immunocompetent individuals.

Treatment and prevention

Effective prevention is available for influenza, which may explain the lower incidence. Health care personnel, family members and visitors are advised to be vaccinated against influenza early in the season. Antiviral therapy is available for influenza virus infection; however, available agents have not been studied systematically in HCT recipients. The M2-inhibitors, amantadine and rimantadine (with a more favorable side-effect profile) are effective against influenza A in prevention and treatment of immunocompetent adults. During treatment, emergence of resistance is common [70]. More recently, neuraminidase inhibitors (zanamivir, oseltamivir) became available [71,72]. Both agents are active against influenza A and B and are potentially useful alone or in combination with rimantadine. Small uncontrolled studies suggest that pre-emptive therapy with either M2 inhibitors or neuraminidase inhibitors (oseltamivir, zanamivir) may be effective in preventing progression to lower tract disease [40,73]. Widespread prophylaxis of susceptible immunosuppressed patients in outbreak situations has been recommended [60]. While rimantadine is presently recommended as agent of choice by the CDC [60], neuraminidase inhibitors are also effective for this indication with fewer side-effects [74]; however, safety of long-term prophylaxis has not been established in HCT recipients (Table 57.3 [75]).

Other community respiratory viruses

Rhinovirus

Rhinovirus is classified as a picornavirus characterized by small naked single-stranded RNA. There are approximately 100 serotypes, which usually cause mild upper respiratory tract symptoms in immunocompetent hosts. Rhinovirus is infrequently reported as a cause of respiratory infection in HCT recipients. However, three reports found the organism in patients with pneumonia. Ghosh *et al.* [31] reported lower tract disease in seven of 22 patients with rhinovirus infection while Bowden *et al.* [69] documented lower tract disease only in one of 29 infected patients. Whether rhinovirus can cause lower tract disease remains controversial. The M.D. Anderson experience would suggest that rhinovirus can cause fatal interstitial pneumonia by itself [31]. However, two analyses from Seattle could not find conclusive evidence [32,69]. In the most recent analysis, of 77 BAL fluids from consecutive HCT recipients with clinical and radiographic pneumonia, eight tested positive for rhinovirus by RT-PCR; however, all patients had significant copathogens [32]. While the fatality rate was high, it is unclear whether rhinovirus contributed to the death in this series [32]. Surveillance studies using RT-PCR will be needed to define more precisely the role of rhinovirus in HCT recipients.

Coronavirus

Human coronavirus is an RNA virus that can cause respiratory infection in immunocompetent individuals. The significance seems to be low compared to RSV, parainfluenza viruses and influenza viruses [76]. One recent study did not find evidence of coronavirus by RT-PCR in 46 consecutive BALs obtained from HCT recipients with pneumonia during the respiratory virus season [32].

Measles virus

Measles virus (rubeola), a paramyxovirus, is a recognized cause of giant-cell pneumonia, developing with and without rash, and severe CNS disease in immunocompromised hosts, including HCT recipients [77,78]. The incidence of measles is extremely low at most centers because of the widespread use of measles immunization. However, an outbreak among HCT recipients has recently been reported from Brazil [79]. During that outbreak among 122 susceptible patients, severe clinical disease occurred in one patient and seven had mild symptoms. Exanthema was present in all these patients, although it was often atypical. Koplik spots could be observed in five patients. All but one patient had fever and nonproductive cough [79]. The use of ribavirin has been reported for measles in two critically ill immunocompromised patients; however, no systematic assessment of this intervention has been made [80].

Human metapneumovirus

Human metapneumovirus is a newly discovered negative-sense nonsegmented RNA paramyxovirus [81]. By age 5 years virtually all children are seropositive. The virus can cause upper and lower tract infection during the winter season [82]. Initial studies suggest that immunosuppressed patients can develop interstitial pneumonia, which can be fatal in some cases [83]. Studies are ongoing to define the significance of human metapneumovirus in HCT recipients.

Table 57.3 Overview of antibody preparations and antiviral agents with *in vitro* activity against other viral infections after hematopoietic cell transplantation (HCT). (See text for details about indications, doses and limitations.)

Virus	Drugs	Clinical use in HCT recipients*	Comment
Adenovirus	Ribavirin (IV)	Adenovirus disease	High rate of failures, possibly because of selection bias
	Cidofovir	Adenovirus disease, pre-emptive therapy	Response to therapy reported, no direct comparison with ribavirin reported
RSV	Ribavirin	RSV pneumonia, pre-emptive therapy for URI	Moderate–strong evidence for pneumonia, pre-emptive therapy with ribavirin under study; combination with immunoglobulin preparations appear to be more effective when RSV-specific preparations are used (Table 57.2)
	RSV-specific immunoglobulin	Combination therapy for RSV pneumonia	
	RSV-specific monoclonal antibodies (palivizumab)	Combination therapy for RSV pneumonia	
	Pooled immunoglobulin	Combination therapy for RSV pneumonia	
Parainfluenza virus	Ribavirin	Parainfluenza virus pneumonia	No apparent effect for pneumonia of either ribavirin or the combination with immunoglobulin; pre-emptive therapy not tested; reduction of immunosuppression may be effective (see text)
	Pooled immunoglobulin	Combination therapy for parainfluenza pneumonia	
Influenza virus	M2-inhibitors (amantadine, rimantadine)	Influenza infection and disease, prophylaxis; combination therapy	M2-inhibitors only effective against influenza A; both groups of drugs extensively studied in immunocompetent subjects; neuraminidase inhibitors appear to have improved toxicity profile, although experience in HCT is limited
	Neuraminidase inhibitors (oseltemavir, zanamivir)	Influenza infection and disease, prophylaxis; combination therapy	
Rhinovirus	Pleconaril	No data	Drug is awaiting FDA approval
HHV-6	Ganciclovir, valganciclovir	HHV-6 CNS disease	Both foscarnet and ganciclovir have been used for the treatment of CNS disease; anti-HHV-6 activity does not appear to be HHV-6 variant-dependent [75]
	Foscarnet	HHV-6 CNS disease	
	Cidofovir	No data	
HHV-7	Foscarnet	No data	
	Cidofovir	No data	
HHV-8	Ganciclovir, valganciclovir	No data	
BK virus	Cidofovir	Hemorrhagic cystitis	Small case series
JC virus	Cidofovir	Multifocal leukoencephalopathy	Case studies only

CNS, central nervous system; FDA, Food and Drug Administration; HHV, human herpesvirus; IV, intravenous; RSV, respiratory syncytial virus; URI, upper respiratory infection.
*All clinical results in HCT recipients are from nonrandomized studies.

Isolation practices

Recommendations for isolation have recently been summarized by the CDC and the American Society for Blood and Marrow Transplantation (ASBMT) [60]. Hand washing is the single most effective way of preventing spread of respiratory viruses and should be performed after each patient contact by all health care personnel and visitors. Respiratory isolation is used for HCT recipients with respiratory virus infections (masks, gowns, gloves and eye protection) [84]. The use of masks among health care workers, family members and asymptomatic patients remains controversial. One nonrandomized study suggests a benefit of masks [58]. However, questions remain on the type of mask, frequency of changing the mask and who should wear masks. Not all transplant centers have a universal mask policy. Recent CDC guidelines recommend using masks during patient transport [60]; however, this recommendation is not based on randomized trials. Another approach that is likely to reduce transmission is to restrict health care workers and family members from patient contact if they have a URI and systemic symptoms such as rhinorhea, watery eyes, sneezing, fever and myalgia [27]. While this is not uniformly done in adult patients, most centers restrict small children from direct patient contact during the respiratory virus season because of their predisposition to URIs and prolonged high-titer shedding [60]. A strategy that restricts access of personnel and other close contacts will only be effective for infections that present with significant drainage and symptoms such as RSV, rhinovirus and influenza infections. Parainfluenza virus infections, which may present with only mild symptoms, may be missed by this approach (see above) [65–67].

Human herpesvirus 6, 7, 8

Human herpesvirus 6

Clinical significance

Human herpesvirus 6 (HHV-6) is a β herpesvirus with similarities to CMV and HHV-7. Several longitudinal studies have examined the role of HHV-6 after HCT [85–88]. Similar to other human herpesviruses, it is ubiquitous, infecting most people by 2 years of age [89]. After primary infection, the virus persists in lymphocytes and salivary glands with 95% of adults having detectable viral DNA in peripheral blood mononuclear cells and saliva [90]. During times of immunosuppression, the virus may reactivate and cause disease. HHV-6 reactivates early after HCT and can be detected in the blood at a median of 20 days after HCT, usually before CMV. Type B is far more common than type A.

Active HHV-6 infection has been documented in 38–46% of patients following HCT [87,91–93]. The search for a clinical syndrome associated with HHV-6 revealed rash, a CNS syndrome consisting of encephalitis, impaired memory and sometimes seizures [94], a possible association with interstitial lung disease [90,95] and the association with delayed platelet engraftment [88]. Secondary graft failure has been documented in case reports [96]. Transplant-related mortality has also been associated with HHV-6 in one small series [97]. The clinical disease that has been most consistently found in prospective studies is HHV-6 CNS disease [88,98].

PCR has been used to diagnose HHV-6-associated encephalitis [94]. Whether monitoring for HHV-6 viremia is useful in predicting these clinical syndromes is not known. In solid organ transplant recipients, there seems to be an interaction between HHV-6 and CMV [99–104]. One study showed a trend toward more CMV infection among patients with >100 copies of HHV-6 DNA/5×10^4 peripheral blood lymphocytes [88] and another study suggests an interaction of HHV-6 and CMV in BAL fluid of HCT recipients [95]. Data in HCT recipients are limited and results are inconclusive. HHV-6 reactivation typically occurs 2–4 weeks after HCT [87,91–93], preceding CMV reactivation which occurs a median of 40–42 days following transplant [105]. An interaction between HHV-6 and CMV may be explained by a generalized immunosuppressive effect of HHV-6 [106–109]. A recent study demonstrates that early HHV-6 reactivation leads to a delay in CMV-specific T-helper immune responses in HCT recipients [110] but the exact mechanism remains unclear.

Treatment and prevention

Currently there is no widely accepted clinical approach to HHV-6 screening or prevention following HCT. *In vitro* studies suggest that HHV-6 is susceptible to foscarnet, cidofovir and ganciclovir while less susceptible to aciclovir [75,111,112]. Foscarnet and ganciclovir have been used to treat HHV-6 associated disease, and a decline in viral load has been documented with therapy [113,114]. No randomized trials have been reported for prophylaxis or pre-emptive therapy [75].

Human herpesvirus 7

HHV-7 is also a β herpesvirus, similar to HHV-6 and CMV. The virus can be detected by PCR [115]. One study found both HHV-6 and HHV-7 in peripheral blood and marrow of healthy subjects [116]. The impact of HHV-7 after HCT has been examined in a longitudinal study but no correlation with clinical disease was found; however, there was a possible association with CMV infection [85]. So far it has not been possible to assign a clinical syndrome to HHV-7, with the exception of one recent report of a CNS infection with myelitis in an unrelated donor transplant recipient [117]. Foscarnet and cidofovir show activity *in vitro* (Table 57.3) [75].

Human herpesvirus 8

HHV-8 is a γ herpesvirus (similar to EBV). HHV-8 is associated with Kaposi's sarcoma in HIV-infected individuals. Two recent case series from areas with high seroprevalence suggested an association of HHV-8 with a febrile syndrome and marrow failure in HCT recipients [118,119]; however, whether HHV-8 causes these clinical syndromes requires further study. HHV-8 can be detected by PCR [112]. While transmission from donor to recipient has been documented in the kidney transplant setting [120], there have been no reports of transmission via stem cells to date. Ganciclovir and cidofovir show activity *in vitro* (Table 57.3) [75].

Papovaviruses

BK virus

BK and JC virus are human polyomaviruses. Both can cause disease in HCT recipients. BK virus is a nonenveloped DNA virus which replicates in the nucleus. Seroprevalence in the population is between 60 and 80%. Primary infection usually occurs during childhood, possibly by the respiratory route. The virus can be detected by PCR [121,122]. BK virus is associated with late post-transplant hemorrhagic cystitis after HCT [123]. After kidney transplantation, BK virus is an important cause of late nephritis [124]. No data exist on BK nephropathy in HCT recipients, although individual cases have been reported (R. Hackman, personal communication, 2003). Although BK virus is often detected in urine by PCR, an association with clinical symptoms may be difficult to prove [125]. Contrary to the renal transplant setting where BK viremia is associated with high risk of nephropathy [122,124], detection in blood was not associated with hemorrhagic cystitis in two studies in HCT recipients [121,126]. High viral load in urine was associated with a higher risk of BK-associated cystitis; however, no threshold was defined [121]. In a study of pediatric HCT recipients, BK virus-associated hemorrhagic cystitis occurred between day 24 and 50 post-transplant in nine of 117 patients. Infection was characterized by a long duration, correlated with use of busulfan and resulted in bladder tamponade in two of nine patients [127]. One case of BK virus-associated pneumonia has been reported [128]. There is no established treatment. Cidofovir has activity *in vitro* but there are only anecdotal treatment results to date [129]. Initial data from renal transplant patients with BK nephropathy suggest that lower doses of cidofovir may be sufficient to treat BK renal disease [130]. Studies are ongoing to define the optimal dose of cidofovir for treatment of BK virus-associated disease.

JC virus

JC virus is a nonenveloped DNA virus classified as polyomavirus. JC virus is the cause of progressive multifocal leukoencephalopathy in immunosuppressed patients. Several cases have been reported after HCT and in patients with hematologic malignancies [131–134]. Overall, this complication seems to be rare. PCR detection of JC virus in the cerebrospinal fluid is used for diagnosis [135]. The optimal treatment is not defined. Cidofovir has activity *in vitro*; however, little is known about its *in vivo* efficacy in HCT recipients [136]. Interleukin 2 (IL-2) has been used in one patient [137].

Human papillomavirus

Human papillomavirus (HPV) is a nonenveploed DNA virus. HPV infections rarely occur after HCT [138,139]. HPV causes cutaneous infections (warts) and there has been an association with cervical carcinoma. In one series, three of 238 allogeneic HCT recipients developed anogenital condylomas associated with HPV [138]. Rapid progression of preexisting warts has been reported [140]. One retrospective study found a higher rate of cervical cytological abnormalities both before and after marrow transplantation when compared to the general population [141]. The clinical significance of these findings is unknown.

Parvovirus B19

Parvoviruses are made of small naked single-stranded DNA. Parvovirus infects a variety of animals, including cats and dogs. In 1975, human parvovirus B19 was isolated from asymptomatic blood donors. Seroepidemiologic studies showed evidence of past infection in approximately

60% of young adults. It is most likely spread by respiratory transmission or by blood. Parvovirus B19 can infect erythroid progenitor cells.

Parvovirus B19 is commonly associated with aplastic crisis in patients with hemolytic anemia. It is also the cause of erythema infectiosum, a self-limiting disease of childhood characterized by fever, fatigue, myalgias, a lace-like rash and a "slapped-cheek" appearance. Parvovirus B19 also is associated with some cases of rheumatoid arthritis.

Immunity to parvovirus B19 is thought to be primarily humoral; neutralizing antibodies to capsid protein have a major role in host defense. IgM antibody detection may be useful in the diagnosis of acute infection in immunocompetent persons. The reliability of serology in HCT recipients is questionable.

In addition to transient marrow failure, parvovirus B19 can cause chronic anemia and, rarely, pancytopenia in HCT recipients [142,143]. PCR is useful as a diagnostic tool [143]. IVIg is effective in treating parvovirus B19 symptomatic infection [144]. Prophylactic IVIg seems to have a protective effect against parvovirus B19, although this has not been established in a randomized study [145].

Enterovirus

Enteroviruses belong to the picornavirus family. They include polioviruses, Coxsackie viruses, echoviruses and other serotypes simply referred to as *enteroviruses*. They are naked virions containing single-stranded RNA that replicate in the cellular cytoplasm. Both tissue culture and molecular methods are used for diagnosis. The virus can be detected in throat washes, stool, cerebrospinal fluid and other body fluids.

Asymptomatic infection is common in normal hosts, and these viruses are most prevalent during the summer and fall months. Infection is usually by fecal–oral route; shedding of the virus from the oropharynx may persist for 1–4 weeks and from the gastrointestinal tract for up to 18 weeks. Viremic spread in the host is common, and can affect a variety of organs.

Infection by enteroviruses in HCT recipients has been reported [11,146,147]. One outbreak of Coxsackie A1-associated diarrhea affected patients in a 13-bed unit over a 3-week period, resulting in death in six of seven infected patients [148]. Coxsackie virus was also identified in stools of four of 78 patients with gastrointestinal infections [8]. All four patients with Coxsackie virus died; two had coinfections with adenovirus and rotavirus [8]. Additional cases of disseminated and life-threatening infection been reported [149–152].

Severe cases of echovirus infections have been reported, including a disseminated infection with pneumonitis and pericarditis [153,154]. Treatment of enterovirus infections is supportive. Plenocaril is active against picornaviruses including entroviruses, however, there are no reports of its use in HCT recipients.

Rotavirus

Rotaviruses consists of double-stranded RNA and have a double-shelled capsid. They infect the duodenum and the jejunum, causing vomiting and diarrhea in normal hosts, occasionally accompanied by low-grade fever. Infection usually occurs in the winter, and transmission is by the oral–fecal route. During one outbreak, contaminated toys in a cancer center playroom were implicated as the mode of transmission [155]; hospital personnel can transmit the virus as well [156]. Diagnosis is by electron microscopy or enzyme-linked immunoabsorbent assay.

Rotavirus is a common cause of diarrhea in HCT recipients, presenting with gastroenteritis [6,8,146,157,158]. Fatalities have been reported [146]. There is no proven specific treatment other than supportive care. Oral IVIg has been used in individual cases [159] but this approach has not been studied in larger series or randomized trials.

Norwalk virus

Norwalk viruses are made of small naked DNA-containing virions that have been associated with outbreaks of diarrhea. There have been no reports of Norwalk virus outbreaks in HCT recipients. Diagnosis is by electron microscopy or PCR. Treatment is supportive care.

Conclusions and future perspective

Major progress has been made in the diagnosis and prevention of viral infections after HCT over the last decade. Perhaps the most impressive example is the prevention of CMV disease by ganciclovir. During the same time period, the significance and our knowledge of other viral infections has increased, especially that of adenovirus, community respiratory viruses and HHV-6. However, important questions remain.

Adenovirus infections are an emerging complication after HCT, especially in recipients of T-cell-depleted grafts or patients with intense post-transplant immunosuppression. Quantitative molecular diagnostic tests could be used for surveillance and to initiate pre-emptive therapy in high-risk patients. However, more information is needed to define who will benefit from such approach given the toxicity of the presently available drugs. Both cidofovir and ribavirin have been used in this setting but no comparative trial has been performed to establish which drug is superior.

Respiratory viruses have been recognized as causes of fatal pneumonia after HCT. RSV, parainfluenza viruses and influenza viruses can cause severe pneumonia. Unfortunately, there are no randomized treatment studies and the relatively low incidence of these cases makes it difficult to conduct clinical trials. For RSV, treatment of pneumonia before the development of respiratory failure is critical. Aerosolized ribavirin with or without RSV-specific immunoglobulin or palivizumab is considered the treatment of choice for RSV pneumonia. Of all respiratory viruses, parainfluenza virus infections are most difficult to control and corticosteroids seem to have a particularly negative effect on outcome. Thus, reduction of steroid dose should be attempted in HCT recipients with parainfluenza virus infection. Improved antiviral agents for parainfluenza viruses are clearly needed. Infection control strategies, including vaccination against influenza of susceptible family members and patient care personnel, are critical for prevention. The role of rhinovirus remains poorly defined in HCT recipients. Although this pathogen can be detected in specimens from the lower respiratory tract, it is unclear whether it is a bystander or pathogen. Virtually no data exist on the role of human metapneumovirus infections.

Human herpesviruses 6–8 have been studied extensively over the past decade; however, no randomized prevention or treatment trial has been performed. This is largely because clinical endpoints remain poorly defined (with the exception of HHV-6 encephalitis) and a lack of non-toxic agents that can be administered safely during the first month after transplant. Additional work is needed to define the impact of HHV-6 on platelet engraftment, pulmonary disease, CMV infection and overall mortality.

BK virus is an emerging pathogen in organ transplantation; however, its significance in HCT recipients remains poorly defined. Although an association with late hemorrhagic cystitis has been demonstrated, extensive studies using quantitative PCR methods in blood and urine have been unable to define threshold levels for disease that would allow treatment and prevention strategies. It is also unclear if BK virus can cause nephritis in HCT recipients, although individual cases have been reported (R. Hackman, personal communication, 2003). In analogy to the solid organ transplant setting, one would expect nephropathy to occur late after transplant in a setting of severe immunosuppression with pre-existing renal injury and BK viremia over months. With improved prevention strategies for CMV and *Aspergillus*, which might lead to long-term survival of such patients, it is possible that BK nephropathy will be diagnosed more frequently in HCT recipients.

Finally, most of the viruses discussed here have a low incidence, yet outcome is often fatal or associated with severe sequelae (e.g. HHV-6). Recognition and the development of management strategies for these viruses have lagged behind for years and there are virtually no randomized intervention trials. The low incidence of these infections requires innovative surveillance and intervention networks among HCT centers. Efforts have started to establish such networks (e.g. the European Group for Blood and Marrow Transplantation [EBMT] Infectious Diseases Working Party and the National Institutes of Health Clinical Trial Network) but more work is needed to obtain surveillance results in a more real-time fashion and to design rational intervention strategies.

References

1 Shenk TE. Adenoviridae: the viruses and their replication. In: Knipe DM, Howley PM, eds. *Fields Virology*, 4th edn. Philadelphia: Lippincott Williams & Wilkins, 2001: 2265–300.

2 Horwitz MS. Adenovirus. In: Knipe DM, Howley PM, eds. *Fields Virology*, 4th edn. Philadelphia: Lippincott Williams & Wilkins, 2001: 2301–26.

3 Shields AF, Hackman RC, Fife KH, Corey L, Meyers JD. Adenovirus infections in patients undergoing bone-marrow transplantation. *N Engl J Med* 1985; **312**: 529–33.

4 Bruno B, Gooley T, Hackman RC, Davis C, Corey L, Boeckh M. Adenovirus infection in hematopoietic stem cell transplantation: effect of ganciclovir and impact on survival. *Biol Blood Marrow Transplant* 2003; **9**: 341–52.

5 Hale GA, Heslop HE, Krance RA *et al*. Adenovirus infection after pediatric bone marrow transplantation. *Bone Marrow Transplant* 1999; **23**: 277–82.

6 van Kraaij MG, Dekker AW, Verdonck LF *et al*. Infectious gastroenteritis: an uncommon cause of diarrhoea in adult allogeneic and autologous stem cell transplant recipients [In process citation]. *Bone Marrow Transplant* 2000; **26**: 299–303.

7 Flomenberg P, Babbitt J, Drobyski WR *et al*. Increasing incidence of adenovirus disease in bone marrow transplant recipients. *J Infect Dis* 1994; **169**: 775–81.

8 Cox GJ, Matsui SM, Lo RS *et al*. Etiology and outcome of diarrhea after marrow transplantation: a prospective study. *Gastroenterology* 1994; **107**: 1398–407.

9 Baldwin A, Kingman H, Darville M *et al*. Outcome and clinical course of 100 patients with adenovirus infection following bone marrow transplantation. *Bone Marrow Transplant* 2000; **26**: 1333–8.

10 Lion T, Baumgartinger R, Watzinger F *et al*. Broad spectrum of adenovirus infections in pediatric patients undergoing allogeneic transplantation: clinical implications of early detection and quantitative monitoring by real-time PCR. *Blood* 2003; **102**: 1114–20.

11 Wasserman R, August CS, Plotkin SA. Viral infections in pediatric bone marrow transplant patients. *Pediatr Infect Dis J* 1988; **7**: 109–15.

12 Howard DS, Phillips IG, Reece DE *et al*. Adenovirus infections in hematopoietic stem cell transplant recipients. *Clin Infect Dis* 1999; **29**: 1494–501.

13 Chakrabarti S, Collingham KE, Fegan CD, Pillay D, Milligan DW. Adenovirus infections following haematopoietic cell transplantation: is there a role for adoptive immunotherapy? [In process citation]. *Bone Marrow Transplant* 2000; **26**: 305–7.

14 Schilham MW, Claas EC, van Zaane W *et al*. High levels of adenovirus DNA in serum correlate with fatal outcome of adenovirus infection in children after allogeneic stem-cell transplantation. *Clin Infect Dis* 2002; **35**: 526–32.

15 Ljungman P, Ribaud P, Eyrich M *et al*. Cidofovir for adenovirus infection after allogeneic hematopoietic stem cell transplantation: a survey by the Infectious Diseases Working Party of the European Group for Blood and Marrow Transplantation. *Bone Marrow Transplant* 2003; **31**: 481–6.

16 Legrand F, Berrebi D, Houhou N *et al*. Early diagnosis of adenovirus infection and treatment with cidofovir after bone marrow transplantation in children. *Bone Marrow Transplant* 2001; **27**: 621–6.

17 Coiras MT, Perez-Brena P, Garcia ML, Casas I. Simultaneous detection of influenza A, B, and C viruses, respiratory syncytial virus, and adenoviruses in clinical samples by multiplex reverse transcription nested-PCR assay. *J Med Virol* 2003; **69**: 132–44.

18 Liles WC, Cushing H, Holt S, Bryan C, Hackman RC. Severe adenoviral nephritis following bone marrow transplantation: successful treatment with intravenous ribavirin [see comments]. *Bone Marrow Transplant* 1993; **12**: 409–12.

19 Chakrabarti S, Collingham KE, Fegan CD, Milligan DW. Fulminant adenovirus hepatitis following unrelated bone marrow transplantation: failure of intravenous ribavirin therapy. *Bone Marrow Transplant* 1999; **23**: 1209–11.

20 Bordigoni P, Carret AS, Venard V, Witz F, Le Faou A. Treatment of adenovirus infections in patients undergoing allogeneic hematopoietic stem cell transplantation. *Clin Infect Dis* 2001; **32**: 1290–7.

21 Gavin PJ, Katz BZ. Intravenous ribavirin treatment for severe adenovirus disease in immunocompromised children. *Pediatrics* 2002; **110**: e9.

22 Hayashi M, Lee C, de Magalhaes-Silverman M, Becker A, Scott S, Gingrich RD. Adenovirus infections in BMT patients successfully treated with cidofovir. *Blood* 2000; **96** (Suppl.): 189a [Abstract].

23 Hoffman JA, Shah AJ, Ross LA, Kapoor N. Adenoviral infections and a prospective trial of cidofovir in pediatric hematopoietic stem cell transplantation. *Biol Blood Marrow Transplant* 2001; **7**: 388–94.

24 Carter BA, Karpen SJ, Quiros-Tejeira RE *et al*. Intravenous cidofovir therapy for disseminated adenovirus in a pediatric liver transplant recipient. *Transplantation* 2002; **74**: 1050–2.

25 Regn S, Raffegerst S, Chen X, Schendel D, Kolb HJ, Roskrow M. *Ex vivo* generation of cytotoxic T lymphocytes specific for one or two distinct viruses for the prophylaxis of patients receiving an allogeneic bone marrow transplant. *Bone Marrow Transplant* 2001; **27**: 53–64.

26 Benjamin DK Jr, Miller WC, Bayliff S, Martel L, Alexander KA, Martin PL. Infections diagnosed in the first year after pediatric stem cell transplantation. *Pediatr Infect Dis J* 2002; **21**: 227–34.

27 Nichols WG, Gooley T, Boeckh M. Community-acquired respiratory syncytial virus and parainfluenza virus infections after hematopoietic stem cell transplantation: the Fred Hutchinson Cancer Research Center experience. *Biol Blood Marrow Transplant* 2001; **7** (Suppl.): 11S–15S.

28 Whimbey E, Vartivarian SE, Champlin RE, Elting LS, Luna M, Bodey GP. Parainfluenza virus infection in adult bone marrow transplant recipients. *Eur J Clin Microbiol Infect Dis* 1993; **12**: 699–701.

29 Whimbey E, Champlin RE, Couch RB *et al*. Community respiratory virus infections among hospitalized adult bone marrow transplant recipients. *Clin Infect Dis* 1996; **22**: 778–82.

30 Ljungman P. Respiratory virus infections in stem cell transplant patients: the European experience. *Biol Blood Marrow Transplant* 2001; **7** (Suppl.): 5S–7S.

31 Ghosh S, Champlin R, Couch R *et al*. Rhinovirus infections in myelosuppressed adult blood and marrow transplant recipients [see comments]. *Clin Infect Dis* 1999; **29**: 528–32.

32 Ison MG, Hayden FG, Kaiser L, Corey L, Boeckh M. Rhinovirus infection in recipients of hematopoietic stem cell transplantation with pneumonia. *Clin Infect Dis* 2003; **36**: 1139–43.

33 Englund JA, Piedra PA, Jewell A, Patel K, Baxter BB, Whimbey E. Rapid diagnosis of respiratory syncytial virus infections in immunocompromised adults. *J Clin Microbiol* 1996; **34**: 1649–53.

34 Hindiyeh M, Hillyard DR, Carroll KC. Evaluation of the Prodesse Hexaplex multiplex PCR assay for direct detection of seven respiratory viruses in clinical specimens. *Am J Clin Pathol* 2001; **116**: 218–24.

35 Zambon MC, Stockton JD, Clewley JP, Fleming DM. Contribution of influenza and respiratory syncytial virus to community cases of influenza-like illness: an observational study. *Lancet* 2001; **358**: 1410–6.

36 Whimbey E, Couch RB, Englund JA *et al*. Respiratory syncytial virus pneumonia in hospitalized adult patients with leukemia. *Clin Infect Dis* 1995; **21**: 376–9.

37 Harrington RD, Hooton TM, Hackman RC *et al*. An outbreak of respiratory syncytial virus in a bone marrow transplant center. *J Infect Dis* 1992; **165**: 987–93.

38 Boeckh M, Gooley T, Bowden RA *et al*. Risk factors for progression from respiratory syncytial virus upper respiratory infection to pneumonia after hematopoietic stem cell transplantation. 39th Interscience Conference on Antimicrobial Agents and Chemotherapy, San Diego, CA. American Society for Microbiology. 1999; **435** [Abstract].

39 Nichols WG, Corey L, Gooley T, Davis C, Boeckh M. Parainfluenza virus infections after hematopoietic stem cell transplantation: risk factors, response to antiviral therapy, and effect on transplant outcome. *Blood* 2001; **98**: 573–8.

40 Nichols WG, Guthrie KA, Corey L, Boeckh M. Influenza infections after stem cell transplanta-

tion: risk factors, mortality, and effect of antiviral therapy. *Biol Blood Marrow Transplant* 2003; **9**: 73–4 [Abstract].

41 Small TN, Casson A, Malak SF et al. Respiratory syncytial virus infection following hematopoietic stem cell transplantation. *Bone Marrow Transplant* 2002; **29**: 321–7.

42 Chakrabarti S, Avivi I, Mackinnon S et al. Respiratory virus infections in transplant recipients after reduced-intensity conditioning with Campath-1H: high incidence but low mortality. *Br J Haematol* 2002; **119**: 1125–32.

43 Lewis VA, Champlin R, Englund J et al. Respiratory disease due to parainfluenza virus in adult bone marrow transplant recipients. *Clin Infect Dis* 1996; **23**: 1033–7.

44 Chakrabarti S, Collingham KE, Holder K, Oyaide S, Pillay D, Milligan DW. Parainfluenza virus type 3 infections in hematopoetic stem cell transplant recipients: response to ribavirin therapy. *Clin Infect Dis* 2000; **31**: 1516–8.

45 Couch RB, Englund JA, Whimbey E. Respiratory viral infections in immunocompetent and immunocompromised persons. *Am J Med* 1997; **102**: 2–9; discussion 25–6.

46 Lujan-Zilbermann J, Benaim E, Tong X, Srivastava DK, Patrick CC, DeVincenzo JP. Respiratory virus infections in pediatric hematopoietic stem cell transplantation. *Clin Infect Dis* 2001; **33**: 962–8.

47 McCarthy AJ, Kingman HM, Kelly C et al. The outcome of 26 patients with respiratory syncytial virus infection following allogeneic stem cell transplantation. *Bone Marrow Transplant* 1999; **24**: 1315–22.

48 Martino R, Ramila E, Rabella N et al. Respiratory virus infections in adults with hematologic malignancies: a prospective study. *Clin Infect Dis* 2003; **36**: 1–8.

49 Khushalani NI, Bakri FG, Wentling D et al. Respiratory syncytial virus infection in the late bone marrow transplant period: report of three cases and review. *Bone Marrow Transplant* 2001; **27**: 1071–3.

50 Adams R, Christenson J, Petersen F, Beatty P. Preemptive use of aerosolized ribavirin in the treatment of asymptomatic pediatric marrow transplant patients testing positive for RSV. *Bone Marrow Transplant* 1999; **24**: 661–4.

51 Ljungman P, Gleaves CA, Meyers JD. Respiratory virus infection in immunocompromised patients. *Bone Marrow Transplant* 1989; **4**: 35–40.

52 Whimbey E, Champlin RE, Englund JA et al. Combination therapy with aerosolized ribavirin and intravenous immunoglobulin for respiratory syncytial virus disease in adult bone marrow transplant recipients. *Bone Marrow Transplant* 1995; **16**: 393–9.

53 Ghosh S, Champlin RE, Englund J et al. Respiratory syncytial virus upper respiratory tract illnesses in adult blood and marrow transplant recipients: combination therapy with aerosolized ribavirin and intravenous immunoglobulin. *Bone Marrow Transplant* 2000; **25**: 751–5.

54 Boeckh M, Berrey MM, Bowden RA, Crawford SW, Balsley J, Corey L. Phase I evaluation of the RSV-specific humanized monoclonal antibody palivizumab (MEDI-493) in hematopoietic stem cell transplant recipients. *J Infect Dis* 2001: 350–4.

55 DeVincenzo JP, Hirsch RL, Fuentes RJ, Top FH Jr. Respiratory syncytial virus immune globulin treatment of lower respiratory tract infection in pediatric patients undergoing bone marrow transplantation: a compassionate use experience. *Bone Marrow Transplant* 2000; **25**: 161–5.

56 Lewinsohn DM, Bowden RA, Mattson D, Crawford SW. Phase I study of intravenous ribavirin treatment of respiratory syncytial virus pneumonia after marrow transplantation. *Antimicrob Agents Chemother* 1996; **40**: 2555–7.

57 Sparrelid E, Ljungman P, Ekelof-Andstrom E et al. Ribavirin therapy in bone marrow transplant recipients with viral respiratory tract infections. *Bone Marrow Transplant* 1997; **19**: 905–8.

58 Raad I, Abbas J, Whimbey E. Infection control of nosocomial respiratory viral disease in the immunocompromised host. *Am J Med* 1997; **102**: 48–52; discussion 53–4.

59 Weinstock DM, Eagan J, Malak SA et al. Control of influenza A on a bone marrow transplant unit [In process citation]. *Infect Control Hosp Epidemiol* 2000; **21**: 730–2.

60 Guidelines for preventing opportunistic infections among hematopoietic stem cell transplant recipients. *Biol Blood Marrow Transplant* 2000; **6**: 659–713.

61 Peck A, Corey L, Boeckh M. Pretransplant RSV infection: impact of a strategy to delay transplantation. *Blood* 2001; **98**: 391a [Abstract].

62 Aslan T, Fassas AB, Desikan R et al. Patients with multiple myeloma may safely undergo autologous transplantation despite ongoing RSV infection and no ribavirin therapy. *Bone Marrow Transplant* 1999; **24**: 505–9.

63 Wendt CH, Hertz MI. Respiratory syncytial virus and parainfluenza virus infections in the immunocompromised host. *Semin Respir Infect* 1995; **10**: 224–31.

64 Cortez K, Murphy BR, Almeida KN et al. Immune-globulin prophylaxis of respiratory syncytial virus infection in patients undergoing stem-cell transplantation. *J Infect Dis* 2002; **186**: 834–8.

65 Cortez KJ, Erdman DD, Peret TC et al. Outbreak of human parainfluenza virus 3 infections in a hematopoietic stem cell transplant population. *J Infect Dis* 2001; **184**: 1093–7.

66 Zambon M, Bull T, Sadler CJ, Goldman JM, Ward KN. Molecular epidemiology of two consecutive outbreaks of parainfluenza 3 in a bone marrow transplant unit. *J Clin Microbiol* 1998; **36**: 2289–93.

67 Nichols WG, Erdman DD, Han A, Zukerman C, Corey L, Boeckh M. Prolonged outbreak of human parainfluenza-3 virus (HPIV3) infection in a stem cell transplant outpatient department: insights from molecular epidemiologic analysis. 42nd Interscience Conference on Antimicrobial Agents and Chemotherapy, San Diego, CA. American Society for Microbiology. 2002: **324** [Abstract K-1227].

68 Ljungman P, Andersson J, Aschan J et al. Influenza A in immunocompromised patients. *Clin Infect Dis* 1993; **17**: 244–7.

69 Bowden RA. Respiratory virus infections after marrow transplant: the Fred Hutchinson Cancer Research Center experience. *Am J Med* 1997; **102**: 27–30; discussion 42–3.

70 Englund JA, Champlin RE, Wyde PR et al. Common emergence of amantadine- and rimantadine-resistant influenza A viruses in symptomatic immunocompromised adults. *Clin Infect Dis* 1998; **26**: 1418–24.

71 Hayden FG, Osterhaus AD, Treanor JJ et al. Efficacy and safety of the neuraminidase inhibitor zanamivir in the treatment of influenza virus infections. GG167 Influenza Study Group [see comments]. *N Engl J Med* 1997; **337**: 874–80.

72 Nicholson KG, Aoki FY, Osterhaus AD et al. Efficacy and safety of oseltamivir in treatment of acute influenza: a randomised controlled trial. Neuraminidase Inhibitor Flu Treatment Investigator Group. *Lancet* 2000; **355**: 1845–50.

73 Johny AA, Clark A, Price N, Carrington D, Oakhill A, Marks DI. The use of zanamivir to treat influenza A and B infection after allogeneic stem cell transplantation. *Bone Marrow Transplant* 2002; **29**: 113–5.

74 Welliver R, Monto AS, Carewicz O et al. Effectiveness of oseltamivir in preventing influenza in household contacts: a randomized controlled trial. *J Am Med Assoc* 2001; **285**: 748–54.

75 De Clercq E, Naesens L, De Bolle L, Schols D, Zhang Y, Neyts J. Antiviral agents active against human herpesviruses HHV-6, HHV-7 and HHV-8. *Rev Med Virol* 2001; **11**: 381–95.

76 Whimbey E, Englund JA, Couch RB. Community respiratory virus infections in immunocompromised patients with cancer. *Am J Med* 1997; **102**: 10–8; discussion 25–6.

77 Kaplan LJ, Daum RS, Smaron M, McCarthy CA. Severe measles in immunocompromised patients. *J Am Med Assoc* 1992; **267**: 1237–41.

78 Nakano T, Shimono Y, Sugiyama K et al. Clinical features of measles in immunocompromised children. *Acta Paediatr Jpn* 1996; **38**: 212–7.

79 Machado CM, Goncalves FB, Pannuti CS, Dulley FL, de Souza VA. Measles in bone marrow transplant recipients during an outbreak in Sao Paulo, Brazil. *Blood* 2002; **99**: 83–7.

80 Mustafa MM, Weitman SD, Winick NJ, Bellini WJ, Timmons CF, Siegel JD. Subacute measles encephalitis in the young immunocompromised host: report of two cases diagnosed by polymerase chain reaction and treated with ribavirin and review of the literature. *Clin Infect Dis* 1993; **16**: 654–60.

81 van den Hoogen BG, de Jong JC, Groen J et al. A newly discovered human pneumovirus isolated from young children with respiratory tract disease. *Nat Med* 2001; **7**: 719–24.

82 Boivin G, Abed Y, Pelletier G et al. Virological features and clinical manifestations associated with human metapneumovirus: a new paramyxovirus responsible for acute respiratory-tract infections in all age groups. *J Infect Dis* 2002; **186**: 1330–4.

83 Pelletier G, Dery P, Abed Y, Boivin G. Respiratory tract reinfections by the new human metapneumovirus in an immunocompromised child. *Emerg Infect Dis* 2002; **8**: 976–8.

84 Guidelines for preventing opportunistic infections among hematopoietic stem cell transplant recipients. Recommendations of CDC, the Infectious Disease Society of America, and the American Society of Blood and Marrow Transplantation. *Morbid Mortal Week Rep* 2000; **49**: 1–128.

85 Wang FZ, Dahl H, Linde A, Brytting M, Ehrnst A, Ljungman P. Lymphotropic herpesviruses in allogeneic bone marrow transplantation. *Blood* 1996; **88**: 3615–20.

86 Cone RW, Huang ML, Corey L, Zeh J, Ashley R, Bowden R. Human herpesvirus 6 infections after bone marrow transplantation: clinical and virologic manifestations. *J Infect Dis* 1999; **179**: 311–8.

87 Kadakia MP, Rybka WB, Stewart JA et al. Human herpesvirus 6: infection and disease following autologous and allogeneic bone marrow transplantation. *Blood* 1996; **87**: 5341–54.

88 Ljungman P, Wang FZ, Clark DA et al. High levels of human herpesvirus 6 DNA in peripheral blood

88 leucocytes are correlated to platelet engraftment and disease in allogeneic stem cell transplant patients. *Br J Haematol* 2000; **111**: 774–81.
89 Okuno T, Takahashi K, Balachandra K et al. Seroepidemiology of human herpesvirus 6 infection in normal children and adults. *J Clin Microbiol* 1989; **27**: 651–3.
90 Cone RW, Hackman RC, Huang ML et al. Human herpesvirus 6 in lung tissue from patients with pneumonitis after bone marrow transplantation [see comments]. *N Engl J Med* 1993; **329**: 156–61.
91 Yoshikawa T, Suga S, Asano Y et al. Human herpesvirus 6 infection in bone marrow transplantation. *Blood* 1991; **78**: 1381–4.
92 Imbert-Marcille BM, Tang XW, Lepelletier D et al. Human herpesvirus 6 infection after autologous or allogeneic stem cell transplantation: a single-center prospective longitudinal study of 92 patients. *Clin Infect Dis* 2000; **31**: 881–6.
93 Yoshikawa T, Asano Y, Ihira M et al. Human herpesvirus 6 viremia in bone marrow transplant recipients: clinical features and risk factors. *J Infect Dis* 2002; **185**: 847–53.
94 Wang FZ, Linde A, Hagglund H, Testa M, Locasciulli A, Ljungman P. Human herpesvirus 6 DNA in cerebrospinal fluid specimens from allogeneic bone marrow transplant patients: does it have clinical significance? *Clin Infect Dis* 1999; **28**: 562–8.
95 Buchbinder S, Elmaagacli AH, Schaefer UW, Roggendorf M. Human herpesvirus 6 is an important pathogen in infectious lung disease after allogeneic bone marrow transplantation [In process citation]. *Bone Marrow Transplant* 2000; **26**: 639–44.
96 Carrigan DR, Knox KK. Bone marrow suppression by human herpesvirus-6: comparison of the A and B variants of the virus. *Blood* 1995; **86**: 835–6 [Letter; comment].
97 Dominietto A, Raiola AM, Van Lint MT et al. Factors influencing haematological recovery after allogeneic haemopoietic stem cell transplants: graft-versus-host disease, donor type, cytomegalovirus infections and cell dose. *Br J Haematol* 2001; **112**: 219–27.
98 Zerr DM, Gooley TA, Yeung L et al. Human herpesvirus 6 reactivation and encephalitis in allogeneic bone marrow transplant recipients. *Clin Infect Dis* 2001; **33**: 763–71.
99 Ward KN, Sheldon MJ, Gray JJ. Primary and recurrent cytomegalovirus infections have different effects on human herpesvirus 6 antibodies in immunosuppressed organ graft recipients: absence of virus cross-reactivity and evidence for virus interaction. *J Med Virol* 1991; **34**: 258–67.
100 Dockrell DH, Prada J, Jones MF et al. Seroconversion to human herpesvirus 6 following liver transplantation is a marker of cytomegalovirus disease. *J Infect Dis* 1997; **176**: 1135–40.
101 DesJardin JA, Gibbons L, Cho E et al. Human herpesvirus 6 reactivation is associated with cytomegalovirus infection and syndromes in kidney transplant recipients at risk for primary cytomegalovirus infection. *J Infect Dis* 1998; **178**: 1783–6.
102 Humar A, Malkan G, Moussa G, Greig P, Levy G, Mazzulli T. Human herpesvirus 6 is associated with cytomegalovirus reactivation in liver transplant recipients. *J Infect Dis* 2000; **181**: 1450–3.
103 Mendez JC, Dockrell DH, Espy MJ et al. Human beta–herpesvirus interactions in solid organ transplant recipients. *J Infect Dis* 2001; **183**: 179–84.
104 Ratnamohan VM, Chapman J, Howse H et al. Cytomegalovirus and human herpesvirus 6 both cause viral disease after renal transplantation. *Transplantation* 1998; **66**: 877–82.
105 Boeckh M, Gooley TA, Myerson D, Cunningham T, Schoch G, Bowden RA. Cytomegalovirus pp65 antigenemia-guided early treatment with ganciclovir versus ganciclovir at engraftment after allogeneic marrow transplantation: a randomized double-blind study. *Blood* 1996; **88**: 4063–71.
106 Flamand L, Gosselin J, D'Addario M et al. Human herpesvirus 6 induces interleukin-1 beta and tumor necrosis factor alpha, but not interleukin-6, in peripheral blood mononuclear cell cultures. *J Virol* 1991; **65**: 5105–10.
107 Kikuta H, Lu H, Tomizawa K, Matsumoto S. Enhancement of human herpesvirus 6 replication in adult human lymphocytes by monoclonal antibody to CD3. *J Infect Dis* 1990; **161**: 1085–7.
108 Flamand L, Gosselin J, Stefanescu I, Ablashi D, Menezes J. Immunosuppressive effect of human herpesvirus 6 on T-cell functions: suppression of interleukin-2 synthesis and cell proliferation. *Blood* 1995; **85**: 1263–71.
109 Knox KK, Carrigan DR. *In vitro* suppression of bone marrow progenitor cell differentiation by human herpesvirus 6 infection. *J Infect Dis* 1992; **165**: 925–9.
110 Wang FZ, Larsson K, Linde A, Ljungman P. Human herpesvirus 6 infection and cytomegalovirus-specific lymphoproliferative responses in allogeneic stem cell transplant recipients. *Bone Marrow Transplant* 2002; **30**: 521–6.
111 Yoshida M, Yamada M, Chatterjee S, Lakeman F, Nii S, Whitley RJ. A method for detection of HHV-6 antigens and its use for evaluating antiviral drugs. *J Virol Meth* 1996; **58**: 137–43.
112 Reymen D, Naesens L, Balzarini J, Holy A, Dvorakova H, De Clercq E. Antiviral activity of selected acyclic nucleoside analogues against human herpesvirus 6. *Antiviral Res* 1995; **28**: 343–57.
113 Tiacci E, Luppi M, Barozzi P et al. Fatal herpesvirus-6 encephalitis in a recipient of a T-cell-depleted peripheral blood stem cell transplant from a 3-loci mismatched related donor. *Haematologica* 2000; **85**: 94–7.
114 Zerr DM, Gupta D, Huang ML, Carter R, Corey L. Effect of antivirals on human herpesvirus 6 replication in hematopoietic stem cell transplant recipients. *Clin Infect Dis* 2002; **34**: 309–17.
115 Zerr DM, Huang ML, Corey L, Erickson M, Parker HL, Frenkel LM. Sensitive method for detection of human herpesviruses 6 and 7 in saliva collected in field studies. *J Clin Microbiol* 2000; **38**: 1981–3.
116 Gautheret-Dejean A, Dejean O, Vastel L et al. Human herpesvirus-6 and human herpesvirus-7 in the bone marrow from healthy subjects. *Transplantation* 2000; **69**: 1722–3.
117 Chan PK, Chik KW, To KF et al. Case report: human herpesvirus 7 associated fatal encephalitis in a peripheral blood stem cell transplant recipient. *J Med Virol* 2002; **66**: 493–6.
118 Luppi M, Barozzi P, Schulz TF et al. Nonmalignant disease associated with human herpesvirus 8 reactivation in patients who have undergone autologous peripheral blood stem cell transplantation [In process citation]. *Blood* 2000; **96**: 2355–7.
119 Luppi M, Barozzi P, Schulz TF et al. Bone marrow failure associated with human herpesvirus 8 infection after transplantation. *N Engl J Med* 2000; **343**: 1378–85.
120 Regamey N, Tamm M, Wernli M et al. Transmission of human herpesvirus 8 infection from renal-transplant donors to recipients. *N Engl J Med* 1998; **339**: 1358–63.
121 Leung AY, Suen CK, Lie AK, Liang RH, Yuen KY, Kwong YL. Quantification of polyoma BK viruria in hemorrhagic cystitis complicating bone marrow transplantation. *Blood* 2001; **98**: 1971–8.
122 Limaye AP, Jerome KR, Kuhr CS et al. Quantitation of BK virus load in serum for the diagnosis of BK virus-associated nephropathy in renal transplant recipients. *J Infect Dis* 2001; **183**: 1669–72.
123 Bedi A, Miller CB, Hanson JL et al. Association of BK virus with failure of prophylaxis against hemorrhagic cystitis following bone marrow transplantation. *J Clin Oncol* 1995; **13**: 1103–9.
124 Hirsch HH, Knowles W, Dickenmann M et al. Prospective study of polyomavirus type BK replication and nephropathy in renal-transplant recipients. *N Engl J Med* 2002; **347**: 488–96.
125 Azzi A, Cesaro S, Laszlo D et al. Human polyomavirus BK (BKV) load and haemorrhagic cystitis in bone marrow transplantation patients. *J Clin Virol* 1999; **14**: 79–86.
126 Bogdanovic G, Ljungman P, Wang F, Dalianis T. Presence of human polyomavirus DNA in the peripheral circulation of bone marrow transplant patients with and without hemorrhagic cystitis. *Bone Marrow Transplant* 1996; **17**: 573–6.
127 Peinemann F, de Villiers EM, Dorries K, Adams O, Vogeli TA, Burdach S. Clinical course and treatment of haemorrhagic cystitis associated with BK type of human polyomavirus in nine paediatric recipients of allogeneic bone marrow transplants. *Eur J Pediatr* 2000; **159**: 182–8.
128 Sandler ES, Aquino VM, Goss-Shohet E, Hinrichs S, Krisher K. BK papova virus pneumonia following hematopoietic stem cell transplantation. *Bone Marrow Transplant* 1997; **20**: 163–5.
129 Held TK, Biel SS, Nitsche A et al. Treatment of BK virus-associated hemorrhagic cystitis and simultaneous CMV reactivation with cidofovir [In process citation]. *Bone Marrow Transplant* 2000; **26**: 347–50.
130 Kadambi PV, Josephson MA, Williams J et al. Treatment of refractory BK virus-associated nephropathy with cidofovir. *Am J Transplant* 2003; **3**: 186–91.
131 Coppo P, Laporte JP, Aoudjhane M et al. Progressive multifocal leucoencephalopathy with peripheral demyelinating neuropathy after autologous bone marrow transplantation for acute myeloblastic leukemia (FAB5). *Bone Marrow Transplant* 1999; **23**: 401–3.
132 Re D, Bamborschke S, Feiden W et al. Progressive multifocal leukoencephalopathy after autologous bone marrow transplantation and alpha-interferon immunotherapy. *Bone Marrow Transplant* 1999; **23**: 295–8.
133 Holzapfel C, Kellinghaus C, Luttmann R et al. [Progressive multifocal leukoencephalopathy (PML) in chronic lymphatic leukemia (CLL): review of the literature and case report]. *Nervenarzt* 2002; **73**: 543–7.
134 Seong D, Bruner JM, Lee KH et al. Progressive multifocal leukoencephalopathy after autologous bone marrow transplantation in a patient with chronic myelogenous leukemia. *Clin Infect Dis* 1996; **23**: 402–3.
135 Taoufik Y, Gasnault J, Karaterki A et al. Prognostic value of JC virus load in cerebrospinal fluid of patients with progressive multifocal leukoencephalopathy. *J Infect Dis* 1998; **178**: 1816–20.

136 Houston S, Roberts N, Mashinter L. Failure of cidofovir therapy in progressive multifocal leukoencephalopathy unrelated to human immunodeficiency virus. *Clin Infectious Dis* 2001; **32**: 150–2.

137 Przepiorka D, Jaeckle KA, Birdwell RR *et al.* Successful treatment of progressive multifocal leukoencephalopathy with low-dose interleukin-2. *Bone Marrow Transplant* 1997; **20**: 983–7.

138 Daneshpouy M, Socie G, Clavel C *et al.* Human papillomavirus infection and anogenital condyloma in bone marrow transplant recipients. *Transplantation* 2001; **71**: 167–9.

139 Barasch A, Eisenberg E, D'Ambrosio JA, Nuki K, Peterson DE. Oral verruca vulgaris in a bone marrow transplant patient: a case report and review of literature. *Eur J Cancer B Oral Oncol* 1996; **32B**: 137–9.

140 Maruyama F, Miyazaki H, Matsui T *et al.* Rapid progression of flat warts in a patient with malignant lymphoma after PBSCT. *Bone Marrow Transplant* 1996; **18**: 1009–11.

141 Sasadeusz J, Kelly H, Szer J, Schwarer AP, Mitchell H, Grigg A. Abnormal cervical cytology in bone marrow transplant recipients. *Bone Marrow Transplant* 2001; **28**: 393–7.

142 Azzi A, Fanci R, Ciappi S, Zakrzewska K, Bosi A. Human parvovirus B19 infection in bone marrow transplantation patients. *Am J Hematol* 1993; **44**: 207–9.

143 Schleuning M, Jager G, Holler E *et al.* Human parvovirus B19-associated disease in bone marrow transplantation. *Infection* 1999; **27**: 114–7.

144 Kurtzman G, Frickhofen N, Kimball J, Jenkins DW, Nienhuis AW, Young NS. Pure red-cell aplasia of 10 years' duration due to persistent parvovirus B19 infection and its cure with immunoglobulin therapy [see comments]. *N Engl J Med* 1989; **321**: 519–23.

145 Frickhofen N, Arnold R, Hertenstein B, Wiesneth M, Young NS. Parvovirus B19 infection and bone marrow transplantation. *Ann Hematol* 1992; **64** (Suppl.): A121–4.

146 Yolken RH, Bishop CA, Townsend TR *et al.* Infectious gastroenteritis in bone-marrow-transplant recipients. *N Engl J Med* 1982; **306**: 1010–12.

147 Chakrabarti S, Collingham KE, Stevens RH, Pillay D, Fegan CD, Milligan DW. Isolation of viruses from stools in stem cell transplant recipients: a prospective surveillance study. *Bone Marrow Transplant* 2000; **25**: 277–82.

148 Townsend TR, Bolyard EA, Yolken RH *et al.* Outbreak of Coxsackie A1 gastroenteritis: a complication of bone-marrow transplantation. *Lancet* 1982; **1**: 820–3.

149 Aquino VM, Farah RA, Lee MC, Sandler ES. Disseminated Coxsackie A9 infection complicating bone marrow transplantation. *Pediatr Infect Dis J* 1996; **15**: 1053–4.

150 Galama JM, de Leeuw N, Wittebol S, Peters H, Melchers WJ. Prolonged enteroviral infection in a patient who developed pericarditis and heart failure after bone marrow transplantation. *Clin Infect Dis* 1996; **22**: 1004–8.

151 Gonzalez Y, Martino R, Badell I *et al.* Pulmonary enterovirus infections in stem cell transplant recipients. *Bone Marrow Transplant* 1999; **23**: 511–3.

152 Fischmeister G, Wiesbauer P, Holzmann HM, Peters C, Eibl M, Gadner H. Enteroviral meningoencephalitis in immunocompromised children after matched unrelated donor-bone marrow transplantation. *Pediatr Hematol Oncol* 2000; **17**: 393–9.

153 Biggs DD, Toorkey BC, Carrigan DR, Hanson GA, Ash RC. Disseminated echovirus infection complicating bone marrow transplantation. *Am J Med* 1990; **88**: 421–5.

154 Schwarer AP, Opat SS, Watson AM, Spelman D, Firkin F, Lee N. Disseminated echovirus infection after allogeneic bone marrow transplantation. *Pathology* 1997; **29**: 424–5.

155 Rogers M, Weinstock DM, Eagan J, Kiehn T, Armstrong D, Sepkowitz KA. Rotavirus outbreak on a pediatric oncology floor: possible association with toys. *Am J Infect Control* 2000; **28**: 378–80.

156 Kruger W, Stockschlader M, Zander AR. Transmission of rotavirus diarrhea in a bone marrow transplantation unit by a hospital worker. *Bone Marrow Transplant* 1991; **8**: 507–8.

157 Troussard X, Bauduer F, Gallet E *et al.* Virus recovery from stools of patients undergoing bone marrow transplantation. *Bone Marrow Transplant* 1993; **12**: 573–6.

158 Yeager AM, Kanof ME, Kramer SS *et al.* Pneumatosis intestinalis in children after allogeneic bone marrow transplantation. *Pediatr Radiol* 1987; **17**: 18–22.

159 Kanfer EJ, Abrahamson G, Taylor J, Coleman JC, Samson DM. Severe rotavirus-associated diarrhoea following bone marrow transplantation: treatment with oral immunoglobulin. *Bone Marrow Transplant* 1994; **14**: 651–2.

58

Simone I. Strasser & George B. McDonald

Gastrointestinal and Hepatic Complications

Introduction

While the incidence of intestinal and liver complications of hematopoietic cell transplantation (HCT) remains high, the severity of these complications is now lower than in the past. The development of more effective strategies to prevent graft-vs.-host disease (GVHD) has had a marked effect on the incidence of severe GVHD. Antiviral agents have almost completely eliminated intestinal and hepatic infections caused by herpes simplex virus (HSV) and cytomegalovirus (CMV). Fungal infections of the intestine and liver have become uncommon since the advent of fluconazole prophylaxis. Transplant centers have altered their regimens of cytoreductive therapy after recognizing that sinusoidal liver injury was dose-limiting. Clinicians have become adept at recognizing unusual presentations of infectious diseases, for example, abdominal pain as a manifestation of varicella-zoster virus (VZV) infection. New challenges, however, have come from the greater use of human leukocyte antigen (HLA)-mismatched and unrelated donors, earlier onset of GVHD, the increase in certain diseases as indications for HCT (e.g. sickle cell disease, renal carcinoma, myeloma, and autoimmune diseases), the older age of patients being considered for HCT and the introduction of nonmyeloablative allogeneic HCT. This chapter is organized by the problems a clinician might encounter in caring for an HCT recipient, in the chronologic order in which these problems are likely to appear.

Problems before the start of cytoreductive therapy

Ulcers and tumors in the intestinal tract

Mucosal ulcerations in the esophagus, stomach and intestine may bleed profusely when platelet counts drop after HCT. Symptoms of esophageal pain, heartburn, dysphagia, epigastric pain, nausea and vomiting should be investigated with upper intestinal endoscopy before HCT. In immunocompromised patients, esophageal, gastric and intestinal ulcers may have an infectious etiology (e.g. CMV, HSV or fungal infection) that requires specific antimicrobial treatment [1]. Identification of *Helicobacter pylori* as the cause of idiopathic gastritis and gastric and duodenal ulcers has led to combination therapy to eradicate this organism and eliminate ulcer recurrences. Ulcers related to acid-peptic juice can be healed with the use of a proton pump inhibitor. Rarely, patients with basophilic leukemia or chronic myeloid leukemia (CML) develop peptic ulcers related to elevated serum histamine levels. Whenever possible, upper intestinal ulcerations should be healed before the start of conditioning therapy.

Patients with inflammatory bowel disease present a more difficult problem, as there is no curative therapy. The goal of pre-HCT therapy in patients with ulcerative colitis or Crohn's disease is to minimize the extent of gross intestinal ulceration to lower the risk of bleeding after HCT. One must also rule out infections as a cause of colonic ulceration. The pathogens that mimic inflammatory bowel disease are CMV, *Entamoeba histolytica* and *Clostridium difficile*. Patients with ulcerative colitis have undergone HCT without incident [2]. Patients with Crohn's disease may represent a greater risk, as they may harbor transmural intestinal inflammation, sinus tracts and abscesses. Patients with Crohn's disease have undergone allogeneic HCT for other indications without complications of bleeding, perforation, or dissemination of microorganisms [3]. Apparent long-term resolution of Crohn's disease was observed in four of five evaluable patients.

Patients who are to undergo HCT for lymphoma, leukemia in relapse, myeloma, or metastatic breast cancer may have intestinal involvement with malignant cells. Cytoreductive therapy results in necrosis of these cells [4,5]. Both large intestinal ulcers and perforation due to tumor lysis have been seen, but the low frequency of this complication (estimated at less than one case in 1000 HCTs) does not warrant screening for intestinal involvement by tumor. Intra-abdominal abscesses and fistulae should be managed surgically before HCT. Patients over the age of 50 years are at risk for the development of colorectal polyps and cancer. These are seldom considerations in younger patients, but the presence of occult blood in stool specimens from patients over 50 years of age should prompt both colonoscopy and upper endoscopy.

Infections of the intestine

Patients with chronic diarrhea should be investigated for organisms that are likely to disseminate during the period of immunosuppression after HCT [6]. Intestinal parasites such as *E. histolytica* and *Strongyloides* can cause death in the immunosuppressed host [7]. *Giardia lamblia*, *E. histolytica* and *Cryptosporidia* may lead to profuse diarrhea post-HCT [8–10]. Diagnosis can usually be made with standard ova and parasite examination of fresh stool specimens, enzyme-linked immunosorbent assay (ELISA) tests for giardia antigen in stool and antibodies to *E. histolytica* in serum. Persistent eosinophilia in a patient from an area where parasites are endemic is also an indication for screening for parasitic disease. Specific therapy is available for amebiasis, strongyloidiasis and giardiasis. Cryptosporidiosis has proven resistant to all therapy except the withdrawal of immunosuppressive medication or the restoration of cellular immunity.

Other treatable causes of diarrhea in patients with hematologic malignancies include clostridial infections (*C. difficile*, *C. perfringens*, *C. septicum*), CMV enterocolitis, rotavirus and adenovirus infections, and overgrowth with *Candida albicans* [11–13]. The patient who has had previous typhlitis during granulocytopenia can present problems if there is persistent fever or tenderness over the cecum. Typhlitis is a syndrome of cecal edema, mucosal friability and ulceration, and fever often associated with polymicrobial sepsis; its cause is usually intestinal clostridial infection, particularly *C. septicum* [14,15]. After appropriate treatment, the risk of post-HCT typhlitis is no different than that of other patients. Pericolic phlegmons and abscesses and persistent colitis caused by *C. difficile* must be treated before the start of conditioning therapy.

Pain in or near the anal canal in a granulocytopenic patient is due to bacterial infection of perianal tissues until proved otherwise [16]. These infections are usually polymicrobial, arising from either anal crypts or tears in the anal canal. Extensive supralevator and intersphincteric abscesses may be present without being apparent on external examination [17]. Peri-anal infections must be dealt with before HCT, as extensive tissue necrosis and septicemia may result from uncontrolled infection [17,18]. Antibiotic treatment should cover anaerobic as well as aerobic bacteria [16]. Perineal HSV infection may also lead to painful ulcerations [19].

Fungal liver infections

HCT candidates with tender hepatomegaly and persistent fever should be evaluated for fungal infection of the liver. Although the differential diagnosis includes malignant involvement of the liver, proving hepatic malignancy is not required if there is evidence of malignancy elsewhere. Diagnosis of active fungal infection is important, as systemic antifungal therapy before and during HCT is indicated [20,21]. The most sensitive imaging modality for fungal liver infection is magnetic resonance imaging (MRI) [22], although all imaging methods are insensitive to tiny fungal lesions [23]. Indirect tests, such as antigen detection and polymerase chain reaction (PCR) for fungal DNA in serum, may be useful [24]. Differentiating active fungal infection in the liver from fibrous remnants of previous fungal infection requires needle (percutaneous, transjugular or transfemoral, laparoscopic) or surgical liver biopsy [25]. *Candida* species are the most common isolates. The choice of antifungal therapy has expanded in recent years, and can now be tailored to the specific fungal species and sensitivity. Patients with invasive fungal infection prior to HCT should be treated aggressively with systemic liposomal

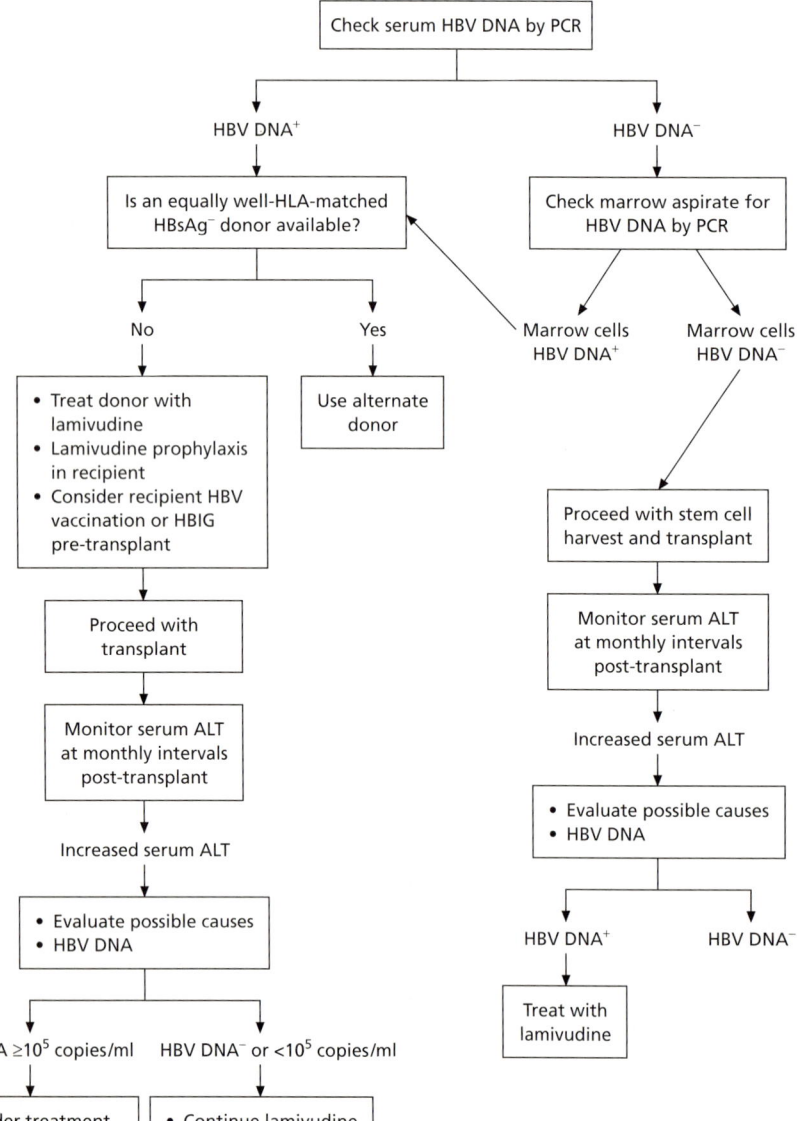

Fig. 58.1 Algorithm for management of a stem cell donor who is either hepatitis B surface antigen-positive or antihepatitis B core antigen-positive. Reproduced with permission from Lau *et al.* [31].

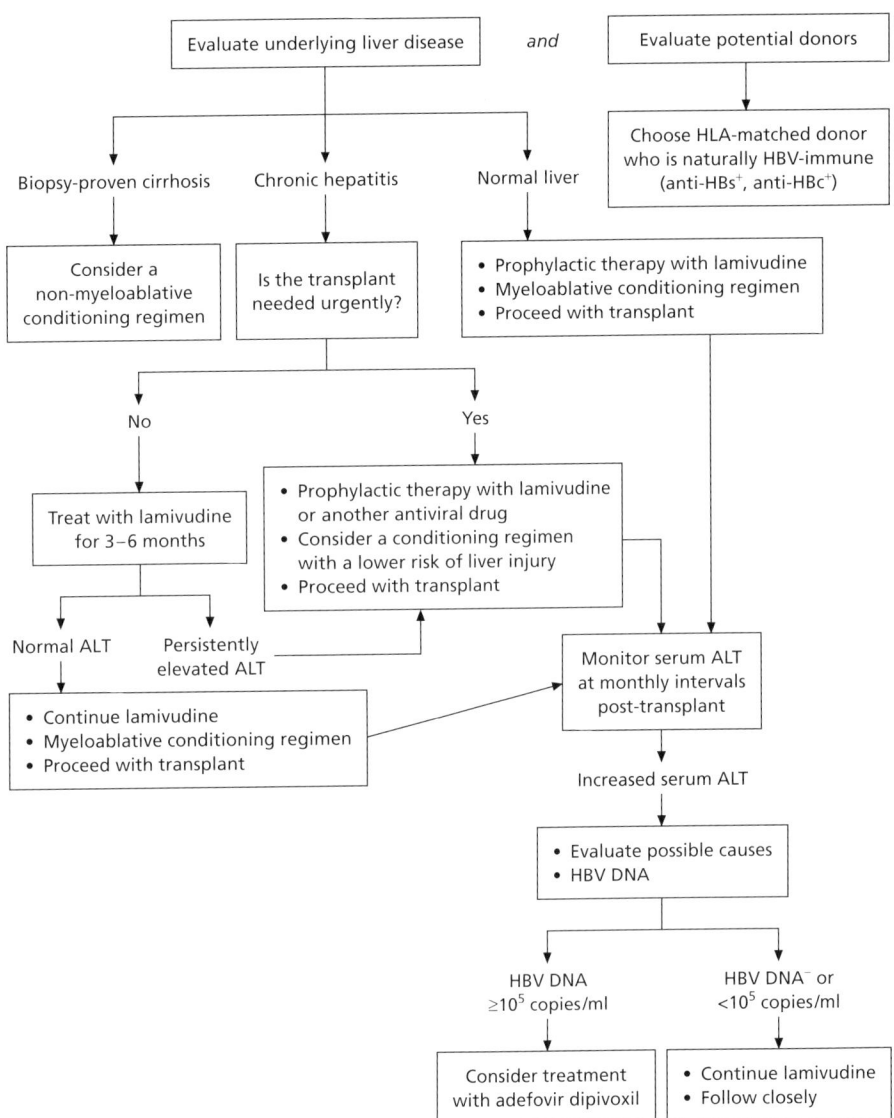

Fig. 58.2 Algorithm for management of a transplant candidate who is hepatitis B surface antigen-positive. Reproduced with permission from Lau *et al.* [31].

amphotericin, voriconazole, or caspifungin [26,27], and then receive ongoing therapy until engraftment is established. With this approach, successful HCT can be performed without fungal dissemination [21,28–30].

Acute and chronic viral hepatitis

Viral hepatitis markers in potential allograft donors [31]

It is not uncommon for potential stem cell donors to have serum markers indicating current or prior infection with hepatitis viruses. Figures 58.1–58.4 provide management guidelines for patients with the most common combinations of serum viral markers in donors and recipients. Note that hepatitis B and C differ in the significance of finding antibodies in the serum: antibodies to hepatitis B virus (HBV) surface antigen (anti-HBs) generally indicate immunity (either following natural infection or vaccination) whereas antibodies to hepatitis C virus (HCV) usually indicate ongoing infection. The risk of donor transmission of hepatitis B or C viruses is best assessed by the presence of HBV DNA or HCV RNA in serum, as determined by PCR. Ideally, when equally HLA-matched donors are available, one should choose the donor who is not infected by hepatitis viruses. When the only available donor, or the most closely HLA-matched donor, has hepatitis virus infection, the risks of passage of the virus, strategies for prevention of infection, and ethical considerations of using that donor are discussed below.

The HBV-infected donor (Fig. 58.1)

Transmission of HBV from an HBV surface antigen-positive donor is not inevitable, having been reported to occur in only 30–44% of cases [32–34]. The explanation for variable transmission is that not all patients with HBV-infected livers have infectious particles in blood or hematopoietic cell precursors. High serum HBV DNA levels and the presence of HBeAg-negative infection (suggesting precore or core promoter mutant infection) are risk factors for transmission [34]. Pre-HCT immunity in the recipient may protect against the development of clinical hepatitis B acquired from the donor [32,35,36]. If the recipient does become infected with HBV from the donor, the risk of severe hepatitis B post-HCT is about 15%. Therefore, regardless of the detection of serum HBV DNA, if an hepatitis B surface antigen (HBsAg)-positive individual is being evaluated as a donor, consideration should be given to treating the donor with antiviral therapy to reduce the risk of passage of virus and to the recipient to reduce the risk of fulminant hepatitis B. Nucleoside analogs, such as lamivudine and adefovir dipivoxil, result in rapid falls in circulating HBV DNA levels within weeks [37–39], which would be expected to

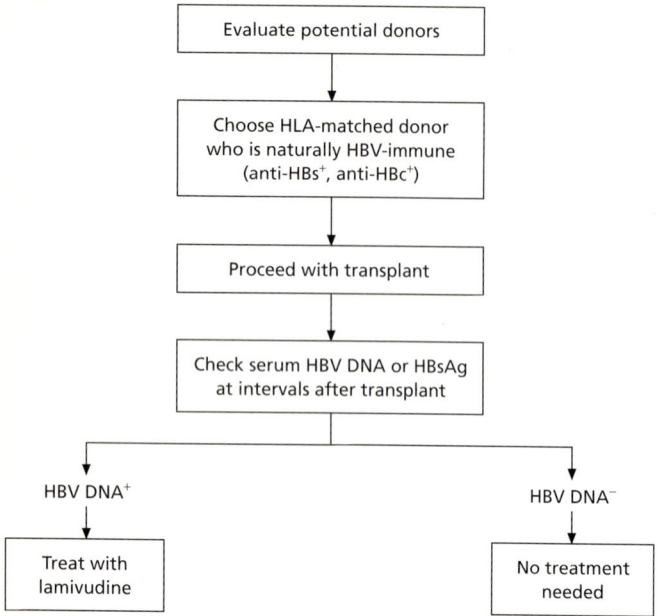

Fig. 58.3 Algorithm for management of a transplant candidate who is antihepatitis B core antigen-positive. Reproduced with permission from Lau *et al.* [31].

a severe hepatitis flare that may be fatal. Data from the prelamivudine era regarding other strategies to modify the risk of transmission, for example, treatment of the recipient with either hepatitis B immunoglobulin or active immunization, are conflicting [32,42,43].

The donor with antibodies to HB core antigen or surface antigen (Fig. 58.1)

Individuals who have serum antibodies to HBV core antigen (hepatitis B core antibodies [anti-HBcs]) in the absence of surface antigen are viremic in <5% of cases [44] and can be used as donors if their serum is HBV DNA-negative by a sensitive PCR assay. An aliquot of hematopoietic cells (a potential extrahepatic reservoir for HBV) can also be tested for HBV DNA. To be certain that passage of HBV has not occurred, recipient serum can be tested at day +25 to +50 for HBV DNA, and lamivudine prescribed if HBV DNA is detected [41].

A donor who is anti-HBs-positive poses no risk of passage of virus, and may be the preferred donor if the recipient is HBsAg-positive or anti-HBc-positive. Serological evidence of immunity can be transferred from both naturally immune donors and donors immunized with hepatitis B vaccine [45–47]. There is convincing evidence that adoptive transfer of immunity to a recipient infected by HBV can effect clearance of virus when the donor had been exposed to HBV naturally, but there is no evidence that anti-HBs acquired via vaccination has this beneficial effect [48,49]. To date, clearance of HBV from 18 infected recipients has been reported; all were related to engraftment of anti-HBs-positive donor marrow [36,47,50–55] at 3–6 months after allogeneic HCT, at the time of tapering of the doses of immunosuppressive drugs and immune reconstitution. Thus, an HBV naturally immune donor is preferred when the recipient is HBV-infected, provided that no better HLA-matched donor is available.

reduce the chance of transmission. Lamivudine will protect the recipient from development of clinical hepatitis if virus is still transmitted [40,41]. Care should be taken when treating an HBV-infected donor for only a short time, as withdrawal of antiviral therapy in this situation can result in

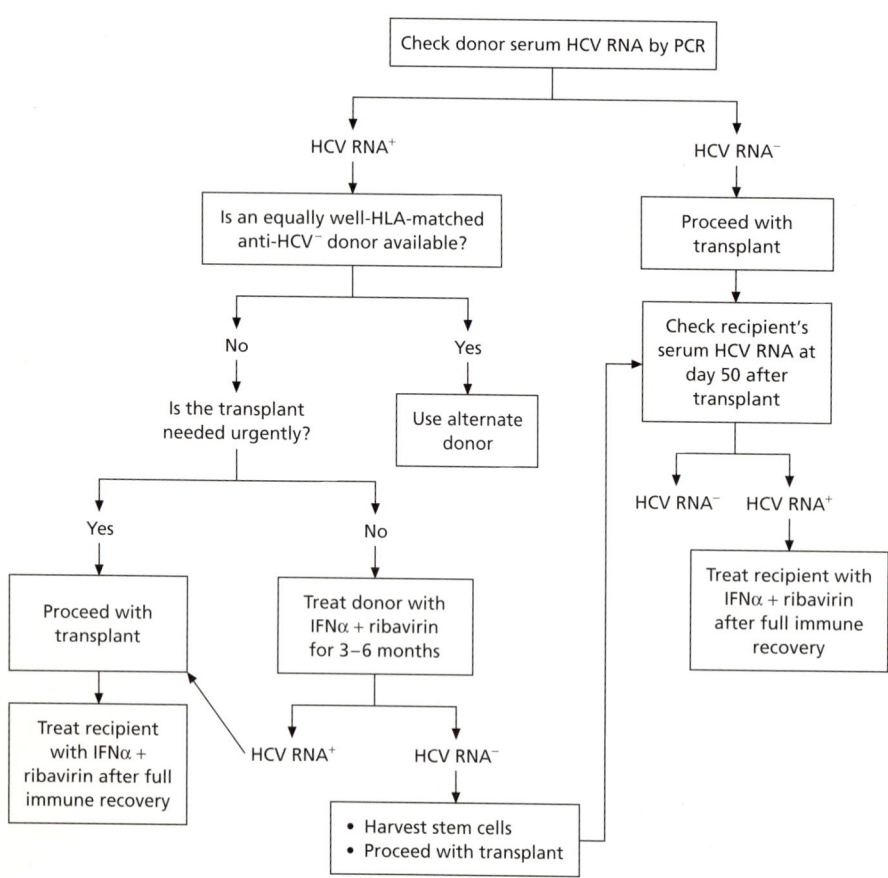

Fig. 58.4 Algorithm for management of an antihepatitis C virus-positive stem cell donor. Reproduced with permission from Lau *et al.* [31].

The HCV-infected donor (Fig. 58.4)

The majority of anti-HCV-positive donors are HCV RNA-positive; transmission of HCV from HCV RNA-positive HSC donors is universal [56]. The use of CD34-selected donor hematopoietic cells does not prevent HCV transmission [57], in keeping with the concept that HCV replicates in peripheral blood mononuclear cells *in vivo* [58]. Attempts have been made to prevent HCV transmission from an infected stem cell donor to a recipient by pretreatment of the donor with interferon-alpha (IFN-α) [59]. However, as antiviral treatment with IFN-α and ribavirin may result in significant side-effects in the donor and would delay HCT by 3–6 months, this strategy is appropriate only if the recipient has a chronic, relatively stable condition, and the donor is agreeable to undergoing antiviral therapy. Antiviral therapy should be stopped at least 1 week prior to stem cell harvest to avoid myelosuppression of donor stem cells and possible engraftment problems in the recipient. In the future, antiviral therapy with an HCV-specific protease inhibitor will likely be useful in this circumstance [60].

When an HCV-infected hematopoietic cell donor is used, recipients become viremic within days of transplantation, but there are no recognizable clinical consequences in the weeks following HCT until immune reconstitution occurs [61]. The likely explanation lies in the pathogenesis of liver injury in HCV infection. It is currently believed that HCV itself does not cause hepatocyte necrosis but, rather, hepatocellular damage is mediated by cellular immune responses, in particular cytotoxic T lymphocytes [62]. Once immune reconstitution occurs, recipients may develop a mild hepatitis. However, morbidity and mortality related to HCV is not increased in the short term or in the first 7–10 years following HCT [61,63]. Thus, the significantly greater short- and medium-term risks of GVHD over hepatitis C support the use of the most closely HLA-matched donor even if that donor is HCV-infected.

Viral hepatitis markers in candidates for HCT (Figs 58.2 & 58.3)

Patients who come to HCT already infected with HBV (HBsAg-positive or HBV DNA-positive, plus some patients who are anti-HBc-positive) or HCV (HCV RNA-positive) may have an increased risk of morbidity and mortality after HCT. HCT candidates with hepatitis B infection are a particular problem in countries where these infections are endemic [36,64,65]. There is approximately a 35% risk of post-HCT reactivation of HBV in patients with isolated anti-HBc antibodies, usually in the setting of immunosuppression for acute GVHD [66–70]. In addition, there are isolated case reports of severe hepatitis in patients with prior immunity to HBV (that is, anti-HBc and anti-HBs-positive) [33,66,71–74] and a single case report of apparent reactivation of occult hepatitis B infection (no serologic markers were positive before transpant) in a patient from an HBV endemic area [75]. The mechanism for reactivation of HBV in patients with natural immunity is related to the presence of low-level replicating virus in the liver many years after the clearance of HbsAg [76,77].

Fortunately, infection with HCV in HCT candidates has become far less frequent than in the past because of the effectiveness of routine screening of blood products. It is, however, important to identify and screen patients at risk for hepatitis virus infection (e.g. those with a history of intravenous drug use, blood transfusion prior to 1991, or birth in a country with high endemic rates). Serological testing for hepatitis C antibodies is inadequate for exclusion of HCV infection among immunocompromised patients, such as those with hematologic malignancy [61,78]; at-risk individuals should be assessed for the presence of HCV RNA. The short-term risks faced by patients with inflammatory liver disease include sinusoidal obstruction syndrome (SOS; also known as veno-occlusive disease [VOD] of the liver) and fulminant viral hepatitis B.

SOS (VOD of the liver) in patients with hepatitis

Sinusoidal injury caused by myeloablative therapy [79] is more frequent and more severe among patients with an active inflammatory hepatitis [61,70,80–82]. The absolute risk of developing fatal SOS when a candidate has an active inflammatory hepatitis and receives a myeloablative conditioning regimen containing cyclophosphamide (CY) is in the 15–25% range [61]. There is no association between HBsAg-positive status and post-HCT sinusoidal liver injury, suggesting that inflammatory hepatitis and fibrosis, rather than HBV itself, confers the risk [64,65]. HCV infection alone is not associated with an increased incidence of liver injury, particularly when lower-dose conditioning regimens are used [61,83–85]. Modifying the conditioning regimen by substituting another drug for CY, or reducing the dose of CY, or using a nonmyeloablative regimen should be considered in a patient with inflammatory hepatitis [86]. If a HCT candidate infected with HBV has an indolent hematological disease, there may be time for antiviral treatment with lamivudine or adevovir dipivoxil to effect a reduction in the necroinflammatory liver process before the start of conditioning therapy.

Fulminant viral hepatitis

In the absence of antiviral prophylaxis, fatal fulminant hepatitis develops in approximately 15% of hepatitis B-infected HCT recipients [32,52–54,67,69,70,87–89]. Because of this risk, all hepatitis B-infected HCT recipients should receive antiviral prophylaxis and, if possible, hematopoietic cells from an HBV naturally immune donor, provided that no better HLA-matched donor is available (Fig. 58.2). Ablation of T cells by conditioning therapy enhances viral replication, leading to increases in serum levels of HBeAg and HBV DNA and infection of naive hepatocytes with HBV [90,91]. Post-HCT prednisone therapy for GVHD also leads to enhanced HBV replication [92–95]. Pre-emptive antiviral therapy has been studied in HBsAg-positive HCT patients and shown to be effective using famciclovir [96] or lamivudine [40]. Lamivudine is a more potent anti-HBV agent than famciclovir [97], and recent studies have shown that primary prophylaxis with lamivudine is effective in reducing the frequency of both chemotherapy-induced HBV exacerbation [98–102] and post-transplant hepatitis B [40]. Lamivudine is continued for a minimum of 1-year post-HCT, and not stopped until after all immunosuppressive drugs have been discontinued and full immunity has returned [40,103]. In HCT candidates whose sole marker of HBV infection is a positive antibody to HBc, a strategy of post-HCT testing of serum ALT or HBV DNA, followed by institution of lamivudine therapy if HBV reactivation is documented, should reduce the risk of fulminant hepatitis B (Fig. 58.3).

Fulminant "immune-rebound" hepatitis C has been reported only rarely following HCT [104]; the usual course is an initial hepatitic flare coincident with post-HCT immune reconstitution, followed by serum aminotransferases fluctuating over the ensuing years, similar to the course of most patients with chronic hepatitis C [61,63,84,105–107].

Hepatic fibrosis and cirrhosis of the liver

Prior to HCT, liver biopsy should be considered if there is a clinical suspicion of cirrhosis or extensive fibrosis, i.e. if there are stigmata of chronic liver disease or portal hypertension, or if risk factors for cirrhosis are present. These risk factors include hepatitis C infection for more than 15 years plus elevated serum aminotransferase levels, or a history of chronic viral hepatitis plus excessive alcohol intake, or iron overload [108–110]. Patients with established cirrhosis or marked hepatic fibrosis should not proceed to standard high-dose myeloablative therapy because of a high risk of fatal SOS (VOD of the liver), multiorgan failure and death [79,82,110,111]. Alternative HCT strategies to avoid fatal liver toxicity in patients with well-compensated cirrhosis or extensive fibrosis include using a nonmyeloablative regimen [112], or a conditioning regimen that does not contain high-doses of CY or doses of total body irradiation (TBI) >13.2 Gy [86], or substituting a nonliver toxic drug for CY. Patients with cirrhosis and portal hypertension may also develop variceal bleeding and hepatic decompensation after HCT when they develop additional liver pathology such as GVHD [112].

Gallbladder and bile duct stones

Patients may present for HCT with gallstones or sludge-like material in the gallbladder, the cystic duct, or the common bile duct. These conditions are asymptomatic in most cases but can cause postprandial nausea, recurrent pain, sepsis, or a flu-like illness from bacterial cholangitis, without symptoms referable to the biliary tree. Symptomatic patients with gallstones in either the gallbladder or bile ducts should be considered for cholecystectomy before HCT, because of the risk for major sepsis when granulocytopenic. Endoscopic retrograde cholangiopancreatography (ERCP) with sphincterotomy and removal of common bile duct stones is an alternative to surgery. HCT candidates with asymptomatic gallstones (incidentally discovered during a computerized tomography [CT] scan or ultrasound) have a low rate of complications and do not require operative intervention [113].

Iron overload

HCT candidates with diseases such as thalassemia or aplastic anaemia commonly come to HCT with marked hepatic siderosis. Patients with hematologic malignancies may also have significant iron overload, with over 25% of patients having grades 3 or 4 siderosis [114]. As ferritin is an acute phase protein, an elevated serum level in an HCT candidate with malignancy or active infection may not accurately predict the degree of hepatic iron overload. In patients with thalassemia and extreme iron overload, effective pre-HCT chelation therapy improves post-HCT survival [115]. While some studies suggest an association between excess tissue iron stores and regimen-related toxicity [116], others have failed to demonstrate that either excess liver iron or circulating free iron are causes of early post-HCT morbidity [117,118]. In general, the quantification of tissue iron stores can be deferred until after recovery from HCT unless there is evidence of significant end-organ damage (see Iron overload in the Problems in long-term survivors of HCT section, below).

Problems in the first 6 months after HCT

Nausea, vomiting and anorexia

Conditioning therapy makes most patients nauseated and anorexic until after day +10 to day +15. After this period, persistent symptoms are usually caused by acute GVHD, herpesvirus infections, or medications. Inability to eat after HCT is currently a major reason for prolonged hospitalization and parenteral nutrition.

Conditioning therapy

Chemotherapy and TBI cause vomiting and anorexia by several mechanisms. One is related to the effects of chemotherapy on mid-brain vomiting centers, causing symptoms during conditioning therapy [119]. The intensity of vomiting tends to be worse with higher dose regimens, but serotonin-antagonist drugs are very effective in dampening the severity of symptoms. Elevated serum cytokine levels are also a possible explanation for persistent anorexia in this early phase [120]. Another cause of nausea and anorexia is oral mucositis, which has its onset a few days before HCT and reaches a peak 10–14 days later [119,121]. Mucositis causes swelling, pain and in severe cases sloughing of the oropharyngeal epithelium that may be worsened by superinfection and methotrexate (MTX) therapy [122,123]. Mucosal involvement can extend into the hypopharynx and esophagus, causing intense gagging, an inability to swallow, vomiting, retrosternal pain and airway obstruction. Opioid therapy is effective in relieving the pain of mucositis but it can lead to gastric stasis, intestinal ileus, anorexia and vomiting. The intestinal mucosa is similarly damaged by myeloablative conditioning therapy, but mucosal regeneration is nearly complete by day +16 post-HCT [124]. After most regimens of conditioning therapy, by day +20 there has been increased appetite and food intake and decreased symptoms of nausea and satiety [125]. Some regimens, notably those that contain cytarabine, etoposide (VP16), high-dose melphalan, or multiple alkylating agents, seem to cause unusually severe intestinal mucosal necrosis and delay the return of eating behavior [126,127].

Acute GVHD

One of the earliest manifestations of acute GVHD involving the intestine is loss of appetite followed by nausea and vomiting. These symptoms can be overlooked when diarrhea and abdominal pain dominate the clinical picture. In this era of more effective prophylaxis against GVHD, over 80% of patients with intractable anorexia, nausea, or vomiting will have GVHD affecting the stomach and duodenum as the sole explanation [128–131]. In the 1980s, HSV and CMV infection were also common causes of upper-gut symptoms [132], but these infections have become increasingly uncommon [128]. Immunosuppressive therapy using prednisone 1–2 mg/kg is effective in treating these symptoms, particularly when they are the only manifestation of GVHD [128]. Oral beclomethasone dipropionate, a potent topically active corticosteroid delivered in capsules, is also effective in treating the symptoms of upper intestinal GVHD [133,134]. Although some patients who present with nausea and vomiting progress to grade III–IV GVHD, most do not. Instead they have persistent problems with lack of appetite, early satiety and inability to eat adequate calories [131,134]. Anorexia, nausea and vomiting may also recur as the only symptom when immunosuppressive agents are tapered after successful treatment of GVHD. Endoscopy of the stomach and duodenum with gastric biopsy is often needed to confirm the diagnosis of upper intestinal GVHD. The diagnosis is based on the endoscopic appearance (edema of the gastric antral mucosa, patchy erythema, bilious fluid in the stomach) and histologic demonstration of epithelial cell apoptosis and drop-out, often with localized lymphocytic infiltrates [129,130,135]. Endoscopy also serves to rule out intestinal infection with herpesviruses, bacteria, and fungi.

Recipients of autologous grafts may also develop a syndrome of anorexia, nausea and vomiting, which is associated with diffuse gastric edema and erythema. Biopsy specimens from the stomach show histologic abnormalities that are identical to those in allogeneic graft recipients with GVHD; that is, apoptosis of epithelial cells in the crypts, lymphocytic infiltration and epithelial cell drop-out [136]. Symptoms respond to a 10-day course of prednisone 1 mg/kg/day in over 80% of cases. While some patients with this gastric lesion improve over time without therapy, in most patients a short course of prednisone is warranted.

Medications and parenteral nutrition

Oral nonabsorbable antibiotics (particularly nystatin), cyclosporine (CSP), mycophenolate mofetil (MMF), trimethoprim-sulfamethoxazole (TMP-SMX), intravenous amphotericin and high-dose opioids are frequent causes of nausea and occasionally protracted vomiting. A temporal association between dosing and symptoms is often present, but not always, especially for TMP-SMX. Parenteral infusions of fat, glucose and amino acid solutions reduce food intake in human volunteers, slow the rate of gastric emptying, and cause nausea [137]. Even after total parenteral nutrition (TPN) has been stopped, appetite suppression may linger for 1–3 weeks. The importance of TPN as an appetite suppressant was demonstrated in a trial in HCT patients who were randomized to either TPN or intravenous hydration after hospital discharge [138]. The time to resumption of adequate oral intake was 16 days in the TPN group compared to 10 days in the hydration group, a significant difference.

Infections

CMV infection of the esophagus and upper intestine was found in 38% of HCT patients with unexplained nausea and vomiting in one prospective study during the pregancyclovir era [132]. These infections were diagnosed a mean of 54 days post-HCT. Although esophageal ulcers were present in almost all of these cases, esophageal symptoms were frequently absent. HSV esophagitis may present similarly [132,139]. CMV and HSV esophagitis are now rare, owing to the use of prophylactic antiviral therapy; for example, a recent study found CMV or HSV infection in only three of 78 consecutive patients with anorexia and nausea [128]. Most current cases of CMV enteritis represent either infections that antedate HCT or CMV infections that appear first in the intestine, thus evading bloodstream surveillance strategies. Intravenous ganciclovir is highly effective in eliminating CMV from upper intestinal lesions, but symptoms and the endoscopic appearance are only minimally improved by 2 weeks of therapy [140]. Factors contributing to persistence of symptoms and ulceration include the large size of CMV ulcers, acid-peptic reflux and the recurrence of CMV after ganciclovir is stopped. The current practice is to continue ganciclovir for an additional 2 weeks at a reduced dosage.

Fungal esophagitis can cause anorexia but not the incessant vomiting often seen with herpesvirus infections [141]. Bacterial esophagitis, phlegmonous gastritis, fungal gastritis and VZV gastritis may also present with anorexia and nausea [139,142–146]. Anorexia and vomiting may also be manifestations of diseases of the central nervous system (e.g. subdural hematoma, sagittal sinus thrombosis, intracerebral bleeding or infections with Aspergillus, Toxoplasma or viruses). Other neurologic signs and symptoms usually dominate the clinical picture with these disorders. Systemic bacterial infection (bacteremia or focal abscesses), cholecystitis, pneumonia, acute pancreatitis and acute viral hepatitis may also present with anorexia and vomiting, particularly in children.

Gastric motility disorders

Studies of gastric emptying and myoelectric activity in HCT patients have shown that symptoms of nausea and vomiting are frequently accompanied by retention of radionuclide meals and disordered electrical activity [147–149]. Promotility agents, such as metaclopramide, domperidone and low-dose erythromycin, are occasionally useful, but in those patients with presistent symptoms, endoscopic evaluation for GVHD and infection should come before empiric promotility therapy. GVHD commonly leads to gastric stasis; diagnosis is made by biopsy of edematous antral mucosa that shows apoptotic cells [129,130]. CMV and VZV are the infections most likely to cause gastric stasis.

Jaundice, hepatomegaly and abnormal liver tests

The development of jaundice following HCT is an ominous prognostic sign, with an increased nonrelapse mortality noted in patients whose total serum bililrubin peaks exceed 4 mg/dL (Table 58.1) [150]. The relationship between jaundice and mortality applies to patients who received either myeloablative or nonmyeloablative regimens, and appears to be independent of when the jaundice develops and the exact causes [112,150]. In many jaundiced patients, several different hepatobiliary problems contribute to the level of hyperbilirubinemia, and it is often challenging to identify the dominant cause [111].

Table 58.1 Non-relapse mortality following myeloablative conditioning therapy and allogeneic HCT as a function of total serum bilirubin at several time points after transplant. The numbers in each cell are the percent of patients alive at that time who died of nonrelapse causes before day +200, based on a prospective study of 1419 consecutive patients. Reproduced with permission from McDonald et al. [150].

Total serum bilirubin (mg/dL)	At day +10 (%)	At day +30 (%)	At day +60 (%)
1–4	25	19	15
4–7	51	51	55
7–10	55	75	70
>10	73	83	88
>19	80	87	100

Sinusoidal obstruction syndrome (SOS) (VOD of the liver)

Definition and change in nomenclature

In the 1950s, investigators coined the term "veno-occlusive disease" (VOD) to describe obliterative fibrosis within small hepatic venules, a feature readily observed by light microscopy, in patients who had ingested certain toxins [151,152]. The term VOD was then used to describe the clinical syndrome of tender hepatomegaly, fluid retention and weight gain, and elevated serum bilirubin that followed high-dose myeloablative therapy [153–155]. However, 20–30% of HCT cases with occluded venules at autopsy were without clinical symptoms [156,157] and several perivenular lesions were correlated with signs of sinusoidal obstruction in the absence of venular occlusion [156,158]. With the recognition that the injury is initiated by changes in the hepatic sinusoid [79,159,160,161] and that involvement of hepatic venules is not essential to development of clinical signs and symptoms [158,162], the name of this clinical syndrome has been changed to sinusoidal obstruction syndrome (SOS) [111].

Incidence

The reported incidence of SOS after HCT varies from 0% to 50%, largely due to differences in conditioning regimens [157,163–167]. There is no obvious SOS from nonmyeloablative conditioning regimens, e.g. fludarabine plus low-dose TBI [112,168], but regimens of CY and TBI >13.2 Gy may cause SOS in half of patients [163]. A major contributor to development of SOS after CY-based conditioning regimens is individual variability in drug metabolism [86]. Overall, the frequency and severity of SOS have fallen dramatically over the last few years for several reasons: (i) physicians have retreated from the strategy of dose escalation of conditioning regimens; (ii) a major risk factor for severe SOS, chronic hepatitis C [61], has almost disappeared from cohorts of patients presenting for HCT; and (iii) drugs that increase the risk of SOS (e.g. norethisterone [169]) have been removed from HCT care protocols.

Clinical presentation and diagnosis

The diagnosis of SOS rests on the findings of tender hepatomegaly, weight gain and jaundice following conditioning therapy in the absence of other explanations for these signs and symptoms (Table 58.2) [157,163]. The onset of SOS is heralded by an increase in liver size, right upper quadrant tenderness, renal sodium retention and weight gain, occurring 10–20 days after the start of CY-based cytoreductive therapy [163] and later after other myeloablative regimens [167,170,171]. Patients then develop hyperbilirubinemia, usually before day 20 [163]. Some authors have described a syndrome of "late VOD" following conditioning with busulfan (BU)-containing regimens, where signs of liver disease are first

Table 58.2 Clinical features of patients with sinusoidal obstruction syndrome according to severity of disease. Reproduced with permission from McDonald et al. [163].

	Mild	Moderate	Severe
Weight gain (% increase)	7.0 ± 3.5%	10.1 ± 5.3%	15.5 ± 9.2%
Maximum total serum bilirubin before day +20 (mg/dL)	4.7 ± 2.9	7.9 ± 6.6	26.0 ± 15.2
Percent of patients with peripheral edema	23%	70%	85%
Percent of patients with ascites	5%	16%	48%
Platelet transfusion requirements to day +20	53.8 ± 27.6	83.6 ± 35.0	118.3 ± 51.8
Day +100 mortality (all causes)	3%	20%	98%

recognized after day +30 [167,171]. After HCT, treatment of relapsed acute myeloid leukemia (AML) with gemtuzumab ozogamicin (Mylotarg™) may also result in SOS [162].

Laboratory tests

Measurement of total serum bilirubin is a sensitive test for SOS but not a specific one, as there are many causes of jaundice after HCT [111]. Elevations of serum aspartate aminotransferase (AST) and alanine aminotransferase (ALT) can occur in the course of SOS and probably reflect ischemic hepatocyte necrosis, as peak AST/ALT levels are seen weeks after toxin exposure [156,172]. Serum AST levels over 750 U/L in patients with SOS is one marker of a poor prognosis [156,172]. Several plasma proteins have been reported to be abnormally high in patients with SOS, including endothelial cell markers (hyaluronic acid, von Willebrand factor, plasminogen activator inhibitor 1 [PAI-1], tissue plasminogen activator), thrombopoietin, cytokines (tumor necrosis factor-alpha [TNF-α], transforming growth factor-β [TGF-β], interleukin 1 [IL-1], IL-2, IL-6 and IL-8, soluble IL-2 receptor), vascular endothelial growth factor (VEGF) and procollagen peptides [120,173–186]. Some laboratory tests are abnormally low in patients with SOS, including the anticoagulant proteins, protein C and antithrombin III [187,188], and platelet counts [163,189]. It is not clear whether any of these tests have diagnostic or prognostic utility beyond the clinical criteria of weight gain, jaundice and hepatomegaly, although levels of PAI-1 and IL-8 have been proposed for this role [182,184,190]. Serum levels of collagen peptides, however, appear to reflect the extent of sinusoidal fibrosis, an important prognostic variable [158].

Ultrasound, CT and MRI

Imaging studies of the liver are useful for demonstrating hepatomegaly, ascites and attenuated hepatic venous flow consistent with SOS [191–194], as well as excluding biliary dilation or infiltrative lesions in the liver and hepatic veins that might also explain hepatomegaly and jaundice [195]. Other abnormal ultrasound findings that have been reported more frequently in patients with SOS, compared to post-HCT controls, include gallbladder wall thickening, splenomegaly, visualization of a paraumbilical vein, enlarged portal vein diameter, slow or reversed portal vein flow, high congestion index, portal vein thrombosis and increased resistive index to hepatic artery flow [192,196–201]. Unfortunately, ultrasound findings very early in the course of SOS do not appear to add to the information provided by clinical criteria [191,202]. Later in the course of SOS, especially in patients with severe disease, ultrasound evidence of altered liver blood flow, particularly reversal of portal flow and portal vein thrombosis, is more common [193,199,201]. There may be some value in following vascular parameters as indices of improvement in sinusoidal blood flow.

Liver biopsy and measurement of the hepatic venous pressure gradient

In cases where the cause of liver dysfunction is unclear, a transvenous approach that allows both biopsy and hepatic venous pressure measurements is the most accurate diagnostic test [203,204]. Percutaneous or laparoscopic needle biopsy are alternative methods of obtaining liver tissue but pose a high risk of bleeding in the thrombocytopenic patient [205] whereas transvenous biopsy methods can be done safely with platelet counts as low as 30,000/mm^3. In HCT patients, a hepatic venous pressure gradient (using an occlusive balloon technique) above 10 mm Hg is highly specific for SOS [203,204]. The histology of injury to hepatic sinusoids, hepatocytes and venules caused by conditioning therapy may be rapidly progressive. The first recognizable histologic changes of SOS, which occur 6–8 days after the start of conditioning therapy, are the dilation and engorgement of sinusoids, the extravasation of red cells through the space of Disse, necrosis of perivenular hepatocytes, and the widening of the subendothelial zone between the basement membrane and the adventitia of central veins and sublobular veins. These findings often appear much more widespread and severe than the extent of occlusion within hepatic venules [156,158,206,207]. In patients with severe SOS, the extent of injury to sinusoidal cells and perivenular hepatocytes is closely tied to clinical prognosis [158]. Color photomicrographs of these histological findings have been published recently (see Chapter 23 and Plate 23.5, *facing p. 296*) [79]. One morphological consequence of sinusoidal obstruction, ischemia, elevated sinusoidal pressures and fragmentation of hepatocyte cords is the dislodgement of clusters of hepatocytes that may flow retrograde into portal veins or embolize through disrupted pores into lumina of damaged central veins. Immunohistology studies have demonstrated the deposition of fibrinogen and factor VIII/von Willebrand factor, but not platelet antigens, in the perivenular zone and in the widened subendothelial space of venules, but not within the venular lumina, corresponding to the clogging of pores that drain sinusoids into hepatic venules [207]. Electron microscopy studies show closure of fenestrae in sinusoidal endothelial cells and accumulation of extracellular material in sinusoidal pores [206]. Within 2 weeks of the onset of clinical signs of SOS, curvilinear deposits of extracellular matrix can be seen in sinusoids and subendothelial spaces. Immunostaining for activated stellate cells with alpha-smooth actin antibodies have demonstrated a marked increase in the number of stellate cells lining the sinusoids [79,208,209] that are clogged by types I, III and IV collagen [207]. The later stages of fatal SOS (that is, beyond day +50 following CY-based regimens, or earlier, following gemtuzumab ozogamicin infusions [162,210]) are characterized by extensive collagenization of sinusoids and venules. In some cases, there is coalescence of extinguished perivenular zones with fibrous bridging between the central veins, simulating cardiac cirrhosis [79].

Differential diagnosis

Other causes of post-HCT jaundice seldom lead to renal sodium avidity, rapid weight gain and hepatomegaly before the onset of jaundice [111,211]. There are patients who present with jaundice and weight gain that can be confused with SOS [195,212]. The most common combinations of illnesses that mimic SOS are: (i) sepsis syndrome requiring large volumes of crystalloid, followed by renal insufficiency and sepsis-related cholestasis; (ii) cholestatic liver disease, hemolysis and congestive heart failure; and (iii) hyperacute GVHD and sepsis syndrome. SOS may also coexist with these disease processes.

Clinical course and prognosis

The severity of SOS has been classified as mild (SOS that is clinically obvious, requires no treatment and resolves completely), moderate (SOS that causes signs and symptoms requiring treatment, such as diuretics or pain medications, but that resolves completely), or severe (SOS that requires treatment but that does not resolve before death or day +100) [157,163,166,213]. There is a range of clinical and laboratory findings that correspond to these operational definitions of disease severity (Table 58.2) [163]. Some patients have subclinical liver damage, evinced by histological signs of liver toxicity in the absence of clinical signs and symptoms [156]. Published case fatality rates for SOS after HCT range from 0% to 67% [157,163,165–167,214]. These figures are dependent on the definition of both SOS and what constitutes fatal SOS. Recovery from SOS was seen in over 70% of patients whose SOS followed CY-containing regimens and in 84% when SOS was caused by other alkylating agents [163,166,170]. Despite deep jaundice, patients with severe SOS seldom die of liver failure but rather from renal and cardiopulmonary failure [157,163,215–217]. A clinically useful model has been developed that predicts the outcome of SOS after CY-based regimens, derived from rates of increase of both bilirubin and weight in the first 2 weeks following HCT [218]. In some patients, there is a bimodal presentation of SOS; that is, clinical signs of SOS appear in the first 2 weeks post HCT, then wane and then reappear later. This pattern is associated with a worse prognosis [170]. In some cases, signs of SOS resolve, but ascites later recurs following development of inflammatory liver disease (e.g. GVHD). A poor prognosis correlates with higher serum AST and ALT values, higher wedged hepatic venous pressure gradient, development of portal vein thrombosis, doubling of the baseline serum creatinine and falling oxygen saturation [172,201,203,204,219].

Pathogenesis of SOS: insights from animal models

Although clinical investigation and histology of liver specimens from patients who have developed SOS after HCT have given insight into risk factors for sinusoidal injury, the use of animal and *in vitro* models have clarified the cellular mechanisms of sinusoidal injury (reviewed in [79]). *In vitro* studies have shown that sinusoidal endothelial cells are more susceptible than hepatocytes to drugs that cause SOS in patients [159,220,221], a finding that led to the observation that CY is the primary sinusoidal toxin in patients conditioned with CY/TBI [86]. An animal model of SOS that uses the toxin monocrotaline has the same histological characteristics as the human disease, as well as the same "clinical features"; that is, hyperbilirubinemia, hepatomegaly and ascites formation. In this model the first morphological change is loss of sinusoidal endothelial cell fenestration, appearance of gaps in the sinusoidal endothelial cell barrier, rounding up of sinusoidal endothelial cells and penetration of red cells into the space of Disse [161]. Sloughed sinusoidal lining cells, i.e. Kupffer cells, sinusoidal endothelial cells and stellate cells, embolize downstream and obstruct sinusoidal flow [222]. By the time hepatocyte necrosis is observed, there is extensive denudation of the sinusoidal lining. Liver histology from patients in the early stages of SOS shows similar changes [79,158]. A number of biochemical changes have also been observed in the experimental studies. Drugs and toxins that cause SOS profoundly deplete sinusoidal endothelial cell glutathione prior to cell death and support of sinusoidal endothelial cell glutathione prevents cell death [220,221,223,224]. Continuous infusion of glutathione or *N*-acetylcysteine into the portal vein prevents the morphologic changes of SOS observed by light microscopy, electron microscopy and *in vivo* microscopy, as well as the "clinical features" of SOS. Infusion of glutathione 24 h after treatment with monocrotaline attenuated, but did not prevent, SOS lending credence to clinical anecdotes of glutathione repletion using *N*-acetylcysteine in patients with SOS post-HCT [225]. The benefit of glutathione is consistent with improved survival after administration of monocrotaline in rats treated with glutathione monoethyl ester [226]. One possible explanation for the rounding up of sinusoidal endothelial cells may be increased activity of matrix metalloproteinases (MMPs) [227], as inhibition of MMP activity completely prevents SOS in animal models. Although SOS is defined as a nonthrombotic obstruction of sinusoidal blood flow, the issue of clotting has been a recurring topic of research interest, based largely on plasma studies in patients with SOS [228] and an immunohistological study [207]. However, electron microscopy of pyrrolizidine alkaloid-induced SOS in humans did not detect clotting [229], and sequential observations during the development of SOS in an animal model have not demonstrated any evidence of clotting [161]. In patients with SOS, it is not clear whether intrasinusoidal thrombosis is a cause of either hepatic injury or clinical signs and symptoms.

Pathogenesis of SOS: clinical studies

The most important predictors of who will develop fatal SOS are the conditioning regimen that is chosen (some regimens contain more liver toxins than others), the metabolism of CY (which is highly variable), the dose of TBI and whether the patient has underlying liver inflammation and fibrosis. Two observations about SOS in patients provide clues as to the mechanism of disease. First, unlike other intrinsic liver diseases, the signs and symptoms of portal hypertension precede evidence of parenchymal damage. In SOS, disruption of the liver circulation is the cause and not the consequence of the parenchymal disease. Second, involvement of the hepatic veins is not essential to the development of the clinical picture: 45% of patients with mild or moderate disease and 25% of patients with severe SOS did not have occluded hepatic venules at autopsy [158]. Occlusion of central veins of the liver lobule is associated with more severe disease and the development of ascites [158,230]. This finding suggests that occlusive lesions involving the central veins, a later development, may exacerbate the acute circulatory impairment that occurs at the level of the sinusoid.

Chemotherapy drugs CY is common to the conditioning regimens with the highest incidence of fatal SOS [163]. The metabolism of CY is highly variable; patients who generate a greater quantity of toxic metabolites are more likely to develop severe SOS following conditioning with CY and TBI [86]. The liver toxin generated by CY metabolism is acrolein (a metabolite formed simultaneously along with the desired metabolite, phosphoramide mustard) via mechanisms dependent upon glutathione [220,226,231,232]. Exposure to one CY metabolite (carboxyethyl phosphoramide mustard) was significantly related to SOS, bilirubin elevation, nonrelapse mortality and survival in patients receiving conditioning with CY/TBI, but there was no relationship to either engraftment or tumor relapse [86]. These data suggest that a strategy that targets the dose of CY on the basis of a patient's metabolism will substantially reduce the risk of fatal SOS without jeopardizing engraftment.

BU is another component of regimens with a high frequency of SOS. A relationship between BU exposure (measured by area-under-the-curve or average steady-state concentration, $\bar{C}_{ss,Bu}$) following oral dosing and the toxicity of conditioning therapy has been reported [233–237]. However, in adults with CML in chronic phase and in children with acute leukemia, there is no correlation between BU exposure and SOS [235,238–240]. BU may contribute to liver injury by inducing oxidative stress, reducing glutathione levels in hepatocytes and sinusoidal endothelial cells [241] and by altering CY metabolism [242]. When CY is given before BU, a lower frequency of SOS results, suggesting that BU predisposes patients to CY toxicity [243]. Most HCT centers now dose oral BU according to its metabolism or give intravenous doses of BU, with more predictable kinetics and somewhat less overall toxicity [244–248].

One retrospective study has reported a lower frequency of fatal SOS when BU was given intravenously compared to oral dosing in a historical comparison group [248], but the groups were not comparable in terms of BU exposure. Intravenous BU appears to be at least as safe as oral BU and may be easier to monitor [249]. SOS has also been described as dose-limiting for regimens that contain high-dose nitrosourea (1,3-bis(2-chloroethyl)-1-nitrosourea [BCNU]), carboplatin, or cytarabine [214].

Total body irradiation (TBI) The doses of TBI given in the setting of HCT are in the range of 10–16 Gy, far less that the dose of liver irradiation that causes radiation-induced liver disease [250,251]. In combination with CY, however, there is a clear relationship between the total dose of TBI and the frequency of severe SOS [86,163,252]. The synergism between CY and TBI in causing sinusoidal injury may be due to sublethal damage to sinusoidal endothelial cells caused by CY metabolites followed by irradiation damage. An alternate mechanism involved the depletion of reduced glutathione in hepatocytes and sinusoidal endothelial cells by CY, leaving sinusoidal endothelial cells more vulnerable to irradiation. In animals exposed to hepatic irradiation or CY, or monocrotaline, liver damage is enhanced by glutathione depletion and lessened by repletion [220,224,226,253,254]. The relation of irradiation technique (fractionated vs. hyperfractionated) to SOS is controversial, with one study showing such a relationship [255] and three studies showing no association [163,256,257].

Gemtuzumab ozogamicin (Mylotarg™) Gemtuzumab ozogamicin utilizes monoclonal antibody technology to specifically target leukemia cells expressing the CD33 receptor by means of a humanized antibody conjugated to a modified cytotoxic agent, calicheamicin [258,259]. Gemtuzumab ozogamicin may cause sinusoidal liver injury when used to treat patients with AML [210,259–261]. In patients who received gemtuzumab ozogamicin followed by myeloablative therapy and HCT, the reported frequency of a post-HCT SOS was six of 38 (16%), with three fatal cases in one series [262] and eight of nine (89%) in another [263]. When gemtuzumab ozogamicin is part of a dose-intensive conditioning therapy, fatal SOS may result. When gemtuzumab ozogamicin is given at full dose to patients with relapses of AML following HCT, the frequency of sinusoidal liver injury may be as high as 50% [162]. The mechanism of liver injury in these cases is probably related to delivery of calicheamicin to CD33+ cells that reside in the sinusoids of the liver; that is, Kupffer cells [264,265], leukemia cells [114] and possibly sinusoidal endothelial cells [266] and stellate cells. The clinical presentation is one of acute portal hypertension, elevations of serum AST/ALT and moderate jaundice, with histology showing intense sinusoidal fibrosis and centrilobular hepatocyte necrosis [162].

Intrahepatic coagulation Some see SOS as a disease of disordered coagulation, in which damage to endothelium in the sinusoids and central veins leads to exposure of tissue factor and initiation of the coagulation cascade, a process abetted by low circulating levels of the natural anticoagulants protein C and antithrombin III, elaboration of cytokines that stimulate coagulation, high plasma levels of tissue plasminogen activator and reduced fibrinolysis (reflected by elevated plasma levels of PAI-1) [182,188,267–271]. However, heparin and antithrombin III infusions are ineffective in preventing fatal SOS and thrombolytic therapy effects improvement in only a minority of patients [166,219,272–278]. Genetic disorders predisposing to coagulation (factor V Leiden and prothrombin gene *20210 G-A*) have weak or no associations with SOS after HCT [279,280]. Current evidence suggests that disordered coagulation in SOS is an epiphenomenon secondary to widespread centrilobular damage, not a cause of sinusoidal injury.

Stellate cells and sinusoidal fibrosis Several series have documented the early appearance of a procollagen peptide in serum of patients who develop more severe SOS, along with inhibitors of fibrolysis [176,177,181,281], consistent with the intense fibrosis in centrilobular sinusoids and venular walls that is common in fatal SOS [79,158,162,210]. The stimuli for stellate cell activation and proliferation in the HCT setting have not been identified; candidates include centrilobular hypoxia, endotoxemia, Kupffer cell damage, loss of sinusoidal endothelial cells, and a melange of circulating growth factors and cytokines (platelet derived growth factor, TGF-β, TNF-α, IL-8 and soluble IL-2 receptor) [120,174,183,184,225,282,283]. Sinusoidal fibrosis is particularly intense following gemtuzumab ozogamicin-caused sinusoidal injury [162].

Vasoactive mediators Serum levels of endothelin-1 are elevated in patients with SOS [284,285]. Low plasma levels of nitrate are also seen during conditioning therapy [284,285]. These data are consistent with the hypothesis that endothelin-1 is a mediator of hepatic sinusoidal constriction, unopposed by a vasorelaxant effect of endothelial nitric oxide.

Renal pathophysiology in SOS Falling fractional excretion of sodium occurs just before the clinical signs of SOS become apparent, reflecting both sinusoidal hypertension [203,204] and renal tubular injury caused by metabolites of CY [286]. Plasma levels of nitrate rise sharply during the period of fluid accumulation in patients who develop moderate to severe SOS [285].

Prevention of SOS in patients receiving myeloablative therapy

In patients with no identifiable risk factors who receive a CY-based myeloablative regimen, fatal SOS develops in ~7% of cases following CY/TBI and in ~5% of cases following targeted oral BU and CY [86,287]. In patients who come to HCT with risk factors for fatal SOS—for example, chronic hepatitis C, hepatic fibrosis, cirrhosis, nonalcoholic steatohepatitis and systemic bacterial or viral infection before the start of cytoreductive therapy—CY-based regimens are more likely to result in mortality [61,82,110,163]. Previous radiation therapy that involved the liver, recent therapy with gemtuzumab ozogamicin and a previous HCT procedure are also predisposing factors [169,170,288]. The relative risk of fatal SOS is ~10-fold in patients with chronic hepatitis C, compared to patients without liver disease, which translates to ~20% absolute risk [61]. Without the benefit of studies of patients who undergo liver biopsy before HCT for malignancy, it is more difficult to define the absolute risk of fatal SOS in cohorts of patients who have extensive hepatic fibrosis or cirrhosis. Anecdotal experience suggests that fatal SOS develops in >70% of patients with cirrhosis. The only certain way to prevent fatal SOS, particularly among patients at risk, is to avoid giving doses of conditioning therapy that are known to damage hepatic sinusoidal cells. Based on studies in experimental animals, it may also be possible to cytoprotect sinusoidal cells, but these strategies have not been proved in the clinical setting and may pose a risk of cytoprotecting tumor cells [79].

Alterations of conditioning therapy The use of nonmyeloablative regimens that contain no liver toxins, followed by allogeneic HCT, may be the only method of avoiding SOS in patients with underlying hepatic fibrosis [168]. However, eliminating liver damage from the conditioning regimen does not eliminate liver-related mortality in patients with marginally compensated cirrhosis, as hepatic failure may occur after development of cholestatic liver disorders such as GVHD or cholangitis lenta [112]. Altering myeloablative conditioning regimens has been reported to lessen the risk of SOS; for example, adjusting oral doses of BU in individual patients based on BU disposition [233,289], or giving BU as an intravenous preparation [245,245,290]. However, other studies of BU dosing based on plasma BU levels targeted to average steady-state concentrations of 900 ng/ml have not shown benefit in preventing SOS [238–240,291]. Giving intravenous BU along with CY does not eliminate fatal SOS, lending credence to CY as the more important liver toxin in this regimen [245,290]. Administering CY before BU has been shown to decrease the frequency of SOS [243]. The likely explanation for this effect is that BU alters CY metabolism (more toxic metabolites are produced) and lowers levels of reduced glutathione in hepatocytes and sinusoidal endothelial cells (lowering CY metabolite detoxification). Giving lower irradiation doses (e.g. 10 Gy TBI at 2–4 cGy/min) with CY may result in a lower incidence of SOS [166,292,169]. Shielding the liver during TBI will lessen liver injury but leads to relapse of underlying hematological disease [293]. Another approach for conditioning a patient who has risk factors for fatal SOS is to choose a regimen that does not contain CY, a component of regimens with the highest frequency of SOS. A recent study has shown that increased exposure to toxic metabolites of CY leads to increased liver toxicity and nonrelapse mortality and lower overall survival after HCT, but that patients were not at risk from either graft rejection or relapse from decreased exposure to toxic CY metabolites [86]. There are two implications of this study: (i) a CY dose of 120 mg/kg, when combined with either TBI = 12 Gy, or BU targeted at 800–900 ng/ml, is excessive and can probably be reduced without jeopardizing either engraftment or relapse rate; and (ii) a strategy to target doses of CY based on its metabolism is likely to substantially reduce regimen-related nonrelapse mortality. Studies of metabolism-based CY dosing are being conducted. In the interim, when faced with patients who have risk factors for fatal SOS and for whom a CY-based regimen is the most appropriate, clinicians might opt for empirically reducing the dose of CY by 10–20%; giving intravenous BU targeted to an average steady-state concentration of 800–900 ng/ml, or not exceeding a TBI dose of 12 Gy; giving CY before BU; and employing one or more of the strategies for cytoprotection of hepatic sinusoidal cells.

Anticoagulant or antithrombin infusions Anticoagulation with heparin can be given safely if the partial thromboplastin time is monitored carefully [294–296]. Two randomized studies have reported a reduction in nonfatal SOS with heparin, but had little power to demonstrate a benefit in preventing fatal SOS [295,297]. Four additional studies of anticoagulation in unselected patients could find no benefit [166,169,294,298]. Nonetheless, some centers routinely use heparin infusions or low molecular weight heparin subcutaneously [296,299,300]. Prophylactic antithrombin III infusions effect no reduction in the frequency or severity of SOS despite restoring plasma antithrombin III levels to normal [272]. There is little in the published literature to recommend anticoagulation as a strategy to prevent fatal SOS.

Defibrotide infusions Patients receiving myeloablative regimens have received defibrotide at 800–2400 mg/day to day +28 as prophylaxis, with the observation that there was a lower frequency of SOS, compared to historical controls [301,302].

Other medical prophylaxis Ursodeoxycholic acid (ursodiol) has been reported to reduce the severity of post-HCT SOS in two randomized trials [303,304], but was without effect in a large randomized Scandinavian study [305]. Ursodiol probably lessens the impact of cholestasis but not toxic liver injury. A combination of ursodiol, heparin and glutamine has also been used as prophylaxis in uncontrolled studies [306]. Two trials have administered prostaglandin E_1 by continuous infusion with no evidence that the frequency of fatal SOS was affected [307,308]. Because some studies have reported elevated levels of cytokines (including TNF-α) in association with SOS [120], anticytokine strategies have been studied. Several placebo-controlled, randomized trials have shown pentoxifylline, an inhibitor of TNF-α release, to be ineffective in preventing SOS [309,310].

Prophylaxis directed at hepatic sinusoidal cells Studies in animals suggests that it may be possible to protect sinusoidal endothelial cells from toxic injury by pretreating with reduced glutathione, or with a nitric oxide donor into the portal vein, or with an MMP inhibitor (reviewed in [79]). There are also data that suggest that production of collagen by activated stellate cells can be down-regulated [282]. Clinical trials of these strategies have not been reported, but this approach may allow myeloablative regimens to be given without causing sinusoidal injury.

Treatment of patients with SOS following myeloablative therapy

As 70–85% of patients recover spontaneously, treatment of SOS involves management of sodium and water balance with diuretics and repeated paracenteses for ascites that is associated with discomfort or pulmonary compromise [163]. Renal and pulmonary failure in patients with severe SOS have been managed with hemodialysis and mechanical ventilation, albeit with little impact on outcome [163,215–217]. In severely ill HCT patients with SOS and organ failure, there are guidelines that have defined futility of treatment, allowing patients and their physicians to eschew life-support measures when appropriate, or to consider a liver transplant in extremely rare circumstances [217]. There is no completely satisfactory treatment for severe SOS, but the literature describes these approaches as outlined below.

Thrombolytic therapy Tissue plasminogen activator (60 mg given in divided doses over 2–4 days) and heparin (150 U/kg/day over 10 days) infusions show evidence of efficacy in less than one-third of patients with severe SOS [219,273–278,311]. In one large series, there were no responses when patients had either renal or pulmonary failure [219]. Thrombolytic therapy is further limited by the risk of fatal intracerebral and pulmonary bleeding [219,278,312,313]. Thrombolytic therapy might be considered for treatment of patients with SOS whose prognostic indices [218] point to a higher than 20% estimated risk of fatality provided that renal and pulmonary function is intact.

Defibrotide Defibrotide, a single stranded polydeoxyribonucleotide drug derived from animal tissue, has antithrombotic, anti-ischemic and thrombolytic properties [314]. Uncontrolled trials with defibrotide (at 20–60 mg/kg/day for 14–20 days) in over 150 patients with moderate to severe SOS showed complete resolution in 35–60% of patients and no evidence of serious toxicity [315–319]. Recovery of patients with severe SOS and multiorgan failure is unusual, lending credence to reports of complete recovery following defibrotide infusion.

Other medical therapies Three patients with clinical evidence of moderate to severe SOS have been treated with intravenous N-acetylcysteine at a dose of 50–150 mg/kg/day for 2–4 weeks, during which serum bilirubin and inflammatory markers improved [225]. Patients with SOS have been treated with infusions of human antithrombin III concentrate or activated protein C [272,320,321], without clear evidence of efficacy. There are also anecdotal reports of improvement after therapy with prostaglandin E_1 [322], prednisone [323], topical nitrate [324], and vitamin E plus glutamine therapy [325]. Use of a liver assist device has been associated with recovery of patients with SOS and extreme jaundice (total serum bilirubin >50 mg/dL), suggesting that recovery from severe sinusoidal injury is possible.

Transjugular intrahepatic portosystemic shunt (TIPS) Transhepatic shunts have been placed in patients with SOS after HCT [326–329]. TIPS placement reduces portal pressure and appears effective in mobilizing ascites but does not have an effect on either serum bilirubin levels or patient outcomes [328–330]. In one case, TIPS led to acute respiratory distress syndrome that was fatal [331].

Surgical approaches Two patients with SOS underwent successful portosystemic shunts for persistent ascites but liver dysfunction had resolved long before these shunts were placed [332,333]. Peritoneovenous shunts for intractable ascites have been unsuccessful. Eleven patients have received liver transplants for severe SOS [313,334–340], four of whom survived over a year [334,337,339,340]. When severe SOS develops in a patient with a benign condition (a rare event) or in a patient with a favorable outcome post-HCT (e.g. CML in chronic phase), liver transplantation should be considered.

Cholestasis caused by CSP and tacrolimus

CSP inhibits canalicular bile transport at pharmacologic levels in a dose-related manner and commonly causes mild increases in serum bilirubin [341,342]. High blood CSP levels lead to correspondingly higher total serum bilirubin values [342]. Patients with acute liver GVHD may have impaired elimination of CSP, with increased blood levels of some CSP metabolites, which may further exacerbate liver dysfunction [343]. If CSP blood levels are in the therapeutic range, bilirubin levels >4 mg/dL cannot be attributed solely to CSP. Very high CSP exposure may result in elevated serum aminotransferase enzyme levels and evidence of hepatocellular injury. Tacrolimus also appears to cause cholestasis at high doses [344], but this effect appears to be less clinically significant than cholestasis caused by CSP [345].

Cholangitis lenta (cholestasis of sepsis)

Sepsis-associated cholestasis is an important contributor to hyperbilirubinemia in the first few weeks after HCT. The cholestatic effects of bacterial infection are mediated directly by endotoxins [346,347], as well as by endotoxin-induced cytokines [348–350]. The usual presentation is of mild-to-moderate elevations of bilirubin in a febrile patient [351]. In some non-HCT patients with infection-related cholestasis, the serum bilirubin level may be as high as 15 mg/dL and serum alkaline phosphatase may increase. Histologic abnormalities due to cholangitis lenta alone are usually minimal, particularly in cases of short duration. In those patients with severe, prolonged cholestasis, biopsy may reveal intrahepatic cholestasis, with dilation and stasis of bile in cholangioles or ducts of Hering [352]. The diagnosis of cholangitis lenta is based entirely on clinical criteria. However, because of the multitude of processes impacting the liver of patients in the weeks following HCT, particularly SOS (VOD of the liver) and GVHD, jaundice in septic patients may be progressive and severe, the prognosis very poor [150] and the contribution of sepsis-associated cholestasis to the level of jaundice difficult to discern. With appropriate antibiotic therapy, a fall in bilirubin level is usually seen, although it may be delayed.

Acute GVHD

The pathophysiology of acute GVHD is discussed in Chapter 27. In the liver, alloreactive T cells recognize foreign major and minor histocompatibility antigens as well as adhesion molecules expressed on biliary epithelial cells [353]. In patients receiving immunosuppressive prophylaxis, the onset is usually after day +15 and coincides with hematopoietic engraftment. As hematologic recovery is more rapid following HCT using blood hematopoietic cells compared to marrow derived cells [354–356], it is apparent that acute GVHD also occurs earlier. Hepatic GVHD usually follows manifestations of cutaneous and/or intestinal GVHD, and is heralded by a gradual rise in serum bilirubin, alkaline phosphatase levels up to 20 times the upper limit of normal and aminotransferases up to 10-times normal [357]. Although elevations of serum alkaline phosphatase have been proposed as a sensitive diagnostic test for GVHD [357], progressive jaundice is the most common presenting feature. Elevated levels of plasma cytokines, particularly IL-6, in patients with acute GVHD may lead to cholestasis by a mechanism similar to that of cholangitis lenta [348–350]. In allograft recipients whose immunosuppressive therapy is being tapered, GVHD may present as an acute hepatitis, with serum aminotransferase levels over 1000 U/L [358]. A cholestatic condition identical to GVHD in allograft recipients has been reported in autologous HCT recipients; histology shows injury to small bile ducts and there is usually a prompt response to corticosteroids [359].

Cholestatic liver abnormalities in an allograft recipient with clinical or biopsy evidence of cutaneous or intestinal GVHD are usually attributable to hepatic GVHD, and a biopsy is frequently not required, particularly as treatment will already be dictated by disease in other organs. Liver biopsy to confirm the presence of GVHD may be required in a patient with concurrent disease processes, such as SOS or sepsis, where it may be impossible to determine clinically the contribution of GVHD to the liver dysfunction. Liver biopsy may also be important in excluding other treatable causes of liver dysfunction, such as viral or fungal infection. Characteristic liver biopsy findings in GVHD include lymphocytic infiltration of small bile ducts with nuclear pleomorphism and epithelial cell dropout. Because these patients are frequently pancytopenic and immunosuppressed, inflammatory infiltrates may be minimal [360,361]. Parenchymal changes include scattered acidophilic bodies, lobular disarray and centrilobular cholestasis, but these findings are less specific for GVHD. In the first 1–2 weeks after the onset of GVHD, liver biopsy may be nondiagnostic because characteristic cholestasis and disrupted septal and interlobular bile duct epithelia are not as florid as in patients who have undergone several weeks of epithelial necrosis [360,361]. Intrahepatic peribiliary glands may also be involved [362]. Abnormalities of small bile ducts have also been described in patients with cholangitis lenta, chronic HCV infection, and extrahepatic obstruction, but the extent of apoptosis and dropout of cells serves to distinguish acute GVHD from these entities [360,361]. In advanced cases of hepatic GVHD, it may be difficult to identify small bile ducts on routinely stained sections because they have been destroyed. In this situation, specialized cytokeratin stains can be used to better demonstrate the paucity of small bile ducts (see Chapter 23).

Treatment of acute GVHD of the liver usually involves the addition of prednisone at a dose of 2 mg/kg/day to the prophylactic regimen. In a large retrospective series, only 30% of patients with liver GVHD had resolution of liver abnormalities after initial treatment, and response in a further 32% was not evaluable because of the presence of other liver diseases [363]. Of patients with liver GVHD who fail primary treatment, secondary treatment results in improvement or resolution of liver disease in only 25% [364]. Approaches to the treatment of acute GVHD that has failed to respond to initial therapy are discussed in Chapter 50. If patients can take oral medications, ursodeoxycholic acid (ursodiol) (15–30 mg/kg/day) is useful adjunctive therapy in patients with acute or chronic GVHD of the liver [305,365,366]. Ursodeoxycholic acid (ursodiol) is well tolerated, ameliorates cholestasis and has immunomodulatory and antiapoptotic properties that may have a beneficial effect on the pathogenic processes in GVHD [367,368]. The *prophylactic* use of ursodiol has been shown to reduce the frequency of cholestasis in general and GVHD-related cholestasis specifically, compared to placebo, and, in view of its safety and efficacy, should be given routinely through day +80 in allograft recipients [305,366]. Over 50% of patients with acute liver GVHD will develop chronic GVHD, which may be seen as early as 40–50 days post-HCT (see Chapter 50).

Drug- and TPN-induced liver injury

In the first few weeks following HCT, patients receive a multitude of drugs, including CSP or tacrolimus, MTX, antibacterials, antifungals, antivirals and growth factors. Although many of these agents have hepatotoxic potential, severe liver abnormalities in this clinical setting are rarely due to drugs and are usually caused by SOS, GVHD or sepsis. MTX, when given for GVHD prophylaxis, is rarely hepatotoxic in the doses commonly used, but a transient rise in AST or ALT may be encountered [369]. Liposomal amphotericin and granulocyte macrophage colony-stimulating factor (GM-CSF) may rarely lead to hepatic injury [370,371]. TPN is commonly implicated in causing mild elevations of bilirubin, transaminases and alkaline phosphatase after HCT, but occasionally marked hyperbilirubinemia may be seen, particularly in the presence of sepsis or hemolysis [372]. Histologic abnormalities due to TPN include steatosis, steatohepatitis and cholestasis. These hepatic abnormalities usually reverse promptly with cessation of TPN. TPN may contribute to biliary sludge, gallstone development and "acalculous" cholecystitis after HCT. If TPN is considered to be causing progressive liver abnormalities in an individual patient, consideration should be given to ceasing or reducing therapy, changing the solution composition, or changing the timing of administration [373].

Viral infections

Herpes simplex virus (HSV) (see Chapter 54)

With the routine use of acyclovir in the immediate post-HCT period, cases of acute hepatitis due to HSV are now rare [374,375]. However, fulminant hepatic failure due to HSV type 2 has been reported despite acyclovir prophylaxis [376]. Presenting features of HSV hepatitis include rapidly rising serum aminotransferases and onset of liver failure with coagulopathy and progressive jaundice. The onset of liver dysfunction may be associated with abdominal pain and fever, and herpetic lesions involving the mouth, esophagus, or skin. Typical herpetic skin lesions, however, may be absent [374]. Characteristic liver biopsy findings include foci of parenchymal necrosis, surrounded by a zone of hepatocytes containing lightly basophilic intranuclear inclusions. Immunohistochemistry using specific antibodies to HSV type 1 and type 2, or *in situ* hybridization using specific anti-HSV probes, is required for definitive diagnosis [377]. Hepatic CT scan may reveal multiple necrotizing lesions resembling pyogenic or fungal abscesses [378], but is usually not helpful. Liver biopsy (usually via the transjugular or transfemoral route) should be performed as soon as possible so that the diagnosis can be confirmed [204,379]. Therapy with high-dose acyclovir should be considered at presentation, before biopsy confirmation, in any HCT recipient developing an acute hepatitis, particularly as HSV hepatitis may be clinically indistinguishable from VZV hepatitis [375,377], and other causes of acute hepatic dysfunction such as GVHD [358]. HSV hepatitis may be fatal if left untreated.

Varicella-zoster virus (VZV) (see Chapter 55)

VZV is one of the most common late infections among both allogeneic and autologous HCT recipients, developing in 17–50% of patients [380–382]. The majority of infections occur within the first 18 months, usually from 4–7-months post-HCT [380,383,384]. While routine acyclovir prophylaxis is effective in preventing clinical VZV infection at the time of its administration, it has no impact on the occurrence of this late presentation [381,385]. Visceral dissemination has been reported in 13% of allograft and 5% of autograft recipients [383,384], and clinical presentation can vary from an isolated severe hepatitis to an abdominal presentation with pain and distention [145,386,387]. Clinical disease due to VZV, particularly disseminated disease, is more common among patients with GVHD than among those without presumably related to prolonged immune suppression. Therapy with high-dose acyclovir should be started in any HCT patient whose serum AST or ALT is over 800–1000 U/L or rapidly rising, before any diagnostic tests are undertaken. Histologic features of VZV hepatitis include widespread hepatocyte necrosis, variable lobular inflammatory cell infiltrate and multinucleated giant cells with intranuclear inclusions. Immunohistochemistry using monoclonal antibodies and *in situ* hybridization using specific anti-VZV probes are essential for prompt diagnosis [377]. Specific VZV PCR may be applied to blood or liver and may rapidly diagnose infection [388]. Intravenous acyclovir at 10–30 mg/kg/day (500 mg/m^2 three times daily) should be given for 7–10 days or until resolution of clinical symptoms [389]. Foscarnet should be used to treat acyclovir-resistant VZV infections [390].

Human herpesvirus-8 (HHV-8) and human herpesvirus-6 (HHV-6) (see Chapter 57)

HHV-8 has been implicated in the development of Kaposi's sarcoma in solid-organ transplant recipients [391]. Recently HHV-8 reactivation has been associated with the development of fever, rash and hepatitis in an HCT recipient [392]. Of note, this syndrome was not prevented by the prophylactic use of acyclovir. PCR assay may be required for diagnosis. HHV-6 has been associated with fever, skin rash, delayed platelet engraftment and the development of encephalitis and pneumonitis after HCT. It has also rarely been implicated in hepatitis occurring after allogeneic HCT [393,394]. As with HHV-8, prophylactic acyclovir does not prevent HHV-6 reactivation [395]. Ganciclovir, foscarnet and GM-CSF have been used effectively in treatment.

Cytomegalovirus (CMV) (see Chapter 53)

Because of antiviral strategies, disseminated CMV disease has become increasingly uncommon in HCT patients except among recipients of HCT from unrelated donors [396], T-cell-depleted grafts [397,398], or in those with severe GVHD. Liver involvement with CMV virtually always accompanies disseminated disease, almost never appears as an isolated liver disease and only rarely results in significant liver dysfunction [399–401]. Histologic findings are usually sparse and include scattered microabscesses, bile duct abnormalities and intranuclear and intracytoplasmic inclusion bodies [399]. Many of these features are nonspecific and may be found in other viral infections and in GVHD. The most sensitive test for the detection of CMV in liver biopsy specimens is PCR [401,402]. However, because PCR of liver tissue for CMV DNA cannot differentiate among viremia, latent infection and true hepatic infection, there is a role for *in situ* hybridization, viral culture, immunohistochemistry using monoclonal antibodies directed against viral proteins and the presence of typical nuclear inclusion bodies in the diagnosis of CMV hepatitis. As CMV hepatitis often accompanies disseminated disease, patients are usually already on specific antiviral therapy, and changes in therapy are dictated by responses in other organs. CMV enteritis, with involvement of the ampulla of Vater, may contribute to liver dysfunction by causing biliary obstruction [403,404].

Adenovirus (see Chapter 57)

An increase in severe disease and mortality due to adenoviral infection after HCT has been noted recently [405]. In immunocompromised patients, adenovirus infection may result in hemorrhagic enterocolitis, interstitial pneumonitis, myocarditis, hemorrhagic cystitis and nephritis, renal failure, meningoencephalitis and fulminant hepatitis [405–408]. However, the majority of adenovirus isolates from patients with diarrhea do not result in disseminated infection. Liver necrosis is heralded by rapidly rising AST and ALT and rapid deterioration of liver function that leads to coagulopathy and encephalopathy. Liver biopsy performed early in the course of adenoviral hepatitis should be diagnostic. Discrete foci of coagulative necrosis surrounded by rims of hepatocytes containing intranuclear inclusions can be seen on stained sections [409]. Immunohistochemistry of liver sections, and viral culture of liver biopsy samples are essential for the precise identification of adenovirus infection. PCR for the identification of viral DNA in tissue samples, blood, sputum, urine or diarrheal stool may be helpful in diagnosis [410–413]. Electron microscopy, while of little use in the clinical setting because of low sensitivity, may show typical findings of adenovirus infection, with intranuclear ring-like inclusions and paracrystalline arrays [409]. The most effective treatments at present are cidofovir or donor leukocyte infusions [414,415]. Cidofovir, however, has significant renal toxicity [416] that can be minimized by use of probenecid and hydration [417]. Intravenous ribavirin has been reported to result in clinical improvement and viral clearance in both single organ and disseminated adenoviral infection [418–422] but ribavirin is not always effective, particularly in the setting of fulminant hepatic failure [414,423].

Echoviruses (see Chapter 57)

Echovirus has been identified in the liver of a patient with disseminated echovirus infection after allogeneic HCT [424]. However, echovirus hepatitis has not been described in this setting. Fatal acute hepatitis due to this virus has been seen in the perinatal period and virus has been isolated from the liver of an infant with marrow hypoplasia [425]. Hepatitis and pneumonia due to echovirus has also been reported in immunocompetent adults [426].

Parvovirus (see Chapter 57)

Infection with human parvovirus B19 is uncommon after HCT, but when present may produce severe clinical illness. Anemia, leukopenia, thrombocytopenia and engraftment failure are the most commonly observed manifestations; however, hepatic dysfunction, myocarditis, vasculitis and respiratory failure have also been reported [427,428]. While liver biopsy may show hepatocytes with eosinophilic nuclear inclusions and swollen hydropic nuclei [429], diagnosis is usually made by PCR [430].

Hepatitis B virus (HBV)

HBV infections arise in HCT recipients in three ways: (i) HBV infection may be evident prior to HCT (that is, the recipient is HBsAg-positive); (ii) latent or occult HBV (HBsAg-negative prior to HCT) may reactivate; or (iii) *de novo* infection may be acquired from an HBV-infected donor [31]. If donors and recipients are carefully screened prior to HCT, if HBV-infected recipients are treated with prophylactic lamivudine, and if recipients at risk for reactivation of latent HBV are monitored with serum ALT and HBV DNA tests post-HCT, there should be relatively few cases of unanticipated post-HCT hepatitis B [31,40]. Unfortunately, however, some patients with HBV are either not identified prior to HCT, or are not given appropriate prophylaxis, and these patients remain at risk of significant morbidity and mortality from HBV-related liver disease. Rarely, a patient arrives for HCT with occult HBV infection (no serological markers are positive for past HBV infection [431]) and reactivates HBV during prolonged immunosuppression after HCT [75].

In the early post-HCT phase in the absence of antiviral prophylaxis, while hepatitis B-infected patients are immunosuppressed, particularly if receiving CSP and prednisone, HBV DNA levels in blood may rise to very high levels without alteration in serum aminotransferases. During this phase, patients may develop a syndrome called "fibrosing cholestatic hepatitis" in which severe hepatic dysfunction occurs due to a direct cytopathic effect from extremely high levels of intracellular viral antigens [88]. A major risk factor for post-HCT hepatitis B is pre-HCT serum HBV DNA level >10^5 copies/ml (by Digene Hybrid Capture II Assay® or quantitiative PCR) [41]. At the time of immune reconstitution, particularly if immunosuppressive drugs are being tapered, an immune-mediated flare of hepatitis B may ensue. In the absence of anti-HBV prophylaxis, approximately 15% of HBV-infections patients may develop fulminant hepatic failure following HCT [31,68,87]. A diagnostic dilemma may arise in a HCT recipient who develops abnormal AST or ALT at the time of tapering of immunosuppressive drugs, particularly when there is evidence of GVHD in other organs and the presence of HBsAg or HBV DNA in serum. Both hepatic GVHD [358] and an immune-mediated flare of viral hepatitis may present with elevated AST/ALT and jaundice. A liver biopsy is crucial to try to determine the dominant process, although frequently both conditions coexist. If the biopsy does reveal characteristic changes of GVHD, then immunosuppression should be targeted to this disease. It is extremely important that HBsAg-positive patients also be treated with an antiviral agent such as lamivudine, particularly if they are requiring increasing doses of immunosuppressive drugs, in order to prevent the development of fibrosing cholestatic hepatitis or fulminant hepatic failure during immunosuppression withdrawal [31,40]. Alternative antiviral drugs (adefovir dipivoxil [39,433], entecavir [434] and emtricitabine [435]) have also been shown to be effective in suppressing HBV replication. Lamivudine is continued for a minimum of 1-year post-HCT and not stopped until after all immunosuppressive drugs have been discontinued and full immunity has returned [40,103]. Once hepatic failure caused by HBV develops, only one-third of patients respond to lamivudine [436]; early lamivudine therapy in patients with progressive hepatitis B may prevent hepatic failure [437].

As discussed previously, patients at risk for HBV infection (usually patients who are HBsAg-positive prior to HCT) should receive prophylaxis with lamivudine [40,438]. In patients receiving lamivudine, rising levels of AST and ALT following HCT may indicate the development of HBV that has acquired lamivudine resistance. The presence of significant serum HBV viremia in this setting is highly suggestive of lamivudine resistance, although this can be confirmed by analysis of the HBV DNA polymerase genome for the presence of the typical YMDD mutation [439]. The clinical impact of these mutations remains to be determined, however, in one study of patients treated with lamivudine after liver transplantation, "breakthrough" hepatitis associated with a lamivudine-resistant mutant resulted in only mild elevations of ALT levels [440]. YMDD mutants have not been described in the setting of lamivudine use in HCT recipients. Alternative drugs include adefovir dipivoxil, which effectively suppresses HBV replication even in the setting of lamivudine resistance [441] and does not appear to lead to emergence of resistant virus when given for over 1 year [39,442]. Other drugs that can be used in this situation are tenofovir disoproxil [443] and entecavir [434].

Hepatitis C virus (HCV)

Post-HCT HCV infections may arise in three ways: progression of pre-HCT infection or acquisition from an HCV-infected hematopoietic cell donor [56] or, rarely now, HCV-infected blood-products [444]. If patients come to HCT with chronic hepatitis C, serum aminotransferases usually normalize and levels of viremia increase after conditioning therapy. Depending on the level of immunosuppression, an asymptomatic elevation of aminotransferases is commonly seen from days +60 to +120, and frequently coincides with the tapering of the immunosuppressive drugs used for GVHD prophylaxis [56,61,63,85,104,107]. Flares of GVHD can also be seen during this time and it may be difficult to decide whether a flare of hepatitis C or GVHD is responsible for elevated AST and ALT. The differentiation of these two disorders is crucial, as GVHD of the liver usually requires prompt immunosuppression to prevent progressive liver injury [358], while acute exacerbations of hepatitis C are self-limited and do not normally require specific therapy [61]. Unless there is evidence of active GVHD in other organs, a liver biopsy may be required before a therapeutic decision is made. Fulminant "immune-rebound" hepatitis C has been reported only rarely following HCT [104] and in these cases a hepatitic presentation of GVHD may have been responsible. The role of antiviral agents, such as ribavirin and IFN-α, has not been defined for treating recurrent hepatitis C at this time after HCT;

the potential for exacerbation of GVHD and depression of leukocyte and platelet counts dictates caution. In the future, treatment with an HCV-specific serine protease inhibitor may prove to be the treatment of choice [60].

After the initial hepatitis C flare following immune reconstitution, liver enzymes may again normalize but often settle into a pattern of chronic hepatitis that is seen in other patients with HCV infection [61,63,84,106]. Therapy directed at chronic HCV infection should be considered once the patient has ceased all immunosuppressive drugs and shows no evidence of active GVHD. The management of chronic HCV in long-term HCT survivors will be discussed below.

GB virus C

The RNA for GB virus C (also known as hepatitis G virus [HGV]) has been identified in the serum of 31–65% of HCT recipients [445–447]. This is not surprising, considering the high rate of infection in volunteer blood donors and the requirement for multiple blood transfusions during HCT. As in the non-HCT population [283], this agent does not appear to have a role in either acute or chronic liver disease after HCT [445–448], but an association with aplastic anaemia has been reported [449].

Transfusion-transmitted virus (TTV)

Like GB virus C, the prevalence of TTV has been found to be very high in HCT recipients [450]. While there is evidence that certain genotypes may be associated with clinical hepatitis, TTV does not appear to be a cause of liver injury following HCT.

Fungal infections (see also Chapter 52)

Candida species are by far the most common cause of fungal abscesses in the liver [23], but the widespread use of antifungal prophylaxis through day +75 has dramatically reduced the incidence of infections with most *Candida* species. A recent autopsy survey showed almost complete absence of candidal liver infection in patients who received prophylactic fluconazole compared to a 14% prevalence in those who did not [451]. However, infections with *C. krusei* and *Torulopsis glabrata* are still seen [452]. Aspergillosis may involve the liver but is usually associated with clinically apparent infection at other sites, particularly the lungs [23,451,453]. Disseminated infection, often with liver involvement, has been described with a wide range of other fungi, including *Scopulariopsis*, *Trichosporon*, *Pseudallescheria*, *Corniothyrium*, *Fusarium*, *Mucor*, *Absidia* and *Dactylaria* species (see Chapter 52) [23,453].

The signs and symptoms of fungi in the liver are fever, tender hepatomegaly and increased serum alkaline phosphatase levels [20,23]. However, these findings are also common to many liver diseases after HCT. A case-control study performed at autopsy found that patients with and without fungal infection had clinical and laboratory findings during the last weeks of life that were indistinguishable from one another [23]. Diagnosis was further obscured by the insensitivity of imaging tests (18% for CT scan or ultrasound) for small, miliary fungal lesions typically found in HCT patients. MRI may be more sensitive for small fungal lesions [22]. Rarely, fungi can invade vascular structures, resulting in hepatic infarcts or venous obstruction mimicking SOS. Massed fungi causing bile duct obstruction have also been described [454,455], but these presentations have become rare since the advent of fluconazole prophylaxis. The diagnosis of fungal liver infection in a patient with a negative imaging test is largely based on a consistent clinical picture in a patient who had past risk factors (positive blood culture, colonization, severe liver dysfunction) [23]. Confirmation of invasive liver disease is usually not indicated in a patient with evidence of fungal disease in other organs, but liver biopsy with special stains and culture may occasionally be required if the liver is the only accessible site. Patients with visceral fungal infections have traditionally been treated with intravenous amphotericin, although agents such as voriconazole [26] or caspofungin [27,456] may be as effective and associated with less toxicity. Treatment courses may need to be protracted in immunosuppressed patients with visceral fungal infection [457,458]. Restoration of granulocyte counts is the single most important factor in recovery from fungal liver infection. However, smaller size of fungal lesions on liver imaging does not assure that the fungi have been eliminated. For example, patients have been observed whose signs and symptoms of candidal liver infection resolved on amphotericin, only to be reactivated months later when prednisone was given for chronic GVHD.

Bacterial infections (see Chapter 51)

In HCT patients, fevers of undetermined origin and bacteremias are rapidly treated with antibiotics. Probably for this reason, bacterial liver abscesses are rarely seen. Reactivation of latent mycobacterial infection within the liver may occur with prolonged immunosuppressive therapy [459]. Disseminated Bacillus Calmette-Guérin (BCG) infection with marrow, liver and spleen involvement has been reported post-HCT [459,460]. Diagnosis of mycobacterial liver infection requires liver biopsy, cultures and the appropriate stains.

Gallbladder and biliary disease

Biliary sludge syndrome

Biliary sludge, a mixture of bile and soft particulate matter of less than 2 mm diameter, can be demonstrated by ultrasound as low amplitude echogenic material without acoustic shadowing that layers in the gallbladder and shifts with positioning [461]. In HCT recipients conditioned with myeloablative regimens, biliary sludge formation is common, documented by ultrasound in approximately 70% of patients followed prospectively and found at autopsy in 100% of patients [462–464]. The composition of sludge after HCT is not cholesterol, but mostly calcium bilirubinate [465]. Risk factors for sludge formation after HCT include prolonged fasting and TPN [466], ceftriaxone treatment, the administration of narcotics and possibly epithelial injury from conditioning therapy or GVHD. Biliary sludge in HCT patients is usually asymptomatic [462]. However, a distinct biliary sludge syndrome has been described in which patients develop epigastric pain, nausea and abnormal serum liver enzymes when starting oral intake after a period of fasting and TPN. Although sludge can cause biliary obstruction and dilation of the common bile duct [404], most patients recover after a few days of discomfort as bile flow flushes the sand-like material into the duodenum. Endoscopic papillotomy is rarely indicated. Stimulation of maximal bile flow is achieved with oral feedings, use of oral ursodiol, 12–15 mg/kg/day, and avoidance of opioids that increase sphincter pressure. Biliary sludge may be a cause of acute "acalculous" cholecystitis [467], acute pancreatitis [464,468] and may result in nonvisualization of the gallbladder on scintigraphy [462]. Acute bacterial cholangitis due to biliary sludge has also been reported [469]. Disappearance of gallbladder sludge may parallel clinical improvement in patients with hepatic GVHD [470], but it is not known if the presence of biliary sludge exacerbates the cholestasis associated with GVHD.

Disorders of the gallbladder

Acute cholecystitis is uncommonly seen in HCT recipients [462] and, when it does occur, it is frequently not associated with the presence of gallstones [471,472]. "Acalculous" cholecystitis in this setting may be due to leukemic relapse with gallbladder involvement [473], CMV [474] or fungal [475] infection, or biliary sludge. Patients experience right upper quadrant pain and tenderness but may not have associated manifestations such as nausea, vomiting, hyperbilirubinemia, or leukocytosis [472]. Diagnosis is difficult because of the high frequency of gallbladder abnormalities on biliary sonography following HCT [462,472]. Sonographic evidence of pericholecystic fluid, gallbladder wall necrosis, or a localized tenderness when the transducer is pressed over the gallbladder, suggest cholecystitis. If these findings are absent, a radionuclide bile excretion study (HIDA or DECIDA) with morphine infusion can be useful; nonvisualization of the gallbladder suggests cholecystitis [476]. Patients with suspected cholecystitis should be managed with laparoscopic cholecystectomy unless gangrene or perforation is present [477].

Extrahepatic biliary obstruction

Among 7412 consecutive patients receiving marrow HCTs at two institutions, only nine cases (0.12%) of extrahepatic biliary obstruction were identified [404]. This series excluded patients with transient biliary dilation caused by the passage of gallbladder sludge. Causes of obstruction after HCT include lymphoblastic infiltration of the common bile duct and gallbladder in Epstein–Barr virus (EBV) lymphoproliferative disease; CMV-related biliary disease, which may include diffuse strictures of the intra- and extrahepatic ducts or localized obstruction at the ampulla of Vater [403]; dissecting duodenal hematoma complicating endoscopic biopsy; inspissated biliary sludge in the distal common bile duct; and leukemic relapse (chloroma) in the head of pancreas and distal common bile duct [478]. In HCT recipients, it is impossible to distinguish between extrahepatic biliary obstruction and the much more common causes of cholestatic liver disease on clinical and laboratory grounds alone. Thus, ultrasound examination of the gallbladder to exclude bile duct dilation is recommended in any HCT recipient with progressive cholestasis, as biliary decompression will be required if extrahepatic biliary obstruction is identified.

Malignant disorders

EBV-associated lymphoproliferative disorder (see Chapter 56)

EBV-associated lymphoproliferative disorder is most commonly seen in allogeneic HCT recipients, with the highest incidence (up to 25%) in recipients of HLA-mismatched T-cell-depleted grafts [479,480] and in recipients of potent anti-T-cell therapies. It is rarely seen after autologous HCT [481]. The median time to onset is around 70–80 days after HCT and patients commonly present with fever, anorexia, abdominal pain and lymphadenopathy. Liver involvement occurs in over 50%, manifest by abnormal serum alkaline phosphatase and massive hepatosplenomegaly. Diagnosis is usually made by biopsy of involved organs such as lymph nodes, gastrointestinal tract or liver. Liver biopsy typically reveals a portal inflammatory cell infiltrate comprising a mixture of small round lymphocytes, plasmacytic lymphocytes and immunoblasts [479]. Bile duct damage and disruption of the limiting plate may be seen. Confirmatory studies include *in situ* hybridization and immunohistochemistry for EBV-specific markers. Therapeutic options are discussed in the Abdominal pain section, below, and in more detail in Chapters 56 and 70, including therapy based on PCR methods for detection of EBV DNA in blood before tissue invasion by transformed immunoblasts.

Recurrent malignancy

Recurrent cancer in patients transplanted for hematologic malignancy or solid tumors may present within the 1st post-HCT year with abnormal liver enzymes, hepatomegaly or abnormal imaging studies. In the absence of disease elsewhere, fine needle aspiration or needle biopsy will usually be required for definitive diagnosis.

Nodular regenerative hyperplasia (NRH)

NRH is a rare cause of portal hypertension and ascites after either HCT, solid organ transplantation, 6-thioguanine or systemic chemotherapy. In HCT recipients, the clinical presentation is usually after day +100, and it should not be confused with SOS. Histologic evidence of NRH is more common than clinically apparent disease, occurring in 22.5% of a series of 103 marrow HCT patients having liver biopsy or autopsy prior to day 100 [482]. Other investigators see a much lower prevalence of NRH [114,158]. In this setting, NRH most likely represents a histologic endpoint of intrahepatic vascular damage related to cytoreductive therapy [483]. Imaging with MRI, CT or ultrasound may be unremarkable or may reveal multiple small liver lesions that can be confused with metastatic malignancy or fungal abscesses [484]. Needle biopsy of the liver may be normal (frequently wedge biopsy is required for definitive diagnosis) or may show characteristic regenerative hepatocellular nodules on reticulin stain without significant fibrosis [482]. Portal decompression may be required.

Idiopathic hyperammonemia and coma

A syndrome of hyperammonemia and coma, in the absence of severe liver dysfunction, has been described in patients who received high-dose chemotherapy, including conditioning for HCT [485–489]. Patients present with progressive lethargy, confusion, weakness, incoordination, vomiting and hyperventilation. The diagnosis is confirmed when the plasma ammonia exceeds 200 μmol/L and there is no evidence of liver failure. The syndrome is rare, being identified in 0.5% of HCT recipients in a recent series [488], but is associated with a high mortality. The pathogenesis is probably multifactorial, with contributions from a hypercatabolic state related to chemotherapy, sepsis and corticosteroids; high exogenous nitrogen, from TPN, intestinal bleeding and constipation; renal impairment; ammonia-producing metabolites of chemotherapeutic drugs; and, in some cases, inherited defects of urea cycle enzymes [488,490,491]. Rapid recognition and treatment may lead to a favorable outcome [488,489]. Management should focus on limiting exogenous nitrogen loads by withholding TPN and controlling intestinal bleeding, reducing the ammonia level by hemodialysis and ammonia-trapping therapy (intravenous sodium benzoate or sodium phenylacetate) [488].

Gastrointestinal bleeding

Severe gastrointestinal bleeding is infrequent after autologous HCT (incidence <1%) and increasingly uncommon after allogeneic HCT (incidence <2%) [492–494]. Bleeding that is either occult or does not require transfusion is considerably more common, particularly when platelet counts are low [492,493]. The incidence of severe bleeding has fallen over the past decade, largely because of more effective prophylaxis against viruses, fungi and acute GVHD [494]. Mortality from severe intestinal bleeding in HCT recipients, however, has remained around 40% [494].

Mucosal trauma from retching

Retching and vomiting during conditioning therapy, formerly a common cause of bleeding, have been controlled with serotonin antagonist drugs and other antiemetics. Nonetheless, mucosal trauma to the mid-body of the stomach caused by retching is the most common cause of "coffee-ground" emesis following conditioning therapy [132]. More severe bleeding results from Mallory–Weiss tears at the gastroesophageal junction and intramural esophageal hematomas, especially when platelet counts are <35,000/mm^3 [492]. Persistent nausea and vomiting from day 15–60 is usually caused by acute GVHD, CMV infection of the upper gut, or, in patients who have not received antiviral prophylaxis, HSV esophagitis [128,131,132,140]. Endoscopic control of bleeding due to mucosal trauma from retching is seldom needed, as bleeding usually ceases when platelet counts are brought to >60,000/mm^3. Intramural hematomas of the esophagus resolve in 7–14 days and do not require surgery.

Mucosal necrosis caused by conditioning therapy

Occult intestinal bleeding is common after conditioning regimens that cause extensive mucosal necrosis; for example, cytarabine-containing regimens, high-dose melphalan, or multiple alkylating agents (BU-melphalan-thiotepa). Massive bleeding can occur when there is involvement of intestinal mucosa with tumor, where tumor lysis leads to ulcerated mucosa. If severe bleeding occurs in a patient with musocal tumor, an urgent radionuclide blood pool scan should be performed to localize the site of bleeding to guide radiological or surgical therapy.

Esophageal, gastric and duodenal ulcers

Ulcers present in the esophagus, stomach and duodenum before HCT may bleed profusely when platelet counts fall after conditioning therapy, particularly if the ulcer has exposed submucosal blood vessels. These "visible vessels" can lead to exsanguination even when platelet counts are normal. Attempts at endoscopic hemostasis with coagulation, heater probe, or injection therapy are usually futile if patients remain thrombocytopenic. Thus, an endoscopic finding of a visible vessel in a thrombocytopenic patient is an indication for urgent surgery. A similar ulcerating lesion can be seen at the site of mucosal metastasis or chloroma after myeloablative therapy has destroyed tumor cells.

After HCT, patients may develop esophagitis caused by the reflux of acid-peptic juice into the esophagus, an infection, or acute GVHD [128,132,495]. Esophageal infection is now rare [128]. Bleeding from diffuse esophagitis is usually responsive to platelet infusions and control of peptic reflux with proton pump inhibitors such as omeprazole, lansoprazole, or pantoprazole. H_2 receptor antagonists should not be used in this setting because they depress granulocyte production [496,497]. Proton pump inhibitors are very effective in blunting gastric acid production but may lead to colonization of the upper intestine with bacteria and fungi. In contrast to diffuse peptic esophagitis, deep esophageal ulcers caused by HSV or CMV esophagitis may bleed profusely, particularly when platelet counts are low [494].

Ulcers in the stomach and duodenum that develop after HCT are usually caused by acute GVHD or CMV infection [130,140]. Gastroduodenal ulcers caused by CMV can be deep and cause severe bleeding, but since the advent of methods to detect and treat CMV viremia, bleeding CMV ulcers have become uncommon [494]. The commonest causes of gastroduodenal ulceration in the general population, *H. pylori* infection and the use of nonsteroidal anti-inflammatory drugs (NSAIDs), are almost nonexistent after HCT. Rarely, gastric ulcerations are caused by VZV infection, bacterial infection with oropharyngeal flora (phlegmonous gastritis) or by EBV lymphoproliferative disease [143–145]. Endoscopic hemostasis of persistently bleeding gastroduodenal ulcers should be undertaken if platelet counts can be kept >50,000/mm³ for 7–10 days.

Intestinal mucosal infection

As noted in the Diarrhea and Abdominal pain sections, most intestinal infections in HCT patients do not cause extensive mucosal necrosis or severe bleeding. Exceptions are ulcerations caused by CMV, some adenovirus genotypes, some *Rotavirus* species, and clostridial infections (especially *C. septicum*) [402,405,406,494,498–502]. There is no effective therapy for mucosa that is diffusely oozing blood other than raising the platelet count and treating the underlying infection. CMV enteritis, while usually diffuse, can present with focal ulcers or segments of ischemic necrosis that bleed [503]; isolated CMV ulcers that bled have been resected successfully [498,504]. *Candida*, *Aspergillus* and *Rhizopus* infections in the intestine rarely may erode into submucosal blood vessels [505–507]. Prophylaxis with fluconazole has almost entirely eliminated bleeding candidal lesions in the gut [494]. Intestinal ischemic necrosis with severe bleeding and infarction has occurred following *Aspergillus* infiltration of intestinal blood vessels and CMV infection of vascular endothelium [503,508].

Acute GVHD

Prospective studies of severe intestinal bleeding in the 1980s and 1990s showed that intestinal GVHD was the most common cause of severe bleeding in both of these time periods, but the frequency of GVHD as a cause of bleeding had declined from 5.8% to 1.2% [494]. Patients who received HLA-mismatched or unrelated donor grafts comprise about half of all patients with severe bleeding [494]. Bleeding in patients with acute GVHD is usually from extensive areas of mucosal ulceration in the small intestine and cecum [498]. There may be hemorrhagic necrosis of the entire mucosa from esophagus to rectum, resulting in exsanguinating hemorrhage when platelet counts fall below 50,000/mm³. In some patients, bleeding may appear to be coming from specific areas of the mucosa, but when such patients are operated or come to autopsy, diffuse rather than focal mucosal ulceration is the rule [498]. Focal bleeding lesions may also occur when infection with CMV or fungus develops in intestinal mucosa already affected by GVHD, but such superinfections have become increasingly uncommon [494]. The diagnosis of acute GVHD in patients with high-volume diarrhea and bleeding is usually obvious because of skin and liver involvement, but the exact site and nature of the intestinal lesions that are bleeding are often uncertain.

Management of severe bleeding in a patient with acute GVHD is difficult even though bleeding is usually emanating from mucosal capillaries and venules rather than from a submucosal artery. Correcting platelet and coagulation abnormalities may slow the bleeding. Immunosuppressive therapy will limit the extent of apoptosis of epithelial cells, but reepithelialization of the intestinal mucosa affected by GVHD is very slow. If bleeding persists, it is useful to consider bleeding lesions other than GVHD (using mucosal biopsy to rule out vascular esctasia, CMV ulcers, and esophageal infections, for example) and to determine whether the bleeding is coming from a single focus by using endoscopy and technetium radionuclide blood pool scans [99]. Focal lesions can be treated with endoscopic cautery, heater probe or epinephrine intramucosal injection provided platelet counts are adequate. These forms of therapy destroy tissue and lead to ulcers 0.5–2.0 cm in size within a few days. Unless the underlying disease process is eliminated, these endoscopic methods will not cure the bleeding problem. Attempts to resect large segments of diffusely bleeding intestine involved with GVHD have not been successful [498]. Temporary control of GVHD bleeding has been achieved with angiographic embolization of mesenteric blood vessels only rarely.

Gastric antral vascular ectasia (GAVE) and dieulafoy lesion

GAVE is a recently recognized cause of severe upper intestinal bleeding in HCT recipients [509,510]. At endoscopy, diffuse areas of hemorrhage are seen in the gastric antrum and proximal duodenum, but the underlying mucosa appears intact. Similar vascular ectasias can be found throughout the intestinal tract, but they are most prominent in the antrum. Mucosal biopsy is diagnostic, revealing abnormal dilated capillaries, thromboses in these capillaries and fibromuscular hyperplasia in the lamina propria [510]. The cause is not known, but associations with hepatic sinusoidal injury, male gender, and use of BU and growth factors have been noted. Endoscopic laser therapy is the treatment of choice to control bleeding, but multiple laser treatments may be required to obliterate ectatic lesions. One case of bleeding from a Dieulafoy lesion (a vascular malformation in the body of the stomach that becomes ulcerated) has been described [494].

Iatrogenic causes of bleeding

Endoscopic biopsy of duodenal mucosa is often needed to confirm diagnoses of GVHD and mucosal infections, but the incidence of significant bleeding (nonhealing ulceration and intramural hematoma) at the sites of duodenal biopsy is unacceptably high [132,404,511]. Duodenal biopsies should be undertaken with caution, particularly in patients with GVHD; gastric biopsies are a more useful site with fewer complications [130]. When performing endoscopic biopsies, platelet counts should be over 60,000/mm^3 at the time of biopsy and maintained at that level for 3–5 days afterwards.

Dysphagia

Infections of the esophagus, formerly the most common cause of difficulty swallowing, have largely disappeared because of prophylaxis with antiviral and antifungal drugs. Mucositis, acid-peptic esophagitis and pill esophagitis are currently the leading causes of dysphagia.

Mucositis

Painful desquamation of the oral and pharyngeal epithelium caused by conditioning therapy may lead to transfer dysphagia if the mucositis is severe. Patients who have severe mucositis complain of pain on initiating a swallow and cannot move a bolus past the esophageal inlet. Extensive edema of tissues at and above the level of the cricopharyngeal muscle may be seen at endoscopy. Edema and hemorrhage may also involve hypopharyngeal and supraglottic parts of the airway, at times necessitating endotracheal intubation [512,513]. Edema and necrosis of esophageal epithelium have been described as a toxicity of conditioning therapy, resulting in persistent nonhealing ulcerations and dysphagia, but this is not common. Severe mucositis has been implicated in the development of esophageal strictures in two autologous marrow recipients [514]. HSV infections and MTX may contribute to mucositis in the HCT setting [122].

Intramural hematomas

The abrupt onset of severe retrosternal pain, hematemesis and painful swallowing suggests development of a hematoma in the wall of the esophagus [515–517]. Esophageal hematomas can occur after retching or spontaneously, particularly when platelet counts are very low or when patients are over-anticoagulated. Effective antiemetic medication during conditioning therapy has almost eliminated this complication. The diagnosis can be confirmed by an esophageal X-ray with swallowed contrast material (water-soluble contrast at first, then barium if there is no evidence of perforation into the mediastinum) and by a CT scan showing a thickened esophageal wall [517–519]. Total esophageal obstruction may be seen. Endoscopy is relatively contraindicated, as many intramural hematomas represent contained perforations that can be converted into complete perforations by insufflation of air [520]. The course of intramural hematomas in HCT patients is one of slow resolution over 1–2 weeks. Surgery is not necessary unless there is persistent bleeding [521].

Esophageal infections

Esophagitis caused by fungi, herpesviruses and bacteria in HCT patients usually present with nausea, vomiting, malaise, and fever, rather than the abrupt onset of dysphagia.

Fungal infections of the esophagus, now unusual because of prophylaxis with fluconazole [522], were largely due to *C. albicans* and occurred during the period of granulocytopenia following conditioning therapy [139]. Patients receiving prophylaxis with fluconazole may become colonized with fungi that are resistant (e.g. nonalbicans *Candida* [523] and *Aspergillus* [524] species), but esophageal infection with these fungi remains uncommon in the HCT setting. In the granulocytopenic patient, creamy adherent plaques typical of candidiasis are absent. Diagnosis depends on demonstrating branching hyphae or large numbers of yeast forms in material obtained by brushings or biopsies of esophageal lesions [141]. Cultures are not useful for diagnosis as they do not differentiate colonization from tissue infection, but they can be useful in guiding therapy [457]. During periods of granulocytopenia, treatment with an intravenous antifungal drug is indicated [457]. If granulocyte counts are >1000/mm^3 and there are no symptoms of systemic fungal infection, oral fluconazole (100–200 mg daily) is the treatment of choice. Seemingly superficial candidal infections of the mouth and esophagus should not be undertreated in HCT patients, as swallowed yeast forms of Candida readily gain access to the portal venous circulation even through the normal small intestine [525]. Visceral Candida infections after HCT are usually preceded by evidence of superficial mucosal infection and positive blood cultures [23,526,527].

Viruses that infect the esophagus after HCT are HSV, CMV and, rarely, VZV [141]. Before the routine use of antiviral prophylaxis, these infections usually appeared after day 40. Nausea and vomiting are the most common presenting symptoms, but some patients have heartburn, painful swallowing and severe retrosternal pain [128,132,140]. HSV causes small 1–2 mm vesicles in the squamous epithelium of the mid- and distal esophagus [528,529]. HSV-infected epithelial cells slough off, leaving ulcers with reddened, raised borders [528]. With extensive infection, ulcers may coalesce to form large areas of denuded epithelium. As HSV infects only squamous epithelial cells in the esophagus, brushings and biopsy specimens must sample the edges and not the center of ulcers. HSV is identified by typical multinucleate cells with intranuclear inclusions, by immunohistology showing specific staining of inclusions using monoclonal antibodies to HSV antigens, and by viral culture [141]. The diagnosis can be made by endoscopic brushings alone if low platelet counts preclude biopsy. If the epithelium of the entire esophagus has been sloughed because of HSV infection, the diagnosis can be difficult, as no infected squamous cells remain except at the proximal margin of the ulcer and possibly in residual islands of squamous epithelium within the ulcer. Intravenous acyclovir or oral valacyclovir are effective in eliminating virus, but large ulcers may heal slowly [530]. HSV isolates resistant to acyclovir are usually responsive to foscarnet [390]. VZV may produce a clinical and endoscopic picture identical to HSV esophagitis, but there is usually evidence of disseminated VZV infection in the skin and other viscera [531]. Immunohistology of infected epithelial cells will differentiate HSV from VZV in the esophagus. CMV esophagitis differs from HSV and VZV infection in several respects. CMV never infects squamous epithelium but involves endothelial cells and fibroblasts in the submucosal tissues of the esophagus [532,533]. In most cases, CMV infection is systemic, not limited to the esophagus, but there are patients whose intestinal tract is the only site where CMV is found (blood tests for CMV antigen and DNA are negative). The endoscopic appearance is of shallow, serpiginous ulcers with erythematous borders in the distal and mid-esophagus. Ulcers can be large, extending over 10–12 cm of the esophagus, but some normal appearing epithelium is usually visible. Biopsies must be obtained from the ulcer crater, a technique which requires platelet counts >60,000/mm^3 to avoid bleeding. Diagnosis of CMV is best made by placing biopsy material into veal infusion broth for transport to the virology laboratory [533]. Shell-vial centrifugation culture methods provide rapid (24 h) results. Use of standard viral tissue culture for CMV is as accurate as centrifugation culture methods but results are not available as promptly. CMV can also be identified by typical amphophilic intranuclear and intracytoplasmic inclusions in large submucosal cells. Immunohistology using antibodies to early and intermediate CMV antigens and *in situ* DNA hybridization are more sensitive than routine staining since these methods identify infected cells that are neither megaloid nor inclusion bearing [533]. Viral culture methods are about twice as sensitive as immunohistologic methods. Ganciclovir is effective in eliminating CMV from esophageal ulcers, but ulcers are slow to heal and symptoms may persist for weeks [140]. Intravenous ganciclovir is given for 2 weeks at high dose (5 mg/kg twice daily or until clearing of CMV from the bloodstream) and then for 2 or more weeks at a maintenance dose. Foscarnet is an effective alternative therapy [534].

Bacterial esophagitis usually occurs as part of a mixed infection with fungi or viruses in patients with poor marrow function [139,142]. The organisms are usually polymicrobial, derived from the oral flora. Diagnosis is made by finding large numbers of bacteria admixed with necrotic epithelial cells in biopsy specimens stained by tissue Gram stain. Drugs that suppress gastric acid production to low levels (e.g. proton pump inhibitors) lead to bacterial and fungal colonization of the upper gut and may predispose patients to bacterial esophagitis [535,536].

Acute GVHD

The esophagus may be involved with a desquamative process in patients with severe acute GVHD. At endoscopy, there is tissue edema, erythema and a peeling of the squamous epithelium, leaving ulcerations [495]. Biopsy specimens show apoptosis of basal cells and desquamation of epithelium [495,537]. Ulcerations in the distal esophagus may be worsened by continued reflux of gastric contents and may become secondarily infected with bacteria and fungi. Esophageal desquamation, fibrosis and strictures can also be seen in patients with chronic GVHD (see the Problems in long-term survivors of HCT section, below).

Acid-peptic esophagitis

Retrosternal discomfort is the most common symptom of reflux esophagitis, but less common symptoms can dominate the clinical picture after HCT; for example, hiccoughs, hoarseness, water brash, persistent coughing and bronchospasm. Factors contributing to reflux esophagitis after HCT include gastric stasis, the recumbent position and poor salivary bicarbonate flow due to both oral mucositis and acute GVHD. As ulcerations heal slowly, patients with esophageal infection may complain of symptoms related to reflux even when the infection has been eliminated [140]. Treatment of reflux with head-of-bed elevation and proton pump inhibitor medication is effective in relieving esophageal symptoms caused by reflux. Prolonged use of proton pump inhibitors, however, may lead to bacterial and fungal colonization of the upper aerodigestive system. Development of peptic strictures after HCT is rare.

Pill esophagitis

Pills commonly lodge in the esophagus, particularly when taken before sleep with too little water. Some pills cause esophageal damage when taken over a period of days to weeks, and the damage can be severe, resulting in ulceration, edema and perforation [141]. HCT patients are not likely to be ingesting the most dangerous of these pills, but esophagitis has been described with medications that might be used in a HCT setting; for example, phenytoin (dilantin), foscarnet, captopril, quinidine, oral bisphosphonates such as alendronate, ascorbic acid, ciprofloxacin, clindamycin, doxycycline, tetracycline and oral potassium chloride [538]. Dysphagia is the most prominent symptom of pill esophagitis. Endoscopy reveals ulceration with surrounding inflammation, which may be confused with infection. Discontinuation of the offending medication usually leads to complete healing.

Diarrhea

Diarrhea caused by intestinal mucosal damage from myeloablative conditioning therapy is a common complaint in the first few weeks after HCT. Acute GVHD is the most common cause of diarrhea after day +15. In allograft recipients, infectious causes of diarrhea are less common than GVHD. Multiple etiologies for diarrhea may coexist.

Toxicity from the conditioning regimen

Diarrhea in the first few days after HCT is nearly always due to toxicity to the intestinal mucosa and is usually accompanied by anorexia. Histologic findings after high-dose chemoradiotherapy include mucosal crypt aberrations with nuclear atypia, epithelial flattening and cell degeneration [124]. The surface epithelium and villous architecture of the small intestine are also distorted. This mucosal injury results in net fluid secretion by the intestine, peaking 1–2 weeks after the start of conditioning and usually returning to normal by day +12 to day +15 [124,539]. Attempts to use tube feedings or glutamine supplements to lessen the intestinal impact of high-dose conditioning therapy have yielded equivocal data [540–543]. Some regimens produce more intestinal necrosis and more severe, prolonged diarrhea than others, for example, cytarabine-containing regimens, high-dose melphalan and the BU/melphalan/thioTEPA regimen [127,544]. Some patients have more severe enteritis than others despite identical doses of chemotherapy drugs, which is possibly related to variation in the metabolism of these drugs and exposure to higher doses of toxic metabolites [86,545–547]. Other clinical consequences of more severe intestinal damage include persistent fever, abdominal pain, pseudo-obstruction and inability to eat. After most conditioning regimens, mucosal regeneration is complete by day +15 to day +20 provided acute intestinal GVHD or enteric infection does not supervene [124]. If patients have persistent intestinal symptoms and diarrhea after day +15 to day +20, biopsy of colonic mucosa can be useful in assessing whether mucosal regeneration is underway, or whether unsuspected GVHD or infection is present. In some patients with unexpectedly severe enteritis, there may be an absence of regenerating epithelial cells in biopsy specimens taken at day +25 to day +30, suggesting that the conditioning therapy has destroyed epithelial stem cells or that stimuli for epithelial regeneration are absent. Intravenous infusion of octreotide may be effective in patients with severe diarrhea associated with regimen-related toxicity [548,549]. Loperamide at maximum doses of 4 mg orally every 6 hours is also effective [550], but opioid medications must be used cautiously because they may cause colonic pseudo-obstruction or narcotic bowel syndrome (see the Abdominal pain section, below). Opioid/anticholinergic drug combinations, for example, Lomotil, are contraindicated in this setting.

Acute GVHD

Diarrhea is more frequent after allogeneic HCT than after autologous HCT, and GVHD is the most common cause of diarrhea [363,551,552]. The onset of diarrhea can be sudden. Large-volume, secretory diarrhea is characteristic, i.e. watery diarrhea that persists even when there is no oral intake. The diarrheal fluid is watery, green in color, with ropy strands of mucoid material that reflect transmucosal protein loss [553]. There is a rough correlation between the volume of diarrhea, the extent of intestinal involvement, and the severity of abdominal pain, nausea and vomiting. In an allografted patient with skin and liver abnormalities typical of acute GVHD, the diarrheal syndrome described above is almost diagnostic of intestinal GVHD. Supporting evidence for GVHD comes from a falling serum albumin level (from gut protein loss) and negative stool studies for organisms that cause enteritis [551,552]. In countries where intestinal parasitism and bacterial contamination of the water supply are common, the spectrum of infectious causes of diarrhea may be wider than in developed countries [6,554]. CMV is the only common cause of enteritis after HCT that requires an intestinal biopsy for diagnosis [551]. If a CMV-seropositive patient who is not receiving prophylactic ganciclovir develops diarrhea, an intestinal biopsy may be needed to differentiate GVHD from CMV enteritis [555]. Otherwise the predictive value of a negative stool examination for other viruses, bacteria, fungi and parasites is high [551].

Occasionally X-rays of the abdomen are useful, not so much to determine whether or not GVHD is present, but to ascertain the extent of involvement. Abdominal plain X-rays, ultrasound, CT and MRI scans may reveal edema of the intestinal wall, but these findings are usually nonspecific and do not help to differentiate between infection and acute intestinal GVHD [556–560]. Technetium-labeled white cell scans may be abnormal in acute GVHD but they are also not specific [561]. Barium studies of the stomach and small bowel show bowel wall thickening with effacement of mucosal folds, excess luminal fluid and rapid transit [562,563]. Pneumatosis intestinalis, which may be associated with GVHD or CMV enteritis, may also be seen by plain X-ray, CT or MRI [564–568]. Pneumatosis intestinalis in patients with GVHD or CMV enteritis does not confer a worse prognosis, in contrast to pneumatosis that occurs after intestinal ischemia or clostridial infection.

A definitive diagnosis of GVHD in problematic cases usually requires gastrointestinal biopsy. Although the yield from mucosal biopsy is higher with gastric than either duodenal or rectal biopsies [129,130,551,569], sigmoidoscopic rectal biopsy is easier, quicker and less costly than upper endoscopic biopsy. When nausea and vomiting are present, gastric rather than rectal biopsies are indicated to rule out infection and other upper gastrointestinal pathology. In mild cases of intestinal GVHD, gastroduodenal and rectosigmoid mucosa appear grossly normal, but moderately severe GVHD causes diffusely edematous and erythematous mucosa. Severe GVHD may lead to ulcerations and large areas of mucosal sloughing in the stomach, small intestine and colon [130,498,570]. Even when the gross appearance is normal, gastrointestinal biopsies often reveal intestinal crypt cell necrosis and apoptotic bodies diagnostic of acute GVHD [124,129,130,135,571]. Biopsies that contain no epithelial cells present difficulties for the pathologist, as the hallmark of GVHD is epithelial cell apoptosis.

The pathogenesis of diarrhea in patients with GVHD involves several mechanisms. First, the areas of the intestine most affected by GVHD, the ileum and cecum [562], are the segments most involved with retrieval of fluid from the intestinal lumen. A defect in fluid absorption in these areas leads to higher volumes of diarrhea than an absorption defect in the upper intestine or distal colon. Second, the abrupt onset of diarrhea is associated more with mucosal edema than with crypt cell necrosis. It is likely that abrupt protein-losing diarrhea and intestinal edema are caused by local release of cytokines that cause increases in vascular permeability and increased flux of fluid across paracellular pores [572–574]. Third, there is ongoing crypt cell necrosis caused by alloimmune cytotoxic T lymphocytes in acute GVHD [575]. Electron microscopy of rectal mucosa in acute GVHD shows T cells extending pseudopods toward the nuclear membranes of epithelial cells [576]. Crypt cells disintegrate in the process of apoptosis [124]. In severe cases of GVHD, whole crypts are destroyed, then adjacent crypts and, finally, whole segments of intestinal mucosa [498,577]. Ropy material comprising necrotic intestinal epithelial cells may be passed per rectum [577,578]. Intestinal bleeding often accompanies diarrhea in patients with severe GVHD that has resulted in mucosal ulceration [492,494].

Successful treatment of acute GVHD with immunosuppressive therapy results in a dramatic reduction in stool volume, with resolution of accompanying symptoms of abdominal pain, nausea and vomiting. The drugs and biologicals that are used for initial treatment of acute GVHD are discussed in Chapters 16 and 50. The management of patients whose diarrhea and other symptoms of intestinal GVHD persist after 7–14 days of immunosuppressive therapy is unsatisfactory, as the rate of failure of secondary therapy can be as high as 50% [364]. Octreotide, a somatostatin analog that inhibits fluid secretion, enhances sodium and chloride absorption and decreases motility, has been reported to reduce stool volume in patients with mild to moderate intestinal GVHD [579,580]. However, octreotide infusions are ineffective in patients with severe GVHD who have failed high-dose corticosteroid therapy [581]. Mu-opioid antidiarrheal medications should be used cautiously during the edematous phase of acute GVHD, as these drugs may cause ileus and painful abdominal distention from intestinal pseudo-obstruction. If the bowel is extensively denuded of mucosa during the GVHD process, epithelial regeneration and recovery may not be possible, despite subsequent control of the GVHD [498,582]. The failure of intestinal epithelial regeneration in patients whose mucosa has been denuded by GVHD stands in contrast to the rapid recovery of epithelium following high-dose conditioning therapy [124], suggesting that intestinal epithelial stem cells (which lie at the base of crypts) have been destroyed in acute GVHD. Patients with acute GVHD who can tolerate small amounts of food should be encouraged to eat, as luminal nutrients are the major stimuli for epithelial regeneration and supply metabolic fuel to mucosal cells (polyamines for small intestinal mucosa and short chain fatty acids for colonic mucosa) [583].

Enteric infections

Two large prospective studies have found that diarrhea was common after day +20 (affecting about 40% of patients) but that infection as a cause of diarrhea was uncommon, accounting for only 10–15% of diarrheal episodes [551,552]. In these studies, the organisms responsible for diarrhea were viruses (astrovirus, adenovirus, rotavirus, CMV) and bacteria (*C. difficile* and *Aeromonas*). With the exception of CMV infection and possibly adenovirus, almost all intestinal infections can be prevented by a program of handwashing by visitors and medical personnel and by avoidance of food that may contain pathogens. In countries where intestinal parasites and pathogens are endemic, there may be a wide range of diarrhea-causing infectious agents [6]. Patients with acute GVHD may be at higher risk for enteric infection due to the immunologic abnormalities associated with GVHD, immunosuppressive therapy used to treat GVHD and exposure to nosocomial pathogens during prolonged hospitalization [396,584]. In one case, *Salmonella* enteritis mimicked the presentation of acute intestinal GVHD [554].

The incidence of gastrointestinal infection with CMV has declined markedly because of antiviral prophylaxis, but CMV may cause diarrhea with or without gastrointestinal bleeding [494,498,499,551,555,585]. Diffuse intestinal ulceration due to CMV with intestinal edema and protein loss identical to that of GVHD has been reported [563,586–588]. Endoscopic examination with tissue biopsy for culture and immunohistochemistry is necessary for definitive diagnosis [533,555,589]. The use of PCR of stool or colonic tissue for diagnosis of CMV can be problematic when a positive PCR result is not concordant with viral culture, immunohistology, or endoscopic findings; in this circumstance a positive result may represent latent infection, viral excretion, or a false-positive test. The lack of CMV in the blood stream (by antigen detection or PCR) does not mean that CMV is absent in the intestinal mucosa. The endoscopic appearance of discrete ulcerations is highly suggestive of viral involvement; the diagnostic yield is highest if biopsies are taken from the central portion of ulcerations. Treatment with ganciclovir eliminates CMV from tissue but healing of ulcerations can be slow [140]. Astrovirus, one of a number of small enteric viruses, was the most common viral cause of diarrhea in a recent study [551]. Commercial tests are not available for diagnosing astrovirus, calicivirus, picobirnavirus or Norwalk-agent enteritis. Fortunately, diarrhea caused by astrovirus in HCT patients does not appear to be a severe disease. Rotavirus, adenovirus and Coxsackie viruses are causes of sporadic diarrhea that can be readily detected by stool culture or ELISA [501,590,591]. Severe necrotizing enteritis can result from infection by some serotypes of adenovirus [405,406,500,592,593] and rotavirus [501,594]. Most cases of adenovirus infection post-HCT are self-limited [551,593]. HSV infection is usually limited to the esophagus and only rarely causes intestinal disease [498,595]. Treatment of viral enteritis is relevant only for CMV, adenovirus, HSV and, possibly, rotavirus.

Bacterial pathogens responsible for intestinal infections in the normal host (*Salmonella*, *Shigella*, *Campylobacter*) almost never cause diarrhea in hospitalized HCT recipients unless patients arrive for HCT already infected [6,554]. *C. difficile* is the most common bacterial cause of infectious diarrhea after HCT [551,552]. Mean diarrheal volumes from *C. difficile* colitis in HCT patients are lower than with acute GVHD, reflecting the higher volumes caused by small intestinal disease [551]. Diagnosis depends on detection of *C. difficile* toxin in diarrheal fluid; the most accurate test is a cytotoxicity assay using tissue cultured cells, but most laboratories use a combination of *C. difficile* antigen detection and ELISA for toxins A and B to make the diagnosis [596]. Clinicians should be aware that nontissue culture tests for *C. difficile* may be falsely negative in 5–10% of cases. A PCR-based test has been developed to detect bacterial genes that code for clostridial toxin production, a method that may eventually replace current tests. Typical pseudomembranes involving the colonic mucosa may be absent when patients are granulocytopenic. Severe colitis and megacolon are unusual occurrences in HCT patients [551,597–599]. Both vancomycin and metronidazole are effective treatments [596,600]. A proposed treatment for *C. difficile* colitis, i.e. the use of *Saccharomyces boulardii*, may itself reach the bloodstream in patients with immune defects and should be avoided in HCT patients [601]. Overgrowth of other clostridial species may cause typhlitis and focal necrotizing enteritis [11,15]. [602,603]. Overgrowth of aerobic Gram-negative organisms such as *Pseudomonas*, *Acinetobacter* and *Aeromonas* can also cause diarrhea if antibiotic use has reduced the colonization resistance of the normal colonic flora [551,584].

Fungal overgrowth of the intestine is an overlooked cause of watery diarrhea in hospitalized non-HCT patients [604–606] and may contribute to diarrhea post-HCT as well. Large numbers of *Candida* species were found in the stools of 21 of 150 HCT patients with diarrhea, some of whom had no other explanation for diarrhea [551]. Microscopy of stool specimens may be more useful than cultures for the identification of fungi when patients are receiving antifungal drugs. The gross morphology of intestinal candidal infection consists of adherent fungal plaques studding the intestine [607]. These cases may respond to oral antifungal therapy with either oral amphotericin, nystatin, or fluconazole [608,609]. Severe diarrhea due to *Cokeromyces recurvatus* has been reported following HCT [610,611].

Watery diarrhea secondary to intestinal parasite infection (*Cryptosporidium*, *G. lamblia* and *E. histolytica*) has been reported in a small number of HCT patients [8–10,612]. Parasitic infections after HCT are more common in countries where parasites are endemic [6]. In most cases, patients came to HCT already infected, but in some patients poor hand-washing practices and hygiene led to parasite infection. Diagnosis of parasitic infection is usually by microscopy, but commercially available ELISA tests for giardia antigens are more sensitive than microscopy [613–615]. Giardiasis and amebiasis can be effectively treated in the immunosuppressed host [9,616], but there is no effective treatment for cryptosporidiosis other than restoration of immune competence. *Stongyloides* infection has also been described after HCT [617]. Because of the morbidity of the hyperinfection syndrome associated with *Strongyloides* infection in the immunosuppressed host, every effort should be made to screen patients for this infection before HCT, particularly in endemic areas.

Fat and carbohydrate malabsorption

An intestine that is grossly ulcerated cannot absorb nutrients properly. Thus, patients who have GVHD or infection involving the small intestine will have increased diarrhea whenever they eat. More subtle absorption defects can also lead to post-HCT diarrhea. For example, after intestinal injury, brush-border disaccharidase enzyme levels may be decreased, leading to diarrhea after ingestion of lactose, fructose, or sucrose. Patients who are jaundiced because of cholestatic liver or biliary disease may not have adequate bile salts delivered to intestinal fluid, leading to steatorrhea. Acute pancreatitis or papillitis involving the ampulla of Vater may lead to insufficient luminal lipase and steatorrhea. These abnormalities of absorption have led to recommendations for low-lactose, low-fat diets in patients with small intestinal disease after HCT [618]. Patients should not be fasted when they have enteritis, as luminal nutrients are needed for epithelial repair and nutrition [583].

Medications that cause diarrhea

The colonic anaerobic flora normally salvage carbohydrates that are not completely absorbed by the upper intestine and convert them to short chain fatty acids. Both intravenous broad-spectrum antibiotics and oral nonabsorbable antibiotics used in gut decontamination cause diarrhea in patients who are eating because their flora cannot perform this salvage function [619]. Antibiotics may also lead to clostridial colitis; that is, pseudomembranous colitis (*C. difficile*) or typhlitis (usually *C. septicum*). Magnesium salts (given during CSP therapy), tacrolimus (a macrolide that acts as a motilin agonist) and pro-motility agents, such as metaclopramide, cisapride and erythromycin, may contribute to diarrhea.

Abdominal pain

Evaluation of HCT patients with abdominal pain is never an easy process, but knowledge of the illnesses that cause pain and early involvement of consultants with experience in the care of these patients should prevent errors in management. It is extremely important to distinguish patients with abdominal pain as an indicator of a rapidly progressive, potentially fatal illness from the more common scenario of illness with a benign natural history that requires only conservative management.

Toxicity from myeloablative conditioning therapy: enteritis and SOS

It is not unusual for patients to develop crampy abdominal pain of mild to moderate severity during and after conditioning therapy. In most cases, mucosal injury is reversible and does not lead to complications [124]. Rarely, transmural necrosis of the intestinal wall and severe pain may develop [498]. In this setting, patients may develop persistent fevers and sepsis, thought to be related to translocation of luminal bacteria to the portal circulation. The finding of right upper quadrant pain, hyperbilirubinemia and fluid overload is strongly suggestive of SOS [79]. Stretching of the liver capsule by the enlarging liver may produce severe, abrupt pain that mimics a surgical abdomen. The time of onset of SOS ranges from day –3 to day +15 for most conditioning regimens. Intestinal perforation may develop occasionally in the setting of lysis of a transmural lymphoma or metastatic carcinoma after conditioning therapy [4,5].

Intestinal pseudo-obstruction

Dilation of the bowel in the absence of a mechanical obstruction is a common cause of moderate to severe abdominal pain in the first 30–50 days after HCT. Most patients with pseudo-obstruction have an underlying intestinal disease, such as enteritis from conditioning therapy, GVHD, or infection, but frequently the acute presentation is related to increasing use of mu-opioid medications [620]. As in the intensive care setting, acidosis, uremia, electrolyte abnormalities, low cardiac output and ventilator use contribute to colonic distension [621]. Pseudo-obstruction also appears to be more frequent and severe among patients who have lymphoma as an underlying disease, probably a result of intestinal neuropathy from repeated use of vincristine. The diagnosis of pseudo-obstruction is suggested by distension and tympany on abdominal examination and by either gas- or fluid-filled loops of intestine on X-ray. True obstruction, a rare occurrence in HCT patients, can usually be ruled out by review of X-rays and by contrast X-ray studies (such as water-soluble contrast enema) in difficult cases. Initial management of pseudo-obstruction involves correcting abnormal electrolytes, treating sepsis and other metabolic disturbances, discontinuing medications with anticholinergic properties and sharply reducing the doses of opioid medications. Identification and treatment of the underlying disease, particularly GVHD, is obviously important. There is no easy solution to the problem of pain control in a patient who has both intestinal disease and pseudo-obstruction. A nasogastric tube will limit the amount of air reaching the intestine, but will be ineffective in decreasing gas and fluid already in the intestine. Switching from a mu-opioid to a kappa-opioid agonist (e.g. butorphanol) may allow pain relief without affecting colon motility, as there are few kappa-opioid receptors in the colon [622,623]. Neostigmine (2 mg intravenously) has been successfully used in patients with acute colonic pseudoobstruction [624], but care should be taken to exclude mechanical obstruction before such treatment is used. Fortunately, intestinal distension in the HCT population is rarely complicated by perforation.

Viral infections (particularly VZV and CMV) may present with abdominal distension and pain. In visceral VZV infection, abdominal distension, severe pain, fever and rising aminotransferases may precede cutaneous manifestations by up to 10 days [145,386,625–627]. In rare instances, a skin rash never develops [625,627,628]. It is important to recognize this presentation which usually occurs 3–6 months post-HCT, after prophylaxis with acyclovir has been discontinued. A steep rise in serum aminotransferase enzymes (AST, ALT) is a reliable sign of liver infection with VZV in this clinical setting. Acyclovir should be started on clinical suspicion while diagnostic tests are planned; delay in therapy may be associated with a high mortality [387]. Detection of VZV DNA in serum has replaced intestinal mucosal and liver biopsy as the diagnostic procedure of choice [388,627]. CMV enteritis is discussed under the Diarrhea section above; distension has been described in patients who had intestinal neuronal CMV involvement [629] and in a patient with segmental ischemia caused by CMV [503].

Hemorrhagic cystitis

Cystitis is a frequent cause of lower abdominal pain among patients whose conditioning regimen contained CY. Hemorrhagic cystitis may also be due to infection with adenovirus or polyomaviruses [630–632]. Patients usually present with suprapubic pain, dysuria, hematuria and urinary frequency, but symptoms can overlap with those of enteritis, pseudoobstruction, or abdominal wall hematoma. Imaging of the bladder may reveal a diffuse thickening of the wall with protrusion into the lumen, or an intraluminal bulky mass with decreased bladder capacity [633,634].

Acute GVHD

Acute intestinal GVHD usually presents with nausea, anorexia, periumbilical crampy abdominal pain and diarrhea [553,562]. When these symptoms accompany a typical skin rash, the diagnosis of acute GVHD is likely. In some patients the sudden onset of intestinal edema can cause a rigid, board-like abdomen with rebound tenderness preceding the development of a skin rash or diarrhea [498,562]. Intra-abdominal catastrophes, such as perforation and abscess formation, can be ruled out by abdominal X-rays (plain films and CT) [556,558], and endoscopic biopsy of the gastric epithelium can yield the diagnosis of GVHD with minimal risk [129,130]. Surgical exploration should be undertaken only for clear indications, such as abscess or perforation, as little is to be gained from making the diagnosis of acute GVHD at laparotomy [498]. The use of opioid and anticholinergic medication to treat pain and diarrhea may cause intestinal pseudo-obstruction with further exacerbation of pain. Intestinal decompression with a nasogastric or small intestinal sump tube may be needed until opioid medications are cleared from the bloodstream. The decision to treat a patient empirically with prednisone when definitive evidence of GVHD is not at hand can be difficult, but when the pretest probability of GVHD is high (e.g. an HLA-mismatched or unrelated donor; signs of engraftment; a nascent skin rash) and that of perforation or infection is low, empiric treatment is reasonable while the precise diagnosis is sought. The confirmation of intestinal GVHD when a skin rash is absent will usually require endoscopic biopsies.

Biliary and pancreatic pain

The majority of patients receiving prolonged TPN develop gallbladder sludge, a gritty collection of microcrystalline bile composed largely of calcium bilirubinate [463–465]. When patients resume oral intake, gallbladder contraction forces this sludge through the cystic and common bile ducts and the ampulla of Vater. Nausea and epigastric abdominal pain are common symptoms. The common bile duct may be transiently dilated, but this dilation and the discomfort it causes usually resolves after patients have been eating for several days. Cholecystitis is a consequence of obstruction of the cystic duct by gallstones or sludge [635], or infection of the gallbladder mucosa by enteric bacteria, fungi and, rarely, CMV [475,636]. Leukemic relapse in the gallbladder as an exceptional cause of cholecystitis has been reported [473]. The diagnosis of gallbladder disease that requires surgery often must be made on clinical grounds, as the prevalence of gallbladder abnormalities at ultrasound (sludge and increased wall thickness) is high in HCT recipients without cholecystitis. Persistent extrahepatic biliary obstruction has been described in a small number of HCT patients, as noted under "Gallbladder and biliary disease" (p. 783) in the "Jaundice, hepatomegaly and abnormal tests" section (p. 775).

Pancreatitis is an uncommon cause of abdominal pain in HCT patients [637,638] but in a study of 184 autopsied patients the prevalence of acute pancreatitis was 28% [464]. Only 35% of these patients had abdominal pain in the week prior to death. Symptoms of pancreatitis were absent in some patients with florid pancreatitis at autopsy, suggesting that symptoms may have been masked by immunosuppressive drugs. The dominant risk factor for pancreatitis was acute GVHD and prolonged treatment with prednisone, a medication previously associated with acute pancreatitis [639]. Biliary sludge, possibly leading to transient obstruction of the ampulla of Vater, may have had a role in pathogenesis as it was present in all HCT patients who came to autopsy [464]. Pancreatitis due to infection with viruses (CMV, VZV and adenovirus) has also been reported as a manifestation of disseminated disease [409,640–642]. In some cases, severe pancreatitis may be attributable to CSP or tacrolimus used for GVHD prophylaxis [643]. Histological changes of GVHD have also been noted in pancreatic tissue at autopsy, but little relation to acute pancreatitis has been noted [641,644].

Hematomas

Patients with low platelet counts or prolongation of blood clotting may develop spontaneous bleeding into the retroperitoneum, abdominal wall, or intra-abdominal viscera, causing significant pain [645–647]. Retroperitoneal hemorrhage may be asymptomatic but usually presents with lumbar or flank pain and less frequently with abdominal discomfort. A CT scan is required for diagnosis. Rectus sheath and other abdominal wall hematomas often develop spontaneously, but occasionally a history of minimal abdominal wall trauma can be elicited [648]. Pain can be severe due to the rapid engorgement of a confined space. Occasionally an abdominal wall mass can be palpated. The diagnosis is made by ultrasound or CT examination [649]. Intramural hematomas of the small intestine can occur due to local ulceration from CMV or GVHD, or at the site of duodenal biopsies [132,511]. Patients usually present with abdominal pain and intestinal obstruction as the hematoma encroaches on the bowel lumen. The diagnosis is often suggested on CT scan or contrast studies of the intestine. For patients with progressively expanding hematomas in the setting of thrombocytopenia and coagulopathy unresponsive to platelet and fresh frozen plasma, recombinant factor VIIa may offer some benefit, at least in the short term [650].

Intestinal perforation

Perforation may present with only mild to moderate abdominal pain and pneumoperitoneum on plain abdominal X-ray [651]. Although perforation is a catastrophic event, most patients will recover from surgery. Fortunately, perforation in HCT patients is rare, with a prevalence of less than four cases per 1000 patients [651]. The diagnosis is often delayed when granulocytopenia and immunosuppressive drugs mask the initial signs and symptoms. The most common causes of perforation are CMV ulcers, colonic diverticula and, rarely, the lysis of tumor in the intestinal wall. In a large retrospective study, risk factors for perforation were male gender, age over 30 years, allogeneic HCT, and high-dose prednisone therapy for GVHD [651]. Perforation is rare with acute intestinal GVHD [498] despite presentation as an acute abdomen because of bowel wall edema. It should be noted that pneumotosis intestinalis or pneumatosis coli (the presence of gas-filled cysts in the bowel wall) may be observed on plain abdominal X-ray or CT scan following HCT, particularly in the setting of intestinal GVHD or CMV infection [564–566,652,653]. In occasional cases, presumably due to cyst rupture, a pneumoperitoneum or pneumoretroperitoneum may be identified [652,653]. This is usually a benign condition that resolves spontaneously and does not require laparotomy in the absence of signs of an acute abdomen. There are, however, catastrophic processes that present with gas in intra-abdominal tissues, for example, intestinal infarction, bowel obstruction, and clostridial infections, that must be differentiated on clinical, microbiological and, occasionally, surgical grounds from the more benign form of pneumatosis intestinalis [654].

Intestinal mucosal infection

The process of bacterial translocation, where normal luminal bacteria traverse the mucosal barrier to reach intestinal lymphatics and nodes, is probably common after HCT. The primary manifestation of bacterial translocation is blood-culture-negative fever; abdominal pain is often absent. The incidence of post-HCT intestinal infection with known pathogens is remarkably low [551,552] considering the frequency of mucosal necrosis from conditioning therapy and GVHD and the time without musocal immunity. Of the intestinal infections with pathogenic organisms, most do not cause pain as much as diarrhea, for example, enteric viruses (astrovirus, rotavirus), parasites (*Giardia, Cryptosporidia*) and bacteria (*C. difficile, Aeromonas*). Some intestinal infections do present with significant pain (adenovirus, HSV, VZV, rotavirus), usually a result of mucosal ulceration, necrosis, edema and inflammation. CMV enteritis can cause diffuse mucosal edema, abdominal pain and intestinal bleeding, but more commonly patients have loss of appetite, fever, nausea and vomiting, and diarrhea as the dominant symptoms [132,140]. When HCT is done in countries where the water supply may be contaminated, there may be a wider range of bacterial enteric pathogens [6].

C. difficile is the most common bacterial cause of colitis and may cause pain, but it is unusual for severe colitis and toxic megacolon to develop in the HCT setting, perhaps because of limited granulocyte responses [551,597,599]. Other clostridial organisms, however, may cause severe mucosal necrosis, pain and a rapidly downhill course. Typhlitis, an inflammatory disease of the right colon caused by clostridial organisms, is a well-known entity in granulocytopenic patients but is less common after HCT [11,15,502,602,655,656]. Symptoms include fever, right lower quadrant pain, nausea and vomiting, diarrhea, occult blood in stool and shock. Diagnosis of typhlitis is usually made clinically by radiologic studies, but laparotomy is occasionally necessary [657,658]. Ultrasound studies may reveal echogenicity and pseudopolypoid thickening in the cecum while CT scans show thickening of the ileum, cecum and right colic wall with spiculation of the pericolic fat. If typhlitis is a possibility, prompt broad-spectrum antibiotic and antifungal therapy should be implemented, covering both luminal *Clostridia* and fecal flora in the bloodstream. Mortality has been reported to be high in the past despite aggressive medical and surgical therapy [659,660], but recent experience with antibiotics as the cornerstone of therapy suggests that most patients with typhlitis will not require surgical resection [656].

Upper intestinal infections can present with epigastric pain; for example, bacterial, fungal, or viral esophagitis. A rare pyogenic infection of the gastric mucosa, phlegmonous gastritis, is caused by the organisms of the normal oral flora [143]. In HCT patients, this disease causes fever, anorexia, and epigastric pain. Fungal infection (*Candida, Aspergillus,* or mould species) of the upper intestinal tract may result in severe inflammatory gastritis or necrotizing enteritis [146,507,661,662].

Intra-abdominal abscesses

Intraperitoneal abscesses are unusual, probably because of the rarity of intestinal perforation and the prompt use of antibiotics for fever. Fungal abscesses of the liver, kidneys, and spleen may cause abdominal pain, usually localized to the site of involvement [20,23,662]. Diagnosis is extremely difficult because radiologic tests are insensitive, especially in patients with miliary disease [23].

Intestinal infarction

Disseminated *Aspergillus* infection may invade the mesenteric circulation and cause vascular obstruction and intestinal infarction [508]. The clinical manifestations are severe abdominal pain, intestinal obstruction and gastrointestinal bleeding. Intestinal involvement may be the initial manifestation of disseminated *Aspergillus* infection. However, most patients have evidence of pulmonary involvement prior to the onset of intestinal symptoms. Survival is rare. CMV involvement of intestinal arteries may also lead to segmental ischemia [503].

EBV lymphoproliferative disease

EBV lymphoproliferative disease most commonly develops in patients with prolonged immunosuppression for severe GVHD, in recipients of T-cell-depleted grafts or following potent anti-T-cell antibody therapy for GVHD. This condition often presents with abdominal pain and fever with an average onset 10 weeks after HCT [479,481]. Transformed lymphoid cells may infiltrate the bowel wall, liver, spleen and manifest as bleeding, obstruction or painful organomegaly [498,663,664]. Findings on abdominal CT scanning are nonspecific, but massive lymphadenopathy suggests the diagnosis. Diagnosis is usually made by biopsy of stomach, liver or lymph node. Therapeutic options are increasing and include infusion of donor leukocytes, adoptive transfer of EBV-specific, HLA-class I-restricted cytotoxic T-lymphocyte lines and chimeric anti-CD20 monoclonal antibody (rituximab) (see Chapters 56 and 70) [664–666].

Approach to the patient with abdominal pain

A systematic approach in evaluating abdominal pain in these difficult patients is important in excluding rapidly fatal diseases. The following questions should be addressed.

Does the patient need urgent surgery?

Surgery is indicated for intestinal perforation, acute cholecystitis, drainage of abscesses and, in some patients with biliary obstruction, typhlitis and dissecting hematomas. The majority of patients with abdominal pain do not require surgery and in patients who have SOS, general anesthesia may jeopardize liver blood flow and lead to progressive liver failure. SOS presenting as severe abdominal pain can usually be recognized by its timing post-HCT, by the finding of liver tenderness in either the epigastrium or the right lobe, away from the gallbladder fossa, and by an ultrasound that shows no intrahepatic mass lesions. Pneumoperitoneum on upright X-ray or CT scan was present in all Seattle patients with perforation

[651], but this finding can be a manifestation of pneumatosis intestinalis, a more benign process than free perforation [652,653]. Recognition of acute cholecystitis is more difficult, as right upper quadrant pain (usually from SOS) and fever are common in the early post-HCT period, and imaging studies frequently show gallbladder wall thickening and luminal sludge in completely asymptomatic patients [462,463]. A radionuclide study with morphine showing filling of the gallbladder suggests that surgical cholecystitis is not present, but false-positive results (i.e. lack of gallbladder filling) do occur in severely ill patients on TPN [476]. Clinical judgement may lead to surgical exploration or laparoscopy in problematic cases. In the 1970s, HCT patients with "surgical abdomens" were sent to exploratory laparotomy, in order not to miss such conditions as intestinal infarction, appendicitis, intussusception, mechanical obstruction and volvulus. These conditions have proved to be rare and far less common than acute GVHD, SOS, pseudo-obstruction and other causes of pain. Modern imaging tests (ultrasound and helical CT scan) and careful examination should allow the surgeon to be highly selective in choosing candidates for operation.

Is the pain a manifestation of acute GVHD?

Prednisone therapy should be given for severe visceral pain from GVHD (even in circumstances where the diagnosis is still uncertain) when the patient is at high-risk for severe GVHD, the time post-HCT is typical of the onset of GVHD and many other causes of acute pain have been ruled out. Imaging studies of the intestine show wall thickening in acute GVHD, a nonspecific but highly suggestive finding, particularly when CMV infection is unlikely. Although one might withhold prednisone therapy until a definitive biopsy diagnosis has been made, delays in therapy may lead to more extensive mucosal necrosis and morbidity. If the pain later proves to be due to causes other than GVHD, prednisone can be discontinued.

Is visceral VZV infection a possibility?

It is critical to consider disseminated VZV in patients who present with difficult-to-explain abdominal pain 2–6 months after HCT. This presentation is most likely in patients with persistent immunosuppression, who had positive pretransplant VZV serology and who are not currently receiving acyclovir or ganciclovir therapy. Importantly, the abdominal pain may precede typical VZV skin lesions by several days. [145,386,625–627]. Marked hyponatremia due to the syndrome of inappropriate antidiuretic hormone secretion has also been observed in this setting [667,668]. Patients should be started on intravenous acyclovir while a definitive diagnosis is sought via PCR detection of VZV DNA in serum by PCR or by intestinal mucosal and liver biopsy [388,627]. Pain from visceral VZV infection may be poorly localized and the patient may not look particularly unwell at presentation but, if not treated promptly, the disease can follow a rapidly fatal course.

Is the pain due to a treatable infection?

Recent advances in antiviral and antifungal prophylaxis have made intestinal and liver infections unusual causes of abdominal pain [451,494]. Nonetheless, infections of the liver and intestinal tract must be considered in patients with pain. Of particular concern is the recent emergence of amphotericin B-resistant mold infections [662], probably related to the widespread use of antifungal prophylaxis. Stool examination by microscopy and culture may identify infectious causes of abdominal symptoms [6,551,552], although this will not be helpful in diagnosis of CMV infection or invasive *Aspergillus* [146,503,508,533].

Identification of other causes of abdominal pain

Once the diseases that need urgent surgical or medical care have been ruled out, one can assess for other causes of pain and perform directed diagnostic tests. Hemorrhagic cystitis is usually seen in the early post-HCT period but may occur later because of adenovirus or polyomavirus infection; it is always accompanied by hematuria. Hematomas of the abdominal wall or intestine should be suspected in patients with a rapidly expanding anterior abdominal wall mass or obstructive symptoms after intestinal biopsy in the setting of profound thrombocytopenia. Intestinal pseudo-obstruction has many potential causes and patients with other intestinal diseases, such as infection or GVHD, are predisposed to this syndrome. History of prior vincristine therapy or present use of narcotics or medications with anticholinergic side-effects should be sought as contributors to pseudo-obstruction.

Peri-anal pain

Peri-anal pain after HCT can be caused by an anal fissure, a thrombosed external hemorrhoid, cellulitis related to tissue maceration, viral infection, and a number of bacterial and fungal infections. In patients with granulocytopenia, infections in the perineum or peri-anal spaces can lead to fatal sepsis.

Bacterial infection

Peri-anal infections are usually polymicrobial, arising either from anal crypts or from tears in the anal canal [16]. After HCT, these infections can be difficult to recognize because they may not produce abscesses but rather a spreading cellulitis [669]. Extensive supralevator and intersphincteric abscesses may be present without being apparent on external examination. The prevalence of peri-anal infection after HCT was 2% in one large series [18]. The diagnosis is a clinical one, based on appearance and symptoms. Examinations should be done cautiously, as bacteremia may result from manipulation of infected tissues. CT or MRI scans or endoscopic ultrasound can give a clear view of the anatomy involved, particularly if there is pus present [670]. Patients with pain whose etiology remains obscure should be examined by a colorectal surgeon, under anesthesia if necessary. Most patients do not have evidence of soft tissue destruction and can be treated with antibiotics that cover both aerobic and anaerobic organisms [16]. If an obvious abscess is present, surgical drainage and antibiotic treatment are usually successful even in granulocytopenic patients [18]. If there is evidence of tissue necrosis, a more extensive surgical approach may be needed to prevent a fatal outcome [671,672]. When proper antibiotics are given to patients with incipient peri-anal infection, far fewer patients require surgical drainage than in the past [16].

Herpes simplex virus (HSV)

HSV can cause painful chronic cutaneous ulcerations in the perineum of patients with defective T cells [19,673]. This infection is now rare after HCT because of the prophylactic use of acyclovir. The appearance is that of multiple superficial ulcers with raised borders. When these ulcers coalesce and become secondarily infected with bacteria, it may be difficult to recognize them as viral. In contrast to decubitus ulcers, HSV perineal ulcers are painful, have scalloped borders and occur away from pressure points. The diagnosis is made by scraping friable tissue at ulcer borders and by taking rectal swabs for viral culture and immunocytology. Acyclovir/valacyclovir treatment is effective, but secondary bacterial or fungal infection may delay healing.

Problems in long-term survivors of HCT

Liver diseases

The three commonest forms of liver disease in long-term survivors are chronic GVHD, chronic viral hepatitis and iron overload. Liver injury caused by medications can also cause abnormal serum liver enzymes. Iron excess is a potential contributor to liver fibrosis. Extrahepatic biliary obstruction, liver involvement with tumor and cirrhosis of the liver can also be seen.

Chronic GVHD involving the liver

The clinical presentation and management of chronic GVHD are discussed in Chapter 50. Liver involvement is present in 80% of patients with extensive chronic GVHD and frequently follows acute liver GVHD [674–676]. Typically, serum liver function tests reveal a cholestatic picture with elevations of alkaline phosphatase (5–15 times the upper limit of normal), γ-glutamyl transpeptidase (GGT), and bilirubin. Elevations of alkaline phosphatase and GGT usually precede the development of jaundice by many weeks to months. By the time that jaundice has developed, liver biopsy usually shows extensive damage to small bile ducts [358,677]. It is recommended that, in the absence of other evidence of chronic GVHD, allograft recipients with progressive elevations of serum alkaline phosphatase greater than five times the upper limit undergo liver biopsy, particularly if the serum ALT and total serum bilirubin are also elevated. Early treatment of chronic GVHD can prevent extensive ductular damage [358,677]. Serum aminotransferases may also be elevated in chronic GVHD, particularly in patients receiving no doses or tapering doses of immunosuppression. In this situation, chronic liver GVHD may present as an acute hepatitis; that is, with abrupt elevations of aminotransferase levels to over 2000 U/L [358,677]. Liver biopsy is essential to exclude acute viral hepatitis due to a herpesvirus (HSV or VZV) or a hepatitis virus and to make a definitive diagnosis of chronic GVHD. While awaiting a histologic diagnosis, allograft recipients who have sudden development of very high AST or ALT levels should be started on high-dose acyclovir therapy at the same time as appropriate immunosuppressive therapy is reinstituted. Histologic features of chronic liver GVHD are described in detail in Chapter 23 and include lymphocytic infiltration of portal tracts, degeneration and destruction of small bile ducts, periportal fibrosis, cholestasis, piecemeal necrosis and hepatocyte degeneration [360,675]. Some of these features can be seen in chronic viral hepatitis, making definitive histologic diagnosis difficult at times. In long-standing chronic GVHD of the liver, the only histologic abnormality may be the absence of small bile ducts, analogous to ductopenic rejection in liver allografts. Specialized cytokeratin stains of liver biopsies may be required to demonstrate the presence or absence of small bile ducts in this situation.

Immunosuppressive drug treatment of chronic GVHD is successful in 50–80% of patients with extensive multiorgan disease [678]. Even with widespread duct destruction, the institution of appropriate immunosuppression can result in very gradual but complete recovery that may take many months. The addition of ursodeoxycholic acid (ursodiol) (15 mg/kg/day) to the immunosuppressive regimen may result in significant biochemical improvement [365,367], and the immunomodulatory and antiapoptotic properties of this agent may have beneficial impact on the clinical course of hepatic GVHD [368].

Chronic hepatitis C

The prevalence of hepatitis C infection among patients undergoing HCT for hematologic malignancies prior to routine blood donor screening varies widely depending on the background sero-prevalence in the population. In studies, hepatitis C antibody positivity was found in 14 of 20 (70%) Japanese patients, 82 of 230 (36%) Italian patients, 20 of 156 (13%) Finnish patients, 28 of 161 (17.4%) Swedish patients, 62 of 355 (17%) American patients and only two of 42 (4.8%) British patients [61,63,105,679–681]. Additional patients became HCV-infected from donor hematopoietic cell infusion and from blood products given during the HCT process. Because of the high prevalence of infection in most countries, all patients transplanted for hematologic malignancy before 1991 should now be screened for hepatitis C.

Hepatitis C infection in HCT survivors almost always results in chronic hepatitis and fluctuating levels of serum aminotransferases [61]. In the first 10 years of HCV infection after HCT, there is little liver-related morbidity, and survival is identical among HCV-infected and HCV-negative patients [61,63,676]. Cirrhosis of the liver related to chronic HCV infection is rising in frequency among patients transplanted during the 1970s and 1980s [682,683]. HCT survivors with chronic hepatitis C should be evaluated for antiviral therapy, whose response rates to IFN-α and ribavirin are similar to those of other patients with chronic hepatitis C. Antiviral therapy should not be given until patients have been off all immunosuppressive agents for at least 6 months and have no evidence of GVHD or myelosuppression [63,676]. In patients with severe iron overload and chronic hepatitis C, chelation therapy or phlebotomy to reduce hepatic iron stores should be considered prior to IFN therapy and may increase the chance of response [676,684]; mobilization of iron in patients with minimal iron overload may not be necessary [685]. Even in the absence of antiviral therapy, iron reduction therapy in patients with severe iron overload (such as patients transplanted for thalassemia) may result in normalization of liver enzymes and reversal of cirrhosis [686]. Patients with evidence of active hepatitis C (particularly if significant fibrosis is present) should be offered therapy with combination pegylated IFN-α plus ribavirin, currently the most effective available therapy. Pegylated IFNs, with their longer half-lives, however, should be administered with caution in HCT survivors, as some patients experience rapid falls in platelet and granulocyte counts. IFN-α may also activate chronic GVHD [687]. Patients with decompensated liver disease should be considered for liver transplantation.

Chronic hepatitis B

A minority of HCT survivors infected with HBV have progressive inflammatory liver disease leading to liver failure 1–3 years post-HCT (reviewed in [31]). The prevalence of chronic HBV infection among HCT survivors varies widely depending on the country. Most of the series examining the long-term effects of HBV infection originated in Asia and Southern Europe, where the seroprevalence of hepatitis B in the general population is high. The serologic pattern of HBV infection may be atypical in HCT survivors, probably as a consequence of immunosuppression. Clearance of antigenemia is commonly observed and is particularly likely if the donor was anti-HBs-positive because of prior HBV infection [31,54,69]. The long-term prognosis is excellent when patients with chronic hepatitis B have cleared HBsAg [688]. Once they are stable and off all immunosuppression, long-term survivors who remain HBsAg-positive generally exhibit only mild liver disease [53,676]. However, in the presence of chronic GVHD, and a requirement for immunosuppressive drugs, patients with chronic HBV infection remain at risk for acute flares of hepatitis whenever immunosuppression is tapered or ceased [67]. Early use of lamivudine or adefovir dipivoxil should be considered whenever an HBV-infected HCT survivor develops a flare of hepatitis, particularly when the flare is temporally related to discontinuation of immunosuppressive therapy [31]. Rarely, a long-term survivor from a country where HBV is endemic but with negative HBV serology pre-HCT will flare with hepatitis after prolonged immunosuppression, a likely result of activation of occult virus [75,431]. Cirrhosis due to HBV infection has not emerged as a major problem in long-term survivors.

Iron overload

In an autopsy study of patients who died from day +50 to day +99 after HCT, the median liver iron concentration at autopsy was 4307 μg/g dry weight [689]. Thus, it is not surprising that hemosiderosis of the liver is found in approximately 90% of long-term survivors of HCT for hematologic malignancies or aplastic anaemia [690,691]. Iron overload is often particularly severe in thalassemic patients who have undergone HCT [692]. Iron overload in HCT patients is caused by a combination of multiple red cell transfusions and dyserythropoiesis leading to increased iron transport by the intestine. After HCT, when the underlying hematological disease has been cured and transfusions are no longer required, iron accumulation stops and body iron stores fall slowly over time [693]. In stable patients without ongoing disease activity, an elevated serum ferritin level may be a reliable indicator of increased tissue iron stores [694]. In the presence of other disease processes, such as GVHD or viral hepatitis, a liver biopsy may be required to accurately quantify the hepatic iron stores. Noninvasive methods of tissue iron quantification, particularly MRI, may be useful in monitoring iron stores in response to phlebotomy or chelation therapy [694,695].

The consequences of extreme iron overload (defined as liver iron content >15,000 μg/g dry weight) in HCT survivors are primarily those of cardiac and endocrine dysfunction [696–698]. Iron overload may also be a cause of persistent hepatic dysfunction after HCT [676,699,700], due to lipid peroxidation of membranes by free radicals and the effects of intracellular iron accumulation. Studies of heavily transfused patients with thalassemia or hematologic malignancy have documented a high prevalence of portal fibrosis, cirrhosis and hepatocellular carcinoma in association with marked hemosiderosis. Many of these patients were also infected with hepatitis C, which may have been a major contributor to the development of liver disease. In patients with chronic hepatitis C, iron overload may worsen the natural history of the liver disease. In addition, the risk of opportunistic infections may be increased in patients with hepatic iron overload, particularly if they are also immunocompromised. Iron overload may contribute to impaired immune responses by decreasing the generation of T cells and impairing natural killer (NK) and T-helper function [701] as well as decreasing Kuppfer cell production of proinflammatory cytokines [702]. Organisms seen in this setting include *Yersinia enterocolitica* [703], *Listeria monocytogenes* [704], mucormycosis [705,706] and noncholera *Vibrio* species [707].

All HCT survivors should be assessed for iron overload, and phlebotomy or chelation therapy considered in those in whom significant iron overload is documented [676,700], particularly if liver function tests are abnormal or there is evidence of chronic viral hepatitis. Patients with iron overload should also be screened for genetic hemochromatosis [708]. As there is a significant correlation between hepatic iron concentration and total body iron stores [692], iron quantification can be used to direct therapy. Patients with liver iron content >15,000 μg/g dry weight should be treated aggressively with both phlebotomy and chelation; when liver iron content is 7000–15,000 μg/g dry weight, phlebotomy is indicated; when liver iron content is under 7000 μg/g dry weight, treatment is indicated only if there is evidence of liver disease [698]. Mobilization of iron from heavily overloaded patients improves cardiac function, normalizes serum ALT levels and results in improved liver histology [676,696,698]. Recently, reversal of cirrhosis has been demonstrated following iron removal in thalassemic patients cured of their disease by HCT [709].

Liver injury caused by medications and herbal preparations

Fewer medications are prescribed to long-term survivors than to patients immediately after HCT. However, HCT survivors are not exempt from disorders that affect the general population and therefore may require medications such as antihypertensive drugs, lipid lowering agents, hypoglycemic agents, NSAIDs, antidepressants, or antibiotics—many of which may be associated with hepatotoxicity [710,711]. Drug hepatotoxicity should always be suspected in long-term survivors with evidence of liver dysfunction [712]. Some HCT-specific medications used in the long term may also be associated with liver injury. Chronic CSP dosing after organ transplantation has been associated with a high prevalence of biliary and pancreatic disease [713]. Corticosteroids may contribute to steatosis in patients with nonalcoholic steatohepatitis, particularly if insulin resistance related to obesity, diabetes or hyperlipidemia is present [714]. TMP-SMX has been associated with cholestasis, hepatitis and microvesicular fat deposition [715,716]. Azathioprine, occasionally used as a second-line drug for the treatment of chronic GVHD, can cause cholestasis, hepatitis, peliosis hepatis, VOD and NRH when used chronically [717,718]. Multiple vitamins that contain iron should be avoided because most HCT survivors are heavily iron overloaded.

Many individuals in the community take herbal preparations. Use of these products is not limited to traditional medicine practitioners in Asia, Africa and the Middle East, and herbal therapies are increasingly common in Western societies [719]. There are increasing numbers of reports of both acute hepatitis and chronic liver disease attributed to herbal preparations [720,721]. HCT survivors who develop evidence of liver disease without an obvious explanation should be questioned about ingestion of herbal preparations. A particular risk of nonsterile herbal remedies in immunosuppressed individuals is the potential for fungal contamination leading to invasive fungal disease, including liver abscesses [722].

Cirrhosis

Cirrhosis was identified in 19 of 704 (2.7%) patients in Seattle who had survived more than 10 years post-HCT [682]. Similar data has recently been reported from Paris [683]. In both series, HCV infection is the primary risk factor. Additional hepatitis C-infected long-term survivors who were transplanted in Seattle and Paris in the 1970s and 1980s have developed decompensated liver disease and complications of portal hypertension. It is anticipated that with longer duration of follow-up, cirrhosis and its complications will become an increasingly important management issue, with up to 25% of 20-year survivors becoming cirrhotic [683]. HCT survivors infected by HCV may have a more rapid progression to cirrhosis than non-HCT patients but the causes are not known (high viral titers after HCT, sinusoidal injury, immunosuppression, chronic GVHD and iron overload are potential factors) [682,683]. Liver transplantation should be considered in any HCT survivor who is developing liver decompensation. In some cases, the original hematopoietic cell donor could be a potential partial liver donor, in which case immunosuppression after liver transplant would not be needed.

Hepatic malignancy

With increasing duration of survival after HCT, the development of secondary malignancy is becoming a clinical problem (see Chapters 69 and 70). Compared to the general population, patients who survive over 10 years post-HCT have an eightfold risk of developing a new solid malignancy [723]. The risk is increased among patients who received HCTs at a younger age. The risk of liver cancer is particularly elevated, with the reported ratio of observed to expected cases as high as 28 [724]. Risk factors for liver cancer in HCT survivors are not known, but it is likely that chronic hepatitis C, iron overload and fibrosis are important [682]. Long-term survivors with new hepatic abnormalities, such as multiple mass lesions on imaging, should be carefully evaluated for malignancy, regardless of their age. Recurrent malignancy presenting as abnormal liver enzymes or multiple liver lesions may be seen in patients transplanted for solid tumors or hematologic malignancy.

Chronic fungal liver infection

Patients who are receiving immunosuppressive therapy for chronic GVHD may rarely activate dormant fungi within the liver. These foci of infection represent fungal abscesses that have been encapsulated by fibrous tissue. *Candida* species are the most common isolate. The clinical presentation includes liver tenderness, fever, and elevated serum alkaline phosphatase levels [20]. This presentation is now rare, as the prophylactic use of fluconazole has virtually eliminated candidal liver infection in HCT recipients [451].

Gallstones and biliary strictures

There appears to be a higher than expected incidence of gallstones and stone-related biliary problems after HCT than in an age-matched population. It seems likely that gallstone formation is related to formation of biliary sludge in the early post-HCT period, as it is known that sludge formation is a precursor to stones in other patient populations, for example, during pregnancy and periods of fasting. Chronic CSP dosing may also lead to gallstones and biliary symptoms [713]. Biliary strictures have been described 1–2 years post-HCT, probably related to earlier biliary stone passage [404].

Esophageal symptoms

About 6% of patients with extensive chronic GVHD have esophageal involvement [674,725]. The abnormalities include desquamation of the squamous epithelium, webs, submucosal fibrous rings, bullae and long, narrow strictures in the upper and mid-esophagus [726–729]. The most common symptom is dysphagia, but some patients present with insidious weight loss, retrosternal pain and aspiration of gastric contents. The diagnosis is suggested by barium contrast X-rays and confirmed by endoscopic inspection and biopsy of involved mucosa. Recurrent heartburn and pulmonary aspiration at night are probably due to a lack of effective esophageal peristalsis and poor salivary bicarbonate production, a result of salivary gland destruction from GVHD. Although webs can be disrupted easily with dilators, dense strictures are difficult to dilate safely; and an increased risk of esophageal perforation has been described as a complication of dilation in these patients [726]. Advanced esophageal involvement can be prevented by prompt treatment of chronic GVHD at its early stages. Immunosuppressive drug treatment of patients with dense strictures will halt progression but some of the damage is irreversible. Therapy with proton pump inhibitors should be considered if there is uncontrolled acid reflux. Myasthenia gravis may also complicate chronic GVHD and may have dysphagia as its presenting complaint [730].

Sporadic cases of fungal and, rarely, viral esophagitis occur in long-term HCT survivors, particularly those with chronic GVHD who receive immunosuppressive and antibiotic therapy. Benign esophageal strictures have been described as rare sequelae of earlier herpesvirus infection or mucositis caused by conditioning therapy [514]. With increasing length of survival of HCT recipients, solid tumors such as carcinoma of the esophagus may develop; this diagnosis should be considered in any long-term survivor who develops dysphagia [723,731].

Diarrhea, anorexia, nausea and weight loss

The incidence of diarrhea falls sharply after day +100, except for patients with severe GVHD of the intestine that is refractory to treatment [364,498,562] and patients with protracted acute GVHD [732]. The prognosis of patients with severe acute GVHD beyond day +100 that is refractory to treatment is very poor. However, patients with protracted acute GVHD often have less severe symptoms that tend to wax and wane with intensity of immunosuppressive therapy, with each exacerbation similar to the presenting signs of GVHD that occurred earlier after HCT.

Prominent symptoms in patients with protracted acute GVHD include satiety, poor appetite, nausea, episodic diarrhea and weight loss [732]. The endoscopic and histologic appearance of intestinal mucosa is identical to that seen in acute GVHD [130].

There are sporadic cases of infectious enteritis among patients whose immune reconstitution is incomplete and among patients with both protracted acute GVHD and chronic GVHD. The organisms most commonly found are *C. difficile* and, rarely, *G. lamblia* and *Cryptosporidia*. Bacterial and fungal overgrowth in the jejunum of patients with chronic GVHD and diarrhea, probably related to deficiency of secretory immunoglobulin A [733], has been reported [725]. These patients respond to appropriate antibiotic or antifungal therapy.

Diarrhea secondary to pancreatic insufficiency has developed in some long-term HCT survivors [63,734–737]. The presentation is typical of patients with steatorrhea, with foul-smelling stools and weight loss despite adequate caloric intake. Its pathogenesis is unknown, but in view of the frequent finding of acute pancreatitis at autopsy post-HCT [464], the most likely cause is pancreatic acinar atrophy as a result of previous pancreatic necrosis or prolonged corticosteroid use.

Twenty years ago a severe malabsorption syndrome in patients with extensive untreated chronic GVHD was described [577,738]. In these cases the intestine was diffusely involved with submucosal and subserosal collagen deposition. This presentation disappeared after the introduction of immunosuppressive drug therapy for chronic GVHD. Rarely, intestinal involvement with malignant cells causes diarrhea in long-term survivors; for example, after intestinal infiltration with EBV-transformed lymphoblasts [479], or extramedullary leukemic relapse [739].

Conclusions

Careful evaluation of patients before the start of conditioning therapy may prevent some of the intestinal and hepatobiliary complications of transplant. Diagnosis of the causes of gastrointestinal and hepatic complications following HCT can be difficult, particularly when several different disease processes are developing simultaneously. Several strategies can be used to unravel complex clinical situations:

1 A history and physical examination, the most useful part of the evaluation of sick HCT patients, should come before the ordering of imaging tests.
2 Follow the dictum of Goethe ("Was man weiss, man sieht"; "What one knows, one sees") by reading extensively beforehand about the complications that others have described over the years.
3 Use Bayes' Theorem in everyday practice (first pursue diagnoses whose pretest probability is high).
4 Remember that Occam's Razor is often disposable in the setting of HCT; that is, the law of parsimony of diagnosis is often in error in circumstances where many disease processes are present simultaneously.
5 Consider the timing and natural history of the major complications in forming a differential diagnosis. This is particularly important in diagnosis of viral infections, whose onset often follows a predictable pattern.
6 No one has ever regretted having more, rather than less, information in dealing with complex, poorly understood severe illness in a transplant patient; that is, for intestinal and liver problems, tissue biopsy is often useful in defining a diagnosis, and in determining the dominant pathophysiological process.
7 Focus on diagnoses that have specific, effective treatments. Diagnosis of an untreatable complication cannot improve survival.
8 Recognize when treatment of severe complications is futile and communicate this fact to patients and families earlier rather than later.
9 In caring for long-term survivors of HCT, be mindful of subtle causes of morbidity; for example, chronic hepatitis B or C and iron overload.

References

1 Owens MM, McDonald GB. Gastrointestinal infections after hematopoietic stem cell or solid organ transplantation. In: Bowden RA, Ljungman T, Paya CV, eds. *Transplant Infections*, 2nd edn. Philadelphia: Lippincott, Williams & Wilkins, 2003, pp. 198–221.

2 Yin JAL, Jowitt SN. Resolution of immune-mediated diseases following allogeneic bone marrow transplantation for leukaemia. *Bone Marrow Transplant* 1992; **9**: 31–3.

3 Otero Lopez-Cubero S, Sullivan KM, McDonald GB. Course of Crohn's disease after allogeneic marrow transplantation. *Gastroenterology* 1998; **114**: 433–40.

4 List AF, Greer JP, Cousar JC et al. Non-Hodgkin's lymphoma of the gastrointestinal tract: an analysis of clinical and pathologic features affecting outcome. *J Clin Oncol* 1988; **6**: 1125–33.

5 Ferrara JJ, Martin EW Jr, Carey LC. Morbidity of emergency operations in patients with metastatic cancer receiving chemotherapy. *Surgery* 1982; **92**: 605–9.

6 Kang G, Srivastava A, Pulimood AB et al. Etiology of diarrhea in patients undergoing allogeneic bone marrow transplantation in South India. *Transplantation* 2002; **73**: 1247–51.

7 Walzer PD, Genta RM. *Parasitic Infections in the Compromised Host*. New York: Marcel Dekker, Inc., 1989.

8 Bromiker R, Korman SH, Or R et al. Severe giardiasis in two patients undergoing bone marrow transplantation. *Bone Marrow Transplant* 1989; **4**: 701–3.

9 Bavaro P, Di Girolamo G, Di Bartolomeo P et al. Amebiasis after bone marrow transplantation. *Bone Marrow Transplant* 1994; **13**: 213–4.

10 Collier AC, Miller RA, Meyers JD. Cryptosporidiosis after marrow transplantation. Person-to-person transmission and treatment with spiramycin. *Ann Intern Med* 1984; **101**: 205–6.

11 Kornbluth AA, Danzig JB, Bernstein LH. *Clostridium septicum* infection and associated malignancy. Report of two cases and review of the literature. *Medicine (Baltimore)* 1989; **68**: 30–7.

12 Myerowitz RL, Pazin GJ, Allen CM. Disseminated candidiasis. Changes in incidence, underlying diseases, and pathology. *Am J Clin Pathol* 1977; **68**: 29–38.

13 Zahradnik JM, Spencer MJ, Porter DD. Adenovirus infection in the immunocompromised patient. *Am J Med* 1980; **68**: 725–32.

14 Sloas MM, Flynn PM, Kaste SC et al. Typhlitis in children with cancer: a 30-year experience. *Clin Infect Dis* 1993; **17**: 484–90.

15 Anonymous. Clostridium septicum infection and neutropenic enterocolitis [editorial]. *Lancet* 1987; **2**: 608.

16 Glenn J, Cotton D, Wesley R et al. Anorectal infections in patients with malignant disease. *Rev Infect Dis* 1988; **16**: 42–52.

17 Hiatt JR, Kuchenbecker SL, Winston DJ. Perineal gangrene in the patient with granulocytopenia. The importance of early diverting colostomy. *Surgery* 1986; **100**: 912–5.

18 Cohen JS, Paz IB, O'Donnell MR et al. Treatment of perianal infection following bone marrow transplantation. *Dis Colon Rectum* 1996; **39**: 981–5.

19 Kalb RE, Grossman ME. Chronic perianal herpes simplex in immunocompromised hosts. *Am J Med* 1986; **80**: 486–90.

20 Thaler M, Pastakia B, Shawker TH et al. Hepatic candidiasis in cancer patients: the evolving picture of the syndrome. *Ann Intern Med* 1988; **108**: 88–100.

21 Bjerke JW, Meyers JD, Bowden RA. Hepatosplenic candidiasis: a contraindication to marrow transplantation? *Blood* 1994; **84**: 2811–4.

22 Anttila VJ, Lamminen AE, Bondestam S et al. Magnetic resonance imaging is superior to computed tomography and ultrasonography in imaging infectious liver foci in acute leukaemia. *Eur J Haematol* 1996; **56**: 82–7.

23 Rossetti F, Brawner DL, Bowden RA et al. Fungal liver infection in marrow transplant patients: prevalence at autopsy, predisposing factors, and clinical features. *Clin Infect Dis* 1995; **20**: 801–11.

24 Donnelly JP. A strategy for managing fungal infections in haematopoietic stem cell transplantation. *Transpl Infect Dis* 2000; **2**: 88–95.

25 Gordon SC, Watts JC, Veneri RJ et al. Focal hepatic candidiasis with perihepatic adhesions: laparoscopic and immunohistologic diagnosis. *Gastroenterology* 1990; **98**: 214–7.

26 Walsh TJ, Pappas P, Winston DJ et al. Voriconazole compared with liposomal amphotericin B for empirical antifungal therapy in patients with neutropenia and persistent fever. *N Engl J Med* 2002; **346**: 225–34.

27 Mora-Duarte J, Betts R, Rotstein C et al. Comparison of caspofungin and amphotericin B for invasive candidiasis. *N Engl J Med* 2002; **347**: 2020–9.

28 Martino R, Nomdedeu J, Altes A et al. Successful bone marrow transplantation in patients with previous invasive fungal infections: report of four cases. *Bone Marrow Transplant* 1994; **13**: 265–9.

29 Hoover M, Morgan ER, Kletzel M. Prior fungal infection is not a contraindication to bone marrow transplant in patients with acute leukemia. *Med Pediatr Oncol* 1997; **28**: 268–73.

30 Sevilla J, Hernandez-Maraver D, Aguado MJ et al. Autologous peripheral blood stem cell transplant in patients previously diagnosed with invasive aspergillosis. *Ann Hematol* 2001; **80**: 456–9.

31 Lau GKK, Strasser SI, McDonald GB. Hepatitis virus infections in patients with cancer. In: Wingard JR, Bowden RA, eds. *Management of Infection in Oncology Patients*. London: Martin Dunitz, 2003, pp. 321–42.

32 Locasciulli A, Alberti A, Bandini G et al. Allogeneic bone marrow transplantation from HBsAg+ donors: a multicenter study from the Gruppo Italiano Trapianti di Midolio Osseo (GITMO). *Blood* 1995; **86**: 3236–40.

33 Fan FS, Tzeng CH, Yeh HM et al. Reverse serconversion of hepatitis B virus infectious status after allogeneic bone marrow transplantation from a carrier donor. *Bone Marrow Transplant* 1992; **10**: 189–91.

34 Lau GKK, Lie AKW, Kwong YL et al. A case-controlled study on the use of HBsAg-positive donors for allogeneic hematopoietic cell transplantation. *Blood* 2000; **96**: 452–8.

35 Chen PM, Liu JH, Fan FS et al. Liver disease after bone marrow transplantation: the Taiwan Experience. *Transplantation* 1995; **59**: 1139–43.

36 Ustun C, Koc H, Karayalcin S et al. Hepatitis B virus infection in allogeneic bone marrow transplantation. *Bone Marrow Transplant* 1997; **20**: 289–96.

37 Dienstag JL, Schiff ER, Wright TL et al. Lamivudine as initial treatment for chronic hepatitis B in the United States. *N Engl J Med* 1999; **341**: 1256–63.

38 Lai CL, Ching CK, Tung AK et al. Lamivudine is effective in suppressing hepatitis B virus DNA in Chinese hepatitis B surface antigen carriers: a placebo-controlled trial. *Hepatology* 1997; **25**: 241–4.

39 Yang H, Westland CE, Delancy WE et al. Resistance surveillance in chronic hepatitis B patients treated with adefovir dipivoxil for up to 60 weeks. *Hepatology* 2002; **36**: 464–73.

40 Lau GK, He M-L, Fong DYT et al. Preemptive use of lamivudine reduces hepatitis B exacerbation after allogeneic hematopoietic cell transplantation. *Hepatology* 2002; **36**: 702–9.

41 Lau GK, Leung YH, Fong DY et al. High hepatitis B virus (HBV) DNA viral load as the most important risk factor for HBV reactivation in patients positive for HBV surface antigen undergoing autologous hematopoietic cell transplantation. *Blood* 2002; **99**: 2324–30.

42 Rosendahl C, Bender-Goetze C, Deinhardt F et al. Immunization against hepatitis B in BMT and leukemia patients. *Exp Hematol* 1985; **13** (Suppl. 17): 104–11.

43 Daily J, Werner B, Soiffer R et al. IGIV: a potential role for hepatitis B prophylaxis in the bone marrow peritransplant period. *Bone Marrow Transplant* 1998; **21**: 739–42.

44 Silva AE, McMahon BJ, Parkinson AJ et al. Hepatitis B virus DNA in persons with isolated antibody to hepatitis B core antigen who subsequently received hepatitis B vaccine. *Clin Infect Dis* 1998; **26**: 895–7.

45 Ilan Y, Nagler A, Adler R et al. Ablation of persistent hepatitis B by bone marrow transplantation from a hepatitis B immune donor. *Gastroenterology* 1993; **104**: 1818–21.

46 Ilan Y, Nagler A, Adler R et al. Adoptive transfer of immunity to hepatitis B virus after T cell-depleted allogeneic bone marrow transplantation. *Hepatology* 1993; **18**: 246–52.

47 Lok AS, Liang RH, Chung HT. Recovery from chronic hepatitis B. *Ann Intern Med* 1992; **116**: 957–8.

48 Brugger SA, Oesterreicher C, Hofmann H et al. Hepatitis B virus clearance by transplantation of bone marrow from hepatitis B immunised donor [Letter]. *Lancet* 1997; **349**: 996–7.

49 Lau GK, Liang R, Lee CK et al. Is vaccination of donor adequate for clearance of hepatitis B virus after bone-marrow transplantation [Letter]? *Lancet* 1997; **349**: 1626–7.

50 Lau GKK, Lok ASF, Liang RHS et al. Clearance of hepatitis B surface antigen after bone marrow transplantation: role of adoptive immunity transfer. *Hepatology* 1997; **25**: 1497–501.

51 Lau GKK, Liang R, Lee CK et al. Clearance of persistent hepatitis B virus infection in Chinese bone marrow transplant recipients whose donors were anti-hepatitis B core- and anti-hepatitis B surface antibody-positive. *J Infect Dis* 1998; **178**: 1585–91.

52 Chen PM, Fan S, Hsieh RK et al. Liver disease in patients with liver dysfunction prior to bone marrow transplantation. *Bone Marrow Transplant* 1992; **9**: 415–9.

53 Reed EC, Myerson D, Corey L et al. Allogeneic marrow transplantation in patients positive for hepatitis B surface antigen. *Blood* 1991; **77**: 195–200.

54 Locasciulli A, Bacigalupo A, Van Lint MT et al. Hepatitis B virus (HBV) infection and liver disease after allogeneic bone marrow transplantation: a report of 30 cases. *Bone Marrow Transplant* 1990; **6**: 25–9.

55 Lau GK, Suri D, Liang R et al. Resolution of chronic hepatitis B and anti-HBs seroconversion in humans by adoptive transfer of immunity to hepatitis B core antigen. *Gastroenterology* 2002; **122**: 614–24.

56 Shuhart MC, Myerson D, Childs B et al. Marrow transplantation from hepatitis C virus seropositive donors: transmission rate and clinical course. *Blood* 1994; **84**: 3229–35.

57 Tomas JF, Rodriguez-Inigo E, Bartolome J et al. Transplantation of allogeneic CD34-selected peripheral stem cells does not prevent transmission of hepatitis C virus from an infected donor. *Bone Marrow Transplant* 1999; **24**: 109–12.

58 Morsica G, Tambussi G, Sitia G et al. Replication hepatitis C virus B lymphocytes (CD19+) [Letter]. *Blood* 1999; **94**: 1138–9.

59 Vance EA, Soiffer RJ, McDonald GB et al. Prevention of transmission of hepatitis C virus in bone marrow transplantation by treating the donor with α-interferon. *Transplantation* 1996; **62**: 1358–60.

60 Hinrichsen H, Benhamou Y, Reiser M et al. First report on the antiviral efficacy of BILN 2061 a novel oral HCV serine protease inhibitor, in patients with chronic hepatitis C genotype 1. *Hepatology* 2002; **36**: 379a [Abstract].

61 Strasser SI, Myerson D, Spurgeon CL et al. Hepatitis C virus infection after bone marrow transplantation: a cohort study with 10 year follow-up. *Hepatology* 1999; **29**: 1893–9.

62 McCaughan GW, Zekry A. Effects of immunosuppression and organ transplantation on the natural history and immunopathogenesis of hepatitis C virus infection. *Transpl Infect Dis* 2000; **2**: 166–85.

63 Ljungman P, Johansson N, Aschan J et al. Longterm effects of hepatitis C virus infection in allogeneic bone marrow transplant recipients. *Blood* 1995; **86**: 1614–8.

64 Locasciulli A, Alberti A, de Bock R et al. Impact of liver disease and hepatitis infections on allogeneic bone marrow transplantation in Europe: a survey from the European Bone Marrow Transplantation (EBMT) Group: Infectious Diseases Working Party. *Bone Marrow Transplant* 1994; **14**: 833–7.

65 Liang R, Lau GK, Kwong YL. Chemotherapy and bone marrow transplantation for cancer patients who are also chronic hepatitis B carriers: a review of the problem. *J Clin Oncol* 1999; **17**: 394–8.

66 Chen PM, Fan S, Liu JH et al. Reactivation of hepatitis B virus in two chronic GVHD patients after transplant. *Int J Hematol* 1993; **58**: 183–8.

67 Martin BA, Rowe JM, Kouides PA et al. Hepatitis B reactivation following allogeneic bone marrow transplantation: case report and review of the literature. *Bone Marrow Transplant* 1995; **15**: 145–8.

68 Webster A, Brenner MK, Prentice HG et al. Fatal hepatitis B reactivation after autologous bone marrow transplantation. *Bone Marrow Transplant* 1989; **4**: 207–8.

69 Chen PM, Fan S, Liu CJ et al. Changing of hepatitis B virus markers in patients with bone marrow transplantation. *Transplantation* 1990; **49**: 708–13.

70 Lau GKK, Liang R, Chiu EKW et al. Hepatic events after bone marrow transplantation in patients with hepatitis B infection: a case controlled study. *Bone Marrow Transplant* 1997; **19**: 795–9.

71 Dhedin N, Douvin C, Kuentz M et al. Reverse seroconversion of hepatitis B after allogeneic bone marrow transplantation: a retrospective study of 37 patients with pretransplant anti-HBs and anti-HBc. *Transplantation* 1998; **66**: 616–9.

72 Blanpain C, Knoop C, Delforge ML et al. Reactivation of hepatitis B after transplantation in patients with pre-existing anti-hepatitis B surface antigen antibodies: report on three cases and review of the literature. *Transplantation* 1998; **66**: 883–6.

73 Chazouilleres O, Mamish D, Kim M et al. Occult hepatitis B virus as source of infection in liver transplant recipients. *Lancet* 1994; **343**: 142–6.

74 Iwai K, Tashima M, Itoh M et al. Fulminant hepatitis B following bone marrow transplantation in an HBsAg-negative, HBsAb-positive recipient; reactivation of dormant virus during the immunosuppressive period. *Bone Marrow Transplant* 2000; **25**: 105–8.

75 Carpenter PA, Huang ML, McDonald GB. Activation of occult hepatitis B from a seronegative patient after hematopoietic cell transplant: a cautionary tale. *Blood* 2002; **99**: 4245–6.

76 Mason AL, Xu LZ, Guo LS et al. Molecular basis for persistent hepatitis B virus infection in the liver after clearance of serum hepatitis B surface antigen. *Hepatology* 1998; **27**: 1736–42.

77 Lau GK, Wu PC, Liang R et al. Persistence of hepatic hepatitis B virus after serological clearance of HBsAg with autologous peripheral stem cell transplantation. *J Clin Pathol* 1997; **50**: 706–8.

78 Locasciulli A, Alberti A. Hepatitis C virus serum markers and liver disease in children with leukemia. *Leuk Lymphoma* 1995; **17**: 245–9.

79 Deleve LD, Shulman HM, McDonald GB. Toxic injury to hepatic sinusoids: sinusoidal obstruction syndrome (venocclusive disease). *Semin Liver Dis* 2002; **22**: 27–41.

80 Frickhofen N, Wiesneth M, Jainta C et al. Hepatitis C virus infection is a risk factor for liver failure from veno-occlusive disease after bone marrow transplantation. *Blood* 1994; **83**: 1998–2004.

81 Mahmoud HK. Schistosomiasis as a predisposing factor to veno-occlusive disease of the liver following allogeneic bone marrow transplantation. *Bone Marrow Transplant* 1996; **17**: 401–3.

82 Lucarelli G, Clift RA, Galimberti M et al. Marrow transplantation for patients with thalassemia: results in class 3 patients. *Blood* 1996; **87**: 2082–8.

83 Ljungman P, Hagglund H, Lonnqvist B et al. Hepatitis C virus as a risk factor for the development of veno-occlusive disease of the liver [Letter]. *Blood* 1994; **84**: 1349–50.

84 Norol F, Roche B, Saint-Marc Girardin MF et al. Hepatitis C virus infection and allogeneic bone marrow transplantation. *Transplantation* 1994; **57**: 393–7.

85 Locasciulli A, Bacigalupo A, Van Lint MT et al. Hepatitis C virus infection and liver failure in patients undergoing allogeneic bone marrow transplantation. *Bone Marrow Transplant* 1995; **16**: 407–11.

86 McDonald GB, Slattery JT, Bouvier ME et al. Cyclophosphamide metabolism, liver toxicity, and mortality following hematopoietic stem cell transplantation. *Blood* 2003; **101**(5): 2043–8.

87 Pariente EA, Goudeau A, Dubois F et al. Fulminant hepatitis due to reactivation of chronic hepatitis B infection after allogeneic bone marrow transplantation. *Dig Dis Sci* 1988; **33**: 1185–91.

88 McIvor C, Morton J, Bryant A et al. Fatal reactivation of precore mutant hepatitis B virus associated with fibrosing cholestatic hepatitis after bone marrow transplantation. *Ann Intern Med* 1994; **121**: 274–5.

89 Chen YC, Lin KH, Huang WS et al. Bone marrow transplantation in Taiwan: an overview. *Bone Marrow Transplant* 1994; **13**: 705–8.

90 Hoofnagle JH, Dusheiko GM, Schafer DF et al. Reactivation of chronic hepatitis B virus infection by cancer chemotherapy. *Ann Intern Med* 1982; **96**: 447–9.

91 McMillan JS, Shaw T, Angus PW et al. Effect of immunosuppressive and antiviral agents on hepatitis B virus replication in vitro. *Hepatology* 1995; **22**: 36–43.

92 Farza H, Salmon AM, Hadchouel M et al. Hepatitis B surface antigen gene expression is regulated by sex steroids and glucocorticoids in transgenic mice. *Proc Natl Acad Sci U S A* 1987; **84**: 1187–91.

93 Chou CK, Wang LH, Lin HM et al. Glucocorticoid stimulates hepatitis B viral gene expression in cultured human hepatoma cells. *Hepatology* 1992; **16**: 13–8.

94 Lau JY, Bain VG, Smith HM et al. Modulation of hepatitis B viral antigen expression by immunosuppressive drugs in primary hepatocyte culture. *Transplantation* 1992; **53**: 894–8.

95 Tur-Kaspa R, Burk RD, Shaul Y et al. Hepatitis B virus DNA contains a glucocorticoid-responsive element. *Proc Natl Acad Sci U S A* 1986; **83**: 1627–31.

96 Lau GKK, Liang R, Wu PC et al. Use of famciclovir to prevent HBV reactivation in HBsAg-positive recipients after allogeneic bone marrow transplantation. *J Hepatol* 1998; **28**: 359–68.

97 Delaney WE 4th, Edwards R, Colledge D et al. Cross-resistance testing of antihepadnaviral compounds using novel recombinant baculoviruses which encode drug-resistant strains of hepatitis B virus. *Antimicrob Agents Chemother* 2001; **45**: 1705–13.

98 Rossi G, Pelizzari A, Motta M et al. Primary prophylaxis with lamivudine of hepatitis B virus reactivation in chronic HbsAg carriers with lymphoid malignancies treated with chemotherapy. *Br J Haematol* 2001; **115**: 58–62.

99 Persico M, De Marino F, Russo GD et al. Efficacy of lamivudine to prevent hepatitis reactivation in hepatitis B virus-infected patients treated for non-Hodgkin lymphoma. *Blood* 2002; **99**: 724–5.

100 Hamaki T, Kami M, Kusumi E et al. Prophylaxis of hepatitis B reactivation using lamivudine in a patient receiving rituximab. *Am J Hematol* 2001; **68**: 292–4.

101 Shibolet O, Ilan Y, Gillis S et al. Lamivudine therapy for prevention of immunosuppressive-induced hepatitit B virus reactivation in hepatitis B surface antigen carriers. *Blood* 2002; **100**: 391–6.

102 Lim LL, Wai CT, Lee YM et al. Prophylactic lamivudine prevents hepatitis B reactivation and mortality in patients receiving immunosuppression and chemotherapy. *Hepatology* 2000; **35**: 455a [Abstract].

103 Storek J, Dawson MA, Storer B et al. Immune reconstitution after allogeneic marrow transplantation compared with blood stem cell transplantation. *Blood* 2001; **97**: 3380–9.

104 Maruta A, Kanamori H, Fukawa H et al. Liver function tests of recipients with hepatitis C virus

infection after bone marrow transplantation. *Bone Marrow Transplant* 1994; **13**: 417–22.
105 Fujii Y, Kaku K, Tanaka M *et al.* Hepatitis C virus and liver disease after allogeneic bone marrow transplantation. *Bone Marrow Transplant* 1994; **13**: 523–6.
106 Locasciulli A, Testa M, Pontisso P *et al.* Hepatitis C virus genotypes and liver disease in patients undergoing allogeneic bone marrow transplantation. *Bone Marrow Transplant* 1997; **19**: 237–40.
107 Fan FS, Tzeng CH, Hsiao KI *et al.* Withdrawal of immunosuppressive therapy in allogeneic bone marrow transplantation reactivates chronic viral hepatitis C. *Bone Marrow Transplant* 1991; **8**: 417–20.
108 Lemley DE, DeLacy LM, Seeff LB *et al.* Azathioprine induced hepatic veno-occlusive disease in rheumatoid arthritis. *Ann Rheum Dis* 1989; **48**: 342–6.
109 Poynard T, Bedossa P, Opolon P. Natural history of liver fibrosis progression in patients with chronic hepatitis C: the OBSVIRC, METAVIR, CLINIVIR, DOSVIRC Groups. *Lancet* 1997; **349**: 825–32.
110 Lucarelli G, Galimberti M, Polchi P *et al.* Bone marrow transplantation in patients with thalassemia. *N Engl J Med* 1990; **322**: 417–21.
111 Strasser SI, McDonald GB. Hepatobiliary complications of hematopoietic stem cell transplantation. In: Schiff ER, Sorrell MF, Maddrey WC, eds. *Schiff's Diseases of the Liver*, 9th edn. Philadelphia: J.B. Lippencott Co., 2003, pp. 1636–63.
112 Hogan WJ, Maris M, Storer B *et al.* Hepatic injury after nonmyeloablative conditioning followed by allogeneic hematopoietic cell transplantation: A study of 193 patients. *Blood*, in press.
113 Safford SD, Safford KM, Martin P *et al.* Management of cholelithiasis in pediatric patients who undergo bone marrow transplantation. *J Pediatric Surg* 2001; **36**: 86–90.
114 Scheimberg IB, Pollock DJ, Collins PW *et al.* Pathology of the liver in leukaemia and lymphoma. A study of 110 autopsies. *Histopathology* 1995; **26**: 311–21.
115 Lucarelli G, Galimberti M, Polchi P *et al.* Marrow transplantation in patients with thalassemia responsive to iron chelation therapy. *N Engl J Med* 1993; **329**: 840–4.
116 Gordon LI, Brown SG, Tallman MS *et al.* Sequential changes in serum iron and ferritin in patients undergoing high-dose chemotherapy and radiation with autologous bone marrow transplantation: possible implications for treatment related toxicity. *Free Radic Biol Med* 1995; **18**: 383–9.
117 Walters MC, Sullivan KM, O'Reilly RJ *et al.* Bone marrow transplantation for thalassemia. The USA Experience. *Am J Pediatr Hematol Oncol* 1994; **16**: 11–7.
118 Foerder CA, Tobin AA, McDonald GB *et al.* Bleomycin-detectable iron in plasma of bone-marrow transplant patients: its correlation with liver injury. *Transplantation* 1992; **54**: 1120–3.
119 Chapko MK, Syrjala KL, Schilter L *et al.* Chemotherapy toxicity during bone marrow transplantation: time course and variation in pain and nausea. *Bone Marrow Transplant* 1989; **4**: 181–6.
120 Holler E, Kolb HJ, Moller A *et al.* Increased serum levels of tumor necrosis factor-α precede major complications of bone marrow transplantation. *Blood* 1990; **75**: 1011–6.
121 Schubert MM, Williams BE, Lloid ME *et al.* Clinical assessment scale for the rating of oral mucosal changes following bone marrow transplantation. *Cancer* 1992; **69**: 2469–77.
122 Schubert MM, Peterson DE, Flournoy N *et al.* Oral and pharyngeal herpes simplex virus infection after allogeneic bone marrow transplantation: analysis of factors associated with infection. *Oral Surg Oral Med Oral Pathol* 1990; **70**: 286–93.
123 Kolbinson DA, Schubert MM, Flournoy N *et al.* Early oral changes following bone marrow transplantation. *Oral Surg Oral Med Oral Pathol* 1988; **66**: 130–8.
124 Epstein RJ, McDonald GB, Sale GE *et al.* The diagnostic accuracy of the rectal biopsy in graft-versus-host disease: a prospective study of thirteen patients. *Gastroenterology* 1980; **78**: 764–91.
125 Aker SN, Lenssen P. Nutritional support of patients with hematologic malignancies. In: Hoffman R, Benz EJ, Shattil SJ *et al.*, eds. *Hematology: Basic Principles and Practice*, 2nd edn. New York: Churchill Livingstone, 1995: 1473–82.
126 Tjon A, Tham RTO, Vlasveld LT, Willemze R. Gastrointestinal complications of cytosine-arabinoside chemotherapy: findings on plain abdominal radiographs. *Am J Roentgenol* 1990; **154**: 95–8.
127 Schiffman KS, Bensinger WI, Appelbaum FR *et al.* Phase II study of high-dose busulfan, melphalan and thiotepa with autologous peripheral blood stem cell support in patients with malignant disease. *Bone Marrow Transplant* 1996; **17**: 943–50.
128 Wu D, Hockenbery DM, Brentnall TA *et al.* Persistent nausea and anorexia after marrow transplantation: a prospective study of 78 patients. *Transplantation* 1998; **66**: 1319–24.
129 Washington K, Bentley RC, Green A *et al.* Gastric graft-versus-host disease: a blinded histologic study. *Am J Surg Pathol* 1997; **21**: 1037–46.
130 Ponec RJ, Hackman RC, McDonald GB. Endoscopic and histologic diagnosis of intestinal graft-vs.-host disease after marrow transplantation. *Gastrointest Endosc* 1999; **49**: 612–21.
131 Weisdorf DJ, Snover DC, Haake R *et al.* Acute upper gastrointestinal graft-versus-host disease: clinical significance and response to immunosuppressive therapy. *Blood* 1990; **76**: 624–9.
132 Spencer GD, Hackman RC, McDonald GB *et al.* A prospective study of unexplained nausea and vomiting after marrow transplantation. *Transplantation* 1986; **42**: 602–7.
133 Baehr PH, Levine DS, Bouvier ME *et al.* Oral beclomethasone dipropionate for treatment of human intestinal graft-versus-host disease. *Transplantation* 1995; **60**: 1231–8.
134 McDonald GB, Bouvier M, Hockenbery DM *et al.* Oral beclomethasone dipropionate for treatment of intestinal graft-versus-host disease: a randomized, controlled trial. *Gastroenterology* 1998; **115**: 28–35.
135 Snover DC, Weisdorf SA, Vercellotti GM *et al.* A histopathologic study of gastric and small intestine graft-versus-host disease following allogeneic bone marrow transplantation. *Hum Pathol* 1985; **16**: 387–92.
136 Tzung S-P, Hackman RC, Hockenbery DM *et al.* Lymphocytic gastritis resembling graft-vs.-host disease following autologous hematopoietic cell transplantation. *Biol Blood Marrow Transplant* 1998; **4**: 43–8.
137 MacGregor IL, Wiley ZD, Lavigne ME *et al.* Slowed rate of gastric emptying of solid food in man by high caloric parenteral nutrition. *Am J Surg* 1979; **138**: 652–4.
138 Charuhas PM, Fosberg KL, Bruemmer B *et al.* A double-blind randomized trial comparing outpatient parenteral nutrition with intravenous hydration: effect on resumption of oral intake after marrow transplantation. *J Parenter Enteral Nutr* 1997; **21**: 157–61.
139 McDonald GB, Sharma P, Hackman RC *et al.* Esophageal infections in immunosuppressed patients after marrow transplantation. *Gastroenterology* 1985; **88**: 1111–7.
140 Reed EC, Wolford JL, Kopecky KJ *et al.* Ganciclovir for the treatment of cytomegalovirus gastroenteritis in bone marrow transplant patients. A randomized, placebo-controlled trial. *Ann Intern Med* 1990; **112**: 505–10.
141 Kearney D, McDonald GB. Esophageal disorders caused by infection, systemic illness, medications, radiation, and trauma. In: Feldman M, Friedman LS, Sleisenger MH, eds. *Sleisenger and Fordtran's Gastrointestinal and Liver Disease: Pathophysiology/Diagnosis/Management*, 7th edn. Philadelphia: W.B. Saunders & Co., 2002: 623–46.
142 Walsh TJ, Belitsos NJ, Hamilton SR. Bacterial esophagitis in immunocompromised patients. *Arch Intern Med* 1986; **146**: 1345–9.
143 Cohen M, Taylor MB. Phlegmonous gastritis. In: Taylor MB, Gollan JL, Steer ML, Wolfe MM, eds. *Gastrointestinal Emergencies*, 2nd edn. Baltimore, MD: Williams & Wilkins, 1997: 219–23.
144 McCluggage WG, Fox JD, Baillie KE *et al.* Varicella zoster gastritis in a bone marrow transplant recipient. *J Clin Pathol* 1994; **47**: 1054–6.
145 David DS, Tegtmeier BR, O'Donnell MR *et al.* Visceral varicella-zoster after bone marrow transplantation: report of a case series and review of the literature. *Am J Gastroenterol* 1998; **93**: 810–3.
146 Yong S, Attal H, Chejfec G. Pseudomembranous gastritis. A novel complication of *Aspergillus* infection in a patient with a bone marrow transplant and graft versus host disease. *Arch Pathol Lab Med* 2000; **124**: 619–24.
147 Eagle DA, Gian V, Lauwers GY *et al.* Gastroparesis following bone marrow transplantation. *Bone Marrow Transplant* 2001; **28**: 59–62.
148 Brand RE, DiBaise JK, Quigley EM *et al.* Gastroparesis as a cause of nausea and vomiting after high-dose chemotherapy and haemopoietic stem-cell transplantation. *Lancet* 1998; **352**: 1985.
149 DiBaise JK, Brand RE, Lyden E *et al.* Gastric myoelectrical activity and its relationship to the development of nausea and vomiting after intensive chemotherapy and autologous stem cell transplantation. *Am J Gastroenterol* 2001; **96**: 2873–81.
150 McDonald GB, Schoch HG, Gooley T. Liver dysfunction and mortality after allogeneic marrow transplantation: analysis of 1419 consecutive patients. *Hepatology* 1999; **30**: 162a [Abstract].
151 Selzer G, Parker RGF. Senecio poisoning exhibiting as Chiari's syndrome. A report on twelve cases. *Am J Pathol* 1950; **27**: 885–7.
152 Bras G, Jeliffe DB, Stuart KL. Veno-occlusive disease of the liver with non-portal type of cirrhosis occurring in Jamaica. *Arch Pathol* 1954; **57**: 285–300.
153 Vowels M, Lam-Po-Tang R, Zagars G *et al.* Total body irradiation and Budd–Chiari syndrome. *Pathology* 1979; **11**: 306.
154 Berk PD, Popper H, Krueger GRF *et al.* Veno-occlusive disease of the liver after allogeneic bone marrow transplantation. *Ann Intern Med* 1979; **90**: 158–64.
155 Jacobs P, Miller JL, Uys CJ *et al.* Fatal veno-occlusive disease of the liver after chemotherapy, whole-body irradiation and bone marrow transplantation

for refractory acute leukaemia. *S Afr Med J* 1979; **55**: 5–10.
156. Shulman HM, McDonald GB, Matthews D *et al*. An analysis of hepatic venocclusive disease and centrilobular hepatic degeneration following bone marrow transplantation. *Gastroenterology* 1980; **79**: 1178–91.
157. Jones RJ, Lee KS, Beschorner WE *et al*. Venooccusive disease of the liver following bone marrow transplantation. *Transplantation* 1987; **44**: 778–83.
158. Shulman HM, Fisher LB, Schoch HG *et al*. Venocclusive disease of the liver after marrow transplantation: histologic correlates of clinical signs and symptoms. *Hepatology* 1994; **19**: 1171–80.
159. DeLeve LD, Wang X, Kuhlenkamp JF *et al*. Toxicity of azathioprine and monocrotaline in murine sinusoidal endothelial cells and hepatocytes: the role of glutathione and relevance to hepatic venoocclusive disease. *Hepatology* 1996; **23**: 589–99.
160. DeLeve LD. Glutathione defense in non-parenchymal cells. *Semin Liver Dis* 1998; **18**: 403–13.
161. DeLeve LD, McCuskey RS, Wang X *et al*. Characterization of a reproducible rat model of hepatic veno-occlusive disease. *Hepatology* 1999; **29**: 1779–91.
162. Rajvanshi P, Shulman HM, Sievers EL *et al*. Hepatic sinusoidal obstruction following gemtuzumab ozogamicin (Mylotarg™) therapy. *Blood* 2002; **99**: 4245–6.
163. McDonald GB, Hinds MS, Fisher LB *et al*. Venocclusive disease of the liver and multiorgan failure after bone marrow transplantation: a cohort study of 355 patients. *Ann Intern Med* 1993; **118**: 255–67.
164. McDonald GB, Sharma P, Matthews DE *et al*. Venocclusive disease of the liver after bone marrow transplantation: diagnosis, incidence, and predisposing factors. *Hepatology* 1984; **4**: 116–22.
165. Ganem G, Saint-Marc Girardin MF, Kuentz M *et al*. Venocclusive disease of the liver after allogeneic bone marrow transplantation in man. *Int J Radiat Oncol Biol Phys* 1988; **14**: 879–84.
166. Carreras E, Bertz H, Arcese W *et al*. Incidence and outcome of hepatic veno-occlusive disease after blood or marrow transplantation: a prospective cohort study of the European Group for Blood and Marrow Transplantation. *Blood* 1998; **92**: 3599–604.
167. Hasegawa S, Horibe K, Kawabe T *et al*. Venoocclusive disease of the liver after allogeneic bone marrow transplantation in children with hematologic malignancies: incidence, onset time and risk factors. *Bone Marrow Transplant* 1998; **22**: 1191–7.
168. McSweeney PA, Niederwieser D, Shizuru JA *et al*. Hematopoietic cell transplantation in older patients with hematologic malignancies: replacing high-dose cytotoxic therapy with graft-versus-tumor effects. *Blood* 2001; **97**: 3390–400.
169. Hagglund H, Remberger M, Klaesson S *et al*. Norethisterone treatment: a major risk-factor for veno-occlusive disease in the liver after allogeneic bone marrow transplantation. *Blood* 1998; **92**: 4568–72.
170. Lee JL, Gooley T, Bensinger W *et al*. Venocclusive disease of the liver after busulfan, melphalan, and thioTEPA conditioning therapy: incidence, risk factors, and outcome. *Biol Blood Marrow Transplant* 1999; **5**: 306–15.
171. Toh HC, McAfee SL, Sackstein R *et al*. Late onset veno-occlusive disease following high-dose chemotherapy and stem cell transplantation. *Bone Marrow Transplant* 1999; **24**: 891–5.
172. Strasser SI, McDonald SJ, Schoch HG, McDonald GB. Severe hepatocellular injury after hematopoietic cell transplant. Incidence and etiology in 2136 consecutive patients. *Hepatology* 2000; **32**: 299a [Abstract].
173. Blann A, Collins P. Von Willebrand factor, angiotensin converting enzyme and endothelial cell damage in veno-occlusive disease and bone marrow transplantation. *Thromb Res* 1992; **66**: 617–8.
174. Anscher MS, Peters WP, Reisenbichler H *et al*. Transforming growth factor β as a predictor of liver and lung fibrosis after autologous bone marrow transplantation for advanced breast cancer. *N Engl J Med* 1993; **328**: 1592–8.
175. Oh H, Tahara T, Bouvier M *et al*. Plasma thrombopoietin levels in marrow transplant patients with veno-occlusive disease of the liver. *Bone Marrow Transplant* 1998; **22**: 675–9.
176. Eltumi M, Trivedi P, Hobbs J *et al*. Monitoring of veno-occlusive disease after bone marrow transplantation by serum aminopropeptide of type III procollagen. *Lancet* 1993; **342**: 518–21.
177. Rio B, Bauduer F, Arrago JP *et al*. N-terminal peptide of type III procollagen: a marker for the development of hepatic veno-occlusive disease after BMT and a basis for determining the timing of prophylactic heparin. *Bone Marrow Transplant* 1993; **11**: 471–2.
178. Park YD, Yasui M, Yoshimoto T *et al*. Changes in hemostatic parameters in hepatic veno-occlusive disease following bone marrow transplantation. *Bone Marrow Transplant* 1997; **19**: 915–20.
179. Murase T, Jirtle RL, McDonald GB. Transforming growth factor-β plasma concentrations in patients with leukemia and lymphoma receiving chemoradiotherapy and marrow transplantation [Letter]. *Blood* 1994; **83**: 2383.
180. Farrand AL, Bouvier ME, McDonald GB. Plasma levels of the propeptide of type III collagen predict the severity of venocclusive disease of the liver. *Hepatology* 1996; **24**: 508A [Abstract].
181. Heikinheimo M, Halila R, Fasth A. Serum procollagen type III is an early and sensitive marker for venocclusive disease of the liver in children undergoing bone marrow transplantation. *Blood* 1994; **83**: 3036–40.
182. Salat C, Holler E, Kolb HJ *et al*. Plasminogen activator inhibitor-1 confirms the diagnosis of hepatic veno-occlusive disease in patients with hyperbilirubinemia after bone marrow transplantation. *Blood* 1997; **89**: 2184–8.
183. Remberger M, Ringden O. Increased levels of soluble interleukin-2 receptor in veno-occlusive disease of the liver after allogenic bone marrow transplantation. *Transplantation* 1995; **60**: 1293–9.
184. Remberger M, Ringden O. Serum levels of cytokines after bone marrow transplantation: increased IL-8 levels during severe veno-occlusive disease of the liver. *Eur J Haematol* 1997; **59**: 254–62.
185. Iguchi A, Kobayashi R, Yoshida M *et al*. Vascular endothelial growth factor (VEGF) is one of the cytokines causative and predictive of hepatic veno-occlusive disease (VOD) in stem cell transplantation. *Bone Marrow Transplant* 2001; **27**: 1173–80.
186. Fried MW, Duncan A, Soroka S *et al*. Serum hyaluronic acid in patients with veno-occlusive disease following bone marrow transplantation. *Bone Marrow Transplant* 2001; **27**: 635–9.
187. Scrobohaci ML, Drouet L, Monem-Mansi A *et al*. Liver venocclusive disease after bone marrow transplantation. Changes in coagulation parameters and endothelial markers. *Thromb Res* 1991; **63**: 509–19.
188. Faioni EM, Krachmalnicoff A, Bearman SI *et al*. Naturally occurring anticoagulants and bone marrow transplantation: plasma protein C predicts the development of venocclusive disease of the liver. *Blood* 1993; **81**: 3458–62.
189. Rio B, Andreu G, Nicod A *et al*. Thrombocytopenia in venocclusive disease after bone marrow transplantation or chemotherapy. *Blood* 1986; **67**: 1773–6.
190. Lee JH, Lee KH, Lee JH *et al*. Plasminogen activator inhibitor-1 is an independent diagnostic marker as well as severity predictor of hepatic veno-occlusive disease after allogeneic bone marrow transplantation in adults conditioned with busulphan and cyclophosphamide. *Br J Haematol* 2002; **118**: 1087–94.
191. Hommeyer SC, Teffey SA, Jacobson AF *et al*. Venocclusive disease of the liver: prospective study of US evaluation. *Radiology* 1992; **184**: 683–6.
192. Herbetko J, Grigg AP, Buckley AR *et al*. Venoocclusive liver disease after bone marrow transplantation: findings at duplex sonography. *Am J Roentgenol* 1992; **158**: 1001–5.
193. Lassau N, Auperin A, Leclere J *et al*. Prognostic value of doppler-ultrasonography in hepatic veno-occlusive disease. *Transplantation* 2002; **74**: 60–6.
194. Mortele KJ, Van Vlierberghe H, Wiesner W *et al*. Hepatic veno-occlusive disease: MRI findings. *Abdom Imaging* 2002; **27**: 523–6.
195. Costa F, Choy CG, Seiter K *et al*. Hepatic outflow obstruction and liver failure due to leukemic cell infiltration in chronic lymphocytic leukemia. *Leuk Lymphoma* 1998; **30**: 403–10.
196. Brown BP, Abu-Yousef M, Farner R *et al*. Doppler sonography: a noninvasive method for evaluation of hepatic venocclusive disease. *Am J Roentgenol* 1990; **154**: 721–4.
197. Deeg KH, Glockel U, Richter R *et al*. Diagnosis of veno-occlusive disease of the liver by color-coded Doppler sonography. *Pediatr Radiol* 1993; **23**: 134–6.
198. Nicolau C, Bru C, Carreras E *et al*. Sonographic diagnosis and hemodynamic correlation in venoocclusive disease of the liver. *J Ultrasound Med* 1993; **12**: 437–40.
199. Grigg A, Gibson R, Bardy P *et al*. Acute portal vein thrombosis after autologous stem cell transplantation. *Bone Marrow Transplant* 1996; **18**: 949–53.
200. Lassau N, Leclere J, Auperin A *et al*. Hepatic veno-occlusive disease after myeloablative treatment and bone marrow transplantation: value of gray-scale and Doppler US in 100 patients. *Radiology* 1997; **204**: 545–52.
201. Kikuchi K, Rudolph R, Murakami C *et al*. Portal vein thrombosis after hematopoietic cell transplantation: frequency, treatment, and outcome. *Bone Marrow Transplant* 2002; **29**: 329–33.
202. McCarville MB, Hoffer FA, Howard SC *et al*. Hepatic veno-occlusive disease in children undergoing bone-marrow transplantation: usefulness of sonographic findings. *Pediatric Radiol* 2001; **31**: 102–5.
203. Carreras E, Granena A, Navasa M *et al*. Transjugular liver biopsy in bone marrow transplantation. *Bone Marrow Transplant* 1993; **11**: 21–6.
204. Shulman HM, Gooley T, Dudley MD *et al*. Utility of transvenous liver biopsies and wedged hepatic venous pressure measurements in sixty marrow

205 Sharma P, McDonald GB, Banaji M. The risk of bleeding after percutaneous liver biopsy: relation to platelet count. *J Clin Gastroenterol* 1982; **4**: 451–3.
206 Vonnahme F-J. *Die Leber des Menschen. Rasterelektronenmikroskopischer Atlas. The Human Liver. A Scanning Electron Microscopic Atlas*, 1st edn. Freiburg, Germany: S. Karger, 1993.
207 Shulman HM, Gown AM, Nugent DJ. Hepatic veno-occlusive disease after bone marrow transplantation. Immunohistochemical identification of the material within occluded central venules. *Am J Pathol* 1987; **127**: 549–58.
208 Watanabe K, Iwaki H, Satoh M et al. Veno-occlusive disease of the liver following bone marrow transplantation: a clinical-pathological study of autopsy cases. *Artif Organs* 1996; **20**: 1145–50.
209 Sato Y, Asada Y, Hara S et al. Hepatic stellate cells (Ito cells) in veno-occlusive disease of the liver after allogeneic bone marrow transplantation. *Histopathology* 1999; **34**: 66–70.
210 Giles FJ, Kantarjian HM, Kornblau SM et al. Mylotarg™ (gemtuzumab ozogamicin) therapy is associated with hepatic venoocclusive disease in patients who have not received stem cell transplantation. *Cancer* 2001; **92**: 406–13.
211 Zimmerman HJ, Fang M, Utili R et al. Jaundice due to bacterial infection. *Gastroenterology* 1979; **28**: 249–58.
212 Vukelja SJ, Baker WJ, Jeffreys P et al. Nonbacterial thrombotic endocarditis clinically mimicking veno-occlusive disease of the liver complicating autologous bone marrow transplantation. *Am J Clin Oncol* 1992; **15**: 500–2.
213 McDonald GB, Sharma P, Matthews DE et al. The clinical course of 53 patients with venocclusive disease of the liver after marrow transplantation. *Transplantation* 1985; **36**: 603–8.
214 Bearman SI. The syndrome of hepatic venocclusive disease after marrow transplantation. *Blood* 1995; **85**: 3005–20.
215 Wingard JR, Mellits ED, Jones RJ et al. Association of hepatic veno-occlusive disease with interstitial pneumonitis in bone marrow transplant recipients. *Bone Marrow Transplant* 1989; **4**: 685–9.
216 Zager RA, O'Quigley J, Zager BK et al. Acute renal failure following bone marrow transplantation: a retrospective study of 272 patients. *Am J Kidney Dis* 1989; **13**: 210–6.
217 Rubenfeld GD, Crawford SW. Withdrawing life support from mechanically ventilated recipients of bone marrow transplants: a case for evidence-based guidelines. *Ann Intern Med* 1996; **125**: 625–33.
218 Bearman SI, Anderson GL, Mori M et al. Veno-occlusive disease of the liver: development of a model for predicting fatal outcome after marrow transplantation. *J Clin Oncol* 1993; **11**: 1729–36.
219 Bearman SI, Lee JL, Baron AE et al. Treatment of hepatic venocclusive disease with recombinant human tissue plasminogen activator and heparin in 42 marrow transplant patients. *Blood* 1997; **89**: 1501–6.
220 DeLeve LD, Wang XD, Huybrechts MM. Cellular target of cyclophosphamide toxicity in the murine liver: role of glutathione and site of metabolic activation. *Hepatology* 1996; **24**: 830–7.
221 DeLeve LD. Dacarbazine toxicity in murine liver cells. A model of hepatic endothelial injury and glutathione defense. *J Pharmacol Exp Ther* 1994; **268**: 1261–70.
222 DeLeve LD, Ito Y, Machen NW, McCuskey MK, Wang X, McCuskey RS. Embolization by sinusoidal lining cells causes the congestion of hepatic venocclusive disease. *Gastroenterology* 2000; **118**: 1003a [Abstract].
223 DeLeve LD, Wang X. Identification of two distinct mechanisms of busulfan toxicity in isolated murine hepatocytes. *Hepatology* 1996; **24**: 464a [Abstract].
224 Wang X, Kanel GC, DeLeve LD. Support of sinusoidal endothelial cell glutathione prevents hepatic veno-occlusive disease in the rat. *Hepatology* 2000; **31**: 428–34.
225 Ringden O, Remberger M, Lehmann S et al. N-acetylcysteine for hepatic veno-occlusive disease after allogeneic stem cell transplantation. *Bone Marrow Transplant* 2000; **25**: 993–6.
226 Teicher BA, Crawford JM, Holden SA et al. Glutathione monoethyl ester can selectively protect liver from high dose BCNU or cyclophosphamide. *Cancer* 1988; **62**: 1275–81.
227 DeLeve LD, Wang X, Tsai J, Kanel G, Tokes Z. Prevention of hepatic venocclusive disease in the rat by inhibition of matrix metalloproteinases. *Gastroenterology* 2001; **120**: 54a [Abstract].
228 Korte W. Veno-occlusive disease of the liver after bone marrow transplantation: is hypercoagulability really part of the problem? *Blood Coagul Fibrinolysis* 1997; **8**: 367–81.
229 Brooks SE, Miller CG, McKenzie K et al. Acute veno-occlusive disease of the liver. Fine structure in Jamaican children. *Arch Pathol Lab Med* 1970; **89**: 507–20.
230 Rollins BJ. Hepatic veno-occlusive disease. *Am J Med* 1986; **81**: 297–306.
231 Honjo I, Suou T, Hirayama C. Hepatotoxicity of cyclophosphamide in man: pharmacokinetic analysis. *Res Commun Chem Pathol Pharmacol* 1988; **61**: 149–65.
232 Gurtoo HL, Dahms R, Hipkens J et al. Studies of the binding of 3H-chloroethyl-cyclophosphamide and 14C-4-cyclophosphamide to hepatic microsomes and native calf thymus DNA. *Life Sci* 1977; **22**: 45–52.
233 Grochow LB, Piantadosi S, Santos G, Jones R. Busulfan dose adjustment decreases the risk of hepatic veno-occlusive disease in patients undergoing bone marrow transplantation. *Proc Am Assoc Cancer Res* 1992; **33**: 200 [Abstract].
234 Yeager AM, Wagner JE Jr, Graham ML et al. Optimization of busulfan dosage in children undergoing bone marrow transplantation: a pharmacokinetic study of dose escalation. *Blood* 1992; **80**: 2425–8.
235 Demirer T, Buckner CD, Appelbaum FR et al. Busulfan, cyclophosphamide and fractionated total body irradiation for allogeneic marrow transplantation for advanced acute and chronic myelogenous leukemia: phase I dose escalation of busulfan based on targeted plasma levels. *Bone Marrow Transplant* 1996; **17**: 341–6.
236 Dix SP, Wingard JR, Mullins RE et al. Association of busulfan area under the curve with venocclusive disease following BMT. *Bone Marrow Transplant* 1996; **17**: 225–30.
237 Vassal G, Deroussent A, Challine D et al. Is 600 mg/m² the appropriate dosage of busulfan in children undergoing bone marrow transplantation? *Blood* 1992; **79**: 2475–9.
238 Schuler U, Schroer S, Kuhnle A et al. Busulfan pharmacokinetics in bone marrow transplant patients: is drug monitoring warranted? *Bone Marrow Transplant* 1994; **14**: 759–65.
239 Slattery JT, Clift RA, Buckner CD et al. Marrow transplantation for chronic myeloid leukemia: the influence of plasma busulfan levels on the outcome of transplantation. *Blood* 1997; **89**: 3055–60.
240 Shaw PJ, Scharping CE, Brian RJ et al. Busulfan pharmacokinetics using a single daily high-dose regimen in children with acute leukemia. *Blood* 1994; **84**: 2357–62.
241 DeLeve LD, Wang X. Role of oxidative stress and glutathione in busulfan toxicity in cultured murine hepatocytes. *Pharmacology* 2000; **60**: 143–54.
242 Slattery JT, Kalhorn TF, McDonald GB et al. Conditioning regimen-dependent disposition of cyclophosphamide and hydroxycyclophosphamide in human marrow transplantation patients. *J Clin Oncol* 1996; **14**: 1484–94.
243 Meresse V, Hartmann O, Vassal G et al. Risk factors of hepatic venocclusive disease after high-dose busulfan-containing regimens followed by autologous bone marrow transplantation: a study in 136 children. *Bone Marrow Transplant* 1992; **10**: 135–41.
244 Hassan M. The role of busulfan in bone marrow transplantation. *Med Oncol* 1999; **16**: 166–76.
245 Andersson BS, Gajewski J, Donato M et al. Allogeneic stem cell transplantation (BMT) for AML and MDS following i.v. busulfan and cyclophosphamide (i.v. BuCy). *Bone Marrow Transplant* 2000; **25** (Suppl. 2): S35–8.
246 Fernandez HF, Tran HT, Albrecht F et al. Evaluation of safety and pharmacokinetics of administering intravenous busulfan in a twice-daily or daily schedule to patients with advanced hematologic malignant disease undergoing stem cell transplantation. *Biol Blood Marrow Transplant* 2002; **8**: 486–92.
247 Andersson BS, Thall PF, Madden T et al. Busulfan systemic exposure relative to regimen-related toxicity and acute graft-versus-host disease: defining a therapeutic window for i.v. BuCy2 in chronic myelogenous leukemia. *Biol Blood Marrow Transplant* 2002; **8**: 477–85.
248 Kashyap A, Wingard J, Cagnoni P et al. Intravenous versus oral busulfan as part of a busulfan/cyclophosphamide preparative regimen for allogeneic hematopoietic stem cell transplantation: decreased incidence of hepatic venoocclusive disease (HVOD), HVOD-related mortality, and overall 100-day mortality. *Biol Blood Marrow Transplant* 2002; **8**: 493–500.
249 Grochow LB. Commentary: parenteral busulfan. Is therapeutic monitoring still warranted? *Biol Blood Marrow Transplant* 2002; **8**: 465–7.
250 Fajardo LF, Colby TV. Pathogenesis of veno-occlusive liver disease after radiation. *Arch Pathol Lab Med* 1980; **104**: 584–8.
251 Lawrence TS, Robertson JM, Anscher MS et al. Hepatic toxicity resulting from cancer treatment. *Int J Radiat Oncol Biol Phys* 1995; **31**: 1237–48.
252 McDonald GB, Ren S, Bouvier ME et al. Venocclusive disease of the liver and cyclophosphamide pharmacokinetics: a prospective study in marrow transplant patients. *Hepatology* 1999; **30**: 314a [Abstract].
253 Geraci JP, Mariano MS, Jackson KL. Radiation hepatopathy of the rat: microvascular fibrosis and

enhancement of liver dysfunction by diet and drugs. *Radiat Res* 1992; **129**: 322–32.
254 Shulman HM, Luk K, Deeg HJ *et al.* Induction of hepatic venocclusive disease in dogs. *Am J Pathol* 1987; **126**: 114–25.
255 Girinsky T, Benhamou E, Bourhis JH *et al.* Prospective randomized comparison of single-dose versus hyperfractionated total-body irradiation in patients with hematologic malignancies. *J Clin Oncol* 2000; **18**: 981–6.
256 Ozsahin M, Pene F, Touboul E *et al.* Total-body irradiation before bone marrow transplantation. Results of two randomized instantaneous dose rates in 157 patients. *Cancer* 1992; **69**: 2853–65.
257 Belkacemi Y, Ozsahin M, Rio B *et al.* Is veno-occlusive disease incidence influenced by the total-body irradiation technique? *Strahlenther Onkol* 1995; **171**: 694–7.
258 Bernstein ID. Monoclonal antibodies to the myeloid stem cells. Therapeutic implications of CMA-676, a humanized anti-CD33 antibody calicheamicin conjugate. *Leukemia* 2000; **14**: 474–5.
259 Sievers EL, Appelbaum FR, Spielberger RT *et al.* Selective ablation of acute myeloid leukemia using antibody-targeted chemotherapy: a phase I study of an anti-CD33 calicheamicin immunoconjugate. *Blood* 1999; **93**: 3678–84.
260 Sievers EL, Larson RA, Stadtmauer EA *et al.* Efficacy and safety of Mylotarg™ (gemtuzumab ozogamicin) in patients with CD33-positive acute myeloid leukemia in first relapse. *J Clin Oncol* 2001; **19**: 3244–54.
261 Neumeister P, Elbl M, Zinke-Cerwenka W *et al.* Hepatic veno-occlusive disease in two patients with relapsed acute myeloid leukemia treated with anti-CD33 calicheamicin (CMA-676) immunoconjugate. *Ann Hematol* 2001; **80**: 119–20.
262 Sievers EL, Larson RA, Estey E *et al.* Low incidence of hepatic veno-occlusive disease after treatment with gemtuzumab ozogamicin (Mylotarg™, CMA-676): relationship to hematopoietic stem cell transplantation. *Blood* 2000; **96**: 206b [Abstract].
263 Goldberg SL, Ellent D, Shtrambrand D *et al.* Gemtuzumab ozogamicin (Mylotarg™) prior to allogeneic hematopoietic stem cell transplantation increases the risk of hepatic veno-occlusive disease. *Blood* 2002; **100**: 415a [Abstract].
264 Peiper SC, Leboeuf RD, Hughes CB *et al.* Report on the CD33 cluster workshop: biochemical and genetic characterization of gp67. In: Knapp W, Dorken B, Gilks WR *et al.*, eds. *Leucocyte Typing. IV. White Cell Differentiation Antigens*, 1st edn. Oxford, UK: Oxford University Press, 1989: 814–6.
265 Tchilian EZ, Beverley PCL, Young BD *et al.* Molecular clonine of two isoforms of the murine homolog of the myeloid CD33 antigen. *Blood* 1994; **83**: 3188–98.
266 Gao Z, McAlister VC, Williams GM. Repopulation of liver endothelium by bone-marrow-derived cells. *Lancet* 2001; **357**: 932–3.
267 Gordon B, Haire H, Kessinger A *et al.* High frequency of antithrombin 3 and protein C deficiency following autologous bone marrow transplantation for lymphoma. *Bone Marrow Transplant* 1991; **8**: 497–502.
268 Lee JH, Lee KH, Kim S *et al.* Relevance of proteins C and S, antithrombin III, von Willebrand factor, and factor VIII for development of hepatic veno-occlusive disease in patients undergoing allogeneic bone marrow transplantation: a prospective study. *Bone Marrow Transplant* 1998; **22**: 883–8.
269 Lee JH, Lee KH, Choi SJ *et al.* Veno-occlusive disease of the liver after allogeneic bone marrow transplantation for severe aplastic anemia. *Bone Marrow Transplant* 2000; **26**: 657–62.
270 Salat C, Holler E, Kolb HJ *et al.* The relevance of plasminogen activator inhibitor 1 (PAI-1) as a marker for the diagnosis of hepatic veno-occlusive disease in patients after bone marrow transplantation. *Leuk Lymphoma* 1999; **33**: 25–32.
271 Villalon L, Avello AG, Cesar J *et al.* Is veno-occlusive disease a specific syndrome or the exacerbation of physiopathologic hemostatic changes in hematopoietic stem cell transplantation (HSCT)? *Thrombosis Res* 2000; **99**: 439–46.
272 Budinger MD, Bouvier M, Shah A, McDonald GB. Results of a phase I trial of antithrombin III as prophylaxis in bone marrow transplant patients at risk for venocclusive disease. *Blood* 1996; **88**: 172a [Abstract].
273 Baglin TP, Harper P, Marcus RE. Venocclusive disease of the liver complicating ABMT successfully treated with recombinant tissue plasminogen activator. *Bone Marrow Transplant* 1990; **5**: 439–41.
274 Rosti G, Bandini G, Belardinelli A *et al.* Alteplase for hepatic veno-occlusive disease after bone-marrow transplantation [Letter]. *Lancet* 1992; **339**: 1481–2.
275 Laporte JP, Lesage S, Tilleul P *et al.* Alteplase for hepatic veno-occlusive disease complicating bone-marrow transplantation [Letter]. *Lancet* 1992; **339**: 1057.
276 Leahey AM, Bunin NJ. Recombinant human tissue plasminogen activator for the treatment of severe hepatic veno-occlusive disease in pediatric bone marrow transplant patients. *Bone Marrow Transplant* 1996; **17**: 1101–4.
277 Kulkarni S, Rodriguez M, Lafuente A *et al.* Recombinant tissue plasminogen activator (rtPA) for the treatment of hepatic veno-occlusive disease (VOD). *Bone Marrow Transplant* 1999; **23**: 803–7.
278 Yoshimi A, Kato K, Maeda N *et al.* Treatment of hepatic veno-occlusive disease after bone marrow transplantation with recombinant human tissue plasminogen activator (rh-tPA). *Rinsho Ketsueki* 2000; **41**: 103–8 [Japanese].
279 Duggan C, Schmidt M, Lawler M *et al.* The prothrombin gene variant G20210A but not factor V Leiden may be associated with veno-occlusive disease following BMT. *Bone Marrow Transplant* 1999; **24**: 693–9.
280 Chauncey TR, Thompson AR, Stewart L, Gooley T, McDonald GB. No association between activated protein C (APC) resistance and hepatic veno-occlusive disease (VOD) following stem cell transplantation. *Blood* 1997; **90**: 356b–7b [Abstract].
281 Schuppan D, Farrand A, Oesterling C, Gehrmann M, McDonald GB. Circulating markers of hepatic fibrosis predict evolution of venocclusive disease after marrow transplantation. *Hepatology* 1997; **26**: 452a [Abstract].
282 Friedman SL. Molecular regulation of hepatic fibrosis, an integrated cellular resonse to tissue injury. *J Biol Chem* 2000; **275**: 2247–50.
283 Tanaka J, Imamura M, Kasai M *et al.* Rapid analysis of tumor necrosis factor-α mRNA expression during venocclusive disease of the liver after allogeneic bone marrow transplantation. *Transplantation* 1993; **55**: 430–2.
284 Farrand AL, Nash RA, Zager RA, Gmur D, McDonald GB. Pathogenesis of venocclusive disease of the liver. The role of cytokines, NO, endothelin-1, and fibrosis. *Gastroenterology* 1996; **110**: 1189a [Abstract].
285 Rajvanshi R, Farrand A, Bouvier ME, Batchelder A, McDonald GB. Plasma levels of endothelin-1 and nitrate in patients with venocclusive disease of the liver after hematopoietic cell transplantation. *Hepatology* 2000; **32**: 405a [Abstract].
286 Fink J, Cooper M, Burkhart K *et al.* Marked enzymuria following bone marrow transplantation: a correlate of veno-occlusive disease–induced "hepatorenal syndrome." *J Am Soc Nephrol* 1995; **6**: 1655–60.
287 Deeg HJ, Storer B, Slattery JT *et al.* Conditioning with targeted busulfan and cyclophosphamide for hemopoietic stem cell transplantation from related and unrelated donors in patients with myelodysplastic syndrome. *Blood* 2002; **100**: 1201–7.
288 Radich JP, Sanders JE, Buckner CD *et al.* Second allogeneic marrow transplantation for patients with recurrent leukemia after initial transplant with TBI-containing regimens. *J Clin Oncol* 1993; **11**: 304–13.
289 Hassan M, Ehrsson H, Ljungman P. Aspects concerning busulfan pharmacokinetics and bioavailability. *Leuk Lymphoma* 1996; **22**: 395–407.
290 Andersson B, Kashyap A, Gian V *et al.* Conditioning therapy with intravenous busulfan and cyclophosphamide (IV BuCy2) for hematologic malignancies prior to allogeneic stem cell transplantation: a phase II study. *Biol Blood Marrow Transplant* 2002; **8**: 145–54.
291 Demirer T, Buckner CD, Appelbaum FR *et al.* Busulfan, cyclophosphamide and fractionated total body irradiation for autologous or syngeneic marrow transplantation for acute and chronic myelogenous leukemia: phase I dose escalation of busulfan based on targeted plasma levels. *Bone Marrow Transplant* 1996; **17**: 491–5.
292 Locasciulli A, Bacigalupo A, Alberti A *et al.* Predictability before transplant of hepatic complications following allogeneic bone marrow transplantation. *Transplantation* 1989; **48**: 68–72.
293 Anderson JE, Appelbaum FR, Schoch G *et al.* Relapse after allogeneic bone marrow transplantation for refractory anemia is increased by shielding lungs and liver during total body irradiation. *Biol Blood Marrow Transplant* 2001; **7**: 163–70.
294 Bearman SI, Hinds MS, Wolford JL *et al.* A pilot study of continuous infusion heparin for the prevention of hepatic venocclusive disease after bone marrow transplantation. *Bone Marrow Transplant* 1990; **5**: 407–11.
295 Attal M, Huguet F, Rubie H *et al.* Prevention of hepatic veno-occlusive disease after bone marrow transplantation by continuous infusion of low-dose heparin: a prospective, randomized trial. *Blood* 1992; **79**: 1–7.
296 Simon M, Hahn T, Ford LA *et al.* Retrospective multivariate analysis of hepatic veno-occlusive disease after blood or marrow transplantation: possible beneficial use of low molecular weight heparin. *Bone Marrow Transplant* 2001; **27**: 627–33.
297 Rosenthal J, Sender L, Secola R *et al.* Phase II trial of heparin prophylaxis for veno-occlusive disease of the liver in children undergoing bone marrow

transplantation. *Bone Marrow Transplant* 1996; **18**: 185–91.
298 Marsa-Vila L, Gorin NC, Laporte JP *et al*. Prophylactic heparin does not prevent liver venoocclusive disease following autologous bone marrow transplantation. *Eur J Haematol* 1991; **47**: 346–54.
299 Cahn JY, Flesch M, Brion A *et al*. Prevention of veno-occlusive disease of the liver after bone marrow transplantation: heparin or no heparin? *Blood* 1992; **80**: 2149–50.
300 Or R, Nagler A, Shpilberg O *et al*. Low molecular weight heparin for the prevention of veno-occlusive disease of the liver in bone marrow transplantation patients. *Transplantation* 1996; **61**: 1067–71.
301 Chalandon Y, Roosnek E, Helg C, Newton A, Wacker P, Chapuis B. Efficient prophylaxis with defibrotide for hepatic veno-occlusive disease (VOD) after allogeneic stem cell transplantation (SCT). *Blood* 2002; **100**: 111a [Abstract].
302 Joshi R, Kerridge IGS, Ethell M, Potter M. Prophylctic defibrotide for the prevention of hepatic veno-occlusive disease (VOD) in hematopoietic stem cell transplantation (HSCT). *Blood* 2002; **100**: 413a [Abstract].
303 Essell JH, Schroeder MT, Harman GS *et al*. Ursodiol prophylaxis against hepatic complications of allogeneic bone marrow transplantation. A randomized, double-blind, placebo-controlled trial. *Ann Intern Med* 1998; **128**: 975–81.
304 Ohashi K, Tanabe J, Watanabe R *et al*. The Japanese multicenter open randomized trial of ursodeoxycholic acid prophylaxis for hepatic veno-occlusive disease after stem cell transplantation. *Am J Hematol* 2000; **64**: 32–8.
305 Ruutu T, Eriksson B, Remes K *et al*. Ursodeoxycholic acid for the prevention of hepatic complications in allogeneic stem cell transplantation. *Blood* 2002; **100**: 1977–83.
306 Goyal M, Sahdev I, Vlachos A, Focazio B, Lipton JM. A combination of heparin, ursodiol and glutamine prophylaxis for hepatic venoocclusive disease (VOD) after hematopoietic stem cell transplantation (HSCT) in children. *Blood* 2002; **100**: 414a [Abstract].
307 Gluckman E, Jolivet I, Scrobohaci ML *et al*. Use of prostaglandin E$_1$ for prevention of liver veno-occlusive disease in leukaemic patients treated by allogeneic bone marrow transplantation. *Br J Haematol* 1990; **74**: 277–81.
308 Bearman SI, Shen D, Hinds MS *et al*. A phase I/II study of prostaglandin E$_1$ for the prevention of hepatic venocclusive disease after bone marrow transplantation. *Br J Haematol* 1993; **84**: 724–30.
309 Clift RA, Bianco JA, Appelbaum FR *et al*. A randomized controlled trial of pentoxifylline for the prevention of regimen-related toxicities in patients undergoing allogeneic marrow transplantation. *Blood* 1993; **82**: 2025–30.
310 Attal M, Huguet F, Rubie H *et al*. Prevention of regimen-related toxicities after bone marrow transplantation by pentoxifylline: a prospective randomized trial. *Blood* 1993; **82**: 732–6.
311 Bearman SI, Shuhart MC, Hinds MS *et al*. Recombinant human tissue plasminogen activator for the treatment of established severe hepatic venocclusive disease of the liver after bone marrow transplantation. *Blood* 1992; **80**: 2458–62.
312 Ringden O, Wennberg L, Ericzon BG *et al*. Alteplase for hepatic veno-occlusive disease after bone marrow transplantation [Letter]. *Lancet* 1992; **340**: 546–7.
313 Hagglund H, Ringden O, Ericzon BG *et al*. Treatment of hepatic venoocclusive disease with recombinant human tissue plasminogen activator or orthotopic liver transplantation after allogeneic bone marrow transplantation. *Transplantation* 1996; **62**: 1076–80.
314 Palmer KJ, Goa KL. Defibrotide. A review of its pharmacodynamic and pharmacokinetic properties, and its therapeutic use in vascular disorders. *Drugs* 1993; **45**: 259–94.
315 Richardson PG, Elias AD, Krishnan A *et al*. Treatment of severe veno-occlusive disease with defibrotide: compassionate use results in efficacy without significant toxicity in a high risk population. *Blood* 1998; **92**: 737–44.
316 Chopra R, Eaton JD, Grassi A *et al*. Defibrotide for the treatment of hepatic veno-occlusive disease: results of the European compassionate-use study. *Br J Haematol* 2000; **111**: 1122–9.
317 Richardson PG, Murakami C, Wei LJ. *et al*. Multi-institutional use of defibrotide in 88 patients post stem cell transplant with severe veno-occlusive disease and multi-system organ failure; response without significant toxicity in a high risk population and factors predictive of outcome. *Blood* 2002; **100**: 4337–43.
318 Richardson PG, Soiffer R, Antin JH *et al*. Defibrotide (DF) appears effective and safe in a phase II, randomized study of patients (pts) with severe veno-occlusive disease (VOD) and multi-system organ failure (MOF) post stem cell transplantation (SCT). *Blood* 2002; **100**: 112a [Abstract].
319 Corbacioglu S, Greil J, Laws HJ *et al*. Defibrotide for the treatment of veno-occlusive disease in children. *Blood* 2002; **100**: 111a [Abstract].
320 Haire WD, Ruby EI, Stephens LC *et al*. A prospective randomized double-blind trial of antithrombin III concentrate in the treatment of multiple-organ dysfunction syndrome during hematopoietic stem cell transplantation. *Biol Blood Marrow Transplant* 1998; **4**: 142–50.
321 Mertens R, Brost H, Granzen B *et al*. Antithrombin treatment of severe hepatic veno-occlusive disease in children with cancer. *Eur J Pediatr* 1999; **158** (Suppl. 3): S154–8.
322 Ibrahim A, Pico JL, Maraninchi D *et al*. Hepatic venocclusive disease following bone marrow transplantation treated by prostaglandin E$_1$. *Bone Marrow Transplant* 1991; **7** (Suppl. 2): 53.
323 Khoury H, Adkins D, Brown R *et al*. Does early treatment with high-dose methylprednisolone alter the course of hepatic regimen-related toxicity? *Bone Marrow Transplant* 2000; **25**: 737–43.
324 Kajiume T, Yoshimi S, Nagita A *et al*. Application of nitric oxide for a case of veno-occlusive disease after peripheral blood stem cell transplantation. *Paediatr Hematol Oncol* 2000; **17**: 601–4.
325 Nattakom TV, Charlton A, Wilmore DW. Use of vitamin E and glutamine in the successful treatment of severe veno-occlusive disease following bone marrow transplantation. *Nutr Clin Pract* 1995; **10**: 16–8.
326 Smith FO, Johnson MS, Scherer LR *et al*. Transjugular intrahepatic portosystemic shunting (TIPS) for treatment of severe hepatic veno-occlusive disease. *Bone Marrow Transplant* 1996; **18**: 643–6.
327 Fried MW, Connaghan DG, Sharma S *et al*. Transjugular intrahepatic portosystemic shunt for the management of severe venoocclusive disease following bone marrow transplantation. *Hepatology* 1996; **24**: 588–91.
328 Azoulay D, Castaing D, Lemoine A *et al*. Transjugular intrahepatic portosystemic shunts (TIPS) for severe veno-occlusive disease of the liver following bone marrow transplantation. *Bone Marrow Transplant* 2000; **25**: 987–92.
329 Zenz T, Rossle M, Bertz H *et al*. Severe veno-occlusive disease after allogeneic bone marrow or peripheral stem cell transplantation: role of transjugular intrahepatic portosystemic shunt (TIPS). *Liver* 2001; **21**: 31–6.
330 Rajvanshi P, McDonald GB. Expanding the use of transjugular intrahepatic portosystemic shunts for veno-occlusive disease. *Liver Transpl* 2001; **7**: 154–9.
331 Meacher R, Venkatesh B, Lipman J. Acute respiratory distress syndrome precipitated by transjugular intrahepatic porto-systemic shunting for severe hepatic veno-occlusive disease. Is it due to pulmonary leucostasis? *Intensive Care Med* 1999; **25**: 1332–3.
332 Murray JA, LaBrecque DR, Gingrich RD *et al*. Successful treatment of hepatic venocclusive disease in a bone marrow transplant patient with side-to-side portacaval shunt. *Gastroenterology* 1987; **92**: 1073–7.
333 Jacobson BK, Kalayoglu M. Effective early treatment of hepatic venocclusive disease with a central splenorenal shunt in an infant. *J Pediatr Surg* 1992; **27**: 531–3.
334 Nimer SD, Milewicz AL, Champlin RE *et al*. Successful treatment of hepatic venocclusive disease in a bone marrow transplant patient with orthotopic liver transplantation. *Transplantation* 1990; **49**: 819–21.
335 Rapoport AP, Doyle HR, Starzl T *et al*. Orthotopic liver transplantation for life-threatening veno-occlusive disease of the liver after allogeneic bone marrow transplant. *Bone Marrow Transplant* 1991; **8**: 421–4.
336 Salat C, Holler E, Wolf C *et al*. Laboratory markers of veno-occlusive disease in the course of bone marrow and subsequent liver transplantation. *Bone Marrow Transplant* 1997; **19**: 487–90.
337 Schlitt HJ, Tischler HJ, Ringe B *et al*. Allogeneic liver transplantation for hepatic veno-occlusive disease after bone marrow transplantation: clinical and immunological considerations. *Bone Marrow Transplant* 1995; **16**: 473–8.
338 Dowlati A, Honore P, Damas P *et al*. Hepatic rejection after orthotopic liver transplantation for hepatic veno-occlusive disease or graft-versus-host disease following bone marrow transplantation. *Transplantation* 1995; **60**: 106–9.
339 Bunin N, Leahey A, Dunn S. Related donor liver transplant for veno-occlusive disease following T-depleted unrelated donor bone marrow transplantation. *Transplantation* 1996; **61**: 664–6.
340 Rosen HR, Martin P, Schiller GJ *et al*. Orthotopic liver transplantation for bone-marrow transplant-associated veno-occlusive disease and graft-versus-host disease of the liver. *Liver Transplant Surg* 1996; **2**: 225–32.
341 Stockschlaeder M, Storb R, Pepe M *et al*. A pilot study of low dose cyclosporin for graft-versus-host prophylaxis in marrow transplantation. *Br J Haematol* 1992; **80**: 49–54.
342 List AF, Spier C, Greer J *et al*. Phase I/II trial of cyclosporine as a chemotherapy-resistance modifier in acute leukemia. *J Clin Oncol* 1993; **11**: 1652–60.
343 Christians U, Spiekermann K, Bader A *et al*. Cyclosporine metabolite pattern in blood from

patients with acute GVHD after BMT. *Bone Marrow Transplant* 1993; **12**: 27–33.
344 Sanchez-Campos S, Lopez-Acebo R, Gonzalez P *et al.* Cholestasis and alterations of glutathione metabolism induced by tacrolimus (FK506) in the rat. *Transplantation* 1998; **66**: 84–8.
345 Ericzon BG, Eusufzai S, Soderdahl G *et al.* Secretion and composition of bile after human liver transplantation: studies on the effects of cyclosporine and tacrolimus. *Transplantation* 1997; **63**: 74–80.
346 Roelofsen H, van der Veere CN, Ottenhoff R *et al.* Decreased bilirubin transport in the perfused liver of endotoxemic rats. *Gastroenterology* 1994; **107**: 1075–84.
347 Trauner M, Nathanson MH, Rydberg SA *et al.* Endotoxin impairs biliary glutathione and HCO_3^- excretion and blocks the choleretic effect of nitric oxide in rat liver. *Hepatology* 1997; **25**: 1184–91.
348 Green RM, Whiting JF, Rosenbluth AB *et al.* Interleukin-6 inhibits hepatocyte taurocholate uptake and sodium-potassium-adenosinetriphosphatase activity. *Am J Physiol* 1994; **267**: G1094–100.
349 Whiting JF, Green RM, Rosenbluth AB *et al.* Tumor necrosis factor-α decreases hepatocyte bile salt uptake and mediates endotoxin-induced cholestasis. *Hepatology* 1995; **22**: 1273–8.
350 Green RM, Beier D, Gollan JL. Regulation of hepatocyte bile salt transporters by endotoxin and inflammatory cytokines in rodents. *Gastroenterology* 1996; **111**: 193–8.
351 Brooks GS, Zimbler AG, Bodenheimer HC, Jr *et al.* Patterns of liver test abnormalities in patients with surgical sepsis. *Am Surg* 1991; **57**: 656–62.
352 Phillips MJ, Poucell S, Oda M. Mechanisms of cholestasis. *Lab Invest* 1986; **54**: 593–608.
353 Leon MP, Bassendine MF, Gibbs P *et al.* Immunogenicity of biliary epithelium: study of adhesive interaction with lymphocytes. *Gastroenterology* 1997; **112**: 968–77.
354 Powles R, Mehta J, Kulkarni S *et al.* Allogeneic blood and bone-marrow stem-cell transplantation in haematological malignant diseases: a randomised trial. *Lancet* 2000; **355**: 1231–7.
355 Blaise D, Kuentz M, Fortanier C *et al.* Randomized trial of bone marrow versus lenograstim-primed blood cell allogeneic transplantation in patients with early-stage leukemia: a report from the Societe Francaise de Greffe de Moelle. *J Clin Oncol* 2000; **18**: 537–46.
356 Bensinger WI, Martin PJ, Storer B *et al.* Transplantation of bone marrow as compared with peripheral-blood cells from HLA-identical relatives in patients with hematologic cancers. *N Engl J Med* 2001; **344**: 175–81.
357 Yasmineh WG, Filipovich AH, Killeen AA. Serum 5′nucleotidase and alkaline phosphatase-highly predictive liver function tests for the diagnosis of graft-versus-host disease in bone marrow transplant recipients. *Transplantation* 1989; **48**: 809–14.
358 Strasser SI, Shulman HM, Flowers ME *et al.* Chronic graft-vs.-host disease of the liver: presentation as an acute hepatitis. *Hepatology* 2000; **32**: 1265–71.
359 Saunders MD, Shulman HM, Murakami CS *et al.* Bile duct apoptosis and cholestasis resembling acute graft-versus-host disease after autologous hematopoietic cell transplantation. *Am J Surg Pathol* 2000; **24**: 1004–8.
360 Shulman HM, Sharma P, Amos D *et al.* A coded histologic study of hepatic graft-versus-host disease after human marrow transplantation. *Hepatology* 1988; **8**: 463–70.
361 Snover DC, Weisdorf SA, Ramsay AK *et al.* Hepatic graft-versus-host disease: a study of the predictive value of liver biopsy in diagnosis. *Hepatology* 1984; **4**: 123–30.
362 Nakanuma Y. Graft-versus-host disease involves intrahepatic peribiliary glands. *J Clin Gastroenterol* 1988; **10**: 233–4.
363 Martin PJ, Schoch G, Fisher L *et al.* A retrospective analysis of therapy for acute graft-versus-host disease: initial treatment. *Blood* 1990; **76**: 1464–72.
364 Martin PJ, Schoch G, Fisher L *et al.* A retrospective analysis of therapy for acute graft-versus-host disease: secondary treatment. *Blood* 1991; **77**: 1821–8.
365 Fried RH, Murakami CS, Fisher LD *et al.* Ursodeoxycholic acid treatment of refractory chronic graft-versus-host disease of the liver. *Ann Intern Med* 1992; **116**: 624–9.
366 Ruutu T, Remberger M, Remes K *et al.* Improved survival with ursodeoxycholic acid (UDCA) prophylaxis in allogeneic stem cell transplantation: long-term follow-up of a randomized study of the Nordic Bone Marrow Transplantation Group. *Blood* 2002; **100**: 111a [Abstract].
367 Wulffraat NM, Haddad E, Benkerrou M *et al.* Hepatic GVHD after HLA-haploidentical bone marrow transplantation in children with severe combined immunodeficiency: the effect of ursodeoxycholic acid. *Br J Haematol* 1997; **96**: 776–80.
368 Guicciardi ME, Gores GJ. Ursodeoxycholic acid cytoprotection. Dancing with death receptors and survival pathways. *Hepatology* 2002; **35**: 971–3.
369 Essell JH, Thompson JM, Harman GS *et al.* Marked increase in veno-occlusive disease of the liver associated with methotrexate use for graft-versus-host disease prophylaxis in patients receiving busulfan/cyclophosphamide. *Blood* 1992; **79**: 2784–8.
370 Prince HM, Cheng M, Cameron RG *et al.* Severe hepatotoxicity from granulocyte-macrophage colony-stimulating factor administered after autologous bone marrow transplantation. *Bone Marrow Transplant* 1995; **16**: 195–7.
371 Ellis M, Shamoon A, Gorka W *et al.* Severe hepatic injury associated with lipid formulations of amphotericin B. *Clin Infect Dis* 2001; **32**: E87–9.
372 Wagman LD, Burt ME, Brennan MF. The impact of total parenteral nutrition on liver function tests in patients with cancer. *Cancer* 1982; **49**: 1249–57.
373 Briones ER, Iber FL. Liver and biliary tract changes and injury associated with total parenteral nutrition: pathogenesis and prevention. *J Am Coll Nutr* 1995; **14**: 219–28.
374 Johnson JR, Egaas S, Gleaves CA *et al.* Hepatitis due to herpes simplex virus in marrow-transplant recipients. *Clin Infect Dis* 1992; **14**: 38–45.
375 Hayashi M, Takeyama K, Takayama J *et al.* Severe herpes simplex virus hepatitis following autologous bone marrow transplantation: successful treatment with high dose intravenous acyclovir. *Jap J Clin Oncol* 1991; **21**: 372–6.
376 Gruson D, Hilbert G, Le Bail B *et al.* Fulminant hepatitis due to herpes simplex virus-type 2 in early phase of bone marrow transplantation. *Hematol Cell Ther* 1998; **40**: 41–4.
377 Nikkels AF, Delvenne P, Sadzot-Delvaux C *et al.* Distribution of varicella zoster virus and herpes simplex virus in disseminated fatal infections. *J Clin Pathol* 1996; **49**: 243–8.
378 Wolfsen HC, Bolen JW, Bowen JL *et al.* Fulminant herpes hepatitis mimicking hepatic abscesses. *J Clin Gastroenterol* 1993; **16**: 61–4.
379 Papatheodoridis GV, Patch D, Watkinson A *et al.* Transjugular liver biopsy in the 1990s: a 2-year audit. *Aliment Pharmacol Ther* 1999; **13**: 603–8.
380 Han CS, Miller W, Haake R *et al.* Varicella zoster infection after bone marrow transplantation: incidence, risk factors and complications. *Bone Marrow Transplant* 1994; **13**: 277–83.
381 Steer CB, Szer J, Sasadeusz J *et al.* Varicella-zoster infection after allogeneic bone marrow transplantation: incidence, risk factors and prevention with low-dose aciclovir and ganciclovir. *Bone Marrow Transplant* 2000; **25**: 657–64.
382 Koc Y, Miller KB, Schenkein DP *et al.* Varicella zoster virus infections following allogeneic bone marrow transplantation: frequency, risk factors, and clinical outcome. *Biol Blood Marrow Transplant* 2000; **6**: 44–9.
383 Locksley RM, Flournoy N, Sullivan KM *et al.* Infection with varicella-zoster virus after marrow transplantation. *J Infect Dis* 1985; **152**: 1172–81.
384 Schuchter LM, Wingard JR, Piantadosi S *et al.* Herpes zoster infection after autologous bone marrow transplantation. *Blood* 1989; **74**: 1424–7.
385 Perren TJ, Powles RL, Easton D *et al.* Prevention of herpes zoster in patients by long-term oral acyclovir after allogeneic bone marrow transplantation. *Am J Med* 1988; **85**: 99–101.
386 Schiller GJ, Nimer SD, Gajewski JL *et al.* Abdominal presentation of varicella-zoster infection in recipients of allogeneic bone marrow transplantation. *Bone Marrow Transplant* 1991; **7**: 489–91.
387 Yagi T, Karasuno T, Hasegawa T *et al.* Acute abdomen without cutaneous signs of varicella zoster virus infection as a late complication of allogeneic bone marrow transplantation: importance of empiric therapy with acyclovir. *Bone Marrow Transplant* 2000; **25**: 1003–5.
388 de Jong MD, Weel JF, van Oers MH *et al.* Molecular diagnosis of visceral herpes zoster. *Lancet* 2001; **357**: 2101–2.
389 Arvin AM. Varicella-zoster virus. *Clin Microbiol Rev* 1996; **9**: 361–81.
390 Balfour HH Jr, Benson C, Braun J *et al.* Management of acyclovir-resistant herpes simplex and varicella-zoster virus infections. *J Acquir Immune Defic Syndr* 1994; **7**: 254–60.
391 Regamey N, Tamm M, Wernli M *et al.* Transmission of human herpesvirus 8 infection from renal-transplant donors to recipients. *N Engl J Med* 1998; **339**: 1358–63.
392 Luppi M, Barozzi P, Schulz TF *et al.* Nonmalignant disease associated with human herpesvirus 8 reactivation in patients who have undergone autologous peripheral blood stem cell transplantation. *Blood* 2000; **96**: 2355–7.
393 Ljungman P, Wang FZ, Clark DA *et al.* High levels of human herpesvirus 6 DNA in peripheral blood leucocytes are correlated to platelet engraftment and disease in allogeneic stem cell transplant patients. *Br J Haematol* 2000; **111**: 774–81.
394 Tajiri H, Tanaka-Taya K, Ozaki Y *et al.* Chronic hepatitis in an infant in association with human herpesvirus-6 infection. *J Pediatrics* 1997; **131**: 473–5.
395 Cone RW, Huang ML, Corey L *et al.* Human herpesvirus 6 infections after bone marrow transplantation: clinical and virologic manifestations. *J Infectious Dis* 1999; **179**: 311–8.

396 Takenaka K, Gondo H, Tanimoto K et al. Increased incidence of cytomegalovirus (CMV) infection and CMV-associated disease after allogeneic bone marrow transplantation from unrelated donors. Bone Marrow Transplant 1997; **19**: 241–8.

397 Hertenstein B, Hampl W, Bunjes D et al. In vivo/ex vivo T cell depletion for GVHD prophylaxis influences onset and course of active cytomegalovirus infection and disease after BMT. Bone Marrow Transplant 1995; **15**: 387–93.

398 Couriel D, Canosa J, Engler H et al. Early reactivation of cytomegalovirus and high risk of interstitial pneumonitis following T-depleted BMT for adults with hematological malignancies. Bone Marrow Transplant 1996; **18**: 347–53.

399 Snover DC, Hutton S, Balfour HH, Jr et al. Cytomegalovirus infection of the liver in transplant recipients. J Clin Gastroenterol 1987; **9**: 659–65.

400 Rees GM, Sarmiento JI, Myerson D, Coen D, Meyers JD, McDonald GB. Cytomegalovirus hepatitis in marrow transplant patients. Clinical, histologic and histochemical analysis. Gastroenterology 1990; **98**: 470a [Abstract].

401 Einsele H, Waller HD, Weber P et al. Cytomegalovirus in liver biopsies of marrow transplant recipients: detection methods, clinical, histological and immunohistological features. Med Microbiol Immunol (Berl) 1994; **183**: 205–16.

402 Evans MJ, Edwards-Spring Y, Myers J et al. Polymerase chain reaction assays for the detection of cytomegalovirus in organ and bone marrow transplant recipients. Immunol Invest 1997; **26**: 209–29.

403 Cheung AN, Ng IO. Cytomegalovirus infection of the gastrointestinal tract in non-AIDS patients. Am J Gastroenterol 1993; **88**: 1882–6.

404 Murakami CS, Louie W, Chan GS et al. Biliary obstruction in hematopoietic cell transplant recipients: an uncommon diagnosis with specific causes. Bone Marrow Transplant 1999; **23**: 921–7.

405 Blanke C, Clark C, Broun ER et al. Evolving pathogens in allogeneic bone marrow transplantation: increased fatal adenoviral infections. Am J Med 1995; **99**: 326–8.

406 Shields AF, Hackman RC, Fife KH et al. Adenovirus infections in patients undergoing bone marrow transplantation. N Engl J Med 1985; **312**: 529–33.

407 Hale GA, Heslop HE, Krance RA et al. Adenovirus infection after pediatric bone marrow transplantation. Bone Marrow Transplant 1999; **23**: 277–82.

408 Somervaille TC, Kirk S, Dogan A et al. Fulminant hepatic failure caused by adenovirus infection following bone marrow transplantation for Hodgkin's disease. Bone Marrow Transplant 1999; **24**: 99–101.

409 Niemann TH, Trigg ME, Winick N et al. Disseminated adenoviral infection presenting as acute pancreatitis. Hum Pathol 1993; **24**: 1145–8.

410 Matsuse T, Matsui H, Shu CY et al. Adenovirus pulmonary infections identified by PCR and in situ hybridisation in bone marrow transplant recipients. J Clin Pathol 1994; **47**: 973–7.

411 Turner PC, Bailey AS, Cooper RJ et al. The polymerase chain reaction for detecting adenovirus DNA in formalin-fixed, paraffin-embedded tissue obtained post mortem. J Infect 1993; **27**: 43–6.

412 Allard A, Girones R, Juto P et al. Polymerase chain reaction for detection of adenoviruses in stool samples. J Clin Microbiol 1991; **29**: 2683.

413 Echavarria MS, Ray SC, Ambinder R et al. PCR detection of adenovirus in a bone marrow transplant recipient: hemorrhagic cystitis as a presenting manifestation of disseminated disease. J Clin Microbiol 1999; **37**: 686–9.

414 Bordigoni P, Carret AS, Venard V et al. Treatment of adenovirus infections in patients undergoing allogeneic hematopoietic stem cell transplantation. Clin Infect Dis 2001; **32**: 1290–7.

415 Ribaud P, Scieux C, Freymuth F et al. Successful treatment of adenovirus disease with intravenous cidofovir in an unrelated stem-cell transplant recipient. Clin Infect Dis 1999; **28**: 690–1.

416 Vandercam B, Moreau M, Goffin E et al. Cidofovir-induced end-stage renal failure. Clin Infect Dis 1999; **29**: 948–9.

417 Ljungman P, Deliliers GL, Platzbecker U et al. Cidofovir for cytomegalovirus infection and disease in allogeneic stem cell transplant recipients. Blood 2001; **97**: 388–92.

418 McCarthy AJ, Bergin M, De Silva LM et al. Intravenous ribavirin therapy for disseminated adenovirus infection. Pediatr Infect Dis J 1995; **14**: 1003–4.

419 Kapelushnik J, Or R, Delukina M et al. Intravenous ribavirin therapy for adenovirus gastroenteritis after bone marrow transplantation. J Pediatr Gastroenterol Nutr 1995; **21**: 110–2.

420 Sabroe I, McHale J, Tait DR et al. Treatment of adenoviral pneumonitis with intravenous ribavirin and immunoglobulin. Thorax 1995; **50**: 1219–20.

421 Jurado M, Navarro JM, Hernandez J et al. Adenovirus-associated haemorrhagic cystitis after bone marrow transplantation successfully treated with intravenous ribavirin [Letter]. Bone Marrow Transplant 1995; **15**: 651–2.

422 Arav-Boger R, Echavarria M, Forman M et al. Clearance of adenoviral hepatitis with ribavirin therapy in a pediatric liver transplant recipient. Pediatr Infect Dis J 2000; **19**: 1097–100.

423 Chakrabarti S, Collingham KE, Fegan CD et al. Fulminant adenovirus hepatitis following unrelated bone marrow transplantation: failure of intravenous ribavirin therapy. Bone Marrow Transplant 1999; **23**: 1209–11.

424 Schwarer AP, Opat SS, Watson AM et al. Disseminated echovirus infection after allogeneic bone marrow transplantation. Pathology 1997; **29**: 424–5.

425 Ho Yen DO, Hardie R, McClure J et al. Fatal outcome of echovirus 7 infection. Scand J Infect Dis 1989; **21**: 459–61.

426 Schleissner LA, Portnoy B. Hepatitis and pneumonia associated with ECHO virus type 9 infection in two adult siblings. Ann Intern Med 1968; **68**: 1315–9.

427 Broliden K. Parvovirus B19 infection in pediatric solid-organ and bone marrow transplantation. Pediatr Transplant 2001; **5**: 320–30.

428 Schleuning M, Jager G, Holler E et al. Human parvovirus B19-associated disease in bone marrow transplantation. Infection 1999; **27**: 114–7.

429 Liatsos C, Mehta AB, Potter M et al. The hepatologist in the haematologists' camp. Br J Haematol 2001; **113**: 567–78.

430 Soderlund M, Ruutu P, Ruutu T et al. Primary and secondary infections by human parvovirus B19 following bone marrow transplantation: characterization by PCR and B-cell molecular immunology. Scand J Infectious Dis 1997; **29**: 129–35.

431 Brechot C, Thiers V, Kremsdorf D et al. Persistent hepatitis B virus infection in subjects without hepatitis B surface antigen: clinically significant or purely "occult?" Hepatology 2001; **34**: 194–203.

432 Hadziyannis SJ, Tassopoulos NC, Heathcote EJ et al. Adefovir dipivoxil for the treatment of hepatitis B e antigen-negative chronic hepatitis B. N Eng J Med 2003; **348**: 800–7.

433 Marcellin P, Chang TT, Lim SG et al. Adefovir dipivoxil for the treatment of hepatitis B e antigen-positive chronic hepatitis B. N Eng J Med 2003; **348**: 808–16.

434 Lai C-L, Rosmawati M, Lao J et al. Entecavir is superior to lamivudine in reducing hepatitis B virus DNA in patients with chronic hepatitis B infection. Gastroenterology 2002; **123**: 1831–8.

435 Gish R, Leung NWY, Wright TL et al. Anti-hepatitis B virus (HBV) activity and pharmacokinetics of FTC in a 2-month trial in HBV-infected patients. Gastroenterology 1999; **116**: 1216a [Abstract].

436 Tsang SW, Chan HL, Leung NW et al. Lamivudine treatment for fulminant hepatic failure due to acute exacerbation of chronic hepatitis B infection. Aliment Pharmacol Ther 2001; **15**: 1737–44.

437 Tillmann HL, Wedemeyer H, Hadem J et al. Early lamivudine therapy may prevent liver failure in patients with fulminant hepatitis B. Hepatology 2002; **36**: 375a [Abstract].

438 Lau GKK, Yiu HHY, Fung DY et al. "Early" is superior to "deferred" pre-emptive lamivudine therapy for hepatitis B patients undergoing chemotherapy. Gastroenterology, in press.

439 Ling R, Mutimer D, Ahmed M et al. Selection of mutations in the hepatitis B virus polymerase during therapy of transplant recipients with lamivudine. Hepatology 1996; **24**: 711–3.

440 Perrillo R, Rakela J, Dienstag J et al. Multicenter study of lamivudine therapy for hepatitis B after liver transplantation. Hepatology 1999; **29**: 1581–6.

441 Perrillo R, Schiff E, Hann HWW et al. The addition of adefovir dipivoxil to lamivudine in decompensated chronic hepatitis B patients with YMDD variant HBV and reduced response to lamivudine. Preliminary 24 week results. Hepatology 2001; **34**: 349a [Abstract].

442 Marcellin P, Chang TT, Lim SG et al. Adefovir dipivoxil (ADV) 10 mg for the treatment of patients with HBEAG+ chronic hepatitis B. Continued efficacy beyond 48 weeks. Hepatology 2002; **36**: 373a [Abstract].

443 van Bommel F, Wunsche T, Schurmann D et al. Tenofovir treatment in patients with lamivudine-resistant hepatitis B mutants strongly affects viral replication. Hepatology 2002; **36**: 507–8.

444 Shuhart MC, Myerson D, Spurgeon CL et al. Hepatitis C virus infection in bone marrow transplant patients after transfusions from anti-HCV positive donors. Bone Marrow Transplant 1996; **17**: 601–6.

445 Skidmore SJ, Collingham KE, Harrison P et al. High prevalence of hepatitis G virus in bone marrow transplant recipients and patients treated for acute leukemia. Blood 1997; **89**: 3853–6.

446 Rodriguez-Inigo E, Tomas JF, Gomez-Garcia de Soria V et al. Hepatitis C and G virus infection and liver dysfunction after allogeneic bone marrow transplantation: results from a prospective study. Blood 1997; **90**: 1326–31.

447 Maruta A, Tanabe J, Hashimoto C et al. Long-term liver function of recipients with hepatitis G virus

447 infection after bone marrow transplantation. *Bone Marrow Transplant* 1999; **24**: 359–63.
448 Ljungman P, Halasz R, Hagglund H *et al*. Detection of hepatitis G virus/GB virus C after allogeneic bone marrow transplantation. *Bone Marrow Transplant* 1998; **22**: 499–501.
449 Kiem HP, Storb R, McDonald GB. Hepatitis-associated aplastic anemia [Letter]. *N Engl J Med* 1997; **337**: 424–5.
450 Kanda Y, Hirai H. TT virus in hematological disorders and bone marrow transplant recipients. *Leuk Lymphoma* 2001; **40**: 483–9.
451 van Burik JH, Leisenring W, Myerson D *et al*. The effect of prophylactic fluconazole on the clinical spectrum of fungal diseases in bone marrow transplant recipients with special attention to hepatic candidiasis: an autopsy study of 355 patients. *Medicine (Baltimore)* 1998; **77**: 246–54.
452 Momin F, Chandrasekar PH. Antimicrobial prophylaxis in bone marrow transplantation. *Ann Intern Med* 1995; **123**: 205–15.
453 Jantunen E, Ruutu P, Niskanen L *et al*. Incidence and risk factors for invasive fungal infections in allogeneic BMT recipients. *Bone Marrow Transplant* 1997; **19**: 801–8.
454 Magnussen CR, Olson JP, Ona FV *et al*. Candida fungus balls in the common bile duct. Unusual manifestation of disseminated candidiasis. *Arch Intern Med* 1979; **139**: 821–2.
455 Marucci RA, Whitely H, Armstrong D. Common bile duct obstruction secondary to infection with Candida. *J Clin Microbiol* 1978; **7**: 490–2.
456 Valgus JM. Caspofungin. The first class of a new class of antifungal agents. *Cancer Prac* 2001; **9**: 314–6.
457 Rex JH, Walsh TJ, Sobel JD *et al*. Practice guidelines for the treatment of candidiasis. *Clin Infect Dis* 2000; **30**: 662–78.
458 Sallah S, Semelka RC, Wehbie R *et al*. Hepatosplenic candidiasis in patients with acute leukaemia. *Br J Haematol* 1999; **106**: 697–701.
459 Navari RM, Sullivan KM, Springmeyer SC *et al*. Mycobacterial infections in marrow transplant patients. *Transplantation* 1983; **36**: 509–13.
460 Skinner R, Appleton AL, Sprott MS *et al*. Disseminated BCG infection in severe combined immunodeficiency presenting with severe anaemia and associated with gross hypersplenism after bone marrow transplantation. *Bone Marrow Transplant* 1996; **17**: 877–80.
461 Lee SP, Hayashi A, Kim YS. Biliary sludge: curiosity or culprit? *Hepatology* 1994; **20**: 523–5.
462 Jacobson AF, Teefey SA, Lee SP *et al*. Frequent occurrence of new hepatobiliary abnormalities after bone marrow transplantation: results of a prospective study using scintigraphy and sonography. *Am J Gastroenterol* 1993; **88**: 1044–9.
463 Teefey SA, Hollister MS, Lee SP *et al*. Gallbladder sludge formation after bone marrow transplant: sonographic observations. *Abdom Imaging* 1994; **19**: 57–60.
464 Ko CW, Gooley T, Schoch HG *et al*. Acute pancreatitis in marrow transplant patients: prevalence at autopsy and risk factor analysis. *Bone Marrow Transplant* 1997; **20**: 1081–6.
465 Ko CW, Murakami C, Sekijima JH *et al*. Chemical composition of gallbladder sludge in patients after marrow transplantation. *Am J Gastroenterol* 1996; **91**: 1207–10.
466 Fisher RL. Hepatobiliary abnormalities associated with total parenteral nutrition. *Gastroenterol Clin North Am* 1989; **18**: 645–66.
467 Ohara N, Schaefer J. Clinical significance of biliary sludge. *J Clin Gastroenterol* 1990; **12**: 291–4.
468 Lee SP, Nicholls JF, Park HZ. Biliary sludge as a cause of acute pancreatitis. *N Engl J Med* 1992; **326**: 589–93.
469 Grier JF, Cohen SW, Grafton WD *et al*. Acute suppurative cholangitis associated with choledochal sludge. *Am J Gastroenterol* 1994; **89**: 617–9.
470 Frick MP, Snover DC, Feinberg SB *et al*. Sonography of the gallbladder in bone marrow transplant patients. *Am J Gastroenterol* 1984; **79**: 122–7.
471 Pitkaranta P, Haapiainen R, Taavitsainen M *et al*. Acalculous cholecystitis after bone marrow transplantation in adults with acute leukaemia. *Eur J Surg* 1991; **157**: 361–4.
472 Jardines LA, O'Donnell MR, Johnson DL *et al*. Acalculous cholecystitis in bone marrow transplant patients. *Cancer* 1993; **71**: 354–8.
473 Hurley R, Weisdorf DJ, Jessurun J *et al*. Relapse of acute leukemia presenting as acute cholecystitis following bone marrow transplantation. *Bone Marrow Transplant* 1992; **10**: 387–9.
474 Bigio EH, Haque AK. Disseminated cytomegalovirus infection presenting with acalculous cholecystitis and acute pancreatitis. *Arch Pathol Lab Med* 1989; **113**: 1287–9.
475 Valainis GT, Sachitano A, Pankey GA. Cholecystitis due to *Torulopsis glabrata*. *J Infect Dis* 1987; **156**: 244–5.
476 Cabana MD, Alavi A, Berlin JA *et al*. Morphine-augmented hepatobiliary scintigraphy: a meta-analysis. *Nucl Med Commun* 1995; **16**: 1068–71.
477 Yang HK, Hodgson WJ. Laparoscopic cholecystotomy for acute acalculous cholecystitis. *Surg Endosc* 1996; **10**: 673–5.
478 Fleming DR, Slone SP. CML blast crisis resulting in biliary obstruction following BMT. *Bone Marrow Transplant* 1997; **19**: 853–4.
479 Zutter MM, Martin PJ, Sale GE *et al*. Epstein–Barr virus lymphoproliferation after bone marrow transplantation. *Blood* 1988; **72**: 520–9.
480 Shapiro RS, McClain K, Frizzera G *et al*. Epstein–Barr virus associated B cell lymphoproliferative disorders following bone marrow transplantation. *Blood* 1988; **71**: 1234–43.
481 Chao NJ, Berry GJ, Advani R *et al*. Epstein–Barr virus-associated lymphoproliferative disorder following bone marrow transplantation for non-Hodgkin's lymphoma. *Transplantation* 1993; **55**: 1425–8.
482 Snover DC, Weisdorf S, Bloomer J *et al*. Nodular regenerative hyperplasia of the liver following bone marrow transplantation. *Hepatology* 1989; **9**: 443–8.
483 Kondo F. Benign nodular hepatocellular lesions caused by abnormal hepatic circulation. Etiological analysis and introduction of a new concept. *J Gastroenterol Hepatol* 2001; **16**: 1319–28.
484 Clouet M, Boulay I, Boudiaf M *et al*. Imaging features of nodular regenerative hyperplasia of the liver mimicking hepatic metastases. *Abdom Imaging* 1999; **24**: 258–61.
485 Leonard JV, Kay JD. Acute encephalopathy and hyperammonaemia complicating treatment of acute lymphoblastic leukaemia with asparaginase [Letter]. *Lancet* 1986; **1**: 162–3.
486 Sharp RA, Lang CC. Hyperammonaemic encephalopathy in chronic myelomonocytic leukaemia [Letter]. *Lancet* 1987; **1**: 805.
487 Mitchell RB, Wagner JE, Karp JE *et al*. Syndrome of idiopathic hyperammonemia after high-dose chemotherapy: review of nine cases. *Am J Med* 1988; **85**: 662–7.
488 Davies SM, Szabo E, Wagner JE *et al*. Idiopathic hyperammonemia: a frequently lethal complication of bone marrow transplantation. *Bone Marrow Transplant* 1996; **17**: 1119–25.
489 Frere P, Canivet JL, Gennigens C *et al*. Hyperammonemia after high-dose chemotherapy and stem cell transplantation. *Bone Marrow Transplant* 2000; **26**: 343–5.
490 Liaw CC, Liaw SJ, Wang CH *et al*. Transient hyperammonemia related to chemotherapy with continuous infusion of high-dose 5-fluorouracil. *Anticancer Drugs* 1993; **4**: 311–5.
491 Felig DM, Brusilow SW, Boyer JL. Hyperammonemic coma due to parenteral nutrition in a woman with heterozygous ornithine transcarbamylase deficiency. *Gastroenterology* 1995; **109**: 282–4.
492 Kaur S, Cooper G, Fakult S *et al*. Incidence and outcome of overt gastrointestinal bleeding in patients undergoing bone marrow transplantation. *Dig Dis Sci* 1996; **41**: 598–603.
493 Nevo S, Swan V, Enger C. Acute bleeding after bone marrow transplantation (BMT)-incidence and effect on survival. A quantitative analysis in 1402 patients. *Blood* 1998; **91**: 1469–77.
494 Schwartz JM, Wolford JL, Thornquist MD *et al*. Severe gastrointestinal bleeding after marrow transplantation, 1987–97: incidence, causes, and outcome. *Am J Gastroenterol* 2001; **96**: 385–93.
495 Otero Lopez-Cubero S, Sale GE, McDonald GB. Acute graft-versus-host disease of the esophagus. *Endoscopy* 1997; **29**: S35–S36.
496 Fitchen JH, Koeffler HP. Cimetidine and granulopoesis: bone marrow culture studies in normal man and patients with cimetidine-associated neutropenia. *Br J Haematol* 1980; **46**: 361–6.
497 Agura ED, Vila E, Peterson FB *et al*. The use of ranitidine in bone marrow transplantation. *Transplantation* 1988; **46**: 53–6.
498 Spencer GD, Shulman HM, Myerson D *et al*. Diffuse intestinal ulceration after marrow transplantation: a clinical-pathological study of 13 patients. *Hum Pathol* 1986; **17**: 621–33.
499 West JC, Armitage JO, Mitros FA *et al*. Cytomegalovirus cecal erosion causing massive hemorrhage in a bone marrow transplant recipient. *World J Surg* 1982; **6**: 252–5.
500 Charles AK, Caul EO, Porter HJ *et al*. Fatal adenovirus 32 infection in a bone marrow transplant recipient. *J Clin Pathol* 1995; **48**: 779–81.
501 Kanfer EJ, Abrahamson G, Taylor J *et al*. Severe rotavirus-associated diarrhoea following bone marrow transplantation: treatment with oral immunoglobulin. *Bone Marrow Transplant* 1994; **14**: 651–2.
502 Hopkins DG, Kushner JP. Clostridial species in the pathogenesis of necrotizing enterocolitis in patients with neutropenia. *Am J Hematol* 1983; **14**: 289–94.
503 Keates J, Lagahee S, Crilley P *et al*. CMV enteritis causing segmental ischemia and massive intestinal hemorrhage. *Gastrointest Endosc* 2001; **53**: 355–9.
504 Sutherland DE, Chan FY, Fourcar E *et al*. The bleeding cecal ulcer in transplant patients. *Surgery* 1979; **86**: 386–98.
505 Eras P, Goldstein MJ, Sherlock P. Candida infection of the gastrointestinal tract. *Medicine (Baltimore)* 1972; **51**: 367–79.

506 Welsh RA, McClinton LT. Aspergillosis of lungs and duodenum with fatal intestinal hemorrhage. *Arch Pathol* 1954; **57**: 379–82.

507 Foy TM, Hawkins EP, Peters KR *et al.* Colonic ulcers and lower GI bleeding due to disseminated aspergillosis. *J Ped Gastroent Nutrit* 1994; **18**: 399–403.

508 Cohen R, Heffner JE. Bowel infarction as the initial manifestation of disseminated aspergillosis. *Chest* 1992; **101**: 877–9.

509 Marmaduke DP, Greenson JK, Cunningham I *et al.* Gastric vascular ectasia in patients undergoing bone marrow transplantation. *Am J Clin Pathol* 1994; **102**: 194–8.

510 Tobin RW, Hackman RC, Kimmey MB *et al.* Bleeding from gastric antral vascular ectasia in marrow transplant patients. *Gastrointest Endosc* 1996; **44**: 223–9.

511 Lipson SA, Perr HA, Koerper MA *et al.* Intramural duodenal hematoma after endoscopic biopsy in leukemic patients. *Gastrointest Endosc* 1996; **44**: 620–3.

512 Jonas MM, Kelly DA, Mizerski J *et al.* Clinical trial of lamivudine in children with chronic hepatitis B. *N Engl J Med* 2002; **346**: 1706–13.

513 Horak DA, Forman SJ. Critical care of the hematopoietic stem cell patient. *Crit Care Clin* 2001; **17**: 671–95.

514 Stemmelin GR, Pest P, Peters RA *et al.* Severe esophageal stricture after autologous bone marrow transplant [Letter]. *Bone Marrow Transplant* 1995; **15**: 1001–2.

515 Hiller N, Zagal I, Hadas-Halpern I. Spontaneous intramural hematoma of the esophagus. *Am J Gastroenterol* 1999; **94**: 2282–4.

516 Sanaka M, Kuyama Y, Hirama S, Nagayama R, Tanaka H, Yamanaka M. Spontaneous intramural hematoma localized in the proximal esophagus: Truly "spontaneous?" *J Clin Gastroenterol* 1998; **27**: 265–6.

517 Ackert JJ, Sherman A, Lustbader IJ, McCauley DI. Spontaneous intramural hematoma of the esophagus. *Am J Gastroenterol* 1989; **84**: 1325–8.

518 Demos TC, Okrent DM, Studlo JD *et al.* Spontaneous esophageal hematoma diagnosed by computed tomography. *J Comput Assist Tomogr* 1986; **10**: 133–5.

519 Schweiger F, Depew WT. Spontaneous intramural esophageal hematoma. Diagnosis by CT scanning. *J Clin Gastroenterol* 1987; **9**: 546–8.

520 Skillington PD, Matar KS, Gardner MA. Intamural haematoma of oesophagus complicated by perforation. *Aust N Z J Surg* 1989; **59**: 430–2.

521 Folan RD, Smith RE, Head JM. Esophageal hematoma and tear requiring emergency surgical intervention. A case report and literature review. *Dig Dis Sci* 1992; **37**: 1918–21.

522 Goodman JL, Winston DJ, Greenfield RA *et al.* A controlled trial of fluconazole to prevent fungal infections in patients undergoing bone marrow transplantation. *N Engl J Med* 1992; **326**: 845–51.

523 Laing RB, Brettle RP, Leen CL. Clinical predictors of azole resistance, outcome and survival from oesophageal candidiasis in AIDS patients. *Int J STD AIDS* 1998; **9**: 16–20.

524 Choi JH, Yoo JH, Chung IJ *et al.* Esophageal aspergillosis after bone marrow transplant. *Bone Marrow Transplant* 1997; **19**: 293–4.

525 Krause W, Matheis H, Wulf K. Fungaemia and funguria after oral administration of *Candida albicans*. *Lancet* 1969; i: 598–9.

526 Tollemar J, Ringden L, Bostrom L *et al.* Variables predicting deep fungal infections in bone marrow transplant recipients. *Bone Marrow Transplant* 1989; **4**: 635–41.

527 Goodrich JM, Reed EC, Mori M *et al.* Clinical features and analysis of risk factors for invasive candidal infection after bone marrow transplantation. *J Infect Dis* 1991; **164**: 731–40.

528 McBane RD, Gross JB. Herpes esophagitis. Clinical syndrome, endoscopic appearance, and diagnosis in 23 patients. *Gastrointest Endosc* 1991; **37**: 600–3.

529 Silverstein FE, Tytgat GNJ. *Gastrointestinal Endoscopy*, 3rd edn. London: Mosby-Wolfe, 1997.

530 Spruance SL, Stewart JC, Rowe NH *et al.* Treatment of recurrent herpes labialis with oral acycovir. *J Infect Dis* 1990; **161**: 185–90.

531 Sherman RA, Silva J, Gandoor-Edwards R. Fatal varicella in an adult. Case report and review of the gastrointestinal complications of chickenpox. *Rev Inf Dis* 1991; **13**: 424–7.

532 Theise ND, Rotterdam H, Dietrich D. Cytomegalovirus esophagitis in AIDS. Diagnosis by endoscopic biopsy. *Am J Gastroenterol* 1991; **86**: 1123–6.

533 Hackman RC, Wolford JL, Gleaves CA *et al.* Recognition and rapid diagnosis of upper gastrointestinal cytomegalovirus infection in marrow transplant recipients. A comparison of seven virologic methods. *Transplantation* 1994; **57**: 231–7.

534 Nelson MR, Connolly GM, Hawkins DA *et al.* Foscarnet in the treatment of cytomegalovirus infection of the esophagus and colon in patients with the acquired immune deficiency syndrome. *Am J Gastroenterol* 1991; **86**: 876–81.

535 Larner AJ, Hamilton MIR. Review article. Infective complications of therapeutic gastric acid inhibition. *Aliment Pharmacol Ther* 1994; **8**: 579–84.

536 Yeomans ND, Brimblecone RW, Elder J *et al.* Effects of acid suppression on microbial flora of upper gut. *Dig Dis Sci* 1995; **40**: 81S–95S.

537 Iwakuma A, Matsuyoshi T, Arikado T *et al.* Two cases of postoperative erythroderma: clinical and pathological investigation. *J Jpn Assoc Thorac Surg* 1991; **39**: 209–13.

538 Kikendall JW. Pill esophagitis. *J Clin Gastroenterol* 1999; **28**: 298–305.

539 Fegan C, Poynton CH, Whittaker JA. The gut mucosal barrier in bone marrrow transplantation. *Bone Marrow Transplant* 1990; **5**: 373–7.

540 Lenssen P, Bruemmer B, Aker SN *et al.* Nutrient support in hematopoietic cell transplantation. *J Parenter Enteral Nutr* 2001; **25**: 219–28.

541 Ziegler TR. Glutamine supplementation in cancer patients receiving bone marrow transplantation and high dose chemotherapy. *J Nutrition* 2001; **131**: 2578S–84S.

542 Langdana A, Tully N, Molloy E *et al.* Intensive enteral nutrition support in paediatric bone marrow transplantation. *Bone Marrow Transplant* 2001; **27**: 741–6.

543 Coghlin Dickson TM, Wong RM, Offrin RS *et al.* Effect of oral glutamine supplementation during bone marrow transplantation. *J Parenteral Enteral Nutrition* 2000; **24**: 61–6.

544 Slavin RE, Dias MA, Saral R. Cytosine arabinoside induced gastrointestinal toxic alterations in sequential chemotherapeutic protocols. A clinical-pathologic study of 33 patients. *Cancer* 1978; **42**: 1747–59.

545 Slattery JT, Sanders JE, Buckner CD *et al.* Graft-rejection and toxicity following bone marrow transplantation in relation to busulfan pharmacokinetics. *Bone Marrow Transplant* 1995; **16**: 31–42.

546 Gouyette A, Hartmann O, Pico J-L. Phamacokinetics of high-dose melphalan in children and and adults. *Cancer Chemother Pharmacol* 1986; **16**: 184–9.

547 Tranchand B, Ploin YD, Minuit MP *et al.* High-dose melphalan dosage adjustment: possibility of using a test-dose. *Cancer Chemother Pharmacol* 1989; **23**: 95–100.

548 Morton AJ, Durrant ST. Efficacy of octreotide in controlling refractory diarrhea following bone marrow transplantation. *Clin Transpl* 1995; **9**: 205–8.

549 Crouch MA, Restino MS, Cruz JM *et al.* Octreotide acetate in refractory bone marrow transplant-associated diarrhea. *Ann Pharmacother* 1996; **30**: 331–6.

550 Geller RB, Gilmore CE, Dix SP *et al.* Randomized trial of loperamide versus dose escalation of octreotide acetate for chemotherapy-induced diarrhea in bone marrow transplant and leukemia patients. *Am J Hematol* 1995; **50**: 167–72.

551 Cox GJ, Matsui SM, Lo RS *et al.* Etiology and outcome of diarrhea after marrow transplantation: a prospective study. *Gastroenterology* 1994; **107**: 1398–407.

552 van Kraaij MG, Dekker AW, Verdonck LF *et al.* Infectious gastro-enteritis: an uncommon cause of diarrhoea in adult allogeneic and autologous stem cell transplant recipients. *Bone Marrow Transplant* 2000; **26**: 299–303.

553 Weisdorf SA, Salati LM, Longsdorf JA *et al.* Graft-vs.-host disease of the intestine: a protein-losing enteropathy characterized by fecal α_1-antitrypsin. *Gastroenterology* 1983; **85**: 1076–81.

554 Shaikh ZH, Ueno NT, Kontoyiannis DP. Fatal Salmonella group G enteritis mimicking intestinal graft-versus-host disease in a bone marrow transplant recipient. *Transpl Infect Dis* 2001; **3**: 29–33.

555 Einsele H, Ehninger G, Hebart H *et al.* Incidence of local CMV infection and acute intestinal GVHD in marrow transplant recipients with severe diarrhoea. *Bone Marrow Transplant* 1994; **14**: 955–63.

556 Maile CW, Frick MP, Crass JR *et al.* The plain radiograph in acute intestinal graft-versus-host disease. *Am J Roentgenol* 1985; **145**: 289–92.

557 Belli A-M, Williams MP. Graft versus host disease. Findings on plain abdominal radiography. *Clin Radiol* 1988; **39**: 262–4.

558 Jones B, Fishman EK, Kramer SS *et al.* Computed tomography of gastrointestinal inflammation after marrow transplantation. *Am J Roentgenol* 1986; **146**: 691–6.

559 Worawattanakul S, Semelka RC, Kelekis NL *et al.* MR findings of intestinal graft-versus-host disease. *Magn Reson Imaging* 1996; **14**: 1221–3.

560 Klein SA, Martin H, Schreiber-Dietrich D *et al.* A new approach to evaluating intestinal acute graft-versus-host disease by transabdominal sonography and colour Doppler imaging. *Br J Haematol* 2001; **115**: 929–34.

561 Mahendra P, Bedlow AJ, Ager S *et al.* Technetium (^{99m}Tc)-labelled white cell scanning, 51Cr-EDTA and 14C-mannitol-labelled intestinal permeability studies: non-invasive methods of diagnosing acute intestinal graft-versus-host disease. *Bone Marrow Transplant* 1994; **13**: 835–7.

562 Fisk JD, Shulman HM, Greening RR et al. Gastrointestinal radiographic features of human graft-versus-host disease. Am J Roentgenol 1981; **136**: 277–81.

563 Jones B, Kramer SS, Saral R et al. Gastrointestinal inflammation after bone marrow transplantation: graft-versus-host disease or opportunistic infection? Am J Roentgenol 1988; **150**: 277–81.

564 Navari RM, Sharma P, Deeg HJ et al. Pneumatosis cystoides intestinalis following allogeneic marrow transplantation. Transplant Proc 1983; **25**: 1720–4.

565 Yeager AM, Kanof ME, Kramer SS et al. Pneumatosis intestinalis in children after allogeneic bone marrow transplantation. Pediatr Radiol 1987; **17**: 18–22.

566 Day DL, Ramsay NKC, Letourneau JG. Pneumatosis intestinalis after bone marrow transplantation. Am J Roentgenol 1988; **151**: 85–7.

567 Lipton J, Patterson B, Mustard R et al. Pneumatosis intestinalis with free air mimicking intestinal perforation in a bone marrow transplant patient. Bone Marrow Transplant 1994; **14**: 323–6.

568 Hosomi N, Yoshioka H, Kuroda C et al. Pneumatosis cystoides intestinalis: CT findings. Abdom Imaging 1994; **19**: 137–9.

569 Roy J, Snover DC, Weisdorf S et al. Simultaneous upper and lower endoscopic biopsy in the diagnosis of intestinal graft-versus-host disease. Transplantation 1991; **51**: 642–6.

570 Saito H, Oshimi K, Nagasako K et al. Endoscopic appearance of the colon and small intestine of a patient with hemorrhagic enteric graft-versus-host disease. Dis Colon Rectum 1990; **33**: 695–7.

571 Bombi JA, Nadal A, Carreras E et al. Assessment of histopathologic changes in the colonic biopsy in acute graft-versus-host disease. Am J Clin Pathol 1995; **103**: 690–5.

572 Piguet P-F, Grau GE, Allet B et al. Tumor necrosis factor/cachectin is an effector of skin and gut lesions of the acute phase of graft-versus-host disease. J Exp Med 1987; **166**: 1280–9.

573 Madara JL. Loosening tight junctions: lessons from the intestine. J Clin Invest 1989; **83**: 1089–94.

574 Hill GR, Ferrara JLM. The primacy of the gastrointestinal tract as a target organ of acute graft-versus-host disease: rationale for the use of cytokine shields in allogeneic bone marrow transplantation. Blood 2000; **95**: 2754–9.

575 Dilly SA, Sloane JP. Changes in rectal leukocytes after allogeneic bone marrow transplantation. Clin Exp Immunol 1987; **67**: 951–8.

576 Gallucci BB, Sale GE, McDonald GB et al. The fine structure of human rectal epithelium in acute graft-versus-host disease. Am J Surg Pathol 1982; **6**: 293–305.

577 McDonald GB, Sale GE. The human gastrointestinal tract after allogenic marrow transplantation. In: Sale GE, Shulman HM, eds. The Pathology of Bone Marrow Transplantation. New York: Masson, 1984: 77–103.

578 Silva MRR, Henne K, Sale GE. Positive identification of enterocytes by keratin antibody staining of sloughed intestinal tissue in severe GVHD. Bone Marrow Transplant 1993; **12**: 35–6.

579 Ely P, Dunitz J, Rogosheske J et al. Use of a somatostatin analogue, octreotide acetate, in the management of acute gastrointestinal graft-versus-host disease. Am J Med 1991; **90**: 707–10.

580 Bianco JA, Higano C, Singer J et al. The somatostatin analog octreotide in the management of the secretory diarrhea of acute intestinal graft-versus-host disease in patients after bone marrow transplantation. Transplantation 1990; **49**: 1194–5.

581 Singh C, Gooley T, McDonald GB. Octreotide treatment for secretory diarrhea caused by graft-vs.-host disease: a dose escalation study. Gastroenterology 1996; **110**: 1016a [Abstract].

582 Fox RJ, Vogelsang GB, Beschorner WE. Denuded bowel after recovery from graft-versus-host disease. Transplantation 1996; **62**: 1681–4.

583 Rabbani GH, Teka T, Zaman B et al. Clinical studies in persistent diarrhea: dietary management with green banana or pectin in Bangladeshi children. Gastroenterology 2001; **121**: 554–60.

584 Beschorner WE, Yardley JH, Tutschka PJ et al. Deficiency of intestinal immunity with graft-versus-host disease in humans. J Infect Dis 1981; **144**: 38–46.

585 Snover DC. Mucosal damage simulating acute graft-versus-host disease in cytomegalovirus colitis. Transplantation 1985; **39**: 669–70.

586 Underwood JCE, Corbett CL. Persistent diarrhea and hypoalbuminenia associated with cytomegalovirus enteritis. Br Med J 1978; **1**: 1029–30.

587 Tajima T. An autopsy case of primary cytomegalic inclusion enteritis with remarkable hypoproteinemia. Acta Pathol Jpn 1974; **24**: 151–62.

588 Pinho Vaz C, Ibrahim A, Avila Garavito A et al. Protein-losing gastropathy associated with cytomegalovirus: a rare and late complication of allogeneic bone marrow transplantation. Bone Marrow Transplant 1996; **17**: 887–9.

589 Lepinski SM, Hamilton JW. Isolated cytomegalovirus ileitis detected by colonoscopy. Gastroenterology 1990; **98**: 1704–6.

590 Yolken RH, Bishop CA, Townsend TR et al. Infectious gastroenteritis in bone marrow transplant recipients. N Engl J Med 1982; **306**: 1010–2.

591 Townsend TR, Bolyard EA, Yolken RH et al. Outbreak of coxsackie A_1 gastroenteritis: a complication of bone marrow transplantation. Lancet 1982; **1**: 820–3.

592 Flomenberg P, Babbit J, Drobyski WR et al. Increasing incidence of adenovirus disease in bone marrow transplant patients. J Infect Dis 1994; **169**: 775–81.

593 Baldwin A, Kingman H, Darville M et al. Outcome and clinical course of 100 patients with adenovirus infection following bone marrow transplantation. Bone Marrow Transplant 2000; **26**: 1333–8.

594 Willoughby RE, Wee SB, Yolken RH. Non-group A rotavirus infection associated with severe gastroenteritis in a bone marrow transplant patient. Pediatr Infect Dis J 1988; **7**: 133–5.

595 Naik HR, Chandrasekar PH. Herpes simplex virus (HSV) colitis in a bone marrow transplant recipient. Bone Marrow Transplant 1996; **17**: 285–6.

596 Bartlett JG. Pseudomembranous enterocolitis and antibiotic-associated diarrhea. In: Feldman M, Friedman LS, Sleisenger MH, eds. Gastrointestinal and Liver Disease Pathophysiology/Diagnosis/Management, 7th edn. Philadelphia: Saunders & Co., 2002:1914–31.

597 Rampling A, Warren RE, Berry PJ et al. Atypical Clostridium difficile colitis in neutropenic patients [Letter]. Lancet 1982; **2**: 162–3.

598 Gorschluter M, Glasmacher A, Hahn C et al. Clostridium difficile infection in patients with neutropenia. Clin Infect Dis 2001; **33**: 786–91.

599 Schweitzer MA, Sweiss I, Silver DL et al. The clinical spectrum of Clostridium difficile colitis in immunocompromised patients. Am Surg 1996; **62**: 603–7.

600 Wenisch C, Parschalk B, Hasenhundl M et al. Comparison of vancomycin, teicoplanin, metronidazole, and fusidic acid for the treatment of Clostridium difficile-associated diarrhea. Clin Infect Dis 1996; **22**: 813–8.

601 Cesaro S, Chinello P, Rossi L et al. Saccharomyces cerevisiae fungemia in a neutropenic patient treated with Saccharomyces boulardii. Support Care Cancer 2000; **8**: 504–5.

602 Nagler A, Pavel L, Naparstek E et al. Typhilitis occurring in autologous bone marrrow transplantation. Bone Marrow Transplant 1992; **9**: 63–4.

603 Van Kessel LJP, Verbrugh HA, Stringer MF et al. Necrotizing enteritis associated with toxigenic type A Clostridium perfringens. J Infect Dis 1985; **151**: 974–5.

604 Kane JG, Chretien JH, Garagusi VF. Diarrhea caused by Candida. Lancet 1976; **i**: 335–6.

605 Gupta TP, Ehrinpreis MN. Candida-associated diarrhea in hospitalized patients. Gastroenterology 1990; **98**: 780–5.

606 Danna PL, Urban C, Bellin E et al. Role of Candida in pathogenesis of antibiotic-associated diarrhea in elderly patients. Lancet 1991; **337**: 511–4.

607 Prescott RJ, Harris M, Banerjee SS. Fungal infections of the small and large intestine. J Clin Pathol 1992; **45**: 806–11.

608 Hofstra W, de Vries-Hospers HG, van der Waaij D. Concentrations of nystatin in faeces after oral administration of various doses. Infection 1979; **4**: 166–70.

609 Hofstra W, de Vries-Hospers HG, van der Waaij D. Concentrations of amphotericin B in faeces and blood of healthy volunteers after the oral administration of various doses. Infection 1982; **10**: 223–7.

610 Alvarez OA, Maples JA, Tio FO et al. Severe diarrhea due to Cokeromyces recurvatus in a bone marrow transplant recipient. Am J Gastroenterol 1995; **90**: 1350–1.

611 Tsai TW, Hammond LA, Rinaldi M et al. Cokeromyces recurvatus infection in a bone marrow transplant recipient. Bone Marrow Transplant 1997; **19**: 301–2.

612 Manivel C, Filipovich A, Snover DC. Cryptosporidiosis as a cause of diarrhea following bone marrow transplantation. Dis Colon Rectum 1985; **28**: 741–2.

613 Long EG, Christie JD. The diagnosis of old and new gastrointestinal parasites. Clin Laboratory Med 1995; **15**: 307–31.

614 Zimmerman SK, Needham CA. Comparison of conventional stool concentration and preserved-smear methods with Merifluor Cryptosporidium/Giardia direct immunofluorescence assay and ProSPECT Giardia EZ microplate assay for detection of Giardia lamblia. J Clin Microbiol 1995; **33**: 1942–3.

615 Aldeen WE, Hale D, Robison AJ et al. Evaluation of a commercially available ELISA assay for detection of Giardia lamblia in fecal specimens. Diagn Microbiol Infect Dis 1995; **21**: 77–9.

616 Zaat JO, Mank TG, Assendelft WJ. A systematic review on the treatment of Giardiasis. Trop Med Int Health 1997; **2**: 63–82.

617 Aplin MS, Weiner R, Graham Pole J, Hiemenz J, Elfenbein G, Oblon DJ. Enterocolitis in allogeneic marrow transplant patients. Exp Hematol 1990; **18**: 696 [Abstract].

618 Gauvreau JM, Lenssen P, Cheney CL et al. Nutritional management of patients with intestinal graft-versus-host disease. J Am Diet Assoc 1981; **79**: 673–7.

619 Hove H, Tvede M, Mortensen PB. Antibiotic-associated diarrhoea, Clostridium difficile, and short-chain fatty acids. Scand J Gastroenterol 1996; **31**: 688–93.

620 Rogers M, Cerda JJ. The narcotic bowel syndrome. J Clin Gastroenterol 1989; **11**: 132–5.

621 Camilleri M, Phillips SF. Acute and chronic intestinal pseudo-obstruction. Adv Intern Med 1991; **36**: 287–306.

622 Burton MB, Gebhart GF. Effects of kappa-opioid receptor agonists on responses to colorectal distension in rats with and without acute colonic inflammation. J Pharmacol Exp Ther 1998; **285**: 707–15.

623 Gillis JC, Benfield P, Goa KL. Transnasal butorphanol. A review of its pharmacodynamic and pharmacokinetic properties, and therapeutic potential in acute pain management. Drugs 1995; **50**: 157–75.

624 Ponec RJ, Saunders MD, Kimmey MB. Neostigmine for the treatment of acute colonic pseudo-obstruction. N Engl J Med 1999; **341**: 137–41.

625 Stemmer SM, Kinsman K, Tellschow S et al. Fatal noncutaneous visceral infection with varicella-zoster virus in a patient with lymphoma after autologous bone marrow transplantation. Clin Infect Dis 1993; **16**: 497–9.

626 Nomdedeu JF, Nomdedeu J, Martino R et al. Ogilvie's syndrome from disseminated varicella-zoster infection and infarcted celiac ganglia. J Clin Gastroenterol 1995; **20**: 157–9.

627 Rogers SY, Irving W, Harris A et al. Visceral varicella zoster infection after bone marrow transplantation without skin involvement and the use of PCR for diagnosis. Bone Marrow Transplant 1995; **15**: 805–7.

628 Grant RM, Weitzman SS, Sherman CG et al. Fulminant disseminated varicella zoster virus infection without skin involvement. J Clin Virol 2002; **24**: 7–12.

629 Sonsino E, Mouy R, Foucaud P et al. Intestinal pseudoobstruction related to cytomegalovirus infection of myenteric plexus [Letter]. N Engl J Med 1984; **311**: 196–7.

630 Bedi A, Miller CB, Hanson JL et al. Association of BK virus with failure of prophylaxis against hemorrhagic cystitis following bone marrow transplantation. J Clin Oncol 1995; **13**: 1103–9.

631 Leung AY, Suen CK, Lie AK et al. Quantification of polyoma BK viruria in hemorrhagic cystitis complicating bone marrow transplantation. Blood 2001; **98**: 1971–8.

632 Akiyama H, Kurosu T, Sakashita C et al. Adenovirus is a key pathogen in hemorrhagic cystitis associated with bone marrow transplantation. Clin Infect Dis 2001; **32**: 1325–30.

633 Cartoni C, Arcese W, Avvisati G et al. Role of ultrasonography in the diagnosis and follow-up of hemorrhagic cystitis after bone marrow transplantation. Bone Marrow Transplant 1993; **12**: 463–7.

634 McCarville MB, Hoffer FA, Gingrich JR et al. Imaging findings of hemorrhagic cystitis in pediatric oncology patients. Pediatric Radiol 2000; **30**: 131–8.

635 Janowitz P, Kratzer W, Zemmler T et al. Gallbladder sludge: spontaneous course and incidence of complications in patients without stones. Hepatology 1994; **20**: 291–4.

636 Adolph MD, Bass SN, Lee SK et al. Cytomegaloviral acalculous cholecystitis in acquired immunodeficiency syndrome patients. Am Surg 1993; **59**: 679–84.

637 Werlin SL, Casper J, Antonson D et al. Pancreatitis associated with bone marrow transplantation in children. Bone Marrow Transplant 1992; **10**: 65–9.

638 Shore T, Bow E, Greenberg H et al. Pancreatitis post-bone marrow transplantation. Bone Marrow Transplant 1996; **17**: 1181–4.

639 Mallory A, Kern FJ. Drug-induced pancreatitis: a critical review. Gastroenterology 1980; **78**: 813–20.

640 Parenti DM, Steinberg W, Kang P. Infectious causes of acute pancreatitis. Pancreas 1996; **13**: 356–71.

641 Washington K, Gossage DL, Gottfried MR. Pathology of the pancreas in severe combined immunodeficiency and DiGeorge syndrome: acute graft-versus-host disease and unusual viral infections. Hum Pathol 1994; **25**: 908–14.

642 Washington K, Peters W. Pathology of the pancreas in bone marrow transplant patients. Hum Pathol 1993; **24**: 152–9.

643 Nieto Y, Russ P, Everson G et al. Acute pancreatitis during immunosuppression with tacrolimus following an allogeneic umbilical cord blood transplantation. Bone Marrow Transplant 2000; **26**: 109–11.

644 Foulis AK, Farquharson MA, Sale GE. The pancreas in acute graft-versus-host disease in man. Histopathology 1989; **14**: 48a [Abstract].

645 Scott WW, Fishman EK, Siegelman SS. Anticoagulants and abdominal pain. JAMA 1984; **252**: 2053–6.

646 Finnance N, Sullivan KM, Tobin R et al. A female bone marrow recipient with abdominal pain. Physician Assist 1995; **19**: 106–9.

647 Koura T, Itoh T, Motimaru J et al. Rectus hematoma secondary to vomiting: a complication of conditioning regimen for bone marrow transplantation. Intern Med 1995; **34**: 39–41.

648 Titone C, Lipsius M, Krakauer JS. "Spontaneous" hematoma of the rectus abdominus muscle: critical review of 50 cases with emphasis on early diagnosis and treatment. Surgery 1972; **72**: 568–72.

649 Young JR, Cressman M, O'Hara PJ. Rectus sheath hematoma: diagnosis by computed tomography. Arch Intern Med 1981; **141**: 820–2.

650 Blatt SH, Gold SH, Wiley JM et al. Off-label use of recombinant factor VIIa in patients following bone marrow transplantation. Bone Marrow Transplant 2001; **28**: 405–7.

651 Shimoda NT, Chauncey TR, Durtschi M, McDonald GB. Intestinal perforation in marrow transplant patients: incidence, risk factors, and clinical features. Gastroenterology 1994; **106**: 27a [Abstract].

652 de Magalhaes-Silverman M, Simpson J, Ball E. Pneumoperitoneum without peritonitis after allogeneic peripheral blood stem cell transplantation. Bone Marrow Transplant 1998; **21**: 1153–4.

653 Schulenburg A, Herold C, Eisenhuber E. et al. Pneumatosis correction of Pneumocystis cystoides intestinalis with pneumoperitoneum and pneumoretroperitoneum in a patient with extensive chronic graft-versus-host disease. Bone Marrow Transplant 1999; **24**: 331–3. Erratum: Bone Marrow Transplant 2000; **25**: 463.

654 Knechtle SJ, Davidoff AM, Rice RP. Pneumatosis intestinalis. Surgical management and clinical outcome. Ann Surg 1990; **212**: 160–5.

655 King A, Rampling A, Wight DGD et al. Neutropenic enterocolitis due to Clostridium septicum infection. J Clin Pathol 1984; **37**: 335–43.

656 Otaibi AA, Barker C, Anderson R et al. Neutropenic enterocolitis (typhlitis) after pediatric bone marrow transplant. J Pediatric Surg 2002; **37**: 770–2.

657 Teefey SA, Montant MA, Goldfogel GA et al. Sonographic diagnosis of neutropenic typhlitis. Am J Roentgenol 1987; **149**: 731–3.

658 Frick MP, Maile CW, Cras JR et al. Computed tomography of neutropenic colitis. Am J Roentgenol 1984; **143**: 763–5.

659 Kunkel JM, Rossenthal D. Management of the ileocecal syndrome: neutropenic enterocolitis. Dis Colon Rectum 1986; **29**: 196–9.

660 Shamberger RC, Weinstein HJ, Delorey MJ et al. The medical and surgical management of typhlitis in children with acute nonlymphocytic (myelogenous) leukemia. Cancer 1986; **57**: 603–9.

661 Tie ML, Stephens DH. Candida jejunitis: a rare cause of intestinal pneumatosis in the immunocompromised patient. Australas Radiol 2000; **44**: 206–7.

662 Marr KA, Carter RA, Crippa F et al. Epidemiology and outcome of mould infections in hematopoietic stem cell transplant recipients. Clin Infect Dis 2002; **34**: 909–17.

663 Zutter MM, Durnam DM, Hackman RC et al. Secondary T-cell lymphoproliferation after marrow transplantation. Am J Clin Pathol 1990; **94**: 714–21.

664 Faye A, Quartier P, Reguerre Y et al. Chimaeric anti-CD20 monoclonal antibody (rituximab) in post-transplant B-lymphoproliferative disorder following stem cell transplantation in children. Br J Haematol 2001; **115**: 112–8.

665 O'Reilly RJ, Lacerda JF, Lucas KG et al. Adoptive cell therapy with donor lymphocytes for EBV-associated lymphomas developing after allogeneic marrow transplants. In: DeVita VT, Hellman S, Rosenberg SA, eds. Important Advances in Oncology 1996. Philadelphia: Lippincott-Raven, 1996: 149–66.

666 Hoffmann T, Russell C, Vindelov L. Generation of EBV-specific CTLs suitable for adoptive immunotherapy of EBV-associated lymphoproliferative disease following allogeneic transplantation. APMIS 2002; **110**: 148–57.

667 Szabo F, Horvath N, Seimon S et al. Inappropriate antidiuretic hormone secretion, abdominal pain and disseminated varicella-zoster virus infection: an unusual triad in a patient 6 months post mini-allogeneic peripheral stem cell transplant for chronic myeloid leukemia. Bone Marrow Transplant 2000; **26**: 231–3.

668 McIlwaine LM, Fitzsimons EJ, Soutar RL. Inappropriate antidiuretic hormone secretion, abdominal pain and disseminated varicella-zoster virus infection: an unusual and fatal triad in a patient 13 months post rituximab and autologous stem cell transplantation. Clin Lab Haematol 2001; **23**: 253–4.

669 Corfitsen MT, Hansen CP, Christensen TH et al. Anorectal abscesses in immunosuppressed patients. Eur J Surg 1992; **158**: 51–3.

670 Schwartz DA, Harewood GC, Wiersema MJ. EUS for rectal disease. Gastrointest Endosc 2002; **56**: 100–9.

671 Barnes SG, Sattler FR, Ballard JO. Perirectal infections in acute leukemia. Improved survival after incision and debridement. Ann Intern Med 1984; **10**: 515–8.

672 Carroll PR, Cattolica EV, Turzan CW et al. Necrotizing soft-tissue infections of the perineum and genitalia. Etiology and early reconstruction. *West J Med* 1986; **144**: 174–8.

673 Siegal FP, Lopez C, Hammer GS et al. Severe acquired immunodeficiency in male homosexuals manifested by chronic perianal ulcerative herpes simplex lesions. *N Engl J Med* 1981; **305**: 1439–44.

674 Sullivan KM, Shulman HM, Storb R et al. Chronic graft-versus-host disease in 52 patients: adverse natural course and successful treatment with combination immunosuppression. *Blood* 1981; **57**: 267–76.

675 Crawford JM. Graft-versus-host disease of the liver. In: Ferrara JLM, Deeg HJ, Burakoff SJ, eds. *Graft-vs.-Host Disease*, 2nd edn. New York: Marcel Dekker, Inc., 1997: 315–36.

676 Tomas JF, Pinilla I, Garcia-Buey ML et al. Long-term liver dysfunction after allogeneic bone marrow transplantation: clinical features and course in 61 patients. *Bone Marrow Transplant* 2000; **26**: 649–55.

677 Malik AH, Collins RH, Jr, Saboorian MH et al. Chronic graft versus host disease (GVHD) following hematopoietic cell transplantation (HCT) presenting as an acute hepatitis. *Am J Gastroenterol* 2001; **96**: 588–90.

678 Siadak M, Sullivan KM. The management of chronic graft-versus-host disease. *Blood Rev* 1994; **8**: 154–60.

679 Locasciulli A, Bacigalupo A, Van Lint MT et al. Hepatitis C virus infection in patients undergoing allogeneic bone marrow transplantation. *Transplantation* 1991; **52**: 315–8.

680 Kolho E, Ruutu P, Ruutu T. Hepatitis C infection in BMT patients. *Bone Marrow Transplant* 1993; **11**: 119–23.

681 Neilson JR, Harrison P, Skidmore SJ et al. Chronic hepatitis C in long-term survivors of haematological malignancy treated in a single centre. *J Clin Pathol* 1996; **49**: 230–2.

682 Strasser SI, Sullivan KM, Myerson D et al. Cirrhosis of the liver in long-term marrow transplant survivors. *Blood* 1999; **93**: 3259–66.

683 Peffault de Latour R, Levey V, Ades L et al. Long-term follow-up of hepatitis C virus (HCV)-infected allogeneic stem cell transplant (SCT) recipients: high incidence of cirrhosis and cancers. *Blood* 2002; **100**: 114a [Abstract].

684 Bonkovsky HL, Banner BF, Rothman AL. Iron and chronic viral hepatitis. *Hepatology* 1997; **25**: 759–68.

685 Sievert W, Pianko S, Warner S et al. Hepatic iron overload does not prevent a sustained virological response to interferon-α therapy: a long term follow-up study in hepatitis C-infected patients with beta thalassemia major. *Am J Gastroenterol* 2002; **97**: 982–7.

686 Muretto P, Angelucci E, Lucarelli G. Reversibility of cirrhosis in patients cured of thalassemia by bone marrow transplantation. *Ann Intern Med* 2002; **136**: 667–72.

687 Serrano P, Prieto E, Mazarbeitia F et al. Atypical chronic graft-versus-host disease following interferon therapy for chronic myeloid leukaemia relapsing after allogeneic BMT. *Bone Marrow Transplant* 2001; **27**: 85–7.

688 Chen YC, Sheen IS, Chu CM et al. Prognosis following spontaneous HBsAg seroclearance in chronic hepatitis B patients with or without concurrent infection. *Gastroenterology* 2002; **123**: 1084–9.

689 Strasser SI, Kowdley KV, Sale GE et al. Iron overload in bone marrow transplant recipients. *Bone Marrow Transplant* 1998; **22**: 167–73.

690 McKay PJ, Murphy JA, Cameron S et al. Iron overload and liver dysfunction after allogeneic or autologous bone marrow transplantation. *Bone Marrow Transplant* 1996; **17**: 63–6.

691 Iqbal M, Creger RJ, Fox RM et al. Laparoscopic liver biopsy to evaluate hepatic dysfunction in patients with hematologic malignancies: a useful tool to effect changes in management. *Bone Marrow Transplant* 1996; **17**: 655–62.

692 Angelucci E, Brittenham GM, McLaren CE et al. Hepatic iron concentration and total body iron stores in thalassemia major. *N Engl J Med* 2000; **343**: 327–31.

693 Lucarelli G, Angelucci E, Giardini C et al. Fate of iron stores in thalassaemia after bone-marrow transplantation. *Lancet* 1993; **342**: 1388–91.

694 Jensen PD, Jensen FT, Christensen T et al. Evaluation of transfusional iron overload before and during iron chelation by magnetic resonance imaging of the liver and determination of serum ferritin in adult non-thalassaemic patients. *Br J Haematol* 1995; **89**: 880–9.

695 Kornreich L, Horev G, Yaniv I et al. Iron overload following bone marrow transplantation in children: MR findings. *Pediatr Radiol* 1997; **27**: 869–72.

696 Mariotti E, Angelucci E, Agostini A et al. Evaluation of cardiac status in iron-loaded thalassaemia patients following bone marrow transplantation: improvement in cardiac function during reduction in body iron burden. *Br J Haematol* 1998; **103**: 916–21.

697 Angelucci E, Baronciani D, Lucarelli G et al. Liver iron overload and liver fibrosis in thalassemia. *Bone Marrow Transplant* 1993; **12** (Suppl. 1): 29–31.

698 Angelucci E, Muretto P, Lucarelli G et al. Phlebotomy to reduce iron overload in patients cured of thalassemia by bone marrow transplantation. Italian Cooperative Group for the Phlebotomy Treatment of Transplanted Thalassemia Patients. *Blood*, 1997; **90**: 994–8.

699 Mahendra P, Hood IM, Bass G et al. Severe hemosiderosis post allogeneic bone marrow transplantation. *Hematol Oncol* 1996; **14**: 33–5.

700 Harrison P, Neilson JR, Marwah SS et al. Role of non-transferrin bound iron in iron overload and liver dysfunction in long term survivors of acute leukaemia and bone marrow transplantation. *J Clin Pathol* 1996; **49**: 853–6.

701 Kaplan J, Sarnaik S, Gitlin J et al. Diminished helper/suppressor lymphocyte ratios and natural killer activity in recipients of repeated blood transfusions. *Blood* 1984; **64**: 308–10.

702 Olynyk JK, Clarke SL. Iron overload impairs pro-inflammatory cytokine responses by Kupffer cells. *J Gastroenterol Hepatol* 2001; **16**: 438–44.

703 Blei F, Puder DR. *Yersinia enterocolitica* bacteremia in a chronically transfused patient with sickle cell anemia. Case report and review of the literature. *Am J Pediatr Hematol Oncol* 1993; **15**: 430–4.

704 Lee AC, Ha SY, Yuen KY et al. Listeria septicemia complicating bone marrow transplantation for Diamond–Blackfan syndrome. *Pediatr Hematol Oncol* 1995; **12**: 295–9.

705 Maertens J, Demuynck H, Verbeken EK et al. Mucormycosis in allogeneic bone marrow transplant recipients: report of five cases and review of the role of iron overload in the pathogenesis. *Bone Marrow Transplant* 1999; **24**: 307–12.

706 Gaziev D, Baronciani D, Galimberti M et al. Mucormycosis after bone marrow transplantation: report of four cases in thalassemia and review of the literature. *Bone Marrow Transplant* 1996; **17**: 409–14.

707 Bullen JJ, Spalding PB, Ward CG et al. Hemochromatosis, iron and septicemia caused by *Vibrio vulnificus*. *Arch Intern Med* 1991; **151**: 1606–9.

708 Grigg AP, Bhathal PS. Compound heterozygosity for haemochromatosis gene mutations and hepatic iron overload in allogeneic bone marrow transplant recipients. *Pathology* 2001; **33**: 44–9.

709 Muretto P, Angelucci E, Lucarelli G. Reversibility of cirrhosis in patients cured of thalassemia by bone marrow transplantation. *Ann Intern Med* 2002; **136**: 667–72.

710 Chitturi S, George J. Hepatotoxicity of commonly used drugs: nonsteroidal anti-inflammatory drugs, antihypertensives, antidiabetic agents, anticonvulsants, lipid-lowering agents, psychotropic drugs. *Semin Liver Dis* 2002; **22**: 169–83.

711 Brown SJ, Desmond PV. Hepatotoxicity of antimicrobial agents. *Semin Liver Dis* 2002; **22**: 157–67.

712 Nierenberg DW. "Did this drug cause my patient's hepatitis?" and related questions. *Ann Intern Med* 2002; **136**: 480–3.

713 Lorber MI, Van Buren CT, Flechner SM et al. Hepatobiliary and pancreatic complications of cyclosporine therapy in 466 renal transplant recipients. *Transplantation* 1987; **43**: 35–40.

714 Farrell GC. Drugs and steatohepatitis. *Semin Liver Dis* 2002; **22**: 185–94.

715 Munoz SJ, Martinez Hernandez A, Maddrey WC. Intrahepatic cholestasis and phospholipidosis associated with the use of trimethoprim-sulfamethoxazole. *Hepatology* 1990; **12**: 342–7.

716 Kowdley KV, Keeffe EB, Fawaz KA. Prolonged cholestasis due to trimethoprim-sulfamethoxazole. *Gastroenterology* 1992; **102**: 2148–50.

717 Mion F, Napoleon B, Berger F et al. Azathioprine induced liver disease: nodular regenerative hyperplasia of the liver and perivenous fibrosis in a patient treated for multiple sclerosis. *Gut* 1991; **32**: 715–7.

718 Adler M, Delhaye M, Deprez C et al. Hepatic vascular disease after kidney transplantation: report of two cases and review of the literature. *Nephrol Dial Transplant* 1987; **2**: 183–8.

719 De Smet PAGM. Herbal remedies. *N Engl J Med* 2002; **347**: 2046–56.

720 Chitturi S, Farrell GC. Herbal hepatotoxicity: an expanding but poorly defined problem. *J Gastroenterol Hepatol* 2000; **15**: 1093–9.

721 McRae CA, Agarwal K, Mutimer D et al. Hepatitis associated with Chinese herbs. *European J Gastroenterol Hepatol* 2002; **14**: 559–62.

722 Oliver MR, Van Voorhis WC, Boeckh M et al. Hepatic mucormycosis in a bone marrow transplant recipient who ingested naturopathic medicine. *Clin Infect Dis* 1996; **22**: 521–4.

723 Curtis RE, Rowlings PA, Deeg HJ et al. Solid cancers after bone marrow transplantation. *N Engl J Med* 1997; **336**: 897–904.

724 Bhatia S, Louie AD, Bhatia R et al. Solid cancers after bone marrow transplantation. *J Clin Oncol* 2001; **19**: 464–71.

725 Sullivan KM, Agura E, Anasetti C et al. Chronic graft-versus-host disease and other late complications of bone marrow transplantation. *Semin Hematol* 1991; **28**: 250–8.

726 McDonald GB, Sullivan KM, Schuffler MD *et al.* Esophageal abnormalities in chronic graft-versus-host disease in humans. *Gastroenterology* 1981; **80**: 914–21.

727 McDonald GB, Sullivan KM, Plumley TF. Radiographic features of esophageal involvement in chronic graft-versus-host disease. *Am J Roentgenol* 1984; **142**: 501–6.

728 Minocha A, Mandanas RA, Kida M *et al.* Bullous esophagitis due to chronic graft-versus-host disease. *Am J Gastroenterol* 1997; **92**: 529–30.

729 Schima W, Pokieser P, Forstinger C *et al.* Videofluoroscopy of the pharynx and esophagus in chronic graft-versus-host disease. *Abdom Imaging* 1994; **19**: 191–4.

730 Mackey JR, Desai S, Larratt L *et al.* Myasthenia gravis in association with allogeneic bone marrow transplantation: clinical observations, therapeutic implications and review of literature. *Bone Marrow Transplant* 1997; **19**: 939–42.

731 Atree SV, Crilley PA, Conroy JF *et al.* Cancer of the esophagus following allogeneic bone marrow transplantation for acute leukemia. *Am J Clin Oncol* 1995; **18**: 343–7.

732 Patey-Mariaud de Serre N, Reijasse D, Verkarre V *et al.* Chronic intestinal graft-versus-host disease: clinical, histological and immunohistochemical analysis of 17 children. *Bone Marrow Transplant* 2002; **29**: 223–30.

733 Izutsu KT, Sullivan KM, Schubert MM *et al.* Disordered salivary immunoglobulin secretion and sodium transport in human chronic graft-versus-host disease. *Transplantation* 1983; **35**: 441–6.

734 Jurges E, O'Donohoe J, El Tumi M *et al.* Pancreatic insufficiency after bone-marow transplantation. *Lancet* 1991; **338**: 517.

735 Tyden G, Brattstrom C, Ringden O *et al.* Pancreatic insufficiency after bone-marrow transplantation. *Lancet* 1991; **338**: 1088–9.

736 Anderson H, Grimes DS, Morgenstern AR *et al.* Pancreatic insufficiency after bone marrow transplantation [Letter]. *Lancet* 1991; **11**: 1089.

737 Akpek G, Valladares JL, Lee L *et al.* Pancreatic insufficiency in patients with chronic graft-versus-host disease. *Bone Marrow Transplant* 2001; **27**: 163–6.

738 Shulman HM, Sullivan KM, Weiden PL *et al.* Chronic graft-versus-host syndrome in man. A long-term clinicopathologic study of 29 Seattle patients. *Am J Med* 1980; **69**: 204–17.

739 Webb M, Meyer B, Jackson JM *et al.* Localized relapse of chronic myeloid leukaemia post allogeneic bone marrow transplantation. *Br J Haematol* 1993; **84**: 178–9.

59

Harry Openshaw

Neurological Complications of Hematopoietic Cell Transplantation

Introduction

There have been several reviews of neurological complications associated with hematopoietic cell transplantation (HCT), both in adults [1–3] and children [4,5] Published rates of complications varied from 3% in autologous transplants [6] to as high as high as 44% in matched unrelated donor transplants [7]. A monograph published in 1999 discusses this subject with comparisons to liver, kidney and heart-lung transplants [8]. The present chapter classifies neurological complications under standard disease categories of infectious, cerebrovascular, metabolic, immune-mediated and toxic. The last section outlines an approach to neurological differential diagnosis.

Complications from central nervous system (CNS) infection

Survival after transplantation has improved, in part as a consequence of advances in the management of infectious complications [9]. The neurological presentation of CNS infection in HCT recipients is usually an alteration in mental status, delirium, or depression of sensorium, often without meningeal signs or obvious lateralizing neurological signs. A spinal fluid examination is indicated once a mass lesion has been excluded. For a suspected brain abscess, a stereotactic biopsy under appropriate platelet support usually is diagnostic.

The incidence of CNS infection was 5% in a clinical series of allogeneic transplantation from the early 1970s, and in three autopsy series the incidence was 8–15% [1,10–12]. *Aspergillus* spp. accounted for 30–50% of CNS infections in autopsy series and remains a major problem in HCT. Magnetic resonance imaging (MRI) of an aspergillus abcsess is shown in Fig. 59.1a. As noted in Chapter 52, trials with prophylaxis and treatment have been disappointing [13], although occasional patients with CNS aspergillus abscess survive [14] and treatment prospects may improve with the availability of voriconazole [15]. *Candida albicans*, the other serious fungal pathogen encountered after transplantation, infects the CNS in only 3% of transplant patients with systemic candidemia [16], although candida species abscesses accounted for 15% of the CNS infections in a large autopsy series from Brazil [12]. Chronic fungal meningitides, for example from *Cryptococcus neoformans*, so frequent a complication of immunosuppression in other disease processes, is rarely encountered in HCT recipients.

CNS infection with the protozoan *Toxoplasma gondii* is occasionally seen during the early post-transplantation period after engraftment [17,18], particularly in patients who do not receive trimethoprim and sulfamethoxazole prophylaxis. Figure 59.1c,d shows an MRI of a City of Hope National Medical Center patient who developed CNS toxoplasmosis after autologous transplantation and had a good response to pyramethamine and sulfadiazine.

Antimicrobial prophylaxis early in the transplant course is particularly effective for gram-negative organisms, and bacterial meningitis at this stage is now unusual, although at least six reported cases of *Listeria monocytogenes* meningitis occurred in the first 4 months after allogeneic HCT [19,20]. Also unusual, but still a risk, is bacterial meningitis in long-term survivors with chronic graft-vs.-host disease (GVHD). In addition to rare patients with *L. monocytogenes* meningitis, meningitis due to penicillin-resistant *Streptococcus pneumoniae* has been documented in long-term survivors [21]. Meningitis is even rarer after autologous transplantation, although two cases of *L. monocytogenes* and one of *Stomatococcus mucilaginosus* have been reported [20]. A fatal case of *Mycobacterium tuberculosis* CNS infection has been reported [3], but mycobacterial infections are relatively uncommon in transplant patients—only 0.47% of 1486 allogeneic transplantations and 0.25% of 756 autologous transplantations [22].

Recognized manifestations of cytomegalovirus (CMV) infection in transplant patients include pulmonary, hepatic and gastrointestinal involvement (see Chapter 53). For reasons that are uncertain, CMV chorioretinitis, a very common problem in human immunodeficiency virus/acquired immune deficiency syndrome (HIV/AIDS), is rarely diagnosed in HCT recipients [23]. Similarly, CMV encephalitis is recognized at least histopathologically in HIV/AIDS but is rarely diagnosed or documented in marrow transplant recipients [1,24]. A neuropathological review of 28 HCT patients who died after systemic CMV infection noted microglial nodules compatible with CMV infection in seven, all of whom had a clinical course compatible with a nonfocal encephalitis [1]. However, CMV cultures, detection of viral inclusion bodies and immunocytochemical staining for CMV antigens were negative or not done in these patients. It remains to be established whether CMV encephalitis is a clinically important entity in HCT recipients.

Herpes simplex virus, type 1 (HSV-1) reactivates and is shed in the oral secretions of 80% of seropositive patients during the first few weeks after HCT [25]. As described in Chapter 54, acyclovir prophylaxis prevents viral shedding [26] and is used routinely now in many transplant centers. Despite the high incidence of viral reactivation, the clinical diagnosis of herpes simplex encephalitis is rarely made in transplant recipients. In immunocompetent individuals, herpes encephalitis usually occurs without any sign of mucocutaneous infection, and the infection is focal in the temporal lobes, most often presenting with seizures and psychiatric symptoms. Two fatal cases of herpes encephalitis were noted from the transplant unit at Johns Hopkins University [1]. The diagnosis in these patients was confirmed by viral culture and immunohistochemistry, but unlike typical herpes encephalitis in otherwise normal individuals,

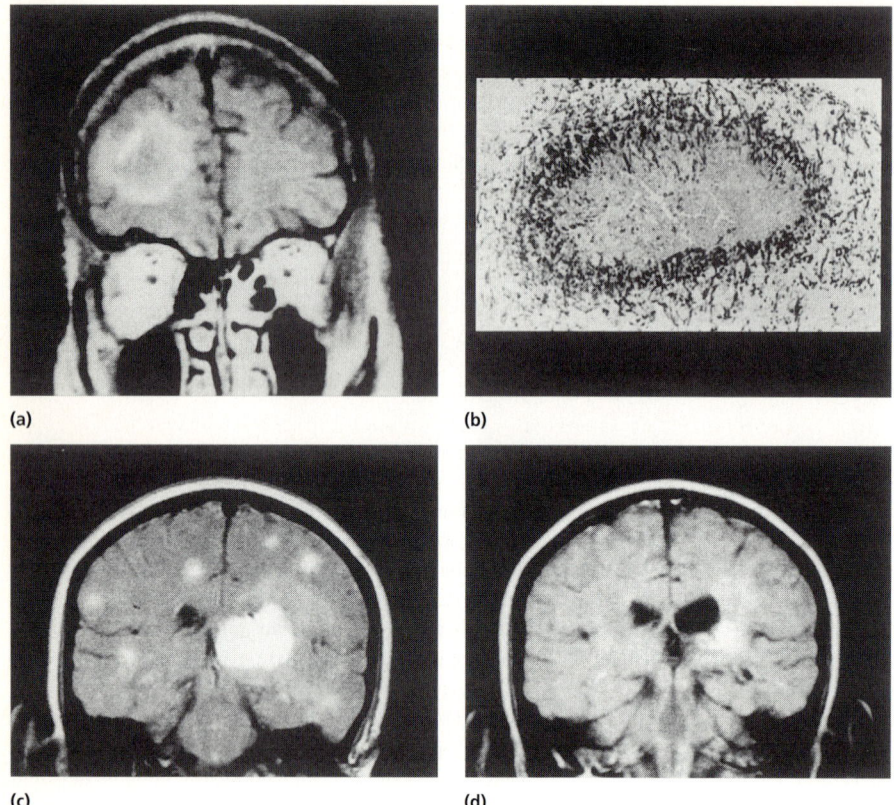

Fig. 59.1 Fungal and parasitic central nervous system (CNS) infections. (a) Magnetic resonance imaging (MRI) of CNS *Aspergillus* infection. A 27-year-old man with Hodgkin's disease developed pulmonary aspergillosis as documented by bronchoscopy 5 months after autologous transplantation. Gadolinium ring-enhanced lesions were documented in the right frontal lobe. CNS aspergillosis was confirmed at autopsy. (b) Post-mortem aspergillus histopathology of a 45-year-old woman who developed a locked-in syndrome, rapidly evolving to coma and death 2 months after allogeneic transplantation for granulocytic sarcoma. Shown is a thrombosed branch of the basilar artery with mural invasion of the arterial wall by branching fungal hyphae (Gormori methanimine silver, ×100). (c) MRI of CNS *Toxoplasma gondii* infection. At 3.5 months after autologous transplantation for Hodgkin's disease, a 21-year-old Hispanic woman developed right-sided upper motor neuron clumsiness with sensory symptoms. The MRI showed multiple gadolinium-enhancing lesions, the largest in the left parietotemporal area. (d) Neurological recovery and almost complete resolution of the lesions on MRI occurred after 6 months of therapy with pyrimethamine and sulfadiazine.

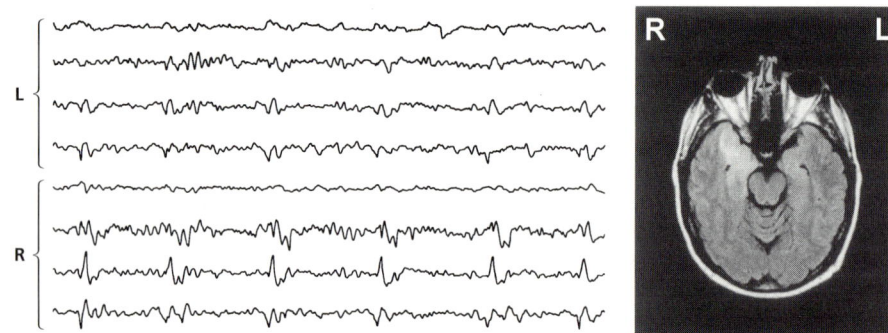

Fig. 59.2 Electroencephalogram (EEG) and brain magnetic resonance imaging (MRI) in herpes simplex encephalitis. A 46-year-old man whose acute myelogenous leukemia relapsed 8 months after autologous stem cell transplant underwent a nonmyeloablative matched unrelated donor transplant with melphalan and fludarabine conditioning. On cyclosporine and prednisone for skin graft-vs.-host disease (GVHD), he developed abrupt confusion with visual agnosias 4 months after allogeneic transplantation. An EEG showed right-sided periodic sharp waves. Right frontotemporal increase signal developed on follow-up brain MRI FLAIR (fluid attenuated inversion recovery) sequence. The cerebrospinal fluid had 44 white blood cells (87% lymphocytes), 11 red blood cells; and herpes simplex type 1 was cultured from the cerebrospinal fluid. Despite therapy with both acyclovir and foscarnet, there was neurological progression with the patient developing an amnestic state, unable to form new memory traces.

the infection in these two patients was diffuse throughout the brain and a subacute, mucocutaneous herpetic infection preceded the onset of CNS symptoms. Fig. 59.2 shows an electroencephalogram (EEG) and MRI of a City of Hope National Medical Center transplant patient who developed typical frontotemporal herpes simplex encephalitis. The EEG is helpful since periodic lateralized epileptiform discharges (as in Fig. 59.2) are characteristic for herpes encephalitis and may precede the MRI abnormality. Although HSV-1 was cultured from the cerebrospinal fluid in the patient shown in Fig. 59.2, viral cultures usually are negative in herpes encephalitis. CSF polymerase chain reaction (PCR) assay of HSV-1 nucleic acid is helpful, but treatment should be initiated and continued in suspicious cases regardless of the PCR result.

Present about half as often as HSV-1, active varicella-zoster virus (VZV) infection occurs later in the transplant course. The greatest incidence is during the 4th and 5th months after allogeneic transplantation (see Chapter 55). In a study from Seattle during the 1970s, 4% of transplant recipients with active zoster or varicella developed clinical encephalitis [27]. This was before the widespread use of antiviral drugs, and a follow-up study showed less morbidity in patients who received antiviral agents [28]. Nevertheless, 25% of the transplant patients with varicella-zoster developed post-herpetic neuralgia. Facial nerve palsy and hearing loss were associated with cranial zoster; arm weakness was associated with cervical zoster; and neurogenic bladder was associated with lumbosacral zoster. In nontransplant patients with zoster, a pleocytosis is present in most who have undergone spinal fluid examination, and it is likely that the occasional motor signs seen with zoster are from involvement of anterior horn cells in the spinal cord or motor nuclei in the brain stem [29]. Hence, in a strict sense, a mild meningoencephalitis with or without motor signs is probably more common with zoster than is usually acknowledged. The designation of varicella-zoster encephalitis is usually reserved for the rare instances of diffuse encephalitis with a decrease in sensorium. Recently HSV-1 and VZV have been shown to be major causes of peripheral facial weakness (Bell's palsy) in normal individuals [30–32]. A course of acyclovir is advisable for any HCT patient who develops Bell's palsy.

Fatal meningoencephalitis due to adenovirus or human herpesvirus type 6 has been documented in marrow transplant recipients [33,34]. Progressive multifocal leukoencephalopathy, the slow virus infection caused by polyomavirus JC, was documented at Johns Hopkins University in only two patients, one of whom had HIV/AIDS [1]. This low incidence is surprising because the related polyomavirus BK is very often cultured from the urine in HCT recipients [25]. More recently, progressive multifocal leukoencephalopathy has been reported after autologous HCT [35,36].

Cerebrovascular complications

Intracranial hemorrhage is most frequently associated with refractory thrombocytopenia and, except for subdural hematomas, large intracranial hemorrhages are usually fatal in HCT recipients. In a large autopsy series from Brazil, hemorrhagic CNS lesions were present in one-third and considered the main cause of death in one-tenth of patients [37]. The characteristic clinical course of large supratentorial hemorrhages is abrupt onset of hemiparesis, or other neurological deficit localized to the cerebral hemispheres, followed by rapid depression of the sensorium and development of brain stem signs from transtentorial herniation (Fig. 59.3a). A cerebellar hemorrhage is more difficult to recognize because of the subtlety of the initial signs—abnormalities of gait and eye movement, which then progress to gaze paresis and coma. Computerized tomography (CT) is preferable to MRI in evaluating patients suspected of having acute intracranial bleeding, because the hyperintense signal of blood is not seen on MRIs until methemoglobin has formed, 12 h or more after the bleed. Treatment of intracranial hemorrhage is the neurosurgical evacuation of the hematoma in those instances where this is feasible [38].

Subdural hematomas characteristically reduce the sensorium with no or mild lateralizing signs. Consequently, they can be overlooked early in the course, particularly in patients who are sedated or encephalopathic for metabolic reasons. In one clinical study, the overall subdural hematoma risk in patients with leukemia refractory to platelet transfusion was 44%, and in this series subdural hematomas occurred more often after autologous than allogeneic transplantation [3]. Nonhemorrhagic subdural fluid collections (hygromas) may develop over the cerebral convexities in patients who have low cerebrospinal fluid pressure as a consequence of repeated lumbar punctures (e.g. patients with acute lymphocytic leukemia undergoing intrathecal treatment or prophylaxis for CNS leukemia). An epidural lumbar blood patch may help decrease the headache and shorten the time for the hygroma to resolve. However, with or without the blood patch, the hygroma may increase in size, as shown in Fig. 59.3b, and surgical drainage may be necessary even if bleeding into the hygroma can be avoided. With or without neurosurgery, this complication may seriously compromise treatment of the leukemia by delaying further intrathecal therapy and the date of HCT.

Ischemic strokes in transplant recipients may be embolic from endocarditis or thrombotic associated with a hypercoagulable state. Cerebral vasospasm leading to ischemic symptoms or stroke has been suspected in rare patients at the time of cryopreserved stem cell transfusion [39].

Thrombotic thrombocytopenic purpura (TTP) has occurred after allogeneic transplantation [40] and could be a cause of seizures or focal neurological signs in transplant patients. Tumor embolization, at least initially, may be clinically indistinguishable from emboli of atheromatous disease or infectious endocarditis. An endarteritis associated with meningeal infection, particularly with *Aspergillus* spp., may occur and be difficult to distinguish clinically from primary cerebrovascular disease (Fig. 59.1b). Bacterial or fungal sphenoid sinusitis in transplant patients may result in a major hemisphere stroke by extension of the infection to the carotid artery in the venous cavernous sinus (Fig. 59.3b). Cavernous sinus syndrome includes orbital and retinal congestion, limited eye movement from involvement of cranial nerves III and VI, and decreased corneal reflex from involvement of the first division of cranial nerve V. It is important that patients with severe sphenoid sinus infections undergo surgery and receive appropriate antibiotic or antifungal therapy to prevent cavernous sinus syndrome.

A prospective study measuring von Willebrand factor, thrombomodulin, and intracellular adhesion molecule 1 (ICAM-1) showed evidence of vascular endothelial damage before transplant conditioning, probably as a result of prior chemotherapy; and additional injury from endothelial activation occurred after transplantation [41]. Levels of the circulating anticoagulant protein C, as well as levels of certain clotting factors, have also been shown to be decreased in breast cancer patients receiving chemotherapy and patients undergoing autologous transplantation for solid tumors [42,43]. There is one report of an ischemic stroke attributed to reduced protein C levels occurring 11 months after allogeneic transplantaion [44]. Nonbacterial thrombotic endocarditis occurs in transplant patients as a consequence of a hypercoagulable state [45,46]. Chemotherapy-induced endothelial damage and circulating immune complexes may also be contributing factors. In an autopsy series of 91 allogeneic transplant patients, there was a single case of bacterial endocarditis (group D streptococcus) with stroke and seven cases of nonbacterial thrombotic endocarditis, with two of these patients having had ischemic strokes. Neither septicemia nor GVHD was shown to be an additional risk factor for nonbacterial thrombotic endocarditis [45]. Prophylactic warfarin may be considered for patients with a hypercoagulable state and repeated episodes of transient cerebral ischemia but, following a stroke, there is a danger of heparin converting a bland infarct to a hemorrhagic infarct, particularly within the first 72 h following the stroke.

Metabolic complications

Metabolic encephalopathy in transplant patients is most often associated with gram-negative sepsis or the use of sedative-hypnotic drugs. Hypoxic encephalopathy, carrying the risk of permanent neurological disability, may occur from interstitial pneumonia or from hypoxemia associated with red blood cell lysis in the hemolytic–uremic syndrome. Hepatic encephalopathy may occur from liver involvement in GVHD or from fulminant hepatic failure in veno-occlusive disease. Renal failure with resultant uremic encephalopathy has been attributed to nephrotoxic drugs, including cyclosporine (CSP), the renal glomerulopathy that is rarely seen as a manifestation of GVHD, radiation nephritis, or the hemolytic–uremic syndrome. Hypomagnesemia, associated with CSP or as a residual from cisplatin nephrotoxicity, may cause convulsions as well as cramps and muscle weakness.

The characteristic clinical features of metabolic encephalopathy are delirium or depression of the sensorium, from lethargy to stupor or coma, usually but not always without lateralizing neurological signs. In hepatic coma particularly, there may be abnormal neurological signs, including hemiplegia and brain stem signs with extensor or flexor posturing to noxious stimuli. Preservation of the pupillary light response and eye

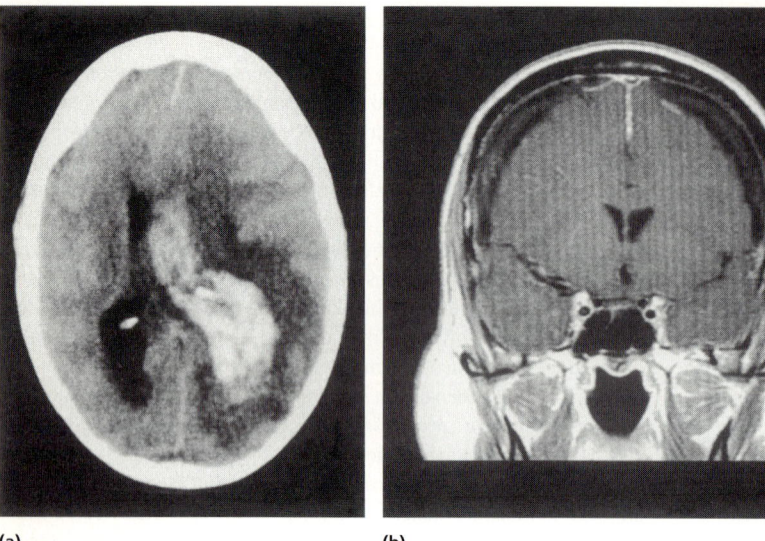 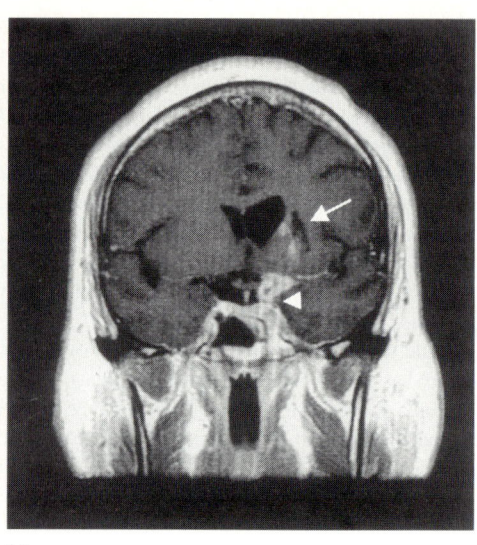

Fig. 59.3 Cerebrovascular disease. (a) Brain computerized tomography (CT) of a fatal intracranial hemorrhage. A 34-year-old woman with biphenotypic leukemia underwent allogeneic bone marrow transplantation and 1.5 months later had a fatal massive left intraparenchymal hemorrhage with rupture into the left lateral ventricle. (b) Brain magnetic resonance imaging (MRI) of bilateral subdural hygromas resulting from multiple lumbar punctures and low cerebrospinal fluid pressure. A 48-year-old man with human immunodeficiency virus (HIV)-associated diffuse large cell lymphoma and leptomeningeal disease underwent three lumbar punctures for intrathecal therapy the week before high dose 1,3-bis(2-chloroethyl)-1-nitrosourea (BCNU; carmustine) and etoposide with autologous stem cell transplantation. Two weeks after transplantation, there was confusion and reduced sensorium. The MRI showed bilateral subdural fluid collections, obliteration of cortical sulci and balanced mass effect. After bilateral surgical drainage of the subdural hygromas, there was improvement in his sensorium. (c) Brain MRI of left sphenoid sinus infection with extension to the cavernous sinus (arrow head) and left hemisphere stroke (arrow). Sphenoid sinusitis developed in a 35-year-old man 5 months after autologous stem cell transplantation for acute myelogenous leukemia. Despite repeated sphenoid surgeries, a left sixth nerve palsy developed followed by right hemiparesis and dysphasia. He was treated with amphotericin B and intraconazole for a presumed fungal infection. The MRI shows sphenoid sinus opacification; a soft tissue mass within the left cavernous sinus occluding or narrowing the carotid artery; and an infarction involving the internal capsule, putamen and head of caudate nucleus.

movements in the face of reflexive posturing argues for a metabolic rather than a structural etiology of coma.

Multiple organ failure in HCT patients, as in other critically ill patients, is a poorly understood but generally fatal entity. Veno-occlusive disease of the liver or pulmonary failure after transplant may herald multiorgan failure, including CNS failure [47,48]. A recent prospective study found that about 50% of HCT patients who develop a decrease in a standardized bedside mental status instrument in the 1st month of transplant go on to develop pulmonary or hepatic involvement and almost two-thirds of these patients do not survive 100 days after transplant [49]. An argument has been advanced that regardless of the initial organ system involved, the course in these patients reflects a systemic inflammatory response, the so-called multiple organ dysfunction syndrome (MODS) [50]. As such, a systemic rather than an organ-specific approach to therapy is needed and such an approach will depend on a better understanding of the pathophysiology and initiating events of MODS and how these may be affected by high dose chemoradiation.

Because of the increased risk of sepsis and shock, neurological complications of critical illness may occur in transplant patients [51,52]. Critical illness polyneuropathy (CIPN) is thought to occur from inadequate perfusion of peripheral nerves and is often associated with encephalopathy, multiorgan failure and prolonged mechanical ventilation. It is a predominantly motor axonal neuropathy with moderate to severe neurological deficit interfering with respiratory weaning [53–55]. Recovery may be partial and slow, with survivors usually requiring months before they can resume ambulation. Another complication that interferes with respiratory weaning and may be confused clinically is acute critical illness myopathy [55–57]. Coincidence of both CIPN and acute critical illness myopathy probably occurs, particularly in patients with multiorgan failure who have received neuromuscular blocking agents and corticosteroids.

Immune-mediated complications

Three immune-mediated diseases, all affecting the peripheral nervous system, can occur after HCT. Most common is polymyositis—a clinical syndrome characterized by proximal muscle weakness, elevated levels of creatine phosphokinase and other muscle enzymes, short-duration (myopathic) motor units on electromyography with signs of acute denervation (fibrillation potentials and positive sharp waves), and necrotic myofibers and mononuclear inflammatory cells on muscle biopsy. Less common, but still well-recognized is myasthenia gravis (MG), an immune-mediated disorder of the neuromuscular junction in which autoantibodies to the post-synaptic acetylcholine receptor produce a characteristic clinical syndrome of ptosis and extraocular muscle weakness, most often with proximal limb and facial muscle weakness. Less well accepted as a complication of HCT is immune-mediated demyelinating polyneuropathy, a condition producing neuropathic weakness, which can be severe, sensory loss and nerve conduction slowing on electrophysiologic tests.

There are several case reports of polymyositis associated with chronic GVHD after allogeneic bone marrow transplantation [58–62]. The largest series reported polymyositis in 3% of 318 patients with chronic GVHD [62]. Onset of weakness occurred 7–24 months after transplantation, and all patients showed improved strength with reinstitution or an increase in the dose of prednisone. Immunohistochemical study of muscle biopsy specimens showed a predominance of $CD8^+$ T cells. There are at least four reported patients in whom polymyositis was the sole manifestation of GVHD [62,63], and there is a case report of polymyositis occurring after autologous transplantation [64]. It is important to exclude infectious causes of polymyositis and to exclude the occasional patient with drug-induced myositis. Zidovudine (AZT) as well as the combination of lovastatin and CSP can cause an inflammatory myopathy, and a fatal case of rhabdomyolysis occurred after a CSP-associated seizure in a transplant patient [65]. Muscle weakness in a patient with GVHD may also be from autoimmune hyperthyroidism [66], or much more commonly, from steroid myopathy. A common treatment dilemma is whether steroids should be increased as therapy for polymyositis or decreased because of presumptive steroid myopathy. Further testing should help in this situation because, unlike polymyositis, patients with steroid or other endocrine myopathies have neither electromyographic evidence of denervation nor inflammatory cells in muscle biopsy specimens.

The prevalence of post-transplantation MG is low, <0.5% of transplant recipients. Only three of 1800 allogeneic transplant recipients have been diagnosed at Seattle, and there is a similar low prevalence at other centers [67–72]. Onset tends to be later than polymyositis. Most patients are diagnosed after immunosuppressant drugs to prevent chronic GVHD have been decreased or discontinued. Patients transplanted for aplastic anemia appear to have a greater risk for acquiring MG; and many post-transplant MG patients have antiplatelet, antismooth muscle, antimitochondrial and antinuclear antibodies as well as antiacetyl choline receptor antibodies. Although antireceptor antibodies without neuromuscular symptoms have been detected after autologous as well as allogeneic transplantation [68], there are no reported cases of MG acquired after autologous transplantation. Thymoma, present in about 15% of patients with idiopathic MG, has not been identified in post-transplant MG. Unlike polymyositis which usually is self-limited, post-transplant MG tends to be a chronic, albeit sometimes fluctuating, problem requiring anticholinesterase drugs to control symptoms. Alternate day low-dose prednisone is generally adequate if immunosuppressants are required. Return to higher dose immunosuppressants or treatment with plasma exchange is generally not necessary or recommended. It may be important to avoid, or use with caution in these patients, drugs that affect neuromuscular transmission, including aminoglycoside antibiotics, certain cardiac antiarrhythmic agents, such as procainamide, and parenteral magnesium.

Because of the known increased risk of Guillain–Barré syndrome in Hodgkin's disease and other disorders with reduced cellular immunity [73], it is not surprising that Guillain–Barré-like neuropathies occasionally occur in transplant recipients [74–78]. Compared to MG and polymyositis, there is a greater clinical heterogeneity in these patients and less certainty as to the pathogenesis. The prevalence has been estimated at only 1% of allogeneic transplantations [79], but these neuropathies produce considerable morbidity because the deficits are predominantly motor and because they occur early after transplantation when patients are medically most vulnerable. Additional recent reports attributed some instances of demyelinating neuropathy in transplant patients to CSP or to prior CMV or *Campylobacter jejuni* infection [80–82]. An immune mechanism is suspected in these neuropathies, but the pathogenesis is uncertain. GVHD is present in most but not all patients, and the neuropathy has been thought to correlate with the course of GVHD in some patients. Necessary for the diagnosis of demyelinating neuropathy is the electrophysiological demonstration of nerve conduction slowing or conduction block. It may be helpful to document cerebrospinal fluid protein elevation and myelin breakdown with reactive macrophages on nerve biopsy [83]. No study of antiGM$_1$ ganglioside antibody or other peripheral nerve antibody in transplant recipients has been reported. Treatment of demyelinating polyneuropathy in these patients has included plasmapheresis with variable success; prednisone, which is effective in nontransplant-associated chronic inflammatory demyelinating polyneuropathy and intravenous gammaglobulin. There may be a need for caution in considering a transplant for hematological malignancy in patients with a pre-existing inflammatory demyelinating neuropathy since abrupt worsening after conditioning therapy involving fractionated total body irradiation has been reported in rare patients [84].

Complications from cyclosporine (CSP) and FK506 (tacrolimus)

CSP causes more neurological problems in transplant patients than any other drug [85–104]. Complications are diverse. Essential tremor is almost always present and headaches of a vascular quality occur in up to 20% of patients. Seizures and encephalopathy are the most common serious complications of CSP. Typically CSP seizures follow complaints of headache, increased tremulousness, mild confusion, asterexis and, sometimes, visual symptoms [85,86,103]. Although usually single and generalized, multiple and partial CSP seizures may also occur and there may be transient post-seizure deficits such as cortical blindness and behavioral abnormality. The newer immunosuppressive drug tacrolimus (FK506) has the same mechanism of action and a similar toxicity profile as CSP [105–108], although the risk of neurotoxicity may be lower with FK506 [109]. Incidence of neurotoxicity from both drugs is highest in the first few months after HCT, occurring in up to 5% of patients [110].

Patients with CSP or FK506 neurotoxicity may have T_2 and FLAIR (fluid attenuated inversion recovery) sequence abnormalities on MRIs with multifocal areas of signal hyperintensity, most often in the occipital lobe white matter with associated occipital blindness (Fig. 59.4a) [109]. Parallels to MRI changes in eclampsia have been made [111,112], and patients who are encephalopathic during CSP therapy usually have elevated blood pressure—although hypertension is not invariably present and often is mild. A less common pattern of MRI abnormality from CSP/FK506 is mixed cortical and subcortical white matter lesions, sometimes associated with punctate cortical gadolinium enhancement (Fig. 59.4d) [113]. There may on rare occasions be intraparenchymal hemorrhages associated with CSP/FK506 MRI abnormalities. These usually are small but there is a report of a fatal hemorrhage associated with CSP/FK506 [114]. Cerebellar and brain stem MRI lesions exceptionally occur and eye movement abnormalities have been reported (Fig. 59.4b,c) [115,116]. CSP/FK506 hardly ever produces lateralized motor or sensory abnormalities. Such signs in transplant patients suggest a structural lesion rather than CSP/FK506 neurotoxicity. Very rarely, CSP-induced edema itself acts as a mass lesion. There is a report of cerebellar swelling producing brain stem compression and requiring decompressive suboccipital craniectomy [117]. There is also a report of fatal respiratory failure from involvement of brain stem respiratory center [118].

CSP/FK506 neurotoxicity is less often detected by CT than by MRI, but marked CT abnormalities can occur as shown in Fig. 59.4e. The reversibility of the CT abnormality on follow-up scans (Fig. 59.4f) argues against cerebral infarction and for vasogenic edema. Damage to vascular endothelium from chemotherapeutic drugs, breakdown of the blood–brain barrier from radiation, or from CSP itself—these may all be contributing factors. CSP leads to the release of endothelins, vasoactive neuropeptides that have been implicated in cerebral vasospasm [119,120]. Endothelin release may be triggered by or may cause microangiopathic hemolytic anaemia, a condition found by multivariate analysis to have the highest correlation with CSP toxicity [85]. Vasospasm, shown to be present on an MR angiogram [113], may explain involvement at junctions of major vessels (watershed areas) or at the distal distribution of major vessels, such as the occipital pole. Neuropathology of CSP toxicity is limited, but reports indicate edema or demyelination. There is one report of vasculitis attributed to FK506 in a liver transplant patient [121].

Although these vascular abnormalities are now well recognized, they probably do not account for all instances of serious CSP/FK506 neurotoxicity. Sometimes there is severe neurotoxicity with encephalopathy prolonged for days, to near-coma, yet the MRI is normal. In other instances, there is relatively mild encephalopathy but with MRI abnormalities on FLAIR or T_2 sequences. In animals, CSP has a direct neurotoxic effect, independent of alterations in blood pressure or renal function

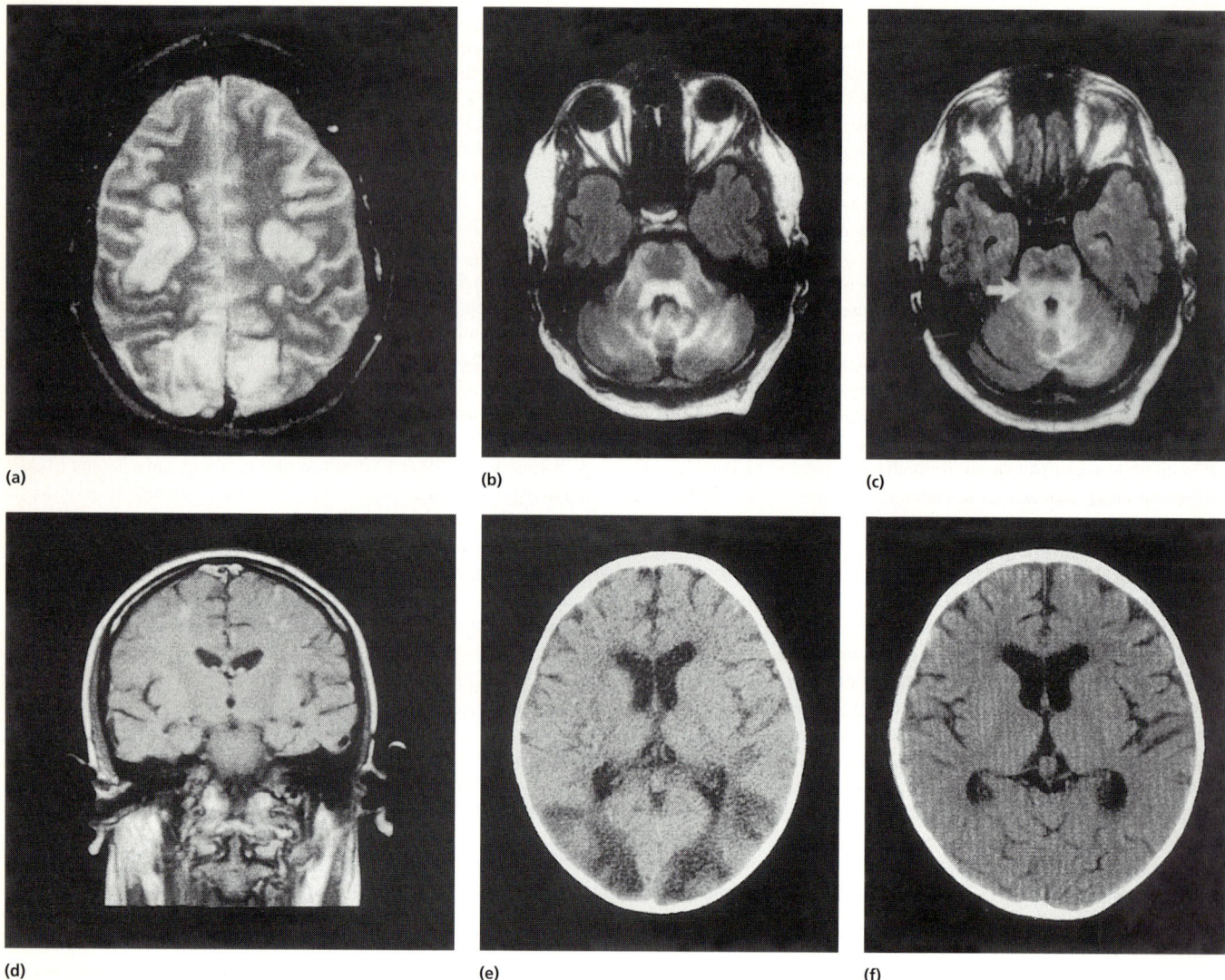

Fig. 59.4 Cyclosporine (CSP)/FK506 neurotoxicity. (a) Brain magnetic resonance imaging (MRI) (T_2 sequence) of a 20-year-old woman 5 weeks after allogeneic transplantation for chronic myeloid leukemia who developed abrupt onset of confusion and headache. Patches of bright signal on T_2-weighted images were present, especially in the parietal and occipital subcortical white matter. Later, a generalized seizure with encephalopathy occurred and CSP was stopped for 4 days and then restarted at a lower dose. A repeat MRI showed resolution of the lesions. (b & c) Brain MRI FLAIR (fluid attenuated inversion recovery) sequence of a 50-year-old man who developed diplopia 2 months after allogeneic transplant for mantle cell lymphoma. The arrow shows signal abnormality included the area of the VI nerve nucleus. Eye movements returned to normal 2 days after CSP was discontinued. Reproduced with permission from Openshaw [116]. (d) MRI (T_1 with gadolinium enhancement) showing punctate cortical gadolinium enhancement (same patient as in panel a). (e & f) Brain computerized tomography (CT) of FK506 leukoencephalopathy in a 2-year-old girl with acute lymphocytic leukemia and liver chronic graft-vs.-host disease (GVHD) who developed seizures and reduced sensorium 1 year after matched unrelated donor transplant. The follow-up scan (panel f), which was done 1 month later, showed almost complete resolution of parieto-occipital edema.

[122]. A cell-culture study showed that CSP can induce neuronal apoptosis and selective oligodendrocyte death [123]. The mechanism probably involves inhibition of the phosphatase activity of calcineurin, the same mechanism whereby CSP inhibits T-cell proliferation (see Chapter 16). CSP is bound by serum lipoproteins, metabolized in the liver cytochrome P450 enzyme system, and excreted in bile. Blood levels may become elevated in patients with hyperbilirubinemia, GVHD of the liver, or veno-occlusive disease [124]. Erythromycin, ketoconazole and calcium channel blockers decrease the hepatic metabolism of CSP [85,89] whereas phenytoin enhances the hepatic metabolism [125]. Hypocholesterolemia is associated with an increased risk of CSP neurotoxicity [94], probably because of an increase in unbound CSP; it is likely the low cholesterol levels in liver disease account at least in part for the twofold greater prevalence of CSP neurotoxicity in liver transplant patients compared to HCT patients. CSP does not penetrate the blood–brain barrier well under normal conditions [110], but damage to the barrier by conditioning agents, particularly irradiation, may increase CSP/FK506 penetration. Despite clinical experience suggesting a direct toxic role of CSP/FK506, neurotoxicity does not always correlate with steady state drug levels. It has been proposed that high peak levels (e.g. at times of intravenous use) may predispose to neurotoxicity [110]. The lower neurotoxicity, at least in liver transplant patients, of the oral microemulsion preparation Neoral® may be explained by a steadier gastrointestinal absorption [126].

A considerable degree of clinical judgement often goes into decisions when to reduce or hold CSP/FK506 to prevent the more serious instances of neurotoxicity. For CSP-associated headache, propranolol often is helpful [127] and there is a report of resolution of a CSP headache by conversion to FK506 [128]. Even mildly encephalopathic patients who have worsening asterexis or develop myoclonus should be considered for supplementary intravenous magnesium, temporary discontinuation of CSP/FK506 regardless of the drug level and, possibly, a loading dose of intravenous phenytoin. Switching from CSP to FK506 and vice versa in patients with neurotoxicity has been studied in liver transplant patients [110]. Clinical experience in HCT suggests that temporary discontinuation of CSP/FK506 and then restarting at a lower dose is usually successful in preventing worsening or recurrence of neurotoxicity. Switching from CSP to FK506 or vice versa is seldom necessary and is not always successful in preventing recurrence of neurotoxicity. In patients with CSP/FK506 seizures, phenytoin is usually used; however, there is no agreement as to how long phenytoin or other anticonvulsants should be continued. Since repeat CSP seizures are rare, some clinicians maintain phenytoin for only a few weeks. Most, however, continue anticonvulsants until high-dose CSP/FK506 is no longer required. There is some rationale for using valproic acid as the long-term anticonvulsant, since valproic acid, unlike phenytoin, does not affect CSP hepatic metabolism [129,130].

Complications from other immunosuppressive drugs

A sense of well-being and even euphoria often accompanies the initiation of corticosteroid treatment. With continued administration, psychotic depression, mania, or delirium may occur [131]. This toxicity is often dose dependent, but when reduction in steroid dose is not feasible neuroleptic or antianxiety medications may be necessary. Proximal muscle weakness due to muscle protein catabolism is experienced by virtually all transplant patients who receive the equivalent of 40 mg/day of prednisone for more than 3 weeks [132,133]. Typical symptoms include difficulty arising from a chair and difficulty washing hair. Muscle cramps and tenderness occur less often with steroid myopathy than with polymyositis. Unlike polymyositis, serum creatine phosphokinase levels are normal or only slightly elevated in steroid myopathy, and electromyography often shows only slight abnormalities with myopathic motor units. Muscle biopsy may reveal type IIB fiber atrophy, but this finding is not specific to steroid myopathy. Treatment consists of switching from the more myotoxic fluorinated steroids, such as dexamethasone, to nonfluorinated agents, such as prednisone or methylprednisolone, tapering the steroids when possible and instituting daily physical therapy. There is anecdotal evidence that regular exercise during corticosteroid treatment may reduce the catabolic effect on muscle. A conditioning program may be of particular value for patients who are sensitive to the muscle toxicity of steroids but will require steroid prophylaxis because of the risk of GVHD.

Recognized in the 1960s soon after thalidomide was introduced as a sedative-hypnotic agent, peripheral neuropathy can become symptomatic after 2 months of therapy at 100 mg/day [134], the starting dose sometimes used for chronic GVHD [135]. Lower-limb numbness and paresthesias occur, often accompanied by burning and hyperesthesia of the feet. With continued exposure, leg cramps and a stocking-glove pattern of sensory loss develop involving superficial sensation more than proprioception or vibration. Patients with severe neuropathy may have muscle weakness. An unusual feature compared to other toxic neuropathies is the preservation of deep tendon reflexes well into the course of the neuropathy. There may be mild elevation of cerebrospinal fluid protein, and nerve conduction tests as well as morphological analysis indicate a large-fiber, "dying-back" sensory neuronopathy (i.e. initial degeneration in the distal region of the axon and progression of the degeneration proximally to the nerve cell body) [136]. The extent of neurological recovery after discontinuation of thalidomide depends on the severity of the symptoms and, possibly, the patient's age and duration of exposure. Motor signs revert more readily and completely than sensory symptoms and, in some patients, distressing sensory complaints may be permanent [137]. In a review of 58 transplant patients who received thalidomide for at least 2 months, 14% of patients discontinued thalidomide because of symptoms and signs of peripheral neuropathy [138]. There was no correlation of neuropathy with age, hematological diagnosis, or the post-transplantation month when thalidomide was started.

Low-dose intravenous methotrexate (MTX), frequently used for GVHD prophylaxis, causes only occasional and minor neurotoxicity—headache, dizziness and, rarely, seizures—when given to the patients with rheumatoid arthritis [139–141]. High-dose MTX (5 g/m^2/cycle) used mainly for osteogenic sarcoma can trigger transient leukoencephalopathy, similar in appearance but usually more extensive than the MRI abnormalities seen with CSP/FK506 [142]. The major progressive and permanent neurological disability from MTX in transplant recipients is the delayed-onset, chronic, often fatal, leukoencephalopathy resulting usually from the combination of intrathecal MTX and whole brain irradiation [143]. The most common neurological signs include dysarthria, ataxia, dysphasia, spasticity and upper motor neuron weakness, seizures, confusion and a decrease in sensorium. The incidence of leukoencephalopathy was as high as 7% in a series of leukemic patients from Seattle who received CNS radiation and intrathecal therapy before transplant and intrathecal MTX after transplant [144]. Onset of leukoencephalopathy was usually 4–5 months after transplantation. Leukoencephalopathy with severe neurological sequelae and death has also been attributed to amphotericin B following total body irradiation (TBI) in a transplant recipient [145].

Complications from conditioning agents

Neurological complications from chemotherapeutic drugs in the conditioning regimen include encephalopathy and seizures, as acute self-limited complications, and peripheral neuropathy, as delayed longer-lasting complications. Busulfan (BU) and 1,3-*bis*(2-chloroethyl)-1-nitrosourea (BCNU; carmustine) are common causes of encephalopathy, and etoposide (VP16) and cisplatinin are common causes of peripheral neuropathy. Granulocyte colony-stimulating factor (G-CSF) may exacerbate autoimmune activity during peripheral blood hematopoietic stem cell mobilization of patients with multiple sclerosis or rheumatoid arthritis [146–148]. Long-term disabilities of conditioning agents that may involve cognition and quality of life are discussed in Chapters 39 and 69, and the long-term risk of primary brain tumors is discussed in Chapter 70 [149,150].

Generalized seizures occur overall in about 10% of patients receiving high-dose BU (4 mg/kg/day for 4 days) [151–154]. BU readily crosses the blood–brain barrier, producing cerebrospinal fluid to plasma drug ratios of 1 or higher and it is presumed that seizures occur as a direct neurotoxic effect [155]. Although myoclonic twitching may be seen shortly before or after the ictus, BU seizures usually are not focal and seldom are they multiple or complicated. Prophylactic anticonvulsant treatment has been recommended when high-dose BU is used in conditioning regimens [154,156]. For such treatment to have value, a therapeutic drug level must be reached before the start of BU and maintained for 2 days after administration of the last BU dose. An oral phenytoin-loading dose of 18 mg/kg is generally adequate for this purpose with a daily maintenance dose of 5 mg/kg. Similar phenytoin prophylaxis has been used for high dose BCNU. Seizures occurred in two of 61 patients receiving autologous transplants for relapsed Hodgkin's disease who were conditioned with 300 mg/m^2 of BCNU in combination with cyclophosphamide and VP16 [157]. Headache with flushing and paresthesias around the lips have been reported during high-dose BCNU infusion [158].

CNS toxicity as manifested by coma was the dose-limiting toxicity of ifosfamide at 24 g/m² given over 6 days in a dose-escalation study with carboplatin and VP16 (ICE) and autologous hematopoietic HCT [159]. At lower doses in this study, CNS toxicity occurred in 8% of 102 patients. A similar incidence of severe CNS toxicity was seen with conventional-dose ifosfamide (5 g/m² given over 36 h) without peripheral stem cell transplantation in patients with advanced malignancies [160]. Neurological manifestations include seizures, acute confusional state, mutism and disordered sensorium. Rare instances of extrapyramidal toxicities with opisthotonos have also been noted [161,162]. The toxicity may be related to a buildup of a chloral hydrate-like compound, chloracetaldehyde, a major breakdown product of ifosfamide. There have been reports of treatment with methylene blue [163]. Other chemotherapeutic drugs in conditioning regimens that may cause encephalopathy are high-dose mechlorethamine used infrequently in the past as a substitute for cyclophosphamide with TBI [164] and fludarabine used now in non-myeloablative allogeneic transplants. An unusual feature of fludarabine neurotoxicity is the delay in onset of the encephalopathy [165]. Seizures and transient encephalopathy have been observed with high-dose cytarabine (cytosine arabinoside; ara-C), although the most common neurological problem is cerebellar, occurring in 10% and leaving permanent ataxia from Purkinje cell dropout in 3% of treated patients [166]. There have also been a few published cases of peripheral neuropathy with high dose ara-C, including patients with clinical and electrophysiological features of acute demyelinating polyneuropathy consistent with the diagnosis of Guillain–Barré syndrome [167–169].

A sensory axonal neuropathy with mild or no motor disability developed in 4% of autologous transplant patients conditioned with high-dose VP16 (60 mg/kg intravenously for hematological malignancy) [170]. Distal symmetrical sensory symptoms began within 2 months of the transplantation and improved slowly over months. One patient had a superimposed autonomic neuropathy and another had a peroneal neuropathy. All patients received vincristine at some point prior to the transplantation. A self-limited sensory neuropathy from VP16 conditioning occurs in allogeneic transplant recipients as well. The delay in sensory symptoms for 1–2 months after VP16 is similar to what is sometimes seen with cisplatin and suggests an abnormality in axonal transport [171].

In a phase I trial with escalating doses of paclitaxel (with fixed dosages of cyclophosphamide and cisplatin), 25 of 26 patients receiving at least 625 mg/m² of paclitaxel developed peripheral neuropathy, usually within 5 days of paclitaxel treatment [172]. Although reported as purely sensory in all affected patients, the neuropathy was sufficiently severe to require a walker in some patients.

Clinical features of cisplatin neuropathy are usually characteristic with large sensory fiber involvement, giving a proprioceptive deficit usually with preserved tactile and pin sensation and without muscle weakness [173]. By contrast, VP16 and paclitaxel neuropathies involve all sensory modalities [170,174]. Cisplatin neuropathy tends to correlate with cumulative dose rather than dose intensity. Symptoms usually occur after a cumulative dose of 300–600 mg/m². Also dose dependent is cisplatin ototoxicity, affecting high-frequency hearing initially and—with continued cisplatin courses—speech frequency hearing, but very seldom producing vestibular toxicity [175]. In terms of cisplatin CNS toxicity, transient Lhermitte phenomenon occurs occasionally from an effect on the dorsal column of the cervical region of the spinal cord [176] and there are rare reports of cortical blindness and seizures [177].

Complications from supportive care and other drugs

Depression of the sensorium occurs very frequently in the 1st week after HCT from sedative-hypnotic drugs or analgesics. What can be especially misleading in these patients is unilateral pupillary dilatation from a scopolamine patch [178] used for drug-associated nausea. Recognition of this anticholinergic effect of scopolamine may prevent a needless break in isolation for a head scan to exclude a cerebral mass lesion.

Many of the antibiotics used after transplantation have been associated with neurological toxicity: for example, seizures from penicillin, piperacillin, metronidazole and imipenem; encephalopathy from penicillin and metronidazole; hearing loss from aminoglycosides and vancomycin; peripheral neuropathy from metronidazole; and a myasthenia-like syndrome from aminoglycosides [179–182]. Since toxicity is often enhanced by renal insufficiency, special caution applies to those patients on CSP/FK506 and at risk for nephrotoxicity.

Much of the clinical experience with antiviral drugs comes from treating HIV/AIDS patients, and it is often difficult to know whether a particular neurotoxicity is drug or disease related. Adenine arabinoside has been associated with tremors, hallucinations and complex motor and behavioral disturbances [183,184], but this agent has been replaced largely by the less toxic acyclovir for herpetic infections. In HCT patients, acyclovir at 1500–3000 mg/m²/day can also cause tremor, agitation, or lethargy, occasionally with EEG epileptiform features [185]. In the setting of renal failure, reversible stupor and coma and occasionally generalized seizures have followed both oral and intravenous administration of acyclovir [186–188]. Delirium, which improved with dose reduction, was seen with ganciclovir treatment given at 10 mg/kg/day for CMV infection in a transplant patient [189]. Similar mental status changes have been noted in up to 5% of HIV/AIDS patients on ganciclovir, with seizures occurring rarely and most often in patients also receiving imipenem [190]. Foscarnet most often causes renal and electrolyte disturbances, and low calcium and magnesium levels from foscarnet have been associated with paresthesias, muscle cramps and, rarely, seizures [191,192].

Problems in the differential diagnosis of neurological complications

It is still unanswered whether GVHD can affect the CNS. Allogeneic stimulation in an animal model has been shown to provoke major histocompatibility complex (MHC) class I and II antigen expression in the brain [193]. Compatible with loss of the immunological privileged status of the CNS with allogeneic stimulation are reports of global neurological signs and chronic inflammatory cells in the brain of patients with systemic GVHD [194,195]. In long-term HCT survivors, the incidence of MRI white matter abnormalities and abnormalities in neuropsychological tests correlated most strongly with GVHD and the requirement for prolonged corticosteroid and CSP use [196]. There are also clinical reports of rare instances of myelitis and optic neuritis after allogeneic HCT and a report of remitting and relapsing cerebral demyelination, analogous to episodes of demyelination in multiple sclerosis [197,198]. Etiological factors other than GVHD, however, are possible in these patients and it remains to be convincingly established that chronic GVHD can trigger immune-mediated CNS disorders.

Weakness is a common symptom in transplant patients. Upper motor neuron weakness carries an ominous prognosis since it is usually caused by a mass lesion in the brain or an epidural deposit with spinal cord compression. Weakness in a segmental distribution (i.e. in the distribution of a spinal nerve root) suggests leptomeningeal disease or an epidural deposit at that particular spinal level. Much less commonly, herpes zoster infection produces weakness in a segmental distribution, as does also subacute motor neuronopathy, rarely seen as a remote effect of lymphoma [29,199]. Weakness of extraocular eye muscles, seen in virtually all patients with post-transplant MG, tends to be a fluctuating weakness with characteristic fatigability and associated ptosis. Clinically, this can be distinguished on repeated neurological examinations and differentiated

Table 59.1 Neurological complications organized by disease categories and the usual stage of occurrence: conditioning, pancytopenia, and chronic GVHD.

Neurological complications	Conditioning	Pancytopenia	GVHD
Infectious		Bacterial meningitis	Fungal abscess Meningoencephalitis Septic embolism, mycotic aneurysm
Cerebrovascular		Intracranial bleed	← Ischemic stroke →
Metabolic		Gram-negative sepsis Sedative-hypnotic drugs Hepatic encephalopathy of veno-occlusive disease	Hypoxic encephalopathy of intersitital pneumonia Hepatic encephalopathy GVHD Uremic encephalopathy
Toxic	Encephalopathy (BCNU, BU, mechloethamine, ifosfamide) Neuropathy (VP16, cisplatin, paclitaxel)	CSP neurotoxicity→ Steriod toxicity→ Leukoencephalopathy→	Thalidomide neuropathy
Immune-mediated			Polymyositis Myasthenia gravis Demyelinating polyneuropathy

BCNU, 1,3-*bis*(2-chloroethyl)-1-nitrosourea (carmustine); BU, busulfan; CSP, cyclosporine; GVHD, graft-vs.-host disease; VP16, etoposide.

from the fixed cranial nerve palsies associated with leptomeningeal disease or with intra-axial brain stem lesions. Ophthalmoplegia is only rarely seen with acute inflammatory demyelinating polyneuropathy, the so-called Miller–Fisher variant of Guillain–Barré syndrome, and ophthalmoplegia has not been reported in those cases of demyelinating polyneuropathy associated with transplantation, although transient ophthalmoplegia with ptosis has been attributed to CSP, possibly in association with ganciclovir [116]. It is not difficult to differentiate polymyositis from MG and polyneuropathy. A potential problem arises when mild polymyositis goes unrecognized and accounts for a slower than usual functional recovery from transplantation.

Clinical features more consistent with polyneuropathy than myopathy include the distal distribution of weakness, the presence of sensory symptoms and the absence of deep tendon reflexes. Clearly the last two features are often not helpful in many transplant patients who have pre-existing neuropathy from vincristine, cisplatin, or other neurotoxic drugs. Muscle tenderness, subcutaneous swelling and rash favor an inflammatory myopathy over the usually milder myopathic weakness associated with disuse, corticosteroids, or other endocrine-metabolic myopathies, such as thyrotoxic myopathy. Cramps—involuntary, painful muscle contractions that occur spasmodically—are sometimes seen in transplant patients, are associated with myopathy or neuropathy [74]. When such cramps occur daily and interfere with rest or ordinary activity, preventative therapy with phenytoin often provides benefit [200].

Pretransplantation neurological screening may identify patients particularly prone for neurological complications and, in some cases, this screening may lead to changes in treatment to minimize these complications. For example, anticonvulsant prophylaxis should be considered in transplant recipients with past seizures or a strong family history of epilepsy when these patients are treated with CSP or other drugs known to lower the seizure threshold. Because of the cumulative toxicity of radiation therapy on the nervous system, it may be prudent to use preparatory regimens without fractionated TBI in brain-damaged patients or in patients with degenerative CNS diseases.

Concluding comment

A practical approach to the transplant patient requires an understanding of which problems are most likely at different times of the transplant course. Neurological complications may occur at three stages of HCT: (i) from the conditioning agents used for marrow ablation; (ii) during post-transplantation pancytopenia; or (iii) from immunosuppressive therapies and GVHD in allogeneic transplant recipients. As a summary, Table 59.1 lists neurological complications that can occur during these three stages and classifies the complications under the standard disease categories of infectious, cerebrovascular, metabolic, toxic and immune-mediated disorders. A CNS relapse of leukemia or lymphoma may masquerade as a late complication of HCT. Also, with transplantation for solid tumors, for inheritable disorders and, experimentally, in autoimmune diseases, the clinician must differentiate neurological manifestations of the original disease from complications of the transplantation. Familiarity with transplantation complications should permit ready recognition of most problems.

References

1 Patchell RA, White CL, Clark AW, Beschorner WE, Santos GW. Neurologic complications of bone marrow transplantation. *Neurology* 1985; **35**: 300–6.

2 Openshaw H, Slatkin NE. Differential diagnosis of neurological complications in bone marrow transplantation. *Neurologist* 1995; **1**(4): 191–206.

3 Graus F, Saiz A, Sierra J *et al*. Neurologic complications of autologous and allogeneic bone marrow transplantation in patients with leukemia: a comparative study. *Neurology* 1996; **46**: 1004–9.

4 Wiznitzer M, Packer RJ, August CS, Burkey ED. Neurological complications of bone marrow transplantation in childhood. *Ann Neurol* 1984; **16**: 569–76.

5 Iguchi A, Kobayashi R, Yoshida M *et al*. Neurological complications after stem cell transplantation in childhood. *Bone Marrow Transplant* 1999; **24**: 647–52.

6 Guerrero A, Perez Simon JA, Gutierrez N *et al*. Neurological complications after autologous stem cell transplantation. *Eur Neurol* 1999; **41**: 48–50.

7 de Brabander C, Cornelissen J, Smitt PA, Vecht CJ, van den Bent MJ. Increased incidence of neurological complications in patients receiving an allogenic bone marrow transplantation from alternative donors. *J Neurol Neurosurg Psychiatry* 2000; **68**: 36–40.

8 Wijdicks EFM. *Neurologic Complications in Organ Transplant Recipients*. Boston; Butterworth–Heinemann, 1999.

9 Wingard JR. Advances in the management of infectious complications after bone marrow transplantation. *Bone Marrow Transplant* 1990; **6**: 371–83.

10 Winston D, Gale R, Meyer D, Young L. Infectious complications of human bone marrow transplantation. *Medicine (Baltimore)* 1979; **58**: 1–31.

11 Mohrmann RL, Mah V, Vinters HV. Neuropathologic findings after bone marrow transplantation: an autopsy study. *Hum Pathol* 1990; **21**: 630–9.

12 Bleggi Torres LF, de Medeiros BC, Werner B et al. Neuropathological findings after bone marrow transplantation: an autopsy study of 180 cases. *Bone Marrow Transplant* 2000; **25**: 301–7.

13 Milliken ST, Powles RL. Antifungal prophylaxis in bone marrow transplantation. *Rev Infect Dis* 1990; **12** (Suppl. 3): S374–9.

14 Khoury H, Adkins D, Miller G, Goodnough L, Brown MR, DiPersio J. Resolution of invasive central nervous system aspergillosis in a transplant recipient. *Bone Marrow Transplant* 1997; **20**: 179–80.

15 Herbrecht R, Denning DW, Patterson TF et al. Voriconazole versus amphotericin B for primary therapy of invasive aspergillosis. *N Engl J Med* 2002; **347**: 408–15.

16 Verfaillie C, Weisdorf D, Haake R, Hostetter M, Ramsay NK, McGlave P. Candida infections in bone marrow transplant recipients. *Bone Marrow Transplant* 1991; **8**: 177–84.

17 Lowenberg B, van Gijn J, Prins E, Polderman AM. Fatal cerebral toxoplasmosis in a bone marrow transplant recipient with leukemia. *Transplantation* 1983; **35**: 30–4.

18 Jehn U, Fink M, Gundlach P et al. Lethal cardiac and cerebral toxoplasmosis in a patient with acute myeloid leukemia after successful allogeneic bone marrow transplantation. *Transplantation* 1984; **38**: 430–3.

19 Long S, Leyland M, Milligan D. Listeria meningitis after bone marrow transplantation. *Bone Marrow Transplant* 1993; **12**: 537–9.

20 Abraham J, Bilgrami S, Dorsky D et al. Stomatococcus mucilaginosus meningitis in a patient with multiple myeloma following autologous stem cell transplantation. *Bone Marrow Transplant* 1997; **19**: 639–41.

21 Antonio D, Di Bartolomeo P, Iacone A et al. Meningitis due to penicillin-resistant Streptococcus pneumoniae in patients with chronic graft-versus-host disease. *Bone Marrow Transplant* 1992; **9**: 299–300.

22 Roy V, Weisdorf D. Mycobacterial infections following bone marrow transplantation: a 20-year retrospective review. *Bone Marrow Transplant* 1997; **19**: 467–70.

23 Palestine AG. Clinical aspects of cytomegalovirus retinitis. *Rev Infect Dis* 1988; **10** (Suppl. 3): S515–21.

24 Cordonnier C, Feuilhade F, Vernant JP, Marsault C, Rodet M, Rochant H. Cytomegalovirus encephalitis occurring after bone marrow transplantation. *Scand J Haematol* 1983; **31**: 248–52.

25 Meyers JD. Infection in recipients of bone marrow transplants. *Curr Clin Top Infect Dis* 1985; **6**: 261–92.

26 Saral R, Burns WH, Laskin OL, Santos GW, Lietman PS. Acyclovir prophylaxis of herpes-simplex-virus infections. *N Engl J Med* 1981; **305**: 63–7.

27 Atkinson K, Meyers JD, Storb R, Prentice RL, Thomas ED. Varicella-zoster virus infection after marrow transplantation for aplastic anemia or leukemia. *Transplantation* 1980; **29**: 47–50.

28 Locksley RM, Flournoy N, Sullivan KM, Meyers JD. Infection with varicella-zoster virus after marrow transplantation. *J Infect Dis* 1985; **152**: 1172–81.

29 Thomas E, Howard F. Segmental zoster paresis: a disease profile. *Neurology* 1971; **173**: 843–5.

30 Furuta Y, Ohtani F, Kawabata H, Fukuda S, Bergstrom T. High prevalence of varicella-zoster virus reactivation in herpes simplex virus-seronegative patients with acute peripheral facial palsy. *Clin Infect Dis* 2000; **30**: 529–33.

31 Ohtani F, Furuta Y, Horal P, Bergstrom T. Rapid strip assay for detection of anti-herpes simplex virus antibodies: application to prediction of varicella-zoster virus reactivation in patients with acute peripheral facial palsy. *J Med Virol* 2000; **62**: 37–41.

32 Sweeney CJ, Gilden DH. Ramsay Hunt syndrome. *J Neurol, Neurosurg, Psychiatry* 2001; **71**: 149–54.

33 Davis D, Henslee PJ, Markesbery WR. Fatal adenovirus meningoencephalitis in a bone marrow transplant patient. *Ann Neurol* 1988; **23**: 385–9.

34 Drobyski WR, Knox KK, Majewski D, Carrigan DR. Brief report: fatal encephalitis due to variant B human herpesvirus-6 infection in a bone marrow-transplant recipient. *N Engl J Med* 1994; **330**: 1356–60.

35 Seong D, Bruner JM, Lee KH et al. Progressive multifocal leukoencephalopathy after autologous bone marrow transplantation in a patient with chronic myelogenous leukemia. *Clin Infect Dis* 1996; **23**: 402–3.

36 Re D, Bamborschke S, Feiden W et al. Progressive multifocal leukoencephalopathy after autologous bone marrow transplantation and α-interferon immunotherapy. *Bone Marrow Transplant* 1999; **23**: 295–8.

37 Bleggi Torres LF, Werner B, Gasparetto EL, de Medeiros BC, Pasquini R, de Medeiros CR. Intracranial hemorrhage following bone marrow transplantation: an autopsy study of 58 patients. *Bone Marrow Transplant* 2002; **29**: 29–32.

38 Rabinstein AA, Atkinson JL, Wijdicks EF. Emergency craniotomy in patients worsening due to expanded cerebral hematoma: to what purpose? *Neurology* 2002; **58**: 1367–72.

39 Hoyt R, Szer J, Grigg A. Neurological events associated with the infusion of cryopreserved bone marrow and/or peripheral blood progenitor cells. *Bone Marrow Transplant* 2000; **25**: 1285–7.

40 Tschuchnigg M, Bradstock KF, Koutts J, Stewart J, Enno A, Seldon M. A case of thrombotic thrombocytopenic purpura following allogeneic bone marrow transplantation. *Bone Marrow Transplant* 1990; **5**: 61–3.

41 Richard S, Seigneur M, Blann A et al. Vascular endothelial lesion in patients undergoing bone marrow transplantation. *Bone Marrow Transplant* 1996; **18**: 955–9.

42 Kaufman PA, Jones RB, Greenberg CS, Peters WP. Autologous bone marrow transplantation and factor XII, factor VII, and protein C deficiencies. Report of a new association and its possible relationship to endothelial cell injury. *Cancer* 1990; **66**: 515–21.

43 Gordon B, Haire W, Kessinger A, Duggan M, Armitage J. High frequency of antithrombin 3 and protein C deficiency following autologous bone marrow transplantation for lymphoma. *Bone Marrow Transplant* 1991; **8**: 497–502.

44 Gordon BG, Saving KL, McCallister JA et al. Cerebral infarction associated with protein C deficiency following allogeneic bone marrow transplantation. *Bone Marrow Transplant* 1991; **8**: 323–5.

45 Patchell RA, White CL, Clark AW, Beschorner WE, Santos GW. Nonbacterial thrombotic endocarditis in bone marrow transplant patients. *Cancer* 1985; **55**: 631–5.

46 Jerman MR, Fick RB. Nonbacterial thrombotic endocarditis associated with bone marrow transplantation. *Chest* 1986; **90**: 919–22.

47 McDonald GB, Hinds MS, Fisher LD et al. Venoocclusive disease of the liver and multiorgan failure after bone marrow transplantation: a cohort study of 355 patients. *Ann Intern Med* 1993; **118**: 255–67.

48 Haire WD, Ruby EI, Gordon BG et al. Multiple organ dysfunction syndrome in bone marrow transplantation. *JAMA* 1995; **274**: 1289–95.

49 Gordon B, Lyden E, Lynch J et al. Central nervous system dysfunction as the first manifestation of multiple organ dysfunction syndrome in stem cell transplant patients. *Bone Marrow Transplant* 2000; **25**: 79–83.

50 Haire WD. The multiple organ dysfunction syndrome in cancer patients undergoing hematopoietic stem cell transplantation. *Semin Thromb Hemost* 1999; **25**: 223–37.

51 Lorin S, Nierman DM. Critical illness neuromuscular abnormalities. *Crit Care Clin* 2002; **18**: 553–68.

52 Openshaw H, Slatkin NE. Critical illness neuropathy in patients with bone marrow transplantation. *Ann Neurol* 1997; **42**: 423a [Abstract].

53 Coakley JH, Nagendran K, Ormerod IE, Ferguson CN, Hinds CJ. Prolonged neurogenic weakness in patients requiring mechanical ventilation for acute airflow limitation. *Chest* 1992; **101**: 1413–6.

54 Witt NJ, Zochodne DW, Bolton CF et al. Peripheral nerve function in sepsis and multiple organ failure. *Chest* 1991; **99**: 176–84.

55 Sandrock A, Cros D, Loius D. A 51-year-old man with chronic obstructive pulmonary disease and generalized muscle weakness. *N Engl J Med* 1997; **336**: 1079–88.

56 Zochodne DW, Ramsay DA, Saly V, Shelley S, Moffatt S. Acute necrotizing myopathy of intensive care: electrophysiological studies. *Muscle Nerve* 1994; **17**: 285–92.

57 Lacomis D, Giuliani MJ, Van Cott A, Kramer DJ. Acute myopathy of intensive care: clinical, electromyographic, and pathological aspects. *Ann Neurol* 1996; **40**: 645–54.

58 Sullivan KM, Shulman HM, Storb R et al. Chronic graft-versus-host disease in 52 patients: adverse natural course and successful treatment with combination immunosuppression. *Blood* 1981; **57**: 267–76.

59 Anderson BA, Young PV, Kean WF, Ludwin SK, Galbraith PR, Anastassiades TP. Polymyositis in chronic graft vs. host disease. A case report. *Arch Neurol* 1982; **39**: 188–90.

60 Reyes MG, Noronha P, Thomas W. Heredia R. Myositis of chronic graft versus host disease. *Neurology* 1983; **33**: 1222–4.

61 Urbano Marquez A, Estruch R, Grau JM et al. Inflammatory myopathy associated with chronic graft-versus-host disease. *Neurology* 1986; **36**: 1091–3.

62 Parker P, Chao NJ, Ben Ezra J et al. Polymyositis as a manifestation of chronic graft-versus-host disease. *Medicine (Baltimore)* 1996; **75**: 279–85.

63 Pier N, Dubowitz V. Chronic graft versus host disease presenting with polymyositis. *Br Med J (Clin Res Ed)* 1983; **286**: 2024.

64 Schmidley JW, Galloway P. Polymyositis following autologous bone marrow transplantation in Hodgkin's disease. *Neurology* 1990; **40**: 1003–4.

65 Volin L, Jarventie G, Ruutu T. Fatal rhabdomyolysis as a complication of bone marrow transplantation. *Bone Marrow Transplant* 1990; **6**: 59–60.

66 Mulligan SP, Joshua D, Joasoo A, Kronenberg H. Autoimmune hyperthyroidism associated with chronic graft-versus-host disease. *Transplantation* 1987; **44**: 463–4.

67 Lefvert AK, Bjorkholm M. Antibodies against the acetylcholine receptor in hematologic disorders. Implications for the development of myasthenia gravis after bone marrow grafting. *N Engl J Med* 1987; **317**: 170.

68 Lefvert AK, Bolme P, Hammarstrom L et al. Bone marrow grafting selectively induces the production of acetylcholine receptor antibodies, immunoglobulins bearing related idiotypes, and anti-idiotypes, and anti-idiotypic antibodies. *Ann N Y Acad Sci* 1987; **505**: 825–7.

69 Bolger GB, Sullivan KM, Spence AM et al. Myasthenia gravis after allogeneic bone marrow transplantation: relationship to chronic graft-versus-host disease. *Neurology* 1986; **36**: 1087–91.

70 Seeley E, Drachman D, Smith B et al. Post bone marrow transplantation (BMT) myasthenia gravis: evidence for acetylcholine receptor AChR0 abnormality. *Blood* 1984; **64**: 221a [Abstract].

71 Smith C, Aarlija J, Biberfeld P et al. Myasthenia gravis after bone marrow transplantation. Evidence of a donor origin. *N Engl J Med* 1983; **309**: 1565–8.

72 Grau JM, Casademont J, Monforte R et al. Myasthenia gravis after allogeneic bone marrow transplantation: report of a new case and pathogenetic considerations. *Bone Marrow Transplant* 1990; **5**: 435–7.

73 Lisak RP, Mitchell M, Zweiman B, Orrechio E, Asbury AK. Guillain–Barré syndrome and Hodgkin's disease: three cases with immunological studies. *Ann Neurol* 1977; **1**: 72–8.

74 Greenspan A, Deeg HJ, Cottler Fox M, Sirdofski M, Spitzer TR, Kattah J. Incapacitating peripheral neuropathy as a manifestation of chronic graft-versus-host disease. *Bone Marrow Transplant* 1990; **5**: 349–52.

75 Granena A, Grau JM, Carreras E et al. Subacute sensorimotor polyneuropathy in a recipient of an allogeneic bone marrow graft. *Exp Hematol* 1983; **11** (Suppl. 113): 10–12.

76 Maguire H, August CS, Sladky J. Chronic inflammatory demyelinating polyneuropathy. A previously unreported complication of bone marrow transplantation. *Neurology* 1989; **39**: 410a [Abstract].

77 Eliashiv S, Brenner T, Abramsky O et al. Acute inflammatory demyelinating polyneuropathy following bone marrow transplantation. *Bone Marrow Transplant* 1991; **8**: 315–7.

78 Amato AA, Barohn RJ, Sahenk Z, Tutschka PJ, Mendell JR. Polyneuropathy complicating bone marrow and solid organ transplantation. *Neurology* 1993; **43**: 1513–8.

79 Openshaw H. Peripheral neuropathy after bone marrow transplantation. *Biol Blood Marrow Transplant* 1997; **3**: 202–9.

80 Liedtke W, Quabeck K, Beelen DW, Straeten V, Schaefer UW. Recurrent acute inflammatory demyelinating polyradiculitis after allogeneic bone marrow transplantation. *J Neurol Sci* 1994; **125**: 110–11.

81 Perry A, Mehta J, Iveson T, Treleaven J, Powles R. Guillain–Barré syndrome after bone marrow transplantation. *Bone Marrow Transplant* 1994; **14**: 165–7.

82 Hagensee ME, Benyunes M, Miller JA, Spach DH. Campylobacter jejuni bacteremia and Guillain–Barré syndrome in a patient with GVHD after allogeneic BMT. *Bone Marrow Transplant* 1994; **13**: 349–51.

83 Asbury AK, Bolis L, Gibbs C. Autoimmune neuropathies: Guillain–Barré syndrome. *Ann Neurol* 1990; **27** (Suppl.): 1–79.

84 Openshaw H, Hinton DR, Slatkin NE, Bierman PJ, Hoffman FM, Snyder DS. Exacerbation of inflammatory demyelinating polyneuropathy after bone marrow transplantation. *Bone Marrow Transplant* 1991; **7**: 411–4.

85 Reece D, Frei Lahr D, Shepherd JD et al. Neurologic complications in allogeneic bone marrow transplant patients receiving cyclosporin. *Bone Marrow Transplant* 1991; **8**: 393–401.

86 Ghany AM, Tutschka PJ, McGhee RB et al. Cyclosporine-associated seizures in bone marrow transplant recipients given busulfan and cyclophosphamide preparative therapy. *Transplantation* 1991; **52**: 310–5.

87 Truwit CL, Denaro CP, Lake JR, DeMarco T. MR imaging of reversible cyclosporin A-induced neurotoxicity. *AJNR Am J Neuroradiol* 1991; **12**: 651–9.

88 Ghalie R, Fitzsimmons WE, Bennett D, Kaizer H. Cortical blindness. A rare complication of cyclosporine therapy. *Bone Marrow Transplant* 1990; **6**: 147–9.

89 Kahan BD. Cyclosporine. *N Engl J Med* 1989; **321**: 1725–38.

90 Atkinson K, Biggs J, Darveniza P, Boland J, Concannon A, Dodds A. Spinal cord and cerebellar-like syndromes associated with the use of cyclosporine in human recipients of allogeneic marrow transplants. *Transplant Proc* 1985; **17**: 1673–5.

91 Kahan BD, Flechner SM, Lorber MI, Golden D, Conley S, Van Buren CT. Complications of cyclosporine-prednisone immunosuppression in 402 renal allograft recipients exclusively followed at a single center for from 1 to 5 years. *Transplantation* 1987; **43**: 197–204.

92 Powell Jackson PR, Carmichael FJ, Calne RY, Williams R. Adult respiratory distress syndrome and convulsions associated with administration of cyclosporine in liver transplant recipients. *Transplantation* 1984; **38**: 341–3.

93 Grigg MM, Costanzo Nordin MR, Celesia GG et al. The etiology of seizures after cardiac transplantation. *Transplant Proc* 1988; **20**: 937–44.

94 de Groen PC, Aksamit AJ, Rakela J, Forbes GS, Krom RA. Central nervous system toxicity after liver transplantation. The role of cyclosporine and cholesterol. *N Engl J Med* 1987; **317**: 861–6.

95 Lane RJ, Roche SW, Leung AA, Greco A, Lange LS. Cyclosporin neurotoxicity in cardiac transplant recipients. *J Neurol Neurosurg Psychiatry* 1988; **51**: 1434–7.

96 Scheinman SJ, Reinitz ER, Petro G, Schwartz RA, Szmalc FS. Cyclosporine central neurotoxicity following renal transplantation. Report of a case using magnetic resonance images. *Transplantation* 1990; **49**: 215–6.

97 Hauser RA, Lacey DM, Knight MR. Hypertensive encephalopathy. Magnetic resonance imaging demonstration of reversible cortical and white matter lesions. *Arch Neurol* 1988; **45**: 1078–83.

98 Wilczek H, Ringden O, Tyden G. Cyclosporine-associated central nervous system toxicity after renal transplantation. *Transplantation* 1985; **39**: 110.

99 Berden JH, Hoitsma AJ, Merx JL, Keyser A. Severe central-nervous-system toxicity associated with cyclosporin. *Lancet* 1985; **1**: 219–20.

100 Lind MJ, McWilliam L, Jip J, Scarffe JH, Morgenstern GR, Chang J. Cyclosporin associated demyelination following allogeneic bone marrow transplantation. *Hematol Oncol* 1989; **7**: 49–52.

101 Rubin AM, Kang H. Cerebral blindness and encephalopathy with cyclosporin A toxicity. *Neurology* 1987; **37**: 1072–6.

102 Noll RB, Kulkarni R. Complex visual hallucinations and cyclosporine. *Arch Neurol* 1984; **41**: 329–30.

103 Appleton RE, Farrell K, Teal P, Hashimoto SA, Wong PK. Complex partial status epilepticus associated with cyclosporin A therapy. *J Neurol Neurosurg Psychiatry* 1989; **52**: 1068–71.

104 Thompson C, Sullivan K, June C, Thomas E. Association between cyclosporin neurotoxocity and hypomagnesaemia. *Lancet* 1984; **2**: 1116–20.

105 Shutter LA, Green JP, Newman NJ, Hooks MA, Gordon RD. Cortical blindness and white matter lesions in a patient receiving FK506 after liver transplantation. *Neurology* 1993; **43**: 2417–8.

106 Fung JJ, Alessiani M, Abu Elmagd K et al. Adverse effects associated wuth the use of FK506. *Transplant Proc* 1991; **23**: 3105–8.

107 Frank B, Perdrizet GA, White HM, Marsh JW, Lemann W, Woodle ES. Neurotoxicity of FK506 in liver transplant recipients. *Transplant Proc* 1993; **25**: 1887–8.

108 Eidelman BH, Abu Elmagd K, Wilson J et al. Neurologic complications of FK506. *Transplant Proc* 1991; **23**: 3175–8.

109 Singh N, Bonham A, Fukui M. Immunosuppressive-associated leukoencephalopathy in organ transplant recipients. *Transplantation* 2000; **69**: 467–72.

110 Wijdicks EF. Neurotoxicity of immunosuppressive drugs. *Liver Transpl* 2001; **7**: 937–42.

111 Porapakkham S. An epidemiologic study of eclampsia. *Obstet Gynecol* 1979; **54**: 26–30.

112 Crawford S, Varner MW, Digre KB, Servais G, Corbett JJ. Cranial magnetic resonance imaging in eclampsia. *Obstet Gynecol* 1987; **70**: 474–7.

113 Bartynski WS, Zeigler Z, Spearman MP et al. Etiology of cortical and white matter lesions in cyclosporin-A and FK-506 neurotoxicity. *AJNR Am J Neuroradiol* 2001; **22**: 1907–14.

114 Mori A, Tanaka J, Kobayashi S et al. Fatal cerebral hemorrhage associated with cyclosporin-A/FK506-related encephalopathy after allogeneic bone marrow transplantation. *Ann Hematol* 2000; **79**: 588–92.

115 Openshaw H, Slatkin NE, Smith E. Eye movement disorders in bone marrow transplant patients on

cyclosporin and ganciclovir. *Bone Marrow Transplant* 1997; **19**: 503–5.
116 Openshaw H. Eye movement abnormally associated with cyclosporin. *J Neurol Neurosurg Psychiatry* 2001; **70**: 809.
117 Nussbaum ES, Maxwell RE, Bitterman PB, Hertz MI, Bula W, Latchaw RE. Cyclosporine A toxicity presenting with acute cerebellar edema and brainstem compression. Case report. *J Neurosurg* 1995; **82**: 1068–70.
118 Gopal AK, Thorning DR, Back AL. Fatal outcome due to cyclosporine neurotoxicity with associated pathological findings. *Bone Marrow Transplant* 1999; **23**: 191–3.
119 Zoja C, Furci L, Ghilardi F, Zilio P, Benigni A, Remuzzi G. Cyclosporin-induced endothelial cell injury. *Lab Invest* 1986; **55**: 455–62.
120 Lerman A, Hildebrand F, Margulies K et al. Endothelin: a new cardiovascular regulatory peptide. *Mayo Clin Proc* 1990; **65**: 1441–9.
121 Pizzolato GP, Sztajzel R, Burkhardt K, Megret M, Borisch B. Cerebral vasculitis during FK506 treatment in a liver transplant patient. *Neurology* 1998; **50**: 1154–7.
122 Famiglio L, Racusen L, Fivush B, Solez K, Fisher R. Central nervous system toxicity of cyclosporine in a rat model. *Transplantation* 1989; **48**: 316–21.
123 McDonald JW, Goldberg MP, Gwag BJ, Chi SI, Choi DW. Cyclosporine induces neuronal apoptosis and selective oligodendrocyte death in cortical cultures. *Ann Neurol* 1996; **40**: 750–8.
124 Jacobson P, Ng J, Ratanatharathorn V, Uberti J, Brundage RC. Factors affecting the pharmacokinetics of tacrolimus (FK506) in hematopoietic cell transplant (HCT) patients. *Bone Marrow Transplant* 2001; **28**: 753–8.
125 Freeman DJ, Laupacis A, Keown PA, Stiller CR, Carruthers SG. Evaluation of cyclosporin–phenytoin interaction with observations on cyclosporin metabolites. *Br J Clin Pharmacol* 1984; **18**: 887–93.
126 Wijdicks EF, Dahlke LJ, Wiesner RH. Oral cyclosporine decreases severity of neurotoxicity in liver transplant recipients. *Neurology* 1999; **52**: 1708–10.
127 Gryn J, Goldberg J, Viner E. Propranolol for the treatment of cyclosporine-induced headaches. *Bone Marrow Transplant* 1992; **9**: 211–2.
128 Rozen TD, Wijdicks EF, Hay JE. Treatment-refractory cyclosporine-associated headache: relief with conversion to FK-506. *Neurology* 1996; **47**: 1347.
129 Fischman MA, Hull D, Bartus SA, Schweizer RT. Valproate for epilepsy in renal transplant recipients receiving cyclosporine. *Transplantation* 1989; **48**: 542.
130 Hillebrand G, Castro L, Van Scheidt W, Beukelman D, Land W, Schmidt D. Valproate for epilepsy in renal transplant recipients receiving cyclosporine. *Transplantation* 1987; **43**: 915–6.
131 Hall RC, Popkin MK, Stickney SK, Gardner ER. Presentation of the steroid psychoses. *J Nerv Ment Dis* 1979; **167**: 229–36.
132 Askari A, Vignos PJ, Moskowitz RW. Steroid myopathy in connective tissue disease. *Am J Med* 1976; **61**: 485–92.
133 Khaleeli AA, Edwards RH, Gohil K et al. Corticosteroid myopathy: a clinical pathological study. 1983; **18**: 155–66.
134 Fullerton P, Kremer M. Neuropathy after intake of thalidomide (Distaval®). *Br Med J* 1961; **2**: 855–8.

135 Vogelsang GB, Farmer ER, Hess AD et al. Thalidomide for the treatment of chronic graft-versus-host disease. *N Engl J Med* 1992; **326**: 1055–8.
136 Fullerton P, O'Sullivan D. Thalidomide neuropathy: a clinical electrophysiological, and histological follow-up study. *J Neurol Neurosurg Psychiatry* 1968; **31**: 543–51.
137 Clemmensen OJ, Olsen PZ, Andersen KE. Thalidomide neurotoxicity. *Arch Dermatol* 1984; **120**: 338–41.
138 Openshaw H, Slatkin NE, Parker P. Thalidomide neuropathy in bone marrow transplantation. *Neurology* 1996; **46**: 332a [Abstract].
139 Weinblatt ME. Toxicity of low dose methotrexate in rheumatoid arthritis. *J Rheumatol* 1985; **12** (Suppl. 12): 35–9.
140 McKendry RJ, Cyr M. Toxicity of methotrexate compared with azathioprine in the treatment of rheumatoid arthritis. A case-control study of 131 patients. *Arch Intern Med* 1989; **149**: 685–9.
141 Wernick R, Smith DL. Central nervous system toxicity associated with weekly low-dose methotrexate treatment. *Arthritis Rheum* 1989; **32**: 770–5.
142 Ebner F, Ranner G, Slavc I et al. MR Findings in methotrexate-induced CNS abnormalities. *AJNR Am J Neuroradiol* 1989; **10**: 959–64.
143 Bleyer WA. Neurologic sequelae of methotrexate and ionizing radiation: a new classification. *Cancer Treat Rep* 1981; **65** (Suppl. 1): 89–98.
144 Thompson CB, Sanders JE, Flournoy N, Buckner CD, Thomas ED. The risks of central nervous system relapse and leukoencephalopathy in patients receiving marrow transplants for acute leukemia. *Blood* 1986; **67**: 195–9.
145 Devinsky O, Lemann W, Evans AC, Moeller JR, Rottenberg DA. Akinetic mutism in a bone marrow transplant recipient following total-body irradiation and amphotericin B chemoprophylaxis. A positron emission tomographic and neuropathologic study. *Arch Neurol* 1987; **44**: 414–7.
146 Openshaw H, Stuve O, Antel JP et al. Multiple sclerosis flares associated with recombinant granulocyte colony-stimulating factor. *Neurology* 2000; **54**: 2147–50.
147 Burt RK, Fassas A, Snowden J et al. Collection of hematopoietic stem cells from patients with autoimmune diseases. *Bone Marrow Transplant* 2001; **28**: 1–12.
148 McGonagle D, Rawstron A, Richards S et al. A phase I study to address the safety and efficacy of granulocyte colony-stimulating factor for the mobilization of hematopoietic progenitor cells in active rheumatoid arthritis. *Arthritis Rheum* 1997; **40**: 1838–42.
149 Witherspoon RP, Fisher LD, Schoch G et al. Secondary cancers after bone marrow transplantation for leukemia or aplastic anemia. *N Engl J Med* 1989; **321**: 784–9.
150 Kolb HJ, Bender Gotze C. Late complications after allogeneic bone marrow transplantation for leukaemia. *Bone Marrow Transplant* 1990; **6**: 61–72.
151 De La Camara R, Tomas JF, Figuera A, Berberana M, Fernandez Ranada JM. High dose busulfan and seizures. *Bone Marrow Transplant* 1991; **7**: 363–4.
152 Hartmann O, Benhamou E, Beaujean F et al. High-dose busulfan and cyclophosphamide with autologous bone marrow transplantation support in advanced malignancies in children: a phase II study. *J Clin Oncol* 1986; **4**: 1804–10.
153 Marcus RE, Goldman JM. Convulsions due to high-dose busulphan. *Lancet* 1984; **2**: 1463.

154 Vassal G, Deroussent A, Hartmann O et al. Dose-dependent neurotoxicity of high-dose busulfan in children: a clinical and pharmacological study. *Cancer Res* 1990; **50**: 6203–7.
155 Hassan M, Ehrsson H, Smedmyr B et al. Cerebrospinal fluid and plasma concentrations of busulfan during high-dose therapy. *Bone Marrow Transplant* 1989; **4**: 113–4.
156 Grigg AP, Shepherd JD, Phillips GL. Busulphan and phenytoin. *Ann Intern Med* 1989; **111**: 1049–50.
157 Jagannath S, Armitage JO, Dicke KA et al. Prognostic factors for response and survival after high-dose cyclophosphamide, carmustine, and etoposide with autologous bone marrow transplantation for relapsed Hodgkin's disease. *J Clin Oncol* 1989; **7**: 179–85.
158 Woo MH, Ippoliti C, Bruton J, Mehra R, Champlin R, Przepiorka D. Headache, circumoral paresthesia, and facial flushing associated with high-dose carmustine infusion. *Bone Marrow Transplant* 1997; **19**: 845–7.
159 Fields KK, Elfenbein GJ, Lazarus HM et al. Maximum-tolerated doses of ifosfamide, carboplatin, and etoposide given over 6 days followed by autologous stem-cell rescue: toxicity profile. *J Clin Oncol* 1995; **13**: 323–32.
160 Meanwell CA, Blake AE, Kelly KA, Honigsberger L, Blackledge G. Prediction of ifosfamide/mesna associated encephalopathy. *Eur J Cancer Clin Oncol* 1986; **22**: 815–9.
161 Anderson N, Tandon D. Ifosfamide extrapyramidal neurotoxicity. *Cancer* 1991; **68**: 72–5.
162 Pallotta MG, Velazco A, Sadler A. Ifosfamide extrapyramidal neurotoxicity. *Cancer* 1992; **70**: 2743–5.
163 Pelgrims J, De Vos F, Van den Brande J, Schrijvers D, Prove A, Vermorken JB. Methylene blue in the treatment and prevention of ifosfamide-induced encephalopathy: report of 12 cases and a review of the literature. *Br J Cancer* 2000; **82**: 291–4.
164 Sullivan KM, Storb R, Shulman HM et al. Immediate and delayed neurotoxicity after mechlorethamine preparation for bone marrow transplantation. *Ann Intern Med* 1982; **97**: 182–9.
165 Spriano M, Clavio M, Carrara P et al. Fludarabine in untreated and previously treated B-CLL patients: a report on efficacy and toxicity. *Haematologica* 1994; **79**: 218–24.
166 Baker WJ, Royer GL, Weiss RB. Cytarabine and neurologic toxicity. *J Clin Oncol* 1991; **9**: 679–93.
167 Openshaw H, Slatkin NE, Stein AS, Hinton DR, Forman SJ. Acute polyneuropathy after high dose cytosine arabinoside in patients with leukemia. *Cancer* 1996; **78**: 1899–905.
168 Vogler WR, Winton EF, Heffner LT et al. Ophthalmological and other toxicities related to cytosine arabinoside and total body irradiation as preparative regimen for bone marrow transplantation. *Bone Marrow Transplant* 1990; **6**: 405–9.
169 Johnson NT, Crawford SW, Sargur M. Acute acquired demyelinating polyneuropathy with respiratory failure following high-dose systemic cytosine arabinoside and marrow transplantation. *Bone Marrow Transplant* 1987; **2**: 203–7.
170 Imrie KR, Couture F, Turner CC, Sutcliffe SB, Keating A. Peripheral neuropathy following high-dose etoposide and autologous bone marrow transplantation. *Bone Marrow Transplant* 1994; **13**: 77–9.

171 Mollman JE, Hogan WM, Glover DJ, McCluskey LF. Unusual presentation of *cis*-platinum neuropathy. *Neurology* 1988; **38**: 488–90.

172 Stemmer SM, Cagnoni PJ, Shpall EJ *et al*. High-dose paclitaxel, cyclophosphamide, and cisplatin with autologous hematopoietic progenitor-cell support: a phase I trial. *J Clin Oncol* 1996; **14**: 1463–72.

173 Mollman JE. Cisplatin neurotoxicity. *N Engl J Med* 1990; **322**: 126–7.

174 Rowinsky EK, Donehower RC. Paclitaxel (Taxol®). *N Engl J Med* 1995; **332**: 1004–14.

175 Pollera CF, Marolla P, Nardi M, Ameglio F, Cozzo L, Bevere F. Very high-dose cisplatin-induced ototoxicity. A preliminary report on early and long-term effects. *Cancer Chemother Pharmacol* 1988; **21**: 61–4.

176 Walther PJ, Rossitch E, Bullard DE. The development of Lhermitte's sign during cisplatin chemotherapy. Possible drug-induced toxicity causing spinal cord demyelination. *Cancer* 1987; **60**: 2170–2.

177 Berman IJ, Mann MP. Seizures and transient cortical blindness associated with *cis*-platinum (II) diamminedichloride (PDD) therapy in a 30-year-old man. *Cancer* 1980; **45**: 764–6.

178 Price B. Anisocoria from scopalamine patches. *JAMA* 1985; **254**: 1720–1.

179 Snavely SR, Hodges GR. The neurotoxicity of antibacterial agents. *Ann Intern Med* 1984; **101**: 92–104.

180 Frytak S, Moertel CH, Childs DS. Neurologic toxicity associated with high-dose metronidazole therapy. *Ann Intern Med* 1978; **88**: 361–2.

181 Eng RH, Munsif AN, Yangco BG, Smith SM, Chmel H. Seizure propensity with imipenem. *Arch Intern Med* 1989; **149**: 1881–3.

182 Kusumi RK, Plouffe JF, Wyatt RH, Fass RJ. Central nervous system toxicity associated with metronidazole therapy. *Ann Intern Med* 1980; **93**: 59–60.

183 Burdge DR, Chow AW, Sacks SL. Neurotoxic effects during vidarabine therapy for herpes zoster. *Can Med Assoc J* 1985; **132**: 392–5.

184 Feldman S, Robertson PK, Lott L, Thornton D. Neurotoxicity due to adenine arabinoside therapy during varicella-zoster virus infections in immunocompromised children. *J Infect Dis* 1986; **154**: 889–93.

185 Wade JC, Meyers JD. Neurologic symptoms associated with parenteral acyclovir treatment after marrow transplantation. *Ann Intern Med* 1983; **98**: 921–5.

186 Spiegal DM, Lau K. Acute renal failure and coma secondary to acyclovir therapy. *JAMA* 1986; **255**: 1882–3.

187 Cohen SM, Minkove JA, Zebley JW, Mulholland JH. Severe but reversible neurotoxicity from acyclovir. *Ann Intern Med* 1984; **100**: 920.

188 Swan SK, Bennett WM. Oral acyclovir and neurotoxicity. *Ann Intern Med* 1989; **111**: 188.

189 Davis CL, Springmeyer S, Gmerek BJ. Central nervous system side effects of ganciclovir. *N Engl J Med* 1990; **322**: 933–4.

190 De Armand B. Safety considerations in the use of ganciclovir in immunocompromised patients. *Transplant Proc* 1991; **23**: 26–9.

191 Jacobsen M, O'Donnell J. Approaches to the treatment of cytomegalovirus retinitis: ganciclovir and foscarnet. *J Acquir Immune Defic Syndr* 1991; **4** (Suppl.): S11–15.

192 Chrisp P, Clissold SP. Foscarnet. A review of its antiviral activity, pharmacokinetic properties and therapeutic use in immunocompromised patients with cytomegalovirus retinitis. *Drugs* 1991; **41**: 104–29.

193 Hickey WF, Kimura H. Graft-vs.-host disease elicits expression of class I and class II histocompatibility antigens and the presence of scattered T lymphocytes in rat central nervous system. *Proc Natl Acad Sci U S A* 1987; **84**: 2082–6.

194 Rouah E, Gruber R, Shearer W, Armstrong D, Hawkins EP. Graft-versus-host disease in the central nervous system. A real entity? *Am J Clin Pathol* 1988; **89**: 543–6.

195 Marosi C, Budka H, Grimm G *et al*. Fatal encephalitis in a patient with chronic graft-versus-host disease. *Bone Marrow Transplant* 1990; **6**: 53–7.

196 Padovan CS, Yousry TA, Schleuning M, Holler E, Kolb HJ, Straube A. Neurological and neuroradiological findings in long-term survivors of allogeneic bone marrow transplantation. *Ann Neurol* 1998; **43**: 627–33.

197 Openshaw H, Slatkin NE, Parker PM, Forman SJ. Immune-mediated myelopathy after allogeneic marrow transplantation. *Bone Marrow Transplant* 1995; **15**: 633–6.

198 Kelly P, Staunton H, Lawler M *et al*. Multifocal remitting-relapsing cerebral demyelination 20 years following allogeneic bone marrow transplantation. *J Neuropathol Exp Neurol* 1996; **55**: 992–8.

199 Schold SC, Cho ES, Somasundaram M, Posner JB. Subacute motor neuronopathy. A remote effect of lymphoma. *Ann Neurol* 1979; **5**: 271–87.

200 Layzer RB, Rowland LP. Cramps. *N Engl J Med* 1971; **285**: 31–40.

60 Margaret R. O'Donnell

Blood Group Incompatibilities and Hemolytic Complications of Hematopoietic Cell Transplantation

The etiologies of hemolytic disorders following hematopoietic cell transplantation (HCT) can be grouped as either immune mediated or mechanical complications of thrombotic microangiopathy syndromes. The majority of immune mediated hemolytic reactions are caused by alloantibodies directed at red cell antigens in blood group incompatible donor–recipient pairs. Autoimmune hemolysis is less common but can be seen following both allogeneic and autologous HCT. In these instances, hemolysis may be related to drugs, infections, recurrent disease (in the case of chronic lymphocytic leukemia and lymphomas) or as a manifestation of chronic graft-vs.-host disease (GVHD). The inciting factors for hemolysis resulting from thrombotic microangiopathy are unclear after either autologous or allogeneic HCT. The supposition has been that endothelial cells are injured by radiation and dose-intensive chemotherapy, cyclosporine (CSP) or cytokine release associated with GVHD. This chapter addresses the issues of prevention, diagnosis and treatment of these disorders in the context of HCT.

Hemolytic complications of ABO incompatibility

The inheritance of blood group antigens (ABO, Rh, Jk, etc.) is independent of that of the human leukocyte antigen (HLA) tissue antigen complex. In most series of sibling allogeneic HCT, there is discordance of ABO groups in 30–40% of donor–recipient pairs; the rate may be somewhat higher in unrelated donor HCTs. While ABO incompatibility may increase the complexity of HCT, it is not an obstacle to a successful HCT. There are two distinct immune mechanisms that can trigger hemolysis early following allogeneic bone marrow transplantation (BMT) or peripheral blood hematopoietic cell (PBHC) transplantation based either on:
1 the presence of pre-existing isohemagglutinins that immediately lyse the target red cell; or
2 generation of new isohemagglutinins as a response to exposure to foreign antigens in the recipient by "passenger lymphocytes" in the graft causing hemolysis 5–14 days after HCT [1–3].

The first type of reaction is most often seen in major or bidirectional ABO mismatches while the second is most often seen after minor mismatch transplants (Table 60.1) [4–6].

In major ABO incompatible HCT, the isohemagglutinins can continue to lyse cells expressing the target antigen as long as the recipient antibody is being produced. As erythroid progenitors acquire blood group antigens early at the level of the burst forming unit-erythroid (BFU-E) in stem cell culture, the antibodies can produce destruction of intramedullary precursors giving rise to pure red cell aplasia (PRCA) [7–9]. In patients receiving myeloablative conditioning, there is no evidence that ABO incompatibility has any impact on myeloid or megakaryocytic engraftment, graft rejection or incidence of GVHD. Several authors have documented delayed red blood cell (RBC) engraftment and increased transfusion requirements in major ABO incompatible HCT [10–14]. Worel et al. [15] reported a median time to reticulocytosis of >3% at 32 days for major mismatches vs. 21 and 22 days for ABO identical or minor mismatches and a twofold increase of RBC transfusions within the first 100 days (12 vs. 6 and 8) ($p = 0.045$). Recently, low-intensity nonmyeloablative HCTs have been introduced to expand the applicability of transplantation to older individuals with a broad number of transfusion-dependent diseases such as myelodysplasia and myeloma [16–18]. The "low-intensity" regimens vary widely but all permit a more protracted coexistence of host and donor hematopoiesis because the strategy is predicated on using the donor's allogeneic response rather than chemotherapy to eradicate the underlying malignancy. A recent report from Bolan et al. [19] indicates that RCB engraftment was delayed beyond 100 days in >60% patients with major ABO incompatible nonmyeloablative HCTs compared with a median of 40 days for the myeloablative transplants with major mismatches. The incidence of PRCA appears to be higher in nonmyeloablative HCTs (16–32%), compared with myeloablative conditioning regimens (5–7%) [19–21]. It is premature to speculate on the impact of ABO major mismatch in graft rejection in these reduced conditioning

Table 60.1 Immunohematologic problems of ABO incompatible hematopoietic cell transplantation (HCT).

Major incompatible (20%)
Example: Recipient O, Donor A, B, AB *or* Recipient A or B, Donor AB
    Immediate hemolysis of RBC infused with graft
    Delayed hemolysis of donor RBCs by persistent recipient isohemagglutinin
    Delayed erythrocyte production
    Pure red cell aplasia

Minor incompatibility (22–24%)
Example: Recipient A, B or AB, Donor O *or* Recipient AB, Donor A or B
    Immediate hemolysis of recipient RBC by donor-derived isohemagglutinin in graft
    Delayed hemolysis of recipient RBC by isohemagglutinin

Bidirectional incompatibility (1–2%)
Example: Donor A, Recipient B *or* vice versa
    Both immediate and delayed hemolysis are possible with isoagglutinins of donor against recipient RBC and recipient antibodies directed against donor RBC

RBC, red blood cell.

Table 60.2 Method of red blood cell (RBC) depletion of hematopoietic cell transplantation (HCT) graft.

Method	Equipment	Residual RBC content (mL)	CFU-GM recovery (%)
Buffy coat preparation	Manual sedimentation over hydroxyethyl starch	4–21 (1 run)	55–75
	Discontinuous flow cell separator	8–38	86
	Continuous flow cell separator	5–10	78–85

CFU-GM, colony-forming unit–granulocyte/macrophage.

regimens as the incidence of autologous recovery varies widely from regimen to regimen even in blood group compatible HCT.

Strategies to prevent acute hemolysis in major ABO incompatible HCTs focus on removal of red cells from the marrow or peripheral blood stem cell (PBSC) product and decreasing the concentration of isohemagglutinins in the recipient plasma. Methods for removing red cells from marrow products are listed in Table 60.2. The techniques for erythrocyte depletion vary in length and labor intensity of process, complexity of equipment required and degree of mononuclear cell loss [22–33]. PBHC products by the nature of the collection method are all relatively red cell depleted (regardless of ABO match). The goal is to infuse a graft product with <10 mL red cell contamination while maintaining sufficient nucleated cells (0.5×10^8 mononuclear or 1×10^6 CD34$^+$ cells/kg recipient weight) to achieve engraftment; this often requires collecting larger volumes of marrow or processing larger volumes of donor blood in mismatched donor–recipient pairs than in matched transplants.

In minor ABO mismatched HCT, donor isohemagglutinins passively transferred with the graft can produce acute hemolysis of recipient erythrocytes, so donor plasma is removed from the product prior to infusion. Rarely, single donor platelet products with high isoagglutinin titers have also been reported to cause severe hemolysis when transfused without volume reduction to an out of group recipient [34].

Delayed hemolytic reactions

In minor ABO mismatched HCT, as well as solid organ transplants, hemolysis, which may be severe and occasionally fatal, can emerge abruptly 5–17 days post-transplant as a result of development of new isohemogglutinins generated by "passenger" B lymphocytes transferred from the donor at the time of transplantation. The incidence of "passenger lymphocyte syndrome" increases with the B-cell contamination of the graft; it is therefore reasonable to expect a higher incidence of hemolysis with PBHC products, as they contain a tenfold increase in CD10$^+$ and CD20$^+$ cells compared to marrow grafts. The use of granulocyte colony-stimulating factors (G-CSF) to mobilize donor PBHC can also modulate T-lymphocyte cytokine production in such a way that promotes antibody production. In solid organ transplants, the incidence of hemolysis ranges from 10% for kidney to 70% for lung or heart–lung recipients. While ABO antigens are the most common targets, hemolysis has also been reported against Rh, Jka, Kidd and Lewis blood group antigens [35–38]. Several factors influence the severity of the hemolysis including rapidity of rise of donor antibody in the recipient post-transplant, secretor status and rapidity of engraftment (i.e. type of graft) [39,40]. Massive hemolysis in which most, if not all, recipient RBCs are lysed over 2–3 days seem to be complement-mediated, analogous to post-transfusion purpura.

Delayed hemolysis can also occur in ABO major mismatched HCT depending on the potency of the recipient isohemagglutinin directed at the newly emerging donor erythrocytes. Even when overt hemolysis is not evident, several series have reported delayed erythroid engraftment of 30–40 days, vs. 20–22 days for ABO identical and minor mismatch grafts, in myeloablative HCT and >3 months in reduced dose intensity conditioning HCT. Persistence of host isohemagglutinins has been associated with PRCA in major ABO incompatible transplants with incidence of 8–16% in myeloablative and up to 30% in a small sample of non-myeloablative HCTs [19]. Several authors have suggested that GVHD prophylaxis regimens using CSP alone or with prednisone create a mileau more likely to allow isohemagglutinin to persist or develop because CSP (and, by inference, tacrolimus [FK506] permits B cells to persist longer than combinations of CSP with methotrexate (MTX) or mycofenalate (MMF)) [41,42]. Recipients who do develop GVHD have been shown to have more rapid clearance of host isohemagglutinins, which gives some credence to a "graft-vs.-plasma cell" effect [43].

Management of ABO and Rh incompatibility

Approach to decreasing risks for hemolysis

The strategies for managing blood product support for these patients are outlined in Table 60.3. In all instances, in the immediate peritransplant period, it is appropriate to use group O cells as they lack target antigens and, when used in non-group O recipients, will serve to dilute the percentage of red cells targeted by donor-generated antibodies. The donor and recipient of ABO or Rh incompatible grafts should have titers of the isohemagglutinin identified before HCT [44,45]. If the donor has high-titer anti-A, for example, a pre-emptive RBC exchange prior to HCT may prevent the abrupt onset of hemolysis from emerging alloantibodies generated by donor B cells in a minor mismatch. If the recipient has high isohemagglutinin titers directed against donor-derived RBC antigen, the titer may be decreased by plasma infusion or exchange [45,46]. This procedure is usually carried out 3–4 days before HCT, after immunosuppressive treatment has been initiated to try to prevent rebound phenomena with the intention of decreasing the antibody titer to <1 : 16. Other strategies include the infusion of donor-type fresh frozen plasma (FFP) to provide a noncellular source of A or B antigen to absorb the recipient isohemagglutinin [46–49]. A rarely used technique is the infusion of small aliquots of donor red blood cells 12–24 h before transplant. This intervention requires forced alkaline diuresis and intensive monitoring for potential hemolytic reaction [50].

Complications associated with these strategies to deplete isohemagglutinin include citrate toxicity, risk of transmission of infection and platelet depletion. There are also risks of febrile transfusion reactions, transfusion-related lung injury and, with FFP infusion, volume overload. Red cell depletion and reduction of isohemagglutinin are quite effective in preventing immediate hemolysis in major mismatches; however, 10% of patients receiving myeloablative transplants with either a marrow or PHSC graft will develop delayed hemolysis.

Following HCT, all patients should be monitored for the emergence of donor-derived erythrocytes, persistence of recipient isohemagglutinin and evidence of hemolysis (using lactic dehydrogenase [LDH], reticulocyte counts and direct agglutinin test (DAT). Early after HCT, a rising bilirubin is a nonspecific marker for hemolysis because hyperbilirubinemia can be triggered by a myriad of other causes including veno-occlusive disease of the liver, drug effects from MTX, CSP, antifungal azols or GVHD. Patients with major mismatches and high isohemagglutinin titers pre-HCT are particularly at risk for delay of RBC engraftment, hemolysis and PRCA. Titers of isohemagglutinins in major mismatches should be monitored at least twice monthly until disappearance. Patients whose titers increase rather than fall over time, and who also have increasing transfusion requirements may merit marrow examination to look for PRCA. Isohemagglutinin

Table 60.3 Management of blood support for ABO incompatible transplant recipients.

	RBC	Plasma
Major mismatch Example: Recipient 0 Donor A	Remove RBC from HCT product	If recipient anti A titer is >1 : 256, consider: 1 Plasma exchange pretransplant 2 Daily infusion of donor type FFP to lower titer to 1 : 1, or lowest stable titer <1 : 16
	Transfuse O cells post-transplant until anti A titer nondetectable and recipient types as group A	Give donor type platelets and plasma or volume reduce all out of donor group products
Minor mismatch Example: Recipient B Donor O	Transfuse group O cells. Red cell exchange with group O cell pre HCT to dilute recipient type RBC down to <30% of RBC volume	1 Remove plasma from HCT graft to prevent immediate hemolysis if titer ≥1 : 128 2 Give platelet and plasma lacking anti-B isohemagglatinin or volume reduce product 3 Monitor Coombs test beginning day 5–20 every 2–3 days to monitor for hemolysis caused by "passenger" lymphocyte syndrome
Bidirectional mismatch Example: Recipient B Donor A	Transfuse O cells Remove RBC from HCT product Red cell exchange with group O cells to deplete percentage of B cells prior to HCT	Plasma deplete donor HCT product before infusions Use group AB plasma and platelet products before and after transplant (or volume reduce out of group products) Consider plasma exchange for high titer (>1 : 256) IgG isohemagglutinin
Rh incompatible Major Minor	Deplete RBC from graft. Use Rh product Use Rh product	Consider prophylactic removal of Rh antibody in patient by red cell exchange Consider Rhogam

titers seem to fall more rapidly in unrelated donor transplants than with sibling donors. Investigators from Seattle examined the rate of fall of isohemagglutinin in 383 major or minor HCT recipients [43]. The time to undetectable titers was significantly shorter (46 vs. 61 days) in unrelated and sibling ablative HCT, respectively. In related donors, those who developed GVHD had a twofold more rapid decline in antibody titers. In this study, ABO incompatibility did not affect the incidence of GVHD or survival. In two other studies, ABO incompatibility did affect survival at day 100 in subgroups of patients (chronic myelogenous leukemia patients in one and acute myeloid leukemia and myelodysplasia in the second) [14,51]. Neither report specified the factors influencing the poorer outcomes for ABO incompatible HCT. One may speculate that more protracted transfusional support required indwelling venous access devices, which placed patients at higher risk of infection. Iron overload would be a potential problem for those patients who developed PRCA but this would not be a factor by day 100. In minor mismatches, the risk for donor-derived antibody-mediated hemolysis begins at 5–16 days post-HCT; the DAT usually is positive and donor-derived antibody can be eluted from the recipient RBCs. Because the isohemagglutinins responsible for hemolysis may be newly generated by passenger B cells, pretransplant titers may not be predictive of the severity of the hemolysis.

Despite immunosuppression, patients can also develop alloimmunization to non-ABO RBC antigens post-HCT; most commonly, involving Rh, Kell or Kidd (Jk) antigens [37,38]. Development of non-ABO antibodies has been reported in high frequency in patients receiving ABO incompatible HCT: 9.6% vs. 1.6% [38]. In a large series from Spain, de la Rubia *et al.* [38] reported a 3.7% incidence of detection of new alloimmunization to Jka, K, M, Le and Rh antigens, usually within the first 30 days post-HCT. In the majority of cases in which the specificity of the antibody was identified by elutriation from RBC, the antibody was directed at antigens, which were not detected in either the donor or recipient at time of HCT. The isohemagglutinins could have been produced by either residual host- or by donor-derived lymphocytes in response to new RBC antigens presented post-HCT. Clinically, the agglutinins that develop in response to antigens which are different from those expressed on either donor or recipient RBC have little hemolysis associated with them as compared to quite severe hemolytic reactions which have been seen with Rh– donor lymphocytes infused into Rh+ recipients. In the Spanish series, the rate of developing non-ABO antibodies was 9.6% in ABO mismatched pairs [38]. There have been two reports of severe hemolysis associated with the Jka system. In both instances, the donor had previously been sensitized to Jka, but the method used for the pretransplantation antibody screen did not detect the Jka antibody. It is not uncommon for an individual with known anti-Jka to have no serologically identifiable serum antibody a few months after the antibody was originally identified, making the risk of a clinically significant hemolytic event higher in Jka+ recipients [37].

Treatment of pure red cell aplasia

The most extreme example of delayed erythroid engraftment following major ABO incompatible HCT is suppression at the intramedullary precursor stage [7]. The mechanism for PRCA is presumed to be persistence of recipient isohemaglutinins that target antigens on donor-derived erythroid precursors in the marrow when all the antigen-presenting cells in the circulation have been removed. As erythroid precursors acquire ABH antigens early after commitment to erythroid differentiation, destruction of these early precursors effectively shuts off red cell production. Usually, erythroid production resumes when the recipient antibody titers (usually anti-A) are no longer detectable. Reports of this severe complication are increasing in number, doubling in the literature in the last 5 years. Incidence varies depending on HCT source (marrow vs. PBHC), conditioning regimen (myeloablative vs. nonmyeloablative) and type of GVHD prophylaxis (CSP or FK506 with or without MTX or T-cell depletion). Duration of aplasia can vary from 3 months to >5 years. There are now at least 56 reported cases of PRCA following ABO incompatible HCT (without evidence of concomitant viral infection) [52–66]. The majority of these patients had received myeloablative transplants with only eight cases reported following a reduced dose intensity transplant. Thirty-six patients received CSP without MTX, 18 received CSP and short course MTX prophylaxis and two received T-cell-depleted grafts. Almost half the patients (24 of 56) recovered without any intervention other than tapering CSP. Many patients received a trial of erythropoietin alone or combined with steroids; eight patients responded. Plasma exchange improved hematopoiesis in 16 patients while two patients received donor lymphocyte infusion: antithymocyte globulin and anti-CD-20 monoclonal antibody (rituximab) were each successfully used in one patient. The incidence of this problem seems to vary from <10% in some large series of myeloablative transplants using CSP/MTX to almost 30% in a recent small series of nonmyeloablative HCT with CSP alone.

In addition to PRCA associated with ABO incompatibility, aplasia has also been reported in conjunction with parvovirus 19 infection in both HCT and solid organ transplantation [67,68]. Most of these patients responded to immunoglobulin administration. On rare occasions, change of FK506 to CSP or discontinuation of MMF was necessary. Two children with renal allografts have been reported to develop PRCA associated with FK506, which resolved when the drug was withdrawn [69].

Non-ABO-related Coombs-positive autoimmune hemolytic anemia (AIHA) can also develop late post-HCT as an autoimmune manifestation of chronic GVHD [70–72]. Drugs such as antibiotics and fludarabine, or infections with mycoplasma may also produce hemolysis. Impaired B-cell regulation may occur as a consequence of functional or quantitative T-cell depletion of the HCT product with a AIHA incidence of 3% in one large series.

Patients who develop AIHA after HCT usually receive the same battery of immunosuppressive agents as nontransplant patients: steroids, immunoglobulin and splenectomy as well as less conventional approaches such as plasma immunoabsorption, vincristine, rituximab or reinfusion of aliquots of donor T cells to exert immunoregulation on the autoreactive T cells.

Hemolysis associated with thrombotic microangiopathy

There is a wide variance in the reported incidences of non-Coombs-positive hemolytic anemia (4–79%) caused by thrombotic microangiopathy (TM) in the post-HCT setting. The vascular endothelium is repeatedly exposed to injury by radiation, chemotherapy and CSP/FK506 as well as infectious agents which may precipitate a cascade of events leading to aggregated platelet thrombi in small capillaries [73–82]. The majority of patients manifest TM by a slight rise in LDH and increase in fragmented RBCs in circulation, while a minority of HCT patients (4–33%) will show several of the symptoms associated with classic thrombotic thrombocytopenic purpura (TTP): thrombocytopenia, microangiopathic hemolysis, fluctuating neurologic abnormalities, fever and renal insufficiency. In the nontransplant setting, TM has been associated with:
1 bacterial infections from *Escherichia coli* strain 0157:H7 in epidemic hemolytic uremic syndrome (HUS);
2 human immunodeficiency virus (HIV) infection;
3 pregnancy; and
4 drugs such as ticlopidine, quinine, oral contraceptives, mitomycin and nitrosureas [83,84].

In the transplant setting, factors related to TM are multiple cycles of high-dose chemotherapy in the autologous setting and radiation-based conditioning, CMV infection and CSP or FK506 for GVHD prophylaxis in allogeneic HCT recipients. In a recent report, French investigators noted severe TM-related organ toxicity in three of 11 patients with relapsed high-risk lymphoma receiving at least three of five planned cycles of high-dose chemotherapy and sequential autologous HCT [85]. Two of three patients with TM had cardiac and pulmonary injury in addition to the usual organ toxicities seen in primary HUS/TTP. The incidence of TM is <5% in autologous HCT, compared with 10–20% in matched sibling donor HCT and up to 30% in unrelated donor allogeneic HCT using myeloablative conditioning. As yet, there is little information on the incidence of TM in reduced-dose conditioning regimens, but it is likely to be similar to the 3–8% incidence reported in solid organ transplants receiving CSP or FK506 as antirejection therapy.

The inciting endothelial injury may differ between primary TTP/HUS and TM in the transplant setting. In primary TTP, there appears to be a decrease in a plasma metalloprotease directed at cleaving unusually large von Willebrand's factor (uLvWF) multimers. The uLvWF multimers bind platelet glycoprotein Ib more efficiently than smaller multimers [86]. The initial binding of uLvWF to the platelet receptor leads to activation of adenosine diphosphate (ADP) dependent platelet aggregation through the glycoprotein IIb–IIIa complex [83,86,87]. The metalloprotease, referred to as ADAMTS-13 (a disintegrin and metalloprotease with thrombospondin-1-like domain) usually cleaves the uLvWF on the surface of the endothelial cell, allowing less thrombogenic smaller multimers into the plasma. In familial TTP, the plasma ADAMTS-13 activity is usually undetectable because of a genetic mutation of the protein [88]. In cases of sporadic, acquired or ticlopidine-related TTP autoantibodies have been detected that prevent binding of ADAMTS-13 to CD36 thrombospondin receptors on the surface of the endothelial cells (Fig. 60.1). In contrast, ADAMTS-13 levels are not usually reduced in patients with TTP/HUS associated with HCT or solid organ transplantation, suggesting that an alternative mechanism for microthrombus generation may be involved [89]. Therapeutic responses may differ based on whether the TM is associated with a deficiency or inhibition of ADAMTS-13 or not [90,91]. In HCT-related TM, endothelial damage caused by chemotherapy and radiation may trigger intravascular platelet aggregation by a mechanism not dependent on the metalloprotease cleavage of vWF multimers, but more analogous to TM associated with Shiga toxin in the *E. coli* infections. The toxin causes release of tumor necrosis factor and interleukins 1 and 6 leading to increased exposure of P selectin, β integrin receptors and platelet endothelial adhesion molecules on cell surfaces as well as causing direct platelet activation [92–96]. Cyclosporine also contributes to prothrombotic changes by release of endothelin, a vasoconstrictive peptide, which leads to high shear conditions in the renal microvasculature as well as increasing thromboxane A_2 and decreasing prostacycline and protein C production [97–100]. Cyclosporine also directly increases platelet aggregation in response to collagen and ADP.

Clinical presentation of TTP

The first descriptions of TTP-like syndrome in BMT recipients were reported in 1980 shortly after CSP was introduced as part of the armamentarium for GVHD prophylaxis [73–77]. High CSP levels in the plasma have been associated with hypertension, mild rise in creatinine and red cell fragmentation, which usually improve with dose reduction. The incidence of clinically significant TTP has been reported to be 0.5–1.0% after autologous HCT and 6–10% following allogeneic HCT in patients who received either CSP or tacrolimus for GVHD prophylaxis [101,102]. The hallmark of microangiopathic hemolysis is RBC fragmentation associated with increased red cell turnover without evidence for either an immunomediated hemolysis or disseminated intravascular

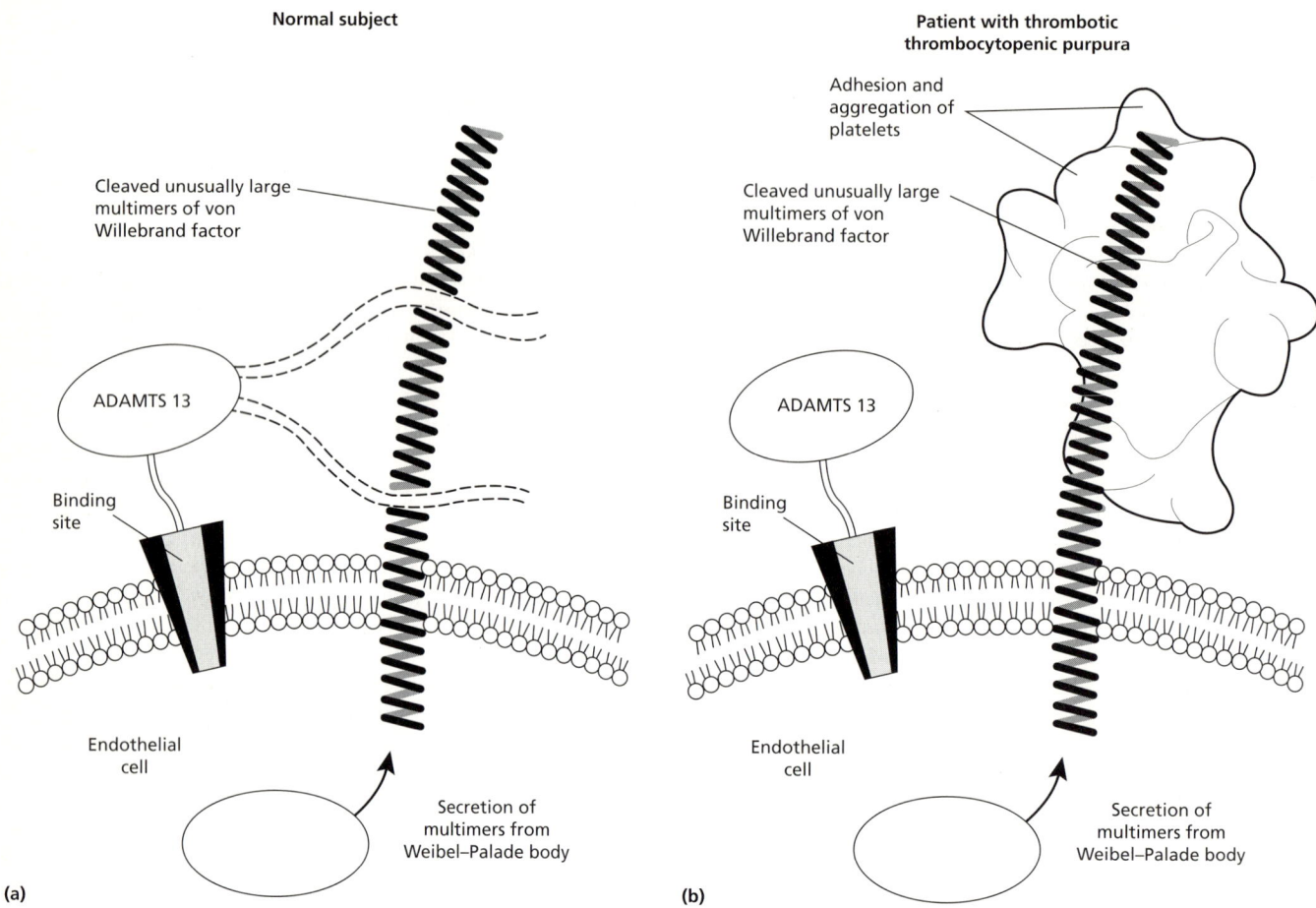

Fig. 60.1 Proposed relation among the absence of ADAMTS-13 activity *in vivo*, excessive adhesion and aggregation of platelets, and thrombotic thrombocytopenia purpura. (a) In normal subjects, ADAMTS-13 (von Willebrand factor-cleaving metalloprotease) molecules attach to binding sites on endothelial cell surfaces and cleave unusually large multimers of von Willebrand's factor as they are secreted by stimulated endothelial cells. The smaller von Willebrand's factor forms that circulate after cleavage do not induce the adhesion and aggregation of platelets during normal blood flow. ADAMTS-13 may use one of its thrombospondin-1-like domains to attach to the surface of endothelial cells. (b) Absent or severely reduced activity of ADAMTS-13 in patients with thrombotic thrombocytopenic purpura prevents timely cleavage of unusually large multimers of von Willebrand's factor as they are secreted by endothelial cells. The uncleaved multimers induce the adhesion and aggregation of platelets in flowing blood. A congenital deficiency of ADAMTS-13 activity, or an acquired defect of ADAMTS-13 (such as that caused by autoantibodies or by a change in the production or survival of the protein) can lead to thrombotic thrombocytopenic purpura. Interference with the attachment of ADAMTS-13 to endothelial cells *in vivo* (e.g. as a result of ADAMTS-13 receptor blockade by other types of autoantibodies) may also cause thrombotic thrombocytopenic purpura in patients with normal ADAMTS-13 activity in plasma.

coagulation (DIC). The clinical manifestations of the vascular injury run the gamut from mild hemolysis to severe anemia, thrombocytopenia, fever, hematuria, altered mental status and renal failure that requires dialysis. The HUS form without neurological signs is seen more commonly in autologous and pediatric allogeneic HCT recipients with clinical similarities to the acute verotoxin (*E. coli* 0157:H7) induced HUS.

While the full constellation of severe TTP-like microangiopathy is relatively uncommon, more subtle evidence of microangiopathic hemolysis (MAHA) is fairly prevalent. Valilis *et al.* [103] prospectively evaluated 82 HCT recipients for evidence of RBC fragmentation, increased LDH and thrombomodulin as markers of endothelial cell injury. Increased RBC fragmentation was seen in 46% of autologous and in 98% of allogeneic graft recipients; >50% of allogeneic recipients had clinically significant mechanical hemolysis (3–7%). The degree of hemolysis was stable or decreased during the 2-month period of observation in the autologous HCT recipients; in the allogeneic recipients all three markers showed progressive rises over the same time span.

In the more overt TTP/HUS-like syndromes, the degree of RBC fragmentation is more severe, with 5–10% of RBC altered; early nucleated erythrocytes may emerge in the circulation. Platelet consumption is more marked but DIC screens show no evidence of increased fibrinogen or factor VIII utilization. Elevated plasma levels of vWF are described but are not pathognomonic for TTP/HUS. Collins *et al.* [81] followed vWF levels serially in both allogeneic and autologous HCT recipients and showed that even in asymptomatic patients vWF levels increased over time and were more markedly elevated in recipients of allogeneic grafts. The highest levels of vWF in patients with microangiopathy were seen 3–4 months after transplantations, the peak time of onset of clinical TTP. The diagnosis of TTP/HUS rests mainly on clinical manifestation of end-organ dysfunction in the setting of "mechanical" hemolytic anemia and thrombocytopenia rather than laboratory findings of abnormal multimers patterns or deficient metalloprotease activity. Several investigators have reported normal plasma activity of the vWF cleaving protease (ADAMTS-13) and variable to normal amounts of vWF multimers [88,89,91]. The predilection for involvement of the vascular beds of kidney and brain rather than other organs such as liver, lung or gastrointestinal tract in both idiopathic and post-transplant TTP/HUS remains unexplained [104]. Schriber and Herzig [105] analyzed the natural

history of untreated TTP/HUS in 124 BMT recipients (82 allogeneic, 42 autologous) reported in the literature up to May 1996, who had been followed for a minimum of 3 months after diagnosis. Sixty-two patients (50%) died within 3 months of diagnosis; mortality was 64% in allogeneic and 21% in autologous HCT recipients. Factors associated with an increased risk of mortality were:
1 onset of TTP/HUS within 120 days of BMT;
2 use of CSP or FK506; and
3 neurologic symptoms.

Mortality was 12% in patients who lacked any of these features, 26% in those with a solitary risk factor and 85% for patients with two or more risk features [105]. Many of the surviving patients still had significant morbidity, usually persistent renal dysfunction, with approximately one-third of survivors requiring dialysis. It is clear that, while the initial endothelial cell injury caused by total body irradiation (TBI) and high-dose chemotherapy may be similar in autologous and allogeneic HCT, factors such as CSP use, acute GVHD with its associated "cytokine storm" and infections, particularly with viruses such as CMV, will perpetuate the injury, creating a much more fertile setting for microthrombotic damage.

Differential diagnosis

There are two forms of CSP toxicity, which can either be considered as prodromes of more severe microangiopathy or mistaken for TTP/HUS.

Isolated microangiopathy

Evidence of RBC fragmentation (1–2% of cells) is seen in most patients who receive CSP or FK506 post-transplant [106]. In patients with toxic serum levels (usually >1500 µg/L for CSP) of these drugs, fragmentation may increase to 3–4% of erythrocytes accompanied by an increase of unconjugated bilirubin and reticulocytosis. Hemolysis and renal abnormalities resolve with reduction of CSP levels to the therapeutic range. Azuma et al. [107] reported improvement in a case of severe post-transplant hemolysis with administration of vitamin E.

A second clinical scenario that occurs within the first 6 months after allogeneic BMT, which can often be confused with thrombotic thrombocytopenic purpura, is CSP-related central nervous system (CNS) dysfunction (see Chapter 59). Patients may present with seizures, altered levels of consciousness including coma, apraxia/ataxia, or cortical blindness [108]. These symptoms are often associated with poorly controlled hypertension and renal dysfunction manifested primarily as renal tubular acidosis and magnesium wasting. White matter abnormalities in the occipitoparietal cortex are seen on magnetic resonance imaging, analogous to eclampsia, in which vasomotor spasms lead to multifocal areas of ischemia and edema [109,110]. The syndrome is thought to be caused by increased release of endothelin, a vasoactive peptide, which can cause cerebral vasospasm. In most instances, the symptoms will resolve within 48–72 h after CSP is withdrawn; radiographic changes require up to 2 weeks for clearing. Therapy requires at least temporary discontinuation of CSP and substitution of an alternate drug for GVHD prophylaxis, control of hypertension, correction of hypomagnesemia and institution of antiepileptic prophylaxis. In patients who have had seizures as the only manifestation of neurological dysfunction, CSP can usually be resumed at a lower dose without recurrent seizure activity or other CNS symptoms. In patients with symptoms such as cortical blindness, speech disturbance or coma, resumption of CSP can lead to recurrence of symptoms; in some instances FK506 can be substituted without problems. Cortical blindness and apraxia/ataxia seem to be more associated with reversible CSP toxicity; behavior disorders, seizures and altered levels of consciousness are common presentations in both CSP toxicity and TTP.

Therapy

In 1991, Rock et al. [111] published results of a Canadian trial that compared plasma infusion to plasma exchange in 102 patients with spontaneous TTP. Treatment was given for 7 of 9 days. After the initial treatment course, 24 of 51 patients who underwent plasma exchange improved, whereas only 13 of 51 plasma infusion patients showed improvement in hematological parameters ($p = 0.25$). Patients in whom plasma infusion failed subsequently received exchange transfusion as well. A 6-month follow-up showed an overall mortality of 28% for the 102 patients. Based on our current understanding that autoantibodies directed at the ADAMTS-13 metalloprotease can be implicated in a high proportion of sporadic idopathic TTP and that a deficiency of a functional metalloprotease exists in familial relapsing TTP, the rationale for plasma exchange to remove the antibodies and replacing it with normal plasma containing a functional enzyme is clear [112]. Usually, the initial event producing the endothelial injury is self-limiting in nontransplant-related TTP and sustained immunosuppression is not often necessary after the autoantibodies have been depleted by 2–3 weeks of exchange and infusion. In 1992, Snyder et al. [113] reported on the treatment of chemotherapy-associated TTP using pheresis in conjunction with a staphylococcal protein A immunoabsorption column; clinical improvement in anemia and thrombocytopenia was seen in 25 of 55 patients (45%) treated. Renal function stabilized but dialysis requirements did not improve from pretreatment levels. More than half of the nonresponding patients died of TTP/HUS-related disease at a median of 17 days. In the post-transplant setting, only a few small series have been published reporting results of therapeutic interventions. Trials of gammaglobulin infusions alone or followed by splenectomy have been employed in the nontransplant TTP setting. Competing medical problems make this approach hazardous in the immediate peritransplant period. Tarantolo et al. [82] described rod-like inclusions in erythrocytes caused by a Bartonella-like organism in 13 patients with clinical post-BMT microangiopathy. Hemolysis reversed with treatment with doxycycline in nine patients. In nine patients with severe TTP/HUS treated with plasma exchange, Sarode et al. [114] attained a hematological response in three patients; two remain alive with chronic renal insufficiency 3 years after HCT. Responses were seen in two of three patients who received cryo-poor plasma and only one of six patients receiving FFP [114]. Roy et al. [115] reported on 17 of 125 allogeneic patients treated for TM within 100 days post-HCT. All had severe thrombocytopenia and MAHA, renal insufficiency was present in 82% and neurolgic abnormality existed in 61%. Only three of 17 patients responded to plasma exchange. Of the remaining patients, two patients failed to respond after 30 exchanges, and eight died within 21 days of starting plasma exchange. Zeigler et al. [116] combined plasma exchange with protein A immunoabsorption in 12 allogeneic HCT recipients who exhibited severe MAHA early (median day 37) after HCT associated with neurological abnormalities in 10 patients. Seven patients had improvement in hemolysis with a 2-week course of cryo-poor pheresis alternating with protein A immunoabsorption. All five nonresponders died of multiorgan failure within 4 weeks. Silva et al. [117] treated eight patients with plasma exchange and vincristine. Four of these individuals showed hematological improvement; unfortunately three of the four succumbed to progressive GVHD and fungal infections within 3 weeks of therapy. The much lower response rate to plasma exchange of TM in the post-transplant setting compared with the spontaneous variety is more understandable when we see that the laboratory markers for active TTP are different in post-HCT TM compared with spontaneous TTP/HUS, suggesting that the mechanism for the pathogenesis of the disease is different [118–120]. In addition, factors such as active GVHD, CMV infection and CSP use perpetuate endothelial injury; many patients die of comorbid conditions even if they show improvement in TM-related hematologic parameters with plasma exchange.

Conclusions

Hemolysis following HCT can arise from either immunomediated or vascular "mechanical" causes. Immunomediated destruction is seen predominantly in the allogeneic setting because discordance of RBC antigens between donor and recipient is a powerful trigger for hemolysis. The potential for acute hemolysis can be identified in the pretransplant setting based on ABO and Rh antigen testing. Prophylactic measures to decrease either the quantity of antigen or antibody can be accomplished either by manipulation of the HCT product or by red cell or plasma exchange, or both. These measures are effective in preventing significant hemolysis in 80–85% of ABO or Rh incompatible transplants.

Hemolysis as a consequence of TM can be seen in both autologous and allogeneic HCTs because the inciting agents (high-dose chemotherapy and/or radiation) that are thought to initiate the endothelial injury are common to both. The incidence of TTP/HUS is higher and onset is usually earlier in allogeneic recipients, presumably because of ongoing endothelial perturbation by CSP and cytokine release associated with GVHD. At the present time, there are no clinically available screening tests to identify patients at risk of TM.

Hemolysis should be considered as a cause of relatively acute anemia, renal insufficiency, and hyperbilirubinemia along with more common entities, such as GVHD, veno-occlusive disease and CSP toxicity. When hemolysis because of ABO or Rh incompatibility is identified, removal of the offending antibody via plasma exchange should be initiated promptly along with supportive care measures to improve renal function. Adequacy of removal can be monitored by following titers of the isohemagglutinins. In the rare instances of persistent high titers with either active hemolysis or RBC aplasia, more aggressive immunosuppressive measures may be warranted. In the case of microangiopathic hemolysis, plasma exchange alone or in combination with immunoabsorption may be helpful in restoring functional metalloprotease activity in 30–40% of allogeneic and 60–70% of autologous recipients although many of the patients with HUS may continue to show evidence of renal dysfunction.

References

1 Buckner CD, Clift RA, Sanders JE, Gray W, Storb R, Thomas ED. ABO incompatible marrow transplants. *Transplantation* 1978; **26**: 233–8.
2 Lasky LC, Warkentin PI, Kersey JH, Ramsay NKC, McGlave PB, McCullough J. Hematology in patients undergoing blood group incompatible bone marrow transplantation. *Transfusion* 1983; **23**: 277–85.
3 Rowley SD, Liang PS, Ulz L. Transplantation of ABO-incompatible bone marrow and peripheral blood stem cell components. *Bone Marrow Transplant* 2000; **26**: 749–57.
4 Salmon JP, Michaux S, Hermanne JP et al. Delayed massive immune hemolysis mediated by minor ABO incompatibility after allogeneic peripheral blood progenitor cell transplantation. *Transfusion* 1999; **39**: 824–7.
5 Sniecinski JK, Petz LD, Oien L, Blume KG. Immunohematologic problems arising from ABO incompatible bone marrow transplantation. *Transplant Proc* 1987; **19**: 4609–11.
6 Warkentin PI, Yomtovian R, Hurd D et al. Severe delayed hemolytic transfusion reaction complicating an ABO-incompatible bone marrow transplantation. *Vox Sang* 1983; **45**: 40–7.
7 Blacklock HA, Katz F, Michalevicz R et al. A and B blood group antigen expression on mixed colony cells and erythroid precursors: relevance for human allogeneic bone marrow transplantation. *Br J Haematol* 1984; **58**: 267–76.
8 Sniecinski IJ, Oien L, Petz LD, Blume KG. Immunohematologic consequences of major ABO-mismatched bone marrow transplantation. *Transplantation* 1988; **45**: 530–4.
9 Benjamin RJ, Connors JM, McGurk S, Churchill WH, Antin JH. Prolonged erythroid aplasia after major ABO-mismatched transplantation for chronic myelogenous leukemia. *Biol Blood Marrow Transplant* 1998; **4**: 151–6.
10 Hows J, Chipping PM, Palmer S, Gordon-Smith EC. Regeneration of peripheral blood cells following ABO incompatible allogeneic bone marrow transplantation for severe aplastic anemia. *Br J Haematol* 1983; **53**: 145–51.
11 Lee JH, Lee KH, Kim S et al. Anti-A isoagglutinin as a risk factor for the development of pure red cell aplasia after major ABO-incompatible allogeneic bone marrow transplantation. *Bone Marrow Transplant* 2000; **25**: 179–84.
12 Marmont AM, Frassoni F, van Lint MT et al. Isohemagglutinin induced pure red cell aplasia following ABO incompatible marrow transplant for severe aplastic anemia: resolution after plasma exchange. *Exp Hematol* 1983; **11** (Suppl. 11): 51.
13 Barge AJ, Johnson G, Witherspoon R, Torok-Storb B. Antibody-mediated marrow failure after allogeneic bone marrow transplantation. *Blood* 1989; **74**: 1477–80.
14 Hows J, Beddow K, Gordon-Smith E et al. Donor derived RBC antibodies and immune hemolysis after allogeneic BMT. *Blood* 1986; **67**: 177–81.
15 Worel N, Greinix HT, Schneider B et al. Regeneration of erythropoiesis after related and unrelated donor BMT or peripheral blood HPC transplantation: a major ABO mismatch means problems. *Transfusion* 2000; **40**: 543–50.
16 Slavin S, Nagler A, Naparstek E et al. Non-myeloablative stem cell transplantation and cell therapy as an alternative to conventional bone marrow transplantation with lethal cytoreduction for treatment of malignant and nonmalignant hematologic diseases. *Blood* 1998; **91**: 756–63.
17 McSweeney P, Niederwieser D, Shiauru J et al. Hematopoietic cell transplantation in older patients with hematologic malignancies: replacing high-dose cytoxic therapy with graft-versus-tumor effects. *Blood* 2001; **97**: 3390–400.
18 Giralt S, Estey E, Albitar M et al. Engraftment of allogeneic hematopoietic progenitor cells with purine analog-containing chemotherapy: harnessing graft-versus-leukemia without myeloablative therapy. *Blood* 1997; **89**: 4531–6.
19 Bolan C, Leitman S, Griffith L et al. Delayed donor red cell chimerism and pure red cell aplasia following major ABO-incompatible nonmyeloablative hematopoietic stem cell transplantation *Blood* 2001; **98**: 1687–94.
20 Badros A, Tricot G, Toor A et al. ABO mismatch may affect engraftment in multiple myeloma patients receiving nonmyeloablative conditioning. *Transfusion* 2002; **42**: 205–9.
21 Peggs K, Morris E, Kottaridis P et al. Outcome of major ABO-incompatible nonmyeloablative hematopoietic stem cell transplantation may be influenced by conditioning regimen. *Blood* 2002; **99**: 4642–3.
22 Dinsmore RE, Reich LM, Kapoor N et al. ABO incompatible bone marrow transplantation: removal of erythrocytes by starch sedimentation. *Br J Haematol* 1983; **54**: 441–9.
23 Ho WG, Champlin RE, Feig SA, Gale RE. Transplantation of ABO incompatible bone marrow: gravity sedimentation of donor marrow. *Br J Haematol* 1984; **57**: 155–62.
24 Brame HG, Sensenbrener LL, Wright SK, Tutschka PJ, Saral R, Santos GW. Bone marrow transplantation with major ABO blood group incompatibility using erythrocyte depletion of marrow prior to infusion. *Blood* 1982; **60**: 420–5.
25 Blacklock HA, Prentice HG, Evans JPM et al. ABO-incompatible bone marrow transplantation: removal of red blood cells from donor marrow avoiding recipient antibody depletion. *Lancet* 1982; **2**: 1061–4.
26 Jin NR, Hill R, Segal G et al. Preparation of red-blood-cell-depleted marrow for ABO-incompatible marrow transplantation by density-gradient separation using the IBM 2991 blood cell processor. *Exp Hematol* 1987; **15**: 93–8.
27 Tsang KS, Li CK, Wong AP et al. Processing of major ABO-incompatible bone marrow for transplantation by using dextran sedimentation. *Transfusion* 1999; **39**: 1212–9.
28 Warkentin PI, Hilden JM, Kersey JH, Ramsay NKC, McCullough J. Transplantation of major ABO-incompatible bone marrow depleted of red cells by hydroxyethyl starch. *Vox Sang* 1985; **48**: 89–104.
29 English D, Lamberson R, Graves V et al. Semi-automated processing of bone marrow grafts for transplantation. *Transfusion* 1989; **29**: 12–16.
30 Smith JW, Halpern LN, Johnson KA et al. Mononuclear cell purification by continuous density gradient separation in the haemonetics V-50. *Bone Marrow Transplant* 1987; **2**: 74–9.
31 Areman EM, Cullis H, Spitzer T, Sacher RA. Automated processing of human bone marrow can result in a population of mononuclear cells capable of achieving engraftment following transplantation. *Transfusion* 1991; **31**: 724–30.
32 Dragani A, Angelini A, Iacone A, D'Antonio D, Torlontano G. Comparison of five methods for concentrating progenitor cells in human marrow transplantation. *Blut* 1990; **60**: 278–81.
33 Wriest DL, Reich LM. Removal of ABO-incompatible red cells from lymphocytapheresis and granulocytapheresis components before transfusion. *Transfusion* 1997; **37**: 144–9.

34 Larsson LG, Welsh VJ, Ladd DJ. Acute intravascular hemolysis secondary to out-of-group platelet transfusion. *Transfusion* 2000; **40**: 902–6.

35 Leo A, Mytilineos J, Voso MT et al. Passenger lymphocyte syndrome with severe hemolytic anemia due to an anti-Jk[a] after allogeneic PBPC transplantation. *Transfusion*; 2000; **40**: 632–6.

36 Franchini M, de Gironcoli M, Gandini G et al. Transmission of an anti-RhD alloantibody from donor to recipient after ABO-incompatible BMT. *Bone Marrow Transplant* 1998; **21**: 1071–3.

37 Young PP, Goodnough LT, Westervelt P, DiPersio JF. Immune hemolysis involving non-ABO/RhD alloantibodies following hematopoietic stem cell transplantation. *Bone Marrow Transplant* 2001; **27**: 1305–10.

38 de la Rubia J, Arriaga F, Andreu R et al. Development of non-ABO RBC alloantibodies in patients undergoing allogeneic HPC transplantation: is ABO incompatibility a predisposing factor? *Transfusion* 2001; **4**: 106–10.

39 Bornhauser M, Ordemann R, Paaz U et al. Rapid engraftment after allogeneic ABO-incompatible peripheral blood progenitor cell transplantation complicated by severe hemolysis. *Bone Marrow Transplant* 1997; **19**: 295–7.

40 Moog R, Melder C, Prumbaum M, Muller N, Schaefer UW. Rapid donor type isoagglutinin production after allogeneic peripheral progenitor cell transplantation. *Beitr Infusionsther Transfusionsmed* 1997; **34**: 150–2.

41 Gajewski J, Petz LD, Calhoun L et al. Hemolysis of transfused group O red blood cells in minor ABO-incompatible unrelated-donor bone marrow transplants in patients receiving cyclosporine without post-transplant methotrexate. *Blood* 1992; **79**: 3076–85.

42 Rosental GJ, Weigand GW, Germolec DR et al. Suppression of 13 cell functions by methotrexate and trimetrexate-evidence for inhibition of purine biosynthesis as a major mechanism of action. *J Immunol* 1988; **141**: 410–6.

43 Mielcarek M, Leisenring W, Torok-Storb B, Storb R. Graft-versus-host disease and donor-directed hemagglutinin titers after ABO-mismatched related and unrelated marrow allografts: evidence for a graft-versus-plasma cell effect. *Blood*; 2000; **96**: 1150–6.

44 Lapierre V, Kuentz M, Tiberghien P. Allogeneic peripheral blood hematopoietic stem cell transplantation: guidelines for red blood cell immunohematological assessment and transfusion practice. Societe Francaise Greffe Moelle. *Bone Marrow Transplant*: 2000; **25**: 507–12.

45 Bensinger WI, Deeg JH. Transfusion support and donor considerations in marrow transplantation. In: Sacher RA, Aubuchon JP, eds. *Marrow Transplantation: Practical and Technical Aspects of Stem Cell Reconstitution*. Bethesda, MD: American Association of Blood Banks, 1992: 157–79.

46 Bensinger WI, Baker DA, Buckner CD, Clift RA, Thomas ED. Immunoadsorption for removal of A and B blood-group antibodies. *N Engl J Med* 1981; **304**: 160–2.

47 Osterwalder B, Gratwohl A, Nissen C, Speck B. Immunoadsorption for removal of anti-A and anti-B blood group antibodies in ABO-incompatible bone marrow transplantation. *Blut* 1986; **53**: 379–90.

48 Tichelli A, Gratwohl A, Wenger R et al. ABO incompatible bone marrow transplantation: *in vivo* adsorption, an old forgotten method. *Transplant Proc* 1987; **19**: 4632–7.

49 Webb IJ, Soiffer RJ, Anderson JW et al. In vivo adsorption of isohemagglutinins with fresh frozen plasma in major ABO-incompatible bone marrow transplantation. *Biol Blood Marrow Transplant* 1997; **3**: 267–72.

50 Nussbaumer W, Schwaighofer H, Gratwohl A et al. Transfusion of donor-type red cells as a single preparative treatment for bone marrow transplants with major ABO incompatibility. *Transfusion* 1995; **35**: 592–5.

51 Benjamin RJ, McGurk S, Ralston MS et al. ABO incompatibility as an adverse risk factor for survival after allogeneic bone marrow transplantation. *Transfusion* 1999; **39**: 179–87.

52 Klumpp TR, Block CC, Caligiuri MA et al. Immune-mediated cytopenia following bone marrow transplantation: case reports and review of the literature. *Medicine* 1992; **71**: 73.

53 Labar B, Bogdanic V, Nemet D et al. Antilymphocyte globulin for treatment of pure red cell aplasia after major ABO incompatible marrow transplant. *Bone Marrow Transplant* 1992; **10**: 471–2.

54 Paltiel O, Cournoyer D, Rybka W. Pure red cell aplasia following ABO-incompatible bone marrow transplantation: response to erythropoietin. *Transfusion* 1993; **33**: 418–21.

55 Ohashi K, Akiyama H, Takamoto S, Tanikawa S, Sakamaki H, Onozawa Y. Treatment of pure red cell aplasia after major ABO-incompatible bone marrow transplantation resistant to erythropoietin. *Bone Marrow Transplant* 1994; **13**: 335–6.

56 Reviron J, Schenmetzler C, Bussel A, Frappaz D, Devergie A, Gluckman E. Obstacle to red cell engraftment due to major ABO incompatibility in allogeneic bone marrow transplants (BMT): quantitative and kinetic aspects in 58 BMTs. *Transplant Proc* 1987; **19**: 4618–22.

57 Bierman PJ, Warkentin P, Hutchins M, Klassen L. Pure red cell aplasia following ABO mismatched marrow transplantation for chronic lymphocytic leukemia: response to antithymocyte globulin. *Leuk Lymphoma* 1990; **9**: 169–71.

58 Volin L, Ruutu T. Pure red-cell aplasia of long duration after major ABO-incompatible bone marrow transplantation. *Acta Haematol* 1990; **84**: 195–7.

59 Or R, Naparsick E, Mani N, Slavin S. Treatment of pure red cell aplasia following major ABO-mismatched T cell-depleted bone marrow transplant. *Transpl Int* 1991; **4**: 99–102.

60 Taniguchi S, Yamasaki K, Shibuya T, Asayama R, Harada M, Niho Y. Recombinant human erythropoietin for long-term persistent anemia after major ABO incompatible bone marrow transplantation. *Bone Marrow Transplant* 1993; **12**: 423.

61 Bar B, Van Dijk BA, Schattenberg A et al. Erythrocyte repopulation after major ABO incompatible transplantation with lymphocyte-depleted bone marrow. *Bone Marrow Transplant* 1995; **16**: 793–9.

62 Fujisawa S, Maruta A, Sakai R et al. Pure red cell aplasia after major ABO incompatible bone marrow transplantation: two case reports of treatment with recombinant human erythropoietin. *Transpl Int* 1996; **9**: 506–8.

63 Santamaria A, Sureda A, Martino R, Domingo-Albos A, Muniz-Diaz E, Brunet S. Successful treatment of pure red cell aplasia after major ABO-incompatible T cell-depleted bone marrow transplantation with erythropoietin. *Bone Marrow Transplant* 1997; **20**: 1105–7.

64 Bavaro P, Di Girolamo G, Olioso P et al. Donor lymphocyte infusion as therapy for pure red cell aplasia following bone marrow transplantation. *B J Haematol* 1999; **104**: 930–1.

65 Roychowdhury DF, Linker CA. Pure red cell aplasia complicating an ABO-compatible allogeneic bone marrow transplantation, treated successfully with antithymocyte globulin. *Bone Marrow Transplant* 1995; **16**: 471–2.

66 Selleri C, Raiola A, De Rosa G et al. CD34[+]-enriched donor lymphocyte infusions in a case of pure red cell aplasia and late graft failure after major ABO-incompatible bone marrow transplantation. *Bone Marrow Transplant* 1998; **22**: 605–7.

67 So B, Chae KM, Lee KK, Lee YJ, Jeong BH. Pure red cell aplasia due to parvovirus B19 infection in a renal transplant patient: a case report. *Transplant Proc* 2000; **32**: 1954–6.

68 Geetha D, Zachary B, Baldardo H, Kronz J, Kraus E. Pure red cell aplasia caused by parvovirus B19 infection in solid organ transplant recipients: a case report and review of literature. *Clin Transplant* 2000; **14**: 586–91.

69 Misra S, Moore T, Ament M, Busuttil R, McDiarmid S. Red cell aplasia in children on tacrolimus after liver transplantation. *Transplantation* 1998; **65**: 575–7.

70 Anasetti C, Rybka W, Sullivan KM et al. Graft-versus-host disease is associated with autoimmune-like thrombocytopenia. *Blood* 1989; **73**: 1054–8.

71 Drobyski WR, Potluri J, Sauer D, Gottschall JL. Autoimmune hemolytic anemia following T cell-depleted allogeneic bone marrow transplantation. *Bone Marrow Transplant* 1996; **17**: 1093–9.

72 Keung YK, Cobos E, Bolanos-Meade J, Issarachai S, Brideau A, Morgan D. Evans syndrome after autologous bone marrow transplant for recurrent Hodgkin's disease. *Bone Marrow Transplant* 1997; **20**: 1099–101.

73 Chappell ME, Keeling DM, Prentice HG, Sweny P. Haemolytic uraemic syndrome after bone marrow transplantation: an adverse effect of total body irradiation? *Bone Marrow Transplant* 1988; **3**: 339–47.

74 Guinan EC, Tarbell NJ, Niemeyer CM et al. Intravascular hemolysis and renal insufficiency after bone marrow transplantation. *Blood* 1988; **72**: 451–5.

75 Rabinowe SN, Soiffer RJ, Tarbell NJ et al. Hemolytic–uremic syndrome following bone marrow transplantation in adults for hematologic malignancies. *Blood* 1991; **77**: 1837–44.

76 Juckett M, Perry EH, Daniels BS, Weisdorf DJ. Hemolytic uremic syndrome following bone marrow transplantation. *Bone Marrow Transplant* 1991; **7**: 405–9. 84

77 Spruce WE, Forman SJ, Blume KG et al. Hemolytic uremic syndrome after bone marrow transplantation. *Acta Haematol* 1982; **67**: 206–10.

78 Pettitt AR, Clark RE. Thrombotic microangiopathy following bone marrow transplantation. *Bone Marrow Transplant* 1994; **14**: 495–504.

79 van der Lelie H, Baars JW, Rodenhuis S et al. Hemolytic uremic syndrome after high dose chemotherapy with autologous stem cell support. *Cancer* 1995; **76**: 2338–42.

80 Holler E, Kolb HJ, Hiller F et al. Microangiopathy in patients on cyclosporine prophylaxis who developed acute graft-versus-host disease after HLA-identical bone marrow transplantation. *Blood* 1989; **73**: 2018–24.

81 Collins PW, Gutteridge A, O'Driscoll A et al. Van Willebrand factor a marker endothelial cell activation following BMT. *Bone Marrow Transplant* 1992; **12**: 499–506.

82 Tarantolo SR, Landmark JD, Hinrichs SH et al. *Bartonella*-like erythrocyte inclusions associated with post-transplant thrombotic microangiopathy: improved survival with doxycycline. *Blood* 1997; **90**: 252a [Abstract].

83 Moake J. Thrombotic microangiopathies. *N Engl J Med* 2002; **34**: 589–600.

84 Kwaan HC, Ganguly P. Thrombotic thrombocytopenic purpura and the hemolytic uremic syndrome. *Semin Hematol* 1997; **34**: 81–148.

85 Vantelon JM, Munck JN, Bourhis JH et al. Thrombotic microangiopathy: a new dose-limiting toxicity of high-dose sequential chemotherapy. *Bone Marrow Transplant* 2001; **27**: 531–6.

86 Tsai H, Lian E. Antibodies to von Willebrand factor-cleaving protease in acute thrombotic thrombocytopenic purpura. *N Engl J Med* 1998; **339**: 1585–94.

87 Furlan M, Robles R, Galbusera M et al. von Willebrand factor-cleaving protease in thrombotic thrombocytopenic purpura and the hemolytic-uremic syndrome. *N Engl J Med* 1998; **339**: 1578–84.

88 Van der Plas RM, Schiphorst M, Huizinga E et al. Von Willebrand factor proteolysis is deficient in classic, but not in bone marrow transplantation-associated, thrombotic thrombocytopenic purpura. *Blood* 1999; **93**: 3798–802.

89 Arai S, Allan C, Streiff M, Hutchins GM, Vogelsang GB, Tsai HM. Von Willegrand factor-cleaving protease activity and proteolysis of von Willbrand factor in bone marrow transplant-associated thrombotic microangiopathy. *Hematol J* 2001; **2**: 292–9.

90 Veyradier A, Obert B, Houllier A, Meyer D, Girma JP. Specific von Willebrand factor-cleaving protease in thrombotic microangiopathies: a study of 111 cases. *Blood* 2001; **98**: 1765–72.

91 Mori Y, Wada H, Cabazza E et al. Predicting response to plasma exchange in patients with thrombotic thrombocytopenic purpura with measurement of vWF-cleaving protease activity. *Transfusion* 2002; **42**: 572–80.

92 Chong BH, Murray B, Berndt MC et al. Plasma P-selectin is increased in thrombotic consumptive platelet disorders. *Blood* 1994; **83**: 1535–41.

93 Wada H, Kaneko T, Ohiwa M et al. Plasma cytokine levels in thrombotic thrombocytopenic purpura. *Am J Hematol* 1992; **40**: 167–70.

94 Asada Y, Sumiyoshi A, Hayashi T et al. Immunohistochemistry of vascular lesions in thrombotic thrombocytopenic purpura, with special reference to factor VIII related antigen. *Thromb Res* 1985; **38**: 469–79.

95 Tandon N, Rock G, Jamieson GA. Anti-CD36 antibodies in thrombotic thrombocytopenic purpura. *Br J Haematol* 1994; **88**: 816–25.

96 Moake JL. Studies in the pathophysiology of thrombotic thrombocytopenic purpura. *Semin Hematol* 1997; **34**: 83–9.

97 Haug C, Duell T, Lenich A, Kolb HJ, Grunert A. Elevated plasma endothelin concentrations in cyclosporine-treated patients after bone marrow transplantation. *Bone Marrow Transplant* 1995; **15**: 191–4.

98 Garcia-Maldonado M, Kaufman CE, Comp PC. Decrease in endothelial celldependent protein C activation induced by thrombomodulin by treatment with cyclosporine. *Transplantation* 1991; **51**: 701–5.

99 Zeigler ZR, Rosenfeld CS, Andrews DF et al. Plasma von Willebrand factor antigen (vWF:AG) and thrombomodulin (TM) levels in adult thrombotic thrombocytopenic purpura/hemolytic uremic syndromes (TTP/HUS) and bone marrow transplant-associated thrombotic microangiopathy (BMT-TM). *Am J Hematol* 1996; **53**: 213–20.

100 Cohen H, Bull HA, Seddon A et al. Vascular endothelial cell function and ultrastructure in thrombotic microangiopathy following allogeneic bone marrow transplantation. *Eur J Haematol* 1989; **43**: 207–14.

101 Lesesne JB, Rothschild N, Erickson B et al. Cancer associated hemolytic uremic syndrome: analysis of 85 cases from a national registry. *J Clin Oncol* 1989; **7**: 781–9.

102 Gharpure VS, Devine SM, Holland HK, Geller RB, O'Toole K, Wingard JR. Thrombotic thrombocytopenic purpura associated with FK506 following bone marrow transplantation. *Bone Marrow Transplant* 1995; **16**: 715–6.

103 Valilis PN, Zeigler ZR, Shadduck RK et al. A prospective study of bone marrow transplant-associated thrombotic microangiopathy (BMT-TM) in autologous (auto) and allogeneic (allo) BMT *Blood* 1995; **86**: 970a [Abstract].

104 Srivastava A, Gottlieb D, Bradstock KE. Diffuse alveolar hemorrhage associated with microangiopathy after allogeneic bone marrow transplantation. *Bone Marrow Transplant* 1995; **15**: 863–7.

105 Schriber JR, Herzig GP. Transplantation-associated thrombotic throbocytopenic purpura and hemolytic uremic syndrome. *Semin Hematol* 1997; **34** (2): 126–33.

106 Akiyama H, Yoshinaga H, Endou M et al. Microangiopathy without hemolysis in a patient following allogeneic bone marrow transplantation. *Bone Marrow Transplant* 1997; **20**: 261–3.

107 Azuma E, Hirayama M, Nakano T et al. Acute hemolysis during cyclosporine therapy successfully treated with vitamin E. *Bone Marrow Transplant* 1995; **16**: 321–2.

108 Reece DE, Frei-Lahr DA, Shepherd JD et al. Neurologic complications in allogeneic bone marrow transplant patients receiving cyclosporin. *Bone Marrow Transplant* 1991; **8**: 393–401.

109 Truwit CL, Denaro CP, Lake JR et al. MR imaging of reversible cyclosporin A-induced neurotoxicity. *Am J Neuroradiol* 1991; **12**: 651–9.

110 Zimmer W, Wang H, Schriber J. Cyclosporine A (CyA) neurotoxicity in allogeneic bone marrow transplantation for hematologic malignancy: magnetic resonance imaging (MRI) and clinical correlation. 34th Procedings of the American Society of Neuroradiologists. *Am J Neuroradiol* 1996; **19**: 73a [Abstract].

111 Rock GA, Shumak KH, Buskard NA et al. Comparison of plasma exchange with plasma infusion in the treatment of thrombotic thrombocytopenic purpura. *N Engl J Med* 1991; **325**: 393–403.

112 Rock GA. Management of thrombotic thrombocytopenic purpura. *Br J Haematol* 2000; **109**: 496–507.

113 Snyder HW, Mittelman A, Oral A et al. Treatment of cancer chemotherapy related thrombotic thrombocytopenic purpura/hemolytic uremic syndrome by protein A immunoadsorption of plasma. *Cancer* 1993; **71**: 1882–92.

114 Sarode R, McFarland JG, Flomenberg N et al. Therapeutic plasma exchange does not appear to be effective in the management of thrombotic thrombocytopenic purpura/hemolytic uremic syndrome following bone marrow transplantation. *Bone Marrow Transplant* 1995; **16**: 271–5.

115 Roy V, Rizvi MA, Vesely SK, George JN. Thrombotic thrombocytopenic purpura-like syndromes following bone marrow transplantation: an analysis of associated conditions and clinical outcomes. *Bone Marrow Transplant* 2001; **27**: 641–6.

116 Zeigler ZR, Shadduck RK, Nath R, Andrews DE. Pilot study of combined cryosupernatant and protein A immunoadsorption exchange in the treatment of grade 3–4 bone marrow transplant-associated thrombotic microangiopathy. *Bone Marrow Transplant* 1996; **17**: 81–6.

117 Silva VA, Frei-Lahr D, Brown RA, Herzig GP. Plasma exchange and vincristine in the treatment of hemolytic uremic syndrome/thrombotic thrombocytopenic purpura associated with bone marrow transplantation. *J Clin Apheresis* 1991; **6**: 16–20.

118 Dua A, Zeigler ZR, Shadduck RK, Nath R, Andrews DF, Agha M. Apheresis in grade 4 bone marrow transplant associated thrombotic microangiopathy: a case series. *J Clin Apheresis* 1996; **11**: 176–84.

119 Llamas P, Romero R, Cabrera R, Sanjuan I, Fores R, Fernandez MN. Management of thrombotic microangiopathy following allogeneic transplantation: what is the role of plasma exchange? *Bone Marrow Transplant* 1997; **20**: 305–6.

120 Milone J, Napal J, Bordone J, Etchegoyen O, Morales V. Complete response in severe thrombotic microangiopathy post bone marrow transplantation (BMT-TM) after multiple plasmapheresis. *Bone Marrow Transplant* 1998; **22**: 1019–21.

61

Jeffrey McCullough

Principles of Transfusion Support before and after Hematopoietic Cell Transplantation

Introduction

An effective blood bank and a transfusion-medicine program are essential for a successful hematopoietic cell transplantation (HCT) program [1]. Patients who are candidates for or are undergoing HCT have unique transfusion requirements. This special consideration is due to the need to minimize the likelihood of alloimmunization, the severe immunosuppression these patients undergo, their temporary inability to produce blood cells, the fact that their blood type may change and they may have temporary or permanent chimera. This chapter includes a brief description of the blood components and derivatives used by HCT patients and the relevant transfusion strategies.

Red blood cell components

Red cells

Red blood cells (RBCs) are the cells that remain after most of the plasma has been removed from whole blood. This blood component is often called "packed red cells" or "packed cells." A unit of red cells has a volume of about 350 mL and will contain about 200 mL red cells with an hematocrit of about 60%. The fluid portion of the unit is primarily the additive preservative solution, although about 20 mL plasma remains from the original unit of whole blood. One unit of red cells will increase the hemoglobin and hematocrit in an average-sized adult (70 kg) by about 1 g/dL or 3%, respectively.

Red cells are the component of choice for any patient with severe anemia. Most patients who require red cell replacement do not also need intravascular volume replacement because anemia has developed slowly. Thus, almost all transfusions given for red cell replacement are packed red cells and whole blood is rarely used.

Red cell transfusions are usually given to HCT patients because of anemia. Most patients with hemoglobins of ≥10 g/dL do not require transfusion, and most patients with a hemoglobin of <7 g/dL will benefit from transfusion [2–9]. Because of the heterogeneity of patients and these clinical situations, there is no single standard indication for red cell transfusion [10]. In deciding whether an individual requires reduced transfusion, the clinical condition of the patient is of primary importance, and patients should not be transfused based only on their hemoglobin level.

When there is sudden acute blood loss, the major threat to the patient is the loss of intravascular volume and resultant cardiovascular collapse. In most "normal" patients the loss of approximately 1000 mL blood can be replaced by colloid or crystalloid solutions alone. An otherwise healthy individual can tolerate the loss of up to half of the red cell mass without need for replacement [11]. Because many patients have some degree of cardiovascular compromise, they will require red cell replacement after smaller volumes of blood loss. If blood loss is judged sufficient to require transfusion, it is not necessary to wait until symptoms such as pallor, diaphoresis, tachycardia, or hypotension develop. Transfusion is with the standard RBC component from the stock supply of the blood bank.

Leukocyte-depleted red cells

Red cell and platelet blood components contain contaminating leukocytes that can alloimmunize transfusion recipients leading to multiple problems (Table 61.1). In order to avoid these problems, leukoreduced red cells have been used for years. Several methods have been employed in the past to prepare leukoreduced red cells, but currently filters are used to remove about 99.9% of the leukocytes leaving $<5 \times 10^6$/U. Filtration can be performed at the bedside, or, preferably, when the red cells are being prepared initially (prestorage leukoreduction), to obtain more consistency and prevent the accumulation of cytokines produced by the contaminating leukocytes.

Contaminating leukocytes also modulate the immune response. It has been known for years that patients who receive blood transfusions have improved renal graft survival. Transfusions may also cause increased postoperative infection and the recurrence of certain malignancies [12–15]. Although some controversy remains about these immunomodulatory effects, many blood centers, blood organizations and countries are implementing universal prestorage leukoreduction. The indications for leukodepleted red cells are:

Table 61.1 Adverse effects of leukocytes in blood components.

Immunologic effects
Alloimmunization:
    Febrile nonhemolytic transfusion (FNHT) reactions
    Refractoriness to platelet transfusion
    Rejection of transplanted organs
Graft-vs.-host disease (GVHD)
Transfusion-related acute lung injury
Immunomodulation
    Increased bacterial infections
    Increased recurrance of malignancy

Infectious disease
Cytomegalovirus
Human T-lymphotrophic virus HTLV-1
Epstein–Barr virus

Table 61.2 Clinical situations in which leukodepleted red cells are recommended.

Bone marrow or peripheral blood stem cell recipients
Acute leukemia
Chronic leukemia
Congenital platelet function abnormalities
Congenital immune deficiency syndrome
Hematologic malignancies potentially treated with stem cell transplantation
Solid tumors potentially treated with stem cell transplantation
Intrauterine transfusions
Exchange transfusion for hemolytic disease of the newborn
Hemoglobinopathy or thalassemia

1 Prevention of alloimmunization to leukocytes and platelets.
2 Prevention of transmission of cytomegalovirus (CMV).
3 Treatment of patients with multiple febrile transfusion reactions.
4 Prevention of immunomodulatory effects of transfusion.

The kinds of patients who should receive leukodepleted red cells include any individuals with a disease that can potentially be treated by HCT and those who will receive multiple transfusions during their life, such as patients with hemoglobinopathies (Table 61.2).

Washed red cells

Washed red cells are red cells suspended in an electrolyte solution. Most plasma, platelets and leukocytes have been removed, although leukocyte removal is not as complete as with frozen deglycerolized red cells. After washing, the red cells can be stored for only 24 h because of the possibility of bacterial contamination. Since the major advantage is the removal of the plasma by washing, washed red cells are indicated for patients who have severe reactions caused by plasma.

Coagulation factor components

Fresh frozen plasma

Fresh frozen plasma (FFP) is plasma separated from whole blood and placed at −18°C or lower within 8 h of collection. The unit of FFP has a volume of about 200–250 mL and contains all of the coagulation factors that are present in fresh blood. FFP is not considered to contain red cells and is usually administered without regard to rhesus (Rh) type. However, occasional rare reports have suggested that units of FFP contain a small amount of red cell stroma that can cause immunization to red cells [16]. Because the plasma contains ABO antibodies, the plasma must be compatible with the recipient's red cells.

The generally accepted indications for FFP [17] are documented coagulation factor deficiencies for which factor concentrates are not available, multiple factor deficiencies and massive transfusion in selected patients. FFP is used as the replacement solution for plasma exchange in patients with thrombotic thrombocytopenic purpura, but it is not indicated for use as a volume expander or a nutritional source [17].

Bleeding due to multiple coagulation factor deficiency can occur in massive transfusion due to dilution of coagulation factors. This occurs because red cell components contain little plasma. If coagulation factor replacement is necessary in these patients, FFP is usually used. Patients who are undergoing massive transfusion may also develop disseminated intravascular coagulopathy (DIC) because of the severity of the underlying problem. Thus, a bleeding diathesis may develop that is a combination of the dilutional coagulopathy of massive transfusion and the "consumption coagulopathy" of DIC.

Treatment of the underlying cause of the DIC is essential since without intervention transfusion of blood components merely adds more substrate for the coagulation process. In mild forms of DIC, transfusion is usually not necessary. However, in the more extreme forms, there is usually a deficiency of factors V and VIII, fibrinogen and platelets. Replacement of coagulation factors in the management of DIC should be based on laboratory abnormalities and not on arbitrary formulas. When replacement is necessary FFP is usually used to replace all factors.

Cryoprecipitate

Cryoprecipitate is the cold-insoluble portion of FFP that has been thawed between 1 and 6°C. It is stored at −18°C or below and can be kept for up to 1 year. Cryoprecipitate contains coagulation factor VIII, fibrinogen [18] and von Willebrand factor. Each bag of cryoprecipitate contains about 250 mg fibrinogen [18] and this is now its major use. Cryoprecipitate is not a suitable source of coagulation factors II, V, VII, IX, X, XI, or XII.

Blood group compatibility of components used to replace coagulation factors

FFP need not be ABO-identical but should be compatible with the recipient's red cells and can be given without regard to Rh type. Red cell compatibility testing is not necessary.

Cryoprecipitate should also be administered as ABO compatible. Although the volume of each unit is small, most therapy involves many units and, thus, the total volume of plasma may be large. Cryoprecipitate can be administered without regard to Rh type. While compatibility testing is not necessary, ABO-incompatible cryoprecipitate and commercial concentrated preparations of factor VIII contain anti-A and anti-B, which may cause a positive direct antiglobulin test [19] or a hemolytic anemia, or both, if massive doses are administered. In addition, the recipient's fibrinogen may become elevated by the fibrinogen contained in cryoprecipitate if many units are given to patients who are not hypofibrinogenemic.

Platelet components

Platelet concentrates prepared from whole blood

Platelet concentrates, often referred to as "random-donor" platelet concentrates, are prepared by centrifugation of whole blood [20,21]. At least 75% of the units of random-donor platelets must contain at least 5.5×10.0^{10} platelets. Although there is no required volume of the random-donor platelet concentrate, the volume is usually about 50 mL to maintain viability and function during the storage period, which is 5 days at 20–24°C. Platelets can also be produced by cytapheresis using blood cell separators.

Platelet concentrates prepared by apheresis

A major advance in the production of blood components and component therapy was the development and large-scale implementation of apheresis. Several different instruments are available for the collection of platelets by apheresis. All of these instruments use the centrifugation principle to separate blood components. The instrument operation is controlled by a microprocessor that regulates the blood flow rate, the anticoagulant added to the whole blood entering the system, the centrifuge conditions, the component separation and recombination of the remaining components, which are then returned to the donor.

The most common use of cytapheresis today is for the production of platelets by apheresis. The official name of this component is "platelets, pheresis" but it is usually called "single-donor platelet" or "plateletpheresis concentrate," which is a suspension of platelets in plasma prepared by cytapheresis. A unit or bag of plateletpheresis concentrate must contain at least 3×10^{11} platelets in a minimum of 75% of the units tested. Plateletpheresis usually requires about 1.5 h and involves processing 4000–5000 mL of the donor's blood through the instrument. Platelets obtained by plateletpheresis are processed, tested and labeled in a manner similar to that for whole blood. This includes ABO and Rh typing and testing for all required transfusion-transmitted diseases. The plateletpheresis concentrates can be stored for 5 days at 20–24°C. The number of platelets contained in each concentrate is determined, although this information may not necessarily be recorded on the label. Each platelet concentrate has a volume of approximately 200 mL and contains very few (<0.5 mL) red cells so that red cell cross-matching is not necessary. The white blood cell content varies depending upon the instrument and technique used for collection. Apheresis procedures involving leukocyte depletion are being implemented so that platelet concentrates produced by apheresis are leukocyte depleted and contain $<5 \times 10^6$ leukocytes per unit.

Platelet storage conditions and duration

Platelets stored at 20–24°C maintain functional effectiveness for several days [22–26]. The variables that affect the quality of platelets during storage [20,27] include the temperature, anticoagulant preservative solution, storage container, type of agitation and volume of plasma. Citrate phosphate dextrose (CPD) and CPD-adenine solutions are satisfactory platelet preservatives [20,28]: undisturbed storage is inferior to gentle agitation and horizontal agitation is preferable to end-over-end agitation [29]. The composition, surface area and size of the storage container influence the ability for carbon dioxide to diffuse out and oxygen to enter the platelet concentrate, and storage containers specifically designed to optimize platelet quality are now used routinely [30,31].

Maintenance of the pH above 6.0 is the crucial factor indicating satisfactory platelet preservation. This combination of storage container, agitation, preservative solution, temperature and the use of about 50 mL plasma provides satisfactory preservation of random-donor platelets for up to 7 days [30,31]. However, several instances of bacterial contamination of platelet concentrates stored for this period were reported [32,33] and the storage time was reduced to the 5 days that are presently the limit [34]. One plateletpheresis unit contains an adequate therapeutic dose of platelets, but usually several whole blood platelet concentrates must be pooled to provide an adequate dose for most patients. For some individuals, the volume of plasma in the final pooled component is too large and plasma must be removed before transfusion. The loss of platelets during this concentration step is reported to be from 15% to as much as 55% [35,36]. Several centrifugation procedures appear to be satisfactory [35,36,38]. Thus, concentration or volume reduction of pooled platelets can be carried out successfully and is often done for small patients or those who are receiving large volumes of blood components or intravenous fluids.

Transfusion of platelets

The decision as to whether to transfuse platelets depends on the clinical condition of the patient, the cause of the thrombocytopenia, the platelet count and the functional ability of the patient's own platelets. The responses to platelet transfusion vary, and the strategies to deal with patients who fail to respond are complex. Most platelets are transfused to patients with transient thrombocytopenia due to chemotherapy for malignancy or those undergoing HCT [37,38]. Most platelet transfusions are used for the prevention of bleeding (prophylactic) rather than the treatment of active bleeding.

Before the availability of platelets for transfusion, hemorrhage was the major cause of death in patients with marrow failure [39]. There is little risk of serious spontaneous hemorrhage when the platelet count is >20,000/μL, but the risk increases with lower platelet counts [40]. Because of ethical concerns, very few controlled studies of prophylactic platelet transfusion were carried out when platelet therapy first became available. Several studies supported the use of prophylactic transfusions [41–44], but other studies were not able to show a benefit of prophylactic platelet transfusion [45,46]. Despite the lack of substantial convincing clinical trial data, it became common practice for physicians to use platelet transfusions to prevent serious bleeding when the platelet count was <20,000/μL, depending on the patient's age, diagnosis, clinical condition, treatment and concomitant medications [47].

In an effort to evaluate the risks of thrombocytopenia, occult blood loss in the stools was quantified using chromium-51 (^{51}Cr)-labeled red cells in patients with different degrees of thrombocytopenia [46,48]. In stable thrombocytopenic patients, no increase occurred in stool blood loss at platelet counts of 10,000/μL and blood loss increased only when the platelet count reached 5000/μL [46,48]. Since the early days of platelet transfusion, considerable experience has been gained in the management of thrombocytopenic patients, which led to improvements in their outcome while maintaining much lower platelet counts than were previously believed to be safe. Serious bleeding usually occurred only when the platelet count was below 10,000/μL [49], and fatal bleeding is unlikely to occur at platelet counts above 5000/μL [49–52]. Gmur et al. [53] found that the threshold for prophylactic platelet transfusion could be 5000/μL in uncomplicated patients, 10,000/μL in individuals with fever or bleeding and 20,000/μL in patients with coagulopathy or bleeding sites. Heckman et al. [54] found no difference in red cell use, days of fever, hospitalization, thrombocytopenia, remission, death, or major bleeding complications when prophylactic transfusion thresholds of 20,000/μL and 10,000/μL were compared. Rebulla et al. [55] reported that in acute leukemia patients undergoing first remission induction there was no difference in deaths, red cell transfusions or severe hemorrhage, but there was a 21.5% reduction in platelet use using a transfusion threshold of 10,000/μL compared to 20,000/μL. Wandt et al. [56], summarizing experiences in 17 centers in Germany, found no difference in bleeding complications when 10,000/μL or 20,000/μL thresholds were used and hemorrhagic deaths actually occurred in two patients with platelet counts of 36,000/μL and 50,000/μL. In stable marrow transplant recipients, lowering the transfusion threshold from 20,000/μL to 10,000/μL did not increase severe bleeding or deaths due to bleeding but it did reduce platelet use by about 25% [57]. Aderka et al. [52] proposed, based on analysis of 196 patients with acute leukemia, that prophylactic platelet transfusion was not necessary when the platelet count is above 10,000/μL. More recently, Zumberg et al. [58] reported no differences in the incidence or severity of bleeding in 159 HCT patients prospectively randomized to receive platelet transfusions at a threshold count of 20,000/μL or 10,000/μL. Establishing the indications for platelet transfusion remains complex because many studies are not powered to show modest differences, most do not use bleeding as the endpoint, and the patient population is heterogenous [59]. A National Institutes of Health (NIH) Consensus Conference recommended that the 20,000/μL-value traditionally used for prophylactic platelet transfusion could be safely lowered for many patients [51]. A more recent summary of the data and recommendation by Beutler [60] began a major shift downward in the indications for prophylactic platelet transfusion, although in a 1995 survey about two-thirds of HCT centers still used a 20,000/μL threshold [61]. Bleeding is more common in allogeneic than autologous transplant recipients [61,62] and the increasing use of peripheral blood hematopoietic cells with more rapid engraftment may further decrease the incidence of bleeding. Now many physicians and hospital guidelines use platelet counts of 10,000 or 5000/μL as the indication for transfusion to uncomplicated patients. However, many HCT recipients are febrile and often have lesions, such as mucositis, and, thus, many of these patients are transfused at platelet counts of about 20,000/μL or higher.

The usual dosage of platelets in a prophylactic platelet transfusion is one whole blood platelet concentrate/10-kg patient weight or 1 plateletpheresis unit per day. It has been suggested that frequent transfusions of a lower dose of platelets will reduce the number of platelets needed [63]. Conversely, when thrombopoietin was given to platelet donors and very large numbers ($15-18 \times 10^{11}$) of platelets were collected and transfused, the time between transfusions was extended suggesting that overall fewer platelets might be needed [64]. Platelet dose studies will probably be carried out in the next few years and may lead to changes in transfusion strategy.

Treatment of active bleeding

Platelet transfusions are not necessary for bleeding patients with a platelet count above 100,000/μL because these patients have a normal bleeding time [65]. With platelet counts below 100,000/μL, the bleeding time is increasingly prolonged [65]. The optimum platelet count to achieve in a bleeding patient is not known. In one study of patients undergoing surgery with platelet counts <100,000/μL, prophylactic platelet transfusions were given to those whose platelet count was <50,000/μL [66]. Bleeding was similar in patients with <50,000/μL who received platelet transfusion compared to those whose platelet count was >50,000/μL but did not receive platelet transfusion. The bleeding did not relate to the platelet count but instead to the severity of the surgical procedure. Thus, in actively bleeding patients, platelet transfusion should be considered in those with a platelet count of less than approximately 75,000/μL. An attempt to achieve a level of above 50,000/μL is recommended. If the patient's platelets are dysfunctional due to causes such as due to drugs or uremia, the bleeding time may be much longer than would be expected based on the degree of thrombocytopenia. In those situations the decision to give a platelet transfusion is made on clinical grounds alone.

Outcome of platelet transfusion

There is a dose–response effect from platelet transfusion [40,51]. Within 1 h after transfusion, the platelet count increases approximately 10,000/μL when 1×10^{11} platelets are transfused into a 70-kg patient [67,68]. Since a platelet transfusion usually contains approximately 4.0×10^{11} platelets, the platelet count should increase by about 40,000/μL in an average-sized adult. The 1-h post-transfusion platelet count is an excellent predictor of an effective platelet transfusion [68]. If a very accurate determination of the response to platelet transfusion is needed, the 1-h corrected count increment (CCI) or the percent recovery can be determined. Today, the CCI is most commonly used. The CCI is calculated as follows:

$$CCI = \frac{(\text{Post-transfusion}-\text{pretransfusion platelet count}) \times (\text{body surface area})}{\text{No. of platelets transfused}}$$

The expected CCI is about 15,000/μL × 10^{11} platelets transfused/m² body-surface area. If the CCI is <5000–7500 the patient is considered to be refractory. If platelet recovery is used as an indicator, the expected result is about 65% because some of the platelets normally are sequestered in the spleen.

ABO(H) and Rh in platelet transfusion

ABO antigens are intrinsic to the platelet and some are adsorbed onto its surface [69]. When ^{51}Cr-labeled group A platelets are transfused to normal group O volunteers, the recovery is reduced [70] and the higher the ABO isoagglutinin titers, the greater the reduction in recovery of transfused platelets. This ABO effect has been substantiated clinically in several studies. There is a reduced recovery when platelets from human leukocyte antigen (HLA)-matched donors are transfused to alloimmunized patients who were ABO incompatible with the donor platelets [71–73], and blood group O patients may be refractory to platelets transfused from group A donors but not from platelets transfused from group O donors [71,74]. All of these studies substantiate the concept that if platelets that contain ABH antigens are transfused into patients with circulating antibody directed against those antigens, the intravascular recovery of the transfused platelets is substantially decreased. Heal et al. [73] also observed an 18% decreased recovery of transfused platelets when the incompatibility involved transfusion of ABO antibody directed against the recipient's ABO antigens (e.g. group O platelets transfused to a group A patient). It is postulated that the ABO effect is due to the formation of circulating immune complexes by soluble ABH substance and ABO antibodies [75,76]. This can occur with the antigen-antibody complexes from either donor or recipient anti-body and donor or recipient ABH substance. Thus, the reduced platelet recovery due to circulating immune complexes can occur when the ABO incompatibility is either the "major" or "minor" type. It now seems clear that ABO incompatibility is associated with reduced posttransfusion platelet recovery [70–78]; however, this is not of a magnitude that would contraindicate transfusion of ABO-mismatched but HLA-matched platelets.

A separate consideration involving the ABO system and platelet transfusion is the potential administration of large volumes of ABO-incompatible plasma if transfusions involve "minor" incompatibility (e.g. group O platelets transfused to group A patients). This plasma may reduce the survival of the transfused platelets, but another concern is the potential for hemolysis when large amounts of ABO-incompatible anti-body are transfused. To avoid these problems it is now common to limit the volume of ABO-incompatible plasma that a patient can receive. This can be in terms of a percentage of the patient's estimated blood volume or an absolute volume limit. Adults can be limited to no more than 1 L of ABO-incompatible plasma per week. It is recognized that a rare unit may have a very high titer, but this approach seems to be satisfactory.

Rh antigens are not present on the platelet surface. However, the few red cells contained in the platelet concentrate can lead to immunization and, thus, Rh must be considered in platelet transfusion. In Rh-negative cancer patients, reported rates of immunization to the D antigen range from 0% to 18% [79–85]. Because oncology patients and HCT recipients receive a large number of platelet transfusions, it is usually not possible to provide Rh-negative platelets for Rh-negative patients. Thus, it is common to provide platelets to these patients without regard to Rh type. Rh immunoglobulin is not administered to prevent alloimmunization. Even when circulating anti-D develops, this antibody does not interfere with the circulation of Rh D-positive platelets [86]. If Rh immunoglobulin (RhIg) is to be administered to prevent alloimmunization, the dose of RhIg can be determined from the number of units of platelets that the patient receives. For instance, since most therapeutic doses of platelets (e.g. 1 single-donor unit or 6 pooled, random-donor units) contain less than 1 mL red cells, one standard dose of 300 μg of RhIg is sufficient.

Lack of response (refractoriness) to platelet transfusion

Many patients do not attain the expected post-transfusion increment in platelet count and are said to be "refractory" to platelet transfusion. Refractoriness to platelet transfusion can be caused by factors related to the patient and factors related to the platelet concentrate.

Factors related to the patient

In patients who have HLA or platelet antibodies, such as those with autoimmune thrombocytopenic purpura or patients who are immunized to antigens of the HLA system, survival of circulating platelets is extremely brief, sometimes only a matter of minutes [46]. Splenomegaly also causes sequestration of platelets and a reduced post-transfusion increment [87]. In a careful study of 941 platelet transfusions administered to 133 patients, Bishop et al. [88] found that the following factors were associated with a poor response to platelet transfusion: DIC, amphotericin administration, palpable spleen, presence of HLA antibody, presence of platelet antibody, status post-HCT and fever. Active bleeding has been thought to be associated with a reduced response to platelet transfusion, but this concept was not substantiated in Bishop et al.'s study [88]. Thus, patients can be refractory due to alloimmunization (HLA and/or platelet antibodies) or nonimmune factors. In one study nonimmune factors were present alone in 67% of refractory patients and were present with immune factors in an additional 21% of patients [89]. In some studies, refractoriness is clearly associated with the presence of HLA antibodies [68,89]; however, many of these patients also have one or more clinical factors present, which could account at least partially for the refractoriness. Thus, in practice it is very difficult to determine whether a patient is refractory due to immune or nonimmune factors and this affects the strategy used to manage these patients.

In the past, the incidence of refractoriness was rather high. In one study, about 38% of patients who received multiple platelet transfusions, such as those with hematological malignancies, became refractory to platelets [90]. This problem occurred after approximately nine transfusions that involved 61 U of platelets. It appears that patients who become refractory do so after relatively few transfusions and that some patients do not become refractory regardless of the number of transfusions [91]. However, the incidence of platelet refractoriness seems to be changing. In a more recent study of newly diagnosed patients with acute myeloid leukemia, only about 15% became refractory after the first 8 weeks of therapy [92]. This decrease may be due to changing transfusion practices, described in the Prevention of alloimmunization and platelet refractoriness section, or to more intensive chemotherapy.

Factors related to the platelet concentrate

ABO incompatibility can reduce the intravascular recovery and survival of transfused platelets. Patients who are refractory to platelet transfusion should receive a trial of at least two ABO identical platelet transfusions. Another cause of reduced recovery of transfused platelets is the transfusion of platelets near the end of their storage period. Lazarus et al. [93] demonstrated that platelets stored for longer than 24 h provided a substantially reduced post-transfusion increment. Although data on this topic are not extensive, it is generally accepted that platelets near the end of their 5-day storage period may provide less of an increment than fresh platelets. Therefore, in determining whether a patient is refractory, at least one transfusion of platelets, about 24-h old, should be provided.

Strategies for managing patients who are refractory to platelet transfusion

HLA matching for platelet transfusion

If the use of ABO-matched platelets of approximately 24-h storage fails to produce a satisfactory increment, transfusion of either HLA-matched or cross-matched platelets can be used. During the 1960s, it was observed that in refractory patients platelets from HLA-identical siblings provided a good response. Later, it was shown that HLA-identical platelets from unrelated donors were also beneficial [94]. The use of HLA-matched platelets became practical when it was shown that good responses could be obtained when the donor platelets were only partially matched [95–97]. Many blood banks also have large files of HLA-typed volunteer donors so that HLA-matched platelets can be provided for most patients. However, most HLA-matched platelets obtained from unrelated donors have some antigens mismatched with the patient. Although the average response to these partially matched transfusions is similar to that from fully matched HLA-identical transfusions, about 30% of HLA-matched transfusions do not provide a satisfactory response [95–98]. Also, since these patients require frequent platelet transfusions, many donors who are matched with the patient must be available to sustain the patient for days or a few weeks.

Platelet cross-matching for platelet transfusion

One approach that should be effective in overcoming the 30% failure of HLA-matched transfusions [96–98] is cross-matching the patient's serum and potential donor's cells. The development of this approach was slow for many years because the platelet antibody detection techniques were complex. Platelet-specific antibodies may sometimes be involved in refractoriness. Because the relative role of platelet-specific vs. HLA antibodies has not been clear, the choice of the optimum method for cross-matching was complicated.

There has been great variability in the experience with platelet cross-matching [99]. The positive predictive value of platelet cross-matching ranged from 73% to 100% and the negative predictive value from 52% to 92% in 10 studies summarized by Heal et al. [73]. Many of these studies were retrospective, and some of the prospective studies did not use fresh platelets [99]. A variety of methods have been reported to be effective. However, none was suitable for general use and none gained wide practical application.

Although platelet refractoriness is often associated with the presence of lymphocytotoxic antibodies in the patient's serum, Moroff et al. [99] were unable to demonstrate such antibodies in 55% of the patients in their study who were refractory to platelet transfusion and had no obvious clinical causes for the refractoriness. HLA matching and platelet cross-matching provided similar degrees of successful 1-h corrected-count increments (40–60%). If only transfusions were used in which four HLA-A, B-locus antigens were identical between donor and recipient (A match) or in which only three HLA-A, B-locus antigens were identified in the donor, HLA matching was superior to platelet cross-matching. However, Moroff et al. [99] concluded that a similar number of successful transfusions could be obtained by either HLA matching or platelet cross-match.

During the past several years, a solid-phase red cell adherence assay was developed specifically for platelet cross-matching [100]. This method has overcome the previous barriers of test complexity and speed of results. In clinical use, the method predicted a successful transfusion outcome in 97% of patients with no clinical factors to cause nonimmune platelet destruction [101]. Successful prediction of transfusion response using the solid phase red cell adherence assay was confirmed by O'Connell et al. [102], and by Friedberg et al. [103] who, in a separate study of 962 single-donor platelet transfusions to 71 refractory patients, showed that the solid-phase red cell adherence assay was superior to HLA matching. This method is now widely used because of its effectiveness and practicality.

Other approaches to the refractory patient

Other strategies that have been attempted but are not usually successful and are not recommended include plasma exchange [104], treatment of the patient's plasma with a staphylococcal protein A (SPA) column [105] and cyclosporine. The use of the SPA column enjoyed brief popularity because of a report that 6–10 patients who were refractory to platelet transfusion responded after receiving SPA-treated plasma [106]. This was not a structured prospective study with appropriate controls and because no such studies have been published subsequently, the use of the SPA column is not an established method for dealing with platelet refractoriness. In refractory patients who are experiencing life-threatening complications, SPA column therapy is sometimes used even in the absence of evidence to support its effectiveness. Case reports have shown a beneficial effect of intravenous immunoglobulin in improving the response to platelet transfusion in alloimmunized refractory patients [107,108], but another larger, more definitive study found no benefit from intravenous immunoglobulin [109] and recommended against its use.

A practical approach to the patient who is refractory to platelet transfusion

The lack of a response to platelet transfusion is often associated with bleeding. These patients are usually quite ill, with problems such as fever, sepsis, DIC, or viral infections. Therefore, clinical factors, such as infection that might cause refractoriness, should be sought and, if they are present, appropriate treatment should be initiated. Depending on the patient's condition and the degree of concern about the platelet count, additional simple steps that can be attempted include the transfusion of ABO identical platelets and platelets less than 48-h old. The techniques for platelet transfusion should be reviewed to be sure the platelets are not being damaged or lost due to improper handling after leaving the blood bank, use of incorrect filters, or improper storage conditions. An additional step is to be certain that the platelet concentrates contain an adequate number of platelets, which can be done by checking the blood bank routine quality control testing. If questions continue, the platelet count and content of the specific concentrates being used for the patient can be determined.

If these measures fail, platelets that are matched to the recipient should be used. This can be accomplished by HLA-matching donor and recipient or by using platelets that are compatible in a cross-match. Most HLA-matched platelets obtained from unrelated donors will not be matched for all four of the HLA-A and B locus antigens and, thus, there will be some degree of antigen mismatch between the patient and donor. Although the average response to these partially matched transfusions is similar to that from fully matched transfusions, about 30% of HLA-matched transfusions do not provide a satisfactory response [95–98]. Also, since these patients require frequent platelet transfusions, many donors who are matched to the patient must be available to sustain the patient for days or a few weeks. For many patients this approach may not be practical. An additional or alternative approach is to cross-match the patient's serum and potential donor's cells. As described above, the success rate is similar to that with HLA-matched transfusions.

Thus, it seems that either HLA matching or platelet cross-matching can be used to obtain about the same effect. One practical difference is that usually cross-matched platelets can be obtained more rapidly than HLA-matched platelets because cross-matching is done on platelets already collected and available in inventory whereas HLA-matched donors must be located and scheduled for donation. A suggested practical strategy for dealing with patients who are refractory to platelet transfusion is as follows:
1 Treat any correctable clinical factors present that may cause platelet refractoriness. Until these factors are eliminated, recognize that any of the steps listed below may not be effective.
2 Ensure that the patient is receiving the correct dose of platelets.
3 Give at least one test transfusion of platelets that are not more than 48-h old.
4 Ensure that platelets being transfused are ABO-identical.
5 If these steps have failed and transfusion is urgently needed, give transfusions of either cross-match compatible or HLA-matched platelets, whichever is available soonest. Give at least one and preferably two or three such transfusions.
6 Continue to use either cross-matched or HLA-matched platelets until the desired increment is obtained.
7 Determine whether the patient has HLA or platelet-specific antibodies, or both. This precaution may be of value in making future decisions about platelet transfusion if the patient does not respond to HLA-matched or cross-matched platelets.
8 Determine whether the patient is receiving medications such as vancomycin that might cause drug-dependent antiplatelet antibodies. If so, carry out a drug-platelet antibody test.

Some patients do not respond to either HLA-matched or cross-matched platelets. Often these are patients in whom marrow grafting has failed, who have graft-vs.-host disease (GVHD), who are septic, or who are experiencing other severe complications of cytopenia. One approach is to increase the dose of platelets to two or even three single-donor or 20–30 random donor units per day. While this may enable physicians to feel that they are doing something helpful, usually the patients fail to achieve a substantial increase in platelet count. It is not known whether the transfusions are helpful despite the lack of increase in circulating platelets.

Prevention of alloimmunization and platelet refractoriness

Because of the difficulty in managing patients who are refractory to platelet transfusion, there is considerable interest in preventing alloimmunization. Immunization may be caused by pregnancy but is also due to the leukocytes contained in the platelet and red cell transfusions [110,111]. Although the exact mechanism of alloimmunization has not been defined, it appears that intact viable leukocytes present HLA class I and II antigens for processing [112,113]. Thus, strategies to modify the transfusion products have been attempted. In general, these strategies have involved limiting the number of donor exposures, removing the leukocytes, or treating the components to render the leukocytes nonimmunogenic. Two studies [114,115] demonstrated that use of non-HLA-matched single-donor platelet concentrates reduced the incidence of alloimmunization (HLA), prolonged the time to immunization, reduced the incidence of refractoriness and prolonged the time to refractoriness. However, because of the role of leukocytes, the expense of single-donor platelet concentrates in some centers and the remarkable improvements in blood filtration systems, leukodepletion has become the major approach to preventing alloimmunization

There is a very substantial body of data that establishes that leukocyte depletion reduces the incidence of alloimmunization and delays and/or reduces the onset of refractoriness [116–121]. Clinical trials are difficult to accomplish perfectly and many of these studies have one or another shortcoming; however, there is little disagreement that leukocyte depletion is effective. This observation has recently been confirmed in the largest prospectively randomized trial reported [92]. In that study of more than 500 newly diagnosed patients with acute leukemia, the use of leukocyte-depleted red cells and platelet concentrates reduced the incidence of alloimmunization. No difference was found between pooled random-donor and single-donor platelet concentrates suggesting that the important factor is the reduction of the leukocyte exposure rather than the number of different donors. Filtration of the components at the time they are produced in the laboratory may be more effective for prevention of alloimmunization [122–124].

Another strategy proposed for the prevention of alloimmunization is the treatment of the platelet concentrates with ultraviolet (UV) light. UV radiation inhibits the ability of lymphocytes to either proliferate or stimulate in a mixed lymphocyte culture [125], but UV-B light does not interfere with platelet function *in vitro* [125,126] or *in vivo* [127] at doses that will abrogate lymphocyte function. In mice, UV-B treatment of platelets reduced the alloantigenicity of transfused leukocyte-depleted platelets [128]. In a recent large study, UV-irradiated platelets reduced the incidence of alloimmunization but no more so than filtered leukodepleted platelets [92]. Thus, although this approach appears to be effective in preventing alloimmunization, it is not presently used and no systems are licensed by the Food and Drug Administration (FDA) for routine blood bank use.

Role of thrombopoietin in platelet transfusion

It was hoped that the long-sought platelet growth factor thrombopoietin (TPO), discovered more than a decade ago, would reduce the need for platelet transfusions [129]. TPO produced primarily in the liver and kidneys causes an increase in the number, size and ploidy of megakaryocytes, speeds the maturation of megakaryocytes into platelets and produces platelets that have normal function *in vitro* and circulation *in vivo* [129–131]. TPO could influence transfusion therapy in HCT patients in at least two ways. It can be given to the patient in hopes of speeding the recovery of platelet production and shortening the period of thrombocytopenia, thus reducing bleeding complications and the need for platelet transfusions. Alternatively, TPO can be given to platelet donors to elevate the donor's platelet count, increase the number of platelets collected and transfused in hopes of increasing the time between transfusions and reducing the number of donor exposures that the patient receives.

Two different agents have undergone clinical evaluation. One is the full TPO molecule and the other is the erythropoietin-like domain coupled with polyethylene glycol (PEG) to provide stability *in vivo*. The former agent is called TPO and the latter agent is called PEG megakaryocyte growth and development factor (MGDF).

In patients with advanced cancer, TPO or MGDF increased the platelet count in a dose-dependent manner by 50–500%, elevated the nadir platelet count, shortened the period of thrombocytopenia and decreased platelet transfusion requirements [132–135]. However, this observation has had little impact on platelet use because these patients do not receive many platelet transfusions. The response to TPO in HCT patients receiving myeloablative therapy is even less impressive. TPO therapy has not shorted the duration of thrombocytopenia or decreased the need for platelet transfusions [130,136,137], possibly because endogenous TPO levels are already very high in these patients [138], TPO receptors may be downgraded [130], or TPO may actually inhibit release of mature platelets from megakaryocytes [130]. Because the many pluripotent functions of TPO have not been well studied, the reasons for its role or lack thereof in the HCT setting are not completely understood.

MGDF can be administered to normal plateletpheresis donors to increase the level of circulating platelets and, thus, the yield of platelets following plateletpheresis increased two to four times. When these high-dose concentrates are used as a single transfusion, they provide a larger increase in platelet count than present transfusions [64], which prolongs the interval between transfusions and reduces the number of donor exposures. However, in separate studies, TPO inhibitors developed in normal subjects [139] and development of MGDF has been discontinued. TPO has not been used in platelet donors.

Granulocyte concentrates and granulocyte transfusion

A series of studies in the 1970s established that granulocyte transfusions provided improved survival in patients with documented gram-negative sepsis who remained granulocytopenic for at least 10 days [140,141]. Some additional data indicate that granulocytes may be helpful in patients with other kinds of documented infections (either gram-positive or gram-negative) and granulocytopenia of more than 10 days' duration [141]. Patients with fever of unknown origin do not experience improvement as a result of granulocyte transfusion [142]. Most clinical trials of granulocyte transfusion involve patients with gram-negative bacteremia [143] and there is little information regarding other organisms. There is also little information that collates the site of infection other than bacteremia with response to granulocyte transfusion [143]. However, today most patients respond to antibiotics and granulocyte transfusion is rarely used for bacterial infections. Prophylactic granulocyte transfusions are also not helpful [144]. There is renewed interest in granulocyte transfusion because hematopoietic growth factors, such as granulocyte colony-stimulating factor (G-CSF), can be used to stimulate granulocyte production in normal blood donors, increasing the level of circulating granulocytes and the yield of granulocytes [145,146]. The minimum dose of granulocytes required for clinical efficacy has not been established. Encouraging results were obtained from the use of approximately 5×10^9 granulocytes/day [140]; however, this number represents less than 5% of the total daily granulocyte production by normal humans. Most physicians believe it is necessary to transfuse at least 1×10^{10} granulocytes/day and this dose is probably suboptimal.

The level of circulating granulocytes can be increased to about 30,000/μL with G-CSF alone [146] and, by combining the use of corticosteroids and G-CSF, the level of circulating granulocytes can be increased to approximately 40,000/μL [147]. It appears that administration of G-CSF to health donors is safe [147–150]. Leukapheresis of these donors results in a dose of up to 7 or 8×10^{10} granulocytes/day in some cases. These doses of granulocytes far exceed those used in the studies of the 1970s and may make transfusions clinically effective. It should be feasible to obtain enough family or community donors to provide a series of transfusions [151]. The major potential role for granulocyte transfusions presently would be for fungal infections. No clinical trials have documented the effectiveness of granulocyte transfusion for fungal infections, although animal [152] and clinical [153] studies support their use.

Transfusion strategies in HCT

Pretransplantation

For pretransplant transfusion strategy, patients can be thought of in three groups: (i) immunocompetent but not requiring transfusion, (ii) immunocompetent and requiring transfusion, and (iii) immunocompromised. An example of the first group is patients with inborn errors of metabolism who rarely require transfusion before HCT. The other two groups of patients have a variable degree of immunocompetence and they may become alloimmunized to leukocytes or platelets following transfusion. Alloimmunization may cause transfusion reactions but, more importantly, may interfere with engraftment in some patients. The presence of HLA antibodies is associated with marrow graft rejection [154]. Pretransplant transfusions are associated with increased graft failure rates [155,156]. For immunocompetent patients, such as those with aplastic anemia, hemoglobinopathies, or myelodysplastic syndrome who require pretransplant transfusions, efforts should be made to prevent alloimmunization. Patients with aplastic anemia should be evaluated quickly and HCT, if indicated, should be performed as soon as possible to minimize the number of pretransplant transfusions. Storb and Weiden [157] have recommended that prophylactic platelets be given only when the platelet count is <5000/μL. For patients, such as those with hemoglobinopathies or myelodysplastic syndrome who require red cell or platelet transfusions before HCT, the following are recommended:

1 Red cells should be depleted of leukocytes.

2 Platelet concentrates should be depleted of leukocytes. This can be done by filtration or by certain apheresis collection procedures.

3 The use of single-donor instead of pooled random-donor platelet concentrates should be considered. However, the largest most recently completed study did not show a difference in the rate of alloimmunization between single-donor and pooled random-donor platelet concentrates [92].
4 Family members should not be used as blood or blood component donors (before transplant) because of the risk of alloimmunization causing an unsuccessful marrow graft [157].

Patients with malignancies who will undergo HCT usually have received multiple transfusions during the initial chemotherapy of their underlying disease. However, the effects of this on subsequent marrow engraftment are not as severe as for patients with aplastic anemia because standard chemotherapy is extremely immunosuppressive. Thus, transfusion therapy for these patients can be that necessitated by their chemotherapy. The increasing use of nonmyeloablative preparative regimens may make engraftment more problematic in heavily alloimmunized patients. Therefore, red cells and platelets should be leukoreduced in order to minimize the possibility of alloimmunization. Transfusions from family members probably should be avoided [157], although one study showed no increase in graft failure in patients with leukemia who received transfusions from family donors [158].

Post-transplantation

Because of the severe immunosuppression caused by the pretransplant preparative regimen, fatal GVHD can occur as a result of transfusion of viable lymphocytes that are present in blood components [159]. Transfusion-related GVHD can be prevented by irradiating all blood components with at least 2500 cGy (see below).

About 10–25 days elapse between HCT and marrow engraftment, although this period is becoming more variable as different sources of stem cells are used. The return of production of different blood cell lines varies so that although the duration of transfusion therapy may range from 2 to 6 weeks, the need for different components varies with different types of transplants. Almost all patients require platelet and red cell transfusions but since HCT does not usually interfere with the production of coagulation factors, transfusion of FFP and cryoprecipitate is necessary only if coagulopathy develops. Although HCT patients are severely neutropenic, granulocyte transfusions are usually not necessary.

Because of their complex situation these patients may place a major demand on the blood bank for blood components, especially platelets. The red cells used can be routine red cell components, although leukocyte-depleted red cells are recommended to minimize the likelihood of inducing alloimmunization. Another unique consideration in the transfusion management of HCT patients is the source of platelets. Either random- or single (apheresis)-donor platelets can be utilized. Leukocyte depletion is also used to prevent alloimmunization. Results of studies of leukocyte-depleted platelet concentrates in situations other than HCT have indicated that this strategy is effective [117–121]. One large study [92] found that leukocyte depletion reduced platelet refractoriness even in patients who were already alloimmunized, but another study [116] showed no benefit from leukocyte-depleted platelets in preventing secondary alloimmunization. Although studies in HCT patients have not been reported, the effectiveness of leukocyte depletion in other situations suggests that this could be helpful and leukocyte-reduced platelets are recommended

If patients become refractory to platelet transfusion, HLA-matched unrelated or family donor platelets can be used. Platelets can be obtained from the marrow donor if the patient is refractory and experiencing serious bleeding problems, but this decision requires considerable thought because of ethical considerations regarding the donor.

Prevention of transfusion-transmitted CMV infection

CMV disease is an important source of post-transplant mortality (see Chapter 53) [160]. Most CMV infections in HCT patients occur in those with CMV antibody and probably are due to reactivation of virus from a previous infection, not to acquisition of a new strain [161]. However, in CMV antibody-negative patients who receive unscreened blood products, the risk of developing CMV infection is approximately 40% [161]. The likelihood of these patients acquiring CMV infection is almost eliminated by the use of CMV antibody-negative blood components [161,162]. Therefore, it is now customary to provide these blood components to CMV antibody-negative HCT recipients whose marrow donor is CMV antibody-negative.

As a substantial portion of blood donors are CMV antibody-positive, providing CMV antibody-negative blood components is sometimes difficult, especially as the indications for CMV-free blood components have increased. Although infectious viral particles cannot be recovered from normal donors previously infected with CMV who have antibodies to CMV, blood from these donors can transmit CMV. Because it is presumed that leukocytes are the reservoir of CMV in these asymptomatic blood donors, prevention of transfusion-transmitted CMV has been attempted using leukocyte-depleted components. Several small studies [163,164] and one large controlled trial [165] have established that leukocyte-depleted components are as effective as antibody-negative components in preventing transfusion-transmitted CMV. Leukocyte-depleted and antibody-negative components can be considered equivalent and used interchangeably depending on logistical considerations of each transfusion service.

The use of CMV antibody-negative blood components in potential HCT patients who are CMV antibody-negative has been suggested. This would prevent these patients from becoming infected with CMV as a result of transfusions received earlier in their disease and before entering an HCT program. This practice is gaining in popularity and the conversion to routine use of leukocyte-depleted blood components makes it more practical.

Other approaches that have been attempted for the prevention of CMV infection include the use of CMV intravenous immunoglobulin [166,167] or ordinary intravenous immunoglobulin [168], although the increasing use of leukodepleted blood products should obviate these other strategies.

Prevention of transfusion-associated GVHD

GVHD from blood transfusion was originally identified in immunodeficient children but the more common situation in which GVHD occurs is HCT [159]; and it is now clear that GVHD can occur in a wide variety of immunocompromised patients and even in some immunocompetent patients. Following HCT, GVHD is caused by the immunocompetent marrow donor cells, while in blood transfusion, viable lymphocytes contained in blood components can cause GVHD in susceptible patients [159].

Irradiation of blood components

Warning

Hematopoietic stem cells are sensitive to irradiation. Marrow, peripheral blood, or cord blood stem cells that are intended for transplantation should not be exposed to irradiation.

To prevent transfusion-associated GVHD, blood components are subjected to irradiation, which interferes with the ability of lymphocytes to proliferate. Gamma irradiation or X-rays damage the lymphocytes by forming electrically charged particles or ions that alter DNA, making lymphocytes unable to proliferate [169]. UV irradiation is not an effective method of damaging lymphocytes to prevent GVHD because the rays cannot penetrate the plastic containers that are used to store blood products. Blood banks that provide large numbers of irradiated products usually irradiate with a dedicated instrument. These instruments use caesium-137 or cobalt-60 as the source of the radioactivity.

The optimal dose of irradiation has evolved over the years. Following early experiences with transfusion-associated GVHD, a dose of 3000 cGy was recommended [170]. The occurrence of transfusion-associated GVHD in several individuals who received blood components supposedly irradiated with at least 1500 cGy [170–172] has focused attention during the past few years on the configuration of the blood containers in the irradiated field, the distribution of irradiation within the field and quality control methods to assure that the desired dose was actually being administered [169]. A survey of irradiation practices revealed that doses range from 1500 to 5000 cGy, with 97% of institutions using 1500–3000 cGy [173].

Gamma irradiation at a dose of only 500 cGy will abolish lymphocyte proliferation in mixed lymphocyte culture [174,175]. Irradiation with 1500–5000 cGy reduces the incorporation of Carbon-14-thymidine into mitogen-stimulated lymphocytes by 85.0–98.5% [176]. Doses of up to 5000 cGy do not have an adverse effect on red cells, platelets, or granulocytes [176,177]. Red cell survival *in vivo* and certain *in vitro* assays are normal afterwards up to 10,000 cGy [177]. Granulocyte chemotaxis may be slightly reduced by even 500 cGy, but this defect does not become significant until above 10,000 cGy [177]. Very high doses, such as 40,000 cGy, are required to interfere with phagocytosis and microbial killing [175,177,178]. *In vitro* platelet function studies have generally been normal following up to a 5000-cGy dose [179]. Studies involving lower doses of irradiation such as 2500 or 3000 cGy showed normal *in vivo* survival [179,180] and post-transfusion increments [181]. Thus, it appears that at the doses of irradiation generally in use there is no interference with platelet function or survival.

One difficulty in selecting an irradiation dose is the lack of a definitive *in vitro* assay to establish a clinically effective dose. During the past few years, the limiting dilution assay (LDA) has been proposed as a good indicator of the effects of irradiation on lymphocytes because LDA detects a 5-$\log_{10}$ reduction in viable T cells, compared to a 1–2-$\log_{10}$ reduction in the mixed lymphocyte culture [169,182,183]. Studies using the LDA showed that 2500 cGy completely eliminated T-lymphocyte growth [184] and, based on this experience, the FDA has recommended a minimum dose of 2500 cGy [184].

Storage of irradiated components

In almost all of the studies of irradiation on blood components the cells were studied shortly after irradiation. As the use of irradiated blood components has increased, interest has developed in irradiating the components after collection and storing them for use days or weeks later. Doses of 2000 or 3000 cGy to units of red cells result in potassium levels that are two and three times normal after storage for 4–5 days [185,186]. This leakage suggests damage to the red cell membrane or the sodium-potassium pump. Some blood banks wash red cells that have been stored for several days after irradiation. However, in a thorough review, Strauss [187] concluded that washing is not necessary for most clinical situations. Based on these studies, red cells can be stored for only 28 days after irradiation. Because there is no reduction in platelet recovery and survival when previously irradiated platelets are stored [180], platelets can be irradiated and stored for the usual 5 days.

Quality control of irradiation

Quality control of blood irradiators is extremely important to ensure that the components receive the expected dose. Moroff *et al.* [169] have proposed the following as appropriate quality control measures for blood irradiation:
1 Use of qualitative indicators to confirm that irradiation was performed as intended.
2 Periodic measurement over the delivered dose using appropriate dosimetric techniques.
3 Periodic surveys to detect isotope leakage.
4 Daily confirmation of timer accuracy.

Leukocyte depletion to prevent GVHD

As blood filters are very effective in removing leukocytes, the question has arisen as to whether blood filtration might be an alternative to irradiation for prevention of GVHD. Although on average filters produce components that contain $<5 \times 10^6$ leukocytes per unit, a small proportion of units may contain considerably more leukocytes [188]. Thus, filtration is not an acceptable approach to prevention of transfusion-associated GVHD.

Autologous bone marrow transplantation

Although there may be some differences in the irradiation and chemotherapy preparation for autologous compared with allogeneic bone marrow transplantation (BMT), patients undergoing autologous BMT are severely immunocompromised for several weeks. The use of irradiated blood components has been adopted for autologous BMT without clinical or laboratory study.

Noncellular blood components

Transfusion-associated GVHD has occurred in patients with congenital immune deficiency following transfusion of fresh liquid plasma [170,189,190] but has not been reported to be caused by previously frozen components, FFP, or cryoprecipitate. These components contain fragments of leukocytes but few, if any, viable lymphocytes. They would not be expected to cause transfusion-associated GVHD. Although irradiation of FFP and cryoprecipitate is probably not necessary, many blood banks do irradiate these components to avoid clerical errors in which a cellular blood component might not be irradiated when necessary.

Transfusion therapy for HCT donors

Patients (autologous donors) or normal allogeneic donors of marrow may require some replacement of red cells. The volume of replacement needed can be predicted from the size of the patient and the donor [191]. It is important to anticipate whether red cell transfusion of the normal allogeneic donor will be necessary and, if so, to take steps to avoid exposure to allogeneic red cells. If red cell replacement is contemplated, the normal donor should provide autologous red cells for transfusion during marrow donation [191]. Usually 2 U of red cells will suffice. Erythropoietin has been used to increase erythropoiesis in autologous blood donors before elective surgery, and this step may be a helpful strategy for allogeneic marrow donors. Donation of autologous peripheral blood hematopoietic cells by apheresis involves much less red cell loss than marrow donation, and usually red cell replacement is not necessary unless the patient is anemic from the disease.

Various strategies using chemotherapy or hematopoietic growth factors are being used to mobilize hematopoietic cells for transplantation from either patients or normal allogeneic donors. G-CSF can be administered to normal allogeneic donors to increase the level of circulating CD34+ cells and leukapheresis used to obtain an adequate dose of cells for transplantation with an acceptable donor side-effect profile [148,192–196]. Thus, HCT can be accomplished without subjecting these donors to general anesthesia, which is necessary for marrow donation. Although these donors do not have transfusion requirements, many other donor-related issues must be considered [197]. These include the effect of the G-CSF on the donors, the methods of vascular access, the optimum apheresis procedures and the effect of the donation of hematopoietic cells on the donor's hematological status. These issues are discussed more fully in Chapters 41, 42, 45 and 46.

Complications of blood transfusion

The complications of transfusion can be categorized as immunological and nonimmunological. Approximately 1–3% of transfusions result in an adverse effect during or shortly after the transfusion, but the incidence of longer-term adverse effects is difficult to establish. As many as 20% of transfusions may result in some kind of adverse effect, but these effects are considered serious in only about 0.5% of transfusions [198]. The most common adverse effects are alloimmunization to leukocytes or platelets, CMV seroconversion and alloimmunization to red cell antigens [198]. The fatality rate immediately surrounding transfusion is estimated to be about 1 in 100,000 patients transfused, or about 35 deaths, annually in the USA [199].

Hemolytic transfusion reactions

Hemolysis can occur as a result of HCT that is incompatible for ABO or other red cell antigens (see Chapter 60), but these are not transfusion complications and will not be considered here. The most common cause (about 41%) of transfusion fatalities reported to the FDA is ABO-incompatible transfusion [200]. Other causes of red cell hemolysis in transfusion recipients, such as improper storage or techniques of administering the blood, are not immunological [201,202]. ABO-incompatible hemolytic transfusion reactions are very dangerous because the patient has preformed ABO antibodies that often are immunoglobulin M (IgM) and bind complement, causing activation of the complement system with associated systemic manifestations and leading to red cell lysis. In addition, cytokines cause important biological effects in hemolytic transfusion reactions. There is substantial production of interleukin (IL)-1, IL-8 and tumor necrosis factor in response to red cell incompatibility [203], and these could act like a final common pathway for both the IgM and IgG red cell incompatible systems [203–205].

The nature and severity of the symptoms do not correlate with the severity or ultimate outcome of a hemolytic transfusion reaction [206,207]. Some patients may experience a severe reaction after only 20 mL of ABO-incompatible red cells, whereas others may tolerate an entire unit without signs or symptoms. The reaction may begin almost immediately upon beginning the transfusion or up to several hours after transfusion. The signs and symptoms that may accompany a hemolytic transfusion reaction are due to complement activation and release of cytokines and include fever, chills, flushing, low back pain, hypotension, dyspnea, abdominal pain, vomiting, diarrhea, chest pain or unexpected bleeding.

A delayed hemolytic transfusion reaction (DHTR) can occur in a patient in whom no red cell antibody was detected at the time of compatibility testing but who experiences accelerated destruction of the transfused red cells after an interval during which reactivation of a previous immune response to the transfused red cells occurs. The interval after transfusion may be as little as 24 h or up to about 1 week. A DHTR may be symptomatic or asymptomatic. When symptomatic, the most common symptom is a decrease in hemoglobin after transfusion [208], the way most DHTRs are identified. A DHTR can appear to be unexplained blood loss if repeat red cell antibody detection testing is not done.

Febrile nonhemolytic transfusion reactions

These reactions occur in association with about 0.5–1.0% of transfusions. It was believed that they are due to leukocyte antibodies present in the patients that react with leukocytes present in the transfused components. The severity of the reaction is directly related to the number of leukocytes in the blood component [209]. Febrile leukocyte reactions can be prevented by removing leukocytes from the blood components [210,211]. These febrile reactions to platelets have been studied more extensively and cytokines play a major role (see Reactions to platelet transfusions, p. 843). In red cell transfusions the relative contribution of leukocyte antibody-antigen reactions vs. cytokines released from contaminating leukocytes during storage is not known. Both mechanisms are probably important, and both can be prevented by the leukoreduction of the red cells shortly after they are collected—known as prestorage leukoreduction. Previously, the use of leukocyte-depleted blood components was not recommended routinely after a first febrile nonhemolytic transfusion (FNHT) reaction because there is only a 12% likelihood that a patient will experience a subsequent reaction [211]. As the use of leukodepleted red cells and platelets has become common for HCT patients, the time to convert to leukodepleted blood has become moot. Many FNHT reactions can also be prevented by the administration of antipyretics, such as acetaminophen, but the increased use of leukodepleted blood should decrease FNHT reactions and the need for antipyretics.

Allergic reactions

Allergic reactions that involve hives only with no other symptoms are probably the most frequent kind of reaction, occurring after 1–2% of transfusions. These reactions involve hives only with no other signs or symptoms. Allergic reactions are the only situation in which the transfusion is stopped and the patient can be given an antihistamine and the transfusion can be restarted after 15–30 min.

Pulmonary reactions—transfusion-related acute lung injury

A very severe type of transfusion reaction is the acute, sometimes fatal, pulmonary reaction that has been termed transfusion-related acute lung injury (TRALI) [212,213]. Patients develop acute respiratory distress, hypoxemia, diffuse pulmonary infiltrates on X-ray and the general clinical presentation of noncardiogenic pulmonary edema. Fever and hypotension may also occur and symptoms begin <6 h after the transfusion is initiated. Many cases have been reported [214], and TRALI has been estimated to occur once in 3000–5000 transfusions [214]. TRALI has been caused by all blood products, but it appears to be related to the plasma since in most cases the blood component contained at least 60 mL [214]. Leukocyte (HLA or granulocyte-specific) antibodies have been thought to be the inciting cause of TRALI, being found in almost 90% of cases [213]. It has been suggested that two events are necessary for TRALI to occur: first, a phenomenon, such as platelet activating factor or cytokines that accumulate in blood during storage [214,215] and cause general activation of neutrophils; and then, second, an insult, such as a leukocyte antibody, leading to pulmonary endothelial adherence and damage. It has been suggested that TRALI is more common than presently believed and that to avoid it, plasma from multiparous donors should not be used [214]. This strategy has not been pursued. The prompt recognition that pulmonary symptoms occurring during or shortly after transfusion could be due to TRALI allows prompt initiation of respiratory supportive therapy. This intervention is important because TRALI is a transient phenomenon that clears usually within 72 h.

Anaphylactic reactions

Patients who are IgA deficient and have anti-IgA antibodies may experience an anaphylactic reaction if they receive blood components that contain IgA [216]. The treatment is the same as for any anaphylactic reaction. The reactions can be prevented by using red cells or platelet concentrates, washed to remove plasma IgA, and using plasma components prepared from IgA-deficient donors.

Reactions to platelet transfusions

Patients with platelet or HLA antibodies may have febrile nonhemolytic reactions, probably due to leukocytes contained in the platelet concentrates. The reactions usually involve chills and fever, but platelets may be trapped in the pulmonary capillaries, causing dyspnea and pulmonary edema. These febrile nonhemolytic reactions occur following 5–30% of platelet transfusions [217]. The reactions have been thought to be due to antibodies to leukocytes and have been considered similar to febrile nonhemolytic reactions from units of red cells. Because these reactions sometimes occur in nontransfused males, are more common when stored platelets are used and are more related to the plasma than the platelets in the platelet concentrates, it has been suggested that some bioactive substance other than leukocyte antibodies might be involved [217]. Leukocytes in the platelet concentrates produce cytokines during storage, and platelet transfusion reactions are correlated with the concentration of IL-1 and IL-6 in the plasma. Thus, a landmark study [217] established that many (if not most) reactions to platelet transfusion are due to cytokines, not antigen-antibody reactions. Removal of the leukocytes soon after collection of the blood prevents the accumulation of cytokines in the platelet concentrate [123,218] and avoids platelet transfusion reactions [218]. Removal of leukocytes by bedside filtration at the time of transfusion does not decrease the incidence of platelet transfusion reactions [219]. Thus, many transplant centers are beginning to use platelet concentrates that are depleted of leukocytes either as part of the apheresis collection procedure or by filtration at the time of production, not later at the time of transfusion.

Allergic reactions can also occur with platelet transfusions. In one study, the IL-6 levels in platelet concentrates were correlated with allergic reactions [220], suggesting that cytokines might be involved in allergic as well as febrile reactions.

Reactions to granulocyte transfusions

Transfusion reactions are common following granulocyte transfusions, especially from random donors who are not HLA matched. Many of these reactions are probably due to the physiological activity of the large dose of leukocytes being administered to infected neutropenic patients or to cytokines contained in the granulocyte concentrate. Since granulocyte concentrates do not undergo a leukocyte cross-match, leukocyte incompatibility may be present in many granulocyte transfusions and may also account for some reactions.

Other immunological complications of transfusion

As a result of exposure to blood, patients may form antibodies to red cells, to lymphocyte, granulocyte or platelet surface antigens, or to plasma proteins. The likelihood of antibody formation depends on the immunogenicity of the antigen and the ability of the individual to mount an antibody response. Each kind of antibody can cause a particular clinical problem later if the patient requires subsequent transfusions, organ or tissue grafts, or becomes pregnant.

Bacterial contamination of units

Bacterial contamination continues to be an important complication of blood transfusion [221,222]. The extent of the problem is difficult to ascertain, but it is estimated that 1/3000–1/22,000 U of platelets are contaminated [223,224], although most of these do not cause a clinical problem. In France, it is estimated deaths due to contaminated platelets is 1/140,000 [225] and in the USA the death rate is estimated to be 1/71,000 apheresis platelet transfusions and 1/16,000 whole blood derived platelet units [226]. The number of deaths due to contaminated blood components reported to the FDA between 1986 and 1991 was twice as high as the number reported in the previous 10 years [227]. The two general types of problems are bacterial contamination of platelet concentrates stored at room temperature and transmission of bacteria, especially *Yersinia enterocolitica*, from red cells stored at refrigerator temperatures [221]. The approaches suggested to prevent transfusion of contaminated blood components include Gram staining, routine leukocyte depletion, the *Limulus* lysate assay for endotoxin, automated culture systems, antigen detection systems, immunological methods and nucleic acid probes, or the visual identification of infected units due to their different color. Although none of these methods is presently licensed by the FDA, blood banks are beginning to screen platelet concentrates for bacterial contamination. Because of the reduction in transmission of viral diseases that has occurred in the last decade, bacterial contamination of blood components is now potentially the most serious complication of transfusion, especially in the immunocompromised recipient.

Nonimmunological complications of blood transfusion

Nonimmunological complications of transfusion [228] include hypothermia from transfusion of large volumes of red cells that have been stored in the refrigerator, citrate toxicity that may manifest itself as hypocalcemia, and a bleeding tendency since red cells suspended in the additive preservative solution do not provide coagulation factor replacement. Proper management of fluid balance can avoid circulatory overload. Iron overload is a complication of patients who receive many transfusions, patients with hemoglobinopathies. It is a problem in HCT for patients with thalassemia major and may require an iron removal program following HCT (see Chapter 103) [229,230]. Air or particulate emboli that were a problem in the early days of transfusion no longer occur if proper techniques are used to administer the blood.

Transfusion-transmitted diseases

The acquired immune deficiency syndrome (AIDS) epidemic has greatly increased the fear of transfusion-transmitted diseases. As a result, there have been great changes in the nature of transfusion practice and the regulation of blood banks by the FDA [231,232]. The risks of transfusion can be reduced by improving donor selection, improving transmissible disease testing, reducing the number of donor exposures and reducing blood use (Tables 61.3 & 61.4). Physicians have become much more conservative in the use of blood by changing the indications for transfusion and by using pharmacological substitutes. The number of donor exposures has been reduced by using autologous blood, and directed-donor and limited-donor programs. Donor eligibility criteria have been changed to reflect the understanding of behavior that places potential donors at risk of transmitting disease. The number of donor screening questions has increased by about 30% and the nature of the questions has changed to become quite specific. These strategies have been remarkably successful.

Table 61.3 Strategies to reduce transfusion-transmitted disease.

Improve donor selection
Improve transmissible disease testing:
    Reduce donor exposure
        Autologous blood
        Directed-donor programs
        Limited-donor programs
Decrease blood use
    Changed indications for transfusion
    Pharmacological stimulation or substitution
Modification of the blood component
Viral and bacterial inactivation
Blood substitutes

Table 61.4 Methods of reducing the infectivity of the blood supply.

Recruitment health criteria
Medical history
Physical examination
Donor deferral registry
Laboratory tests
Donor call back
Confidential unit exclusion

Table 61.5 Estimated risk of transfusion-transmitted infections in the USA. From Glynn et al. [239] and Dodd et al. [240].

	Present FDA licensed tests		Licensed tests plus NAT		
	Risk/10^6 donations	Case/units	Risk/10^6 donations	Case/units	Estimated no. of cases annually*
HIV	0.7	1,400,000	0.5	2,000,000	6
HCV	3.6	280,000	0.5	2,000,000	6
HBV	4.9	204,000	4.0	250,000	48

*Based on 12,000,000 U of whole blood collected annually in the USA. FDA, Food and Drug Administration; HBV, hepatitis B virus; HCV, hepatitis C virus; HIV, human immunodeficiency virus; NAT, nucleic acid amplification test.

agent rather than antibodies to the agent. NAT testing is farthest along in implementation. Screening tests for HIV and hepatitis C virus (HCV) detect antibodies to these viruses and, thus, there is a "window phase" between exposure to the virus and the development of a positive screening test. During this window phase, the blood can be infectious. In order to eliminate these infectious donors, NAT methods have been developed [236–238]. Although these kinds of tests are not yet licensed by the FDA, all blood collected in the USA is presently being screened for HIV and HCV using NAT. It is hoped that this testing strategy will virtually eliminate the window phase of blood donor infectivity. Present estimates of transmission are shown in Table 61.5 [239,240]. A brief review of transfusion-transmitted diseases is presented below.

Syphilis

Transmission of syphilis by blood transfusion was common in the early days of blood transfusion but now it is extremely rare, the last case being reported in 1966 [241,242]. Syphilis testing is still required of all donated blood despite the fact that the test is almost always negative when circulating spirochetes are present. In the early days of the AIDS epidemic, it was believed that testing for syphilis might be a surrogate to identify sexually promiscuous donors who would be at increased risk for transmitting HIV. This assumption has not proved to be correct and syphilis testing today may [242,243] or may not [244] have value but has not yet been eliminated by the FDA.

Hepatitis

Post-transfusion hepatitis is the most common disease transmitted by blood transfusion and is a major public health problem. It can be caused by the hepatitis A virus, hepatitis B virus, hepatitis C virus, CMV, or Epstein–Barr virus, or may be defined as non-A, non-B, or non-C, which means hepatitis due to none of these agents. It is difficult to provide a single estimate of the frequency of occurrence of post-transfusion hepatitis because the incidence depends on the blood donor population, when the studies were done and the type of patients involved. Prospective studies involving the period 1974–81 showed rates of post-transfusion hepatitis that ranged from 5.9% to 21.0% of patients [245]. The incidence of post-transfusion hepatitis was substantially reduced in the USA and other countries in the early 1970s due to the conversion from paid donors to volunteer donors [246].

Hepatitis A

Hepatitis A usually has a short period of viremia, symptoms occur early during the viremic phase and there is no carrier state. Because there is no chronic viremia and symptoms coincide with the acute viremic phase,

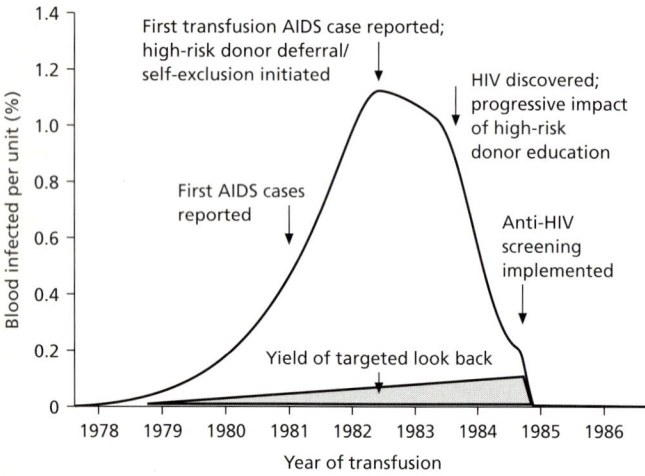

Fig. 61.1 Impact of different donor screening procedures on the estimated infectivity of blood by the human immune deficiency virus (HIV) in San Francisco, California. Adapted from Busch et al. [258] with permission.

For instance, changes in donor selection resulted in a 90% decrease in the human immunodeficiency virus (HIV) infectivity of the blood supply in the San Francisco Bay area even before the introduction of the anti-HIV test (Fig. 61.1). Presently a complex process is used to obtain the safest possible donors.

Laboratory testing of donated blood has also greatly expanded. Starting with the introduction of the test for HIV, the number of routine infectious disease screening tests done on each unit of blood increased from two to eight. These steps have been extremely effective in reducing the risks of blood transfusion [233–235]. The additional strategies being developed to further improve blood safety are: (i) development of blood substitutes that are free of disease; (ii) development of methods of inactivating viruses and bacteria in blood components; and (iii) implementation of nucleic acid amplification tests (NATs) for the actual infectious

infectious donors are usually identified by medical history. Thus, post-transfusion hepatitis A is rare [247,248]. Laboratory testing of blood donors for hepatitis A is not done. Hepatitis A can be transmitted by coagulation factor concentrates or rarely by plasma derivatives. In evaluating a patient with suspected post-transfusion hepatitis, hepatitis A should be considered, but only as a remote possibility.

Hepatitis B

Most people infected with the hepatitis B virus are asymptomatic and, thus, an apparently healthy individual may meet all of the donor medical history criteria and donate a unit of infectious blood. The adoption of routine screening of blood donors for hepatitis B surface antigen reduced the incidence of post-transfusion hepatitis B. Despite testing for transfusion-transmitted hepatitis B, it is now the most common transfusion-transmitted viral infection [240]. This is probably because some infectious carriers have a level of viremia below the limit of detection in the antigen-screening test.

Hepatitis C

In 1989, an RNA virus similar in classification to a togavirus [249] was identified and termed hepatitis C because it appears to account for most post-transfusion non-A and non-B hepatitis [250]. Acute hepatitis C is usually mild, with up to 80% of patients being asymptomatic [251]. However, the long-term effects are more serious because the virus tends to be persistent and the condition develops into chronic liver disease [251,252]. It has been estimated that introduction of hepatitis C testing of blood donors has prevented about 40,000 cases of post-transfusion hepatitis C annually in the USA [251]. Thus, some transfusion-transmitted hepatitis C remains but it is estimated that there is only about 50, or fewer, cases per year in the USA (Table 61.5).

Hepatitis G

Despite the discovery of the hepatitis C virus and implementation of screening donated blood for this virus, a few patients with post-transfusion hepatitis test negative for the known hepatitis viruses [253–255]. A new RNA virus called hepatitis G or GB virus has been identified in some of these patients. From 1% to 4% of normal blood donors are carriers of hepatitis G when polymerase chain reaction (PCR) techniques are used [254,255]. The apparent association of GB virus with hepatitis is probably due to similarities between GB virus and hepatitis C. The designation "hepatitis" virus was premature and GBV is not considered a cause of transfusion-transmitted hepatitis [255]. There is no practical test and no established role of hepatitis G in disease transmission. Presently there is no plan to screen blood donors for the virus.

TT virus

Although the designation of this virus suggests that it is "transfusion-transmitted," the nomenclature signifies the initials of the patient from whom it was isolated. The TT virus was found in a patient with unexplained hepatitis and was thought to be a new viral hepatitis agent [255,256]. Although the TT virus is prevalent in blood donors and can be transmitted to as many as 30% of transfusion recipients, it is not associated with hepatitis [257].

Human immunodeficiency virus (HIV)

Although HIV-1 infection can be transmitted by blood transfusion [258–261], only a very small proportion of AIDS cases are due to transfusion. As was mentioned previously, changes in donor eligibility criteria reduced the infectivity of blood by about 90% in the San Francisco Bay area before the introduction of the laboratory test for the HIV virus [258]. The risk of acquiring HIV infection following transfusion with anti-HIV-1-positive blood is as high as 70–91% [262]. It has been estimated that before the introduction of HIV-1 antibody testing in May 1985 approximately 12,000 patients were infected with HIV-1 by transfusion [263].

Because there is the interval or "window" between infection and development of antibody to the infecting virus, HIV infection can be transmitted by anti-HIV-negative donors if they are in this window period [264,265]. Using reagents currently licensed by the FDA, the window period is estimated to be about 11 days [239]. The screening of blood for the HIV antigen might be an effective way of reducing or eliminating transmission of infection by blood donated during the window phase [266]. Two large studies involving approximately 500,000 donors each did not identify any donors whose serum contained HIV antigen but no HIV antibody [267,268]. Although these studies indicated that HIV antigen testing would not be helpful, the FDA requires the antigen test as an additional approach to reducing the possibility of transfusion-transmitted HIV. Another approach to reducing the window phase includes the use of methods to amplify DNA or RNA sequences, thus making it possible to detect minute amounts of proviral DNA [236]. As mentioned previously, this testing is now underway [237–240].

Human T-lymphotrophic virus (HTLV)-1/2

HTLV-1 is the first retrovirus that has been shown to cause malignancy, adult T-cell leukemia (ATL), in humans [269]. The virus is also associated with a form of myelopathy referred to as HTLV associated myelopathy or tropical spastic paraparesis (TSP) [270]. Donors with a true positive test for HTLV-1/2 have approximately a 1–5% chance of developing ATL during a 70-year life span and another 2% may develop TSP within 5–10 years of initial infection [271]. Although no cases of transfusion-transmitted ATL or TSP have been identified, transmission of the virus by blood transfusion does occur [272]. Approximately 60% of seronegative recipients developed anti-HTLV-1 after transfusion of cellular blood products containing anti-HTLV-1 [270,272]. In the USA, anti-HTLV-1 is found almost exclusively in intravenous drug abusers or persons from areas that are endemic for HTLV-1. Because of the potential for disease transmission, although no cases of transfusion-transmitted ATL have been identified, routine testing of all donated blood for anti-HTLV-1 was initiated in the USA in December 1988 [273]. It is hoped that this step will avoid the potential problem of transfusion-transmitted ALT or TSP.

Parvovirus

The parvovirus B19 has been transmitted by blood transfusion (see Chapter 57) [274,275]. The prevalence of parvovirus in blood donors is estimated to be 1/3300–1/50,000 [274,275]. The low prevelence, combined with the brief period of viremia, makes transmission of parvovirus by blood transfusion rare. When transmission occurs, it usually involves coagulation factor concentrates [275], although a few cases of transmission by single donor components have been reported [275–277].

Epstein–Barr virus (EBV)

Infection with EBV is followed by a lifelong carrier state and most adults have been infected (see Chapter 56). EBV can be transmitted by transfusion [278,279], usually as the "post-perfusion" syndrome, a virus-like illness that occurs after transfusion of fresh blood during open-heart surgery. Transfusion transmission of EBV has not been a major clinical problem in HCT (see Chapter 56), although it can be transmitted to organ recipients [279].

Parasitic diseases

It has been known for years that some parasites are transmitted by transfusion. All species of *Plasmodium* can survive in refrigerated blood and have caused transfusion-transmitted malaria, although most cases involve *P. malariae*. Malaria parasites are still viable and able to induce malaria infection after storage of the blood for a week in a refrigerator. All components, including RBCs, white blood cells, platelet concentrates and fresh plasma can transmit malaria [280]. The prevention of transfusion-transmitted malaria relies on the exclusion of asymptomatic carriers based on residence or travel to an endemic area. However, in most cases of post-transfusion malaria, the interview failed to exclude the infectious donors. Laboratory tests are not used in the USA for screening donors for malaria. Thus, periodic spiking fever in a patient who has recently received a transfusion could be due to malaria, but this is very unlikely in North America because donor selection procedures are designed to identify potentially infectious donors.

Trypanosoma cruzi is endemic in many parts of Central and South America. Many patients with chronic *T. cruzi* infection may be asymptomatic and, thus, could pass the blood donor medical questions. *Trypansoma cruzi* survives in refrigerated blood and can be transmitted by transfusion [281], although this event is rare in the USA [281]. As the number of immigrants from endemic areas increases, transfusion-transmitted *T. cruzi* could become a larger problem. For instance, in the Los Angeles area, which has a large Latin-American population, about 1/1000 donors has antibodies to *T. cruzi* [281,282]. Presently efforts are under way to develop improved antibody detection tests and to design medical history questions to identify donors at risk in hopes of reducing or eliminating the potential of transfusion-transmitted *T cruzi* [283].

Babesia microti and *B. bovi* are protozoa that occasionally infect humans by tick bites. Many infected individuals are asymptomatic and, thus, *B. microti* can be transmitted by blood donated by asymptomatic infected donors [284,285]. The ticks are prevalent in the North-East, mid-Atlantic and upper midwest of the USA. Because no suitable laboratory screening test exists, some blood banks defer individuals from heavily tick-infested areas during the summer months.

Borrelia burgdorferi, the spirochete that causes Lyme disease, is transmitted by ticks to humans. In up to 40% of persons the infection is asymptomatic, and the spirochetes survive in stored blood for up to 45 days [286]. Thus, transmission of *B. burgdorferi* by transfusion is theoretically possible, but this has not been reported [285]. Although a serological test is available, it is not a suitable laboratory test for donor screening and the widespread prevalence of the tick makes it impractical to defer donors from endemic areas.

Creutzfeldt–Jakob disease (CJD)

A variant of CJD that appears to be associated with ingestion of beef from cows affected with bovine spongiform encephalopathy or "mad cow disease" [287] raised the question of whether the variant of CJD could be transmitted by blood transfusion. Since the exact cause of CJD is not known, there is no laboratory test to identify the infectious agent if one exists. CJD has been transmitted by dura, corneas and pituitary growth hormone from CJD patients and electroencephalographic electrodes used on CJD patients [288]. Prions, thought to be involved in CJD, are highly resistant to inactivation with methods currently used in the production of plasma derivatives. Thus, even 1 U of plasma contaminated with the CJD agent could render a large amount of plasma derivatives infectious. There is no evidence of blood-borne transmission or of a recent "outbreak" of CJD in the USA [289]. However, during the past few years several instances have been recognized in which a blood donor subsequently developed CJD. Whether CJD will prove to be a threat to the blood supply and blood safety remains to be learned [290,291].

West Nile virus

This virus, newly arrived in the USA, has epidemiologic characteristics that suggest it could be transmitted by blood transfusion [292]. Mosquitoes are the vector, mosquito bites are common, there is transient viremia shortly after infection and most infected persons are asymptomatic, especially during the period of viremia [293]. Thus, an infected individual could donate blood. Although no cases of transfusion-transmitted West Nile infection have been reported, it seems likely that this problem can occur. Because HCT patients are severely immunosuppressed, such an infection could become quite serious. Blood banks have moved quickly to develop a screening test and as of the summer of 2003, almost all blood is tested by WNV.

Summary of transfusion-transmitted diseases

The diseases of most concern for transmission by blood transfusion have been discussed here. However, there is a concern that emerging pathogens, the mobility of people and continued immigration can alter the situation with transfusion-transmitted diseases. Blood safety depends on many strategies, not just laboratory testing. The donor medical history and the use of volunteer donors are excellent examples. When considering a new screening test, many factors about the infectious agent and the disease must be taken into consideration. Examples are the prevalence of the disease, infectivity of the agent, status of the epidemic and likelihood of a carrier state. Although some of the diseases may be regional in nature, the mobility of the population may make regional screening practices unsuitable. However, when all of the scientific discussion is completed, the issues of social policy and the public expectations of its blood supply remain. The public expects the transfusion medicine community to take steps to achieve the maximum possible safety. In the past, policy makers and politicians have shown little tolerance for failure to take steps that would decrease risks to their constituents regardless of the cost. For instance, the cost of laboratory tests and additional regulations during the past decade have probably increased the cost of blood by 50% and it has been estimated that introduction of NAT testing for HIV and HCV costs $4–11,000 000 for each quality adjusted life year [294]. A more rational approach to blood safety has been sought by many and has been publicly advocated by at least two thoughtful, knowledgeable transfusion medicine professionals [295,296]. However, the decision-making process is still a complex one with no easily discernible structure for these decisions.

Conclusion

The kinds of blood products available for transfusion have become sophisticated and transfusion strategies are complex. Beginning with the diagnosis and treatment of the underlying disease, transfusion therapy is designed to minimize its interference with successful engraftment. Following transplantation, patient transfusion needs can be met effectively. The blood supply is safer than ever and, although some risks of infection remain, most patients can be supported safely and effectively.

Acknowledgment

Portions of this chapter were taken from McCullough, J. Transfusion Medicine, McGraw Hill, New York, NY, 1998.

References

1 McCullough J. The role of the blood bank in transplantation. *Arch Pathol Lab Med* 1991; **115**: 1195–200.

2 National Institutes of Health Consensus Conference: perioperative red blood cell transfusion. *JAMA* 1988; **260**: 2700–3.

3 Robertie PG, Gravlee GP. Safe limits of isovolemic hemodilution and recommendations for erythrocyte transfusion. *Int Anesthesiol Clin* 1990; **28**: 197–204.

4 Welch HG, Meehan KR, Goodnough LT. Prudent strategies for elective red blood cell transfusion. *Ann Intern Med* 1992; **116**: 393–402.

5 American College of Physicians. Practice strategies for elective red blood cell transfusion. *Ann Intern Med* 1992; **116**: 403–6.

6 Carson JL, Herbert PC. Anemia and red cell transfusion. In: Simon TL, Dzik WH, Snyder E *et al*., eds. *Rossi's Principles of Transfusion Medicine*. Philadelphia: Lippincott, Williams & Wilkins, 2002; 149–64.

7 Hebert PC, Wells G, Blajchman MA *et al*. A multicenter, randomized, controlled clinical trial of transfusion requirements in critical care. Transfusion requirements in critical care investigators, Canadian Critical Care Trials Group. *N Engl J Med* 1999; **340**: 409–17.

8 Carson JL, Terrin ML, Barton FB *et al*. A pilot randomized trial comparing symptomatic vs. hemoglobin-level-driven red blood cell transfusions following hip fracture. *Transfusion* 1998; **38**: 522–9.

9 Hebert PC, Wells G, Tweeddale M *et al*. Does transfusion practice affect mortality in critically ill patients? *Am J Resp Crit Care Med* 1997; **155**: 1618–23.

10 Engelfriet CP, Reesink HW, McCullough J *et al*. Perioperative triggers for red cell transfusions. *Vox Sanguinis* 2002; **82**: 215–26.

11 Hillman RS. Acute blood loss anemia. In: Beutler E, Lichtman MA, Coller BS, Kipps TJ, eds. *Williams Hematology*, 5th edn. New York: McGraw-Hill, 1995: 704–8.

12 Dzik S, Aubuchon J, Jeffries L *et al*. Leukocyte reduction of blood components: public policy and new technology. *Transfus Med Rev* 2000; **14**: 34–52.

13 Miller JP, Mintz PD. The use of leukocyte-reduced blood components. *Transfus Med* 1995; **9**: 69–90.

14 Sweeney JD. Universal leukoreduction of cellular blood components in 2001? *Am J Clin Pathol* 2001; **115**: 665–77.

15 Vamvakas EC, Blajchman MA. Universal WBC reduction: the case for and against. *Transfusion* 2001; **41**: 691–712.

16 Ching EP, Poon MC, Neurath D *et al*. Red blood cell alloimmunization complicating plasma transfusion. *Am J Clin Pathol* 1991; **96**: 201–2.

17 National Institutes of Health Consensus Conference. Fresh frozen plasma: indications and risks. *JAMA* 1985; **253**: 551–3.

18 Ness PM, Perkins HA. Cryoprecipitate as a reliable source of fibrinogen replacement. *JAMA* 1979; **241**: 1690–1.

19 Rosati LA, Barnes B, Oberman H, Penner J. Hemolytic anemia due to anti-A in concentrated hemophilia factor preparations. *Transfusion* 1970; **10**: 139–41.

20 Slichter SJ, Harker LA. Preparation and storage of platelet concentrates. II. Storage and variables influence platelet viability and function. *Br J Haematol* 1976; **34**: 403–19.

21 Murphy S, Heaton WA, Rebulla P. Platelet production in the old world—and the new. *Transfusion* 1996; **36**: 751–4.

22 Murphy S, Gardner FH. Platelet preservation—effect of storage temperature on maintenance of platelet viability—deleterious effect of refrigerated storage. *N Engl J Med* 1969; **380**: 1094–8.

23 Murphy S, Sayer SN, Gardner FH. Storage of platelet concentrates at 22°C. *Blood* 1970; **35**: 549–57.

24 Handin RI, Valeri CR. Hemostatic effectiveness of platelets stored at 22°C. *N Engl J Med* 1971; **285**: 538–43.

25 Becker GA, Tucceli MT, Kunicki T, Chalos MK, Aster RH. Studies of platelet concentrates stored at 22°C and 4°C. *Transfusion* 1973; **13**: 61–8.

26 Filip DJ, Aster RH. Relative hemostatic effectiveness of human platelets stored at 4°C and 22°C. *J Lab Clin Med* 1978; **91**: 618–24.

27 Kunicki TJ, Tuccelli M, Becker GA, Aster RH. A study of variables affecting the quality of platelets stored at "room temperature." *Transfusion* 1975; **15**: 414–21.

28 Scott EP, Slichter SJ. Viability and funtion of platelet concentrates stored in CPD-adenine (CPDA-I). *Transfusion* 1980; **20**: 489–97.

29 Holme S, Vaidja K, Murphy S. Platelet storage at 22°C. Effect of type of agitation on morphology, viability, and function *in vitro*. *Blood* 1978; **52**: 425–35.

30 Murphy S, Kahn RA, Holme S *et al*. Improved storage of platelets for transfusion in a new container. *Blood* 1982; **60**: 194–200.

31 Simon TL, Nelson EJ, Murphy S. Extension of platelet concentrate storage to 7 days in second-generation bags. *Transfusion* 1987; **27**: 6–9.

32 Heal JM, Singal S, Sardisco E, Mayer T. Bacterial proliferation in platelet concentrates. *Transfusion* 1986; **26**: 388–90.

33 Braine HG, Kickler TS, Charache P *et al*. Bacterial sepsis secondary to platelet transfusion: an adverse effect of extended storage at room temperature. *Transfusion* 1986; **26**: 391–3.

34 Schiffer CA, Lee EJ, Ness PM, Reilly J. Clinical evaluation of platelet concentrates stored for 1–5 days. *Blood* 1986; **67**: 1591–4.

35 Simon TL, Sierra ER. Concentration of platelet units into small volumes. *Transfusion* 1984; **24**: 173–5.

36 Moroff G, Friedman A, Robkin-Kline L *et al*. Reduction of the volume of stored platelet concentrates for use in neonatal patients. *Transfusion* 1984; **24**: 144–6.

37 McCullough J, Steeper TA, Connelly DP, Jackson B, Huntington S, Scott ER. Platelet utilization in a university hospital. *JAMA* 1988; **259**: 2414–8.

38 McCullough J, Vesole D, Benjamin RJ *et al*. Pathogen inactivated platelets using Helinx technology (INTERCEPT) are hemostatically effective in thrombocytopenic patients: The SPRINT trial. *Blood* 2001; **98**: 450a [Abstract].

39 Hersch EM, Bodey GP, Nies BA, Freireich EJ. Causes of death in acute leukemia: a 10-year study of 414 patients from 1954 to 1963. *JAMA* 1965; **193**: 105–9.

40 Gaydos LA, Freireich EJ, Mantel N. The quantitative relation between platelet count and hemorrhage in patients with acute leukemia. *N Engl J Med* 1962; **266**: 905–12.

41 Roy AJ, Jaffe N, Djerassi I. Prophylactic platelet transfusions in children with acute leukemia: a dose–response study. *Transfusion* 1973; **13**: 283–90.

42 Higby DJ, Cohen E, Holland JF, Sinks L. The prophylactic treatment of thrombocytopenic leukemia patients with platelets: a double blind study. *Transfusion* 1974; **14**: 440–6.

43 Solomon J, Bokufkamp T, Fahey JL *et al*. Platelet prophylaxis in acute nonlymphocytic leukemia. *Lancet* 1978; **1**: 267.

44 Han T, Stutzman L, Cohen E *et al*. Effect of platelet transfusion on hemorrhage in patients with acute leukemia. *Cancer* 1966; **19**: 1937–42.

45 Murphy S, Litwin S, Herring LM *et al*. Indications for platelet transfusion in children with acute leukemia. *Am J Hematol* 1982; **12**: 347–53.

46 Slichter SJ. Controversies in platelet transfusion therapy. *Annu Rev Med* 1980; **31**: 509–40.

47 Pisciotto PT, Benson K, Hume H *et al*. Prophylactic versus therapeutic platelet transfusion practices in hematology and/or oncology patients. *Transfusion* 1995; **35**: 498–502.

48 Slichter S, Harker LA. Thrombocytopenia: mechanisms and management of defects in platelet production. *Clin Haematol* 1978; **7**: 523–9.

49 Patten E. Controversies in transfusion medicine—prophylactic platelet transfusion revisited after 25 years: con. *Transfusion* 1992; **32**: 381–5.

50 Belt RJ, Leite C, Haas CD, Stephens RL. Incidence of hemorrhagic complications in patients with cancer. *JAMA* 1978; **239**: 2571–4.

51 National Institutes of Health Consensus Conference. Platelet transfusion therapy. *JAMA* 1987; **257**: 1777–80.

52 Aderka D, Praff G, Santo M. Bleeding due to thrombocytopenia in acute leukemias and reevaluation of the prophylactic platelet transfusion policy. *Am J Med Sci* 1986; **291**: 147–51.

53 Gmur J, Burger J, Schanz U, Fehr J, Schaffner A. Safety of stringent prophylactic platelet transfusion policy for patients with acute leukaemia. *Lancet* 1991; **338**: 1223–6.

54 Heckman KD, Weiner GJ, Davis CS *et al*. Randomized study of prophylactic platelet transfusion threshold during induction therapy for adult acute leukemia: 10,000/µL versus 20,000/µL. *J Clin Oncol* 1997; **15**: 1143–9.

55 Rebulla P, Finazzi G, Marangoni F *et al*. The threshold for prophylactic platelet transfusions in adults with acute myeloid leukemia. *N Engl J Med* 1997; **337**: 1870–5.

56 Wandt H, Frank M, Ehninger G *et al*. Safety and cost effectiveness of a 10×10^9/L trigger for prophylactic platelet transfusions compared with the traditional 20×10^9/L trigger: a prospective comparative trial in 105 patients with acute myeloid leukemia. *Blood* 1998; **91**: 3601–6.

57 Gil-Fernandez JJ, Alegre A, Fernandez-Villalta MJ *et al*. Clinical results of a stringent policy on prophylactic platelet transfusion: non-randomized comparative analysis in 190 bone marrow transplant patients from a single institution. *Bone Marrow Transplant* 1996; **18**: 931–5.

58 Zumberg MS, del Rosario MLU, Nejame CF *et al*. A prospective randomized trial of prophylactic platelet transfusion and bleeding incidence in hematopoietic stem cell transplant recipients: 10,000/µL versus 20,000/µL trigger. *Biol Blood Marrow Transplant* 2002; **8**: 569–76.

59 Heddle N, Cook RJ, Webert KE, Sigouin C, Rebulla P. Methodological issues in the use of bleeding as an outcome in transfusion medicine studies. *Transfusion* 2003; **43**: 742–52.

60 Beutler E. Platelet transfusions: the 20,000/µL trigger. *Blood* 1993; **81**: 1411–3.

61 Bernstein SHH, Nademanee AP, Vose JM *et al*. A multicenter study of platelet recovery and utilization in patients after myeloablative therapy and hematopoietic stem cell transplantation. *Blood* 1998; **91**: 3509–17.

62 Nemo S, Swan V, Enger C. Acute bleeding after bone marrow transplantation (BMT)—incidence and effect of survival. A quantitative analysis in 1402 patients. *Blood* 1998; **91**: 1469–77.

63 Hersh JK, Hom EG, Brecher ME. Mathematical

modeling of platelet survival with implications for optimal transfusion practice in the chronically platelet transfusion-dependent patient. *Transfusion* 1998; **38**: 637–44.
64 Goodnough LT, Kuter DJ, McCullough J et al. Prophylactic platelet transfusions from healthy normal apheresis platelet donors undergoing treatment thrombopoietin. *Blood* 2001; **98**: 1346–51.
65 Harker LA, Slichter SJ. The bleeding time as a screening test for evaluation of platelet function. *N Engl J Med* 1972; **287**: 155–9.
66 Bishop JF, Schiffer CA, Aisner J, Matthews JP, Wiernik PH. Surgery in acute leukemia. A review of 167 operations in thrombocytopenic patients. *Am J Hematol* 1987; **26**: 147–55.
67 Freireich EJ, Kliman A, Gaydos LA et al. Response to repeated platelet transfusions from the same donor. *Ann Intern Med* 1963; **50**: 277–81.
68 Daly PA, Schiffer CA, Aisner J, Wiernik PH. Platelet transfusion therapy: 1 hour posttransfusion increments are valuable in predicting the need for HLA matched preparations. *JAMA* 1980; **243**: 435–8.
69 Dunstan RA, Simpson MB, Knowles RW, Rosse WE. The origin of ABO antigens on human platelets. *Blood* 1985; **65**: 615–9.
70 Aster RH. Effect of anticoagulant and ABO incompatibility on recovery of transfused human platelets. *Blood* 1965; **26**: 732–43.
71 Duquesnoy RJ, Anderson AJ, Tomasulo PA, Aster RH. ABO compatibility and platelet transfusions of alloimmunized thrombocytopenic patients. *Blood* 1979; **54**: 595–9.
72 Skogen B, Rossebo Hansen B, Husebekk A, Havnes T, Hannestad K. Minimal expression of blood group A antigen on thrombocytes from A_2 individuals. *Transfusion* 1988; **28**: 456–9.
73 Heal JM, Blumberg N, Masel D. An evaluation of crossmatching, HLA, and ABO matching for platelet transfusions to refractory patients. *Blood* 1987; **70**: 23–30.
74 Ogasawara K, Ueki J, Takenaka M, Furihata K. Study on the expression of ABH antigens on platelets. *Blood* 1993; **82**: 993–9.
75 Heal JM, Masel D, Blumberg N. Interaction of platelet Fc and complement receptors with circulating immune complexes involving the ABO system. *Vox Sang* 1996; **71**: 205–11.
76 Heal JM, Masel D, Rowe JM, Blumberg N. Circulating immune complexes involving the ABO system after platelet transfusion. *Br J Haematol* 1993; **85**: 566–72.
77 Lee EJ, Schiffer CA. ABO compatibility can influence the results of platelet transfusion: Results of a randomized trial. *Transfusion* 1989; **29**: 384–9.
78 Murphy S. ABO blood groups and platelet transfusion. *Transfusion* 1988; **28**: 401–2.
79 Goldfinger D, McGinnis MA. Rh incompatible platelet transfusions-risks and consequences of sensitizing immunosuppressed patients. *N Engl J Med* 1971; **284**: 942–4.
80 Lichtiger B, Surgeon J, Rhorer S. Rh-incompatible platelet transfusion therapy in cancer patients. *Vox Sang* 1983; **45**: 139–41.
81 Baldwin ML, Ness PM, Scott D, Braine H, Kickler TS. Alloimmunization to D antigen and HLA in D-negative immunosuppressed oncology patients. *Transfusion* 1988; **28**: 330–3.
82 McLeod BC, Piehl MR, Sassetti RJ. Alloimmunization to RhD by platelet transfusions in autologous bone marrow transplant recipients. *Vox Sang* 1990; **49**: 185–9.

83 Menitove JE. Immunoprophylaxis for D− patients receiving platelet transfusions from D− donors? *Transfusion* 2002; **42**: 136–8.
84 Molnar R, Johnson R, Seat LT, Geiger TL. Absence of D alloimmunization in D− pediatric oncology patients receiving D-incompatible single-donor platelets. *Transfusion* 2002; **42**: 177–82.
85 Cid J, Ortin X, Elies E et al. Absence of anti-D alloimmunization in hematologic patients after D-incompatible platelet transfusions. *Transfusion* 2002; **42**: 173–6.
86 Pfisterer H, Thierfelder S, Kottusch H, Stich W. Untersuchung menschlicher thrombocyten auf Rhesusantigene durch abbaustudien *in vivo* nach 51Cr-markierung. *Klin Wochenschr* 1967; **45**: 5519–22.
87 Aster RJ, Jandl JH. Platelet sequestration in man. II. Immunological and conical studies. *J Clin Invest* 1964; **43**: 869–73.
88 Bishop JF, McGrath K, Wolf MM et al. Clinical factors influencing the efficacy of pooled platelet transfusions. *Blood* 1988; **71**: 383–7.
89 Doughty HA, Murphy MF, Metcalfe P et al. Relative importance of immune and non-immune causes of platelet refractoriness. *Vox Sang* 1994; **66**: 200–5.
90 Dutcher JP, Schiffer CA, Aisner J, Wiernik PH. Alloimmunization following platelet transfusion. The absence of a dose–response relationship. *Blood* 1981; **57**: 395–8.
91 Dutcher JP, Schiffer CA, Aisner J, Wiernik PH. Long-term follow-up of patients with leukemia receiving platelet transfusions: identification of a large group of patients who do not become alloimmunized. *Blood* 1981; **58**: 1007–11.
92 The Trial to Reduce Alloimmunization to Platelets Study Group. Leukocyte reduction and ultraviolet B irradiation of platelets to prevent alloimmunization and refractoriness to platelet transfusions. *N Engl J Med* 1997; **337**: 1861–9.
93 Lazarus HM, Herzig RH, Warm SE, Fishman DJ. Transfusion experience with platelet concentrates stored for 24–72 hours at 22°C. *Transfusion* 1982; **22**(39): 39–43.
94 Yankee RA, Graff KS, Dowling R, Henderson ES. Selection of unrelated compatible platelet donors by lymphocyte HL-A matching. *N Engl J Med* 1973; **288**: 760–4.
95 Lohrman HP, Bull MI, Decter JA et al. Platelet transfusions from HLA compatible unrelated donors to alloimmunized patients. *Ann Intern Med* 1974; **80**: 9–14.
96 Duquesnoy RJ, Filip DJ, Rodey GE et al. Successful transfusion of platelets 'mismatched' for HLA antigens to alloimmunized thrombocytopenic patients. *Am J Hematol* 1977; **2**: 219–23.
97 Duquesnoy RJ, Vieira J, Aster RH. Donor availability for platelet transfusion support of alloimmunized thrombocytopenic patients. *Transplant Proc* 1977; **9**: 519–21.
98 McFarland JG, Anderson AJ, Slichter SJ. Factors influencing the transfusion response to HLA-selected apheresis donor platelets in patients refractory to random platelet concentrates. *Br J Haematol* 1989; **73**: 380–6.
99 Moroff G, Garratty G, Heal JM et al. Selection of platelets for refractory patients by HLA matching and prospective crossmatching. *Transfusion* 1992; **32**: 633–40.
100 Rachel JM, Sinor LT, Tawfik OW et al. A solid-phase red cell adherence test for platelet cross-matching. *Med Lab Sci* 1985; **42**: 194–5.

101 Rachel JM, Summers TC, Sinor LT, Plapp FV. Use of a solid phase red blood cell adherence method for pretransfusion platelet compatibility testing. *Am J Clin Pathol* 1988; **90**: 63–8.
102 O'Connell BA, Lee EJ, Rothko K, Hussein MA, Schiffer CA. Selection of histocompatibility apheresis platelet donors by cross-matching random donor platelet concentrates. *Blood* 1992; **79**: 527–31.
103 Friedberg RC, Donnelly SF, Boyd JC, Gray LS, Mintz PD. Clinical and blood bank factors in the management of platelet refractoriness and alloimmunization. *Blood* 1993; **81**: 3428–34.
104 Bensinger WI, Buckner C, Clift RA, Slichter SJ, Thomas ED. Plasma exchange for platelet alloimmunization. *Transplantation* 1986; **41**: 602–5.
105 Howe RB, Christie DJ. Protein A immunoadsorption treatment in hematology: an overview. *J Clin Apheresis* 1994; **9**: 31–2.
106 Christie DJ, Howe RB, Lennon SS, Sauro SC. Treatment of refractoriness to platelet transfusion by protein A column therapy. *Transfusion* 1993; **33**: 234–42.
107 Kekomaki R, Elfenbein G, Gardner R. Improved response of patients refractory to random-donor platelet transfusions by intravenous γ globulin. *Am J Med* 1984; **73**: 199–203.
108 Junghans RP, Ahn YS. High-dose intravenous γ globulin to suppress alloimmune destruction of donor platelets. *Am J Med* 1994; **73**: 204–8.
109 Schiffer CA, Hogge DE, Aisne J et al. High-dose intravenous gammaglobulin in alloimmunized platelet transfusion recipients. *Blood* 1984; **64**: 937–40.
110 Class FHJ, Smeenk RJT, Schmidt R et al. Alloimmunization against the MHC antigens after platelet transfusions is due to contaminating leukocytes in the platelet suspension. *Exp Hematol* 1981; **9**: 84–9.
111 Meryman HT. Transfusion-induced alloimmunization and immunosuppression and the effects of leukocyte depletion. *Transfus Med Rev* 1989; **3**: 180–3.
112 Schiffer CA. Prevention of alloimmunization against platelets. *Blood* 1991; **77**: 1–4.
113 Semple JW, Freedman J. Recipient antigen-processing pathways of allogeneic platelet antigens: essential mediators of immunity. *Transfusion* 2002; **42**: 958–61.
114 Gmur J, von Felten A, Osterwalder B et al. Delayed alloimmunization using random single donor platelet transfusions: a prospective study in thrombocytopenic patients with acute leukemia. *Blood* 1983; **62**: 473–9.
115 Sintnicolaas K, Vriesendorp HM, Sizoo W et al. Delayed alloimmunization by random single donor platelet transfusions. A randomized study to compare single donor and multiple donor platelet transfusions in cancer patients with severe thrombocytopenia. *Lancet* 1981; **1**: 750–4.
116 Sintnicolaas K, van Marwijk Kooij M, van Prooijen HC et al. Leukocyte depletion of random single-donor platelet transfusions does not prevent secondary human leukocyte antigen-alloimmunization and refractoriness: a randomized prospective study. *Blood* 1995; **85**: 824–8.
117 Sniecinski I, O'Donnell MR, Nowicki B, Hill LR. Prevention of refractoriness and HLA-alloimmunization using filtered blood products. *Blood* 1988; **71**: 1402–7.
118 Novotny VMJ, van Doorn R, Wirvliet MD et al. Occurrence of allogeneic HLA and non-HLA

118. antibodies after transfusion of prestorage filtered platelets and red blood cells: a prospective study. *Blood* 1995; **85**: 1736–41.
119. Andreu G, Dewailly J, Leberre C et al. Prevention of HLA immunization with leukocyte-poor packed red cells and platelet concentrates obtained by filtration. *Blood* 1988; **72**: 964–9.
120. Saarinen UM, Kekomaki R, Siimes MA, Myllyla G. Effective prophylaxis against platelet refractoriness in multitransfused patients by use of leukocyte-free blood components. *Blood* 1990; **75**: 512–7.
121. van Marwijk Kooy M, van Prooijen HC, Moes M et al. Use of leukocyte depleted platelet concentrates for the prevention of refractoriness and primary HLA alloimmunization: a prospective, randomized trial. *Blood* 1991; **77**: 201–5.
122. Williamson LM, Wimperis JZ, Williamson P et al. Bedside filtration of blood products in the prevention of HLA alloimmunization—a prospective randomized study. *Blood* 1994; **83**: 3028–35.
123. Blajchman MA, Bardossy L, Carmen RA et al. An animal model of allogeneic donor platelet refractoriness: the effect of the time of leukodepletion. *Blood* 1992; **79**: 11,371–5.
124. Heddle NM, Blajchman MA. The leukodepletion of cellular blood products in the prevention of HLA-alloimmunization and refractoriness to allogeneic platelet transfusions. *Blood* 1995; **85**: 603–6.
125. Deeg HJ. Transfusions with a tan—prevention of allosensitization by ultraviolet irradiation. *Transfusion* 1989; **29**: 450–5.
126. Kahn RA, Duffy BF, Rodey GG. Ultraviolet irradiation of platelet concentrate abrogates lymphocyte activation with affecting platelet function *in vitro*. *Transfusion* 1985; **25**: 547–50.
127. Deeg HJ, Aprile J, Graham TC, Appelbaum FR, Storb R. Ultraviolet irradiation of blood prevents transfusion-induced sensitization and marrow graft rejection in dogs. *Blood* 1986; **87**: 537–9.
128. Grana NH, Kao KJ. Use of 8-methoxypsoralen and ultraviolet-A pretreated platelet concentrates to prevent alloimmunization against class I major histocompatibility antigens. *Blood* 1991; **77**: 2530–7.
129. Kaushansky K. Thrombopoietin: platelets on demand? *Ann Intern Med* 1997; **126**: 731–3.
130. Kuter DJ. Whatever happened to thrombopoietin? *Transfusion* 2002; **42**: 279–83.
131. Kuter DJ. Thrombopoietin: biology, clinical applications, role in the donor setting. *J Clin Apheresis* 1996; **11**: 149–59.
132. Basser RL, Rasko JEJ, Klarke K et al. Thrombopoietic effects of pegylated recombinant human megakaryocyte growth and development factor (PEG-rHUMGDF) in patients with advanced cancer. *Lancet* 1996; **348**: 1279–81.
133. Fanucchi M, Glaspy J, Crawford J et al. Effects of polyethylene glycol-conjugated recombinant human megakaryocyte growth and development factor on platelet counts after chemotherapy for lung cancer. *N Engl J Med* 1997; **336**: 404–9.
134. Vadhan-Raj S, Verschraegen CF, Bueso-Ramos C. et al. Recombinant human thrombopoietin attenuates carboplatin-induced severe thrombocytopenia and the need for platelet transfusions in patients with gynecologic cancer. *Ann Intern Med* 2000; **132**: 364–8.
135. Basser RL, Rasko JE, Clarke K. et al. Randomized, blinded placebo-controlled phase I trial of pegylated recombinant human megakaryocyte growth and development factor with filgrastim after dose-intensive chemotherapy in patients with advanced cancer. *Blood* 1997; **89**: 3118–28. Erratum: *Blood* 1997; **90**: 2513.
136. Archimbaud E, Ottmann OG, Yin JA et al. A randomized, double-blind, placebo-controlled study with pegylated recombinant human megakaryocyte growth and development factor (PEG-rHuMGDF) as an adjunct to chemotherapy for adults with *de novo* acute myeloid leukemia. *Blood* 1999; **94**: 3694–701.
137. Schiffer CA, Miller K, Larson RA et al. A double-blind, placebo controlled trial of pegylated recombinant human megakaryocyte growth and development factor as an adjunct to induction and consolidation therapy for patients with acute myeloid leukemia. *Blood* 2000; **95**: 2530–5.
138. Nichol JL. Thrombopoietin levels after chemotherapy and in naturally occurring human diseases. *Curr Opin Hematol* 1998; **5**: 203–8.
139. Li J, Yang C, Xia Y et al. Thrombocytopenia caused by the development of antibodies to thrombopoietin. *Blood* 2001; **98**: 3241–8.
140. Graw RH Jr, Herzig G, Perry S, Henderson ES. Normal granulocyte transfusion therapy: treatment of septicemia due to gram-negative bacteria. *N Engl J Med* 1972; **287**: 367–8.
141. Herzig GP, Graw RG Jr. Granulocyte transfusions for bacterial infections. In: Brown EB, ed. *Progress in Hematology*, Vol. 9. New York: Grune & Stratton, 1975: 207–31.
142. Alavi JB, Roat RK, Djerassi I et al. A randomized clinical trial of granulocyte transfusions for infection of acute leukemia. *N Engl J Med* 1977; **296**: 706–11.
143. Strauss RG. Therapeutic granulocyte transfusions in 1993. *Blood* 1993; **81**: 1675–8.
144. Strauss RG, Connett JE, Gale RP et al. A controlled trial of prophylactic granulocyte transfusion during initial induction. *N Engl J Med* 1981; **305**: 597–8.
145. Bensinger WI, Price TH, Dale DC et al. The effects of daily recombinant human granulocyte-colony-stimulating factor administration on normal granulocyte donors undergoing leukapheresis. *Blood* 1993; **81**: 1883–8.
146. Caspar CB, Seger RA, Burger J, Gmur J. Effective stimulation of donors for granulocyte colony-stimulating factor. *Blood* 1993; **81**: 2866–71.
147. Liles WC, Juang JE, Llewellyn C et al. A comparative trial of granulocytecolony-stimulating factor and dexamethasone, separately and in combination, for the mobilization of neutrophils in the peripheral blood of normal volunteers. *Transfusion* 1997; **37**: 182–7.
148. Stroncek DF, Clay ME, Petzoldt ML et al. Treatment of normal individuals with granulocyte-colony-stimulating factor: donor experiences and the effects on peripheral blood CD34+ cell counts and on the collection of peripheral blood stem cells. *Transfusion* 1996; **36**: 601–10.
149. Stroncek DF, Clay ME, Herr G, Smith J, Ilstrup S, McCullough J. Blood counts in healthy donors 1 year after the collection of granulocyte-colony-stimulating factor-mobilized progenitor cells and the results of a second mobilization and collection. *Transfusion* 1997; **37**: 304–8.
150. McCullough J, Clay M, Herr G, Smith J, Stroncek DF. Effects of granulocyte-colony-stimulating factor on potential normal granulocyte donors. *Transfusion* 1999; **39**: 1136–40.
151. Hubel K, Carter RA, Liles WC et al. Granulocyte transfusion therapy for infections in candidates and recipients of hematopoietic stem cell transplantation: a comparative analysis of feasibility and outcome of community donors versus related donors. *Transfusion* 2002; **42**: 1414–21.
152. Ruthe RC, Ansersen BR, Cunningham BL, Epstein RB. Efficacy of granulocyte transfusions in the control of systemic candidiasis in leukopenic host. *Blood* 1978; **52**: 493–8.
153. Raubitschek AA, Levin AS, Stites DP et al. Normal granulocyte infusion therapy for aspergillosis in chronic granulomatous disease. *Pediatrics* 1973; **51**: 230–5.
154. Storb R, Prentice RL, Thomas ED. Marrow transplantation for treatment of aplastic anemia: an analysis of factors associated with graft rejection. *N Engl J Med* 1977; **296**: 61–5.
155. Storb R, Thomas ED, Buckner CD et al. Marrow transplantation in 30 'untransfused' patients with severe aplastic anemia. *Ann Intern Med* 1980; **92**: 30–6.
156. Champlin RE, Horowitz MM, van Bekkum DW et al. Graft failure following bone marrow transplantation for severe aplastic anemia: risk factors and treatment results. *Blood* 1989; **73**: 606–13.
157. Storb R, Weiden PL. Transfusion problems associated with transplantation. *Semin Hematol* 1981; **18**: 163–76.
158. Ho WG, Champlin RE, Winston DJ, Feig SA, Gale RP. Bone marrow transplantation in patients with leukaemia previously transfused with blood products from family members. *Br J Haematol* 1987; **67**: 67–70.
159. Thomas ED, Storb R, Cliff RA et al. Bone-marrow transplantation. *N Engl J Med* 1975; **292**: 832–43 & 895–902.
160. Miller W, Flynn P, McCullough J et al. Cytomegalovirus infection after bone marrow transplantation: an association with acute graft-vs-host disease. *Blood* 1986; **67**: 1162–7.
161. Bowden RA, Sayers M, Flournoy N et al. Cytomegalovirus immune globulin and senonegative blood products prevent primary cytomegalovirus infection after marrow transplantation. *N Engl J Med* 1986; **314**: 1006–15.
162. Miller WJ, McCullough J, Balfour HH et al. Prevention of CMV infection following bone marrow transplantation: a randomized trial of blood product screening. *Bone Marrow Transplant* 1991; **7**: 227–34.
163. Gilbert GL, Hudson IL, Hayes JJ. Prevention of transfusion-acquired cytomegalovirus infection in infants by blood filtration to remove leucocytes. *Lancet* 1989; **1**: 1228–31.
164. Murphy MF, Grint PCA, Hardiman AE, Lister TA, Waters AH. Use of leukocyte-poor blood components to prevent primary cytomegalovirus (CMV) infection in patients with acute leukemia. *Br J Haematol* 1988; **70**: 253–5.
165. Bowden RA, Slichter SJ, Sayers M et al. A comparison of filtered leukocyte reduced and cytomegalovirus (CMV) seronegative blood products for the prevention of transfusion-associated CMV infection after marrow transplant. *Blood* 1995; **86**: 3598–603.
166. Condie RM, O'Reilly RJ. Prevention of cytomegalovirus infection by prophylaxis with an intravenous, hyperimmune, native, unmodified cytomegalovirus globulin. *Am J Med* 1984; **76**: 134–41.
167. Meyers JD, Leszczynski J, Zaia JA et al. Prevention of cytomegalovirus infection by cytomegalovirus immune globulin after marrow transplantation. *Ann Intern Med* 1983; **98**: 442–6.

168 Winston DJ, Ho WG, Lin C et al. Intravenous immunoglobulin for modification of cytomegalovirus infections associated with bone marrow transplantation. *Am J Med* 1984; **76**: 128–33.
169 Moroff G, Leitman SF, Luban NLC. Principles of blood irradiation, dose validation and quality control: a practical approach. *Transfusion* 1997; **37**: 1084–92.
170 Park BH, Good RA, Gate J et al. Fatal graft-versus-host reaction following transfusion of allogeneic blood and plasma in infants with combined immunodeficiency disease. *Transplant Proc* 1974; **6**: 385–7.
171 Lowenthal RM, Challis DR, Griffiths AE et al. Transfusion-associated graft-versus-host disease: report of a case following administration of blood. *Transfusion* 1993; **33**: 524–9.
172 Sproul AM, Chalmers EA, Mills KI et al. Third party mediated graft rejection despite irradiation of blood products. *Br J Haematol* 1992; **80**: 251–2.
173 Anderson KC, Goodnough LT, Sayers M et al. Variation in blood component irradiation practice: implications for prevention of transfusion-associated graft-versus-host disease. *Blood* 1991; **77**: 2096–102.
174 Leitman SF, Holland PV. Irradiation of blood products: indication guidelines. *Transfusion* 1985; **25**: 293–300.
175 Sprent J, Anderson RE, Miller JFAP. Radiosensitivity of T and B lymphocytes. II. Effect of irradiation on response of T cells to alloantigens. *Eur J Immunol* 1974; **4**: 204–10.
176 Valerius NH, Johansen KS, Nielsen OS et al. Effect of in vitro X-irradiation on lymphocyte and granulocyte function. *Scand J Haematol* 1981; **27**: 9–18.
177 Button LN, DeWolf WC, Newburger PE, Jacobson MS, Kevy SV. The effects of irradiation on blood components. *Transfusion* 1981; **21**: 419–26.
178 Holly TR, Van Epps DE, Harvey RL et al. Effect of high doses of radiation on human neutrophil chemotaxis, phagocytosis, and morphology. *Am J Pathol* 1974; **75**: 61–72.
179 Greenberg ML, Chanana AD, Cronkite EP et al. Extracorporeal irradiation of blood in man: radiation resistance of circulating platelets. *Radiat Res* 1968; **35**: 147–54.
180 Read EJ, Kodis C, Carter CS, Leitman SF. Viability of platelets following storage in the irradiated state. A pair-controlled study. *Transfusion* 1988; **23**: 446–50.
181 Duguid JKM, Carr R, Jenkins JA et al. Clinical evaluation of the effects of storage time and irradiation on transfused platelets. *Vox Sang* 1991; **60**: 151–4.
182 Moroff G, Luban NLC. Prevention of transfusion-associated graft-versus-host disease [Editorial]. *Transfusion* 1992; **32**: 101–3.
183 Pelszynski M, Moroff G, Luban N et al. Dose dependent lymphocyte inactivation in red blood cell (RBC) units with gamma irradiation. *Transfusion* 1991; **31** (Suppl.): 17S [Abstract].
184 Center for Biologics Evaluation and Research. *License Amendments and Procedures for Gamma Irradiation of Blood Products*. Bethesda, MD: Food and Drug Administration, 1993.
185 Ramirez AM, Woodfield DG, Scott R, McLachlan J. High potassium levels in stored irradiated blood [Letter]. *Transfusion* 1987; **27**: 444–5.
186 Rivet C, Baxter A, Rock G. Potassium levels in irradiated blood [Letter]. *Transfusion* 1989; **29**: 185.
187 Strauss RG. Routine washing of irradiated red cells before transfusion seems unwarranted. *Transfusion* 1990; **30**: 675–7.
188 Kao KH, Mickel M, Braine HG et al. White cell reduction in platelet concentrates and packed red cells by filtration: a multicenter clinical trial. *Transfusion* 1995; **35**: 13–9.
189 Douglas SD, Fudenberg HH. Graft-versus-host reaction in Wiskott–Aldrich syndrome: antemortem diagnosis of human GVH in an immunologic deficiency disease. *Vox Sang* 1969; **16**: 172–8.
190 Hathaway WE, Githens JH, Blackburn WR et al. Aplastic anemia, histiocytosis and erythrodermia in immunologically deficient children: probable human runt disease. *N Engl J Med* 1965; **271**: 953–4.
191 Thompson HW, McCullough J. Use of blood components containing red cells by donors of allogeneic bone marrow. *Transfusion* 1986; **26**: 98–100.
192 Stroncek DF, Clay ME, Smith J, Ilstrup S, Oldham F, McCullough J. Changes in blood counts following the administration of G-CSF and the collection of peripheral blood stem cells from healthy donors. *Transfusion* 1996; **36**: 596–600.
193 Stroncek DF, McCullough J. Policies and procedures for the establishment of an allogeneic blood stem cell collection program. *Transfus Med* 1997; **7**: 77–87.
194 Stroncek DF, Clay ME, Herr G et al. The kinetics of G-CSF mobilization of CD34+ cells in healthy people. *Transfus Med* 1997; **7**: 19–24.
195 Stroncek DF, Clay ME, Smith J et al. Composition of peripheral blood progenitor cell components collected from healthy donors. *Transfusion* 1997; **37**: 411–7.
196 Stroncek DF, Anderlini P. Mobilized PBPC concentrates: a maturing blood component. *Transfusion* 2001; **41**: 168–71.
197 Stroncek DF, McCullough J. Policies and procedures for the establishment of an allogeneic blood stem cell collection programme. *Transfus Med* 1997; **7**: 77–87.
198 Walker RH. Special report: transfusion risks. *Am J Clin Pathol* 1987; **88**: 374–8.
199 Sazama K. 355 Reports of transfusion-associated deaths. *Transfusion* 1990; **30**: 583–90.
200 Myhre BA. Fatalities from blood transfusion. *JAMA* 1980; **244**: 1333–5.
201 DeCesare WR, Bove JR, Ebaugh FG Jr. The mechanism of the effect of iso- and hyperosmolar dextrose-saline solutions on in vivo survival of human erythrocytes. *Transfusion* 1964; **4**: 237–50.
202 Ryden SE, Oberman HA. Compatibility of common intravenous solutions with CPD blood. *Transfusion* 1975; **15**: 250–5.
203 Davenport RD, Strieter RM, Kunkel SL. Red cell ABO incompatibility and production of tumour necrosis factor-α. *Br J Haematol* 1991; **78**: 540–4.
204 Davenport RD, Strieter RM, Standiford TJ, Kunkel SL. Interleukin-8 production in red blood cell incompatibility. *Blood* 1990; **76**: 22,439–42.
205 Davenport RD, Burdick MD, Strieter RM, Kunkel SL. In vitro production of interleukin-1 receptor antagonist in IgG-mediated red cell incompatibility. *Transfusion* 1994; **34**: 297–303.
206 Pineda AA, Brzica SM, Taswell HE. Hemolytic transfusion reaction: recent experience in a large blood bank. *Mayo Clin Proc* 1978; **53**: 378–88.
207 Honing CL, Bove JR. Transfusion-associated fatalities. Review of bureau of biologics reports 1976–78. *Transfusion* 1980; **20**: 653–61.
208 Vamvakas EC, Pineda AA, Reisner R, Santach PJ, Moore SB. The differentiation of delayed hemolytic and delayed serologic transfusion reactions: incidence and predictors of hemolysis. *Transfusion* 1995; **35**: 26–32.
209 Perkins HA, Payne R, Ferguson J et al. Nonhemolytic febrile transfusion reactions: quantitative effects of blood components with emphasis on isoantigenic incompatibility of leukocytes. *Vox Sang* 1966; **11**: 578–82.
210 Brittingham TE, Chaplin H. Febrile transfusion reactions caused by sensitivity to donor leukocytes and platelets. *JAMA* 1957; **165**: 819–21.
211 Menitove JE, McElligott MC, Aster RH. Febrile transfusion reaction: what blood component should be given next. *Vox Sang* 1982; **42**: 318–21.
212 Popovsky MA, Moore SB. Diagnostic and pathogenetic considerations in transfusion-related acute lung injury. *Transfusion* 1985; **25**: 573–7.
213 Popovsky MA, Chaplin HC, Moore SB. Transfusion-related acute lung injury: a neglected, serious complication of hemotherapy. *Transfusion* 1992; **32**: 589–92.
214 Popovsky MA, Davenport RD. Transfusion-related acute lung injury: femme fatale? *Transfusion* 2001; **41**: 312–5.
215 Silliman CC, Paterson AJ, Dickey WO et al. The association of biologically active lipids with the development of transfusion-related acute lung injury: a retrospective study. *Transfusion* 1997; **37**: 719–26.
216 Vyas GN, Holmdahl L, Perkins HA, Fudenberg HH. Serologic specificity of human anti-IgA and its significance in transfusion. *Blood* 1969; **34**: 573–81.
217 Heddle NM, Klama L, Singer J et al. The role of the plasma from platelet concentrates in transfusion reactions. *N Engl J Med* 1994; **331**: 625–8.
218 Bordin JO, Heddle NM, Blajchman MA. Biologic effects of leukocytes present in transfused cellular blood products. *Blood* 1994; **84**: 1703–21.
219 Goodnough LT, Riddell J, Lazarus H et al. Prevalence of platelet transfusion reactions before and after implementation of leukocyte-depleted platelet concentrates by filtration. *Vox Sang* 1993; **65**: 103–7.
220 Muylle L, Wouters E, Peetermans ME. Febrile reactions to platelet transfusion: the effect of increased interleukin 6 levels in concentrates prepared by the platelet-rich plasma method. *Transfusion* 1996; **36**: 886–90.
221 Klein HG, Dodd MY, Ness PM, Fratantoni JA, Nemo GJ. Current status of microbial contamination of blood components: summary of a conference. *Transfusion* 1997; **37**: 95–101.
222 Morrow JF, Braine HG, Kickler TS, Ness PM, Dick JD, Fuller AK. Septic reactions to platelet transfusions—a persistent problem. *JAMA* 1991; **266**: 555–8.
223 Blajchman MA. Bacterial contamination of blood products and the value of pre-transfusion testing. *Immunol Invest* 1995; **24**: 163–70.
224 Goldman M, Blajchman MA. Blood product-associated bacterial sepsis. *Transfus Med Rev* 1991; **5**: 73–83.
225 Perez P, Salmi LR, Follea G et al. Determinants of transfusion-associated bacterial contamination: results of the French BACTHEM case control study. *Transfusion* 2001; **41**: 862–72.
226 Ness P, Braine H, King K et al. Single-donor platelets reduce the risk of septic platelet transfusion reactions. *Transfusion* 2001; **41**: 857–61.

227 Sazama K. Bacteria in blood for transfusion—a review. *Arch Pathol Lab Med* 1994; **118**: 350–65.
228 McCullough J. Complications of transfusion. In: *Transfusion Medicine*. New York: McGraw-Hill, 1998: 337–59.
229 Lucarelli G, Angelucci E, Giardini C et al. Fate of iron stores in thalassemia after bone marrow transplantation. *Lancet* 1993; **342**: 1388–91.
230 Angelucci E, Baronciani D, Giardini C et al. Iron removal in ex-thalassemics after BMT. Preliminary results from the phlebotomy program. *Bone Marrow Transplant* 1993; **1** (Suppl.): 105–7.
231 McCullough J. The nation's changing blood supply system. *JAMA* 1993; **269**: 2239–45.
232 McCullough J. The continuing evolution of the nation's blood supply system. *Am J Clin Pathol* 1996; **105**: 689–95.
233 Dodd RY. The risk of transfusion-transmitted infection [Editorial]. *N Engl J Med* 1992; **327**: 419–22.
234 Lackritz EM, Satten GA, Aberle-Grasse J et al. Estimated risk of transmission of the human immunodeficiency virus by screened blood in the United States. *N Engl J Med* 1995; **333**: 1721–5.
235 Schreiber GB, Busch MP, Kleinman SH. The risk of transfusion-transmitted viral infections. *N Engl J Med* 1996; **334**: 1685–90.
236 Hewlett IK, Epstein JS. Food and Drug Administration conference on the feasibility of genetic technology to close the HIV window in donor screening. *Transfusion* 1997; **37**: 346–51.
237 Report of the Interorganizational Task Force on Nucleic Acid Amplification Testing of Blood Donors. Nucleic acid amplification testing of blood donors for transfusion-transmitted infectious diseases. *Transfusion* 2000; **40**: 143–59.
238 Stramer SL, Caglioti C, Strong DM. NAT of the United States and Canadian blood supply. *Transfusion* 2000; **40**: 1165–8.
239 Glynn DA, Kleinman SH, Wright DJ, Busch MP. International application of the incidence rate/window period model. *Transfusion* 2002; **42**: 966–72.
240 Dodd RY, Notari EP, Stramer SL. Current prevalence of incidence of infectious disease markers and estimated window-period risk in the American Red Cross blood donor population. *Transfusion* 2002; **42**: 975–9.
241 Schmidt PJ. Syphilis: a disease of direct transfusion. *Transfusion* 2001; **41**: 1069–71.
242 Greenwalt TJ, Rios JA. To test or not to test for syphilis: a global problem. *Transfusion* 2001; **41**: 976.
243 Cable R. Evaluation of syphilis testing of blood donors. *Transfus Med Rev* 1996; **10**: 296–302.
244 NIH Consensus Development Panel on infectious disease testing for blood transfusions. Infectious disease testing for blood transfusion. *JAMA* 1995; **274**: 1374–9.
245 Bove JR. Transfusion-associated hepatitis and AIDS: what is the risk? *N Engl J Med* 1987; **317**: 242–5.
246 Alter HJ, Holland PV, Purcell RH et al. Posttransfusion hepatitis after exclusion of commercial and hepatitis-B antigen-positive donors. *Ann Intern Med* 1972; **77**: 691–9.
247 Hollinger FB, Khan NC, Oefinger PA et al. Posttransfusion hepatitis type A. *JAMA* 1983; **250**: 2313–7.
248 Noble RC, Kane MA, Reeves SA, Roeckel I. Posttransfusion hepatitis A in a neonatal intensive care unit. *JAMA* 1984; **252**: 2711–21.
249 Choo QL, Kuo G, Weiner AJ et al. Isolation of a cDNA derived from a blood-borne non-A, non-B viral hepatitis genome. *Science* 1989; **244**: 359–61.
250 Alter HJ, Purcell RH, Shih JW et al. Detection of antibody to hepatitis C virus in prospectively followed transfusion recipients with acute and chronic non-A, non-B hepatitis. *N Engl J Med* 1989; **321**: 1494–500.
251 Alter HJ. To C or not to C: these are the questions. *Blood* 1995; **85**: 1681–95.
252 Tong MJ, El-Farra NS, Reikes AR, Co RL. Clinical outcomes after transfusion-associated hepatitis C. *N Engl J Med* 1995; **332**: 1463–6.
253 Alter HJ, Nakatsuji Y, Melpolder J et al. The incidence of transfusion-associated hepatitis G virus infection and its relation to liver disease. *N Engl J Med* 1997; **336**: 747–54.
254 Alter HJ. G-pers creepers, where'd you get those papers? A reassessment of the literature on the hepatitis G virus. *Transfusion* 1997; **37**: 569–72.
255 Mosley JW, Rakela J. Foundling viruses and transfusion medicine. *Transfusion* 1999; **39**: 1041–4.
256 Nishizawa T, Okamoto H, Konishi K et al. A novel DNA virus (TTV) associated with elevated transaminase levels in posttransfusion hepatitis of unknown etiology. *Biochem Biophys Res Commun* 1997; **241**: 92–7.
257 Wang JT, Lee CZ, Kao JH, Sheu JC, Wang TH, Chen DS. Incidence and clinical presentation of posttransfusion TT virus infection in prospectively followed transfusion recipients: emphasis on its relevance to hepatitis. *Transfusion* 2000; **40**: 596–601.
258 Busch MP, Young MJ, Samson SJ et al. Risk of human immunodeficiency virus (HIV) transmission by blood transfusions before the implementation of HIV-I antibody screening. *Transfusion* 1991; **31**: 4–11.
259 Peterman TA, Jaffe HW, Feorino PM et al. Transfusion-associated acquired immunodeficiency syndrome in the United States. *JAMA* 1985; **254**: 2913–7.
260 Jaffe HW, Sarngadharan MG, DeVico AL et al. Infection with HTLV-III/LAV and transfusion-associated acquired immunodeficiency syndrome: serologic evidence of an association. *JAMA* 1985; **254**: 770–3.
261 Feorino PM, Jaffe HW, Palmer E et al. Transfusion-associated acquired immunodeficiency syndrome: evidence for persistent infection in blood donors. *N Engl J Med* 1985; **312**: 1293–6.
262 Menitove JE. Status of recipients of blood from donors subsequently found to have an antibody to HIV. *N Engl J Med* 1986; **315**: 1095–6.
263 Centers for Disease Control (CDC). Human immunodeficiency virus infection in transfusion recipients and their family members. *Morb Mortal Wkly Rep* 1987; **36**: 137–8.
264 Roberts CS, Longfield JN, Platte RC et al. Transfusion-associated human immunodeficiency virus type I from screened antibody-negative blood donors. *Arch Pathol Lab Med* 1994; **118**: 1188–92.
265 Cohen ND, Munoz A, Reitz BA et al. Transmission of retroviruses by transfusion of screened blood in patients undergoing cardiac surgery. *N Engl J Med* 1989; **320**: 1172–6.
266 Irani MS, Dudley AW, Lucco LJ. Case of HIV-I transmission by antigen-positive, antibody negative blood [Letter]. *N Engl J Med* 1991; **325**: 1174–5.
267 Busch MP, Taylor PE, Lenes BA et al. Screening of selected male blood donors for p24 antigen of human immunodeficiency type 1. Transfusion Safety Study Group. *N Engl J Med* 1990; **323**: 1308–12.
268 Alter HJ, Epstein JS, Swenson SG et al. Prevalence of human immunodeficiency virus type I p24 antigen in US blood donors—an assessment of the efficacy of testing in donor screening. HIV-antigen study group. *N Engl J Med* 1990; **323**: 1312–7.
269 Hollsberg P, Hafler DA. Pathogenesis of diseases induced by human lymphotropic virus type I infection. *N Engl J Med* 1993; **328**: 1173–82.
270 Shih JWK, Lee HH, Falchek M et al. Transfusion-transmitted HTLV-I/II infection in patients undergoing open-heart surgery. *Blood* 1990; **75**: 5466–9.
271 Holland PV. Notification and counseling of blood donors. *Vox Sang* 1996; **70**: 46–9.
272 Okochi K, Sato H. Adult T-cell leukemia virus, blood donors and transfusion: experience in Japan. *Prog Clin Biol Res* 1985; **182**: 245–9.
273 Williams AE, Fang CT, Slamon DJ et al. Seroprevalence and epidemiologic correlates of HTLV-I infection in US blood donors. *Science* 1988; **240**: 643–6.
274 Lefrere JJ, Mariotti M, de la Croix I et al. Albumin batches and B19 parvovirus DNA. *Transfusion* 1995; **35**: 389–91.
275 Brown KE, Young NS, Alving BM, Barbosa LH. Parvovirus B19: implications for transfusion medicine. *Transfusion* 2001; **41**: 130–5.
276 Cohen BJ, Beard S, Knowles WA et al. Chronic anemia due to parvovirus B19 infection in a bone marrow transplant patient after platelet transfusion. *Transfusion* 1997; **37**: 947–52.
277 Zanell A, Rossi F, Cesana C et al. Transfusion-transmitted human parvovirus B19 infection in thalassemic patients. *Transfusion* 1995; **35**: 769–72.
278 Henle W, Henle G, Scriba M et al. Antibody responses to the Epstein–Barr virus and cytomegalovirus after open-heart and other surgery. *N Engl J Med* 1970; **282**: 1068–74.
279 Alfieri C, Tanner J, Carpentier L et al. Epstein–Barr virus transmission from a blood donor to an organ transplant recipient with recovery of the same virus stain from the recipient's blood and oropharynx. *Blood* 1996; **87**: 812–7.
280 Mungai M, Tegtmeier G, Chamberland M, Parise M. Transfusion-transmitted malaria in the United States from 1963 through 1999. *N Engl J Med* 2001; **344**: 1973–8.
281 Leiby DA, Herron RM, Read EJ et al. Trypanosoma cruzi in Los Angeles and Miami blood donors: impact of evolving donor demographics on seroprevalence and implications for transfusion transmission. *Transfusion* 2002; **42**: 549–55.
282 Shulman IA, Appleman MD, Saxena S, Hiti AL, Kirchhoff LV. Specific antibodies to *Trypansoma cruzi* among blood donors in Los Angeles, California. *Transfusion* 1997; **37**: 727–31.
283 Galel S, Kirchhoff LV. Risk factors for *Trypanosoma cruzi* infection in California blood donors. *Transfusion* 1996; **36**: 227–31.
284 Linden JV, Wong SJ, Chu FK, Schmidt GB, Bianco C. Transfusion-associated transmission of babesiosis in New York State. *Transfusion* 2000; **40**: 285–90.
285 McQuiston JH, Childs JE, Chamberland ME, Tabor E. Transmission of tick-borne agents of disease by blood transfusion: a review of known and potential risks in the United States. *Transfusion* 2000; **40**: 274–84.
286 Badon SJ, Fister RD, Cable RG. Survival of *Borrelia burgdorferi* in blood products. *Transfusion* 1989; **29**: 581–3.

287 World Health Organization consultation on public health issues related to bovine spongiform encephalopathy and the emergence of a new variety of Creutzfeldt–Jakob disease. *MMWR* 1996; **45**: 295–303.

288 Surveillance for Creutzfeldt–Jakob disease—United States. *MMWR* 1996; **45**: 665–8.

289 Evatt B, Austin H, Barnhart E *et al.* Surveillance for Creutzfeldt–Jakob disease among persons with hemophilia. *Transfusion* 1998; **38**: 817–20.

290 Dodd RY, Busch MP. Animal models of bovine spongiform encephalopathy and vCJD infectivity in blood: two swallows do not a summer make. *Transfusion* 2002; **42**: 509–12.

291 Brown P. Transfusion medicine and spongiform encephalopathy. *Transfusion* 2001; **41**: 433–6.

292 Hollinger B, Kleinman S. Potential for transfusion-transmission of West Nile virus. *Transfusion*, in press.

293 Biggerstaff BJ, Petersen LR. Estimated risk of West Nile virus transmission through blood transfusion during an epidemic in Queens, New York City. *Transfusion* 2002; **42**: 1019–26.

294 Jackson BR, Busch MP, Stramer SL, AuBuchon JP. The cost-effectiveness of nucleic acid testing for HIV, HCV and HBV in whole blood donations. *Transfusion* 2003; **43**: 721–9.

295 Alter HJ. G-pers creepers, where'd you get those papers? A reassessment of the literature on the hepatitis G virus. *Transfusion* 1997; **37**: 569–72.

296 Dodd RY. Scaling the heights. *Transfusion* 1995; **35**: 186–7.

62

Robertson Parkman & Kenneth I. Weinberg

Immune Reconstitution following Hematopoietic Cell Transplantation

Hematopoietic cell transplant (HCT) recipients are characterized by an immunodeficiency of varying severity and duration. Initially, immune evaluations following HCT were used to document the success of HCT as treatment for infants with severe combined immunodeficiency syndrome (SCID) and the immune deficits associated with chronic graft-vs.-host disease (GVHD) [1–3]. The clinical importance of post-HCT immunodeficiency in allogeneic HCT recipients without chronic GVHD was not realized until the mid-1990s when the high rate of opportunistic infections in the adult recipients of unrelated HCT without chronic GVHD or of T-cell-depleted (TCD) HCT were documented [4,5]. These observations established that the lack of protective immune function is a major problem following allogeneic HCT. This chapter reviews the present understanding of the biology of and attempts to improve post-HCT immune reconstitution.

The reconstitution of the immune system following HCT is characterized by:
1 a recapitulation of normal lymphoid ontogeny;
2 reduced thymic function;
3 the effects of pretransplant chemoradiotherapy; and
4 the effects of acute and chronic GVHD and their therapies.

Other factors that can influence immune reconstitution include the donor–recipient relationship (autologous, syngeneic, allogeneic [histocompatible or unrelated donor]), recipient age and intervening infections, etc.

Transfer of donor immunity

When ablative pretransplant chemoradiotherapy is given, all normal recipient hematopoiesis, T-lymphocyte immunity and the majority of B-lymphocyte immunity are eliminated. When unmanipulated sources of hematopoietic stem cells (HSCs) are transplanted, either autologous or allogeneic, donor-derived antigen-specific T and B lymphocytes are infused with the HSC, which may contribute to the recipient's post-HCT immunocompetence.

T-lymphocyte immunity

Currently, multiple sources of HSC are used for transplantation. The ratio of mature T lymphocytes to HSC varies depending upon the HSC source, with the number of mature T lymphocytes being greatest in mobilized peripheral blood cells (PBCs) and least in bone marrow (BM). In cord blood the proportion of T lymphocytes is intermediate but their immunological maturity is limited. When patients receive TCD or CD34 selected HSC, the number of T lymphocytes is markedly reduced. Throughout this chapter an effort is made to state clearly what the characteristics of the HSC product is when evaluating post-HCT immunological function.

Antigen-specific T-lymphocyte immunity is necessary for the clinical control of DNA and RNA viral, protozoan and fungal infections. Through their control of specific antibody production by B lymphocytes, T lymphocytes are also necessary for the control of infections with encapsulated respiratory bacteria. Assessments of the transfer of donor T-lymphocyte immunity have failed to detect clinically significant transfer in the recipients of allogeneic BM [6–12]. Following HCT with allogeneic BM, recipients are at high risk of infections with DNA viruses to which the recipients had pretransplant immunity. *In vitro* evaluations for the presence of antigen-specific T-lymphocyte proliferation early following HCT with BM have failed to detect antigen-specific T-lymphocyte immunity to DNA viral antigens, which is usually not detected until viral reactivation (either clinical or subclinical) occurs, resulting in the production of new antigen-specific T-lymphocytes.

Although antigen-specific T lymphocytes are not detectable following the transplantation of BM, the transfer of antigen-specific T lymphocytes can be detected in the recipients of PBC [13]. PBC contain 1–1.5 logs more T lymphocytes than BM. Thus, the quantitative increase in the number of T lymphocytes transferred at the time of HCT may contribute to post-HCT immunity. Clinical data have demonstrated that the transfusion of antigen-specific T lymphocytes in PBC can result in clinical protection against opportunistic infections. Recipients of autologous HSC, who received CD34-selected PBC (void of significant numbers of mature T lymphocytes) have a higher rate of infection with DNA viruses than those who received unfractionated PBC, indicating that the infused T lymphocytes provided protection against cytomegalovirus (CMV) infection [14,15]. Drugs, especially methotrexate (MTX), used as prophylaxis for acute GVHD, can selectively destroy the transferred antigen-specific T lymphocytes that are stimulated *in vivo* by specific antigen. Because PBC contains many more antigen-specific T lymphocytes than BM, significant numbers of antigen-specific T lymphocytes may persist in the recipients of PBC but not of BM. However, analysis of infections after allogeneic PBC transplantation as compared to BM has shown no differences in the rate of fatal infections [16].

B-lymphocyte immunity

Whereas donor-derived T-lymphocyte immunity is variably present following HCT, donor-derived antibody production can be readily detected early following HCT after immunization with a variety of antigens (tetanus toxoid, diphtheria toxoid, poliovirus, hepatitis virus) [17–21]. Increased antibody levels have been detected when either the donor or recipient was immunized prior to HCT. The maximal antibody response

was obtained when both the donor and recipient were immunized [19]. If recipients were not immunized, antibody production was not maintained, and in most cases clinically significant antibody levels were no longer detectable 1 year following HCT. The temporary transfer of donor-derived salivary IgA antibody has been reported following transplantation [22]. The evaluation of the transfer of B-lymphocyte immunity has been confounded by the fact that studies to detect antibody production following HCT have not used immunoglobulin allotyping to determine the source of the antibodies, i.e. donor or recipient B lymphocytes [21]. Because nondividing antibody-producing B lymphocytes and plasma cells are resistant to the cytoablative effects of many of the chemoradiotherapeutic agents used as preparation for HCT, antibody production by host cells occurred when recipients were immunized immediately following HCT. Increased post-transplant antibody production following donor and recipient immunization can be a result of the transfer of:
1 immune donor B lymphocytes;
2 antigen-primed donor antigen-presenting cells; or
3 immune donor T lymphocytes that cooperate with either donor or recipient antigen-specific B lymphocytes.

Both the transferred donor and residual recipient nondividing antibody-producing B lymphocytes can persist for their normal lifespan, at the end of which time a decline in antibody production is detected.

The routine administration of intravenous immunoglobulin (IVIg) to HCT recipients negates the need for antibody production early following HCT [23]. HCT recipients are incapable of normal antibody production to the capsular polysaccharide antigens of encapsulated respiratory bacteria for a prolonged period following HCT and no difference between the autologous recipients of BM and PBC was seen [3,24–27]. When immunoglobulin replacement therapy ceases, patients can develop recurrent pyogenic infections if they do not receive prophylactic antibiotics.

Normal lymphoid ontogeny

Although significant numbers of antigen-specific donor-derived T lymphocytes are transplanted into recipients who received PBC, there is a lack of detectable antigen-specific donor T lymphocytes when TCD or CD34 selected HSCs are used. If a nonsignificant number of donor-derived T lymphocytes are infused at the time of HCT, then the only source of recipient T lymphocytes is the differentiation of the transplanted donor HSC or common lymphoid progenitor cells (CLP) under the control of the recipient thymus [28,29]. Decreased thymic function brought about by age, pretransplant chemoradiotherapy, GVHD or post-transplant immunosuppression can all reduce the capacity of the recipient thymus to support the differentiation of donor HSC or CLP.

Lymphoid ontogeny can be characterized in terms of both cellular and molecular differentiation. The progeny of HSC that are first restricted to lymphoid differentiation (CLP) express CD34 and CD7 as their first distinctive surface antigens and are found in the fetal yolk sac and liver [29]. As CLP migrate to the thymus, the receptors for IL-7 and stem cell factor (c-kit) can be detected. The CLP become thymocytes, which express only the IL-7 receptor, but not CD3, CD4 or CD8 (triple negative [TN] thymocytes) [30]. Cytoplasmic CD3$^+$ cells can be detected at 8–9 weeks of fetal life in the thymus followed by the surface expression of CD2 (Fig. 62.1). Concurrent with the surface expression of CD3, the surface expression of rearranged T-cell receptor (TCR) genes can be detected with both TCR-αβ and TCR-γδ expressing cells present [31–36]. Initially, the TCR-αβ$^+$ cells express low levels of surface TCR and CD3 but not CD4 or CD8 (double negative [DN] thymocytes) which then traverse a stage of CD8^{low} expression to become CD3^{low}, CD4$^+$, CD8$^+$ double positive (DP) thymocytes.

Central to normal thymic lymphoid differentiation is the role of IL-7. Patients with defective IL-7 receptors (X-linked SCID) have markedly decreased numbers of T lymphocytes [37]. IL-7 has both stimulatory and antiapoptotic effects at the triple negative stage of thymocyte differentiation [38]. Positive and negative selection occurs at the double positive thymocyte stage [39–41]. Positive selection is a result of interactions between the TCR-αβ receptor and the thymic epithelium, resulting in the proliferation and clonal expansion of T lymphocytes with specificity for exogenous (nonself) antigens. Following their positive selection, the double positive thymocytes differentiate into CD3$^+$, CD4$^+$, TCR-αβ or

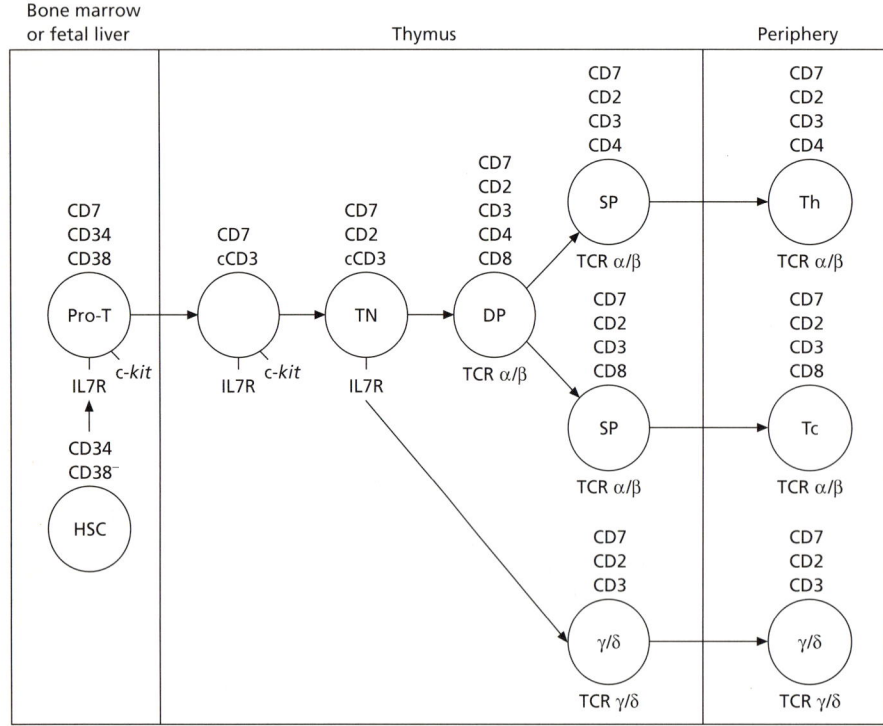

Fig. 62.1 Schema for T-lymphocyte differentiation.

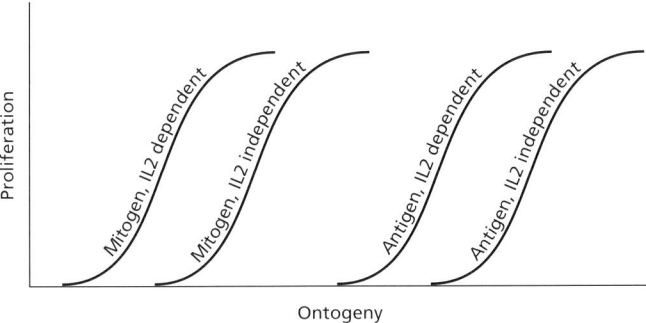

Fig. 62.2 Schematic representation of ontogeny of T-lymphocyte proliferation.

CD3+, CD8+, TCR-αβ single positive thymocytes, which are exported to the peripheral circulation as mature peripheral blood T lymphocytes, either CD4+ helper T lymphocytes (Th) or CD8+ cytotoxic T lymphocytes (Tc). Negative selection also occurs at the double positive thymocyte stage. The interaction of double positive TCR-αβ thymocytes with self-antigens expressed on BM-derived dendritic cells present in the thymus results in an apoptotic signal, the death of the cell and the clonal deletion of cells with specificity for self-antigens.

In early fetal life the frequency of TCR-γδ thymocytes is equal to that of TCR-αβ cells [32]. The development of TCR-γδ cells is characterized by rearrangements of the δ variable and joining regions. Different joining regions are used in fetal as opposed to adult differentiation. Most TCR-γδ thymocytes do not express significant surface CD4 or CD8 but do express CD1. Following their export from the thymus, TCR-γδ T lymphocytes selectively migrate to epithelial organs including skin, uterus and gut. The mechanisms involved in the positive and negative selection of TCR-γδ thymocytes are imperfectly understood.

In addition to the surface and molecular changes that occur during T-lymphocyte differentiation, a series of functional changes occur which can be measured by proliferation. The first proliferative responses that can be demonstrated in thymocytes following phytohemagglutan A (PHA) stimulation require the presence of exogenous cytokine IL-2 [33]. The requirement for exogenous cytokines demonstrates that thymocytes capable of expressing cytokine receptors (IL-2R) are present earlier in ontogeny than cells capable of cytokine production. In normal lymphoid ontogeny, PHA-responsive IL-2-dependent cells are followed by the appearance of PHA-responsive IL-2-producing cells. Later in ontogeny, thymocytes capable of responding to allogeneic lymphocytes can be identified. Following their export to the peripheral circulation, T lymphocytes can be sensitized after exposure to specific antigen. Antigen-specific *in vitro* proliferation is first detected only in the presence of exogenous IL-2 followed by normal proliferation without exogenous IL-2, demonstrating that antigen-specific IL-2-dependent T lymphocytes develop before antigen-specific IL-2-producing T lymphocytes (Fig. 62.2).

Early B-lymphocyte ontogeny is T-lymphocyte independent. The differentiation of HSC to CLP and then to pre-B cells does not require the presence of T lymphocytes or T-lymphocyte-derived cytokines. However, at the pre-B cell stage, interaction with T lymphocytes through CD40–CD40 ligand is required for the terminal differentiation of the pre-B cells into mature B lymphocytes, which can then enter the lymph nodes and become antibody-secreting plasma cells [42]. Thus, defects in T-lymphocyte differentiation can result in the inability of pre-B cells to terminally differentiate, resulting in a decreased primary antibody response and an absence of significant immunoglobulin class switching.

Phenotypic analysis of HCT recipients

The recipients of autologous HSC recover their CD3+ T-lymphocyte count by 6–8 weeks following HCT, while allogeneic recipients normalize their CD3+ T-lymphocyte counts by 12 weeks. Acute GVHD has no effect on the recovery of CD3+ T lymphocytes. Recipients of unmanipulated autologous HSC achieve an absolute lymphocyte count of 500/µL more rapidly than do recipients of untreated histocompatible HSC (15 vs. 27–30 days) [43,44]. The delay in normalization of the absolute lymphocyte count in allogeneic recipients may be caused in part by the routine administration of post-transplant MTX as prophylaxis against acute GVHD [45]. The normalization of the percentage and absolute number of CD8+ T lymphocytes is more rapid than that of CD4+ T lymphocytes [43,45–48]. CD8+ T lymphocytes reach normal values by 4 months following HCT with allogeneic BM, while significant deficits in CD4+ T lymphocytes exist for the first 6 months following HCT. The more rapid normalization of CD8+ T-lymphocyte levels in conjunction with the reduced CD4+ levels results in an inversion of the normal CD4/CD8 ratio, which does not normalize until 6–9 months following HCT. Natural killer cells (CD16+, CD8^{dim}) reappear early post-HCT and during the first month represent the major lymphoid population [49]. The presence of natural killer cells in addition to the CD8+, CD3+ T lymphocytes further increases the total number of CD8+ lymphocytes and contributes to the inversion of the CD4/CD8 ratio.

In addition to the presence of mature CD3+ single positive T lymphocytes, phenotypic T lymphocytes, which are normally found in the peripheral circulation only during fetal life or in the adult thymus during postnatal life, can be present [50]. CD3^{dim} double negative and CD3+, CD4+, CD8+ (double positive) T lymphocytes can be detected. In addition, T lymphocytes expressing CD1, normally found only on thymocytes, are present in the peripheral circulation [51]. Some patients have the sustained presence of increased numbers of TCR-γδ T lymphocytes. These findings are consistent with a recapitulation of lymphoid ontogeny occurring after HCT.

Central to the production of mature T lymphocytes from the engrafted donor HCT or CLP is the recipient thymus. Two assays permit an assessment of normal and dysfunctional thymopoiesis:
1 the immunophenotypic characterization of recent thymic emigrants; and
2 the quantification of T-cell receptor excision circle (TREC) positive cells [52,53].

In normal individuals CD4+ recent thymic emigrants express the RA isoform of CD45 (CD4+, CD45RA+). The absolute number of new CD4+, CD45RA+ T lymphocytes is inversely correlated with transplant recipient age [54,55]. Thus, older recipients have a reduced capacity to produce new CD4+ T lymphocytes, secondary to decreased thymic function. Recent thymic emigrants contain TREC; as they proliferate, the TREC DNA does not duplicate and the frequency of TREC-positive cells decreases. In normal individuals the frequency of TREC-positive cells decreases with age, indicating that thymopoiesis decreases with age [53].

The number of B lymphocytes as determined by either the presence of surface immunoglobulin or CD20 expression returns to normal levels by 1–2 months following HCT and is unaffected by T-cell depletion [45]. Analysis of the variable heavy chain (VH) genes present in circulating B lymphocytes early following transplantation demonstrated VH usage similar to that seen in fetal B lymphocytes, indicating that a recapitulation of B-lymphocyte ontogeny occurs [56]. B lymphocytes expressing CD5 occur at increased frequency following transplantation, suggesting that post-HCT B lymphocytes are predisposed to autoantibody production or are activated [49]. Defects in mucosal IgA production exist for 6 months following HCT [57]. Without replacement IVIg transplant recipients have reduced levels of IgG, IgA and IgM for the first 6 months following BMT. Patients without chronic GVHD normalize their IgG levels by 8–9 months, their IgM levels by 9–12 months and their IgA levels by 2–3 years [2]. Patients with chronic GVHD may have elevated levels of IgM and IgG starting 6–9 months following HCT (Fig. 62.3).

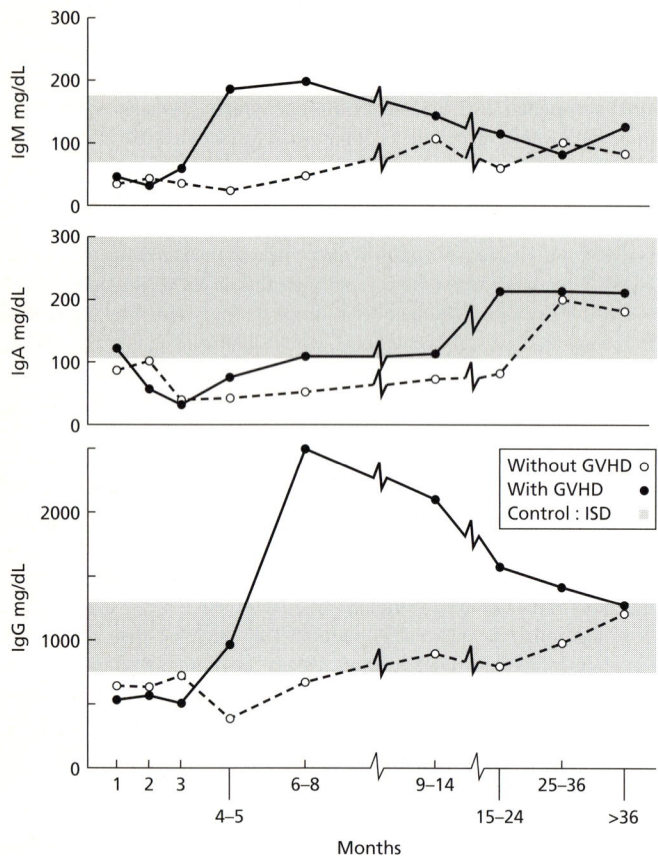

Fig. 62.3 Median values of serum IgG, IgA and IgM in patients after marrow transplantation. Shaded area represents values of marrow donors. Reproduced with permission from [2].

Functional analysis of T-lymphocyte reconstitution

The recovery of T-lymphocyte function following HCT can be assayed in terms of the response to either mitogenic stimuli (PHA, anti-CD3 antibody) or specific antigenic stimulation (tetanus toxoid, herpes virus antigens). Recipients of non-TCD BM show decreased proliferation to stimulation with PHA or anti-CD3 antibody for the first 1–2 months following HCT [45]. By the third month the addition of exogenous IL-2 can normalize the proliferative response to PHA stimulation when the proliferation is corrected for the percentage of $CD3^+$ T lymphocytes [58,59]. By 4–6 months proliferative responses to mitogenic stimulation are normal without the addition of exogenous IL-2, suggesting that a normal capacity to produce IL-2 is present. The addition of exogenous IL-1 rarely improves the proliferative response to mitogenic stimulation, demonstrating that normal IL-1 production by monocytes and other antigen-presenting cells is present following HCT.

Direct measurement of IL-2 following HCT demonstrates decreased IL-2 production. Recipients of histocompatible BM have decreased IL-2 production early after HCT as do long-term recipients with chronic GVHD [59]. When $CD4^+$ T lymphocytes are isolated early after HCT, IL-2 production is relatively normal on a per cell basis, suggesting that the decreased IL-2 production is caused in part by the quantitative decrease in the number of $CD4^+$ T lymphocytes in addition to the recapitulation of lymphoid ontogeny.

The T lymphocytes present following HCT can be derived from either the mature T lymphocytes in the HSC inoculum or the transplanted HSC. The most accurate assessment of T-lymphoid ontogeny following HSC can be observed in the recipients of TCD HSC where there is no significant contribution by the mature donor-derived T lymphocytes to post-HCT immune function.

Significant differences exist between the immune reconstitution of infants and adults following TCD haploidentical HCT [45,60,61]. Recipients who receive TCD haploidentical BM for severe combined immunodeficiency have no phenotypic T lymphocytes for 2–3 months following HCT, at which time $CD3^{dim}$ T lymphocytes first appear [60]. Three months after HCT a proliferative response to PHA stimulation in the presence of exogenous IL-2 can be first detected. The proliferative response to PHA in the absence of exogenous IL-2 normalizes by 4–6 months following HCT if no immunosuppression (cyclosporine [CSP]/steroids) is administered. The time course of responsiveness to mitogenic stimulation and the need for exogenous IL-2 parallels the time course of normal lymphoid ontogeny (Fig. 62.2). The capacity of T lymphocytes from the adult recipients of TCD HSC is markedly delayed, with PHA responses without exogenous IL-2 not being detectable until 9–12 months post-HCT.

T-lymphocyte immunity is characterized by antigen-specific responses. Recipient immunological response to specific antigens can be determined after either herpes virus reactivation/infection or specific immunization (phage ϕX174, tetanus toxoid). Protection against infection with opportunistic organisms does not correlate with mitogen-induced proliferation but with the reconstitution of antigen-specific T-lymphocyte function, which includes cytotoxic T lymphocytes (CTL), cytokine production (IL-2, IL-4, γ-interferon) and cooperation with B lymphocytes in specific antibody production.

Herpes viruses that are latent in HCT recipients are a potential source of infection following HCT. The acquisition of antigen-specific T-lymphocyte reactivity to herpes virus antigens following HCT is common and can be used to assess the reconstitution of post-HCT antigen-specific T-lymphocyte function. T-lymphocyte proliferation responses to herpes simplex (HSV), varicella zoster (VZV) and cytomegalovirus (CMV) are rarely detected during the first month following allogeneic HCT with BM, regardless of the immune status of the donor. By 40 days post-HCT a T-lymphocyte proliferation response to HSV can be detected, followed by the acquisition of responses to VZV and CMV [11,12]. The sequential acquisition of immunological responsiveness parallels the time course of viral reactivation (HSV < VZV < CMV). The routine administration of acyclovir delays the appearance of antigen-specific proliferation to HSV and VZV by inhibiting viral reactivation. The acquisition of antigen-specific T-lymphocyte proliferation, however, does not mean that normal T-lymphocyte function is present. Assessment of cytokine production has demonstrated decreased γ-interferon production following herpes virus antigen stimulation in the presence of normal proliferation [62]. When CTL function was assessed against VZV- and CMV-infected autologous fibroblasts, absence of a CTL response was noted in some patients even though normal proliferation was present, suggesting that the reconstitution of CTL activity lags behind the acquisition of antigen-specific proliferation [10,63].

The increased number of T lymphocytes present in PBC has been shown to provide clinical protection against infections with DNA viruses following autologous HCT; no reduction in the incidence of fatal infections has been seen in the allogeneic setting [16].

Functional analysis of B-lymphocyte reconstitution

Specific antibody production requires the interaction of antigen-specific T and B lymphocytes. Therefore defective antibody production can be caused by defects in either T or B lymphocytes. B-lymphocyte function can be determined following either mitogenic stimulation, which does not require antigen-specific T lymphocytes, or antigen-specific stimulation, which requires immunocompetent T lymphocytes. The proliferative

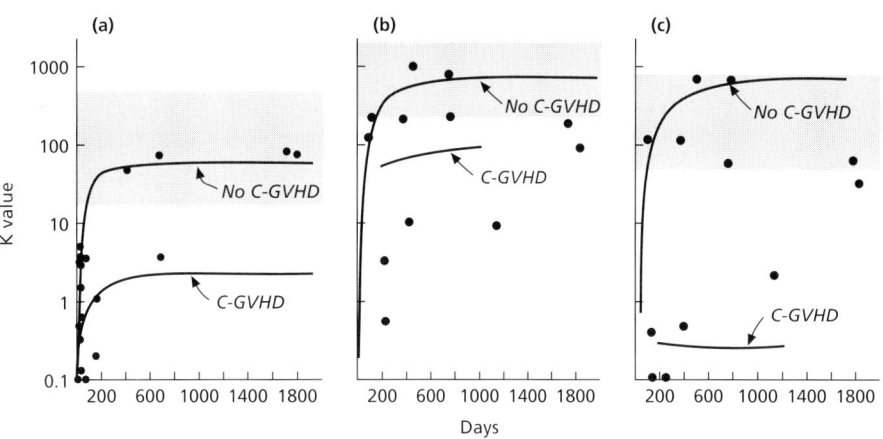

Fig. 62.4 Maximum antibody activity following (a) primary and (b) secondary φX174 phage injection in normal subjects and allogeneic and syngeneic marrow transplant recipients. (c) The IgG antibody activity of the secondary response. Hatched area represents 5th–95th percentile response for normal subjects. The curves represent the estimated means for data from allogeneic recipients with or without chronic graft-vs.-host disease (GVHD). The dots represent individual data points from syngeneic recipients. Reproduced with permission from [75].

response of B lymphocytes to mitogenic stimulation (*Staphylococcus aureus* Cowan strain A or cross-linked anti-IgM antibodies [antiμ]) returns to normal by 2 months after HCT, regardless of the type of transplant, and parallels the recovery of phenotypic B lymphocytes [45]. Thus, the functional capacity of B lymphocytes to respond to mitogenic stimulation normalizes early following HCT.

Because specific antibody production requires T–B lymphocyte interaction, *in vitro* immunoglobulin production following polyclonal T-lymphocyte stimulation is a more accurate assessment of B-lymphocyte immunocompetence than mitogenic stimulation. *In vitro* stimulation of T and B lymphocytes with pokeweed mitogen and nonmitogenic doses of *Staphylococcus aureus* Cowan strain A has revealed markedly reduced IgM and IgG production for the first 3 months following HCT [64–66]. Histocompatible recipients of BM have normal IgM production after 4–6 months. Recipients of unmodified BM have normal IgG production by 7–9 months, while recipients of TCD BM do not normalize their IgG production until 1 year. The normal production of IgM without IgG production 4–6 months post-HCT represents defective immunoglobulin switching (IgM → IgG), which is secondary to defects in T-lymphocyte function [45].

Specific antibody production *in vivo* can be assessed by the evaluation of antibody-positive recipients who receive BM from antibody-negative donors and of antibody-negative recipients who are transplanted from antibody-positive donors. Antibody-positive recipients have detectable antibody early after HCT but sustained antibody production is not present 1 year following the transplantation of BM. Antibody-negative recipients who receive BM from antibody-positive donors have detectable antibody post-HCT, but the antibody production is not sustained. Thus, without antigenic stimulation following HCT, sustained antibody production does not occur [19]. When antibody-positive recipients are immunized immediately (0–14 days) following HCT, a transient rise in antibody titer can be observed. Immunization later in the post-HCT period does not result in specific antibody production unless new antigen-specific T lymphocytes are generated.

Immunization with new antigens such as keyhole limpet hemocyanin (KLH) or phage φX174, to which neither the donor nor the recipient has been immunized, provide the most accurate assessment of the recipient's capacity to produce specific antibody [3]. Primary immunization during the first 2–3 months following HCT of either allogeneic or syngeneic BM results in absent or minimal IgM antibody production. Primary immunization more than 3 months following HCT produces a heterogeneous response; recipients without chronic GVHD have normal primary IgM responses, while recipients with chronic GVHD have markedly reduced primary responses. Repeat immunization to determine the recipient's secondary antibody response and the capacity to switch from IgM to IgG antibody production varies with the chronic GVHD status of the recipient. Patients without chronic GVHD have a normal secondary response and normal immunoglobulin switching, while patients with chronic GVHD have a reduced secondary antibody response which remains primarily IgM (Fig. 62.4). Thus, patients with chronic GVHD have a reduced capacity to make specific antibodies to new antigens and an inability to switch from IgM to IgG antibody production.

Transplant recipients are similar to normal newborns, who can respond to protein antigens but not to polysaccharide antigens [67,68]. Thus, the reconstitution of B-lymphocyte function following HCT, like that of T lymphocytes, recapitulates normal lymphoid ontogeny. The reconstitution of the capacity to produce antibody to polysaccharide antigens is delayed in allogeneic recipients without chronic GVHD as compared to their capacity to respond to protein antigens. The recipients of autologous HCT and the majority of histocompatible HCT recipients without chronic GVHD have a normal ontogeny of their antibody responses to bacterial polysaccharide antigens (normal antibody levels by 2–3 years following HCT) [69]. The recipients of unrelated HCT, who do not have clinically evident GVHD, have a sustained inability to produce anticarbohydrate antibodies to *Haemophilus influenzae* type b, which may be the basis for the observed increase in their incidence of infections with encapsulated respiratory bacteria. Because the defects in anticarbohydrate antibody production have persisted for more than a decade in some patients, it is possible that many recipients of unrelated HCT will have a lifelong inability to produce protective levels of anticarbohydrate antibodies requiring the long-term administration of prophylactic antibiotics and/or IVIg.

Effect of GVHD on immunologic reconstitution

Acute GVHD following histocompatible HCT has little effect on the tempo of lymphoid reconstitution as measured by absolute lymphocyte count or the absolute number of $CD3^+$ T lymphocytes. Transient depression of the absolute lymphocyte count and $CD3^+$ T-lymphocyte counts occurs following the administration of antithymocyte globulin (ATG) and anti-T-lymphocyte monoclonal antibodies. In the absence of antibody therapy the tempo of recovery of T- and B-lymphocyte numbers is unaffected by acute GVHD. The presence of acute GVHD and/or its treatment with ATG is associated with a decreased primary antibody response to KLH even if patients do not develop chronic GVHD [3]. Thus, acute GVHD may result in a sustained immunodeficiency in the absence of chronic GVHD, presumably because of thymic damage [70,71].

Transient elevation of IgE levels and the production of specific IgE antibodies have been demonstrated early following HCT (14–28 days) and correlate with the presence of acute GVHD [72,73]. IgE production is normally stimulated by IL-4 and suppressed by γ-interferon, suggesting that imbalances in these cytokines occur early following HCT.

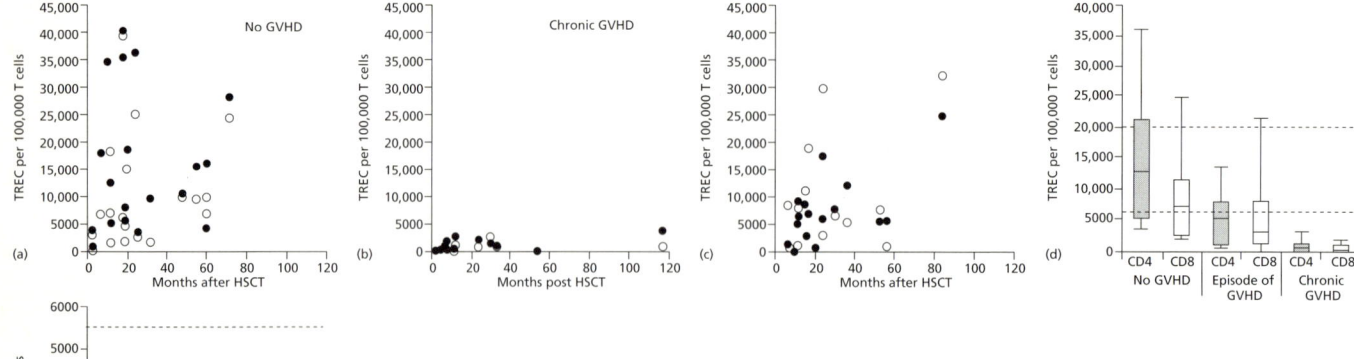

Fig. 62.5 Cross-sectional analysis of TREC levels in relationship to GVHD. (a) Individual $CD4_1$ (●) and $CD8_1$ (○) T-cell TREC levels are shown for a cross-section of patients through years of age with no history of GVHD. (b) Patients through 25 years of age with chronic GVHD. (c) Patients through 25 years of age with a history of GVHD. (d) A composite box plot for TREC levels is shown for all 3 groups. The top, bottom, and line through the middle of the box correspond to the 75th, 25th, and 50th percentile (median) respectively. The whiskers on the bottom and top extend from the 10th percentile and top 90th percentile, respectively. (e) Individual $CD4_1$ (closed symbols) and $CD8_1$ (open symbols) T-cell TREC levels are shown for a cross-section of patients older than 25 years of age with no history of GVHD (squares), with chronic GVHD (triangles), and with a history of GVHD (circles). Normal range of TREC levels for individuals of ages in groups studied are shown lying between the dashed lines.

The most apparent immune abnormalities caused by GVHD are seen in chronic GVHD. Patients with chronic GVHD have a decreased capacity to develop an antigen-specific T-lymphocyte response and to produce specific antibodies, particularly to polysaccharide antigens, while having an increased incidence of autoantibodies (anti-DNA, erythrocyte, thyroid, etc.) [74]. Immunization of patients with chronic GVHD with recall antigens such as tetanus and diphtheria toxoids or neoantigens such as KLH has revealed sustained defects in antibody production, including decreased primary antibody production, decreased immunoglobulin switching and decreased secondary antibody production (Fig. 62.4) [3,75]. Analysis of the infectious complications of chronic GVHD recipients before the routine administration of prophylactic antibiotics and IVIg showed an increased incidence of infections with encapsulated respiratory bacteria, including sepsis, pneumonitis and sinusitis [76,77]. The routine administration of prophylactic antibiotics and IVIg has markedly reduced these infection complications. However, the inability of patients with chronic GVHD to produce protective antibodies to bacterial polysaccharide antigens remains. Conjugated polysaccharide vaccines can immunize normal infants at 2–6 months of age, a time when they are unable to respond to nonconjugated polysaccharide vaccines [77]. Similar efficiency with conjugated polysaccharide vaccine has been shown in HCT recipients [78]. However, the ability of HCT recipients to respond successfully to conjugated polysaccharide vaccines does not mean that they can respond to wild type bacterial polysaccharide antigens.

In vitro analysis of the cellular basis of the immunodeficiency present in chronic GVHD patients has demonstrated a variety of cellular defects. Decreases in the number and function of $CD4^+$ helper T lymphocytes have been described in addition to the presence of activated $CD4^+$ and $CD8^+$ suppressor T lymphocytes [79,80]. Patients with chronic GVHD have a reduced capacity to produce new $CD4^+$ T lymphocytes [54,55]. Limiting dilution analysis has identified a decrease in the frequency of helper T-lymphocyte precursors early after HCT in all recipients and a sustained decrease in the frequency of CTL and helper T-lymphocyte precursors in patients with chronic GVHD [81]. Intrinsic B-lymphocyte defects that result in a lack of normal responsiveness to T-lymphocyte stimulation have been identified [82,83].

The absolute number of new $CD4^+$ T lymphocytes predicts the capacity of HCT recipients to respond to immunization [55]. Thus, recipients who are unable to produce new $CD4^+$ T lymphocytes have difficulty in responding to antigenic stimuli. Thus, much of the immunocompetence of older HCT recipients may be derived from mature T lymphocytes infused at the time of HCT. From murine experiments it is still unclear what the antigenic repetitive of such T lymphocytes will be, especially their responses to new antigens to which the donor had not previously been exposed [84].

Evaluation of recent thymic immigrants by both immunophenotyping and TREC analysis has demonstrated that there is an age-dependent decline in the ability of HCT recipients who do not have chronic GVHD to produce new T lymphocytes [54,55,85,86]. The capacity to produce new T lymphocytes was found to be predictive of the ability of recipients to respond to reimmunization with a recalled antigen (tetanus toxoid). Of particular importance is the observation that a history of acute GVHD, even in recipients who do not have chronic GVHD, results in a sustained inability of the recipient to produce new T lymphocytes (Fig. 62.5) [87]. Because the thymopoietic capacity of older autologous HCT recipients (over the age of 40 years) is adequate to produce new T lymphocytes and the effects of pretransplant chemoradiotherapy without the allogeneic effects of GVHD do not result in a sustained inability to produce new T lymphocytes, the impact of GVHD on thymic function appears to be central to post-HCT immunodeficiency. If HCT recipients with a history of acute GVHD have a limited capacity to produce new $CD4^+$ T lymphocytes, they must depend upon the clonal expansion of donor-derived T lymphocytes for their immunocompetence. The spectrum of antigens to which such T lymphocytes can respond may be limited and this may explain the increased incidence of opportunistic infections found in older recipients of unrelated HSC.

CSP can inhibit the differentiation of double positive thymocytes into $CD3^+$ single positive thymocytes [88]. The combined effects of thymic damage and CSP may result in defects in both positive and negative thymic selection. Defective positive thymic selection results in a reduction in the frequency of mature T lymphocytes with specificity for exogenous antigens, while reduced negative selection results in an increased frequency of autoreactive T lymphocytes involved in the pathogenesis of chronic GVHD.

Therapies to improve post-HCT immune function

Based upon research in murine models, approaches to improve post-HCT immune function have been identified and are entering phase 1 studies. The attempts to improve post-HCT immunological function can be divided into:
1 thymic protection;
2 thymic replacement;
3 CLP transfer; and
4 adoptive therapy with antigen-specific cells.

Table 62.1 Immunization following hematopoietic cell transplantation (HCT).

Vaccine	Patients without chronic GVHD	Patients with chronic GVHD
Diphtheria–tetanus toxoid	3–6 months	3–6 months
Oral polio virus (Sabin)	Not recommended	Not recommended
Inactivated polio virus (Salk)	6–12 months	Not indicated if on IVIg
Hepatitis B	6–12 months	6–12 months
Measles–mumps–rubella	1–2 years	Not recommended
Varicella	2 years	Not recommended

GVHD, graft-vs.-host disease; IVIg, intravenous immunoglobulin.

Keratinocyte growth factor (KGF) can protect epithelial cells, including the thymic epithelium, from the toxic effects of pretransplant chemoradiotherapy. The protection of thymic epithelial cells can result in improved immunologic function following the transplantation of both autologous and allogeneic HSC [89].

The first successful attempt to improve post-HCT immune function was the administration of IL-7 following HCT. IL-7 is a central cytokine in early thymic differentiation where it has both proliferative and anti-apopotic effects on thymocytes. Murine studies have showed that the post-transplant administration of IL-7 enhances immune reconstitution but a parallel increase in acute GVHD has been observed in some studies [90–92].

Recently, CLP has immunophenotypically been identified in humans [29]. The differentiation of CLP is restricted to cells of lymphoid origin. Preclinical studies in mice have shown that the infusion of CLP into animals receiving only purified HSC results in improved post-HCT immunologic function when challenged with CMV [93]. The determination of conditions that would support the *in vitro* expansion of CLP would mean that it would be possible to infuse large numbers of naive CLP into HCT recipients; CLP would then undergo differentiation through the recipient thymus—giving rise to the appropriate antigen-specific T lymphocytes.

During the last decade several investigators have shown that the infusion of antigen-specific CD4+ or CD8+ T lymphocytes with specificity for viral pathogens such as CMV and EBV can have both therapeutic and prophylactic effects [94,95]. The problem associated with the administration of antigen-specific T lymphocytes is that no protective immunity to other pathogens is generated.

Transfer of immunologically mediated diseases following HCT

The chemoradiotherapy that HCT recipients receive ablates all their T-lymphocyte and the majority of their B-lymphocyte immunity. The transplantation of a donor immune system with a genetically determined predilection to produce autoimmune or IgE antibodies results in recipients with autoimmune or allergic diseases. When nonallergic recipients were transplanted with HSC from skin test positive donors who have had clinical allergies, skin test reactivity was detected in 8 of 11 long-term recipients; 7 recipients developed clinical allergic rhinitis; and 2 developed clinical asthma without a prior history of the disease [96]. Thus, the clinical transfer of IgE-mediated hypersensitivity can occur following HCT.

One recipient transplanted with BM from a donor who produced an antiplatelet antibody developed thrombocytopenia that ultimately resolved but had persistent autoantibody production [97]. The transfer of antiacetylcholine receptor antibody production from a donor with myasthenia gravis resulted in clinical myasthenia gravis in the recipient [98].

Immunization

Immunization with protein antigens in the immediate post-HCT period can result in short-lived increases in antibody levels. However, sustained anti-body production following immunization with protein antigens can occur only when adequate T-lymphocyte immunocompetence has been established. Therefore, immunization with protein antigen during the first 1–2 months after HCT does not result in sustained antibody production. The onset of antigen-specific T-lymphocyte function in patients without chronic GVHD occurs 3–6 months following BMT. Recipients reimmunized with tetanus and diphtheria toxoids during this period routinely develop antigen-specific T-lymphocyte proliferation and the *in vivo* production of specific antibody (Table 62.1). Immunization with unconjugated poly-saccharide vaccines during the same period rarely results in the production of protective antibody lines although immunization with conjugated poly-saccharide vaccines results in protective antibody. Most recipients with chronic GVHD are unable to develop protective T- or B-lymphocyte immunity even after repeated immunizations. The routine administration of IVIg to patients with chronic GVHD abrogates the need for these patients to receive routine immunization with protein or polysaccharide antigens.

Because of potential defects in the production of antibodies to viral proteins, the use of inactivated polio virus vaccine is preferable to the use of live oral polio vaccine for HCT recipients [99,100]. Transplant recipients without chronic GVHD can be immunized with inactivated polio vaccine 6–12 months after BMT. Because of the risks associated with the administration of live attenuated viral vaccines, immunization with the measles–mumps–rubella and varicella vaccines is not advocated in patients without chronic GVHD until 1–2 years following HCT unless the social environment demands early immunization [99–101]. Patients with chronic GVHD who are receiving IVIg are not at risk of infection because they have passive antibody protection. Indeed, vaccination with a live viral vaccine in the presence of IVIg replacement therapy is ineffective. The efficacy of immunization can be confirmed by the measurement of specific antibody levels.

References

1 Parkman R, Gelfand EW, Rosen FS, Sanderson A, Hirschhorn R. Severe combined immunodeficiency and adenosine deaminase deficiency. *N Engl J Med* 1975; **292**: 714–9.
2 Noel DR, Witherspoon RP, Storb R *et al*. Does graft-versus-host disease influence the tempo of immunologic recovery after allogeneic human marrow transplantation? An observation on 56 long-term survivors. *Blood* 1978; **51**: 1087–105.
3 Witherspoon RP, Storb R, Ochs HD *et al*. Recovery of antibody production in human allogeneic marrow graft recipients: influence of time posttransplantation, the presence or absence of chronic graft-versus-host disease, and antithymocyte globulin treatment. *Blood* 1981; **58**: 360–8.
4 Ochs L, Shu XO, Miller J *et al*. Late infections after allogeneic bone marrow transplantations: comparison of incidence in related and unrelated

donor transplant recipients. *Blood* 1995; **86**: 3979–86.
5 Small TN, Papadopoulos EB, Boulad F *et al.* Comparison of immune reconstitution after unrelated and related T-cell depleted bone marrow transplantation: effect of patient age and donor leukocyte infusions. *Blood* 1999; **93**: 467–80.
6 Meyers JD, Flournoy N, Thomas ED. Cytomegalovirus infection and specific cell-mediated immunity after marrow transplant. *J Infect Dis* 1980; **142**: 816–24.
7 Meyers JD, Flournoy N, Thomas ED. Cell-mediated immunity to varicella-zoster virus after allogeneic marrow transplant. *J Infect Dis* 1980; **141**: 479–87.
8 Meyers JD, Flournoy N, Thomas ED. Infection with herpes simplex virus and cell-mediated immunity after marrow transplant. *J Infect Dis* 1980; **142**: 338–46.
9 Wade JC, Day LM, Crowley JJ, Meyers JD. Recurrent infection with herpes simplex virus after marrow transplantation: role of the specific immune response and acyclovir treatment. *J Infect Dis* 1980; **149**: 750–6.
10 Quinnan GV, Kirmani N, Rook AH *et al.* Cytotoxic cells in cytomegalovirus infection: HLA-restricted T-lymphocyte and non-T-lymphocyte cytotoxic responses correlate with recovery from cytomegalovirus infection in bone marrow transplant recipients. *N Engl J Med* 1982; **307**: 7–13.
11 Ljungman P, Wilczek H, Gahrton G *et al.* Long-term acyclovir prophylaxis in bone marrow transplant recipients and lymphocyte proliferation responses to herpes virus antigens *in vitro*. *Bone Marrow Transplant* 1986; **1**: 185–92.
12 Gratama JW, Verdonck LF, Van Der Linden JA *et al.* Cellular immunity to vaccinations and herpes-virus infections after bone marrow transplantation. *Transplantation* 1986; **41**: 719–24.
13 Ottinger HD, Beelen DW, Scheulen B, Schaefer UW, Gross-Wilde H. Improved immune reconstitution after allotransplantation of peripheral blood stem cells instead of bone marrow. *Blood* 1996; **88**: 2775–9.
14 Holmberg LA, Boeckh M, Hooper H *et al.* Increased incidence of cytomegalovirus disease after autologous CD34-selected peripheral blood stem cell transplantation. *Blood* 1999; **94**: 4029–35.
15 Crippa F, Holmbertg L, Carter RA *et al.* Infectious complications after autologous CD34-selected peripheral blood stem cell transplantation. *Biol Blood Marrow Transplant* 2002; **8**: 281–9.
16 Storek J, Dawson MA, Storer B *et al.* Immune reconstitution after allogeneic marrow transplantation compared with blood stem cell transplantation. *Blood* 2001; **97**: 3380–9.
17 Lum LG, Seigneuret MC, Storb R. The transfer of antigen-specific humoral immunity from marrow donors to marrow recipients. *J Clin Immunol* 1986; **6**: 389–96.
18 Lum LG, Munn NA, Schanfield MS, Storb R. The detection of specific antibody formation to recall antigens after human bone marrow transplantation. *Blood* 1986; **67**: 582–7.
19 Wimperis JZ, Brenner MK, Prentice HG *et al.* Transfer of a functioning humoral immune system in transplantation of T-lymphocyte-depleted bone marrow. *Lancet* 1986; **1**: 339–43.
20 Wahren B, Gahrton G, Linde A *et al.* Transfer and persistence of viral antibody-producing cells in bone marrow transplantation. *J Infect Dis* 1984; **150**: 358–65.
21 Witherspoon RP, Schanfield MS, Strob R, Thomas ED, Giblett ER. Immunoglobulin production of donor origin after marrow transplatation for acute leukemia or aplastic anemia. *Transplantation* 1978; **26**: 407–8.
22 Chaushu S, Chaushu G, Garfunkel A *et al.* Salivary immunoglobulins in recipients of bone marrow grafts. II. Transient secretion of donor-derived salivary IgA following transplantation of T-cell-depleted bone marrow. *Bone Marrow Transplant* 1994; **14**: 925–8.
23 Sullivan KM, Kopecky KJ, Jocom J *et al.* Immunomodulatory and antimicrobial efficacy of intravenous immunoglobulin in bone marrow transplantation. *N Engl J Med* 1990; **323**: 705–12.
24 Winston DJ, Gale RP, Meyer DV, Young LS, The UCLA Bone Marrow Transplantation Group. Infectious complications of human bone marrow transplantation. *Medicine* 1979; **58**: 1–31.
25 Winston DJ, Ho WG, Schiffman G *et al.* Pneumococcal vaccination of recipients of bone marrow transplant. *Arch Intern Med* 1983; **143**: 1735–7.
26 Parkkali T, Kayhty H, Ruutu T *et al.* A comparison of early and late vaccination with *Haemophilus influenzae* type b conjugate and pneumococcal polysaccharide vaccines after allogeneic BMT. *Bone Marrow Transplant* 1996; **18**: 961–7.
27 Gandhi MK, Egner W, Sizer L *et al.* Antibody responses to vaccinations given within the first 2 years after transplant are similar between autologous peripheral blood stem cell and bone marrow transplant recipients. *Bone Marrow Transplant* 2001; **28**: 775–81.
28 Kondo M, Weissman IL, Akashi K. Identification of clonogenic common lymphoid progenitors in mouse bone marrow. *Cell* 1997; **91**: 661–72.
29 Hao QL, Zhu J, Price MA *et al.* Identification of a novel, human multilymphoid progenitor in cord blood. *Blood* 2001; **97**: 3683–90.
30 Haynes BF, Denning SM, Singer KH, Kurtzberg J. Ontogeny of T-cell precursors: a model for the initial stages of human T-cell development. *Immunol Today* 1989; **10**: 87–91.
31 Sudo T, Nishikawa S, Ohno N *et al.* Expression and function of the interleukin 7 receptor in murine lymphocytes. *Proc Natl Acad Sci U S A* 1993; **90**: 9125–9.
32 Ferrick DA, Ohashi PS, Wallace V, Schilham M, Mak TW. Thymic ontogeny and selection of $\alpha\beta$ and $\gamma\delta$ T cells. *Immunol Today* 1989; **10**: 403–7.
33 Toribio ML, Alonso JM, Barcena A *et al.* Human T-cell precursors: involvement of the IL-2 pathway in the generation of mature T cells. *Immunol Rev* 1988; **104**: 55–79.
34 Haynes BF, Martin ME, Kay HH, Kurtzberg J. Early events in human T cell ontogeny. *J Exp Med* 1988; **168**: 1061–80.
35 Campana D, Janossy G, Coustan-Smith E *et al.* The expression of T cell receptor-associated proteins during T cell ontogeny in man. *J Immunol* 1989; **142**: 57–66.
36 Haynes BF, Singer KH, Dennings SM, Martin ME. Analysis of expression of CD2, CD3 and T cell antigen receptor molecules during early human fetal thymic development. *J Immunol* 1988; **141**: 3776–84.
37 Noguchi M, Yi H, Rosenblatt HM, Filipovich AH *et al.* Interleukin-2 receptor gamma chain mutation results in X-linked severe combined immunodeficiency in humans. *Cell* 1993; **73**: 147–57.
38 Akashi K, Kondo M, von Freeden-Jeffry U, Murray R, Weissman IL. Bcl-2 rescues T lymphopoiesis in interleukin-7 receptor-deficient mice. *Cell* 1997; **89**: 1033–41.
39 Marrack P, Lo D, Brinster R *et al.* The effect of thymus environment on T cell development and tolerance. *Cell* 1988; **53**: 627–34.
40 Sha WC, Nelson CA, Newberry RD *et al.* Positive and negative selection of an antigen receptor on T cells in transgenic mice. *Nature* 1988; **336**: 73–6.
41 Zuniga-Pflucker JC, Longo DL, Kruisbeek AM. Positive selection of CD4–8$^+$ T cells in the thymus of normal mice. *Nature* 1989; **338**: 338–76.
42 Fluckiger AC, Sanz E, Garcia-Lloret M *et al.* In vitro reconstitution of human B-cell ontogeny: from CD34 ($^+$) multipotent progenitors to Ig-secreting cells. *Blood* 1998; **92**: 4509–20.
43 Atkinson K. Reconstitution of the haemopoietic and immune systems after marrow transplantation. *Bone Marrow Transplant* 1990; **5**: 209–26.
44 Linch DC, Knott LJ, Thomas RM *et al.* T cell regeneration after allogeneic and autologous bone marrow transplantation. *Br J Haematol* 1983; **53**: 451–8.
45 Keever CA, Small TN, Flomenberg N *et al.* Immune reconstitution following bone marrow transplantation: comparison of recipients of T-cell depleted marrow with recipients of conventional marrow grafts. *Blood* 1989; **73**: 1340–50.
46 Friedrich W, O'Reilly RJ, Koziner B *et al.* T-lymphocyte reconstitution in recipients of bone marrow transplants with and without GVHD: imbalances of T-cell subpopulations having unique regulatory and congnitive functions. *Blood* 1982; **59**: 696–701.
47 Forman SJ, Nocker P, Gallagher M *et al.* Pattern of T cell reconstitution following allogeneic bone marrow transplantation for acute hematological malignancy. *Transplantation* 1982; **34**: 96–8.
48 Atkinson K. T cell sub-populations defined by monoclonal antibodies after HLA-identical sibling marrow transplantation. II. Activated and fuctional subsets of the helper-inducer and the cytotoxic-suppressor sub-populations defined by two colour fluorescence flow cytometry. *Bone Marrow Transplant* 1986; **1**: 121–32.
49 Ault KE, Antin JH, Ginsburg D *et al.* Phenotype of recovering lymphoid cell populations after marrow transplantation. *J Exp Med* 1985; **161**: 1483–502.
50 Gratama JW, Fibbe WE, Visser JW *et al.* CD3$^+$, 4$^+$ and/or 8$^+$ T cells and CD3$^+$, 4$^-$, 8$^-$ T cells repopulate at different rates after allogeneic bone marrow transplantation. *Bone Marrow Transplant* 1989; **4**: 291–6.
51 Rappeport JM, Dunn MJ, Parkman R. Immature T lymphocytes in the peripheral blood of bone marrow transplant recipients. *Transplantation* 1983; **36**: 674–80.
52 Mackall CL, Fleisher TA, Brown MR *et al.* Age, thymopoiesis, and CD4$^+$ T-lymphocyte regeneration after intensive chemotherapy. *N Engl J Med* 1995; **332**: 143–9.
53 Douek DC, McFarland RD, Keiser PH *et al.* Changes in thymic function with age and during the treatment of HIV infection. *Nature* 1998; **396**: 690–5.
54 Storek J, Witherspoon RP, Storb R. T cell reconstitution after bone marrow transplantation into adult patients does not resemble T cell development in

55. Weinberg K, Annett GM, Kashyap A et al. The effect of thymic function on immunocompetence following bone marrow transplantation. *Biol Blood Marrow Transplant* 1995; **1**: 18–23.
56. Storek J, King L, Ferrara S et al. Abundance of a restricted fetal B cell repertoire in marrow transplant recipients. *Bone Marrow Transplant* 1994; **14**: 783–90.
57. Chaushu S, Chaushu G, Garfunkel AA et al. Salivary immunoglobulins in recipients of bone marrow grafts. I. A longitudinal follow-up. *Bone Marrow Transplant* 1994; **14**: 871–6.
58. Roosnek EE, Brouwer MC, Vossen JM et al. The role of interleukin-2 in proliferative responses *in vitro* of T cells from patients after bone marrow transplantation. *Transplantation* 1987; **43**: 855–60.
59. Welte K, Liobanu N, Moore MAS et al. Defective interleukin-2 production in patients after bone marrow transplantation and *in vitro* restoration of defective T-lymphocyte proliferation by highly purified interleukin 2. *Blood* 1984; **64**: 380–5.
60. O'Reilly RJ, Keever CA, Small TN, Brochstein J. The use of HLA-non-identical T-cell-depleted marrow transplants for correction of severe combined immunodeficiency disease. *Immunodeficiency Rev* 1989; **1**: 273–309.
61. Aversa F, Tabilio A, Velardi A et al. Treatment of high-risk acute leukemia with T-cell depleted stem cells from related donors with one fully mismatched HLA haplotype. *N Engl J Med* 1998; **339**: 1186–93.
62. Levin MJ, Parkman R, Oxman MN et al. Proliferative and interferon responses following transplantation in man. *Infect Immunol* 1997; **20**: 678–84.
63. Reusser P, Riddell SR, Meyers JD, Greenberg PD. Cytotoxic T-lymphocyte response to cytomegalovirus after human allogeneic bone marrow transplantation. Pattern of recovery and correlation with cytomegalovirus infection and disease. *Blood* 1991; **78**: 1373–80.
64. Witherspoon RP, Lum LG, Storb R, Thomas ED. *In vitro* regulation of immunoglobulin synthesis after human marrow transplantation. II. Deficient T and non-T-lymphocyte function within 3–4 months of allogeneic, syngeneic, or autologous marrow grafting for hematologic malignancy. *Blood* 1982; **59**: 844–50.
65. Ringden O, Witherspoon R, Storb R, Ekelund E, Thomas ED. B cell function in human marrow transplantation recipients assessed by direct and indirect haemolysis-in gel. *J Immunol* 1979; **123**: 2729–34.
66. Witherspoon RP, Goehle S, Kretschmer M, Storb R. Regulation of immunoglobulin production after human marrow grafting: the role of helper and suppressor T cells in acute graft-versus-host disease. *Transplantation* 1986; **41**: 328–35.
67. Peltola H, Kayhta H, Sivonen A, Makela PH. *Haemophilus influenzae* type B capsular polysaccharide vaccine in children. A double-blind field study of 100 000 vaccinees 3 months to 5 years of age in Finland. *Pediatrics* 1977; **60**: 730–3.
68. Wilkens J, Wehrle PF. Further characterization of responses of infants and children to meningococcal polysaccharide vaccine. *J Pediatr* 1979; **94**: 828–32.
69. Kapoor N, Chan R, Weinberg KI, Burotto F, Parkman R. Defective anticarbohydrate antibody responses to naturally occurring bacteria following bone marrow transplantation. *Biol Blood Marrow Transplant* 1999; **5**: 46–50.
70. Seddik M, Seemayer TA, Lapp WS. T cell functional defect associated with thymic epithelial cell injury induced by a graft-versus-host reaction. *Transplantation* 1980; **29**: 61–6.
71. Seddik M, Seemayer TA, Lapp WS. The graft-versus-host reaction and immune function. *Transplantation* 1984; **37**: 281–6.
72. Saryan JA, Rappeport J, Leung DY, Parkman R, Geha RS. Regulation of human immunoglobulin E synthesis in acute graft-versus-host disease. *J Clin Invest* 1983; **71**: 556–64.
73. Ringden O, Persson U, Johansson SG et al. Markedly elevated serum IgE levels following allogeneic and syngeneic bone marrow transplantation. *Blood* 1983; **61**: 1190–5.
74. Graze PR, Gale RP. Chronic graft versus host disease. A syndrome of disordered immunity. *Am J Med* 1979; **66**: 611–20.
75. Witherspoon RP, Kopecky K, Storb RF et al. Immunological recovery in 48 patients following syngeneic marrow transplantation for hematological malignancy. *Transplantation* 1982; **33**: 143–9.
76. Atkinson K, Storb R, Prentice RL et al. Analysis of late infections in 89 long-term survivors of bone marrow transplantation. *Blood* 1979; **53**: 720–31.
77. Anderson PW, Pichichero ME, Insel RA et al. Vaccines consisting of periodate-cleaved oligosaccharides from the capsule of *Haemophilus influenzae* type b coupled to a protein carrier: structural and temporal requirements for priming the human infant. *J Immunol* 1986; **137**: 1181–6.
78. Vance E, George S, Guinan EC et al. Comparison of multiple immunization schedules for *Haemophilus influenzae* type b-conjugate and tetanus toxoid vaccines following bone marrow transplantation. *Bone Marrow Transplant* 1998; **22**: 735–41.
79. Reinherz EL, Parkman R, Rappeport J, Rosen FS, Schlossman SF. Aberrations of suppressor T cells in human graft-versus-host disease. *N Engl J Med* 1979; **300**: 1061–8.
80. Lum LG, Seigneuret MC, Storb RF, Witherspoon RP, Thomas ED. *In vitro* regulation of immunoglobulin synthesis after marrow transplantation. I. T-cell and B-cell deficiencies in patients with and without chronic graft-versus-host disease. *Blood* 1981; **58**: 431–9.
81. Rozans MK, Smith BR, Burakoff SJ, Miller RA. Long-lasting deficit of functional T cell precursors in human bone marrow transplant recipients revealed by limiting dilution methods. *J Immunol* 1986; **136**: 4040–8.
82. Lum LG, Seigneuret MC, Oreutt-Thordarson N et al. The regulation of immunoglobulin synthesis after HLA-identical bone marrow transplantation. VI. Differential rates of maturation of distinct functional groups within lymphoid subpopulations in patients after human marrow grafting. *Blood* 1985; **65**: 1422–33.
83. Storek J, Saxon A. Reconstitution of B cell immunity following bone marrow transplantation. *Bone Marrow Transplant* 1992; **9**: 395–408.
84. Fry TJ, Christensen BL, Komschlies KL, Gress RE, Mackall CL. Interleukin-7 restores immunity in athymic T-cell depleted hosts. *Blood* 2001; **97**: 1525–33.
85. Douek DC, Vescio RA, Betts MA et al. Assessment of thymic output in adults after hematopoietic stem-cell transplantation and prediction of T-cell reconstitution. *Lancet* 2000; **355**: 1875–81.
86. Storek J, Joseph A, Dawson MA, Douek DC, Storer B, Maloney DG. Factors influencing T-lymphopoiesis after allogeneic hematopoietic cell transplantation. *Transplantation* 2002; **73**: 1154–8.
87. Weinberg K, Blazar BR, Wagner JE et al. Factors affecting thymic function after allogeneic hematopoietic stem cell transplantation. *Blood* 2001; **97**: 1458–66.
88. Jenkins MK, Schwartz RH, Pardoll DM. Effects of cyclosporine A on T cell development and clonal deletion. *Science* 1988; **241**: 1655–8.
89. Min D, Taylor PA, Panoskaltisis-Mortari A et al. Protection from thymic epithelial cell injury by keratinocyte growth factor: a new approach to improve thymic and peripheral T-cell reconstitution after bone marrow transplantation. *Blood* 2002; **99**: 4592–600.
90. Bolotin E, Smorgorzewska M, Smith S, Widmer M, Weinberg K. Enhancement of thymopoiesis after bone marrow transplant by *in vivo* interleukin-7. *Blood* 1996; **88**: 1887–94.
91. Alpdogan O, Schmaltz C, Muriglan SJ et al. Administration of interleukin-7 after allogeneic bone marrow transplantation improves immune reconstitution without aggravating graft-versus-host disease. *Blood* 2001; **98**: 2256–65.
92. Mackall CL, Fry TJ, Bare C et al. IL-7 increases both thymic-dependent and thymic-independent T-cell regeneration after bone marrow transplantation. *Blood* 2001; **97**: 1491–7.
93. Brown JM, BitMansour A, Mocarski ES, Akashi K, Weissman IL. Immune protection from lethal murine common lymphocyte progenitors or lymph node cells with hematopoietic stem cells. *Biol Blood Marrow Transplant* 1999; **5**: 98–104.
94. Walter EA, Greenberg PD, Gilbert MJ et al. Reconstitution of cellular immunity against cytomegalovirus in recipients of allogeneic bone marrow by transfer of T-cell clones from the donor. *N Engl J Med* 1995; **333**: 1038–44.
95. Koehne G, Smith KM, Ferguson TL et al. Quantification, selection, and functional characterization of Epstein–Barr virus-specific and alloreactive T-cells detected by intracellular interferon-gamma production and growth of cytotoxic precursors. *Blood* 2002; **99**: 1730–40.
96. Agosti JM, Sprenger JD, Lum LG et al. Transfer of allergen-specific IgE-mediated hypersensitivity with allogeneic bone marrow transplantation. *N Engl J Med* 1988; **319**: 1623–8.
97. Minchinton RM, Waters AH, Kendra J, Barrett AJ. Autoimmune thrombocytopenia acquired from an allogeneic bone-marrow graft. *Lancet* 1982; **1**: 627–9.
98. Smith CIE, Aarli JA, Biberfeld P et al. Myasthenia gravis after bone-marrow transplantation. *N Engl J Med* 1983; **309**: 1565–8.
99. Ljungman P, Duraj V, Magnius L. Response to immunization against polio after allogeneic marrow transplantation. *Bone Marrow Transplant* 1991; **7**: 89–93.
100. Engelhard D, Handsher R, Naparstek E et al. Immune response to polio vaccination in bone marrow transplant recipients. *Bone Marrow Transplant* 1991; **8**: 295–300.
101. Ljungman P, Fridell E, Lonnqvist B et al. Efficacy and safety of vaccination of marrow transplant recipients with a live attenuated measles, mumps, and rubella vaccine. *J Infect Dis* 1989; **159**: 610–5.

63

Clare A. Dykewicz

Vaccination of Hematopoietic Cell Transplant Recipients

Antibody titers to vaccine-preventable diseases (e.g. tetanus, polio, measles, mumps, rubella and encapsulated organisms) decline during the first 4 years after allogeneic or autologous hematopoietic cell transplantation (HCT) if the recipient is not revaccinated [1–8].

There is controversy about whether HCT recipients with and without graft-vs.-host disease (GVHD) lose the same amount of antibodies to vaccine preventable diseases. For example, Ljungman et al. [1,6] found that allogeneic bone marrow transplant recipients with chronic GVHD lost antibodies to tetanus toxoid, measles, mumps and rubella to the same degree as those patients without GVHD. However, Lum wrote that patients with chronic GVHD lost immunoglobulin G (IgG) antibodies to tetanus toxoid, diphtheria toxoid and measles at a higher rate than did patients without chronic GVHD [9]. Hammarström et al. [10] reported that HCT patients with chronic GVHD lost pneumococcal antibodies at a higher rate than did HCT patients without chronic GVHD. But both allogeneic and autologous bone marrow transplant recipients lose serologic evidence of immunity to measles, mumps and rubella at a faster rate than normal persons [7,11], supporting the need to revaccinate HCT recipients.

The clinical relevance of decreased antibodies to vaccine-preventable diseases among HCT recipients is not immediately apparent because a limited number of cases of vaccine-preventable diseases are reported among HCT recipients. According to a search of Medline listings from 1966–mid-2002, tetanus, diphtheria, poliomyelitis, pertussis and rubella have not been reported to date in HCT recipients. Lum suggested that herd immunity and transferred specific immunity are the reasons that vaccine preventable diseases do not occur more commonly in HCT recipients [12].

Development of vaccine-preventable diseases in HCT recipients

Measles occurs rarely in HCT recipients, but has caused interstitial pneumonia [13,14]. Mumps is also rare in HCT recipients, but it has been reported to cause fatal meningoencephalitis post-HCT [15]. Hepatitis B infection in HCT recipients has been associated with an increased prevalence of veno-occlusive disease, GVHD and graft failure [16]. Four vaccine preventable diseases that most commonly infect HCT recipients are Streptococcus pneumoniae, Haemophilus influenzae type b, influenza and varicella zoster [17–20].

One center reported that from 1973 to 1977, seven (27%) of 26 HCT recipients developed pneumococcal infections >7 months after transplantation, during which time none were receiving immunosuppressive therapy [21]. Increased risk of pneumococcal disease is associated with impaired serum opsonic activity and low serum antibody levels to S. pneumoniae. Winston et al. [21] concluded that HCT recipients have an increased susceptibility to pneumococcal infection late post-transplant and should be immunized post-transplant against pneumococcal disease.

At one center in Germany, 20 of the 54 (37%) allogeneic HCT recipients with chronic GVHD transplanted from 1979 to 1996 developed S. pneumoniae infections. The infections occurred a median of 2.2 years post-transplant (range 6 months to 5 years), and incidence was not related to use of corticosteroids or cyclosporin [22]. In the United Kingdom, pneumococcal infection was the most commonly documented bacterial infection following autologous and allogeneic HCT recipients from 1986 to 1990; in this series, pneumococcal infections occurred at a median of 11 month post-transplant (range 4–72 months), although none of these patients was neutropenic [23].

A European Bone Marrow Transplantation survey done from July 1994 to December 1997 found that the incidence of invasive pneumococcal infection was significantly higher in allogeneic compared to autologous HCT recipients (12.20/1000 vs. 4.60/1000, $p <0.01$). In addition, the incidence of invasive pneumococcal infection among allogeneic patients was significantly higher among those with GVHD compared to those without GVHD (18.85/1000 vs. 8.25/1000, $p = 0.015$). The predisposition of HCT recipients with GVHD to developing pneumococcal disease has been suggested to be due to multiple factors including functional hyposplenism from total body irradiation and chronic GVHD, and decreased IgG_2 and pneumococcal antibody production after allogeneic HCT [24,25].

In the early 1980s, a French group reported that H. influenzae type b (Hib) infection was a major cause of morbidity and mortality post-HCT [26]. At that time, Hib was the main cause of pneumonia occurring after the 3rd month post-HCT; Hib pneumonia accounted for 35% of pneumonias of known etiology and 19% of all pneumonias [27]. More recent data on Hib incidence in HCT recipients have not been reported.

During a 1991 community and nosocomial outbreak of influenza in Houston, TX, Whimbey et al. [18] at M.D. Anderson noted that 68 HCT recipients were hospitalized during the outbreak. Of these, 28 developed an acute respiratory infection and eight (29%) of 28 had documented influenza. Influenza occurred in five (28%) of 18 autologous and three (33%) of 10 allogeneic HCT recipients with acute respiratory infections. Five (63%) of the eight influenza infections occurring in inpatient HCT recipients were nosocomially acquired. Risk factors for severe influenza disease include infection after HCT just before engraftment or chronic

GVHD. Six (75%) of all eight influenza cases during this outbreak were associated with pneumonia. Influenza pneumonia mortality was one (17%) of six [18].

Locksley et al. [19] reported that 231 (16.6%) of 1394 HCT recipients treated from 1969 to 1982 in Seattle, WA, developed infection with varicella-zoster virus (VZV). Eighty percent of the VZV infections occurred within 9 months of HCT [19]. Risk factors for VZV infection were allogeneic transplantation, acute or chronic GVHD, age between 10 and 29 years, a diagnosis other than chronic myelogenous leukemia and post-transplant use of antithymocyte globulin [19]. In another cohort, Han et al. [20] in Minneapolis, MN, reported that 216 (18%) of 1186 HCT recipients from 1974 to 1989 developed VZV infection from 4 days to 10.8 years after HCT. A total of 135 (62%) of the 216 VZV infections resulted in dermatomal zoster (shingles) [20]. Unlike Locksley's study, Han's series showed that allogeneic and autologous HCT recipients had similar rates of VZV infection. In Han's study, age ≥10 years and radiation in the preparatory regimen were risk factors for VZV infection [20]. In a more recent series, Koc et al. [28] found that 41% of patients undergoing allogeneic HCT from 1992 to 1997 developed VZV reactivation at a median of 227 days (range 45–346 days) post-HCT. In some series, VZV infection incidence has ranged as high as 52% [29]. Clearly, VZV infection causes significant morbidity in HCT recipients.

Vaccine-preventable diseases still pose risks to the overall US population. Therefore, HCT recipients should be routinely revaccinated with the routine childhood vaccines after HCT so that they can develop immunity to the same vaccine-preventable diseases as others. In 1995, US transplantation centers performing allogeneic HCTs were surveyed to determine the patterns of vaccine use after HCT. The survey found that most centers administered vaccines to HCT recipients, but schedules varied widely; HCT center personnel used 3–11 different vaccination schedules per vaccine [30]. Consequently, the study authors requested national guidelines for doses and timing of vaccines after HCT to eliminate confusion among HCT center personnel.

Response to vaccination in healthy persons

Infection or vaccination may result in the production of memory T and B cells that recognize a specific antigen. These memory cells may last for years and upon a second exposure to the same antigen, they develop into effector cells which may secrete antibodies or cytokines, or become cytotoxic T lymphocytes (CTLs), which eliminate cells infected with the pathogen. This secondary response, an anamnestic immune response, produces a more intense and rapid immune response to the antigen than during the initial exposure at the time of vaccination or initial infection [31].

Successful vaccination causes the development of: (i) high-affinity antibodies, which neutralize the specific pathogen; and/or (ii) a high concentration of memory effector T cells [32]. The goal of vaccination against bacterial pathogens is to create a high enough titer of antigen-specific antibodies so that the infecting organism is neutralized, the infection becomes subclinical or resolves, and disease is averted [32]. Antibody can also be involved in the cellular response such as antibody-dependent cell-mediated cytotoxicity (ADCC). However, antibody may not be essential for recovery from viral infections, since agammaglobulinemic persons recover from some viral infections [32]. Viruses replicate inside host cells, and therefore are not always accessible to neutralizing antibodies. For extracellular pathogens (e.g. some bacteria), the humoral immune response is more important, for intracellular pathogens (e.g. viruses), the cell mediated immune response is paramount.

During viral infections, the virus infected host cell presents viral antigens on the cell surface bound to the major histocompatibility complex (MHC) Class I receptors and thereby becomes an antigen-presenting cell (APC). These APC may be monocyte/macrophages or B cells. $CD8^+$ cells become activated CTLs that recognize the antigens presented on the APCs as foreign. The activated CTLs, with help from $CD4^+$ cells, release substances which lyse the APCs, thereby killing the infecting virus [31]. Other possible mechanisms of immune protection against intracellular infections include phagocytosis by macrophages activated by the T helper cell-derived cytokine, interferon-gamma (IFN-γ), natural killer (NK) cells, and opsonization of antigens by antibodies [31]. Cytokines such as IFN-γ can also have antiviral properties or can up-regulate MHC Class I expression.

Response to vaccination in HCT patients

In general, the literature on vaccine studies in HCT recipients are limited by small numbers of patients and a paucity of data on vaccinations in autologous, T-cell depleted and peripheral HCT.

The bulk of the literature indicates that the polysaccharide pneumococcal vaccine is less immunogenic in HCT recipients than other vaccines. For example, in 1983, Winston et al. [33] wrote that the 14-valent pneumococcal vaccine was poorly immunogenic in allogeneic HCT recipients when given early after HCT (e.g. less than 7 months post-HCT) and when given to patients receiving corticosteroids. They predicted that HCT recipients not receiving corticosteroids would achieve normal responses to pneumococcal vaccine at 3.5 years post-HCT.

A second group vaccinated allogeneic HCT recipients with 14-valent pneumococcal vaccine at 12 months post-HCT. Of the 29 patients who lost pneumococcal antibodies after HCT and were subsequently vaccinated against pneumococcus, 11 (38%) did not respond to vaccination, eight (28%) had an increase in IgG_1 (immature response) and 10 (34%) had an increase in IgG_2 (mature response). However, even patients with an "immature" response may be protected against pneumococcal disease. Of note, six (75%) of eight HCT patients with chronic GVHD did not respond to the 14-valent pneumococcal vaccination [10]. A third group of researchers found that HCT recipients had a poor response to vaccination with a 23-valent polysaccharide pneumococcal vaccines, even when given at 12 and 24 months post-HCT [34].

A fourth group found that when 53 pediatric allogeneic and autologous HCT recipients were given 23-valent polysaccharide pneumococcal vaccine, all children who were vaccinated at least 2 years post-transplant had a significant rise in serum antibody titers [35]. Univariate analysis showed that lapse of time from bone marrow transplantation (BMT) to vaccination, female sex, and chronic GVHD influenced the response rate to pneumococcal polysaccharide vaccine; however, multivariate analysis showed that only time elapsed between marrow transplant and immunization was significant [35]. This study's researchers calculated that 50% of BMT recipients would respond to polysaccharide pneumococcal vaccine at 14–16 months post-transplant [35]. Since some HCT recipients may benefit from vaccination with the 23-valent pneumococcal vaccine 1 year post-HCT, administration of polysaccharide pneumococcal vaccine to HCT recipients is recommended, although immune response is not optimal for all serotypes. In addition, the gradual increase in penicillin-resistant S. pneumoniae strains make it increasingly important to try to effectively vaccinate HCT recipients against S. pneumoniae.

Based on the hypothesis that administering a polysaccharide protein-conjugate vaccine may be more immunogenic in HCT recipients than a polysaccharide vaccine, a 7-valent polysaccharide-protein conjugate pneumococcal vaccine was injected into nine HCT recipients at 1 year post-transplant. Their IgG responses were compared to six HCT

Table 63.1 Evidence-based rating system used to determine the strength of recommendations. Adapted from CDC/USPHS/IDSA [50].

Category	Definition	Recommendation
A	Strong evidence for efficacy and substantial benefit	Strongly recommended
B	Strong or moderate evidence for efficacy, but only limited clinical benefit	Generally recommended
C	Insufficient evidence for efficacy; or efficacy does not outweigh possible adverse consequences (e.g. drug toxicity or interaction or cost of chemoprophylaxis or alternative approaches)	Optional
D	Moderate evidence against efficacy or for adverse outcome	Generally not recommended
E	Strong evidence against efficacy or of adverse outcome	Never recommended

Table 63.2 Evidence-based rating system used to determine quality of evidence supporting recommendations. Adapted from CDC/USPHS/IDSA [50].

Category	Definition
I	Evidence from at least one well-executed randomized, controlled trial
II	Evidence from at least one well-designed clinical trial without randomization; cohort or case-controlled analytic studies (preferably from more than one center); multiple time-series studies, or dramatic results from uncontrolled experiments
III	Evidence from opinions of respected authorities based on clinical experience, descriptive studies, or reports of expert committees

recipients who received the 23-valent polysaccharide pneumococcal vaccine. Overall, the IgG response was similar in these two groups of patients, but numbers of patients may have been too small to detect a significant difference between the two groups [36]. Further studies are indicated to determine whether a 7-valent polysaccharide-protein conjugate pneumococcal vaccine will be more immunogenic than the 23-valent polysaccharide vaccine in HCT recipients.

A Hib capsular polysacccharide vaccine conjugated to a tetanus protein was more immunogenic in allogeneic HCT recipients than a Hib capsular polysaccharide vaccine.

Consequently, Barra *et al.* [27] recommend three doses of conjugated Hib vaccine for allogeneic HCT recipients. Parkkali *et al.* [37] vaccinated 45 adult allogeneic HCT recipients with a Hib capsular polysaccharide vaccine conjugated to a tetanus protein and found that those with chronic GVHD retained Hib antibodies the same as those without chronic GVHD.

One center investigated immunizing donors using a polysaccharide-conjugate Hib vaccine, a 23-valent pneumococcal vaccine and tetanus toxoid before HCT donation. Results were promising for the Hib and tetanus toxoid vaccines but not for the 23-valent pneumococcal vaccine. However, data were limited [8,38].

Inactivated influenza vaccine is not effective when given within the first 6 months post-HCT, but it has been shown to be safe and immunogenic in HCT recipients when given after the first 6 months post-HCT [39]. Influenza vaccination of family members and close or household contacts is strongly recommended during each influenza season (i.e. October–May) starting the season before HCT and continuing >24 months after HCT to prevent influenza exposure among the recipients or candidates. All family members and close or household contacts of HCT recipients who remain immunocompromised >24 months after HCT should continue to be vaccinated annually as long as the HCT recipient's immunocompromise persists. Seasonal influenza vaccination is strongly recommended for all health care workers (HCWs) of HCT recipients.

If HCWs, family members or other close contacts of HCT recipients receive influenza vaccination during an influenza A outbreak, they should receive amantadine or rimantadine chemoprophylaxis for 2 weeks after influenza vaccination while they develop an immunologic response to the vaccine. Such a strategy is likely to prevent transmission of influenza A to HCWs and other close contacts of HCT recipients, which could prevent influenza A transmission to HCT recipients themselves. However, if a nosocomial outbreak occurs with an influenza A strain that is not contained in the available influenza vaccine, all healthy family members, close and household contacts, and HCWs of HCT recipients and candidates should be given influenza A chemoprophylaxis with amantadine or rimantadine until the end of the outbreak.

In 1999, two neuroaminidase inhibitors (zanamivir and oseltamivir) were approved for treatment of uncomplicated influenza. HCWs, family members or other close contacts can be offered a neuroaminidase inhibitor if: (a) rimantadine or amantadine cannot be tolerated; (b) the outbreak strain of influenza A is amantadine or rimantadine-resistant; or (c) the outbreak strain is influenza B [40].

Life-long seasonal influenza vaccination is recommended for all HCT candidates and recipients, beginning during the influenza season before HCT and resuming >6 months after HCT [40]. Neither amantadine nor rimantadine is effective against influenza B. Additionally, antiviral-resistant strains of influenza can emerge during treatment with amantadine or rimantadine, and drug resistant strains of influenza can be transmitted from person-to-person. Therefore, clinicians must be vigilant in identifying the type of influenza and in monitoring patients for the development of drug resistance.

The licensed, live varicella vaccine is contraindicated in HCT recipients because of the concern that this may result in disseminated infection with vaccine strain VZV. However, three doses of an investigational heat-inactivated varicella vaccine were given to allogeneic and autologous HCT recipients at 1, 2, and 3 months after HCT [41]. Varicella zoster prevalence was not significantly different between the vaccinated and unvaccinated HCT recipients, but severity of zoster was much less among the vaccinated HCT recipients. In a follow-up study, the inactivated varicella vaccine was administered to autologous HCT recipients with Hodgkin's or non-Hodgkin's lymphoma within 30 days before transplantation and at 1, 2, and 3 months after transplantation. Zoster developed in only seven (13%) of 53 vaccinated HCT recipients, compared to 19 (33%) of 58 unvaccinated HCT recipients ($p = 0.01$) [42]. Furthermore, the heat-inactivated vaccine was found to be safe in autologous HCT recipients. No formal recommendation for use of the inactivated varicella vaccine can be given because it remains investigational, but it holds promise for decreasing zoster incidence in autologous HCT recipients within the first 12.5 months post-HCT.

Successful tetanus immunization was achieved in HCT recipients after three doses of tetanus toxoid vaccine regardless of whether GVHD was present or not. Therefore, Ljungman et al. [1] recommended three doses of tetanus toxoid post-HCT. In a separate study, Parkkali et al. [43] concluded that HCT recipients with chronic GVHD responded to tetanus toxoid immunization and should be vaccinated. Storek and Saxon hypothesized that, since more than one dose of tetanus toxoid must be administered to attain a lasting serum IgG antibody level, that virgin and not memory B cells are stimulated [44].

No information was available on loss of pertussis antibodies post-HCT or of immunogenicity after HCT. Although pertussis containing vaccine (DTP) has been commonly used for HCT recipients <7 years of age, there have been no significant adverse events reported [30]. Pertussis continues to be reported in the US and [45], therefore, pertussis immunization is recommended for HCT recipients <7 years of age. The acellular pertussis vaccine is preferred over the whole cell vaccine [46].

In 1989, Ljungman et al. [6] reported that although seroconversions to measles–mumps–rubella (MMR) were not as high in HCT recipients as in controls, MMR vaccination appeared immunogenic and safe in allogeneic HCT recipients vaccinated 2-years post-transplant when they did not have active chronic GVHD or immunosuppressive therapy at the time of vaccination. In 1991, Ljungman et al. [47] wrote that reimmunization of allogeneic HCT recipients with polio vaccination is necessary post-HCT, and a three-dose schedule is needed.

A prospective study of hepatitis B vaccination looked at eight pairs of HCT donors and recipients of T-cell-depleted HCT. The donors were all negative for antibody to hepatitis B core and surface antigen (anti-HBc, anti-HBs) and negative to hepatitis B surface antigen itself (HBsAg). The donors were immunized against hepatitis B using a recombinant vaccine once at 11–30 days prior to marrow harvest. The HCT recipients all seroconverted to anti-HBs. HCT recipients were then boosted with recombinant hepatitis B vaccination on day 30, 60, and 150 post-HCT. No significant adverse events were noted in HCT recipients after hepatitis B vaccination [16]. Therefore, hepatitis B vaccination can be safely administered post-HCT.

Smallpox vaccine is contraindicated in the immunocompromised because it is a live virus vaccine and there is concern that the vaccine strain virus may cause disseminated disease. Consequently, smallpox vaccine is contraindicated in allogeneic HCT recipients within the first 2 years of transplantation, and in HCT recipients who are ≥2-years post-transplant but who have GVHD or are taking immunosuppressive drugs, or who have disease relapse. No data are available on the safety, immunogenicity or efficacy of vaccinia (smallpox) vaccine in HCT recipients. In addition, smallpox vaccination is contraindicated in the household contacts of immunocompromised HCT recipients because of the concern that they may transmit vaccine-strain vaccinia virus to the immunocompromised HCT recipient [48]. (HCT recipients are presumed immunocompetent at ≥24 months after HCT if they are not on immunosuppressive therapy and do not have GVHD.)

Vaccine recommendations

To address the need for a national vaccination schedule for HCT recipients, an interim schedule was drafted by the Hematopoietic Stem Cell Transplant Guidelines Immunization Working Group in collaboration with partner organizations, including Centers for Disease Control's (CDC's) Advisory Committee on Immunization Practices [40]. The purpose of the vaccination schedule is to provide guidance for HCT centers. Limited data were found regarding safety and immunogenicity (e.g. serologic studies of antibody titres after vaccination) among HCT recipients, and no data were found regarding vaccine efficacy among HCT recipients (e.g. which determine whether vaccinated HCT recipients have decreased attack rates of disease compared with unvaccinated HCT recipients), except for the investigational heat-inactivated varicella zoster vaccine. However, the working group believes that the benefits of reimmunizing HCT recipients post-HCT outweigh the potential adverse events following vaccination.

For most killed vaccines, except for the influenza vaccine, the first dose is given at 12 months post-HCT because this is the time at which immune reconstitution has occurred sufficiently to allow an adequate seroconversion to the vaccination which is comparable to that of non-HCT recipient controls [44, 49]. The reconstitution of B-cell immunity post-HCT resembles the development of immunity in the normal infant [7]. For a description of immune recovery post-HCT, please see Chapter 62.

Even though B-cell mediated immunity reconstitution is delayed in persons with chronic GVHD [7], the working group recommends that patients with chronic GVHD be immunized according to the same schedule as patients without GVHD, except for administration of live vaccines (e.g. MMR vaccine). Lum suggested that titres to antigens should be checked in patients with active chronic GVHD who have been vaccinated to verify seroconversion [9]; however, the working group made no recommendation regarding this. Antigen specific serum IgG levels will be unreliable in patients receiving intravenous immunoglobulin.

For all recommendations, prevention strategies are rated by the strength of the recommendation (Table 63.1 (p. 864) [50]) and the quality of the evidence (Table 63.2 (p. 864) [50]) supporting the recommendation. The principles of this rating system were developed by the Infectious Diseases Society of America and the US Public Health Service for use in the guidelines for preventing opportunistic infections among human immunodeficiency virus (HIV)-infected persons [50–52]. This rating system allows for assessments of recommendations to which adherence is critical.

Because certain HCT recipients have faster immune system recovery after HCT than others, researchers have proposed that different vaccination schedules be recommended for recipients of different types of HCT. However, currently data are too limited to do so. Therefore, the same vaccination schedule is recommended for all HCT recipients (e.g. allogeneic, autologous and bone marrow, peripheral blood, or umbilical cord blood grafts) until additional data become available. In the tables, vaccines have only been recommended for use among HCT recipients if evidence exists of safety and immunogenicity for those recipients (Table 63.3 (pp. 866–7)) [40]. Vaccination of family members, household contacts and HCWs are also recommended to minimize exposure of vaccine-preventable diseases among HCT recipients (Table 63.4 (p. 868)) [40]. Recommendations for vaccinations for HCT recipients traveling to areas endemic for selected vaccine-preventable diseases are given in Table 63.5 (p. 869) [40]. Recommendations for use of passive immunization for HCT recipients are given in Table 63.6 (p. 870) and a summary of recommendations for HCT recipients is given in Table 63.7 (p. 871) [40].

Table 63.3 Recommended vaccinations for hematopoietic cell transplantation* (HCT) recipients, including both allogeneic and autologous recipients. For these guidelines, HCT recipients are presumed immunocompetent at ≥24 months after HCT if they are not on immunosuppressive therapy and do not have graft-vs.-host disease (GVHD). Adapted from Centers for Disease Control and Prevention [40].

Vaccine or toxoid	Time after HSCT			Rating
	12 months	14 months	24 months	
Inactivated vaccine or toxoid				
Diphtheria, tetanus, acellular pertussis				
Children aged <7 years*	Diphtheria toxoid–tetanus toxoid–acellular pertussis vaccine (DTaP) or diphtheria toxoid–tetanus toxoid (DT)†	DTaP or DT	DTaP or DT	BIII
Children aged ≥7 years‡	Tetanus–diphtheria toxoid (Td)	Td	Td	BII
Haemophilus influenzae type B (Hib) conjugate§	Hib conjugate	Hib conjugate	Hib conjugate	BII
Hepatitis (HepB)¶	HepB	HepB	HepB	BIII
23-valent pneumococcal polysaccharide (PPV23)**	PPV23	—	PPV23	BIII
Hepatitis A††	Routine administration not indicated			Not rated because of limited data
Inactivated influenza‡‡	Lifelong, seasonal administration, beginning before HCT and resuming at ≥6 months after HCT			BII
Meningococcal§§	Routine administration not indicated			Not rated because of limited data
Inactivated polio (IPV)¶¶	IPV	IPV	IPV	BII
Rabies***	Routine administration not indicated			Not rated because of limited data
Live-attenuated vaccine				
measles–mumps–rubella (MMR)†††	—	—	MMR	BIII
Varicella vaccine‡‡‡	Contraindicated for HCT recipients			EIII

*Studies report that an HCT recipient can be primed if the donor has had primary vaccination series. Studies also report that a recipient's antibody titer before HCT might affect the titer 1 year after HCT [9]. No data were found regarding safety and immunogenicity of pertussis vaccination among HCT recipients.
†DT should be used whenever a contraindication exists to pertussis vaccination.
‡HCT recipients should be revaccinated with tetanus–diphtheria toxoids every 10 years, as routinely recommended for all adolescents and adults [53,54].
§Hib conjugate vaccine is recommended for HCT recipients of any age [54,55].

¶ Hepatitis B vaccination is recommended for all susceptible persons aged ≤18 years and for adults who have risk factors for hepatitis B virus infection [56,57]. Advisory Committee on Immunization Practices (ACIP) hepatitis B vaccination recommendations indicate that high doses (40 μg/dose) are recommended for adult dialysis patients and other immunocompromised adults [57]. No data were found regarding immunocompromised children and their response to higher doses of vaccine. Post-vaccination testing for antibody to hepatitis B surface antigen is recommended 1–2 months after the third vaccine dose to ensure protection among immunocompromised persons [57]. Persons who do not respond to the primary vaccine series should complete a second three-dose series.

** The 23-valent pneumococcal polysaccharide vaccine might not be protective against pneumococcal infection among HCT recipients. The second dose of vaccine is not a booster dose, but provides a second chance for immunologic response among persons who failed to respond to the first dose [34]. Adjunctive antibiotic prophylaxis against encapsulated organisms, including pneumococcal disease, is recommended for allogeneic recipients with chronic GVHD [58]. Little data were found regarding safety and immunogenicity of the seven-valent conjugate pneumococcal vaccine among HCT recipients; therefore, no recommendation regarding use of this vaccine can be made.

†† No data were found regarding immunogenicity, safety and efficacy of hepatitis A vaccine among HCT recipients. Researchers report that hepatitis A vaccination can be used for investigational use among HCT recipients aged ≥24 months at ≥12 months after HCT and who are at increased risk for hepatitis A or its adverse consequences (e.g. persons with chronic liver disease, including chronic GVHD, and children living in areas with consistently elevated hepatitis A incidence) [59].

‡‡ Children aged ≥6 months and <9 years receiving influenza vaccination for the first time require two doses spaced at least one month apart. Children aged ≤12 years should receive only split-virus influenza vaccine. ACIP's and the American Academy of Pediatrics' dosing schedule should be used [60,61]. For optimal influenza prevention, both vaccination and influenza chemoprophylaxis should be used among HCT recipients. Only inactivated influenza vaccine should be administered to HCT recipients.

§§ Administration of meningococcal vaccine should be evaluated for HCT recipients who live in endemic areas or areas experiencing outbreaks [62]. However, meningococcal vaccine immunogenicity and efficacy among HCT recipients have not been studied.

¶¶ Inactivated polio virus vaccine is immunogenic among HCT recipients, although no data were found regarding optimal methods and timing of immunization [30,63].

*** Clinicians can administer preexposure rabies vaccine to HCT recipients with potential occupational exposures to rabies [64]. However, the safety and immunogenicity of rabies vaccination among HCT recipients has not been studied. Preexposure rabies vaccination should probably be delayed until 12–24 months after HCT. Post-exposure administration of rabies vaccine with human rabies immunoglobulin can be administered anytime after HCT as indicated. Existing ACIP and American Academy of Pediatrics guidelines for post-exposure human rabies immunoglobulin and vaccine administration should be followed, which include administering five doses of rabies vaccine administered on days 0, 3, 7, 14, and 28 post-exposure [64,65].

††† The first dose of MMR vaccine should be administered ≥24 months after HCT if the HCT recipient is presumed immunocompetent. The second MMR dose is recommended 6–12 months later (BIII); however, the benefit of a second dose among HCT recipients has not been evaluated. During outbreaks, the second dose can be administered 4 weeks after the first dose [54].

The half-life of intravenous immunoglobulin is decreased among HCT recipients, but its effect on vaccine immunogenicity has not been evaluated. ACIP's and the American Academy of Pediatrics' recommendations regarding intervals between administration of immunoglobulin preparations for various indications and vaccines containing live measles virus should be used [66–68]. Further research is needed to determine the safety, immunogenicity, and efficacy of varicella vaccine among HCT recipients.

‡‡‡ To protect HCT recipients from varicella exposure, all varicella-susceptible health care workers (HCWs), family members and close contacts of the recipient should be vaccinated against varicella [70].

Additional notes: All indicated nonlive vaccines should be administered to HCT recipients regardless of HCT type or presence of GVHD. Live-attenuated vaccines (e.g. MMR, varicella, Bacillus Calmette-Guérin, yellow fever, and oral typhoid vaccines) should not be administered to any HCT recipient with active GVHD or immunosuppression [71]. To date, no adverse events have been reported (e.g. exacerbation of GVHD) among vaccinated HCT recipients. However, data regarding immunization among HCT recipients are limited and further studies are needed to evaluate safety, efficacy and immunogenicity of the proposed HCT immunization schedule. Use of combination vaccines is encouraged [72]. No contraindications to simultaneous administration of any vaccines exist, except cholera and yellow fever. Adverse events after vaccination should be reported promptly to the Vaccine Adverse Event Reporting System (VAERS), P.O. Box 1100, Rockville, MD 20849–1100. Forms and information can be obtained from VAERS ([800] 822–7967). If the HCT recipient has lapsed immunizations after HCT (i.e. has missed one or more vaccine doses), the immunization schedule does not have to be restarted. Instead, the missing vaccine dose should be administered as soon as possible or during the next scheduled clinic appointment.

Table 63.4 Vaccinations for family, close contacts and health care workers (HCWs) of hematopoietic cell transplantation (HCT) recipients.* Adapted from Centers for Disease Control and Prevention [40].

Vaccine	Recommendations for use	Rating
Hepatitis A	Routine vaccination is recommended for persons at increased risk for hepatitis A or its adverse consequences (e.g. persons with chronic liver disease or persons traveling to hepatitis A-endemic countries) and for children aged ≥24 months living in areas with consistently elevated hepatitis A incidence [49]	BII
Influenza[†]	Household contacts—vaccination is strongly recommended during each influenza season (i.e. October–May) beginning in the season before the transplant and continuing to ≥24 months after HCT. All household contacts of immunocompromised HCT recipients should be vaccinated annually as long as these conditions persist. HCWs and home caregivers—annual vaccination is strongly recommended during each influenza season	AI
Polio[‡]	Vaccination is not routinely recommended for adults but should be administered when polio vaccination is indicated according to published Advisory Committee on Immunization Practices guidelines; when polio vaccine is administered, inactivated polio vaccine should be used	AI
Measles–mumps–rubella (MMR)[§]	Vaccination is recommended for all persons who are aged ≥12 months and who are not pregnant or immunocompromised	AI
Varicella[¶]	Vaccination should be administered to all susceptible HCWs, household contacts, and family members who are aged ≥12 months and who are not pregnant or immunocompromised. When varicella vaccination is administered to persons aged ≥13 years, two doses are required, administered 4–8 weeks apart	AIII

*This vaccination schedule refers only to vaccine-preventable diseases that are spread person-to-person.

†Children aged ≥6 months and <9 years receiving influenza vaccination for the first time require two doses spaced at least one month apart. Children aged ≤12 years should receive only split-virus influenza vaccine. [61]. If HCWs, family members or other close contacts of HCT recipients receive influenza vaccination during an influenza A outbreak, they should also receive amantadine or rimantadine chemoprophylaxis for 2 weeks after the influenza vaccination (BI) while the vaccinee develops an immunologic response to the vaccine. However, if a nosocomial outbreak occurs with an influenza A strain that is not contained in the available influenza vaccine, HCWs, family members and other close contacts of HCT recipients and candidates should be administered influenza A chemoprophylaxis with amantadine or rimantadine until the end of the outbreak [61] (BIII). HCWs, family members or other close contacts can be offered a neuroaminidase inhibitor (e.g. zanamivir or oseltamivir) using the same strategies outlined previously, if one or more of the following exists: (a) rimantadine or amantadine cannot be tolerated; (b) the outbreak strain of influenza A is amantadine- or rimantadine-resistant; or (c) the outbreak strain is influenza B [73–76]. Zanamivir can be administered to persons aged ≥7 years and oseltamivir can be administered to persons aged ≥1 year.

‡Caution: vaccine-strain polio virus in oral polio vaccine can be transmitted person-to-person; therefore, oral polio vaccine administration is contraindicated among household contacts of immunocompromised persons. If oral polio vaccine is inadvertently administered to a household contact of an HCT recipient, Advisory Committee on Immunization Practices' (ACIP's) and the American Academy of Pediatrics' recommendations should be followed to minimize close contact with the immunocompromised person for 4–6 weeks after vaccination [63,77,78]. Although vaccine-associated paralytic poliomyelitis has not been reported among HCT recipients after exposure to household contacts inadvertently vaccinated with oral polio vaccine, inactivated polio vaccine should be used among family members, close contacts and HCWs to avoid person-to-person transmission of vaccine-strain polio virus [63].

§No evidence exists that live-attenuated vaccine-strain viruses in the MMR vaccine have ever been transmitted from person-to-person, except for rubella vaccine virus from a nursing mother to her infant [67].

¶HCWs, family members, close contacts and visitors who do not have a documented history of varicella-zoster infection or who are seronegative should receive this vaccination before being allowed to visit or have direct contact with an HCT recipient (AIII). Ideally, varicella-zoster-susceptible HCWs, family members, household contacts and potential visitors of immunocompromised HCT recipients should be vaccinated as soon as the decision to perform an HCT is made. The vaccination dose or doses should be completed ≥4 weeks before the conditioning regimen begins or ≥6 weeks (42 days) before contact with the HCT recipient is planned (BIII). If a varicella vaccinee develops a post-vaccination rash within 42 days of vaccination, the vaccinee should avoid contact with HCT recipients until all rash lesions are crusted or the rash has resolved [69,77].

References

1. Ljungman P, Wiklund-Hammarsten M, Duraj V et al. Response to tetanus toxoid immunization after allogeneic bone marrow transplantation. *J Infect Dis* 1990; **162**: 496–500.
2. Hammarström V, Pauksen K, Björkstrand B, Simonsson B, Öberg G, Ljungman P. Tetanus immunity in autologous bone marrow and blood stem cell transplant recipients. *Bone Marrow Transplant* 1998; **22**: 67–71.
3. Ljungman P, Cordonnier C, de Bock R et al. Immunizations after bone marrow transplantation: results of a European survey and recommendations from the infectious diseases working party of the European Group for Blood and Marrow Transplantation. *Bone Marrow Transplant* 1995; **15**: 455–60.
4. Volti SL, Mauro L, DiGregorio F et al. Immune status and immune response to diphtheria-tetanus and polio vaccines in allogeneic bone marrow-transplanted thalassemic patients. *Bone Marrow Transplant* 1994; **14**: 225–7.
5. Parkkali T, Ruutu T, Stenvik M et al. Loss of protective immunity to polio, diphtheria and *Haemophilus influenzae* type b after allogeneic bone marrow transplantation. *APMIS* 1996; **104**: 383–8.
6. Ljungman P, Fridell E, Lönnqvist B et al. Efficacy and safety of vaccination of marrow transplant recipients with a live attenuated measles, mumps, and rubella vaccine. *JID* 1989; **159**: 610–5.
7. Ljungman P, Lewensohn-Fuchs I, Hamarsström V et al. Long term immunity to measles, mumps, and rubella after allogeneic bone marrow transplantation. *Blood* 1994; **84**: 657–63.
8. Molrine DC, Guinan EC, Antin JH et al. Haemo-

Table 63.5 Vaccinations for hematopoietic cell transplantation (HCT) recipients traveling to areas endemic for selected vaccine-preventable diseases. Adapted from Centers for Disease Control and Prevention [40].

Vaccine	Recommendations for use	Rating
Bacillus of Calmette and Guérin (BCG) (live-attenuated vaccine)	Use of live-attenuated vaccine is contraindicated among HCT recipients at <24 months after HCT and among all persons who are immunocompromised [71]. No data were found regarding use among HCT recipients	EIII
Cholera	Vaccination is not indicated. No data were found regarding safety and immunogenicity among HCT recipients [79]	DIII
Hepatitis A	No data were found regarding immunogenicity, safety, or efficacy of hepatitis A vaccine among HCT recipients; therefore, intramuscular immunoglobulin use is preferred for hepatitis A prophylaxis among hematopoietic stem cell (HSC) transplant recipients. However, administration of intramuscular immunoglobulin does not replace avoidance behaviors (e.g. careful selection of food and water) [59]. Researchers recommend that hepatitis A vaccination be evaluated for investigational use among HCT recipients aged ≥24 months; however, no recommendation can be made because of limited data	Not rated because of limited data
Japanese B encephalitis	No data were found regarding safety, immunogenicity, or efficacy among HCT recipients [80]	Not rated because of limited data
Meningococcal vaccine	Vaccine should be administered to HCT recipients traveling to endemic areas or to areas experiencing outbreaks [62]. However, meningococcal vaccine immunogenicity and efficacy have not been studied among HCT recipients	Not rated because of limited data
Polio (inactivated polio vaccine only)	Booster dose can be administered as indicated [63]	CIII
Rabies	Researchers recommend that administration of a preexposure series be evaluated for persons at ≥12 months after HCT if they anticipate travel to endemic areas [64]. However, no data were found regarding safety, immunogenicity or efficacy among HCT recipients	Not rated because of limited data
Typhoid, oral (live-attenuated vaccine)	Use of oral typhoid vaccine (live-attenuated strain) is contraindicated among HCT recipients at <24 months after HCT and among those who are immunocompromised [81]. No data were found regarding safety, immunogenicity or efficacy among HCT recipients	EIII
Typhoid (intramuscular)	No data were found regarding safety, immunogenicity, or efficacy among HCT recipients	Not rated because of limited data
Yellow fever (live-attenuated vaccine)	Use of live-attenuated vaccine is contraindicated among HCT recipients at <24 months after HCT and among all immunocompromised persons [82]. No data were found regarding safety, immunogenicity, or efficacy among HCT recipients	EIII

Note: Specific advice for international travelers, including information regarding endemic diseases by country, is available through the internet at http://www.cdc.gov and by file transfer protocol at ftp.cdc.gov.

philus influenzae type b (Hib)-conjugate immunization before bone marrow harvest in autologous bone marrow transplantation. *Bone Marrow Transplant* 1996; **17**: 1149–55.

9 Lum LG. The kinetics of immune reconstitution after human marrow transplantation. *Blood* 1987; **69**: 369–80.

10 Hammarström V, Pauksen K, Azinge J, Öberg G, Ljungman P. Pneumococcal immunity and response to immunization with pneumococcal vaccine in bone marrow transplant patients: the influence of graft versus host reaction. *Support Care Cancer* 1993; **1**: 195–9.

11 Pauksen K, Duraj V, Ljungman P et al. Immunity to and immunization against measles, rubella and mumps in patients after autologous bone marrow transplantation. *Bone Marrow Transplant* 1992; **9**: 427–32.

12 Lum LG. Immune recovery after bone marrow transplantation. *Hematology/Oncol Clinics North Am* 1990; **4**: 659–75.

13 Machado CM, Goncalves FB, Pannuti CS, Dulley FL, de Souza VA. Measles in bone marrow transplant recipients during an outbreak in Sao Paulo. Brazil *Blood* 2002; **99**(1): 83–7.

14 Storek J. Measles in bone marrow transplant recipients. *Blood* 2002; **99**: 3070.

15 Bakshi N, Lawson J, Hanson R, Ames C, Vinters HV. Fatal mumps meningoencephalitis in a child with severe combined immunodeficiency after bone marrow transplantation. *J Child Neurol* 1996; **11**: 159–62.

16 Ilan Y, Nagler A, Adler R et al. Adoptive transfer of immunity to hepatitis B virus after T cell-depleted allogeneic bone marrow transplantation. *Hepatology* 1993; **18**: 146–32.

17 Atkinson K, Storb R, Prentice RL et al. Analysis of late infections in 89 long-term survivors of bone marrow transplantation. *Blood* 1979; **52**: 720–31.

18 Whimbey E, Elting LS, Cough RB et al. Influenza A virus infections among hospitalized adult bone marrow transplant recipients. *Bone Marrow Transplant* 1994; **13**: 437–40.

19 Locksley RM, Flournoy N, Sullivan KM, Meyers JD. Infection with varicella-zoster virus after marrow transplantation. *J Infect Dis* 1985; **152**: 1172–81.

20 Han CS, Miller W, Haake R, Weisdorf D. Varicella zoster infection after bone marrow transplantation. Incidence, risk factors and complications. *Bone Marrow Transplant* 1994; **13**: 277–83.

21 Winston DJ, Schiffman G, Wang DC et al. Pneumococcal infections after human bone-marrow transplantation. *Ann Intern Med* 1979; **91**: 835–41.

22 Guenther C, Holler E, Muth A et al. Incidence of *Streptococcus pneumoniae* infection after allogeneic bone marrow transplantation. *Blood* 1997; **90** (Suppl. 1): 368b [Abstract 4405].

23 Hoyle C, Goldman JM, on behalf of 18 UK Bone Marrow Transplant Teams. Life-threatening infections occurring more than 3 months after BMT. *Bone Marrow Transplant* 1994; **14**: 247–52.

24 Engelhard D, Cordonnier C, Shaw PJ et al. Early and late invasive pneumococcal infection following stem cell transplantation: a European Bone Marrow

Table 63.6 Use of passive immunization for hematopoietic cell transplantation (HCT) recipients. Adapted from Centers for Disease Control and Prevention [40].

Vaccine	Recommendations for use	Rating
Cytomegalovirus immunoglobulin	Not recommended for prophylaxis among HCT recipients because of its lack of efficacy [83]	DI
Hepatitis B immunoglobulin	Immunocompromised persons who have percutaneous or permucosal exposure to hepatitis B virus should receive two doses administered 1 month apart. For immunocompetent persons, the need for post-exposure prophylaxis depends on the vaccination history and antibody to hepatitis B surface antigen response status of the exposed person [73]	CIII
Human rabies immunoglobulin	Should be administered with rabies vaccine at any time after HCT as indicated for post-exposure rabies prophylaxis. Existing Advisory Committee on Immunization Practices guidelines for post-exposure should be followed, with five doses of rabies vaccine administered on days 0, 3, 7, 14, and 28 post-exposure [64,65]	CIII
Respiratory syncytial virus immunoglobulin	Because of high rates of case fatality from respiratory syncytial virus pneumonia among HCT recipients, HCT physicians can administer HCT recipients with upper or lower respiratory infection preemptive therapy with a high titre of neutralizing antibodies to prevent severe disease and death until controlled trials can be performed*	CIII
Respiratory syncytial virus monoclonal antibody	Physicians can use respiratory syncytial virus monoclonal antibody investigationally as preemptive therapy [84]	Not rated because of limited data
Tetanus immunoglobulin	Post-exposure vaccination should be administered with or without tetanus immunoglobulin as indicated for tetanus exposure that occurs anytime after HCT [53]	CIII
Varicella-zoster immunoglobulin[†]	Ideally, should be administered to HCT recipients ≤96 h after close contact with a person with varicella or shingles if the HCT recipient is at (a) <24 months after HCT, or (b) ≥24 months after HCT and still immunocompromised. Administration can extend the varicella incubation period from 10–21 days to 10–28 days. If the HCT recipient experiences a varicella-zoster (VZV)-like rash after contact with or exposure to a person with varicella or herpes zoster, antiviral drug therapy should be administered until ≥2 days after all lesions have crusted [69]	AII
Intramuscular immunoglobulin	Should be administered to hepatitis A-susceptible HCT recipients who anticipate hepatitis A exposure (e.g. during travel to endemic areas) and for post-exposure prophylaxis as indicated [59]. Should also be administered after measles exposure among HCT recipients who were not vaccinated against measles after HCT [67,85]	BIII
Intravenous immunoglobulin[‡]	Can be administered to HCT recipients with severe hypogammaglobulinemia (immunoglobulin G [Ig G] <400 mg/dL) ≤100 days after HCT to prevent bacterial infections [86,87]	CIII

*Researchers recommend substituting respiratory syncytial virus immunoglobulin for intravenous immunoglobulin for hematopoietic stem cell (HSC) transplant recipients on replacement intravenous immunoglobulin therapy during respiratory syncytial virus season (i.e. November–April) [88] (CIII). However, no data were found demonstrating safety and efficacy of respiratory syncytial virus immunoglobulin use among HSC transplant recipients.
†If intravenous immunoglobulin replacement therapy (>250 mg/kg) has been administered <2 weeks before varicella or zoster rash exposure, varicella-zoster immunoglobulin administration is probably not required. Varicella-zoster immunoglobulin is distributed by the American Red Cross, except in Massachusetts, where it is distributed by the Massachusetts Public Health Biologic Laboratories (now a unit of the University of Massachusetts) [69].
‡When administered, serum Ig G levels should be monitored regularly (e.g. every 2 weeks).
Additional notes: Intravenous immunoglobulin can be obtained from the American Red Cross Blood Services, although shortages occasionally occur. Physicians who have difficulty obtaining urgently needed intravenous immunoglobulin and other immunoglobulin products are advised to contact any of the following:
- American Red Cross Customer Service Center (800) 261–5772
- Alpha Therapeutic Corporation (800) 421–0008
- Baxter Healthcare Corporation (847) 940–5955
- Bayer Pharmaceutical Division (800) 288–8370
- Aventis Behring Customer Support (800) 683–1288
- Novartis Pharmaceuticals Corporation (973) 781–8300, or the Intravenous Immunoglobulin Emergency Hotline (888) 234–2520, or the Immune Deficiency Foundation (800) 296–4433.

Patients with Ig E anti-immunoglobulin A antibodies are at high risk for experiencing anaphylaxis from immunoglobulin administration [89]. Therefore, persons with Ig A deficiency should not be administered standard immunoglobulin preparations (DIII). However, researchers report that use of Ig A-depleted immunoglobulin preparations can be used with caution in these persons [89–91].

Molrine and colleagues showed that administration of 3 doses of the 7-valent pneumococcal conjugate vaccine (PCV7) at 3, 6, and 12 months post-HCT was safe and immunogenic. Efficacy data have not been collected, and further studies are needed to determine the role of this vaccine in HCT [92].

Table 63.7 Summary of vaccinations for hematopoietic cell transplantation (HCT) recipients.

Vaccine	When administered post-HCT
DTaP or Td	12, 14, and 24 months
IPV	12, 14, and 24 months
Hib	12, 14, and 24 months
23-valent pneumococcal vaccine	12 and 24 months
Inactivated influenza vaccine	Annually, beginning at 6 months
MMR	24 months only if immunocompetent (e.g. no active chronic GVHD, no immunosuppressive drugs)

DTaP, diphtheria toxoid–tetanus toxoid–acellular pertussis; GVHD, graft-vs.-host disease; Hib, *H. influenzae* type b; IPV, inactivated polio; MMR, measles–mumps–rubella; Td, tetanus–diphtheria toxoid.

References (continued from p. 869)

Transplantation survey. *Br J Haematol* 2002; **117**: 444–50.

25 Giebink GS, Warkentin PI, Ramsay NKC, Kersey JH. Titers of antibody to pneumococci in allogeneic bone marrow transplant recipients before and after vaccination with pneumococcal vaccine. *J Infect Dis* 1986; **154**: 590–6.

26 Cordonnier C, Bernaudin JF, Bierling P, Huet Y, Vernant JP. Pulmonary complications occurring after allogeneic bone marrow transplantation. A study of 130 consecutive transplanted patients. *Cancer* 1986; **58**: 1047–54.

27 Barra A, Cordonnier C, Preziosi MP et al. Immunogenicity of *Haemophilus influenzae* type b conjugate vaccine in allogeneic bone marrow recipients. *JID* 1992; **166**: 1021–8.

28 Koc Y, Miller KB, Schenkein DP et al. Varicella zoster virus infections following allogeneic bone marrow transplantation: frequency, risk factors, and clinical outcome. *Biol Blood Marrow Transplant* 2000; **6**: 44–9.

29 Arvin AM. Varicella-zoster virus. Pathogenesis, immunity, and clinical management in hematopoietic cell transplant recipients. *Biol Blood Marrow Transplant* 2000; **6**: 219–30.

30 Henning KJ, White MH, Sepkowitz KA, Armstrong D. National survey of immunization practices following allogeneic bone marrow transplantation. *JAMA* 1997; **277**: 1148–51.

31 Zane HD. *Immunology. Theoretical and Practical Concepts in Laboratory Medicine.* Philadelphia: W.B. Saunders Co., 2001.

32 Ada G, Ramsay A. *Vaccines, Vaccination and the Immune Response.* Philadelphia: Lippincott-Raven, 1997.

33 Winston DJ, Ho WG, Schiffman G, Champlin RE, Feig SA, Gale RP. Pneumococcal vaccination of recipients of bone marrow transplants. *Arch Intern Med* 1983; **143**: 1735–7.

34 Guinan EC, Molrine DC, Antin JH et al. Polysaccharide conjugate vaccine responses in bone marrow transplant patients. *Transplantation* 1994; **57**: 677–84.

35 Avanzini MA, Carra AM, Maccario R et al. Antibody response to pneumococcal vaccine in children receiving bone marrow transplantation. *J Clin Immunol* 1995; **15**: 137–44.

36 Storek J, Mendelman PM, Witherspoon RP, McGregor BA, Storb R. IgG response to pneumococcal polysaccharide-protein conjugate appears similar to IgG response to polysaccharide in bone marrow transplant recipients and healthy adults. *CID* 1997; **25**: 1253–5.

37 Parkkali T, Käyhty H, Ruutu T, Volin L, Eskola J, Ruutu P. A comparison of early and late vaccination with *Haemophilus influenzae* type b conjugate and pneumococcal polysaccharide vaccines after allogeneic BMT. *Bone Marrow Transplant* 1996; **18**: 961–7.

38 Molrine DC, Guinan EC, Antin JH et al. Donor immunization with *Haemophilus influenzae* type b (Hib)–conjugate vaccine in allogeneic bone marrow transplantation. *Blood* 1996; **87**: 3012–8.

39 Engelhard D, Nagler A, Hardan I et al. Antibody response to a two-dose regimen of influenza vaccine in allogeneic T cell-depleted and autologous BMT recipients. *Bone Marrow Transplant* 1993; **11**: 1–5.

40 CDC. Guidelines for preventing opportunistic infections among hematopoietic stem cell transplant recipients: recommendations of CDC, the Infectious Disease Society of America, and the American Society of Blood and Marrow Transplantation. *MMWR* 2000; **49** (no. RR-10): 1–125; and *Biol Blood and Marrow Transplant* 2000; **6**(6a): 659–734.

41 Redman RL, Nader S, Zerboni L et al. Early reconstitution of immunity and decreased severity of herpes zoster in bone marrow transplant recipients immunized with inactivated varicella vaccine. *J Infect Dis* 1997; **176**: 578–85.

42 Hata A, Asanuma H, Rinki M et al. Use of an inactivated varicella vaccine in recipients of hematopoietic-cell transplants. *New Engl J Med* 2002; **347**: 26–34.

43 Parkkali T, Ölander R-M, Ruutu T et al. A randomized comparison between early and late vaccination with tetanus toxoid vaccine after allogeneic BMT. *Bone Marrow Transplant* 1997; **19**: 933–8.

44 Storek J, Saxon A. Reconstitution of B cell immunity following bone marrow transplantation. *Bone Marrow Transplant* 1992; **9**: 395–408.

45 CDC. Pertussis: United States, 1997–2000. *MMWR* 2002; **51**: 73–6.

46 CDC. Pertussis vaccination. Use of acellular pertussis vaccines among infants and young children: recommendations of the Advisory Committee on Immunization Practices (ACIP). *MMWR* 1997: **46** (no. RR-7): 1–25.

47 Ljungman P, Duraj V, Magnius L. Response to immunization against polio after allogeneic marrow transplantation. *Bone Marrow Transplant* 1991; **7**: 89–93.

48 CDC. Vaccinia (smallpox) vaccine. Recommendations of the Advisory Committee on Immunization Practices (ACIP). *MMWR* 2001; **50** (no. RR-10): 1–25.

49 King SM, Saunders EF, Petric M, Gold R. Response to measles, mumps and rubella vaccine in paediatric bone marrow transplant recipients. *Bone Marrow Transplant* 1996; **17**: 633–6.

50 CDC/USPHS/IDSA. Guidelines for the prevention of opportunistic infections in persons infected with human immunodeficiency virus. *MMWR* 1999; **48** (no. RR-10): 1–66.

51 CDC/USPHS/IDSA. Guidelines for the prevention of opportunistic infections in persons infected with human immunodeficiency virus: a summary. *MMWR* 1995; **44** (no. RR-8): 1–34.

52 CDC/USPHS/IDSA. Guidelines for the prevention of opportunistic infections in persons infected with human immunodeficiency virus. *MMWR* 1997; **46** (no. RR-12): 1–46.

53 CDC. Diphtheria, tetanus, and pertussis: recommendations of vaccine use and other preventive measures: recommendations of the Advisory Committee on Immunization Practices (ACIP). *MMWR* 1991; **40** (no. RR-10): 1–28.

54 CDC. Use of vaccines and immunoglobulin in persons with altered immunocompetence: recommendations of the Advisory Committee on Immunization Practices (ACIP). *MMWR* 1993; **42** (no. RR-4): 1–18.

55 CDC. Recommendations for use of *Haemophilus* b conjugate vaccines and a combined diphtheria, tetanus, pertussis, and *Haemophilus* b vaccine: recommendations of the Advisory Committee on Immunization Practices (ACIP). *MMWR* 1993; **42** (no. RR-13): 1–15.

56 CDC. Hepatitis B virus. A comprehensive strategy for eliminating transmission in the United States through universal childhood vaccination: recommendations of the Immunization Practices Advisory Committee (ACIP). *MMWR* 1991; **40** (no. RR-13): 1–25.

57 CDC. Notice to readers: update. Recommendations to prevent hepatitis B virus transmission, United States. *MMWR* 1995; **44**: 574–5.

58 Bortin MM, Horowitz MM, Gale RP et al. Changing trends in allogeneic bone marrow transplantation for leukemia in the 1980s. *JAMA* 1992; **268**: 607–12.

59 CDC. Prevention of hepatitis A through active or passive immunization: recommendations of the Advisory Committee on Immunization Practices (ACIP). *MMWR* 1999; **48** (no. RR-12): 1–37.

60 American Academy of Pediatrics. Influenza. In: Pickering LK, ed. *Red Book: Report of the Committee on Infectious Diseases*, 26th edn. Elk Grove Village, IL: American Academy of Pediatrics, 2003: 382–91.

61 CDC. Prevention and control of influenza: recommendations of the Advisory Committee on Immunization Practices. *MMWR* 2003; **52** (no. RR-8): 1–36.

62 CDC. Control and prevention of meningococcal disease and control and prevention of serogroup C meningococcal disease: evaluation and management of suspected outbreaks. *MMWR* 1997; **46** (no. RR-5): 1–21.

63 CDC. Poliomyelitis prevention in the United States. Introduction of a sequential vaccination schedule of inactivated poliovirus vaccine followed by oral poliovirus vaccine: recommendations of the Advisory Committee on Immunization Practices (ACIP). *MMWR* 1997; **46** (no. RR-3): 1–25.

64 CDC. Human rabies prevention: United States, 1999. Recommendations of the Advisory Committee on Immunization Practices (ACIP). *MMWR* 1999; **48** (no. RR-1): 1–21. Erratum: 48 (no. RR-1): 16.

65 American Academy of Pediatrics. Rabies. In: Pickering LK, ed. *Red Book: Report of the Committee on Infectious Diseases*, 26th edn. Elk Grove Village, IL: American Academy of Pediatrics, 2003: 514–21.

66 American Academy of Pediatrics. Measles. In: Pickering LK, ed. *Red Book: Report of the Committee on Infectious Diseases*, 26th edn. Elk Grove Village, IL: American Academy of Pediatrics, 2003: 419–29.

67 CDC. Measles, mumps, and rubella-vaccine use and strategies for elimination of measles, rubella, and congenital rubella syndrome and control of mumps: recommendations of the Advisory Committee on Immunization Practices (ACIP). *MMWR* 1998; **47** (no. RR-8): 1–48.

68 CDC. General recommendations on immunization: recommendations of the Advisory Committee on Immunization Practices (ACIP) and the American Academy of Family Physicians (AAFP). *MMWR* 2002; **52** (no. RR-2): 1–35.

69 CDC. Prevention of varicella: recommendations of the Advisory Committee on Immunization Practices (ACIP). *MMWR* 1996; **45** (no. RR-11): 1–36.

70 American Academy of Pediatrics. Varicella-zoster infections. In: Pickering LK, ed. *Red Book: Report of the Committee on Infectious Diseases*, 26th edn. Elk Grove Village, IL: American Academy of Pediatrics, 2003: 672–86.

71 CDC. Role of BCG (Bacillus of Calmette and Guérin) vaccine in the prevention and control of tuberculosis in the United States: a joint statement by the Advisory Council For the Elimination of Tuberculosis and the Advisory Committee on Immunization Practices. *MMWR* 1996; **45** (no. RR-4): 1–18.

72 CDC. Combination vaccines for childhood immunization: recommendations of the Advisory Committee on Immunization Practices (ACIP), the American Academy of Pediatrics (AAP), and the American Academy of Family Physicians (AAFP). *MMWR* 1999; **48** (no. RR-5): 1–15.

73 Monto AS, Robinson DP, Herlocher ML, Hinson JM Jr, Elliott MJ, Crisp A. Zanamivir in the prevention of influenza among healthy adults: a randomized controlled trial. *JAMA* 1999; **282**: 31–5.

74 Hayden FG, Atmar RL, Schilling M *et al*. Use of the selective oral neuraminidase inhibitor oseltamivir to prevent influenza. *New Engl J Med* 1999; **341**: 1336–43.

75 Hayden FG, Gubareva L, Klein T *et al*. Inhaled zanamivir for preventing transmission of influenza in families [Abstract LB-2]. In: *Final Program, Abstracts and Exhibits Addendum, 38th Interscience Conference on Antimicrobial Agents and Chemotherapy*. Washington, DC: American Society for Microbiology, 1991: 1.

76 CDC. Neuraminidase inhibitors for treatment of influenza A and B infections. *MMWR* 1999; **48** (no. RR-14): 1–10.

77 CDC. Immunization of health care workers: recommendations of the Advisory Committee on Immunization Practices (ACIP) and the Hospital Infection Control Practices Advisory committee. *MMWR* 1997; **46** (no. RR-18): 1–42.

78 American Academy of Pediatrics. Poliovirus infections. In: Pickering LK, ed. *Red Book: Report of the Committee on Infectious Diseases*, 26th edn. Elk Grove Village, IL: American Academy of Pediatrics, 2003: 505–9.

79 CDC. Recommendations of the Immunization Practices Advisory Committee: cholera vaccine. *MMWR* 1988; **37**(40): 617–8; 623–4.

80 CDC. Inactivated Japanese encephalitis virus vaccine. Recommendations of the Advisory Committee on Immunization Practices (ACIP). *MMWR* 1993; **42** (no. RR-1): 1–15.

81 CDC. Typhoid immunization. Recommendations of the Advisory Committee on Immunization Practices (ACIP). *MMWR* 1994; **43** (no. RR-14): 1–7.

82 CDC. Yellow fever vaccine. Recommendations of the Advisory Committee on Immunization Practices (ACIP) *MMWR* 2002; **51** (no. RR-17): 1–11.

83 Boeckh M, Bowden R. Cytomegalovirus infection in marrow transplantation. In: Buckner CD, ed. *Technical and Biological Components of Marrow Transplantation*. Boston, MA: Kluwer Academic Publishers, 1995: 97–136.

84 Boeckh M, Berrey MM, Bowden RA, Crawford SW, Balsley J, Corey L. Phase 1 evaluation of the respiratory syncytial virus-specific monoclonal antibody palivizumab in recipients of hematopoietic stem cell transplants. *J Infect Dis* 2001; **184**: 350–4.

85 Eibl MM, Wedgwood RJ. Intravenous immunoglobulin: a review. *Immunodeficiency Rev* 1989; **1**: 1–42.

86 Antman KH, Rowlings PA, Vaughn WP *et al*. High-dose chemotherapy with autologous hematopoietic stem cell support for breast cancer in North America. *J Clin Oncol* 1997; **15**: 1870–9.

87 Wolff SN, Fay JW, Herzig RH *et al*. High-dose weekly intravenous immunoglobulin to prevent infections in patients undergoing autologous bone marrow transplantation or severe myelosuppressive therapy. *Ann Intern Med* 1993; **118**: 937–42.

88 American Academy of Pediatrics. Respiratory syncytial virus. In: Pickering LK, ed. *Red Book: Report of the Committee on Infectious Diseases*, 26th edn. Elk Grove Village, IL: American Academy of Pediatrics, 2003: 523–8.

89 Burks AW, Sampson HA, Buckley RH. Anaphylactic reactions after gamma globulin administration in patients with hypogammaglobulinemia. *New Engl J Med* 1986; **314**(9): 560–4.

90 Gunn V, Nechyba C. *Harriet Lane Handbook: a Manual for Pediatric House Officers*, 16th edn. Philadelphia, PA: Mosby Inc, 2002: 311–717.

91 Stiehm ER. Human intravenous immunoglobulin in primary and secondary antibody deficiencies (review). *Pediatr Infect Dis* 1997; **16**: 696–707.

92 Molrine DC, Antin JH, Guinan EC *et al*. Donor immunization with pneumococcal conjugate vaccine and early protective antibody responses following allogeneic hematopoietic cell transplantation. *Blood* 2003; **101**(3): 831–6.

64

David A. Horak

Pulmonary Complications after Hematopoietic Cell Transplantation

Over the last 20 years, there has been an exponential increase in the volume of hematopoietic cell transplant (HCT) recipients being treated for an expanding array of underlying malignant and nonmalignant diseases. Consequently, the need for utilization of the intensive care unit (ICU) for life-threatening complications also has increased dramatically. Depending on the type of transplant, patient age, conditioning regimen and underlying disease, between 7% and 40% of patients require ICU care for hemodynamic and cardiac monitoring, mechanical ventilation, hemodialysis or other specialized treatment [1]. The approach to critical care of the HCT patient varies at different transplant centers, some advocating bringing monitoring and life-support equipment as well as trained personnel to the transplant unit, and other institutions transferring unstable patients to the ICU. At the City of Hope National Medical Center (COHNMC), we utilize the latter approach, transferring HCT patients to a combined medical–surgical ICU.

Recently, there has been much debate in the literature suggesting that transitioning from an "open" to a "closed", intensivist-run ICU results in more rational and efficient resource utilization, decreased length of stay, fewer days of mechanical ventilation, lower costs and better outcomes [2–9]. However, these studies were largely carried out in medical–surgical ICUs and the applicability of their conclusions to the HCT population is not certain. At COHNMC, we have found that optimal management of the critically ill HCT recipient involves a multidisciplinary team approach. Team leadership is provided by the primary hematologist/oncologist and the adult or pediatric pulmonary intensivist. Depending on the patient's illness, other physician services should be immediately available including cardiology, gastroenterology, nephrology, infectious diseases, transfusion medicine, psychiatry, general surgery, neurosurgery and otolaryngology. Equally important are the nonphyszcian members of the team including critical care nurses with experience in oncology and HCT, and representatives from respiratory therapy, dietary, pharmacy, social services, physical and occupational therapy and pastoral care. At COHNMC, daily bedside rounds are made on all ICU patients by the entire multidisciplinary team allowing close communication and multifaceted assessment and treatment of these complex patients.

Spectrum of critical care complications

Many of the critical care complications in HCT recipients are similar to those occurring in other immunocompromised patient populations, such as septic shock, systemic inflammatory response syndrome (SIRS), multiorgan dysfunction syndrome (MODS), pancytopenia, drug toxicity and bleeding. Problems unique to HCT recipients include specific organ toxicities from high-dose myeloablative chemotherapy or "regimen-related toxicity" (RRT), and graft-vs.-host disease (GVHD). Complications with critical care implications are outlined in Table 64.1. Although critical injury to all organ systems potentially can occur in the HCT recipient, this chapter focuses primarily on pulmonary complications. Other areas of critical toxicity and organ dysfunction are covered thoroughly elsewhere in this text.

Pretransplant assessment

In order to assess a patient's suitability for HCT, to anticipate potential complications and to stratify risk, most transplant centers perform a rigorous pretransplant evaluation. Especially important is recognition of pre-existing organ system compromise, assessment of cardiopulmonary reserve and identification of any occult nidus of infection that could potentially reactivate following myeloablative therapy. At COHNMC, the routine pretransplant evaluation is as listed in Table 64.2.

Pulmonary function testing

It is generally acknowledged that HCT recipients typically experience some decline in pulmonary function parameters such as forced expiratory volume in 1 s (FEV-1), forced vital capacity (FVC), diffusion capacity for carbon monoxide (DLCO) and lung volumes [10–16]. This tends to create a pattern of restrictive physiology in the early post-transplant period, which usually improves over the subsequent 12–24 months. These abnormalities have been attributed to HCT-related pulmonary infections, cytotoxic chemoradiotherapy, fibrosis and scarring.

The ability of pre-HCT pulmonary fuction tests (PFTs) to predict complications accurately is somewhat more controversial, with some small studies suggesting that flow rates and diffusion capacity can predict interstitial pneumonitis [16–18]. In a larger study by Crawford and Fisher [19] of 1297 patients undergoing HCT at the Fred Hutchinson Cancer Research Center (FHCRC), decreased DLCO and elevated (A-a) P_{O_2} were the only pulmonary function parameters predictive of mortality. Most authorities concur that poor performance on pre-HCT PFTs by itself should not absolutely contraindicate HCT. A DLCO of <70% has been said to predict an increased risk of fatal veno-occlusive disease (VOD) [1].

Radiographic imaging

Other than limited chest computerized tomography (CT) scanning for total body irridiation (TBI) dosimetry planning, pre-HCT CT screening is not routinely performed. There have been multiple reports of invasive

Table 64.1 Critical care complications of hematopoietic cell transplantation (HCT).

Pulmonary	*Renal*
Pulmonary edema	Acute tubular necrosis
ARDS	Hepatorenal syndrome
Pneumonia	
Aspiration	*Gastrointestinal*
Bacterial	Hepatic insufficiency/failure
Fungal	Veno-occlusive disease
Viral	GVHD
Protozoal	Drug toxicity
Other	Hepatitis
Idiopathic pneumonia syndrome	Hepatic abscess
Diffuse alveolar hemorrhage	Upper/lower GI hemorrhage
Engraftment syndrome	Typhlitis
Pleural disease	Pancreatitis
Pulmonary fibrosis	
Obstructive lung disease	*Neuromuscular*
Pulmonary vascular disease	CNS bleed/infarct
Pulmonary cytolytic thrombi	CNS infection
Upper airway obstruction/mucositis	Metabolic encephalopathy
Sinusitis	Seizures
	Polyneuropathy
Cardiovascular	Myopathy
Cardiomyopathy	
Arrhythmias	*Infection*
Heart block	Sepsis
Pericardial effusions/tamponade	Bacterial
Constrictive pericarditis	Fungal
	Candida
Hematologic/oncologic	*Aspergillus*
Graft failure	Viral
Pancytopenia	CMV
Relapsed malignancy	HSV
DIC	VZV
Reaction to HCT infusion	RSV
TTP/HUS	Influenza
GVHD	Parainfluenza
	HHV-6

ARDS, acute respiratory distress syndrome; CMV, cytomegalovirus; CNS, central nervous system; DIC, disseminated intravascular coagulopathy; GI, gastrointestinal; GVHD, graft-vs.-host disease; HHV, human herpesvirus; HSV, herpes simplex virus; HUS, hemolytic uremic syndrome; RSV, respiratory syncytial virus; TTP, thrombotic thrombocytopenic purpura; VZV, varicella-zoster virus.

Table 64.2 Pretransplant assessment.

Complete history/physical examination
Chest radiograph
Pulmonary function test
Electrocardiogram
Two-dimensional echocardiogram
Cardiac stress testing (over age 50)
HIV, HSV, CMV, hepatitis serologies
Immunoglobulin levels
24 h urine for creatinine clearance
Pregnancy testing (women)
Sperm banking (men)
Dental exam
Dietary evaluation
Psychosocial assessment

CMV, cytomegalovirus; HIV, human immunodeficiency virus; HSV, herpes simplex virus.

fungal disease discovered on CT scan before HCT which have been successfully treated with combined surgical resection and antifungal therapy [20–24]. At COHNMC, routine surveillance chest X-rays are obtained weekly during the early post-HCT period, and frequently disclose otherwise unsuspected pulmonary infections. The utility of the practice may be greater in allogeneic than autologous HCT recipients [25]. Standard postero-anterior and lateral view chest radiographs do not exclude pneumonia in the symptomatic or febrile HCT patient and high-resolution CT scanning has been advocated in this setting [26].

Diagnostic approaches to pulmonary infiltrates

Radiographic patterns are sometimes helpful in establishing a differential diagnosis but are rarely pathognomonic. Diffuse bilateral pulmonary infiltrates, especially in the presence of cardiomegaly, pleural effusions and clinical signs of left- or right-sided heart failure are suggestive of cardiogenic edema, but at times the radiographic appearance may be confused with noncardiogenic edema, idiopathic pneumonia syndrome (IPS), diffuse alveolar hemorrhage (DAH), engraftment syndrome (ES), adult respiratory distress syndrome (ARDS) or viral infection. As a practical point, patients are often given a trial of diuretics, the X-ray is repeated and bronchoalveolar lavage (BAL) is performed if there is no improvement.

Focal pulmonary infiltrates are usually infectious in nature. Nodular disease, especially with the "halo" sign is typical of fungal infection, particularly aspergillosis. However, bacterial infection, Legionnaire's disease, *Nocardia* and noninfectious etiologies such as bronchiolitis obliterans with organizing pneumonia (BOOP) can also have a similar radiographic appearance.

BAL is usually the procedure of choice for attempting to establish a specific pulmonary diagnosis, both for diffuse and focal disease, and is safe and well-tolerated, even in patients with severe thrombocytopenia and immunosuppression. Yeasts in BAL specimens may represent upper airway contamination and are rarely clinically significant, especially if only a few organisms are seen. BAL positivity for *Aspergillus* has a high predictive value for true infection, making treatment with amphotericin-B advisable [27–32]. Technologic advances in microbiologic testing now permit rapid and accurate detection in BAL fluid of cytomegalovirus (CMV) (shell vial methodology), influenza A and B, parainfluenza 1–3, adenovirus, respiratory syncytial virus (RSV) and *Legionella pneumophila* by direct fluorescent monoclonal antibody staining (DFA). Transbronchial lung biopsy increases the risk of bleeding and rarely improves the yield over BAL, although it may occasionally disclose a diagnosis of BOOP treatable with steroids [33,34].

CT-guided aspiration needle biopsy (ANB) is usually reserved for patients with a nondiagnostic BAL, progressive disease, pleural-based lesions, adequate pulmonary reserve to tolerate a potential pneumothorax and an acceptable platelet count with blood product support. At COHNMC, ANB is typically performed with placement of an 18 G coaxial needle into the target lesion under CT monitoring. Approximately three to five 20-G core biopsies are then obtained through the guide needle. Patients are monitored for 4 h with chest radiograph 2 and 4 h after the procedure. Over the past 2 years at COHNMC, a total of 88 CT-guided needle lung biopsies (HCT and non-HCT patients) were

Table 64.3 Time frame of pulmonary complications after blood and marrow transplantation. Adapted from [36], with permission.

	Early (<30 days)	Middle (+30 to +100 days)	Late (>100 days)
Infectious			
	Bacteria	Cytomegalovirus	Bacteria
	Fungi (*Candida, Aspergillus*)	Human herpesvirus 6	Filamentous fungi (*Aspergillus* and others)
	Viruses (non-CMV)	*Pneumocystis carinii*	*Nocardia*
	Aspiration	Atypical bacteria	Viruses
		Aspergillus	Mycobacteria
			Pneumocystis carinii
Non-infectious			
	Cardiac dysfunction	Idiopathic pneumonia syndrome	Obstructive airways disease
	Hypervolemia	Diffuse alveolar hemorrhage	Bronchiolitis obliterans
	Capillary-leak syndrome		Relapsed disease
	Veno-occlusive disease		
	Engraftment syndrome		

performed by our radiology division. The pneumothorax rate was 29.5%, including pneumothoraces seen only on postbiopsy CT scan, with 6.8% of patients requiring tube thoracostomy (M. Hogan, personal communication, 2002).

Open lung biopsy has historically been considered the "gold standard" for the diagnosis and management of pulmonary infiltrates in the immunocompromised host [35]. In recent years, with the advent of rapid and specific virologic tests available for analysis of BAL fluid and with technologic advances in diagnostic video-assisted thoracoscopy, formal open lung biopsy is seldom performed.

Time course of pulmonary complications following HCT

Pulmonary complications following HCT tend to conform to a fairly predictable temporal sequence and this pattern often aids the clinician in establishing a differential diagnosis. This phenomenon is related to the evolution of immunologic changes following myeloablative chemoradiotherapy with sequential pancytopenia and gradual reconstitution of the immune system occurring with engraftment (Table 64.3).

The first 30 days or "early period" is characterized by pancytopenia and is dominated by the effects of myeloablative chemoradiotherapy (RRT). The pulmonary edema syndromes, both cardiogenic and noncardiogenic, are especially common during this period. Cardiac dysfunction has been reported to occur in 5–40% of HCT patients [37–39]. Prior treatment with anthracyclines, and conditioning with fractionated TBI, cyclophosphamide and melphalan have all been implicated in cardiotoxicity [40]. Hertenstein *et al*. [37], in a prospective study of 170 patients undergoing HCT, found that a baseline reduced left ventricular ejection refraction as ascertained by radionuclide ventriculography did predict cardiotoxic events, but life-threatening events could not reliably be predicted in individual patients, thereby limiting its value as a screening tool. Iatrogenic fluid overload may also contribute to pulmonary edema as a result of large volumes of blood products, antibiotics and total parenteral nutrition (TPN). Capillary-leak syndrome resulting from ARDS, ES or hepatic VOD may also have a role. Fluid overload in these settings usually responds well to diuretic therapy.

Other complications during the "early period" include oropharyngeal mucositis leading to aspiration pneumonia, particularly in the dependent lung regions such as the posterior segments of the upper lobes and the superior and posterior segments of the lower lobes. Infectious etiologies during the first 30 days include bacterial and fungal infection as well as herpes simplex virus (HSV) disease.

The "middle period" corresponds to approximately the time of engraftment (days 15–30) until day 100 (the traditional cutoff point between acute and chronic GVHD), and is characterized by relative decreased risk of bacterial infection and increase in viral and fungal disease. During the "late period", beyond 100 days following HCT, further recovery of the immune system occurs, except in patients with chronic GVHD. Infectious etiologies during this phase include bacteria, fungi, *Nocardia*, viruses, Mycobacteria and *Pneumocystis carinii*.

Although this temporal sequence provides some clues in establishing differential diagnosis, there is considerable overlap of complications occurring during the three periods and therefore more specific diagnostic tests are usually required, especially when empiric and supportive therapies fail. Moreover, the use of prophylactic broad-spectrum antibiotics and antifungal therapy, pre-emptive ganciclovir therapy and liberal use of multiple empiric antibiotics in suspected infection greatly obfuscates the classic temporal sequence of infection, as outlined above.

Specific pulmonary diseases

Pulmonary complications occur in 40–60% of HCT patients and have a higher mortality than any other organ dysfunction [1,36,41]. Primary lung infections from bacterial, fungal and viral etiologies as well as acute lung injury (ALI) and ARDS secondary to sepsis are amongst the most frequent causes for requests for consultation by the pulmonary intensivist. Other noninfectious pulmonary complications include DAH, IPS and ES. Complications from RRT, mucositis, pleural disease and pulmonary vascular diseases may also have critical care implications which will be addressed here.

Infectious complications

As specific infections are described in great detail in Chapters 51–57, only brief mention is made here. Bacterial infections occur in the early, middle and late periods following HCT, although most commonly in the first month. Historically, gram-negative bacteria have predominated in the neutropenic phase, with the major offenders being *Escherichia coli*, *Klebsiella*, *Pseudomonas*, *Enterobacter*, *Acinetobacter* and *Xanthomonas* species. Access portals include intravenous and urinary catheters, mucositis, gastrointestinal disease and skin breakdown. More recently, with the widespread use of prophylactic gram-negative antibiotics such as quinolones, the bacterial spectrum has shifted more towards gram-positive bacteria such as *Staphylococcus aureus* (including methacillin-resistant organisms), coagulase-negative *Staphylococcus*, *Streptococcus viridans* and *Enterococcus*.

Despite the progress in recent years in prophylactic, pre-emptive and therapeutic antibiotic strategies, fungal disease continues to be a major cause of post-transplant morbidity and mortality, with *Candida* and *Aspergillus* species remaining the most common organisms. *Candida* species normally colonize mucous membranes of the mouth, gastrointestinal and urinary tracts. Disruption of these mucosal barriers by RRT and GVHD, overgrowth of *Candida* resulting from broad-spectrum antibiotics and immunosuppression all contribute to *Candida* infection.

Aspergillus species are ubiquitous in the environment with over 300 species having been described. The classic presentation of pulmonary aspergillosis consists of fever, pleuritic chest pain, dyspnea and hemoptysis with nodular or cavitating infiltrates on imaging studies, including the "halo sign" on chest CT, although such manifestations are frequently absent. Tracheobronchial aspergillosis can present bronchoscopically as a yellowish-white to gray pseudomembrane comprised of necrotic material tightly adherent to the bronchial mucosa [42]. *Aspergillus* has a vasotropic tendency, increasing the risk of bleeding when performing bronchial and transbronchial biopsies. *Aspergillus* sinusitis in the HCT patient is usually fatal [43].

Viral infections in the HCT recipient include CMV, HSV, varicella-zoster virus (VZV), adenovirus, RSV, influenza, parainfluenza and human herpesvirus 6 (HHV-6). With no effective treatment available, CMV interstitial pneumonia in the 1970s and 1980s had a mortality rate approaching 100%. Perhaps one of the most significant advances in management of the HCT patient over the last two decades has been the development of sensitive tests for early detection of CMV infection including DFA, shell vial cultures and polymerase chain reaction (PCR) assays, accompanied by the development of prophylactic and pre-emptive strategies using ganciclovir and immunoglobulin leading to substantial reduction in both incidence and mortality of CMV infection [44–47]. Foscarnet is an alternate anti-CMV agent in patients with ganciclovir marrow toxicity or resistant infection. HSV and VZV infection usually occur as a result of reactivation of dormant disease. HSV frequently occurs in the oral cavity and genitalia but may also present as bronchitis or pneumonia.

VZV may or may not present with the classic vesicular rash and may cause pneumonia, hepatitis and encephalitis. Acyclovir remains the treatment of choice for both. Adenovirus usually presents as a nonspecific diffuse pulmonary infiltrate with respiratory compromise and is treated primarily with supportive care. RSV is treatable with aerosolized ribavirin when it is detected in the early nasopharyngeal phase, but patients with respiratory failure resulting from RSV pneumonia have an extremely high morbidity despite either aerosolized or intravenous ribavirin.

Pneumocystis carinii pneumonia (PCP) may occur because of reactivation of latent organisms or person–person transmission. Presenting symptoms are usually dyspnea, cough and fever with mild pulmonary signs on physical examination and bilateral pulmonary infiltrates on chest X-ray. Minimal to absent X-ray findings are reported in up to 15% of patients [48]. BAL is positive in most patients but occasionally transbronchial lung biopsy is required [49,50]. Because of the effectiveness of PCP prophylactic strategies, BAL-diagnosed PCP has become less common in recent years [51]. Prophylaxis is recommended for allogeneic HCT recipients for the period between 1 and 2 weeks prior to transplant (e.g. days −14 to −2) and from engraftment until termination of immunosupressive therapy [52]. Long-term prophylaxis beyond 1 year is recommended in patients with severe chronic GVHD [53]. Trimethoprim-sulfamethoxazole (TMP-SMX) 2–3 days a week is the recommended prophylaxis, although myelosuppression and hypersensitivity are potential adverse effects. Aerosolized pentamidine 300 mg via Respirgard II™ nebulizer (Marquest, Englewood, CO) every 3–4 weeks is an alternative agent, but is significantly less effective [54–56]. Dapsone 100 mg/day or atovaquone 1500 mg/day by mouth have also been utilized [57,58] and are the preferred alternatives to TMP-SMX at COHNMC. For proven PCP infection with moderate to severe hypoxemia, high-dose TMP-SMX with adjuvant glucocorticoid administration remains the treatment of choice.

Idiopathic pneumonia syndrome

Historically, HCT patients with interstitial pulmonary infiltrates were classified as having either "early" (within 100 days following HCT) or "late" (occurring over 100 days following HCT) interstitial pneumonitis [59–62]. Most disease occurred during the first 100 days, with the median time of onset being the seventh week following HCT. Etiologies were heterogeneous and included CMV, *Pneumocystis*, other infections, RRT and "idiopathic" pneumonia. In order to define the term "idiopathic" more narrowly, in 1991 a National Heart, Lung and Blood Institute (NHLBI) workshop was held in Bethesda, Maryland [63]. The workshop defined the syndrome termed idiopathic pneumonia syndrome (IPS). The definition included cases with evidence of widespread alveolar injury, as manifested by cough, dyspnea, crackles, hypoxemia, restrictive physiology and multilobar pulmonary infiltrates on imaging studies, in the absence of evidence of lower respiratory tract infection. The proposed definition specified that BAL must be negative on bacterial, viral and fungal cultures, shell vial CMV culture and cytology including special stains. A second confirmatory BAL was recommended 2–14 days following the initial negative study. Postulated etiologies of IPS include occult infection, RRT and cell-mediated immunity. Suspected cytokine mediators include tumor necrosis factor (TNF) and interleukin 8 (IL-8). Advanced IPS is sometimes characterized by progression to pulmonary fibrosis.

Crawford and Hackman [64] at FHCRC reviewed a case series of 41 allogeneic HCT recipients who underwent open lung biopsy for the evaluation of diffuse interstitial pulmonary infiltrates showing no evidence of infection between 1983 and 1988. Disease occurred 11–133 days following HCT (mean 35 days) and the hospital mortality was approximately 70%. Less than one-third of the patients died from progressive respiratory failure alone, with subsequent infection and liver failure being important contributors to mortality. In 1997, this same Seattle group [65] updated their description of IPS in a case series review of 1165 consecutive HCT recipients between 1988 and 1991. IPS was documented in 85 patients (7.3%), with no significant difference in incidence between autologous and allogeneic HCT recipients (5.7% and 7.6%, respectively). The median time to disease onset was 21 days and hospital mortality was 74%. The authors concluded that the spectrum of IPS had changed with a decreasing incidence, earlier onset and stronger association with RRT and immunologically induced multisystem organ failure. Treatment for IPS remains primarily supportive, and although steroids are frequently utilized their value has not been proven.

Diffuse alveolar hemorrhage

DAH is an idiopathic syndrome characterized by diffuse pulmonary infiltrates, dyspnea, cough and hypoxemia, with or without overt hemoptysis. Initial radiographic abnormalities are usually bilateral but may be unilateral, and are more often interstitial than alveolar [66]. The classic finding on BAL is increasingly bloody return on serially instilled and aspirated saline aliquots, with fluid analysis showing red blood cells, hemosiderin-laden macrophages if blood has been present for more than 2–3 days and negative microbiologic studies. Possible etiologies for this syndrome include nonspecific RRT, occult infection and immunologic abnormalities related to engraftment. It is unclear whether DAH is a subset of IPS.

Although previously described in non-HCT immunocompromised patients, one of the early descriptions of the syndrome was by Robbins et al. [67] in Omaha, who in 1989 published a series of 29 patients from a total of 141 consecutive autologous HCT recipients undergoing BAL for evaluation of pulmonary infiltrates. Risk factors for DAH were found to include age >40 years, underlying solid tumor, fever >39°C, severe mucositis, evidence of engraftment and renal insufficiency. Interestingly, platelet counts were not lower in the DAH group nor did any patients present initially with hemoptysis. Mortality was in the 80% range.

Chao et al. [68] from Stanford in 1991 reported four patients who developed DAH in a series of 77 undergoing autologous HCT for lymphoma. The treatment regimen consisted of high-dose methylprednisolone amounting to 1 g/day IV for 3 days, 500 mg/day for the next 3 days, 250 mg/day for an additional 3 days, then 60 mg/day with subsequent taper over the next 2 months. All four patients in this small series survived and the authors indicated that there were no infectious complications attributable to the high-dose steroids.

Metcalf et al. [69] from Omaha in 1994 retrospectively studied 65 episodes of DAH in 608 consecutive patients undergoing either autologous or allogeneic HCT. Survival to discharge was significantly higher in the "high-dose" steroid-treated group (defined as ≥30 mg/day methylprednisolone) compared to the "low-dose" (<30 mg/day methylprednisolone) and nonsteroid groups. Additional studies have reported DAH in allogeneic HCT patients with similar results [70–73]. The sensitivity and specificity of BAL in diagnosing DAH is controversial, because most patients never undergo pulmonary biopsy. Agustí et al. [70] reviewed postmortem data in 47 patients who had undergone allogeneic HCT, 21 of whom had a BAL within 7 days before death with negative microbiologic findings. Eight of the 21 patients had autopsy-proven DAH, but only four of these had hemorrhagic BAL fluid. Conversely, of the 13 patients without DAH at autopsy, seven patients did have bloody BAL fluid.

Engraftment syndrome

In recent years there have been multiple reports of pulmonary infiltrates occurring in association with stem cell engraftment, particularly during the phase of steep neutrophil recovery [74–78]. Although the term engraftment syndrome (ES) has been coined, it has no specific histopathologic or biochemical markers and there is controversy in the transplant community as to whether this indeed represents a distinct clinical entity or only a manifestation of early acute GVHD in the setting of underlying RRT-related epithelial and endothelial damage. As with IPS and DAH, therapy for ES is primarily supportive. Although unproven, steroids are often utilized.

Pleural disease

Pleural effusions occur fairly commonly in the post-transplant period and are usually related to fluid overload, RRT, VOD or pulmonary infection. Parapneumonic effusions are much more common than empyemas. Effusions have also been described in association with a polyserositis-type picture in patients with acute and chronic GVHD [79]. Recurrence of underlying malignancy is a less frequent etiology. If either infection or malignancy is suspected, diagnostic thoracentesis is performed, usually with platelet support and ultrasonic guidance.

HCT-related obstructive airway disease

It has been estimated that obstructive airway disease (OAD) develops in approximately 10% of HCT recipients, with a mortality of approximately 50% [80–89]. Those patients who have undergone lung biopsy most commonly exhibit findings consistent with constrictive bronchiolitis obliterans (BO). This is to be differentiated from BOOP, which usually presents more as a focal infiltrate with restrictive physiology, responsiveness to steroids and a much better prognosis. BO occurs primarily in allogeneic HCT recipients, but has also been described following autologous HCT [81]. The typical presentation is one of gradual onset of dyspnea and dry cough, occurring 3–12 months following HCT, with wheezing on examination and nonbronchodilator responsive obstructive physiology with hyperinflation and reduced DLCO on pulmonary function testing. Thin-section CT scan usually reveals bronchial dilatation, mosaic pattern attenuation and evidence of air trapping on expiration [82]. Transbronchial biopsies do not contain sufficient volume of tissue to make a definitive diagnosis so thoracoscopic biopsy is usually required. Often, the diagnosis of BO is made presumptively on the basis of clinical, imaging and spirometric findings without a tissue biopsy. Clarke et al. [83,84] in Seattle have reported an association between extensive chronic GVHD and prolonged methotrexate administration and immunoglobulin deficiency in OAD. Response to bronchodilators and steroids is generally poor [85–87], and azathioprine and cyclosporine also have been utilized with equivocal results.

Lung transplantation offers some promise in treating patients with refractory advanced OAD [88]. In our experience at COHNMC, we have had one 38-year-old male patient with advanced oxygen-dependent chronically hypercapneic OAD who successfully underwent bilateral cadaveric lung transplantation. The FEV-1 of 0.5 L before lung transplant improved to 3.26 L, with resolution of hypoxemia and hypercapnea, and the patient continues to do well from a pulmonary point of view 1.5 years post-transplant.

Pulmonary vascular disease

The incidence of clinically documented venous thromboembolism in HCT recipients is quite low [40]. However, in an autopsy series, eight of nine allogeneic HCT patients were found to have widespread intravascular fat deposits within the lungs, the clinical significance of which was unclear [90]. Pulmonary VOD following HCT has been reported in association with a conditioning regimen consisting of BCNU, etoposide and cyclophosphamide [91]. Disease responded favorably to therapy with high-dose steroids. There have also been isolated case reports of pulmonary hypertension with histopathology showing occlusion of small muscular pulmonary arteries, with 100% mortality [92,93]. Woodard et al. [94] from Minneapolis have recently described a syndrome characterized by fever and pulmonary nodules which they term "pulmonary cytolytic thrombi" (PCT). They retrospectively reviewed 13 PCT cases in which lung biopsy showed necrotic basophilic thromboemboli with amphorous debris and negative cultures. Empiric therapy included steroids and amphotericin, with nine patients surviving. Eleven of the 13 patients had either acute or chronic GVHD and one patient had BO.

Upper airway complications

Oropharyngeal mucositis has emerged in recent years as a major nonhematologic cause of dose-limiting RRT, occurring in up to 50% patients receiving high-dose chemotherapy [95–100]. Although oral complications are covered in more detail in Chapter 67, focus here is placed on pulmonary and critical care implications of severe mucositis.

Patients present with oral pain, swelling, dysphagia and odynophagia, and these constitute some of the most distressing complications of HCT from the patient's point of view. On examination, mucositis may progress from erythema to edema, ulceration, bleeding, necrosis, desiccation and sloughing of tissue with frank upper airway obstruction and stridor.

Table 64.4 "COH-TEAM" orders.

1. Initiate "COH-TEAM" Intensive Mouth Care (**C**ritical **O**ral **H**ygiene for Treatment of **E**dematous **A**ggressive **M**ucositis). Call respiratory therapist assigned to unit.
2. If formal pulmonary consultation requested, please Fax consult requisition.
3. Therapist to discuss with nurse previous mouth care regimen.
4. Baseline analgesia _____ drip @ _____ (rate). (Titrate dose down or hold if patient drowsy.)
5. All treatments to be performed by respiratory therapist (*frequency*).
6. Pulse oximetry. Record saturation on vital sign sheet every shift.
7. Oxygen (*FiO$_2$*) via (*appliance*).
8. Benzonatate 400 mg (4–100 mg perles). Dissolve contents in 30 mL sterile H$_2$O, swish for 60 s and spit out.
9. Swish, gargle, rinse and spit with 30 mL Biotene (Laclede Inc., Rancho Dominguez, CA) to remove secretions from posterior pharynx.
10. Administer racemic epinephrine 0.25 mL via hand-held nebulizer. Call physician if heart rate ≥140 beats/min before or after epinephrine. Check first with MD if medical record indicates any history of heart disease/arrythmias.
11. Administer dexamethasone 4 mg in 2 mL normal saline via hand-held nebulizer. (optional).
12. Spray affected areas of mucosa, especially the posterior tongue, soft palate and faucial pillars with fluticasone (44, 110, 220 mcg/actuation) metered-dose inhaler totaling six puffs.
13. Nystatin 5 mL, swish and spit.
14. Call pulmonary MD if increased respiratory distress.
15. Apply lidocaine 2% jelly to lips every 2 h as necessary.
16. Endotracheal intubation/emergency cricothyrotomy kits at bedside (optional).
17. Heliox at bedside (optional).

Physician's signature _____ Date _____

Anterior oral mucositis can be very painful to the patient but is less worrisome than posterior mucositis with supraglottic and glottic edema potentially compromising the airway. Particularly problematic is the fact that patients are often in too much pain to cooperate with mouth hygiene measures. Instead, they are usually treated with systemic narcotics, which may result in sedation and obtundation, in turn predisposing to both aspiration and further accumulation of inspissated secretions. Mucositis usually begins within the first week following HCT, but at times may either coincide with or even antedate stem cell infusion. Disruption of the oral mucosa during this neutropenic phase often predisposes to systemic infection.

Therapies have included a wide variety of mouth rinses with antiseptic, antifungal, anti-inflammatory, vaso-constrictive and/or mucolytic properties. These include hydrogen peroxide, glycerin, epinephrine, chlorhexidine, glutamine, steroids in various forms, benzydamine, lidocaine and dyclonine. Capsaicin has also been advocated as a desensitizer of the pain receptors [96]. Bioadhesive cellular films have been utilized [97], as have beta-carotene [98] and vitamin E [99], with variable results.

Mucositis usually improves around the time of engraftment, suggesting that there may be a role for granulocyte/granulocyte macrophage colony-stimulating factor (G/GM-CSF) in accelerating neutrophil recovery and hence reducing mucositis. Cytokines such as transforming growth factor beta (TGF-β), keratinocyte growth factor (KGF) and IL-11 have also been investigated.

At COHNMC, we have developed a standardized intensive mouth care protocol utilizing readily available medications having topical anesthetic, mucolytic and anti-inflammatory properties (Table 64.4). This regimen, together with meticulous attention to mouth hygiene including careful débridement of sloughed tissue by a consulting pulmonologist when indicated, has decreased the need for endotracheal intubation, emergency cricothyrotomy and tracheostomy in patients at our institution with severe oropharyngeal mucositis (unpublished data).

Prognosis of the critically ill HCT recipient

Although predictive models for ICU mortality have been available for years, until recently there had been few data specific for cancer patients requiring critical care services. In 1998, Groeger *et al.* [101] pooled prospective data obtained from ICUs at five participating cancer centers (Memorial Sloan-Kettering Cancer Center [MSKCC], New York, NY; Mount Sinai Medical Center, New York, NY; University of Texas M.D. Anderson Cancer Center, Houston, TX; COHNMC, Duarte, CA; and Johns Hopkins Medical Institutions, Baltimore, MD). A preliminary model was derived from 1483 cancer patients admitted to ICU and then validated on an additional 230 patients. Using multivariant logistical regression, 16 easily available variables were found to have high specificity and sensitivity in predicting cancer ICU outcome. The overall observed ICU cancer mortality rate was 42%. In a subset of 782 patients requiring mechanical ventilation, the mortality rate increased to 76% with no difference between the five cancer centers [102]. The mortality in HCT patients was in the 80–90% range, corroborating earlier data from Rubenfeld and Crawford [103] at FHCRC as well as data from other transplant centers [104–106].

In 2001, Bach *et al.* [107] at MSKCC performed a systematic review of the literature to assess prognostic factors associated with outcome in mechanically ventilated HCT patients. Fifteen evaluable studies were identified and a validation cohort was drawn from the five aforementioned cancer centers [101]. This study confirmed earlier data from FHCRC indicating that the presence of simultaneous elevation of bilirubin >4 mg/dL and creatinine >2 mg/dL in the ventilated HCT patient carries an estimated mortality in the 98–100% range. These data must be interpreted with great caution because such predictive models only apply to patient population aggregates and not to individual patients [108]. For example, predictive rules previously summarized by Crawford [1] would seem to indicate only a 0–0.2% chance of survival in HCT patients with certain combinations of lung injury, hypotension, hepatic and renal dysfunction (Table 64.5). At COHNMC over the past 2 years, five patients who met these criteria for "fatal prognosis" were nevertheless treated very aggressively. All five survived their acute episodes, and four are still living at the time of this writing (unpublished data), as demonstrated in Table 64.6. Strict application of the prognostic algorithm in these survivors may have led to erroneous decision-making and potential withdrawal of seemingly "futile" life-sustaining support.

As a practical point, at COHNMC our approach to respiratory failure in the HCT patient usually entails aggressive treatment for at least several days because most patients who are going to survive will show some improvement within this time frame. Occasionally, patients, families and surrogates insist on "absolutely everything being done" despite clear evidence of progressive multisystem organ failure with obvious futility of continued aggressive life support. Patients and their loved ones are increasingly medically sophisticated, and occasionally try to control patient care by insisting on mechanical ventilation and hemodialysis, against the advise of the attending physician. Frequent family conferences with multidisciplinary attendance by the primary physician, consultants, nursing staff, social services and pastoral care as well as ethics committee consultations are sometimes helpful in reassuring the family that "everything appropriate and feasible has been done" and that there is no realistic chance of recovery. Despite the fact that cardiopulmonary resuscitation in the ventilated critically ill HCT patient has uniformly

Table 64.5 Probability of survival after mechanical ventilation following hematopoietic cell transplantation (HCT). Mechanical ventilation excludes intubation <24 h after surgery. (Adapted from [1], with permission.)

Risk factors for mortality in the hospital in patients receiving mechanical ventilation after BMT:
- Severe lung injury (FiO_2 = 0.6 or PEEP >5 cm H_2O after first 24 h)
- Hypotension requiring vasopressor support for more than 4 h
- Combined hepatic and renal dysfunction (bilirubin >4 mg/dL and creatinine >2 mg/dL)

Risk factor(s) present	Probability of survival (%)
None	27
Hepatic and renal dysfunction only	16
Hypotension only	1.5
Any two	0.2
All three	0

BMT, bone marrow transplantation; FiO_2, fraction of inspired oxygen; PEEP, positive end-expiratory pressure.

been found to have a dismal prognosis, convincing the occasional recalcitrant family remains a daunting challenge for the health care team. Although discussing end of life issues with patients while they are still well prior to transplant carries the potential disadvantage of creating an atmosphere of pessimism, this step often proves invaluable in later deciding on the appropriate course of therapy when the family and surrogate decision-makers are struggling with these end of life issues.

Conclusions

The increasing frequency of HCT as a modality for treatment of an enlarging spectrum of malignant and nonmalignant diseases will almost certainly lead to greater ICU utilization for managing life-threatening complications in these patients. It is hoped that this trend will be mitigated by the development of less toxic conditioning regimens (e.g. nonmyeloablative transplants), improvement in GVHD prophylaxis, greater understanding of the pathophysiology of IPS, DAH and ES, more effective antibiotics, broader utilization of "lung protection" ventilator strategies and wiser decision-making in determining the point of futility despite highly aggressive critical care management.

Table 64.6 Outcome of multisystem organ dysfunction in selected hematopoietic cell transplantation (HCT) recipients.

UPN	Diagnosis	HCT	Conditioning regimen	"Fatal prognosis"	Outcome
2355	NHL	05/04/00 URD allo HCT	TBI/CY	06/09/00 Ventilated × 17 days Severe lung injury Cr 1.9 T. bili 8.9	Alive 07/21/03
1433	HD	11/28/00 allo HCT	5-FU/Melph	12/23/00 Ventilated × 3 days Severe lung injury Cr 2.7 T. bili 11.3	Alive 07/21/03
6785	NHL	11/28/01 auto HCT	TBI/VP16/CY	12/07/01 Ventilated × 2 days Severe lung injury Cr 3.5 T. bili 4.1	Discharged 01/22/02 Deceased 02/04/02
6795	AML	12/31/01 auto HCT	TBI/VP16/BU	01/11/02 Ventilated × 3 days Severe lung injury Pressors × 6 days Cr 1.9 T. bili 3.9	Alive 07/21/03
2475	MPD	07/02/02 URD allo HCT	5-FU/Melph	07/12/02 Ventilated × 4 days Pressors × 4 days Cr 3.7 T. bili 56.3	Alive 07/21/03

allo, allogeneic; AML, acute myelogenous leukemia; auto, autologous; BU, busulfan; Cr, serum creatinine; CY, cyclophosphamide; 5-FU, fludarabine; HD, Hodgkin's disease; Melph, melphalan; MPD, myeloproliferative disease; NHL, non-Hodgkin's lymphoma; T. bili, total bilirubin; TBI, total body irradiation; UPN, unique patient number; URD, unrelated donor; VP16, etoposide.

References

1 Crawford SW. Critical care and respiratory failure. In: Thomas ED, Blume KG, Forman SJ, eds. *Hematopoietic Cell Transplantation*, 2nd edn. Malden, MA: Blackwell Science, 1999: 712–22.
2 Multz AS, Chalfin DB, Samson IM *et al.* A "closed" medical intensive care unit (MICU) improves resource utilization when compared with an "open" MICU. *Am J Respir Crit Care Med* 1998; **157**: 1468–73.
3 Manthous CA, Amoateng-Adjepong Y, Al-Kharrat T *et al.* Effects of a medical intensivist on patient care in a community teaching hospital. *Mayo Clin Proc* 1997; **72**: 391–9.
4 Brilli RJ, Spevetz A, Branson RD *et al.* Critical care delivery in the intensivist care unit: defining clinical roles and the best practice model. *Crit Care Med* 2001; **29**: 2007–19.
5 Reynolds HN, Haupt MT, Thill-Baharozian MC *et al.* Impact of critical care physician staffing on patients with septic shock in a university hospital medical intensive care unit. *J Am Med Assoc* 1988; **260**: 3446–50.
6 Li TCM, Phillips MC, Shaw L *et al.* On-site physician staffing in a community hospital intensive care unit. *J Am Med Assoc* 1984; **252**: 2023–7.
7 Carson SS, Stocking C, Podsadecki T *et al.* Effects of organizational change in the medical intensive care unit of a teaching hospital: a comparison of "open" and "closed" formats. *J Am Med Assoc* 1996; **276**: 322–8.
8 Dimick JB, Pronovost PJ, Heitmiller RF *et al.* Intensive care unit physician staffing is associated with decreased length of stay, hospital cost, and complications after esophageal resection. *Crit Care Med* 2001; **29**: 753–8.
9 Hanson CW, Deutschman CS, Anderson HL. *et al.* Effects of an organized critical care service on outcomes and resource utilization: a cohort study. *Crit Care Med* 2000; **27**: 270–4.
10 Depledge MH, Barrett A, Powles RL. Lung function after bone marrow grafting. *Radiat Oncol Biol Phys* 1983; **9**: 145–51.
11 Link H, Reinhard U, Blaurock M *et al.* Lung function changes after allogenic bone marrow transplantation. *Thorax* 1986; **41**: 508–12.
12 Prince DS, Wingard JR, Sarol R *et al.* Longitudinal changes in pulmonary function following bone marrow transplantation. *Chest* 1989; **96**: 301–6.
13 Sutedja TG, Apperley JF, Hughes JM *et al.* Pulmonary function after bone marrow transplantation for chronic myeloid leukaemia. *Thorax* 1988; **43**: 163–9.
14 Sorensen PG, Ernst P, Panduro J *et al.* Reduced lung function in leukaemia patients undergoing bone barrow transplantation. *Scand J Haematol* 1984; **32**: 253–7.
15 Springmeyer SC, Silvestri RC, Flournoy N *et al.* Pulmonary function of marrow transplant patients. I. Effects of marrow infusion, acute graft-versus-host disease, and interstitial pneumonitis. *Exp Hematol* 1984; **12**: 805–10.
16 Serota FT, August CS, Koch PA *et al.* Pulmonary function in patients undergoing bone marrow transplantation. *Med Pediatr Oncol* 1984; **12**: 137–43.
17 Milburn HJ, Prentice HG, du Bois RM. Can lung function measurements be used to predict which patients will be at risk of developing interstitial pneumonitis after bone marrow transplantation? *Thorax* 1992; **47**: 421–5.
18 Horak DA, Schmidt GM, Zaia JA *et al.* Pretransplant pulmonary function predicts cytomegalovirus-associated interstitial pneumonia following bone marrow transplantation. *Chest* 1992; **102**: 1484–90.
19 Crawford SW, Fisher L. Predictive value of pulmonary function tests before bone marrow transplantation. *Chest* 1992; **101**: 1257–64.
20 Hoover M, Morgan ER, Kletzel M. Prior fungal infection is not a contraindication to bone marrow transplant in patients with acute leukemia. *Med Pediatr Oncol* 1997; **28**: 268–73.
21 Leleu X, Sendid B, Fruit J *et al.* Combined antifungal therapy and surgical resection as treatment of pulmonary zygomycosis in allogeneic bone marrow transplantation. *Bone Marrow Transplant* 1999; **24**: 417–20.
22 Martino R, Nomdedéu J, Altés A *et al.* Successful bone marrow transplantation in patients with previous invasive fungal infections: report of four cases. *Bone Marrow Transplant* 1994; **13**: 265–9.
23 Lupinetti FM, Behrendt DM, Giller RH *et al.* Pulmonary resection for fungal infection in children undergoing bone marrow transplantation. *Thorac Cardiovasc Surg* 1992; **104**: 684–7.
24 Reichenberger F, Habicht J, Kaim A *et al.* Lung resection for invasive pulmonary aspergillosis in neutropenic patients with hematologic diseases. *Am J Respir Crit Care Med* 1998; **158**: 885–90.
25 Roy V, Ali LI, Selby GB. Routine chest radiography for the evaluation of febrile neutropenic patients after autologous stem cell transplantation. *Am J Hematol* 2000; **64**: 170–4.
26 Heussel CP, Kauczor HU, Heussel GE *et al.* Pneumonia in febrile neutropenic patients and in bone marrow and blood stem-cell transplant recipients: use of high-resolution computed tomography. *J Clin Oncol* 1999; **17**: 796–805.
27 Kahn FW, Jones JM, England DM. The role of bronchoalveolar lavage in the diagnosis of invasive pulmonary aspergillosis. *Am J Clin Pathol* 1986; **86**: 518–23.
28 Yu VL, Muder RR, Poorsattar A. Significance of isolation of aspergillus from the respiratory tract in diagnosis of invasive pulmonary aspergillosis. *Am J Med* 1986; **81**: 249–54.
29 Levy H, Horak DA, Tegtmeier BR *et al.* The value of bronchoalveolar lavage and bronchial washings in the diagnosis of invasive pulmonary aspergillosis. *Respir Med* 1992; **86**: 243–8.
30 Stover DE, Zaman MB, Hajdu JI *et al.* Bronchoalveolar lavage in the diagnosis of diffuse pulmonary infiltrates in the immunocompromised host. *Ann Intern Med* 1984; **101**: 1–7.
31 McWhinney PH, Kibbler CC, Hamon MD *et al.* Progress in the diagnosis and management of aspergillosis in bone marrow transplantation: 13 years' experience. *Clin Infect Dis* 1993; **17**: 397–404.
32 Reichenberger F, Habicht J, Matt P *et al.* Diagnostic yield of bronchoscopy in histologically proven invasive pulmonary aspergillosis. *Bone Marrow Transplant* 1999; **24**: 1195–9.
33 Feinstein MB, Mokhtari M, Ferreiro R *et al.* Fiberoptic bronchoscopy in allogeneic bone marrow transplantation: findings in the era of serum cytomegalovirus antigen surveillance. *Chest* 2001; **120**: 1094–100.
34 Dunn JC, West KW, Rescorla FJ *et al.* The utility of lung biopsy in recipients of stem cell transplantation. *J Pediatr Surg* 2001; **36**: 1302–3.
35 Crawford SW, Hackman RC, Clark JG. Open lung biopsy diagnosis of diffuse pulmonary infiltrates after bone marrow transplantation. *Chest* 1988; **94**: 949–53.
36 Shanholtz C. Respiratory complications of blood and marrow transplantation. *Clin Pulm Med* 1999; **6**: 254–62.
37 Hertenstein B, Stefanic M, Schmeiser T *et al.* Cardiac toxicity of bone marrow transplantation: predictive value of cardiologic evaluation before transplant. *J Clin Oncol* 1994; **12**: 998–1004.
38 Eames GM, Crosson J, Steinberger J *et al.* Cardiovascular function in children following bone marrow transplant: a cross-sectional study. *Bone Marrow Transplant* 1997; **19**: 61–6.
39 Kupari M, Volin L, Suokas A *et al.* Cardiac involvement in bone marrow transplantation: serial changes in left ventricular size, mass and performance. *J Intern Med* 1990; **227**: 259–66.
40 Pihkala J, Saarinen UM, Lundström U *et al.* Effects of bone marrow transplantation on myocardial function in children. *Bone Marrow Transplant* 1994; **13**: 149–55.
41 Krowka MJ, Rosenow EC, Hoagland HC. Pulmonary complications of bone marrow transplantation. *Chest* 1985; **87**: 237–46.
42 Machida U, Kami M, Kanda Y *et al.* Aspergillus tracheobronchitis after allogeneic bone marrow transplantation. *Bone Marrow Transplant* 1999; **24**: 1145–9.
43 Verschraegen CF, Van Besien KW, Dignani C *et al.* Invasive aspergillus sinusitis during bone marrow transplantation. *Scand J Infect Dis* 1997; **29**: 436–8.
44 Goodrich JM, Bowden RA, Fisher L *et al.* Ganciclovir prophylaxis to prevent cytomegalovirus disease after allogeneic marrow transplant. *Ann Intern Med* 1993; **118**: 173–8.
45 Schmidt GM, Horak DA, Niland JC *et al.* A randomized, controlled trial of prophylactic ganciclovir for cytomegalovirus pulmonary infection in recipients of allogeneic bone marrow transplants. *N Engl J Med* 1991; **324**: 1005–11.
46 Winston DJ, Ho WG, Bartoni K *et al.* Ganciclovir prophylaxis of cytomegalovirus infection and disease in allogeneic bone marrow transplant recipients: results of a placebo-controlled, double-blind trial. *Ann Intern Med* 1993; **118**: 179–84.
47 Goodrich JM, Mori M, Gleaves CA *et al.* Early treatment with ganciclovir to prevent cytomegalovirus disease after allogeneic marrow transplantation. *N Engl J Med* 1991; **325**: 1601–7.
48 Tuan IZ, Dennison D, Weisdorf DJ. *Pneumocystis carinii* pneumonitis following bone marrow transplantation. *Bone Marrow Transplant* 1992; **10**: 267–72.
49 Huaringa AJ, Leyva FJ, Signes-Costa J *et al.* Bronchoalveolar lavage in the diagnosis of pulmonary complications of bone marrow transplant patients. *Bone Marrow Transplant* 2000; **25**: 975–9.
50 Leroy X, Copin MC, Ramon P *et al.* Nodular granulomatous *Pneumocystis carinii* pneumonia in a bone marrow transplant recipient: case report. *APMIS* 2000; **108**: 363–6.
51 Feinstein MB, Mokhtari M, Ferreiro R *et al.* Fiberoptic bronchoscopy in allogeneic bone marrow transplantation: findings in the era of serum cytomegalovirus antigen surveillance. *Chest* 2001; **120**: 1094–100.

52. Centers for Disease Control and Prevention. Guidelines for preventing opportunistic infections among hematopoietic stem cell transplant recipients: recommendations of CDC, the Infectious Disease Society of America, and the American Society of Blood and Marrow Transplantation. *Morb Mortal Wkly Rep* 2000; **49** (RR-10): 25–6; 106.
53. Lyytikainen O, Ruutu T, Volin L et al. Late onset *Pneumocystis carinii* pneumonia following allogeneic bone marrow transplantation. *Bone Marrow Transplant* 1996; **17**: 1057–9.
54. Link H, Vöhringer H-F, Wingen F et al. Pentamadine aerosol prophylaxis of *Pneumocystis carinii* pneumonia after BMT. *Bone Marrow Transplant* 1993; 11: 403–6.
55. Vasconcelles MJ, Bernardo MV, King C et al. Aerosolized pentamidine as *Pneumocystis* prophylaxis after bone marrow transplantation is inferior to other regimens and is associated with decreased survival and an increased risk of other infections. *Biol Blood Marrow Transplant* 2000; **6**: 35–43.
56. Marras TK, Sanders K, Lipton JH et al. Aerosolized pentamidine prophylaxis for *Pneumocystis carinii* pneumonia after allogeneic marrow transplantation. *Transpl Infect Dis* 2002; **4**: 66–74.
57. Souza JP, Boeckh M, Gooley TA et al. High rates of *Pneumocystis carinii* pneumonia in allogeneic blood and marrow transplant recipients receiving dapsone prophylaxis. *Clin Infect Dis* 1999; **29**: 1467–71.
58. Colby C, McAfee S, Sackstein R et al. A prospective randomized trial comparing the toxicity and safety of atovaquone with trimethoprim/sulfamethoxazole as *Pneumocystis carinii* pneumonia prophylaxis following autologous peripheral blood stem cell transplantation. *Bone Marrow Transplant* 1999; **24**: 897–902.
59. Wingard JR, Santos GW, Saral R. Late-onset interstitial pneumonia following allogeneic bone marrow transplantation. *Transplantation* 1985; 39: 21–3.
60. Meyers JD, Flournoy N, Thomas ED. Nonbacterial pneumonia after allogeneic marrow transplantation: a review of 10 years' experience. *Rev Infect Dis* 1982; **4**: 1119–32.
61. Neiman PE, Reeves W, Ray G et al. A prospective analysis of interstitial pneumonia and opportunistic viral infection among recipients of allogeneic bone marrow grafts. *J Infect Dis* 1977; **136**: 754–67.
62. Weiner RS, Bortin MM, Gale RP et al. Interstitial pneumonitis after bone marrow transplantation. *Ann Intern Med* 1986; **104**: 168–75.
63. Clark JG, Hansen JA, Hertz MI et al. Idiopathic pneumonia syndrome after bone marrow transplantation. *Am Rev Respir Dis* 1993; **147**: 1601–6.
64. Crawford SW, Hackman RC. Clinical course of idiopathic pneumonia after bone marrow transplantation. *Am Rev Respir Dis* 1993; **147**: 1393–400.
65. Kantrow SP, Hackman RC, Boeckh M et al. Idiopathic pneumonia syndrome. *Transplantation* 1997; **63**: 1079–86.
66. Witte RJ, Gurney JW, Robbins RA et al. Diffuse pulmonary alveolar hemorrhage after bone marrow transplantation: radiographic findings in 39 patients. *Am J Roentgenol* 1991; **157**: 461–4.
67. Robbins RA, Linder J, Stahl MG et al. Diffuse alveolar hemorrhage in autologous bone marrow transplant recipients. *Am J Med* 1989; **87**: 511–8.

68. Chao NJ, Duncan SR, Long GD et al. Corticosteroid therapy for diffuse alveolar hemorrhage in autologous bone marrow transplant recipients. *Ann Intern Med* 1991; **114**: 145–6.
69. Metcalf JP, Rennard SI, Reed EC et al. Corticosteroids as adjunctive therapy for diffuse alveolar hemorrhage associated with bone marrow transplantation. *Am J Med* 1994; **96**: 327–34.
70. Agustí G, Ramirez J, Picado C et al. Diffuse alveolar hemorrhage in allogeneic bone marrow transplantation. *Am J Respir Crit Care Med* 1995; **151**: 1006–10.
71. Schmidt-Wolf I, Schwerdtfeger R, Schwella N et al. Diffuse pulmonary alveolar hemorrhage after allogeneic bone marrow transplantation. *Ann Hematol* 1993; **67**: 139–41.
72. Raptis A, Mavroudis D, Suffredini AF et al. High-dose corticosteroid therapy for diffuse alveolar hemorrhage in allogeneic bone marrow stem cell transplant recipients. *Bone Marrow Transplant* 1999; **24**: 879–83.
73. Srivastava A, Gottlieb D, Bradstock KF. Diffuse alveolar hemorrhage associated with microangiopathy after allogeneic bone marrow transplantation. *Bone Marrow Transplant* 1995; **15**: 863–7.
74. Ravoet C, Feremans W, Husson B et al. Clinical evidence for an engraftment syndrome associated with early and steep neutrophil recovery after autologous blood stem cell transplantation. *Bone Marrow Transplant* 1996; **18**: 943–7.
75. Cahill RA, Spitzer TR, Mazumder A. Marrow engraftment and clinical manifestations of capillary leak syndrome. *Bone Marrow Transplant* 1996; **18**: 177–84.
76. Lee C-K, Gingrich RD, Hohl RJ et al. Engraftment syndrome in autologous bone marrow and peripheral stem cell transplantation. *Bone Marrow Transplant* 1995; **16**: 175–82.
77. Capizzi SA, Kumar S, Huneke NE et al. Peri-engraftment respiratory distress syndrome during autologous hematopoietic stem cell transplantation. *Bone Marrow Transplant* 2001; **27**: 1299–303.
78. Spitzer TR. Engraftment syndrome following hematopoietic stem cell transplantation. *Bone Marrow Transplant* 2001; **27**: 893–8.
79. Seber A, Khan SP, Kersey JH. Unexplained effusions. association with allogeneic bone marrow transplantation and acute or chronic graft-versus-host disease. *Bone Marrow Transplant* 1996; **17**: 207–11.
80. St. John RC, Gadek JE, Tutschka PJ et al. Analysis of airflow obstruction by bronchoalveolar lavage following bone marrow transplantation: implications for pathogenesis and treatment. *Chest* 1990; **98**: 600–7.
81. Paz HL, Crilley P, Patchefsky A et al. Bronchiolitis obliterans after autologous bone marrow transplantation. *Chest* 1992; **101**: 775–8.
82. Worthy SA, Flint JD, Müller NL. Pulmonary complications after bone marrow transplantation: high resolution CT and pathologic findings. *Radiographics* 1997; **17**: 1359–71.
83. Clark JG, Schwartz DA, Flournoy N et al. Risk factors for airflow obstruction in recipients of bone marrow transplants. *Ann Intern Med* 1987; **107**: 648–56.
84. Clark JG, Crawford SW, Madtes DK et al. Obstructive lung disease after allogeneic marrow transplantation. *Ann Intern Med* 1989; **111**: 368–76.
85. Ostrow D, Buskard N, Hill RS et al. Bronchiolitis obliterans complicating bone marrow transplantation. *Chest* 1985; **87**: 828–30.

86. Wyatt SE, Nunn P, Hows JM et al. Airways obstruction associated with graft-versus-host disease after bone marrow transplantation. *Thorax* 1984; **39**: 887–94.
87. Kurzrock R, Zander A, Kanojia M et al. Obstructive lung disease after allogeneic bone marrow transplantation. *Transplantation* 1984; **37**: 156–60.
88. Calhoon JH, Levine S, Anzueto A et al. Lung transplantation in a patient with a prior bone marrow transplant. *Chest* 1992; **102**: 948.
89. Crawford SW, Clark JG. Bronchiolitis associated with bone marrow transplantation. *Clin Chest Med* 1993; **14**: 741–9.
90. Paradinas FJ, Sloane JP, Depledge MH et al. Pulmonary fat embolisation after bone marrow transplantation. *Lancet* 1983; **1**: 715–6.
91. Hackman RC, Madtes DK, Petersen FB et al. Pulmonary venoocclusive disease following bone marrow transplantation. *Transplantation* 1989; **47**: 989–92.
92. Seguchi M, Hirabayashi N, Fujii Y et al. Pulmonary hypertension associated with pulmonary occlusive vasculopathy after allogeneic bone marrow transplantation. *Transplantation* 2000; **69**: 177–9.
93. Selby DM, Rudzki JR, Bayever ES et al. Vasculopathy of small muscular arteries in pediatric patients after bone marrow transplantation. *Hum Pathol* 1999; **30**: 734–40.
94. Woodard JP, Gulbahce E, Shreve M et al. Pulmonary cytolytic thrombi: a newly recognized complication of stem cell transplantation. *Bone Marrow Transplant* 2000; **25**: 293–300.
95. Karthaus M, Rosenthal C, Ganser A. Prophylaxis and treatment of chemo- and radiotherapy-induced oral mucositis: are there new strategies? *Bone Marrow Transplant* 1999; **24**: 1095–108.
96. Berger A, Henderson M, Nadoolman W et al. Oral capsaicin provides temporary relief for oral mucositis pain secondary to chemotherapy/radiation therapy. *J Pain Symptom Manage* 1995; **10**: 243–8.
97. Le Veque FG, Parzuchowski JB, Farinacci GC et al. Clinical evaluation of MGI 209, an anesthetic, film-forming agent for relief from painful oral ulcers associated with chemotherapy. *J Clin Oncol* 1992; **10**: 1963–8.
98. Mills EE. The modifying effect of beta-carotene on radiation and chemotherapy induced oral mucositis. *Br J Cancer* 1988; **57**: 416–7.
99. Wadleigh RG, Redman RS, Graham ML et al. Vitamin E in the treatment of chemotherapy-induced mucositis. *Am J Med* 1992; **92**: 481–4.
100. Rapoport AP, Miller Watelet LF, Linder T et al. Analysis of factors that correlate with mucositis in recipients of autologous and allogeneic stem-cell transplants. *J Clin Oncol* 1999; **17**: 2446–53.
101. Groeger JS, Lemeshow S, Price K et al. Multicenter outcome study of cancer patients admitted to the intensive care unit: a probability of mortality model. *J Clin Oncol* 1998; **16**: 761–70.
102. Groeger JS, White P, Nierman DM et al. Outcome for cancer patients requiring mechanical ventilation. *J Clin Oncol* 1999; **17**: 991–7.
103. Rubenfeld GD, Crawford SW. Withdrawing life support from mechanically ventilated recipients of bone marrow transplants: a case for evidence-based guidelines. *Ann Intern Med* 1996; **125**: 625–33.
104. Afessa B, Tefferi A, Clark Hoagland H et al. Outcome of recipients of bone marrow transplants who require intensive-care unit support. *Mayo Clin Proc* 1992; **67**: 117–22.

105 Denardo SJ, Oye RK, Bellamy PE. Efficacy of intensive care for bone marrow transplant patients with respiratory failure. *Crit Care Med* 1989; **17**: 4–6.
106 Paz HL, Crilley P, Weinar M *et al.* Outcome of patients requiring medical ICU admission following bone marrow transplantation. *Chest* 1993; **104**: 527–31.
107 Bach PB, Schrag D, Nierman DM *et al.* Identification of poor prognostic features among patients requiring mechanical ventilation after hematopoietic stem cell transplantation. *Blood* 2001; **98**: 3234–40.
108 Schuster DP. Everything that should be done-not everything that can be done. *Am Rev Respir Dis* 1992; **145**: 508–9.

65

Sally Weisdorf-Schindele & Sarah Jane Schwarzenberg

Nutritional Support of Hematopoietic Cell Recipients

Introduction

Diverse requirements for supportive care

Supportive care, specifically nutrition support, of hematopoietic cell transplantation (HCT) recipients has become as varied as the types of HCT now being utilized. The broadening of indications for HCT has also led to diversity in the need for supportive care. Much of this widening of the spectrum of supportive care is due to developments in the use of hematopoietic and tissue growth factors [1]. Cytokine therapy has had a major impact in autologous transplantation and is being used to reduce complications of allogeneic transplantation as well [2,3]. Colony-stimulating factors and tissue growth factors are used to stimulate hematopoietic cell graft function and gastrointestinal tissue repair. This decreases the period of time that HCT recipients are cytopenic with impaired mucosal barriers to infection [4,5] Mucositis and infection often limit a recipient's ability to maintain or resume adequate oral nourishment.

At the same time, other types of HCT have been developed which have decreased the toxicity of conditioning regimens [6]. The use of peripheral blood cells as hematopoietic progenitors has increased the use of both autologous and allogeneic transplantation [7]. Other types of allogeneic transplantation have been developed which decrease the incidence and severity of graft-vs.-host disease (GVHD). Specifically, allogeneic cord blood cell transplantation [8,9] to date appears to have a lower incidence of GVHD [10,11]. Intestinal GVHD often results in use of chronic parenteral nutrition (PN) after HCT because patients are unable to eat, secondary to nausea and vomiting, or are unable to absorb nutrients. Unrelated allogeneic donor transplantation, on the other hand, has increased the intensity of supportive care [12,13]. These recipients tend to require more intensive support, including nutrition support due to the higher incidence and severity of infection and GVHD.

The use of new sources of hematopoietic cells and the use of cytokines has impacted transplantation such that both autologous marrow and peripheral blood hematopoietic cell transplantation can now be done in the outpatient setting, particularly for nonhematological malignancies [14,15]. Recipients are admitted to the hospital for any complications, which can include nutritional depletion.

The benefits of maintaining nutritional intake during allogeneic bone marrow transplantation (BMT) were established in the 1980s [16] and are not necessarily applicable to other types of HCT. In a randomized, controlled study, which the authors carried out at the University of Minnesota, there was a clear long-term survival advantage for allogeneic BMT recipients who received prophylactic nutrition support in the form of PN compared to control recipients who were fed *ad libitum* with intravenous

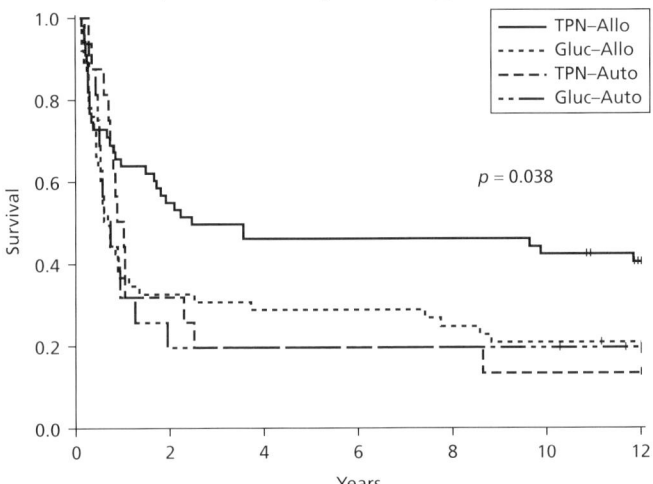

Fig. 65.1 Overall survival for 71 patients given prophylactic total parenteral nutrition (TPN) vs. 66 control patients not receiving prophylactic TPN in a prospective, randomized trial ($p = 0.035$). Separate curves are shown for allogeneic and autologous transplantation patients. Reproduced with permission from Schwarzenberg and Weisdorf-Schindele [139].

supplementation of minerals and vitamins until nutritional depletion was documented (Fig. 65.1). Thirty-two of 137 subjects had autologous transplants. They were randomized and analyzed separately from the 104 allogeneic recipients, showing no difference in survival. Because the allogeneic recipients also had a lower incidence of relapse ($p = 0.001$), we concluded that their improved survival may have been due to a nutritional effect on graft function, such as graft-vs.-tumor activity, as was suggested by early murine studies [17].

In our trial the control group was fed orally until four of six standard nutritional assessment measures fell below the 10th percentile values. Sixty-one percent of control patients met these criteria for nutritional depletion at a median of day 21 post-transplant. These patients had significantly longer hospitalizations than the PN patients. However, the other 39% of control patients who were able to maintain adequate oral nutrition had significantly shorter hospitalization periods than PN patients.

In another study published in the same year, intensive dietary counseling with use of both nasogastric feedings and intravenous protein supplementation, meant nutritional support was maintained without a prolonged course of PN in a majority (~75%) of BMT recipients without adverse effects on graft function [18]. At the time these two studies were done the population of BMT recipients was much more homogenous than HCT populations are now. Hematopoietic cell sources, cytoreduction, GVHD prophylaxis and the availability of agents to reduce regimen-related toxicities were more limited. Since the publication of these two studies there have been no further studies published with control HCT recipients who do not receive some parenteral or enteral nutritional support. In both these studies, patients generally met the criteria for initiation of PN after several weeks of profound neutropenia, often with infection.

Therefore, reducing the period of time following cytoreduction during which recipients are neutropenic and have tissue injury with use of less toxic conditioning, growth factors and alternate prophylaxis for GVHD has reduced the requirement to use PN for all patients throughout the course of HCT. The resolution of mucositis and the ability of HCT recipients to resume oral intake frequently coincides with the appearance of circulating neutrophils. While nutrition support remains an essential aspect of supportive care, the range of nutrition support options is now as varied as the settings for HCT. Nutrition support recommendations are now based on the nutrition status of the individual patient and PN is no longer indicated for all HCT recipients [19].

Changes during transplantation

This chapter outlines the metabolic support of HCT recipients through the complex progression of medical events that may occur in the course of HCT. The provision of nutrition support to HCT recipients requires an integrated approach between physicians with expertise in nutritional/metabolic requirements of stressed patients and physicians with expertise in management of the rapidly changing physiology of patients recovering from high-dose chemotherapy and radiation, often with infectious complications. The nutrition support consultant must anticipate and avoid complications, including weight gain or loss, fluid and electrolyte imbalance, sugar and protein overload and liver dysfunction [20]. The overriding goal is to enable the recipient to recover the ability to nourish him/herself normally, i.e. orally, as quickly as possible following transplantation.

The course of transplantation can be divided into three periods, each presenting distinct metabolic challenges [21]. These are (i) cytoreduction and tissue damage; (ii) pancytopenia and tissue repair; and (iii) engraftment, which can be complicated by GVHD, graft rejection or return of the primary disease process. Specific organ failure, such as of liver, kidney, heart or lung can confound nutritional requirements during any of these sequential periods. These organ failure syndromes can be due to veno-occlusive disease [22], biliary obstruction, recurrence of pre-existing hepatitis [21], drug toxicity and GVHD when there is hepatic dysfunction [23]. They can include renal insufficiency or renal failure with fluid and electrolyte imbalance [24,25], cardiac failure due to drug toxicity [26], compounded by fluid and electrolyte imbalance [27], or pulmonary failure due to drug toxicity, infection, GVHD and fluid imbalance [28]. Multiple organ failure due to the systemic inflammatory response can supervene in these settings, often temporally related to sepsis.

Cytoreduction

The first barrier to oral nutrition during cytoreduction is the central nervous system effect of chemotherapy and radiation, causing severe vomiting [29]. Cytoreductive therapy also causes painful mucositis in the oral pharynx and esophagus [30]. Taste sensation is altered; both hypogeusia and dysgeusia are reported [31]. Intestinal dysmotility due to narcotic analgesics can exacerbate vomiting. The normal growth and repair of oral and gastrointestinal mucosal epithelium is disrupted. Histologic changes attributable to standard, high-dose cytoreductive conditioning therapy have been found to persist up to day 21 after HCT [32]. The loss of functioning intestinal epithelium results in malabsorption and reversal of salt and water absorption. The result is typically an interval of watery diarrhea in the 1st week following chemo/radiotherapy [33]. Stool sodium transiently increases to 50–80 meq/L. There is usually enough mucosal disruption to cause a transient rise in exudative protein loss into the feces [34], with concomitant loss of zinc and failure to absorb minerals and vitamins. At the same time that patients are unable to ingest and absorb nutrients adequately, protein breakdown is occurring, due both to direct tissue damage and to relative immobilization of the patient. Nitrogen losses have been documented in a number of studies [35–38]. The massive increased waste nitrogen must be processed by the liver via the urea cycle, which increases the energy demands of the liver and, consequently, of the whole patient [39].

Cytopenia

As a result of cytoreduction, HCT recipients may be profoundly pancytopenic for 12–21 days. Growth factors are used to minimize the duration of this effect [40,41]. However, there remains a high risk of bacterial infection, treatment of which increases the risk of fungal invasion [42]. The damaged intestine may serve as a portal of entry for such infection or can itself be affected with bacterial or fungal overgrowth [43]. In a recent study of lisofylline, it was suggested that this modulator of the pro-inflammatory cytokine response could reduce infection via stabilization of their intestinal mucosal barrier [44]. Narcotic pain therapy can cause intestinal stasis, predisposing to intestinal bacterial overgrowth, which leads to further mucosal damage. Bacterial deconjugation of bile acids promotes fat malabsorption. Passage of bile acid into the colon results in secretory diarrhea by the direct toxic effect that bile salts exert on colonic mucosa. Systemic effects of infection, such as fever, have appetite-suppressant effects as well. Tissue damage and nitrogen mobilization from protein breakdown can be exacerbated by infection, with altered nutrient utilization resulting from the cytokines and hormones elaborated during systemic infection. At this point in transplant, cytokines and modulators of inflammation can be applied with the goal of reducing some of these effects. During the same time that neutropenia is maximum, tissue repair is occurring, and adequate nutrient intake to support tissue repair is also indicated.

Engraftment

After engraftment, mucosal lesions heal and patients are often able to resume some oral intake. The absence of enteral nutrients, even with parenteral support, and the consequent lack of the neuroendocrine trophic factors that are stimulated in the intestine by nutrients, may affect absorption by delaying epithelial cell regeneration. When diarrhea occurs during this time, the differential diagnosis includes GVHD and infection [21,34]. Acute GVHD of the intestine can involve the entire intestinal tract [32,45,46]. Intestinal GVHD is a lesion that directly damages mucosa and varies in intensity from scattered cell necrosis to complete epithelial denudation [47]. Clinically, GVHD diarrhea is similar to that resulting from cytoreduction, but is often more severe and prolonged. It has been characterized by massive protein loss in the stool [47] and can cause a profound decrease in nitrogen balance [48]. The protein exudation is accompanied by large stool zinc losses, due to the disruption of its entero-pancreatic circulation. Decreased zinc stores are reflected clinically in low levels of serum alkaline phosphatase, noted even in patients whose elevated bilirubin and 5′-nucleotidase indicate obvious cholestasis. Stool sodium rises to approximately 70–100 meq/L. Other symptoms of GVHD that can interfere with oral nutrient intake include persistent nausea, with or without vomiting, and anorexia [49].

Nutrition support during HCT

Parenteral therapy

Guidelines for the prescription of PN have been published in the context of studies done with varied aims. The purpose of some of these studies was to determine optimal nutritional support for HCT recipients [16,18,50–54]. Other studies were aimed at determining nutritional outcomes of support [36–38,55–58]. The guidelines are similar from center to center in their prescription of energy intake for HCT recipients. The prescribed energy intake includes protein calories in some, but only nonprotein caloric intake in others. The Harris–Benedict equations [59] are used to estimate basal energy expenditure (BEE) in the majority of these reports, and ideal body weight was used in these calculations. There is a trend to lower estimation of initial energy requirements in the more recent studies, based on more accurate measurements of actual energy expenditure. The use of fat as an energy source was varied, depending on the goal of the study. In the study that actually compared different levels of fat intake, lipid was shown to be helpful in maintaining energy balance without significant complications [51]. Fat-free TPN can be complicated by hepatic steatosis and glycogenosis, causing increased transaminases and increased serum triglyceride; thus, a balanced caloric intake (using both fat and carbohydrate) is recommended. Electrolytes, minerals, vitamins and trace elements are added to the total parenteral nutrition (TPN) according to the recommended daily allowance (RDA) and individual needs. Standard trace element solutions contain chromium, zinc, copper, manganese and selenium.

One study compared two levels of energy and protein intake and found that the lower intakes supported nutritional status with fewer metabolic complications [37]. In this study, nitrogen balance was not different between the groups. Although fluid intake was similar in both groups, body weight was lower, serum albumin was higher and serum sodium was more often in the normal range in the group with the lower protein/calorie intake. All of these factors suggest less water retention in these patients. An earlier study of body composition showed that there was a fluid shift from the intracellular compartment to the extracellular compartment [60]. This study used protein and energy intakes similar to the high-intake group [37]. This shift may account for the apparent fluid overload, without an actual increase in total body water. In contrast, another recent study compared a standard protein prescription to a high-protein prescription with the same total energy intake [38]. These authors reported an improvement in nitrogen balance with this approach. They also reported that measured energy expenditure was lower than they had predicted [38]. Other studies have examined specialized nutrition therapy [53,54] and these are discussed below.

Adjusting PN during HCT

For adequately nourished patients, a graded approach is recommended based on the protocols described in the studies listed in Table 65.1. Calorie counts are initiated at the start of cytoreduction. At the University

Table 65.1 Calorie and protein intake prescribed in studies of total parenteral nutrition (TPN) in bone marrow transplantation (BMT).

Institution	n	Caloric intake	Protein intake	Lipid (% kcal)	NPC : N	Starting Day	Oral intake	Study duration (days)	Reference
City of Hope [36]	10	150% BEE	1.4 g/kg	–	170 : 1	+1	Yes	28–60	36
FHCRC [50]	7	160% BEE	1.5 g/kg	0/25/50		–6	Yes	25	50
FHCRC	20	160% (adult) 170% (child)	1.5 g/kg 2.0 g/kg	0/25/50		–1	Yes	37	51
Johns Hopkins Univ.	31	35 kcal/kg	1.4 g/kg	–		–1	Yes	30	18
Univ. of MN	71	150% BEE	1.0 (adult) 2.0 (child)	33	150 : 1 200 : 1	–6	Yes	35	16
FHCRC	40	160% BEE	1.5 g/kg	25–30		–6	Yes	35	55
Groningen Univ.	11	3400 kcal/day	148 g/day	40		–3	Yes	21	52
Basel Univ.	6	35 kcal/kg	1.8 g/kg	33	125 : 1	0	No	7	56
McGill Univ.	10 5	150% BEE 100% BEE	1.4 g/kg 0.8 g/kg	2×/week		+1	No	24	37
Ohio State Univ.	14 14	40 kcal/kg	1.1 g/kg 2.2 g/kg	–	120 : 1 100 : 1	–1	not noted	18	38
Univ. of Milan	25	90 kcal/kg (infant) 68 kcal/kg (toddler) 55 kcal/kg (older)	2.5–3.0 g/kg 1.5–2.5 g/kg	–	150 : 1	–7	Yes	26	57
Brigham & Women's	45	150% BEE	1.5 g/kg	30	165 : 1	+1	Yes	28	53
Univ. of Rome	16	35 kcal/kg	1.4 g/kg	40		+1		16	58
Brigham & Women's	45	150% BEE	1.5 g/kg	23	165 : 1	+1	Yes	PRN	54

BEE, basal energy expenditure; FHCRC, Fred Hutchinson Cancer Research Center; MN, Minnesota; NPC : N, nonprotein calorie to nitrogen ratio; PRN, as needed.

of Minnesota, PN is initiated when intake is <50% BEE (based on the Harris–Benedict equation, modified as necessary for small children) for 2–3 days. Some patients with minimal or no cytoreduction may not need PN at all. Charuhas *et al.* compared intravenous hydration alone to PN in a group of outpatient HCT patients and showed that, compared to PN, intravenous hydration resulted in no increase in hospital admissions or survival but a more rapid return to oral intake [61].

However, when mucositis, vomiting and nausea reduce intake below accepted levels, a high-energy formula is prescribed (120–130% BEE). Protein calories are included in this total and 30–40% of total calories are given as lipid over 18 h on a daily basis. Protein is administered at or slightly above RDA: 1.0–1.5 g/kg/day in adults and 1.5–2.5 g/kg/day in children. An amino acid solution containing taurine (TrophAmine®) is used for children under 1 year of age. During cytoreduction, tissue damage occurs, resulting in an increased endogenous nitrogen burden; exogenous nitrogen is prescribed only for maintenance of lean body mass. This maintenance formula is similar to those prescribed after surgery or trauma in patients who are unable to eat for at least 1 week.

Generally, HCT recipients are not good candidates for complete enteral alimentation by feeding tube because of the mucositis, neutropenia and vomiting associated with cytoreduction. Many patients can often continue to consume small quantities of oral intake throughout HCT. Even small amounts of enteral intake may reduce infection rates and/or hepatic complications of PN. In a study in which a predominantly enteral feeding program was compared with a predominantly parenteral feeding program, it was suggested that a very aggressive enteral feeding program could support HCT recipients. This study randomized patients to two different nutritional support protocols during HCT; 30 to an individualized enteral program using intensive counseling and (in some patients) tube feedings, and 27 to PN. Of the 30 enteral alimentation patients, 73% required supplemental intravenous amino acids for adequate nutritional support and 23% were crossed over to PN because of failure to achieve adequate total enteral intake. The study showed that the parenterally nourished group had more days of diuretic use, more hyperglycemia and more catheter complications, but had fewer episodes of hypomagnesaemia. There was no difference between the groups in length of stay, hematopoietic recovery, or survival. The authors point out the high cost of PN and suggest that PN be utilized for patients who are enteral alimentation failures [18]. This study introduced an important treatment option, which is the use of combined parenteral and enteral alimentation to take advantage of both the mucosal-preserving aspects of enteral alimentation and the nutritional support of PN [52].

About 7 days after transplant, the energy intake is decreased to 100–110% BEE and protein intake is increased to compensate for negative nitrogen balance, hypoproteinemia and tissue repair. This recommendation anticipates the additional protein required for tissue repair and regrowth.

At engraftment, recovery of enteral intake is anticipated and the PN caloric intake is decreased further, usually by decreasing lipid infusion from seven to three times per week. Enteral intake is vigorously supported. PN is cycled if electrolytes and glucose are normal to increase the opportunity for ambulation and social interaction. Two types of patients require further therapeutic modifications of nutrition support: patients who are malnourished at the time of hospitalization for HCT and patients in whom hypermetabolism develops as a result of stress.

Enteral therapy

The complications in patients receiving allogeneic HCT transplantation with high-dose cytoreduction has made PN the dominant nutritional modality [16,34,61]. Many HCT protocols now involve less cytoreduction, less immunosuppression and, subsequently, fewer gastrointestinal complications. Many patients with HCT may not require PN, or may transition very early to enteral nutrition. The case has been made that the more heterogeneous nature of HCT demands that enteral nutrition now be considered as an option for patients undergoing these procedures [1].

There are substantial theoretical reasons for preferring enteral nutrition to PN in ill and critically ill individuals. PN is associated with cholestasis, hyperlipidemia, line sepsis and other complications. Meta-analysis of studies comparing enteral nutrition to PN in adults (non-HCT patients) showed a lower risk of infection in those patients on enteral nutrition [62]. Lowered costs and improved immune status are also seen with enteral nutrition compared to PN [63]. Unfortunately, current data do not permit a conclusion regarding superiority of enteral nutrition vs. PN in HCT [64]. Carefully designed controlled trials comparing groups with similar primary disease and type of HCT are essential to assess the feasibility of enteral nutrition in these patients. Currently the selection of nutritional modality is individualized on a case-by-case basis.

Two methods are available to provide enteral calories and protein to patients after HCT: nasogastric/nasojejunal feedings and gastrostomy feedings. In the late 1980s, two groups examined nasogastric tube feedings in small numbers of HCT patients, with evidence of poor tolerance of the tubes, increased bacterial infections, and the need to rely on intravenous support for the majority of calories and protein [18,52]. Gastroparesis, a known complication of HCT [65], was a major problem in achieving full nasogastric feedings.

A recent pilot study demonstrated the feasibility of using nasojejunal feedings after HCT [66]. Transpyloric feedings reduce problems with gastroparesis and vomiting. In this study, tubes were placed before cytoreduction, to avoid placement during the peak of mucositis. Of the 15 patients in the pilot group, eight were nourished with tube feedings alone without the need to replace the tube prior to engraftment. The other seven patients received partial enteral nutrition via the tube. Another group, working with children during HCT, used nasogastric tubes and continuous infusions to nourish 42 HCT patients, but replaced vomited tubes multiple times during the therapy [67]. Both groups of investigators emphasize the need for a dedicated team to support enteral nutrition in these complex patients; an observation made in studies of adults with trauma or sepsis nourished enterally [68]. In many cases, protocol-driven enteral nutrition succeeds better than individual management of patients. The protocols prevent unnecessary halting of the enteral feeds and hasten the increases necessary to achieve full feedings.

Gastrostomy feedings have been used in patients with HCT. Percutaneous endoscopic gastrostomy placement may be done before cytoreduction, to avoid neutropenia and esophageal mucositis during placement. Alternatively, radiographic ("push") gastrostomy placement may be done if the patient has mucositis. In the latter method, no bumper is pulled through the esophagus, reducing the risk of esophageal bleeding or rupture in patients with mucositis. Traction removal of the initial tube should be avoided until well-after full engraftment to reduce infection and dehiscence at the site. While several investigators have shown that, in principle, gastrostomy placement is possible during HCT [69,70], it is unclear if any real advantage accrues to the patient. Most patients require tube feedings for only a short period before returning to oral intake. The risks associated with gastrostomy placement [71] may not be outweighed by the small increase in comfort associated with the absence of a nasogastric or nasojejunal tube. While the authors would recommend using a pre-existing gastrostomy tube during HCT, we do not recommend routine placement of such a device.

In patients who have received PN, oral intake can resume when mucositis subsides and narcotic therapy is reduced. The initial foods desired by HCT recipients are usually cold and very sweet. Taste sensation is altered after HCT, with a deceased threshold for sweet and salt that may last for more than 1 year [31]. Continuing parenteral amino acid

Table 65.2 Nutrition support monitoring studies.

Daily	Biweekly	Weekly
Weight, urine glucose	Glucose, urea, creatinine, electrolytes, Ca, Mg, phosphorus	Triglyceride
Calorie/protein intake		Albumin, transferrin
Electrolytes, glucose, urea, creatinine (first 3 days)	Transaminases 5′-nucleotidase, bilirubin, alkaline phosphatase	Nitrogen balance
		Zinc

Ca, calcium; Mg, magnesium.

administration may be necessary, even in patients consuming adequate calories, because protein-containing foods are often refused. A dietitian trained in post-HCT management is essential to counsel patients regarding appropriate food choices and to encourage patients to keep retrying foods [72]. As appetite improves, a previously requested food may become more acceptable. The dietary kitchen must be flexible and, if possible, a kitchen on the HCT ward or in communal family quarters should be available. Patients may respond better to familiar dishes or ethnic foods.

Dietary prescriptions at some institutions include complex, highly restrictive diets, eliminating vegetables and requiring the autoclaving of foods. Lactose intake may not be tolerated during the 1st year after HCT. Many institutions use some aspect of a low-bacteria diet [73,74], but the exact degree of restriction necessary to reduce infection in neutropenic patients is unclear [75]. Most institutions teach some aspect of safe food handling, and restrict unwashed fruits and vegetables, raw or unpasteurized milk products, raw or undercooked protein sources (e.g. meat and eggs) and unpasteurized fermented or aged products [74]. Patients with intestinal GVHD may benefit from the protocol of Gauvreau and colleagues, which utilizes a phased dietary restoration plan [76].

GVHD, malignant relapse, or infection may lead to temporary dependence on PN. Some patients leave the hospital on PN, and children are often resistant to oral intake until in familiar surroundings. If there is no organic cause of prolonged refusal of enteral intake, nasogastric or nasojejunal feedings can be used to promote intestinal recovery, thus stimulating appetite. With prolonged food refusal, food aversion should be suspected and behavioral modification therapy can be sought.

Monitoring nutrition support

To individualize therapy, certain nutritional/metabolic parameters need to be monitored. It is somewhat arbitrary to distinguish between monitoring schema to follow nutrition therapy and to follow the overall medical status of the patient. Certain laboratory tests are indicated to anticipate and correct potential metabolic problems that can be caused by PN, or metabolic problems of other causes which can be treated with the PN solution. These laboratory tests, however, may not accurately reflect an individual patient's nutritional status [58]. From the studies listed in Table 65.1 a consensus can be derived which is shown in Table 65.2.

Weight is followed primarily to judge hydration status, which is also reflected by electrolytes, blood urea nitrogen (BUN), creatinine and albumin. Acid–base imbalances can be detected with these routine studies [77]. Glucose tolerance can vary in this setting and needs to be monitored. There is an association between hyperglycemia and Candida sepsis [78]; thus, awareness of changing glucose tolerance can be helpful in anticipating infectious complications as well as metabolic complications. Liver function abnormalities may result from TPN, or liver dysfunction from other causes may require modification of the TPN formula (see Complications of nutrition support section, below). A particularly difficult, and as yet poorly understood, occurrence in HCT patients is hyperammonemia [79,80]. This abnormality is not frequent enough to require routine laboratory monitoring, but an awareness of the potential for hyperammonemia should be kept in mind when evaluating liver function and level of nutrition, particularly protein, support. Patients with hyperammonemia may exhibit classic symptoms of hepatic encephalopathy, but these may be obscured by the effects of complications and medications used in HCT. A high index of suspicion is thus warranted.

Parenteral and enteral protein and caloric intake are recorded daily to allow for the reduction of parenteral intake as enteral intake increases. Measurement of electrolytes, major minerals and zinc is needed to adjust a patient's TPN formula. Ascribing abnormalities in serum albumin to protein nutrition does not seem to be reliable in this setting. Serum albumin is helpful in assessment of fluid status and as a guide to albumin replacement therapy for the maintenance of intravascular volume. Transferrin seems more reflective of amino acid intake for visceral protein synthesis [16]. Parallel low T_3 with nonthyroidal illness has been associated with low transferrin reflecting poor nutritional status [81]. The authors have found that prealbumin levels reflect caloric, rather than protein, intake and should not be used to adjust protein intake. Although nitrogen balance is helpful, attempting to maintain positive balance is unrealistic and could result in an increased demand on the liver to process ammonia. An additional study that assists in individualizing therapy and anticipating complications is measurement of resting energy expenditure (REE) and respiratory quotient (RQ), based on oxygen consumption and carbon dioxide (CO_2) production. The quantity and appropriate mix of energy producing substrate can be optimized with these data [38].

Complications of nutrition support

There are risks in both parenteral and enteral nutritional support. Contributing factors to complications with PN include the length of time PN is given, malnutrition of the recipient prior to HCT and the presence of organ failure during HCT, particularly hepatic or renal failure. Enteral feeding tube placement and maintenance are associated with risks of formula aspiration, bleeding, diarrhea, sinusitis and bowel perforation. Some of the more common problems encountered in nutritional support of HCT recipients are reviewed below.

Catheter-related complications

The availability of large bore, multiple-port, right atrial silicone catheters for venous access is a significant improvement over the less stable access systems previously used [82]. Central venous access catheters remain a major source of complications in HCT recipients. The incidence of central catheter sepsis is high, despite the use of strict aseptic technique for blood draws, infusions and tubing changes, as well as daily site cleaning and dressing changes [5]. In a prospective study of 143 Hickman catheter placements in 111 HCT recipients, 44% of the patients had positive blood cultures during the lifetime of the catheter [83]. Of these infections, 40 of the 63 were coagulase-negative *Staphylococcus*, suggestive of primary line sepsis rather than catheter contamination from a blood-borne enteric source. The majority of these infections are treated with antibiotics, not

Table 65.3 Treatment options for rising liver enzymes in patients on parenteral nutrition (PN). Reproduced with permission from Weisdorf and Schwarzenberg [139].

---

1 Evaluate the patient for other causes of liver disease (other than PN), including: infection: bacterial (particularly gram-negative bacteria), viral, fungal; recurrence of malignancy; veno-occlusive disease; medications causing cholestasis (e.g. methotrexate, furosemide); allergic response to medication; graft-vs.-host disease [131]
2 Cycle PN over 12–20 h rather than 24 h [132,133]. This has reduced hepatic steatosis. Ideally, this should be an early intervention [134]
3 Initiate small enteral feeds to provide a protective effect on the liver during PN [87]
4 Modify PN to avoid overnutrition and/or micronutrient deficiency. Decrease the total calorie intake empirically by 10–15% to reduce the nonprotein calorie to nitrogen ratio and to provide a balanced caloric intake [87]. PN toxicity has been associated with various micronutrients, particularly in long-term PN: choline [135], carnitine [136,137] and taurine [138]. Taurine is found in TrophAmine® (Kendall McGaw, Inc., Irvine, CA) that some hepatologists suggest is the most appropriate amino acid source for patients with evidence of PN-related liver disease [86]
5 Treat with ursodeoxycholic acid, 20–30 mg/kg/day orally divided into four doses, to decrease cholestasis and transaminases. There is no evidence that this chemical modification of blood parameters is indicative of improved hepatic histopathology [86]
6 Treat with enteral metronidazole to decrease enteral gram-negative bacteria and, thus, endotoxin formation

---

with catheter removal [83,84]. In Ulz *et al.* [83], mechanical obstruction occurred in 38% of the catheters, and more than once in some. Approximately half of these episodes required no intervention, whereas the others responded to heparin, urokinase, or required catheter replacement [83]. Other complications, including dislodgement or leakage, occurred in small numbers.

Hepatic enzyme elevations

Hepatic injury in PN has been attributed to enteric stasis with translocation of endotoxin into portal venous blood, deficiencies in micronutrients, and with administration of high nonprotein-calorie-to-nitrogen ratios. Hepatic complications occur in only a subset of PN recipients. The initial manifestation is an elevation of transaminase levels approximately 1–2 weeks after the start of PN infusion. Bilirubin elevations and elevations of canalicular enzymes (alkaline phosphatase, 5′-nucleotidase) may occur 2–3 weeks into therapy. The transaminase level elevations often resolve spontaneously. Hepatic steatosis may occur without enzyme elevation. Liver biopsy may show steatosis, glycogenosis, intrahepatic cholestasis and nonspecific portal infiltrate.

Minor adjustments to the PN formula may reduce enzymes (Table 65.3), and no hepatic dysfunction or long-term injury results if PN is short-term (<3 months). If PN therapy is prolonged, functional abnormalities may develop. Steatonecrosis and fibrosis may occur and may progress to cirrhosis, with complications of hepatic dysfunction and portal hypertension. The time course for development of this lesion is variable and can depend on the age of the patient (adults are more resistant to necrotic changes associated with PN than children) and the presence of other hepatotoxic factors. Some studies have shown fibrosis with as little as 6 months of PN. Finally, acalculous cholecystitis or gallstone formation can occur during administration of PN [85–87].

Diagnosis of PN-related hepatic disease must include consideration of other hepatic complications of HCT (see Chapter 58). Prevention of hepatic complications of PN includes choosing this therapy only in those patients who need and are likely to benefit from it, and providing a high standard of oversight when using this therapy. Table 65.3 shows the treatment options for patients with elevated liver enzymes and/or cholestasis while on PN.

Metabolic abnormalities/vitamin deficiencies

The potential disruption of normal electrolyte, mineral and vitamin balance exists in any critically ill patient and certainly in HCT recipients. As treatment protocols have become more complicated, interactions of medications and PN in ways not previously anticipated have resulted in serious complications, as recently reported in a patient who developed serious electrolyte imbalance while receiving the combination of foscarnet and PN [88]. Zinc deficiency is now a well-described complication of HCT, more common in younger patients and in patients with diarrhea. Anorexia, diarrhea and rash may be seen in zinc-deficient patients. Low alkaline phosphatase may be a good indicator of zinc deficiency in these patients, as serum zinc levels may be misleading [89].

While brief shortages of the multivitamins used in PN have occurred from time to time, a recent long-term shortage of both the adult and pediatric formulations of multivitamin preparation resulted in severe deficiencies in water-soluble vitamins. Clinicians saw the manifestations of vitamin deficiencies previously known only through texts and history of medicine lectures [77]. As there is no reason to believe that similar shortages will not occur in the future, we suggest that those monitoring PN be alert to changes in the availability of components.

PN can be associated with episodes of hyperlipidemia and hyperglycemia. Essential fatty acid deficiency is a problem in parenterally nourished patients who do not receive lipids [90] and in enterally nourished patients with cholestasis. Extrapyramidal symptoms resembling Parkinson's disease were reported in a HCT patient with elevated serum manganese during cholestasis [91]. Trace element supplementation should be reviewed in any patient with hepatic or renal dysfunction.

Complications of enteral feeding

Potential complications of enteral nutrition include aspiration, tube displacement, due to vomiting, loss of fluid and electrolytes, due to diarrhea, and sinusitis. HCT patients receiving tube feedings frequently require slow drip feeds to maximize tolerance. This commits patients to prolonged periods on a feeding pump. Some patients, particularly children, have an aversion to tube feedings. Diarrhea is a complication commonly mentioned with tube feedings. If loose stools do not cause excessive loss of water or electrolytes, and are not associated with skin breakdown in the perineum, they may not be clinically significant. Addition of fiber (7–14 g/L of formula) to the feedings may be helpful [92]. Thus, while enteral feeds provide significant advantages, recognition of potential complications and a flexible approach is important.

Adjusting nutrition support during HCT

Malnourished patients

Baseline nutritional assessment will identify patients who are malnourished prior to HCT [93]. Malnutrition is more likely to occur in children with multiply relapsed acute lymphoblastic leukemia, any patient on long-term steroid therapy, patients with a history of multiple infections (immunodeficiency patients) and patients with metabolic disorders associated with neurological impairment. There is a particularly high incidence of malnutrition in patients with solid tumors [94]. These patients require restorative rather than maintenance nutritional therapy. Restorative therapy uses lower total energy intake and higher protein intake. Greater attention is paid to micronutrient shifts, particularly of potassium, phosphorus, magnesium and zinc. Body stores of these elements are low in chronic malnutrition, although serum levels are initially normal. With increased calorie intake, serum stores of these elements are utilized and can decrease precipitously. Fluid overload is also a frequent complication of intensive nutritional therapy in chronically undernourished patients [95].

Systemic inflammatory response

The systemic inflammatory response is a complex metabolic reaction to elevated cytokine levels that leads to vascular endothelial damage with impairment of multiple organs. The inciting injury may be sepsis, multiple trauma [96], acute pancreatitis [97], or other catabolic events, including cytokine elevations from cytoreduction during HCT or severe GVHD [98,99]. Sepsis is the most common stress associated with hypermetabolism in HCT recipients. Subsequent to the initial perfusion deficit, stability may be restored for 48–72 h, but thereafter a hypermetabolic state develops, which is associated with pulmonary injury. The hypermetabolic state may resolve over 7–10 days or it may persist, with progressive kidney and liver dysfunction. These final stages constitute multiple-organ failure syndrome, which has a mortality rate in excess of 50% [97].

The systemic inflammatory response is characterized by profound loss of body protein, in distinction to simple starvation, in which lean body mass is preserved. Protein catabolism is accounted for, in part, by utilization of amino acids from skeletal muscle in areas of wound healing or in acute phase response protein synthesis. However, in the hypermetabolic state, amino acids are also utilized for gluconeogenesis, and branched chain amino acids may be oxidized outside the liver for energy. The net result is a dramatic shift to negative nitrogen balance. These changes cannot be corrected with glucose infusions, exogenous amino acids, or insulin. Despite increased gluconeogenesis, glucose oxidation and uptake do not increase. Fat metabolism is also altered, lipid stores are mobilized and lipid oxidation increases. In the progression from sepsis to multisystem organ failure with development of liver dysfunction, hepatic lipogenesis increases, triglyceride clearance is impaired and utilization of lipids by peripheral tissues declines. Thus, lipid clearance becomes macrophage-dependent, possibly limiting these cells' phagocytic capacity [97,100].

In patients with a systemic inflammatory response, the initial goals are to restore fluid and electrolyte balance. Thereafter, the goals are to administer adequate calories to prevent starvation and minimize, to whatever degree possible, the breakdown of endogenous protein. Protein is administered initially at increased levels (up to 1.5–2.0 g/kg/day in adults and up to 2.5–3.0 g/kg/day in children) to attempt to compensate for urinary nitrogen loss and restore lean body mass. Development of azotemia is common and frequently limits protein intake. Glucose administration should not exceed 4–5 mg/kg/min and fat intake should not exceed 1.0 g/kg/day in adults [100,101]. Ideally, one would like to support ongoing inflammation-associated protein synthesis and allow for improved nitrogen balance, which has been associated with increased survival [97]. However, in clinical practice, this is very difficult. In addition, it is unclear whether improved nitrogen balance is the cause of improved survival, or if those patients who were less ill were capable of utilizing exogenous protein. Improved nitrogen balance in response to exogenous protein may thus be a marker for less severe disease.

Frequent adjustments of PN are required. Severe azotemia (BUN >60 mg/dL) requires decreasing protein intake or dialysis to permit increased protein support. Because stress hypermetabolism utilizes a mixed fuel source, the RQ should range from 0.80 to 0.85. Excess carbohydrate intake is associated with increased CO_2 production and an RQ >1.0. Patients with respiratory difficulty may benefit from decreasing their CO_2 production by decreasing the percentage of their calories given as glucose. Indirect calorimetry can indicate if caloric intake is too high. Excess energy intake does not preserve lean body mass or restore the patient to health more quickly, but it does promote hyperglycemia, lipogenesis, hypertriglyceridemia and hepatic steatosis. Fluid overload in stressed patients is an indication to concentrate PN, which decreases free water and corrects hyponatremia. Correction of significant electrolyte abnormalities can be done separately from the PN, avoiding the need for frequent PN reformulation. Recommended allowances of trace elements and vitamins may not be adequate in severely stressed patients, particularly for zinc, copper and vitamin K. Patients with renal or hepatic dysfunction may require further modification of the PN. In the ill patient requiring PN for longer than 1 month, weekly serum trace element monitoring can anticipate chromium toxicity or excessive manganese and copper supplementation [100,102].

Graft-vs.-host disease (GVHD)

Several specific nutritional effects result from GVHD treatment and prophylaxis. Newer agents are being tested, most often in combination with the established therapies used in GVHD prophylaxis, namely cyclosporine (CSP), methotrexate and corticosteroids [103]. Corticosteroids promote muscle breakdown and hepatic gluconeogenesis from amino acid, and thus increase urea cycle activity to dispose of nitrogen. The alteration of energy metabolism can be manifest as hyperglycemia and hypertriglyceridemia, which has also been reported as a complication of CSP therapy [104]. The hypoproteinemia that results can be compounded further by fluid overload from the simultaneous use of fluid resuscitation and nephrotoxic agents, including CSP, tacrolimus and antibiotics. Renal sodium wasting is common at this time, added to fecal sodium losses. Attempts to correct serum sodium levels may result in increased total body sodium and fluid retention, leading to the use of diuretic agents that may exacerbate the nephrotoxicity. Renal magnesium wasting is caused by CSP, tacrolimus and diuretics [105]. Mycophenolate mofetil can result in leukopenia and diarrhea in HCT recipients with GVHD [106,107].

GVHD and its therapy can be a major challenge to maintaining good nutrition support. In severe intestinal GVHD, diarrhea and bleeding limit enteral nutrition and the majority of a patient's calories and protein are provided parenterally. If hepatic GVHD is present, cholestasis and consequent fat malabsorption may further complicate oral nutrition [108]. Basal caloric needs are given, in a balanced formulation, with 30% of the calories from lipid. Because GVHD is associated with protein-losing enteropathy and consequent hypoalbuminemia, these patients require increased protein administration, sometimes up to 3 g/kg/day, to improve nitrogen balance and to maintain lean body mass [34,39]. Although PN may be needed to provide the majority of nutrition, if possible, some enteral nutrition should be maintained. Enteral nutrition stimulates gallbladder function, thus reducing cholestatic complications, and has a trophic effect on the intestine, thus reducing bacterial translocation into the blood stream.

Experimental modifications

Experimental alterations in nutritional support formulation and adjunctive therapy may ultimately improve the ability to nourish HCT recipients safely and effectively. Glutamine is being studied intensively in the HCT population and is discussed in detail below. More controversial are the immunomodulatory formulas, which are also reviewed below.

Glutamine

Glutamine, while generally considered a nonessential amino acid, is an essential amino acid under conditions of stress and hypermetabolism. Glutamine has a crucial role in nitrogen transport as a scavenger of ammonia and is a precursor for nucleotide synthesis. Intestinal mucosa utilizes large amounts of glutamine in nucleotide synthesis to support its rapid regeneration. In the enterocyte, metabolism of glutamine produces α-ketoglutarate, which enters the tricarboxylic acid cycle, and ammonia, citrulline, alanine and proline. Alanine is utilized by the liver for gluconeogenesis, whereas citrulline is used in the urea cycle to synthesize arginine. Critical illness has been associated with plasma glutamine depletion, which impairs normal maintenance of intestinal mucosal integrity. Loss of the mucosal barrier can result in increased bacterial translocation with increased episodes of sepsis due to enteric organisms [109,110].

Glutamine has been studied in patients with a wide spectrum of catabolic states to improve nutrition support. It may improve outcome and reduce the systemic inflammatory response to injury [109]. Trials of glutamine in HCT patients have been done, using both enteral and parenteral glutamine supplementation. Wide variation in glutamine dosing and study design has precluded clear indications for clinical use of glutamine, but the data suggest it may be effective in both forms [64].

Glutamine in doses up to 0.57 g/kg/day in a balanced PN solution has been shown to be safe in humans, both in normal volunteers and in a group of HCT patients [111]. Glutamine supplementation of PN was studied in a double-blind, randomized, controlled trial of allogeneic HCT recipients. The PN was identical in calorie and nitrogen content; one group received standard amino acids and the other group received glutamine (0.57 g/kg/day) and standard amino acid solution to the same total nitrogen content as the control group. The group receiving glutamine demonstrated improved nitrogen balance (-1.4 ± 0.5 g/day compared to -4.2 ± 1.2, $p = 0.002$) and decreased morbidity. The number of bacterial infections and the length of hospital stay were less in the glutamine group (three in one glutamine group compared to nine in the control group, $p = 0.041$) [53]. This therapy appeared to result in significant reduction in morbidity and hospital stay, with cost savings to the hospital (hospital stay of 29 ± 1 day in the glutamine group compared with 36 ± 2 day, $p = 0.017$) [112].

A subsequent small trial of glutamine supplementation of PN also supported the conclusion that glutamine decreases hospital stay [113]. There are also small studies suggesting that glutamine may protect the liver during HCT or be effective (with vitamin E) in the treatment of veno-occlusive disease [114,115]. Studies thus far have used varying outcomes measures, HCT populations and glutamine doses [64]. Although promising, recommendation of this addition to PN requires large-scale clinical trials.

A randomized, double-blind, placebo controlled trial of oral glutamine to reduce opiate use for mucositis demonstrated improvement in patients with autologous, but not allogeneic, HCT with glutamine [116]. In this study, glutamine was given as a "swish and swallow" preparation. Another study using a similar protocol confirmed these results [117]. Studies in which glutamine is administered intravenously or orally as a nutritional supplement demonstrate no impact on mucositis [53,113,118,119]. Again, because of problems with the published trials, further studies are necessary before recommending glutamine as a preventive for mucositis [64].

Few studies have examined enteral glutamine as a nutritional supplement. Two small studies have shown no effect of enteral glutamine on engraftment, diarrhea, PN use, or length of stay [113,119].

Immunomodulatory formulas

Data from animal studies and clinical studies indicate that some nutrients improve immune function independent of alternations in general nutrition or nitrogen balance. Function of T lymphocytes and macrophages is affected specifically by arginine, ω3 polyunsaturated fatty acids (fish oil) and purine/pyrimidines. In addition, ω3 fatty acids reduce inflammation in several clinical conditions. Unlike ω6 fatty acids, ω3 fatty acids do not serve as precursors to inflammatory eicosanoids (e.g. prostaglandins E_2 and I_2, thromboxane A_2 and tetrainoic leukotrienes) [120].

Clinical studies in critically ill patients after sepsis, trauma, or complex surgery have suggested that formulas supplemented with arginine, RNA and fish oil (ω3 fatty acids) improve immune function, thus reducing the number of infections and length of hospital stay [120,121]. Limited studies of these agents or formulas have been performed in HCT patients [122]. There are theoretical considerations that may make their use inadvisable in this population; in particular, the stimulation of the immune system in patients at risk for GVHD. Thus, while these formulas hold the promise of decreasing infectious complications, careful trial in HCT populations will be necessary before they are used.

Long-term nutrition support considerations

Discharge from the hospital does not end the need for nutritional care in HCT recipients. Malnutrition was common in a study of 192 children and adults evaluated 1 year after HCT [123]. Approximately 16% of patients were 10% or more below their ideal body weight, and significant weight loss seemed associated with discharge from the transplant center. In a study to evaluate weight recovery and complications of HCT impacting nutrition, Iestra *et al.* found that 66% of patients had eating difficulties 50 days post-transplantation [124]. More than 50% of patients conditioned with total body irradiation remained below their ideal body weight 1 year after HCT. Anorexia, xerostomia, altered taste, nausea and tiredness were cited by the patients as the causes of poor intake. It is clear that HCT recipients require specific, intensive post-hospitalization observation and long-term management of nutrition.

Long-term follow-up of patients with chronic GVHD is beginning to define nutritional problems specific to this complication. In a study of nine adults with chronic GVHD, Stern *et al.* demonstrated them to be at significant risk for osteoporosis. Further studies are necessary to determine optimal intervention strategies [125]. Nausea and anorexia [49] and painful mouth sores [126] may limit oral intake in patients with GVHD. Information on the long-term nutritional status of patients after HCT is somewhat spotty. More data have been collected on children than on adults. Growth after HCT has been a particular concern in children. Growth failure was felt to be common and frequently related to total body irradiation and consequent growth hormone deficiency or dysregulation of the growth hormone-insulin-like growth factor I axis [127,128]. Corticosteroid therapy and the impact of the primary disease are also important factors.

The European Group for Blood and Marrow Transplantation examined data on children undergoing HCT at age <15 years who survived more than 5 years after transplantation [129]. Irradiation was correlated with height decrease. Body mass index was normal or slightly above normal for this group of children. The conclusion of the authors was that linear growth was affected by multiple factors during HCT, predominantly irradiation, while nutrition itself was not a long-term problem [129]. In a study of muscle mass in children 1 year out from HCT, return of skeletal muscle protein reserve occurred late after HCT (>6 months) and was not complete at 1 year in patients receiving allogeneic transplants [130]. This would suggest that children may obtain normal weight for height after HCT, but the weight normalization may not reflect normal muscle mass.

In summary, HCT patients experience a long nutritional recovery period after hospital discharge. Clinicians should be aware of factors impacting recovery, such as chronic GVHD. Weight and, for children, height should be monitored over the subsequent years. This is not, however, enough to ensure optimal strength and function for these patients. In many cases, measurement of muscle mass (either by anthropometrics or by ultrasound) or strength measurement will uncover unsuspected deficiencies. Dual-energy X-ray absorptiometry (DEXA) scan to assess bone mineralization may be of benefit in some HCT subpopulations. All patients should consume a daily multivitamin after discharge (the availability of liquid formulations for patients with swallowing difficulties is important). Frequent clinical evaluation of nutrition is a valuable adjunctive therapy for these patients, even for those patients with normal weight for height. This would insure the detection of micronutrient deficiencies and allow for the monitoring of muscle mass.

References

1 Lenssen P, Bruemmer B, Aker SN, McDonald GB. Nutrient support in hematopoietic cell transplantation. *J Parenter Enteral Nutr* 2001; **25**: 219–28.

2 Appelbaum FR. Allogeneic marrow transplantation and the use of hematopoietic growth factors. *Stem Cells* 1995; **13**: 344–50.

3 Singer JW. Use of recombinant hematopoietic growth factors in bone marrow transplantation. *Am J Pediatr Hematol Oncol* 1993; **15**: 175–84.

4 Appelbaum FR. The use of colony stimulating factors in marrow transplantation. *Cancer* 1993; **72** (Suppl.): 3387–92.

5 Marena C, Zecca M, Carenini ML et al. Incidence of, and risk factors for, nosocomial infections among hematopoietic stem cell transplantation recipients, with impact on procedure-related mortality. *Infect Control Hosp Epidemiol* 2001; **22**: 510–7.

6 Vindelov L. Allogeneic bone marrow transplantation with reduced conditioning (RC-BMT). *Eur J Haematol* 2001; **66**: 73–82.

7 Lickliter JD, McGlave PB, DeFor TE et al. Matched-pair analysis of peripheral blood stem cells compared to marrow for allogeneic transplantation. *Bone Marrow Transplant* 2000; **26**: 723–8.

8 Wagner JE. Allogeneic umbilical cord blood transplantation. *Cancer Treat Res* 1997; **77**: 187–216.

9 Gluckman E. Umbilical cord blood transplant in human. *Bone Marrow Transplant* 1996; **18** (Suppl. 2): S166–70.

10 Mogul MJ. Unrelated cord blood transplantation vs. matched unrelated donor bone marrow transplantation. The risks and benefits of each choice. *Bone Marrow Transplant* 2000; **25** (Suppl. 2): S58–60.

11 Fauser AA, Basara N, Blau IW, Kiehl MG. A comparative study of peripheral blood stem cell vs. bone marrow transplantation from unrelated donors (MUD): a single center study. *Bone Marrow Transplant* 2000; **25** (Suppl. 2): S27–31.

12 Davies SM, Wagner JE, Shu XO et al. Unrelated donor bone marrow transplantation for children with acute leukemia. *J Clin Oncol* 1997; **15**: 557–65.

13 Sierra J, Storer B, Hansen JA et al. Unrelated donor marrow transplantation for acute myeloid leukemia: an update of the Seattle experience. *Bone Marrow Transplant* 2000; **26**: 397–404.

14 Jassak PF, Riley MB. Autologous stem cell transplant: an overview. *Cancer Pract* 1994; **2**: 141–5.

15 Ruiz Arguelles GJ. Oupatient programs of myeloablative chemotherapy, autologous and allogeneic bone marrow transplantation. *Haematologica* 2000; **85**: 1233–4.

16 Weisdorf SA, Lysne J, Wind D et al. Positive effect of prophylactic total parenteral nutrition on long-term outcome of bone marrow transplantation. *Transplantation* 1987; **43**: 833–8.

17 Stuart RK, Sensenbrenner LL. Adverse effects of nutritional deprivation on transplanted hematopoietic cells. *Exp Hematol* 1979; **7**: 435–42.

18 Szeluga DJ, Stuart RK, Brookmeyer R, Utermohlen V, Santos GW. Nutritional support of bone marrow transplant recipients: a prospective, randomized clinical trial comparing total parenteral nutrition to an enteral feeding program. *Cancer Res* 1987; **47**: 3309–16.

19 Herrmann VM, Petruska PJ. Nutrition support in bone marrow transplant recipients. *Nutr Clin Pract* 1993; **8**: 19–27.

20 Rollins CJ. Role of clinical pharmacy specialist in nutrition management of bone marrow transplant patient. *Nutrition* 1993; **9**: 313–22.

21 McDonald GB, Shulman HM, Sullivan KM, Spencer GD. Intestinal and hepatic complications of human bone marrow transplantation, I and II. *Gastroenterol* 1986; **90**: 460–77 & 770–84.

22 McDonald GB, Sharma P, Matthews DE, Shulman HM, Thomas ED. Venocclusive disease of the liver after bone marrow transplantation: diagnosis, incidence, and predisposing factors. *Hepatology* 1984; **4**: 116–22.

23 Kim BK, Chung KW, Sun HS et al. Liver disease during the first post-transplant year in bone marrow transplantation recipients: retrospective study. *Bone Marrow Transplant* 2000; **26**: 193–7.

24 Zager RA, O'Quigley J, Zager BK et al. Acute renal failure following bone marrow transplantation: a retrospective study of 272 patients. *Am J Kidney Dis* 1989; **13**: 210–6.

25 Cohen EP. Renal failure after bone-marrow transplantation. *Lancet* 2001; **357**: 6–7.

26 Nicolini B, Rovelli A, Uderzo C. Cardiotoxicity in children after bone marrow transplantation. *Pediatr Hematol Oncol* 2000; **17**: 203–9.

27 Kupari M, Volin L, Suokas A, Timonen T, Hekali P, Ruutu T. Cardiac involvement in bone marrow transplantation. Electrocardiographic changes, arrhythmias, heart failure and autopsy findings. *Bone Marrow Transplant* 1990; **5**: 91–8.

28 Springmeyer SC, Silvestri RC, Flournoy N et al. Pulmonary function of marrow transplant patients. I. Effects of marrow infusion, acute graft-versus-host disease, and interstitial pneumonitis. *Exp Hematol* 1984; **12**: 805–10.

29 Abbott B, Ippoliti C, Hecth D, Bruton J, Whaley B, Champlin R. Granisetron (Kytril®) plus dexamethasone for antiemetic control in bone marrow transplant patients receiving highly emetogenic chemotherapy with or without total body irradiation. *Bone Marrow Transplant* 2000; **25**: 1279–83.

30 Wardley AM, Jayson GC, Swindell R et al. Prospective evaluation of oral mucositis in patients receiving myeloablative conditioning regimens and haemopoietic progenitor rescue. *Br J Haematol* 2000; **110**: 292–9.

31 Mattsson T, Arvidson K, Heimdahl A, Ljungman P, Dahllöf G, Ringdén O. Alterations in taste acuity associated with allogeneic bone marrow transplantation. *J Oral Pathol Med* 1992; **21**: 33–7.

32 Sale GE, Shulman HM, McDonald GB, Thomas ED. Gastrointestinal graft-versus-host disease in man. A clinicopathologic study of the rectal biopsy. *Am J Surg Pathol* 1979; **3**: 291–9.

33 Bearman SI, Appelbaum FR, Buckner CD et al. Regimen-related toxicity in patients undergoing bone marrow transplantation. *J Clin Oncol* 1988; **6**: 1562–8.

34 Weisdorf SA, Salati LM, Longsdorf JA, Ramsay NK, Sharp HL. Graft-versus-host disease of the intestine: a protein losing enteropathy characterized by fecal α_1-antitrypsin. *Gastroenterology* 1983; **85**: 1076–81.

35 Cheney CL, Lenssen P, Aker SN et al. Sex differences in nitrogen balance following marrow grafting for leukemia. *J Am Coll Nutr* 1987; **6**: 223–30.

36 Schmidt GM, Blume KG, Bross KJ, Spruce WE, Waldron JC, Levine R. Parenteral nutrition in bone marrow transplant recipients. *Exp Hematol* 1980; **8**: 506–11.

37 Taveroff A, McArdle AH, Rybka WB. Reducing parenteral energy and protein intake improves metabolic homeostasis after bone marrow transplantation. *Am J Clin Nutr* 1991; **54**: 1087–92.

38 Geibig CB, Owens JP, Mirtallo JM, Bowers D, Nahikian-Nelms M, Tutschka P. Parenteral nutrition for marrow transplant recipients. Evaluation of an increased nitrogen dose. *J Parenteral Enteral Nutr* 1991; **15**: 184–8.

39 Papadopoulou A, Lloyd DR, Williams MD, Darbyshire PJ, Booth IW. Gastrointestinal and nutritional sequelae of bone marrow transplantation. *Arch Dis Child* 1996; **75**: 208–13.

40 Baron F, Sautois B, Baudoux E, Matus G, Fillet G, Beguin Y. Optimization of recombinant human erythropoietin therapy after allogeneic hematopoietic stem cell transplantation. *Exp Hematol* 2002; **30**: 546–54.

41 Levine JE, Boxer LA. Clinical applications of hematopoietic growth factors in pediatric oncology. *Curr Opin Hematol* 2002; **9**: 222–7.

42 Winston DJ, Ho WG, Champlin RE. Current approaches to management of infections in bone marrow transplants. *Eur J Cancer Clin Oncol* 1989; **25** (Suppl. 2): S25–35.

43 King CE, Toskes PP. Breath tests in the diagnosis of small intestine bacterial overgrowth. *Crit Rev Clin Lab Sci* 1984; **21**: 269–81.

44 List AF, Maziarz R, Stiff P et al. A randomized placebo-controlled trial of lisofylline in HLA-identical, sibling-donor, allogeneic bone marrow transplant recipients. The Lisofylline Marrow Transplant Study Group. *Bone Marrow Transplant* 2000; **25**: 283–91.

45 Snover DC, Weisdorf SA, Vercellotti GM, Rank B, Hutton S, McGlave P. A histopathologic study of gastric and small intestinal graft-versus-host disease following allogeneic bone marrow transplantation. *Hum Pathol* 1985; **16**: 387–92.

46 Roy J, Snover D, Weisdorf S, Mulvahill A, Filipovich A, Weisdorf D. Simultaneous upper and lower endoscopic biopsy in the diagnosis of

intestinal graft-versus-host disease. *Transplantation* 1991; **51**: 642–6.

47 Snover DC. Graft-versus-host disease of the gastrointestinal tract. *Am J Surg Pathol* 1990; **14** (Suppl. 1): 101–8.

48 Szeluga DJ, Stuart RK, Brookmeyer R, Utermohlez V, Santos GW. Energy requirements of parenterally fed bone marrow transplant recipients. *J Parenter Enteral Nutr* 1985; **9**: 139–43.

49 Wu D, Hockenberry DM, Brentnall TA *et al.* Persistent nausea and anorexia after marrow transplantation: a prospective study of 78 patients. *Transplantation* 1998; **66**: 1319–24.

50 Hutchinson ML, Clemans GW, Springmeyer SC, Flournoy N. Energy expenditure estimation in recipients of marrow transplants. *Cancer* 1984; **54**: 1734–8.

51 Hutchinson ML, Clemans GW. Prospective trial of Liposyn® 20% in patients undergoing bone marrow transplantation. *Clin Nutr* 1984; **3**: 5–9.

52 Mulder PO, Bouman JG, Gietema JA *et al.* Hyperalimentation in autologous bone marrow transplantation for solid tumors. Comparison of total parenteral versus partial parenteral plus enteral nutrition. *Cancer* 1989; **64**: 2045–52.

53 Ziegler TR, Young LS, Benfell K *et al.* Clinical and metabolic efficacy of glutamine-supplemented parenteral nutrition after bone marrow transplantation: a randomized, double-blind, controlled study. *Ann Int Med* 1992; **116**: 821–8.

54 Young LS, Bye R, Scheltinga M, Ziegler TR, Jacobs DO, Wilmore DW. Patients receiving glutamine-supplemented intravenous feedings report an improvement in mood. *J Parenter Enteral Nutr* 1993; **17**: 422–7.

55 Lenssen P, Cheney CL, Aker SN *et al.* Intravenous branched chain amino acid trial in marrow transplant recipients. *J Parenter Enteral Nutr* 1987; **11**: 112–8.

56 Keller U, Kraenzlin ME, Gratwohl A *et al.* Protein metabolism assessed by 1–13C leucine infusions in patients undergoing bone marrow transplantation. *J Parenter Enteral Nutr* 1990; **14**: 480–4.

57 Uderzo C, Rovelli A, Bonomi M, Fomia L, Pirovano L, Masera G. Total parenteral nutrition and nutritional assessment and leukaemic children undergoing bone marrow transplantation. *Eur J Cancer* 1991; **27**: 758–62.

58 Muscaritoli M, Conversano L, Cangiano C *et al.* Biochemical indices may not accurately reflect changes in nutritional status after allogeneic bone marrow transplantation. *Nutrition* 1995; **11**: 433–6.

59 Harris JA, Benedict FG. *Standard Basal Metabolism Constants for Physiologists and Clinicians: a Biometric Study of Basal Metabolism.* Philadelphia: J.B. Lippincott, 1919.

60 Cheney CL, Abson KG, Aker SN *et al.* Body composition changes in marrow transplant recipients receiving total parenteral nutrition. *Cancer* 1987; **59**: 1515–9.

61 Charuhas PM, Fosberg KL, Bruemmer B *et al.* A double-blind randomized trial comparing outpatient parenteral nutrition with intravenous hydration: effect on resumption of oral intake after marrow transplantation. *J Parenter Enteral Nutr* 1997; **21**: 157–61.

62 Braunschweig CL, Levy P, Sheean PM, Wang X. Enteral compared with parenteral nutrition: a meta-analysis. *Am J Clin Nutr* 2001; **74**: 534–42.

63 Mercadante S. Parenteral versus enteral nutrition in cancer patients: indications and practice. *Support Care Cancer* 1998; **6**: 85–93.

64 Murray SM, Pindoria S. Nutrition support for bone marrow transplant patients. *Cochrane Database Syst Rev* 2002; **2**: CD002920.

65 Eagle DA, Gian V, Lauwers GY *et al.* Gastroparesis following bone marrow transplantation. *Bone Marrow Transplant* 2001; **28**: 59–62.

66 Sefcick A, Anderton D, Byrne JL, Teahon K, Russell NH. Naso-jejunal feeding in allogeneic bone marrow transplant recipients. Results of a pilot study. *Bone Marrow Transplant* 2001; **28**: 1135–9.

67 Langdana A, Tully N, Molloy E, Bourke B, O'Meara A. Intensive enteral nutrition support in paediatric bone marrow transplantation. *Bone Marrow Transplant* 2001; **27**: 741–6.

68 Spain DA, McClave SA, Sexton LK *et al.* Infusion protocol improves delivery of enteral tube feeding in the critical care unit. *J Parenter Enteral Nutr* 1999; **23**: 288–92.

69 Roberts SR, Miller JE. Success using PEG tubes in marrow transplant recipients. *Nutr Clin Prac* 1998; **13**: 74–8.

70 Barron MA, Duncan DS, Green GJ *et al.* Efficacy and safety of radiologically placed gastrostomy tubes in paediatric haematology/oncology patients. *Med Pediatr Oncol* 2000; **34**: 177–82.

71 Fox VL, Abel SD, Malas S, Duggan C, Leichtner AM. Complications following percutaneous endoscopic gastrostomy and subsequent catheter replacement in children and young adults. *Gastrointest Endosc* 1997; **45**: 64–71.

72 Gauvreau-Stern JM, Cheney CL, Aker SN, Lenssen P. Food intake patterns and foodservice requirements on a marrow transplant unit. *J Am Diet Assoc* 1989; **89**: 367–72.

73 French MR, Levy-Milne R, Zibrik D. A survey of the use of low microbial diets in pediatric bone marrow transplant programs. *J Am Diet Assoc* 2001; **101**: 1194–8.

74 Rust DM, Simpson JK, Lister J. Nutritional issues in patients with severe neutropenia. *Semin Oncol Nurs* 2000; **16**: 152–62.

75 Driedger L, Burstall CD. Bone marrow transplantation. Dietitian's experience and perspective. *J Am Diet Assoc* 1987; **87**: 1387–8.

76 Gauvreau JM, Lenssen P, Cheney CL, Aker SN, Hutchinson ML, Barale KV. Nutritional management of patients with intestinal graft-versus-host disease. *J Am Diet Assoc* 1981; **79**: 673–7.

77 Sawada M, Tsurumi H, Hara T *et al.* Graft failure of autologous peripheral blood stem cell transplantation due to acute metabolic acidosis associated with total parenteral nutrition in a patient with relapsed breast cancer. *Acta Haematol* 1999; **102**: 157–9.

78 Curry CR, Quie PG. Fungal septicemia in patients receiving parenteral hyperalimentation. *N Engl J Med* 1971; **285**: 1221–5.

79 Mitchell RB, Wagner JE, Karp JE *et al.* Syndrome of idiopathic hyperammonemia after high-dose chemotherapy: review of nine cases. *Am J Med* 1988; **85**: 662–7.

80 Davies SM, Szabo E, Wagner JE, Ramsay NK, Weisdorf DJ. Idiopathic hyperammonemia. A frequently lethal complication of bone marrow transplantation. *Bone Marrow Transplant* 1996; **17**: 1119–25.

81 Schulte C, Reinhardt W, Beelen D, Mann K, Schaefer U. Low T_3 syndrome and nutritional status as prognostic factors in patients undergoing bone marrow transplantation. *Bone Marrow Transplant* 1998; **22**: 1171–8.

82 Aker SN, Cheney CL, Sanders JE, Lenssen PL, Hickman RO, Thomas ED. Nutritional support in marrow graft recipients with single versus double lumen right atrial catheters. *Exp Hematol* 1982; **10**: 732–7.

83 Ulz L, Petersen FB, Ford R *et al.* A prospective study of complications in Hickman right-atrial catheters in marrow transplant patients. *J Parenter Enteral Nutr* 1990; **14**: 27–30.

84 Petersen FB, Clift RA, Hickman RO *et al.* Hickman catheter complications in marrow transplant recipients. *J Parenter Enteral Nutr* 1986; **10**: 58–62.

85 Kelly DA. Liver complications of pediatric parenteral nutrition: epidemiology. *Nutrition* 1998; **14**: 153–7.

86 Kaufman SS. Prevention of parenteral nutrition-associated liver disease in children. *Pediatr Transplant* 2002; **6**: 37–42.

87 Sax HC, Bower RH. Hepatic complications of total parenteral nutrition. *J Parenter Enteral Nutr* 1988; **12**: 615–8.

88 Matarese LE, Speerhas R, Seidner DL, Steiger E. Foscarnet-induced electrolyte abnormalities in a bone marrow transplant patient receiving parenteral nutrition. *J Parenter Enteral Nutr* 2000; **24**: 170–3.

89 Papadopoulou A, Nathavitharana K, Williams MD, Darbyshire PJ, Booth IW. Diagnosis and clinical associations of zinc depletion following bone marrow transplantation. *Arch Dis Child* 1996; **74**: 328–31.

90 Clemans GW, Yamanaka W, Flournoy N *et al.* Plasma fatty acid patterns of bone marrow transplant patients primarily supported by fat-free parenteral nutrition. *J Parenter Enteral Nutr* 1981; **5**: 221–5.

91 Fredstrom S, Rogosheske J, Gupta P, Burns LJ. Case report. Extrapyramidal symptoms in a BMT recipient with hyperintense basal ganglia and elevated manganese. *Bone Marrow Transplant* 1995; **15**: 989–92.

92 Reese JL, Means ME, Hanrahan K, Clearman B, Colwill M, Dawson C. Diarrhea associated with nasogastric feedings. *Oncol Nurs Forum* 1996; **23**: 59–66; discussion 66–8.

93 Layton PB, Gallucci BB, Aker SN. Nutritional assessment of allogeneic bone marrow recipients. *Cancer Nurs* 1981; **4**: 127–34.

94 Tyc VL, Vallelunga L, Mahoney S, Smith BF, Mulhern RK. Nutritional and treatment-related characteristics of pediatric oncology patients referred or not referred for nutritional support. *Med Pediatr Oncol* 1995; **25**: 379–88.

95 Apovian CM, McMahon MM, Bistrian BR. Guidelines for refeeding the marasmic patient. *Crit Care Med* 1990; **18**: 1030–3.

96 Wilmore DW. Catabolic illness: stratagies for enhancing recovery. *N Engl J Med* 1991; **325**: 695–702.

97 Barton R, Cerra FB. The hypermetabolism–multiple organ failure syndrome. *Chest* 1989; **96**: 1153–60.

98 Hill GR, Crawford JM, Cooke KR, Brinson YS, Pan L, Ferrara JL. Total body irradiation and acute graft-versus-host disease: the role of gastrointestinal damage and inflammatory cytokines. *Blood* 1997; **90**: 3204–13.

99 Takatsuka H, Takemoto Y, Yamada S *et al.* Complications after bone marrow transplantation are manifestations of systemic inflammatory response

99. syndrome. *Bone Marrow Transplant* 2000; **26**: 419–26.
100. Wesley JR. Nutrient metabolism in relation to the systemic stress response. In: Zimmerman JJ, ed. *Pediatric Critical Care*, 2nd edn. St Louis: Mosby, 1998: 799–819.
101. Ziegler TR, Gatzen C, Wilmore DW. Strategies for attenuating protein-catabolic responses in the critically ill. *Ann Rev Med* 1994; **45**: 459–80.
102. Cochran EB, Kamper CA, Phelps SJ, Brown RO. Parenteral nutrition in the critically ill patient. *Clin Pharm* 1989; **8**: 783–99.
103. Simpson D. Drug therapy for acute graft-versus-host disease prophylaxis. *J Hematother Stem Cell Res* 2000; **9**: 317–25.
104. Carreras E, Villamor N, Reverter JC, Sierra J, Grañena A, Rozman C. Hypertriglyceridemia in bone marrow transplant recipients. Another side effect of cyclosporine A. *Bone Marrow Transplant* 1989; **4**: 385–8.
105. June CH, Thompson CB, Kennedy MS, Nims J, Thomas ED. Profound hypomagnesemia and renal magnesium wasting associated with the use of cyclosporine for marrow transplantation. *Transplantation* 1985; **39**: 620–4.
106. Basara N, Blau WI, Kiehl MG et al. Efficacy and safety of mycophenolate mofetil for the treatment of acute and chronic GVHD in bone marrow transplant recipient. *Transplant Proc* 1998; **30**: 4087–9.
107. Basara N, Blau WI, Kiehl MG et al. Mycophenolate mofetil for the prophylaxis of acute GVHD in HLA-mismatched bone marrow transplant patients. *Clin Transplant* 2000; **14**: 121–6.
108. Wolford JL, McDonald GB. A problem-oriented approach to intestinal and liver disease after marrow transplantation. *J Clin Gastroenterol* 1988; **10**: 419–33.
109. Boelens PG, Nijveldt RJ, Houdijk AP, Meijer S, van Leeuwen PA. Glutamine alimentation in catabolic state. *J Nutr* 2001; **131** (Suppl.): S2569–77; discussion S2590.
110. van der Hulst RR, von Meyenfeldt MF, Soeters PB. Glutamine: an essential amino acid for the gut. *Nutrition* 1996; **12** (Suppl. 11–12): S78–81.
111. Alverdy JC. Effects of glutamine-supplemented diets on immunology of the gut. *J Parenter Enteral Nutr* 1990; **14** (Suppl.): S109–13.
112. MacBurney M, Young LS, Ziegler TR, Wilmore DW. A cost-evaluation of glutamine-supplemented parenteral nutrition in adult bone marrow transplant patients. *J Am Diet Assoc* 1994; **94**: 1263–6.
113. Schloerb PR, Skikne BS. Oral and parenteral glutamine in bone marrow transplantation: a randomized, double-blind study. *J Parenter Enteral Nutr* 1999; **23**: 117–22.
114. Brown SA, Goringe A, Fegan C et al. Parenteral glutamine protects hepatic function during bone marrow transplantation. *Bone Marrow Transplant* 1998; **22**: 281–4.
115. Goringe AP, Brown S, O'Callaghan U et al. Glutamine and vitamin E in the treatment of hepatic veno-occlusive disease following high-dose chemotherapy. *Bone Marrow Transplant* 1998; **21**: 829–32.
116. Anderson PM, Ramsay NK, Shu XO et al. Effect of low-dose oral glutamine on painful stomatitis during bone marrow transplantation. *Bone Marrow Transplant* 1998; **22**: 339–44.
117. Cockerham MB, Weinberger BB, Lerchie SB. Oral glutamine for the prevention of oral mucositis associated with high-dose paclitaxel and melphalan for autologous bone marrow transplantation. *Ann Pharmacother* 2000; **34**: 300–3.
118. Ziegler TR. Glutamine supplementation in cancer patients receiving bone marrow transplantation and high dose chemotherapy. *J Nutr* 2001; **131** (Suppl.): S2578–84; discussion S2590.
119. Coghlin Dickson TM, Wong RM, Offrin RS et al. Effect of oral glutamine supplementation during bone marrow transplantation. *J Parenter Enteral Nutr* 2000; **24**: 61–6.
120. Suchner U, Kuhn KS, Furst P. The scientific basis of immunonutrition. *Proc Nutr Soc* 2000; **59**: 553–63.
121. Heys SD, Walker LG, Smith I, Eremin O. Enteral nutritional supplementation with key nutrients in patients with critical illness and cancer: a meta-analysis of randomized controlled clinical trials. *Ann Surg* 1999; **229**: 467–77.
122. Takatsuka H, Takemoto Y, Iwata N et al. Oral eicosapentaenoic acid for complications of bone marrow transplantation. *Bone Marrow Transplant* 2001; **28**: 769–74.
123. Lenssen P, Sherry ME, Cheney CL et al. Prevalence of nutrition-related problems among long-term survivors of allogeneic marrow transplantation. *J Am Diet Assoc* 1990; **90**: 835–42.
124. Iestra JA, Fibbe WE, Zwinderman AH, van Staveren WA, Kromhout D. Body weight recovery, eating difficulties and compliance with dietary advice in the first year after stem cell transplantation: a prospective study. *Bone Marrow Transplant* 2002; **29**: 417–24.
125. Stern JM, Chesnut CH 3rd, Bruemmer B et al. Bone density loss during treatment of chronic GVHD. *Bone Marrow Transplant* 1996; **17**: 395–400.
126. Franca CM, Domingues-Martins M, Volpe A, Pallotta Filho RS, Soares de Araujo N. Severe oral manifestations of chronic graft-vs.-host disease. *J Am Dent Assoc* 2001; **132**: 1124–7.
127. Brauner R, Adan L, Souberbielle JC et al. Contribution of growth hormone deficiency to the growth failure that follows bone marrow transplantation. *J Pediatr* 1997; **130**: 785–92.
128. Bozzola M, Giorgiani G, Locatelli F et al. Growth in children after bone marrow transplantation. *Horm Res* 1993; **39**: 122–6.
129. Cohen A, Duell T, Socie G et al. Nutritional status and growth after bone marrow transplantation (BMT) during childhood: EBMT Late-Effects Working Party retrospective data. *Bone Marrow Transplant* 1999; **23**: 1043–7.
130. Taskinen M, Saarinen UM. Skeletal muscle protein reserve after bone marrow transplantation in children. *Bone Marrow Transplant* 1996; **18**: 937–41.
131. Liatsos C, Mehta AB, Potter M, Burroughs AK. The hepatologist in the haematologists' camp. *Br J Haematol* 2001; **113**: 567–78.
132. Reed MD, Lazarus HM, Herzig RH et al. Cyclic parenteral nutrition during bone marrow transplantation in children. *Cancer* 1983; **51**: 1563–70.
133. Maini B, Blackburn GL, Bistrian BR et al. Cyclic hyperalimentation: an optimal technique for preservation of visceral protein. *J Surg Res* 1976; **20**: 515–25.
134. Hwang TL, Lue MC, Chen LL. Early use of cyclic TPN prevents further deterioration of liver functions for the TPN patients with impaired liver function. *Hepatogastroenterology* 2000; **47**: 1347–50.
135. Buchman AL, Dubin MD, Moukarzel AA et al. Choline deficiency: a cause of hepatic steatosis during parenteral nutrition that can be reversed with intravenous choline supplementation. *Hepatology* 1995; **22**: 1399–403.
136. Dahlstrom KA, Ament ME, Moukarzel A, Vinton NE, Cederblad G. Low blood and plasma carnitine levels in children receiving long-term parenteral nutrition. *J Pediatr Gastroenterol Nutr* 1990; **11**: 375–9.
137. Helms RA, Whitington PF, Mauer EC, Catarau EM, Christensen ML, Borum PR. Enhanced lipid utilization in infants receiving oral L-carnitine during long-term parenteral nutrition. *J Pediatr* 1986; **109**: 984–8.
138. Meehan JJ, Georgeson KE. Prevention of liver failure in parenteral nutrition-dependent children with short bowel syndrome. *J Pediatr Surg* 1997; **32**: 473–5.
139. Schwarzenberg SJ, Weisdorf-Schindele S. Cancer treatment. In: Walker W, Watkins J, Duggan C, eds. *Nutrition in Pediatrics: Basic Science and Clinical* Applications, 3rd edn. Hamilton, ON: BC Decker, 2003: 709–21.

66 Pain Management

Jonathan R. Gavrin & F. Peter Buckley

Patients who receive hematopoietic cell transplantation (HCT) may suffer pain of varying etiologies and severity (Table 66.1). This chapter defines the neurophysiology and pharmacology of pain; what is meant by "pain"; what factors lead a patient to experience and suffer pain; what physical, psychologic, environmental and pharmacologic factors influence the amount of pain and suffering; how this compendium of pain and suffering can be evaluated; and the different means by which pain and suffering can be relieved in the HCT recipient.

Table 66.1 Common sources of pain in bone marrow transplantation (BMT).

Etiology	Example
Infiltration from primary disease	Bone pain
	Fractures
	Soft tissue of visceral pain
Hematopoietic stem cell mobilization	Bone or joint aching
Chemotherapy or irradiation	Mucositis
	Cutaneous burns
	Peripheral neuropathies
Graft-vs.-host disease	Skin irritation
	Gut cramps
	Oropharyngeal pain
Immunosuppressive drugs	Peripheral neuropathies
	Joint aching
	Long bone pain
	Osteopenic bone fractures
Infection or viral activation	Shingles from herpes zoster
	Postherpetic neuralgia
	Cytomegalovirus gut pain
Diagnostic and surgical procedures	Bone marrow aspiration
	Lumbar puncture
	Post-lumbar puncture headache
	Line placement
	Tissue biopsies
Pains unrelated to disease	Headache
	Low back pain
	Myalgias from inactivity

Anatomy and physiology of pain

Classically, pain begins with tissue damage (nociception), the type and location detected by peripheral nerves and then signaled to the brain. Our understanding of the neurophysiology and neurochemistry of nociceptive damage detection, transmission to the central nervous system (CNS), and CNS processing to produce the clinical phenomenon of pain, is far from perfect. Our understanding of how the CNS may be influenced by pharmacologic or nonpharmacologic means to suppress nociception and reduce pain is also imperfect. A summary of the known neurophysiology and neuropharmacology of nociception and pain is helpful in understanding clinical management of the HCT patient.

Ascending nociceptive systems

All body tissues possess nociceptors (neural structures that detect tissue damage) that are activated by physical stimuli or by algogenic (pain producing) substances released when there is tissue injury. Alternatively, nociceptors may be sensitized by algogenic substances, resulting in noxious activation by normally innocuous stimuli, e.g. light touch in the presence of inflammation. Nociceptors signal to the spinal cord through fast-conducting A delta fibers, or slow-conducting C fibers in peripheral nerves, which enter the neuraxis and synapse through dorsal horn cells (Fig. 66.1). Dorsal horn cell axons cross the midline and ascend cephalad in the spinothalamic tracts. Information from the fast A delta fibers ascends rapidly, with no intermediate synapses, to the thalamus and hence to the cerebrum. Information from the slow C fibers ascends through a number of different synapses, notably to the limbic system, before reaching the thalamus and cerebrum. The C fiber/limbic system synapses initiate the emotional responses to pain [1].

Modulation of nociceptive traffic

Afferent nociceptive transmission is not "hard wired"—signals do not progress to the cerebrum unimpeded and unimpedable. With evolving neurophysiologic knowledge it has been recognized that afferent transmission may be modulated, as hypothesized in the "gate control theory" of pain [2,3]. This theory states that there are various "gates" within the nervous system that may be opened, or closed, to nociceptive transmission by a variety of processes. The "gating" concept is a useful tool when teaching patients and relatives about pain relief techniques. A basic understanding of this physiology helps patients and family members understand that active interventions, pharmacologic and nonpharmacologic, are essential to obtain optimal pain relief.

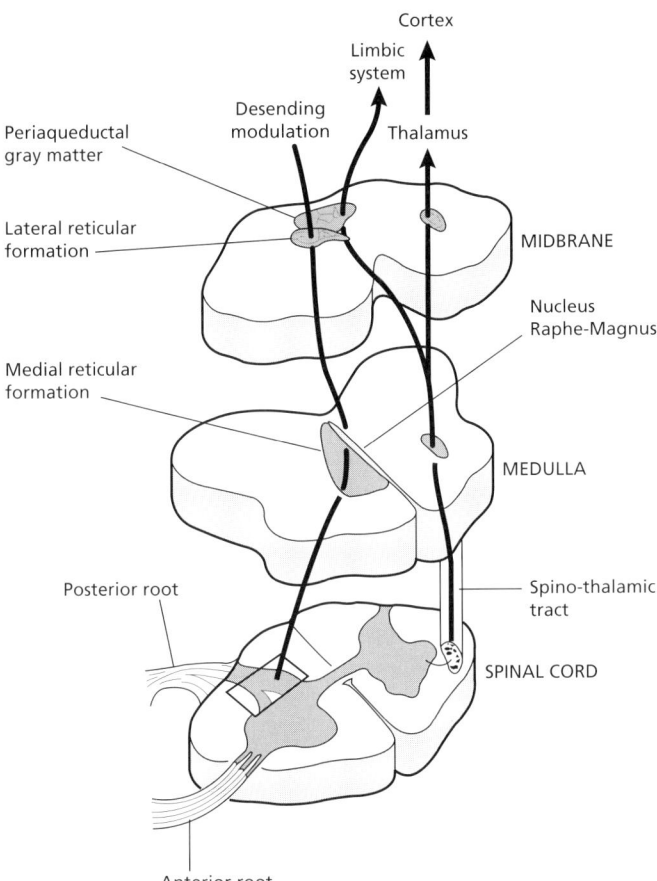

Fig. 66.1 Nociceptive information is carried to the spinal cord in A delta and C fibers. The nerves enter the dorsal horn, where they synapse with second-order neurons that cross the midline of the cord at about the entry level and ascend in the spinothalamic tracts. The A delta-derived information goes on a fast track directly to the thalamus. The C fiber-derived information reaches the thalamus later, having synapsed in the limbic system. The descending nociceptive afferent modulating system originates in the periaqueductal gray matter. It projects through the nucleus raphe magnus down to the posterior horn, where it has a modulatory effect on the afferent nociceptive traffic.

Afferent nociceptive transmission can be enhanced or, more importantly, inhibited by:
1 Modification of the peripheral nociceptor signaling. Algogenic substances (prostaglandins, serotonin) can activate or sensitize peripheral nociceptors; anti-inflammatory medications (aspirin and other non-steroidal anti-inflammatory drugs [NSAIDs]) can oppose such effects.
2 Inhibition of nociceptive transmission in the dorsal horn by nonnoxious peripheral stimulation. Rubbing, heat, cold or electric stimulation peripherally activates sensory afferent fibers that synapse with dorsal horn cells to inhibit nociceptive transmission.
3 Inhibition of dorsal horn nociceptive transmission by the descending nociceptive modulating system. This process originates in the periaqueductal gray matter of the hindbrain (Fig. 66.1). The neurotransmitters of this system include serotonin, norepinephrine and endogenous opioid (morphine-like) substances. The descending modulatory system can be activated to produce pain relief by learned behavioral or cognitive strategies or by pharmacologic agents that either mimic endogenous neurotransmitters (e.g. opioids) or that stimulate activity of the system (e.g. tricyclic antidepressants) [4].

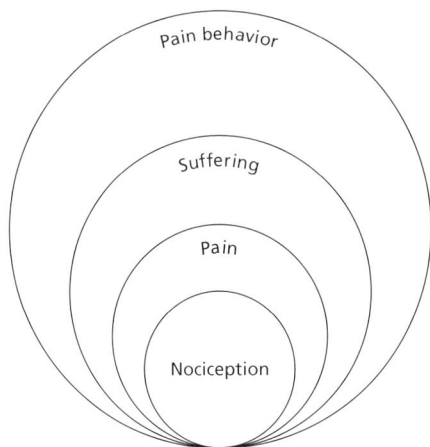

Fig. 66.2 A schema of the various aspects of the human pain experience.

The clinical phenomenon of pain

The neurophysiology and neuropharmacology described so far deal only with physiologically demonstrable phenomena. The experience of pain clearly is more than neurophysiology, encompassing the subjective interpretation and expression of the neurophysiologic phenomenon.

What is pain?

Pain is defined as a multidimensional experience [5]. The degree to which an individual feels pain, suffers from pain and complains of pain is influenced by a number of factors in addition to tissue damage/nociception. The model depicted in Fig. 66.2 [6] is helpful in conceptualizing these components. Nociception is the detection of tissue damage by sensory transducers and the signaling of this information to brain. Processing of nociceptive information by the CNS results in the human experience of pain, which is both sensory and affective (feeling). Suffering, the negative cognitive and emotional responses to pain, can be heightened by pain-independent emotional factors, such as fear, anxiety and depression, that may impact the HCT patient [7]. The compendium of nociception, pain and suffering, which are subjective, personal and unmeasurable, emerge to be expressed as pain behaviors. Observations of pain behaviors, including report of pain and inhibition of activity, constitute the raw data that enable diagnosis of the source of pain and estimation of the magnitude of suffering.

Pain and suffering in the HCT patient

When an HCT patient complains of pain, the most common circumstance is one of obvious tissue damage (e.g. oral mucositis). Patients may also complain of pain with little evidence of tissue damage (e.g. neuropathy). Irrespective of its source, nociceptive information is processed identically by the CNS and in all cases the patient feels pain, suffers and exhibits pain behaviors.

Some patients have obvious tissue damage, such as an erythematous and ulcerated mucosa in the mouth, but complain of little pain and appear to suffer little. Other patients have little or no evidence of tissue damage yet complain of much pain and suffer a great deal. What can a clinician make of these two disparate situations? Is the first patient really in pain and really suffering, but not telling anyone? Is the second patient imagining or faking pain? Both explanations are plausible, but unlikely. The relationship between nociception, pain, suffering and pain behaviors is not a fixed one. A number of correlates, in addition to physiologic and pharmacologic factors, influence how much patients feel, suffer and complain of pain. Among these correlates are the following.

1 *The meaning of the pain.* Pain from a known or predictable source often results in less suffering and fewer complaints than pain from an unknown, potentially threatening source.

2 *The circumstances in which the pain occurs.* A simple pain problem, such as toothache, may result in more suffering and complaints in a patient undergoing HCT than the same pain experienced in normal circumstances.

3 *The patient's style of coping with adversity.* This style is influenced by social and cultural factors. At one end of the spectrum are those who tough it out and never call for help, at the other end are those who call for help at the first sign of adversity.

4 *Emotional state.* Fear or anxiety can lead patients to be hyperattentive to sensations. Similarly, depression often reduces activities and increases attention to discomforts.

5 *Previous experience with pain.* Experience with chemotherapy may serve to reassure patients that current experience is "normal" and will resolve. An inexperienced patient may be thinking, "How can I feel so bad and possibly be doing OK?"

6 *Previous exposure to CNS active pharmacologic agents* (analgesics, anxiolytics, alcohol). These agents may directly influence CNS processing of nociception. If a patient is opioid-tolerant or has extensive exposure to alcohol, opioid dosing needs may be higher than average. Usage patterns may also reflect the patient's style of coping with adversity, perhaps to escape into a "pharmacologic fog".

It is well to remember that, regardless of the source, all patients have cognitive and processing components to their pain. Remember the phrase "no brain, no pain": if it is not processed in the brain, it is not felt. The vast majority of HCT patients have a nociceptive source of their pain onto which the cognitive and processing components are grafted.

Assessment of pain and treatment efficacy

History

Some patients will have histories suggesting they are at risk of having significant pain problems or may have difficulty obtaining pain relief. Significant historical factors include the following.

1 Active pain problems related or unrelated to the patient's disease or therapies.
2 Previous severe pain after surgery or trauma.
3 Difficulty in obtaining satisfactory pain control during events in items 1 and 2.
4 Nonpharmacologic pain-relieving strategies that the patient uses.
5 Analgesics the patient has used and any problems with them.
6 Previous or current significant emotional or affective disorders.
7 Previous or current CNS active substance use (alcohol, opioids, anxiolytics).
8 The patient's understanding of the current pain, its significance and likely duration.
9 The patient's preferred mode of dealing with pain (both nonpharmacologic and pharmacologic).

Pain measurement and monitoring

How is one to assess what the HCT patient is experiencing? Much of the system of nociceptive transmitting, processing and suffering is subjective and not directly observable (Fig. 66.2). It is possible to observe and quantify the system's output (complaints of pain) and use that as an approximation. In clinical practice, an HCT patient's pain is what the patient says hurts, in the amount the patient says it hurts. Those caring for HCT patients should accept pain complaints as real, genuine, worthy of attention and deserving alleviation.

In practice, pain and its impact are monitored by subjective pain scores and observational function scores. The indices used to monitor pain, the effects and side-effects of therapies and medication use should be observed and recorded frequently using a pain assessment tool. Far from feeling burdened by reporting pain and other symptoms on a daily or per shift basis, patients are often relieved that staff are aware of their symptoms. Consistent evaluation assures patients that their experience is recognized and that evaluation is routine and therefore normal. Uncertainty and unpredictability about what will happen causes the greatest distress for the greatest number of HCT patients [8–10]. Knowledge that the pain is expected, how it is likely to feel and how long it is likely to last can help patients to endure even extremely difficult circumstances.

Cancer and HCT patients are reluctant to complain and do not know what experiences are "normal" or what should be reported. They will often answer "fine" or "OK" if asked only "How are you feeling?" Pain scores and ratings can be used as "objective" quality assurance tools to determine need for further evaluation or change in treatment. Pain above the equivalent to a score of 3 or 4 indicates a need to improve pain treatment because the pain will substantially disrupt function [11]. Even temporary pain should not exceed 6 on a scale from 0 to 10 without mandating further evaluation or additional pain treatment methods [11–13].

Pain scales

Adults and children from about the age of 7 years can report with scales as seen in Figs 66.3 and 66.4.

1 Numeric rating scores from 0 = "no pain" to 10 = "pain as bad as can be". It can be helpful the first time with a patient to use a few familiar

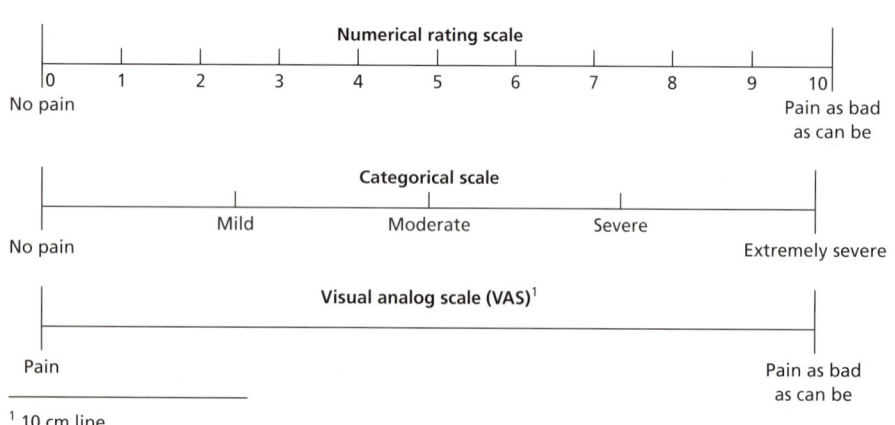

Fig. 66.3 Self-report scales for assessing pain in adults. The numerical rating scale is used most frequently.

[1] 10 cm line

Fig. 66.4 A "faces" scale used to monitor pain and pain management efficacy in children between ages 3 and 7 years.

examples such as: "When you think of a headache you have had in your lifetime, can you remember how it felt?" (Help the person think of a pain he or she remembers.) "When you think of that pain, where would it be on a scale from no pain, which is a 0, to pain as bad as anyone could possibly have, which is a 10? Further help can be offered by saying: "Many people think of 1, 2 or 3 as milder pain; of 4, 5 or 6 as moderate pain; of 7, 8 or 9 as severe pain; and 10 as being the most extreme pain anyone could ever have." If the patient is still unable to use the scale, or sometimes for patients from other cultures, the addition of the faces, as in Fig. 66.4, can be helpful when added to the scale above the numbers. Numeric scales can be given orally or on paper as seen in Fig. 66.3. In general, these numeric scales are easy to use and record. This scale is favored by clinicians and researchers [12,14].

2 Categoric scales using descriptive words from "no pain" to "extremely severe pain". Such scales are well understood by patients but are difficult to record or to use to track pain and treatment success.

3 Visual analog scales. These are 10 cm lines anchored at one end with "no pain" and at the other end with "pain as bad as can be". Patients make a mark at any point along the scale to indicate pain intensity. These scales require measurement of the line in millimeter increments after the patient completes the written scale.

Children below the age of 7 years usually cannot use the above scales. From ages 3 to 7 children can usually indicate their pain using one of a variety of "faces" scales (Fig. 66.4) [15]. Children below the age of 3–4 years cannot use such scales and observation scales from nurses or family members may be used.

Ability to function

The provision of adequate pain control is essential not only for humane reasons, but also to preserve the patient's ability to provide self-care and to maintain health. Function may be directly observed, based on specific behaviors necessary to participate in HCT (bathing, exercise, mouth care). Pain behaviors may be noted, such as request for medication, grimacing or refusal to move the affected area of the body [16].

Medication use and side-effects

Analgesics reduce the sensation of pain and can improve function, but can also produce unacceptable side-effects. The magnitude of drug consumption and the occurrence of common side-effects should be monitored and recorded on the same scale format and on the same assessment sheets as pain scores.

Pain diagnostics and therapy selection

A clear diagnosis of the cause of a pain is essential in selecting therapies. To be effective, therapies must be aimed at the specific issues that contribute to the patient's problem. For pain with a large nociceptive contribution from tissue damage (e.g. mucositis), antinociceptive agents (analgesics) are appropriate. For pain with a nociceptive component originating from neural tissue, different agents are appropriate (e.g. anticonvulsants). For pain complaints that are concurrent with strong emotional or environmental components, treatments aimed at those components, in addition to pharmacologic agents, are appropriate. The first step in intervention is usually education as described below. Pharmacologic therapies should be pursued in a rational pharmacokinetic and pharmacodynamic fashion, for a period of time that will give the therapies a reasonable trial.

Treating the patient with difficult pain management problems

Pain can be alleviated by a variety of methods that can be initiated and used effectively by the staff caring for the patient. Sometimes, the magnitude of the problem may be beyond abilities of the primary caregivers. In these circumstances, the assistance of personnel with special expertise in pain management (nurses, neurologists, anesthesiologists, psychologists, psychiatrists) may be helpful. The assistance can be provided in a variety of forms, ranging from occasional consultations to weekly "pain rounds", or the presence of a formal pain consultation team.

Nonpharmacologic techniques in pain management

When HCT patients report pain, analgesic medications are appropriately considered as a first line of treatment. Concurrent nonpharmacologic methodologies are almost always incorporated into the treatment of the patient, whether these interventions are intended or not [17]. Even with optimal opioid and other analgesic methods, HCT patients with mucositis may receive only 50–60% reductions in pain with analgesics [18,19].

Mechanisms of nonpharmacologic techniques

The broad goal of nonpharmacologic methods is to close the "gate" on pain messages or to impede transmission of pain messages and facilitate transmission of nonpain messages. In general, this is done by disrupting afferent pain pathways through the addition of competing sensory inputs or by modifying descending pathways through changes in thoughts and responses to the sensory messages received.

A number of nonpharmacologic methods seem to operate mechanically, modulating transmission of ascending nociceptive messages by sending competing sensory messages from the body surface or limbs. Putting these mechanical methods into operation requires activity. Patients must increase their physical activity, increase thoughts not focused on pain and achieve an emotional calmness through a sense of control over some aspects of functioning. Lying in bed in a dark quiet room without outside stimuli does not permit the activation of these mechanical methods and can lead patients to focus on the dominant sensory input—pain.

Staff and family members can assist patients by preparing structured activities and statements that facilitate attention to stimuli other than the pain. These need not be complex. Indeed, patients have limited attention span and often have disruptions in fine motor control. Simple conversation, walking outside the room or movement in the room and simple games all serve to distract the mind from discomfort.

Education of patients and families, except in rare instances, provides reassurance and enhances the ability to cope with unfamiliar and uncomfortable situations. Autonomic nervous system activity decreases as anxieties and fears are allayed. Resultant reductions in serotonin and norepinephrine availability help patients as they prepare to guard against worsening symptoms. Adaptive thoughts are those that reassure or calm the patient and relax the autonomic nervous system.

Emotions are closely tied to and influenced by thoughts. Cognitive–behavioral methodologies for treating depression and anxiety [20,21] successfully have been adapted specifically for cancer and HCT patients [17,19,22]. Patients who are more distressed pretransplant report greater

Table 66.2 Pain-related education needs of hematopoietic cell transplantation (HCT) patients and their families.

Question	Usual information offered
Why treat pain?	Pain is harmful to your physical health
	There is no benefit to proving you can stand pain without treatment, but there are serious negative health effects from suffering unnecessary pain
What treatments are common?	Most HCT patients need strong pain medications (opioids) at some time
When are treatments used:	
How often?	When pain is constant, scheduled doses provide better relief than waiting until pain is severe to take medication
How much at a time?	Your doctor will only prescribe safe levels of medication; let your nurse or doctor know if:
	You are too sleepy during the day
	Nausea increases when you take medication
	You have other symptoms that are new
	You have a new pain
How do you know when more is needed?	Pain medication should be used to keep pain under control, rather than waiting until pain is intolerable
Is addiction a concern?	HCT patients with no history of overusing drugs or alcohol have no cravings for the medication when the pain stops. Even people who need high doses of medication do not become addicts
Do people become tolerant to the drugs so that they stop working if pain gets really bad?	If you use the medication to keep the pain under control, the medication will not stop working when the pain increases, or if pain continues longer than expected
What if the medication does not work or makes a person sick?	There are many pain treatments. Tell your doctor or nurse if pain is out of control or if a medication makes you feel bad—numerous treatment options are available in these cases

pain during transplant [9,19]. Over time, unrelieved pain can engender feelings of helplessness and hopelessness. Introduction of alternative experiences of joy or self-control counter these feelings. When any of us feels more in control, we are better able to manage difficulties and feel less discomfort and less distress [8–10,23].

Strategies used in normal medical or nursing practice influence the thoughts patients have about their situation. Information, education and "reframing" techniques can facilitate coping. Other behaviors that are particularly useful in influencing both the ascending and descending modulatory systems include physical methods such as the use of ice or heat, rest when appropriate, transcutaneous nerve stimulation and physical positioning (see [24] for details on use of ice, heat and massage).

Information

Information that can be helpful to patients includes the following.
1 Time frame information. When is something likely to happen, how long will it last. It is helpful to break events into the smallest time frames possible.
2 Procedural information. What will be done, what comfort measures will be used.
3 Sensory information to prepare patients for specific discomforts.

Education

Education empowers patients to participate in their medical care and to modify their own behaviors. In addition to facts, patients must have the opportunity for dialogue to fit their own situation. Increasingly, patients and families administer their own pain medication and participate actively in medical treatment. To adhere to treatments, patients must understand them and not be frightened by the potential side-effects.

The common barriers to willingness to use available pain treatments are well-established [25,26]. Patients, family members and medical staff frequently fear opioids and are reluctant to identify when treatment is inadequate. Specific areas where HCT patients and their families need education are listed in Table 66.2. Problems with resistance to medications or lack of understanding about pain are routinely prevented by conducting a brief assessment and education session with patients and families prior to the start of treatment. This session serves the double purpose of identifying those patients who may experience difficulties achieving comfort.

Education alone can significantly reduce pain, reduce length of hospitalization, decrease complications and improve overall outcomes [27–29]. Information and education do not cause anxiety where none exists and they are not harmful [30,31].

Other cognitive–behavioral strategies

Reframing, active distraction and relaxation are all techniques that can be valuable adjuncts to the use of analgesic medications. To the degree possible, speak about events in positive terms, give patients a sense of control (including participation in clinical decisions), involve patients in activities (if only as an observer at times), provide a calm and caring environment. Research has shown that more specialized techniques, such as imagery and hypnosis, can be helpful but rarely eliminate the need for analgesic medications [19,22,32]. More widely available and simple techniques, such as progressive muscle relaxation, deep breathing and concentrating on pleasant thoughts and places, also are helpful adjuncts to pain relief [33,34].

Pediatric considerations

Most of these methods need little adaptation for use with children. Age-appropriate information is important for children. As with adults, this information should reinforce areas over which the child has some control, such as asking for medication or understanding rewards for self-care activities. Children can plan for their own active distractions and can be engaged in play even when quite ill. Story telling, art projects and play are effective imagery and distraction methods for children with pain.

It is crucially important to be aware that many children will withdraw from socializing when they are in pain. Their quiet demeanor should not be confused with comfort. Socialization and playfulness are often the best indicators of effective pain relief.

Nonopioid pharmacologic management of pain

NSAIDs and acetaminophen

Many nonopioid analgesics, both over-the-counter and prescription, are available. Two major groups are NSAIDs and phenacetin derivatives—acetaminophen being the only clinically used drug. All of these analgesics exhibit a "ceiling effect". Efficacy will increase with increasing doses up to a particular level; dosing beyond that point will not improve analgesia but will expose the patient to dose-related side-effects.

Other than the distinction that NSAIDs suppress inflammation and acetaminophen has few anti-inflammatory effects, there are few hard data on the comparable efficacy of the various agents as analgesics. Different agents offer varying durations of action, degree of side-effects and individual patient tolerance. These actions tend to be quite idiosyncratic so it would be unwise to recommend any specific medication regimen. It is essential to tailor therapy on an individual basis.

Nonopioid analgesics are suitable for use in mild to moderate nociceptive and inflammatory pain. Alone they provide inadequate analgesia for moderate to severe nociceptive pain but, if used in conjunction with opioids, may improve the quality of analgesia and demonstrate an "opioid-sparing effect", reducing the dose of opioid necessary to produce a given level of analgesia, thus reducing the potential for side-effects.

Nonopioid analgesics in the management of neuropathic pain currently are under study. Emerging data suggest only a limited role.

Pharmacology of NSAIDs and acetaminophen

The pharmacologic effect of NSAIDs is to inhibit the enzyme cyclo-oxygenase, part of the arachidonic acid cascade, reducing production of prostaglandins, one of the algogenic agents released by injured tissue (others are bradykinin, histamine, hydroxytryptamine [5-HT]) that stimulate or sensitize nociceptors. Consistent with their anti-inflammatory efficacy, the primary effect of NSAIDs classically has been believed to be peripheral. However, prostaglandins also have a role in the CNS transmission of pain [35–38]. Newer medications that selectively inhibit cyclo-oxygenase-2 (COX-2 inhibitors) and offer lower side-effect profiles have become available in recent years.

Acetaminophen produces similar analgesia to NSAIDs, but unlike NSAIDs has only minor anti-inflammatory effects. Acetaminophen is as potent as aspirin in inhibiting prostaglandin synthesis in the CNS, but has little effect on prostaglandin metabolism peripherally [39–43]. Analgesic effects of acetaminophen and NSAIDs appear to be additive [44–46].

Side-effects of NSAIDs and acetaminophen

Nonopioids have a variety of side-effects that are of significance for, and limit their use in the HCT patient.
1 *Interference with platelet function*. This lasts for days after stopping the drug in the case of aspirin, or for shorter periods with other NSAIDs. Although COX-2 inhibitors have little or no effect on platelet aggregation, the authors caution against their use until more is known. Acetaminophen has virtually no hematologic effects.
2 *Gastric irritation and occult upper gastrointestinal (GI) bleeding*. This is a feature of virtually all NSAIDs to some degree, even the COX-2 inhibitors. Acetaminophen is benign to the gut.

3 *Renal effects*. In high dosage NSAIDs have direct renal toxic effects. The effect of moderate NSAID dose upon already compromised renal function is not clear. Acetaminophen has virtually no renal effects.
4 *Hepatic effects*. In high dosage acetaminophen is severely hepatotoxic.

Use of NSAIDs and acetaminophen in HCT

The role of NSAIDs for pain management in the acute phase of HCT is limited by the fact that they are available only in oral form, except ketorolac, by their hematologic and GI side-effects, and by the fact that they may suppress pyrexia. Oral acetaminophen is recommended until these potential confounding effects are of no significant clinical concern. Table 66.3 includes dosing data for acetaminophen and the NSAIDs [47].

Tricyclic antidepressants

Tricyclic antidepressants (TCAs) classically are used to treat depression. They have analgesic effects independent of their antidepressant effect, providing pain relief in the nondepressed patient or providing pain relief, without affecting mood, in the depressed patient [48–50]. Moreover, the analgesic effects of many TCAs occur at lower dose and blood levels of drug than those which produce antidepressant effects.

Tricyclic antidepressants are thought to relieve pain by altering the serotonin (5-HT) and norepinephrine (NE) levels in the descending antinociceptive modulating system. Animal studies suggest that 5-HT specificity is important in producing analgesia, but this may not be the case in humans [46] where both 5-HT and NE enhancement are effective [51–53].

TCA administration in HCT

There is considerable concern about the use of TCAs in the HCT patient, as many TCAs appear to have marrow suppressant effects [54]. Clinical experience indicates that up to 25% of HCT patients will have significant marrow suppression in the early engraftment period with either TCAs or the newer selective serotonergic reuptake inhibitors (SSRIs). If TCAs are used, it is desirable to begin with a low dose, e.g. 10 mg amitriptyline, and titrate upwards against side-effects, which often are the limiting factors. A useful tactic is to have the patient take the drug at bedtime so that sedation and other side-effects are less problematic or can even be useful in helping sleep. All TCAs have long elimination half-lives. The analgesic effects of TCAs can occur within days or weeks, making it necessary to monitor clinical and hematologic function frequently.

TCAs for neuropathic pain

An extensive literature on TCAs for neuropathic pain exists (see the section on Neuropathic pain below for details).

Opioids in the management of pain

Drugs that produce analgesia by stimulating morphine-accepting CNS receptors are colloquially referred to as narcotic analgesics. It is more appropriate to refer to these drugs as "opioids", rather than "narcotics". Semantically, this term associates the drugs with opium, the source of the prototype drug, morphine. "Narcotic" is a legislative, administrative or legal word, which is applied to a number of psychoactive drugs with abuse potential. In the current social and legislative atmosphere, the word "narcotic" should be avoided in medical settings.

The avoidance of the use of opioids by patients or health care professionals in circumstances where they could be used safely and appropriately is a grave disservice to those suffering from treatable pain. Opioids are not without liabilities, but the incidence and severity are often overstated. Pain relief is integral to humane treatment and, indeed, has been shown to attenuate disease in animals [55,56].

Table 66.3 Dosing data for acetaminophen and nonsteroidal anti-inflammatory drugs (NSAIDs). (Adapted and modified from [47].)

Drug	Usual dose for adults and children >50 kg body weight	Usual dose for children* and adults† <50 kg body weight
Acetaminophen‡	650 mg/4 h	10–15 mg/kg/4 h
	975 mg/6 h	15–20 mg/kg/4 h (rectal)
Aspirin§	650 mg/4 h	10–15 mg/kg/4 h
	975 mg/4 h	15–20 mg/kg/4 h (rectal)
Carboprofen	100 mg TID	
Choline magnesium trisalicylate¶	1000–1500 mg TID	25 mg/kg TID
Choline salicylate¶	870 mg/3–4 h	
Diflunisal‖	500 mg/12 h	
Etodolac	200–400 mg/6–8 h	
Fenoprofen calcium	300–600 mg/6 h	
Ibuprofen	400–600 mg/6 h	10 mg/kg/6–8 h
Ketoprofen	25–60 mg/6–8 h	
Ketorolac tromethamine oral**	10 mg/4–6 h (to a maximum of 40 mg/day)	
Ketorolac tromethamine intravenous**††	30 mg initially, then 15 mg/8 h	
Magnesium salicylate	650 mg/4 h	
Meclofenamate‡‡	50–100 mg/6 h	
Naproxen	250–275 mg/6–8 h	5 mg/kg/8 h
Naproxen sodium	275 mg/6–8 h	
Sodium salicylate	325–650 mg/3–4 h	
Celecoxib§§	200 mg/day	
Rofecoxib§§	12.5–25 mg/day	

*Only drugs that are Food and Drug Administration approved as an analgesic for use in children are included.
†Acetaminophen and NSAID dosages for adults weighing less than 50 kg should be adjusted for weight.
‡No antiplatelet activity.
§The standard against which other NSAIDs are compared. May inhibit platelet aggregation for more than 1 week and may cause bleeding. Aspirin is contraindicated in children with fever or other viral disease because of its association with Reye's syndrome.
¶May have minimal antiplatelet activity.
‖Administration with antacids may decrease absorption.
**For short-term use (less than 5 days).
††Has the same gastointestinal toxicities as oral NSAIDs.
‡‡Coombs-positive autoimmune hemolytic anemia has been associated with prolonged use.
§§Cyclo-oxygenase-2 inhibitors.

Opioid pharmacology

Opioids act at a number of different levels of the CNS to produce analgesia.
1 They inhibit the transmission of nociceptive input in the dorsal horn of the spinal cord (Fig. 66.1).
2 They activate descending inhibitory systems in the basal ganglia (Fig. 66.1), which modulate peripheral nociceptive input at the spinal cord level.
3 They affect the limbic system, altering the emotional response to pain, thereby making it more bearable.

Opioids bind primarily to mu and kappa receptors in the CNS. Agonists, such as morphine, activate inhibitory pain pathways in both supraspinal and spinal regions. Antagonists, such as naloxone, competitively inhibit the analgesic effects of opioid agonists. Some opioid drugs exhibit both an antagonistic action (at mu receptors) and an agonist action (at kappa receptors); these "mixed agonist antagonists", such as nalbuphine and butorphanol, have clinical efficacy in HCT patients who experience a wide variety of GI syndromes, especially those associated with cramping. Medications with mixed effects can precipitate an abstinence syndrome in people already taking opioid pain relievers so they must be used with vigilance.

Opioid pharmacokinetics

A schema of opioid pharmacokinetics with various modes of administration is given in Fig. 66.5. As with many drugs, the blood levels of opioids that result can be measured and interpreted to yield a number of "half-lives". Within individual patients opioid pharmacokinetics and half-lives are very consistent. This is true to the extent that the blood levels resulting from a single dose of opioid may be used in sophisticated pharmacokinetic analyses to calculate infusion regimens that hold blood levels of opioid very close to a predetermined level [57]. However, opioid pharmacokinetics are highly variable from patient to patient, with half-lives and rates of elimination varying two- to fourfold.

Opioid pharmacodynamics

Opioids exhibit dose-dependent effects in many realms of activity. The analgesic dose–response curve of opioids is not a straight line; they have

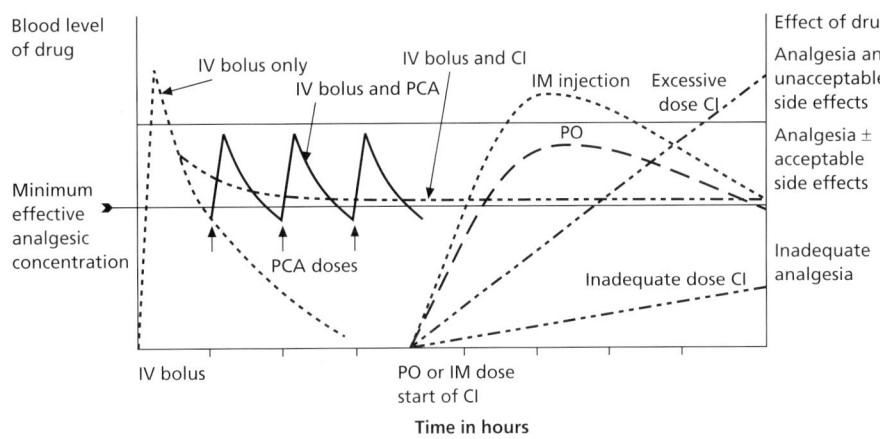

Fig. 66.5 Pharmacokinetics of opioids with various routes of administration. The "therapeutic window" of opioids is the range of blood levels of opioid within which they produce satisfactory pain relief without unacceptable side-effects. CI, continuous infusion; IM, intramuscular; IV, intravenous; PCA, patient-controlled analgesia; PO, oral. Following administration by various routes, plasma levels of opioids rise, according to the mode of administration, and then fall, depending on the speed of redistribution or elimination. As a general rule, as plasma levels of opioids rise they will reach the minimum effective analgesic concentration (MEAC) and enter the drug's therapeutic window. Rises in plasma level of drug beyond this therapeutic window produce some improvements in analgesia but large increases in the incidence and magnitude of opioid side-effects.

a threshold of efficacy and a narrow "therapeutic window" and among individuals there is a wide range of effective analgesic blood levels of drug.

A useful concept is the minimum effective analgesic concentration (MEAC), the blood level of opioid at which a patient reports satisfactory pain relief (Figure 66.5) [58]. For an individual patient with a specific pain, the MEAC is quite consistent. However, amongst individual patients with similar pains MEACs vary over a five- to sixfold range, e.g. mean morphine MEAC is 16 ng/mL (range 6–33 ng/mL) and mean meperidine MEAC is 455 ng/mL (range 94–754 ng/mL) [59].

The variability of individual MEAC, in conjunction with the individually variable drug half-lives and speeds of elimination, results in a wide range of opioid regimens necessary to maintain analgesic blood levels. The practical manifestation is that opioid regimens must be individualized, based on the effects of the drug, which in practice are derived from patient report of pain relief and occurrence of side-effects.

Opioid side-effects

Opioids have a wide variety of side-effects, many of which will abate or disappear with exposure over a several day period.

Gastrointestinal effects

Opioids slow gastric emptying and intestinal transit. They change the motor activity of the gut to magnify the individual peristaltic waves but reduce their frequency. Constipation, nausea, vomiting and a sense of fullness are the most common problems.

Genitourinary effects

Increased tone and contractility of ureters and increased detrusor tone may lead to urinary retention.

Sedation

Sedation is an almost universal side-effect of opioids. Typically, the sedation will resolve within 72 h of initiating opioid therapy. In the HCT patient receiving opioids, not all sedation is caused by opioids; other culprits include CNS active drugs (antiemetics, anxiolytics, antihistamines, cyclosporine), metabolic derangements (renal dysfunction, hypo- or hypernatremia), fatigue (sleep deprivation, disturbed biorhythms) and the prodrome of sepsis. If sedation does not spontaneously resolve, and the opioids are providing good pain control, small doses of methylphenidate (5–10 mg two or three times daily) will reverse this side-effect (avoid giving methylphenidate after mid afternoon).

Euphoria

Opioid euphoria is rare in the HCT patient.

Dysphoria

If dysphoria occurs, it is usually early during opioid exposure and progressively declines with more prolonged exposure.

Nausea and vomiting

Opioids cause nausea and vomiting in about 20% of patients either by direct stimulation of the chemotactic trigger zone (CTZ) or by sensitizing the vestibular apparatus (patients with a history of motion sickness are especially vulnerable). If nausea and vomiting are caused by opioids, they usually occur early in the course of treatment and are temporally related to an opioid dose change. Management strategies include changing opioid, using smaller doses given more frequently or adding antiemetics.

Confusion, hallucinations and delusions

These CNS symptoms, more accurately called "delirium", occur in 10–15% of HCT patients receiving opioids. The most common manifestations are conversations with people who are not present or beliefs that something has been seen or done that others do not know about. Surprisingly, these often do not upset or scare the patient and nothing needs to be done except to assure the patient and family that these are common experiences with the medication and will resolve quickly as medication is tapered with pain resolution. When these hallucinations or delusions take on a frightening quality, factors other than the opioid likely are contributing. For patients in whom symptoms are disturbing or threaten safety, treatment strategies include changing opioid or adding small doses of an antipsychotic such as haloperidol to the regimen, e.g. 1–2 mg intravenously every 4–6 h. If symptoms fail to abate, or if excessively large doses are required (more than 4 mg of haloperidol every 4 h), every effort should be made to look for a metabolic cause to the delirium, including sepsis or impending organ failure.

Respiratory depression

When monitored by sensitive indices, all opioids blunt the respiratory drive in a dose-dependent fashion. In the dose range that produces analgesia, respiratory depression (defined as $Paco_2 > 42$ torr) is uncommon. Patients with pre-existing respiratory disease, sleep apnea-like symptoms and those receiving other CNS active drugs, especially benzodiazepines, are most at risk of respiratory depression. The degree of

Table 66.4 Dose equivalents and starting doses for opioid analgesics. (Adapted and modified from [47].)

Drug	Approximate equi-analgesic dose (mg)		Usual starting dose			
			>50 kg	>50 kg	<50 kg	<50 kg
	Oral	Parenteral	Oral	Parenteral	Oral	Parenteral
Morphine	30	10	30 mg/3–4 h	10 mg/3–4 h	0.3 mg/kg/3–4 h	0.1 mg/kg/3–4 h
Hydromorphone	7–15	1.5–3.5	6 mg/3–4 h	1.5 mg/3–4 h	0.06 mg/kg/3–4 h	0.015 mg/kg/3–4 h
Oxycodone	30	N/A	10 mg/3–4 h	N/A	0.2 mg/kg/3–4 h	N/A
Hydrocodone	30	N/A	10 mg/3–4 h	N/A	0.2 mg/kg/3–4 h	N/A
Methadone	10–20	10	10–20 mg/6–8 h	10 mg/6–8 h	0.1–0.2 mg/kg/6–8 h	0.1 mg/kg/6–8 h
Levorphanol	2	1	4 mg/6–8 h	2 mg/6–8 h	0.04 mg/kg/6–8 h	0.02 mg/kg/6–8 h
Meperidine	100	100	N/R	100 mg/2–3 h	N/R	0.75 mg/kg/2–3 h
Codeine	200	130	60 mg/3–4 h	60 mg/2–3 h	0.5–1 mg/kg/6–8 h	N/R
Sufentanil	N/A	0.01	N/A	10 μg/10 min	N/A	0.1 μg/kg/10 min
Fentanyl	0.2 (transmucosal)	0.1	200–400 μg/h	50 μg/10 min	2–4 μg/kg/h	1–2 μg/kg/10 min

N/A, not available; N/R, not recommended.

respiratory depression parallels slowing respiratory rate and degree of sedation; these signs can be monitored if respiratory depression is a concern.

Tolerance

Tolerance is the progressively decreasing effect (analgesic or other effects) of a given dose of drug when that dosage is administered repetitively. Tolerance may be seen when a patient who has been achieving satisfactory analgesia with a given dosage of drug progressively fails to achieve analgesia without evidence of an increase in nociception. If it occurs in the HCT patient, tolerance may be overcome by increasing the dosage of drug or changing to a different opioid. Tolerance is a drug-related effect only and has little or no relation to addiction.

Incomplete cross-tolerance

When changing from one opioid to another, it often takes less than an equi-analgesic dose of the second opioid (Table 66.4). This phenomenon is observed frequently; the mechanisms are not completely understood. If there is a need to switch opioid medications, a good rule of thumb is to give approximately two-thirds of an equi-analgesic dose and provide liberal amounts of breakthrough medication until a new equilibrium is established. Although most opioid-related side-effects dissipate spontaneously after a few days, a change can provide analgesia at "lower" dosage of the second drug and, perhaps, with a lower side-effect profile.

Physical dependence

Physical dependence is characterized by the occurrence of an abstinence syndrome (yawning, lacrimation, sneezing, agitation, tremors, fever, tachycardia and other signs of sympathetic arousal) if the opioid abruptly is withdrawn. Like tolerance, dependence is a drug characteristic not a patient characteristic, and is a separate entity from addiction. Few patients who are opioid-dependent are addicts (see below). Abstinence syndromes can be avoided by slow reduction of opioid dosage (10–20% every day or every other day) or by using adrenergic alpha 2 agonists such as clonidine, which mask some of the peripheral adrenergic symptoms [47]. Using the strategies described below (see section on Opioid tapering, p. 904), it is rare to get a true abstinence syndrome when opioids are used with HCT patients.

Psychologic dependence (addiction)

This complication is characterized by an abnormal pattern of drug use; of drug craving for effects other than pain relief; by an overwhelming involvement with procuring and consuming the drug, even when such activity is contrary to the individual's best interests; and with a tendency to relapse into drug use after tapering off the drug. Addiction is the conjunction of genetic, psychologic, social and cultural factors that affect an individual. Unlike tolerance and physical dependence, psychologic dependence is a patient issue, not a drug issue.

Patients with no previous history of substance abuse who receive opioids therapeutically have an extremely low incidence of iatrogenic addiction, of the order of 1/2000–4000 [60]. Therefore, in patients with no history of substance abuse, fear of psychologic dependence should not be a concern.

Opioids commonly used in the HCT patient

Table 66.4 includes a list of opioids, their approximate equi-analgesic doses and dosage intervals for oral or intravenous use. The choice of agent should be limited to opioid agonists. The following are commonly used opioids in the HCT patient and some of their specific complications.

Morphine

The prototypical opioid agonist morphine can be given by any route but has low oral bioavailability (Table 66.4). Oral duration of effect is 3–5 h, which can be extended to 6–12 h by the use of sustained release preparations. Morphine is conjugated in the liver to two major metabolites, 3-glucuronide and 6-glucuronide, which may produce unintended side-effects (sedation, confusion). Glucuronidation is a high-capacity conjugative pathway in the liver so morphine is relatively safe to use in patients with moderate degrees of hepatic failure. Because both glucuronides are excreted by the kidneys, morphine should be used cautiously in patients with any degree of renal impairment. On initial use, morphine has a 15–25% incidence of pruritus, or nausea and vomiting, which often diminish with use over a few days.

Meperidine (Demerol)

This opioid agonist has about one-tenth of the potency of morphine.

Meperidine is metabolized to normeperidine, a renally excreted metabolite, which has pronounced excitatory and convulsive effects. In patients with normal renal function, normeperidine levels do not become problematic until relatively large doses of the parent drug have been administered over a prolonged period of time, e.g. 800–900 mg/day over about 5–7 days. However, if used as an analgesic, this meperidine dosage could be met or exceeded in the HCT patient. Thus, patients with normal renal function should be restricted to short-term low-dose use, e.g. for chills and premedication before platelet transfusions. In patients with abnormal renal function, meperidine should be avoided, or its use greatly restricted.

Hydromorphone (Dilaudid)

This agonist has a spectrum of effects similar to morphine. Hydromorphone is thought to be 5–8 times more potent than morphine, although data from the HCT population support a dose equivalency of about 3 [47,61]. It is generally believed to have fewer side-effects than morphine; this belief is not substantiated by double blind studies [62]. It is metabolized to a number of renally excreted metabolites, which appear to be pharmacologically inert. Hence, hydromorphone is a good choice of opioid in patients with impaired renal function or those with unacceptable side-effects with morphine. In some countries, sustained release preparations are available for ambulatory patients with persistent pain syndromes who are able to swallow.

Fentanyl

This is a classic agonist with a spectrum of effects similar to morphine. It is 100 times more potent than morphine and has a faster onset of effect. In short-term use it has a relatively short duration of effect, but in longer term use its duration of effect is similar to hydromorphone. Fentanyl is metabolized to a number of pharmacologically inert metabolites and is a good choice of opioid in a patient with impaired renal function or those with unacceptable side-effects with morphine or hydromorphone. Fentanyl is predominantly administered intravenously. It is also available as an oral transmucosal product, which is useful in some HCT patients. Transdermal fentanyl (Duragesic), is a useful alternative to intravenous opioids for patients needing long-term stable dosage, in the absence of fever and with intact skin. It should be noted that the patch takes 16–24 h to achieve stable plasma levels of drug and, conversely, when the patch is removed it takes 16–24 h for plasma levels of drug to fall.

Butorphanol

This is a mixed agonist–antagonist with marked kappa agonist effect and moderate mu antagonist effect. It is a useful drug for HCT patients in treating the pain from graft-vs.-host disease (GVHD) of the gut. Compared to mu agonists, it is believed to impair visceral nociceptive transmission more and yet cause less gut stasis. Butorphanol may be given intravenously or by nasal inhalation. It is not recommended for moderate to severe pain syndromes because it has a relatively low analgesic ceiling and can precipitate abstinence syndrome if a patient is on other opioids [47].

Nalbuphine

This is another mixed kappa agonist–mu antagonist opioid. It effectively treats opioid-induced pruritus without reversing analgesia. Additionally, clinical experience has demonstrated efficacy in treating pruritus associated with cholestasis [63,64].

Tramadol

This is a centrally acting synthetic analgesic. It has weak opioid activity and inhibits reuptake of both serotonin and norepinephrine. The side-effect profile is similar to opioids; respiratory depression may occur with overdose and an abstinence syndrome can occur with abrupt withdrawal.

Opioid use in clinical practice

The basic precept in providing analgesia with opioids is to raise and maintain the patient's plasma level of opioid above the patient's MEAC and within the therapeutic window. Consult Fig. 66.5 to help understand the following paragraphs.

Oral administration

Opioids are readily absorbed by the gut but undergo extensive first-pass metabolism by the liver so that to produce a given blood level the oral dose may be 3–6 times the parenteral dose (Table 66.4). After oral administration, blood levels rise slowly, reach the effective range in 30–45 min, and stay within the therapeutic window for about 3–4 h; hence 3–4-hourly dosing is necessary, except with methadone which is effective taken every 6 h. Slow release preparations extend this dosing schedule to 8–12 h.

Rectal administration

This route should be avoided in the HCT patient because of the bacterial shower produced by inserting a suppository.

Intramuscular and subcutaneous opioids

Intramuscular (IM) and subcutaneous (SC) opioids are rarely used in the HCT population as frequent doses may be necessary and the mixture of IM/SC injections and thrombocytopenia results in hematoma formation.

Intravenous bolus

Intravenous bolus dosing rapidly raises the plasma level of a drug. However, the drug is then rapidly redistributed and metabolized, and blood levels fall quickly. Consequently, therapeutic levels above MEAC are maintained for only a short period of time, less than 30 min. Intravenous bolus administration is widely used in the HCT population as most patients have indwelling venous access. The drug reliably and rapidly reaches its targets.

Fixed rate (continuous) infusion

Infusions of opioid take a long time to raise plasma levels to the effective range, leaving the patient in pain. Moreover, to choose an infusion rate that will maintain an effective plasma level of opioid, the rate at which the individual patient metabolizes and excretes the opioid must be known. Chosen infusion rates can be excessive, leading to plasma levels of drug rising into the toxic range, or inadequate, leading to plasma levels falling into the poor analgesia range (Fig. 66.5).

Intravenous bolus followed by a fixed rate infusion

An intravenous bolus will rapidly raise plasma levels of drug to therapeutic levels which then can be sustained with continuous infusion. Patient report will determine the initial effective bolus (loading) dose. An hourly infusion rate equal to approximately 20% of the effective loading dose usually provides good relief. Intensive nurse monitoring is necessary to guarantee relief and avoid overdose.

Patient controlled analgesia

In the early 1970s the revolutionary concept that patients might be capable of acting as their own "sensor" of pain relief and analgesic need was advanced. The concept held that if patients were given as-needed access to opioids, they would titrate their dose to keep plasma concentrations at analgesic levels, close to MEAC, thereby achieving satisfactory analgesia and would not over or under use the opioid, even when the drug was taken over long periods of time. This concept reached clinical reality with the advent of computerized pumps which enable patients to self-administer

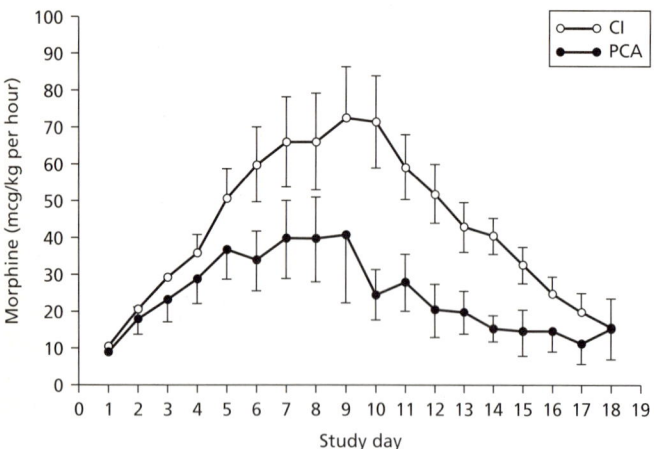

Fig. 66.6 Daily mean morphine dose for adolescents with mucositis pain during HCT. Morphine delivered by physician-prescribed continuous infusion (CI) or by PCA (patient-controlled anagesia). As the apin worsened the PCA patients delivered more drug, and as the mucositis healed they automatically tapered their dosage. Note also the lesser amount of drug used by the PCA patients, even though pain scores were very similar in the two groups. Reproduced with permission from Mackie *et al.* [65]. (Results have been the same in adults [18].)

small doses of opioids at frequent intervals, the clinical technique of patient controlled analgesia (PCA).

The plasma levels of drug, which result from a loading dose plus PCA, are shown in Fig. 66.5. By individualizing the dosage of opioid, allowing the patient to titrate to effect, PCA circumvents the problems posed by other modes of administration: variations in MEAC; pharmacokinetic differences; changes in degree of nociception. Virtually all adult patients have the cognitive and discriminative ability to use PCA. PCA can be used reliably by children down to at least the age of 12 years [65] and may even be safely and successfully used in some children down to the age of 4 or 5 years [66]. Current clinical practice is to offer PCA to younger children, provided they are able to grasp the concept and use the technique. If a child can play a video game, he or she can probably use a PCA.

In HCT patients the classical instance of PCA use is for mucositis pain. As the mucositis pain becomes worse patients use more drug and then, as their mouth and throat heal and the pain lessens, they naturally taper their opioid dose (Fig. 66.6). In randomized controlled clinical trials, testing patients with PCA vs. continuous infusions of opioid for mucositis pain, patients using PCA tend to have lower pain scores and use less drug over shorter periods of time, hence a tendency to have fewer side-effects [67]. PCA pumps have various parameters that must be defined for safe and effective use. When used effectively, PCA can decrease nursing time, provide more timely pain relief and involve the patient importantly in symptom relief.

PCA bolus dose

Initial bolus sizes are 0.5–2 mg morphine (10–30 µg/kg) in adults and 10–20 µg/kg in children, or equivalent doses of other drugs. As nociception and pain worsen, bolus size should be increased; if nociception and pain become less, dose size should be decreased. Experience has shown that the optimal bolus size is one that permits the patient's 24-h drug need, obtained from the nursing records or the PCA pump memory, delivered in 25–40 doses.

PCA lock-out interval

After a bolus of opioid has been delivered, the pump will not deliver another dose for this set interval—usually 6–10 min. This is a safety feature as it prevents the administration of a further dose of drug until after the patient has had the opportunity to experience the effects (analgesia, sedation) of the previous dose.

PCA plus fixed infusion

PCA alone has some disadvantages. If a patient sleeps or is disconnected from the intravenous drip and does not self-administer opioid, blood levels of drug will fall. The patient may then have difficulty in self-administering sufficient drug to raise the blood level of opioid back into analgesic range. To circumvent this problem, PCA pumps have a constant infusion option. This option should not be used until a patient has established his or her individual dose requirement, i.e. by opioid use via the PCA alone. For example, a patient has used 84 mg morphine in the previous 24 h. This averages 3.5 mg/h morphine. It is advised that the infusion be set at not greater than 30–50% of the expected opioid need with some day/night variability as needed—in this case 1.0–1.8 mg/h. In addition to helping with sleep, the addition of an infusion means that the blood levels of opioid fall more slowly after each PCA dose, giving the patient a longer period between the need for repeat PCA doses. Studies in postoperative patients using PCA for 24–48 h have not shown a marked improvement in analgesia by the addition of an infusion to PCA [68,69]. None the less, there is a strong body of opinion that the addition of an infusion to a PCA improves the quality of analgesia in HCT patients when pain persists over days, and can help with sleep.

Opioid tapering

Some HCT patients have pain problems of extended duration, which necessitate opioid therapy for long periods of time. Usually, as the pain problem diminishes, a patient's PCA or oral self-administered opioid dosage is gradually reduced and ultimately eliminated. However, with relatively long-term use (10–14 days) a patient may be physically dependent on the opioid; abrupt cessation of opioid intake may precipitate an abstinence syndrome. In the HCT patient, these symptoms can be confused with stress reactions or can be attributed to infectious or symptoms of GVHD. It is important that both the physician and patient understand that these symptoms are entirely unrelated to addiction (see sections on Physical dependence and Psychologic dependence above [47]); and that even if an abstinence syndrome does occur it is rarely physically dangerous and does not have sinister long-term implications, although it is most unpleasant. The onset of these symptoms can occur within 6–12 h after an opioid dose reduction and peak at 24–72 h. For both humanitarian and treatment success reasons, any tapering process should be designed to minimize the possibility of an abstinence syndrome, and if an abstinence syndrome occurs, it should be treated by using small doses of opioid until symptoms dissipate.

Practical realities of tapering

All patients should be watched closely for abstinence symptoms because they may not be aware that their experiences are related to opioid dose changes. If an abstinence syndrome does occur, an intravenous infusion or PCA dosing schedule that eliminates symptoms is the first intervention. This dose is then reduced by about 10–20% a day, assuming the pain or abstinence syndrome does not reappear [58].

For ambulatory patients, continuous monitoring for symptoms by medical staff is not possible and therefore a slower taper is advised. One simple method is the "pill count". The patient is prescribed the usual opioid in a tablet preparation and is instructed to take it on a time contingent basis (consistent with the duration of effect of the opioid) rather than as needed. Reductions of 10–20% of the dose are successively made until the patient is taking no drug. Immediate-release opioid preparations usually provide greater dosage flexibility than do sustained release preparations, which cannot be divided. Peripheral adrenergic symptoms during the taper can be avoided or masked by using adrenergic alpha-2-agonists such as clonidine [47].

For more complex patients, such as those who are overly focused on the dose or number of tablets, an alternative to the pill count method is to use "pain cocktail" [70,71]. In this strategy the patient's mean daily intake of opioid is combined into a fixed volume of a taste-masked liquid vehicle, e.g. cherry syrup, and the volume is split into regularly scheduled doses appropriate to the expected duration of action of the drug. When reducing the opioid content the total daily volume stays stable, but the milligram opioid content is reduced 10–20%.

Clinical pain management in the HCT patient

Pretransplant

Approaching and entering a transplantation program is an exceedingly stressful experience for patients and may result in more vulnerability than usual to a variety of stresses, including pain. This is also a time of peak motivation to understand and participate actively in anything that will improve treatment comfort or success. Patients and families should be assured that symptom management, including pain, will be treated effectively, safely and in a timely manner. In particular, education about the appropriate and safe use of opioids in HCT is important so that fears of addiction may be dispelled prior to the need for these medications. The pretransplant period is the ideal time to learn, practice and perfect non-pharmacologic pain-relieving skills.

As the time of the transplant gets closer, analgesic drugs that may be contraindicated during the transplant (e.g. TCAs, SSRIs and NSAIDs) should be stopped and safer substitutes (e.g. opioids or shorter-acting anxiolytics, such as clonazepam) begun.

Inpatient peritransplant period

This is the most vulnerable time for the patient. Pain management measures used are those least likely to impede engraftment or to interfere with the patient's ability to function. Analgesic drugs are usually given intravenously, as patients are frequently unable to take oral medication, and intramuscular injections are contraindicated.

It is more difficult to evaluate and treat patients who use nonprescription psychoactive drugs. In these individuals, who are likely to be opioid tolerant, analgesic use is usually greater than normal, and the clinician evaluating the success of therapy may have to rely on external observable criteria rather than the usual patient report criteria. Contracts may need to be set to outline explicit behaviors that must be adhered to by the patient to ensure that drug delivery is maintained or increased. Expected behaviors can include all the self-care activities necessary, along with appropriate interactions with staff in relation to anger control, manipulations, inappropriate drug-seeking activities and number of requests for medications. When the nociceptive phase of the transplant is over, it may be necessary to impose an externally derived, relatively rigid opioid tapering schedule, rather than allowing the patient to self-taper as is normally done.

Pseudoaddiction

Care must be taken not to underdose patients who have previous—licit or illicit—experience with opioids, or who simply have high opioid requirements because of idiosyncrasies associated with the drugs. Persistent underdosing of patients leaves them in pain and often sets up a nasty cycle in which the patient continually asks for medication and the staff, frustrated, begin to deny medication or label the patient as a "drug-seeker". These behaviors can lead to accusations of addiction when it is the failure to provide adequate pain relief that is at fault.

Patients with prior history of substance abuse

Patients who have a history of substance abuse (tobacco, alcohol, illicit drugs, opioids or sedatives) may present management problems in the peri-transplant period, especially with opioid tapering. It is essential to identify these at-risk patients prior to transplant, provide adequate analgesia (see Pseudoaddiction above), set clear guidelines for acceptable behavior and be cognizant of increased opioid requirements. Opioid withdrawal may be made easier by providing time contingent medications, rather than "as needed" dosage, removing a layer of control from the patient.

The following are the most common pain problems and their management approaches.

Oropharyngeal mucositis

The chemoradiotherapeutic regimens used in HCT produce oropharyngeal muscositis (OPM), which usually begins to be painful from 2 to 7 days post-HCT. OPM generally peaks at about 9–13 days post-HCT and begins to resolve a few days after the last dose of methotrexate or when the transplant shows signs of engraftment. The pain from OPM parallels the severity of tissue damage [9]; indeed, a diminution in oropharyngeal pain will often herald the arrival of the graft. In the most aggressive conditioning regimens, the pain from OPM is sufficiently severe that 90% of patients require opioid analgesics at some point [9,72; see Chapter 13]. The duration of analgesic need may be from a few days to many (20+) days in the case of delayed engraftment. Coincident with engraftment, pain and opioid needs usually resolve over a few days to a week. If oral GVHD develops, this may significantly delay the resolution of mucositis and pain.

Topical measures are helpful. Irrespective of the extent of OPM and pain, meticulous and frequent rinsing with saline is critical to pain relief and oropharyngeal hygiene. In the early stages of OPM, the use of topical anesthetic agents (e.g. viscous lidocaine or Dyclone [chlorobutanol 0.5% solution]) may be helpful, and capsaicin also has shown efficacy [73]. As OPM increases in severity most patients stop using these agents because they burn and do not offer adequate relief. Some patients report that ice slush or chips help numb sensation and keep the oral mucosa moist. Patients also wrap small ice packs externally around the throat and jaw.

When topical measures cease to provide adequate pain relief, systemic opioids are started. Oral opioids are of limited use as patients find them difficult to swallow, nausea and vomiting are frequent, and absorption from the gut is uncertain. The systemic management of mucositis is usually accomplished by intravenous opioids, with intravenous push in the first instance and, when frequent doses are required, by PCA opioids with or without infusion in adults and children who can manage PCA, and opioid continuous infusion in young children plus bolus dosing when needed. Opioids are usually effective in relieving oral pain, less effective in relieving pharyngeal pain at rest and may have little effect on swallowing pain.

Patient controlled analgesia normally begins with 1–2 mg (20–40 µg/kg) bolus doses of morphine (or equivalent doses of other opioids) in adults and 10–20 µg/kg in children. Adjust PCA dose such that patients will have to self-administer 25–40 doses to match the previous day's opioid use. As opioid use declines, adjust PCA bolus dose down so that again patients receive the previous 24 h use in 25–40 doses (further specifics on PCA use are described above in the sections on Opioid use in clinical practice and Medication tapering).

Conditioning regimen-related cutaneous skin toxicity

In HCT this complication occurs predominantly in the hands, feet, groin and axillae but also may be localized to the genitals. The magnitude of skin disruption varies from mild erythema to frank lesions similar to second-degree burns. These will usually heal by 6–10 days post-engraftment. The skin lesions may require treatment with silver-containing creams or biologic dressings, e.g. pig skin. For mild toxicity, cold packs often supply adequate pain control. For more severe pain, opioids, as used for OPM, are appropriate.

Neuropathic-type burning pain associated with immunosuppressive drugs

A burning neuropathic-type pain in the hands and feet is classically associated with intravenous cyclosporine, but has also been observed with FK-506, VP16 and thiotepa. Pain severity is often associated with high blood levels of drug, and changing the duration of intravenous administration to 24 h continuous infusion is helpful. This pain may persist into the immediate post-transplant period. In milder cases, cooling with water, fans and ice packs is useful. If the pain becomes severe, a trial of opioids—pushing the dose until limited by side-effects—is worthwhile although this pain often does not respond to opioids. For severe cases, a trial of intravenous lidocaine to achieve "cardiac" blood levels of drug (1–2 µg/mL) is sometimes helpful.

Hepatic capsule distension

Veno-occlusive disease (VOD) of the liver may cause liver engorgement with capsular distension. Intravenous or PCA opioids as for OPM are appropriate. Patients with VOD will tolerate and metabolize opioids normally until either the VOD becomes severe (bilirubin >20 mg/dL), hepatic failure ensues (rising ammonia) or renal dysfunction occurs. It is essential to remember that the high-capacity hepatic degradation pathways may overwhelm a mildly dysfunctional kidney, leading to accumulation of degradation products, particularly important with meperidine and morphine.

Pain associated with hematopoietic growth factors

Hematopoietic growth factors may produce severe pain of rapid onset, occurring some 2–4 h after their administration. The usual sites are lower abdominal, distal femur and proximal tibia. Between these episodes patients are typically pain-free. Treatment is intravenous or PCA opioids in doses sufficiently large to abort the rapid and severe onset of this type of pain. Outpatients should have access to ample "as needed" doses of a rapid-onset oral opioid, e.g. morphine (also available in sublingual preparations), hydromorphone, oxycodone or hydrocodone, often in combination with acetaminophen.

Post-engraftment

Graft-vs.-host disease

Patients who receive allogeneic transplants are at risk for GVHD, despite prophylaxis with immunosuppressive drugs and steroids. The following are commonly occurring sites of GVHD that tend to have accompanying pain.

Oral GVHD

Oral GVHD sometimes overlaps mucositis and the pain from mucositis merges into GVHD pain. Persisting oral pain after adequate engraftment should raise suspicions of GVHD or infection. Treatment is to ensure good hygiene, use topical analgesics and oral or systemic opioids titrated to effect.

Skin GVHD

Skin GVHD pain responds to opioids. Itch is often a problem—try oral hydroxyzine or intravenous nalbuphine, as there are suspicions that itch may be mediated through systems that are opioid-sensitive [63,74].

Gut GVHD

Gut GVHD can cause pain for a variety of reasons. Bowel wall inflammation and hepatic engorgement can cause pain at rest and with movement. Vigorous peristalsis of inflamed gut can cause episodic cramping pain that is not responsive to opioids. Indeed, opioids may make the pain worse by contributing to bowel dysmotility. Clinical experience strongly suggests that kappa agonist opioids such as butorphanol produce better pain relief and less gut atony than mu agonist opioids. There may be a place for the use of invasive analgesic techniques, such as epidural analgesia, which provide potent analgesia with low-dose drug use in this circumstance. Chronic GVHD is a difficult pain management problem and long-term opioids or one of the invasive analgesic techniques should be considered.

In circumstances in which opioids are not very helpful, and pain is unpredictable and brief, as in chronic GVHD gut cramping, patients can use an image that counteracts the physical sensation combined with deep breathing. For example, a patient with a cramping pain might imagine a tight fist that progressively relaxes as he or she blows out each slow deep breath. Or, in the case of burning pain, the patient might imagine breathing arctic air through the hot body part and watching as the red turns to orange and cools to green or blue. Both adults and children have used this method to shorten the duration of pain.

Pain associated with steroid tapering

This usually occurs at the time that steroids are being tapered slowly. Typically, the pain is severe, of rapid onset and short duration, usually occurs in the distal femur and proximal tibia in the small hours of the morning. This pain is usually responsive to opioids—but doses need to be large enough to abort the pain episode (compare with pain caused by growth factors).

Pain associated with herpes zoster

The acute episode is painful in some 75% of cases. Pain may persist beyond the acute episode and, if this persists beyond about 1 month after the onset of symptoms, it may be caused by peripheral nerve damage and is therefore termed post-herpetic neuralgia (PHN). In the acute episode, nonopioids and opioid analgesics are appropriate and effective. For PHN, nonopioid and opioid analgesics are relatively ineffectual. With PHN three types of pain, which respond to differing therapeutic modalities, occur.

1 Severe skin sensitivity with pain to the slightest touch (allodynia). Try EMLA cream (a 2.4% lidocaine/2.5% prilocaine mixture applied topically) or newer preparations such as lidocaine patches [75]. Effective systemic drugs include anticonvulsants and TCAs (see section below on Neuropathic pain).
2 Episodic shooting pain best thought of as an epileptiform discharge from damaged dorsal horn neurons. Treat with the anticonvulsants phenytoin or gabapentin.
3 Background burning pain, which is the most common form of PHN. This responds best to TCAs [52,53] and occasionally to opioids.

Prevention of PHN has been the subject of various studies. The early suggestion that corticosteroids might prevent PHN [76] has not been confirmed [77]. More recent studies strongly suggest that early use of antiviral medications may reduce the incidence and duration of PHN [78,79]. Even more exciting is gathering evidence that early sympathetic blockade (e.g. by using epidural analgesia) shortens the acute phase and reduces incidence, duration and severity of PHN [80,81]. Combined with antiviral therapy, this would now appear to be the intervention of choice, especially in patients over 50 years.

Neuropathic pain

Damage to parts of the nervous system lacking specialized nociceptors can create neuropathic pain. Such pain typically is out of proportion to the stimulus intensity and primarily involves activity of large A fibers. Neuropathic pain often is associated with sensory or autonomic nervous system dysfunction, described as "burning", "raw", "gnawing", "aching" or "tightness", and also is associated with shooting shock-like pain. Common causes include exposure to chemotherapeutic agents, particularly vinca alkaloids, damage to large neural plexi by radiation or surgery, spinal cord compression or nerve root infiltration in conditions such as herpes zoster.

TCAs for neuropathic pain

Many HCT patients will have neuropathic pain. There have been no clinical trials of TCA analgesic efficacy in these conditions, but it is probably reasonable to extrapolate data from the available trials of TCA analgesic efficacy, usually diabetic neuropathy or PHN models, to the HCT population [82]. Compared to placebo, amitriptyline, imipramine and desipramine produce benefits in neuropathic pain when administered in either low dose or high dose [49,51,53,83,84]. Benefits appear after about 2 weeks; a frank correlation between blood level of drug and analgesic efficacy has not been established. Amitriptyline is probably the drug of choice but desipramine is a good alternative with similar efficacy and possibly fewer side-effects [52,53]. Evidence thus far does not support a similar analgesic efficacy for the SSRIs, although studies are still underway [53].

Anticonvulsants for neuropathic pain

A wide variety of anticonvulsants, including carbamazepine, phenytoin, valproic acid and clonazepam, have been used to treat neuropathic pain, with some success [82,85]. The more recently developed anticonvulsant gabapentin, however, appears to be more effective, safer and better tolerated by cancer patients [86,87].

Topical preparations for neuropathic pain

Topical application of lidocaine patches [88,89] and capsaicin [90,91] have successfully been used to control peripheral neuropathic pain. Topical capsaicin has been used to treat mucocutaneous neuropathic pain, such as oral mucositis [73], although it is recommended only for early or mild cases because capsaicin can cause severe pain by releasing substance P.

Opioid treatment of neuropathic pain

The historical dogma that opioids are ineffective in the treatment of neuropathic pain has been shown to be false [92–94]. Neuropathic pain does respond to opioid treatment, but may require higher doses than in treatment of nociceptive pain. Furthermore, adjunctive treatments may enhance and complement analgesia provided by opioids in the setting of neuropathic cancer pain [95]. It is often helpful to treat neuropathic pain with opioids until the effect plateaus or unacceptable side-effects emerge.

Pain associated with diagnostic or therapeutic maneuvers

Post-lumbar puncture headache

Post-lumbar puncture headache (PLPHA) is believed to be caused by a continuing leak of cerebrospinal fluid through the hole in the dura created by the lumbar puncture (LP). This leak causes a low-pressure headache or pressure or traction on the base of brain structures as they migrate distally through the foramen magnum. LPs should be performed with the smallest needles possible, certainly no bigger than 22 G, and preferably 25 G. With a 22 G needle the incidence of PLPHA is 20–30% in 20–30-year-olds but only 2–3% in those over 60 years.

A classic PLPHA is an occiput to frontal headache that occurs after an LP and which is exquisitely sensitive to positional changes. It may be associated with photophobia, nausea, vomiting, tinnitus, diplopia and changes in auditory and visual acuity. Not all headaches post-LP are PLPHAs. Patients with a history of headaches are more likely to get a headache post-lumbar puncture, but whether these are PLPHAs is often debatable.

Prophylactic measures to minimize the incidence of PLPHA include:
- using small needles, preferably those with noncutting "pencil point" tips, such as Whitacre or Sprotte needles;
- single punctures; and
- lying flat after the LP, presumably allowing the dural hole to heal. A 1-h initial period followed by as much time as possible recumbent for 24 h is advised.

Once a headache has occurred a variety of treatments can be used.
- Bed rest, mild analgesics and copious fluids.
- Caffeine infusion, 500 mg in 500–1000 mL over 1–2 h, repeated twice.
- Wearing an abdominal binder while out of bed. This increases intra-abdominal pressure, increases epidural blood flow, and reduces transdural pressure gradients thus reducing cerebrospinal fluid loss.
- Epidural blood patch. This is achieved by carrying out an epidural puncture at the site of the LP and then instilling 10–15 mL of the patient's own blood into the epidural space at the site of the previous puncture. The blood either decreases the transdural pressure gradient, allowing the hole to heal, or acts as "physiologic glue", sealing the hole. Epidural blood patches should be used with caution in the HCT patient because of the risk of creating an epidural hematoma in the coagulation-impaired patient and of introducing a perfect bacterial culture medium close to the neuraxis in an immunocompromised patient.

Surgical pain

HCT patients often undergo a number of procedures, ranging from the simple, with little postoperative pain (e.g. indwelling central line placement), to the complex and painful (e.g. lung biopsy). The management of postoperative pain in HCT patients should be aggressive. Invasive techniques, such as epidural catheters for administration of spinal opioids and local anesthetics, should be weighed carefully. After thoracic and abdominal surgery, epidural analgesia can aid pulmonary function and overall activity but there is a small risk of infection at the catheter site [96,97].

Analgesia/sedation for painful and unpleasant procedures

HCT patients have to undergo a number of different painful, unpleasant and anxiety-provoking procedures. In small children, the only way these can be accomplished is under deep sedation or general anesthesia. Preprocedure fears and intraprocedure discomforts can be managed in a variety of ways.

Nonpharmacologic management of procedures

Cognitive–behavioral and physical methods can be effective for both pre-procedural anxiety and for active distraction during procedures [98]. These methods require patients to be alert; even moderate sedation with benzodiazepines disrupts effectiveness of these methods. Relaxation and imagery can effect cognitive distraction and reduce physical stress.

Pharmacologic management of procedures

Pharmacologic management can take a variety of forms, depending on the procedure, the patient and local resources. Adults will often tolerate procedures with local anesthetic and a minimum of CNS active drug. Children are likely to need more CNS active drugs. In increasing order of complexity and invasiveness, the following techniques can be used.

Cutaneous local anesthetic

A 1-h cutaneous application of EMLA cream will produce dense skin anesthesia. Infiltration of skin and deep structures with percutaneous local anesthetic is highly efficacious. Local anesthetics do not work instantaneously and it is good practice to leave the local anesthetic in place for about 5 min before attempting any potentially painful maneuver. The addition of 2–3 mL standard sterile sodium bicarbonate solution into a 30-mL vial of 1% lidocaine reduces or eliminates the stinging pain of injection.

Premedication

Small doses of an anxiolytic (e.g. midazolam) and a short-acting opioid (e.g. fentanyl) prior to the procedure makes injection of local anesthetic more pleasant for patients. Patients will often have no recollection of the procedure but recall the experience pleasantly, even when there were difficulties or the patient expressed discomfort.

Conscious sedation

Conscious sedation is achieved with short-acting opioids and sedatives, given in doses such that patients remain responsive to verbal stimuli and are able to protect their airway and breath spontaneously. Only qualified nurses and physicians should provide conscious sedation because of the potential need, albeit small, for airway support.

Deep sedation and general anesthesia

The continuum from conscious sedation to deep sedation, when the patient is virtually unarousable, to general anesthesia, when the patient is rendered unconscious, is indistinct. Whereas well-trained nurses can administer conscious sedation safely, only those providers who are highly skilled in airway management and interventions for cardiovascular instability should provide deep sedation and general anesthesia. The American Society of Pediatrics has provided practice guidelines for such situations [99].

Invasive analgesic techniques in the HCT patient

In the non-HCT population, patients whose longer term nociceptive pain is poorly managed by systemic analgesics are candidates for one of a number of potent but invasive analgesic techniques. In HCT patients, these techniques have been used infrequently because of the risks of hematoma and infection. Post-HCT, there are patients with severe pain problems that are not responsive to systemic analgesics, e.g. chronic gut GVHD or pathologic fractures, who should be considered for these potent techniques. Examples of the techniques, their potential indications in the HCT patient and potential complications are as follow.
1 Peripheral nerve blocks with local anesthetic for pain in well-circumscribed anatomic distributions; e.g. intercostal blocks may be appropriate for fractured ribs, chest tube placement or following thoracotomy.
2 Sympathetic nerve blocks with local anesthetic in conditions that have a sympathetic nervous system mediated component; e.g. stellate ganglion blocks may be appropriate for head and neck herpes zoster.
3 Neurodestructive sympathetic nerve blocks for pain that is likely to be long-standing and resistant to other analgesics; e.g. neurodestructive celiac plexus block may sometimes be considered for pain associated with intra-abdominal candidiasis.
4 Neuraxial (epidural or subarachnoid) blocks with either opioids or local anesthetic. The techniques may be used on a short-term basis; e.g. for postoperative pain after thoracic or abdominal surgery, via percutaneously inserted catheters. For pain of likely longer duration (e.g. gut GVHD), more complex and expensive implanted systems may be considered.

Analgesia and sedation in dying patients

In providing pharmacologic relief of discomfort in the dying, the choice of the most effective and least burdensome route of drug delivery is often a problem. Choosing the route of drug administration in the HCT patient is simplified by the fact that most have indwelling central venous catheters. The fundamental drug in providing comfort care is an opioid. The choice of opioid may be suggested by what has been used effectively earlier in the patient's course. Both continuous infusion of opioids and PCA have a part to play, although as the patient's condition deteriorates he or she will less likely be able to use PCA effectively. If patients are not receiving any opioid, one should start with either PCA or continuous infusion as for mucositis and adjust dosage upwards based on response. If patients are receiving opioids, dosage should be adjusted up to achieve comfort. It is often necessary to use high doses of opioid to obtain comfort, and the usual dose increases may be inadequate. In these circumstances, a bolus dose of 1-h worth of opioid, followed by an increase of 25–50%, may be necessary. The occurrence of unwanted side-effects, such as nausea, delirium, agitation, tremulousness or other CNS phenomena, can be treated by changing to an equi-analgesic dose of another opioid or by the addition of further CNS active drugs, including low-dose (0.5–1 mg/kg) ketamine once or twice a day [100].

In the event opioids do not provide adequate comfort, especially with inadequate control of anxiety or tremulousness, sedative drugs such as benzodiazepines or barbiturates should be considered. Initial benzodiazepine regimens would be 1–2 mg/h midazolam or 1–2 mg/h lorazepam; dose increases of 25–50% are appropriate. As with opioids, substantial doses may be needed. A further useful category of drug is the butyrophenones, such as haloperidol and droperidol. These can be used to treat delirium and confusion, and in association with opioids may produce a calm neuroleptic-like state. Specimen regimens would be 0.25–1.0 mg/kg haloperidol or 0.1–0.2 mg droperidol IV every 4–6 h. In the terminal stages agitation may require the use of classical CNS depressants such as barbiturates (1–2 mg/kg bolus and continuous infusion 1–5 mg/kg/h pentobarbital) or propofol (50–200 µg/kg/min) [101]. In some instances, comfort measures can shorten a patient's life. The Doctrine of Double Effect, which invokes the axiom that intervening on the patient's behalf may incur risks, including the possibility of death, is a well-accepted ethical principle; it protects the practitioner legally and permits extreme comfort measures in dying patients.

Conclusions

This chapter outlines the neurophysiology and pharmacology of pain, and describes the common sources of discomfort in patients undergoing HCT. The chapter provides practical guidelines for the evaluation and pharmacologic treatment of pain in HCT. Most HCT patients can be managed effectively by the oncology team. In situations where continued inadequate or ineffective analgesia prevails, it is strongly recommended that a multidisciplinary expert pain relief team be consulted and involved.

References

1 Terman G, Bonica J. Spinal mechanisms and their modulation. In: Loeser J, ed. *Bonica's Management of Pain*, 3rd edn. Philadelphia: Lippincott Williams & Wilkins, 2001: 110–25.

2 Melzack R, Wall PD. Pain mechanisms: a new theory. *Science* 1965; **150**: 971.

3 Melzack R, Wall PD. *The Challenge of Pain*. New York: Basic Books, 1982.

4 Terman G, Bonica J. Spinal mechanisms and their modulation. In: Loeser J, ed. *Bonica's Management of Pain*, 3rd edn. Philadelphia: Lippincott Williams & Wilkins, 2001: 125–40.

5 International Association for the Study of Pain. Pain terms: a list with definitions and notes on usage. *Pain* 1979; **6**: 249.

6 Loeser J. Concepts of pain. In: Stanton-Hicks M, Boas R, eds. *Chronic Low Back Pain*. New York: Raven Press, 1982, 146.

7 Chapman C, Gavrin J. Suffering: the contributions of persisting pain. *Lancet* 1999; **26**: 2233–7.

8 Mishel M. Perceived uncertainty and stress in illness. *Res Nurs Health* 1984; **7**: 163–71.

9 Syrjala K, Chapko M. Evidence for a biopsychosocial model of cancer treatment-related pain. *Pain* 1995; **61**: 69–79.

10 Thompson S. Will it hurt less if I can control it? A complex answer to a simple question. *Psychol Bull* 1981; **90**: 89–101.

11 Serlin R, Mendoza T, Nakamura Y, Edwards K, Cleeland C. When is cancer pain mild, moderate or severe? Grading pain severity by its interference with function. *Pain* 1995; **61**: 277–84.

12 Cleeland C, Syrjala K. How to assess cancer pain. In: Turk D, Melzack R, eds. *Handbook of Pain Assessment*. New York: Guilford Press, 1992: 362–87.

13 Cleeland C, Gonin R, Hatfield A et al. Pain and its treatment in outpatients with metastatic cancer. *N Engl J Med* 1994; **330**: 592–6.

14 Jensen M, Karoly P. Self-report scales and procedures for assessing pain in adults. In: Turk D, Melzack R, eds. *Handbook of Pain Assessment*. New York: Guilford Press, 1992: 135–51.

15 Whaley L, Wong D. *Nursing Care of Infants and Children*. New York: CV Mosby, 1987.

16 Chapko M, Syrjala K, Schilter L, Cummings C, Sullivan K. Chemoradiotherapy toxicity during bone marrow transplantation: time course and variation in pain and nausea. *Bone Marrow Transplant* 1989; **4**: 181–6.

17 Syrjala K, Roth-Roemer S. Non-pharmacologic approaches to pain. In: Berger A, Levy M, Portenoy R, Weissman D, eds. *Principles and Practice of Supportive Oncology*. Philadelphia: JB Lippincott, 1998: 77–91.

18 Hill H, Chapman C, Kornell J et al. Self-administration of morphine in bone marrow transplant patients reduces drug requirement. *Pain* 1990; **40**: 121–9.

19 Syrjala K, Donaldson G, Davis M, Kippes M, Carr J. Relaxation and imagery and cognitive–behavioral training reduce pain during cancer treatment: a controlled clinical trial. *Pain* 1995; **63**: 189–98.

20 Beck A, Rush A, Shaw B, Emergy G. *Cognitive Therapy of Depression*. New York: Guilford Press, 1979.

21 Turk D, Meichenbaum D, Genest M. *Pain and Behavioral Medicine: a Cognitive–Behavioral Perspective*. New York: Guilford Press, 1983.

22 Syrjala K, Cummings C, Donaldson G. Hypnosis or cognitive–behavioral training for the reduction of pain and nausea during cancer treatment: a controlled clinical trial. *Pain* 1992; **48**: 137–46.

23 Lazarus R, Folkman S. *Stress, Appraisal and Coping*. New York: Springer-Verlag, 1984.

24 McCaffrey M, Wolff M. Pain relief using cutaneous modalities, positioning, and movement. In: Turk D, Feldman C, eds. *Non-Invasive Approaches to Pain Management in the Terminally Ill*. New York: Haworth Press, 1992: 121–52.

25 Von Roenn J, Cleeland C, Gonin R, Hatfield A, Pandya K. Physician attitudes and practice in cancer pain management: a survey from the Eastern Cooperative Oncology Group. *Ann Intern Med* 1993; **119**: 121–6.

26 Ward S, Goldberg N, Miller-McCauley V et al. Patient related barriers to management of cancer pain. *Pain* 1993; **52**: 319–24.

27 Devine E, Westlak S. The effects of psychoeducational care provided to adults with cancer: meta-analysis of 116 studies. *Oncol Nurs Forum* 1995; **22**: 1369–77.

28 Hathaway D. Effect of preoperative instruction on postoperative outcome: a meta-analysis. *Nurs Res* 1986; **35**: 269–75.

29 Syrjala K, Abrams J, Cowan J et al. Is educating patients and families the route to relieving cancer pain?. *8th World Congress on Pain* 1996, 167.

30 Howland J, Baker M, Poe T. Does patient education cause side effects? A controlled trial. *J Fam Pract* 1990; **31**: 62–4.

31 Wilson J. Behavioral preparation for surgery: benefit or harm? *J Behav Med* 1981; **4**: 79–102.

32 Fernandez E, Turk D. The utility of cognitive coping strategies for altering pain perception: a meta-analysis. *Pain* 1989; **38**: 123–35.

33 Bernstein D, Borkevic T. *Progressive Relaxation Training*. Champaign, IL: Research Press, 1973.

34 Syrjala K. Relaxation technique. In: Bonica J, Chapman C, Fordyce W, Loeser J, eds. *The Management of Pain*, 2nd edn. Philadelphia: Lea & Febiger, 1990.

35 Devoghel J. Small intrathecal doses of lysine acetylsalicylate relieve intractable pain in man. *J Intern Med Res* 1983; **11**: 90–1.

36 Ramwell P, Shaw J, Jessup R. Spontaneous and evoked release of prostaglandins from frog spinal cord. *Am J Physiol* 1966; **211**: 998–1104.

37 Willer J, De Brouke T, Bussel B et al. Central analgesic effect of ketoprofen in humans: electrophysiologic evidence for a supraspinal mechanism in a double-blind cross-over study. *Pain* 1989; **38**: 1–7.

38 Yaksh T. Central and peripheral mechanisms for the antialgesic action of acetylsalicic acid. In: Barnett H, Hirsh J, Mustard J, eds. *Acetylsalicylic Acid: New Uses for an Old Drug*. New York: Raven Press, 1982: 137–51.

39 Carlsson K, Jurna I. Central analgesic effects of paracetamol manifested by depression of nociceptive activity in thalamic neurons of the rat. *Neurosci Lett* 1987; **77**: 339–43.

40 Flower R, Moncada S, Vane J. Analgesics: antipyretics and anti-inflammatory agent. Drugs used in the treatment of gout. In: Goodman L, et al. eds. *Pharmacological Basis of Therapeutics*, 7th edn. New York: Macmillan, 1985: 674–715.

41 Hunskaar S, Fasmer O, Hole K. Acetylsilicilic acid, paracetamol and morphine inhibit behavioral responses to intrathecally administered substance P or capsaicin. *Life Sci* 1985; **37**: 1835–41.

42 Piletta P, Porchet H, Dayer P. Distinct central nervous system involvement of paracetamol and salicylate. In: Bond M, Charlton J, Woolf C, eds. *Proceedings of the VI World Congress on Pain*. New York: Elsevier, 1991: 181–4.

43 Taio Y. Prostaglandins inhibit endogenous pain control mechanisms by blocking transmission at spinal noradrenergic synapses. *J Neurosci* 1988; **8**: 1346–9.

44 Dahl V, Raeder J. Non-opioid postoperative analgesia. *Acta Anaesthesiol Scand* 2000; **44** (10): 1191–203.

45 Dionne R. Additive analgesia without opioid side-effects. *Compend Contin Educ Dent* 2000; **21** (7): 572–4; 576–7.

46 Hyllested M, Jones S, Pedersen J, Kehlet H. Comparative effect of paracetamol, NSAIDs or their combination in postoperative pain management: a qualitative review. *Br J Anaesth* 2002; **88**: 199–214.

47 Agency for Health Care Policy and Research. *Clinical Practice Guidelines No. 9. The Management of Cancer Pain*. Public Health Service, Rockville, MD, 1992.

48 Magni G. The use of antidepressants in the treatment of chronic pain. *Drugs* 1991; **42**: 730–48.

49 Max M, Culnane M, Schafer S, et al. Amitriptyline relieves diabetic neuropathy pain in patients with normal or depressed mood. *Neurology* 1987; **37**: 589–96.

50 Monks R. Psychotropic drugs. In: Bonica J, ed. *The Management of Pain*, 2nd edn. Philadelphia: Lea & Febiger, 1990: 1676–89.

51 Kishore-Kumar R, Max M, Schafer S et al. Desipramine relieves post-herpetic neuralgia. *Clin Pharmacol Ther* 1990; **47**: 305–12.

52 Max M, Kishore-Kumar R, Schafer S et al. Efficacy of desipramine in painful diabetic neuropathy: a placebo controlled trial. *Pain* 1991; **45**: 3–9.

53 Max M, Lynch S, Muir J et al. Effects of desipramine, amitriptyline and fluoxetine on pain in diabetic neuropathy. *N Engl J Med* 1992; **326**: 1250–6.

54 Bacon R, Berchiou R. Hematologic side-effects of psychotropic drugs. *Psychosomatics* 1986; **27**: 119–27.

55 Page G. The medical necessity of adequate pain management. *Pain Forum* 1996; **5**: 227–33.

56 Page G, Ben-Eliyahu S, Liebeskind J. The role of LGL/NK cells in surgery-induced promotion of metastasis and its attenuation by morphine. *Brain Behav Immun* 1994; **8**: 241–50.

57 Hill H, Jacobson R, Coda B, Mackie A. A computer based system for controlling plasma opioid concentration according to patient need for analgesia. *Clin Pharmacokinet* 1991; **20**: 319–30.

58 Austin K, Stapleton J, Mather L. Relationship of meperidine concentration and analgesic response: a preliminary report. *Anesthesiology* 1980; **53**: 460–6.

59 Bennedetti C. Acute pain: a review of its effects and therapy with systemic opioids. In: Bennedetti C, Chapman C, Giron G, eds. *Advances in Pain Research and Therapy*. New York: Raven Press, 1990: 367–424.

60 Porter J, Jick H. Addiction rare in patients treated with narcotics. *N Engl J Med* 1980; **302**: 123–8.

61 Dunbar P, Buckley F, Gavrin J. Clinical analgesic equivalence for morphine and hydromorphone with prolonged PCA. *Pain* 1996; **68**: 256–70.

62 Coda B, O'Sullivan B, Donaldson G, Bohl S, Chapman C, Shen D. Comparative efficacy of patient-controlled administration of morphine, hydromorphone, or sufentanil for the treatment of oral mucositis pain following bone marrow transplantation. *Pain* 1997; **72**: 333–46.

63 Jones E, Neuberber J, Bergasa N. Opiate antagonist therapy for the pruritus of cholestasis: the avoidance of opioid withdrawal-like reactions. *Q J Med* 2002; **95**: 547–52.

64 Schmelz M. Itch: mediators and mechanisms. *J Dermatol Sci* 2002; **28**: 91–6.

65 Mackie A, Coda B, Hill H. Adolescents use patient controlled analgesia effectively for relief from prolonged oropharyngeal pain. *Pain* 1991; **46**: 265–9.

66 Dunbar P, Buckley F, Gavrin J. Use of PCA for pain control for children receiving a bone marrow transplant. *J Pain Symptom Manage* 1995; **10**: 606–11.

67 Hill H, Mackie A, Coda B. Patient controlled analgesic infusion. In: Max M, Portenoy R, Laska E, eds. *Advances in Pain Research and Therapy*. New York: Raven Press, 1991: 507–23.

68 Owen H, Szekely S, Plummer J et al. Variables of patient controlled analgesia. II. Concurrent infusion. *Anaesthesia* 1989; **44**: 11–13.

69 Parker R, Holtman B, White P et al. Efficacy of a nighttime opioid infusion with PCA therapy on patient comfort and analgesic requirements after hysterectomy. *Anesthesiology* 1991; **76**: 362–7.

70 Buckley F, Sizemore W, Charlton J. Medication management in patients with chronic non-malignant pain: a review of the use of a drug withdrawal protocol. *Pain* 1986; **26**: 153–65.

71 Halpern L. Psychotropic drugs and the management of chronic pain. In: Bonica J, eds. *Advances in Neurology*. New York: Raven Press, 1975: 539–45.

72 Schubert M, Williams B, Lloid M, Donaldson G, Chapko M. Clinical assessment for the rating of oral mucosal changes following bone marrow transplantation. *Cancer* 1992; **69**: 2469–77.

73 Berger A, Henderson M, Nadoolman W et al. Oral capsaicin provides temporary relief for oral mucositis pain secondary to chemotherapy/radiation therapy. *J Pain Symptom Manage* 1995; **10** (3): 243–8.

74 Heyer G, Dotzer M, Diepgen T, Handwerker H. Opiate and H1 antagonist effects on histamine induced pruritus and allokinesis. *Pain* 1997; **73**: 239–43.

75 Argoff C. New analgesics for neuropathic pain: the lidocaine patch. *Clin J Pain* 2000; **16**: S62–6.

76 Keczkes K, Basheer A. Do corticosteroids prevent post-herpetic neuralgia? *Br J Dermatol* 1980; **102**: 551–5.

77 Finn R. Prednisolone does not prevent post-herpetic neuralgia. *Lancet* 1987; **2**: 126–9.

78 Crooks R, Jones D, Fiddian A. Zoster-associated chronic pain: an overview of clinical trials with acyclovir. *Scand J Infect Dis Suppl* 1991; **80**: 62–8.

79 Johnson R. Herpes zoster: predicting and minimizing the impact of post-herpetic neuralgia. *J Antimicrob Chemother* 2001; **47** (Suppl. T1): 1–8.

80 Pasqualucci A, Pasqualucci V, Galla F et al. Prevention of post-herpetic neuralgia: acyclovir and prednisolone versus epidural local anesthetic and methylprednisolone. *Acta Anaesthesiol Scand* 2000; **44**: 910–18.

81 Winnie A, Hartwell P. Relationship between time of treatment of acute herpes zoster with sympathetic blockade and prevention of post-herpetic neuralgia: clinical support for a new theory of the mechanism by which sympathetic blockade provides therapeutic benefit. *Reg Anesth Pain Med* 1993; **18**: 277–82.

82 McQuay H. Pharmacologic treatment of neuralgic and neuropathic pain. *Cancer Surv* 1988; **7**: 141–59.

83 Kvinesdal B, Molin J, Froland A, Gram L. Imipramine treatment of painful diabetic neuropathy. *J Am Med Assoc* 1984; **251**: 1727–30.

84 Sindrup S, Ejlertsen B, Froland A et al. Imipramine treatment in diabetic neuropathy relief of subjective symptoms without changes in peripheral and autonomic nerve function. *Eur J Clin Pharmacol* 1989; **37**: 151–3.

85 McQuay H, Carroll D, Jadad A, Wiffen P, Moore A. Anticonvulsant drugs for management of pain: a systematic review. *Br Med J* 1995; **311**: 1047–52.

86 Caracini A, Zecca E, Martini C, DeConno F. Gabapentin as an adjuvant to opioid analgesia for neuropathic cancer pain. *J Pain Symptom Manage* 1999; **17**: 441–5.

87 Rowbotham M, Harden N, Stacey B, Bernstein P, Magnus-Miller L. Gabapentin for the treatment of postherpetic neuralgia: a randomized controlled study. *J Am Med Assoc* 1998; **280**: 1837–42.

88 Galer B, Jensen M, Ma T, Davies P, Rowbotham M. The lidocaine patch 5% effectively treats all neuropathic pain qualities: results of a randomized, double-blind, vehicle-controlled, 3-week efficacy study with use of the neuropathic pain scale. *Clin J Pain* 2002; **18**: 297–301.

89 Rowbotham M, Davies P, Fields H. Topical lidocaine gel relieves postherpetic neuralgia. *Ann Neurol* 1995; **37**: 246–53.

90 Lynn B. Capsaicin: actions on nociceptive C-fibers and therapeutic potential. *Pain* 1990; **40**: 61–9.

91 Watson C. Topical capsaicin as an adjuvant analgesic. *J Pain Symptom Manage* 1994; **9**: 425–33.

92 Cherney N, Thaler H, Friedlander-Klar H et al. Opioid responsiveness of cancer pain syndromes caused by neuropathic or nociceptive mechanisms. *Neurology* 1994; **44**: 857–61.

93 Dellemijin P, van Duijn H, Vanneste J. Prolonged treatment with transdermal fentanyl in neuropathic pain. *J Pain Symptom Manage* 1998; **16**: 220–9.

94 Watson C, Babul N. Efficacy of oxycodone in neuropathic pain: a randomized trial in postherpetic neuralgia. *Neurology* 1998; **50**: 1837–41.

95 Mercadante S, Portenoy R. Opioid poorly responsive cancer pain. II. Basic mechanisms that could shift dose–response for analgesia. *J Pain Symptom Manage* 2001; **21**: 255–64.

96 Cicala RS, Voeller GR, Fox T, Fabian TC, Kudsk K, Mangiante EC. Epidural analgesia in thoracic trauma: effects of lumbar morphine and thoracic bupivacaine on pulmonary function. *Crit Care Med* 1990; **18**: 229–31.

97 Wisner DH. A stepwise logistic regression analysis of factors affecting morbidity and mortality after thoracic trauma: effect of epidural analgesia. *J Trauma* 1990; **30**: 799–804.

98 Jay S, Elliot C, Katz E, Siegel S. Cognitive–behavioral and pharmacologic interventions for children's distress during painful medical procedures. *J Consult Clin Psychol* 1987; **55**: 860–5.

99 American Society of Pediatrics. Guidelines for monitoring and management of pediatric patients during and after sedation for diagnostic or therapeutic purposes. *Pediatrics* 1992; **89**: 1110–5.

100 Gavrin J, Chapman C. Clinical management of dying patients. *West J Med* 1995; **163**: 266–77.

101 Gavrin J. Anesthesia and palliative care. *Anesthesiol Clin North Am* 1999; **17**: 467–77.

Mark M. Schubert, Douglas E. Peterson & Michele E. Lloid

Oral Complications

Introduction

Advances in stem cell biology in the past five years have fostered new clinical practices in hematopoietic cell transplantation (HCT). Similarly, new basic science knowledge relative to selected oral toxicities is now providing the basis for novel translational research strategies administered by a multiprofessional oncology team. For example, oropharyngeal mucositis historically has been a frequent, often serious toxicity of HCT. New molecular models developed during the past 5 years relative to mucosal injury in cancer have translated into a considerable number of phase I, II and III clinical trials at present. The recent research base for oral mucosal injury in HCT patients as well as potential clinical applications will be reviewed in this chapter.

Assessment and management methodologies for other oral toxicities, including oral pain, local and systemic infection arising from the dentition/periapices and periodontium, and salivary hypofunction continue to be based on National Institutes of Health (NIH) Consensus Development Guidelines published in 1990 [1], as well as recommendations delineated on the National Cancer Institute (NCI) Physician Data Query (PDQ®) website [2].

Implementation of prevention and treatment of the oral sequelae of HCT often requires a multidisciplinary approach to be maximally effective. Optimal, evidenced-based management can in turn directly benefit the patient's overall clinical course, including reduced morbidity, mortality and cost of care as well as improved quality of life. This chapter will review the current state of knowledge of oral complications in the HCT cohort, with emphasis on recent research advances relative to this clinical practice.

Correlations with the phases of transplantation

Oral complications can occur in all phases of transplantation. It is important to prevent these complications whenever possible and to promptly and efficiently manage those that do occur. Oral complications generally are a reflection of the general condition of the patient. Specific complications can be correlated with the phases of transplantation (Table 67.1).

Phase I: pretransplantation

Oral complications encountered during the pretransplantation phase essentially represent those related to: (i) current systemic and oral health; (ii) oral manifestations of underlying disease; and (iii) oral complications of recent cancer or medical therapy. During this period, dental disease (dental decay, periodontal infections and pulpal/endodontic disease) and sources of potential trauma should be identified and eliminated. Additionally, patients should be educated regarding the range and management of oral complications that can occur with HCT and be provided instructions for oral hygiene.

Phase II: conditioning/neutropenic phase

During this period, oral complications arise primarily from the acute toxicities associated with the conditioning regimens, the type of graft-vs.-host-disease (GVHD) prophylaxis and other medical therapies. These oral sequelae are caused both by direct damage to oral tissues (e.g. mucositis, xerostomia) and indirectly secondary to systemic toxicity (e.g. myelosuppression, thrombocytopenia, and anaemia). This phase is associated with the predictably most frequent and intense oral complications. Oral mucositis is noted generally between days 2 and 18 after transplantation. Oral infections (viral, fungal and bacterial) are potentially problematic, with the incidence varying significantly depending on whether prophylactic regimens (fungal and viral) are used, the patient's oral health coming into transplantation and the duration and severity of neutropenia (i.e. rate of engraftment). With resolution of mucositis and neutrophil engraftment, the frequency of infections declines notably but they still occur. Xerostomia and taste dysfunction may occur early after conditioning but generally will resolve in 2–3 months.

Phase III: initial engraftment to hematopoietic reconstitution

The intensity and severity of oral complications typically begin to decrease approximately 3–4 weeks after transplantation as oral tissues recover from the direct toxicity of the conditioning regimen and as initial engraftment and an increase in peripheral blood cell counts (especially neutrophils) occur. For allogeneic graft recipients, oral GVHD also becomes a concern. The risk for oral infections gradually decreases as local and systemic immune function recovers. Oral fungal infections, especially candidiasis, and herpes simplex virus (HSV) infection are most notable.

Phase IV: immune reconstitution/late post-transplantation

Oral complications noted during this phase are predominantly related to the chronic toxicity associated with the conditioning regimen and include

Table 67.1 Oral complications of hematopoietic stem cell transplantation.

Phase I: pretransplantation
Oral infections
Dental caries
Endodontic infections
Periodontal disease: gingivitis, periodontitis
Mucosal infections: viral, fungal, bacterial
Gingival leukemic infiltrates
Metastatic cancer
Oral bleeding
Oral ulceration: aphthous, erythema multiforme
Temporomandibular dysfunction (TMD)

Phase II: conditioning/neutropenic phase
Oropharyngeal mucositis
Oral infections
Mucosal infections: viral, fungal, bacterial
Periodontal infections
Hemorrhage
Xerostomia
Taste dysfunction
Neurotoxicity
Dental pain
Muscle tremor: jaws, tongue, etc.
Temporomandibular dysfunction (TMD)
Jaw pain/headache/myositis/temporomandibular joint pain
Jaw locking

Phase III: engraftment/hematopoietic recovery
Oral mucosal infections-viral, fungal, bacterial*
Acute GVHD
Hemorrhage
Xerostomia
Neurotoxicity
Dental pain (thermal sensitivity)
Muscle tremor: jaws, tongue, etc.
TMD
Jaw pain
Headache
Joint pain
Granulomas/gingival hyperplasia

Phase IV: immune reconstitution/late post-transplantation
Oral mucosal infections-viral, fungal, bacterial†
Chronic GVHD
Dental/skeletal growth and development alterations
Xerostomia
Relapse-related oral lesions: hematologic malignancies
Second malignancies: squamous cell carcinomas, lymphoproliferative disorders, other

*Mucosal bacterial infections during this phase become increasingly uncommon unless engraftment is slow or if the patient has acute GVHD or is on GVHD therapy.
†Mucosal bacterial infections are rare unless patient has severe chronic GVHD, especially when on intensive therapy for GVHD.
GVHD, graft-vs.-host disease; TMD, temporomandibular dysfunction.

salivary gland dysfunction, craniofacial growth and development abnormalities in pediatric cohorts, and late viral infections. Oral manifestations of chronic GVHD, relapse, graft failure and second malignancies can also develop.

Table 67.2 Medical and dental information pertinent to pretransplantation oral and dental stabilization.

Medical information to be provided to dental team
Underlying disease:
    Cancer: type, stage, prognosis
    Aplastic anaemia
    Other
Type of transplant:
    Autologous
    Allogeneic
    Related: matched, mismatched
    Unrelated: matched, mismatched
    Syngeneic
    Non myeloblative
Planned date of transplantation
Conditioning regimen chemotherapy, total body irradiation (TBI)
Current hematological values
Complete blood cell count differential
Medications
Other medical considerations
Splenectomy
Cardiac disease (including murmur)
Indwelling venous access line

Dental information to be provided to oncology team
Dental caries
Number of teeth requiring restorations
Endodontic disease
Teeth with pulpal infection
Teeth requiring endodontic treatment
Periodontal disease status
Number of teeth requiring extraction
Other urgent care required
Time to complete stabilization

Pretransplantation oral evaluation and stabilization

The initial prevention or risk reduction of oral complications in patients receiving HCT requires stabilizing or eliminating oral disease prior to initiation of transplant or myeloablative regimens [1–8]. Upon becoming a transplant candidate, the patient should be advised to promptly seek oral evaluation and treatment if indicated.

It is prudent to have the patient's dental practitioner involved with the initial management whenever possible, but the dentist and hygienist must clearly understand the goals and objectives of pretransplant stabilization and provide appropriate and realistic care. To maximize outcomes of oral management, the oncology team should advise the community dentist as to the patient's medical status (Table 67.2). The overall goal is to complete a comprehensive oral care plan that eliminates or stabilizes oral diseases and conditions that could otherwise produce acute clinical complications during recovery from HCT. Elimination of these conditions will reduce oral toxicities during and following admission for transplantation, thereby reducing risk for systemic sequelae, improving the quality of life, and reducing the cost of patient care [3,9–13]. If the patient is unable to receive the necessary care in the private community, the oncology team should immediately evaluate and coordinate the oral management before and during HCT [14–16].

Dental treatment

It is imperative that dental treatment does not needlessly delay the transplant procedure or induce complications (e.g. nonhealing extraction sites). If time permits, it may be expedient also to provide less urgent dental care since elective dentistry will need to be postponed until immunologic recovery has occurred, which may take at least 9–12 months after transplantation if chronic GVHD is present [17]. For patients whose medical condition prohibits dental treatment, medically noninvasive care should be implemented until routine care can be performed.

Management of dental decay and endodontic disease

Dental decay and periodontal disease are the two most common oral conditions requiring stabilization prior to transplantation [5,18–20]. If decay progresses and causes pulpal infection while the patient is immunocompromised, the resulting endodontic infection could be life threatening. Thus, risk for pulpal infection and pain determines which carious lesions should be treated: the more extensive the caries, the higher the risk of infectious complications. While it is usually desirable to restore teeth permanently, the use of durable temporary or intermediate restorative materials is valid when time or costs necessitates.

Whenever the potential for pulpal infection exists, it is important to definitively determine the vitality of the teeth. Pulpal and endodontic infections can seriously compromise the medical status of the patient and can be difficult to manage in the initial months after transplantation. Teeth that are nonvital or for which the pulpal status is questionable should be either endodontically treated or extracted. Both direct and indirect pulpal exposures should be aggressively treated to eliminate the risk of subsequent infection. The cause of periapical lesions associated with previously endodontically treated teeth should be determined. Radiographic radiolucencies can be caused by a number of diverse factors including pulpal infections, inflammatory reactions, apical scars, cysts and malignant lesions. Recent reviews have clearly established the need to treat pulpally infected and symptomatic nonvital teeth [5,21]. In cases in which a periapical radiolucency is associated with an endodontically treated tooth and there are no signs or symptoms of infection, retreatment or extraction is not typically necessary since the radiolucency is most likely due to an apical scar [21]. However, if risk exists for endodontic infection or treatment failure after transplantation, extractions should be performed expeditiously.

Periodontal disease stabilization

Of the dental diseases commonly encountered in HCT candidates, inflammatory periodontal diseases—gingivitis and periodontitis—pose the most significant infectious disease risk for the immunocompromised post-transplant patient [22]. Periodontal disease is commonly encountered in patients presenting for transplantation and ranges from mild marginal gingivitis to severe chronic periodontitis with periodontal pocketing and bone loss, acute and chronic abscesses and tooth mobility. Sulcular tissues (i.e. the unattached gingival tissues lining the periodontal pockets) are generally infected and ulcerated, and can result in local, regional and systemic infection and increased risk of bleeding. Gingival bleeding after transplantation predominantly results from pre-existing periodontal disease leading to ulcerated and inflamed mucosal surfaces and is not solely due to low platelet counts. Healthy gingival tissue does not typically bleed unless significantly traumatized. Teeth with severe periodontal involvement and with which there is significant bone loss, furcation involvement (i.e. loss of supporting bone and attachment between the roots of multirooted teeth), or mobility should generally be extracted. Combined antimicrobial (topical or systemic or both) therapy and curettage techniques, followed by effective dental bacterial plaque removal, can render mild to moderate infections as "low risk" relative to both transplantation and bleeding diathesis. The key to reducing risk of significant gingival associated infections and bleeding is to perform intense periodontal disease-stabilizing procedures in advance of myeloablation and maintain excellent oral hygiene throughout and following myeloablation until recovery of immune function [3]. This strategy will generally lead to a reduction in microbial flora and aid in the healing of chronically infected periodontal tissues.

Debate exists as to the management of unerupted or partially erupted third molars (i.e. "wisdom teeth") prior to transplantation. Some authors have suggested that all third molars that are not fully erupted should be extracted prior to HCT [5]. The authors favor a more conservative approach that supports the extraction of third molars that are either at risk for pulpal infection or at significant risk for periodontal infections (e.g. pericoronitis, cellulitis involving the gingival tissue surrounding an incompletely erupted tooth and/or periodontal abscesses) that are not able to be maintained with routine oral hygiene measures.

Dental extractions

Dental extractions should be performed as atraumatically as possible, with primary closure if clinically achievable. It is difficult to define a minimal time to allow for healing of extractions sites before conditioning can be initiated, based on the literature. Ideally, every effort should be made to allow for epithelialization of the extraction site and resolution of any edema and inflammation in order to reduce the risk of local infection, bacteremia, distant infection and bleeding [23]. The amount of time necessary for initial healing generally increases when the teeth being extracted are infected teeth (periodontal and/or endodontic infections) or if it is necessary to lay gingival flaps and remove bone. A simple extraction of a noninfected tooth followed by full primary closure will generally epithelialize in 5–7 days. In contrast, extraction of an impacted mandibular third molar can require as long as 14–21 days to resolve swelling and edema and heal incisions. The more time that can be afforded for healing of extraction site the better—which, again, supports having dental evaluations and treatment completed as soon as a patient becomes a candidate for transplant.

Techniques and strategies to promote healing and reduce risk of residual infection are highly recommended, including minimizing trauma to tissues during surgery, primary closure of extraction sites and use of appropriate antibiotics.

Dentures and orthodontic appliances

Removable prostheses (e.g. full or partial dentures) should be examined thoroughly and adjusted as needed prior to myeloablation. Realignment or adjustment not only can improve the patient's ability to eat and talk but also can reduce the risk of mucosal trauma, as described below. During the period of conditioning and for the first several weeks post-transplantation, dentures should be worn for minimal periods of time (e.g. just for eating) to reduce risk of mucosal injury and secondary infection. Antimicrobial soaking solutions are strongly recommended when dentures are being stored (Table 67.3).

All oral prosthetic devices can cause tissue trauma and may harbor potentially infectious organisms. Thus, they represent a source of oral infection in immunocompromised cancer patients [24,25]. Poor-fitting appliances can abrade oral mucosa that has been injured by the cytotoxic effects of chemotherapy. This mechanical irritation can exacerbate mucosal ulceration and increase the risk of microbial invasion. Additionally, denture soaking cups can readily become colonized with a variety of pathogens, including *Pseudomonas aeruginosa*, *Escherichia coli*, *Enterobacter* species, *Staphylococcus aureus*, *Klebsiella* species, *Torulopsis glabrata* and *Candida albicans*. Adjustment of dentures prior to the start of chemotherapy and ensuring that appropriate soaking solutions are changed daily are important components of preventing infection.

Patients requiring extraction of remaining teeth immediately prior to transplantation can receive prosthetic care once engraftment has occurred

Table 67.3 Use and care of dentures and oral appliances.

Minimize use during first 3–4 weeks after transplantation
Wear only when eating
Leave out at all other times
Clean twice a day with a soft brush and rinse well
Soak in antimicrobial solutions when not being worn
Perform routine oral mucosal care procedures with the oral appliances out 3–4 times a day
Leave appliances out of mouth at night and during periods of significant mouth soreness
Dentures may be used to hold medications needed for oral care (e.g. antifungals)

Orthodontic appliances (brackets, wires, retainers, etc.)
Remove prior to conditioning
Discontinue use of removable appliances (until oral mucositis has healed).

and the medical condition has stabilized. Either transitional or permanent dentures are typically feasible under these circumstances.

Orthodontic bands and fixed appliances, with the exception of fixed mandibular lingual arch retainers, should be removed before treatment is started. These appliances can significantly exacerbate the mucositis during the first several weeks after transplantation due to the significant mucosal trauma they cause. Additionally, it is possible that for patients conditioned with total body irradiation (TBI), back-scatter radiation can be produced from dental restorative materials and orthodontic appliances which will intensify mucosal damage for tissues overlying the metal surfaces [26,27]. In situations in which TBI is to be utilized and the patient's dentition has been restored with multiple or large metallic dental restorations, or metal orthodontic hardware in place, protective splints can be made to gently displace tissues 3–4 mm away from the metal surfaces. This approach can thus prevent the increased radiation damage [28]. Removable orthodontic retainers may be of value until orthodontic care can be resumed post-transplantation. If orthodontic bands and brackets cannot be removed, custom vinyl mouth guards or orthodontic wax should be utilized to help reduce tissue trauma.

Temporomandibular dysfunction

Patients with a history of temporomandibular dysfunction (TMD), especially those with a myofascial pain component, should be identified prior to transplant. Parafunctional habits including cheek or lip chewing, clenching and bruxism (tooth grinding) should be noted and efforts should be instituted to modify or eliminate these behaviors. Patients can be instructed to utilize physical therapy modalities of moist heat/cold packs, massage and stretching to the involved muscles and cold packs for painful joints. Muscle relaxants (or possibly tricyclic antidepressants) can be useful for managing many of the acute muscle-based TMD signs and symptoms should they occur. Selected patients may benefit from use of an appropriately fitted vinyl mouth guard (athletic mouthpiece), flat-plane acrylic occlusal mouth guard or splint.

Other oral disease

All oral mucosal or osseous lesions should be assessed and diagnosed; X-rays are essential for this documentation. Lesions could include infections, drug reactions or allergies, or neoplasia. Clinical and radiographic examinations should be augmented with appropriate tests. For example, microbiology testing (bacterial, fungal or viral direct examinations, cultures or immunofluorescence tests) for lesions, special tissue tests (such as toluidine blue and exfoliative cytology) and tissue biopsy maybe indicated. Clinical presentations can be nonspecific, with several conditions existing simultaneously. It is important to correlate the patient's systemic health status with any oral lesions noted.

Prophylactic antibiotics

The need for prophylactic antibiotics prior to any dental procedures escalates as risk for bacteremia and infection increases. However, there are no clear guidelines for the use of prophylactic antibiotics for dental treatment prior to HCT. Prudent clinical practice suggests that prophylactic antimicrobials may well be of benefit for patients with low absolute neutrophil counts or who are immunologically compromised [16]. Some authors have recommended antibiotic prophylaxis to reduce bacteremia and potential catheter colonization by oral bacteria prior to dental procedures for patients who have central venous access [29]. This recommendation was generally empiric or based on anecdotal experience and not evidenced-based analysis. The policy endorsed by the authors (established in collaboration with the input from infectious disease consultants) recommends the following. (a) Patients who are at increased risk of infection due to poor immune status be given appropriate antibiotics prior to dental treatment and, as the risk of infection increases, the intensity of therapy needs to be increased. (b) For patients who have central venous access catheters in place, patients should be given antibiotics to prevent colonization of the catheter following dental treatment-induced bacteremia in accordance with the American Heart Association's prophylactic antibiotics' guidelines for patients at risk for infectious endocarditis. However, the risk vs. benefit of this latter recommendation should be considered, as the inappropriate use of prophylactic antibiotics can possibly lead to bacterial resistance [30]. Additional research is thus clearly needed. Patients at risk for endocarditis (e.g. patients with mitral valve prolapse with regurgitation or other valvular defects) should be given prophylactic antibiotics according to American Heart Association guidelines. The role of prophylactic antibiotics when dentally treating splenectomized patients is controversial [31–33].

Post-HCT oral complications

Oral complications of HCT can be classified based on whether they result directly from the toxic effects of the conditioning regimens on oral tissues (direct toxicities) or indirectly from the toxicities of therapies involving nonoral tissues (indirect toxicities). Historically, direct oral toxicities have been linked principally to turnover kinetics of replicating oral mucosa [34,35]. For example, oral epithelium exhibiting rapid replacement times has been considered at greater risk for ulcerative lesions as compared with epithelium with less rapid replacement times. It is now becoming apparent that this model, while valid, is not exclusively responsible for explaining ulcerative oral mucositis [36–38]. Derangements in mucosal immune systems, including cytokines, neutrophil recovery and degree of epithelial permeability, may also contribute to the expression of mucositis [39]. Clinical expression of ulcerative oral mucositis thus represents the combined effect of these and related interactions.

Direct toxicities of conditioning regimens also include salivary gland dysfunction, taste dysfunction, neurotoxicities and damage to developing craniofacial structures in children [16,40–42]. As with ulcerative oral mucositis, these conditions are multivariate in causation. They emerge clinically to varying degrees depending on the severity of injury and compromise of host response.

Table 67.4 Routine oral hygiene care.

Toothbrushing
Soft/ultra-soft nylon-bristle (two or three rows) brush
Electric and ultrasonic toothbrushes with soft bristles are acceptable (patient must be able to use without causing trauma and irritation)
Brush 2–3 times daily with Bass sulcular scrub method
Rinse frequently

Dentifrice
Patient preference/tolerated
Fluoride recommended with increased risk of dental caries (especially with xerostomia)
Use 0.9% saline, solution or water if toothpaste causes irritation.

Flossing
Floss once daily
Atraumatic technique with modifications as needed

Foam toothbrushes
Use only when impossible to use regular toothbrush
Use *with* antimicrobial rinses when possible
Brush teeth and mucosal surfaces 2–3 times a day
Rinse frequently

Bland rinses
0.9% saline solution (3/4 tsp of NaCl in a quart of water)
Sodium bicarbonate solution (2 tbsp of sodium bicarbonate in a quart of water)
0.9% saline solution plus sodium bicarbonate (2 tbsp of sodium bicarbonate in a quart of 0.9% saline)
  180–240 mL rinsed, held and spit out
  Repeat every 1–4 h or prn for pain

Topical fluoride
1.1% neutral sodium fluoride gel
0.4% stannous fluoride gel
Brush on for 2–3 min
Spit-out and rinse mouth once gently
Apply once a day

Topical antimicrobial rinses
0.12–0.20% chlorhexidine oral rinse
Rinse, hold 1–2 min and spit out
Repeat 2–4 times a day depending on severity of periodontal disease

Oral care protocols

Oral care protocols are based on two levels of intervention: nonmedicated vs. medicated strategies. The nonmedicated oral care protocol focuses on topical therapy and emphasizes frequent (e.g. every 1–3 h) rinsing with 0.9% saline or sodium bicarbonate solutions. Additional interventions may include tooth brushing with toothpaste, dental flossing, sucking on ice chips, application of external ice packs and rinsing with 0.12% chlorhexidine digluconate, or hydrogen peroxide (Table 67.4). Because of limited data defining the efficacy of these various practices to improved oral health during HCT, oral care interventions across institutions have tended to vary significantly [30,43–46]. The intensity and backgrounds of personnel monitoring compliance with these practices also vary. In some centers, the primary responsibility for monitoring rests with the nurses, while in other centers a comprehensive, research-based team that includes physicians, dentists, dental hygienists and nurses is responsible.

Interventions incorporating systemic medications (e.g. antibacterials and antifungals) have been based on clinical and laboratory trials. These interventions are specifically adapted to each institution's profile of toxicities associated with HCT. For example, use of antimicrobial drugs that can impact oral status (e.g. vancomycin, nystatin, fluconazole) must be considered in light of the microbial epidemiology of the infections associated with HCT and the potential complications (e.g. vancomycin resistant enterococcus, emergence of resistant fungi). The degree and duration of marrow ablation as well as the risk for resistant organisms additionally influence decisions. Protocols incorporating antimicrobial agents are not necessarily targeted specifically for oral infection prevention but can positively influence oral colonization and infection. The antimicrobial component of oral care protocols is in need of continual reevaluation based on changes in infection profiles over time in the HCT population.

Compliance with oral care protocols during periods of marrow suppression is critical to reducing the risk for acute complications. The patient must understand the rationale for the oral hygiene program, as well as the potential side-effects of the cancer chemotherapy and radiation therapy. Effective oral hygiene is important throughout the entire course of transplantation recovery, beginning during the pretransplantation phase with emphasis on control of dental plaque levels [1,9,20,47]. Mechanical techniques (including brushing and dental flossing) and antimicrobial oral rinses can be used [1,20,30,47].

Toothbrushing

Dental plaque is a key factor related to gingival and periodontal disease [20,30]; it can also contribute to acute soft-tissue infections with systemic sequelae during myeloablation. Toothbrushing and flossing represent the most biologically and cost-effective approach to plaque control measures relative to the prevention of gingivitis and periodontal disease. It is unfortunate that policy at selected institutions mandates that patients discontinue brushing and flossing when peripheral blood components (notably platelets) decrease below defined thresholds, based on the concept that these interventions will induce bleeding. Mechanical plaque control not only promotes gingival health, but also may decrease the risk of exacerbation of oral mucositis secondary to microbial colonization of damaged mucosal surfaces [36,48,49].

Patients should brush with a soft nylon bristled toothbrush two to three times a day using techniques that specifically focus on keeping the gingival one-third of the tooth and periodontal sulcus free of bacterial plaque. Rinsing the toothbrush in hot water frequently while brushing will soften the bristles and reduce the potential for trauma. Rinsing with water or saline solution three to four times while brushing will aid in removal of dental plaque initially dislodged by the brushing. Proper technique for dental brushing should be reviewed with the patient in advance of the conditioning regimen, and reviewed again on a daily basis throughout the hospital course to assure effectiveness and compliance. Fluoride toothpaste can be used if desired, but during periods of mucositis it can be discontinued and water or saline solution substituted [30,46,49]; when mucositis resolves, toothpaste can be reinstituted. Brushes should be air-dried between interventions. While disinfectants have been suggested, their routine use to clean brushes has not been proven of value. Electric and ultrasonic toothbrushes may be substituted for manual brushes if patients are properly trained in their use.

Foam toothbrushes are not effective in removing dental plaque [30,47,48] unless they are used in conjunction with a topical antimicrobial solution [50,51]. If the patient with mucositis is unable to tolerate the toothbrushing, foam brushes (without toothpaste/toothpowder) may be substituted to clean the teeth and mucosal surfaces. Additionally, these brushes may be used to remove debris from soft tissues and eliminate accumulation of mucous secretions. However, it must be cautioned that foam brushes can rub and abrade mucosal surfaces and potentially promote mucosal breakdown during periods of times when patients are at risk for mucositis (primarily from the start of conditioning until approximately day 14 post-transplant). The use of soft-nylon bristled toothbrushes should be resumed as soon as oral mucosal lesions improve [24,52,53]. The dental team may specify additional oral hygiene aids for mechanical removal of plaque.

Flossing

If patients are skilled at flossing without traumatizing gingival tissues, it is reasonable to have them continue flossing throughout the HCT course. As with the other oral care interventions, including dental brushing, it is important that daily monitoring of the efficacy and side-effects be conducted by the professional staff [53,54].

Antimicrobial rinses

Antimicrobial agents are available to control oral bacterial surface colonization and formation of dental plaque. The most commonly utilized is chlorhexidine oral rinse [20,55,56]. This agent augments mechanical cleaning for patients with gingivitis and mild to moderate periodontal disease but is especially effective when patients are unable to brush and floss. Initial studies regarding the use of chlorhexidine by HCT patients indicated a significant decrease in oral mucositis and oral candidiasis [30,57]. However, several subsequent studies have not reproduced these results relative to prevention or treatment of this lesion [20,58–62]. Other potentially useful agents currently under study include a topical defensin, tetracycline-related agents, and cetylpyridinium chloride [63,64].

Topical fluorides

Patients at increased risk for dental decay secondary to xerostomia should receive topical fluoride therapy. Prescription-strength neutral sodium fluorides (>1.1%) or stannous fluorides (>0.4%) should be used. A brush-on application is the most convenient technique, thus making patients more compliant [30,53,65]. A flavorless or colorless neutral sodium fluoride gel (e.g. Thera-flur-N®) is recommended when patients develop mucositis. Use of prescription topical fluorides with or without desensitizing dentifrices may promote reduction in the thermal tooth sensitivity that some HCT patients experienced (Table 67.4).

Oral mucosal care

In addition to dental hygiene care, interventions directed to maintaining oral mucosal health should be utilized on a daily basis. Bland oral rinses and lip care not only promote patient comfort but also help maintain moisturization/lubrication of the oral epithelial barriers and thus reduce risk of secondary infection.

Bland rinses

In addition to contributing to tissue integrity, bland rinses can be useful for managing mild mucositis neutralizing acidity and reducing the volume of thick mucous secretions [52,61,62]. Frequent rinsing with 0.9% saline solution, sodium bicarbonate solution or saline-sodium bicarbonate solution can help relieve mucosal discomfort and provide moisturization (Table 67.4). These solutions do not generally need to be sterile, unless the patient is in laminar airflow isolation. Care must be taken in the preparation of these solutions. If the solutions are too concentrated, they can cause mucosal discomfort as well as alter the pH of the oral cavity [31]. It may also be beneficial to use "iced" bland rinses where the solution containers are placed in an ice water bath. This step can enhance the pain relief experienced by some patients. Additionally, care must be taken to ensure that the solutions and containers do not become colonized with bacteria or fungal organisms.

Hydrogen peroxide rinses should not be used as a routine mouth rinse because of the tendency to cause tissue dryness and inhibit wound healing [1,20,50,66–69]. However, a mixture of 3% hydrogen peroxide and 0.9% saline solution (1 : 1 to 1 : 3 by volume) can aid in the removal of blood clots or tenacious mucous accumulation. Lemon glycerin swabs also should not be used for extended periods because citric acid can reduce the pH of the oral cavity and contribute to enamel decalcification. Additionally, glycerin can cause mucosal drying [65,70,71]. Commercial mouthwashes are not generally recommended because the alcohol, flavoring agents and other chemicals they contain can cause tissue irritation and increase dryness.

Lip care

Lip dryness and chapping can be a significant problem for HCT recipients. Conditioning regimens and GVHD can contribute to epithelial thinning and desiccation. While lip care products containing petroleum-based oils and waxes can be helpful, lanolin-based creams and ointments are typically more effective in moisturizing and protecting against damage.

Patient education

Patient education is one of the most important elements of the oral care plan. Individual patient needs must be addressed in developing oral care regimens. Instructions should be given clearly and concisely. Demonstrations or diagrams should be used when appropriate. Written materials offering additional information are often helpful. Motivation and compliance with oral care procedures can have considerable impact on the transplantation course [50,53,72,73].

In addition to oral hygiene care instructions, patients must be educated as to potential oral complications of HCT, such as mucositis, oral bleeding, oral infections, GVHD and pain. Patients need to be motivated to accept responsibility for self-care protocols and should understand that their efforts can have a positive impact on their clinical course [47,66,72]. A systematic approach based on written protocol is essential to maximizing uniformity of the approach. It should be noted that the systematic performance of oral hygiene may be more effective than the specificity of the agents used, and that consistent instruction and frequent reinforcement will help promote patient compliance [20,20,49].

Oropharyngeal mucositis

Oral mucositis is a frequent, serious toxicity of phase II of HCT therapy. It occurs in virtually all HCT patients who receive myeloablative preparative conditioning regimens to varying degrees and is of multifactorial origin. It can produce significant pain and bleeding and can increase risk of systemic infection. When oropharyngeal mucositis is severe, it can also compromise the upper airway such that endotracheal intubation is required. In these situations, it may become necessary to modify treatment. In some centers, for instance, when patients are conditioned for HCT with regimens with a high rate of stomatotoxicity (e.g. allogeneic HCT utilizing TBI and cyclophosphamide or etoposide [VP16] conditioning followed by four doses of methotrexate), the day 11 dose of methotrexate may need to be held if mucositis is severe and there is evolving airway embarrassment. The use of total parenteral nutrition is often necessary because of the patient's inability to receive enteral nutrition. Mucositis thus typically exerts a profound influence on the overall course of the patient in the early post-transplant period.

Understanding the structure and function of normal oral mucosa is necessary to define the clinical significance of cancer therapy associated oral mucositis (see Chapter 13). The oral mucosa is a complex physical and chemical barrier that, when functioning normally, provides critical defense against pathogens and other challenges [35,36,74]. Mucosal immune systems are becoming increasingly recognized as a critical component of host defense mechanisms, including those in HCT patients. Relationships between cancer therapy-induced compromise of systemic immune constituents and functionally distinct mucosal immune com-

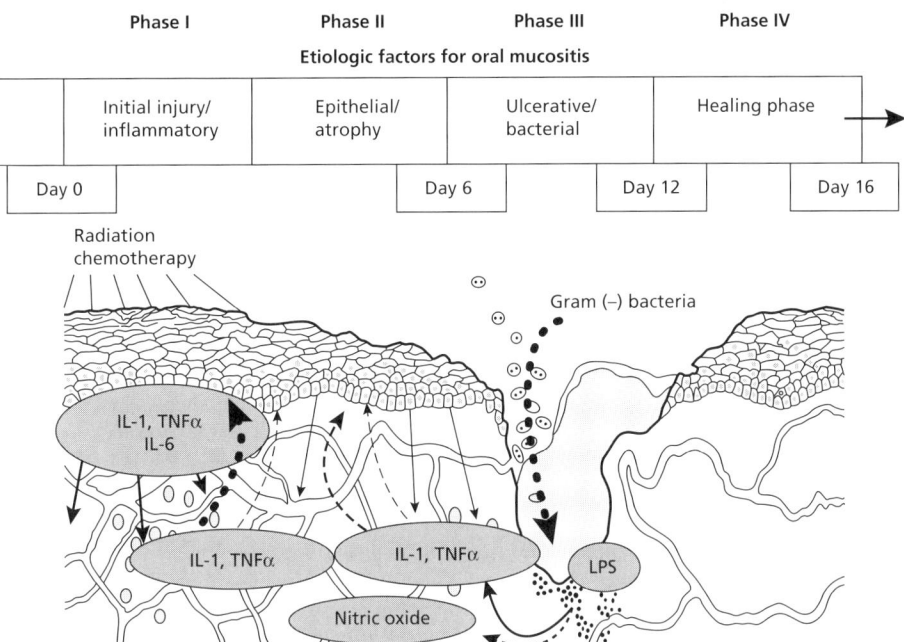

Fig. 67.1 The phases of mucositis following exposure of mucosa to radiation or chemotherapy.
Phase I: inflammatory/vascular phase. Epithelial cells release cytokines (interleukin 1 [IL-1], tumor necrosis factor alpha [TNF-α] and, possibly, IL-6) following damage resulting from exposure to cancer chemotherapy or radiation. Cytokine damage causes further local tissue damage. IL-1 increases submucosal cellularity, which may result in further concentration of chemotherapy drugs in local tissues.
Phase II: epithelial phase. Direct cytotoxicity of chemotherapy and radiation on basal epithelium results in atrophy and ulceration of oral mucosa. Trauma and further cytokine release increase damage to epithelial surface.
Phase III: ulcerative/bacterial phase. With atrophy and ulceration of mucosal surfaces, fibrin-exudate pseudomembranes form. They can become colonized by bacteria by mixed oral flora, which unfortunately is usually during the period of most profound neutropenia. Included in invading organisms are gram negative bacteria that can release endotoxins (lipopolysaccharide [LPS]) which cause further release of cytokines from surrounding tissue.
Phase IV: healing phase. With recovery of the basal layer mucosal epithelial cells, the mucosal surface is renewed and ulcerations are healed. The return of circulating white blood cells (especially neutrophils) aids in clearing bacteria from tissue. Adapted from Sonis [75].

ponents are not well understood. Additionally, the role of cytokines and oral mucosal lymphocyte subsets in this model has not been investigated systematically. Evidence now supports the impact of derangements in tumor necrosis factor, interleukin 1 (IL-1), and monocytes as possible key contributors to the development of oral mucositis (Fig. 67.1) [75]. Understanding these mechanisms and related processes may delineate preventive or therapeutic strategies at the clinical level.

Clinical oral mucosal changes typically emerge 5–10 days after initiation of myeloablative chemotherapy or TBI [76]. Initially, mucosal atrophy and erythema occur, notably on nonkeratinized oral mucosa. Atrophy of the mucosa then progresses to ulceration, which becomes most severe approximately 7–11 days after HCT (see Plates 22.2 & 22.3, facing p. 296). The mucosa then gradually heals over the next 2 weeks. The oral mucosal sites most commonly affected include the lateral and ventral aspects of the tongue and buccal and labial mucosa [77]. Severity of lesions is primarily related to the type of conditioning regimen utilized as well as the degree of genetic match between the donor and patient (e.g. syngeneic, autologous, allogeneic, and unrelated donors). For example, oral hemorrhage and emerging oral acute GVHD can significantly confound clinical presentation of conditioning regimen-related mucositis [78].

Mucosal injury can be accentuated by a number of factors including but not limited to:
1 Salivary gland dysfunction, with resulting derangements in lubricatory and antimicrobial functions of saliva.
2 Mucosal trauma, including that resulting from normal oral function.
3 Infection or irritation caused by indigenous oral flora, acquired pathogens and reactivation of latent organisms including herpes group viruses (HSV, cytomegalovirus [CMV] and varicella-zoster virus [VZV]). Additionally, these conditions can substantially elevate the risk for infection of oral mucosa.

Management

Mucositis management can be challenging for the clinician and patient. Until new strategies for mucositis prevention or reduction are developed via research, management will be centered on supportive care approaches. Appropriate management is based on the severity of tissue damage and symptoms, infection prevention and therapy, nutritional support and use of standardized pain decision matrices ("pain management ladders") to determine need for analgesics and narcotics (Table 67.5) [76,77,79].

Most oral mucositis regimens should incorporate a combination of different agents that collectively serve to coat and anesthetize the mucosa, as well as reduce the risk for mucosal infection [76]. Saline and/or sodium bicarbonate rinses can provide symptomatic relief for mild mucositis. Mucosal coating agents, such as antacid and kaolin solutions, can also be used. As mucosal breakdown and pain increase, agents that provide topical anesthetics are utilized. A wide variety of agents is available and range from antihistamines (e.g. diphenhydramine), anesthetics (e.g. lidocaine, benzocaine) and analgesics (e.g. benzydamine, doxepin, capsaicin) [80–86].

Topical, local application of anesthetic agents allows the patient to concentrate the anesthetic effect to the most symptomatic oral sites. While some authors have raised concern about central nervous system depression or excitation that may follow excessive absorption of topical anesthetic agents, research does not identify this risk [84]. However, sedation may clearly result following systemic absorption of antihistamines when they are swished and swallowed. Generalized oral rinsing

Table 67.5 Mucositis management.

Bland rinses
0.9% saline solution
Sodium bicarbonate solution
0.9% saline solution and sodium bicarbonate solution

Topical anesthetics
Lidocaine: viscous, ointment, sprays
Benzocaine: sprays, gels
Diphenhydramine solution

Mucosal coating agents
Aluminum hydroxide (Amphojel®), Kaolin-pectin (Kaopectate®)
Hydroxypropylcellulose film-forming agents (Zilactin®)

Analgesics
Topical agents: benzydamine hydrochloride, doxepin rinse
Opioid drugs: oral, intravenous (bolus, continuous infusion, patient-controlled analgesia)
Transdermal patches, oral transmucosal

Experimental agents under investigation
Protegrins/defensins
Cytokines and growth factors: KGF, G-CSF, GM-CSF, TGF-β_3
Low-energy laser therapy (helium-neon, aluminum-gallium-arsenide, gallium-arsenide)
Antimicrobials
Other: glutamine

G-CSF, granulocyte colony-stimulating factor; GM-CSF, granulocyte macrophage colony-stimulating factor; KGF, keratinocyte growth factor (a.k.a. FGF-7); TGF, transforming growth factor.

---

or gargling with anesthetics also carries the risk of impairing the gag reflex due to oropharyngeal anesthesia, which can result in aspiration and pneumonia. Therefore, local application to areas of ulceration may be more appropriate than extensive oral rinsing. The most common problem is inadvertent mucosal damage due to trauma and irritation because the oral mucosal neurosensory function is dulled. Hydroxypropylcellulose film forming agents can be used to cover and protect smaller areas of ulceration or areas prone to trauma [87].

Historically, studies of either 0.12% or 0.20% topical chlorhexidine to reduce bacterial colonization and infection have produced mixed results. The drug has been reported to reduce the severity or duration of mucositis in cancer patients [88] or have no benefit or exacerbated mucositis [60–62,89]. While the benefits of chlorhexidine are generally clear regarding its use to treat gingivitis prior to HCT, these conflicting reports prevent the development of any care guidelines relative to its use to prevent oral mucositis.

Systemic pain medications can be given concurrently with topical anesthetics. Oral mucositis typically results in gradually increasing pain that peaks 7–10 days after HCT. Use of a comprehensive, research based approach to assessment and intervention can significantly reduce pain and disability [90] (see Chapter 66). Systemic pain medications, especially narcotics, are usually indicated when topical oral interventions fail to produce sufficient pain relief [76,90–93]. Morphine has generally been the most frequently utilized agent and has been found to be extremely effective when administered with patient controlled analgesia. Opiates including hydromorphone hydrochloride (Dilaudid®), meperidine and time-release oral or intravenous morphine and fentanyl (intravenous, transdermal patches, and more recently oral transmucosal) are also used [94].

Even though systemic approaches are typically required during the most severe phase of mucositis, the patient should be encouraged to continue to perform systematic oral care. This basic wound care remains targeted to reducing the risk of microbial colonization and infection of damaged mucosal surfaces, which can delay healing of oral tissues and lead to systemic infection of oral origin [3]. Since oral mucositis occurs during the period of most profound thrombocytopenia, oral bleeding or oozing can be problematic. Mucosal breakdown can expose submucosal vascular beds that can result in hemorrhage that ranges from slow oozing to frank bleeding. The accumulation of clots can compromise oral function and in some cases potentially obstruct the oral airway (see below) [95].

Many centers utilize oral rinses that are compounded by combining a number of agents empirically [96]. These rinses will generally include topical anesthetic agents (lidocaine, diphenhydramine, etc.), a coating agent (milk of magnesia or antacid solutions) and an antifungal (nystatin solution). While these multiagent rinses may be able to reduce symptoms, a recent study appears to indicate that they are not any more efficacious than single agent rinses [62]. Before prescribing these combinations, other aspects that need to be considered include:

1 *Necessity of agents.* Is the agent efficacious for the condition being treated? For instance, topical antifungals (e.g. nystatin solution) are often added. However, several studies have demonstrated that topical antifungals are not effective for prophylaxis and yeast organisms do not necessarily contribute to the severity of mucositis. A topical coating agent or single topical anesthetic may suffice.

2 *Patient tolerance.* Is the agent provided in a form that is tolerated by the patient? For example, diphenhydramine elixir contains alcohol, a coloring agent and a flavoring agent, all of which can sting and irritate damaged mucosal surfaces. On the other hand, the injectable diphenhydramine can be used in the rinse instead of the elixir form and thus provide anesthesia without irritation from the additional components found in the elixir.

3 *Specific dosing.* Has the correct dose for each agent been provided to the patient, with the specified volume dispensed at each dosing? The components must be administered in correct concentration with appropriate dosing levels achieved by the patient.

4 *Cost-benefit.* Has the most cost-effective approach relative to desired biological effect been selected? Multiagent therapy is typically substantially more costly than mono agent regimens. Biological efficacy must be reconciled against the cost of each type of intervention.

The currently available agents have only a minimal ability to prevent mucositis or lead to more rapid healing. Most strategies only reduce symptoms. Prevention of ulcerative mucositis during HCT course might ultimately provide the setting for escalating the intensity of chemotherapy, leading to more durable remissions or increased patient survival. There are significant clinical research efforts underway to identify medications and agents capable of actually reducing or eliminating oral tissue damage that result in mucositis. The role of biological response modifiers in the prevention and treatment of oral mucosal damage is currently receiving intense investigation. For example, research is being directed toward epithelial cell mitogens, inhibitors of epithelial cell cycling and modulators of the immune response. Cytokines that have been studied include tumor necrosis factor, IL-1 and IL-11, transforming growth factor (TGF) P3, keratinocyte growth factor (KGF) (KGF-2 [repifermin]) and epidermal growth factor (EGF) [75]. Despite initially encouraging animal studies, a recently terminated clinical escalating dose trial of IL-11 has shown no benefit (unpublished results). Early human trials utilizing intravenous KGF (KGF-2 [repifermin]) to reduce HCT toxicities have shown promising results [79]. Future research will be influenced by the ability to develop new laboratory models. Various therapies and agents that may have the potential to actually reduce or prevent mucosal breakdown and inflammation include: (i) low-energy helium-neon (HeNe) laser [97]; (ii) cytokines (TGF-β_3), interferon-alpha (IFN-α) and KGF (KGF-2 [repifermin]) [63,79,98–100]; (iii) protegrins [10]; and (iv) lisofylline (see Chapter 13) [75,76,79]. The sponsor of a recently completed phase III study on the use of iseganan hydrochloride, a protegrin with broad-spectrum antimicrobial activity, reported that the agent failed to reduce the incidence or severity of ulcerative oral mucositis in HCT patients. Topical application of GM-CSF to aid management of mucositis has shown mixed results [101,102]. While the use of oral glutamine or the addition of glutamine to intravenous nutritional supplements has been shown to decrease the severity and duration of oral mucositis in some clinical trials, other studies have been unable to show promising results [102,103].

Obviously, considerably more research needs to be done in this area. It is very possible that given the fact that mucositis appears to result from a number of different factors, that it will be necessary to combine a number of different agents to effect truly effective prevention of mucositis. For instance, it may prove useful to: (a) initially administer agents to increase mucosal thickness prior to conditioning KGF (KGF-2 [repifermin]); (b) next administer agents to take epithelial cells out of cycle to reduce cytotoxicity during conditioning (TGF-β_3) along with anti-inflammatory agents (benzydamine, misoprostol) and antimicrobial agents or growth factors to speed engraftment and recovery of neutrophils; and, finally, (c) agents given following conditioning to speed recovery of normal mucosal thickness (KGF, EGF, etc.).

Early oral infections

HCT associated myeloablation is directly associated with increased risks for both acute oral infection and acute systemic infection of oral origin [76,104]. The types of organisms causing acute oral infections are primarily related to the colonizing oral microflora, the degree and duration of immunocompromise, and the specific systemic and mucosal immune components that are affected.

The multiple protective functions associated with normal oral mucosa directly affect acute infection acquisition. Intact oral mucosa serves to (i) reduce levels of oral microorganisms colonizing the mucosa by means of shedding of the surface layer, and (ii) limit penetration of many compounds into the epithelium by maintaining a chemical barrier [74]. Recently, a number of proteins secreted by mucosal epithelium, referred to as defensins, have been identified. These molecules are capable of lethal activity against bacteria and some fungal organisms [105,106]. If alterations in salivary gland function develop secondary to cancer or its therapy, interactions of salivary immune mediators with oral mucosa may be diminished, further increasing the risk for acute infection [107].

The frequency and causes of oral infections observed in HCT patients have been similar to those seen in immunosuppressed patients receiving high-dose cancer therapy without transplantation [108]. In the 1980s and early 1990s, pseudomembranous candidiasis was common. Fortunately, use of prophylactic fluconazole during the past several years reduced the incidence of oral and associated disseminated candidal infection. HCT patients are at risk for reactivation of HSV and CMV infection in the early period after marrow transplantation. However, prophylaxis with acyclovir for HSV and ganciclovir for CMV, along with the use of CMV-negative blood products, has significantly reduced the occurrence of infection. The risk of oral bacterial infection has been reduced over the past 10 years in the setting of increasingly sophisticated oral hygiene protocols as well as improved bacterial prophylaxis and treatment interventions. Opportunistic gram-negative pathogens, such as *P. aeruginosa*, *Neisseria* species and *E. coli*, as well as gram-positive cocci, such as *Staphylococci* and *Streptococci*, however, remain of substantial concern.

Fungal infections

Candidiasis is the most frequent oral infection seen in HCT patients [109]. The risk for oral *Candida* infection increases as the severity and duration of immunosuppression increases. While numerous *Candida* species can be isolated from immunosuppressed patients, *C. albicans* is considered to be the most pathogenic and most frequently associated with oral infection; although there is increasing evidence of infection caused by other species as well, including *C. krusei*, *C. tropicalis*, *C. glabrata* and *C. dubliniensis* (see Chapter 52) [110–113]. At the same time, epidemiological data support consideration of *C. albicans* as a component of the normal oral flora. Thus, identification of *C. albicans* in culture specimens from oropharyngeal mucosa may only indicate colonization, not infection, unless recovered in high numbers. It is important to correlate clinical findings of mucosal atrophy, erythema and/or pseudomembranous plaques with the results of laboratory tests to identify yeasts to determine both the need to treat these infections as well as judge their response to therapy.

Acute oral pseudomembranous candidiasis is the most common clinical presentation for oral candidiasis. The clinical appearance of acute oral candidiasis in the cancer patient varies, but is frequently described as white lesions that can be wiped off, typically involving the tongue, the mucosa and the lip commissures. The risk of oral candidiasis is highest during phase II and the first half of phase III. The most prominent risk factors for this infection are increasing neutropenia, GVHD, GVHD therapy (especially steroids), salivary gland dysfunction and the use of broad-spectrum antibiotics.

Atrophic candidiasis is less commonly seen and presents with the mucosal surfaces appearing atrophic and erythematous. The most frequently involved sites are the dorsal region of the tongue and the hard and soft palate. There can be "moderate to heavy" colonization that does not produce clinically apparent oral lesions but can cause increased pain and irritation for mucositis or oral GVHD.

Mucosal and food debris, fibrin exudates, mucous secretions and hyperkeratotic striae related to GVHD may cause white changes that can be misinterpreted as representing pseudomembranous candidiasis. Consequently, it is reasonable to utilize direct examination (potassium hydroxide or gram-stained smears of oral lesions) to identify fungal elements and cultures to identify the type of fungus. Final diagnosis must incorporate all relevant features of the history, risk factors, and clinical and laboratory examinations.

A variety of topical antifungal strategies are available when localized oral candidiasis is present. Nystatin (oral solutions, pastilles, powder), clotrimazole (troches, cream) or amphotericin B solution can be used to control acute oral candidiasis. Systemic agents, such as ketoconazole, fluconazole and itraconazole, can help control oropharyngeal candidiasis.

Other oral fungal infections that can complicate the post-HCT course include aspergillosis and mucormycosis [110,114–117]. Systemic prophylaxis can reduce the risk of invasive fungal infection. Topical treatment of oral invasive fungal infections is not effective and treatment depends on systemic therapy.

HCT patients are also at risk for many other invasive fungal organisms. The tendency for aggressive local invasion and systemic spread, often with lethal outcome, is a major concern. Diagnosis of these infections often requires histopathological examinations and culture of tissue specimens. Therapy requires selection of appropriate systemic agents.

Viral infections

The HCT patient is at high risk for acute viral infections originating in oropharyngeal tissues [118–123]. During phase II and early phase III, oral viral lesions are predominately caused by HSV, although VZV and CMV infections can also emerge. Infections caused by Epstein–Barr virus (EBV), Coxsackie virus, adenovirus and human herpesvirus 6 are less common (see Chapters 53–57).

Herpes group viruses
Herpes group viruses cause significant oral disease in patients receiving cancer therapy [118–124]. HSV, VZV, CMV and EBV have all been recognized as being capable of causing oral lesions in cancer patients [122–124]. Most HSV, VZV and EBV infections represent reactivation of latent virus, while CMV infections can result from either reactivation of latent virus or newly acquired virus.

Herpes simplex virus (HSV) Reactivation of intraoral HSV lesions in phase II tends to result in hemorrhagic, ulcerative lesions involving extensive mucosal surfaces [124]. HSV-induced mucositis can be confused easily with severe oropharyngeal mucositis secondary to mucosal damage caused by HCT conditioning regimens. As immune responsiveness recovers, HSV lesions occur as more focal ulcerations, often involving the attached gingiva and hard palate. Extraoral HSV lesions usually present at commissures and vermilion borders of the lips or on the philtrum, and follow a clinical course similar to that seen with intraoral herpes infection.

For patients not receiving prophylactic or therapeutic doses of acyclovir, early diagnosis of HSV infection in immunosuppressed HCT patients is important: if not treated promptly, infection can disseminate with serious sequelae. Diagnostic approaches include viral culture (including shell vial testing) as the gold standard, or immunofluorescent staining. Other techniques, including immunoassay for HSV antigens, may provide more rapid alternatives to the clinician. Biopsy may be valuable in selected cases. Prophylactic systemic acyclovir for HSV-seropositive patients has dramatically reduced the incidence of HSV reactivation during phase II [119]. HSV resistance to acyclovir is uncommon. Failures in prophylaxis or treatment often represent inadequate dosing or absorption of oral acyclovir (see Chapter 54).

Varicella-zoster virus (VZV) Reactivation of VZV in HCT patients usually results in zoster-like patterns of lesions, although multiple dermatomes can be involved. Infection tends to occur during mid-to-late phase III and phase IV. Lesions are characterized as vesicular eruptions following a single dermatomal distribution. In severe cases, dissemination can occur, representing a life-threatening complication [122]. In susceptible patients, primary VZV infection can occur with skin lesions typical of chickenpox. The infection can be fatal, depending on the degree of immunosuppression.

Cytomegalovirus (CMV) CMV has become recognized only in the past several years as capable of causing oral lesions in immunosuppressed patients [123]. The risk of infection is highest during phase II and early phase III. CMV lesions have a nonspecific appearance, with a tendency for shallow to moderate depth irregular ulcerations covered with pseudomembranous fibrin exudate. In severe cases, lesions can be extensive and involve large areas of mucosa [124,125]. Surface swab cultures may yield false-negative results, perhaps due to the virus's propensity for infecting endothelial cells and fibroblasts with resulting low levels of free virus. Shell vial cultures can improve the possibility of detecting CMV, but examination using immunohistochemical tissue stains specific for CMV and biopsy materials is the most reliable technique to diagnose this disease. Ganciclovir and its prodrug form, valganciclovir, are the drugs of choice for treatment (see Chapter 53).

Epstein–Barr virus (EBV) EBV-related hairy leukoplakia lesions have been observed occasionally in immunosuppressed patients other than human immunodeficiency virus (HIV) infected patients, including solid-organ and HCT recipients who are chronically immunosuppressed [122]. These lesions have no apparent clinical significance. On the other hand, EBV-related lymphomas are associated with head and neck lymphadenopathy, generally in phases III and IV. This disease can be fatal if not diagnosed and treated promptly (see Chapters 56 & 70).

Bacterial infections
Bacterial infections in the HCT patient can be caused by indigenous oral flora or nosocomial pathogens (see Chapter 51). Organisms typically classified as being of low virulence in immunocompetent patients can produce both local and systemic infections in HCT patients [107,126,127]. Examples include gram-positive organisms such as *Streptococcus viridans* and *Streptococcus mutans* [128].

The risk of viridans group streptococcal bacteremia and infection in patients with severe mucositis is heightened in those individuals receiving oral, nonabsorbable quinolone antibiotics [23,115,128–132]. In addition, a number of pathogens including *P. aeruginosa*, *S. aureus* and *E. coli* can be acquired. These highly pathogenic organisms can cause serious morbidity and can be fatal. Infection management strategies should involve preventive or therapeutic regimens that target these microbes. Microbiological documentation of causative organisms is essential, given the nonspecific presentation of bacterial infections. It is important to recognize that secondary bacterial infection can occur with all types of oral lesions in immunosuppressed HCT patients.

Immunocompromised HCT patients with chronic periodontal disease may develop acute periodontal infections with associated systemic sequelae. Although not frequent in HCT patients, these lesions can occur in subtle fashion as in other myelosuppressed cancer populations [133]. Erythema and other inflammatory signs are typically suppressed. Dental plaque can significantly increase the risk of periodontal and associated systemic infections. Broad-spectrum antibiotic therapy should be considered while culture results are pending for periodontal infections. Local therapy can be augmented with: (i) irrigation with effervescent (peroxide) agents that are toxic to anaerobic bacteria colonizing the periodontal pocket, as well as (ii) gentle mechanical plaque removal (dental brushing and flossing).

Late oral infections

The oral cavity can remain at risk for a variety of infections as immunological recovery progresses (late phase III and IV), although the risk of infection decreases with immune recovery. Most significant oral infections during these phases are caused by viral and fungal organisms [121,123,134]. Serious oral bacterial infections are less common, with most developing secondary to periodontal or dental infections.

The most common fungal infection during these later phases is candidiasis, commonly presenting with pseudomembranous white plaques and striae; however, atrophic oral candidiasis can also occur. Since the appearance of oral GVHD and even oral mucosal debris can be similar to that of candidiasis (see Plate 23.56, *facing p. 296*), it is important that the specimen recovered from lesions be subjected to direct microbiological examinations to document candidiasis.

In phase III, oral HSV infections can range from herpetic stomatitis in severely immunosuppressed patients with widespread oral ulcerations to relatively minor herpes labialis lesions in patients as immune function recovers. CMV lesions are associated with more compromised immune status and can be difficult to diagnose [121,122]. It is reasonable to consider obtaining material from chronic painful oral ulcerations for viral cultures, especially in patients who are CMV antibody positive. EBV infections are relatively rare.

Post-transplantation patients are at increased risk for oral human papillomavirus (HPV) infections, especially in immunocompromised patients, especially those on high-dose therapy for GVHD. It appears that most cases represent the reactivation of latent virus with patients reporting hand or genital lesions at times prior to transplant. The presentations of these oral lesions can vary from exophytic oral verrucous vulgaris-like masses to more flat condyloma acuminata-like appearance. Attached gingival surfaces have been the most frequently noted surfaces involved, although lips, tongue and soft palate have also been noted as involved when immune recovery is slow. While laser therapy, surgery, or cryotherapy are the most commonly utilized techniques for the removal of oral HPV lesions, intralesional injections of IFN-α may prove effective for recurrent lesions.

Oral hemorrhage

Hemorrhage from oral tissues in patients receiving cancer therapy can occur for multiple reasons. Hematological factors include thrombocytopenia and loss of coagulation factors due to disseminated intravascular coagulation or liver disease. Spontaneous gingival bleeding can be an early clinical indicator of impaired marrow function resulting from neoplastic involvement. The oral bleeding usually occurs in the setting of pre-existing periodontal disease. Spontaneous mucosal petechiae can be observed when the platelet count falls below 20–30,000/μL; spontaneous gingival bleeding can be a problem when the platelet count drops below 10–15,000/μL. As noted previously, it is important to encourage patients to perform thorough but careful oral hygiene. There is an increased risk of gingival hemorrhage if plaque is allowed to accumulate. Trauma or infections that damage mucosal tissues also increase the risk of bleeding.

Oral hemorrhage associated with thrombocytopenia is rarely a serious complication, although its occurrence can be frustrating as well as alarming. Local measures are directed to decreasing the flow of blood along with promoting adequate clot formation, followed by protecting the clot until healing has occurred [76]. Topically applied vasoconstrictors, such as epinephrine or cocaine, can be used to reduce the loss of blood, though rebound vasodilation can occur as the drug effect subsides. Direct pressure applied via gauze soaked in topical thrombin can be used as needed. Clot forming agents, especially hemostatic collagen products (avetine, instat) can also be used to organize and stabilize clots.

Salivary gland hypofunction

Normal salivary function is essential to preserving oral health. In addition to its lubricating properties, saliva normally contains numerous antimicrobial factors that contribute to host defense. These components include mucins that inhibit microbial adherence to mucosa, secretory immunoglobulin A, lactoferrin, lactoperoxidase, transferrin and other proteins that additionally affect microbial colonization and proliferation [135–138].

Salivary gland hypofunction is frequently associated with HCT [107,139,140]. Patients may report various degrees of oral dryness ("xerostomia") in relation to these changes. The etiology may include toxicity associated with conditioning regimens, GVHD, or use of anticholinergic medications [107,141]. Correlation of clinical symptoms and medical events will often reveal the likely cause. For example, ionizing radiation is the component of the transplant-conditioning regimen most likely to induce salivary disturbances. Chemotherapy can also cause salivary gland damage. Numerous other drugs or interventions may alter salivary function. For example, anticholinergic antiemetic drugs or tricyclic antidepressants can reduce the saliva output. Oral dryness can be exacerbated by the desiccating effect of mouth breathing or oxygen administration. In contrast, however, drug-induced salivary hyperfunction is generally rare. Most instances of apparent sialorrhea are related to dysphagia and inadequate clearance due to painful oral mucositis and pharyngitis.

Table 67.6 Management of post-transplantation xerostomia-associated decay.

Plaque removal
Toothbrushing
Flossing
Other oral hygiene aids

Remineralization
Topical high-concentration fluorides*
Children: topical and systemic†
Adults: topical fluorides
Calcium/phosphate remineralizing solutions

Topical antimicrobials
Chlorhexidine solutions (rinses)
Tetracycline oral rinses

Sialogogues
Pilocarpine
Cevimeline
Taste stimulants: sugar-free candies (especially lemon flavored), mints, gum

*Prescription-strength fluorides should be used; nonprescription fluoride preparations are inadequate in the face of moderate to high dental caries risk.
†If drinking water does not have adequate fluoride content to prevent tooth decay, then oral fluoride (drops, vitamins, etc.) should be provided.

The symptom of xerostomia can significantly compromise the quality of life for patients post-HCT. In addition, salivary hypofunction can lead to oral lesions caused by trauma or the colonizing microflora. Techniques to manage xerostomia include frequent sipping of water, rinsing with bland oral rinses (0.9% saline or sodium bicarbonate rinses) and use of artificial saliva and oral moisturizers. These strategies can promote mucosal lubrication and hygiene.

Stimulation of salivary flow can also be of benefit. Sugarless lemon drops, mints, and gums can also transiently increase salivary flow rates. Sialogogues such as pilocarpine (5 or 10 mg every 6–8 h), bethanechol (25–50 mg every 6–8 h) and cevimeline hydrochloride (30 mg every 6–8 h) can be used to stimulate the salivary glands and improve oral moisturization [142]. Recent evidence suggests that pilocarpine administration during cancer chemotherapy or radiation therapy, including HCT conditioning, can prevent or reduce the severity of mucositis. However, the mechanism has not been delineated [71,143].

Salivary gland function may improve during the first 3–6 months after transplantation. In some instances, however, damage may be permanent. GVHD induced salivary gland dysfunction clinically resembles Sjögren syndrome and results from injury caused by donor lymphocytes reacting against ductal and acinar tissue (see Plate 23.57, *facing p. 296*). Mucoceles can occur in association with oral GVHD, with labial and soft palate mucosae being the most frequently involved sites. These mucoceles can often be confused with HSV vesicles, although pain is not a prominent feature of salivary gland GVHD.

Patients with xerostomia are at increased risk of dental decay and should be placed on appropriate regimens to minimize dental plaque and provide for enamel remineralization via topical fluorides, remineralizing solutions, or both (Table 67.6) [144].

Oral GVHD

GVHD represents an immune-mediated disease principally occurring after allogeneic transplantation, although cases of autologous GVHD have been described (see Chapters 30 & 50) [145]. Oral GVHD mimics a

Table 67.7 Management of oral chronic graft-versus-host disease (GVHD).

Topical agents
Steroids: dexamethasone (rinses), fluocinonide/clobetasol/halobetasol/
Beclomethasone (creams, gels, atomizers, inhalers)
Other immunosuppressants: azathioprine (rinses), FK506 (tacrolimus), cyclosporine (CSP)

Antifungals
Topical preparations: nystatin, clotrimazole, amphotericin
Systemic agents: fluconazole, itraconazole, amphotericin, voriconazole

Sialogogues
Pilocarpine, cevimeline
Topical anesthetics: lidocaine, benzocaine diphenhydramine, benzydamine (rinses, gels)

Dental decay prevention
Oral hygiene (dental plaque removal)
Fluorides,* remineralizing solutions

*If drinking water does not have acceptable fluoride levels for fluoride supplementation for developing teeth to reduce risk of tooth decay, oral fluoride (drops, vitamins, etc.) should be provided to children under the age of 12.

---

number of naturally occurring autoimmune disorders, including lichen planus, lupus and scleroderma [146–150]. Symptoms of mouth dryness and sensitivity are often associated with evolving GVHD. The clinical presentation of oral GVHD is similar in both acute and chronic GVHD, with mucosal erythema, atrophy, pseudomembranous ulcerations and hyperkeratotic striae, plaques and papules consistent with oral lichen planus as classic components (see Plate 23.56, *facing p. 296*). The buccal and labial mucosae and lateral and ventral regions of the tongue are the most commonly involved sites [151].

In allogeneic HCT, acute GVHD appears within 2–3 weeks after transplantation and most often involves the skin, liver, oral cavity and gastrointestinal tract. Chronic oral GVHD presents in similar fashion to acute GVHD, and becomes apparent between 100 and 500 days after HCT. False oral GVHD reactions have been noted occasionally in autologous HCT recipients, with lichenoid reactions being the most recognizable clinical manifestations [151]. As noted above, GVHD can injure major and minor salivary glands, with resulting xerostomia and mucoceles (see Plate 23.57, *facing p. 296*). With extensive chronic GVHD, the extent and severity of oral lesions can become more disabling. Mucosal lesions can cause significant pain and produce an increased risk of oral infection. Sclerodermatous changes can result in perioral fibrosis that decreases oral opening and interferes with oral function. Oral secondary infections caused by HSV, CMV, *Candida* species, or trauma, can exacerbate oral GVHD lesions and confound the diagnosis [78,151].

Symptoms associated with oral GVHD generally require systemic immunosuppressive therapy. Several approaches to the local management of oral GVHD may be considered, including topical application of steroids (rinses and creams), cyclosporine (CSP), azathioprine, FK506 (tacrolimus) and oral psoralen and ultraviolet light A (PUVA) therapy (Table 67.7) [147,152,153]. While these interventions can reduce the symptoms and severity of oral lesions (especially pseudomembranous ulcerations), none produces definitive resolution. Additionally, there are technical problems with the local administration of ultraviolet A light due to lack of ultraviolet A light sources that can directly illuminate oral tissues with appropriate intensity and field size. Ultraviolet A light sources used to cure dental composite restorative materials have been successfully used [152]. Extracorporeal photochemotherapy (ECP), typically used to treat cutaneous T-cell lymphoma, has recently been shown to reduce the oral signs and symptoms in patients with treatment resistant GVHD [154–156]. Additional investigations to examine the effectiveness of this therapy are ongoing.

Xerostomia and salivary hypofunction associated with oral GVHD not only impacts quality of life for patients but also can have a negative effect on oral and dental health. Lack of saliva interferes with eating and talking and can lead to symptoms of burning and general irritation. With the loss of salivary proteins that help control oral flora, there can be a significant shift to a predominance of dental decay-causing bacteria, which if not appropriately addressed can result in rampant caries [144]. This type of decay can advance very rapidly; every effort should be made to prevent this problem. Patients need to be able to carry out extremely efficient oral hygiene (brushing and flossing) along with daily topical fluoride applications and, possibly, antibacterial mouth rinses. Attempts to use sialogogues to increase resting salivary gland flow rates have not only improved patient comfort, but may actually help improve oral health as well [157–160].

Taste dysfunction

Taste dysfunction is a neurosensory problem often associated with cancer chemotherapy and ionizing radiation [161]. While taste dysfunction has long been reported by patients following HCT, the nature and patterns of taste dysfunction have not been extensively studied in HCT patients [162–164]. The taste receptor cell is derived from neuroepithelium. With a turnover rate of approximately 10 days, it can regenerate if not irreversibly damaged [164]. It is thus conceptually possible that the number of functional taste receptor cells will decrease to a level insufficient for detecting chemical stimuli, with resultant ageusia reported by the patient. In addition to damage to taste receptors, the potential for alteration or damage to olfactory receptor cells must be considered. Patients receiving cancer chemotherapy will occasionally describe symptoms consistent with dysgeusia (disordered or persistent bad taste) resulting from diffusion of drug into the oral cavity as well as venous taste phenomena [165].

Taste dysfunction in HCT patients is not preventable; management initially consists of supportive care including alteration of enteral diet. Total parenteral nutrition typically becomes necessary for several days post-transplant, due to painful ulcerative oral mucositis. During this time, oral dietary intake is usually highly restricted. The symptoms associated with taste dysfunction generally persist for several months post-transplant [164]. However, unlike selected head/neck cancer patients with radiation-induced irreversible salivary hypofunction and associated dysgeusia, normal taste function typically returns between 90 and 120 days following hospital discharge.

Neurotoxicity and orofacial pain

Frequently patients will report dental hypersensitivity, especially to thermal stimuli between 2 and 4 months after HCT. The mechanism is not understood, though it would seem to be associated with conditioning regimen toxicity. Symptoms usually resolve spontaneously within a few months. Topical brush-on fluorides or desensitizing toothpaste will generally reduce or eliminate symptoms.

Oral neuromuscular complications resulting from medication-induced neurotoxicity have been noted with a number of agents including cyclophosphamide, CSP and FK506 (see Chapter 59) [166,167]. Tongue and jaw muscle tremors have been associated with high-dose CSP therapy. Reducing drug doses usually promotes resolution. Similar neurotoxicity problems have been associated with thalidomide.

TMD may present as facial pain, headache, muscle spasms, or joint dysfunction, with occasional ear or pharyngeal pain. In most instances of recent onset TMD, patients are prone to increased clenching or bruxing as a result of stress, sleep dysfunction, or, occasionally, central nervous system toxicity of selected medications. Masticatory muscle tenderness on palpation, temporomandibular joint dysfunction, and pain radiating to the ear are hallmark findings. The short-term use of muscle relaxants or anxiety reducing agents plus physical therapy (moist heat applications, massage and gentle stretching) will often resolve these symptoms. Occlusal splints may be indicated for patients to utilize while sleeping to reduce clenching or bruxing diatheses.

Nonmyeloablative transplantation

Research experience with nonmyeloablative transplantation is providing promising results (see Chapters 85 & 86). While there have been no detailed research reports relative to oral complications of this form of hematopoietic transplant, the Seattle group has had the opportunity to follow a large number of these patients for several years. With the use of a markedly less toxic conditioning regimen, there is essentially no oropharyngeal mucositis. Additionally, there is minimal salivary gland toxicity and patients rarely report any alterations in sense of taste. During the first several weeks post-transplant there is a period of significant neutropenia during which neutropenic mucosal ulcerations have been noted. These lesions have generally shown no identifiable association with any bacterial, fungal, or viral organisms and have responded to topical antibacterial rinses (e.g. 2–4 mg/mL tetracycline, 25–30 mL swished/held for 1–2 min, spat out four times per day). Prophylactic antifungal and antiviral therapy will generally prevent oral fungal and viral infections. We have noted the emergence of oral signs and symptoms of GVHD 6–8 weeks after transplant when immunosuppression is withdrawn with the clinical presentation and course similar to that seen in "standard" allogeneic transplant patients.

Day 100 and long-term follow-up oral assessment

Evaluation of the oral cavity approximately 80–100 days after transplantation can provide useful information as part of day 100 studies [168,169], as well as provide a basis for recommendations for oral care for the next year. Clinical evaluations should be directed to determining the overall oral health (especially oral infections) and the presence or risk for oral chronic GVHD. Similarly, at later times after HCT, oral examinations and oral biopsies can provide information useful for the diagnosis of chronic GVHD.

Oral examination

The day 100 oral examination to reassess the general oral and dental health should look to detect the presence or risk for dental, pulpal/endodontic and periodontal disease. Patients should be encouraged to continue careful and thorough oral hygiene. Brush-on fluorides should be prescribed for patients with xerostomia or active decay. Additionally, chlorhexidine rinses used once or twice a week can further help reduce the risk for dental caries [170]. Patients with high risk for tooth decay should be managed comprehensively with both topical fluorides and topical antimicrobial agents [171,172].

Sialogogues, such as pilocarpine and cevimeline, can be used to increase baseline salivary flow rates and improve patient comfort. While it is suspected that improved flow rates will improve oral health, no studies have substantiated this relationship [160]. This strategy may have particular benefit in reducing xerostomia decay. However, even if patients respond to these agents and have reduced salivary dysfunction, systematic follow-up and aggressive strategies to prevent dental caries and periodontal disease are required.

Patients should not resume routine dental treatment until adequate immunological reconstitution, including recovery from chronic GVHD, has occurred. Patients generally can receive routine clinical and radiographic dental examinations to detect dental disease after discharge from the transplant center. However, other dental treatment, including dental cleanings and soft tissue curettage, should not be performed without assessing the patient's risk for local and systemic infection. The authors have received reports of instances of aspiration pneumonia developing in HCT patients receiving dental scaling and polishing carried out prior to 6 months post-HCT, presumably due to aspiration of bacteria and debris aerosolized by dental instruments and water sprays. Furthermore, since bacteremias resulting from dental treatment are essentially unavoidable, there is an additional risk of systemic infection to be considered. If dental treatment is imperative, it is important that the dentist and physician determine what supportive medical care is necessary, including antibiotics, immunoglobulin G administration, adjustment of steroid doses and platelet transfusions. Dentists should also utilize techniques to reduce the risk of aspiration (use of rubber dams and high volume suction), in addition to reducing the complexity of treatments and shortening treatment times.

Clinical assessment for oral GVHD

Oral examinations should be performed to delineate the presence of GVHD. Both oral labial mucosal biopsy and clinical examination can provide data supporting the diagnosis of GVHD as a component of day +80 assessments [168,173]. Oral mucosal changes including erythema, atrophy, lichenoid hyperkeratotic striae and pseudomembranous ulcerations are associated with oral GVHD (see Plate 23.56, *facing p. 296*) [78]. Patients with clearly evident oral GVHD mucosal changes will generally not require biopsy to confirm oral mucosal and minor salivary gland involvement by GVHD. When oral changes are less diagnostic, oral biopsies can provide important diagnostic information. Histopathological diagnosis of oral GVHD can be made from specimens obtained by labial mucosa biopsies. Following anesthesia for the mental branch of the inferior alveolar nerve, a small (3–4-mm × 4–6-mm) elliptical wedge containing epithelium and minor salivary gland lobules is removed. Closure of the biopsy site with chromic gut sutures enhances healing and reduces the risks of infection and bleeding. The presence of a lymphocytic infiltrate (grade I) with epithelial cell necrosis (grade II) provides the diagnostic basis for oral GVHD [147,174].

Orofacial/dental growth and development

Children younger than 16 years who undergo HCT are at risk for the development of abnormalities in developing dental and/or skeletal structures [175–177]. Conditioning regimens, in addition to cancer therapy prior to transplantation, can damage tooth buds with sequelae including enamel hypoplasia and root-growth alterations (root tapering and blunting, agenesis with premature apical closure, complete agenesis). While permanent teeth are most commonly involved, some children who have undergone transplantation before the age of 1 year have developed both primary and permanent tooth malformations. Delayed dental eruption following HCT is common. Altered skeletal development for craniofacial bones can result in orthognathic changes. Decreased tooth length can result in shortened alveolar processes, while damage to growth centers for the maxilla and mandible or decreased growth hormone secretion can result in decreased jaw size and arch length. It is useful to note that these skeletal changes appear to occur in a symmetrical manner such that the child does not appear to have obviously hypoplastic jaws with corresponding esthetic changes and, essentially, the face appears smaller but is relatively in proportion to the child's overall stature due to general retardation in growth.

Oral granulomatous lesions and gingival hyperplasia

Late in phase II through to the middle of phase III, exophytic soft tissue masses have been noted to occasionally form on the lateral and ventrolateral surfaces of the tongue and buccal mucosa [178–180]. These painless hypertrophic lesions can range from several millimeters to several centimeters in length and can be up to 1.5 cm in height. While usually covered with normal appearing mucosa, they can occasionally be covered by a pseudomembranous fibrin exudate or have a granulomatous appearing surface. Histological examination reveals granulation tissue. Studies have not identified any associated infectious organisms and there is evidence to support the clinical impression that trauma initially causes mucosal damage; then as the granulation tissue forms, persistent trauma and irritation promote growth of the lesions. Due to the highly vascularized nature of these lesions, they can bleed easily when traumatized.

Primary therapy focuses on preventing recurrent trauma to the lesions and the reduction in inflammation through the use of topical steroids. Patients have reported that their polyps regressed and "fell off" spontaneously when protected from trauma and treated with steroids (immune status recovery probably plays a role in this process). Treatment of persistent or enlarging granulomas usually requires surgical removal followed by careful primary closure [178,179]. The Seattle group has additionally managed several cases with carbon dioxide laser with good results.

Gingival hyperplasia is not a frequent complication of HCT and usually represents a reaction induced by medications. Given the dose levels and duration of therapy, the incidence of CSP-induced hyperplasia is relatively uncommon. Patients with persistent high-blood level doses appear to be at higher risk for this problem. The use of calcium channel blockers to manage CSP-related hypertension, especially nifedipine, is also associated with gingival hypertrophy. The risk of gingival hypertrophy appears to be highest when CSP and nifedipine are used in combination.

The gingival hyperplasia is related to excessive production of collagen by gingival fibroblasts. Mild cases may not need to be treated, but more extensive involvement generally requires gingivectomy using either surgical excision or surgical laser therapy.

Relapse

As with primary hematological malignancies, relapse of leukemia or lymphoma after day +100 may present with oral signs and symptoms. Classically, oral bleeding and infections (especially periodontal) are the most frequently encountered oral changes associated with leukemia. However, generally with the close medical monitoring of recovering HCT patients, these signs are rarely the initial presenting problem indicating relapse. Additionally, gingival infiltrates can be noted with patients with acute myeloid leukemia. Oral and head or neck lesions, including oral lesions and enlarged lymph nodes, can also be associated with lymphomas.

Second malignancy

As more patients become long-term survivors, the risk for the development of oral malignancies following HCT has become increasingly apparent. Pretransplantation exposure to chemotherapy and radiation, regimens and alterations in immune function, GVHD and GVHD therapy all contribute to the risk for second malignancy. Lishner *et al.* [180] reported an association between GVHD and the development of secondary oral malignancies. Squamous cell carcinomas are the most common type of solid secondary oral malignancy (see Chapter 70) [182–185].

Lymphoproliferative disorders have been noted to have head and neck presentations, including enlarged submandibular and cervical lymph nodes [186]. New hematological neoplasms, such as lymphoma and leukemia, can potentially present with oral manifestations that may be the first clinical sign of disease. Consequently, because of an increased risk of secondary oral malignancy, any suspicious oral lesion noted in long-term HCT survivors must be aggressively diagnosed. In most instances, the prognosis of secondary oral malignancy is poor: early diagnosis and timely treatment can potentially improve outcome.

Long-term survivors of HCT should be instructed to monitor oral lesions appropriately—most common oral lesions (trauma, irritation, aphthous ulcers, etc.) will heal in 7–10 days. Lesions persisting longer than 2–3 weeks should be carefully assessed and considered for biopsy.

Conclusions

The oral cavity is highly susceptible to the direct and indirect toxic effects of the chemo-radiotherapy used in HCT protocols. Assessment of oral status and stabilization of oral disease patterns prior to HCT admission are critical to overall patient care. Oral complications can have a profound influence on the course and outcome of cancer treatment, including the interruption of cancer therapy or the development of a life-threatening infection. Oral care should be both preventive and therapeutic as indicated to minimize the risks for oral and associated systemic complications. Multidisciplinary approaches to research and treatment are essential to providing the highest standard of care possible.

Development of new technologies to prevent conditioning induced oral mucositis could substantially reduce the risk for systemic infection, the pain and the number of hospital days. Both improvements in quality of life and reductions in hospital costs could emerge. As important, the prevention of oral mucositis could provide the setting in which new classes of chemotherapeutic drugs utilized at increased doses could be considered, with possible improvements in cancer cure rates and durability of disease remissions.

References

1 National Institutes of Health. Consensus Development Conference on Oral Complications of Cancer Therapies. Prevention and Treatment. *NCI Monogr* 1990; **9**: 1–84.

2 National Cancer Institute. Oral complications of chemotherapy and head/neck radiation. PDQ® Cancer Information Summaries: Supportive Care August 2000. Cancer Net: http://www.cancer.gov/cancer_information/pdq/.

3 Peterson DE. Pretreatment strategies for infection prevention in chemotherapy patients. *NCI Monogr* 1990; **9**: 61–71.

4 Epstein JB. Infection prevention in bone marrow transplantation and radiation patients. *NCI Monogr* 1990; **9**: 73–95.

5 Woo SB, Matin K. Off-site dental evaluation program for prospective bone marrow transplant recipients. *J Am Dent Assoc* 1997; **128**: 189–93.

6 Peters E, Monopoli M, Woo SB, Sonis S. Assessment of the need for treatment of postendodontic asymptomatic periapical radiolucencies in bone marrow transplant recipients. *Oral Surg Oral Med Oral Pathol* 1993; **76**: 45–8.

7 Pistorius A, Krahwinkel T, Willershausen B, Kolbe K. Research for corresponding dental therapy for patients undergoing bone marrow and peripheral blood stem-cell transplantation. *Eur J Med Res* 2000; **5**: 318–22.

8 Bocca M, Coscia D, Bottalico L, De Stefano R. Orodental management in patients with malignant hematologic diseases who are waiting for bone marrow transplantation. *Minerva Stomatol* 1999; **48**: 615–9.

9 Daeffler R. Oral hygiene measures for patients with cancer. *Cancer Nurs* 1981; **4**: 29–35.

10 Sonis ST, Woods PD, White BA. Oral complications of cancer therapies. Pretreatment oral assessment. *NCI Monogr* 1990; **9**: 29–32.

11 Bellm LA, Epstein JB, Rose-Ped A, Martin P,

Fuchs HJ. Patient reports of complications of bone marrow transplantation. *Support Care Cancer* 2000; **8**: 33–9.

12 Sonis ST, Oster G, Fuchs H et al. Oral mucositis and the clinical and economic outcomes of hematopoietic stem-cell transplantation. *J Clin Oncol* 2001; **19**: 2201–5.

13 Sonis ST, Fey EG. Oral complications of cancer therapy. *Oncology (Huntingt)* 2002; **16**: 680–6; discussion 686, 691–2, 695.

14 Garfunkel AA, Tager N, Chatisu S, Chausu G, Haze C, Galili D. Oral complications in bone marrow transplantation patients: recent advances. *Isr J Med Sci* 1994; **30**: 120–4.

15 Sums S, Kunz A. Impact of improved dental services on the frequency of oral complication of cancer therapy for patients with non head and neck malignancy. *Oral Med Oral Surg Oral Pathol* 1988; **65**: 19–22.

16 National Institutes of Health Consensus Development Panel. Consensus statement: oral complications of cancer therapies. *NCI Monogr* 1990; **9**: 1–8.

17 Fujimaki K, Maruta A, Yoshida M et al. Immune reconstitution assessed during five years after allogeneic bone marrow transplantation. *Bone Marrow Transplant* 2001; **27**: 1275–81.

18 Peterson DE, Minah GE, Reynolds MA et al. Effect of granulocytopenia on oral microbial relationships in patients with acute leukemia. *Oral Surg Oral Med Oral Pathol* 1990; **70**: 720–3.

19 Barker GJ. Current practices in the oral management of the patient undergoing chemotherapy or bone marrow transplantation. *Support Care Cancer* 1999; **7**: 17–20.

20 Solomon CS, Amenah BS, Arendorf TM. An efficacious oral health care protocol for immunocompromised patients. *Spec Care Dentist* 1995; **15**: 228–33.

21 Peters E, Monopoli M, Woo SB, Sums S. Assessment of the need for treatment of post endodontic asymptomatic periapical radiolucencies in bone marrow transplant recipients. *Oral Surg Oral Med Oral Pathol* 1993; **76**: 45–8.

22 Epstein JB, Stevenson-Moore P. Periodontal disease and periodontal management in patients with cancer. *Oral Oncol* 2001; **37**: 613–9.

23 Graber CJ, de Almeida KN, Atkinson JC et al. Dental health and viridans streptococcal bacteremia in allogeneic hematopoietic stem cell transplant recipients. *Bone Marrow Transplant* 2001; **27**: 537–42.

24 Krishnasamy M. Oral problems in advanced cancer. *Eur J Cancer Care (Engl)* 1995; **4**: 173–7.

25 Peterson DE. Oral complications associated with hematologic neoplasms and their treatment. In: Peterson DE, Elias EG, Sonis ST, eds. *Head and Neck Management of the Cancer Patient*. Boston: Martinus-Nijhoff, 1986: 351–61.

26 Farman AG, Sharma S, George DI et al. Backscattering from dental restorations and splint materials during therapeutic radiation. *Radiology* 1985; **156**: 523–6.

27 Farahani M, Eichmiller FC, McLaughlin WL. Measurement of absorbed doses near metal and dental material interfaces irradiated by X- and gamma-ray therapy beams. *Phys Med Biol* 1990; **35**: 369–85.

28 Reitemeier B, Reitemeier G, Schmidt A et al. Evaluation of a device for attenuation of electron release from dental restorations in a therapeutic radiation field. *J Prosthet Dent* 2002; **87**: 323–7.

29 Spuller RL. The central indwelling venous catheter in the pediatric patient: dental treatment considerations. *Spec Care Dentist* 1988; **8**: 74–6.

30 Kite K, Pearson L. A rationale for mouth care. The integration of theory with practice. *Intensive Crit Care Nurs* 1995; **11**: 71–6.

31 da F, Hirsch A. Dental care of the pediatric patient with splenic dysfunction. *Pediatr Dent* 2002; **24**: 57–63.

32 De Rossi SS, Glick M. Dental considerations in asplenic patients. *J Am Dent Assoc* 1996; **127**: 1359–63.

33 Llibre JM, Cucurull J, Aloy A, Hernandez JA. Antimicrobial prophylaxis for dental extractions after splenectomy. *Lancet* 1991; **337**: 1485–6.

34 Squier CA. Oral complications of cancer therapies. Mucosal alterations. *NCI Monogr* 1990; **9**: 169–72.

35 Squier CA, Kremer MJ. Biology of oral mucosa and esophagus. *J Natl Cancer Inst Monogr* 2001; **29**: 7–15.

36 Sonis S, Clark J. Prevention and management of oral mucositis induced by antineoplastic therapy. *Oncology* 1991; **5**: 11–22.

37 Sonis ST, Lindquist L, Van Vogt A et al. Prevention of chemotherapy-induced ulcerative mucositis by transforming growth factor β_3. *Cancer Res* 1994; **54**: 1135–8.

38 Sonis S, Muska A, O'Brien J et al. Alteration in the frequency, severity and duration of chemotherapy-induced mucositis in hamsters by interleukin-11. *Eur J Cancer B Oral Oncol* 1995; **31**(B): 261–6.

39 Sonis ST, Peterson DE, McGuire DB, Williams DA. Mucosal injury in cancer patients: new strategies for research and treatment. *J Natl Cancer Inst Monogr* 2001; **29**: 1–54.

40 Dahllof G, Bagesund M, Ringden O. Impact of conditioning regimens on salivary function, caries-associated microorganisms and dental caries in children after bone marrow transplantation. A 4-year longitudinal study. *Bone Marrow Transplant* 1997; **20**: 479–83.

41 Majorana A, Schubert MM, Porta F, Ugazio AG, Sapelli PL. Oral complications of pediatric hematopoietic cell transplantation: diagnosis and management. *Support Care Cancer* 2000; **8**: 353–65; comment 347–8.

42 Peterson DE. Research advances in oral mucositis. *Curr Opin Oncol* 1999; **11**: 261–6.

43 McGuire DB. Mucosal injury in cancer therapy. More than mucositis and a mouthwash. *Cancer Pract* 2002; **10**: 179–91.

44 Yeager KA, Webster J, Crain M, Kasow J, McGuire DB. Implementation of an oral care standard for leukemia and transplantation patients. *Cancer Nurs* 2000; **23**: 40–7.

45 Patton LL, White BA, Field MJ. State of the evidence base for medically necessary oral health care. *Oral Surg Oral Med Oral Pathol Oral Radiol Endod* 2001; **92**: 272–5.

46 Stiefel KA, Damron S, Sowers NJ, Velez L. Improving oral hygiene for the seriously ill patient: implementing research-based practice. *Med Surg Nurs* 2000; **9**: 40–3; 46.

47 Armstrong TS. Stomatitis in the bone marrow transplant patient. An overview and proposed oral care protocol. *Cancer Nurs* 1994; **17**: 403–10.

48 Miaskowski C. Oral complications of cancer therapies. Management of mucositis during therapy. *NCI Monogr* 1990; **9**: 95–8.

49 Dudjak LA. Mouth care for mucositis due to radiation therapy. *Cancer Nurs* 1997; **10**: 131–40.

50 Bavier AR. Nursing management of acute oral complications of cancer. *NCI Monogr* 1990; **9**: 123–8.

51 Ransier A, Epstein JB, Lunn R, Spinelli J. A combined analysis of a toothbrush, foam brush, and a chlorhexidine-soaked foam brush in maintaining oral hygiene. *Cancer Nurs* 1995; **18**: 393–6.

52 Borowski B, Benhaurnou JL, Pico JL, Laplanche A, Margainaue JP, Hayat M. Prevention of oral mucositis in patients treated with high-dose chemotherapy and bone marrow transplantation: a randomized controlled trial comparing two protocols of dental care. *Eur J Cancer B Oral Oncol* 1994; **30**(B): 93–7.

53 Lloid ME. Oral medicine concerns of the BMT patient. In: Buchsel PC, Whedon MB, eds. *Transplantation Administrative and Clinical Strategies*. Boston: Jones and Bartlett, 1995: 257–76.

54 Dodd MJ, Miaskowski C, Shiba GH et al. Risk factors for chemotherapy-induced oral mucositis: dental appliances, oral hygiene, previous oral lesions, and history of smoking. *Cancer Invest* 1999; **17**: 278–84.

55 Domingo MA, Farrales MS, Loya RM, Pura MA, Uy H. The effect of 1% povidone iodine as a pre-procedural mouthrinse in 20 patients with varying degrees of oral hygiene. *J Philipp Dent Assoc* 1996; **48**: 31–8.

56 Balbuena L, Stambaugh KI, Ramirez SG, Yeager C. Effects of topical oral antiseptic rinses on bacterial counts of saliva in healthy human subjects. *Otolaryngol Head Neck Surg* 1998; **118**: 625–9.

57 Ferretti GA, Ash RC, Brown AT et al. Chlorhexidine for prophylaxis against oral infections and associated complications in bone marrow transplant patients. *J Am Dent Assoc* 1987; **114**: 461–7.

58 Raether D, Walker PO, Bostrum B et al. Effectiveness of oral chlorhexidine for reducing stomatitis in a pediatric bone marrow transplant population. *Pediatr Dent* 1989; **11**: 37–42.

59 Spijkervet FKL, Van Saene HKF, Panders AK et al. Effect of chlorhexidine rinsing on the oropharyngeal ecology in patients with head and neck cancer who have irradiation mucositis. *Oral Surg Oral Med Oral Pathol* 1989; **67**: 154–61.

60 Epstein JB, Vickars L, Spinelli J, Reece D. Efficacy of chlorhexidine and nystatin rinses in prevention of oral complications in leukemia and bone marrow transplantation. *Oral Surg Oral Med Oral Pathol* 1992; **73**: 682–9.

61 Dodd MJ, Larson PJ, Dibble SL et al. Randomized clinical trial of chlorhexidine versus placebo for prevention of oral mucositis in patients receiving chemotherapy. *Oncol Nurs Forum* 1996; **3**: 21–7.

62 Dodd MJ, Dibble SL, Miaskowski C et al. Randomized clinical trial of the effectiveness of three commonly used mouthwashes to treat chemotherapy-induced mucositis. *Oral Surg Oral Med Oral Pathol Oral Radiol Endod* 2000; **90**: 39–47.

63 Giles FJ, Redman R, Yazji S, Bellm L. Iseganan HCl: a novel antimicrobial agent. *Expert Opin Investig Drugs* 2002; **11**: 1161–70.

64 Jenkins S, Addy M, Wade W, Newcombe RG. The magnitude and duration of the effects of some mouthrinse products on salivary bacterial counts. *J Clin Periodontol* 1994; **21**: 397–401.

65 Dose AM. The symptom experience of mucositis, stomatitis and xerostomia. *Semin Oncol Nurs* 1995; **11**: 248–55.

66 Thombes MB, Galluci B. The effects of hydrogen peroxide rinses on the normal oral mucosa. *Nurs Res* 1993; **42**: 332–7.

67 Takahashi A, Aoshiba K, Nagai A. Apoptosis of wound fibroblasts induced by oxidative stress. *Exp Lung Res* 2002; **284**: 275–84.
68 Bennett LL, Rosenblum RS, Perlov C, Davidson JM, Barton RM, Nanney LB. An *in vivo* comparison of topical agents on wound repair. *Plast Reconstr Surg* 2001; **108**: 675–87.
69 O'Toole EA, Goel M, Woodley DT. Hydrogen peroxide inhibits human keratinocyte migration. *Dermatol Surg* 1996; **22**: 525–9.
70 Daeffler R. Oral hygiene measures for patients with cancer, II. *Cancer Nurs* 1980; **3**: 427–32.
71 Davies AN. The management of xerostomia: a review. *Eur J Cancer Care (Engl)* 1997; **6**: 209–14.
72 Caniner LG, Sandell IL, Sarhed G. The role of patient involvement in oral hygiene compliance. *Br Clin Psychol* 1994; **33**: 379–90.
73 Tedesco LA, Keffer MA, Davis EL, Christersson LA. Effect of a social cognitive intervention on oral health status, behavior reports, and cognitions. *J Periodontol* 1992; **63**: 567–75.
74 Squier CA. Barrier functions of oral epithelia. In: Mackenzie IC, Squier CA, Dabelsteen E, eds. *Oral Mucosal Diseases: Biology, Etiology and Therapy.* Copenhagen: Laegeforeningens Forlag, 1987: 7–9.
75 Sonis ST. Mucositis as a biological process. A new hypothesis for the development of chemotherapy-induced stomatotoxicity. *Oral Oncol* 1998; **34**: 39–43.
76 Schubert MM. Oro-pharyngeal mucositis. In: Atkinson K, ed. *Clinical Bone Marrow Transplantation: a Reference Textbook*, 2nd edn. Cambridge, UK: Cambridge University Press, 2003, in press.
77 Walter EA, Bowden PA. Infection in the bone marrow transplant recipient. *Infect Dis Clin North Am* 1995; **9**: 823–47.
78 Schubert MM, Williams BE, Lloid ME *et al.* Clinical assessment scale for the rating of oral mucosal changes associated with bone marrow transplantation. *Cancer* 1992; **69**: 2469–77.
79 Stiff P. Mucositis associated with stem cell transplantation: current status and innovative approaches to management. *Bone Marrow Transplant* 2001; **2** (Suppl.): S1–11.
80 Carnel SB, Blakeslee DB, Oswald SG, Barnes M. Treatment of radiation and chemotherapy-induced stomatitis. *Otolaryngol Head Neck Surg* 1990; **102**: 326–30.
81 Epstein JB, Schubert MM. Management of orofacial pain in cancer patients. *Eur J Cancer B Oral Oncol* 1993; **29**(B4): 243–50.
82 Berger A, Henderson M, Nadoolman W *et al.* Oral capsaicin provides temporary relief for oral mucositis pain secondary to chemotherapy/radiation therapy. *J Pain Symptom Manage* 1995; **10**: 243–8. Erratum: *J Pain Symptom Manage* 1996; **11**: 331.
83 Epstein JB, Schubert MM. Oral mucositis in myelosuppressive cancer therapy. *Oral Surg Oral Med Oral Pathol Oral Radiol Endod* 1999; **88**: 273–6.
84 Elad S, Cohen G, Zylber-Katz E *et al.* Systemic absorption of lidocaine after topical application for the treatment of oral mucositis in bone marrow transplantation patients. *J Oral Pathol Med* 1999; **28**: 170–2.
85 Epstein JB, Truelove EL, Oien H, Allison C, Le ND, Epstein MS. Oral topical doxepin rinse: analgesic effect in patients with oral mucosal pain due to cancer or cancer therapy. *Oral Oncol* 2001; **37**: 632–7.

86 Epstein JB, Silverman S Jr, Paggiarino DA *et al.* Benzydamine HCl for prophylaxis of radiation-induced oral mucositis: results from a multicenter, randomized, double-blind, placebo-controlled clinical trial. *Cancer* 2001; **15**: 875–85.
87 LeVeque FG, Parzuchowski JB, Farinacci GC *et al.* Clinical evaluation of MGI 209, an anesthetic film-forming agent for relief from painful oral ulcers associated with chemotherapy. *J Clin Oncol* 1992; **10**: 1963–8.
88 Ferretti GA, Ash RC, Brown AT, Parr MD, Romond EH, Lillich TT. Control of oral mucositis and candidiasis in marrow transplantation: a prospective, double blind trial of chlorhexidine digluconate oral rinse. *Bone Marrow Transplant* 1988; **3**: 483–93.
89 Weisdorf DJ, Bostrom B, Raether D *et al.* Oropharyngeal mucositis complicating bone marrow transplantation: prognostic factors and the effect of chlorhexidine mouth rinse. *Bone Marrow Transplant* 1989; **4**: 89–95.
90 Practice guidelines for cancer pain management. A report by the American Society of Anesthesiologists Task Force on Pain Management. Cancer Pain Section. *Anaesthesia* 1996; **84**: 1243–57.
91 Dunbar PJ, Chapman CR, Buckley FP, Gavrin JR. Clinical analgesic equivalence for morphine and hydromorphone with prolonged PCA. *Pain* 1996; **68**: 265–70.
92 Chapman CR, Donaldson GW, Jacobson RC, Hautman B. Differences among patients in opioid self-administration during bone marrow transplantation. *Pain* 1997; **71**: 213–23.
93 Coda BA, O'Sullivan B, Donaldson G, Bohl S, Chapman CR, Shen DD. Comparative efficacy of patient-controlled administration of morphine, hydromorphone, or sufentanil for the treatment of oral mucositis pain following bone marrow transplantation. *Pain* 1997; **72**: 333–46.
94 Payne R, Coluzzi P, Hart L *et al.* Long-term safety of oral transmucosal fentanyl citrate for breakthrough cancer pain. *J Pain Symptom Manage* 2001; **22**: 575–83.
95 Connolly SF, Lockhart PB, Sonis ST. Severe oral hemorrhage and sepsis following bone marrow transplant failure. *Oral Surg Oral Med Oral Pathol* 1983; **56**: 483–6.
96 Turhal NS, Erdal S, Karacay S. Efficacy of treatment to relieve mucositis-induced discomfort. *Support Care Cancer* 2000; **8**: 55–8.
97 Cowen D, Tardieu C, Schubert M *et al.* Low energy helium-neon laser in the prevention of oral mucositis in patients undergoing bone marrow transplant: results of a double blind randomized trial. *Int J Radiat Oncol Bio Phys* 1997; **38**: 697–703.
98 Sonis ST, Costa JW, Evitts SM *et al.* Effect of epidermal growth factor on ulcerative mucositis in hamsters that receive cancer chemotherapy. *Oral Surg Oral Med Oral Pathol* 1992; **74**: 749–55.
99 Farrell CL, Rex KL, Kaufman SA *et al.* Effects of keratinocyte growth factor in the squamous epithelium of the upper aerodigestive tract of normal and irradiated mice. *Int J Radiat Biol* 1999; **75**: 609–20.
100 Farrell CL, Rex KL, Chen JN *et al.* The effects of keratinocyte growth factor in preclinical models of mucositis. *Cell Prolif* 2002; **35**: 78–85.
101 Carl W, Haven J. The cancer patient with severe mucositis. *Curr Rev Pain* 2000; **4**: 197–202.
102 van der Lelie H, Thomas BL, van Oers RH *et al.* Effect of locally applied GM-CSF on oral mucositis after stem cell transplantation: a prospective placebo-controlled double-blind study. *Ann Hematol* 2001; **80**: 150–4.
103 Cockerham MB, Weinberger BB, Lerchie SB. Oral glutamine for the prevention of oral mucositis associated with high-dose paclitaxel and melphalan for autologous bone marrow transplantation. *Ann Pharmacother* 2000; **34**: 300–3.
104 McGuire DB, Altomonte V, Peterson DE *et al.* Patterns of mucositis and pain in patients receiving preparative chemotherapy and bone marrow transplantation. *Oncol Nurs Forum* 1993; **20**: 1493–502.
105 Ganz T, Lehrer RI. Defensins. *Curr Opin Immunol* 1994; **6**: 584–9.
106 Kelly KJ. Using host defenses to fight infectious diseases. *Nat Biotech* 1996; **14**: 587–90.
107 Schubert MM, Izutsu KT. Iatrogenic causes of salivary gland dysfunction. *J Dent Res* 1987; **66**: 680–8.
108 Rolston KVI, Bodey GP. Infections in patients with cancer. In: Bast RC, Kufe DW, Pollock RE *et al.*, eds. *Cancer Medicine*, 5th edn. Hamilton, Ontario: BC Decker, 2002: 2407–32.
109 Eisen D, Essell J, Broun ER. Oral cavity complications of bone marrow transplantation. *Semin Cutan Med Surg* 1997; **16**: 265–72.
110 Marr KA, Bowden RA. Fungal infections in patients undergoing blood and marrow transplantation. *Transpl Infect Dis* 1999; **1**: 237–46.
111 Redding SW. The role of yeasts other than *Candida albicans* in oropharyngeal candidiasis. *Curr Opin Infect Dis* 2001; **14**: 673–7.
112 Calderone RA, Fonzi WA. Virulence factors of *Candida albicans*. *Trends Microbiol* 2001; **9**: 327–35.
113 Schaller M, Mailhammer R, Grassl G, Sander CA, Hube B, Korting HC. Infection of human oral epithelia with *Candida* species induces cytokine expression correlated to the degree of virulence. *J Invest Dermatol* 2002; **118**: 652–7.
114 Schubert MM, Peterson DE, Meyers JD, Hackman R, Thomas ED. Head and neck aspergillosis in patients undergoing bone marrow transplantation. Report of four cases and review of the literature. *Cancer* 1986; **57**: 1092–6.
115 Schiodt I, Bergmann OJ, Johnsen HE, Hansen NE. Early infections after autologous transplantation for haematological malignancies. *Med Oncol* 1998; **15**: 103–8.
116 Bow EJ. Invasive aspergillosis in cancer patients. *Oncology (Huntingt)* 2001; **15**: 1035–9; discussion 1040, 1042–4, 1047.
117 Bodey GP, Mardani M, Hanna HA *et al.* The epidemiology of *Candida glabrata* and *Candida albicans* fungemia in immunocompromised patients with cancer. *Am J Med* 2002; **112**: 380–5.
118 Saral R. Oral complications of cancer therapies: management of acute viral infections. *NCI Monogr* 1990; **9**: 107–10.
119 Bustamante CI, Wade JC. Herpes simplex virus infection in the immunocompromised cancer patient. *J Clin Oncol* 1991; **9**: 1903–15.
120 Machado CM, Vilas Boas LS, Dulley FL *et al.* Herpes simplex virus shedding in bone marrow transplant recipients during low-dose oral acyclovir prophylaxis. *Braz J Infect Dis* 1997; **1**: 27–30.
121 Kawasaki H, Takayarna J, Chita M. Herpes zoster infection after bone marrow transplantation in children. *J Pediatr* 1996; **128**: 353–6.

122. Schubert MM. Oral manifestations of viral infections in immunocompromised patients. *Curr Opin Dent* 1991; **1**: 384–97.
123. Lloid ME, Schubert MM, Myerson D et al. Cytomegalovirus infection in the tongue following marrow transplantation. *Bone Marrow Transplant* 1994; **14**: 99–104.
124. Schubert MM, Epstein JB, Lloid ME, Cooney E. Oral infection due to cytomegalovirus in immunocompromised patients. *J Oral Pathol Med* 1993; **22**: 268–73.
125. Gomez RS, Carneiro MA, Souza LN et al. Oral recurrent human herpes virus infection and bone marrow transplantation survival. *Oral Surg Oral Med Oral Pathol Oral Radiol Endod* 2001; **91**: 552–6.
126. Kusne S, Krystofiak S. Infection control issues after bone marrow transplantation. *Curr Opin Infect Dis* 2001; **14**: 427–31.
127. Lark RL, McNeil SA, VanderHyde K, Noorani Z, Uberti J, Chenoweth C. Risk factors for anaerobic bloodstream infections in bone marrow transplant recipients. *Clin Infect Dis* 2001; **33**: 338–43.
128. Villablanca JG, Steiner M, Kersey J et al. The clinical spectrum of infections with *Viridans streptococci* in bone marrow transplant patients. *Bone Marrow Transplant* 1990; **5**: 387–93.
129. Steiner M, Villablanca J, Kersey J et al. Viridans streptococcal shock in bone marrow transplantation patients. *Am J Hematol* 1993; **42**: 354–8.
130. Offidani M, Corvatta L, Olivieri A et al. Infectious complications after autologous peripheral blood progenitor cell transplantation followed by G-CSF. *Bone Marrow Transplant* 1999; **24**: 1079–87.
131. Marron A, Carratala J, Gonzalez-Barca E, Fernandez-Sevilla A, Alcaide F, Gudiol F. Serious complications of bacteremia caused by *Viridans streptococci* in neutropenic patients with cancer. *Clin Infect Dis* 2000; **31**: 1126–30.
132. Shenep JL. Viridans-group streptococcal infections in immunocompromised hosts. *Int J Antimicrob Agents* 2000; **14**: 129–35.
133. Peterson DE, Minah GE, Overholser CD et al. Microbiology of acute periodontal infection in myelosuppressed cancer patients. *J Clin Oncol* 1987; **5**: 1461–8.
134. Ochs L, Shu XO, Miller J et al. Late infections after allogeneic bone marrow transplantation: Comparison of incidence in related and unrelated donor transplant recipients. *Blood* 1995; **86**: 3979–86.
135. Garfunkel AA, Tager N, Chausu S, Chausu G, Haze C, Galili D. Oral complications in bone marrow transplantation patients: recent advances. *Isr J Med Sci* 1994; **81**: 120–4.
136. Chaushu S, Chaushu G, Garfunkel AA, Slavin S, Or R, Yefenof E. Salivary immunoglobulins in recipients of bone marrow grafts. A longitudinal follow-up. *Bone Marrow Transplant* 1994; **14**: 871–6.
137. Chaushu S, Chaushu G, Garfunkel AA, Slavin S, Or R, Yefenof E. Salivary immunoglobulins in recipients of bone marrow grafts. II. Transient secretion of donor-derived salivary IgA following transplantation of T cell-depleted bone marrow. *Bone Marrow Transplant* 1994; **14**: 925–8.
138. Chaushu S, Chaushu G, Garfunkel AA, Slavin S, Or R, Yefenof E. Salivary immunoglobulins in recipients of bone marrow grafts. III. A longitudinal follow-up of CMV specific antibodies. *Bone Marrow Transplant* 1996; **17**: 237–41.
139. Peterson DE. Oral problems in supportive care: no longer an orphan topic? *Support Care Cancer* 2000; **8**: 347–8.
140. Oneschuk D, Hanson J, Bruera E. A survey of mouth pain and dryness in patients with advanced cancer. *Support Care Cancer* 2000; **8**: 372–6.
141. Epstein JB, Tsang AHF, Warkentin D, Ship JA. The role of salivary function in modulating chemotherapy-induced oropharyngeal mucositis: a review of the literature. *Oral Surg Oral Med Oral Pathol Oral Rad Endod* 2002; **94**: 39–44.
142. Singhal S, Powles R, Treleaven J, Rattenbury H, Mehta J. Pilocarpine hydrochloride for symptomatic relief of xerostomia due to chronic graft-versus-host disease or total-body irradiation after bone-marrow transplantation for hematologic malignancies. *Leuk Lymphoma* 1997; **24**: 539–43.
143. Leveque F. Use of concurrent oral pilocarpine to treat mucositis during bone marrow transplant: a pilot study. *Proc ASCO* 1997; **6**: 108 [Abstract].
144. Dens E, Boogaerts M, Boute P et al. Caries-related salivary microorganisms and salivary flow rate in bone marrow recipients. *Oral Surg Oral Med Oral Pathol Oral Radiol Endod* 1996; **81**: 38–43.
145. Martin RW, Farmer ER, Altomonte VL, Vogelsang GB, Santos GW. Lichenoid graft-vs-host disease in an autologous bone marrow transplant recipient. *Arch Dermatol* 1995; **131**: 333–5.
146. Nakamura S, Hiroki A, Shinohara M et al. Oral involvement in chronic graft-versus-host disease after allogeneic bone marrow transplantation. *Oral Surg Oral Med Oral Pathol Oral Radiol Endod* 1996; **82**: 556–63.
147. Woo SB, Lee SJ, Schubert MM. Graft-vs-host disease. *Crit Rev Oral Biol Med* 1997; **8**: 201–16.
148. Ratanatharathorn V, Ayash L, Lazarus HM, Fu J, Uberti JP. Chronic graft-versus-host disease. Clinical manifestation and therapy. *Bone Marrow Transplant* 2001; **28**: 121–9.
149. Nicolatou-Galitis O, Kitra V, Van Vliet-Constantinidou C et al. The oral manifestations of chronic graft-versus-host disease (cGVHD) in paediatric allogeneic bone marrow transplant recipients. *J Oral Pathol Med* 2001; **30**: 148–53.
150. Demarosi F, Bez C, Sardella A, Lodi G, Carrassi A. Oral involvement in chronic graft-vs.-host disease following allogeneic bone marrow transplantation. *Arch Dermatol* 2002; **138**: 842–3.
151. Schubert MM, Sullivan KM. Recognition, incidence, and management of oral graft-versus-host disease. *NCI Monogr* 1990; **9**: 135–44.
152. Redding SW, Callander NS, Haveman CW, Leonard DL. Treatment of oral chronic graft-versus-host disease with PUVA therapy: case report and literature review. *Oral Surg Oral Med Oral Pathol Oral Radiol Endod* 1998; **86**: 183–7.
153. Epstein JB, Nantel S, Sheoltch SM. Topical azathioprine in the combined treatment of chronic oral graft-versus-host disease. *Bone Marrow Transplant* 2000; **25**: 683–7.
154. Child FJ, Ratnaval R, Watkins P et al. Extracorporeal phototpheresis (ECP) in the treatment of chronic graft-versus-host disease (GVHD). *Bone Marrow Transplant* 1991; **23**: 881–7.
155. Greinix HT, Bolc-Platzer B, Kahls P, Fischer G et al. Extracorporeal photochemotherapy in the treatment of severe steroid-refractory acute graft versus host disease: a pilot study. *Blood* 2000; **96**: 2426–31.
156. Foss FM, Gorgun G, Miller KB. Extracorporeal photopheresis in chronic graft-versus-host disease. *Bone Marrow Transplant* 2002; **29**: 719–25.
157. Nagler RM, Nagler A. Major salivary gland involvement in graft-versus-host disease: considerations related to pathogenesis. The role of cytokines and therapy. *Cytokines Cell Mol Ther* 1999; **5**: 227–32.
158. Nagler RM, Nagler A. Pilocarpine hydrochloride relieves xerostomia in chronic graft-versus-host disease: a sialometrical study. *Bone Marrow Transplant* 1999; **23**: 1007–11.
159. Jenke A, Renner U, Richte M et al. Pharmacokinetics of intravenous mycophenolate mofetil after allogeneic blood stem cell transplantation. *Clin Transplant* 2001; **15**: 176–84.
160. Nagler RM, Nagler A. The effect of pilocarpine on salivary constituents in patients with chronic graft-versus-host disease. *Arch Oral Biol* 2001; **46**: 689–95.
161. Bartosbuk LM. Chemosensory alterations and cancer therapies. *NCI Monogr* 1990; **9**: 179–84.
162. Barale K, Aker SN, Martinsen CS. Primary taste thresholds in children with leukemia undergoing marrow transplantation. *J Parenter Enteral Nutr* 1982; **6**: 287–90.
163. Boock CA, Reddick JE. Taste alterations in bone marrow transplant patients. *J Am Diet Assoc* 1991; **91**: 1121–2.
164. Marinone MG, Rizzom D, Ferremi P, Rossi G, Izzi T, Brusotti C. Late taste disorders in bone marrow transplantation. Clinical evaluation with taste solutions in autologous and allogeneic bone marrow recipients. *Heamotologica* 1991; **76**: 519–22.
165. Mattsson T, Arvidson K, Heimdahl A, Ljungman P, Dahllof G, Ringden O. Alterations in taste acuity associated with allogeneic bone marrow transplantation. *Oral Pathol Med* 1992; **21**: 33–7.
166. Antonini G, Ceschin V, Morino S et al. Early neurologic complications following allogeneic bone marrow transplant for leukemia: a prospective study. *Neurology* 1998; **50**: 1441–5.
167. Bartynski WS, Zeigler Z, Spearman MP, Lin L, Shadduck RK, Lister J. Etiology of cortical and white matter lesions in cyclosporin-A and FK-506 neurotoxicity. *Am J Neuroradiol* 2001; **22**: 1901–14.
168. Flowers MED, Sullivan KM. Preadmission procedures, transplant hospitalization, and post-transplant outpatient monitoring. In: Atkinson K, ed. *Clinical Bone Marrow Transplantation: a Reference Textbook*. Cambridge, UK: Cambridge University Press 2003, in press.
169. Wagner JL, Flowers ME, Longton G, Storb R, Schubert M, Sullivan KM. The development of chronic graft-versus-host disease: an analysis of screening studies and the impact of corticosteroid use at 100 days after transplantation. *Bone Marrow Transplant* 1998; **22**: 139–46.
170. Marsh PD. Antimicrobial strategies in the prevention of dental caries. *Caries Res* 1993; **27** (Suppl. 1): 72–6.
171. Giertsen E, Scheie AA. *In vivo* effects of fluoride, chlorhexidine and zinc ions on acid formation by dental plaque and salivary mutans streptococcus counts in patients with irradiation-induced xerostomia. *Eur J Cancer B Oral Oncol* 1993; **29**B: 307–12.
172. Whelton H, O'Mullane D. The use of combinations of caries preventive procedures. *J Dent Educ* 2001; **65**: 1110–3.
173. Loughran TP, Sullivan K, Morton T et al. Value of day 100 screening studies for predicting the development of chronic graft-versus-host disease

174 Sale G, Shulman H, Schubert M *et al*. Oral and ophthalmic pathology of graft-versus-host disease in man: predictive value of the lip biopsy. *Hum Pathol* 1981; **12**: 1022–30.

175 Dahllof G, Heimdahl A, Blome P, Lonnquist B, Ringden O. Oral condition in children treated with bone marrow transplantation. *Bone Marrow Transplant* 1988; **3**: 43–51.

176 Dahllof G, Forseberg CM, Ringden O. Facial growth and morphology in longterm survivors after bone marrow transplantation. *Eur J Orthod* 1989; **11**: 332–40.

177 Uderzo C, Fraschini D, Balduzzi A *et al*. Long-term effects of bone marrow transplantation on dental status in children with leukaemia. *Bone Marrow Transplant* 1997; **20**: 865–9.

178 Schubert MM, Sullivan KM, Truelove EL. Head and neck complications of bone marrow transplantation. In: Peterson DE, Sonis ST, Elias EC, eds. *Head and Neck Management of the Cancer Patient*. Boston: Martinus-Nijhoff, 1986: 429–52.

179 Woo SB, Allen CM, Orden A, Porter D, Antin JH. Non-gingival soft tissue growths after allogeneic marrow transplant. *Bone Marrow Transplant* 1996; **17**: 1127–32.

180 Kanda Y, Arai C, Chizuka A *et al*. Pyogenic granuloma of the tongue early after allogeneic bone marrow transplantation for multiple myeloma. *Leuk Lymphoma* 2000; **37**: 445–9.

181 Lishner M, Patterson R, Kandel R *et al*. Cutaneous and mucosal neoplasms in bone marrow transplant recipients. *Cancer* 1990; **65**: 473–6.

182 Witherspoon RP, Deeg HJ, Storb R. Secondary malignancies after marrow transplantation for leukemia or aplastic anemia. *Transplant Sci* 1994; **4**: 33–41.

183 Millen FJ, Rainey MG, Hows JM, Burton PA, Irvine GH, Swirsky D. Oral squamous cell carcinoma after allogeneic bone marrow transplantation for Fanconi anaemia. *Br J Haematol* 1997; **99**: 410–4.

184 Otsubo H, Yokoe H, Miya T *et al*. Gingival squamous cell carcinoma in a patient with chronic graft-versus-host disease. *Oral Surg Oral Med Oral Pathol Oral Radiol Endod* 1997; **84**: 171–4.

185 Abdelsayed RA, Sumner T, Allen CM, Treadway A, Ness GM, Penza SL. Oral precancerous and malignant lesions associated with graft-versus-host disease: report of two cases. *Oral Surg Oral Med Oral Pathol Oral Radiol Endod* 2002; **93**: 75–80.

186 Raut A, Huryn J, Pollack A, Zlotolow I. Unusual gingival presentation of post-transplantation lymphoproliferative disorder: a case report and review of the literature. *Oral Surg Oral Med Oral Pathol Oral Radiol Endod* 2000; **90**: 436–41.

68

Jean E. Sanders

Growth and Development after Hematopoietic Cell Transplantation

High-dose marrow ablative chemotherapy or chemoradiotherapy followed by hematopoietic cell infusion for children and young adults with malignant and nonmalignant disorders has resulted in an ever-increasing number of long-term disease-free survivors. Nonmyeloablative transplant preparative regimens are also resulting in an increasing number of long-term survivors. An understanding of the late effects resulting from agents used in hematopoietic cell transplantation (HCT) preparative regimens is necessary to appreciate and anticipate the effects on growth and development after transplantation. Because the preparative regimens are designed to use various agents not only to suppress the patient's immune system but also to eradicate abnormal cells, the doses of the agents administered are not limited by marrow toxicity. The most common regimens utilize high-dose cyclophosphamide (CY) given alone or in combination with busulfan (BU) or other chemotherapy agents, and given with or without total body irradiation (TBI). Other chemotherapy agents that have been used in preparative regimens include high-dose carmustine (BiCNU), melphalan, etoposide (VP-16), fludarabine and thiotepa. Other irradiation regimens include thoracoabdominal irradiation (TAI) and total lymphoid irradiation (TLI). The myeloablative doses of TBI are usually 8–14.0 Gy, whereas the doses of TBI used for nonmyeloablative transplant preparative regimens range from 2 to 6 Gy. Chapter 13 presents complete descriptions of various myeloablative and nonmyeloablative transplant preparative utilized.

Both high-dose chemotherapy and irradiation are known to affect the function of the neuroendocrine system, and therefore growth and development [1]. Endocrine gland secretions act as catalysts to promote normal growth, and normal growth and development require balanced endocrine gland function. Growth- and maturation-promoting hormones include growth hormone (GH), thyroid hormones, androgens and estrogens. The adrenal glucocorticoids are antagonistic to growth.

This chapter reviews the effects observed to date of agents used in HCT myeloablative preparative regimens on endocrine function and the subsequent effects on growth and development of children and young adults that have been described to date. Chapter 69 presents other delayed complications observed after transplantation.

Thyroid function

Normal thyroid hormone production is necessary for normal linear height growth in young children. Consequently, subnormal thyroid hormone production contributes to decreased growth in height. Thyroid function is not impaired following conventional chemotherapy, but irradiation to the thyroid gland has been associated with development of compensated hypothyroidism, overt hypothyroidism, thyroiditis and thyroid neoplasms [2]. Irradiation of the thyroid causes subsequent hyperplasia and induction of nodules and malignancies. Following irradiation, thyroid dysfunction onset usually begins as asymptomatic compensated hypothyroidism with elevated thyroid-stimulating hormone (TSH) and normal thyroid hormone production within the first year and may progress to overt hypothyroidism with elevated TSH and subnormal thyroid hormone production over the next several decades. Hypothyroidism contributes to diminished linear growth in young children. Reports indicate that 40–90% of survivors of Hodgkin's disease, non-Hodgkin's lymphoma, brain tumors and head and neck tumors develop overt or compensated hypothyroidism within 6 years of receiving radiotherapy doses of 30–60 Gy [3]. Children with acute lymphoblastic leukemia (ALL) who did not receive central nervous system (CNS) irradiation have not developed thyroid abnormalities, but up to 9% of those receiving 18–24 Gy CNS irradiation have developed compensated hypothyroidism [4]. Among 1677 patients treated with 7.5–44 Gy mantle field radiotherapy for Hodgkin's disease, the actuarial risk for development of thyroid disease at 20 years after irradiation exposure was 52%, and 67% at 26 years [3]. The risk for development of thyroid malignancies was 1.7% beyond 19 years, which was significantly greater than the expected risk of 0.07% in nonirradiated age-matched normal control subjects [3]. Another study reported a 45.6% (21 of 46 patients) incidence of clinical or biochemical thyroid abnormalities in children evaluated at a median of 10.5 years (2–21 years) after thyroid irradiation of 20 Gy to more than 30 Gy for Hodgkin's disease [5]. The incidence of compensated hypothyroidism was 21%, overt hypothyroidism 8.7%, Graves' disease 2.2% and other abnormality 13%. In this study age was not a contributing factor. Irradiation increases the risk of thyroid neoplasia, and many other factors have been implicated in the etiology of radiation-induced thyroid cancer in survivors of pediatric cancer. The identified risk factors include female gender, younger age at irradiation and longer elapsed time since irradiation [6]. The incidence of thyroid neoplasia is dose dependent, but is increased with exposures as small as 0.05 cGy [7].

Physical examination is often unreliable in detecting thyroid nodules. Fluctuations in serum thyroxine (T_4) or triiodothyronine (T_3) levels do not distinguish benign from malignant disease [3]. Ultrasonography detected thyroid abnormalities in 42 of 96 (44%) survivors of childhood cancer who received head and neck irradiation, compared to 14% with palpable lesions [3]. Thyroid nodules were detected by ultrasonography in 22 of the 96 patients (23%) and were significantly more frequent in patients whose thyroid exposure was more than 31 Gy. Another study of 47 children with Hodgkin's disease who received 22.5–40 Gy to the neck found that 39% developed a focal lesion on ultrasound by 10 years after radiotherapy and 71% developed a focal lesion by 15 years [8]. Three of the 47 developed thyroid carcinoma between 11 and 20 years after radiotherapy, which is an incidence in excess of the expected incidence of 1/400. Some

Table 68.1 Thyroid function following irradiation.

	Preparative regimen				
	CY (%)	BUCY (%)	CY + TLI (%)	7–10 Gy S-TBI (%)	12–15.75 Gy FTBI (%)
No. patients evaluated	100	94	28	143	351
Follow-up (median in years)	9	2	5	6	4
TSH					
normal	99 (99%)	86 (91%)	26 (93%)	95 (66%)	298 (85%)
elevated	1 (1%)	8 (8.5%)	2 (7%)	48 (34%)	53 (15%)
Thyroxine					
normal	99 (99%)	88 (94%)	27 (96%)	129 (90%)	336 (96%)
abnormal	1 (1%)	6 (6.4%)	1 (4%)	14 (10%)	15 (4%)
Reference	[16]	[17–22]	[21,23]	[16,23–25]	[16,21–24]

BU, busulfan; CY, cyclophosphamide; FTBI, fractionated exposure total body irradiation; S-TBI, single-exposure total body irradiation; TLI, total lymphoid irradiation; TSH, thyroid-stimulating hormone.

report thyroid neoplasia occurring between 1.5 and 6.0 years after radiotherapy, whereas other reports suggest a latency period for up to 40 years with a peak incidence occurring 15–25 years after irradiation exposure of 2–5 Gy [9,10].

While the prevalence of thyroid neoplasia in irradiated survivors of pediatric cancer is unknown, a 1991 epidemiological investigation of 9170 patients who survived childhood cancer at least 2 years reported a 53-fold increased risk of thyroid neoplasia [11]. Doses less than 2 Gy were associated with a 13-fold increased risk. Other studies suggest a radiation dose–response relationship as well as a relationship to patient age at time of exposure with younger age patients at highest risk [4,10,12]. Epidemiology studies of thyroid malignancies among individuals exposed to irradiation from the 1986 Chernobyl accident have suggested an age-associated incidence of thyroid cancer. Among children <15 years of age one case of thyroid cancer was observed prior to the Chernobyl accident (rate = 0.5/year/million children), but 21 cases were observed 1986–90 (rate = 10.5) and 143 cases during 1991–94 (rate = 97) [13]. At the time of the accident, their average age was 3.8 years (± 2.4 years), and their average age at time of diagnosis was 9.4 years (± 2.8) years. More than 90% of children were less than 6 years of age and three were *in utero* at the time of the accident. This observation is in contrast to results observed among 1984 men who were Chernobyl cleanup workers where 201 (10.2%) developed thyroid nodules whose biopsies indicated benign nodular disease, two cases of papillary carcinoma and three of benign follicular neoplasms [14]. Thus, the susceptibility of the thyroid to carcinogenetic effects of irradiation is particularly apparent in younger individuals, and suggests that children who have received TBI, TAI or TLI in their HCT preparative regimens are at risk for development of thyroid abnormalities. Because no single historical factor, physical finding or clinical laboratory result is pathognomonic of thyroid neoplasia, use of ultrasound to detect subtle architectural changes in the thyroid gland may be useful as a screening tool to detect asymptomatic nodules.

Preparative regimens consisting of chemotherapy only

After HCT, thyroid function has usually been evaluated with TSH and T_4 and T_3 plasma levels. Abnormal values often prompt further study with free T_4, T_3, resin T_3 uptake (RT_3U) and TSH response to thyrotropin-stimulating hormone. The majority of results from reported studies (Table 68.1) show that chemotherapy regimens including CY, BU plus CY, and other chemotherapy agents plus CY have not resulted in thyroid function abnormalities in the majority of patients [15–21]. Idiopathic thyroiditis developed at age 14 (10 years after HCT) in one child of 100 transplanted for severe aplastic anaemia after a preparative regimen of CY (200 mg/kg) [15], an incidence that is not different from the expected 1% observed in a normal population of school-aged children. Children given BUCY preparative regimens and marrow transplantation for acute myeloid leukemia (AML) have shown a 9% incidence of hypothyroidism occurring at 6 years, suggesting that patients who received BUCY must be considered at risk for development of hypothyroidism and careful post-transplant evaluation of thyroid function is necessary [19]. While thyroid malignancies have not yet been observed after BUCY, longer follow-up is needed to be able to determine whether thyroid malignancies will occur.

Preparative regimens containing irradiation

Compensated hypothyroidism and overt hypothyroidism have often occurred following TBI or TLI preparative regimens [4,20–25]. Among 171 children given 7.5 Gy single-exposure TLI or 7.8–10.0 Gy single-exposure TBI, compensated hypothyroidism developed in 35% and overt hypothyroidism developed in 8.7% (see Table 68.1). These findings are in contrast to a 12% incidence of compensated hypothyroidism and 4.2% incidence of overt hypothyroidism observed among 351 children after 12.0–15.74 Gy fractionated TBI. The incidence of compensated hypothyroidism reported after BUCY preparative regimen is 8.5% and of overt hypothyroidism is 6.4% among children with malignant disease. The patients in these longitudinal studies where single-exposure TBI was administered were followed more than 8 years after irradiation exposure, whereas those given fractionated exposure TBI were followed a median of 4–6 years after irradiation exposure. Although fractionated TBI appears to result in a lower incidence of thyroid abnormalities, data from nontransplant irradiation studies have shown that a risk for development of thyroid dysfunction and thyroid malignancies may be delayed several decades. The development of thyroid dysfunction has not been associated with sex, age at transplantation or acute or chronic graft-vs.-host disease

(GVHD). Detailed evaluations of the hypothalamic–pituitary–thyroid neuroendocrine axis with free thyroxine, RT_3U, thyrotropin-stimulating hormone and microsomal and thyroglobulin antibody has demonstrated that the major effect of irradiation is at the level of the thyroid gland and not at the level of the hypothalamus or pituitary gland [18].

Treatment

All patients in whom overt hypothyroidism develops should receive treatment with T_4, but the benefit of thyroid replacement in patients with compensated hypothyroidism is controversial. Although the carcinogenic potential of thyroid irradiation has been well documented, the ability of thyroid replacement to reduce the incidence of radiation-associated thyroid carcinoma remains unproven [2,26]. Recommendations from pediatric endocrinologists vary with respect to treatment of compensated hypothyroidism after irradiation therapy. Among patients in whom benign thyroid nodules developed after conventional irradiation therapy, treatment with T_4 decreases the risk of recurrence of these nodules but does not decrease the risk of thyroid carcinoma [27]. Papillary carcinoma, toxic goiter and an adenoma have been observed between 4 and 14 years in six children after 10.0 Gy single-exposure TBI and in at least five after exposure to 12–15.75 Gy fractionated TBI. All of these children had abnormal thyroid function and none had received thyroid hormone therapy prior to discovery of the thyroid mass. The adenoma was found at autopsy, but the other patients were treated successfully with thyroidectomy or radioactive iodine thyroid ablation. Thus, all patients who have received TBI, TLI or TAI should be examined annually with physical examinations and tests of thyroid function and perhaps ultrasound.

Growth

Linear growth is a continuous and finely regulated phenomenon that is the result of the interaction of genetic makeup, nutritional factors, hormones, metabolism and cerebrocortical influences. The importance of each major factor varies with different periods of growth. Growth in infancy is largely determined by nutrition and metabolic factors. Growth in childhood is largely influenced by GH and in puberty by the synergistic action of GH and sex steroids [1]. Thus, GH has a major role in the growth process. Conventional chemotherapy may result in subnormal growth as a result of the effect of chemotherapy on the GH–somatomedin–condrocyte axis and/or related to cranial or cranial spinal irradiation. The impact of GH deficiency on subsequent growth in this population is difficult to determine because GH studies have not been performed consistently. Data are difficult to interpret as to whether intensive chemotherapy regimens with or without CNS irradiation are associated with persistent growth impairment because often only growth rates are reported [28–32]. Some studies suggest that the intensity and duration of combination antineoplastic therapy as well as CNS irradiation and age at diagnosis influence patterns of growth [33–35]. The younger the child is at the time of CNS irradiation, the greater the loss of growth during puberty.

Three studies have compared growth outcome for children treated with conventional chemotherapy with or without cranial irradiation and HCT. One study of children with AML concluded that patterns of growth were similar between those who were treated with chemotherapy and those treated with HCT [36]. Follow-up for the 26 patients in the chemotherapy group was 7.4 (1.8–15.5) years and follow-up for the 26 patients in the HCT group was 5.6 (2.0–15.4) years. None of the patients had GH testing performed, and 11 chemotherapy patients had received 18–24 Gy cranial irradiation and nine HCT patients had received TBI. The change in height from time of diagnosis to last follow-up was –0.43 SD for chemotherapy patients and –0.48 for HCT patients. A second comparison study included 10 patients given chemotherapy, 18 patients given chemotherapy plus 18.0–24.0 Gy cranial irradiation and 15 given chemotherapy plus 12–15 Gy TBI and HCT [37]. Change in height SD was –0.21 for the chemotherapy group, –1.26 for the chemotherapy plus cranial irradiation group ($p = 0.0001$) and –1.33 for the HCT group ($p = 0.0008$). All patients had GH testing performed and the only patients with GH deficiency were in the HCT group ($p = 0.003$). The third study evaluated infants less than 1 year of age diagnosed with AML and ALL [38]. Ten were treated with chemotherapy only, 17 received chemotherapy plus cranial irradiation and seven received HCT (six with TBI). Median change in height SD at 5 years after diagnosis was 0.9 for the chemotherapy group, –1.0 for the chemotherapy plus cranial irradiation group ($p = 0.07$) and –2.3 for the HCT group ($p = 0.01$). Further follow-up for a small number suggested that height continued to decline with increasing time after diagnosis. These studies suggest that recipients of chemotherapy only without cranial irradiation have height losses that are substantially less than observed after HCT using TBI-containing regimens.

Because GH secretion is episodic, determination of GH levels involves use of a stimulus to enhance pituitary GH secretion followed by multiple venous blood samplings. Commonly used stimuli include exercise, sleep or pharmacologic agents such as clonidine, levodopa, arginine and insulin. Failure to attain a normal circulating GH level after two different stimuli tests accompanied by decreased growth rates or height SD score (height minus mean height for age and sex divided by the SD of height for age and sex) defines classic GH deficiency. Children who have received cranial irradiation have had variable responses to the provocative stimuli used, which may be because of the use of different pharmacological agents, variations in the interval between irradiation and testing, or neurosecretory defects [39–41]. Although the 24-h spontaneous pulsatile GH secretion test is considered by many to be the most physiologic assessment of GH secretion, it is impractical because of the large volumes of blood required (5 mL every 20 min for 24 h) [42,43]. The 12-h overnight sampling schedule has been shown to be well tolerated, reliable and reproducible, but is less frequently used because of the inconvenience of overnight hospitalization and extensive blood sampling [44]. After TBI, different results between spontaneous GH production tests and stimulated GH response tests often make interpretation of GH data and diagnosis of GH deficiency difficult. This is particularly challenging when one or both GH responses are normal despite decreased growth rates [45,46]. Repeating these tests 1 or 2 years later will often clarify GH production responses. The standard utilized by pediatric endocrinologists today is two different GH tests to assure the diagnosis of biochemical GH deficiency. Most investigators utilize two different tests of GH stimulation, such as the clonidine and arginine stimulation tests. Subnormal results accompanied by decreased growth rates indicate GH deficiency.

Central nervous system irradiation has been associated with the development of GH deficiency, which appears to be related to the child's age at time of irradiation, the irradiation dose received and the length of time lapsed after completion of irradiation [39]. Many children, especially those with ALL, referred for bone marrow transplantation (BMT) have received 18–24 Gy CNS irradiation as part of their initial treatment prior to referral for BMT. When TBI is included in their preparative regimen, their total CNS irradiation dose usually exceeds 30 Gy, the estimated threshold for development of GH deficiency [47]. GH deficiency may be expected to develop in the majority of patients who received this total dose of CNS irradiation 2–3 years after initial irradiation, whereas GH deficiency may not develop in patients who receive lower doses of CNS irradiation for up to 5–10 years after irradiation. Thus, it may be anticipated that nearly all children who have received CNS irradiation in addition to TBI are likely to develop GH deficiency, but GH deficiency may not develop in those who receive only TBI until just prior to or after their growth period, depending on their age at TBI.

Preparative regimens containing chemotherapy

Following preparative regimens with high-dose CY only, normal growth rates and height SD were observed in 91 children [48]. When tested, normal levels of GH were detected. Some children with chronic GVHD treated with corticosteroids had decreased growth velocity during the time chronic GVHD was active and while being treated with corticosteroid therapy. Once chronic GVHD was controlled and corticosteroid therapy discontinued, catch-up growth occurred prior to growth rates returning to normal for age. Final height achieved for 26 girls and 25 boys was at a median of the 25th percentile (range 5th–90th) for girls and the 50th percentile (range 5th–95th) for boys. The European Group for Blood and Marrow Transplantation (EBMT) reported that mean final height SD among 26 patients prepared with CY only was -0.15 ± 1.68 [49].

BU, an alkylating agent frequently combined with CY in preparative regimens, is an agent that affects dividing cells as well as nondividing cells, and it crosses the blood–brain barrier [50,51]. The effect of BU on growth has been reported for children prepared with 14 mg/kg BU and 200 mg/kg CY prior to BMT for thalassemia major [16,52]. Both studies found an effect of patient age at the time of HCT on subsequent growth. Younger patients ($\leq$7 years [52] and <10 years [16]) have growth that was consistent over time after HCT. Among 47 patients evaluable for final adult height, the 26 patients $\leq$7 years at HCT had final adult height that correlated positively with the height of their mother and father, whereas the 21 patients >7 years at HCT had final adult height that showed no relation with either parent's height as these patients failed to achieve their full genetic height potential [52]. Among children prepared with 16 mg/kg BU and 120 mg/kg or 200 mg/kg CY prior to BMT for AML, similar data are emerging. Data among the AML children who had not received prior CNS irradiation have generally demonstrated normal growth velocity [18,19,49,53–56]. Recent studies show that height SD improves following HCT. One study of 23 children found no significant difference between height SD at HCT and yearly height SD from 1 to 5 years post-HCT with mean height at HCT of –0.38 SD to mean height at 5 years of +0.11 [55]. The EBMT group reported final adult height to be -0.38 ± 1.16 for 10 children [49]. The impact of chronic illness on height growth has been demonstrated in one report of 30 children evaluated at 3 years after HCT. The 12 children with no post-HCT complications had change in height from HCT to 3 years of –0.2 SD whereas the 18 children with complications (mainly chronic GVHD) had change in height of –1.7 SD ($p = 0.001$), demonstrating that factors other than the preparative regimen have significant impact on the child's growth [56].

Irradiation containing preparative regimens

Growth rates

Growth impairment after TBI has been well documented [18,19,21,45,48,49,53,54,57–66]. Children given single-exposure TBI have the highest incidence of growth rate impairment, which has also been associated with decreased GH production. Fractionated TBI was initially thought to have a growth "sparing" effect, but these children have demonstrated decreased growth rates and decreased height SD scores [46,59,67,68]. One study comparing height SD scores for 26 patients given 9–10 Gy single-exposure TBI with those for 23 patients given 12–14.40 Gy fractionated-exposure TBI found that all had decreased height SD scores. The patients with single fraction TBI had height SD scores change from –0.29 to –0.90 ($p = 0.0001$) between 1 and 3 years, whereas the height SD scores for patients who received fractionated TBI changed from –0.09 to –0.22 ($p = 0.02$) between 1 and 3 years after HCT [59]. Children who had received cranial irradiation before either single fraction TBI or fractionated TBI had height SD scores less than those who had not received cranial irradiation [61]. A second study reported the mean cumulative height change during the first 3 years after TBI among prepubertal children not given cranial irradiation. These height changes were significantly worse for the 11 given 10 Gy single-exposure TBI ($p = 0.001$) (mean height change –1.4 SD) compared to seven children given 12 Gy fractionated TBI (p = NS; mean cumulative height change –0.4 SD) [46]. A third study reported no differences in height SD at 8 years after single-exposure TBI for 81 children (whose mean cumulative height changes were –1.25 at 3 years and –1.80 at 8 years after TBI) [68]. The mean height changes for 237 children who had not received cranial irradiation prior to 12.0–15.75 Gy fractionated TBI were –1.0 at 3 years and –1.3 at 6 years, and among the 79 who received cranial irradiation and fractionated TBI, the mean height changes were –1.4 SD at 3 years and –1.7 SD at 6 years. Prior cranial irradiation and years post-transplant were the only factors found to significantly influence subsequent height SD scores. Children who had cranial irradiation were significantly shorter at the time of TBI compared to those who had not ($p = 0.02$). A similar effect of cranial irradiation on growth during the first 4 years after TBI has been observed by others [45,53,54,57,62].

Based on height at the time of transplantation and parental height, the impact of these children's decreasing height SD scores on adult height is a final height that is lower than that predicted [64]. Several investigators have reported that patients who received cranial irradiation in addition to TBI have lower height than those who received TBI without prior cranial irradiation (Table 68.2) [49,63,64,68]. The final adult height of 14 children who received cranial irradiation and 10 children who did not was less than –2.0 SD, or within the range of what is considered to be normal height [64]. These patients were 6.3–14.6 (median 10.8) years at time of transplant. Patient age at transplant has been found to be a significant factor in predicting final adult height [49,64,65,68]. These studies have shown that children less than 6–8 years of age at time of transplant have the greatest risk for growth failure and significantly decreased final adult height. Patient gender has also been found to have a significant influence on final adult height with boys at greater risk of growth failure compared to girls [64,65].

Growth hormone

Growth hormone stimulates growth of epiphyseal cartilage and subsequent bone growth directly via the action of insulin-like growth factor I (IGF-I). When insufficient GH is secreted, growth velocity and bone maturation are usually delayed, and the divergence of the growth rate from normal increases with age unless replacement therapy is initiated. Studies of children with hypopituitarism have shown that the final adult height achieved is related to the height at the start of treatment [69]. The total height gained from GH therapy is inversely related to patient age at the start of treatment and positively related to the duration of therapy. Treatment with GH before the child's height decreased to below the third percentile ($\geq$–1.8 SD) results in the greatest final height response to

Table 68.2 Growth hormone deficiency and treatment [49,63–65,68].

	CNS irradiation		
	No	Yes	Total
No. patients tested	304	147	451
Growth hormone			
normal	104 (32%)	26 (18%)	130 (29%)
deficient	207 (68%)	120 (82%)	327 (73%)
No. patients treated with growth hormone	102 (49%)	90 (75%)	192 (59%)

Table 68.3 Response to growth hormone (GH) therapy.

Reference	No. patients	Pre-GH SD score	1-year GH SD score	2-year GH SD score
[60]	9	−2.7	+1.2	−
[54]	23	−2.20	−1.1	−0.78
[62]	5	−1.56	+0.7	−
[61]	17	−1.2	−1.2	−
[68]	16*	−1.6	−1.1	−1.1
	32†	−1.8	−1.4	−1.3

*16 patients <10 years of age at hematopoietic cell transplantation (HCT).
†32 patients ≥10 years of age at HCT.

treatment. Because growth before puberty is the major determinant of final height, treatment with GH during the prepubertal period needs to be optimized. Among nontransplant children who received cranial irradiation, GH deficiency may develop in those with previously normal GH secretion at the time of puberty because of an inability of the pituitary to increase production of GH in an amount to produce the growth spurt [34,70]. At puberty, normal production of gradually increasing doses of sex hormones contributes to the growth spurt. Many HCT patients have the problem of impaired sex hormone production, especially if the transplant preparative regimen included BU or TBI. The failure of the gonad to produce appropriate sex hormone contributes to their decreased height velocity. These individuals with primary gonadal failure may have improved height velocity from the additional use of gradually increasing doses of sex hormone therapy administered by the pediatric endocrinologist after the child achieves the age of 12–13 years of age [71].

Growth hormone has additional beneficial effects for the growing child in addition to height growth. Children with GH deficiency are at risk for decreased bone mineral density because of reduced osteoblastic activity leading to decreased bone mineral accrual and decreased bone mineral density [72–74]. Studies in children with GH deficiency have shown that GH deficiency-associated reduced bone turnover is reversed with GH therapy [75]. Because the foundation for skeletal health is established in childhood, prevention of decreased bone mineral density begins by optimizing gains in bone mineral acquisition throughout childhood. Children with decreased bone mineral density are at significant risk for decreased bone mineral density as an adult [63,76]. Bone health among children following HCT has not been well studied. One study evaluating bone mineral density found that among the 23 GH-deficient patients bone mineral density z-scores for the hip (−1.25) and spine (−0.41) were less than the bone mineral density z-scores for the hip (0.72) and spine (0.83) among 20 transplant patients with normal GH levels ($p = 0.003$ and $p = 0.04$, respectively) [77].

Growth hormone deficient children have been reported to have behavior and cognitive disturbances including immaturity, anxiety, academic underachievement and problems with social skills [78]. A study of psychological morbidity of childhood GH deficiency suggests that GH replacement therapy results in improved behavior observed after 3 years of GH therapy [79]. There are no data reported among HCT children. GH also contributes to body mass and those who are GH deficient have reduced lean body mass, omental obesity hyperlipidemia and a threefold increase in cardiovascular mortality [80]. Treatment with GH has resulted in improved lean body mass and decreased hyperlipidemia among non-HCT children.

The incidence of GH deficiency after TBI and HCT varies from 20% to 85% depending upon differences in time of testing after HCT, differences in preparative regimens received, inclusion of patients with and without cranial irradiation, and use of different methods of GH testing [57,60,66,81–86]. Even though GH deficiency has been observed, less than half have received GH therapy (Table 68.2) [81]. Retrospective studies have shown that height SD is significantly lower than predicted based on height at HCT and mid-parental height (Table 68.3) [49,63,64]. Authors concluded that GH therapy was not needed because final height SD was not more than 2 SD below the mean, or because GH-treated children did not have significantly improved growth [49,64]. Others have reported, based on a retrospective study, that GH therapy does not benefit children, but most of the children had received less than 1 year of GH therapy [65]. One study reported 13 children, eight of whom received prophylactic cranial irradiation, who were given GH, which restored normal height velocity but without "catch-up" growth. The final height SD scores remained impaired. In these children a mean of 3.2 years had elapsed between TBI and initiation of GH therapy, which began at a mean age of 12.2 (range 5.8–18.2) years of age. The poor response to GH therapy has been attributed to factors such as spinal irradiation, early puberty, suboptimal GH dosing schedules and older age of most patients when GH therapy was initiated. Recent data suggest that improvements in growth and final height can be achieved with contemporary dosing regimens that utilize daily doses of 0.04 mg/kg, increasing to 0.06 mg/kg at puberty [60,62,87,88].

Final height as measured when the child has reached 15–16 years of age or at a time with no further height growth is achieved is an important measure of the impact of the preparative regimen on the child's growth. As shown in Table 68.4, all studies demonstrate decrease in height growth between HCT and final height achieved. All authors observed a significant decrease in height, ranging from −0.5 SD to as much as −2.07 SD. Most authors concluded that treatment with GH was of little value. We have observed that the interval change in height SD score between transplant and diagnosis of GH deficiency was −0.2 SD and an additional −0.2 SD decrement occurred during the median 8-months' interval between the diagnosis of GH deficiency and initiation of GH treatment. Children who received GH therapy subsequently maintained height SD scores while untreated children experienced a further −0.9 SD decrement in height by the time final adult height was reached (Fig. 68.1). Factors predictive of improved final height after GH therapy were prior cranial irradiation, age ≥10 years and height SD above −1.5 at time of GH deficiency. Further loss in height SD was prevented in younger children whose height SD was −1.5 or below. The final height SD in GH treated children was +0.52 SD more compared to untreated children ($p = 0.003$) in a multiple linear regression model adjusted for gender, age at transplant and height SD at time of GH deficiency diagnosis (J. Sanders, unpublished data, 2002).

Initially, treatment with human GH was restricted because of the limited supply of the drug, but with the availability of recombinant GH, access is no longer a problem. Reports of leukemia occurring in patients treated with human GH raised concern that there might be a causal relationship between GH therapy and development of leukemia [85,89–91]. The Lawton Wilkins Pediatric Endocrine Society and the Human Growth Foundation of the USA convened a workshop in 1988 to review known

Table 68.4 Final adult height SD scores for children transplanted with total body irradiation preparative regimens.

Reference	Regimen	No. patients	Height SD at HCT	Final height SD	Height SD change	p-value
[64]	TBI	14	0.25 (−2.6 to +2.3)	−0.66 (−1.7 to +0.6)	−0.91	0.02
	CRT + TBI	11	0.44 (−1.3 to +2.4)	−1.02 (−2.14 to +1.4)	−1.46	0.0002
[65]	TBI	16	−0.2 (±0.79)	−1.77 (±1.03)	−1.57 (±0.94)	0.0001
[63]	TBI	6	0.8 (0.5–2.3)	0.3 (0.7–1.1)		0.02
	CRT + TBI	8	−0.4 (−1.9 to +1.9)	−1.0 (−1.5 to +0.4)		0.02
[49]	CRT + S-TBI	13			−2.07 (±0.91)	
	S-TBI	39			−1.37 (±1.06)	
	CRT + FTBI	34			−1.11 (±1.61)	
	FTBI	39			−0.88 (±1.25)	

CRT, cranial irradiation; FTBI, fractionated-exposure total body irradiation; HCT, hematopoietic cell translplantation; S-TBI, single-exposure total body irradiation; TBI, total body irradiation.

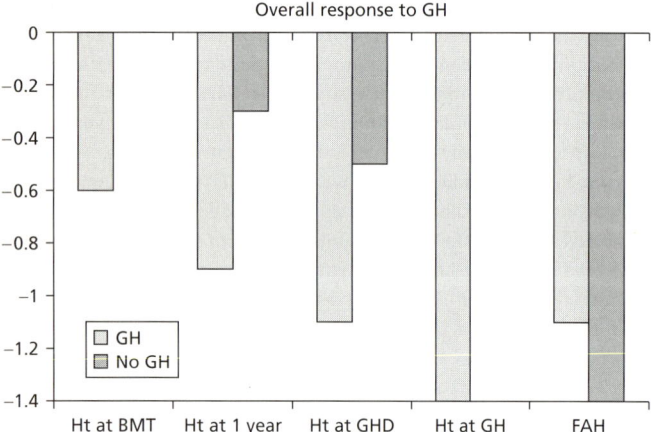

Fig. 68.1 Height SD scores of growth hormone (GH) deficient children pretransplant and following fractionated total body irradiation (FTBI) and hematopoietic cell transplantation (HCT) at noted time intervals to final adult height (FAH). Forty-two patients received GH therapy (light bars) and 48 did not receive GH therapy (dark bars) ($p = 0.003$ at FAH).

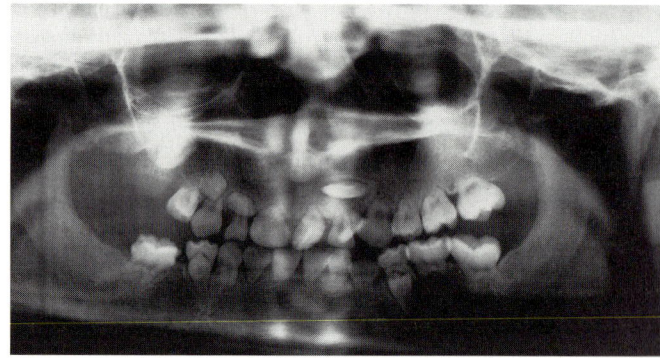

Fig. 68.2 Post-transplant dental Panorex demonstrating shortened root structure on primary teeth, secondary tooth agenesis (multiple teeth), and globular or conical crowns in this child who was less than 6 years of age at total body irradiation (TBI).

leukemia cases in 22,000 GH-treated patients in Europe, North America, Japan and Australia since 1959 [92]. Of 15 cases of leukemia, four occurred after a brief period of GH therapy or there were compelling reasons to suspect another cause for the leukemia. The 11 suspect cases developed during 150,000 patient-years of risk, including periods of treatment and follow-up, so that the incidence of leukemia was approximately 1/21,000 patient-years at risk. The expected annual leukemia incidence among hypopituitary patients treated was estimated to be 1/42,000 patient-years. After review of all available data, workshop participants concluded that there may be a small increase in leukemia incidence associated with GH treatment of GH-deficient patients; however, it was not clear that this incidence was directly related to GH therapy. In absolute terms, a current estimate of individual risk, assuming a 10-year GH treatment course, would be 1/2400 (0.042%), which is not different from the surveillance and end results (SEER) estimate of new cases of leukemia reported in the USA (1/2400/year). Thus, treatment of GH-deficient children after BMT should not contribute to an increased risk of leukemia occurrence. To date, there have been no reported or known cases of leukemia occurring in GH-treated children after TBI. Among a group of 106 children given more than 1 year of GH therapy, none have developed recurrent leukemia or other secondary malignancy. These children received a total of 269 patient-years of GH therapy (J. Sanders, unpublished data, 2002).

Orofacial growth

Irradiation to bone produces epiphyseal, metaphyseal and diaphyseal injury that affects subsequent bone growth [93]. The effect is related to patient age at the time of irradiation as well as the site irradiated, the dose schedule and the total dose of irradiation [94]. Young children, especially children less than 6 years of age at the time of irradiation to the head and neck, have the greatest risk for development of subsequent craniofacial and dental abnormalities [95–98]. Enamel and dentin formation are disturbed by TBI because of destruction of cells during mitotic phase. Chemotherapy drugs are selectively toxic to actively proliferating cells by disruption of DNA synthesis and replication, RNA transcription and cytoplasmic transport mechanisms [99]. Chemotherapy and irradiation effects on dental development include tooth agenesis, complete or partial arrest of root development with thin tapered roots, early apical closure, globular and conical crowns, dentin and enamel opacities and defects, microdontia, enlarged pulp chambers, taurodontism and abnormal occlusion (Fig. 68.2) [97,100,101]. Hence, the development of secondary teeth is often affected, with delayed or arrested tooth formation, shortening and blunting of tooth roots, incomplete calcification, premature closure of apices and dental caries. However, some children with hematologic malignancies who received preparative regimens with chemotherapy alone do not have abnormalities in dental maturity or eruption of their permanent dentition [102].

Reduction in lower face height in HCT patients correlated with impaired dental development [98]. Vertical condyle growth and the alveolar and molar heights were adversely affected by pretransplant preparative regimens. Cephalometric measurements of facial bones to evaluate facial growth before and after 10 Gy TBI and HCT have resulted in a significant reduction in the maxilla length and mandible growth compared with healthy age-matched nontransplant children. These differences were most pronounced in mandibular growth [98]. Compared with the control group, the children and adolescents in the HCT group also had significantly reduced mouth opening capacity with reduced translation movement of the condyles diagnosed in 53% of children treated with TBI, compared with 5% in the control group [96]. Signs of craniomandibular dysfunction were found in 84% of children in the HCT children, compared with 58% in the control group. The long-term alterations in connective and muscle tissues result in changes in tissue inflammation and eventually fibrosis.

An evaluation of craniofacial development in 16 prepubertal children (age range 1.7–11.0 years) with growth failure and GH deficiency following CY plus 10.0 Gy TBI and HCT demonstrated a significant positive effect on growth among the nine GH-treated patients compared to seven non-GH-treated patients [95]. Another study demonstrated improvement in vertical growth of the condyles, suggesting that condylar cartilage is the most likely site of mandibular growth activity [103]. These observations support the hypothesis that GH most likely encourages longitudinal bone growth both directly, by stimulating differentiation of epiphyseal growth plate precursor cells, and indirectly, by increasing the responsiveness to IGF-I [104]. Treatment with GH, however, did not improve the disturbed root development of the teeth. Thus, there does not appear to be a stimulating effect of dental development on growth of the alveolar process.

Few data are available for the use of orthodontic treatment for children who have dental growth disturbances after TBI and HCT. A retrospective study of 10 children has demonstrated that orthodontic treatment plans were modified to reflect the patient's medical condition but, in general, the orthodontic treatment did not produce any harmful side-effects, even though most treated children exhibited severe pre-existing disturbances in dental development [105]. Nine of the 10 patients had severe disturbances in dental development with short V-shaped roots, premature apical closure, enamel disturbances, microdontia and aplasia. The most severe disturbances were found in children less than 5 years of age at the time of 10 Gy TBI. The strategies used to cope with the severe problems of dental growth disturbances included using appliances that minimized the risk of root resorption, using weaker forcers, terminating treatment earlier than normal and choosing the simplest method for treatment needs. In general, the lower jaw was not treated. The treatment was judged as unsatisfactory in four of the 10 patients.

Puberty

Puberty, a transitional stage from a sexually immature to a mature sexual state, is accompanied by significant changes in gonadal and growth hormonal activity, development of secondary sexual characteristics and increased growth velocity. There is considerable variation in the timing and sequence of pubertal events which make it difficult to assess a child's pubertal development based only on chronological age. In the normal individual, pubertal development is usually closely related with osseous maturation as measured by bone age. An intact hypothalamic–pituitary–gonadal axis is required for initiation and completion of puberty. The normal pubertal growth rate is 1.5–2 times greater than prepubertal growth rates [106]. In the absence of pubertal sex hormone secretion, the increased growth velocity associated with the pubertal growth spurt is substantially blunted, and development of secondary sexual characteristics is delayed or absent. Gonadal hormone production and germ-cell viability are affected by high doses of alkylating agents and irradiation, with variables related to patient age, sex, and type and dose of therapy [107]. Azoospermia develops in prepubertal boys who have received a cumulative dose of more than 350 mg/kg CY, whereas doses of 200 mg/kg or less result in minimal alteration of spermatogenesis. The total dose of BU impacting future developmental potential for the prepubertal testes is not known. Irradiation to the prepubertal testes results in damage to the germinal epithelium that does not become apparent until after puberty [108]. Boys who have received more than 24 Gy testicular irradiation have delayed or arrested development of secondary sexual characteristics, with elevated gonadotropin and low testosterone values. Primary ovarian failure usually occurs following total cumulative doses of more than 500 mg/kg CY to prepubertal girls [107]. No data are available regarding BU or irradiation on the prepubertal ovary.

Sex hormones indirectly stimulate linear growth by increasing endogenous GH secretion [109]. This stimulation leads to increasing circulating and tissue levels of IGF-I, which activates growth at the level of bone and cartilage. Treatment with low to moderate doses of sex hormones promotes increased linear growth, but physiologic adult doses of sex hormones result in a greater influence on skeletal maturation with resultant compromise in final adult height via the mechanism of premature epiphyseal closure. Children with idiopathic GH deficiency usually have a late but normal pubertal growth spurt. Children with hypogonadotropic hypogonadism have an absence of sex hormone production, delayed puberty, delayed pubertal growth spurt and an increase in final adult height [71]. Thus, interruption in either production of pubertal GH or sex hormone production is likely to result in both delayed pubescence and decreased linear height.

Preparative regimens containing only chemotherapy

Following 200 mg/kg CY and BMT for aplastic anaemia, 31 of 32 girls and 28 of 31 boys who were prepubertal at time of administration of CY have now been followed long enough to be more than 12 years of age and evaluable for pubertal development [48,81,110,111]. Nearly all of these children demonstrated normal age-appropriate progression through puberty (Tables 68.5 and 68.6). The three girls with delayed pubertal development all had Fanconi's syndrome and eventually developed normal secondary sexual characteristics and normal lutenizing hormone (LH), follicle-stimulating hormone (FSH) and estradiol. Among the 26 girls with normal age-appropriate development, menarche occurred at a median of 12.5 years of age (range 11–16) and the three with delayed development had menarche occur between 16 and 19 years of age. Twenty-one of these formerly prepubertal girls have given birth to 36 normal children [111; J. Sanders, unpublished data, 2002]. The three boys with delayed pubertal development had chronic GVHD and ultimately developed normal secondary sexual characteristics with normal LH, FSH and testosterone. Eighteen of these formerly prepubertal boys have fathered 36 normal children.

Gonadal function after 14 mg/kg BU plus 200 mg/kg CY and allogeneic BMT for thalassemia has been reported for 30 prepubertal patients (15 girls, 15 boys) who ranged in age from 9.3 to 17.2 years [81,112]. Thirteen girls had evidence of primary ovarian failure, with elevated gonadotropin levels, and two patients had hypogonadotropic hypogonadism. All girls had low estradiol levels both before and after transplantation. Among the 15 boys, post-transplant LH and FSH concentrations were within normal limits. However, after gonadotropin-releasing hormone stimulation, three had normal responses, two had elevated FSH responses, and 10 had low responses. These gonadal function results must be interpreted with caution, however, because patients with thalassemia treated with chelation and transfusion therapy frequently show delayed or absent puberty.

Pubertal development has been evaluated among children transplanted for malignancy who received 16 mg/kg BU plus 120–200 mg/kg CY

Table 68.5 Pubertal development in girls.

		Preparative regimen			
		CY*	BUCY†	10.0 Gy TBI‡	12–15.75 Gy TBI§
Current age	≥12 years	31	39	24	77
Development	Normal	26 (84%)	7 (18%)	7 (29%)	39 (50%)
	Delayed	5 (16%)	32 (82%)	17 (71%)	38 (50%)
LH	Prepubertal	5	–	–	–
	Normal	26	7	7	39
	Elevated	–	32	17	38
FSH	Prepubertal	5	–	–	–
	Normal	26	7	7	39
	Elevated	–	32	17	38
Estradiol	Normal	26	7	7	39
	Low	5	32	17	38
Pregnancies	No. girls	21	–	3	20
	No. live births	36	–	2	10

BU, busulphan; CY, cyclophosphamide; FSH, follicle-stimulating hormone; LH, lutenizing hormone; TBI, total body irradiation.
*References [48,112].
†Reference [155; J. Sanders, unpublished data, 2002].
‡References [48,67,111,156; J. Sanders, unpublished data, 2002].
§References [48,67,111,156; J. Sanders, unpublished data, 2002].

Table 68.6 Pubertal development in boys.

		Preparative regimen			
		CY*	BUCY†	10.0 Gy TBI‡§	12–15.75 Gy TBI‡¶
Current age	≥12 years	28	25	32	77
Development	Normal	24 (86%)	8 (32%)	6 (19%)	32 (42%)
	Delayed	4 (14%)	17 (68%)	26 (81%)	45 (58%)
LH	Prepubertal	4	–	–	–
	Normal	24	8	6	32
	Elevated	–	17	26	45
FSH	Prepubertal	4	–	–	–
	Normal	21	8	6	32
	Elevated	–	17	26	45
Testosterone	Normal	24	8	6	32
	Low	4	17	26	45
Children fathered	No. men	18	–	–	7
	No. live births	36	–	–	6

BU, busulphan; CY, cyclophosphamide; FSH, follicle-stimulating hormone; LH, lutenizing hormone; TBI, total body irradiation.
*References [48,112].
†References [155; J. Sanders, unpublished data, 2002].
‡No additional testicular irradiation.
§References [48,67,111,156; J. Sanders, unpublished data, 2002].
¶References [48,67,111,156; J. Sanders, unpublished data, 2002].

[19,81,113; J. Sanders, unpublished data, 2002]. Sixty-three children have now been followed long enough to be evaluable for development of spontaneous pubertal development (Tables 68.5 and 68.6). Thirty-one of 39 (79%) evaluable girls and 17 of 24 (71%) evaluable boys have developed normally through puberty and have normal LH, FSH and sex hormone production. These data demonstrate that BU is highly toxic to the prepubertal gonad and that these children must be carefully followed with gonadal function evaluation beginning about 12 years of age.

Table 68.7 Pubertal development in boys given testicular irradiation (J. Sanders, unpublished data, 2002).

		Testicular irradiation	
		4.0 Gy	≥10 Gy
Current age	≥12 years	25	30
Development	Normal	13 (52%)	2 (6%)
	Delayed	12 (48%)	28 (94%)

Supplementation with appropriate gonadal hormones administered in gradually increasing doses under supervision of a pediatric endocrinologist is needed for these children to develop secondary sexual characteristics.

Preparative regimens containing irradiation

Development of secondary sexual characteristics among children who were prepubertal at the time of TBI administration but more than 12 years of age at follow-up was evaluated in 24 girls and 31 boys after 10 Gy single fraction TBI and 77 girls and 77 boys after 12–15.75 Gy fractionated exposure TBI (Tables 68.5 and 68.6). Following 10.0 Gy single-exposure TBI, 71% of girls and 83% of boys had delayed development of secondary sexual characteristics and elevated LH, FSH and low sex hormone levels. After fractionated exposure TBI, 49% of girls and 58% of boys had delayed development. The majority of these girls and boys have received appropriate sex hormone therapy for promotion of secondary sexual characteristic development. As larger numbers of prepubertal children are becoming evaluable for pubertal development, the amount of testicular irradiation received and patient age at the time of TBI are emerging as important factors in subsequent normal spontaneous pubertal development (Table 68.7). Twenty-eight of 30 (93%) boys who had received more than 10 Gy testicular irradiation for testicular leukemia in addition to 12–15.75 Gy TBI have primary gonadal failure and require testosterone therapy to promote development of secondary sexual characteristics. However, about half of the boys who receive 400 cGy prophylactic testicular irradiation in addition to fractionated TBI develop normally through puberty [33; J. Sanders, unpublished data, 2002]. Among children receiving 14.40 Gy fractionated TBI, one study reported that among 17 boys evaluated, those with increased levels of LH were significantly younger at BMT (5.4 ± 0.8 vs. 7.8 ± 0.8 years; $p = 0.024$) but, among the 16 girls evaluated, those with ovarian failure were significantly older at time of TBI than those with spontaneous puberty (8.6 ± 2.3 vs. 6.1 ± 1.8 years; $p = 0.03$) [33]. Another study did not observe an effect of age with all eight children less than 9 years, but neither girl and seven of the eight boys more than 9 years at time of 12.0–14.40 Gy fractionated TBI had normal FSH [59]. A third analysis suggested that an effect of age may be linked to the total dose of TBI [81]. Among 30 evaluable children given 12.0 Gy TBI, 15 of 16 (94%) less than 10 years of age and 11 of 14 (78%) more than 10 years of age developed normally. However, among the 46 evaluable children given 14.40–15.75 Gy TBI, 23 of 30 (77%) less than 10 years of age and three of 16 (19%) more than 10 years of age developed normally. Larger numbers of patients are needed to draw firm conclusions regarding the impact of patient age and total dose of TBI administered on development of puberty.

It is recommended that the development of secondary sexual characteristics be monitored carefully after patients reach 10–11 years of age and that Tanner Developmental Scores be determined annually. Because production of sex hormones is necessary for promotion of the pubertal growth spurt in addition to promoting sexual maturation, children with evidence of gonadal failure and delayed development of secondary sexual characteristics may benefit from supplemental hormones. This supplementation should be administered under the guidance of a pediatric endocrinologist and doses of sex hormone treatment should begin low with gradual increase to simulate natural hormone production and to prevent premature advancement of bone age and to promote the pubertal growth spurts. Patients with normal pubertal development, normal gonadotropins and sex hormone production should receive appropriate sexual behavior counseling as pregnancy may occur.

Gonadal function after puberty

Alkylating agent therapy administered to adult women may impair reproductive function [114]. Ovarian atrophy has been observed following treatment with BU [115]. After CY therapy, examination of ovarian biopsy specimens demonstrated loss of ova, which suggests that CY acts directly on the oocyte [116]. The reversibility of this loss of ova is related to patient age and the total dose of CY received. Because CY acts by first-order kinetics and the number of oocytes normally decreases steadily with increasing age, equivalent drug doses in older patients whose ova are more depleted than those of younger patients may explain why the likelihood of infertility is increased in older women. A cumulative total dose of 5.2 Gy CY given to a 40-year-old woman results in ovarian failure, whereas a cumulative total dose of 20 g given to a 25-year-old woman is needed to produce ovarian failure [116].

Impairment of ovarian function following irradiation to the ovary is related to the age of the woman at the time of irradiation; more precisely, the number of oocytes remaining at the time of irradiation [117]. In women less than 40 years old, doses of 800 cGy result in 70% of the women becoming permanently sterilized. Fractionated irradiation doses of up to 20.0 Gy result in more than 50% of women 20–30-year-olds developing ovarian failure [107].

The predominant gonadal lesion after alkylating agent therapy in adult men is localized to the germinal epithelium [118]. Examination of testicular biopsy specimens from men treated with CY demonstrated Sertoli cell damage, with germinal aplasia and absent spermatogonia and spermatozoa [119,120]. This level of damage is usually reflected in an elevated FSH level and azoospermia. Leydig cell function is spared, as evidenced by normal LH and testosterone levels. The degree of testicular function compromise is related to total dose of CY, but age does not appear to be a factor. Azoospermia develops in patients who receive more than a cumulative total dose of 18 Gy CY, but oligospermia develops in those who receive less than 250 mg/kg CY given as low doses of CY for short periods. This condition is often reversible. Recovery of spermatogenesis may occur after a period of a year or more.

Studies of the irradiated adult male have demonstrated that the magnitude and duration of suppression of spermatogenesis are dependent on the dose administered [107,121]. As little as 0.3 Gy to the testes has resulted in germinal epithelial damage, decreased sperm counts and increased FSH levels. Leydig cell function is usually spared, with normal LH and testosterone levels. Leydig cell damage usually does not occur until higher doses of irradiation, and even then the testosterone levels remain normal. After doses of 200–300 cGy, FSH levels and sperm counts return to normal after 3 years, but after doses of 400–600 cGy, testicular function does not return to normal until 5 years or later. When irradiation is administered in fractionated exposures, the effect may be more profound than when it is administered as a single exposure. The total irradiation doses above which recovery never occurs has not been firmly established, but few patients have been documented to have recovered above doses of 800 cGy.

Table 68.8 Ovarian function in post-pubertal women.

	Preparative regimen			
	CY*	BUCY†	CY + TAI/TLI‡	CY + TBI§
No. evaluated	145	93	9	562
Age at BMT (years)	13–48	14–47	15–22	13–50
Follow-up (years)	1–17	1–6	1–5	1–14
No. ovarian recovery	98	2	9	83
	(68%)	(2%)	(100%)	(15%)
No. pregnant	28+	0	1	32
No. live births	44+	0	1	13+
No. abortions	12+	0	0	10+

CY, cyclophosphamide; BU, busulfan; TAI, thoracoabdominal irradiation; TBI, total body irradiation; TLI, total lymphoid irradiation.
+ The number of additional pregnancies and live births not reported in reference [157].
*References [110,111,122–128].
†References [110,111,130].
‡References [128,132,133].
§References [110,111,122,128,134–138].

Table 68.9 Testicular function in post-pubertal men.

	Preparative regimen		
	CY*	BUCY†	CY + TBI‡
No. evaluated	128	98	498
Age at BMT (years)	13–52	13–56	11–62
Follow-up (years)	1–19	1–12	1–19
No. testicular recovery	86	48	107
	(68%)	(49%)	(21%)
No. partners pregnant	28+	9	34
No. live births	44+	12	8+
No. abortions	12	1	8+

+ The number of additional pregnancies and live births not reported in reference [157].
*References [110,111,122,127,128].
†References [110,111,130].
‡References [110,111,122,128].

Preparative regimens containing chemotherapy only

Women

Ovarian function has been evaluated in 145 women who were between ages 13 and 48 years at the time of receiving 200 mg/kg CY and BMT for aplastic anaemia [110,111,122–128]. All women had normal menstrual periods prior to CY administration, and therefore were considered as having normal ovarian function. Follow-up studies with measurements of LH, FSH and estradiol as well as histories of menstruation, constitutional symptoms related to menopause and hormone replacement therapy administered were obtained (Table 68.8). All women developed amenorrhea for varying lengths of time after CY administration. Ovarian function recovered in 54% at a median of 9 (range 3–36) months with a return of normal gonadotropin and estrogen levels and normal spontaneous menstruation. Forty women with ovarian function recovery have been reported by the EBMT, but what proportion of the population these 40 represent was not able to be determined [128]. Patient age at the time of receiving CY appears to be an important factor with nearly all women less than 26 years of age having evidence of ovarian function recovery. Those who do not recover normal estradiol levels benefit from receiving estrogen/progesterone cyclic hormone supplementation. Chronic GVHD was not a factor associated with ovarian recovery, but may be a factor in normal sexual function because of dry vaginal mucosa [129]. At 20 years post-transplant, the probability that a female patient would become pregnant was 47% (range 26% in patients with acute and chronic GVHD to 61% among patients with *de novo* chronic GVHD). It is not possible to determine precisely the number of patients who had attempted to have children [127].

Ninety-three women have been evaluated for return of ovarian function following receiving BU plus CY preparative regimen (Table 68.8) [110,130]. Two of these women had return of normal gonadotropin and estradiol levels and menstruation. The remainder had primary ovarian failure with LH and FSH levels elevated in the menopausal range and have low estradiol levels. Many of these women had symptoms of ovarian failure, which may be controlled with cyclic estrogen/progesterone therapy. Two of the women have had children using fertilized ova from their sisters [130].

Men

Testicular function has been evaluated in 128 men between 13 and 52 years of age when given 200 mg/kg CY and BMT (Table 68.9) [110,111,127,128]. Follow-up studies demonstrated that Leydig cell function was normal in more than 95% with normal LH and normal testosterone values. Sertoli cell function was normal in 61% with normal FSH levels suggesting normal spermatogenesis. The probability of spermatogenesis and quality of the sperm was not able to be evaluated as a result of lack of specimen submission. In the 12% who did submit semen for analysis, sperm motility was normal as were sperm counts. The EBMT reported 19 men who recovered testicular function following preparative regimens with CY only, but the total number of men evaluated was not reported, making the proportion of men who recovered impossible to determine [128]. The probability of fathering a child was 50% (range 29% among those with acute and chronic GVHD to 62% among patients with neither acute of chronic GVHD) [127]. It was not possible to determine what proportion of patients had attempted to have children.

Following a preparative regimen of 16 mg/kg BU and 120 or 200 mg/kg CY, 98 men had testicular function evaluated between 1 and 12 years after BMT [110,130,131]. Leydig cell function was normal for the majority with normal LH and testosterone levels, but Sertoli cell function was impaired with elevated FSH levels and azoospermia for 65%. Forty-eight men had return of testicular function defined as high normal FSH levels and low normal sperm counts. A fine needle testicular biopsy carried out in one of the azoospermic patients with chronic GVHD demonstrated that all seminiferous tubules were reduced in diameter, with moderate peritubular fibrosis. No germ cells were identified in any of 30 tubules present in the biopsy [130]. Data from two patients with serial semen analyzed suggest that sperm counts increase with increasing years post-transplant [130].

Preparative regimens containing thoracoabdominal irradiation

Women

Nine women who were 15–36 years of age at time of TAI administration have had ovarian function reported [128,132,133]. All had evidence for primary ovarian failure for at least the first 3 years after TAI with elevated

LH, FSH and low estradiol levels. One woman followed for more than 3 years recovered ovarian function approximately 4 years after TAI.

Men

Three men have been noted to have recovery of testicular function following TAI. No details are included regarding recovery [128].

Preparative regimens containing total body irradiation

Women

A total of 562 women who were between 13 and 50 years of age at the time of exposure to 10 Gy TBI in a single setting or 12–15.75 Gy fractionated TBI had ovarian function evaluated from 1 to 14 years (median 4) after BMT [110,111,122,128,134–138]. All of these women were menstruating prior to initiation of the preparative regimen. After TBI, all women developed primary ovarian failure with elevated LH and FSH levels, low estradiol levels and amenorrhea. Between 3 and 7 years (median 5 years) after TBI, 83 women demonstrated ovarian recovery with spontaneous return of normal LH, FSH and estradiol levels and spontaneous menstruation. Chronic GVHD did not influence recovery of ovarian function. More than half of the women with primary ovarian failure experienced symptoms of menopause with vasomotor instability, insomnia, osteoporosis, vaginitis and vaginal atrophy [122,129]. In addition, women with chronic GVHD are at risk for development of vaginal strictures and vaginal web formation secondary to vaginal mucosal involvement with chronic GVHD. Vaginal dilation and systemic control of chronic GVHD are necessary, in addition to systemic cyclic estrogen/progesterones, to control symptoms. In order to minimize the contribution of lack of estrogen to osteoporosis and to control systemic symptoms, it is recommended that all women receive cyclic hormone therapy beginning approximately 3 months after TBI.

Men

A total of 498 men were evaluated for return of testicular function between 1 and 12 years after HCT with TBI-containing preparative regimens [110,111,128]. In general, Leydig cell function was preserved, with normal LH and testosterone levels, but Sertoli cell function was damaged as evidenced by elevated FSH levels in the majority of men. A high incidence of sexual dysfunction following TBI for malignancy was reported in 51 men, more than half of whom had chronic GVHD [139]. Among 16 men, 75% reported normal interest in sexual activities, 87.5% reported normal erectile function, but four of 16 reported moderate loss of interest in sexual activities and another two reported frequent loss of erectile function [140]. Decreased testosterone levels correlated with a moderate or total loss of libido ($p = 0.008$). Gynecomastia with hypergonadotropic hypogonadism and Leydig cell insufficiency has been reported in three men who received TBI preparative regimen [141]. A total of 463 men have been evaluated for return of testicular function between 1 and 12 years after HCT with TBI-containing preparative regimens [110,111]. In general, Leydig cell function was preserved, with normal LH and testosterone levels, but Sertoli cell function was damaged as evidenced by elevated FSH levels in the majority of men. Among the 71 men evaluated after 10 Gy TBI, 14 recovered testicular function as did 37 of those given 12.0 Gy TBI and 30 of the 166 given 14–15.75 Gy TBI. A high incidence of sexual dysfunction following TBI for malignancy, in 51 men, was reported in more than half of whom had chronic GVHD (68).

Pregnancies

Both alkylating agents and irradiation are mutagenic with the potential of injury to germ cell chromosomes. Fertility is reduced when alkylating agents are combined with irradiation below the diaphragm [142–144].

Thus, children born to patients who recover gonadal function after TBI may be at increased risk for the development of genetic diseases and congenital anomalies [145,146]. However, children born to long-term survivors of conventional chemotherapy for childhood cancer do not have an increased incidence of congenital anomalies, but survivors who received abdominal irradiation have a higher risk of spontaneous abortions and the babies tend to have lower birth weights [143–147]. Irradiation may reduce the elasticity of the uterine musculature or produce uterine vascular damage, which could partially explain the higher spontaneous abortion rates and lower birth weights [148,149].

Initially, reports of pregnancies occurring among patients who have received marrow transplantation were limited individual cases that included limited information regarding the actual pregnancy and few details other than a live birth [123–126,132–138]. Two analyses of a large number of pregnancies following HCT have now been reported: one from a single-center study and one from the EBMT [110,128]. The single-center analysis reported 41 women who had 72 pregnancies and 35 men whose partners had 63 pregnancies. This study showed that women who had undergone HCT, especially those who received TBI, were at high risk for spontaneous abortion, preterm labor and delivery of low-birthweight infants [110]. The data from the EBMT indicated a frequency of pregnancy complications that was significantly increased in female patients who received allogeneic but not autologous HCT. This group also noted a significantly higher than normal rate of preterm delivery and low-birthweight babies in female recipients of allogeneic HCT who had received TBI. Minor congenital anomalies were observed in two (4.5%) of 44 infants of CY-treated female patients (ventricular septal defect and congenital nevi), six of 51 (11.8%) infants of partners of CY-treated male patients (ventricular septal defect, congenital hip disease, eczema at birth) and none of the infants of TBI-treated patients [110]. The EBMT reported that seven of 209 (3%) infants had congenital anomalies (cerebral palsy, patent ductus arteriosus, dislocation of the hip, congenital hemangioma, everted feet) [128]. This incidence is not different from that of minor congenital anomalies identified at birth in the general population (3.8–14.8%), nor the 8.7% and the 11% frequencies observed among children of parents treated for childhood cancer [147,150]. These data regarding congenital anomalies in the offspring born to former HCT patients are limited by the relatively small numbers of children born. The few observed congenital anomalies may not permit the observance of a biologically significant change in the germ-line mutation rate.

An evaluation of the effects of irradiation, specifically gamma irradiation and neutron irradiation, on the frequency of mutations among Japanese children exposed to atomic bombs in Hiroshima and Nagasaki showed no immediate evidence of an effect [151]. Mutation injury was identified many years after exposure to gamma or neutron radiation in adult cancer patients treated with irradiation therapy, chemotherapy, or both [152–154]. HCT patients have been evaluated for a relatively short time after irradiation exposure (<30 years) and so it may be that these and the prepubertal patients who develop normal gonadal function after TBI are at high risk for the occurrence of germ cell mutational injury. Further longitudinal studies are needed in young children, adolescents and young adults who received HCT to determine if any late mutational injury that will affect their offspring can be detected. The children born to HCT patients must also continue to be followed to define any late sequelae developing as a result of parental therapy.

Conclusions

Evaluations of endocrine function following HCT demonstrate that the occurrence of abnormalities that may influence subsequent growth and development are related to the type of HCT preparative regimen received. Children who receive CY only usually do not have endocrine function abnormalities. These children have normal thyroid function, normal growth rates and normal development through puberty. In postpubertal adolescents and adults, gonadal function usually returns to normal. Individuals who develop normally through puberty or in whom gonadal function returns to normal may be fertile. Offspring of these patients, in general, do not differ from the general population.

Children who receive BU plus CY preparative regimens have normal thyroid function and the majority have normal prepubertal growth rates. Pubertal growth may be affected, but the small number of evaluable patients precludes definitive conclusions regarding the pubertal growth spurt. Data from the patients evaluable for pubertal development suggest that a substantial portion of these children may not develop secondary sexual characteristics at a normal age. Postpubertal patients and young adults rarely have return of gonadal function and should be appropriately counseled regarding the high probability of infertility.

In contrast, multiple endocrine function abnormalities that affect normal growth and development frequently occur after HCT regimens that contain TBI. Patients are at risk for development of thyroid function abnormalities for many years after TBI. These patients are also at risk for development of thyroid malignancy. Growth rates are usually blunted, especially if the child has received prior CNS irradiation. GH deficiency, which frequently occurs, and growth failure should be diagnosed and treated with synthetic GH early for best response. Without GH treatment, young children have significantly compromised final adult heights. Gonadal function damage results in a significant fraction of prepubertal patients having delayed pubertal development and frequently results in early primary gonadal failure among postpubertal adolescents and adults. Children with delayed development of secondary sexual characteristics may benefit from careful administration of appropriate sex hormone therapy. Young women with early primary gonadal failure benefit from cyclic hormone therapy. Children who do develop normally through puberty and have normal gonadal function as well as those postpubertal patients who recover normal gonadal function are potentially fertile. Girls who have received TBI are at high risk for spontaneous abortions, premature labor and delivery of low-birthweight babies. The infants of these individuals, however, do not appear to be at higher risk for congenital anomalies than the general population, although the small number of babies born, the few congenital anomalies observed and the relatively short follow-up suggest that these observations must be regarded with caution.

All patients who receive HCT should continue to undergo long-term follow-up evaluations. Similarly, the children of former HCT patients should also be identified and followed for subsequent development of abnormalities that may be related to therapy received by their parent.

References

1 Lowrey GJ. *Growth and Development of Children*, 8th edn. Chicago: Year Book Medical Publishers, 1986.

2 Fleming ID, Black TL, Thompson EI, Pratt C, Rao B, Hustu O. Thyroid dysfunction and neoplasia in children receiving neck irradiation for cancer. *Cancer* 1985; **55**: 1190–4.

3 Crom DB, Kaste SC, Tubergen DG, Greenwald CA, Sharp GB, Hudson MM. Ultrasonography for thyroid screening after head and neck irradiation in childhood cancer survivors. *Med Pediatr Oncol* 1997; **28**: 15–21.

4 Neglia JP, Nesbit ME Jr. Care and treatment of long-term survivors of childhood cancer. *Cancer* 1993; **71**: 3386–91 [Review].

5 Atahan IL, Yildiz F, Ozyar E, Uzal D. Thyroid dysfunction in children receiving neck irradiation for Hodgkin's disease. *Radiat Med* 1998; **16**: 359–61.

6 Viswanathan K, Gierlowski TC, Schneider AB. Childhood thyroid cancer: characteristics and long-term outcome in children irradiated for benign conditions of the head and neck. *Arch Pediatr Adolesc Med* 1994; **148**: 260–5.

7 Ron E, Lubin JH, Shore RE et al. Thyroid cancer after exposure to external radiation: a pooled analysis of seven studies. *Radiat Res* 1995; **141**: 259–77.

8 Shafford EA, Kingston JE, Healy JC, Webb JA, Plowman PN, Reznek RH. Thyroid nodular disease after radiotherapy to the neck for childhood Hodgkin's disease. *Br J Cancer* 1999; **80**: 808–14.

9 Shore RE, Woodard E, Hildreth N, Dvoretsky P, Hempelmann L, Pasternack B. Thyroid tumors following thymus irradiation. *J Natl Cancer Inst* 1985; **74**: 1177–84.

10 DeGroot LJ. Clinical review 2. Diagnostic approach and management of patients exposed to irradiation to the thyroid. *J Clin Endocrinol Metab* 1989; **69**: 925–8.

11 Tucker MA, Jones PH, Boice JD Jr. et al. Therapeutic radiation at a young age is linked to secondary thyroid cancer. The Late Effects Study Group. *Cancer Res* 1991; **51**: 2885–8.

12 Schneider AB, Ron E, Lubin J, Stovall M, Gierlowski TC. Dose–response relationships for radiation-induced thyroid cancer and thyroid nodules: evidence for the prolonged effects of radiation on the thyroid. *J Clin Endocrinol Metab* 1993; **77**: 362–9.

13 Antonelli A, Miccoli P, Derzhitski VE, Panasiuk G, Solovieva N, Baschieri L. Epidemiologic and clinical evaluation of thyroid cancer in children from the Gomel region (Belarus). *World J Surg* 1996; **20**: 867–71.

14 Inskip PD, Hartshorne MF, Tekkel M et al. Thyroid nodularity and cancer among Chernobyl cleanup workers from Estonia. *Radiat Res* 1997; **147**: 225–35.

15 Sanders JE, Buckner CD, Sullivan KM et al. Growth and development after bone marrow transplantation. In: Buckner CD, Gale RP, Lucarelli G, eds. *Advances and Controversies in Thalassemia Therapy: Bone Marrow Transplantation and Other Approaches*. New York: Alan R. Liss, 1989: 375–82.

16 Manenti F, Galimberti M, Lucarelli G et al. Growth and endocrine function after bone marrow transplantation for thalassemia. In: Buckner CD, Gale RP, Lucarelli G, eds. *Advances and Controversies in Thalassemia Therapy: Bone Marrow Transplantation and Other Approaches*. New York: Alan R. Liss, 1989: 273–80.

17 Urban C, Schwingshandl J, Slavc I et al. Endocrine function after bone marrow transplantation without the use of preparative total body irradiation. *Bone Marrow Transplant* 1988; **3**: 291–6.

18 Sanders JE & The Long-Term Follow-Up Team. Endocrine problems in children after bone marrow transplant for hematologic malignancies. *Bone Marrow Transplant* 1991; **8**: 2–4.

19 Michel G, Socié G, Gebhard F et al. Late effects of allogeneic bone marrow transplantation for children with acute myeloblastic leukemia in first complete remission: the impact of conditioning regimen without total-body irradiation: a report from the Societe Francaise de Greffe de Moelle. *J Clin Oncol* 1997; **15**: 2238–46.

20 Legault L, Bonny Y. Endocrine complications of bone marrow transplantation in children. *Pediatr Transplant* 1999; **3**: 60–6.

21 Cohen A, Rovelli R, Zecca S et al. Endocrine late effects in children who underwent bone marrow transplantation: review. *Bone Marrow Transplant* 1998; **21** (Suppl. 2): S64–S67 [Review].

22 Katsanis E, Shapiro RS, Robison LL, Haake RJ, Kim T, Pescovitz OH. Thyroid dysfunction following bone marrow transplantation: long-term follow-up of 80 pediatric patients. *Bone Marrow Transplant* 1990; **5**: 335–40.

23 Sklar CA, Kim TH, Ramsay NKC. Thyroid dysfunction among long-term survivors of bone marrow transplantation. *Am J Med* 1982; **73**: 688–94.

24 Borgstrom B, Bolme P. Thyroid function in children after allogeneic bone marrow transplantation. *Bone Marrow Transplant* 1994; **13**: 59–64.

25 Boulad F, Bromley M, Black P et al. Thyroid dysfunction following bone marrow transplantation using hyperfractionated radiation. *Bone Marrow Transplant* 1995; **15**: 71–6.

26 Hancock SL, Cox RS, McDougall R. Thyroid diseases after treatment of Hodgkin's disease. *N Engl J Med* 1991; **325**: 599–606.

27 Ferrebee JW, Thomas ED. Factors affecting the survival of transplanted tissues. *Am J Med Sci* 1958; **235**: 369–86.

28 Robinson LL, Nesbit ME Jr, Sather HN, Meadows AT, Ortega JA, Hammond GD. Height of children successfully treated for acute lymphoblastic leukemia: a report from the late effects study committee of Children's Cancer Study Group. *Med Pediatr Oncol* 1985; **13**: 14–21.

29 Berry DH, Elders MJ, Crist W et al. Growth in children with acute lymphocytic leukemia: a Pediatric Oncology Group study. *Med Pediatr Oncol* 1983; **11**: 39–45.

30 Kirk JA, Raghupathy P, Stevens MM et al. Growth failure and growth-hormone deficiency after treatment for acute lymphoblastic leukaemia. *Lancet* 1987; **1**: 190–3.

31 Wells RJ, Foster MB, D'Ercole AJ, McMillan CW. The impact of cranial irradiation on the growth of children with acute lymphocytic leukemia. *Am J Dis Child* 1983; **137**: 37–9.

32 Starceski PJ, Lee PA, Blatt J, Finegold D, Brown D. Comparable effects of 1800- and 2400-rad (18- and 24-Gy) cranial irradiation on height and weight in children treated for acute lymphocytic leukemia. *Am J Dis Child* 1987; **141**: 550–2.

33 Wallace WH, Kelnar CJ. Late effects of antineoplastic therapy in childhood on growth and endocrine function. *Drug Saf* 1996; **15**: 325–32 [Review].

34 Moëll C, Marky I, Hovi L et al. Cerebral irradiation causes blunted pubertal growth in girls treated for acute leukemia. *Med Pediatr Oncol* 1994; **22**: 375–9.

35 Friedlaender GE, Tross RB, Dogannis AC, Kirkwood JM. Effects of chemotherapeutic agents on bone. *J Bone Joint Surg* 1984; **66**: 602–6.

36 Leahey AM, Teunissen H, Friedman DL, Moshang T, Lange BJ, Meadows AT. Late effects of chemotherapy compared to bone marrow transplantation in the treatment of pediatric acute myeloid leukemia and myelodysplasia. *Med Pediatr Oncol* 1999; **32**: 163–9.

37 Leung W, Hudson MM, Strickland DK et al. Late effects of treatment in survivors of childhood acute myeloid leukemia. *J Clin Oncol* 2000; **18**: 3273–9.

38 Leung W, Hudson M, Zhu Y et al. Late effects in survivors of infant leukemia. *Leukemia* 2000; **14**: 1185–90.

39 Shalet SM. Irradiation-induced growth failure. *Clin Endocrinol Metab* 1986; **15**: 591–606.

40 Romshe CA, Zipf WB, Miser A, Miser J, Sotos JF, Newton WA. Evaluation of growth hormone release and human growth hormone treatment in children with cranial irradiation-associated short stature. *J Pediatr* 1984; **104**: 177–81.

41 Bercu BB, Damond FB Jr. Growth hormone neurosecretory dysfunction. *Clin Endocrinol Metab* 1986; **15**: 537–90.

42 Albertsson-Wikland K, Rosberg S. Analyses of 24-hour growth hormone profiles in children: relation to growth. *J Clin Endocrinol Metab* 1988; **67**: 493–500.

43 Saggese G, Cesaretti G, Cinquanta L et al. Evaluation of 24-hour growth hormone spontaneous secretion: comparison with a nocturnal and diurnal 12-hour study. *Horm Res* 1991; **35**: 25–9.

44 Richards GE, Cavallo A, Meyer WJI. Diagnostic validity of 12-hour integrated concentration of growth hormone. *Am J Dis Child* 1987; **141**: 553–5.

45 Ryalls M, Spoudeas HA, Hindmarsh PC et al. Short-term endocrine consequences of total body irradiation and bone marrow transplantation in children treated for leukemia. *J Endocrinol* 1993; **136**: 331–8.

46 Brauner R, Fontoura M, Zucker JM et al. Growth and growth hormone secretion after bone marrow transplantation. *Arch Dis Child* 1993; **68**: 458–63.

47 Shalet SM, Clayton PE, Price DA. Growth and pituitary function in children treated for brain tumours or acute lymphoblastic leukaemia. *Horm Res* 1988; **30**: 53–61.

48 Sanders JE, Buckner CD, Sullivan KM et al. Growth and development in children after bone marrow transplantation. *Horm Res* 1988; **30**: 92–7.

49 Cohen A, Rovelli A, Bakker B et al. Final height of patients who underwent bone marrow transplantation for hematological disorders during childhood: a study by the Working Party for Late Effects-EBMT. *Blood* 1999; **93**: 4109–15.

50 Hassan M, Oberg G, Ehrsson H. Pharmacokinetic and metabolic studies of high-dose busulphan in adults. *Eur J Clin Pharmacol* 1989; **36**: 525–30.

51 Spruyt LL, Glennie MJ, Beyers AD, Williams AF. Signal transduction by the CD2 antigen in T cells and natural killer cells: requirement for expression of a functional T-cell receptor or binding of antibody Fc to the Fc receptor, Fc gamma RIIIA (CD16). *J Exp Med* 1991; **174**: 1407–15.

52 De Simone M, Verrotti A, Lughetti L et al. Final height of thalassemic patients who underwent bone marrow transplantation during childhood. *Bone Marrow Transplant* 2001; **28**: 201–5.

53 Wingard JR, Plotnick LP, Freemer CS et al. Growth in children after bone marrow transplantation: busulfan plus cyclophosphamide versus cyclophosphamide plus total body irradiation. *Blood* 1992; **79**: 1068–73.

54 Giorgiani G, Bozzola M, Locatelli F et al. Role of busulfan and total body irradiation on growth of prepubertal children recieving bone marrow transplantation and results of treatment with recombinant human growth hormone. *Blood* 1995; **86**: 825–31.

55 Afify Z, Shaw PJ, Clavano-Harding A, Cowell CT. Growth and endocrine function in children with acute myeloid leukaemia after bone marrow transplantation using busulfan/cyclophosphamide. *Bone Marrow Transplant* 2000; **25**: 1087–92.

56 Adan L, de Lanversin ML, Thalassinos C, Souberbielle JC, Fischer A, Brauner R. Growth after bone marrow transplantation in young children conditioned with chemotherapy alone. *Bone Marrow Transplant* 1997; **19**: 253–6.

57 Hovi L, Rajantie J, Perkkiö M, Sainio K, Sipilä I, Siimes MA. Growth failure and growth hormone deficiency in children after bone marrow transplantation for leukemia. *Bone Marrow Transplant* 1990; **5**: 183–6.

58 Sanders JE, Pritchard S, Mahoney P et al. Growth and development following marrow transplantation for leukemia. *Blood* 1986; **68**: 1129–35.

59 Thomas BC, Stanhope R, Plowman PN, Leiper AD. Growth following single fraction and fractionated total body irradiation for bone marrow transplantation. *Eur J Pediatr* 1993; **152**: 888–92.

60 Huma Z, Boulad F, Black P, Heller G, Sklar CA. Growth in children after bone marrow transplantation for acute leukemia. *Blood* 1995; **86**: 819–24.

61 Thomas BC, Stanhope R, Plowman PN, Leiper AD. Endocrine function following single fraction and fractionated total body irradiation for bone marrow transplantation in childhood. *Acta Endocrinol* 1993; **128**: 508–12.

62 Bozzola M, Giorgiani G, Locatelli F et al. Growth in children after bone marrow transplantation. *Horm Res* 1993; **39**: 122–6.

63 Holm K, Nysom K, Rasmussen MH et al. Growth, growth hormone and final height after BMT: possible recovery of irradiation-induced growth hormone insufficiency. *Bone Marrow Transplant* 1996; **18**: 163–70.

64 Cohen A, Rovelli A, Van-Lint MT et al. Final height of patients who underwent bone marrow transplantation during childhood. *Arch Dis Child* 1996; **74**: 437–40.

65 Clement-De Boers A, Oostdijk W, Van Weel-Sipman MH, Van den Broeck J, Wit JM, Vossen JM. Final height and hormonal function after bone marrow transplantation in children. *J Pediatr* 1996; **129**: 544–50.

66 Brauner R, Adan L, Souberbielle JC et al. Contribution of growth hormone deficiency to the growth failure that follows bone marrow transplantation. *J Pediatr* 1997; **130**: 785–92.

67 Sanders JE. Bone marrow transplantation in pediatric oncology. In: Pizzo PA, Poplack DG, eds. *Principles and Practice of Pediatric Oncology*. Philadelphia: Lippincott-Raven, 1997: 357–73.

68 Sanders J, Flowers M, Siadak M, McGuire T. Negative impact of prior central nervous system (CNS) irradiation on growth and neuropsychological function (NPsF) after total body irradiation (TBI) and bone marrow transplant (BMT). *Blood* 1994; **84** (Suppl. 1): 250A [Abstract].

69 Joss E, Zuppinger K, Schwartz HP, Roten H. Final height of patients with pituitary growth failure and changes in growth variables after long-term hormonal therapy. *Pediatr Res* 1983; **17**: 676–9.

70 Mauras N, Blizzard RM, Link K, Johnson ML, Rogol AD, Veldhuis JD. Augmentation of growth hormone secretion during puberty: evidence for a pulse amplitude-modulated phenomenon. *J Clin Endocrinol Metab* 1987; **64**: 596–601.

71 Bourguignon J-P. Linear growth as a function of age at onset of puberty and sex steroid dosage: therapeutic implications. *Endocr Rev* 1988; **9**: 467–88.

72 Ohlsson C, Bengtsson BA, Isaksson OG, Andreassen TT, Slootweg MC. Growth hormone and bone. *Endocr Rev* 1998; **19**: 55–79 [Review].

73 Bachrach LK. Acquisition of optimal bone mass in childhood and adolescence [Review]. *Trends Endocrinol Metab* 2001; **12**: 22–8.

74 Biller BMK. Efficacy of growth hormone-replacement therapy: body composition and bone density. *Endocrinologist* 1998; **8** (Suppl. 1): 15S–21S.

75 Baroncelli GI, Bertelloni S, Ceccarelli C, Cupelli D, Saggese G. Dynamics of bone turnover in children with GH deficiency treated with GH until final height. *Eur J Endocrinol* 2000; **142**: 549–56.

76 Hui SL, Slemenda CW, Johnston CC Jr. The contribution of bone loss to postmenopausal osteoporosis. *Osteoporos Int* 1990; **1**: 30–4.

77 Mauseth RS, Kelly BE, Sanders JE. Bone mineral density (BMD) in pediatric marrow transplant patients. *Pediatr Res* 2001; **49** (2): 82A [Abstract].

78 Rotnem D, Genel M, Hintz RL, Cohen DJ. Personality development in children with growth hormone deficiency. *J Am Acad Child Psychiatry* 1977; **16**: 412–26.

79 Stabler B, Siegel PT, Clopper RR, Stoppani CE, Compton PG, Underwood LE. Behavior change after growth hormone treatment of children with short stature. *J Pediatr* 1998; **133**: 366–73.

80 Vance ML, Mauras N. Growth hormone therapy in adults and children. *N Engl J Med* 1999; **341**: 1206–16 [Review].

81 Sanders JE. Growth and development after hematopoietic cell transplantation. In: Thomas ED, Blume KG, Forman SJ, eds. *Hematopoietic Cell Transplantation*, 2nd edn. Malden, MA: Blackwell Science, 1999: 764–75.

82 Papadimitriou A, Urena M, Hamill G, Stanhope R, Leiper AD. Growth hormone treatment of growth failure secondary to total body irradiation and bone marrow transplantation. *Arch Dis Child* 1991; **66**: 689–92.

83 Borgström B, Bolme P. Growth and growth hormone in children after bone marrow transplantation. *Horm Res* 1988; **30**: 98–100.

84 Ogilvy-Stuart AL, Clark DJ, Wallace WH et al. Endocrine deficit after fractionated total body irradiation. Arch Dis Child 1992; 67: 1107–10.

85 Olshan JS, Willi SM, Gruccio D, Moshang T Jr. Growth hormone function and treatment following bone marrow transplant for neuroblastoma. Bone Marrow Transplant 1993; 12: 381–5.

86 Shalet SM, Toogood A, Rahim A, Brennan BM. The diagnosis of growth hormone deficiency in children and adults. Endocr Rev 1998; 19: 203–23 [Review].

87 Ogilvy-Stuart AL, Shalet SM. Growth and puberty after growth hormone treatment after irradiation for brain tumours. Arch Dis Child 1995; 73: 141–6.

88 MacGillivray MH, Baptista J, Johanson A. Outcome of a four-year randomized study of daily versus three times weekly somatropin treatment in prepubertal naive growth hormone-deficient children. Genentech Study Group. J Clin Endocrinol Metab 1996; 81: 1806–9.

89 Endo M, Kaneko Y, Shikano T, Minami H, Chino J. Possible association of human growth hormone treatment with an occurrence of acute myeloblastic leukaemia with an inversion of chromosome 3 in a child with pituitary dwarfism. Med Pediatr Oncol 1988; 16: 45–7.

90 Sasaki U, Hara M, Watanabe S. Occurrence of acute lymphoblastic leukemia in a boy treated with growth hormone for growth retardation after irradiation to the brain tumor. J Clin Oncol 1988; 18: 81–4.

91 Delemarre-Van De Waal HA, Odink RJH, De Grauw TJ, De Waal FC. Leukaemia in patients treated with growth hormone. Lancet 1988; 1: 1159 [Letters].

92 Fisher DA, Job J-C, Preece M, Underwood LE. Leukaemia in patients treated with growth hormone. Lancet 1988; 1: 1159–60.

93 Parker RG, Berry HC. Late effects of therapeutic irradiation on the skeleton and bone marrow. Cancer 1976; 37: 1162–71.

94 Lochte HL Jr, Kasakura S, Karetzky M, Ferrebee JW, Thomas ED. Infusion of marrow in the mouse and dog after Thio-TEPA. Blood 1963; 21: 424–8.

95 Dahllöf G, Forsberg CM, Borgstrom B. Changes in craniofacial development induced by growth hormone therapy in children treated with bone marrow transplantation. Acta Paediatr 1994; 83: 1165–9.

96 Dahllöf G, Krekmanova L, Kopp S, Borgstrom B, Forsberg CM, Ringden O. Craniomandibular dysfunction in children treated with total-body irradiation and bone marrow transplantation. Acta Odontol Scand 1994; 52: 99–105.

97 Rosenberg SW, Kolodney H, Wong GY, Murphy ML. Altered dental root development in long-term survivors of pediatric acute lymphoblastic leukemia. Cancer 1987; 59: 1640–8.

98 Dahllöf G, Forsberg CM, Ringden O et al. Facial growth and morphology in long-term survivors after bone marrow transplantation. Eur J Orthod 1989; 11: 332–40.

99 da Fonseca MA. Long-term oral and craniofacial complications following pediatric bone marrow transplantation. Pediatr Dent 2000; 22: 57–62 [Review].

100 Dahllöf G, Barr M, Bolme P et al. Disturbances in dental development after total body irradiation in bone marrow transplant recipients. Oral Surg Oral Med Oral Pathol 1988; 65: 41–4.

101 Dahllöf G, Heimdahl A, Bolme P, Lönnqvist B, Ringdén O. Oral condition in children treated with bone marrow transplantation. Bone Marrow Transplant 1988; 3: 43–51.

102 Dahllof G, Nasman M, Borgstrom A et al. Effect of chemotherapy on dental maturity in children with hematological malignancies. Pediatr Dent 1989; 11: 303–6.

103 Dahllöf G, Forsberg C-M, Näsman M et al. Craniofacial growth in bone marrow transplant recipients treated with growth hormone after total body irradiation. Scand J Dent Res 1991; 99: 44–7.

104 Green H, Morikawa M, Nixon T. A dual effector theory of growth-hormone action. Differentiation 1985; 29: 195–8 [Review].

105 Eisen D, Essell J, Broun ER. Oral cavity complications of bone marrow transplantation. Semin Cutan Med Surg 1997; 16: 265–72 [Review].

106 Cutter GB, Cassosta FG, Ross JR. Pubertal growth: physiology and pathophysiology. Recent Prog Horm Res 1986; 42: 443–70.

107 Ray H, Mattison D. How radiation and chemotherapy affect gonadal function. Contemp Ob Gyn 1985; 109: 106–15.

108 Shalet SM, Beardwell CG, Jacobs HS, Pearson D. Testicular function following irradiation of the human prepubertal testes. Clin Endocrinol 1978; 9: 483–90.

109 Pescovitz OH. The endocrinology of the pubertal growth spurt. Acta Paediatr Scand Suppl 1990; 367: 119–25.

110 Sanders JE, Hawley J, Levy W et al. Pregnancies following high-dose cyclophosphamide with or without high-dose busulfan or total-body irradiation and bone marrow transplantation. Blood 1996; 87: 3045–52.

111 Sanders JE and the Seattle Marrow Transplant Team. The impact of marrow transplant preparative regimens on subsequent growth and development. Semin Hematol 1991; 28: 244–9.

112 De Sanctis V, Galimberti M, Lucarelli G, Polchi P, Ruggiero L, Vullo C. Gonadal function after allogeneic bone marrow transplantation for thalassaemia. Arch Dis Child 1991; 66: 517–20.

113 Teinturier C, Hartmann O, Valteau-Couanet D, Benhamou E, Bougneres PF. Ovarian function after autologous bone marrow transplantation in childhood: high-dose busulfan is a major cause of ovarian failure. Bone Marrow Transplant 1998; 22: 989–94.

114 Uldall PR, Kerr DNS, Tacchi D. Amenorrhea and sterility. Lancet 1972; 1: 693–4.

115 Belohorsky B, Siracky J, Sandor L, Klauber E. Comments on the development of amenorrhea caused by Myleran in cases of chronic myelosis. Neoplasia 1960; 4: 397–402.

116 Warne GL, Fairley KF, Hobbs JB, Martin FIR. Cyclophosphamide-induced ovarian failure. N Engl J Med 1973; 289: 1159–62.

117 Lushbaugh CC, Casarett GW. The effects of gonadal irradiation in clinical radiation therapy: a review. Cancer 1976; 37: 1111–20.

118 Shalet SM. Effects of cancer chemotherapy on gonadal function of patients. Cancer Treat Rev 1980; 7: 131–52.

119 Etteldorf JN, West CD, Pitcock JA, Williams DL. Gonadal function, testicular histology, and meiosis following cyclophosphamide therapy in patients with nephrotic syndrome. J Pediatr 1976; 88: 206–12.

120 Fairley KF, Barrie JU, Johnson W. Sterility and testicular atrophy related to cyclophosphamide therapy. Lancet 1972; 1: 568–9.

121 Shapiro E, Kinsella TJ, Makuch RW et al. Effects of fractionated irradiation on endocrine aspects of testicular function. J Clin Oncol 1985; 3: 1232–9.

122 Sanders JE, Buckner CD, Amos D et al. Ovarian function following marrow transplantation for aplastic anemia or leukemia. J Clin Oncol 1988; 6: 813–8.

123 Card RT, Holmes IH, Sugarman RG, Storb R, Thomas ED. Successful pregnancy after high dose chemotherapy and marrow transplantation for treatment of aplastic anemia. Exp Hematol 1980; 8: 57–60.

124 Jacobs P, Dubovsky DW. Bone marrow transplantation followed by normal pregnancy. Am J Hematol 1981; 11: 209–12.

125 Deeg HJ, Kennedy MS, Sanders JE, Thomas ED, Storb R. Successful pregnancy after marrow transplantation for severe aplastic anemia and immunosuppression with cyclosporine. J Am Med Assoc 1983; 250: 647.

126 Schmidt H, Ehninger G, Dopfer R, Waller HD. Pregnancy after bone marrow transplantation for severe aplastic anemia. Bone Marrow Transplant 1987; 2: 329–32.

127 Deeg HJ, Leisenring W, Storb R et al. Long-term outcome after marrow transplantation for severe aplastic anemia. Blood 1998; 91: 3637–45.

128 Salooja N, Szydlo RM, Socie G et al. Pregnancy outcomes after peripheral blood or bone marrow transplantation: a retrospective survey. Lancet 2001; 358: 271–6.

129 Schubert MA, Sullivan KM, Schubert MM et al. Gynecological abnormalities following allogeneic bone marrow transplantation. Bone Marrow Transplant 1990; 5: 425–30.

130 Grigg AP, McLachlan R, Zaja J, Szer J. Reproductive status in long-term bone marrow transplant survivors receiving busulfan-cyclophosphamide (120 mg/kg). Bone Marrow Transplant 2000; 26: 1089–95.

131 Tura S, Mazza P, Gherlinzoni F et al. High-dose therapy followed by autologous bone marrow transplantation (ABMT) in previously untreated non-Hodgkin's lymphoma. Scand J Haematol 1986; 37: 347–52.

132 Hinterberger-Fischer M, Kier P, Kalhs P et al. Fertility, pregnancies and offspring complications after bone marrow transplantation. Bone Marrow Transplant 1991; 7: 5–9.

133 Calmard-Oriol P, Dauriac C, Vu Van H, Lacroze M, Landriot B, Guyotat D. Successful pregnancy following allogeneic bone marrow transplantation after conditioning by thoraco-abdominal irradiation. Bone Marrow Transplant 1991; 8: 229–30.

134 Russell JA, Hanley DA. Full-term pregnancy after allogeneic transplantation for leukemia in a patient with oligomenorrhea. Bone Marrow Transplant 1989; 4: 579–80.

135 Buskard N, Ballem P, Hill R, Fryer C. Normal fertility after total body irradiation and chemotherapy in conjunction with a bone marrow transplantation for acute leukemia. 15th Annual Meeting of the EBMT, Badgastein, Austria 1989, February 26–March 2, 76. [Abstract].

136 Milliken S, Powles R, Parikh P et al. Successful pregnancy following bone marrow transplantation for leukaemia. Bone Marrow Transplant 1990; 5: 135–7.

137 Giri N, Vowels MR, Barr AL, Mameghan H. Successful pregnancy after total body irradiation and bone marrow transplantation for acute

138 Lipton JH, Derzko C, Fyles G, Meharchand J, Messner HA. Pregnancy after BMT: three case reports. *Bone Marrow Transplant* 1993; **11**: 415–8.

139 Baruch J, Benjamin S, Treleaven J, Wilcox AH, Barron JL, Powles R. Male sexual function following bone marrow transplantation. *Bone Marrow Transplant* 1991; **7** (Suppl. 2): 52.

140 Schimmer AD, Ali V, Stewart AK, Imrie K, Keating A. Male sexual function after autologous blood or marrow transplantation. *Biol Blood Marrow Transplant* 2001; **7**: 279–83.

141 Harris E, Mahendra P, McGarrigle HH, Linch DC, Chatterjee R. Gynaecomastia with hypergonadotrophic hypogonadism and Leydig cell insufficiency in recipients of high-dose chemotherapy or chemo-radiotherapy. *Bone Marrow Transplant* 2001; **28**: 1141–4.

142 Aisner J, Wiernik PH, Pearl P. Pregnancy outcome in patients treated for Hodgkin's disease. *J Clin Oncol* 1993; **11**: 507–12.

143 Li FP, Gimbrere K, Gelber RD *et al*. Outcome of pregnancy in survivors of Wilms' tumor. *J Am Med Assoc* 1987; **257**: 216–9.

144 Ortin TTS, Shostak CA, Donaldson SS. The Stanford gonadal status and reproductive function following treatment for Hodgkin's disease in childhood: The Stanford experience. *Int J Radiat Oncol Biol Phys* 1990; **19**: 873–80.

145 Byrne J, Mulvihill JJ, Myers MH *et al*. Effects of treatment on fertility in long-term survivors of childhood or adolescent cancer. *N Engl J Med* 1987; **317**: 1315–21.

146 Mulvihill JJ. Sentinel and other mutational effects in offspring of cancer survivors. *Prog Clin Biol Res* 1990; **340C**: 179–86.

147 Green DM, Zevon MA, Lowrie G, Seigelstein N, Hall B. Congenital anomalies in children of patients who received chemotherapy for cancer in childhood and adolescence. *N Engl J Med* 1991; **325**: 141–6.

148 Hopewell JW. The importance of vascular damage in the development of late radiation effects in normal tissues. In: Meyn RE, Withers HR, eds. *Radiation Biology in Cancer Research*. New York: Raven Press, 1980: 449–59.

149 Critchley HOD, Wallace WHB, Shalet SM, Mamtora H, Higginson Y, Anderson DC. Abdominal irradiation in childhood: the potential for pregnancy. *Br J Obstet Gynaecol* 1992; **99**: 392–4.

150 Marden PM, Smith DW, McDonald MJ. Congenital anomalies in the newborn infant, including minor variations. *J Pediatr* 1964; **64**: 357–71.

151 Neel JV, Satoh C, Goriki K *et al*. Search for mutations altering protein charge and/or function in children of atomic bomb survivors: final report. *Am J Hum Genet* 1988; **42**: 663–76.

152 Albertini RJ. Somatic gene mutations *in vivo* as indicated by the 6-thioguanine-resistant T-lymphocytes in human blood. *Mutat Res* 1985; **150**: 411–22.

153 Hakoda M, Akiyama M, Kyoizumi S, Ava AA, Yamakido M, Otake N. Increased somatic mutant frequency in atomic bomb survivors. *Mutat Res* 1988; **201**: 39–48.

154 Kyoizumi S, Nakamura N, Hakoda M, Awa AA, Bean MA, Jensen RH. Detection of somatic mutations at the glycophorin A locus in erythrocytes of atomic bomb survivors using a single beam flow sorter. *Cancer Res* 1989; **49**: 581–8.

155 Shull RM, Breider MA, Constantopoulos GC. Long-term neurological effects of bone marrow transplantation in a canine lysosomal storage disease. *Pediatr Res* 1988; **24**: 347–52.

156 Sarafoglou K, Boulad F, Gillio A, Sklar C. Gonadal function after bone marrow transplantation for acute leukemia during childhood. *J Pediatr* 1997; **130**: 210–6.

157 Fann JR, Roth-Roemer S, Burington BE, Katon WJ, Syrjala KL. Delirium in patients undergoing hematopoietic stem cell transplantation: incidence and pre transplantation risk factors. *Cancer* 2002; **95**: 1971–81.

69

Mary E.D. Flowers & H. Joachim Deeg

Delayed Complications after Hematopoietic Cell Transplantation

Introduction

Transplantation of marrow or blood derived hemopoietic stem cells (hematopoietic cell transplantation [HCT]) is intended to be curative and to offer the patient a normal life span. Current data show, indeed, that patients transplanted for aplastic anemia and patients without chronic graft-vs.-host disease (GVHD) have life expectancies similar to age-matched controls. Patients with advanced malignant diseases, however, and those who develop chronic GVHD after transplant may experience late disease recurrence or incur delayed complications that may prove fatal [1]. With the increase in numbers of transplants over the past three decades and the considerable improvement in early post-transplant survival (Fig. 69.1) an increasing population of survivors is at risk of developing late complications (Fig. 69.2) [2–4].

Etiology and spectrum of delayed complications

Major complications are listed in Table 69.1. Chronic GVHD and the associated immunodeficiency are the most frequent complications and are directly transplant related. However, it is currently impossible to separate the contributions of genetic predisposition, original disease, or pretransplant therapy to post-transplant complications from transplant-related factors. Late complications also develop in patients given high-dose therapy who are not transplanted, and a typical transplant-related complication such as GVHD is affected by the patient's primary disease and the intensity of the conditioning regimen [5]. Infertility and cataract development are dependent upon the type of the treatment regimen. Other complications are related to the prolonged use of corticosteroids (loss of bone mass) and other immunosuppressive drugs, and many are multifactorial in etiology (e.g. chronic pulmonary disease, secondary malignancies). Some delayed complications are due directly to therapy-induced trauma and scar formation (e.g. destruction of skeletal growth plates; bladder dysfunction), others are related to immunological graft–host interactions (e.g. lymphoproliferative disorders). Side-effects of the treatment of acute complications early after HCT may also contribute. Nearly all organ systems can be affected. (Table 69.2).

Follow-up is too short to determine to what extent delayed complications differ in patients prepared with the more recently developed reduced-intensity or nonmyeloablative transplant regimens.

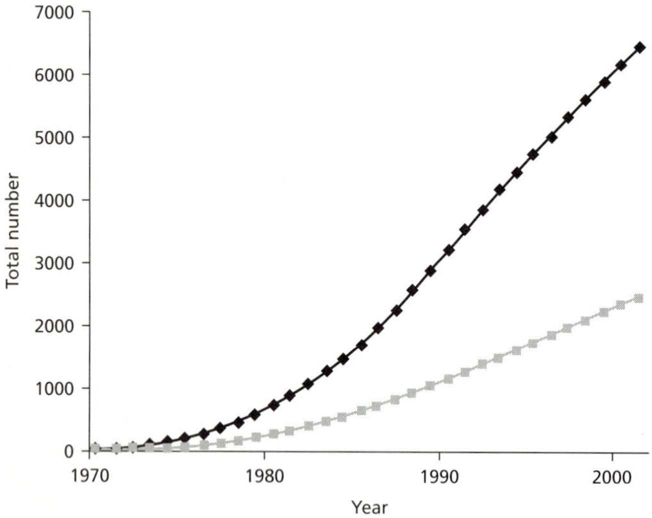

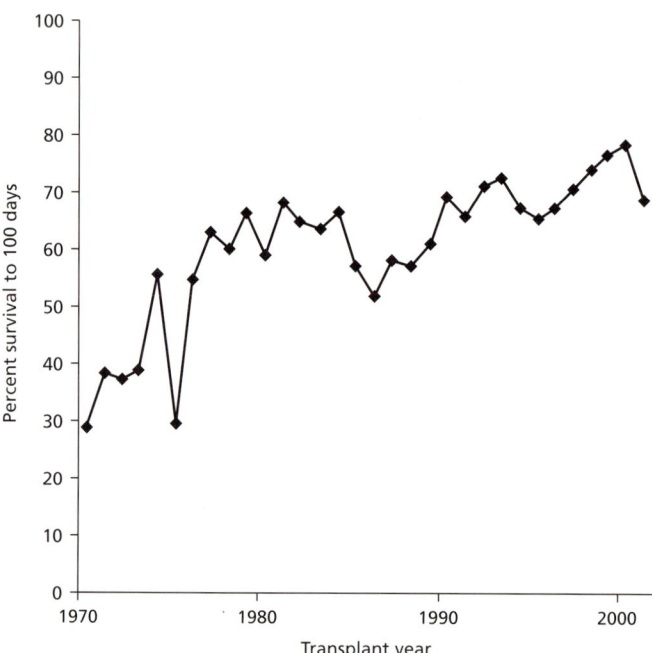

Fig. 69.1 Allogeneic hematopoietic transplants at the Fred Hutchinson Cancer Research Center (FHCRC) (■) and the total number of allogeneic transplant recipients surviving beyond 1 year (▓).

Fig. 69.2 Proportion of patients given an allogeneic hematopoietic transplant at the Fred Hutchinson Cancer Research Center (FHCRC) who survived at least 100 days post-transplant.

Table 69.1 Delayed complications after hematopoietic cell transplantation (HCT).

Chronic graft-vs.-host disease (GVHD)
Immunodeficiency and infections
Airway and pulmonary disease
Autoimmune disorders
Neuroendocrine dysfunction
Impairment of growth and development
Infertility
Cardiac disease
Ocular problems
Musculoskeletal disease
Dental problems
Dysfunction of the genitourinary tract
Gastrointestinal and hepatic complications
Post-transplant malignancies
Central and peripheral nervous system impairment
Psychosocial effects

Table 69.2 Organs affected by late complications according to etiology.

Organ	RRT	Chronic GVHD	Infections
Skin	●	●	●
Eyes	●	●	●
Sinuses	●	●	●
Gastrointestinal tract	●	●	●
Liver	●	●	●
Lungs	●	●	●
Muscles	●	●	
Connective tissues		●	
Bones	●		
Endocrine glands	●	●	
Gonads	●		
Kidneys	●		

GVHD, graft-vs.-host disease; RRT, regimen-related toxicity.

Chronic GVHD

The most significant cause of delayed morbidity and mortality after allogeneic HCT is chronic GVHD and toxicities related to its treatment (see Chapter 50). A three-step grading scale (mild, moderate and severe) has been developed to help quantify the morbidity of chronic GVHD at the time of diagnosis of chronic GVHD, at any time when changes in therapy to control GVHD occur (i.e. due to an increase in the dose of corticosteroid ≥1 mg/kg/every-other-day, the substitution of one therapy to another, or additional therapy) at 1 year after transplant and yearly thereafter if manifestations of GVHD persist or immunosuppressive treatment continues [6]. A morbidity scale used at the Fred Hutchinson Cancer Research Center (FHCRC) is shown in Table 69.3.

Infections

Late infections, due to bacterial, viral and fungal organisms occur most commonly in patients with chronic GVHD. Antibiotic prophylaxis given early post-transplant may impact on late infections. For example, prophylaxis with acyclovir or preemptive therapy of cytomegalovirus (CMV) with ganciclovir has resulted in an increased incidence of late CMV infections. Conversely, short-term administration of fluconazole early after transplantation has led to a significant decline in candida infections, even late post-transplant. It is standard practice to give prophylaxis for infections caused by *Pneumocystis carinii*, varicella zoster and encapsulated bacteria during the 1st year post-transplant, or longer, for patients with chronic GVHD.

Hepatitis B and C virus may result in chronic hepatitis and cirrhosis (see Gastrointestinal and hepatic complications, p. 952). Transfusion-related human immunodeficiency virus (HIV) infections have been extremely rare in recent years. Other latent infections including malaria have been transmitted from the transplant donor [7].

A detailed discussion of infections is provided in Chapters 51–57.

Airway and pulmonary disease

Airways and lungs are sensitive to cytotoxic therapy, but are also prominent targets of infections. Mucositis early post-transplant interferes with mucociliary clearance and leads to mucous retention and inflammation in the lower airways. This process can be aggravated by sinus drainage and postnasal drip.

Lung injury occurs in the interstitium and in the alveolar space and may be associated with hemorrhage and edema. Scarring of the interstitial space interferes with effective gas exchange, respiratory dynamics and kinetics. The conditioning regimen, in particular the dose of irradiation, is a contributing factor [8]. The bronchial tree may also be involved by GVHD [9]. Chronic pulmonary complications affect at least 15–20% of patients after HCT, and pulmonary dysfunction is an important indicator for long-term outcome (see below).

Late onset pneumonitis

Interstitial pneumonitis is characterized by thickening of the interstitial space due to cellular infiltrates, fluid and fibrous deposits. Patients generally experience dyspnea or shortness of breath. The physical examination may not be remarkable, but chest X-rays typically show a pattern of diffuse infiltrates. Late onset interstitial pneumonitis usually occurs in patients with chronic GVHD [10]. Most require therapy with immunosuppressive agents also for other manifestations of chronic GVHD; treatment with bronchodilators is usually ineffective. Prolonged prophylaxis with ganciclovir, as stated above, has led to an increase in late CMV infections, including pneumonitis, which are observed in 10–15% of patients 1 year or later after HCT [11]. In other patients, no organisms are isolated.

A recent analysis of results in 1359 patients transplanted at the FHCRC in 1992–97 shows that late pneumonias occur also in the absence of GVHD and even after autologous transplantation in patients who did not previously have pulmonary disease [12]. The incidence at 4 years was 31% overall [12]. The prognosis was generally good with bacterial etiology, but mortality reached 80% with fungal or polymicrobial pneumonia [12]. Diagnostic bronchoalveolar lavage is recommended in patients who develop pulmonary infiltrates to rule out infection and provide guidance for treatment.

Restrictive pulmonary disease

Earlier analyses showed that patients with pretransplant abnormal pulmonary function tests (PFTs), in particular decreased diffusing capacity (DLCO) and increased oxygen gradient ($P_{A-a}O_2$) have a higher mortality after transplantation than patients with normal tests. In one study the relative risk of death was 1.43 for patients with a DLCO of <80% and 1.28 for patients with a ($P_{A-a}O_2$) of ≥20 mmHg [13]. Importantly, however, excess mortality was due to miscellaneous causes and only in part to respiratory failure.

Table 69.3 Morbidity scale used for follow-up in patients with chronic GVHD.*

Patient:_____   Date:_____

Performance	☐ Asymptomatic and fully active (ECOG 0; KPS/Lansky 100%)
Score	☐ Symptomatic, fully ambulatory, restricted only in physically strenuous activity (ECOG 1, KPS 80–90%)
	☐ Symptomatic, ambulatory, capable of self-care, >50% of waking hours out of bed (ECOG 2, KPS 60–70%)
PS _____	☐ Symptomatic, limited self care, >50% of waking hours in bed (ECOG 3–4, KPS <60%)
Skin	☐ No cutaneous changes caused by chronic GVHD
	☐ <18% BSA rash (erythema, pigment change, ichthyosis or lichenoid) **or** any scleroderma (pockets of normal skin)
	☐ 18–50% BSA rash **or** any scleroderma (no pockets of normal skin but not hidebound)
___% BSA	☐ >50% BSA rash, **or** any scleroderma (hidebound, unable to pinch) **or** interference with ADL due to impaired mobility or ulceration
involved	☐ abnormality present but not thought to represent GVHD

Clinical features: ☐ erythematous macular papular   ☐ lichenoid changes   ☐ erythema
                   ☐ hyperpigmentation   ☐ pruritis   ☐ scleroderma
                   ☐ hypopigmentation   ☐ ichthyosis

Mouth	☐ Asymptomatic, no physical manifestations of chronic GVHD
	☐ Oral symptoms (dryness, food sensitivity or oral pain) **or** physical manifestations (erythema, hyperkeratosis, lichenoid or ulceration), no interference with oral intake
	☐ Oral symptoms or physical manifestations with partial limitation of oral intake
	☐ Oral symptoms or physical manifestations with major limitation of oral intake
	☐ Abnormality present but not thought to represent GVHD
Eyes	☐ Asymptomatic, no keratitis
	☐ Asymptomatic keratitis **or** symptomatic ocular sicca not affecting ADL
Tear test	☐ Symptomatic keratoconjunctivitis due to ocular sicca without vision impairment but requiring frequent use of moisturizers (>3 times per day)
OD___mm	☐ Loss of vision caused by pseudomembranes, corneal ulceration or requiring special glasses (such as goggles) to relieve pain/discomfort
OS___mm	☐ Abnormality present but not thought to represent GVHD
Gut	☐ No GI symptoms (anorexia, nausea, vomiting or diarrhea), weight stable
	☐ GI symptoms, not requiring parenteral fluids or nutrition, weight stable
	☐ GI symptoms requiring parenteral fluids or nutrition, weight stable
	☐ GI symptoms requiring complete parenteral nutrition **or** weight loss ≥15% not due to other causes
	☐ Abnormality present but not thought to represent GVHD
Liver	☐ Total bilirubin <1.6, alkaline phosphatase (AP) <130
	☐ Total bilirubin 1.6–3.0, AP 130–260
	☐ Total bilirubin 3.1–6.0, AP 261–520
	☐ Abnormal liver function tests not due to other causes with total bilirubin >6.0, AP >5 × normal, AST or ALT >3 × normal
	☐ Abnormality present but not thought to represent GVHD
Lungs	☐ Asymptomatic or normal PFTs
	☐ 51–75% FEV1, FEV1/FVC <65% **or** decrease of FEV1/FVC by >12% within <1 year **or** dyspnea with moderate exertion not explained by infection or other causes
	☐ 25–50% FEV1 **or** dyspnea with mild exertion **or** desaturation with exercise not explained by infection or other causes
	☐ <25% FEV1 **or** dyspnea at rest **or** requirement for supplemental oxygen during exercise or rest not explained by infection or other causes
	☐ Abnormality present but not thought to represent GVHD
Joints and	☐ Full range of motion (ROM)
Fasciae	☐ Tightness limited to arms **or** tightness limited to legs
	☐ Contractures that do not affect activity of daily living (ADL) **or** tightness involving both upper and lower extremities
	☐ Contractures that interfere with ADL
	☐ Abnormality present but not thought to represent GVHD
Genital tract	☐ Asymptomatic
	☐ Physical manifestations (atrophy, erythema, lichenoid changes or edema) not explained by estrogen deficiency and not interfering with intercourse or ADL
	☐ Physical manifestations causing coital symptoms without affecting any other ADL
	☐ Physical manifestations affecting ADL
	☐ Abnormality present but not thought to represent GVHD

Severe complications or other signs of chronic GVHD

☐ Weight loss	☐ Bronchiolitis obliterans (BO)	☐ Bronchiolitis obliterans organizing pneumonia (BOOP)
☐ Eosiophilia (>0.4 × 10³/μL)	☐ Esophageal stricture or web	☐ Malabsorption ☐ Fasciitis
☐ Myositis	☐ Serositis	☐ Other: _____ ☐ None

Platelets <100,000	☐ Yes	☐ No	**Organ system(s) biopsied:** _____
Biopsy obtained	☐ Yes	☐ No	
GVHD confirmed by histology	☐ Yes	☐ No	

*At time of diagnosis of chronic GVHD, at any time when changes in therapy occurs (i.e., due to increase in the dose of corticosteroids ≥1 mg/kg/q.o.d., substitution of one therapy to another, or additional therapy), at one year after transplant, and yearly thereafter if manifestation of GVHD persists or if treatment with immunosuppressive continues.

More recent studies indicate that post-transplant PFTs similarly have predictive value for HCT outcome [14]. At 3 months after HCT PFTs frequently show declines in total lung capacity (TLC) and DLCO. Restrictive defects, defined as a decrease in TLC to <80% of predicted values, are present in one-third of all patients studied. In one study, such a defect (or a loss of ≥15% of TLC) was associated with a twofold increase in nonrelapse mortality related to respiratory failure but was not significantly associated with chronic GVHD. The effect was most pronounced at over 1 year post-transplant.

Restrictive pulmonary changes are not correlated with the type of conditioning regimen or with chronic GVHD and generally do not produce severe symptoms. However, since they are associated with an increase in late mortality, routine evaluation of lung function after HCT is warranted (Table 69.3). Aggressive bronchial hygiene and prophylaxis and prompt therapy of infection may be useful in reducing severe complications and in slowing disease progression [15].

Obstructive pulmonary disease

The pathogenesis of air flow obstruction (AFO) after HCT is not fully understood [16]. AFO, defined as decreased expiratory airflow—in particular, a decrease in the proportion of air that can be exhaled over the 1st second of expiration—may represent sequelae to extensive restrictive changes in the small airways. Alternatively, as in obstructive bronchiolitis, it may be related to small airway destruction. Recurrent aspirations, possibly associated with GVHD of the esophagus or purulent sinus secretions (postnasal drip), contribute to airway inflammation and the development of obstructive lung disease.

A recent study analyzed AFO in 1049 patients who received an allogeneic HCT between 1990 and 2000 at the FHCRC (J. Chien et al., unpublished data). There were 257 patients (25%) with significant AFO as defined by a decline in pFEV$_1$ (FEV$_1$: forced expiratory volume in 1 s) by over 5% per year. In multivariate logistic regression analysis, advanced age (relative risk [RR] 1.03, 95%CI 1.02–1.04), male donor–female recipient (RR 1.5, 95%CI 1.1–2.0), patients with quiescent (RR 1.5, 95%CI 1.2–1.7) or progressive onset (RR 2.5, 95%CI 1.4–3.1) of chronic GVHD were associated with an increased risk of developing AFO. Among patients with chronic GVHD, those with AFO had a higher risk of mortality (HR 1.9, $p = 0.002$) than patients without AFO. The AFO attributable adjusted mortality rate was 13% at 3 years, 17% at 5 years and 29% at 10 years. These data suggest that using the rate of decline in pFEV$_1$ definition, the incidence of new onset AFO in patients after HCT was higher than previously estimated. Both acute and chronic GVHD were important risk factors for AFO, and AFO had a significant independent effect on long-term survival.

In this setting, AFO generally shows no response to bronchodilator treatment. Only 30–40% of patients improve on glucocorticoids, given alone or in combination with cyclosporine (CSP). Few patients with end-stage disease have been treated successfully with cadaveric lung transplants [17,18]. Single-lobe transplantation from the original marrow donor has also been reported [19].

Bronchiolitis obliterans

Progressive bronchiolitis obliterans, the narrowing or occlusion of small airways that may also lead to air trapping, has been reported to occur in 10% of all patients with chronic GVHD [20,21] from 3 months to 2 years after HCT. Clinical and pathological findings (Table 69.4) are similar to those seen after lung or heart–lung transplants [21,22]. Chest X-rays may show hyperinflation of the lungs and flattening of the diaphragm, but abnormalities are best identified by high resolution computerized axial tomography (CAT) scans (inspiratory and expiratory cuts). Recurrent pneumothoraces and pneumomediastinum [23] have been observed. PFTs show a reduction in forced mid-expiratory flow to 10% or 20% of predicted values and moderate to severe reduction in forced vital capacity. The DLCO is usually normal. Pulmonary ventilation scans show decreased activity patterns corresponding to areas of obliteration of bronchiolar walls along with atelectatic areas. Histological changes are thought to be due to a graft-vs.-host reaction, possibly aggravated by infections. Pulmonary infections develop in over 20% of allogeneic HCT recipients without GVHD and in over 60% of patients with chronic GVHD, where they represent a significant cause of morbidity and mortality.

Table 69.4 Manifestation of bronchiolitis obliterans organizing pneumonia (BOOP) compared to bronchiolitis obliterans (BO).

Feature	BOOP	BO
Symptoms	Dyspnea, fever, cough	Cough, dyspnea
Signs	Crackles >>> wheezes	Wheezes >>> crackles
Chest X-ray	Abnormal	Normal
PFTs	Reduced DLCO and volumes	Reduced spirometry
Pathology	Alveoli and alveolar ducts	Proximal bronchioles

DLCO, diffusion capacity; PFTs, pulmonary function tests.

The clinical course of bronchiolitis varies from mild, with slow deterioration, to diffuse necrotizing fatal bronchiolitis. Severe disease may not respond to glucocorticoids, but corticosteroids in combination with calcineurin inhibitors can stabilize PFTs and improve outcome. Combination therapy with glucocorticoids and CSP and FK506 (tacrolimus) or, possibly, azathioprine is indicated, despite concerns about the myelosuppressive and possibly mutagenic effects of azathioprine [24]. It is of note that a randomized trial examining the effect of intravenous immunoglobulin (IVIg) on chronic GVHD and bronchiolitis showed a marked decrease in the incidence of obliterative bronchiolitis in all patients such that an effect of IVIg was not apparent [25]. It is possible that changes in prophylactic and therapeutic management of infections in recent years are factors for the decline of obliterative bronchiolitis.

Lung transplantation is an option for patients with far advanced disease [18,26,27]; however, since the process is at least in part immunologically mediated, it is not certain that a lung transplant will be curative, since the transplanted organ may also serve as a target of the graft-vs.-host reaction. On the other hand, it is possible that the graft-vs.-host reaction is directed at a polymorphic antigen that is not expressed in the transplanted lung, in which case a propagation of the disease in the lung might not occur.

Bronchiolitis obliterans organizing pneumonia (BOOP) histologically shows polypoid masses of granulation tissue in the bronchioles and alveolar sacs as well as infiltration of alveolar septa by mononuclear cells. The disease may be patchy. It has been associated with infections, drugs, collagen vascular diseases and transplantation. A recent analysis of results in 6523 patients transplanted at the FHCRC revealed 51 cases of BOOP and all but two were after allogeneic transplants [28]. BOOP was diagnosed at 5–2819 days (median 108) after HCT. The chest X-ray was abnormal in 47 patients. Most patients presented with fever, dyspnea, or cough, but 23% were asymptomatic (Table 69.4). Sixty percent of patients had abnormal PFT (restrictive ≥ obstructive). The disease was significantly associated with acute and chronic GVHD. The disease progressed in 22% of patients and resolved or was stable in the remaining patients. Infections were uncommon [28]. Most patients respond to glucocorticosteroids (1–2 mg/kg) (M.E.D. Flowers, unpublished data), which often must be continued for 6 months or longer [28,29].

Late respiratory failure has also been reported in patients transplanted for dyskeratosis congenita, where it may be related to the underlying disease [30].

Dysregulation of immunity

All currently used conditioning regimens are associated with immunosuppression of the transplant recipient. Even with autologous HCT there is a period of several months of slow recovery of cellular immunity that, to a large extent, reflects a recapitulation of ontogeny [31]. The typical pattern of Ig recovery after HCT follows the same sequence as in ontogeny: IgM, IgG_1 and IgG_3 with IgG_2, IgG_4 and IgA lagging behind. However, antibodies observed early after HCT are to a large extent mono- or oligoclonal and, with the exception of autoreactivity, have irrelevant specificities. With lengthening of the post-transplant interval there is generally a rise of specific titers to infectious antigens, particularly to those to which the donor is immune and to which the patient is exposed. Nonspecific IgE elevations have also been reported [32]. A recent study by Storek et al. [33] in patients surviving over 20 years after HCT showed basically normal immunity. Patients transplanted as adults had an insignificant deficiency of de novo generated $CD4^+$ T cells. The average rate of infection was 0.07 infections per patient year (one every 14 years).

Allogeneic donor-derived cells recognize recipient antigens as nonself (alloreactivity) [34]. However, once donor-derived cells are established in the recipient, these cells, by generating the new immune system of the recipient, basically express "autoreactivity" if they exhibit humoral or cellular reactivity against host tissue. The presence of thymic damage, due to conditioning (and GVHD), would be expected to interfere with the negative selection of autoreactive cells and thereby facilitate the development of cellular and, via $CD4^+$ cells, humoral autoreactivity [35,36]. Conditioning-induced thymic damage is also present in autologous transplant recipients, where it may have an effect similar to that observed after allogeneic HCT [37].

Autoantibodies are observed frequently after HCT, particularly with chronic GVHD, but correlation with GVHD activity is uncertain. Most commonly detected are rheumatoid factor, antinuclear, antismooth muscle and antimitochondrial antibodies [38,39]. Generally no therapy is needed. However, patients with antiacetylcholine receptor antibodies and myasthenia gravis, typically 1–2 years after HCT, will require therapy as given for other patients with myasthenia. The antiacetylcholine receptor antibodies are donor-derived as shown by Ig allotyping [40]. Consistent with that concept, patterns of abnormal immune reactivity of the donor are also transferred to the recipients [31]. Such a transfer has been reported for atopic asthma, psoriasis and food allergies, albeit inconsistently [41–44]. Antibodies to interferon-alpha (IFN-α) may contribute to the patients' susceptibility to infection [45].

Hematologic problems

Hematological problems include immune thrombocytopenia, anemia and neutropenia; presumably autoimmune mediated [46,47]. Marrow can be a target of GVHD, and persistent thrombocytopenia is a poor prognostic factor in chronic GVHD [48]. Immunosuppressive treatment of GVHD often is successful [49]. However, immune-mediated thrombocytopenia has also been observed after syngeneic and autologous transplants and, in these instances, should be treated like idiopathic thrombocytopenic purpura. The use of high-dose IVIg is successful in some patients [50]. Immune-mediated neutropenia is less frequent and, if spontaneous recovery does not occur, therapy with steroids is warranted. Patients transplanted from ABO-incompatible donors may experience hemolysis and severe anemia for months or even years after HCT until long-lived host cells have been eliminated. An occasional patient developing classical pure red cell aplasia has been treated successfully with immunosuppressive therapy [51,52]. Recent data suggest that CD34-enriched donor lymphocyte infusion may be beneficial [53].

Some reports on patients followed for as long as 30 years after HCT suggest an accelerated shortening of telomeres in the first few years post-transplant [54,55]. While this view is not undisputed, individual cases of "late graft failure" have been reported, and several cases of myelodysplasia in donor cells have been observed (see Hematologic malignancies p. 953).

Neuroendocrine dysfunction

Cytotoxic therapy and gamma irradiation damage endocrine glands [56]. Thus, intensive therapy given before transplantation and the conditioning regimens used in preparation for HCT have the potential of causing endocrine insufficiency. A detailed description of the effects on growth and development as well as fertility is provided in Chapter 68.

Thyroid

Overt or compensated hypothyroidism and the "euthyroid sick syndrome" (ETS; low free triiodothyronine, free thyroxine, or both, along with normal or low thyroid-stimulating hormone [TSH]) are the most frequent thyroid abnormalities. In one study, the incidence of thyroid dysfunction after total body irradiation (TBI) was 57% at 3 months and 29% at 14 months, suggesting some spontaneous recovery [57]. Thyroid dysfunction was less frequent in patients who had not received TBI (14% at 3 and 14 months). Of note in this study was that ETS was associated with a significantly lower survival than observed in patients not affected by ETS (34.5% vs. 96.2%; $p < 0.0001$). Among pediatric patients prepared with TBI, an incidence of thyroid dysfunction as high as 85% has been reported [58], although others have observed a substantially lower incidence [59]. The incidence of hypothyroidism was about three times higher in patients given single dose than in those patients given fractionated irradiation [60,61]. The risk is further enhanced in patients who received pre-transplant cranial irradiation or irradiation to the neck (e.g. for Hodgkin's disease [HD]) [62]. Hypothyroidism may be diagnosed rather early post-transplant, but it may also become manifest only years after HCT [63]. The incidence is highest in children and lowest in adults (see Chapter 68).

Patients may also develop benign (adenoma) or malignant (carcinoma) thyroid tumors related directly to radiation exposure and to enhanced TSH stimulation [64,65]. All patients who have received irradiation (including TBI) to the thyroid should be followed for life with annual physical evaluation and thyroid function studies as indicated [62]. Patients with thyroid nodules should be referred to an endocrinologist. Patients with hypothyroidism require replacement therapy; however, since some patients show spontaneous recovery, intermittent trials off therapy are indicated.

Adrenal glands

Many HCT patients receive glucocorticoid therapy in the pre-, peri- or post-transplant period and show the classic side-effects of steroid therapy, including Cushingoid features, myopathy and bone loss. Endogenous cortisol production is suppressed, and any superimposed stress may cause a relative adrenal insufficiency. For the same reason, prolonged glucocorticoid therapy for GVHD should be given on alternate days and must be tapered very gradually. Nausea and fatigue are common after discontinuation of prolonged use of corticosteroids and can be misdiagnosed as exacerbation of GVHD of the gastrointestinal (GI) tract. Cortisol stimulation tests are recommended in this setting to rule out adrenal insufficiency (cortisol levels checked pre- and 30-min after 1 μg IV cosyntropin).

One study in 78 patients showed 24% to have subnormal 11-deoxycortisol levels following discontinuation of glucocorticoid therapy at 1–8 years post-transplant. No patient was symptomatic, and the proportion of patients affected did not increase with time post-transplant [63,66]. However, recent data suggest that the incidence of adrenal insufficiency may have been underestimated in the past (J.E. Sanders, unpublished data). Subnormal stimulated cortisol levels are also observed in patients given cranial irradiation and a central (primary) effect may play a role in patients post-transplant [67]. One report described a patient who developed Addison disease, apparently of an autoimmune nature, 10 years after HCT for Wiskott–Aldrich syndrome [67].

Hypothalamic–pituitary axis

Cranial irradiation, with or without TBI, may have severe effects on the pituitary gland [68–70]. Thyrotropin-releasing hormone (TRH) may be low early post-transplant, and TRH-induced TSH responses may be subnormal and delayed [68]. Release of gonadotropin in response to luteinizing hormone-releasing hormone (LHRH) may be elevated [68]. Prolactin secretion and the pituitary-adrenal axis are usually intact. Growth hormone levels are decreased after cranial irradiation (±TBI), and deficiency becomes apparent earlier with younger age at transplant [63,69]. Details of growth and development are discussed in Chapter 68.

Gonadal function, puberty and fertility

Chemotherapy and TBI regimens used prior to hematopoietic transplantation usually cause gonadal failure, dependent upon the intensity and type of the regimen and the age of the patient at transplant (see Chapter 68). Annual assessment of gonadal function is recommended in patients after HCT, including determination of blood levels of free and total testosterone in men and estradiol levels in women. Puberty and menarche are markedly delayed or may not occur, and fertility is rarely regained in either men or women (see Chapter 68).

In men, decreased libido, reduced bone mineral and low testosterone levels after transplant are indications for testosterone replacement unless contraindicated for other reasons. Treatment with testosterone transdermal patch (60 cm^2 containing 328 mg testosterone) with either Androderm® 5 mg/day or Testododerm® 5 mg/day (applied to the skin of the arms, back or buttocks) represents an adequate regimen for men with hypogonadism. Androgel is less convenient than transdermal formulations, and the scrotal transdermal formulation appears to be poorly tolerated (M.E.D. Flowers, unpublished data). Another effective formulation is androgen injections using prolonged action formulations such as testosterone cypionate (Andro-Cyp®, Dep-Ando®, Depo-testosterone®, Duratest®) or testosterone enanthate (Ando LA 200®, Andryl 200®, Delatestryl®) given as 50–200 mg every 2–4 weeks (deep into the gluteal muscle). Prolonged use of high-dose androgens has been associated with development of peliosis hepatitis and hepatic neoplasms. Men treated with testosterone may be at increased risk for prostate hypertrophy and prostate carcinoma. Benefits and risks of testosterone replacement must be discussed with each patient and its benefit/risk ratio reassessed periodically. Testosterone blood levels should be monitored periodically and the dose adjusted according to levels and side-effects. Digital prostate examination, prostate specific antigen (PSA) levels, liver test panel, lipid profile and hemoglobin should be evaluated prior to initiation of testosterone and should be repeated periodically. Gynecomastia, edema, male baldness, nausea, tachycardia, increased cholesterol and cholestatic liver enzyme abnormalities are some of the side-effects associated with testosterone.

Permanent ovarian failure invariably occurs in women who receive busulfan and cyclophosphamide (BU/CY) pretransplant, while recovery of ovarian function has been observed after transplant in 54% of younger patients (<26 years) conditioned with CY only, and in 10% of younger patients who received over 1000 cGy TBI with CY (see Chapter 68).

Appropriate management of menopausal symptoms, bone loss and growth and development in children can improve the quality of life of HCT recipients (see Chapter 68). Hormone replacement therapy (HRT) with estrogen alone (for patients without a uterus) or combined with progestin (for patients with a uterus) is effective after HCT for management of hot flashes, relief of vaginal and vulvar symptoms (menopausal symptoms) and to decrease bone loss. The positive effect on cognitive function claimed by many women taking estrogen remains to be confirmed. Unfortunately, combined estrogen and progestin were recently found to increase the risk of cardiovascular disease (venous thrombosis, strokes, pulmonary emboli) and to increase the risk of invasive breast cancer after 3 years of therapy in post-menopausal nontransplanted women, but no effect on survival was observed [71]. A trial of estrogen replacement therapy alone for post-menopausal women without a uterus is in progress. While premature menopausal symptoms and bone loss are common complications observed in the 1st year after transplant, the increased risk of developing a secondary malignancy becomes significant at about 5 years after transplant. The benefit of administration of estrogen combined with progestin (for adult patients with a uterus) or estrogen alone (for adult patients without a uterus) during the first 2–3 years after transplant in women with gonadal failure after HCT might offset its risks in this setting. Whether combined HRT may contribute to increased risk of secondary cancers, in particular, breast cancer after stem cell transplantation, is difficult to establish. Thus, HRT after transplant should be individualized and its associated risks reviewed and discussed carefully with each patient before initiation of therapy, and reassessed at least yearly if continued beyond 1 year. HRT should not be used in patients with history of cardiovascular diseases (i.e. venous thrombosis, pulmonary embolism, strokes, hypercoagulation disorders, breast cancer, or liver disease). Non-hormonal strategies for alternative management of menopausal symptoms and bone loss should be provided to all patients. Topical estrogen HRT can relieve local vaginal/vulvar symptoms caused by gonadal insufficiency and may allow for the use of lower doses of systemic estrogen. Gynecologic evaluation at yearly intervals, self-breast examination at monthly intervals and mammograms between 35 and 40 years of age (baseline for women on HRT) and yearly thereafter are recommended in all women after transplantation.

Cardiovascular disease

Cardiac insufficiency and coronary artery disease have been recognized as complications of intensive cytotoxic therapy, in particular high-dose anthracycline, and mediastinal irradiation [72]. Cardiac insufficiency may also be seen in patients conditioned with CY 200 mg/kg, usually early, sometimes before conditioning is completed, although the overall incidence is low [73]. Rather typical for CY-induced cardiac toxicity is a loss of voltage on the electrocardiogram, followed by clinical decompensation. Pretransplant determination of ejection fraction has not been a reliable tool in predicting this complication. It has been suggested that cardiac toxicity can be avoided if CY is administered at doses up to 6.2 g/m^2 over 4 days or if two divided doses (rather than a single dose) are given daily [74,75].

Late cardiomyopathy has been treated successfully by orthotopic cardiac transplantation [76]. Coronary artery disease and thrombotic events have been reported at various time intervals after HCT [77,78]. Hyperlipidemia and hyperglycemia (common in patients treated with calcineurin inhibitors, rapamycin and glucocorticosteroids), treatment with estrogen/progesterone and inactivity due to fatigue or other causes are potential risk factors for the development of coronary disease in long-term survivors of HCT. General recommendations include monitoring lipid profiles at least yearly, encourage patients to engage in a routine exercise activity (20 min 4–5 times/week), adjust GVHD drug levels as applicable, and avoid prolonged use (>3 years) of standard dose estrogen and progesterone in post-menopausal women. Anticoagulation, at least for a limited duration, may be indicated in high-risk patients, especially in those with previous episodes of thrombotic events.

A syndrome of endothelial damage in patients with Dyskeratosis congenita 2–8 years after HCT leading to severe microangiopathy with renal and hepatic failure has been reported [79]. A relationship to the transplant *per se* is difficult to prove.

Ocular problems

The most common problems affecting the eyes after HCT are cataracts and ocular sicca, usually caused by chronic GVHD.

Cataracts

Glucocorticoids and gamma irradiation are the primary causes of cataracts after HCT. After TBI, posterior capsular cataracts are noticed approximately 1 year after HCT [80]. Following single-dose TBI (usually 920–1000 cGy), the incidence of cataracts is 60–80% at 5–6 years [81]. After fractionated TBI, the incidence is approximately 50% at cumulative doses above 1200 cGy, 30–35% at doses of 1200 cGy and as low as 10% in patients given hyperfractionated TBI (over six fractions) or treated a low exposure rates (0.04 cGy/min) [81–84]. Eye shielding might prevent cataracts, but relapse of malignancy in the ocular bulb can occur.

Among patients who have not received TBI or cranial irradiation, the incidence of cataracts is in the range of 10–20%, almost exclusively due to glucocorticosteroids [4,80]. The incidence of cataracts overall is higher in patients who also received cranial irradiation.

Approaches to cataract prevention in the setting of HCT are experimental. Preclinical studies suggest that the administration of a pantothenic acid derivative in the peri-irradiation period protects against cataract development, apparently by preventing macromolecular phase separation in the lens [85]. This approach has not been tested clinically. One report suggests that heparin given, for example, in patients with veno-occlusive disease, has a protective effect [81].

The treatment of choice of cataracts is lens extraction and implantation of artificial lenses. Contact lenses can be used but may be difficult to wear in patients with ocular sicca due to chronic GVHD. Although surgery should be done preferably after discontinuation of all systemic immunosuppressive treatment, procedures have been performed while patients received prednisone (<0.25 mg/kg). Improved quality of modern lenses has allowed successful implants also in children [82].

Ocular sicca and other problems

Dry eyes (ocular sicca) are frequently due to chronic GVHD and are often irreversible (see Chapter 50) [86]. Chronic GVHD involving the eyes can result in scar formation (e.g. in the tarsus) and lead to synechiae, ectropion, corneal damage and, potentially, perforation if not treated meticulously and aggressively. Keratoconjunctivitis sicca also occurs in patients without chronic GVHD, although the possibility that it represents a sequel of prior GVHD or a form fruste of GVHD must be considered [3,86]. Long-term management includes artificial tears and ointments at night, punctual plugs or ligation of cannaliculas that normally drain the lacrimal fluid. Moisture chamber eyeglasses (prosthetic device coupled to the eyeglasses) can significantly improve the symptoms of dry eyes [87].

Obstruction of the nasolacrimal duct, related either to GVHD or conditioning-induced fibrosis, has been infrequently observed [88]. Transplantation of limbal epithelial cells, as reported for other conditions [89], has been performed in some patients (using the original donor cells) with mixed results (R. Bensinger and M.E.D. Flowers, unpublished data).

Musculofascial problems

The most common muscular complication is corticosteroid-induced myopathy. Since patients frequently lack energy and initiative, muscle weakness further adds to inactivity and loss of muscle and bone mass. It is important therefore to maintain and gradually increase the level of physical activity to counter a progressive decline in physical function.

Occasionally, patients with chronic GVHD have involvement of muscle, fascia and serous membranes, including the synovia [90]; joint effusions may occur in patients without any other sign of GVHD. Diagnostic procedures and management are discussed in Chapter 50. Involvement of fascia or tendons by an eosinophilic infiltrate (early) or fibrosis (late) frequently preceded by edema and often resulting in joint contractures of the wrists (most common), fingers, shoulders, elbows, ankles and, occasionally, knees may be manifestations of chronic GVHD. Because of the significant morbidity associated with joint contractures, range of motion assessment, including the extension of hands and wrists (i.e. palms together with the elbows extended, referred to by the author as the "Buddha pray position") is necessary when examining allogeneic transplant recipients to rule out fibrotic fasciitis, panniculitis or tendinitis. Patients with limitations of wrist extension often use the back of the hands (rather than the palms of their hands) to e.g. stand up. Some patients may be misdiagnosed as having carpal tunnel syndrome (Table 69.3).

Stretching exercises are important to improve range of motion of affected joints and restore functions of daily living. Physiotherapy and deep myofascial massage (Heller works) are critically important in the management of joint contractures.

Skeletal complications

Osteoporosis/osteopenia

Bone loss after HCT is related to several factors including irradiation, glucocorticoid therapy, inactivity and iatrogenic hypogonadism [91–97]. Dual-energy X-ray absorptiometry (DEXA), a semiquantitative method to assess bone mineral density (BMD), is a validated method commonly used to detect osteoporosis (T-score of ≤ –2.5 SD below age-related mean BMD) and osteopenia (T-score of –1.0 to 2.4 SD below age-related mean BMD). Reduction of bone mass using DEXA has been reported in approximately 40% of men and women at 1 year after HCT [94]. In another BMD study, osteopenia was reported in 33% and osteoporosis in 18% of women after HCT [91]. The bone alkaline phosphatase may be elevated, particularly in women, as may be the C-terminal propeptide. Increased urinary excretion of hydroxyproline can also be used to assess bone loss and response to treatment [98].

In women, supplementation with estrogens and medroxyprogesterone can increase bone mass after HCT [99,100]. A recent large randomized Women's Health Initiative study found an increase in the risks of cardiovascular diseases and breast cancer in post-menopausal women (with intact uterus) given conjugated equine estrogen (0.625 with medroxyprogesterone [2.5 mg]) [71]. HCT recipients are known to be at risk for secondary malignancies late after transplantation even without hormone replacement. However, osteoporosis and osteopenia are far more common and occur early after HCT. Thus, the overall risk and benefits of hormone replacement must be discussed individually before starting therapy and again at yearly intervals. Lower doses of estrogen alone (after hysterectomy) or combined with progestin (with uterus intact) have been used for the management of bone loss in other patient populations [101]. Since hormone replacement >3 years [71] may add to the already increased risk of breast cancers in long-term HCT survivors [102], the decision to continue therapy beyond 3 years must be carefully reassessed.

Estrogen-only therapy in another trial for post-menopausal women after hysterectomy so far has not shown an increase in breast cancer after 4 years [71].

All patients on hormone replacement must be follow by a gynecologist (yearly) and should perform monthly self-breast examinations. They should have mammograms at baseline at 35–40 years of age, and yearly after 40 years of age.

All patients should also have adequate intake of vitamin D (400 IU/day or 800 IU/day for patients on corticosteroids) and calcium (1200 mg/day or 1500 mg/day for patients on corticosteroids), should pursue an exercise program that combines aerobic weight-bearing and resistive exercises (20–30 min five times per week) and should follow fall prevention strategies (conditioning, removing trip hazards from home, eye examination and correction of vision). Also patients should stop smoking and limit their alcohol consumption.

Medications, such as alendronate (Fosamax®), risedronate (Actonel®), raloxifene (Evista®), calcitonin (Miacalcin®), pamidronate (Aredia®) and zoledronic acid (Zometa®) may be useful. However, the safety and efficacy in HCT recipients remains to be determined. Whenever possible, glucocorticoids should be tapered or discontinued.

Avascular necrosis

Avascular necrosis, especially in weight-bearing joints, is a classic side-effect of glucocorticoid therapy and has been reported in 4–10% of allogeneic HST survivors at a median of 12 months (range: 2–132) after transplant [93,103,104]. The hip is the joint most frequently affected (two-thirds of all cases). In most patients more than one joint is affected. In addition to glucocorticoid therapy, male gender (RR 4.2) and age ≥16 years (RR 3.8) were risk factors. One-third of patients required joint replacement at 2–42 months. A multi-institutional study from France, which included 4388 patients, found 77 patients with avascular necrosis for a 5-year incidence of 4.3% [103]. Symptoms developed at 2–132 months and 1–7 joints (mean 1.9) were affected. The hip joint was affected in 88% of cases, and 48% of these patients required joint replacement. Older age, a diagnosis of aplastic anemia or acute leukemia as opposed to other diagnoses, an irradiation-based conditioning regimen, the type of GVHD prophylaxis and acute or chronic GVHD were associated with an increased risk of avascular necrosis. In a case–control study of 87 patients with avascular necrosis, post-transplant glucocorticoid use and TBI given in preparation for HCT were significant risk factors [93]. CSP, shown by others to stimulate osteoclasts, was not a significant risk factor in that study. Thus, avascular necrosis occurs in about 4–8% of patients as early as 2 months and as late as 10 years post-transplant. The major risk factor is glucocorticoid use. Once avascular necrosis has developed, the only satisfactory treatment, particularly in weight-bearing joints, is joint replacement.

Dental problems

An oral sicca syndrome related to conditioning therapy or chronic GVHD may lead to poor oral hygiene with recurrent infection and periodontitis. Dental decay occurs because of a lack of cleansing by saliva, which is of altered consistency, and reduced volume [105]. Also, the mouth is painful and patients are hesitant to take care of their teeth and mucosa. One study [106] found that the incidence of dental caries was not higher in children after HCT than in children given chemotherapy only, suggesting that these problems are mostly regimen rather than transplant related [107]. The management is similar to that in nontransplant patients who have received head or neck irradiation, and includes diligent hygiene, fluoride treatment, artificial saliva, capping of teeth and other supportive measures.

In children, irradiation interferes with dental and facial development [106]. There may be poor calcification, micrognathia, mandibular hypoplasia, root blunting and apical closure [106,108]. The changes are most severe in children <7 years of age at the time of HCT. While chemotherapy mostly results in qualitative disturbances of dentine and enamel, irradiation induces both quantitative and qualitative alterations [109]. No effective prophylactic measures are currently available; careful planning (and, where possible, timing) of the preparative regimen may minimize these side-effects.

A detailed discussion of oral complications is provided in Chapter 67.

Genitourinary dysfunction

Bladder

Cystitis with microscopic or macroscopic hematuria occurs in 10–15% of patients [110]. The CY metabolite acrolein causes inflammation of the bladder mucosa, which can be particularly severe in patients who also receive BU [111,112]. In most patients, cystitis is an acute problem. However, some patients will have protracted hematuria, and scarring of the bladder wall with volume loss may present a chronic problem manifested by urinary frequency and, occasionally, hydronephrosis. Prophylaxis of hemorrhagic cystitis includes the use of mesna, forced hydration and diuresis, as well as continuous bladder irrigation with saline. Mesna is given concurrently with CY and at the same dose as CY [113]. Treatment consists in bladder irrigation, cystoscopic fulguration and, in extreme cases, in cystectomy with the construction of an artificial bladder from a bowel loop. A recent report indicates efficacy of hyperbaric oxygen [114]. In patients with severe scarring, antispasmodic treatment may be beneficial.

Viral infections with adenovirus, polyomavirus, BK virus, or other viruses may also be responsible for hematuria. Adenovirus strains with a tropism for the genitourinary organs also involve ureters and kidneys and may cause renal failure. Late onset cystitis associated with the polyoma virus has been treated successfully with vidarabine infusion [115].

Patients receiving immunosuppressive therapy for chronic GVHD, particularly women with GVHD of the vagina, are at risk for recurrent urinary tract infections which require prompt antibiotic therapy.

Kidneys

Renal failure related to antibiotic therapy, CSP, FK506, or chemotherapy given before HCT occurs frequently in the early post-transplant period [116]. Late failure, in contrast to observations in solid-organ transplant recipients, is less frequent. However, particularly in patients treated aggressively with nephrotoxic chemotherapy (e.g. with platinum compounds) or irradiaton before transplant, renal insufficiency has been observed in as many as 20–25% of patients by 2 years post-HCT [117–119], although other investigators disagree with this assessment [67]. The term "marrow transplant nephropathy" has been coined for this syndrome, which comprises of azotemia, hypertension and a disproportionate degree of anemia [118,120]. Some patients may also show features of a hemolytic uremic syndrome. Renal biopsies show changes of radiation nephritis including mesangial and endothelial drop-out, expansion of the glomerular basement membrane and widening of the glomerular capillary loops.

Analysis of clinical data and animal studies indicates that TBI can lead to long-term renal function impairment, as determined by creatinine levels, blood urea nitrogen (BUN), Chromium-51-ethylene diamine tetraacetic acid (^{51}Cr-EDTA) residual activity, proteinuria or hematocrit changes [121]. In one clinical study, renal dysfunction was strongly related to total TBI dose delivered and to the dose per fraction: the presence of GVHD was another risk factor [122]. These authors suggest that renal shielding should be used for TBI doses >1200 cGy [122]. In preclinical studies, fractionation or hyperfractionation had a protective effect [119]. The use of angiotensin converting enzyme inhibitors such as captopril may be beneficial [123]. Once nephropathy has developed, control of hypertension is the mainstay of therapy. At least one experimental study showed exacerbation of radiation nephropathy by retinoic acid [124].

Renal failure associated with hemolytic uremic syndrome or microangiopathic hemolytic anemia can occur in patients who are not heavily pretreated and are not conditioned with TBI. The mechanism is not fully understood. The syndrome may become manifest either during or following discontinuation of therapy with CSP [125]; similar observations have been made in FK506-treated patients. The mechanism involves altered pathways of prostaglandin synthesis, which, in conjunction with endothelial damage, might interfere with coagulation homeostasis. Plasmapheresis and discontinuation of the presumptive causative agent, as well as the use of glucocorticoids, have been suggested as therapeutic options [126]. In some patients, the disease stabilizes upon blood pressure control.

Genital organs

Complications related to chronic GVHD may also involve the genital organs, in particular the glans penis and vagina. Vaginitis may be severe and cause considerable distress and dyspareunia. Prolonged treatment with topical estrogens and with glucocorticoids, is indicated to prevent the development of atrophic vaginitis and adhesions. The vulva has also been a site of post-transplant malignancies (see Post-transplant malignancies, on this page). Post-transplant reproductive function is discussed in Chapter 68.

Gastrointestinal and hepatic complications

Gastrointestinal (GI) tract

The GI tract is a frequent target of acute transplant-related complications. Chronic problems are less common and generally related to GVHD. Involvement of the esophagus by chronic GVHD may lead to strictures and web formation [127–129]. Prolonged dilator treatment is required to allow for normal food intake. Chronic GVHD of the small bowel may result in malabsorption. Oral enzyme supplementation is often useful.

Pneumatosis cystoides intestinalis has been described in patients post-transplant generally while receiving glucocorticoid therapy [127,128]. The diagnosis is usually made 2–3 months post-transplant. No specific therapy is available, and the bowel normalizes spontaneously or with the resolution of other underlying problems.

Diarrhea may occur for various reasons. In many instances it is related to an "irritable bowel," but other causes, in particular infections, must be ruled out.

A potential problem is the late occurrence of viral disease. As viral infections are being controlled very successfully in the early post-transplant period, as many as 15% of patients experience late onset (12–18 months) CMV esophagitis or enteritis [130]. Apparently, the early suppression by appropriate prophylaxis delays the development of patient immunity to the disease, thereby allowing for delayed disease manifestations.

Liver

As discussed in Chapter 58, liver function abnormalities related to the conditioning regimen, and GVHD or infections, in particular viral infections, are frequent in the early post-transplant period. At 3 or more months after transplant the most frequent cause for enzyme or bilirubin elevation is chronic GVHD. However, viral hepatitis has to be considered at any time after HCT. Hepatitis may be due to hepatitis B or C (or other) viruses and may be transmitted from transplant or transfusion donors or occur by reactivation of the host virus. Some cases of hepatitis after HCT were diagnosed upon the tapering of immunosuppressive drugs given for GVHD prophylaxis or therapy [131]. There is evidence that treatment with IFN is useful, but the optimum regimen has not been determined [132,133]. In an occasional patient, liver function abnormalities may be related to the varicella-zoster virus, which may cause hepatitis without showing cutaneous manifestations. Prompt institution of therapeutic doses of acyclovir is indicated [134].

Of considerable concern are the late sequelae of hepatitis (i.e. cirrhosis, related to the hepatitis C virus (HCV), and hepatoma, related to the hepatitis B virus). A recent report by the transplant team in Pesaro, Italy, summarizes the effects of iron overload and HCV on liver fibrosis in patients transplanted for thalassemia [135]. Among 211 patients followed for a median of over 5 years, 46 (22%) showed progressive fibrosis of the liver. The risk was related to median hepatic iron concentration, high hepatic iron content and HCV positivity. None of the HCV-negative patients with an iron content of <16 mg/g dry weight showed progression, whereas all patients who were HCV-positive and had iron >22 mg/g progressed. Thus, attempts should be made at treating both iron overload (with phlebotomy and chelation) and HCV (with IFN and antiviral antibiotics). Several hepatic malignancies, including unusual fibrous histiocytomas, have been observed [136].

Anecdotal cases of hemosiderosis of the liver have occurred post-transplant and are thought to be related to altered iron absorption [127,128,137,138].

Post-transplant malignancies

Chromosomal instability (e.g. Fanconi anemia), immunosuppression or chronic antigenic stimulation (both resulting in disruption of normal regulatory mechanisms) and viral infections (e.g. Epstein–Barr virus [EBV])—all factors relevant to groups of patients undergoing HCT [139]—have been associated with the development of malignancies. In addition, patients are treated with potentially mutagenic agents. There are three major categories of secondary malignancies as illustrated schematically in Fig. 69.3 (see also Chapter 70).

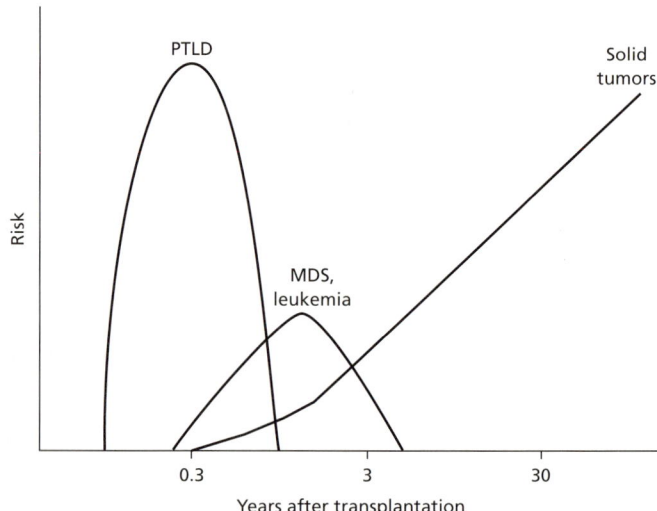

Fig. 69.3 Time course and relative risk (arbitrary scale) of major categories of secondary malignancies after hematopoietic cell transplantation (HCT). PTLD, post-transplant lymphoproliferative disorders.

Lymphoid malignancies

Lymphoproliferative disorders after HCT (post-transplant lymphoproliferative disease [PTLD]), generally of B-cell lineage, occur mostly in allogeneic transplant recipients [140–145]. T-cell PTLD, non-Hodgkin's lymphoma (NHL) and Hodgkin's disease (HD) have also been reported.

B-cell PTLD

Results in 18,014 allogeneic transplant recipients followed for up to 25 years revealed 78 cases of PTLD. In agreement with an earlier review by Cohen [141], 82% were diagnosed within 1 year of transplantation, with peak occurrence (120 cases/10,000 patients/year) at 2–5 months [146], and a decline to <5 cases/10,000/year among 1-year survivors. The incidence at 4–10 years was 1–2%, although figures of 0.6–10.0% have been reported. The incidence is highest in patients transplanted for immunodeficiency disorders.

Clinically and morphologically, B-cell PTLDs are heterogeneous, usually associated with EBV and developing in a milieu of T-cell dysfunction after any type of organ transplant [147–150]. B-cell PTLDs after allogeneic HCT are almost always of donor origin, and associated with EBV-genomic DNA integration. Histopathology ranges from diffuse large-cell lymphomas to aggressive immunoblastic lymphoma [144,151–153]. Most PTLDs after HCT are oligoclonal or monoclonal [144,154–156]. PTLDs express the full array of latent EBV antigens [144,157–159]. There is no strong correlation between clonality and morphology [153].

Numerous studies have identified risk factors for PTLD [152,160]: use of antithymocyte globulin (RR 6.4) or anti-CD3 monoclonal antibody (RR 43.2) for acute GVHD prophylaxis (RR 5.9), or in the preparative regimen (RR 3.1); use of TBI in the conditioning regimen (RR 2.9); use of T-cell depletion of donor marrow (RR 12.7) [161]; unrelated donor or human leukocyte antigen (HLA)-nonidentical related donor (RR 4.1; 8.9); primary immune deficiency disease (RR 2.5); acute GVHD (grades III–IV) (RR 1.9); and treatment of acute GVHD with antithymocyte globulin or monoclonal anti-T-cell antibody. In patients transplanted with marrow depleted of T cells with specific anti-CD3 monoclonal antibodies, the incidence of EBV plus PTLD ranged from 11% to 25%, while the incidence was <1% with techniques removing both T and B lymphocytes (e.g. soybean agglutinin or Campath-1), which presumably reflects the 2–3 log reduction in B lymphocytes associated with these procedures. The risk of PTLD is particularly high in EBV-negative patients transplanted from EBV-positive donors. The impact of risk factors is additive (or synergistic). The role of HLA-mismatching in the pathogenesis of B-cell PTLD probably relates to chronic antigenic stimulation or delayed immune reconstitution [162]. Increasing the intensity of post-transplant immunosuppression in patients who are otherwise at low risk significantly increases the incidence of PTLD [144].

Limiting dilution analysis has been used to quantify anti-EBV specific cytotoxic T-lymphocyte precursor (CTLp) frequencies in recipients of unmodified or T-cell-depleted grafts from EBV-positive donors [163]. At 3 months (interval of peak incidence of B-cell PTLD), only 20% of patients had EBV CTLp frequencies in the range of seropositive controls, while at 6 months 70% were normal. Infusion of unirradiated donor leukocytes (1.0×10^6 CD3$^+$ T cells/kg) induced complete histologic and clinical responses but also chronic GVHD [164]. Gene-marked EBV-specific cytotoxic T lymphocytes persisted *in vivo*, restored cellular immunity against EBV and responded to *in vivo* or *ex vivo* challenge with the virus for as long as 18 months.

Rising titers of EBV DNA in patient plasma are useful as a criterion to institute pre-emptive therapy with anti-CD20 antibodies or EBV-specific T-cell clones in high-risk patients [165]. Herpes simplex virus thymidine kinase (HSV-tk) gene-modified polyclonal donor lymphocytes have been reported to be effective [165–167].

The possibility of treating B-cell PTLD in hematopoietic stem cell transplantation recipients with IFN-α or B-cell-specific monoclonal or polyclonal antibodies has also been explored. A combination of IFN-α and IVIg was reported to be effective in inducing remissions in patients with B-cell PTLD [168].

Among 19 marrow transplant recipients with B-cell PTLDs treated with anti-CD21 and anti-CD24 antibodies, 10 achieved complete remissions and six, all with oligoclonal disease, survived at a median follow-up of 20 months [169,170]. Based on *in vitro* data showing antitumor effects of anti-interleukin-6 (IL-6) antibody (disrupting the IL-6-dependent proliferative loop) [171,172], neutralization of IL-6 may also be a strategy worth exploring. Chemotherapy and irradiation as well as surgical resection have been useful in selected cases, but generally only in solid organ recipients [141,148].

The best approach currently is close monitoring and pre-emptive therapy with anti-CD20 monoclonal antibody (325 mg) in patients with rising EBV titers. Additional doses of anti-CD20 antibody can be given if high EBV titers persist.

T-cell lymphoproliferative disorders

Rare T-cell proliferative disorders with or without EBV association have been reported [173,174]. None was associated with human T-cell lymphotropic virus 1 (HTLV-1), HIV, or human herpesvirus 6 (HHV-6) infection.

Hodgkin's disease (HD) and other lymphomas

Several cases of late occurring lymphomas have been reported [139,175–178], some linked to EBV infection (just as early onset PTLD) and others associated with T-cell depletion of the graft.

A study of 18,531 transplant recipients (covering over 42,000 patient years) identified eight cases of HD at 2.9–9.1 years after HCT (observed/expected ratio 6.2) [179]. Five cases (67%) showed mixed cellularity subtype and five of six cases studied contained the EBV genome [175]. Two patients were also positive for HIV. Risk factors identified for early PTLDs were generally absent. Patients with HD were more likely than matched controls to have acute GVHD and to require therapy for chronic GVHD (in one study RR 4.0). These data add support to the theory which links overstimulation of cellular immunity and exposure to EBV to various subtypes of HD [180].

Hematologic malignancies

After allogeneic HCT

Lymphoblastic leukemias in donor cells, with the donors remaining healthy, were recognized 30 years ago [181–183] but molecular studies indicate that this is an infrequent event [184]. Transformation of donor cells via antigenic stimulation by host tissue [185,186], a leukemogenic host environment [181] and fusion of normal cells with leukemic cells [187–189] have all been proposed as possible mechanisms. Recent work suggests that transplanted donor HSCs are subjected to increased "replicative stress" after transplantation, resulting in accelerated telomere shortening, which in turn would lead to chromosomal instability and increased probability of myelodysplastic syndrome (MDS) or leukemia [54,55]. This concept has remained controversial. Nevertheless, several cases of MDS/acute myeloid leukemia (AML) in donor cells presenting 5 year, 10 years, or even later after HCT have been observed (J. Deeg, unpublished data). Some patients have been treated with second transplants using myeloablative or nonmyeloablative protocols.

New leukemias in patient cells, i.e. leukemias of a different morphology or lineage than the patient's primary disease have also been described [190].

In addition, cases of leukemia or MDS transplanted from the donor into the patient have been reported [191,192].

After autologous HCT

"Secondary" MDS and AML occur after conventional chemotherapy with or without radiotherapy for HD, NHL or solid tumors [193–196], as well as after autologous HCT [139,197–200].

In four studies involving over 1200 patients the incidence of MDS was 4–18% at 3–6 years, with the post-transplant interval ranging from 2.5 to 8.5 years [191,201–203]. A case–control study revealed 12 cases of MDS/AML in 511 patients after autologous transplants for HD ($n = 249$) or NHL ($n = 262$) for a cumulative incidence of 4% at 5 years. Another report showed clonal chromosomal abnormalities in 10 of 275 patients 1.8–6.5 years after chemotherapy and 0.5–3.1 years after autologous transplant for HD or NHL [204], but only five patients had morphological evidence of MDS or AML. The cumulative probability of developing clonal chromosomal abnormalities reached 9% ± 4.7% at 3 years after transplantation. In several studies the risk was higher with peripheral blood cell transplants [205], in patients over 35 years of age at transplantation (RR 3.5) and with the use of TBI [206].

A case–control study under the auspices of the US National Cancer Institute analyzed data on 56 patients who developed MDS/AML and 168 controls within a cohort of 2739 patients with HD or NHL transplanted at 12 institutions (K. Metayer et al. unpublished data). MDS/AML was significantly correlated with the intensity of pretransplant chemotherapy, specifically mechlorethamine (RR 2.0; 4.3 for doses of ≤ 50 mg/m^2) and chlorambucil (RR 3.8; 8.4 for duration ≤ 10 months; $p = 0.0009$) compared to CY. Also, higher doses of TBI (>1200 cGy) used for transplant conditioning tended to carry a higher risk (RR 4.7). The difference between marrow and peripheral blood stem cells was not significant in this analysis.

It is controversial whether MDS/AML arises from infused hematopoietic stem cell or from residual cells in the patient. However, post-transplant MDS/AML clearly is a clonal disorder, and in most patients cytogenetic abnormalities (e.g. –7, +8, 7q-, 20q-, 11q23, etc.) are present, even if they were not detected in cells used for transplantation. In some female patients without cytogenetic abnormalities clonality has been documented by X-inactivation based clonality assays [207] and mutations of *RAS*, *FLT3*, *AML1* and *CBF* among others have been recognized (reviewed in [208]). According to current thinking, more than one mutagenic/leukemogenic event is required for MDS or AML to develop. Gene fusion products recognized as leukemogenic (e.g. *BCR/ABL*, *TEL/AML1*) are detectable even in normal individuals with the use of sensitive PCR technology. Thus, such clones may exist in patients pretransplant and a "second hit" might occur during or after transplantation. It has also been argued that many patients may not have MDS but rather "disordered engraftment" [200].

Taken together the data suggest that pretransplant exposure to chemotherapy, in particular alkylating agents, topoisomerase inhibitors and irradiation, should be minimized and the duration of therapy should be limited in patients who are candidates for transplantation [209]. Possibly alkylators and topoisomerase inhibitors should not be used for stem cell mobilization. If cytogenetics are abnormal at the time of stem cell harvest, an allogeneic transplant should be considered. In addition to standard cytogenetics, interphase fluorescence *in situ* hybridization (FISH), determination of loss of heterozygosity or point mutations and X-inactivation-based clonality assays can be used to detect a clonal population of cells. Once MDS/AML has evolved, the options are limited. Chemotherapy is often not well tolerated, and remissions are of short duration. Allogeneic HCT with standard or reduced intensity conditioning is a realistic option for a proportion of patients [210].

Solid tumors

After allogeneic HCT

Three single institution studies showed a spectrum of tumors including glioblastoma, melanoma, squamous cell carcinoma, adenocarcinoma, hepatoma and basal cell carcinoma, and found an incidence of about 5% at 10–15 years [160,161,211].

A recent collaborative study analyzed results in 19,220 patients (97.2% allogeneic recipients; 2.8% syngeneic recipients) transplanted between 1964 and 1992 [136]. There were 80 solid tumors for an observed/expected (O/E) ratio of 2.7 ($p < 0.001$). In 10-year survivors, the risk was increased eightfold. The tumor incidence was 2.2% at 10 years and 6.7% at 15 years. The risk was increased significantly for melanoma (O/E 5.0), cancers of the oral cavity (O/E 11.1), liver (O/E 7.5), central nervous system (CNS) (O/E 7.6), thyroid (O/E 6.6), bone (O/E 13.4) and connective tissue (O/E 8.0). The risk was highest for the youngest patients and declined with age.

The updated cohort now comprises 28,874 patients (<1–72 years of age, 74% with leukemia, 76% transplanted from an HLA-identical sibling, 59% given TBI was part of the conditioning regimen) transplanted from 1964 to 1996 (J. Deeg et al. unpublished data). Among 5-year survivors there were 161 solid tumors for an O/E ratio of 2.2. The highest ratios, ranging from 10.0 to 4.1, were observed for bone, buccal cavity, connective tissue, liver, brain, thyroid and melanoma (in that order). Among 10-year survivors, the O/E ratios were 26.5 for buccal cavity, 32.3 for liver, 18.3 for thyroid, 6.0 for melanoma and 3.3 for breast cancer. The rates of excess cancers/10,000/year were highest in patients <17 years (O/E 16.06) and lowest for patients >40 years of age (O/E 2.42).

Preliminary data from an ongoing nested case–control study in this same updated cohort suggest that duration of chronic GVHD >2 years and prolonged therapy are risk factors, in particular for the development of squamous cell carcinoma (J. Deeg et al. unpublished data).

After autologous HCT

A French study in 4322 patients with HD found 18 new malignancies in 467 patients who had received autologous HCT (8.9% at 5 years; $p = 0.039$ in comparison to nontransplanted patients) [205]. Another study found seven solid tumors in 750 autotransplant recipients for an incidence of 5.6% at 13 years [161]. In a third analysis among 625 autologous transplant recipients who survived at least 3 years after HCT, 14 developed second neoplasms at 4–116 months; 10 of these had received TBI [212]. The types of tumors observed were similar to those seen with allogeneic transplants. As with MDS/AML, the incidence was particularly increased in patients over 35 years of age and in recipients of peripheral blood (rather than marrow) hematopoietic stem cell.

Pathogenesis of solid tumors

Interactions of various factors play a role in the etiology and pathogenesis of secondary solid tumors. Socie et al. [213] identified human papillomavirus (HPV) 13, 15, or 16 in three of eight squamous cell carcinomas; human herpesvirus 8 was present in one. Further, the pattern of p53 expression suggested mutations of this gene in all eight tumors studied. Mutations might be induced by cytotoxic therapy, and suppressed immunity would interfere with normal surveillance. There is also evidence that polymorphism at position 72 in p53 (in particular homozygosity for arginine) may confer unusual susceptibility of p53 to inactivation by HPV. Chronic inflammation and impaired DNA repair are other factors. Observations in autologous patients will be of interest because etiologic factors, such as chronic allogeneic stimulation and GVHD are absent. It is also important to note that patients with a malignant disease are more likely to develop another (secondary) malignancy than the population at large. This increased probability is presumably due to genetic predisposition (xenobiotic polymorphism). Finally, even patients who receive cytotoxic therapy but do not undergo HCT are at an increased risk of developing a new malignancy.

Prophylaxis and therapy

Omission of (high-dose) irradiation from the conditioning regimen should be beneficial, in particular for the prevention of melanomas, thyroid carcinomas, carcinomas of the buccal cavity and breast cancer. Prevention (or different therapy) of chronic GVHD should have an effect on the development of oral carcinomas.

Surgical resection, whenever possible, is the front line therapy for solid tumors. Selective immunostimulation and measures aimed at scavenging free radicals have yielded some promising results in experimental studies.

Nervous system

Chronic or delayed neurological complications are known to occur after intensive chemoradiotherapy in patients who do not undergo HCT. The conditioning regimens used in preparation for HCT and the immunocompromise in the post-transplant period further contribute to these problems.

A severe syndrome is leukoencephalopathy [214]. Damage to the white matter of the brain is due to extensive intrathecal chemotherapy, in particular methotrexate alone or combined with cranial irradiation (1800–2400 cGy or even higher doses) and the use of TBI. Leukoencephalopathy has been observed predominantly in pediatric patients who often lose higher cortical functions and may be left in a vegetative state. Recovery is uncommon. Leukoencephalopathy has been diagnosed less frequently in recent years, conceivably due to a more judicious use of intrathecal therapy, brain shielding where appropriate, or omission of cranial irradiation whenever possible. Anecdotal reports have also described multifocal cerebral demyelination, inflammatory demyelinating polyneuropathy, immune-mediated myelopathy and encephalopathy [215–217].

The possibility of CNS involvement by GVHD has been debated but generally rejected. However, HCT results in patients with Hurler's disease show that the patient's microglia is being replaced by donor cells and, hence, donor/host interactions might take place in the CNS [218]. Others have described cerebellar and pyramidal signs correlating with GVHD activity [219]. In addition, Padovan et al. [220] and Takatsuka et al. [221] described periventricular white matter lesions and vasculitis or an angiitis-like syndrome that they attributed to GVHD in several patients. Some patients improved on treatment with CY or glucocorticoids.

Several clearly documented cases of peripheral neuropathy with reduced nerve conduction velocity related to chronic GVHD have been reported [222,223]. Destruction of Schwann cells seems to be responsible for this phenomenon, and patients respond to glucocorticoid therapy.

Infections of the CNS usually occur during the first few weeks after HCT. However, infections, e.g. with toxoplasma gondii, have occurred 6–8 months after transplantation [224]. In particular, patients with chronic GVHD are prone to develop septicemia and meningitis caused by encapsulated organisms [225]. Patients with chronic GVHD who receive immunosuppressive therapy should therefore also be given prophylactic antibiotics. In one autopsy study of 180 patients, only 17 had normal CNS findings [226].

As discussed in Chapters 59 and 68, patients may have impaired memory, shortened attention span and defects in verbal fluency [227]. Children, particularly those who also received cranial irradiation, are likely to score lower than controls in visual–motor processing tasks and various IQ tests [228].

Psychosocial effects and rehabilitation

Long-term adjustments and rehabilitation after HCT depend strongly on pretransplant conditions and events along the way. Considerable insights have been gained in recent years (see Chapters 38 & 39) [229–231].

Several studies have compared the quality of life of patients who received HCT to that of patients with comparable diagnoses who were given maintenance chemotherapy [232,233]. In regards to symptoms of depression, multifocal psychiatric symptomatology and scores according to several quality-of-life instruments no significant differences between the two groups were found. An estimated 75% of patients were back to pretransplant physical function by 1-year post-transplant [234,235]. However, at least in one study, 20% of HCT recipients had failed to return to full-time employment 40 months after transplantation [233], whereas another group reported that only 9% of 4-year survivors had failed to return to full-time occupation [236].

Not knowing what the future will bring, thoughts of dying, feeling tired, reduced attention span, short-term memory deficit, depression, inability to attain sexual satisfaction, low self-esteem because of reduced physical functioning and worrying about being a burden all contribute to psychosocial morbidity [233,237,238]. Pretransplant family conflict, nonmarried status and lack of social support are predictive of post-transplant problems. The development of chronic GVHD after transplant predicts a delay in physical recovery.

Changes in body image due to skin disfigurement, weight loss and weakness, in addition to medications, especially glucocorticoids or CSP and their side-effects, weigh heavily on patients. Patients with joint contractures or pulmonary disease may be crippled for years. Realistic and open pretransplant communication about potential long-term complications and pretransplant identification of patients at high risk for post-transplant physical and psychosocial morbidity will help to deal successfully with these problems as they arise.

Problems in obtaining employment and insurance coverage are frequent. Even patients without chronic GVHD and autologous HCT recipients may experience discrimination. This issue requires extensive counseling of both the patient and insurance carrier and continuing analysis of long-term results to provide detailed information on survival.

Effects of conditioning and HCT on growth and development of pediatric and adolescent patients are discussed elsewhere (see Chapter 68). Early detection of potential problems and health maintenance are important, possibly for several decades. The desire to be equal to their peers may cause severe problems with compliance in this age group, and problems with self-esteem, body image and sexuality may be particularly severe. A multidisciplinary approach involving adolescent medicine physicians and endocrinologists along with group therapy is most promising. Rehabilitation must begin at the time of diagnosis and should involve a long-term treatment plan [239].

Recent developments

Long-term follow-up is important and necessary to identify, prevent, or treat late complications after HCT (see Table 69.5).

Considerable effort has gone into the development of reduced-intensity/nonmyeloablative transplant regimens in an attempt to lessen toxicity early post-transplant, thereby enhancing recovery and preventing

Table 69.5 General long-term follow-up recommendations for adult patients after hematopoietic stem cell transplantation.*

- Routine oncologic evaluation at yearly intervals is recommended due to increased risk of secondary malignancy after HCT. Annual oncologic screening includes a history and complete physical examination, PAP smears and mammogram (women starting age ≥35 years), prostate exam and PSA (men taking testosterone or age ≥45 years) and testing for occult blood in stool. Baseline colonoscopy at age 45–50 years is also recommended. Oral examination by a dentist should be done yearly. The skin, head and neck are the most common sites of secondary malignancies. Secondary malignancy occurring before 2 years after transplant are rare, but the risk of developing cancer increases progressively after 5 years

- In patients transplanted for CML or Ph$^+$ ALL, routine monitoring for *BCR/abl* transcripts by nested PCR testing of a blood sample is recommended every 6 months for the first 2 years after transplant and yearly thereafter if results of the PCR test remain negative. If *BCR/abl* is positive by RT-PCR in blood, bone marrow testing is recommended for conventional cytogenetic analysis, morphology, molecular studies for the *BCR/abl* by both FISH and quantitative RT-PCR, and chimerism testing by DNA (if sex-matched patient/donor pair) or by Y and X chromosome probes by FISH (sex-mismatched patient/donor pair)

- Measures to prevent osteoporosis in patients receiving long-term treatment with corticosteroids include:
  - Calcium 1500 mg/day in the diet or in supplements to meet daily requirements
  - Vitamin D 800 IU/day in the diet or in supplements to meet daily requirements
  - Daily weight-bearing exercise for 20–60 min
  - Bone density test annually
  - Sex hormone replacement therapy if levels are low and if benefits offset the risks

The benefits and potential toxicity of treatment with bisphosphonates for prevention of osteoporosis or bone fractures have not been studied in a systematic manner after HCT. Patients should be encouraged to participate in clinical trials for prevention or treatment of bone loss after HCT

- Antibiotic prophylaxis should be maintained for 6 months after discontinuing all immunosuppressive medications in patients who have had chronic GVHD. Herbal medications and naturopathic remedies should not be administered to immunocompromised patients

- Pulmonary function should be tested at 1, 5 and 10 years after transplant and annually in patients receiving treatment for chronic GVHD

- Thyroid function should be tested at annual intervals, especially in patients given prior irradiation

- Ophthalmologic examination, Schirmer's test and the slit-lamp examination should be done at annual intervals

- Immunizations: see Chapter 51

*These follow-up guidelines represent generally accepted practices for medical care after hematopoietic stem cell transplantation at the Fred Hutchinson Cancer Research Center and the Seattle Cancer Care Alliance (FHCRC/SCCA). These guidelines should be implemented in a way that accounts for the specific situation of each individual patient.
ALL, acute lymphoblastic leukemia; CML, chronic myeloid leukemia; FISH, fluorescence *in situ* hybridization; GVHD, graft-vs.-host disease; HCT, hematopoietic cell transplantation; PCR, polymerase chain reaction; Ph$^+$, Philadelphia chromosome positive; PSA, prostate specific antigen; RT-PCR, reverse transcription-polymerase chain reaction.

long-term complications. These strategies are discussed in detail elsewhere (see Chapters 85 & 86). Available data show a low rate of mortality early post-transplant. However, GVHD requiring therapy occurs in about half of the patients and further observation is needed for a more definitive assessment, particularly of long-term complications.

Summary

Most patients who recover from the immediate post-transplant problems become healthy long-term survivors and return to normal activities of life. Some patients, however, develop chronic or delayed complications. Major factors contributing to these problems are pretransplant therapy, intensive conditioning regimens and chronic GVHD. Ongoing studies are expected to provide a better understanding of the psychosocial adjustment of patients. Effective therapy or preemptive treatment for some complications is available. Thus, systematic yearly long-term follow-up is recommended for all post-transplant patients (Table 69.5). Further refinement of conditioning regimens, prevention of GVHD, especially in its chronic form, and accelerated immunoreconstitution should reduce complications and improve the quality of life of HCT recipients.

References

1 Socie G, Stone JV, Wingard JR *et al*. Long-term survival and late deaths after allogeneic bone marrow transplantation. Late Effects Working Committee of the International Bone Marrow Transplant Registry. *N Engl J Med* 1999; **341**: 14–21.

2 Flowers MED, Parker PM, Johnston LJ *et al*. Comparison of chronic graft-versus-host disease after transplantation of peripheral blood stem cells versus bone marrow in allogeneic recipients: long

term follow up of a randomized trial. *Blood* 2002; **100**: 415–9.
3 Duell T, Van Lint MT, Ljungman P *et al*. Health and functional status of long-term survivors of bone marrow transplantation. EBMT Working Party on Late Effects and EULEP Study Group on Late Effects. *Ann Intern Med* 1997; **126**: 184–92.
4 Deeg HJ, Leisenring W, Storb R *et al*. Long-term outcome after marrow transplantation for severe aplastic anemia. *Blood* 1998; **91**: 3637–45.
5 Deeg HJ, Cottler-Fox M, Cahill R, Lynch M, Spitzer TR. Ineffective *in vivo* prophylaxis of graft-versus-host disease due to conditioning induced organ toxicity. *Bone Marrow Transplant* 1989; **4**: 96–101.
6 Lee SJ, Klein JP, Barrett AJ *et al*. Severity of chronic graft-versus-host disease: association with treatment-related mortality and relapse. *Blood* 2002; **100**: 406–14.
7 Dharmasena F, Gordon-Smith EC. Transmission of malaria by bone marrow transplantation [letter]. *Transplantation* 1986; **42**: 228.
8 Gopal R, Ha CS, Tucker SL *et al*. Comparison of two total body irradiation fractionation regimens with respect to acute and late pulmonary toxicity. *Cancer* 2001; **92**: 1949–58.
9 Madtes DK, Crawford SW. Lung injuries associated with graft-versus-host reactions. In: Ferrara JLM, Deeg HJ, Burakoff SJ, eds. *Graft-vs.-Host Disease*, 2nd edn. New York: Marcel Dekker, Inc., 1997: 425–46.
10 Kantrow SP, Hackman RC, Boeckh M, Myerson D, Crawford SW. Idiopathic pneumonia syndrome. Changing spectrum of lung injury after marrow transplantation. *Transplantation* 1997; **63**: 1079–86.
11 Boeckh M. Management of cytomegalovirus infections in blood and marrow transplant recipients. In: Mills J, Volberding PA, Corey L, eds. *Antiviral Chemotherapy 5: New Directions for Clinical Application and Research*. New York: Kluwer Academic/Plenum Publishers, 1999: 89–109.
12 Chen CS, Boeckh M, Seidel K *et al*. Incidence, risk factors and mortality of pneumonia developing late after hematopoietic stem cell transplantation. *Bone Marrow Transplant*, in press.
13 Crawford SW, Fisher L. Predictive value of pulmonary function tests before marrow transplantation. *Chest* 1992; **101**: 1257–64.
14 Crawford SW, Pepe M, Lin D, Benedetti F, Deeg HJ. Abnormalities of pulmonary function tests after marrow transplantation predict nonrelapse mortality. *Am J Respir Crit Care Med* 1995; **152**: 690–5.
15 Crawford SW. Respiratory infections following organ transplantation. *Curr Opin Pulmonary Med* 1995; **1**: 209–15.
16 Clark JG, Schwartz DA, Flournoy N, Sullivan KM, Crawford SW, Thomas ED. Risk factors for airflow obstruction in recipients of bone marrow transplants. *Ann Intern Med* 1987; **107**: 648–56.
17 Boas SR, Noyes BE, Kurland G, Armitage J, Orenstein D. Pediatric lung transplantation for graft-versus-host disease following bone marrow transplantation. *Chest* 1994; **105**: 1584–6.
18 Spray TL, Mallory GB, Canter CB, Huddleston CB. Pediatric lung transplantation. Indications, techniques, and early results. *J Thorac Cardiovasc Surg* 1994; **107**: 990–9; discussion 999–10.
19 Svendsen UG, Aggestrup S, Heilmann C *et al*. Transplantation of a lobe of lung from mother to child following previous transplantation with maternal bone marrow. *Eur Resp J* 1995; **8**: 334–7.
20 Sullivan KM, Mori M, Sanders JE *et al*. Late complications of allogeneic and autologous marrow transplantation (Review). *Bone Marrow Transplant* 1992; **10**: 127–34.
21 Philit F, Wiesendanger T, Archimbaud E, Mornex JF, Brune J, Cordier JF. Post-transplant obstructive lung disease ('bronchiolitis obliterans'): a clinical comparative study of bone marrow and lung transplant patients. *Eur Resp J* 1995; **8**: 551–8.
22 Sharples LD, Tamm M, McNeil K, Higenbottam TW, Stewart S, Wallwork J. Development of bronchiolitis obliterans syndrome in recipients of heart–lung transplantation: early risk factors. *Transplantation* 1996; **61**: 560–6.
23 Kumar S, Tefferi A. Spontaneous pneumomediastinum and subcutaneous emphysema complicating bronchiolitis obliterans after allogeneic bone marrow transplantation: case report and review of literature [Review]. *Ann Hematol* 2001; **80**: 430–5.
24 Deeg HJ, Socié G, Schoch G *et al*. Malignancies after marrow transplantation for aplastic anemia and Fanconi anemia: a joint Seattle and Paris analysis of results in 700 patients. *Blood* 1996; **87**: 386–92.
25 Sullivan KM, Storek J, Kopecky KJ *et al*. A controlled trial of long-term administration of intravenous immunoglobulin to prevent late infection and chronic graft-vs.-host disease after marrow transplantation: clinical outcome and effect on subsequent immune recovery. *Biol Blood Marrow Transplant* 1996; **2**: 44–53.
26 Heath JA, Kurland G, Spray TL *et al*. Lung transplantation after allogeneic marrow transplantation in pediatric patients: the Memorial Sloan-Kettering experience. *Transplantation* 2001; **72**: 1986–90.
27 Rabitsch W, Deviatko E, Keil F *et al*. Successful lung transplantation for bronchiolitis obliterans after allogeneic marrow transplantation. *Transplantation* 2001; **71**: 1341–3.
28 Freudenberger T, Madtes DK, Hackman RC. Characterization of bronchiolitis obliterans organizing pneumonia in a hematopoietic stem cell transplant population. *Am J Respir Crit Care Med* 2000; **161**: 890a [Abstract].
29 Palmas A, Tefferi A, Myers JL *et al*. Late-onset noninfectious pulmonary complications after allogeneic bone marrow transplantation. *Br J Haematol* 1998; **100**: 680–7.
30 Langston AA, Sanders JE, Deeg HJ *et al*. Allogeneic marrow transplantation for aplastic anaemia associated with dyskeratosis congenita. *Br J Haematol* 1996; **92**: 758–65.
31 Storek J, Witherspoon RP. Immunologic reconstitution after hematopoietic stem cell transplantation. In: Atkinson K, ed. *Clinical Bone Marrow and Blood Stem Cell Transplantation*. Cambridge, UK: Cambridge University Press, 2000: 111–46.
32 Wernet D, Weiss B, Schmidt H, Northoff H. Antigen-independent reactivation of anti-E years after allogeneic bone marrow transplantation: a case report. *Br J Haematol* 1995; **91**: 758–60.
33 Storek J, Joseph A, Espino G *et al*. Immunity of patients surviving 20–30 years after allogeneic or syngeneic bone marrow transplantation (Plenary Paper). *Blood* 2001; **98**: 3505–12.
34 Billingham RE. The biology of graft-versus-host reactions. *The Harvey Lectures*. New York: Academic Press, 1966: 21–78.
35 Hakim FT, Mackall CL. The immune system: effector and target of graft-versus-host disease. In: Ferrara JLM, Deeg HJ, Burakoff SJ, eds. *Graft-vs.-Host Disease*, 2nd edn. New York: Marcel Dekker, Inc., 1997: 257–90.
36 Hess AD. The immunobiology of syngeneic/autologous graft-versus-host disease. In: Ferrara JLM, Deeg HJ, Burakoff SJ, eds. *Graft-vs.-Host Disease*, 2nd edn. New York: Marcel Dekker, Inc., 1997: 561–86.
37 Lambertenghi-Deliliers GL, Annaloro C, Della Volpe A, Oriani A, Pozzoli E, Soligo D. Multiple autoimmune events after autologous bone marrow transplantation. *Bone Marrow Transplant* 1997; **19**: 745–7.
38 Rouquette-Gally AM, Boyeldieu D, Prost AC, Gluckman E. Autoimmunity after allogeneic bone marrow transplantation. *Transplantation* 1988; **46**: 238–40.
39 Muro Y, Kamimoto T, Hagiwara M. Anti-mitosin antibodies in a patient with chronic graft-versus-host disease after allogeneic bone marrow transplantation. *Bone Marrow Transplant* 1997; **19**: 951–3.
40 Smith CIE, Aarli JA, Biberfeld P *et al*. Myasthenia gravis after bone-marrow transplantation. Evidence for a donor origin. *N Engl J Med* 1983; **309**: 1565–8.
41 Bellou A, Kanny G, Fremont S, Moneret-Vautrin DA. Transfer of atopy following bone marrow transplantation. *Ann Allergy Asthma Immunol* 1997; **78**: 513–6.
42 Snowden JA, Heaton DC. Development of psoriasis after syngeneic bone marrow transplant from psoriatic donor: further evidence for adoptive autoimmunity. *Br J Dermatol* 1997; **137**: 130–2.
43 Snowden JA, Atkinson K, Kearney P, Brooks P, Biggs JC. Allogeneic bone marrow transplantation from a donor with severe active rheumatoid arthritis not resulting in adoptive transfer of disease to recipient. *Bone Marrow Transplant* 1997; **20**: 71–3.
44 Sturfelt G, Lenhoff S, Sallerfors B, Nived O, Truedsson L, Sjoholm AG. Transplantation with allogenic bone marrow from a donor with systemic lupus erythematosus (SLE). Successful outcome in the recipient and induction of an SLE flare in the donor. *Ann Rheum Dis* 1996; **55**: 638–41.
45 Prummer O, Bunjes D, Wiesneth M *et al*. Antibodies to interferon-α: a novel type of autoantibody occurring after allogeneic bone marrow transplantation. *Bone Marrow Transplant* 1996; **17**: 617–23.
46 Sivakumaran M, Hutchinson RM, Pringle H *et al*. Thrombocytopenia following autologous bone marrow transplantation: evidence for autoimmune aetiology and B cell clonal involvement. *Bone Marrow Transplant* 1995; **15**: 531–6.
47 De Lord C, Marsh JC, Smith JG, Singer CR, Gordon-Smith EC. Fatal autoimmune pancytopenia following bone marrow transplantation for aplastic anaemia. *Bone Marrow Transplant* 1996; **18**: 237–9.
48 Wingard JR, Piantadosi S, Vogelsang GB *et al*. Predictors of death from chronic graft-versus-host disease after bone marrow transplantation. *Blood* 1989; **74**: 1428–35.
49 Sullivan KM, Witherspoon RP, Storb R *et al*. Alternating-day cyclosporine and prednisone for treatment of high-risk chronic graft-versus-host disease. *Blood* 1988; **72**: 555–61.

50 Lee SJ, Churchill WH, Konugres A, Gilliland DG, Antin JH. Idiopathic thrombocytopenic purpura following allogeneic bone marrow transplantation: treatment with anti-D immunoglobulin. *Bone Marrow Transplant* 1997; **19**: 173–4.

51 Ohashi K, Akiyama H, Takamoto S, Tanikawa S, Sakamaki H, Onozawa Y. Treatment of pure red cell aplasia after major ABO-incompatible bone marrow transplantation resistant to erythropoietin. Bone Marrow Transplantation Team. *Bone Marrow Transplant* 1994; **13**: 335–6.

52 Roychowdhury DF, Linker CA. Pure red cell aplasia complicating an ABO-compatible allogeneic bone marrow transplantation, treated successfully with antithymocyte globulin. *Bone Marrow Transplant* 1995; **16**: 471–2.

53 Selleri C, Raiola A, De Rosa G et al. CD34+-enriched donor lymphocyte infusions in a case of pure red cell aplasia and late graft failure after major ABO-incompatible bone marrow transplantation. *Bone Marrow Transplant* 1998; **22**: 605–7.

54 Mathioudakis G, Storb R, McSweeney PA et al. Polyclonal hematopoiesis with variable telomere shortening in human long-term allogeneic marrow graft recipients (Brief Report). *Blood* 2000; **96**: 3991–4.

55 Wynn RF, Cross MA, Hatton C et al. Accelerated telomere shortening in young recipients of allogeneic bone-marrow transplants. *Lancet* 1998; **351**: 178–81.

56 Constine LS, Donaldson SS, McDougall IR, Cox RS, Link MP, Kaplan HS. Thyroid dysfunction after radiotherapy in children with Hodgkin's disease. *Cancer* 1984; **53**: 878–83.

57 Toubert ME, Socié G, Gluckman E et al. Short- and long-term follow-up of thyroid dysfunction after allogeneic bone marrow transplantation without the use of preparative total body irradiation. *Br J Haematol* 1997; **98**: 453–7.

58 Borgstrom B, Bolme P. Thyroid function in children after allogeneic bone marrow transplantation. *Bone Marrow Transplant* 1994; **13**: 59–64.

59 Thomas O, Mahe M, Campion L et al. Long-term complications of total body irradiation in adults. *Int J Radiat Oncol Biol Phys* 2001; **49**: 125–31.

60 Thomas BC, Stanhope R, Plowman PN, Leiper AD. Endocrine function following single fraction and fractionated total body irradiation for bone marrow transplantation in childhood. *Acta Endocrinol (Copenh)* 1993; **128**: 508–12.

61 Boulad F, Bromley M, Black P et al. Thyroid dysfunction following bone marrow transplantation using hyperfractionated radiation. *Bone Marrow Transplant* 1995; **15**: 71–6.

62 Neglia JP, Nesbit ME Jr. Care and treatment of long-term survivors of childhood cancer [Review]. *Cancer* 1993; **71**: 3386–91.

63 Sanders JE. Growth and development after hematopoietic cell transplantation. In: Thomas ED, Blume KG, Forman SJ, eds. *Hematopoietic Cell Transplantation*, 2nd edn. Malden, MA: Blackwell Science, 1999: 764–75.

64 Uderzo C, Van Lint MT, Rovelli A et al. Papillary thyroid carcinoma after total body irradiation. *Arch Dis Child* 1994; **71**: 256–8.

65 Lupoli G, Cascone E, Vitale G et al. Risk factors and prevention of thyroid carcinoma [Review]. *Minerva Endocrinol* 1996; **21**: 93–100.

66 Sierra J, Bjerke J, Hansen J et al. Marrow transplants from unrelated donors as treatment for acute leukemia. *Leuk Lymphoma* 2000; **39**: 495–507.

67 Kumar M, Kedar A, Neiberger RE. Kidney function in long-term pediatric survivors of acute lymphoblastic leukemia following allogeneic bone marrow transplantation. *Pediatr Hematol Oncol* 1996; **13**: 375–9.

68 Kubota C, Shinohara O, Hinohara T et al. Changes in hypothalamic–pituitary function following bone marrow transplantation in children. *Acta Paediatr Jpn* 1994; **36**: 37–43.

69 Brauner R, Adan L, Souberbielle JC et al. Contribution of growth hormone deficiency to the growth failure that follows bone marrow transplantation. *J Pediatr* 1997; **130**: 785–92.

70 Clement-De Boers A, Oostdijk W, Van Weel-Sipman MH, Van den Broeck J, Wit JM, Vossen JM. Final height and hormonal function after bone marrow transplantation in children. *J Pediatr* 1996; **129**: 544–50.

71 Risks and benefits of estrogen plus progestin in healthy postmenopausal women. *JAMA*, 2002; **288**: 321–33.

72 Yahalom J. Re-visiting the role of radiation therapy in Hodgkin's disease [Review]. *Isr J Med Sci* 1995; **31**: 137–43.

73 Murdych T, Weisdorf DJ. Serious cardiac complications during bone marrow transplantation at the University of Minnesota 1977–97. *Bone Marrow Transplant* 2001; **28**: 283–7.

74 Braverman AC, Antin JH, Plappert MT, Cook EF, Lee RT. Cyclophosphamide cardiotoxicity in bone marrow transplantation. A prospective evaluation of new dosing regimens. *J Clin Oncol* 1991; **9**: 1215–23.

75 Goldberg MA, Antin JH, Guinan EC, Rappeport JM. Cyclophosphamide cardiotoxicity. An analysis of dosing as a risk factor. *Blood* 1986; **68**: 1114–8.

76 Ramrakha PS, Marks DI, O'Brien SG, Yacoub M, Schofield JB, Goldman JM. Orthotopic cardiac transplantation for dilated cardiomyopathy after allogeneic bone marrow transplantation. *Clin Transplant* 1994; **8**: 23–6.

77 Kakavas PW, Ghalie R, Parrillo JE, Kaizer H, Barron JT. Angiotensin converting enzyme inhibitors in bone marrow transplant recipients with depressed left ventricular function. *Bone Marrow Transplant* 1995; **15**: 859–61.

78 Hochster H, Wasserheit C, Speyer J. Cardiotoxicity and cardioprotection during chemotherapy [Review]. *Curr Opin Oncol* 1995; **7**: 304–9.

79 Rocha V, Devergie A, Socie G et al. Unusual complications after bone marrow transplantation for dyskeratosis congenita. *Br J Haematol* 1998; **103**: 243–8.

80 Benyunes MC, Sullivan KM, Deeg HJ et al. Cataracts after bone marrow transplantation: long-term follow-up of adults treated with fractionated total body irradiation. *Int J Radiat Oncol Biol Phys* 1995; **32**: 661–70.

81 Belkacemi Y, Labopin M, Vernant JP et al. Cataracts after total body irradiation and bone marrow transplantation in patients with acute leukemia in complete remission: a study of the European Group for Blood and Marrow Transplantation. *Int J Radiat Oncol Biol Phys* 1998; **41**: 659–68.

82 Belkacemi Y, Ozsahin M, Pene F et al. Cataractogenesis after total body irradiation. *Int J Radiat Oncol Biol Phys* 1996; **35**: 53–60.

83 Fife K, Milan S, Westbrook K, Powles R, Tait D. Risk factors for requiring cataract surgery following total body irradiation. *Radiother Oncol* 1994; **33**: 93–8.

84 van Kempen-Harteveld ML, Belkacemi Y, Kal HB, Labopin M, Frassoni F. Dose-effect relationship for cataract induction after single-dose total body irradiation and bone marrow transplantation for acute leukemia. *Int J Radiat Oncol Biol Phys* 2002; **52**: 1367–74.

85 Clark JI, Livesey JC, Steele JE. Delay or inhibition of rat lens opacification using pantethine and WR-77913. *Exp Eye Res* 1996; **62**: 75–84.

86 Tichelli A, Duell T, Weiss M et al. Late-onset keratoconjunctivitis sicca syndrome after bone marrow transplantation: incidence and risk factors. European Group or Blood and Marrow Transplantation (EBMT) Working Party on Late Effects. *Bone Marrow Transplant* 1996; **17**: 1105–11.

87 Hart DE, Simko M, Harris E. How to produce moisture chamber eyeglasses for the dry eye patient. *J Am Optom Assoc* 1994; **65**: 517–22.

88 Hanada R, Ueoka Y. Obstruction of nasolacrimal ducts closely related to graft-versus-host disease after bone marrow transplantation. *Bone Marrow Transplant* 1989; **4**: 125–6.

89 Tsai RJ, Li LM, Chen JK. Reconstruction of damaged corneas by transplantation of autologous limbal epithelial cells. *N Engl J Med* 2000; **343**: 86–93.

90 Cutler C, Giri S, Jeyapalan S, Paniagua D, Viswanathan A, Antin JH. Acute and chronic graft-versus-host disease after allogeneic peripheral-blood stem-cell and bone marrow transplantation: a meta-analysis. *J Clin Oncol* 2001; **19**: 3685–91.

91 Castaneda S, Carmona L, Carvajal I, Arranz R, Diaz A, Garcia-Vadillo A. Reduction of bone mass in women after bone marrow transplantation. *Calcif Tissue Int* 1997; **60**: 343–7.

92 Grigsby PW, Roberts HL, Perez CA. Femoral neck fracture following groin irradiation. *Int J Radiat Oncol Biol Phys* 1995; **32**: 63–7.

93 Fink JC, Leisenring WM, Sullivan KM, Sherrard DJ, Weiss NS. Avascular necrosis following bone marrow transplantation: a case–control study. *Bone* 1998; **22**: 67–71.

94 Stern JM, Sullivan KM, Ott SM et al. Bone density loss after allogeneic hematopoietic stem cell transplantation: a prospective study. *Biol Blood Marrow Transplant* 2001; **7**: 257–64.

95 Kashyap A, Kandeel F, Yamauchi D et al. Effects of allogeneic bone marrow transplantation on recipient bone mineral density: a prospective study. *Biol Blood Marrow Transplant* 2000; **6**: 344–51.

96 Valimaki MJ, Kinnunen K, Volin L et al. A prospective study of bone loss and turnover after allogeneic bone marrow transplantation: effect of calcium supplementation with or without calcitonin. *Bone Marrow Transplant* 1999; **23**: 355–61.

97 Weilbaecher KN. Mechanisms of osteoporosis after hematopoietic cell transplantation [Review]. *Biol Blood Marrow Transplant* 2000; **6**: 165–74.

98 Withold W, Wolf HH, Kollbach S, Heyll A, Schneider W, Reinauer H. Monitoring of bone metabolism after bone marrow transplantation by measuring two different markers of bone turnover. *Eur J Clin Chem Clin Biochem* 1996; **34**: 193–7.

99 Castelo-Branco C, Rovira M, Pons F et al. The effect of hormone replacement therapy on bone mass in patients with ovarian failure due to bone marrow transplantation. *Maturitas* 1996; **23**: 307–12.

100 Bellati U, Iammarrone E, Bavaro P et al. Efficacy of estrogen-progestin replacement therapy after

bone marrow transplantation. *Minerva Ginecol* 1996; **48**: 351–4.
101 Lindsay R, Gallagher JC, Kleerekoper M, Pickar JH. Effect of lower doses of conjugated equine estrogens with and without medroxyprogesterone acetate on bone in early postmenopausal women. *JAMA* 2002; **287**: 2668–76.
102 Rizzo J, Curtis R, Deeg H *et al*. Solid cancers in survivors of allogeneic bone marrow transplantation (BMT). *Blood* 2000; **96**(1): 557a [Abstract].
103 Socié G, Cahn JY, Carmelo J *et al*. Avascular necrosis of bone after allogeneic bone marrow transplantation: analysis of risk factors for 4388 patients by the Societe Francaise de Greffe de Moelle (SFGM). *Br J Haematol* 1997; **97**: 865–70.
104 Fletcher BD, Crom DB, Krance RA, Kun LE. Radiation-induced bone abnormalities after bone marrow transplantation for childhood leukemia. *Radiology* 1994; **191**: 231–5.
105 Izutsu KT, Sullivan KM, Schubert MM *et al*. Disordered salivary immunoglobulin secretion and sodium transport in human chronic graft-versus-host disease. *Transplantation* 1983; **35**: 441–6.
106 Nasman M, Forsberg CM, Dahllof G. Long-term dental development in children after treatment for malignant disease. *Eur J Orthod* 1997; **19**: 151–9.
107 Pajari U, Ollila P, Lanning M. Incidence of dental caries in children with acute lymphoblastic leukemia is related to the therapy used. *ASDC J Dent Child* 1995; **62**: 349–52.
108 Nasman M, Bjork O, Soderhall S, Ringden O, Dahllof G. Disturbances in the oral cavity in pediatric long-term survivors after different forms of antineoplastic therapy. *Pediatr Dent* 1994; **16**: 217–23.
109 Dahllof G, Rozell B, Forsberg CM, Borgstrom B. Histologic changes in dental morphology induced by high dose chemotherapy and total body irradiation. *Oral Surg Oral Med Oral Pathol* 1994; **77**: 56–60.
110 Yang CC, Hurd DD, Case LD, Assimos DG. Hemorrhagic cystitis in bone marrow transplantation. *Urology* 1994; **44**: 322–8.
111 Stella F, Battistelli S, Marcheggiani F *et al*. Urothelial cell changes due to busulfan and cyclophosphamide treatment in bone marrow transplantation. *Acta Cytol* 1990; **34**: 885–90.
112 Vela-Ojeda J, Tripp-Villanueva F, Sanchez-Cortes E *et al*. Intravesical rhGM-CSF for the treatment of late onset hemorrhagic cystitis after bone marrow transplant. *Bone Marrow Transplant* 1999; **24**: 1307–10.
113 Vose JM, Reed EC, Pippert GC *et al*. Mesna compared with continuous bladder irrigation as uroprotection during high-dose chemotherapy and transplantation: a randomized trial. *J Clin Oncol* 1993; **11**: 1306–10.
114 Hattori K, Yabe M, Matsumoto M *et al*. Successful hyperbaric oxygen treatment of life-threatening hemorrhagic cystitis after allogeneic bone marrow transplantation. *Bone Marrow Transplant* 2001; **27**: 1315–7.
115 Vianelli N, Renga M, Azzi A *et al*. Sequential vidarabine infusion in the treatment of polyoma virus-associated acute haemorrhagic cystitis late after allogeneic bone marrow transplantation. *Bone Marrow Transplant* 2000; **25**: 319–20.
116 Zager RA. Acute renal failure in the setting of bone marrow transplantation. *Kidney Int* 1994; **46**: 1443–58.
117 Tarbell NJ, Guinan EC, Niemeyer C, Mauch P, Sallan SE, Weinstein HJ. Late onset of renal dysfunction in survivors of bone marrow transplantation. *Int J Radiat Oncol Biol Phys* 1988; **15**: 99–104.
118 Cohen EP, Lawton CA, Moulder JE. Bone marrow transplant nephropathy: radiation nephritis revisited [Review]. *Nephron* 1995; **70**: 217–22.
119 Safwat A, Nielsen OS, el-Badawy S, Overgaard J. Late renal damage after total body irradiation and bone marrow transplantation in a mouse model: effect of radiation fractionation. *Eur J Cancer* 1995; **31**A: 987–92.
120 Cohen EP, Lawton CA, Moulder JE, Becker CG, Ash RC. Clinical course of late-onset bone marrow transplant nephropathy. *Nephron* 1993; **64**: 626–35.
121 Niemer-Tucker MM, Sluysmans MM, Bakker B, Davelaar J, Zurcher C, Broerse JJ. Long-term consequences of high-dose total-body irradiation on hepatic and renal function in primates. *Int J Radiat Biol* 1995; **68**: 83–96.
122 Miralbell R, Bieri S, Mermillod B *et al*. Renal toxicity after allogeneic bone marrow transplantation: the combined effects of total-body irradiation and graft-versus-host disease. *J Clin Oncol* 1996; **14**: 579–85.
123 Cohen EP, Moulder JE, Fish BL, Hill P. Prophylaxis of experimental bone marrow transplant nephropathy. *J Lab Clin Med* 1994; **124**: 371–80.
124 Moulder JE, Fish BL, Regner KR, Cohen EP, Raife TJ. Retinoic acid exacerbates experimental radiation nephropathy. *Radiat Res* 2002; **157**: 199–203.
125 Arai S, Allan C, Streiff M, Hutchins GM, Vogelsang GB, Tsai HM. Von Willebrand factor-cleaving protease activity and proteolysis of von Willebrand factor in bone marrow transplant-associated thrombotic microangiopathy. *Hematol J* 2001; **2**: 292–9.
126 Kaplan AA. Therapeutic apheresis for cancer related hemolytic uremic syndrome [Review]. *Ther Apher* 2000; **4**: 201–6.
127 Strasser SI, Sullivan KM, Myerson D *et al*. Cirrhosis of the liver in long-term marrow transplant survivors. *Blood* 1999; **93**: 3259–66.
128 Strasser SI, McDonald GB. Gastrointestinal and hepatic complications. In: Thomas ED, Blume KG, Forman SJ, eds. *Hematopoietic Cell Transplantation*, 2nd edn. Malden, MA: Blackwell Science, 1999: 627–58.
129 Strasser SI, McDonald GB. Hepatobiliary complications of hematopoietic cell transplantation. In: Schiff ER, Sorrell MF, Maddrey WC, eds. *Schiff's Diseases of the Liver*, 9th edn. Philadelphia: J.B. Lippincott & Co., 2003: 1636–63.
130 Boeckh M, Riddell SR, Cunningham T, Myerson D, Flowers M, Bowden RA. Increased risk of late CMV infection and disease in allogeneic marrow transplant recipients after ganciclovir prophylaxis is due to a lack of CMV-specific T cell responses. *Blood* 1996; **88** (Suppl. 1): 302a [Abstract].
131 Mertens T, Kock J, Hampl W *et al*. Reactivated fulminant hepatitis B virus replication after bone marrow transplantation: clinical course and possible treatment with ganciclovir. *J Hepatol* 1996; **25**: 968–71.
132 Tong MJ, Reddy KR, Lee WM *et al*. Treatment of chronic hepatitis C with consensus interferon: a multicenter, randomized, controlled trial. Consensus Interferon Study Group. *Hepatology* 1997; **26**: 747–54.
133 Papatheodoridis GV, Katsoulidou A, Touloumi G, Delladetsima JK, Hatzakis A, Tassopoulos NC. Biochemical and virological response of chronic hepatitis C after treatment with interferon-α for 6 or 12 months: predictors of sustained remission. *Eur J Gastroenterol Hepatol* 1996; **8**: 469–75.
134 Steer CB, Szer J, Sasadeusz J, Matthews JP, Beresford JA, Grigg A. Varicella-zoster infection after allogeneic bone marrow transplantation. Incidence, risk factors and prevention with low-dose aciclovir and ganciclovir. *Bone Marrow Transplant* 2000; **25**: 657–64.
135 Angelucci E, Muretto P, Nicolucci A *et al*. Effects of iron overload and hepatitis C virus positivity in determining progression of liver fibrosis in thalassemia following bone marrow transplantation. *Blood* 2002; **100**: 17–21.
136 Curtis RE, Rowlings PA, Deeg HJ *et al*. Solid cancers after bone marrow transplantation. *N Engl J Med* 1997; **336**: 897–904.
137 Mahendra P, Hood IM, Bass G, Patterson P, Marcus RE. Severe hemosiderosis post allogenic bone marrow transplantation. *Hematol Oncol* 1996; **14**: 33–5.
138 Gabutti V, Borgna-Pignatti C. Clinical manifestations and therapy of transfusional haemosiderosis [Review]. *Bailliere's Clin Haematol* 1994; **7**: 919–40.
139 Deeg HJ, Socié G. Malignancies after hematopoietic stem cell transplantation: many questions, some answers. *Blood* 1998; **91**: 1833–44.
140 Shepherd JD, Gascoyne RD, Barnett MJ, Coghlan JD, Phillips GL. Polyclonal Epstein–Barr virus-associated lymphoproliferative disorder following autografting for chronic myeloid leukemia. *Bone Marrow Transplant* 1995; **15**: 639–41.
141 Cohen JI. Epstein–Barr virus lymphoproliferative disease associated with acquired immunodeficiency [Review]. *Medicine* 1991; **70**: 137–60.
142 Okada S, Nagayoshi K, Nakauchi H, Nishikawa S, Miura Y, Suda T. Sequential analysis of hematopoietic reconstitution achieved by transplantation of hematopoietic stem cells. *Blood* 1993; **81**: 1720–5.
143 Socié G, Henry-Amar M, Devergie A *et al*. Malignant diseases after allogeneic bone marrow transplantation: an updated overview [Review]. *Nouv Rev Fr Hematol* 1994; **36** (Suppl. 1): S75–7.
144 O'Reilly RJ, Lacerda JF, Lucas KG, Rosenfield NS, Small TN, Papadopoulos EB. Adoptive cell therapy with donor lymphocytes for EBV-associated lymphomas developing after allogeneic marrow transplants. In: DeVita VT Jr, Hellman S, Rosenberg SA, eds. *Important Advances in Oncology*. Philadelphia: J.B. Lippincott & Co., 1996: 149–66.
145 Witherspoon RP, Deeg HJ, Storb R. Secondary malignancies after marrow transplantation for leukemia or aplastic anemia. *Transplantation* 1994; **57**: 1413–8.
146 Curtis RE, Travis LB, Rowlings PA *et al*. Risk of lymphoproliferative disorders after bone marrow transplantation: a multi-institutional study. *Blood* 1999; **94**: 2208–16.
147 Leblond V, Sutton L, Dorent R *et al*. Lymphoproliferative disorders after organ transplantation: a report of 24 cases observed in a single center. *J Clin Oncol* 1995; **13**: 961–8.
148 Swinnen LJ, Mullen GM, Carr TJ, Costanzo MR, Fisher RI. Aggressive treatment for postcardiac transplant lymphoproliferation. *Blood* 1995; **86**: 3333–40.

149 Morrison VA, Dunn DL, Manivel JC, Gajl-Peczalska KJ, Peterson BA. Clinical characteristics of post-transplant lymphoproliferative disorders. *Am J Med* 1994; **97**: 14–24.

150 Wilkinson AH, Smith JL, Hunsicker LG *et al.* Increased frequency of posttransplant lymphomas in patients treated with cyclosporine, azathioprine, and prednisone. *Transplantation* 1989; **47**: 293–6.

151 Simon M, Bartram CR, Friedrich W *et al.* Fatal B-cell lymphoproliferative syndrome in allogeneic marrow graft recipients. A clinical, immunobiological and pathological study. *Virchows Arch* 1991; **60**: 307–19.

152 Shapiro RS, McClain K, Frizzera G *et al.* Epstein–Barr virus associated B cell lymphoproliferative disorders following bone marrow transplantation. *Blood* 1988; **71**: 1234–43.

153 Orazi A, Hromas RA, Neiman RS *et al.* Posttransplantation lymphoproliferative disorders in bone marrow transplant recipients are aggressive diseases with a high incidence of adverse histologic and immunobiologic features. *Am J Clin Pathol* 1997; **107**: 419–29.

154 Seiden MV, Sklar J. Molecular genetic analysis of post-transplant lymphoproliferative disorders [Review]. *Hematol Oncol Clin North Am* 1993; **7**: 447–65.

155 Knowles DM, Cesarman E, Chadburn A *et al.* Correlative morphologic and molecular genetic analysis demonstrates three distinct categories of posttransplantation lymphoproliferative disorders. *Blood* 1995; **85**: 552–65.

156 Chadburn A, Suciu-Foca N, Cesarman E, Reed E, Michler RE, Knowles DM. Post-transplantation lymphoproliferative disorders arising in solid organ transplant recipients are usually of recipient origin. *Am J Pathol* 1995; **147**: 1862–70.

157 Suhrbier A, Burrows SR, Fernan A, Lavin MF, Baxter GD, Moss DJ. Peptide epitope induced apoptosis of human cytotoxic T lymphocytes. Implications for peripheral T cell deletion and peptide vaccination. *J Immunol* 1993; **150**: 2169–78.

158 McKnight JL, Cen H, Riddler SA *et al.* EBV gene expression, EBNA antibody responses and EBV+ peripheral blood lymphocytes in post-transplant lymphoproliferative disease [Review]. *Leuk Lymphoma* 1994; **15**: 9–16.

159 Randhawa PS, Jaffe R, Demetris AJ *et al.* Expression of Epstein–Barr virus-encoded small RNA (by the *EBER-1* gene) in liver specimens from transplant recipients with post-transplantation lymphoproliferative disease. *N Engl J Med* 1992; **327**: 1710–4.

160 Witherspoon RP, Fisher LD, Schoch G *et al.* Secondary cancers after bone marrow transplantation for leukemia or aplastic anemia. *N Engl J Med* 1989; **321**: 784–9.

161 Bhatia S, Ramsay NK, Steinbuch M *et al.* Malignant neoplasms following bone marrow transplantation. *Blood* 1996; **87**: 3633–9.

162 Kernan NA, Bartsch G, Ash RC *et al.* Analysis of 462 transplantations from unrelated donors facilitated by The National Marrow Donor Program. *N Engl J Med* 1993; **328**: 593–602.

163 Lucas KG, Small TN, Heller G, Dupont B, O'Reilly RJ. The development of cellular immunity to Epstein–Barr virus after allogeneic bone marrow transplantation. *Blood* 1996; **87**: 2594–603.

164 Papadopoulos EB, Small T, Ladanyi M *et al.* Current results of donor leukocyte infusions for treatment of Epstein–Barr virus associated lymphoproliferative disorders following related and unrelated T cell depleted bone marrow transplant. *Blood* 1996; **88**: 681a [Abstract].

165 Heslop HE, Ng CY, Li C *et al.* Long-term restoration of immunity against Epstein–Barr virus infection by adoptive transfer of gene-modified virus-specific T lymphocytes. *Nat Med* 1996; **2**: 551–5.

166 Rooney CM, Smith CA, Ng CY *et al.* Use of gene-modified virus-specific T lymphocytes to control Epstein–Barr-virus-related lymphoproliferation. *Lancet* 1995; **345**: 9–13.

167 Bonini C, Ferrari G, Verzeletti S *et al. HSV-TK* gene transfer into donor lymphocytes for control of allogeneic graft-versus-leukemia. *Science* 1997; **276**: 1719–24.

168 Shapiro RS, Chauvenet A, McGuire W *et al.* Treatment of B-cell lymphoproliferative disorders with interferon α and intravenous γ globulin [letter]. *N Engl J Med* 1988; **318**: 1334.

169 Benkerrou M, Durandy A, Fischer A. Therapy for transplant-related lymphoproliferative diseases [Review]. *Hematol Oncol Clin North Am* 1993; **7**: 467–75.

170 Fischer A, Blanche S, Le Bidois J *et al.* Anti-B-cell monoclonal antibodies in the treatment of severe B-cell lymphoproliferative syndrome following bone marrow and organ transplantation. *N Engl J Med* 1991; **324**: 1451–6.

171 Durandy A, Emilie D, Peuchmaur M *et al.* Role of IL-6 in promoting growth of human EBV-induced B-cell tumors in severe combined immunodeficient mice. *J Immunol* 1994; **152**: 5361–7.

172 Tanner JE, Menezes J. Interleukin-6 and Epstein–Barr virus induction by cyclosporine A: potential role in lymphoproliferative disease. *Blood* 1994; **84**: 3956–64.

173 Hanson MN, Morrison VA, Peterson BA *et al.* Posttransplant T-cell lymphoproliferative disorders: an aggressive, late complication of solid-organ transplantation. *Blood* 1996; **88**: 3626–33.

174 van Gorp J, Doornewaard H, Verdonck LF, Klopping C, Vos PF, van den Tweel JG. Posttransplant T-cell lymphoma. Report of three cases and a review of the literature [Review]. *Cancer* 1994; **73**: 3064–72.

175 Meignin V, Devergie A, Brice P *et al.* Hodgkin's disease of donor origin after allogeneic bone marrow transplantation for myelogenous chronic leukemia [Review]. *Transplantation* 1998; **65**: 595–7.

176 Verschuur A, Brousse N, Raynal B *et al.* Donor B cell lymphoma of the brain after allogeneic bone marrow transplantation for acute myeloid leukemia. *Bone Marrow Transplant* 1994; **14**: 467–70.

177 O'Riordan JM, Molloy K, O'Briain DS *et al.* Localized, late-onset, high-grade lymphoma following bone marrow transplantation: response to combination chemotherapy. *Br J Haematol* 1994; **86**: 183–6.

178 Schouten HC, Hopman AH, Haesevoets AM, Arends JW. Large-cell anaplastic non-Hodgkin's lymphoma originating in donor cells after allogenic bone marrow transplantation. *Br J Haematol* 1995; **91**: 162–6.

179 Rowlings PA, Curtis RE, Passweg JR *et al.* Increased incidence of Hodgkin's disease after allogeneic bone marrow transplantation. *J Clin Oncol* 1999; **17**: 3122–7.

180 Mueller NE. Hodgkin's disease. In: Schottenfeld D, Fraumeni JF, eds. *Cancer Epidemiology and Prevention*. New York: Oxford University Press, 1996: 893–919.

181 Fialkow PJ, Thomas ED, Bryant JI, Neiman PE. Leukaemic transformation of engrafted human marrow cells *in vivo. Lancet* 1971; **1**: 251–5.

182 Thomas ED, Bryant JI, Buckner CD *et al.* Leukaemic transformation of engrafted human marrow cells *in vivo. Lancet* 1972; **1**: 1310–3.

183 Boyd CN, Ramberg RE, Thomas ED. The incidence of recurrence of leukemia in donor cells after allogeneic bone marrow transplantation. *Leuk Res* 1982; **6**: 833–7.

184 Radich J. Detection of minimal residual disease in acute and chronic leukemias. *Curr Opin Hematol* 1996; **3**: 310–4.

185 Cornelius EA. Rapid viral induction of murine lymphomas in the graft-versus-host reaction. *J Exp Med* 1972; **136**: 1533–44.

186 Schwartz RS. Immunoregulation, oncogenic viruses, and malignant lymphomas. *Lancet* 1972; **1**: 1266–9.

187 Martin GM, Sprague CA. Parasexual cycle in cultivated human somatic cells. *Science* 1969; **166**: 761–3.

188 Cornelius EA. Rapid immunological induction of murine lymphomas: evidence for a viral etiology. *Science* 1972; **177**: 524–5.

189 de Klein A, van Kessel AG, Grosveld G *et al.* A cellular oncogene is translocated to the Philadelphia chromosome in chronic myelocytic leukaemia. *Nature* 1982; **300**: 765–7.

190 Deeg HJ, Witherspoon RP. Risk factors for the development of secondary malignancies after marrow transplantation. *Hematol Oncol Clin North Am* 1993; **7**: 417–29.

191 Niederwieser DW, Appelbaum FR, Gastl G *et al.* Inadvertent transmission of a donor's acute myeloid leukemia in bone marrow transplantation for chronic myelocytic leukemia. *N Engl J Med* 1990; **322**: 1794–6.

192 Mielcarek M, Bryant E, Loken M, Torok-Storb B, Storb R. Haemopoietic reconstitution by donor-derived myelodysplastic progenitor cells after haemopoietic stem cell transplantation. *Br J Haematol* 1999; **105**: 361–5.

193 Travis LB, Curtis RE, Stovall M *et al.* Risk of leukemia following treatment for non-Hodgkin's lymphoma. *J Natl Cancer Inst* 1994; **86**: 1450–7.

194 Thirman MJ, Larson RA. Therapy-related myeloid leukemia [Review]. *Hematol Oncol Clin North Am* 1996; **10**: 293–320.

195 Bennett JM. Secondary acute myeloid leukemia [Editorial]. *Leuk Res* 1995; **19**: 231–2.

196 Travis LB, Weeks J, Curtis RE *et al.* Leukemia following low-dose total body irradiation and chemotherapy for non-Hodgkin's lymphoma. *J Clin Oncol* 1996; **14**: 565–71.

197 Chao NJ, Nademanee AP, Long GD *et al.* Importance of bone marrow cytogenetic evaluation before autologous bone marrow transplantation for Hodgkin's disease. *J Clin Oncol* 1991; **9**: 1575–9.

198 Kumar L. Secondary leukaemia after autologous bone marrow transplantation. *Lancet* 1995; **345**: 810–2.

199 Rohatiner A. Myelodysplasia and acute myelogenous leukemia after myeloablative therapy with autologous stem-cell transplantation [Editorial]. *J Clin Oncol* 1994; **12**: 2521–3.

200 Stone RM. Myelodysplastic syndrome after autologous transplantation for lymphoma. The price of progress? *Blood* 1994; **83**: 3437–40.

201 Philip T, Guglielmi C, Hagenbeek A *et al*. Autologous bone marrow transplantation as compared with salvage chemotherapy in relapses of chemotherapy-sensitive non-Hodgkin's lymphoma. *N Engl J Med* 1995; **333**: 1540–5.

202 Stone RM, Neuberg D, Soiffer R *et al*. Myelodysplastic syndrome as a late complication following autologous bone marrow transplantation for non-Hodgkin's lymphoma. *J Clin Oncol* 1994; **12**: 2535–42.

203 Miller JS, Arthur DC, Litz CE, Neglia JP, Miller WJ, Weisdorf DJ. Myelodysplastic syndrome after autologous bone marrow transplantation. An additional late complication of curative cancer therapy. *Blood* 1994; **83**: 3780–6.

204 Traweek ST, Slovak ML, Nademanee AP, Brynes RK, Niland JC, Forman SJ. Myelodysplasia and acute myeloid leukemia occurring after autologous bone marrow transplantation for lymphoma [Review]. *Leuk Lymphoma* 1996; **20**: 365–72.

205 Andre M, Henry-Amar M, Blaise D *et al*. Treatment-related deaths and second cancer risk after autologous stem-cell transplantation for Hodgkin's disease. *Blood* 1998; **92**: 1933–40.

206 Darrington DL, Vose JM, Anderson JR *et al*. Incidence and characterization of secondary myelodysplastic syndrome and acute myelogenous leukemia following high-dose chemoradiotherapy and autologous stem-cell transplantation for lymphoid malignancies. *J Clin Oncol* 1994; **12**: 2527–34.

207 Mach-Pascual S, Legare RD, Lu D *et al*. Predictive value of clonality assays in patients with non-Hodgkin's lymphoma undergoing autologous bone marrow transplant: a single institution study. *Blood* 1998; **91**: 4496–503.

208 Gilliland DG, Gribben JG. Evaluation of the risk of therapy-related MDS/AML after autologous stem cell transplantation. *Biol Blood Marrow Transplant* 2002; **8**: 9–16.

209 Govindarajan R, Jagannath S, Flick JT *et al*. Preceding standard therapy is the likely cause of MDS after autotransplants for multiple myeloma. *Br J Haematol* 1996; **95**: 349–53.

210 Witherspoon RP, Deeg HJ, Storer B, Anasetti C, Storb R, Appelbaum FR. Hematopoietic stem-cell transplantation for treatment-related leukemia or myelodysplasia. *J Clin Oncol* 2001; **19**: 2134–41.

211 Kolb HJ, Duell T, Socié G *et al*. New malignancies in patients surviving more than 5 years after marrow transplantation. *Blood*, 1825; **1995**(86): 460a [Abstract].

212 Deeg HJ. Long-term complications after high-dose therapy and hematopoietic cell transplantation. In: Lorigan PC, Vandenberghe E, eds. *An Introduction to High Dose Chemotherapy*. London: Harwood Academic, 2002: 249–66.

213 Socie G, Scieux C, Gluckman E *et al*. Squamous cell carcinomas after allogeneic bone marrow transplantation for aplastic anemia: further evidence of a multistep process. *Transplantation* 1998; **66**: 667–70.

214 Thompson CB, Sanders JE, Flournoy N, Buckner CD, Thomas ED. The risks of central nervous system relapse and leukoencephalopathy in patients receiving marrow transplants for acute leukemia. *Blood* 1986; **67**: 195–9.

215 Griggs JJ, Commichau CS, Rapoport AP, Griggs RC. Chronic inflammatory demyelinating polyneuropathy in non-Hodgkin's lymphoma. *Am J Hematol* 1997; **54**: 332–4.

216 Kelly P, Staunton H, Lawler M *et al*. Multifocal remitting-relapsing cerebral demyelination twenty years following allogeneic bone marrow transplantation. *J Neuropathol Exp Neurol* 1996; **55**: 992–8.

217 Openshaw H, Slatkin NE, Parker PM, Forman SJ. Immune-mediated myelopathy after allogeneic marrow transplantation. *Bone Marrow Transplant* 1995; **15**: 633–6.

218 Unger ER, Sung JH, Manivel JC, Chenggis ML, Blazar BR, Krivit W. Male donor-derived cells in the brains of female sex-mismatched bone marrow transplant recipients; a Y-chromosome specific *in situ* hybridization study. *J Neuropathol Exp Neurol* 1993; **52**(5): 460–70.

219 Solaro C, Murialdo A, Giunti D, Mancardi G, Uccelli A. Central and peripheral nervous system complications following allogeneic bone marrow transplantation. *Eur J Neurol* 2001; **8**: 77–80.

220 Padovan CS, Bise K, Hahn J *et al*. Angiitis of the central nervous system after allogeneic bone marrow transplantation? *Stroke* 1999; **30**: 1651–6.

221 Takatsuka H, Okamoto T, Yamada S *et al*. New imaging findings in a patient with central nervous system dysfunction after bone marrow transplantation. *Acta Haematol* 2000; **103**: 203–5.

222 Amato AA, Barohn RJ, Sahenk Z, Tutschka PJ, Mendell JR. Polyneuropathy complicating bone marrow and solid organ transplantation [Review]. *Neurology* 1993; **43**: 1513–8.

223 Greenspan A, Deeg HJ, Cottler-Fox M, Sirdofski M, Spitzer TR, Kattah J. Incapacitating peripheral neuropathy as a manifestation of chronic graft-versus-host disease. *Bone Marrow Transplant* 1990; **5**: 349–52.

224 Slavin MA, Meyers JD, Remington JS, Hackman RC. *Toxoplasma gondii* infection in marrow transplant recipients: a 20-year experience. *Bone Marrow Transplant* 1994; **13**: 549–57.

225 Sullivan KM, Wade JC, Bowden RA, Reed EC. Management of the immunocompromised host. In: Schrier SL, McArthur JR, eds. *Hematology*. St Louis, MO: American Society of Hematology, 1993: 163–74.

226 Bleggi-Torres LF, de Medeiros BC, Werner B *et al*. Neuropathological findings after bone marrow transplantation: an autopsy study of 180 cases. *Bone Marrow Transplant* 2000; **25**: 301–7.

227 Sanders JE. Late effects following hematopoietic stem cell transplantation. *Turk J Haem* 1999; **16**: 103–15.

228 Chou RH, Wong GB, Kramer JH *et al*. Toxicities of total-body irradiation for pediatric bone marrow transplantation. *Int J Radiat Oncol Biol Phys* 1996; **34**: 843–51.

229 Meyers CA, Weitzner M, Byrne K, Valentine A, Champlin RE, Przepiorka D. Evaluation of the neurobehavioral functioning of patients before, during, and after bone marrow transplantation. *J Clin Oncol* 1994; **12**: 820–6.

230 Wingard JR, Curbow B, Baker F, Piantadosi S. Health, functional status, and employment of adult survivors of bone marrow transplantation. *Ann Intern Med* 1991; **114**: 113–8.

231 Bush NE, Haberman M, Donaldson G, Sullivan KM. Quality of life of 125 adults surviving 6–18 years after bone marrow transplantation. *Soc Sci Med* 1995; **40**: 479–90.

232 Wellisch DK, Centeno J, Guzman J, Belin T, Schiller GJ. Bone marrow transplantation vs. high-dose cytarabine-based consolidation chemotherapy for acute myelogenous leukemia. A long-term follow-up study of quality-of-life measures of survivors. *Psychosomatics* 1996; **37**: 144–54.

233 Molassiotis A, van den Akker OBA, Milligan DW *et al*. Quality of life in long-term survivors of marrow transplantation: comparison with a matched group receiving maintenance chemotherapy. *Bone Marrow Transplant* 1992; **17**: 249–58.

234 Syrjala KL, Dikmen S, Roth-Roemer S *et al*. Neuropsychological function after marrow or stem cell transplant: prospective longitudinal result. *Psychooncology* 1998; **7** (Suppl.): 1 [Abstract].

235 Bush NE, Donaldson GW, Haberman MH, Dacanay R, Sullivan KM. Conditional and unconditional estimation of multidimensional quality of life after hematopoietic stem cell transplantation: a longitudinal follow-up of 415 patients. *Biol Blood Marrow Transplant* 2000; **6**: 576–91.

236 Syrjala KL, Chapko MK, Vitaliano PP, Cummings C, Sullivan KM. Recovery after allogeneic marrow transplantation. Prospective study of predictors of long-term physical and psychosocial functioning. *Bone Marrow Transplant* 1993; **11**: 319–27.

237 Leigh S, Wilson KC, Burns R, Clark RE. Psychosocial morbidity in bone marrow transplant recipients: a prospective study. *Bone Marrow Transplant* 1995; **16**: 635–40.

238 Baker F, Wingard JR, Curbow B *et al*. Quality of life of bone marrow transplant long-term survivors. *Bone Marrow Transplant* 1994; **13**: 589–96.

239 Gillis TA, Donovan ES. Rehabilitation following bone marrow transplantation [Review]. *Cancer* 2001; **92**: 998–1007.

70

Smita Bhatia & Ravi Bhatia

Secondary Malignancies after Hematopoietic Cell Transplantation

During the past three decades, the number of patients undergoing hematopoietic cell transplantation (HCT) for malignant or nonmalignant disorders has increased steadily. Improvement in survival after HCT and extended follow-up of this growing population of HCT survivors has resulted in an increasing focus on issues related to long-term complications (see Chapter 69). An important and potentially devastating complication of HCT is the occurrence of secondary malignancies.

Secondary malignancies are a known complication of conventional chemotherapy and radiation treatment [1–13], and are now being increasingly recognized as a complication among HCT recipients [14–26]. The magnitude of risk of secondary malignancies after HCT has ranged from fourfold [16,21] to 11-fold [15] that of the general population. The estimated actuarial incidence is reported to be 3.5% at 10 years, increasing to 12.8% at 15 years among recipients of allogeneic HCT (Table 70.1) [16].

Risk factors associated with the development of secondary malignancies include exposure to chemotherapy and radiation prior to HCT, use of total body irradiation (TBI) and high-dose chemotherapy for myeloablation, infection with viruses such as Epstein–Barr virus (EBV) and hepatitis B and C viruses (HBV and HCV), immunodeficiency after HCT aggravated by the use of immunosuppressive drugs for prophylaxis and treatment of graft-vs.-host disease (GVHD), including monoclonal and polyclonal antibodies, human leukocyte antigen (HLA) nonidentity, T-cell depletion, type of transplant (autologous vs. allogeneic), type of hematopoietic stem cell (HSC) and the primary malignancy [15,16,18,21,23]. However, assessment of risk factors for all secondary malignancies in aggregate is somewhat artificial because of the heterogeneous nature of the secondary malignancies, with differing clinicopathologic features, distinct pathogenesis and hence very distinct risk factors associated with their development.

It has become conventional practice to classify secondary malignancies after HCT into three distinct groups [18]:
1 myelodysplasia and acute myeloid leukemia;
2 lymphoma, including other lymphoproliferative disorders; and
3 solid tumors.

Table 70.1 Risk factors for all subsequent neoplasms after hematopoietic cell transplantation.

Study [reference]	Size of cohort	Length of follow-up (median yr)	No. of SMN	Age at HCT (median yr)	Year to SMN (median)	Incidence	RR	Risk factors	Outcome (% alive)
Kolb et al. [16]*	1036	10.7	53	21	–	11.5% (15 year)	3.8	Older age at transplant Cyclosporine	81
Bhatia et al. [15][†]	2150	3.1	53	20	–	9.9% (13 year)	11.6		32
Lowsky et al. [21]*	557	–	10	17–55	5 (means)	12% (11 year)	4.2	TBI Acute GVHD (≥grade II) Chronic GVHD (for skin tumors)	30
Witherspoon et al. [18][†]	2245	–	35	–	1		6.7	Antithymocyte globulin, anti-CD3 monoclonal antibody TBI	14
Deeg et al. [23]*	700 (SAA)	–	23	18	7.6	14% (20 year)	9.1	Fanconi's anemia Azathioprine Irradiation	–

GVHD, graft-vs.-host disease; HCT, hematopoietic cell transplantation; RR, relative risk; SAA, severe aplastic anemia; SMN, secondary malignant neoplasm; TBI, total body irradiation.
*Allogeneic HCT only.
[†]Allogeneic and autologous HCT.

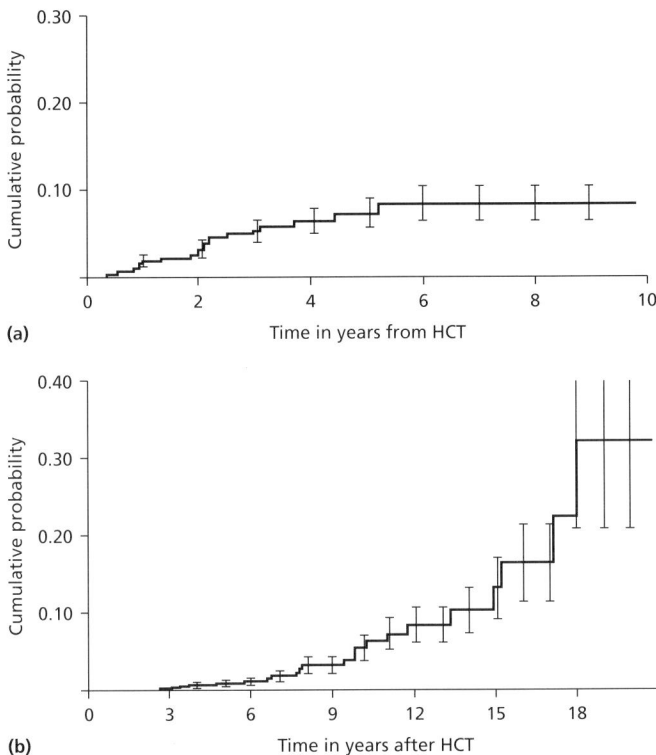

Fig. 70.1 (a) Cumulative probability of therapy-related myelodysplasia and acute myeloid leukemia (t-MDS/t-AML) in a cohort of 612 patients undergoing autologous hematopoietic cell transplantation (HCT) for Hodgkin's disease and non-Hodgkin's lymphoma. (Adapted from [27] with permission). (b) Cumulative probability of solid malignancies after HCT in 2129 patients. (Adapted from [28] with permission from the American Society of Clinical Oncology.)

Leukemias and lymphomas develop relatively early in the post-transplant period. On the other hand, solid cancers have a longer latency period and are being increasingly described because of improved survival after HCT and longer follow-up (Fig. 70.1a,b). In this chapter, we discuss the three types of secondary malignancies seen among patients undergoing HCT. The emphasis is on clinical presentation of these malignancies, the magnitude of risk and risk factors associated with their development, insights into their pathogeneses and the treatment options and outcome of patients with these malignancies.

Myelodysplasia and acute myeloid leukemia after autologous stem cell transplantation

Autologous HCT has become the treatment of choice for patients with Hodgkin's disease (HD) and non-Hodgkin's lymphoma (NHL) who have a suboptimal response to initial therapy, those with refractory or relapsed disease or for those at high risk for relapse after conventional therapy. Autologous HCT is also being increasingly used in specific clinical situations among patients with multiple myeloma, breast cancer and advanced stage germ-cell tumors. With improvement in survival following autologous HCT, therapy-related myelodysplasia (t-MDS) and therapy-related acute myeloid leukemia (t-AML) are emerging as serious long-term complications [15,27,29–37]. The cumulative probability of t-MDS/t-AML reported in the literature has ranged from 1.1% at 20 months [38] to 24.3% at 43 months after autologous HCT [39]. The median time to development of t-MDS/t-AML is 12–24 months after HCT (range 4 months to 6 years). t-MDS/t-AML has also been observed after conventional chemotherapy and to a lesser extent radiotherapy for HD and NHL

Table 70.2 Clinical presentation of therapy-related myelodysplasia and acute myeloid leukemia.

Property	Alkylating agents	Epipodophyllotoxins
Presentation	Myelodysplasia	Abrupt, no preleukemia
Cytogenetic abnormalities	Loss of genetic material, often from chromosomes 5 and 7	Balanced translocations (often include 11q23)
Age	Typically older patients	Younger patients
Outcome	Poor	Poor

[1,3–13,40–43]. The incidence of t-MDS/t-AML following conventional chemotherapy or radiation therapy ranges from 0.8% at 30 years to 6.3% at 20 years. The median time to development of t-MDS/t-AML has been reported to be 3–5 years, with the risk decreasing markedly after the first decade. It therefore appears that the magnitude of risk of t-MDS/t-AML is higher after HCT when compared with conventional chemotherapy and radiation therapy. In addition, the time to development of t-MDS/t-AML is shorter after HCT, as compared to that after conventional chemoradiotherapy. However, the difference in the magnitude of risk may, in part, be because there are fewer long-term survivors of conventional therapy who have been exposed to multiple salvage therapies.

Clinicopathologic syndromes

Two types of t-AML and t-MDS are recognized in the World Health Organization (WHO) classification (Table 70.2) depending on the causative therapy: an alkylating agent/radiation-related type and a topoisomerase II inhibitor-related type [44].

Alkylating agent/radiation-related t-MDS/t-AML

Alkylating agents kill cancer cells by transferring alkyl groups to cellular molecules. Mutagenicity is related to the ability of alkylating agents to form crosslinks and/or transfer alkyl groups to form monoadducts in DNA. The most significant site of alkylation in DNA in terms of cytotoxicity is probably the formation of a covalent bond between the drug and the N^7 group of guanine in DNA, although the O^6-alkylguanine position is also favored. Alkylation results in inaccurate base pairing during replication and single and double strand breaks in the double helix as the alkylated bases are repaired. Expressed mutations involve different base substitutions, including all kinds of transitions and transversions [45–47].

Alkylating agent-related t-MDS/t-AML usually appears 4–7 years after exposure to the mutagenic agent. Approximately two-thirds of patients present with MDS and the remainder with AML with myelodysplastic features [48–50]. Patients frequently present with cytopenias, often pancytopenia. Multilineage dysplasia is often present. There is a high frequency of the multidrug-resistance phenotype. In addition, there is a high incidence of abnormalities involving chromosomes 5 (-5/del[5q]) and 7 (-7/del[7q]).

Topoisomerase II inhibitor-related AML

DNA topoisomerase II catalyzes the relaxation of supercoiled DNA by covalently binding and transiently cleaving and re-ligating both strands of the DNA helix. DNA topoisomerase II inhibitors stabilize the enzyme–DNA covalent intermediate, decrease the religation rate and cause chromosomal breakage. These events initiate apoptosis, required for antineoplastic activity [51,52]. On the other hand, repair of chromosomal damage results in chromosomal translocations, leading to leukemogenesis [51,53–56]. Most of the translocations disrupt a breakpoint cluster region between exons 5 and 11 of the band 11q23 and fuse mixed lineage leukemia (*MLL*) with a partner gene [57–61]. A comprehensive study of chromosomal abnormalities among patients with therapy-related leukemia indicates that translocations to 11q23 predominate following therapy with epipodophyllotoxins, whereas patients with translocations to 21q22, inv(16), t(15,17), and t(9,22) most often occur following therapies with anthracyclines [62].

In contrast to alkylating agent-related t-MDS/t-AML, AML secondary to topoisomerase II inhibitors often does not have a preceding myelodysplastic phase, and presents as overt acute leukemia, often with a prominent monocytic component [63,64]. The latency period between the initiation of treatment with topoisomerase II inhibitors and the onset of leukemia is brief, ranging from 6 months to 5 years, with a median of 2–3 years [64]. Most often, this type of t-AML is associated with balanced translocations involving chromosome bands 11q23 or 21q22 [64]. Other translocations including inv(18)(p13q22) or t(17,19)(q22;q12) have been reported [63,65].

When used in combination with the DNA topoisomerase II inhibitor doxorubicin, cisplatin may be associated with acute leukemias with t(8,21), typically observed in DNA topoisomerase II inhibitor-related cases [66]. Cisplatin forms N^7-alkyl intrastrand adducts on adjacent deoxyguanosines or deoxyguanosine and deoxyadenosine, monoadducts and interstrand crosslinks [67].

Clinical diagnosis

Cytopenias and dysplastic changes on marrow examination can often be seen in isolation in many patients after autologous HCT, many of whom may not subsequently develop t-MDS/t-AML. Therefore, the Dana-Farber Cancer Institute group has proposed [68] that the diagnosis of t-MDS/t-AML after HCT be based on the presence of:
1 significant marrow dysplasia in at least two cell lines;
2 peripheral cytopenias without alternative explanations; and
3 blast counts in marrow defined by French–American–British (FAB) classification.

However, many patients may not have an increase in blasts. The presence of a clonal cytogenetic abnormality in addition to morphologic criteria of dysplasia may aid in making this diagnosis in these cases.

Risk factors for t-MDS/t-AML after HCT

Factors associated with an increased risk of t-MDS/t-AML include host factors (older age at HCT) [15,34], pretransplantation therapy with alkylating agents, topoisomerase II inhibitors and radiation therapy [27,33,37,39,68–70], method of stem cell mobilization (use of peripheral blood hematopoietic cells, priming with etoposide for hematopoietic cell mobilization) [15,27,32] and transplantation conditioning with TBI (Table 70.3) [33,69]. Some other factors reported recently include a lower number of CD34+ cells infused at HCT [71] and a history of multiple transplants [69]. Therefore, t-MDS/t-AML appears to be related to pretransplant chemotherapy and radiotherapy, transplant-related factors such as the stem cell priming and transplant conditioning regimens or the cumulative effect of all these exposures.

The significant impact of primary chemotherapy and radiotherapy on the risk of t-MDS and t-AML after HCT [27,29,36,37,39,68,70,72] points toward an origin of events prior to HCT. Moreover, the nature of the pretransplant cytotoxic exposure (alkylating agent vs. topoisomerase II inhibitor) has a significant impact on the type of t-MDS/t-AML that evolves post-transplant, reinforcing this observation. A role for pretransplant exposures is further supported by the observation that specific cytogenetic abnormalities observed post-transplantation have also been observed in the pretransplant marrow or peripheral blood graft among patients who develop t-MDS/t-AML after HCT [73,74]. Abruzzese et al. [74] reported that nine of 12 cases of t-MDS/t-AML studied demonstrated abnormal cells in pretransplant bone marrow samples using fluorescence in situ hybridization (FISH). Lillington et al. [73] reported that significant levels of clonally abnormal cells could be detected in samples obtained prior to high-dose therapy in 20 of 20 patients with t-MDS/t-AML using single-locus specific FISH probes to detect loss of chromosomal material from 5q31, 7q22 and 13q14. In comparison, only three of 24 patients who had not developed t-MDS/t-AML had abnormal clones in pretreatment samples. These studies support a role for genetic abnormalities induced by prior cytotoxic chemotherapy in the etiology of t-MDS/t-AML. However, prospective studies of larger groups of patients are warranted to determine the significance of these observations.

The use of TBI in the conditioning regimen has been reported to be associated with an increased risk of t-MDS/t-AML after autologous HCT [69], although other studies fail to confirm this association [27,68]. A recent report suggests that transplant conditioning regimens that included TBI at doses ≤12 Gy did not appear to elevate leukemia risk compared with non-TBI regimens; whereas a statistically significant increased risk was found for TBI doses of 13.2 Gy [75]. An association of TBI with increased risk for t-MDS/t-AML raises the possibility that the disease may arise from residual stem cells that persist in the patient despite myeloablative treatment, rather than from reinfused stem cells, although it is also possible that TBI-induced alteration in the hematopoietic microenvironment may contribute to the development of t-MDS/t-AML. Therefore, it is unclear whether t-MDS/t-AML arises from the graft, from residual cells in the patient or as a result of a damaged microenvironment.

A higher risk of t-MDS/t-AML has been demonstrated among recipients of CD34-enriched cells isolated from peripheral blood after chemotherapy priming and growth factors, as compared to autologous transplantation using CD34+ cells from the bone marrow without pretreatment [15,27,32]. Potential explanations offered for this observation include harvesting of hematopoietic precursor cells damaged by chemotherapy at a time before they have completed DNA repair or an over-representation of damaged cells in the mobilized product [76]. Supporting this hypothesis is the study by Krishnan et al. [27] demonstrating an increased risk of t-AML with 11q23 abnormalities among patients with HD and NHL mobilized with high doses of etoposide for collection of stem cells prior to autologous HCT.

Friedberg et al. [71] reported an increased risk of t-MDS among patients who received a significantly smaller number of cells reinfused per kilogram of body weight. In the setting of low stem cell numbers, reconstitution of bone marrow clearly may result in a great proliferative stress, which may increase susceptibility to irreversible DNA damage associated with t-MDS. These findings are consistent with in vitro data suggesting an increased proliferative stress placed upon committed progenitors at the expense of the primitive progenitors, as shown later in the chapter [77]. Alternatively, reduced ability to harvest cells could indicate an existing defect in marrow function.

It therefore seems that in addition to the important role of pretransplant exposure to cytotoxic agents, the transplant process itself may also potentiate the risk of t-MDS/t-AML through several mechanisms, including stem cell mobilization, collection and storage, chemotherapy and radiation used for myeloablation, and the stress on hematopoietic precursors of engraftment and hematopoietic regeneration [76–78].

Pathogenesis of t-MDS/t-AML

t-MDS/t-AML are clonal hematologic disorders that are the consequence of an acquired somatic mutation induced by cytotoxic therapy in hematopoietic stem cells which confers a proliferative and/or survival advantage. Improved understanding of the molecular pathogenesis of t-MDS/t-AML may allow development of strategies to identify populations at risk and modify therapies in order to decrease the morbidity and

Table 70.3 Risk factors for therapy-related myelodysplasia/acute myeloid leukemia after autologous hematopoietic cell transplantation.

Study	Size of cohort	Primary Diagnosis	No. of SMN	Year to SMN (median)	Incidence	Risk factors	Outcome (% alive)
Krishnan et al. [27]	612	HD, NHL	22	1.9 year	8.6% (6 year)	VP-16 (Stem cell priming) Peripheral blood stem cell transplant Pre-transplant radiation	32%
Traweek et al. [30]	275	HD, NHL	10	1.4 year	6.4% (2 year)	None described	60%
Stone et al. [29]	262	NHL	20	2.6 year	18% (6 year)	Number of chemotherapy regimens Previous radiation Age >38 year Low platelet counts Prolonged interval between diagnosis, transplant	—
Miller et al. [32]	206	HD, NHL	9	2.8 year	14.5% (5 year)	Peripheral blood stem cell transplant	20%
Darrington et al. [33]	511	HD, NHL	12	3.7 year	4% (5 year)	Age at transplant (>40 year) TBI	—
Bhatia et al. [15]	258	HD, NHL	10	3.0 year	13.5% (6 year)	Peripheral blood stem cell transplant Age >35 year at transplant	20%
Friedberg et al. [71]	552	NHL	41		19.8% (10 year)	Fewer no. of cells infused	17%
Wheeler et al. [70]	300	HD, NHL	6	—	4.2% (5 year)	Prior relapses Prior radiotherapy	—
Andre et al. [34]	467	HD	8		4.3% (5 year)	Splenectomy Peripheral blood stem cell transplant	13%
Harrison et al. [72]	595	HD	8		3.1% (5 year)	Quantity of prior therapy MOPP Lomustine Age at transplantation	—
Milligan et al. [69]	4998	HD, NHL	66		4.6% at 5 year (HD) 3.0% at 5 year for NHL	Age at transplantation TBI Number of transplants Years from diagnosis to transplantation	—

HD, Hodgkin disease; MOPP, mecloethamine, vincristine, procarbazine, prednisone; NHL, non-Hodgkin lymphoma; TBI, total body irradiation; VP-16, etoposide.

mortality associated with this complication. Furthermore, t-MDS/t-AML offers a unique perspective on mutagen-induced carcinogenesis and the role of genetic susceptibility to cancer in humans.

t-MDS/t-AML after autologous HCT appears to result from genetic damage to the stem cell from pretransplant cytotoxic treatment, which may be potentiated by the transplant process itself through several mechanisms, including hematopoietic cell mobilization, collection and storage, chemotherapy and radiation used for myeloablation, and the stress of engraftment and hematopoietic regeneration on the hematopoietic precursors. A hypothetical schema for the sequence of events leading to the development of t-MDS/t-AML after autologous HCT is shown in Fig. 70.2.

Genetic lesions associated with t-MDS/t-AML

Loss of chromosome 5 or del(5q) and loss of chromosome 7 and del(7q) are recurring abnormalities in t-MDS/t-AML. These abnormalities are also seen in AML evolving from MDS and *de novo* AML in elderly subjects. This has led to a search for candidate tumor suppressor genes in these regions. Several groups have attempted to identify commonly deleted segments and to derive transcript maps of these segments [79,80]. The majority of patients with 5q deletions exhibit losses at the 5q31

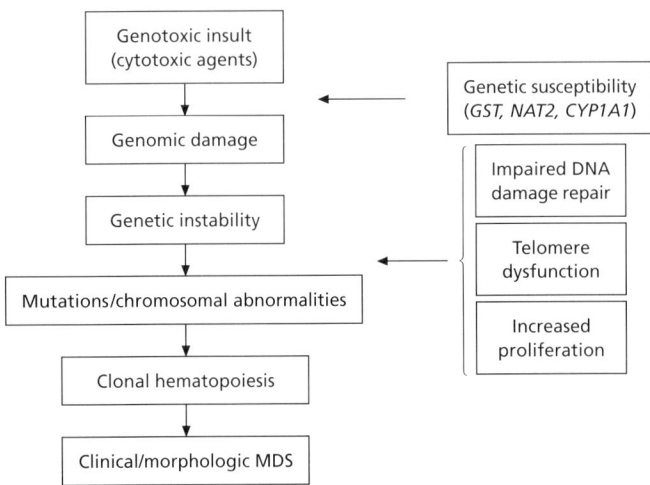

Fig. 70.2 Proposed pathogenesis of t-MDS/t-AML after autologous HCT.

locus, with deletions in 5q33 being seen in some patients. Chromosomal segment 7q22 is a common site of chromosome 7 deletions. Such studies may assist in cloning of a putative myeloid tumor suppressor gene thought to be located in this region. Although several known and unknown genes have been identified in these regions, including a number of key genes that regulate hematopoietic cell growth and differentiation, identification of a commonly deleted tumor suppressor gene has been elusive thus far. However, it has been hypothesized that haploinsufficiency and reduced gene dosage for critical genes involved in hematopoiesis may sufficiently alter the balance between growth and differentiation to induce dysplastic hematopoiesis [81]. Chromosomal engineering technologies are being used to induce these segmental deletions in mouse models. This approach may be combined with retrovirus-mediated insertional mutagenesis to generate new models and aid in gene discovery [82].

Another possibility is that these chromosomal abnormalities may be secondary events important for disease progression rather than initiation. Alternatively, these chromosomal abnormalities may be simply a manifestation of this disorder, but may not play a significant pathogenetic part. Abnormalities in chromosome 7 are also associated with myeloid leukemias in genetically predisposed individuals, such as Fanconi's anemia or neurofibromatosis type 1 [83,84]. This observation raises the possibility that similar predisposition may be present in patients with t-MDS/t-AML with loss of chromosome 7. 5q and 7q deletions in familial platelet disorder with leukemia are associated with mutations or deletions of a single *AML1* allele [85]. Balanced translocations involving the *AML1* gene have also been associated with t-MDS/t-AML in patients exposed to topoisomerase II inhibitors [86,87]. Transgenic expression of *AML1-ETO* leads to immortalization of murine myeloid progenitors but not overt leukemia; additional mutations are required for leukemogenesis [88,89]. Therefore, altered *AML1* function may have a major role in dysregulation of hematopoietic growth and genomic instability and predispose to leukemia through a multistep process. The *MLL* gene located at chromosome band 11q23, which is frequently involved in translocations associated with topoisomerase II inhibitors, has a major role in developmental regulation [90]. Altered *MLL* function, as with *AML1*, may dysregulate hematopoietic growth and genomic instability and predispose to leukemia through a multistep process. The long latency period to onset of leukemia in the knock-in mouse suggests that additional genetic changes are required for evolution of t-AML [91]. The role of *MLL* and *AML1* mutations as early events in the development of t-MDS/t-AML merits further investigation.

Genetic susceptibility: polymorphisms in drug-metabolizing enzymes

Underlying genetic characteristics interacting with treatment might be associated with an increased risk of therapy-related leukemia. An example of such an interaction is the presence of a polymorphism in a drug-metabolizing enzyme such as thiopurine *S*-methyltransferase (TPMT). TPMT catalyzes the *S*-methylation of thiopurines, including 6-mercaptopurine and 6-tioguanine. TPMT activity exhibits genetic polymorphism, with about 1/300 individuals inheriting TPMT deficiency as an autosomal recessive trait. There is emerging evidence that TPMT genotype might influence the risk of AML [92]. Several other genetic polymorphisms of enzymes capable of metabolic activation or detoxification of anticancer drugs, such as NAD(P)H:quinone oxidoreductase (NQO1), glutathione-*S*-transferase (GST) -M1, -T1 and -P1, and CYP3A4, have been examined for their role in the development of therapy-related leukemia or myelodysplasia [93–101]. An NQO1 polymorphism has been shown to be significantly associated with the genetic risk of t-MDS/t-AML [98]. Recently, Allan *et al.* [96] reported data suggesting that inheritance of at least one *Val* allele at GSTP1 codon 105 confers a significantly increased risk of developing t-AML after chemotherapy, but not after radiotherapy. In addition, individuals with CYP3A4-W genotype may be at increased risk of treatment-related leukemia, by increasing the production of reactive intermediates that might damage DNA [94]. Although all these studies report patients treated with conventional chemotherapy and radiation therapy, the gene–environment interactions could potentially be applicable to patients undergoing HCT, and therefore merit further exploration.

Genetic instability

Genetic instability is hypothesized to be an early event in the development of malignancy, allowing accumulation of multiple mutations in the same cell over time and evolution of a clonal malignant population. T cells from patients who have received chemotherapy for acute lymphoblastic leukemia demonstrate increased frequency of mutations in the hypoxanthine-guanine phosphoribosyltransferase (*HPRT*) reporter gene [102,103]. Further characterization of *HPRT* mutant isolates indicated that multiple mutations were present in individually isolated mutant T-cell clones from four of 15 individuals with high frequency of *HPRT* mutations, consistent with genetic instability [103]. Therefore treatment with cytotoxic agents can lead to genetic instability in some individuals, which could contribute to the induction of t-MDS/t-AML. The mechanism underlying genetic instability could be related to altered expression or function of cell cycle, apoptosis or DNA repair regulatory genes.

Defective DNA repair mechanisms

DNA repair mechanisms have a major role in maintaining genomic integrity. The major repair pathways include mismatch repair, base excision repair, nucleotide excision repair and DNA double strand break repair [104]. Defects in repair proteins and proteins associated with the regulation of repair are connected to many different types of cancer, including therapy-related leukemia. In 1996, Ben-Yehuda *et al.* [105] showed a 94% incidence of microsatellite instability (MSI) in t-MDS/t-AML, suggesting that patients with therapy-related leukemia may have an inherited defect of a DNA mismatch repair gene leading to accelerated DNA instability in other oncogenes or tumor suppressor genes occurring as a consequence of treatment for a primary malignancy. In another study, Sheikhha *et al.* [106] reported MSI in eight of 17 patients with t-AML studied. However, an analysis of 132 patients with AML, including 62 patients with t-AML, failed to demonstrate MSI in a single case [107]. Therefore, although MSI and defective DNA mismatch repair are seen in some patients, they do not appear to be a common feature among patients with t-MDS/t-AML.

p53 gene mutations

The p53 gene has a critical role in DNA damage response signaling, affecting cell cycle, cell death and DNA repair pathways. Abnormal p53 activity could lead to reduced ability to repair DNA damage, resulting in genomic instability and increased susceptibility to leukemogenesis. In patients with *de novo* MDS and AML, p53 mutations are seen in <10% of patients. However, p53 mutations may be more common in patients with t-MDS/t-AML. Ben-Yehuda *et al.* [105] evaluated 21 patients with t-MDS/t-AML for p53 mutations using polymerase chain reaction (PCR) and single strand conformation polymorphism (SSCP) analysis and identified mutations in 38% of patients. Mutations were nongermline and restricted to leukemic cells, and differed from p53 mutations seen in the original tumors of individual patients. Horiike *et al.* [108] identified p53 mutations in six of 12 patients with t-MDS chromosome 5 and/or 7 losses, but did not observe any p53 mutations in nine other patients without chromosome 5 and/or 7 involvement. Christiansen *et al.* [109] observed mutations in p53 in 21 of 77 patients (27%) with t-MDS or t-AML, 19 of whom had received alkylating agents. Fifteen patients demonstrated loss of heteozygosity [85] of p53. p53 mutations were associated with deletion or loss of 5q and a complex karyotype, were more common in elderly patients and were associated with an extremely poor prognosis [109]. These studies indicate that p53 mutations may be observed in certain cytogenetic and prognostic subsets of patients with t-MDS/t-AML, but do not identify a clear role for p53 mutations in the pathogenesis of this disorder.

Telomeric shortening

Telomeres are noncoding regions of DNA that provide a cap at the ends of chromosomes and prevent dicentric fusion and other chromosomal aberrations [110]. Each somatic cell division is associated with a loss of telomere length. Cumulative telomere shortening can impose a limit on cell divisions and lead to cell senescence. Telomere shortening is also associated with genetic instability [111]. In hematopoietic tissues, there is progressive shortening of telomere length through life, with considerable variability between age-matched individuals [112]. Following HCT, the increased replicative demand on stem cells associated with hematopoietic regeneration can lead to accelerated telomere shortening. Several studies have shown that telomere length of cells in the marrow of recipients of allogeneic transplantation is considerably shorter than the telomere length of cells from the donor [113–116]. Most of this decrease occurs in the first year after transplantation [117]. The extent of telomere shortening correlates with the number of cells transplanted. In most studies, the degree of shortening did not reach levels that would compromise marrow function, although two cases were recently described in which telomere shortening may have contributed to late graft failure after allogeneic HCT [118]. However, in autologous HCT this could be an important issue, especially when telomere length in the transplanted cells is already short because of prior chemotherapy [119], older age at HCT, increased replicative stress on the stem cells because of a small number of cells transplanted or other unknown causes.

Hematopoietic abnormalities

Autologous HCT for lymphoma and HD has been reported to be associated with hematopoietic abnormalities including marked and possibly permanent reduction in primitive progenitor long-term culture initiating cells (LTC-IC) and committed progenitor colony-forming cell (CFC) numbers, altered progenitor expansion potential and microenvironmental defects [120–126]. These abnormalities may be related in part to damage to hematopoietic cells from pretransplant chemotherapy because hematopoietic defects can also be seen in pretransplant samples [123,125–127]. Although committed progenitors recover to pretransplant levels, primitive progenitor capacity is further depleted and does not show evidence of recovery for up to 2 years after HCT, consistent with extensive proliferation and differentiation of the committed progenitors and subsequent depletion of primitive progenitors during hematopoietic regeneration post-HCT [126]. A recent study has shown that CD34$^+$ cells in the graft from lymphoma patients also show reduced migration compared to normal CD34$^+$ cells. *In vitro* migratory capacity of CD34$^+$ cells in the graft correlated with the speed of hematopoietic recovery after transplantation [128]. Therefore, pretransplant chemotherapy may also lead to reduced engraftment potential of primitive progenitor cells. This observation is consistent with experimental data showing that exposure to chemotherapeutic agents results in long-lasting damage to repopulating ability of HSC as measured in competitive repopulating unit (CRU) assays in mice [129]. Autologous or allogeneic HCT may also be associated with defects in the marrow hematopoietic microenvironment, including reduction in stromal precursor growth and reduced capacity to support growth of myeloid progenitors and B progenitors [124,127,130,131]. These microenvironmental defects may contribute to hematopoietic abnormalities post-transplantation.

Marked and prolonged reduction in primitive progenitors is also seen after allogeneic HCT [132]. Extensive proliferation of stem cells bearing genotoxic damage post-transplant may have a role in establishment and amplification of an abnormal clone. Alternatively, the numerous replication cycles imposed on HSCs after HCT may result in excessive shortening of telomeres in descendent cells (as discussed above). Telomeric shortening may be associated with genomic instability and chromosomal abnormalities and could contribute to the pathogenesis of t-MDS/t-AML [111].

Gene expression profiling

Yeoh *et al.* [133] reported that the gene expression profile of acute lymphoblastic leukemia cells at diagnosis was predictive of therapeutic outcomes including the risk of development of t-MDS/t-AML. Qian *et al.* [134] performed gene expression profiling of CD34$^+$ hematopoietic progenitor cells from t-AML patients. This analysis identified different subtypes of t-AML with characteristic gene expression patterns. Common to each subgroup were gene expression patterns characteristic of arrested differentiation in early progenitor cells. Extension of such studies may enhance our understanding of the molecular pathways involved in t-AML.

Outcome of patients with t-MDS/t-AML after autologous HCT

The prognosis of t-MDS after autologous HCT is uniformly poor, with a median survival of 6 months. Because of the poor response to conventional chemotherapy, allogeneic HCT has been attempted with an actuarial survival ranging from 0% to 24% at 3 years [71,135–138]. Friedberg *et al.* [71] reported outcome of 41 patients who developed MDS after HCT for NHL. Twenty-nine of 33 evaluable patients had del(7) or complex chromosomal abnormalities. The median survival from diagnosis of MDS was 9.4 months. Thirteen patients underwent allogeneic HCT as treatment for MDS, and all died of bone marrow transplantation (BMT)-related complications (11 patients) or relapse (two patients), with a median survival of only 1.8 months.

Some lessons may be derived from reviewing the results of treatment of t-MDS/t-AML that develops in a nonautologous HCT setting. The response to chemotherapy of t-MDS/t-AML is lower than that seen in *de novo* leukemia, with an average complete remission (CR) rate between 35% and 40%, and the overall long-term survival is poor (reviewed in [139]), although a subgroup of patients with favorable cytogenetics appear to have better outcomes [140]. As a result, allogeneic transplantation has been evaluated as a therapeutic modality for t-MDS/t-AML. Witherspoon *et al.* [141] reviewed data from patients transplanted for t-MDS/t-AML developing in a nonautologous HCT setting, with the aim of identifying patient characteristics that are associated with a better long-term disease-free survival after an allogeneic transplant. The probability of survival after transplantation for all patients was 13%, and by stage of disease was 33% for refractory anemia, 20% for refractory anemia with excess blasts, and 8% for refractory anemia with excess blasts in transformation or acute leukemia. The overall probability of non-relapse mortality was 78%, divided equally among infection or organ failure-related cause of death [135]. In a subsequent report, results of related or unrelated HCT in 111 patients with treatment-related leukemia or myelodysplasia performed consecutively at the Fred Hutchinson Cancer Research Center between December 1971 and June 1998 were reviewed, and the results of different conditioning regimens analyzed. The 5-year disease-free survival was 8% for TBI, 19% for busulphan and cyclophosphamide (BU/CY) and 30% for BU/CY-t (targeted dose BU/CY) conditioning regimens. The 5-year cumulative incidence of relapse was 40% for secondary AML, 40% for refractory anemia with excess blasts in transformation (RAEB-T), 26% for refractory anemia with excess blasts (RAEB) and 0% for refractory anemia or refractory anemia with ringed sideroblasts (RARS). The 5-year cumulative incidence of nonrelapse mortality after TBI was 58%, after BU/CY 52%, and after BU/CY-t 42% [141]. Yakoub-Agha et al. [136] analyzed the predictors of survival, relapse and treatment-related mortality among 70 patients with t-MDS/t-AML undergoing allogeneic HCT. Older age (>37 years), male sex, positive recipient cytomegalovirus (CMV) serology, absence of CR at HCT and intensive conditioning schedules were independently associated with poor outcome. These studies indicate that in spite of the significant treatment-related mortality, the disease-free survival was better when transplantation was performed earlier in the evolution of disease because it resulted in a lower relapse rate.

Anderson et al. [138] described the results of allogeneic HCT as initial treatment for 46 patients with secondary AML, which included 17 t-AML patients who had not received remission induction chemotherapy. Five-year actuarial disease-free survival was 24.4%, and the cumulative incidences of relapse and nonrelapse mortality were 31.3% and 44.3%, respectively. Lower peripheral blood blast count was associated with a lower risk of relapse and shorter time from AML diagnosis to HCT was associated with a lower risk of nonrelapse mortality and improved disease-free survival. Patients with t-AML tended to have lower disease-free survival (8.3%) and a higher relapse rate (43%) than patients whose leukemia was not therapy-related. There was no statistically significant difference in outcome in the results of these previously untreated patients compared to 20 patients (12 therapy-related, eight myelodysplasia-related) transplanted with chemosensitive disease after induction chemotherapy [136,138,141].

These analyses of the results of allogeneic transplantation for t-MDS/t-AML developing after conventional therapy may have implications for treatment of t-MDS/t-AML developing after HCT. For t-MDS/t-AML developing after HCT, an additional consideration is the very high rate of nonrelapse mortality associated with allogeneic HCT performed after an initial autologous HCT, especially in adult patients [142]. Treatment of t-MDS/t-AML should include consideration of likelihood of success of achieving induction of remission with chemotherapy and, depending on the availability of an appropriate donor, the likelihood of a successful outcome with an allogeneic transplant approach. The few patients with favorable cytogenetics may have a better chance of remission induction with chemotherapy. However, patients with unfavorable cytogenetics without a high peripheral blast count may be considered for immediate transplant [138]. It is important to follow patients at risk for development of t-MDS closely to identify the early development of myelodysplasia. Prompt transplantation should be considered after diagnosis of secondary AML or, if possible, high-risk myelodysplasia, particularly in patients with low peripheral blast counts. Innovative transplant strategies are needed to reduce the high risks of relapse and nonrelapse mortality seen in this patient population. Because the poor outcomes of allogeneic transplant for t-MDS/t-AML are related in part to the high risk of treatment-related mortality, it will be of interest to evaluate the role of reduced intensity conditioning approaches in this setting. Preliminary reports suggest that allogeneic HCT using reduced-intensity conditioning is feasible and may result in improved outcomes in patients who have failed a previous autologous HCT compared to conventional allogeneic HCT [143,144].

Prediction of risk of t-MDS/t-AML

Because of the poor prognosis associated with t-MDS/t-AML, attempts are being made to identify predictors or early biomarkers to decrease the morbidity associated with this disease. Several studies have attempted to correlate identification of genetically abnormal clones with subsequent risk of development of t-MDS/t-AML and are discussed below. Assessment of risk of t-MDS/t-AML after autologous HCT is complicated by the lack of a single underlying genetic abnormality. The development of MDS or AML appears to require the acquisition of more than one mutation. Moreover, t-MDS/t-AML is a heterogeneous disorder with multiple subtypes characterized by different genetic abnormalities. Therefore, the identification of a single genetic abnormality may not necessarily have predictive value for development of t-MDS/t-AML.

Standard cytogenetics and FISH

Abnormal clones are frequently detected on cytogenetic analysis after autologous HCT for lymphoma. Traweek et al. [30] reported the risk of developing a clonal cytogenetic abnormality typical of MDS to be 9% at 3 years. Five of 10 patients with the abnormal clone developed t-MDS. Stone et al. [29] reported that 50% of sporadically tested post-transplant patients who were hematologically normal had clonal cytogenetic abnormalities. However, <30% of these patients developed t-MDS [68]. Evaluation by FISH may enhance sensitivity of detection of chromosomal abnormalities. Significant levels of clonally abnormal cells could be detected by FISH prior to high-dose therapy in samples obtained from 20 of 20 patients who developed t-MDS/t-AML but only three of 24 patients who had not developed t-MDS/t-AML [73]. However, this technique is locus-specific and requires prior selection of markers for analysis. The predictive value of clonal cytogenetic abnormalities for subsequent development of t-MDS/t-AML requires to be systematically studied in a prospective fashion.

Clonality analysis

The predictive value of clonal bone marrow hematopoiesis for the development of t-MDS/t-AML was investigated in a group of patients undergoing autologous HCT for NHL at the Dana-Farber Cancer Institute. An X-inactivation based clonality assay at the human androgen receptor locus (HUMARA) was used. A total of 104 female patients were evaluated. At the time of HCT, the prevalence of skewed X-inactivation pattern (XIP) was 20% and of clonal hematopoiesis was 3%. Of the 78 patients followed for at least 18 months, 53 continue to demonstrate polyclonal hematopoiesis, 15 developed skewed XIP and 10 either had clonal hematopoiesis at the time of transplant or developed clonal hematopoiesis after BMT. t-MDS/t-AML developed in two of 53 patients with polyclonal hematopoiesis, and four of 10 with clonal hematopoiesis. Clonal hematopoiesis at the time of transplant or after transplant was predictive of the development of t-MDS/t-AML [145]. Five of seven patients with clonal hematopoiesis also had a clonal cytogenetic abnormality involving 50% or more metaphases. This assay is limited by its low sensitivity, requiring a high proportion of monoclonal cells to be present prior to reaching the threshold for detection, and is applicable only to female patients. However, if proven to predict t-MDS/t-AML in prospective studies, it could potentially be a useful method to detect patients at risk for this complication.

Loss of heterozygosity analysis and PCR assays for point mutations

Other tests that may be useful for detection of evolution of clonal genetic abnormality after HCT are loss of heterozygosity (LOH) analysis and PCR assays for point mutations [85]. In LOH analysis, loss of one allele at a particular locus is evaluated, most commonly by PCR analysis. This method is specific and can be adapted to high-throughput strategies, but is relatively insensitive and requires prior selection of loci. This method has not been validated as being a useful predictor of t-MDS/t-AML.

PCR for point mutations and chromosomal translocations is another potentially useful tool. Mutations in genes such as *MLL* or *AML1* or gene rearrangements involving 11q23 gene may be useful markers for risk of subsequent t-MDS/t-AML. This method is highly sensitive, but is locus-specific, and the specificity and predictive value of such assays is unknown at present. This test may be most helpful if performed using quantitative techniques that would allow assessment of increasing levels of abnormality [68].

Reducing risk of t-MDS/t-AML after autologous HCT

It is possible to consider potential strategies to reduce the risk of t-MDS/t-AML, based on our understanding of the risk factors and pathogenesis of t-MDS/t-AML. Such strategies may include minimizing pretransplant cytotoxic exposure, possibly by bringing high-risk patients to HCT earlier in the course of disease, prior to exposure to multiple treatment regimens. Alteration in autologous hematopoietic cell procurement regimens and the conditioning regimens could be considered to eliminate factors associated with increased risk of this complication. If strategies to develop predictors for patients at high risk prior to HCT are realized, alternative treatment approaches such as allogeneic transplantation or nontransplant modalities may be worth considering for patients identified to be at increased risk of this complication. Finally, strategies for chemoprevention may be worth exploring in this population.

Acute leukemia after allogeneic HCT

t-MDS/t-AML seen typically after autologous HCT has occurred extremely infrequently after allogeneic HCT, with only four cases observed in 4749 patients [reviewed in [146]].

Donor-derived acute leukemia has been reported in rare patients receiving allogeneic HCT for AML, acute lymphoblastic leukemia or chronic myelogenous leukemia [14,22]. Conditioning regimens in these patients had consisted of chemotherapy alone or chemotherapy combined with TBI. The diagnosis of recurrent leukemia in donor cells was made 6 months to 3 years after HCT. It has been suggested that these leukemias are the result of transfection of a dominant oncogene from the DNA of degenerating host leukemic cells to developing donor cells, in which the oncogene is later expressed as leukemia. Another hypothesis is that a transmissible agent or environmental factor might first transform the host cells, persist and later also transform the donor cells [25]. Recent studies using variable number tandem repeat analysis to determine the origin (host vs. donor) of normal or abnormal cells in patients post-HCT indicate that disease reappearance in donor-derived cells is infrequent [147].

Lymphomas

Post-transplantation lymphoproliferative disorder

Lymphoproliferative disorders are the most common secondary malignancy in the first year after allogeneic T-cell depleted HCT. Most of these cases are related to compromised immune function and EBV infection. The large majority of the post-transplantation lymphoproliferative disorders (PTLDs) have a B-cell origin, although some T-cell PTLD has been described.

B-cell post-transplant lymphoproliferative disorder

B-cell PTLD was first described among patients receiving solid organ transplants [148]. B-cell PTLD is a clinically and morphologically heterogeneous group of diseases. B-cell PTLD usually develops within the first 6 months after HCT, with most of the events occurring within the first 3 months. The cumulative incidence of PTLD has been reported to range from 1.0% to 2.0% at 10 years [2,18,149,150]. The incidence is highest in the first 5 months after HCT (120 cases/10,000/year), with a steep decline thereafter to <5 cases/10,000/year among HCT recipients surviving 1 year or longer.

Risk factors for B-cell PTLD

Risk factors found to be independently associated with an increased risk for the development of PTLD include *in vitro* T-cell depletion of the donor marrow, unrelated or HLA-mismatched related donor, use of antithymocyte globulin or anti-CD3 monoclonal antibody for acute GVHD prophylaxis or in the preparative regimen, TBI and primary immunodeficiency (Table 70.4) [2,24]. Patients transplanted for congenital immunodeficiency are at a particularly high risk for PTLD, because of both the underlying immunodeficiency and the use of T-cell depletion of the donor graft [2,18,149,152]. Moreover, the risk of PTLD also depends on the method of T-cell depletion, being considerably higher where specific monoclonal antibodies are used for T-cell depletion (11–25%) rather than in patients where techniques removing both T and B lymphocytes, such as soybean agglutinin or Campath-1 (<1%), are used [149,152]. However, the incidence of PTLD is higher in the latter group (6–18%) after exposure to immunosuppressive therapy such as steroids or antithymocyte globulins. The more recent use of nonmyeloablative therapy coupled with highly immunosuppressive therapy needs close observation for the development of PTLD [153].

Pathogenesis of B-cell PTLD

B-cell PTLD is commonly associated with T-cell dysfunction, occurs in the presence of EBV infection and is thought to develop because of a combination of depressed EBV-specific cellular immunity and the inherent transforming capacities of EBV. EBV is a ubiquitous herpesvirus that infects 95% of individuals by adulthood (see Chapter 56). The virus persists as a latent infection in B lymphocytes, where reactivation and replication occur intermittently [154]. The latent membrane protein 1 (LMP-1) is one of the EBV-encoded proteins believed to have an important role in B-cell immortalization by inducing the expression of *bcl-2*, which inhibits programmed death of the infected cells. *LMP-1* is also considered to be an oncogene and deletions near the 3′ end of the *LMP-1* gene, in a region that affects the half-life of the LMP-1 protein have been reported in some lymphoproliferative disorders [155,156]. Infection of B cells by EBV also induces high levels of cytokines such as interleukin 1 (IL-1), IL-5, IL-6, IL-10, CD23 and tumor necrosis factor (TNF). Some of these factors have been shown to act as autocrine growth factors, stimulating the proliferation of EBV-transformed B cells and inhibiting their susceptibility to apoptosis [152].

Studies exploring susceptibility to EBV-PTLD have shown that cytotoxic T-lymphocyte precursor frequencies are low at 3 months after allogeneic HCT, but appear to normalize at 9–12 months, thus correlating with the time-period when B-cell PTLD is most frequently observed. Moreover, the EBV-specific cytotoxic T lymphocytes home preferentially and induce selective regression of autologous EBV-induced B-cell lymphoproliferative lesions in xenografted severe combined immunodeficiency syndrome (SCID) mice [157]. These studies have formed the basis for clinical trials using adoptive transfer of EBV-specific cytotoxic T lymphocytes [158]. The studies demonstrated long-term persistence of gene-marked EBV-specific cytotoxic T lymphocytes *in vivo*, which not only restore cellular immunity against EBV but also provide a population of cytotoxic T-lymphocyte precursors that respond to *in vivo* and *ex vivo* challenges with the virus for as long as 18 months [159]. It has also been demonstrated in the xenografted SCID mouse model that lack of natural killer (NK) cell function may have a role in the pathogenesis of PTLD [160]. These studies have demonstrated that a combination of granulocyte macrophage colony-stimulating factor (GM-CSF) and low-dose IL-2 therapy can prevent the immunodeficiency that leads to fatal EBV-lymphoproliferative disease in xenografted SCID mice depleted of murine NK cells, and thus support a critical role for several human cellular subsets in mediating this protective effect.

Table 70.4 Risk factors for lymphoma after allogeneic hematopoietic cell transplantation.

Study	Size of cohort	Length of follow-up (median)	No. of SMN	Age at HCT (median)	Year to SMN (median)	Incidence	RR	Risk factors	Outcome (% alive)
EBV-associated post-transplant lymphoproliferative disorder (PTLD)									
Socie et al. [24]	3182	3.6 year	20	8.2 year	1.5 year	1% (5 year)	182	HLA mismatch T-cell depletion of donor marrow Antithymocyte globulin (prophylaxis/ treatment of Acute GVHD) Chronic GVHD	0%
Bhatia et al. [15]	2150	3.1 year	22	20 year	0.2 year	1.6% (4 year)	105.6	Primary diagnosis of immunodeficiency Antithymocyte globulin (preparative regimen or GVHD prophylaxis) T-cell depletion of donor marrow Unrelated donor transplantation HLA mismatch	9%
Curtis et al. [149]	18,014	42,349 (person-years at risk)	78	60% of patients less than 40 years of age	0.4 year	1% (10 year)	51.5	HLA mismatch Unrelated donor transplantation T-cell depletion of donor marrow Antithymocyte globulin Ant-CD3 monoclonal antibody TBI Acute GVHD (grades II to IV) Chronic GVHD (extensive)	15%
Hodgkin disease after transplantation									
Rowlings et al. [151]	18,531	8.1 year	8	26 year	4.2 year		6.2	Acute GVHD (grade II to IV) Chronic GVHD	75%

GVHD, graft-versus-host disease; HCT, hematopoietic cell transplant; HLA, human leukocyte antigen; RR, relative risk; SMN, secondary malignant neoplasm; TBI, total body irradiation.

Prediction of risk of B-cell PTLD

Quantitative competitive polymerase chain reaction (Q-PCR) has been demonstrated to be an effective technique in allowing frequent monitoring of the DNA load to predict the development of PTLD. Rapid increases in peripheral blood EBV DNA load predicted PTLD [161,162]. EBV-specific T lymphocytes can be monitored through tetramer technology which allows detection of small quantities of antigen-specific T cells. Thus, it has been demonstrated that EBV-specific CD8 T cells are rapidly established following unmanipulated matched sibling allogeneic HCT, and HLA class I tetramers complexed with viral peptides can provide direct and rapid assessment of pathogen-specific immunity. In contrast, patients undergoing T-cell-depleted or unrelated cord blood transplantation have undetectable EBV-specific T cells, even in the presence of Epstein–Barr viremia [163].

Treatment of B-cell PTLD

Patients considered to be at an increased risk for development of PTLD (primary immunodeficiency, HLA-mismatched HCT, GVHD prophylaxis) should be monitored closely, so that appropriate therapy can be instituted early, prior to the development of overt disease. Therapeutic approaches that have been used include alpha interferon, B-cell specific monoclonal antibodies and cellular therapy. A combination of alpha interferon and intravenous immunoglobulin was reported to be effective in one study [164] but, with the advent of more effective therapies such as monoclonal antibodies and cellular therapy, interferon no longer remains the treatment of choice.

Several investigators have reported the efficacy of anti-CD20 monoclonal antibody (rituximab) in the treatment of PTLD [165–167]. All the studies indicate that the drug is well-tolerated by all age groups and is more efficacious in patients without mass lesions. This observation forms the basis for recommendations to initiate treatment at an early stage, based on increasing EBV load, and before the development of lymphomatous lesions. However, large multicenter trials followed longitudinally would address the efficacy and safety of this approach.

EBV-associated lymphoproliferative disorder developing after HCT has been shown to result from T-cell dysfunction. Reconstitution of "at-risk" patients with EBV-specific cytotoxic T-lymphocyte (CTL) lines that have been reactivated and expanded *in vitro* should prevent the development of PTLD or treat pre-existing disease. The CTL-reconstituted cellular immune responses to EBV have been shown to persist for up to 80 months. Cytotoxic T-cell therapy has been shown to be efficacious in controlling PTLD, with a decrease in the EBV DNA concentrations and remission of clinical signs and symptoms [168–170].

Thus, over the past few years, the administration of *in vitro*-generated EBV-specific cytotoxic T cells or anti-B-cell monoclonal antibodies have provided effective options for the prophylaxis or treatment of PTLD. Advances in quantitative PCR-based assays allow both the precise measurement of EBV load in peripheral blood samples and the identification of high-risk patients for early initiation of therapy. Recommendations need to be refined for the indications for pre-emptive treatment, based upon the significance of an elevated EBV load post-transplantation.

T-cell lymphoproliferative disorders

A few cases of T-cell lymphoproliferative disorders have been reported after HCT [171]. There is no association with EBV, human T-cell lymphotropic virus 1 (HTLV1), human immunodeficiency virus (HIV) or human herpesvirus 6 (HHV6). The T-cell lymphoproliferative disorders tend to occur much later than the EBV-associated B-cell PTLD.

Late-onset lymphoma

Several cases of late-occurring lymphoma have been reported in the literature [25,172–175]. It is believed that these late-occurring lymphomas represent an entity that is distinct from the early occurring B-cell PTLD. In a large study of 18,000 HCT recipients, the only risk factor associated with the development of the late-occurring lymphoma was extensive chronic GVHD [149].

Hodgkin's disease developing among HCT recipients has also been described [151]. The HCT recipients followed as part of a large cohort were at a sixfold increased risk of developing HD when compared with the general population. Most of the reported cases were of the mixed cellularity subtype, and most of the cases contained the EBV genome. These cases differed from the EBV-associated PTLD by the absence of risk factors commonly associated with EBV-associated PTLD, by a later onset (>2.5 years) and relatively good prognosis. The increased incidence of HD among HCT recipients could possibly be explained by exposure to EBV and overstimulation of cell-mediated immunity.

Solid tumors

Solid tumors have been described after syngeneic, allogeneic and autologous HCT. The magnitude of the increased risk of solid tumors has ranged from 2.1-fold [28] to 2.7-fold [176] when compared to an age- and sex-matched general population. The risk increased with increasing follow-up and, among those who survived ≥10 years after transplantation, was reported to be 8.3 times as high as expected in the general population. Types of solid tumors reported in excess among HCT recipients, when compared to the general population, are those typically associated with exposure to radiation therapy and include melanoma, cancers of the oral cavity and salivary glands, brain, liver, uterine cervix, thyroid, breast, bone and connective tissue [176,178]. Although most studies have focused on allogeneic HCT recipients, there is emerging evidence for an increased incidence of new solid malignancies among patients conditioned with TBI and receiving autologous HCT [34,175]. There is therefore a need to follow this cohort of patients long-term in order to describe the risk of new solid malignancies with precision.

A relatively small number of HCT recipients have been followed for ≥10 years, limiting the ability to estimate the risk of subsequent malignancies among long-term survivors. Rizzo et al. [177] have maintained continued surveillance of 28,884 HCT survivors to determine whether solid cancer risk changed beyond 10 years after transplantation. Average age at transplantation of this cohort of patients was 27 years, and 67% of the patients had received TBI. The cumulative incidence of invasive solid cancers for all patients was 2.2% at 10 years, 5% at 15 years and 8.1% at 20 years. Compared to an age- and sex-matched general population, transplant recipients were at a twofold increased risk of developing new invasive solid cancers. Risk increased with time since transplantation, with the 10-year survivors being at a fivefold increased risk of developing invasive solid tumors. Sites with significantly increased risks of second cancers included the oral cavity, salivary glands, liver, skin, brain, thyroid, breast, bone and connective tissues. TBI was associated with an increased risk of secondary solid cancers in the univariate analysis, and the risk diminished with increasing age at transplantation.

Thus, the risk of solid tumors increases sharply over time, and has been reported to be higher among children who underwent HCT at <10 years of age [176]. TBI is associated with an increased risk of solid tumors. The risk of solid tumors rises with the dose of radiation, with three to four times the risk at the highest dose levels, as compared with those who did not receive radiation therapy (Table 70.5) [176].

Pathogenesis of solid tumors after HCT

Little is known about the pathogenesis of solid tumors after HCT. An interaction of cytotoxic therapy, genetic predisposition, viral infection and GVHD with the consequent antigenic stimulation and use of immunosuppressive therapy, all seem to have a role in the development of new solid tumors.

Radiogenic cancers generally have a long latent period, and the risk of such cancers is frequently high among patients undergoing irradiation at a young age [24,179]. A large series reported an increased risk of brain and thyroid cancers after TBI as part of myeloablative conditioning, although most of these patients had received cranial irradiation prior to transplantation [24,148,176]. Both thyroid cancer and brain tumors have been reported after exposure to radiation to the craniospinal axis and the neck used as part of the conventional therapy for childhood acute lymphoblastic leukemia [77,180], Hodgkin's disease [2,181] and other primary brain tumors [181]. Similarly, osteogenic sarcoma and other connective tissue tumors have been reported as secondary malignancies developing among patients receiving radiation therapy as part of conventional therapy for other primary malignancies such as retinoblastoma and other bone tumors [182–184]. These studies indicated the presence of a strong dose–response relationship for radiation exposure, in addition to an increased risk with increasing exposure to alkylating agents [182,183]. The increased risk of thyroid, breast, brain, bone and soft tissue cancers seen after HCT appear to be related to cumulative doses of radiation exposure, both as a result of the pretransplant treatment regimen and the conditioning regimen used for transplant.

Immunologic alterations may predispose patients to squamous-cell carcinoma of the buccal cavity, particularly in view of the association with chronic GVHD. Patients transplanted for aplastic anemia have been reported to be at an increased risk of solid tumors, predominantly tumors of the buccal cavity and skin. The risk of these tumors was significantly increased after the administration of azathioprine for chronic GVHD [23]. In immunosuppressed patients, oncogenic viruses such as human papillomaviruses (HPVs) may contribute to squamous-cell cancers of the skin and buccal mucosa after transplantation [185,186]. The observation of the excess risk of squamous-cell cancers of the buccal cavity and skin in males is unexplained, but may be indicative of an interaction between ionizing radiation, immunodeficiency and other risk factors more prevalent among men than women [28,176].

The increased risk of new solid tumors after HCT is thus likely related to TBI used for pretransplant myeloablation, altered immune function in association with viral infections (HBV, HCV or HPV), and prior treatment for the primary disease (Table 70.5; Fig. 70.3) [22,28,176,187,188].

Genetic susceptibility

Patients with a family history of early-onset cancers have been shown to be at an increased risk for developing a secondary cancer. In one study, 159 3-year survivors of childhood soft-tissue sarcoma, treated with conventional therapy, and their relatives were surveyed to determine the frequency of secondary malignancies among the patients and history of cancer in their relatives [189]. A highly significant cancer excess was observed in the relatives of cancer survivors who developed a second cancer. The tumor types occurring in excess in close relatives were also observed as second cancers in patients (cancers of the breast, bone, joint

Table 70.5 Risk factors for solid tumors after hematopoietic cell transplantation.

Study	Size of cohort	Length of follow-up (median)	No. of SMN	Age at HCT (median)	Year to SMN (median)	Incidence	RR	Risk factors	Outcome (% alive)
Socie et al.* [24]	3182	3.6 year	25	8.2 year	6 year	11% (15 year)	34	TBI Younger age at transplant Chronic GVHD (decreased risk)	52%
Curtis et al. [176]*	19,229	3.5 year	80	25.5 year	—	6.7% (15 year)	2.7	TBI Younger age at transplant Chronic GVHD (squamous cell cancer) Male sex (squamous cell cancer)	55%
Bhatia et al. [28]†	2129	3.3 year	29	33.9		6.1% (10 year)	2.0	Younger age at transplant	90%
Socie, 1991 [178]*	147 (SAA)	5.3 (mean)	4	17 year (mean)	7 year	22% (8 year)	41	No risk factors identified	75%
Bhatia et al. [15]†	2150	3.1 year	17	20 year	4 year	5.6% (13 year)	3.2	TBI	60%

*Allogeneic HCT only.
†Allogeneic and autologous HCT.
GVHD, graft-versus-host disease; HCT, hematopoietic cell transplant; RR, relative risk; SAA, severe aplastic anemia; SMN, secondary malignant neoplasm; TBI, total body irradiation.

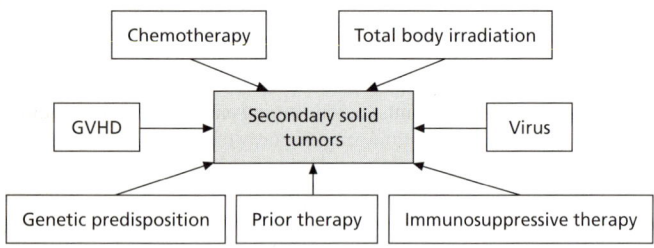

Fig. 70.3 Proposed pathogenesis of solid malignancies after HCT.

or soft tissue), indicating that the risk of second cancers is associated with a familial predisposition. In another study, members of families with Li–Fraumeni syndrome—a hereditary susceptibility to several cancers that is usually caused by mutation of the *TP53* tumor suppressor gene—were reported to be at increased risk of multiple subsequent cancers compared with the general population [190]. The highest risk was observed among survivors of childhood cancer. Moreover, the excess risk was mainly for cancers characteristic of Li–Fraumeni syndrome. It therefore appears that germline mutations in tumor suppressor genes, as occur in Li–Fraumeni syndrome, might interact with therapeutic exposures to result in an increased risk of secondary cancers.

Genetic susceptibility and gene–environment interaction

Genetic predisposition also has a substantial impact on risk of secondary cancers, e.g. sarcomas in patients with hereditary retinoblastoma. This risk is further increased by radiation treatment and increases with the total dose of radiation delivered [184].

Mutational analysis of the ataxia telangiectasia (*ATM*) gene, which is mutated in individuals with the recessive hereditary cancer syndrome, ataxia-telangiectasia [2], has been performed in cohorts of patients with radiation-associated secondary cancers. ATM protein—a protein kinase—plays an important part in regulation of the G1/S cell cycle checkpoint.

ATM phosphorylates p53, resulting in its stabilization following ionizing radiation. *In vitro* studies have shown that cells from ataxia-telangiectasia patients and obligate heterozygotes have an increased sensitivity to ionizing radiation, and there is epidemiologic evidence that ataxia-telangiectasia carriers are at an increased risk of radiation-induced breast cancer [191,192]. The studies conducted so far have failed to support the hypothesis that ataxia-telangiectasia carriers account for a significant fraction of radiation-induced secondary cancers [193,194], although there is some evidence that missense mutations in *ATM* are more common in primary breast cancer cases selected for family history and young age at diagnosis [195].

Underlying genetic characteristics interacting with treatment might be associated with an increased risk of certain secondary cancers. An example of such an interaction is the presence of a polymorphism in a drug-metabolizing enzyme such as TPMT. There is emerging evidence that *TPMT* genotype might influence the risk of secondary brain tumors [196].

Studies exploring genetic predisposition and gene–environment interactions have focused thus far on patients exposed to nontransplant conventional therapy for cancer. Future studies are needed in the transplant population to understand how the interaction of genetic predisposition with myeloablative chemotherapy, TBI and the attendant post-transplant immunosuppression have a role in the development of secondary solid tumors.

Treatment of patients with solid tumors after HCT

Treatment strategies for patients developing solid tumors after transplantation are not well-defined. Small case series indicate both ends of the spectrum: favorable outcomes and hence a recommendation for an intensive approach [197] and aggressive tumor growth and early relapse after standard therapy [198]. A comprehensive study of a large number of patients with second solid tumors will help determine the nature of these tumors and their outcomes as compared to *de novo* tumors. Until then, patients with solid tumors developing after transplant should be treated with the best available therapy for that tumor, unless there is compelling evidence that they will not be able to tolerate that therapy.

Screening for solid tumors after HCT

Extending the follow-up of HCT recipients to 20 years post-transplantation will help clarify the risks of radiation-associated cancers such as breast, lung and colon cancers. These epithelial cancers typically develop at a median of 15–20 years after exposure to radiation therapy and are now beginning to emerge among cancer survivor populations treated with conventional therapy [2,199]. These data indicate that HCT survivors face an increasing risk of solid cancers with time from HCT, thus supporting the need for life-long surveillance.

Preventive measures that need to be considered include programs to educate clinicians and survivors about the risk of secondary malignancies, and measures taken to decrease the morbidity associated with secondary malignancies, such as adopting healthy lifestyle choices. Other measures include intervention programs for smoking cessation, periodic and aggressive screening for breast, lung, skin, colorectal, prostate, thyroid and cervical cancers, chemoprevention for specific cancers, and avoidance of unnecessary exposure to sunlight, especially among patients who have received radiation [200]. Health counseling should include guidance about smoking cessation, diet and physical activity. By understanding the risk factors for secondary malignancies, and taking measures to avoid them, it may be possible to decrease the incidence of the most devastating consequences of surviving cancer while maintaining the high cure rates in this population.

Evidence-based guidelines for screening for early detection of cancer in HCT survivors are not available at present, but guidelines published by the American Cancer Society (ACS) [201] and the National Comprehensive Cancer Network (NCCN) Practice Guidelines in Oncology [202] present a reasonable framework for the physicians taking care of this high-risk population. The recommended frequency and the age at onset are based on the ACS recommendations for individuals identified to be at increased risk for the development of these cancers. Colon cancer screening should include colonoscopy with biopsy for dysplasia every 1–2 years beginning 10 years after TBI. Cervical screening is recommended annually, beginning at age 18 years, until the age of 45 years, and should be performed with conventional cervical cytology smears. The prostate specific antigen (PSA) test and digital rectal examination should be offered annually beginning at age 45. For female patients receiving radiation to the chest and/or TBI, screening recommendations include monthly breast self-examination, beginning at age 20 (or earlier, if the patients have received radiation to the chest at an earlier age), and clinical breast examination, beginning at age 20 (or earlier if needed), performed yearly until age 25, and then every 6 months. The NCCN guidelines also recommend a baseline mammogram at 8 years after exposure to radiation, or at the attained age of 40, whichever occurs first, and then annually. In addition, certain screening recommendations may be based on specific risk factors. For example, patients with a history of transfusions prior to 1993 should be screened for viral hepatitis. An examination for cancerous and precancerous lesions of the oral cavity should be in the periodic health examination of patients with oral chronic GVHD.

Conclusions

HCT offers curative therapy for many patients with otherwise incurable disease. Currently, 45,000–50,000 transplants are performed annually (see Chapter 2) and most patients who do not experience a recurrence of their underlying disease within 1 or 2 years of transplantation do well and lead productive lives. However, some complications do occur, and among those that have been described after HCT, malignant diseases are of particular clinical concern, because increasing numbers of patients survive the early phase after transplantation and remain free of their original disease. The incidence of post-transplant malignancies appears to be low, although reliable estimates of the overall risk will require a much longer follow-up. Despite the lack of randomized studies, the benefit of HCT, as compared with conventional therapy alone, in certain clinical situations outweighs the risk of late secondary malignancies. However, it is imperative to follow this population of HCT recipients closely in order to screen them for the development of subsequent malignancies, and thus decrease the morbidity and mortality associated with this complication. Longitudinal clinical and genetic monitoring of patients at multiple time points (before, during and after HCT) is required to evaluate risk factors, study the evolution of genetic lesions and identify biomarkers for secondary malignancies. Improved understanding of risk factors may allow future modification of pretransplant and transplant-related therapeutic exposures to minimize risk for these complications. A better understanding of the pathogenesis of secondary malignancies will allow for more effective screening to identify patients at risk prior to the HCT procedure, and allow more effective monitoring to detect early evolution of the malignancy post-transplantation. This may, in turn, allow for improved therapeutic decision-making while evaluating patients for HCT, and early institution of treatments directed at preventing and treating secondary malignancies in patients at risk after HCT.

References

1 Boivin JF, Hutchison GB, Zauber AG. Incidence of second cancers in patients treated for Hodgkin's disease. *J Natl Cancer Inst* 1995; **87**: 732.

2 Bhatia S, Robison LL, Oberlin O *et al*. Breast cancer and other second neoplasms after childhood Hodgkin's disease. *N Engl J Med* 1996; **334**: 745.

3 Meadows AT, Obringer AC, Marrero O *et al*. Second malignant neoplasms following childhood Hodgkin's disease: treatment and splenectomy as risk factors. *Med Pediatr Oncol* 1989; **17**: 477–84.

4 Pedreson-Bjergaard J, Larsen S. Incidence of acute nonlymphocytic, preleukemia, and acute myeloproliferative syndrome up to 10 years after the treatment of Hodgkin's disease. *N Engl J Med* 1982; **307**: 965.

5 van Leeuwen FE, Chorus AM, van den Belt-Dusebout AW *et al*. Leukemia risk following Hodgkin's disease: relation to cumulative dose of alkylating agents, treatment with teniposide combinations, number of episodes of chemotherapy, and bone marrow damage. *J Clin Oncol* 1994; **12**: 1063.

6 Valagussa P, Santoro A, Fossati-Bellani F, Banfi A, Bonadonna G. Second acute leukemia and other malignancies following treatment for Hodgkin's disease. *J Clin Oncol* 1986; **4**: 830.

7 Tucker MA, Coleman CN, Cox RS, Varghese A, Rosenberg SA. Risk of second cancers after treatment for Hodgkin's disease. *N Engl J Med* 1988; **318**: 76.

8 Cimino G, Papa G, Tura S *et al*. Second primary cancer following Hodgkin's disease: updated results of an Italian multicentric study. *J Clin Oncol* 1991; **9**: 432.

9 Andrieu JM, Ifrah N, Payen C *et al*. Increased risk of secondary acute nonlymphocytic leukemia after extended-field radiaton therapy combined with MOPP chemotherapy for Hodgkin's disease. *J Clin Oncol* 1990; **8**: 1148.

10 Kaldor JM, Day NE, Clarke EA *et al*. Leukemia following Hodgkin's disease. *N Engl J Med* 1990; **322**: 7.

11 Lavey RS, Eby NL, Prosnitz LR. Impact on second malignancy risk of the combined use of radiation and chemotherapy for lymphomas. *Cancer* 1990; **66**: 80.

12 Sankila R, Garwicz S, Olsen JH *et al*. Risk of subsequent malignant neoplasms among 1641 Hodgkin's disease patients diagnosed in childhood and adolescence: a population-based cohort study in the five Nordic countries. Association of the Nordic Cancer Registries and the Nordic Society of Pediatric Hematology and Oncology. *J Clin Oncol* 1996; **14**: 1442.

13 Travis LB, Curtis RE, Glimelius B et al. Second cancers among long-term survivors of non-Hodgkin's lymphoma. J Natl Cancer Inst 1993; **85**: 1932.

14 Deeg HJ, Sanders J, Martin P et al. Secondary malignancies after marrow transplantation. Exp Hematol 1984; **12**: 660.

15 Bhatia S, Ramsay NKC, Steinbuch M et al. Malignant neoplasms following bone marrow transplantation. Blood 1996; **87**: 3633.

16 Kolb HJ, Socie G, Duell T et al. Malignant neoplasms in long-term survivors of bone marrow transplantation. Ann Intern Med 1999; **131**: 738–44.

17 Witherspoon RP, Deeg H, Storb R. Secondary malignancies after marrow transplantation for leukemia or aplastic anemia. Transplant Sci 1994; **4**: 33–41.

18 Witherspoon RP, Fisher LD, Schoch G et al. Secondary cancers after bone marrow transplantation for leukemia or aplastic anemia. N Engl J Med 1989; **321**: 784–9.

19 Socie G. Secondary malignancies. Curr Opin Hematol 1996; **3**: 466–70.

20 Ades L, Guardiola P, Socie G. Second malignancies after allogeneic hematopoietic stem cell transplantation: new insight and current problems. Blood Rev 2002; **16**: 135–46.

21 Lowsky R, Lipton J, Fyles G, Minden M et al. Secondary malignancies after bone marrow transplantation in adults. J Clin Oncol 1994; **12**: 2187–92.

22 Deeg HJ, Socie G. Malignancies after hematopoietic stem cell transplantation: many questions, some answers. Blood 1998; **91**: 1833–44.

23 Deeg HJ, Socie G, Schoch G et al. Malignancies after marrow transplantation for aplastic anemia and Fanconi anemia: a joint Seattle and Paris analysis of results in 700 patients. Blood 1996; **87**: 386–92.

24 Socie G, Curtis RE, Deeg J et al. New malignant disease after allogeneic marrow transplantation for childhood acute leukemia. J Clin Oncol 2000; **18**: 348–57.

25 Socie G, Kolb HJ, Ljungman P. Malignant disease after allogeneic bone marrow transplantation: the case for assessment of risk factors. Br J Haematol 1992; **80**: 427–30.

26 Deeg H, Witherspoon RP. Risk factors for the development of secondary malignancies after marrow transplantation. Hematol Oncol Clin North Am 1993; **7**: 417–29.

27 Krishnan A, Bhatia S, Slovak ML et al. Predictors of therapy-related leukemia and myelodysplasia following autologous transplantation for lymphoma: an assessment of risk factors. Blood 2000; **95**: 1588–93.

28 Bhatia S, Louie AD, Bhatia R et al. Solid cancers after bone marrow transplantation. J Clin Oncol 2001; **19**: 464–71.

29 Stone RM, Neuberg D, Soiffer R et al. Myelodysplastic syndrome as a late complication following autologous bone marrow transplantation for non-Hodgkin's lymphoma. J Clin Oncol 1994; **12**: 2535.

30 Traweek ST, Slovak ML, Nademanee AP et al. Clonal karyotypic hematopoietic cell abnormalities occurring after autologous bone marrow transplantation for Hodgkin's disease and non-Hodgkin's lymphoma. Blood 1994; **84**: 957.

31 Marolleau JP, Brice P, Morel P, Gisselbrecht C. Secondary acute myeloid leukemia after autologous bone marrow transplantation for malignant lymphoma. J Clin Oncol 1991; **11**: 590.

32 Miller JS, Arthur DC, Litz CE et al. Myelodysplastic syndrome after autologous bone marrow transplantation: an additional late complication of curative cancer therapy. Blood 1994; **83**: 3780.

33 Darrington DL, Vose JM, Anderson JR et al. Incidence and characterization of secondary myelodysplastic syndrome and acute myelogenous leukemia following high-dose chemoradiotherapy and autologous stem cell transplantation for lymphoid malignancies. J Clin Oncol 1994; **12**: 2527.

34 Andre M, Henry-Amar M, Blaise D et al. Treatment-related deaths and second cancer risk after autologous stem cell transplantation for Hodgkin's disease. Blood 1998; **92**: 1933.

35 Laughlin MJ, McGaughey DS, Crews JR et al. Secondary myelodysplasia and acute leukemia in breast cancer patients after autologous bone marrow transplant. J Clin Oncol 1998; **16**: 1008–12.

36 Kollmannsberger C, Beyer J, Droz J-P et al. Secondary leukemia following cumulative doses of etoposide in patients treated for advanced germ cell tumors. J Clin Oncol 1998; **16**: 3386.

37 Govindarajan R, Jagannath S, Flick JT et al. Preceding standard therapy is the likely cause of MDS after autotransplants for multiple myeloma. Br J Haematol 1996; **95**: 349–53.

38 Taylor PRA, Jackson GH, Lennard AL, Hamilton PJ. Low incidence of myelodysplastic syndrome following transplantation using autologous non-cryopreserved bone marrow. Leukemia 1997; **11**: 1650.

39 Pedersen-Bjergaard J, Pedersen M, Myhre J, Geisler C. High risk of therapy-related leukemia after BEAM chemotherapy and autologous stem cell transplantation for previously treated lymphomas is mainly related to primary chemotherapy and not to BEAM-transplantation procedure. Leukemia 1997; **11**: 1654.

40 Tucker MA, Meadows AT, Boice JD et al. Leukemia after therapy with alkylating agents for childhood cancer. J Natl Cancer Inst 1987; **78**: 459–64.

41 Curtis RE, Boice JD, Stovall M et al. Risk of leukemia after chemotherapy and radiation treatment for breast cancer. N Engl J Med 1992; **326**: 1745.

42 Pui C-H, Ribiero RC, Hancock ML et al. Acute myeloid leukemia in children treated with epipodophyllotoxins for acute lymphoblastic leukemia. N Engl J Med 1991; **325**: 1682.

43 Winick NJ, McKenn RW, Shuster JJ et al. Secondary acute myeloid leukemia in children with acute lymphoblastic leukemia treated with etoposide. J Clin Oncol 1993; **11**: 209.

44 Vardiman JW, Harris NL, Brunning RD. The World Health Organization (WHO) classification of the myeloid neoplasms. Blood 2002; **100**: 2292–302.

45 Sanderson BJ, Shield AJ. Mutagenic damage to mammalian cells by therapeutic alkylating agents. Mutat Res 1996; **355**: 41–57.

46 Tew KD, Clovin M, Chabner BA. Alkylating agents. In: Chabner BA, Longo DL, eds. Cancer Chemotherapy and Biotherapy: Principles and Practice, Vol. 1. New York: Lippincott-Raven, 1996: 297–32.

47 Chabner BA, Myers CE. Clinical pharmacology of cancer chemotherapy. In: DeVita VT, Hellman S, Rosenberg SA, eds. Principles and Practice of Oncology, 3rd edn. Philadelphia: JB Lippincott, 1989: 349–95.

48 Le Beau MM, Albain KS, Larson RA et al. Clinical and cytogenetic correlations in 63 patients with therapy-related myelodysplastic syndromes and acute nonlymphocytic leukemia: further evidence for characteristic abnormalities of chromosomes 5 and 7. J Clin Oncol 1986; **4**: 325–45.

49 Karp JE, Sarkodee-Adoo CB. Therapy-related acute leukemia. Clin Lab Med 2000; **20**: 71–9.

50 Michels SD, McKenna RW, Arthur DC, Brunning RD. Therapy-related acute myeloid leukemia and myelodysplastic syndrome: a clinical and morphologic study of 65 cases. Blood 1985; **65**: 1364–72.

51 Felix CA. Secondary leukemias induced by topoisomerase targeted drugs. Biochim Biophys Acta 1998; **1400**: 233–5.

52 Corbett AH, Osheroff N. When good enzymes go bad: conversion of topoisomerase II to a cellular toxin by antineoplastic drugs. Chem Res Toxicol 1993; **6**: 585–97.

53 Lovett B, Strumberg D, Blair I. et al. Etoposide metabolites enhance DNA topoisomerase II cleavage near leukemia-associated MLL translocation breakpoints. Biochemistry 2001; **40**: 1159–70.

54 Super HJG, McCabe NR, Thirman MJ et al. Rearrangements of the MLL gene in therapy-related acute myeloid leukemia in patients previously treated with agents targeting DNA topoisomerase II. Blood 1993; **82**: 3705–11.

55 Megonigal M, Cheung N-K, Rappaport E et al. Detection of leukemia-associated MLL-GAS7 translocation early during chemotherapy with DNA topoisomerase II inhibitors. Proc Natl Acad Sci U S A 2000; **97**: 2814–9.

56 Atlas M, Head D, Behm F. et al. Cloning and sequence analysis of four t(9;11) therapy-related leukemia breakpoints. Leukemia 1998; **12**: 1895–902.

57 Felix CA, Winick NJ, Negrini M et al. Common region of ALL-1 gene disrupted in epipodophyllotoxin-related secondary acute myeloid leukemia. Cancer Res 1993; **53**: 2954–6.

58 Felix C, Lange B, Hosler M, Fertala J, Bjornsti M-A. Chromosome band 11q23 translocation breakpoints are DNA topoisomerase II cleavage site. Cancer Res 1995; **55**: 4287–92.

59 Hunger SP, Tkachuk DC, Amylon MD et al. HRX involvement in de novo and secondary leukemias with diverse chromosome 11q23 abnormalities. Blood 1993; **81**: 3197–203.

60 Bower M, Parry P, Gibbons B et al. Human trithorax gene rearrangements in therapy-related acute leukemia after etoposide treatment. Leukemia 1994; **8**: 226–9.

61 Broeker PLS, Super HG, Thirman MJ et al. Distribution of 11q23 breakpoints within the MLL breakpoint cluster region in de novo acute leukemia and therapy-related acute myeloid leukemia: correlation with scaffold attachment regions and topoisomerase II consensus binding sites. Blood 1996; **87**: 1912–22.

62 Andersen MK, Johansson B, Larsen SO, Pedersen-Bjergaard J. Chromosomal abnormalities in secondary MDS and AML: relationship to drugs and radiation with specific emphasis on the balanced rearrangements. Haematologica 1998; **83**: 438–8.

63 Pedersen-Bjergaard J, Andersen MK, Christiansen DH, Nerlov N. Genetic pathways in therapy-related myelodysplasia and acute myeloid leukemia. Blood 2002; **99**: 1909–12.

64 Pedersen-Bjergaard J, Philip P. Balanced translocation involving chromosome bands 11q23 and 21q22 are highly characteristic of myelodysplasia and leukemia following therapy with cytostatic agents targeting at DNA-topoisomerase II. Blood 1991; **78**: 1147–8.

65 Rowley JD, Olney HJ. International workshop on the relationship of prior therapy to balanced chromosome aberrations in therapy-related leukemia and myelodysplastic syndromes and acute leukemia: overview report. *Genes Chromosomes Cancer* 2002; **33**: 331–45.
66 Jeha S, Jaffe N, Robertson R. Secondary acute non-lymphoblastic leukemia in two children following treatment with a *cis*-diamminechloroplatinum-II-based regimen for osteosarcoma. *Med Pediatr Oncol* 1992; **20**: 71–4.
67 Greene MH. Is cisplatin a human carcinogen? *J Natl Cancer Inst* 1992; **84**: 306–12.
68 Gilliland DG, Gribben JG. Evaluation of the risk of therapy-related MDS/AML after autologous stem cell transplantation: biology of blood and marrow transplantation. 2002; **8**: 9–16.
69 Milligan DW, Ruiz De Elvira MC, Kolb H-J *et al.* Secondary leukemia and myelodysplasia after autografting for lymphoma: results from the EBMT. *Br J Haematol* 1999; **106**: 1020.
70 Wheeler C, Khurshid A, Ibrahim J *et al.* Incidence of post-transplant myelodysplasia/acute leukemia in non-Hodgkin's lymphoma patients compared with Hodgkin's disease patients undergoing autologous transplantation following cyclophosphamide, carmustine, and etoposide (CBV). *Leuk Lymphoma* 2001; **40**: 499–509.
71 Friedberg JW, Neuberg D, Stone RM *et al.* Outcome of patients with myelodysplastic syndrome after autologous bone marrow transplantation for non-Hodgkin's lymphoma. *J Clin Oncol* 1999; **17**: 3128.
72 Harrison CN, Gregory W, Hudson GV *et al.* High-dose BEAM chemotherapy with autologous haemopoietic stem cell transplantation for Hodgkin's disease is unlikely to be associated with a major increased risk of secondary MDS/AML. *Br J Cancer* 1999; **81**: 476–83.
73 Lillington DM, Micallef IN, Carpenter E *et al.* Detection of chromosome abnormalities pre-high-dose treatment in patients developing therapy-related myelodysplasia and secondary acute myelogenous leukemia after treatment for non-Hodgkin's lymphoma. *J Clin Oncol* 2001; **19**: 2472–81.
74 Abruzzese E, Radford JE, Miller JS *et al.* Detection of abnormal pretransplant clones in progenitor cells of patients who developed myelodysplasia after autologous transplantation. *Blood* 1999; **94**: 1814–9.
75 Metayer C, Curtis RE, Vose J *et al.* Myelodysplastic syndrome and acute myeloid leukemia after autotransplantation for lymphoma: a multicenter case–control study. *Blood* 2002; **95**: 3273–9.
76 Pedersen-Bjergaard J, Andersen MK, Christiansen DH. Therapy-related acute myeloid leukemia and myelodysplasia after high-dose chemotherapy and autologous stem cell transplantation. *Blood* 2000; **95**: 3273–9.
77 Bhatia S, Sather HN, Pabustan OB *et al.* Low incidence of second neoplasms among children diagnosed with acute lymphoblastic leukemia after 1983. *Blood* 2002; **99**: 4257–64.
78 Stone RM. Myelodysplastic syndrome after autologous transplantation for lymphoma: the price of progress? *Blood* 1994; **83**: 3437.
79 Lai F, Godley LA, Joslin J *et al.* Transcript map and comparative analysis of the 1.5-Mb commonly deleted segment of human 5q31 in malignant myeloid diseases with a del(5q). *Genomics* 2001; **71**: 235–45.
80 Kratz CP, Emerling BM, Donovan S *et al.* Candidate gene isolation and comparative analysis of a commonly deleted segment of 7q22 implicated in myeloid malignancies. *Genomics* 2001; **77**: 171–80.
81 Karp JE. Molecular pathogenesis and targets for therapy in myelodysplastic syndrome (MDS) and MDS-related leukemias. *Curr Opin Oncol* 1998; **10**: 3–9.
82 Shannon KM, Le Beau MM, Largaespada DA, Killeen N. Modeling myeloid leukemia tumor suppressor gene inactivation in the mouse. *Semin Cancer Biol* 2001; **11**: 191–200.
83 Luna-Fineman S, Shannon KM, Lange BJ. Childhood monosomy 7: epidemiology, biology, and mechanistic implications. *Blood* 1995; **85**: 1985–99.
84 Shannon KM, Turhan AG, Chang SS *et al.* Familial bone marrow monosomy 7: evidence that the predisposing locus is not on the long arm of chromosome 7. *J Clin Invest* 1989; **84**: 984–9.
85 Song WJ, Sullivan MG, Legare RD *et al.* Haploinsufficiency of CBFA2 causes familial thrombocytopenia with propensity to develop acute myelogenous leukaemia. *Nat Genet* 1999; **23**: 166–75.
86 Nucifora G, Birn DJ, Espinosa R 3rd *et al.* Involvement of the AML1 gene in the t(3;21) in therapy-related leukemia and in chronic myeloid leukemia in blast crisis. *Blood* 1993; **81**: 2728–34.
87 Roulston D, Espinosa R 3rd, Nucifora G *et al.* CBFA2 (AML1) translocations with novel partner chromosomes in myeloid leukemias: association with prior therapy. *Blood* 1998; **92**: 2879–85.
88 Higuchi M, O'Brien D, Lenny N *et al.* Expression of AML1-ETO immortalizes myeloid progenitors and cooperates with secondary mutations to induce granulocytic sarcoma/acute myeloid leukemia. *Blood* 2000; **96**: 222A.
89 Downing JR. AML1/CBFbeta transcription complex: its role in normal hematopoiesis and leukemia. *Leukemia* 2001; **15**: 664–5.
90 Djabali M, Selleri L, Parry P *et al.* A trithorax-like gene is interrupted by chromosome 11q23 translocations in acute leukaemias. *Nat Genet* 1992; **2**: 113–8.
91 Corral J, Lavenir I, Impey H *et al.* An *Mll-AF9* fusion gene made by homologous recombination causes acute leukemia in chimeric mice: a method to create fusion oncogenes. *Cell* 1996; **85**: 853–61.
92 Relling MV, Yanishevski Y, Nemec J *et al.* Etoposide and antimetabolite pharmacology in patients who develop secondary acute myeloid leukemia. *Leukemia* 1998; **12**: 346–52.
93 Woo MH, Shuster JJ, Chen CL *et al.* Glutathione S-transferase genotypes in children who develop treatment-related acute myeloid malignancies. *Leukemia* 2000; **14**: 226–31.
94 Felix CA, Walker AH, Lange BJ *et al.* Association of CYP3A4 genotype with treatment-related leukemia. *Proc Natl Acad Sci U S A* 1998; **95**: 13176–81.
95 Chen H, Sandler DP, Taylor JA *et al.* Increased risk for myelodysplastic syndromes in individuals with glutathione transferase theta 1 (GSTT1) gene defect. *Lancet* 1996; **347**: 295–7.
96 Allan JM, Wild CP, Rollinson S *et al.* Polymorphism in glutathione S-transferase P1 is associated with susceptibility to chemotherapy-induced leukemia. *Proc Natl Acad Sci U S A* 2001; **98**: 11592–7.
97 Hayes JD, Pulford DJ. The glutathione S-transferase supergene family: regulation of GST and the contribution of the isoenzymes to cancer chemoprotection and drug resistance. *Crit Rev Biochem Mol Biol* 1995; **30**: 445–600.
98 Naoe T, Takeyama K, Yokozawa T *et al.* Analysis of genetic polymorphism in NQO1, GST-M1, GST-T1, and CYP3A4 in 469 Japanese patients with therapy-related leukemia/myelodysplastic syndrome and *de novo* acute myeloid leukemia. *Clin Cancer Res* 2000; **6**: 4091–5.
99 Smith G, Stanley LA, Sim E, Strange RC, Wolf CR. Metabolic polymorphisms and cancer susceptibility. *Cancer Surv* 1995; **25**: 27–65.
100 Wrighton S, Stevens J. The human hepatic cytochromes P450 involved in drug metabolism. *Crit Rev Toxicol* 1992; **22**: 1–21.
101 Raunio H, Husgafvel-Pursianen K, Anttila S *et al.* Diagnosis of polymorphisms in carcinogen-activating and inactivating enzymes and cancer susceptibility. *Gene* 1995; **159**: 113–21.
102 Albertini RJ, Nicklas JA, O'Neill J, P. *et al. In vivo* somatic mutations in humans: measurement and analysis. *Ann Rev Genet* 1990; **24**: 305–26.
103 Finette BA, Homans AC, Albertini RJ. Emergence of genetic instability in children treated for leukemia. *Science* 2000; **288**: 514–7.
104 Das-Gupta EP, Seedhuse CH, Russell NH. DNA repair mechanisms and acute myeloblastic leukemia. *Hematol Oncol* 2000; **18**: 99–110.
105 Ben-Yehuda D, Krichevsky S, Caspi O *et al.* Microsatellite instability and p53 mutations in therapy-related leukemia suggest mutator phenotype. *Blood* 1996; **88**: 4296–303.
106 Sheikhha MH, Tobal K, Liu Yin JA. High level of microsatellite instability but not hypermethylation of mismatch repair genes in therapy-related and secondary acute myeloid leukaemia and myelodysplastic syndrome. *Br J Haematol* 2002; **117**: 359–65.
107 Rimsza LM, Kopecky KJ, Ruschulte J *et al.* Microsatellite instability is not a defining genetic feature of acute myeloid leukemogenesis in adults: results of a retrospective study of 132 patients and review of the literature. *Leukemia* 2000; **14**: 1044–51.
108 Horiike S, Misawa S, Kaneko H *et al.* Distinct genetic involvement of the TP53 gene in therapy-related leukemia and myelodysplasia with chromosomal losses of Nos 5 and/or 7 and its possible relationship to replication error phenotype. *Leukemia* 1999; **13**: 1235–42.
109 Christiansen DH, Andersen MK, Pedersen-Bjergaard J. Mutations with loss of heterozygosity of p53 are common in therapy-related myelodysplasia and acute myeloid leukemia after exposure to alkylating agents and significantly associated with deletion or loss of 5q, a complex karyotype, and a poor prognosis. *J Clin Oncol* 2001; **19**: 1405–13.
110 Blackburn EH. Structure and function of telomeres. *Nature* 1991; **266**: 569.
111 Hackett JA, Feldser DM, Greider CW. Telomere dysfunction increases mutation rate and genomic instability. *Cell* 2001; **106**: 275–86.
112 Vaziri H, Dragowska W, Allsopp RC *et al.* Evidence for a mitotic clock in human hematopoietic stem cells: loss of telomeric DNA with age. *Proc Natl Acad Sci U S A* 1994; **91**: 9857–60.
113 Akiyama M, Hoshi Y, Sakurai S *et al.* Changes of telomere length in children after hematopoietic stem cell transplantation. *Bone Marrow Transplant* 1998; **21**: 167–71.
114 Lee J, Kook H, Chung I *et al.* Telomere length changes in patients undergoing hematopoietic stem

cell transplantation. *Bone Marrow Transplant* 1999; **24**: 411–5.

115 Seligman SJ. Telomere shortening in recipients of bone-marrow transplants. *Lancet* 1998; **351**: 1287–8.

116 Wynn RF, Cross MA, Hatton C et al. Accelerated telomere shortening in young recipients of allogeneic bone-marrow transplants. *Lancet* 1998; **351**: 178–81.

117 Rufer N, Brummendorf TH, Chapuis B et al. Accelerated telomere shortening in hematological lineages is limited to the first year following stem cell transplantation. *Blood* 2001; **97**: 575–7.

118 Awaya N, Baerlocher GM, Manley TJ et al. Telomere shortening in hematopoietic stem cell transplantation: a potential mechanism for late graft failure? *Biol Blood Marrow Transplant* 2002; **8**: 597–600.

119 Engelhardt M, Ozkaynak MF, Drullinsky P et al. Telomerase activity and telomere length in pediatric patients with malignancies undergoing chemotherapy. *Leukemia* 1998; **12**: 13–24.

120 Domenech J, Gihana E, Dayan A et al. Haemopoiesis of transplanted patients with autologous marrows assessed by long-term marrow culture. *Br J Haematol* 1994; **88**: 488–96.

121 Domenech J, Linassier C, Gihana E et al. Prolonged impairment of hematopoiesis after high-dose therapy followed by autologous bone marrow transplantation. *Blood* 1995; **85**: 3320–7.

122 del Canizo C, Lopez N, Cabalerro D et al. Haematopoietic damage persists 1 year after autologous peripheral blood stem cell transplantation. *Bone Marrow Transplant* 1999; **23**: 901–5.

123 Novitzky N, Mohammed R. Alterations in the progenitor cell population follow recovery from myeloablative therapy and bone marrow transplantation. *Exp Hematol* 1997; **25**: 471–7.

124 Novitzky N, Mohamed R. Alterations in both the hematopoietic microenvironment and the progenitor cell population follow the recovery from myeloablative therapy and bone marrow transplantation. *Exp Hematol* 1995; **23**: 1661–6.

125 Soligo DA, Lambertenghi Deliliers G, Sevida F et al. Hematopoietic abnormalities after autologous stem cell transplantation for leukemia. *Bone Marrow Transplant* 1998; **21**: 15–22.

126 Bhatia S, Van Heijzen K, Palmer A et al. Hematopoietic damage persists 2 years after autologous peripheral stem cell transplantation (aPBSCT) for lymphoma. *Blood* 2002; **100**: 850A.

127 Gilabert R, Ayats R. Human long-term bone marrow culture as a prognostic factor for hematopoietic reconstitution in autologous transplantation. *Bone Marrow Transplant* 1994; **13**: 635–40.

128 Voermans C, Kooi ML, Rodenhuis S et al. In vitro migratory capacity of $CD34^+$ cells is related to hematopoietic recovery after autologous stem cell transplantation. *Blood* 2001; **97**: 799–804.

129 Gardner RV, Astle CM, Harrison DE. Hematopoietic precursor cell exhaustion is a cause of proliferative defect in primitive hematopoietic stem cells (PHSC) after chemotherapy. *Exp Hematol* 1997; **25**: 495–501.

130 Dittel BN, LeBien TW. Reduced expression of vascular cell adhesion molecule-1 on bone marrow stromal cells isolated from marrow transplant recipients correlates with a reduced capacity to support human B lymphopoiesis in vitro. *Blood* 1995; **86**: 2833–41.

131 Domenech J, Roingeard F, Herault O et al. Changes in the functional capacity of marrow stromal cells after autologous bone marrow transplantation. *Leuk Lymphoma* 1998; **29**: 533–46.

132 Selleri C, Maciejewski JP, De Rosa G et al. Long-lasting decrease of marrow and circulating long-term culture initiating cells after allogeneic bone marrow transplant. *Bone Marow Transplant* 1999; **23**: 1029–37.

133 Yeoh E-J, Williams K, Patel S et al. Expression profiling of pediatric acute lymphoblastic leukemia (ALL) blasts at diagnosis accurately predicts both the risk of relapse and of developing therapy-induced acute myelogenous leukemia (AML). *Blood* 2001; **98**: 433A.

134 Qian Z, Fernald AA, Godley LA, Larson RA, Le Beau MM. Expression profiling of $CD34^+$ hematopoietic stem/progenitor cells reveals distinct subtypes of therapy-related acute myeloid leukemia. *Proc Natl Acad Sci U S A* 2002; **99**: 14925–30.

135 Witherspoon RP, Deeg HJ. Allogeneic bone marrow transplantation for secondary leukemia or myelodysplasia. *Haematologica* 1999; **84**: 1085–7.

136 Yakoub-Agha I, de La Salmoniere P, Ribaud P et al. Allogeneic bone marrow transplantation for therapy-related myelodysplastic syndrome and acute myeloid leukemia: a long-term study of 70 patients. Report of the French society of bone marrow transplantation. *J Clin Oncol* 2000; **18**: 963–71.

137 Ballen KK, Gilliland DG, Guinan EC et al. Bone marrow transplantation for therapy-related myelodysplasia: comparison with primary myelodysplasia. *Bone Marrow Transplant* 1997; **20**: 737.

138 Anderson JE, Gooley TA, Schoch G et al. Stem cell transplantation for secondary acute myeloid leukemia: evaluation of transplantation as initial therapy or following induction chemotherapy. *Blood* 1997; **89**: 2578–85.

139 Appelbaum FR, LeBeau MM, Willman CL. *Secondary Leukemia: Hematology*. Education Program, American Society of Hematology. 1996; 33–47.

140 Quesnel B, Kantarjian H, Bjergaard JP et al. Therapy-related acute myeloid leukemia with t(8;21), inv(16), and t(8;16): a report on 25 cases and review of the literature. *J Clin Oncol* 1993; **11**: 2370–9.

141 Witherspoon RP, Deeg HJ, Storer B et al. Hematopoietic stem-cell transplantation for treatment-related leukemia or myelodysplasia. *J Clin Oncol* 2001; **19**: 2134–41.

142 Radich JP, Gooley T, Sanders JE et al. Second allogeneic transplantation after failure of first autologous transplantation. *Biol Blood Marrow Transplant* 2000; **6**: 272–9.

143 Cohen S, Fung H, Stein A et al. Reduced intensity allogeneic stem cell transplantation for patients who have failed a prior autologous stem cell transplant. *Blood* 2002; **100**: 157A.

144 Feinstein LC, Sandmaier BM, Maloney DG. et al. Allografting after nonmyeloablative conditioning as a treatment following failed conventional hematopoietic cell transplant. *Biol Blood Marrow Transplant* 2003; **9**: 266–72.

145 Mach-Pascual S, Legare RD, Lu D et al. Predictive value of clonality assays in patients with non-Hodgkin's lymphoma undergoing autologous bone marrow transplant: a single institution study. *Blood* 1998; **91**: 4496.

146 Kollmannsberger C, Hartmann JT, Kanz L, Bokemeyer C. Risk of secondary myeloid leukemia and myelodysplastic syndrome following standard-dose chemotherapy or high-dose chemotherapy with stem cell support in patients with potentially curable malignancies. *J Cancer Res Clin Oncol* 1998; **124**: 207–14.

147 Radich J. Detection of minimal residual disease in acute and chronic leukemias. *Curr Opin Hematol* 1996; **3**: 310.

148 Cohen JL. Epstein–Barr virus lymphoproliferative disease associated with acquired immunodeficiency. *Medicine* 1991; **70**: 137–60.

149 Curtis RE, Travis LB, Rowlings PA et al. Risk of lymphoproliferative disorders after bone marrow transplantation: a multi-institutional study. *Blood* 1999; **94**: 2208.

150 Kernan NA, Bartsch G, Ash RC et al. Analysis of 462 transplantations from unrelated donors facilitated by the National Marrow Donor Program. *N Engl J Med* 1993; **328**: 593–602.

151 Rowlings PA, Curtis RE, Passweg JR et al. Increased incidence of Hodgkin's disease after allogeneic bone marrow transplantation. *J Clin Oncol* 1999; **17**: 122–7.

152 O'Reilly RJ, Lacerda JF, Lucas KG et al. Adoptive cell therapy with donor lymphocytes for EBV-associated lymphomas developing after allogeneic marrow transplants. In: De Vita TD, Hellman S, Rosenberg SA, eds. *Important Advances in Oncology 1996*. Philadelphia: Lippincott-Raven, 1996: 149–66.

153 Milpied N, CosteBurel M, Accard F et al. Epstein–Barr virus associated B-cell lymphoproliferative disease after non-myeloablative allogeneic stem cell transplantation. *Bone Marrow Transplant* 1999; **23**: 629–30.

154 Klein G. Epstein–Barr virus strategy in normal and neoplastic B cells. *Cell* 1997; **77**: 791–3.

155 Kingma DW, Weiss WB, Jaffe ES et al. Epstein–Barr virus latent membrane protein-1 oncogene deletions: correlation with malignancy in Epstein–Barr virus-associated lymphoproliferative disorders and malignant lymphomas. *Blood* 1996; **88**: 242–51.

156 Klein C, Rothenberger S, Niemeyer C et al. EBV-associated lymphoproliferative syndrome with a distinct 69 base-pair detetion in the LMP-1 oncogene. *Br J Haematol* 1995; **91**: 938–40.

157 Lacerda JF, Ladanyi M, Louie DC et al. Epstein–Barr virus (EBV) specific cytotoxic T lymphocytes home preferentially to and induce selective regressions of autologous EBV-induced B cell lymphoproliferations in xenografted C.B-17 SCID/SCID mice. *J Exp Med* 1996; **183**: 1215–28.

158 Heslop HE, Ng CY, Li C et al. Long-term restoration of immunity against Epstein–Barr virus infection by adoptive transfer of gene-modified virus-specific T lymphocytes. *Nat Med* 1996; **2**: 551–5.

159 Rooney CM, Smith CA, Ng CYC et al. Use of gene-modified virus-specific T lymphocytes to control Epstein–Barr virus-related lymphoproliferation. *Lancet* 1996; **345**: 9–13.

160 Baiocchi RA, Ward JS, Carrodeguas L et al. GM-CSF and IL-2 induce specific cellular immunity and provide protection against Epstein–Barr virus lymphoproliferative disorder. *J Clin Invest* 2001; **108**: 887–94.

161 Van Esser JW, Van Der HB, Meijer E et al. Epstein–Barr virus (EBV) reactivation is a frequent event after allogeneic stem cell transplantation (SCT) and quantitatively predicts EBV-lymphoproliferative disease following T-cell-depleted SCT. *Blood* 2001; **98**: 972–8.

162 Van Esse JW, Niesters HG, Thijsen SF *et al.* Molecular quantification of viral load in plasma allows for fast and accurate prediction of response to therapy of Epstein–Barr virus-associated lymphoproliferative disease after allogeneic stem cell transplantation. *Br J Haematol* 2001; **113**: 814–21.

163 Marshall NA, Howe JG, Formica R *et al.* Rapid reconstitution of Epstein–Barr virus-specific T lymphocytes following allogeneic stem cell transplantation. *Blood* 2000; **96**: 2814–21.

164 Shapiro RS, Chauvenet A, McGuire W *et al.* Treatment of B-cell lymphoproliferative disorders with interferon alpha and intravenous gammaglobulin. *N Engl J Med* 1988; **318**: 1334–5.

165 Kuehnle I, Huls MH, Liu Z *et al.* CD20 monoclonal antibody (rituximab) for therapy of Epstein–Barr virus lymphoma after hemopoietic cell transplantation. *Blood* 2000; **95**: 1502–5.

166 Milpied N, Vasseur B, Parquet N *et al.* Humanized anti-CD20 monoclonal antibody (rituximab) in post-transplant B-lymphoproliferative disorder: a retrospective analysis on 32 patients. *Ann Oncol* 2000; **11** (Suppl. 1): S113–6.

167 Faye A, Quartier P, Reguerre Y *et al.* Chimeric anti-CD20 monoclonal antibody (rituximab) in post-transplant B-lymphoproliferative disorder following stem cell transplantation in children. *Br J Haematol* 2001; **115**: 112–8.

168 Rooney CM, Smith CA, Ng CYC *et al.* Use of gene-modified virus-specific T lymphocytes to control Epstein–Barr virus-related lymphoproliferation. *Lancet* 1995; **345**: 9–13.

169 Papadopoulos EB, Ladanyi M, Emmanuel D *et al.* Infusions of donor leukocytes to treat Epstein–Barr virus-associated lymphoproliferative disorders after allogeneic bone marrow transplantation. *N Engl J Med* 1994; **330**: 1185–91.

170 Liu Z, Savaldo B, Huls H *et al.* Epstein–Barr virus (EBV)-specific cytotoxic T lymphocytes for the prevention and treatment of EBV-associated post-transplant lymphomas. *Recent Results Cancer Res* 2002; **159**: 123–33.

171 Zutter MM, Durnam DM, Hackman RC *et al.* Secondary T-cell lymphoproliferation after marrow transplantation. *Am J Clin Pathol* 1990; **94**: 714–21.

172 Verschuur A, Brousse N, Raynal B *et al.* Donor B cell lymphoma of the brain after allogeneic bone marrow transplantation for acute myeloid leukemia. *Bone Marrow Transplant* 1994; **14**: 467–70.

173 Meignin V, Devergie A, Brice P *et al.* Hodgkin's disease of donor origin after allogeneic bone marrow transplantation for myelogenous chronic leukemia. *Transplantation* 1998; **65**: 595–7.

174 Schouten HC, Hopman AHN, Haesevoets AM, Arends JW. Large-cell anaplastic non-Hodgkin's lymphoma originating in donor cells after allogeneic bone marrow transplantation. *Br J Haematol* 1995; **91**: 162–6.

175 Trimble MS, Waye JS, Walker IR, Brain MC, Leber BF. B-cell lymphoma of recipient origin 9 years after allogeneic bone marrow transplantation for T-cell acute lymphoblastic leukemia. *Br J Haematol* 1993; **85**: 99–102.

176 Curtis RE, Rowlings PA, Deeg J *et al.* Solid cancers after bone marrow transplantation. *N Engl J Med* 1997; **336**: 897–904.

177 Rizzo J, Curtis R, Deeg H *et al.* Long-term follow-up of allogeneic blood stem cell and bone marrow transplantation: a collaborative study of EBMT and IBMTR. *Blood* 2001; **98**: 774A.

178 Socie G, Henry-Amar JM, Cosset A *et al.* Increased risk of solid malignant tumors after bone marrow transplantation for severe aplastic anemia. *Blood* 1991; **78**: 277–9.

179 United Nations Scientific Committee on the Effects of Atomic Radiation (UNSCEAR). *Sources and Effects of Ionizing Radiation*. New York: United Nations, 1994. United Nations Publications no. E.94IX.11.

180 Neglia JP, Meadows AT, Robison LL *et al.* Second neoplasms after acute lymphoblastic leukemia in childhood. *N Engl J Med* 1991; **325**: 1330–6.

181 Neglia JP, Friedman DL, Yasui Y *et al.* Second malignant neoplasms in 5-year survivors of childhood cancer: childhood cancer survivor study. *J Natl Cancer Inst* 2001; **93**: 618–29.

182 Tucker MA, D'Angio GJ, Boice JDJ *et al.* Bone sarcomas linked to radiotherapy and chemotherapy in children. *N Engl J Med* 1987; **317**: 588–93.

183 Hawkins MM, Wilson LM, Burton HS *et al.* Radiotherapy, alkylating agents, and risk of bone cancer after childhood cancer. *J Natl Cancer Inst* 1996; **88**: 270–8.

184 Wong FL, Boice JDJ, Abramson DH *et al.* Cancer incidence after retinoblastoma: radiation dose and sarcoma risk. *J Am Med Assoc* 1997; **278**: 1262–7.

185 Kinlen LJ. Immunologic factors, including AIDS. In: Schottenfeld D, Fraumeni JF Jr, eds, *Cancer Epidemiology and Prevention*, 2nd edn. New York: Oxford University Press, 1996: 532–45.

186 Vittorio CC, Schiffman MH, Weinstock MA. Epidemiology of human papillomaviruses. *Dermatol Clin* 1995; **13**: 561–74.

187 Daneshpouy M, Socie G, Clavel C *et al.* Human papilloma virus infection and anogenital condyloma in bone marrow recipients. *Transplantation* 2001; **71**: 167–9.

188 Socie G, Scieux C, Gluckman E *et al.* Squamous cell carcinomas after allogeneic bone marrow transplantation for aplastic anemia. *Transplantation* 1998; **66**: 667–70.

189 Strong LC, Stine M, Norsted TL. Cancer in survivors of childhood soft tissue sarcoma and their relatives. *J Natl Cancer Inst* 1987; **79**: 1213–20.

190 Hisada M, Garber JE, Fung CY, Fraumeni JF Jr, Li FP. Multiple primary cancers in families with Li–Fraumeni syndrome. *J Natl Cancer Inst* 1998; **90**: 606–11.

191 Swift M, Morrell D, Massey RB, Chase CL. Incidence of cancer in 161 families affected by ataxia-telangiectasia. *N Engl J Med* 1991; **325**: 1831–6.

192 Swift M. Public health burden of cancer in ataxia-telangiectasia heterozygotes. *J Natl Cancer Inst* 2001; **93**: 84–5.

193 Shafman TD, Levitz S, Nixon AJ *et al.* Prevalence of germline truncating mutations in ATM in women with a second breast cancer after radiation therapy for a contralateral tumor. *Genes Chromosomes Cancer* 2000; **27**: 124–9.

194 Nichols KE, Levitz S, Shannon KE *et al.* Heterozygous germline ATM mutations do not contribute to radiation-associated malignancies after Hodgkin's disease. *J Clin Oncol* 1999; **17**: 1259.

195 Teraoka SN, Malone KE, Doody DR *et al.* Increased frequency of ATM mutations in breast carcinoma patients with early onset disease and positive family history. *Cancer* 2001; **92**: 479–87.

196 Relling MV, Rubnitz JE, Rivera GK *et al.* High incidence of secondary brain tumours after radiotherapy and antimetabolites. *Lancet* 1999; **354**: 34–9.

197 Favre-Schmuziger G, Hofer S, Passweg J *et al.* Treatment of solid tumors following allogeneic bone marrow transplantation. *Bone Marrow Transplant* 2000; **25**: 895–8.

198 Socie G, Henry-Amar M, Devergie A *et al.* Poor clinical outcome of patients developing malignant solid tumors after bone marrow transplantation for severe aplastic anemia. *Leuk Lymphoma* 1992; **7**: 419–23.

199 Hancock SL, Hoppe RT. Long-term complications of treatment and causes of mortality after Hodgkin's disease. *Semin Radiat Oncol* 1996; **6**: 225–42.

200 Kaste SC, Hudson MM, Jones DJ *et al.* Breast masses in women treated for childhood cancer: incidence and screening guidelines. *Cancer* 1998; **82**: 784–92.

201 Smith RA, Cokkinides V, von Eschenbach AC *et al.* American Cancer Society guidelines for the early detection of cancer. *CA Cancer J Clin* 2002; **52**: 8–22.

202 National Comprehensive Cancer Network. *Practice Guidelines in Oncology*, Version 2001. 2002.

Section 5

Allogeneic Transplantation for Acquired Diseases

71

George E. Georges & Rainer Storb

Allogeneic Hematopoietic Cell Transplantation for Aplastic Anemia

Aplastic anemia (AA) is a rare disease with an incidence of three cases per million per year in the USA and western Europe and about 15 cases per million per year in East Asia [1,2]. When treated with supportive care including blood transfusions and antibiotics, only about 28% of patients are alive 2 years after diagnosis [3]. More than 50% of patients with severe aplastic anemia (SAA) may die within 6 months of diagnosis without definitive therapy [4]. Effective therapies for AA consist of either immunosuppressive therapy (IST) with agents such as antithymocyte globulin (ATG) or allogeneic hematopoietic cell transplantation (HCT).

The disease is characterized by pancytopenia and marrow parenchyma that is lacking hematopoietic elements. Typically, the marrow cavities are filled with fat, and the aspirates show mainly lymphocytes, plasma cells and fibroblasts. The differential diagnosis of a marrow aspirate with this appearance includes myelodysplastic syndrome (MDS), T-cell clonal disorders and AA associated with paroxysmal nocturnal hemoglobinuria (PNH). One of the most difficult entities to distinguish from AA is hypocellular myelodysplasia (see Chapter 79), but the difference is important as the two disease entities are treated differently. The conditioning regimen for HCT for MDS often contains busulfan (BU) or total body irradiation (TBI) as for acute leukemias, whereas conditioning regimens without radiation are preferred for patients with AA (see later discussion). Cytogenetic analysis of marrow is sometimes useful in distinguishing between hypocellular MDS and AA. Marrow cytogenetics are normal in AA in contrast to MDS and, in contrast to hypocellular myelodysplasia, developing blood cells are usually normal in appearance. Occasionally, there may be dysplastic erythroid cells in AA [5]. However, the presence of dyshematopoiesis in nonerythroid cell lines is more consistent with MDS [5].

Severe aplastic anemia is defined as marrow cellularity ≤25% with at least two of the following:
1 absolute neutrophil count less than 0.5×10^9/L;
2 platelet count less than 20×10^9/L; and
3 absolute reticulocyte count less than 40×10^9/L [6].

Very severe AA is defined by a neutrophil count less than 0.2×10^9/L and at least one other peripheral blood criterion of SAA and marrow features consistent with SAA.

Aplastic anemia may be the result of a variety of causes, including ionizing radiation, benzene and chemotherapeutic agents [7,8]. Drugs causing idiosyncratic marrow injury include chloramphenicol, phenylbutazone, sulfonamides, gold and anticonvulsants such as felbamate (reviewed in [5]). Rarely, AA is associated with viral diseases such as non-A, non-B, non-C hepatitis, parvovirus (pure red cell aplasia) or Epstein–Barr virus, and autoimmune disorders such as eosinophilic fasciitis [5]. Some cases of AA result from congenital or hereditary disorders, including Diamond–Blackfan anemia and Fanconi's anemia. In most patients the disease etiology is unknown (idiopathic or primary AA).

Possible pathophysiologic mechanisms of AA include quantitative and/or qualitative deficiencies of hematopoietic stem cells (HSCs), a defective marrow microenvironment, impairment of cellular interactions needed to sustain hematopoiesis and immunologic suppression of marrow function. The result is a reduction in morphologically recognizable precursor cells in the marrow aspirate [1].

The variable response of SAA to therapy and the diverse evolution of the disease with time are perhaps a reflection of the multiple pathophysiologic mechanisms. The observation that the infusion of syngeneic marrow without prior immunosuppressive conditioning results in cure of the disease in approximately 50% of patients suggests that a defect in stem cells is a likely cause in these patients [9–12]. While most patients with AA have normally functioning stromal cells [9,11], there are a few cases where defects in the marrow microenvironment have been thought to have a role in the pathogenesis of their disease [13]. Immunologic mechanisms may cause AA as suggested by therapeutic responses to infusions of ATG and also by the fact that patients with certain immunodeficiencies may develop marrow aplasia after receiving marrow or blood products containing viable histoincompatible lymphocytes [14,15].

This chapter summarizes the results of marrow HCT for SAA over the past 30 years. Early reports of marrow HCT for SAA identified three major transplant related problems:
1 graft rejection;
2 acute graft-vs.-host disease (GVHD); and
3 chronic GVHD [16–18].

The incidence of graft rejection has decreased in part because of the use of more effective immunosuppressive conditioning regimens and in part because of changes in transfusion practices (see below). The incidence of acute GVHD has also decreased owing to improved GVHD prevention protocols. The incidence and mortality of chronic GVHD may also have declined slightly. These changes, in turn, have resulted in significant improvement in survival. With longer follow-up, late sequelae including impaired growth and development among children [19] and secondary malignancies [20] have become better understood.

Syngeneic grafts

Patients with syngeneic donors were among the first to receive marrow HCTs. Six of 12 patients in Seattle showed complete and sustained marrow recovery after HCT without preceding immunosuppression. In the other six patients, second marrow infusions were performed after conditioning with 200 mg/kg cyclophosphamide (CY). In one of the six patients the second transplant also failed after more than 1 year, and a third transplant was carried out following conditioning with CY and TBI. Three years after the third transplant this patient developed pure red cell aplasia, required multiple transfusions and died from the consequences of iron overload 9 years after the first marrow infusion. The other five recipients of a second graft had complete and sustained engraftment after conditioning with CY alone, although one patient died 7 years after HCT from complications of diabetes mellitus (unrelated to the transplant). Thus, 10 of 12 patients are alive with an overall survival of 83% and follow-up ranging from 1.5 to 30 years [21]. The International Bone Marrow Transplant Registry (IBMTR) recently reviewed data on 40 syngeneic transplants worldwide. Twenty-three patients did not receive an initial conditioning regimen, and eight of the 23 had full hematologic recovery, while 15 required second transplants that were preceded by conditioning regimens. Twelve of 17 patients whose initial HCT was preceded by conditioning had full hematologic recovery. Four of these 17 patients died within 20 days of transplantation: one from fungal pneumonia, one from acute respiratory distress syndrome and two from diffuse alveolar hemorrhage. One patient required a second transplant with conditioning for a full hematologic recovery. While initial sustained engraftment was higher in patients who had transplants with conditioning, their 10-year survival was lower (70%) than that of patients who did not require conditioning initially (87%) [22].

These observations suggest that syngeneic HCT can be attempted without conditioning and, if the graft fails, a second marrow infusion with a conditioning regimen is usually successful without compromising overall survival. The results of syngeneic HCTs are consistent with the concept that some cases of AA are caused by a defect in HSCs that can be corrected by simple intravenous infusion of syngeneic marrow. However, there are other cases in which the infused twin marrow HCT either fails to engraft or is rejected following a period of transient recovery of hematopoietic function. The etiology of the aplasia in these cases may be immune or be the result of unknown factors whereby the dysfunction of marrow can be overcome by conditioning with CY and a second marrow infusion [23].

HLA-identical related bone marrow transplants

The largest number of transplants for SAA performed to date have been from human leukocyte antigen (HLA) matched sibling donors. In preparation for allogeneic HLA-identical HCT, recipients have been treated by intensive immunosuppression to prevent rejection of the grafts. Immunosuppressive agents have included CY given either alone at a dosage of 50 mg/kg/day intravenously on each of 4 successive days or combined with ATG. In other patients, CY at a dosage of 60 mg/kg/day for 2 days has been combined with TBI or limited field radiation (LFR), such as total lymphoid irradiation (TLI) or thoracoabdominal irradiation (TAI).

Table 71.1 summarizes reports on outcome since 1983. The median ages of patients reported in all studies has been approximately 25 years or less with ranges of 1–59 years. The conditioning regimens and agents used for GVHD prophylaxis varied widely, even within studies. Most transplanted patients have been previously transfused, a variable that has been shown to adversely affect transplant outcome by increasing the risk of graft rejection. The survival rates have improved with time in part because of decreased incidences of graft rejection, the result of changes in transfusion policies, improved conditioning programs [21] and in part because of a decreased incidence of acute GVHD owing to the introduction of cyclosporine (CSP) [24] and the combination of methotrexate (MTX) and CSP [25].

Graft rejection

Graft rejection occurs because of genetic disparity between donor and recipient. Two forms of graft rejection may be seen. Primary rejection is

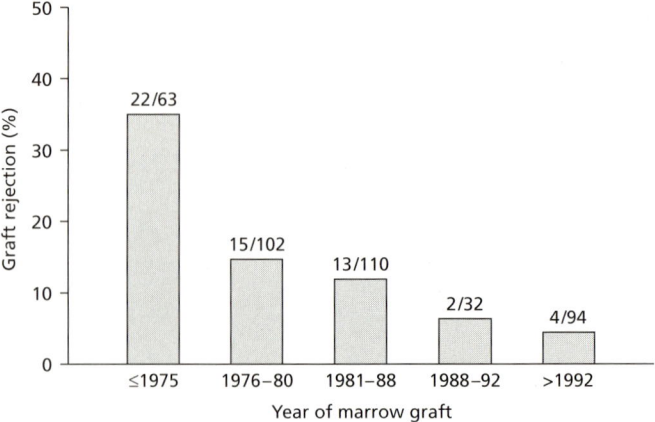

Fig. 71.1 The incidence of graft rejection vs. year of transplantation for patients in Seattle and collaborating transplant centers receiving marrow from human leukocyte antigen (HLA) identical siblings. All patients were conditioned with cyclophosphamide-containing regimens. The numbers above the bars indicate the number of rejections per number of patients transplanted. (Updated from Storb et al. [21,50].)

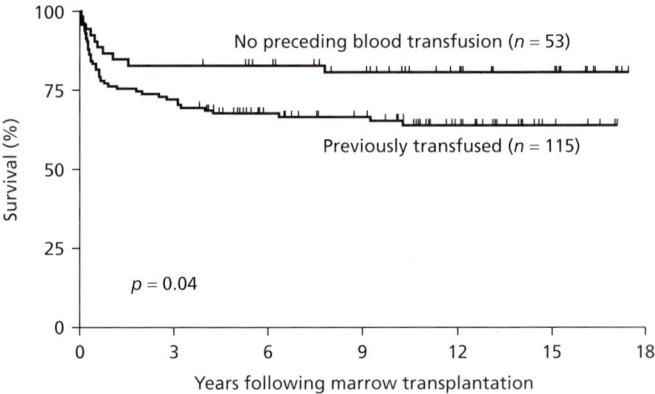

Fig. 71.2 The effect of transfusion status on actuarial survival. Tick marks denote censoring times of surviving patients. The p-values were calculated using the log–rank test and are two-sided. (Adapted from Doney et al. [33].)

defined by the absence of any sign of hematologic function of the graft, and late rejection is defined as graft loss after initial graft function. Patients with primary or late graft rejection can often be rescued with a second HCT [26].

Graft rejection was formerly a frequent problem among patients who received CY alone for conditioning. As can be seen from Fig. 71.1, graft rejection at the Fred Hutchinson Cancer Research Center (FHCRC) was seen in over 35% of patients transplanted in the early 1970s [21]. A report from the European Group for Blood and Bone Marrow Transplantation (EBMT) showed a rejection incidence of 32% among patients transplanted before 1980 [27].

A major factor associated with graft rejection has been sensitization to histocompatibility antigens through previous blood product transfusions as shown by extensive animal studies and confirmed in clinical trials [28–32]. Figure 71.2 shows that previously transfused patients have a lower overall survival compared to untransfused patients [33], mainly because of complications of graft rejection.

Data in animals have shown dendritic cells in the transfusion product to play an important part in sensitizing recipients to disparate minor histocompatibility antigens of the transfusion (and marrow) donor [34]. Exposing blood products to 2000 cGy of gamma irradiation in vitro before transfusion almost eliminated sensitization to minor histocompatibility

Table 71.1 Human leukocyte antigen (HLA) identical HCT for SAA: summary of results.

Transplant team	Year of report	Year of transplant	Number of patients	Age range in years (median)	Conditioning program*	Prevention of GVHD[†]	Rejection (%)[‡]	GVHD (%) Acute	GVHD (%) Chronic	Survival (%)	Range of follow-up (years) (median)
UCLA [104]	1983	1977–81	46	2–44 (19)	CY + 300 cGy TBI	MTX	2	70	—	63	0.75–4.5 (2)
Boston [158]	1985	1977–84	40	2–35 (17)	PAPAPA-CY	MTX	10	53	>35	61	<0.8–11 (5)
Seattle [159]	1986	1971–81	81	2–17 (13)	CY	MTX	18	30	30	71	10–20
Seattle# [31,32]	1986	1972–84	50	3–32 (17)	CY	MTX	10	23	37	82	1–12 (7)
Minneapolis [160,161]	1983, 1987	1977–86	58	2–45 (18)	CY + 750 cGy TLI	MTX, MTX + ATG + PSE	5	38	12–54	70	<0.05–8
EBMT [63]	1988	1981–88	218	1–50	CY ± TLI, TAI or TBI	MTX or CSP	—	—	—	63	<1–6
Seattle [39,80]	1982, 1988	1976–81	42	1–49 (20)	CY	MTX	14	36	60	67	7–11
London [24]	1989	1979–85	49	3–47 (22)	CY	CSP	17	50	37	69	1.8–7.8 (5.8)
IBMTR [162]	1989	1978–86	625	—	CY / CY + TLI or TAI / CY + TBI	MTX or CSP	20 / 9 / 5	—	—	—	—
UCLA [101]	1990	1984–88	29	0.7–41 (19)	CY + 300 cGy TLI	MTX + CSP	23	22	—	78	0.6–5 (2)
EBMT [102]	1990	1970–88	171	1–15	CY ± TLI, TAI or TBI	MTX or CSP	—	—	—	63	0.08–15 (4.5)
Seattle [21,61]	1991, 1992	1981–90	35	1–18 (10)	CY	MTX + CSP	24	15	30	94	1–10.5 (5)
Paris [163]	1991	1980–89	107	5–46 (19)	CY + 600 cGy TAI	MTX, CSP or MTX + CSP	3	32	55	62	1–10 (3.75)
IBMTR [60]	1992	1980–87	595	1–<40	CY ± TLI, TAI or TBI	MTX, CSP or MTX + CSP	10	40	45	63	>2–>7
Seattle [21]	1992	1988–91	29	2–46 (24)	CY + ATG	MTX + CSP	3	15	30	93	0.5–3.5 (2)
Seattle [47,83]	1994, 1997 (update)	1988–93	39	2–52 (24.5)	CY + ATG	MTX + CSP	5	15	34	92	3.2–8.2 (5.2)
Vancouver [82]	1995	1982–92	16	2–40 (15)	CY ± ATG ± TBI	MTX, MTX + CSP	6	36	31	75	2.1–11 (6)

Table 71.1 *(cont'd)*

Institution	Year	N	Age range (median)	Conditioning	GVHD prophylaxis	Graft failure (%)	Acute GVHD (%)	Chronic GVHD (%)	Survival (%)	Follow-up (years)
Memorial Sloan Kettering [100]	1994	23	2.5–32 (13)	CY + TLI	CSP + PSE, MTX + CSP, others	14	27	18	60	3.2–10.4 (5.7)
Hamburg [165]	1995	9	7–30 (25)	CY + ATG	MTX + CSP	0	0	0	87	1.6–3.1 (2.5)
Children's Hospital of Philadelphia [76]	1996	11	1.5–16 (3)	CY + ATG	CSP	0	—	0	100	0.6–4.6 (2.2)
Hopkins [178]	1993	24	4–53 (21)	CY	CSP	29	5	0	79	—
Helsinki [78]	1995	11	0.6–17.3 (9.3)	CY ± TLI	Varied	9	—	0	73	2–19
UCLA/Sloan-Kettering/MD Anderson [151]	1995	55	—	CY ± TBI or ± TLI	MTX, MTX + CSP		9	45	38	52 (6)
Japan [77]	1997	10	1.5–14 (8)	CY + ATG	MTX + CSP	0	0	10	100	0.6–3.4
IBMTR [81]	1997	186	2–56 (19)	CY, CY + TBI, CY + LFR	Varied	20	39	37	48	(6)
		648	1–57 (20)	CY, CY + TBI, CY + LFR	Varied	11	37	47	61	(6)
		471	1–51 (20)	CY, CY + LFR, CY + ATG	Varied	16	19	32	66	(5)
Seattle/Stanford/City of Hope§ [50]	2001	94	2–59 (26)	CY + ATG	MTX + CSP	4	29	32	88	0.5–11.6 (6.0)
GITMO/EBMT [51]	2000	71	4–46 (19)	CY	CSP vs. MTX + CSP	8	33	35	86¶	0.6–7.8 (4.0)
IBMTR [98]	2000	874	1–20	—	—	—	—	—	75 ± 3	0.2–5.0
		696	20–40	—	—	—	—	—	68 ± 4	
		129	>40						35 ± 18	
EBMT** [99]	2000	583 }	1–50 (18)	—	—	—	—	—	54	0.2–5.0
	1974–90 1991–96								77	0.2–5.0

EBMT, European Group for Blood and Marrow Transplantation; CY, cyclophosphamide; GITMO, Gruppo Italiano Trapianti di Midolio Osseo; IBMTR, International Bone Marrow Transplant Registry; UCLA, University of California at Los Angeles.

*ATG, antithymocyte globulin; CY, cyclophosphamide; LFR, limited field irradiation (either TLI or TAI); PAPAPA, alternating procarbazine and antithymocyte globulin; TAI, thoracoabdominal irradiation; TBI, total body irradiation; TLI, total lymphoid irradiation; — Data not reported.

†CSP, cyclosporine; MTX, methotrexate; PSE, prednisone.

‡Graft failure with first transplant.

§Includes 39 patients previously reported [83].

¶5-year Kaplan–Meier survival estimate for CSP patients 78%, for MTX + CSP 94% [51].

**Additional interactive Cox survival model analysis for transplant outcome based on EBMTR data of neutrophil count, age and year of transplant is available at the following website: http://www.ebmt.org/4Registry/registry5.html

In all series the majority of patients were previously transfused except those designated with a pound sign (#).

Table 71.2 Hematopoietic grafts from dog leukocyte antigen (DLA) identical littermates after 9.2 Gy TBI.*

Group	Preceding blood product transfusion on days −24, −17, −10[†]	2000 cGy *in vitro* gamma irradiation	Total no. of dogs studied	No. of dogs with sustained engraftment (%)[‡]	Statistical significance
A	None	Not applicable	62	61 (95%)	
B	From marrow donor	Yes	20	17 (85%)	*p*-value <0.001
		No	27	0 (0%)	
C	From two different unrelated dogs on each of the 3 successive days	Yes	16	15 (94%)	*p*-value = 0.001
		No	27	10 (37%)	
D	Leukocyte poor red blood cell transfusions from the donor	No	14	9 (64%)	*p*-value = 0.001 (compared to Group A) *p*-value <0.001 (compared to Group B with no irradiation)
E	Leukocyte-poor platelet transfusions from the donor	No	15	8 (53%)	*p*-value <0.001 (compared to Group A and Group B with no irradiation)

*All received donor buffy coat infusions in addition to marrow for 21 dogs which did not receive any preceding transfusions and 12 dogs who received unirradiated blood from their marrow donors or unrelated dogs. Adapted from [28,30,35,166,167].
[†]Approximately 50 mL of heparinized blood per transfusion.
[‡]The *p*-values were calculated using Fisher's exact text.

antigens and prevented rejection of dog leukocyte antigen (DLA) identical marrow grafts (see Table 71.2) [35,36]. Other factors reducing rejection in the canine model included the use of platelet and red blood cell transfusions that were leukocyte depleted (see Table 71.2) [30]. These data strongly suggested that human patients with AA who are candidates for HCT should be managed with irradiated leukocyte-poor blood products [37].

While early transplantation before transfusion has reduced graft rejection, less than 15% of patients were untransfused prior to transplant. Given that fact, other methods have been developed to overcome marrow graft rejection. At FHCRC, an inverse relation was observed between the number of donor marrow cells infused and the risk of graft rejection in patients conditioned with CY [38]. A low incidence of graft rejection was seen with a high ($>3 \times 10^8$ cells/kg) marrow cell dose and vice versa. On the basis of that observation, an attempt was made to increase the number of HSCs transplanted by infusing unirradiated donor buffy coat cells in addition to the marrow [39]. While effective in reducing the incidence of graft rejection and improving survival compared to patients given marrow alone, the infusion of donor buffy coat cells increased the risk of *de novo* chronic GVHD [40,41]. Therefore, one current strategy to decrease the rate of graft rejection without increasing the risk of chronic GVHD has been to maximize the amount of marrow cells infused by harvesting $\geq 3.5 \times 10^8$ cells/kg and deleting buffy coat cell infusions [41,42].

Other attempts to overcome graft rejection have included intensifying the conditioning regimen, e.g. using CY combined with TBI or LFR. While effective in reducing the incidence of rejection, radiation-based regimens have been associated with a higher rate of transplant related mortality (TRM) and may cause cancer and problems with growth, development and fertility (see later discussion and Chapters 68 and 69).

Recently there has been interest in the use of granulocyte colony-stimulating factor (G-CSF) mobilized peripheral blood stem cells (G-PBSC) as the source of HSCs for allogeneic transplantation. G-PBSC contains an increased number of CD34[+] stem cells and an approximately 10-fold increased numbers of T cells compared to marrow [43]. With the infusion of a larger number of donor cells, G-PBSC could potentially decrease the risk of graft rejection in patients with SAA. EBMT registry data indicate that approximately 20% of HLA-identical sibling transplants for SAA in the years 1998–99 used G-PBSC as the stem cell source (EBMT website, 2002). However, it is prudent to refrain from the use of G-PBSC for patients with SAA because of concerns of the significantly increased long-term risk of development of chronic GVHD [44]. Furthermore, in AA there is no compensatory benefit of a graft-vs.-leukemia effect provided by PBSC.

Animal studies have shown synergistic immunosuppressive effects between ATG and alkylating agents such as procarbazine and CY as assessed by the criteria of skin graft prolongation and of overcoming marrow graft rejection [45,46]. On the basis of these experimental animal data, the regimen of CY and ATG was developed and used to rescue patients who had rejected their first graft. Fifteen of 19 previously transplanted patients who were reconditioned with CY and ATG had successful second marrow grafts, and 50% became long-term survivors [47]. Over the past 15 years, survival of patients after second HCT increased to 83% at FHCRC, a result not significantly different from survival after first transplant [26].

Because of the success of CY and ATG in second transplants, the combination was chosen as a conditioning regimen for first transplants beginning in 1988. Figure 71.3 shows the comparison of results in 39 historical patients conditioned with CY and ATG and 39 patients conditioned with CY alone, 24 of whom received supplemental buffy coat infusions. Patients in both groups received marrow grafts from HLA-identical family members. The incidences of graft rejection and acute GVHD were similar in both groups, but overall survival was significantly higher in patients conditioned with CY and ATG (Fig. 71.3) owing to a significantly lessened incidence of and morbidity from chronic GVHD, the result of the omission of buffy coat cell infusions.

While changes in transfusion policies and improved conditioning regimens before transplant have led to significant decreases in graft rejection [27], it has been suggested that post-grafting immunosuppression aimed at controlling GVHD may also have a role in controlling host-vs.-graft (HVG) reactions. A retrospective analysis by the EBMT group suggested that the use of CSP as GVHD prophylaxis has decreased the rejection rate compared to MTX [27], but a randomized prospective study from Seattle failed to show differences in rejection [21,25] when long-term MTX was compared to a short course of MTX combined with CSP. Studies in animals showed MTX and CSP to be superior to CSP alone, not only in controlling GVHD but also in suppressing HVG reactions thereby enhancing

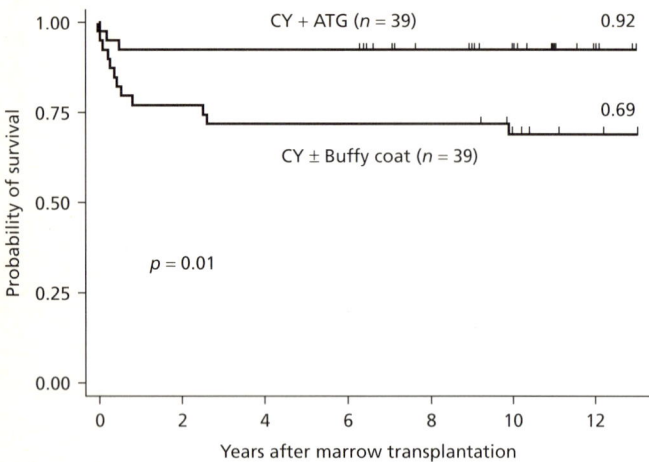

Fig. 71.3 Kaplan–Meier estimates of survival in the patients with severe aplastic anemia given human leukocyte antigen (HLA) identical hematopoietic cell transplantation and graft-vs.-host disease (GVHD) prophylaxis with methotrexate (MTX) and cyclosporine (CSP). Data for 39 historical patients are shown conditioned with cyclophosphamide (CY) alone, 62% of whom were given additional donor buffy coat infusions compared with 39 patients conditioned with CY and antithymocyte globulin (ATG). There was a statistically significant higher rate of survival among patients conditioned with CY and ATG vs. those who received CY with or without buffy coat infusions. The p-values were calculated using the log–rank test. The data are current as of July 2002. (Adapted from Storb et al. [83].)

engraftment [48]. More recent data demonstrated that a novel combination of mycophenolate mofetil (MMF) and CSP provided even better control of HVG reactions than MTX and CSP [48,49]. Thus, postgrafting immunosuppression used for GVHD prevention also has to be considered when evaluating new conditioning regimens for their efficacy in decreasing the risk of graft rejection.

Updated results from a multicenter study of CY and ATG for patients with SAA confirmed that graft rejection had become a minor problem (Fig. 71.4a). Of the 94 consecutive patients enrolled, 87 had received multiple transfusions and 38 had failed immunosuppressive therapy. The ages of the patients ranged from 2 to 59 years. After transplantation, 89 patients received MTX and CSP for GVHD prophylaxis. There was a 4% incidence of graft rejection between 2 and 7 months after transplantation (Fig. 71.4a). Of the four patients with graft rejection, three were alive following successful second HSC transplantation. With a median follow-up of 6.0 years (range 0.5–11.6 years), the overall survival rate was 88% [50].

Some transplant centers have continued to use CY without ATG as the conditioning regimen for younger patients receiving marrow HCT from HLA-identical siblings. Results from a prospective randomized multicenter trial sponsored by the Gruppo Italiano Trapianti di Midolio Osseo (GITMO) and the EBMT that compared CSP alone vs. MTX and CSP for GVHD prophylaxis in 71 patients with SAA showed the overall incidence of graft rejection was 8% [51]. Several factors may explain why the GITMO/EBMT results with CY conditioning alone were superior to the historic data from the Seattle group in the 1980s. Since the initial Seattle report there has been increased awareness in the medical community of the benefit of leukodepleted and irradiated blood products for patients with SAA. Seventy of 71 patients in the GITMO/EBMT study had been transfused with a median of 6 units of blood products prior to transplantation. Although not specifically addressed in the GITMO/EBMT study, the widespread use of irradiated and leukodepleted blood products for transfusion support prior to transplantation for patients with AA may have contributed to the lower incidence of graft rejection seen in the

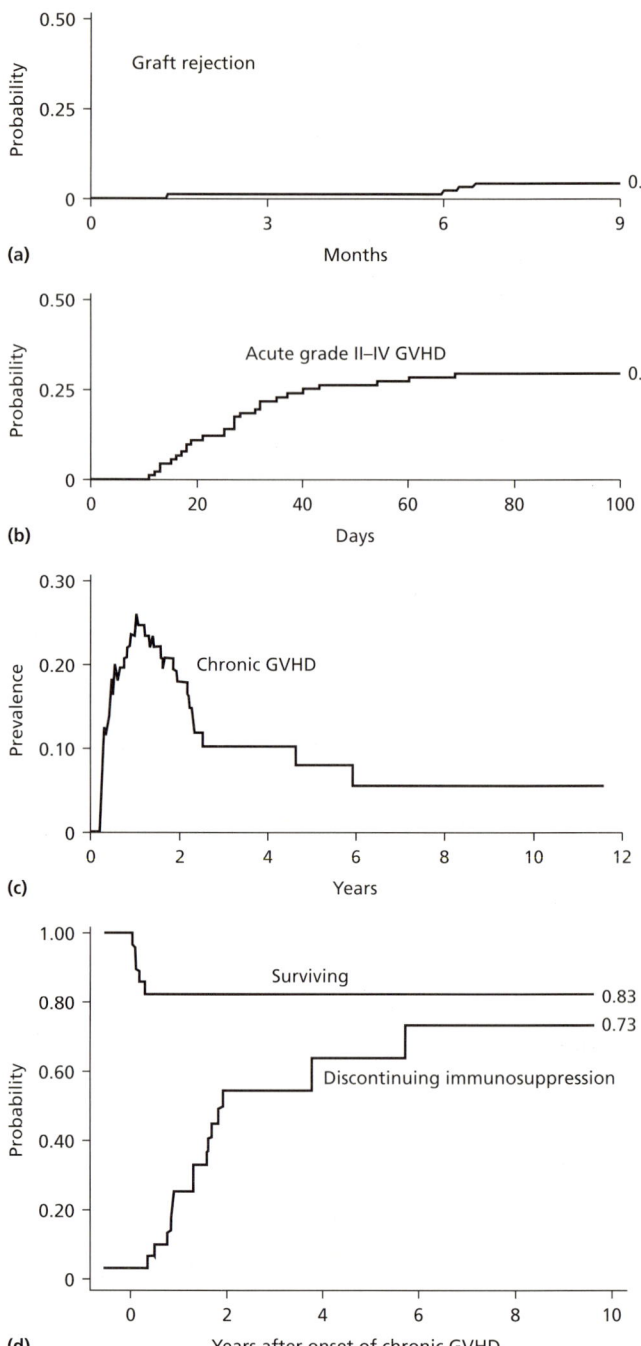

Fig. 71.4 Cumulative incidences of (a) graft rejection and (b) developing acute grade II–IV graft-vs.-host disease (GVHD) in 94 consecutive patients with aplastic anemia given human leukocyte antigen (HLA) identical marrow grafts following cyclophosphamide (CY) and antithymocyte globulin (ATG) conditioning and GVHD prophylaxis with methotrexate (MTX) and cyclosporine (CSP). (c) Prevalence of chronic GVHD. (d) Probability of surviving among the 29 patients with chronic GVHD and probability of discontinuing immunosuppression given for chronic GVHD. (Reproduced with permission from Storb et al. [50].)

1980s. The GITMO/EBMT study included predominantly younger patients, many of whom were not treated with a trial of immunosuppression prior to proceeding to allogeneic HSC transplant. In contrast, the updated multicenter trial of CY and ATG included older, heavily transfused patients whose prior treatment with immunsuppressive therapy had failed [50].

In addition to CY and ATG for conditioning following first graft rejection, there have been other anecdotal reports for treating graft failure. One patient at the FHCRC was successfully retransplanted using the anti-CD3 antibody BC3 and high-dose corticosteroids [52]. Another regimen included Campath I-G, a monoclonal antibody that reportedly eliminates radiation-resistant and CY-resistant host T cells [53]. One case report described the use of G-PBSC without reconditioning [54], and another center has employed the use of rabbit ATG [55] to overcome graft failure.

In summary, results from clinical trials to date indicate that combined CY and ATG conditioning followed by MTX and CSP as post-grafting immunosuppression is the most effective and reliable regimen to prevent marrow graft rejection following HLA-identical HCT for SAA. Similar survival might be obtained without ATG in younger, relatively untransfused patients. The use of the least toxic transplant regimen associated with the lowest incidence of graft rejection avoids the need for having to deal with this potentially life-threatening complication after transplant. For first transplants, the use of G-PBSC is not appropriate given the increased risk of chronic GVHD. Treatment guidelines for SAA include uniform adherence to the following:
1 the use of irradiated and leukodepleted blood products before transplant;
2 the well-established and well-tolerated conditioning regimen of CY and ATG;
3 infusion of $\geq 3.5 \times 10^8$ donor marrow cells/kg; and
4 combined MTX and CSP post-grafting immunosuppression.

Mixed donor–host hematopoietic chimerism

Transient mixed chimerism is common in patients after marrow allografts for AA. In one study almost 60% of patients had mixed chimerism in peripheral blood or bone marrow after HCT, and two-thirds of these eventually converted to complete donor-type hematopoiesis while the remainder rejected their grafts [56]. One other study showed that T-cell mixed chimerism in two patients conditioned with CY predated late graft failure [57]. In a larger study of 116 patients with AA transplanted from sex-mismatched HLA-identical siblings, 54% were mixed chimeras detected in either blood or marrow. While patients with mixed chimerism appeared to have a higher incidence of graft rejection (14%) than those who were complete chimeras (9%), this difference was not statistically significant [58]. Among patients who received MTX and CSP for GVHD prophylaxis there was no association between the presence of mixed chimerism and acute GVHD nor survival. T-cell chimerism can now be routinely determined after HCT. Whether chimerism analysis is useful to predict future graft rejection is yet unknown, but it is certainly an indispensable tool to monitor the kinetics of engraftment and the ultimate fate of the graft.

Acute graft-vs.-host disease (see Chapter 50)

Once engraftment has been accomplished acute GVHD may develop, usually within the first 6 weeks after HCT. Grade II–IV acute GVHD has a strong adverse effect on survival in patients transplanted for SAA. Early Seattle data showed an actuarial probability of survival at 11 years of 45% for SAA patients with preceding grade II–IV acute GVHD compared to 80% survival among patients with grades 0 and I acute GVHD [59]. Similarly, subsequent IBMTR data showed a 31% 5-year actuarial probability of survival for SAA patients with grades II–IV acute GVHD compared to 80% among patients with no or mild acute GVHD [60]. During the 1970s, MTX was the most commonly used agent given after HCT to prevent acute GVHD, and 35% of MTX-treated SAA patients developed grades II–IV acute GVHD [59].

Because of the high mortality associated with acute GVHD, a number of studies were carried out in the 1980s to investigate whether the incid-

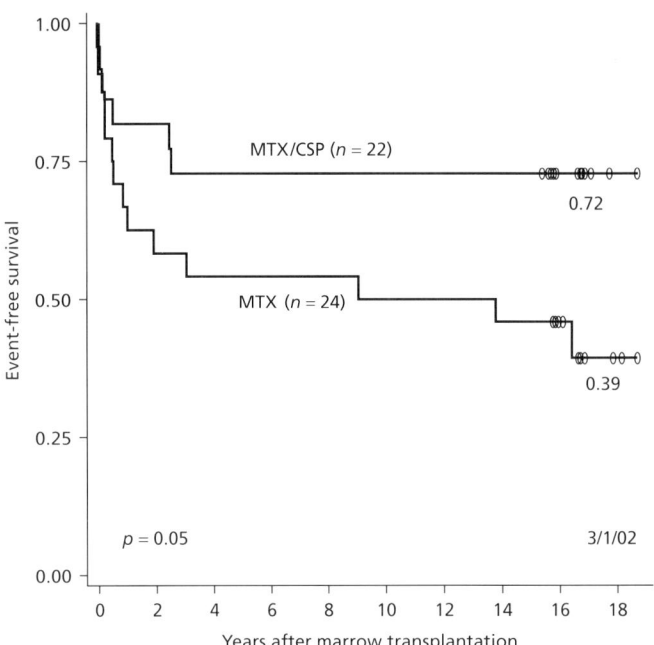

Fig. 71.5 Survival of patients given marrow grafts from human leukocyte antigen (HLA) identical siblings after conditioning with cyclophosphamide (CY). Shown are the results of a randomized prospective trial comparing methotrexate (MTX) alone vs. MTX and cyclosporine (CSP) for graft-vs.-host disease (GVHD) prophylaxis. Most of the patients enrolled in the trial were adults because of Food and Drug Administration restrictions. The data are current as of March 2002.

ence of this complication could be reduced and survival improved. CSP was initially studied as a single agent to prevent acute GVHD. Retrospective analyses showed that CSP favorably influenced survival of more recently transplanted SAA patients compared to historical control patients given MTX alone [61–65]. However, results of several controlled prospective randomized trials showed no significant differences in incidence of acute GVHD or in survival among leukemia patients given CSP compared to those given MTX as single agent prophylaxis [66,67].

A number of transplant centers combined prednisone (PSE) and CSP in hopes of improving control of acute GVHD. A recent randomized prospective study of patients with high-risk lymphohematopoietic malignancies has shown that the combination of CSP and PSE was only marginally better than CSP alone in preventing acute GVHD, but this came at the expense of a significant increase in chronic GVHD [68,69]. Another study of patients with leukemia or lymphoma found a combination of MTX, CSP and PSE more effective in preventing acute GVHD than CSP and PSE [70].

Encouraging data in experimental animals led, in 1981, to the introduction in the clinic of a combination of a short course of MTX (given on days 1, 3, 6 and 11 after HCT) combined with CSP. One randomized trial from Seattle showed a significant reduction in incidence and severity of acute GVHD in 22 SAA patients given the combination vs. 24 patients receiving MTX alone [25], and overall survival was higher in patients who received the combination of drugs (Fig. 71.5) [25,71]. Similar findings were made in patients with leukemia where the combination of MTX and CSP was found to be superior to CSP alone in preventing acute GVHD [72]. In a later nonrandomized retrospective analysis of IBMTR data from 595 patients with SAA who had received HCTs from matched siblings, patients who received either CSP alone or CSP with MTX compared to MTX alone had a statistically significant improved survival rate of 69% vs. 56%, respectively [60]. Importantly, no grade IV acute

GVHD was seen in patients given MTX and CSP. The reduction in acute GVHD resulted in improved survival, a finding that was especially impressive among pediatric patients with SAA [61]. One retrospective analysis suggested that optimal doses of both MTX and CSP were important in controlling acute GVHD [73]. Because of the success of the combination of MTX and CSP, a randomized study was carried out to compare MTX and CSP to CSP, MTX and PSE for patients with hematologic malignancies and SAA. Among patients with HLA-identical donors, the addition of PSE increased the risk of acute and chronic GVHD unless the PSE was administered after the completion of a short course of MTX [74]. A subsequent randomized trial of MTX and CSP vs. MTX, CSP and "late PSE" was completed in patients with leukemia which showed improved survival in the MTX and CSP arm ($p = 0.1$) [75].

The recently completed prospective randomized study by GITMO/EBMT confirmed the initial Seattle report and showed that the combination of MTX and CSP resulted in superior 5-year estimated survival compared to the use of CSP alone for SAA patients transplanted with an HLA-identical sibling marrow graft. The incidence of acute GVHD in the MTX and CSP group vs. CSP alone was 30% and 38%, respectively. The advantage in the observed survival, however, could not be ascribed to a reduction in the incidence of acute or chronic GVHD [51].

The updated results of the multicenter study with the Seattle regimen consisting of CY and ATG, HLA-identical marrow followed by combined MTX and CSP immunosuppression in 94 consecutive patients showed that the cumulative incidence of grades II–IV acute GVHD was 29% (Fig. 71.4b) [50]. The severity of GVHD observed was grade II (21%), grade III (7%) and grade IV (1%). Thus, despite the increased age of patients in the Seattle regimen study compared to the GITMO/EBMT study, the overall incidence of acute GVHD was equivalent in both studies. This finding suggests that the incorporation of ATG in the conditioning regimen may be effective in preventing acute GVHD, particularly in the older patient age groups. ATG may have an effect on deletion or depletion of the infused donor T cells.

Chronic graft-vs.-host disease (see Chapter 50)

While significant progress has been made in reducing the incidences of graft rejection and acute GVHD, chronic GVHD continues to be a major complication of marrow grafting for AA. Unlike the graft-vs.-leukemia effect associated with chronic GVHD that can improve survival of patients with leukemia, there is no benefit of chronic GVHD in patients transplanted with AA. Historically, the incidence of chronic GVHD varied depending on the patient groups studied. A few small series of children transplanted from HLA-identical siblings reported incidences of 0–25% [76–79], whereas the incidence was as high as 40–60% among other series that included adult patients and those who received supplemental buffy coat infusions [80,81]. In most current series of matched sibling transplants that included adults the incidence of chronic GVHD was around 30% [81–83] (see Table 71.1).

Early studies identified a history of acute GVHD as the most important risk factor for chronic GVHD [40,84]. Older patients also experienced more chronic GVHD. *De novo* chronic GVHD occurs without preceding acute GVHD. Besides donor buffy coat infusions, other risk factors including increased patient age and preceding corticosteroid therapy have been associated with *de novo* chronic GVHD development [40,85].

G-CSF mobilized PBSC appears to increase the risk of chronic GVHD which is more protracted and less responsive to treatment compared to bone marrow [44]. Because of the excellent overall survival of SAA patients after allogeneic marrow HCT, it will be very unlikely for future studies to demonstrate any significant benefit of utilizing T-cell-depleted or CD34-enriched PBSC over HLA-identical bone marrow as stem cell source. Therefore, for patients with SAA, bone marrow with a target cell dose of at least 3.5×10^8 nucleated cells per kilogram body weight remains the preferred source of stem cells.

Chronic GVHD is associated with significant morbidity and requires prolonged IST, although ultimately immunosuppression can be discontinued in most patients as chronic GVHD resolves [86]. Up to one-third of affected patients may die, often from infections. PSE, azathioprine, CY, procarbazine, CSP, thalidomide, MMF, tacrolimus (FK-506), extracorporeal photopheresis given either alone or in combination have all been used for treatment of chronic GVHD beginning in a systematic manner in 1976 (see Chapter 50) [86–91].

Recent evidence suggests that chronic GVHD is a risk factor for the development of solid tumors late after transplant. In addition, in the recent Seattle survey of long-term survivors after allogeneic transplantation for AA, chronic GVHD was a major risk factor for development of cataracts, lung disease, bone and joint disease and depression [92]. In the Seattle experience, since the introduction of the CY and ATG conditioning regimen and the discontinuation of added buffy coat cell infusions, the prevalence of chronic GVHD has significantly decreased. Chronic GVHD was not only less frequent but also appeared to be more responsive to therapy in patients conditioned with CY and ATG and given marrow alone compared to historical control patients treated with CY and marrow plus buffy coat. In the updated multicenter study report using the Seattle transplant regimen with HLA-identical sibling marrow grafts consisting of CY and ATG followed with MTX and CSP, the cumulative incidence of chronic GVHD observed was 32% (Fig. 71.4c) [50]. In most patients chronic GVHD responded to therapy with complete responses. Of the patients with chronic GVHD, 83% survived long-term (Fig. 71.4d). At a median of 2.6 years (range 1.5–10 years) after transplantation, 8% of patients still required IST for chronic GVHD.

The incidences of chronic GVHD in the GITMO/EBMT trial with CY conditioning and post-grafting immunosuppression with either CSP alone vs. MTX and CSP were 30% and 44%, respectively [51]. This difference in incidence of chronic GVHD was not significant. The majority of patients with chronic GVHD had limited disease of the skin; the overall incidence of extensive chronic GVHD was 9% [51]. Most of the patients in the GITMO/EBMT study were children, who have a lower incidence of chronic GVHD compared with adults.

Prompt diagnosis of chronic GVHD combined with aggressive initiation of IST with the combination of CSP and PSE has resulted in an apparent decrease in the duration of time needed for inducing remission of chronic GVHD and the overall response to treatment has improved over time. However, this improvement has not been associated with a significant increase in survival for patients with SAA who develop chronic GVHD [88,93]. Thus, mortality associated with chronic GVHD remains a significant problem for patients following allogeneic HCT. Figure 71.6 shows that the mortality rates after diagnosis of chronic GVHD did not change significantly over four different time periods among patients transplanted in Seattle.

These observations suggest that improvements in the prevention of chronic GVHD must be sought to further improve patient survival. Perhaps prompt diagnosis and treatment of chronic GVHD may help improve response to treatment and overall survival. However, in a randomized prospective study comparing CSP continued at "therapeutic levels" for 24 months vs. 6 months after HCT for patients at highest risk of developing chronic GVHD, e.g. those with preceding acute GVHD, corticosteroid therapy and older patients, there was no difference in overall survival between the two groups [89].

Taken together, current evidence indicates that the Seattle regimen of CY and ATG conditioning followed by HLA-identical marrow transplantation and combined MTX and CSP post-grafting immunosuppression appears to provide the lowest risks of graft rejection, acute and chronic GVHD compared to other transplantation regimens.

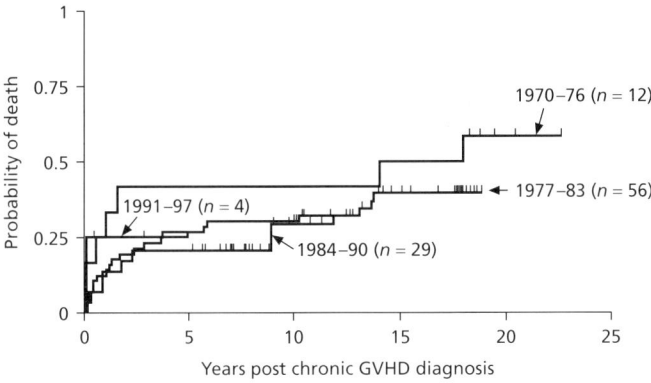

Fig. 71.6 Probability of death after diagnosis of chronic graft-vs.-host disease (GVHD) following human leukocyte antigen (HLA) identical marrow grafts conditioned with cyclophosphamide (CY) in Seattle over four different time periods. Tick marks indicate censoring times.

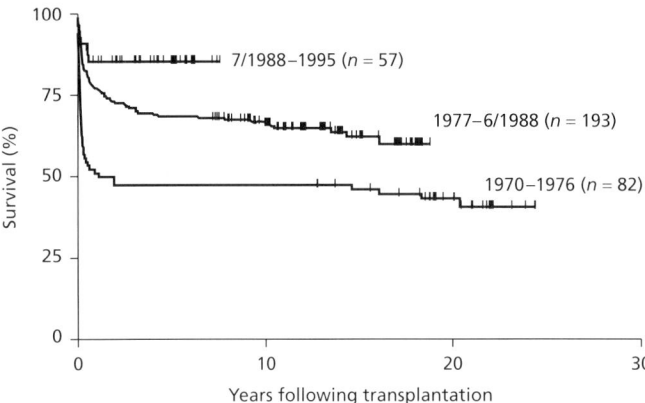

Fig. 71.7 Hematopoietic cell transplantation from human leukocyte antigen (HLA) identical family members after cyclophosphamide (CY). Overall survival indicated by transplant year cohort. The combination of methotrexate and cyclosporine was used for graft-vs.-host disease (GVHD) prophylaxis in some patients since 1981 and in all patients since 1985. Patients transplanted since July 1988 were conditioned with CY and antithymocyte globulin (ATG) without supplemental buffy coat cell infusions.

Interstitial pneumonia

The incidence of interstitial pneumonia occurring after transplantation in patients with SAA has decreased over time. In 1989, Weiner et al. [94] reviewed IBMTR data from 547 patients with AA receiving HLA-identical marrow grafts for the risk of interstitial pneumonia. They found an overall incidence of interstitial pneumonia of 17%. Cytomegalovirus (CMV) pneumonia affected 37% of patients, 22% had pneumonia from other organisms and in 41% of cases no organisms were identified. The case fatality rate was 64%. At that time, four factors predicted the development of interstitial pneumonia:
1 the use of MTX rather than CSP after HCT;
2 moderate to severe acute GVHD;
3 TBI compared to CY in the preparative regimen; and
4 increased patient age.

Results from 329 patients treated for SAA in Seattle from 1974 to 1990 showed the overall incidence of interstitial pneumonia was 16%. Forty-four percent of affected patients had CMV pneumonia, 37% had pneumonia resulting from a variety of other infectious organisms and 19% had pneumonia of unknown etiology. The overall mortality was 7%. TBI and acute GVHD were significant risk factors for the development of interstitial pneumonia, but there was no adverse influence of patient age or of MTX prophylaxis on the development of interstitial pneumonia [21]. More recent studies confirmed that grade II–IV acute GVHD was the major risk factor for the development of interstitial pneumonitis [95]. A recent study of idiopathic lung disease after transplant found that patients with AA conditioned with CY had a significantly lower incidence (less than 5%) than those transplanted for malignant diseases who were conditioned with TBI or BU-containing regimens (especially compared to malignancies such as non-Hodgkin's lymphoma) [96]. The case mortality rate for this study and an earlier Seattle study, both of which contained large numbers of patients with malignant diseases, was 71–74% [95,96]. Over time, avoidance of TBI, improved prophylaxis for acute GVHD with MTX and CSP, and improved supportive care including the prompt treatment of CMV antigenemia, have all contributed to the decreased incidence of interstitial pneumonitis. In the recent update of the patients with SAA treated with the Seattle regimen, two of 94 patients died of idiopathic interstitial pneumonia [50].

Survival

Overall survival has increased over the last 30 years. During the 1970s, survival rates of 40–60% were commonly seen, whereas the survival rates now range from 60 to 100% [16,97] (see Table 71.1). Figure 71.7 shows improved survival among Seattle patients transplanted after July 1988 (87%) compared to patients transplanted before 1977 (41%) and compared to patients transplanted between 1977 and 1988 (61%). All patients transplanted since 1985 received MTX and CSP for GVHD prophylaxis, and since 1988 all were conditioned with CY and ATG rather than CY alone. Updated results of the multicenter trial at Seattle, City of Hope National Medical Center, and Stanford University, employing the Seattle transplant regimen (CY and ATG conditioning, HLA-identical marrow HCT with combined MTX and CSP post-grafting immunosuppression) confirmed that with a median follow-up of 6 years (range 0.5–11.6 years), the survival rate was 88% [50]. In this study of 94 consecutive SAA patients, the median age was 26 and the range was 2–59 years.

The recently reported randomized GITMO/EBMT trial comparing CSP alone vs. combined MTX and CSP for patients conditioned with CY alone showed estimated 5-year 94% survival in the MTX and CSP group and 78% for those in the CSP alone group [51]. The difference in survival between the two groups was statistically significant. This study confirmed the initial Seattle results demonstrating the superiority of combined MTX and CSP post-grafting immunosuppression.

Analysis of transplant registry data has been helpful to identify important trends influencing survival over time. The reported results are in general less favorable than the optimal conditioning regimens reported by some transplant centers because multiple conditioning regimens are used by registry members some of which may be suboptimal. A retrospective multicenter multiregimen IBMTR study reported that 5-year survival after HLA-identical sibling transplants had increased from 48% in 1976–80 to 66% in 1988–92 [81]. Because of the introduction of CSP for GVHD prophylaxis, the risk of GVHD decreased. Improved long-term survival was because of decreased mortality in the first 3 months post-transplant. The incidence of reported graft failure did not significantly change, ranging from 20% in 1976–80 to 16% in 1988–92. However, only 9% of reported transplants in 1988–92 included CY and ATG conditioning.

Updated IBMTR data for 1699 patients receiving HLA-identical sibling transplants for SAA between 1991 and 1997 showed a 5-year probability of survival (95% confidence intervals) of 75% ± 3% for 874 patients ≤20 years of age, 68% ± 4% for 696 who were 21–39 years and 35% ± 18% for 129 who were 40 years or older [98]. Survival was highest in untransfused patients transplanted early in the course of their disease and who were without active infection at the time of transplant. Despite the demonstrated improvement in outcome with the Seattle regimen, only a minority of patients reported to the registry received CY and ATG conditioning with combined MTX and CSP post-grafting immunosuppression. It is likely that the recent IBMTR results were inferior to data from centers using the Seattle regimen because relatively few of the IBMTR centers had yet to adopt treatment with CY and ATG conditioning with combined MTX and CSP post-grafting immunosuppression.

EBMT data for 1799 patients receiving HLA-identical sibling transplant between 1971 and 1998 confirmed the IBMTR results. The year of the transplant and the age of the patient predicted outcome after HSC transplant. There has been a striking improvement in 5-year survival rates comparing patients transplanted before or after 1990. In the years 1990–98 actuarial survival was 77% for patients aged 16 years or less, 68% for those 17–40 years and 54% for patients older than 40 years. CY alone as conditioning and CSP with or without MTX for GVHD prophylaxis were given to 551 patients and their survival rate was 69%. Based on the EBMT registry data, antilymphocyte globulin (ALG) was added to the conditioning regimen in 28 patients and their survival was 87% [99].

Previously transfused patients aged 2–52 years (median 24.5 years) undergoing allogeneic HCT in Seattle between 1988 and 1993 who were conditioned with CY and ATG and who received MTX and CSP for GVHD prophylaxis had 5% graft failure, 15% acute GVHD (no grade IV GVHD), 34% chronic GVHD [83] and 92% survival at 3–8.2 years (median 5.2 years) (see Fig. 71.3). Three other studies found a survival of more than 85% of patients conditioned with CY and ATG [76,77,165]. In contrast, reports of patients conditioned with CY and irradiation had survival rates ranging from 60 to 78% [100,101], although follow-up on some of these reported studies was short. Pediatric patients (younger than 19 years) generally fared better than adult patients in four studies [21,61,76,77] with survival rates of 94–100% while another study [78] and an EBMT report [102] showed 73 and 63% survivals, respectively, among children.

Radiation-containing regimens were widely used in the late 1970s and 1980s because of their better immunosuppressive properties resulting in a decreased incidence of graft rejection. However, the use of radiation has been associated with the risks of interstitial pneumonia, growth impairment, development of secondary solid tumors (see later discussion) and lower overall survival compared to CY and ATG. Radiation is no longer recommended as an initial preparative component for patients with HLA-matched sibling donors.

Influence of etiology of aplastic anemia on the outcome of the marrow grafts

It is now well established that HCT can cure AA resulting from causes other than an idiopathic etiology. This finding has included patients with hepatitis-associated AA, Fanconi's anemia and dyskeratosis congenita. For hepatitis-associated AA, there was concern that liver damage caused by hepatitis might lead either to increased liver damage from CY or that the damaged liver might not be able to enzymatically activate CY. Neither of these concerns proved valid [103,104]. Marrow grafts were successful, even when CY was administered at times of highly abnormal liver function tests. Also, there were no long-term sequelae related to the HCT procedure in these patients. Survival was in excess of 80% [103].

Fanconi's anemia is covered in detail in Chapter 109, but is often included in reports describing patients with SAA. Fanconi's anemia is an autosomal recessive disease with progressive pancytopenia, chromosomal fragility and hypersensitivity to DNA cross-linking agents that can progress to acute leukemia. Currently, the only successful treatment for marrow failure in patients with Fanconi's anemia is HCT. Conditioning regimens used in the past to prepare Fanconi's anemia patients for transplantation have been associated with considerable toxicity and transplant-related mortality [105,106]. In addition, irradiation and high-dose CY are associated with a very high risk of secondary malignancies [107]. It has recently been recognized that unlike other AA patients, those with Fanconi's anemia can be conditioned with lower doses of CY than conventionally used because of their unusual sensitivity to toxicity from alkylating agents [108,109]. Results from Curitiba, Brazil and Seattle show that patients with Fanconi's anemia can be transplanted successfully without incorporation of irradiation into the conditioning regimen with substantially lower doses of CY than used in the past. Sixteen patients transplanted with 100 mg/kg CY and HLA-identical marrow with MTX and CSP post-grafting immunosuppression had 88% survival at 37 months and sustained donor engraftment in 94% of patients [110]. More recently, further dosage reduction of CY to 20 mg/kg/day given for 4 consecutive days has been successful in achieving durable donor engraftment accompanied with decreased toxicity and improved survival without decreased engraftment. An ongoing trial of step-wise CY dose reduction offers the possibility of further improvement in long-term outcome. Thus, the optimal dosage of CY that will allow sustained engraftment with minimal toxicity has yet to be determined.

Dyskeratosis congenita is a rare inherited syndrome of ectodermal dysplasia that is associated with AA in 50% of cases [111]. Eight patients with AA associated with dyskeratosis congenita received allogeneic HCT, but only one of four who survived beyond 50 days remained alive. Three patients died of pulmonary fibrosis, suggesting that while the AA can be corrected with HCT, the other disease manifestations are not [112]. Among the four patients who died before day 50, three died of fungal infections while neutropenic and one died of refractory GVHD [112].

HCT has also been used to treat SAA resulting from PNH and Diamond–Blackfan syndrome (see Chapter 72) [113–115]. Among nine patients transplanted for PNH, six were alive without evidence of disease 2–20 years after HCT [114]. Of four patients with Diamond–Blackfan syndrome, three were alive with normal hematopoiesis 3–10 years after HCT [115].

Late effects

Long-term survival

The long-term outcome among 212 patients transplanted for SAA has recently been reported [92]. Ninety-three percent of patients were conditioned with CY with or without ATG, and 89% were given transplants from HLA identical siblings (8% had mismatched related donors, 2% had unrelated donors and 1% had syngeneic donors). The 20-year survival among patients without chronic GVHD ($n = 125$) was 89% compared to 69% among those with chronic GVHD ($n = 86$). Of the 17 patients who died between 2.5 and 20.4 years after transplant, 13 had chronic GVHD while four did not [92]. Among the 13 patients with chronic GVHD, two died of human immunodeficiency virus (HIV) disease, five died of pulmonary failure (one from pulmonary complications of dyskeratosis congenita), three died of septicemia and three died of squamous cell carcinoma. Among the four patients who died without chronic GVHD, one died of suicide, one in an automobile accident, one of HIV disease and one of pulmonary complications from dyskeratosis congenita. All of the cases of HIV disease occurred before blood transfusion testing for HIV antibodies had become standard. Nearly all of the patients who survived beyond 2 years returned to a fully functional life [92].

Gonadal function and fertility (see Chapters 68 and 69)

Gonadal function in patients conditioned only with CY often returns to normal. Among 65 women between the ages of 13 and 25 years who received CY, all had evidence of recovery of ovarian function, whereas among women aged 26–38 years 37% developed primary ovarian failure [19,116–119]. These data suggested that older age was a risk factor for ovarian failure. Testicular function had returned to normal in most men aged 14–41 years who received CY only for conditioning [19]. Many successful pregnancies had been reported after conditioning regimens containing CY only. At 20 years post-transplant the probability that a female patient would become pregnant after transplantation for SAA was 47% and the probability that a male patient would father a child was 50% [92]. In contrast, pregnancy or fathering a child after conditioning with TBI were rare events [19].

Growth and development (see Chapter 68)

A recent study of hormonal function and growth after HCT found that children conditioned with CY only had normal height, normal thyroid and adrenal function, and no GH deficiency. However, in children given TBI as part of the conditioning, while prepubertal growth in the first 3 years after transplant was normal, the final height was lower than target height [120]. Therefore, TBI-containing regimens should be avoided in children if possible. Both children and adults treated with TBI-containing regimens were also more likely to develop thyroid dysfunction after transplantation [19], and these patients should be monitored with yearly thyroid function tests.

Secondary malignancies (see Chapter 70)

Since the first patients have been transplanted successfully for AA over 27 years ago, data have been accumulated on the incidence and types of secondary malignancies resulting from HCT. Generally, secondary malignancies following HCT are uncommon but they may be fatal. Deeg et al. [107] described results in 700 patients with AA who had an estimated 14% incidence of secondary malignancies at 20 years. The cancer risk among transplanted patients was ninefold higher than that among the general population [107]. Overall, 18 of 621 patients (excluding those with Fanconi's anemia) developed secondary malignancies a median of 91 months post-transplant. Of the tumors, five were lymphoid malignancies seen a median of 3 months after transplant, and 13 were solid tumors occurring a median of 99 months after transplant. Nine of the solid tumors were squamous cell carcinomas of the head and neck and most of these patients were cured following surgical resection. All of the patients with lymphoid malignancies have died, whereas only 46% of those with solid tumors have died. Significant risk factors for the development of secondary malignancies in this series included the use of azathioprine for chronic GVHD treatment, increased age and use of irradiation in the conditioning regimen [107]. With regimens not containing irradiation there was a cumulative incidence of secondary cancers at 10 years of 1.4% [121] compared to a 22% ($\pm$ 11%) incidence at 8 years [122] with radiation-containing regimens. Other studies have also implicated irradiation-based conditioning regimens as risk factors for late malignancies [20,123] and so these regimens should be avoided in HLA-identical HCT candidates.

Chronic GVHD is also a risk factor for the development of solid tumors after transplant for AA with an estimated 30% probability at 20 years for patients with both acute and chronic GVHD [92]. Carcinomas of the oropharyngeal mucosa developed in patients with a history of chronic GVHD. These findings were also confirmed in a larger study of 19,229 patients who had undergone transplantation between 1964 and 1992 that showed chronic GVHD was associated with a significantly increased risk of squamous cell carcinoma of the buccal cavity and skin [124]. The severity of chronic GVHD and duration of IST for chronic GVHD appear to be risk factors for secondary malignancy. These findings emphasize the importance of avoiding infusion of buffy coat or PBSC to prevent chronic GVHD in patients with SAA.

Nonmyeloablative conditioning regimens

Considerable interest has been generated recently with the development of nonmyeloablative or reduced intensity conditioning regimens which can decrease transplant-related mortality and permit successful allogeneic HCT of older or medically infirm patients with hematologic malignancies, renal cell cancer or inborn errors of metabolism (see Chapter 85) [49,125–129]. The current standard CY/ATG regimen for SAA is nonmyeloablative, although it is a more intensive conditioning regimen compared with the nonmyeloablative Seattle regimen of 90 mg/m^2 fludarabine and 2 Gy TBI. Whether or not an alternative conditioning regimen such as fludarabine or reduced-dose CY could be less toxic or better tolerated and yet as effective as CY/ATG for SAA patients remains to be determined. Given the historical experience with high rates of graft rejection for transfusion-sensitized SAA patients, the potential benefit of a slight reduction in conditioning regimen toxicity must be carefully balanced against the increased risk of complications associated with graft rejection. Recent experimental studies in the dog have emphasized the important role of post-grafting immunosuppression, not only for preventing GVHD but also for suppressing HVG reactions, thereby improving the rate of engraftment. In a canine model of nonmyeloablative conditioning and allogeneic HCT, the combination of MMF and CSP was superior to MTX and CSP in enhancing engraftment [48]. Thus, enhanced post-grafting immunosuppression may allow reduction in the intensity and toxicity of conditioning regimens in future years.

Grafts from alternative marrow donors

Transplantation of marrow obtained from unrelated or mismatched related donors has been less successful than the use of grafts from HLA-identical siblings. There are probably two major reasons for this discrepancy:
1 there is an increased risk of transplant-related complications because of the greater genetic disparity between donors and recipients; and
2 patients are not considered candidates for HCT from alternative donors until they have failed attempts at IST.

By this time, these patients are often refractory to platelet transfusions, have received multiple antibiotics because of life-threatening infections and are often severely infected at the time of transplantation. Perhaps, in order to improve patient survival, transplantation from alternative donors should be considered at earlier time points before patients become severely ill. Earlier transplantation from one HLA-antigen mismatched related and from unrelated donors in patients with chronic myeloid leukemia, for example, has resulted in long-term survival that may be comparable to that seen with HLA-identical sibling grafts (see Chapter 73) [130].

HLA nonidentical related donors (see Chapter 82)

Table 71.3 summarizes the results from patients who received marrow grafts from genotypically HLA nonidentical relatives. Data from Seattle and the EBMT group indicate that patients with HLA phenotypically matched related donors have better overall survival ranging from 64 to 100% than patients with HLA-mismatched related donors whose survival is generally 50% or less [131,132]. For patients with phenotypically HLA-matched donors, irradiation proved not to be a necessary component of the conditioning regimen, and survival of CY conditioned patients was similar to that of patients with HLA-identical siblings donors [131].

For patients with mismatched related donors conditioning with CY with or without ATG did not provide sufficient immunosuppression to prevent graft rejection in most patients, and none of the patients achieved long-term survival. High rates of acute and chronic GVHD occurred

Table 71.3 Hematopoietic cell transplantation from human leukocyte antigen (HLA) nongenotypically matched relatives.

Transplant team, reference	Year of report	Year of transplantation	Number of patients	Age range in years (median)	Conditioning regimen	GVHD prophylaxis	HLA match*	Graft failure (%)	GVHD (%) Acute grade II–IV	GVHD (%) Chronic	Survival (%)	Range of follow-up (years) (median)
Seattle [131]	1996	1970–93	8	2–30 (11)	CY + ATG	MTX, MTX + CSP, others	=	22	33	38	100	3–16 (10)
Seattle [131]	1996	1970–93	15	4–44 (18)	CY ± ATG	MTX, MTX + CSP, others	≠	71	16	100	0	(All died by 1 year)
Seattle [131]	1996	1970–93	16	3–29 (12)	CY + TBI	MTX, MTX + CSP, others	≠	14	78	25	50	2–9.5 (4.5)
Taipei [168]	1996	1991–95	6	6–38 (26)	CY + 8 Gy TBI	MTX + CSP	≠	0	66	0	66	0.7–4.0 (2.5)
Vancouver [82]	1995	1982–92	3	9, 14, 25	CY ± TBI or ± TLI	Varied	≠	0	0	100	33	2 (Duration of follow-up for 1 surviving patient)
Italy [169]	1993	1989	2	3, 5	CY + TAI + AraC + ALG	CSP	≠	0	0	0	100	2.3 (Duration of follow-up for both patients)
Milwaukee [170]	1989	—	9	2–12 (6)	CY ± TBI ± AraC	CSP + PSE, MTX, CSP, T-cell depletion	≠	33	0	50	44	0.08–5.4 (3)
EBMT†‡ [132]	1991	1970–89	11	<19	CY ± TBI ± ATG ± other	Varied	=	29	0	38	64	—
EBMT†‡ [132]	1991	1970–89	23	<15	CY ± TBI ± other	Varied	≠				4	—

AraC, cytosine arabinoside; ATG, antithymocyte globulin; CSP, cyclosporine; CY, cyclophosphamide; EBMT, European Bone Marrow Transplant Group; GVHD, graft-vs.-host disease; HLA, human leucocyte antigen; MTX, methotrexate; PSE, prednisone; TAI, thoracoabdominal irradiation; TBI, total body irradiation;
*=, HLA phenotypic match; ≠, HLA mismatched.
†Data for reference [132] also includes six patients with unrelated donors.
‡GVHD and graft failure from both HLA phenotypic matched and mismatched patient groups combined.
— Data not reported.

among those few patients who did engraft (see Table 71.3) [131]. For subsequently transplanted patients with HLA-mismatched related donors, the use of CY combined with TBI decreased the incidence of graft failure and increased survival, but pre- and peri-transplant infections and post-transplant GVHD have remained major problems [131]. The optimal dose of TBI for these patients to prevent rejection with a minimal amount of regimen-related toxicity is not known.

In some series there was the suggestion that increasing HLA disparity can adversely affect transplant outcome [131,132], consistent with findings in patients transplanted for leukemia [133,134]. Earlier reports also suggested that the greater the HLA disparity, the poorer the overall survival [135]. EBMT surveys showed 25% projected survival for one HLA-locus mismatched HCT, whereas Seattle data showed 50% survival for these patients [131,132]. Three studies indicated a less than 20% survival for two or more HLA-loci mismatched recipients [63,65,135]. In the Seattle study patients with more than one HLA-locus mismatch also had poor survival [131].

Unrelated donors (see Chapter 83)

Patients with AA who do not have suitably HLA-matched related donors receive IST as the first-line treatment of choice. They are considered candidates for unrelated donor HSC transplantation only if they fail to respond to IST. Historically, rates of transplant-related morbidity and mortality have been high. In a National Marrow Donor Program (NMDP) retrospective analysis of 141 patients transplanted between 1988 and 1995, the overall survival at a median of 36 months after transplant was 36% [136]. Eighty-six percent of these patients received a radiation-containing conditioning regimen, 74% received HLA-matched marrow while 26% received marrow mismatched for at least one HLA-A, -B or -DR antigen; 32% received T-cell-depleted marrow and all but 13% received a CSP-containing regimen to prevent GVHD. Eighty-nine percent achieved sustained engraftment, and 52% of patients developed grade II–IV acute GVHD.

In a pilot study, five patients received unrelated donor transplants following CY and ATG conditioning as used for recipients of HLA-identical donor marrow. Three patients experienced graft failure and only one patient survived long-term [137]. Other groups reported that high-dose irradiation regimens, although effective in achieving engraftment, resulted in an increased incidence of fatal organ toxicity without increasing the probability of survival.

A collaborative multicenter prospective NMDP-sponsored study was undertaken to define the minimum effective dose of TBI sufficient to achieve engraftment for patients with AA transplanted with unrelated donor marrow [138]. The starting dose of TBI was 6 Gy given after three doses of 30 mg/kg/day ATG, combined with four consecutive infusions of 50 mg/kg/day CY. The TBI dose was to be escalated in increments of 2 Gy if graft failure occurred in the absence of prohibitive toxicity, and de-escalated for toxicity in the absence of graft failure.

A total of 50 patients were enrolled: 38 patients received HLA-A, B- and DR-phenotypically matched marrow transplants and 12 patients received marrow from donors that differed by one HLA-antigen. The ages of the patients ranged from 1.3 to 46.5 years with a median age of 14.4 years. The time intervals from diagnosis to transplantation were 2.8–264 months with a median of 14.5 months. All patients had received multiple transfusions and a median of four courses of IST. All 20 patients treated with 6 or 4 Gy TBI, CY, ATG and HLA-matched marrow engrafted, and survival was 50%. Of the 13 patients receiving 2 Gy TBI, CY, ATG and HLA-matched marrow, one rejected and eight were alive. Severe pulmonary toxicity occurred in eight of 30 patients conditioned with 6 or 4 Gy TBI and in two of 13 patients conditioned with 2 Gy TBI. The incidence of acute GVHD was 61%, with three deaths attributable to

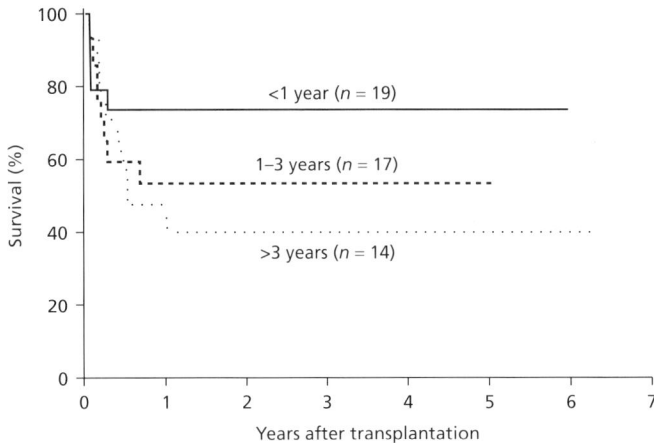

Fig. 71.8 Survival by pretransplantation disease duration for patients with aplastic anemia who underwent human leukocyte antigen (HLA) matched unrelated donor transplantation. The survival rate was 73% with a pretransplantation disease duration of <1 year (—), 53% for 1–3 years (- - -) and 39% for >3 years (·····) ($p = 0.32$). (Reproduced with permission from Deeg et al. [138].)

GVHD and infection. Chronic GVHD requiring therapy developed in 37% of evaluable patients [138].

Patients who underwent transplantation within 1 year of diagnosis had a 73% probability of survival, while patients who delayed transplantation beyond 3 years after initial diagnosis had 39% survival (Fig. 71.8). Age was an important risk factor for survival. Patients who were under the age of 20 years at the time of transplantation had a 67% survival compared with 43% for patients over 20 years old [138].

A phase 2 study with the conditioning regimen of 2 Gy TBI, CY and ATG is currently underway. Preliminary results confirm that 2 Gy TBI is sufficient to sustain engraftment from unrelated donors who are either HLA-matched or one minor HLA-antigen (non-Creg) mismatched without incurring excessive organ toxicity (H.J. Deeg, personal communication, June 2002).

The IBMTR data for unrelated donor HCT show that among 288 patients transplanted with unrelated donor marrow between 1991 and 1997, the 5-year survival probability was 44% ± 8% for those ≤20 years of age and 35% ± 12% for those 21–40 years of age [98]. As multiple suboptimal preparative regimens were used, the results are inferior to the new regimen identified by Deeg et al. for unrelated donor HCT. Most unrelated donor transplants were performed late in the course of disease after failure to respond to one or more courses of immunosuppression. Furthermore, in the near future it is anticipated that the widespread adoption of improved molecular techniques for HLA-typing will result in better outcomes for recipients of HLA-matched unrelated donor HCT [139].

Table 71.4 summarizes the marrow transplant results of patients who received marrow grafts from HLA-matched unrelated donors. In these studies, patients who were younger than 20 years had better survival. As with transplants using HLA-mismatched related donors, nonradiation-containing conditioning regimens provided insufficient immunosuppression to prevent rejection among patients receiving unrelated marrow grafts [137]. Although graft rejection was prevented with TBI doses of 10–14 Gy, the incidence of fatal toxicity diminished enthusiasm for these intensive regimens. Even with the use of TBI to prevent graft rejection, infections and GVHD still pose formidable risks for this group of patients. More recent studies have endeavored to achieve engraftment with less intensive TBI doses [138,140,141].

In summary, the NMDP-sponsored study reported by Deeg et al. showed improved outcome of patients transplanted less than 1 year after

Table 71.4 Hematopoietic cell transplantation (HCT) from unrelated donors.

Transplant team, reference	Year of report	Year of transplantation	Number of patients	Age range in years (median)	Conditioning regimen	GVHD prophylaxis	Graft failure (%)	GVHD (%) Acute grade II–IV	GVHD (%) Chronic	Survival (%)	Range of follow-up (years)* (median)
Milwaukee [171]	1996	1986–94	28	0.75–24 (8.5)	AraC ± CY ± 13.3–14 Gy TBI ± T-cell depletion	CSP	10	28	52	54	1.1–8.4 (2.75)
Seattle [137]	1996	—	5	17–23 (19)	CY + ATG	CSP + MTX	25	50	0	20†	1
IMUST [172]	1992	1981–90	40	1–41 (19)	CY ± TBI, CY ± TLI ± T-cell depletion	CSP + MTX, others	18	86	—	28	0.7–10.7
Seattle‡ [173]	1995	1985–94	34	4–47 (20.5)	CY + ATG, CY + TBI ± ATG	—	20	72	56	29	0.25–7.3
NMDP [174]	1993	1987–90	31	3–37.8 (21.1)	—	—	—	—	—	32§	(2.7)
London¶ [175]	1986	1981–86	8	11–32 (22)	CY ± ALG, CY ± TBI	CSP ± T-cell depletion	43	100	100	25	0.6–4.6
IBMTR [98]	2000	1991–97	298	0–40	—	—	—	—	—	44% ≤ 20 year. 35% age 21–40	0.2–5.0 (—)
NMDP** [138]	2001	1994–99	50	1.3–46 (14)	2–6 Gy TBI + CY + ATG	MTX + CSP	2	61	37	58††	1.0–6.3 (3.25)
Nagoya [140]	2001	1993–2000	15	3–19 (11)	5 Gy TBI + CY + ATG	MTX + CSP/FK-506	0	33	7	100	0.2–7.2 (4.25)
London/Bristol [141]	2001	1995–2000	8	0.6–15 (7.2)	Campath IG + CY + 3 Gy TBI	MTX + CSP	0	25	0	100	0.9–5.9 (1.4)
JMDP‡‡ [176]	2002	1993–2000	154	1–46 (17)	TBI/LFI + CY ± ATG	MTX + CSP/FK-506	11	29.3%	30%	56	0.25–6.8 (2.4)

AraC, cytosine arabinoside; ALG, antilymphocyte antigen; ATG, antithymocyte globulin; CSP, cyclosporine; CY, cyclophosphamide; GVHD, graft-vs.-host disease; IBMTR, International Bone Marrow Transplant Registry; IMUST, International Marrow Unrelated Search and Transplant study (includes some Seattle patients); JMDP, Japanese Marrow Donor Program; LFI, limited field irradiation; MTX, methotrexate; NMDP, National Marrow Donor Program; TBI, total body irradiation.

*Single time points represent survivals at that instance.
†All survivors with marrow aplasia or hypoplasia.
‡Includes patients in [137].
§Four of 10 survivors are transfusion dependent.
¶Six out of eight patients were transplanted from HLA-mismatched unrelated donors.
**Includes 12 HLA-mismatched unrelated donors.
††89% of patients aged <20 years transplanted within 1 year of diagnosis are surviving.
‡‡79 donor pairs matched at HLA-A, -B, -DRB1 loci by DNA-typing, 75 mismatched (DNA typing showed 51 mismatched at one HLA-locus, 12 at two or more loci)
— Data not reported.

diagnosis and identified a conditioning regimen of 2 Gy TBI, CY and ATG that achieved reliable engraftment with significantly decreased organ toxicity [138]. These results combined with the recent advances in molecular HLA-typing suggest that patients who have unrelated donors fully HLA-matched for class I and II, including HLA-C, by high-resolution DNA-based typing may have superior long-term outcome with HCT over IST. If a high-resolution HLA-matched donor is identified, then unrelated donor HCT should be considered early in the course of treatment of patients with SAA. Because of the time interval involved in the donor search, unrelated donor HCT is unlikely to be used as first-line therapy for acquired SAA. However, patients could proceed to unrelated donor HCT within 4 months if response to IST was unsatisfactory. As with the HLA-identical sibling setting, transfusion with leukodepleted irradiated blood products pretransplant is critical to decrease the risk of graft rejection. Although confirmatory data are lacking, younger patients (≤35 years of age) with 1-HLA antigen minor mismatched donors could also proceed to bone marrow transplantation if treatment with one or possibly more optimal IST regimens had failed [138].

Nontransplant therapy

The value of immunosuppressive agents for the treatment of AA was first described by Mathé et al. in Paris in 1970 [142]. They observed recovery of autologous hematopoiesis in patients conditioned with ALG administered in preparation for transplants of marrow from HLA-mismatched donors. Later prospective studies showed that the mismatched marrow graft did not contribute to the responsiveness, and subsequently ALG or ATG were used alone to treat patients with AA. More recently, CSP with or without corticosteroids was added to ATG or ALG [143]. A combination of ATG, CSP and G-CSF has shown promising results [144,145].

In a study of 100 patients with SAA treated with a combination of ALG, CSP, PRE and G-CSF as first-line therapy, trilineage hematopoietic recovery was seen in 77 patients after one or more courses of ALG treatment. Fifty percent of patients responded to one course of IST. The actuarial probability of discontinuing CSP was 38%, which indicated that most patients remained dependent on CSP at a median follow-up period of 3.9 years. Cytogenetic abnormalities were seen in 11% of patients and relapse of marrow aplasia in 9%. Actuarial survival at 5 years was 87%: 76% for patients with neutrophil counts $<0.2 \times 10^9$/L at the time of treatment and 98% for patients with neutrophil counts $>0.2 \times 10^9$/L. The 19 patients who did not achieve a white blood cell count of 5×10^9/L during G-CSF treatment had a low probability of responding to IST and had a mortality rate of 42%. The results suggested that poor response to G-CSF was an important predictor of early mortality with IST and that those patients warranted early transplantation from alternative HSC donors [145].

The role of G-CSF in the nontransplant treatment of SAA remains uncertain. In a recent study, children treated with ATG, CSP, danazol and G-CSF identified duration of G-CSF therapy greater than 120 days and failure of response to therapy at 6 months as a risk factor for subsequent progression to MDS or AML [146].

Alternative treatment to ATG or ALG and CSP has also been explored. In a study that extended over 9 years, 10 patients were treated with a high dose of 180 mg/kg CY without marrow rescue, and seven patients responded with increases in peripheral blood counts so that they no longer met the criteria for SAA. Six patients were alive and without relapse or clonal disorders with a median follow-up of 10.8 years [147]. A more recent study of 19 patients treated with 50 mg/kg/day CY for 4 consecutive days without CSP but with G-CSF support reported an 84% probability of 2-year survival and a 65% probability of complete remission at 4 years [148]. Recovery of neutrophil counts was delayed and the median time to independence from transfusion of red blood cells and platelets was 11 months. However, a randomized trial conducted at the National Institutes of Health (NIH) that compared high-dose CY with ATG (both treatment groups included CSP) was terminated early because of excessive infectious mortality in the CY group [149]. In the NIH study, CY induced prolonged pancytopenia, particularly in patients with a pretreatment absolute neutrophil counts greater than 0.5×10^9/L, which contributed to the increased risk of infectious deaths. The authors concluded that high-dose CY without allogeneic HSC transplantation was a dangerous choice for treatment of AA. In a subsequent report of late complications, relapse of disease and clonal evolution of cytogenetic abnormalities occurred in both ATG and CY treatment groups [150]. Given these results, high-dose CY alone without subsequent HSC transplant is unlikely to become a widely used alternative IST regimen for the treatment of SAA.

Several reports have compared the effectiveness of conventional IST to HCT. Table 71.5 summarizes the results of six of these studies. In the two largest studies, there was a clear survival benefit for patients who underwent HCT, especially for those under 40 years of age [33,64]. In a third study there was a survival advantage of HCT compared to IST for patients transplanted in the last 5 years of the study, but not for patients transplanted in the earlier years of the study [151]. Two studies that examined survival by age group did not demonstrate an advantage of HCT or IST for older patients [33,64]. In a long-term study of 100 consecutive children under the age of 17 years with SAA, the Nagoya transplant team confirmed that HCT was superior to IST [152].

Figure 71.9 demonstrates the survival of 168 HCT patients compared to 227 IST patients from Seattle. In this study, as in most others, many of the patients treated with HCT already had failed initial IST [33]. Overall survival in this study at 15 years was 69% for the HCT patients and 38% for patients receiving IST ($p < 0.001$) [33]. The higher overall survival with HCT compared to IST is seen in all groups of patients under 40 years of age (Fig. 71.10). For patients over 40 years of age the long-term survival with IST or HCT was less than 40% and there was no statistical difference ($p > 0.2$), although the number of patients in this age group treated with HCT was small and many of these older patients were transplanted prior to the development of the CY plus ATG conditioning regimen [33].

In contrast to the results from Seattle, a retrospective survival analysis was completed based on initial treatment offered to patients with SAA reported to the EBMT registry from 1974 to 1996 [99]. Outcome was primarily affected by neutrophil counts at the time of treatment and patient age. Patients up to age 20 had consistently superior 5-year survival with HCT. Adults between the ages of 20–40 years with neutrophil counts below 0.3×10^9/L had better 5-year survival with HCT. For patients with neutrophil counts greater than 0.3×10^9/L, the predicted 5-year survival was comparable to HCT or slightly superior with IST. For patients over 40 years, IST offered a better survival advantage than HCT at 5 years of follow-up. However, this recommendation carries the caveat that the majority of patients reported to the registry database did not receive what is now considered the optimal transplant regimen, CY and ATG conditioning with infusion of HLA-identical bone marrow and combined MTX and CSP post-grafting immunosuppression. As suggested by the more recent Seattle studies, it is very likely that older patients over age 40 have long-term survival benefit from allogeneic HCT if treated with the optimal transplant regimen. In Seattle, patients up to age 65 with SAA and an HLA-identical marrow donor are considered potential candidates for HCT.

One important difference between IST and HCT is that immunosuppression may not correct the underlying marrow abnormality. About 30% of IST patients may relapse, i.e. have a return of their marrow aplasia, and a substantial proportion may develop clonal abnormalities including MDS and acute myeloid leukemia (AML) [23,153,154]. In a recent

Table 71.5 Immunosuppressive therapy (IST) vs. hematopoietic cell transplantation (HCT) survival.

Transplant team, reference	Number of patients		Timepoint at which survival was measured (years)	IST (%)	BMT (%)
	IST	BMT			
Toronto [177]*	22	9	5	82	80
Seattle (overall) [33]	227	168	15	38	69
age <6 years	25	12	15	51	100
age 6–19 years	62	63	15	38	75
age 20–39 years	73	82	15	44	65
age ≥40 years	67	11	15	36	25
UCLA, Sloan-Kettering, MD Anderson [151]†	146	55	6	49	52
EBMT [64]‡					
age ≤20 years	115	134	6	38	64
age ≥20 years	130	77	6	82	62
Nagoya [152]					
age ≤17 years	63	37	10–14	55	97

EBMT, European Group for Blood and Marrow Transplantation; UCLA, University of California at Los Angeles.

*In this study all patients were initially treated with corticosteroids and antithymocyte globulin (ATG) and some later with cyclosporine before receiving a matched sibling transplant if a donor was available. In all other studies only a proportion of patients who received BMT initially failed immunosuppression with ATG.

†For patients treated with BMT in the last 5 years of the study, there was a statistically significant improvement in the outcome of BMT compared to IST. Some of the patients treated with IST had moderate aplastic anemia (AA) while all patients treated with BMT had severe aplastic anemia (SAA) or very severe AA.

‡Updated EBMT data available with interactive statistical survival models at the following website: http://www.ebmt.org/4Registry/registry5.html

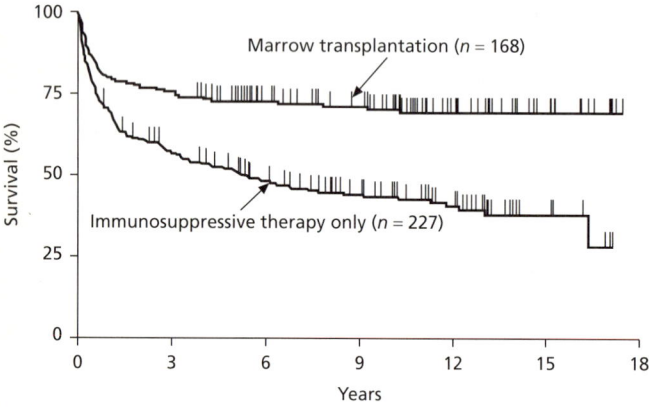

Fig. 71.9 Actuarial survival after therapy for aplastic anemia. Survival of 168 patients who received marrow hematopoietic cell transplantation (HCT) from human leukocyte antigen (HLA) matched related donors compared to 227 patients who received immunosuppressive therapy (IST). Tick marks indicate censoring times of surviving patients. (Adapted from Doney et al. [33].)

report of 50 children treated with a combination of G-CSF and CSP, 22% developed MDS or AML [155]. In another study of immunosuppression with ATG and CSP, survival was 72% at 2 years but 10% of patients had developed PNH [156]. One study by Socié et al. [154] compared the incidence of secondary malignancies among patients with HCT vs. IST. Forty-two malignancies were noted in 860 patients receiving IST while nine were reported in 748 patients who received HCTs. Overall, the 10-year cumulative incidence of cancer was 18.8% after IST while the rate was 3.1% after HCT. In this study, MDS and acute leukemia were seen exclusively in patients treated with IST while the incidence of solid tumors after IST vs. HCT was similar [154]. The relatively high incidence of malignancies after IST was in agreement with earlier work by Tichelli et al. [157] who reported an incidence of PNH, MDS and acute leukemia as high as 57% at 8 years after treatment. Thus, long-term survival curves after IST have as yet not become stable in distinction to those after HCT.

Conclusions

There are at least two reasons for the improved survival of patients with AA who were treated by HLA-identical HCT. One is the decreased incidence of graft rejection. The decline in rejection has resulted from the more judicious use of transfusions before HCT, the removal of sensitizing white blood cells from transfusion products, and improvements in the immunosuppressive qualities of the conditioning programs used to prepare patients for transplantation. Irradiation-based programs have been effective but at the price of more transplant-related complications, and the CY and ATG combination is just as successful in preventing rejection with better long-term survival. With regard to transfusions before HCT, in vitro irradiation of all blood products may further reduce the risk of sensitization to minor histocompatibility antigens in the future [28,30]. The second reason for improved survival has been a decrease in the incidence and severity of acute GVHD through the introduction of

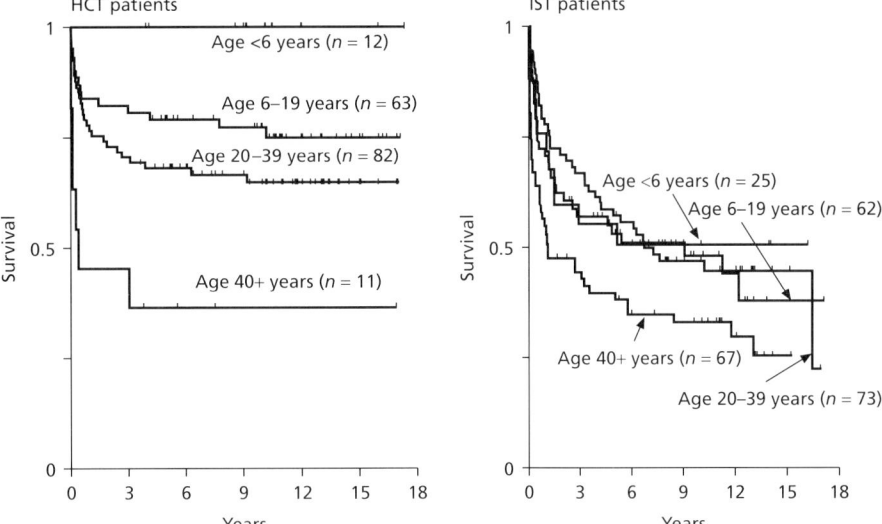

Fig. 71.10 The effect of age on actuarial survival by treatment group. The p-values for survival of patients treated with marrow hematopoietic cell transplantation (HCT) vs. immunosuppressive therapy (IST) are as follows: age <6 years ($p = 0.006$), ages 6–19 years ($p = 0.001$), ages 20–39 years ($p = 0.04$) and age >40 ($p > 0.2$). p-Values were calculated using the log–rank test and are two-sided. Tick marks indicate censoring times of surviving patients. (Adapted from Doney et al. [33].)

better GVHD prevention regimens, e.g. combined MTX and CSP. The incidence of chronic GVHD may be decreasing, but mortality from it has not changed much despite prompt therapy. Therefore, better ways of preventing chronic GVHD are necessary. As more patients become long-term survivors, the problem of long-term sequelae from the initial conditioning programs and from certain post-grafting immunosuppressive agents, e.g. azathioprine, must be considered, in particular secondary cancer. In future studies, perhaps less toxic conditioning programs can be developed. Radiation-based regimens should not be used in HLA-identical recipients because of the higher likelihood of inducing secondary cancer, the deleterious effect on fertility, and the potential detrimental effects on growth and development for pediatric patients.

For patients without HLA-matched sibling donors, transplantation from HLA-mismatched related donors or unrelated donors should be considered. Prompt initiation of an unrelated donor search is needed after diagnosis of SAA in case there is failure to respond to IST within 4 months. Radiation appears to be an essential part of the currently used conditioning regimen for patients with alternative donors to prevent rejection. Recent results with unrelated donor marrow transplantation indicate that 2 Gy TBI, CY and ATG conditioning and combined MTX and CSP post-grafting immunosuppression is sufficient to prevent graft rejection and avoid TBI-induced organ toxicity [138]. The use of molecular-based methods for identifying optimally HLA-matched unrelated donors appears to be critical to further improve survival after transplant.

References

1 Jandl JH. *Blood Textbook of Hematology*, 2nd edn. Boston: Little, Brown, 1996.
2 Szklo M, Sensenbrenner L, Markowitz J, Weida S, Warm S, Linet M. Incidence of aplastic anemia in metropolitan Baltimore: a population-based study. *Blood* 1985; **66**: 115–9.
3 Camitta BM, Thomas ED, Nathan DG et al. A prospective study of androgens and bone marrow transplantation for treatment of severe aplastic anemia. *Blood* 1979; **53**: 504–14.
4 Camitta B, O'Reilly RJ, Sensenbrenner L et al. Anti-thoracic duct lymphocyte globulin therapy of severe aplastic anemia. *Blood* 1983; **62**: 883–8.
5 Fonseca R, Tefferi A. Practical aspects in the diagnosis and management of aplastic anemia. *Am J Med Sci* 1997; **313**: 159–69.
6 Khatib Z, Wilimas J, Wang W. Outcome of moderate aplastic anemia in children. *Am J Ped Hematol Oncol* 1994; **16**: 80–5.
7 International Agranulocytosis and Aplastic Anemia Study. Incidence of aplastic anemia: the relevance of diagnostic criteria. *Blood* 1987; **70**: 1718–21.
8 Yardley-Jones A, Anderson D, Parke DV. The toxicity of benzene and its metabolism and molecular pathology in human risk assessment. *Br J Indust Med* 1991; **48**: 437–44 [Review].
9 Thomas ED, Phillips JH, Finch CA. Recovery from marrow failure following isogenic marrow infusion. *J Am Med Assoc* 1964; **188**: 1041–3.
10 Champlin RE, Feig SA, Sparkes RS, Gale RP. Bone marrow transplantation from identical twins in the treatment of aplastic anemia: implication for the pathogenesis of the disease. *Br J Haematol* 1984; **56**: 455–63.
11 Pillow RP, Epstein RB, Buckner CD, Giblett ER, Thomas ED. Treatment of bone-marrow failure by isogeneic marrow infusion. *N Engl J Med* 1966; **275**: 94–7.
12 Thomas ED, Rudolph RH, Fefer A, Storb R, Slichter S, Buckner CD. Isogeneic marrow grafting in man. *Exp Hematol* 1971; **21**: 16–8.
13 Holmberg LA, Seidel K, Leisenring W, Torok-Storb B. Aplastic anemia: analysis of stromal cell function in long-term marrow cultures. *Blood* 1994; **84**: 3685–90.
14 Hathaway WE, Fulginiti VA, Pierce CW et al. Graft-vs.-host reaction following a single blood transfusion. *J Am Med Assoc* 1967; **201**: 1015–20.
15 Parkman R, Mosier D, Umansky I, Cochran W, Carpenter CB, Rosen FS. Graft-versus-host disease after intrauterine and exchange transfusions for hemolytic disease of the newborn. *N Engl J Med* 1974; **290**: 359–63.
16 Storb R, Thomas ED, Buckner CD et al. Allogeneic marrow grafting for treatment of aplastic anemia. *Blood* 1974; **43**: 157–80.
17 Storb R, Thomas ED, Weiden PL et al. Aplastic anemia treated by allogeneic bone marrow transplantation: a report on 49 new cases from Seattle. *Blood* 1976; **48**: 817–41.
18 Thomas ED, Buckner CD, Storb R et al. Aplastic anemia treated by marrow transplantation. *Lancet* 1972; **1**: 284–9.
19 Sanders JE and the Seattle Marrow Transplant Team. The impact of marrow transplant preparative regimens on subsequent growth and development. *Semin Hematol* 1991; **28**: 244–9.
20 Witherspoon RP, Fisher LD, Schoch G et al. Secondary cancers after bone marrow transplantation for leukemia or aplastic anemia. *N Engl J Med* 1989; **321**: 784–9.
21 Storb R, Longton G, Anasetti C et al. Changing trends in marrow transplantation for aplastic anemia. *Bone Marrow Transplant* 1992; **10**: 45–52 [Review].
22 Hinterberger W, Rowlings PA, Hinterberger-Fischer M et al. Results of transplanting bone marrow from genetically identical twins into patients with aplastic anemia. *Ann Intern Med* 1997; **126**: 116–22.
23 Thomas ED, Storb R. Acquired severe aplastic anemia: progress and perplexity. *Blood* 1984; **64**: 325–8.
24 Hows JM, Marsh JC, Yin JL et al. Bone marrow transplantation for severe aplastic anemia using cyclosporin: long-term follow-up. *Bone Marrow Transplant* 1989; **4**: 11–6.
25 Storb R, Deeg HJ, Farewell V et al. Marrow transplantation for severe aplastic anemia: methotrexate alone compared with a combination of methotrexate and cyclosporine for prevention of acute graft-versus-host disease. *Blood* 1986; **68**: 119–25.

26 Stucki A, Leisenring W, Sandmaier BM, Sanders J, Anasetti C, Storb R. Decreased rejection and improved survival of first and second marrow transplants for severe aplastic anemia (a 26-year-old retrospective analysis). *Blood* 1998; **92**: 2742–9.

27 McCann SR, Bacigalupo A, Gluckman E et al. Graft rejection and second bone marrow transplants for acquired aplastic anemia: a report from the Aplastic Anemia Working Party of the European Bone Marrow Transplant Group. *Bone Marrow Transplant* 1994; **13**: 233–7.

28 Storb R, Raff RF, Appelbaum FR, Schuening FW, Sandmaier BM, Graham TC. The influence of transfusions from unrelated DLA-matched or mismatched donors upon marrow grafts between DLA-identical canine littermates. *Transplantation* 1988; **46**: 334–6 [Brief communication].

29 Storb R, Epstein RB, Rudolph RH, Thomas ED. The effect of prior transfusion on marrow grafts between histocompatible canine siblings. *J Immunol* 1970; **105**: 627–33.

30 Storb R, Deeg HJ. Failure of allogeneic canine marrow grafts after total body irradiation: allogeneic "resistance" vs. transfusion induced sensitization. *Transplantation* 1986; **42**: 571–80.

31 Storb R, Thomas ED, Buckner CD et al. Marrow transplantation in thirty "untransfused" patients with severe aplastic anemia. *Ann Intern Med* 1980; **92**: 30–6.

32 Anasetti C, Doney KC, Storb R et al. Marrow transplantation for severe aplastic anemia: long-term outcome in fifty "untransfused" patients. *Ann Intern Med* 1986; **104**: 461–6.

33 Doney K, Leisenring W, Storb R, Appelbaum FR, for the Seattle Bone Marrow Transplant Team. Primary treatment of acquired aplastic anemia: outcomes with bone marrow transplantation and immunosuppressive therapy. *Ann Intern Med* 1997; **126**: 107–15.

34 Kalhs P, White JS, Gervassi A, Storb R, Bean MA. *In vitro* recall of proliferative and cytolytic responses to minor histocompatibility antigens by dendritic cell enriched canine peripheral blood mononuclear cells. *Transplantation* 1995; **59**: 112–8.

35 Bean MA, Storb R, Graham T et al. Prevention of transfusion-induced sensitization to minor histocompatibility antigens on DLA-identical canine marrow grafts by gamma irradiation of marrow donor blood. *Transplantation* 1991; **52**: 956–60.

36 Bean MA, Graham T, Appelbaum FR et al. Gamma radiation of blood products prevents rejection of subsequent DLA-identical marrow grafts: tolerance vs. abrogation of sensitization to non-DLA antigens. *Transplantation* 1996; **61**: 334–5.

37 Schuening F, Bean MA, Deeg HJ, Storb R. Prevention of graft failure in patients with aplastic anemia. *Bone Marrow Transplant* 1993; **12**: S48–S49.

38 Storb R, Prentice RL, Thomas ED. Marrow transplantation for treatment of aplastic anemia: an analysis of factors associated with graft rejection. *N Engl J Med* 1977; **296**: 61–6.

39 Storb R, Doney KC, Thomas ED et al. Marrow transplantation with or without donor buffy coat cells for 65 transfused aplastic anemia patients. *Blood* 1982; **59**: 236–46.

40 Storb R, Prentice RL, Sullivan KM et al. Predictive factors in chronic graft-versus-host disease in patients with aplastic anemia treated by marrow transplantation from HLA-identical siblings. *Ann Intern Med* 1983; **98**: 461–6.

41 Niederwieser D, Pepe M, Storb R, Loughran TP Jr, Longton G, for the Seattle Marrow Transplant Team. Improvement in rejection, engraftment rate and survival without increase in graft-versus-host disease by high marrow cell dose in patients transplanted for aplastic anemia. *Br J Haematol* 1988; **69**: 23–8.

42 Deeg HJ, Self S, Storb R et al. Decreased incidence of marrow graft rejection in patients with severe aplastic anemia: changing impact of risk factors. *Blood* 1986; **68**: 1363–8.

43 Korbling M, Anderlini P. Peripheral blood stem cell versus bone marrow allotransplantation: does the source of hematopoietic stem cells matter? *Blood* 2001; **98**: 2900–8.

44 Flowers MED, Parker PM, Johnston LJ et al. Comparison of chronic graft-versus-host disease after transplantation of peripheral blood stem cells versus bone marrow in allogeneic recipients: long-term follow-up of a randomized trial. *Blood* 2002; **100**: 415–9.

45 Storb R, Floersheim GL, Weiden PL et al. Effect of prior blood transfusions on marrow grafts: abrogation of sensitization by procarbazine and antithymocyte serum. *J Immunol* 1974; **112**: 1508–16.

46 Weiden PL, Storb R, Slichter S, Warren RP, Sale GE. Effect of six weekly transfusions on canine marrow grafts: tests for sensitization and abrogation of sensitization by procarbazine and antithymocyte serum. *J Immunol* 1976; **117**: 143–50.

47 Storb R, Etzioni R, Anasetti C et al. Cyclophosphamide combined with antithymocyte globulin in preparation for allogeneic marrow transplants in patients with aplastic anemia. *Blood* 1994; **84**: 941–9.

48 Storb RYuC, Wagner JL et al. Stable mixed hematopoietic chimerism in DLA-identical littermate dogs given sublethal total body irradiation before and pharmacological immunosuppression after marrow transplantation. *Blood* 1997; **89**: 3048–54.

49 McSweeney PA, Niederwieser D, Shizuru JA et al. Hematopoietic cell transplantation in older patients with hematologic malignancies: replacing high-dose cytotoxic therapy with graft-versus-tumor effects. *Blood* 2001; **97**: 3390–400.

50 Storb R, Blume KG, O'Donnell MR et al. Cyclophosphamide and antithymocyte globulin to condition patients with aplastic anemia for allogeneic marrow transplantations: the experience in four centers. *Biol Blood Marrow Transplant* 2001; **7**: 39–44.

51 Locatelli F, Bruno B, Zecca M et al. Cyclosporin A and short-term methotrexate versus cyclosporin A as graft versus host disease prophylaxis in patients with severe aplastic anemia given allogeneic bone marrow transplantation from an HLA-identical sibling: results of a GITMO/EBMT randomized trial. *Blood* 2000; **96**: 1690–7.

52 Bjerke JW, Lorenz J, Martin PJ, Storb R, Hansen JA, Anasetti C. Treatment of graft failure with anti-CD3 antibody BC3, glucocorticoids and infusion of donor hematopoietic cells. *Blood* 1995; **86**: 107a [Abstract].

53 Or R, Mehta J, Kapelushnik J et al. Total lymphoid irradiation, anti-lymphocyte globulin and Campath 1-G for immunosuppression prior to bone marrow transplantation for aplastic anemia after repeated graft rejection. *Bone Marrow Transplant* 1994; **13**: 97–9.

54 Redei I, Waller EK, Holland HK, Devine SM, Wingard JR. Successful engraftment after primary graft failure in aplastic anemia using G-CSF mobilized peripheral stem cell transfusions. *Bone Marrow Transplant* 1997; **19**: 175–7.

55 Yoshida Y, Ichinoe T, Dodo M et al. Successful bone marrow transplantation with rabbit anti-human thymocyte globulin in aplastic anemia: report of a case previously treated with equine anti-human lymphocyte globulin. *Int J Hematol* 1994; **60**: 79–83.

56 Hill RS, Petersen FB, Storb R et al. Mixed hematologic chimerism after allogeneic marrow transplantation for severe aplastic anemia is associated with a higher risk of graft rejection and a lessened incidence of acute graft-versus-host disease. *Blood* 1986; **67**: 811–6.

57 Casado LF, Steegmann JL, Pico M et al. Study of chimerism in long-term survivors after bone marrow transplantation for severe acquired aplastic anemia. *Bone Marrow Transplant* 1996; **18**: 405–9.

58 Huss R, Deeg HJ, Gooley T et al. Effect of mixed chimerism on graft-versus-host disease, disease recurrence, and survival after HLA-identical marrow transplantation for aplastic anemia or chronic myelogenous leukemia. *Bone Marrow Transplant* 1996; **18**: 767–76.

59 Storb R, Prentice RL, Buckner CD et al. Graft-versus-host disease and survival in patients with aplastic anemia treated by marrow grafts from HLA-identical siblings: beneficial effect of a protective environment. *N Engl J Med* 1983; **308**: 302–7.

60 Gluckman E, Horowitz MM, Champlin RE et al. Bone marrow transplantation for severe aplastic anemia: influence of conditioning and graft-versus-host disease prophylaxis regimens on outcome. *Blood* 1992; **79**: 269–75.

61 Storb R, Sanders JE, Pepe M et al. Graft-versus-host disease prophylaxis with methotrexate/cyclosporine in children with severe aplastic anemia treated with cyclophosphamide and HLA-identical marrow grafts. *Blood* 1991; **78**: 1144–5 [Letter].

62 Hows J, Palmer S, Gordon-Smith EC. Cyclosporine and graft failure following bone marrow transplantation for severe aplastic anemia. *Br J Haematol* 1985; **60**: 611–7.

63 Bacigalupo A, Van Lint MT, Congiu M, Marmont AM. Bone marrow transplantation (BMT) for severe aplastic anemia (SAA) in Europe: a report of the EBMT-SAA Working Party. *Bone Marrow Transplant* 1988; **3**: 44–5.

64 Bacigalupo A, Hows J, Gluckman E et al. Bone marrow transplantation (BMT) versus immunosuppression for the treatment of severe aplastic anemia (SAA): a report of the EBMT SAA Working Party. *Br J Haematol* 1988; **70**: 177–82.

65 Bacigalupo A, Hows J, Gordon-Smith EC et al. Bone marrow transplantation for severe aplastic anemia from donors other than HLA identical siblings: a report of the BMT Working Party. *Bone Marrow Transplant* 1988; **3**: 531–5.

66 Storb R, Deeg HJ, Fisher LD et al. Cyclosporine vs. methotrexate for graft-v-host disease prevention in patients given marrow grafts for leukemia: long-term follow-up of three controlled trials. *Blood* 1988; **71**: 293–8.

67 Ringden O, Backman L, Lonnqvist B et al. A randomized trial comparing use of cyclosporin and methotrexate for graft-versus-host disease

67. prophylaxis in bone marrow transplant recipients with hematologic malignancy. *Bone Marrow Transplant* 1986; **1**: 41–51.
68. Deeg HJ, Lin D, Leisenring W *et al*. Cyclosporine or cyclosporine plus methylprednisolone for prophylaxis of graft-versus-host disease: a prospective, randomized trial. *Blood* 1997; **89**: 3880–7.
69. Deeg HJ, Flowers MED, Leisenring W, Appelbaum FR, Martin PJ, Storb RF. Cyclosporine (CSP) or CSP plus methylprednisolone for graft-versus-host disease prophylaxis in patients with high-risk lymphohemopoietic malignancies: long-term follow-up of a randomized trial. *Blood* 2000; **96**: 1194–5 [Letter].
70. Chao NJ, Schmidt GM, Niland JC *et al*. Cyclosporine, methotrexate, and prednisone compared with cyclosporine and prednisone for prophylaxis of acute graft-versus-host disease. *N Engl J Med* 1993; **329**: 1225–30.
71. Storb R, Leisenring W, Deeg HJ *et al*. Long-term follow-up of a randomized trial of graft-versus-host disease prevention by methotrexate/cyclosporine versus methotrexate alone in patients given marrow grafts for severe aplastic anemia. *Blood* 1994; **83**: 2749–50 [Letter].
72. Storb R, Deeg HJ, Whitehead J *et al*. Methotrexate and cyclosporine compared with cyclosporine alone for prophylaxis of acute graft versus host disease after marrow transplantation for leukemia. *N Engl J Med* 1986; **314**: 729–35.
73. Nash RA, Pepe MS, Storb R *et al*. Acute graft-versus-host disease: analysis of risk factors after allogeneic marrow transplantation and prophylaxis with cyclosporine and methotrexate. *Blood* 1992; **80**: 1838–45.
74. Storb R, Pepe M, Anasetti C *et al*. What role for prednisone in prevention of acute graft-versus-host disease in patients undergoing marrow transplants? *Blood* 1990; **76**: 1037–45.
75. Chao NJ, Snyder DS, Jain M *et al*. Equivalence of two effective graft-versus-host disease prophylaxis regimens: results of a prospective double-blind randomized trial. *Biol Blood Marrow Transplant* 2000; **6**: 254–61.
76. Bunin N, Leahey A, Kamani N, August C. Bone marrow transplantation in pediatric patients with severe aplastic anemia: cyclophosphamide and anti-thymocyte globulin conditioning followed by recombinant human granulocyte-macrophage colony stimulating factor. *J Pediatr Hematol Oncol* 1996; **18**: 68–71.
77. Azuma E, Kojima S, Kato K *et al*. Conditioning with cyclophosphamide/antithymocyte globulin for allogeneic bone marrow transplantation from HLA-matched siblings in children with severe aplastic anemia. *Bone Marrow Transplant* 1997; **19**: 1085–7.
78. Makipernaa A, Saarinen UM, Siimes MA. Allogeneic bone marrow transplantation in children: single institution experience from 1974 to 1992. *Acta Paediatr* 1995; **84**: 683–8.
79. Sanders JE, Storb R, Anasetti C *et al*. Marrow transplant experience for children with severe aplastic anemia. *Am J Pediatr Hematol Oncol* 1994; **16**: 43–9.
80. Anasetti C, Storb R, Longton G *et al*. Donor buffy coat cell infusion after marrow transplantation for aplastic anemia. *Blood* 1988; **72**: 1099–100 [Letter].
81. Passweg JR, Socié G, Hinterberger W *et al*. Bone marrow transplant for severe aplastic anemia: has outcome improved? *Blood* 1997; **90**: 858–64.
82. Cuthbert RJ, Shepherd JD, Nantel SH *et al*. Allogeneic bone marrow transplantation for severe aplastic anemia: the Vancouver experience. *Clin Invest Med* 1995; **18**: 122–30.
83. Storb R, Leisenring W, Anasetti C *et al*. Long-term follow-up of allogeneic marrow transplants in patients with aplastic anemia conditioned by cyclophosphamide combined with antithymocyte globulin. *Blood* 1997; **89**: 3890–1 [Letter].
84. Atkinson K, Horowitz MM, Gale RP *et al*. Risk factors for chronic graft-versus-host disease after HLA-identical sibling bone marrow transplantation. *Blood* 1990; **75**: 2459–64.
85. Niederwieser D, Pepe M, Storb R, Witherspoon R, Longton G, Sullivan K. Factors predicting chronic graft-versus-host disease and survival after marrow transplantation for aplastic anemia. *Bone Marrow Transplant* 1989; **4**: 151–6.
86. Sullivan KM, Agura E, Anasetti C *et al*. Chronic graft-versus-host disease and other late complications of bone marrow transplantation. *Semin Hematol* 1991; **28**: 250–9.
87. Furlong T, Leisenring W, Storb R *et al*. Psoralen and ultraviolet A irradiation (PUVA) as therapy for steroid-resistant cutaneous acute graft-versus-host disease. *Biol Blood Marrow Transplant* 2002; **8**: 206–12.
88. Koc S, Leisenring W, Flowers MED *et al*. Therapy for chronic graft-versus-host disease: a randomized trial comparing cyclosporine plus prednisone versus prednisone alone. *Blood* 2002; **100**: 48–51.
89. Kansu E, Gooley T, Flowers MED *et al*. Administration of cyclosporine for 24 months compared with 6 months for prevention of chronic graft-versus-host disease: a prospective randomized clinical trial. *Blood* 2001; **98**: 3868–70 [Brief report].
90. Koc S, Leisenring W, Flowers MED *et al*. Thalidomide for treatment of patients with chronic graft-versus-host disease. *Blood* 2000; **96**: 3995–6.
91. Nash RA, Furlong T, Storb R *et al*. Mycophenolate mofetil (MMF) as salvage treatment for graft-versus-host-disease (GVHD) after allogeneic hematopoietic stem cell transplantation (HSCT): safety analysis. *Blood* 1997; **90** (Suppl. 1): 105a [Abstract].
92. Deeg HJ, Leisenring W, Storb R *et al*. Long-term outcome after marrow transplantation for severe aplastic anemia. *Blood* 1998; **91**: 3637–45.
93. Goerner M, Gooley T, Flowers MED *et al*. Morbidity and mortality of chronic GVHD after hematopoietic stem cell transplantation from HLA-identical siblings for patients with aplastic or refractory anemias. *Biol Blood Marrow Transplant* 2002; **8**: 47–56.
94. Weiner RS, Horowitz MM, Gale RP *et al*. Risk factors for interstitial pneumonia following bone marrow transplantation for severe aplastic anemia. *Br J Haematol* 1989; **71**: 535–43.
95. Crawford SW, Longton G, Storb R. Acute graft-versus-host disease and the risks for idiopathic pneumonia after marrow transplantation for severe aplastic anemia. *Bone Marrow Transplant* 1993; **12**: 225–31.
96. Kantrow SP, Hackman RC, Boeckh M, Myerson D, Crawford SW. Idiopathic pneumonia syndrome: changing spectrum of lung injury after marrow transplantation. *Transplantation* 1997; **63**: 1079–86.
97. Bortin MM, Rimm AA. Treatment of 144 patients with severe aplastic anemia using immunosuppression and allogeneic marrow transplantation: a report from the International Bone Marrow Registry. *Transplant Proc* 1981; **13**: 227–33.
98. Horowitz MM. Current status of allogeneic bone marrow transplantation in acquired aplastic anemia. *Semin Hematol* 2000; **37**: 30–42 [Review].
99. Bacigalupo A, Brand R, Oneto R *et al*. Treatment of acquired severe aplastic anemia: bone marrow transplantation compared with immunosuppressive therapy. The European Group for Blood and Marrow Transplantation experience. *Semin Hematol* 2000; **37**: 69–80 [Review].
100. Castro-Malaspina H, Childs B, Laver J *et al*. Hyperfractionated total lymphoid irradiation and cyclophosphamide for preparation of previously transfused patients undergoing HLA-identical marrow transplantation for severe aplastic anemia. *Int J Radiat Oncol Biol Phys* 1994; **29**: 847–54.
101. Champlin RE, Ho WG, Nimer SD *et al*. Bone marrow transplantation for severe aplastic anemia: effect of a preparative regimen of cyclophosphamide-low-dose total-lymphoid irradiation and post-transplant cyclosporine–methotrexate therapy. *Transplantation* 1990; **49**: 720–4.
102. Locasciulli A, van't Veer L, Bacigalupo A *et al*. Treatment with marrow transplantation or immunosuppression of childhood acquired severe aplastic anemia: a report from the EBMT SAA Working Party. *Bone Marrow Transplant* 1990; **6**: 211–7.
103. Witherspoon RP, Storb R, Shulman H *et al*. Marrow transplantation in hepatitis-associated aplastic anemia. *Am J Hematol* 1984; **17**: 269–78.
104. Feig SA, Champlin R, Arenson E *et al*. Improved survival following bone marrow transplantation for aplastic anemia. *Br J Haematol* 1983; **54**: 509–17.
105. Hows J, Chappel M, Marsh JCW, Durrane S, Yin JL, Swirsky D. Bone marrow transplantation for Fanconi's anemia: the Hammersmith experience. *Bone Marrow Transplant* 1989; **4**: 629–34.
106. Gluckman E, Devergie A, Dutreix J. Bone marrow transplantation for Fanconi anemia. In: Schroeder-Kurth TM, Auerbach AD, Obe G, eds. *Fanconi Anemia: Clinical, Cytogenetic and Experimental Aspects*. Berlin, Heidelberg: Springer-Verlag, 1989: 60–7.
107. Deeg HJ, Socié G, Schoch G *et al*. Malignancies after marrow transplantation for aplastic anemia and Fanconi anemia: a joint Seattle and Paris analysis of results in 700 patients. *Blood* 1996; **87**: 386–92.
108. Flowers MED, Zanis J, Pasquini R *et al*. Marrow transplantation for Fanconi anemia: conditioning with reduced doses of cyclophosphamide without radiation. *Br J Haematol* 1996; **92**: 699–706.
109. Flowers MED, Doney KC, Storb R *et al*. Marrow transplantation for Fanconi anemia with or without leukemic transformation: an update of the Seattle experience. *Bone Marrow Transplant* 1992; **9**: 167–73.
110. Medeiros C, Zanis-Neto J, Pasquini R. Bone marrow transplantation for patients with Fanconi anemia: reduced doses of cyclophosphamide without irradiation as conditioning. *Bone Marrow Transplant* 1999; **24**: 849–52.
111. Trowbridge AA, Sirinavin C, Linman JW. Dyskeratosis congenita: hematologic evaluation of a sibship and review of the literature. *Am J Hematol* 1977; **3**: 143–52.
112. Langston AA, Sanders JE, Deeg HJ *et al*. Allogeneic marrow transplantation for aplastic anemia associated with dyskeratosis congenita. *Br J Haematol* 1996; **92**: 758–65.

113 Szer J, Deeg HJ, Witherspoon RP et al. Long-term survival after marrow transplantation for paroxysmal nocturnal hemoglobinuria with aplastic anemia. *Ann Intern Med* 1984; **101**: 193–5.

114 Kawahara K, Witherspoon RP, Storb R. Marrow transplantation for paroxysmal nocturnal hemoglobinuria. *Am J Hematol* 1992; **39**: 283–8.

115 Greinix HT, Storb R, Sanders JE et al. Long-term survival and cure after marrow transplantation for congenital hypoplastic anemia (Diamond–Blackfan syndrome). *Br J Haematol* 1993; **84**: 515–20.

116 Sanders JE, Buckner CD, Amos D et al. Ovarian function following marrow transplantation for aplastic anemia or leukemia. *J Clin Oncol* 1988; **6**: 813–18.

117 Jacobs P, Dubovsky DW. Bone marrow transplantation followed by normal pregnancy. *Am J Hematol* 1981; **11**: 209–12.

118 Hinterberger-Fischer M, Kier P, Kalhs P et al. Fertility, pregnancies and offspring complications after bone marrow transplantation. *Bone Marrow Transplant* 1991; **7**: 5–9.

119 Schmidt H, Ehninger G, Dopfer R, Waller HD. Pregnancy after bone marrow transplantation for severe aplastic anemia. *Bone Marrow Transplant* 1987; **2**: 329–32.

120 Clement-De Boers A, Oostdijk W, Van Weel-Sipman MH, Van den Broeck J, Wit JM, Vossen JM. Final height and hormonal function after bone marrow transplantation in children. *J Pediatr* 1996; **129**: 544–50.

121 Witherspoon RP, Storb R, Pepe M, Longton G, Sullivan KM. Cumulative incidence of secondary solid malignant tumors in aplastic anemia patients given marrow grafts after conditioning with chemotherapy alone. *Blood* 1992; **79**: 289–92 [Letter].

122 Socié G, Henry-Amar M, Cosset JM, Devergie A, Girinsky T, Gluckman E. Increased incidence of solid malignant tumors after bone marrow transplantation for severe aplastic anemia. *Blood* 1991; **78**: 277–9.

123 Pierga JY, Socié G, Gluckman E et al. Secondary solid malignant tumors occurring after bone marrow transplantation for severe aplastic anemia given thoraco-abdominal irradiation. *Radiother Oncol* 1994; **30**: 55–8.

124 Curtis RE, Rowlings PA, Deeg HJ et al. Solid cancers after bone marrow transplantation. *N Engl J Med* 1997; **336**: 897–904.

125 Giralt S, Estey E, Albitar M et al. Engraftment of allogeneic hematopoietic progenitor cells with purine analog-containing chemotherapy: harnessing graft-versus-leukemia without myeloablative therapy. *Blood* 1997; **89**: 4531–6.

126 Slavin S, Nagler A, Naparstek E et al. Nonmyeloablative stem cell transplantation and cell therapy as an alternative to conventional bone marrow transplantation with lethal cytoreduction for the treatment of malignant and nonmalignant hematologic diseases. *Blood* 1998; **91**: 756–63.

127 Sykes M, Preffer F, McAfee S et al. Mixed lymphohaemopoietic chimerism and graft-versus-lymphoma effects after nonmyeloablative therapy and HLA-mismatched bone-marrow transplantation. *Lancet* 1999; **353**: 1755–9.

128 Childs R, Chernoff A, Contentin N et al. Regression of metastatic renal-cell carcinoma after nonmyeloablative allogeneic peripheral-blood stem-cell transplantation. *N Engl J Med* 2000; **343**: 750–8.

129 Kottaridis PD, Milligan DW, Chopra R et al. In vivo CAMPATH-1H prevents graft-versus-host disease following nonmyeloablative stem cell transplantation. *Blood* 2000; **96**: 2419–25.

130 Hansen JA, Gooley TA, Martin PJ et al. Bone marrow transplants from unrelated donors for patients with chronic myeloid leukemia. *N Engl J Med* 1998; **338**: 962–8.

131 Wagner JL, Deeg HJ, Seidel K et al. Bone marrow transplantation for severe aplastic anemia from genotypically HLA-nonidentical relatives: an update of the Seattle experience. *Transplantation* 1996; **61**: 54–61.

132 Locasciulli A, van't Veer L, Hows J et al. Bone marrow transplantation (BMT) in children with severe aplastic anemia (SAA) from donors other than HLA identical siblings. EBMT Working Party on Severe Aplastic Anemia. *Bone Marrow Transplant* 1991; **7** (Suppl. 3): 90–1.

133 Beatty PG, Clift RA, Mickelson EM et al. Marrow transplantation from related donors other than HLA-identical siblings. *N Engl J Med* 1985; **313**: 765–71.

134 Anasetti C, Amos D, Beatty PG et al. Effect of HLA compatibility on engraftment of bone marrow transplants in patients with leukemia or lymphoma. *N Engl J Med* 1989; **320**: 197–204.

135 Beatty PG, Di Bartolomeo P, Storb R et al. Treatment of aplastic anemia with marrow grafts from related donors other than HLA genotypically matched siblings. *Clin Transplant* 1987; **1**: 117–24.

136 Deeg HJ, Seidel K, Casper J et al. Marrow transplantation from unrelated donors for patients with severe aplastic anemia who have failed immunosuppressive therapy. *Biol Blood Marrow Transplant* 1999; **5**: 243–52.

137 Deeg HJ, Anasetti C, Petersdorf E et al. Cyclophosphamide plus ATG conditioning is insufficient for sustained hematopoietic reconstitution in patients with severe aplastic anemia transplanted with marrow from HLA-A, B, DRB matched unrelated donors. *Blood* 1994; **83**: 3417–8 [Letter].

138 Deeg HJ, Amylon MD, Harris RE et al. Marrow transplants from unrelated donors for patients with aplastic anemia: minimum effective dose of total body irradiation. *Biol Blood Marrow Transplant* 2001; **7**: 208–15.

139 Petersdorf EW, Hansen JA, Martin PJ et al. Major-histocompatibility-complex class I alleles and antigens in hematopoietic-cell transplantation. *N Engl J Med* 2001; **345**: 1794–800.

140 Kojima S, Inaba J, Yoshimi A et al. Unrelated donor marrow transplantation in children with severe aplastic anemia using cyclophosphamide, anti-thymocyte globulin and total body irradiation. *Br J Haematol* 2001; **114**: 706–11.

141 Vassiliou GS, Webb DK, Pamphilon D, Knapper S, Veys PA. Improved outcome of alternative donor bone marrow transplantation in children with severe aplastic anemia using a conditioning regimen containing low-dose total body irradiation, cyclophosphamide and Campath. *Br J Haematol* 2001; **114**: 701–5.

142 Mathé G, Amiel JL, Schwarzenberg L et al. Bone marrow graft in man after conditioning by antilymphocytic serum. *Br Med J* 1970; **2**: 131–6.

143 Frickhofen N, Kaltwasser JP, Schrezenmeier H et al. Treatment of aplastic anemia with antilymphocyte globulin and methylprednisolone with or without cyclosporine. *N Engl J Med* 1991; **324**: 1297–304.

144 Bacigalupo A, Broccia G, Corda G et al. Anti-lymphocyte globulin, cyclosporin, and granulocyte colony-stimulating factor in patients with acquired severe aplastic anemia (SAA): a pilot study of the EBMTT SAA working party. *Blood* 1995; **85**: 1348–53.

145 Bacigalupo A, Bruno B, Saracco P et al. Anti-lymphocyte globulin, cyclosporine, prednisolone, and granulocyte colony-stimulating factor for severe aplastic anemia: an update of the GITMO/EBMT study on 100 patients. European Group for Blood and Marrow Transplantation (EBMT) Working Party on Severe Aplastic Anemia and the Gruppo Italiano Trapianti di Midolio Osseo (GITMO). *Blood* 2000; **95**: 1931–4.

146 Kojima S, Ohara A, Tsuchida M et al. Risk factors for evolution of acquired aplastic anemia into myelodysplastic syndrome and acute myeloid leukemia after immunosuppressive therapy in children. *Blood* 2002; **100**: 786–90.

147 Brodsky RA, Sensenbrenner LL, Jones RJ. Complete remission in severe aplastic anemia after high-dose cyclophosphamide without bone marrow transplantation. *Blood* 1996; **87**: 491–4.

148 Brodsky RA, Sensenbrenner LL, Smith BD et al. Durable treatment-free remission after high-dose cyclophosphamide therapy for previously untreated severe aplastic anemia. *Ann Intern Med* 2001; **135**: 477–83.

149 Tisdale JF. Dunn DE, Geller N et al. High-dose cyclophosphamide in severe aplastic anemia: a randomised trial. *Lancet* 2000; **356**: 1554–9.

150 Tisdale JF, Maciejewski JP, Nuñez O, Rosenfeld SJ, Young NS. Late complications following treatment for severe aplastic anemia (SAA) with high-dose cyclophosphamide (Cy): follow-up of a randomized trial. *Blood* 2002; **100**: 4668–70.

151 Paquette RL, Tebyani N, Frane M et al. Long-term outcome of aplastic anemia in adults treated with antithymocyte globulin: comparison with bone marrow transplantation. *Blood* 1995; **85**: 283–90.

152 Kojima S, Horibe K, Inaba J et al. Long-term outcome of acquired aplastic anemia in children: comparison between immunosuppressive therapy and bone marrow transplantation. *Br J Haematol* 2000; **111**: 321–8.

153 Schrezenmeier H, Marin P, Raghavachar A et al. Relapse of aplastic anemia after immunosuppressive treatment: a report from the European Bone Marrow Transplantation Group SAA Working Party. *Br J Haematol* 1993; **85**: 371–7.

154 Socié G, Henry-Amar M, Bacigalupo A et al. Malignant tumors occurring after treatment of aplastic anemia. *N Engl J Med* 1993; **329**: 1152–7.

155 Ohara A, Kojima S, Hamajima N et al. Myelodysplastic syndrome and acute myelogenous leukemia as a late clonal complication in children with acquired aplastic anemia. *Blood* 1997; **90**: 1009–13.

156 Rosenfeld SJ, Kimball J, Vining D, Young NS. Intensive immunosuppression with antithymocyte globulin and cyclosporine as treatment for severe acquired aplastic anemia. *Blood* 1995; **85**: 3058–65.

157 Tichelli A, Gratwohl A, Wursch A, Nissen C, Speck B. Late haematological complications in severe aplastic anemia. *Br J Haematol* 1988; **69**: 413–8.

158 Smith BR, Guinan EC, Parkman R et al. Efficacy of a cyclophosphamide-procarbazine-antithymocyte serum regimen for prevention of graft rejection following bone marrow transplantation for

159 Sanders JE, Whitehead J, Storb R et al. Bone marrow transplantation experience for children with aplastic anemia. *Pediatrics* 1986; **77**: 179–86.

160 Ramsay NK, Kim TH, McGlave P et al. Total lymphoid irradiation and cyclophosphamide conditioning prior to bone marrow transplantation for patients with severe aplastic anemia. *Blood* 1983; **62**: 622–6.

161 McGlave PB, Haake R, Miller W, Kim T, Kersey J, Ramsay NKC. Therapy of severe aplastic anemia in young adults and children with allogeneic bone marrow transplantation. *Blood* 1987; **70**: 1325–30.

162 Champlin RE, Horowitz MM, van Bekkum DW et al. Graft failure following bone marrow transplantation for severe aplastic anemia: risk factors and treatment results. *Blood* 1989; **73**: 606–13.

163 Gluckman E, Socié G, Devergie A, Bourdeau-Esperou H, Traineau R, Cosset JM. Bone marrow transplantation in 107 patients with severe aplastic anemia using cyclophosphamide and thoraco-abdominal irradiation for conditioning: long-term follow-up. *Blood* 1991; **78**: 2451–5.

164 Buckley JD, Chard RL, Baehner RL et al. Improvement in outcome for children with acute nonlymphocytic leukemia. A report from the Childrens Cancer Study Group. *Cancer* 1989; **63**: 1457–65.

165 Horstmann M, Stockschlaeder M, Kruger W et al. Cyclophosphamide/antithymocyte globulin conditioning of patients with severe aplastic anemia transfused patients with aplastic anemia. *Transplantation* 1985; **39**: 671–3.

for marrow transplantation from HLA-matched siblings: preliminary results. *Ann Hematol* 1995; **71**: 77–81.

166 Storb R, Weiden PL, Deeg HJ et al. Rejection of marrow from DLA-identical canine littermates given transfusions before grafting: antigens involved are expressed on leukocytes and skin epithelial cells but not on platelets and red blood cells. *Blood* 1979; **54**: 477–84.

167 Bean MA, Graham T, Appelbaum FR et al. Gamma-irradiation of pretransplant blood transfusions from unrelated donors prevents sensitization to minor histocompatibility antigens on dog leukocyte antigen-identical canine marrow grafts. *Transplantation* 1994; **57**: 423–6.

168 Tzeng CH, Chen PM, Fan S, Liu JH, Chiou TJ, Hsieh RK. CY/TBI-800 as a pretransplant regimen for allogeneic bone marrow transplantation for severe aplastic anemia using HLA-haploidentical family donors. *Bone Marrow Transplant* 1996; **18**: 273–7.

169 Locatelli F, Porta F, Zecca M et al. Successful bone marrow transplantation in children with severe aplastic anemia using HLA-partially matched family donors. *Am J Hematol* 1993; **42**: 328–33.

170 Camitta B, Ash R, Menitove J et al. Bone marrow transplantation for children with severe aplastic anemia: use of donors other than HLA-identical siblings. *Blood* 1989; **74**: 1852–7.

171 Margolis D, Camitta B, Pietryga D et al. Unrelated donor bone marrow transplantation to treat severe aplastic anemia in children and young adults. *Br J Haematol* 1996; **94**: 65–72.

172 Hows JM, Szydlo R, Anasetti C, Camitta B, Gajewsky J, Gluckman E. Unrelated donor marrow transplants for severe acquired aplastic anemia. *Bone Marrow Transplant* 1992; **10**: 102–6.

173 Camitta B, Deeg HJ, Castro-Malaspina H, Ramsay NKC. Unrelated or mismatched bone marrow transplants for aplastic anemia: experience at four major centers. In: Gluckman E, Coulombel L, eds. *Ontogeny of Hematopoiesis Aplastic Anemia*. Montrouge, France: John Libbey Eurotext, 1995: 325–30.

174 Kernan NA, Bartsch G, Ash RC et al. Analysis of 462 transplantations from unrelated donors facilitated by the National Marrow Donor Program. *N Engl J Med* 1993; **328**: 593–602.

175 Hows JM, Yin JL, Marsh J et al. Histocompatible unrelated volunteer donors compared with HLA nonidentical family donors in marrow transplantation for aplastic anemia and leukemia. *Blood* 1986; **68**: 1322–8.

176 Kojima S, Matsuyama T, Kato S et al. Outcome of 154 patients with severe aplastic anemia who received transplants from unrelated donors: the Japan Marrow Donor Program. *Blood* 2002; **100**: 799–803.

177 Crump M, Larratt LM, Maki E et al. Treatment of adults with severe aplastic anemia: primary therapy with antithymocyte globulin (ATG) and rescue of ATG failures with bone marrow transplantation. *Am J Med* 1992; **92**: 596–602.

178 May WS, Sensenbrenner LL, Burns WH et al. BMT for severe aplastic anemia using cyclosporine. *Bone Marrow Transplant* 1993; **11**: 459–64.

72 Robert P. Witherspoon

Allogeneic Transplantation for Paroxysmal Nocturnal Hemoglobinuria

Paroxysmal nocturnal hemoglobinuria (PNH) is an acquired clonal disorder that has a varied spectrum of clinical presentations [1,2]. Patients may present with intermittent hemolysis, thrombotic events or pancytopenia initially indistinguishable from idiopathic aplastic anemia. Rarely, it may appear in association with other hematopoietic diseases, such as myelodysplasia, acute myelogenous leukemia or T-cell leukemia [3]. PNH may also develop following immunosuppressive therapy for aplastic anemia [4,5]. Some patients present with only mild symptoms while others have life-threatening complications of thrombosis, hemolysis or marrow failure with infection from neutropenia or bleeding from thrombocytopenia. The disease often has a waxing and waning course, sometimes as long as 15 or more years, and it is difficult to predict when a life-threatening complication will occur [6].

Pathogenesis

In the past 10 years a number of studies have elucidated the molecular basis for PNH. The abnormal clone of cells has a defect in the formation of the phosphatidyl inositol glycans that are part of the anchor proteins on the cell surface which protect red blood cells from lysis by complement. The defect is caused by an acquired somatic mutation in the phosphatidyl inositol glycan-A (*PIG-A*) gene on the X chromosome [7,8]. The *PIG-A* gene is responsible for directing the protein synthesis of enzymes that enable the biosynthesis of the PIG anchor proteins. The anchor proteins are identified on the surface of red cells and blood mononuclear cells by CD14, CD16, CD24, CD55, CD59 and CD66b and can be detected by flow cytometry. The acquired mutations result in loss of expression of the anchor proteins and a failure to detect the anchor proteins by flow cytometry [9,10]. The extent to which cells bearing the defect circulate in the blood of affected individuals is dependent on several factors including:
1 the stage of differentiation of the progenitor cell containing the mutation;
2 the type of *PIG-A* mutation which may cause either deletion or alteration in quantity of the enzyme needed for biosynthesis of the anchor proteins; and
3 the often simultaneous presence of normal unaffected cells in the circulation [11].

Although studies of PNH have primarily focused on the red cell, it is now clear that the clone affects other cell lines as well [10,11].

The PNH clone expands through a selective advantage of resisting apoptosis. This notion is supported by the finding that cell lines from PNH patients have decreased apoptosis induced by irradiation [12]. Restoration of gene activity at the *PIG-A* mutation site in cell lines has been associated with restoration of CD59 expression on the cell surface, and a return of the normal apoptosis pattern [12].

The pathogenesis of thrombotic events associated with PNH has been better elucidated in recent years. Complement-mediated hemolysis, impairment of the fibrinolytic system and platelet activation are thought to be responsible for the thrombotic complications of PNH [13,14]. Membrane microparticles may act as procoagulants in the blood of PNH patients and predispose them to thromboses. These circulating particles are platelet derived and can be detected in patients with PNH and patients with aplastic anemia with a PNH clone, but not in patients with aplastic anemia without a PNH clone [13]. These findings indicate that platelet activation results in procoagulant phospholipid particles in the blood of PNH patients. If such markers in the blood correlate with an increased risk of thrombosis, they would be of value clinically in identifying patients who are at risk for life-threatening thromboses and who therefore would be candidates for early transplantation.

Clinical diagnosis of PNH

A diagnosis of PNH should be considered when a patient presents with nonautoimmune hemolytic anemia or aplastic anemia. It should also be included in the differential diagnosis of individuals presenting with a life-threatening thrombosis or recurrent thromboses. PNH is somewhat of a misnomer because the hemolysis is not necessarily nocturnal or paroxysmal. In fact, patients may recognize a low level of continuous hemolysis only with urination in the morning after free hemoglobin has accumulated overnight in the urine.

As the abnormal PNH clone expands as a result of the selective resistance to apoptosis, the hemolytic events can be expected to occur more frequently. The time-honored tests to diagnose patients in whom the diagnosis of PNH is suspected have been sugar water hemolysis and Ham's tests. However, these tests are positive only when abnormal cells remain in circulation after a major hemolytic episode. In recent years, the recognition of the loss of the anchor proteins associated with CD59 has revolutionized the diagnosis by making it possible to quantify the percentage of red cells affected. The recognition of the abnormalities of expression of other anchor proteins including CD14 and CD55 on affected monocytes, the expression of anchor proteins CD16, CD24, CD59 and CD66b on neutrophils, and CD24 and CD59 on lymphocytes makes it possible to establish the diagnosis by flow cytometry of cells that remain in circulation and are unaffected by the presence or absence of hemolysis [10,11]. Flow cytometry has become the standard screening test to diagnose patients earlier in the course of PNH.

PNH and idiopathic aplastic anemia are closely related disorders [15]. Occasionally, patients who appear to have idiopathic aplastic anemia are found by flow cytometry to have small percentages of cells in circulation that do not express CD14, CD16 or CD59 [16]. More sensitive tests have been developed that raise questions about the relationship between the two different diseases [17]. Aerolysin is a toxin that binds to cells by the anchor proteins directed by the *PIG-A* gene. Because PNH red cells cannot bind the toxin, they survive in an aerolysin-based assay. Using this assay, residual PNH cells can be detected in samples from PNH patients, but not in cells from patients with myelodysplasia or normal control samples. However, as many as 60% of the cells obtained from patients who have idiopathic aplastic anemia and not PNH by flow cytometry before treatment with the aerolysin toxin show characteristics of PNH after treatment [17]. This sensitive test indicates that previously undetectable PNH cells of different lineages circulate in patients with untreated aplastic anemia, and raises the possibility of a feature of clonality in the early stages of aplastic anemia.

Transplantation for PNH

Hematopoietic cell transplantation (HCT) from an human leukocyte antigen (HLA) identical sibling for a patient with PNH was first reported in 1973 [18]. This patient was found to have PNH at the time of presentation of severe aplastic anemia and had a positive sucrose hemolysis or Ham's test. In subsequent reports, most patients had life-threatening disease from marrow aplasia, and hemolysis played a less important part [19–22]. More recently, patients with hemolysis or thrombosis were evaluated for transplantation. Overall, the number of individuals who have been transplanted is small (Table 72.1).

The experience in Seattle with transplantation for nine patients was summarized in 1992 [23]. Subsequently, 14 additional patients have been transplanted, and the results are updated in Table 72.2. Among the total of 23 patients, nine presented with the severe aplastic anemia phase of PNH and had severely hypocellular marrows. The remaining 14 patients presented with hemolysis or thrombosis and had moderately cellular to hypercellular marrows.

Conditioning for grafting of the patients with aplastic anemia who had HLA identical sibling donors consisted of 200 mg/kg cyclophosphamide (CY) with or without antithymocyte globulin (ATG) in five patients, and 16 mg/kg busulfan (BU) with 60 mg/kg CY in two patients. One of these patients with aplastic anemia received two grafts from the same donor. The patient with aplastic anemia and the haploidentical parental graft had 120 mg/kg CY and 1200 cGy total body irradiation (TBI). The syngeneic recipient with aplastic anemia received an infusion of marrow without conditioning.

The conditioning regimens for the HLA identical siblings with thrombotic or hemolytic presentations of PNH consisted of BUCY plus ATG in five patients, BUCY in two patients and CY in one patient. The recipients of the parental donor graft and the child donor graft received BUCY and ATG, or BUCY, respectively. Two recipients of unrelated donor marrow were conditioned with BUCY and ATG, and one CY ATG and 1350 cGy TBI for an unrelated umbilical cord blood graft. The syngeneic marrow recipient did not receive conditioning.

Twelve of the 23 patients developed acute graft-vs.-host disease (GVHD) (seven grade II, three grade III and two grade IV) and eight subsequently developed clinically extensive chronic GVHD. PNH recurred 9–17 years after transplant in both syngeneic recipients, and 2.7 years after transplantation in one allogeneic recipient [23]. Nine patients died. The causes of death included GVHD complicated by infection in two patients, fungal pneumonia in two patients and a gastrointestinal bleed in one patient. The latter patient had thromboses of the portal and splenic veins from PNH, which led to bleeding varices. One patient rejected the haploidentical parental graft and died of pulmonary hemorrhage shortly after a second transplant from another haploidentical family member. One patient died of a post-transplant lymphoproliferative disorder (PTLD) 169 days after an unrelated umbilical cord blood transplant. Two patients who were alive at the time of the previous report have died: one from human immunodeficiency virus (HIV) infection 9.3 years after transplantation, and the second, a syngeneic recipient, 25.4 years after transplantation as a result of complications from hepatitis C and subsequent liver transplant. Fourteen patients are surviving 105 days to 29 years (median 4.3 years) after transplantation. Nine of these individuals are well, and five have clinically extensive chronic GVHD.

These results show that patients with the aplastic anemia presentation of PNH do well because none of the seven patients who received HLA identical sibling grafts died from the complications of transplantation,

Table 72.1 Published reports of transplantation for PNH.

Author	No. of patients	Type of donor and number of each	Conditioning regimen	PNH after transplant
Storb *et al.* [18]	1	Allogeneic 1	Yes	No
Fefer *et al.* [20]	1	Syngeneic 1	No	Yes
Kolb *et al.* [21]	2	Allogeneic 1	Yes	No
		Syngeneic 1	No	Yes
Antin *et al.* [19]	4	Allogeneic 4	Yes	No
Szer [22]	4	Allogeneic 3	Yes	No
		Syngeneic 1	No	Yes
Kawahara *et al.* [23]*	9	Allogeneic 7	Yes	No[†]
		Syngeneic 2	No	Yes
Saso *et al.* [24]	57	Allogeneic 55	Yes	No
		Syngeneic 2	No/Yes	Yes
Bemba *et al.* [25]	16	Allogeneic 16	Yes	No
Raiola *et al.* [26]	7	Allogeneic 7	Yes	No
Graham *et al.* [27]	1	Syngeneic 1	Yes	No
Hershko *et al.* [28]	1	Syngeneic 1	No	Yes
Endo *et al.* [29]	1	Syngeneic 1	No	Yes
Woodard *et al.* [30]	3	Allogeneic 3	Yes	No

*Reference [23] contains cases previously reported in references [18,20,22].
[†]One allogeneic recipient had return of the PNH clone 2.7 years after transplant.

Table 72.2 Patients in the Seattle transplantation program.

Patient number	Age (years)	Marrow donor	PNH presentation	Conditioning regimen	GVHD acute grade/chronic	Status	Survival days or years post-transplant	Cause of death
1	23	HLA ID SIB	A	CY	0/No	A	>29.0 years	
2	19	Syngeneic	A	None	0/No	D	25.2 years	Hepatitis C
3	14	HLA ID SIB	A	PAPAPA BC CY BUCY	II/Limited	A	>28.0 years	
4	16	HLA ID SIB	A	CY	0/NA	A	>21.1 years	
5	29	Syngeneic	H	None	0/0	A	>20.2 years	
6	38	HLA ID SIB	A	BC CY	II/Clin ext	D	9.3 years	HIV
7	20	Haplo parent/haplo SIB	A	CY TBI ATG BC CY	No/NA	D	39 days	Pulmonary hemorrhage
8	37	HLA ID SIB	T	CY	0/Clin ext	A	>11.9 years	
9	22	HLA ID SIB	H	BU CY	II/No	A	>13.2 years	
10	25	HLA ID SIB	H	BU CY	II/NA	D	105 days	Fungal pneumonia
11	32	HLA ID SIB	H	ATG BU CY	IV/Clin ext	D	83 days	GVHD infection
12	29	Matched unrel	H	ATG BU CY	IV/NA	D	58 days	GVHD infection
13	33	1Ag MM parent	T, H	ATG BU CY	III/NA	D	81 days	Fungal pneumonia
14	21	HLA ID SIB	A	ATG BU CY	II/No	A	>5.4 years	
15	42	HLA ID SIB	T	ATG BU CY	0/NA	D	11 days	Bleeding varices
16	39	HLA ID SIB	H	ATG BU CY	0/Subclin	A	>105 days	
17	41	1Ag MM child	H	BUCY	II/Clin ext	A	>2.6 years	
18	19	MM SIB	H	ATG BU CY	III/Clin ext	A	>3.3 years	
19	21	HLA ID SIB	H	ATG BU CY	0/Subclin	A	>3.1 years	
20	35	Unrel cord blood	T	ATG CY TBI 1350	III/Clin ext	D	169 days	PTLD
21	36	Matched unrel	T	ATG BU CY	II/Clin ext	A	>2.1 years	
22	33	HLA ID SIB	A	ATG CY	/Limited	A	>1.1 years	
23	18	HLA ID SIB	A	ATG BU CY	/Clin ext	A	>0.9 year	

Abbreviations: A, aplastic anemia; 1ag, 1 antigen; ATG, antithymocyte globulin; BC, donor buffy coat; BU CY, busulfan cyclophosphamide; Clin ext, clinical extensive; CY, cyclophosphamide; GVHD, graft-vs.-host disease; H, hemolysis; haplo, haploidentical; HIV, human immunodeficiency virus; HLA ID SIB, HLA identical sibling; NA, not applicable; MM, mismatched; PA, procarbazine + ATG; PTLD, post-transplant lymphoproliferative disorder; Subclin, subclinical; T, thrombosis; TBI 1350, 1350 cGy total body irradiation; Unrel, unrelated.
Status: A, alive, D, dead.

and only one of these died later from HIV infection. In contrast, only eight of the 14 patients who received transplants for the hemolytic or thrombotic presentations of PNH survived. These patients died of the complications of grafting from GVHD with nonfungal infection, fungal infection, variceal bleeding or PTLD.

The International Bone Marrow Transplant Registry has reported the results of 57 patients with PNH who were transplanted at 31 different centres [24]. Thirty-nine of these patients presented with PNH as the only diagnosis. Sixteen evolved from PNH into an aplastic anemia presentation by the time of transplantation, and two developed PNH syndrome after initially presenting with aplastic anemia. The donors were HLA identical siblings in 48 cases, syngeneic donors in two cases, a haploidentical family member in one case and HLA phenotypically identical unrelated donors in six cases. These patients received conditioning consisting of BUCY for 30 patients, CY/TBI for 12, limited field irradiation/CY for 11 and CY alone for three patients. One identical twin recipient did not receive any pretransplant conditioning. GVHD prophylaxis consisted of methotrexate or cyclosporine plus methotrexate in 39 patients, and cyclosporine plus corticosteroids in 11 patients. Six patients received T-depleted grafts and one identical twin recipient did not receive prophylaxis. Graft failure occurred in 11 of 48 patients evaluable for engraftment. Of those with engraftment, 34% developed grade II or greater acute GVHD and 33% of patients surviving beyond 90 days developed chronic GVHD. Overall, 27 of the 57 patients survived. Among those 48 patients receiving HLA identical sibling grafts, 26 (56%) survived compared to one survivor among seven patients (14%) receiving HLA nonidentical family member or unrelated donor grafts.

One report describes three patients with the aplastic anemia presentation of PNH given unrelated donor bone marrow grafts following T-cell depletion of marrow. The post-transplant course was complicated by an Epstein–Barr virus (EBV) lymphoproliferative disorder that responded to EBV-specific cytotoxic T-cell therapy. Another had veno-occlusive disease (VOD) and another had severe hemolytic uremic syndrome and hemorrhagic cystitis. However, they all recovered and are alive without PNH 2.5–5.1 years after transplantation [30].

These data suggest that survival after transplantation for the aplastic phase of PNH using HLA identical sibling donors is quite good. However, transplantation is successful in only about half of the cases for the nonaplastic presentations of PNH using HLA identical sibling donors. Results using partially matched family member donors are poor. Finally, there are too few transplant procedures using matched unrelated donors to draw any conclusions about the results of unrelated donor transplantation.

Nonmyeloablative transplants

Reports of nonmyeloablative transplantation for PNH are beginning to appear [31]. The lack of toxicity with a nonmyeloablative or less-intensive conditioning regimen is an appealing approach. One patient had long-standing hemolysis and an episode of acute renal failure from hemolysis and infection. He received hematopoietic stem cells from an HLA identical sibling donor after conditioning with 8 mg/kg BU, 0.66 mg/kg cladribine and 5 mg/kg ATG with cyclosporine for GVHD prophylaxis. Although the follow-up after transplant was short, 6 months after transplant the recipient had sustained engraftment and no detectable PNH-positive cells. The dosage of BU in this case was the dosage used in myeloablative regimens, and one could argue that this case was not a typical nonmyeloablative transplant because of the intensity of the conditioning regimen.

Another center reported four PNH patients given allogeneic stem cells after conditioning with extracorporeal phototherapy, 2′-deoxycoformycin and 600 cGy TBI. All four patients are alive and well 2 years after transplantation (K. Miller, unpublished observations, 2002). Similar to the report above, this dose of TBI is actually myeloablative. The lower dose nonmyeloablative conditioning regimens often used in reports other than these two may be insufficient for sustained donor engraftment in patients with nonaplastic presentations because even those syngeneic recipients of marrow for the aplastic phase of PNH required conditioning regimens to achieve sustained donor engraftment [20,21,23,24,27–29,32].

Furthermore, sufficient conditioning, perhaps in combination with GVHD, may be necessary to eliminate the PNH clone because syngeneic recipients who did not receive pretransplant conditioning eventually had return of PNH disease years later [22,23]. Except for one patient, recipients of allogeneic stem cells had sustained elimination of the disease (Table 72.1) [23]. These results suggest that a graft-vs.-PNH type of effect in either a myeloablative or nonmyeloablative allogeneic transplant procedure makes an important contribution toward eliminating the PNH clone. In this regard, five patients with PNH, one with aplastic anemia and four with the nonaplastic presentation received nonmyeloablative transplants from matched unrelated donors after conditioning with 90 mg/kg fludarabine and 200 cGy TBI. These patients achieved complete donor chimerism by day 56 and lost all signs of the PNH clone by flow cytometry. Unfortunately, two patients died of treatment-related complications: one from acute pancreatitis and one from infection during treatment for chronic GVHD. Three patients are alive with follow-up ranging from 1 to 2 years after transplantation (U. Hegenbart, unpublished observations, 2003). Further studies of the nonmyeloablative approach are warranted, especially for patients who cannot undergo conventional transplantation because of an increased risk of transplant-related mortality as a result of pretransplant organ dysfunction.

Autologous transplantation for PNH

An interesting hypothesis has been put forward by Musto *et al.* [33]. They demonstrated that flow cytometry could select $CD34^+/CD59^+$ cells from PNH patients who had a mixed population of circulating normal and abnormal cells. If these cells do not bear the mutation in the *PIG-A* gene, a rationale to mobilize and select autologous normal HSC for autotransplantation exists, although at the time of publication no autologous transplant cases have been reported [34].

Nontransplant treatment of PNH

Immunosuppressive therapy has been reported in the treatment of PNH, most often when the presentation was that of aplastic anemia. However, the use of cyclosporine, granulocyte-colony stimulating factor and ATG has generally not eradicated the abnormal clone and patients continue to be symptomatic from the disease [34–37]. In a small number of patients, high-dose CY without marrow infusion has resulted in autologous marrow recovery without persistence of the PNH clone [38].

Conclusions

The diagnosis of PNH alone should not be the sole indication for transplantation therapy. Defining the risk of a fatal complication in an individual PNH patient is still the most important determination to make before recommending transplantation. Risk factors for a poor outcome in the natural history of PNH are thrombosis at initial presentation, evolution to pancytopenia and aplastic anemia, thrombocytopenia at diagnosis, evolution to myelodysplasia or leukemia and age over 55 years at diagnosis. Patients with infection at diagnosis are at greater risk for thrombosis [6]. When the patient has a life-threatening presentation with aplastic anemia and an HLA identical sibling or identical twin donor is available, transplantation is recommended. Unrelated donors have been used to achieve successful grafts in patients with idiopathic aplastic anemia, and transplantation with a matched unrelated donor for the life-threatening aplastic phase of PNH is warranted, although the experience is small [30,39]. Nonmyeloablative transplantation should be explored further, especially for patients with severe PNH who cannot tolerate a full myeloablative transplant because of comorbid medical conditions. In all other phases of disease the care should be supportive, and transplantation should be performed when the disease becomes life-threatening, or reliable predictors are developed to identify which patients with the nonaplastic phases of PNH are at particularly high risk of death from PNH.

References

1. Rosse WF, Parker CJ. Paroxysmal nocturnal haemoglobinuria. *Clin Haematol* 1985; **14**: 105–25.
2. Rotoli B, Luzzatto L. Paroxysmal nocturnal hemoglobinuria. *Semin Hematol* 1989; **26**: 201–7.
3. Karadimitris A, Li K, Notaro R *et al.* Association of clonal T-cell large granular lymphocyte disease and paroxysmal nocturnal haemoglobinuria (PNH): further evidence for a pathogenetic link between T cells, aplastic anemia and PNH. *Br J Haematol* 2001; **115**: 1010–4.
4. de Planque MM, Bacigalupo A, Wursch A *et al.* Long-term follow-up of severe aplastic anemia patients treated with antithymocyte globulin. Severe Aplastic Anemia Working Party of the European Cooperative Group for Bone Marrow Transplantation (EBMT). *Br J Haematol* 1989; **73**: 121–6.
5. Tichelli A, Gratwohl A, Wursch A, Nissen C, Speck B. Late haematological complications in severe aplastic anemia. *Br J Haematol* 1988; **69**: 413–8.
6. Socié G, Mary JY, de Gramont A *et al.* Paroxysmal nocturnal haemoglobinuria: long-term follow-up and prognostic factors. French Society of Haematology. *Lancet* 1996; **348**: 573–7.
7. Bessler M, Mason PJ, Hillmen P *et al.* Paroxysmal nocturnal haemoglobinuria (PNH) is caused by somatic mutations in the *PIG-A* gene. *EMBO J* 1994; **13**: 110–7.
8. Yeh ETH, Rosse WF. Paroxysmal nocturnal hemoglobinuria and the glycosylphosphatidylinositol anchor. *J Clin Invest* 1994; **93**: 2305–10.
9. Rotoli B, Bessler M, Alfinito F, Del Vecchio L. Membrane proteins in paroxysmal nocturnal haemoglobinuria. *Blood Rev* 1993; **7**: 75–86.
10. van der Schoot CE, Huizinga TW, van't Veer-Korthof ET, Wijmans R, Pinkster J, von dem Borne AE. Deficiency of glycosyl-phosphatidylinositol-linked membrane glycoproteins of leukocytes in paroxysmal nocturnal hemoglobinuria, description of a new diagnostic cytofluorometric assay. *Blood* 1990; **76**: 1853–9.
11. Alfinito F, Del Vecchio L, Rocco S, Boccuni P, Musto P, Rotoli B. Blood cell flow cytometry in paroxysmal nocturnal hemoglobinuria: a tool for measuring the extent of the PNH clone. *Leukemia* 1996; **10**: 1326–30.
12. Brodsky RA, Vala MS, Barber JP, Medof ME, Jones RJ. Resistance to apoptosis caused by *PIG-A* gene mutations in paroxysmal nocturnal hemoglobinuria. *Proc Natl Acad Sci U S A* 1997; **94**: 8756–60.
13. Hugel B, Socie G, Vu T *et al.* Elevated levels of circulating procoagulant microparticles in patients with paroxysmal nocturnal hemoglobinuria and aplastic anemia. *Blood* 1999; **93**: 3451–6.

14 Wiedmer T, Hall SE, Ortel TL, Kane WH, Rosse WF, Sims PJ. Complement-induced vesiculation and exposure of membrane prothrombinase sites in platelets of paroxysmal nocturnal hemoglobinuria. *Blood* 1993; **82**: 1192–6.
15 Rosse WF. Paroxysmal nocturnal haemoglobinuria in aplastic anemia. *Clin Haematol* 1978; **7**: 541–53.
16 Mukhina GL, Buckley JT, Barber JP, Jones RJ, Brodsky RA. Multilineage glycosylphosphatidylinositol anchor-deficient haematopoiesis in untreated aplastic anemia. *Br J Haematol* 2001; **115**: 476–82.
17 Mukhina GL, Buckley T, Brodsky RA. A rapid spectrophotometric screening assay for paroxysmal nocturnal hemoglobinuria. *Acta Haematol* 2002; **107**: 182–4.
18 Storb R, Evans RS, Thomas ED et al. Paroxysmal nocturnal haemoglobinuria and refractory marrow failure treated by marrow transplantation. *Br J Haematol* 1973; **24**: 743–50.
19 Antin JH, Ginsburg D, Smith BR, Nathan DG, Orkin SH, Rappeport JM. Bone marrow transplantation for paroxysmal nocturnal hemoglobinuria: eradication of the PNH clone and documentation of complete lymphohematopoietic engraftment. *Blood* 1985; **66**: 1247–50.
20 Fefer A, Freeman H, Storb R et al. Paroxysmal nocturnal hemoglobinuria and marrow failure treated by infusion of marrow from an identical twin. *Ann Intern Med* 1976; **84**: 692–5.
21 Kolb HJ, Holler E, Bender-Götze Ch et al. Myeloablative conditioning for marrow transplantation in myelodysplastic syndromes and paroxysmal nocturnal hemoglobinuria. *Bone Marrow Transplant* 1989; **4**: 29–34.
22 Szer J, Deeg HJ, Witherspoon RP et al. Long-term survival after marrow transplantation for paroxysmal nocturnal hemoglobinuria with aplastic anemia. *Ann Intern Med* 1984; **101**: 193–5.
23 Kawahara K, Witherspoon RP, Storb R. Marrow transplantation for paroxysmal nocturnal hemoglobinuria. *Am J Hematol* 1992; **39**: 283–8.
24 Saso R, Marsh J, Cevreska L et al. Bone marrow transplants for paroxysmal nocturnal haemoglobinuria. *Br J Haematol* 1999; **104**: 392–6.
25 Bemba M, Guardiola P, Garderet L et al. Bone marrow transplantation for paroxysmal nocturnal haemoglobinuria. *Br J Haematol* 1999; **105**: 366–8.
26 Raiola AM, Van Lint MT, Lamparelli T et al. Bone marrow transplantation for paroxysmal nocturnal hemoglobinuria. *Haematologica* 2000; **85**: 59–62.
27 Graham ML, Rosse WF, Halperin EC, Miller CR, Ware RE. Resolution of Budd–Chiari syndrome following bone marrow transplantation for paroxysmal nocturnal haemoglobinuria. *Br J Haematol* 1996; **92**: 707–10.
28 Hershko C, Ho WG, Gale RP, Cline MJ. Cure of aplastic anemia in paroxysmal nocturnal haemoglobinuria by marrow transfusion from an identical twin: failure of peripheral-leukocyte transfusion to correct marrow aplasia. *Lancet* 1979; **2**: 945.
29 Endo M, Beatty PG, Vreeke TM, Wittwer CT, Singh SP, Parker CJ. Syngeneic bone marrow transplantation without conditioning in a patient with paroxysmal nocturnal hemoglobinuria: *in vivo* evidence that the mutant stem cells have a survival advantage. *Blood* 1996; **88**: 742–50.
30 Woodard P, Wang W, Pitts N et al. Paroxysmal nocturnal haemoglobinuria: successful unrelated donor bone marrow transplantation for paroxysmal nocturnal haemoglobinuria. *Bone Marrow Transplant* 2001; **27**: 589–92.
31 Suenaga K, Kanda Y, Niiya H et al. Successful application of nonmyeloablative transplantation for paroxysmal nocturnal hemoglobinuria. *Exp Hematol* 2001; **29**: 639–42.
32 Champlin RE, Feig SA, Sparkes RS, Gale RP. Bone marrow transplantation from identical twins in the treatment of aplastic anemia: implication for the pathogenesis of the disease. *Br J Haematol* 1984; **56**: 455–63.
33 Musto P, D'Arena G, Cascavilla N, Carotenuto M. Normal G-CSF-mobilized CD34[+] peripheral blood stem cells in paroxysmal nocturnal hemoglobinuria: a perspective for autologous transplantation. *Leukemia* 1997; **11**: 890–2.
34 Schubert J, Scholz C, Geissler RG, Ganser A, Schmidt RE. G-CSF and cyclosporin induce an increase of normal cells in hypoplastic paroxysmal nocturnal hemoglobinuria. *Ann Hematol* 1997; **74**: 225–30.
35 Paquette RL, Yoshimura R, Veiseh C, Kunkel L, Gajewski J, Rosen PJ. Clinical characteristics predict response to antithymocyte globulin in paroxysmal nocturnal haemoglobinuria. *Br J Haematol* 1997; **96**: 92–7.
36 Stoppa AM, Vey N, Sainty D et al. Correction of aplastic anemia complicating paroxysmal nocturnal haemoglobinuria: absence of eradication of the PNH clone and dependence of response on cyclosporin A administration. *Br J Haematol* 1996; **93**: 42–4.
37 van Kamp H, van Imhoff GW, de Wolf JT, Smit JW, Halie MR, Vellenga E. The effect of cyclosporine on haematological parameters in patients with paroxysmal nocturnal haemoglobinuria. *Br J Haematol* 1995; **89**: 79–82.
38 Brodsky RA, Sensenbrenner LL, Smith BD et al. Durable treatment-free remission after high-dose cyclophosphamide therapy for previously untreated severe aplastic anemia. *Ann Intern Med* 2001; **135**: 477–83.
39 Deeg HJ, Amylon MD, Harris RE et al. Marrow transplants from unrelated donors for patients with aplastic anemia: minimum effective dose of total body irradiation. *Biol Blood Marrow Transplant* 2001; **7**: 208–15.

73

Frederick R. Appelbaum

Allogeneic Transplantation for Chronic Myeloid Leukemia

Chronic myeloid leukemia (CML) is a malignant disorder of hematopoiesis resulting from the clonal expansion of a primitive hematopoietic cell that, for a variable period of time, retains the capacity to differentiate, leading to marked marrow hyperplasia and increased numbers of myeloid cells and platelets in the peripheral blood. The natural history of untreated CML is a relatively benign chronic phase (CP) lasting on average approximately 3 years followed by an accelerated phase (AP) lasting several months and then eventually terminating in a rapidly fatal blast crisis (BC). CML was the first malignant disease found to be consistently associated with a specific cytogenetic abnormality, the Philadelphia (Ph) chromosome, and continues to be a disease that is particularly instructive to our understanding of the malignant process and the development of new therapeutic approaches.

Incidence and epidemiology

With an annual incidence of 1.6 cases per 100,000 per year, CML represents 14% of all new leukemias in the USA [1]. The median age at diagnosis is 67 years according to Surveillance, Epidemiology and End Results (SEER) data, and the incidence seems to increase almost exponentially with age [2]. There is a slight male predominance and very little geographic variation. Exposure to ionizing radiation, as in survivors of the atomic bomb, is a risk factor [3], but essentially no other genetic or environmental risk factors are known.

Molecular biology

Nowell and Hungerford in 1960 [4] described the presence of a small chromosome in metaphase preparations of marrow from patients with CML. This abnormal chromosome, termed the Philadelphia chromosome after the city where it was discovered, was later shown by Rowley to be the result of a translocation between chromosomes 9 and 22 [t(9;22)(q34;q11)] [5]. The result of this translocation is the fusion of the *BCR* (breakpoint cluster region) gene on chromosome 22 to the *ABL* (Abelson leukemia virus) gene on chromosome 9. The translocation results in the production of an abnormal BCR fusion protein, which is a constitutively active cytoplasmic tyrosine kinase [6–9]. The exact size of the fusion protein varies depending on the site of the breakpoint in the *BCR* gene. Virtually all patients with typical chronic phase CML express a 210-kDa BCR-ABL protein, whereas patients with Ph-positive acute lymphoblastic leukemia (ALL) express either a 190-kDa BCR-ABL protein or a 210-kDa BCR-ABL protein indistinguishable from that found in CML. A larger 230-kDa BCR-ABL fusion protein has recently been described in a small subgroup of patients with CML presenting with lower white cell counts and slower progression to blast crisis [10]. In any individual patient, the translocation is found in cells of myeloid, erythroid, megakaryocytic and B-lymphoid origin, demonstrating the stem cell nature of the disease. As the disease accelerates and enters blast crisis, additional cytogenetic abnormalities develop including duplication of the Ph chromosome and trisomy 8 [11].

Laboratory studies demonstrate that the BCR-ABL translocation is both necessary and sufficient to cause CML. Transgenic expression of the 190-kDa BCR-ABL protein in mice causes acute leukemia at birth [12]. Retroviral transfer of the *BCR-ABL* gene into hematopoietic stem cells of normal mice leads to the development of a variety of acute and chronic myeloid leukemias depending on the strain of mice studied [13,14]. The BCR-ABL protein transforms hematopoietic cells so that their growth *in vitro* becomes cytokine independent [15], protects hematopoietic cells from apoptotic responses to DNA damage [16] and increases adhesion of hematopoietic cells to extracellular matrix proteins [17].

The normal ABL protein is a nonreceptor tyrosine kinase with important roles in signal transduction and the regulation of cell growth [18]. The BCR-ABL protein, unlike normal ABL, is constitutively active and has increased kinase activity. The persistent and increased activity results in the continuous activation of a number of cytoplasmic and nuclear signal transduction pathways involved in the growth and survival of hematopoietic cells including STAT, RAS, JUN kinase, MYC and phosphatidylinositol-3 kinase [8]. Loss of the tyrosine kinase activity of BCR-ABL, either through mutation or pharmacologic blockade, blocks its leukemogenic activity [19].

Clinical description

At diagnosis, most patients (>90%) are in chronic phase, and estimates are that up to 50% of patients are diagnosed incidentally during routine screening. Symptoms, when present, usually include fatigue, weight loss, bony aches and abdominal discomfort from splenomegaly. Typically, patients exhibit leukocytosis, thrombocytosis and anaemia at presentation. The marrow is virtually always hypercellular and, on cytogenetic analysis, the Ph chromosome is found in 90% of patients. In the remaining 10%, cryptic or complex translocations detected by fluorescence *in situ* hybridization (FISH) or polymerase chain reaction (PCR) assays can be found.

After a variable period of time, CML evolves from a chronic to an accelerated phase and eventually to blast crisis. In approximately 25% of patients, there is no intervening accelerated phase between chronic phase and blast crisis. Various definitions of accelerated phase have been developed. Two of the more commonly employed are those of Sokal *et al.* [20] and the International Bone Marrow Transplant Registry (IBMTR) [20] (Table 73.1). In general, accelerated phase is characterized by symptoms of fever, night sweats, weight loss and bone pain, difficulty in controlling

Table 73.1 Definition of accelerated phase chronic myeloid leukemia.

Sokal criteria [20]	IBMTR criteria [46]
Peripheral blood or marrow blasts ≥5%	Leukocyte count difficult to control with conventional therapy
Basophils >20%	Rapid doubling time of leukocytes (<5 days)
Platelet count ≥1000 × 10^9/L despite adequate therapy	Peripheral blood or marrow blasts ≥10%
Karyotype evolution	Peripheral blood or marrow blasts plus promyelocytes ≥20%
Frequent Pelger–Huet-like neutrophils; nucleated erythrocytes, megakaryocytic nuclear fragments	Peripheral blood basophils and eosinophils ≥20%
Marrow collagen fibrosis	Anemia or thrombocytopenia unresponsive to therapy
Anemia or thrombocytopenia unrelated to therapy	Persistent thrombocytosis
Progressive splenomegaly	Karyotypic evolution
Leukocyte doubling time <5 days	Progressive splenomegaly
Fever not otherwise explained	Development of chloromas or myelofibrosis

IBMTR, International Bone Marrow Transplant Registry.

counts using conventional therapy, increased numbers of blasts and early myeloid cells in marrow and peripheral blood, and evidence of karyotypic evolution. The most common cytogenetic changes associated with disease evolution are an additional Ph chromosome, trisomy 8, isochrome i(17q) and trisomy 19 [21]. Blast crisis is defined as having more than 30% blasts and promyelocytes in the bone marrow or peripheral blood, or the development of extramedullary blastic infiltrates [20]. In approximately two-thirds of patients, the blasts have a myeloid or undifferentiated-like phenotype while in the remaining third the blasts appear more lymphoid-like [22]. In the third of patients with lymphoid blast crisis, the blasts are characterized by expression of CD19, CD20, CD10 and terminal deoxynucleotidyl transferase, and patients temporarily respond to treatment with regimens active in the treatment of ALL.

The natural history of CML, determined more than 75 years ago, suggests a median survival from diagnosis of approximately 3 years [23]. A number of prognostic scoring systems have been developed with the goal of predicting the length of chronic phase in individual patients. While Tura et al. [24] described one of the first, the study published by Sokal et al. in 1984 [25] has become one of the best known and widely used. An algorithm was developed based on the outcome of a training population of 361 patients and applied to a test population of 317 patients. Spleen size, percentage of circulating blasts, platelet count and age were identified as prognostic factors and Sokal's system allowed chronic phase patients to be assigned to three prognostic groups with median survivals of 2.5, 4 and 5 years. The patients in Sokal's study received out-of-date therapies by today's standards, including busulfan (BU) and splenectomy. When patients treated with interferon were analyzed, the power of the Sokal model diminished and accordingly newer prognostic scoring systems were proposed [26,27]. Whether these systems have any relevance to the current era dominated by imatinib and transplantation is unknown.

Nontransplant therapies

Palliative chemotherapy

Prior to the introduction of interferon alfa (IFN) in the late 1980s, palliative low-dose chemotherapy was the standard treatment of CML. Busulfan was introduced as therapy for CML in 1953 [28] and was the most commonly used agent until surpassed by hydroxyurea in the 1980s. Busulfan is generally given at 0.1 mg/kg/day until the white count decreases by 50%, with the dose then being reduced by 50%. Once the white count is reduced to 20,000/mm^3, patients are maintained with repeat courses of 2–8 mg/day for 5–10 days. With this regimen, white count, platelet count and splenomegaly can be controlled in the majority of patients, but cytogenetic responses are rare. While generally well tolerated, busulfan can be associated with a number of serious side-effects including infertility, lung fibrosis and marrow aplasia.

Hydroxyurea was first reported as a therapy for CML in 1963 [29] and gradually gained favor over busulfan based on excellent tolerability and wide therapeutic index. Like busulfan, hydroxyurea provides an excellent method to control white counts, platelets and splenomegaly in most patients but does not generally affect the percentage of Ph-positive cells in the marrow. Hydroxyurea has few side-effects, and is administered orally, generally at a dosage of around 40 mg/kg/day with the dosage adjusted to maintain a white count of 5000–10,000/mm^3. In randomized trials, hydroxyurea was shown to prolong survival of patients with CML chronic phase compared to busulfan [30,31].

Interferon alfa

Interferon alfa was first reported to have activity in chronic phase CML in 1986 [32]. The mechanisms by which IFN work in CML are not understood, but it has been hypothesized that IFN controls proliferation or adhesion of the malignant progenitor in CML or that it functions by stimulating an immune response to CML. IFN is administered subcutaneously at a dosage of 3 million units (Mu)/m^2/day and at that dosage hematologic remissions can be achieved in 70–80% of cases. However, unlike busulfan or hydroxyurea, partial or complete cytogenetic responses (defined as having less than 34% Ph-positive cells in the marrow) are seen in 20–30% of patients. A series of randomized controlled trials have compared IFN to either busulfan or hydroxyurea. A meta-analysis of the seven largest randomized trials reported an improvement in 5-year survival from 42 to 57% with the use of IFN [33]. Interferon responses were highest in younger good-risk patients treated within 1 year of diagnosis. A higher rate of hematologic and cytogenetic responses have been reported with higher dosage (5 Mu/m^2/day), if tolerable. The optimal length of therapy is unknown. Unlike busulfan and hydroxyurea, side-effects are common with IFN and include fatigue, myalgia, arthralgia, weight loss, depression, memory changes and autoimmune disorders. In fact, 14–25% of patients on the randomized trials included in the meta-analysis discontinued IFN as a result of side-effects. In an effort to improve response rates and duration, several investigators have combined low-dose cytarabine with IFN. While a benefit was suggested in one study, the results looked less promising in a second [34,35]. In both trials, the addition of cytarabine substantially increased gastrointestinal and hematologic toxicity.

Imatinib mesylate

Imatinib mesylate, formerly called STI 571, is a small molecule inhibitor of several protein tyrosine kinases including the ABL tyrosine kinase. A drug screen conducted by chemists at Ciba-Geigy identified two phenylaminopyrimidine compounds as inhibitors of certain tyrosine kinases. Subsequent modifications of these compounds produced imatinib, a compound with particular activity against the tyrosine kinases ABL, C-KIT and PDGF. Druker et al. [19] subsequently found that imatinib specifically inhibited or killed proliferating myeloid cell lines containing BCR-ABL but had no effect on normal cells. A phase 1 trial was initiated in 1998 testing imatinib in patients with chronic phase CML who had failed therapy with IFN [36]. Of 54 patients who received oral doses of imatinib of 300 mg/day or more, 53 had a complete hematologic response, usually within 4 weeks of starting the drug. In addition, cytogenetic responses were seen in 54% of patients. In a companion study, 58 patients with CML in myeloid or lymphoid blast crisis or Ph-positive ALL in relapse were studied [37]. Partial or complete responses were seen in 60% of patients with CML in myeloid blast crisis and 70% of patients with CML in lymphoid blast crisis or recurrent Ph-positive ALL had partial or complete responses. Unfortunately, most of the responses in patients with CML and all of the responses in patients with ALL were brief, usually less than 4 months. The toxicity profile of imatinib in these phase 1 studies suggests that it is more toxic than hydroxyurea but far easier to take than IFN. Nausea, edema and muscle cramps were seen in approximately 50% of patients with diarrhea, vomiting, rash and headache seen in one-third [38].

The initial phase 1 results were confirmed in broader phase 2 studies of imatinib and, based on these results, the drug was approved by the US Food and Drug Administration in May 2001 for treatment of CML in chronic phase refractory to IFN, accelerated phase and blast crisis. Subsequently, 1106 patients were entered onto a phase 3 study comparing imatinib with IFN plus cytarabine for the treatment of previously untreated chronic phase CML [39]. At 6 months, major and complete cytogenetic responses were seen in 63 and 40% of the imatinib treated patients vs. 10 and 2% with IFN. Disease progression was seen in 1.4% of the imatinib group vs. 10.3% of the IFN patients. Crossovers as a result of intolerance occurred in 1% of imatinib and 19% of IFN patients. Based primarily on a higher rate of disease progression with IFN plus cytarabine, the study was closed by the study's independent monitoring board with the conclusion that imatinib is the initial nontransplant treatment of choice for patients with newly diagnosed chronic phase CML.

While imatinib is a highly effective therapy for CML, both de novo and acquired resistance have been seen. In those cases where it has been studied, resistance has been associated with BCR-ABL gene amplification in some, and mutations in BCR-ABL that prevent imatinib from inhibiting the kinase in others [40]. In some patients, point mutations in BCR-ABL can be found at diagnosis and, with imatinib treatment, cells bearing these mutations may undergo positive selection [41].

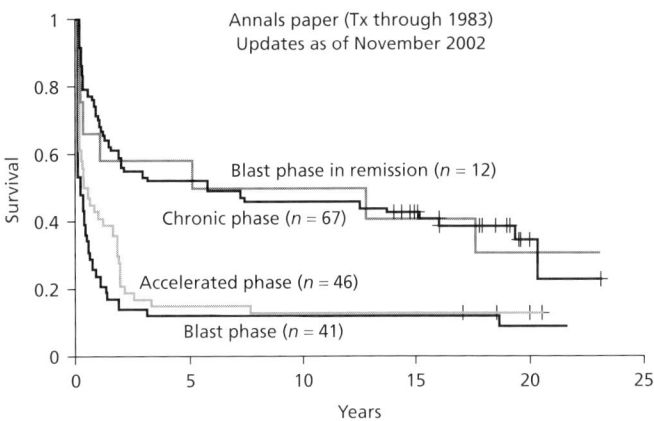

Fig. 73.1 Kaplan–Meier probabilities of survival by phase at the time of transplantation for 166 patients with chronic myeloid leukemia who received transplants through 1983 from human leukocyte antigen (HLA) identical siblings, first published in 1986 [45]. The results are updated as of November 2002.

Hematopoietic cell transplantation

Syngeneic hematopoietic cell transplantation

In 1979, Fefer et al. [42] published results of identical twin transplants in four patients with chronic phase CML treated with dimethyl busulfan, cyclophosphamide (CY), and a single 920 cGy exposure of total body irradiation (TBI). All four recovered with Ph-negative normal hematopoiesis. In 1982, the same group reported on 22 CML recipients of twin transplants, including 12 treated in chronic phase [43]. As of August 2002, seven of the 12 chronic phase patients are alive 20.8–26.3 years after transplant, of whom five are in their initial complete remission, one is alive in remission after a second transplant and one is alive in relapse. These data demonstrate that a high-dose preparative regimen can, in some cases, cure CML even without the benefit of an allogeneic graft-vs.-leukemia (GVL) effect.

Allogeneic hematopoietic cell transplantation from matched siblings

Chronic phase

Based on the results from twin studies, the Seattle team began studying human leukocyte antigen (HLA) matched sibling transplants as therapy for chronic phase CML in 1979 and in 1982 reported initial results from 10 patients [44]. As of November 2002, four of these patients remain alive without detectable CML between 20 and 23 years after transplant. These results and other early reports prompted increased study of allogenic transplantation for CML. In 1986, the Seattle group published the first moderately large study when they reported the outcome of 167 patients transplanted through 1983 from matched siblings [45]. These results have been updated through November 2002, as shown in Figs 73.1 and 73.2. The long-term follow-up demonstrates that approximately 40% of patients transplanted in chronic phase more than 17 years ago are surviving, and also demonstrates the importance of disease phase on survival (Fig. 73.1) and relapse (Fig. 73.2). Since these early results, large numbers of patients with chronic phase CML have been treated with allogeneic transplants. Data from 4267 recipients of matched-sibling transplants reported to the IBMTR between 1994 and 1999 show a probability of survival of 69 ± 2% for 2876 patients transplanted within the first year from diagnosis, and 57 ± 3% for 1391 patients transplanted more than 1 year from diagnosis (Fig. 73.3) [46]. Results from selected

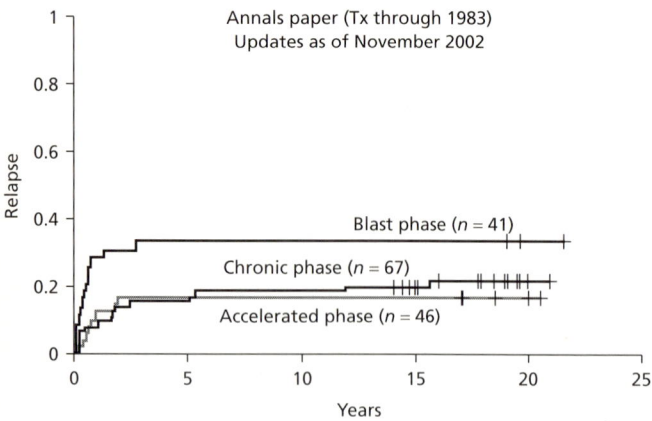

Fig. 73.2 Cumulative evidence of cytogenetic relapse by phase at the time of transplantation for 166 patients with chronic myeloid leukemia who received transplants through 1983 from HLA-identical siblings, first published in 1986 [45]. The results are updated as of November 2002.

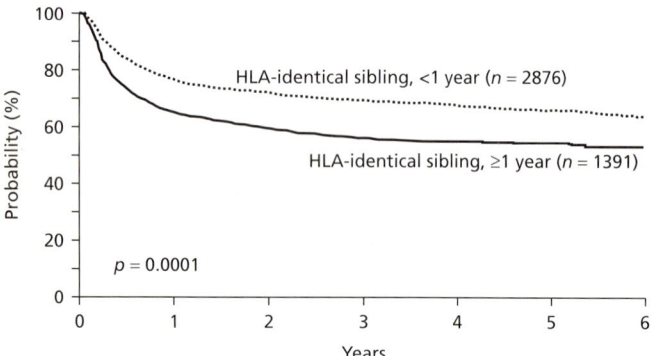

Fig. 73.3 Probability of survival after allogeneic transplants for patients with chronic myeloid leukemia in chronic phase transplanted between 1994 and 1999 and reported to the International Bone Marrow Transplant Registry, by disease duration [46].

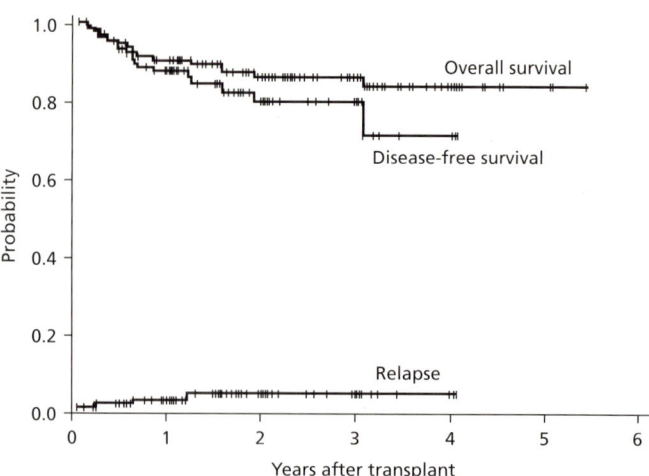

Fig. 73.4 Kaplan–Meier probabilities of survival and disease-free survival and the cumulative incidence of relapse among 131 patients with chronic myeloid leukemia in chronic phase transplanted from matched siblings following a preparative regimen of targeted busulfan and cyclophosphamide [47].

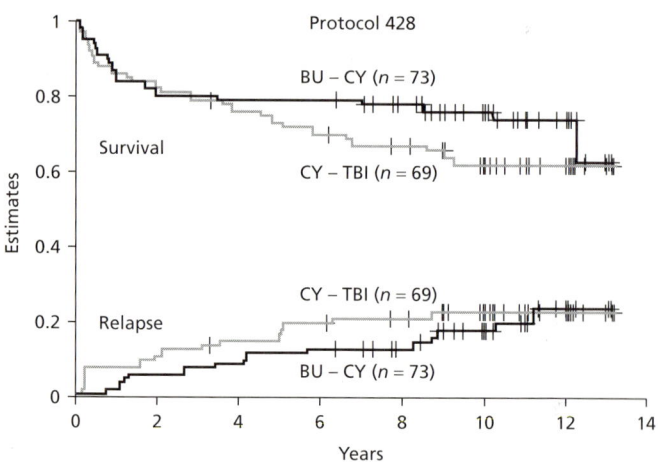

Fig. 73.5 Kaplan–Meier probabilities of survival and the cumulative incidences of relapse among 142 patients with chronic myeloid leukemia in chronic phase transplanted from matched siblings following a preparative regimen of either busulfan plus cyclophosphamide or cyclophosphamide plus total body irradiation. Results of this randomized trial were originally published in 1994 and are here updated as of November 2002.

single institutions exceed those of the registry. The Seattle group has recently reported on their most recent trial using a preparative regimen of targeted busulfan (BU) plus CY and cyclosporine plus methotrexate for graft-vs.-host disease (GVHD) prevention in 131 consecutive patients. Survival 3 years post-transplant was 86%, and 87% of surviving patients were molecularly negative for BCR-ABL mRNA by PCR analysis (Fig. 73.4) [47].

A number of different factors may possibly influence the outcome of transplantation for CP CML, including the preparative regimen, the source of stem cells, the form of GVHD prophylaxis, patient age, interval from diagnosis to transplant, prior therapy and the gender of the donor and patient. The majority of patients treated in the early 1980s received a preparative regimen of 120 mg/kg CY, followed by TBI. In the initial series reported by Thomas *et al.* [45], the TBI dose was 2.0 Gy on each of 6 successive days. A randomized trial conducted in Seattle asked whether an increase in the TBI dose from 12 Gy in six exposures to 15.75 Gy in seven exposures would decrease post-transplant relapse and improve survival. This study found that the relapse rate was, in fact, decreased with the increased TBI dose, but because of an increase in nonrelapse mortality neither survival nor disease-free survival were improved with the higher TBI dose [48]. In 1987, Tutschka *et al.* [49] described the use of a preparative regimen consisting of 16 mg/kg BU administered over 4 days combined with 60 mg/kg CY on each of 2 successive days, reporting excellent results in a limited number of patients with myeloid malignancies. Similar results were noted by others [50], and in 1988 a randomized trial was initiated in Seattle comparing the BU-CY regimen with CY plus 12 Gy TBI. At the time of the initial report, there were no differences between the CY-TBI and BU-CY treatment groups in survival at 3 years (80% for both), relapse (13% for both) or event-free survival (68% for CY-TBI and 71% for BU-CY) [51]. The BU-CY regimen was better tolerated with more rapid engraftment, shorter hospitalization and less GVHD making it the preferred regimen of the two. An update of this study was published in 1999 [52] and a further update in 2002 shows overall survival of 78% at 10 years with BU-CY vs. 64% with CY-TBI (Fig. 73.5).

The absorption and subsequent metabolism of busulfan varies from patient to patient. Accordingly, the group in Seattle began measuring the concentration of busulfan in plasma of patients transplanted for CML using a standard BU-CY regimen. These studies showed that patients who had a steady state busulfan concentration of less than 917 ng/mL, the median value found in the originally studied cohort, had a significantly higher risk of disease recurrence and worse overall survival than those with levels above 917 ng/mL [53]. These investigators also found that by measuring the metabolism of busulfan on the first day of therapy, it was possible to adjust subsequent dosing to keep steady state busulfan concentrations between 900 and 1200 ng/mL. A subsequent report of 131 consecutive patients transplanted for CML chronic phase from HLA-identical relatives, showed a 3-year survival of 86%, a relapse rate of only 8% and nonrelapse mortality rate of 14% [47]. The median age of this group of patients was 43 years with 30 of the patients being above age 50 (the oldest was aged 66). Although there have been no randomized comparisons, other preparative regimens have also been reported to provide excellent disease control with acceptable toxicities in the treatment of CML chronic phase including the regimen of TBI plus etoposide, reported by the groups from City of Hope National Medical Center and Stanford University [54] and the use of CY plus 500 cGy TBI given as a single dose at high dose rate [55].

Because CML chronic phase is so often associated with splenomegaly, a number of investigators have asked whether therapy directed specifically towards the spleen should be considered. A retrospective analysis found no benefit of splenectomy prior to transplantation [56]. A prospective randomized trial of the addition of splenic irradiation to the conditioning regimen found no overall advantage for irradiation [57]. A retrospective subgroup analysis of this randomized trial suggested a possible reduction in relapse in poor-risk patients with high basophil counts.

Bone marrow has served as the source of stem cells for the large majority of patients transplanted for CML chronic phase from matched siblings. Two separate large randomized trials involving patients with a variety of hematologic malignancies receiving transplants from matched siblings have been published demonstrating that use of filgrastim [granulocyte-colony stimulating factor (G-CSF)] mobilized peripheral blood hematopoietic cells, when compared to bone marrow, leads to more rapid myeloid and platelet recovery, no significant difference in acute or chronic GVHD and an overall survival advantage. These studies were not prospectively designed to address the role of peripheral blood vs. bone marrow for individual disease states. In the studies by Bensinger et al. [58] and Couban et al. [59] there was a trend towards improved survival in CML patients with the use of peripheral blood. In the study by Couban et al. among 109 CML patients, survival at 3 years was 80% with peripheral blood vs. 65% with bone marrow. Both of these studies used conventional GVHD prophylaxis. A third randomized trial comparing filgrastim mobilized peripheral blood vs. bone marrow used a GVHD regimen with reduced dosage of methotrexate (MTX) and found more rapid engraftment with peripheral blood, an increase in GVHD with peripheral blood and no impact on survival [60]. No analysis restricted to CML was presented.

The form of GVHD prophylaxis used in the treatment regimens also influences the outcome of transplantation for CML in chronic phase. Prior to 1984, most patients were given either single agent MTX or single agent cyclosporine (CSP) as GVHD prophylaxis, and randomized trials demonstrated the relative equivalence of the two approaches [61]. In 1986, the Seattle group published results of a randomized trial showing that a regimen combining four doses of MTX with CSP was superior to single agent CSP prophylaxis in reducing the incidence of GVHD and in improving overall survival for patients transplanted for CML chronic phase [62]. A number of variations from the standard MTX-CSP regimen have been explored, including adding prednisone or substituting FK506 for CSP. While each of these variations has also provided excellent GVHD prophylaxis for matched siblings with CML undergoing transplantation during chronic phase, none has shown an overall survival advantage. Prevention of GHVD by removing T cells from the donor marrow was explored in a number of transplant studies in the 1980s. Although successful in reducing the incidence of GVHD, T-cell deple-

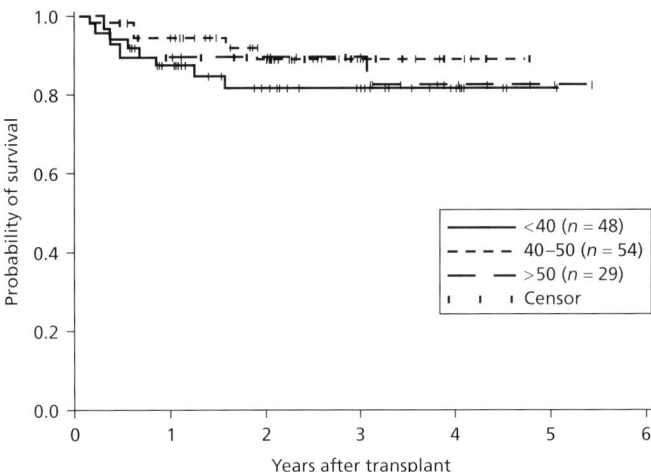

Fig. 73.6 Kaplan–Meier probabilities of survival according to age among 131 patients with chronic myeloid leukemia in chronic phase transplanted from matched siblings following a preparative regimen of targeted busulfan and cyclophosphamide [47].

tion in CML was associated with high rates of graft failure and relapse leading to poorer disease-free and overall survival [63]. These findings illustrated the critical role of the GVL effect in eradicating CML following allogeneic transplantation. Because of these observations, T-cell depletion was largely abandoned as a method to control GVHD in CML transplants. However, there has been renewed interest in the possibility of preventing GVHD without loss of a GVL effect by combining T-cell depletion with an intensified conditioning regimen and delayed reinfusion of viable donor lymphocytes [64].

Initial studies of transplantation for CML in chronic phase from HLA-matched siblings suggested that results might deteriorate with increasing patient age. Given the median age of patients with CML at diagnosis, these observations significantly limited the proportion of patients who were candidates for transplantation. As methods for GHVD prophylaxis and supportive care were improved, the impact of age on outcome appeared to diminish. In 1993, the Seattle group published results of 33 patients with CML in chronic phase, aged 50–60 years, and reported an 85% survival at 5 years [65]. The relative lack of effect of age up to age 65 on outcome of matched sibling transplantation for CML in chronic phase has been reconfirmed in the most recent Seattle experience utilizing the targeted BU-CP preparative regimen (Fig. 73.6).

An unanticipated finding that emerged from an analysis of the original cohort of 167 patients transplanted in Seattle was that an increased interval from diagnosis to transplant was associated with a worse transplant outcome, even for patients remaining in chronic phase at the time of transplant. This finding, which was at first controversial, has since been confirmed by others and is evident in the most recent IBMTR data (Fig. 73.3) [66,67]. Reasons for the effect of delay on outcome are not readily apparent. No single cause of failure is markedly increased with delay; rather there is a modest effect of delay on multiple outcomes including a slightly higher relapse rate and a slight increase in nonrelapse mortality. None the less, the aggregate effect of delay on outcome is readily apparent and, as discussed below, is a major factor in developing an optimal strategy for the management of patients with CML in chronic phase.

One hypothesis for the effect of delay on outcome focused on the effects of prior therapy. An early report from the IBMTR strongly suggested that exposure to low-dose busulfan led to a worse outcome with subsequent transplantation [66]. Some reports suggested that exposure to IFN might worsen the outcome of unrelated donor transplant, but data on the effect of IFN on matched sibling transplantation were less clear. In a recent German report of 856 patients randomized to hydroxyurea, busulfan or interferon, 197 went on to transplant. Although there was no overall difference in transplant outcome according to the initial treatment, the 5-year survival from transplant was only 46% for the 50 patients who received IFN within the last 90 days before transplant, but was 71% for the 36 who did not ($p = 0.0057$) [68]. These observations suggest that IFN should be avoided, if possible, in the months immediately preceding allogeneic hematopoietic cell transplantation. There are no data as yet as to the effect of prior exposure to imatinib on the outcome of subsequent transplantation.

There appears to be a complex interaction between donor and recipient gender in the outcome of transplantation for CML in chronic phase. In the European Group for Blood and Marrow Transplant (EBMT) experience, being a male recipient of a female donor was associated with a worse outcome compared to all other gender combinations. The Seattle experience also shows a worse outcome in male recipients with female donors, and in addition shows a superior outcome in female recipients of female donors.

Other factors that have been hypothesized to influence outcomes of HLA-matched sibling transplants for CML in chronic phase include cytomegalovirus (CMV) seropositivity of patient and donor, and patient spleen size. In general, these have not remained as significant factors in multivariate analyses after taking into account patient age, interval from diagnosis to transplant, and the gender combination of donor and recipient.

Accelerated phase

As noted in Fig. 73.1, and other studies, the outcomes of matched sibling transplants for accelerated phase CML are generally worse than seen in chronic phase [69,70]. However, the term accelerated phase encompasses a wide spectrum of patients. In a Seattle analysis of 58 patients with accelerated phase CML transplanted from HLA-identical siblings, the 4-year probabilities of survival and event-free survival were 49 and 43%, and the actual probability of relapse, censoring for other causes of death, was 12% [71]. Of particular interest was the observation that the probability of survival was 66% for those who were declared to be in accelerated phase solely because of cytogenetic progression but only 34% if factors other than or in addition to cytogenetic progression were the reasons for declaring disease progression ($p < 0.01$). Further analyses of this cohort of patients showed that a shorter interval from diagnosis to transplant and age 37 years or less (the median age of the group) appeared to be significant predictors of favorable outcome in univariate analysis. In multivariate analysis, only age and the reason for declaring progression (cytogenetics only vs. other) remained significant.

Blast phase

In virtually all studies, the outcome of transplantation for patients in blast phase is very poor, both because of a high risk of disease recurrence and a high incidence of transplant-related deaths [45,50,63]. The Seattle team had performed transplants for 100 patients in blast phase before 1993, with event-free survivals of 43, 18 and 11% at 100 days, 1 year and 3 years, respectively. Although these results are disappointing, the small but definite percentage of patients cured (see Fig. 73.1) still provides a justification for transplantation because there is no other curative therapy available for such patients.

Prior to the development of imatinib, only a small proportion of patients with blast phase CML could achieve a hematologic remission when treated with chemotherapy. These were largely patients with lymphoid blast phase, where short-term remissions with ALL-like therapy can be attained in up to 60% [72]. In myeloid blast crisis, complete response rates to regimens used to treat acute myeloid leukemia (AML) are rarely higher than 15% [73]. As shown in Fig. 73.1, transplantation for patients with CML in remission after a previous blast phase results in cure rates not substantially worse than seen in chronic phase patients.

These results have since been confirmed in a further analysis of 35 patients transplanted from matched siblings in Seattle for CML in remission after blast crisis. The survival updated to November 2002 shows a probability of 44% at 10 years, with a probability of recurrence of 20%. Others have also documented the importance of achieving a second chronic phase before proceeding to transplant [74].

Response rates of patients with CML in blast phase to imatinib are considerably higher than seen with conventional chemotherapy. However, as with most conventional chemotherapy regimens, these responses tend to be short, particularly in the setting of lymphoid blast crisis. There are, as yet, almost no data on the outcome of transplantation for patients with previous blast crisis back in remission following treatment with imatinib.

Allogeneic hematopoietic cell transplantation from alternative donors

Because only approximately one-third of patients have HLA-matched family members to serve as donors, considerable research into the use of alternative donors for transplantation in CML has been conducted. In Chapter 83, details concerning the use of unrelated donors for transplantation in CML are presented. As discussed in that chapter, while early results with matched unrelated donor transplantation in CML suggested results somewhat poorer than seen with matched siblings [75], advances in donor selection, GVHD prophylaxis and supportive care have resulted in continued improvements in outcome so that now selected single institutions are reporting results almost equivalent to those seen with matched siblings, and registry data are showing 65% survival at 5 years among younger patients transplanted within a year of diagnosis [76–78]. Details about the use of mismatched related donors are presented in Chapter 82, and use of cord-blood transplants are included in Chapter 43. The experience with autologous transplantation in CML is detailed in Chapter 91.

Graft-vs.-leukemia effect in CML

While evidence for a GVL effect can be found in many settings, nowhere is it as strong as in the setting of allogeneic transplantation for CML. Evidence in support of such an effect includes, first, the higher rates of relapse following syngeneic and T-cell depleted transplants compared to nonmodified allogeneic transplants [63,79]. Second, following non-T-cell depleted transplants there is a close association between the development of acute and chronic GVHD and freedom from relapse [80,81]. Third, response rates to donor lymphocyte infusions to treat post-transplant relapse range from 50 to 100% in various reports, higher than in any other malignancy [82,83]. While the mechanisms underlying the GVL effect in CML are not entirely understood, the markedly increased relapse rates seen with T-cell depletion argue that it is largely a T-cell mediated process. The targets of T cells might include minor histocompatibility antigens shared by most cells in the body, thus accounting for the association of GVL with GVHD. Alternatively, there may be polymorphic minor histocompatibility antigens with expression limited to hematopoietic tissue. A number of such antigens have been identified [84,85] and their role as targets for GVL could explain the observation that relapse rates are less following non-T-cell depleted transplants than with T-cell depleted transplants even in patients who develop no signs of GVHD. A third possible category of targets for the GVL effect in CML are overexpressed self-antigens. For example, PR3 is a neutral serine proteinase with expression largely restricted to very immature myeloid cells. In a very provocative paper, Molldrem et al. [86] detected $CD8^+$ cytotoxic T-cells specific for PR3 in the blood of CML patients who had been treated successfully with allogeneic transplantation or with interferon alfa. When patients recurred, these responses were lost. Finally, it is possible that T-cell responses could be directed at the tumor-specific peptides spanning the BCR-ABL fusion region, but there is little evidence for the presence of high numbers of T cells with specificity against BCR-ABL in patients successfully transplanted for CML. Understanding the cells and their targets responsible for the potent GVL effect seen in CML will be critical to the development of more effective, less toxic transplant-based therapies in the future.

Even without a clear understanding of the cell populations mediating the GVL effect following standard transplantation for CML, investigators have begun to study reduced intensity or nonablative transplant approaches in an attempt to avoid the toxicities of high-dose preparative regimens while retaining the potentially powerful GVL effects. These approaches, which are discussed in more detail in Chapter 85, are of particular relevance for patients with CML given that their median age at diagnosis is 67 years. While the results of these studies are still in the early stages, some of the early observations are intriguing. For example, using a preparative regimen consisting only of 200 cGy TBI and GVHD prophylaxis using CSP and mycophenolate mofetil, McSweeney et al. [87] reported complete molecular responses in five of nine patients transplanted for CML in chronic phase ($n = 6$) or accelerated phase ($n = 3$). The other four patients rejected their grafts. By adding 30 mg/m^2 × 3 fludarabine pretransplant, these investigators report that graft rejection has been eliminated as a problem following matched sibling transplantation. Or et al. [88] have recently reported similar encouraging results using a preparative regimen of fludarabine, low-dose busulfan and antithymocyte globulin. Thus, nonablative allogeneic hematopoietic cell transplantation may offer a safe and effective way to treat CML in chronic phase.

Monitoring minimal residual disease

The fact that CML is always associated with the BCR-ABL translocation coupled with the development of PCR techniques capable of detecting and quantitating extraordinarily small numbers of abnormal cells among a large population of normal ones makes CML an ideal setting to test the capabilities of minimal residual disease monitoring to provide insight into the disease and direct therapies. Details about minimal residual disease detection are provided in Chapter 22. With nonquantitative PCR techniques it is possible to detect a single CML cell in a population of 10^5–10^6 cells. Using such an assay, Radich et al. [89] studied 346 patients after transplantation and found that in over 40% of patients PCR assays were positive for residual disease at 3 months post-transplant but that this finding was not predictive of outcome, suggesting that eradication of the CML clone post-transplant takes an extended period of time. In contrast, at 6 or 12 months post-transplant, the risk of being PCR positive dropped to 27%, and by this time the assay had become a powerful predictor of outcome, with only 3% of PCR-negative patients eventually relapsing compared to 42% of PCR-positive patients ($p < 0.0001$). Subsequently, Radich et al. have found that the predictive power of PCR among longer term survivors is somewhat weaker. When studied at 18 months or more post-transplant, only 1% of 289 BCR-ABL negative patients subsequently relapsed compared to 14% of 90 BCR-ABL positive patients [90]. It is of interest that some PCR-negative patients relapse and perhaps somewhat surprising that such a small proportion of PCR-positive patients do so. Chomel et al. [91] have suggested BCR-ABL rearrangements may exist in nonproliferating cells detectable by FISH but undetectable by PCR.

While a positive nonquantitative PCR assay does not inevitably lead to relapse, some have used it as a marker for disease. Elmaagacli et al. [92] reported that the probability of becoming PCR negative was higher in chronic phase CML patients transplanted using peripheral blood as opposed to marrow as the source of stem cells.

While qualitative PCR testing has been revealing, the amount of information gained is still limited, with some PCR-negative patients relapsing and many PCR-positive patients remaining in remission. Accordingly, attempts have been made to develop quantitative PCR assays and apply them to the post-transplant CML setting. Olavarria et al. [93] studied 138 patients who received allografts, using a quantitative reverse transcription polymerase chain reaction (RT-PCR) assay performed at 3–5 months post-transplant, and were able to define patients as having a low risk (16%) of relapse, an intermediate risk (43%) or a high risk (86%) based on the quantification of the PCR signal [92]. Others have also demonstrated that PCR quantification of BCR-ABL is feasible [93], but no head-to-head comparison of utility and practicality of qualitative vs. quantitative PCR monitoring has yet been published. None the less, monitoring of minimal residual disease after transplantation for CML offers an obvious opportunity for early intervention for patients with residual or recurring disease.

Treatment of post-transplant relapse

The pace of disease progression after post-transplant relapse is variable. Indeed, if relapse is defined at a molecular (PCR) level, some patients may never progress, or at least may not progress for a very long time. Similarly, patients whose only evidence of relapse is detection of low levels of Ph-positive metaphases may remain stable for many years, and even patients with clinical relapse may not progress rapidly. The EBMT retrospectively studied 130 patients who relapsed after transplant before 1990 [at a time prior to the use of donor lymphocyte infusions (DLIs) or imatinib] and noted that post-relapse survival was significantly affected by disease phase at relapse, time from transplant to relapse and patient gender [94]. An update of that study including an additional 370 newer cases has since been published [95]. In this broader retrospective study, stage at transplant and relapse, time from diagnosis to transplantation and from transplantation to relapse, and type of donor (matched sibling vs. volunteer) all affected survival. Specifically, recipients of matched sibling grafts for chronic phase disease with a short interval from diagnosis to transplant but a long interval from transplant to relapse did particularly well, with a likelihood of being alive 10 years after post-transplant relapse of 42%. An appreciation of the likely tempo of progression is necessary when considering treatment interventions.

An increasing number of potential interventions are available to the patient who has relapsed after allogeneic transplantation for CML. Treatment with IFN can produce both clinical and cytogenetic remissions in patients who have relapsed after transplantation [96,97]. Results with IFN appear better if treatment is initiated at the time of cytogenetic relapse instead of waiting until hematologic relapse. In fact, if used to treat cytogenetic relapse, IFN induces molecular remissions in some individuals. Based on these results, the Seattle group completed a phase 2 study of IFN for patients who were PCR positive at 6–12 months post-transplant. The large majority of patients have become PCR negative and compared to historical controls, the proportion of patients who have progressed to hematologic relapse (10%) is less than previously seen [47]. This study thus suggests that early interventions based on PCR monitoring may be clinically beneficial for some patients.

Since the initial description of DLI as treatment of post-transplant relapse, experience with this approach has grown considerably and is detailed in Chapter 84. There are now a large number of studies demonstrating cytogenetic complete response rates of 50–100% in patients treated for clinically relapsed chronic phase CML (reviewed in [83]). Response rates tend to be higher for patients treated earlier at the time of cytogenetic relapse and lower for patients in accelerated phase. There is a trend towards improved response rates in patients treated within 2 years after transplantation [98]. Whether the higher response rate in early relapses reflects treatment at a time of less disease burden or some other biologic principle is unknown. The two major complications of DLI are transient marrow failure and the development of GVHD. Marrow failure only occurs in patients treated in hematologic relapse and likely reflects clearance of host hematopoiesis before donor hematopoiesis recovers, and thus is of particular concern for patients in full-blown hematologic relapse with no evidence of residual donor hematopoiesis [99]. Treatment earlier in the course of relapse can avoid this complication. The overall incidence of GVHD following DLI ranges around 50% in most series. Although complete remissions can be achieved in the absence of GVHD, with currently used approaches there is a close correlation between development of GVHD and achievement of complete responses to DLI [98]. Most early studies of DLI involved a single infusion of a relatively large number of donor T cells. In a dose escalation study conducted in patients who had recurrent CML after T-depleted transplants, Mackinnon et al. [100] found that 5×10^7/kg T cells were necessary to control CML, but that the incidence of GVHD also increased with higher T-cell doses. Dazzi et al. [101] have since reported that large numbers of T cells are tolerated with less GVHD if administered in a fractionated fashion rather than as a single bulk dose. A recent report from the EBMT provides further support for starting at lower doses of lymphocytes and escalating dosage as required. In their retrospective study of 298 patients, they found that beginning with a lower initial cell dose was associated with less GVHD, less myelosuppression, equal response rates and better survival [102]. They recommend an initial cell dose no higher than 0.2×10^8/kg.

Given its dramatic activity as initial therapy for CML, it is hardly surprising that imatinib mesylate should also be active as post-transplant therapy [103]. In a recent report of 28 patients who were treated with imatinib for post-transplant relapse, an overall response rate of 79% was seen, with complete hematologic response seen in 100% of patients in chronic phase, 83% in accelerated phase and 43% in blast crisis. Complete cytogenetic responses were seen in 29% of patients. Recurrence of GVHD disease was seen in 18% and granulocytopenia requiring dose adjustments of imatinib developed in 43% of patients. Because imatinib has only recently become available, almost all of the reported cases treated with imatinib for post-transplant relapse had never been treated with the drug previously. How pretransplant exposure and particularly demonstration of pretransplant resistance to imatinib will influence the activity of imatinib as post-transplant therapy is untested.

Second transplants have been used to treat patients who have developed recurrent CML following a first transplant. In general, preparative regimens based on chemotherapy only have been used for patients previously exposed to TBI and TBI-based regimens have been used when the first regimen relied only on chemotherapy. The Seattle group previously reported on 17 chronic phase patients treated with a second transplant for recurrent CML and three became long-term survivors [104]. Cullis et al. [105] reported on 16 patients who relapsed after T-cell depleted transplants and eight were alive a median of 424 days after a second transplant. With the availability of IFN, DLI, and now imatinib, the use of second transplants has diminished substantially.

Management of the newly diagnosed CML patient in the imatinib era

Imatinib mesylate has become the initial nontransplant treatment of choice for patients with CML. For patients diagnosed in accelerated phase or blast crisis, initial treatment with imatinib results in better responses than seen with other nontransplant therapies, but these responses in general tend to be short lived. Therefore, all such patients should be evaluated for transplantation and, if found to be appropriate candidates with suitable donors, should proceed to transplantation as soon as possible. For patients diagnosed during chronic phase, the decision about whether to first attempt a trial of imatinib and consider transplantation only if imatinib fails or whether to move directly to transplantation is a very difficult one. There are a number of arguments favoring early transplantation. First, transplantation is the only therapy known to truly cure patients of CML with large numbers of patients alive in hematologic, cytogenetic and molecular complete remission now more than two decades after transplantation. Second, with current approaches, the outcome of transplantation is reasonably good if carried out early in the disease course with 86% survival at 3 years in patients up to age 65 transplanted from matched siblings, and in patients up to age 50 transplanted from unrelated donors at selected centres [47,77]. Third, the outcome of transplantation is considerably worse if delayed until patients evolve into accelerated phase or blast crisis. Fourth, even if patients stay in chronic phase, delay from diagnosis to time of transplant has a decidedly negative effect on subsequent transplant outcome.

There are also a number of arguments in favor of initial therapy with imatinib mesylate. The overwhelming argument is quite straightforward; why subject a patient to a potentially life-threatening procedure when a relatively nontoxic oral medication achieves hematologic control in virtually all patients and cytogenetic responses in the majority? The essential problem facing the physician and patient is that we simply do not have enough information yet to make this choice intelligently. While we know that initially all patients achieve a hematologic response to imatinib and the majority achieve a cytogenetic response, we know little about the likely duration of these responses. While we know that the majority of transplant survivors have not even molecular evidence of disease, we know comparatively little about what happens with imatinib. Early results suggest that very few patients treated with imatinib become PCR negative, but this proportion could grow with time or if imatinib were combined with other drugs. We do not know if patients failing imatinib will recur with slowly progressing disease in chronic phase allowing for salvage transplantation or if patients will present with rapidly accelerating disease. Nor do we know how prior extensive therapy with imatinib might affect transplant outcomes.

In most settings, therapies that are proven to result in cures are recommended over newer therapies without such track records. Thus, many physicians and patients will choose early transplantation, particularly if patients have an HLA-matched sibling or are under age 50 with a perfectly matched unrelated donor. However, given the considerably different toxicity profiles of the two approaches, many patients and their physicians will opt for an initial trial of imatinib therapy. Recent data on the use of allogeneic transplantation reflect this trend [106]. If imatinib is chosen as initial therapy, those patients require careful monitoring so that, if required, transplantation can be scheduled and conducted in a timely manner. In this regard, it is important to remember that it takes, on average, 3 months to complete an unrelated donor search and schedule the transplant procedure. At present, monitoring patients on imatinib involves frequent assays of peripheral blood counts and intermittent assessment of marrow cytogenetics. While it is unproven that a complete cytogenetic response to imatinib is required for long-term control of the disease, it would seem prudent to consider transplantation in any patient who is a candidate for that treatment and who has not achieved at least a major cytogenetic response after 1 year of imatinib therapy, with continual fall in the number of Ph-positive metaphases. Semi-quantitative PCR assays will almost certainly be used to help guide therapy in the future.

Conclusions

CML serves as an excellent model for how insights into the molecular basis of a malignant disease and the body's response to that disease can be translated into powerful diagnostic tools and highly effective therapies. While the simultaneous development of imatinib and improvements in transplant techniques have made it harder to advise patients on which initial therapeutic path to take, both paths are superior to anything that could previously be offered to these patients.

References

1 Greenlee RT, Murray T, Bolden S, Wingo PA. Cancer statistics, 2000. *CA Cancer J Clin* 2000; **50**: 7–33.
2 National Cancer Institute. *Surveillance, Epidemiology, and End Results (SEER) Program.* National Cancer Institute, DCPC, Surveillance Program, Cancer Statisitics Branch: Bethesda, MD, USA 1997; Public use CD-ROM 1973–94 released October 1997 based on the August 1996 submission.
3 Heyssel R, Brill AB, Woodbury LA et al. Leukemia in Hiroshima atomic bomb survivors. *Blood* 1960; **15**: 313–31.
4 Nowell PC, Hungerford DA. A minute chromosome in human granulocytic leukemia. *Science* 1960; **132**: 1497.
5 Rowley JD. A new consistent chromosomal abnormality in chronic myelogenous leukemia. *Nature* 1973; **243**: 290–3.
6 Faderl S, Talpaz M, Estrov Z, O'Brien S, Kurzrock R, Kantarjian HM. The biology of chronic myeloid leukemia. *N Engl J Med* 1999; **341**: 164–72 [Review].
7 Faderl S, Talpaz M, Estrov Z, Kantarjian HM. Chronic myelogenous leukemia: biology and therapy. *Ann Intern Med* 1999; **131**: 207–19 [Review].
8 Sawyers CL. Chronic myeloid leukemia. *N Engl J Med* 1999; **340**: 1330–40 [Review].
9 Lee SJ. Chronic myelogenous leukaemia. *Br J Haematol* 2000; **111**: 993–1009 [Review].
10 Pane F, Frigeri F, Sindona M et al. Neutrophilic-chronic myeloid leukemia: a distinct disease with a specific molecular marker (BCR/ABL with C3/A2 junction). *Blood* 1996; **88**: 2410–14. [Erratum appears in *Blood* 1997; **89**: 4244.]
11 Bernstein R. Cytogenetics of chronic myelogenous leukemia. *Semin Hematol* 1988; **25**: 20–34 [Review].
12 Heisterkamp N, Jenster G, ten Hoeve J, Zovich D, Pattengale PK, Groffen J. Acute leukaemia in bcr/abl transgenic mice. *Nature* 1990; **344**: 251–3.
13 Daley GQ, van Etten RA, Baltimore D. Induction of chronic myelogenous leukemia in mice by the p210 bcr/abl gene of the Philadelphia chromosome. *Science* 1990; **247**: 824–30.
14 Kelliher MA, McLaughlin J, Witte ON, Rosenberg N. Induction of a chronic myelogenous leukemia-like syndrome in mice with v-abl and BCR/ABL. *Proc Natl Acad Sci U S A* 1990; **87**: 6649–53. [Erratum appears in *Proc Natl Acad Sci U S A* 1990; **87**: 9072.]
15 McLaughlin J, Chianese E, Witte ON. In vitro transformation of immature hematopoietic cells by the P210 BCR/ABL oncogene product of the Philadelphia chromosome. *Proc Natl Acad Sci U S A* 1987; **84**: 6558–62.
16 Evans CA, Owen-Lynch PJ, Whetton AD, Dive C. Activation of the Abelson tyrosine kinase activity is associated with suppression of apoptosis in hemopoietic cells. *Cancer Res* 1993; **53**: 1735–8.
17 Bazzoni G, Carlesso N, Griffin JD, Hemler ME. Bcr/Abl expression stimulates integrin function in hematopoietic cell lines. *J Clin Invest* 1996; **98**: 521–8.
18 Wang JY. Abl tyrosine kinase in signal transduction and cell-cycle regulation. *Curr Opin Genet Dev* 1993; **3**: 35–43 [Review].
19 Druker BJ, Tamura S, Buchdunger E et al. Effects of a selective inhibitor of the Abl tyrosine kinase on the growth of Bcr-Abl positive cells. *Nat Med* 1996; **2**: 561–6.
20 Sokal JE, Baccarani M, Russo D, Tura S. Staging and prognosis in chronic myelogenous leukemia. *Semin Hematol* 1988; **25**: 49–61 [Review].
21 Mitelman F. The cytogenetic scenario of chronic myeloid leukemia. *Leuk Lymphoma* 1993; **11** (Suppl. 1): 11–5 [Review].
22 Griffin JD, Todd RF, Ritz J et al. Differentiation patterns in the blastic phase of chronic myeloid leukemia. *Blood* 1983; **61**: 85–91.
23 Minot GR, Buckman TE, Isaacs R. Chronic myelogenous leukemia. *N Engl J Med* 1924; **82**: 1489–95.
24 Tura S, Baccarani M, Corbelli G, The Italian Cooperative Study Group in CML. Staging of chronic myeloid leukaemia. *Br J Haematol* 1981; **47**: 105–19.
25 Sokal JE, Cox EB, Baccarani M et al. Prognostic discrimination in 'good-risk' chronic granulocytic leukemia. *Blood* 1984; **63**: 789–99.
26 Hehlmann R, Ansari H, Hasford J et al. Comparative analysis of the impact of risk profile and of drug therapy on survival in CML using Sokal's index and a new score: German chronic myeloid leukaemia (CML) Study Group. *Br J Haematol* 1997; **97**: 76–85.
27 Hasford J, Pfirrmann M, Hehlmann R et al. A new prognostic score for survival of patients with chronic myeloid leukemia treated with interferon alfa. Writing Committee for the Collaborative CML Prognostic Factors Project Group. *J Natl Cancer Inst* 1998; **90**: 850–8.
28 Haddow A, Timmis GM. Myleran in chronic myeloid leukaemia: chemical constitution and biological action. *Lancet* 1953; **1**: 207–8.
29 Krakoff IH, Murphy ML, Savelk H. Preliminary trials of hydroxyurea in neoplastic disease in man. *Proc Am Assoc Cancer Res* 1963; **4**: 35.
30 Hehlmann R, Heimpel H, Hasford J et al. Randomized comparison of busulfan and hydroxyurea in chronic myelogenous leukemia: prolongation of survival by hydroxyurea. *Blood* 1993; **82**: 398–407.
31 Hehlmann R, Heimpel H, Hasford J et al. Randomized comparison of interferon-α with busulfan and hydroxyurea in chronic myelogenous leukemia. *Blood* 1994; **84**: 4064–77.
32 Talpaz M, Kantarjian HM, McCredie K, Trujillo JM, Keating MJ, Gutterman JU. Hematologic remission and cytogenetic improvement induced by recombinant human interferon alpha$_A$ in chronic myelogenous leukemia. *N Engl J Med* 1986; **314**: 1065–9.
33 Chronic Myeloid Leukemia Trialists' Collaborative Group. Interferon alfa versus chemotherapy for chronic myeloid leukemia: a meta-analysis of seven randomized trials. *J Natl Cancer Inst* 1997; **89**: 1616–20.
34 Guilhot F, Chastang C, Michallet M et al. Interferon alfa-2b combined with cytarabine versus interferon alone in chronic myelogenous leukemia. *N Engl J Med* 1997; **337**: 223–9.
35 Tura S. Cytarabine increases karyotypic response in alpha-IFN treated chronic myeloid leukemia patients: results of a national prospective randomized trial. *Blood* 1998; **92**: 317a [Abstract].
36 Druker BJ, Talpaz M, Resta DJ et al. Efficacy and safety of a specific inhibitor of the BCR-ABL tyrosine kinase in chronic myeloid leukemia. *N Engl J Med* 2001; **344**: 1031–7.
37 Druker BJ, Sawyers CL, Kantarjian H et al. Activity of a specific inhibitor of the BCR-ABL tyrosine kinase in the blast crisis of chronic myeloid leukemia and acute lymphoblastic leukemia with the Philadelphia chromosome. *N Engl J Med* 2001; **344**: 1038–42.
38 Savage DG, Antman KH. Imatinib mesylate: a new oral targeted therapy. *N Engl J Med* 2002; **346**: 683–93 [Review].
39 Druker BJ. STI571 (Gleevec/Glivec, imatinib) versus interferon (IFN) + cytarabine as initial therapy for patients with CML: results of a randomized study (Plenary Presentation). *Program/Proc Am Soc Clin Oncology* 2002; **21**: 1a [Abstract].
40 Gorre ME, Sawyers CL. Molecular mechanisms of resistance to STI571 in chronic myeloid leukemia. *Curr Opin Hematol* 2002; **9**: 303–7.
41 Roche-Lestienne C, Soenen-Cornu V, Grardel-Duflos N et al. Several types of mutations of the Abl gene can be found in chronic myeloid leukemia patients resistant to STI571, and they can pre-exist to the onset of treatment. *Blood* 2002; **100**: 1014–18.
42 Fefer A, Cheever MA, Thomas ED et al. Disappearance of Ph[1]-positive cells in four patients with chronic granulocytic leukemia after chemotherapy, irradiation and marrow transplantation from an identical twin. *N Engl J Med* 1979; **300**: 333–7.
43 Fefer A, Cheever MA, Greenberg PD et al. Treatment of chronic granulocytic leukemia with chemoradiotherapy and transplantation of marrow from identical twins. *N Engl J Med* 1982; **306**: 63–8.
44 Clift RA, Buckner CD, Thomas ED et al. Treatment of chronic granulocytic leukaemia in chronic phase by allogeneic marrow transplantation. *Lancet* 1982; **2**: 621–3.
45 Thomas ED, Clift RA, Fefer A et al. Marrow transplantation for the treatment of chronic myelogenous leukemia. *Ann Intern Med* 1986; **104**: 155–63.
46 International Bone Marrow Transplant Registry. http://wwwibmtrorg2002
47 Radich JP, Gooley T, Bensinger W et al. Matched-related transplantation for chronic myeloid leukemia in chronic phase using a targeted busulfan and cyclophosphamide preparative regimen. *Blood*, in press.
48 Clift RA, Buckner CD, Appelbaum FR et al. Allogeneic marrow transplantation in patients with chronic myeloid leukemia in the chronic phase: a randomized trial of two irradiation regimens. *Blood* 1991; **77**: 1660–5.
49 Tutschka PJ, Copelan EA, Klein JP. Bone marrow transplantation for leukemia following a new busulfan and cyclophosphamide regimen. *Blood* 1987; **70**: 1382–8.
50 Biggs JC, Szer J, Crilley P et al. Treatment of chronic myeloid leukemia with allogeneic bone marrow transplantation after preparation with BuCy2. *Blood* 1992; **80**: 1090–3.
51 Clift RA, Buckner CD, Thomas ED et al. Marrow transplantation for chronic myeloid leukemia: a randomized study comparing cyclophosphamide and total body irradiation with busulfan and cyclophosphamide. *Blood* 1994; **84**: 2036–43.

52 Clift RA, Radich J, Appelbaum FR *et al.* Long-term follow-up of a randomized study comparing cyclophosphamide and total body irradiation with busulfan and cyclophosphamide for patients receiving allogeneic marrow transplants during chronic phase of chronic myeloid leukemia. *Blood* 1999; **94**: 3960–2 [Letter].

53 Slattery JT, Clift RA, Buckner CD *et al.* Marrow transplantation for chronic myeloid leukemia: the influence of plasma busulfan levels on the outcome of transplantation. *Blood* 1997; **89**: 3055–60.

54 Snyder DS, Negrin RS, O'Donnell MR *et al.* Fractionated total body irradiation and high dose etoposide as a preparatory regimen for bone marrow transplantation for 94 patients with chronic myelogenous leukemia. *Blood* 1994; **84**: 1672–9.

55 Fyles GM, Messner HA, Lockwood G *et al.* Long-term results of bone marrow transplantation for patients with AML, ALL and CML prepared with single dose total body irradiation of 500 cGy delivered with a high dose rate. *Bone Marrow Transplant* 1991; **8**: 453–63.

56 Gratwohl A, Gluckman E, Goldman J, Zwaan F. Effect of splenectomy before bone marrow transplantation on survival in chronic granulocytic leukaemia. *Lancet* 1985; **2**: 1290–1.

57 Gratwohl A, Hermans J, van Biezen A *et al.* Splenic irradiation before bone marrow transplantation for chronic myeloid leukaemia. Chronic Leukaemia Working Party of the European Group for Blood and Marrow Transplantation (EBMT). *Br J Haematol* 1996; **95**: 494–500.

58 Bensinger WI, Martin PJ, Storer B *et al.* Transplantation of bone marrow as compared with peripheral-blood cells from HLA-identical relatives in patients with hematologic cancers. *N Engl J Med* 2001; **344**: 175–81.

59 Couban S, Simpson DR, Barnett MJ *et al.* A randomized multicenter comparison of bone marrow and peripheral blood in recipients of matched sibling allogeneic transplants for myeloid malignancies. *Blood* 2002; **100**: 1525–31.

60 Schmitz N, Beksac M, Hasenclever D *et al.* Transplantation of mobilized peripheral blood cells to HLA-identical siblings with standard-risk leukemia. *Blood* 2002; **100**: 761–7.

61 Storb R, Deeg HJ, Thomas ED *et al.* Marrow transplantation for chronic myelocytic leukemia: a controlled trial of cyclosporine versus methotrexate for prophylaxis of graft-versus-host disease. *Blood* 1985; **66**: 698–702.

62 Storb R, Deeg HJ, Whitehead J *et al.* Methotrexate and cyclosporine compared with cyclosporine alone for prophylaxis of acute graft versus host disease after marrow transplantation for leukemia. *N Engl J Med* 1986; **314**: 729–35.

63 Goldman JM, Gale RP, Horowitz MM *et al.* Bone marrow transplantation for chronic myelogenous leukemia in chronic phase: increased risk of relapse associated with T-cell depletion. *Ann Intern Med* 1988; **108**: 806–14.

64 Drobyski WR, Hessner MJ, Klein JP *et al.* T-cell depletion plus salvage immunotherapy with donor leukocyte infusions as a strategy to treat chronic-phase chronic myelogenous leukemia patients undergoing HLA-identical sibling marrow transplantation. *Blood* 1999; **94**: 434–41. [Erratum appears in *Blood* 2000; **95**: 1137.]

65 Clift RA, Appelbaum FR, Thomas ED. Treatment of chronic myeloid leukemia by marrow transplantation. *Blood* 1993; **82**: 1954–6 [Review].

66 Goldman JM, Szydlo R, Horowitz MM *et al.* Choice of pretransplant treatment and timing of transplants for chronic myelogenous leukemia in chronic phase. *Blood* 1993; **82**: 2235–8.

67 Enright H, Daniels K, Arthur DC *et al.* Related donor marrow transplant for chronic meyloid leukemia: patient characteristics predictive of outcome. *Bone Marrow Transplant* 1996; **17**: 537–42.

68 Hehlmann R, Hochhaus A, Kolb HJ *et al.* Interferon-alpha before allogeneic bone marrow transplantation in chronic myelogenous leukemia does not affect outcome adversely, provided it is discontinued at least 90 days before the procedure. *Blood* 1999; **94**: 3668–77.

69 Martin PJ, Clift RA, Fisher LD *et al.* HLA-identical marrow transplantation during accelerated phase chronic myelogenous leukemia: analysis of survival and remission duration. *Blood* 1988; **72**: 1978–84.

70 Devergie A, Reiffers J, Vernant JP *et al.* Long-term follow-up after bone marrow transplantation for chronic myelogenous leukemia: factors associated with relapse. *Bone Marrow Transplant* 1990; **5**: 379–86. [Erratum appears in *Bone Marrow Transplant* 1990; **6**: 282.]

71 Clift RA, Buckner CD, Thomas ED *et al.* Marrow transplantation for patients in accelerated phase of chronic myeloid leukemia. *Blood* 1994; **84**: 4368–73.

72 Janossy G, Woodruff RK, Pippard MJ *et al.* Relation of "lymphoid" phenotype and response to chemotherapy incorporating vincristine-prednisolone in the acute phase of Ph1 positive leukemia. *Cancer* 1979; **43**: 426–34.

73 List AF, Kopecky KJ, Willman CL *et al.* Cyclosporine inhibition of P-glycoprotein in chronic myeloid leukemia blast phase. *Blood* 2002; **100**: 1910–2.

74 Visani G, Rosti G, Bandini G *et al.* Second chronic phase before transplantation is crucial for improving survival of blastic phase chronic myeloid leukaemia. *Br J Haematol* 2000; **109**: 722–8.

75 Kernan NA, Bartsch G, Ash RC *et al.* Analysis of 462 transplantations from unrelated donors facilitated by the National Marrow Donor Program. *N Engl J Med* 1993; **328**: 593–602.

76 Hansen JA, Gooley TA, Martin PJ *et al.* Bone marrow transplants from unrelated donors for patients with chronic myeloid leukemia. *N Engl J Med* 1998; **338**: 962–8.

77 Morton AJ, Gooley T, Hansen JA *et al.* Association between pretransplant interferon-α and outcome after unrelated donor marrow transplantation for chronic myelogenous leukemia in chronic phase. *Blood* 1998; **92**: 394–401.

78 McGlave PB, Shu XO, Wen W *et al.* Unrelated donor marrow transplantation for chronic myelogenous leukemia: 9 years' experience of the National Marrow Donor Program. *Blood* 2000; **95**: 2219–25.

79 Marmont AM, Horowitz MM, Gale RP *et al.* T-cell depletion of HLA-identical transplants in leukemia. *Blood* 1991; **78**: 2120–30.

80 Gratwohl A, Hermans J, Apperley J *et al.* Acute graft-versus-host disease: grade and outcome in patients with chronic myelogenous leukemia. Working Party Chronic Leukemia of the European Group for Blood and Marrow Transplantation. *Blood* 1995; **86**: 813–8 [Review].

81 van Rhee F, Szydlo RM, Hermans J *et al.* Long-term results after allogeneic bone marrow transplantation for chronic myelogenous leukemia in chronic phase: a report from the Chronic Leukemia Working Party of the European Group for Blood and Marrow Transplantation. *Bone Marrow Transplant* 1997; **20**: 553–60.

82 Kolb HJ, Mittermüller J, Clemm Ch *et al.* Donor leukocyte transfusions for treatment of recurrent chronic myelogenous leukemia in marrow transplant patients. *Blood* 1990; **76**: 2462–5.

83 Dazzi F, Szydlo RM, Goldman JM. Donor lymphocyte infusions for relapse of chronic myeloid leukemia after allogeneic stem cell transplant: where we now stand. *Exp Hematol* 1999; **27**: 1477–86 [Review].

84 Goulmy E. Human minor histocompatibility antigens: new concepts for marrow transplantation and adoptive immunotherapy. *Immunol Rev* 1997; **157**: 125–40 [Review].

85 Warren EH, Greenberg PD, Riddell SR. Cytotoxic T-lymphocyte-defined human minor histocompatibility antigens with a restricted tissue distribution. *Blood* 1998; **91**: 2197–207.

86 Molldrem JJ, Lee PP, Wang C *et al.* Evidence that specific T lymphocytes may participate in the elimination of chronic myelogenous leukemia. *Nat Med* 2000; **6**: 1018–23.

87 McSweeney PA, Niederwieser D, Shizuru JA *et al.* Hematopoietic cell transplantation in older patients with hematologic malignancies: replacing high-dose cytotoxic therapy with graft-versus-tumor effects. *Blood* 2001; **97**: 3390–400.

88 Or R, Shapira MY, Resnick I *et al.* Nonmyeloablative allogeneic stem cell transplantation for the treatment of chronic myeloid leukemia in first chronic phase. *Blood* 2003; **101**: 441–5.

89 Radich JP, Gehly G, Gooley T *et al.* Polymerase chain reaction detection of the *BCR-ABL* fusion transcript after allogeneic marrow transplantation for chronic myeloid leukemia: results and implications in 346 patients. *Blood* 1995; **85**: 2632–8.

90 Radich JP, Gooley T, Bryant E *et al.* The significance of *bcr-abl* molecular detection in chronic myeloid leukemia patients "late", 18 months or more after transplantation. *Blood* 2001; **98**: 1701–7.

91 Chomel JC, Brizard F, Veinstein A *et al.* Persistence of BCR-ABL genomic rearrangement in chronic myeloid leukemia patients in complete and sustained cytogenetic remission after interferon-alpha therapy or allogeneic bone marrow transplantation. *Blood* 2000; **95**: 404–8.

92 Elmaagacli AH, Beelen DW, Opalka B, Seeber S, Schaefer UW. The risk of residual molecular and cytogenetic disease in patients with Philadelphia-chromosome positive first chronic phase chronic myelogenous leukemia is reduced after transplantation of allogeneic peripheral blood stem cells compared with bone marrow. *Blood* 1999; **94**: 384–9.

93 Olavarria E, Kanfer E, Szydlo R *et al.* Early detection of *BCR-ABL* transcripts by quantitative reverse transcriptase-polymerase chain reaction predicts outcome after allogeneic stem cell transplantation for chronic myeloid leukemia. *Blood* 2001; **97**: 1560–5.

94 Arcese W, Goldman JM, D'Arcangelo E *et al.* Outcome for patients who relapse after allogeneic bone marrow transplantation for chronic myeloid leukemia. *Blood* 1993; **82**: 3211–9.

95 Guglielmi C, Arcese W, Hermans J *et al.* Risk assessment in patients with Ph+ chronic myelogen-

ous leukemia at first relapse after allogeneic stem cell transplant: an EBMT retrospective analysis. The Chronic Leukemia Working Party of the European Group for Blood and Marrow Transplantation. *Blood* 2000; **95**: 3328–34.

96 Higano CS, Raskind W, Singer JW. Use of alpha interferon for the treatment of relapse of chronic myelogenous leukemia in chronic phase after allogeneic bone marrow transplantation. *Blood* 1992; **80**: 1437–42.

97 Higano C, Raskind W, Flowers M. Alpha interferon (IFN) results in high complete cytogenetic response rate in patients with cytogenetic-only relapse of chronic myelogenous leukemia (CML) after marrow transplantation (BMT). *Blood* 1993; **82**: 669a [Abstract].

98 Collins RHJ, Shpilberg O, Drobyski WR *et al*. Donor leukocyte infusions in 140 patients with relapsed malignancy after allogeneic bone marrow transplantation. *J Clin Oncol* 1997; **15**: 433–44.

99 Keil F, Haas OA, Fritsch G *et al*. Donor leukoctye infusion for leukemic relapse after allogeneic marrow transplantation: lack of residual donor hematopoiesis predicts aplasia. *Blood* 1997; **89**: 3113–7.

100 Mackinnon S, Papadopoulos EB, Carabasi MH *et al*. Adoptive immunotherapy evaluating escalating doses of donor leukocytes for relapse of chronic myeloid leukemia after bone marrow transplantation: separation of graft-versus-leukemia responses from graft-versus-host disease. *Blood* 1995; **86**: 1261–8.

101 Dazzi F, Szydlo RM, Craddock C *et al*. Comparison of single-dose and escalating-dose regimens of donor lymphocyte infusion for relapse after allografting for chronic myeloid leukemia. *Blood* 2000; **95**: 67–71.

102 Guglielmi C, Arcese W, Dazzi F *et al*. Donor lymphocyte infusion for relapsed chronic myelogenous leukemia: prognostic relevance of the initial cell dose. *Blood* 2002; **100**: 397–405.

103 Kantarjian HM, O'Brien S, Cortes JE *et al*. Imatinib mesylate therapy for relapse after allogeneic stem cell transplantation for chronic myelogenous leukemia. *Blood* 2002; **100**: 1590–5.

104 Thomas ED, Clift RA. Allogeneic transplantation for chronic myeloid leukemia. In: Thomas ED, Blume KG, Forman SJ, eds. *Hematopoietic Cell Transplantation*, 2nd edn. Boston: Blackwell Science, 1999: 807–16.

105 Cullis JO, Schwarer AP, Hughes TP *et al*. Second transplants for patients with chronic myeloid leukaemia in relapse after original transplant with T-depleted marrow: feasibility of using busulphan alone for re-conditioning. *Br J Haematol* 1992; **80**: 33–9.

106 Gratwohl A, Baldomero H, Horisberger B *et al*. Current trends in hematopoietic stem cell transplantation in Europe. *Blood* 2002; **100**: 2374–86.

74

Robert A. Krance

Hematopoietic Cell Transplantation for Juvenile Myelomonocytic Leukemia

There is no specific molecular feature to identify patients with juvenile myelomonocytic leukemia (JMML). Rather the diagnosis of JMML rests on a compilation of physical and laboratory findings. Recently the International JMML Working Group and the European Working Group (EWOG) on childhood myelodysplastic syndrome have established criteria necessary to the diagnosis of JMML (Table 74.1) [1]. These consensus criteria are inclusive of children previously classified as having chronic myelomonocytic leukemia (CMML) or the infantile monosomy 7 syndrome. JMML replaces the older terminology of juvenile chronic myelogenous leukemia (JCML). The consensus criteria provide a framework within which to compare patients and treatment efficacy.

Clinical manifestations and laboratory findings

Past efforts to categorize JMML among the hematopoietic diseases had been made difficult because this disease exhibits features of myelodysplasia and myeloproliferation. A recently developed classification system for hematologic malignancies has established a category for myelodysplastic/myeloproliferative disease, which includes JMML, adult CMML and atypical chronic myeloid leukemia (CML) [2,3].

Reports suggest that the incidence of myelodysplastic/myeloproliferative diseases may range from 1% up to 17% of childhood hematologic malignancies [4–6]. This rather wide range may be explained by the inclusion in some reports of patients whose disease has evolved to acute myeloid leukemia (AML) [5,6]. Among all children with myelodysplastic/myeloproliferative disease, a sizeable portion will have JMML. Contemporary studies, which use the consensus criteria to define JMML, find that JMML comprises between 17% and 36% of childhood myelodysplastic/myeloproliferative disease; further, if patients classified as monosomy 7 syndrome and CMML are included, JMML may be the most common pediatric myelodysplastic/myeloproliferative disease [7,8].

JMML is primarily a disease of infants and young children with the median age of onset less than 2 years [9,10]. More than a third of patients are diagnosed during the 1st year of life, and almost every patient presents before age 5 years [10,11]. Boys are affected approximately twice as often as girls [9,10].

As defined by the consensus criteria, the presenting signs and symptoms of JMML reflect the failure of one or more hematopoietic lineages accompanied by widespread infiltration of viscera by malignant cells. Pallor, bleeding, fever and infection, often involving the respiratory system, can occur alone or in combination in half the patients. Splenomegaly, often massive, appears in more than 90% of patients and is a hallmark of the disease. Hepatomegaly occurs almost as frequently, while lymphadenopathy is found in 25–75% of patients [10,12–15]. Besides petechiae and ecchymoses, cutaneous manifestations of JMML may include xanthomas and eczematoid lesions.

Approximately 10–14% of children with JMML have neurofibromatosis type 1 (NF-1); the incidence of NF-1 in children with JMML exceeds

Table 74.1 Criteria for the diagnosis of juvenile myelomonocytic leukemia (JMML)* Adapted from Niemeyer et al. [1].

Category	Item
Suggestive clinical features	Hepatosplenomegaly
	Lymphadenopathy
	Pallor
	Fever
	Skin rash
Minimal laboratory criteria (all three have to be fulfilled)	No Ph$^+$ chromosome, no *bcr-abl* rearrangement
	Peripheral blood monocytes count $>1 \times 10^9$/L
	Bone marrow blasts <20
Criteria requested for definite diagnosis (at least two)	Hb F increased for age
	Myeloid precursors on peripheral blood smear
	White blood count $>10 \times 10^9$/L
	Clonal abnormality (including monosomy 7)
	GM-CSF hypersensitivity of myeloid progenitors *in vitro*

GM-CSF, granulocyte macrophage colony-stimulating factor; Hb, hemoglobin.

that in normal children by 200–300-fold [7,10,16,17]. Patients with JMML and NF-1 tend to present at a later age (median age >5 years) compared to patients without NF-1 [10]. Younger children with JMML may have café-au-lait spots, suggestive of NF-1 but insufficient to establish the diagnosis [18].

The presence of the Philadelphia (Ph) chromosome precludes the diagnosis of JMML; otherwise the laboratory findings of JMML are largely nonspecific (Table 74.1) [1,9–11]. Although leukocytosis may be profound, for the majority of patients the initial white count does not exceed 50×10^9/L, usually ranging from 25 to 50×10^9/L. An absolute monocytosis, $\geq 1.0 \times 10^9$/L, is a requisite to the diagnosis. Thrombocytopenia is almost invariably present at diagnosis and, as splenomegaly increases, patients become unresponsive to platelet transfusions. The blood smear may show nucleated red cells, immature myeloid cells, and 1–2% blast forms. Increased hemoglobin (Hb) F concentration occurs in two-thirds of patients. Finally, bone marrow examination demonstrates myelodysplastic findings similar to CMML. Most pathologists make no distinction between the marrow findings of JMML and CMML.

Monosomy 7 is the most common cytogenetic abnormality of JMML occurring in 25–30% of patients; another 10% of cases feature non-specific cytogenetic abnormalities [9–11,19]. The majority of children with JMML have a normal karyotype [9,10,20,21]. For some patients with monosomy 7, distinction between JMML and another entity, the infant monosomy 7 syndrome, has posed a problem [20,22]. Although many features of the infant monosomy 7 syndrome and JMML overlap, differences between the two, for example the concentration of Hb F or the response to chemotherapy, have led some to consider them as different entities. When larger patient cohorts are studied, it is not certain that the infant monosomy 7 syndrome is distinct from JMML [10,23]. The International JMML Working Group recommends that these disorders be approached from a common treatment scheme [7].

Biology of JMML

One feature used to define JMML is the exuberant *in vitro* growth from blood of almost pure monocyte colonies; normal colony growth is largely absent [24,25]. Efforts to identify the source of this peculiar growth pattern have shown that blood and marrow myeloid precursors from patients with JMML exhibit exaggerated and largely exclusive sensitivity to granulocyte macrophage colony-stimulating factor (GM-CSF) [26]. Hypersensitivity of the JMML cells to GM-CSF underlies the pathogenesis of the proliferative process [26,27]. What constitutes this hypersensitivity to GM-CSF is unclear. No activating mutations have been defined for the GM-CSF cell receptor, nor has excess production of GM-CSF production from paracrine or apocrine sources been shown [28,29]. Rather most clinical and experimental evidence suggest that GM-CSF hypersensitivity arises from disordered regulation of the intracellular GM-CSF signaling pathways.

The association between JMML and NF-1, which is caused by a mutation of the *NF1* gene, a tumour suppressor gene encoding the protein neurofibromin, has provided insight into JMML leukemogenesis [10,30,31]. Beyond the 15% coincidence of JMML and NF-1, an additional 15% of JMML patients without clinical findings of NF-1 have now been shown to have *NF1* mutations [18]. Bone marrow cells from patients with JMML and NF-1 demonstrate loss of heterozygosity in which the normal *NF1* allele is lost [32]. Neurofibromin, a GTPase-activating protein (GAP), negatively regulates the active state of Ras proteins, and loss of functional neurofibromin in JMML is associated with elevated levels of activated Ras protein [33]. Ras proteins serve a pivotal role in membrane signal transduction and increased activation is relevant to cellular proliferation [34]. A mouse model for JMML transplants allogeneic fetal liver hematopoietic cells homozygous for loss of the murine homologue of *NF1*. This induces a myeloproliferative disease similar to human JMML in which engrafted cells exhibit enhanced GM-CSF sensitivity mediated through the Ras pathway [35]. Mutations in *RAS* genes have been identified in an additional 20–30% of patients with JMML [36,37]. When found in patients, mutations in *RAS* or *NF1* occur exclusive of each other. Taken together more than 60% of children with JMML show genetic mutations that involve Ras signaling [18,38].

If activated Ras signaling is critical to the pathogenesis of JMML, then agents, which target this pathway, may prove therapeutically useful. Compounds which inhibit membrane signaling through the GM-CSF receptor, such as E21R, an antagonist of GM-CSF, or a fusion complex of diphtheria toxin and the GM-CSF receptor, have been shown to inhibit the growth of JMML cells in model systems [39,40]. Intracellularly, for Ras to be functional it must be linked to a farnesyl group. This reaction is catalyzed by the enzyme farenesyl-protein transferase. *In vitro*, inhibitors of farnesyl-transferase have prevented spontaneous colony growth of JMML cells [41]. The activity of these pharmacologic measures strengthen the likelihood for a pathogenetic role of RAS pathway in JMML [39,42].

Beyond the mechanisms underlying the GM-CSF hypersensitivity of JMML, the derivation of the malignant cell within the hematopoietic hierarchy remains uncertain. The cellular proliferation of JMML involves the macrophage/monocytic compartment; however, anemia and thrombocytopenia reflect a primary rather than secondary manifestation of disease. Patterns of X-chromosome inactivation and *NF1* allelic loss establish that the clonal nature of JMML originates among the most primitive hemopoietic progenitor cells [43,44]. While $CD34^+$ selected cells from JMML marrow or spleen recapitulate the aberrant growth pattern typical of JMML, these cells have the capacity to generate erythroid colonies under erythropoietin stimulation [45–48]. Other observations suggest that JMML has the capacity to differentiate along lymphoid pathways [43,49–52]. If true, the malignant cell of JMML must emanate at a point close to the true 'stem cell.' Therapies other than allogeneic hematopoietic stem cell (HSC) transplantation are unlikely to be curative.

Treatment of JMML

Although progressive in most patients, the course of JMML may be indolent or protracted, and a number of prognostic systems have been created to predict the likelihood of progression and survival [10–13,20]. Higher Hb F concentration and lower platelet count have been associated with shorter survival in some systems. Younger patients tended to live longer, but the discriminate age has ranged from 6 months to 4 years. Cytogenetic findings have been considered a factor in the disease course. At least one scoring system separated infant monosomy 7 syndrome from JMML and reported superior outcome for the former [20]. Other reports do not find JMML cytogenetic changes influential in regards to prognosis [8–10]. Part of the difficulty with these systems has been the lack of consistent diagnostic criteria. Differences between patient groups hinder comparison of treatments and outcomes. It is anticipated that adoption of the consensus criteria will reduce concerns over patient selection. The consensus criteria notwithstanding, the diagnosis of JMML rests upon signs and symptoms that are largely nonspecific. A number of reports illustrate the difficulty in distinguishing JMML from viral infections, such as cytomegalovirus, parvovirus, human herpesvirus 6, and Epstein–Barr virus [53–56]. That the diagnostic criteria of JMML remain imprecise is underscored by an infant with human herpesvirus 6 infection, whose bone marrow cells displayed GM-CSF hypersensitivity [55]. Ultimately, a molecular definition for JMML is needed [7].

The earliest reports of treatment of JMML document poor response to chemotherapy. Investigators employed low dose drug schedules that minimized drug regimen-related toxicity [13,57]. Treatment did not

Table 74.2 Results following hematopoietic stem cell (HSC) transplantation for children with juvenile myelomonocytic leukemia (JMML).

Author [ref.]	Pts (donor type)	Interval of accrual	BMT preparatory treatment	GVHD prophylaxis	Pts alive (EFS or DFS)	DFS duration	Relapse
Locatelli et al. [70]	43: 23 (MRD); 2 (1 Ag MMRD) 14 (MMRD); 4 (MMUD)	87–95	22 (TBI + CY ± other) 6 (BU/CY) 8 (BU/CY/VP16) 7 (BU/CY/MEL)	8 (CSP A) 8 (MTX) 16 (MTX/CSP A) 12 (MTX/CSP A/ATG); 1 (TCD)	14 EFS (31%) (38%) (21%)	~30 months median (9–66 months)	22
Donadieu et al. [71]	12: 6 (MRD) 5 (MMRD); 1 (MUD)	82–93	5 (BU/CY/VP16) 4 (TBI + chemotherapy) 3 (Other chemotherapy)	CSP A ± MTX TCD/CSP A	5 4 1	35 months median (3–128 months)	6 2 4
Smith et al. [72]	27: 10 (MRD) 14 (1, 2, or 3 Ag MMRD) 3 (MUD)	76–93	9 (dimethyl BU/CY/TBI) 2 (BU/CY/TBI) 15 (TBI/CY) 1 (BU/CY)	9 (MTX/CSP A/ATG) 8 (MTX/CSP A) 8 (MTX) 2 (MTX/prednisone)	5 25% DFS	7.3 year median (2.7–10 year)	10
Bunin et al. [73]	12: 7 (MUD) 2 (MMUD) 1 (MRD) 2 (MMRD)	90–97	7 (BU/AC/CY/TBI) 1 (VP16/TBI) 1 (BU/CY) 3 (CY/VP16/TBI)	5 (TCD/CSP A) 7 (MTX/CSP A)	8 64%	30 months median (11–56 months)	2
Matthes-Martin et al. [74]	11: 6 (MUD) 4 (MRD) 1 (MMRD)	90–98	3 (CY/VP16/TBI) 1 (CY/VP16/TBI/ATG) 5 (BU/CY/MEL ± ATG) 1 (BU/CY/ATG) 1 (MTX/CSP A)	9 (MTX/CSP A) 2 (MTX)	4 37% DFS	52 months median (9–107 months)	4
Locatelli et al. [75]	71: 36 (MRD) 35 (MUD or MMUD)	90–97	71 (BU/CY/MEL)	CSP A (MRD) MTX/CSP A/ATG (MUD)	44 DFS 61% MRD DFS 52% MUD or MMUD	20 months median (3–67 months)	18
Manabe et al. [76]	27: 12 (MRD) 10 (MUD) 4 (MMRD) 1 (MMUD)	90–97	18 (TBI-based); 9 (BU-based)	15 (MTX/CSP A); 12 (Other)	17 54% EFS	27 months median	7
Smith et al. [77]	46: 29 (MUD) 17 (1 or 2 Ag MMUD)	90–97	35 (TBI-based); 11 (Chemo-based)	15 (TCD); 31 (no TCD) 13 (CSP A+); 30 (MTX+); 3 (other)	12	24% DFS	26
Lutz et al. [61]	18: 11 (MRD) 2 (MMRD) 5 (MUD)	78–93	12 (TBI-based); 6 (Chemo-based)	3 (TCD); 15 (MTX/CSP A)	8 32% EFS	65 months	

AC, cytosine arabinoside (ARA-C); Ag, HLA antigen; ATG, antithymocyte globulin; BU, busulfan; CSP A, cyclosporine A; CY, cyclophosphamide; DFS, disease-free survival; EFS, event-free survival; GVHD, graft-vs.-host disease; MEL, melphalan; MMRD, mismatched-related donor; MMUD, mismatched-unrelated donor; MRD, matched-related donor; MUD, matched-unrelated donor; MTX, methotrexate; TBI, total body irradiation; TCD, T-cell depletion; VP16, etoposide.

affect survival although some patients experienced transient benefit, e.g. improved blood count or diminished extramedullary disease. This observation led to trials in which patients received intensive, AML-like therapy that produced clinical remissions but did not eradicate the JMML-characteristic colony formation [58]. One report, which reviewed the outcome for 57 children with JMML treated at several pediatric hospitals between 1975 and 1995, found 34% ± 16% actuarial survival for patients treated with diverse but mostly high-dose chemotherapy compared to 31% ± 9% survival for patients undergoing HSC transplantation [9]. However, most studies report very poor outcome for patients treated with chemotherapy alone. The EWOG on Myelodysplastic Diseases in Children noted 6% ± 4% 10 years actuarial survival for 72 patients with JMML treated with chemotherapy between 1975 and 1994 [10]. For 38 patients undergoing HSC transplantation survival was 39% ± 10%. Chemotherapy treatment was not uniform, with approximately one-third of the patients receiving intensive therapy, but survival for these patients did not exceed that for children treated less intensively. In part, the long interval of patient accrual and the lack of uniform diagnostic criteria and treatment make it difficult to reconcile the differences in outcome between these two retrospective studies. Other reports which consider the efficacy of intensive chemotherapy find survival rates less than 10% [11,59–61]. In the end, the cumulative experience of intensive chemotherapy does not support its use as the sole treatment for JMML.

Based upon its activity in Ph^+ CML, interferon-alpha (IFN-α) therapy underwent trial in JMML patients. Although disease stabilized temporarily in some patients, treatment was largely ineffective and toxic [12,62–65]. Interferon gave way to 13-*cis*-retinoic acid (retinoic acid) when *in vitro* studies showed that addition of retinoic acid to JMML colony assays at concentrations achievable with oral administration inhibited spontaneous growth [66]. In a phase II study, 22 patients, 19 of whom showed *in vitro* growth characteristic of JMML, were treated with retinoic acid and five achieved a complete response, i.e. normal white count and absence of organomegaly [67]. Culture of blood or marrow cells from some of the responding patients showed inhibition of spontaneous proliferation and loss of GM-CSF hypersensitivity. Treatment with retinoic acid was largely nontoxic; but while a few patients had sustained responses (up to 54 months), disease progression occurred, and more than half of the patients did not respond. The efficacy of 13-*cis*-retinoic acid (retinoic acid) in treating JMML still remains uncertain and clinical trials are ongoing.

Potentially effective therapy may be found in agents that specifically antagonize or interfere with GM-CSF hypersensitivity and/or the Ras pathway. One target is the GM-CSF membrane receptor. The previously mentioned analog to GM-CSF (E21R) and a compound, which fuses a truncated diphtheria toxin to GM-CSF (DT388-GM-CSF), have both shown *in vitro* activity against JMML cells [39,40,68]. Other promising drugs act on the intracellular signaling pathways believed critical to JMML propagation. These include inhibitors of farnesyl-protein transferase and DNA enzymes that degrade the protein kinase Raf-1 [41,42]. Thus far, clinical experience treating patients with these agents has been limited. Transient but clinically important activity was seen in one patient treated with E21R after having failed transplantation and multiple chemotherapies [69]. While unlikely to be curative, these agents may prove beneficial in controlling JMML prior to initiating curative therapy. Alternatively the use of these agents in an adjuvant setting, e.g. post marrow transplantation, may increase the cure rate.

Hematopoietic cell transplantation (HCT)

Allogeneic HCT is the only proven curative therapy for JMML [61,70–77]. The first JMML patient to undergo allogeneic HCT survived disease-free for 17 years but died of a secondary malignancy [72,78]. Subsequent

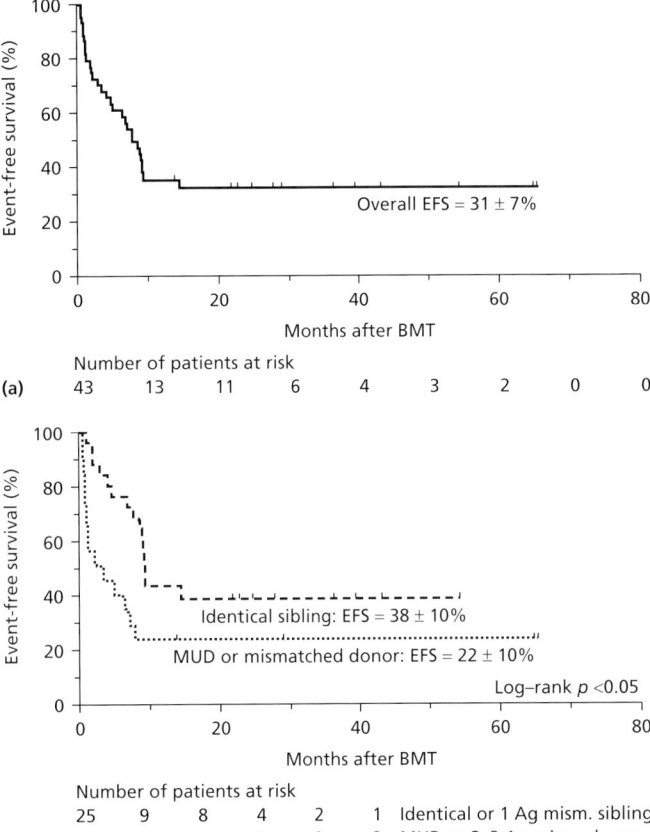

Fig. 74.1 Overall probability of event-free survival (EFS) for the entire cohort of patients (a) and for the children transplanted using a human leukocyte antigen (HLA)-identical sibling/one antigen-disparate relative or a matched unrelated donor (MUD)/two–three antigen-disparate relative (b). Adapted from Locatelli [70].

experience has confirmed the curative potential for HCT but has also underscored its limitations [70,72,73]. Recurrent disease is the major cause of failure. In an effort to improve outcome and reduce relapse, investigators have questioned the value of pretransplantation treatment, including splenectomy, the role for total body irradiation (TBI) as part of the transplant conditioning therapy, and the contribution of graft-vs.-host disease (GVHD)/graft-vs.-leukemia (GVL) to the maintenance of remission.

Between 1987 and 1995, 43 patients underwent allogeneic HCT ($n = 23$ from human leukocyte antigen (HLA) identical siblings (matched-related donor [MRD]); $n = 2$ from one antigen mismatched family member (mismatched-related donor [MMRD]); $n = 4$ from greater than one antigen MMRD; $n = 14$ from matched unrelated donor (MUD) (Table 74.2 [70–77]) [70]. Treatment prior to transplant was classified as either "AML-type" or other. For transplant preparation, 21 patients received busulfan (BU) and cyclophosphamide (CY), either alone or with etoposide (VP16) or melphalan, while 22 patients received regimens that included TBI and CY. No patient relapsed after 18 months, and the probability of event-free survival (EFS) was 31% at 5-years. EFS was superior for patients transplanted from six of six or five of six MRDs vs. that for other patient/donor combinations, 38% vs. 22% (Fig. 74.1 [70]). Regardless of donor type, the probability of relapse was 58%. Noteworthy, five of 18 patients transplanted from alternative donors failed to engraft and four of these relapsed early post-transplantation. Univariate analysis indicated that EFS was superior for patients treated with chemotherapy-based preparatory regimens, as opposed to TBI-based (EFS 48%

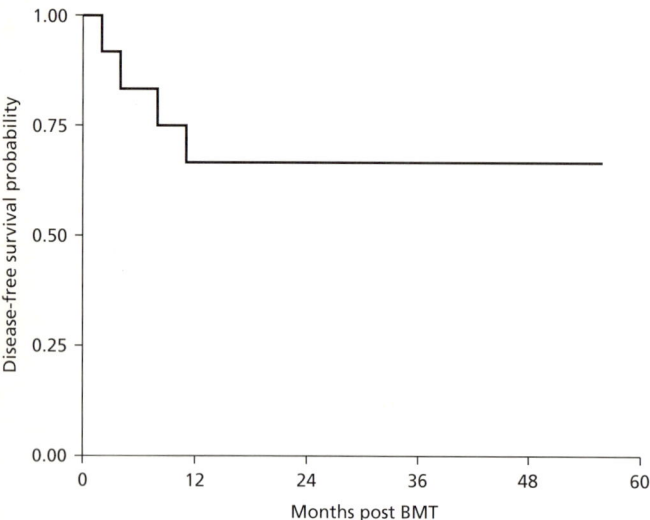

Fig. 74.2 Kaplan–Meier estimate shows the probability of disease-free survival (DFS) for patients with juvenile myelomonocytic leukemia (JMML) who received alternative donor transplants. Adapted from Bunin [73].

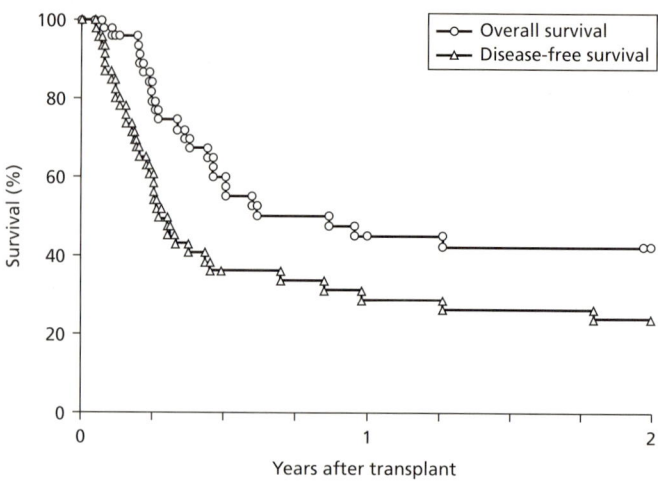

Fig. 74.3 Survival and disease-free survival (DFS) for patients with juvenile myelomonocytic leukemia (JMML) following unrelated donor hematopoietic stem cell (HSC) transplantation. Adapted from Smith [77].

vs. 15%). Compared to the combination of methotrexate (MTX) and cyclosporine (CSP) (±antithymocyte globulin [ATG]), the relapse rate was lowest and EFS was highest when either MTX or CSP was used alone for GVHD prevention (EFS 56% vs. 20%). Neither splenectomy nor pretransplant therapy effected outcome.

The ongoing EWOG on Myelodysplastic Diseases in Children trial has enrolled 71 children with JMML [75]. All patients receive BU, CY and melphalan as conditioning therapy. This regimen was chosen because of prior favourable experience in treating children with JMML and AML; furthermore alkylating agents in combination were considered to be advantageous against malignant cells not in active replication [79]. CSP was administered for GVHD prevention to the majority of 36 patients undergoing MRD transplant, and CSP, MTX and ATG to most of the 36 patients transplanted from six of six or five of six MUDs. Eighteen patients have relapsed; the probability of relapse is 36% with no significant difference between related and unrelated donor transplantation. Median follow up is 20 months (3–93 months); the probability of EFS is 61% and 52% for recipients of related and unrelated HCT ($P < 0.5$). Primary or secondary graft failure occurred in four patients transplanted from unrelated donors. EFS for patients diagnosed after 2 years of age appeared inferior. As in the prior study, pretransplant splenectomy did not confer an advantage. These preliminary findings, if sustained, will represent a major improvement in outcome.

Similar outcomes have been reported for 12 children with JMML transplanted from unrelated or MMRDs ($n = 8$ fully matched; $n = 4$, one or two antigen mismatched) [73]. In contrast to the EWOG approach, all but one patient received TBI, CY and other chemotherapy. For GVHD prevention, T-cell depletion was combined with CSP ($n = 5$) or MTX and CSP. Eight patients are alive and disease free (64% EFS); four patients died, two following relapse and two from regimen-related mortality (Fig. 74.2 [73]). The role for splenectomy ($n = 9$) and/or aggressive chemotherapy prior to transplant ($n = 10$) could not be evaluated; however, neither adversely impacted EFS. All patients developed GVHD ($n = 3$ >grade II), and nine developed chronic GVHD.

Data from National Marrow Donor Program for 46 children with JMML transplanted from unrelated donors showed 96% engraftment rate, 24% EFS and 58% relapse rate at 2-years post-transplant (Fig. 74.3) [77]. Treatment was heterogeneous and outcome could not be related to the type of conditioning or GVHD preventive therapies. Neither the intensity of treatment prior to transplantation nor splenectomy was a factor in outcome. For evaluable patients, the cumulative incidence of acute GVHD = grade II was 54% and, importantly, acute GVHD >grade II (33% cumulative incidence) adversely effected survival. Conversely, chronic GVHD (34% cumulative incidence) was associated with enhanced EFS and lower relapse rate. This observation supports a GVL effect arising from allogeneic transplantation.

As these and other reports document, relapse of JMML remains the principal cause of failure for patients undergoing bone marrow transplantation (BMT) [70,71,80]. Second transplants for relapse have been performed but rarely do these achieve a satisfactory outcome [71,74,80–83]. An uncommon patient has had autologous marrow recovery without evidence of disease [61,84]. GVL activity against JMML has been surmised based upon several reports in which withdrawal of immunosuppressives in relapsed patients led to an increase in donor chimerism and disease remission [85–87]. Halting immunosuppressives or adding donor lymphocyte infusions and/or chemotherapy have become widely adopted in managing relapse [77]. Presumably if GVL activity is important to control or eradicate JMML, withdrawal of immunosuppression at the earliest indication of recurrent or resistant disease is justified. And to that end, chimerism determination is the likely earliest indicator for disease relapse, presaging the reappearance of GM-CSF hypersensitivity [88].

Conclusion

HCT is the only proven curative therapy for JMML. Several recent studies suggest that the outcome following transplantation is improving with EFS now at 50% for both related and unrelated donors. Nevertheless, treatment is not optimal with relapse rates exceeding 30% even in the best circumstances. Further improvement may be expected when it is determined whether there is a role for pretransplant therapy, including splenectomy, and which stem cell preparative regimen is optimal. Perhaps more important will be an effective means to incite a post-transplant immune response against residual disease. Alternatively, implementation of treatments that interfere with the pathogenesis of JMML may be useful. Agents that block GM-CSF sensitivity or interfere with Ras-signaling in leukemic cells may offer the benefit of disease specificity with acceptable toxicity. These agents may be used to reduce the burden of disease pretransplantation or to contribute to a combined immunologic and pharmacologic approach against residual disease post-transplantation.

JMML is, fortunately, a very uncommon disease, but this makes the development of the optimal treatment approach difficult. Studies conducted by large cooperative groups such as the EWOG on Myelodysplastic Diseases in Children and the Children's Oncology Group attempt to address several of these dilemmas. Adoption of the International JMML Working Group and the EWOG on Myelodysplastic Diseases in Children consensus criteria for the diagnosis of JMML will allow more meaningful comparison between patients and treatment approaches. The years ahead offer promise in the struggle to cure children with JMML.

References

1 Niemeyer CM, Fenu S, Hasle H, Mann G, Stary J, van Wering E. Differentiating juvenile myelomonocytic leukemia from infectious diseases. *Blood* 1998; **91**: 365–7.
2 Harris NL, Jaffe ES, Diebold J *et al*. World Health Organization classification of neoplastic diseases of the hematopoietic and lymphoid tissues: report of the Clinical Advisory Committee meeting, Airlie House, Virginia, November 1997. *J Clin Oncol* 1999; **17**: 3835–49.
3 Vardiman JW, Harris NL, Brunning RD. The World Health Organization (WHO) classification of the myeloid neoplasms. *Blood* 2002; **100**: 2292–302.
4 Jackson GH, Carey PJ, Cant AJ, Bown NP, Reid MM. Myelodysplastic syndromes in children. *Br J Haematol* 1993; **84**: 185–6.
5 Hasle H. Myelodysplastic syndromes in childhood-classification, epidemiology, and treatment. *Leukemia Lymphoma* 1994; **13**: 11–26.
6 Blank J, Lange B. Preleukemia in children. *J Pediatr* 1981; **98**: 565–8.
7 Emanuel PD. Myelodysplasia and myeloproliferative disorders in childhood: an update. *Br J Haematol* 1999; **105**: 852–63.
8 Woods WG, Barnard DR, Alonzo TA *et al*. Prospective study of 90 children requiring treatment for juvenile myelomonocytic leukemia or myelodysplastic syndrome: a report from the Children's Cancer Group. *J Clin Oncol* 2002; **20**: 434–40.
9 Luna-Fineman S, Shannon KM, Atwater SK *et al*. Myelodysplastic and myeloproliferative disorders of childhood: a study of 167 patients. *Blood* 1999; **93**: 459–66.
10 Niemeyer CM, Arico M, Biondi A *et al*. Chronic myelomonocytic leukemia in childhood: a retrospective analysis of 110 cases. *Blood* 1997; **89**: 3534–43.
11 Arico M, Biondi A, Pui CH. Juvenile myelomonocytic leukemia. *Blood* 1997; **90**: 479–88.
12 Arico M, Bossi G, Schiro R *et al*. Juvenile chronic myelogenous leukemia: report of the Italian registry. *Haematologica* 1993; **78**: 264–9.
13 Castro-Malaspina H, Schaison G, Passe S *et al*. Subacute and chronic myelomonocytic leukemia in children (juvenile CML). *Cancer* 1984; **54**: 675–86.
14 Owen G, Lewis IJ, Morgan M, Robinson A, Stevens RF. Prognostic factors in juvenile chronic granulocytic leukaemia. *Br J Cancer* 1992; **66** (Suppl. 18): S68–71.
15 Freedman MH, Estrov Z, Chan HSL. Juvenile chronic myelogenous leukemia. *The Am J Pediatric Hematology/Oncology* 1988; **10**: 261–7.
16 Stiller CA, Chessells JM, Fitchett M. Neurofibromatosis and childhood leukemia/lymphoma: a population-based UKCCSG study. *Br J Cancer* 1994; **70**: 969–72.
17 Bader JL, Miller RW. Neurofibromatosis and childhood leukemia. *Pediatrics* 1997; **92**: 925–9.
18 Side LE, Emanuel PD, Taylor B *et al*. Mutations of the *NF1* gene in children with juvenile myelomonocytic leukemia without clinical evidence of neurofibromatosis, type 1. *Blood* 1998; **92**: 267–72.
19 Luna-Fineman S, Shannon KM, Lange BJ. Childhood monosomy 7: epidemiology, biology, and mechanistic implications. *Blood* 1995; **85**: 1985–99.
20 Passmore SJ, Hann IM, Stiller CA *et al*. Pediatric myelodysplasia: a study of 68 children and a new prognostic scoring system. *Blood* 1995; **85**: 1742–50.
21 Gadner H, Haas O. Experiences in pediatric myelodysplastic syndromes. *Hematology/Oncol Clinics North Am* 1992; **6**: 655–72.
22 Butcher M, Frenck R, Emperor J *et al*. Molecular evidence that childhood monosomy 7 syndrome is distinct from juvenile chronic myelogenous leukemia and other childhood myeloproliferative disorders. *Genes, Chromosome Cancer* 1995; **12**: 50–7.
23 Hasle H, Arico M, Basso G *et al*. Myelodysplastic syndrome, juvenile myelomonocytic leukemia, and acute myeloid leukemia associated with complete or partial monosomy 7. European Working Group on MDS in Childhood (EWOG-MDS). *Leukemia* 1999; **13**: 376–85.
24 Altman A, Palmer CG, Baehner R. Juvenile 'chronic granulocytic' leukemia: a panmyelopathy with prominent monocytic involvement and circulating monocyte colony-forming cells. *Blood* 1974; **43**: 341–50.
25 Estrov Z, Grunberger T, Chan HSL, Freedman MH. Juvenile chronic myelogenous leukemia: characterization of the disease using cell cultures. *Blood* 1986; **67**: 1382–7.
26 Emanuel PD, Bates LJ, Castleberry RP, Gualtieri RJ, Zuckerman KS. Selective hypersensitivity to granulocyte-macrophage colony-stimulating factor by juvenile chronic myeloid leukemia hematopoietic progenitors. *Blood* 1991; **77**: 925–9.
27 Emanuel PD, Shannon KM, Castleberry RP. Juvenile myelomonocytic leukemia: molecular understanding and prospects for therapy. *Mol Med Today* 1996; **2**: 468–74.
28 Freeburn RW, Gale RE, Wagner HM, Linch DC. Analysis of the coding sequence for the GM-CSF receptor α and β chains in patients with juvenile chronic myeloid leukemia (JCML). *Exp Hematol* 1997; **25**: 306–11.
29 Emanuel PD, Bates LJ, Zhu SW, Castleberry RP, Gualtieri RJ, Zuckerman KS. The role of monocyte-derived hemopoietic growth factors in the regulation of myeloproliferation in juvenile chronic myelogenous leukemia. *Exp Hematol* 1991; **19**: 1017–24.
30 Gutmann DH, Aylsworth A, Carey JC *et al*. The diagnostic evaluation and multidisciplinary management of neurofibromatosis 1 and neurofibromatosis 2. *JAMA* 1997; **278**: 51–7.
31 Boguski MS, McCormick F. Proteins regulating Ras and its relatives. *Nature* 1993; **366**: 643–54.
32 Shannon KM, O'Connell P, Martin G *et al*. Loss of the normal NF1 allele from the bone marrow of children with type 1 neurofibromatosis and malignant myeloid disorders. *N Engl J Med* 1994; **330**: 597–601.
33 Bollag G, Clapp DW, Shih S *et al*. Loss of NF1 results in activation of the Ras signaling pathway and leads to aberrant growth in haematopoietic cells. *Nature Genet* 1996; **12**: 144–8.
34 Satoh T, Nakafuku M, Miyajima A, Kaziro Y. Involvement of Ras p21 protein in signal-transduction pathways from interleukin 2, interleukin 3, and granulocyte/macrophage colony-stimulating factor, but not from interleukin 4. *Proc Natl Acad Sci U S A* 1991; **88**: 3314–8.
35 Largaespada DA, Brannan CI, Jenkins NA, Copeland NG. NF1 deficiency causes Ras-mediated granulocyte/macrophage colony stimulating factor hypersensitivity and chronic myeloid leukemia. *Nature Genet* 1996; **12**: 137–43.
36 Miyauchi J, Asada M, Sasaki M, Tsunematsu Y, Kojima S, Mizutani S. Mutations of the *N-RAS* gene in juvenile chronic myelogenous leukemia. *Blood* 1994; **83**: 2248–54.
37 Flotho C, Valcamonica S, Mach-Pascual S *et al*. Ras mutations and clonality analysis in children with juvenile myelomonocytic leukemia (JMML). *Leukemia* 1999; **13**: 32–7.
38 Kalra R, Paderanga D, Olson K, Shannon KM. Genetic analysis is consistent with the hypothesis that NF1 limits myeloid cell growth through $p21^{ras}$. *Blood* 1994; **84**: 3435–9.
39 Frankel AE, Lilly M, Kreitman R *et al*. Diphtheria toxin fused to granulocyte-macrophage colony-stimulating factor is toxic to blasts from patients with juvenile myelomonocytic leukemia and chronic myelomonocytic leukemia. *Blood* 1998; **92**: 4279–86.
40 Iversen PO, Lewis ID, Turczynowicz S *et al*. Inhibition of granulocyte-macrophage colony-stimulating factor prevents dissemination and induces remission of juvenile myelomonocytic leukemia in engrafted immunodeficient mice. *Blood* 1997; **90**: 4910–7.
41 Emanuel PD, Snyder RC, Wiley T, Gopurala B, Castleberry RP. Inhibition of juvenile myelomonocytic leukemia cell growth *in vitro* by farnesyltransferase inhibitors. *Blood* 2000; **95**: 639–45.
42 Iversen PO, Emanuel PD, Sioud M. Targeting *Raf-1* gene expression by a DNA enzyme inhibits juvenile myelomonocytic leukemia cell growth. *Blood* 2002; **99**: 4147–53.
43 Miles DK, Freedman MH, Stephens K *et al*. Patterns of hematopoietic lineage involvement in children with neurofibromatosis type 1 and malignant myeloid disorders. *Blood* 1996; **88**: 4314–20.
44 Busque L, Gilliland DG, Prchal JT *et al*. Clonality in juvenile chronic myelogenous leukemia. *Blood* 1995; **85**: 21–30.
45 Cambier N, Menot ML, Fenaux P, Wattel E, Baruchel A, Chomienne C. GM-CSF hypersensitivity in CD34+ purified cells in juvenile and adult chronic myelomonocytic leukemia: effect of retinoids. *Blood* 1995; **86** (Suppl. 1): 791a [Abstract].
46 Lapidot T, Cohen A, Grunberger T, Dick JE, Freedman MH. Aberrent growth properties of juvenile chronic myelogenous leukemia CD34+ cells *in vitro* and *in vivo* using SCID mouse assays. *Blood* 1993; **82** (Suppl. 1): 197a [Abstract].

47 Freedman MH, Hitzler JK, Bunin N, Grunberger T, Squire J. Juvenile chronic myelogenous leukemia multilineage CD34+ cells: aberrant growth and differentiation properties. *Stem Cells* 1996; **14**: 690–701.

48 Lapidot T, Grunberger T, Vormoor J et al. Identification of human juvenile chronic myelogenous leukemia stem cells capable of initiating the disease in primary and secondary SCID mice. *Blood* 1996; **88**: 2655–64.

49 Lau RC, Squire J, Brisson L et al. Lymphoid blast crisis of B-lineage phenotype with monosomy 7 in a patient with juvenile chronic myelogenous leukemia (JCML). *Leukemia* 1994; **8**: 903–8.

50 Cooper LJ, Shannon KM, Loken MR, Weaver M, Stephens K, Sievers EL. Evidence that juvenile myelomonocytic leukemia can arise from a pluripotential stem cell. *Blood* 2000; **96**: 2310–3.

51 Nakazawa T, Koike K, Agematsu K et al. Cytogenetic clonality analysis in monosomy 7 associated with juvenile myelomonocytic leukemia: clonality in B and NK cells, but not in T cells. *Leuk Res* 1998; **22**: 887–92.

52 Monti F, Longoni D, Sainati L, Basso G, Sacchini P, Vecchi V. A case of juvenile myelomonocytic leukemia presenting with a B-lymphoblastic immunophenotype. *Haematologica* 2001; **86**: 875–6.

53 Herrod HG, Dow LW, Sullivan JL. Persistent Epstein–Barr virus infection mimicking juvenile chronic myelogenous leukemia: immunological and hematologic studies. *Blood* 1983; **61**: 1098–104.

54 Pinkel D. Differentiating juvenile myelomonocytic leukemia from infectious disease. *Blood* 1998; **91**: 365–7.

55 Lorenzana A, Lyons H, Sawaf H, Higgins M, Carrigan D, Emanuel PD. Human herpesvirus 6 infection mimicking juvenile myelomonocytic leukemia in an infant. *J Pediatr Hematol Oncol* 2002; **24**: 136–41.

56 Yetgin S, Cetin M, Yenicesu I, Ozaltin F, Uckan D. Acute parvovirus B19 infection mimicking juvenile myelomonocytic leukemia. *Eur J Haematol* 2000; **65**: 276–8.

57 Lilleyman JS, Harrison JF, Black JA. Treatment of juvenile chronic myeloid leukemia with sequential subcutaneous cytarabine and oral mercaptopurine. *Blood* 1977; **49**: 559–62.

58 Chan HSL, Estrov Z, Weitzman S, Freedman MH. The value of intensive combination chemotherapy for juvenile chronic myelogenous leukemia. *J Clin Oncol* 1987; **5**: 1960–7.

59 Festa RS, Shende A, Lanzkowsky P. Juvenile chronic myelocytic leukemia: experience with intensive combination chemotherapy. *Med Pediatric Oncol* 1990; **18**: 311–6.

60 Brandwein JM, Horsman DE, Eaves AC et al. Childhood myelodysplasia: suggested classification as myelodysplastic syndromes based on laboratory and clinical findings. *The Am J Pediatric Hematology/Oncology* 1990; **12**: 63–70.

61 Lutz P, Zix-Kieffer I, Souillet G et al. Juvenile myelomonocytic leukemia: analyses of treatment results in the EORTC Children's Leukemia Co-operative Group (CLCG). *Bone Marrow Transplant* 1996; **18**: 1111–6.

62 Maybee D, Dubowy R, Krischner J et al. Unusual toxicity of high dose alpha interferon (αIFN) in the treatment of juvenile chronic myelocytic leukemia (JCML). *Proc Am Soc Clin Oncol* 1992; **11**: 285a [Abstract].

63 Mutz ID, Zoubek A. Transient response to alpha-interferon in juvenile chronic myelomonocytic leukemia. *Pediatric Hematol Oncol* 1988; **5**: 71–5.

64 Toraldo R, Pistoia V, Tolone C, Canino G, D'Avanzo M, Iafusco F. Interferon alpha therapy in an infant with juvenile chronic myelogenous leukemia. *Pediatric Hematol Oncol* 1995; **12**: 189–94.

65 Hazani A, Barak Y, Berant M, Bar-Maor A. Congenital juvenile chronic myelogenous leukemia: therapeutic trial with interferon alpha-2. *Med Pediatric Oncol* 1993; **21**: 73–6.

66 Castleberry RP, Emanuel PD, Zuckerman KS et al. A pilot study of isotretinoin in the treatment of juvenile chronic myelogenous leukemia. *N Engl J Med* 1994; **331**: 1680–4.

67 Castleberry RP, Chang M, Maybee D, Emanuel PD. A phase II study of 13-cis-retinoic acid in juvenile myelomonocytic leukemia. A Pediatric Oncology Group study. *Blood* 1997; **90** (Suppl. 1): 346a [Abstract].

68 Iversen PO, Rodwell RL, Pitcher L, Taylor KM, Lopez AF. Inhibition of proliferation and induction of apoptosis in juvenile myelomonocytic leukemic cells by the granulocyte-macrophage colony-stimulating factor analogue E21R. *Blood* 1996; **88**: 2634–9.

69 Bernard F, Thomas C, Emile JF et al. Transient hematologic and clinical effect of E21R in a child with end-stage juvenile myelomonocytic leukemia. *Blood* 2002; **99**: 2615–6.

70 Locatelli F, Niemeyer CM, Angelucci E et al. Allogeneic bone marrow transplantation for chronic myelomonocytic leukemia in childhood: a report from the European Working Group on myelodysplastic syndrome in childhood. *J Clin Oncol* 1997; **15**: 566–73.

71 Donadieu J, Stephan JL, Blanche S et al. Treatment of juvenile chronic myelomonocytic leukemia by allogeneic bone marrow transplantation. *Bone Marrow Transplant* 1994; **13**: 777–82.

72 Smith FO, Sanders JE, Robertson KA, Gooley T, Sievers EL. Allogeneic marrow transplantation for children with juvenile chronic myelogenous leukemia. *Blood* 1994; **84** (Suppl. 1): 201a [Abstract].

73 Bunin N, Saunders F, Leahey A, Doyle J, Calderwood S, Freedman MH. Alternative donor bone marrow transplantation for children with juvenile myelomonocytic leukemia. *J Pediatr Hematol Oncol* 1999; **21**: 479–85.

74 Matthes-Martin S, Mann G, Peters C et al. Allogeneic bone marrow transplantation for juvenile myelomonocytic leukaemia: a single centre experience and review of the literature. *Bone Marrow Transplant* 2000; **26**: 377–82.

75 Locatelli F, Noellke P, Zecca M et al. Allogeneic stem cell transplantation in children with juvenile myelomonocytic leukemia: results of a prospective study of the EWOG-MDS/EBMT groups. *Blood* 2001; **98** (Suppl. 1): 848a [Abstract].

76 Manabe A, Okamura J, Yumura-Yagi K et al. Allogeneic hematopoietic stem cell transplantation for 27 children with juvenile myelomonocytic leukemia diagnosed based on the criteria of the International JMML Working Group. *Leukemia* 2002; **16**: 645–9.

77 Smith FO, King R, Nelson G et al. Unrelated donor bone marrow transplantation for children with juvenile myelomonocytic leukaemia. *Br J Haematol* 2002; **116**: 716–24.

78 Sanders J, Buckner C, Stewart P, Thomas ED. Successful treatment of juvenile chronic granulocytic leukemia with marrow transplantation. *Pediatrics* 1979; **63**: 44–6.

79 Locatelli F, Pession A, Comoli P et al. Role of allogeneic bone marrow transplantation from an HLA-identical sibling or a matched unrelated donor in the treatment of children with juvenile chronic myeloid leukaemia. *Br J Haematol* 1996; **92**: 49–54.

80 Chown SR, Potter MN, Cornish J et al. Matched and mismatched unrelated donor bone marrow transplantation for juvenile chronic myeloid leukaemia. *Br J Haematol* 1996; **93**: 674–6.

81 Urban C, Schwinger W, Slavc I et al. Busulfan/cyclophosphamide plus bone marrow transplantation is not sufficient to eradicate the malignant clone in juvenile chronic myelogenous leukemia. *Bone Marrow Transplant* 1990; **5**: 353–6.

82 Mattot M, Ninane J, Vermylen C, Cornu G. Second bone marrow transplant in eight children. *Pediatric Hematol Oncol* 1992; **9**: 353–7.

83 MacMillan ML, Davies SM, Orchard PJ, Ramsay NK, Wagner JE. Haemopoietic cell transplantation in children with juvenile myelomonocytic leukaemia. *Br J Haematol* 1998; **103**: 552–8.

84 Suttorp M, Schmitz N, Prange E et al. Remission of juvenile chronic myeloid leukemia following graft failure of an unrelated marrow transplant and autologous recovery of marrow function promoted by GM-CSF and IL-3. *Leukemia* 1991; **5**: 723–5.

85 Veys P, Saunders F, Calderwood S et al. The role of graft-versus-leukemia in bone marrow transplantation for juvenile chronic myeloid leukemia. *Blood* 1994; **84** (Suppl. 1): 337a [Abstract].

86 Rassam SMB, Katz F, Chessells JM, Morgan G. Successful allogeneic bone marrow transplantation in juvenile CML. Conditioning or graft-versus-leukaemia effect? *Bone Marrow Transplant* 1993; **11**: 247–50.

87 Orchard PJ, Miller JS, McGlennen R, Davies SM, Ramsay NK. Graft-versus-leukemia is sufficient to induce remission in juvenile myelomonocytic leukemia. *Bone Marrow Transplant* 1998; **22**: 201–3.

88 Wagner JE, Broxmeyer HE, Byrd RL et al. Transplantation of umbilical cord blood after myeloablative therapy: analysis of engraftment. *Blood* 1992; **79**: 1874–81.

75

Keith E. Stockerl-Goldstein & Karl G. Blume

Allogeneic Hematopoietic Cell Transplantation for Adult Patients with Acute Myeloid Leukemia

Introduction

Acute myeloid leukemia (AML) remains a fatal disease with a rapid progression if untreated. The history of leukemic therapy has been recently recounted [1]. Although the majority of adults currently diagnosed with AML will enter a complete remission (CR) with standard chemotherapy regimens, most will suffer a relapse of their disease despite the use of consolidation regimens. Prognostic factors help to identify good risk patients who may enjoy prolonged disease-free survival (DFS) following induction-consolidation regimens. However, most adults fall into an intermediate or poor prognosis group. Unfortunately, most studies using standard induction-consolidation regimens report long-term DFS at less than 40%, even for patients under 60 years of age [2]. The role of hematopoietic cell transplantation (HCT) for AML has progressed from early reports of syngeneic marrow transplantation [3], to the extensive data now available on allogeneic HCT from matched-sibling donors with evidence of a beneficial graft-vs.-leukemia (GVL) effect [4].

In this chapter we will explore the role of allogeneic HCT for adult patients with AML in first CR, during second CR or in early first relapse, and also for patients with more advanced or refractory disease. A review of data regarding the optimal treatment of patients with *de novo* AML in first CR will be presented. The use of hematopoietic cells from matched-related donors (MRDs) and from unrelated donors, from placental cord blood and from haplo-identical donors will also be discussed. In addition, the expanding information of nonmyeloablative regimens for treating patients with AML will be presented and the future of allogeneic HCT will be considered.

Allogeneic HCT for AML in first CR

The early use of HCT for AML was for patients with advanced stages of disease, usually while in relapse, in second or subsequent remission, or with resistant disease [5–8]. As nonrelapse mortality of the allografting procedure decreased, the use of allogeneic HCT from matched-sibling donors for adults with AML in first CR increased. These studies performed in first CR patients yielded survival data significantly better than the outcomes reported with standard dose chemotherapy during the same period [7,9,10].

Prognostic factors at presentation

One of the early reports of allogeneic transplantation for AML in first CR described the outcome of 69 patients, including 49 adults, treated with matched-sibling donor grafts [11]. DFS was 48% for the adult patients with 41% dying of causes other than relapse, predominantly related to graft-vs.-host disease (GVHD). There was no association between pre-transplant factors including age, white blood cell count (WBC) at diagnosis, FAB subtype, length of time before achieving remission or time from diagnosis until transplantation and transplant outcome.

Another report described the outcome of 220 adults and children, age range 1–53 years, with AML who received matched-sibling donor transplants [12]. Fifteen clinical and laboratory variables were studied in relation to the transplant result to determine prognostic factors predictive of outcome. DFS for this group of patients was 45%. Improved overall survival (OS) was associated with younger age and female gender as well as lower peripheral blast count, no prior hepatitis and shorter duration of symptoms at the time of presentation.

Another group of investigators described the outcome of 32 adults with projected 7-year DFS of 62% [13]. This report included a multivariate analysis of diagnostic characteristics and the post-transplant events in 32 adults and 41 children. Development of acute GVHD or interstitial pneumonia and a presenting WBC of >20,000/μL were independent variables associated with poor DFS.

The outcome of patients treated with allogeneic HCT has also been reported as part of a cooperative European transplant trial [14]. The median follow-up was 41 months for the 169 patients allografted during first CR with an actuarial 3-year DFS rate of 60%, a relapse rate of 23% and treatment-related mortality (TRM) at 2 years of 22%. A univariate analysis demonstrated improved DFS for patients who required only one course of induction therapy to achieve CR, shorter time to attain CR and a lower WBC at presentation.

The French HCT group representing the Société Française de Greffe de Moelle investigated the relationship between the time from diagnosis to allogeneic HCT in 109 patients transplanted in first CR of AML [15]. Actuarial 5-year leukemia-free survival was 55% for the whole group, with TRM of 25% and a relapse rate of 26%. Leukemia-free survival was significantly better in patients transplanted within 120 days from diagnosis, while patients transplanted at a later time had a higher risk for relapse as well as TRM, although these variables were not statistically significant.

The role of cytogenetics in the prognosis of *de novo* AML has become recognized by many groups evaluating patients who received standard chemotherapy regimens [16–19]. Although slight differences between the prognostic factors are reported by several investigators, certain groupings of karyotypic abnormalities seem to be observed consistently. The good prognosis group associated with long-term DFS in excess of 50% includes patients with t(8;21), t(15;17) or inv(16) or other abnormalities of chromosome 16 including t(16;16) or del(16) [18]. The utility of cytogenetic risk stratification has been applied to allogeneic transplantation in evaluating outcomes following HCT to determine which patients might benefit from transplantation vs. standard chemotherapy. One group evaluated 118 patients with AML who achieved CR with induction chemotherapy [20]. These patients underwent human leukocyte antigen (HLA)-identical allogeneic HCT if a matched-sibling donor was available. If no donor was found, an autologous HCT was recommended. The cytogenetics groups evaluated were based on those proposed by Keating *et al.* [16]. The outcomes for all patients, regardless of type of treatment received demonstrated that those in the good prognosis group had the best outcome with 65% leukemia-free survival, and those with the poor prognosis group had a low leukemia-free survival of 10%. There was no difference in outcome for patients in the different cytogenetic groups that received allogeneic HCT suggesting that this treatment approach may overcome the poor prognosis seen in these patients when they are treated with standard chemotherapy regimens.

Data from the International Bone Marrow Transplant Registry (IBMTR) have been analyzed in a group of 708 patients with cytogenetic information who received allogeneic HCT from matched-sibling donors [21]. Patients were stratified into good, intermediate and poor risk cytogenetics as well as normal karyotype. The leukemia-free survival was not statistically different in the normal, good or intermediate prognosis groups, ranging from 50% to 56%. The poor prognosis group had a significantly worse leukemia-free survival of only 24% due to a higher risk of relapse.

A report from the European Group for Blood and Marrow Transplantation (EBMT) described 500 patients transplanted with AML in first CR who received an allogeneic HCT from a matched-sibling donor [22]. Patients with good or intermediate risk cytogenetics had a similar outcome with DFS of 67% and 57%, respectively. However, the poor risk group had DFS of only 29%. Cytogenetics remained a significant predictor of DFS, relapse and death on multivariate analysis as well.

A cytogenetic analysis of the British Medical Research Council (MRC) "AML 10 Trial" found that patients with favorable or intermediate risk cytogenetics receiving an allogeneic HCT in first CR attained a better outcome than patients in the adverse cytogenetic group [19].

Karyotypic analysis of an American Intergroup phase III study of post-remission therapy for adults with AML has also been described [23]. This study used four cytogenetic groups adopted by the Southwest Oncology Group (SWOG) with risk groups considered either favorable, intermediate, unfavorable or unknown. The investigators also analyzed outcomes using the cytogenetic coding adopted by the MRC trial [19]. OS for all patients regardless of therapy was 55% for the favorable group and 38% and 11%, respectively, for the intermediate and unfavorable cytogenetic groups. Figure 75.1 demonstrates the outcome of patients in this trial with unfavorable cytogenetic abnormalities and based on assigned therapy [23]. The 5-year OS estimates were 44% for the allogeneic HCT arm, 13% for the autologous HCT arm and 15% for the chemotherapy arm. The *p*-value for this analysis was not significant (0.11), probably due to small numbers of patients in each group. When combining the autologous and chemotherapy arms and comparing those patients with unfavorable cytogenetics to those patients in the allogeneic HCT arm, the *p*-value decreased to 0.043.

More recently, an analysis of 93 patients with AML transplanted in first CR was reported, with 82 receiving a related donor transplant and 11 receiving an unrelated donor graft [24]. Karyotypic abnormalities were classified using the MRC trial criteria [19]. Nineteen percent of patients were classified as favorable risk cytogenetics, 70% as intermediate risk, and 11% as adverse risk. This study found no differences in DFS, OS or TRM among the three groups. These observations suggest again that allogeneic HCT may improve the impact of unfavorable cytogenetics demonstrated with standard chemotherapy and that patients with these risk factors who have an HLA-matched-sibling donor should be considered for allogeneic HCT during first CR.

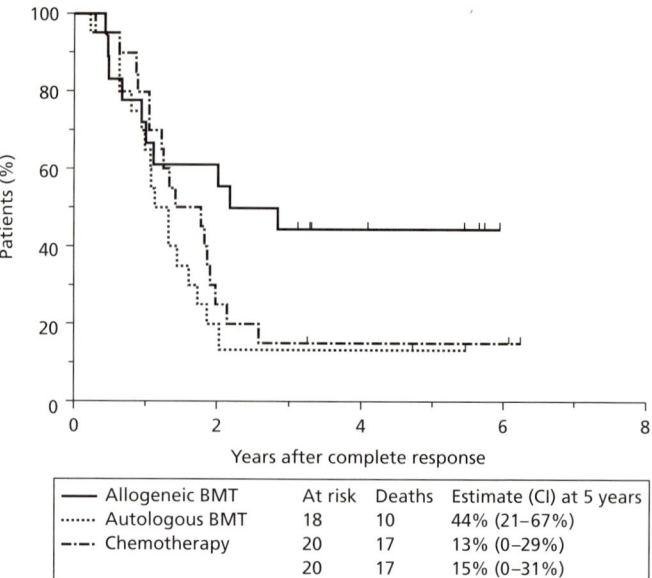

Fig. 75.1 Kaplan–Meier estimate of overall survival (OS) of 58 patients with acute myeloid leukemia (AML) in first complete remission (CR) with unfavorable cytogenetics based on treatment arm. Reproduced with permission from Slovak *et al.* [23].

Investigations of the cytogenetic abnormalities associated with AML have led to important advances in the understanding of the molecular characteristics of AML. These findings include the involvement of the retinoic acid receptor associated with the t(15;17) translocation of acute promyelocytic leukemia [25] and the association of the *AML1* and *CBF*α genes that are part of the AML1-CBFα transcription factor seen in the t(8;21) and inv(16) cytogenetic abnormalities, respectively [26–28]. The importance of the Flt3 ligand in AML is also being explored [29–31], and the role of immunophenotyping has been investigated in determining the prognosis of patients with newly diagnosed AML. Factors that have an adverse influence on outcome for *de novo* AML include low expression of CD98 [32], expression of CD10 or CD14 [33], and no expression of CD33 [34]. In a more recent report of 177 patients with AML, patients with blasts expressing CD13, CD33, CDw65, CD117 and myeloperoxidase had a poor prognosis [35]. The investigators proposed a prognostic scoring system, which includes this panmyeloid phenotype as well as age, performance status and permeability glycoprotein activity to stratify patients with AML. As the data on the impact of immunophenotyping, molecular diagnosis and measurement of minimal residual disease grow, this information, along with cytogenetic studies, may help to determine which patients are not in need of an allogeneic HCT procedure during first remission.

The effect of consolidation therapy

A discussion of the type of induction-consolidation chemotherapy for treatment of patients with AML is beyond the scope of this chapter. Several studies have addressed the dose intensity of cytarabine used for consolidation or even the need for consolidation chemotherapy before patients proceed to allogeneic HCT in first CR. An analysis from the IBMTR evaluated the role of post-remission chemotherapy prior to matched-sibling donor HCT in first CR of AML patients [36]. This review of registry data compared patients receiving no consolidation chemotherapy (*n* = 62) to patients treated with standard dose cytarabine (*n* = 222) or those treated with high-dose cytarabine (*n* = 147). There were no differences in OS, DFS or relapse rate among the three groups of patients. As shown in Fig. 75.2, DFS for the groups receiving no

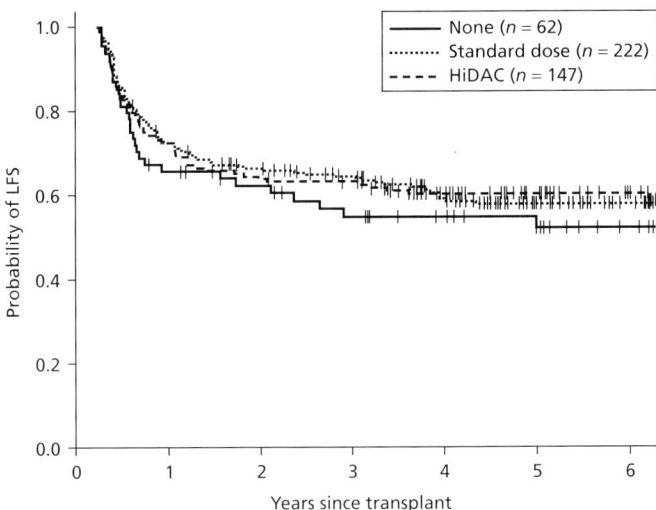

Fig. 75.2 Kaplan–Meier estimate of event-free survival (EFS) of 431 patients with acute myeloid leukemia (AML) in first remission following allogeneic transplantation based upon post-remission therapy received prior to hematopoietic cell transplantation (HCT), i.e. no post-remission therapy, standard dose cytarabine therapy or high-dose cytarabine therapy. Reproduced with permission from Tallman et al. [36].

consolidation, standard dose cytarabine or high-dose cytarabine were 50%, 56% and 59%, respectively, and were not statistically different from each other [36]. A review of data from EBMT also indicates no difference in outcome for 826 patients allografted in first CR from matched-sibling donors who had received the standard dose, intermediate-dose or high-dose cytarabine [37].

The influence of the preparatory regimen

The question of which preparative regimen is optimal for patients with AML undergoing allogeneic HCT in first CR has also been investigated. One group reported no significant differences in outcome in 84 patients receiving cyclophosphamide (CY) with either single fraction total body irradiation (TBI) or fractionated TBI in which the radiation regimen was determined by year of transplant and not in a randomized fashion [38]. Another analysis also reported no significant differences in survival of 63 patients with AML in first remission prospectively randomized to receive either a preparatory regimen of CY/TBI or melphalan/TBI [39]. An additional study demonstrated no difference in relapse-free survival comparing two different irradiation regimens [40]. There were significantly higher incidences of severe GVHD and transplant-related mortality in patients treated with higher doses of TBI although these patients also had a lower risk of relapse.

A retrospective analysis performed by EBMT involving 536 patients with AML who received an allogeneic transplant using either busulfan (BU)/CY or CY/TBI was reported [41]. No differences in acute or chronic GVHD, relapse or survival were noted. A randomized trial of BU/CY and CY/TBI was performed by the Nordic Bone Marrow Transplantation Group, which included 51 patients with AML in first CR and demonstrated no difference in leukemia-free survival [42]. This report described an increase in chronic GVHD and obstructive bronchiolitis associated with the BU/CY regimen when patients with all disease types and disease status were included. One group of investigators described a high incidence of extramedullary relapse in AML patients treated with the BU/CY regimen [43]. In this report, 10 of 22 patients who relapsed following allografting had extramedullary involvement with six of the 10 suffering an isolated extramedullary relapse.

The Société Française de Greffe de Moelle performed a randomized study of CY/TBI with BU/CY in 101 patients with AML in first remission with a uniform GVHD prophylaxis regimen [44]. This trial was recently updated and with extended follow-up demonstrates the BU/CY regimen to be significantly inferior to CY/TBI [45]. These data are contrary to other studies evaluating BU-containing preparatory regimens in chronic myeloid leukemia, and it is not apparent whether the differences observed were related to poor BU absorption in the BU/CY regimen or whether the use of TBI is really superior to BU for AML [46,47]. These data supporting a lower risk of relapse [40,45] with TBI-containing regimens provide additional rationale for trials using radioimmunotherapy to deliver radiation to sites of disease while hopefully limiting toxicity [48,49].

The effect of HCT source

The use of peripheral blood progenitor cells from matched-sibling donors as the source of allogeneic HCT is becoming increasingly more common as studies have demonstrated equivalent or improved outcomes when compared to bone marrow grafts [50,51]. Data from one study demonstrated that patients with advanced leukemias had superior survival when receiving peripheral blood HCT compared with bone marrow [51]. A report of 21 patients with AML in first CR transplanted with peripheral blood progenitor cells demonstrated a 3-year DFS of 60% [52] and was similar to reports using bone marrow [9,11,53]. A more recent randomized trial compared HCT using peripheral blood vs. bone marrow [54]. The total of 228 patients with hematologic malignancies included 82 patients with AML, predominantly in first CR. All patients received BU/CY with cyclosporine (CSP)/methotrexate (MTX) for GVHD prophylaxis and received grafts from matched-sibling donors. There was no difference in the incidence of acute or chronic GVHD or relapse between the two groups, although OS was improved in the group receiving peripheral blood grafts.

The effect of GVHD prophylaxis

GVHD remains a significant problem contributing to the morbidity and mortality associated with myeloablative therapy followed by allogeneic HCT for patients with AML. Numerous studies have compared different regimens of GVHD prophylaxis, with some evidence that these manipulations can affect DFS of patients with AML transplanted in first CR. A report of 184 patients treated with TBI/CY followed by GVHD prophylaxis with CSP, MTX or CSP plus MTX demonstrated an increase in the relapse rate of patients who received CSP plus MTX. DFS of this group, however, was not significantly different from the other regimens [55]. Another group of investigators evaluated the effect of low-dose CSP (1–2 mg/kg/day) vs. high-dose CSP (5 mg/kg/day) in 91 patients with AML allografted in first CR [56]. This study indicated that patients treated with high-dose CSP had inferior OS and higher risk of relapse, but no difference in TRM.

An alternative approach to GVHD prophylaxis involves the use of T-cell-depleted grafts, a technique that is discussed in further detail in Chapter 17. A number of reports of the outcomes of this approach have been published. A report from Memorial Sloan Kettering Cancer Center (MSKCC) provides the outcome data of 31 adults with AML who received allogeneic HCT in first remission with T-cell-depleted grafts utilizing a soybean-lectin/sheep red blood cell agglutination separation technique and demonstrated a 45% 3-year DFS rate with 13% relapse and 15% graft rejection [57]. Six years later, this same group reported an additional group of 31 patients with AML transplanted during first CR who received an intensified preparative regimen followed by T-cell-depleted allogeneic grafts [58]. No cases of grade II–IV acute GVHD were observed, and only two patients developed chronic GVHD. The 4-year DFS was 77.4% with a median follow-up of 56.2 months. Another report describes 15 patients who received T-cell-depleted allografts with 11 patients surviving free of disease with a median follow-up of 76 months and only one relapse [59]. Investigators at the Dana-Farber Cancer Institute described the outcome of 28 adults with AML who received T-cell-depleted allogeneic grafts using a monoclonal antibody depletion method of $CD6^+$ T cells [60]. The report indicated a 5% transplant-related mortality with 4-year DFS of 63% and OS of 71%. The relapse risk, however, was increased to 25%, and the incidence of GVHD was 15%, with one patient failing to engraft and two patients developing late graft failure. It is difficult to assess the benefit of the lower toxicity and decreased GVHD in T-cell-depleted transplants for AML with the increased risk of relapse and graft rejection. A randomized study is needed to determine if T-cell-depleted is superior for this group of patients.

Allogeneic HCT vs. autologous HCT vs. standard dose chemotherapy for patients with AML in first remission

The clinical phase II trials reported in the literature since 1979 suggest that allogeneic HCT is the superior therapy for patients with AML in first remission who have HLA-matched-sibling donors and no contraindications to proceed to transplantation. Based on the improved outcomes reported in the early publications, many investigators have performed studies to compare the results of standard chemotherapy regimens to allogeneic or autologous HCT [10,61–80]. In most of the study designs, the allocation to allogeneic HCT was determined by a "genetic randomization", i.e. patients who had an appropriately matched-sibling donor would proceed to allogeneic HCT and those without a suitable donor would receive the alternative therapy.

Although numerous studies have addressed this issue, the landmark study performed prospectively by the European Organization for Research and Treatment of Cancer (EORTC) and Gruppo Italiano Malattie Ematologiche Maligne dell' Adulto (GIMEMA) was the first large randomized, controlled prospective study reported [76]. This trial compared allogeneic HCT, autologous HCT or intensive consolidation chemotherapy for patients with AML in first remission. The analysis included 168 patients, mostly adults, allocated to receive allogeneic HCT, 128 patients to autologous HCT and 126 patients to consolidation chemotherapy. The 4-year estimates of DFS were 55%, 48% and 30%, respectively, and demonstrated a statistically significant improvement in DFS for allogeneic HCT (Fig. 75.3 [76]). The relative relapse risk was significantly lower in the allogeneic HCT group compared to either autologous HCT or consolidation chemotherapy. No significant advantage in OS for allogeneic or autologous transplantation vs. standard chemotherapy was observed.

Table 75.1 summarizes the results of 16 clinical trials comparing allogeneic HCT with alternative therapies for patients with AML in first remission [61–69,71–76,79,80]. The conclusion from these 16 studies can be summarized as follows:
1 In all trials, the relapse rates were the lowest for the allograft recipients compared to those who received autologous transplants or further chemotherapy. In seven of the 11 reports in which the relapse rates were analyzed, the difference was significantly superior for patients who were transplanted from histocompatible siblings as compared to those receiving the alternative therapies.
2 Allogeneic transplantation from a matched-related donor resulted in significantly superior DFS in five of the 14 trials in which this important outcome was reported. None of the studies demonstrated an advantage for any of the alternative modalities (autografting or further chemotherapy) as compared to allogeneic transplantation.

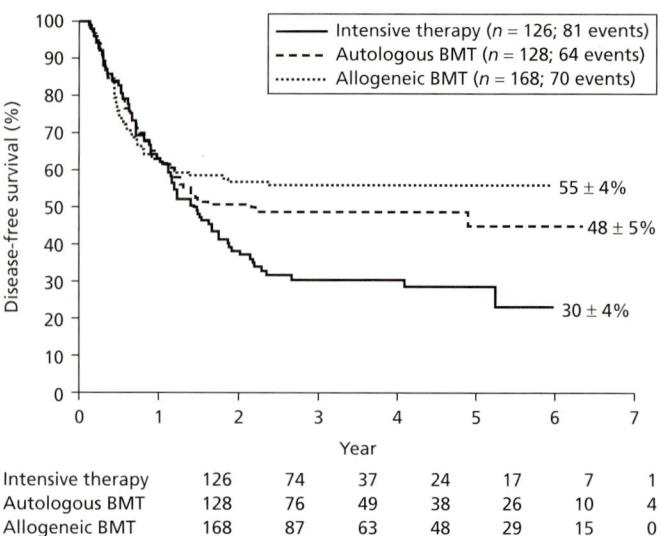

Fig. 75.3 Kaplan–Meier estimates of disease-free survival (DFS) for patients with acute myeloid leukemia (AML) in first complete remission (CR) assigned to allogeneic bone marrow transplantation (BMT) (- - - n = 168), autologous BMT (– – – n = 128) or intensive consolidation chemotherapy (—— n = 126). Percentages represent estimated DFS rates ± SE. Reproduced with permission from Zittoun et al. [76].

3 OS was described for 10 of the 16 studies and was statistically superior in favor of allografting in one trial and in favor of chemotherapy in another study. Seven trials were described as showing no significant difference, or no analysis of OS was included in the publication. It is also important to recognize that patients who received chemotherapy or even autologous transplantation in these trials and subsequently relapsed often received salvage therapy involving allogeneic HCT. Thus, the equivalence of OS in some trials may reflect the ability of an allogeneic transplant procedure to salvage patients in first relapse or second CR.

It is unlikely that another large prospective study will answer in a clear way the important question regarding the optimal therapy for patients with AML in first CR. In general, these trials have treated AML as a single disease, without stratification based upon recognized prognostic factors. Unfortunately, so called meta-analyses tend to generalize from individual trial data and may result in misleading information and, thus, erroneous recommendations. A shortcoming in the recent prospective randomized trials is the failure of many patients to remain on trial with less than 70% of those enrolled completing trials after attaining a CR.

Allogeneic HCT for AML in untreated first relapse or during second CR

Although the results of allogeneic matched-sibling donor HCT in first CR indicate an overall improved outcome compared with chemotherapy, many patients do not undergo transplantation while in first CR based on either favorable disease characteristics and/or patient or physician preference. In early reports from Seattle, the outcomes of patients receiving an allograft in second CR were similar to those of patients transplanted in untreated first relapse with similar DFS of 24% and 26%, respectively [81,82]. A subsequent evaluation compared 17 patients receiving allogeneic HCT in untreated first relapse with 25 patients who were transplanted in second CR [8]. The decision to proceed to transplantation in untreated first relapse was based upon bed availability and on physician recommendation. This study also analyzed a third group of patients who did not enter a second remission with reinduction chemotherapy. The survival of patients transplanted in untreated first relapse was 29% and of

Table 75.1 Allogeneic bone marrow transplantation (BMT) vs. autologous BMT vs. chemotherapy for AML in first remission.

	Treatment	No. of pts	DFS (%)	p value	OS (%)	p value	Relapse (%)	p value
*Royal Marsden [61]	AlloBMT	53	54	p <0.005				
	ChemoRx	51	21					
Seattle [62,65]	*AlloBMT	33	48	p <0.05				
	*ChemoRx	43	21					
	†AlloBMT	43	40	p = 0.07				
	†ChemoRx	43	21					
†UCLA [63]	AlloBMT	23			40	p = n.s.	40	p <0.01
	ChemoRx	44			27		71	
*Genova [64]	AlloBMT	19	64	p <0.05	70	p = n.r.		
	ChemoRx	18	13		21			
*MD Anderson [67]	AlloBMT	11			36	p = n.s.	9	p <0.01
	ChemoRx	27			15		85	
*Spain [66]	AlloBMT	14	70	p = n.s.			10	p <0.005
	ChemoRx	25	10				88	
*France [68]	AlloBMT	20	66				18	
	AutoBMT	12	41	p <0.004			50	p <0.0002
	ChemoRx	20	16				83	
*Netherlands [69]	AlloBMT	23	51	p = n.s.	66	p = 0.05	34	p = 0.03
	AutoBMT	32	35		37		60	
*UCLA [72]	AlloBMT	42	45	p = n.s.	45	p = n.s.	32	p = 0.05
	ChemoRx	28	38		53		60	
†ECOG [71]	AlloBMT	54	42	p = n.s.	43	p = n.s.		
	ChemoRx	29	30		42			
†France [73]	AlloBMT	27	41	p = n.s.	41	p = n.s.	43	p = 0.1
	ChemoRx	31	27		46		67	
Boston [75]	*AlloBMT	23	62	p = n.s.			0	p = Sgnfct
	*AutoBMT	27	62				38	
	†AlloBMT	31	56	p = n.s.			20	p = 0.04
	†AutoBMT	53	45				50	
*SWOG [74]	AlloBMT	34	38	p = n.s.				
	ChemoRx	110	28					
†EORTC/GIMEMA [76]	AlloBMT	168	55		59		27	
	AutoBMT	128	48	p = Sgnfct	56	p = n.r.	41	p = n.r.
	ChemoRx	126	30		46		57	
*GOELAM [79]	AlloBMT	73	50		55		37	
	AutoBMT	75	48	p = n.r.	52	p = n.r.	45	p = n.r.
	ChemoRx	71	43		59		55	
US Intergroup [80]	†AlloBMT	113	43		46	p = 0.04‡	29	
	†AutoBMT	116	35	p = n.s.	43	p = 0.05§	48	p = n.r.
	†ChemoRx	117	35		52		62	
	*AlloBMT	92	47	p = n.r.	48	p = n.r.		
	*AutoBMT	63	45		55			

*Patients assigned to transplantation based on availability of matched siblings, or to chemotherapy and analyzed according to treatment received.
†Patients assigned to transplantation based on availability of matched siblings, or to chemotherapy and analyzed according to intent-to-treat.
‡p value reflects comparison of alloBMT and chemotherapy.
§p value reflects comparison of autoBMT and chemotherapy.
alloBMT, allogeneic bone marrow transplantation; AML, acute myeloid leukemia; autoBMT, autologous bone marrow transplantation; chemoRx, chemotherapy; DFS, disease-free survival; n.r., not reported; n.s., not significant; OS, overall survival; Sgnfct, significant.

those transplanted in second CR was 22%, which was not statistically different. The group of patients in refractory relapse fared worse with OS of 10%. A larger review from Seattle provided an update of 126 patients with AML transplanted during untreated first relapse using a variety of different preparative and GVHD prevention regimens [83]. Actuarial DFS was 23% with a nonrelapse mortality of 44% and a relapse rate of 57%. This comparison of the different treatment conditions indicated that those patients who had received the CY/TBI regimen in combination with single agent MTX had attained the best outcome with respect to relapse and survival.

The North American Marrow Transplant Group reported the outcome of 40 patients transplanted following a regimen of etoposide (VP16), CY and TBI while in untreated first relapse [84]. DFS at 44 months was 29%. Similar outcomes have been reported by other HCT centers as well [85,86]. The use of T-cell-depleted grafts has been examined in a small group of patients transplanted in second CR resulting in 50% DFS, a relapse rate of 12.5% and nonrelapse mortality of 37.5% [58].

A small study comparing allogeneic vs. autologous HCT for patients with AML in second remission demonstrated a 40% DFS after allogeneic HCT without significant differences in outcome compared to autologous HCT [87]. There was a lower relapse rate in the patients receiving an allograft. However this gain was balanced by an increase in TRM. The IBMTR reported the results of allogeneic HCT for 257 patients with AML in second remission compared with a cohort of 244 patients treated with chemotherapy alone [88]. This study showed a 3-year DFS of 26% for patients receiving an allograft vs. 17% for those treated with chemotherapy alone. Another retrospective analysis from IBMTR and the Autologous Blood and Marrow Transplant Registry—North America (ABMTR) compared 106 patients with AML in second remission who received an autologous HCT and 163 patients who underwent an allogeneic HCT [89]. This analysis showed 3-year DFS of 27% and 43%, respectively. Finally, the EBMT group reported a retrospective analysis of 98 patients allografted in second remission and compared them with 190 patients who received an autologous HCT [78]. The relapse rate was significantly lower for patients who received an allogeneic HCT, but DFS (55% and 42%, respectively) was again not statistically different.

The currently available data suggest that patients with AML who are in untreated first relapse can expect a similar outcome following allogeneic HCT from a matched-sibling donor as those patients proceeding to transplantation during second CR. Moreover, many patients in first relapse will never achieve a second CR. A prospective, randomized study would be required to determine if this interpretation is correct. The current results may be based on selection factors, such as extent of disease at relapse, immediate donor availability and insurance-related issues. Given these confounding circumstances, it is unlikely that such a study could ever be completed. It is therefore reasonable to proceed to myeloablative allogeneic HCT in untreated first relapse in situations in which the patient is diagnosed in early relapse with a limited disease burden.

Allogeneic transplantation for patients with primary induction failure or in second or subsequent relapse

Three decades ago, allogeneic transplantation for AML was first tested in patients with multiply recurrent or refractory relapse [5]. The transplant outcome for patients with induction failure or resistant relapse AML, or for those with extramedullary disease treated with standard-dose chemotherapy has been and remains quite poor. Although the results are less than satisfactory, there is still a role for allogeneic HCT for patients with advanced AML. However, relapsed AML involving extramedullary sites (chloromas or central nervous system infiltration) may be associated with particularly poor prognosis. Investigators at City of Hope National Medical Center (COHNMC) described 10 patients with extramedullary involvement of AML who underwent allogeneic HCT and reported only one patient to be alive and in continued CR 2 years following transplantation [90]. The investigators at MSKCC compared the outcome following allogeneic HCT of 13 patients with AML and leukemia cutis to 189 patients with AML but without skin involvement [91]. Although they found no difference in relapse rate, the incidence of extramedullary relapse was significantly higher in the patients with leukemia cutis.

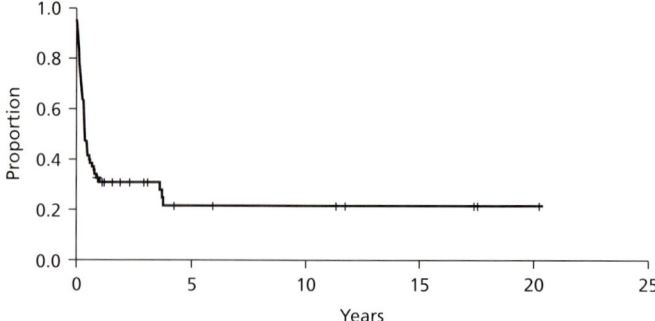

Fig. 75.4 Kaplan–Meier estimates of disease-free survival (DFS) of 71 patients with refractory acute myeloid leukemia (AML) who received an allogeneic hematopoietic cell transplantation (HCT) from a matched-sibling donor. Updated from Fung *et al.* [95].

The investigators at the M.D. Anderson Cancer Center reported the outcomes of 14 patients with primary refractory AML who received matched-sibling donor HCT with five of the patients surviving for 98–1790 days post-transplant at the time of the report [92]. The outcome of 16 patients with AML who were refractory to at least two cycles of induction chemotherapy was reported from COHNMC [93]. Ninety percent of these patients achieved a remission after HCT and with a minimum follow-up of 18 months, eight of the 16 patients were alive and in continuous CR. The IBMTR reported data for 88 patients, adults and children, with AML who had not achieved CR with chemotherapy [94]. The 3-year relapse rate for this group of patients was 63%, 3-year DFS was 21% and nonrelapse mortality was 44%.

More recently, the investigators from COHNMC reported their extended experience with 71 patients with refractory AML who were treated with allogeneic HCT during a period of 22 years with 82% receiving grafts from matched-sibling donors [95]. The median age of these patients was 37 years (range 2–62 years) and the median follow-up was 1 year. Three-year DFS was 29% with a relapse rate of 54% (Fig. 75.4 [95]). These results are similar to earlier reports [5]. Cytogenetic data were available in 51 of the patients treated at COHNMC. Using the cytogenetic prognostic criteria of SWOG [23], three patients had favorable, 27 had intermediate and 21 had unfavorable cytogenetics. Those patients with favorable or intermediate cytogenetics had DFS of 44% vs. only 18% in those with unfavorable cytogenetic features, again demonstrating the powerful effect of cytogenetics on the outcome in AML.

Studies evaluating patients who receive an allogeneic bone marrow transplantation (BMT) in second or subsequent relapse, or third or later remissions following standard therapy have demonstrated very few long-term survivors. In one early study, there were no survivors in a group of 16 patients with end-stage AML and only one patient of four in third or subsequent relapse was alive for 27 months, with relapse of his disease at the time of the report [96].

In one report, 127 patients, including 33 patients with disease resistant to chemotherapy, second or subsequent relapse or with secondary AML, received a preparatory regimen of BU/CY and a matched-sibling donor HCT [86]. Three-year DFS was 24.2% for the 33 patients with advanced disease. The actuarial relapse rate was significantly higher in this advanced

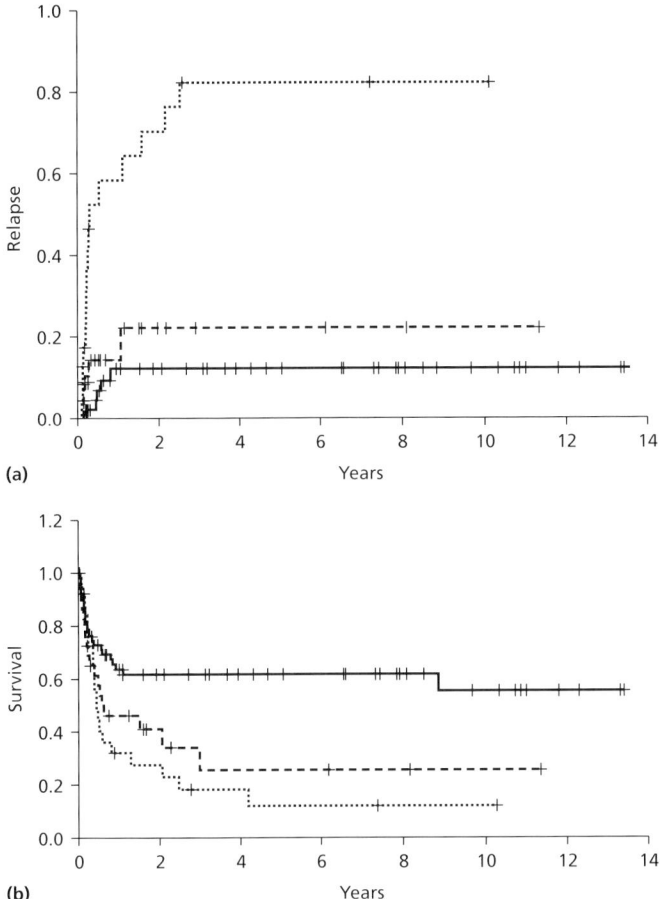

Fig. 75.5 Effect of remission status at the time of hematopoietic cell transplantation (HCT) on relapse (a) and survival (b) after allogeneic transplantation from matched-sibling donors for 115 adults with acute myeloid leukemia (AML) treated at the Stanford University Medical Center from 1988 to 2001. —— first complete remission (CR) ($n = 60$); – – – second CR or first relapse ($n = 29$); - - - advanced disease ($n = 26$).

group (61%) compared to patients in first remission and patients in first relapse/remission, 14.1% and 40.6%, respectively. Data from Stanford University, CA, also demonstrate the influence of disease status on outcome following allogeneic transplantation for *de novo* AML. A comparison of 115 patients receiving a myeloablative regimen followed by allogeneic HCT from HLA-matched-sibling donors transplanted with various stages of AML is presented in Fig. 75.5. Sixty patients were transplanted in first CR, 29 in second CR or untreated first relapse and 26 patients with more advanced disease, including induction failure. Actuarial 5-year relapse rate was 12% for patients in first CR compared with 22% for patients in second CR or first relapse and 82% for patients with more advanced disease ($p < 0.0001$). The actuarial 5-year OS was 62% for patients in first CR compared with 26% for second CR or first relapse and 12% for those with advanced disease ($p = 0.0013$). This analysis confirms the findings of other groups of investigators demonstrating the importance of early referral for transplantation [86,97].

Alternative cell sources for allogeneic transplantation for patients with AML

Approximately two-thirds of patients with AML do not have an appropriately matched-sibling donor available for allogeneic HCT. Although these patients may receive alternative therapies, such as autologous transplantation, for those patients with resistant or refractory disease, this approach is not a viable option. Data reported for the outcome of patients treated with autografting for high-risk AML demonstrated that this is a poor treatment choice for this group of patients [98,99]. Consequently, as prophylaxis and treatment of GVHD improved and manipulations of the donor graft became more feasible, the use of partially matched-related donors (PMRD) has been investigated.

The initial reports using PMRD showed some promise [100,101], although the survival of patients who received PMRD allografts with acute leukemia in relapse was lower than for a similar group of patients who received HLA-identical sibling grafts [102]. More recently, reports using various donor cell manipulations have demonstrated improved outcomes following mismatched transplants (see Chapter 82 for a more detailed discussion) [103–105].

For those patients who do not have an adequately MRD, the use of alternative sources of hematopoietic cells has been investigated for adults with AML, including the use of volunteer unrelated donor cells, umbilical cord blood units or grafts obtained from haplo-identical related donors.

The use of unrelated donor cells

Bone marrow transplants from unrelated donors were initially reported 20 years ago and were facilitated by local blood banks and histocompatability laboratories [106,107]. Those smaller registries were limited in the number of patients for whom they were able to identify a donor because of the relatively low numbers of volunteers. The establishment of the National Marrow Donor Program (NMDP) evolved from the dauntless efforts of many in 1986 to establish a national resource in the USA to locate donors for patients in need [108] and similar efforts have taken place on almost every continent (see Chapter 49 for details).

An analysis of 70 patients with AML who received unrelated donor BMT demonstrated a 2-year DFS of 45% for patients in first or second remission and 19% for patients with more advanced disease [109]. In a study of patients with advanced acute leukemia, the actuarial 2-year DFS was 23% following unrelated donor transplantation [110]. GVHD and relapse remain significant barriers to long-term survival. The largest experience of outcomes of matched-unrelated donor (MUD) transplants for AML is based on 161 HCT recipients ranging in age from 1 year to 55 years [111]. Most patients were predominantly treated with a CY/TBI preparatory regimen with CSP/MTX used for GVHD prophylaxis. DFS was 50% for patients transplanted in first CR and 28% for patients treated in second CR. Patients with more advanced disease, including those with primary induction failure, had worse outcomes. The relapse rates were significantly lower in patients transplanted in CR than when in relapse or with refractory disease. Patients receiving a higher bone marrow cell dose ($>3.5 \times 10^8$) and those who were cytomegalovirus seronegative had superior outcomes. Rates of acute and chronic GVHD were 77% and 65%, respectively. These outcomes for DFS are comparable to those reported with matched-sibling donor transplants, although the risk of GVHD appears higher in these patients.

The outcomes of 1755 adults transplanted from MUD facilitated by the NMDP using myeloablative preparatory regimens are presented in Fig. 75.6. These survival curves demonstrate the importance of performing unrelated donor transplants early in the course of disease, as evidenced by the survival of less than 10% for patients transplanted in third or subsequent CR, or in relapse.

These data suggest that the use of MUD transplants for patients with AML is an appropriate therapy for those patients with high-risk disease in first or second remission while those with resistant or relapsed disease fare poorly.

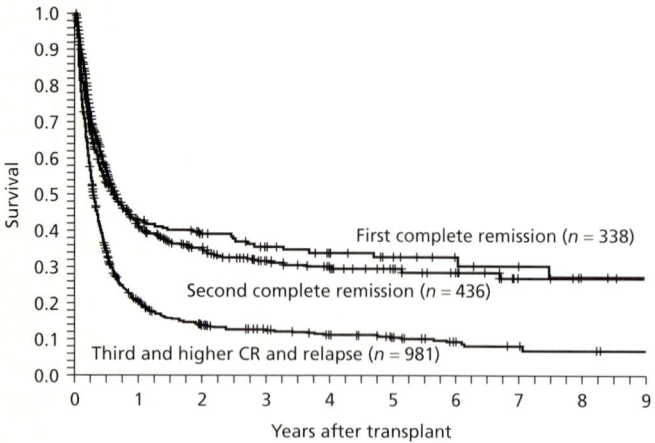

Fig. 75.6 Kaplan–Meier estimates of survival following unrelated donor hematopoietic cell transplantation (HCT) for acute myeloid leukemia (AML) facilitated by the National Marrow Donor Program (NMDP) for 1755 adults 17 years of age or older in first complete remission (CR), second CR, or third or higher CR or relapse. This figure was kindly provided by the National Marrow Donor Program, Minneapolis, MN.

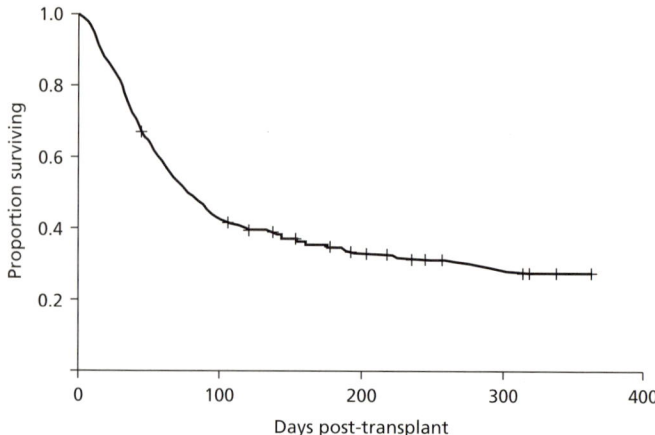

Fig. 75.7 Kaplan–Meier estimates of survival following unrelated umbilical cord blood (UCB) transplantation facilitated by the New York Blood Center for 79 patients 17 years of age or older. This figure was kindly provided by Dr Pablo Rubenstein and colleagues from the New York Blood Center, New York.

The use of umbilical cord blood

Umbilical cord blood (UCB) contains hematopoietic progenitor cells similar to those found in bone marrow. In fact, there is evidence that cord blood progenitor cells have some proliferation advantages compared to cells in marrow or peripheral blood. In addition, it is postulated that the immaturity of the T cells obtained from the umbilical cord might be associated with decreased GVHD and may allow mismatching of HLA loci between the graft and the transplant recipient (see Chapter 43).

The largest report of UCB transplants describes the outcome of 562 unrelated UCB transplants facilitated by the Placental Blood Program at the New York Blood Center [112]. The majority of transplants were performed for children; only 18% of patients were ≥18 years of age. One-hundred and twenty-four patients had AML. The relapse rate was 30% at 1 year for the patients with AML. Another report of 68 adults who received mismatched transplants included 19 patients with AML [113]. Evaluation of all patients included in this study demonstrated 26% DFS at 40 months following transplantation.

The outcome of 79 patients over the age of 16 years transplanted for AML with UCB grafts is presented in Fig. 75.7. As shown in this analysis, over 60% of patients died within 100 days of transplant from all causes and, so far, only limited long-term data are available (data courtesy of Dr Pablo Rubenstein and colleagues, the New York Blood Center, New York).

These data regarding the use of UCB for transplants are encouraging for selected patients but must be viewed in the appropriate context. Most importantly, the follow-up information regarding relapse is limited and there must be consideration that the decreased risk of GVHD seen after UCB, presumably due to immaturity of the donor lymphocytes, may also be associated with a decreased GVL effect. In addition, this type of graft still is of limited utility in adults based on recipient body weight and cell dose-related factors. Current investigations into expanding cells from cord blood units may help alleviate this issue, but the concerns regarding GVL activity of these UCB cells and the high nonrelapse mortality still make this approach a high-risk procedure.

The use of haplo-identical related donors

One alternative method to performing transplants in patients who do not have a fully MRD is the use of HCT from a haplo-identical donor, if one is available. This approach increases the likelihood of identifying a related donor since the patient will have a haplotype match with both parents as well as a 50% chance of sharing a single haplotype match with any sibling. In addition, it is also fairly likely that close relatives could be identified who share a haplotype with the patient and all of the patient's children will have one haplotype in common with the patient. Haplo-identical HCT will involve major HLA mismatches that are associated with GVHD, so adequate graft manipulation and/or immunosuppression is required to allow a safer outcome (see Chapter 82 for details).

In a recently published study, a group of 43 patients with high-risk acute leukemia, including 20 patients with AML, were transplanted from haplo-identical donors after no appropriate unrelated donor could be identified [114]. The patients were treated with a preparatory regimen of TBI plus thiotepa, antithymocyte globulin (ATG) and fludarabine. The hematopoietic cell grafts consisted of T-cell-depleted peripheral blood hematopoietic cells with or without T-cell-depleted marrow, and no post-transplant immunosuppression was given. Remarkably, even with major HLA incompatability, no evaluable patients developed acute or chronic GVHD. Only two of the 20 patients with AML had relapsed at the time of the report with a 1.5-year DFS of 36%. An additional report from this group of investigators described the influence of natural killer (NK) cell reactivity and outcome in 57 patients with AML and 35 patients with acute lymphoblastic leukemia (ALL) who received a graft from a haplo-identical donor [115]. As shown in Table 75.2, patients who received a graft with killer immunoglobulin-like receptors (KIR) reactivity in the GVH direction had no rejection or grade II–IV acute GVHD compared with 15.5% and 13.7%, respectively, for those without such reactivity. When evaluating patients with AML, there was a relapse rate of 0% for those with KIR reactivity in the GVH direction vs. a 75% relapse rate for patients without reactivity. Also notable is the lack of effect of KIR reactivity on relapse in patients with ALL.

Ongoing studies of haplo-identical transplants continue to expand on these early trials. Further investigations into the effect of NK reactivity and outcome are necessary as are methods of decreasing the incidence of infectious complications to decrease the risks associated with this maneuver, and to make it more acceptable and successful for patients with AML.

Reduced intensity regimens for AML

Myeloablative preparatory regimens for allogeneic HCT are designed to eradicate the malignant clone of cells while also causing immunosup-

Table 75.2 Outcome of haploidentical transplants for acute leukemia.

KIR ligand incompatibility in GVH direction	No	Yes
Number of transplants	58	34
Donors displaying antirecipient NK clones	1/58	34/34*
Disease		
ALL	21	14
AML	37	20
Transplantation outcomes		
Rejection	15.5%	0%*
Acute GVHD, ≥ grade II	13.7%	0%*
Probability of relapse at 5 years		
ALL	90%	85%
AML	75%	0%**

*$p \leq 0.01$.
**$p < 0.0008$ [22].
ALL, acute lymphoblastic leukemia; AML, acute myeloid leukemia; GVH, graft-versus-host; GVHD, graft-versus-host disease; KIR, killer Ig-like receptors; NK, natural killer.

pression of the host to reduce the risk of graft rejection. The myeloablative maneuver was also felt to be necessary in order to create space in the marrow for the hematopoietic cell graft. It was subsequently detected that some patients were not full hematopoietic chimeras as expected but, rather, had attained a status of mixed hematopoietic chimerism with both host and donor hematopoietic cells present [116,117]. Initially, there were concerns that the identification of residual host hematopoietic cells would be indicative of subsequent relapse and of a failure of the transplant procedure to cure the patient. However, studies in animals as well as human clinical long-term follow-up data suggested otherwise. In fact, a large retrospective analysis even demonstrated that patients who developed some degree of mixed chimerism had a decreased incidence of GVHD and improved leukemia-free survival [118].

Animal studies were undertaken to develop a nonmyeloablative regimen that would intentionally result in mixed chimerism, at least transiently. This approach might allow tolerance to host tissues to develop with a decrease in GVHD and hopefully not interfere with the desired GVL effect. The potential of these transplants to treat a variety of conditions, even for patients unable to tolerate the rigors of a myeloablative regimen, has been developed and reviewed (see Chapter 85) [119].

The use of a low-dose TBI preparatory regimen studied in a collaboration between researchers at the Fred Hutchinson Cancer Research Center (FHCRC) Seattle, WA, Stanford University, CA, and the University of Leipzig, Germany, has been reported [120]. This protocol used low-dose TBI in a single 200 cGy dose with post-transplant immunosuppression using CSP and mycophenolate mofetil. Patients ($n = 45$) included in this study were not considered candidates for a standard allogeneic transplant due to age or comorbid conditions. Fifty-three percent of the patients completed the procedure entirely in an outpatient setting. Grade II–III acute GVHD occurred in 47% of patients and nonfatal graft rejection was encountered in 20% of patients. TRM was 6.7% and survival was 73.3% with a median follow-up of 244 days. Fifty percent of patients with sustained donor engraftment attained a CR. The addition of fludarabine to the TBI regimen drastically decreased the incidence of graft rejection while still providing a nonmyelosuppressive outpatient procedure.

A larger collaborative effort using this new regimen is ongoing, and increasing numbers of patients with AML have been treated with this combination [121,122]. Newer data are presented in Table 75.3 [122]. Thirty-four patients have received a nonmyeloablative allogeneic HCT from a matched-sibling donor. Twenty of the patients on this study were in first CR and 14 were beyond first CR. Four patients died of transplant-related causes and 14 patients are alive and in CR. In addition, 41 patients have received the same nonmyeloablative fludarabine/TBI regimen and grafts from closely MUDs. This group of patients included 11 in first CR and 30 beyond first CR. A higher percentage of patients died of nonrelapse causes in this group, predominantly in patients with more advanced disease. Nineteen of the 41 patients are alive and in CR.

Other studies using nonmyeloablative regimens have been described with fewer numbers of AML patients [123,124]. Although this approach has demonstrated decreased morbidity and mortality than seen with myeloablative regimens, long-term data from ongoing studies are required to determine the full impact of such chimerism-induced immunotherapy for patients with AML.

Relapse following allogeneic HCT for AML

Relapse remains the major cause of treatment failure following allogeneic HCT for AML with over 50% of patients with advanced disease suffering a relapse, most commonly within the first 2 years after transplantation. The optimal therapy for these patients is indeterminate with most therapies being of only limited utility. One report describes the outcome of 95 patients who relapsed with AML following allogeneic HCT [125]. Sixty-two patients received additional therapy for treatment of their disease, the majority treated with chemotherapy, and 13 patients received a second HCT. There was a 34% response rate to chemotherapy and 43% of the patients treated with chemotherapy who had relapsed within 100 days of HCT died of treatment-related complications. Only four of the 95 patients in this report experienced prolonged survival.

The use of repeat allogeneic HCT has been reported with increasing frequency since the early reports demonstrating the feasibility of a second

Table 75.3 Outcome of patients receiving a nonmyeloablative allogeneic transplant for acute myeloid leukemia (AML).

	Related donors					Unrelated donors				
Disease status	Total	Alive	Alive in CR	NRM	Relapse	Total	Alive	Alive in CR	NRM	Relapse
CR1	20	10	8	2	8	11	9	9	0	2
CR2	9	5	4	1	3	10	6	6	2	2
Beyond CR2	5	2	2	1	2	20	5	4	9	6
Total	34	17	14	4	13	41	20	19	11	10

Updated from Hegenbart et al. [122].
AML, acute myeloid leukemia; CR, complete remission; CR1, first complete remission; CR2, second complete remission; NRM, nonrelapse mortality.

marrow transplant attempt [126]. EBMT described the outcome of 75 second transplants for patients with relapsed leukemia and reported an 11.5% survival when evaluating all patients [127]. Patients who relapsed more than 1 year following autologous transplantation had a 35% survival, while all those who relapsed within 1 year died. Another report of second transplants for recurrent acute leukemia demonstrated a 34% DFS if the transplant procedure was performed during another chemotherapy-induced remission but only 2% for patients with resistant disease [128].

In an attempt to induce a GVL effect in patients who relapsed following allogeneic transplantation, the amount of immunosuppression may be reduced. This approach was first successfully tried in a single patient [129]. A subsequent report included 13 patients with AML with three entering CR following withdrawal of CSP [130]. However, there was only a 10% probability of achieving and maintaining a CR at 3 years. The reduction or cessation of immunosuppression for the development of a GVL effect seems to be of limited utility for patients with AML. Another approach to exploit a GVL effect for relapsed leukemia following allogeneic BMT uses donor lymphocyte infusion (DLI) (see Chapter 84). One study reported four patients who had suffered a relapse of AML following allogeneic BMT treated with DLI with three patients developing severe GVHD and one patient surviving in remission for over 1 year [131]. The EBMT group reported results for 135 patients with hematologic diseases [132]. Significant complications of DLI included a 41% incidence of grade II–IV GVHD with 14 deaths attributed to this complication and/or severe pancytopenia. Twenty-one of the 135 patients had recurrent AML treated with induction chemotherapy followed by DLI or DLI alone. Five of these patients achieved a CR.

A 2002 study prospectively evaluated the outcome of patients with myeloid malignancies who relapsed following allogeneic HCT and then were subsequently treated with chemotherapy followed by granulocyte colony-stimulating factor (G-CSF) mobilized hematopoietic cells obtained from their matched-sibling donor [133]. This study included 47 patients with AML and 18 patients with other myeloid malignancies. The OS for the cohort was only 19% with patients entering a CR following the cytoreductive chemotherapy having an improved outcome. Although outcomes for the different disease types were not reported separately in the publication however, the authors found no statistical difference in outcomes for AML vs. CML or myelodysplasia.

Efforts are underway to optimize DLI doses to separate the GVL effect from significant GVHD. However, the use of DLI remains a viable option for selected patients with AML in relapse after allogeneic HCT (see Chapter 84) [134,135].

Allogeneic HCT for patients relapsing after autologous transplantation

The use of a second transplant for patients who have failed an initial syngeneic or allogeneic transplant has been attempted for almost 3 decades with the goal to cure these unfortunate patients [126]. The use of second allogeneic transplants for patients who have failed an allogeneic transplant has largely been supplanted by the use of DLI. However, the use of allogeneic transplants from matched or unmatched donors has been utilized with increasing frequency in patients who have failed an autograft for AML. A report from EBMT included the outcome of 35 patients who had failed an autograft for AML and subsequently underwent an allogeneic HCT [136]. The relapse rate at 2 years was 15% but DFS for the AML patients was not reported. Overall, the 2-year TRM for the 62 patients who received allografts in this study was 51% and the 2-year DFS was 27%.

A report from the FHCRC described 59 patients who received a myeloablative allogeneic HCT after relapsing following an autologous transplant, including 24 patients with AML [137]. Two-year DFS in this group was 46% with a nonrelapse mortality of 30% and a relapse rate of 25%. A statistical analysis demonstrated that pediatric patients had a significantly better outcome when all 59 patients were analyzed. However, the relationship between age, disease and preparatory regimen confounded the analysis making it difficult to draw conclusions about which patients might derive the most benefit from this approach.

Seventeen patients who relapsed after autologous transplantation for AML received a T-cell-depleted transplant from a PMRD [138]. The majority of these grafts were mismatched for two or more HLA antigens, and the median age of transplant recipients included in this report was 26 years. Ten of the 17 patients died of nonrelapse mortality, two patients relapsed and 29% were surviving in remission for a median of 68 months after transplantation.

These studies demonstrate the potential of a GVL effect to cure a minority of patients who have failed an autograft. However, this gain comes at the expense of a high morbidity and mortality. The excessive toxicity reported in these studies may be abrogated with the use of non-myeloablative regimens, [139] although the role of these transplants for relapse following an autograft remains to be investigated.

Conclusions and future directions

The survival of adults with newly diagnosed AML over the past 3 decades has improved with refinements in induction and consolidation chemotherapy, advances in supportive care and the increasing use of allogeneic HCT, especially in earlier stages of this disease. The crucial predictive role of cytogenetic abnormalities in determining chemotherapy response, prognosis and treatment outcome make it imperative that all patients with newly diagnosed AML have bone marrow cytogenetic studies performed at initial presentation and again to confirm cytogenetic remissions. In addition, the increasing need of allogeneic transplantation for adults with AML requires that all patients and their siblings undergo HLA typing early after diagnosis to determine if a matched-sibling donor is available and to allow for the possiblility of unrelated donor or UCB searches. Additionally, referral of all patients for a transplant evaluation should be considered early, even for those with good-prognosis cytogenetics to allow rapid transition towards transplantation in those patients who are likely to benefit from allografting at the time of relapse following best available chemotherapy.

The most important advance in AML over the past decade has been the recognition of the crucial role of cytogenetic abnormalities in determining prognosis. The stratification of patients based on cytogenetic features has been recommended by leukemia experts as a key factor to determine the timing of transplantation [140]. A proposed treatment algorithm for patients with newly diagnosed AML is presented in Fig. 75.8. The initial approach for patients should be determined by cytogenetic risk factors, availability of an HLA-matched-sibling donor and response to induction chemotherapy. Patients with cytogenetic features associated with a good prognosis who achieve a CR with induction followed by consolidation chemotherapy should be observed without immediate transplantation, although HLA typing of these patients and their siblings is warranted at diagnosis. Patients with intermediate or poor cytogenetics who achieve a CR with induction/consolidation chemotherapy should undergo an allogeneic HCT procedure early during first CR if a histocompatible donor is available. For those patients who do not enter a CR or who relapse after standard therapy, an allogeneic HCT from a sibling donor or a closely MUD should be performed sooner rather than later. The transplant approach should be individualized for all patients based on remission status, performance status and coexisting medical problems, i.e. high-dose myeloablative or dose-intensity reduced preparatory regimens.

Studies evaluating different preparative regimens for adults with AML do not demonstrate a clear advantage of one specific regimen, although

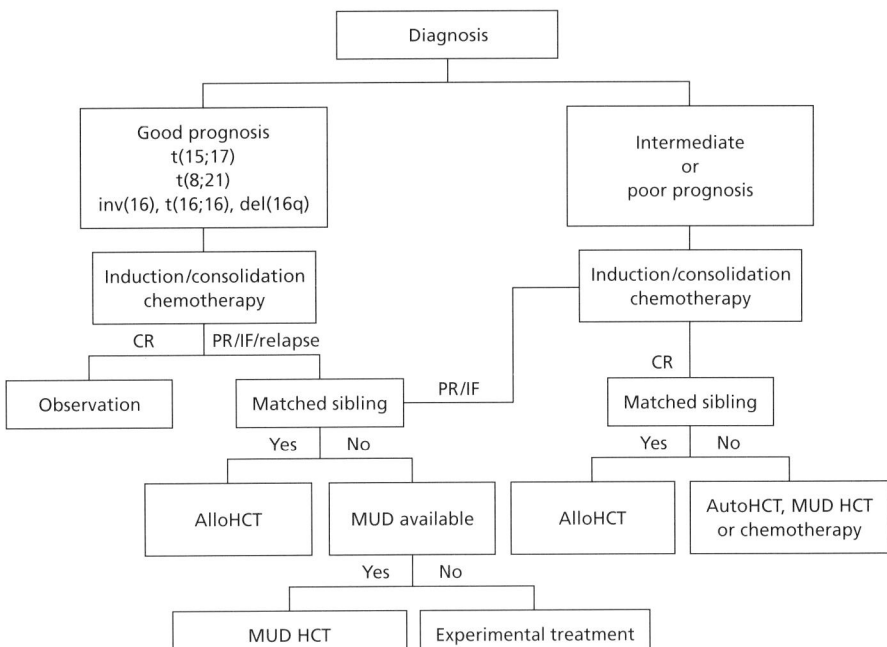

Fig. 75.8 Proposed algorithm for treatment of adult patients newly diagnosed with acute myeloid leukemia (AML). Prognosis refers to the cytogenetic abnormalities proposed by Keating et al. [16]. alloHCT, allogeneic hematopoietic cell transplantation; autoHCT, autologous hematopoietic cell transplantation; CR, complete remission; IF, induction failure; MUD, matched-unrelated donor; PR, partial remission.

recent reports suggest the BU/CY combination may be less effective than the TBI/CY regimen for AML. Although there is evidence of increased toxicity with higher doses of TBI, the data demonstrate a lower relapse rate in these trials [40,45]. These results provide the rationale for trials using radioimmunoconjugates to allow the delivery of radiation to tumor, while hopefully limiting toxicity [48,49]. In addition, recent studies suggest that the use of peripheral blood progenitor cells rather than bone marrow from matched-sibling donors is associated with improved outcome without an increase in acute GVHD [51,141,142]. The use of alternative sources of hematopoietic cells for allografting such as haplo-identical grafts or UCB units are being investigated. However, there are only limited data at this time to consider these types of transplants outside of well-organized prospective clinical trials, especially for patients with early stage AML.

The numerous studies that address the question of optimal therapy for patients with AML in first remission have yielded mixed results, although the trend for improved DFS and lower relapse rate with allografting compared to chemotherapy is clearly evident. These studies suffer from high drop-out rates and low percentages of patients completing their assigned therapy, making it increasingly difficult to detect differences among the various treatments using intent-to-treat analyses. The optimal timing of allogeneic transplantation is still undetermined, although consistent reports of DFS of 45–65% for patients allografted in first CR with relapse rates of <20% would suggest that earlier transplantation is most successful. A significant proportion of patients allografted during second CR or in early first relapse are also being cured of AML, but whether more patients are curable with allogeneic HCT in first CR vs. allogeneic HCT in second CR/first relapse remains unclear. Although a controlled trial has the potential to answer this important question, the sample size necessary and the length of time to complete such a trial makes it unlikely ever to be performed.

The results of allogeneic BMT for patients with advanced AML are consistently poor, and all patients with poor prognostic features at initial presentation who are eligible for allografting should receive their transplant early during the clinical course of their disease, whether from a matched-sibling donor or a MUD. It is essential that all adults with AML be referred to a transplant center as early as possible given the superior outcomes demonstrated for those transplanted earlier in their disease course and to allow adequate time to identify donors for those patients who do not have suitably matched siblings.

The treatment outcome of patients who have suffered a relapse of AML following allogeneic BMT remains poor. Additional chemotherapy and second transplants are associated with exceptionally high morbidity and mortality and have generally resulted in short remissions. Unfortunately, the results of DLI for relapse of AML after allogeneic BMT have been less satisfactory than for patients with early signs of relapse of CML. Nonmyeloablative allogeneic HCT is now being investigated, and it is likely that these reduced intensity regimens will play an increasing role in the treatment of AML, especially in older or medically infirm patients.

It is only through continued prospective trials that these unresolved issues regarding the optimal timing of allogeneic BMT, the ideal GVHD regimen and the use of alternative sources of hematopoietic cells and alternative methods of transplantation will be resolved. It is important that the economic constraints increasingly imposed on investigators by insurers and medical centers do not deter us from continuing our studies to increase the proportion of patients cured of AML [143].

References

1 Beutler E. The treatment of acute leukemia: past, present and future. *Leukemia* 2001; **15**: 658–61.
2 Mayer RJ, Davis RB, Schiffer CA et al. Intensive postremission chemotherapy in adults with acute myeloid leukemia. Cancer Leukemia Group B. *N Engl J Med* 1994; **331**: 896–903.
3 Fefer A, Einstein AB, Thomas ED et al. Bone-marrow transplantation for hematologic neoplasia in 16 patients with identical twins. *N Engl J Med* 1974; **290**: 1389–93.
4 O'Reilly RJ. Allogenic bone marrow transplantation: current status and future directions. *Blood* 1983; **62**: 941–64.
5 Thomas ED, Buckner CD, Banaji M et al. One hundred patients with acute leukemia treated by chemotherapy, total body irradiation, and allogeneic marrow transplantation. *Blood* 1977; **49**: 511–33.
6 Stewart PS, Buckner CD, Clift RA et al. Allogeneic marrow grafting for acute leukemia: a follow-up of long-term survivors. *Exp Hematol* 1979; **7**: 509–18.

7 Blume KG, Beutler E, Bross KJ et al. Bone-marrow ablation and allogeneic marrow transplantation in acute leukemia. N Engl J Med 1980; 302: 1041–6.
8 Appelbaum FR, Clift RA, Buckner CD et al. Allogeneic marrow transplantation for acute non-lymphoblastic leukemia after first relapse. Blood 1983; 61: 949–53.
9 Thomas ED, Buckner CD, Clift RA et al. Marrow transplantation for acute nonlymphoblastic leukemia in first remission. N Engl J Med 1979; 301: 597–9.
10 Powles RL, Morgenstern G, Clink HM et al. The place of bone-marrow transplantation in acute myelogenous leukaemia. Lancet 1980; 1: 1047–50.
11 Forman SJ, Krance RA, O'Donnell MR et al. Bone marrow transplantation for acute nonlymphoblastic leukemia during first complete remission. An analysis of prognostic factors. Transplantation 1987; 43: 650–3.
12 Tallman MS, Kopecky KJ, Amos D et al. Analysis of prognostic factors for the outcome of marrow transplantation or further chemotherapy for patients with acute nonlymphocytic leukemia in first remission. J Clin Oncol 1989; 7: 326–37.
13 McGlave PB, Haake RJ, Bostrom BC et al. Allogeneic bone marrow transplantation for acute nonlymphocytic leukemia in first remission. Blood 1988; 72: 1512–7.
14 Keating S, Suciu S, de Witte T et al. Prognostic factors of patients with acute myeloid leukemia (AML) allografted in first complete remission: an analysis of the EORTC-GIMEMA AML 8A trial. Bone Marrow Transplant 1996; 17: 993–1001.
15 Jourdan E, Maraninchi D, Reiffers J et al. Early allogeneic transplantation favorably influences the outcome of adult patients suffering from acute myeloid leukemia. Société Française de Greffe de Moelle (SFGM). Bone Marrow Transplant 1997; 19: 875–81.
16 Keating MJ, Smith TL, Kantarjian H et al. Cytogenetic pattern in acute myelogenous leukemia: a major reproducible determinant of outcome. Leukemia 1988; 2: 403–12.
17 Bloomfield CD, Lawrence D, Arthure DC, Berg DT, Schiffer CA, Mayer RJ. Curative impact of intensification with high-dose cytarabine (HiDAC) in acute myeloid leukemia (AML) varies by cytogenetic group. Blood 1994; 84: 111a [Abstract].
18 Bloomfield CD, Lawrence D, Byrd JC et al. Frequency of prolonged remission duration after high-dose cytarabine intensification in acute myeloid leukemia varies by cytogenetic subtype. Cancer Res 1998; 58: 4173–9.
19 Grimwade D, Walker H, Oliver F et al. The importance of diagnostic cytogenetics on outcome in AML. analysis of 1612 patients entered into the MRC AML 10 trial. The Medical Research Council Adult and Children's Leukaemia Working Parties. Blood 1998; 92: 2322–33.
20 Ferrant A, Doyen C, Delannoy A et al. Karyotype in acute myeloblastic leukemia: prognostic significance in a prospective study assessing bone marrow transplantation in first remission. Bone Marrow Transplant 1995; 15: 685–90.
21 Gale RP, Horowitz MM, Weiner RS et al. Impact of cytogenetic abnormalities on outcome of bone marrow transplants in acute myelogenous leukemia in first remission. Bone Marrow Transplant 1995; 16: 203–8.
22 Ferrant A, Labopin M, Frassoni F et al. Karyotype in acute myeloblastic leukemia: prognostic significance for bone marrow transplantation in first remission: a European Group for Blood and Marrow Transplantation study. Acute Leukemia Working Party of the European Group for Blood and Marrow Transplantation (EBMT). Blood 1997; 90: 2931–8.
23 Slovak ML, Kopecky KJ, Cassileth PA et al. Karyotypic analysis predicts outcome of preremission and postremission therapy in adult acute myeloid leukemia: a Southwest Oncology Group/Eastern Cooperative Oncology Group Study. Blood 2000; 96: 4075–83.
24 Chalandon Y, Barnett MJ, Horsman DE et al. Influence of cytogenetic abnormalities on outcome after allogeneic bone marrow transplantation for acute myeloid leukemia in first complete remission. Biol Blood Marrow Transplant 2002; 8: 435–43.
25 Grimwade D, Solomon E. Characterisation of the PML/RAR alpha rearrangement associated with t(15;17) acute promyelocytic leukaemia. Curr Top Microbiol Immunol 1997; 220: 81–112.
26 Miyoshi H, Shimizu K, Kozu T, Maseki N, Kaneko Y, Ohki M. t(8;21) breakpoints on chromosome 21 in acute myeloid leukemia are clustered within a limited region of a single gene, AML1. Proc Natl Acad Sci U S A 1991; 88: 10,431–4.
27 Erickson P, Gao J, Chang KS et al. Identification of breakpoints in t(8;21) acute myelogenous leukemia and isolation of a fusion transcript, AML1/ETO, with similarity to Drosophila segmentation gene, runt. Blood 1992; 80: 1825–31.
28 Liu P, Tarle SA, Hajra A et al. Fusion between transcription factor CBF beta/PEBP2 beta and a myosin heavy chain in acute myeloid leukemia. Science 1993; 261: 1041–4.
29 Kondo M, Horibe K, Takahashi Y et al. Prognostic value of internal tandem duplication of the FLT3 gene in childhood acute myelogenous leukemia. Med Pediatr Oncol 1999; 33: 525–9.
30 Stirewalt DL, Kopecky KJ, Meshinchi S et al. FLT3, RAS, and TP53 mutations in elderly patients with acute myeloid leukemia. Blood 2001; 97: 3589–95.
31 Thiede C, Steudel C, Mohr B et al. Analysis of FLT3-activating mutations in 979 patients with acute myelogenous leukemia: association with FAB subtypes and identification of subgroups with poor prognosis. Blood 2002; 99: 4326–35.
32 Nikolova M, Guenova M, Taskov H, Dimitrova E, Staneva M. Levels of expression of CAF7 (CD98) have prognostic significance in adult acute leukemia. Leuk Res 1998; 22: 39–47.
33 Bene MC, Bernier M, Casasnovas RO et al. Acute myeloid leukaemia M0: haematological, immunophenotypic and cytogenetic characteristics and their prognostic significance: an analysis in 241 patients. Br J Haematol 2001; 113: 737–45.
34 de Nully Brown P, Jurlander J, Pedersen-Bjergaard J, Victor MA, Geisler CH. The prognostic significance of chromosomal analysis and immunophenotyping in 117 patients with de novo acute myeloid leukemia. Leuk Res 1997; 21: 985–95.
35 Legrand O, Perrot JY, Baudard M et al. The immunophenotype of 177 adults with acute myeloid leukemia: proposal of a prognostic score. Blood 2000; 96: 870–7.
36 Tallman MS, Rowlings PA, Milone G et al. Effect of postremission chemotherapy before human leukocyte antigen-identical sibling transplantation for acute myelogenous leukemia in first complete remission. Blood 2000; 96: 1254–8.
37 Cahn JY, Labopin M, Sierra J et al. No impact of high-dose cytarabine on the outcome of patients transplanted for acute myeloblastic leukaemia in first remission. Acute Leukaemia Working Party of the European Group for Blood and Marrow Transplantation (EBMT). Br J Haematol 2000; 110: 308–14.
38 Kim TH, McGlave PB, Ramsay N et al. Comparison of two total body irradiation regimens in allogeneic bone marrow transplantation for acute non-lymphoblastic leukemia in first remission. Int J Radiation Oncol, Biology, Physics 1990; 19: 889–97.
39 Helenglass G, Powles RL, McElwain TJ et al. Melphalan and total body irradiation (TBI) versus cyclophosphamide and TBI as conditioning for allogeneic matched sibling bone marrow transplants for acute myeloblastic leukaemia in first remission. Bone Marrow Transplant 1988; 3: 21–9.
40 Clift RA, Buckner CD, Appelbaum FR et al. Allogeneic marrow transplantation in patients with acute myeloid leukemia in first remission: a randomized trial of two irradiation regimens. Blood 1990; 76: 1867–71.
41 Ringden O, Labopin M, Tura S et al. A comparison of busulphan versus total body irradiation combined with cyclophosphamide as conditioning for autograft or allograft bone marrow transplantation in patients with acute leukaemia. Acute Leukaemia Working Party of the European Group for Blood and Marrow Transplantation (EBMT). Br J Haematol 1996; 93: 637–45.
42 Ringden O, Remberger M, Ruutu T et al. Increased risk of chronic graft-versus-host disease, obstructive bronchiolitis, and alopecia with busulfan versus total body irradiation: long-term results of a randomized trial in allogeneic marrow recipients with leukemia. Nordic Bone Marrow Transplantation Group. Blood 1999; 93: 2196–201.
43 Simpson DR, Nevill TJ, Shepherd JD et al. High incidence of extramedullary relapse of AML after busulfan/cyclophosphamide conditioning and allogeneic stem cell transplantation. Bone Marrow Transplant 1998; 22: 259–64.
44 Blaise D, Maraninchi D, Archimbaud E et al. Allogeneic bone marrow transplantation for acute myeloid leukemia in first remission: a randomized trial of a busulfan–cytoxan versus cytoxan–total body irradiation as preparative regimen: a report from the Group d'Etudes de la Greffe de Moelle Osseuse. Blood 1992; 79: 2578–82.
45 Blaise D, Maraninchi D, Michallet M et al. Long-term follow-up of a randomized trial comparing the combination of cyclophosphamide with total body irradiation or busulfan as conditioning regimen for patients receiving HLA-identical marrow grafts for acute myeloblastic leukemia in first complete remission. Blood 2001; 97: 3669–71.
46 Clift RA, Buckner CD, Thomas ED et al. Marrow transplantation for chronic myeloid leukemia: a randomized study comparing cyclophosphamide and total body irradiation with busulfan and cyclophosphamide. Blood 1994; 84: 2036–43.
47 Ringden O, Ruutu T, Remberger M et al. A randomized trial comparing busulfan with total body irradiation as conditioning in allogeneic marrow transplant recipients with leukemia: a report from the Nordic Bone Marrow Transplantation Group. Blood 1994; 83: 2723–30.
48 Matthews DC, Appelbaum FR, Eary JF et al. Phase I study of ^{131}I-anti-CD45 antibody plus cyclophos-

phamide and total body irradiation for advanced acute leukemia and myelodysplastic syndrome. *Blood* 1999; **94**: 1237–47.
49 Bunjes D, Buchmann I, Duncker C et al. Rhenium 188-labeled anti-CD66 (a, b, c, e) monoclonal antibody to intensify the conditioning regimen prior to stem cell transplantation for patients with high-risk acute myeloid leukemia or myelodysplastic syndrome: results of a phase I–II study. *Blood* 2001; **98**: 565–72.
50 Schmitz N, Bacigalupo A, Hasenclever D et al. Allogeneic bone marrow transplantation vs. filgrastim-mobilised peripheral blood progenitor cell transplantation in patients with early leukaemia: first results of a randomised multicentre trial of the European Group for Blood and Marrow Transplantation. *Bone Marrow Transplant* 1998; **21**: 995–1003.
51 Bensinger WI, Martin PJ, Storer B et al. Transplantation of bone marrow as compared with peripheral-blood cells from HLA-identical relatives in patients with hematologic cancers. *N Engl J Med* 2001; **344**: 175–81.
52 Fung HC, Snyder D, Smith D et al. Allogeneic peripheral-blood cells transplantation for patients with acute leukemia in first remission. *Blood* 2001; **98**: 409a–10a [Abstract].
53 Forman SJ, Spruce WE, Farbstein MJ et al. Bone marrow ablation followed by allogeneic marrow grafting during first complete remission of acute nonlymphocytic leukemia. *Blood* 1983; **61**: 439–42.
54 Couban S, Simpson DR, Barnett MJ et al. A randomized multicenter comparison of bone marrow and peripheral blood in recipients of matched sibling allogeneic transplants for myeloid malignancies. *Blood* 2002; **100**: 1525–31.
55 Weaver CH, Clift RA, Deeg HJ et al. Effect of graft-versus-host disease prophylaxis on relapse in patients transplanted for acute myeloid leukemia. *Bone Marrow Transplant* 1994; **14**: 885–93.
56 Fagioli F, Bacigalupo A, Frassoni F et al. Allogeneic bone marrow transplantation for acute myeloid leukemia in first complete remission: the effect of FAB classification and GVHD prophylaxis. *Bone Marrow Transplant* 1994; **13**: 247–52.
57 Young JW, Papadopoulos EB, Cunningham I et al. T-cell-depleted allogeneic bone marrow transplantation in adults with acute nonlymphocytic leukemia in first remission. *Blood* 1992; **79**: 3380–7.
58 Papadopoulos E, Carabasi M, Castro-Malaspina H et al. T cell-depleted allogeneic bone marrow transplantation as post-remission therapy for acute myelogenous leukemia: freedom from relapse in the absence of graft-versus-host disease. *Blood* 1998; **91**: 1083–90.
59 Aversa F, Terenzi A, Carotti A et al. Improved outcome with T-cell-depleted bone marrow transplantation for acute leukemia. *J Clin Oncol* 1999; **17**: 1545–50.
60 Soiffer RJ, Fairclough D, Robertson M et al. CD6-depleted allogeneic bone marrow transplantation for acute leukemia in first complete remission. *Blood* 1997; **89**: 3039–47.
61 Powles RL, Watson JG, Morgenstern GR, Kay HE. Bone-marrow transplantation in leukaemia remission. *Lancet* 1982; **1**: 336–7.
62 Appelbaum FR, Dahlberg S, Thomas ED et al. Bone marrow transplantation or chemotherapy after remission induction for adults with acute non-lymphoblastic leukemia. A prospective comparison. *Ann Intern Med* 1984; **101**: 581–8.
63 Champlin RE, Ho WG, Gale RP et al. Treatment of acute myelogenous leukemia. A prospective controlled trial of bone marrow transplantation versus consolidation chemotherapy. *Ann Intern Med* 1985; **102**: 285–91.
64 Marmont A, Bacigalupo A, Van Lint MT, Frassoni F, Carella A. Bone marrow transplantation versus chemotherapy alone for acute nonlymphoblastic leukemia. *Exp Hematol Supplement* 1985; **17**: 40.
65 Appelbaum FR, Fisher LD, Thomas ED. Chemotherapy v marrow transplantation for adults with acute nonlymphocytic leukemia: a five-year follow-up. *Blood* 1988; **72**: 179–84.
66 Conde E, Iriondo A, Rayon C et al. Allogeneic bone marrow transplantation versus intensification chemotherapy for acute myelogenous leukaemia in first remission: a prospective controlled trial. *Br J Haematol* 1988; **68**: 219–26.
67 Zander AR, Keating M, Dicke K et al. A comparison of marrow transplantation with chemotherapy for adults with acute leukemia of poor prognosis in first complete remission. *J Clin Oncol* 1988; **6**: 1548–57.
68 Reiffers J, Gaspard MH, Maraninchi D et al. Comparison of allogeneic or autologous bone marrow transplantation and chemotherapy in patients with acute myeloid leukaemia in first remission: a prospective controlled trial. *Br J Haematol* 1989; **72**: 57–63.
69 Lowenberg B, Verdonck LJ, Dekker AW et al. Autologous bone marrow transplantation in acute myeloid leukemia in first remission: results of a Dutch prospective study. *J Clin Oncol* 1990; **8**: 287–94.
70 Ferrant A, Doyen C, Delannoy A et al. Allogeneic or autologous bone marrow transplantation for acute non-lymphocytic leukemia in first remission. *Bone Marrow Transplant* 1991; **7**: 303–9.
71 Cassileth PA, Lynch E, Hines JD et al. Varying intensity of postremission therapy in acute myeloid leukemia. *Blood* 1992; **79**: 1924–30.
72 Schiller GJ, Nimer SD, Territo MC, Ho WG, Champlin RE, Gajewski JL. Bone marrow transplantation versus high-dose cytarabine-based consolidation chemotherapy for acute myelogenous leukemia in first remission. *J Clin Oncol* 1992; **10**: 41–6.
73 Archimbaud E, Thomas X, Michallet M et al. Prospective genetically randomized comparison between intensive postinduction chemotherapy and bone marrow transplantation in adults with newly diagnosed acute myeloid leukemia. *J Clin Oncol* 1994; **12**: 262–7.
74 Hewlett J, Kopecky KJ, Head D et al. A prospective evaluation of the roles of allogeneic marrow transplantation and low-dose monthly maintenance chemotherapy in the treatment of adult acute myelogenous leukemia (AML): a Southwest Oncology Group study. *Leukemia* 1995; **9**: 562–9.
75 Mitus AJ, Miller KB, Schenkein DP et al. Improved survival for patients with acute myelogenous leukemia. *J Clin Oncol* 1995; **13**: 560–9.
76 Zittoun RA, Mandelli F, Willemze R et al. Autologous or allogeneic bone marrow transplantation compared with intensive chemotherapy in acute myelogenous leukemia. European Organization for Research and Treatment of Cancer (EORTC) and the Gruppo Italiano Malattie Ematologiche Maligne dell'Adulto (GIMEMA) Leukemia Cooperative Groups. *N Engl J Med* 1995; **332**: 217–23.
77 Gale RP, Büchner T, Zhang MJ et al. HLA-identical sibling bone marrow transplants vs. chemotherapy for acute myelogenous leukemia in first remission. *Leukemia* 1996; **10**: 1687–91.
78 Gorin NC, Labopin M, Fouillard L et al. Retrospective evaluation of autologous bone marrow transplantation vs. allogeneic bone marrow transplantation from an HLA identical related donor in acute myelocytic leukemia. A study of the European Cooperative Group for Blood and Marrow Transplantation (EBMT). *Bone Marrow Transplant* 1996; **18**: 111–7.
79 Harousseau JL, Cahn JY, Pignon B et al. Comparison of autologous bone marrow transplantation and intensive chemotherapy as postremission therapy in adult acute myeloid leukemia. The Groupe Ouest Est Leucemies Aigues Myeloblastiques (GOELAM). *Blood* 1997; **90**: 2978–86.
80 Cassileth P, Harrington D, Appelbaum F et al. Chemotherapy compared with autologous or allogeneic bone marrow transplantation in the management of acute myeloid leukemia in first remission. *N Engl J Med* 1998; **339**: 1649–56.
81 Buckner CD, Clift RA, Thomas ED et al. Allogeneic marrow transplantation for patients with acute non-lymphoblastic leukemia in second remission. *Leukemia Res* 1982; **6**: 395–9.
82 Buckner CD, Clift RA, Thomas ED et al. Allogeneic marrow transplantation for acute non-lymphoblastic leukemia in relapse using fractionated total body irradiation. *Leukemia Res* 1982; **6**: 389–94.
83 Clift RA, Buckner CD, Appelbaum FR et al. Allogeneic marrow transplantation during untreated first relapse of acute myeloid leukemia. *J Clin Oncol* 1992; **10**: 1723–9.
84 Brown RA, Wolff SN, Fay JW et al. High-dose etoposide, cyclophosphamide, and total body irradiation with allogeneic bone marrow transplantation for patients with acute myeloid leukemia in untreated first relapse: a study by the North American Marrow Transplant Group. *Blood* 1995; **85**: 1391–5.
85 Bortin MM, Gale RP, Kay HE, Rimm AA. Bone marrow transplantation for acute myelogenous leukemia. Factors associated with early mortality. *JAMA* 1983; **249**: 1166–75.
86 Copelan EA, Biggs JC, Thompson JM et al. Treatment for acute myelocytic leukemia with allogeneic bone marrow transplantation following preparation with BuCy2. *Blood* 1991; **78**: 838–43.
87 Tomas F, Gomez-Garcia de Soria V, Lopez-Lorenzo JL et al. Autologous or allogeneic bone marrow transplantation for acute myeloblastic leukemia in second complete remission. Importance of duration of first complete remission in final outcome. *Bone Marrow Transplant* 1996; **17**: 979–84.
88 Gale RP, Horowitz MM, Rees JK et al. Chemotherapy versus transplants for acute myelogenous leukemia in second remission. *Leukemia* 1996; **10**: 13–9.
89 Keating A, Rowlings PA, Zhang MJ, Horowitz MM, Klein JP. Autologous versus HLA-identical sibling bone marrow transplantation for acute myelogenous leukemia (AML). *Proc Am Soc Clin Oncology* 1995; **14**: 965 [Abstract].
90 Spruce WE, Forman SJ, Krance RA et al. Outcome of bone marrow transplantation in patients with extramedullary involvement of acute leukemia. *Blut* 1983; **48**: 75–9.
91 Michel G, Boulad F, Small TN et al. Risk of extramedullary relapse following allogeneic bone marrow transplantation for acute myelogenous

91 leukemia with leukemia cutis. *Bone Marrow Transplant* 1997; **20**: 107–12.
92 Zander AR, Dicke KA, Keating M et al. Allogeneic bone marrow transplantation for acute leukemia refractory to induction chemotherapy. *Cancer* 1985; **56**: 1374–9.
93 Forman SJ, Schmidt GM, Nademanee AP et al. Allogeneic bone marrow transplantation as therapy for primary induction failure for patients with acute leukemia. *J Clin Oncol* 1991; **9**: 1570–4.
94 Biggs JC, Horowitz MM, Gale RP et al. Bone marrow transplants may cure patients with acute leukemia never achieving remission with chemotherapy. *Blood* 1992; **80**: 1090–3.
95 Fung HC, O'Donnell M, Popplewell L et al. Allogeneic stem cell transplantation (SCT) for patients with primary refractory acute myelogenous leukemia (AML): impact of cytogenetic risk group on the transplant outcome. *Blood* 2001; **98**: 483a [Abstract].
96 Santos GW, Tutschka PJ, Brookmeyer R et al. Marrow transplantation for acute nonlymphocytic leukemia after treatment with busulfan and cyclophosphamide. *N Engl J Med* 1983; **309**: 1347–53.
97 Clift RA, Buckner CD, Thomas ED et al. The treatment of acute non-lymphoblastic leukemia by allogeneic marrow transplantation. *Bone Marrow Transplant* 1987; **2**: 243–58.
98 Linker CA, Ries CA, Damon LE et al. Autologous stem cell transplantation for acute myeloid leukemia in first remission. *Biol Blood Marrow Transplant* 2000; **6**: 50–7.
99 Linker CA, Damon LE, Ries CA, Navarro WA, Case D, Wolf JL. Autologous stem cell transplantation for advanced acute myeloid leukemia. *Bone Marrow Transplant* 2002; **29**: 297–301.
100 Clift RA, Hansen JA, Thomas ED et al. Marrow transplantation from donors other than HLA-identical siblings. *Transplantation* 1979; **28**: 235–42.
101 Powles RL, Morgenstern GR, Kay HE et al. Mismatched family donors for bone-marrow transplantation as treatment for acute leukaemia. *Lancet* 1983; **1**: 612–5.
102 Beatty PG, Clift RA, Mickelson EM et al. Marrow transplantation from related donors other than HLA-identical siblings. *N Engl J Med* 1985; **313**: 765–71.
103 Aversa F, Tabilio A, Terenzi A et al. Successful engraftment of T-cell-depleted haploidentical "three-loci" incompatible transplants in leukemia patients by addition of recombinant human granulocyte colony-stimulating factor-mobilized peripheral blood progenitor cells to bone marrow inoculum. *Blood* 1994; **84**: 3948–55.
104 Munn RK, Henslee-Downey PJ, Romond EH et al. Treatment of leukemia with partially matched related bone marrow transplantation. *Bone Marrow Transplant* 1997; **19**: 421–7.
105 Soiffer RJ, Mauch P, Fairclough D et al. CD6+ T cell depleted allogeneic bone marrow transplantation from genotypically HLA nonidentical related donors. *Biol Blood Marrow Transplant* 1997; **3**: 11–7.
106 O'Reilly RJ, Dupont B, Pahwa S et al. Reconstitution in severe combined immunodeficiency by transplantation of marrow from an unrelated donor. *N Engl J Med* 1977; **297**: 1311–8.
107 Hansen JA, Clift RA, Thomas ED, Buckner CD, Storb R, Giblett ER. Transplantation of marrow from an unrelated donor to a patient with acute leukemia. *N Engl J Med* 1980; **303**: 565–7.
108 McCullogh J, Hansen J, Perkins H, Stroncek D, Bartsch G. Establishment of the National Bone Marrow Donor Registry. In: Gale RP, Champlin R, eds. *Bone Marrow Transplantation: Current Controversies*. New York: Alan R. Liss, 1989: 641–58.
109 Kernan NA, Bartsch G, Ash RC et al. Analysis of 462 transplantations from unrelated donors facilitated by the National Marrow Donor Program. *N Engl J Med* 1993; **328**: 593–602.
110 Schiller G, Feig SA, Territo M et al. Treatment of advanced acute leukaemia with allogeneic bone marrow transplantation from unrelated donors. *Br J Haematol* 1994; **88**: 72–8.
111 Sierra J, Storer B, Hansen JA et al. Unrelated donor marrow transplantation for acute myeloid leukemia: an update of the Seattle experience. *Bone Marrow Transplant* 2000; **26**: 397–404.
112 Rubinstein P, Carrier C, Scaradavou A et al. Outcomes among 562 recipients of placental-blood transplants from unrelated donors. *N Engl J Med* 1998; **339**: 1565–77.
113 Laughlin MJ, Barker J, Bambach B et al. Hematopoietic engraftment and survival in adult recipients of umbilical-cord blood from unrelated donors. *N Engl J Med* 2001; **344**: 1815–22.
114 Aversa F, Tabilio A, Velardi A et al. Treatment of high-risk acute leukemia with T-cell-depleted stem cells from related donors with one fully mismatched HLA haplotype. *N Engl J Med* 1998; **339**: 1186–93.
115 Ruggeri L, Capanni M, Urbani E et al. Effectiveness of donor natural killer cell alloreactivity in mismatched hematopoietic transplants. *Science* 2002; **295**: 2097–100.
116 Branch DR, Gallagher MT, Forman SJ, Winkler KJ, Petz LD, Blume KG. Endogenous stem cell repopulation resulting in mixed hematopoietic chimerism following total body irradiation and marrow transplantation for acute leukemia. *Transplantation* 1982; **34**: 226–8.
117 Hill RS, Petersen FB, Storb R et al. Mixed hematologic chimerism after allogeneic marrow transplantation for severe aplastic anemia is associated with a higher risk of graft rejection and a lessened incidence of acute graft-versus-host disease. *Blood* 1986; **67**: 811–6.
118 Petz LD, Yam P, Wallace RB et al. Mixed hematopoietic chimerism following bone marrow transplantation for hematologic malignancies. *Blood* 1987; **70**: 1331–7.
119 McSweeney PA, Storb R. Mixed chimerism. Preclinical studies and clinical applications. *Biol Blood Marrow Transplant* 1999; **5**: 192–203.
120 McSweeney PA, Niederwieser D, Shizuru JA et al. Hematopoietic cell transplantation in older patients with hematologic malignancies: replacing high-dose cytotoxic therapy with graft-versus-tumor effects. *Blood* 2001; **97**: 3390–400.
121 Feinstein LC, Sandmaier BM, Hegenbart U et al. Nonmyeloablative allografting from HLA-identical sibling donors for treatment of acute myeloid leukemia in first complete remission. *Br J Haematol* 2002; **120**: 281–8.
122 Hegenbart U, Sandmaier B, Lange T et al. Followup of allogeneic hematopoietic stem cell transplants (HSCT) from related and unrelated donors following minimal conditioning in patients with acute myelocytic leukemia (AML). *Blood* 2002; **11**: 769a [Abstract].
123 Giralt S, Estey E, Albitar M et al. Engraftment of allogeneic hematopoietic progenitor cells with purine analog-containing chemotherapy: harnessing graft-versus-leukemia without myeloablative therapy. *Blood* 1997; **89**: 4531–6.
124 Slavin S, Nagler A, Naparstek E et al. Nonmyeloablative stem cell transplantation and cell therapy as an alternative to conventional bone marrow transplantation with lethal cytoreduction for the treatment of malignant and nonmalignant hematologic diseases. *Blood* 1998; **91**: 756–63.
125 Mortimer J, Blinder MA, Schulman S et al. Relapse of acute leukemia after marrow transplantation: natural history and results of subsequent therapy. *J Clin Oncol* 1989; **7**: 50–7.
126 Wright SE, Thomas ED, Buckner CD et al. Experience with second marrow transplants. *Exp Hematol* 1976; **4**: 221–6.
127 Barrett AJ, Helenglass G, Treleaven J, Gratwohl A. Second transplants in leukaemia: The EBMT experience. *Bone Marrow Tranplant* 1989; **4** (Suppl. 2): 11a [Abstract].
128 Mrsic M, Horowitz MM, Atkinson K et al. Second HLA-identical sibling transplants for leukemia recurrence. *Bone Marrow Transplant* 1992; **9**: 269–75.
129 Higano CS, Brixey M, Bryant EM et al. Durable complete remission of acute nonlymphocytic leukemia associated with discontinuation of immunosuppression following relapse after allogeneic bone marrow transplantation. A case report of a probable graft-versus-leukemia effect. *Transplantation* 1990; **50**: 175–7.
130 Elmaagacli AH, Beelen DW, Trenn G, Schmidt O, Nahler M, Schaefer UW. Induction of a graft-versus-leukemia reaction by cyclosporin A withdrawal as immunotherapy for leukemia relapsing after allogeneic bone marrow transplantation. *Bone Marrow Transplant* 1999; **23**: 771–7.
131 Szer J, Grigg AP, Phillips GL, Sheridan WP. Donor leucocyte infusions after chemotherapy for patients relapsing with acute leukaemia following allogeneic BMT. *Bone Marrow Transplant* 1993; **11**: 109–11.
132 Kolb HJ, Schattenberg A, Goldman JM et al. Graft-versus-leukemia effect of donor lymphocyte transfusions in marrow grafted patients. European Group for Blood and Marrow Transplantation Working Party for Chronic Leukemia. *Blood* 1995; **86**: 2041–50.
133 Levine JE, Braun T, Penza SL et al. Prospective trial of chemotherapy and donor leukocyte infusions for relapse of advanced myeloid malignancies after allogeneic stem-cell transplantation. *J Clin Oncol* 2002; **20**: 405–12.
134 Mackinnon S, Papadopoulos EB, Carabasi MH et al. Adoptive immunotherapy evaluating escalating doses of donor leukocytes for relapse of chronic myeloid leukemia after bone marrow transplantation: separation of graft-versus-leukemia responses from graft-versus-host disease. *Blood* 1995; **86**: 1261–8.
135 Slavin S, Naparstek E, Nagler A, Ackerstein A, Kapelushnik J, Or R. Allogeneic cell therapy for relapsed leukemia after bone marrow transplantation with donor peripheral blood lymphocytes. *Exp Hematol* 1995; **23**: 1553–62.
136 Ringden O, Labopin M, Frassoni F et al. Allogeneic bone marrow transplant or second autograft in patients with acute leukemia who relapse after an autograft. Acute Leukaemia Working Party of the European Group for Blood and Marrow

Transplantation (EBMT). *Bone Marrow Transplant* 1999; **24**: 389–96.
137 Radich JP, Gooley T, Sanders JE, Anasetti C, Chauncey T, Appelbaum FR. Second allogeneic transplantation after failure of first autologous transplantation. *Biol Blood Marrow Transplant* 2000; **6**: 272–9.
138 Godder KT, Metha J, Chiang KY *et al.* Partially mismatched related donor bone marrow transplantation as salvage for patients with AML who failed autologous stem cell transplant. *Bone Marrow Transplant* 2001; **28**: 1031–6.
139 Feinstein LC, Sandmaier BM, Maloney DG *et al.* Nonmyeloablative allografting as a treatment following a failed conventional hematopoietic stem cell transplant. *Br J Haematol* 2002. In press.
140 Gale RP, Park RE, Dubois RW *et al.* Delphi-panel analysis of appropriateness of high-dose therapy and bone marrow transplants in adults with acute myelogenous leukemia in first remission. *Leuk Res* 1999; **23**: 709–18.
141 Flowers ME, Parker PM, Johnston LJ *et al.* Comparison of chronic graft-versus-host disease after transplantation of peripheral blood stem cells versus bone marrow in allogeneic recipients: long-term follow-up of a randomized trial. *Blood* 2002; **100**: 415–9.
142 Schmitz N, Beksac M, Hasenclever D *et al.* Transplantation of mobilized peripheral blood cells to HLA-identical siblings with standard-risk leukemia. *Blood* 2002; **100**: 761–7.
143 Freireich EJ. Can we afford to treat acute leukemia? *N Engl J Med* 1980; **302**: 1084–5.

76

David A. Margolis & James T. Casper

Allogeneic Transplantation for Acute Myeloid Leukaemia in Children

Introduction

Acute myeloid leukemia (AML) is the most common type of myeloid malignancy of childhood. The annual incidence of AML in the USA is approximately 6/1,000,000 and it accounts for 15–20% of leukemias in individuals under the age of 20 years [1]. The incidence of childhood AML varies with age, with the highest rates in the first 2 years of life followed by a slow decline to a nadir at the age of 9 years and slowly increasing rates during the adolescent years [2]. In the USA, the incidence of AML is similar in white and black children for all age groups.

AML is a clonal disorder due to an acquired somatic mutation in a hematopoietic progenitor cell. It is a heterogenous disease showing variability in the degree of commitment and differentiation of the cell lineage involved [3]. While the exact cause of AML has not been elucidated, a number of risk factors may predispose a child to the development of AML. Known risk factors include genetic predispositions as well as environmental factors. Down syndrome, Fanconi anemia, Shwachman syndrome, Kostmann granulocytopenia and neurofibromatosis are examples of genetic conditions associated with a known increased risk of AML [2]. More recently, a familial AML syndrome with monosomy 7 has been reported [4]. Also, patients with severe aplastic anemia treated with granulocyte colony-stimulating factor (G-CSF) for a prolonged period of time may be at risk for development of AML [5]. Exposure to specific chemotherapy agents, such as alkylating agents or epidodophyllotoxins, has been associated with an increased risk of childhood AML [2]. Parental exposure to benzene and to pesticides and maternal alcohol consumption are factors for which causal evidence is suggestive but not conclusive [2].

The French–American–British (FAB) Cooperative Group has developed the most comprehensive morphologic-histochemical classification system for AML. This classification system categorizes AML into subtypes called M0–M7 [6–9]. M0 does not show localized differentiation, M1–M3 are more myeloid in nature, M4 and M5 myelomonocytic-monocytic, M6 erythroid and M7 megakaryocytic. Fifty to sixty percent of children with AML can be classified as having M1, M2, M3, M6, or M7 subtypes; approximately 40% have M4 or M5 subtypes [10]. The distribution between the groups is similar between adults and children except for M5, which may be increased in infants, and M6, which rarely occurs in children [11]. Cell surface phenotype analysis is also employed and at least one of the myeloid markers (CD33, CD13, CD15, CD11b, CD14, CD36, CD117) is seen in the vast majority of cases [12,13]. Type M7 (megakaryocytic) is classified based on its expression of the platelet glycoprotein antigens IIb/IIIa or Ib [14].

More recently, and with increasingly recognized prognostic significance, the cytogenetic systems have been utilized based on the clonal chromosomal abnormality observed [3]. Conventional chromosome studies performed by skilled personnel can identify nonrandom clonal aberration in at least 60–80% of patients with AML [15]. Multiple studies and groups of investigators have verified the link between cytogenetic classification and prognosis for childhood AML [16–19]. In summary, these studies find that t(15;17) patients have an excellent prognosis while patients with t(8;21) and inversion of chromosome 16 (inv16) are notable in that they have a better than average prognosis. On the other hand, AML with deletions of chromosome 5 or 7 are associated with a poor prognosis.

Further molecular characterization has shown that those children whose AML blasts have an internal tandem repeat of a tyrosine kinase gene (*FLT3/ITD*) have a significantly worse prognosis [20]. The World Health Organization (WHO) has proposed a new classification system linking the previous morphologic determinants with the biologic and genetic information to define a nomenclature with clinical relevance [21]. Gene expression profiling is rapidly becoming another method to subclassify AML [22]. Clearly, the classification of AML and prognostic characteristics continues to be a work in progress.

The clinical presentation of the child with AML varies, but it usually includes pallor, infection and bruising, reflecting production problems of the normal hematopoietic cells. Severe hemorrhagic problems can be seen in patients with the promyelocytic (M3) type of disease. Infiltration of the skin is often seen in neonates with monocytic (M5) leukemia. The white blood cell count (WBC) is >100,000/mL in about a quarter of the patients and is a negative prognostic factor.

Historical background

The goal of treating the child who presents with AML is to attain a complete remission (CR) and cure while maintaining a reasonable quality of life. Over the past 25 years, survival rates for children with AML have remained lower than those for children with acute lymphoblastic leukemia (ALL), but these rates continue to improve [2]. Initial attempts at alleviating AML in children were chemotherapy based and are summarized in Table 76.1 [23–32]. An important observation is the improvement in survival outcome for children treated with highly intensive chemotherapy regimens [31,33].

Because of the poor results obtained with chemotherapy in the 1970s, other treatment options were pursued. It was during this time that E.D. Thomas and his colleagues in Seattle demonstrated the curative effect of bone marrow transplantation (BMT) in a small number of patients with refractory leukemia [34]. As the remission induction chemotherapy regimens for childhood AML improved, investigators applied BMT to children and young adults with AML who achieved a remission and had a matched sibling donor. In the early 1980s, BMT groups in Seattle, Minneapolis and Baltimore reported disease-free survival (DFS) of

Table 76.1 Chemotherapy trials for childhood acute myeloid leukemia (AML) reported from large multi-institutional studies. Reproduced with permission from Lie et al. [30].

	CCG 251	CCG 213	POG 8498	CCG 2861	AIEOP	BFM 83	BFM 87	NOPHO 84	NOPHO 88	MRC 10	CCG 2891
Year of report	1994	1994	1991	1993	1993	1990	1993	1996	1996	1998	1996
Ref.	23	24	25	26	27	28	29	30	30	31	32
Years entered	1979–83	1986–89	1984–88	1986–89	1987–90	1985–86	1986–91	1984–88	1988–92	1989–95	1989–93
No. evaluable	490	591	285	142	161	173	210	105	118	341	589
Death in aplasia (%)	10	6	7	13	7	7	5	8	12	5	7
Resistant disease (%)	12	15	8	11	14	13	17	14	3	4	18
CR (%)	78	77	85	76	79	80	78	78	85	91	74
pDFS (%)	40	39	45	40	31	61	52	43	56	51	46

AIEOP, Associazione Italiano Emotologia ed Oncologia Pediatricia; BFM, Berlin–Frankfurt–Münster; CCG, Children's Cancer Group; CR, complete remission; MRC, Medical Research Council; NOPHO, Nordic Society of Pediatric Hematology Oncology; pDFS, probability of disease-free survival; POG, Pediatric Oncology Group.

approximately 65% for children with AML in first complete remission (CR1) [35–37]. Figure 76.1 illustrates the DFS and incidence of relapse for 38 children with AML in CR1 who received a BMT from human leukocyte antigen (HLA)-matched sibling donors in Seattle [35]. The conditioning regimen consisted of fractionated total body irradiation (TBI) to a dose of 1200 cGy and cyclophosphamide (CY) 60 mg/kg/day × 2. Methotrexate (MTX) was used for graft-vs.-host disease (GVHD) prophylaxis. This regimen, with the addition of cyclosporine (CSP) and the use of only four doses of MTX, remains a standard treatment regimen more than 20 years later. The success of BMT contrasted with DFS rates of <50% for patients treated with conventional chemotherapy during this same time period [38–43]. For this reason, many groups incorporated BMT into their AML treatment strategies if an HLA-matched sibling was available. Similar results were reported during the 1980s (Table 76.2) [35,44–48]. Relapse rates post-BMT ranged from 0% to 30%. Only one study reported a DFS <50%. The conditioning regimen used most often was similar to the Seattle TBI/CY regimen described above. GVHD prophylaxis usually consisted of MTX and CSP, alone or in combination. In all these studies, BMT appeared to be superior to chemotherapy for the treatment of childhood AML. However, one must be cautious when interpreting these results. Most of these studies were not prospectively designed and, as a result, allowed for selection bias of patients. For example, some patients with a matched sibling donor may have been excluded from transplant because of therapy-related toxicity or early relapse. More recent data are based on large, and in most cases, prospective multi-institutional trials. These late trials have demonstrated DFS >70% in most studies (Tables 76.3 [23,24,33,48–51] and 76.4 [27,31,52–57]. Because of advances in standard treatment regimens, hematopoietic

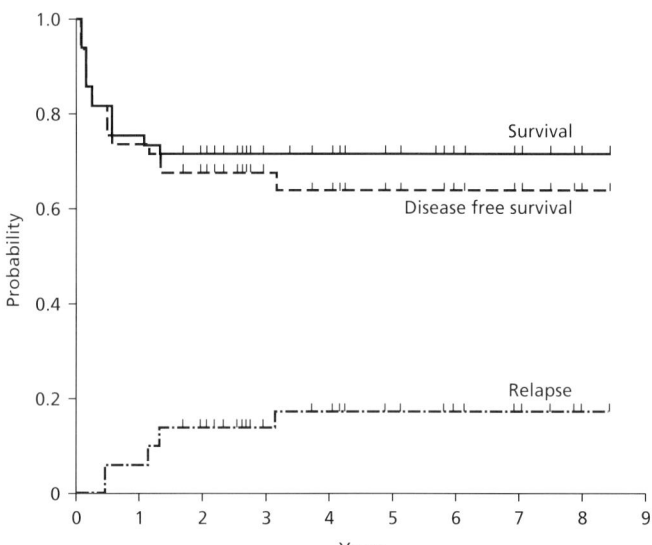

Fig. 76.1 Kaplan–Meier product limit estimates for probability of survival (——), disease-free survival (DFS) (– – –) and relapse (- · · · -) of children who received transplants for acute myeloid leukemia (AML) in first remission. The tick marks indicate living patients. Reproduced with permission from Sanders et al. [35].

Table 76.2 Single institution reports of matched sibling allogeneic bone marrow transplantation (BMT) for children with acute myeloid leukemia (AML) in first complete remission (CR1).

Center (year)	No. of patients	Conditioning	GVHD prophylaxis	DFS (%)	Relapse (%)	Ref.
Seattle (1985)	38	CY/TBI	MTX or CSP	64	13	35
Sloan Kettering (1987)	24	CY/TBI	MTX	66	0	44
Minnesota (1988)	41	CY/TBI	MTX ± ATG	61	15	45
City of Hope (1987)	20	CY/TBI ± ARA-C	PSE + MTX or CSP	56	30	46
Sweden (1989)	11	CY/TBI	MTX	100	0	47
St Jude (1990)	19	CY/TBI	MTX or CSP	43	26	48

ARA-C, cytosine arabinoside; ATG, antithymocyte globulin; CSP, cyclosporine; CY, cyclophosphamide (60 mg/kg/day × 2); DFS, disease-free survival; GVHD, graft-vs.-host disease; MTX, methotrexate; PSE, prednisone: TBI, total body irradiation (720–1320 cGy).

Table 76.3 Prospective comparisons of allogeneic bone marrow transplantation (BMT) vs. chemotherapy and/or autologous BMT in children with newly diagnosed acute myeloid leukemia (AML). Reproduced with permission from Chen et al. [72].

Study	Design***	Age (yrs)	n* Allo	n* Auto	n* Chemo	DFS or EFS Allo	DFS or EFS Auto	DFS or EFS Chemo	F/u†	p‡	OS Allo	OS Auto	OS Chemo	F/u§	p‡	Ref.
CCG 251 (1994)	P/I	0–21	79/89		242/252	45		33	5 D	0.05	50		36	5	0.04	23
AML 80 (1990)	P/I	0–19	15/19		42	43		31	6 D	0.33						48
CCG 213 (1994)	P/I	0–21	83/113		297	46 + 10		38 + 6	5 D	0.06	52 + 10		46 + 10	5	0.13	24
ANZC CSG (1992)	P/C	0–15	15	42	15	86 + 13	58 + 9		13 B							50
RAHC ANZ CCSG (1994)	P¶/C	0–15	11/13	23/24		81	57		3 B							51
POG 8821 (1996)	PR/I	0–20	89	71/115	113/117	52 + 8	38 + 6	36 + 6	3 E	0.01** 0.06	~62	40 + 6	44 + 6	3	0.77** 0.15	49
CCG 2891 (2001)	PR/I	0–20	164/181	137/177	171/179	55 + 9	42 + 8	47 + 8	8 D	0.001** 0.01	60 + 9	48 + 8	53 + 8	8	0.002** 0.05	33

*Numerator is the number treated as allocated and denominator is the number of patients allocated to the arm.
†Years follow-up.
‡p-value for allo versus chemo, except as noted.
§Years of follow-up from end of induction.
¶Retrospectively defined subset for analysis from prospectively designed study.
**Allo vs. auto.
***Prospectively assigned to BMT if matched sibling available.
A, analysis as treated; ANZC CSG, Australia and New Zealand Childhood Cancer Study Group; C, analysis restricted to patients treated correctly as assigned; B, event-free survival from BMT; CCG, Children's Cancer Group; D, disease-free survival from end of induction; E, event-free survival from diagnosis; I, intent-to-treat analysis; POG, Pediatric Oncology Group; R, randomized consolidation arms; RAHC, Royal Alexandra Hospital for Children.

cell source (cord blood and peripheral blood) and prognostication, the questions at this time are who should receive an HLA-matched sibling hematopoietic cell transplantation (HCT) during CR1 and what is the role and timing of alternative donor transplants?

Determining the appropriateness of any medical treatment rests in answering the pertinent question: what are the risks and benefits of the treatment proposed compared to other treatments? With that in mind, the purpose of this chapter is to evaluate the current role for HCT in caring for the child with AML. The following questions will be addressed. (i) What is the role and timing of matched sibling HCT? (ii) What is the role for alternative donor HCT? (iii) How does one treat the child who has relapsed after a HCT? (iv) What are the long-term consequences related to HCT? By evaluating the data and answering these questions, an algorithm to help in the decision process can be constructed. Figure 76.2 is a proposed algorithm outlining our approach to the treatment of childhood AML. This chapter presents the data addressing the above questions and concludes with the rationale behind the algorithm illustrated.

Treatment options for newly diagnosed patients

HCT vs. chemotherapy

The treatment of choice for the child with AML after attaining a first remission has been the central question in a number of multi- and single institution studies as well as analyses by the International Bone Marrow Transplant Registry (IBMTR) and the National Marrow Donor Program (NMDP) over the past 20 years [23,24,27,30,33,49,51,55,58–63]. Treatment options include allogeneic HCT using an HLA-matched sibling, intensive chemotherapy with or without a maintenance phase, or autologous HCT with or without purging of the marrow inoculum. However, there is a growing body of data which looks at the use of alternative donor transplants—specifically unrelated donor marrow and unrelated cord blood grafts. For pediatric patients, many institutions consider a well matched unrelated donor equivalent to a matched sibling [64–68]. The role of an alternative donor transplant in a pediatric patient with AML will be addressed in Alternative donor HCT for AML (p. 1046).

Because only about 30% of children have an HLA-matched sibling, studies that have compared allogeneic-matched sibling HCT to other treatments often have used the presence or absence of an HLA-matched sibling as a basis for "biologic randomization." Thus, if an HLA-matched sibling were available, the patient would not be randomized but would undergo HCT. The remaining patients would be treated using a different plan with survival and relapse rates compared between the HCT group and other treatment modalities.

Tables 76.3 and 76.4 summarize the European, North American and Australian studies that have been conducted using the concept of "biologic randomization" over the past 15 years. Since various induction and conditioning regimens were used, direct comparisons of the outcomes between studies are difficult. For example, the induction regimen used in most of the studies was daunomycin, cytosine arabinoside and thioguanine,

Table 76.4 Results according to post-remission treatment: the European experience. Reproduced with permission from Creutzig and Reinhardt [154].

Study group (year)	Treatment given	n	Percent of total CR group	Relapse n	Relapse %	TRM n	TRM %	pDFS (SE) %	Ref.
AIEOP/LAM 87 (1993)	Allo MRD SCT	24	19	9	38	0	0	51 + 13	27
n = 161	Auto SCT	35	29	25	71	1	3	21 + 8	
	Chth	37	27	22	59	3	8	27 + 8	
	Nonrandomized	31	24	11	35	5	16	34 + 10	
AML-BFM 93 (2001)	Allo MRD	31	8	8	26	3	10	65 + 9	52 & 53
n = 471	Other SCT*	17	4	6		4			
	Chth	339	88	112	33	13	4	61 + 3	
EORTC (1996)	Allo MRD SCT	13	15					n.g.	54
n = 108	Auto SCT	2	2					n.g.	
	Chth	69	82					(52% total group)	
MRC AML 10 (1998)	Allo MRD SCT	61	19			8	13	70 (donor)	31
n = 341	Allo MUD SCT	4				2			
	Auto SCT	60	19			1	2	68	
	Stop Chth (randomized)	50	16			4		46	
	No SCT (nonrandomized)†	144	46						
LAME (1996)	Allo MRD SCT	33	22			1	3	72 + 15 (71 + 15)	55
n = 171	Chth	116	78			8	8	48 + 10 (55 + 10)	
NOPHO 93 (2001)	Allo MRD SCT	24	19			4	14	79 + 8	56
n = 127‡	Allo MUD SCT	4	3						
	Auto SCT	15	12					60 + 13	
	Chth	73	57			1		47 + 7	
Spain (1998)	Allo MRD SCT (incl. 2 PR)	16	31			2		81 + 13	57
n = 51	Auto SCT	31	69			0		80 + 12	

*Other SCT: MUD (n = 7), haploidentical SCT (n = 4), auto-SCT (n = 6).
†One hundred and forty-four patients not eligible for randomization because of TRM (n = 19); early relapse, elected by parents/clinicians (n = 127).
‡Down syndrome excluded.
AIEOP, Associazione Italiano Emotologia ed Oncologia Pediatricia; allo, allogeneic; AML, acute myeloid leukemia; auto, autologous; BFM, Berlin–Frankfurt–Münster; Chth, chemotherapy; CR, complete remission; EORTC, European Organization for Research and Treatment of Cancer; LAM, leukaemia acute mieloide; LAME, French Cooperative AML Group; MRD, matched related donor; MUD, matched unrelated donor; n.g., not given; NOPHO, Nordic Society of Pediatric Hematology Oncology; pDFS, probability of disease-free survival; PR, partial remission; SCT, stem cell transplantation; SE, standard error; TRM, treatment-related mortality.

but this was not uniform. As demonstrated by study CCG 2891 from the Children's Cancer Group, post-remission outcomes are influenced by the therapy utilized to induce remission [32]. The CCG 2891 study found superior outcomes in patients who received intensive timed induction therapy irrespective of the post-remission therapy to which they were allocated. The authors of this study point out that without controlling for the type of induction therapy, results of various studies are difficult to compare.

As detailed in Tables 76.3 and 76.4, patients were enrolled into various treatment arms, including allogeneic HCT, autologous HCT and intensive chemotherapy [27,30,31,33,49]. Each of these studies were collaborative group studies, providing larger numbers of patients than single institution studies. Despite the use of different treatments and randomization strategies, examining the outcomes in these studies provides clues as to how to approach the child with AML in CR1. In none of these trials did autologous BMT show significantly improved survival over intensive post-remission chemotherapy alone. Figure 76.3 illustrates the CCG 2891 data, which led the authors to conclude that allogeneic BMT in CR1 is the treatment of choice for children with a matched sibling donor [33]. Their conclusion has fueled debate over this issue [69–71]. One reason for this debate is that as outcomes with intensive chemotherapy improve, one can ask whether children should be exposed to the potential morbidity associated with allogeneic HCT. As seen in Fig. 76.4, improving outcome for the nontransplant modality diminishes the survival advantage for children who have a matched sibling donor available [71]. With the improving ability to predict outcome by incorporating cytogenetic data, current studies, especially in Europe, should help resolve whether transplantation should be recommended only in CR1 for patients with high-risk biologic features [69]. There is also the argument that patients who fail chemotherapy could be successfully transplanted in relapse or in second complete remission (CR2). Using this "salvage" approach a group of patients would not be exposed to transplant-related mortality (TRM) and

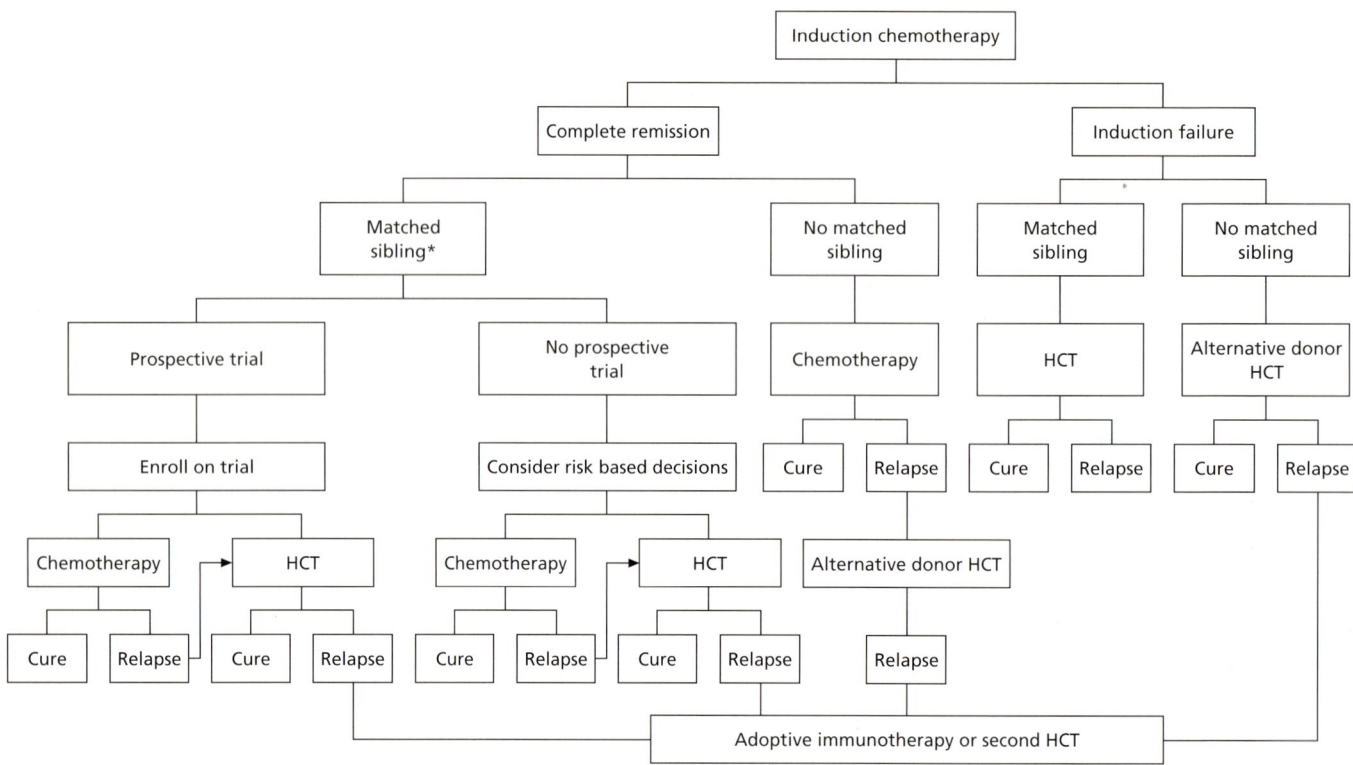

*Patients with t(15;17) or Down Syndrome would be treated with conventional therapy

Fig. 76.2 An algorithm for the management of the child with acute myeloid leukemia (AML).

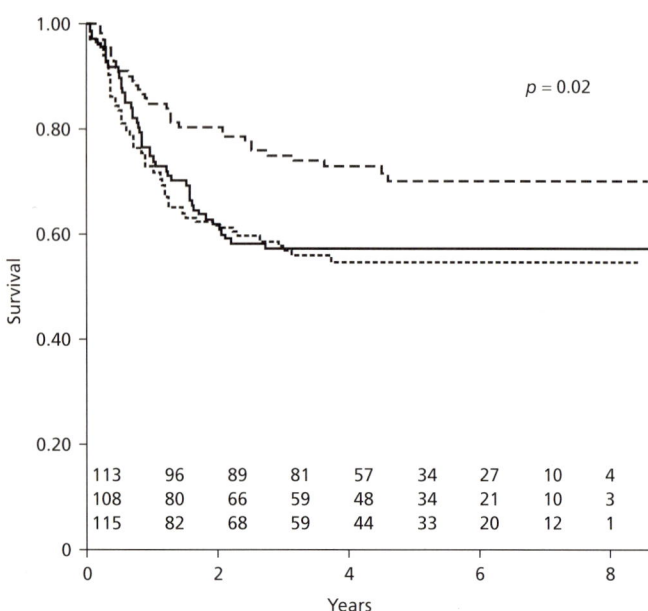

Fig. 76.3 Actuarial survival from acute myeloid leukemia (AML) remission for the CCG 2891 patients who received intensive-timing induction therapy, comparing the three post-remission regimens. Numbers are patients at risk at yearly intervals; rows are in the same order as the curves. *p*-value is for homogeneity. – – – indicates allogeneic bone marrow transplantation (BMT); ——— intensive nonmarrow-ablative chemotherapy; ······· autologous BMT. Reproduced with permission from Woods *et al*. [33].

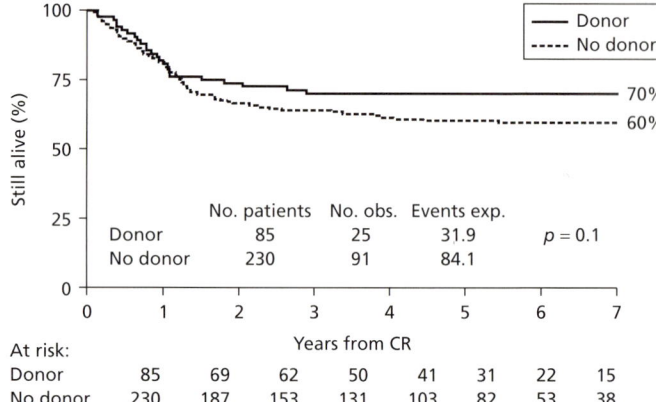

Fig. 76.4 Survival from complete remission (CR) by tissue typing status in the Medical Research Council (MRC) 10 trial. ——— indicates patients with matched sibling donors; – – – indicates patients without matched sibling donors. Obs. is the observed number of deaths in each arm and Exp. is the expected number (from log-rank analysis). Reproduced with permission from Stevens *et al*. [31].

Role of the preparatory regimen

The preparatory regimen is but one aspect of the overall "transplant package" which also includes the type of hematopoietic cell graft (related, unrelated, matched, unmatched) and nature of GVHD prophylaxis. The choice of a preparatory regimen must take into account antileukemic efficacy as well as the risks of rejection, end-organ damage and late effects. The effect that a preparatory regimen has on the outcome of an allogeneic transplant performed during CR1 may be significant. Most myeloablative conditioning regimens used for AML have consisted either of chemotherapy-based busulfan and cyclophosphamide (BU/CY) regimens or TBI with one or more chemotherapeutic agents [65,73].

harmful late effects. However, Chen *et al*. [72] conclude that overall survival is superior among those assigned to allogeneic HCT in first remission, even after accounting for successful HCT after chemotherapy failure.

Table 76.5 Probability of relapse, transplant-related mortality (TRM) and event-free survival (EFS) according to conditioning regimen. Reproduced with permission from Michel et al. [59].

Regimen	Relapse	TRM	EFS
BU/CY 120	54% ± 24%	0% ± 11%	46% ± 24%
BU/CY 200	13% ± 17%	5% ± 11%	82% ± 18%
TBI	10% ± 11%	10% ± 11%	80% ± 14%

Data are Kaplan–Meier estimates. In the multivariate analysis, BU/CY 120 was associated with a significantly higher relapse risk ($p = 0.02$) and with a statistical trend for lower EFS ($p = 0.07$).
BU, busulfan; CY, cyclophosphamide; TBI, total body irradiation.

Historically, the use of BU in children has been considered problematic because of the difficulty in having young children reliably ingest and retain BU pills as well as the variable metabolism of BU in young children [74]. The emergence of BU pharmacokinetics and intravenous BU holds promise for overcoming inconsistent oral BU dosing. By combining test doses of BU (0.5 mg/kg) with follow-up pharmacokinetic sampling, two groups of investigators have reported dose adjustment of oral BU leading to individualized BU dosing with improved engraftment rates and decreased risk of veno-occlusive disease (VOD) [75–77]. Intravenous BU may be advantageous for a number of reasons. First, there is no need to rely on the compliance of the child to ingest the pills. Also, if the child has an emesis shortly afterwards, it is often difficult to assess how, or if, the oral dose should be repeated. Second, intravenous BU is noted to have higher intrapatient pharmacokinetic consistency when compared to oral BU. It also may be possible to give intravenous BU as a single daily dose, allowing for outpatient treatment [78]. Thus, the combination of intravenous BU and individualized pharmacokinetic dose adjustments may permit maximum drug delivery without excessive toxicity [79].

Michel et al. [59] tried to address the issue of the preparatory regimen in an analysis of children reported to the French registry who received either BU/CY 120, BU/CY 200, or a TBI containing regimen. Except for the BU/CY 200 group, which had a mean WBC that was higher than that of the TBI group, the patient characteristics, including age, were not statistically different. The outcomes with regard to relapse, TRM and event-free survival (EFS) are summarized in Table 76.5. These data suggest that patients treated with a more intense conditioning regimen had better EFS with only a slight increase in TRM. However, one must be careful in evaluating this study in view of the small number of patients in each treatment arm, its retrospective nature and the lack of BU kinetics.

TBI has proven to be an excellent treatment modality for AML. Higher doses are associated with less relapse but these benefits are counterbalanced by an increase in regimen-related toxicity [80]. Several groups are using radioisotopes conjugated to monoclonal antibodies (CD33, CD45) present on hematopoietic tissue and AML blasts to deliver the radiation dose in a more targeted and, hopefully, less toxic manner [81,82].

Nonmyeloablative regimens have been developed primarily for use in older adults who cannot tolerate the regimen-related toxicity associated with standard myeloablative conditioning [83]. While this strategy is showing promise in certain adult patient groups, no data on its use in pediatric AML are available at this time.

GVHD and graft-vs.-leukemia (GVL)

The fine line between the benefit of an allogeneic immune response against the leukemia (GVL) and the risk of an alloresponse against other tissues (GVHD) is aptly illustrated by studies comparing overall survival and the incidence of leukemic relapse in patients with acute GVHD (see Chapter 28) [84,85]. The role of GVHD/GVL reactions to the cure of a particular disease can be assessed, in part, by examining how modulation of the GVHD prophylaxis affects outcome. For example, in a multicenter, prospective, randomized trial, the effect of altering the dose of CSP on outcomes for children with leukemia who receive matched sibling BMT was examined [86]. This is one of the few studies of the GVHD/GVL relationship that is limited to children. The patient cohort included a total of 59 children with either ALL ($n = 47$) or AML ($n = 12$). There was no difference in the incidence of chronic GVHD and overall survival was not statistically different between the two CSP treatment groups.

Whether a GVL effect can be separated from GVHD remains a point of intense study and beyond the scope of this chapter (see Chapters 28 & 29). Strategies to separate GVL and GVHD include the use of antigen-specific T-cell immunotherapy for leukemia [87] as well as utilizing delayed and/or modified donor leukocyte infusions (DLIs) [88,89]. Clinical GVHD may not be necessary for a GVL effect. For AML patients who receive donor marrow from an identical twin, there is a significantly higher incidence of relapse compared to patients who receive marrow from a matched sibling but who did not develop clinical GVHD [90,91]. These data are consistent with IBMTR reports evaluating the incidence of acute leukemia relapse in patients receiving either an autograft, identical-twin graft or HLA-matched sibling graft without developing clinical GVHD [92]. The implication is that there is a GVL effect in patients receiving HLA-matched sibling grafts without clinical signs of GVHD.

Patients who may benefit from chemotherapy alone

Because of the excellent outcome of children with Down syndrome using conventional chemotherapy [49], matched sibling HCT in CR1 is generally not recommended for this group of children. Similarly, because of the significant response seen with the targeted therapy of acute promyelocytic leukemia (APML) using all-*trans*-retinoic-acid and arsenic trioxide, patients with this subtype of AML are not offered matched sibling HCT in CR1 [93].

Another subgroup of children whose outcome may be improving without HCT are infants with AML. The presence of the mixed lineage leukemia (*MLL*) gene rearrangements does not correlate with treatment response in infants with AML [94,95]. Using an intensive chemotherapy regimen, Kawasaki et al. [96] have reported a 72% EFS at 3 years in a cohort of 35 infants with AML.

As previously discussed, the improved outcomes seen in children with AML who receive intensive chemotherapy alone have fueled the debate as to when to recommend a matched sibling allogeneic HCT in CR1 for the child with AML [33,69–71]. Controversy exists in determining whether children with favorable cytogenetics defined as t(8;21) and inv16 should receive a HCT in CR1 [97]. While t(8;21) has been considered a good prognostic variant, Nguyen et al. [98] defined subgroups of patients with this translocation based on the WBC index which takes into account the peripheral blood WBC and the percent of blasts in the marrow. Patients with a high WBC index fare worse and consideration should be given to transplant in CR1. A prospective trial of patients with good risk features comparing a group that receives HCT in CR1 to chemotherapy with HCT reserved until first relapse or CR2 is warranted [72].

Treatment of patients with AML beyond CR1

Management of the patient who fails conventional chemotherapy is complex. If relapse occurs, especially for patients on therapy, the chance of cure with alternate chemotherapy remains poor. Only 30–50% of children who experience a first relapse will achieve a second CR, and these remissions are usually not durable [99]. An HCT procedure with a matched sibling or an alternative donor offers the best chance for survival. If the relapse is in an early stage, proceeding to HCT without attempting to attain a second remission is probably the best option [100]. Although there is no standard for assessing minimal residual disease (MRD) for childhood AML, improvements in MRD technology could help in making the decision to transplant early, i.e. before the standard definition of relapse (>5% blasts in the marrow) is met. Flow cytometry and DNA-based techniques such as fluorescence *in situ* hybridization (FISH) and polymerase chain reaction (PCR) have been used to identify MRD in AML (see Chapter 22) [101–105]. If relapse is extensive and a search for an alternative donor must be done, then an attempt at inducing a second remission, or at least decreasing the leukemic burden, may be required to provide time for identifying the best alternative donor. Gemtuzumab, a humanized anti-CD33 monoclonal antibody conjugated to a modified cytotoxic agent, calicheamicin, has been effective in decreasing the leukemic burden and, in some cases, inducing a remission in patients with AML whose cells express CD33 [106]. Data on its use in children are limited [107]. The use of gemtuzumab in the post-transplant setting is associated with increased toxicity, specifically with VOD [108,109]. Whether this agent increases regimen-related toxicity in the pretransplant setting has not been established, but VOD has been seen in the absence of HCT in these heavily treated patients [110]. Approximately 15–20% of AML patients have refractory disease and do not attain a remission after gemtuzumab or other therapeutic options. HCT has been used successfully to cure a significant proportion of these refractory AML patients [111,112].

Alternative donor HCT for AML

Our goal for this section is to make the reader aware of the treatment options available for the child who needs an alternative donor HCT for AML. The concepts of alternative donor transplants are reviewed in more detail in Chapters 82 and 83.

Expanding the donor options, if an HLA-matched sibling is unavailable, has been a significant advancement for the field of HCT. Alternative donor transplants for AML include (i) unrelated donor HCT utilizing bone marrow, peripheral blood or cord blood grafts and (ii) the use of partially matched or haploidentical related hematopoietic cell donors [65,66,113–117]. There have been no collaborative group prospective studies evaluating the efficacy of alternative donor transplants for AML in children. However, there are data from individual centers and the NMDP that show alternative donor transplants for pediatric AML are successful (Fig. 76.5).

Alternative donor transplants generally are associated with higher complication rates than matched sibling donor transplants due to the greater risks of graft rejection and GVHD [118]. Recipients of alternative donor transplants have delayed immune reconstitution and are at increased long-term risk for infections because of the increased and prolonged immune suppression needed to prevent rejection and prevent and/or treat GVHD [119]. Consequently, alternative donor transplants are often reserved for patients who are considered to be at higher risk for, or have already failed, conventional therapy. For children with AML, this includes patients who (i) never enter a remission, (ii) relapse after conventional therapy or autologous HCT, (iii) develop AML after myelodysplasia, or (iv) develop therapy related AML. Additional factors also may be used to identify children with AML in CR1 whose outcome with intensive chemotherapy is likely to be inferior to the published outcomes for alternative donor transplants for children with AML [72]. For example, in the United Kingdom (UK) Medical Research Council 10 (MRC-10) trial, children classified as poor-risk (i.e. not entering CR or partial remission after one course of chemotherapy or with adverse cytogenetic abnormalit-

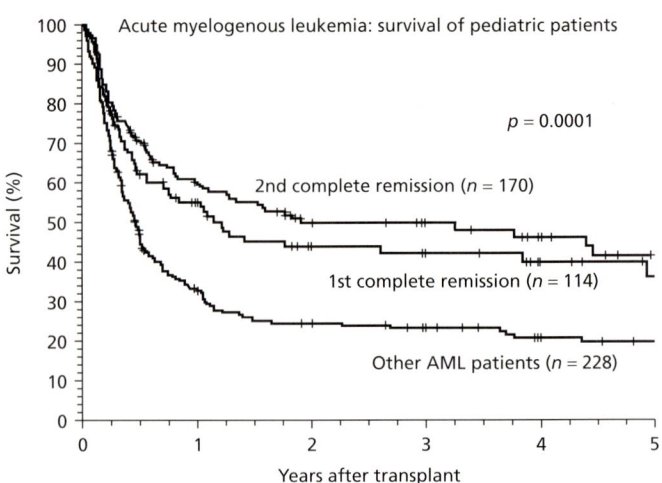

Fig. 76.5 Probability of survival for pediatric patients with acute myeloid leukemia (AML) based on transplants done between 1987 and February 2001 using donors from the National Marrow Donor Program (NMDP). Data kindly provided by NMDP.

ies, such as monosomy of chromosomes 5 or 7; del(5q), or abnormalities of 3q, or a complex karyotype defined as more than four abnormalities) had a significantly inferior DFS of 32% at 7 years [31]. No child in this high-risk group who relapsed after having attained a remission and then relapsed survived [31]. The hypothesis that these children would fare better with an alternative donor transplant in CR1 deserves further study.

Bone marrow

The role of T-cell depletion (TCD) to prevent GVHD in unrelated donor transplants has not been established [120]. There is no question that the incidence of severe (grade III–IV) GVHD is lower in the T-cell depleted setting compared to the T-replete group (5–10% vs. 30–40%). However, whether this lower rate of GVHD will translate into a DFS advantage is still not clear.

Data on the use of T-cell replete HCT for pediatric AML comes from the Fred Hutchinson Cancer Research Center [121]. Of the 135 AML patients in this report, 26 were under the age of 18 years. The primary conditioning regimen was CY/TBI. MTX/CSP was used for GVHD prevention. An important observation from the entire cohort is the relationships between overall survival and leukemic relapse based on the disease status of the patient (Fig. 76.6). Patients transplanted with higher risk disease had an increased risk of failure due to relapse. The cohort of 16 patients receiving an alternative donor graft in CR1 suggests data to consider when evaluating the use of unrelated donor transplants for high-risk AML patients. All of these individuals had adverse features, such as delayed achievement of remission or high-risk cytogenetics. Their DFS was about 50%, which compares very favorably to high-risk patients who are treated with chemotherapy only (DFS ~30%) [31].

Data for T-cell depleted HCT for AML come from the transplant group in Bristol, UK [117]. Of 39 AML patients treated, 33 were under the age of 19 years. Twenty-five of 39 patients were transplanted in CR2, with a median time of 3 months from relapse to transplantation. Fourteen individuals were transplanted in CR1 with major adverse prognostic features, such as failed remission induction ($n = 5$), antecedent myelodysplastic syndrome (MDS) ($n = 2$), infantile leukemia with 11q23 abnormality ($n = 22$) and for other reasons. The Bristol approach primarily involved CY/TBI conditioning combined with Campath-1G *in vivo* and *ex-vivo* for TCD together with CSP for GVHD prevention. The survival rate for this cohort is shown in Fig. 76.7. No patient in this study developed Grade

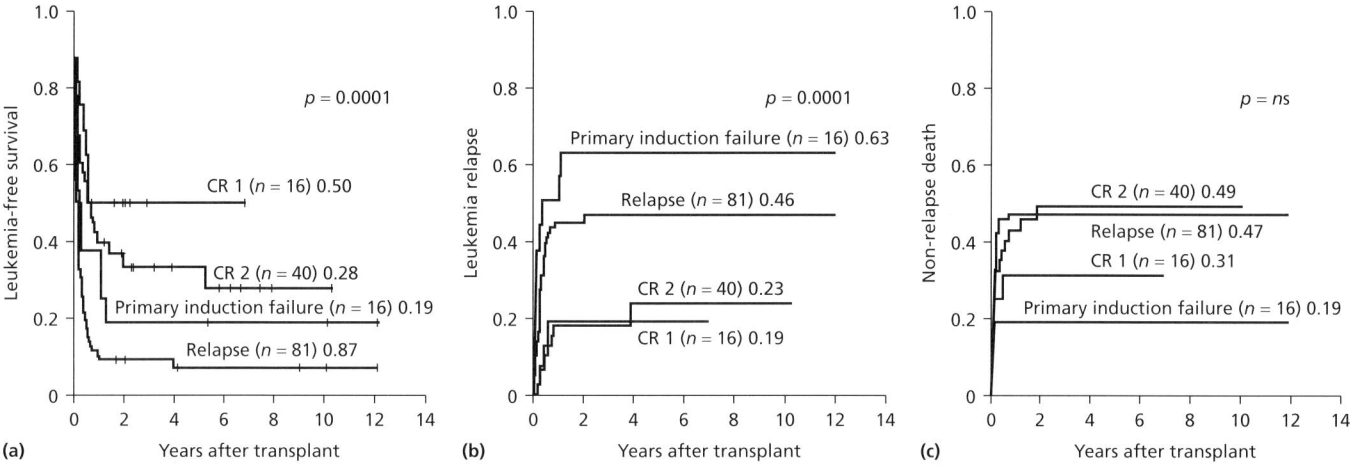

Fig. 76.6 Outcome of unrelated bone marrow transplantation (BMT) for acute myeloid leukemia (AML) according to disease status ($n = 161$); leukemia-free survival (a), leukemia (b) and cumulative incidence of nonrelapse death (c). Reproduced with permission from Sierra et al. [121].

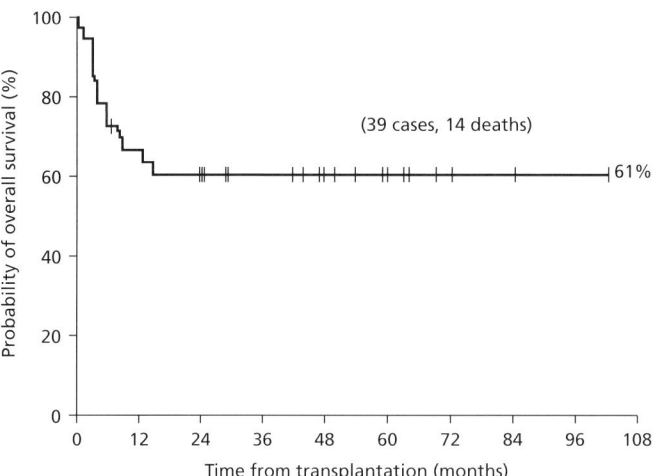

Fig. 76.7 Probability of overall survival in 39 patients who received unrelated donor bone marrow transplantations (BMTs) for acute myeloid leukemia (AML) in remission using T-cell-depleted marrow. Reproduced with permission from Marks et al. [117].

III or IV GVHD; however, there were five cases of chronic GVHD (four extensive, one limited). The total incidence of relapse was 13%. Infection related complications were frequent and severe. There were 20 viral infections documented, with 12 of the 20 infections considered to be serious or life threatening. In the surviving cohort, the performance status is excellent. Similar to the Seattle report [121], the results for the group with high-risk features transplanted in CR1 seem to suggest that TCD may also be feasible for these individuals.

Analysis of data from the NMDP does not clearly define if TCD results in superior outcomes compared to non-TCD strategies. Wagner et al. reported on 4938 transplants facilitated through the NMDP from 1987 to 1998 [122]. Children accounted for 1318 of the patients and, of these, 279 had AML. TCD, using various methods, was performed in 113 patients while 166 patients received a T-replete transplant with MTX and CSP or FK506 (tacrolimus) for GVHD prophylaxis. While the survival at 5 years was better for the TCD group, it was not statistically different from that of the T-replete group. Similarly, a prospective, randomized study comparing unrelated donor BMT using TCD plus CSP with T-replete grafts with MTX/CSP has shown equivalent DFS between the T-replete and T-deplete arms [123]. Of note, TCD was associated with less GVHD but not an increase in relapse for patients with chronic myeloid leukemia (CML).

Umbilical cord blood

An alternative source of hematopoietic cell for transplantation of a child with AML is cryopreserved unrelated cord blood. Several studies have demonstrated that unrelated cord blood is a reasonable option for children lacking a suitably matched unrelated marrow donor (see Chapter 43) [124,125]. The Minnesota group has demonstrated that key variables in determining outcome for patients receiving UCB transplants are $CD34^+$ cell dose and HLA disparity [126]. Based on their data, an unrelated cord blood graft should have at least a $CD34^+$ cell dose of 1.7×10^5 $CD34^+$ cells/kg. There appears to be interplay between the cell dose and HLA disparity. For each degree of HLA disparity, there appears to be a critical infused cell dose below which survival is significantly impaired, particularly in recipients of unrelated cord blood with ≥2-HLA disparities. Hence, they argue, based on their data, that the choice of unrelated cord blood graft should be based primarily on CD34 cell dose and secondarily on degree of HLA disparity. In this data set, there were 26 individuals with AML (one in CR1, 14 in CR2, 1 in >CR2 and 10 in relapse). The survival rate was two of four patients in the standard-risk group and 33% (95%CI 12–54%) for high-risk patients. A significant obstacle to survival in the AML cohort was relapse.

Recently, Michel et al. reported the experience for EUROCORD and the use of unrelated cord blood for children with AML [127]. Ninety-five children were analyzed. The median age was 6 years and the median weight was 21 kg. Twenty children were in CR1, 47 in CR2, five in CR3 and 23 were not in remission. Forty-one had ≥2-HLA disparities. TRM was significantly lower for children who received a cell dose >4.4 $\times 10^7$/kg. The 2-year probabilities of survival and DFS were $45 \pm 5\%$ and $42 \pm 5\%$, respectively. DFS was not associated with the number of HLA disparities. Notably, the results were particularly promising, even in CR2 patients who experienced an early relapse and for children with poor risk karyotypes.

Haploidentical family donors

Another potentially exciting modality for treatment of children with AML is the use of a graft from a related haploidentical donor. Haploidentical transplants are attractive because most patients have a donor readily available and can proceed to transplant quickly. Godder and colleagues have reported data on 67 children treated for acute leukemia utilizing a partially matched family member [115]. The treatment plan included a partially TCD product with post-transplant immune suppression including antithymocyte globulin, CSP and glucocorticoids. In this cohort, 24 of the 67 patients had AML; 75% of the AML patients had peripheral blasts. Donor–recipient pairs were mismatched in the GVHD direction for either three antigens ($n = 10$), two antigens ($n = 8$) or one antigen ($n = 6$). The estimated probability of survival at 3 years was 26%, and was similar for patients with ALL and AML. In the AML cohort, 39% of the transplants failed because of relapse. In particular, patients with circulating blasts had a very high risk of relapse. Neither GVHD nor rejection were common causes of failure. In the multivariate statistical analysis, use of a younger donor (age <30 years) as well as absence of blasts at the time of HCT were found to be associated with better outcomes. This study demonstrated that HCT from a partially matched family member is feasible for children with AML.

In contrast to the transplant protocol utilized by Godder and colleagues, other centers are exploring the use of megadose $CD34^+$/low $CD3^+$ haploidentical transplants as originally described by the transplant group in Perugia, Italy [128,129]. Hematopoietic cells are collected by apheresis from donors who have been stimulated with G-CSF. The apheresis cells are positively selected on an immunomagnetic column resulting in a relatively pure population of $CD34^+$ cells. The number of T cells remaining is usually less than 50,000/kg. The theory underlying this strategy is that the megadose $CD34^+$ infusion with low $CD3^+$ cells permits engraftment across haplotype barriers without the development of GVHD, even though no post-transplant immune suppression is used. The Tübingen transplant group in Germany has published the largest pediatric series to date using this approach [116]. Few pediatric AML patients have been treated using this modality, but the overall low risk of GVHD observed to date is encouraging. Thus far, the major barriers to survival have been infection and relapse. For patients with AML, this transplant approach may take advantage of the unique role that alloreactive natural killer (NK) cells play in mediating GVL effect. The data in adults with AML receiving megadose $CD34^+$/low $CD3^+$ haploidentical transplants is provocative with a very low incidence of AML relapse, perhaps because of alloreactive NK cells [130].

Relapse after HCT

Despite the intensity of conditioning and the GVL effect, relapse of AML after either matched sibling or alternative donor HCT is not uncommon and often leads to death. The propensity for AML to recur despite intense conditioning points to the need for innovative therapies for the child who relapses after HCT.

Second myeloablative transplant procedure

One option is a second myeloablative HCT procedure. If the original donor was a matched sibling, the data suggest that a second transplant may result in salvage of about one-third of patients [131]. A study from the Sociéte Francaise de Greffe de Moelle evaluated the use of second transplants in 150 individuals with leukemia (AML = 61), combining both adult and pediatric patients [132]. Although recipients of grafts from unrelated donors were included in this study, the vast majority of the patients received grafts from matched sibling donors. For the pediatric cohort, univariate statistical analysis showed the 2-year post-second transplant overall survival was 50% ± 18%, DFS was 47% ±16% with TRM at 20% ± 18%. In the multivariate analysis, the factors that were associated with better prognosis were age <16 years and disease recurrence more than 1 year after the original transplant. Therefore, children whose disease recurs more than a year after the initial transplant should be considered for a second transplant procedure, especially if the original donor is again available.

The Italian cooperative group, Gruppo Italiano Trapianti di Midolio Osseo (GITMO), has reported similar results in 38 patients receiving a second allogeneic BMT procedure [133]. Twenty-one of the 38 patients had AML, and the youngest was 2 years old. Median age was 23 years. Interestingly, they observed a better outcome for patients with AML as compared to ALL. The incidence of acute and chronic GVHD was not different between the AML and ALL cohorts; therefore, GVHD differences do not explain the outcome disparity.

Adoptive immunotherapy

In addition to second myeloablative transplant regimens, adoptive immunotherapy, with or without chemotherapy, has been used to treat or prevent post-transplant relapse (see Chapter 84) [134–137]. Following the success seen with DLI for CML, there are case reports and retrospective reviews describing DLI for AML in adults and children [138–143]. These series vary as to whether chemotherapy and/or biologic response modifiers, such as interferon and/or interleukin 2, were used as an adjunct to DLI therapy. Occasionally patients attain durable responses, while others either relapse with their diseases and/or develop GVHD. Kolb and the European Group for Blood and Marrow Transplantation (EBMT) have reported the largest number of AML patients treated with DLI at multiple institutions [142]. Five of 21 evaluable AML patients had achieved prolonged leukemia-free survival at the time of the publication.

Following the success of MRD directed DLI for CML [144,145], it was hypothesized that improved identification of MRD also would lead to better responses after DLI for AML. Bader *et al.* [136,137] have utilized increasing levels of host chimerism as an indication for withdrawing CSP and/or using low dose DLI for children with acute leukemia or MDS. Although the number of observations are small (12 children; three with AML and four with MDS), this pediatric study suggests that prophylactic immunotherapy may play a role in children with acute leukemia who exhibit increasing host chimerism.

There has been one prospective study to evaluate the role of chemotherapy cytoreduction coupled with DLI to treat myeloid malignancies in patients who relapsed after HCT [134]. This multi-institutional study had 50 AML patients within a total cohort of 65 individuals. The age range was 2–59 years. The study utilized chemotherapy followed by G-CSF mobilized DLI with a goal of delivering 1×10^8 $CD3^+$ cells/kg along with $CD34^+$ cells. The study objective was to transfuse DLI to confer a GVL effect as well as $CD34^+$ cells to minimize aplasia after chemotherapy. For the entire cohort, the 2-year survival was 19% (95%CI = 11–33%). Patients whose disease relapsed beyond 6 months from the initial transplant had a statistically higher probability of survival as compared to those whose relapse occurred within 6 months of BMT (Fig. 76.8 [134]). The major barriers to survival in this study were early failures due to the ineffective induction of remission with the debulking doses of chemotherapy as well as a 23% chance of TRM. This study provides evidence that nonmyeloablative conditioning with DLI can be efficacious for patients who relapse beyond 6 months post-HCT.

A recently described phenomenon that raises concerns about the efficacy of adoptive immunotherapy for AML, is the occurrence of extra-medullary relapse after HCT and DLI [146–148]. At the Medical College of Wisconsin, we have observed this phenomenon in four children who received an allogeneic HCT procedure for AML. The relapses occurred as chloromas in skin ($n = 2$), sinus ($n = 1$) and central nervous system ($n = 1$). Interestingly, at the time of extra-medullary relapse, the bone marrow in each case was 100% donor origin with no evidence of leukemia. While DLI and/or second transplant have been attempted, together with radiotherapy for local control, systemic leukemic relapse leading to death occurred in three of the four patients. The pathophysiology of these observations remains unclear, but relapses in extra-medullary sites, while the bone marrow is initially unaffected, suggests that the GVL effect may be compartmentalized [147].

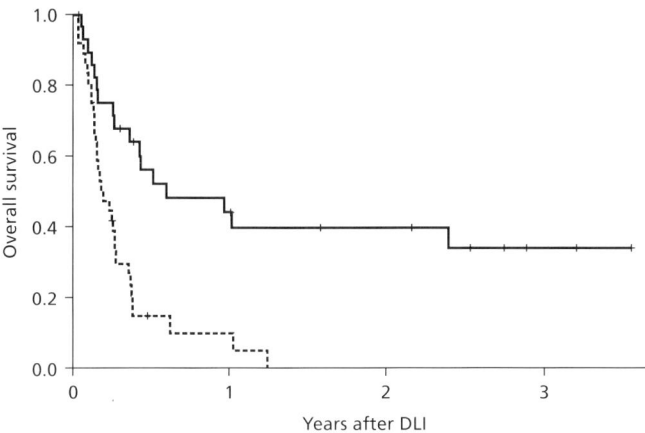

Fig. 76.8 Overall survival rates. ------ indicate relapse after bone marrow transplantation (BMT) within 6 months. ──── indicate relapse after BMT after 6 months. Reproduced with permission from Levine et al. [134].

Late effects associated with HCT

When assessing the risks and benefits of different treatment plans, the long-term risks of each treatment option are of obvious relevance. Increasing numbers of children are surviving AML, and the long-term effects of treatment are becoming better appreciated. The late complications associated with HCT are reviewed in more detail specifically in Chapters 68, 69 and 70.

The choice between transplant and chemotherapy for the child with AML who has a matched sibling is controversial, in part because of concerns that transplantation is associated with more profound late sequelae. Investigators at Children's Hospital of Philadelphia (CHOP) have examined the question of late effects for 52 survivors treated for AML, comparing chemotherapy regimens ($n = 26$) with transplants ($n = 26$). Most of the HCT recipients (17 out of 26) had not received TBI [149]. They found that the two treatment modalities had similar effects on growth, and renal and cardiac function. Their data suggest an increased risk of infertility in the HCT group. Liesner and colleagues likewise compared chemotherapy and transplant cohorts and found that the risk of infertility was higher in the transplant group [150]. In contrast to the study from CHOP, Liesner et al. observed more growth retardation in the transplant cohort as compared to the chemotherapy group.

Because of the similar antileukemia efficacy in AML of BU/CY 200 with TBI-based regimens [59], many centers utilize a non-TBI-based regimen. In a cohort of 45 children with AML comparing late effects using BU/CY vs. CY/TBI, Michel et al. [151] have reported that the TBI group had more frequent decreases in height standard deviation scores, hypothyroidism and cataracts. A concern for pediatricians, *vis a vis* TBI, has been the worry that TBI will have a negative effect on cognitive functioning. This concern has been the focus of research done at the Medical College of Wisconsin [152]. Kupst and colleagues have prospectively evaluated the cognitive and psychosocial functioning of 153 children and adolescents [152]. Patients were evaluated pretransplant as well as at 1-year and 2-years post-HCT. One hundred and forty-two patients had received TBI. The data demonstrated that IQ tests, as a measure of cognitive function, remained stable over time and were not adversely affected by TBI. The strongest predictor of cognitive outcome was pre-HCT functioning.

The range of the late effects reported in the literature point to the need for comprehensive follow-up for the survivors of AML, regardless of the treatment received. Children need to be monitored consistently for growth and sexual development, thyroid dysfunction, cataracts, second malignancies and neuropsychological late effects. Close monitoring will then facilitate appropriate treatment.

Conclusion

According to the Surveillance, Epidemiology and End Results (SEER) database, survival for children with AML has improved from 14%, from 1974 to 1976, to 45%, from 1992 to 1997 [153]. We now have even more successful chemotherapy protocols, several different donor sources for HCT and adoptive cellular therapies, as well as targeted monoclonal antibody and molecular therapies. As more children survive their primary disease, we need to pay more attention to long-term side-effects and second malignancies. Nevertheless, the current 45% survival rate clearly indicates that the cure of childhood AML is work in progress.

The data reviewed in this chapter provide a basis for decision-making when the physician evaluates a child with AML. The algorithm in Fig. 76.2 should be used as a framework, not a rigid plan. The results with chemotherapy have improved but, in most instances, HCT from a matched sibling leads to improved DFS. However, there remains an ongoing controversy regarding the interpretation of the data concerning HCT for AML in CR1. The European groups, due to their excellent results in children with AML employing chemotherapy alone, currently advocate HCT with a matched sibling in CR1 only for those patients with high-risk features of AML [154]. Data from the North American pediatric AML trials completed to date suggest that the long-term survival is superior for children assigned to allogeneic HCT in CR1 [72]. The reasons for this discrepancy are unclear, but the North American patients were comprised of a more heterogeneous ethnic background and included older patients [71]. Notably, Davies et al. [155] report that African-American children with AML enrolled on CCG 2891 did significantly worse when treated with chemotherapy compared to Caucasian children. However, there was no difference for children of different race who underwent HCT [155]. It is crucial that we continue to stratify patients based on the same risk parameters so that comparisons between treatment strategies are not biased. The advent of microarray technology along with the escalating information with regard to genetic markers should allow investigators to more precisely define AML based on biologic parameters. This information should at least lead to standardization and agreement as to risk assignment. If results with chemotherapy improve, or if TRM decreases, the algorithm in Fig. 76.2 could change.

The argument has been made that patients who fail on the current chemotherapy protocols could proceed to HCT in early relapse or CR2. However, as conventional chemotherapy protocols for AML may have reached their toxicity limit, the patients who fail chemotherapy may not be as responsive to a myeloablative HCT [156].

Strategies designed to employ molecular techniques to identify patients who continue to have leukemia cells early on (i.e. before they develop a clinical relapse) are well underway. This concept could potentially allow for transplantation before the patient is refractory and in poor condition secondary to intense but ineffective treatment. Unfortunately, the molecular profile of AML blasts at diagnosis may not be the same at relapse [157–159]. The assumption is that patients whose AML blasts express *FLT3/ITD* at diagnosis will do so at relapse. However, two recent reports demonstrate that this marker is not always reliable, as a subset of patients did not express *FLT3/ITD* at relapse [158,159]. Nevertheless, for those patients who can accurately be diagnosed with a molecular relapse or residual disease, moving quickly to HCT might be a potential strategy.

It is important to ascertain at the time of AML diagnosis whether the patient has an HLA-matched sibling. If a matched sibling is available, and the patient has high-risk AML, as discussed earlier, we would recommend proceeding to transplant in CR1. Conversely, children with Down syndrome or APML should not be transplanted in CR1, as the current treatment results for those patients are excellent. Ideally, patients with an HLA-matched sibling and standard risk AML would be randomized in an international, multi-institutional trial to a transplant or chemotherapy arm. In the absence of a randomized clinical trial, discussions with the patient and family regarding relative risks and benefits (as framed by the expertise of the physician) will need to guide the decision.

If a child does not have a matched sibling, then the usual treatment plan includes primary intensive conventional chemotherapy. Alternative donor HCT may be considered in CR1 for high-risk cases or when the patient relapses during or soon after conventional therapy. The source of the alternative donor hematopoietic cells will depend on a number of factors which includes the underlying diagnosis and stage of disease, degree of mismatch for the various potential hematopoietic cell sources and cell dose available based on the size of the patient.

Future directions

It is clear that, especially in the pediatric population, hematopoietic cells from an unrelated individual can be lifesaving. In fact, many institutions have reported no significant difference between outcomes for a well-matched unrelated donor and an HLA-matched sibling [64–68]. The challenge remains as to how best to manipulate the hematopoietic cell inoculum, conditioning regimens and GVHD strategies to ensure a successful outcome.

For the proponents of unrelated cord blood HCT, the major challenges are securing an adequate cell dose in order to ensure engraftment and shorten the period of pancytopenia. Investigators are currently evaluating *ex vitro* expansion of cells [160], the addition of mesenchymal cells [161] and the transplantation of multiple cord blood units [162].

The major challenges facing unrelated donor HCT are GVHD in the setting of a T-cell-replete graft, and infection and relapse in a T-cell-depleted strategy. When the donor and recipient are HLA-mismatched, these problems are magnified. The use of peripheral blood compared to bone marrow as a source of HCs in children is under investigation [163]. The development of reproducible methods to deliver a defined number of both $CD34^+$ cells and T cells may alleviate some of the obstacles. Studies on the generation of cytotoxic T lymphocytes targeted to specific viruses [164] or to minor histocompatibility antigens [165] and leukemia antigens [166] are well underway.

In the future, HCT is likely to advance toward a selective component therapy in order to become a less toxic and more effective treatment for a broader range of patients [167]. Because tumor cells use multiple mechanisms of immune evasion, a combination of several approaches, rather than a single treatment, will be necessary.

References

1 Linet MS, Ries LA, Smith MA, Tarone RE, Devesa SS. Cancer surveillance series. Recent trends in childhood cancer incidence and mortality in the United States. *J Natl Cancer Inst* 1999; **91**: 1051–8.

2 Smith MA, Ries LA, Gurney JG *et al.*, eds. *Cancer Incidence and Survival Among Children and Adolescents: United States SEER Program 1975–95.* Bethesda, MD: National Institutes of Health, 1999: 17–34.

3 Bernasconi P, Boni M, Cavigliano PM *et al.* Molecular genetics of acute myeloid leukemia. *Ann N Y Acad Sci* 2002; **963**: 297–305.

4 Kwong YL, Ng MH, Ma SK. Familial acute myeloid leukemia with monosomy 7. Late onset and involvement of a multipotential progenitor cell. *Cancer Genet Cytogenet* 2000; **116**: 170–3.

5 Kojima S, Ohara A, Tsuchida M *et al.* Risk factors for evolution of acquired aplastic anemia into myelodysplastic syndrome and acute myeloid leukemia after immunosuppressive therapy in children. *Blood* 2002; **100**: 786–90.

6 Bennett JM, Catovsky D, Daniel MT *et al.* Proposals for the classification of the acute leukaemias. French–American–British (FAB) cooperative group. *Br J Haematol* 1976; **33**: 451–8.

7 Bennett JM, Catovsky D, Daniel MT *et al.* Proposed revised criteria for the classification of acute myeloid leukemia. A report of the French–American–British Cooperative Group. *Ann Intern Med* 1985; **103**: 620–5.

8 Bennett JM, Catovsky D, Daniel MT *et al.* Criteria for the diagnosis of acute leukemia of megakaryocyte lineage (M7). A report of the French–American–British Cooperative Group. *Ann Intern Med* 1985; **103**: 460–2.

9 Bennett JM, Catovsky D, Daniel MT *et al.* Proposal for the recognition of minimally differentiated acute myeloid leukaemia (AML-MO). *Br J Haematol* 1991; **78**: 325–9.

10 *Childhood Acute Myeloid Leukemia/Other Malignancies PDQ® Treatment. Health Professionals Version*. National Cancer Institute, 2002. http://cancer.gov/cancerinfo/pdq/treatment/child AML/healthprofessional#Section_10

11 Creutzig U, Schaaff A, Ritter J, Jobke A, Kaufmann U, Schellong G. Acute myelogenous leukemia in children under 2 years of age: studies and treatment results in 23 children in the AML therapy study BFM-78. *Klin Padiatr* 1984; **196**: 130–4.

12 Griffin JD, Ritz J, Nadler LM, Schlossman SF. Expression of myeloid differentiation antigens on normal and malignant myeloid cells. *J Clin Invest* 1981; **68**: 932–41.

13 Ball ED, Fanger MW. The expression of myeloid-specific antigens on myeloid leukemia cells: correlations with leukemia subclasses and implications for normal myeloid differentiation. *Blood* 1983; **61**: 456–63.

14 Betz SA, Foucar K, Head DR, Chen IM, Willman CL. False-positive flow cytometric platelet glycoprotein IIb/IIIa expression in myeloid leukemias secondary to platelet adherence to blasts. *Blood* 1992; **79**: 2399–403.

15 Rowley JD. The role of chromosome translocations in leukemogenesis. *Semin Hematol* 1999; **36**: 59–72.

16 Wells RJ, Arthur DC, Srivastava A *et al.* Prognostic variables in newly diagnosed children and adolescents with acute myeloid leukemia: Children's Cancer Group Study 213. *Leukemia* 2002; **16**: 601–7.

17 Chang M, Raimondi SC, Ravindranath Y *et al.* Prognostic factors in children and adolescents with acute myeloid leukemia (excluding children with Down syndrome and acute promyelocytic leukemia): univariate and recursive partitioning analysis of patients treated on Pediatric Oncology Group (POG) Study 8821. *Leukemia* 2000; **14**: 1201–7.

18 Grimwade D, Walker H, Oliver F *et al.* The importance of diagnostic cytogenetics on outcome in AML. Analysis of 1612 patients entered into the MRC AML 10 trial. The Medical Research Council Adult and Children's Leukaemia Working Parties. *Blood* 1998; **92**: 2322–33.

19 Raimondi SC, Chang MN, Ravindranath Y *et al.* Chromosomal abnormalities in 478 children with acute myeloid leukemia: clinical characteristics and treatment outcome in a cooperative pediatric oncology group study-POG 8821. *Blood* 1999; **94**: 3707–16.

20 Zwaan CM, Meschinchi S, Radich J *et al.* FLT3 internal tandem duplication in childhood acute myeloid leukemia: prognostic significance and relation to cellular drug resistance. *Blood* 2002; **100**: 33a [Abstract].

21 Vardiman JW, Harris NL, Brunning RD. The World Health Organization (WHO) classification of the myeloid neoplasms. *Blood* 2002; **100**: 2292–302.

22 Schoch C, Kohlmann A, Schnittger S *et al.* Acute myeloid leukemias with reciprocal rearrangements can be distinguished by specific gene expression profiles. *Proc Natl Acad Sci U S A* 2002; **99**: 10,008–13.

23 Nesbit ME Jr, Buckley JD, Feig SA *et al.* Chemotherapy for induction of remission of childhood acute myeloid leukemia followed by marrow transplantation or multiagent chemotherapy: a report from the Children's Cancer Group. *J Clin Oncol* 1994; **12**: 127–35.

24 Wells RJ, Woods WG, Buckley JD *et al.* Treatment of newly diagnosed children and adolescents with acute myeloid leukemia: a Children's Cancer Group study. *J Clin Oncol* 1994; **12**: 2367–77.

25 Ravindranath Y, Steuber CP, Krischer J *et al.* High-dose cytarabine for intensification of early therapy of childhood acute myeloid leukemia: a Pediatric Oncology Group Study. *J Clin Oncol* 1991; **9**: 572–80.

26 Woods WG, Kobrinsky N, Buckley J *et al.* Intensively timed induction therapy followed by autologous or allogeneic bone marrow transplantation for children with acute myeloid leukemia or myelodysplastic syndrome: a Children's Cancer Group pilot study. *J Clin Oncol* 1993; **11**: 1448–57.

27 Amadori S, Testi AM, Arico M *et al.* Prospective comparative study of bone marrow transplantation

and postmission chemotherapy for childhood acute myelogenous leukemia. The Associazione Italiana Ematologia ed Oncologia Pediatrica Co-operative Group. *J Clin Oncol* 1993; **11**: 1046–54.

28. Creutzig U, Ritter J, Schellong G. Identification of two risk groups in childhood acute myelogenous leukemia after therapy intensification in study AML-BFM-83 as compared with study AML-BFM-78. AML-BFM Study Group. *Blood* 1990; **75**: 1932–40.

29. Creutzig U, Ritter J, Zimmermann M, Schellong G. Does cranial irradiation reduce the risk for bone marrow relapse in acute myelogenous leukemia? Unexpected results of the Childhood Acute Myelogenous Leukemia Study BFM-87. *J Clin Oncol* 1993; **11**: 279–86.

30. Lie SO, Jonmundsson G, Mellander L, Siimes MA, Yssing M, Gustafsson G. A population-based study of 272 children with acute myeloid leukaemia treated on two consecutive protocols with different intensity: best outcome in girls, infants, and children with Down's syndrome. Nordic Society of Paediatric Haematology and Oncology (NOPHO). *Br J Haematol* 1996; **94**: 82–8.

31. Stevens RF, Hann IM, Wheatley K, Gray RG. Marked improvements in outcome with chemotherapy alone in paediatric acute myeloid leukemia. Results of the United Kingdom Medical Research Council's 10th AML Trial. MRC Childhood Leukaemia Working Party. *Br J Haematol* 1998; **101**: 130–40.

32. Woods WG, Kobrinsky N, Buckley JD *et al.* Timed-sequential induction therapy improves postremission outcome in acute myeloid leukemia: a report from the Children's Cancer Group. *Blood* 1996; **87**: 4979–89.

33. Woods WG, Neudorf S, Gold S *et al.* A comparison of allogeneic bone marrow transplantation, autologous bone marrow transplantation, and aggressive chemotherapy in children with acute myeloid leukemia in remission. *Blood* 2001; **97**: 56–62.

34. Thomas ED, Storb R, Clift RA *et al.* Bone-marrow transplantation. *N Engl J Med* 1975; **292**: 832–43; 895–902.

35. Sanders JE, Thomas ED, Buckner CD *et al.* Marrow transplantation for children in first remission of acute nonlymphoblastic leukemia: An update. *Blood* 1985; **66**: 460–2.

36. Kersey JH, Ramsay NK, Kim T *et al.* Allogeneic bone marrow transplantation in acute nonlymphocytic leukemia: a pilot study. *Blood* 1982; **60**: 400–3.

37. Santos GW, Tutschka PJ, Brookmeyer R *et al.* Marrow transplantation for acute nonlymphocytic leukemia after treatment with busulfan and cyclophosphamide. *N Engl J Med* 1983; **309**: 1347–53.

38. Weinstein HJ, Mayer RJ, Rosenthal DS, Coral FS, Camitta BM, Gelber RD. Chemotherapy for acute myelogenous leukemia in children and adults: VAPA update. *Blood* 1983; **62**: 315–9.

39. Lie SO, Slordahl SH. Long-term relapse-free survival in childhood acute nonlymphocytic leukemia. *Semin Oncol* 1987; **14**: 7–11.

40. Hurwitz CA, Mounce KG, Grier HE. Treatment of patients with acute myelogenous leukemia: review of clinical trials of the past decade. *J Pediatr Hematol Oncol* 1995; **17**: 185–97.

41. Buckley JD, Chard RL, Baehner RL *et al.* Improvement in outcome for children with acute nonlymphocytic leukemia. A report from the Children's Cancer Study Group. *Cancer* 1989; **63**: 1457–65.

42. Krischer JP, Steuber CP, Vietti TJ *et al.* Long-term results in the treatment of acute nonlymphocytic leukemia: a Pediatric Oncology Group Study. *Med Pediatr Oncol* 1989; **17**: 401–8.

43. Kalwinsky D, Mirro J Jr, Schell M, Behm F, Mason C, Dahl GV. Early intensification of chemotherapy for childhood acute nonlymphoblastic leukemia: improved remission induction with a five-drug regimen including etoposide. *J Clin Oncol* 1988; **6**: 1134–43.

44. Brochstein JA, Kernan NA, Groshen S *et al.* Allogeneic bone marrow transplantation after hyperfractionated total-body irradiation and cyclophosphamide in children with acute leukemia. *N Engl J Med* 1987; **317**: 1618–24.

45. McGlave PB, Haake RJ, Bostrom BC *et al.* Allogeneic bone marrow transplantation for acute nonlymphocytic leukemia in first remission. *Blood* 1988; **72**: 1512–7.

46. Forman SJ, Krance RA, O'Donnell MR *et al.* Bone marrow transplantation for acute nonlymphoblastic leukemia during first complete remission. An analysis of prognostic factors. *Transplantation* 1987; **43**: 650–3.

47. Ringden O, Bolme P, Lonnqvist B, Gustafsson G, Kreuger A. Allogeneic bone marrow transplantation versus chemotherapy in children with acute leukemia in Sweden. *Pediatr Hematol Oncol* 1989; **6**: 137–44.

48. Dahl GV, Kalwinsky DK, Mirro J Jr *et al.* Allogeneic bone marrow transplantation in a program of intensive sequential chemotherapy for children and young adults with acute nonlymphocytic leukemia in first remission. *J Clin Oncol* 1990; **8**: 295–303.

49. Ravindranath Y, Yeager AM, Chang MN *et al.* Autologous bone marrow transplantation versus intensive consolidation chemotherapy for acute myeloid leukemia in childhood. Pediatric Oncology Group. *N Engl J Med* 1996; **334**: 1428–34.

50. Vowels M, Stevens M, Tiedemann K, Brown R. Autologous and allogeneic bone marrow transplantation for childhood acute nonlymphoblastic leukemia. *Transplant Proc* 1992; **24**: 184–5.

51. Shaw PJ, Bergin ME, Burgess MA *et al.* Childhood acute myeloid leukemia: outcome in a single center using chemotherapy and consolidation with busulfan/cyclophosphamide for bone marrow transplantation. *J Clin Oncol* 1994; **12**: 2138–45.

52. Creutzig U, Ritter J, Zimmermann M *et al.* Idarubicin improves blast cell clearance during induction therapy in children with AML. Results of study AML-BFM 93. AML-BFM Study Group. *Leukemia* 2001; **15**: 348–54.

53. Creutzig U, Ritter J, Zimmermann M *et al.* Improved treatment results in high-risk pediatric acute myeloid leukemia patients after intensification with high-dose cytarabine and mitoxantrone: results of the Study of Acute Myeloid Leukemia, Berlin–Frankfurt–Münster 93. *J Clin Oncol* 2001; **19**: 2705–13.

54. Behar C, Suciu S, Benoit Y *et al.* Mitoxantrone-containing regimen for treatment of childhood acute leukemia (AML) and analysis of prognostic factors: results of the EORTC Children Leukemia Cooperative Study 58872. *Med Pediatr Oncol* 1996; **26**: 173–9.

55. Michel G, Leverger G, Leblanc T *et al.* Allogeneic bone marrow transplantation vs. aggressive post-remission chemotherapy for children with acute myeloid leukemia in first complete remission. A prospective study from the French Society of Pediatric Hematology and Immunology (SHIP). *Bone Marrow Transplant* 1996; **17**: 191–6.

56. Lie SO, Jonmundsson G, Mellander L, Siimes M, Gustafsson G. Early response to therapy is the strongest prognostic factor in childhoood AML. *Haematol Blood Transfus* 2001; **40**: 499–507.

57. Ortega JJ, Olive T. Haematopoietic progenitor cell transplant in acute leukaemias in children. Indications, results and controversies. *Bone Marrow Transplant* 1998; **21** (Suppl. 2): S11–6.

58. Dini G, Boni L, Abla O *et al.* Allogeneic bone marrow transplantation in children with acute myelogenous leukemia in first remission. Associazione Italiana di Ematologia e Oncologia Pediatrica (AIEOP) and the Gruppo Italiano per il Trapianto di Midollo Osseo (GITMO). *Bone Marrow Transplant* 1994; **13**: 771–6.

59. Michel G, Gluckman E, Esperou-Bourdeau H *et al.* Allogeneic bone marrow transplantation for children with acute myeloblastic leukemia in first complete remission: Impact of conditioning regimen without total-body irradiation: a report from the Sociéte Francaise de Greffe de Moelle. *J Clin Oncol* 1994; **12**: 1217–22.

60. Perel Y, Auvrignon A, Leblanc T *et al.* Impact of addition of maintenance therapy to intensive induction and consolidation chemotherapy for childhood acute myeloblastic leukemia: results of a prospective randomized trial, LAME 89/91. Leucamie Aique Myeloide Enfant. *J Clin Oncol* 2002; **20**: 2774–82.

61. Cesaro S, Meloni G, Messina C *et al.* High-dose melphalan with autologous hematopoietic stem cell transplantation for acute myeloid leukemia: results of a retrospective analysis of the Italian Pediatric Group for Bone Marrow Transplantation. *Bone Marrow Transplant* 2001; **28**: 131–6.

62. Bonetti F, Zecca M, Pession A *et al.* Total-body irradiation and melphalan is a safe and effective conditioning regimen for autologous bone marrow transplantation in children with acute myeloid leukemia in first remission. The Italian Association for Pediatric Hematology and Oncology—Bone Marrow Transplantation Group. *J Clin Oncol* 1999; **17**: 3729–35.

63. Locatelli F, Labopin M, Ortega J *et al.* Factors influencing outcome and incidence of long-term complications in children given autologous stem cell transplantation for acute myeloid leukemia in 1st complete remission. *Blood* 2003; **101**(4): 1611–9.

64. Hongeng S, Krance RA, Bowman LC *et al.* Outcomes of transplantation with matched-sibling and unrelated-donor bone marrow in children with leukaemia. *Lancet* 1997; **350**: 767–71.

65. Casper J, Camitta B, Truitt R *et al.* Unrelated bone marrow donor transplants for children with leukemia or myelodysplasia. *Blood* 1995; **85**: 2354–63.

66. Balduzzi A, Gooley T, Anasetti C *et al.* Unrelated donor marrow transplantation in children. *Blood* 1995; **86**: 3247–56.

67. Oakhill A, Pamphilon DH, Potter MN *et al.* Unrelated donor bone marrow transplantation for children with relapsed acute lymphoblastic leukaemia in second complete remission. *Br J Haematol* 1996; **94**: 574–8.

68. Heslop HE. Haemopoietic stem cell transplantation from unrelated donors. *Br J Haematol* 1999; **105**: 2–6.

69. Creutzig U, Reinhardt D, Zimmermann M, Klingebiel T, Gadner H. Intensive chemotherapy

70 Horan J, Korones D. Intensive chemotherapy and bone marrow transplantation for children with acute myeloid leukemia. *Blood* 2001; **97**: 3672–3.

71 Pinkel D, Woods G, Lange B. Treatment of children with acute myeloid leukemia. *Blood* 2001; **97**: 3673–5.

72 Chen AR, Alonzo TA, Woods WG, Arceci RJ. Current controversies: Which patients with acute myeloid leukaemia should receive a bone marrow transplantation? An American view. *Br J Haematol* 2002; **118**: 378–84.

73 Amylon MD, Co JP, Snyder DS, Donaldson SS, Blume KG, Forman SJ. Allogeneic bone marrow transplant in pediatric patients with high-risk hematopoietic malignancies early in the course of their disease. *J Pediatr Hematol Oncol* 1997; **19**: 54–61.

74 Yeager AM, Wagner JE Jr, Graham ML, Jones RJ, Santos GW, Grochow LB. Optimization of busulfan dosage in children undergoing bone marrow transplantation: a pharmacokinetic study of dose escalation. *Blood* 1992; **80**: 2425–8.

75 Bolinger AM, Zangwill AB, Slattery JT et al. An evaluation of engraftment, toxicity and busulfan concentration in children receiving bone marrow transplantation for leukemia or genetic disease. *Bone Marrow Transplant* 2000; **25**: 925–30.

76 Bolinger AM, Zangwill AB, Slattery JT et al. Target dose adjustment of busulfan in pediatric patients undergoing bone marrow transplantation. *Bone Marrow Transplant* 2001; **28**: 1013–8.

77 Bleyzac N, Souillet G, Magron P et al. Improved clinical outcome of paediatric bone marrow recipients using a test dose and Bayesian pharmacokinetic individualization of busulfan dosage regimens. *Bone Marrow Transplant* 2001; **28**: 743–51.

78 Schuler US, Renner UD, Kroschinsky F et al. Intravenous busulphan for conditioning before autologous or allogeneic human blood stem cell transplantation. *Br J Haematol* 2001; **114**: 944–50.

79 Tran H, Madden T, Worth L et al. Pharmacokinetic (PK) guided dose adjustment of intravenous busulfan (IVBU) (Busulfex™) in pediatric patients receiving busulfan-based preparative regimen for stem cell transplantation (SCT). *Blood* 2001; **98**: 198a [Abstract].

80 Clift RA, Buckner CD, Appelbaum FR et al. Allogeneic marrow transplantation in patients with chronic myeloid leukemia in the chronic phase: a randomized trial of two irradiation regimens. *Blood* 1991; **77**: 1660–5.

81 Perentesis JP, Sievers EL. Targeted therapies for high-risk acute myeloid leukemia. *Hematol Oncol Clin North Am* 2001; **15**: 677–701.

82 Matthews DC, Appelbaum FR, Eary JF et al. Phase I study of ^{131}I-anti-CD45 antibody plus cyclophosphamide and total body irradiation for advanced acute leukemia and myelodysplastic syndrome. *Blood* 1999; **94**: 1237–47.

83 Storb RF, Champlin R, Riddell SR, Murata M, Bryant S, Warren EH. Non-myeloablative transplants for malignant disease. *Hematology (Am Soc Hematol Educ Program)* 2001; 375–91.

84 Weiden PL, Flournoy N, Thomas ED et al. Antileukemic effect of graft-versus-host disease in human recipients of allogeneic-marrow grafts. *N Engl J Med* 1979; **300**: 1068–73.

85 Weiden PL, Sullivan KM, Flournoy N, Storb R, Thomas ED. Antileukemic effect of chronic graft-versus-host disease: contribution to improved survival after allogeneic marrow transplantation. *N Engl J Med* 1981; **304**: 1529–33.

86 Locatelli F, Zecca M, Rondelli R et al. Graft versus host disease prophylaxis with low-dose cyclosporine-A reduces the risk of relapse in children with acute leukemia given HLA-identical sibling bone marrow transplantation: results of a randomized trial. *Blood* 2000; **95**: 1572–9.

87 Riddell SR, Murata M, Bryant S, Warren EH. T-cell therapy of leukemia. *Cancer Control* 2002; **9**: 114–22.

88 Schaap N, Schattenberg A, Bar B et al. Induction of graft-versus-leukemia to prevent relapse after partially lymphocyte-depleted allogeneic bone marrow transplantation by pre-emptive donor leukocyte infusions. *Leukemia* 2001; **15**: 1339–46.

89 Link CJ Jr, Traynor A, Seregina T, Burt RK. Adoptive immunotherapy for leukemia: donor lymphocytes transduced with the herpes simplex thymidine kinase gene. *Cancer Treat Res* 1999; **101**: 369–75.

90 Horowitz MM, Gale RP, Sondel PM et al. Graft-versus-leukemia reactions after bone marrow transplantation. *Blood* 1990; **75**: 555–62.

91 Gale RP, Horowitz MM, Ash RC et al. Identical-twin bone marrow transplants for leukemia. *Ann Intern Med* 1994; **120**: 646–52.

92 Ringden O, Labopin M, Gorin NC et al. Is there a graft-versus-leukaemia effect in the absence of graft-versus-host disease in patients undergoing bone marrow transplantation for acute leukaemia? *Br J Haematol* 2000; **111**: 1130–7.

93 Nabhan C, Mehta J, Tallman MS. The role of bone marrow transplantation in acute promyelocytic leukemia. *Bone Marrow Transplant* 2001; **28**: 219–26.

94 Pui CH, Ribeiro RC, Campana D et al. Prognostic factors in the acute lymphoid and myeloid leukemias of infants. *Leukemia* 1996; **10**: 952–6.

95 Satake N, Maseki N, Nishiyama M et al. Chromosome abnormalities and MLL rearrangements in acute myeloid leukemia of infants. *Leukemia* 1999; **13**: 1013–7.

96 Kawasaki H, Isoyama K, Eguchi M et al. Superior outcome of infant acute myeloid leukemia with intensive chemotherapy: results of the Japan Infant Leukemia Study Group. *Blood* 2001; **98**: 3589–94.

97 Arceci RJ. Progress and controversies in the treatment of pediatric acute myelogenous leukemia. *Curr Opin Hematol* 2002; **9**: 353–60.

98 Nguyen S, Leblanc T, Fenaux P et al. A white blood cell index as the main prognostic factor in t(8;21) acute myeloid leukemia (AML): a survey of 161 cases from the French AML Intergroup. *Blood* 2002; **99**: 3517–23.

99 Dahl GV, Lacayo NJ, Brophy N et al. Mitoxantrone, etoposide, and cyclosporine therapy in pediatric patients with recurrent or refractory acute myeloid leukemia. *J Clin Oncol* 2000; **18**: 1867–75.

100 Appelbaum FR, Clift RA, Buckner CD et al. Allogeneic marrow transplantation for acute non-lymphoblastic leukemia after first relapse. *Blood* 1983; **61**: 949–53.

101 Campana D, Coustan-Smith E. Detection of minimal residual disease in acute leukemia by flow cytometry. *Cytometry* 1999; **38**: 139–52.

102 Buonamici S, Ottaviani E, Testoni N et al. Real-time quantitation of minimal residual disease in inv(16)-positive acute myeloid leukemia may indicate risk for clinical relapse and may identify patients in a curable state. *Blood* 2002; **99**: 443–9.

103 Tobal K, Newton J, Macheta M et al. Molecular quantitation of minimal residual disease in acute myeloid leukemia with t(8;21) can identify patients in durable remission and predict clinical relapse. *Blood* 2000; **95**: 815–9.

104 Okoshi Y, Shimizu S, Kojima H et al. Detection of minimal residual disease in a patient having acute myelogenous leukemia with t(16;21) (p11;q22) treated by allogeneic bone marrow transplantation. *Acta Haematol* 2001; **105**: 45–8.

105 Venditti A, Buccisano F, Del Poeta G et al. Level of minimal residual disease after consolidation therapy predicts outcome in acute myeloid leukemia. *Blood* 2000; **96**: 3948–52.

106 Sievers EL, Larson RA, Stadtmauer EA et al. Efficacy and safety of gemtuzumab ozogamicin in patients with CD33-positive acute myeloid leukemia in first relapse. *J Clin Oncol* 2001; **19**: 3244–54.

107 Sievers E, Arceci R, Franklin J et al. Preliminary report of an ascending dose study of gemtuzumab ozogamicin (Mylotarg™, CMA-676) in pediatric patients with acute myeloid leukemia. *Blood* 2000; **96**: 320a [Abstract].

108 Bastie JN, Suzan F, Garcia I et al. Veno-occlusive disease after an anti-CD33 therapy (gemtuzumab ozogamicin). *Br J Haematol* 2002; **116**: 924.

109 Rajvanshi P, Shulman HM, Sievers EL, McDonald GB. Hepatic sinusoidal obstruction after gemtuzumab ozogamicin (Mylotarg™) therapy. *Blood* 2002; **99**: 2310–4.

110 Sievers E, Larson R, Estey EF et al. Final report of prolonged disease-free survival in patients with acute myeloid leukemia in first relapse treated with gemtuzumab ozogamicin followed by hematopoietic stem cell transplantation. *Blood* 2002; **100**: 89a [Abstract].

111 Biggs JC, Horowitz MM, Gale RP et al. Bone marrow transplants may cure patients with acute leukemia never achieving remission with chemotherapy. *Blood* 1992; **80**: 1090–3.

112 Forman SJ, Schmidt GM, Nademanee AP et al. Allogeneic bone marrow transplantation as therapy for primary induction failure for patients with acute leukemia. *J Clin Oncol* 1991; **9**: 1570–4.

113 Davies SM, Wagner JE, Shu XO et al. Unrelated donor bone marrow transplantation for children with acute leukemia. *J Clin Oncol* 1997; **15**: 557–65.

114 Kurtzberg J, Laughlin M, Graham ML et al. Placental blood as a source of hematopoietic stem cells for transplantation into unrelated recipients. *N Engl J Med* 1996; **335**: 157–66.

115 Godder KT, Hazlett LJ, Abhyankar SH et al. Partially mismatched related-donor bone marrow transplantation for pediatric patients with acute leukemia: younger donors and absence of peripheral blasts improve outcome. *J Clin Oncol* 2000; **18**: 1856–66.

116 Handgretinger R, Klingebiel T, Lang P et al. Megadose transplantation of purified peripheral blood $CD34^+$ progenitor cells from HLA-mismatched parental donors in children. *Bone Marrow Transplant* 2001; **27**: 777–83.

117 Marks DI, Bird JM, Vettenranta K et al. T cell-depleted unrelated donor bone marrow transplantation for acute myeloid leukemia. *Biol Blood Marrow Transplant* 2000; **6**: 646–53.

118 Kernan NA, Bartsch G, Ash RC et al. Analysis of 462 transplantations from unrelated donors facil-

versus bone marrow transplantation in pediatric acute myeloid leukemia. A matter of controversies. *Blood* 2001; **97**: 3671–2.

itated by the National Marrow Donor Program. *N Engl J Med* 1993; **328**: 593–602.
119 Keever-Taylor CA. Immune reconstitution following allogeneic transplantation. In: Soiffer RJ, ed. *Hematopoietic Stem Cell Transplantation*. Totowa, NJ: Humana Press, Inc., 2003, in press.
120 Ho VT, Soiffer RJ. The history and future of T-cell depletion as graft-versus-host disease prophylaxis for allogeneic hematopoietic stem cell transplantation. *Blood* 2001; **98**: 3192–204.
121 Sierra J, Storer B, Hansen JA et al. Unrelated donor marrow transplantation for acute myeloid leukemia: an update of the Seattle experience. *Bone Marrow Transplant* 2000; **26**: 397–404.
122 Wagner JE, King R, Kollman C et al. Unrelated donor bone marrow transplantation in 5075 patients with malignant and non-malignant disorders: impact of marrow T cell depletion. *Blood* 1998; **92**: 686a [Abstract].
123 Wagner JE, Thompson JS, Carter S, Jensen L, Kernan NA. Impact of graft-versus-host disease (GVHD) prophylaxis on 3-year disease-free survival (DFS): results of a multi-center, randomized phase II–III trial comparing T cell depletion/cyclosporine (TCD) and methotrexate/cyclosporine (M/C) in 410 recipients of unrelated donor bone marrow (BM). *Blood* 2002; **100**: 75a [Abstract].
124 Rocha V, Cornish J, Sievers EL et al. Comparison of outcomes of unrelated bone marrow and umbilical cord blood transplants in children with acute leukemia. *Blood* 2001; **97**: 2962–71.
125 Barker JN, Davies SM, DeFor T, Ramsay NK, Weisdorf DJ, Wagner JE. Survival after transplantation of unrelated donor umbilical cord blood is comparable to that of human leukocyte antigen-matched unrelated donor bone marrow: results of a matched-pair analysis. *Blood* 2001; **97**: 2957–61.
126 Wagner JE, Barker JN, DeFor TE et al. Transplantation of unrelated donor umbilical cord blood in 102 patients with malignant and nonmalignant diseases: influence of CD34 cell dose and HLA disparity on treatment-related mortality and survival. *Blood* 2002; **100**: 1611–8.
127 Michel G, Rocha V, Arcese W et al. Unrelated cord blood transplantation for childhood AML. *Blood* 2002; **100**: 41a [Abstract].
128 Aversa F, Tabilio A, Velardi A et al. Treatment of high-risk acute leukemia with T-cell-depleted stem cells from related donors with one fully mismatched HLA haplotype. *N Engl J Med* 1998; **339**: 1186–93.
129 Aversa F, Terenzi A, Carotti A et al. Improved outcome with T-cell-depleted bone marrow transplantation for acute leukemia. *J Clin Oncol* 1999; **17**: 1545–50.
130 Ruggeri L, Capanni M, Urbani E et al. Effectiveness of donor natural killer cell alloreactivity in mismatched hematopoietic transplants. *Science* 2002; **295**: 2097–100.
131 Chiang KY, Weisdorf DJ, Davies SM et al. Outcome of second bone marrow transplantation following a uniform conditioning regimen as therapy for malignant relapse. *Bone Marrow Transplant* 1996; **17**: 39–42.
132 Michallet M, Tanguy ML, Socie G et al. Second allogeneic haematopoietic stem cell transplantation in relapsed acute and chronic leukaemias for patients who underwent a first allogeneic bone marrow transplantation: a survey of the Sociéte Francaise de Greffe de Moelle (SFGM). *Br J Haematol* 2000; **108**: 400–7.

133 Bosi A, Bacci S, Miniero R et al. Second allogeneic bone marrow transplantation in acute leukemia: a multicenter study from the Gruppo Italiano Trapianto Di Midollo Osseo (GITMO). *Leukemia* 1997; **11**: 420–4.
134 Levine JE, Braun T, Penza SL et al. Prospective trial of chemotherapy and donor leukocyte infusions for relapse of advanced myeloid malignancies after allogeneic stem-cell transplantation. *J Clin Oncol* 2002; **20**: 405–12.
135 de Lima M, Bonamino M, Vasconcelos Z et al. Prophylactic donor lymphocyte infusions after moderately ablative chemotherapy and stem cell transplantation for hematological malignancies: high remission rate among poor prognosis patients at the expense of graft-versus-host disease. *Bone Marrow Transplant* 2001; **27**: 73–8.
136 Bader P, Klingebiel T, Schaudt A et al. Prevention of relapse in pediatric patients with acute leukemias and MDS after allogeneic SCT by early immunotherapy initiated on the basis of increasing mixed chimerism: a single center experience of 12 children. *Leukemia* 1999; **13**: 2079–86.
137 Bader P, Beck J, Schlegel PG, Handgretinger R, Niethammer D, Klingebiel T. Additional immunotherapy on the basis of increasing mixed hematopoietic chimerism after allogeneic BMT in children with acute leukemia: is there an option to prevent relapse? *Bone Marrow Transplant* 1997; **20**: 79–81.
138 Mehta J, Powles R, Kulkarni S, Treleaven J, Singhal S. Induction of graft-versus-host disease as immunotherapy of leukemia relapsing after allogeneic transplantation: single-center experience of 32 adult patients. *Bone Marrow Transplant* 1997; **20**: 129–35.
139 Sica S, Di Mario A, Salutari P et al. Chemotherapy and recombinant human granulocyte colony-stimulating factor primed donor leukocyte infusion for treatment of relapse after allogeneic bone marrow transplantation. *Bone Marrow Transplant* 1995; **16**: 483–5.
140 Buzyn-Veil A, Belanger C, Audat F et al. Sustained complete cytologic and molecular remission induced by donor leucocyte infusions alone in an acute myeloblastic leukaemia in relapse after bone marrow transplantation. *Br J Haematol* 1996; **92**: 423–5.
141 Pati AR, Godder K, Lamb L, Gee A, Henslee-Downey PJ. Immunotherapy with donor leukocyte infusions for patients with relapsed acute myeloid leukemia following partially mismatched related donor bone marrow transplantation. *Bone Marrow Transplant* 1995; **15**: 979–81.
142 Kolb HJ, Schattenberg A, Goldman JM et al. Graft-versus-leukemia effect of donor lymphocyte transfusions in marrow grafted patients. European Group for Blood and Marrow Transplantation Working Party Chronic Leukemia. *Blood* 1995; **86**: 2041–50.
143 Collins RH Jr, Shpilberg O, Drobyski WR et al. Donor leukocyte infusions in 140 patients with relapsed malignancy after allogeneic bone marrow transplantation. *J Clin Oncol* 1997; **15**: 433–44.
144 Drobyski WR, Hessner MJ, Klein JP et al. T-cell depletion plus salvage immunotherapy with donor leukocyte infusions as a strategy to treat chronic-phase chronic myelogenous leukemia patients undergoing HLA-identical sibling marrow transplantation. *Blood* 1999; **94**: 434–41.
145 Drobyski WR, Endean DJ, Klein JP, Hessner MJ. Detection of *BCR/ABL* RNA transcripts using the polymerase chain reaction is highly predictive for relapse in patients transplanted with unrelated marrow grafts for chronic myelogenous leukaemia. *Br J Haematol* 1997; **98**: 458–66.
146 Szomor A, Passweg JR, Tichelli A, Hoffmann T, Speck B, Gratwohl A. Myeloid leukemia and myelodysplastic syndrome relapsing as granulocytic sarcoma (chloroma) after allogeneic bone marrow transplantation. *Ann Hematol* 1997; **75**: 239–41.
147 Seo S, Kami M, Honda H et al. Extramedullary relapse in the so-called 'sanctuary' sites for chemotherapy after donor lymphocyte infusion. *Bone Marrow Transplant* 2000; **25**: 226–7.
148 Bekassy AN, Hermans J, Gorin NC, Gratwohl A. Granulocytic sarcoma after allogeneic bone marrow transplantation: a retrospective European multicenter survey. Acute and Chronic Leukemia Working Parties of the European Group for Blood and Marrow Transplantation. *Bone Marrow Transplant* 1996; **17**: 801–8.
149 Leahey AM, Teunissen H, Friedman DL, Moshang T, Lange BJ, Meadows AT. Late effects of chemotherapy compared to bone marrow transplantation in the treatment of pediatric acute myeloid leukemia and myelodysplasia. *Med Pediatr Oncol* 1999; **32**: 163–9.
150 Liesner RJ, Leiper AD, Hann IM, Chessells JM. Late effects of intensive treatment for acute myeloid leukemia and myelodysplasia in childhood. *J Clin Oncol* 1994; **12**: 916–24.
151 Michel G, Socie G, Gebhard F et al. Late effects of allogeneic bone marrow transplantation for children with acute myeloblastic leukemia in first complete remission: the impact of conditioning regimen without total-body irradiation. A report from the Sociéte Francaise de Greffe de Moelle. *J Clin Oncol* 1997; **15**: 2238–46.
152 Kupst MJ, Penati B, Debban B et al. Cognitive and psychosocial functioning of pediatric hematopoietic stem cell transplant patients: a prospective longitudinal study. *Bone Marrow Transplant* 2002; **30**: 609–17.
153 Jemal A, Thomas A, Murray T, Thun M. Cancer statistics, 2002. *CA Cancer J Clin* 2002; **52**: 23–47.
154 Creutzig U, Reinhardt D. Current controversies: which patients with acute myeloid leukaemia should receive a bone marrow transplantation? A European view. *Br J Haematol* 2002; **118**: 365–77.
155 Davies SM, Alonzo TA, Lange B et al. Reduced survival in black children with acute myeloid leukemia. A Children's Cancer Group Study. *Blood* 2002; **100**: 35a [Abstract].
156 Gibson B, Webb D, de-Graf S, Wheatley K. Improved outcome in MRC AML 12 paediatrics: has the limit of conventional chemotherapy been reached? *Blood* 2002; **100**: 35a [Abstract].
157 Gilliland DG. Murky waters for MRD detection in AML. Flighty *FLT3/ITD*s. *Blood* 2002; **100**: 2277b [Abstract].
158 Shih LY, Huang CF, Wu JH et al. Internal tandem duplication of *FLT3* in relapsed acute myeloid leukemia: a comparative analysis of bone marrow samples from 108 adult patients at diagnosis and relapse. *Blood* 2002; **100**: 2387–92.
159 Kottaridis PD, Gale RE, Langabeer SE, Frew ME, Bowen DT, Linch DC. Studies of *FLT3* mutations in paired presentation and relapse samples from patients with acute myeloid leukemia: implications for the role of *FLT3* mutations in leukemogenesis, minimal residual disease detection, and possible therapy with *FLT3* inhibitors. *Blood* 2002; **100**: 2393–8.

160 Lewis ID, Almeida-Porada GJ, Du J et al. Umbilical cord blood cells capable of engrafting in primary, secondary, and tertiary xenogeneic hosts are preserved after *ex vivo* culture in a noncontact system. *Blood* 2001; **97**: 3441–9.

161 Kim DW, Oh IH, Chung YJ et al. Cotransplantation of mesenchymal stem cells suppress donor-deviated engraftment in mixed double cord transplantion using two unrelated donors. *Blood* 2002; **100**: 172a [Abstract].

162 Barker JN, Weisdorf D, DeFor T, McGlave P, Wagner JE. Multiple unit unrelated donor umbilical cord blood transplantation in high risk adults with hematologic malignancies. Impact on engraftment and chimerism. *Blood* 2002; **100**: 41a [Abstract].

163 Eapen M, Klein JP, Champlin R et al. Increased chronic graft versus host disease and mortality after peripheral blood stem cell transplantation in older children and adolescents with acute leukemia. *Blood* 2002; **100**: 145a [Abstract].

164 Keever-Taylor CA, Margolis D, Konings S et al. Cytomegalovirus-specific cytolytic T-cell lines and clones generated against adenovirus-pp65-infected dendritic cells. *Biol Blood Marrow Transplant* 2001; **7**: 247–56.

165 Mutis T, Goulmy E. Hematopoietic system-specific antigens as targets for cellular immunotherapy of hematological malignancies. *Semin Hematol* 2002; **39**: 23–31.

166 Ostankovitch M, Buzyn A, Bonhomme D et al. Antileukemic HLA-restricted T-cell clones generated with naturally processed peptides eluted from acute myeloblastic leukemia blasts. *Blood* 1998; **92**: 19–24.

167 Munker R, Gunther W, Kolb HJ. New concepts about graft-versus-host and graft-versus-leukaemia reactions. A summary of the 5th International Symposium held in Munich, 21 and 22 March 2002. *Bone Marrow Transplant* 2002; **30**: 549–56.

77

Stephen J. Forman

Allogeneic Hematopoietic Cell Transplantation for Acute Lymphoblastic Leukemia in Adults

Acute lymphoblastic leukemia (ALL) is a hematologic malignancy characterized by rapid proliferation and subsequent accumulation of immature lymphocytes. ALL accounts for 20% of all acute leukemias seen in adults over 20 years of age and affects approximately two persons per 100,000 in the USA annually. Over the past decade, there has been substantial improvement in the management of adult patients with ALL [1]. The success of therapy for children with ALL fueled the quest for a similar success rate in adults with this disease utilizing intensive remission induction therapy and the concept of post-remission consolidation and maintenance therapies.

Recent laboratory and clinical studies have contributed greatly to the understanding of the biology of ALL and its prognostic features. This insight has led to more precise classification of the disease and the development of individualized treatment programs, as well as improvement in the means of assessing the success of therapy (measurement of minimal residual disease [MRD]). Despite documented improvements in the long-term survival of adult patients with certain phenotypes of ALL, the results have not been as good as those achieved in children. Several large studies have shown that complete remissions can now be achieved in 80–90% of newly diagnosed adult patients under the age of 60 years [2–5]. With modern intensive chemotherapy, approximately 30% of adult patients can achieve a cure of the disease [1–5]. Over the past 30 years, high-dose chemoradiotherapy followed by allogeneic hematopoietic cell transplantation (HCT) has resulted in long-term disease-free survival (DFS) in some patients with advanced or relapsed disease and has also been successfully utilized in patients with high-risk disease transplanted in first remission. This chapter reviews the biology of adult ALL, the relationship of specific disease characteristics to the natural history and treatment of adult ALL and the role of allogeneic HCT in the management of adult patients with this disease.

Diagnosis, classification and biology of adult ALL

Morphology

Similar to the molecular diversity of acute myeloid leukemia (AML), ALL also comprises a heterogeneous group of disorders based on morphologic, immunologic and, most importantly, cytogenetic characteristics. These features also have emerged as important prognostic indicators and therefore have become highly relevant in the decision-making about the timing of allogeneic HCT. Classically, the French–American–British (FAB) morphologic classification has defined three types of leukemic blasts: L1, L2 and L3 [6,7]. This classification is based on the spectrum of microscopic appearances of these cells. In childhood ALL, 85% of the patients have L1 morphology while adult ALL patients more commonly display L2 features. With the exception of distinguishing the L3 morphology and its associated cytogenetic and clinical behavior, morphology has not been useful in the treatment of adult patients with ALL.

Immunophenotyping

Immunophenotyping by flow cytometry has become an important part of the diagnostic evaluation of a patient with an acute lymphoid malignancy [8–10]. In the initial assessment of acute leukemia patients, a limited panel of monoclonal antibodies (MABs) allows patients to be divided into those with ALL derived from either B lymphocytes (B lineage) or T lymphocytes (T lineage) and to distinguish patients with ALL from patients with AML [10–12]. The precise immunologic characterization of the blasts also allows distinction between minimally differentiated AML (M0 by FAB) and acute undifferentiated leukemia. Both of these forms of acute leukemia lack lymphoid surface markers. Table 77.1 shows the immunologic and morphologic classification of ALL [10,13].

Occasional patients may have hybrid acute leukemia where the blast cells express both myeloid and lymphoid cell surface antigens [10,14,15]. The leukemias may be either bilineal where such features are seen on separate cell populations, or biphenotypic where antigens are detected on the same cell. In general, when there is more than one population of cells, therapy is usually directed at the predominant cell type in a mixed population. Approximately 20% of cases of ALL in adults express both myeloid and lymphoid antigens. This occurs more commonly in B-lineage than T-lineage ALL. There has been some controversy as to whether the coexpression of myeloid antigens on cells of an ALL phenotype confer a poor prognosis [14,15]. However, it appears that recent improvements in the treatment of adult ALL have overcome the poor prognosis formerly associated with myeloid antigen expression in adult patients who have ALL [1,5].

Except for those leukemias with FAB L3 morphology whose cells express surface immunoglobulin, a marker of more mature B lineage, most cases of ALL are strongly positive for the terminal deoxynucleotidyl transferase (TdT) enzyme.

Cytogenetics

As with cases of AML, cytogenetic analysis has emerged as a very important part of the classification and therapeutic decision making for patients with ALL. In two studies, clonal chromosomal aberrations could be detected in cells from 62% to 85% of adult patients with ALL [16,17]. The most predictable clinical outcomes for patients with ALL have been in patients who have been classified according to their specific cytogenetic abnormality. The major cytogenetic abnormalities in ALL are the

Table 77.1 Immunologic classification of adult acute lymphoblastic anemia (ALL) [13].

Leukemia subtype	Most important surface markers	Frequency (%)	Frequent cytogenetic aberrations
B-lineage	HLA-DR+, TdT+, CD19+	76	
Early pre-B	CD10−	11	t(4;11)
Common	CD10+	51	t(9;22)
			9p aberr
			12p aberr
			Hyperdiploid
Pre-B	CD10±, cyIgM+	10	t(1;19)
			t(9;22)
			Hyperdiploid
Mature B	TdT±, CD10±, sIgM+	4	t(8;14)
			t(8;22)
			t(2;8)
T-lineage	TdT+, cyCD3+, CD7+	24	
Early T	CD2−, sCD3−, CD1a−	6	t(11;14)
Thymic T	sCD3±, CD1a+	12	t(10;14)
Mature T	sCD3+, CD1a−	5	9p aberr

IgM, immunoglobulin M; TdT, terminal deoxynucleotidyl transferase.

Table 77.2 Chromosomal abnormalities in adult acute lymphoblastic anemia (ALL) [16–18].

	Frequency (%) (n = 793)
Clonal abnormalities	68–85
Normal diploid	15–34
Numerical aberrations	
Hypodiploid	4–8
Hyperdiploid (47–50)	7–15
Hyperdiploid (>50)	7–8
Near tri/tetraploid	3–5
Structural aberrations	
t(9;22)	11–29
t(4;11)	3–4
t(8;14)	5
t(1;19)	2–3
t(10;14)	3
9p abnormalities	5–15
6q abnormalities	4–6
12p abnormalities	4–5

clonal translocations t(9;22), t(4;11), t(1;19) or t(8;14) and other structural abnormalities (9p, 6q or 12p). The leukemic cell can also be classified by the modal number of chromosomes in the cell (Table 77.2).

The most common cytogenetic abnormality in adult ALL is the Philadelphia (Ph) chromosome, which results from a reciprocal translocation between the long arms of chromosomes 9 and 22, t(9;22) and (q34;q11). This translocation occurs in >95% of patients with chronic myeloid leukemia (CML) and up to 30% of adult patients with ALL with a frequency increasing with age [18–20]. Molecular analyses have established that the Ph translocation results in the joining of the 3′ sequences of the tyrosine kinase c-abl proto-oncogene on chromosome 9 to the 5′ sequences of the bcr gene on chromosome 22. In CML and some ALL cases, the Ph breakpoint occurs within a 5.8-kb region on chromosome 22 known as the major breakpoint cluster region (m-bcr) of the bcr gene.

This bcr-abl transcript encodes the chimeric p210 protein; however, in >50% of Ph chromosome positive ALL cases, the breakpoint in the bcr gene occurs 5′ to the m-bcr region and the subsequent rearrangement with the abl gene yields a shorter version (7.0 kb) of the bcr-abl mRNA with expression producing 190 kDa fusion protein. Like the chimeric RNA associated with CML, both the p210 and p190 chimeric RNAs can be detected by polymerase chain reaction (PCR) and thus are useful both in the diagnosis and follow-up of patients with this subtype of ALL (see Chapter 22) [21].

The second most common translocation is between chromosomes 4 and 11, t(4;11), q21;q23. Most of these patients have an L2 morphology. This type of ALL is often associated with a high white blood cell count (WBC) and occurs frequently in children under the age of 1 year [22–24]. Abnormalities of the long arm of chromosome 11 involving band q23 have been reported to occur frequently in a wide range of hematologic malignancies. Most ALL patients with abnormalities of chromosome 11 have the t(4;11) translocation. It is found in approximately 6% of adult ALL cases and is usually confined to the B-lineage group. The cells often show coexpression of myeloid antigen, and the median presenting WBC is very high, often >100,000/mL.

Mature B-cell ALL is a rare ALL subtype that compromises only 2–4% of patients. As noted above, these cases have L3 morphology, express monoclonal surface immunoglobulin and a specific nonrandom chromosomal translocation (8;14) (see below).

Prognostic features

Many studies of ALL have examined prognostic factors present at diagnosis to determine the intensity and type of therapy including allogeneic HCT that should be administered to the patient. Utilizing morphologic criteria, most studies have found no difference in remission rate or DFS in L1 or L2 morphologies. Initially, data in the L3 subtype suggested that these patients had lower remission rates, shorter durations of remission and a high incidence of central nervous system (CNS) leukemia, similar to Burkitt's lymphoma [25]. However, more recent studies have shown improved outcome of adult B-cell ALL when patients receive treatment with a shorter but more intensive chemotherapy strategy utilizing a regimen that includes high-dose methotrexate (MTX) and fractionated higher

Table 77.3 Treatment outcome with T-cell acute lymphoblastic anemia (ALL).

Trial	Reference	No. patients (%)	Probability CCR CR (%)	Median survival Percent (yr)	(months)
CALGB 8811	[3]	39 (28)	38 (97)	63 (3)	>40
UCSF/SU/COH	[2]	19 (21)	18 (95)	59 (5)	NR
LALA87	[30]	150 (26)	122 (81)	48 (3)*	25
GMALLO1	[4]	50 (22)	41 (82)	55 (5)	NR

CALGB, Cancer and Leukemia Group B; CCR, continuous complete remission; CR, complete remission; GMALLO1, German Multicenter Study Group for Treatment of Adult Acute; LALA87, French Group on Therapy for Adult Acute Lymphoblastic Leukemia; NR, not reported; UCSF/SU/COH, University of California San Francisco, Stanford University, City of Hope National Medical Center.
*Disease-free survival.

doses of cyclophosphamide (CY) or ifosfamide [26,27]. Reports from Frankfurt, Germany indicate a complete remission rate of 74% and a DFS of 71% with a major decrease in CNS relapses, most likely attributable to the high dose MTX and triple drug intrathecal therapy. DFS in these patients with L3 subtype was influenced by the initial WBC with patients with <50,000/mL having a 71% DFS vs. 29% for those with the high WBC numbers. Patients who required more than one cycle of therapy to achieve a remission also fared poorly [26].

Increasing age is an adverse prognostic factor for complete remission (CR) rate and survival in patients with adult ALL [28]. Most modern chemotherapy studies show that, for patients <30 years old, the CR rate can increase to 95% but falls with increasing age. A WBC count >30,000/mL is a negative prognostic factor that affects the duration of remission in patients with B-lineage ALL but not in T-cell ALL [13,29].

Studies in adults utilizing combination chemotherapy suggests that T-cell ALL, which formerly had a very poor prognosis in children and adults, is now considered the most favorable subgroup [2]. This phenotype, which accounts for 25% of patients with adult ALL, often presents with an increased WBC and a mediastinal mass. Table 77.3 shows the treatment outcome for T-cell ALL in the four large series reported to date [2–4,31,32]. A high initial WBC is not as clearly associated with a poor prognosis in patients with T-ALL lineage. The presence of a mediastinal mass, which is often found in patients with T-cell ALL, also correlates with long remission duration and survival, probably related to the T-cell phenotype. With the exception of T-cell ALL, the WBC count at presentation influences the remission rate as well as the duration of remission.

Several studies have indicated that the rate of achievement of remission (i.e. disappearance of blasts in the marrow) has a significant impact on the long-term DFS. Those patients who require more than one cycle of therapy to achieve remission have a poor prognosis regardless of the absence of other factors [2–4]. Table 77.4 lists the adverse prognostic features in adult ALL. Table 77.5 shows the impact of four of these adverse features on the outcome of treatment of ALL in two studies from the Cancer and Leukemia Group B (CALGB 8811/9111) [29,33]. Table 77.5 also demonstrates that a large number of adult patients with ALL have features of their disease at diagnosis that would predict for a DFS <50% [29,33].

The presence of specific cytogenetic abnormalities influences more the duration of rather than the rate of remission. Those with a particularly poor prognosis include those patients with the Ph chromosome or translocations involving t(4;11). These karyotypes represent independent adverse risk factors regardless of age, immune phenotype or initial WBC. Some investigators have hypothesized that the poor long-term outcome of pre-B common ALL in adults is explained by the higher frequency of the 9;22 translocation and the relative resistance to chemotherapy of this type of ALL [2].

Table 77.4 Adverse prognostic features in adult acute lymphoblastic anemia (ALL).

1. Age above 50 years
2. WBC >30,000 µL
3. Pre-B, early T, mature T
4. Lack of mediastinal adenopathy
5. Poor performance status at diagnosis
6. t(9;22) or *bcr-abl* rearrangement
7. t(4;11), t(1;19), t(8;14)
8. More than 4 weeks of induction therapy to achieve remission

WBC, white blood cell count.

Table 77.5 Impact of four adverse features on the outcome of treatment of acute lymphoblastic anemia (ALL) [3].

| No. adverse features | No. patients | Adverse features | | | | Estimated survival at 3 years (95%CI) |
		Age ≥60 year	WB ≥30,000/mL	Absence of mediastinal mass	Laboratory features*	
0	22	0	0	0	0	91% (66–98%)
1	83	1	16	63	3	64% (51–75%)
2	146	12	25	145	110	49% (36–61%)
3	89	25	68	89	85	21% (12–35%)
4	13	13	13	13	13	0

*Adverse laboratory features include L3 morphology or B/B-myeloid immunophenotype or Ph+/*bcr-abl*+ genetics.

Table 77.6 Survival of adult ALL by cytogenetic subset [33]. (Adapted from Cancer and Leukemia Group B.)

Karyotype	No.	Overall survival		
		Median (year)	5-year (%)	p*
Normal	79	2.9	37	
t(9;22)	67	1.3	11	<0.001
+8	23	1.3	12	0.004
t(4;11)	17	0.8	18	<0.001
–7	14	1.3	14	0.01
+21	32	1.5	26	0.06
del(9p) or t(9p)	28	1.3	38	0.58
del(12p) or t(12p)	11	6.8	82	0.10
t(14q11)	9	7.4	78	0.04

*p value from the log–rank test for the difference in survival for each cytogenetic subset compared with patients with a normal karyotype.

Table 77.6 shows patient survival in clinical trials of adult ALL by cytogenetic subset. Compared to patients with normal cytogenetics, many of the specific chromosomal abnormalities predict for poor survival despite intensive post-remission chemotherapy [34].

Allogeneic HCT for patients with ALL

An early demonstration of the potential of HCT in the treatment of advanced ALL occurred in 1959 when a child with relapsed ALL underwent high-dose total body irradiation (TBI) followed by marrow from an identical twin. Hematological recovery was rapid and a CR was achieved that lasted 6 months without maintenance therapy (see Chapter 1). In 1974, Fefer et al. [35] reported 16 patients with advanced leukemia who received marrow grafts from identical twins following chemotherapy and TBI. Three were alive and well 30 years later. In 1977, Thomas et al. [36] reported 100 patients with advanced leukemia treated with TBI-containing regimens and marrow from matched sibling donors. Six of 46 with ALL achieved unmaintained remissions of >5 years, two of whom were alive and well 29 and 28 years later, respectively. Almost all relapses occurred during the first 5 years after HCT and late deaths were brought about by complications of graft-vs.-host disease (GVHD) or hepatitis, the latter presumably related to multiple blood transfusions before blood donor screening became available. These results in end-stage patients with leukemia provided the basis for examination of the role of allogeneic HCT in other clinical circumstances.

In 1979, the investigators from Seattle also reported 22 patients with ALL who underwent bone marrow transplantation (BMT) in second or subsequent remission and were compared with a concurrent group of 26 patients receiving transplants in relapse utilizing an identical conditioning regimen [37]. The results showed that patients in remission had a lower incidence of recurrent leukemia, a lower death rate from nonleukemic causes and improved survival. Of those patients transplanted in remission, more than half were alive and in remission 1–3 years after marrow grafting.

Allogeneic HCT for adult patients with ALL beyond first remission

Although remarkable strides have been made in the primary therapy of newly diagnosed adult patients with ALL, many will suffer a relapse following successful induction of remission. The primary cause of failure following chemotherapy is recurrence of leukemia with relapses occurring in the marrow or in extramedullary sites such as the testes or the CNS. Treatment of relapse usually employs standard doses of chemotherapy to achieve a second remission. Although in earlier trials, the rate of second remission was higher than 50%, the current intensive chemotherapy regimens utilized to achieve long-term DFS also selects cells for chemotherapy resistance. Currently, when a patient suffers a leukemic relapse, the ability to achieve a second remission of ALL is less than it was in the 1980s and is related to the duration of the first remission. Even in those patients who achieve a second remission, its duration is usually <6 months and nearly all patients succumb to their disease. In the adult patient, except for those unusual patients who have very late relapses off chemotherapy, allogeneic HCT from a histocompatible sibling donor offers the best chance for DFS.

The experience of allogeneic HCT for patients in second remission is summarized in Table 77.7. In some of these studies, the data for adults and children are reported together. Allogeneic HCT for ALL patients with advanced disease results in DFS of approximately 20–40%, superior to any other form of therapy [38–47]. Recent results from the International Bone Marrow Transplant Registry (IBMTR) on 388 patients >20 years who were in second remission and underwent transplantation from a matched sibling show a probability of survival at 5 years of 30% [48]. Thus, although HCT could be performed at a later time, there does not appear to be any reason to delay transplantation until another relapse has occurred in the adult patients with recurrent ALL. Not surprisingly, the main cause of failure after HCT in this group of patients is leukemic recurrence. Figure 77.1 shows the impact of remission status on subsequent relapse and survival in 182 patients who underwent allogeneic transplant in Seattle [49].

A difficult clinical decision for a patient suffering leukemic relapse who has a histocompatible sibling donor is whether to attempt reinduction therapy or proceed directly to HCT. In addition to the difficulty in achieving a second remission, patients have a risk for acquiring secondary complications such as fungal infections that complicate the use of potential curative therapy such as HCT. The current experience with patients with ALL suggests that those patients who relapse early while on chemotherapy should probably proceed directly to allogeneic HCT, whereas those patients who relapse either late on maintenance therapy or off therapy after a long first remission could benefit from reinduction therapy in order to potentially improve the outcome after HCT [48].

Unrelated HCT for advanced ALL

In general, for patients suffering a relapse of ALL, HCT from a human leucocyte antigen (HLA) matched sibling is the best therapeutic approach. However, given the poor outcome for adult patients with ALL suffering a relapse, if a family member cannot be identified who is either matched or mismatched at only a single class I or class II antigen, then a search for an unrelated donor should be pursued. While unrelated donor grafts are often associated with more GVHD and other complications, the compensatory decrease in relapse rates *plus* recent innovations in supportive care have narrowed the gap between the two hematopoietic stem cell sources for most patient groups including ALL. Recent single institution or group studies dealing with both children and adults have reported outcomes using unrelated donors that are very similar to those seen with matched sibling transplants. The Nordic Transplant Group has reported similar outcomes utilizing matched siblings and unrelated donors in both children and adults [50]. A summary reported by the IBMTR involving 4441 patients transplanted for ALL reported a DFS of 44% utilizing matched unrelated donor transplants in first remission vs. 52% for patients in first remission undergoing transplantation from matched sibling donors [48]. When the analysis was conducted on those patients in

Table 77.7 Hematopoietic cell transplantation (HCT) for acute lymphoblastic anemia (ALL) patients in second remission.

Institution	n (children)*	Preparative regimen(s)	Follow-up in years (median)	Disease-free survival (%)	Relapse (%)	Reference
Patients in CR2						
Leiden, Westminster, Basel	96 (NS)	CY/TBI	3 (1)	34	34	[38]
Seattle	48 (0)	CY/TBI	9 (2)	10	65	[39]
Johns Hopkins	36 (NS)	CY/TBI	8.9 (4.9)	43	26	[40]
City of Hope	30 (NS)	Ara-C/CY/TBI, FTBI/CY	5 (2.7)	46	30	[41]
Memorial Sloan Kettering	28 (NS)	TBI/CY	2.4 (1.2)	65	NS	[42]
Genova	25 (NS)	CY/TBI	2 (NS)	32	NS	[43]
Kiel, Ulm.Leiden (NB. CR2; >CR2)	18 (NS)	FTBI/VP16	2.9 (.6)	63	12	[44]
Westminster	11 (5)	CY/TBI (VP)	2.6 (1)	10	NS	[45]
Greinix	27	–	3.0	14	78	[46]
Michallet	47		5.0	30	44	[47]

Ara-C, cytosine arabinoside; CY, cyclophosphamide; FTBI, fractionated total body irradiation; NS, not specified; P, prednisone; TBI, total body irradiation; V, vincristine.
*Number in parenthesis represents the subgroup of children from the total number of patients.

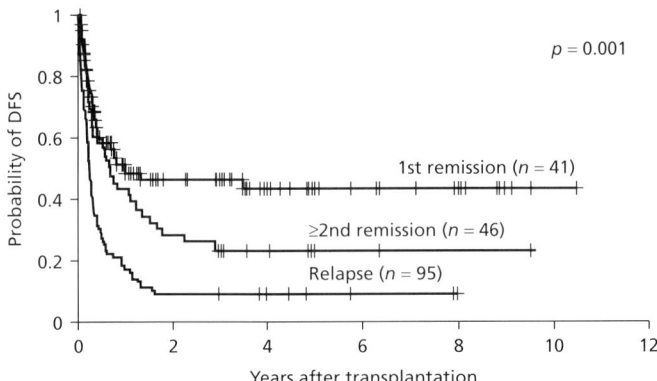

Fig. 77.1 Impact of remission status on subsequent relapse and long-term survival in 182 patients with acute lymphoblastic anemia (ALL) who underwent allogeneic transplantation. The result demonstrates a higher relapse rate for those patients transplanted after first remission and the inferior relapse-free survival in those patients with more advanced disease [49].

second remission, 35% of those patients undergoing matched unrelated donor transplants vs. 42% for patients who had a sibling donor were cured of their disease. Although there are issues related to patients surviving long enough to undergo an unrelated donor transplant, the potentially curative therapy in a patient with relapsed disease is well-documented and should be pursued for a patient with relapsed disease lacking a related donor.

Allogeneic HCT for ALL in first CR

Hoelzer et al. [4] first proposed a risk classification of adult ALL based on age, WBC, immunophenotype, cytogenetics or time to achievement of CR. This simple classification identified patients who had either good long-term DFS or poor outcome because of relapse of disease. One implication of this analysis was that it might be possible to identify patients during first remission who might benefit from early HCT from a histocompatible sibling donor when the disease burden was at a lower level and thus possibly reduce the chances of relapse. Several studies have

Table 77.8 Allogeneic hematopoietic cell transplantation (HCT) in acute lymphoblastic anemia (ALL) in first remission.

Author, year	Reference	No.	Median age (year, range)	% Disease-free survival (years)
Blume et al. (1987)	[51]	39	23 (1–41)	63
Vernant et al. (1988)	[52]	27	25 (15–44)	59
Wingard et al. (1990)	[40]	18	24 (5–36)	42
Blaise et al. (1990)	[53]	25	22 (4–36)	71
Carey et al. (1991)	[54]	15	19 (15–40)	34
Chao et al. (1991)	[55]	53	28 (1–45)	61
Doney et al. (1991)	[39]	41	22 (18–50)	21 (5 year)
Horowitz et al. (1991)	[56]	234	15–45	44
Sebban et al. (1994)	[57]	116	26 (16–45)	48 (5 year)
DeWitte et al. (1994)	[58]	22	NS	63 (5 year)
Vey et al. (1994)	[59]	29	24 (16–41)	62 (8 year)
Attal et al. (1995, 2000)	[30]	41	33	46 (10 year)
Oh et al. (1998)	[60]	87	>30	30 (5 year)
Oh et al. (1998)	[60]	127	<30	53 (5 year)
Rowe et al. (1999)	[61]	173	14–60	58
Thiebaut et al. (2000)	[62]	116	15–40	46 (10 year)
Forman et al. (2003)	[63]	117	27	64 (6 year)

investigated this approach in patients with high-risk ALL who were treated with myeloablative therapy followed by allogeneic HCT while in first CR. Table 77.8 summarizes the various reports of allogeneic HCT for ALL during first remission [30,39,51–63]. The data reported in these phase 2 and 3 trials suggest DFS for patients with high-risk ALL ranging from 30 to 63%. In one updated series of 117 patients from the City of Hope National Medical Center and Stanford University (median age 27 years; range 1–59 years), the selection criteria for transplant included WBC >25,000/mL, chromosomal translocations t(9;22), t(4;11) or t(8;14), age >30 years, extramedullary disease at diagnosis or time to achieve a CR >4 weeks [55]. Two-thirds of the patients had at least one risk factor and the remaining patients had two or more high-risk features

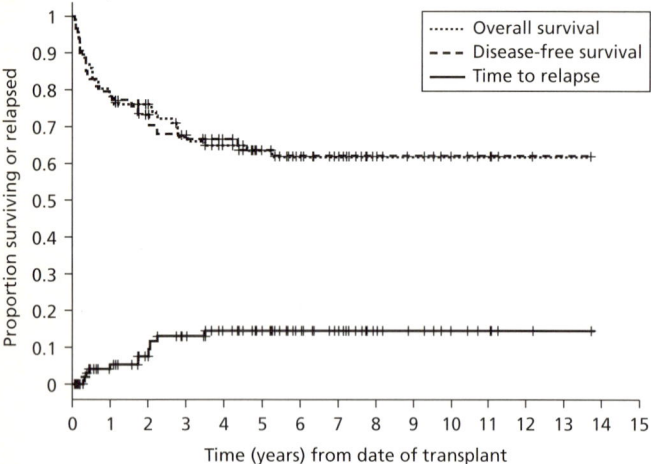

Fig. 77.2 Disease-free survival and time to relapse in 117 adult patients with high-risk acute lymphoblastic anemia (ALL) who underwent human leucocyte antigen (HLA) matched sibling non-T-cell-depleted transplant following a preparatory regimen of fractionated total body irradiation and VP16 [63].

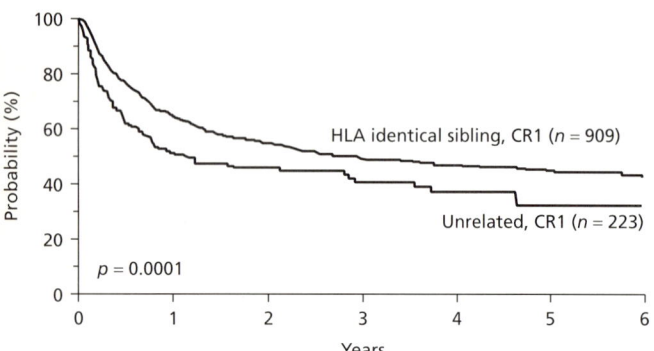

Fig. 77.3 Results of allogeneic transplantation for related or unrelated transplant for adult patients with acute lymphoblastic anemia (ALL) who underwent allogeneic transplantation in first remission [12].

Table 77.9 French Protocol LALA 87 [30,62]. Allogeneic trial $n = 257$.

	BMT		Chemotherapy		
	n	10-year survival (%)	n	10-year survival (%)	p
All	116	46	141	31	0.04
High-risk	41	44	55	11	0.009
Standard-risk	75	49	86	43	n.s.

n.s., not significant.

at presentation. The majority of these patients underwent HCT in the first 4 months after achieving a CR. As shown in Fig. 77.2, HCT in first remission led to prolonged DFS in this patient population who would otherwise have been expected to fare poorly. With a median follow-up of more than 6 years, the actual DFS was 64% with a relapse rate of 19%.

Figure 77.3 shows the results as reported from the IBMTR for allogeneic transplantation for adult ALL in patients receiving an allogeneic transplant in first remission from either an HLA identical sibling donor or an unrelated donor [48].

Although these trials present encouraging data for patients with high-risk ALL, a few randomized trials have been performed that have compared allogeneic transplant to nontransplant approaches. The French Group on Therapy for Adult ALL conducted a prospective study of post-remission therapy (allogeneic BMT, autologous BMT or chemotherapy) in 572 patients with ALL who achieved a first remission, which has now been updated [30,62]. Those with matched sibling donors were treated with allogeneic HCT, randomizing those without donors to either autologous HCT or chemotherapy. The 5-year overall DFS for the allogeneic transplant group was 46% compared to 31% for the other two groups ($p = 0.04$). In this study, there was no significant difference between chemotherapy and autologous HCT. In an analysis of specific risk groups, the advantage of allogeneic HCT was particularly striking for those patients who had high-risk disease, defined as having Ph+, null or undifferentiated ALL, patient age >35 years, WBC >30,000/mL or requiring more than 4 weeks to achieve CR. The analysis of this group of patients shows that the 10-year survival was 44% following allogeneic HCT vs. 11% for chemotherapy ($p = 0.009$). Table 77.9 shows the overall survival in this trial of the patients with ALL who underwent allogeneic HCT or continued chemotherapy during first CR. Table 77.9 shows the relative efficacy of allogeneic HCT, particularly for patients with high-risk disease.

The MRC UKALL/ECOG Trial is an international effort to prospectively define the role of allogeneic HCT, autologous HCT and chemotherapy in adult patients with ALL in first remission. The study was initiated in 1993 and over 1100 patients have now been enrolled. Based on the data presented in 1999, 173 patients received an allogeneic stem cell transplant and 426 received chemotherapy or autologous transplant [61]. The overall event-free survival for the allogeneic stem cell transplant group was 58% vs. 39% for the chemotherapy or autologous BMT group. When patients were stratified into high vs. standard risks, the difference in event-free survival became more dramatic in the high-risk subset, with allogeneic BMT showing 57% vs. chemotherapy/autologous BMT of 32%. Therefore, for patients with poor prognostic features at diagnosis and who have a histocompatible sibling donor, HCT is a very reasonable therapeutic approach to achieve cure of adult ALL.

Allogeneic HCT for patients with Philadelphia chromosome positive ALL

Ph+ ALL is a variant of ALL that carries an exceptionally poor prognosis. Although many patients can achieve a CR, the median duration is <1 year. Studies have been conducted to determine the effectiveness of allogeneic HCT for these patients and whether long-term DFS can be achieved. In one report, 27 patients with Ph+ ALL received allogeneic HCT [64]. Six of 10 patients transplanted in first CR were alive with a median follow-up of 2.4 years. Analysis of the first CR patients demonstrated an actuarial DFS of 44% with a relapse rate of 20%. Four of 17 patients transplanted with more advanced disease were alive with a median follow-up of 2 years. Figure 77.4 shows the survival curve for 23 patients with Ph+ ALL transplanted in first CR from histocompatible sibling donors [65]. The median age was 25 years. The DFS for this group of patients is 60% with a 9% incidence of relapse. This report, as well as summary data from the IBMTR, indicate that allogeneic HCT is very effective therapy for patients with Ph+ ALL, particularly while in first CR.

The poor prognosis of patients with Ph+ ALL and the optimistic results from allogeneic HCT from sibling donors have led to studies exploring the effectiveness of HCT from unrelated donors for patients who do not have a histocompatible sibling. The development of international registries of volunteer donors has facilitated this approach (see Chapter 49). A report from Seattle described the outcome of 18 patients with Ph+ ALL who underwent an allogeneic HCT from unrelated donors [66]. The median age was 25 years (range 1.1–51 years). Six patients were in first CR, one in second remission and three in first relapse. The remaining

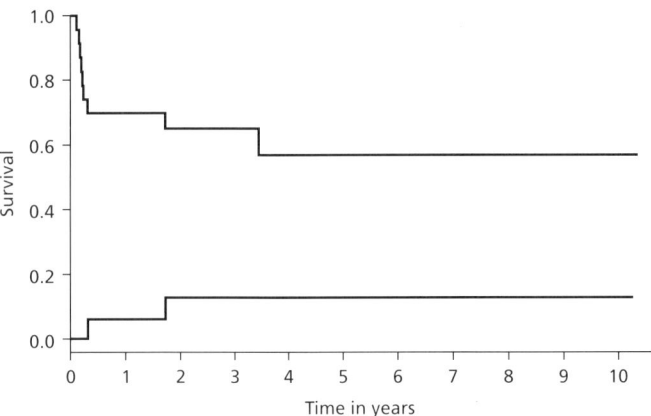

Fig. 77.4 Disease-free survival for 23 patients with Philadelphia chromosome positive acute lymphoblastic anemia (ALL) who underwent transplantation in first remission of their disease [65].

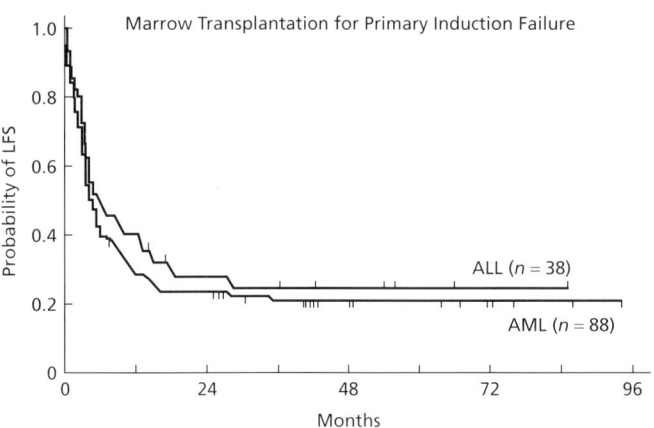

Fig. 77.5 Results of transplantation for patients with acute lymphoblastic anemia (ALL) or acute myeloid leukemia (AML) who failed to achieve a remission with initial induction therapy and then went on to allogeneic transplantation [48,110].

seven had more advanced or chemotherapy-refractory disease at the time of transplant. All were treated with cyclophosphamide (CY) and TBI followed by marrow transplantation from closely HLA matched unrelated donors. Six patients transplanted in first remission, two in first relapse and one in second remission remained alive and leukemia-free with a median follow-up of 17 months (range 9–73 months). The probability of leukemia-free survival at 2 years was 49%. These data indicate that unrelated donor HCT is an effective treatment option for patients with early stage Ph+ ALL without a related donor. Given that the duration of remission of this disease is short, an unrelated donor search should be initiated soon after diagnosis.

Allogeneic HCT for patients with ALL who do not achieve a first remission

Despite improved remission rates for patients with ALL, a small proportion of patients (10–30%) will not achieve CR, even with the best available combination chemotherapy. Often, these patients have one or more defined poor prognostic factors at presentation. After failing to enter a remission with first-line chemotherapy, these patients are usually treated again with second- or third-line regimens but these attempts are most often unsuccessful. Even when a remission is finally achieved, very few, if any, of these patients treated with chemotherapy will go on to become long-term disease-free survivors.

Allogeneic HCT has been utilized as an approach for the patient who fails induction therapy in an attempt to achieve both a remission and a cure. In a study from the City of Hope National Medical Center and Stanford University of 22 patients with primary induction failure (five of whom had ALL), all were treated with high-dose preparatory regimens followed by allogeneic HCT from a histocompatible donor [67]. Despite the poor prognosis of this patient population, all patients achieved a remission following HCT and 38% of the whole group became long-term disease-free survivors.

A report from the IBMTR on the outcome of patients undergoing transplant as treatment for primary induction failure, suggests that approximately 20% of such patients with ALL can be cured by transplantation [48]. Figure 77.5 shows a summary from the IBMTR of the results of marrow transplantation for primary induction failure in a group of patients with ALL and AML, showing a similar result for those patients with either disease who fail to achieve a remission. Thus, strong consideration should be given to tissue typing a patient at the time of diagnosis so that transplantation can be utilized both to achieve a remission as well as to achieve long-term cure of the disease in this clinical situation.

Management of the central nervous system

In general, the development of a CNS relapse in patients with ALL portends a poor prognosis both for the effect it has on the CNS and because it is a harbinger of systemic relapse. Most patients with ALL have had some form of CNS prophylaxis with radiation or chemotherapy prior to their first systemic relapse. Although children with an isolated CNS relapse can still do well with the treatment of CNS and systemic reinduction therapy, adults with an isolated CNS relapse fare poorly [68]. Patients who relapse in the CNS require additional therapy to control the disease prior to HCT. Previous prophylactic intrathecal therapy and CNS radiation does not necessarily preclude the use of TBI in the preparation for HCT. Usually, it is unnecessary to irradiate again the patient's brain or the spinal cord prior to HCT as this may lead to more neurotoxicity following transplantation. In general, these patients can be managed with either intrathecal MTX or the combination of MTX, cytosine arabinoside and hydrocortisone until there is clearing of leukemic cells from the spinal fluid. Following HCT, such patients receive five intrathecal MTX injections during the first 100 days followed by one monthly injection for 18 months. This approach, designed in Seattle, can result in control of the leukemia without substantially increasing the risk of leukoencephalopathy [69]. The risk of CNS damage caused by cranial radiation, intrathecal chemotherapy and high-dose chemotherapy has been documented and is related to the amount of intrathecal chemotherapy following the HCT procedure [69]. Currently, a common approach for patients with ALL undergoing first induction therapy without any evidence of CNS disease is to administer intrathecal MTX as prophylaxis for a total of five times prior to the HCT procedure. Cranial radiation is not necessary if the patient then receives a transplant preparatory regimen containing fractionated TBI.

Management of relapse after allogeneic HCT for patients with ALL

Once patients with ALL relapse after HCT, the prognosis is very poor. Similar to the approach in patients with AML and CML, manipulation of the antitumor effect mediated by the donor graft is often employed as a treatment strategy. Unfortunately, in patients with ALL, this therapy has not been as effective as it has been for patients with CML (see Chapter 84). A report from 25 North American BMT programs of 140 patients who received donor lymphocyte infusion (DLI) showed that the CR rate was 60% in CML with the responses being higher in patients with cytogenetic and chronic phase relapse compared to those with accelerated phase or blastic phase (75, 33 and 16%, respectively) [70]. The CR rates in relapsed AML and ALL are 15% and 18%, similar to the blastic phase of CML. In that study, the development of acute and chronic GVHD following DLI was highly correlated with disease response. In a report from Europe, 40 patients with ALL received DLI as treatment for relapse and of 29 evaluable patients, only one achieved CR [71]. Therefore, DLI as a sole therapy appears to have low potential for contributing to a remission and long-term control of disease in patients with relapsed ALL and, if considered, should be a component of a chemotherapy-based treatment program. For those patients with Ph+ ALL, STI 571 (Gleevec®), either alone or with chemotherapy, is effective in helping some patients achieve another remission, although the duration of the remission is often quite short and DLI should be performed before another relapse occurs [72].

Role of graft-vs.-leukemia effect in patients with ALL

The low response rate in patients with ALL following DLI has led to questions about the significance of the graft-vs.-leukemia (GVL) effect on preventing relapse. The GVL effect (see Chapter 28) is derived from observations of a higher relapse after autologous or syngeneic HCT compared to allogeneic HCT, lower incidence of relapse in patients who had GVHD, as well as increased relapse rates in recipients of T-cell-depleted marrow grafts. The most compelling argument for a strong GVL effect in ALL comes from both single institution and registry data [73,74]. These studies show consistent decrease in relapse rates in patients who develop GVHD compared to those patients who do not. Table 77.10 shows the rate of relapse after HCT for ALL in first CR and the correlation with GVHD. The occurrence of acute, chronic or both forms of GVHD correlated with the best DFS. In a study of 192 patients with ALL, most of whom were transplanted in second remission, Doney *et al.* [39] evaluated the probability of relapse among patients without or with GVHD. Relapse was significantly higher in the group that had less grade II GVHD. In fact, in patients without significant GVHD, the actuarial risk of relapse approached 80% vs. 40% in those who developed grade II or more. A study by Weisdorf *et al.* [75] confirmed this observation for both relapse and overall DFS. A recent evaluation of 1132 patients with T- or B-lineage ALL supports the observation that both acute and chronic GVHD are associated with a decreased risk of relapse in both of the major immunophenotypes of adult ALL [76].

Although the data support the importance of GVL effect in mediating a clinically useful antileukemic response in patients with ALL, the reasons for the limited beneficial effect for patients with relapsed ALL treated with DLI is not clear. The different outcomes may reflect differences in the ability of ALL cells to present as antigen targets, the frequency of T-cell precursors reactive with minor antigens presented by ALL cells, the susceptibility of ALL targets to lysis or kinetic differences in the way leukemic cells grow after HCT. Thus, cytoreduction with chemotherapy prior to infusion of DLI is a better strategy for patients with relapsed ALL. Studies focused on developing antigen-specific T-cell immunotherapy for ALL may help augment the GVL activity of donor T cells [77–81].

Regimen development for allogeneic HCT for ALL

Sequential studies from many BMT centers around the world have led to improvements in the prevention and treatment of transplant-related complications including GVHD and cytomegalovirus (CMV) associated interstitial pneumonia (see Chapters 50 and 53). Although this progress could translate into improved DFS, leukemic relapse is still the most significant problem, particularly for those patients transplanted for advanced disease.

The most commonly used regimen for transplantation of patients with ALL is CY plus TBI. Several different preparative regimens have been described, each based on substituting a different chemotherapeutic agent for CY in combination with TBI for patients with ALL. High-dose fractionated TBI in combination with high-dose cytosine arabinoside (Ara-C) has been employed by several centers and, with the exception of a small series of pediatric patients at Case Western Reserve, there has been no significant improvement in DFS with this regimen in recipients of allogeneic HCT from sibling donors [82,83].

Investigators at Johns Hopkins University approached the problem by substituting busulfan (BU) for TBI in order to decrease the long-term side-effects of TBI and determine the efficacy of high-dose combined alkylating therapy in eliminating leukemic cells [84,85]. These nonradiation-dependent regimens have shown activity in the treatment of advanced ALL, suggesting that TBI is not an absolute requirement for successful treatment of ALL by HCT. A retrospective analysis from the IBMTR found that a conventional CY/TBI regimen was superior to a non-TBI-containing regimen of BU plus CY, with a 3-year survival of 55% vs. 40% for BU/CY [86]. However, despite these differences in survival, the risk of relapse was similar.

The group at the City of Hope National Medical Center studied the substitution of etoposide (VP16) for CY in combination with fractionated TBI (13.2 Gy) followed by allogeneic HCT [87]. A phase 1–2 trial indicated that a VP16 dose of 60 mg/kg is the maximum tolerated dose when combined with TBI. In that study, 36 patients with ALL were treated, 20 of whom were in relapse. The actual DFS was 57% with a 32% relapse rate, suggesting that the regimen had significant activity in patients with advanced ALL, a result confirmed in a subsequent trial from the South-West Oncology Group [88]. A study from City of Hope/Stanford showed a 64% DFS for adult patients undergoing transplantaton with this regimen in first CR (see section on Allogeneic transplant for ALL in first remission). Currently, the MRC UKALL XII/ECOG 2993 Trial, a comparative study of chemotherapy, autologous and allogeneic stem cell transplantation, is utilizing this regimen for patients in first CR. An interim report of overall event-free survival for the allogeneic stem cell transplantation group was 58% vs. 39% for the chemotherapy or autologous stem cell transplantation group [61].

Studies in AML have shown lower relapse rates with higher doses of TBI suggesting that methods that can selectively deliver radiation to sites of leukemia without increasing systemic toxicity might be of benefit to the patient. The use of tumor-reactive MAB conjugated with local acting radionucleotides such as iodine-131 (^{131}I) or yttrium-90 (^{90}Y) are being explored to accomplish the goal of decreased relapse. Initial studies conducted in Seattle in an animal model showed the feasibility of this novel approach, and subsequent phase 1 and 2 studies in patients have been initiated. These studies (see Chapter 15) have demonstrated that initial targeting of marrow and other sites of leukemia could be accomplished

Table 77.10 Relapse after transplantation for acute lymphoblastic anemia (ALL) in first complete remission [73,74].

Group	Probability of relapse at 3 years (%)
Allogeneic, non-T-cell-depleted	
No GVHD	44 ± 17
Acute only	17 ± 9
Chronic only	20 ± 19
Both	15 ± 10
Syngeneic	41 ± 32
Allogeneic, T-cell-depleted	34 ± 13

utilizing ^{131}I-conjugated MABs. The most recent studies have focused on a MAB reactive with CD45, an antigen that is found in leukemic cells as well as hematopoietic tissue and, unlike CD33, does not internalize after antibody binding. A phase 1 trial of ^{131}I anti-CD45 MAB plus CY and TBI for advanced leukemia was completed [89]. This study focused on the biodistribution and toxicity of escalating doses of targeted radiation combined with 120 mg/kg CY and 12 Gy TBI followed by matched related HCT or autologous BMT. Among 44 patients, five had ALL in relapse or refractory disease and five were in second or third CR of ALL. Eighty-four percent of the patients had a favorable biodistribution of antibody with a higher estimated radiation absorbed dose to marrow and spleen than in normal tissues. Thirty-four patients received a therapeutic dose of ^{131}I labeled with 76–612 mg ^{131}I designed to deliver an estimated radiation absorbed dose to liver of 3.5–12.25 Gy. In the group of nine patients treated for ALL, six of whom underwent allogeneic and three autologous HCT, two died of infection, four relapsed and three survived 10, 45 and 57 months after transplantation. This study demonstrated that ^{131}I anti-CD45 antibody can deliver appreciable supplemental doses of radiation to the marrow (approximately 24 Gy) and spleen when combined with conventional fractionated TBI. Estimation of the ultimate benefit to DFS and improved safety of the regimen will await larger phase 2 studies in patients with ALL undergoing transplantation either in remission or in relapse.

Hematopoietic cell source

Although bone marrow has traditionally been the source of the graft for patients undergoing allogeneic HCT for most diseases, a series of phase 2 studies published in the mid-1990s both from single institutions and comparative trials, suggested that the use of granulocyte colony-stimulating factor (G-CSF) mobilized peripheral blood hematopoietic cells (PBHC) leads to rapid engraftment without an apparent increase in GVHD [90,91]. A prospective randomized trial confirmed that the use of PBHC led to faster engraftment, a similar rate of acute GVHD and improved survival [92]. The study was not designed to evaluate individual diseases but was divided into those patients with either good- or poor-risk disease. The advantage of PBHC transplants was more obvious in those patients with high risk of relapse and complications. Thus, for patients with advanced disease, it would appear that peripheral blood would be the optimal stem cell source from the matched related donor. There are few published data on the use of this stem cell source for those patients in first remission. In addition, there are fewer data concerning the use of mobilized PBHC in the unrelated donor setting, although phase 2 data seem very consistent with what has been described in the matched sibling setting, namely faster engraftment without a clear increase in acute GVHD [93]. Trials are currently being planned through the National Marrow Donor Program to study this question.

For those patients lacking either a related or unrelated donor, the use of cryopreserved unrelated cord blood offers an alternative stem cell source [94]. As described in Chapter 43, the potential advantages include the rapid availability of the cord blood and because of decreased T-cell content and function, the use of a mismatched cord is possible. The clinical result of transplant using this stem cell source is influenced by the number of nucleated cells per kilogram infused and the underlying disease, age and degree of match with the recipient. Transplantation of patients utilizing haploidentical matches is also being tested (see Chapter 82) [95]. Studies of these transplants, which rely upon a high CD34 cell number, T-cell-depletion strategy to achieve engraftment with little risk of GVHD, are showing effectiveness in some trials. However, advanced ALL stands out as having a poorer outcome after transplantation, particularly when compared to those patients undergoing transplantation for AML. The reasons for this are unclear and studies are continuing, particularly in children with relapsed ALL.

Post-transplant monitoring of patients

The development of molecular techniques both to diagnose and monitor small amounts of ALL cells have been utilized to determine the risk of relapse in patients undergoing either standard therapy or HCT. A number of transplant studies have reported the clinical significance of detection of Ph+ metaphases or positive PCR signals for *bcr-abl* gene fusion in patients with CML (see Chapters 22 and 23). Treatment with either interferon or DLI has been utilized to treat disease prior to clinical relapse and has achieved long-term control of the disease in many patients.

Several studies have indicated that testing for MRD both pre- and post-transplant for patients with ALL may also be useful [96–100]. In general, these studies show relapse was higher in patients who showed a positive assay before BMT or within the first year after HCT compared to those who showed no PCR positivity. A study in Ph+ ALL also noted the significance of the particular translocation for the chimeric mRNA (p190 vs. p210) [96,101]. The relapse rate was higher in those patients who expressed the p190 *bcr-abl* gene compared to those who expressed only p210. The relapse rate of patients with a positive PCR post-HCT compared to negative PCR was 5.7. Those patients with p190 *bcr-abl* had an 88% relapse rate when compared to 12% for those patients expressing the p210 transcript. This study suggests the expression of p190 *bcr-abl* may portend an especially aggressive ALL and implies that there may be a difference in clinical and biologic behavior between p190 and p210 *bcr-abl* in patients with ALL. This finding is consistent with animal model data indicating that *bcr-abl* p210 and p190 cause distinct leukemias in transgenic mice [102].

The same molecular principle for detection of Ph+ ALL also applies to the detection of MRD in other patients with ALL after HCT. Similar to Ph_1+ ALL, the detection of IGHV-D-G-J in the first 100 days of transplant is associated with a higher incidence of relapse compared to PCR negative patients [103,104]. Taken together, these observations suggest that possible pre-emptive therapeutic interventions for patients who test positive for these leukemia-specific gene products after HCT may be warranted to prevent relapse [105]. This approach could include withdrawal of immunosuppression, the infusion of donor leukocytes or possibly Gleevec® (for Ph+ ALL) to treat MRD before its full expression as clinical relapse [106]. The median time interval between detection of MRD and relapse is approximately 3 months, providing a window of opportunity to intervene prior to florid hematologic relapse [105,106]. More importantly, an analysis of MRD in conventionally treated patients with ALL without obvious high-risk features may identify those at greater risk for relapse and for whom transplant prior to overt relapse may be beneficial [107–109]. A number of studies have been conducted, particularly in pediatric ALL, which show that the quantitative analysis of MRD following chemotherapy can identify patients at high risk for relapse [107–109].

Conclusions

The improvements in the treatment and understanding of adult ALL have had a significant impact on defining the role of allogeneic HCT in the management of the disease. Although most patients will achieve CR, those patients who fail to achieve CR or are delayed in their achievement of CR should be considered for allogeneic HCT early in the course of their disease. For those patients who achieve a remission, a decision concerning the timing of allogeneic HCT can be derived from analysis of the pretreatment prognostic factors; most importantly, the WBC, age of the patient, leukemic phenotype and the rapidity of the response to initial therapy. For patients with poor-risk features, particularly those with the Ph chromosome, allogeneic HCT is the therapy most likely to lead to long-term DFS. For those patients who relapse, allogeneic HCT offers the only chance for long-term DFS.

References

1 Laport GF, Larson RA. Treatment of adult acute lymphoblastic leukemia. *Semin Oncol* 1997; **24**: 70–82.

2 Linker CA, Levitt LJ, O'Donnell M et al. Treatment of adult acute lymphoblastic leukemia with intensive cyclical chemotherapy: a follow-up report. *Blood* 1991; **78**: 2814–22.

3 Larson RA, Dodge RK, Burns CP et al. A five-drug remission induction regimen with intensive consolidation for adults with acute lymphoblastic leukemia. Cancer and Leukemia Group B Study 8811. *Blood* 1995; **85**: 2025–37.

4 Hoelzer D, Thiel E, Loffler T et al. Prognostic factors in a multicentric study for treatment of acute lymphoblastic leukemia in adults. *Blood* 1988; **71**: 123–31.

5 Hoelzer D, Gokbuget N. New approaches to acute lymphoblastic leukemia in adults: where do we go? *Semin Oncol* 2000; **27**: 540–59.

6 Bennett JM, Catousky D, Daniel MT. Proposals for the classification of acute leukemias. *Br J Haematol* 1976; **33**: 451–7.

7 Brearley RL, Johnson S, Lister TA. Acute lymphoblastic leukemia in adults: clinicopathological correlations with the French–American–British (FAB) cooperative group classification. *Eur J Cancer* 1979; **15**: 909–14.

8 Foon KA, TR. Immunologic classification of leukemia and lymphoma. *Blood* 1986; **68**: 1–31.

9 Greaves MF, Lister TA. Prognostic importance of immunologic markers in adult acute lymphoblastic leukemia. *N Engl J Med* 1981; **304**: 119–20.

10 Ludwig W-D, Haferlach T, Schoch C. Classification of acute leukemias. Perspective 1. In: Pui C-H, ed. *Treatment of Acute Leukemias: New Directions for Clinical Research*. Totowa, NJ: Humana Press, 2003: 3–41.

11 Korsmeyer SJ, Arnold A, Bakhshi A et al. Immunoglobulin gene rearrangement and cell surface antigen expression in acute lymphocytic leukemias of T cell and B cell precursor origins. *J Clin Invest* 1983; **71**: 301–13.

12 Melnick SJ. Acute lymphoblastic leukemia. *Clin Lab Med* 1999; **19**: 169–86.

13 Hoelzer D, Gokbuget N. Treatment of adult acute lymphoblastic leukemia. Perspective 2. In: Pui C-H, ed. *Treatment of Acute Leukemias: New Directions for Clinical Research*. Totowa, NJ: Humana Press, 2003: 143–57.

14 Mirro J, Zipf T, Pui CH. Acute mixed lineage leukemia: clinicopathologic correlations and prognostic significance. *Blood* 1985; **66**: 1115–23.

15 Sobol RE, Mick R, Royston I et al. Clinical importance of myeloid antigen expression in adult acute lymphoblastic leukemia. *N Engl J Med* 1987; **316**: 1111–7.

16 Secker-Walker LM, Prentice HG, Durrant J et al. Cytogenetics adds independent prognostic information in adults with acute lymphoblastic leukaemia on MRC trial UKALL XA. *Br J Haematol* 1997; **96**: 601–10.

17 Charrin C. Cytogenetic abnormalities in adult acute lymphoblastic leukemia: correlations with hematologic findings and outcome. Collaborative study of the Groupe Francais de Cytogénétique Hématologique. *Blood* 1996; **87**: 3135–42.

18 Secker-Walker LM, Craig JM, Hawkins JM et al. Philadelphia positive acute lymphoblastic leukemia in adults: age distribution, BCR breakpoint and prognostic significance. *Leukemia* 1991; **5**: 196–9.

19 Westbrook CA, Hooberman AL, Spino C et al. Clinical significance of the *BCR-ABL* gene in adult acute lymphoblastic leukemia: a Cancer and Leukemia Group B study (8762). *Blood* 1992; **80**: 2983–90.

20 Preti HA, O'Brien S, Giralt S et al. Philadelphia-chromosome-positive adult acute lymphocytic leukemia: characteristics, treatment results, and prognosis in 41 patients. *Am J Med* 1994; **97**: 60–5.

21 Maurer J, Janssen JW, Thiel E et al. Detection of chimeric *BCR-ABL* genes in acute lymphoblastic leukemia by the polymerase chain reaction. *Lancet* 1991; **337**: 1055–8.

22 Pui C-H, Frankel LS, Carroll AJ et al. Clinical characteristics and treatment outcome of childhood acute lymphoblastic leukemia with the t(4;11) (q21;q23): a collaborative study of 40 cases. *Blood* 1991; **77**: 440–7.

23 Schardt C, Ottmann OG, Hoelzer D et al. Acute lymphoblastic leukemia with the (4;11) translocation: combined cytogenetic, immunological and molecular genetic analyses. *Leukemia* 1992; **6**: 370–4.

24 Heerema NA, Arthur DC, Sather H et al. Cytogenetic features of infants less than 12 months of age at diagnosis of acute lymphoblastic leukemia: impact of the 11q23 breakpoint on outcome: a report of the Children's Cancer Group. *Blood* 1994; **83**: 2274–84.

25 Hoelzer D. Treatment of acute lymphoblastic leukemia. *Semin Hematol* 1994; **31**: 1–15.

26 Hoelzer D, Ludwig WD, Thiel D et al. Improved outcome in adult B-cell acute lymphoblastic leukemia. *Blood* 1996; **87**: 495–508.

27 Soussain C, Patte C, Ostronoff M et al. Small non-cleaved cell lymphoma and leukemia in adults: a retrospective study of 65 adults treated with the LMB pediatric protocols. *Blood* 1995; **85**: 664–74.

28 Copelan EA, McGuire EA. The biology and treatment of acute lymphoblastic leukemia in adults. *Blood* 1995; **85**: 1151–68.

29 Larson RA, Dodge RK, Bloomfield CD et al. Treatment of biologically determined subsets of acute lymphoblastic leukemia in adults. Cancer and Leukemia Group B studies. In: Buchner T, Hiddeman W, Wormann B, et al. eds. *Acute Leukemias VI: Prognostic Factors and Treatment Strategies*. Berlin: Springer-Verlag, in press.

30 Attal M, Blaise D, Marit G et al. Consolidation treatment of adult acute lymphoblastic leukemia: a prospective, randomized trial comparing allogeneic versus autologous bone marrow transplantation and testing the impact of recombinant interleukin-2 after autologous bone marrow transplantation. *Blood* 1995; **86**: 1619–28.

31 Fiere D, Lepage E, Sebban C et al. Adult acute lymphoblastic leukemia: a multicenter randomized trial testing bone marrow transplantation as post-remission therapy. *J Clin Oncol* 1993; **11**: 1990–2001.

32 Boucheix C, David B, Sebban C et al. Immunophenotype of adult acute lymphoblastic leukemia, clinical parameters and outcomes: an analysis of a prospective trial, including 562 tested patients (LALA87). *Blood* 1994; **84**: 1603–12.

33 Kebriaei P, Stock W. Allogeneic stem cell transplantation for adult acute lymphoblastic leukemia. In: Laughlin MJ, Lazarus HM, eds. *Allogeneic Stem Cell Transplantation: Clinical Research and Practice*. Totowa, NJ: Humana Press, 2003: 29–46.

34 Cataland SR, Larson RA. Treatment of adult acute lymphoblastic leukemia. Perspective 1. In: Pui C-H, ed. *Treatment of Acute Leukemias: New Directions for Clinical Research*. Totowa, NJ: Humana Press, 2003: 131–41.

35 Fefer A, Einstein AB, Thomas ED et al. Bone marrow transplantation for hematologic neoplasia in 16 patients with identical twins. *N Engl J Med* 1974; **290**: 1389–93.

36 Thomas ED, Buchner CD, Banaji M et al. One hundred patients with acute leukemia treated by chemotherapy, total body irradiation, and allogeneic marrow transplantation. *Blood* 1977; **49**: 511–33.

37 Thomas ED, Sanders JE, Flournoy N et al. Marrow transplantation for patients with acute lymphoblastic leukemia in remission. *Blood* 1979; **54**: 468–76.

38 Zwaan FE, Hermans J, Barrett AJ, Speck B. Bone marrow transplantation for acute lymphoblastic leukaemia: a survey of the European Group for Bone Marrow Transplantation (EGBMT). *Br J Haematol* 1984; **58**: 33–42.

39 Doney K, Fisher LD, Appelbaum FR et al. Treatment of adult acute lymphoblastic leukemia with allogeneic bone marrow transplantation: multivariate analysis of factors affecting acute graft-versus-host disease, relapse, and relapse-free survival. *Bone Marrow Transplant* 1991; **7**: 453–9.

40 Wingard JR, Piantadosi S, Santos GW et al. Allogeneic bone marrow transplantation for patients with high-risk acute lymphoblastic leukemia. *J Clin Oncol* 1990; **8**: 820–30.

41 Blume KG, Forman SJ, Krance RA, Henke M, Findley DO, Hill LR. Bone marrow transplantation for acute leukemia. *Hematol Blood Transfusion* 1985; **29**: 39–41.

42 Shank B, O'Reilly RJ. Allogeneic marrow transplantation for acute lymphoblastic leukemia in remission: the importance of early transplantation. *Transplant Proc* 1983; **15**: 1397–400.

43 Van Lint M, Bacigalupo A, Frassoni F et al. Bone marrow transplantation (BMT) for acute lymphoblastic leukemia (ALL) in remission. *Haematology* 1986; **71**: 135–8.

44 Schmitz N, Gassman W, Rister M et al. Fractionated total body irradiation and high dose VP16-213 followed by allogeneic bone marrow transplantation in advanced leukemias. *Blood* 1988; **72**: 1567–73.

45 Barrett A, Dendra JR, Lucas CF et al. Bone marrow transplantation for acute lymphoblastic leukemia. *Br J Hematol* 1982; **52**: 181–8.

46 Greinix HT, Reiter E, Keil F et al. Leukemia-free survival and mortality in patients with refractory or relapsed acute leukemia given marrow transplants from sibling and unrelated donors. *Bone Marrow Transplant* 1998; **21**: 673–8.

47 Michallet M, Tanguy ML, Socie G. Second allogeneic hematopoietic stem cell transplantation in relapsed acute and chronic leukemias for patients who underwent a first allogeneic bone marrow transplantation: a survey of the Societe Francaise de Greffe de Moelle (SFGM). *Br J Haematol* 2000; **108**: 400–7.

48 International Bone Marrow Transplant Registry. http://www.ibmtr.org

49 Doney K, Hägglund H, Leisenring W, Chauncey T, Appelbaum FR, Storb R. Predictive factors for outcome of allogeneic hematopoietic cell transplantation for adult acute lymphoblastic leukemia. *Biol Blood Marrow Transplant* 2003; **9**: 472–81.

50 Cornelissen JJ, Carston M, Kollman C et al. Unrelated marrow transplantation for adult patients with poor-risk acute lymphoblastic leukemia: strong graft-versus-leukemia effect and risk factors determining outcome. *Blood* 2001; **97**: 1572–7.

51 Blume KG, Forman SJ, Snyder DS et al. Allogeneic bone marrow transplantation for acute lymphoblastic leukemia during first complete remission. *Transplantation* 1987; **43**: 389–92.

52 Vernant JP, Marit G, Maraninchi D et al. Allogeneic bone marrow transplantation in adults with acute lymphoblastic leukemia in first complete remission. *J Clin Oncol* 1988; **6**: 227–31.

53 Blaise D, Gespard MH, Stoppa AM et al. Allogeneic or autologous bone marrow transplantation for acute lymphoblastic leukemia in first complete remission. *Bone Marrow Transplant* 1990; **5**: 7–12.

54 Carey PJ, Proctor SJ, Taylor P et al. Autologous bone marrow transplantation for high-grade lymphoid malignancy using melphalan-irradiation conditioning without marrow purging or cryopreservation. *Blood* 1991; **77**: 1593–8.

55 Chao NJ, Forman SJ, Schmidt GM et al. Allogeneic bone marrow transplantation for high-risk acute lymphoblastic leukemia during first complete remission. *Blood* 1991; **78**: 1923–7.

56 Horowitz MM, Messerer D, Hoelzer D et al. Chemotherapy compared with bone marrow transplantation for adults with acute lymphoblastic leukemia in first remission. *Ann Intern Med* 1991; **115**: 13–8.

57 Sebban C, Lepage E, Vernant JP et al. Allogeneic bone marrow transplantation in adult acute lymphoblastic leukemia in first complete remission: a comparative study. *J Clin Oncol* 1994; **12**: 2580–7.

58 DeWitte T, Awwad B, Boezeman J et al. Role of allogeneic bone marrow transplantation in adolescent or adult patients with acute lymphoblastic leukemia or lymphoblastic lymphoma in first remission. *Bone Marrow Transplant* 1994; **14**: 767–74.

59 Vey N, Blaise D, Stoppa AM et al. Bone marrow transplantation in 63 adult patients with acute lymphoblastic leukemia in first complete remission. *Bone Marrow Transplant* 1994; **14**: 383–8.

60 Oh H, Gale R, Zhang M et al. Chemotherapy vs. HLA-identical sibling bone marrow transplant for adults with acute lymphoblastic leukemia in first remission. *Bone Marrow Transplant* 1998; **22**: 253–7.

61 Rowe JM, Richards S, Wienik PH et al. Allogeneic bone marrow transplantation (BMT) for adults with acute lymphoblastic leukemia (ALL) in first complete remission (CR): early results from the International ALL Trial (MRC UKALL/ECOG 2993). *Blood* 1999; **94**: 168a.

62 Thiebaut A, Vernant JP, Degos L. Adult acute lymphocytic leukemia study testing chemotherapy and autologous and allogeneic transplantation: a follow-up report of the French protocol LALA 87. *Hematol Oncol Clin North Am* 2000; **14**: 1353–65.

63 Forman SJ, Smith D, Negrin R. Allogeneic hematopoietic cell transplantation for high risk ALL in adults with fractionated total body irradiation and VP-16. Submitted, in press.

64 Forman SJ, O'Donnell MR, Nademanee AP et al. Bone marrow transplantation for patients with Philadelphia chromosome-positive acute lymphoblastic leukemia. *Blood* 1987; **70**: 587–8.

65 Snyder DS. Allogeneic stem cell transplantation for Philadelphia chromosome-positive acute lymphoblastic leukemia. *Biol Blood Marrow Transplant* 2000; **6**: 597–603.

66 Sierra J, Radich J, Hansen JA et al. Marrow transplants from unrelated donors for treatment of Philadelphia chromosome-positive acute lymphoblastic leukemia. *Blood* 1997; **90**: 1410–4.

67 Forman SJ, Schmidt GM, Nademanee AP et al. Allogeneic bone marrow transplantation as therapy for primary induction failure for patients with acute leukemia. *J Clin Oncol* 1991; **9**: 1570–4.

68 van Besien K, Przepiorka D, Mehra R et al. Impact of pre-existing CNS involvement on the outcome of bone marrow transplantation in adult hematologic malignancies. *J Clin Oncol* 1996; **14**: 3036–42.

69 Thompson CB, Sanders JE, Flournoy N, Buckner CD, Thomas ED. The risks of central nervous system relapse and leukoencephalopathy in patients receiving marrow transplants for acute leukemia. *Blood* 1986; **67**: 195–9.

70 Collins RH, Shpilberg O, Drobyski WR et al. Donor leukocyte infusions in 140 patients with relapsed malignancy after allogeneic bone marrow transplantation. *J Clin Oncol* 1997; **15**: 433–44.

71 Kolb HJ, Schattenberg A, Goldman JM et al. Graft-versus-leukemia effect of donor lymphocyte transfusions in marrow grafted patients. European Group for Blood and Marrow Transplantation Working Party Chronic Leukemia. *Blood* 1995; **86**: 2041–50.

72 Wassmann B, Pfeifer H, Scheuring U et al. Therapy with imatinib mesylate (Glivec) preceding allogeneic stem cell transplantation (SCT) in relapsed or refractory Philadelphia-positive acute lymphoblastic leukemia (Ph+ ALL). *Leukemia* 2002; **16**: 2358–65.

73 Horowitz MM, Gale RP, Sondel PM et al. Graft-versus-leukemia reactions after bone marrow transplantation. *Blood* 1990; **75**: 555–62.

74 Appelbaum FR. Graft versus leukemia (GVL) in the therapy of acute lymphoblastic leukemia (ALL). *Leukemia* 1997; **11**: S15–S17.

75 Weisdorf DJ, Billett AL, Hannan P et al. Autologous versus unrelated donor allogeneic marrow transplantation for acute lymphoblastic leukemia. *Blood* 1997; **90**: 2962–8.

76 Passweg JR, Tiberghien P, Cahn J-Y et al. Graft-versus-leukemia effects in T lineage and B lineage acute lymphoblastic leukemia. *Bone Marrow Transplant* 1998; **21**: 153–8.

77 Appelbaum FR. Hematopoietic cell transplantation as immunotherapy. *Nature* 2001; **411**: 385–9.

78 Mutis T, Verdijk R, Schrama E, Esendam B, Brand A, Goulmy E. Feasibility of immunotherapy of relapsed leukemia with ex vivo-generated cytotoxic T lymphocytes specific for hematopoietic system-restricted minor histocompatibility antigens. *Blood* 1999; **93**: 2336–41.

79 Warren EH, Greenberg PD, Riddell SR. Cytotoxic T-lymphocyte-defined human minor histocompatibility antigens with a restricted tissue distribution. *Blood* 1998; **91**: 2197–207.

80 Jensen MC, Clarke P, Tan G et al. Human T lymphocyte genetic modification with naked DNA. *Mol Ther* 2000; **1**: 49–55.

81 Cooper LJ, Topp MS, Serrano LM et al. T-cell clones can be rendered specific for CD19: toward the selective augmentation of the graft-versus-B-lineage leukemia effect. *Blood* 2003; **101**: 1637–44.

82 Coccia PF, Strandjord SE, Warkentin PI et al. High-dose cytosine arabinoside and fractionated total-body irradiation: an improved preparative regimen for bone marrow transplantation of children with acute lymphoblastic leukemia in remission. *Blood* 1988; **71**: 888–93.

83 Champlin R, Jacobs A, Gale RP et al. High-dose cytarabine in consolidation chemotherapy or with bone marrow transplantation for patients with acute leukemia: preliminary results. *Semin Oncol* 1985; **12**: 190–5.

84 Santos GW, Tutschka PJ, Brookmeyer R et al. Marrow transplantation for acute nonlymphocytic leukemia after treatment with busulfan and cyclophosphamide. *N Engl J Med* 1983; **309**: 1347–53.

85 Tutschka PJ, Copelan EA, Klein JP. Bone marrow transplantation for leukemia following a new busulfan and cyclophosphamide regimen. *Blood* 1987; **70**: 1382–8.

86 Davies SM, Ramsay NKC, Klein JP et al. Comparison of preparative regimens in transplants for children with acute lymphoblastic leukemia. *J Clin Oncol* 2000; **18**: 340–7.

87 Blume KG, Forman SJ, O'Donnell MR et al. Total body irradiation and high-dose etoposide: a new preparatory regimen for bone marrow transplantation in patients with advanced hematologic malignancies. *Blood* 1987; **69**: 1015–20.

88 Blume KG, Kopecky KJ, Henslee-Downey JP et al. A prospective randomized comparison of total body irradiation–etoposide versus busulfan–cyclophosphamide as preparatory regimens for bone marrow transplantation in patients with leukemia who were not in first remission: a South-West Oncology Group study. *Blood* 1993; **81**: 2187–93.

89 Matthews DC, Appelbaum FR, Eary JF et al. Phase I study of 131I-anti-CD45 antibody plus cyclophosphamide and total body irradiation for advanced acute leukemia and myelodysplastic syndrome. *Blood* 1999; **94**: 1237–47.

90 Bensinger WI, Weaver CH, Appelbaum FR et al. Transplantation of allogeneic peripheral blood stem cells mobilized by recombinant human granulocyte colony-stimulating factor. *Blood* 1995; **85**: 1655–8.

91 Korbling M, Przepiorka D, Huh YO et al. Allogeneic blood stem cell transplantation for refractory leukemia and lymphoma: potential advantage of blood over marrow allografts. *Blood* 1995; **85**: 1659–65.

92 Bensinger WI, Martin PJ, Storer B et al. Transplantation of bone marrow as compared with peripheral blood cells from HLA-identical relatives in patients with hematologic malignancies. *N Engl J Med* 2001; **344**: 175–81.

93 Remberger M, Ringden O, Blau IW et al. No difference in graft-versus-host disease, relapse, and survival comparing peripheral stem cells to bone marrow using unrelated donors. *Blood* 2001; **98**: 1739–45.

94 Rubinstein P, Carrier C, Scaradavou A et al. Outcomes among 562 recipients of placental-blood transplants from unrelated donors. *N Engl J Med* 1998; **339**: 1565–77.

95 Aversa F, Tabilio A, Velardi A et al. Treatment of high-risk acute leukemia with T-cell-depleted stem cells from related donors with one fully mismatched HLA haplotype. *N Engl J Med* 1998; **339**: 1186–93.

96 Radich J, Gehly G, Lee A et al. Detection of *bcr-abl* transcripts in Philadelphia chromosome-positive

acute lymphoblastic leukemia after marrow transplantation. *Blood* 1997; **89**: 2602–9.
97 Knechtli CJ, Goulden NJ, Hancock JP *et al.* Minimal residual disease status before allogeneic bone marrow transplantation is an important determinant of successful outcome for children and adolescents with acute lymphoblastic leukemia. *Blood* 1998; **92**: 4072–9.
98 Uzunel M, Mattsson J, Jaksch M, Remberger M, Ringden O. The significance of graft-versus-host disease and pretransplantation minimal residual disease status to outcome after allogeneic stem cell transplantation in patients with acute lymphoblastic leukemia. *Blood* 2001; **98**: 1982–4.
99 Sanchez J, Serrano J, Gomez P *et al.* Clinical value of immunological monitoring of minimal residual disease in acute lymphoblastic leukaemia after allogeneic transplantation. *Br J Haematol* 2002; **116**: 686–94.
100 Bader P, Hancock J, Kreyenberg H *et al.* Minimal residual disease (MRD) status prior to allogeneic stem cell transplantation is a powerful predictor for post transplant outcome in children with ALL. *Leukemia* 2002; **16**: 1668–72.
101 Stirewalt DL, Guthrie KA, Beppu L *et al.* Predictors of relapse and overall survival in Philadelphia chromosome-positive acute lymphoblastic leukemia after transplantation. *Biol Blood Marrow Transplant* 2003; **9**: 206–12.
102 Voncken JW, Kaartinen V, Pattengale PK, Germeraad WTV, Groffen J, Heisterkamp N. BCR/ABL P210 and P190 cause distinct leukemia in transgenic mice. *Blood* 1995; **86**: 4603–11.
103 Radich J, Ladne P, Gooley T. PCR-based detection of unique immunoglobulin V-D-J gene rearrangements in acute lymphoblastic leukemia predicts relapse after allogeneic bone marrow transplantation. *Biol Blood Marrow Transplant* 1995; **1**: 24–7.
104 Miglino M, Berisso G, Grasso R *et al.* Allogeneic bone marrow transplantation (BMT) for adults with acute lymphoblastic leukemia (ALL): predictive role of minimal residual disease monitoring on relapse. *Bone Marrow Transplantation* 2002; **30**: 579–85.
105 Jandula BM, Nomdedeu J, Marin P, Vivancos P. Rituximab can be useful as treatment for minimal residual disease in *bcr-abl*-positive acute lymphoblastic leukemia. *Bone Marrow Transplant* 2001; **27**: 225–7.
106 Baron F, Frere P, Fillet G, Beguin Y. Treatment of leukemia relapse after allogeneic hematopoietic stem cell transplantation by donor lymphocyte infusion and STI-571. *Haematologica* 2001; **86**: 993–4.
107 Brisco MJ, Condon J, Highes E *et al.* Outcome prediction in childhood acute lymphoblastic leukaemia by molecular quantification of residual disease at the end of induction. *Lancet* 1994; **343**: 196–200.
108 Mortuza FY, Papaioannou M, Moreira IM *et al.* Minimal residual disease tests provide an independent predictor of clinical outcome in adult acute lymphoblastic leukemia. *J Clin Oncol* 2002; **20**: 1094–104.
109 Foroni L, Coyle LA, Papaioannou M *et al.* Molecular detection of minimal residual disease in adult and childhood acute lymphoblastic leukaemia reveals differences in treatment response. *Leukemia* 1997; **11**: 1732–41.
110 Biggs JC, Horowitz MM, Gale RP *et al.* Bone marrow transplants may cure patients with acute leukemia never achieving remission with chemotherapy. *Blood* 1992; **80**: 1090–3.

78

Stella M. Davies, Norma K.C. Ramsey & John H. Keresy

Allogeneic Transplantation for Acute Lymphoblastic Leukemia in Children

Acute lymphoblastic leukemia (ALL) of childhood represents a heterogeneous group of disorders, each with differing molecular genetic abnormalities and clinical behavior. Significant advances in chemotherapy regimens have been made over the last 50 years, such that more than 70% of children with ALL are now cured with chemotherapy [1]. The remarkable progress achieved in the treatment of ALL is the result of series of large-scale clinical studies conducted by cooperative clinical trials groups. In addition, biologic investigations have led to improvements in risk group identification and allowed administration of risk-assigned therapy, improving the results of clinical trials. These advances in chemotherapy treatment have occurred in parallel with important changes in transplant techniques, donor availability and supportive care in hematopoietic cell transplantation (HCT). Together, these events have lead to changes over time in indications for and outcome of HCT for childhood ALL. The indications for HCT in childhood ALL are likely to continue to change in future years as advances are made in chemotherapy, HCT and biology.

This chapter reviews the genetic characteristics of childhood ALL, which are central to accurate risk assessment, and discusses the biologic differences between childhood and adult ALL. Outcomes of sibling donor HCT are reviewed, followed by a discussion of the selection of conditioning regimens. For the majority of patients who have no available sibling hematopoietic cell donor the use of alternative hematopoietic cell sources are an important therapeutic option, and outcomes of mismatched related, unrelated marrow and umbilical cord blood (UCB) donor transplants are reviewed. Two particular pediatric populations, infants with ALL and children with Down's syndrome and ALL, require special consideration and the appropriate use of HCT in these cases is discussed. Finally, data regarding the effectiveness of management of post-transplant relapse with a second transplant are presented.

Diagnosis and classification of ALL in childhood

The last 20 years have seen an explosion in our knowledge of the phenotypic and genotypic characteristics of childhood ALL. The advent of monoclonal antibodies allowed the characterization of cell surface phenotypes of childhood ALL, and now categorization of leukemia according to cell of origin is routine. Immunophenotyping demonstrates that most cases of childhood ALL are B-lineage, while the remainder is T-lineage (Table 78.1) [1]. B-lineage leukemias generally arise early in B-lymphocyte development before the maturation of surface immunoglobulin, and are termed "B precursor ALL". Cases with cytoplasmic immunoglobulin are termed "pre-B ALL". Cases with similar pre-B surface markers that do not express cytoplasmic immunoglobulin are termed "early pre-B ALL" [2]. Some mixed lineage phenotypes (expressing lymphoid and myeloid markers) have been observed. The association of B-cell and monocyte markers is especially important in childhood leukemia because it is seen frequently in the high-risk leukemias that arise in infants [3].

While immunophenotyping allows categorization of ALL by cell of origin, the development of molecular genetics has allowed a finer classification of ALL into prognostically important subgroups on the basis of acquired genetic abnormalities. A large number of specific genetic alterations, commonly but not always associated with specific chromosomal translocations, have been described (summarized in Table 78.1), and are important predictors of outcome of chemotherapy. Some genetic abnormalities appear to be the consequence of mistakes in the normal process of DNA rearrangement used to generate immunologic diversity in lymphoid progenitor cells, as shown in Table 78.1. Examples include leukemias that involve immunoglobulin (Ig) or T-cell receptor (TCR) rearrangements. The functional result of such rearrangements is usually a fusion between the immunoglobulin or T-cell receptor gene and a "caretaker gene" or proto-oncogene, such as *MYC*, resulting in dysregulation of cellular proliferation.

The most frequent genetic abnormalities in childhood ALL are translocations that result in fusion of two genes that are important in regulation of gene transcription in hematopoietic cells such as *TEL*, *AML1*, *MLL* or *AF4*. The fused genes produce a chimeric or fusion gene protein product that alters normal cellular function, frequently through regulation of signal transduction or transcriptional pathways [4,5].

It is important to note that the major genotypic forms of childhood ALL cannot be distinguished by morphology in most cases, and even by cytogenetics in some cases. An excellent example is the *TEL-AML1* fusion that is generally cryptic in cytogenetic analysis and is important to identify by molecular analysis because of the excellent prognosis of these leukemias when treated with chemotherapy [6]. In contrast, the *BCR-ABL* rearrangement, and rearrangements of the *MLL* gene in infants, are associated with markedly inferior outcomes with chemotherapy [7–12]. Rapid identification of molecular abnormalities that can importantly affect prognosis of ALL has allowed risk-adjusted therapy assignment in many cases. Despite advances in molecular diagnosis, cytogenetic studies in addition remain important for identifying leukemias with hyperdiploidy, confirming the results of molecular analyses and guiding the development of molecular assays to detect specific rearrangements.

Biologic differences between pediatric and adult ALL

Chemotherapy outcomes in adults with ALL are notably inferior to results achieved in children. With intensive combination chemotherapy, more than 70% of children with ALL will be cured of their disease, while

Table 78.1 Cellular genotype defines major forms of childhood acute lymphoblastic leukemia (ALL).

Molecular genetic abnormality	Translocation	Biochemical defect	Associated features	Recommended timing for blood or marrow stem cell transplantation
B-cell lineage leukaemia				
TEL-AML1 (CBFα) fusion	t(12;21) cryptic	Transcription	Good prognosis with chemotherapy	Following relapse
BCR-ABL fusion (p 185)	t(9;22)(q34;q11)	Signal transduction	Poor prognosis with chemotherapy	Early in disease as treatment of choice
E2A-PBX fusion	t(1;19)(q23;p13)	Transcription	Pre-B phenotype, intermediate response to intensive chemotherapy	Following relapse
MLL-AF4 fusion	t(4;11)(q21;q23)	Transcription	Infants have poor prognosis	Early using research protocol
			Noninfants have intermediate prognosis	Following relapse
MLL-ENL fusion	t(11;19)(q23;p13)	Transcription	Hyperleukocytosis	Not determined
IGH-MYC fusion	t(8;14)(q24;q32)	Transcription	FAB L3, extramedullary disease	Following relapse
Igκ-MYC fusion	t(2;8)(p12;q24)	Transcription	FAB L3, extramedullary disease	Following relapse
Igλ-MYC fusion	t(8;22)(q24;q11)	Transcription	FAB L3, extramedullary disease	Following relapse
Hyperdiploidy	None	Unknown	Good prognosis with chemotherapy	Following relapse
Hypodiploidy (less than 45)	None	Unknown	Poor prognosis with chemotherapy	Early in disease
T-cell lineage leukaemia				
TAL1 (SCL) deletion	None	Transcription	Extramedullary disease, $CD2^+$, $CD10^-$	Following relapse
TCRδ-TAL1 (SCL) fusion	t(1;14)(p32;q11)	Transcription	Extramedullary disease, $CD2^+$, $CD10^-$	Following relapse
TCRβ-TAL1 (SCL) fusion	t(1;7)(p32;q35)	Transcription	Extramedullary disease, $CD2^+$, $CD10^-$	Following relapse
TCRα-MYC fusion	t(8;14)(q24;q11)	Transcription	Extramedullary disease	Following relapse
TCRδ-RBTN1 fusion	t(11;14)(p15;q11)	Transcription	Extramedullary disease	Following relapse
TCRδ-RBTN2 fusion	t(11;14)(p13;q11)	Transcription	Extramedullary disease	Following relapse
TCRδ-HOX11 fusion	t(10;14)(q24;q11)	Transcription	Extramedullary disease	Following relapse
TCRβ-LCK fusion	t(1;7)(p32;q35)	Signal transduction	Extramedullary disease	Following relapse

results in adult studies indicate survival rates of 30–40%, despite adoption of similar treatment strategies [1,13]. Biologic differences between adult and pediatric ALL are likely to influence response to chemotherapy and include age-dependent differences in immunophenotype and in cytogenetic and molecular genetic characteristics [14].

While the incidence of ALL increases in the elderly, there is also a marked peak in incidence in children between the ages of 2 and 5 years of age. The leukemias occurring within this peak are generally of B-precursor origin, express CD10 surface antigen and are hyperdiploid, all features associated with an excellent response to therapy [15]. Interestingly, occurrence of this peak appears to be related to improvements in socioeconomic status, as it did not occur in the early years of this century and does not currently occur in developing countries [16]. Worldwide, the lowest rates of childhood ALL are reported in black African children ($4/10^6$ annually), with rates approximately 10-fold higher in white children [17–20]. These epidemiologic characteristics may indicate that this subset of leukemias specific to childhood has a unique etiology. Experimental studies indicate that at least two molecular events are required for leukemogenesis and the age of the children in this peak suggests that the first of these events take place *in utero* [21,22]. The nature of the later events that trigger overt leukemia have been the subject of speculation on possible infectious etiologies, perhaps related to delayed exposure to common viruses leading to an abnormal immune response [16–18,23,24].

The majority of adult and childhood ALL cases are derived from B-lineage cells (70–75% of adult and 85% of pediatric cases). Approximately two-thirds of childhood ALL cases express early pre-B-cell markers, in contrast to 50% of adult cases [25–29]. This phenotype is associated with the best response to chemotherapy, regardless of patient age, perhaps because lymphocytes in this developmental stage are particularly susceptible to apoptosis and so to killing by glucocorticoids and antimetabolites. Approximately 15% of pediatric and 25% of adult ALL cases express T-lineage markers [27,29]. Although some early studies indicated that T-lineage ALL was associated with poor outcome, treatment of these patients with intensive multidrug regimens has improved prognosis such that T-cell phenotype is no longer an adverse risk factor in adults or children [30–34].

Approximately one-third of childhood leukemia early pre-B cases are hyperdiploid (>50 chromosomes) in contrast to less than 5% of adults. Hyperdiploidy is associated with a particularly favorable response to chemotherapy, perhaps because of the ability to accumulate high levels of methotrexate polyglutamates [35–37]. Probably the most frequent structural rearrangement in childhood ALL, present in 20–30% of cases, is the translocation t(12;21)(p13;q22), which encodes a chimeric fusion product of the *TEL* and *AML1* genes [38–42]. In addition to formation of the chimeric protein the nontranslocated *TEL* allele is deleted in many cases. Loss of *TEL* activity is clearly a secondary event in some cases, occurring in a subclone of leukemia. This observation suggests that loss of *TEL* expression gives an additional proliferative advantage to the malignant cells, possibly because the normal *TEL* gene product can interact with the TEL-AML fusion protein in a dominant negative fashion [41]. The *TEL-AML1* translocation seems to define a subgroup of childhood ALL characterized by age 1–10 years, a nonhyperdiploid karyotype and an excellent prognosis [40]. The *TEL-AML1* translocation occurs at a low frequency (<5%) in adult leukemia, which likely contributes to the poorer prognosis of adult ALL [43–46].

The Philadelphia (Ph) chromosome t(9;22)(q34;q11) also results in production of a chimeric fusion protein derived from fusion of the *BCR* and *ABL* genes. In contrast to *TEL-AML1* the Philadelphia chromosome is frequent in adult leukemias (25–30%), infrequent in childhood leukemias (3–5%), and is associated with a reduced prognosis regardless of age; Ph-positive leukemia often proves resistant to even the most intensive chemotherapy regimens [1,47,48].

The biologic characteristics described here indicate that the majority of children with leukemia have disease likely to be responsive to current chemotherapy regimens with acceptable toxicity, e.g. early pre-B disease with either hyperdiploidy or the cryptic *TEL-AML1* fusion transcript. In contrast, adult patients commonly have biologic features associated with drug-resistant disease, e.g. Ph chromosome and less favorable immunophenotypes. The biologic differences between adult and pediatric ALL lead to important differences in the appropriate indications for transplantation for children with ALL compared with adults.

Outcome of sibling donor transplant in children with ALL

Transplant in first remission

Children with ALL with unfavorable biologic features, e.g. *BCR-ABL* or *MLL* gene rearrangement have poor outcomes with chemotherapy and may benefit from HCT in first remission. Results of HCT for childhood ALL in first remission are summarized in Table 78.2. An early report from a group in France evaluated the role of sibling donor HCT in first remission for a group of high-risk patients defined by a white blood cell count (WBC) above 100,000/μL, structural chromosomal abnormalities or resistance to initial induction therapy [49]. The relapse rate was very low in this group of patients, with an actuarial relapse rate of only 3.5%. Disease-free survival (DFS) was 84.4% with median follow-up of 30 months. These authors also reported a retrospective multicenter study evaluating the outcome of HCT using a chemotherapy-based conditioning regimen in children under 4 years old with ALL [50]. Sixteen of the 21 patients were transplanted in first complete remission and five in second remission or relapse, and 4-year DFS was 61.1%. There was no peritransplant mortality and the relapse rate was 38.1% (13.5–67.2%CI) for the patients transplanted in first remission.

Investigators from the Nordic bone marrow transplantation (BMT) group reported on 22 children with high-risk ALL transplanted in first complete remission [51]. Criteria for high-risk ALL in this study included WBC $>50 \times 10^9$/L, central nervous system (CNS) disease at diagnosis, T-cell ALL, a mediastinal mass, or specific chromosomal translocations t(9;22) or t(4;11). These 22 patients were matched on prognostic criteria with 44 control patients who received conventional chemotherapy during the same time. Control cases must have survived event-free for at least as long as the time taken for the case patient to receive transplantation to be included in the analysis. DFS at 10 years for transplanted patients was 73% vs. 50% in the matched control patients receiving chemotherapy. The improved outcome was because of a low relapse rate of 9% in transplant recipients.

Taken together, these studies demonstrate that a low toxic death rate and a low relapse rate can be achieved for children with ALL in first remission. It is important to note that some of the criteria used to define high risk in each of these studies (e.g. T-cell ALL and mediastinal mass) are no longer associated with inferior outcomes with modern chemotherapy and would not currently be considered an indication for HCT in first remission. Indications for early HCT will continue to change over time as risk group classification improves and survival with chemotherapy increases.

Outcomes of transplant in second or subsequent remission

There are a number of single and multi-institution studies describing the outcome of HCT for patients with recurrent ALL. Many of the studies combine data for children and adults. In this chapter, where possible, the data from children are highlighted. A summary of results of sibling donor HCT for children with ALL in second or subsequent remission in single institution and multi-institutional studies is presented in Tables 78.3 and

Table 78.2 Single institution studies of sibling donor bone marrow transplantation (BMT) for children with acute lymphoblastic leukemia (ALL).

Transplant group/reference	Years of HCT	No. of patients	Remission status (n)		Preparative regimen	Follow-up (years)*	DFS (%)	Relapse (%)
Seattle [52]	1973–85	57	CR2	57	CY/TBI	NS (1.4–10.4)	40	NS
Memorial Sloan-Kettering [53]	1979–85	59	CR2	31	TBI/CY	CR2 5.1 (2.7–6.9)	64	13
			CR3	12		CR3 5.3 (3.9–6.5)	42	25
			CR4/rel	16		CR4/rel 6.2 (1.5–7.0)	23	64
Minnesota [54]	1978–80	15	≥CR2	15	CY/TBI	4	43	NS
Minnesota [55]	1979–91	123 (85 <18 year)	CR1	19	CY/TBI (80)	7.8 (1.0–12.7)	29	56
			CR2	68	TBI/AraC (15)			
			CR3	36	TBI/CY (28)			
Boston [56]	1986–92	17	CR2	14	CY/AraC/TBI	4.6 (3.0–7.3)	53	31
			CR3	3	CY/Etop/TBI			
Australia [57]	1988–93	26	CR1	2	BU/CY/Mel	4.8 (2.5–6.2)	27	4
			CR2	22				
			≥CR3	2				
Memorial Sloan-Kettering [58]	1979–92	37	CR2	37	TBI/CY	NS	62	19
Australia [59]	1990–97	20	CR2	17	TBI/CY	6.3 (4.5–8.5)	55	NS
			CR3	1				
			Relapse	2				

AraC, cytosine arabinoside; BU, busulfan; CY, cyclophosphamide; DFS, disease-free survival; Etop, etoposide; Mel, melphalan; NS, not stated; TBI, total body irradiation; VCR, vincristine.
*Median and range.

Table 78.3 Bone marrow transplantation (BMT) for children with acute lymphoblastic leukemia (ALL) in first complete remission (CR).

Transplant group [reference]	Year of report	No. of patients	Remission status (n)		Preparative regimen	Follow-up (years)*	DFS (%)	Relapse (%)
France [49]	1980–87	32	CR1	32	TBI/CY	2.5 (0.6–6.8)	84.4	3.5
France [50]	1982–92	21	CR1	16	BU + other chemotherapy	3.9 (1.8–6.4)	61.1	38.9
			CR2	5				
Nordic [51]	1981–91	22	CR1	22	CY/TBI	>2	73	9

BU, busulfan; CY, cyclophosphamide; DFS, disease-free survival; TBI, total body irradiation.
*Median and range.

78.4. Reported DFS ranges from 23% for patients with advanced disease, to 35–64% for cases transplanted in second remission [52–63]. The report from Memorial Sloan Kettering Cancer Center (MSKCC) describes 59 children in second, third and subsequent remission, transplanted between 1979 and 1985, who received a then novel conditioning regimen of hyperfractionated total body irradiation (TBI) followed by cyclophosphamide [53]. This study is one of the few that has demonstrated superior survival for patients in second remission compared with patients transplanted in third remission or later, and overall survival was improved compared to earlier reports. An update of this experience continues to show encouraging results [58]. Overall, studies from other single and multi-institution studies show quite comparable survival, perhaps varying depending on patient mix.

The large size of the registry report from the International Bone Marrow Transplant Registry (IBMTR) allows analysis of prognostic factors [66]. In this report, use of busulfan and cyclophosphamide as a conditioning regimen was associated with a significantly higher risk of treatment failure (lower probability of leukemia-free survival) than use of cyclophosphamide and TBI. Other factors associated with lower leukemia-free survival in multivariate analysis were transplantation while not in remission, presence of the t(4;11) translocation, short duration of first remission and use of combined methotrexate and cyclosporine for graft-vs.-host disease (GVHD) prophylaxis.

Timing of transplantation in childhood ALL

An important goal of treatment of childhood ALL is to accurately identify children likely to be cured with chemotherapy alone, and to offer HCT early (in first remission) to those with a low chance of cure with chemotherapy. Cooperative children's cancer therapy groups worldwide have successfully investigated the role of chemotherapy in the treatment of childhood ALL for over 30 years [68–76]. Considerable effort has been directed towards identifying subsets of children with inferior prognoses so that additional or alternative therapies can be targeted to these children, and the use of risk-adapted therapies has been one of the major achievements in the management of childhood ALL. Over time, approaches to risk classification have become more complex and more effective in predicting prognosis. The simplest level of ALL risk classification is the use of National Cancer Institute (NCI)/Rome standard criteria (age and WBC at diagnosis) to broadly categorize leukemias, as high risk (WBC ≥50,000/µL or age ≥10 years) or standard risk (WBC <50,000/µL and age 1–9.99 years) [77]. These criteria are widely used to assign therapy for children with B-lineage ALL, but are less effective in categorization of children with T-lineage disease [77,78]. The molecular genetics of the ALL blasts and the response of the disease to initial therapy (rapid or slow early response) are now routinely also used in risk classification and intensified chemotherapy is given to children in poor prognostic groups [68,71,79,80].

Typically, only a minority of children with ALL is considered for HCT in first remission. In an effort to identify children with very high-risk ALL who should be considered for HCT in first remission, the Children's Cancer Group (CCG) studied outcomes among 5122 children enrolled on CCG risk-adjusted trials between 1989 and 1995 [81]. The very high-risk group was defined as those with presenting features that predicted 5-year event-free survival (EFS) of <45%, a level at which equivalent or superior survival with sibling donor HCT would be predicted. The analysis indicated poor survival in those with a Philadelphia chromosome t(9;22) (5-year EFS 9.1%), hypodiploidy (<45 chromosomes) (5-year EFS 29%), balanced t(1;9) (5-year EFS 42%), t(4;11) in infants <1 year old (5-year EFS 11%) and all infants <6 months of age (5-year EFS 22%). These data are in agreement with reports from other cooperative study groups from the USA and Europe that report significantly inferior outcomes in childhood ALL with t(9;22), hypodiploidy and infants [69–76,82]. These data support the early use of HCT in children with ALL falling into these categories, as outcomes with chemotherapy are clearly unsatisfactory.

The small number of high-risk cases has limited ability to determine the effectiveness of early HCT in increasing survival. In an effort to circumvent this limitation, data from a number of international study groups have been pooled to examine therapy outcomes for children with ALL carrying a Philadelphia chromosome [47]. Data on 326 children and young adults treated by 10 study groups were analyzed. The analysis showed that HCT from a matched sibling donor is superior to other types of transplantation, and to intensive chemotherapy alone in prolonging initial complete remission (Fig. 78.1). These data support the common clinical practice of offering HCT in first remission to children with Philadelphia chromosome positive ALL and a matched sibling donor. However, for the majority of children without a matched sibling donor, there is less clear consensus on optimum management. The report from Arico et al. [47] included 21 children treated with unrelated donor HCT, and showed no improvement in survival in these cases compared with those treated with chemotherapy. A report of 15 children with Ph-positive ALL (nine in CR1, six beyond CR1) treated with a T-cell-depleted unrelated donor HCT at a single center reported 2-year overall survival of 44% and DFS of 37% [83]. A report from Seattle, addressing children and adults with Ph-positive ALL, describes six of seven patients surviving after unrelated donor HCT in CR1 [84].

The multicenter report by Arico et al. [47] was the first with sufficient cases for analysis of multiple prognostic factors within the Ph-positive subgroup. There were important differences in outcomes in children with Ph-positive ALL treated with chemotherapy, according to modified Rome/NCI criteria, suggesting that chemotherapy may be an adequate treatment for those with the most favorable characteristics. Children 10 years old or younger with a WBC <50,000/mm^3 at diagnosis had a 5-year DFS of 49%; however, children of any age with a WBC >100,000/mm^3 at diagnosis had a 5-year DFS of 20%. Continued investigation of the role

Table 78.4 Multi-institutional studies of sibling donor BMT for children with acute lymphoblastic leukemia (ALL).

Transplant group [reference]	Years of HCT	No. of patients	Remission status (n)		Preparative regimen	Follow-up (years)*	DFS (%)	Relapse (%)
German [60]	NS	51	CR2	51	CY/TBI Etop/TBI	2.5 (0.1–5.6)	5	NS
Multiple in USA [61]	1981–89	213	CR1	25	AraC + TBI	NS	38	NS
			CR2	119				
			CR3	32				
IBMTR [62]	1983–91	255	CR2	255	Multiple	NS	40	45
France [63]	1983–93	42	CR2	42	Multiple	3 (0.1–6.0)	53	17
Italy [64]	1986–93	46	CR2	46	High dose VCR/TBI/CY	2.8 (0.8–7.5)	58.2	30
Spain [65]	1980–88	21	CR2	21	Multiple	14.5 (11.1–18.5)	42.8	40
IBMTR [66]	1988–95	627	CR1	51	BU/CY (176)		35	41
			CR2	73				
			CR ≥3	27				
			Relapse	25				
			CR1	134	CY/TBI (451)		50	35
			CR2	194				
			CR ≥3	51				
			Relapse	72				
Spain [67]	1995–99	67	PBSC	34	BU/CY	Median follow-up of 25 months	53	28.7
			CR1	9	CY/TBI			
			CR2	15				
			≥CR3 or relapse	10				
			BMT	33				
			CR1	9			54.9	27.1
			CR2	195				
			≥CR3 or relapse					

AraC, cytosine arabinoside; BU, busulfan; CY, cyclophosphamide; DFS, disease-free survival; Etop, etoposide; Mel, melphalan; NS, not stated; TBI, total body irradiation; VCR, vincristine.
*Median and range.

of unrelated donor HCT in first remission for the children in this poorer prognosis group is justified.

Children with severe hypodiploidy (<45 chromosomes) have poor outcomes (<40% survival) with chemotherapy [82]. Twenty-nine children with hypodiploid ALL transplanted in first or second remission with a matched sibling donor between 1990 and 2001 have been reported to the IBMTR. Three-year survival was 65% (95%, 45–80%CI), supporting the use of early HCT in this small subgroup (M. Eapen, personal communication, 2002).

Cooperative group studies have contributed the important observation that initial response of childhood ALL to therapy is a strong indicator of long-term outcome, with better outcomes in rapid early responders [74,75]. Additionally, it has been shown that a proportion of slow responders (whether measured by clearance of peripheral blasts after 7 days of prednisone or marrow examination after 7 or 14 days of induction chemotherapy) can be subsequently rescued by intensification of therapy [79,80]. Intensification of chemotherapy improves survival to around 70% in poor responders, so these children do not generally require transplantation in first remission. However, a small subset of slow responders fail to achieve remission after 28 days of chemotherapy, and for those children, if they do achieve remission, only 40% will survive, suggesting that early transplantation once remission is achieved might be of benefit [81].

Newer technologies are being developed to better assess response to therapy in childhood ALL, as early response is such a powerful prognostic indicator. The detection of minimal residual disease using immunophenotyping or molecular detection of residual cells is increasingly being applied to clinical trials of chemotherapy for ALL [85–90; Chapter 22]. These studies have the potential to identify children who have an inadequate response to therapy or show early predictors of relapse, and might benefit from early intervention with HCT.

Two studies have compared outcomes of children with ALL thought to be very high risk transplanted in first remission with matched chemotherapy-treated controls. Both studies showed superior outcomes

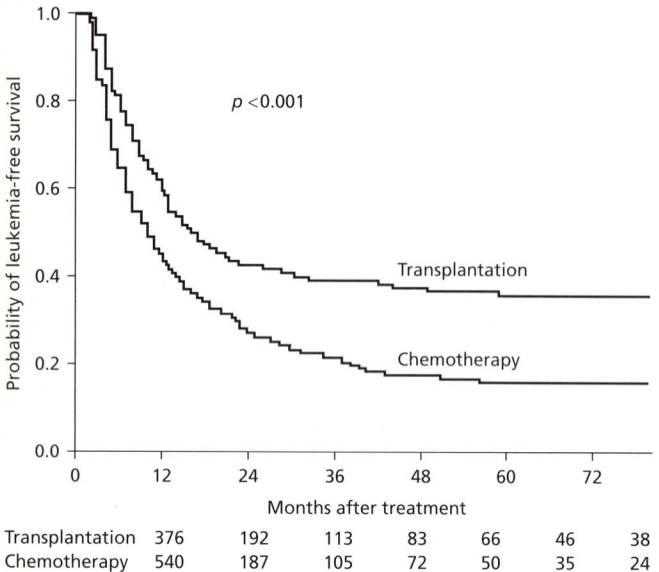

Fig. 78.1 Estimates of disease-free and overall survival (± SE) in 267 patients with Philadelphia chromosome-positive acute lymphoblastic leukemia (ALL) treated with transplantation of bone marrow from human leukocyte antigen (HLA) matched related donors or chemotherapy alone: $p = 0.002$ for the comparison of the two treatments with respect to overall survival; $p <0.001$ for the comparison with respect to disease-free survival.

in the transplanted cases [51,91]. In contrast, two consecutive Medical Research Council (MRC) protocols identified cases considered to be very high risk for relapse (survival expected to be <40%), and offered sibling donor HCT to those with available donors [92]. The data showed a small benefit of 4.6% improvement in 10-year EFS in transplanted patients. However, when patients with an HLA-matched donor were compared with those without, regardless of treatment received (intent-to-treat analysis), patients with a donor had adjusted EFS 10.7% lower than those without a donor. These studies illustrate some of the challenges of transferring excellent single center outcomes to cooperative group studies. Difficulties in group studies include heterogeneous populations, noncompliance with assigned therapy leading to selection bias and transplantation at multiple smaller centers. Transplantation at centers with higher annual numbers of transplants and longer experience has been associated with improved outcomes [93,94]. Continuing investigation of the role of HCT in first remission will require careful attention to optimization of statistical and clinical trial design, and the evaluation of newer transplant strategies, including newer hematopoietic cell sources and reduced intensity conditioning regimens.

The majority of children with ALL are only considered as candidates for transplantation if they relapse despite receiving chemotherapy. Survival rates are typically poor with chemotherapy when relapse has occurred early (first remission duration less than 3 years) [68,95]. However, a proportion of children with later relapses can be long-term survivors after retreatment with chemotherapy [48,96–98]. The appropriate use of HCT or chemotherapy alone for children with relapsed ALL remains a controversial topic, and there have been no successful randomized studies to compare transplantation in second remission with further chemotherapy. In the absence of randomized studies, retrospective comparisons can provide useful guidance to therapy choices. In the largest such study reported, 376 children with second remission ALL treated with sibling donor transplant, reported to the IBMTR, were compared to 540 similar children treated with chemotherapy by the Pediatric Oncology Group [62]. In this comparison, the probability of leukemia-free survival (LFS) was superior in HCT patients when compared to either a matched cohort of 255 chemotherapy-treated patients or to the entire cohort of 540 chemotherapy-treated patients (Fig. 78.2). The mean probability of relapse at 5 years was significantly lower among the transplant recipients (45 ± 4%) vs. the chemotherapy recipients (80 ± 3%; $p <0.001$). LFS after transplantation was 40% compared with 17% ± 3% after chemotherapy ($p <0.001$). This superior outcome was not dependent on the duration of initial remission. Patients who had a short or long (defined as shorter than or longer than 36 months) initial remission benefited from marrow transplantation.

In a smaller single center study, investigators at MSKCC compared HLA-matched sibling donor transplantation using hyperfractionated TBI and cyclophosphamide ($n = 38$) with chemotherapy ($n = 37$) for children with ALL in second remission [58]. DFS was 62% in the transplantation group compared to 26% in the chemotherapy group at 5 years ($p = 0.03$). The relapse rate was 19% in the transplanted group and 67% in the chemotherapy group ($p = 0.01$). Of note, an advantage for HCT was again seen in those with both short and long first remissions. This analysis was conducted with considerable care to adjust statistically for possible bias, although it remains possible that undetected biases existed in determining selection for HCT.

The Italian Bone Marrow Transplant group reported on 57 children who received allogeneic transplant for ALL in second remission and compared them to 230 patients who received chemotherapy following their relapse [98]. They demonstrated that patients who had an early first relapse (<30 months) had significantly longer DFS following allogeneic transplant than treatment with chemotherapy. However, in patients with a later relapse (>30 months following diagnosis) this advantage was lost.

A comparison of allogeneic BMT vs. chemotherapy for ALL in second remission children was reported from Spanish investigators, first in 1989 and updated in 1999 [65]. DFS in children undergoing transplantation was superior compared to the group of children receiving chemotherapy (43% vs. 10%; $p = 0.001$), with notably long follow-up median 14.5 years (range 11.1–18.5 years).

The German pediatric cooperative groups (BFM and COALL) reported 51 children with second remission ALL, all treated with similar initial chemotherapy, receiving matched sibling donor transplant after

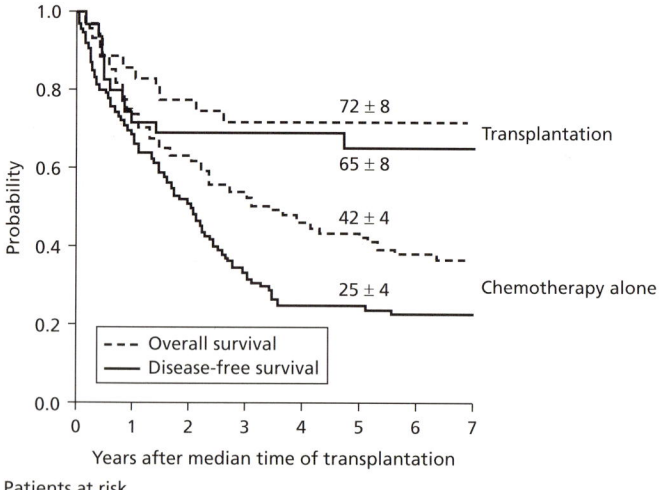

Fig. 78.2 Actuarial probability of leukemia-free survival in matched cohorts of children with acute lymphoblastic leukemia (ALL) in second remission receiving chemotherapy or undergoing transplantation. The numbers below the figure indicate the numbers of children at risk.

Table 78.5 Indications for transplantation in childhood acute lymphoblastic leukemia (ALL).

Stage of leukemia at time of BMT	Donor type	
	Matched sibling or 1 Ag mismatched family member	Unrelated marrow or cord blood
CR1, Philadelphia chromosome +ve	Indicated; poor results with chemotherapy [1,47], transplant studies suggest improved outcome [47,87,88,103–105]	Indicated for those with NCI high-risk characteristics. Children with NCI good risk characteristics may achieve equivalent results with chemotherapy [47]. Data should be contributed to registries to allow evaluation of outcomes
CR1, t(4;11) or other *MLL* rearrangement in infant <1 year old at diagnosis	Indicated; poor results with chemotherapy [11–15]. Reported results suggesting improved outcome with BMT [106–110] involve small numbers and not all studies report benefit; careful prospective evaluation needed	Poor results with chemotherapy, no data to show improved outcome with unrelated donor stem cells available. Data should be contributed to registries/group studies to allow evaluation of outcomes
CR1, >28 days to achieve CR	Transplant may be offered; limited data available comparing outcome with outcome of chemotherapy [63,76]	Transplant may be offered, particularly in cases with other high-risk features; data not available comparing outcome with outcome of chemotherapy
CR2, relapse with CR1 <36 months	Indicated. Outcome improved in transplant recipients in case-control comparison [74,82,84,85]	Indicated; good outcomes reported in significant series of cases [111–115]; however, careful case–control comparison still needed to confirm improved outcome. Single and multicenter studies suggest outcomes can be equivalent to related donor BMT using URD matched at HLA A,B and -DRB1 [116–119]
CR2, relapse with CR1 >36 months	Transplant typically offered; chemotherapy can also cure a proportion of cases [48,58,120,121]	Transplant may be offered if high-risk features are present. Single and multicenter studies suggest outcomes can be equivalent to related donor BMT using URD matched at HLA A,B and -DRB1 [116–119]
CR3 and higher	Transplant indicated, cure with chemotherapy unlikely	Transplant indicated, cure with chemotherapy unlikely
Relapse	Results poor; transplant not generally offered unless in context of investigation of new BMT strategies	Results poor; transplant not generally offered unless in context of investigation of new BMT strategies
Isolated extramedullary relapse	Controversial: transplant may be offered if CNS relapse occurs early (<18 months from diagnosis) [121] and on therapy as outcomes with chemotherapy are poor in some reports [121]; not generally offered for testicular relapse or for CNS relapse occurring after end of therapy which can respond well to chemotherapy [121]	Transplant not generally offered unless associated with marrow relapse

BMT, bone marrow transplantation; CNS, central nervous system; HLA, human leukocyte antigen; URD, unrelated donor.

a relapse [60]. The 7-year EFS was 52% for the transplanted group, with a median follow-up of 3.4 years. Comparison of HCT results with outcomes in children treated with chemotherapy for a bone marrow relapse showed that patients with an initial remission longer than 18 months had comparable survival whether treated with chemotherapy or bone marrow transplant. Patients who had a very early relapse (first remission less than 18 months) or a relapse of T-ALL had a minimal chance of surviving following chemotherapy, and survival rates were significantly improved by allogeneic HCT.

Outcomes of 56 children with relapsed ALL were reported in a single institution study from Australia [59]. All patients with a matched family donor ($n = 20$) received transplant and the other patients received chemotherapy ($n = 32$) or alternative donor transplants ($n = 2$). EFS at 8 years was 55% in children with an available family donor compared with 9.2% in patients without a matched family donor ($p = 0.002$).

These data indicate that HCT from a matched family donor is usually the best option for a child with relapsed ALL, especially when relapse is early. Data are currently insufficient to determine whether similar benefit can be achieved with alternative donor HCT. At the time of relapse a careful reassessment of the morphologic, cytogenetic and molecular genetic characteristics of the leukemia is essential to confirm that this is a recurrence of the original disease and not a new secondary leukemia, perhaps related to the use of chemotherapy. Reinduction chemotherapy is successful in achieving remission in 70–90% of children with relapsed ALL. The problem of how to manage a patient when attempts at chemotherapy reinduction fail is not resolved. In some centers such patients will be considered for allogeneic transplantation even in relapse. There are currently insufficient published data to predict outcomes accurately in these patients, although experience suggests extremely high treatment-related mortality and a high post-transplant relapse rate because of resistant leukemic cells.

When considering the role of HCT in children with ALL, it is important to recognize that there has been continuous progressive improvement in chemotherapy outcomes, and that HCT can be associated with significant late morbidity [99–102]. Comparisons of HCT and chemotherapy outcomes must be ongoing to allow appropriate therapeutic choices. Table 78.5 summarizes current approaches to indications for HCT for children with ALL.

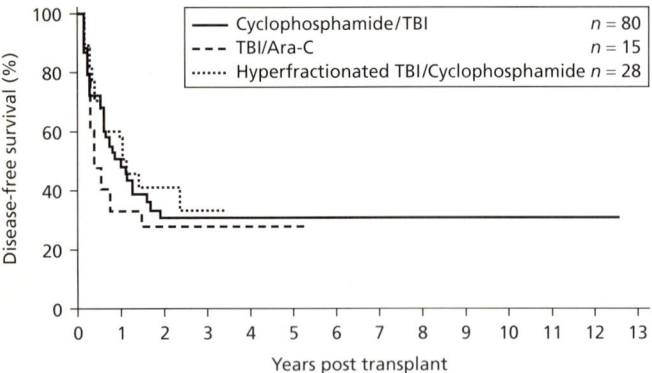

Fig. 78.3 Comparison of three conditioning regimens used for allogeneic hematopoietic cell transplantation (HCT) for acute lymphoblastic leukemia (ALL): disease-free survival is shown. Follow-up after bone marrow transplantation (BMT) differs because the cyclophosphamide/total body irradiation (TBI) (single dose and fractionated) regimens were used 1979–83 (———); TBI/AraC 1984–87 (– – –); and hyperfractionated TBI/cyclophosphamide 1987–91 (· · · ·).

Selection of conditioning regimens

The conditioning regimen used to prepare a patient for a myeloablative HCT for childhood ALL is expected to provide sufficient immunosupression to facilitate donor cell engraftment, and cytotoxicity to assist in the eradication of residual leukemic cells. In the early years of transplantation, most regimens included TBI given in a single fraction. More recently, TBI has typically been administered in multiple fractions to reduce toxicity. Hyperfractionated TBI combined with cyclophosphamide, now considered a standard regimen, was first introduced for the treatment of children with leukemia by investigators at MSKCC [53]. After the original reports of the use of cyclophosphamide and TBI, several investigators added other chemotherapeutic agents to the regimen, or substituted other drugs for cyclophosphamide in an attempt to improve outcomes. Although studies with some of these other combinations, such as TBI and Ara-C showed initial promise [122], additional toxicity often occurred and the long-term outcome was often not appreciably changed. To specifically address the value of Ara-C in conditioning, data were combined from 14 centers that used a TBI and Ara-C regimen in a total of 213 allogeneic HCT recipients with ALL [61]. This study included children and adults, although 89% of cases were less than 25 years of age. The overall 3-year DFS was 38% (31–45%CI), similar to that reported with other regimens. In this study younger patients and those in first remission had superior outcomes. The authors noted an increase in toxic deaths with this regimen, particularly in older patients, similar to a single-institution study that also reported an increased toxic death rate with Ara-C and TBI [123].

Figure 78.3 demonstrates the similarity in outcome among the different conditioning regimens utilized for patients transplanted at the University of Minnesota between 1979 and 1991. Investigators at the University of Minnesota analyzed the results of four different regimens tested sequentially over 12 years using histocompatible related donor marrow grafts [55]. A total of 123 patients with ALL were treated and 92 were less than 20 years of age, with a median follow-up of 7.8 years. The regimens studied included cyclophosphamide plus single dose TBI ($n = 35$), cyclophosphamide plus fractionated TBI ($n = 45$), TBI plus high-dose Ara-C ($n = 15$) and hyperfractionated TBI plus cyclophosphamide ($n = 28$). Outcomes of all the regimens were similar, with 29 + 8% DFS. The most frequent cause of failure with all regimens was leukemic relapse. The only notable difference among the regimens was that the regimen using TBI/Ara-C was associated with greater treatment-associated mortality, in agreement with other reports. In this comparison, the regimen originally reported from MSKCC using hyperfractionated TBI and cyclophosphamide was no more effective in prevention of leukemic recurrence and offered no substantial advantage over the prior regimens.

Investigators at the Hopital Saint-Louis in Paris, France evaluated 42 children with ALL in second remission following allogeneic transplantation to address the value of multiple different conditioning regimens [63]. Thirty-eight of these patients received marrow from HLA-identical siblings. The actuarial relapse rate was lower than many other reported studies at 17%; however, the 4-year EFS rate was 53%, similar to that of other reports. In this study it was noted that there were no post-transplant relapses in children receiving the conditioning regimen of TBI, Ara-C and melphalan (TAM). The authors suggested a possible advantage of using the TAM conditioning regimen in the eradication of ALL, although differences in outcomes by conditioning regimen did not reach statistical significance in this small study. Investigators in Italy have evaluated the feasibility of high-dose vincristine (4 mg/m^2 over 4 days) with fractionated TBI and cyclophosphamide as a conditioning regimen for allogeneic bone marrow transplant [64]. Thirty-three of 46 patients had had a bone marrow relapse and 13 an isolated extramedullary relapse prior to transplant. The 3-year EFS rate was 58.2% (range 40–76%) and the relapse rate was 30% (range 12–49%).

More encouraging data come from investigators at the City of Hope National Medical Center and in Kiel, Germany, who have studied the substitution of VP16 for cyclophosphamide in the treatment of ALL patients receiving HCT [124,125]. Their studies suggested that VP16 and TBI are associated with a decreased relapse rate following transplant for ALL, although data from a prospective randomized comparison are not available. Other investigators in Germany also used VP16 and fractionated TBI in 23 children with ALL in second remission [60]. Their data also suggested a reduced relapse rate in these patients compared with those receiving cyclophosphamide and TBI, with or without Ara-C. A VP16 and TBI conditioning regimen has been tested in high-risk patients, primarily adults, undergoing bone marrow transplant during a first complete remission with good outcomes [126]. These data support further investigation of the use of VP16 to reduce post-transplant relapse.

Investigators from MSKCC have described the use of hyperfractionated TBI, thiotepa and cyclophosphamide as conditioning regimen for children with ALL receiving T-cell-depleted grafts from related or unrelated donors [127]. Preliminary reports suggest excellent outcomes with 87% DFS at 3 years in 11 related marrow recipients and 73% DFS in 23 unrelated donor marrow recipients, all transplanted in first or second remission.

Concerns about the late effects of TBI in children have lead to a number of studies of conditioning regimens using chemotherapy only. Early studies of busulfan and cyclophosphamide as a conditioning regimen focused on treatment of myeloid malignancies, and data indicated that the regimen was adequate to achieve donor cell engraftment [128,129]. The use of a radiation-free conditioning regimen is an attractive option for young children if equivalent survival can be demonstrated as fewer late adverse effects on growth, endocrine and cognitive function might be expected. A study from Australia evaluated a conditioning regimen combining busulfan and cyclophosphamide with single dose melphalan in 25 patients with ALL, the majority in second remission [57]. Toxicity with this regimen was unacceptable, with 42% of the patients dying of regimen-related toxicity. There was a 50% incidence of interstitial pneumonitis and 35% of the patients had severe hemorrhagic cystitis. Because of the severe toxicity, the outcome was not improved over that of a historical control group transplanted earlier using cyclophosphamide and TBI, despite a low relapse rate.

An IBMTR analysis of children with ALL receiving HLA-identical sibling donor HCT compared outcomes with conditioning regimes of cyclophosphamide and TBI ($n = 451$) or busulfan and cyclophosphamide

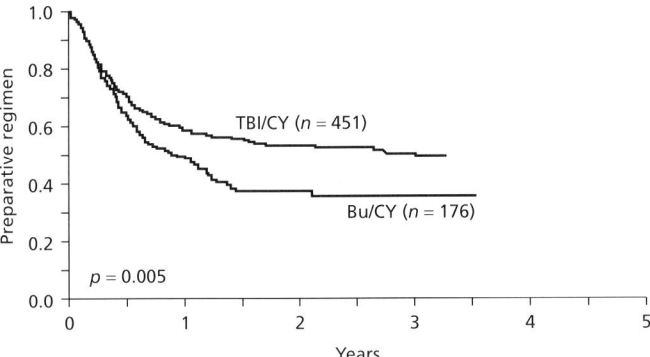

Fig. 78.4 Leukemia-free survival after human leukocyte antigen (HLA) identical sibling donor transplant for childhood acute lymphoblastic leukemia (ALL) according to conditioning regimen used.

($n = 176$) [66]. Patients from 144 institutions, transplanted between 1988 and 1995 were included, and patients were in first, second or subsequent remission or relapse at the time of transplantation. The 3-year probability of LFS was significantly higher in the group receiving cyclophosphamide and TBI compared to the group receiving busulfan and cyclophosphamide (Fig. 78.4). The risk of relapse was similar in the two groups, but treatment-related mortality was higher in children receiving busulfan and cyclophosphamide. Other factors associated with lower survival rates were transplantation not in remission, short duration of first remission (for transplants performed after first relapse), presence of a t(4;11) translocation in leukemic blasts, and use of T-cell-depletion or combined methotrexate and cyclosporine compared with cyclosporine or methotrexate alone for GVHD prophylaxis.

Together these reports indicate that in the past modification of conditioning regimens for children with ALL has had limited success in improving outcomes. Inclusion of additional chemotherapeutic agents has, in some instances, led to increased morbidity and mortality without significant improvement in long-term DFS. In addition, current data suggest reduced survival with radiation-free regimens. However, a number of recent studies indicate that use of TBI and VP16, instead of TBI and cyclophosphamide, or the addition of thiotepa to TBI and cyclophosphamide might reduce post-transplant relapse and improve outcome [60,127–130]. These are important areas for future investigation.

Alternative donor HCT for children with ALL

Mismatched family member transplants in children with ALL

Many of the problems of hematopoietic cell donor availability could be addressed using one, two or three antigen mismatched family member donors, who are available for almost every patient [129]. Early studies of highly mismatched related donor transplants reported high rates of graft failure and GVHD, limiting enthusiasm for this approach [130,131]. Although newer transplant approaches have shown improvement in outcomes, experience with transplantation using mismatched family member donors remains limited. There are few data regarding the use of these transplants for uniform patient populations, although there are several series summarizing overall experience at single institutions. In reports of heterogeneous patient groups, a number of authors have shown that results using a one-antigen mismatched family member as a donor can be comparable to those achieved using a matched sibling donor, while risk of treatment failure increases incrementally with increasing HLA-disparity [132–135]. In keeping with this, a report of a series of 82 patients with leukemia (adults and children) treated with marrow grafts T-cell-depleted *ex vivo* with the monoclonal antibody T10B9 described survival of 31% for the entire cohort [136]. It should be noted, however, that only one of 20 patients receiving a three-antigen disparate graft was surviving at the time of reporting.

Studies of the use of a high degree of T-cell-depletion together with infusion of a high dose of haploidentical CD34$^+$ cells to overcome the problems of GVHD and graft failure have been pioneered by investigators in Perugia, Italy [137]. These authors demonstrated that donor vs. recipient natural killer cell alloreactivity can eliminate leukemia relapse and graft rejection and protect patients against GVHD in cases with AML. Unfortunately, activity against leukemia cells appeared to be specific for AML and not ALL blasts, and outcomes were not satisfactory in ALL cases. A pediatric study has been performed assessing HLA-mismatched HCT from HLA-mismatched parents for children who lack an otherwise suitable donor. "Megadoses" of purified positively selected mobilized peripheral blood CD34$^+$ progenitor cells were used as a stem cell source in a report from Germany [138]. Thirty-nine children were transplanted, 16 for the treatment of ALL. Rapid engraftment was observed in 36 patients, and three patients did not engraft. In two additional patients rejection occurred following primary engraftment. After further immunosuppression and transplantation of purified CD34$^+$ from the same donor all but one patient permanently engrafted. Only five of 38 evaluable patients experienced acute GVHD grade I and one patient had grade II GVHD. DFS was 46% for the 10 ALL patients transplanted in remission. The six patients transplanted in relapse all died less than 1 year following transplant. This transplant strategy continues to be investigated by a number of groups.

Unrelated donor HCT

Donor selection

The use of phenotypically matched unrelated donors has increased markedly in the last decade. The remarkable growth of national and international registries of HLA-typed potential bone marrow donors such as the National Marrow Donor Program in the USA has greatly facilitated the process of donor identification and marrow acquisition [139,140]. Additionally, refinements in HLA-typing technologies have allowed for more accurate matching at class I and class II loci [141]. Despite these improvements, donor identification can still be a logistical challenge, particularly for patients in whom remissions are likely to be short such as those with ALL beyond first remission. An analysis of consecutive referrals to the University of Minnesota between September 1991 and August 1993 showed that an unrelated donor was identified in 37% of searches a median of 10 weeks after search initiation [142]. Although considerable efforts were made to expedite donor identification, 19% of patients died prior to transplantation. However, more recent data indicate a median time to donor identification of 49 days, suggesting that strategies by registries and transplant centers to reduce search times have been effective [143].

The use of less closely matched grafts can increase the pool of available donors, and data indicate that young patients can tolerate greater degrees of HLA mismatch than adult patients. A study of 211 consecutive unrelated donor marrow transplants performed at the University of Minnesota showed that in younger recipients (<18 years) survival was not significantly different after matched (HLA-A, -B and -DRB1) or major mismatched (HLA-A or -B locus) donor HCT ($p = 0.4$; survival 53% vs. 41% at 3 years) [144]. In contrast, for adults survival after matched unrelated donor HCT was significantly better than that with mismatched donors ($p < 0.01$; survival 30% vs. 10% at 3 years). These data were confirmed in a study of 50 children with ALL in second remission who received T-depleted unrelated donor grafts performed in Bristol, UK [109]. In this study, 15 of 50 patients received marrow with a single locus

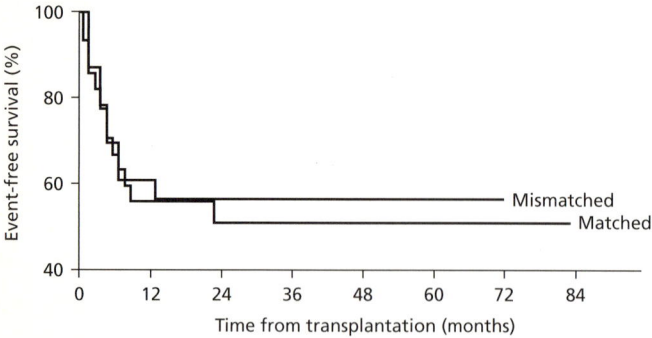

Fig. 78.5 Event-free survival after unrelated donor hematopoietic cell transplantation (HCT) in children with acute lymphoblastic leukemia (ALL) according to the degree of patient–donor matching at human leukocyte antigen (HLA) -A, -B, -DR and -DQ. Donors were fully matched in 27 cases and mismatched in 23. No significant difference was seen in event-free survival between the two groups (51% vs. 57%).

mismatch at HLA-A, -B or -DRB1 and there was no significant difference in EFS between the matched and mismatched groups ($p = 0.73$; 51% vs. 57%). An update of this experience indicated an increased frequency of graft failure in recipients of HLA-mismatched T-cell-depleted grafts (11.8%; $n = 52$), but still no reduction in LFS compared with recipients of matched grafts ($p = 0.65$; 45% vs. 40%) (Fig. 78.5) [113].

Outcomes

Initial reports of the results of unrelated donor transplants necessarily included small heterogeneous groups of patients. As donor availability has improved, larger single center experiences and registry studies are now reported. Table 78.6 summarizes outcomes reported in published series including more than 25 children with ALL. Outcomes from different centers show some variability, which may reflect heterogeneous patient populations or differing treatment strategies and provision of supportive care. Taken together, DFS for children transplanted in first and second remission is generally in the range of 40–50%, and outcomes are not markedly different from those reported for related donor HCT (compare with Tables 78.4 and 78.5).

A number of single center studies of pediatric HCT have demonstrated that in children equivalent results can be achieved using matched (HLA-A, -B and -DRB1) unrelated donors and sibling donors, although the majority of these studies included heterogeneous diagnoses, not just children with ALL [114–117]. In agreement with these reports, data regarding 69 children with ALL in second remission receiving allogeneic HCT at the University of Minnesota indicate 5-year DFS of 41% for recipients of sibling donor grafts and 52% for recipients of HLA-A, -B, -DRB1 matched unrelated donor grafts (N.K.C. Ramsay, unpublished data). Similar to the experience with chemotherapy, length of first remission influenced outcome of HCT regardless of donor source, with DFS of 28% in children with a first remission of less than 1 year, compared to 58% for those with a first remission of 1–2 years. Further studies support the belief that at least equivalent outcomes can be achieved with sibling donor and unrelated donor grafts in children with ALL. A multicenter study of 65 children with ALL in second remission showed 5-year EFS of 39% in sibling donor HCT recipients and 54% in unrelated donor HCT recipients [117]. A single center study from the Hospital for Sick Children, Toronto, Canada, including 62 children with ALL in first, second or third remission or relapse also showed similar outcomes in sibling and unrelated donor HCT recipients [116].

Taken together, these data indicate that in children good outcomes can be achieved with well-matched (typically HLA-A, -B, -DRB1) unrelated donor HCT, and that this graft source can be regarded as equivalent to matched sibling donor BMT. Despite this, the translation of these single center observations into improved survival for the overall population of children with relapsed ALL remains challenging. Well-matched donors are not available for all children, results from single large centers might not be transferable to multiple smaller centers, and children who do not achieve remission or die of early chemotherapy toxicity cannot benefit from HCT. The performance of a randomized trial comparing unrelated donor HCT with chemotherapy to try to translate reports from single centers into a proven therapy has been difficult to achieve, despite a number of attempts. Such a study requires randomization to one of two conceptually very different therapies (HCT vs. chemotherapy) which can be difficult for families to accept. In addition, there has been perhaps a lack of universal acceptance among physicians that equipoise exists in asking this question, with some physicians strongly favoring HCT and some strongly favoring chemotherapy. In the MRC UKALLR1 study of relapsed ALL, children with no matched family donor were randomized to continuation chemotherapy or intensification with autologous HCT. Only 9% of patients eligible for randomization were actually randomized, and even fewer received assigned therapy [146]. As a consequence of these difficulties, there are no available large-scale randomized trials comparing HCT and chemotherapy in childhood ALL. In a small descriptive study, Feig et al. [118] reported a Children's Cancer Group comparison of chemotherapy ($n = 43$) vs. transplant ($n = 12$ allogeneic, $n = 7$ autologous) and showed improved survival in the transplant group overall. In contrast, an MRC report described the outcome of 489 children with relapsed ALL [119]. EFS at 5 years for children who relapsed in the marrow within 2 years of diagnosis was 3%, irrespective of the type of postrelapse treatment (HCT or chemotherapy), suggesting that HCT from any donor source was not able to rescue this very high-risk group. These studies all indicate the need for continuing efforts to improve the efficacy of HCT in children with early relapse of ALL. The most effective way to do this might be further development of tools to identify high-risk cases likely to fail with chemotherapy, who should be transplanted in first remission, avoiding the need for later HCT.

As larger series of unrelated donor HCTs are being reported, it is now possible to evaluate prognostic factors influencing outcome of unrelated donor HCT for children with ALL. An analysis of transplants facilitated by the National Marrow Donor Program for children with ALL in second remission showed improved LFS associated with longer duration of first remission, HLA match and age less than 15 years [145]. Similarly, longer duration of first remission predicted better LFS for children in second remission in the studies from Bristol, UK [113] and Seattle, USA [110]. The Seattle study reported that age younger than 10 years and T-cell phenotype were associated with improved LFS. A report from Toronto, Canada showed reduced LFS in patients with more advanced disease status prior to HCT and the occurrence of a higher grade of acute GVHD [116].

These data indicate that unrelated donor transplantation can offer a cure for some children with ALL who are unlikely to be cured with chemotherapy. Challenges that remain include the time needed to acquire donor marrow and the high rate of treatment-related mortality associated with GVHD (particularly in unmanipulated grafts) and early and late infections (particularly in T-cell-depleted grafts) and relapse.

Umbilical cord blood transplantation for children with ALL

The establishment of banks of cryopreserved UCB for use in transplantation has been an important development in the treatment of children with ALL [147–151; Chapter 43]. Potential advantages of UCB include immediate availability of stored units for transplantation once identified (particularly valuable for patients in whom remissions are likely to be short) and reduced GVHD, a major reason for treatment failure in recipients of unrelated donor marrow. The median time needed to identify

Table 78.6 Outcome of unrelated donor bone marrow transplantation (BMT) for children with acute lymphoblastic leukemia (ALL).

Transplant group [reference]	Years of HCT	No. of patients	Remission status (n)		Preparative regimen	Follow-up (months)*	DFS (%)		Relapse (%)	
Single institution series										
Bristol, England [113]	1988–97	137	CR1 CR2 >CR2	(24) (88) (25)	CAMPATH 1-G, CY, TBI	38 (6–181)	CR1 CR2 >CR2 at 5 years	42% 45% 26%	36.5% overall at 5 years	
Seattle, USA [110]	1983–99	88	CR1 CR2 CR3 Relapse	(10) (34) (10) (34)	CY/TBI	NS	CR1 CR2 CR3 BMT in relapse at 3 years	67% 47% 20% 9%	CR1 CR2 CR3 BMT in relapse at 3 years	11% 33% 20% 50%
Minnesota, USA [112]	1985–94	35	CR1 CR2 CR3 Relapse	(4) (15) (11) (3)	CY/TBI ± VP16	25 (12–88)	CR1/CR2 >CR2 at 2 years	21% 42%	4 of 35 cases	
Milwaukee, USA [111]	1986–91	25	CR1 CR2 >CR2 Relapse	(4) (8) (7) (6)	CY/TBI/AraC/ ± BU	49 (27–85)	CR1 CR2 >CR2	3 of 4 5 of 8 2 of 13	4 of 25	
Toronto, Canada [116]	1990–98	26	CR1 CR2 CR3 Relapse	(8) (12) (5) (1)	TBI/VP16	38 (3–97)	49% overall at 3 years		28%	
Multi-institutional series										
National Marrow Donor Program, USA [145]	1988–2000	363	CR2		Multiple; 90% include TBI	29 (0–125)	36% at 5 years		22%	
Nordic Society of Pediatric Hematology and Oncology [115]	1990–97	28	CR2		Multiple	54 (24–174)	54% at 5 years		40%	

AraC, cytosine arabinoside; BU, busulfan; CY, cyclophosphamide; DFS, disease-free survival; NS, not stated; TBI, total body irradiation; VP16, etoposide.
*Median and range.

a suitably matched UCB graft at the University of Minnesota in 2001 was 13.5 days, significantly shorter than the 49 days needed to identify a compatible unrelated marrow donor [143]. Initial reports of outcomes of UCB transplant procedures have been limited to relatively small series, although larger single center experiences and registry series are now being reported.

The report of successful use of UCB from sibling donors was the basis for development of unrelated donor UCB banks [152]. The first report of 44 sibling donor UCB transplants included eight children with ALL receiving 0–1 antigen HLA-mismatched grafts and four receiving 2–3 antigen HLA-mismatched grafts. Two patients with ALL died of graft failure (one transplanted in fifth relapse and one in fourth remission). Actuarial EFS overall for patients with malignant disease was 46% with median follow-up of 1.6 years. The probability of relapse was 49%.

Investigators at the New York Blood Center have pioneered the cryopreservation and distribution of unrelated donor UCB grafts. These investigators have reported outcomes of 562 UCB transplants performed with UCB cryopreserved by their Placental Blood Program [153]. In this series, 177 patients had ALL and 20 were reported to relapse after transplantation. Survival and EFS for the ALL subgroup was not described.

A registry report from the European Eurocord group described 143 UCB transplantations from related and unrelated donors performed at 45 different centers [154]. This series included 24 children with ALL receiving related donor UCB transplant and 16 receiving unrelated donor UCB. Survival was 63% overall at 1 year for recipients of related donor UCB and 29% at 1 year for recipients of unrelated donor grafts; separate outcomes were not reported for ALL cases. Relapse was reported in five of 24 related donor UCB transplant recipients and three of 16 unrelated donor UCB transplant recipients.

In a single center report, Wagner et al. [155] described 102 patients receiving unrelated donor UCB transplants at the University of Minnesota. Twenty-eight patients had ALL and survival was 0.55 (range 0.23–0.87) for standard risk and 0.32 (range 0.06–0.59) for high risk recipients (defined as short first remission for patients in second remission, or patients beyond second remission).

As experience with UCB transplants has increased it has become possible to compare outcomes of UCB transplants with other graft sources to assist physicians in donor selection. A registry comparison of unrelated donor marrow (T-depleted and T-replete analyzed separately) and UCB transplants in children with leukemia indicated equivalent survival between the three categories. Acute GVHD was reduced in UCB recipients compared with recipients of T-replete marrow [156]. Similarly, a single center matched pair comparison of unrelated donor UCB and either unmanipulated or T-cell-depleted marrow grafts also indicated at least equivalent survival in UCB recipients [157].

Studies that have indicated reduced frequencies of acute GVHD with UCB compared with marrow grafts have raised concern about the possibility of a reduced graft-vs.-leukemia effect if UCB is used in place of marrow. Current data do not indicate a major difference in relapse frequencies between UCB and marrow grafts in recipients with acute leukemias [156,157]. However, larger numbers of cases will be needed to address this concern in a more rigorous fashion in the future. In addition, while UCB transplantation is used infrequently in recipients with CML in whom a graft-vs.-leukemia effect might be most evident, careful analysis those cases that are transplanted cases might cast light on this issue as numbers increase.

Special pediatric considerations

Transplantation of infants with ALL

Treatment of infant ALL presents particular challenges because of variability in outcomes between the various genetic subtypes, and the susceptibility of very young children to adverse long-term consequences of therapy. Using standard chemotherapy, some children with infant ALL have a reasonable prognosis (those with biologic characteristics similar to older children), while others have possibly the most disappointing outcomes in childhood leukemia [108]. As a result, transplantation decisions are especially critical in infants.

Molecular rearrangements that involve the *MLL* gene occur in a high proportion of leukemias arising in infants less than 1 year of age (see Table 78.1). The most frequent of these is a fusion between the *MLL* gene and the *AF4* gene as a consequence of a t(4;11)(q21;q23) translocation. *MLL* gene-rearranged infant leukemias frequently have marked leukocytosis and a mixed lineage (expressing both early B-cell and monocyte markers) phenotype [158]. Prognosis in *MLL*-rearranged ALL in infants is very poor with current chemotherapy, with generally less than 20% 5-year EFS [8–12,108].

Because of the poor response to chemotherapy, infants with *MLL*-rearranged ALL are often considered as candidates for early transplantation. Unfortunately, there are no prospective series of HCT for infants, and outcomes are difficult to compare with those achieved with chemotherapy because of lack of uniform criteria for transplantation eligibility, varying donor sources and the relatively small numbers of patients transplanted. Long-term survivors following transplantation for high-risk infant ALL have been reported from the University of Minnesota in Minneapolis, the Fred Hutchinson Cancer Research Center (FHCRC) in Seattle and other centers. A consensus has developed that survival is generally poor in infants who are transplanted in relapse or late in their disease course. In contrast, an update of the Seattle experience demonstrates that 13 of 17 infants transplanted in first remission are alive 1–13 years (median 3.9 years) after HCT (J. Sanders, unpublished data). This series included 11 infants with cytogenetic evidence of high-risk disease including those with *MLL* 11q23 abnormalities, t(9;22) or hypodiploidy.

The use of unrelated donor marrow or UCB grafts plays an important part in infant leukemia, as most infants do not have a suitable family donor. Largely because of greatly increased availability and the need for a lesser degree of HLA-matching, the use of unrelated donor UCB as a source of stem cells is increasing. At Duke University, a total of 18 patients with infant ALL have been transplanted using UCB as a stem cell source and busulfan and cyclophosphamide as conditioning regimen (J. Kurtzberg, unpublished data). One-year EFS for this group was 71% (95%, 38–100%CI) for seven infants transplanted in first remission, 69% (95%, 32–100%CI) for seven infants transplanted in second remission and 25% (95%, 0–67%CI) for infants transplanted in relapse. Fourteen of the 18 infants transplanted had high-risk disease as defined by *MLL* 11q23 abnormality. The long-term results from this group of patients remain to be determined.

Establishing without doubt that HCT can improve outcome compared with chemotherapy in high-risk infants requires a randomized study, and such a trial is unlikely to take place because of the rarity of this disease and the logistic challenges of performing such studies. A retrospective analysis of outcomes of chemotherapy ($n = 103$) and transplant ($n = 28$) in infants with leukemia carrying t(4:11) from 11 institutions concluded that hematopoietic transplantation did not improve clinical outcome [108]. Similarly, Chessells *et al.* [158] reported the experience with infant treatment protocols in the UK. The most recent study (Infant 92) reports 4-year EFS of 33% overall, compared with 22.5% in the prior study (Infant 87). The Infant 92 study allowed BMT in first remission and 12 infants were transplanted (three sibling donors, nine unrelated donors), five of whom survive. Notably, the main reason for failure in the transplanted patients was relapse ($n = 6$), with only one death from toxicity in a recipient of a sibling donor graft. This outcome was not statistically different from that achieved with chemotherapy. While data from these two multicenter reports are perhaps the best available, interpretation is limited by the small number of patients transplanted, multiple donor types, the lack of prospective enrollment, absence of standardized eligibility requirements and absence of standardized treatments.

There is a clear need for a prospective study to define the role of HCT in infants with genetically defined leukemias that are at high risk for treatment failure. Such studies will need to be multi-institutional and possibly multinational, as infant leukemia is rare. Studies should include evaluation of the late consequences of therapy in survivors, as morbidity can be significant in young children.

Transplantation of children with Down syndrome and ALL

Children with Down syndrome have an approximately 20-fold increased risk of leukemia and now represent around 2% of children enrolled onto phase 3 cooperative group studies for ALL [159,160]. Initial clinical reports of chemotherapy treatment of leukemia in children with Down syndrome indicated increased toxicity in these patients [161]. In support of this, *in vitro* data indicated increased cellular sensitivity to chemotherapeutic agents in cells from children with Down syndrome [162]. However, more recent studies have shown chemotherapy outcomes as good as those seen in children with ALL without Down syndrome [163].

The suggestion of increased therapy-related toxicity with chemotherapy in children with Down syndrome may have led to reluctance to transplant these children in earlier years. The first report of transplant in four children with Down syndrome indicated poor outcome because of increased toxicity [164]. However, a number of more recent reports have described successful transplantation of children with Down syndrome and leukemia using both related and unrelated donor grafts, indicating that these children should be considered as candidates for transplantation [165–168]. Rubin *et al.* [168] reported 27 patients with Down syndrome (18 collected from a survey of BMT centers and nine from the literature). Sixteen received a graft from an HLA-matched sibling, two from nonsibling family members, four from unrelated donors and five received autologous grafts. This study included 14 children with ALL, nine in second remission and five in third remission. Five of the 14 ALL patients were surviving 9–60 months post-transplant. The authors did identify a high rate of regimen-related toxicity in these patients (39% cumulative risk of death in remission at 3 years). A high frequency of airway problems and lung problems were noted, perhaps associated with the use of methotrexate. Despite the significant toxicity, relapse-free survival for the whole group was 44% at 3 years, results that are comparable to those seen in children with ALL without Down syndrome.

Occasionally, the clinical need arises to consider the use of an HLA-matched sibling who has Down syndrome as a bone marrow donor. Although data are limited, Barquinero et al. [169] have described four transplants from matched sibling donors with Down syndrome. In only one of these cases was sustained engraftment achieved. This poor graft function may have been related to poor quality of donor stem cells and suggest that donors with Down syndrome should not be used for transplantation.

Role of second transplant procedures for post-transplant relapse

The most important cause of treatment failure following transplantation for childhood ALL is recurrent leukemia. Additional chemotherapy can induce further remission in a proportion of patients, although very few will survive long term. Experience with the use of second transplants following relapse after bone marrow transplantation is limited. The IBMTR reported on 114 recipients of HLA-identical sibling grafts who received a second allogeneic HCT for treatment of relapse between 1978 and 1989 [170]. Twenty-nine of these patients had ALL. LFS for all the ALL cases was 21% (range 14–30%); however, outcomes were extremely poor in patients who had relapsed less than 6 months after their first transplant, in whom LFS was only 7% (range 2–19%). High rates of treatment-related mortality were seen in those relapsing less than 6 months from initial transplant. Patients with long remissions after their first transplant, those with good performance status and those achieving remission after their initial post-transplant relapse had the best outcomes. Three single center series of second transplant procedures, each including small numbers of ALL cases, also report high early transplant mortality and poor long-term survival [171–173]. A common theme of these reports is the importance of length of remission after transplant, with poor survival after a second HCT in those experiencing early relapse [174,175]. While these procedures remain challenging, some success can be achieved in those with a long remission after the first HCT with careful patient selection.

Conclusions

Overall, the treatment of childhood ALL with chemotherapy has been a story of remarkable success, with survival rates in excess of 70% in the majority of studies. This success is counterbalanced by the fact that current chemotherapy is still inadequate for the 30% of cases who will relapse. As ALL is the most frequent malignancy in children, relapsed ALL remains one of the most frequent causes of death from malignant disease in childhood. Determining the appropriate role for HCT in childhood ALL has been a dynamic process, as success with chemotherapy has increased and additional stem cell sources have become available. Improvements with chemotherapy have been achieved through serial, large scale, essentially population-based randomized studies. Application of a similar rigorous approach to evaluation of the role of HCT has not proved possible so significant uncertainty remains in some areas. Access to HCT has been improved by increased availability and selection of unrelated hematopoietic cell donors and the development of unrelated donor UCB as a hematopoietic cell source. Indeed, outcomes with unrelated donor HCT have improved such that results are now equivalent to sibling donor HCT in well-matched cases.

Future improvements in outcome and applicability of HCT for childhood ALL may result from the development of methodologies to identify at the earliest possible time children who are destined to relapse, allowing HCT in first remission when outcomes are superior. The detection of minimal residual disease in children receiving chemotherapy, either as a harbinger of relapse or as a measure of inadequate early response to therapy, will allow early referral for HCT as intensification therapy [91–95; Chapter 22]. A report describing the use of microarray expression profiling to examine ALL blasts at diagnosis indicated extraordinary accuracy in predicting relapse, if supported by other studies, would allow immediate referral of children with ALL destined to relapse for HCT in first remission [176]. Improved strategies for donor selection using molecular methods of HLA-typing, or examination of non-HLA loci that influence HCT also have potential to improve outcomes [177–179]. Inclusion of chemotherapy agents such as VP16 or thiotepa in the conditioning regimen may reduce relapse and improve survival. Targeting of conditioning therapy with radioimmunoconjugates offers the possibility of reducing radiation toxicity while maintaining the therapeutic effect [180].

References

1 Pui CH. Childhood leukemias. *N Engl J Med* 1995; **332**: 1618–30.

2 van Dongen JJM, Adriaansen HJ. Immunobiology of leukemia. In: Henderson ES, Lister TA, Greaves MF, eds. *Leukemia*, 6th edn. Philadelphia, PA: WB Saunders, 1996: 83–130.

3 Stong RC, Korsmeyer SJ, Parkin JL, Arthur DC, Kersey JH. Human acute leukemia cell line with the t(4;11) chromosomal rearrangement exhibits B-lineage and monocytic characteristics. *Blood* 1985; **65**: 21–31.

4 Rabbitts TH. Chromosomal translocations in human cancer. *Nature* 1994; **372**: 143–9.

5 Kersey JH. Commentary on 50 years of studies of the biology and therapy of childhood leukemia. *Blood* 1998; **92**: 1838.

6 Rubnitz JE, Downing JR, Pui CH et al. TEL gene rearrangement in acute lymphoblastic leukemia: a new genetic marker with prognostic significance. *J Clin Oncol* 1997; **15**: 1150–7.

7 Suryanarayan K, Hunger SP, Kohler S. et al. Consistent involvement of the bcr gene by 9;22 breakpoints in pediatric acute leukemias. *Blood* 1991; **77**: 324–30.

8 Chen CS, Sorensen HB, Domer H et al. Molecular rearrangements on chromosome 11q23 predominate in infant acute lymphoblastic leukemia and are associated with specific biologic variable and poor outcome. *Blood* 1993; **81**: 2386–93.

9 Pui CH, Behm FG, Downing JR et al. 11q23/MLL rearrangement confers a poor prognosis in infants with acute lymphoblastic leukemia. *J Clin Oncol* 1994; **12**: 909–15.

10 Cimino G, Rapanotti MC, Rivolta A et al. Prognostic relevance of ALL-1 gene rearrangement in infant acute leukemias. *Leukemia* 1995; **9**: 391–5.

11 Pui CH, Ribeiro RC, Campana D et al. Prognostic factors in the acute lymphoid and myeloid leukemias of childhood. *Leukemia* 1996; **10**: 952–6.

12 Taki T, Ida K, Bessho F et al. Frequency and the clinical significance of the MLL gene rearrangements in infant acute leukemia. *Leukemia* 1996; **10**: 1303–7.

13 Copelan EA, McGuire EA. The biology and treatment of acute lymphoblastic leukemia in adults. *Blood* 1995; **85**: 1151–68.

14 Perentesis JP. Why is age such an important prognostic factor in acute lymphoblastic leukemia? *Leukemia* 1997; Suppl. 4: S4–S7.

15 Greaves MF, Pegram SM, Chan LC. Collaborative group study of epidemiology of acute lymphoblastic leukemia subtypes: background and first report. *Leuk Res* 1985; **9**: 715–33.

16 Greaves MF, Alexander FE. An infectious etiology for common acute lymphoblastic leukemia. *Leukemia* 1993; **7**: 349–60.

17 Parkin DNM, Stiller CA, Draper GJ, Bieber CA. The international incidence of cancer. *Int J Cancer* 1988; **42**: 511–20.

18 Linet MS, Devesa SS. Descriptive epidemiology of childhood leukemia. *Br J Cancer* 1991; **63**: 424–9.

19 Williams CKO, Folami AO, Laditan AAO, Ukaejiofo EO. Childhood acute leukemia in a tropical population. *Br J Cancer* 1982; **46**: 89–94.

20 Fleming AF. Epidemiology of the leukemias in Africa: an overview. *Leuk Res* 1985; **9**: 735–40.

21 Land H, Parada LF, Weinberg RA. Tumorigenic conversion of primary embryo fibroblasts requires at least two cooperating oncogenes. *Nature* 1983; **304**: 596–602.

22 Graf T. Leukemia as a multi-step process: studies with avian retroviruses containing two oncogenes. *Leukemia* 1988; **2**: 127–31.
23 Alexander FA, Ricketts JT, McKinney PA, Cartwright RA. Community lifestyle characteristics and risk of acute lymphoblastic leukemia in children. *Lancet* 1990; **336**: 1461–5.
24 Kinlen LJ, Clarke K, Hudson C. Evidence from population mixing in British new towns 1946–85 of an infective basis for childhood leukemia. *Lancet* 1990; **339**: 557–82.
25 Crist WM, Grossi CE, Pullen DJ, Cooper MD. Immunologic markers in childhood acute lymphocytic leukemia. *Semin Oncol* 1985; **12**: 105–21.
26 Crist W, Pullen J, Boyett J et al. Acute lymphoid leukemia in adolescents: clinical and biologic features predict a poor prognosis: a Pediatric Oncology Group study. *J Clin Oncol* 1988; **6**: 34–43.
27 Pui CH, Behm FG, Crist WM. Clinical and biological relevance of immunologic marker studies in childhood acute lymphoblastic leukemia. *Blood* 1993; **82**: 343–62.
28 Hoelzer D, Thiel T, Loffler H et al. Intensified therapy in acute lymphoblastic and acute undifferentiated leukemia in adults. *Blood* 1984; **64**: 38–47.
29 Clarkson B, Ellis S, Little C et al. Acute lymphoblastic leukemia in adults. *Semin Oncol* 1985; **12**: 160–79.
30 Bowman WP, Melvin SL, Aur RJ, Mauer AM. A clinical perspective on cell markers in acute lymphocytic leukemia. *Cancer Res* 1981; **41**: 4794–801.
31 Greaves MF, Janossy G, Peto J, Kay H. Immunologically defined subclasses of acute lymphoblastic leukemia in children: their relationship to presentation features and prognosis. *Br J Hematol* 1981; **48**: 179–97.
32 Gingrich RD, Burns GCP, Armitage JO et al. Long term relapse-free survival in adult acute lymphoblastic leukemia. *Cancer Treatment Res* 1985; **69**: 153–60.
33 Bloomfield CD, Foon KA, Levine EG. Leukemias. In: Calabresi P, Schein PS, eds. *Medical Oncology*, 2nd edn. New York: McGraw-Hill, 1993.
34 Uckun FM, Steinherz PG, Sather H et al. CD2 antigen expression on leukemic cells as a predictor of event-free survival after chemotherapy for T-lineage acute lymphoblastic leukemia: a Children's Cancer Group Study. *Blood* 1996; **88**: 4288–95.
35 Kaspers GJ, Smets LA, Pieters R, Van Zantwijk CH, Van Wering ER, Veerman AJP. Favorable prognosis of hyperdiploid common acute lymphoblastic leukemia may be explained by sensitivity to antimetabolites and other drugs: results of an *in vitro* study. *Blood* 1995; **85**: 751–6.
36 Trueworthy R, Shuster J, Look T et al. Ploidy of lymphoblasts is the strongest predictor of treatment outcome in B-progenitor cell acute lymphoblastic leukemia of childhood: a Pediatric Oncology Group Study. *J Clin Oncol* 1992; **10**: 606–13.
37 Whitehead VM, Vucich MJ, Lauer SJ et al. Accumulation of high levels of methotrexate polyglutamates in lymphoblasts from children with hyperdiploid (greater than 50 chromosomes) B-lineage acute lymphoblastic leukemia: a Pediatric Oncology Group Study. *Blood* 1992; **80**: 1316–23.
38 Golub TR, Barker GF, Bohlander SK et al. Fusion of the TEL gene on 12p13 to the AML1 gene on 21q22 in acute lymphoblastic leukemia. *Proc Natl Acad Sci U S A* 1995; **92**: 4917–21.
39 Romana SP, Mauchaffe M, Le Coniat M. et al. The t(12;21) of acute lymphoblastic leukemia results in a TEL–AML-1 gene fusion. *Blood* 1991; **85**: 3662–70.
40 Shurtleff SA, Buijs A, Behm FG et al. TEL-AML.1 fusion resulting from a cryptic t(12;21) is the most common genetic lesion in pediatric ALL and defines a subgroup of patients with an excellent prognosis. *Leukemia* 1995; **9**: 1985–9.
41 Raynaud S, Cave H, Baens M. et al. The 12;21 translocation involving TEL and deletion of the other TEL allele: two frequently associated alterations found in childhood acute lymphoblastic leukemia. *Blood* 1996; **87**: 2891–9.
42 McClean TW, Ringold S, Neuberg D et al. TEL-AML1 dimerizes and is associated with a favorable outcome in childhood acute lymphoblastic leukemia. *Blood* 1996; **88**: 4252–8.
43 Shih LY, Chou TB, Liang DC. et al. Lack of TEL-AML1 fusion transcript resulting from a cryptic t(12;21) in adult B lineage acute lymphoblastic leukemia in Taiwan. *Leukemia* 1996; **10**: 1456–8.
44 Raynaud S, Mauvieux L, Cayuela JM et al. TEL/AML1 fusion gene is a rare event in adult acute lymphoblastic leukemia. *Leukemia* 1996; **10**: 1529–30.
45 Aguiar RC, Sohal J, van Rhee F et al. TEL–AML1 fusion in acute lymphoblastic leukemia of adults. MRC Adult Leukemia Working Party. *Br J Hematol* 1996; **95**: 673–7.
46 Kantarjian HM. Adult acute lymphocytic leukemia: critical review of current knowledge. *Am J Med* 1994; **97**: 176–84.
47 Aricò M, Grazia Valsecchi M, Camitta B et al. Outcome of treatment in children with Philadelphia chromosome-positive acute lymphoblastic leukemia. *N Engl J Med* 2000; **342**: 998–1006.
48 Rivera GK, Hudson MM, Liu Q et al. Effectiveness of intensified rotational combination chemotherapy for late hematologic relapse of childhood acute lymphoblastic leukemia. *Blood* 1996; **88**: 831–7.
49 Bordigoni P, Vernant JP, Souillet G et al. Allogeneic marrow transplantation for children with acute lymphoblastic leukemia in first remission: a cooperative study of the Groupe d'Etude de al Greffe de Moelle Osseuse. *J Clin Oncol* 1989; **7**: 747–53.
50 von Bueltzingsloewen A, Esperou-Bourdeau H, Souillet G et al. Allogeneic bone marrow transplantation following a busulfan-based conditioning regimen in young children with acute lymphoblastic leukemia: a cooperative study of the Societe Francaise de Greffe de Moelle. *Bone Marrow Transplant* 1995; **16**: 521–7.
51 Saarinen UM, Mellander L, Nysom K et al. Allogeneic bone marrow transplantation in first remission for children with very high risk acute lymphoblastic leukemia: a retrospective case–control study in the Nordic countries. Nordic Society for Pediatric Hematology and Oncology (NOPHO). *Bone Marrow Transplant* 1996; **17**: 357–63.
52 Sanders JE, Thomas ED, Buckner CD, Doney K. Marrow transplantation for children with acute lymphoblastic leukemia in second remission. *Blood* 1987; **70**: 324–6.
53 Brochstein JA, Kernan NA, Groshen S et al. Allogeneic bone marrow transplantation after hyperfractionated total body irradiation and cyclophosphamide in children with acute leukemia. *N Engl J Med* 1987; **317**: 1618–24.
54 Woods WG, Nesbit ME, Ramsay NK et al. Intensive therapy followed by bone marrow transplantation for patients with acute lymphocytic leukemia in second or subsequent remission: determination of prognostic factors (a report from the University of Minnesota Bone Marrow Transplantation Team). *Blood* 1983; **61**: 1182–9.
55 Weisdorf DJ, Woods WG, Nesbit ME et al. Allogeneic bone marrow transplantation for acute lymphoblastic leukaemia: risk factors and clinical outcome. *Br J Haematol* 1994; **86**: 62–9.
56 Parsons SK, Castellino SM, Lehmann LE et al. Relapsed acute lymphoblastic leukemia: similar outcomes for autologous and allogeneic marrow transplantation in selected children. *Bone Marrow Transplant* 1996; **17**: 763–8.
57 Carpenter PA, Marshall GM, Giri N, Vowels MR, Russell SJ. Allogeneic bone marrow transplantation for children with acute lymphoblastic leukemia conditioned with busulfan, cyclophosphamide and melphalan. *Bone Marrow Transplant* 1996; **18**: 489–94.
58 Boulad F, Steinherz P, Reyes B et al. Allogeneic bone marrow transplantation versus chemotherapy for the treatment of childhood acute lymphoblastic leukemia in second remission: a single-institution study. *J Clin Oncol* 1999; **17**: 197–207.
59 Bleakley M, Shaw PJ, Nielsen JM. Allogeneic bone marrow transplantation for childhood relapsed acute lymphoblastic leukemia: comparison of outcome in patients with and without a matched family donor. *Bone Marrow Transplant* 2002; **30**: 1–7.
60 Dopfer R, Henze G, Bender-Gotze C et al. Allogeneic bone marrow transplantation for childhood acute lymphoblastic leukemia in second remission after intensive primary and relapse therapy according to the BFM and CoALL protocols. Results German Cooperative Study. *Blood* 1991; **78**: 2780–4.
61 Weyman C, Graham-Pole J, Emerson S et al. Use of cytosine arabinoside and total body irradiation as conditioning for allogeneic marrow transplantation in patients with acute lymphoblastic leukemia: a multicenter survey. *Bone Marrow Transplant* 1993; **11**: 43–50.
62 Barrett AJ, Horowitz MM, Pollock BH et al. Bone marrow transplants from HLA-identical siblings as compared with chemotherapy for children with acute lymphoblastic leukemia in a second remission. *N Engl J Med* 1994; **331**: 1253–8.
63 Moussalem M, Esperou Bourdeau H, Devergie A et al. Allogeneic bone marrow transplantation for childhood acute lymphoblastic leukemia in second remission: factors predictive of survival, relapse and graft-versus-host disease. *Bone Marrow Transplant* 1995; **15**: 943–7.
64 Uderzo C, Rondelli R, Dini G et al. High-dose vincristine, fractionated total-body irradiation and cyclophosphamide as conditioning regimen in allogeneic and autologous bone marrow transplantation for childhood acute lymphoblastic leukaemia in second remission: a 7-year Italian multicentre study. *Br J Haematol* 1995; **89**: 790–7.
65 Torres A, Alvarez MA, Sanchez J et al. Allogeneic bone marrow transplantation vs. chemotherapy for the treamtent of acute lymphoblastic leukaemia in second complete remission (revisited 10 years on). *Bone Marrow Transplant* 1999; **23**: 1257–60.
66 Davies SM, Ramsay NKC, Klein JP et al. Comparison of preparative regimens in transplants for children with acute lymphoblastic leukemia. *J Clin Oncol* 2000; **18**: 340–7.
67 Vicent MG, Madero L, Martinez A et al. Matched-pair analysis comparing allogeneic PBPCT and

BMT from HLA-identical relatives in childhood acute lymphoblastic leukemia. *Bone Marrow Transplant* 2002; **30**: 9–13.
68 Coccia PF, Strandjord SE, Warkentin PI *et al*. High-dose cytosine arabinoside and fractionated total body irradiation: an improved preparative regimen for bone marrow transplantation of children with acute lymphoblastic leukemia in remission. *Blood* 1988; **71**: 888–93.
69 Woods WG, Ramsay NKC, Weisdorf DJ *et al*. Bone marrow transplantation for acute lymphocytic leukemia utilizing total body irradiation followed by high doses of cytosine arabinoside: lack of superiority over cyclophosphamide-containing conditioning regimens. *Bone Marrow Transplant* 1990; **6**: 9–16.
70 Maloney KW, Shuster JJ, Murphy S, Pullen J, Camitta BA. Long-term results of treatment studies for childhood acute lymphoblastic leukemia: Pediatric Oncology Group studies from 1986–1994. *Leukemia* 2000; **14**: 2276–85.
71 Gaynon PS, Qu RP, Chappell RJ *et al*. Survival after relapse in childhood acute lymphoblastic leukemia: impact of site and time to first relapse—the Children's Cancer Group experience. *Cancer* 1998; **82**: 1387–95.
72 Buhrer C, Hartmann R, Fengler R *et al*. Peripheral blast counts at diagnosis of late isolated bone marrow relapse of childhood acute lymphoblastic leukemia predict response to salvage chemotherapy and outcome. Berlin-Frankfurt-Munster Relapse Study Group. *J Clin Oncol* 1996; **14** (10): 2812–7.
73 Camitta BM, Pullen J, Murphy S. Biology and treatment of acute lymphocytic leukemia in children. *Semin Oncol* 1997; **24**: 83–91.
74 Uderzo C, Valsecchi MG, Bacigalupo A *et al*. Treatment of childhood acute lymphoblastic leukemia in second remission with bone marrow transplantation and chemotherapy: ten year experience of the Italian Bone Marrow Transplantation Group and the Italian Pediatric Hematology Oncology Association. *J Clin Oncol* 1995; **134**: 352–8.
75 Gustafsson G, Schmiegelow K, Forestier E *et al*. Improving outcome through two decades in childhood ALL in the Nordic countries: the impact of high-dose methotrexate in the reduction of CNS irradiation. *Leukemia* 2000; **14**: 2267–75.
76 Vilmer E, Suciu S, Ferster A. *et al*. Long-term results of three randomized trials (58831, 58832, 58881) in childhood acute lymphoblastic leukemia: A CLCG–EORTC report. *Leukemia* 2000; **14**: 2257–66.
77 Silverman LB, Declerck L, Gelber RD *et al*. Results of Dana-Farber Cancer Institute protocols for children with newly diagnosed acute lymphoblastic leukemia (1981–95). *Leukemia* 2000; **14**: 2247–56.
78 Kamps WA, Veerman AJJP, van Wering ER, van Weerden JF, Slater R, van der Does-van den Berg A. Long-term follow-up of Dutch Childhood Leukemia Study Group (DCLSG) protocols for children with acute lymphoblastic leukemia, 1984–91. *Leukemia* 2000; **14**: 2240–6.
79 Harms DO, Janka-Schaub GE, on behalf of the COALL Study Group. Co-operative study group for childhood acute lymphoblastic leukemia (COALL): long-term follow-up of trials 82, 85, 89 and 92. *Leukemia* 2000; **14**: 2234–9.
80 Gaynon PS, Trigg ME, Heerema NA *et al*. Children's Cancer Group trials in childhood acute lymphoblastic leukemia: 1983–95. *Leukemia* 2000; **14**: 2223–33.

81 Schrappe M, Reiter A, Zimmermann M *et al*. Long-term results of four consecutive trials in childhood ALL performed by the ALL-BFM study group from 1981 to 1995. *Leukemia* 2000; **14**: 2205–22.
82 Conter V, Aricò M, Valsecchi MG *et al*. Long-term results of the Italian Association of Pediatric Hematology and Oncology (AIEOP) Acute Lymphoblastic Leukemia Studies, 1982–95. *Leukemia* 2000; **14**: 2196–204.
83 Smith M, Arthur D, Camitta B *et al*. Uniform approach to risk classification and treatment assignment for children with acute lymphoblastic leukemia. *J Clin Oncol* 1996; **14**: 18–24.
84 Pullen J, Shuster JJ, Link M *et al*. Significance of commonly used prognostic factors differs for children with T cell acute lymphocytic leukemia (ALL), as compared to those with B-precursor ALL: a Pediatric Oncol Group (POG) study. *Leukemia* 1999; **13**: 1696–707.
85 Schultz KR, Bostrom B, Cairo M. *et al*. Very high risk features in childhood acute lymphoblastic leukemia in recent Children's Cancer Group therapeutic studies. SIOP-ASPH/O Meeting Abstract, O-100. *Med Ped Oncol* 1999; **33**: 169.
86 Heerema NA, Nachman JB, Sather HN *et al*. Hypodiploidy with less than 45 chromosomes confers adverse risk in childhood acute lymphoblastic leukemia: a report from the Children's Cancer Group. *Blood* 1999; **94**: 4036–46.
87 Marks DI, Bird JM, Cornish JM *et al*. Unrelated donor bone marrow transplantation for children and adolescents with Philadelphia-positive acute lymphoblastic leukemia. *J Clin Oncol* 1998; **16**: 931–6.
88 Sierra J, Radich J, Hansen JA *et al*. Marrow transplants from unrelated donors for treatment of Philadelphia chromosome-positive acute lymphoblastic leukemia. *Blood* 1997; **90**: 1410–4.
89 Nachman JB, Sather HN, Sensel MG *et al*. Augmented post-induction therapy for children with high-risk acute lymphoblastic leukemia and a slow response to initial therapy. *N Engl J Med* 1998; **388**: 1663–71.
90 Aricò M, Grazia Valsecchi M, Conter V *et al*. for the Associazione Italiana di Ematologia ed Oncologia Pediatrica. Improved outcome in high-risk childhood acute lymphoblastic leukemia defined by prednisone-poor response treated with double Berlin-Frankfurt-Muenster protocol II. *Blood* 2002; **100**: 420–6.
91 Nyvold C, Madsen HO, Ryder LP *et al*. on behalf of the Nordic Society for Pediatric Hematology and Oncology. Precise quantification of minimal residual disease at day 29 allows identification of children with acute lymphoblastic leukemia and an excellent outcome. *Blood* 2002; **99**: 1253–8.
92 Dworzak MN, Fröschi G, Printz D *et al*. for the Austrian Berlin-Frankfurt-Münster Study Group. Prognostic significance and modalities of flow cytometric minimal residual disease detection in childhood acute lymphoblastic leukemia. *Blood* 2002; **99**: 1952–8.
93 Tarusawa M, Yashima A, Endo M, Maesawa C. Quantitative assessment of minimal residual disease in childhood lymphoid malignancies using an allele-specific oligonucleotide real-time quantitative polymerase chain reaction. *Int J Hematol* 2002; **75**: 166–73.
94 Willemse MJ, Seriu T, Hettinger K *et al*. Detection of minimal residual disease identifies differences in treatment response between T-ALL and precursor B-ALL. *Blood* 2002; **99**: 4386–93.

95 Coustan-Smith E, Sancho J, Behm FG *et al*. Prognostic importance of measuring early clearance of leukemic cells by flow cytometry in childhood acute lymphoblastic leukemia. *Blood* 2002; **100**: 52–8.
96 Van Der Velden VH, Jacobs DC, Wijkhuijs AJ *et al*. Minimal residual disease levels in bone marrow and peripheral blood are comparable in children with T-cell acute lymphoblastic leukemia (ALL), but not in precursor-B-ALL. *Leukemia* 2002; **16**: 1432–6.
97 Uderzo C, Valsecchi MG, Balduzzi A *et al*. Allogeneic bone marrow transplantation versus chemotherapy in high-risk childhood acute lymphoblastic leukaemia in first remission. Associazone Italiana di Ematologia ed Oncologia Pediatrica (AIEOP) and the Gruppo Italiano Trapianto di Midollo Osseo (GITMO). *Br J Haemtol* 1997; **96**: 387–94.
98 Wheeler KA, Richards SM, Bailey CC *et al*. for the Medical Research Council Working Party on Childhood Leukaemia. Bone marrow transplantation versus chemotherapy in the treatment of very high-risk childhood acute lymphoblastic leukaemia in first remission: Results from Medical Research Council UKALL X and XI. *Blood* 2000; **96**: 2412–8.
99 Horowitz MM, Przepiorka D, Champlin RE *et al*. Should HLA-identical sibling bone marrow transplants for leukemia be restricted to large centers? *Blood* 1992; **79**: 2771–4.
100 Frassoni F, Labopin M, Powles R *et al*. Effect of centre on outcome of bone-marrow transplantation for acute myeloid leukaemia. Acute Leukaemia Working Party of the European Group for Blood and Marrow Transplantation. *Lancet* 2000; **355**: 1393–8.
101 Duell T, van Lint MT, Ljungman P *et al*. Health and functional status of long-term survivors of bone marrow transplantation. EBMT Working Party on Late Effects and EULEP Study Group on Late Effects. European Group for Blood Marrow Transplantation. *Ann Intern Med* 1997; **126**: 184–92.
102 Cerveri I, Zoia MC, Fulgoni P *et al*. Late pulmonary sequelae after childhood bone marrow transplantation. *Thorax* 1999; **54**: 131–5.
103 Grigg AP. Approaches to the treatment of Philadelphia-positive acute lymphoblastic leukemia. *Bone Marrow Transplant* 1993; **12**: 431–3.
104 Stockschlader M, Hegewisch-Becker S, Kruger W *et al*. Bone marrow transplantation for Philadelphia-chromosome-positive acute lymphoblastic leukemia. *Bone Marrow Transplant* 1995; **16**: 663–7.
105 Chao NJ, Blume KG, Forman SJ, Snyder DS. Long term follow-up of allogeneic bone marrow recipients for Philadelphia chromosome-positive acute lymphoblastic leukemia. *Blood* 1995; **85**: 3353–6.
106 Emminger W, Emminger-Schmidmeier W, Haas OA *et al*. Treatment of infant leukemia with busulfan, cyclophosphamide +/− etoposide and bone marrow transplantation. *Bone Marrow Transplant* 1992; **9**: 313–8.
107 Blume KG, Forman SJ, Snyder DS *et al*. Allogeneic bone marrow transplantation for acute lymphoblastic leukemia during first complete remission. *Transplantation* 1987; **43**: 389–92.
108 Amylon MD, Co JP, Snyder DS *et al*. Allogeneic bone marrow transplantation in pediatric patients with high risk hematopoietic malignancies early in the course of their disease. *J Pediatr Hematol Oncol* 1997; **19**: 54–61.

109 Hilden JM, Frestedt JL, Moore RO. et al. Molecular analysis of infant acute leukemia: MLL gene rearrangement and reverse transcriptase-polymerase chain reaction for t(4;11)(q21;q23). *Blood* 1995; **86**: 3876–82.

110 Pui C-H, Gaynon PS, Boyett JM et al. Outcome of treatment in childhood acute lymphoblastic leukaemia with rearrangements of the 11q23 chromosomal region. *Lancet* 2002; **359**: 1909–15.

111 Oakhill A, Pamphilon DH, Potter MN et al. Unrelated donor bone marrow transplantation for children with relapsed acute lymphoblastic leukaemia in second complete remission. *Br J Haematol* 1996; **94**: 574–8.

112 Woolfrey AE, Anasetti C, Storer B et al. Factors associated with outcome after unrelated marrow transplantation for treatment of acute lymphoblastic leukemia in children. *Blood* 2002; **99**: 2002–8.

113 Casper J, Camitta B, Truitt R et al. Unrelated bone marrow donor transplants for children with leukemia or myelodysplasia. *Blood* 1995; **85**: 2354–63.

114 Davies SM, Wagner JE, Shu XO et al. Unrelated donor bone marrow transplantation for children with acute leukemia. *J Clin Oncol* 1997; **15**: 557–65.

115 Green A, Clarke E, Hunt L et al. Children with acute lymphoblastic leukemia who receive T-cell-depleted HLA mismatched marrow allografts from unrelated donors have an increased incidence of primary graft failure but a similar overall transplant outcome. *Blood* 1999; **94**: 2236–46.

116 Hongeng S, Krance RA, Bowman LC et al. Outcomes of transplantation with matched-sibling and unrelated-donor bone marrow in children with leukaemia. *Lancet* 1997; **350**: 767–71.

117 Saarinen-Pihkala UM, Gustafsson G, Ringdén O et al. for the Nordic Society of Pediatric Hematology and Oncology. No disadvantage in outcome of using matched unrelated donors as compared with matched sibling donors for bone marrow transplantation in children with acute lymphoblastic leukemia in second remission. *J Clin Oncol* 2001; **19**: 3406–14.

118 Al-Kasim FA, Thornley I, Rolland M et al. Single-centre experience with allogeneic bone marrow transplantation for acute lymphoblastic leukaemia in childhood: similar survival after matched-related and matched-unrelated donor transplants. *Br J Haematol* 2002; **116**: 483–90.

119 Davies SM, DeFor TE, McGlave PB et al. Equivalent outcomes in patients with chronic myelogenous leukemia after early transplantation of phenotypically matched bone marrow from related or unrelated donors. *Am J Med* 2001; **110**: 339–46.

120 Feig SA, Harris RE, Sather HN. Bone marrow transplantation versus chemotherapy for maintenance of second remission of childhood acute lymphoblastic leukemia: a study of the Children's Cancer Group (CCG-1884). *Med Pediatr Oncol* 1997; **29**: 534–40.

121 Wheeler K, Richards S, Bailey C, Chessells J, for the Medical Research Council Working Party on Childhood Leukaemia. Comparison of bone marrow transplant and chemotherapy for relapsed childhood acute lymphoblastic leukaemia. The MRC UKALL X Experience. *Br J Haematol* 1998; **101**: 94–103.

122 Schroeder H, Garwicz S, Kristinsson J et al. Outcome after first relapse in children with acute lymphoblastic leukemia: a population-based study of 315 patients from the Nordic Society of Pediatric Hematology and Oncology (NOPHO). *Med Ped Oncol* 1995; **25**: 372–8.

123 Borgmann A, Hartmann R, Schmid H et al. Isolated extramedullary relapse in children with acute lymphoblastic leukemia: a comparison between treatment results of chemotherapy and bone marrow transplantation. BFM Relapse Study Group. *Bone Marrow Transplant* 1995; **15**: 515–21.

124 Blume KG, Forman SJ, O'Donnell MR et al. Total body irradiation and high-dose etoposide: a new preparatory regimen for bone marrow transplantation in patients with advanced hematologic malignancies. *Blood* 1987; **69**: 1015–20.

125 Schmitz N, Gassmann W, Rister M et al. Fractionated total body irradiation and high-dose VP 16-213 followed by allogeneic bone marrow transplantation in advanced leukemias. *Blood* 1988; **72**: 1567–73.

126 Snyder DS, Chao NJ, Amylon MD et al. Fractionated total body irradiation and high-dose etoposide as a preparatory regimen for bone marrow transplantation for 99 patients with acute leukemia in first complete remission. *Blood* 1993; **82**: 2920–8.

127 Kernan NA, Boulad F, Small TN et al. Improved outcome with T-cell depleted (SBA_E_) marrow transplants from related and unrelated donors for children with acute leukemia transplanted in first or second remission. *Blood* 2001; **98**: 2821.

128 Tutschka PJ, Copelan EA, Klein JP. Bone marrow transplantation for leukemia following a new busulfan and cyclophosphamide regimen. *Blood* 1987; **70**: 1382–8.

129 Henslee-Downey PJ, Abhyankar SH, Parrish RS et al. Use of partially mismatched related donors extends access to allogeneic marrow transplant. *Blood* 1997; **89**: 3864–72.

130 Filipovich AH, Ramsay NK, Arthur DC, McGlave PB, Kim T, Kersey JH. Allogeneic bone marrow transplantation with related donors other than HLA MLC-matched siblings, and the use of antithymocyte globulin, prednisone and methotrexate for prophylaxis of graft-versus-host disease. *Transplantation* 1985; **39**: 282–5.

131 Bozdech MJ, Sondel PM, Trigg ME et al. Transplantation for haploidentical T-cell-depleted marrow for leukemia: addition of cytosine arabinoside to the pretransplant conditioing prevents rejection. *Exp Hematol* 1985; **13**: 1201–10.

132 Beatty PG, Clift RA, Mickelson EM et al. Marrow transplantation from related donors other than HLA-identical siblings. *N Engl J Med* 1985; **313**: 765–71.

133 Anasetti C, Amos D, Beatty PG et al. Effect of HLA compatibility on engraftment of bone marrow transplants in patients with leukemia or lymphoma. *N Engl J Med* 1989; **320**: 197–204.

134 Ash RC, Horowitz MM, Gale RP et al. Bone marrow transplantation from related donors other than HLA-identical siblings: effect of T-cell depletion. *Bone Marrow Transplant* 1991; **7**: 443–52.

135 Szydlo R, Goldman JM, Klein JP et al. Results of allogeneic bone marrow transplants for leukemia using donors other than HLA-identical siblings. *J Clin Oncol* 1997; **15**: 1767–77.

136 Munn RK, Henslee-Downey PJ, Romond EH et al. Treatment of leukemia with partially matched related bone marrow transplantation. *Bone Marrow Transplant* 1997; **19**: 421–7.

137 Ruggeri L, Campanni M, Urbani E et al. Effectiveness of donor natural killer cell alloreactivity in mismatched hematopoietic transplants. *Science* 2002; **295**: 2097–100.

138 Handgretinger H, Klingebiel T, Lang P et al. Megadose transplantation of purified peripheral blood $CD34^+$ progenitor cells from HLA-mismatched parental donors in children. *Bone Marrow Transplant* 2001; **27**: 777–83.

139 Beatty PG, Kollman C, Howe CW. Unrelated-donor marrow transplants. the experience of the National Marrow Donor Program. *Clin Transpl* 1995: 271–7.

140 Stroncek DF, Holland PV, Bartsch G et al. Experiences of the first 493 unrelated marrow donors in the National Marrow Donor Program. *Blood* 1993; **81**: 1940–6.

141 Schreuder GM, Hurley CK, Marsh SG et al. The HLA Dictionary: a summary of HLA-A, -B, -C, -DRB1/3/4/5 and -DQB1 alleles and their association with serologically defined HLA-A, -B, -C, -DR and DQ antigens. *Eur J Immunogenet* 2001; **28**: 565–96.

142 Davies SM, Ramsay NKC, Weisdorf DJ. Feasibility and timing of unrelated donor identification for patients with ALL. *Bone Marrow Transplant* 1996; **17**: 737–40.

143 Barker JN, Krepski TP, Davies SM et al. Searching for unrelated donor hematopoietic stem cells: availability and speed of umbilical cord blood versus bone marrow. *Biol Blood Marrow Transplant* 2002; **8**: 257–60.

144 Davies SM, Shu XO, Blazar BR et al. Unrelated donor bone marrow transplantation: influence of HLA A and B incompatibility on outcome. *Blood* 1995; **86**: 1636–42.

145 Bunin N, Carston M, Wall D et al. 7 and the National Marrow Donor Program Working Group. Unrelated marrow transplantation for children with acute lymphoblastic leukemia in second remission. *Blood* 2002; **99**: 3151–7.

146 Lawson SE, Harrison G, Richards S et al. on behalf of the MRC Childhood Leukaemia Working Party. The UK experience in treating relapsed childhood acute lymphoblastic leukaemia: a report on the Medical Research Council UKALLR1 study. *Br J Haematol* 2000; **108**: 531–43.

147 Rubinstein P, Dobrila L, Rosenfield RE et al. Processing and cryopreservation of placental/umbilical cord blood for unrelated bone marrow reconstitution. *Proc Natl Acad Sci U S A* 1995; **92**: 10119–22.

148 Rubinstein P, Taylor PE, Scaradavou A et al. Unrelated placental blood for bone marrow reconstitution: organization of the placental blood program. *Blood Cells* 1994; **20**: 587–96.

149 Harris DT. Experience in autologous and allogeneic cord blood banking. *J Hematother* 1996; **5**: 123–8.

150 Lazzari L, Corsini C, Curioni C et al. The Milan Cord Blood Bank and the Italian Cord Blood Network. *J Hematother* 1996; **5**: 117–22.

151 Gluckman E, Thierry D, Traineau R. Blood banking for hematopoietic stem cell transplantation. *J Hematother* 1993; **2**: 269–70.

152 Wagner JE, Kernan NA, Steinbuch M, Broxmeyer HE, Gluckman E. Allogeneic sibling umbilical-cord-blood transplantation in children with malignant and nonmalignant disease. *Lancet* 1995; **346**: 214–9.

153 Rubinstein P, Carrier C, Scaradavou A et al. Outcomes among 562 recipients of placental-blood transplants from unrelated donors. *N Engl J Med* 1998; **339**: 1565–77.

154 Gluckman E, Rocha V, Boyer-Chammard A *et al.* for the Eurocord Transplant Group and the European Blood and Marrow Transplantation Group. Outcome of cord-blood transplantation from related and unrelated donors. *N Engl J Med* 1997; **337**: 373–81.

155 Wagner JE, Barker JN, DeFor TE *et al.* Transplantation of unrelated donor umbilical cord blood in 102 patients with malignant and nonmalignant diseases: influence of CD34 cell dose and HLA disparity on treatment-related mortality and survival. *Blood* 2002; **100**: 1611–8.

156 Rocha V, Cornish J, Sievers EL *et al.* Comparison of outcomes of unrelated bone marrow and umbilical cord blood transplants in children with acute leukemia. *Blood* 2001; **97**: 2962–71.

157 Barker JN, Davies SM, DeFor T, Ramsay NKC, Weisdorf DJ, Wagner JE. Survival after transplantation of unrelated donor umbilical cord blood is comparable to that of human leukocyte antigen-matched unrelated bone marrow: results of a matched-pair analysis. *Blood* 2001; **97**: 2957–61.

158 Chessells JM, Harrison CJ, Watson SL, Vora AJ, Richards SM, for the Medical Research Council Working Party on Childhood Leukaemia. Treatment of infants with lymphoblastic leukaemia. Results UK Infant Protocols 1987–99. *Br J Haematol* 2002; **117**: 306–14.

159 Robison LL, Nesbit ME, Sather HN *et al.* Down syndrome and acute leukemia in children: a 10 year retrospective survey from Children's Cancer Study Group. *J Pediatr* 1984; **105**: 235–42.

160 Ragab AH, Abdel-Mageed A, Shuster JJ *et al.* Clinical characteristics and treatment outcome of children with acute lymphoblastic leukemia and Down's syndrome: a Pediatric Oncology Group study. *Cancer* 1991; **67**: 1057–63.

161 Blatt J, Albo V, Prin W *et al.* Excessive chemotherapy-related toxicity in children with Down syndrome and acute lymphoblastic leukemia. *Lancet* 1986; **2**: 914 [Letter].

162 Peeters MA, Poon A. Down syndrome and leukemia: unusual clinical aspects and unexpected methotrexate sensitivity. *Eur J Pediatr* 1987; **146**: 416–22.

163 Garre ML, Relling MV, Kalwinsky D *et al.* Pharmacokinetics and toxicity of methotrexate in children with Down syndrome and acute lymphoblastic leukemia. *J Pediatr* 1987; **111**: 606–12.

164 Rubin CM, O'Leary M, Koch PA *et al.* Bone marrow transplantation for children with acute leukemia and Down syndrome. *Pediatics* 1986; **78**: 688–91.

165 Arensen EB, Forde MD. Bone marrow transplantation for acute leukemia and Down syndrome: Report of a successful case and results of a national survey. *J Pediatr* 1989; **114**: 69–72.

166 Pawlowska AB, Davies SM, Orchard PJ, Wagner JE, Ramsay NKC. Unrelated donor transplantation for children with Down syndrome. *Bone Marrow Transplant* 1996; **18**: 435–55.

167 Conter V, D'Angelo P, Rizzari C *et al.* High-dose cytosine arabinoside and fractionated total body irradiation as a preparative regimen for the treatment of children with acute lymphoblastic leukemia and Down syndrome. *Bone Marrow Transplant* 1996; **17**: 287–9.

168 Rubin CM, Mick R, Johnson FL. Bone marrow transplantation for the treatment of hematological disorders in Down's syndrome: toxicity outcome. *Bone Marrow Transplant* 1996; **18**: 533–40.

169 Barquinero J, Witherspoon R, Sanders J *et al.* Allogeneic marrow grafts from donors with congenital chromosomal abnormalities in marrow cells. *Br J Haematol* 1995; **90**: 595–601.

170 Mrsic M, Horowitz MM, Atkinson K *et al.* Second HLA-identical sibling transplants for leukemia recurrence. *Bone Marrow Transplant* 1992; **9**: 269–75.

171 Wagner JE, Vogelsang GB, Zehnbauer BA, Griffin CA, Shah N, Santos GW. Relapse of leukemia after bone marrow transplantation: effect of second myeloablative therapy. *Bone Marrow Transplant* 1992; **9**: 205–9.

172 Radich JP, Sanders JE, Buckner CD *et al.* Second allogeneic marrow transplantation for patients with recurrent leukemia after initial transplant with total-body irradiation-containing regimens. *J Clin Oncol* 1993; **11**: 304–13.

173 Chiang K-Y, Weisdorf DJ, Davies SM *et al.* Outcome of second bone marrow transplantation following a uniform conditioning regimen as therapy for malignant relapse. *Bone Marrow Transplant* 1996; **17**: 39–42.

174 Kumar L. Leukemia: management of relapse after allogeneic bone marrow transplantation. *J Clin Oncol* 1994; **12**: 1710–7.

175 Giralt SA, Champlin RE. Leukemia relapse after allogeneic bone marrow transplantation: a review. *Blood* 1994; **84**: 3603–12.

176 Yeoh E-J, Ross ME, Shurtleff SA *et al.* Classification, subtype discovery, and prediction of outcome in pediatric acute lymphoblastic leukemia by gene expression profiling. *Cancer Cell* 2002; **1**: 133–43.

177 Sasazuki T, Juji T, Morishima Y *et al.* Effect of matching of class I HLA alleles on clinical outcome after transplantation of hematopoietic stem cells from an unrelated donor. Japan Marrow Donor Program. *N Engl J Med* 1998; **339**: 1177–85.

178 Cavet J, Middleton PG, Segall M, Noreen H, Davies SM, Dickinson AM. Recipient tumor necrosis factor-alpha and interleukin-10 gene polymorphisms associate with early mortality and acute graft-versus-host disease severity in HLA-matched sibling bone marrow transplants. *Blood* 1999; **94**: 3941–6.

179 Rocha V, Franco RF, Porcher R *et al.* Host defense and inflammatory gene polymorphisms are associated with outcomes after HLA-identical sibling bone marrow transplantation. *Blood* 2002; **100** (12): 3908–18.

180 Matthews DC, Appelbaum FR, Eary JF *et al.* Phase I study of (131)-anti-CD45 antibody plus cyclophosphamide and total body irradiation for advanced acute leukemia and myelodysplastic syndrome. *Blood* 1999; **94**: 1237–47.

79

Jeanne E. Anderson

Allogeneic Transplantation for Myelodysplastic and Myeloproliferative Disorders

The myelodysplastic and myeloproliferative disorders include a wide spectrum of clonal hematopoietic diseases. The major distinction between the myelodysplastic and myeloproliferative diseases is that in myelodysplasia clonal proliferation is generally ineffective, resulting in the development of progressive cytopenias, whereas in the myeloproliferative disorders increased peripheral counts are generally the rule, at least until late stages of the disease. An important similarity among these disorders is that they all arise from neoplastic transformation of an early hematopoietic stem cell. Studies have shown that the myeloid cells in these disorders are clonal in origin [1–10]. However, whether or not B and T lymphocytes are also derived from the same neoplastic clone is controversial, as in some studies lymphocytes have been found to be nonclonal in origin, at least at the time of study [5,6,9]. Another marked similarity between the myelodysplastic and myeloproliferative disorders is the increased risk of developing acute myeloid leukemia (AML). The observation of clonality in early hematopoietic stem cells may explain why these disorders are incurable with conventional therapies. Only with complete eradication of the marrow and replacement using stem cells from a normal donor have cures been achieved. However, because of the variable natural history of these diverse disorders, optimal management of any patient, particularly the timing of hematopoietic cell transplantation (HCT), requires both an understanding of the natural history of these specific syndromes and knowledge of the current results obtainable with HCT.

Myelodysplasia

Disease definition

Myelodysplastic syndrome (MDS) includes a group of clonal hematopoietic stem cell disorders characterized by impaired maturation of hematopoietic cells, progressive peripheral cytopenias and a tendency to progress into AML. The pathogenesis of MDS is complex and incompletely understood, but includes clonal transformation of an early hematopoietic stem cell, progressive genetic events [1,11,12], enhanced apoptosis of hematopoietic progenitor cells and dysregulated cytokine environment [12–14]. The French–American–British (FAB) Cooperative Group recognizes five distinct forms of pathology in MDS:
1 refractory anemia (RA);
2 refractory anemia with ringed sideroblasts (RARS);
3 refractory anemia with excess blasts (RAEB);
4 refractory anemia with excess blasts in transformation (RAEB-T); and
5 chronic myelomonocytic leukemia (CMML) (Table 79.1) [15–17].

The World Health Organization (WHO) has developed a new classification system in which:

1 CMML is reclassified as a disorder with mixed myelodysplastic and myeloproliferative features;
2 RAEB is divided into two categories based on marrow blast count (5–10% and 11–20%);
3 RAEB-T is eliminated and >20% blasts is categorized as AML; and
4 several other unique categories are now defined [18–21].
However, in this chapter, the FAB system has been used because of the data available from published transplant studies on MDS.

The incidence of MDS ranges from 3.5 to 12.6 cases/100,000 patient population/year [22–24] and increases dramatically with age, with one study finding an incidence of 4.9/100,000 population in patients 50–70 years of age and 22.8/100,000 population in patients over 70 years of age [22]. The median age at diagnosis is approximately 65–70 years. Although uncommon in the young, MDS can occur in children [25–27].

The etiology of MDS is unknown in the majority of cases. However, an increasing proportion of patients diagnosed with MDS have developed their disease following treatment with chemotherapy or ionizing radiation, or the combination of both. Alkylating agents are the most common drugs associated with development of therapy-related MDS, which typically occurs 4–5 years following the inciting agent, and in ≥90% of cases is associated with chromosome abnormalities most commonly involving chromosome 5 and 7 [28]. With increasing intensity of chemotherapy for malignancies, such as autologous HCT for lymphoma, and increasing cure rate for some malignancies, there appears to be an increasing incidence of therapy-related MDS [29].

In this chapter, therapy-related MDS is defined as MDS that develops after exposure to chemotherapy or radiation. Other predisposing factors to MDS include antecedent hematologic disorders such as aplastic anemia and paroxysmal nocturnal hemoglobinuria, congenital chromosome fragility states such as Fanconi's anemia, ataxia telangiectasia and occupational exposure to benzene.

The International Prognostic Scoring System (IPSS) currently offers the best system for determining prognosis for patients with MDS [30]. This scoring system considers the number of cytopenias, marrow blast percentage and karyotype, and differentiates patients into four distinct risk groups with significant differences in both survival and likelihood of evolving to AML (Table 79.2). Patients with therapy-related MDS were not included in this prognostic scoring system, and most experience suggests that patients with secondary MDS have a worse prognosis than those with primary MDS.

Patients with MDS usually die either from disease progression to AML or from complications of pancytopenia. Patients with complex cytogenetic abnormalities or blast count ≥10% have a greater likelihood of progressing to AML than other patients [30]. Infection and hemorrhage associated with low peripheral blood counts are the most common

Table 79.1 French–American–British (FAB) Cooperative Group Classification of myelodysplastic syndrome (MDS). (Data from [16].)

Classification	Marrow blasts (%)	Peripheral blood blasts (%)	Auer rods	Ring sideroblasts (>15%)	Monocytes (>1000/µL)
RA	<5	<1	–	–	–
RARS	<5	<1	–	+	–
RAEB	5–20	≤5	–	±	–
RAEB-T	21–30 or	>5 or	+	±	±
CMML	≤20	<5	–	±	+

+ always present; – always absent; ± variable.
CMML, chronic myelomonocytic leukemia; RA, refractory anemia; RAEB, refractory anemia with excess blasts; RAEB-T, refractory anemia with excess blasts in transformation; RARS, refractory anemia with ringed sideroblasts.

Table 79.2 International Prognostic Scoring System for myelodysplastic syndrome (MDS). (With permission from Greenberg et al. [30].)

Risk group	Score*	Median survival (years)		Time to 25% risk of AML evolution (years)	
		All patients	≤60 years	All patients	≤60 years
Low	0	5.7	11.8	9.4	>9.4
Intermediate-1	0.5–1.0	3.5	5.2	3.3	6.0
Intermediate-2	1.5–2.0	1.2	1.8	1.1	0.7
High	≥2.5	0.4	0.3	0.2	0.2

*Total score is based on sum of individual scores for marrow blast percentage, karyotype and peripheral cytopenias. For marrow blast percentage, a score of 0 is given for blasts <5%; 0.5 for 5–10%; 1.5 for 11–20%; and 2.0 for 21–30%. For karyotype, a score of 0 is given for normal; -Y, del(5q) or del(20q); 1.0 for ≥3 abnormalities or chromosome 7 anomalies; and 0.5 for other abnormalities. For peripheral cytopenias, a score of 0 is given for none or one cytopenia and 0.5 for two or three cytopenias. A cytopenia is defined as neutrophil count <1800/µL, hemoglobin <10 g/dL or platelet count <100,000/µL.

immediate causes of death in MDS, accounting for 35–50% of all deaths [31,32]. Because this disease occurs predominantly in the elderly, non-hematologic deaths account for 10–20% of deaths [31,32].

The majority of patients with MDS, because of their advanced age, are generally managed solely with supportive care. Supportive care includes transfusional support, antimicrobial therapy and, on occasion, iron chelation [33]. Other treatments that have been evaluated in patients with MDS include steroids, differentiating agents, hematopoietic growth factors, immunosuppressive therapy, hypomethylating agents, low-dose chemotherapy and intensive induction chemotherapy [33–38]. There are some data, although controversial, to suggest that in the rare young individual with RAEB or RAEB-T and normal cytogenetics, treatment with intensive chemotherapy may result in cure [38]. However, all other nontransplant treatment for MDS is palliative at best, and not curative. Although restrictions based on patient age and donor availability limit the use of HCT to a small number of patients with MDS, the potential for cure has encouraged extensive investigation of this therapeutic option.

Hematopoietic cell transplantation

Allogeneic HCT was initially attempted in the treatment of patients with MDS based on incurability of the disease with conventional measures, and the observation that HCT could cure patients with other forms of incurable hematologic malignancies. Several early studies in the 1980s established the feasibility of such treatment [39–44].

General results

Numerous single center and registry studies have reported results of patients with MDS undergoing allogeneic HCT [45–60]. Some of these reports included a small number of patients with MDS-related AML (generally defined as patients with a history of MDS and subsequent progression into AML). Although there was a wide variety of patient characteristics and transplantation procedures, the major endpoints of relapse and death were relatively similar between these studies. Most studies report a disease-free survival (DFS) rate of 30–40% (range 23–63%), nonrelapse mortality (NRM) rate of 40–45% (range 35–68%) and relapse rate of approximately 20% (range 0–58%). Representative results of outcome from the International Bone Marrow Transplant Registry (IBMTR) [46] and Seattle [48] are shown in Figs 79.1 and 79.2.

Outcome based on disease morphology and cytogenetics

The two most important independent variables associated with the incidence of relapse and, thereby, DFS are disease morphology and cytogenetic group. Most studies have demonstrated that with increasing blast percentage or advanced disease morphology (i.e. RAEB or RAEB-T compared with RA or RARS) there is a higher risk of relapse post-transplant and a shorter DFS (Fig. 79.1) [45–51,58,60,61]. DFS rates for RA and RARS range from 50 to 75% (partly dependent on patient age and donor source), with relapse rates ranging from 0 to 13% [45,46,62]. On the other hand, DFS rates for RAEB and RAEB-T are generally 25–30%, with relapse rates of 20–50% [45,46,56,61]. Similar to the other disease subtypes, patients with CMML have an overall DFS rate of 39%, and a relapse rate that is dependent on the presence or absence of excess blasts [63].

Approximately 40% of patients with primary MDS have a clonal cytogenetic abnormality [30,64]. The IPSS classifies good risk karyotype as no abnormality or a single abnormality consisting of del(5q), del(20q) or -Y [30]. Poor-risk karyotype comprises complex (≥3) or chromosome 7 abnormalities and intermediate-risk karyotype comprises all other abnormalities. Several studies have shown that karyotype, classified either by the IPSS or other systems, is predictive of the natural history of MDS [30,64]. Although early transplant studies yielded conflicting results on outcome following HCT based on karyotype [51,53,54,58,59,61,62], several recent studies using the IPSS cytogenetic classification system have shown unequivocally the prognostic importance of the cytogenetic grouping [48,52,56,65]. The results of 250 patients transplanted in Seattle ($n = 77$ poor risk, $n = 53$ intermediate risk, $n = 110$ good risk cytogenetics) showed a significantly higher

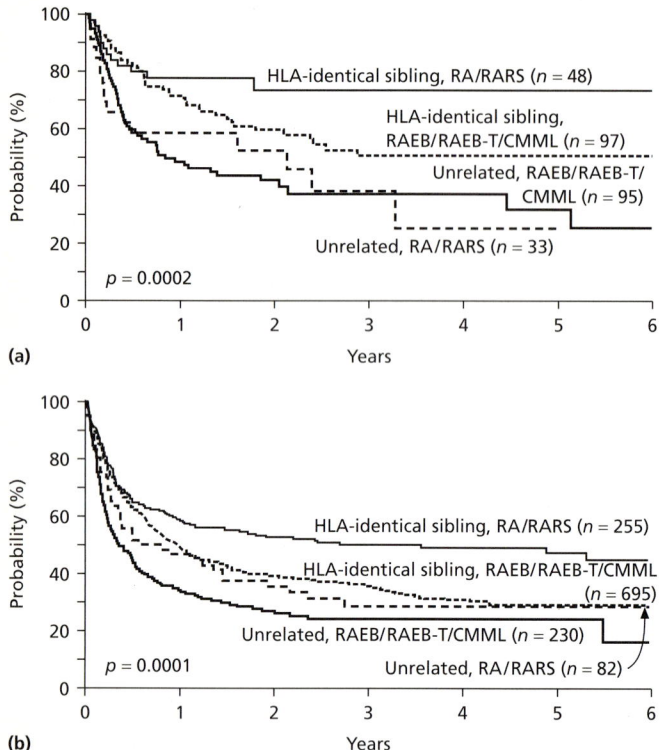

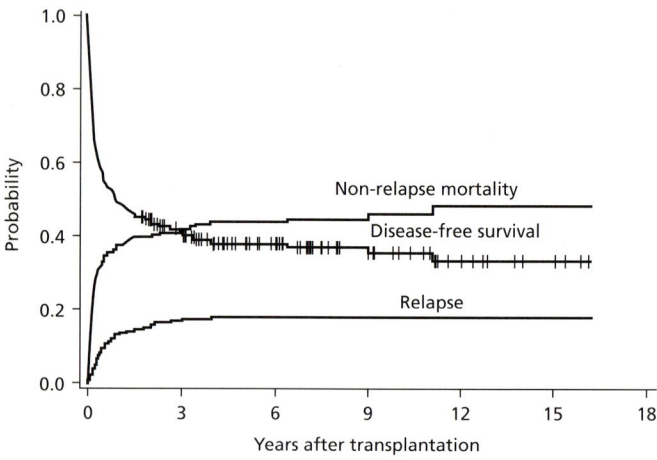

Fig. 79.1 Probability of survival after hematopoietic cell transplantation (HCT) for patients with myelodysplastic syndrome (MDS) by French–Amercan–British (FAB) Cooperative Group classification and age (a) ≤20 years or (b) >20 years from the International Bone Marrow Transplant Registry (IBMTR), 1994–9.

Fig. 79.2 Actuarial disease-free survival (DFS) and cumulative incidences of relapse and nonrelapse mortality (NRM) for 250 patients with myelodysplastic syndrome (MDS) after hematopoietic cell transplantation (HCT) in Seattle between 1981 and 1996.

relapse rate for poor risk (32%) vs. intermediate or good risk (12%) and lower DFS (28% vs. 43%, respectively) (Fig. 79.3) [48]. Both disease morphology and karyotype are independent predictive factors for both relapse and DFS [48].

Outcome by patient age

For MDS, as for many other diseases, there is an increase in NRM and, often, a decrease in DFS with increasing patient age [45,47,48,50,55,58,62]. Two studies have also found, unexpectedly, older age to be associated with an increased risk of relapse [48,51]. The difference in DFS by age is most striking for patients <20 years of age, compared with patients 20 years and older. In this younger age range, the DFS rates are generally about 20% higher than for the older age range [46,48]. Although the median age at diagnosis of MDS is approximately 65 years, the toxicity of allogeneic HCT has discouraged most transplant centers from transplanting MDS patients over the age of 50 years. One study reported the results of 55 patients with MDS between 55 and 66 years of age (median 59 years) who underwent HCT [65]. For patients at risk, 77% developed acute grades II–IV graft-vs.-host disease (GVHD) (16% grades III–IV) and 62% developed chronic GVHD. The actuarial DFS was 42% and the cumulative incidence of relapse was 19%. Among the 22 survivors, at time of last contact, the Karnofsky performance score was 100% for 11, 90–95% for six and <90% for five patients. Similar to data for younger patients, patients with poor-risk karyotype, increased blasts, high-risk IPSS and therapy-related MDS had a worse outcome [65].

Outcome for therapy-related MDS

A number of reports on bone marrow transplantation (BMT) for MDS and secondary AML have included patients with therapy-related MDS and therapy-related AML [44,49,52,53,55,58–60,66–69]. With complete survival data on 263 of the 275 reported patients with therapy-related MDS or AML, 73 patients (28%) were disease-free survivors, 64 (24%) relapsed, 125 (48%) died of transplant-related causes and one died of the primary disease. The largest of these studies reported a 6-year DFS rate of 13%, relapse rate of 47% and NMR rate of 78% for all 99 patients [66]. By FAB subtype, the DFS was 33% for 12 RA/RARS patients, 20% for 18 RAEB patients and 8% for 67 RAEB-T or AML patients [66].

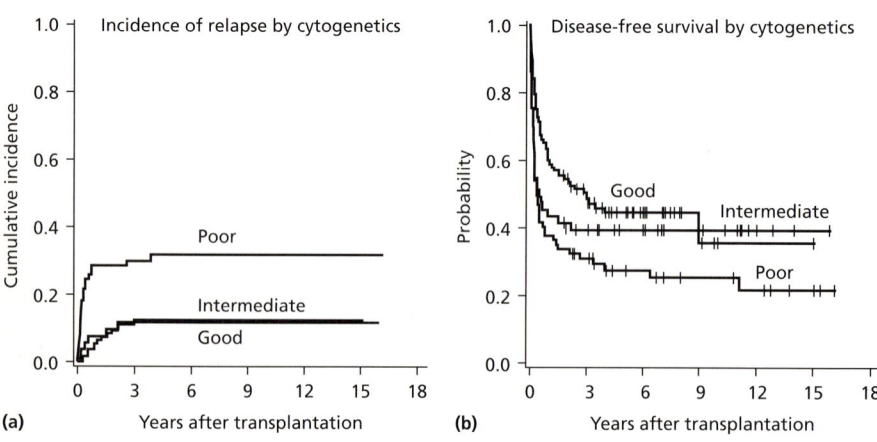

Fig. 79.3 Cumulative incidence of (a) relapse and (b) actuarial disease-free survival (DFS) based on cytogenetic risk group for 240 patients with myelodysplastic syndrome (MDS) after hematopoietic cell transplantation (HCT) in Seattle between 1981 and 1996.

These data suggest that HCT is a feasible treatment option for therapy-related myeloid malignancies, but do not address the question of whether the results are different from those seen with patients with *de novo* MDS. A study of 18 patients with therapy-related MDS was compared to 25 patients with primary MDS who were transplanted at the same institution [53]. The 3-year DFS rates were 24% for therapy-related and 43% for primary MDS, a difference that was suggestive but did not reach statistical significance [53]. In a study of the first 250 patients with MDS who underwent HCT in Seattle, the 5-year DFS for 35 patients with therapy-related MDS was 20%, compared to 41% for the remaining patients [48]. In multivariable analysis, there was a significantly shorter DFS because of a higher incidence of NMR among these 35 patients compared with the remaining patients, and there was no difference in relapse rate [48]. This finding of worse survival as a result of greater NMR, after adjustment for other factors known to influence outcome, may be caused by the cumulative toxicity associated with treatment for the prior malignancy and toxicity associated with HCT. However, a study restricted to MDS patients transplanted from unrelated donors found a similar outcome for 396 patients with idiopathic MDS (4-year DFS 29%) and 70 patients with therapy-related MDS (4-year DFS 24%) [47]. Finally, a study restricted to human leukocyte antigen (HLA) identical sibling donor transplantation also found no difference in outcome for patients with idiopathic MDS or "therapy" MDS/AML [45]. However, in this latter study, the interpretation is confounded because "therapy"-related disease also included prior immunosuppressive treatment or prior hematologic condition.

Outcome by hematopoietic cell source

In this section, outcome by hematopoietic cell source is analyzed separately using available data for patients undergoing unrelated donor HCT [45,47,50,70], nonidentical related donor HCT [45,71], related donor peripheral blood hematopoietic cell transplantation (PBHCT) vs. BMT [72] or autologous HCT [45,71,73]. There are insufficient data on cord blood HCT for MDS or MDS-related AML to discuss in detail in this chapter [74].

The largest report on transplantation for MDS using unrelated donor HCT is a registry report of 510 patients using data from the National Marrow Donor Program (NMDP) [47]. In this study, the median age was 38 years (range <1–62 years), and a variety of transplant methods were used. The incidences of primary and secondary graft failure were 5% and 8%, respectively. Grades II–IV acute GVHD and chronic GVHD were reported in 47% and 27% of patients, respectively. The 2-year rates of DFS, NRM and relapse were 29%, 54% and 14%, respectively. Patients with RAEB-T and MDS-related AML had a significantly higher risk of relapse and lower DFS. Additional factors associated with lower DFS were acute GVHD, lower nucleated cell dose infused, positive patient cytomegalovirus serology, disease duration over 9 months and earlier year of transplantation. Factors associated with higher NRM were acute GVHD, HLA mismatch, positive patient cytomegalovirus serology, and older patient and donor age. Registry data from the European Group for Blood and Marrow Transplantation (EBMT) ($n = 198$) reported a 3-year DFS rate of 25%, NRM rate of 58% and relapse rate of 41% [45,50]. In this study, increasing patient age was associated with higher NRM and lower DFS [45,50]. The IBMTR results suggest that survival after unrelated donor HCT is worse than after HLA-identical sibling donor HCT, particularly for the subset of patients with early phase disease (Fig. 79.1) [46]. The most favorable outcome for unrelated donor HCT comes from a single-center experience in Seattle [70,75]. Of note, this group reported a 56% 3-year survival for 40 patients with RA [75], results that are similar to the outcome for HLA-identical sibling results for RA reported to the IBMTR database [46]. These favorable results may in part be caused by transplant technique, such as allele-level matching and/or preparative regimen using targeting of busulfan (BU) levels [75].

There are few data on the outcome for MDS patients undergoing genotypically nonidentical related donor HCT [45,71]. Data from the EBMT on 79 patients showed a 3-year DFS of 31%, NRM 62% and relapse rate of 16% [71]. Not surprisingly, recipients of phenotypically identical HSC had a better survival and lower NRM than recipients of mismatched HSC. Although age was not a predictive factor, early stage disease (RA, RARS or first complete remission) was a favorable factor in the DFS analysis.

For patients who have a HLA-identical sibling donor, there are data available comparing the use of peripheral blood hematopoietic cells (PBHCs) with bone marrow hematopoietic cells (BMHCs), based on a retrospective comparison of 234 patients with MDS [72]. In this study, 132 patients received BMHC and 102 received granulocyte colony-stimulating factor-mobilized PBHC. The use of PBHC resulted in shorter durations of neutropenia and thrombocytopenia. Acute GVHD was similar between the two different hematopoietic cell sources, but chronic GVHD was more common among recipients of PBHC. The 2-year event-free survival was 50% for recipients of PBHC vs. 39% for recipients of BMHC. In multivariate analysis, patients with RA and patients with poor-risk cytogenetics had a better outcome when transplanted using PBHC rather than BMHC. Patients with poor-risk cytogenetics transplanted using PBHC had a particularly high NRM, resulting in a low DFS, an outcome that is not readily explained. Importantly, patients with advanced disease (based on either excess blasts or on intermediate-2 or high-risk IPSS) had a better outcome with use of PBHC because of lower relapse rate, compared to use of BMHC.

The use of autologous cells in transplantation for MDS is dependent on the ability to collect nonclonal hematopoietic cells. The finding that some MDS patients treated with induction chemotherapy can achieve a complete morphologic and cytogenetic remission [35] suggests polyclonal hematopoiesis can be achieved. X-linked clonality studies in females with MDS have shown residual polyclonal hematopoietic cells either at steady state [76] or after chemotherapy [77,78]. PBHC collections following chemotherapy have been shown in some patients to be polyclonal based on X-chromosome inactivation patterns [79] or to be cytogenetically normal [80]. A number of reports from Europe have demonstrated the feasibility of autologous HCT for MDS patients [45,73,80–84]. Engraftment after autologous HCT is slow: in a study of 35 patients, the median time to neutrophil recovery was 48 days and to platelet recovery was 85 days [73]. However, preferential use of PBHC rather than BMHC may results in more rapid engraftment [84]. The largest study reported a 3-year DFS rate of 33% for 126 patients with MDS who were transplanted after achieving a first complete remission with conventional chemotherapy [45]. Results with autologous HCT are dependent, at least in part, on age, karyotype and ability to achieve a complete remission [45,73].

Use of induction chemotherapy prior to HCT

Because of the high rate of relapse among patients with RAEB-T and MDS-related AML, many physicians have chosen to administer intensive induction chemotherapy to these patients before allogeneic HCT. This treatment is usually given for one or more of three reasons:
1 life-threatening peripheral cytopenias are present, which will improve if remission is obtained;
2 the ability to proceed rapidly to HCT is not readily available; and
3 there is the perception that if a patient achieves remission, the outcome with allogeneic HCT will be improved because of a reduced risk of relapse.

Conversely, there are several reasons to suggest that induction chemotherapy before HCT may not improve or may actually worsen long-term survival:
1 if HCT is readily available cytopenias will improve as quickly with HCT as with chemotherapy;
2 complete remission rate with chemotherapy is only 50–60%;
3 the patient may die of toxicity during chemotherapy, thereby preventing HCT altogether;

4 the patient may develop a complication during chemotherapy, such as a fungal infection, that may increase the risk of death with HCT; and
5 the risk of relapse may be equally high for remission patients vs. untreated patients, after accounting for karyotype and blast percentage.

Unfortunately, there have been no prospective comparative studies of immediate HCT vs. induction chemotherapy followed by HCT. Furthermore, retrospective comparisons of patients transplanted without attempt at remission induction therapy or after such treatment have resulted in contradictory results [45,47,51,52,85–87]. The two largest studies that provide data on this topic are registry reports from the EBMT on HLA-identical sibling HCT [45] and from the NMDP on unrelated donor HCT [47]. For HLA-identical sibling HCT, 111 patients transplanted with previously untreated RAEB-T or MDS-related AML had a 28% DFS, 32% NRM and 43% relapse rate; 230 patients transplanted in first complete remission had a 44% DFS, 37% NRM and 30% relapse rate; and 440 patients transplanted after chemotherapy but not in first remission had a 32% DFS, 45% NRM and 42% relapse rate [45]. For unrelated donor HCT, the relapse rate and DFS for patients transplanted in first complete remission or second phase of RA was similar to the outcome for patients transplanted with untreated RA/RAEB patients and was more favorable than the outcome for patients transplanted with active RAEB-T and AML [47]. These data would suggest that patients transplanted in first complete remission might have a better outcome than patients transplanted with active advanced disease. However, these data do not take into account how many patients receive induction chemotherapy but die before transplant.

A study from Seattle of 46 patients with MDS-related AML and therapy-related AML who underwent HCT without attempt at induction chemotherapy reported a 24% 5-year DFS, which was not statistically significantly different from the 15% 5-year DFS of 20 patients who underwent HCT after induction chemotherapy (while in first or second complete remission or first untreated relapse) [85]. A retrospective review of 51 children with advanced MDS who underwent HCT found a trend towards improved event-free survival among the patients who did not receive prior induction chemotherapy compared to those who did (61% vs. 47%, $p = 0.08$) [86]. Other smaller studies also argue against a benefit of induction chemotherapy. A study by Nevill et al. [52] included 19 patients who received induction chemotherapy before HCT, only four of whom were disease-free survivors after HCT: three of four patients transplanted while in first complete remission and one of 15 transplanted without achieving remission or in relapse. A study by Copelan et al. [57] included 19 patients with MDS-related AML, 11 of whom received induction chemotherapy before HCT. There were more disease-free survivors after HCT among patients who did not receive pre-HCT induction chemotherapy (five of eight patients) vs. patients who did receive such therapy (two of 11 patients). These studies help demonstrate that the difficulty in accounting for patients who receive chemotherapy but do not go to subsequent HCT, may confound our ability to make accurate comparisons.

Assuming a complete remission rate of approximately 50%, and a DFS of approximately 50% after HCT for patients transplanted in first complete remission, the overall long-term DFS for patients intended to receive induction chemotherapy followed by HCT, would be predicted to be only 25% (although this rate may be higher because of some success with salvage HCT after induction failure). This 25% DFS rate is similar to the outcome after HCT for patients with previously untreated RAEB-T and MDS-related AML and patients with *de novo* AML transplanted in first relapse [46]. Therefore, one should not assume that induction chemotherapy prior to HCT is mandatory. Only prospective studies or large retrospective studies that account for all patients receiving remission induction chemotherapy (including those who die during such treatment or become ineligible for HCT) will be able to address the use of such pretransplant therapy definitively.

Preparative regimens in HCT for MDS

Innovative HCT approaches are needed to reduce the risk of relapse in patients with excess blasts and poor-risk cytogenetics and to reduce the risk of NRM in all MDS patients, especially older patients and recipients of unrelated donor HSC. Preliminary results from a number of different approaches are summarized in this section; however, none has conclusively shown a superior outcome to standard approaches. Many studies have evaluated preparative regimens that intensify or modify the standard BU/cyclophosphamide (CY) or CY/total body irradiation (TBI) regimens. One abstract describing the use of BU/CY/cytarabine reported a favorable DFS (52%) and low relapse rate (16%), despite 63% of patients having advanced morphology [87]. The Seattle group has sequentially studied a BU/CY/TBI regimen and then a BU/TBI regimen among patients with MDS with excess blasts and MDS-related AML [56,61]. In these latter two studies there appeared to be a lower relapse rate but higher NRM, resulting in no improvement in DFS (approximately 25%), compared with historical controls. A study performed in Houston using BU/CY/thiotepa reported a 17% 3-year survival among 12 patients with MDS [88]. Therefore, nonspecifically intensified preparative regimens do not appear to be beneficial. Another ongoing approach to reducing relapse without increasing toxicity is to target radiation specifically to hematopoietic tissues using radiolabeled monoclonal antibodies (see Chapter 15).

The reason for the high NRM rate (approximately 40%) seen in patients with MDS treated with HCT is not well understood, but may be because of the prolonged period of marrow failure preceding HCT. Studies using T-cell depletion among 22 patients with RA undergoing HLA-matched sibling donor HCT [89,90] have reported DFS rates of 75–80%, which are similar to select reports of similar patients receiving non-T depleted marrow [51,62]. However, there appears to be a much lower incidence of GVHD with the use of T-cell depletion, which may reduce long-term morbidity and mortality. The use of T-cell depletion techniques among patients with advanced MDS or MDS-related AML resulted in poor results in one study [90] and favorable results in another [91]. The use of targeting BU to avoid "toxic" levels is also an attractive way to reduce toxicity. The results from this approach in 109 patients are encouraging (16% 100-day NRM and 31% 3-year NRM); however, the heterogeneity in the patient population and hematopoietic cell source complicates definitive conclusions [92]. Finally, administration of BU intravenously rather than orally may also improve outcome after transplantation, but results in MDS patients are limited [93].

Another approach designed to reduce toxicity of conventional HCT is the use nonmyeloablative preparative regimens (discussed in Chapter 85). However, data available specifically on patients with MDS are very preliminary [94–98]. One study compared the outcome of 20 MDS patients who received a nonmyeloablative regimen (fludarabine, BU, and Campath or fludarabine, idarubicin and cyarabine) to the outcome of 26 MDS patients who received a myeloablative regimen (BU/CY or BU/CY/TBI/Campath) [94]. The patients received nonmyeloablative regimens because of advanced age and/or comorbid conditions. The nonmyeloablative regimen was associated with a lower day 100 mortality compared to the myeloablative regimen (5% vs. 23%). At the time of this report, three of 20 in the nonmyeloablative and one of 26 in the myeloablative arm had relapsed and the 3-year survival rates were 49% and 54%, respectively [94]. Another study detailed the outcome of 18 patients with MDS or MDS-related AML, who had a median age of 61 years [95]. These patients received a nonmyeloablative preparative regimen of 200 cGy TBI with or without fludarabine. At the time this study was presented, three patients had died of nonrelapse causes, five had died of disease progression and two had either stable disease or partial remission. Eight of the 18 patients were in continuous complete remission at a median of 246 days (range 120–445 days) post-transplant: three of six with RA, one of two with RAEB, none of three with RAEB-T, one of two with CMML and three of five with MDS-related AML (these five AML patients were in partial or complete remission prior to administration of the of preparative regimen) [95]. A third study reported on 12 patients with high-risk MDS (seven unrelated donor recipients) who received fludarabine/BU/antithymocyte globulin (ATG) [96]. Four patients died of non-relapse causes and the 2-year DFS was only 12% [96]. Two other studies presented data on patients with MDS and acute leukemia and found that results were worse among patients with advanced disease and among patients with chemotherapy-refractory disease [97,98]. These preliminary data on nonmyeloablative regimens suggest that, in comparison to standard ablative regimens, this treatment can be safely administered to a greater proportion of patients with MDS (i.e. those with increased age and/or comorbid conditions). However, the total number of reported patients is small and the follow-up is short, so that the rate of durable DFS for any phase of MDS is not yet known.

When to transplant?

As described earlier, the risk of relapse in patients with low blast count and good or intermediate risk cytogenetics is lower than in patients with more advanced disease, thereby resulting in improved DFS in less advanced patients. These results would suggest that transplantation should strongly be considered in these early disease patients before a poor risk karyotype or progressive blast count develops.

Consideration of disease duration is also important in determining the appropriate timing of HCT for MDS, not only because the disease may progress in blast percentage or karyotype during an observation period, but also because longer disease duration may result in greater transplant-related toxicity. Patients with MDS have a particularly high rate of NRM compared to patients with other "chronic" diseases, such as chronic myeloid leukemia. If the pretransplant period of marrow failure in MDS patients results in complications such as iron overload, HLA alloimmunization and fungal colonization or infection, then one might expect that prolonged disease duration would result in an inferior outcome after HCT. However, studies that have evaluated the relationship between disease duration and post-transplant outcome have not yielded consistent results [45,47–52,61,62]. This discrepancy may be caused by differences in disease duration categories, disease subsets, pretransplant treatment of patients or difficulty in determining the exact time of MDS diagnosis. However, the data supporting a lower NRM and, in some studies, a better DFS for patients transplanted soon after diagnosis (within approximately 1 year) [47–50,62], are sufficient to warrant strong consideration for early transplantation. Parenthetically, some studies show a lower risk of relapse among patients with longer disease duration [45,48], which is a finding that is difficult to explain and may be caused by patient selection and decision-making on timing of transplantation.

Another approach to determining the appropriate timing for HCT is to compare the outcome with HCT to the outcome without HCT. The IPSS (Table 79.2) [30] has been applied to 241 patients who underwent HCT in Seattle [48]. Because of insufficient detail on marrow blast percentage, the score for marrow blasts was modified to be 0 for RA or RARS, 1.0 for RAEB and 2.0 for RAEB-T. There were 94 patients in the intermediate-1, 68 in the intermediate-2, and 77 in the high-risk groups (two patients in the low-risk group were not further analyzed). There were no statistically significant differences in NRM rates by IPSS. However, there were significant differences in relapse rates (cumulative incidence of 2% for intermediate-1, 17% for intermediate-2 and 38% for high risk groups; $p = 0.0001$) and in 5-year DFS rates (56% for intermediate-1, 32% for intermediate-2 and 24% for high-risk groups; $p = 0.0003$) (Fig. 79.4). The main drawback to comparing these HCT results with the natural history results reported by Greenberg et al. [30] is that the IPSS was not designed to evaluate prognosis at a delayed time after diagnosis, as

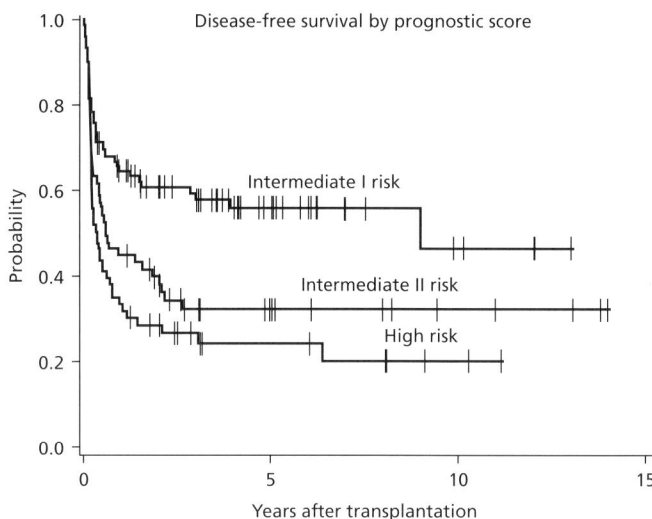

Fig. 79.4 Actuarial disease-free survival (DFS) for 239 patients with myelodysplastic syndrome (MDS), by International Prognostic Scoring System (IPSS) after hematopoietic cell transplantation (HCT) in Seattle between 1981 and 1996.

used in the HCT analysis [48]. None the less, the long-term DFS in the intermediate-1, intermediate-2 and high-risk groups appears to be better in the transplanted group than nontransplanted group, thus supporting a decision of immediate HCT for eligible patients within these IPSS risk groups. These data do not address the routine use of HCT for patients in the low-risk group. However, it is appropriate to consider early transplantation in select situations of very young patients or those with a life-threatening single cytopenia. Clearly, because of the lack of randomized trials proving a survival benefit of transplantation over less intensive therapy, the decision to proceed to HCT must rest on careful discussion with the patient about individualized risks and benefits.

Myeloproliferative disorders

The myeloproliferative disorders are a group of diseases that classically include chronic myeloid leukemia (CML), polycythemia vera (PV), essential thrombocythemia (ET) and agnogenic myeloid metaplasia with myelofibrosis (AMM). These diseases are characterized by the slow but relentless progressive expansion of a clone of hematopoietic cells generally limited to a single myeloid lineage and, with varying frequencies, eventuate in a myeloid blast crisis similar to AML. A proportion of patients with ET, however, appear to have a nonclonal disorder and a more indolent course than patients with clonal hematopoiesis [99]. One of the myeloproliferative disorders, CML, is dealt with in Chapter 73 and will not be discussed here.

Polycythemia vera and essential thrombocythemia

Disease definition

PV is a rare disorder that occurs with an annual incidence of approximately 1–2/100,000 population. PV is characterized by an expansion of the total red cell mass and is often accompanied by splenomegaly and an increase in granulopoiesis and thrombopoiesis. Additional diagnostic findings include low serum erythropoietin levels and autonomous growth of erythroid colonies [100]. Cytogenetic abnormalities occur in 10–15% of patients at diagnosis and commonly include trisomy 8, trisomy 9 and 20q- [101]. The median age at onset is 60 years, but approximately 7% of patients are younger than 40 years with rare reports of PV occurring in children [102]. If left untreated, the median survival of patients with PV is 2 years, mostly as a result of death from thrombotic events. However, with use of current nontransplant therapies, the median survival is approximately 15 years [103]. The initial objective of therapy for most patients is to reduce the hematocrit to normal levels using phlebotomy [100,104,105]. Additional therapeutic options include myelosuppression with hydroxyurea, interferon-α or, less commonly ^{32}P [100,104–106]. The use of aspirin is controversial for thrombotic prophylaxis, but is helpful for treatment of erythromelalgia. Eventually, with time, most patients with PV fail treatment. Causes of failure include life-threatening thrombotic complications, AML or post-polycythemic myeloid metaplasia with myelofibrosis with progressive pancytopenia and splenomegaly.

ET is characterized by the isolated expansion of the megakaryocytic lineage. The reported annual incidence is 2–3/100,000 population [107]. Revised criteria for the diagnosis primarily include criteria used to exclude the other myeloproliferative and myelodysplastic disorders and nonmalignant disorders associated with thrombocytosis [108]. The median age at diagnosis is approximately 70 years, with up to 20% being younger than 40 years at diagnosis [107]. The median survival of patients with ET is at least 10 years [103,107,108] and appears to be similar to that of age- and sex-matched normal nonaffected individuals [103] or slightly worse [107]. Most disease-related deaths are a result of thrombotic or bleeding complications, but some patients progress to post-thrombocythemic myeloid metaplasia with myelofibrosis or to AML. Although it is clear that patients with symptomatic bleeding or thrombosis require treatment to normalize the platelet count, it is controversial whether asymptomatic patients should be treated regardless of the platelet count. Treatment options for lowering the platelet count include hydroxyurea, anagrelide and interferon-α [105].

HCT for PV and ET

The role of HCT in PV and ET is more hypothetical than actual. Given that PV and ET are diseases of hematopoietic stem cells, one would expect them to be curable with allogeneic HCT. However, because the average survival is measured in decades and the average age at onset of the disease is 60 years or older, HCT has been virtually untested as a treatment for PV or ET. A total of 22 patients with PV ($n = 13$) and ET ($n = 9$) have been reported to have received allogeneic HCT [109–113]. One 16-year-old female with PV was transplanted because of persistent neurologic symptoms despite treatment with phlebotomy and hydroxyurea [109]. At time of the case report, this patient was disease-free 15 months after HCT [109]. Two other case reports describe two cases of successful HCT for post-polycythemic myelofibrosis [110,111]. One of these patients required post-transplant splenectomy before donor engraftment was established [111]. The remaining 19 patients (10 PV, nine ET) were reported in a single series from Seattle, and were transplanted because of progression to myeloid metaplasia with myelofibrosis ($n = 10$), MDS ($n = 3$) or AML ($n = 6$) [113]. The median age was 43 years (range 18–59 years) and seven had undergone splenectomy prior to HCT. All six patients with AML had received prior remission-induction chemotherapy, three of whom were in remission at time of HCT. All 19 patients received myeloablative regimens, followed by related (10 HLA-identical, one single antigen mismatched) or unrelated (seven HLA-matched, one single antigen mismatched) HCT. Twelve patients survive a median of 41 months (range 5–116 months) after HCT, one of whom is a mixed chimera on interferon therapy. The underlying malignant clone appears to have been eradicated in all the remaining surviving patients. Seven patients died of transplant-related complications; one of 10 transplanted for myeloid metaplasia with myelofibrosis, one of two transplanted for MDS and five of six transplanted for AML.

From these limited data, and our knowledge of the natural history of PV and ET, it appears reasonable to consider HCT in younger patients with appropriate donors who have failed first-line therapy and have severe symptomatic hemorrhagic or thrombotic complications or who have progressed into a myelofibrotic state. The usefulness of HCT if the disease has progressed into AML is not established by these data.

Agnogenic myeloid metaplasia

Disease definition

AMM (also known as idiopathic or primary myelofibrosis) is a chronic myeloproliferative disorder characterized by marrow fibrosis, splenomegaly, peripheral blood leukoerythroblastosis and extramedullary hematopoiesis [114]. Although fibrosis is a reactive process of nonclonal fibroblasts, the HSC responsible for the disease is clonal in origin [7]. The diagnosis of AMM requires exclusion of other disorders associated with marrow fibrosis, including myeloid malignancies, lymphoproliferative disorders, metastatic carcinoma, rheumatologic disorders and infections [114]. An elevated absolute content of CD34$^+$ cells in the peripheral blood may also be used to help diagnose AMM over other disorders [115]. The incidence of AMM is approximately 1/100,000 population. The median age at diagnosis is approximately 65 years, and approximately 20% are 55 years of age or younger [106,114,116]. Although survival after diagnosis varies from 1 to 30 years, it is generally short (median 4–5 years), and is considerably lower than age- and sex-matched controls [103,107]. Patients commonly die from heart failure, complications of marrow failure or leukemic transformation [114–118]. Factors associated with shortened survival include hemoglobin <10 g/dL, leukocyte count <4000/μL or >30,000/μL, the presence of constitutional symptoms, abnormal cytogenetics, absolute peripheral blood CD34$^+$ count >300 × 10^6/L, and the presence of ≥1% circulating blasts or >10% circulating leukocyte precursors (blasts + promyelocytes + myelocytes) [114–118]. A study of 121 patients with AMM under 56 years of age created a useful prognostic scoring system, which includes hemoglobin <10 g/dL, the presence of constitutional symptoms and the presence of circulating blasts ≥1% [116]. In this study, patients with none or one of these three adverse prognostic factors had a median survival of 176 months, and patients with two or three factors had a median survival of only 33 months [116].

Conventional therapy for AMM is palliative and primarily aimed at reducing symptoms related to cytopenias, organomegaly, hypercatabolic state and myeloid metaplasia. Standard treatments include transfusional support, androgens, corticosteroids, hydroxyurea, splenectomy and splenic irradiation [114]. Additional therapies currently under investigation include erythropoietin and thalidomide.

HCT for AMM

Allogeneic HCT

Because of the shortened life expectancy of patients with AMM, which is more akin to CML and MDS, there is more extensive experience with HCT for AMM than for PV and ET. However, there was early hesitation to recommend transplantation to AMM patients because of concern that fibrosis in the marrow was a barrier to successful engraftment. An early report on the use of HCT for myelofibrotic disorders suggested that engraftment was prompt in patients with mild or moderate fibrosis (two out of 32 patients; 6%), but failed in a larger percentage of patients with severe fibrosis (five of 15; 33%) [119]. However, a larger retrospective case–control comparison of 203 patients with hematologic disorders and marrow fibrosis who underwent either autologous or allogeneic HCT reported no statistically significant difference in engraftment endpoints between patients with or without fibrosis [120]. Among 33 patients in this analysis who had severe fibrosis, there was a 7-day delay to reach platelet transfusion independence and a 2-day delay to reach red cell

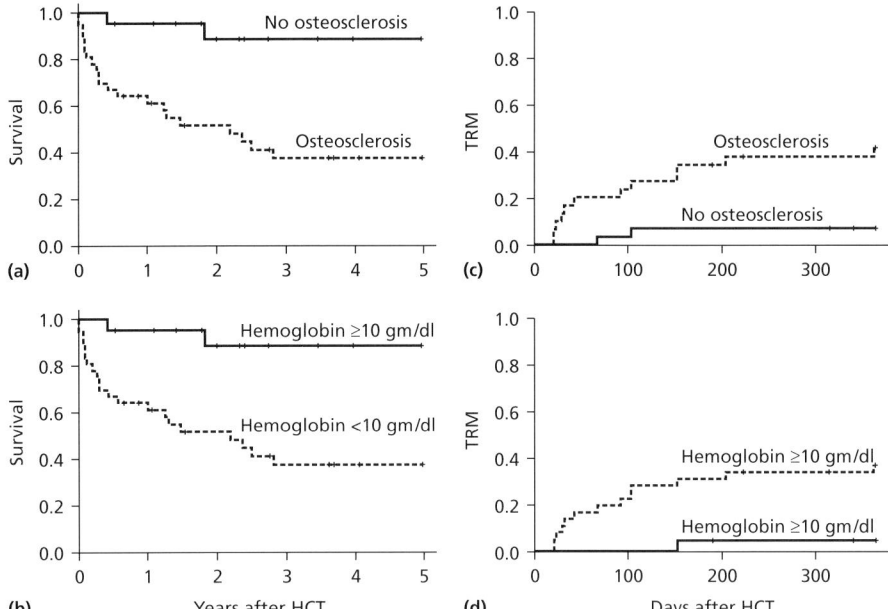

Fig. 79.5 (a,b) Survival and (c,d) transplant-related mortality (TRM) for 55 patients with agnogenic myeloid metaplasia (AMM) by (a,c) presence or absence of osteosclerosis and (b,d) by hemoglobin < or ≥10 g/dL. (From P. Guardiola, with permission.)

independence compared to the matched controls without fibrosis, but the differences were not statistically significant [120]. These latter results, in a heterogeneous group of patients, suggested that fibrosis does not influence engraftment rates after transplantation. However, when analyzing associations between the degree of fibrosis and engraftment, it is important to note the histologic grading system used. In the initial study [119], assessment of degree of reticulin fibrosis and presence or absence of collagen fibrosis was scored [121]. In the second study [120] only the degree of reticulin fibrosis was assessed [122]. A third scoring system takes into account the presence of osteosclerosis [123] and was used in the largest study reported on HCT for AMM [124,125], as discussed in detail below.

The largest report on transplantation for AMM was an international collaborative study from 28 centers worldwide, which initially included 55 patients [124] and was then updated with 11 additional patients [125]. This study included data from earlier small single-center reports [112,126–132]. Patients with acute leukemic transformation were excluded. Median age was 42 years (range 4–57 years); median time from diagnosis to transplant was 19 months (range 2–266 months). Pretransplant, 50% had undergone splenectomy, 65% had received red cell transfusions, 36% had high-risk disease by the Dupriez scoring system [117] and 48% had grade III fibrosis (defined as osteomyelosclerosis with hypocellular marrow). Cytogenetic abnormalities were detected in 14 of 53 assessable karyotypes. There was no uniformity in transplant techniques used, although all patients received myeloablative preparative regimens. Donor and recipient were HLA-matched related in 56 cases and HLA-mismatched or unrelated in 10 cases.

Neutrophil engraftment occurred in 86% and 97% of patients by day 30 and day 50 post-HCT, respectively. Independent variables associated with delayed engraftment were osteosclerosis, no prior splenectomy, lower number of nucleated cells infused and pre-HCT hemoglobin <10 g/dL. The probability of developing acute GVHD was 60%, with osteosclerosis and use of TBI identified as risk factors for this complication. The risk of disease recurrence was dependent on increased patient age, longer time from diagnosis to transplant, presence of cytogenetic abnormalities and use of T-cell depletion. Survival at 5-years post-HCT was 48% for all 66 patients and 59% for 50 recipients of unmanipulated grafts from HLA-identical siblings. Factors associated with a lower survival included osteosclerosis, pre-HCT hemoglobin <10 g/dL and age ≥45 years. For patients undergoing unmanipulated HLA-identical sibling HCT, 5-year survival was 40% for patients with osteosclerosis vs. 68% for patients without osteosclerosis ($p = 0.015$) and 5-year survival was 35% for patients with hemoglobin at HCT <10 g/dL vs. 88% for patients with hemoglobin ≥10 g/dL ($p = 0.001$) (P. Guardiola, personal communication; Fig. 79.5). The corresponding 1-year transplant-related mortality was 42% vs. 7% for patients with vs. without osteosclerosis ($p = 0.003$) and 37% vs. 5% for patients with hemoglobin <10 g/dL vs. ≥10 g/dL ($p <0.001$) (P. Guardiola, personal communication; Fig. 79.5).

The largest single-center results on transplantation for myelofibrosis are from the Seattle group [133–135]. These data comprise 51 patients, for whom the underlying diagnosis was AMM in 36, postpolycythemic or post-thrombocythemic myelofibrosis in 13 and not defined in four. The 3-year relapse-free survival was 66% for patients transplanted from related donors ($n = 35$) and 48% for patients transplanted from unrelated donors ($n = 16$) [135]. Patients who received the targeted BU/CY regimen ($n = 31$) had the most favorable outcome: 78% relapse-free survival. Compared to the international experience [124,125], these survival data are similar for HLA-identical siblings, but more encouraging for unrelated donors. Also, these survival data for patients ≥45 years of age are more favorable ($n = 23$; 5-year DFS 50%) [133] than that reported with the international experience ($n = 23$; 5-year survival 14%) [125]. This marked difference in outcome by age between the two reports is not readily explained, but may in part be brought about by differences in preparative regimens used. The Seattle group has also addressed the question of whether pre-HCT splenectomy influences outcome after HCT. Similar to the international experience [125], there was a delay in neutrophil engraftment among nonsplenectomized patients but no difference in incidence of GVHD, relapse or survival (Fig. 79.6) [134].

As with MDS, because allogeneic HCT currently offers the only curative therapy for AMM, it should be discussed with any young (e.g. under 55 years of age) physiologically fit patient with a suitable donor. Based on the natural history of the disease and the reported outcome with HCT, the following guidelines can be offered. For patients who present with two or more poor risk factors according to either the Cervantes score (hemoglobin <10 g/dL, constitutional symptoms or circulating blasts ≥1%) [116] or the Dupriez score (hemoglobin <10 g/dL, white blood count <4000 or >30,000) [117], immediate transplantation should be considered. For most patients with zero or one poor-risk factor, observation followed by transplantation when two factors develop, or hemoglobin is

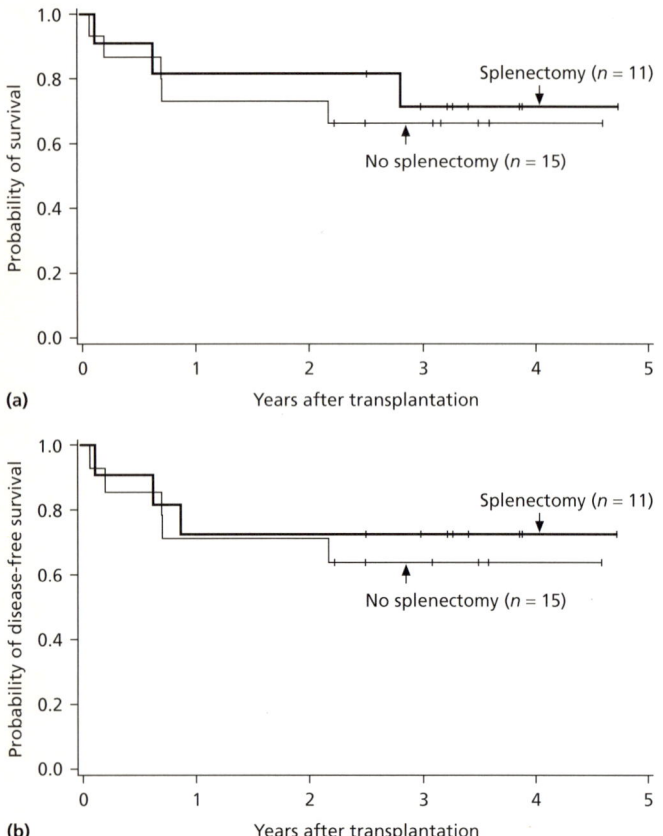

Fig. 79.6 Probability of (a) survival and (b) disease-free survival for 26 patients with myelofibrosis based on splenectomy status at time of hematopoietic cell transplantation (HCT).

<10 g/dL, or when red cell transfusion dependence is imminent can be considered. Strong consideration for early transplantation should be given to patients with isolated white blood count >30,000 or cytogenetic abnormality because such patients have a higher risk of leukemic transformation [117]. Ideally, transplantation should be performed before progression towards acute leukemia because of the increased risk of relapse and nonrelapse mortality. The transplant results described earlier would suggest that:

1 pre-HCT splenectomy is not necessary, but that infusion of a large number of nucleated cell dose at time of HCT [125] might help reduce delayed engraftment in nonsplenectomized patients; and
2 the most favorable outcome after HCT appears to be with the use of targeting BU levels with CY as a preparative regimen.

As with MDS, the use of nonmyeloablative allogeneic HCT for AMM is theoretically an attractive approach to reduce toxicity of conventional HCT. However, data available specifically on patients with AMM are anecdotal, with only six cases being reported [135,136]. These cases, plus a report on the successful use of donor leukocyte infusions in a patient with AMM after a myeloablative HCT [137], suggest that a "graft-vs.-myelofibrosis" effect may exist. Research on the nonmyeloablative approach for AMM is ongoing.

Autologous HCT

Because some patients with AMM are not eligible for allogeneic HCT, the use of autologous HCT has been evaluated [138]. Such treatment is not designed to be curative because means to purge clonal hematopoietic cells from the graft are not available. The rationale for autologous HCT is that myelofibrosis, splenomegaly and myeloid metaplasia are reversible following cytotoxic therapy and allogeneic HCT and that the high number of circulating progenitor cells in AMM may allow for autologous PBHC collection. In a multicenter study, 27 patients with myelofibrosis secondary to AMM, PV or ET underwent PBHC collection and 21 underwent BU-only myeloablation followed reinfusion of PBHCs [138]. The median time to platelet and neutrophil recovery were both 21 days. One patient died within 100 days from transplant-related complications. Clinically significant responses were seen in 10 of 17 patients with anemia, four of eight patients with thrombocytopenia and seven of 10 patients with symptomatic splenomegaly. Despite these early encouraging results [138], the study was subsequently closed when occurrence of graft failure was found to be excessive, five of 27 patients (J.E. Anderson, personal communication). The investigators of this study have hypothesized that the high graft failure rate may have been a result of collection of PBHCs late in the disease course. Currently, some transplant centers are investigating the potential of collecting PBHCs early in the disease course in both AMM (J.E. Anderson, personal communication) and PV [139].

Conclusions

Myelodysplasia and the myeloproliferative disorders are clonal hematopoietic cell diseases that demonstrate varying degrees of aberrant peripheral blood counts and risk of progression to AML, and are incurable with nontransplant therapies. It is critical that the transplant physician understands the prognostic factors and the natural history of the different subtypes of these diseases, given their wide heterogeneity. There is a minimal role for HCT for most patients with PV and ET, who generally have a long survival and respond to nontransplant therapies. In contradistinction, most patients with MDS and AMM live significantly shorter than age-adjusted controls, despite use of modern nontransplant therapies. Such patients who are physiologically fit for allogeneic transplantation should be considered for HCT. Results of HCT for MDS are heavily dependent on karyotype, marrow blast percentage and, consequently, risk category according to the IPSS. Less clear-cut factors that influence outcome after HCT include patient age, disease duration, disease etiology, donor HC source and preparative regimen used. Results of HCT for AMM are less well-defined because of relatively minimal data. However, progressive anemia, red cell transfusion dependency, osteosclerosis, and perhaps increased age, impact adversely on outcome after HCT. Significant improvements in outcome after HCT for MDS and AMM have been made over the past two decades; however, further refining transplant techniques and patient selection to minimize relapse and NRM rates are needed.

References

1 Prchal JT, Throckmorton DW, Carroll AJ III, Fuson EW, Gams RA, Prchal JF. A common progenitor for human myeloid and lymphoid cells. *Nature* 1978; **274**: 590–1.
2 Raskind WH, Tirumali N, Singer J, Fialkow PJ. Evidence for a multistep pathogenesis of a myelodysplastic syndrome. *Blood* 1984; **63**: 1318–23.
3 Tefferi A, Thibodeau SN, Solberg LA Jr. Clonal studies in the myelodysplastic syndrome using X-linked restriction fragment length polymorphisms. *Blood* 1990; **75**: 1770–3.
4 Janssen JWG, Buschle M, Layton M *et al*. Clonal analysis of myelodysplastic syndromes: evidence of multipotent stem cell origin. *Blood* 1989; **73**: 248–54.
5 van Kamp H, Fibbe WE, Jansen RP *et al*. Clonal involvement of granulocytes and monocytes, but

not of T and B lymphocytes and natural killer cells in patients with myelodysplasia: analysis by X-linked restriction fragment length polymorphisms and polymerase chain reaction of the phosphoglycerate kinase gene. *Blood* 1992; **80**: 1774–80.
6. Abrahamson G, Boultwood J, Madden J et al. Clonality of cell populations in refractory anaemia using combined approach of gene loss and X-linked restriction fragment length polymorphism-methylation analyses. *Br J Haematol* 1991; **79**: 550–5.
7. Jacobson RJ, Salo A, Fialkow PJ. Agnogenic myeloid metaplasia: a clonal proliferation of hematopoietic stem cells with secondary myelofibrosis. *Blood* 1978; **51**: 189–94.
8. Lucas GS, Padua RA, Masters GS, Oscier DG, Jacobs A. The application of X-chromosome gene probes to the diagnosis of myeloproliferative disease. *Br J Haematol* 1989; **72**: 530–3.
9. Anger B, Janssen JW, Schrezenmeier H, Hehlmann R, Heimpel H, Bartram CR. Clonal analysis of chronic myeloproliferative disorders using X-linked DNA polymorphisms. *Leukemia* 1990; **4**: 258–61.
10. Fialkow PJ, Faguet GB, Jacobson RJ, Vaidya K, Murphy S. Evidence that essential thrombocythemia is a clonal disorder with origin in a multipotent stem cell. *Blood* 1981; **58**: 916–9.
11. Jacobs A. Genetic lesions in preleukaemia. *Leukemia* 1991; **5**: 277–82.
12. Gallagher A, Darley RL, Padua RA. The molecular basis of myelodysplastic syndromes. *Haematologica* 1997; **82**: 191–204.
13. Rajapaksa R, Ginzton N, Rott LS, Greenberg PL. Altered oncoprotein expression and apoptosis in myelodysplastic syndrome marrow cells. *Blood* 1996; **88**: 4275–87.
14. Raza A, Mundle S, Shetty V et al. A paradigm shift in myelodysplastic syndromes. *Leukemia* 1996; **10**: 1648–52.
15. Bennett JM, Catovsky D, Daniel MT et al. Proposals for the classification of the acute leukaemias. French–American–British (FAB) Cooperative Group. *Br J Haematol* 1976; **33**: 451–8.
16. Bennett JM, Catovsky D, Daniel MT et al. Proposals for the classification of the myelodysplastic syndromes. *Br J Haematol* 1982; **51**: 189–99.
17. Bennett JM, Catovsky D, Daniel MT et al. Proposed revised criteria for the classification of acute myeloid leukemia. A report of the French–American–British Cooperative Group. *Ann Intern Med* 1985; **103**: 626–9.
18. Harris NL, Jaffe ES, Diebold J et al. World Health Organization classification of neoplastic diseases of the hematopoietic and lymphoid tissues. Report of Clinical Advisory Committee Meeting, Airlie House, Virginia, November 1997. *J Clin Oncol* 1999; **17**: 3835–49.
19. Rosati S, Mick R, Xu F et al. Refractory cytopenia with multilineage dysplasia: further characterization of an 'unclassifiable' myelodysplastic syndrome. *Leukemia* 1996; **10**: 20–6.
20. Kouides PA, Bennett JM. Morphology and classification of the myelodysplastic syndromes and their pathologic variants. *Semin Hematol* 1996; **33**: 95–110.
21. Rosati S, Anastasi J, Vardiman J. Recurring diagnostic problems in the pathology of the myelodysplastic syndromes. *Semin Hematol* 1996; **33**: 111–26.
22. Aul C, Gattermann N, Schneider W. Age-related incidence and other epidemiological aspects of myelodysplastic syndromes. *Br J Haematol* 1992; **82**: 358–67.
23. Williamson PJ, Kruger AR, Reynolds PJ, Hamblin TJ, Oscier DG. Establishing the incidence of myelodysplastic syndrome. *Br J Haematol* 1994; **87**: 743–5.
24. Radlund A, Thiede T, Hansen S, Carlsson M, Engquist L. Incidence of myelodysplastic syndromes in a Swedish population. *Eur J Haematol* 1995; **54**: 153–6.
25. Hasle H. Myelodysplastic syndromes in childhood: classification, epidemiology, and treatment. *Leuk Lymphoma* 1994; **13**: 11–26.
26. Locatelli F, Zecca M, Pession A, Maserati E, De Stefano P, Severi F. Myelodysplastic syndromes: the pediatric point of view. *Haematologica* 1995; **80**: 268–79.
27. Kumar T, Mandla SG, Greer WL. Familial myelodysplastic syndrome with early age of onset. *Am J Hematol* 2000; **64**: 53–8.
28. Pedersen-Bjergaard J, Pedersen M, Roulston D, Philip P. Different genetic pathways in leukemogenesis for patients presenting with therapy-related myelodysplasia and therapy-related acute myeloid leukemia. *Blood* 1995; **86**: 3542–52.
29. Pedersen-Bjergaard J, Klarskov Andersen M, Christiansen DH. Therapy-related acute myeloid leukemia and myelodysplasia after high-dose chemotherapy and autologous stem cell transplantation. *Blood* 2000; **95**: 3273–9.
30. Greenberg P, Cox C, LeBeau MM et al. International scoring system for evaluating prognosis in myelodysplastic syndromes. *Blood* 1997; **89**: 2079–88.
31. Sanz GF, Sanz MA, Vallespí T et al. Two regression models and a scoring system for predicting survival and planning treatment in myelodysplastic syndromes: a multivariate analysis of prognostic factors in 370 patients. *Blood* 1989; **74**: 395–408.
32. Aul C, Gattermann N, Heyll A, Germing U, Derigs G, Schneider W. Primary myelodysplastic syndromes: analysis of prognostic factors in 235 patients and proposals for an improved scoring system. *Leukemia* 1992; **6**: 52–9.
33. Cazzola M, Anderson JE, Ganser A, Hellstrom-Lindberg E. A patient-oriented approach to treatment of myelodysplastic syndromes. *Haematologica* 1998; **83**: 910–35.
34. Silverman LR, Demakos EP, Peterson BL et al. Randomized controlled trial of azacitidine in patients with the myelodysplastic syndrome: a study of the Cancer and Leukemia Group B. *J Clin Oncol* 2002; **20**: 2429–40.
35. De Witte T, Suciu S, Peetermans M et al. Intensive chemotherapy for poor prognosis myelodysplasia (MDS) and secondary acute myeloid leukemia (sAML) following MDS of more than 6 months duration. A pilot study by the Leukemia Cooperative Group of the European Organisation for Research and Treatment in Cancer (EORTC-LCG). *Leukemia* 1995; **9**: 1805–11.
36. Ruutu T, Hanninen A, Jarventie G et al. Intensive chemotherapy of poor prognosis myelodysplastic syndromes (MDS) and acute myeloid leukemia following MDS with idarubicin and cytarabine. *Leuk Res* 1997; **21**: 133–8.
37. Hasle H, Kerndrup G, Yssing M et al. Intensive chemotherapy in childhood myelodysplastic syndrome: a comparison with results in acute myeloid leukemia. *Leukemia* 1996; **10**: 1269–73.
38. Bernstein SH, Brunetto VL, Davey FR et al. Acute myeloid leukemia-type chemotherapy for newly diagnosed patients without antecedent cytopenias having myelodysplastic syndrome as defined by French–American–British criteria: a Cancer and Leukemia Group B study. *J Clin Oncol* 1996; **14**: 2486–94.
39. Appelbaum FR, Storb R, Ramberg RE et al. Allogeneic marrow transplantation in the treatment of preleukemia. *Ann Intern Med* 1984; **100**: 689–93.
40. Appelbaum FR, Storb R, Ramberg RE et al. Treatment of preleukemic syndromes with marrow transplantation. *Blood* 1987; **69**: 92–6.
41. O'Donnell MR, Nademanee AP, Snyder DS et al. Bone marrow transplantation for myelodysplastic and myeloproliferative syndromes. *J Clin Oncol* 1987; **5**: 1822–6.
42. Bèlanger R, Gyger M, Perreault C, Bonny Y, St-Louis J. Bone marrow transplantation for myelodysplastic syndromes. *Br J Haematol* 1988; **69**: 29–33.
43. Kolb HJ, Holler E, Bender-Götze C et al. Myeloablative conditioning for marrow transplantation in myelodysplastic syndromes and paroxysmal nocturnal haemoglobinuria. *Bone Marrow Transplant* 1989; **4**: 29–34.
44. Bunin NJ, Casper JT, Chitambar C et al. Partially matched bone marrow transplantation in patients with myelodysplastic syndromes. *J Clin Oncol* 1988; **6**: 1851–5.
45. de Witte T, Hermans J, Vossen J et al. Haematopoietic stem cell transplantation for patients with myelodysplastic syndromes and secondary acute myeloid leukaemias: a report on behalf of the Chronic Leukaemia Working Party of the European Group for Blood and Marrow Transplantation (EBMT). *Br J Haematol* 2000; **110**: 620–30.
46. Horowitz MM. Report on state of the art in blood and marrow transplantation. *IBMTR/ABMTR Newsletter* 2002; **9**: 1–12.
47. Castro-Malaspina H, Harris RE, Gajewski J et al. Unrelated donor marrow transplantation for myelodysplastic syndromes: outcome analysis in 510 transplants facilitated by the National Marrow Donor Program. *Blood* 2002; **99**: 1943–51.
48. Anderson JE. Bone marrow transplantation for myelodysplasia. *Blood Rev* 2000; **14**: 63–77.
49. Runde V, de Witte T, Arnold R et al. Bone marrow transplantation from HLA-identical siblings as first-line treatment in patients with myelodysplastic syndromes: early transplantation is associated with improved outcome. *Bone Marrow Transplant* 1998; **21**: 255–61.
50. Arnold R, de Witte T, van Biezen A et al. Unrelated bone marrow transplantation in patients with myelodysplastic syndromes and secondary acute myeloid leukemia: an EBMT survey. *Bone Marrow Transplant* 1998; **21**: 1213–6.
51. Sutton L, Chastang C, Ribaud P et al. Factors influencing outcome in *de novo* myelodysplastic syndromes treated by allogeneic bone marrow transplantation: a long-term study of 71 patients Societe Française de Greffe de Moelle. *Blood* 1996; **88**: 358–65.
52. Nevill TJ, Fung HC, Shepherd JD et al. Cytogenetic abnormalities in primary myelodysplastic syndrome are highly predictive of outcome after allogeneic bone marrow transplantation. *Blood* 1998; **92**: 1910–7.
53. Ballen KK, Gilliland DG, Guinan EC et al. Bone marrow transplantation for therapy-related

myelodysplasia: comparison with primary myelodysplasia. *Bone Marrow Transplant* 1997; **20**: 737–43.
54 Locatelli F, Niemeyer C, Angelucci E et al. Allogeneic bone marrow transplantation for chronic myelomonocytic leukemia in childhood: a report from the European Working Group on Myelodysplastic Syndrome in Childhood. *J Clin Oncol* 1997; **15**: 566–73.
55 Yakoub-Agha I, de La Salmoniere P, Ribaud P et al. Allogeneic bone marrow transplantation for therapy-related myelodysplastic syndrome and acute myeloid leukemia: a long-term study of 70 patients. Report of the French Society of Bone Marrow Transplantation. *J Clin Oncol* 2000; **18**: 963–71.
56 Jurado M, Deeg HJ, Storer B et al. Hematopoietic stem cell transplantation for advanced myelodysplastic syndrome after conditioning with busulfan and fractionated total body irradiation is associated with low relapse rate but considerable nonrelapse mortality. *Biol Blood Marrow Transplant* 2002; **8**: 161–9.
57 Copelan EA, Penza SL, Elder PJ et al. Analysis of prognostic factors for allogeneic marrow transplantation following busulfan and cyclophosphamide in myelodysplastic syndrome and after leukemic transformation. *Bone Marrow Transplant* 2000; **25**: 1219–22.
58 O'Donnell MR, Long GD, Parker PM et al. Busulfan/cyclophosphamide as conditioning regimen for allogeneic bone marrow transplantation for myelodysplasia. *J Clin Oncol* 1995; **13**: 2973–9.
59 Ratanatharathorn V, Karanes C, Uberti J et al. Busulfan-based regimens and allogeneic bone marrow transplantation in patients with myelodysplastic syndromes. *Blood* 1993; **81**: 2194–9.
60 Demuynck H, Verhoef GE, Zachee P et al. Treatment of patients with myelodysplastic syndromes with allogeneic bone marrow transplantation from genotypically HLA-identical sibling and alternative donors. *Bone Marrow Transplant* 1996; **17**: 745–51.
61 Anderson JE, Appelbaum FR, Schoch G et al. Allogeneic marrow transplantation for myelodysplastic syndrome with advanced disease morphology: a phase II study of busulfan, cyclophosphamide, and total-body irradiation and analysis of prognostic factors. *J Clin Oncol* 1996; **14**: 220–6.
62 Anderson JE, Appelbaum FR, Schoch G et al. Allogeneic marrow transplantation for refractory anemia: a comparison of two preparative regimens and analysis of prognostic factors. *Blood* 1996; **87**: 51–8.
63 Zang DY, Deeg JH, Gooley T et al. Treatment of chronic myelomonocytic leukaemia by allogeneic marrow transplantation. *Br J Haematol* 2000; **110**: 217–22.
64 Morel P, Hebbar M, Lai J-L et al. Cytogenetic analysis has strong independent prognostic value in de novo myelodysplastic syndromes and can be incorporated in a new scoring system: a report on 408 cases. *Leukemia* 1993; **7**: 1315–23.
65 Deeg HJ, Shulman HM, Anderson JE et al. Allogeneic and syngeneic marrow transplantation for myelodysplastic syndrome in patients 55–66 years of age. *Blood* 2000; **95**: 1188–94.
66 Witherspoon RP, Deeg HJ. Allogeneic bone marrow transplantation for secondary leukemia or myelodysplasia. *Haematologica* 1999; **84**: 1085–7.
67 Le Maignan C, Ribaud P, Maraninchi D et al. Bone marrow transplantation for mutagen-related leukemia or myelodysplasia. *Exper Hematol* 1990; **18**: 660 [Abstract].
68 Bandini G, Rosti G, Calori E, Albertazzi L, Tura S. Allogeneic bone marrow transplantation for secondary leukaemia and myelodysplastic syndrome. *Br J Haematol* 1990; **75**: 442–3.
69 De Witte T. Response to 'Allogeneic bone marrow transplantation for secondary leukaemia and myelodysplastic syndrome'. *Br J Haematol* 1990; **75**: 443–4.
70 Anderson JE, Anasetti C, Appelbaum FR et al. Unrelated donor marrow transplantation for myelodysplasia (MDS) and MDS-related acute myeloid leukaemia. *Br J Haematol* 1996; **93**: 59–67.
71 de Witte T, Pikkemaat F, Hermans J et al. Genotypically nonidentical related donors for transplantation of patients with myelodysplastic syndromes: comparison with unrelated donor transplantation and autologous stem cell transplantation. *Leukemia* 2001; **15**: 1878–84.
72 Guardiola P, Runde V, Bacigalupo A et al. Retrospective comparison of bone marrow and granulocyte colony-stimulating factor-mobilized peripheral blood progenitor cells for allogeneic stem cell transplantation using HLA identical sibling donors in myelodysplastic syndromes. *Blood* 2002; **99**: 4370–8.
73 de Witte T, Suciu S, Verhoef G et al. Intensive chemotherapy followed by allogeneic or autologous stem cell transplantation for patients with myelodysplastic syndromes (MDSx) and acute myeloid leukemia following MDS. *Blood* 2001; **98**: 2326–31.
74 Ooi J, Iseki T, Nagayama H et al. Unrelated cord blood transplantation for adult patients with myelodysplastic syndrome-related secondary acute myeloid leukaemia. *Br J Haematol* 2001; **114**: 834–6.
75 Bjerke J, Anasetti C, Gooley T et al. Unrelated donor (URD) bone marrow transplantation (BMT) for refractory anemia (RA). *Blood* 1998; **92**: 142a.
76 Busque L, Kohler S, DeHart D et al. High incidence of polyclonal granulocytopoiesis in myelodysplastic syndromes (MDS). *Blood* 1993; **82**: 196a [Abstract].
77 Ito T, Ohashi H, Kagami Y, Ichikawa A, Saito H, Hotta T. Recovery of polyclonal hematopoiesis in patients with myelodysplastic syndromes following successful chemotherapy. *Leukemia* 1994; **8**: 839–43.
78 Culligan DJ, Bowen DT, May A, White D, Padua RA, Burnett AK. Refractory anaemia with preleukaemic polyclonal haemopoiesis and the emergence of monoclonal erythropoiesis on disease progression. *Br J Haematol* 1995; **89**: 675–7.
79 Delforge M, Demuynck H, Vandenberghe P et al. Polyclonal primitive hematopoietic progenitors can be detected in mobilized peripheral blood from patients with high-risk myelodysplastic syndromes. *Blood* 1995; **86**: 3660–7.
80 Carella AM, Dejana A, Lerma E et al. In vivo mobilization of karyotypically normal peripheral blood progenitor cells in high-risk MDS, secondary or therapy-related acute myelogenous leukaemia. *Br J Haematol* 1996; **95**: 127–30.
81 Demuynck H, Delforge M, Verhoef GE et al. Feasibility of peripheral blood progenitor cell harvest and transplantation in patients with poor-risk myelodysplastic syndromes. *Br J Haematol* 1996; **92**: 351–9.
82 Wattel E, Solary E, Caillot D et al. Autologous bone marrow (ABMT) or peripheral blood stem cell (ABSCT) transplantation after intensive chemotherapy in myelodysplastic syndromes (MDS). *Leuk Res* 1997; **21** (Suppl. 1): S52 [Abstract].
83 Oberg G, Simonsson B, Smedmyr B et al. Is haematological reconstitution seen after ABMT in MDS patients? *Bone Marrow Transplant* 1989; **4** (Suppl. 2): 52 [Abstract].
84 Boogaerts MA, Demuynck H, De Witte T et al. Repopulation after autologous bone marrow versus peripheral blood progenitor cell transplantation in younger patients with high risk myelodysplastic syndromes in complete remission after intensified induction therapy: a joint EORTC/EBMT study. *Blood* 1995; **86**: 101a [Abstract].
85 Anderson JE, Gooley TA, Schoch G et al. Stem cell transplantation for secondary acute myeloid leukemia: evaluation of transplantation as initial therapy or following induction chemotherapy. *Blood* 1997; **89**: 2578–85.
86 Niemeyer C, Duffner U, Bender-Gotze C et al. AML-type intensive chemotherapy prior to stem cell transplantation (SCT) does not improve survival in children and adolescents with primary myelodysplastic syndromes (MDS). *Blood* 2000; **96**: 521a.
87 Karanes C, Abella E, Du W et al. Allogeneic bone marrow transplantation (alloBMT) in myelodysplastic syndromes (MDS). *Blood* 1998; **92**: 659a [Abstract].
88 Bibawi S, Abi-Said D, Fayad L et al. Thiotepa, busulfan, and cyclophosphamide as a preparative regimen for allogeneic transplantation for advanced myelodysplastic syndrome and acute myelogenous leukemia. *Am J Hematol* 2001; **67**: 227–33.
89 Mattijssen V, Schattenberg A, Schaap N, Preijers F, De Witte T. Outcome of allogeneic bone marrow transplantation with lymphocyte-depleted marrow grafts in adult patients with myelodysplastic syndromes. *Bone Marrow Transplant* 1997; **19**: 791–4.
90 Castro-Malaspina H, Childs B, Papadopoulos E et al. T-cell depleted (SBA-E-) bone marrow transplantation for myelodysplastic syndromes. *Leuk Res* 1997; **21** (Suppl. 1): S51 [Abstract].
91 O'Donnell PV, Noga SJ, Grever M, Vogelsang GB, Jones RJ. Using engineered allografts to improve transplant outcome in myelodysplastic syndrome (MDS). *Blood* 1997; **90**: 229a [Abstract].
92 Deeg HJ, Storer B, Slattery JT et al. Conditioning with targeted busulfan and cyclophosphamide for hemopoietic stem cell transplantation from related and unrelated donors in patients with myelodysplastic syndrome. *Blood* 2002; **100**: 1201–7.
93 Andersson BS, Gajewski J, Donato M et al. Allogeneic stem cell transplantation (BMT) for AML and MDS following i.v. busulfan and cyclophosphamide (i.v. BU/CY). *Bone Marrow Transplant* 2000; **25** (Suppl. 2): S35–8.
94 Parker JE, Shafi T, Mijovic A et al. Allogeneic stem cell transplantation (SCT) in MDS: interim results of outcome following nonmyeloablative conditioning compared to standards preparative regimens. *Blood* 2000; **96**: 554a [Abstract].
95 Cao TM, McSweeney PA, Niederwieser D et al. Nonmyeloablative allogeneic hematopoietic cell transplantation (AHCT) for patients with myelodysplastic syndromes (MDS) and myeloproliferative disorders (MPD). *Blood* 2000; **96**: 170a.
96 Kroger N, Schetelig J, Zabelina T et al. A fludarabine-based dose-reduced conditioning regimen

followed by allogeneic stem cell transplantation from related or unrelated donors in patients with myelodysplastic syndrome. *Bone Marrow Transplant* 2001; **28**: 643–7.

97 Rezvani K, Lalancette M, Szydlo R *et al.* Nonmyeloablative stem cell transplant (NMSCT) in AML, ALL, and MDS: disappointing outcome for patients with advanced phase disease. *Blood* 2000; **96**: 479a [Abstract].

98 Shimoni A, Khouri I, Donato M *et al.* Allogeneic transplantation with nonmyeloablative or reduced intensity conditioning: the intensity of the conditioning regimen is related to outcome in patients with active disease but not in those in remission at the time of transplantation. *Blood* 2000; **96**: 199a.

99 Harrison CN, Gale RE, Machin SJ, Linch DC. A large proportion of patients with a diagnosis of essential thrombocythemia do not have a clonal disorder and may be at lower risk of thrombotic complications. *Blood* 1999; **93**: 417–24.

100 Streiff MB, Smith B, Spivak JL. The diagnosis and management of polycythemia vera in the era since the Polycythemia Vera Study Group: a survey of American Society of Hematology members' practice patterns. *Blood* 2002; **99**: 1144–9.

101 Diez-Martin JL, Graham DL, Petitt RM, Dewald GW. Chromosome studies in 104 patients with polycythemia vera. *Mayo Clin Proc* 1991; **66**: 287–99.

102 Gruppo Italiano Studio Policitemia. Polycythemia vera: the natural history of 1213 patients followed for 20 years. *Ann Intern Med* 1995; **123**: 656–64.

103 Rozman C, Giralt M, Feliu E, Rubio D, Cortes MT. Life expectancy of patients with chronic nonleukemic myeloproliferative disorders. *Cancer* 1991; **67**: 2658–63.

104 Spivak JL. The optimal management of polycythaemia vera. *Br J Haematol* 2002; **116**: 243–54.

105 Tefferi A, Solberg LA, Silverstein MN. A clinical update in polycythemia vera and essential thrombocythemia. *Am J Med* 2000; **109**: 141–9.

106 Najean Y, Rain JD. Treatment of polycythemia vera: use of ^{32}P alone or in combination with maintenance therapy using hydroxyurea in 461 patients greater than 65 years of age. The French Polycythemia Study Group. *Blood* 1997; **89**: 2319–27.

107 Mesa RA, Silverstein MN, Jacobsen SJ, Wollan PC, Tefferi A. Population-based incidence and survival figures in essential thrombocythemia and agnogenic myeloid metaplasia: an Olmsted County study, 1976–95. *Am J Hematol* 1999; **61**: 10–5.

108 Murphy S, Peterson P, Iland H, Laszlo J. Experience of the Polycythemia Vera Study Group with essential thrombocythemia: a final report on diagnostic criteria, survival, and leukemic transition by treatment. *Semin Hematol* 1997; **34**: 29–39.

109 Stobart K, Rogers PCJ. Allogeneic bone marrow transplantation for an adolescent with polycythemia vera. *Bone Marrow Transplant* 1994; **13**: 337–9.

110 de Revel T, Giraudier S, Nedellec G *et al.* Allogeneic bone marrow transplantation for postpolycythemic myeloid metaplasia with myelofibrosis: a case report. *Bone Marrow Transplant* 1995; **16**: 187–9.

111 Richard S, Isola L, Scigliano E *et al.* Syngeneic stem cell transplant for spent-phase polycythaemia vera: eradication of myelofibrosis and restoration of normal haematopoiesis. *Br J Haematol* 2002; **117**: 245–6.

112 Anderson JE, Sale G, Appelbaum FR, Chauncey TR, Storb R. Allogeneic marrow transplantation for primary myelofibrosis and myelofibrosis secondary to polycythemia vera or essential thrombocytosis. *Br J Haematol* 1997; **98**: 1010–6.

113 Jurado M, Deeg HJ, Gooley T *et al.* Haemopoietic stem cell transplantation for advanced polycythaemia vera or essential thrombocythaemia. *Br J Haematol* 2001; **112**: 392–6.

114 Tefferi A. Myelofibrosis with myeloid metaplasia. *N Engl J Med* 2000; **342**: 1255–65.

115 Barosi G, Viarengo G, Pecci A, Rosti V, Piaggio G, Marchetti M. Diagnostic and clinical relevance of the number of circulating CD34$^+$ cells in myelofibrosis with myeloid metaplasia. *Blood* 2001; **98**: 3249–55.

116 Cervantes F, Barosi G, Demory JL *et al.* Myelofibrosis with myeloid metalasia in young individuals: disease characteristics, prognostic factors and identification of risk groups. *Br J Haematol* 1998; **102**: 684–90.

117 Dupriez B, Morel P, Demory JL *et al.* Prognostic factors in agnogenic myeloid metaplasia: a report on 195 cases with a new scoring system. *Blood* 1996; **88**: 1013–8.

118 Visani G, Finelli C, Castelli U *et al.* Myelofibrosis with myeloid metaplasia: clinical and haematological parameters predicting survival in a series of 133 patients. *Br J Haematol* 1990; **75**: 4–9.

119 Rajantie J, Sale GE, Deeg HJ *et al.* Adverse effect of severe marrow fibrosis on hematological recovery after chemoradiotherapy and allogeneic bone marrow transplantation. *Blood* 1986; **67**: 1693–7.

120 Soll E, Massumoto C, Clift RA *et al.* Relevance of marrow fibrosis in bone marrow transplantation: a retrospective analysis of engraftment. *Blood* 1995; **86**: 4667–73.

121 Bauermeister DE. Quantitation of bone marrow reticulin: a normal range. *Am J Clin Pathol* 1971; **56**: 24.

122 Dekmezian R, Kantarjian HM, Keating MJ *et al.* The relevance of reticulin stain-measured fibrosis at diagnosis in chronic myelogenous leukemia. *Cancer* 1987; **59**: 1739.

123 Sultan C. *Histopathologie de la Moelle Osseuse: Indications et Interprétation de la Biopsie Médullaire*. Paris: Masson, 1991.

124 Guardiola P, Anderson JE, Bandini G *et al.* Allogeneic stem cell transplantation for angogenic myeloid metaplasia: a European Group for Blood and Marrow Transplantation, Société Française de Greffe de Moelle, Gruppo Italiano per il Trapianto del Midollo Osseo and Fred Hutchinson Cancer Research Center collaborative study. *Blood* 1999; **93**: 2831–8.

125 Guardiola P, Anderson JE, Gluckman E. Allogeneic stem cell transplantation (SCT) in myelofibrosis with myeloid metaplasia (MMM). *N Engl J Med* 2000; **343**: 659.

126 Rossbach H-C, Grana NH, Chamizo W, Barrios NJ, Barbosa JL. Successful allogeneic bone marrow transplantation for agnogenic myeloid metaplasia in a 3-year-old boy. *J Pediatr Hematol Oncol* 1996; **18**: 213–5.

127 Singhal S, Powles R, Treleaven J, Pollard C, Lumley H, Mehta J. Allogeneic bone marrow transplantation for primary myelofibrosis. *Bone Marrow Transplant* 1995; **16**: 743–6.

128 Creemers GJ, Lowenberg B, Hagenbeek A. Allogeneic bone marrow transplantation for primary myelofibrosis. *Br J Haematol* 1992; **82**: 772–3.

129 Schmitz N, Suttorp M, Schlegelberger B, Weber-Matthiesen K, Tiemann M, Sonnen R. The role of the spleen after bone marrow transplantation for primary myelofibrosis. *Br J Haematol* 1992; **81**: 616–8.

130 Ifrah N, Gardembas-Pain M, Hunault M, Saint-Andre JP, Foussard C, Boasson M. Allogeneic bone marrow transplantation for primary myelofibrosis. *Br J Haematol* 1989; **73**: 575–6.

131 Dokal I, Jones L, Deenmamode M, Lewis SM, Goldman JM. Allogeneic bone marrow transplantation for primary myelofibrosis. *Br J Haematol* 1989; **71**: 158–60.

132 Guardiola P, Esperou H, Cazals-Hatem D *et al.* Allogeneic bone marrow transplantation for agnogenic myeloid metaplasia. *Br J Haematol* 1997; **98**: 1004–9.

133 Deeg HJ, Appelbaum FR. Stem cell transplantation for myelofibrosis. *N Engl J Med* 2001; **344**: 775–6.

134 Li Z, Gooley T, Appelbaum FR, Deeg HJ. Splenectomy and hemopoietic stem cell transplantation for myelofibrosis. *Blood* 2001; **97**: 2180–1.

135 Deeg J, Platzbecker U, Sale GE *et al.* Allogeneic hemopoietic stem cell transplantation for myelofibrosis. *Blood* 2001; **98**: 856a [Abstract].

136 Devine SM, Hoffman R, Verma A *et al.* Allogeneic blood cell transplantation following reduced-intensity conditioning is effective therapy for older patients with myelofibrosis with myeloid metaplasia. *Blood* 2002; **99**: 2255–8.

137 Byrne JL, Beshti H, Clark D *et al.* Induction of remission after donor leucocyte infusion for the treatment of relapsed chronic idiopathic myelofibrosis following allogeneic transplantation: evidence for a "graft vs. myelofibrosis" effect. *Br J Haematol* 2000; **108**: 430–3.

138 Anderson JE, Tefferi A, Craig F *et al.* Myeloablation and autologous peripheral blood stem cell rescue results in hematologic and clinical responses in patients with myeloid metaplasia with myelofibrosis. *Blood* 2001; **98**: 586–93.

139 Skerrett D, Fruchtman S, Scigliano E, Zangari M, Isola L. Autologous progenitor cell collections in polycythemia vera. *Blood* 1998; **92**: 123a [Abstract].

80

David G. Maloney & Gösta Gahrton

Allogeneic Hematopoietic Cell Transplantation for Multiple Myeloma

Multiple myeloma (MM) occurs with a 4–5/100,000 incidence in the USA and Europe and patients present at a median age of 65–70 years, with only a minority of patients (approximately 7%) presenting before the age 55 years [1,2]. Myeloma is more frequent in men than women and more common in black than white people. While sensitive to chemotherapy, the disease is not curable with conventional therapy with median survival of approximately 3 years [3]. High-dose therapy and autologous hematopoietic cell transplantation (HCT) provides higher remission rates, and prolonged survival when compared to standard chemotherapy [4] and may be used in patients to the age of 70 or above (see Chapter 92) [5]. Several trials, including the Intergroupe Francais Myeloma (IFM) 94 study, suggest that tandem autologous HCTs are superior to treatment with a single transplant [6]. However, even with single or tandem transplants, the median event-free survival was only 31 and 37 months, respectively. At 6 years, event-free survival was 19% vs. 28% and overall survival 26% vs. 46% for single vs. tandem autologous HCT, respectively. In subsequent trials, 200 mg/m^2 melphalan has emerged as the preferred conditioning for autologous HCT [7]. Failure following autologous HCT is likely caused by the inability of the preparative regimen to eliminate all of the tumor cells in the patient or possibly the reinfusion of tumor cells collected with the supportive hematopoietic cells. The former is more likely as attempts to "purge" tumor cells from hematopoietic cell grafts have not decreased the risk of relapse [8–10] and may cause prolonged immunodeficiency [11]. Relapses are also frequently observed following syngeneic transplantation [12], although a case matched series from the European Group for Blood and Marrow Transplantation (EBMT) demonstrated a lower risk of relapse than autologous HCT [13].

Allogeneic hematopoietic cell transplantation

Advantages of allogeneic HCT include a source of hematopoietic cells that is myeloma free and provides graft-vs.-myeloma (GVM) immune responses as a result of minor antigen differences between host and donor. Direct evidence for GVM has been demonstrated by the activity of donor lymphocyte infusion (DLI) for patients who have relapsed following allogeneic HCT [14–17] and inferred by the higher rates of relapse associated with T-cell-depleted grafts observed in patients transplanted for leukemia [18]. The largest experience using allogeneic HCT for myeloma has been following conditioning with myeloablative chemotherapy with or without total body irradiation (TBI). In early studies, a high transplant-related mortality (TRM) of 20–50% was observed (Table 80.1). This poor outcome was primarily a result of regimen-related toxicities, infections and graft-vs.-host disease (GVHD) or its treatment, limiting this approach to medically fit patients <50–60 years. More recently, reduced intensity or nonmyeloablative conditioning regimens with augmented immunosuppression have been developed that reliably allow allogeneic engraftment and shift the burden of tumor reduction from the preparative regimen to the GVM activity of the donor immune system. Although this approach reduces the early TRM, risks of GVHD and its complications remain. The lower intensity of the conditioning regimen provides less disease cytoreduction and early disease control, prompting evaluation of this approach in patients in remission or with low tumor burden. A third approach has been to use an initial autologous HCT procedure to cytoreduce the disease, followed by allogeneic HCT with nonmyeloablative or reduced intensity conditioning. This sequence provides tumor reduction with a low TRM from the autologous HCT followed by a tumor-free graft and GVM effects of the allogeneic HCT. These three approaches are discussed below.

Myeloablative conditioning and allogeneic HCT

As outlined in Table 80.1, multiple studies have evaluated the effects of high-dose therapy and allogeneic HCT for patients with myeloma using either bone marrow or mobilized peripheral blood stem cells (PBSCs). This topic has been the subject of many recent reviews [1,19,30,31]. The high early TRM (20–50% by day 100) observed in the majority of these studies has restricted this approach to younger patients. Series of patients have been reported from single institutions and collective data reported by the EBMT and the International Blood and Marrow Transplant Registry (IBMTR). There is considerable overlap from some of these sources, while results from other groups, including Seattle, the Dana Farber Cancer Center and the University of Arkansas have to date not been included in the transplant registries.

Multiple myeloablative conditioning regimens have been used, with the most common being cyclophosphamide (CY) with total body irradiation (CY/TBI) or busulfan with CY (BU/CY) and melphalan in combinations with TBI (MEL/TBI) (reviewed in [1]). While randomized studies have not been conducted, none of the combinations appear greatly superior to CY/TBI. However, the outcome of small trials has been strongly influenced by patient selection and their pretransplant characteristics. With myeloablative conditioning, complete remissions (CR) have been observed in 20–70% of patients (Table 80.1). Complicating this analysis are the variable definitions of CR that have been used. Recent criteria for CR include negative serum and urine electrophoresis and immunofixation and no morphologic evidence of myeloma cells on bone marrow biopsy [32]. In most trials approximately 50% of patients with chemosensitive disease will achieve a CR (Tables 80.1 and 80.2). The median onset of CR is approximately 3 months, but sometimes requires months to years following transplant. In contrast to autologous HCT, molecular remissions are frequent and occur in up to 50% of CR patients

Table 80.1 Single institutional reports of myeloablative therapy followed by allogeneic transplantation for myeloma.

Study [Reference] Years of HCT	n	Age (range)	TRM	CR (%)	OS % (mo)	RFS % (mo)	% sensitive	Dx-HCT (mo)	Notes
Seattle [19,20] 1987–99	136	43–48 <60	48% day 100 63% 1 year	34	22 (60)	14 (60)	21		16% URD
Montreal [21] 1990–2000	37	47 (25–53)	22%	57	32 (40)		>67	9.3	46% CR at HCT 50% PBHCT
Toronto [22] 1983–95	22	43 (25–53)	27% day 90 59%	~50	32 (36)	22 (36)	73	16	
Michigan [23] 1989–95	24	43 (31–56)	25%		40 (36)	40 (36)		~12	
Bologna [24] 1989–92	19	43 (36–50)	37%	42	26 (48)	21 (48)	37	19	
Surrey [25] 1981–98	33	38 (30–53)	54%	37	36 (36)	39 (36)	24	14	42% prior auto 10/12 died TRM
Torino [26] 1995–97	10	45 (35–53)	20%	71	80 (18)	60 (18)	60	8	PBSCT, 30% in CR at HCT
Arkansas [27] 1992–96	42	45 (29–59)	43%	41	29 (36)	20 (36)			Persistent/progressive disease post 1 Auto HCT
Boston [28] 1996–99	24	46 (36–54)	10%		55 (24)	42 (24)	100	10	CD6 depleted BM and CD4+ DLI
Vancouver [29] 1988–93	26	43 (29–55)	19% day 100	62	47 (36)	40 (14)	81	4	4 URD

CR, complete remission; DLI, donor lymphocyte infusion; Dx-HCT, time from diagnosis to hematopoietic cell transplantation; OS, overall survival; PBHCT, peripheral blood hematopoietic cell transplantation; PBSCT, peripheral blood stem cell transplantation; RFS, relapse-free survival; TRM, transplant-related mortality; URD, unrelated donor.

Table 80.2 European Group for Blood and Marrow Traansplantation (EBMT) registry data on allogeneic hematopoietic cell transplantation (HCT) for myeloma [33].

Cohort	n	Age	Dx-HCT (mo)	TRM (%) 6 month	TRM (%) 2 year	CR (%) 6 month	PFS mo	OS mo	OS (%) 2 year	OS (%) 3 year
BMT 1983–93	334	43	14	38	46	53	7	10	40	35
BMT 1994–98	223	44	10	21	30	54	19	50	57	55
PBHCT 1994–98	133	46	10	25	37	50	15	50+	57	57

BMT, bone marrow transplantation; CR, complete remission; Dx-HCT, time from diagnosis to hematopoietic cell transplantation; OS, overall survival; PBHCT, peripheral blood hematopoietic cell transplantation; PFS, progression-free survival; TRM, transplant-related mortality.

following allogeneic HCT and may be prolonged, suggesting cure of MM in some patients [34–36]. Despite the higher molecular remission rate, late relapses do occur, and in most series only 10–25% of patients remain disease-free at 10 years. Analysis of EBMT registry data suggest that survival has recently improved by reductions in TRM through better supportive care and patient selection (Table 80.2) [33].

As shown in Table 80.1, the majority of trials of allogeneic HCT have been performed in younger patients, with median ages of 38–47 years. Even in these younger patients, the reported early TRM from these trials ranges from 20 to 50% with an additional 10–30% late deaths from TRM brought about by complications of GVHD or its treatment. The reason for the high TRM associated with allogeneic HCT for MM is not clear. Possible factors include myeloma effects on baseline renal function that alter drug handling and disposition and underlying immunodeficiency, both predisposing to transplant complications. The largest single center experience is from Seattle as reviewed by Bensinger et al. [19,20]. In total, 136 patients (median ages 43–48 years, all <60 years) were treated between 1987 and 1999. Most of the patients were heavily pretreated, with only 21% with chemosensitive disease responsive to initial chemotherapy, while the remainder were beyond first response or had chemotherapy-resistant disease. The majority of patients received BU/CY with or without TBI, followed by cyclosporine (CSP) and methotrexate (MTX) for GVHD prophylaxis and matched related allografts (16% unrelated donors). The day 100 TRM was 48% with an additional 15% TRM at 1 year as a result of GVHD and infections. For the entire group, the 5-year survival was 22% with relapse-free survival (RFS) of 14%. For the 34% who achieved a CR, survival and RFS at 5 years was 48% and 37%, respectively. Overall, 13% of patients died from acute or chronic GVHD. In subset analysis, the early TRM was lower (approximately 20%) for patients with responsive disease who were transplanted <1 year from diagnosis [20].

The impact of patient selection and better supportive care on the outcome of myeloablative allogeneic HCT is best demonstrated in the analysis of the EBMT registry data using outcomes from 690 myeloma allografts as presented by Gahrton et al. [33] (Table 80.2). In this analysis, patients receiving BMT between 1983–93 were compared to BMT in later years (1994–98) and with a smaller cohort who received HCT using peripheral blood hematopoietic cells (PBHCs) in the later years. The TRM at 6 months and at 2 years was significantly lower in patients transplanted between 1994–98, 38% vs. 21% and 46% vs. 30%, respectively. The decrease in TRM appeared to be because of better treatment of infections and fewer pulmonary complications. This reduction in TRM has led to improved outcome, with median overall survival increasing from 10 to 50 months. Overall survival at 3 years increased from 35% to 55%. Median progression-free survival improved from 7 to 19 months. Interestingly, the cohort of patients receiving PBHC had an identical outcome, although there was a trend toward higher incidence of chronic GVHD. Overall survival in this group of patients was 57% at 3 years. Other significant factors influencing the improved outcome of recent conventional allogeneic transplants included earlier transplantation (median of 10 months from diagnosis) and less prior therapy. The median ages in these cohorts ranged from 43 to 46 years.

Multiple small studies have reported high TRM with only a minority of patients attaining long-term disease-free survival (Table 80.1). Investigators in Vancouver and Toronto used conditioning with BU/CY with or without melphalan or with CY/TBI and observed a early TRM of 16–27%, a CR rate of 42–58% and progression-free survival at 3 years of 22–40% [22,29]. Additional small series suggest improvement in patients with responsive disease (chemosensitive) who are treated early in the disease course. The use of PBHC following BU/MEL conditioning led to 80% survival and 60% event-free survival at 18 months in 10 patients (60% chemosensitive) transplanted a median of 8 months from diagnosis [26]. Altogether, these trials support the concept that allogeneic HCT may benefit a minority of younger patients with matched sibling donors, and that long-term cure is possible.

Graft-vs.-host disease

Acute GVHD is one of the most important complications of allogeneic HCT following myeloablative and reduced intensity regimens with grade II–IV disease occurring in 20–60% of patients transplanted with non-T-depleted allografts. The incidence of GVHD increases with a number of factors including the use of unrelated or mismatched donors, patient age and multiparous female donors (see Chapter 50). The development of GVHD may be reduced by treatment with CSP and MTX, or similar drugs, or by T-cell depletion of the graft (see below). It is clear that advanced GVHD (grades III–IV) is associated with inferior survival; however, GVHD has also been associated with decreased risk of disease relapse [14]. In an analysis of EBMT data, there have not been changes in the management of GVHD that have yet translated into significant survival advantages compared to other methods [1]. Overall, 14% of patients transplanted with non-T-depleted grafts developed grade III–IV GVHD compared with 9% of patients receiving T-depleted BMT [37]. As discussed below, GVHD and its treatment remain the most significant risk of allogeneic HCT following reduced intensity or nonmyeloablative conditioning.

Prognostic factors

In the Seattle series, the day 100 TRM was influenced by the pretransplant serum albumin level (albumin <3.0 g/dL, relative risk 1.7) which replaced the earlier observed correlation with shorter time from diagnosis to transplant [19,20]. A higher risk of relapse or progression was associated with male donors (relative risk 4.3) and the extent of prior chemotherapy (>6 cycles, relative risk 4.2). Patients with female donors had a lower risk of relapse, but progression-free survival was offset by more severe GVHD. Progression-free survival was worsened by Durie stage III disease (relative risk 1.9) and overall survival worsened by chemotherapy resistance at the time of allogeneic HCT (relative risk 2.2). Analysis of the EBMT data found that favorable pretransplant factors were to be female, to have received only one treatment regimen, a low β_2-microglobulin and chemosensitive disease [1,33,37]. Donor gender was also important and was the lowest risk for female patients with female donors and the highest risk for male patients with female donors. In recent analyses a shorter time from diagnosis to transplant was also correlated with improved outcome, and likely related to degree of prior therapy [33]. Many of these factors are closely interrelated, as patients transplanted with chemosensitive disease are usually early in the course of their disease and have not had multiple prior therapies, do not have high β_2-microglobulin or adverse cytogenetics (chromosome 13 abnormalities).

Source of allogeneic cells

The majority of early data on allografting for MM utilized bone marrow grafts. More recently there has been a shift to utilizing growth factor mobilized PBHC for patients with matched sibling donors. For patients requiring unrelated donor collection, the availability of PBHC has been more restricted. Similar to the observations made following autologous HCT, the use of PBHC has been associated with significantly more rapid engraftment [38–42]. There are significant differences in graft composition between bone marrow and PBHC, the most notable being a ~10-fold increase in the number of T cells in granulocyte colony-stimulating factor (G-CSF) mobilized peripheral blood (reviewed in [39] and Chapter 46). There are also phenotypic and biologic differences in PBHC including the expression of more lineage-specific antigens, less metabolically active cells and a polarization toward a Th2 cell type (reviewed in [43]). Surprisingly, there is not a greater incidence or severity of acute GVHD [38]. The effect on chronic GVHD is more uncertain, as several studies have suggested higher rates of chronic GVHD in recipients of PBHC, and a meta-analysis of available trials concluded that there was a 1.5-fold increase in chronic GVHD risk (reviewed in [39]). A prospective randomized study in patients with a variety of hematologic malignancies (few patients with MM) by the Fred Hutchinson Cancer Research Center, Stanford University and the City of Hope National Medical Center found more rapid engraftment and superior 3-year disease-free survival associated with the use of PBHC [38]. In this trial, the incidence of chronic GVHD was not different; however, the number of successive treatments needed to control chronic GHVD and the duration of glucocorticoid treatment were longer following the use of PBHC [44].

In MM, several small series have suggested a lower TRM associated with HCT using PBHC (Table 80.1 and [23,26]). In contrast, analysis of the EBMT data for transplants performed between 1994 and 1998 has not shown any difference in TRM, or disease-free and overall survival in patients receiving PBHC compared with BMT (Fig. 80.1 and [33]). However, there was a trend toward greater chronic GVHD in the PBSC recipients. As the follow-up is still short it is not clear what the ultimate impact of PBHC transplantation will be, as chronic GVHD has been also associated with a decreased risk of relapse.

In contrast, nearly all trials utilizing reduced intensity or nonmyeloablative conditioning have utilized PBHC as the preferred source of hematopoietic cells. Recent analyses of patients with hematological malignancies treated with matched unrelated donor HCT following fludarabine and 200 cGy TBI demonstrated increased risk of graft rejection associated with the use of bone marrow (Chapter 85), likely because

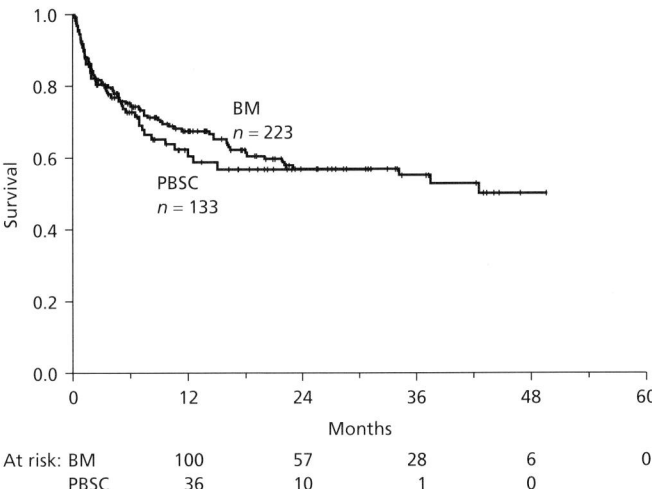

Fig. 80.1 Overall actuarial survival after transplantation performed 1994–8 according to the type of graft. The Kaplan–Meier curves show a similar survival among patients who received bone marrow (BM) cells as among those who received peripheral blood stem cells (PBSCs). (From Gahrton et al. [33].)

of the fewer number of T cells or hematopoietic cells in the marrow vs. PBHC harvests [39].

T-cell-depleted transplants

GVHD can be nearly eliminated by efficient T-cell depletion of the donor PBHC or bone marrow graft. While specific experience in MM is limited, it appears consistent with what has been observed in other hematologic malignancies, showing a greater risk of graft rejection and of disease relapse [18]. Several approaches have been used to partially T-cell deplete the graft, allowing engraftment yet limiting the risk of GVHD. One such approach is to use T-cell depletion with anti-CD6 monoclonal antibodies or by the use of the monoclonal antibody Campath (alemtuzumab) treatment "in the bag" or systemically prior to transplantation.

Investigators in Boston have used CY/TBI as a preparatory regimen followed by HCT with a CD6-depleted bone marrow graft for patients with MM. To attain GVM, the investigators infused CD4 positive donor lymphocytes (DLI) after [28]. In 24 patients, the incidence of grade II–III GVHD was 21% (only one patient with grade III) and the TRM was 10%. Only one patient achieved a CR at 6 months without the addition of DLI. Fourteen patients (58%) received DLI with responses in 10, although seven developed acute or chronic GVHD. The 2-year overall survival and progression-free survival were 55% and 42%, respectively. This study was performed in "good prognosis" patients with a median age of 46 years, all had chemosensitive disease and were transplanted a median of 10 months from diagnosis. DLI could not be given to 42% of patients, either as a result of GVHD or because of transplant-related complications. Comparison with a reference group suggested that the administration of DLI was associated with improved outcome. This study points out the important role of donor T cells in achieving CR and the need to supplement T-depleted grafts with DLI to provide immunologic GVM activity.

Campath has also been used to reduce the incidence of GVHD, either by *ex vivo* treatment of the collected bone marrow or by the infusion of antibody prior to the conditioning regimen (as reviewed in [45]). When used at a total dose of 100 mg/m^2 in the pretransplant conditioning, significant levels of antibody persisted through day +28 to affect the allogeneic graft [46]. Campath has been used with myeloablative conditioning with clear reductions in severity of GVHD. The major risks associated with the use of this antibody have been the increase of opportunistic infections because of removal of donor immune cells and the increased requirement to utilize DLI to provide adequate antitumor effects. Details on reduced intensity regimens using Campath as part of conditioning are presented below.

Donor lymphoctye infusions

The most compelling data for the existence of GVM activity associated with allogeneic HCT stem from the use of DLI for patients who have persistent or relapsed disease following allogeneic HCT [47]. The infusion of lymphocytes, collected from the original graft donor, may induce remissions in up to 50% of relapsed patients, including remissions of long duration (reviewed in [14]). However, this therapy is often associated with clinical GVHD and many of the responses are only partial and temporary. Lokhorst et al. [15,16] reported on the use of DLI in 27 patients receiving 52 infusions of DLI for relapsed MM. Thirteen patients received reinduction chemotherapy resulting in partial remission (PR) in eight patients prior to the administration of DLI. The response rate to DLI was 52% with 22% CR. Five patients responded only following escalated doses of lymphocytes. Five patients remained in remission more than 30 months following DLI, including two patients in sustained molecular remission, indicating that responses can be prolonged in a minority of patients. Acute GVHD was observed in 55%, and chronic GVHD in 26% of patients and represented the most significant toxicity. Median survival of the group was 18 months and was only 11 months in nonresponders and was not yet reached in responding patients. Important factors that were correlated with response to DLI were the infusion of >1 × 10^8 cells/kg, response to reinduction therapy and chemosensitive disease prior to the HCT.

Analysis of 25 patients receiving DLI in 15 transplant centers for relapsed or progressive MM was reported by Salama et al. [17]. Only two of 22 patients responded to the initial DLI infusion alone, while five of nine given additional infusions responded, resulting in two CR and three PR. All three patients given chemotherapy before the DLI responded. All responders developed acute GVHD and 11 of 21 patients developed chronic GVHD. Four patients had responses lasting for >1 year and three ongoing with <1 year of follow-up. Three of 15 patients who did not respond to DLI nevertheless had significant GVHD.

New approaches that may decrease the toxicity of DLI, while retaining the GVM activity, are needed (see Chapter 84). Possible solutions include the use of cloned T cells against minor antigens expressed on tumor but not host tissues, the use of CD8-depleted DLI [48,49], and the use of suicide gene-transduced T cells that could be ablated should severe GVHD without GVM develop [50,51].

Myeloablative HCT following failed autologous HCT

Myeloablative conditioning and autologous HCT is currently considered the standard of care for patients under the age of 70 years who are able to tolerate treatment with 200 mg/m^2 melphalan. However, even with a single or tandem transplant, there is an almost continuous risk of relapse, with only 10–20% of patients remaining disease-free at 7 years [6]. Thus, an increasingly common problem is the number of patients who have relapsed following one or two prior autologous HCT who are being considered for salvage allogeneic HCT. The use of conventional myeloablative allografts in this setting has been associated with prohibitive TRM. Analysis of the Seattle data by Radich et al. [52] for second myeloablative allografts following failed conventional transplants for patients with a variety of hematologic malignancies indicated a 2-year incidence of nonrelapse mortality of 51% with 26% relapse mortality resulting in only 23% 2-year survival. All surviving patients had acute myeloid or lymphoblastic leukemia. Only three patients had myeloma and, of those, two died of nonrelapse causes and one of disease progression.

The impact of a failed prior autologous HCT on outcome following myeloablative conditioning and allogeneic HCT was also observed in the experience at the Royal Marsden Hospital using CY/TBI conditioning. The 2-year event-free survival was 48% vs. 17% for those patients without or with a prior autologous HCT, respectively [27]. The University of Arkansas HCT group treated 42 MM patients with persistent or progressive disease following prior autologous HCT with myeloablative conditioning and allogeneic HCT and observed a 43% TRM, 41% CR rate but only 29% survival and 20% relapse-free survival at 3 years [53]. These observations have prompted the evaluation of reduced intensity conditioning regimens and allogeneic HCT as consolidation of autologous HCT prior to disease progression and is described below.

Reduced intensity or nonmyeloablative conditioning

A major recent change in allogeneic HCT is based on the observation that myeloablation is not required for allogeneic engraftment. As discussed in Chapter 85, this approach shifts the burden of tumor control and eradication of host hematopoiesis to the donor immune response against antigens expressed on host cells. However, the reduced intensity regimens provide less immediate antimyeloma effect, risking progression of disease prior to the emergence of GVM activity. An increasing number of regimens have been developed that achieve allogeneic engraftment with reduced intensity or even nonmyeloablative conditioning and have been applied to the treatment of patients with MM (Table 80.3). The lower early TRM associated with reduced intensity conditioning allows treatment of patients not fit for myeloablative regimens because of age or comorbid medical conditions. Many of these regimens were first evaluated in the setting of patients who had failed autologous HCT.

Clinical trials at the M.D. Anderson Cancer Center demonstrated that the addition of fludarabine to intermediate-dose melphalan (140–180 mg/m^2) was sufficient to allow engraftment from both human leukocyte antigen (HLA) matched sibling and unrelated donors [53]. In heavily pretreated patients with myeloma (median five prior regimens, nine patients with failed autologous HCT), the day 100 TRM was 19%. The CR rate was 32%; however, the estimated 2-year survival was only 30% with progression-free survival of 19%. A similar approach using Campath *in vivo* prior to hematopoietic cell infusion (to control both host-vs.-graft and GVHD reactions) and melphalan (140 mg/m^2) was evaluated in 12 patients with myeloma following a failed autologous HCT [55]. At a median follow-up of 14 months, one patient was in CR and four patients had detectable but stable disease. DLI was given to three patients with progressive disease with one PR. One patient received DLI for persistent disease and has achieved an ongoing CR.

The same regimen was used for the treatment of 17 patients as consolidation therapy following chemotherapy [46]. The TRM was only 12%; however, only 6% achieved a CR from the initial transplant and 10 patients required subsequent DLI. The 18-month overall survival was 80% and progression-free survival 53%. Conditioning with the FLU/MEL regimen in patients with chronic lymphoproliferative diseases using either Campath/cyclosporine (CSA) vs. CSA/MTX for GVHD prophylaxis demonstrated that the *in vivo* antibody was associated with a lower incidence of acute (22% vs. 45%) and chronic GVHD (5% vs. 67%) [57]. However, it was also associated with a higher incidence of cytomegalovirus (CMV) reactivation, and a lower rate of CR + PR at 3 months after transplantation (21% vs. 68%), requiring DLI to be given for disease control. The end result was a similar overall and progression-free survival, but with less GVHD in the Campath-treated cohort. This study clearly demonstrates the effect of T-cell depletion to decrease GVHD and GVM responses in association with subsequent DLI for disease control.

The University of Arkansas HCT group has also used intermediate melphalan (100 mg/m^2) alone followed by allogeneic HCT from HLA matched siblings or combined with fludarabine and 250 cGy TBI for HCT from unrelated allografts [57,58]. In a recent report of 31 patients, all with poor-risk features, 89% attained full engraftment and two patients experienced autologous reconstitution. The CR rate was 61%, with three patients (10%) having early TRM. However, an additional six patients died of late TRM (including five who died from infections complications resulting from treatment for GVHD) resulting in a 1-year survival of 71% and event-free survival of 55%. Patients treated following a

Table 80.3 Selected trials of reduced intensity or nonmyeloablative conditioning for allogeneic hematopoietic cell transplantation (HCT) in myeloma.

Author [Reference]	n	Age (range)	TRM (%)	CR (%)	OS % (mo)	PFS % (mo)	Chemo sens (%)	Dx-HCT, (mo)	Regimen/notes
As salvage to chemotherapy									
Maloney et al. [46]	17	48 (NA)	12	6	80 (18)	53 (18)	100	NA	Campath/FLU/MEL, no prior auto, 10 DLI
Giralt et al. [54]	22	51 (46–64)	19 @ day 100 40 @ 1 year	32	30 (24)	19 (24)	41	36	FLU/MEL, heavily pretreated, 9 failed auto
As salvage for failed autologous HCT									
Garban et al. [54]	12	53 (45–61)	42	33	33 (13)	33 (13)	NA	NA	FLU/BU/ATG
Branson et al. [55]	12	NA	~20	8	NA	42 (14)	NA	NA	Campath/FLU/MEL
Badros et al. [57,58]	31	56 (38–69)	10 @ day 100 29 @ 1 year	61	71 (12)	55 (12)	45	29	MEL, better outcome for pts with 1 vs. 2 prior auto HCT
Kröger et al. [59]	21	50 (32–61)	10 @ day 100 26 @ 1 year	40	74 (24)	53 (24)	43	33	FLU/MEL/ATG, all URD 9 planned auto/allo
Planned tandem autologous followed by allogeneic HCT									
Maloney et al. [46]	52	52 (29–71)	15	52	79 (18)	64 (18)	52	10	Auto: MEL Allo (200 cGy TBI)
Kröger et al. [60]	17	51 (32–64)	11 @ day 100	73	74 (24)	56 (24)	70	13	Auto: MEL, Allo: FLU/MEL/ATG, URD = 8

Allo, allogeneic; ATG, antithymocyte globulin; Auto, autologous; BU, busulfan; CR, complete remission; DLI, donor lymphocyte infusion; Dx-HCT, time from diagnosis to hematopoietic cell transplantation; FLU, fludarabine; MEL, melphalan; OS, overall survival; PFS, progression-free survival; TRM, transplant-related mortality; URD, unrelated donor.

planned single autologous HCT (without relapse prior to allogeneic HCT) had a improved outcome, with overall and event-free survivals of 86% and 86% vs. 48% and 31% at 1-year for patients with one vs. two prior autologous HCT, respectively. Grades II–IV acute GVHD was observed in 58% of patients. Eighteen (58%) of patients received subsequent DLI either for disease or mixed chimerism, complicated by increased risk of GVHD [57,58]. Compared to a group of similar patients treated with myeloablative conditioning (but with fewer poor-risk features), the reduced intensity regimen was associated with a lower early TRM (10% vs. 29%) and a better survival at 1 year (71% vs. 45%), respectively. However, the median follow-up was only 6 months and there did not appear to be a plateau of the event-free survival curve. The ability to salvage patients with refractory myeloma who have relapsed post-autologous HCT by the use of an allogeneic HCT appears limited.

Planned tandem autologous/allogeneic HCT

As demonstrated above, the outcome following reduced intensity regimens is better for patients who have not failed autologous HCT. For patients who have not had a prior HCT, an alternative approach is to use tandem transplants. High-dose therapy with autologous HCT is used first to cytoreduce the disease (with a low TRM), followed by reduced intensity or nonmyeloablative conditioning and allogeneic HCT to provide GVM effects, with the goal of eradicating the malignancy and preventing relapse, all with a lower overall TRM.

This approach has been undertaken by several groups of investigators. In a series of patients treated in a consortium of institutions coordinated through the Fred Hutchinson Cancer Research Center in Seattle, including the City of Hope National Medical Center, Stanford University, the University of Colorado, the University of Torino, Italy, and the University of Leipzig, Germany, 54 patients with advanced myeloma have been treated using a planned "tandem auto/allo" approach as shown in Fig. 80.2(a). Newly diagnosed patients with stage II–III disease requiring therapy were recommended to have induction chemotherapy with vincristine, adriamycin, dexamethasone (VAD) chemotherapy (3–4 cycles) followed by autologous PBHC harvesting using high-dose cyclophosphamide (with or without Taxol) and G-CSF. Relapsed or refractory patients were also eligible, as long as sufficient autologous PBHC could be collected to support HCT. High-dose therapy with single agent melphalan (200 mg/m^2) was used for tumor cytoreduction followed by autologous PBSC support. Following recovery from transplant toxicities, 40–120 days later, patients underwent allografting following nonmyeloablative conditioning using a single fraction of 200 cGy TBI administered at a low dose rate (Fig. 80.2b). Matched sibling donor PBHC, harvested from two aphereses following stimulation with G-CSF were infused immediately following TBI. Patients received postgrafting immunosuppression with cyclosporine and mycophenolate mofetil (MMF).

Updated results include the treatment of 54 patients with this planned tandem approach [46]. Toxicity following the autologous HCT included medians of 6 days of neutropenia and 7 days of hospitalization. One patient (of the first five) who had received CD34 selected graft died from CMV pneumonia. Fifty-two of the 54 patients proceeded to the planned allograft procedure with a median time between autologous and allogeneic transplant of 62 days. The allografts were well-tolerated with a median of 0 days of hospitalization, and only mild neutropenia and thrombocytopenia. The granulocyte and platelet nadirs were 760 cells/μL and 95,000 cells/μL, respectively. All patients developed donor engraftment with medians of 90% donor T-cell chimerism by day +28 which increased to 96% by day +84. One patient died before day 100 from disease progression. Acute GVHD was seen in 38% of patients and was grade II in all but four cases. Forty-six percent of patients developed chronic GHVD requiring therapy. Tumor responses occurred slowly and thus far 57% of patients not in CR at the time of treatment have achieved CR and 26% PR. Of 28 patients with responsive disease at study entry, three have died from transplant-related complications and two have relapsed. Sixteen remain in continuous CR, five in ongoing PR and two patients have stable disease. Patients with relapsed/refractory disease have had greater TRM, with five of 26 patients dying from complications of acute and chronic GVHD or infections. In this group, 11 of 26 patients achieved CR and four of 26 patients are in PR following the allograft. One responding patient has relapsed. Three additional patients have died from myeloma ($n = 2$) or lung cancer. With a median follow-up of 18 months, 79% of patients are alive (Fig. 80.3).

This study has been used to plan a comparative trial in the BMT Clinical Trials Network (BMT-CTN) that will evaluate the use of this approach in a multicentre setting for the treatment of patients with stage II–III myeloma within 9 months of initiation of chemotherapy. The current plans for this trial include the treatment of patients with HLA

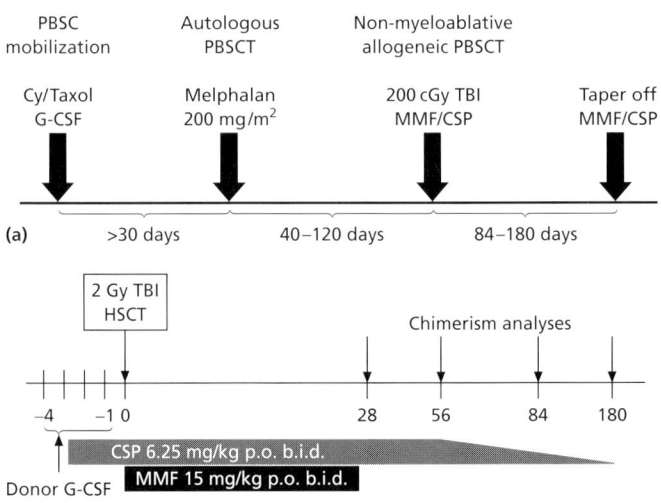

Fig. 80.2 Timeline and Seattle conditioning regimen for "tandem auto/allo" hematopoietic cell transplantation (HCT).

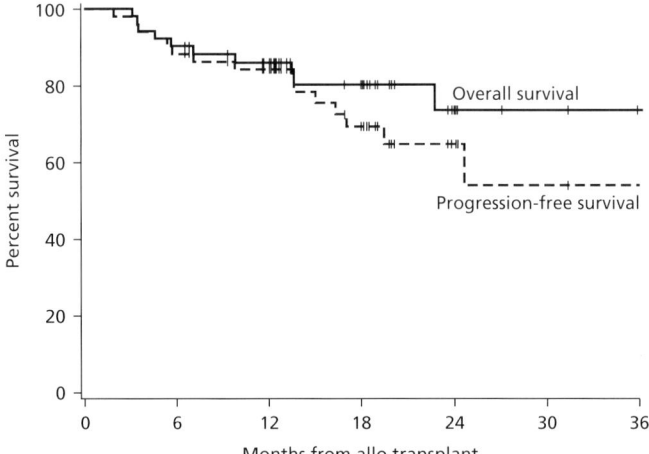

Fig. 80.3 Overall and progression-free survival of 52 myeloma patients treated with autologous followed by allogeneic HCT using nonmyeloablative conditioning in the Seattle Consortium. Median follow-up is 18 months.

matched sibling donors with the "auto/allo approach" compared to the use of tandem autografts with or without post-transplant therapy (dexamethasone and thalidomide) for patients without HLA identical sibling donors. Within the EBMT group, a nearly identical study is comparing the treatment of MM patients with stage II and III disease at diagnosis, using autologous HCT alone (single or tandem HCT using conditioning with 200 mg/m^2 melphalan) vs. treatment with the "tandem auto/allo" approach. The conditioning regimen for the nonmyeloablative allogeneic HCT is with fludarabine and 200 cGy TBI. To be eligible for the EBMT study patients must have at least one potential sibling donor. Patients are assigned to treatment regimens using "genetic randomization" based on having an available matched sibling donor. Patients with donors receive the "tandem auto/allo" approach, while patients without donors receive either a single or tandem autologous HCT. While the EBMT trial and the BMT-CTN trial are not true randomized trials, and they may have confounding imbalances in prognostic factors, they should provide a reasonable test to evaluate the contribution of a consolidative allogeneic HCT using nonmyeloablative conditioning as a treatment for MM.

A similar approach using a more aggressive allogeneic conditioning regimen has been reported by Kröger et al. [60] in myeloma patients with stable disease or better following induction or salvage chemotherapy (12 patients in PR). Seventeen patients, median age 51 years (range 32–64 years) received melphalan (200 mg/m^2) and autologous HCT. At a median of 119 days post-autologous HCT (range 60–210 days) patients underwent conditioning with fludarabine (180 mg/m^2), melphalan (100 mg/m^2) and antithymocyte globulin (ATG) (30 mg/kg) followed by allogeneic HCT. Eight of the patients received matched unrelated grafts. GVHD prophylaxis was with CSP and MTX. The allograft regimen did lead to at least 8 days of neutropenia (median time to leukocyte >1 × 10^9/L was 16 days, range 11–24 days). All patients required red blood cell and platelet transfusions. All patients developed full donor chimerism by day 30–40. The day 100 mortality was 11%. Acute GVHD (38%) included four cases with grade II and three with grade III disease. Forty percent of patients developed chronic GVHD, but only one case was extensive requiring further therapy. Overall 18% of patients attained a CR following the autograft and 73% a CR following the allograft. With a median follow-up of 13 months following the allogeneic HCT, 13 patients were alive and 12 free of progression or relapse. The estimated 2-year overall survival was 74% and disease-free survival 56%. Two patients relapsed following allogeneic HCT. None of the patients entering the study with less than a PR from their prior therapy (prior to the autologous HCT) had a CR following the allogeneic HCT. Longer follow-up is required to determine if this regimen, which appeared better tolerated than a fully ablative regimen, will ultimately result in long-term DFS.

Although promising, longer follow-up is needed to assess the risk of relapse and of the long-term risks of GVHD and its treatment. There will likely be a higher early TRM associated with the "tandem auto/allo" approach compared with tandem autologous HCT, and it remains to be determined if this will be compensated for by a lower risk of relapse. It is not clear which patients will benefit the most from such an approach. The use of prognostic factors important in autologous HCT outcome, such as β$_2$-microglobulin, chromosome 13 abnormalities or elevated LDH, has been able to identify patients likely to have a shorter event-free survival following tandem autologous HCT; however, it is not yet clear that these patients will benefit from nonmyeloablative conditioning and allogeneic HCT more than patients with lower risk disease. Other studies ongoing in Europe are evaluating this approach ("tandem auto/allo") only in patients with adverse prognostic features such as high β$_2$-microglobulin or chromosome 13 abnormalities on cytogenetics.

Future directions

Although progress has been made with the reduction in TRM associated with both conventional and reduced intensity conditioning for allogeneic HCT for myeloma, only a minority of patients appear to be cured. Tumor progression remains the most significant issue, even with the use of DLI. Treatment of patients earlier in their disease course, prior to the development of chemotherapy resistance improves outcome, but will remain difficult until the late complications of GVHD and infections can be decreased. Separation of GVT immune reactions from GVHD would allow more specific tumor targeting with less toxicity, and may be possible through vaccination or the use of antigen-specific T-cell clones. Additional approaches that render the donor tolerant to host tissues, but allow sensitization to tumor antigens are being explored. The use of more tumor-specific agents in conditioning regimens by marrow-directed treatments or monoclonal antibodies may provide more specific tumor kill. The incorporation of new agents with high single-agent activity such as thalidomide analogs or PS-341 may further improve the outcome of allogeneic HCT for myeloma by providing more effective cytoreduction.

Conclusions

These studies suggest that there will be a renewed interest in the use of allogeneic HCT for patients with myeloma because of the shift from ablative high-dose conditioning and allogeneic HCT to the immunologic manipulation of allogeneic engraftment and establishment of an initial mixed chimeric state by reduced intensity regimens. This goal can clearly be accomplished with a lower early TRM. However, complications related to GVHD or its treatment remain serious causes of late morbidity and mortality. GVM activity has been closely associated with GVHD and reduction of GVHD by global T-cell depletion is associated with increased risk of graft rejection, immunodeficiency and tumor relapse, often requiring subsequent DLI for tumor control. The use of cytoreductive therapy and autologous HCT followed by a nonmyeloablative regimen and allogeneic HCT may allow the benefits of both high-dose therapy and GVM effects with a lower TRM. However, much longer follow-up is required to determine whether the remissions will be durable and to determine the ultimate consequences of chronic GVHD. The future lies with a better understanding of the nature of the targets of GVHD- and GVM-associated immune responses and subsequent manipulation of these phenomena.

References

1 Gahrton G, Bjorkstrand B. Progress in haematopoietic stem cell transplantation for multiple myeloma. *J Intern Med* 2000; **248**: 185–201.

2 Jemal A, Thomas A, Murray T et al. Cancer statistics, 2002. *CA Cancer J Clin* 2002; **52**: 23–47.

3 Kyle RA. Current therapy of multiple myeloma. *Intern Med* 2002; **41**: 175–80.

4 Attal M, Harousseau JL, Stoppa AM et al. A prospective, randomized trial of autologous bone marrow transplantation and chemotherapy in multiple myeloma. Intergroupe Francais Myelome. *N Engl J Med* 1996; **335**: 91–7.

5 Badros A, Barlogie B, Siegel E et al. Autologous stem cell transplantation in elderly multiple myeloma patients over the age of 70 years. *Br J Haematol* 2001; **114**: 600–7.

6 Anderson KC, Shaughnessy JD Jr, Barlogie B et al. Multiple myeloma. *Hematology* (Am Soc Hematol Educ Program) 2002: 214–40.

7 Moreau P, Facon T, Attal M et al. Comparison of 200 mg/m^2 melphalan and 8 Gy total body irradiation plus 140 mg/m^2 melphalan as conditioning regimens for peripheral blood stem cell transplantation in patients with newly diagnosed multiple myeloma: final analysis of the Intergroupe Francophone du Myelome 9502 randomized trial. *Blood* 2002; **99**: 731–5.

8 Anderson KC, Barut BA, Ritz J et al. Monoclonal antibody-purged autologous bone marrow transplantation therapy for multiple myeloma. *Blood* 1991; **77**: 712–20.

9. Schiller G, Vescio R, Freytes C et al. Transplantation of CD34+ peripheral blood progenitor cells after high-dose chemotherapy for patients with advanced multiple myeloma. Blood 1995; 86: 390–7.
10. Stewart AK, Vescio R, Schiller G et al. Purging of autologous peripheral-blood stem cells using CD34 selection does not improve overall or progression-free survival after high-dose chemotherapy for multiple myeloma: results of a multicenter randomized controlled trial. J Clin Oncol 2001; 19: 3771–9.
11. Holmberg LA, Boeckh M, Hooper H et al. Increased incidence of cytomegalovirus disease after autologous CD34-selected peripheral blood stem cell transplantation. Blood 1999; 94: 4029–35.
12. Bensinger WI, Demirer T, Buckner CD et al. Syngeneic marrow transplantation in patients with multiple myeloma. Bone Marrow Transplant 1996; 18: 527–31.
13. Gahrton G, Svensson H, Bjorkstrand B et al. Syngeneic transplantation in multiple myeloma: a case-matched comparison with autologous and allogeneic transplantation. European Group for Blood Marrow Transplantation. Bone Marrow Transplant 1999; 24: 741–5.
14. Mehta J, Singhal S. Graft-versus-myeloma. Bone Marrow Transplant 1998; 22: 835–43.
15. Lokhorst HM, Schattenberg A, Cornelissen JJ et al. Donor leukocyte infusions are effective in relapsed multiple myeloma after allogeneic bone marrow transplantation. Blood 1997; 90: 4206–11.
16. Lokhorst HM, Schattenberg A, Cornelissen JJ et al. Donor lymphocyte infusions for relapsed multiple myeloma after allogeneic stem-cell transplantation: predictive factors for response and long-term outcome. J Clin Oncol 2000; 18: 3031–7.
17. Salama M, Nevill T, Marcellus D et al. Donor leukocyte infusions for multiple myeloma. Bone Marrow Transplant 2000; 26: 1179–84.
18. Horowitz MM, Gale RP, Sondel PM et al. Graft-versus-leukemia reactions after bone marrow transplantation. Blood 1990; 75: 555–62.
19. Bensinger WI, Maloney D, Storb R. Allogeneic hematopoietic cell transplantation for multiple myeloma. Semin Hematol 2001; 38: 243–9.
20. Bensinger WI, Buckner CD, Anasetti C et al. Allogeneic marrow transplantation for multiple myeloma: an analysis of risk factors on outcome. Blood 1996; 88: 2787–93.
21. Le Blanc R, Montminy-Metivier S, Belanger R et al. Allogeneic transplantation for multiple myeloma: further evidence for a GVHD-associated graft-versus-myeloma effect. Bone Marrow Transplant 2001; 28: 841–8.
22. Couban S, Stewart AK, Loach D et al. Autologous and allogeneic transplantation for multiple myeloma at a single centre. Bone Marrow Transplant 1997; 19: 783–9.
23. Varterasian M, Janakiraman N, Karanes C et al. Transplantation in patients with multiple myeloma: a multicenter comparative analysis of peripheral blood stem cell and allogeneic transplantation. Am J Clin Oncol 1997; 20: 462–6.
24. Cavo M, Bandini G, Benni M et al. High-dose busulfan and cyclophosphamide are an effective conditioning regimen for allogeneic bone marrow transplantation in chemosensitive multiple myeloma. Bone Marrow Transplant 1998; 22: 27–32.
25. Kulkarni S, Powles RL, Treleaven JG et al. Impact of previous high-dose therapy on outcome after allografting for multiple myeloma. Bone Marrow Transplant 1999; 23: 675–80.
26. Majolino I, Corradini P, Scime R et al. Allogeneic transplantation of unmanipulated peripheral blood stem cells in patients with multiple myeloma. Bone Marrow Transplant 1998; 22: 449–55.
27. Mehta J, Tricot G, Jagannath S et al. Salvage autologous or allogeneic transplantation for multiple myeloma refractory to or relapsing after a first-line autograft? Bone Marrow Transplant 1998; 21: 887–92.
28. Alyea E, Weller E, Schlossman R et al. T-cell-depleted allogeneic bone marrow transplantation followed by donor lymphocyte infusion in patients with multiple myeloma: induction of graft-versus-myeloma effect. Blood 2001; 98: 934–9.
29. Reece DE, Shepherd JD, Klingemann HG et al. Treatment of myeloma using intensive therapy and allogeneic bone marrow transplantation. Bone Marrow Transplant 1995; 15: 117–23.
30. Gahrton G. Allogeneic bone marrow transplantation in multiple myeloma. Pathol Biol (Paris) 1999; 47: 188–91.
31. Bensinger WI. Allogeneic hematopoietic cell transplantation for multiple myeloma. Biomed Pharmacother 2002; 56: 133–8.
32. Blade J, Samson D, Reece D et al. Criteria for evaluating disease response and progression in patients with multiple myeloma treated by high-dose therapy and haemopoietic stem cell transplantation. Myeloma Subcommittee of the European Group for Blood Marrow Transplantation. Br J Haematol 1998; 102: 1115–23.
33. Gahrton G, Svensson H, Cavo M et al. Progress in allogenic bone marrow and peripheral blood stem cell transplantation for multiple myeloma: a comparison between transplants performed 1983–93 and 1994–98 at European Group for Blood and Marrow Transplantation centres. Br J Haematol 2001; 113: 209–16.
34. Corradini P, Voena C, Tarella C et al. Molecular and clinical remissions in multiple myeloma: role of autologous and allogeneic transplantation of hematopoietic cells. J Clin Oncol 1999; 17: 208–15.
35. Martinelli G, Terragna C, Zamagni E et al. Polymerase chain reaction-based detection of minimal residual disease in multiple myeloma patients receiving allogeneic stem cell transplantation. Haematologica 2000; 85: 930–4.
36. Martinelli G, Terragna C, Zamagni E et al. Molecular remission after allogeneic or autologous transplantation of hematopoietic stem cells for multiple myeloma. J Clin Oncol 2000; 18: 2273–81.
37. Gahrton G, Tura S, Ljungman P et al. An update of prognostic factors for allogeneic bone marrow transplantation in multiple myeloma using matched sibling donors. European Group for Blood Marrow Transplantation. Stem Cells 1995; 13 (Suppl. 2): 122–5.
38. Bensinger WI, Martin PJ, Storer B et al. Transplantation of bone marrow as compared with peripheral-blood cells from HLA-identical relatives in patients with hematologic cancers. N Engl J Med 2001; 344: 175–81.
39. Cutler C, Antin JH. Peripheral blood stem cells for allogeneic transplantation: a review. Stem Cells 2001; 19: 108–17.
40. Blaise D, Kuentz M, Fortanier C et al. Randomized trial of bone marrow versus lenograstim-primed blood cell allogeneic transplantation in patients with early-stage leukemia: a report from the Societe Francaise de Greffe de Moelle. J Clin Oncol 2000; 18: 537–46.
41. Champlin RE, Schmitz N, Horowitz MM et al. Blood stem cells compared with bone marrow as a source of hematopoietic cells for allogeneic transplantation. IBMTR Histocompatibility and Stem Cell Sources Working Committee and the European Group for Blood and Marrow Transplantation (EBMT). Blood 2000; 95: 3702–9.
42. Schmitz N, Bacigalupo A, Hasenclever D et al. Allogeneic bone marrow transplantation vs. filgrastim-mobilised peripheral blood progenitor cell transplantation in patients with early leukaemia: first results of a randomised multicentre trial of the European Group for Blood and Marrow Transplantation. Bone Marrow Transplant 1998; 21: 995–1003.
43. Gyger M, Stuart RK, Perreault C. Immunobiology of allogeneic peripheral blood mononuclear cells mobilized with granulocyte-colony stimulating factor. Bone Marrow Transplant 2000; 26: 1–16.
44. Flowers ME, Parker PM, Johnston LJ et al. Comparison of chronic graft-versus-host disease after transplantation of peripheral blood stem cells versus bone marrow in allogeneic recipients: long-term follow-up of a randomized trial. Blood 2002; 100: 415–9.
45. Hale G, Jacobs P, Wood L et al. CD52 antibodies for prevention of graft-versus-host disease and graft rejection following transplantation of allogeneic peripheral blood stem cells. Bone Marrow Transplant 2000; 26: 69–76.
46. Maloney DG, Sandmaier BM, Mackinnon S et al. Non-myeloablative transplantation. Hematology (Am Soc Hematol Educ Program) 2002: 392–421.
47. Slavin S, Morecki S, Weiss L et al. Donor lymphocyte infusion: the use of alloreactive and tumor-reactive lymphocytes for immunotherapy of malignant and nonmalignant diseases in conjunction with allogeneic stem cell transplantation. J Hematother Stem Cell Res 2002; 11: 265–76.
48. Giralt S, Hester J, Huh Y et al. CD8-depleted donor lymphocyte infusion as treatment for relapsed chronic myelogenous leukemia after allogeneic bone marrow transplantation. Blood 1995; 86: 4337–43.
49. Alyea EP, Soiffer RJ, Canning C et al. Toxicity and efficacy of defined doses of CD4+ donor lymphocytes for treatment of relapse after allogeneic bone marrow transplant. Blood 1998; 91: 3671–80.
50. Bordignon C, Bonini C, Verzeletti S et al. Transfer of the HSV-tk gene into donor peripheral blood lymphocytes for in vivo modulation of donor anti-tumor immunity after allogeneic bone marrow transplantation. Hum Gene Ther 1995; 6: 813–9.
51. Tiberghien P. Use of suicide genes in gene therapy. J Leukoc Biol 1994; 56: 203–9.
52. Radich JP, Gooley T, Sanders JE et al. Second allogeneic transplantation after failure of first autologous transplantation. Biol Blood Marrow Transplant 2000; 6: 272–9.
53. Giralt S, Aleman A, Anagnostopoulos A et al. Fludarabine/melphalan conditioning for allogeneic transplantation in patients with multiple myeloma. Bone Marrow Transplant 2002; 30: 367–73.
54. Garban F, Attal M, Rossi JF et al. Immunotherapy by non-myeloablative allogeneic stem cell transplantation in multiple myeloma: results of a pilot study as salvage therapy after autologous transplantation. Leukemia 2001; 15: 642–6.
55. Branson K, Chopra R, Kottaridis PD et al. Role of nonmyeloablative allogeneic stem-cell transplantation after failure of autologous transplantation in patients with lymphoproliferative malignancies. J Clin Oncol 2002; 20: 4022–31.

56 Perez-Simon JA, Kottaridis PD, Martino R *et al.* Nonmyeloablative transplantation with or without alemtuzumab: comparison between two prospective studies in patients with lymphoproliferative disorders. *Blood* 2002; **100**: 3121–7.

57 Badros A, Barlogie B, Morris C *et al.* High response rate in refractory and poor-risk multiple myeloma after allotransplantation using a nonmyeloablative conditioning regimen and donor lymphocyte infusions. *Blood* 2001; **97**: 2574–9.

58 Badros A, Barlogie B, Siegel E *et al.* Improved outcome of allogeneic transplantation in high-risk multiple myeloma patients after nonmyeloablative conditioning. *J Clin Oncol* 2002; **20**: 1295–303.

59 Kröger N, Sayer HG, Schwerdtfeger R *et al.* Unrelated stem cell transplantation in multiple myeloma after a reduced-intensity conditioning with pretransplantation antithymocyte globulin is highly effective with low transplantation-related mortality. *Blood* 2002; **100**: 3919–24.

60 Kröger N, Schwerdtfeger R, Kiehl M *et al.* Autologous stem cell transplantation followed by a dose-reduced allograft induces high complete remission rate in multiple myeloma. *Blood* 2002; **100**: 755–60.

81

Issa Khouri & Richard Champlin

Allogeneic Transplantation for Lymphoma and Chronic Lymphocytic Leukemia

Allogeneic blood and marrow transplants have been extensively evaluated for the treatment of acute leukemias and chronic myelogenous leukemia. Over the last few years, more data became available regarding their use for chronic lymphocytic leukemia (CLL) and lymphomas, indicating efficacy in patients with advanced disease. These data indicate existence of a potent graft-vs.-malignancy effect against many lymphoid malignancies. The precise indications and role of allogeneic transplants in these disorders are not well-defined. Allotransplantation is an effective, potentially curative approach for these disorders. Treatment with high-dose myeloablative chemoradiotherapy has, however, been associated with a substantial risk of treatment-related mortality. Preliminary data involving less toxic, nonmyeloablative preparative regimens have demonstrated a significant reduction of mortality, while retaining efficacy in producing durable complete remissions. Further studies are clearly warranted.

Lymphoid malignancies encompass a broad range of neoplasms from indolent to highly aggressive natural histories. A number of classification systems have been proposed to separate these disorders into clinically meaningful prognostic groups [1]. The World Health Organization (WHO) identifies two major categories of lymphomas: B cell and T cell/NK cell. Each major category has indolent (including small lymphocytic/CLL and follicular), aggressive, leukemic-like and viral-induced subtypes of lymphoma. Considerations of the role and timing of transplantation-based therapies requires analysis of treatment alternatives throughout the natural history of each disorder. There has been considerable progress in defining the immunophenotypic, cytogenetic and molecular abnormalities associated with each lymphoid malignancy. These disorders are associated with a characteristic rearrangement of immunoglobulin and/or T-cell receptor genes [2–4]. Characteristic cytogenetic and molecular abnormalities also occur [5–8]. These clonal genetic abnormalities provide molecular markers that can be assessed by sensitive techniques for detection of minimal residual disease and early relapse following therapy.

Considerations for allogeneic bone marrow transplantation: graft-vs.-malignancy effects

Lymphomas and CLL have characteristics that make them attractive targets for high-dose chemoradiotherapy and allogeneic hematopoietic transplantation. Lymphomas and CLL are sensitive to alkylating agents and radiation, the cornerstones of high-dose preparative regimens, and exhibit a steep dose–response effect. Investigational approaches to improve cytoreduction of high-dose therapy are under study for lymphoid malignancies, including evaluation of new anticancer drugs, and the incorporation of monoclonal anti-B-cell antibodies into the treatment regimen. Anti-B-cell monoclonals have been studied either as native antibodies [9,10] or targeted radiotherapy to the malignant cells, partially sparing normal tissues [11,12].

Allogeneic bone marrow transplantation (BMT) was originally proposed as a means to escalate the doses of myelotoxic chemotherapy and radiation with BMT to restore hematopoiesis [13]. Considerable evidence indicates that the high-dose preparative regimen does not completely eradicate the malignancy in most patients and an immune-mediated graft-vs.-leukemia/lymphoma (GVL) effect is important to prevent relapse [14–21]. Allogeneic transplants are associated with a lower risk of relapse than syngeneic or purged autologous transplants [21–23]. Some patients with lymphoma who have relapsed post-allogeneic transplantation have achieved remissions after withdrawal of immunosuppressive therapy without additional therapy; van Besien reported two complete remissions and two partial remissions in nine relapsed patients treated with immunosuppression withdrawal [24]. The most direct demonstration of the GVL effect is the reinduction of complete remission by infusion of donor lymphocytes in patients who had relapsed after allogeneic marrow transplantation [14,25]. After donor lymphocyte infusion, responses generally take several months to occur and presumably require engraftment and expansion of the relevant effector cells [26].

The target antigens of graft-vs.-malignancy likely overlap with those involved with graft-vs.-host disease (GVHD). Recipient derived lymphoid cells are targets of GVHD; and graft-vs.-malignancy may involve reactivity against lymphohematopoietic restricted antigens shared by normal lymphoid tissues and lymphoid malignancies [15,27].

Indolent lymphoid malignancies such as CLL, mantle cell lymphoma and follicular lymphomas appear highly sensitive to graft-vs.-malignancy effects. Allogeneic transplants for CLL and low-grade lymphoma are associated with a substantially lower rate of relapse than autologous transplants using purged bone marrow [14,21]. Allotransplants have been effective to produce durable remission in patients with refractory bone marrow involvement who have no other effective treatment options [28,29]. Conversion from polymerase chain reaction (PCR) positivity to PCR-negativity was observed to occur spontaneously several months after an allogeneic transplant, whereas most patients with PCR positivity post-autologous transplant relapse [30]. In patients relapsing post-allotransplantation, reinduction of complete remission may occur with reduction of immunosuppressive therapy [31], development of GVHD [32] or following donor lymphocyte infusion [16,33].

Published studies of allogeneic bone marrow transplantation for lymphoma and CLL

Most studies have been small institutional trials, which generally included a variety of lymphoid malignancies. Most studies involved a younger patient population. Most patients had advanced disease at the time of BMT [18,28,34,35], but some studies included patients with high-grade lymphoma in first remission [36]. Total body irradiation (TBI) containing regimens were most commonly used for conditioning [37–40], but some studies involved busulfan/cyclophosphamide combinations [41,42] or BCNU-based regimens, particularly in patients with contraindications to radiation [43]. No single preparative regimen has been demonstrated to be superior. Treatment-related mortality after myeloablative preparative regimens is <20% in patients undergoing allogeneic transplants in first remission, but 30–45% for patients with more advanced disease. The European Bone Marrow Transplant Registry (EBMT) reported a case–control study of patients undergoing allogeneic vs. autologous BMT [22]. The majority of patients had high-grade lymphomas. A lower relapse rate was seen with allogeneic transplants, but this was offset by a higher rate of treatment-related mortality. A prospective study by Ratanatharathorn et al. [44] compared allogeneic with autologous BMT and reported a significantly decreased recurrence rate and a trend toward improved disease-free survival with allogeneic transplantation. Similar results were reported by Jones et al. [45]. Other studies have confirmed the relatively low relapse rate with allogeneic transplants, but found the benefit offset by higher rates of treatment-related mortality [46–48].

Results of myeloablative allogeneic transplants have varied markedly among the histologic subtypes of lymphoma. Sixty-four patients with advanced non-Hodgkin's lymphoma (NHL) were treated at the M.D. Anderson Cancer Center, accrued between 1981 and 1994 [37]. A major difference in disease-free and overall survival according to histologic subtype was detected. Allogeneic BMT was most effective in low-grade lymphoma; actuarial survival was 65% ± 13%. Two patients with recurrent disease responded to cyclosporine withdrawal. In contrast, patients with intermediate- or high-grade lymphomas had relatively poor results, with high rates of treatment-related mortality as well as relapse. Only one of 14 patients with intermediate-grade lymphoma survived for an actuarial survival 21%. Four of 25 patients with lymphoblastic lymphoma were alive (actuarial survival 21%). One of 10 patients with diffuse small non-cleaved cell (DSNCC) lymphoma is a long-term disease-free survivor (actuarial survival 10%).

The EBMT group performed a retrospective analysis of 764 allogeneic transplants as treatment for lymphoma [46]. Lymphoma subtype was low grade in 113 patients, 272 intermediate–high grade, 222 lymphoblastic, 53 Burkitt's and 104 Hodgkin's disease. Human leukocyte antigen (HLA) identical siblings donors were used in 86% of cases. The actuarial rate of treatment-related mortality at 2 years varied by histology: Burkitt's lymphoma 19%; intermediate–high grade 30%; lymphoblastic 31%; low grade 38%; and Hodgkin's disease 40%. The overall survival and progression-free survival at 4 years were low grade 42% and 50%; intermediate–high grade 43% and 50%; lymphoblastic 38% and 42%; Burkitt's 44% and 39% and Hodgkin's disease 20% and 25%, respectively. The only prognostic factor for survival identified in multivariate analysis was disease status for the intermediate- and high-grade histologies. These patients were compared with 9488 lymphoma patients receiving autologous transplants in the EBMT registry by multivariate analysis using the Cox regression model for prognostic factors influencing relapse rate and overall survival. Allogeneic transplantation produced a lower relapse rate in low-grade lymphoma ($p = 0.0005$) and high–intermediate grade lymphoma ($p = 0.0006$). Autologous transplants had a lower relapse rate than allografts for Hodgkin's disease ($p = 0.044$). Because of the higher treatment-related mortality with allogeneic transplants, autologous transplants produced superior survival for most histologies: low grade ($p < 0.001$); high–intermediate ($p = 0.0173$) ($p = 0.0085$); and Hodgkin's disease ($p = 0.0002$). No significant difference was detected for Burkitt's lymphoma.

Retrospective studies examining the role of allogeneic transplants vs. alternative treatments are largely limited by patient selection. In most centers, there has been a preference to perform autologous transplants, if feasible, for patients with recurrent or high-risk lymphomas. Allogeneic transplants are typically reserved for patients with very poor prognostic factors, including high-level bone marrow involvement or resistance to chemotherapy. Multivariate analysis cannot completely account for important differences in patient selection and prospective controlled trials are necessary to define the relative role of allogeneic BMT.

Indications for allogeneic hematopoietic transplantation

Recommendations regarding the use of BMT need to consider disease characteristics and results of therapeutic alternatives. Each disease category needs to be considered separately.

Chronic lymphocytic leukaemia

CLL is a lymphoid malignancy that typically has an indolent natural history [49–52]. CLL is a clonal disorder of B cells, characterized by the accumulation of small mature-appearing lymphocytes, although rare T-cell variants also occur. CLL is more common in males than females, and typically occurs in older individuals. The etiology of CLL is unknown and has not been related to occupational or environmental factors.

Chromosomal aberrations are detectable in over 80% of cases with CLL using interphase fluorescence in situ hybridization [53–56]. Unlike some other hematologic malignancies, B-CLL is characterized by the chromosomal loss or gain of genetic material but not by translocations. In a study by Dohner et al. [57] the most frequent was a deletion in chromosome 13q (55% of patients). This is associated with low $CD38^+$ expression and mutation of immunoglobulin genes, both of which are markers of good prognosis [58].

Patients with CLL frequently develop autoimmune hematopoietic disorders, most commonly autoimmune hemolytic anemia and immune thrombocytopenic purpura [59]. Much less frequently, patients may develop pure red blood cell aplasia or neutropenia secondary to the development of autoantibodies against marrow hematopoietic progenitor cells. Non-hematopoietic autoimmune diseases are uncommon. Patients with CLL have an acquired immunodeficiency and are at increased risk for infection. Most develop hypogammaglobulinemia during the advanced stages of their disease [60,61]. Cellular immune defects also occur. Some of these features may be becauese of production of transforming growth factor beta (TGF-β) an inhibitor of T- and B-cell proliferation [62].

The diagnosis of CLL is based upon peripheral blood lymphocytosis with an absolute lymphocyte count of >5000/mm^3, with morphologically mature-appearing cells [49], with cells expressing CD5 and at least one B-cell marker ($CD19^+$, $CD20^+$, $CD23^+$) and negative for other pan-T-cell markers. The malignant cells are clonal, expressing low density, surface immunoglobulin with either a kappa or lambda light chain. The bone marrow aspirate is generally normo- or hypercellular with >30% lymphocytes. Diffuse lymphoid infiltration in the marrow biopsy is associated with a poorer prognosis than an interstitial pattern.

CLL must be distinguished from prolymphocytic leukemia in which the differential is >55% prolymphocytes and/or >15,000/mm^3 absolute count of prolymphocytes in the blood. Mantle-cell lymphoma with leukemic manifestations can appear similar to CLL; the malignant cells are also $CD5^+$ B cells, but the immunophenotype is $CD23^-$ and lymph node histology is characteristic [63]. Other disorders in the differential diagnosis include hairy cell leukemia, large granular lymphocytosis, leukemic phase of follicular center-cell lymphoma. Sezary syndrome and adult T-cell leukemia/lymphoma can be distinguished by morphology and their immunophenotype.

The Rai and the Binet systems separate CLL patients into prognostic groups [50,51]. The National Cancer Institute-sponsored Working Group (NCI-WG) recommends usage of the "three-risk group" modification of the original five-stage Rai staging system [49]:
Low-risk group (stage 0) with only lymphocytosis (blood and marrow);
Intermediate-risk group with lymphocytosis and enlarged nodes (stage I) and/or enlarged spleen/liver (stage II);
High-risk group. Lymphocytosis with anemia, defined as hemoglobin <11 gm/dl (stage III) and/or platelets <100,000/mm^3 (stage IV).

The median survival of the low-risk group is >10 years, 8 years for the intermediate-risk group and 4 years for the high-risk group. The NCI-WG recommends chemotherapy treatment if the disease causes impaired performance or produces disease-related symptoms. These include systemic symptoms such as fatigue, fever, weight loss, sweats, anemia or thrombocytopenia, autoimmune cytopenia (not responding to corticosteroids), massively enlarged nodes or spleen, rapid increase in blood lymphocyte count or repeated infections with or without hypogammaglobulinemia.

Chemotherapy has been palliative and is generally used for control of disease symptoms. Chlorambucil has been the standard of care for the last 4 decades and is useful to control leukocytosis and lymphadenapathy. Fludarabine has recently been demonstrated to be a highly active agent [64–66], producing complete and partial remissions in the majority of previously untreated patients. However, these remissions are transient and overall survival has not been substantially improved. There are no long-term disease-free survivors. Radiation therapy is effective for local management of symptomatic lymphoid masses. Splenectomy is warranted for hypersplenism and/or immune-mediated cytopenias.

Over the last decade, major advancements in our understanding of CLL and its variants have occurred. It has become apparent that there is diversity in types of CLL including those patients that do or do not have hypermutation of immunoglobulin genes [67]. Unmutated genes confer an unfavorable prognosis. The prognosis is poorer once disease progression occurs after initial chemotherapy. For previously treated CLL patients under the age of 60 years (and hence potentially eligible for transplantation-based therapies), fludarabine treatment resulted in complete remission or nodular complete remission in 41% of patients and partial remission in 21% [68]. The median time to progression for the complete responders was 117 weeks, 92 weeks for the nodular complete remissions and 88 weeks for the partial remissions. The overall survival of the complete remission patients, nodular complete and partial remission patients was 44, 36 and 30 months, respectively. This provides justification for evaluation of innovative strategies for these patients, including autologous and allogeneic BMT to intensify complete remissions in patients with previously treated CLL.

High-dose chemotherapy with purged autologous bone marrow or blood stem cell transplantation has been studied as cytoreductive treatment for CLL [23,30,69–71]. These trials have used the preparative regimen of cyclophosphamide 120 mg/kg and TBI (10–12 Gy). Use of autologous transplantation is limited by involvement of the blood and bone marrow as a part of the natural history of these diseases as well as the inability of even high-dose chemoradiotherapy to eradicate systemic disease. Reports have had disparate results. Khouri et al. [23] and Pavletic et al. [71] reported transient remissions in heavily pretreated patients. Rabinowe et al. [69] and Provan et al. [70] at the Dana Farber Cancer Center reported more encouraging results, focusing on patients early in the course of their disease. Although extended complete remissions were achieved in approximately 80% of patients, it is not clear that cure is possible and whether long-term survival will be improved. There is concern regarding the risk of myelodysplasia or other secondary malignancies in these patients with a relatively long natural history [72,73].

Because of the advanced age of patients, allogeneic hematopoietic transplantation was not widely explored. Selected patients with CLL have been treated with allogeneic BMT [29,30,69,74–76], with approximately 20–55% achieving extended disease-free survival. This approach is capable of producing long-term disease-free survival in patients with advanced disease. In a series of 28 patients with advanced disease and heavily pretreated patients at M.D. Anderson Cancer Center, the progression-free survival rates at 5 years were 78% for the chemosensitive and 26% for those who were refractory to conventional chemotherapy at the time of transplantation ($p = 0.03$) [77]. The EBMT and the International Bone Marrow Transplant Registry (IBMTR) reported that patients with lower stage chemotherapy-responsive disease had improved survival [74]. In a study at the University of Texas, M.D. Anderson Cancer Center, in 15 advanced CLL patients having progressive disease despite a median of three prior chemotherapy regimens, allotransplantation has superior 3-year disease-free survival rates compared with purged autologous transplants (57% vs. 24%) [77]. Overall, 3-year survival is 57% vs. 33%. This additional benefit of allogeneic transplant is likely related to the GVL effect, and donor lymphocyte infusion has been successful in reinducing remission in a patient relapsing post-transplant [78]. Further studies are necessary to assess the feasibility and treatment-related morbidity of this approach in this older, often debilitated, patient group.

It is uncertain when in the prolonged course of CLL should allogeneic transplantation be considered. The potential efficacy of allogeneic transplantation must be balanced against its risks and the natural history using alternative therapies. First-line treatment using alkylating agents and fludarabine-based chemotherapy is generally effective in controlling disease symptoms for a number of years. Although autologous transplants appear most effective early in the course of CLL, this has not been convincingly demonstrated with allogeneic transplants, which may be successful even with advanced leukemia. Results of allogeneic transplants appear to be superior in patients sensitive to chemotherapy compared to those with refractory disease or with Richter's transformation. It is our policy to recommend allogeneic BMT to patients after initial failure or relapse after fludarabine-based therapy.

Low-grade lymphoma

The low-grade lymphomas (small lymphocytic lymphoma, follicular small cleaved cell lymphoma and follicular mixed cell lymphoma) are indolent diseases, but incurable with standard forms of chemotherapy. Follicular small cleaved cell lymphoma and follicular mixed cell lymphoma are the most common categories included among low-grade lymphomas; these diseases are associated with the t(14;18) resulting in rearrangement of the *bcl*-2 gene [5]. *Bcl*-2 is overexpressed and acts to prevent apoptosis, resulting in expansion of the malignant clone.

Low-grade lymphomas have a prolonged natural history with median survival of 7–9 years [79]. A number of patient and disease characteristics contribute to prognosis [80–82]. The major factors include stage, lactate dehydrogenase (LDH) and beta-2-microglobulin level. Patients may remain stable for years and a policy of delaying chemotherapy until disease progression has produced similar long-term survival as initiating chemotherapy at diagnosis [83]. Chemotherapy using intensive combination chemotherapy regimens, such as cyclophosphamide, doxorubicin, vincristine and prednisone (CHOP), results in complete and partial response rates of 50–70% but no consistent improvement in survival over use of a single alkylating agent or other conservative approaches. More recently, higher responses have been obtained by combining CHOP or fludarabine with rituximab [84]. Following progression after initial chemotherapy, the prognosis worsens [80,85]. Active chemotherapy regimens include ESHAP (etoposide, cytarabine, cisplatin and corticosteroids), MINE (methotrexate, ifosfamide, mitoxantrone and etoposide) [86] and FND (fludarabine, mitoxantrone and dexamethasone) [87], and radioimmunotherapy with yttrium-90 ibritumomab tiuxetan [11].

High-dose chemotherapy with autologous bone marrow or blood stem cell transplantation has been widely employed as cytoreductive treatment for low-grade lymphoma, producing rates of complete remission >80%. Patients receiving marrow or blood stem cell autografts effectively depleted of malignant cells using anti-B-cell monoclonal antibodies may achieve prolonged remissions [70,88,89]. However, there is controversy whether purging improves clinical outcome [90] and whether autologous transplantation provides an advantage in long-term survival compared to conservative forms of standard-dose chemotherapy [91]. Use of autologous transplantation is limited by involvement of the blood and bone marrow as a part of the natural history of these diseases as well as the inability of even high-dose chemoradiotherapy to eradicate systemic disease in most patients. In addition, there has been a high rate of secondary myelodysplasia in long-term survivors after autotransplants in this disease [72,92,93].

Allogeneic BMT has generally been reserved for far advanced patients with low-grade lymphoma. Van Besien *et al*. [94,95] reported encouraging results with extended disease-free survival in 12 of 15 heavily pretreated patients. Other groups have also reported a high fraction of long-term remissions [35,44,45,76,96,97]. Relapse rates after allogeneic transplants have been substantially lower than with transplantation of purged autologous transplants, most likely as a result of the graft-vs.-lymphoma effect [21,98].

Figure 81.1 summarizes results of a prospective study at the M.D. Anderson Cancer Center in which patients with resistant or relapsed low-grade lymphoma were treated with high-dose etoposide (1500 mg/m^2), cyclophosphamide (120 mg/kg) and TBI (10.6–12 Gy) with allogeneic marrow transplantation if a matched sibling was available or otherwise with an autologous transplant. For the autologous transplant group the bone marrow was depleted of malignant cells by treatment with anti-CD19 monoclonal antibody and immunomagnetic separation. Forty-four patients received allogeneic BMT and 68 an autologous transplant. The allogeneic transplant group has a higher risk of treatment-related mortality of 34% vs. 6%, but a lower risk of relapse and improved disease-free survival. In the allogeneic group the median follow-up time was 53 months, and the overall survival and disease-free survival were 49% and 45%, respectively. After treatment and a median follow-up time of 71 months in the autologous group, the overall survival and disease-free survival rates were 34% and 17%, respectively. The probability of disease progression was significantly higher in the autologous group than in the allogeneic group (74% vs. 19%, $p = 0.003$). Late relapses were uncommon after allotransplantation.

Verdonck *et al*. [99] published a similar study in 28 patients comparing results with allogeneic vs. autologous transplants in patients with advanced low-grade lymphoma. The patients had received 2–5 prior conventional chemotherapy regimens. Eighteen patients, all with chemosensitive disease, received autologous BMT and 15 patients underwent allogeneic transplantation. A common conditioning regimen, cyclophosphamide plus TBI was used for all patients. With a median follow-up time of 25 months in the allogeneic group, the 3-year probabilities of overall survival and event-free survival were both 70%, and the relapse rate was 0%. In the autologous group, the 3-year probability of overall survival and event-free survival were 33% and 22%, respectively. The relapse rate in the autologous group was 78%.

The IBMTR recently analyzed results of allogeneic BMT from HLA identical sibling donors in 113 patients transplanted by 50 teams [28]. Median age was 38 years (range 15–61 years). The median interval from diagnosis to transplant was 24 months and the median number of prior chemotherapy regimens was two. At transplantation, 18% of the patients had small lymphocytic lymphoma, 46% had follicular small cleaved cell

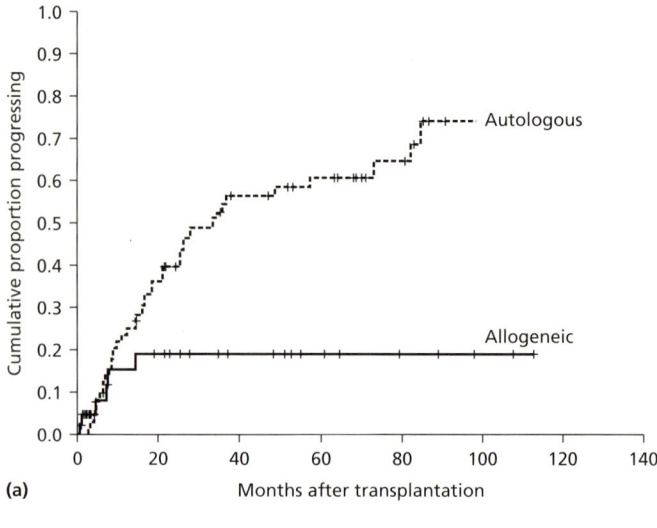

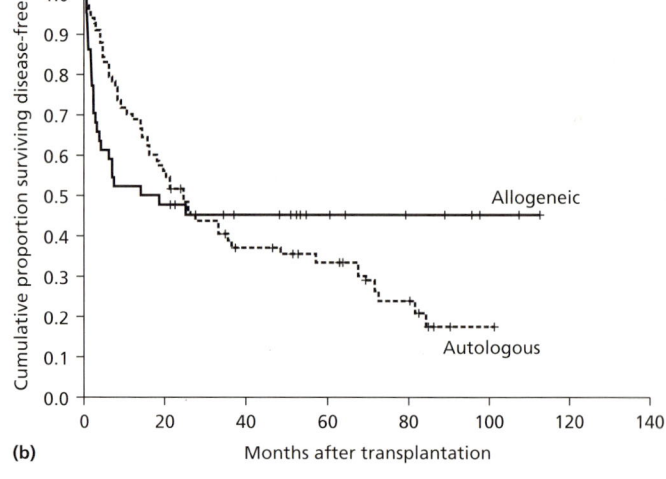

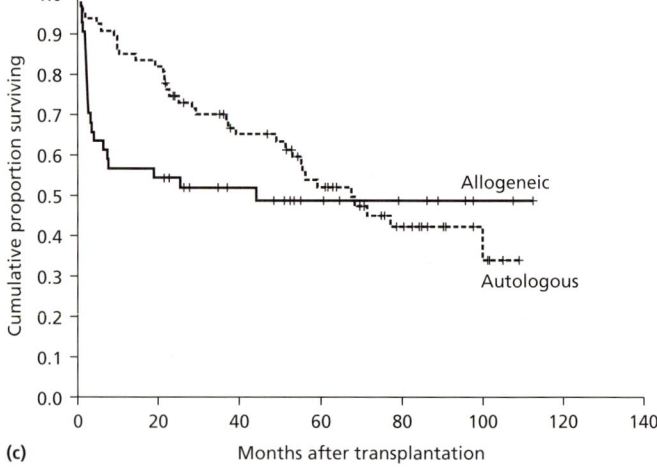

Fig. 81.1 (a) Actuarial progression. (b) Progressive-free survival. (c) Overall survival for allogeneic and autologous transplants for patients with relapsed low-grade lymphoma.

lymphoma and 36% had follicular mixed cell lymphoma. At diagnosis, 81% of the patients had stage IV disease, most commonly resulting from the presence of bone marrow involvement. At transplant, 14% of the patients were in complete remission and 71% continued to have stage IV disease. Sixty-three percent of patients had chemosensitive disease and

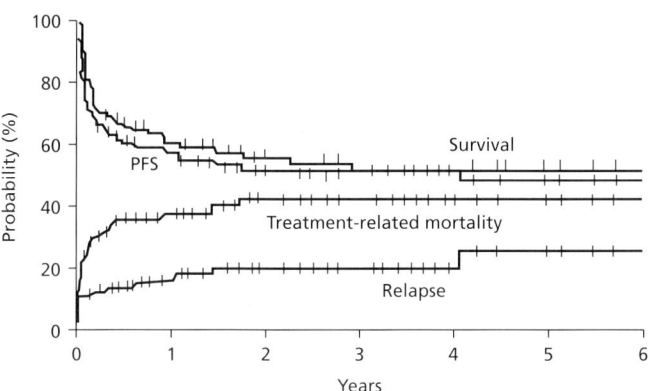

Fig. 81.2 International Bone Marrow Transplant Registry (IBMTR) data for allogeneic bone marrow transplantation for low-grade lymphoma [28].

37% were considered chemoresistant. Twenty-nine percent of the patients had a performance status ≤80%. The conditioning regimen contained TBI in 82% of the patients. T-cell-depleted transplants were undertaken in 22% of patients. Cyclosporine alone or in combination with other agents was used as GVHD prophylaxis in almost all other cases. Median follow-up for surviving patients was 22 months after transplantation. Three-year probability of disease-free survival was 49% (95%CI, 39–59) and the probability of disease recurrence was 16% (95%CI, 9–27) (Fig. 81.2). The probability of treatment-related mortality was 28% (95%CI, 19–39). A decreased Karnofsky score, presence of chemotherapy-resistant disease and the use of a non-TBI regimen were independent predictors for shorter survival.

Attal et al. [47] performed a retrospective case–control analysis of 216 patients reported to the French Bone Marrow Transplant Group Registry from 1986 to 1996. Seventy-two allogeneic transplants were matched with 144 autologous grafts on the basis of age, disease status and conditioning regimen. Patient characteristics were comparable for sex, age (median 40 years), stage, interval from diagnosis to transplant (33 months) and number of prior chemotherapy regimens (2). At transplantation, 53% of patients were refractory to chemotherapy. The conditioning regimen was TBI-based in 75% of patients. Median follow-up was 34 months. A comparable initial complete response rate occurred after allogeneic or autologous transplantation: 86% and 78%, respectively. Allogeneic transplants had a significantly lower relapse rate of 12% at 60 months with a plateau after 15 months, in contrast to 55% with autologous transplantation without an apparent plateau ($p < 0.001$). Transplant-related mortality was 30% after allogeneic BMT vs. 4% with autotransplantation ($p < 0.001$). However, event-free survival at 4 years was not significantly improved (53% for allogeneic BMT and 45% for autologous transplantation), because the improved control of the malignancy was offset by the higher rate of treatment-related mortality.

Collectively, these studies indicate that high-dose chemoradiotherapy and allogeneic BMT is potentially curative for patients with advanced low-grade lymphoma. Unlike the case with autologous transplants, there have been very few relapses after 2 years from transplantation, presumably because of a graft-vs.-lymphoma effect or the lack of malignant cells in an allograft.

At what point in the course of low-grade lymphomas should allogeneic transplantation be considered? The potential efficacy of allogeneic transplantation must be balanced against its risks and the long natural history using conservative therapy. As a general rule, allogeneic transplants are most successful when performed early in the course of a disease, before development of resistance and while a patient is in good general medical condition, and best able to tolerate the procedure. These disorders may undergo transformation to a more aggressive histology, associated with a poorer prognosis to any therapy. On the other hand, these disorders can generally be controlled for a number of years by relatively nontoxic treatment and transplants have been successful in many patients with far advanced disease. Patients responding to initial therapy have a median remission duration of 3–5 years and generally do well until relapse [81,82,85]. After recurrence, median progression-free survival is <18 months with salvage therapy. Given these considerations, there is presently no clear consensus regarding when transplantation should be considered in the course of low-grade lymphomas, so this decision needs to be individualized for each patient.

The current data are inconsistent regarding the relative role of allogeneic vs. autologous BMT. All studies report a lower relapse rate with allotransplantation, presumably because of graft-vs.-lymphoma effects. The EBMT data suggested that this benefit was offset by a higher rate of treatment-related mortality. The M.D. Anderson study and IBMTR study had somewhat better survival favoring allogeneic transplantation.

At the M.D. Anderson Cancer Center, we generally recommend hematopoietic transplantation for patients after failure of initial chemotherapy or relapse. Patients with low-grade lymphoma in a second remission or with a low tumor bulk and a marrow collection free of malignant cells by PCR analysis have had relatively good results with autologous transplantation. We prefer allotransplantation for other categories of patients if an HLA-identical sibling donor is available. There is little experience with transplants from matched unrelated donors for lymphoid malignancies. Given the durability of complete remissions achieved, it is generally our policy to recommend allogeneic transplants for patients with matched sibling donors rather than autologous transplantation.

Intermediate- and high-grade lymphomas

Intermediate- and high-grade lymphomas are aggressive malignancies with a short natural history in the absence of effective therapy. These disorders are responsive to combination chemotherapy and a fraction of patients achieve durable remissions. Chemotherapy for large cell lymphoma with the CHOP combination was developed in the 1970s resulting in a cure in approximately 40% of patients with intermediate-grade lymphoma [100]. Addition of other active agents to the core of alkylating agents and anthracyclines led to the design of second- and third-generation regimens with more promising results in phase 2 studies. Recent multicenter randomized studies failed to demonstrate superiority of any of these regimens compared to CHOP [101,102]. More recently, the addition of rituximab to CHOP chemotherapy resulted in significant improvement of both overall and disease-free survival in elderly patients [9].

High-dose chemotherapy and autologous transplantation have long been felt to result in improved cure rates for patients with recurrent large cell lymphoma who respond to salvage chemotherapy [103,104]. Despite these successes, relapse is common and autologous transplantation will only lead to long-term disease-free survival in <50% of patients. Whether high-dose chemotherapy also contributes to improved survival when used in the initial treatment of patients with aggressive NHL remains uncertain. A number of staging systems have been proposed to identify prognostic groups for patients with intermediate-grade lymphoma [105–109]. The international index has been the most widely accepted system [110]. A revised European–American (REAL) classification has been proposed which incorporates immunophenotype as well as morphologic criteria [111]. Autologous BMT has been studied in several prospective randomized studies; none have shown benefit in patients with low-risk disease, but two of which indicate a potential benefit to high-dose chemotherapy in specific high-risk subgroups of patients [112–114].

High-dose chemotherapy with autologous bone marrow or blood stem cell transplantation has been effective for patients with recurrent intermediate-grade lymphoma. A randomized trial comparing cisplatin, cytarabine and decadron (DHAP) chemotherapy vs. DHAP followed by high-dose BCNU, etoposide, cytarabine and cyclophosphamide (BEAC) chemotherapy with autologous marrow transplantation resulted in a significant improvement in 5-year disease-free survival of 46% vs. 12% as well as improved overall survival (53 vs. 32%). Results with autologous transplants are better for patients in first relapse, with low lactate dehydrogenase levels and low bulk chemotherapy-responsive disease [115,116]. Patients with chemoresistant disease and those with multiple relapses have considerably poorer results, with <20% durable remissions.

High-dose therapy with allogeneic transplantation has been examined in a number of phase 1 and 2 studies in patients with intermediate- or high-grade lymphoma [40,43,44,96–98,117–120,120]. Most were in young patients with advanced disease. A number of studies examined allografts for Burkitt's lymphoma or lymphoblastic lymphoma in first remission [121,122]. Results are difficult to interpret without concurrent controls given the impact of eligibility criteria and patient selection on outcome. Chopra et al. [22] reported a case–control study comparing allogeneic vs. autologous transplants in 100 patients, primarily with intermediate- and high-grade lymphomas. Although relapse rates were lower with allogeneic transplants, treatment-related mortality was higher and there was no significant advantage with allogeneic transplants. A subsequent retrospective study by the EBMT compared allogeneic and autologous transplants. They also reported a lower risk of relapse by allotransplantation, but generally inferior event-free survival and overall survival because of excessive treatment-related mortality.

A major problem with allogeneic transplantation for recurrent intermediate- and high-grade lymphomas is the high rate of treatment-related mortality in these heavily pretreated patients. The use of peripheral blood stem cell transplantation has been studied as an alternative approach for allogeneic transplantation. Studies indicate accelerated hematopoietic recovery and potentially reduced early treatment-related morbidity [123,124]. Studies at M.D. Anderson Cancer Center demonstrated encouraging results in 30 patients with recurrent or resistant large cell lymphoma; 43% of patients had refractory disease and 42% survive disease-free beyond 2 years [43]. Further study of allogeneic blood progenitor transplants is warranted.

The role of allogeneic transplantation for aggressive lymphomas is controversial. Unlike the case for low-grade lymphomas, high-dose chemotherapy with autologous transplantation is effective and potentially curative in patients with partial responses to induction chemotherapy, chemosensitive first relapse [103,115,125]. Patients with recurrent large cell lymphoma with elevated LDH levels, multiple relapses and chemotherapy-insensitive disease have a relatively poor prognosis with autologous transplants [116]. A fraction of these far advanced patients achieve prolonged remission with allogeneic transplantation. The additional graft-vs.-lymphoma effect suggests a role in these high-risk categories and further evaluation of allogeneic transplantation is warranted.

Mantle cell lymphoma is a newly recognized entity that composes approximately 2–11% of newly diagnosed NHL [126]. The entity appears to combine the aggressive behavior of intermediate- and high-grade lymphomas with the lack of curability associated with low-grade lymphoma. Median survival is approximately 3–4 years. A series of 16 allogeneic transplants for mantle cell lymphoma were reported from our institution [18]. Fourteen received high-dose chemotherapy and two patients received nonmyeloablative preparative regimens. Overall and progression-free survival were both 55% at 3 years. Survival was significantly better for patients with chemosensitive disease.

There is a paucity of data with respect to the use of allogeneic transplantation in T-cell lymphomas. Anecdotal cases have been described of cutaneous T-cell lymphoma responding to GVHD [127]. In a retrospective study at the M.D. Anderson Cancer Center, seven patients with relapsed peripheral T-cell lymphoma were treated with high-dose chemotherapy and allogeneic transplantation [119]. The 3-year probability of survival was 29% (95%CI, 9–92%).

There is considerable controversy regarding the relative role of allogeneic vs. autologous transplants in each category of lymphoid malignancy. The lower risk or treatment-related morbidity and mortality with autologous transplants needs to be balanced against the risk of marrow and blood involvement by malignancy and a lack of a graft-vs.-malignancy effect; treatment recommendations depend on disease and patient characteristics.

Induction of GVL using nonmyeloablative preparative regimen and donor lymphocyte infusion

Allogeneic blood and marrow transplantation is associated with a substantial risk of treatment-related morbidity, primarily because of the toxicity of high-dose therapies, acute and chronic GVHD and associated infections. Advances in supportive care have allowed transplants to be performed for older recipients; many centers now perform myeloablative therapy with autologous transplants for patients up to age 75 years and with allogeneic transplants for recipients up to age 65 years [19,128,129], but treatment-related mortality exceeds 40% in these heavily pretreated patients.

The benefits of high-dose myeloablative therapy with allogeneic hematopoietic transplantation for CLL and lymphomas are largely offset by the high rate of treatment-related mortality, exceeding 40% in many studies. Risks increase with comorbidities, advanced age, histocompatibility and disease-related prognostic factors. CLL and lymphomas are generally diseases of older, often debilitated, patients and only a minority have been considered eligible for high-dose myeloablative transplantation therapies.

Given the potential efficacy of graft-vs.-malignancy effects against many lymphoid malignancies, we evaluated an alternative strategy of utilizing less toxic, nonmyeloablative preparative regimens with allogeneic hematopoietic transplantation. The goal of the preparative regimen is to achieve sufficient immunosuppression to prevent graft rejection. The nonmyeloablative preparative regimen produces little or no cytoreduction of the malignancy; this approach is designed to exploit the graft-vs.-malignancy effects of allogeneic transplantation as the primary therapy.

As a working definition, a truly nonmyeloablative regimen should allow relatively prompt autologous hematopoietic recovery (within 28 days) without a transplant and, upon engraftment, mixed chimerism should occur. These regimens do not eradicate recipient immunity and depend on the activity of donor T cells to achieve engraftment. Success of the nonmyeloablative procedure also requires development of an effective graft-vs.-malignancy effect before the underlying disease can progress. Therefore, the pretransplant regimen or prior induction therapy must cytoreduce the lymphoma sufficiently to prevent any marked early progression.

At the M.D. Anderson Cancer Center we studied nonmyeloablative hematopoietic transplantation in patients with CLL and lymphoma. In an initial study, CLL patients received 30 mg/m^2/day fludarabine and 300 mg/m^2/day cyclophosphamide for 3 days, a regimen that is nonmyeloablative and well-tolerated without transplantation [130]. For patients with aggressive lymphoid histologies, the combination of cisplatin, fludarabine and cytosine arabinoside (Ara-C) was used; this regimen produces reversible myelosuppression and has established activity against transformed lymphomas as a salvage chemotherapy regimen without transplantation. In vitro, fludarabine enhances the cytotoxicity of both Ara-C and cisplatin, increasing Ara-C incorporation into DNA and inhibiting repair of cisplatin/DNA-adducts. This regimen is sufficiently immunosuppressive to allow engraftment of HLA compatible allografts

[131]. These regimens were followed by allogeneic transplantation from an HLA compatible donor. Six of nine patients with advanced CLL, which had relapsed or was resistant to fludarabine-based therapy, had engraftment with complete chimerism and four achieved complete remission. One additional patient with bulky residual lymphadenopathy achieved a complete remission after a donor lymphocyte infusion. These preliminary data demonstrate achievement of engraftment following "standard dose" nonablative conditioning and marked antitumor responses related to GVL, suggesting the potential efficacy of this approach in older and medically infirm patients with CLL or transformed lymphomas.

In a separate trial, patients with indolent lymphoma received 25 mg/m^2/day fludarabine administered intravenously (IV) on days –6 to –2 before transplantation and 1000 mg/m^2/day cyclophosphamide, given IV on days –3 and –2 before transplantation [19]. Rituximab was also added to improve short-term control of the malignancy with no overlapping toxicity [20]. A relatively high dose of rituximab (375–1000 mg/m^2/week for 4 weeks) was used based upon studies from our institution, which demonstrated a dose–response relationship against CLL. Transformed lymphoma patients received a combination of cisplatin, fludarabine and cytarabine (PFA). Patients received unfractionated bone marrow or peripheral blood progenitor cell transplants and post-transplant treatment with cyclosporine or tacrolimus with short course methotrexate for GVHD prevention. Patients generally continued immunosuppression for 100 days, but immunosuppression was withdrawn earlier if disease progression occurred.

Forty-nine patients with HLA-identical donors were included. Forty-five received related donors and four were from HLA-A, -B, -DR matched unrelated donors. The patients ranged in age from 21 to 68 years (median 55 years). Twenty patients had follicular lymphoma, 15 had transformed or *de novo* diffuse large cell lymphoma and 14 patients had mantle cell lymphoma. All patients were previously treated and had advanced recurrent disease. The number of prior chemotherapy regimens received by each patient ranged from 1 to 4 (median 4). Eight patients had failed a prior autologous transplant. At the time of transplantation, 35 (71%) had chemosensitive and 14 (29%) had chemorefractory disease.

All patients had prompt hematopoietic recovery. The median percentage of donor cells at 1 month after transplantation was 80% (range 0–100%). One patient had primary graft failure. Three additional patients had a secondary graft failure in the setting of disease progression (one patient) or viral infection (two patients). All patients with graft failure were in the group who received the PFA regimen and patients recovered autologous hematopoiesis promptly.

Eleven patients had early withdrawal of immunosuppression because of persistent or progressive disease after transplantation and five received donor lymphocyte infusion of 10^7–10^8 CD3+ cells/kg. Four of these patients also received rituximab with their immuno-manipulation. Rituximab was given weekly for 4 weeks, with a first dose of 375 mg/m^2 body-surface area and subsequent doses of 1000 mg/m^2 body-surface area. Six patients were reinduced into durable complete remission. The two patients who had secondary graft failure were still in complete remission at the time of this analysis, at 20+ and 24+ months after transplant. These two patients never had complete remission with any form of conventional chemotherapy prior transplantation. The median follow-up period was 19 months (range 5–52 months). Actuarial overall survival was 79% (95%CI, 61–89%) (Fig. 81.3). Current progression-free survival for the indolent, diffuse or transformed large cell and mantle cell patients were 85%, 60% and 68%, respectively [19,64].

The cumulative incidence of acute grade II–IV GVHD was 20%. Only two patients developed grade III GVHD. The cumulative incidence of extensive chronic GVHD was 36%. One patient (2%) died within 100 days. Seven other patients died secondary to relapse (four patients), chronic GVHD (two patients), multiorgan failure (one patient) and secondary malignancy (one patient). Patients who died of relapse had refractory disease at the time of transplantation.

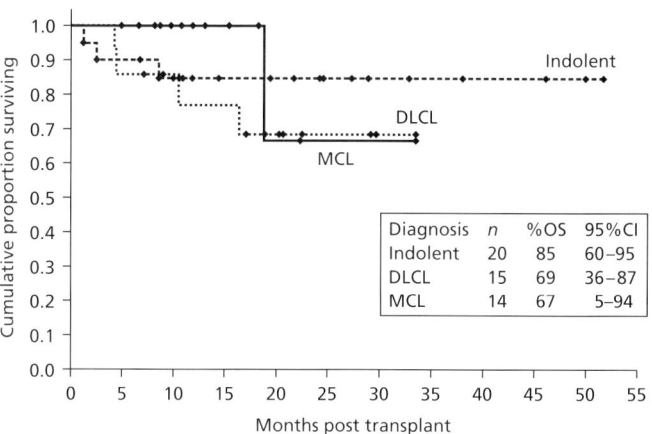

Fig. 81.3 Survival after nonmyeloablative allogeneic transplantation for chemosensitive patients with relapsed indolent (low-grade) lymphoma, mantle cell lymphoma (MCL) or diffuse large cell lymphoma (DLCL).

Similar data have been reported from other groups [132–139], although most are small studies with limited follow-up time. Many studies have utilized reduced intensity ablative regimens, such as intermediate-dose busulfan and fludarabine [135], and it is unclear whether the additional myelosuppression provides any benefits compared to the truly nonablative regimens.

These data indicate that the use of nonmyeloablative preparative regimens has reduced the risks of early treatment-related mortality and allows treatment of older patients as well as those with comorbidities who would not be considered eligible for high-dose myeloablative regimens. Durable remissions have been induced related to the graft-vs.-lymphoma effects of allogeneic hematopoietic transplantation. The reduction of treatment-related mortality makes allogeneic transplantation a more attractive option for patients with recurrent disease. Controlled trials comparing nonablative allogeneic transplants vs. autologous hematopoietic transplants or alternative forms of treatment are warranted. In our center, we offer clinical trials involving nonablative allogeneic transplantation to patients with an HLA compatible donor who have chemosensitive relapse of CLL or indolent and aggressive lymphomas.

The major barrier to this approach is the risk of acute and chronic GVHD. A number of investigational approaches have been proposed to separate graft-vs.-malignancy effects from GVHD, including generation of antigen-specific T cells reactive with the malignancy [140] or thymidine kinase transduced donor lymphocytes that can be ablated by ganciclovir in patients developing GVHD [141].

Conclusions

In conclusion, allogeneic blood stem cell and bone marrow transplantation is an effective treatment for CLL and lymphoma. The benefits related to high-dose chemotherapy and the immune GVL effect must be weighed against the risk of treatment-related morbidity and mortality. Treatment decisions must be individualized with consideration for the natural history of these disorders and the efficacy of less toxic treatment modalities. The use of nonmyeloablative regimens and other advances improving the therapeutic index of allogeneic transplantation make this an increasingly attractive option, offering a curative potential for patients with advanced lymphoid malignancies. Future directions must focus on the fundamental problems of separating graft-vs.-malignancy effects from GVHD and preventing associated infections.

References

1 International Non-Hodgkin's Lymphoma Prognostic Factors Project. A predictive model for aggressive non-Hodgkin's lymphoma. *N Engl J Med* 1993; **329**: 987–94.

2 Arnold A, Cossman J, Bakhshi A, Jaffe ES, Waldmann TA, Korsmeyer SJ. Immunoglobulin-gene rearrangements as unique clonal markers in human lymphoid malignancies. *N Engl J Med* 1983; **309**: 1593–8.

3 Tkachuk DC, Griesser H, Takihara Y et al. Rearrangement of T-cell delta locus in lymphoproliferative disorders. *Blood* 1988; **72**: 353–7.

4 Waldmann TA, Davis MM, Bongiovanni KF, Korsmeyer SJ. T cell antigen receptor gene rearrangements serve as markers of lineage and clonality in human lymphoid neoplasms. *N Engl J Med* 1985; **313**: 776–83.

5 Croce CM. Molecular biology of lymphomas. *Semin Oncol* 1993; **20** (Suppl. 5): 31–46.

6 Chaganti RSK, Nanjangud G, Schmidt H, Teruya-Feldstein J. Recurring chromosomal abnormalities in non-Hodgkin's lymphoma: biologic and clinical significance. *Semin Hematol* 2000; **37**: 396–411.

7 Cuneo A, Bigoni R, Rigolin GM et al. Cytogenetic profile of lymphoma of follicle mantle lineage: correlation with clinicobiologic features. *Blood* 1999; **93**: 1372–80.

8 Korsmeyer SJ. Chromosomal translocations in lymphoid malignancies reveal novel protooncogenes. *Annu Rev Immunol* 1992; **10**: 785–807.

9 Coiffier B, Lepage E, Briäre J et al. CHOP chemotherapy plus rituximab compared with CHOP alone in elderly patients with diffuse large B-cell lymphoma. *N Engl J Med* 2002; **346** (4): 235–42.

10 McLaughlin P, Grillo-L'pez AJ, Link BK et al. Rituximab chimeric Anti-CD20 monoclonal antibody therapy for relapsed indolent lymphoma: half of patients respond to a four-dose treatment program. *J Clin Oncol* 1998; **16**: 2825–33.

11 Witzig TE, Gordon LI, Cabanillas F et al. Randomized controlled trial of yttrium-90-labeled ibritumomab tiuxetan radioimmunotherapy vs. rituximab immunotherapy for patients with relapsed or refractory low-grade, follicular, or transformed B-cell non-Hodgkin's lymphoma. *J Clin Oncol* 2002; **20**: 2453–63.

12 Kaminski MS, Estes J, Zasadny KR et al. Radioimmunotherapy with iodine ^{131}I tositumomab for relapsed or refractory B-cell non-Hodgkin lymphoma: updated results and long-term follow-up of the University of Michigan experience. *Blood* 2000; **96**: 1259–66.

13 Thomas ED. The role of bone marrow transplantation for eradication of malignant disease. *Cancer* 1969; **10**: 1963–9.

14 Van Besien KW, De Lima M, Giralt SA et al. Management of lymphoma recurrence after allogeneic transplantation: the relevance of graft-versus-lymphoma effect. *Bone Marrow Transplant* 1997; **19**: 977–82.

15 Mutis T, Goulmy E. Hematopoietic system-specific antigens as targets for cellular immunotherapy of hematological malignancies. *Semin Hematol* 2002; **39**: 23–31.

16 Mandigers CMPW, Meijerink JPP, Raemaekers JMM, Schattenberg AVMB, Mensink EJBM. Graft-versus-lymphoma effect of donor leukocyte infusion shown by real-time quantitative PCR analysis of t(14;18). *Lancet* 1998, **352** (9139): 1522–3.

17 Kwak LW, Campbell MJ, Zelenetz AD, Levy R. Transfer of specific immunity to B-cell lymphoma with syngeneic bone marrow in mice: a strategy for using autologous marrow as an anti-tumor therapy. *Blood* 1991; **78**: 2768–72.

18 Khouri I, Lee M-S, Romaguera J et al. Allogeneic hematopoietic transplantation for mantle-cell lymphoma: molecular remissions and evidence of graft-versus-malignancy. *Ann Oncol* 1999; **10**: 1293–9.

19 Khouri I, Keating M, Korbling M et al. Transplant Lite: induction of graft-versus-leukemia using fludarabine-based nonablative chemotherapy and allogeneic blood progenitor cell transplantation as treatment for lymphoid malignancies. *J Clin Oncol* 1998; **16**: 2817–24.

20 Khouri I, Saliba R, Giralt S et al. Nonablative allogeneic hematopoietic transplantation as adoptive immunotherapy for indolent lymphoma: low incidence of toxicity, graft-vs.-host disease and treatment-related mortality. *Blood* 2001; **98**: 3595–9.

21 Verdonck LF, Dekker AW, Lokhorst HM, Petersen EJ, Nieuwenhuis HK. Allogeneic versus autologous bone marrow transplantation for refractory and recurrent low-grade non-Hodgkin's lymphoma. *Blood* 1997; **90**: 4201–5.

22 Chopra R, Goldstone AH, Pearce R et al. Autologous versus allogeneic bone marrow transplantation for non-Hodgkin's lymphoma: a case–controlled analysis of the European Bone Marrow Transplant Group registry data. *J Clin Oncol* 1992; **10**: 1690–5.

23 Khouri IF, Keating MJ, Vriesendorp HM et al. Autologous and allogeneic bone marrow transplantation for chronic lymphocytic leukemia: preliminary results. *J Clin Oncol* 1994; **12**: 748–58.

24 Van Besien KW, De Lima M, Giralt SA et al. Management of lymphoma recurrence after allogeneic transplantation: the relevance of graft-versus-lymphoma effect. *Bone Marrow Transplant* 1997; **19** (10): 977–82.

25 Rondon G, Giralt S, Huh Y et al. Graft-versus-leukemia effect after allogeneic bone marrow transplantation for chronic lymphocytic leukemia. *Bone Marrow Transplant* 1996; **18**: 669–72.

26 Kolb HJ, Schattenberg A, Goldman JM et al. Graft-vs.-leukemia effect of donor lymphocyte transfusions in marrow grafted patients. *Blood* 1995; **86**: 2041–50.

27 Champlin R, Khouri I, Shimoni A et al. Harnessing graft-versus-malignancy: non-myeloablative preparative regimens for allogeneic haematopoietic transplantation, an evolving strategy for adoptive immunotherapy. *Br J Haematol* 2000; **111**: 18–29.

28 Van Besien K, Sobocinski K, Rowlings PA et al. Allogeneic bone marrow transplantation for low-grade lymphoma. *Blood* 1998; 92 (5): 1832–6.

29 Khouri IF, Przepiorka D, Van Besien K et al. Allogeneic blood or marrow transplantation for chronic lymphocytic leukaemia: timing of transplantation and potential effect of fludarabine on acute graft-versus-host disease. *Br J Haematol* 1997; **97**: 466–73.

30 Esteve J, Villamor N, Colomer D et al. Stem cell transplantation for chronic lymphocytic leukemia: different outcome after autologous and allogeneic transplantation and correlation with minimal residual disease status. *Leukemia* 2001; **15**: 445–51.

31 DeMagalhaes-Silverman M, Donnenberg A, Hammert L et al. Induction of graft-versus-leukemia effect in a patient with chronic lymphocytic leukemia. *Bone Marrow Transplant* 1997; **20**: 175–7.

32 Mehta J, Powles R, Singhal S, Iveson T, Treleaven J, Catovsky D. Clinical and hematologic response of chronic lymphocytic and prolymphocytic leukemia persisting after allogeneic bone marrow transplantation with the onset of acute graft-versus-host disease: possible role of graft-versus-leukemia. *Bone Marrow Transplant* 1996; **17**: 371–5.

33 Dey BR, McAfee S, Sackstein R et al. Successful allogeneic stem cell transplantation with non-myeloablative conditioning in patients with relapsed hematologic malignancy following autologous stem cell transplantation. *Biol Blood Marrow Transplant* 2001; **7** (11): 604–12.

34 Dhedin N, Giraudier S, Gaulard P et al. Allogeneic bone marrow transplantation in aggressive non-Hodgkin's lymphoma (excluding Burkitt and lymphoblastic lymphoma): a series of 73 patients from the SFGM database. *Br J Haematol* 1999; **107**: 154–61.

35 Lundberg JH, Hansen RM, Chitambar CR et al. Allogeneic bone marrow transplantation for relapsed and refractory lymphoma using genotypically HLA-identical and alternative donors. *J Clin Oncol* 1991; **9**: 1848–59.

36 Nademanee A, Forman SJ, Schmidt GM et al. Allogeneic bone marrow transplantation for high risk non-Hodgkin's lymphoma during first complete remission. *Blut* 1987; **55**: 11–8.

37 Van Besien KW, Mehra RC, Giralt SA et al. Allogeneic bone marrow transplantation for poor-prognosis lymphoma: response, toxicity and survival depend on disease histology. *Am J Med* 1996; **100** (3): 299–307.

38 Long GD, Amylon MD, Stockerl-Goldstein KE et al. Fractionated total-body irradiation, etoposide, and cyclophosphamide followed by allogeneic bone marrow transplantation for patients with high-risk or advanced-stage hematological malignancies. *Biol Blood Marrow Transplant* 1997; **3** (6): 324–30.

39 Bierman PJ. Allogeneic bone marrow transplantation for lymphoma. *Blood Rev* 2000; **14**: 1–13.

40 Appelbaum FR, Sullivan KM, Buckner CD et al. Treatment of malignant lymphoma in 100 patients with chemotherapy, total body irradiation and marrow transplantation. *J Clin Oncol* 1987; **5**: 1340–7.

41 Fernandez HF, Tran HT, Albrecht F, Lennon S, Caldera H, Goodman MS. Evaluation of safety and pharmacokinetics of administering intravenous busulfan in a twice-daily or daily schedule to patents with advanced hematologic malignant disease undergoing stem cell transplantation. *Biol Blood Marrow Transplant* 2002; **8** (9): 486–92.

42 Copelan EA, Kapoor N, Gibbins B et al. Allogeneic marrow transplantation in non-Hodgkin's lymphoma. *Bone Marrow Transplant* 1990; **5**: 47–50.

43 Przepiorka D, Van Besian K, Khouri I et al. Carmustine, etoposide, cytarabine and melphalan as a preparative regimen for allogeneic transplantation for high-risk malignant lymphoma. *Ann Oncol* 1999; **10**: 527–32.

44 Ratanatharathorn V, Uberti J, Karanes C et al. Prospective comparative trial of autologous versus allogeneic bone marrow transplantation in patients with non-Hodgkin's lymphoma. *Blood* 1994; **84**: 1050–5.

45 Jones RJ, Ambinder RF, Piantadosi S, Santos GW. Evidence of a graft-versus-lymphoma effect associated with allogeneic bone marrow transplantation. *Blood* 1991; **77**: 649–53.

46 Peniket AJ, Ruiz de Elvira MC, Taghipour G et al. Allogeneic transplantation for lymphoma produces a lower relapse rate than autologous transplantation but survival has not risen because of higher treatment-related mortality: a report of 764 cases from the EBMT lymphoma registry. *Blood* 1997; **93**:1124a.

47 Attal M, SociÇG, Molina L et al. Allogeneic bone marrow transplantation for refractory and recurrent follicular lymphoma: a case-matched analysis with autologous transplantation from the French bone marrow transplant group registry data. *Blood* 1997; **93**: 1120a.

48 Van Besien K, Champlin RE. Non-Hodgkin's lymphoma: allogeneic and autologous blood and marrow transplantation. *Adv Oncol* 2000; **16**: 3–16.

49 Cheson BD, Bennett JM, Grever M et al. National Cancer Institute-sponsored Working Group guidelines for chronic lymphocytic leukemia: revised guidelines for diagnosis and treatment. *Blood* 1996; **87**: 4990–7.

50 Rai KR, Sawitsky A, Cronkite EP et al. Clinical staging of chronic lymphocytic leukemia. *Blood* 1975; **46**: 219–34.

51 Binet JL, Catovsky D, Chandra P et al. Chronic lymphocytic leukemia: proposals for a revised prognostic staging system. *Br J Haematol* 1981; **48**: 365–7.

52 Geisler C, Hansen MM, Yeap BY et al. Chemotherapeutic options in chronic lymphocytic leukemia: a meta-analysis of the randomized trials. *J Natl Cancer Inst* 1999; **91** (10): 861–8.

53 Dohner H, Stilgenbauer S, James MR et al. 11q deletions identify a new subset of B-cell chronic lymphocytic leukemia characterized by extensive nodal involvement and inferior prognosis. *Blood* 1997; **89**: 2516–22.

54 Brito-Babapulle V, Garcia-Marco J, Maljaie SH et al. The impact of molecular cytogenetics on chronic lymphoid leukaemia. *Acta Haematol* 1997; **98** (4): 175–86.

55 Crossen PE. Genes and chromosomes in chronic B-cell leukemia. *Cancer Genet Cytogenet* 1997; **94**: 44–51.

56 Juliusson G, Merup M. Cytogenetics in chronic lymphocytic leukemia. *Semin Oncol* 1998; **25**: 19–26.

57 Dohner H, Stilgenbauer S, Benner A et al. Genomic aberrations and survival in chronic lymphocytic leukemia. *N Engl J Med* 2000; **343**: 1910–6.

58 Hamblin TJ, Orchard JA, Ibbotson RE et al. CD38 expression and immunoglobulin variable region mutations are independent prognostic variables in chronic lymphocytic leukemia, but CD38 expression may vary during the course of the disease. *Blood* 2002; **99**: 1023–9.

59 Kipps TJ, Carson DA. Autoantibodies in chronic lymphocytic leukemia and related systemic autoimmune diseases. *Blood* 1993; **81**: 2475–87.

60 Jurlander J, Hartmann Geisler C, Hansen MM. Treatment of hypogammaglobulinaemia in chronic lymphocytic leukaemia by low-dose intravenous gammaglobulin. *Eur J Haematol* 1994; **53**: 114–8.

61 Bunch C. Intravenous immunoglobulin for the prevention of infection in chronic lymphocytic leukemia: a randomized, controlled clinical trial. *N Engl J Med* 1988; **319**: 902–7.

62 Lagneaux L, Delforge A, Dorval C, Bron D, Stryckmans P. Excessive production of transforming growth factor by bone marrow stromal cells in B-cell chronic lymphocytic leukemia inhibits growth of hematopoietic precursors and interleukin-6 production. *Blood* 1993; **82**: 2379–85.

63 Majlis A, Pugh WC, Rodriguez MA, Benedict WF, Cabanillas F. Mantle cell lymphoma: correlation of clinical outcome and biologic features with three histologic variants. *J Clin Oncol* 1997; **15**: 1664–71.

64 Gandhi V, Kemena A, Keating MJ, Plunkett W. Cellular pharmacology of fludarabine triphosphate in chronic lymphocytic leukemia cells during fludarabine therapy. *Leuk Lymphoma* 1993; **10**: 49–56.

65 Fenaux P, Binet JL, Leporrier M et al. Multicentre prospective randomised trial of fludarabine versus cyclophosphamide, doxorubicin, and prednisone (CAP) for treatment of advanced-stage chronic lymphocytic leukaemia. *Lancet* 1996; **347** (9013): 1432–8.

66 Keating MJ, O'Brien S, Kantarjian H et al. Long-term follow-up of patients with chronic lymphocytic leukemia treated with fludarabine as a single agent. *Blood* 1993; **81**: 2878–84.

67 Hamblin TJ, Davis Z, Gardiner A, Oscier DG, Stevenson FK. Unmutated Ig VH genes are associated with a more aggressive form of chronic lymphocytic leukemia. *Blood* 1999; **94**: 1848–54.

68 Seymour JF, Robertson LE, O'Brien S, Lerner S, Keating MJ. Survival of young patients with chronic lymphocytic leukemia failing fludarabine therapy: a basis for the use of myeloablative therapies. *Leuk Lymphoma* 1995; **18**: 493–6.

69 Rabinowe SN, Soiffer RJ, Gribben JG et al. Autologous and allogeneic bone marrow transplantation for poor prognosis patients with B-cell chronic lymphocytic leukemia. *Blood* 1993; **82**: 1366–76.

70 Provan D, Bartlett-Pandite L, Zwicky C et al. Eradication of polymerase chain reaction-detectable chronic lymphocytic leukemia cells is associated with improved outcome after bone marrow transplantation. *Blood* 1996; **88**: 2228–35.

71 Pavletic Z, Bierman P, Vose J et al. Long-term outcome of autologous stem cell transplantation for chronic lymphocytic leukemia or small lymphocytic lymphoma (B-CLL). *Blood* 1997; **97**: 234a.

72 Traweek ST, Slovak ML, Nademanee AP, Brynes RK, Niland JC, Forman SJ. Clonal karyotypic hematopoietic cell abnormalities occurring after autologous bone marrow transplantation for Hodgkin's disease and non-Hodgkin's lymphoma. *Blood* 1994; **84**: 957–63.

73 Armitage JO. Myelodysplasia and acute leukemia after autologous bone marrow transplantation. *J Clin Oncol* 2000; **18**: 945–6.

74 Michallet M, Archimbaud E, Bandini G et al. HLA-identical sibling bone marrow transplantation in younger patients with chronic lymphocytic leukemia. *Ann Intern Med* 1996; **124**: 311–5.

75 Flinn IW, Vogelsang G. Bone marrow transplantation for chronic lymphocytic leukemia. *Semin Oncol* 1998; **25**: 60–4.

76 Toze CL, Shepherd JD, Connors JM et al. Allogeneic bone marrow transplantation for low-grade lymphoma and chronic lymphocytic leukemia. *Bone Marrow Transplant* 2000; **25**: 605–12.

77 Khouri I, Keating M, Saliba R, Champlin RE. Long-term follow-up of patients with chronic lymphocytic leukemia treated with allogeneic hematopoietic transplantation. *Cytotherapy* 2001; **4**: 217.

78 Rondon G, Giralt S, Huh Y et al. Graft-versus-leukemia effect after allogeneic bone marrow transplantation for chronic lymphocytic leukemia. *Bone Marrow Transplant* 1996; **18**: 669–72.

79 Horning SJ. Natural history of and therapy for the indolent non-Hodgkin's lymphomas. *Semin Oncol* 1993; **20** (Suppl. 5): 75–88.

80 Coiffier B, Bastion Y, Berger F, Felman P, Bryon PA. Prognostic factors in follicular lymphomas. *Semin Oncol* 1993; **20** (Suppl. 5): 89–95.

81 Lopez-Guillermo A, Montserrat E, Bosch F, Terol MJ, Campo E, Rozman C. Applicability of the International Index for aggressive lymphomas to patients with low-grade lymphoma. *J Clin Oncol* 1994; **12**: 1343–8.

82 Romaguera JE, McLaughlin P, North L et al. Multivariate analysis of prognostic factors in stage IV follicular low-grade lymphoma: a risk model. *J Clin Oncol* 1991; **9**: 762–9.

83 Portlock CS. Management of the low-grade non-Hodgkin's lymphomas. *Semin Oncol* 1990; **17**: 51–9.

84 Czuczman MS, Fallon A, Mohr A et al. Rituximab in combination with CHOP or fludarabine in low-grade lymphoma. *Semin Oncol* 2002; **29**: 36–40.

85 Weisdorf DJ, Andersen JW, Glick JH, Oken MM. Survival after relapse of low-grade non-Hodgkin's lymphoma: implications for marrow transplantation. *J Clin Oncol* 1992; **10**: 942–7.

86 Rodriguez MA, Cabanillas FC, Velasquez W et al. Results of a salvage treatment program for relapsing lymphoma: MINE consolidated with ESHAP. *J Clin Oncol* 1995; **13**: 1734–41.

87 McLaughlin P, Hagemeister FB, Romaguera JE et al. Fludarabine, mitoxantrone, and dexamethasone: an effective new regimen for indolent lymphoma. *J Clin Oncol* 1996; **14**: 1262–8.

88 Rohatiner AZS, Johnson PWM, Price CGA et al. Myeloablative therapy with autologous bone marrow transplantation as consolidation therapy for recurrent follicular lymphoma. *J Clin Oncol* 1994; **12**: 1177–84.

89 Negrin RS, Kusnierz-Glaz CR, Still BJ et al. Transplantation of enriched and purged peripheral blood progenitor cells from a single apheresis product in patients with non-Hodgkin's lymphoma. *Blood* 1995; **85**: 3334–41.

90 Bierman PJ, Vose JM, Anderson JR, Bishop MR, Kessinger A, Armitage JO. High-dose therapy with autologous hematopoietic rescue for follicular low-grade non-Hodgkin's lymphoma. *J Clin Oncol* 1997; **15**: 445–50.

91 Johnson PWM, Rohatiner AZS, Whelan JS et al. Patterns of survival in patients with recurrent follicular lymphoma: a 20-year study from a single center. *J Clin Oncol* 1995; **13**: 140–7.

92 Stone RM, Neuberg D, Soiffer R et al. Myelodysplastic syndrome as a late complication following autologous bone marrow transplantation for non-Hodgkin's lymphoma. *J Clin Oncol* 1994; **12**: 2535–42.

93 Darrington DL, Vose JM, Anderson JR et al. Incidence and characterization of secondary myelodysplastic syndrome and acute myelogenous leukemia following high-dose chemoradiotherapy and autologous stem-cell transplantation for lymphoid malignancies. *J Clin Oncol* 1994; **12**: 2527–34.

94 Van Besien KW, Khouri IF, Giralt SA et al. Allogeneic bone marrow transplantation for refractory and recurrent low-grade lymphoma: the case for aggressive management. *J Clin Oncol* 1995; **13**: 1096–102.

95 Van Besien KW, Mehra RC, Giralt SA et al. Allogeneic bone marrow transplantation for poor-prognosis lymphoma: response, toxicity, and survival depend on disease histology. *Am J Med* 1996; **100**: 299–307.

96 Dann EJ, Daugherty CK, Larson RA. Allogeneic bone marrow transplantation for relapsed and refractory Hodgkin's disease and non-Hodgkin's lymphoma. *Bone Marrow Transplant* 1997; **20** (5): 369–74.

97 Shepherd JD, Barnett MJ, Connors JM et al. Allogeneic bone marrow transplantation for poor-prognosis non-Hodgkin's lymphoma. *Bone Marrow Transplant* 1993; **12**: 591–6.

98 Van Besien K, Thall P, Korbling M et al. Allogeneic transplantation for recurrent or refractory non-Hodgkin's lymphoma with poor prognostic features after conditioning with thiotepa, busulfan and cyclophosphamide: experience in 44 consecutive patients. *Biol Blood Marrow Transplant* 1997; **3**: 150–6.

99 Verdonck LF. Allogeneic versus autologous bone marrow transplantation for refractory and recurrent low-grade non-Hodgkin's lymphoma: updated results of the Utrecht experience. *Leuk Lymphoma* 1999; **34**: 129–36.

100 Armitage JO. Drug therapy: treatment of non-Hodgkin's lymphoma. *N Engl J Med* 1993; **328**: 1023–30.

101 Gordon LI, Harrington D, Andersen J et al. Comparison of a second-generation combination chemotherapeutic regimen (m-BACOD) with a standard regimen (CHOP) for advanced diffuse non-Hodgkin's lymphoma. *N Engl J Med* 1992; **327**: 1342–9.

102 Fisher RI, Gaynor ER, Dahlberg S et al. Comparison of a standard regimen (CHOP) with three intensive chemotherapy regimens for advanced non-Hodgkin's lymphoma. *N Engl J Med* 1993; **328**: 1002–6.

103 Philip T, Guglielmi C, Hagenbeek A et al. Autologous bone marrow transplantation as compared with salvage chemotherapy in relapses of chemotherapy-sensitive non-Hodgkin's lymphoma. *N Engl J Med* 1995; **333** (23): 1540–5.

104 Philip T, Biron P. High-dose chemotherapy and autologous bone marrow transplantation in diffuse intermediate- and high-grade non-Hodgkin's lymphoma. *Crit Rev Oncol Hematol* 2002; **41**: 213–23.

105 Coiffier B, Gisselbrecht C, Vose JM et al. Prognostic factors in aggressive malignant lymphomas: description and validation of a prognostic index that could identify patients requiring a more intensive therapy. *J Clin Oncol* 1991; **9**: 211–9.

106 Engelhard M, Brittinger G, Huhn D et al. Subclassification of diffuse large B-cell lymphomas according to the Kiel classification: distinction of centroblastic and immunoblastic lymphomas is a significant prognostic risk factor. *Blood* 1997; **89**: 2291–7.

107 Coiffier B, Lepage E. Prognosis of aggressive lymphomas: a study of five prognostic models with patients included in the LNH-84 regimen. *Blood* 1989; **74**: 558–64.

108 Shipp MA. Prognostic factors in aggressive non-Hodgkin's lymphoma: who has 'high-risk' disease. *Blood* 1994; **83**: 1165–73.

109 Rodriguez J, Cabanillas F, McLaughlin P et al. A proposal for a simple staging system for intermediate grade lymphoma and immunoblastic lymphoma based on the 'tumor score'. *Ann Oncol* 1992; **3**: 711.

110 Project TIN-HsLPF. A predictive model for aggressive non-Hodgkin's lymphoma. *N Engl J Med* 1993; **329**: 987–95.

111 Harris NL, Jaffe ES, Stein H et al. A revised European–American classification of lymphoid neoplasms: a proposal from the International Lymphoma Study Group. *Blood* 1994; **84**: 1361–92.

112 Haioun C, Lepage E, Gisselbrecht C et al. Comparison of autologous bone marrow transplantation with sequential chemotherapy for intermediate-grade and high-grade non-Hodgkin's lymphoma in first complete remission: a study of 464 patients. *J Clin Oncol* 1994; **12**: 2543–51.

113 Verdonck LF, Van Putten WLJ, Hagenbeek A et al. Comparison of CHOP chemotherapy with autologous bone marrow transplantation for slowly responding patients with aggressive non-Hodgkin's lymphoma. *N Engl J Med* 1995; **332**: 1045–51.

114 Gianni AM, Bregni M, Siena S et al. High-dose chemotherapy and autologous bone marrow transplantation compared with MACOP-B in aggressive B-cell lymphoma. *N Engl J Med* 1997; **336**: 1290–7.

115 Philip T, Armitage JO, Spitzer G et al. High-dose therapy and autologous bone marrow transplantation after failure of conventional chemotherapy in adults with intermediate grade or high-grade non-Hodgkin's lymphoma. *N Engl J Med* 1987; **316**: 1493–8.

116 Van Besien K, Tabocoff J, Rodriguez M et al. High-dose chemotherapy with BEAC regimen and autologous bone marrow transplantation for intermediate grade and immunoblastic lymphoma: durable complete remissions, but a high rate of regimen-related toxicity. *Bone Marrow Transplant* 1995; **15**: 549–55.

117 Blume KG, Long GD, Negrin RS, Chao NJ, Kusnierz-Glaz C, Amylon MD. Role of etoposide (VP-16) in preparatory regimens for patients with leukemia or lymphoma undergoing allogeneic bone marrow transplantation. *Bone Marrow Transplant* 1994; **14** (Suppl. 4): S9–S10.

118 Demirer T, Weaver CH, Buckner CD et al. High-dose cyclophosphamide, carmustine, and etoposide followed by allogeneic bone marrow transplantation in patients with lymphoid malignancies who had received prior dose-limiting radiation therapy. *J Clin Oncol* 1995; **13**: 596–602.

119 Rodriguez J, Munsell M, Yajis S et al. Impact of high-dose chemotherapy on peripheral T-cell lymphomas. *J Clin Oncol* 2001; **19**: 3766–70.

120 Phillips GL, Herzig RH, Lazarus HM, Fay JW, Griffith R, Herzig GP. High-dose chemotherapy, fractionated total-body irradiation, and allogeneic marrow transplantation for malignant lymphoma 1986; **4**: 480–8.

121 de Witte T, Awwad B, Boezeman J et al. Role of allogeneic bone marrow transplantation in adolescent or adult patients with acute lymphoblastic leukaemia or lymphoblastic lymphoma in first remission. *Bone Marrow Transplant* 1994; **14**: 767–74.

122 Troussard X, Leblond V, Kuentz M et al. Allogeneic bone marrow transplantation in adults with Burkitt's lymphoma or acute lymphoblastic leukemia in first complete remission. *J Clin Oncol* 1990; **8**: 809–12.

123 Przepiorka D, Anderlini P, Ippoliti C et al. Allogeneic blood stem cell transplantation in advanced hematologic cancers. *Bone Marrow Transplant* 1997; **19**: 455–60.

124 Champlin RE, Schmitz N, Horowitz MM et al. Blood stem cells versus bone marrow as a source of hematopoietic cells for allogeneic transplantation. *Blood* 2000; **95**: 3702–9.

125 Philip T, Hartman O, Brian P et al. High-dose therapy and autologous bone marrow transplantation in partial remission after first line induction therapy for diffuse non-Hodgkin's lymphoma. *J Clin Oncol* 1988; **8**: 784–91.

126 Velders GA, Kluin-Nelemans JC, De Boer CJ et al. Mantle-cell lymphoma: a population-based clinical study. *J Clin Oncol* 1996; **14**: 1269–74.

127 Guitaret J, Wickless SC, Omaya Y et al. Long-term remission after allogeneic hematopoietic stem cell transplantation for refractory autogeneous T-cell lymphoma. *Arch Dermatol* 2002; **138**: 1355–65.

128 Badros A, Barlogie B, Siegel E et al. Autologous stem cell transplantation in elderly multiple myeloma patients over the age of 70 years. *Br J Haematol* 2001; **114**: 600–7.

129 Jantunen E, Mahlamnki E, Nousiainen T. Feasibility and toxicity of high-dose chemotherapy supported by peripheral blood stem cell transplantation in elderly patients (≥60 years) with non-Hodgkin's lymphoma: comparison with patients <60 years treated within the same protocol. *Bone Marrow Transplant* 2000; **26**: 737–41.

130 Gandhi V, Robertson LE, Keating MJ, Plunkett W. Combination of fludarabine and arabinosylcytosine for treatment of chronic lymphocytic leukemia: clinical efficacy and modulation of arabinosylcytosine pharmacology. *Cancer Chemother Pharmacol* 1994; **34**: 30–6.

131 Khouri I, Champlin RE. Non-myeloablative stem cell transplantation for lymphoma. *Scand Oncol*; in press.

132 Grigg A, Bardy P, Byron K, Seymour JF, Szer J. Fludarabine-based non-myeloablative chemotherapy followed by infusion of HLA-identical stent cells for relapsed leukaemia and lymphoma. *Bone Marrow Transplant* 1999; **23**: 107–10.

133 Carella AM, Cavaliere M, Lerma E et al. Autografting followed by nonmyeloablative immunosuppressive chemotherapy and allogeneic peripheral-blood hematopoietic stem-cell transplantation as treatment of resistant Hodgkin's disease and non-Hodgkin's lymphoma. *J Clin Oncol* 2000; **18**: 3918–24.

134 Mohty M, Fegueux N, Exbrayat C et al. Enhanced graft-versus-tumor effect following dose-reduced conditioning and allogeneic transplantation for refractory lymphoid malignancies after high-dose therapy. *Bone Marrow Transplant* 2001; **28**: 335–9.

135 Nagler A, Slavin S, Varadi G, Naparstek E, Samuel S, Or R. Allogeneic peripheral blood stem cell transplantation using a fludarabine-based low intensity conditioning regimen for malignant lymphoma. *Bone Marrow Transplant* 2000; **25**: 1021–8.

136 Robinson SP, MacKinnon S, Goldstone AH et al. Higher than expected transplant-related mortality and relapse following non-myeloablative stem cell transplantation for lymphoma adversely effects progression free survival. *Blood* 2000; **96** (Suppl. 1): 554a.

137 Sykes M, Preffer F, McAfee S et al. Mixed lymphohaemopoietic chimerism and graft-versus-lymphoma effects after non-myeloablative therapy and HLA-mismatched bone-marrow transplantation. *Lancet* 1999; **353** (9166): 1755–9.

138 Barrett J, Childs R. Non-myeloablative stem cell transplants. *Br J Haematol* 2000; **111**: 6–17.

139 McSweeney PA, Niederwieser D, Shizuru JA et al. Hematopoietic cell transplantation in older patients with hematologic malignancies: replacing high-dose cytotoxic therapy with graft-versus-tumor effects. *Blood* 2001; **97**: 3390–400.

140 Kwak LW, Campbell MJ, Czerwinski DK, Hart S, Miller RA, Levy R. Induction of immune responses in patients with B-cell lymphoma against the surface-immunoglobulin idiotype expressed by their tumors. *N Engl J Med* 1992; **327**: 1209–15.

141 Bonini C, Ferrari G, Verzeletti S et al. HSV-TK gene transfer into donor lymphocytes for control of allogeneic graft-versus-leukemia. *Science* 1997; **276** (5319): 1719–24.

82

Claudio Anasetti & Andrea Velardi

Hematopoietic Cell Transplantation from HLA Partially Matched Related Donors

Hematopoietic cell transplantation (HCT) from human leukocyte antigen (HLA) matched siblings has become the treatment of choice for many hematologic diseases, but fewer than 40% of patients will have an HLA-matched sibling [1]. Registries of HLA-typed volunteers have been established worldwide to provide HLA-matched unrelated donors for HCT transplantation (see Chapter 83). The chance of finding an unrelated donor matched for HLA-A, -B and -DR depends on the HLA diversity of the population and varies with race, ranging from 75% in white people to less than 50% for US ethnic minorities (www.marrow.org). A limitation in the use of unrelated donors derives from the long duration of the search which may allow disease progression in patients who urgently need transplantation, such as those with acute leukemia. For these reasons, HCT from an HLA-matched sibling or unrelated donor is not feasible for many patients, and other sources of hematopoietic stem cells (HSCs) are sought.

Umbilical cord blood offers the advantages of easy procurement, no risk to the donors, low risk of transmissible infections and immediate availability of the cryopreserved graft (see Chapter 43). However, engraftment is a major concern when the harvested cord blood contains an average or low number of mononuclear cells. Patient age over 10 years and HLA disparity are poor risk factors for engraftment and survival [2,3].

An alternative source of hematopoietic cells is from relatives who are partially matched for HLA. Almost all patients have at least one HLA partially matched family member, parent, sibling or child, who is immediately available as donor. Transplants of T-replete marrow or growth factor-mobilized peripheral blood hematopoietic cells (PBHC) from relatives mismatched for a single HLA-A, -B or -DR antigen have met with acceptable success rates using standard protocols commonly employed for transplants from HLA-identical siblings [4,5]. Conversely, transplants of T-replete marrow from donors mismatched for two or three HLA-A, -B and -DR antigens have resulted in an extremely high incidence of severe acute graft-vs.-host disease (GVHD) [4,6]. Marrow T cell-depletion has been associated with increased risk of graft rejection, but the use of T-depleted PBHC has enhanced the probability of engraftment despite donor mismatch for two or three HLA antigens and carries low incidences of acute and chronic GVHD [7,8].

In this chapter, we first present principles for the selection of related donors with the least degree of HLA disparity for use in conventional transplants, and later present recent developments in the field of T-depleted PBHC transplants from donors mismatched for two or three HLA-A, -B and -DR antigens.

Donor selection

Function and polymorphism of HLA

The HLA system (described in detail in Chapter 4) includes at least 12 genetic sites, named HLA loci, located on the short arm of human chromosome 6. Each HLA locus is highly polymorphic because it is occupied by multiple alternative forms of an HLA gene, designated HLA alleles, any of which may be carried by a given individual. HLA alleles encode class I HLA-A, -B and -C antigens, and class II HLA-DR, -DQ and -DP antigens. Class I HLA antigens are expressed on the surface of all nucleated cells in the body, while class II HLA antigens are expressed on the surface of antigen-presenting cells such as dendritic cells, monocytes, B cells and activated T cells. It is the function of HLA molecules to bind antigenic peptides and activate the immune response in a specific manner. In order to accommodate the need for the binding of ever changing environmental and microbial antigens, HLA molecules have evolved through gene duplication, gene conversion, recombination and point mutation to acquire an enormous degree of polymorphism, most evident across different ethnic groups (see Chapter 5).

Class I HLA molecules present antigenic peptides and activate cytotoxic $CD8^+$ T cells, while class II HLA molecules present antigenic peptides and activate helper $CD4^+$ T cells. Both classes of HLA molecules lead to T cell activation through the binding of specific T cell antigen receptors. In the case of HLA-incompatible HCT, donor and recipient differ not only for one or more types of HLA molecule, but also for the thousands of antigenic peptides that each mismatched HLA molecule can bind and present to foreign T cells [9]. By this process, HCT leads to the activation of an enormous number of both donor and host T cells that mount a response, its strength depending on the degree of HLA mismatch. T cell recognition of antigenic peptides presented by mismatched HLA molecules can result both in graft rejection and GVHD.

HLA class I molecules also bind and activate specific receptors on natural killer (NK) cells. Recent developments on the role of NK cells in transplantation are presented later in this chapter, in the section on T-depleted grafts. HLA class I and II molecules also function as antigens by eliciting antibody responses by B cells. It is thought that anti-HLA antibodies can mediate a hyperacute rejection of allogenic HCTs [10].

HLA haplotypes and segregation in families

The HLA antigens inherited together from one chromosome of each parent are referred to as an HLA haplotype (Fig. 82.1). When a family study is performed in search of an HLA-identical sibling donor, parents should also be typed for HLA-A, -B and -DR, and each of the four parental HLA

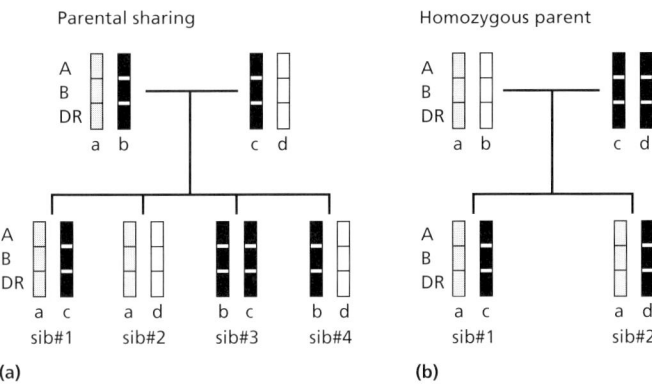

Fig. 82.1 Segregation of human leukocyte antigen (HLA) haplotypes and partial sharing of HLA antigens within a family. (a) The two parental haplotypes "b" and "c" are identical, so that sibling 1 (haplotypes "a" and "c") is compatible with one of these parents (haplotypes "a" and "b"). (b) One parent is HLA homozygous (haplotype "c" and "d" are identical), so that sibling 1 (haplotypes "a" and "c") and sibling 2 (haplotypes "a" and "d") are compatible.

haplotypes identified. Parental haplotypes can segregate among the offspring in four different combinations, and the chance that any one sibling is HLA identical with another is 25%. If an HLA-identical sibling is not found, it is possible to find family members who are partially matched for HLA, even though they have not inherited the same two haplotypes, because certain HLA antigens and haplotypes are frequent. The parental haplotypes should be reviewed for homozygosity or sharing of antigens. The parents, siblings and children, and other relatives who share a haplotype with the patient may have a second haplotype that is partially matched with the patient. Figure 82.1(a) illustrates a family in which the parents have matching haplotypes, "b" and "c". The patient (sib 1, "a/c") has a unique HLA type, and none of the siblings are HLA identical with the patient. However, the patient and the father ("a/b") share the paternal "a" haplotype and are matched for the HLA-A, -B and -DR antigens of their unshared haplotypes ("b" and "c"). Figure 82.1(b) illustrates a family in which the mother ("c/d") is HLA homozygous. The patient (sib 1, "a/c") and sib 2 ("a/d") share the paternal "a" haplotype and each has inherited one of the two maternal haplotypes ("c" and "d"). Because of the serendipitous similarity of the maternal "c" and "d" haplotypes, sib 1 and sib 2 are HLA matched.

Donor and recipient matching

Potential donors are those relatives who share by inheritance one HLA haplotype with the patient and are variably mismatched for 0, 1, 2 or 3 HLA-A, -B and -DR loci of the unshared haplotype. A more precise classification of matching, useful in predicting the risk of rejection and GVHD after HLA-incompatible T-replete transplants, takes into consideration the vector of incompatibility in situations where donor or recipients are homozygous at one of the mismatched loci (Table 82.1) [6]. If recipient and donor are overall incompatible for one HLA locus but the recipient is homozygous at the mismatched locus, the mismatch does not contribute a risk for GVHD. Conversely, if recipient and donor are overall incompatible for one HLA locus but the donor is homozygous at the mismatched locus, the mismatch does not contribute a risk for graft rejection.

Originally, some of the polymorphisms of HLA class I and II antigens were defined serologically by typing with alloantisera obtained from women with history of pregnancy. The development of genetic typing has demonstrated that few HLA antigens represent unique alleles. For example, HLA-A2 is defined as an antigen by serology, but DNA sequencing has determined that as many as 59 distinct HLA-A*0201–0259 alleles may exist, each with unique sequence but all recognized by the same anti-HLA-A2 antibody [11]. Distinction between the variants of polymorphic HLA antigens appears to be functionally relevant because, for example, each of the seven B27 antigen variants can be distinguished by specific cytotoxic T cell clones [12].

The clinical importance of HLA-A, -B and -C allelic differences that cannot be distinguished by serological typing was first suggested by a study in which a significant increase in the risk of graft rejection was found in unrelated donor transplants mismatched for multiple HLA-A, -B or -C alleles as defined by DNA sequencing [13]. Matching between donor and recipients for HLA-A, -B or -C alleles was also associated with decreased GVHD and improved survival [14–17]. The role of matching for -DRB1 alleles, which are subtypes of serologically defined -DR antigens, was demonstrated in studies of unrelated donor HCTs where DRB1 allele matching was associated with decreased GVHD and improved survival [18,19]. The relevance of donor disparity for -DQB1 or -DPB1 on transplant outcome remains disputed [20–23].

In the process of donor selection, we must consider that many recipients and donor pairs, who have not inherited the same HLA haplotypes but are assumed HLA identical on the basis of serological typing alone, would be reclassified as mismatched for one or more HLA alleles using modern DNA typing technology.

Crossmatching

Patients may be alloimmunized by pregnancy or blood transfusions, and sensitization to donor alloantigens increases the risk of graft failure

Table 82.1 Mismatching according to vector of genetic disparity for human leukocyte antigen (HLA)-A, -B and -DR.

Example	Haplotype	Recipient	Donor*	Vector[†]		
				Overall	Rejection	GVHD
I. Heterozygous Recipient and donor	Mismatched Shared*	**A2, B44, DR7**[‡] A1, B8, DR3	**A3, B7, DR2** A1, B8, DR3	3	3	3
II. Homozygous recipient	Mismatched Shared	A1, B35, DR1 A1, B8, DR3	**A3**, B35, DR1 A1, B8, DR3	1	1	0
III. Homozygous donor	Mismatched Shared	**A2, B44**, DR4 A1, B8, DR3	A1, B8, DR4 A1, B8, DR3	2	0	2

*Recipient and donor are related and share HLA haplotype.
†Number of mismatches at HLA-A, -B or -DR loci.
‡Incompatible antigens are represented in bold.

[10,24]. Crossmatch testing can determine if the recipient has been sensitized to HLA antigens of the donor, and is indicated before the selection of an HLA-mismatched donor for HCT. Standard assays for crossmatching the patient's serum with donor lymphocytes include complement-dependent microcytotoxicity, and multicolor flow microfluorimetry [25,26].

Probability of identifying an HLA partially compatible family donor

One report from Germany found that the probability of identifying an HLA-matched sibling was 40.7%, a matched relative 4.0%, a one HLA-A, -B or -DR locus mismatched sibling 3.1% and a one-locus mismatched relative 10.4% [1]. The best chance of finding a donor for patients without an HLA-matched or a one-locus mismatched sibling is an unrelated donor search, because this is currently successful in up to 75% of the cases. If the initial search identifies one or more HLA-A, -B and -DR matched unrelated donors, there is no obvious justification to undertake an extended family search beyond siblings, because not only the probability of finding a suitable donor would be lower, but also the donor typing effort and the cost of finding donors would be greater [1]. Computer programs have recently been developed that can calculate the probability of finding a suitable related or unrelated donor based on patient typing [1,27–29]. Results of such programs can be utilized to define the best search strategy for an individual patient. Candidates for allogeneic HCT with no suitably matched donor and a short life expectancy might be better served by immediate transplantation from a relative mismatched for one entire HLA haplotype than by a lengthy search for a completely matched donor.

Transplantation of T-replete marrow grafts

Transplant outcome

The relevance of HLA incompatibility between donor and recipient has been analyzed in patients with hematologic disorders who received HCTs of T-replete marrow grafts. The patient and related donor shared one HLA haplotype but differed to a variable degree for the HLA-A, -B and -DR antigens of the unshared haplotype. The results of these transplants have shown the effect of HLA incompatibility on graft failure, GVHD and survival, formally demonstrating that HLA antigens constitute the major histocompatibility complex (MHC) in humans.

Graft failure

Clinical presentation

Primary graft failure is likely to occur if severe granulocytopenia persists for 21 days after transplantation, but secondary graft failure may also occur after the initial take [10]. Studies of chimerism (see Chapter 19) are necessary to assess the presence of donor cells. Functional studies in patients with graft failure have demonstrated that residual host T lymphocytes are cytotoxic against donor alloantigens, or the patient's serum may be active in the antibody-dependent cell-mediated cytotoxicity test against donor cells [30,31]. These findings have been interpreted to indicate alloimmune-mediated rejection as the predominant mechanism for graft failure after HCT from HLA-incompatible donors. If a myeloablative conditioning regimen is administered, either primary or secondary graft failure is usually associated with persistent aplasia. In certain patients, recovery of autologous myeloid cells can occur, especially if the patient is treated with granulocyte macrophage colony-stimulating factor (GM-CSF) or granulocyte colony-stimulating factor (G-CSF) [32]. If there is no recovery of myeloid function despite growth factor therapy, a second transplant from the same or a different donor can be attempted, but the success of second transplants has been limited [10].

Risk factors

HLA mismatch. The relevance of HLA compatibility to sustained engraftment was first analyzed in 269 patients with hematologic neoplasms who underwent marrow transplantation from a family member who shared one HLA haplotype with the patient but differed to a variable degree for the HLA-A, -B and -DR antigens of the unshared haplotype [10]. These 269 patients were compared with 930 patients who received marrow from siblings with an identical HLA genotype. All patients were treated with cyclophosphamide (CY) and total body irradiation (TBI) followed by infusion of unmodified donor marrow cells. The incidence of graft failure was 12.3% among recipients of marrow from an HLA partially matched donor as compared with 2.0% among recipients of marrow from an HLA-matched sibling ($p < 0.0001$) (Table 82.2). The incidence of graft failure correlated with the degree of HLA incompatibility in the host-vs.-graft direction. Graft failure occurred in three of 43 transplants (7%) from donors who were matched with their recipient for HLA-A, -B and -DR, in 11 of 121 donors (9%) incompatible for one HLA locus, in 18 of 86 (21%) incompatible for two loci, and in 1 of 19 (5%) incompatible for three loci ($p = 0.028$). Therefore, donor HLA incompatibility is a significant risk factor for graft failure.

The reasons for the apparently lower incidence of graft failure with a transplant incompatible for three loci compared to two loci reported in that study are not obvious [10]. Transplants with the highest degree of mismatch were conducted predominantly in children who received a higher marrow cell dose. It is also possible that the higher degree of mismatch led to a more rapid and intense graft-vs.-host reaction that blunted host immune responses that mediate graft rejection.

An update of that study later found an additional effect of HLA disparity in particular donor and recipient combinations [33]. When the recipient is homozygous at a mismatched HLA locus, the degree of HLA disparity is greater in the direction of rejection than the direction of GVHD (Table 82.1). Transplants in recipients homozygous at one or more mismatched loci had a significantly higher incidence of graft failure than transplants in heterozygous recipients. Graft failure after a transplant mismatched for one or more HLA loci occurred in 11 of 76 (15%) homozygous recipients compared to 22 of 350 (6%) heterozygous recipients. The effect of the vector of incompatibility on graft failure was significant

Table 82.2 Effect of human leukocyte antigen (HLA) incompatibility on marrow graft failure. (Modified from Anasetti *et al.* [10].)

	No. of patients (%)		
	HLA nonidentical donor ($n = 269$)	HLA genotype identical donor ($n = 930$)	*p* value
Failure of engraftment	23 (8.5%)	15 (1.6%)	$p < 0.0001$
Late graft failure	10 (4.1%)	4 (0.4%)	$p < 0.0001$
All failures	33 (12.3%)	19 (2.0%)	$p < 0.0001$

in a multivariable analysis ($p = 0.0054$). The association between recipient homozygosity for the mismatched locus and increased graft failure has been confirmed in a subsequent study of HLA-mismatched unrelated donor transplants [34]. These results are consistent with the concept that the graft-vs.-host reaction (GVHR) protects from graft failure. Presumably, the GVHR is directed against residual immune cells of the recipient that are responsible for graft failure. In cases where the degree of disparity in the donor exceeds the degree of disparity in the host, the GVHR is less and the risk of graft failure is increased.

Recipient sensitization. Prior patient immunization to donor HLA antigens has a profound effect on engraftment. In a study of marrow transplants from HLA-incompatible relatives, graft failure occurred in 13 of 21 (62%) patients with a positive pretransplant crossmatch of patient serum reactive against donor T or B lymphocytes, compared with 31 of 501 (7%) patients with a negative crossmatch ($p = 7.8$, E-10) [10,33]. Among all the microcytotoxicity assays, the antiglobulin crossmatch and the B-cell crossmatch at 22°C or 37°C correlated best with graft failure [26]. Autoreactive antibodies were observed in four patients who were all successfully engrafted. Alloimmunized patients who tested positive for anti-HLA antibodies by screening against a random cell panel but were crossmatched negative with the donor did not demonstrate an increased risk of graft failure [26]. A recent study by Ottinger et al. [24] also found that positive serum crossmatch is a predictor for graft failure and poor survival after peripheral blood hematopoietic transplantation (PBHT) from an HLA-mismatched donor. In the presence of a positive antidonor crossmatch, graft failure is likely the result of alloimmune rejection mediated both by sensitized radioresistant host T cells and by antibody-dependent cell-mediated killing. Removal of antidonor antibody through a plasma exchange followed by CY (120 mg/kg) and TBI (1200–1575 cGy), the addition of total lymphoid irradiation (600 cGy in four fractions over 2 days) or antithymocyte globulin (10 mg/kg/day, day –2 to day +3) to the standard regimen of CY and TBI has not resulted in consistent marrow engraftment [10,33].

Patient diagnosis. The risk of graft failure is low in patients who are immunodeficient by virtue of a congenital disorder or as result of prior cytotoxic or immunosuppressive therapy provided as treatment for the underlying disease. Some patients with severe combined immunodeficiency lacking both T and NK cells have been engrafted with HLA-incompatible HCT despite receiving neither pretransplant conditioning nor post-transplant immunosuppression [35]. Patients with leukocyte adhesion deficiency (see Chapter 108), a congenital defect resulting in failure to express the leukointegrin β_2 chain on white cells including T and NK cells, demonstrate low resistance to engraftment with T-depleted transplants from HLA-incompatible donors [36]. Thus, β_2 leukointegrins have a critical role in the rejection of HLA-incompatible HCTs.

Patients with chronic myeloid leukemia (CML) have a higher risk of graft failure than patients with acute myeloid leukemia (AML) or acute lymphoblastic leukemia (ALL). The incidence of graft failure was examined in non-T-depleted marrow grafts from HLA partially matched relatives in patients treated with the same conditioning regimen of CY (120 mg/kg) plus hyperfractionated TBI (1320–1440 cGy) followed by post-transplant immunosuppression by cyclosporine (CSP) and a short course of methotrexate (MTX). Graft failure occurred in 11 of 84 (13%) patients with CML compared to five of 133 (4%) patients with other diagnoses (odds ratio = 3.5, 95%CI, range 1.1–10.5, multivariate $p = 0.03$) (P. Servida, unpublished data). Patients with acute leukemia may be at lower risk for graft failure because of the immunodeficiency induced by repeated treatment with chemotherapy agents [37].

Conditioning regimen. Increasing the intensity of the pretransplant conditioning regimen can minimize the incidence of immunomediated rejection. Pretransplant immunosuppression with CY alone (200 mg/kg for 4 days) allowed sustained engraftment in only four of 11 patients with severe aplastic anemia transplanted from donors incompatible for one HLA-A, -B or -DR locus, and none of three patients transplanted from a two-locus incompatible donor [38]. The addition of thiotepa (15 mg/kg) and thymoglobulin (15 mg/kg) to CY (150 mg/kg) allowed sustained engraftment of marrow or blood HCT in all 17 patients transplanted from a one-locus mismatched donor, and six of seven patients transplanted from a two-locus mismatched donor [39].

Conditioning with busulfan (BU) (13–16 mg/kg over 4 days) in addition to CY (120–200 mg/kg over 2–4 days) was used for 11 patients with myelodysplastic syndrome (MDS), lymphoma or myeloma. Nine patients transplanted from one HLA locus incompatible donors and one of two transplanted from two HLA locus incompatible donors engrafted, suggesting that BU adds to the immunosuppression produced by CY alone [40; C. Anasetti, unpublished data]. However, BU/CY was less effective in allowing engraftment of marrow from HLA-mismatched donors in patients with thalassemia: sustained grafts were achieved in eight of 15 patients mismatched at one HLA locus, two of five patients mismatched at two loci, and none of three mismatched at three loci [41]. Thalassemia patients are not only more immunocompetent than leukemia patients but are also sensitized to histocompatibility antigens by multiple blood cell transfusions. The addition of thiotepa to BU/CY has decreased significantly the risk of graft failure in thalassemia patients transplanted from HLA partially compatible unrelated donors [42].

Pretransplant conditioning with CY (120 mg/kg over 2 days) and TBI (920–1575 cGy) allowed engraftment in 88% of 269 patients transplanted from HLA partially matched relatives [10]. The rate of graft failure was 17% in patients conditioned with 1200 cGy TBI over 6 days, 12% in patients conditioned with 1575 cGy, 9% in patients conditioned with 1320–1440 cGy (120 cGy three times a day for 11–12 doses) and 5% in patients conditioned with 1000 cGy in a single dose. A more effective regimen was developed for T-depleted transplants: CY was replaced by antithymocyte globulin (ATG), fludarabine and thiotepa, agents that contributed immunosuppressive activity without additional toxicity (see below) [43].

Post-transplant immunosuppression. Post-transplant immunosuppression can decrease the incidence of graft failure. Patients transplanted from HLA partially matched donors had a graft failure rate of 5% when treated with CSP plus short MTX, but 9% when treated with MTX alone ($p = 0.03$) [33]. This observation is consistent with the report from the International Bone Marrow Transplant Registry (IBMTR) showing that in T-depleted marrow transplants from HLA-identical sibling donors, the use of post-transplant immunosuppression with CSP plus MTX was associated with a lower risk of graft failure than CSP alone [44].

Graft-vs.-host disease

Clinical presentation of acute GVHD

Acute GVHD occurs early after HLA-incompatible transplants. The median onset of acute GVHD was 14 days after HLA-incompatible transplants, compared to 22 days after HLA-identical sibling transplants [4]. Acute GVHD after HLA-incompatible transplants can be associated with a hyperacute syndrome characterized by fever 7–10 days after transplantation, fluid retention, low central venous pressure, low serum albumin, pulmonary edema and renal failure (see Chapter 50). If the syndrome cannot be reversed promptly by the use of immunosuppressive agents, the patient may die from respiratory failure [45].

Risk factors

HLA mismatch. The incidence and severity of acute GVHD correlates with the degree of HLA incompatibility. In the initial report when patients received MTX as single agent for GVHD prophylaxis, the incidence of grades II–IV GVHD was 34% for recipients of HLA-identical

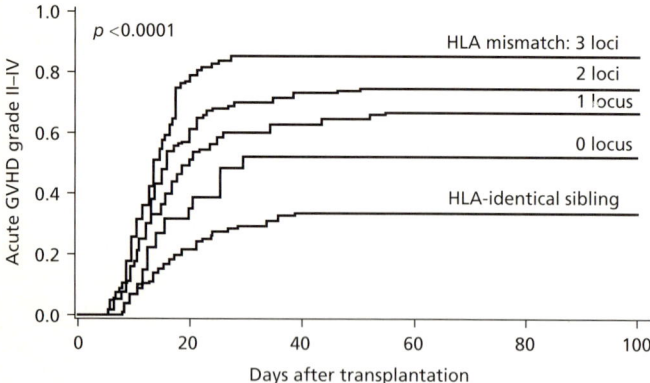

Fig. 82.2 Effect of donor and recipient human leukocyte antigen (HLA) mismatch on acute graft-vs.-host disease (GVHD). Probability of grades II–IV acute GVHD according to the degree of matching for HLA-A, -B and -D/DRB1 in patients transplanted from a haploidentical relative or an HLA genotype identical sibling. Patients received unmodified marrow and methotrexate plus cyclosporine for GVHD prophylaxis.

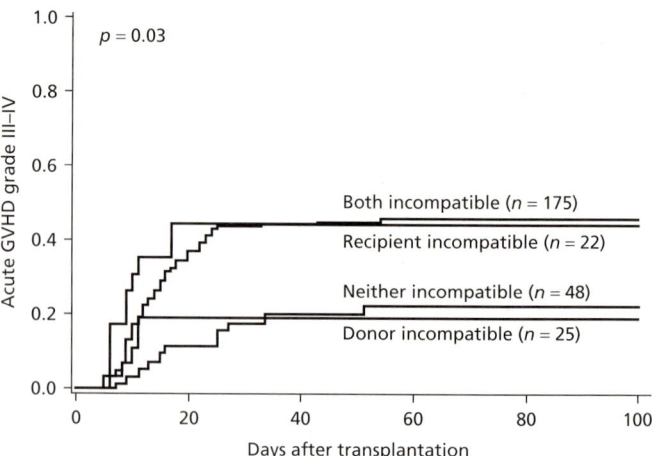

Fig. 82.3 Effect of the vector of human leukocyte antigen (HLA) mismatch on acute graft-vs.-host disease (GVHD). Probability of grades III–IV acute GVHD in patients who received a marrow transplant from a haploidentical relative. Transplants incompatible for one HLA-A, -B or -D/DRB1 locus are classified as "donor incompatible" in the case of homozygous recipients where mismatch is only in the direction of graft-vs.-host, as "recipient incompatible" in the case of homozygous donors where mismatch is only in the direction of host-vs.-graft, or as "both incompatible" in the case where donor and recipient are both heterozygous. Transplants from a haploidentical relative whose unshared haplotype is matched to the patient's are classified as "neither incompatible".

sibling marrow and increased progressively up to 84% for recipients of a three-locus incompatible marrow [4]. Despite post-transplant immunosuppression with CSP and MTX, HLA incompatibility has remained an important risk factor for GVHD (Fig. 82.2) [6]. In patients transplanted from HLA nonidentical donors, acute GVHD is not only more frequent in the skin, but also in the gastrointestinal tract and liver. Among patients transplanted for CML, the incidence of gastrointestinal involvement was 10% in HLA-identical sibling transplants and 22% in a one HLA locus incompatible transplant. The incidence of liver involvement was 13% in HLA-identical sibling transplants compared to 36% in a one HLA locus incompatible transplant [46].

The vector of HLA incompatibility affects the risk of acute GVHD. Because HLA homozygous recipients are matched with their donors in the direction of GVHD, transplants incompatible for one HLA locus in homozygous recipients are associated with lower incidence of acute GVHD than in heterozygous recipients ($p = 0.03$) (Fig. 82.3) [6]. The incidence of acute GVHD for homozygous recipients of one-locus incompatible transplants is similar to that seen in HLA-matched transplants. Conversely, HLA homozygosity in the donor does not affect the incidence of GVHD.

Post-transplant immunosuppression. Initial transplants from HLA-incompatible related donors were performed in patients receiving MTX as the only immunosuppressive agent. When it became apparent that the combination of CSP and MTX was superior to either agent alone in HLA sibling transplants the same regimen was adopted for HLA partially matched transplants. In a multivariate analysis of 474 patients who received CSP and MTX or MTX alone and achieved sustained engraftment, HLA incompatibility was a significant risk factor for acute GVHD (relative risk [RR] = 1.95 per HLA locus; $p < 0.0001$) [6,33]. The risk of severe acute GVHD of grade III–IV was significantly less and the time of onset was delayed by the use of CSP and MTX (RR = 0.35; $p < 0.0001$). The incidence of severe grade III–IV acute GVHD was decreased from 53 to 28% in one-locus incompatible recipients and from 63 to 47% in two-locus incompatible recipients. Recipients incompatible for one HLA-A or -B locus had a significantly lower incidence of acute GVHD when receiving CSP and MTX rather than MTX alone, but there was no apparent benefit from CSP and MTX in patients incompatible for one HLA-DR locus. Thus, the addition of CSP to a regimen of MTX was most effective in transplants incompatible for HLA-A or -B. The major remaining problem is to overcome HLA disparity for HLA-DR, either alone or in combination with HLA-A or -B. Not even substituting CSP with tacrolimus was adequate to prevent GVHD after transplantation from HLA-DR incompatible relatives [47].

Patient age. Patient age does not appreciably affect the risk of grades II–IV acute GVHD after HLA-incompatible transplants, but younger age is associated with a decreased risk of acute GVHD grades III–IV (RR = 1.23; 95%CI, 1.05–1.44 per decade of patient age; $p = 0.04$) [6]. Post-transplant immunosuppression with CSP and MTX has not resulted in improved outcome for patients of any age after transplants incompatible at two or three HLA loci [6].

Chronic GVHD

Marrow transplants from HLA partially matched family members have been associated with a higher probability for developing clinical extensive chronic GVHD (49% vs. 33%) and an earlier median day of onset (159 vs. 201 days) compared with transplants from HLA-identical siblings [48]. Consistent results have been found by the IBMTR [49]. A detailed description of the clinical manifestations of chronic GVHD and the duration of the disease following HLA partially matched related donor transplants have not yet been reported.

Graft-vs.-leukemia effect

Relapse of leukemia after HLA-identical sibling transplants is less frequent in patients who develop clinically significant GVHD compared to syngenic or allogenic transplant recipients without GVHD (see Chapter 28). Patients with ALL after transplant from HLA partially matched donors in whom GVHD developed also had a lower risk of relapse than patients without GVHD [6]. However, the probability of leukemic relapse in patients without clinically significant GVHD was the same whether the marrow donor was an HLA-identical sibling or an HLA partially matched relative. These data suggested that HLA disparity in absence of acute GVHD has no obvious antileukemic effect. In one analysis, chronic but not acute GVHD was associated with a lower relapse rate in patients with AML or CML [6]. Because recipients of one HLA locus incompatible transplants have a higher incidence of acute GVHD than recipients of HLA-identical sibling transplants, one would expect to see a lower incidence of leukemic relapse. A study from the IBMTR comparing the outcome of 1222 HLA-identical sibling transplants to the outcome of 238 transplants from one HLA locus incompatible donors failed to detect different rates of relapse [7]. One study found an association of donor mismatch for one HLA antigen with a lower incidence of leukemic relapse in patients transplanted from unrelated volunteers [50]. The use of T-replete grafts of G-CSF-mobilized PBHC from one HLA antigen mismatched related or an unrelated donors has been associated with a lower risk of post-transplant relapse in CML patients [51]. The apparent increase in antitumor effect with PBHC compared to marrow is perhaps related to the number of donor T cells transplanted [52].

Immune reconstitution

After transplantation, new T cells derive from donor HSCs following positive and negative selection within the host thymus. T lymphocytes recognize immunogenic peptides presented by self- HLA but not by allogenic HLA molecules, a phenomenon defined as HLA restriction (see Chapter 5). Positive T cell selection is facilitated by HLA molecules expressed on thymic epithelial cells, whereas negative selection is controlled predominantly by HLA molecules expressed on marrow-derived antigen-presenting cells [53]. Thus, new T cells that are positively selected on thymic epithelium can optimally recognize antigen in the context of marrow-derived antigen-presenting cells in peripheral tissues only if there is sharing of HLA antigens between donor and recipient [54]. Mature T cells transplanted into an HLA-disparate recipient may not recognize antigens presented by host antigen-presenting cells, thereby failing to help immune reconstitution. These premises justify why donor and recipient matching for at least one HLA haplotype is the minimal requisite for donor selection.

Extrathymic pathways of immune reconstitution after transplantation are predominant in adults as thymus function begins to decline relatively early in life, usually before the age of 20 years. Therefore, T cells that repopulate adult transplant recipients derived predominantly from the relatively small number of mature donor T cells infused with the marrow innoculum [55]. Immunosuppressive regimens should be developed that are effective in preventing GVHD, while sparing donor T cells that do not recognize host alloantigen and contribute to long-term immune reconstitution. Both acute and chronic GVHD also contribute to immunodeficiency.

Because adult patients have very poor thymic function, marrow T cell-depletion has been associated with severe and prolonged post-grafting immunodeficiency [56]. Recent data on T cell receptor excision circles as a marker for recent thymus emigrants has demonstrated that the human thymus continues to function at low levels until late in life, providing hope that effective treatment can be developed to restore immunity quickly in T cell-deficient adults [57]. Preclinical data on interleukin 7 (IL-7) and keratinocyte growth factor are promising for this application [58,59].

Survival

Effect of HLA mismatch

Studies from Seattle in patients receiving HCT for AML, ALL, CML, MDS or lymphoma have evaluated the role of HLA-A, -B and -D/DR incompatibility on survival after T-replete marrow transplants. HLA-DR subtypes, termed HLA-D, were defined by functional testing with homozygous typing cells and utilized in the definition of a match. Survival in patients receiving post-transplant immunosuppression with MTX alone was similar after transplantation from an HLA-identical sibling or a one HLA-antigen incompatible family donor. However, survival was lower in patients transplanted from a family donor incompatible for two or three HLA loci [4]. Subsequent studies of patients whose post-transplant immunosuppression consisted of CSP and MTX also showed that the

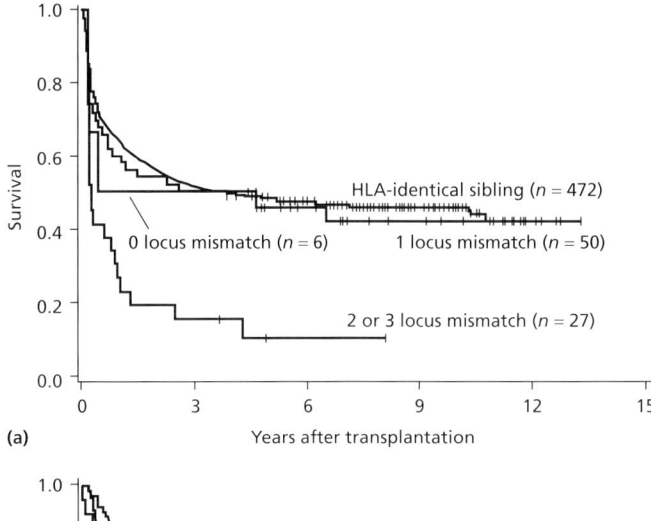

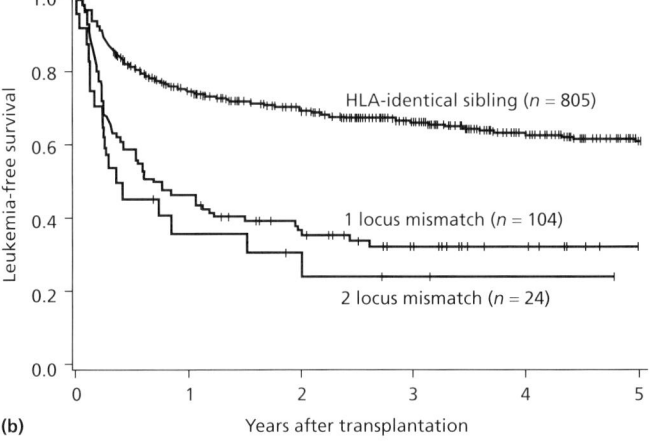

Fig. 82.4 Effect of donor and recipient human leukocyte antigen (HLA) mismatch on survival after marrow transplantation. Probability of survival in patients with chronic myeloid leukemia in chronic phase, acute myeloid leukemia in first remission or acute lymphoblastic leukemia in first or second remission, according to the degree of donor and recipient HLA incompatibility. (a) Results from a single center study. (Reprinted with permission from Anasetti *et al.* [6].) (b) Results from a study of the International Bone Marrow Transplant Registry. (Reprinted with permission from Szydlo *et al.* [49].)

degree of overall HLA incompatibility is inversely correlated with the probability of survival (Fig. 82.4a). Survival was predicted more precisely by matching classified according to the degree of overall incompatibility than incompatibility for each vector alone, presumably because the degree of overall incompatibility best reflects both the risks of graft rejection and GVHD. In a multivariate proportional hazard regression analysis, the factors associated with lower survival were leukemia in marrow relapse at time of transplant and the degree of overall HLA incompatibility between donor and recipient. Post-transplant immunosuppression with CSP and MTX compared to MTX alone did not have a beneficial effect on survival.

A large study from the IBMTR compared the outcomes of marrow transplants from HLA-identical siblings, HLA partially matched related donors and unrelated donors for treatment of leukemia [49]. The definition of donor and recipient histocompatibility differed from the Seattle criteria because matching for the -DR locus was based exclusively on serological data but not on cellular or DNA typing data. The probability of leukemia-free survival for patients transplanted for early stage leukemia, CML in chronic phase, AML or ALL in first remission is presented in Fig. 82.4(b). A multivariable analysis of transplant-related mortality showed an increase in risk with the use of a one HLA locus mismatched relative compared to an HLA-identical sibling, and for the use of a two HLA locus incompatible relative compared to a one HLA locus incompatible relative. Results of matched unrelated donor transplants were similar to results of one-antigen mismatched related donor transplants, while results of one-antigen mismatched unrelated donors transplants were similar to results of two-antigen mismatched related donor transplants [49]. A large proportion of patient and donor pairs serologically compatible at -DR are mismatched for one or two -DRB1 subtypes [18], and mismatching for -DRB1 correlates with allele mismatching at HLA-B and -DQB1 (see Chapters 4 and 83). Therefore, transplants assessed as mismatched for only one HLA locus in the IBMTR report are expected to be more genetically disparate than transplants assessed as mismatched for one-HLA locus in the Seattle report. Taken together, these data demonstrate that a limited degree of HLA disparity between donor and recipient can be tolerated with T-replete marrow in transplants for hematologic malignancies, but a higher degree of donor HLA disparity reduces survival.

A single center study from Milwaukee compared transplantation outcomes in patients with hematologic malignancies who received marrow grafts from either HLA-matched unrelated, one-antigen mismatched unrelated or highly mismatched family donors [60]. All patients received a standardized conditioning regimen and a uniform GVHD prophylaxis schedule with the exception of mismatched related recipients, who received ATG as additional post-grafting immunosuppression. There was a higher probability of survival for matched unrelated transplants (58%) than either mismatched unrelated (34%; $p = 0.01$) or mismatched related transplants (21%; $p = 0.002$). This study supports that patients lacking an HLA-matched family donor be offered a matched unrelated donor, if available. With the limitations imposed by the low degree of HLA typing resolution and the small sample sizes, the IBMTR and Milwaukee studies both found no detectable advantage to using a one HLA-A, -B or -DR antigen mismatched unrelated vs. a more HLA-disparate family donor.

Transplantation of T-depleted hematopoietic cell grafts

Risk of graft failure

Numerous clinical trials have demonstrated that extensive *ex vivo* depletion of T cells from the marrow graft without post-transplant immunosuppression prevents acute and chronic GVHD and associated morbidity (see Chapter 17) [44,61–63]. Unfortunately, depletion of T cells from the donor marrow is associated with an increased rate of graft failure that is proportional to the degree of donor HLA incompatibility. A study from the IBMTR on transplantation from donors incompatible for two or three HLA-A, -B and -DR antigens found an incidence of graft failure of 42% with T-depleted marrow compared to 28% in non-T-depleted marrow ($p < 0.03$) [7]. In a small series of patients with leukemia transplanted from a two or three HLA antigen mismatched donor at Memorial Sloan Kettering Cancer Center in New York, the use of T-depletion was also associated with an incidence of graft failure approaching 50% [64]. Resistance to engraftment is mediated primarily by host T lymphocytes [30]. We presume that with T-depleted marrow grafts, the balance between competing host and donor T cells shifts in favor of the host, resulting in unopposed host-vs.-graft reaction [65,66].

Partial marrow T cell depletion

One method to limit the degree of host resistance to HLA-mismatched transplants is to deplete a subset of T cells rather than all T cells in the marrow graft. Soiffer *et al.* [67] transplanted 27 adults from HLA-mismatched donors, in 10 cases mismatched for two HLA loci. Grafts were T-depleted with anti-CD6 monoclonal antibody T12, and no post-transplant immunosuppression was given. Conditioning included total lymphoid irradiation, fractionated TBI and standard dose CY. Twenty-four of the 27 (88%) patients engrafted, and 40% developed grade II–IV acute GVHD. The survival of HLA-mismatched patients was 56% at 2 years, and was not affected by the degree of HLA disparity. The 2-year disease-free survival was 69% for early disease patients and 20% for those with more advanced disease. The mechanism for immunologic tolerance after infusion of CD6⁻ T cells is unclear.

Removal of less than 2 logs T cells from the donor marrow requires, in general, administration of post-transplant immunosuppression for prevention of GVHD [68]. Henslee-Downey *et al.* [68] achieved partial T cell depletion by *ex vivo* treatment of donor marrow with anti-T cell receptor monoclonal antibody T10B9 and rabbit complement. The CD5-specific immunotoxin H65-RTA and ATG were administered *in vivo* after transplantation to deplete both host and donor T cells. In a study of 72 patients, most of whom received two or three HLA antigen-mismatched grafts, the probability of engraftment was 88%, and the incidence of grade II–IV acute GVHD was 16%. The probability of 2-year survival was 55% in low-risk patients vs. 27% in high-risk patients ($p = 0.048$) [69]. This study demonstrated that partial T cell depletion can be used to prevent GVHD after transplantation of marrow from donors mismatched for one HLA haplotype, and the risk of graft failure is low if post-grafting immunosuppression is administered.

The anti-CD3 monoclonal antibody OKT3 has been tested for T depletion of HLA-mismatched marrow grafts in one study of 67 pediatric patients. The engraftment rate was as high as 97% and the probability of grade II–IV acute GVHD was 24%. The 3-year survival was 26%, better with low blood blast count at transplant and with donors under 30 years of age [70]. In patients with acute leukemia refractory to primary induction chemotherapy, the 3-year disease-free survival was 14–19% [71,72]. These studies indicate that techniques for partial T cell depletion of highly mismatched marrow grafts vary in safety and efficacy. Some of these techniques are clearly associated with high incidence of GVHD and poor outcomes and are inadequate for crossing the HLA barrier safely.

Selective *ex vivo* depletion or tolerization of alloreactive T cells in the graft

An alternative approach to *ex vivo* partial T cell depletion for the prevention of GVHD involves the coincubation of T-replete donor bone marrow with recipient antigen-presenting cells in the presence of agents that can selectively eliminate or inactivate host-reactive T cells. Donor T cells were exposed *ex vivo* to recipient alloantigen and treated with an immunotoxin specific for the IL-2 receptor alpha chain. This approach was effective in selectively eliminating alloreactive T cells but not T cells reactive to third-party antigens. Reinfusion of nonalloreactive T cells into patients previously transplanted with T-depleted grafts from HLA-mismatched donors led to immune reconstitution without GVHD [73].

Extensive preclinical data demonstrated that antigen presentation in the absence of CD28 costimulation induces a state of T cell unresponsiveness to antigen restimulation [74,75]. Based on these preclinical data, one clinical trial employed host antigen-presenting cells and soluble CTLA-4-Ig to present host alloantigen to donor T cells while blocking the CD28 costimulatory pathways. This approach resulted in *ex vivo* donor T cell unresponsiveness to the HLA-mismatched cells of the recipient [76]. Transplantation of marrow replete with alloantigen unresponsive T cells led to primary engraftment in nine of the 12 children, and three cases of acute GVHD despite post-transplant immunosuppressive therapy. No other clinical studies have yet been reported using the same principle of *ex vivo* costimulation blockade for tolerance induction.

Conditioning regimen

Research in animal models showed that recipient immune cells survive after supralethal doses of TBI, but their response can be suppressed by increasing the dose of TBI [77] or by combining the standard dose of TBI with selective anti-T cell reagents with low nonhematologic toxicity [78]. Engraftment is also enhanced when alkylating drugs, such as busulfan, dimethyl-busulfan or thiotepa, are administered in combination with TBI [79,80]. However, a regimen of ATG, thiotepa, CY and single dose TBI did not ensure engraftment after transplant of T-depleted marrow cells from HLA haplotype mismatched donors in patients with leukemia [81].

Hematopoietic cell dose and use of PBHC

Murine studies

Animal models showed that the barrier to engraftment of MHC-mismatched HCT could be overcome without GVHD by transplanting high doses of T-depleted marrow cells. When purified HSCs were transplanted in irradiated mice, stable hematopoietic chimeras were generated in all cases, but 10–60 times the number of HSCs were required for survival of mice transplanted across MHC disparities as compared to Ly-5 congenic (nonallogenic) disparities [82].

Cell dose escalation allowed full donor cell engraftment even in mice that had been presensitized by donor lymphocytes [83], in mice whose immune system had been partially reconstituted with the infusion of small numbers of host T cells before the allogenic transplant, and in mice pretreated with sublethal doses of TBI low enough to spare recipient T lymphocytes [79].

Human studies

A major advance in HCT from donors incompatible for a full HLA haplotype derives from the higher probability of engraftment achieved by increas-ing the dose of hematopoietic cells. This goal has been reached thanks to the recent availability of hematopoietic growth factors. Treatment of normal donors with G-CSF leads to the mobilization of HSC from marrow to blood (see Chapter 46). Collection of blood cells through leukapheresis yields more hematopoietic progenitors than an average marrow graft.

Transplant outcome

Studies in Perugia

Graft characteristics

In 1993, the hypothesis that escalation of the hematopoietic cell dose could facilitate engraftment of T-depleted HLA-mismatched transplants was first tested in patients with advanced leukemia [8]. Donor and recipients were incompatibile for two or three HLA-A, -B and -DR antigens of the unshared haplotype. Donor marrow was supplemented with G-CSF-mobilized PBHC and both components were depleted of T lymphocytes by soybean agglutination and E-rosetting [84]. The dose of T cells in the graft was in the range of $1–2 \times 10^5$/kg recipient body weight. The average dose of colony forming unit granulocyte-macrophage in the PBHC products was 7–10-fold greater than the dose in the marrow. Grafts contained a median of approximately 10×10^6 CD34$^+$ cells/kg. Patients received G-CSF after transplantation until engraftment occurred. Of the 36 adults in the trial 80% achieved primary sustained engraftment. Although no post-transplant immunosuppressive therapy was used as prophylaxis, the incidence of GVHD was significantly lower (20% vs. >80%) than in T-replete mismatched transplants [6]. These data compared favorably with historical experience using an identical T-depletion technique and

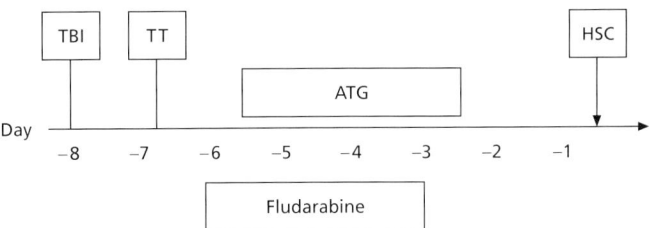

Fig. 82.5 Conditioning regimen used for transplantation of T-depleted peripheral blood hematopoietic transplantation (PBHT) in Perugia since 1995. Total body irradiation (TBI) is administered at the dose of 800 cGy in a single fraction at 16 cGy/min. Thiotepa (TT) is administered in a single dose of 10 mg/kg. Rabbit antihuman thymocyte globulin (ATG) (Fresenius, Bad Homburg, Germany) is administered at 5 mg/kg/day for 4 days. Fludarabine is administered at 40 mg/sqm/day for 4 days.

marrow from donors mismatched for two or three HLA-A, -B and -DR loci, in which the incidence of graft failure approached 50% [7,64].

A hypothesis to explain how the large dose of CD34$^+$ cells overcomes the immune barrier of residual donor-specific cytotoxic T-lymphocyte precursors (CTLp) of the host after an immunoablative and myeloablative conditioning is that CD34$^+$ cells exert "veto" activity. "Veto" cells neutralize CTLp directed against their antigens [85]. The veto activity of human CD34$^+$ cells, like other veto cells, appears to be mediated by apoptosis of antigen-specific T cells [86]. This hypothesis has been recently challenged by data demonstrating that G-CSF-mobilized CD34$^+$ cells induce cytolytic activity of alloreactive CTL [87].

Transplant protocols

The Perugia protocol for transplantation of HLA haplotype incompatible grafts evolved over time. In 1995, fludarabine was substituted for cyclophosphamide in the conditioning regimen in order to minimize nonhematologic toxicity (Fig. 82.5) and the number of CD3$^+$ cells in the graft was reduced to a median of 2.0×10^4/kg recipient body weight (range $1–3 \times 10^4$) by means of CD34$^+$ cell positive selection procedures with the aim of eliminating GVHD [43]. Since 1999, CD34$^+$ cells have been selected in a one-step procedure using the Clinimacs device (Miltenyi Biotech, Bergisch Gladbach, Germany). Furthermore, post-transplant G-CSF was no longer administered because experimental data suggested that it induces immunosuppression [88].

Infections

The high incidence of infection-related deaths in mismatched transplants has emerged as a major clinical issue. In the Perugia experience, approximately 1 in 4 transplant recipients dies of infection. Common fatal infections are from cytomegalovirus (CMV), fungi (*Aspergillus*) and yeasts (*Candida*), followed by bacteria (*Pseudomonas* and *Staphylococcus*) and occasionally protozoa (*Pneumocystis carinii* and *Toxoplasma*). Infections with Epstein–Barr virus (EBV) and EBV-associated lymphoproliferative disorders rarely occur when the graft is depleted not only of T cells but also of B cells, because B cells harbour latent EBV (see Chapter 56). In Perugia, all patients transplanted from a T-depleted HLA haplotype mismatched donor are treated according to the following protocol. For CMV-positive recipients, prophylaxis of reactivation consists of ganciclovir (10 mg/kg/day) from day –9 to day –2 and foscarnet (90 mg/kg/day) from day +4 to day +20. If CMV reactivates, patients receive ganciclovir (10 mg/kg/day) or foscarnet (180 mg/kg/day) until resolution. Antifungal prophylaxis includes amphotericin B (0.7 mg/kg/day in continuous infusion) or AmBisome (1 mg/kg/day) from day –9 to day +30, and itraconazole oral solution (400 mg/day) from day +31 to +120. Patients are treated with cyprofloxacin for selective gut decontamination, trimethoprim-sulfamethoxazole for *Pneumocystis carinii* prophylaxis,

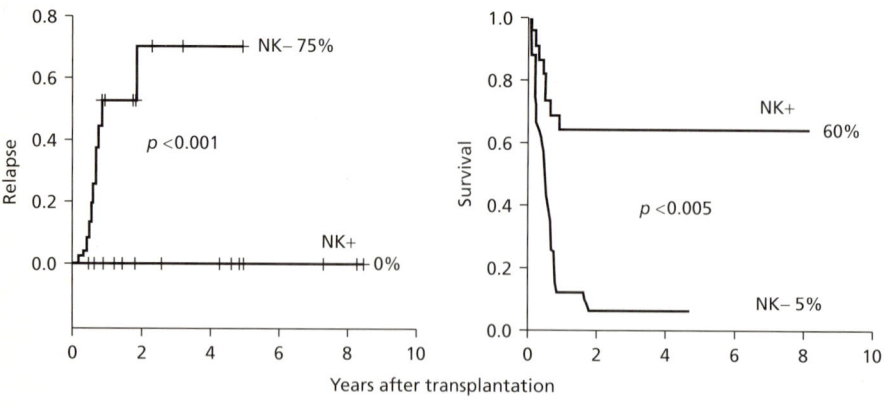

Fig. 82.6 Outcomes of human leukocyte antigen (HLA) haplotype-mismatched transplants for acute myeloid leukemia (AML) according to donor ability to mount natural killer (NK) alloreactivity against recipient targets. Such ability was characterized by the absence of recipient HLA class I alleles recognized by donor killer immunoglobulin-type receptors (KIRs), as defined in Table 82.6. Outcomes of 57 patients was classified on the basis of whether ($n = 20$) or not ($n = 37$) they had received a graft from donors with NK alloreactivity against the recipient. (Data from Ruggeri et al. [95].)

and intravenous immunoglobulins for replacement therapy. Patients are usually discharged 4–6 weeks after transplant. Careful monitoring on an outpatient basis is crucial for the following 6 months to detect and promptly treat infections at an early stage.

Immunodeficiency

Several mechanisms are responsible for patient immunodeficiency after transplantation. In adults, early immune recovery stems from expansion of mature T cells in the graft, and several months later from *de novo* production of naive T cells [89,90]. Intense conditioning regimens induce tissue damage that prevents T cell homing to peripheral lymphoid tissues, where generation and maintenance of T cell memory take place [91]. In HLA-mismatched transplants, the number of T cells in the graft must be sufficiently low to prevent GVHD. ATG or other anti-T cell antibodies administered in the conditioning regimen have a long half-life and inhibit T cell expansion after transplantation. Administration of G-CSF after transplantation is also immunosuppressive. G-CSF blocks IL-12 production in antigen-presenting cells (APCs) and decreases T cell responses to pathogens *in vitro* and *in vivo* after transplantation [88]. Since administration of G-CSF after transplantation was suspended in Perugia trials, engraftment rates have remained unchanged, and recovery rates of immune parameters including APC production of IL-12, $CD4^+$ cell numbers and type-1 helper function have markedly improved [88].

Survival

The revised transplant protocol including fludarabine was used to treat an initial series of 43 adult patients with high-risk acute leukemia [43]. Primary sustained engraftment was achieved in 41 of the 43 (95%) cases. Two patients rejected the first graft but engrafted after second transplants. Hematopoietic recovery was rapid with neutrophil counts reaching $1 \times 10^9/L$ and platelet counts $25 \times 10^9/L$ at a median of 12 (range 8–19) days and 18 (range 12–84) days, respectively. Analysis of DNA polymorphism documented complete donor-type chimerism in both peripheral blood and marrow cells of all evaluable patients. The incidence of grade II–IV GVHD was less than 5%. Twelve of the 43 (28%) patients were alive, leukemia-free, and with a Karnofsky score of 100 after a median follow-up of 18 months (range 8–30 months). The 2-year disease-free survival was $36 \pm 11\%$ for the 20 patients with AML and $17 \pm 7\%$ for the 23 patients with ALL ($p = 0.052$).

The status of leukemia and the length and intensity of chemotherapy before transplant influences patient outcome by selecting for resistant leukemia, and decreasing the patient tolerance to transplant therapies and complications. Because only patients with advanced disease have initially been offered transplantation from HLA haplotype mismatched donors, those pre-existing risks have undoubtedly confounded the interpretation of clinical results [43,92–94]. Inclusion of patients with less advanced leukemia in clinical trials has allowed analysing results according to disease risk at transplantation. A yet unpublished analysis of 65 patients transplanted in Perugia between January 1999 and September 2002 confirmed the very high engraftment rate and low incidence of GVHD achieved with the same transplant protocol in use since 1995. Patients had a median follow-up of 22 months (range 3–45 months). In ALL, disease-free survival was $40 \pm 16\%$ for 12 patients transplanted in remission and $13 \pm 11\%$ for 10 patients transplanted in relapse. In AML, disease-free survival was $60 \pm 11\%$ for 26 patients transplanted in remission and $10 \pm 8\%$ for 17 transplanted in relapse. By multivariable analysis, a new prognostic parameter has emerged as the most significant risk factor for the clinical outcome: lack of donor-vs.-recipient NK cell alloreactivity (see below) was associated with a hazard ratio of 6.1 (95%CI, range 2.6–14.9). AML patients who received transplants from donors with NK alloreactivity against recipient cells had a 2-year disease-free survival of 60% vs. 5% of those without such donors (Fig. 82.6) [95].

Studies in Tubingen

Thirty-nine children with high-risk acute leukemia were conditioned with chemotherapy or TBI-based regimens, and transplanted with PBHC grafts containing a median of 20×10^6 $CD34^+$ cells. Sustained engraftment was achieved in 38 (97%) cases, in four after second transplants from the same donors. The 1-year disease-free survival was 39% for 17 patients transplanted in remission, 13% for 14 patients in relapse and 75% for eight patients with nonmalignant disorders [94]. GVHD prevention was by *ex vivo* T-depletion, using the Clinimacs system to select for $CD34^+$ cells, and post-grafting immunosuppression with OKT3 and prednisone. The graft T cell content was less than $1 \times 10^4/kg$, a threshold dose below which GVHD was consistently prevented in patients with severe combined immunodeficiency syndrome transplanted from HLA-mismatched donors [35]. OKT3 administered after transplant may have contributed to T cell depletion *in vivo*, thereby reducing the incidence of GVHD. We believe that the critical component to facilitate engraftment of T-depleted HLA haplotype mismatched grafts without TBI, was the large number of hematopoietic cells transplanted.

Studies in Japan

A transplant trial of $CD34^+$ cells selected with the Isolex device (Nexell, Irvine, CA) enrolled 135 children, 64 of whom received two HLA locus mismatched grafts and 43 three locus mismatched grafts [92]. The median $CD34^+$ cell dose was $3.2 \times 10^6/kg$ for patients receiving marrow only, $5.5 \times 10^6/kg$ for those receiving PBHC only and $4.9 \times 10^6/kg$ for those receiving both marrow and PBHC. The median T cell doses were 6.0, 9.4 and $12.1 \times 10^4/kg$ for the three groups, respectively. Thus, the $CD34^+$ cell doses were lower than in the studies in Perugia, while the T cell doses were higher. Most patients received post-transplant immunosuppression for GVHD prevention. Graft failure occurred in 13% of patients with hematologic malignancies and 40% of patients with nonmalignant disease. The incidence of GVHD was 10% when ATG was included in the conditioning and 27% when it was not included. Disease-free survival at 5 years was 39% in standard-risk patients and 5% in high-risk patients. Results of this study support the hypothesis that standard doses of CD34+ cells are inadequate for consistent engraftment of HLA haplotype mismatched transplants, and that a moderate degree of T-depletion is inadequate to prevent GVHD without post-grafting immunosuppression.

Immunology of NK cells in T-depleted grafts from HLA-mismatched donors

T cell-mediated host-vs.-graft and graft-vs.-host reactions can be controlled to a large extent by a conditioning regimen of appropriate immunosuppressive intensity to prevent graft rejection, and extensive T-depletion of the graft to prevent GVHD. With T-depletion, NK cell alloreactivity has been recently appreciated as an important biologic phenomenon unique to HLA-mismatched transplants. Donor NK cells react against HLA-mismatched cells of the host and impact greatly on clinical outcomes of the transplant [reviewed in 96].

Killer cell immunoglobulin-like receptors

NK cell function is negatively regulated by inhibitory receptors for MHC class I molecules on target cells. Research in mice initially established that MHC class I molecules are inhibitory for specific NK cells, leading to the formulation of the "missing self" hypothesis [97]. Thus, NK cells kill target cells expressing decreased levels or no self-MHC class I molecules, such as some tumors or virally infected cells, and certain allogeneic cells [98]. Host NK cells can reject MHC class I-incompatible hematopoietic grafts in rodents [99].

In humans, inhibitory control of NK cell function is exerted by two families of receptors specific for HLA class I molecules, i.e. killer cell immunoglobulin-like receptors (KIRs) and the CD94/NKG2A receptor [reviewed in 100,101]. KIRs bind specific amino acid sequences shared only by certain groups of class I alleles. The best characterized KIRs include the following: KIR 2DL1 specific for HLA-Cw2 related alleles (group 1); KIR 2DL2/3 specific for HLA-Cw1 related alleles (group 1); and KIR 3DL1 specific for HLA-B antigens sharing the Bw4 supertype. KIRs are clonally distributed on NK cells. Although multiple receptors may be coexpressed on the same cell, there are cells in the repertoire that express a single KIR and which are blocked only by a specific (self) HLA class I molecule. Missing expression of the correct inhibitory class I molecule on allogeneic targets triggers NK cell alloreactivity [102–106]. CD94-NKG2A expression is regulated so that it fills the holes in the KIR repertoire, being expressed primarily in NK cells that do not express an inhibitory KIR for self-HLA class I. Alloreactive NK cells are not found among CD94-NKG2A positive NK cells because HLA-E, the ligand for this receptor, is expressed on cells from all individuals [107–109]. Thus, in any given individual, KIR-bearing NK cells make up a discrete repertoire, which is tolerant of self because it is blocked by the self class I molecules but may give rise to alloreactions when confronted with allogeneic targets failing to express its inhibitory class I.

KIR genes are part of the leukocyte receptor complex on chromosome 19p13.4 and are inherited independently of HLA genes on chromosome 6 [110]. During development, the HLA genotype dictates which KIR gene products are to be used as inhibitory receptors for self-HLA. In European populations most individuals have a full complement of KIR genes encoding inhibitory receptors [111,112], and can thus make an NK repertoire which is as diverse as the individual's HLA class I, the KIR ligands. Consequently, every donor may be expected to possess NK cells that are specific for each one of the KIR ligands he or she expresses.

Table 82.3 Human leukocyte antigen (HLA) class I specificity of well-characterized inhibitory killer immunoglobulin-like receptors (KIRs) expressed by human natural killer (NK) cells.*

KIR genes†	Encoded protein	HLA specificity‡
KIR 2DL1	P58.1 receptor	HLA-C group 2 i.e. Cw2 Sequence: Asn77, Lys80
KIR 2DL2/3	P58.2 receptor	HLA-C group 1 i.e. Cw1 Sequence: Ser77, Asn80
KIR 3DL1	P70/NKB1 receptor	HLA-Bw4-associated i.e. B27
KIR 3DL2	P140 receptor	HLA-A3/11

*Additional KIR genes include the following: KIR 2DL4 encodes for an inhibitory receptor specific for HLA-G, and KIR 2DS1, KIR 2DS2 and KIR 2DS4 encode for activating receptors P50.1, P50.2 and P50.3, respectively.
†KIR 2D refer to receptor molecules with two immunoglobulin-like domains whereas KIR 3D to those displaying three immunoglobulin-like domains. Receptors having a long inhibitory cytoplasmic tail are designated as L (long), whereas those having a short activating tail are termed S (short).
‡Two groups of HLA-C alleles can be distinguished on the basis of alternative amino acid sequence motif at position 77 and 80 of the α1 helix.

Two distinct allelic groups of HLA-C molecules are distinguished by KIRs on the basis of alternative amino acid sequence motifs at position 77 and 80 of the α 1 helix [106,113–115] (Table 82.3). Thus, NK cells expressing KIR 2DL1 are specific for HLA-C group 2 alleles, and they will kill cells expressing HLA-C group 1 but not group 2 alleles [116]. Vice versa, NK cells expressing either one of the two inhibitory receptors (KIR 2DL2 or KIR 2DL3) are specific for HLA-C group 1 alleles, and will kill target cells expressing HLA-C group 2 but not group 1 alleles (Fig. 82.7) [117]. NK cells coexpressing inhibitory receptors for both HLA-C groups are not alloreactive, presumably because every individual expresses alleles from either one or both HLA-C groups. Cells expressing the Bw4-specific, KIR 3DL1 receptor are also alloreactive and kill Bw4− (Bw6+) cells, but not cells expressing Bw4. Table 82.4 shows HLA-Bw4-associated antigens, and HLA-C group 1 and group 2 alleles, along with the amino acid sequences that are the basis of the group classification. As new HLA-C alleles are discovered, they are grouped according to their amino acid sequence. There was a high frequency of alloreactive NK clones in all 95 donors against recipients mismatched for one HLA-C group, and all 50 such donors tested for the KIR genotype were positive for the predicted KIR 2DL1, KIR 2DL2Q2 or KIR 2DL3 gene. Conversely, only 19 of 29 HLA-BW4+ donors had alloreactive NK clones against HLA-Bw4− recipients, although 49 of 50 HLA-Bw4+ donors were positive for the HLA-Bw4 receptor KIR 3DLI gene (Andrea Velerdi, unpublished data). Based on these studies, we surmise that HLA-C typing predicts with good approximation the donor's potential to exert NK alloreactivity against a given recipient, while NK alloreactivity against HLA-Bw4− recipients cannot be predicted by HLA typing alone and has to be tested.

NK cell triggering receptors

When a target cell does not express HLA class I ligands for the inhibitory receptors (e.g. allogeneic cells), the effector function of NK cells may be induced by a series of NK receptors that are involved in triggering NK-mediated cytotoxicity and cytokine/chemokine release. KIR genes KIR 2DS1, KIR 2DS2, KIR 2DS3, KIR 2DS4 and KIR 3DS1 encode for activating receptors [118,119]. While KIR 2DS1 binds HLA-C alleles, the ligands for other activating KIRs are unknown and so is their function.

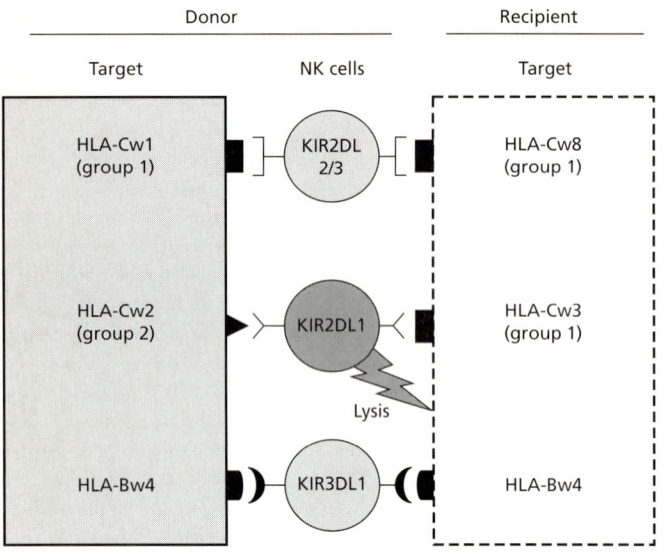

Fig. 82.7 Donor-vs.-recipient natural killer (NK) cell alloreactivity in human leukocyte antigen (HLA) mismatched transplants. This figure illustrates the example of a donor–recipient pair with a combination of mismatched HLA-C antigens, resulting in donor NK cell alloreactivity against recipient targets. The top donor NK cell expresses KIR 2DL2/3 and is blocked by HLA-C group 1 antigens, -Cw1 on donor cells and -Cw8 on recipient cells. The bottom donor NK cell expresses KIR 3DL1 that is blocked by Bw4 on both recipient and donor cells. The middle donor NK cell expresses KIR 2DL1 that is blocked by donor (self)-HLA-Cw2 (an HLA-C group 2 antigen), but not by the recipient HLA-Cw3 (an HLA-C group 1 antigen). Consequently, this NK cell is alloreactive and lyses recipients' cells (lightning bolt). When donors and recipients were mismatched for HLA-Bw4 or an HLA-C group allele so that donor KIRs were not blocked, as in this example, 100% of the donors tested had alloreactive NK cells in their repertoires. On the other hand, when donors and recipients were matched for HLA-Bw4 and both HLA-C groups, no donors' alloreactive NK cells were found [95].

The triggering NK receptors have recently included a heterogeneous family of NK specific immunoglobulin-like molecules termed natural cytotoxicity receptors (NCR), including NKp30, NKp46 and NKp44 [119], and by NKG2D, a member of the lectin superfamily which is shared by NK and cytolytic T cells [119–121]. The cellular ligands for NCR remain to be determined, while the class I-like molecules MICA/B [122] and ULBP [123] are the ligands for NKG2D. Both NCR and NKG2D transduce activating signals because of their physical association with immunoreceptor tyrosine-based activating motives (ITAM) containing polypeptides.

The function of NK cell triggering receptors is normally counterbalanced by that of the HLA-specific inhibitory receptors. However, this balance is rapidly altered as soon as the magnitude of the inhibitory signals is decreased by an insufficient engagement of the HLA-specific inhibitory receptors. Conversely, certain tissues, even when they fail to express inhibitory HLA class I molecules, display no susceptibility to NK-mediated cytotoxicity. In this case the level of expression of adhesion molecules and/or ligands recognized by the triggering receptors may be insufficient to induce NK cell activation. This may explain why ALL cells are resistant to killing by alloreactive NK cells, and why NK cells do not mediate GVHD [95,124; also see below].

Impact of donor-vs.-recipient NK cell alloreactivity in transplantation

Because NK cells distinguish groups of HLA class I molecules, HLA-incompatible transplants can be classified in at least two categories.

Table 82.4 Human leukocyte antigen (HLA)-C group 1 and group 2 alleles and HLA-Bw4-associated antigens.

HLA-C group 1 (Ser 77, Asn 80)		HLA-C group 2 (Asn 77, Lys 80)		HLA-Bw4-associated antigens
Antigens	Alleles	Antigens	Alleles	
Cw1	C*0102–9			B5
		Cw2	C*0202–5	B5102
Cw3	C*0302–6	Cw3	C*0307	B5103
	C*0308–9		C*0310	B13
	C*0310–14		C*0315	B17
	C*0316			B27
		Cw4	C*0401	B37
			C*0403–10	B38
		Cw5	C*0501–6	B44
		Cw6	C*0602–8	B47
				B49
Cw7	C*0701–6	Cw7	C*0707	B51
	C*0708		C*0709	B52
	C*0710–17			B53
Cw8	C*0801–9			B57
				B58
Cw12	C*1202–3	Cw12	C*1204–5	B59
	C*1206			B63
	C*1208			B77
Cw14	C*1402–3			
	C*1405			
Cw15	C*1507	Cw15	C*1502–6	
			C*1508–11	
Cw16	C*1601	Cw16	C*1602	
	C*1604			
		Cw17	C*1701–3	
		Cw18	C*1802	

C*0310 (Ser 77, Lys 80) belongs to both HLA-C group 1 and group 2, i.e. it blocks natural killer (NK) cells expressing any HLA-C-specific receptor, but it does not block NK cells expressing the Bw4-specific receptor [106]. Patients who express C*0310 should be considered to express both HLA-C groups. C*1404 (Asn 77, Asn 80) does not belong to either HLA-C group 1 or group 2, i.e. it does not block NK cells expressing either class of HLA-C specific receptors [106]. Expression of C*1404 in a patient behaves with respect to NK cell recognition, as if the patient does not express that HLA-C allele. C*1207 Gly 77, Asn 80, cannot be assigned to either group based on its amino acid sequence, and still needs to be tested functionally.

1 "NK alloreactive" transplants in which grafted NK cells do not recognize the class I alleles of the host and can kill host targets.
2 "NK nonalloreactive" transplants in which donor-vs.-recipient NK alloreactivity does not occur because all grafted NK cells recognize the HLA class I alleles of the host, and are blocked (Table 82.5).

Role of donor NK cells in MHC-incompatible grafts in rodents

Experimental evidence suggests that donor NK cells attack hematopoietic cells of the host including leukemia cells, while sparing other tissues [95]. In mice, activated donor NK cells ablated the host immune system, thereby allowing engraftment of marrow transplants mismatched for one MHC haplotype, despite recipient conditioning with low-intensity regimens. Donor alloreactive NK cells protected mice from GVHD by

Table 82.5 Donor–recipient combinations predicting donor natural killer (NK) cell alloreactivity against the recipient.

Recipient HLA type*			HLA type of NK alloreactive donor†
HLA-C group 1	HLA-C group 2	HLA-Bw4	
+	+	+	None found
+	+	−	HLA-Bw4
+	−	+	HLA-C group 2
−	+	+	HLA-C group 1
+	−	−	HLA-C group 2 and/or HLA-Bw4
−	+	−	HLA-C group 1 and/or HLA-Bw4

*One additional rare mismatch associated with possible NK alloreactivity is between the HLA-A3/11 negative recipient and HLA-A3/A11 positive donor. In the study by Ruggeri et al. [95], the HLA-A3/A11 mismatch was never found alone but always in conjunction with HLA-C group mismatches. Therefore, no prediction can be made on the association between mismatch for HLA-A3/11 and donor NK alloreactivity against the recipient.
†Donor NK cells are blocked specifically by the HLA group(s) indicated in the donor column and are alloreactive against recipients that do not express this HLA group.

ablating recipient APCs that are responsible for initiating GVHD [125]. Thus, NK conditioning allowed the safe infusion of otherwise lethal doses of allogeneic T cells. Finally, human alloreactive NK clones cleared human leukemia in immunodeficient mice [95]. These preclinical data in mice demonstrated that donor NK cells inhibit graft rejection, GVHD and leukemia relapse in MHC-incompatible recipients.

Human NK cell clones isolated from recipients of HLA-mismatched grafts

After transplantation of T-depleted PBHC from NK alloreactive donors, Ruggeri et al. [124] observed that the engrafted cells give rise to an NK cell wave of donor origin. Alloreactive NK clones of donor origin were isolated in high frequency, and showed the ability to kill host lymphocytes. Killing could be blocked only by targets expressing the donor HLA class I allele that was missing in the recipient. Alloreactive NK clones killed all AML and CML cells tested, but only a rare example of ALL. ALL resistance to killing was associated with the lack of expression of leukocyte function-associated-1, a leukocyte adhesion receptor. These data suggested, for the first time, that donor alloreactive NK cells could enhance the probability of cure for patients with myeloid leukemia.

Donor-vs.-recipient NK cell alloreactivity and outcome of HLA-mismatched transplants

Ruggeri et al. [95] evaluated the impact of donor NK cell alloreactivity against recipient targets on rejection, GVHD, relapse and survival in 92 patients with high-risk leukemia, who had received hematopoietic transplants from HLA haplotype mismatched relatives. Transplants were classified according to the presence of recipient HLA-B or -C alleles recognized by donor inhibitory receptors, as predicted by donor HLA typing. Donors were also evaluated for NK alloreactivity by screening their NK repertoire by the analysis of NK clones. Isolation of donor NK clones able to kill recipient targets correlated closely with the recipient lacking HLA-B or -C alleles recognized by the donor inhibitory KIRs. Transplantation from NK alloreactive donors totally protected from rejection, GVHD and AML relapse (Table 82.6). In AML ($n = 57$), disease-free survival after a median follow-up of 5 years (range 1–8 years) was 60% with NK alloreactive donors vs. 5% ($p < 0.0005$) (Fig. 82.6). A multivariable analysis, which considered variables affecting transplantation outcome, such as age, status of disease at transplant, conditioning regimens and numbers of CD34$^+$ cells and T cells in the graft, showed that

Table 82.6 Outcomes of human leukocyte antigen (HLA) haplotype mismatched transplants according to donor natural killer (NK) mismatch against recipient targets. Mismatch was characterized by the absence of recipient HLA class I alleles recognized by donor killer immunoglobulin-like receptors (KIRs), as defined in Tables 82.3–82.5 and Fig. 82.6. Twenty-six pairs (11 in acute lymphoblastic leukemia [ALL] and 15 in acute myeloid leukemia [AML]) were mismatched for HLA-C groups, and eight (three in ALL and five in AML) were mismatched for the HLA-Bw4 group. (Reprinted with permission from Ruggeri et al. [95].)

Donor NK mismatch against recipient targets	No	Yes
Number of transplants	58	34
Donors displaying anti-recipient NK clones	1/58	34/34*
Disease:		
ALL	21	14
AML	37	20
Transplantation outcomes:		
Rejection	16%	0%*
Acute GVHD, grade II	14%	0%*
Probability of relapse at 5 years:		
ALL	90%	85%
AML	75%	0%**

*$p = 0.01$; **$p < 0.0008$.

the presence of patient HLA-B or -C alleles recognized by the predicted donor inhibitory receptors was the only independent factor associated with poor outcome in AML (hazard ratio 0.33, 95%CI, range 0.11–0.94; $p < 0.04$) but had no effect on ALL (Table 82.6). Since this report was published, another 20 patients with AML have received HLA haplotype mismatched transplants in Perugia. With a follow-up of 0.25–9.75 years, an analysis of 77 transplants for AML confirms the striking survival advantage of transplantation from NK alloreactive donors with a probability of survival of 56% vs. 5% ($p < 0.001$).

Based on these results, the Perugia transplant team has revised the criteria for the selection of HLA-mismatched donors for transplantation of T-depleted grafts. Donor selection should involve a deliberate search for the "perfect mismatch" at HLA class I to drive donor-vs.-recipient NK cell alloreactivity [126]. Selection for NK mismatched donors should be based on high-resolution HLA class I typing of parents and siblings and, if necessary, other family members such as aunts, uncles and cousins or, perhaps, unrelated donors. Such an extended search would raise the chance of finding an NK alloreactive donor from 30% for the use of any random donor, to approximately 60%. About 30% of the population express class I alleles belonging to one or more of the three major HLA class I groups (HLA-C group 1, HLA-C group 2 and HLA-Bw4-associated antigens) and will therefore block all known NK cell patterns of reactivity from every donor. For these individuals, it would be unlikely to find an NK alloreactive donor. Conversely, recipients who express HLA alleles belonging to one or two of these three HLA class I groups, have a good chance of finding NK alloreactive donors. In this case, the donor search should proceed to find the relative who expresses any one of the alleles in the HLA class I group not expressed by the patient.

Other studies on the outcome of HLA-mismatched transplants according to predicted donor NK cell alloreactivity

Approximately half of unrelated donor HCT compatible for HLA-A, -B and -DR antigens are mismatched for one or more HLA-A, -B or -C alleles. Therefore, donor NK cell alloreactivity may also occur with unrelated donor HCT, if the recipient lacks the appropriate ligand for donor inhibitory KIRs. In a study of 130 unrelated donor HCTs by Giebel et al. [127], all patients received GVHD prophylaxis including CSP/MTX and pretransplant ATG. Twenty patients lacked the appropriate ligand for donor KIRs and fared better that the other 110 patients with the appropriate KIR ligand: grade III–IV acute GVHD was 0% vs. 15% ($p = 0.08$), relapse was 6% vs. 21% ($p = 0.07$), nonrelapse mortality was 6% vs. 40% ($p = 0.01$), survival at 4.5 years was 87% vs. 48% ($p = 0.006$); and disease-free survival was 87% vs. 39% ($p = 0.007$). Albeit preliminary, these results support the model of NK alloreactivity proposed by Ruggeri et al. [95].

Outcome of HLA-incompatible HCT did not correlate in every study with the presence or absence of appropriate recipient ligands for donor inhibitory KIRs. Davies et al. [128] reported the results of unrelated donor HCT mismatched for at least one HLA class I locus in 175 patients with a variety of diseases. GVHD prophylaxis included CSP with partial T-cell depletion in one-third of patients, and CSP/MTX with no T-depletion in the others. There were no apparent advantages for the patients whose HLA class I alleles were recognized by donor inhibitory KIRs [128]. In a study of unrelated donor HCT in 122 CML patients, patients mismatched for HLA-C alleles recognized by donor inhibitory KIRs had longer survival and disease-free survival than patients mismatched for HLA-C alleles not recognized by donor KIRs [129]. De Santis et al. [130] studied 56 patients transplanted from HLA haplotype mismatched donors: engraftment was 90% in the presence of recipient HLA-C alleles recognized by donor inhibitory KIRs, and 55% in their absence ($p = 0.034$). Among patients with engraftment, GVHD was 82% and 40% ($p = 0.02$), and among all patients survival was 28% and 7%, respectively ($p = 0.05$). While the methods for GVHD prophylaxis were not provided in the report, the high incidence of GVHD suggested an insufficient degree of T-cell depletion. Of interest, the presence of four or more activating KIRs in the donor genome was associated with GVHD ($p = 0.007$) [130].

How can we reconcile these apparently conflicting results? On average, T-replete marrows used in the studies discussed above contain 4 log more T cells than T-depleted PBHTs utilized for the studies in Perugia. It is possible that the expansion of alloreactive T cells in the donor graft and the resulting GVHD may exert such a strong influence on clinical outcomes to obscure the effects of donor stem cell-derived alloreactive NK cells. Further, T-replete grafts depend on post-transplant immunosuppression to control GVHD and this treatment may inhibit NK cell repopulation and function. ATG causes in vivo depletion of recipient T cells favoring engraftment, and donor T cells reducing the incidence of acute and chronic GVHD. Thus, ATG used in the study by Giebel et al. may have caused depletion of donor T cells in vivo and may have permitted NK alloreactions to manifest. The numbers of hematopoietic cells in the graft influence the transplant outcome. In the study by Giebel et al. the mean marrow cell dose was 4.4×10^8/kg, more than twice the number in the report by Davies et al., where the dose was 2×10^8/kg. We surmise that the clinical effects of donor alloreactive NK cells may only become apparent after a T-depleted graft, where no post-grafting immunosuppression is administered, and that pretransplant ATG achieves an adequate degree of T-depletion and low incidence of GVHD for the effects of NK cells to become appreciable. Prospective protocols are needed to assess the potential benefits of NK cell alloreactivity on transplant outcome.

The KIR genomic region displays extensive diversity through variation in gene content and allelic polymorphism within individual KIR genes [110]. Diversity by gene content alone gives rise to at least 20 different KIR haplotypes that vary for their content of inhibitory and activating KIRs. The study by De Santis et al. [130] suggests that the donor KIR genotype may affect outcome of transplantation. These effects may not be mediated by NK cells because some memory T cells also express KIRs [131]. KIR genotypes enriched for activating KIRs have been associated with rheumatoid arthritis and progression of acquired immune deficiency syndrome (AIDS) [132,133]. In addition to genomic diversity, KIR allelic polymorphism imposes extensive individual variability, the relevance of which remains to be explored. Thus, the correlation between transplant outcome and donor NK alloreactivity directed to the biallelic polymorphism at the HLA-C locus may represent the initial step in our understanding of a much more complex immune regulatory system.

Conclusions

Transplant results have demonstrated that increasing degree of donor HLA incompatibility is associated with a proportionally increased risk of graft failure, GVHD and transplant-related mortality. Initial studies utilizing T-replete marrow transplants found that donor incompatibility for two or three HLA antigens represented a formidable barrier to success, did not allow sufficient control of GVHD and led to unacceptably low patient survival. As post-transplant immunosuppression protocols have failed to control GVHD from highly mismatched donors, great effort has been invested to test the use of T-depleted marrow grafts. Such studies showed a decrease in acute and chronic GVHD, but at the expense of increased graft failure and leukemia relapse, and impaired immune reconstitution, leading to no advantage in survival. The most recent advance in HLA-mismatched HCT has been the use of hematopoietic growth factors to mobilize PBHC. Transplantation from a full HLA haplotype mismatched family member is nowadays a viable option for patients with acute leukemia at high risk of relapse who urgently need a transplant and who do not have a matched unrelated donor. The mismatched transplant relies for its success on the combined action of:

1 high-intensity conditioning regimens to ensure the lowest possible residual leukemia burden and maximal degree of immunosuppression;
2 very high doses of hematopoietic cells to ensure engraftment across the HLA barrier;
3 extensive T-cell depletion of the graft to prevent GVHD;
4 no post-transplant immunosuppression to ensure undisturbed immune reconstitution; and
5 donor-vs.-recipient NK cell alloreactivity to facilitate engraftment, prevent GVHD and exert antileukemia effects.

Exploiting NK cell alloreactivity may enhance the efficacy and safety of HLA-mismatched transplants.

References

1 Ottinger H, Grosse-Wilde M, Schmitz A, Grosse-Wilde H. Immunogenetic marrow donor search for 1012 patients: a retrospective analysis of strategies, outcome and costs. *Bone Marrow Transplant* 1994; **14** (Suppl 4): S34–S38.

2 Rubinstein P, Carrier C, Scaradavou A et al. Outcomes among 562 recipients of placental-blood transplants from unrelated donors. *N Engl J Med* 1998; **339**: 1565–77.

3 Laughlin MJ, Barker J, Bambach B et al. Hematopoietic engraftment and survival in adult recipients of umbilical-cord blood from unrelated donors. *N Engl J Med* 2001; **344**: 1815–22.

4 Beatty PG, Clift RA, Mickelson EM et al. Marrow transplantation from related donors other than HLA-identical siblings. *N Engl J Med* 1985; **313**: 765–71.

5 Beelen DW, Ottinger HD, Elmaagacli A et al. Transplantation of filgrastim-mobilized peripheral blood stem cells from HLA-identical sibling or alternative family donors in patients with hematologic malignancies: a prospective comparison on clinical outcome, immune reconstitution, and hematopoietic chimerism. *Blood* 1997; **90**: 4725–35.

6 Anasetti C, Beatty PG, Storb R et al. Effect of HLA incompatibility on graft-versus-host disease, relapse, and survival after marrow transplantation for patients with leukemia or lymphoma. *Hum Immunol* 1990; **29**: 79–91.

7 Ash RC, Horowitz MM, Gale RP et al. Bone marrow transplantation from related donors other than HLA-identical siblings: effect of T-cell depletion. *Bone Marrow Transplant* 1991; **7**: 443–52.

8 Aversa F, Tabilio A, Terenzi A et al. Successful engraftment of T-depleted haploidentical "three-loci" incompatible transplants in leukemia patients by addition of recombinant human granulocyte colony-stimulating factor-mobilized peripheral blood progenitor cells to bone marrow inoculum. *Blood* 1994; **84**: 3948–55.

9 Benichou G, Tam RC, Soares LR, Fedoseyeva EV. Indirect T-cell allorecognition: perspectives for peptide-based therapy in transplantation. *Immunol Today* 1997; **18**: 67–71.

10 Anasetti C, Amos D, Beatty PG et al. Effect of HLA compatibility on engraftment of bone marrow transplants in patients with leukemia or lymphoma. *N Engl J Med* 1989; **320**: 197–204.

11 Schreuder GM, Hurley CK, Marsh SG et al. The HLA dictionary 2001: a summary of HLA-A, -B, -C, -DRB1/3/4/5, -DQB1 alleles and their association with serologically defined HLA-A, -B, -C, -DR and -DQ antigens. *Tissue Antigens* 2001; **58**: 109–40.

12 Choo SY, Fan LA, Hansen JA. A novel HLA-B27 allele maps B27 allospecificity to the region around position 70 in the alpha 1 domain. *J Immunol* 1991; **147**: 174–80.

13 Petersdorf EW, Longton GM, Anasetti C et al. Association of HLA-C disparity with graft failure after marrow transplantation from unrelated donors. *Blood* 1997; **89**: 1818–23.

14 Petersdorf EW, Gooley TA, Anasetti C et al. Optimizing outcome after unrelated marrow transplantation by comprehensive matching of HLA class I and II alleles in the donor and recipient. *Blood* 1998; **92**: 3515–20.

15 Sasazuki T, Juji T, Morishima Y et al. Effect of matching of class I alleles on clinical outcome after transplantation of hematopoietic stem cells from an unrelated donor. *N Engl J Med* 1998; **339**: 1177–85.

16 Flomenberg N, Baxter-Lowe LA, Confer D et al. Impact of HLA class I and class II high resolution matching on outcomes of unrelated donor BMT. *Blood* 2001; **98**: 813 [Abstract].

17 Morishima Y, Sasazuki T, Inoko H et al. The clinical significance of human leukocyte antigen (HLA) allele compatibility in patients receiving a marrow transplant from serologically HLA-A, HLA-B, and HLA-DR matched unrelated donors. *Blood* 2002; **99**: 4200–6.

18 Petersdorf EW, Longton GM, Anasetti C et al. The significance of HLA-DRB1 matching on clinical outcome after HLA-A, B, DR identical unrelated donor marrow transplantation. *Blood* 1995; **86**: 1606–13.

19 Petersdorf EW, Kollman C, Hurley CK et al. Effect of HLA class II gene disparity on clinical outcome in unrelated donor hematopoietic cell transplantation for chronic myeloid leukemia: the US National Marrow Donor Program Experience. *Blood* 2001; **98**: 2922–9.

20 Petersdorf EW, Longton GM, Anasetti C et al. Definition of HLA-DQ as a transplantation antigen. *Proc Natl Acad Sci U S A* 1996; **93**: 15358–63.

21 Petersdorf EW, Smith AG, Mickelson EM et al. The role of HLA-DPB1 disparity in the development of acute graft-versus-host disease following unrelated donor marrow transplantation. *Blood* 1993; **81**: 1923–32.

22 Varney MD, Lester S, McCluskey J et al. Matching for HLA DPA1 and DPB1 alleles in unrelated bone marrow transplantation. *Hum Immunol* 1999; **60**: 532–8.

23 Petersdorf EW, Gooley T, Malkki M et al. The biological significance of HLA-DP gene variation in haematopoietic cell transplantation. *Br J Haematol* 2001; **112**: 988–94.

24 Ottinger HD, Rebmann V, Pfeiffer KA et al. Positive serum crossmatch as predictor for graft failure in HLA-mismatched allogeneic blood stem cell transplantation. *Transplantation* 2002; **73**: 1280–5.

25 National Institutes of Health lymphocyte microcytotoxicity technique. In: *NIAID Manual of Tissue Typing Techniques*. DHEW Publication No. [NIH] 80–545. Atlanta: National Institute of Allergy and Infectious Disease, 1979: 39.

26 Anasetti C. The role of the immunogenetics laboratory in marrow transplantation. *Arch Pathol Lab Med* 1991; **115**: 288–92.

27 Kaufman R. HLA prediction model for extended family matches. *Bone Marrow Transplant* 1995; **15**: 279–82.

28 Schipper RF, D'Amaro J, Oudshoorn M. The probability of finding a suitable related donor for bone marrow transplantation in extended families. *Blood* 1996; **87**: 800–4.

29 Mori M, Graves M, Milford EL, Beatty PG. Computer program to predict likelihood of finding and HLA-matched donor: methodology, validation, and application. *Biol Blood Marrow Transplant* 1996; **2**: 134–44.

30 Kernan NA, Flomenberg N, Dupont B, O'Reilly RJ. Graft rejection in recipients of T-depleted HLA-nonidentical marrow transplants for leukemia: identification of host-derived antidonor allocytotoxic T lymphocytes. *Transplantation* 1987; **43**: 842–7.

31 Barge AJ, Johnson G, Witherspoon R, Torok-Storb B. Antibody-mediated marrow failure after allogeneic bone marrow transplantation. *Blood* 1989; **74**: 1477–80.

32 Nemunaitis J, Singer JW, Buckner CD et al. Use of recombinant human granulocyte-macrophage colony-stimulating factor in graft failure after bone marrow transplantation. *Blood* 1990; **76**: 245–53.

33 Anasetti C, Hansen J. Bone marrow transplantation from HLA-partially matched related donors and unrelated volunteer donors. In: Forman SJ, Blume KG, Thomas ED, eds. *Bone Marrow Transplantation*. Boston: Blackwell Science, 1994: 665–79.

34 Petersdorf EW, Hansen JA, Martin PJ et al. Major-histocompatibility-complex class I alleles and antigens in hematopoietic-cell transplantation. *N Engl J Med* 2001; **345**: 1794–800.

35 O'Reilly RJ, Keever CA, Small TN, Brochstein J. The use of HLA-non-identical T-depleted marrow transplants for correction of severe combined immunodeficiency disease. *Immunodeficiency Rev* 1989; **1**: 273–309.

36 Le DF, Blanche S, Keable H et al. Successful HLA nonidentical bone marrow transplantation in three patients with the leukocyte adhesion deficiency. *Blood* 1989; **74**: 512–6.

37 Mackall CL, Fleisher TA, Brown MR et al. Lymphocyte depletion during treatment with intensive chemotherapy for cancer. *Blood* 1994; **84**: 2221–8.

38 Beatty PG, Di Bartolomeo P, Storb R et al. Treatment of aplastic anemia with marrow grafts from related donors other than HLA genotypically matched siblings. *Clin Transpl* 1987; **1**: 117–24.

39 Lamparelli T, van Lint MT, Gualandi F et al. Alternative donor transplants for patients with advanced hematologic malignancies, conditioned with thiotepa, cyclophosphamide and antithymocyte globulin. *Bone Marrow Transplant* 2000; **26**: 1305–11.

40 Slattery JT, Sanders JE, Buckner CD et al. Graft-rejection and toxicity following bone marrow transplantation in relation to busulfan pharmacokinetics. *Bone Marrow Transplant* 1995; **16**: 31–42.

41 Gaziev D, Galimberti M, Lucarelli G et al. Bone marrow transplantation from alternative donors for thalassemia: HLA-phenotypically identical relative and HLA-nonidentical sibling or parent transplants. *Bone Marrow Transplant* 2000; **25**: 815–21.

42 La Nasa G, Giardini C, Argiolu F et al. Unrelated donor bone marrow transplantation for thalassemia: the effect of extended haplotypes. *Blood* 2002; **99**: 4350–6.

43 Aversa F, Tabilio A, Velardi A et al. Treatment of high-risk acute leukemia with T-depleted stem cells from related donors with one fully mismatched HLA haplotype. *N Engl J Med* 1998; **339**: 1186–93.

44 Marmont AM, Horowitz MM, Gale RP et al. T-cell depletion of HLA-identical transplants in leukemia. *Blood* 1991; **78**: 2120–30.

45 Powles RL, Morgenstern GR, Kay HE et al. Mismatched family donors for bone marrow transplantation as treatment for acute leukaemia. *Lancet* 1983; **1**: 612–5.

46 Servida P, Gooley T, Hansen JA. Improved survival of haploidentical related donor marrow

46 transplants mismatched for HLA-A or B versus HLA-DR. *Blood* 1996; **88**: 484 [Abstract].
47 Przepiorka D, Khouri I, Ippoliti C *et al*. Tacrolimus and minidose methotrexate for prevention of acute graft-versus-host disease after HLA-mismatched marrow or blood stem cell transplantation. *Bone Marrow Transplant* 1999; **24**: 763–8.
48 Sullivan KM, Agura E, Anasetti C *et al*. Chronic graft-versus-host disease and other late complications of bone marrow transplantation. *Semin Hematol* 1991; **28**: 250–9.
49 Szydlo R, Goldman JM, Klein JP *et al*. Results of allogeneic bone marrow transplants for leukemia using donors other than HLA-identical siblings. *J Clin Oncol* 1997; **15**: 1767–77.
50 Sierra J, Storer B, Hansen JA *et al*. Transplantation of marrow cells from unrelated donors for treatment of high-risk acute leukemia: the effect of leukemic burden, donor HLA-matching, and marrow cell dose. *Blood* 1997; **89**: 4226–35.
51 Elmaagacli AH, Beelen DW, Opalka B, Seeber S, Schaefer UW. The risk of residual molecular and cytogenetic disease in patients with Philadelphia-chromosome positive first chronic phase myelogenous leukemia is reduced after transplantation of allogeneic peripheral blood stem cells compared with bone marrow. *Blood* 1999; **94**: 384–9.
52 Appelbaum FR. Choosing the source of stem cells for allogeneic transplantation: no longer a peripheral issue. *Blood* 1999; **94**: 381–3.
53 Anderson G, Moore NC, Owen JJ, Jenkinson EJ. Cellular interactions in thymocyte development. *Annu Rev Immunol* 1996; **14**: 73–99.
54 Katz DH, Skidmore BJ, Katz LR, Bogowitz CA. Adaptive differentiation of murine lymphocytes. I. Both T and B lymphocytes differentiating in F1 transplanted to parental chimeras manifest preferential cooperative activity for partner lymphocytes derived from the same parental type corresponding to the chimeric host. *J Exp Med* 1978; **148**: 727–45.
55 Mackall CL, Gress RE. Pathways of T-cell regeneration in mice and humans: implications for bone marrow transplantation and immunotherapy. *Immunol Rev* 1997; **157**: 61–72.
56 Albi N, Ruggeri L, Aversa F *et al*. Natural killer (NK) cell function and antileukemic activity of a large population of $CD3^+/CD8^+$ T-cells expressing NK receptors for major histocompatibility complex class I after "three-loci" HLA-incompatible bone marrow transplantation. *Blood* 1996; **87**: 3993–4000.
57 Douek DC, Vescio RA, Betts MR *et al*. Assessment of thymic output in adults after haematopoietic stem-cell transplantation and prediction of T-cell reconstitution. *Lancet* 2000; **355**: 1875–81.
58 Fry TJ, Mackall CL. Interleukin-7: from bench to clinic. *Blood* 2002; **99**: 3892–904.
59 Min D, Taylor PA, Panoskaltsis-Mortari A *et al*. Protection from thymic epithelial cell injury by keratinocyte growth factor: a new approach to improve thymic and peripheral T-cell reconstitution after bone marrow transplantation. *Blood* 2002; **99**: 4592–600.
60 Drobyski WR, Klein J, Flomenberg N *et al*. Superior survival associated with transplantation of matched unrelated versus one-antigen-mismatched unrelated or highly human leukocyte antigen-disparate haploidentical family donor marrow grafts for the treatment of hematologic malignancies: establishing a treatment algorithm for recipients of alternative donor grafts. *Blood* 2002; **99**: 806–14.

61 Reisner Y, Kapoor N, Kirkpatrick D *et al*. Transplantation for severe combined immunodeficiency with HLA-A, -B, -D, -DR incompatible parental marrow cells fractionated by soybean agglutinin and sheep red blood cells. *Blood* 1983; **61**: 341–8.
62 Prentice HG, Janossy G, Price-Jones L *et al*. Depletion of T lymphocytes in donor marrow prevents significant graft-versus-host disease in matched allogeneic leukemic marrow transplant recipients. *Lancet* 1984; **1**: 472–6.
63 Hale G, Cobbold S, Waldmann H. T-cell depletion with Campath-1 in allogeneic bone marrow transplantation. *Transplantation* 1988; **45**: 753–9.
64 O'Reilly RJ, Keever C, Kernan NA *et al*. HLA nonidentical T-depleted marrow transplants: a comparison of results in patients treated for leukemia and severe combined immunodeficiency disease. *Transplant Proc* 1987; **19**: 55–60.
65 Gale RP, Reisner Y. Graft rejection and graft-versus-host disease: mirror images. *Lancet* 1986; **1**: 1468–70.
66 Martin PJ, Hansen JA, Torok-Storb B *et al*. Graft failure in patients receiving T-depleted HLA-identical allogeneic marrow transplants. *Bone Marrow Transplant* 1988; **3**: 445–56.
67 Soiffer RJ, Mauch P, Fairclough D *et al*. $CD6^+$ T-depleted allogeneic bone marrow transplantation from genotypically HLA nonidentical related donors. *Biol Blood Marrow Transplant* 1997; **3**: 11–17.
68 Henslee-Downey PJ, Parrish RS, MacDonald JS *et al*. Combined *in vitro* and *in vivo* T lymphocyte depletion for the control of graft-versus-host disease following haploidentical marrow transplant. *Transplantation* 1996; **61**: 738–45.
69 Henslee-Downey PJ, Abhyankar SH, Parrish RS *et al*. Use of partially mismatched related donors extends access to allogeneic marrow transplant. *Blood* 1997; **89**: 3864–72.
70 Godder KT, Hazlett LJ, Abhyankar SH *et al*. Partially mismatched related donor bone marrow transplantation for pediatric patients with acute leukemia: younger donors and absence of peripheral blast improve outcome. *J Clin Oncol* 2000; **18**: 1856–66.
71 Chiang KY, Van Rhee F, Godder K *et al*. Allogeneic bone marrow transplantation from partially mismatched related donors as therapy for primary induction failure acute myeloid leukemia. *Bone Marrow Transplant* 2001; **27**: 507–10.
72 Singhal S, Powles R, Henslee-Downey PJ *et al*. Allogeneic transplantation from HLA-matched sibling or partially HLA-mismatched related donors for primary refractory acute leukemia. *Bone Marrow Transplant* 2002; **29**: 291–5.
73 Andre-Schmutz I, Le Deist F, Hacein-Bey-Abina S *et al*. Immune reconstitution without graft-versus-host disease after haemopoietic stem-cell transplantation: a phase 1–2 study. *Lancet* 2002; **360**: 130–7.
74 Tan P, Anasetti C, Hansen JA *et al*. Induction of alloantigen-specific hyporesponsiveness in human T lymphocytes by blocking interaction of CD28 with its natural ligand B7/BB1. *J Exp Med* 1993; **177**: 165–73.
75 Gribben JG, Guinan EC, Boussiotis VA *et al*. Complete blockade of B7 family-mediated costimulation is necessary to induce human alloantigen-specific anergy: a method to ameliorate graft-versus-host disease and extend the donor pool. *Blood* 1996; **87**: 4887–93.
76 Guinan EC, Boussiotis VA, Neuberg D *et al*. Transplantation of anergic histoincompatible bone marrow allografts. *N Engl J Med* 1999; **340**: 1704–14.
77 Schwartz E, Lapidot T, Gozes D *et al*. Abrogation of bone marrow allograft resistance in mice by increased total body irradiation correlates with eradication of host clonable T-cells and alloreactive cytotoxic precursors. *J Immunol* 1987; **138**: 460–5.
78 Cobbold SP, Martin G, Quin S *et al*. Monoclonal antibodies to promote marrow engraftment and tissue graft tolerance. *Nature* 1986; **323**: 164–6.
79 Lapidot T, Terenzi A, Singer TS *et al*. Enhancement by dimethyl myleran of donor type chimerism in murine recipients of bone marrow allografts. *Blood* 1989; **73**: 2025–32.
80 Terenzi A, Lubin I, Lapidot T *et al*. Enhancement of T-depleted bone marrow allografts in mice by thiotepa. *Transplantation* 1990; **50**: 717–20.
81 Reisner Y, Martelli MF. Bone marrow transplantation across HLA barriers by increasing the number of transplanted cells. *Immunol Today* 1995; **16**: 437–40.
82 Shizuru JA, Jerabek L, Edwards CT, Weissman IL. Transplantation of purified hematopoietic stem cells: requirements for overcoming the barriers of allogeneic engraftment. *Biol Blood Marrow Transplant* 1996; **2**: 3–14.
83 Bachar-Lusting E, Rachamim N, Li HW *et al*. Megadose of T-depleted bone marrow overcomes MHC barriers in sublethally irradiated mice. *Nat Med* 1995; **1**: 1268–73.
84 Reisner Y, Kapoor N, Kirkpatrick D *et al*. Transplantation for acute leukaemia with HLA-A and B nonidentical parental marrow cells fractionated with soybean agglutinin and sheep red blood cells. *Lancet* 1981; **2**: 327–31.
85 Rachamin N, Gan J, Segall R *et al*. Tolerance induction by "megadose" hematopoietic transplants: donor-type human CD34 stem cells induce potent specific reduction of host anti-donor cytotoxic T lymphocyte precursors in mixed lymphocyte culture. *Transplantation* 1998; **65**: 1386–93.
86 Gur H, Krauthgamer R, Berrebi A *et al*. Tolerance induction by megadose hematopoietic progenitor cells: expansion of veto cells by short-term culture of purified human $CD34^+$ cells. *Blood* 2002; **99**: 4174–81.
87 Arpinati M, Terragna C, Chirumbolo G *et al*. Human $CD34^+$ blood cells induce T-cell unresponsiveness only under costimulatory blockade. *Exp Hematol* 2003; **31**: 31–8.
88 Volpi I, Perruccio K, Tosti A *et al*. Post-grafting granulocyte colony-stimulating factor administration impairs functional immune recovery in recipients of HLA haplotype-mismatched hematopoietic transplants. *Blood* 2001; **97**: 2514–21.
89 Dumont-Girard F, Roux E, van Lier RA *et al*. Reconstitution of the T-cell compartment after bone marrow transplantation: restoration of the repertoire by thymic emigrants. *Blood* 1998; **92**: 4464–71.
90 Heitger A, Greinix H, Mannhalter C *et al*. Requirement of residual thymus to restore normal T-cell subsets after human allogeneic bone marrow transplantation. *Transplantation* 2000; **69**: 2366–73.
91 Sallusto F, Lenig D, Forster R *et al*. Two subsets of memory T lymphocytes with distinct homing potentials and effector functions. *Nature* 1999; **401**: 708–12.
92 Kato S, Yabe H, Yasui M *et al*. Allogeneic hematopoietic transplantation of $CD34^+$ selected cells from an HLA haplo-identical related donor. A

long-term follow-up of 135 patients and a comparison of stem cell source between the bone marrow and the peripheral blood. *Bone Marrow Transplant* 2000; **26**: 1281–90.

93 Aversa F, Velardi A, Tabilio A, Reisner Y, Martelli MF. Haploidentical stem cell transplantation HCT in leukemia. *Blood Rev* 2001; **15**: 111–9.

94 Handgretinger R, Klingebiel T, Lang P et al. Megadose transplantation of purified peripheral blood CD34+ progenitor cells from HLA-mismatched parental donors in children. *Bone Marrow Transplant* 2001; **27**: 777–83.

95 Ruggeri L, Capanni M, Urbani E et al. Effectiveness of donor natural killer cell alloreactivity in mismatched hematopoietic transplants. *Science* 2002; **295**: 2097–100.

96 Parham P, McQueen KL. Alloreactive killer lymphocytes: hindrance and help to hematopoietic stem cell transplantation. *Nat Rev Immunol* 2003; **3**: 108–22.

97 Kärre K, Ljunggren HG, Piontek G et al. Selective rejection of H-2 deficient lymphoma variants suggests alternative immune defence strategy. *Nature* 1986; **319**: 675–8.

98 Herberman RB, Nunn ME, Lavrin DH. Natural cytotoxic reactivity of mouse lymphoid cells against syngeneic and allogeneic tumors. I. Distribution of reactivity and specificity. *Int J Cancer* 1975; **16**: 216–29.

99 George T, Yu YY, Liu J et al. Allorecognition by murine natural killer cells: lysis of T-lymphoblasts and rejection of bone-marrow grafts. *Immunol Rev* 1997; **155**: 29–40.

100 Farag SS, Fehniger TA, Ruggeri L et al. Natural killer cell receptors: new biology and insights into the graft versus leukemia effect. *Blood* 2002; **100**: 1935–47.

101 Velardi A, Ruggeri L, Moretta A, Moretta L. NK cells: a lesson from mismatched hematopoietic transplantation. *Trends Immunol* 2002; **23**: 438–44.

102 Ciccone E, Viale O, Pende D et al. Specific lysis of allogeneic cells after activation of CD3-lymphocytes in mixed lymphocyte culture. *J Exp Med* 1988; **168**: 2403–8.

103 Ciccone E, Pende D, Viale O et al. Evidence of a natural killer (NK) cell repertoire for (allo) antigen recognition: definition of five distinct NK determined allospecificities in humans. *J Exp Med* 1992; **175**: 709–18.

104 Ciccone E, Pende D, Viale O et al. Involvement of HLA class I alleles in natural killer (NK) cell-specific functions: expression of HLA-Cw3 confers selective protection from lysis by alloreactive NK clones displaying a defined specificity (specificity 2). *J Exp Med* 1992; **176**: 963–71.

105 Colonna M, Borsellino G, Falco M et al. HLA-C is the inhibitory ligand that determines dominant resistance to lysis by NK1- and NK2-specific natural killer cells. *Proc Natl Acad Sci U S A* 1993; **90**: 1200–4.

106 Colonna M, Brooks EG, Falco M et al. Generation of allospecific natural killer cells by stimulation across a polymorphism of HLA-C. *Science* 1993; **260**: 1121–4.

107 Moretta A, Moretta L. HLA class I specific inhibitory receptors. *Curr Opinion Immunol* 1997; **9**: 964–71.

108 Valiante NM, Lienert K, Shilling HG et al. Killer cell receptors: keeping pace with MHC class I evolution. *Immunol Rev* 1997; **155**: 155–64.

109 Lanier LL. NK cell receptors. *Ann Rev Immunol* 1998; **16**: 359–93.

110 Hsu KC, Chida S, Dupont B, Geraghty DE. The killer cell immunoglobulin-like receptor (KIR) genomic region: gene-order, haplotypes and allelic polymorphism. *Immunol Rev* 2002; **190**: 40–52.

111 Uhrberg M, Valiante NM, Shum BP et al. Human diversity in killer cell inhibitory receptor genes. *Immunity* 1997; **7**: 753–60.

112 Shilling H, Young N, Guethlein LA et al. Genetic control of human NK cell repertoire. *J Immunol* 2002; **169**: 239–47.

113 Ciccone E, Pende D, Vitale M et al. Self Class I molecules protect normal cells from lysis mediated by autologous natural killer cells. *Eur J Immunol* 1994; **24**: 1003–6.

114 Biassoni R, Falco M, Cambiaggi A et al. Amino acid substitution can influence the NK mediated recognition of HLA-C molecules: role of serine-77 and lysine-80 in the target T-cell protection from lysis mediated by "group 2" or "group 1" NK clones. *J Exp Med* 1995; **182**: 605–9.

115 Winter CC, Long EO. A single amino acid in the p58 killer cell inhibitory receptor controls the ability of natural killer cells to discriminate between the two groups of HLA-C allotypes. *J Immunol* 1997; **158**: 4026–8.

116 Moretta A, Bottino C, Pende D et al. Identification of four subset of human CD3-CD16+ NK cells by the expression of clonally distributed functional surface molecules: correlation between subset assignment of NK clones and ability to mediate specific alloantigen recognition. *J Exp Med* 1990; **172**: 1589–98.

117 Moretta A, Vitale M, Bottino C et al. P58 molecules as putative receptors for MHC class I molecules in human natural killer (NK) cells. Anti-p58 antibodies reconstitute lysis of MHC class I-protected cells in NK clones displaying different specificities. *J Exp Med* 1993; **178**: 597–604.

118 Moretta A, Biassoni R, Bottino C et al. Natural cytotoxicity receptors that trigger human NK mediated cytolysis. *Immunol Today* 2000; **21**: 228–34.

119 Moretta A, Bottino C, Vitale M et al. Activating receptors and coreceptors involved in human natural killer cell-mediated cytolysis. *Annu Rev Immunol* 2001; **19**: 197–223.

120 Cerwenka A, Lanier LL. Ligands for natural killer cell receptors: redundancy or specificity. *Immunol Rev* 2001; **181**: 158–69.

121 Diefenbach A, Raulet DH. Strategies for target cell recognition by natural killer cells. *Immunol Rev* 2001; **181**: 170–84.

122 Bauer S, Groh V, Wu J et al. Activation of NK cells and T-cells by NKG2D, a receptor for stress-inducible MICA. *Science* 1999; **285**: 727–9.

123 Sutherland CL, Chalupny NJ, Cosman D. The UL16-binding proteins, a novel family of MHC class I-related ligands for NKG2D, activate natural killer cell functions. *Immunol Rev* 2001; **181**: 185–92.

124 Ruggeri L, Capanni M, Casucci M et al. Role of natural killer cell alloreactivity in HLA-mismatched hematopoietic stem cell transplantation. *Blood* 1999; **94**: 333–9.

125 Shlomchik WD, Couzens MS, Tang CB et al. Prevention of graft versus host disease by inactivation of host antigen-presenting cells. *Science* 1999; **285**: 412–5.

126 Kärre K. A perfect mismatch. *Science* 2002; **295**: 2029–31.

127 Giebel S, Locatelli F, Lamparelli T et al. Survival advantage with KIR ligand incompatibility in hematopoietic stem cell transplantation from unrelated donors. *Blood* 2003; **102**: 814–9.

128 Davies SM, Ruggieri L, DeFor T et al. Evaluation of KIR ligand incompatibility in mismatched unrelated donor hematopoietic transplants. *Blood* 2002; **100**: 3825–7.

129 Schaffer M, Remberger M, Ringden O, Olerup O. Role of HLA-C incompatibilities in unrelated donor hematopoietic stem cell transplantation. *Tissue Antigens* 2002; **S59**: 18 [Abstract].

130 De Santis D, Witt C, Nagler A, Brautbar C, Christiansen F, Bishara A. HLA-C KIR ligands and donor recipient KIR genotypes influence outcome of haploidentical HCT. *Hum Immunol* 2002; **S63**: 17 [Abstract].

131 Mingari MC, Ponte M, Vitale C, Bellomo R, Moretta L. Expression of HLA class I-specific inhibitory receptors in human cytolytic T lymphocytes: a regulated mechanism that controls T-cell activation and function. *Hum Immunol* 2000; **61**: 44–50.

132 Yen JH, Moore BE, Nakajima T et al. Major histocompatibility complex class I-recognizing receptors are disease risk genes in rheumatoid arthritis. *J Exp Med* 2001; **193**: 1159–67.

133 Martin MP, Gao X, Lee JH et al. Epistatic interaction between KIR3DS1 and HLA-B delays the progression to AIDS. *Nat Genet* 2002; **31**: 429–34.

83

Effie W. Petersdorf

Hematopoietic Cell Transplantation from Unrelated Donors

Introduction

Hematopoietic cell transplantation (HCT) from unrelated donors is a curative modality for hematologic malignancies. The success of unrelated donor HCT has closely paralleled discoveries about the genes and function of the human leukocyte antigen (HLA) system, the major histocompatibility complex (MHC) in humans. Availability of robust typing methods and the continued growth of registries of HLA-typed volunteer donors have allowed the identification of suitable donors for increasing numbers of patients. The clinical results of unrelated donor HCT have greatly improved as a consequence of more complete understanding of the immunogenetic barriers that give rise to host-vs.-graft (HVG) and graft-vs.-host (GVH) reactions, and to the development of less toxic transplant regimens, advances in the prevention and treatment of graft-vs.-host disease (GVHD) and in the supportive care of the transplant recipient.

The HLA barrier

In unrelated donor HCT, the major challenge to successful outcome is the need to overcome the HVG and GVH immunogenetic reactions that give rise to graft failure and GVHD, respectively. The importance of understanding the HLA system in allogeneic transplantation also extends to the development of tolerance, immune reconstitution, and in the promotion of graft-vs.-leukemia effect (GVLE). Comprehensive donor–recipient allele matching decreases risks of graft failure and GVHD and promotes optimal immune reconstitution of immune function. Leveraging control of leukemia through GVLE requires some incompatibility between the donor and recipient, although the optimal degree of disparity for HLA and/or non-HLA genes that can produce GVLE is not known.

HLA-matched siblings share the same two extended haplotypes and therefore are identical for all genes residing within the MHC. In unrelated donor HCT, phenotypic identity for serologically defined antigens does not guarantee allele (sequence) identity; furthermore, the haplotypes of an unrelated donor are unknown. As a surrogate for matching for the two HLA haplotypes, allele typing and matching for the classical HLA genetic loci has been undertaken under the assumption that comprehensive and precise genotyping will more closely approximate the matching that is achieved between siblings.

This chapter will focus on the immunogenetic variables that influence outcome after unrelated donor HCT, as it is the HLA barrier that distinguishes related from unrelated transplantation. Understanding the clinical influence of class I and class II gene products on HVG and GVH reactions requires an appreciation of the historical development of typing technology (see Chapter 4). Over the last 15 years, the introduction of polymerase chain reaction (PCR)-based technology for the class II *HLA-DR* and *-DQ* genes and more recently for the class I *HLA-A*, *-C* and *-B* genes necessarily created a continuum of improved resolution for a greater number of HLA genes over time. In turn, as information on HLA matching and its effects on transplant outcome became available, donor selection criteria were refined. Today, the definition of a "matched" donor requires information on the loci tested and level of typing performed at each locus.

An appreciation of the challenges of HLA research in clinical transplantation is also important. As discussed in the "HLA polymorphism and linkage disequilibrium: impact on donor matching and clinical outcome" section below, the extensive diversity of HLA genes and the high degree of nonrandom association of alleles (linkage disequilibrium [LD]) influence the probability of identifying matched donors. Ethnogeographic differences in HLA gene and haplotype frequencies give rise to qualitative differences in HLA mismatches between racially diverse unrelated transplant candidates. As discussed in the "Clinical relevance of HLA matching" section below, knowledge of the sequence disparity may hold the key to understanding permissibility of HLA mismatching. In this chapter the basic concepts of HLA matching and clinical outcome in myeloablative unrelated donor HCT for adults are presented. The reader is directed to the following chapters for specialized topics within unrelated donor HCT: Histocompatibility (Chapter 4), Peripheral Blood Hematopoietic Cells for Allogeneic Transplantation (Chapter 46), Hematopoietic Cell Donor Registries (Chapter 49) and unrelated donor HCT for the treatment of marrow disorders in children (Chapters 76 & 78).

A historical review of donor–recipient matching

The importance of matching for MHC antigens was initially demonstrated in experimental models [1,2] and applied clinically in 1968 with the first successful human allogeneic marrow transplants [3,4]. At that time, the HLA system was poorly defined and genes encoding HLA antigens had not been identified. Typing was performed with serological methods using panels of alloantisera detecting polymorphic specificities that segregated as distinct clusters. Initially two groups of antigens were identified, HLA-A and -B; a third group was identified in 1970 and named the HLA-C locus [5].

In addition to alloantigens inducing antibody responses, the HLA complex was shown to control determinants responsible for T-cell activation in the mixed lymphocyte culture (MLC). Studies in HLA recombinant families showed that MLC-stimulating determinants could segregate as a locus distinct from the class I *HLA-A*, *-B* and *-C* genes [6]. The MLC-stimulating locus, also known as the *HLA-D* region, could not be defined by the available typing sera. A modified MLC assay was developed to type for "Dw" specificities using lymphocytes from HLA homozygous donors as stimulator cells (also known as homozygous typing cells or HTC) [7,8]. During the late 1970s knowledge of the class II HLA-D region progressed rapidly. Studies with alloantisera, which had been absorbed with platelets to remove antibodies to the class I HLA-A, -B and -C antigens, identified a new family of alloantigens expressed on B-cells and monocytes similar to the tissue restricted Ia antigens identified in mice [9]. A correlation was found between these "Ia-like" specificities and the T-cell-defined "Dw" allotypes determined by MLC typing [6,7]. Eventually the human "Ia" antigens were shown to be encoded by three distinct loci named HLA-DR, -DQ and -DP [5,10].

The concept of selecting HLA-matched donors from outside the family by serology and MLC was first applied by Speck et al. [11] for a patient with severe aplastic anemia using marrow cells from an HLA-A, -B-matched and MLC-compatible unrelated donor. Antilymphocyte serum (ALS) was given before transplantation, but the patient failed to engraft. An unrelated donor transplant procedure was attempted for a second patient with aplastic anemia by Lohrmann et al. [12] and this patient also failed to achieve sustained engraftment despite conditioning with cyclophosphamide (CY). Horowitz et al. [13] transplanted marrow cells from an HLA-B and MLC compatible but HLA-A mismatched unrelated donor for a patient with severe combined immunodeficiency syndrome (SCID). Unfortunately the patient died on day 30 from interstitial pneumonia before immunological reconstitution could be adequately assessed. L'Esperance et al. [14] also attempted an unrelated donor marrow transplant for a SCID patient. The donor was matched for HLA-B, -C and MLC, but HLA-A mismatched. The initial graft failed to take, but sustained engraftment was eventually achieved following conditioning with CY [15]. Although immune reconstitution was demonstrated, the patient developed chronic GVHD and died from metastatic squamous cell carcinoma 10 years following HCT. Enthusiasm for unrelated donor transplants waned after these initial attempts until 1979 when the Seattle group undertook an HLA-matched unrelated donor transplant for a 10-year-old patient with acute lymphoblastic leukemia (ALL) in second complete remission (CR2). An HLA family study was performed, but none of the three siblings or parents was an adequate match. It was recognized, however, that the patient had the two most common HLA haplotypes found in North America (HLA-A1, -B8, -DR3 and HLA-A3, -B7, -DR2). A potential match was found by searching a local donor research file. The unrelated individual agreed to a donation of marrow cells and HCT was performed [16]. Complete donor engraftment was documented and there was no evidence of acute or chronic GVHD. Unfortunately, the patient relapsed and died with resistant leukemia approximately 2 years following HCT. Although the procedure ultimately was not successful, the very positive short-term observation clearly established the feasibility of matched unrelated donor HCT.

Development of donor registries

The Anthony Nolan Appeal, established in London in 1975, was the first effort to demonstrate the feasibility of donor recruitment and fund raising was sufficient to finance the cost of HLA typing [17]. The Anthony Nolan Appeal, now known as the Anthony Nolan Research Centre, was also the first donor registry to promote access to HLA-matched marrow donors for patients around the world. Similar projects were begun in the USA, initially through the efforts of individual centers [18]. As public interest in unrelated donor transplants grew, the US Congress amended the Transplant Act of 1984 to authorize the creation of a national registry comprising of a network of donor centers, transplant centers and a national coordinating center. In 1986, a federal contract to establish a national registry was awarded to the National Marrow Donor Program (NMDP) ([19]; http://www.nmdp.org). Throughout the 1980s, marrow donor registries were organized in several countries. In an effort to facilitate donor searches at the international level, the Europdonor Foundation in the Netherlands, under the direction of Professor Jon J. van Rood, began collecting HLA phenotype data from several national registries and combined these into a new database known as Bone Marrow Donors Worldwide (BMDW) [20]. Participating transplant centers from around the world can perform preliminary searches by accessing BMDW through the Internet (http://www.bmdw.org). Requests for specific donors, however, are directed to the individual donor registries (see Chapter 49).

HLA polymorphism and linkage disequilibrium (LD): impact on donor matching and clinical outcome

HLA diversity in donors and transplant recipients

The successful unrelated donor search for the patient described above was fortuitous because the patient's genotype consisted of two very common haplotypes [16]. The HLA typing technology available in 1979 was not adequate for detecting the allelic variants that occur between the majority of haplotypes despite apparent or phenotypic identity as defined by serologic typing. Many of the unrelated donor–patient transplant pairs initially matched for HLA-A, -B, and -DR by serology and MLC are now known to be mismatched for *HLA-A, -C, -B, -DR, -DQ* and *-DP* alleles [21–42]. Importantly, allele mismatching occurs to a variable degree depending on the haplotypes and ethnic composition of the population being tested [43–50].

Detection of class I allelic disparity among phenotypically matched unrelated donor–recipient pairs has been described in several large studies [25,37–39,41]. Hurley et al. [41] used molecular methods to define the *HLA-DRB1, -DRB3, -DRB5, -DQA1, -DQB1, -DPA1* and *-DPB1* alleles in 1250 serologically matched donor–recipient transplant pairs. Only 9.4% of this study population were allele-matched for all seven loci. When *HLA-DRB1* was examined, 79.4% of pairs were matched but only 13.2% of pairs were identical for both alleles. Scott et al. [38] uncovered a high percentage (35%) of mismatching at the HLA-C locus among pairs who were selected on the basis of HLA-A and -B serological identity at the time of transplant. This study demonstrates that HLA-A/B matching does not predict HLA-C matching; furthermore, molecular methods are required for accurate typing of this locus. In Caucasian transplant populations, donor–recipient allele disparity is frequent for common phenotypes including A2, B27, B35, B39 and DR4 [37,39]. The overall frequency of allele mismatching is lower if the recipient has a common haplotype [39].

The frequencies of HLA alleles, antigens and haplotypes reflect the ethnicity and race of the transplant recipient and donor. As a consequence, the specific donor–recipient HLA mismatches can be ethno-geographically distinct [35,37,51,52]. A side-by-side analysis of two large transplant populations illustrates the complex patterns of HLA mismatching among unrelated pairs and also the unique HLA mismatches that characterize them [51]. The class I and II allele frequencies among 440 Japanese transplants reported by Sasazuki et al. [52] for the Japan Marrow Donor Program (JMDP) and 300 Caucasian transplants reported by Petersdorf et al. [37] were compared. The two transplant populations shared similar degrees of disparity at *HLA-A, -B* and *-DR* loci among serologically matched pairs. Mismatching was most frequent for the *HLA*-C locus, and reflects the early donor selection criteria, which did not require matching for this gene. The distribution of mismatches was noteworthy in that both transplant populations exhibited very complex patterns of multiple mismatches: single locus mismatches comprised <50% of the mismatched pairs (Table 83.1).

The Japanese and the Caucasian transplant populations differed in the frequency of HLA alleles and, accordingly, the specific donor–recipient

Table 83.1 Distribution of allele mismatches according to HLA locus.*

					Number of mismatched donor–recipient pairs	
A	B	C	DRB1	DQB1	JMDP†	Seattle data‡
X	X	X	X	X	5	1
X	X	X	=	X	3	2
X	X	X	=	=	11	9
X	=	X	X	X	9	1
X	=	X	X	=	3	1
X	=	X	=	X	1	3
X	=	X	=	=	25	6
X	=	=	X	X	8	0
X	X	=	X	=	1	3
X	X	=	=	X	1	0
X	X	=	=	=	1	2
X	=	=	X	=	1	0
X	=	=	=	X	4	0
X	=	=	=	=	44	21
=	X	X	X	X	4	4
=	X	X	=	X	2	3
=	X	X	X	=	7	5
=	X	X	=	=	22	14
=	X	=	X	X	5	0
=	X	=	X	=	1	2
=	X	=	=	X	2	2
=	X	=	=	=	5	11
=	=	X	X	X	12	3
=	=	X	X	=	5	1
=	=	X	=	X	10	7
=	=	X	=	=	51	25
=	=	=	X	X	16	6
=	=	=	X	=	2	9
=	=	=	=	X	4	16
					265	157

Donor–recipient pairs were retrospectively typed using molecular methods. Allele disparities (donor–recipient mismatches that were detectable only through the use of molecular methods) were identified among serologically matched donor and recipients.
*Overall mismatching between donor and recipient.
†$n = 437$ patients total. At least 172 (39%) pairs were matched; however, HLA-C-locus typing was not available for three pairs.
‡$n = 300$ patients total; 143 (48%) pairs were matched.
JMDP, Japan Marrow Donor Program. "X" indicates mismatched and "=" indicates matched.

Table 83.2 HLA-A allele mismatching among donor–recipient pairs from two transplant populations.

HLA-A mismatch	JMDP data* No. (%)	Seattle data† No. (%)
*0201/0205	0	8 (25)
*0201/0206	25 (56)	2 (6)
*0201/0207	5 (11)	0
*0201/0210	3 (7)	0
*0201/0211	0	2 (6)
*0201/0225	0	1 (3)
*0206/0210	3 (7)	0
*0301/0302	0	4 (13)
*2402/2403	0	2 (6)
*2402/2407	0	1 (3)
*2601/6601	0	1 (3)
*2601/2602	3 (7)	0
*2601/2603	4 (8)	0
*2602/2603	2 (4)	0
*2901/2902	0	3 (9)
*3001/3002	0	4 (13)
*3301/3303	0	1 (3)
*6801/6802	0	2 (6)
Total	**45 (100)**	**32 (100)**

The number of times each allele mismatch combination was observed in the JMDP and Seattle datasets is shown [37,52]. As described more fully in the text, these two transplant populations differed from one another by the specific allele mismatch combinations. The A*0201/0206 mismatch combination was observed in both populations; the remaining mismatches were unique to each transplant group.
*166 donor–recipient pairs; 27% mismatched for HLA-A.
†300 donor–recipient pairs; 18% mismatched for HLA-A.
JMDP, Japan Marrow Donor Program.

allele mismatch combinations. Using the *HLA-A* locus as an example, mismatching for HLA-A*02 alleles within the HLA-A2 antigen was the most frequent mismatch in each population occurring in 80% of Japanese pairs and in 41% of Caucasian pairs (Table 83.2). However, the most common mismatch involved A*0201 vs. 0206 (56%) in Japanese pairs, and A*0201 vs. 0205 (25%) in Caucasian pairs. The two populations were distinguished by nonoverlapping mismatches for HLA-A*0201/0207; 0201/0210; 0206/0210; 2601/2602; 2601/2603; 2602/2603 which were present in the Japanese but not in the Caucasian dataset. Conversely, HLA-A*0201/0205; 0201/0211; 0201/0225; 0301/0302; 2402/2403; 2402/2407; 2601/6601; 2901/2902; 3001/3002; 3301/3303 and 6801/6802 were observed exclusively in the Caucasian transplant pairs. Overall survival for the Japanese and Caucasian patients was the same, however, *HLA-A* allele disparity was associated with better survival among the Caucasian patients than the Japanese patients and the risk of acute GVHD was lower among *HLA-A* mismatched Caucasian patients than Japanese patients (Fig. 83.1 & Table 83.3). These data indicate that qualitative differences in the sequence of the mismatched alleles may be an important determinant of the permissibility of a mismatch. Association of HLA matching and clinical outcome in large numbers of unrelated transplant recipients representing all racial populations is under active investigation by the International Histocompatibilty Working Group in Hematopoietic Cell Transplantation (www.ihwg.org).

The transition from serological phenotyping to DNA-based genotyping has introduced a need for refined HLA nomenclature for the purpose of donor matching. To maintain consistency in nomenclature, the results of intermediate-level DNA-based typing are transformed into serological equivalents. It is important to note that not all DNA-derived typing results can be uniformly translated to serotypes. Furthermore, some of the novel class I HLA alleles cannot be clearly defined by serology. Dictionaries of HLA alleles and antigen-equivalents have become a necessary tool to bridge the transition from primarily serological data to genotype data [34,53].

The introduction of molecular typing methods to the donor search

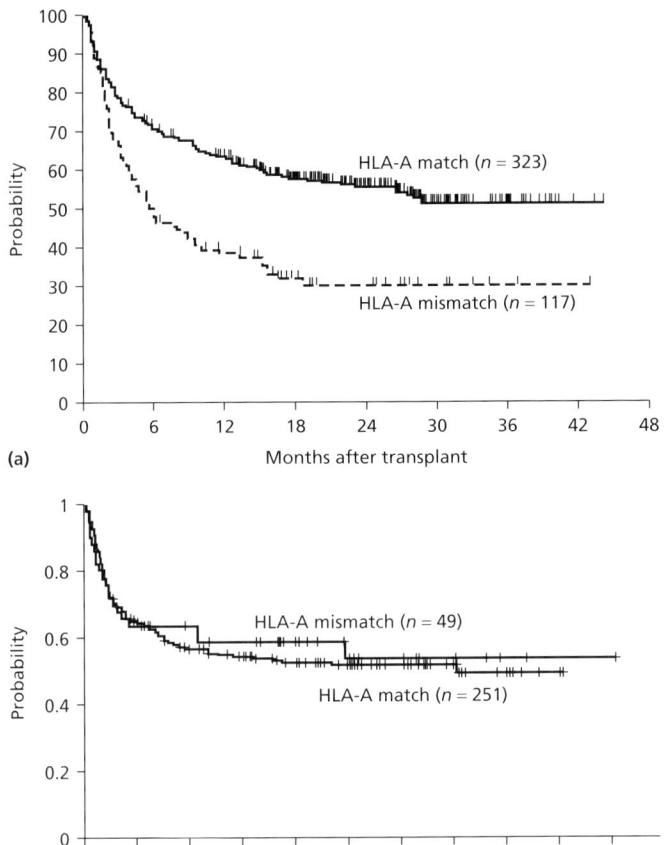

Fig. 83.1 Probability of survival for JMDP (a) and Seattle (b) patients according to donor-recipient matching at HLA-A [51]. A total of 440 patients underwent unrelated HCT as described by Sasazuki et al. for a variety of hematologic malignancies, hereditary disease or severe aplastic anemia [52]. The 300 patients described by Petersdorf et al. carried the diagnosis of CML [37]. As such, the recipients of these two populations differed with respect to age, transplant regimens and disease stage at diagnosis.

The development of informatic networks to effectively interpret and use molecular typing data has been a necessary resource for implementation of DNA typing methods for donor search and selection [57,58].

Linkage disequilibrium (LD): impact on donor identification and HLA matching

As of March 2002, over 209 *HLA-A*, 414 *HLA-B*, 101 *HLA-C*, 273 *HLA-DRB1* and 45 *HLA-DQB1* alleles have been defined in diverse human populations [59]. Assuming that any combination of these alleles can be expressed in an individual, the total estimated number of possible five-locus *HLA-A*, *-B*, *-C*, *-DRB1* and *-DQB1* genotypes is 3.6×10^{20}. If inheritance of HLA alleles were indeed random, then the odds of identifying two individuals with the same genotype would be an impossible task. Clinical experience demonstrates that some patients have been able to find a matched donor even in a relatively small file of unrelated donors. Donor identification is successful because HLA alleles are found in association with each other at an observed frequency that exceeds their expected frequency, a phenomenon known as linkage disequilibrium (LD) [60,61]. Furthermore, donor matching for patients with relatively common HLA haplotypes is likely to occur when donors share similar ethnic background to the patient. The *HLA-A1*, *-B8*, *-DR3* and *HLA-A3*, *-B7*, *-DR2* haplotypes are two of the most common haplotypes found in Caucasians occurring with a frequency of 5.2% and 2.6%, respectively, and both demonstrate significant positive linkage disequilibrium [45]. The number of common haplotypes, however, is relatively limited. Among North American Caucasians there are only seven haplotypes which occur with frequencies exceeding 1% [45].

The HLA gene and haplotype frequencies of donor registries worldwide and the probability of identifying suitable donors have been extensively evaluated [43–50,55,62–65]. Information on HLA allele, gene and haplotype frequencies from donor registries is important not only for estimating the probability of a successful search, but also for estimating optimal registry size and composition.

Analysis of donor–recipient HLA matching and clinical outcome: methodologic considerations

Substantial information on the role of donor compatibility in unrelated donor HCT has emerged over the last decade [21,27,29,30,32,37,52,66–95]. The majority of information on HLA matching and outcome has process led to the establishment of guidelines for histocompatiblity testing by donor registries and transplant centers worldwide [54–56].

Table 83.3 Analysis of grade III–IV acute graft-vs.-host disease (GVHD) according to human leukocyte antigen (HLA) matching in chronic myeloid leukemia (CML) patients.

	JMDP data (n = 166)*				Seattle data (n = 300)*			
HLA	Matched	Mismatched	Hazard ratio (*p*-value)†	Hazard ratio (*p*-value)‡	Matched	Mismatched	Hazard ratio (*p*-value)†	Hazard ratio (*p*-value)‡
A	18%	38%	2.4 (0.008)	2.3 (0.030)	39%	39%	1.0 (0.9800)	1.0 (0.890)
B	21%	39%	2.2 (0.040)	2.3 (0.060)	38%	45%	1.3 (0.3000)	1.0 (0.900)
C	20%	30%	1.5 (0.260)	1.0 (0.950)	36%	48%	1.5 (0.0400)	1.3 (0.230)
DRB1	21%	36%	1.8 (0.090)	4.5 (0.007)	37%	60%	1.8 (0.0100)	1.5 (0.120)
DQB1	24%	21%	0.9 (0.710)	0.3 (0.080)	35%	62%	2.1 (0.0005)	1.8 (0.007)

Data from the JMDP and Seattle CML transplant populations are summarized [37,52]. Multivariable model adjusted for mismatching at all other loci. The risk of acute GVHD was increased for HLA-A, HLA-B and HLA-DR among Japanese patients; HLA-DQ conferred risk among the Caucasian patients.
*Cumulative incidence of GVHD in patients matched for HLA-A, -B, -C, -DRB1 and -DQB1 was 11% and 32% in Japanese and Caucasian patients, respectively.
†Univariate analysis.
‡Multivariable analysis.
JMDP, Japan Marrow Donor Program.

emerged from retrospective analysis of donor–recipient transplant pairs. Many studies have retyped donor–recipient pairs using DNA methods to redefine the degree of allele compatibility, often including information for HLA loci that were not routinely evaluated at the time of donor selection. As described in the previous section, undetected mismatching between phenotypically identical pairs can be uncovered by newer DNA methods thereby leading to highly complex patterns of donor–recipient matching (Table 83.1). In order to define the relative risk of HLA mismatching to the clinical endpoint of interest comparison groups are established. Adjustment for non-HLA variables that influence the clinical endpoints is made in multivariable analysis. Two different approaches can be taken to examine the HLA variable. One approach (Method 1) is to define a matched group and a mismatched group for each HLA locus [90,92,95]. In Method 1, donor–recipient pairs may be variably mismatched for the other HLA loci, the presence of which is adjusted in multivariable analysis. For example, to test the hypothesis that donor–recipient matching at HLA-A is associated with a lower risk of acute GVHD compared to mismatching at HLA-A in a study population of 100 pairs, two comparison groups are identified: HLA-A matched pairs ($n = 60$) and HLA-A mismatched pairs ($n = 40$). The 60 HLA-A matched pairs may be variably mismatched at other HLA loci, the effect of which is controlled in multivariable analysis. Method 1 assumes that the association of mismatching at the locus in question is approximately the same across all other loci. Method 1 allows the effect of mismatching at a particular locus to be examined among the entire study population. An alternative approach (Method 2) is to define nonoverlapping groups of donor–recipient pairs based on match/mismatch at every HLA locus [37,93]. In Method 2, mutually exclusive comparison groups are defined on the basis of matching information at all loci simultaneously. Using the example described above for 100 pairs, potential comparison groups could include the following: HLA-A, -B, -DR matched ($n = 50$); HLA-A matched and HLA-B, -DR mismatched ($n = 10$); HLA-A mismatched and HLA-B, -DR matched ($n = 30$); HLA-A, -B mismatched and HLA-DR matched ($n = 5$) and HLA-A, -B, -DR mismatched ($n = 5$). Method 2 allows comparison of each group to all others. In this way, there is no potential confounding effect of other loci to the locus under examination. Because each group is mutually exclusive, a limitation of Method 2 may be smaller numbers of observations in each group.

HLA studies of unrelated transplant populations can differ by the HLA loci under examination as well as the resolution of typing for those loci. Hence, comparison of results between studies that are not comparable for the specific loci typed, or the definition of a "match" can be difficult if not impossible. Finally, the composition of the study population (diagnosis and stage of disease at the time of transplant), the conditioning regimen (T-cell depleted vs. T-replete; total body irradiation (TBI) vs. no TBI), the stem cell source and the immunosuppressive regimen are all important factors to consider in interpreting the results of the HLA associations on post-transplant complications [82]. The presence or absence of HLA disparity may be linked to the specific conditioning regimen and immunosuppressive agents used after transplantation; hence, the level of HLA disparity (serologically detectable mismatch vs. allele mismatch in serologically matched donor) as well as the number of HLA mismatches may be quite different in a T-cell-depleted transplant population than in a population receiving unmanipulated marrow.

Clinical relevance of HLA matching

The long-term goal of establishing HLA matching criteria should be threefold: (i) maximize *safety*; (ii) maximize *efficacy*; and (iii) increase *availability* of unrelated donor HCT for patients who have no other therapeutic option. Given the extreme polymorphism of the HLA system, it is not likely that allele matching can be achieved for most patients. If donor selection criteria are "maximized" to require allele identity then the number of patients eligible for transplantation will be limited. Exhaustive efforts to find the best match may theoretically increase the success of transplantation, however, a prolonged donor search may only delay transplantation and increase cost without necessarily increasing the benefit to the patient. The likelihood of patients reaching transplantation would increase if matching requirements were "minimized"; however, a greater degree of mismatching may compromise safety and decrease the probability of survival. To achieve optimal matching for individual patients it may be necessary to adjust the guidelines according to disease-specific criteria that appropriately reflect patient diagnosis, patient age, clinical urgency and the potential benefit of GVHD. GVLE may contribute significantly to the prevention of post-transplant relapse in patients with high-risk leukemia, however, GVHD will only increase the risk of transplant-related mortality (TRM) in patients undergoing HCT for a non-malignant disorder.

Currently, there is worldwide consensus that high-resolution typing is desirable to identify (and thereby avoid) donors with multiple mismatches as the effects of mismatching are additive. The use of molecular typing tools for donor searching and matching should not be viewed simply to identify "perfectly matched" donors, but to also identify and avoid donors who have multilocus hidden mismatches, as the negative impact of cumulative HLA mismatches on engraftment, GVHD and mortality are significant. As described in detail below, many studies demonstrate that in the absence of an allele-matched donor, selection of the least mismatched donor may lower risks of graft failure, GVHD and mortality. The locus at which mismatching may be allowed, however, differs according to the demographics of the study population, the transplant procedure, and non-HLA factors that affect overall outcome.

Data support a new model for optimal HLA matching of unrelated donors in which both *quantitative* (the total number of mismatched alleles) and *qualitative* (alleles vs. antigens) measures of donor–recipient disparity are considered. Three variables define the acceptability of an HLA mismatch: (i) the HLA genetic *locus* (or loci) that is (are) mismatched; (ii) the *number* of HLA allele mismatches; and (iii) the specific nucleotide *sequence* of the mismatch. The following section summarizes sentinel work in immunogenetics and unrelated donor HCT (Table 83.4). These studies provide a basis for the current selection for unrelated donors and focus on identification of deleterious mismatches (i.e. to improve safety and efficacy of unrelated donor HCT) as well as tolerable mismatches (i.e. to increase the number of suitable donors for more patients).

Graft failure

Early studies identified donor HLA mismatching to be a risk factor for graft failure [68]. Several non-HLA factors have been associated with an increased risk of graft failure including the transplantation of a lower marrow cell dose [96], the use of T-cell-depleted marrow [97] and the transplantation of marrow from a cross-match positive donor (presence of anti-donor lymphocyte antibodies in the patient's serum pretransplant) [77].

HLA genes involved in graft failure

Class I HLA-*A*, -*C* and -*B* and class II HLA-*DR* are important in engraftment [29,37,70,83,86,87,94]. In an analysis of 5246 transplants facilitated by the NMDP, the incidence of primary graft failure was 4% [86]. Multivariable analysis revealed HLA-matched marrow, higher cell dose, younger recipient age and recipients of non-African-American background to be favorable factors for engraftment. Factors favoring platelet engraftment included higher marrow cell dose, donor *HLA-DRB1* identity, recipient cytomegalovirus (CMV) seronegativity, donor identity for HLA-A and -B antigens, and the use of male donors. Among patients who initially achieved engraftment, secondary graft failure was observed in 10% of whom 18% are surviving. In a separate analysis of 1423

Table 83.4 Clinical significance of donor–recipient HLA matching in unrelated HCT in adults using myeloablative conditioning regimens.

	Observations		
Clinical endpoint	Genetic loci involved	Quantitative (tally) effect	Qualitative (sequence) effect
Graft failure	**Class I** Fleischhauer et al. (1990) [70] Nagler et al. (1996) [29] Petersdorf et al. (1997) [83] Petersdorf et al. (1998) [37] Petersdorf et al. (2001) [94] **Class I and II** Davies et al. (2000) [86] McGlave et al. (2000) [87]	**Class I** Petersdorf et al. (1998) [37] Petersdorf et al. (2001) [94] **Class I and II** Morishima et al. (2002) [95]	**Class I** Petersdorf et al. (2001) [94]
GVHD	**Class I** Flomenberg et al. (2001) [90] Ferrara et al. (2001) [89] Sasazuki et al. (1998) [52] Nagler et al. (1996) [29] Morishima et al. (2002) [95] **Class I and II** Pawlec et al. (1986) [66] Al-Daccak et al. (1990) [21] Kato et al. (1991) [73] Petersdorf et al. (1993) [76] Nademanee et al. (1995) [27] Petersdorf et al. (1995) [80] Petersdorf et al. (1996) [30] Gajewski et al. (1997) [81] Petersdorf et al. (1998) [37] Przepiorka et al. (1999) [84] Varney et al. (1999) [85] McGlave et al. (2000) [87] Przepiorka et al. (2000) [88] Keever-Taylor et al. (2001) [67] Flomenberg et al. (2001) [90] Loiseau et al. (2001) [91] Petersdorf et al. (2001) [92] Petersdorf et al. (2001) [93]	**Class I** Petersdorf et al. (1998) [37] Sasazuki et al. (1998) [52] Flomenberg et al. (2001) [90] Morishima et al. (2002) [95] **Class II** Petersdorf et al. (1996) [30] Petersdorf et al. (1998) [37] Przepiorka et al. (1999) [84] Keever-Taylor et al. (2001) [67] Petersdorf et al. (2001) [93] **Class I and II** Petersdorf et al. (1998) [37] Sasazuki et al. (1998) [52] Flomenberg et al. (2001) [90] Morishima et al. (2002) [95]	**Class I** Ferrara et al. (2001) [89] Flomenberg et al. (2001) [90] Wade et al. (2001) [117]
Relapse	**Class I** Sasazuki et al. (1998) [52] Morishima et al. (2002) [95]		
Mortality	**Class I** Davies et al. (1995) [79] Nagler et al. (1996) [29] Petersdorf et al. (1998) [37] Sasazuki et al. (1998) [52] McGlave et al. (2000) [87] Ferrara et al. (2001) [89] Petersdorf et al. (2001) [94] Morishima et al. (2002) [95] **Class II** Nademanee et al. (1995) [27] Petersdorf et al. (1995) [80] Petersdorf et al. (1996) [30] Gajewski et al. (1997) [81] Przepiorka et al. (1999) [84]	**Class I** Petersdorf et al. (1998) [37] Sasazuki et al. (1998) [52] Flomenberg et al. (2001) [90] Petersdorf et al. (2001) [94] Morishima et al. (2002) [95] **Class II** Petersdorf et al. (1998) [37] Przepiorka et al. (1999) [84] Keever-Taylor et al. (2001) [67]	**Class I** Davies et al. (1995) [79] Ferrara et al. (2001) [89] Flomenberg et al. (2001) [90] Petersdorf et al. (2001) [94] Wade et al. (2001) [117]

(Continued on p. 1138)

Table 83.4 (cont'd)

Clinical endpoint	Observations		
	Genetic loci involved	Quantitative (tally) effect	Qualitative (sequence) effect
	Varney et al. (1999) [85]		
	Keever-Taylor et al. (2001) [67]		
	Flomenberg et al. (2001) [90]		
	Loiseau et al. (2001) [91]		
	Petersdorf et al. (2001) [92]		
	Petersdorf et al. (2001) [93]		
	Class I and II	**Class I and II**	
	Speiser et al. (1996) [32]	Petersdorf et al. (1998) [37]	
	Petersdorf et al. (1998) [37]	Sasazuki et al. (1998) [52]	
	Sasazuki et al. (1998) [52]	Keever-Taylor et al. (2001) [67]	
	Davies et al. (2000) [86]	Flomenberg et al. (2001) [90]	
	McGlave et al. (2000) [87]	Shaw et al. (2001) [115]	
	Flomenberg et al. (2001) [90]	Morishima et al. (2002) [95]	
	Shaw et al. (2001) [115]		
	Morishima et al. (2002) [95]		
	Drobyski et al. (2002) [116]		

patients transplanted for chronic myeloid leukemia (CML), a lower risk of primary graft failure was associated with TBI dose, transplantation in the first chronic phase (CP), the use of HLA identical donors and a marrow cell dose of at least 2.1×10^8 total nucleated cells (TNC)/kg recipient body weight [87]. Late graft failure was found to be significantly decreased if the transplant was performed in the first CP.

HLA-A, -C, -B class I allele disparity is a risk factor for graft failure. One of the first descriptions of graft failure in class I mismatched unrelated transplantation was made by Fleischhauer et al. [70] who isolated a cytotoxic T lymphocyte (CTL) clone reactive with an *HLA-B44* variant that was undetectable by serology (the donor was B*4402 and the patient was B*4403). The Seattle program identified *HLA-C* as a risk factor for graft failure in CML unrelated donor HCT using a matched case–control study design [83]. Graft failure occurred in 21 (3.8%) of 521 evaluable transplants. Retrospective allele typing of donors and recipients was performed for the 21 graft failure cases and 42 controls who did not have graft failure. The controls were matched to the cases for variables known to influence engraftment. Only 2 (10%) of the 21 cases were fully matched for *HLA-A, -B* and *-C* alleles compared to 19 (45%) of the controls. Mismatching for *HLA-A* and/or *-B* alleles occurred in 19% of cases compared to 21% of controls. Mismatching for at least one *HLA-C* locus allele, however, occurred in 71% of cases compared to 33% of controls. Multivariable analysis revealed that the odds ratio (OR) of graft failure given an *HLA-C* mismatch was 4.0 ($p = 0.03$). There was a trend towards an increased OR of graft failure with *HLA-A* and/or *-B* mismatching (OR 3.1, $p = 0.09$), low marrow cell dose (the median cell dose was 2.7×10^8 TNC/kg in the graft failure group compared to 3.3×10^8 TNC/kg in the control group, $p = 0.03$) and primary disease diagnosis (6% for patients with CML, 6% for patients with aplastic anemia and 0.7% for patients with acute leukemia).

Effect of the number of HLA mismatches on risk of graft failure

The risk of graft failure increases in parallel with the number of HLA disparities. Morishima et al. [95] examined the impact of allele disparity on engraftment in 1298 patients. The overall incidence of graft failure increased with increasing numbers of mismatched HLA loci (1.7% matched; 4.8%, 4.1%, 4.8% of single *HLA-A/B*, *HLA-C* and *HLA-DR/DQ*, respectively; 10.4%, 8.9%, 6% in two-locus *HLA-A/B* plus *-C*, *HLA-A/B* plus *-DR/DQ* and *HLA-C* plus *-DR/DQ*, respectively; and 10.6% of three-locus incompatible transplants). In a study by the Seattle program, the dose effect of allele mismatches was evaluated in 300 patients who underwent unrelated donor HCT for the treatment of CML [37]. A single allele mismatch at *HLA-A, -B* or *-C* did not increase the risk of graft failure compared to matched recipients (2%); however, multiple *HLA-A, -B* and/or *-C* allele mismatches were associated with a 29% incidence of graft failure.

Importance of the HLA sequence

With the availability of molecular methods to define the HLA genetic sequences of transplant recipients and donors, it is now possible to evaluate the impact of the primary nucleotide sequence disparity on clinical outcome. New information implies the importance of the location and the number of amino acid residues mismatched in class I molecules, and recipient homozygosity in defining risk of graft failure [94]. Recipient homozygosity for alleles or antigens was significantly associated with graft failure among patients with a single class I mismatch ($p < 0.001$). Among pairs mismatched for a single *allele*, graft failure occurred in one of two homozygous recipients and in none of 47 heterozygous recipients ($p = 0.04$). Among pairs mismatched for a single *antigen*, graft failure occurred in four of five homozygous recipients and in seven of 51 heterozygous recipients ($p = 0.004$). The presence of recipient disparity in the heterozygous recipient may have induced an antirecipient T-cell response in the donor cells, which eliminated host cells that could cause graft failure. This counterbalancing mismatch was absent in the homozygous recipients. The allele and antigen mismatches differed in the number of nonsynonymous substitutions and in the location of the mismatch in the α1 and α2 domains of the molecule; the distribution of mismatched amino acid residues was not random (Fig. 83.2; see also Plate 83.1, *facing p. 296*). Specifically, donor–recipient pairs with a single class I allele disparity encoded from 0–11 mismatched residues implicated in peptide binding, and zero to one residue involved in T-cell receptor contact. In contrast, single antigen mismatched pairs had involvement of 0–16 residues involved in peptide repertoire and 0–9 substitutions involved in T-cell receptor contact. These data suggest that multiple mismatches for residues that affect peptide binding and T-cell receptor contact might have been instrumental in evoking T-cell responses that led to graft failure in these patients.

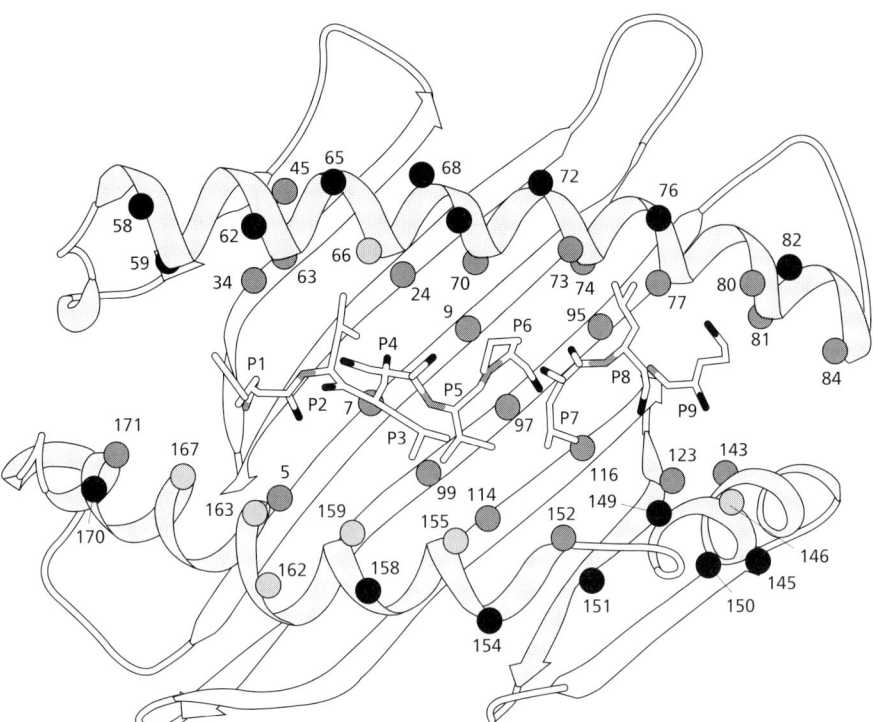

Fig. 83.2 Ribbon diagram of the HLA-A2 molecule showing α-carbon backbone of the α1 and α2 domains and the β-pleated sheet. Residues are colored according to their putative role in peptide repertoire (dark grey), TCR contact (black) or both (light grey) [174,175]. The bound peptide is labeled (P1–P9). Residues implicated in peptide-binding are: 5,7,9,24,25,34,45,63,67,70, 73,74,77,80,81,84,95,97,99,113,114,116,123,143, 147,152,156,160, and 171. Residues implicated in TCR contact are: 58,62,65,68,69,72,76,82,145, 149,150,151,154,158,166, and 170. Residues involved in both peptide and TCR contact are: 59,66,146,155,159,162,163 and 167. (*See also Plate 83.1, facing p. 296.*)

Graft-vs.-host disease (GVHD)

The risk of acute GVHD remains a major limitation of unrelated donor HCT. Historical observations in haplo-identical related transplantation demonstrated that HLA mismatching increases the incidence and severity of acute GVHD [98], the effect of which is higher with class II than with class I mismatching [99]. Early clinical experience in mismatched related transplantation uncovered the tally effect on GVHD risk. In one clinical study, grades II–IV GVHD was observed in 75% of single-locus, 78% of two-locus and 80% of three-locus mismatches [77].

Early studies of patients receiving HLA serologically matched MLC-compatible unrelated donor HCT uniformly reported a relatively high incidence of acute GVHD compared to that in HLA identical siblings [69,71,72,74]. The rates of TRM were also higher for unrelated transplant recipients, consistent with the higher incidence of acute and chronic GVHD. The likelihood of undetected HLA disparity in these early cases matched only by serology gave impetus to the hypothesis that the safety and success of unrelated donor transplants could be improved by further advances in HLA typing and donor matching.

The HLA class II genes: *HLA-DRB1*, *-DQB1* and *-DPB1*

Studies of allele matching initially focused on *HLA-DR*. In a study of 364 patients with hematological malignancy transplanted from an *HLA-A*, *-B*, *-DR* serologically matched unrelated donor there was a significant increase in severe acute GVHD and decreased survival in cases mismatched for an *HLA-DRB1* allele [80]. This study did not take into account *HLA-DQ*, a locus in strong positive linkage disequilibrium with *HLA-DR*. An expanded dataset later permitted evaluation of both *HLA-DRB1* and *-DQB1* genes and uncovered a synergistic effect of two-locus mismatching [30]. Among 449 *HLA-A*, *-B* and *-DR* serologically matched pairs, allele typing for *HLA-DRB1* and *-DQB1* alleles revealed that 335 (75%) were *HLA-DRB1* and *-DQB1* matched, 41 (9%) were *HLA-DRB1* matched but *-DQB1* mismatched, 48 (11%) were *HLA-DRB1* mismatched but *-DQB1* matched and 25 (6%) were mismatched at both *HLA-DRB1* and *-DQB1*. The conditional probabilities of grades III–IV acute GVHD were 0.42, 0.61, 0.55 and 0.71, respectively. In multivariable analysis, *HLA-DQB1* mismatching conferred a significantly increased relative risk (RR 1.8; $p = 0.01$) for grades II–IV acute GVHD demonstrating that *HLA-DQ* gene products function as transplantation determinants.

Recently, several large studies of unrelated transplants confirm and extend the findings of *HLA-DR* and *-DQ* disparity and risk of clinically significant acute GVHD [81,84,88,90,92]. In an NMDP analysis of 831 CML transplants, *HLA-DRB1* allele mismatching was associated with increased risk of grades III–IV acute GVHD [92]. The effects were significant when class II allele matching was evaluated in a good-risk subset of patients who received transplants during the first CP from class I serologically matched unrelated donors. Expanding the clinical population to include other hematologic malignancies, Flomenberg *et al*. [90] have reported the findings of 1874 transplants in whom *HLA-DRB1* mismatching was associated with a RR of 1.26 (95%CI 1.0–1.6, $p = 0.05$). Przepiorka *et al*. [84] found a pronounced effect of two-locus *HLA-DRB1*, *-DQB1* mismatching on the risk of grades III–IV acute GVHD (22% matched; 43% single locus; 64% two-locus mismatches). Gajewski *et al*. [81] compared the risk of grades III–IV GVHD among 44 *HLA-A*, *-B* and *-DR* serologically matched unrelated pairs who received unmodified grafts. Patients and donors were typed for *HLA-DRB1* and *-DQB1* using oligonucleotide probe methods. Matching for both *HLA-DRB1* and *-DQB1* reduced the rate of GVHD from 73% (any mismatch) to 38% (matched for both genes, $p = 0.02$).

The role of HLA-DP as a transplantation alloantigen has recently come into focus [21,66,73,76,85,90,91,93]. Population studies have shown that the *HLA-DP* locus is unique among the class I and class II genes because there is very weak LD between *HLA-DP* and *HLA-A*, *-B*, *-DR* and *-DQ*. Consequently, <20% of *HLA-A*, *-B*, *-DRB1*, *-DQB1*-matched unrelated donor pairs are also matched for *HLA-DP*. Retrospective examination of *HLA-DP* has required very large transplant populations so that sufficient numbers of *HLA-DP*-matched pairs can be compared to mismatched pairs. Analysis of *HLA-DP* has furthermore required information about class I gene disparity and function so as to control for confounding effects of mismatching at other HLA loci.

No significant effect of matching for *HLA-DP* was identified in an early report of 129 unrelated donor transplants matched for HLA-A, -B antigens and -*DRB1* and -*DQB1* alleles [76]. The relatively small number of *HLA-DPB1* matched cases and the lack of information on class I allele matching limited the power of this study. A follow-up study by the Seattle program restricted the study population to HLA-A, -C, -B, -*DRB1* and -*DQB1* allele matched CML transplants [93]. Patients who were mismatched for two *HLA-DPB1* alleles had an increased risk of clinically significant acute GVHD compared to pairs who were matched or mismatched for a single allele (OR 2.2, 1.2–4.1; $p = 0.01$). Varney et al. [85] found an increased risk of grades III–IV acute GVHD associated with *HLA-DPB1* disparity compared to the matched situation ($p = 0.04$). Loiseau et al. [91] reported *HLA-DPB1* disparity to be an independent risk factor for severe acute GVHD. An analysis of *HLA-DPB1* conducted by the NMDP confirms a trend towards increased acute GVHD in the setting of donor–recipient *HLA-DP* incompatibility [72].

Interestingly, two large studies by the JMDP have not confirmed a role for *HLA-DP* as a transplantation determinant [52,95]. If *HLA-DPB1* typing and matching is attempted, the clinical challenge is the relative lack of *HLA-DPB1*-identical donors despite comprehensive matching for other class I and II genes. Therefore, the selection of donors might include consideration for this gene when the search process identifies several potential HLA-A, -C, -B, -DR, -DQ matched donors and when the patient's clinical course affords sufficient time to evaluate donor compatibility for this gene.

The HLA class I genes: *HLA-A*, *-C* and *-B*

The recent availability of molecular methods for the class I region genes has enabled investigators to evaluate the potential contribution of *HLA-A*, *-C* and *-B* to GVHD risk. Analysis of HLA-A, -B serologically matched pairs demonstrates a high degree of nonidentity for *HLA-A*, *-C* and *-B* alleles. Retrospective studies on clinical outcome have uncovered a complex interaction of class I and class II allele disparity on GVHD risk.

In an early report by Keever et al. [78] donor-derived CTL were isolated and exclusively recognized a different *HLA-B44* allele in the patient (B*4402 vs. B*4403). These results suggested that class I allele differences may evoke donor-antihost responses which may correlate with the development of acute GVHD. The JMDP published the first large study describing the effect of class I on GVHD risk [52]. *HLA-A* and *HLA-C* allele disparity were each independent risk factors for severe acute GVHD; interestingly, no contribution from class II was found. In a recent update of the JMDP experience, *HLA-A*, *-C*, *-B* and *-DRB1* were each found to be independent risk factors for grades III–IV acute GVHD ([1.58 HR (hazard ratio); 1.2–2.1]; $p = 0.001$]; [1.85HR; 1.4–2.4; $p < 0.001$]; [1.43HR; 1.0–2.0; $p = 0.04$] and [1.42HR; 1.1–1.9; $p = 0.02$], respectively) [95]. *HLA-A* allele mismatching was also found to be a risk factor of severe GVHD in the NMDP analysis by Flomenberg et al. [90] (RR 1.33; 1.0–1.7; $p = 0.04$), however, *HLA-B* and *HLA-C* allele mismatches did not appear to contribute. These studies may have come to different conclusions regarding the relative contributions of class I and class II mismatching because of different allele and antigen mismatches between patients and donors.

Tally effects

Quantitative effects of multiple class I, multiple class II or simultaneous class I and II mismatching can be discerned for acute GVHD risk [37,52,67,84,90,93,95]. Additive *HLA-DRB1* and *-DQB1* effects can readily be measured [37,67,84]. In all three studies, the risk of clinically significant acute GVHD was increased in the presence of multiple class II mismatches. Additive effects of multilocus mismatching on GVHD risk were evaluated in the recent JMDP update [95]. Not only were multiple class I disparities a risk factor for GVHD but *HLA-C* disparity in the presence of mismatching at any other HLA locus (class I and/or class II) was

Table 83.5 Incidence of grades III–IV acute graft-vs.-host disease (GVHD) according to number of mismatched class I and class II alleles.*

	0 class I	1 class I	≥2 class I	Total
0 class II	77/237 (32%)	28/94 (30%)	21/59 (36%)	126/390 (32%)
1 class II	13/29 (45%)	4/14 (29%)	11/20 (55%)	28/63 (44%)
≥2 class II	6/9 (67%)	2/3 (67%)	6/7 (86%)	14/19 (74%)
Total	96/275 (34%)	34/111 (31%)	38/86 (44%)	168/472 (36%)

*This summary is restricted to 472 patients who underwent myeloablative conditioning and unrelated bone marrow transplantation for the treatment of chronic myeloid leukemia (CML) and had acute GVHD grading information available. The number of mismatched class I and class II alleles is displayed so that the effect of increasing numbers of class I alleles on GVHD incidence can be viewed within a fixed number of class II mismatches. Similarly, the effect of increasing numbers of class I mismatches can be compared to a fixed number of class I mismatches.

associated with significantly increased incidence of grades II–IV GVHD (60.9%, 55.7% and 64.3% for *HLA-C* plus *-A/B*; *HLA-C* plus *-DR/DQ* and *HLA-C* plus *-A/B* and *-DR/DQ*, respectively) compared to matched (34.5%), *HLA-A/B* mismatched (54.9%), *HLA-C* mismatched (42.7%) or *HLA-DR/DQ* mismatched (34.4%).

The effect of tally has been evaluated by the Seattle program (Table 83.5). When the data are stratified by the number of mismatched *HLA-DPB1* alleles (zero, one or two), the relative associations of class I and class II disparities with GVHD appear to be unaffected. In a logistic regression model that adjusted for the presence of zero, one or two *HLA-DPB1* allele mismatches, patients who were matched at *HLA-DRB1* and *-DQB1* tolerated a single class I *HLA-A* or *-B* or *-C* mismatch (OR 0.8; 0.5–1.4; $p = 0.47$). Among patients who were matched at class I, the presence of multiple class II mismatches was associated with increased risk of GVHD (OR 4.7; 1.1–19.6; $p = 0.03$), as were single class II mismatches (OR 1.8; 0.8–4.0; $p = 0.15$). Multiple class I mismatches were well tolerated provided there was no *HLA-DRB1* or *-DQB1* mismatch (OR 1.2; 0.7–2.2; $p = 0.57$). However, the combinations of class I disparities with class II disparities were associated with significantly increased GVHD risk (OR 11.6; 1.4–99.5; $p = 0.03$). These data suggest that single disparities for class I are in general better tolerated than those for class II with respect to GVHD. Identification of two-locus mismatches that do not increase GVHD risk may provide a means to allow patients who lack a matched donor the option for a transplant.

Impact of HLA sequence on GVHD risk

As the studies described above illustrate, the relative risk conferred by specific HLA loci to GVHD differs from population to population. How can these observations be reconciled? Examination of qualitative differences between the specific HLA antigens and alleles that are encoded in these transplant populations may help to explain why the studies found different associations. As described above, differences in GVHD risk are apparent between the Japanese and Caucasian populations [37,52,95]. Although Japanese and Caucasian donor–recipient pairs encoded a similar degree of disparity for *HLA-A*, *-B* and *-DRB1* alleles, they differed in the specific combinations of allele mismatches [51]. There was little overlap in the *HLA-A*, *-B*, *-C*, *-DRB1* and *-DQB1* allele mismatches in these two populations. These data imply that the specific mismatched residues may play a role in defining risk to GVHD.

Ferrara et al. [89] have carried the concept of residue (mis)matching one step further (Fig. 83.2). The investigators analyzed a total of 100 unrelated donor–recipient pairs, of which 40 were class-I sequence matched and 60 encoded one or more mismatches. Among class I mismatched pairs, substitutions at residue 116 were associated with a significantly increased risk of GVHD and TRM compared to transplants without substitutions at residue 116 (58% vs. 28%, $p = 0.001$). This is the first study to implicate the importance of the HLA sequence disparity and its position within the class I heavy chain. Involvement of residue 116 is predicted to participate in peptide binding (residue P9 of the peptide) (Fig. 83.2). These results provide a basis for future investigation of how the nature of amino acid substitutions at critical positions in the class I molecule may define peptide binding or involve interaction with the TCR to define alloreactivity. Together with the data from the JMDP and the Seattle programs, these studies point to the need to examine large ethnically diverse transplant populations in order to better understand how qualitative differences in the primary sequence of the HLA alloantigen confer biological effects.

Data on the effect of mismatching for class I alleles or antigens provide information in support of the hypothesis that the nature of the sequence disparity influences GVHD risk. Flomenberg et al. [90] compared the RR of grades III–IV acute GVHD between patients with an antigen ("low" level) and allele ("high" level) mismatch at HLA-A, -B and -DR genes. Multivariable analysis showed that mismatching at any class I locus was associated with a significantly higher incidence of grades III–IV acute GVHD and mortality compared to matching for HLA-A, -C, and -B. The associations were even stronger when the mismatch was defined at the antigen level compared to allele level. Furthermore, among HLA-A, -B antigen-matched, -DRB1 allele-matched recipients, 5-year survival was significantly inferior if additional allele disparities at HLA-A, -C, and/or -B were detected.

Relapse

HLA incompatibility is associated with GVLE. Elimination of recipient leukemia cells by GVLE mechanisms can provide a therapeutic advantage particularly for patients with a high risk of relapse after transplantation. The most comprehensive analysis of donor matching and post-transplant relapse has been conducted by the JMDP in five-locus allele-typed donor–recipient pairs [52,95]. Mismatching at the HLA-C locus in combination with mismatching at HLA-A/B and/or DR/DQ was associated with a lower 3-year relapse rate compared to complete matching or mismatching at HLA-A/B alone [52].

CML is very sensitive to GVLE. In 1990, Kolb et al. [100] described the use of donor lymphocyte infusion (DLI) to treat post-transplant relapse of CML. DLI has been shown to be effective in salvaging relapsed patients, but its limitations include GVHD and aplasia [101–106]. Efforts to decrease toxicity have led to refinements in the DLI procedure [107,108].

Survival

Risk factors for mortality after unrelated donor HCT include patient age (>50 years), HLA disparity, more than 3 years from the time of diagnosis of CML to transplantation, increased body weight index, CMV serostatus of the recipient and dose of infused nucleated cells [86–88,109–114]. Donor–recipient HLA matching for HLA-A, -B antigens and -DRB1 alleles correlates with improved survival and platelet recovery [86,87]. Among patients with CML, survival is improved with younger patient age, transplantation during the first CP, transplantation within 1 year of diagnosis and absence of severe acute GVHD [87]. Survival was significantly better at 3 years post-transplant in patients who recovered platelets by day 30, intermediate for patients who recovered between days 31 and 100, and lowest for patients whose platelet counts recovered after day 100. For patients undergoing unrelated donor HCT for the treatment of CML, TRM was associated with transplantation of $<3.65 \times 10^8$ TNC/kg [114]. For acute myeloid leukemia (AML) patients a higher marrow cell

Table 83.6 Hazard ratio for mortality according to class I and class II match status.*

	0 class I	1 class I	≥2 class I	Total
0 class II	1.0 ($n = 231$)	1.4 ($n = 96$)	1.9 ($n = 64$)	**1.0 ($n = 391$)**
1 class II	1.1 ($n = 33$)	3.0 ($n = 12$)	1.8 ($n = 23$)	**1.3 ($n = 68$)**
≥2 class II	1.5 ($n = 9$)	4.3 ($n = 3$)	4.4 ($n = 7$)	**2.1 ($n = 19$)**
Total	**1.0 ($n = 273$)**	**1.5 ($n = 111$)**	**1.6 ($n = 94$)**	

*This study population is identical to that described in Table 83.5 except that patients are not required to have acute graft-vs.-host disease (GVHD) grading information available. Hazard ratios reflect adjustments for stage of disease, age at transplant, time from diagnosis to transplant and use of cytomegalovirus (CMV) and fungal prophylaxis.

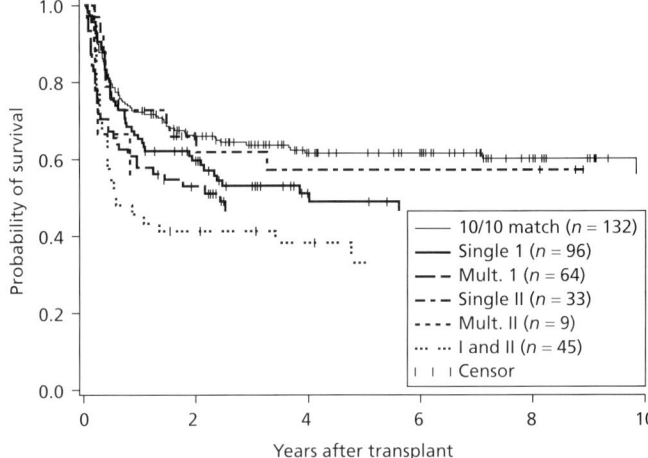

Fig. 83.3 Survival of patients with CML in CP transplanted from an unrelated donor according to HLA-A, -B, -C, -DRB, -DQB1 allele match status. Patients were conditioned with CY/TBI and received MTX/CSP for post-grafting immunosuppression using unmanipulated marrow. Donor–recipient matching for a total of 10 alleles is possible. Mismatched groups are non-overlapping and designed as follows: "Single 1" (one class I allele); "Multi 1" (two or more class I alleles); "Single II" (one class II allele); "Multi II" (two or more class II alleles); "I and II" (at least one class I and one class II alleles).

dose is associated with improved leukemia-free survival (LFS) of 54% at 5 years [112].

Comprehensive matching of HLA class I and II genes is associated with improved survival [27,32,37,52,67,84,89,90,92,93,95,115,116]. In a recent update of CML unrelated donor HCT by the Seattle program, synergistic effects of class I and II allele mismatches were found to strongly influence mortality (Table 83.6 & Fig. 83.3). A single class II allele mismatch appears to be well tolerated. The combination of at least one class II with any number of class I mismatches, however, is associated with significantly increased mortality.

Does the nucleotide sequence of the mismatch predict survival? The difference between antigen and allele mismatches parallels the results for graft failure and GVHD [70,72,90]. The importance of residue 116 mismatching and mortality was demonstrated by Ferrara et al. [89]. Flomenberg et al. [90] found poorer outcome in recipients with antigen mismatches at HLA-A and -B compared to recipients with allele mismatches at the same loci. Wade et al. [117] examined the effect of serologically defined HLA-A and -B antigens according to whether the mismatches occurred within crossreactive antigen groups (CREGs; refer to Chapter 4 for definition) or were defined outside of CREGs ("major" mismatches).

CREG and non-CREG antigen mismatches conferred equivalent outcomes with respect to engraftment, acute and chronic GVHD and survival, suggesting that certain HLA antigen mismatches may be tolerable. In this regard, Elsner and Blasczyk [118] have proposed a structure-based system for rating HLA alleles and antigens as a means to incorporate information on HLA structure (i.e. primary sequence) with function. The extent to which antigen mismatches are tolerable may be influenced by other non-HLA factors. Davies et al. [79] demonstrated that younger patients tolerate antigen disparity better than older patients can.

Role of HLA class I ligands and NK-KIR receptors in transplantation

When it is feasible, comprehensive donor matching can optimize transplantation. Critical to overall success of unrelated donor HCT, however, is the efficiency of the search process and the need to balance the desire to identify matched donors against the time required for extensive typing of multiple donors. Furthermore, complete allele matching can realistically only be achieved for a minority of patients. This is a particularly important issue for patients with high-risk leukemia in whom transplantation during optimal control of the underlying disease is a powerful predictor of overall survival. The identification of tolerable HLA mismatches would enable patients to benefit from mismatched unrelated donor HCT without compromising the overall success of the transplant procedure. Permissible mismatches include HLA molecules that mediate HVG and GVH allorecognition by T cells, but may also include class I allotypes that serve as ligands for natural killer (NK) cell-mediated recognition of host cells.

In contrast to the HLA restriction of T-cell allorecognition, NK cells interact with HLA class I molecules through inhibitory receptors termed killer immunoglobulin-like receptors (KIRs) and CD94/NKG2 (see Chapter 82 for a comprehensive review). Lack of expression of the correct inhibitory HLA class I ligands by the recipient can trigger donor NK cell alloreactivity and thereby lead to killing of recipient cells, including leukemic cells. Destruction of recipient antigen-presenting cells (APCs) removes the target of GVHD; destruction of host tumor cells leads to decreased potential for post-transplant relapse. The recipient's *HLA-C* genotype (specifically, residues 77 and 80) and *HLA-B* genotype (presence of the Bw4 epitope) can predict the pattern of donor KIR recognition. Therefore it is theoretically possible to determine whether potential unrelated donors might be KIR matched (not desirable because the donor NK cells will not be activated) or KIR mismatched (desirable because donor NK cells will kill recipient target cells).

In a landmark paper by Ruggeri et al. [119] the concept of donor NK-mediated killing of recipient APCs was shown in a cohort of 92 patients who underwent haplo-identical mismatched transplantation for high-risk AML or ALL. These patients received T-cell-depleted grafts, a high CD34-postive cell dose, and no postgrafting immunosuppression. This regimen promotes rapid NK recovery [120]. AML patients transplanted from KIR-mismatched donors had significantly improved 5-year survival compared to patients who received KIR-matched transplants (60% vs. 5%, $p < 0.0005$). KIR mismatching was associated with no graft failure, no acute GVHD, and a 0% 5-year probability of relapse. In contrast, KIR matching was an independent risk factor for poor transplant outcome (15.5% incidence of graft failure, 13.7% incidence of acute GVHD and 75% 5-year probability of relapse). Patients carrying the diagnosis of ALL were not protected against relapse with the use of KIR-mismatched donors (90% in KIR-matched donors vs. 85% in KIR-mismatched donors at 5 years).

Can the use of KIR-mismatched unrelated donors leverage the effects of donor NK killing to decrease the risks of acute GVHD and relapse for patients with high-risk myeloid malignancies? Davies et al. [121] provided the first look at this potential. In this retrospective study, 175 patients who received unrelated donor HCT from class I allele mismatched donors were identified as KIR matched or mismatched according to the same classification scheme used in the Ruggeri analysis [119]. Patients received either T-cell-depleted or unmanipulated grafts with cyclosporine (CSP)-based immunosuppression. Conditioning regimens used either TBI or non-TBI regimens with busulfan and CY. Among the 72 patients with a myeloid malignancy, no difference in graft failure, acute GVHD or relapse was observed. Survival of KIR-matched recipients was superior to that of the KIR-mismatched recipients (38% vs. 13%, $p < 0.01$). Several methodologic differences between the haplo-identical transplant regimen used by Ruggeri et al. [119] and the unrelated transplants performed by Davies et al. [121] might help explain the lack of association of KIR and outcome in the unrelated transplants. Ruggieri's study [119] employed extensive T-cell-depleted, high CD34-positive cell dose and no post-transplant immunosuppression in haplo-identical transplants, whereas Davies et al. [121] reported on the use of either unmanipulated or T-cell-depleted grafts with post-transplant immunosuppression for the unrelated transplants. Whether the conditioning regimens used in the unrelated transplants promoted higher numbers of alloreactive T cells, thereby obscuring any NK effect, still remains to be examined in more extensive analyses of haplo-identical and unrelated transplant situations.

Functional assays for donor selection

Several *in vitro* approaches to testing donor immune responses to host alloantigen have been evaluated as a means for predicting prior to transplantation the risk of GVHD and survival. These tests could be very helpful in situations in which there is more than one otherwise equally matched donor. Functional assays could also prove useful in testing the hypothesis that certain HLA incompatibilities may be less likely to activate donor cells and therefore classified as permissive mismatches. *In vitro* tests have included the MLC assay and limiting dilution assays (LDAs) to determine the frequency of donor antihost cytotoxic T-lymphocyte precursors (CTLps) and helper T-lymphocyte precursors (HTLps). These tests have also been proposed as a means for uncovering the presence of otherwise undetected HLA allele mismatching when high-resolution DNA-based typing is not available [122].

The standard one-way MLC assay has proven to be poorly predictive of GVHD in both haplo-identical related and phenotypically matched unrelated donor transplants [123–125]. Mickelson et al. [123] found no significant correlation between the donor-vs.-recipient MLC reaction and the probability of acute GVHD in 157 haplo-identical related transplant recipients who were phenotypically matched for HLA-A and -B, and variably mismatched for HLA-DR. In an analysis of 435 unrelated donor transplants, including 208 matched for HLA-A, -B and -DRB1 and 191 incompatible for one HLA-A, -B or -DR antigen mismatch, donor-vs.-recipient MLC responses were broadly reactive ranging from negative to strongly positive, and the overlap in MLC responses between cases matched and mismatched for *HLA-DRB1* alleles was extensive [124]. Using optimally defined cut-offs of 4% and 16% relative response, there was no correlation with risk of developing acute GVHD ($p = 0.6$ and 0.5, respectively). Even among 208 recipients known to be matched for *HLA-DRB1* alleles, the MLC response (reactive in 45% of cases with a relative response >4%) did not correlate with GVHD.

Given the failure of the conventional MLC assay to predict GVHD, the use of alternative quantitative measurements of CTL and HTL responses by LDA have been used to analyze the donor-vs.-recipient response [126–135]. LDAs have the potential advantage of detecting minor histocompatibility antigens; high precursor frequencies might identify alloimmunized donors whose T cells could have an increased ability to cause GVHD. High CTLp frequencies have been observed with class I donor–recipient mismatching; HTLp has been shown to detect class II disparity [127,128,132]. O'Shea et al. [132] assessed CTLp frequencies in a two-center study. High CTLp were associated with donor–recipient pairs mismatched for class I but matched for class II. The CTLp assay predicted those pairs whose genes encoded allele mismatches that were previously undetectable using standard methods for donor typing. Oudshoorn et al. [135] examined CTLp frequencies in 211 HLA-A, -B, -C allele typed donor–recipient pairs. The presence of class I mismatching correlated with high CTLp frequencies ($p < 0.001$). Exceptions were noted in 14% of HLA-A, -B, -C allele matched pairs who displayed high CTLp frequencies and in 7% of HLA mismatched pairs who displayed low frequencies. Among HLA-C mismatched pairs, disparity at residues 97, 99, 113, 114 and 116 were associated with high CTLp frequencies. This study demonstrates that the CTLp assay is capable of identifying donor–recipient disparity for residues that influence peptide binding.

Several studies have identified an association between the donor-vs.-recipient CTLp frequency and risk of acute GVHD after unrelated donor HCT [126,129,131,133,134]. Most of the patients in these studies received *ex vivo* or *in vivo* T-cell depletion for GVHD prophylaxis. In other studies where T-cell depletion was not used, significant association between CTLp frequency and acute GVHD could not be identified [136–138]. These findings are consistent with the interpretation that the risk of GVHD is related to the total number of transplanted donor T cells that recognize recipient alloantigens. The number of host-reactive T cells in an unmodified graft might often be sufficient to initiate GVHD regardless of the donor antirecipient CTLp frequency, while the number of specific T cells remaining in a T-cell-depleted graft might not be sufficient to initiate GVHD when the CTLp frequency is low. Other explanations could also account for discrepancies between the results of *in vitro* assays and clinical outcome. Antigens that generate a CTL response *in vitro* might not evoke GVHD because of inappropriate tissue distribution *in vivo*, low TCR affinity (which might be sufficient to generate a response *in vitro* but not *in vivo*) [139], or an inadequate helper T-cell response *in vivo* [140]. Likewise, antigens that generate HTL responses might not evoke GVHD in the absence of a CTL response [141]. Finally, the development of GVHD in the apparent absence of a CTL response could reflect the lack of appropriate peptide expression by target cells used for the *in vitro* assay.

Outcome of unrelated donor transplantation for selected hematologic malignancies

Chronic myeloid leukemia (CML)

Of all the clinical indications for allogeneic transplantation, more is understood of the molecular biology and therapeutic role of HCT for CML than for any other hematopoietic malignancy (see Chapters 22 & 73). The favorable success rate of sibling transplantation has given strong impetus for seeking unrelated donors for patients lacking a matched sibling. Factors important in successful outcome from unrelated-donor HCT have now been delineated and include the age of the patient, disease phase at transplantation, HLA match status of the donor and recipient, duration of CP prior to HCT, CMV serostatus of the donor and recipient, and donor gender [82,86,87,111,142]. Efforts to optimize the clinical results for unrelated-donor HCT for CML have focused on improved donor–recipient matching using molecular methods, development of less toxic transplant conditioning regimens, more effective prevention and treatment of GVHD, and improved supportive care of the patient (including prevention and treatment of bacterial, fungal and CMV infection) [143–148]. These efforts have led to survival rates that begin to compare favorably with those seen after HCT from matched-sibling donors, especially if transplantation can be performed from HLA allele matched unrelated donors for young patients with CML during the early course of their disease.

The recent introduction of tyrosine kinase inhibitors has provided clinicians with a powerful chemotherapy for up-front therapy of CML (see Chapter 73). Long-term toxicity and efficacy data on this agent are needed, however, to fully understand how this drug can be optimally used along side transplantation. Until such clinical data become available, allogeneic HCT is the only curative modality for CML. The long-term efficacy of nonmyeloablative transplant regimens on disease-free survival (DFS) in unrelated-donor HCT will become better defined in the near future (see Chapter 85), and may represent an option for older patients with CML.

Initial results from the NMDP reported by McGlave et al. [149] on 196 patients demonstrated 45% DFS at 2 years for CP patients transplanted within 1 year, 36% for patients transplanted more than 1 year from diagnosis, 27% for patients transplanted in accelerated phase (AP) and 0% for patients transplanted in blast phase (BP). Three recent analyses by the NMDP show significantly improved survival for CML after HCT from unrelated donors attributable to the use of transplantation early in the course of disease with improved donor HLA matching. Among 1423 patients evaluated by McGlave, graft failure occurred in 9.9% of patients and grades III–IV acute GVHD in 33% [87]. Among patients receiving HCT in CP, 5.7% developed hematologic relapse at 3 years post-transplant. Factors identified as associated with improved DFS included disease phase (CP) at transplantation, transplantation within 1 year of diagnosis, recipient age below 35 years, CMV-negative recipient and development of no or mild acute GVHD. Such patients had a 63% DFS at 3 years. To better understand the implications of donor matching on outcome of HCT for CML from unrelated donors, the NMDP evaluated 831 donor–recipient pairs using molecular techniques for polymorphic class I loci [92]. Survival for HLA-A, -B serologically matched transplants was significantly better with *HLA-DRB1* allele matching of the donor compared to *HLA-DRB1* mismatching (mismatching conferred a RR of 1.53 for mortality; 95%CI 1.09–2.16, $p = 0.01$). Spencer et al. [150] reported unrelated donor transplant results from a single institution for CML patients receiving antilymphocyte monoclonal antibody (Campath) to achieve T-cell depletion *in vivo*. The probability of graft failure was 16%, probability of grades III–IV acute GVHD was 24%, and probability of clinical extensive chronic GVHD at 1 year was 38%. Clinical relapse occurred in 20% of patients transplanted in first CP. Survival and DFS were 52% and 41% at 3 years for patients transplanted in CP, and 28% and 26% for patients transplanted in AP. CP patients under 40 years of age transplanted from HLA-matched donors had survival and DFS rates of 73% and 49%, respectively.

The Seattle program reported results of 336 transplants for CML of whom 196 were transplanted in CP, 83 in AP, 38 in BP and 19 in a second CP following blast phase (BP/CP2) [111]. All patients received unmodified marrow following conditioning with CY/TBI. CSP and methotrexate (MTX) were given for GVHD prophylaxis. The estimated cumulative incidence of clinical or cytogenetic relapse at 5 years was 10% for patients transplanted in CP. Overall 3-year survival for CP, AP, BP and BP/CP2 patients transplanted from an HLA-A, -B, -*DRB1*-matched donor was 62%, 34%, 9% and 27%, respectively. The probability of surviving 5 years among patients under 50 years of age transplanted from an HLA-A, -B, -*DRB1*-matched donor <1 year or >3 years from diagnosis was 74% and 50%, respectively. A more detailed analysis of GVHD among the 196 patients transplanted in CP shows that 152 (77%) of these cases were matched for HLA-A and -B antigens and -*DRB1* alleles, 19 (10%) were incompatible for one HLA-A or -B CREG antigen mismatch and 20 (10%) were incompatible for one serologically detectable HLA-DR mismatch. Acute GVHD was significantly higher after HCT across an HLA-DR serological mismatch, and there was a trend for a higher incidence of grades II–IV acute GVHD following HCT across an HLA-A or -B CREG antigen mismatch. Mismatching for *HLA-DRB1* was also associated with a significant delay in the recovery of platelets. The cumulative incidence of clinically extensive chronic GVHD was 67% among patients surviving disease-free more than 100 days; there was no significant difference in the risk of clinically extensive chronic GVHD between HLA-matched and HLA-mismatched cases.

Two-year survival rates of 77% have been achieved for patients ≤35 years old in early CP [151]. Similar results have been reported recently by the NMDP in a case-matched comparison of unrelated- and matched-sibling transplantation [148]. When unrelated-donor HCT is performed in CP, within 1 year from diagnosis, 5-year DFS of unrelated- vs. matched-sibling donors are 61% and 68% for patients <30 years; 57% and 67% for patients 30–40 years; and 46% and 57% for patients >40 years.

New developments in supportive care favorably influence survival. The use of fluconazole for prevention of fungal infection [152] and ganciclovir given at engraftment or onset of CMV antigenemia for the prevention of CMV disease [153] have been shown to improve the safety and success of marrow allografts, including unrelated-donor transplants. Since the routine introduction of these two agents in 1991–92, the 3-year survival rates for CML CP patients <50 years of age transplanted from an HLA-matched unrelated donor <1 year from diagnosis ($n = 30$) and >3 years from diagnosis ($n = 20$) has increased to 90% and 65%, respectively [111].

With the availability of chemotherapeutic agents capable of producing clinical and cytogenetic remissions of CML, the choice of the most appropriate treatment option can be very difficult, especially for newly diagnosed patients. Lee et al. [154] applied analytical decision techniques and quality-adjusted life expectancy data to compare interferon and transplantation. The results of this analysis supported early unrelated-donor transplantation for most CML patients. As described above, once data on the efficacy and toxicity of tyrosine kinase inhibitors have matured, similar evaluation of quality of life will be needed to develop appropriate recommendations for first-line therapy of this disease for both low-risk and high-risk patients.

Acute leukemia

Several different approaches have been explored for treating the high-risk patient with AML or ALL (see Chapters 75 and 77). For patients with high-risk acute leukemia achieving a complete remission (CR) after high-dose chemotherapy, autologous HCT has been used as a form of consolidation therapy [155,156]. The success of autologous HCT is limited in theory by the contamination of the reinfused stem cells with malignant progenitor cells and by lack of GVLE. As an alternative therapy for high-risk patients, successful allogeneic HCT from unrelated donors has been achieved by many transplant centers. A retrospective analysis comparing contemporaneous autologous and unrelated-marrow HCT for advanced acute leukemia found that patients in CR transplanted from an unrelated donor had lower relapse rates compared to autologous recipients (27% vs. 55%, $p = 0.8$). However, DFS for the two groups was comparable (33% for unrelated and 25% for autologous recipients, $p = 0.45$) [157]. In a more recent analysis comparing autologous with unrelated-donor HCT for patients with high-risk or recurrent ALL, transplantation from unrelated donors was associated with lower relapse rates but higher TRM [158]. DFS was superior for adults in CR2 transplanted from an unrelated donor compared to autologous transplants (42% vs. 20%, $p = 0.02$). These early data indicate that unrelated-donor HCT may be more effective than autologous HCT for eradicating ALL in selected high-risk patients.

The decline in the overall donor search time, together with ever improving clinical results in CML, have propelled the use of unrelated-donor HCT for the treatment of AML and ALL. Several factors have been identified which can optimize the overall outcome of unrelated-donor HCT for high-risk acute leukemia. DFS is highest when HCT is performed for patients in remission or in early first relapse [74,109,157–161]. Of 18 patients with Philadelphia chromosome-positive ALL studied by Sierra et al. [161] six of seven patients transplanted in first remission and two of three patients transplanted in first relapse were alive and disease-free at a median follow-up of 17 months. Among patients transplanted in relapse with AML or ALL, the presence of circulating blasts in the peripheral blood, as opposed to marrow involvement only, and the presence of >30% blasts in the marrow have both been associated with poor outcome [109]. These data have recently been updated for high-risk AML patients [112]. For CMV seronegative recipients in any CR who receive a marrow cell dose of at least 3.5×10^8 TNC/kg, 5-year LFS of 54% is observed [112]. Outcome of unrelated-donor HCT for Japanese patients has recently been reported [162,163]. For patients with ALL in CR1, CR2, CR3 and no CR, the DFS was 56%, 33%, 22% and 12%, respectively. For AML, those DFS were 71%, 55%, 43% and 12%, respectively [162]. DFS for AML and ALL approaches 75% at 2 years [163]. Greinix et al. [164] reported the findings of 40 patients receiving unrelated-donor HCT for AML. They found that lower TRM was defined by four variables: (i) CR1 disease status; (ii) patient age <46 years; (iii) transplantation performed after 1995; (iv) and absence of acute GVHD. Increased LFS was associated with the use of bone marrow, transplantation in CR1, and presence of chronic GVHD. Overall survival was improved with transplantation after 1995, disease phase CR1, presence of chronic GVHD and absence of grades III–IV acute GVHD. In a report by Marks et al. describing 39 patients transplanted using a T-cell-depletion (Campath-1M) conditioning regimen, DFS was 57% and overall survival was 61% [165].

Two recent analyses of unrelated-donor HCT for ALL demonstrate low post-transplant rates of relapse [166,167]. Patients transplanted in CR1 had DFS of 37%, albeit high TRM [166]. Weisdorf et al. [167] examined 517 unrelated-donor transplant procedures performed in CR1 or CR2. For patients <50 years, TRM was 42%; 14% relapse was observed for patients transplanted in CR1 and 25% if transplantation was carried out in CR2 [167]. Three-year survival was 51% for CR1 and 40% for CR2. Factors identified as predictive of better DFS included younger patient age, >1 year of CR1 if transplantation was performed in CR2, presenting total white blood cell count of $<50 \times 10^9$/L and transplantation after 1995.

Taken together, these studies demonstrate that HCT from unrelated donors should be considered as soon as possible after the diagnosis of high-risk leukemia is made and an unrelated-donor search should be initiated if a suitable family donor is not identified. If an HLA-matched unrelated donor is found transplantation should be carried out during remission or early in relapse. The selection of well-matched unrelated donors is associated with better overall clinical outcomes and is related to decreased risk of acute GVHD. In the absence of an HLA-A, -B, -DRB1, -DQB1-matched donor, the use of donors with limited HLA mismatches has been shown to be acceptable and, furthermore, is associated with decreased leukemic relapse post-transplant indicating the presence of GVLE. HCT from mismatched donors may be associated with decreased relapse rates but higher rates of acute GVHD, which obviates any advantages for survival [161].

Myelodysplastic syndrome (MDS)

Early clinical experience showed feasibility in the use of unrelated-donor HCT as a treatment modality for MDS [74,159,168–170]. Anderson et al. [170] reported on the outcome of 52 patients transplanted for MDS or MDS-related AML. Transplant outcome was related to disease morphology, patient age, disease duration, CMV sero status, blast count and neutrophil count. No relapses were observed among patients transplanted for refractory anemia (RA), refractory anemia with excess blasts (RAEB) or chronic myelomonocytic leukemia (CMML). In contrast, among patients transplanted for RAEB in transformation (RAEB-T), untreated AML or AML, 51% relapsed at 2 years post-transplant. There was a trend for better 2-year DFS for patients with RA, RAEB, RAEB-T, or CMML compared to patients with AML.

Since the early transplant experience, clinical research has focused on efforts to decrease TRM through the use of less toxic conditioning regimens and through a better understanding of disease and other variables that influence transplant outcome for MDS [171–173]. The association of longer disease duration and lower neutrophil count at the time of HCT with increased risk of nonrelapse mortality may be linked to complications resulting from iron overload and alloimmunization from transfusions. Updated data from Deeg et al. [172] found 3-year relapse-free survival of 59%, 11% relapse and 13% nonrelapse mortality at 100 days. Relapse correlated with the International Prognostic Scoring System stage at transplantation, the presence of poor-risk cytogenetics and therapy-related MDS. Improved relapse-free survival is associated with good-risk cytogenetic markers and shorter disease duration [173]. Given the average unrelated donor search time, consideration of HCT should be made for patients with RAEB or RAEB-T at the time of diagnosis because of the short median survival and high incidence of transformation to AML among patients with blasts. When a matched unrelated donor cannot be identified, the use of mismatched family donors is an option [171].

Concluding remarks

More complete understanding of the HLA system together with improvements in post-transplant care have contributed to an improved outcome of HCT from unrelated donors. Both quantitative and qualitative characteristics of donor–recipient HLA matching play a role in defining post-transplant risks of graft failure, GVHD and mortality. Of primary concern is the exclusion of patients from transplantation due to overly stringent HLA selection criteria, or delays in the donor search process in an effort to identify the ideally matched donor. The future of immunogenetics research in clinical HCT requires definition of mismatches that are well tolerated. As more genetic information becomes available from clinically diverse populations, it is anticipated that donor HLA selection criteria will be refined for disease-specific and regimen-specific applications of unrelated-donor HCT.

References

1 Uphoff DE, Law LW. Genetic factors influencing irradiation protection by bone marrow. II. The histocompatibility-2 (H-2) locus. *J Natl Cancer Inst* 1958; **20**: 617–24.

2 Epstein RB, Bryant J, Thomas ED. Cytogenetic demonstration of permanent tolerance in adult outbred dogs. *Transplantation* 1967; **5**: 267–72.

3 Gatti RA, Meuwissen HJ, Allen HD, Hong R, Good RA. Immunological reconstitution of sex-linked lymphopenic immunological deficiency. *Lancet* 1968; **2**: 1366–9.

4 Thomas ED, Storb R, Fefer A et al. Aplastic anemia treated by marrow transplantation. *Lancet* 1972; **1**(745): 284–9.

5 Bodmer WF. HLA. A super supergene. In: *The Harvey Lectures*. New York: Academic Press, 1978; **72**: 7291–138.

6 Dupont B, Hansen JA, Yunis EJ. Human mixed-lymphocyte culture reaction. Genetics, specificity, and biological implications. *Adv Immunol* 1976; **23**: 107–202.

7 Dupont B, Braun DW, Yunis EJ, Carpenter CB. HLA-D by cellular typing In: Terasaki PI, ed. *Histocompatibility Testing 1980*. University California: Los Angeles, 1980: 229–67.

8 Hansen JA, Mickelson EM, Choo SY et al. Clinical bone marrow transplantation: donor selection and recipient monitoring. In: Rose NR, DeMacario EC, Fahey JL, Friedman H, Penn GM, eds. *Manual of Clinical Laboratory Immunology*, 4th edn. Washington DC: American Society for Microbiology, 1992: 850–66.

9 van Rood JJ, van Leeuwen A, Keuning JJ, van Oud Alblas AB. The serological recognition of the human MLC determinants using a modified cytotoxicity technique. *Tissue Antigens* 1975; **5**: 73–9.

10 Terasaki P, Park MS, Bernoco D, Opelz G, Mickey MR. Overview of the 1980 International Histocompatibility Workshop. In: Terasaki PI, ed. *Histocompatibility Testing*. Los Angeles, CA: UCLA Tissue Typing Laboratory, 1980: 1–17.

11 Speck B, Zwaan FE, van Rood JJ, Eernisse JG. Allogeneic bone marrow transplantation in a patient with aplastic anemia using a phenotypically HLA-identical unrelated donor. *Transplantation* 1973; **16**: 24–8.

12 Lohrmann H-P, Dietrich M, Goldmann SF et al. Bone marrow transplantation for aplastic anemia from a HL-A and MLC-identical unrelated donor. *Blut* 1975; **31**: 347–54.

13 Horowitz SD, Bach FH, Groshong T, Hong R, Yunis EJ. Treatment of severe combined immunodeficiency with bone marrow from an unrelated, mixed-leukocyte culture nonreactive donor. *Lancet* 1975; **2**: 431–3.

14 L'Esperance P, Hansen JA, Jersild C et al. Bone-marrow donor selection among unrelated four-locus identical individuals. *Transplant Proc* 1975; **1**: 823–31.

15 O'Reilly R, Dupont B, Pahwa S et al. Successful hematologic and immunologic reconstitution of severe combined immunodeficiency and secondary aplasia by transplantation of bone marrow from an unrelated HLA-D compatible donor. *N Engl J Med* 1977; **297**: 1311–8.

16 Hansen JA, Clift RA, Thomas ED, Buckner CD, Storb R, Giblett ER. Transplantation of marrow from an unrelated donor to a patient with acute leukemia. *N Engl J Med* 1980; **303**: 565–7.

17 Cleaver S. The Anthony Nolan Research Centre and other matching registries. In: Treleaven BJ, ed. *Bone Marrow Transplantation in Practice*. Edinburgh, Scotland: Churchill Livingstone, 1992: 361–6.

18 McCullough J. Bone marrow transplantation from unrelated voluntary donors. Summary of a conference on scientific, ethical, legal, financial and practical issues. *Transfusion* 1982; **22**: 78–81.

19 McCullough J, Hansen J, Perkins H, Stroncek D, Bartsch G. The National Marrow Donor Program: how it works, accomplishments to date. *Oncology* 1989; **3**: 63–74.

20 Oudshoorn M, Leeuwen A, Zanden HGM, van Rood JJ. Bone Marrow Donors Worldwide: a successful exercise in international cooperation. *Bone Marrow Transplant* 1994; **14**: 3–8.

21 Al-Daccak R, Loiseau P, Rabian C et al. HLA-DR, DQ, and/or DP genotypic mismatches between recipient–donor pairs in unrelated bone marrow transplantation and transplant clinical outcome. *Transplantation* 1990; **50**: 960–4.

22 Baxter-Lowe LA, Eckels DD, Ash R, Casper J, Hunter JB, Gorski J. Future directions in selection of donors for bone marrow transplantation: role of oligonucleotide genotyping. *Transplant Proc* 1991; **23**: 1699–700.

23 Petersdorf EW, Smith AG, Mickelson EM, Martin PJ, Hansen JA. Ten HLA-DR4 alleles defined by sequence polymorphisms within the DRB1 first domain. *Immunogenetics* 1991; **33**: 267–75.

24 Tiercy JM, Morel C, Freidel AC et al. Selection of unrelated donors for bone marrow transplantation is improved by HLA class II genotyping with oligonucleotide hybridization. *Proc Natl Acad Sci U S A* 1991; **88**: 7121–5.

25 Santamaria P, Reinsmoen NL, Lindstrom AL et al. Frequent HLA class I and DP sequence mismatches in serologically (HLA-A, HLA-B, HLA-DR) and molecularly (HLA-DRB1, HLA-DQA1, HLA-DQB1) HLA-identical unrelated bone marrow transplant pairs. *Blood* 1994; **83**: 280–7.

26 Fernández-Viña MA, Lazaro AM, Sun Y, Miller S, Forero L, Stastny P. Population diversity of B-locus alleles observed by high-resolution DNA typing. *Tissue Antigens* 1995; **45**: 153–68.

27 Nademanee A, Schmidt GM, Parker P et al. The outcome of matched unrelated donor bone marrow transplantation in patients with hematological malignancies using molecular typing for donor selection and graft-versus-host disease prophylaxis regimen of cyclosporine, methotrexate, and prednisone. *Blood* 1995; **86**: 1228–34.

28 Martinelli G, Farabegoli P, Buzzi M et al. Fingerprinting of HLA class I genes for improved selection of unrelated bone marrow donors. *Eur J Immunogenet* 1996; **23**: 55–65.

29 Nagler A, Brautbar C, Slavin S, Bishara A. Bone marrow transplantation using unrelated and family related donors: the impact of HLA-C disparity. *Bone Marrow Transplant* 1996; **18**: 891–7.

30 Petersdorf EW, Longton GM, Anasetti C et al. Definition of HLA-DQ as a transplantation antigen. *Proc Natl Acad Sci U S A* 1996; **93**: 15358–63.

31 Pursall MC, Clay TM, Bidwell JL. Combined PCR-heteroduplex and PCR-SSCP analysis for matching of HLA-A, B and C allotypes in marrow transplantation. *Eur J Immunogenet* 1996; **23**: 41–53.

32 Speiser DE, Tiercy JM, Rufer N et al. High resolution HLA matching associated with decreased

mortality after unrelated bone marrow transplantation. *Blood* 1996; **87**: 4455–62.

33 Grundschober C, Rufer N, Sanchez-Mazas A *et al*. Molecular characterization of HLA-C incompatibilities in HLA-A-B-DR-matched unrelated bone marrow donor–recipient pairs. Sequence of two new Cw alleles (Cw*02023 and Cw*0707) and recognition by cytotoxic lymphocytes. *Tissue Antigens* 1997; **6**: 612–23.

34 Hurley CK, Schreuder GMT, Marsh SGE, Lau M, Middleton D, Noreen H. The search for HLA-matched donors. A summary of HLA-A*-B*-DRB1/3/4/5* alleles and their association with serologically defined HLA-A-B-DR antigens. *Tissue Antigens* 1997; **50**: 401–18.

35 Szmania S, Keever-Taylor CA, Baxter-Lowe LA. Automated nucleotide sequencing reveals substantial disparity between the *HLA-A2* genes of bone marrow transplant recipients and donors. *Hum Immunol* 1997; **56**: 77–83.

36 Arguello R, Avakian H, Goldman JM *et al*. A novel method for simultaneous high-resolution identification of HLA-A, HLA-B and HLA-Cw alleles. *Nat Genet* 1998; **18**: 192–4.

37 Petersdorf EW, Gooley TA, Anasetti C *et al*. Optimizing outcome after unrelated marrow transplantation by comprehensive matching of HLA class I and II alleles in the donor and recipient. *Blood* 1998; **92**: 3515–20.

38 Scott I, O'Shea J, Bunce M *et al*. Molecular typing shows a high level of HLA class I incompatibility in serologically well matched donor/patient pairs: implications for unrelated bone marrow donor selection. *Blood* 1998; **12**: 4864–71.

39 Prasad VK, Kernan NA, Heller G, O'Reilly RJ, Yang SY. DNA typing for HLA-A and HLA-B identifies disparities between patients and unrelated donors matched by HLA-A and HLA-B serology and HLA-DRB1. *Blood* 1999; **93**: 399–409.

40 Zanone-Ramseier R, Gratwohl A, Gmur J, Roosnek E, Tiercy J-M. Sequencing of two HLA-A blank alleles: implications in unrelated bone marrow donor matching. *Transplantation* 1999; **67**: 1336–41.

41 Hurley CK, Baxter-Lowe LA, Begovich AB *et al*. The extent of HLA class II allele level disparity in unrelated bone marrow transplantation: analysis of 1259 National Marrow Donor Program donor–recipient pairs. *Bone Marrow Transplant* 2000; **25**: 385–93.

42 Sayer D, Whidborne R, Brestovac B, Trimboli F, Witt C, Christiansen F. *HLA-DRB1* DNA sequencing based typing: an approach suitable for high throughput typing including unrelated bone marrow registry donors. *Tissue Antigens* 2002; **57**: 46–54.

43 Beatty PG, Mori M, Milford E *et al*. Impact of racial genetic polymorphism on the probability of finding an HLA-matched donor. *Transplantation* 1995; **60**: 778–83.

44 Lonjou C, Clayton J, Cambon-Thomsen A, Raffoux C. HLA-A-B-DR haplotype frequencies in France. Implications for recruitment of potential bone marrow donors. *Transplantation* 1995; **60**: 375–83.

45 Mori M, Beatty PG, Graves M, Boucher KM, Milford EL. HLA gene and haplotype frequencies in the North American population. The National Marrow Donor Program Donor Registry. *Transplantation* 1997; **64**: 1017–27.

46 Oudshoorn M, Cornelissen JJ, Fibbe WE *et al*. Problems and possible solutions in finding an unrelated bone marrow donor. Results of consecutive searches for 240 Dutch patients. *Bone Marrow Transplant* 1997; **20**: 1011–7.

47 Schipper RF, D'Amaro J, Bakker JT, Van Rood JJ, Oudshoorn M. HLA gene and haplotype frequencies in Bone Marrow Donors Worldwide registries. *Hum Immunol* 1997; **52**: 54–71.

48 Oh HB, Kim SI, Park MH, Akaza T, Juji T. Probability of finding HLA-matched unrelated marrow donors for Koreans and Japanese from the Korean and Japan Marrow Donor Programs. *Tissue Antigens* 1999; **53**: 347–9.

49 Velickovic ZM, Carter JM. Feasibility of finding an unrelated bone marrow donor on international registries for New Zealand patients. *Bone Marrow Transplant* 1999; **23**: 291–4.

50 Brown J, Poles A, Brown CJ, Contreras M, Vavarrete CV. HLA-A-B and -DR antigen frequencies of the London Cord Blood Bank units differ from those found in established bone marrow donor registries. *Bone Marrow Transplant* 2000; **25**: 475–81.

51 Hansen JA, Yamamoto K, Petersdorf E, Sasazuki T. The role of HLA matching in hematopoietic cell transplantation. *Rev Immunogenet* 1999; **1**: 359–73.

52 Sasazuki T, Juji T, Morishima Y *et al*. Effect of matching of class I HLA alleles on clinical outcome after transplantation of hematopoietic stem cells from an unrelated donor. *N Engl J Med* 1998; **339**: 1177–85.

53 Schreuder GM, Hurley CK, Marsh SG *et al*. The HLA dictionary: a summary of HLA-A-B-C-DRB1/3/4/5 and -DQB1 alleles and their association with serologically defined HLA-A-B-C-DR and -DQ antigens. *Eur J Immunogenet* 2001; **6**: 565–96.

54 Hurley CK, Wade JA, Oudshoorn M *et al*. Histocompatibility testing guidelines for hematopoietic stem cell transplantation using volunteer donors: report from The World Marrow Donor Association. Quality assurance and Donor Registries Working Groups of the World Marrow Donor Association. *Bone Marrow Transplant* 1999; **24**: 119–21.

55 O'Shea J, Cleaver S, Little A-M, Madrigal A. Searching for an unrelated haemopoietic stem cell donor: a United Kingdom perspective. In: Cecka M, Terasaki P, eds. *Clinical Transplants 1999*. Los Angeles: UCLA Immunogenetics, 2000. pp. 129–37.

56 Ottinger HD, Muller CR, Goldmann SF *et al*. Second German consensus on immunogenetics donor search for allotransplantation of hematopoietic stem cells. *Ann Hematol* 2001; **80**: 706–14.

57 Maiers M, Hurley CK, Capp K *et al*. A system for periodic reinterpretation of intermediate resolution DNA-based HLA types in a bone marrow registry. *Hum Immunol* 1998; **59** (Suppl. 1): 98 [Abstract].

58 Helmberg W, Hegland J, Hurley CK *et al*. Going back to the roots: effective utilization of HLA typing information for bone marrow registries requires full knowledge of the DNA sequences of the oligonucleotide reagents used in the testing. *Tissue Antigens* 2000; **56**: 99–102.

59 Marsh SG, Bodmer JG, Albert ED *et al*. Nomenclature for factors of the HLA system. *Tissue Antigens* 2000; **57**: 236–8.

60 Piazza A. Haplotype and linkage disequilibrium from the three-locus phenotypes. In: Kissmeyer-Nielsen F, ed. *Histocompatibility Testing 1975*. Copenhagen: Munksgaard, 1975: 923–7.

61 Begovich AB, McClure GR, Suraj VC *et al*. Polymorphism, recombination, and linkage disequilibrium within the HLA class II region. *J Immunol* 1992; **148**: 249–58.

62 Takahashi K, Juji T, Miyazaki H. Determination of an appropriate size of unrelated donor pool to be registered for HLA-matched bone marrow transplantation. *Transfusion* 1989; **29**: 311–3.

63 Schipper RF, D'Amaro J, Oudshoorn M. The probability of finding a suitable related donor for bone marrow transplantation in extended families. *Blood* 1996; **87**: 800–4.

64 Beatty PG, Boucher KM, Mori M, Milford EL. Probability of finding HLA-mismatched related or unrelated marrow or cord blood donors. *Hum Immunol* 2000; **61**: 834–40.

65 Tiercy J-M, Bujan-Lose M, Chapuis B *et al*. Bone marrow transplantation with unrelated donors: what is the probability of identifying an HLA-A/B/Cw/DRB1/B3/B5/DQB1-matched donor? *Bone Marrow Transplant* 2000; **26**: 437–41.

66 Pawlec G, Ehninger G, Schmidt H, Wernet P. HLA-DP matching and graft-versus-host disease in allogeneic bone marrow transplantation. *Transplantation* 1986; **42**: 558–60.

67 Keever-Taylor CA, Bredeson C, Loberiza FR *et al*. Analysis of risk factors for the development of GVHD after T cell-depleted allogeneic BMT. Effect of HLA disparity, ABO incompatibility, and method of T-cell depletion. *Biol Blood Marrow Transplant* 2001; **7**: 620–30.

68 Anasetti C, Amos D, Beatty PG *et al*. Effect of HLA compatibility on engraftment of bone marrow transplants in patients with leukemia or lymphoma. *N Engl J Med* 1989; **320**: 197–204.

69 Ash RC, Casper JT, Chitambar CR *et al*. Successful allogeneic transplantation of T-cell-depleted bone marrow from closely HLA-matched unrelated donors. *N Engl J Med* 1990; **322**: 485–94.

70 Fleischhauer K, Kernan NA, O'Reilly RJ, Dupont B, Yang SY. Bone marrow-allograft rejection by T lymphocytes recognizing a single amino acid difference in HLA-B44. *N Engl J Med* 1990; **323**: 1818–22.

71 Gajewski JL, Ho WG, Feig SA *et al*. Bone marrow transplantation using unrelated donors for patients with advanced leukemia or bone marrow failure. *Transplantation* 1990; **50**: 244–9.

72 Beatty PG, Hansen JA, Longton GM *et al*. Marrow transplantation from HLA-matched unrelated donors for treatment of hematologic malignancies. *Transplantation* 1991; **51**: 443–7.

73 Kato Y, Mitsuishi Y, Cecka M *et al*. HLA-DP incompatibilities and severe graft-versus-host disease in unrelated bone marrow transplants. *Transplantation* 1991; **52**: 374–6.

74 Kernan NA, Bartsch G, Ash RC *et al*. Analysis of 462 transplantations from unrelated donors facilitated by the National Marrow Donor Program. *N Engl J Med* 1993; **328**: 593–602.

75 Marks DI, Cullis JO, Ward KN *et al*. Allogeneic bone marrow transplantation for chronic myelogenous leukemia using sibling and volunteer unrelated donors: a comparison of complications in the first 2 years. *Ann Intern Med* 1993; **119**: 207–12.

76 Petersdorf EW, Smith AG, Mickelson EM *et al*. The role of HLA-DPB1 disparity in the development of acute graft-versus-host disease following unrelated donor marrow transplantation. *Blood* 1993; **81**: 1923–32.

77 Anasetti C, Hansen JA. Effect of HLA incompatibility in marrow transplantation from unrelated and HLA-mismatched related donors. *Transfus Sci* 1994; **15**: 221–30.

78 Keever CA, Leong N, Cunningham I et al. HLA-B44-directed cytotoxic T cells associated with acute graft-versus-host disease following unrelated bone marrow transplantation. Bone Marrow Transplant 1994; 14: 137–45.

79 Davies SM, Shu XO, Blazar BR et al. Unrelated donor bone marrow transplantation: influence of HLA-A and -B incompatibility on outcome. Blood 1995; 86: 1636–42.

80 Petersdorf EW, Longton GM, Anasetti C et al. The significance of HLA-DRB1 matching on clinical outcome after HLA-A, B, DR identical unrelated donor marrow transplantation. Blood 1995; 86: 1606–13.

81 Gajewski J, Gjertson D, Cecka M et al. The impact of T-cell depletion on the effects of HLA-DRB1 and DQB allele matching in HLA serologically identical unrelated donor bone marrow transplantation. Biol Blood Marrow Transplant 1997; 3: 76–82.

82 Madrigal JA, Scott I, Arguello R, Szydlo R, Little AM, Goldman JM. Factors influencing the outcome of bone marrow transplants using unrelated donors. Immunol Rev 1997; 157: 153–66.

83 Petersdorf EW, Longton GM, Anasetti C et al. Association of HLA-C disparity with graft failure after marrow transplantation from unrelated donors. Blood 1997; 89: 1818–23.

84 Przepiorka D, Petropoulos D, Mullen C et al. Tacrolimus for prevention of graft-versus-host disease after mismatched unrelated donor cord blood transplantation. Bone Marrow Transplant 1999; 23: 1291–5.

85 Varney MD, Lester S, McCluskey J, Gao X, Tait BD. Matching for HLA-DPA1 and DPB1 alleles in unrelated bone marrow transplantation. Hum Immunol 1999; 60: 532–8.

86 Davies SM, Kollman C, Anasetti C et al. Engraftment and survival after unrelated-donor bone marrow transplantation: a report from the National Marrow Donor Program. Blood 2000; 96: 4096–102.

87 McGlave PB, Shu XO, Wen W et al. Unrelated donor marrow transplantation for chronic myelogenous leukemia: 9 years' experience of the National Marrow Donor Program. Blood 2000; 95: 2219–25.

88 Przepiorka D, Saliba R, Cleary K et al. Tacrolimus does not abrogate the increased risk of acute graft-versus-host disease after unrelated-donor marrow transplantation with allelic mismatching at HLA-DRB1 and HLA-DQB1. Biol Blood Marrow Transplant 2000; 6: 190–7.

89 Ferrara GB, Bacigalupo A, Lamparelli T et al. Bone marrow transplantation from unrelated donors: the impact of mismatches with substitutions at position 116 of the human leukocyte antigen class I heavy chain. Blood 2001; 98: 3150–5.

90 Flomenberg N, Baxter-Lowe LA, Confer D et al. Impact of HLA-class I and class II high resolution matching on outcomes of unrelated donor BMT. Blood 2001; 98: 813 [Abstract].

91 Loiseau P, Esperou H, Busson M et al. DPB1 disparities contribute to severe GVHD and reduced patient survival after unrelated donor bone marrow transplantation. Blood 2001; 7: 660 [Abstract].

92 Petersdorf EW, Kollman C, Hurley CK et al. Effect of HLA class II gene disparity on clinical outcome in unrelated donor hematopoietic cell transplantation for chronic myeloid leukemia. The US National Marrow Donor Program Experience. Blood 2001; 98: 2922–9.

93 Petersdorf EW, Gooley T, Malkki M et al. The biological significance of HLA-DP gene variation in haematopoietic cell transplantation. Br J Haematol 2001; 112: 988–94.

94 Petersdorf EW, Hansen JA, Martin PJ et al. Major histocompatibility complex class I alleles and antigens in hematopoietic cell transplantation. N Engl J Med 2001; 345: 1794–800.

95 Morishima Y, Sasazuki T, Inoko H et al. The clinical significance of human leukocyte antigen (HLA) allele compatibility in patients receiving a marrow transplant from serologically HLA-A, HLA-B and HLA-DR matched unrelated donors. Blood 2002; 99: 4200–6.

96 Storb R, Prentice RL, Thomas ED. Marrow transplantation for treatment of aplastic anemia. An analysis of factors associated with graft rejection. N Engl J Med 1977; 296: 61–6.

97 Martin PJ, Hansen JA, Torok-Storb B et al. Graft failure in patients receiving T cell-depleted HLA-identical allogeneic marrow transplants. Bone Marrow Transplant 1988; 3: 445–56.

98 Beatty PG, Clift RA, Mickelson EM et al. Marrow transplantation from related donors other than HLA-identical siblings. N Engl J Med 1985; 313: 765–71.

99 Servida P, Gooley T, Hansen JA et al. Improved survival of haploidentical related donor marrow transplants mismatched for HLA-A or B versus HLA-DR. Blood 1996; 88(1): 484 [Abstract].

100 Kolb HJ, Mittermüller J, Clemm CH et al. Donor leukocyte transfusions for treatment of recurrent chronic myelogenous leukemia in marrow transplant patients. Blood 1990; 76: 2462–5.

101 Horowitz MM, Gale RP, Sondel PM et al. Graft-versus-leukemia reactions after bone marrow transplantation. Blood 1990; 75: 555–62.

102 Drobyski W, Keever C, Roth M et al. Salvage immunotherapy using donor leukocyte infusions as treatment for relapsed chronic myelogenous leukemia after allogeneic bone marrow transplantation: efficacy and toxicity of a defined T-cell dose. Blood 1993; 82: 2310–8.

103 Porter DL, Roth MS, McGarigle C, Ferrara JLM, Antin JH. Induction of graft-versus-host diseases immunotherapy for relapsed chronic myeloid leukemia. N Engl J Med 1994; 330: 100–6.

104 Van Rhee F, Lin F, Cullis JO et al. Relapse of chronic myeloid leukemia after allogeneic bone marrow transplant: the case for giving donor leukocyte transfusions before the onset of hematologic relapse. Blood 1994; 83: 3377–83.

105 Kolb HJ, Schattenberg A, Goldman JM et al. Graft-versus-leukemia effect of donor lymphocyte transfusions in marrow grafted patients. Blood 1995; 86: 2041–50.

106 Collins RH Jr, Shilberg O, Drobyski WR et al. Donor leukocyte infusions in 140 patients with relapsed malignancy after allogeneic bone marrow transplantation. J Clin Oncol 1997; 15: 433–44.

107 Dazzi F, Szydlo RM, Cross NC et al. Durability of responses following donor lymphocyte infusions for patients who relapse after allogeneic stem cell transplantation for chronic myeloid leukemia. Blood 2000; 96: 2712–6.

108 Guglielmi C, Arcese W, Dazzi F et al. Donor lymphocyte infusion for relapsed chronic myelogenous leukemia: prognostic relevance of the initial cell dose. Blood 2002; 100: 397–405.

109 Sierra J, Storer B, Hansen JA et al. Transplantation of marrow cells from unrelated donors for treatment of high-risk acute leukemia: the effect of leukemic burden, donor HLA-matching, and marrow cell dose. Blood 1997; 89: 4226–35.

110 Gratwohl A, Hermans J, Goldman JM et al. Chronic Leukemia Working Party of the European Group for Blood and Marrow Transplantation. Risk assessment for patients with chronic myeloid leukaemia before allogeneic blood or marrow transplantation. Lancet 1998; 352: 1087–92.

111 Hansen JA, Gooley T, Martin PJ et al. Bone marrow transplants from unrelated donors for patients with chronic myeloid leukemia. N Engl J Med 1998; 338: 962–8.

112 Sierra J, Storer B, Hansen JA et al. Unrelated donor marrow transplantation for acute myeloid leukemia: an update of the Seattle experience. Bone Marrow Transplant 2000; 26: 397–404.

113 Craddock C, Szydlo RM, Dazzi F et al. CMV serostatus is a major determinant of outcome after T-depleted unrelated donor transplant in patients with chronic myeloid leukaemia: the case for tailored GVHD prophylaxis. Br J Haematol 2001; 112: 228–36.

114 Pocock C, Szydlo R, Davis J et al. Stem cell transplantation for chronic myeloid leukaemia: the role of infused marrow cell dose. Hematol J 2001; 2: 265–71.

115 Shaw BE, Pay AL, Mayor N et al. High resolution molecular typing to ensure allele level matching for six highly polymorphic HLA antigens increases the overall survival in volunteer donor stem cell transplantation, however, "perfect" matches are found in only 10% of pairs. Blood 2001; 98: 668 [Abstract].

116 Drobyski WR, Klein J, Flomenberg N et al. Superior survival associated with transplantation of matched unrelated versus one-antigen-mismatched unrelated or highly human leukocyte antigen-disparate haploidentical family donor marrow grafts for the treatment of hematologic malignancies: establishing a treatment algorithm for recipients of alternative donor grafts. Blood 2002; 99: 806–14.

117 Wade JA, Takemoto SK, Thompson F et al. No deleterious effect of HLA-mismatching outside cross-reactive groups (CREG) compared to within CREG mismatches following unrelated donor bone marrow transplant. Biol Blood Marrow Transplant 2001; 7: 96 [Abstract].

118 Elsner HA, Blasczyk R. Sequence similarity matching: proposal of a structure-based rating system for bone marrow transplantation. Eur J Immunogenet 2002; 29: 229–36.

119 Ruggeri L, Capanni M, Urbani E et al. Effectiveness of donor natural killer cell alloreactivity in mismatched hematopoietic transplants. Science 2002; 20: 97–100.

120 Aversa F, Tabilio A, Velardi A et al. Successful engraftment of T-cell depleted haploidentical "three-loci" incompatible transplants in leukemia patients by addition of recombinant human granulocyte colony-stimulating factor-mobilized peripheral blood progenitor cells to bone marrow inoculum. Blood 1994; 84: 3948–55.

121 Davies SM, Ruggeri L, DeFor T et al. An evaluation of KIR ligand incompatibility in mismatched unrelated donor hematopoietic transplants. Blood 2002; 100: 3825–7.

122 Baxter-Lowe LA, Eckels DD, Ash R, Casper J, Hunter JP, Gorski J. The predictive value of HLA-DR oligotyping for MLC responses. Transplantation 1992; 53: 1352–7.

123 Mickelson EM, Guthrie LA, Etzioni R, Anasetti C, Martin PJ, Hansen JA. Role of the mixed

lymphocyte culture (MLC) reaction in marrow donor selection: matching for transplants from related haploidentical donors. *Tissue Antigens* 1994; **44**: 83–92.
124 Mickelson EM, Longton G, Anasetti C *et al.* Evaluation of the mixed lymphocyte culture (MLC) assay as a method for selecting unrelated donors for marrow transplantation. *Tissue Antigens* 1996; **47**: 27–36.
125 Segall M, Noreen H, Edwins L, Haake R, Shu XO, Kersey J. Lack of correlation of MLC reactivity with acute graft-versus-host disease and mortality in unrelated donor bone marrow transplantation. *Hum Immunol* 1996; **49**: 49–55.
126 Kaminski E, Hows J, Man S *et al.* Prediction of graft versus host disease by frequency analysis of cytotoxic T cells after unrelated donor bone marrow transplantation. *Transplantation* 1989; **48**: 608–13.
127 Zhang L, Rinke de Wit TF, Li S *et al.* Subtypes of HLA-A1 defined on the basis of CTL precursor frequencies. *Hum Immunol* 1990; **27**: 80–9.
128 Kaminski E, Hows JM, Bridge J *et al.* Cytotoxic T lymphocyte precursor (CTLp) frequency analysis in unrelated donor bone marrow transplantation: two case studies. *Bone Marrow Transplant* 1991; **8**: 47–50.
129 Roosnek E, Hogendijk S, Zawadynski S *et al.* The frequency of pretransplant donor cytotoxic T cell precursors with anti-host specificity predicts survival of patients transplanted with bone marrow from donors other than HLA-identical siblings. *Transplantation* 1993; **56**: 691–6.
130 Arguello R, Scott I, O'Shea J *et al.* Cytotoxic T lymphocyte precursor frequency (CTLpf) analysis highlights the need for better matching in the selection of unrelated bone marrow donors. *Bone Marrow Transplant* 1995; **15**: 248: S57 [Abstract].
131 Spencer A, Brookes PA, Kaminski E *et al.* Cytotoxic T lymphocyte precursor frequency analyses in bone marrow transplantation with volunteer unrelated donors. Value in donor selection. *Transplantation* 1995; **59**: 1302–8.
132 O'Shea J, Madrigal A, Davey N *et al.* Measurement of cytotoxic T lymphocyte precursor frequencies reveals cryptic HLA class I mismatches in the context of unrelated donor bone marrow transplantation. *Transplantation* 1997; **64**: 1353–6.
133 Kassar NE, Legouvello S, Joseph CM *et al.* High resolution HLA class I and II typing and CTLp frequency in unrelated donor transplantation: a single-institution retrospective study of 69 BMTs. *Bone Marrow Transplant* 2001; **27**: 35–43.
134 Dolezalova L, Vrana M, Dobrovolna M *et al.* Cytotoxic T lymphocyte precursor frequency analysis in the selection of HLA matched unrelated donors for hematopoietic stem cell transplantation: the correlation of CTLp frequency with HLA class I genotyping and aGVHD development. *Neoplasma* 2002; **49**: 26–32.
135 Oudshoorn M, Doxiadis IIN, van den Berg-Loonen PM *et al.* Functional versus structural matching: can the CTLp test be replaced by HLA allele typing? *Hum Immunol* 2002; **63**: 176–84.
136 Fussell ST, Donnellan M, Cooley MA, Farrell C. Cytotoxic T lymphocyte precursor frequency does not correlate with either the incidence or severity of graft-versus-host disease after matched unrelated donor bone marrow transplantation. *Transplantation* 1994; **57**: 673–6.
137 Schwarer AP, Jiang YZ, Deacock S *et al.* Comparison of helper and cytotoxic anti-recipient T cell frequencies in unrelated bone marrow transplantation. *Transplantation* 1994; **58**: 1198–203.
138 Pei JI, Martin PJ, Longton G *et al.* Evaluation of pretransplant donor anti-recipient cytotoxic and helper T lymphocyte responses as correlates of acute graft-versus-host disease and survival after unrelated marrow transplantation. *Biol Blood Marrow Transplant* 1997; **3**: 142–9.
139 Rosenberg AS, Singer A. Cellular basis of skin allograft rejection: an *in vivo* model of immune-mediated tissue destruction. *Ann Rev Immunol* 1992; **10**: 333–58.
140 Sprent J, Hurd M, Schaefer M, Heath W. Split tolerance in spleen chimeras. *J Immunol* 1995; **154**: 1198–206.
141 Braun MY, Lowin B, French L, Acha-Orbea H, Tschopp J. Cytotoxic T cells deficient in both functional Fas ligand and perforin show residual cytolytic activity yet lose their capacity to induce lethal acute graft-versus-host disease. *J Exp Med* 1996; **183**: 657–61.
142 Goldman JM. Chronic myeloid leukemia. *Curr Opin Hematol* 1997; **4**: 277–85.
143 Drobyski WR, Pelz C, Kabler-Babbitt C, Hessner M, Baxter-Lowe LA, Keever-Taylor CA. Successful unrelated marrow transplantation for patients over the age of 40 with chronic myelogenous leukemia. *Biol Blood Marrow Transplant* 1998; **4**: 3–12.
144 Reiter E, Greinix HT, Keil F *et al.* Long-term follow-up of patients after related- and unrelated-donor bone marrow transplantation for chronic myelogenous leukemia. *Ann Hematol* 1999; **78**: 507–13.
145 Carreras E, Tomas J-F, Sanz G *et al.* Unrelated donor bone marrow transplantation as treatment for chronic myeloid leukemia: the Spanish experience. *Haematologica* 2000; **85**: 530–8.
146 Davies SM, DeFor TE, McGlave PB *et al.* Equivalent outcomes in patients with chronic myelogenous leukemia after early transplantation of phenotypically matched bone marrow from related or unrelated donors. *Am J Med* 2001; **110**: 339–46.
147 Elmaagacli AH, Basoglu S, Peceny R *et al.* Improved disease-free-survival after transplantation of peripheral blood stem cells as compared with bone marrow from HLA-identical unrelated donors in patients with first chronic phase chronic myeloid leukemia. *Blood* 2002; **99**: 1130–5.
148 Weisdorf DJ, Anasetti C, Antin JH *et al.* Allogeneic bone marrow transplantation for chronic myelogenous leukemia: comparative analysis of unrelated versus matched sibling donor transplantation. *Blood* 2002; **99**: 1971–7.
149 McGlave P, Bartsch G, Anasetti C *et al.* Unrelated donor marrow transplantation therapy for chronic myelogenous leukemia: initial experience of the National Marrow Donor Program. *Blood* 1993; **81**: 543–50.
150 Spencer A, Szydlo RM, Brookes PA *et al.* Bone marrow transplantation for chronic myeloid leukemia with volunteer unrelated donors using *ex vivo* or *in vivo* T-cell depletion: major prognostic impact of HLA class I identity between donor and recipient. *Blood* 1995; **86**: 3590–7.
151 Barker JN, Davies SM, DeFor TE *et al.* Determinants of survival after human leucocyte antigen-matched unrelated donor bone marrow transplantation in adults. *Br J Haematol* 2002; **118**: 101–7.
152 Slavin MA, Osborne B, Adams R, Levenstein MJ, Schoch HG. Efficacy and safety of fluconazole for fungal infections after marrow transplant—a prospective, randomized, double-blind study. *J Infect Dis* 1995; **171**: 1545–52.
153 Goodrich JM, Bowden RA, Fisher L *et al.* Ganciclovir prophylaxis to prevent cytomegalovirus disease after allogeneic marrow transplant. *Ann Intern Med* 1993; **118**: 173–8.
154 Lee SJ, Kuntz KM, Horowitz MM *et al.* Unrelated donor bone marrow transplantation for chronic myelogenous leukemia: a decision analysis. *Ann Intern Med* 1997; **127**: 1080–8.
155 Gorin NC, Aegerter P, Auvert B *et al.* Autologous bone marrow transplantation for acute myelocytic leukemia in first remission: a European survey of the role of marrow purging. *Blood* 1990; **75**: 1606–14.
156 Doney K, Buckner CD, Fisher L *et al.* Autologous bone marrow transplantation for patients with acute lymphoblastic leukemia. *Bone Marrow Transplant* 1993; **12**: 315–21.
157 Busca A, Anasetti C, Anderson J *et al.* Unrelated donor or autologous marrow transplantation for treatment of acute leukemia. *Blood* 1994; **83**: 3077–84.
158 Weisdorf DJ, Billett AL, Hannan P *et al.* Autologous versus unrelated donor allogeneic marrow transplantation for acute lymphoblastic leukemia. *Blood* 1997; **90**: 2962–8.
159 Schiller G, Feig SA, Territo M *et al.* Treatment of advanced acute leukaemia with allogeneic bone marrow transplantation from unrelated donors. *Br J Haematol* 1994; **88**: 72–8.
160 Casper J, Camitta B, Truitt R *et al.* Unrelated bone marrow donor transplants for children with leukemia or myelodysplasia. *Blood* 1995; **85**: 2354–63.
161 Sierra J, Radich J, Hansen JA *et al.* Marrow transplants from unrelated donors for treatment of Philadelphia chromosome-positive acute lymphoblastic leukemia. *Blood* 1997; **90**: 1410–4.
162 Kodera Y, Morishima Y, Kato S *et al.* Analysis of 500 bone marrow transplants from unrelated donors (UR-BMT) facilitated by the Japan Marrow Donor Program: confirmation of UR-BMT as a standard therapy for patients with leukemia and aplastic anemia. *Bone Marrow Transplant* 1999; **24**: 995–1003.
163 Ooi J, Iseki T, Takahashi S *et al.* A clinical comparison of unrelated cord blood transplantation and unrelated bone marrow transplantation for adult patients with acute leukaemia in complete remission. *Br J Haematol* 2002; **118**: 140–3.
164 Greinix HT, Nachbaur D, Krieger O *et al.* Factors affecting long-term outcome after allogeneic haematopoietic stem cell transplantation for acute myelogenous leukaemia: a retrospective study of 172 adult patients reported to the Austrian Stem Cell Transplantation Registry. *Br J Haematol* 2002; **117**: 914–23.
165 Marks DI, Bird JM, Vettenranta K *et al.* T cell-depleted unrelated donor bone marrow transplantation for acute myeloid leukemia. *Biol Blood Marrow Transplant* 2000; **6**: 646–53.
166 Cornelissen JJ, Carston M, Kollman C *et al.* Unrelated marrow transplantation for adult patients with poor-risk acute lymphoblastic leukemia: strong graft-versus-leukemia effect and risk factors determining outcome. *Blood* 2001; **97**: 1572–7.
167 Weisdorf D, Bishop M, Dharan B *et al.* Autologous versus allogeneic unrelated donor transplantation for acute lymphoblastic leukemia: comparative toxicity and outcomes. *Biol Blood Marrow Transplant* 2002; **8**: 213–20.

168 Alessandrino EP, Bernasconi P, Bonfichi M et al. Bone marrow transplantation from unrelated donors in myelodysplastic syndromes. *Bone Marrow Transplant* 1993; **11**: 71–3.

169 Ratanatharathorn V, Karanes C, Uberti J et al. Busulfan-based regimens and allogeneic bone marrow transplantation in patients with myelodysplastic syndromes. *Blood* 1993; **81**: 2194–9.

170 Anderson JE, Anasetti C, Appelbaum FR et al. Unrelated donor marrow transplantation for myelodysplasia (MDS) and MDS-related acute myeloid leukaemia. *Br J Haematol* 1996; **93**: 59–67.

171 De Witte T, Pikkemaat F, Hermans J et al. Genotypically nonidentical related donors for transplantation of patients with myelodysplastic syndromes: comparison with unrelated donor transplantation and autologous stem cell transplantation. *Leukemia* 2001; **15**: 1878–84.

172 Deeg HJ, Storer B, Slattery JT et al. Conditioning with targeted busulfan and cyclophosphamide for hemopoietic stem cell transplantation from related and unrelated donors in patients with myelodysplastic syndrome. *Blood* 2002; **100**: 1201–7.

173 Jurado M, Deeg HJ, Strorer B et al. Hematopoietic stem cell transplantation for advanced myelodysplastic syndrome after conditioning with busulfan and fractionated total body irradiation is associated with low relapse rate but considerable nonrelapse mortality. *Biol Blood Marrow Transplant* 2002; **8**: 161–9.

174 Bjorkman PJ, Saper MA, Samraoui B, Bennett WS, Strominger JL, Wiley DC. The foreign antigen binding site and T cell recognition regions of class I histocompatibility antigens. *Nature* 1987; **329**: 512–8.

175 Garboczi DN, Ghosh P, Utz U, Fan QR, Biddison WE, Wiley DC. Structure of the complex between human T-cell receptor, viral peptide and HLA-A2. *Nature* 1996; **384**: 134–41.

84

Robert H. Collins, Jr

Management of Relapse after Allogeneic Transplantation

Introduction

Until approximately a decade ago management of patients with relapsed malignancy after allogeneic hematopoietic cell transplantation (HCT) was limited for the most part to chemotherapy, which was viewed as palliative, and/or a second transplantation, which was viewed as a risky, low-yield procedure. However, the increasing appreciation of graft-vs.-leukemia (GVL) as a potent clinical phenomenon led to attempts to harness it in relapsed patients, through discontinuation of immunosuppression or donor lymphocyte infusion (DLI). It is now well understood that DLI is effective in many patients with post-transplant relapse, and the procedure is probably the most commonly employed approach in this setting. While the usefulness of DLI in certain diseases, in particular chronic myeloid leukemia (CML), has become increasingly clear, continued clinical studies have illuminated its deficiencies as well, in terms of toxicity and limited activity in certain diseases. These problems have led to the investigation of various modifications of DLI and to the testing of different approaches, in particular imatinib mesylate (STI571, Gleevec®) for relapsed CML. As the field continues to evolve it is probably safe to say that there is no standard therapy for any given situation, although current data allow a rational assessment of the various options. This chapter will cover current approaches to relapsed malignancy after allogeneic HCT, with an emphasis on harnessing GVL, as the bulk of research has been in this area, but with discussion of several other traditional and more recently introduced approaches as well (Table 84.1).

Types of relapse

Relapse has been reported rarely in donor cells [1–6]; the mechanisms underlying this important phenomenon are uncertain. However, most relapses occur in patient cells, with the relapse derived from the original malignant clone [7]. Acute leukemia relapses are usually systemic and may be heralded by an unexplained drop in blood counts. The course is usually aggressive but may be smoldering. Relapse limited to extramedullary sites occurs in approximately 13% of acute myelogenous leukemia (AML) relapses and 24% of acute lymphoblastic leukemia (ALL) relapses [8,9]. These relapses commonly occur in the central nervous system (CNS) or testis but may occur at virtually any site [10,11]. Extramedullary relapses tend to occur later in the post-transplant phase than systemic relapses and almost always progress to systemic relapse. CML may relapse in chronic, accelerated or blast phase, regardless of the phase at the time of transplantation. Some patients with CML have no evidence of relapse other than the reappearance of cells containing the Philadelphia chromosome. In most instances this cytogenetic relapse predicts subsequent development of hematologic relapse [12–14]. However, cases have been observed in which the recurrence of the Philadelphia chromosome was only transient and hematologic relapse did not occur. For example, in one study, four of 26 patients with CML and cytogenetic relapse had apparently transient relapses [14]. However, two of these patients subsequently did progress to relapse, and the other two at the time of the report were still strongly positive for bcr-abl transcripts.

Various investigators have studied methods of minimal residual disease (MRD) detection in the post-transplant setting, including polymerase chain reaction (PCR), fluorescence in situ hybridization (FISH) and immunophenotypic analysis by multiparameter flow cytometry [15,16]. The disease most studied is CML. Detection of bcr-abl transcripts by qualitative PCR usually predicts relapse after T-cell-depleted bone marrow transplantation (BMT) [17,18]. However, qualitative PCR positivity may or may not predict relapse after non-T-cell-depleted BMT [19,20]. Positivity at 6 months is associated with a 42% probability of relapse [20], but with increased time post-transplant a positive qualitative PCR test is less predictive of relapse [21]. Quantitative PCR by competitive or real-time techniques may allow better prediction of relapse, with a progressive increase in bcr-abl transcripts in serial samples identifying patients who will relapse; persistently low or decreasing levels of bcr-abl transcripts identify patients who will stay in remission [22]. Preliminary studies suggest that MRD detection may be of value in predicting relapse in several other settings as well but further study is required (see Chapter 22 for detailed discussion) [15,23–26]. If techniques of MRD detection can reliably predict relapse, then earlier therapeutic intervention might result in improved efficacy and lessened toxicity.

Table 84.1 Approaches to relapse after allogeneic transplantation.

Donor leukocyte infusions
Discontinuation of immunosuppression
Second transplants
Cytotoxic chemotherapy
Interferon-alpha (IFN-α)
Interleukin 2 (IL-2)
Granulocyte colony-stimulating factor (G-CSF)
Imatinib mesylate (STI571, Gleevec®)
Irradiation
Palliation

Treatment of relapse

Donor lymphocyte infusion (DLI)

Background

Barnes et al. first showed an antitumor effect of allogeneic immune cells in classic experiments carried out in the 1950s [27]. In these studies, leukemic mice were treated with total body irradiation (TBI) followed by either allogeneic or syngeneic BMT; animals receiving allogeneic marrow were much less likely to relapse than those receiving syngeneic marrow. Subsequent animal studies over the ensuing decades have expanded on these findings, clearly demonstrating a graft-vs.-leukemia (GVL) effect of allogeneic BMT and, in many instances, shedding light on mechanisms of the effect (see Chapter 28) [28]. Clinical observations in the 1970s and 1980s suggested a GVL effect of human BMT: relapse rates were higher in recipients of syngeneic as opposed to allogeneic transplantations [29]; among recipients of allogeneic transplantations, the relapse rates were much lower in patients who developed graft-vs.-host disease (GVHD) [30,31]; T-cell depletion, while decreasing the incidence of GVHD, also significantly increased the incidence of leukemic relapse [32]. Horowitz et al. [33] confirmed these findings in a large analysis of International Bone Marrow Transplant Registry (IBMTR) data.

Based on an appreciation of the power of the GVL effect, several investigators began attempts to harness it [34,35]. These investigators treated patients with recurrent or persistent malignancy after allogeneic BMT with infusions of additional lymphocytes obtained from the original donor, without the cover of immunosuppressive agents. It was anticipated that donor lymphocytes would be effective in this setting because they were not inhibited by immunosuppressive agents and because they had not been inhibited by the tumor escape mechanisms that may have led to the relapse. Complete responses in a significant percentage of patients led to broad application of this approach [36–45].

Most DLIs are given to patients who have relapsed after standard fully myeloablative HCTs and most of the data discussed in this chapter are derived from studies in this setting. However, the appreciation that GVL can be harnessed by DLI has led to a new approach to HCT called nonmyeloablative HCT (see Chapter 85) [46–50]. In this type of transplantation, patients receive relatively low doses of chemotherapy and/or radiation, which are nevertheless immunosuppressive enough to allow donor cell engraftment. Engrafted lymphocytes, it is hoped, will then mediate GVL effects. In some instances, additional DLIs are given after nonmyeloablative HCT to enhance GVL. Although the current published data regarding this approach are relatively limited, these results to some extent have shed light on which diseases might be especially sensitive to GVL.

Chronic myeloid leukemia (CML)

Most reported DLI administrations have been for patients with CML. Several small case series, two large retrospective analyses of European and North American registries, and several publications involving modifications of DLI allow fairly solid conclusions about optimal DLI usage in this disease [34,36–43,51–53].

Antitumor activity

Kolb [34] reported the first three patients with CML successfully treated by DLI. Additional studies have confirmed the pronounced sensitivity of CML to DLI (Table 84.2) [36–43,51,53]. The likelihood of response varies by the extent of disease at the time of DLI. Response rates in chronic phase relapse are approximately 75%, whereas responses in more advanced disease range from 12.5% to 29.0%. Responses are better in

Table 84.2 Donor lymphocyte infusion (DLI) for chronic myeloid leukemia (CML).

	European*	North American[†]
Number of patients	84	56
Mononuclear cell (MNC) dose × 10⁸/kg. Median (range)	3.0 (0.25–12.30)	4.59 (0.79–11.39)
Interferon-α	60 (76%)	31 (55%)
Complete remission[‡]		
Cytogenetic relapse	14/17 (82%)	3/3 (100%)
Hematologic relapse	39/50 (78%)	25/34 (73.5%)
Transformed relapse	1/8 (12.5%)	5/18 (28%)

*Data from Kolb et al. [42].
[†]Data from Collins et al. [43].
[‡]Of assessable patients.

cytogenetic relapse (82–100%) and molecular relapse (eight of eight patients in one study [53]), although the number of DLI patients reported from these categories is relatively low. In the majority of patients with complete remission (CR) defined by cytogenetics, there is no evidence of bcr-abl transcript by PCR analysis [42,43,53]. The time to CR can be quite long, with a median time of 3–4 months and a range of 1–11 months or more. Molecular remissions follow cytogenetic remissions by several weeks. Close monitoring with sensitive techniques can define a "critical switch period" of 4–5 weeks during which recipient cell numbers suddenly decrease associated with a sharp decrease in bcr-abl transcripts [54]. Other patients manifest a slower, more gradual decline in bcr-abl transcripts [55].

The most important pre-DLI predictor of response is disease status at the time of DLI [42,43,53]. It is unclear whether advanced disease is more resistant because of rapid growth, excessive tumor cell numbers for the number of T cells infused, or intrinsic resistance of tumor cells to GVL mechanisms. Other potential predictive factors have not been consistent from study to study, including prior GVHD and time from BMT to DLI. T-cell depletion of the initial BMT was not an important factor in separate multivariate analyses [42,43].

GVHD and response

GVHD is closely correlated with response. In the North American registry study, 42 of 45 assessable complete responders developed acute GVHD and 36 of 41 assessable complete responders developed chronic GVHD following DLI [43]. The correlation of acute and chronic GVHD with CR was highly statistically significant ($p < 0.00001$). In this study, of 23 patients who did not develop either acute or chronic GVHD, only three attained CR. However, it is important to point out that many responders have been reported in the literature who did not develop clinically detectable GVHD. For example, although the European registry analysis reported a high response rate in CML patients who developed GVHD or myelosuppression (91%), they also reported that 45% of patients without any GVHD or myelosuppression had responses (however, it should be noted that this group did not report data regarding chronic GVHD) [42]. Almost all reports of DLI have included at least a small number of patients who responded without GVHD, and in some studies this number has been fairly high [42,51,53,56]. Thus, while GVHD is usually associated with response in patients receiving standard DLI, the observation of apparent GVL without GVHD in some patients is encouraging and has led to a variety of approaches aimed at separating the two phenomena.

Duration of remission

Remissions appear to be durable in most complete responders who had early phase relapse at the time of DLI. In one study with a median follow-up time of 39 months, only two of 32 (6%) complete responders treated for early phase disease relapsed compared to three of seven (43%) with advanced-phase relapse [57]. Another study with median follow-up of 29 months reported relapse in only four of 44 (9%) patients who attained molecular remissions [52]. Many patients are now more than 5 years out from DLI and remain in remission [44,57], and one group has reported 30 patients whose remission duration after DLI exceeds the remission duration after the initial transplantation [52]. It is unknown whether ongoing molecular remissions are due to the tumor being completely eradicated or to immune surveillance. Surveillance by infused T cells can occur in some settings, as shown by the proliferation of gene-marked Epstein–Barr virus-specific T cells in response to a flare of Epstein–Barr virus months after initially controlling the disease [58].

Long-term survival

Kolb *et al.* [44] reported long-term survival data after DLI for CML. With median follow-up of approximately 2 years, 80% of patients treated in cytogenetic relapse were alive compared to approximately 55% of patients treated in chronic phase relapse and approximately 20% of patients treated in transformed phase. Porter *et al.* [57] reported long-term follow-up for 39 CML patients who had attained a CR after DLI. The event-free survival at 3 years was 73%. Seven of 32 patients treated for early phase disease had died—two of disease, two of GVHD and three from other causes. Six of the seven advanced-phase disease patients had died—two of disease, two of GVHD and two of other causes.

Interferon-alpha (IFN-α)

IFN-α conceivably might increase GVL activity by increasing expression of cell-surface molecules necessary for effector and target cell interaction [59,60], or it may have direct antitumor effects. Therefore, many patients have received IFN-α along with DLI. Although occasional patients have seemed to respond to DLI only after the addition of IFN-α [45], multivariate analyses of large numbers of CML patients suggest that IFN-α is not required for response to occur [42,43]. However, only a randomized controlled trial would answer this question definitively.

Cell dose

Most early DLIs have involved large cell doses, generally on the order of 1×10^8 T cells/kg; GVHD is commonly observed after infusion of these doses. Several groups have studied lower doses to determine if there might be a dose at which GVL occurs but GVHD does not. Mackinnon *et al.* [51] treated 22 CML patients with escalating doses of T cells at intervals of 4–33 weeks with eight dose levels between 1×10^5 and 5×10^8/kg. Nineteen patients achieved remission, with eight remissions occurring at a dose of 1×10^7/kg and the other responders requiring doses of $\geq 5 \times 10^7$/kg. Only one of the eight patients who attained remission at 1×10^7/kg developed GVHD, while eight of the 11 responders who received higher doses developed GVHD.

Others have also reported patients treated with escalating doses of T cells. Dazzi *et al.* [53] reported that patients treated with an escalating-dose regimen were as likely to respond as patients treated with a single "bulk" dose; however, the incidence of GVHD was much lower in the group receiving escalating doses (10% vs. 44%) (Fig. 84.1). This difference in GVHD incidence between escalating and "bulk" dose appeared to hold up even if the total dose infused was the same. The mechanisms underlying this observation are unknown; it should be noted that this subset analysis involved relatively small numbers of patients.

A retrospective analysis of 298 CML patients treated with DLI gives

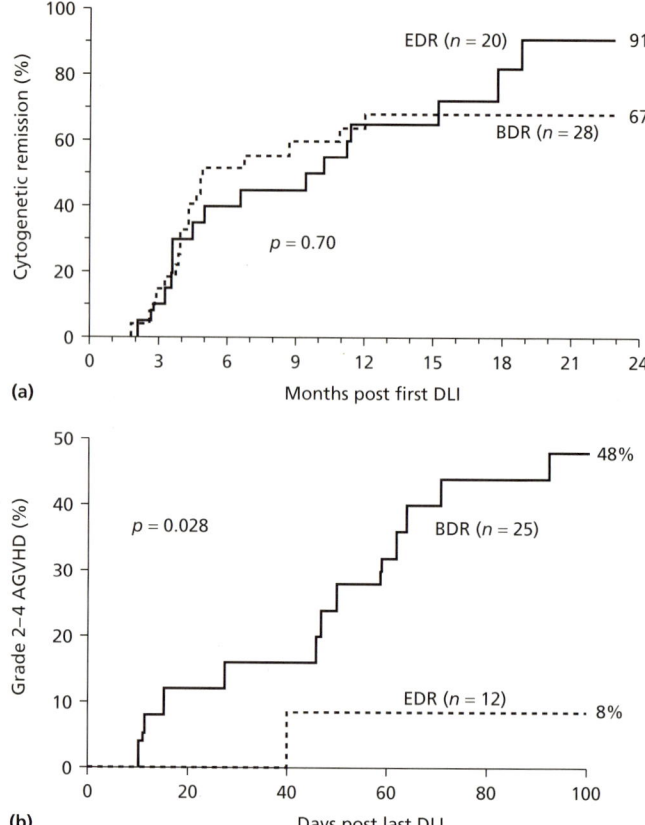

Fig. 84.1 Escalating vs. "bulk" doses of T cells in chronic myeloid leukemia (CML). Disease response is the same (a) but graft-vs.-host disease (GVHD) incidence is less (b) with escalating doses compared to patients who received "bulk" doses of T cells. BDR, bulk-dose regimen. EDR, escalation-dose regimen.

further support to the idea of initiating DLI with lower cell doses for this disease [61]. In this study, patients receiving an initial cell dose of $\leq 0.2 \times 10^8$ mononuclear cells (MNC)/kg (with 62% going on to receive additional infusions) had much less GVHD (26%) than patients receiving initial cell doses of $>0.2 \times 10^8$/kg (58%). The lower GVHD incidence was associated with a lower DLI-related mortality (5% vs. 20%). Moreover, response rates were similar and 3 years overall survival was better with the lower initial cell dose (84% vs. 60%). However, it should be understood that this study was not randomized and that there were significant differences in important pre-DLI characteristics between the three groups that likely contributed in part to different outcomes. Lower cell doses are probably less likely to be effective in patients with more advanced or fast-growing relapses.

Strategy of monitoring for early relapse and treating with low cell doses

Some investigators have argued that DLI's success in salvaging early relapse of CML after allogeneic BMT suggests an alteration of the general transplantation strategy for this disease. These investigators have suggested that patients first receive a T-cell-depleted transplantation; patients curable with high-dose therapy alone will be cured and will incur much less risk of GVHD. Those patients who require GVL effects for cure would be detected by close monitoring after BMT. At an early stage of relapse DLI could be given at a lower dose with less risk of GVHD. One study of this general approach reports a 4% treatment-related mortality and an 80% 5-year survival rate [62]. This survival rate is similar to that achieved by some groups without T-cell depletion; however, groups advocating the T-cell-depleted approach might argue that the incidence of GVHD would be less with their approach. A randomized trial would be needed to settle the question.

Summary of DLI for CML

In summary, DLI is very effective for CML in chronic phase, cytogenetic or molecular relapse. The optimal strategy for this disease probably involves close monitoring post-HCT for *bcr-abl* transcripts by quantitative PCR and treating early relapse (as defined by rising transcript numbers) with low cell doses (approximately 10^7 CD3$^+$ cells/kg for matched siblings). Patients may be given higher cell doses (at approximately half-log increments) if responses are not attained with the initial dose. Patients should be observed for an adequate period of time (at least 3–4 months) before dose-escalation since responses typically take several weeks to evolve. DLI for CML in advanced relapse—accelerated or blast phase—does not generally result in long-term remission; such patients should be considered for novel approaches.

Acute myeloid leukemia (AML) and myelodysplastic syndrome (MDS)

AML: disease activity

DLI is much less active in AML than in CML. The bulk of the data evaluating DLI in this disease are from the European and North American registry studies. The European study reported CR in five of 17 AML patients treated with DLI as sole therapy [42], and the North American study reported CR in six of 39 patients treated in this manner [43]. The median time to remission was 34 days [43]. Ongoing remissions are uncommon in patients with hematologic relapse treated with DLI alone [44]; one of 34 such patients remained in remission at 6 months post-treatment in an unpublished analysis of the North American database. It seems likely that earlier relapses, such as molecular or cytogenetic relapses, are more responsive than hematologic relapses to DLI alone but there are very few data specifically addressing this issue. Thus, DLI as sole therapy in AML patients has very limited efficacy.

AML: pre-DLI chemotherapy

Analysis of CML patients has shown that GVL effects typically require several weeks to months to evolve [42–44,53]. Thus, diseases such as AML in hematologic relapse may advance too fast for GVL effects to develop. If so, then debulking tumor with chemotherapy before DLI might be advantageous [63,64]. A recent prospective study evaluated this approach [64]. Sixty-five patients in hematologic relapse of advanced myeloid malignancy following human leukocyte antigen (HLA)-matched sibling BMT were treated with cytarabine-based chemotherapy followed by granulocyte colony-stimulating factor (G-CSF) primed DLI; prophylactic immunosuppression was not given. The complete response rate was 47%, but the treatment-related mortality was 23% and 2-year survival for the entire cohort was only 19%. The most important predictive factor in this study was relapse within 6 months of BMT, with very few such patients surviving at 1 year (Fig. 84.2). Post-DLI GVHD was not associated with improved event-free survival. Although these results appear to be superior to those seen with DLI alone, they remain far from satisfactory. Long-term follow-up data from the European registry, which include patients receiving DLI with or without chemotherapy, confirm the poor results in AML, with 3-year survival rates of only approximately 20% [44].

An interesting pattern of relapse has been reported in AML patients treated with DLI, with some patients recurring in extramedullary sites, while the bone marrow remains free of disease [65]. This observation suggests that appropriate homing is likely a critical component of successful DLI, with lymphocytes homing to certain areas (and not others) based on the expression of certain cell-surface molecules [66].

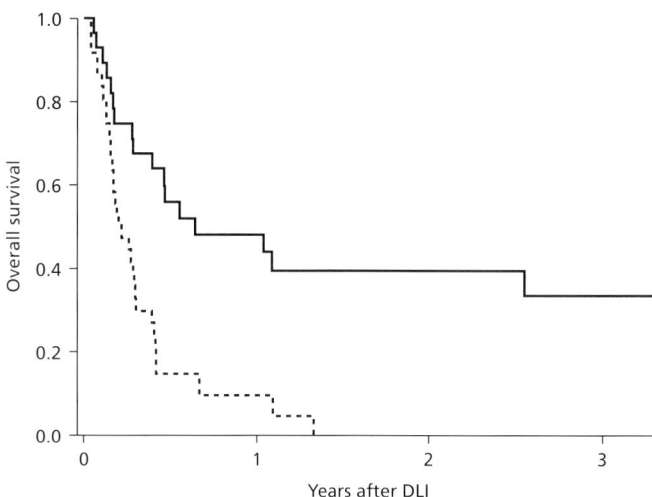

Fig. 84.2 Overall survival of patients with advanced myeloid malignancy who received chemotherapy plus donor lymphocyte infusion (DLI). Dashed lines, relapse after bone marrow transplantation (BMT) within 6 months; solid lines, relapse after BMT after 6 months.

MDS: disease activity

Data are limited regarding DLI in MDS [42,43,67]. From published reports it is often difficult to separate MDS from AML patients and the two diseases are often grouped together for analysis. A series of 20 patients with MDS (17 patients) or myeloproliferative disorder (three patients) treated with nonmyeloablative HCT suggests a GVL effect in these disorders as 50% of patients conditioned with TBI, 2 Gy, with or without fludarabine, achieved CR at a median of 84 days post-transplant [68]. Additional reports have described CR in myelofibrosis patients receiving DLI or nonmyeloablative HCT [69,70].

Summary of DLI for AML and MDS

DLI has only modest activity in AML compared to CML. Patients with hematologic relapse and a relatively long interval between initial HCT and relapse might benefit from combined chemotherapy and DLI, although comparative trials of this approach vs. others have not been done. Patients with short intervals between HCT and hematologic relapse (<6 months) are unlikely to benefit from DLI with or without chemotherapy and should be palliated or considered for investigational approaches. Data regarding DLI for MDS are relatively scanty. Conceivably, AML or MDS patients with molecular or cytogenetic relapses might benefit from DLI but adequate data are not available.

Acute lymphoblastic leukemia (ALL)

Disease activity

The large IBMTR registry analysis of GVL by Horowitz *et al.* [33] showed a GVL effect in ALL that was associated largely with GVHD. Thus, one might suspect that it could be possible to harness GVL in ALL through DLI. Probably the first successful DLI was in a patient with florid relapse of ALL shortly after HCT [35] and additional anecdotal reports have shown clear responses to DLI in patients with this disease [71,72]. However, analyses of larger patient groups have shown that the efficacy of DLI in ALL is quite limited. The European registry includes 43 patients with ALL, with survival at 2 years close to 0% [44]. The North American registry analyzed DLI in 44 ALL patients [73]. Of the 15 patients who received no pre-DLI chemotherapy, two achieved CR, lasting 2 and 3 years. Of 29 patients who received DLI either as consolidation of remission or in the nadir period after chemotherapy, only one had

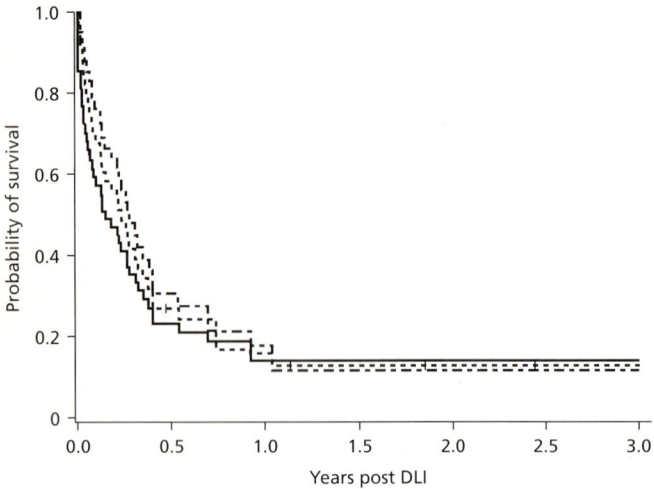

Fig. 84.3 Actuarial survival with 95%CI in 44 acute lymphoblastic leukemia (ALL) patients treated with donor lymphocyte infusion (DLI).

Table 84.3 Donor lymphocyte infusion (DLI) for multiple myeloma (MM).

	Lokhorst *et al.* [83]	Salama *et al.* [84]
Number of patients	27	25
Responses		
CR to DLI	6 (22%)	4 (18%)*
CR to DLI + chemo	–	3 (100%)†
PR to DLI	8 (30%)	3 (14%)*
Overall	14 (52%)	10 (40%)‡
Required >1 DLI to respond	6/14 (43%)	5/10 (50%)
Outcome of responders		
Relapse	4/14 (29%)	4/10 (40%)
Died, toxicity	2/14 (14%)	1/10 (10%)
Ongoing CR or PR	8/14 (57%)	5/10 (50%)
No GVHD/responses	6/14 (43%)	0/10 (0%)
Median duration of remission	~15 months	~6 months

*Of 22 assessable patients.
†Of three assessable patients.
‡Of the total 25 patients.
chemo, chemotherapy; CR, complete remission; DLI, donor lymphocyte infusion; GVHD, graft-vs.-host disease; PR, partial remission.

ongoing remission. The overall survival at 3 years was 13% (Fig. 84.3). Conceivably, ALL would be more sensitive to DLI if treated in earlier relapse. Several case reports or small series have suggested that this approach may be useful in both Philadelphia chromosome-positive and negative disease but additional study is needed [74–76].

Summary of DLI for ALL

DLI has limited activity in ALL. Patients in hematologic relapse should be palliated or considered for investigational studies. Intervention in earlier stage disease might have utility but additional study is needed.

Multiple myeloma

Disease activity

Numerous case reports and small series have documented a graft-vs.-myeloma effect that can be harnessed by DLI [41,77–82]. However, responses in myeloma are somewhat difficult to interpret, as chemotherapy is often given beforehand, and corticosteroids, given for GVHD, have pronounced activity in myeloma as well. Most reports have suggested that the response is usually associated with significant GVHD. Two larger series have reported results of DLI for relapsed multiple myeloma (Table 84.3 [83,84]). The response rates in these two studies were 40–52%, with 22–28% of patients having CR; however, some patients also had received chemotherapy before DLI. In both studies, remissions often did not occur until relatively high total cell doses had been given by multiple DLI. In one study response was highly correlated with GVHD [84] but in the other it was not [83]. The median duration of remission was approximately 15 months in one study [83] and 6 months in the other [84]. Alyea *et al.* [85] reported 14 patients who received CD4+ DLI 6–9 months after T-cell-depleted HCT; three patients were in remission and 11 had persistent disease. Ten of the 11 patients with persistent disease responded, with six complete responses. Six of the seven patients who developed GVHD had disease response.

In addition, nonmyeloablative transplantation studies have suggested a graft-vs.-myeloma effect, with responses to DLI given as part of the transplantation strategy, and with low relapse rates after nonmyeloablative transplantations given as a consolidation strategy after autologous transplantation [86–88].

Lastly, as in AML, extramedullary relapses have been reported in patients with multiple myeloma who previously responded to DLI [89,90].

In summary, there is clearly a graft-vs.-myeloma effect that can be harnessed with DLI. However, the overall response rates are generally not as high as those seen in CML and responses seem to be less durable, with relapse rates of 29–40% in the two larger studies cited above. Most, but not all, observations to date suggest that a relatively high cell dose is required for response. In addition, most, but not all, studies suggest that response is closely correlated with GVHD. The overall utility of DLI in multiple myeloma requires further study.

Non-Hodgkin's lymphoma, chronic lymphocytic leukemia and Hodgkin's lymphoma

The possibility of a graft-vs.-lymphoma has been suggested by the lower relapse rate of lymphoma patients treated with allogeneic compared to autologous transplantations [91–93], and large analyses of follicular lymphoma allograft recipients, which show an apparently flat disease-free survival (DFS) curve [94]. The current published data regarding DLI for these diseases are relatively limited, but small series and case reports have reported CR to DLI in follicular lymphoma, chronic lymphocytic leukemia (CLL), mantle cell lymphoma, diffuse large B-cell lymphoma and lymphoblastic lymphoma [95–102]. Additional information about a potential graft-vs.-lymphoma effect is accumulating from reports of non-myeloablative HCT, most of which are still in abstract form as of this writing (see Chapter 85) [99,103–112].

Solid tumors

Data regarding DLI in solid tumors are very preliminary. Childs and colleagues have treated renal cell cancer patients with DLI and observed clear responses [113]. Additional studies in renal cell cancer patients are ongoing. Conversely, DLI have not been successful in melanoma (R. Childs, personal communication). Limited observations suggest the possibility of a graft-vs.-breast cancer effect [114–116].

Toxicity of DLI

Graft-vs.-host disease (GVHD)

GVHD is the most significant complication of DLI [42,43]. Approximately 60% of patients develop acute GVHD a median of 32 days post-DLI. The incidence of grade II–IV acute GVHD is approximately 46% and that of grade III–IV acute GVHD is approximately 22%. The incidence of chronic GVHD is approximately 60%, with 55% of these patients having extensive disease. Factors predictive of GVHD in the European registry study were IFN-α treatment and T-cell depletion of the grafts for the initial BMT procedure [42]. IFN-α was also predictive of GVHD in the North American registry study, as was post-BMT chronic GVHD; however, T-cell depletion of the initial BMT was not predictive of GVHD in this study [43].

The likelihood of GVHD after DLI depends on several additional factors as well, especially cell dose, histocompatibility of the donor and recipient, and time from HCT to DLI. Most of the patients reported above received DLI from HLA-identical siblings at a T-cell dose of roughly 1×10^8/kg. However, the dose-escalation studies discussed previously have shown that GVHD is less likely to occur at lower T-cell doses. Exactly what the threshold for GVHD is probably depends on the particular minor histocompatiblity differences for a given donor–recipient pair [117], as well as the length of time between HCT and DLI. Animal studies and clinical observations have shown that a given cell dose is much more likely to cause GVHD if infused soon after an intensive preparative regimen rather than later [118–120]. In human BMT, the threshold T-cell dose for inducing GVHD in HLA-matched siblings is 1×10^5/kg at the time of transplantation [121]. Mackinnon et al. [51] have shown that up to 1×10^7 T cells/kg can be given without causing GVHD when infused 9 months to several years after the initial transplantation. Lastly, as discussed below, a given cell dose from an HLA-incompatible donor is much more likely to cause GVHD than the same dose from an HLA-compatible donor.

It should be noted that most patients treated with DLI have not had active GVHD at the time of DLI and have had host immunosuppressive drugs discontinued before DLI. Data are insufficient at this point to answer various questions about immunosuppressive drugs and DLI, such as whether patients with active GVHD could receive DLI if they were maintained on immunosuppresion, or whether evolution of GVL would be inhibited by immunosuppressive drugs, used to treat or prevent GVHD.

Pancytopenia

Pancytopenia occurs in approximately 20% of patients given DLI [42,43]. The likelihood of pancytopenia depends on the status of the disease. It occurs in as many as 50% of CML patients in hematologic relapse but is very infrequent in patients with cytogenetic or molecular relapse [40,53]. Pancytopenia correlates with a low level of donor-derived hematopoiesis at the time of DLI [122]. This observation supports the hypothesis that pancytopenia results when donor lymphocytes ablate recipient cells but donor stem cells are inadequate to allow recovery of hematopoiesis. Patients may recover with observation alone, with a course of G-CSF, or with infusion of bone marrow or peripheral blood hematopoietic cells [42,43]. If pancytopenia is due to insufficient donor stem cells, then infusing donor hematopoietic stem cells along with lymphocytes (most easily accomplished by collecting the DLI after mobilization with G-CSF) might lessen the likelihood of pancytopenia. However, one nonrandomized study suggests that this approach does not prevent aplasia [123], suggesting that some patients may have failure of hematopoiesis from other, as yet undefined, mechanisms. Probably the best way to avoid pancytopenia is to treat the patient early in the course of relapse.

Treatment-related mortality

In the European and American registry studies the probability of death not related to malignancy was 14% at 1 year and 18% at 2 years, with the majority of deaths due to GVHD, myelosuppression, or infection [42,43].

DLI from donors other than HLA-matched siblings

Unrelated donors

One recent analysis has specifically assessed the response to DLIs from unrelated donors [124]. The complete response rates for evaluable patients were 46% for CML, 42% for AML and 50% (two out of four) for ALL. DFS at 1 year after CR was 65% for CML, 23% for AML and 30% for ALL. Interestingly, the incidence and severity of acute and chronic GVHD did not appear to be worse than that seen in DLI from matched siblings. A possible explanation for this finding is that patients who relapse after unrelated donor BMT may be a selected group with a lower risk of GVHD; the most susceptible patients to severe GVHD may have died of GVHD after the initial transplantation or have had severe enough GVHD after BMT that they were deemed to be poor candidates for DLI. Patients treated within 1 year of DLI had an increased incidence of disease-related death, probably because patients relapsing and requiring treatment earlier have more aggressive disease. Another interesting aspect of this study was that cell dose did not correlate with response, survival, or GVHD. Because there was no association between cell dose and GVHD, the authors of this study recommended $0.1–1.0 \times 10^8$ MNC/kg as a reasonable dose in unrelated DLI. However, another group has reported that eight of 11 patients who had nonmyeloablative HCTs using fludarabine, melphalan and Campath and then (≥6 months later) received unrelated DLI at T-cell doses of $\leq 1 \times 10^7$/kg developed GVHD (five with grade III–IV) [125]. Thus, additional study is required to determine the safe DLI cell dose in the unrelated donor setting.

Haploidentical donors

Haploidentical donors have a much higher frequency of alloreactive T cells than HLA-identical donors; therefore, a given DLI cell dose from a haploidentical donor is much more likely to cause GVHD than a similar dose from a matched donor. However, there are relatively few published data addressing the safe haploidentical cell dose [126,127]. One abstract has reported a dose-finding study [127]. CD3$^+$ cell doses of 1×10^4/kg given beginning 1 month after the transplant and subsequent monthly infusions for 3 months were tolerated without causing GVHD; higher doses in this time frame were associated with GVHD. When given more than 3 months after BMT, CD3$^+$ doses of up to 5×10^5/kg were tolerated without causing GVHD. Additional studies of the issue of safe cell dose in the haploidentical setting are required.

Modifications of DLI

Several modifications of the DLI approach are under investigation, which aim to either lessen toxicity of the procedure (by decreasing GVHD or pancytopenia), or increase antitumor activity, or both (Table 84.4). Several of these approaches are discussed elsewhere in this chapter, including giving cells in an escalating dose scheme, collecting donor leukocytes after mobilization with G-CSF, giving chemotherapy before DLI and giving DLI in the MRD state.

CD8$^+$-depleted DLI

Animal and clinical studies have suggested that depletion of CD8$^+$ T cells from the bone marrow inoculum may reduce the incidence of GVHD [128,129]. Based on these observations, two groups have investigated DLI depleted of CD8$^+$ cells [56,130,131]. In the first study, 13 of 15 early phase CML patients (87%) achieved complete responses, but only one of 11 with more advanced relapse responded [56,131]. Acute GVHD occurred in 8% of the patients and extensive chronic GVHD in 11%. Remissions were durable, with only one patient relapsing after 4.2 years median follow-up. In the second study, 40 patients with hematologic malignancies (CML, 25 patients; MM, seven patients; other, eight patients) received targeted doses of CD4$^+$ T cells [130]. Six of 27 patients

Table 84.4 Modifications of donor lymphocyte infusion (DLI).

Attempts to improve treatment efficacy
Pre-DLI chemotherapy
Administration in the minimal residual disease (MRD) state
DLI + interleukin 2 (IL-2) or interferon-alpha (IFN-α)
T-cell lines and clones
Immunization of the donor

Attempts to lessen toxicity
Escalating doses
CD8+ T-cell depletion
Selective depletion of alloreactive cells
T-cell lines and clones
Suicide gene-transduced T cells
Irradiated DLI
Granulocyte colony-stimulating factor (G-CSF) mobilization

(22%) who received 0.3×10^8 CD4+ cells/kg developed GVHD compared with six of 11 patients (55%) who received $\geq 1.0 \times 10^8$ CD4+ cells/kg. All patients in this trial who developed GVHD also had a response; however, 48% of responding patients did not develop GVHD. A randomized study of this approach showed a decreased incidence of acute GVHD (0% vs. 67%) in patients receiving CD8+-depleted DLI and improved DFS at 2 years (86% vs. 52%) [132]. In this study infusions were adjusted so that all patients received 1×10^7 CD4+ cells/kg. Patients randomized to CD8+ depletion received a median of 0.7×10^5 vs. 32.0×10^5 CD8+ cells/kg in the unmanipulated cohort.

Selective T-cell depletion

Alloreactive donor T cells can be selectively depleted from a donor T-cell inoculum by targeting cells that have been activated in a one-way mixed lymphocyte reaction. Activated cells can be targeted using immunotoxins or immunomagnetic beads directed against activation antigens such as CD25 or CD69 [133–136], or by photodynamic therapy taking advantage of dye-exclusion properties of activated T cells [137]. One group of investigators has reported infusion of selectively depleted T cells in 15 haploidentical or matched unrelated transplant patients [136]. Four patients developed grade I–II acute GVHD and one developed limited chronic GVHD. Immune reconstitution appeared to be accelerated compared to historical controls. Whether the selective depletion process will also deplete cells responsible for mediating GVL is unknown.

Cell lines and clones

Antigen-specific T-cell lines and clones represent the most rational way to deliver specific immunity while avoiding GVHD (see Chapter 29). However, relatively few groups have applied to the clinic the difficult technology involved in growing large numbers of these cells. This approach is most feasible when viruses are the targets of immunotherapy and two groups have reported fairly large series of patients treated with CMV-specific T-cell clones or Epstein–Barr virus specific cytotoxic T-cell lines [138–140]. The study of leukemia-reactive cytotoxic T-cell lines has been more limited. Falkenburg *et al.* [141] and Smit *et al.* [142] reported a patient with CML in accelerated phase after allogeneic BMT who had a suboptimal response to an unmanipulated DLI but then had a complete molecular remission after infusion of cytotoxic leukemia-reactive T-cell lines generated from her HLA-identical BMT donor using a modification of a limiting dilution assay. Other investigators are exploring the use of cytotoxic T-cell lines directed against hematopoietic tissue-restricted minor histocompatibility antigens, but clinical results have not yet been reported [143].

Suicide gene-transduced donor T cells

Cycling T cells transduced with the herpes simplex virus, type 1 (HSV1) thymidine kinase (HSV-tk) are susceptible to killing by ganciclovir [144–149]. Thus, conceivably, GVH reactions initiated by HSV-tk-transduced T cells might be ameliorated by administration of ganciclovir. Bonini *et al.* [145] reported eight patients with relapsed malignancy post-BMT who received escalating doses of HSV-tk transduced lymphocytes from their original HLA-matched sibling donor. Gene modified cells were detected repeatedly in blood, marrow and tissue biopsies in all but one patient. Five patients attained disease-responses and three developed GVHD. Two patients with acute GVHD had complete resolution of all signs of GVHD after treatment with ganciclovir and a third patient with chronic GVHD had a partial response to ganciclovir. The two patients with complete disease responses who received ganciclovir for GVHD remained in CR. Tiberghien [148] *et al.* treated 12 patients with HSV-tk transduced T cells, given concomitantly with a T-cell-depleted BMT. Three of four patients who developed GVHD responded to treatment with ganciclovir.

Thus, this area of research has promise. However, potential obstacles should be appreciated. First, the technical challenges of vector design and optimal cell transduction, expansion and selection are formidable. In addition, even if technical issues are completely solved, potential theoretical challenges remain. Even if all transduced T cells are eliminated, it is conceivable that a downstream cascade of secondary effectors involved in GVHD will be initiated that cannot be stopped. If GVHD is completely abrogated, it is conceivable that GVL will be abrogated as well. Further, as the suicide gene is a foreign protein, it may induce an immune response resulting in elimination of transduced cells [150]. Alternative suicide gene designs are under development that might avoid the problem of immunogenicity [151].

Irradiated DLI

Irradiated T cells retain cytotoxic activity against tumor cells. Because these cells are not able to proliferate, their ability to cause GVHD should be limited. Waller and Boyer [152] and Waller *et al.* [153] demonstrated in an animal model that irradiated donor T cells facilitate engraftment and mediate GVL. Early clinical trials assessing this approach are under way. Success of this approach will be limited if significant proliferation of T cells is required for optimal GVL.

DLI plus interleukin 2 (IL-2)

Several patients have received IL-2 with DLI [35,154]. Slavin *et al.* [35] reported a strategy of allogeneic cell therapy involving, first, escalating doses of unmanipulated DLI, followed by, in nonresponders, DLI plus IL-2, followed by, in patients who still do not respond, donor leukocytes activated *in vitro* with IL-2 and given along with IL-2. Ten of 17 patients with acute and chronic leukemia in relapse achieved CR. Four patients with cytogenetic relapses responded to DLI alone, whereas five of six patients with overt hematologic relapse responded only after additional activation of cells with IL-2. Since responses to DLI can take several weeks to occur, it is possible that responses to DLI plus IL-2 were actually responses to previous DLI.

Immunization of the donor with tumor-specific protein before DLI

The immunoglobulin idiotype serves as a tumor-specific protein in myeloma and B-cell lymphomas. Clinical experience with this approach is limited, but encouraging findings have included the detection of idiotype-specific T-cell responses *in vivo* after BMT and a complete and prolonged remission after DLI in one patient [155,156].

Mechanisms of GVL

Our current understanding of the mechanisms of human GVL is relatively limited (see Chapter 28 for more thorough discussion of GVL mechanisms). It is likely that the mechanisms of GVL vary among different diseases and even among different individuals with the same disease. Possible target antigens include antigens expressed only by leukemic cells (true GVL targets), antigens expressed by both leukemia cells and normal nonhematopoietic cells (GVH targets) and antigens which are expressed by both normal and malignant hematopoietic tissue [157]. Additional possible target antigens are antigens shared between donor and host, in effect autoantigens. T cells with high affinity for self-antigens are deleted in the thymus and to some extent in the periphery but T cells with low affinity for self-antigens can persist and become pathogenic under certain circumstances. Potential effectors in GVL reactions include T cells with $\alpha\beta$ T-cell receptors, T cells with $\gamma\delta$ receptors and natural killer (NK) cells. In addition, it is possible that various cytokines released in a dysregulated fashion as part of an exuberant immune reaction could affect leukemia cells nonspecifically [158]. Recent findings suggest that hematopoietic tissue-restricted antigens can be the targets of GVL reactions [159–161].

Most supposition about GVL mechanisms derives from extrapolation from animal models or from after-the-fact inferences about clinical events. However, DLI represents a unique opportunity to study GVL mechanisms by allowing careful study of patients during the evolution of actual tumor responses [82,162–169]. For example, one group of investigators has studied the T-cell repertoire of several CML and myeloma patients during response to DLI [162,163]. In each responding patient, these investigators were able to identify the expansion of at least one $V\beta$ gene subfamily that occurred simultaneously with cytogenetic response. In one patient, further study showed that the $V\beta$ gene subfamily expansion was associated with the appearance of clonal T cells. This clone was further characterized by direct sequencing of the CDR3 region. Similarly, Smit et al. [167] developed assays to look specifically at antihost progenitor cell activity and showed that the GVL effect in responding CML patients was associated with T cells recognizing leukemic CD34$^+$ progenitor cells. A study by Wu et al. [164] has used SEREX technology to show that antibodies specific for certain proteins are temporally asso-ciated with the response to DLI. More sophisticated assays of antigen-specific T cells will likely shed further light on the nature and specificity of immune cells mediating GVL [170–173].

A relatively little studied aspect of DLI involves the sensitivity of tumor tissue to potential GVL effectors. An effective immune response requires not only appropriate effector cells but also proper antigen processing, presentation of antigen in the presence of costimulatory molecules by tumor cells or professional antigen-presenting cells, expression of adhesion molecules by tumor cells and intact pathways allowing the target cell to undergo apoptosis. Deficiency in any one of these components would impair GVL reactivity [174]. Conceivably, the study of patients relapsing from previous DLI-induced responses might lead to insights into mechanisms of resistance. Along these lines, Dermime et al. [175] studied patients who relapsed after transplantation and showed that many critical cell surface molecules involved in immune responses had been down-regulated in leukemia cells at the time of relapse compared to pretransplant cells. This phenomenon was associated with a decrease in responsiveness to lysis by cytotoxic T cells and NK cells.

Discontinuation of immunosuppression

Discontinuation of immunosuppression, in particular cyclosporine, allows expansion of donor immune cells with GVL capability. Scattered case reports have described patients in post-HCT relapse with a variety of malignancies, including AML, CML, ALL and Burkitt's lymphoma, who responded to this approach [176–181]. However, systematic study of this concept has been limited. Elmaagacli et al. [181] reported 20 patients with relapsed CML who were treated with this maneuver. Ten patients with accelerated or blast phase disease did not respond but one chronic phase patient and all nine patients with cytogenetic relapses had complete responses within a median of 53 days; all patients developed GVHD regardless of response. Remissions were durable in seven of the 10 responders. Since many DLI patients at the time of relapse are on immunosuppressive drugs, which are then discontinued shortly before DLI, it seems likely that many patients apparently responding to DLI are responding as well to discontinuation of immunosuppression. (This potential explanation for response should always be considered for patients responding to any other post-transplant intervention as well.) Discontinuation of immunosuppression might be reasonable as a first step for patients with relatively slow growing malignancies that are thought to be susceptible to GVL effects.

Second transplantation procedures

Several studies have evaluated second transplantation procedures using intensive myeloablative regimens [182–185]. In general, since the first procedures have commonly involved TBI, the second procedures have used non-TBI containing regimens, such as bulsulfan and cyclophosphamide, bulsulfan and etoposide, busulfan alone, or carmustine, etoposide and cyclophosphamide. Treatment-related mortality is approximately 40%, relapse rates are approximately 70%, and DFS ranges from 14% to 20%. However, certain factors predict for a better outcome from second transplantation, in particular younger age, longer interval between first and second transplantation procedures, and CML as the underlying disease. Myeloablative transplantations are sometimes performed for patients who have failed nonmyeloablative transplantations (and vice versa) but data at this point are scanty.

Thus, in general, second transplantations are not a good option for management of post-HCT patients, but might be considered in highly selected individuals who are younger and have a long time interval between initial HCT and relapse. With regard to CML, it is likely that the majority of patients cured by second transplantations are actually cured by the GVL effects associated with the second transplantation procedure. A reasonable strategy for CML patients is to first attempt a less toxic approach, e.g. escalating doses of DLI, before resorting to the toxicity associated with a second transplantation.

Cytotoxic chemotherapy

Retrospective surveys have assessed cytotoxic chemotherapy in the management of patients with relapsed acute leukemia after HCT [8,186,187]. Patients with AML are generally treated with standard regimens containing cytosine arabinoside and anthracyclines, and ALL patients are treated with regimens containing vincristine and prednisone with or without other agents such as methotrexate and asparaginase. Patients with AML or ALL who relapse early after transplantation (before day 100) are unlikely to benefit from chemotherapy, experiencing excessive toxicity from the treatment and low remission rates (approximately 7%). Patients who relapse later are more likely to achieve remission; for example, 65% of AML patients in relapse more than a year after transplantation achieved remission in one study [8]. However, long-term DFS is only approximately 2% in relapsed acute leukemia patients treated with chemotherapy alone. The activity of chemotherapy in other diseases has not been systematically evaluated but is not considered to have curative potential. Since the great majority of patients receiving chemotherapy-alone do not have long-term survival, this approach should probably be viewed simply as a stepping-stone, to allow disease control in preparation for application of more definitive approaches.

Interferon-alpha (IFN-α)

IFN-α has well-described activity in CML and has been used to manage post-HCT relapse [188–190]. The mechanism of action is unknown. Possibilities include a direct antiproliferative effect, an alteration in adhesion molecule expression that restores normal interaction between CML stem cells and marrow stroma [191] and an increase in T cells with anti-CML activity. This last possibility is supported by observations of an increase in T cells with specificity for a myeloid-associated antigen, PR-1, in patients responding to IFN-α [161]. In patients with hematologic relapse, IFN-α induces hematologic remissions in approximately 50% and cytogenetic remissions in 25%. Results appear to be better in patients with cytogenetic relapse. Higano et al. [189] reported CR in 12 of 14 patients with cytogenetic relapse treated with IFN-α at doses starting at 1–3 million U/m^2/day, and adjusted as needed to maintain modest cytopenia. The treatment was generally well tolerated, with only one patient stopping therapy because of toxicity. CR occurred at a median of 7.5 months, and eight patients (57%) remained in remission with follow-up ranging from 10+ to 54+ months. The use of IFN-α in management of relapsed AML and ALL patients is less studied.

In summary, IFN-α has significant activity in CML in cytogenetic relapse but, in the absence of controlled trials, it is difficult to tell what its role should be vs. DLI or imatinib mesylate (discussed below).

Interleukin 2 (IL-2)

Interleukin 2 (IL-2) probably works by expanding NK and cytotoxic T lymphocytes. IL-2 has modest activity as a single agent in AML [192,193] but there is minimal experience with it in the management of post-transplant relapse. As noted in DLI plus interleukin 2 (IL-2) (p. 1156), IL-2 has been used in conjunction with adoptive immunotherapy, with some patients appearing to benefit from the addition of IL-2 to donor leukocytes [35].

Granulocyte colony-stimulating factor (G-CSF)

Giralt et al. [194] observed a complete disease response in a patient with relapsed CML who had been treated with G-CSF for neutropenia. This observation led to evaluation of the treatment in six additional patients. Two of these six patients had complete responses, one a patient with AML and the other a patient with refractory anemia with excess blasts. Remissions in the three patients occurred within 10–21 days of beginning treatment with G-CSF. Bishop et al. [195] treated 14 relapsed patients with G-CSF and observed remissions in six patients (CML, four patients; AML, one patient; CLL, one patient) within 1–3 months of beginning treatment. The mechanism of response in these patients is not certain. However, several patients who responded had cyclosporine discontinued at about the time G-CSF was started. This circumstance, and the fact that the majority of the complete responders developed GVHD, suggests that most of the responses may have been due to evolution of GVL effects rather than to an effect of G-CSF. Another possible explanation could be that if G-CSF preferentially stimulated normal cells then malignant cells might appear to decrease in number when in fact they were only diluted by normal marrow expansion [196]. These possibilities, however, cannot explain all of the responses and thus additional study is warranted. However, at this point this treatment should probably not be considered a standard approach to post-HCT relapse.

Imatinib mesylate (STI571, Gleevec®)

Imatinib mesylate has pronounced activity in CML, resulting in a high rate of hematologic and cytogenetic remissions [197,198]. Early studies suggest activity of imatinib mesylate in the management of CML in relapse after allogeneic HCT [199,200]. In a recent study of 28 patients in relapse treated with imatinib mesylate, complete hematologic remissions occurred in 100% of five chronic-phase patients, 83% of 15 accelerated-phase patients and 43% of eight blast-phase patients [200]. Complete cytogenetic remissions occurred in 42% of patients with chronic or accelerated disease. With a median follow-up time of 16 months, 20 patients (68%) were alive, nine with no evidence of disease. Five patients developed acute GVHD (three with grade III and two with grade I–II). Reversible severe granulocytopenia developed in 43% of patients and thrombocytopenia in 27%. Additional studies will likely compare DLI to imatinib mesylate. Another strategy under discussion has been the use of this agent to "debulk" CML before DLI. Because complete response rates are so high with this agent, lower DLI cell doses would likely be sufficient, with a reduced risk of GVHD. If, however, CML cells presenting antigens are required for GVL, then debulking CML below a certain level with imatinib mesylate might prevent GVL effects from developing.

Irradiation

Radiation is effective therapy for localized extramedullary relapses, whether in sanctuary sites like the testis or CNS, or elsewhere [201]. However, as extramedullary relapses are usually followed by systemic relapse, systemic therapy should be employed as well.

Palliation

After the prolonged battle of the transplantation process, many physicians and patients are not inclined to "throw in the towel." However, a realistic and honest assessment of certain clinical situations, for example florid relapse of acute leukemia within a few weeks after transplantation, should lead to the rational understanding that additional aggressive measures are no longer warranted. Under these circumstances the patient will benefit from a shift in efforts that makes sure that physical, emotional and spiritual concerns are met.

Conclusions

The optimal management of patients in relapse post-HCT for the most part remains uncertain. The best success is achieved in patients with CML and appropriate treatments could include tapering of immunosuppression, DLI (preferably in low doses for patients in molecular or cytogenetic relapse), imatinib mesylate and, if in cytogenetic relapse, IFN-α. Controlled trials are needed in CML and should incorporate recently developed risk assessment systems [202]. DLI seems encouraging in lymphoma but it should be noted that extensive published data are still lacking. Similarly, additional data are needed in myeloma: although clear-cut responses are encouraging, it must be emphasized that many patients do not respond and many who do respond subsequently relapse again, and responses seem to be infrequently observed without significant GVHD.

Very few patients with acute leukemia benefit from any of the approaches discussed in this chapter and should probably more often than not be given palliative care. If therapy is to be attempted it should be in the context of well-designed clinical trials assessing novel agents or new immunologic strategies.

Research over the next few years will define better which malignancies are or are not responsive to immunologic antitumor effects. GVL mechanisms will become better understood and immune-sensitive malignancies will be treated with more sophisticated DLI approaches that enhance disease activity while minimizing GVHD. Malignancies that are resistant to GVL will need to be treated by entirely different approaches, or by approaches that increase their inherent sensitivity to immunologic maneuvers.

References

1 Fialkow PJ, Thomas ED, Bryant JI, Neiman PE. Leukaemic transformation of engrafted human marrow cells *in vivo*. *Lancet* 1971; **1**: 251–5.
2 Thomas ED, Bryant JI, Buckne r CD *et al*. Leukaemic transformation of engrafted human marrow cells *in vivo*. *Lancet* 1972; **1**: 1310–3.
3 Goh K, Klemperer MR. *In vivo* leukemic transformation. cytogenetic evidence of *in vivo* leukemic transformation of engrafted marrow cells. *Am J Hematol* 1977; **2**: 283–90.
4 Elfenbein GJ, Brogaonkar DS, Bias WB *et al*. Cytogenetic evidence for recurrence of acute myelogenous leukemia after allogeneic bone marrow transplantation in donor hematopoietic cells. *Blood* 1978; **52**: 627–36.
5 Newburger PE, Latt SA, Pesando JM *et al*. Leukemia relapse in donor cells after allogeneic bone-marrow transplantation. *N Engl J Med* 1981; **304**: 712–4.
6 Marmont A, Frassoni F, Bacigalupo A *et al*. Recurrence of Ph-positive leukemia in donor cells after marrow transplantation for chronic granulocytic leukemia. *N Engl J Med* 1984; **310**: 903–6.
7 Lapidot T, Sirard C, Vormoor J *et al*. A cell initiating human acute myeloid leukaemia after transplantation into SCID mice. *Nature* 1994; **367**: 645–8.
8 Mortimer J, Blinder MA, Schulman S *et al*. Relapse of acute leukemia after marrow transplantation: natural history and results of subsequent therapy. *J Clin Oncol* 1989; **7**: 50–7.
9 Doney K, Fisher LD, Appelbaum FR *et al*. Treatment of adult acute lymphoblastic leukemia with allogeneic bone marrow transplantation. Multivariate analysis of factors affecting acute graft-versus-host disease, relapse, and relapse-free survival. *Bone Marrow Transplant* 1991; **7**: 453–9.
10 Bekassy AN, Hermans J, Gorin NC, Gratwohl A. Granulocytic sarcoma after allogeneic bone marrow transplantation: a retrospective European multicenter survey. Acute and Chronic Leukemia Working Parties of the European Group for Blood and Marrow Transplantation. *Bone Marrow Transplant* 1996; **17**: 801–8.
11 Chong G, Byrnes G, Szer J, Grigg A. Extramedullary relapse after allogeneic bone marrow transplantation for haematological malignancy. *Bone Marrow Transplant* 2000; **26**: 1011–5.
12 Zaccaria A, Rosti G, Sessarego M *et al*. Relapse after allogeneic bone marrow transplantation for Philadelphia chromosome positive chronic myeloid leukemia: cytogenetic analysis of 24 patients. *Bone Marrow Transplant* 1988; **3**: 413–23.
13 Arthur CK, Apperley JF, Guo AP, Rassool F, Gao LM, Goldman JM. Cytogenetic events after bone marrow transplantation for chronic myeloid leukemia in chronic phase. *Blood* 1988; **71**: 1179–86.
14 Lin F, Kirkland MA, van Rhee FV *et al*. Molecular analysis of transient cytogenetic relapse after allogeneic bone marrow transplantation for chronic myeloid leukaemia. *Bone Marrow Transplant* 1996; **18**: 1147–52.
15 Foroni L, Hoffbrand V. Minimal residual disease investigation in haematological malignancies. *Best Prac Res Clin Haematol* 2002; **15**: 1–222.
16 Yin JA, Grimwade D. Minimal residual disease evaluation in acute myeloid leukaemia. *Lancet* 2002; **360**: 160–2.
17 Mackinnon S, Barnett L, Heller G. Polymerase chain reaction is highly predictive of relapse in patients following T cell-depleted allogeneic bone marrow transplantation for chronic myeloid leukemia. *Bone Marrow Transplant* 1996; **17**: 643–7.
18 Drobyski WR, Endean DJ, Klein JP, Hessner MJ. Detection of *BCR/ABL* RNA transcripts using the polymerase chain reaction is highly predictive for relapse in patients transplanted with unrelated marrow grafts for chronic myelogenous leukaemia. *Br J Haematol* 1997; **98**: 458–66.
19 Cross NC, Hughes TP, Feng L *et al*. Minimal residual disease after allogeneic bone marrow transplantation for chronic myeloid leukaemia in first chronic phase: correlations with acute graft-versus-host disease and relapse. *Br J Haematol* 1993; **84**: 67–74.
20 Radich JP, Gehly G, Gooley T *et al*. Polymerase chain reaction detection of the *BCR-ABL* fusion transcript after allogeneic marrow transplantation for chronic myeloid leukemia: results and implications in 346 patients. *Blood* 1995; **85**: 2632–8.
21 Radich JP, Gooley T, Bryant E *et al*. The significance of *bcr-abl* molecular detection in chronic myeloid leukemia patients "late", 18 months or more after transplantation. *Blood* 2001; **98**: 1701–7.
22 Cross NC, Lin F, Chase A *et al*. Competitive polymerase chain reaction to estimate the number of *BCR-ABL* transcripts in chronic myeloid leukemia after bone marrow trasplantation. *Blood* 1993; **82**: 1929–36.
23 Perez-Simon JA, Caballero D, Diez-Campelo M *et al*. Chimerism and minimal residual disease monitoring after reduced intensity conditioning (RIC) allogeneic transplantation. *Leukemia* 2002; **16**: 1423–31.
24 Knechtli CJ, Goulden NJ, Hancock JP *et al*. Minimal residual disease status before allogeneic bone marrow transplantation is an important determinant of successful outcome for children and adolescents with acute lymphoblastic leukemia. *Blood* 1998; **92**: 4072–9.
25 Radich J, Gehly G, Lee A *et al*. Detection of *bcr-abl* transcripts in Philadelphia chromosome-positive acute lymphoblastic leukemia after marrow transplantation. *Blood* 1997; **89**: 2602–9.
26 San Miguel JF, Vidriales MB, Lopez-Berges C *et al*. Early immunophenotypical evaluation of minimal residual disease in acute myeloid leukemia identifies different patient risk groups and may contribute to postinduction treatment stratification. *Blood* 2001; **98**: 1746–51.
27 Barnes D, Loutit J, Neal F. Treatment of murine leukemia with X-rays and homologous bone marrow. *Bri Med J* 1956; **2**: 626–30.
28 Truitt RL, Johnson BD. Principles of graft-vs.-leukemia reactivity. *Biol Blood Marrow Transplant* 1995; **1**: 61–8.
29 Gale RP, Champlin RE. How does bone-marrow transplantation cure leukaemia? *Lancet* 1984; **2**: 28–30.
30 Weiden PL, Flournoy N, Thomas ED *et al*. Antileukemic effect of graft-versus-host disease in human recipients of allogeneic-marrow grafts. *N Engl J Med* 1979; **300**: 1068–73.
31 Weiden PL, Sullivan KM, Flournoy N, Storb R, Thomas ED. Antileukemic effect of chronic graft-versus-host disease: contribution to improved survival after allogeneic marrow transplantation. *N Engl J Med* 1981; **304**: 1529–33.
32 Mitsuyasu RT, Champlin RE, Gale RP *et al*. Treatment of donor bone marrow with monoclonal anti-T-cell antibody and complement for the prevention of graft-versus-host disease. A prospective, randomized, double-blind trial. *Ann Intern Med* 1986; **105**: 20–6.
33 Horowitz MM, Gale RP, Sondel PM *et al*. Graft-versus-leukemia reactions after bone marrow transplantation. *Blood* 1990; **75**: 555–62.
34 Kolb HJ, Mittermuller J, Clemm C *et al*. Donor leukocyte transfusions for treatment of recurrent chronic myelogenous leukemia in marrow transplant patients. *Blood* 1990; **76**: 2462–5.
35 Slavin S, Naparstek E, Nagler A *et al*. Allogeneic cell therapy with donor peripheral blood cells and recombinant human interleukin-2 to treat leukemia relapse after allogeneic bone marrow transplantation. *Blood* 1996; **87**: 2195–204.
36 Bar BM, Schattenberg A, Mensink EJ *et al*. Donor leukocyte infusions for chronic myeloid leukemia relapsed after allogeneic bone marrow transplantation. *J Clin Oncol* 1993; **11**: 513–9.
37 Drobyski WR, Keever CA, Roth MS *et al*. Salvage immunotherapy using donor leukocyte infusions as treatment for relapsed chronic myelogenous leukemia after allogeneic bone marrow transplantation: efficacy and toxicity of a defined T-cell dose. *Blood* 1993; **82**: 2310–8.
38 Hertenstein B, Wiesneth M, Novotny J *et al*. Interferon-α and donor buffy coat transfusions for treatment of relapsed chronic myeloid leukemia after allogeneic bone marrow transplantation. *Transplantation* 1993; **56**: 1114–8.
39 Porter DL, Roth MS, McGarigle C, Ferrara JL, Antin JH. Induction of graft-versus-host disease as immunotherapy for relapsed chronic myeloid leukemia. *N Engl J Med* 1994; **330**: 100–6.
40 van Rhee F, Lin F, Cullis JO *et al*. Relapse of chronic myeloid leukemia after allogeneic bone marrow transplant: the case for giving donor leukocyte transfusions before the onset of hematologic relapse. *Blood* 1994; **83**: 3377–83.
41 Collins RH Jr, Pineiro LA, Nemunaitis JJ *et al*. Transfusion of donor buffy coat cells in the treatment of persistent or recurrent malignancy after allogeneic bone marrow transplantation. *Transfusion* 1995; **35**: 891–8.
42 Kolb HJ, Schattenberg A, Goldman JM *et al*. Graft-versus-leukemia effect of donor lymphocyte transfusions in marrow grafted patients. European Group for Blood and Marrow Transplantation Working Party for Chronic Leukemia. *Blood* 1995; **86**: 2041–50.
43 Collins RH Jr, Shpilberg O, Drobyski WR *et al*. Donor leukocyte infusions in 140 patients with relapsed malignancy after allogeneic bone marrow transplantation. *J Clin Oncol* 1997; **15**: 433–44.
44 Kolb HJ. Donor leukocyte transfusions for treatment of leukemic relapse after bone marrow transplantation. EBMT Immunology and Chronic Leukemia Working Parties. *Vox Sang* 1998; **74**: 321–9.
45 MacKinnon S. Who may benefit from donor leucocyte infusions after allogeneic stem cell transplantation? *Br J Haematol* 2000; **110**: 12–7.
46 Little MT, Storb R. The future of allogeneic hematopoietic stem cell transplantation: minimizing

pain, maximizing gain. *J Clin Invest* 2000; **105**: 1679–81.

47 Carella AM, Champlin R, Slavin S, McSweeney P, Storb R. Mini-allografts: ongoing trials in humans. *Bone Marrow Transplant* 2000; **25**: 345–50.

48 Slavin S, Nagler A, Naparstek E *et al.* Nonmyeloablative stem cell transplantation and cell therapy as an alternative to conventional bone marrow transplantation with lethal cytoreduction for the treatment of malignant and nonmalignant hematologic diseases. *Blood* 1998; **91**: 756–63.

49 McSweeney P, Niederwieser D, Shizuru JA *et al.* Hematopoietic cell transplantation in older patients with hematologic malignancies: replacing highdose cytotoxic therapy with graft-versus-tumor effects. *Blood* 2001; **97**: 3390–400.

50 Michallet M, Bilger K, Garban F *et al.* Allogeneic hematopoietic stem-cell transplantation after nonmyeloablative preparative regimens: impact of pretransplantation and posttransplantation factors on outcome. *J Clin Oncol* 2001; **19**: 3340–9.

51 Mackinnon S, Papadopoulos EB, Carabasi MH *et al.* Adoptive immunotherapy evaluating escalating doses of donor leukocytes for relapse of chronic myeloid leukemia after bone marrow transplantation: separation of graft-versus-leukemia responses from graft-versus-host disease. *Blood* 1995; **86**: 1261–8.

52 Dazzi F, Szydlo RM, Cross NC *et al.* Durability of responses following donor lymphocyte infusions for patients who relapse after allogeneic stem cell transplantation for chronic myeloid leukemia. *Blood* 2000; **96**: 2712–6.

53 Dazzi F, Szydlo RM, Craddock C *et al.* Comparison of single-dose and escalating-dose regimens of donor lymphocyte infusion for relapse after allografting for chronic myeloid leukemia. *Blood* 2000; **95**: 67–71.

54 Baurmann H, Nagel S, Binder T, Neubauer A, Siegert W, Huhn D. Kinetics of the graft-versusleukemia response after donor leukocyte infusions for relapsed chronic myeloid leukemia after allogeneic bone marrow transplantation. *Blood* 1998; **92**: 3582–90.

55 Raanani P, Dazzi F, Sohal J *et al.* The rate and kinetics of molecular response to donor leucocyte transfusions in chronic myeloid leukaemia patients treated for relapse after allogeneic bone marrow transplantation. *Br J Haematol* 1997; **99**: 945–50.

56 Giralt S, Hester J, Huh Y *et al.* CD8-depleted donor lymphocyte infusion as treatment for relapsed chronic myelogenous leukemia after allogeneic bone marrow transplantation. *Blood* 1995; **86**: 4337–43.

57 Porter DL, Collins RH Jr, Shpilberg O *et al.* Longterm follow-up of patients who achieved complete remission after donor leukocyte infusions. *Biol Blood Marrow Transplant* 1999; **5**: 253–61.

58 Heslop HE, Ng CY, Li C *et al.* Long-term restoration of immunity against Epstein–Barr virus infection by adoptive transfer of gene-modified virus-specific T lymphocytes. *Nat Med* 1996; **2**: 551–5.

59 Balkwill FR. Interferons. *Lancet* 1989; **1**: 1060–3.

60 Upadhyaya G, Guba SC, Sih SA *et al.* Interferon-α restores the deficient expression of the cytoadhesion molecule lymphocyte function antigen-3 by chronic myelogenous leukemia progenitor cells. *J Clin Invest* 1991; **88**: 2131–6.

61 Guglielmi C, Arcese W, Dazzi F *et al.* Donor lymphocyte infusion for relapsed chronic myelogenous leukemia: prognostic relevance of the initial cell dose. *Blood* 2002; **100**: 397–405.

62 Drobyski WR, Hessner MJ, Klein JP *et al.* T-cell depletion plus salvage immunotherapy with donor leukocyte infusions as a strategy to treat chronicphase chronic myelogenous leukemia patients undergoing HLA-identical sibling marrow transplantation. *Blood* 1999; **94**: 434–41.

63 Pawson R, Potter MN, Theocharous P *et al.* Treatment of relapse after allogeneic bone marrow transplantation with reduced intensity conditioning (FLAG ± Ida) and second allogeneic stem cell transplant. *Br J Haematol* 2001; **115**: 622–9.

64 Levine JE, Braun T, Penza SL *et al.* A prospective trial of chemotherapy and donor leukocyte infusions for relapse of advanced myeloid malignancies following allogeneic stem cell transplantation. *J Clin Oncol* 2002; **20**: 405–12.

65 Berthou C, Leglise MC, Herry A *et al.* Extramedullary relapse after favorable molecular response to donor leukocyte infusions for recurring acute leukemia. *Leukemia* 1998; **12**: 1676–81.

66 Butcher EC, Picker LJ. Lymphocyte homing and homeostasis. *Science* 1996; **272**: 60–6.

67 Porter DL, Roth MS, Lee SJ, McGarigle C, Ferrara JL, Antin JH. Adoptive immunotherapy with donor mononuclear cell infusions to treat relapse of acute leukemia or myelodysplasia after allogeneic bone marrow transplantation. *Bone Marrow Transplant* 1996; **18**: 975–80.

68 Cao TM, McSweeney PA, Niederwieser D *et al.* Non-myeloablative allogeneic hematopoietic cell transplantation (AHCT) for patients with myelodysplastic syndromes (MDS) and myeloproliferative disorders (MPD). *Blood* 2000; **96**: 170a [Abstract].

69 Cervantes F, Rovira M, Urbano-Ispizua A, Rozman M, Carreras E, Montserrat E. Complete remission of idiopathic myelofibrosis following donor lymphocyte infusion after failure of allogeneic transplantation: demonstration of a graft-versus-myelofibrosis effect. *Bone Marrow Transplant* 2000; **26**: 697–9.

70 Devine SM, Hoffman R, Verma A *et al.* Allogeneic blood cell transplantation following reduced-intensity conditioning is effective therapy for older patients with myelofibrosis with myeloid metaplasia. *Blood* 2002; **99**: 2255–8.

71 Yazaki M, Andoh M, Ito T, Ohno T, Wada Y. Successful prevention of hematological relapse for a patient with Philadelphia chromosome-positive acute lymphoblastic leukemia after allogeneic bone marrow transplantation by donor leukocyte infusion. *Bone Marrow Transplant* 1997; **19**: 393–4.

72 Atra A, Millar B, Shepherd V *et al.* Donor lymphocyte infusion for childhood acute lymphoblastic leukaemia relapsing after bone marrow transplantation. *Br J Haematol* 1997; **97**: 165–8.

73 Collins RH Jr, Goldstein S, Giralt S *et al.* Donor leukocyte infusions in acute lymphocytic leukemia. *Bone Marrow Transplant* 2000; **26**: 511–6.

74 Matsue K, Tabayashi T, Yamada K, Takeuchi M. Eradication of residual *bcr-abl*-positive clones by inducing graft-versus-host disease after allogeneic stem cell transplantation in patients with Philadelphia chromosome-positive acute lymphoblastic leukemia. *Bone Marrow Transplant* 2002; **29**: 63–6.

75 Sanchez J, Serrano J, Gomez P *et al.* Clinical value of immunological monitoring of minimal residual disease in acute lymphoblastic leukaemia after allogeneic transplantation. *Br J Haematol* 2002; **116**: 686–94.

76 Lewalle P, Soree A, Jacquy C *et al.* Molecular evidence of a GVL effect in allogeneic transplant for acute lymphoblastic leukemia restricted to Ph-negative leukemia: post-transplant immunomodulation performed according to molecular follow-up seems efficient only in this subset of patients. *Blood* 2001; **98**: 387a [Abstract].

77 Verdonck LF, Lokhorst HM, Dekker AW, Nieuwenhuis HK, Petersen EJ. Graft-versus-myeloma effect in two cases. *Lancet* 1996; **347**: 800–1.

78 Tricot G, Vesole DH, Jagannath S, Hilton J, Munshi N, Barlogie B. Graft-versus-myeloma effect. Proof of principle. *Blood* 1996; **87**: 1196–8.

79 Lokhorst HM, Schattenberg A, Cornelissen JJ, Thomas LL, Verdonck LF. Donor leukocyte infusions are effective in relapsed multiple myeloma after allogeneic bone marrow transplantation. *Blood* 1997; **90**: 4206–11.

80 van der Griend R, Verdonck LF, Petersen EJ, Veenhuizen P, Bloem AC, Lokhorst HM. Donor leukocyte infusions inducing remissions repeatedly in a patient with recurrent multiple myeloma after allogeneic bone marrow transplantation. *Bone Marrow Transplant* 1999; **23**: 195–7.

81 Mehta J, Singhal S. Graft-versus-myeloma. *Bone Marrow Transplant* 1998; **22**: 835–43.

82 Orsini E, Alyea EP, Schlossman R *et al.* Changes in T cell receptor repertoire associated with graftversus-tumor effect and graft-versus-host disease in patients with relapsed multiple myeloma after donor lymphocyte infusion. *Bone Marrow Transplant* 2000; **25**: 623–32.

83 Lokhorst HM, Schattenberg A, Cornelissen JJ *et al.* Donor lymphocyte infusions for relapsed multiple myeloma after allogeneic stem-cell transplantation: predictive factors for response and long-term outcome. *J Clin Oncol* 2000; **18**: 3031–7.

84 Salama M, Nevill T, Marcellus D *et al.* Donor leukocyte infusions for multiple myeloma. *Bone Marrow Transplant* 2000; **26**: 1179–84.

85 Alyea E, Weller E, Schlossman R *et al.* T-celldepleted allogeneic bone marrow transplantation followed by donor lymphocyte infusion in patients with multiple myeloma: induction of graft-versusmyeloma effect. *Blood* 2001; **98**: 934–9.

86 Peggs K, D'SaS, Kyriakou CA *et al.* Nonmyeloablative allogeneic transplantation as frontline treatment for multiple myeloma: response rates to conditioning and subsequent donor lymphocyte infusions. *Blood* 2001; **98**: 419a [Abstract].

87 Maloney DG, Sahebi F, Stockerl-Goldstein KE *et al.* Combining an allogeneic graft-vs.-myeloma effect with high-dose autologous stem cell rescue in the treatment of multiple myeloma. *Blood* 2001; **98**: 434a [Abstract].

88 Badros A, Barlogie B, Siegel E *et al.* Improved outcome of allogeneic transplantation in high-risk multiple myeloma patients after nonmyeloablative conditioning. *J Clin Oncol* 2002; **20**: 1295–303.

89 Zomas A, Stefanoudaki K, Fisfis M, Papadaki T, Mehta J. Graft-versus-myeloma after donor leukocyte infusion. Maintenance of marrow remission but extramedullary relapse with plasmacytomas. *Bone Marrow Transplant* 1998; **21**: 1163–5.

90 Grigg AP. Multiply recurrent extramedullary plasmacytomas without marrow relapse in the context of extensive chronic GVHD in a patient with myeloma. *Leuk Lymphoma* 1999; **34**: 635–6.

91 Jones RJ, Ambinder RF, Piantadosi S, Santos GW. Evidence of a graft-versus-lymphoma effect associated with allogeneic bone marrow transplantation. *Blood* 1991; **77**: 649–53.

92 Ratanatharathorn V, Uberti J, Karanes C *et al.* Prospective comparative trial of autologous versus allogeneic bone marrow transplantation in patients with non-Hodgkin's lymphoma. *Blood* 1994; **84**: 1050–5.

93 Chopra R, Goldstone AH, Pearce R *et al.* Autologous versus allogeneic bone marrow transplantation for non-Hodgkin's lymphoma: a case-controlled analysis of the European Bone Marrow Transplant Group Registry data. *J Clin Oncol* 1992; **10**: 1690–5.

94 van Besien K, Sobocinski KA, Rowlings PA *et al.* Allogeneic bone marrow transplantation for low-grade lymphoma. *Blood* 1998; **92**: 1832–6.

95 Rondon G, Giralt S, Huh Y *et al.* Graft-versus-leukemia effect after allogeneic bone marrow transplantation for chronic lymphocytic leukemia. *Bone Marrow Transplant* 1996; **18**: 669–72.

96 van Besien KW, de Lima M, Giralt SA *et al.* Management of lymphoma recurrence after allogeneic transplantation: the relevance of graft-versus-lymphoma effect. *Bone Marrow Transplant* 1997; **19**: 977–82.

97 Mandigers CM, Meijerink JP, Raemaekers JM, Schattenberg AV, Mensink EJ. Graft-versus-lymphoma effect of donor leucocyte infusion shown by real-time quantitative PCR analysis of t(14;18). *Lancet* 1998; **352**: 1522–3.

98 Mandigers CM, Verdonck L, Meijerink JP, Schattenberg A, Tonnissen E, Raemaekers JM. Graft-versus-lymphoma effect of donor leukocyte infusion in indolent lymphomas relapsed after T-cell depleted allogeneic stem cell transplantation, substantiated by real-time PCR quantitation and immunophenotyping. *Blood* 2001; **98**: 369b [Abstract].

99 Khouri IF, Keating M, Korbling M *et al.* Transplant-lite: induction of graft-versus-malignancy using fludarabine-based nonablative chemotherapy and allogeneic blood progenitor-cell transplantation as treatment for lymphoid malignancies. *J Clin Oncol* 1998; **16**: 2817–24.

100 Sykes M, Preffer F, McAfee S *et al.* Mixed lymphohaemopoietic chimerism and graft-versus-lymphoma effects after non-myeloablative therapy and HLA-mismatched bone-marrow transplantation. *Lancet* 1999; **353**: 1755–9.

101 Khouri IF, Lee MS, Romaguera J *et al.* Allogeneic hematopoietic transplantation for mantle-cell lymphoma: molecular remissions and evidence of graft-versus-malignancy. *Ann Oncol* 1999; **10**: 1293–9.

102 Sohn SK, Baek JH, Kim DH *et al.* Successful allogeneic stem-cell transplantation with prophylactic stepwise G-CSF primed-DLIs for relapse after autologous transplantation in mantle cell lymphoma: a case report and literature review on the evidence of GVL effects in MCL. *Am J Hematol* 2000; **65**: 75–80.

103 Khouri I, Saliba RM, Giralt S *et al.* Prolonged failure free survival and molecular responses with nonablative allogeneic hematopoietic transplantation as adoptive immunotherapy for indolent lymphoma. *Blood* 2001; **98**: 744a [Abstract].

104 Flowers CR, Maloney DG, Sandmaier BM *et al.* Allogeneic hematopoietic stem cell transplantation with nonmyeloablative conditioning for patients with chronic lymphocytic leukemia. *Blood* 2001; **98**: 418a [Abstract].

105 Hou JW, Fowler DH, Wilson W *et al.* Potent graft-versus-lymphoma effect after non-myeloablative stem cell transplant in refractory non-Hodgkin's lymphoma. The role of rapid complete donor chimerism. *Blood* 2001; **98**: 404a [Abstract].

106 Garcia-Marco JA, Cabrera R, Perez-Sanz N *et al.* Analysis of graft-versus-malignancy effect following nonmyeloablative stem cell transplantation in chronic lymphocytic leukemia (CLL) and non-Hodgkin lymphoma. *Blood* 2001; **98**: 365b [Abstract].

107 Kyriakou CA, Milligan D, Chopra R *et al.* Outcome of non-myeloablative stem cell transplantation for NHL is dependent on histology: good for patients with low grade disease and poor for those with high grade lymphoma. *Blood* 2001; **98**: 414a [Abstract].

108 Khouri I, Saliba RM, Giralt S *et al.* Long term remission and low mortality achieved with cisplatin, fludarabine, cytarabine nonablative preparative regimen and allogeneic stem transplantation (AST) for histologically aggressive non-Hodgkin's lymphoma (NHL). *Blood* 2001; **98**: 190a [Abstract].

109 Spitzer TR, McAfee S, Dey BR *et al.* Durable progression free survival (PFS) following non-myeloablative bone marrow transplantation (BMT) for chemorefractory diffuse large B cell lymphoma (B-LCL). *Blood* 2001; **98**: 672a [Abstract].

110 Carella AM, Beltrami G, Scalzuli P, Carella AM, Greco M, Corsetti MT. Autografting followed by nonmyeloablative allografting for advanced lymphoma. A higher than expected remission rate of disease control. *Blood* 2001; **98**: 743a [Abstract].

111 Carella AM, Cavaliere M, Lerma E *et al.* Autografting followed by nonmyeloablative immunosuppressive chemotherapy and allogeneic peripheral-blood hematopoietic stem-cell transplantation as treatment of resistant Hodgkin's disease and non-Hodgkin's lymphoma. *J Clin Oncol* 2000; **18**: 3918–24.

112 Kottaridis PD, Milligan DW, Chopra R *et al.* Non-myeloablative transplantation for patients with Hodgkin's disease limited transplant-related mortality and possible evidence of graft versus Hodgkin's effect. *Blood* 2001; **98**: 416a [Abstract].

113 Childs R, Chernoff A, Contentin N *et al.* Regression of metastatic renal-cell carcinoma after nonmyeloablative allogeneic peripheral-blood stem-cell transplantation. *N Engl J Med* 2000; **343**: 750–8.

114 Eibl B, Schwaighofer H, Nachbaur D *et al.* Evidence for a graft-versus-tumor effect in a patient treated with marrow ablative chemotherapy and allogeneic bone marrow transplantation for breast cancer. *Blood* 1996; **88**: 1501–8.

115 Ueno NT, Rondon G, Mirza NQ *et al.* Allogeneic peripheral-blood progenitor-cell transplantation for poor-risk patients with metastatic breast cancer. *J Clin Oncol* 1998; **16**: 986–93.

116 Bregni M, Dodero A, Peccatori J *et al.* Non-myeloablative conditioning followed by hematopoietic cell allografting and donor lymphocyte infusions for patients with metastatic renal and breast cancer. *Blood* 2002; **99**: 4234–6.

117 Goulmy E, Schipper R, Pool J *et al.* Mismatches of minor histocompatibility antigens between HLA-identical donors and recipients and the development of graft-versus-host disease after bone marrow transplantation. *N Engl J Med* 1996; **334**: 281–5.

118 Johnson BD, Drobyski WR, Truitt RL. Delayed infusion of normal donor cells after MHC-matched bone marrow transplantation provides an anti-leukemia reaction without graft-versus-host disease. *Bone Marrow Transplant* 1993; **11**: 329–36.

119 Johnson BD, Truitt RL. Delayed infusion of immunocompetent donor cells after bone marrow transplantation breaks graft-host tolerance allows for persistent antileukemic reactivity without severe graft-versus-host disease. *Blood* 1995; **85**: 3302–12.

120 Johnson BD, Becker EE, Truitt RL. Graft-vs.-host and graft-vs.-leukemia reactions after delayed infusions of donor T-subsets. *Biol Blood Marrow Transplant* 1999; **5**: 123–32.

121 Kernan NA, Collins NH, Juliano L, Cartagena T, Dupont B, O'Reilly RJ. Clonable T lymphocytes in T cell-depleted bone marrow transplants correlate with development of graft-v-host disease. *Blood* 1986; **68**: 770–3.

122 Keil F, Haas OA, Fritsch G *et al.* Donor leukocyte infusion for leukemic relapse after allogeneic marrow transplantation: lack of residual donor hematopoiesis predicts aplasia. *Blood* 1997; **89**: 3113–7.

123 Flowers ME, Leisenring W, Beach K *et al.* Granulocyte colony-stimulating factor given to donors before apheresis does not prevent aplasia in patients treated with donor leukocyte infusion for recurrent chronic myeloid leukemia after bone marrow transplant. *Biol Blood Marrow Transplant* 2000; **6**: 321–6.

124 Porter DL, Collins RH Jr, Hardy C *et al.* Treatment of relapsed leukemia after unrelated donor marrow transplantation with unrelated donor leukocyte infusions. *Blood* 2000; **95**: 1214–21.

125 Peggs K, Kottaridis PD, Morris ME *et al.* Escalating dose donor lymphocyte infusions following non-myeloablative allogeneic transplantation are associated with minimal toxicity with sibling donors but a significant risk of severe GVHD with unrelated donors. *Blood* 2001; **98**: 672a [Abstract].

126 Pati AR, Godder K, Lamb L, Gee A, Henslee-Downey PJ. Immunotherapy with donor leukocyte infusions for patients with relapsed acute myeloid leukemia following partially mismatched related donor bone marrow transplantation. *Bone Marrow Transplant* 1995; **15**: 979–81.

127 Lewalle P, Triffet A, Delforge A *et al.* Donor lymphocytes infusion in adult haplo-identical transplant: a dose finding study. *Blood* 2001; **98**: 123a [Abstract].

128 Sprent J, Korngold R. T cell subsets controlling graft-v-host disease in mice. *Transplant Proc* 1987; **19**: 41–7.

129 Nimer SD, Giorgi J, Gajewski JL *et al.* Selective depletion of CD8+ cells for prevention of graft-versus-host disease after bone marrow transplantation. A randomized controlled trial. *Transplantation* 1994; **57**: 82–7.

130 Alyea EP, Soiffer RJ, Canning C *et al.* Toxicity and efficacy of defined doses of CD4+ donor lymphocytes for treatment of relapse after allogeneic bone marrow transplant. *Blood* 1998; **91**: 3671–80.

131 Shimoni A, Gajewski JA, Donato M *et al.* Long-term follow-up of recipients of CD8-depleted donor lymphocyte infusions for the treatment of chronic myelogenous leukemia relapsing after allogeneic progenitor cell transplantation. *Biol Blood Marrow Transplant* 2001; **7**: 568–75.

132 Soiffer R, Alyea E, Canning C *et al.* A randomized trial of CD8+ T cell depletion to prevent

graft-vs.-host disease (GVHD) associated with donor lymphocyte infusions. *Blood* 2001; **98**: 856a [Abstract].

133 Mavroudis DA, Dermime S, Molldrem J et al. Specific depletion of alloreactive T cells in HLA-identical siblings: a method for separating graft-versus-host and graft-versus-leukaemia reactions. *Br J Haematol* 1998; **101**: 565–70.

134 Montagna D, Yvon E, Calcaterra V et al. Depletion of alloreactive T cells by a specific anti-interleukin-2 receptor p55 chain immunotoxin does not impair *in vitro* antileukemia and antiviral activity. *Blood* 1999; **93**: 3550–7.

135 Michalek J, Vitetta ES, Collins RH. The effect of different immunotoxin enhancers on selective T cell depletion using an anti-CD25 immunotoxin for prophylaxis of GVHD. *Blood* 2000; **96**: 312b [Abstract].

136 Andre-Schmutz I, Le Deist F, Hacein-Bey-Abina S et al. Immune reconstitution without graft-versus-host disease after haemopoietic stem-cell transplantation: a phase 1/2 study. *Lancet* 2002; **360**: 130–7.

137 Guimond M, Balassy A, Barrette M, Brochu S, Perreault C, Roy DC. P-glycoprotein targeting: a unique strategy to selectively eliminate immunoreactive T cells. *Blood* 2002; **100**: 375–82.

138 Rooney CM, Smith CA, Ng CY et al. Use of gene-modified virus-specific T lymphocytes to control Epstein–Barr-virus-related lymphoproliferation. *Lancet* 1995; **345**: 9–13.

139 Rooney CM, Smith CA, Ng CY et al. Infusion of cytotoxic T cells for the prevention and treatment of Epstein–Barr virus-induced lymphoma in allogeneic transplant recipients. *Blood* 1998; **92**: 1549–55.

140 Walter EA, Greenberg PD, Gilbert MJ et al. Reconstitution of cellular immunity against cytomegalovirus in recipients of allogeneic bone marrow by transfer of T-cell clones from the donor. *N Engl J Med* 1995; **333**: 1038–44.

141 Falkenburg JH, Wafelman AR, Joosten P et al. Complete remission of accelerated phase chronic myeloid leukemia by treatment with leukemia-reactive cytotoxic T lymphocytes. *Blood* 1999; **94**: 1201–8.

142 Smit WM, Rijnbeek M, van Bergen CA, Willemze R, Falkenburg JH. Generation of leukemia-reactive cytotoxic T lymphocytes from HLA-identical donors of patients with chronic myeloid leukemia using modifications of a limiting dilution assay. *Bone Marrow Transplant* 1998; **21**: 553–60.

143 Mutis T, Verdijk R, Schrama E, Esendam B, Brand A, Goulmy E. Feasibility of immunotherapy of relapsed leukemia with *ex vivo*-generated cytotoxic T lymphocytes specific for hematopoietic system-restricted minor histocompatibility antigens. *Blood* 1999; **93**: 2336–41.

144 Bordignon C, Bonini C, Verzeletti S et al. Transfer of the HSV-tk gene into donor peripheral blood lymphocytes for *in vivo* modulation of donor antitumor immunity after allogeneic bone marrow transplantation. *Hum Gene Ther* 1995; **6**: 813–9.

145 Bonini C, Ferrari G, Verzeletti S et al. HSV-TK gene transfer into donor lymphocytes for control of allogeneic graft-versus-leukemia. *Science* 1997; **276**: 1719–24.

146 Bonini C, Ciceri F, Marktel S, Bordignon C. Suicide-gene-transduced T-cells for the regulation of the graft-versus-leukemia effect. *Vox Sang* 1998; **74**: 341–3.

147 Tiberghien P, Reynolds CW, Keller J et al. Ganciclovir treatment of herpes simplex thymidine kinase-transduced primary T lymphocytes: an approach for specific *in vivo* donor T-cell depletion after bone marrow transplantation? *Blood* 1994; **84**: 1333–41.

148 Tiberghien P, Ferrand C, Lioure B et al. Administration of herpes simplex-thymidine kinase-expressing donor T cells with a T-cell-depleted allogeneic marrow graft. *Blood* 2001; **97**: 63–72.

149 Kuhlcke K, Ayuk FA, Li Z et al. Retroviral transduction of T lymphocytes for suicide gene therapy in allogeneic stem cell transplantation. *Bone Marrow Transplant* 2000; **25** (Suppl. 2): S96–8.

150 Riddell SR, Elliott M, Lewinsohn DA et al. T-cell mediated rejection of gene-modified HIV-specific cytotoxic T lymphocytes in HIV-infected patients. *Nat Med* 1996; **2**: 216–23.

151 Thomis DC, Marktel S, Bonini C et al. A Fas-based suicide switch in human T cells for the treatment of graft-versus-host disease. *Blood* 2001; **97**: 1249–57.

152 Waller EK, Boyer M. New strategies in allogeneic stem cell transplantation: immunotherapy using irradiated allogeneic T cells. *Bone Marrow Transplant* 2000; **25** (Suppl. 2): S20–4.

153 Waller EK, Ship AM, Mittelstaedt S et al. Irradiated donor leukocytes promote engraftment of allogeneic bone marrow in major histocompatibility complex mismatched recipients without causing graft-versus-host disease. *Blood* 1999; **94**: 3222–33.

154 Mehta J, Powles R, Singhal S, Tait D, Swansbury J, Treleaven J. Cytokine-mediated immunotherapy with or without donor leukocytes for poor-risk acute myeloid leukemia relapsing after allogeneic bone marrow transplantation. *Bone Marrow Transplant* 1995; **16**: 133–7.

155 Kwak LW, Taub DD, Duffey PL et al. Transfer of myeloma idiotype-specific immunity from an actively immunised marrow donor. *Lancet* 1995; **345**: 1016–20.

156 Cabrera R, Diaz-Espada F, Barrios Y et al. Infusion of lymphocytes obtained from a donor immunised with the paraprotein idiotype as a treatment in a relapsed myeloma. *Bone Marrow Transplant* 2000; **25**: 1105–8.

157 Barrett AJ, Malkovska V. Graft-versus-leukaemia. Understanding and using the alloimmune response to treat haematological malignancies. *Br J Haematol* 1996; **93**: 754–61.

158 Ferrara JL, Levy R, Chao NJ. Pathophysiologic mechanisms of acute graft-vs.-host disease. *Biol Blood Marrow Transplant* 1999; **5**: 347–56.

159 Fontaine P, Roy-Proulx G, Knafo L, Baron C, Roy DC, Perreault C. Adoptive transfer of minor histocompatibility antigen-specific T lymphocytes eradicates leukemia cells without causing graft-versus-host disease. *Nat Med* 2001; **7**: 789–94.

160 Dazzi F, Simpson E, Goldman JM. Minor antigen solves major problem. *Nat Med* 2001; **7**: 769–70.

161 Molldrem JJ, Lee PP, Wang C et al. Evidence that specific T lymphocytes may participate in the elimination of chronic myelogenous leukemia. *Nat Med* 2000; **6**: 1018–23.

162 Orsini E, Alyea EP, Chillemi A et al. Conversion to full donor chimerism following donor lymphocyte infusion is associated with disease response in patients with multiple myeloma. *Biol Blood Marrow Transplant* 2000; **6**: 375–86.

163 Claret EJ, Alyea EP, Orsini E et al. Characterization of T cell repertoire in patients with graft-versus-leukemia after donor lymphocyte infusion. *J Clin Invest* 1997; **100**: 855–66.

164 Wu CJ, Yang XF, McLaughlin S et al. Detection of a potent humoral response associated with immune-induced remission of chronic myelogenous leukemia. *J Clin Invest* 2000; **106**: 705–14.

165 Bunjes D, Theobald M, Hertenstein B et al. Successful therapy with donor buffy coat transfusions in patients with relapsed chronic myeloid leukemia after bone marrow transplantation is associated with high frequencies of host-reactive interleukin 2-secreting T helper cells. *Bone Marrow Transplant* 1995; **15**: 713–9.

166 Jiang YZ, Cullis JO, Kanfer EJ, Goldman JM, Barrett AJ. T cell and NK cell mediated graft-versus-leukaemia reactivity following donor buffy coat transfusion to treat relapse after marrow transplantation for chronic myeloid leukaemia. *Bone Marrow Transplant* 1993; **11**: 133–8.

167 Smit WM, Rijnbeek M, van Bergen CA, Fibbe WE, Willemze R, Falkenburg JH. T cells recognizing leukemic CD34+ progenitor cells mediate the antileukemic effect of donor lymphocyte infusions for relapsed chronic myeloid leukemia after allogeneic stem cell transplantation. *Proc Natl Acad Sci U S A* 1998; **95**: 10,152–7.

168 Kircher B, Stevanovic S, Urbanek M et al. Induction of HA-1-specific cytotoxic T-cell clones parallels the therapeutic effect of donor lymphocyte infusion. *Br J Haematol* 2002; **117**: 935–9.

169 Bellucci R, Wu CJ, Munshi N, Alyea E, Anderson K, Ritz J. Identification of target antigens associated with graft-vs.-myeloma response after allogeneic bone marrow transplantation and donor lymphocyte infusion. *Blood* 2001; **98**: 405a [Abstract].

170 Mutis T, Gillespie G, Schrama E, Falkenburg JH, Moss P, Goulmy E. Tetrameric HLA class I-minor histocompatibility antigen peptide complexes demonstrate minor histocompatibility antigen-specific cytotoxic T lymphocytes in patients with graft-versus-host disease. *Nat Med* 1999; **5**: 839–42.

171 Maino VC, Picker LJ. Identification of functional subsets by flow cytometry: intracellular detection of cytokine expression. *Cytometry* 1998; **34**: 207–15.

172 Picker LJ. Proving HIV-1 immunity: new tools offer new opportunities. *J Clin Invest* 2000; **105**: 1333–4.

173 Michalek J, Collins RH, Hill BJ, Brenchley JM, Douck DC. Identification and monitoring of graft-versus-host specific T-cell clone in stem cell transplantation. *Lancet* 2003; **361**: 1183–5.

174 Guinan EC, Gribben JG, Boussiotis VA, Freeman GJ, Nadler LM. Pivotal role of the B7: CD28 pathway in transplantation tolerance and tumor immunity. *Blood* 1994; **84**: 3261–82.

175 Dermime S, Mavroudis D, Jiang YZ, Hensel N, Molldrem J, Barrett AJ. Immune escape from a graft-versus-leukemia effect may play a role in the relapse of myeloid leukemias following allogeneic bone marrow transplantation. *Bone Marrow Transplant* 1997; **19**: 989–99.

176 Collins RH Jr, Rogers ZR, Bennett M, Kumar V, Nikein A, Fay JW. Hematologic relapse of chronic myelogenous leukemia following allogeneic bone marrow transplantation: apparent graft-versus-leukemia effect following abrupt discontinuation of immunosuppression. *Bone Marrow Transplant* 1992; **10**: 391–5.

177 Higano CS, Brixey M, Bryant EM et al. Durable complete remission of acute nonlymphocytic leukemia associated with discontinuation of immunosuppression following relapse after allogeneic bone marrow transplantation. A case report of a probable graft-versus-leukemia effect. *Transplantation* 1990; **50**: 175–7.

178 Odom LF, August CS, Githens JH *et al.* Remission of relapsed leukaemia during a graft-versus-host reaction. A "graft-versus-leukaemia reaction" in man? *Lancet* 1978; **2**: 537–40.

179 Peterson FB, Appelbaum FR, Bigelow CL *et al.* High-dose cytosine arabinoside, total body irradiation and marrow tranplantation for advanced malignant lymphoma. *Bone Marrow Transplant* 1989; **4**: 483–8.

180 Brandenburg U, Gottlieb D, Bradstock K. Antileukemic effects of rapid cyclosporin withdrawal in patients with relapsed chronic myeloid leukaemia after allogeneic bone marrow transplantation. *Leuk Lymphoma* 1998; **31**: 545–50.

181 Elmaagacli AH, Beelen DW, Schaefer UW. A retrospective single centre study of the outcome of five different therapy approaches in 48 patients with relapse of chronic myelogenous leukaemia after allogeneic bone marrow transplantation. *Bone Marrow Transplant* 1997; **20**: 1045–55.

182 Mrsic M, Horowitz MM, Atkinson K *et al.* Second HLA-identical sibling transplants for leukemia recurrence. *Bone Marrow Transplant* 1992; **9**: 269–75.

183 Mehta J, Powles R, Treleaven J *et al.* Outcome of acute leukemia relapsing after bone marrow transplantation: utility of second transplants and adoptive immunotherapy. *Bone Marrow Transplant* 1997; **19**: 709–19.

184 Radich JP, Sanders JE, Buckner CD *et al.* Second allogeneic marrow transplantation for patients with recurrent leukemia after initial transplant with total-body irradiation-containing regimens. *J Clin Oncol* 1993; **11**: 304–13.

185 Blau IW, Basara N, Bischoff M *et al.* Second allogeneic hematopoietic stem cell transplantation as treatment for leukemia relapsing following a first transplant. *Bone Marrow Transplant* 2000; **25**: 41–5.

186 Frassoni F, Barrett AJ, Granena A *et al.* Relapse after allogeneic bone marrow transplantation for acute leukaemia: a survey by the EBMT 117 cases. *Br J Haematol* 1988; **70**: 317–20.

187 Bostrom B, Woods WG, Nesbit ME *et al.* Successful reinduction of patients with acute lymphoblastic leukemia who relapse following bone marrow transplantation. *J Clin Oncol* 1987; **5**: 376–81.

188 Higano CS, Raskind WH, Singer JW. Use of a interferon for the treatment of relapse of chronic myelogenous leukemia in chronic phase after allogeneic bone marrow transplantation. *Blood* 1992; **80**: 1437–42.

189 Higano CS, Chielens D, Raskind W *et al.* Use of α_{2a}-interferon to treat cytogenetic relapse of chronic myeloid leukemia after marrow transplantation. *Blood* 1997; **90**: 2549–54.

190 Pigneux A, Devergie A, Pochitaloff M *et al.* Recombinant α-interferon as treatment for chronic myelogenous leukemia in relapse after allogeneic bone marrow transplantation: a report from the Societe Francaise de Greffe de Moelle. *Bone Marrow Transplant* 1995; **15**: 819–24.

191 Bhatia R, McCarthy JB, Verfaillie CM. Interferon-α restores normal negative regulation of mediated proliferation inhibition. *Blood* 1987; **87**: 3883–91.

192 Soiffer RJ, Murray C, Cochran K *et al.* Clinical and immunologic effects of prolonged infusion of low-dose recombinant interleukin-2 after autologous and T-cell-depleted allogeneic bone marrow transplantation. *Blood* 1992; **79**: 517–26.

193 Foa R, Meloni G, Tosti S *et al.* Treatment of acute myeloid leukaemia patients with recombinant interleukin 2: a pilot study. *Br J Haematol* 1991; **77**: 491–6.

194 Giralt S, Escudier S, Kantarjian H *et al.* Preliminary results of treatment with filgrastim for relapse of leukemia and myelodysplasia after allogeneic bone marrow transplantation. *N Engl J Med* 1993; **329**: 757–61.

195 Bishop MR, Tarantolo SR, Pavletic ZS *et al.* Filgrastim as an alternative to donor leukocyte infusion for relapse after allogeneic stem-cell transplantation. *J Clin Oncol* 2000; **18**: 2269–72.

196 Collins RH Jr, Fay JW. Treatment of leukemia in relapse after bone marrow transplantation. *N Engl J Med* 1994; **330**: 645; discussion 645–6.

197 Druker BJ, Lydon NB. Lessons learned from the development of an *abl* tyrosine kinase inhibitor for chronic myelogenous leukemia. *J Clin Invest* 2000; **105**: 3–7.

198 Druker BJ, Talpaz M, Resta DJ *et al.* Efficacy and safety of a specific inhibitor of the *BCR-ABL* tyrosine kinase in chronic myeloid leukemia. *N Engl J Med* 2001; **344**: 1031–7.

199 Olavarria E, Craddock C, Dazzi F *et al.* Imatinib mesylate (STI571) in the treatment of relapse of chronic myeloid leukemia after allogeneic stem cell transplantation. *Blood* 2002; **99**: 3861–2.

200 Kantarjian H, O'Brien S, Cortes J *et al.* Results of imatinib mesylate (STI571) therapy in patients (pts) with chronic myelogenous leukemia (CML) in relapse after allogeneic stem cell transplantation (allo SCT). *Blood* 2001; **98**: 137a [Abstract].

201 Chak LY, Sapozink MD, Cox RS. Extramedullary lesions in non-lymphocytic leukemia. Results of radiation therapy. *Int J Radiat Oncol Biol Phys* 1983; **9**: 1173–6.

202 Guglielmi C, Arcese W, Hermans J *et al.* Risk assessment in patients with Ph+ chronic myelogenous leukemia at first relapse after allogeneic stem cell transplant: an EBMT retrospective analysis. The Chronic Leukemia Working Party of the European Group for Blood and Marrow Transplantation. *Blood* 2000; **95**: 3328–34.

85

Brenda M. Sandmaier & Rainer Storb

Nonmyeloablative Therapy and Hematopoietic Cell Transplantation for Hematologic Disorders

Allogeneic hematopoietic cell transplantation (HCT) has an important role in the treatment of a wide variety of malignant and nonmalignant hematological diseases. Successful allogeneic HCT must overcome two primary and opposing immunologic barriers: the graft-vs.-host (GVH) and host-vs.-graft (HVG) alloimmune responses. The conventional strategy to overcome this bidirectional barrier has relied upon three elements. First, an intensive conditioning regimen is delivered with the dual purposes of immunoablation and disease eradication. For these purposes, conventional regimens have employed otherwise supralethal doses of irradiation and/or chemotherapy. Second, donor hematopoietic cells are given to rescue patients from lethal myeloablation. Third, T-cell depletion or post-grafting immunosuppression is used to control graft-vs.-host disease (GVHD) and to establish long-term graft–host tolerance.

Complications related to the conditioning regimen are a major limitation in the application of conventional HCT. Regimens can be intensified to prevent disease relapse but at the cost of increasing the risks for severe organ toxicities and mortality. Pancytopenia caused by conventional regimens sets the stage for life-threatening infections. Organ toxicities, especially to liver and kidneys, often impair the ability to deliver the doses of immunosuppression necessary for control of GVHD. For these reasons, conventional allogeneic HCTs have been carried out in highly specialized hospital wards and their use restricted to relatively young patients at most transplant centers.

The concept that conditioning dose intensification itself is the only approach for eradication of malignancy came under question early in the history of HCT. Findings in the late 1970s and early 1980s drew attention to graft-vs.-tumor (GVT) effects, as evidenced by the observations that better relapse-free survival was associated with both acute and chronic GVHD [1–6]. Additional evidence supporting the GVT effects included lower relapse rates among patients who received allogeneic HCT as compared with autologous grafts [7,8], a greater incidence of relapse in patients who received syngeneic grafts [9] or T-cell-depleted allografts [6], and the ability to induce durable remissions by using donor lymphocyte infusions (DLI) to treat relapse after allogeneic HCT [10–15]. These observations emphasized the potent role of donor immune cells in the eradication of malignancy and the achievement of cure and led to the hypothesis that GVT effects might be exploited in patients who could not tolerate high-dose conditioning regimens. To expand treatment options for patients, including those thought to be too old or medically infirm to qualify for conventional HCT, several groups of investigators have developed regimens that reduce the toxicities of the conditioning therapy in order to minimize the regimen-related toxicities while relying on the GVT effects for the treatment of the underlying malignancies. While some of the regimens are merely reduced-intensity conventional regimens, others rely on pre- and post-transplant immunosuppression to establish the allografts.

For the latter regimens, it is important to remember that both HVG and GVH reactions are mediated by T cells of host and donor origin, respectively, when transplants are carried out across minor histocompatibility barriers. From these facts follows the hypothesis that some of the HVG reactions can be controlled through novel and effective agents that serve to control GVHD. Consequently, most of the toxic high-dose pretransplant therapy previously employed for HVG control can be replaced by relatively nontoxic immunosuppression. Once established, grafts would create marrow space through subclinical GVH reactions, and cytotoxic and myeloablative doses of total body irradiation (TBI) or busulfan (BU) would not be needed for that purpose. Ideally, control of HVG and GVH reactions results in mutual graft–host tolerance and mixed donor–host hematopoietic chimerism. Mixed chimerism is likely to correct phenotypic expression of certain genetic diseases and, in patients with malignant diseases, can serve as a platform for adoptive immunotherapy through GVT effects. Thus, novel transplantation programs can be designed that are safer than "conventional" high-dose regimens and have the potential to be administered in the ambulatory care setting rather than on intensive care wards. This chapter discusses the results of clinical studies using nonmyeloablative conditioning, including the preclinical studies that served as their basis.

Preclinial studies

Murine studies

A number of successful preclinical studies have involved inbred strains of mice. Most have included *in vivo* depletion of host T cells using antibodies, followed by TBI at high but, at least for mice, sublethal doses and dose rates. In other cases, TBI was delivered along with thymic irradiation and post-grafting cyclosporine (CSP) or high-dose cyclophosphamide (CY). A murine study by Cobbold *et al.* [16] combined pretransplant treatment with anti-CD4 and anti-CD8 monoclonal antibodies (MABs) for *in vivo* T-cell depletion with 600–850 cGy TBI delivered at 35 cGy/min. In other studies, nonobese diabetic (NOD) mice received ≥750 cGy TBI followed by infusion of very large numbers of allogeneic marrow cells, $\geq 30 \times 10^6$/mouse ($\geq 1.5 \times 10^9$/kg) for successful engraftment [17,18]. In one report, mice were conditioned for successful allografts with 500 cGy TBI and given additional immunosuppression with 200 mg/kg CY after transplantation [19].

Other investigators combined anti-CD4 and anti-CD8 MABs with 300 cGy TBI and 700 cGy thymic irradiation to ensure engraftment [20]. These investigators reported that the need for thymic irradiation could be avoided by additional anti-CD4 and anti-CD8 MAB injections after transplantation, thereby depleting host T cells [21,22]. TBI could be

Table 85.1 Marrow toxicity of total body irradiation (TBI) in dogs not rescued by marrow infusion.

TBI dose (cGy)*	No. dogs surviving/No. dogs studied
400—myeloablative and supralethal	1/28
300	7/21
200—sublethal	18/19
100	12/12

* Delivered at 7 cGy/min.

Table 85.2 Total body irradiation (TBI) doses needed for engraftment of DLA-identical marrow in the absence of post-grafting immunosuppression.

TBI dose (cGy)*	No. dogs studied	Sustained engraftment (%)	Autologous recovery (%)
920—immunosuppressive	21	95	0
800	5	80	0
700	5	60	0
600	23	52	17
450—myeloablative and supralethal	39	41	36

* Delivered at 7 cGy/min.

eliminated by pretreatment with anti-CD4 and CD8 MABs, thymic irradiation and the injection of the equivalent of 8.7×10^9 marrow cells/kg, suggesting that the role of TBI was for immunosuppression [23]. Yet another study, using A/J→B10 and B10.A→B10 murine marrow grafts, showed persistent chimerism when recipients were given anti-CD4 and anti-CD8 MABs and 300 cGy TBI administered at 100 cGy/min before and antibodies against natural killer (NK) cells after transplantation for up to 16 weeks, demonstrating the role of NK cells in engraftment [24]. Thymic irradiation could be replaced by injection of one costimulatory blocker (anti-CD154 or CTLA4Ig) [25], whereas both thymic irradiation and host T-cell-depleting MABs could be eliminated by single injections each of anti-CD154 and CTLA4Ig [26].

Koch et al. [27] obtained prolonged chimerism in major histocompatibility complex (MHC) mismatched murine allograft recipients when a synthetic CD4-CDR3 peptide analog was used for immunosuppression in combination with TBI. In mice sensitized to donor cells, treatment with the peptide was more effective than anti-CD4 MAB therapy for enhancing donor chimerism, suggesting this approach may be valuable in obviating rejection after MHC-mismatched HCT. Seledtsov et al. [28] used 200 mg/kg CY to condition mice bearing P815 leukemia for allografts and observed mixed chimerism and prolonged survival compared to syngeneic controls, raising the possibility of using nonlethal cytoreductive therapy in combination with allogeneic cells for a GVT effect.

Canine studies

MHC matched grafts

A clinically successful protocol employing 200 cGy TBI pre- and post-grafting immunosuppression with mycophenolate mofetil (MMF)/CSP after HCT has been developed in a canine model. The following describes the development of the regimen.

Marrow toxicity of TBI

Given the importance of TBI for the studies on mixed chimerism, Table 85.1 shows marrow toxicity of various doses of TBI in dogs given intensive supportive care but no "rescue" by HCT [29]. TBI at 200 cGy was sublethal, and 18 of 19 dogs survived with spontaneous hematopoietic recovery. Hematopoietic recovery was complete by day 50. TBI at 400 cGy was lethal with only one of 28 dogs surviving with spontaneous marrow recovery. We used the model to answer questions about the usefulness of post-grafting immunosuppressive agents in enhancing allogeneic engraftment after suboptimal conditioning.

TBI doses needed for engraftment

Table 85.2 shows results of unmodified dog leukocyte antigen (DLA) identical marrow allografts following increasing single doses of TBI delivered at 7 cGy/min [30]. At the myeloablative and supralethal dose of 450 cGy, only 13% of dogs showed all-donor type engraftment and 28% were stable mixed donor–host chimeras. Most dogs rejected grafts and either died of marrow aplasia (23%) or survived with eventual autologous recovery of hematopoiesis (36%). Survival of the latter dogs was probably because of the extended hematopoietic support provided by the transient allograft. Immunosuppression sufficient for sustained engraftment of 95% of dogs was not achieved until 920 cGy TBI.

Mixed chimerism after low-dose TBI before and immunosuppressive drug treatment after transplantation of unmodified marrow

The first experiments tested whether allogeneic engraftment could be improved in dogs conditioned with 450 cGy TBI [31]. Two drugs were investigated that had been widely used in GVHD prevention: CSP and prednisone. Post-grafting immunosuppression in this and all subsequent experiments was discontinued at the latest by day 35. CSP was given orally twice a day. Prednisone was administered in extremely high doses patterned along a regimen initially used by Kernan et al. [32] along with antithymocyte globulin (ATG) to condition patients for second marrow grafts. All dogs given CSP were stably engrafted and none developed GVHD. This result was significantly better than that seen in controls and was consistent with the theory that post-grafting immunosuppression could control both HVG and GVH reactions. A comparable rate of engraftment in dogs that were not given post-grafting CSP was seen only after conditioning with 920 cGy (Table 85.2). Given that the TBI dose used here was 450 cGy, it follows that the immunosuppression accomplished by post-grafting CSP was similar to that achieved by 470 cGy TBI. In contrast, high-dose prednisone proved ineffective in this setting, and none of the dogs studied had sustained engraftment.

In subsequent experiments, the TBI dose was decreased to the sublethal range [33]. At 200 cGy, CSP alone proved ineffective; all four dogs treated rejected their allografts after 4 weeks but survived with autologous recovery. Six dogs were given methotrexate (MTX) along with CSP, a drug combination previously shown to be synergistic in preventing GVHD both in dogs and humans [34,35]. Three of five evaluable dogs became stable mixed chimeras, and two rejected their grafts. MMF, whose metabolite, mycophenolic acid, blocks de novo purine synthesis by binding to inosine monophosphate dehydrogenase and interferes with lymphocyte replication, was next combined with CSP. The two drugs had been found to be synergistic and superior to MTX/CSP for GVHD prevention [36]. Only one of 12 dogs rejected the allograft at week 12, while 11 dogs remained stable mixed chimeras for up to 130 weeks after HCT without clinical evidence of GVHD. Further reducing the TBI dose to 100 cGy resulted in only transient engraftment in MMF/CSP-treated dogs, suggesting a delicate balance of host and donor immunities.

While the establishment of stable mixed hematopoietic chimerism following nonmyeloablative and relatively nontoxic conditioning programs has remained a difficult goal in large random-bred animal species, these results show that it is achievable with MHC-identical grafts using novel short-term pharmacological immunosuppression after transplantation, which serves to curb both HVG and GVH reactions. Once established, HVG tolerance and GVH tolerance have persisted indefinitely as manifested by stable mixed donor–host chimerism and absence of GVHD, without further need for immunosuppression.

Marrow space vs. immunosuppression

The preceding experiments did not definitely answer the question of whether the low-dose TBI before transplantation served to create marrow space or to provide added host immunosuppression to prevent rejection. To address that question, six canine recipients were given 450 cGy (200 cGy/min) pretransplant irradiation to the cervical, thoracic and upper abdominal lymph node chain, DLA-identical littermate marrow grafts, and MMF/CSF post-transplant [37]. In all six, mixed chimerism was present in peripheral blood granulocytes, T cells and monocytes and nonirradiated marrow and lymph node spaces. Two of the six eventually rejected their grafts after 8 and 18 weeks and four showed sustained engraftment. When, more than 1 year after HCT, T cells from the marrow donors were infused which had been sensitized to recipient minor antigens, conversion to all donor chimerism occurred. While other explanations are possible, results seem consistent with the hypothesis that pretransplant irradiation provides host immunosuppression and grafts can create their own marrow space. Therefore, it is conceivable that the small doses of either lymphoid radiation or TBI that are currently used for establishing mixed chimerism can ultimately be replaced by more specific and less toxic means of inducing HVG anergy, including MABs to T-cell surface determinants. These efforts are prompted by concerns that even low doses of radiation or chemotherapy may increase the risk of secondary malignancies.

A subsequent study showed that the equivalent of 100 cGy TBI could be replaced by costimulatory signal blockade with CTLA4Ig [38]. Recipient T cells were activated with intravenous injections of donor peripheral blood mononuclear cells (PBMCs) before 100 cGy TBI, with concurrent administration of the fusion peptide CTLA4Ig which blocks T-cell costimulation through the B7:CD28 signal pathway. Most dogs so treated showed mixed chimerism lasting for the observation period of 2 years. The control dogs not given CTLA4Ig showed transient mixed chimerism lasting for 3–12 weeks when graft rejection occurred. Data support the hypothesis that stable marrow allografts can be established by combining specific nonmyeloablative pretransplant host immunosuppression with post-transplant host and donor immunosuppression by MMF/CSP.

Radiolabeled MAB

We investigated radioimmunotherapy with an alpha-emitting radionuclide, bismuth-213 (Bi-213) and MABs to TCRαβ and CD45, respectively, before and MMF/CSP after HCT. Alpha-emitters are an attractive alternative to beta-emitting radionuclides for targeting hematopoietic cells given that their high energy is deposited over only a few cell diameters (40–90 μm), sparing surrounding normal tissue. Bi-213 has a $t_{1/2}$ of 46 min and delivers a short-range high energy radiation, leading to a high relative biologic effectiveness.

Studies showed that Bi-213 labeled to an anti-TCRαβ MAB resulted in stable engraftment of DLA-identical littermate marrow [39]. Selectively ablating T cells in this way allowed transplantation with very low toxicity, making it especially suitable for patients with nonmalignant hematologic diseases where the risk of secondary malignancies is more of a concern. Similarly, Bi-213, when conjugated to an anti-CD45 MAB, obviated the need for 200 cGy TBI conditioning and enabled stable mixed hematopoietic chimerism [40]. The use of an MAB against the panhematopoietic marker CD45 would be suitable for use in patients with hematologic malignancies or in patients with MHC-nonidentical donors where additional host immune cells, such as NK, play a major part in graft rejection.

MHC mismatched grafts

The barriers to engraftment are more complex and difficult to overcome in the MHC-nonidentical setting. A nonmyeloablative HCT regimen for MHC-haploidentical recipients would allow extending treatment to include those patients who lack HLA-matched donors. In addition to T cells, NK cells are very important effectors of graft rejection in the MHC-nonidentical setting. In a canine model of unrelated DLA-nonidentical marrow transplantation, engraftment was uniformly seen after conditioning of recipients with 1800 cGy TBI (600 cGy × 3), rarely occurred after 920 cGy, and was not seen at all with lower TBI doses [41]. When marrow grafts were supplemented with PBMC or thoracic duct lymphocytes or when granulocyte colony-stimulating factor (G-CSF) mobilized peripheral blood hematopoietic cells (PBHC) were substituted for marrow, consistent allogeneic engraftment was seen after 920 cGy in DLA-haploidentical littermates [42] and DLA-mismatched unrelated dogs [41,43]. The enhanced engraftment was likely because of larger numbers of transplanted T cells. However, when the conditioning dose of TBI was lowered to the still supralethal level of 450 cGy, PBHC from DLA-mismatched donors failed to engraft [44]. In order to target the cells responsible for graft rejection, we developed an MAB, S5, which recognized an epitope of CD44, a cellular adhesion molecule expressed on both hematopoietic and nonhematopoietic cells [45,46]. When given before 920 cGy TBI, the MAB promoted engraftment of marrow in DLA-mismatched unrelated dogs given no additional immunosuppression. When MAB S5 was given before 450 cGy TBI and HCT from DLA-haploidentical littermates, sustained engraftment was seen in none of the recipients. By combining MAB S5 and 450 cGy TBI before with MMF/CSP after HCT, 10 of 12 dogs showed sustained engraftment [44]. When the TBI dose was further reduced to 200 cGy, all dogs displayed initial mixed donor–host chimerism. Within 5–16 weeks after HCT, recipients either reverted to complete host hematopoiesis by rejecting their grafts (68% of dogs) or converted to complete and sustained donor chimerism (32% of dogs). This result indicated that yet better immunosuppression is required to ensure uniform success in this MHC-mismatched model.

Based on results in both the murine and large animal models, clinical studies have been initiated in patients both with malignant and nonmalignant diseases. Data from ongoing preclinical studies will allow us to refine future approaches for our patients.

Clinical results

Two principal approaches have been used to reduce regimen-related toxicities while exploiting GVT effects. The first approach consists of reduced-intensity regimens in which drugs are chosen with proven activities against the targeted malignancies for disease control while waiting for GVT effects to occur. The cytotoxic conditioning also serves to suppress the HVG reactions. These regimens retain some of the regimen-related toxicities that are characteristic of the conventional high-dose transplants. The second approach employs immunosuppressive conditioning regimens that are minimally myelosuppressive. Engraftment is ensured by innovative post-grafting immunosuppression that also controls GVHD. Other differences between these two broad categories of transplants include the degrees of marrow aplasia and the tempo of establishing complete donor chimerism. In the reduced-intensity regimens, recipients uniformly become severely hypoplastic before graft function occurs. Complete donor engraftment occurs rapidly. In contrast, recipients of an immunosuppressive regimen show only moderate declines of

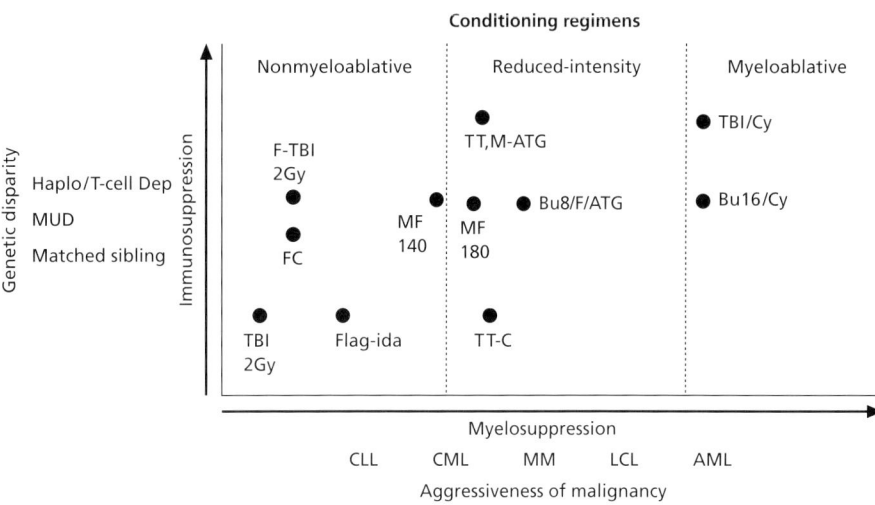

Fig. 85.1 Commonly used nonmyeloablative or reduced-intensity conditioning regimens in relation to their immunosuppressive and myelosuppressive properties. AML, acute myelogenous leukemia; BU, busulfan; CLL, chronic lymphocytic leukemia; CML, chronic myelogenous leukemia; CY, cyclophosphamide; FC, fludarabine/cyclophosphamide; Flag-ida, fludarabine/cytosine arabinoside/idarubicin; F-TBI, fludarabine/TBI; Haplo T Cell Dep, haploidentical T-cell depleted; LCL, large cell lymphoma; MF, melphalan/fludarabine; MM, multiple myeloma; MUD, HLA-matched unrelated donor; TBI, total body irradiation; TT-C, thiotepa/cyclophosphamide; TT-M-ATG, thiotepa/melphalan/antithymocyte globulin. (Adapted from [47]. Copyright the American Society of Hematology, used by permission.)

peripheral blood cell counts before recoveries are seen, and all patients are initially mixed donor–host hematopoietic chimeras. In these patients, it may take 6–12 months before donor engraftment is complete. The comparative benefit of a reduced-intensity regimen vs. a minimally myelosuppressive regimen may depend on the underlying diseases, stage of diseases and clinical status of the patients. In diseases presumed to be more sensitive to GVT effects, such as chronic myelogenous leukemia (CML), chronic lymphocytic leukemia (CLL) and low-grade lymphomas, immunosuppressive regimens may be sufficient to ensure engraftment because there is time for GVT effects to become operative. In rapidly progressive diseases or diseases where GVT is less potent or less able to keep ahead of growth of the underlying malignancy, such as high-grade lymphomas, Hodgkin's disease, multiple myeloma and acute myelogenous leukemia (AML) beyond first remission, a certain amount of cytoreduction may be necessary to minimize residual disease. Figure 85.1 outlines the commonly used nonmyeloablative and reduced-intensity regimens in relation to their immunosuppressive and myelo-suppressive effects. In this chapter, we discuss both strategies of nonmyeloablative transplants, with a review of the initial results and current approaches with a focus on minimally myelosuppressive TBI-based regimens.

Hematologic malignancies

HLA-matched related HCT

While many studies of nonmyeloablative hematopoietic transplants have been performed in elderly and medically infirm patients unable to tolerate a myeloablative preparative regimen, some studies have included younger patients who were otherwise eligible for conventional high-dose transplants with standard eligibility criteria. These differences in patient selection generally preclude meaningful comparison among regimens.

Initial studies at M.D. Anderson Cancer Center in Houston, Texas, utilized purine nucleoside analog-based regimens for treatment of both myeloid and lymphoid malignancies. Giralt et al. [48] combined fludarabine with idarubicin and cytarabine (Ara-C) or melphalan, or cladribine and Ara-C before HCT from HLA-identical or single HLA antigen mismatched sibling donors for treatment of AML or myelodysplastic syndromes (MDS) (Table 85.3). Of 15 patients treated, four failed to engraft, and one treatment-related death occurred before HCT. With a median follow-up of 100 days, six patients were alive, and two were disease-free. Khouri et al. [49], also at M.D. Anderson, treated 15 patients with lymphoid malignancies using a regimen of fludarabine/cyclophosphamide or fludarabine/Ara-C/cisplatin. Eleven of 15 patients attained durable engraftment, and eight of 11 engrafted patients achieved complete remissions. Three nonrelapse deaths occurred. With a median follow-up of 180 days, five of six patients with chemosensitive disease were alive compared to two of nine with refractory or untreated malignancies. Giralt et al. [50] subsequently reported on a study combining purine analogs (fludarabine or cladribine) with melphalan in patients with hematologic malignancies. It was hypothesized that these drug combinations would have enhanced abilities to achieve remissions given the antitumor effects of high-dose melphalan and the observation that purine analogs have been shown to inhibit DNA repair after alkylator-induced damage. Seventy-eight of 86 patients received fludarabine in combination with high-dose melphalan, and eight received cladribine/melphalan. The day 100 nonrelapse mortality was 37% for the fludarabine/melphalan combination and 88% for the cladribine/melphalan combination. Both regimens were sufficiently immunosuppressive to allow for engraftment of both HLA-matched unrelated and related, and 1-HLA-antigen mismatched related donor grafts. Fifty-seven percent of patients achieved complete remissions, illustrating the beneficial effect of the cytoreductive conditioning therapy. Two-year overall and disease-free survivals were 28% and 23%, respectively.

Slavin et al. [51] at Hadassah University in Israel used a regimen that consisted of fludarabine, busulfan (8 mg/kg) and ATG in a younger group of patients (median 34 years; range 1–61 years) with both hematologic malignancies and genetic diseases. All patients achieved either partial or complete donor chimerism with this regimen, with four patients developing moderate to severe hepatic veno-occlusive disease suggesting that this regimen was still quite toxic. This same regimen was used in another group of heavily treated high-risk lymphoma patients with grafts from HLA-matched related and unrelated donors [52]. Again, there was consistent engraftment with disease-free survival of 40% at 37 months. Childs et al. [53] at the National Cancer Institute combined cyclophosphamide and fludarabine to treat patients both with hematologic malignancies and solid tumors. One of 15 patients rejected the graft, and two patients died of transplant-related causes. Ten of 14 patients surviving more than 30 days had disease regression, suggesting GVT effects. The observation was made that full donor T-cell chimerism preceded both acute GVHD and disease regression. Investigators at the Massachusetts General Hospital in Boston evaluated the use of cyclophosphamide, ATG and thymic irradiation (among patients without previous mediastinal radiotherapy) in patients given HLA-matched transplants [54]. Eighteen of 20 evaluable patients developed persistent mixed hematopoietic chimerism. Ten of the 20 received prophylactic DLI to convert mixed to full donor chimerism and to optimize GVL effects. Six of 8 patients receiving prophylactic DLI converted to full donor chimerism. Transplant

Table 85.3 Nonmyeloablative conditioning regimens for patients with hematologic malignancies.

Transplant center [Reference]	Patients studied (n)	Median age, years (range)	Donor	Stem cell source	Diagnosis	Conditioning regimen	Postgraft immunosuppression	Rejections (%)	GVHD* (%) Acute grade II–IV	GVHD* (%) Chronic	Outcome(s)
Houston [48]	15	59 (27–71)	MRD 5/6 RD	PBHC BM	AML MDS	F+I+A F+I+M 2-CDA+A	CSP+MP	27	20	0	OS: 40% DFS: 13% Median F/U: 100 days
Houston [49]	15	55 (47–71)	MRD	PBHC BM	CLL NHL	F+CY F+C+A	±T±MTX	27	7	13	OS: 47% DFS: 33% Median F/U: 180 days
Houston [50]	86	52 (22–70)	MURD MRD 5/6 RD	BM PBHC	HM	F+M 2-CDA+M	T+MTX T+MP CSP+MP	2	40	24	2-yr OS: 28% 2-yr DFS: 23% 2-yr NRM: 45%
Jerusalem [51]	26	34 (1–61)	MRD	PBHC	HM GD	F+B+ATG	CSP	0	38	27	OS: 85% DFS: 81% Median F/U 240 days
Jerusalem [52]	23	41 (13–63)	MRD	PBHC	L	F+B+ATG	CSP	0	35	9	OS: 43% DFS: 43% Median F/U: 675 days
NIH [53]	15	50 (23–68)	MRD	PBHC	HM ST	F+CY	CSP	7	60	27	OS: 53% PFS: 53% Median F/U: 200 days
Boston [54]	21	44 (22–62)	MRD	BM	HM	CY+ATG±TI	CSP	24	29	NA	OS: 52% DFS: 33% Median F/U: 445 days
Seattle [55]	253	54 (18–73)	MRD	PBHC	HM	200 cGY TBI±F	MMF+CSP	5	46	41	2-yr OS: TBI: 55% F/TBI: 39% Auto/Allo: 66%

Study	N	Age	Donor	Source	Disease	Conditioning	GVHD prophylaxis				Outcomes
London [56]	44	41 (18–56)	MRD MURD	PBHC BM	HM	F+M +Campath	CSP±MTX	2	5	2	OS: 82% PFS: 75% Median F/U: 270 days
Boston [57]	5	30 (20–51)	Haplo	BM	NHL	CY+ATG±TI	CSP	0	100	NA	OS: 40% DFS: 20% Median F/U: 103 days
Jerusalem [58]	16	17 (8–48)	MURD	BM	HM	F+B+ATG	CSP	0	44	0	3-yr OS: 75% 3-yr DFS: 60%
Dresden [59]	42	47 (16–65)	MURD MMURD	PBHC BM	HM	F+B+ATG	CSP+MMF CSP±MTX	21	26	38	OS: 36% DFS: 26% Median F/U: 390 days
London [60]	47	44 (18–62)	MURD MMURD	BM	HM	F+M +Campath	CSP	4	21	6	1-yr OS: 75.5% 1-yr PFS: 61.5%
Leipzig [61]	52	48 (6–65)	MURD MMURD	BM PBHC	HM	200 cGy TBI+F	CSP+MMF	12	63	25	OS: 35% DFS: 25% Median F/U: 570 days
Seattle [62]	89	53 (4–69)	MURD	BM PBHC	HM	200 cGy TBI+F	CSP+MMF	21	52	37	1-yr OS: PBHC: 57%; BM: 33% 1-yr PFS: PBHC: 44%; BM: 17%

A, ara-C; AML, acute myelogenous leukemia; ATG, antithymocyte globulin; B, busulfan; BM, bone marrow; C, cisplatin; Campath, alemtuzumab; 2-CDA, cladribine; CLL, chronic lymphocytic leukemia; CSP, cyclosporine; CY, cyclophosphamide; DFS, disease-free survival; F, fludarabine; F/U, follow-up; GD, genetic diseases; Haplo, haploidentical related donor; HM, hematologic malignancies; I, idarubicin; L, lymphoma; M, melphalan; MDS, myelodysplastic syndrome; MMURD, mismatched unrelated donor; MRD, matched related donor; MTX, methotrexate; MURD, matched unrelated donor; NA, not available; NHL, non-Hodgkin's lymphoma; NRM, nonrelapse mortality; OS, overall survival; PBHC, peripheral blood hematopoietic cells; PFS, progression-free survival; RD, related donor; ST, solid tumors; T, tacrolimus; TBI, total body irradiation; TI, thymic irradiation.

*Graft-vs.-host disease before donor lymphocyte infusion.

complications included cyclophosphamide-induced cardiac toxicity. One patient died from transplant complications and one patient died from GVHD after two prophylactic DLIs. Overall, 11 of 21 patients survived; four had continued complete responses with a median follow-up of 14.6 months. In an attempt to reduce the incidence of GVHD, Campath MAB was added to fludarabine and melphalan conditioning, in recipients of both HLA-matched sibling and unrelated donor grafts [56]. Forty-two of 43 evaluable patients had sustained engraftment. Eighteen of 31 patients studied were full donor chimeras, while 13 patients were mixed chimeras. The regimen prevented grade III–IV acute GVHD, and only two patients developed grade II GVHD. At a median follow-up of 9 months, 33 of the 44 patients remained alive either in complete remission or without disease progression.

While the chemotherapy-based reduced-intensity and nonmyeloablative regimens had significantly less toxicities as compared to conventional high-dose allogeneic HCT, patients still experienced significant cytopenias, and most required hospitalizations of a duration that was similar to that of conventional transplants.

In order to further reduce the regimen-related toxicities and thereby perform allogeneic HCT in the outpatient setting, the low-dose (200 cGy) TBI conditioning regimen developed in the dog model was evaluated in a multi-institutional clinical study [55,63]. TBI of 200 cGy was given as a single fraction on day 0, with post-grafting immunosuppression of CSP (6.25 mg/kg given orally twice a day from day –1 to day 35) and MMF (15 mg/kg given orally twice a day from day 0 to 27). G-CSF mobilized PBHC collected over 2 days from HLA-identical related donors were used as a source of stem cells. Trial eligibility criteria required patients to be either too old to be eligible for a "conventional" transplant, or, if younger, to have significant medical contraindications to "conventional" HCT. Overall, the HCT regimen was well-tolerated with the majority of eligible patients having their transplants in the outpatient clinic setting. Most patients did not develop severe neutropenia or thrombocytopenia (Fig. 85.2). While all patients had initial donor engraftment, nine (20%) of the first 45 patients experienced graft rejection between 2 and 4 months after transplant that coincided with discontinuation of the MMF/CSP immunosuppression [63]. Lack of intensive preceding chemotherapy before HCT predicted rejections, and rejecting patients had low-level donor T-cell chimerism on day 28. The rejections were nonfatal, and all patients had autologous reconstitution of peripheral blood counts. To prevent graft rejection, the conditioning regimen was modified by adding 30 mg/m^2/day fludarabine on days –4, –3 and –2 to the 200 cGy TBI. Additionally, CSP administration was prolonged through day 56 with a subsequent taper because some patients developed GVHD after CSP was discontinued on day 35.

A recent update summarized the results of 253 patients with hematologic malignancies (inclusive of the first 45 patients), with a median age of 54 years, who received PBHC transplants from HLA-matched related donors [55]. Of the 253 patients, 58 were conditioned with 200 cGy TBI only, 118 were given fludarabine in addition to the TBI, while 77 patients, all with advanced non-Hodgkin's lymphoma (NHL) or multiple myeloma, received cytoreductive autografts before the nonmyeloablative allografts (auto/allo). The median percentages of donor T-cell chimerisms on days 28, 56 and 84 were significantly higher in both the fludarabine/TBI and the auto/allo patients, as compared to the group of patients given TBI only ($p \leq 0.005$ for TBI vs. fludarabine/TBI and TBI vs. auto/allo). Figure 85.3 illustrates the donor chimerism in marrow and peripheral blood T cells and granulocytes in the overall group of patients. Additionally, the incidences of graft rejection were significantly lower in the fludarabine/TBI (3%) and auto/allo (0%) groups compared to patients given 200 cGy TBI alone (17%) ($p = 0.001$ and 0.0001, respectively). Grades II, III and IV acute GVHD occurred in 31%, 10% and 5% of engrafted patients, respectively, with no statistically significant differences among patients

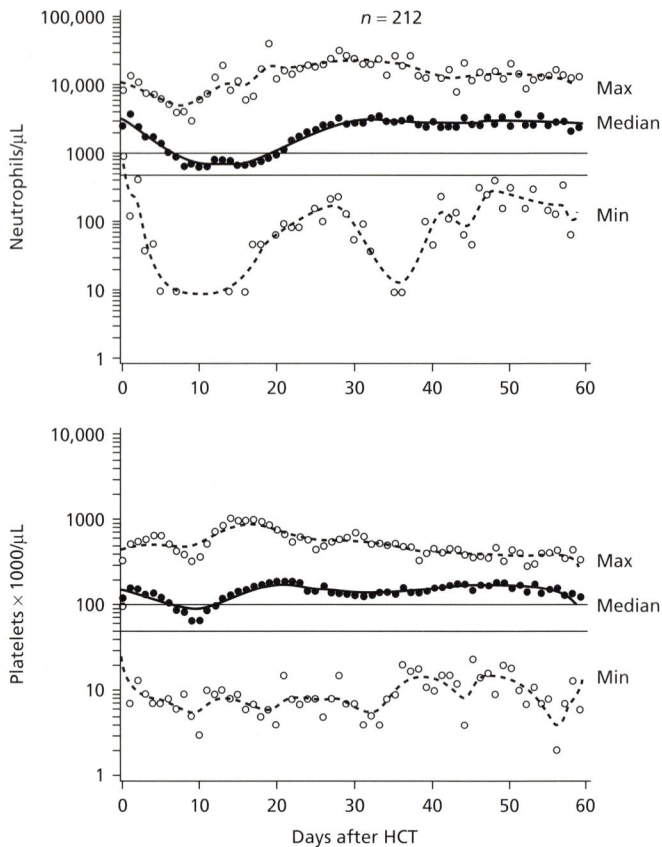

Fig. 85.2 Neutrophil and platelet changes among 212 patients given 200 cGy total body irradiation (TBI) ± fludarabine before and mycophenolate mofetil/cyclosporine (MMF/CSP) after human leukocyte antigen (HLA) matched related hematopoietic cell transplantation (HCT) (From [64]. Reprinted with permission of the American Society of Clinical Oncology.)

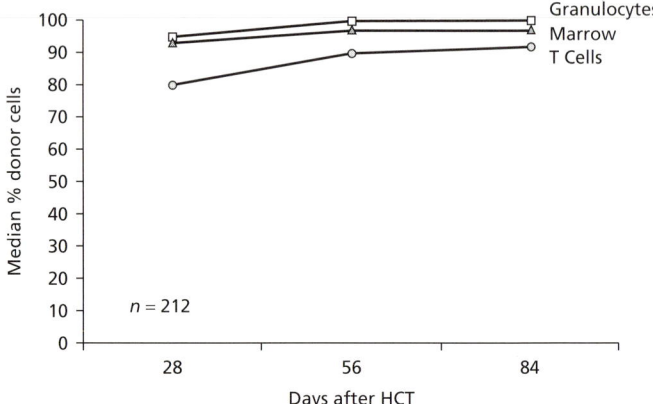

Fig. 85.3 Donor chimerism results in patients given 200 cGy TBI ± fludarabine before and MMF/CSP after HLA-matched related HCT (From [64]. Reprinted with permission of the American Society of Clinical Oncology.)

in the three groups (Fig. 85.4). The 100-day mortality was 9%, with 5% of patients dying from disease progression and 4% from nonrelapse causes. The 2-year overall survival rates were TBI 55%, fludarabine/TBI 39% and auto/allo 66%. Remissions have been seen in virtually all disease categories including molecular remissions. Remissions occurred slowly over time periods ranging from 3 to 24 months. Figures 85.5 and 85.6 show examples of molecular remissions in patients with CLL and CML, respectively, which took 6–7 months to be complete.

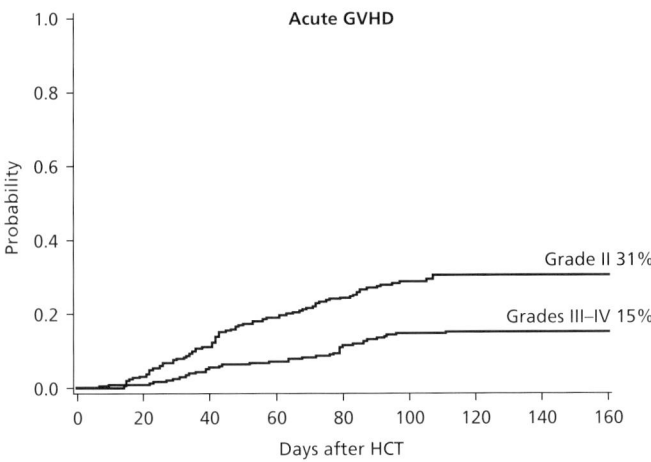

Fig. 85.4 Acute graft-vs.-host disease (GVHD) in the first 253 patients given 200 cGy TBI ± fludarabine before and MMF/CSP after HLA-matched related HCT.

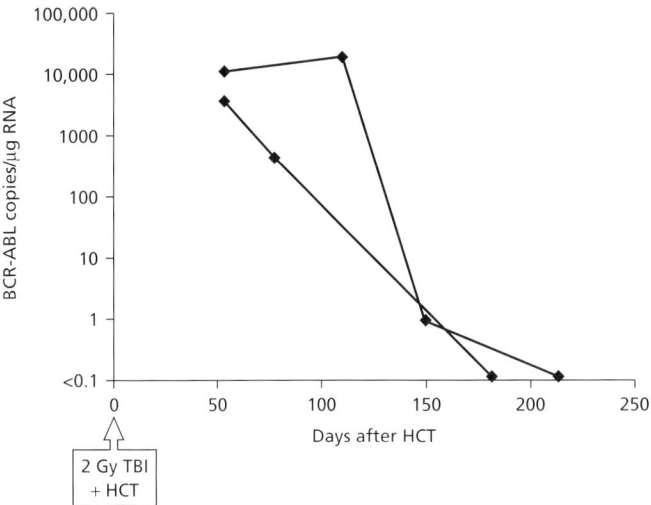

Fig. 85.6 Examples of declines in *bcr/abl* RNA levels in two patients with CML (From [47]. Copyright the American Society of Hematology, used by permission.)

A retrospective analysis was carried out comparing the GVHD incidence in recipients of nonmyeloablative vs. "conventional" myeloablative conditioning. The cumulative incidence of grades II–IV acute GVHD was lower in nonmyeloablative HCT (64% vs. 85%; $p = 0.001$), resulting in the use of fewer systemic immunosuppressants during the first 3 months after transplant [65]. In another retrospective cohort study, recipients of nonmyeloablative conditioning had significantly reduced transfusion requirements compared to conventional HCT recipients with only 23% of the patients requiring platelet transfusions and 63% requiring red blood cell transfusions ($p \leq 0.0001$ as compared to conventional HCT recipients). Patients who received nonmyeloablative HCT had significantly fewer numbers of platelet and red blood cell transfusions ($p \leq 0.0001$) [66].

Recipients of nonmyeloablative conditioning had shorter periods of neutropenia than recipients of myeloablative conditioning ($p < 0.0001$), and this was associated with fewer episodes of bacteremia during the first 30 days ($p = 0.01$) [67]. Similarly, there was a trend to less cytomegalovirus (CMV) antigenemia, viremia and disease in nonmyeloablative HCT recipients as compared to recipients of myeloablative conditioning with a significant reduction when more serious manifestations (CMV viremia and disease) were combined during the first 100 days ($p = 0.01$) [68]. The cumulative incidence of proven or probable invasive mold infections (IMI) in the first year after nonmyeloablative HCT was 15%, which was similar to myeloablative recipients [67,69]. Severe acute GVHD and CMV disease were the primary risk factors associated with IMI after nonmyeloablative conditioning, with high-dose corticosteroid therapy at IMI diagnosis being associated with an increased risk for IMI-related death. The incidence of idiopathic pneumonia syndrome was significantly lower following nonmyeloablative conditioning compared to "conventional" conditioning regimens (2.2% vs. 8.4%; $p = 0.003$) [70].

HLA-mismatched related and HLA-matched and mismatched unrelated donor allografting

In a report by Sykes *et al.* [57], five patients with refractory NHL underwent marrow transplantation from HLA-haploidentical related donors, sharing at least one HLA-A, -B or -DR allele on the mismatched haplotypes after conditioning with high-dose cyclophosphamide, 700 cGy thymic irradiation and ATG. Four evaluable patients showed engraftment with predominantly donor lymphoid cells and varying degrees of myeloid donor chimerism. All five patients developed grades II–III acute GVHD, with three patients dying between days 12 and 108 from pulmonary hemorrhage, progressive lymphoma and aspergillosis. At the time of the report, one patient was alive at day 103 with partial response, and one was alive at day 416 in continuous complete remission.

Nagler *et al.* [58] reported on the results of HLA-matched unrelated marrow transplantation following conditioning with fludarabine and

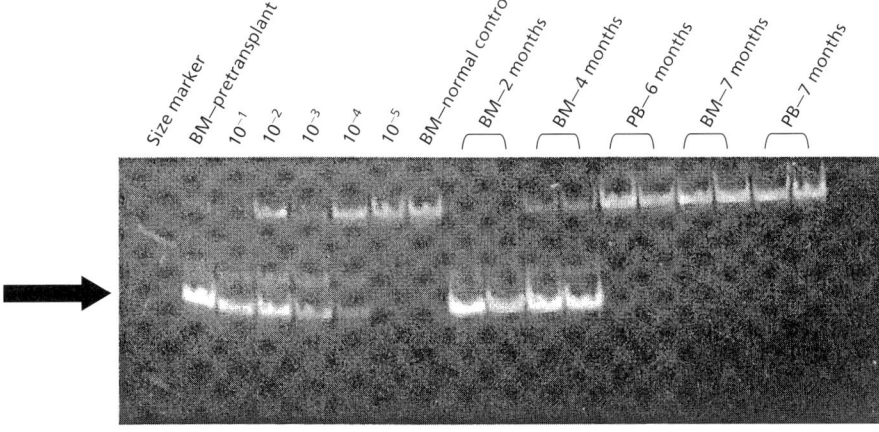

Fig. 85.5 Polymerase chain reaction to detect tumor-specific immunoglobulin H (IgH) rearrangements in a patient with chronic lymphocytic leukemia (CLL) (From [63]. Copyright American Society of Hematology, used by permission.)

busulfan (8 mg/kg) and ATG. Fifteen of 16 patients achieved 100% donor chimerism, and one patient became a mixed chimera. Seven patients developed grades II–IV acute GVHD, with one patient dying from complications related to acute GVHD. The overall and disease-free survival estimates at 36 months were 75% and 60%, respectively, with this reduced-intensity conditioning regimen in a relatively young population of patients (median age 17; range 8–48 years). Using a similar regimen of fludarabine, busulfan and ATG, Bornhauser et al. [59] treated 42 patients with hematologic malignancies with HLA-matched or single HLA-antigen mismatched unrelated donor grafts. In this older population group (median 47 years; range 16–65 years), the disease-free survival was 64% for patients with lymphoid malignancies, 38% for patients with standard-risk leukemias and 14% for patients with high-risk diseases. Nine patients (21%) had either primary or secondary graft failures. In patients with stable engraftment, the probability of acute GVHD grades II–IV was 32%, with one patient dying from grade IV GVHD. In a similarly aged group of patients with hematologic malignancies using a different conditioning regimen consisting of Campath MAB, fludarabine and melphalan [60], 47 patients received HLA-matched or mismatched unrelated donor transplants. Primary graft failure occurred in two patients, and three patients developed grades III–IV acute GVHD. The overall and progression-free survivals at 1 year were 75.5% and 61.5%, respectively.

Using the low-dose TBI (200 cGy) and fludarabine conditioning regimen, Niederwieser et al. [61] reported on 52 patients (median age 48; range 6–65 years) with advanced hematologic malignancies given unrelated grafts. Seventy-one percent were HLA-matched at the antigen (serologic) level and 29% were one HLA antigen mismatched. Additionally, 15 patients had allele level mismatches for class I HLA antigens. Durable donor engraftment was attained in 88% of patients. Grades II–IV acute GVHD occurred in 63% of patients, with 9% of patients having fatal GVHD. With a median follow-up of 19 months, 35% of the patients were alive and 25% were in remissions of their underlying malignancies. In a subsequent study, Maris et al. [62] reported on 89 patients with unrelated grafts. Early data on 22 of the patients were included in the report by Niederwieser et al. [61]. Eligibility criteria for this trial included serological matching for HLA-A, -B and -C, and allele level matching for HLA-DRB1 and HLA-DQB1. The median patient age was 53 years (range 5–69 years). While the preferred source of stem cells was PBHC, these were available in only 71 patients while 18 patients received marrow. Initial donor T-cell engraftment was documented in 89% of patients, with median donor T-cell chimerisms on days 28, 56 and 84 being higher in PBHC recipients than marrow recipients ($p = 0.02, 0.01$ and 0.08, respectively). The peripheral blood granulocyte and marrow donor chimerism values were not significantly different between the two groups of recipients at the various time points. Sustained donor engraftment occurred in 79% of patients. By multivariate analysis, graft rejection was more frequent in marrow recipients ($p = 0.003$) and in patients without preceding chemotherapy ($p = 0.003$). Donor T-cell chimerism values <50% on day 28 were highly associated with eventual graft rejection ($p = 0.001$). Preceding conventional HCT or preceding chemotherapy reduced the risk of rejection, presumably because the prior cytotoxic therapy increased pretransplant immunosuppression of the host. Of the 85 patient–donor pairs with complete 10/10 HLA antigen sequencing, HLA class I allele level mismatch (16 of 85 pairs) was associated with a trend towards increased risk of graft rejection ($p = 0.13$). With a median follow-up of 13 months (range 0.6–28 months), the cumulative probabilities of transplant-related mortality were 11% at 100 days and 16% at 1 year, respectively. The Kaplan–Meier estimates for 1-year survival were 57% vs. 33%, and for progression-free survival were 44% vs. 17% for recipients of PBHC vs. marrow, respectively. A high degree of day 28 CD3 chimerism (>50%) was associated with less relapse ($p = 0.05$) and a trend towards improved progression-free survival ($p = 0.10$). By multivariate analysis,

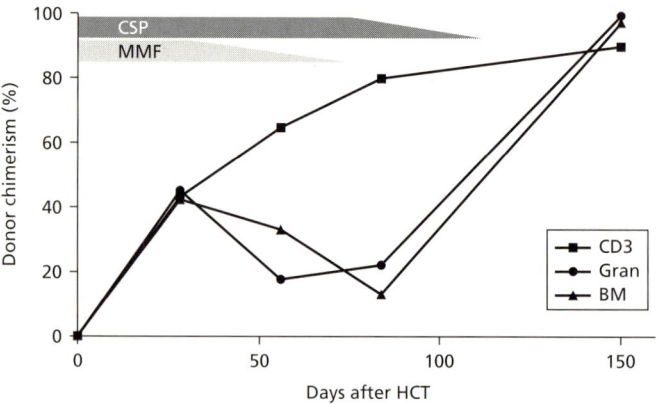

Fig. 85.7 Donor chimerism (fluorescence *in situ* hybridization, FISH) in a patient with Philadelphia (Ph1) negative myeloproliferative disorder after unrelated donor (URD) HCT.

better survival was conferred to patients with low-risk diseases ($p = 0.04$), with no prior transfusions ($p = 0.003$) with <5% blast cells in the marrow before HCT ($p = 0.002$), HCT from female donor ($p = 0.01$) and with CD3$^+$ cell dose greater than or equal to the median ($p = 0.0006$). Better progression-free survival was identified in a multivariate analysis in patients with <5% blasts in the marrow prior to HCT ($p = 0.0001$) and those who received PBHC as a hematopoietic stem cell source ($p = 0.006$).

Figure 85.7 illustrates the donor chimerism changes in a 67-year-old patient with Philadelphia chromosome (Ph1) negative myeloproliferative disorder whose disease was characterized by high white blood cell counts, very high platelet counts (>1 million/μL) and high basophil counts. The patient's T-cell chimerism increased to 80% by day 84 whereas the marrow and granulocyte donor chimerism declined from 40% to 45% on day 28 to 10% in the marrow on day 84. Clinically, the patient's platelet and basophil counts increased to 900,000/μL and 1500/μL, respectively, consistent with disease progression after an initial response. CSP was rapidly tapered to induce a GVT response. The marrow and granulocyte donor chimerism rose to nearly 100% by day 150, and both basophilia and thrombocytosis resolved. The patient also developed mild signs of chronic GVHD which responded to CSP. The patient is surviving close to 3 years after HCT with complete donor engraftment and no evidence of recurrent myeloproliferative disorder. This clinical case illustrates the relationship between post-grafting immunosuppression, GVHD and GVT effects. It also emphasizes the importance of lineage-specific chimerism evaluations in monitoring patients.

The study suggested that PBHC was the preferred source of grafted hematopoietic cells in unrelated transplantation with this low-dose conditioning regimen. Given the importance of post-grafting immunosuppression to both facilitate engraftment and reduce the risk of GVHD, our attention was drawn to another finding of the study, the short (3.5 h) serum half-life of the active metabolite of MMF, mycophenolic acid. This finding resulted in a modification of the post-transplant immunosuppression, an increase in the dosage of MMF to three times daily in the hope of minimizing the risk of late graft rejections. Early results with this dose modification have been promising.

Nonmyeloablative allografting after failed conventional transplants

Use of conventional high-dose conditioning for allografts following failed autologous or allogeneic HCT has resulted in a poor outcome in adult patients, primarily related to early fatal regimen-related toxicities [71]. A number of investigators have therefore evaluated reduced-intensity regimens to condition patients for second HCT. Investigators in Jerusalem conditioned patients with fludarabine, busulfan and ATG, and they received CSP as GVHD prophylaxis [72]. Among 12 patients transplanted (median age 33 years; range 8–63 years), only one nonrelapse death occurred and six patients were disease-free with a median follow-up of 23 months. Actuarial overall and disease-free survivals were 56% and 50%, respectively, at 34 months. Investigators at Massachusetts General Hospital described their results with 13 patients who relapsed following autologous HCT and received HLA-matched related donor allografts following conditioning with cyclophosphamide and ATG with or without thymic irradiation [73]. DLI was administered at 5–6 weeks post-transplant to facilitate full donor chimerism. Only one nonrelapse death occurred and 2-year estimates of overall and disease-free survivals were 45% and 38%, respectively.

Investigators at City of Hope Cancer Center described their results in 28 patients who failed a previous autologous transplant or developed MDS after autografts [74]. The median interval from the failed autologous HCT and allogeneic HCT was 15 months. The median age of the patients was 47 years and patients were treated with either fludarabine *plus* melphalan ($n = 24$) or fludarabine *plus* 200 cGy TBI ($n = 4$). Patients received HCT from either HLA-matched related ($n = 14$) or unrelated ($n = 14$) donors. The day 100 mortality and nonrelapse mortality were 25% and 21%, respectively. With a median follow-up of 16 months, 46% of the patients were alive and in complete remission.

Using the 200 cGy TBI-based regimen (with or without fludarabine), 48 patients who failed conventional autologous ($n = 43$), allogeneic ($n = 4$) or syngeneic ($n = 1$) HCT subsequently received HLA-matched related ($n = 29$) or unrelated ($n = 19$) donor allografts [75]. Patients received the nonmyeloablative HCT a median of 22 months (range 4–26 months) from conventional HCT. The day 100 nonrelapse mortality was 6%, and overall nonrelapse mortality was 15% with a median follow-up of 8.4 months (range 0.6–31.5 months). The Kaplan–Meier estimates of overall survival, progression-free survival and nonrelapse mortality were 52%, 30% and 13%, respectively. In NHL patients, who have particularly poor outcomes with second conventional HCT, the Kaplan–Meier estimate of overall survival was 58% at 1 year, with a transplant-related mortality of 23%, primarily as a result of multiorgan failure, infection and/or GVHD.

Nonmalignant disorders

The rationale for developing nontoxic nonmyeloablative regimens for HCT in patients with nonmalignant disorders includes the risk for short-term and long-term toxicities and even mortality resulting from myeloablative regimens. Thus, "conventional" HCT has been reserved for treatment of life-threatening disorders. The transplant procedure often will be delayed until the development of significant disease complications in order to avoid a high-risk procedure in less-affected patients. Furthermore, the long-term side-effects associated with conventional regimens, including infertility, hormonal dysfunction, growth failure and secondary malignancies, deter patients and families from seeking a curative treatment early in the disease course.

The potential for reversal of disease symptoms with partial chimerism has been demonstrated in a number of studies [76–78]. Persistent and stable mixed chimerism has been reported after conventional HCT, and has been associated with full or partial correction of disease manifestations. Effectiveness of partial chimerism also can be inferred from studies of carriers of X-linked disorders, in which women rarely have symptomatic disease even when Lyonization results in low numbers of unaffected cells.

Immunodeficiency disorders

"Conventional" HCT for treatment of severe combined immunodeficiency (SCID) using HLA-matched sibling donors has generally not required the need for conditioning regimens, given the patients' profound underlying immunodeficiencies (see Chapter 105). Patients with less profound immunodeficiency are able to generate alloreactive responses to donor cells; therefore, the "conventional" approach has been to employ intensive conditioning regimens to prevent graft rejection. Recently, several studies have been initiated to examine the efficacy of establishing mixed chimerism using reduced-intensity or minimal-toxicity regimens. Theoretically, achievement of partial donor chimerism in the appropriate cell lineages should be sufficient to reverse most immunodeficiency syndromes. A reduced-intensity regimen investigated by Amrolia *et al.* [79] used fludarabine, melphalan and antilymphocyte globulin for two SCID patients and six patients with other immunodeficiencies, given transplants from HLA-matched related or unrelated donors. Severe hepatotoxicity was observed in three patients, which was not surprising given that five of eight patients had antecedent liver disease (sclerosing cholangitis, chronic hepatitis B). The regimen established donor chimerism in all patients, which correlated with improvement of T-cell number and function in all evaluable patients. Seven of eight patients are reportedly surviving 8–17 months after HCT. Horwitz *et al.* [80] investigated the ability of a reduced-intensity regimen to establish T-cell-depleted HLA-matched related allografts in patients with chronic granulomatous disease (CGD). Ten patients were conditioned with cyclophosphamide, fludarabine and ATG, and given HLA-matched related PBHC that were T-cell depleted and contained approximately 1×10^5 CD3$^+$ cells/kg of recipient weight. In order to improve the level of donor chimerism, patients received subsequently planned infusions of donor lymphocytes. Eight of 10 patients developed donor chimerism in neutrophils ranging between 33% and 100%, and two patients rejected their grafts. Three patients developed grades II–IV acute GVHD, all occurring in adult patients. Seven patients remained alive with a median follow-up of 17 months.

The Seattle group has studied a minimal-toxicity regimen in severely ill patients with SCID ($n = 2$) and other immunodeficiency syndromes ($n = 7$) who were given HLA-matched related or unrelated marrow grafts [81,82]. One SCID and one non-SCID patient received only post-transplant MMF and CSP, while the remaining patients were given 200 cGy TBI with or without fludarabine depending on the extent of T-cell dysfunction. Five patients developed grades II–III acute GVHD, and four patients developed extensive chronic GVHD. Donor chimerism was established in all patients and ranged from 5% to 100% donor in T cells, B cells and granulocytes. Evidence for both T- and B-cell reconstitution was shown for six of seven evaluable patients including an X-SCID patient with donor B-cell engraftment following an unrelated graft. Among patients with >6 months of follow-up, five of seven have survived with stable donor chimerism ranging from 1 to 5 years after transplant. Together, these studies demonstrated the potential for achieving effective levels of donor chimerism with less toxic regimens in severely ill patients with life-threatening immunodeficiency disorders.

Congenital bone marrow failure syndromes

The development of effective HCT regimens for treatment of Fanconi anemia exemplifies the evolution of the nonmyeloablative approach (see Chapter 109). In the 1970s and 1980s, an unusually high degree of toxic deaths were observed to be associated with conventional intensive conditioning regimens. Subsequent studies demonstrated that engraftment could be achieved with successively lower doses of cyclophosphamide alone without the need for irradiation. The minimal dose of cyclophosphamide required for engraftment has been examined in a dose-reduction study by the Curitiba and Seattle groups. At a total dose of 80 mg/kg cyclophosphamide, engraftment was achieved in seven of seven treated patients, and six of seven survived long-term. The preliminary results using 60 mg/kg appear equally promising [83]. Unfortunately, it has been more difficult to develop a lower toxicity regimen for transplantation of cells from alternative donors. Studies of lower doses of TBI combined with lower doses of cyclophosphamide have not demonstrated an equivalently high rate of survival for patients receiving unrelated donor grafts. More recently, reduced-intensity regimens that have incorporated fludarabine have shown early promise. Boulad et al. [84] report the combination of fludarabine with cyclophosphamide with and without 450 cGy TBI for conditioning prior to transplantation of haploidentical CD34+ selected PBHC in two patients, respectively, which resulted in donor engraftment and survival >1 year. Kurre et al. [85] reported successful engraftment of HLA-matched unrelated PBHC and long-term survival in patients with Fanconi anemia conditioned with 200 cGy TBI and given MMF/CSP after HCT.

Patients with Shwachman–Diamond syndrome (SDS) are also at relatively high risk for mortality with conventional HCT. The Seattle consortium has used the fludarabine/low-dose TBI regimen to treat one patient with SDS who received HLA-matched related PBHC with promising results. High-level donor chimerism was achieved without significant toxicity, and the patient has survived >1 year following HCT [85].

Metabolic storage disorders

"Conventional" marrow transplantation has been shown to achieve favorable long-term outcomes with continuing cognitive development among other physiologic improvements in certain lysosomal acid hydrolase deficiencies and leukodystrophies (see Chapter 107) [86,87]. None the less, there has been significant mortality associated with "conventional" HCT, particularly following transplantation of unrelated donor grafts. While there is great potential to reduce mortality, establishment of normal enzyme levels is likely to be more challenging in these disorders using reduced-intensity or nonmyeloablative regimens, given that significant rates of graft failure have been reported even with conventional regimens. Recently, Slavin et al. [51] reported 100% donor chimerism without GVHD using fludarabine, busulfan and ATG for treatment of Gaucher's syndrome. The Seattle consortium has studied fludarabine and 200 cGy TBI in two patients with Hurler syndrome and one patient with metachromic leukodystrophy given PBHC from unrelated donors. One patient rejected the graft and achieved full chimerism following a second transplant with a conventional regimen, and two achieved partial or full chimerism and normal enzyme levels.

Sickle cell diseases and thalassemia

"Conventional" HCT using HLA-matched related marrow grafts for treatment of severe sickle cell disease has resulted in long-term overall survival of >90% (see Chapter 104) [88]. Similar results have been obtained for good-risk patients with thalassemia [89]. The rationale for studying nonmyeloablative transplantation is based on reports of disease amelioration with stable mixed chimerism observed occasionally following "conventional" transplantation, a finding which suggested a biologic advantage for normal erythroid cells in these settings [78]. Furthermore, while the results of "conventional" transplant regimens have been excellent, the long-term complications related to busulfan, particularly female infertility, have decreased enthusiasm for myeloablative regimens. However, these patients pose a particular challenge for developing a successful nonmyeloablative regimen, as most have been alloimmunized through multiple blood product transfusions and therefore are likely to be at greater risk for graft rejection. Several groups of investigators have studied reduced-intensity regimens that employed fludarabine, busulfan and ATG, with or without total lymphoid irradiation. Results have been encouraging; however, late effects have as yet not been assessed [78]. Studies of minimal-toxicity regimens that have the potential of avoiding late effects have been disappointing thus far. These regimens have resulted in transient donor engraftment and disease amelioration of 6–18 months' duration. Given the excellent results with "conventional" HCT in patients with hemoglobinopathies, nonmyeloablative HCT should be reserved for patients with risk factors for higher mortality given the anecdotal information indicating that stable long-term engraftment has been difficult to achieve.

Conclusions

The use of reduced-intensity or minimally myelosuppressive preparative regimens has resulted in durable donor engraftment, and the development of GVT effects in the setting of underlying malignant diseases. The regimens have been relatively nontoxic in older patients and have been successfully applied to younger patients with comorbid conditions that precluded them from receiving conventional high-dose HCT. The optimal regimen may ultimately be defined by the nature of the disease being treated. In aggressive lymphomas, acute leukemias not in remission or other fast-growing malignancies, cytoreduction by either preceding chemotherapy or by a reduced-intensity regimen with disease-specific chemotherapy may be necessary to allow time for adequate GVT responses to develop. For low-grade lymphomas, acute leukemias in first complete remission, chronic leukemias and other more indolent diseases, truly nonmyeloablative regimens may be sufficient, allowing the donor T cells to generate sufficient GVT responses to eradicate the underlying malignancies. In nonmalignant diseases, mixed chimerism may be sufficient to correct disease manifestations while conversion to full donor chimerism is required for most malignant conditions. The role of DLI for the achievement of full donor chimerism and specific GVT effects needs to be explored, and current ongoing research is aimed toward those goals (see Chapter 29).

Other current issues include minimizing GVHD, which may result in prolonged immunosuppression, thereby placing patients at risk for infections that, in turn, contribute significantly to nonrelapse mortality in all regimens. Additionally, prolonged immunosuppression may blunt optimal GVT effects. Ultimately, nonmyeloablative HCT may be used to establish mixed donor–host chimerism that can serve as a platform for adoptive immunotherapy with infusion of tumor-specific cytotoxic T cells which would exert GVT effects without causing GVHD.

In the future, nonmyeloablative transplants may become the procedure of choice also for younger patients with either malignant or nonmalignant diseases. Towards that end, phase 3 studies are needed to determine both immediate- and long-term outcomes in different disease categories and age groups.

References

1 Weiden PL, Flournoy N, Thomas ED et al. Antileukemic effect of graft-versus-host disease in human recipients of allogeneic-marrow grafts. *N Engl J Med* 1979; **300**: 1068–73.

2 Weiden PL, Sullivan KM, Flournoy N, Storb R, Thomas ED and the Seattle Marrow Transplant Team. Antileukemic effect of chronic graft-versus-host disease: contribution to improved survival after allogeneic marrow transplantation. *N Engl J Med* 1981; **304**: 1529–33.

3 Sullivan KM, Fefer A, Witherspoon R et al. Graft-versus-leukemia in man: relationship of acute and chronic graft-versus-host disease to relapse of acute leukemia following allogeneic bone marrow transplantation. In: Truitt RL, Gale RP, Bortin MM, eds. *Cellular Immunotherapy of Cancer*. New York: Alan R. Liss, 1987: 391–9.

4 Sullivan KM, Weiden PL, Storb R et al. Influence of acute and chronic graft-versus-host disease on relapse and survival after bone marrow transplantation from HLA-identical siblings as treatment of acute and chronic leukemia. *Blood* 1989; **73**: 1720–8.

5 Ringden O, Horowitz MM. Graft-versus-leukemia reactions in humans. *Transplant Proc* 1989; **21**: 2989–92.

6 Horowitz MM, Gale RP, Sondel PM *et al*. Graft-versus-leukemia reactions after bone marrow transplantation. *Blood* 1990; **75**: 555–62.

7 Zittoun RA, Mandelli F, Willemze R *et al*. Autologous or allogeneic bone marrow transplantation compared with intensive chemotherapy in acute myelogenous leukemia. *N Engl J Med* 1995; **332**: 217–23.

8 Gorin NC, Labopin M, Fouillard L *et al*. Retrospective evaluation of autologous bone marrow transplantation vs allogeneic bone marrow transplantation from an HLA identical related donor in acute myelocytic leukemia. *Bone Marrow Transplant* 1996; **18**: 111–7.

9 Fefer A, Sullivan KM, Weiden P *et al*. Graft versus leukemia effect in man: the relapse rate of acute leukemia is lower after allogeneic than after syngeneic marrow transplantation. In: Truitt RL, Gale RP, Bortin MM, eds. *Cellular Immunotherapy of Cancer*. New York: Alan R. Liss, 1987: 401–8.

10 Drobyski WR, Keever CA, Roth MS *et al*. Salvage immunotherapy using donor leukocyte infusions as treatment for relapsed chronic myelogenous leukemia after allogeneic bone marrow transplantation: efficacy and toxicity of a defined T-cell dose. *Blood* 1993; **82**: 2310–8.

11 van Rhee F, Lin F, Cullis JO *et al*. Relapse of chronic myeloid leukemia after allogeneic bone marrow transplant: the case for giving donor leukocyte transfusions before the onset of hematologic relapse. *Blood* 1994; **83**: 3377–83.

12 Porter DL, Roth MS, McGarigle C, Ferrara JLM, Antin JH. Induction of graft-versus-host disease as immunotherapy for relapsed chronic myeloid leukemia. *N Engl J Med* 1994; **330**: 100–6.

13 Kolb HJ, Schattenberg A, Goldman JM *et al*. Graft-versus-leukemia effect of donor lymphocyte transfusions in marrow grafted patients. European Group for Blood and Marrow Transplantation Working Party Chronic Leukemia. *Blood* 1995; **86**: 2041–50.

14 Mackinnon S, Papadopoulos EB, Carabasi MH *et al*. Adoptive immunotherapy evaluating escalating doses of donor leukocytes for relapse of chronic myeloid leukemia after bone marrow transplantation: separation of graft-versus-leukemia responses from graft-versus-host disease. *Blood* 1995; **86**: 1261–8.

15 Collins RH Jr, Shpilberg O, Drobyski WR *et al*. Donor leukocyte infusions in 140 patients with relapsed malignancy after allogeneic bone marrow transplantation. *J Clin Oncol* 1997; **15**: 433–44.

16 Cobbold SP, Martin G, Qin S, Waldmann H. Monoclonal antibodies to promote marrow engraftment and tissue graft tolerance. *Nature* 1986; **323**: 164–6.

17 Li H, Kaufman CL, Boggs SS, Johnson PC, Patrene KD, Ildstad ST. Mixed allogeneic chimerism induced by a sublethal approach prevents autoimmune diabetes and reverses insulitis in nonobese diabetic (NOD) mice. *J Immunol* 1996; **156**: 380–8.

18 Colson YL, Li H, Boggs SS, Patrene KD, Johnson PC, Ildstad ST. Durable mixed allogeneic chimerism and tolerance by a nonlethal radiation-based cytoreductive approach. *J Immunol* 1996; **157**: 2820–9.

19 Colson YL, Wren SM, Schuchert MJ *et al*. A nonlethal conditioning approach to achieve durable multilineage mixed chimerism and tolerance across major, minor, and hematopoietic histocompatibility barriers. *J Immunol* 1995; **155**: 4179–88.

20 Sharabi Y, Abraham VS, Sykes M, Sachs DH. Mixed allogeneic chimeras prepared by a non-myeloablative regimen: requirement for chimerism to maintain tolerance. *Bone Marrow Transplant* 1992; **9**: 191–7.

21 Tomita Y, Sachs DH, Khan A, Sykes M. Additional monoclonal antibody (mAB) injections can replace thymic irradiation to allow induction of mixed chimerism and tolerance in mice receiving bone marrow transplantation after conditioning with anti-T cell mABs and 3-Gy whole body irradiation. *Transplantation* 1996; **61**: 469–77.

22 Tomita Y, Khan A, Sykes M. Mechanism by which additional monoclonal antibody (mAB) injections overcome the requirement for thymic irradiation to achieve mixed chimerism in mice receiving bone marrow transplantation after conditioning with anti-T cell mABs and 3-Gy whole body irradiation. *Transplantation* 1996; **61**: 477–85.

23 Sykes M, Szot GL, Swenson KA, Pearson DA. Induction of high levels of allogeneic hematopoietic reconstitution and donor-specific tolerance without myelosuppressive conditioning. *Nat Med* 1997; **3**: 783–7.

24 Lee LA, Sergio JJ, Sykes M. Natural killer cells weakly resist engraftment of allogeneic, long-term, multilineage-repopulating hematopoietic stem cells. *Transplantation* 1996; **61**: 125–32.

25 Wekerle T, Sayegh MH, Ito H *et al*. Anti-CD154 or CTLA4Ig obviates the need for thymic irradiation in a non-myeloablative conditioning regimen for the induction of mixed hematopoietic chimerism and tolerance. *Transplantation* 1999; **68**: 1348–55.

26 Wekerle T, Sayegh MH, Hill J *et al*. Extrathymic T-cell deletion and allogeneic stem cell engraftment induced with costimulatory blockade is followed by central T cell tolerance. *J Exp Med* 1998; **187**: 2037–44.

27 Koch U, Korngold R. A synthetic CD4-CDR3 peptide analog enhances bone marrow engraftment across major histocompatibility barriers. *Blood* 1997; **89**: 2880–90.

28 Seledtsov VI, Seledtsova GV, Avdeev EV, Samarin DM, Kozlov VA. Induction of mixed allogeneic chimerism for leukemia. *Leuk Res* 1997; **21**: 907–9.

29 Storb R, Raff RF, Graham T *et al*. Marrow toxicity of fractionated versus single dose total body irradiation is identical in a canine model. *Int J Radiat Oncol Biol Phys* 1993; **26**: 275–83.

30 Storb R, Raff RF, Appelbaum FR *et al*. Comparison of fractionated to single-dose total body irradiation in conditioning canine littermates for DLA-identical marrow grafts. *Blood* 1989; **74**: 1139–43.

31 Yu C, Storb R, Mathey B *et al*. DLA-identical bone marrow grafts after low-dose total body irradiation: effects of high-dose corticosteroids and cyclosporine on engraftment. *Blood* 1995; **86**: 4376–81.

32 Kernan NA, Bordignon C, Heller G *et al*. Graft failure after T-cell-depleted human leukocyte antigen identical marrow transplants for leukemia. I. Analysis of risk factors and results of secondary transplants. *Blood* 1989; **74**: 2227–36.

33 Storb R, Yu C, Wagner JL *et al*. Stable mixed hematopoietic chimerism in DLA-identical littermate dogs given sublethal total body irradiation before and pharmacological immunosuppression after marrow transplantation. *Blood* 1997; **89**: 3048–54.

34 Deeg HJ, Storb R, Weiden PL *et al*. Cyclosporin A and methotrexate in canine marrow transplantation: engraftment, graft-versus-host disease, and induction of tolerance. *Transplantation* 1982; **34**: 30–5.

35 Storb R, Deeg HJ, Whitehead J *et al*. Methotrexate and cyclosporine compared with cyclosporine alone for prophylaxis of acute graft versus host disease after marrow transplantation for leukemia. *N Engl J Med* 1986; **314**: 729–35.

36 Yu C, Seidel K, Nash RA *et al*. Synergism between mycophenolate mofetil and cyclosporine in preventing graft-versus-host disease among lethally irradiated dogs given DLA-nonidentical unrelated marrow grafts. *Blood* 1998; **91**: 2581–7.

37 Storb R, Yu C, Barnett T *et al*. Stable mixed hematopoietic chimerism in dog leukocyte antigen-identical littermate dogs given lymph node irradiation before and pharmacologic immunosuppression after marrow transplantation. *Blood* 1999; **94**: 1131–6.

38 Storb R, Yu C, Zaucha JM *et al*. Stable mixed hematopoietic chimerism in dogs given donor antigen, CTLA4Ig, and 100 cGy total body irradiation before and pharmacologic immunosuppression after marrow transplant. *Blood* 1999; **94**: 2523–9.

39 Bethge WA, Wilbur DS, Storb R *et al*. Selective T-cell ablation with bismuth-213 labeled anti-TCRαβ as nonmyeloablative conditioning for allogeneic canine marrow transplantation. *Blood* 2003; **101**: 5068–75.

40 Sandmaier BM, Bethge WA, Wilbur DS *et al*. Bismuth 213-labeled anti-CD45 radioimmunoconjugate to condition dogs for nonmyeloablative allogeneic marrow grafts. *Blood* 2002; **100**: 318–26.

41 Storb R, Deeg HJ. Failure of allogeneic canine marrow grafts after total body irradiation: allogeneic "resistance" vs. transfusion induced sensitization. *Transplantation* 1986; **42**: 571–80.

42 Sandmaier BM, Storb R, Santos EB *et al*. Allogeneic transplants of canine peripheral blood stem cells mobilized by recombinant canine hematopoietic growth factors. *Blood* 1996; **87**: 3508–13.

43 Deeg HJ, Storb R, Weiden PL *et al*. Abrogation of resistance to and enhancement of DLA-nonidentical unrelated marrow grafts in lethally irradiated dogs by thoracic duct lymphocytes. *Blood* 1979; **53**: 552–7.

44 Sandmaier BM, Fukuda T, Gooley T, Yu C, Santos EB, Storb R. Dog leukocyte antigen-haploidentical stem cell allografts after anti-CD44 therapy and reduced-intensity conditioning in a preclinical canine model. *Exp Hematol* 2003; **31**: 168–75.

45 Schuening F, Storb R, Goehle S *et al*. Facilitation of engraftment of DLA-nonidentical marrow by treatment of recipients with monoclonal antibody directed against marrow cells surviving radiation. *Transplantation* 1987; **44**: 607–13.

46 Sandmaier BM, Storb R, Appelbaum FR, Gallatin WM. An antibody that facilitates hematopoietic engraftment recognizes CD44. *Blood* 1990; **76**: 630–5.

47 Storb RF, Champlin R, Riddell SR, Murata M, Bryant S, Warren EH. Non-myeloablative transplants for malignant disease. In: Schechter GP, Broudy VC, Williams ME, eds. *Hematology 2001: American Society of Hematology Education Program Book*. Washington, DC: American Society of Hematology, 2001: 375–391.

48 Giralt S, Estey E, Albitar M *et al*. Engraftment of allogeneic hematopoietic progenitor cells with purine analog-containing chemotherapy: harnessing graft-versus-leukemia without myeloablative therapy. *Blood* 1997; **89**: 4531–6.

49 Khouri IF, Keating M, Körbling M *et al*. Transplant-lite: induction of graft-versus-malignancy using

fludarabine-based nonablative chemotherapy and allogeneic blood progenitor-cell transplantation as treatment for lymphoid malignancies. *J Clin Oncol* 1998; **16**: 2817–24.
50. Giralt S, Thall PF, Khouri I *et al.* Melphalan and purine analog-containing preparative regimens: reduced-intensity conditioning for patients with hematologic malignancies undergoing allogeneic progenitor cell transplantation. *Blood* 2001; **97**: 631–7.
51. Slavin S, Nagler A, Naparstek E *et al.* Non-myeloablative stem cell transplantation and cell therapy as an alternative to conventional bone marrow transplantation with lethal cytoreduction for the treatment of malignant and nonmalignant hematologic diseases. *Blood* 1998; **91**: 756–63.
52. Nagler A, Slavin S, Varadi G, Naparstek E, Samuel S, Or R. Allogeneic peripheral blood stem cell transplantation using a fludarabine-based low intensity conditioning regimen for malignant lymphoma. *Bone Marrow Transplant* 2000; **25**: 1021–8.
53. Childs R, Clave E, Contentin N *et al.* Engraftment kinetics after nonmyeloablative allogeneic peripheral blood stem cell transplantation: full donor T-cell chimerism precedes alloimmune responses. *Blood* 1999; **94**: 3234–41.
54. Spitzer TR, McAfee S, Sackstein R *et al.* Intentional induction of mixed chimerism and achievement of antitumor responses after nonmyeloablative conditioning therapy and HLA-matched donor bone marrow transplantation for refractory hematologic malignancies. *Biol Blood Marrow Transplant* 2000; **6**: 309–20.
55. Sandmaier BM, Maloney DG, Gooley TA *et al.* Low dose TBI conditioning for hematopoietic stem cell transplants (HSCT) from HLA-matched related donors for patients with hematologic malignancies: influence of fludarabine or cytoreductive autografts on outcome. *Blood* 2002; **100**: 145a [Abstract].
56. Kottaridis PD, Milligan DW, Chopra R *et al. In vivo* Campath-1H prevents graft-versus-host disease following nonmyeloablative stem cell transplantation. *Blood* 2000; **96**: 2419–25.
57. Sykes M, Preffer F, McAfee S *et al.* Mixed lymphohaemopoietic chimerism and graft-versus-lymphoma effects after non-myeloablative therapy and HLA-mismatched bone-marrow transplantation. *Lancet* 1999; **353**: 1755–9.
58. Nagler A, Aker M, Or R *et al.* Low-intensity conditioning is sufficient to ensure engraftment in matched unrelated bone marrow transplantation. *Exp Hematol* 2001; **29**: 362–70.
59. Bornhauser M, Thiede C, Platzbecker U *et al.* Dose-reduced conditioning and allogeneic hematopoietic stem cell transplantation from unrelated donors in 42 patients. *Clin Cancer Res* 2001; **7**: 2254–62.
60. Chakraverty R, Peggs K, Chopra R *et al.* Limiting transplantation-related mortality following unrelated donor stem cell transplantion by using a nonmyeloablative conditioning regimen. *Blood* 2002; **99**: 1071–8.
61. Niederwieser D, Maris M, Shizuru JA *et al.* Low-dose total body irradiation (TBI) and fludarabine followed by hematopoietic cell transplantation (HCT) from HLA-matched or mismatched unrelated donors and postgrafting immunosuppression with cyclosporine and mycophenolate mofetil (MMF) can induce durable complete chimerism and sustained remissions in patients with hematological diseases. *Blood* 2003; **101**: 1620–9.
62. Maris MB, Niederwieser D, Sandmaier BM *et al.* HLA-matched unrelated donor hematopoietic cell transplantation after nonmyeloablative conditioning for patients with hematologic malignancies. *Blood* prepublished online June 5, 2003: DOI 10.1182/blood-2003-02-0482.
63. McSweeney PA, Niederwieser D, Shizuru JA *et al.* Hematopoietic cell transplantation in older patients with hematologic malignancies: replacing high-dose cytotoxic therapy with graft-versus-tumor effects. *Blood* 2001; **97**: 3390–400.
64. Storb R. Hematopoietic cell transplantation as immunotherapy for hematologic malignancy. In: Perry MC, ed. *ASCO 2002 Educational Book*. Alexandria, VA: ASCO, 2002: 81.
65. Mielcarek M, Martin PJ, Leisenring W *et al.* Graft-versus-host disease after nonmyeloablative versus conventional hematopoietic stem cell transplantation. *Blood* 2003; **102**: 756–62.
66. Weissinger F, Sandmaier BM, Maloney DG, Bensinger WI, Gooley T, Storb R. Decreased transfusion requirements for patients receiving nonmyeloablative compared with conventional peripheral blood stem cell transplants from HLA-identical siblings. *Blood* 2001; **98**: 3584–8.
67. Junghanss C, Marr KA, Carter RA *et al.* Incidence and outcome of bacterial and fungal infections following nonmyeloablative compared with myeloablative allogeneic hematopoietic stem cell transplantation: a matched control study. *Biol Blood Marrow Transplant* 2002; **8**: 512–20.
68. Junghanss C, Boeckh M, Carter RA *et al.* Incidence and outcome of cytomegalovirus infections following nonmyeloablative compared with myeloablative allogeneic stem cell transplantation: a matched control study. *Blood* 2002; **99**: 1978–85.
69. Fukuda T, Boeckh M, Carter RA *et al.* Risks and outcomes of invasive fungal infections in recipients of allogeneic hematopoietic stem cell transplants after nonmyeloablative conditioning. *Blood* 2003; **102**: 827–33.
70. Fukuda T, Hackman RC, Guthrie KA *et al.* Risks and outcomes of idiopathic pneumonia syndrome after nonmyeloablative compared to conventional conditioning regimens for allogeneic hematopoietic stem cell transplantation. *Blood* prepublished online July 10, 2003; DOI 10.1182/blood-2003-05-1597.
71. Radich JP, Gooley T, Sanders JE, Anasetti C, Chauncey T, Appelbaum FR. Second allogeneic transplantation after failure of first autologous transplantation. *Biol Blood Marrow Transplant* 2000; **6**: 272–9.
72. Nagler A, Or R, Naparstek E, Varadi G, Slavin S. Second allogeneic stem cell transplantation using nonmyeloablative conditioning for patients who relapsed or developed secondary malignancies following autologous transplantation. *Exp Hematol* 2000; **28**: 1096–104.
73. Dey BR, McAfee S, Sackstein R *et al.* Successful allogeneic stem cell transplantation with nonmyeloablative conditioning in patients with relapsed hematologic malignancy following autologous stem cell transplantation. *Biol Blood Marrow Transplant* 2001; **7**: 604–12.
74. Cohen S, Fung H, Stein A *et al.* Reduced intensity allogeneic stem cell transplantation for patients who have failed a prior autologous stem cell transplant. *Blood* 2002; **100**: 177a [Abstract].
75. Feinstein LC, Sandmaier BM, Maloney DG *et al.* Allografting after nonmyeloablative conditioning as a treatment following a failed conventional hematopoietic cell transplant. *Biol Blood Marrow Transplant* 2003; **9**: 266–72.
76. van Leeuwen JE, van Tol MJ, Joosten AM *et al.* Relationship between patterns of engraftment in peripheral blood and immune reconstitution after allogeneic bone marrow transplantation for (severe) combined immunodeficiency [Review]. *Blood* 1994; **84**: 3936–47.
77. Fischer A, Landais P, Friedrich W *et al.* Bone marrow transplantation (BMT) in Europe for primary immunodeficiencies other than severe combine immunodeficiency: a report from the European Group for BMT and the European Group for Immunodeficiency. *Blood* 1994; **83**: 1149–54.
78. Walters MC, Patience M, Leisenring W *et al.* Stable mixed hematopoietic chimerism after bone marrow transplantation for sickle cell anemia. *Biol Blood Marrow Transplant* 2001; **7**: 665–73.
79. Amrolia P, Gaspar HB, Hassan A *et al.* Nonmyeloablative stem cell transplantation for congenital immunodeficiencies. *Blood* 2000; **96**: 1239–46.
80. Horwitz ME, Barrett AJ, Brown MR *et al.* Treatment of chronic granulomatous disease with nonmyeloablative conditioning and a T-cell-depleted hematopoietic allograft. *N Engl J Med* 2001; **344**: 881–8.
81. Woolfrey AE, Nash RA, Frangoul HA *et al.* Nonmyeloablative transplant regimen used for induction of multi-lineage allogeneic hematopoietic mixed donor-host chimerism in patients with T-cell immunodeficiency. *Blood* 1998; **92** (Suppl. 1): 520a [Abstract].
82. Woolfrey AE, Nash RA, Sanders JE, Ochs HD, Thomson B, Storb R. A nonmyeloablative regimen for induction of multi-lineage hematopoietic mixed donor-host chimerism in nonmalignant disorders. *Blood* 2000; **98**: 784a [Abstract].
83. Flowers MED, Zanis-Neto J, Medeiros CR *et al.* Reduced dose cyclophosphamide (Cy) before HLA-matched related bone marrow transplantation (BMT) in patients with Fanconi anemia (FA). *Blood* 1999; **94** (Suppl. 1): 382b [Abstract].
84. Boulad F, Gillio A, Small TN *et al.* Stem cell transplantation for the treatment of Fanconi anaemia using a fludarabine-based cytoreductive regimen and T-cell-depleted related HLA-mismatched peripheral blood stem cell grafts. *Br J Haematol* 2000; **111**: 1153–7.
85. Kurre P, Pulsipher M, Woolfrey A *et al.* Reduced toxicity and prompt engraftment following minimal conditioning of a patient with Fanconi anemia undergoing hematopoietic stem cell transplantation from an HLA-matched unrelated donor. *J Pediatr Hematol Oncol* 2003; **25**: 581–3.
86. Peters C, Balthazor M, Shapiro EG *et al.* Outcome of unrelated donor bone marrow transplantation in forty children with Hurler syndrome. *Blood* 1996; **87**: 4894–902.
87. Peters C, Shapiro EG, Anderson J *et al.* Hurler syndrome. II. Outcome of HLA-genotypically identical sibling and HLA-haploidentical related donor bone marrow transplantation in fifty-four children. Storage Disease Collaborative Study Group. *Blood* 1998; **91**: 2601–8.
88. Walters MC, Storb R, Patience M *et al.* Impact of bone marrow transplantation for symptomatic sickle cell disease: an interim report. *Blood* 2000; **95**: 1918–24.
89. Lucarelli G, Galimberti M, Polchi P *et al.* Marrow transplantation in patients with thalassemia responsive to iron chelation therapy. *N Engl J Med* 1993; **329**: 840–4.

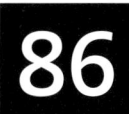

86

Richard W. Childs & Ramaprasad Srinivasan

Allogeneic Hematopoietic Cell Transplantation for Solid Tumors

Our perception of the mechanisms through which malignant cells are eradicated following allogeneic hematopoietic cell transplantation (HCT) has evolved substantially over the past four decades. No longer merely thought of as a means to rescue hematopoietic function following myeloablative conditioning, allogeneic transplantation is now known to be a powerful type of immunotherapy capable of curing patients with otherwise fatal malignant diseases. This conceptual evolution has translated into a diversification of the indications for allotransplants and led to the development of reduced intensity transplant approaches whose beneficial antineoplastic effects occur as a consequence of the transplanted donor immune system. Recently, investigators have begun to test whether nonhematologic malignancies might likewise be susceptible to allogeneic immune attack. In this chapter, we highlight the work that has improved our awareness and understanding of the graft-vs.-tumor (GVT) effect, and discuss the preliminary results of its application as an investigational therapeutic modality in the treatment of metastatic solid tumors.

Allogeneic transplantation as immunotherapy: the graft-vs.-leukemia effect

Acute leukemias have traditionally been viewed as "chemosensitive" malignancies. The inability to "cure" the majority of adults with leukemia following conventional chemotherapeutic regimens was attributed, at least in part, to a failure to deliver high enough doses of antineoplastic agents that would be required to eradicate all malignant cells. Dose-limiting toxicities including prolonged delays in lymphohematopoietic recovery or even lethal "myeloablation" significantly hindered efforts to intensify such regimens. Pioneering work by E.D. Thomas and others led to the development of allogeneic HCT as a method to allow for accelerated recovery of lymphohematopoietic function following the administration of high-dose chemotherapy [1,2].

For the next two decades, allogeneic HCT became increasingly used as a therapeutic option to treat patients with a variety of different treatment-resistant hematologic malignancies. Initially, the curative potential of the procedure was ascribed solely to the cytotoxic effects of the conditioning regimen, be it chemotherapy alone or in conjunction with total body radiation. It was not until decades following its inception that investigators first documented the very important and powerful immune mechanisms that contributed to the curative potential of the approach in humans.

Throughout the 1980s, several landmark observations provided insight into this phenomenon known as the graft-vs.-leukemia (GVL) effect. First, in an analysis of >200 patients with hematologic malignancies undergoing a human leukocyte antigen (HLA) matched HCT from a sibling donor, investigators noted that patients who experienced moderate to severe acute graft-vs.-host disease (GVHD) or chronic GVHD had a significantly lower incidence of leukemic relapse compared with patients with little or no GVHD [3]. Similar benefits in disease-free survival were observed in recipients of HLA-identical (nontwin) sibling donor allografts compared to those receiving syngeneic allografts [4], as well as in recipients of T-replete grafts vs. those receiving T-cell-depleted transplants [4–7]. These observations suggested a very important role for donor T cells in mediating this effect and also implicated the targets of GVL as falling outside the realm of antigens encoded by the major histocompatibility complex (MHC). Definitive evidence that GVL effects were clinically meaningful came from studies in patients with chronic myelogenous leukemia (CML) who relapsed post-transplant and were subsequently induced back into remission following a donor lymphocyte infusion (DLI) [8]. Over the last decade, numerous investigators have successfully exploited GVL effects against a variety of malignancies of hematopoietic origin, including both acute and chronic leukemias, lymphomas, multiple myeloma and Epstein–Barr virus-related lymphoproliferative disorder [9–17]. The efficacy of GVL in terms of its ability to induce remission varies among these malignancies, with the critical determining factors dictating neoplastic susceptibility to GVL not entirely understood.

The immune system and solid tumors

Tumors such as metastatic melanoma and renal cell carcinoma (RCC), with their occasional spontaneous regressions or prolonged periods of stable disease, have long fascinated investigators and led to the concept that the immune system might have a role in the regulation or control of malignant cells. Indeed, the first spontaneous regression of metastatic RCC after nephrectomy was described in 1928 and was attributed to an antibody-mediated immune response [18]. The propensity of nude (athymic) mice to develop lymphoreticular tumors and the increased incidence of malignancies in patients with congenital or acquired immunodeficient states lent credence to the immune system having a role in the control of cancer [19–21]. The development of immune-based therapeutic strategies against metastatic solid tumors was a logical consequence of these observations.

At the National Cancer Institute (NCI), pilot immunotherapy trials in patients with advanced solid tumors—particularly metastatic RCC and metastatic melanoma—were conducted in the early 1980s by Rosenberg *et al.* [22]. The earliest trials were intended to nonspecifically stimulate innate immune responses against tumors using cytokines such as interleukin 2 (IL-2). In their preliminary experience using IL-2 in patients with either metastatic RCC or melanoma, overall response rates of 20% (RCC) and 17% (melanoma) were observed. Importantly, some patients achieved complete and durable remission of disease, providing valuable proof of the concept of the therapeutic potential of immune-based therapy. Subsequent studies conducted at the NCI as well as by the Cytokine Working Group (CWG) employed adoptive transfer of lymphokine-activated killer (LAK) cells or *ex vivo* expanded tumor-infiltrating lymphocytes (TIL) in conjunction with IL-2. Although response rates in some trials approached 35%, it remains unclear if TIL therapy provided any therapeutic benefit over cytokine treatment alone [23–29]. The low response rate and significant morbidity that was frequently associated with such therapy (particularly high-dose IL-2) provided the impetus for the exploration and development of immune strategies which would selectively target the tumor.

The foundation for tumor-specific cellular immunotherapy was laid following the identification of a number of different tumor-associated antigens (TAA) in melanoma and other solid tumors [30–32]. Several clinical trials that are currently active are evaluating the safety and efficacy of cancer vaccines designed to enhance immune responses to TAA. This remains a dynamic area of investigation that holds promise for the future. Although immune correlative studies have shown that some vaccines significantly expand TAA-reactive T-cell populations *in vivo*, early clinical results from such trials have thus far been disappointing.

Several factors likely contribute to the poor clinical efficacy of conventional vaccine strategies designed to enhance "self" immunity against TAA. To date, the vast majority of trials have used an MHC class I restricted peptide-based approach. As a consequence, resultant immune responses are limited to a single antigenic epitope devoid of a critical CD4+ helper T-cell component [33]. Furthermore, such vaccine strategies may promote for the selection of tumor cells lacking the targeted antigen, a phenomenon described as "antigen escape". Modifying this approach by simultaneously immunizing with multiple tumor antigens that are both MHC class I and II restricted or by using the tumor itself as a vaccine (i.e. tumor lysates, tumor apoptotic bodies, etc.) may minimize this risk [34]. It has also been suggested that tumors may evade cytotoxic T lymphocyte (CTL) eradication by downregulating expression of accessory molecules required by CTL to mediate lysis. Perhaps one of the greatest limitations of conventional immunotherapy is that the immune system it attempts to enhance has intrinsic functional compromise. A number of lines of evidence support this concept. First, the host immune system is often rendered incompetent by prior chemotherapy and/or by tumor-related factors. Second, long-standing immune tolerance to tumor antigens, including TAA targeted by conventional cancer vaccines, may exist. Theoretically, these limitations could be circumvented by allogeneic HCT, a procedure that ultimately culminates in complete immune replacement. Perhaps more importantly, an allogeneic immune system would have the capacity to mount immune responses to polymorphic variants of tumor-specific or broadly expressed minor histocompatibility antigens (mHA), a phenomenon that cannot occur from innate host immunity [35–37].

Solid tumors as a GVT target

Animal models exploring graft-vs.-solid tumor effects

The notion that immune responses following allogeneic HCT can be directed against solid tumors was first tested in animal models in the early 1980s. Using a mouse model, Moscovitch and Slavin [38] showed that the high incidence of spontaneous lymphosarcomas in NZB/W hybrids could be significantly diminished by transplantation of allogeneic hematopoietic stem cells (HSCs) from BALB/c mice. Subsequently, this group demonstrated the ability of minor and major histocompatibility antigen-mismatched transplants to protect mice from developing metastatic disease following mouse mammary adenocarcinoma (4T1) tumor challenge [39,40]. These experiments showed that alloimmune responses against mHAs that were expressed on tumors could be generated following HSC transplantation.

Early clinical data suggesting graft-vs.-solid tumor effects in humans

Compelling clinical evidence supporting the therapeutic utility of the graft-vs.-leukemia effect in hematologic malignancies largely prompted investigators to explore allogeneic HCT as a therapeutic tool against metastatic solid tumors. The first report suggesting a possible GVT effect against a tumor of epithelial origin noted the incidental regression of a metastatic breast adenocarcinoma lesion following allogeneic HCT for relapsed acute myelogenous leukemia [41]. Subsequently, Eibl *et al.* [42] reported tumor regression coincident with acute GVHD in a patient with chemoresistant metastatic breast cancer following a myeloablative transplant from an HLA-identical sibling. The ability to expand mHA-specific cytotoxic T lymphocytes (obtained from patient at the time of clinical response) which killed breast cancer cell lines *in vitro* lent credence to the argument that the tumor regression was at least in part alloimmune-mediated. Investigators at the M.D. Anderson Cancer Center reported their experience in 10 patients with metastatic breast cancer who received an allogeneic HCT from an HLA-matched sibling following myeloablative conditioning [43]. One complete response (CR) and five partial responses (PRs) were noted. GVT effects were implicated in at least two patients whose tumors regressed in temporal relationship to acute GVHD and withdrawal of immunosuppression. Delayed regression of metastatic lesions following myeloablative allogeneic HCT in a woman with ovarian cancer offered further evidence that some tumors of epithelial origin were indeed susceptible to GVT effects [44].

Use of nonmyeloablative conditioning in allogeneic transplantation for solid tumors

By the late 1990s, there was sufficient interest in investigating for GVT effects against solid tumors based on available preclinical and clinical data. The major factor limiting the initiation of pilot trials was the significant morbidity and mortality associated with conventional allogeneic HCT. Dose-intensive conditioning used to provide both tumor cytoreduction and a means to allow donor engraftment contributed in part to the morbidity and mortality associated with HCT. Subsequently, it was recognized that reducing the intensity of the conditioning regimen might translate to a reduction in the risk of procedure-related morbidity and mortality.

In the late 1990s, transplant regimens using nonmyeloablative or reduced intensity conditioning were designed by a number of investigators and were evaluated for their engraftment potential and toxicity profile [45–49]. Two major factors impacted on the design and development of these dose-reduced conditioning regimens. First, the recognition that GVL effects alone may be sufficient to eradicate some hematologic malignancies in the absence of dose-intensive therapy. Second, the realization that the primary role of the conditioning regimen could be limited to preparing the recipient for engraftment by inducing adequate host immunosuppression. Thus, nonmyeloablative conditioning regimens were designed using agents that would induce adequate immunosuppression to facilitate donor immune engraftment while maintaining a low toxicity profile. Such "low-intensity" regimens were first evaluated in hematologic malignancies known to be responsive to allogeneic HCT. Pilot trials utilizing nonmyeloablative HCT (NMHCT) demonstrated that such regimens were generally well-tolerated, having a decreased incidence of transplant-related morbidity and mortality while achieving sufficient donor immune engraftment to induce sustained remissions of some hematologic malignancies [45–49]. One of the major contributions of nonmyeloablative conditioning was that it allowed for the extension of allogeneic HCT to debilitated and older patients who, because of the risk for treatment-related mortality (TRM) with a myeloablative transplant, would ordinarily have been denied the benefit of a procedure with curative potential. Importantly, investigators anticipated that the overall risk of TRM would be lower with a nonmyeloablative approach, a notion which emboldened investigators to explore for GVT effects against solid tumors.

Clinical results of NMHCT in solid tumors

Renal cell carcinoma: NIH experience

The current worldwide clinical experience of NMHCT for solid tumors is limited, with <200 cases reported in the literature. Because there existed no convincing evidence to support the existence of a GVT effect in solid tumors, pilot trials have been restricted primarily to terminally ill patients with advanced treatment-refractory metastatic disease. At present, RCC remains the solid tumor in which allogeneic antitumor responses have been best characterized. The following factors provided an incentive to study the susceptibility of this malignancy to a GVT effect. First, metastatic RCC is a uniformly fatal cancer in which the majority of patients succumb to disease within a year of diagnosis. Second, therapeutic options are extremely limited, with conventional chemotherapy and radiotherapy being largely ineffective [50]. Third, RCC is considered an "immunoresponsive" tumor based on its susceptibility to cytokine therapy [22,51,52], history of occasional spontaneous regression [18,53] and existence of tumor-infiltrating T lymphocytes in regressing metastatic lesions [23,25]. These considerations led to the development of a clinical protocol at the National Institutes of Health (NIH) that sought to test the safety and efficacy of NMHCT in patients with cytokine-refractory metastatic RCC [48,54].

The primary considerations in the design of the allogeneic HCT trial for patients with metastatic kidney cancer were the following.
1 Devising a conditioning regimen that would ensure maximal host immunosuppression to favor rapid and complete donor immune engraftment with relative sparing of recipient myeloid progenitors.
2 Devising a post-transplant immunosuppressive approach that would provide optimal prophylaxis for GVHD without precluding the ability to initiate a donor immune-mediated GVT effect.
3 Judicious use of donor lymphocyte infusions to break donor tolerance to host antigens for the promotion of a GVT effect.
4 Appropriate patient selection: choosing patients with cytokine refractory metastatic disease who would be anticipated to survive at least as long as would be required for a delayed GVT effect to occur (i.e. 4–6 months).

Therefore, the presence of evaluable metastatic disease, a good performance status (Eastern Cooperative Oncology Group [ECOG] 0–1), adequate organ function and a life expectancy of at least 3 months were made prerequisites for patient enrollment.

Cyclophosphamide and fludarabine have profound immunosuppressive effects and are well-tolerated when given in combination to treat patients with low-grade lymphoproliferative disorders [55,56]. Accordingly, we devised a NMHCT approach in which patients received a conditioning regimen consisting of 60 mg/kg cyclophosphamide for 2 days and 25 mg/m² fludarabine for 5 days, followed by infusion of an unmanipulated granulocyte colony-stimulating factor (G-CSF) mobilized peripheral blood hematopoetic cell graft from a 6/6 or 5/6 HLA-matched sibling donor (Fig. 86.1). Lineage-specific engraftment of donor myeloid (CD14⁺/CD15⁺) and T cells (CD3⁺) was quantified from post-transplant peripheral blood lymphocyte (PBL) samples using a polymerase chain reaction (PCR)-based analysis of either variable number tandem repeats (VNTRs) or short tandem repeats (STRs) polymorphic between patient and donor (Fig. 86.2).

Based primarily on animal data showing a decreased risk of GVHD following NMHCT, we chose to use single agent cyclosporine (CSP) as GVHD prophylaxis in our initial patient cohort. Much to our surprise, a high probability of grade II–IV acute GVHD (actuarial probability 56%) was observed in the first 25 RCC patients treated (lethal in three cases). As a consequence, mycophenolate mofetil (MMF) was added to CSP as GVHD prophylaxis in the second cohort of RCC patients. Gradual withdrawal of CSP/MMF was initiated on day +30 or +60, with the timing and rapidity of immunosuppression taper being dictated by the rate of tumor progression, degree of donor T-lymphoid chimerism and the presence or absence of GVHD. One or more dose-escalated donor lymphocyte infusions were administered to all patients with mixed T-cell chimerism, progressive disease or partial remissions in the absence of acute or chronic GVHD. Because interferon has been shown to upregulate MHC expression on RCC tumor cells *in vitro* (Fig. 86.3), we hypothesized that treating with this cytokine post-transplant might make the tumor a better target for a GVT effect. As a consequence, patients without GVHD who failed to respond to DLI were eligible to receive post-transplant cytokine therapy with interferon alfa, either alone or in combination with IL-2.

The initial experience of NMHCT in metastatic RCC was recently published [48]. Ten of the first 19 patients treated with this transplant

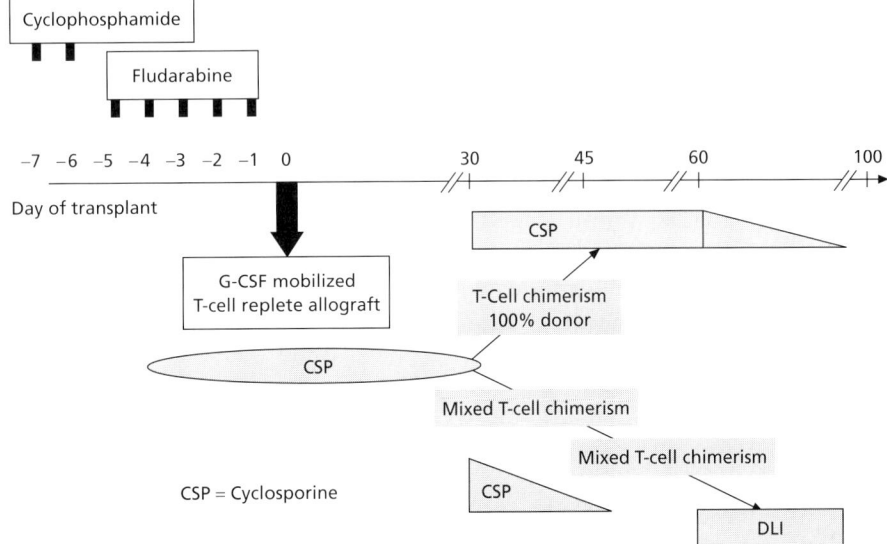

Fig. 86.1 Cyclophosphamide- and fludarabine-based nonmyeloablative hematopoietic cell transplantation (NMHCT) protocol for renal cell carcinoma (RCC).

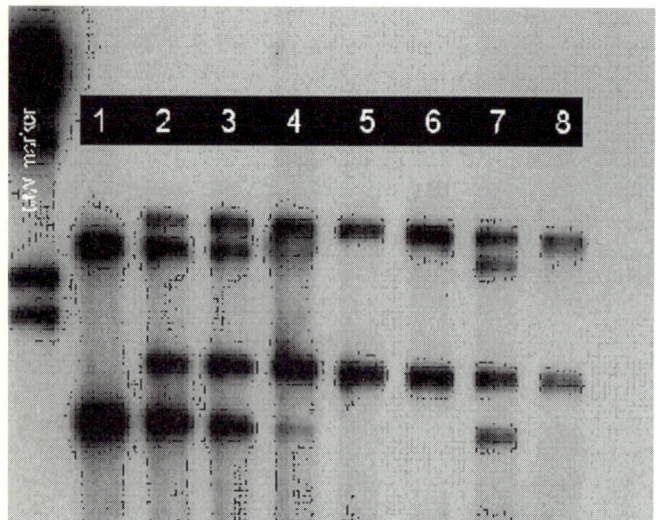

Fig. 86.2 Example of polymerase chain reaction (PCR) based analysis of two different minisatellites polymorphic between patient and donor. Patient (lane 1) and donor (lane 5) lanes show two patient-specific and two donor-specific bands. Control mixtures of donor into patient DNA representing 30% (lane 2), 50% (lane 3) and 90% (lane 4) donor chimerism. Post-transplant blood sample sorted into lineages using magnetic beads showing 100%, 60% and 99% donor chimerism in $CD2^+/CD3^-$ natural killer (NK) cell (lane 6), $CD14^+/CD15^+$ myeloid cell (lane 7) and $CD3^+$ T-cell (lane 8) fractions, respectively.

approach had tumor shrinkage including three who had a CR and seven patients who had a PR. At present, more than 55 patients have undergone NMHCT for RCC at the NIH. Of the 50 patients who are currently evaluable for outcome, 49 engrafted fully and achieved 100% donor T-cell chimerism by day 100 post-transplant. Twenty-two of 50 (44%) patients have had a disease response including four CRs and 18 PRs. Five patients who were deemed "nonresponders" had radiographic evidence for a mixed response. Disease regression was associated with acute and chronic GVHD and was typically delayed in onset and did not occur until CSP was tapered, consistent with an alloimmune-mediated GVT effect. Several patients have proven to have a durable disease response including the first complete responder who remains without evidence of metastatic disease nearly 5 years post-transplant (Fig. 86.4). Regression of disease in multiple metastatic foci has been observed although pulmonary responses appear to occur most frequently. On occasion, disease responses have been dramatic and have included complete resolution of large pulmonary metastases with bulky adenopathy (Fig. 86.5).

Preliminary data would suggest that disease response following NMHCT is a clinically meaningful phenomenon because regression of metastatic RCC appears to be associated with a trend towards improved survival. Survival in nonresponders has been <6 months, in contrast to those achieving a partial response who have survived a median 2 years post-transplant. Median survival has not yet been reached in those patients who have achieved a CR.

In general, patients with metastatic kidney cancer have tolerated this

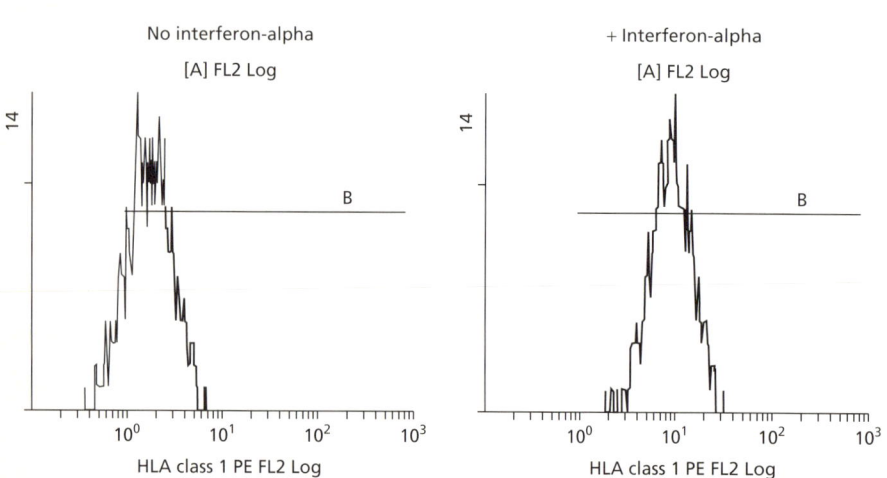

Fig. 86.3 Upregulation of human leukocyte antigen (HLA) class I expression (both percentage positive and mean channel fluorescence) on renal cell carcinoma cells 24 h after exposure to interferon alfa (10,000 units/mL).

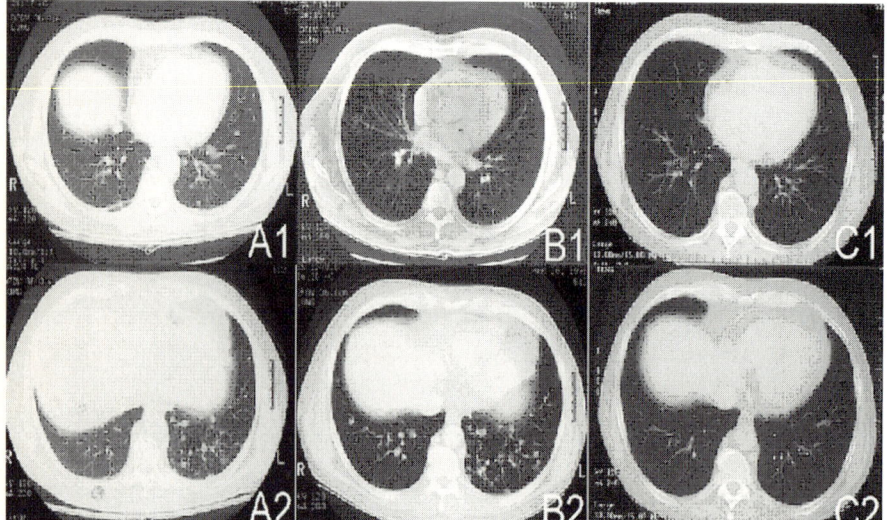

Fig. 86.4 Renal cell carcinoma (RCC) metastatic to the lungs (pretransplant images A1 and A2). No change in metastatic disease 30 days following conditioning (B1 and B2). Following CSP withdrawal, metastases regressed completely by 110 days post-transplant (C1 and C2). The patient remains without evidence of disease nearly 5 years after transplantation.

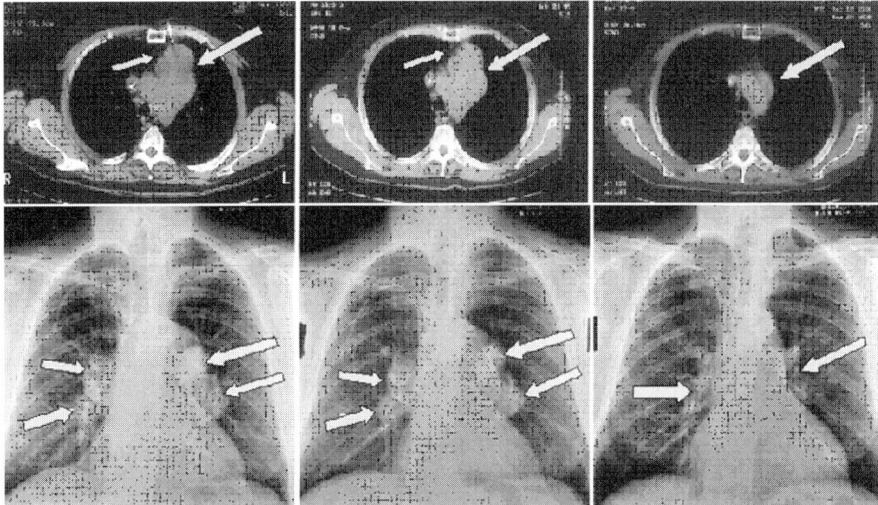

Fig. 86.5 Delayed regression of renal cell carcinoma (RCC). Pretransplant images showing bulky anterior mediastinal (A1) and hilar (A2) adenopathy. Stable disease seen 6 months post-transplant (B1 and B2). Regression of bulky adenopathy was observed 9 months post-transplant (C1 and C2).

conditioning well. Although virtually all patients have developed febrile neutropenia, we observed no veno-occlusive disease (VOD) of the liver or chemotherapy-associated mucositis. Thirty-four percent of patients developed cytomegalovirus (CMV) antigenemia with only one case of CMV disease (esophagitis), which was responsive to ganciclovir therapy. Mortality associated with transplant-related complications occurred in seven of 50 (14%) patients, with either infection or acute or chronic GVHD being the major cause of TRM. Because kidney cancer frequently metastasizes to the lungs, some RCC patients may be at high risk for the development of post-obstructive pneumonia following transplantation. Such a complication occurring in the profoundly immunocompromised can lead to disastrous infectious sequelae, as was observed in two of our RCC patients who died from bacterial sepsis related to obstructive bronchial pneumonia.

Acute GVHD has been the greatest contributor to morbidity and mortality in our RCC patients undergoing NMHCT. Because MMF is a potent inhibitor of inosine monophosphate and has been shown *in vitro* to block proliferative responses of cytotoxic T cells, we added MMF to CSP as prophylaxis for GVHD in our second cohort of RCC patients. Unfortunately, an interim analysis of the first 30 patients treated with both drugs revealed no difference in the incidence of grade II–IV or grade III–IV acute GVHD between the CSP alone and the CSP/MMF cohorts (actuarial probability of acute grade II–IV GVHD, 56% and 61%, respectively). Of equal concern, complete responses were only observed in those patients who did not receive MMF (four of 25 patients in the CSP alone cohort had a CR vs. none of 30 patients in the CSP/MMF cohort). Based on these observations, we have withdrawn MMF from the transplant regimen and are currently investigating the effect of adding low-dose methotrexate to CSP as GVHD prophylaxis.

Assessment of donor chimerism following NMHCT is important not only to document the establishment of donor engraftment, but also to allow for post-transplant manipulation of the donor immune system to optimize the chances of inducing a GVT effect. In our experience, GVT effects following NMHCT typically do not occur until the immune system has converted from mixed to predominantly donor T-cell chimerism. As a consequence, detailed serial measurements of donor engraftment in both lymphoid and myeloid lineages are performed on all patients undergoing this approach. Representative lineage-specific engraftment profiles and their relationship to clinical outcome are shown in Fig. 86.6.

Although donor T-cell engraftment typically precedes myeloid engraftment using cyclophosphamide- and fludarabine-based conditioning, engraftment patterns may vary considerably among individual pati-

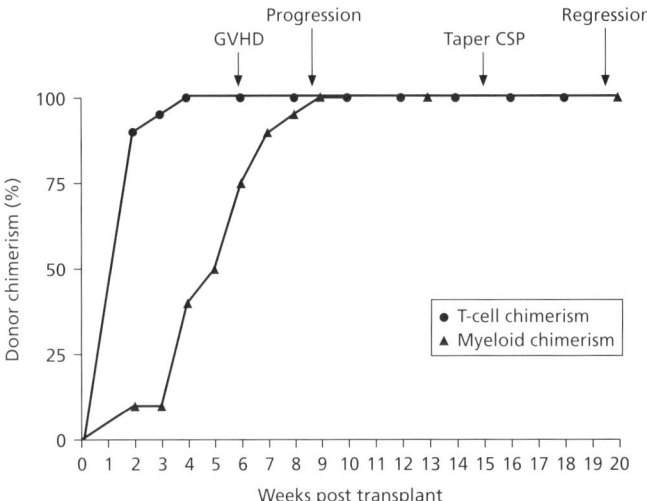

Fig. 86.6 Representative lineage-specific engraftment profile following cyclophosphamide- and fludarabine-based conditioning. The percentage donor chimerism in T cells (circles) and myeloid cells (triangles) are shown in a patient who had a disease response 17 weeks post-transplant.

ents [57]. Several factors influence the degree and rapidity of donor engraftment including the agents used in the conditioning regimen, the prevailing state of host immunity and allograft cell doses. In a recent multivariate analysis of 36 patients with metastatic solid tumors who underwent a NMHCT at the NIH, pretransplant exposure to chemotherapy and increased allograft CD34$^+$ cell dose were found to significantly facilitate the engraftment of donor myeloid and T cells [58]. Therefore, tailoring the intensity of nonmyeloablative conditioning in solid tumor patients based on prior chemotherapy exposure would seem worthy of exploration.

While the exact mechanisms underlying the regression of metastatic RCC following allogeneic HCT are yet to be unraveled, several observations (both laboratory and clinical) would suggest that an alloimmune effect mediated at least in part by donor T cells is at work (Table 86.1) [48]. The majority of patients who ultimately achieved a disease response showed early tumor growth in the first few months after transplantation, a time period when the newly engrafted donor immune system was kept in check by immunosuppressive therapy or when mixed T-cell chimerism prevailed leading to "tolerance" of host tissues (including the tumor). Tumor regression was typically delayed (4–8 months) and followed

Table 86.1 Tumor response patterns consistent with a graft-vs.-tumor effect after nonmyeloablative hematopoietic cell transplantation (NMHCT).

Delayed onset of response (>100 days post-transplant)
Response following withdrawal of immunosuppression
Response following or concomitant with GVHD
Response following donor lymphocyte infusions
Prolonged duration of response in tumors previously treatment-refractory

GVHD, graft-vs.-host disease.

conversion to predominantly donor T-cell chimerism after immunosuppression had been withdrawn or was being tapered. These observations highlight the importance of utilizing a transplant approach that favors rapid donor T-cell engraftment and institutes judicious and timely withdrawal of GVHD prophylaxis. As had previously been described in patients with hematologic malignancies, a prior history of acute GVHD was associated with an increased probability of having a tumor response. One might speculate that disease regression in this setting could be the consequence of alloreactive T cells targeting mHAs that are broadly expressed on both normal tissues and tumor cells. Importantly, however, tumor shrinkage has also been observed to occur in the absence of or temporally distant from GVHD, an observation that might imply that tumor cells are particularly sensitive to allogeneic immune attack or that tumor-specific immune effectors might be involved in mediating RCC regression in some patients.

Finally, regression of RCC following DLI or after treatment with low-dose subcutaneous interferon alfa has also been observed. Disease regression after DLI suggests the mediators of the GVT effect may be analogous to those mediating leukemia regression. Interestingly, some patients who had failed to respond to interferon alfa before transplantation had disease regression when the drug was given post-transplant. This observation suggests that the mechanism by which interferon alfa promotes tumor regression in the post-transplant setting relates to the ability of the drug to make the tumor a better target or enhance the allogeneic immune system rather than to a direct antineoplastic effect.

Emerging role of NMHCT for RCC

Although allogeneic HCT is clearly an investigational approach for the treatment of metastatic RCC, several other investigators have recently begun to report promising results in this disease (Table 86.2). Investigators at the University of Chicago transplanted 15 patients with a fludarabine- and cyclophosphamide-based regimen [59,60]. The first four patients treated were conditioned with an extremely low-intensity regimen consisting of 90 mg/m^2 fludarabine and 2 g/m^2 cyclophosphamide, given at doses that failed to achieve adequate levels of host immunosuppression. As a consequence, three or four (75%) patients failed to achieve stable donor T-cell engraftment and ultimately rejected the transplant. Subsequent patients received higher doses of the same conditioning agents (150 mg/m^2 fludarabine and 4 g/m^2 cyclophosphamide) and achieved successful and sustained donor engraftment. Of their 12 patients who engrafted and were evaluable for a disease response, four (33%) had radiographically documented disease regression consistent with a partial response including one patient who had tumor regression in his primary kidney tumor.

As with other trials of NMHCT for solid tumors, a dominant donor immune system (determined by T-cell chimerism studies) was a prerequisite for the generation of a meaningful GVT effect. Only those patients who had stable and predominantly donor immune engraftment demonstrated a disease response. In fact, one patient with graft rejection (a nonresponder) underwent a second transplant with the intensified conditioning regimen, achieved complete donor engraftment and subsequently had a partial response. Only two of 12 (17%) patients experienced grade ≥II acute GVHD, perhaps the consequence of a more gradual termination of GVHD prophylaxis. Whether delaying the withdrawal of post-transplant immunosuppression will decrease the incidence of acute GVHD without negating beneficial GVT effects will need to be determined from larger studies.

Recently, a group of Italian investigators reported their experience in seven RCC patients undergoing NMHCT using a fludarabine- and thiotepa-based conditioning regimen (Table 86.2) [61]. This regimen was reported to result in rapid and complete donor immune engraftment and to be well-tolerated. In association with CSP withdrawal and GVHD, delayed disease regression consistent with a GVT effect was documented in four of seven (57%) patients.

Toxicities and limitations of NMHCT in metastatic RCC

Although ample evidence to support the susceptibility of metastatic RCC to an allogeneic GVT effect now exists, there are a number of potentially life-threatening toxicities of NMHCT that currently limit the broader application of this approach (Table 86.3). While the incidence of early TRM appears to be less with reduced intensity conditioning, overall 5–20% of patients will ultimately succumb to a transplant-related cause. Indubitably, infection and complications related to acute GVHD are the greatest risks associated with the procedure. In fact, three of the first 25 patients with RCC transplanted at the NIH died from GVHD-related causes [48]. Unfortunately, the addition of MMF to CSP did not reduce the incidence of grade II–IV or grade III–IV acute GVHD. However, new second-line therapies for severe steroid-refractory GVHD such as daclizumab (monoclonal antibody directed against the alpha chain of the IL-2 receptor) and infliximab (monoclonal antibody directed against the TNF-α receptor) have shown early promise [64,65]. Our preliminary experience suggests these monoclonal antibodies are effective in reducing mortality from steroid-refractory GVHD, particularly when given with lipid complexed amphotericin B as *Aspergillus* prophylaxis, concomitant with a rapid reduction in corticosteroid dose once steroid-resistance is apparent [66]. Larger studies will be required to determine whether these agents will ultimately result in a reduction in the risk of GVHD-related mortality without compromising the ability to generate a GVT effect.

Careful patient selection, with particular attention to performance status, medical comorbidities and tumor growth kinetics, may further improve transplant-related outcome. The importance of patient selection is apparent in a recent pilot study of NMHCT in patients with treatment-refractory malignancies that included seven patients with metastatic RCC [62]. All six patients with a poor performance status (ECOG performance status 2–3) experienced severe transplant-related toxicities (grade ≥3) and succumbed within the first 100 days to complications related to the transplant or rapid disease progression. In contrast, the 11 patients who had a good performance status (ECOG performance status 0–1) did relatively well, with only one transplant-related death before day 100. Although the use of NMHCT for solid tumors is presently limited, preliminary clinical experience provides insight into patient characteristics that would be expected to impact favorably on transplant outcome (Table 86.4).

NMHCT in melanoma

Few tumors are associated with a more abysmal prognosis than metastatic melanoma. At present, because of a paucity of efficacious treatments, there exists no accepted "standard therapy" for those who have developed

Table 86.2 Summary of clinical trials of nonmyeloablative hematopoietic cell transplantation (NMHCT) in metastatic renal cell carcinoma and other solid tumors.

Investigators	Conditioning agents	GVHD prophylaxis	Comments	Response	Median time to response	GVHD/TR
Childs et al. [48 and unpublished data]	Cyclophosphamide 120 mg/kg Fludarabine 125 mg/m²	CSP (First 25 patients) CSP + MMF (subsequent patients)	Decisions regarding CSP taper/DLI infusion based on T-cell chimerism and disease progression	Overall RR 44% (22/50) CR 8% (4/50) PR 36% (18/50)	5 months	7/50 died of transplant-related causes including deaths from acute or chronic GVHD
Rini et al. [59,60]	Cyclophosphamide 2 gm/m² Fludarabine 90 mg/m²	FK506 + MMF	High incidence of graft rejection (3/4 patients treated) Cyclophosphamide subsequently increased to 4 gm/m²/fludarabine increased to 150 mg/m²	Overall RR 33% (4/12) All PRs	>100 days	Acute II–IV GVHD 17% (2/12) Chronic GVHD (6/12) Delayed immunosuppression withdrawal (FK506 tapered after day 90) may explain low incidence of acute GVHD
Bregni et al. [61]	Thiotepa 5 mg/kg Fludarabine 60 mg/m² Cyclophosphamide 60 mg/kg	CSP + methotrexate	Decisions regarding CSP tapering based on disease status	Overall PR 57% (4/7) for RCC Overall RR 33% (2/6) for breast cancer	>100 days	Acute II–IV GVHD 85% (6/7) Also noted tumor regression in one patient with ovarian carcinoma
Pedrazzoli et al. [62]	Cyclophosphamide 60 mg/kg Fludarabine 120 mg/m²	CSP and methotrexate	8/8 RCC patients died by day 110 as a consequence of disease progression or TRM Poor PS and rapidly advancing disease may have contributed to poor patient outcome	Overall RR 0% (0/8)	NA	Acute GVHD 0% (0/7 evaluable) Chronic GVHD 0% (0/1 evaluable)
Bay et al. [63]	1 patient received myeloablative conditioning 4/5 patients received fludarabine/busulfan/ATG	CSP	Possible immune mediated regression in patient with ovarian carcinoma who underwent myeloablative HCT Partial responses in 75% patients who underwent nonmyeloablative HCT probably related to chemotherapy	Overall RR 80% (4/5)	NA	One death from progressive disease on day +6 emphasizes need for appropriate patient selection Longer follow-up required to determine if responses in nonmyeloablative group are mediated by GVT effects

ATG, antithymocyte globulin; CR, complete response; CSP, cyclosporine; MMF, mycophenolate mofetil; NA, not available; PR, partial response; PS, performance status; RR, response rate; TRM, treatment-related mortality.

Table 86.3 Limitations of nonmyeloablative hematopoietic cell transplantation (NMHCT) in solid tumors.

	Incidence (%)
HLA-matched sibling donor available	25–30
Acute GVHD	30–60
Chronic GVHD	40–70
CMV reactivation	20–40
Graft rejection	5–10
TRM	10–20

CMV, cytomegalovirus; GVHD, graft-vs.-host disease; HLA, human leukocyte antigen; TRM, transplant-related mortality.

Table 86.4 Patient characteristics likely to predict a favorable outcome after nonmyeloablative hematopoietic cell transplantation (NMHCT) for solid tumors.

- Good performance status (ECOG 0–1)
- Younger patient age (<65 years)
- Small tumor volume
- Slow tumor growth kinetics
- Absence of CNS metastatic disease
- Evidence (clinical or *in vitro*) that tumor is susceptible to immune-mediated attack

CNS, central nervous system; ECOG, Eastern Cooperative Oncology Group.

metastatic disease. Nevertheless, along with kidney cancer, malignant melanoma has long shared the reputation of being an "immunoresponsive" tumor. In fact, more immunotherapy trials have been targeted at melanoma than any other solid tumor. It would seem logical therefore to investigate whether this tumor might be a target for a GVT effect following allogeneic HCT. Unfortunately, and rather surprisingly, the results of NMHCT for melanoma at the NIH and at other centers worldwide have been far from inspiring.

We recently reviewed the outcome of 25 patients with metastatic melanoma treated at four different institutions using one of three different NMHCT conditioning regimens: 120 mg/kg cyclophosphamide/125 mg/m^2 fludarabine ($n = 18$); 8 mg/kg busulfan/150 mg/m^2 fludarabine/antithymocyte globulin (ATG) ($n = 5$); or 200 cGy TBI/90 mg/m^2 fludarabine ($n = 2$) (Childs *et al.*, unpublished data). Engraftment was documented in 24 of 25 patients. Twelve patients (48%) developed grade II–IV acute GVHD, including 11 who had GVHD involving the skin. Eleven patients (92%) responded to immunosuppressive therapy while one died from grade IV steroid-refractory liver GVHD. Five patients (20%) had radiographically documented disease regression consistent with a disease response (all partial responses); four responses occurred in the immediate post-transplant period, likely the consequence of a chemotherapy effect, while one response was delayed in onset and occurred in association with chronic skin GVHD consistent with a GVT effect. None of the disease responses were durable with melanoma progression occurring within 1–3 months in all responders. Six patients were treated with DLI for tumor progression without evidence for a response. Unfortunately, none of the 25 patients transplanted survive. Two (8%) died from transplant-related complications (acute GVHD and idiopathic encephalitis) and 23 (92%) died from progression of metastatic disease. Median survival was only 100 days (range 7–660 days) with no survival difference seen between the five responding patients (median survival 114 days) and the 20 non-responding patients (median survival 93 days).

The disappointing outcome of NMHCT in this tumor is perplexing, particularly when clinically meaningful GVT effects in RCC have been demonstrated. Rapid tumor kinetics and bulky metastatic disease may explain, at least in part, why some patients failed to manifest a GVT effect. However, of more concern was the observation that some patients appeared to have acceleration in the pace of tumor growth in the immediate post-transplant period following NMHCT (D. Niederweiser, personal communication). While the description of this phenomenon is admittedly subjective and could simply reflect the natural evolution of the growth kinetics of the tumor, it is alluring to speculate that transplant-induced immunosuppression could promote tumor progression as a consequence of the destruction of innate host immune surveillance. These preliminary data demonstrate that transient conditioning-related regression of metastatic melanoma may occur following NMHCT, although the likelihood of a clinically meaningful GVT effect appears low. The high risk of death from rapid disease progression has discouraged investigators from pursing similar NMHCT studies in melanoma patients. Preclinical studies of "tumor targeted" allogeneic transplant approaches are needed and, if successful, could lead to future "second generation" NMHCT trials in metastatic melanoma.

NMHCT in other solid tumors

The collective global experience of NMHCT in solid tumors other that RCC and melanoma is limited to a handful of publications, all with small patient numbers. However, the important observation of GVT effects in patients with RCC will likely lead to a rapid rise in the number of experimental transplants conducted for other types of treatment-refractory solid tumors. Indeed, GVT effects against metastatic breast carcinoma following a fully myeloablative HCT have been described in some patients in association with acute GVHD [42,43]. The high prevalence of breast carcinoma in the general population as well as the recent disappointing results of autologous transplantation trials has inspired a number investigators to explore NMHCT in patients with this malignancy. Bregni *et al.* [61] treated six patients with metastatic breast cancer with NMHCT following conditioning with cyclophosphamide, fludarabine and thiotepa. Two patients had a partial response that was delayed and did not occur until several months following transplantation. In both cases, responses were preceded by DLIs and GVHD, consistent with a GVT effect.

A small number of NMHCTs have also been performed in patients with advanced ovarian cancer (Table 86.2). One group reported delayed tumor regression in a patient with metastatic ovarian carcinoma who received an HLA-matched transplant from her sibling donor [44]. A small series of patients ($n = 5$) with treatment-refractory ovarian carcinoma who underwent HCT following either myeloablative (one of five) or nonmyeloablative (four of five) conditioning was recently reported [63]. Three patients had regression of metastasis and/or a decrease in disease-related serum markers (i.e. CA 125) early in the post-transplant period. The proximity of tumor shrinkage to chemotherapeutic conditioning makes it unclear whether these responses were truly related to an alloimmune effect. Longer follow-up and additional patients should clarify whether this tumor is indeed responsive to a GVT effect.

Another group reported the results of a NMHCT that used either cladribine or fludarabine in combination with busulfan and ATG in seven patients with variety of different solid tumors [67]. Partial disease regression ascribed to a GVT effect was reported in a patient with osteosarcoma and two patients with RCC.

In summary, insufficient data are available at this time to comment on the efficacy of NMHCT in the vast majority of solid tumors. Interpreting these limited data is made even more difficult as it is often not clear whether disease regression is related to chemotherapeutic agents in the conditioning regimen or is truly the sequelae of a donor immune mediated GVT effect. Strict adherence to criteria such as those outlined in Table 86.1 may help substantiate that a GVT effect has indeed occurred and should minimize the risk of inadvertent overinterpretation of clinical data.

The efficacy of GVL in terms of its ability to induce remission varies among these malignancies, with the critical determining factors dictating neoplastic susceptibility to GVL not entirely understood.

Mechanisms underlying GVT effects in solid tumors

Disease regression following allotransplantation in some patients with treatment-refractory RCC has stimulated researchers' interest in exploring the mechanisms through which GVT effects occur. A better understanding of both the targets and effectors of the GVT response could lead to the development of safer and more efficacious transplant regimens. Based on clinical data as well as our knowledge of the mediators of the GVL effect, T lymphocytes (both CD8+ and CD4) as well as natural killer (NK) cells probably have a role in mediating immune responses against solid tumors [68–72]. The observation that disease regression is (i) associated with an increase in the percentage of circulating CD8+ T cells with an activated phenotype (DR+/CD38+/CD57+); (ii) does not occur until T-cell chimerism is predominantly donor; and (iii) sometimes follows a DLI provide strong evidence to support this hypothesis [48,73].

What, if any, role allogeneic NK cells have in mediating GVT effects in solid tumors is currently unknown. Researchers have shown that NK cells may play a critical part in mediating GVL effects in patients with acute and chronic myelogenous leukemia undergoing transplants from haploidentical donors with killer immunoglobulin-like receptor (KIR) incompatibility in the GVHD direction (i.e. patient Cw allele mismatched to donor and therefore unable to function as a ligand for donor NK cell KIR) [74,75]. Recently, we have conducted *in vitro* experiments which show NK cell clones generated from KIR mismatched allogeneic donors can kill both melanoma and RCC tumor cells preferentially through KIR incompatibility (T. Igarashi, J. Wynberg & R. Childs, unpublished data). Although not yet explored, these preliminary data would suggest that the antitumor effects seen against acute myeloid leukemia following KIR incompatible allotransplantation might also occur against select solid tumors in the setting of haplotransplantation.

The target antigens involved in GVT effects have not yet been determined, although recent findings suggest that both lineage-restricted and broadly expressed mHAs are potential targets. In an attempt to clarify the role of mHA in alloimmune T-cell responses against RCC, previously characterized mHA-specific CTL clones were tested for cytotoxicity against Epstein–Barr virus transformed B cells (EBV-LCL; HLA matched for the appropriate mHA restricting allele) to first identify RCC patients expressing the relevant antigen. Subsequently, CTL recognizing patients' EBV-LCL were then tested for their ability to recognize mHA present on patients' RCC cells. In the majority of cases, CTL recognizing patients' EBV-LCL also recognized patients' RCC cells, suggesting that broadly expressed mHA could serve as targets for immune mediated tumor regression in the setting of acute GVHD [76].

Preliminary data obtained from patients with RCC regressing after allogeneic transplantation suggest that the target antigens may differ in those who experience tumor regression in the context of GVHD as opposed to those without. T-cell clones that specifically lysed patients' RCC cells or both RCC and patients' hematopoetic cells were isolated and expanded from one responder where a GVT effect occurred in the absence of GVHD. In contrast, we could only expand T-cell clones that reacted against both tumor and hematopoetic cells in a patient who had disease regression that occurred in the setting of acute GVHD [73]. Thus, it is conceivable that cellular immune responses directed against antigens shared by tumor and normal tissues would result in GVHD as well as GVT, while GVT without GVHD would be expected to occur in those having a cellular immune response against tumor-restricted antigens (Fig. 86.7).

The identity of antigens that serve as targets for a GVT effect, specifically those which appear to be restricted to the tumor, could provide clues to the intricate mechanisms of GVT and provide valuable insight that might aid in the development of future tumor-targeted immunotherapeutic approaches. At present, responses following NMHCT have only been observed in patients presenting with the common clear cell form of RCC. Because clear cell RCC is typically associated with a mutation in the von Hippel–Lindau (VHL) tumor suppressor gene, mutant VHL protein or antigens which are up regulated as a consequence of the absence of functional VHL protein (MN/CA9, PDGF, VEGF, etc.) have received considerable scrutiny as possible tumor-associated antigens. Whether

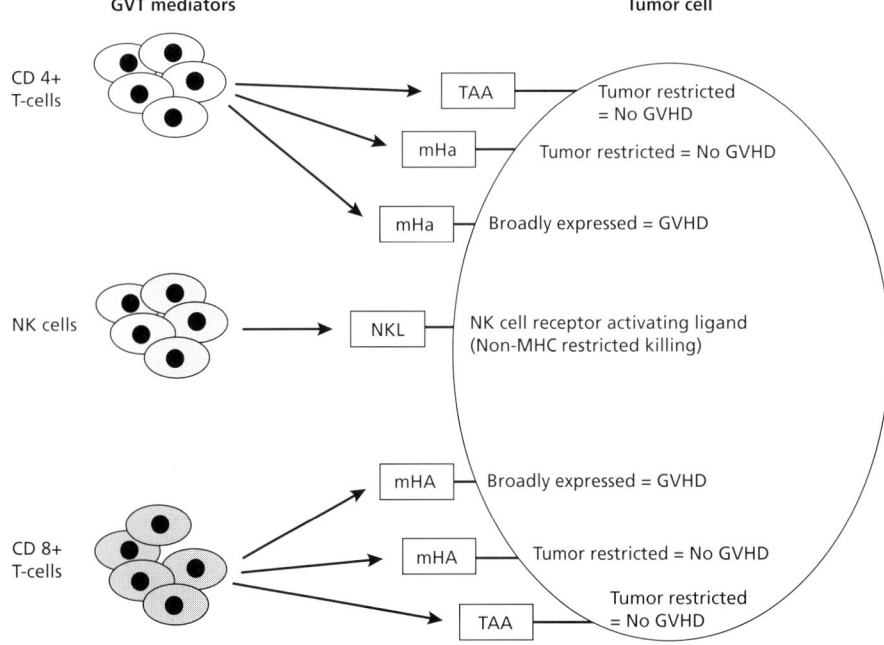

Fig. 86.7 Immune populations hypothesized to contribute to graft-vs.-tumor (GVT) effects following nonmyeloablative hematopoietic cell transplantation (NMHCT). TAA, tumor-associated antigen; mHA, minor histocompatibility antigen either restricted to the tumor (green) or broadly expressed on normal and malignant tissues (red). Tumor cells need to express a dominant natural killer (NK) cell receptor activating ligand (i.e. MIC A) to initiate NK cell-mediated killing.

any of these antigens are targets for the GVT effect in RCC has not yet been elucidated.

Future directions

The lack of efficacy of chemotherapeutics, radiotherapy and cytokine-based immunotherapy for many patients with metastatic cancer has catalyzed, at least in part, enthusiasm for exploring allogeneic-based immunotherapy against solid tumors. While there is little doubt about the potential for its application in oncology, extensive use of NMHCT in the treatment of solid tumors will likely remain limited until both the safety and efficacy of the approach are improved. Further progress in the fields of tumor vaccination and adoptive "tumor targeted" T-cell infusion are needed to address these problems. Recently, murine models have demonstrated that tumor-specific immunity can be boosted following post-transplant tumor immunization. In an MHC-matched but mHA-disparate allotransplant model, immunization of the recipient post-transplant against either leukemia or fibrosarcoma resulted in enhanced antitumor activity without exacerbating GVHD [77]. A similar strategy could be used in humans for those patients who fail to achieve a complete response after NMHCT. Likewise, adoptive transfer of *ex vivo* expanded tumor-specific CTL that are generated from the donor could be used to enhance a GVT effect.

Acute GVHD is undoubtedly the greatest contributor to transplant-related mortality following NMHCT. Allografts that have undergone selective immunodepletion of alloreactive T-cell populations have been studied in murine transplant models and appear to decrease the incidence of GVHD [78–80]. A similar approach is currently under investigation at the NIH for patients with hematologic malignancies. This and similar approaches hold the potential to decrease the toxicity associated with NMHCT and could provide a platform that would enable a method to prevent GVHD without negating GVT effects.

References

1 Thomas ED, Lochte HL Jr, Cannon JH, Sahler OD, Ferrebee JW. Supralethal whole body irradiation and isologous marrow transplantation in man. *J Clin Invest* 1959; **38**: 1709–16.

2 Mathe G, Amiel JL, Schwarzenberg L, Catton A, Schneider M. Adoptive immunotherapy of acute leukemia: experimental and clinical results. *Cancer Res* 1965; **25**: 1525–31.

3 Weiden P, Flournoy N, Thomas E *et al*. Antileukemic effects of graft-versus-host disease in human recipients of allogeneic marrow grafts. *N Engl J Med* 1979; **300**: 1068–73.

4 Horowitz M, Gale RP, Sondel P *et al*. Graft-versus-leukemia reactions after bone marrow transplantation. *Blood* 1990; **75**: 552–62.

5 Apperley JF, Jones L, Hale G *et al*. Bone marrow transplantation for patients with chronic myeloid leukemia: T-cell depletion with Campath-1 reduces the incidence of graft-versus-host disease but may increase the risk of leukemic relapse. *Bone Marrow Transplant* 1986; **1**: 53–68.

6 Goldman JM, Gale RP, Bortin MM *et al*. Bone marrow transplantation for chronic myelogenous leukemia in chronic phase: increased risk of relapse associated with T-cell depletion. *Ann Intern Med* 1988; **108**: 806–14.

7 Marmont AM, Horowitz MM, Gale RP *et al*. T-cell depletion of HLA-identical transplants in leukemia. *Blood* 1991; **78**: 2120–30.

8 Kolb HJ, Mittermueller J, Clemm C *et al*. Donor leukocyte transfusions for treatment of recurrent chronic myelogenous leukemia in marrow transplant patients. *Blood* 1990; **76**: 2462–5.

9 van Besien KW, de Lima M, Giralt SA *et al*. Management of lymphoma recurrence after allogeneic transplantation: the relevance of graft-versus-lymphoma effect. *Bone Marrow Transplant* 1997; **19**: 977–82.

10 Verdonck L, Lokhorst H, Dekker A *et al*. Graft-versus-myeloma effect in two cases. *Lancet* 1996; **347**: 800–1.

11 Tricot G, Vesole D, Jagannath S, Hilton J, Munshi N, Barlogie B. Graft-versus myeloma effect: proof of principle. *Blood* 1996; **87**: 1196–8.

12 Lokhorst HM, Schattenberg A, Cornelissen JJ, Thomas LLM, Verdonck LF. Donor leukocyte infusions are effective in relapsed multiple myeloma after allogeneic bone marrow transplantation. *Blood* 1997; **90**: 4206–11.

13 Jones RJ, Ambinder RF, Piantadosi S, Santos GW. Evidence of a graft-versus-lymphoma effect associated with allogeneic bone marrow transplantation. *Blood* 1991; **77**: 649–53.

14 Kolb H-J, Schattenberg A, Goldman JM *et al*. Graft-versus-leukemia effect of donor lymphocyte transfusions in marrow grafted patients. *Blood* 1995; **86**: 2041–7.

15 Heslop HE, Brenner MK, Rooney CM *et al*. Donor T cells to treat EBV-associated lymphoma. *N Engl J Med* 1994; **331**: 679–80.

16 Papadopoulos EB, Ladanyi M, Emanuel D *et al*. Infusions of donor leukocytes to treat EBV associated lymphoproliferative disorders after allogeneic bone marrow transplantation. *N Engl J Med* 1994; **330**: 1185–91.

17 Mehta J, Powles R, Singhal S, Iveson T, Treleaven J, Catovsky D. Clinical and hematologic response of chronic lymphocytic and prolymphocytic leukemia persisting after allogeneic bone marrow transplantation with the onset of acute graft-versus-host disease: possible role of graft-versus-leukemia. *Bone Marrow Transplant* 1996; **17**: 371–5.

18 Bumpus HC. The apparent disappearance of pulmonary metastasis in a case of hypernephroma following nephrectomy. *J Urol* 1928; **20**: 185.

19 Holland JM, Mitchell TJ, Gipson LC, Whitaker MS. Survival and cause of death in aging germfree athymic nude and normal inbred C3Hf/He mice. *J Natl Cancer Inst* 1978; **61**: 1357–61.

20 Kinlein LJ. Immunologic factors including AIDS. In: Schottenfeld D, Fraumeni JF Jr, eds. *Cancer Epidemiology and Prevention*. New York: Oxford University Press, 1996: 532–45.

21 Servilla KS, Burnham DK, Daynes RA. Ability of cyclosporine to promote the growth of transplanted ultraviolet radiation-induced tumors in mice. *Transplantation* 1987; **44**: 291–5.

22 Rosenberg SA, Yang JC, Topalian SL *et al*. Treatment of 283 consecutive patients with metastatic melanoma or renal cell carcinoma using high-dose bolus interleukin-2. *J Am Med Assoc* 1994; **271**: 907–13.

23 Rosenberg SA, Speiss P, Lafreniere R. A new approach to the adoptive immunotherapy of cancer with tumor-infiltrating lymphocytes. *Science* 1986; **233**: 1318–21.

24 Rosenberg SA, Lotze MT, Muul LM *et al*. A progress report on the treatment of 157 patients with advanced cancer using lymphokine-activated killer cells and interleukin-2 or high-dose interleukin-2 alone. *N Engl J Med* 1987; **316**: 889–97.

25 Belldegrun A, Muul LM, Rosenberg SA. Interleukin 2 expanded tumor-infiltrating lymphocytes in human renal cell cancer: isolation, characterization, and antitumor activity. *Cancer Res* 1988; **48**: 206–14.

26 Topalian SI, Solomon D, Avis FP *et al*. Immunotherapy of patients with advanced cancer using tumor-infiltrating lymphocytes and recombinant interleukin-2: a pilot study. *J Clin Oncol* 1988; **6**: 839–53.

27 Rosenberg SA. The immunotherapy and gene therapy of cancer. *J Clin Oncol* 1992; **10**: 180–99.

28 Rosenberg SA, Lotze MT, Yang JC *et al*. Prospective randomized trial of high-dose interleukin-2 alone or in conjunction with lymphokine-activated killer cells for the treatment of patients with advanced cancer. *J Natl Cancer Inst* 1993; **85**: 622–32.

29 Atkins MB, Dutcher J, Weiss G *et al*. Kidney cancer: the Cytokine Working Group experience, 1986–2001. *Med Oncol* 2001; **18** (3): 197–207.

30 Ada G. The coming of age of tumour immunotherapy. *Immunol Cell Biol* 1999; **77**: 180–5.

31 Rosenberg SA. A new era for cancer immunotherapy based on the genes that encode cancer antigens. *Immunity* 1999; **10**: 281–7.

32 Boon T, Coulie PG, Van den Eynde B. Tumor antigens recognized by T cells. *Immunol Today* 1997; **18**: 267–8.

33 Rosenberg SA, Yang JC, Schwartzentruber DJ *et al*. Immunologic and therapeutic evaluation of a synthetic peptide vaccine for the treatment of patients with metastatic melanoma. *Nature Med* 1998; **4**: 321.

34 Nouri-Shirazi M, Banchereau J, Bell D *et al*. Dendritic cells capture killed tumor cells and present their antigens to elicit tumor-specific immune responses. *J Immunol* 2000; **165**: 3797–803.

35 Goulmy E. Human minor histocompatibility antigens. *Curr Opin Immunol* 1996; **8**: 75–81.

36 De Buerger M, Bakker A, Van Rood JJ, Van der Woude F, Goulmy E. Tissue distribution of minor histocompatibility antigens. *J Immunol* 1992; **149**: 1788–94.

37 Warren EH, Greenberg PD, Riddell SR. Cytotoxic T-lymphocyte-defined human minor histocompatibility antigens with a restricted tissue distribution. *Blood* 1998; **91**: 2197–207.

38. Moscovitch M, Slavin S. Antitumor effects of allogeneic bone marrow transplantation in (NZB X NZW) F1 hybrids with spontaneous lymphosarcoma. *J Immunol* 1984; **132**: 997–1003.
39. Morecki S, Moshel Y, Gelfand Y, Pugatsch T, Slavin S. Induction of graft vs. tumor effect in a murine model of mammary carcinoma. *Int J Cancer* 1997; **71**: 59–63.
40. Morecki S, Yacovlev E, Diab A, Slavin S. Allogeneic cell therapy for murine mammary carcinoma. *Cancer Res* 1998; **58**: 3891–5.
41. Ben-Yosef R, Or R, Nagler A, Slavin S. Graft-versus-tumour and graft-versus-leukaemia effect in patient with concurrent breast cancer and acute myelocytic leukaemia. *Lancet* 1996; **348**: 1242–3.
42. Eibl B, Schwaighofer H, Nachbaur D et al. Evidence of a graft-versus-tumor effect in a patient treated with marrow ablative chemotherapy and allogeneic bone marrow transplantation for breast cancer. *Blood* 1996; **88**: 1501–8.
43. Ueno NT, Rondon G, Mirza NQ et al. Allogeneic peripheral-blood progenitor-cell transplantation for poor-risk patients with metastatic breast cancer. *J Clin Oncol* 1998; **16**: 986–93.
44. Bay JO, Choufi B, Pomel C et al. Potential allogeneic graft-versus-tumor effect in a patient with ovarian cancer. *Bone Marrow Transplant* 2000; **25** (6): 681–2.
45. Khouri IF, Keating M, Korbling M et al. Transplant-lite: induction of graft versus malignancy using fludarabine-based nonablative chemotherapy and allogeneic blood progenitor-cell transplantation as treatment for lymphoid malignancies. *J Clin Oncol* 1998; **16**: 2817–24.
46. Giralt S, Estey E, Albitar M et al. Engraftment of allogeneic hematopoietic progenitor cells with purine analog-containing chemotherapy: harnessing graft versus leukemia without myeloablative therapy. *Blood* 1997; **89**: 4531–6.
47. Slavin S, Nagler A, Naparastak E et al. Nonmyeloablative stem cell transplantation and cell therapy as an alternative to conventional bone marrow transplantation with lethal cytoreduction for the treatment of malignant and nonmalignant hematologic diseases. *Blood* 1998; **91**: 756–63.
48. Childs R, Chernoff A, Contentin N et al. Regression of metastatic renal-cell carcinoma after nonmyeloablative allogeneic peripheral-blood stem-cell transplantation. *N Engl J Med* 2000; **343** (11): 750–8.
49. McSweeney PA, Niederwieser D, Shiruzu JA. Hematopoietic cell transplantation in older patients with hematologic malignancies: replacing high-dose cytotoxic therapy with graft-versus-tumor effects. *Blood* 2001; **97** (11): 3390–400.
50. Motzer RJ, Bander NH, Nanus DM. Renal-cell carcinoma. *N Engl J Med* 1996; **335** (12): 865–75.
51. Quesada JR, Swanson DA, Trindade A. Renal cell carcinoma: anti-tumor effects of leukocyte interferon. *Cancer Res* 1983; **43**: 940.
52. Negrier S, Escudier B, Lasset C et al. Recombinant human interleukin-2, recombinant human interferon alfa 2a, or both in metastatic renal-cell carcinoma. *N Engl J Med* 1998; **338**(18): 1272–8.
53. Fairlamb DJ. Spontaneous regression of metastases of renal cancer: a report of two cases including the first recorded regression following irradiation of a dominant metastasis and review of the world literature. *Cancer* 1981; **47**: 2102–6.
54. Childs R, Clave E, Tisdale J et al. Successful treatment of metastatic renal cell carcinoma with a nonmyeloablative allogeneic peripheral blood progenitor cell transplant: evidence for a graft-versus-tumor effect. *J Clin Oncol* 1999; **17**: 2044–51.
55. Hochster H, Oken M, Bennett J et al. Efficacy of cyclophosphamide (CYC) and fludarabine (FAMP) as first line therapy of low-grade non-Hodgkin's lymphoma (NHL): ECOG 1491. *Blood* 1994; **84**: 383a [Abstract].
56. Flinn IW, Byrd JC, Morrison C et al. Fludarabine and cyclophosphamide with filgrastim support in patients with previously untreated indolent lymphoid malignancies. *Blood* 2000; **96**: 71–5.
57. Childs R, Clave E, Contentin N et al. Engraftment kinetics after nonmyeloablative allogeneic peripheral blood stem cell transplantation: full donor T-cell chimerism preceded alloimmune responses. *Blood* 1999; **94**: 3234–41.
58. Carvallo C, Kurlander R, Geller N, Griffith L, Linehan WM, Childs R. Prior chemotherapy facilitates donor engraftment following nonmyeloablative allogeneic stem cell transplantation. *Blood* 2002; **100** (11): 620a.
59. Rini BI, Zimmerman T, Stadtler WM et al. Allogeneic stem-cell transplantation of renal cell cancer after nonmyeloablative chemotherapy: feasibility, engraftment, and clinical results. *J Clin Oncol* 2002; **20**: 2017–24.
60. Rini B, Zimmerman TM, Gajewski TF et al. Allogeneic peripheral blood stem cell transplantation for metastatic renal cell carcinoma. *J Urol* 2001; **165**: 1208–9.
61. Bregni M, Dodero A, Peccatori J et al. Nonmyeloablative conditioning followed by hematopoietic cell allografting and donor lymphocyte infusions for patients with metastatic renal and breast cancer. *Blood* 2002; **99**: 4234–1.
62. Pedrazzoli P, Da Prada GA, Giogiani G et al. Allogeneic blood stem cell transplantation after a reduced-intensity preparative regimen: a pilot study in patients with refractory malignancies. *Cancer* 2002; **94**: 2409–15.
63. Bay JO, Fleury J, Choufi B et al. Allogeneic hematopoietic stem cell transplantation in ovarian carcinoma: results of five patients. *Bone Marrow Transplant* 2002; **30** (2): 95–102.
64. Przepiorka P, Kernan NA, Ippoliti C et al. Daclizumab, a humanized anti-interleukin-2 receptor alpha chain antibody, for treatment of acute graft-versus-host disease. *Blood* 2000; **95**: 83–9.
65. Anderlini P, Andersson B, Champlin R et al. Infliximab for the treatment of graft-versus-host disease in allogeneic transplant recipients. *Proc Am Soc Hematol* 1999; **52a**: 200.
66. Srinivasan R, Geller N, Chakrabarti S et al. High response rate and improved survival in patients with steroid-refractory acute graft-vs.-host disease treated with daclizumab with or without infliximab. *Blood* 2002; **100** (11): 173a.
67. Makimoto A, Mineishi S, Tanosaki R et al. Non-myeloablative stem cell transplantation (NST) for refractory solid tumors. *Proc Am Soc Clin Oncol* 2001; **20**: 44.
68. Truitt RL, Atasoylu AA. Contribution of CD4[+] and CD8[+] T cells to graft versus host disease and graft versus leukemia reactivity after transplantation of MHC-compatible bone marrow. *Bone Marrow Transplant* 1991; **8**: 51–8.
69. Faber LM, Van Luxemburg-Heijs SAP, Willemze R et al. Generation of leukemia-reactive cytotoxic T lymphocyte clones from the HLA-identical bone marrow donor of a patient with leukemia. *J Exp Med* 1992; **176**: 1283–9.
70. Jiang Y-Z, Barrett AJ. Cellular and cytokine mediated effects of CD4-positive lymphocyte lines generated *in vitro* against chronic myelogenous leukemia. *Exp Hematol* 1995; **23**: 1167–72.
71. Jiang Y-Z, Mavroudis D, Dermime S et al. Alloreactive CD4[+] T lymphocytes can exert cytotoxicity to chronic myeloid leukemia cells processing and presenting exogenous antigen. *Br J Hematol* 1996; **93**: 606–12.
72. Jiang Y-Z, Barrett AJ, Goldman JM et al. Association of natural killer cell immune recovery with a graft versus leukemia effect independent of graft versus host disease following allogeneic bone marrow transplantation. *Ann Hematol* 1997; **74**: 1–6.
73. Mena O, Igarashi T, Srinivasan R et al. Immunologic mechanisms involved in the graft versus tumor effect in renal cell carcinoma (RCC) following nonmyeloablative allogeneic peripheral blood stem cell transplantation. *Blood* 2001; **98**: 356a.
74. Ruggeri L, Cappani M, Martelli MF, Velardi A. Cellular therapy: exploiting NK cell alloreactivity in transplantation. *Curr Opin Hematol* 2001; **8** (6): 355–9.
75. Ruggeri L, Cappani M, Urbani E et al. Effectiveness of donor natural killer cell alloreactivity in mismatched hematopoietic transplants. *Science* 2002; **295**: 2097–100.
76. Childs RW, Mena OJ, Tykodi S, Riddell S, Warren E. Minor histocompatibility antigens (mHA) are expressed on renal cell carcinoma (RCC) cells and are potential targets for a graft-vs.-tumor effect (GVT) following allogeneic blood stem cell transplantation (SCT). *Proc Am Soc Clin Oncol* 2002; **21**: 433a.
77. Anderson AD, Savary CA, Mullen CA. Immunization of allogeneic bone marrow transplant recipients with tumor cell vaccines enhances graft-versus-tumor activity without exacerbating graft-versus-host disease. *Blood* 2000; **95**: 2426–33.
78. Koh MB, Prentice HG, Lowdell MW. Selective removal of alloreactive cells from haematopoietic stem cell grafts: graft engineering for GVHD prophylaxis. *Bone Marrow Transplant* 1999; **23**: 1071–9.
79. Montagna D, Yvon E, Calcaterra V et al. Depletion of alloreactive T cells by a specific anti-interleukin-2 receptor p55 chain immunotoxin does not impair *in vitro* antileukemia and antiviral activity. *Blood* 1999; **93**: 3550–7.
80. Cavazzana-Calvo M, Stephan JL, Sarnacki S et al. Attenuation of graft-versus-host disease and graft rejection by *ex vivo* immunotoxin elimination of alloreactive T cells in an H-2 haplotype disparate mouse combination. *Blood* 1994; **83**: 288–98.

Section 6

Autologous Transplantation for Acquired Diseases

87

Philip J. Bierman & Auayporn Nademanee

Autologous and Allogeneic Hematopoietic Cell Transplantation for Hodgkin's Disease

It is estimated that there were approximately 7000 new cases of Hodgkin's disease (HD) in the USA in 2002 and that 1400 people died with this diagnosis [1]. The first effective combination chemotherapy for HD was developed approximately 40 years ago, and this accomplishment ranks as one of the greatest achievements in modern medicine. More than 50% of patients with advanced HD can be cured with initial combination chemotherapy regimens [2,3], but unfortunately a significant number of patients will fail to attain a complete remission or will relapse after achieving an initial remission. The results of conventional-dose salvage chemotherapy for this group of patients are disappointing.

The poor results of conventional salvage therapy for relapsed and refractory HD has led to the use of high-dose therapy followed by autologous bone marrow transplantation (BMT) and peripheral blood hematopoietic cell (PBHC) transplantation for these patients. This approach is based on the steep dose–response curves exhibited by several drugs, as well as radiation therapy, against HD. In the 1950s the first attempts at using autologous bone marrow to reduce myelosuppression following radiation and chemotherapy were documented [4,5]. Later, techniques for bone marrow harvesting and cryopreservation were refined and the first series of patients undergoing autologous BMT for HD were reported [6–8].

The use of high-dose therapy followed by autologous hematopoietic cell transplantation (HCT) for HD has increased dramatically and has become accepted therapy in certain situations. More than 1200 autologous HCTs for HD were reported to the Autologous Blood and Marrow Transplant Registry (ABMTR) in 2000, and it is estimated that this total represents approximately 60% of the transplants being performed for this indication in North and South America [9]. Similar indications for transplantation are noted in Europe, where 1226 autologous HCTs were reported to the European Group for Blood and Marrow Transplantation (EBMT) in 2000 [10]. This value represents approximately 10% of the volume of autologous HCTs performed for all indications during this period. Over the last 15 years autologous HCT has become easier, safer and less expensive. Several groups of investigators have documented dramatic improvements in transplant outcome over this time period [11–15]. These improvements are related to increased experience at individual institutions, improved patient selection criteria, the routine use of hematopoietic growth factors and the near-universal use of PBHC transplantation. Autologous HCT is commonly performed by community oncologists and outpatient transplants are now common [16,17].

Results of autologous hematopoietic cell transplantation

The results of several series of autologous HCT for HD are displayed in Table 87.1. Results cannot be directly compared because of differences in selection criteria, patient characteristics, high-dose therapy regimens and supportive care. In addition, the length of follow-up varies considerably and some reports include patients transplanted before the routine use of PBHC transplantation and hematopoietic growth factors. Furthermore, these reports may have differences in the definition of important variables, such as early mortality and other outcomes. Nevertheless, these results demonstrate that a significant proportion of patients can achieve long-term disease-free survival following HCT, and that HCT can be accomplished with low early mortality. It must also be noted that results of autologous HCT for HD may change as more effective primary chemotherapy regimens are utilized [3,37].

The results of autologous HCT for patients with relapsed and refractory HD appear better than those reported with conventional-dose salvage chemotherapy. However, conventional-dose salvage chemotherapy may also yield prolonged disease-free survival in some situations [38]. Even in the best situations, >30% of transplant candidates may never proceed to transplantation, and it has been suggested that superior results in transplanted patients may be related to selection bias [39,40].

Two randomized trials have compared the results of conventional salvage chemotherapy with autologous HCT for relapsed and refractory HD. A British National Lymphoma Investigation (BNLI) trial randomized patients with relapsed and refractory HD to receive either treatment with mini-BEAM (carmustine, etoposide, cytarabine, melphalan) conventional-dose salvage chemotherapy or to treatment with BEAM (same drugs at higher doses) followed by autologous BMT [41]. This study design tested the role of dose-intensity in the treatment of HD because the same drugs were used in each treatment arm. The 3-year event-free survival was estimated to be 53% in transplanted patients, as compared with 10% in the group that received mini-BEAM (Fig. 87.1). The risk of progression was also significantly lower in transplanted patients, although no significant differences in overall survival were observed. Some of the participants preferred treatment with autologous BMT and refused randomization, and the study was terminated early. The German Hodgkin's Lymphoma Study Group (GHSG) and the EBMT conducted the second randomized trial [42]. This study was also closed early because of low accrual. Patients were randomized and then received two courses of salvage chemotherapy with Dexa-BEAM (dexamethasone, carmustine, etoposide, cytarabine, melphalan). Responding patients then received either two additional courses of Dexa-BEAM, or high-dose BEAM followed by autologous HCT. At a median follow-up of 39 months, the freedom from treatment failure at 3 years was estimated to be 55% for patients given high-dose BEAM with autologous HCT, as compared with 34% for those who received Dexa-BEAM alone ($p = 0.019$) (Fig. 87.2). Despite this difference, overall survival rates were estimated to be 71% and 65%, respectively ($p = 0.331$).

Table 87.1 Results of autologous hematopoietic cell transplantation for Hodgkin's disease.

Reference	n	Rescue source	Regimen	Median follow-up	Early mortality (%)	Outcome
[18]	50	BM	CBV	NS	4	12 (24%) CCR (9–32 month)
[19]	26	BM	CY + TBI	3.8 year	23	27% PFS
[20]	56	BM	CBV	3.5 year	21	47% 5-year EFS
[21]	35	BM	BEP	13 month	3	16 (46%) CCR (10–52 month)
[22]	21	BM	CBV + Plat	NS	10	29% 3-year DFS
[23]	73	BM, PB	VP16 + Mel	30 month	4	39% 4-year DFS
[24]	25	PB	CY + TBI + MTX + VP16 + Mel	67 month	NS	48% PFS
[25]	47	BM	CY + VP16 + TLI	40 month	17%	50% DFS
[26]	58	BM, PB	CBV ± Plat	2.3 year	5	64% PFS
[27]	155	BM	BEAM	NS	10	50% 5-year DFS
[28]	128	BM, PB	CBV	77 month	9	25% 4-year FFS
[29]	85	BM, PB	CY + VP16 + TBI or CBV	28 month	8	58% 2-year EFS
[30]	62	BM, PB	CBV	NS	0	38% 3-year DFS
[31]	42	BM, PB	BEAM	33 month	2	74% 2-year EFS
[32]	119	BM, PB	Various	40 month	5	48% 4-year EFS
[33]	102	BM, PB	CBV	4.1 year	12	42% 3-year PFS
[34]	280	BM, PB	Various	36 month	6	60% 4-year PFS
[12]	70	BM, PB	BEAC	3.6 year	13	32% 5-year EFS
[35]	414	BM, PB	Various	46 month	7	63% 3-year OS
[36]	40	PB	BEAM	28 month	3	69% 3-year PFS
[13]	56	PB	CY + VP16 + TBI or CBV	43 month	4	68% 3-year EFS
[14]	494	BM, PB	Various	30.5 month	9	45% 5-year EFS
[15]	104	BM, PB	Various	5.1 year	16	26% 10-year EFS

BEAM, carmustine, etoposide, cytarabine, melphalan; BEP, carmustine, etoposide, cisplatin; BM, bone marrow; CBV, cyclophosphamide, carmustine, etoposide; CCR, continuous complete remission; DFS, disease-free survival; EFS, event-free survival; FFS, failure-free survival; Mel, melphalan; MTX, methotrexate; NS, not stated; OS, overall survival; PB, peripheral blood; PFS, progression-free survival; Plat, cisplatin; TBI, total body irradiation; TLI, total lymphoid irradiation.

Autologous HCT has also been compared with conventional salvage chemotherapy in nonrandomized trials. A French–Belgian study retrospectively analyzed treatment results in 187 HD patients after first relapse [43]. Overall survival and freedom from second failure were projected to be 55% and 37%, respectively, for patients who were treated with conventional salvage chemotherapy regimens. Among patients treated with high-dose therapy and autologous HCT, the overall survival and freedom from second failure were projected to be 69% and 57%, respectively (p = n.s.). A trend in favor of better overall survival and freedom from second progression in transplanted patients was noted in the subset with adverse prognostic characteristics, but differences were not statistically significant. Investigators at Stanford University retrospectively analyzed results of autologous HCT in HD patients with primary refractory disease or in first relapse [44]. The outcome was compared with the results of conventional salvage therapy in historical controls. At 4 years, the event-free survival was estimated to be 53% following transplantation, as compared with 27% for patients who received conventional salvage therapy (p <0.01). Nevertheless, overall survival rates were 54% and 47%, respectively (p = 0.25). A French case–control study compared the results of autologous HCT and conventional therapy for HD patients with induction failure [45]. The overall survival rate at 6 years was estimated to be 38% following transplantation, as compared with 29% for conventionally treated patients (p = 0.058). The Groupe d'Etude des Lymphomes de l'Adulte (GELA) retrospectively analyzed results of salvage therapy for HD in patients who failed to attain a complete response on its H89 trial [46]. The 5-year overall survival was estimated at 71% for patients treated with autologous HCT, as compared to 32% for the 48 patients treated without HCT (p = 0.0001). A multivariate analysis revealed that the use of autologous HCT was associated with improved failure-free survival and overall survival in this population of patients (p = 0.02).

These studies have consistently demonstrated that high-dose therapy and autologous HCT improves failure-free survival for patients with relapsed and refractory HD. These studies have also shown trends in favor of improved overall survival, although statistically significant advantages in favor of high-dose therapy and autologous HCT have not been conclusively demonstrated in randomized trials.

Prognostic factors

A large number of variables associated with outcome following autologous HCT for HD have been identified. Several prognostic models have been developed for predicting outcome following transplantation. Reece et al. [26] examined the role of several factors among patients undergoing autologous BMT for HD in first relapse. A model was developed based upon the presence of systemic symptoms or extranodal disease at relapse, and initial remission duration <12 months. The 3-year progression-free survival was estimated at 100%, 81%, 40% and 0% for patients with 0, 1, 2 or 3 risk factors, respectively. In a more recent study, investigators from Memorial Sloan-Kettering Cancer Center validated this model in a group of 57 patients who received autologous HCT for HD [13]. A similar model for patients transplanted with relapsed or refractory HD was developed at Stanford University [32]. The presence of bone marrow or pulmonary involvement, systemic symptoms at relapse and more than minimal disease (>75% reduction in a bulky mass or no nodes >2 cm and

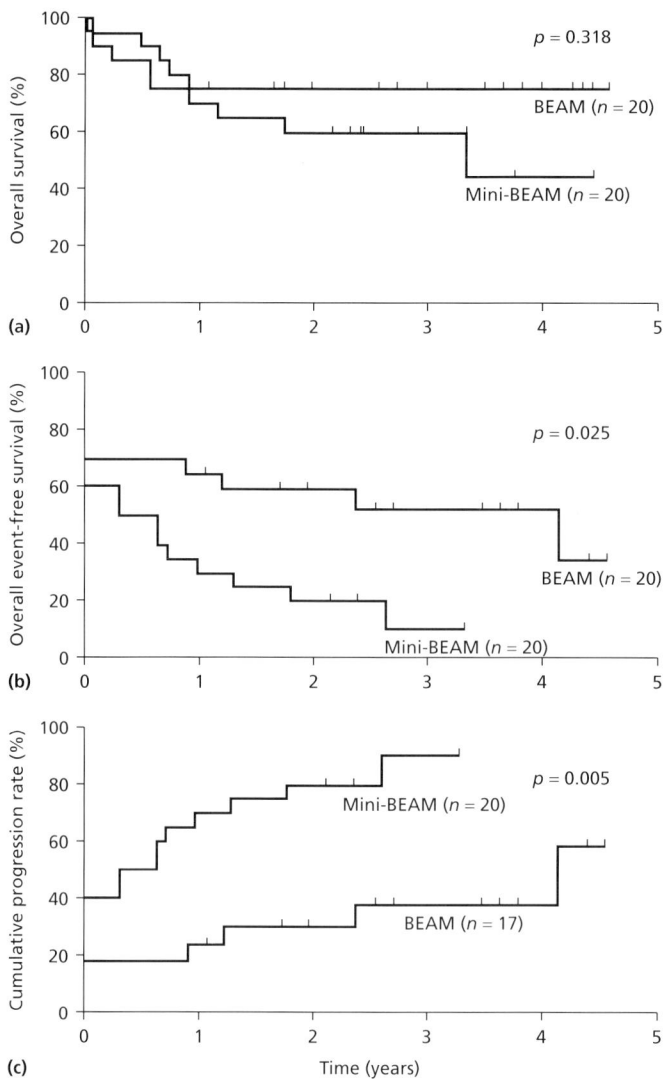

Fig. 87.1 Overall survival, event-free survival, and cumulative progression rate in carmustine, etoposide, cytarabine and melphalan (BEAM) plus autologous bone marrow transplant (ABMT) and mini-BEAM groups. (Reprinted from [41].)

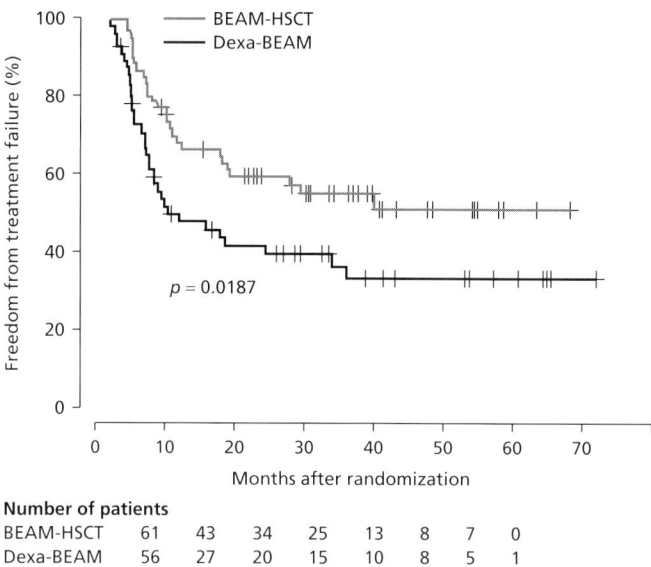

Fig. 87.2 Freedom from treatment failure for patients with relapsed chemosensitive Hodgkin's disease. (Reprinted from [42].)

Table 87.2 Adverse prognostic factors: autologous hematopoietic cell transplantation for Hodgkin's disease.

Prognostic factor	Reference
Bulky or "nonminimal" disease at transplant	[12,23,27,30,32,51,52]
Extensive therapy before transplant	[14,27–29,53,54]
Poor performance status	[19,20,22,28,33,35]
Short initial remission	[26,27,34,39,40,43,55]
Extranodal disease at relapse or at transplant	[26,29,32–34,39]
Systemic symptoms at relapse	[26,30,32,44]
Chemotherapy resistance	[12,14,15,34–36,40,46,56]
Female gender	[27]
Age	[49]
Advanced stage at relapse	[36,43]
Progressive disease at transplant	[33]
Elevated LDH level at transplant	[31,35]
Anemia at relapse or transplant	[39,49]
Hypoalbuminemia at transplant	[49]

LDH, lactate dehydrogenase.

<10% marrow involvement) at HCT were associated with significantly worse overall survival, event-free survival and freedom from progression. Actuarial freedom from progression at 3 years was estimated to be 85%, 57%, 41% and <20% for patients with 0, 1, 2 and 3 risk factors, respectively. Wheeler *et al.* [33] developed a prognostic index based upon the presence of progressive disease at time of HCT, more than one extranodal site of disease at relapse and reduced performance status. The 3-year actuarial survival was 82%, 56% and 19% for patients with 0, 1 or ≥2 risk factors, respectively. Brice *et al.* [34] noted that overall survival was significantly worse for patients who relapsed within 12 months of completing therapy for HD and for patients with extranodal relapse. The 4-year overall survival was estimated to be 93%, 59% and 43%, for patients with 0, 1 or 2 risk factors, respectively.

Josting *et al.* [47] analyzed patients who relapsed after treatment with GHSG protocols and identified short remission, advanced stage at relapse and anemia at relapse as adverse prognostic factors. An index based upon the presence of 0, 1, 2 or 3 of these risk factors was able to identify groups with significantly different rates of survival following autologous HCT ($p<0.0001$). Investigators at the University of Nebraska analyzed whether the prognostic factors used in the International Prognostic Factors Project Score for advanced HD [48] would also be useful for patients undergoing HCT [49]. Low serum albumin, anemia, age and lymphocytopenia were associated with inferior outcomes. The estimated 10-year overall survival rates were 48%, 35%, 27% and 20% for patients with 0, 1, 2 or ≥3 risk factors, respectively. Other indices have also been described [50].

Risk factors associated with adverse outcome following autologous HCT for HD are displayed in Table 87.2. It should be noted that individual prognostic factors have significance in some studies, but not others. These differences are likely related to differences in patient characteristics, selection bias and sample size. Nevertheless, most studies show that extensive therapy prior to transplant, poor performance status, chemotherapy resistance and active disease at the time of transplant are predictive of poor outcome after autologous HCT.

Pretransplant "debulking" therapy

Most patients with relapsed non-Hodgkin's lymphoma (NHL) are first treated with conventional salvage chemotherapy to reduce tumor burden prior to autologous HCT. Sensitivity to conventional therapy administered prior to high-dose therapy may be the most important prognostic factor for NHL patients who are treated with autologous HCT [57]. Most patients with relapsed HD are also treated with a brief course of conventional salvage chemotherapy prior to the administration of high-dose therapy [56,58,59], and most studies show that sensitivity to chemotherapy is an extremely important prognostic factor for these patients (Table 87.2). The potential role of pretransplant conventional salvage chemotherapy was shown in an analysis from the ABMTR where the actuarial 3-year overall survival was 58% for HD patients who received autologous HCT in first relapse, as compared with 75% for patients transplanted in second remission ($p < 0.001$) [35].

Investigators from the University of Rochester reported that 5-year event-free survival was projected to be 46% for patients with minimal disease (all areas ≤2 cm) at the time of HCT, as compared with 10% for those with bulky disease ($p = 0.0002$) [12]. An analysis of autologous HCT results from the Grupo Español de Linfomas/Transplante Autólogo de Médula Ósea (GEL/TAMO) Spanish cooperative group revealed that the 5-year time to treatment failure was projected to be 63.2% following HCT for HD patients transplanted in complete remission, as compared with 32.2% for those with measurable disease [14]. Crump et al. [23] reported that 4-year actuarial disease-free survival was 68% for HD patients who had no evidence of disease at the time of transplant, 26% for patients transplanted with nonbulky disease and 0% for those with bulky disease ($p = 0.0002$). Investigators from Stanford University also reported a significantly higher risk of disease progression among patients with a large tumor burden at the time of transplant [32]. These results suggest that cytoreduction with conventional therapy prior to transplantation is beneficial, although it is possible that the absence of "bulk" is simply a surrogate for chemotherapy sensitivity.

A significant fraction of patients with relapsed and refractory HD fail to respond to conventional salvage therapy and never proceed to transplantation. For this reason a comprehensive two-step transplant regimen was developed at Memorial Sloan-Kettering Cancer Center [13]. This program consists of two cycles of ifosfamide, carboplatin and etoposide (ICE), followed by accelerated fractionation involved-field radiation, and then high-dose therapy and autologous HCT. Eighty-eight percent of patients responded to ICE and the overall survival and event-free survival at a median of 43 months were projected to be 73% and 58%, respectively, for all patients, including those who were never transplanted. This type of intent-to-treat analysis gives a more realistic assessment of the role of transplantation for HD. However, it is possible that pretransplant "debulking" chemotherapy may not be necessary for all patients, and potential disadvantages of this approach for patients with NHL have been described [60]. It is known, for example, that the outcome of allogeneic BMT for acute myeloid leukemia (AML) is similar when patients in early first relapse and those in second remission are compared [61]. A similar situation may exist when autologous HCT for HD is considered. At University College Hospital of London the 5-year progression-free survival was estimated to be 78% in a cohort of patients with HD who were transplanted in "untested" relapse [27]. At the University of Nebraska, the actuarial 5-year overall survival was 100% for patients transplanted without additional therapy after relapse, as compared with 45% for patients who received debulking chemotherapy before transplantation ($p = 0.048$) [55]. A retrospective EBMT analysis showed no significant differences in overall survival or progression-free survival when HD patients in untested relapse and those receiving conventional salvage therapy prior to HCT were compared [51]. Another analysis from the Spanish registry showed that actuarial 5-year progression-free survival was 57% for HD patients transplanted in untested relapse [14].

Patients who are transplanted in untested relapse may do well simply because they have minimal tumor burden at the time of relapse. Furthermore, there is evidence that the use of debulking therapy prior to transplantation for NHL may be beneficial [62]. Nevertheless, it is unknown whether conventional salvage therapy is necessary before transplantation for all patients, especially those with minimal tumor burden at relapse, or those without evidence of disease after biopsy of the site of relapse. However, the vast majority of patients probably benefit from pretransplant chemotherapy, particularly those who have significant tumor burdens. On rare occasions, surgical "debulking" prior to transplantation has also been used [30,63].

Pre- and post-transplant involved-field radiation

Radiation therapy provides effective local control of HD. Because most relapses after autologous HCT for HD occur at sites of prior disease, radiation is frequently used prior to HCT to reduce tumor burden or as consolidative therapy after HCT. There are many unanswered questions regarding the potential advantages and disadvantages of each approach. Pretransplant involved-field radiation can provide effective cytoreduction, and usually does not delay the start of high-dose therapy. This approach also ensures that radiation is delivered, because transplant-related complications can sometimes make it impossible to administer post-transplant irradiation. Numerous institutions have used pretransplant involved-field radiation for patients undergoing autologous HCT for HD, although it has been difficult to demonstrate definite survival advantages associated with this approach and randomized trials have not been performed [19,23,25,29,30,32,64,65]. Investigators at Memorial Sloan-Kettering Cancer Center have utilized a regimen of 1800–3600 cGy accelerated fractionation involved-field radiation administered twice daily over a 5–10-day period prior to HCT [13].

Use of pretransplant involved-field radiation has been associated with improved relapse-free survival, although overall survival advantages have not been demonstrated [64–66]. However, this approach may be associated with increased post-transplant complications such as esophagitis and pulmonary toxicity, especially for those who have received mediastinal irradiation [64,65,67]. In addition, there is evidence from patients undergoing autologous HCT for NHL that the use of radiation therapy as part of initial treatment, or immediately prior to transplantation, may increase the risk of secondary AML or myelodysplasia (MDS) [14,68].

At some institutions post-transplant consolidative radiation has been used routinely following autologous HCT for HD to consolidate areas of prior disease in an attempt to decrease the incidence of relapse [12,14,42]. Delaying radiation until after transplant may decrease the incidence of transplant-related complications and may avoid delays in starting high-dose therapy from toxicities of pretransplant radiation. Post-transplant irradiation can occasionally convert a partial remission after transplantation into a durable complete remission [28,64,69].

A retrospective analysis from the University of Rochester demonstrated that actuarial 5-year event-free survival was 44% for HD patients who received post-transplant consolidative radiotherapy, as compared with 26% for patients who did not receive radiation ($p = 0.0056$) [12]. Potential advantages attributed to post-transplant radiation therapy have been seen in other analyses, although randomized trials have not been conducted [64,66,70,71]. Post-transplant radiation may also lead to significant hematologic and nonhematologic toxicity [72]. Issues relating to selection bias make it difficult to evaluate the advantages of this approach, because patients with early relapse, poor performance status and delayed engraftment may not be able to receive radiation. In addition, the use of radiation therapy with primary therapy makes many patients ineligible for additional radiotherapy. A randomized trial may be necessary to conclusively demonstrate the benefits of pre- and post-transplant radiotherapy and there are numerous unresolved issues regarding the timing and schedule of treatment, treatment fields and radiation dosage.

Post-transplant therapy

In addition to post-transplant involved-field radiation therapy, several investigators have conducted phase 1–2 trials with interferon, interleukin 2 (IL-2), and IL-2 with lymphokine-activated killer cells after autologous HCT for HD [73–76]. Investigators from Israel administered IL-2 in combination with interferon following autologous HCT for HD [77]. The 4-year disease-free survival was estimated to be 88%, as compared with 60% for historical controls who did not receive immunotherapy after transplant ($p < 0.042$). An interim analysis of a randomized trial to test this immunotherapy combination after HCT for HD demonstrated a relapse rate of 16% for patients receiving post-transplant immunotherapy, as compared with 43% for controls [78]. In addition, a retrospective analysis from the Polish Lymphoma Research Group demonstrated that the use of similar immunotherapy following autologous HCT for primary refractory HD was associated with significantly better progression-free survival and overall survival [79]. The use of allogeneic lymphocyte infusions from matched sibling donors following autologous HCT for HD has also been reported [80].

Timing of transplantation

Perhaps the most important issue dealing with autologous HCT for HD relates to the appropriate time to perform transplantation during the course of disease. Although outcomes are improving, transplantation is still expensive and may be associated with morbidity and mortality. Patients with relapsed HD may sometimes be cured with conventional salvage chemotherapy or radiotherapy, and some physicians have elected to delay transplantation until after these approaches fail. Conversely, transplantation should not be delayed until chemotherapy resistance develops and poor performance status makes cure unlikely with any approach. Although decision analysis techniques have been used to determine the optimal timing of transplantation, the assumptions used in these analyses may be invalidated by improved results of transplantation or technology changes that make transplants safer or less expensive [81]. Potential times when autologous HCT for HD can be performed are displayed in Table 87.3. Although data from randomized trials are lacking, results in each situation can be compared to results of conventional salvage therapy.

Failure to attain initial complete remission

Hodgkin's disease patients who do not achieve complete remissions with

Table 87.3 Potential timing of autologous hematopoietic cell transplantation for Hodgkin's disease.

Failure to attain initial complete remission
    Primary refractory
    First partial remission
First relapse
    Short vs. long initial remission
    Initial 4-drug vs. 7- or 8-drug regimen
Second or subsequent relapse
First remission

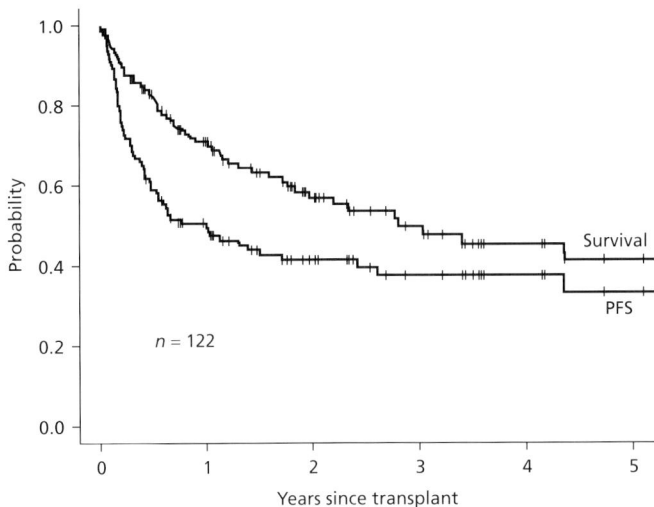

Fig. 87.3 Probability of overall survival and progression-free survival after autotransplantation for Hodgkin's disease in patients never achieving remission. (Reprinted from [83].)

initial chemotherapy have a poor prognosis. At the National Cancer Institute the median survival for patients who did not achieve a complete remission with initial chemotherapy was 16 months, and none of these patients were projected to be alive at 8 years from the time of diagnosis [82]. Bonfante et al. [38] reported that no patients with induction failure were free of disease progression after 8 years and that overall survival at 8 years was estimated to be only 8% for these patients.

Several cooperative groups and single institutions have reported results of high-dose therapy and autologous HCT for primary refractory HD. The ABMTR examined results of autologous HCT in 122 HD patients who had never achieved complete remission [83]. The 3-year actuarial overall survival and progression-free survival were 50% and 38%, respectively (Fig. 87.3). Systemic symptoms at diagnosis and poor performance status at transplant were adverse prognostic factors. The mortality at day 100 was estimated to be 12%. These results are comparable to results of a similar analysis from the EBMT [84]. In this report, the actuarial 5-year overall survival and progression-free survival were 36% and 32%, respectively, in a cohort of 175 patients with primary refractory HD. The early transplant-related mortality was 14%. Other reports of autologous HCT for primary refractory HD are displayed in Table 87.4.

There are no randomized studies comparing high-dose therapy and autologous HCT to conventional salvage therapy in primary refractory HD. At Stanford University, results of autologous HCT for HD patients who failed induction therapy were compared with historical controls who received conventional salvage therapy [44]. The 4-year event-free survival rates were projected to be 52% and 19%, respectively ($p = 0.01$). However, there were no significant differences in overall survival rates (44% vs. 38%, respectively; $p = 0.32$). A case–control study of HD patients with induction failure showed that overall survival 6 years from the time of diagnosis was 38% for transplanted patients, as compared with 29% for patients who received conventional salvage therapy ($p = 0.058$) [45]. A retrospective analysis from Cologne examined outcomes in 67 patients with primary progressive HD [90]. The mean survival was 56.2 months for patients who were treated with autologous HCT, as compared with 11.2 months for those who received conventional salvage therapy. The actuarial 5-year overall survival rates were 53% and 0%, respectively.

Interpretation of results is hampered by confusion regarding the definition of "primary refractory" and "induction failure" in different series. These definitions have included patients with disease progression during

Table 87.4 Results of autologous hematopoietic cell transplantation for Hodgkin's disease patients who fail to attain remission with primary therapy.

Reference	n	Outcome	
[84]	175	32% 5-year PFS	36% 5-year OS
[83]	122	38% 3-year PFS	50% 5-year OS
[45]	86	25% 5-year EFS	35% 5-year OS
[85]	70	31% 5-year PFS	43% 5-year OS
[79]	65	36% 3-year PFS	55% 3-year OS
[14]	49	13% 5-year PFS	
[27]	46	33% 5-year PFS	
[86]	42		49% 4-year OS*
[87]	30	42% 5-year PFS	60% 5-year OS
[88]	30	34% 3-year EFS	51% 3-year OS
[25]	28	33% 4-year DFS	
[89]	28	26% 3-year EFS	34% 5-year OS
[44]	13	52% 4-year PFS	44% 4-year OS
[24]	7	31% 6-year PFS	42% 6-year OS
[29]	6	67% 2-year DFS	

DFS, disease-free survival; EFS, event-free survival; OS, overall survival; PFS, progression-free survival.
*Estimated from survival curve. Some patients received two transplants.

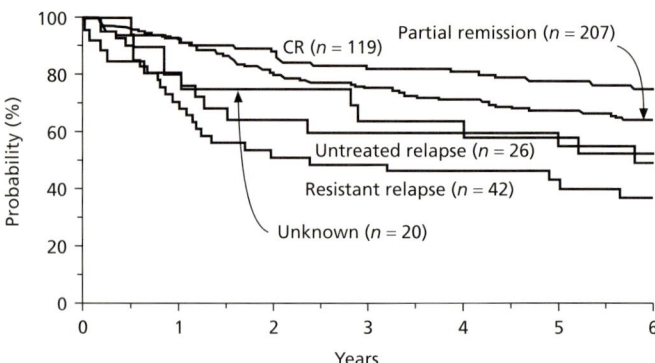

Fig. 87.4 Probability of survival after autotransplant for Hodgkin's disease in second complete remission or first relapse, according to sensitivity to salvage chemotherapy. (Reprinted from [35].)

initial therapy, stable disease after initial therapy, progression within 90 days of completing initial therapy, and partial remission with initial therapy. It would seem that patients who progress on primary therapy, and those who have no response, are likely to have a different prognosis than patients who have a partial remissions or near-complete remission. This concept is supported by French registry data demonstrating significantly worse overall survival and progression-free survival when transplant results for primary refractory patients were compared with results from patients in first partial remission [89].

Interpretation of results is also hampered by the fact that many patients do not have biopsy-proven residual disease before transplantation. It is possible that some patients in these series may have had residual radiographic abnormalities without actually having persistent disease [91]. Inclusion of patients who were actually in remission would improve the results of series reporting results of autologous HCT for primary refractory disease, although this problem would be encountered with any treatment. Finally, it is important to note that a significant proportion of patients with primary refractory disease are not able to undergo autologous HCT and therefore transplanted patients may be highly selected [85]. Nevertheless, the results in Table 87.4 appear superior to those attainable with conventional salvage chemotherapy.

Transplantation appears to be the best option for HD patients who fail to attain complete remission with primary therapy. Additional chemotherapy or radiation may be considered prior to high-dose therapy for patients with significant tumor burden, while other patients with minimal disease persisting after primary therapy may be candidates for immediate transplantation [84]. Despite the improved outcome with high-dose treatment, only a minority of patients with primary refractory HD can achieve prolonged remission, therefore new treatment strategies need to be explored. The French Cooperative Group and GELA are conducting a phase 2 trial of intensified cytoreductive chemotherapy followed by tandem high-dose therapy in HD patients with induction failure.

First relapse

Transplantation for HD is usually considered when patients relapse following their initial chemotherapy-induced complete remission. Several reports of autologous HCT in this situation have been published and allow comparison with results of conventional salvage therapy.

A report from the ABMTR examined results of autologous HCT for HD in first relapse [35]. Outcomes in relation to chemotherapy sensitivity following relapse were examined (Fig. 87.4). The 3-year overall survival rate was projected to be 58%. Reece *et al.* [26] reported that 4-year progression-free survival was estimated to be 64% for patients with HD who were transplanted after their initial relapse. Analyses from the French registry and the EBMT noted progression-free survival rates of 57% and 45%, respectively, following autologous HCT in first relapse [43,51]. Similar results have been reported in other series [24,27,46,55,92,93].

These results appear to be better than those reported for conventional salvage therapy although prospective trials have not been reported. Furthermore, comparable results with conventional salvage chemotherapy have sometimes been described, especially when the duration of initial remission is >12 months [38]. Results of autologous HCT for HD may also be superior when transplantation is preceded by a longer initial remission (Table 87.5). However, the length of initial remission has not influenced outcome in all series [33,51,92,93].

Patients were stratified on the basis of early and late relapse in the randomized GHSG study [42]. Among HD patients with initial remissions lasting <1 year, the 3-year time to treatment failure was estimated to be 41% for transplanted patients, as compared with 12% for patients who continued to receive conventional salvage chemotherapy ($p = 0.008$). However, overall survival was estimated at 43% and 40%, respectively ($p = 0.623$). The actuarial 3-year time to treatment failure for patients with longer first remissions was 75% following autologous HCT, as compared with 44% for patients who received conventional salvage chemotherapy ($p = 0.025$). Overall survival rates were 93% and 75%, respectively ($p = 0.088$). A Stanford University analysis compared transplant results with historical controls for patients in first relapse [44]. The 4-year event-free survival for patients with initial remissions of ≤12 months was estimated to be 56% for transplanted patients, as compared with 19% for those who received conventional salvage chemotherapy ($p < 0.01$). Overall survival rates were 58% and 38%, respectively ($p = 0.15$). No significant differences in overall survival or event-free survival were seen in patients with longer initial remissions.

It has also been suggested that patients who relapse after treatment with a four-drug regimen may have a prognosis that is different than those who relapse after regimens containing seven or eight drugs [81]. A retrospective analysis from the Spanish cooperative group noted that 5-year failure-free survival following HCT for HD was estimated at 40.3% for patients who were initially treated with a regimen containing

Table 87.5 Results of autologous hematopoietic cell transplantation for Hodgkin's disease in first relapse.

Reference	n	Progression-free survival			Overall survival		
		CR <1 year	CR >1 year	p	CR <1 year	CR >1 year	p
[55]	85	32% 5-year	47% 5-year	0.16	44% 5-year	59% 5-year	0.17
[26]	58	48% 4-year	85% 4-year	0.016			
[27]	52	41% 5-year	57% 5-year	0.039			
[34]	280				54% 4-year	73% 4-year	0.05
[14]	284	39% 5-year	52% 5-year	0.003			
[42]	93	41% 3-year	75% 3-year		43% 3-year	93% 3-year	

seven or eight drugs, as compared with 50.2% for those treated with other regimens ($p = 0.05$) [14]. An analysis from the ABMTR showed that patients relapsing after mechlorethamine, vincristine, procarbazine and prednisone (MOPP) had inferior outcomes [35]. However, other analyses have failed to show that transplant outcome is influenced by choice of initial therapy [33,55].

Although overall survival advantages have not been demonstrated, most investigators would recommend autologous HCT for HD patients who relapse within 1 year of attaining remission with initial chemotherapy. There is more controversy regarding management of patients with longer remission because a significant proportion may achieve prolonged second remissions with conventional salvage therapy. It may be reasonable to delay transplantation until second relapse in some patients, although transplantation regardless of length of initial remission has been advocated [42,51,94].

Second or subsequent relapse

Prolonged disease-free survival is unusual following treatment with third-line chemotherapy regimens for HD. No significant differences in time to treatment failure or overall survival were identified when autologous HCT and conventional salvage chemotherapy were compared in patients with multiple relapses in the randomized GHSG trial [42]. However, only 11 patients were transplanted and most investigators would recommend transplantation for HD patients following a second relapse from chemotherapy. Autologous HCT is rarely curative in patients who have experienced multiple relapses. Nevertheless, this treatment is probably the only treatment option for these patients.

First remission

Prospective randomized trials have demonstrated that certain patients with NHL may benefit from consolidation with autologous HCT in first remission [95]. There is less experience with early autologous HCT for HD, although a number of variables have been identified that might be used to identify candidates for this approach [48,96].

Carella et al. [97] reported results of high-dose chemotherapy followed by autologous HCT in 15 HD patients with adverse prognostic characteristics who achieved complete remission following treatment with MOPP/doxorubicin, bleomycin, vinblastine and dacarbazine (MOPP/ABVD). Outcome was compared to concurrently treated patients who also achieved complete remission but were not transplanted. At a median follow-up of 36 months, 87% of transplanted patients were alive and in remission, as compared with 33% of nontransplanted patients who were followed for a median of 42 months (Fig. 87.5). Follow-up data on a larger cohort of 22 patients transplanted in first remission indicated that 77% were in unmaintained remission with a median follow-up of 86 months [98]. A matched-pair analysis from the EBMT and GHSG compared pati-

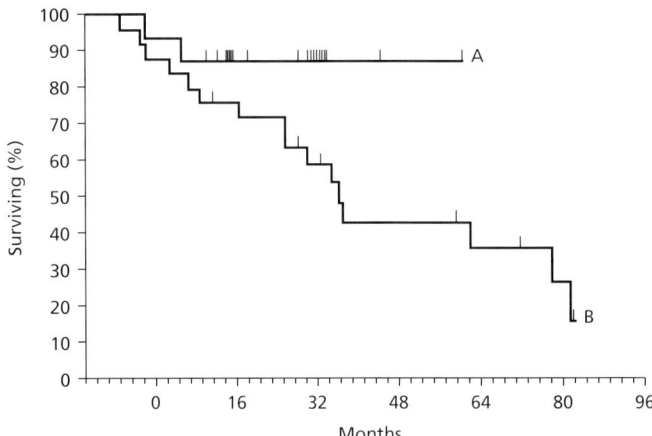

Fig. 87.5 Disease-free survival time in poor-risk Hodgkin's disease patients intensified with autologous bone marrow transplant (ABMT) in (a) first remission; or (b) historical group. (Reprinted from [97].)

Table 87.6 Results of autologous hematopoietic cell transplantation for Hodgkin's disease in first remission.

Reference	n	Outcome
[9]	184	81% 3-year OS
[14]	57	70% 5-year FFS
[89]	45	70% 5-year EFS
[98]	22	77% CCR (34–114 months)
[100]	20	100% CCR (13.2–149.2 months)*
[101]	16	87% 5-year DFS
[102]	13	77% 5-year DFS

CCR, continuous complete remission; DFS, disease-free survival; EFS, event-free survival; FFS, failure-free survival; OS, overall survival.
*Some patients in first partial remission.

ents transplanted in first remission with patients who achieved complete remission with standard therapy [99]. The time to relapse was significantly longer in patients who were consolidated with early autologous HCT, although no significant differences in overall survival were identified.

Results of trials examining autologous HCT for patients with HD in first remission are displayed in Table 87.6. The limited data suggest that time to progression may be prolonged by early transplantation for poor-prognosis HD. However, there is little evidence that overall survival is prolonged, because transplantation or other salvage therapies can be used at relapse. In addition, most series only report outcomes for the selected poor-prognosis patients who are able to be transplanted. It is likely that many patients with adverse prognostic features do not attain remission or may not be transplanted for other reasons, and this "denominator" is rarely reported [102]. Until prospective trials demonstrate significant advantages for patients undergoing autologous HCT for HD in first remission, this approach should not be considered standard therapy.

Autologous HCT for pediatric patients

The prognosis for children with HD is better than for adults. The majority of pediatric HD patients are cured with combination chemotherapy administered alone, or combined with low-dose radiotherapy. Nevertheless, approximately 10–15% of pediatric HD patients fail to achieve a complete response or subsequently relapse. The results of salvage therapy are poor and the use of high-dose therapy and autologous HCT has been extended to the pediatric population.

The results of high-dose therapy and autologous HCT for relapsed or refractory HD in pediatric patients are similar to those reported in adults. A case-matching study from the EBMT compared the results of autologous HCT in 81 HD patients under the age of 16 with results from 81 adults [103]. With a median follow-up of 36 months, the progression-free survival for pediatric patients was estimated at 39%, as compared with 48% in adults who had a median follow-up of 34 months ($p = 0.64$). The patterns of relapse and the incidence of transplant-related toxicities were also similar. Of interest is the fact that male gender was associated with significantly better outcome.

Baker et al. [104] reported results of high-dose therapy and autologous HCT in 53 children and adolescents (age ≤21 years) with relapsed and refractory HD. The actuarial 5-year failure-free survival and overall survival were 43% and 31%, respectively. No significant differences in outcome were observed when younger pediatric patients were compared with adolescents, and no significant differences in outcome were observed when these patients were compared to a historical control group of patients over the age of 21 from the same institution. The 5-year disease-free survival and overall survival were estimated to be 67% and 76%, respectively, in a group of 34 pediatric (≤21 years) patients treated with autologous HCT for relapsed and refractory HD at Stanford University [105]. Inferior outcomes were seen in children with extranodal disease and bulky disease at relapse.

However, somewhat poorer results of HCT were observed in a Children's Cancer Group trial [106]. Children under the age of 21 with relapsed HD received salvage chemotherapy with dexamethasone, etoposide, cisplatin, cytarabine, L-asparaginase (DECAL), which was followed by additional conventional salvage chemotherapy or HCT. There was no survival benefit for the patients with responsive disease who underwent transplant, although this study was not a randomized trial, transplantation protocols were not standardized and some patients received allogeneic HCT.

Long-term failure-free survival can be seen following autologous HCT for children with HD and results appear to be similar to those observed in adults, although the risk of short-term and delayed toxicity is concerning. Although no post-transplant growth and development abnormalities were observed in the Nebraska series, two cases of MDS/AML were encountered [104]. In the Stanford series, 15 children (44%) developed idiopathic diffuse lung injury and four children (12%) died of pulmonary complications [105]. A history of pre-existing atopy was highly predictive of post-transplant pulmonary complications. Late interstitial pneumonitis was also observed in the series from the EBMT [103].

Transplantation for elderly patients

Autologous HCT for various conditions is now routinely performed for patients beyond the age of 60 years. Retrospective series have demonstrated that mortality rates may be somewhat higher and EFS may be lower in elderly patients, although long-term disease-free survival can be observed in this population [107,108]. Although exceptions have been noted [49], most series have failed to identify age as an important variable for patients who undergo autologous HCT for HD. This may relate to the fact that the median age of HD patients in most transplant series is approximately 30 years and few elderly patients are included. Nevertheless, age alone should not exclude an otherwise eligible patient for HCT.

Transplantation for HIV-associated Hodgkin's disease

Early therapeutic approaches to human immunodeficiency virus (HIV) associated lymphoma focused on reduction of chemotherapy dose intensity to reduce the risk of infection and worsening of immune function. Highly active antiretroviral therapy (HAART) has changed the natural history of HIV infection by improving immune function in infected patients. It is now possible for patients with HIV-related NHL to receive the same treatment as HIV-negative individuals, and HIV-infected patients with HD can also be treated aggressively [109].

There are now scattered reports of autologous HCT for HIV-associated HD. Gabarre et al. [110] reported the results of autologous HCT in four patients with relapsed HIV-associated HD. All patients received HAART for a median of 24 months before transplantation and were continued on HAART during hematopoietic cell collection, during transplantation and after transplantation. Three patients achieved a complete response and were alive in complete remission at 4, 13 and 15 months after transplant. One patient died from progressive disease 3 months after HCT. Krishnan et al. [111] described two patients who were treated with autologous HCT for acquired immune deficiency syndrome (AIDS) associated HD. Both patients were alive and in remission following HCT.

The results from these two studies suggest that PBHCs can be successfully collected in HIV-infected individual on HAART, and that autologous HCT can be performed in selected individuals with HIV-associated HD. Whenever possible, candidates for transplant should be entered on clinical trials or referred to centers with experience in this population of patients.

Kang et al. [112] described a case of nonmyeloablative allogeneic transplantation in an HIV-infected patient with HD. A complete response was seen, but the patient died of progressive disease 12 months after transplantation.

Late events

There are increasing numbers of people who are long-term survivors after autologous HCT for HD and other hematologic malignancies. Unfortunately, long-term follow-up data on large numbers of patients are lacking. There are several reports on quality of life after HCT for lymphoma and solid tumors, although no reports have dealt exclusively with outcomes following autologous HCT for HD by itself.

Most surveys indicate that the majority of patients are able to return to a normal functional status and that most are employed or attending school when surveyed beyond 6–12 months after transplant [113–116]. Patients from Stanford University reported that quality of life was 8.9 on a 10.0 scale at 1 year after autologous HCT for HD [115]. A similar survey from Dartmouth-Hitchcock Medical Center indicated that mean global quality of life score was 8.17 on a 10.0 point scale in a cohort of long-term survivors of HCT [116]. Fatigue [116,117] and sexual dysfunction [114,117] appear to be relatively common delayed side-effects.

Patients who undergo autologous HCT for HD are at risk for late relapse. Although some series have not reported late relapses, others have demonstrated that patients continue to be at risk of relapse for at least several years following transplantation. Reports of relapse >6 years following transplantation have been documented [28,118], and relapse nearly 8 years after HCT has been reported [14]. These results indicate that life-long follow-up is necessary after autologous HCT for HD.

There is increasing concern regarding the risk of second malignancies following autologous HCT for HD and NHL. These secondary malignancies are thought to be a consequence of damage induced by radiation or chemotherapy administered prior to HCT or from high-dose therapy regimens themselves. Several series have described the risks of AML and MDS following autologous HCT for HD. The 5-year cumulative risk of developing AML or MDS following autologous HCT for HD was 4.3% in a study from the French Registry [119], 4.6% in an EBMT analysis [120] and 3.1% in an analysis from University College Hospital at London and from BNLI [121]. Other studies have shown a risk of developing AML or MDS that ranges between 4% and 15% within 5 years of autologous HCT for HD [122–125]. This complication may appear within months of the transplant, although MDS/AML may appear several years after the HCT [124].

Several risk factors for the development of post-transplant MDS/AML have been identified. The use of autologous PBHC transplantation, as compared with autologous BMT has been associated with a higher risk of secondary leukemia [119,122,123,126] although this observation may be related to confounding variables. Other risk factors associated with MDS/AML after autologous HCT for HD include older age [14,120], use of total body irradiation (TBI) conditioning or use of radiation with prior chemotherapy [14], pretransplant priming with etoposide [125], splenectomy [119], female gender [120] and time interval from diagnosis to transplant [120].

Several lines of evidence suggest that secondary MDS/AML is related to HD treatment administered prior to transplant rather than the high-dose conditioning regimen itself. Chao et al. [127] detected cytogenetic abnormalities prior to bone marrow harvest and in cryopreserved bone marrow harvests of HD patients who relapsed but had not been transplanted. Investigators have also used fluorescence in situ hybridization (FISH) analysis to demonstrate that the same cytogenetic abnormalities present in post-transplant MDS/AML can be detected in stored pretransplant blood or marrow samples from patients with HD [128]. These observations have led to the recommendation that cytogenetic analysis should be performed in all patients prior to hematopoietic cell collection. In addition, most studies of post-transplant MDS/AML have identified abnormalities of chromosomes 5 and 7 that are associated with typical alkylating agent based therapy administered prior to HCT. The short latency period between autologous HCT and development of MDS/AML in many cases also suggests that malignancy results from prior therapy and not the high-dose chemotherapy regimen.

A French case-matching analysis compared transplanted and nontransplanted HD patients and failed to find that autologous HCT was a significant risk factor for the development of MDS/AML [119]. An analysis from Denmark examined the incidence of secondary MDS/AML from the time of HD diagnosis and also failed to find a higher risk of this complication in transplanted patients [129]. Harrison et al. [121] analyzed results from 4576 HD patients in the BNLI and University College Hospital databases for risk factors associated with the development of secondary MDS or AML. The risk of these complications was related to the extent of prior therapy and to prior exposure to MOPP and lomustine chemotherapy, whereas high-dose chemotherapy was not itself a risk factor. A case–control analysis from the ABMTR also showed that the risk of MDS and leukemia following autologous HCT for HD was primarily related to the use of pretransplant mechlorethamine and chlorambucil [126]. A multivariate analysis from the EBMT found that the risk of secondary MDS/AML following autologous HCT for HD was not signifi-cantly different than the risk of similar patients who were not transplanted [120]. Wheeler et al. [130] noted that the incidence of MDS/AML was higher in HD patients who received high-dose cyclophosphamide, carmustine and etoposide (CBV) before autologous HCT, than patients with NHL who received the same high-dose regimen. The increased risk in patients with HD appeared to be related to the fact that these patients had received more conventional chemotherapy and radiation prior to HCT.

These results suggest that the risk of MDS/AML is primarily related to the type and duration of pretransplant chemotherapy and it appears that the high-dose chemotherapy is associated with less risk than previously feared. Some investigators have used this information to support the recommendation that autologous HCT should be performed early in the course of disease.

The occurrence of solid tumors has also been described following autologous HCT for HD [14], although some institutions have reported a low incidence of this complication [131]. An analysis of data from the French registry indicated that the cumulative risk of developing a solid tumor following HCT was 3.7% at 5 years, and that the administration of high-dose therapy was a risk factor for the development of this complication [119].

Other late complications of autologous transplantation for HD have included delayed infections [14,27,35,51], cardiac complications [27,29] and pulmonary complications [14,29,30,35,118]. Almost all women will develop amenorrhea following autologous HCT for HD, although return of ovarian function is not unusual [132]. Successful pregnancies, both assisted and unassisted, have been described following autologous HCT for HD [27,28,133,134] and patients should be counseled about the need for contraception. Men who undergo autologous HCT for HD may have decreased levels of testosterone and may have an increased risk of sexual dysfunction [135].

Management of relapse

Although many patients appear to be cured, a significant fraction of patients will relapse following autologous HCT for HD. The median survival following disease progression after autologous HCT is <12 months [136,137]. Nevertheless, some patients who progress after transplantation may survive for long periods of time [136–138]. Bolwell et al. [138] noted that median survival was 8 months in patients who relapsed within the first 6 months following autologous HCT, whereas median survival was 30 months for patients who relapsed later ($p = 0.0008$). Investigators from Detroit also noted that time to progression after HCT was associated with outcome [137].

Treatment must be individualized, and options are frequently limited because of prior therapy, low blood counts and poor performance status. Radiation therapy should be considered for patients with localized relapse. High response rates and occasional long-term remissions have been noted with single-agent vinblastine [139], and investigators have reported success with other chemotherapy regimens [140,141]. Surgical resection is occasionally useful and some cases can be managed with a watch-and-wait approach.

Some patients may be candidates for second transplants. The EBMT reported that 50% of selected HD patients were alive and in remission 2 years after a second transplant: 11 autologous, one allogeneic [142]. Others have reported similar results [143]. Mortality rates for allogeneic HCT following failure of autologous HCT for HD are extremely high, although successful transplants have been reported [144]. Freytes et al. [145] analyzed IBMTR results of allogeneic HCT in 114 patients who relapsed after autologous HCT for lymphoma. All patients received myeloablative conditioning, although some patients received unrelated or mismatched transplants. The 3-year cumulative incidence of relapse was 75% and the actuarial 3-year disease-free survival was 33%. Outcomes for patients with HD and NHL were similar. The use of nonmyeloablative allogeneic stem cell transplantation for these patients is being explored (see below).

Peripheral blood hematopoietic cell transplantation

More than 95% of autologous transplants performed in North America and Europe are now being performed using PBHCs, rather than bone marrow [9,10]. A sufficient quantity of cells can frequently be collected with a single apheresis [146]. Hematopoietic recovery is more rapid following PBHC transplantation and this approach allows cells to be collected without the use of general anesthesia. Most important, PBHC can be collected from patients whose marrow cannot be harvested because of tumor involvement or prior radiation.

Retrospective comparisons of autologous BMT and PBHC transplantation in cohorts with HD and NHL have generally failed to show significant differences in overall survival and failure-free survival, although more rapid hematopoietic recovery and shorter hospital stays were seen in patients who were transplanted with PBHCs [147–149].

Three prospective trials in patients with both HD and NHL also compared outcomes following autologous BMT and PBHC transplantation [150–154]. No significant differences in survival were noted, although more rapid engraftment, shorter hospital stays, lower costs and improved quality of life were seen in patients who received PBHC transplants.

Several retrospective analyses in cohorts containing only HD patients have also failed to identify significant survival differences between autologous BMT and PBHC transplants [34,51,63,155]. A univariate analysis from the Spanish registry indicated that transplantation with PBHCs was associated with improved overall survival, although this difference was not seen in the multivariate analysis [14].

An EBMT matched-pair analysis showed that actuarial 4-year progression-free survival was 52% for HD patients who were treated with autologous BMT, as compared with 38% for those who received PBHC transplantation ($p = 0.008$) [156]. A retrospective analysis from the City of Hope National Medical Center also noted that transplantation with PBHCs was associated with a significantly higher risk of treatment failure [92]. However, a single-center matched-pair analysis from University College Hospital at London showed no significant differences in progression-free survival when results of autologous HCT with marrow or blood were compared [157]. The 3-year overall survival rates were 69% and 78%, respectively ($p = 0.078$).

Although transplantation with PBHCs has not been associated with definite survival advantages, this approach is now preferred because of secondary advantages associated with ease of collection and engraftment rate. Reports of inferior results following transplantation of PBHCs will need confirmation [92,156], as will reports of increased risk of secondary MDS/AML [119,122,123,126]. It should also be recognized that enhanced rates of engraftment are associated with the use of *mobilized* PBHC transplants. There is evidence to suggest that hematopoietic recovery may be accelerated when autologous marrow is collected after cytokine administration [158–160], and this technique might negate some of the advantages associated with the use of PBSCs.

Allogeneic HCT for HD

In 2000, approximately 5% of HCTs for HD in North America and Europe used allogeneic donors [9,10]. Allogeneic HCT may be considered for patients with inadequate autologous hematopoietic cell collections, for patients with dysplastic marrow or with cytogenetic abnormalities in the marrow [127]. It has also been suggested that allogeneic HCT might correct the lifelong immunologic defects seen in HD patients [161]. Finally, the use of allogeneic HCT may also result in a graft-vs.-Hodgkin disease

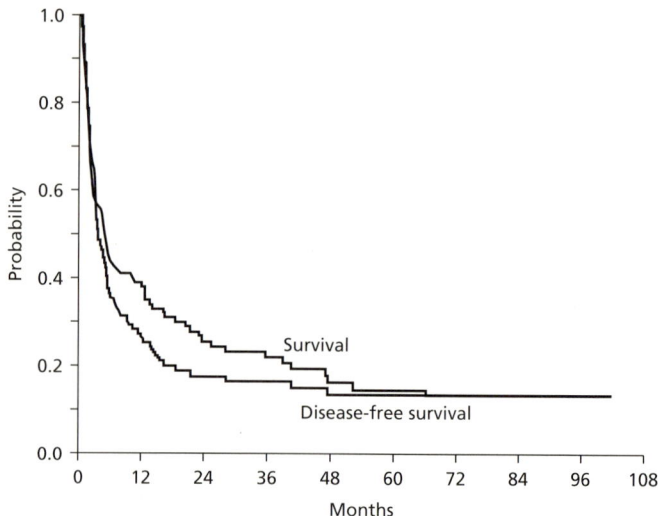

Fig. 87.6 Probability of survival and disease-free survival after human leukocyte antigen (HLA) identical sibling bone marrow transplantation for Hodgkin's disease. (Reprinted from [164].)

effect similar to the graft-vs.-leukemia effect observed after allogeneic HCT for leukemia [162].

The use of allogeneic donors also eliminates the risks of reinfusing malignant cells, although it is unknown whether infused Reed–Sternberg cells are clonogenic. Results of autologous HCT for HD in patients with involved marrow are poor, although this may simply reflect the presence of advanced or refractory disease at transplant [30,155]. Most relapses following autologous HCT occur at sites of prior disease [18,19,26,27,32,64,69], and this outcome suggests that disease progression is a result of high-dose therapy failure and not from reinfusion of malignant cells. The clonogenicity of Reed–Sternberg cells can also be questioned on the basis of reports of long-term disease-free survival following autologous BMT with marrow that was known to contain evidence of HD at the time of harvest [163].

Prolonged disease-free survival has been observed following allogeneic HCT for HD, although transplant-related mortality is extremely high. The actuarial 3-year disease-free survival was 15% in a series of 100 patients from the IBMTR who were treated with allogeneic BMT for HD (Fig. 87.6) [164]. The 3-year risk of treatment-related mortality was 61%. Factors associated with treatment failure included older age, poor performance status and recent infection. In an EBMT analysis, the 4-year actuarial progression-free survival and nonrelapse-mortality were 15% and 48%, respectively, following allogeneic HCT in a series of 45 HD patients [165]. The results of several series of allogeneic HCT for HD are displayed in Table 87.7.

The EBMT analysis showed no significant differences in outcome when autologous and allogeneic HCT results were compared with a case-matching approach [165]. An EBMT multivariate analysis demonstrated that the use of allogeneic HCT for HD was associated with significantly worse overall survival in comparison with autologous HCT [166]. At Johns Hopkins University Oncology Center patients with relapsed and refractory HD were preferentially assigned to receive allogeneic HCT if they had a matched sibling donor and were under the age of 56 years [15]. Otherwise patients were treated with autologous HCT and a retrospective comparison revealed no significant differences in relapse, event-free survival or overall survival between groups.

Although no clear evidence of a graft-vs.-Hodgkin's disease effect has been demonstrated, some studies suggest that the rate of relapse is lower after allogeneic HCT for HD when compared with autologous HCT

Table 87.7 Results of allogeneic hematopoietic cell transplantation for Hodgkin's disease.

Reference	n	Mortality (%)	Outcome
[166]	104	40	20% 4-year PFS
[164]	100	61	15% 3-year DFS
[15]	53	43	27% 10-year EFS
[165]	45	31	15% 4-year PFS
[167]	44	53	26% 5-year EFS
[168]	8	63	2 CCR 38+, 39+ months
[169]	8	50	1 CCR 29+ months
[170]	6	NS	2 CCR (17–20 months)
[171]	6	17	3 CCR (19–42 months)

CCR, continuous complete remission; DFS, disease-free survival; EFS, event-free survival; NS, not stated; PFS, progression-free survival.

[15,167]. There is also evidence that relapse rates may be lower in patients with HD who develop graft-vs.-host disease (GVHD) [165]. Finally, responses to donor leukocyte infusion have been described following allogeneic HCT for HD [172,173].

The high mortality rate following allogeneic HCT for HD and the frequent lack of donor availability limits the applicability of this approach. It is unknown whether this toxicity is disease-related or whether the high mortality results from adverse characteristics of patients selected for this form of treatment [164,165]. Autologous HCT recipients who were matched to allogeneic recipients in the EBMT analysis had a relatively poor outcome [165]. This study supports the hypothesis that the poor results of allogeneic HCT for HD may be largely related to the poor prognosis of patients selected for this treatment [165]. Results of allogeneic HCT for HD may be better if performed earlier in the course of disease, although it is not known which patients are candidates for this procedure.

Nonmyeloablative (reduced-intensity) regimens followed by allogeneic HCT

Recent studies have shown that donor lymphocyte infusions (DLI) can eradicate some malignancies that recur after conventional allogeneic HCT. These observations confirm the existent of a graft-vs.-tumor (GVT) effect. Although evidence for graft-vs.-Hodgkin's disease effects are limited [15,165,167,173], several investigators have explored the use of nonmyeloablative (reduced-intensity) conditioning regimens followed by allogeneic HCT to exploit potential GVT effects and to reduce nonrelapse mortality [174–176]. These studies have shown the feasibility of this approach in patients who have relapsed after autologous HCT and in patients who are not candidates for allogeneic HCT using conventional myeloablative regimens.

The largest series of reduced-intensity allogeneic HCT for HD was reported by the EBMT [177]. Fifty-two patients were conditioned with a wide variety of regimens, although the majority received fludarabine-based treatments. The 2-year overall survival and progression-free survival were estimated to be 56.3% and 42%, respectively. The 1-year transplant-related mortality was 17.3%. Patients with HD had better outcomes than those with high-grade NHL or mantle cell lymphoma.

Several other investigators have reported results of nonmyeloablative allogeneic HCT in cohorts containing small numbers of patients with HD. Anderlini et al. [178] used fludarabine-based conditioning regimens followed by allogeneic HCT in six patients with advanced and refractory HD who had failed multiple chemotherapy regimens including autologous HCT. Two patients (33%) died within 100 days of transplant and three remained alive and in remission between 6 and 26 months post-transplant. Nagler et al. [174] included four HD patients in a series of patients transplanted with a regimen of fludarabine, busulfan and anti-T-lymphocyte globulin. Two were alive at 17 and 25 months post-transplant. Kottaridis et al. [179] transplanted 10 HD patients with a regimen combining Campath-1H, fludarabine and melphalan. Seven patients had relapsed after autologous HCT. Eight remained alive and progression-free between 3 and 22 months after transplant. Porter et al. [172] conducted a series of studies of nonmyeloablative allogeneic HCT in 14 patients (11 with HD) who had relapsed after autologous HCT. Eight patients with HD received fludarabine and cyclophosphamide and three received unstimulated donor leukocyte infusions. Four patients attained a complete remission, although only one was alive and in remission at 33 weeks. McSweeney et al. [175] utilized low-dose (200 cGy) TBI followed by a combination of mycophenolate mofetil and cyclosporine to allow stable engraftment in 45 patients with hematologic malignancies. One of four HD patients remained in remission >1 year after transplant. Dey et al. [180] performed nonmyeloablative allogeneic HCT in four HD patients who were conditioned with cyclophosphamide, peritransplant antithymocyte globulin and thymic irradiation. One patient remained alive and in remission 21 months after transplant.

The results from these studies provide additional evidence to support the existence of a graft-vs.-Hodgkin's disease effect. Nonmyeloablative conditioning can be associated with GVHD and other significant toxicity and long-term follow-up is not available. Current results appear better than those reported with full-intensity myeloablative allogeneic conditioning, especially for patients who have been treated with a prior autologous HCT. Additional studies are required to compare results with more traditional approaches, determine the appropriate timing of transplantation, develop optimal reduced-intensity regimens and design strategies to decrease toxicity.

Several investigators are also studying the strategy of autologous HCT followed by allogeneic immunotherapy for HD. This approach would allow administration of allogeneic HCT to patients who have achieved a minimal disease state after high-dose therapy. Carella et al. [181] have shown that this approach is feasible and associated with acceptable toxicity. Ten patients with relapsed and refractory HD received high-dose therapy with BEAM chemotherapy followed by autologous HCT. At a median of 84 days after autologous HCT, patients underwent allogeneic HCT after conditioning with fludarabine and cyclophosphamide. Five patients were alive between 210 and 430 days after the second transplant. These results are encouraging; however, additional studies in a larger number of patients with longer follow-up are required to assess the curative potential of this approach.

High-dose therapy regimens

A wide variety of high-dose therapy regimens have been used with autologous HCT for HD (Table 87.1). No prospective trials have been performed, although regimens have been compared in retrospective analyses. Regimens are frequently divided into those that use TBI and those that contain only drugs. The prior use of radiation eliminates the possibility of using TBI in many patients.

Investigators from Seattle examined a cohort of HD patients who were treated with both autologous and allogeneic HCT [167]. No significant differences in event-free survival were observed when TBI-containing and drug-only regimens were compared, although 5-year overall survival rates were 28% and 14%, respectively ($p = 0.08$). At City of Hope National Medical Center, patients received a regimen of TBI, etoposide and cyclophosphamide, or else carmustine, etoposide and cyclophosphamide if they had received prior radiation therapy [29]. No significant differences in response rate, disease-free survival, overall survival or toxicity were observed. At Stanford University, patients received TBI, etoposide and cyclophosphamide, or regimens where carmustine or lomustine were substituted for TBI [32]. No significant differences in overall survival, progression-free survival or event-free survival were noted. Similarly, the choice of high-dose therapy did not influence outcome in EBMT analyses of patients treated in first relapse or with primary refractory disease [51,84], in French registry data [34] or in an ABMTR analysis [35].

The use of TBI may be associated with increased pulmonary toxicity, particularly in patients who have received mediastinal irradiation in the past [19]. The use of TBI should be avoided in patients who have received mantle irradiation, although TBI and total-lymphoid irradiation [25] can be used in selected patients who have not been previously irradiated [29,32].

One of the most common high-dose chemotherapy regimens for HD patients is the cyclophosphamide, carmustine and etoposide (CBV) regimen developed at the M.D. Anderson Cancer Center [182]. This regimen has been highly modified and individual institutions have used widely differing schedules, with total doses of cyclophosphamide between 4800 and 7200 mg/m^2, total carmustine doses between 300 and 600 mg/m^2 and doses of etoposide between 750 and 2400 mg/m^2. No prospective trials have examined whether variations in the CBV regimen lead to different outcomes, although poorer results have been observed in trials where lower doses of etoposide were used [18,28,30]. The CBV regimen has been modified by the addition of cisplatin, but it is unknown whether this modification improves outcome [22,26]. A retrospective EBMT analysis noted significantly better progression-free survival in HD patients who received high-dose BEAM, as compared with patients who received CBV [183]. A higher likelihood of pulmonary toxicity has been seen in patients with prior chest irradiation who have been treated with CBV [184]. Several investigators have also noted a significantly higher risk of interstitial pneumonitis with carmustine doses of 600 mg/m^2, as compared with lower doses [167,184,185].

Gianni et al. [24] have used a novel regimen consisting of rapid sequential administration of high-dose cyclophosphamide, methotrexate, etoposide and TBI plus melphalan, followed by reinfusion of peripheral blood stem cells collected after cyclophosphamide administration. A similar regimen has been used for patients with NHL [186]. The use of radiolabeled antibodies in combination with high-dose chemotherapy has also been tested [187].

It is unclear from existing data that any high-dose therapy regimen is superior for patients with HD. It is likely that prospective trials will be required to prove the superiority of any regimen and it is difficult to recommend any single regimen, although TBI and higher doses of carmustine should be avoided in patients with pulmonary disease or a history of chest irradiation.

Several institutions have tested the use of double (tandem) autologous HCT for HD. This approach is feasible and good outcomes are possible, although a significant fraction of patients are not able to receive the second planned transplant [86,188–190].

Conclusions and future directions

Autologous HCT for HD has become easier and safer and is accepted therapy in certain situations. Nevertheless, only two prospective randomized trials have been reported for this condition. Accrual could not be completed in either trial and overall survival advantages were not observed. Autologous HCT is still associated with significant morbidity for some patients, although transplant-related mortality rates are extremely low at most institutions. Important questions relating to issues such as timing have not been completely resolved. More effective preparative regimens are needed and the role of post-transplant therapy has not been adequately explored. Reduced-intensity nonmyeloablative allogeneic transplants are beginning to be explored and mature data on the results of this approach are awaited. The role of autologous HCT for HD will continue to evolve as more effective primary treatments are developed.

References

1 Jemal A, Thomas A, Murray T, Thum M, Landis SH, Thun M. Cancer Statistics 2002. *CA Cancer J Clin* 2002; **52**: 23–47.

2 Canellos GP, Anderson JR, Propert KJ et al. Chemotherapy of advanced Hodgkin's disease with MOPP, ABVD, or MOPP alternating with ABVD. *N Engl J Med* 1992; **327**: 1478–84.

3 Horning SJ, Hoppe RT, Breslin S et al. Stanford V and radiotherapy for locally extensive and advanced Hodgkin's disease: mature results of a prospective clinical trial. *J Clin Oncol* 2002; **20**: 630–7.

4 McFarland W, Granville NB, Dameshek W. Autologous bone marrow infusion as an adjunct in therapy of malignant disease. *Blood* 1959; **14**: 503–21.

5 Kurnick NB. Autologous and isologous bone marrow storage and infusion in the treatment of myelosuppression. *Transfusion* 1962; **2**: 178–87.

6 Carella AM, Santini G, Santoro A et al. Massive chemotherapy with non-frozen autologous bone marrow transplantation in 13 cases of refractory Hodgkin's disease. *Eur J Cancer* 1985; **21**: 607–13.

7 Philip T, Dumont J, Teillet F et al. High dose chemotherapy and autologous bone marrow transplantation in refractory Hodgkin's disease. *Br J Cancer* 1986; **53**: 737–42.

8 Jagannath S, Dicke KA, Armitage JO et al. High-dose cyclophosphamide, carmustine, and etoposide and autologous bone marrow transplantation for relapsed Hodgkin's disease. *Ann Intern Med* 1986; **104**: 163–8.

9 Summary slides 2002. *IBMTR/ABMTR Newsletter* 2002; **9**: 1–11.

10 Gratwohl A, Baldomero H, Horisberger B et al. Current trends in hematopoietic stem cell transplantation in Europe. *Blood* 2002; **100**: 2374–86.

11 Bennett CL, Armitage JL, Armitage GO et al. Costs of care and outcomes for high-dose therapy and autologous transplantation for lymphoid malignancies: results from University of Nebraska 1987–91. *J Clin Oncol* 1995; **13**: 969–73.

12 Lancet JE, Rapoport AP, Brasacchio R et al. Auto-transplantation for relapsed or refractory Hodgkin's disease: long-term follow-up and analysis of prognostic factors. *Bone Marrow Transplant* 1998; **22**: 265–71.

13 Moskowitz CH, Nimer SD, Zelenetz AD et al. A two-stem comprehensive high-dose chemoradiotherapy second-line program for relapsed and refractory Hodgkin disease: analysis by intent to treat and development of a prognostic model. *Blood* 2001; **97**: 616–23.

14 Sureda A, Arranz R, Iriondo A et al. Autologous stem-cell transplantation for Hodgkin's disease: results and prognostic factors in 494 patients from the Grupo Español de Linfomas/ Trasplante Autólogo de Médula Ósea Spanish Cooperative Group. *J Clin Oncol* 2001; **19**: 1395–404.

15 Akpek G, Ambinder RF, Piantadosi S et al. Long-term results of blood and marrow transplantation for Hodgkin's lymphoma. *J Clin Oncol* 2001; **19**: 4314–21.

16 Weaver CH, Schwartzberg LS, Hainsworth J et al. Treatment-related mortality in 1000 consecutive patients receiving high-dose chemotherapy and peripheral blood progenitor cell transplantation in community cancer centers. *Bone Marrow Transplant* 1997; **19**: 671–8.

17 Meisenberg BR, Miller WE, McMillan R et al. Outpatient high-dose chemotherapy with autologous stem-cell rescue for hematologic and non-hematologic malignancies. *J Clin Oncol* 1997; **15**: 11–17.

18 Carella AM, Congiu AM, Gaozza E et al. High-dose chemotherapy with autologous bone marrow transplantation in 50 advanced resistant Hodgkin's disease patients: an Italian study group report. *J Clin Oncol* 1988; **6**: 1411–16.

19 Phillips GL, Wolff SN, Herzig RH et al. Treatment of progressive Hodgkin's disease with intensive chemoradiotherapy and autologous bone marrow transplantation. *Blood* 1989; **73**: 2086–92.

20 Reece DE, Barnett MJ, Connors JM et al. Intensive chemotherapy with cyclophosphamide, carmustine, and etoposide followed by autologous bone marrow transplantation for relapsed Hodgkin's disease. *J Clin Oncol* 1991; **9**: 1871–9.

21 Lazarus HM, Crilley P, Ciobanu N et al. High-dose carmustine, etoposide, and cisplatin and autologous bone marrow transplantation for relapsed and

22. Spinolo JA, Jagannath S, Velásquez et al. Cisplatin-CBV with autologous bone marrow transplantation for relapsed Hodgkin's disease. *Leuk Lymphoma* 1993; **9**: 71–7.
23. Crump M, Smith AM, Brandwein J et al. High-dose etoposide and melphalan, and autologous bone marrow transplantation for patients with advanced Hodgkin's disease: importance of disease status at transplant. *J Clin Oncol* 1993; **11**: 704–11.
24. Gianni AM, Siena S, Bregni M et al. High-dose sequential chemo-radiotherapy with peripheral blood progenitor cell support for relapsed or refractory Hodgkin's disease: a 6-year update. *Ann Oncol* 1993; **4**: 889–91.
25. Yahalom J, Gulati SC, Toia M et al. Accelerated hyperfractionated total-lymphoid irradiation, high-dose chemotherapy, and autologous bone marrow transplantation for refractory and relapsing patients with Hodgkin's disease. *J Clin Oncol* 1993; **11**: 1062–70.
26. Reece DE, Connors JM, Spinelli JJ et al. Intensive therapy with cyclophosphamide, carmustine, etoposide ± cisplatin, and autologous bone marrow transplantation for Hodgkin's disease in first relapse after combination chemotherapy. *Blood* 1994; **83**: 1193–9.
27. Chopra R, McMillan AK, Linch DC et al. The place of high-dose BEAM therapy and autologous bone marrow transplantation in poor-risk Hodgkin's disease: a single-center eight-year study of 155 patients. *Blood* 1993; **81**: 1137–45.
28. Bierman PJ, Bagin RG, Jagannath S et al. High-dose chemotherapy followed by autologous hematopoietic rescue in Hodgkin's disease: long-term follow-up in 128 patients. *Ann Oncol* 1993; **4**: 767–73.
29. Nademanee A, O'Donnell MR, Snyder DS et al. High-dose chemotherapy with or without total body irradiation followed by autologous bone marrow and/or peripheral blood stem cell transplantation for patients with relapsed and refractory Hodgkin's disease: results in 85 patients with analysis of prognostic factors. *Blood* 1995; **85**: 1381–90.
30. Burns LJ, Daniels KA, McGlave PB et al. Autologous stem cell transplantation for refractory and relapsed Hodgkin's disease: factors predictive of prolonged survival. *Bone Marrow Transplant* 1995; **16**: 13–18.
31. Lumley MA, Milligan DW, Knechtli CJC, Long SG, Billingham LJ, McDonald DF. High lactate dehydrogenase level is associated with an adverse outlook in autografting for Hodgkin's disease. *Bone Marrow Transplant* 1996; **17**: 383–8.
32. Horning SJ, Chao NJ, Negrin RS et al. High-dose therapy and autologous hematopoietic progenitor cell transplantation for recurrent or refractory Hodgkin's disease: analysis of the Stanford University results and prognostic indices. *Blood* 1997; **89**: 801–13.
33. Wheeler C, Eickhoff C, Elias A et al. High-dose cyclophosphamide, carmustine, and etoposide with autologous transplantation in Hodgkin's disease: a prognostic model for treatment outcome. *Biol Blood Marrow Transplant* 1997; **3**: 98–106.
34. Brice P, Bouabdallah R, Moreau P et al. Prognostic factors for survival after high-dose therapy and autologous stem cell transplantation for patients with relapsing Hodgkin's disease: analysis of 280 patients from the French registry. *Bone Marrow Transplant* 1997; **20**: 21–6.
35. Lazarus HM, Loberiza FR, Zhang M-J et al. Autotransplants for Hodgkin's disease in first relapse or second remission: a report from the Autologous Blood and Marrow Transplant Registry (ABMTR). *Bone Marrow Transplant* 2001; **27**: 387–96.
36. Argiris A, Seropian S, Cooper DL. High-dose BEAM chemotherapy with autologous peripheral blood progenitor-cell transplantation for unselected patients with primary refractory or relapsed Hodgkin's disease. *Ann Oncol* 2000; **11**: 665–72.
37. Engel C, Loeffler M, Schmitz S et al. Acute hematologic toxicity and practicability of dose-intensified BEACOPP chemotherapy for advanced stage Hodgkin's disease. *Ann Oncol* 2000; **11**: 1105–14.
38. Bonfante V, Santoro A, Viviani S et al. Outcome of patients with Hodgkin's disease failing after primary MOPP-ABVD. *J Clin Oncol* 1997; **15**: 528–34.
39. Josting A, Kàtay I, Rueffer U et al. Favorable outcome of patients with relapsed or refractory Hodgkin's disease treated with high-dose chemotherapy and stem cell rescue at the time of maximal response to conventional salvage therapy (Dexa-BEAM). *Ann Oncol* 1998; **9**: 289–95.
40. Ribrag V, Nasr F, Bouhris JH et al. VIP (etoposide, ifosfamide and cisplatinum) as a salvage intensification program in relapsed or refractory Hodgkin's disease. *Bone Marrow Transplant* 1998; **21**: 969–74.
41. Linch DC, Winfield D, Goldstone AH et al. Dose intensification with autologous bone-marrow transplantation in relapsed and resistant Hodgkin's disease: results of a BNLI randomised trial. *Lancet* 1993; **341**: 1051–4.
42. Schmitz N, Pfistner B, Sextro M et al. Aggressive conventional chemotherapy compared with high-dose chemotherapy with autologous haemopoietic stem-cell transplantation for relapsed chemosensitive Hodgkin's disease: a randomised trial. *Lancet* 2002; **359**: 2065–71.
43. Brice P, Bastion Y, Divine M et al. Analysis of prognostic factors after the first relapse of Hodgkin's disease in 187 patients. *Cancer* 1996; **78**: 1293–9.
44. Yuen AR, Rosenberg SA, Hoppe RT, Halpern JD, Horning SJ. Comparison between conventional salvage therapy and high-dose therapy with autografting for recurrent or refractory Hodgkin's disease. *Blood* 1997; **89**: 814–22.
45. André M, Henry-Amar M, Pico J-L et al. Comparison of high-dose therapy and autologous stem-cell transplantation with conventional therapy for Hodgkin's disease induction failure: a case–control study. *J Clin Oncol* 1999; **17**: 222–9.
46. Fermé C, Mounier N, Diviné M et al. Intensive salvage therapy with high-dose chemotherapy for patients with advanced Hodgkin's disease in relapse or failure after initial chemotherapy: results of the Groupe d'Études des Lymphomes de l'Adulte H89 trial. *J Clin Oncol* 2002; **20**: 467–75.
47. Josting A, Franklin J, May M et al. New prognostic score based on treatment outcome of patients with relapsed Hodgkin's lymphoma registered in the database of the German Hodgkin's Lymphoma Study Group. *J Clin Oncol* 2001; **20**: 221–30.
48. Hasenclever D, Diehl V. A prognostic score for advanced Hodgkin's disease. *N Engl J Med* 1998; **339**: 1506–14.
49. Bierman PJ, Lynch JC, Bociek RG et al. The International Prognostic Factors Project score for advanced Hodgkin's disease is useful for predicting outcome of autologous hematopoietic stem cell transplantation. *Ann Oncol* 2002; **13**: 1370–7.
50. O'Brien MER, Milan S, Cunningham D et al. High-dose chemotherapy and autologous bone marrow transplantation in relapsed Hodgkin's disease: a pragmatic prognostic index. *Br J Cancer* 1996; **73**: 1272–7.
51. Sweetenham JW, Taghipour G, Milligan et al. High-dose therapy and autologous stem cell rescue for patients with Hodgkin's disease in first relapse after chemotherapy: results from the EBMT. *Bone Marrow Transplant* 1997; **20**: 745–52.
52. Bolwell BJ, Kalaycio M, Goormastic M et al. Progressive disease after ABMT for Hodgkin's disease. *Bone Marrow Transplant* 1997; **20**: 761.
53. Jagannath S, Armitage JO, Dicke KA et al. Prognostic factors for response and survival after high-dose cyclophosphamide, carmustine, and etoposide with autologous bone marrow transplantation for relapsed Hodgkin's disease. *J Clin Oncol* 1989; **7**: 179–85.
54. Armitage JO, Bierman PJ, Vose JM et al. Autologous bone marrow transplantation for patients with relapsed Hodgkin's disease. *Am J Med* 1991; **91**: 605–11.
55. Bierman PJ, Anderson JR, Freeman MB et al. High-dose chemotherapy followed by autologous hematopoietic rescue for Hodgkin's disease patients following first relapse after chemotherapy. *Ann Oncol* 1996; **7**: 151–6.
56. Rodriguez J, Rodriguez MA, Fayad L et al. ASHAP: a regimen for cytoreduction of refractory or recurrent Hodgkin's disease. *Blood* 1999; **93**: 3632–6.
57. Philip T, Armitage JO, Spitzer G et al. High-dose therapy and autologous bone marrow transplantation after failure of conventional chemotherapy in adults with intermediate-grade or high-grade non-Hodgkin's lymphoma. *N Engl J Med* 1987; **316**: 1493–8.
58. Brandwein JM, Callum J, Sutcliffe SB, Scott JG, Keating A. Evaluation of cytoreductive therapy prior to high dose treatment with autologous bone marrow transplantation in relapsed and refractory Hodgkin's disease. *Bone Marrow Transplant* 1990; **5**: 99–103.
59. Colwill R, Crump M, Couture F, Danish R et al. Mini-BEAM as salvage therapy for relapsed or refractory Hodgkin's disease before intensive therapy and autologous bone marrow transplantation. *J Clin Oncol* 1995; **13**: 396–402.
60. Phillips GL, Reece DE, Wolff SN, Goldie JH. The use of conventional salvage chemotherapy before dose-intensive cytotoxic therapy and autologous transplantation for aggressive-histology lymphoma: a case for re-evaluation. *Leuk Lymphoma* 1997; **26**: 507–13.
61. Clift RA, Buckner CD, Thomas ED et al. The treatment of acute non-lymphoblastic leukemia by allogeneic marrow transplantation. *Bone Marrow Transplant* 1987; **2**: 243–58.
62. Bosly A, Sonet A, Salles G et al. Superiority of late over early intensification in relapsing/refractory aggressive non-Hodgkin's lymphoma: a randomized study from the GELA: LNH RP 93. *Blood* 1997; **90** (Suppl. 1): 594a.
63. Rapoport AP, Rowe JM, Kouides PA et al. One hundred autotransplants for relapsed or refractory Hodgkin's disease and lymphoma: value of

pretransplant disease status for predicting outcome. *J Clin Oncol* 1993; **11**: 2351–61.
64 Mundt AJ, Sibley G, Williams S *et al.* Patterns of failure following high-dose chemotherapy and autologous bone marrow transplantation with involved field radiotherapy for relapsed/refractory Hodgkin's disease. *Int J Radiat Oncol Biol Phys* 1995; **33**: 261–70.
65 Pezner RD, Nademanee A, Niland JC, Vora N, Forman SJ. Involved field radiation therapy for Hodgkin's disease autologous bone marrow transplantation regimens. *Radiother Oncol* 1995; **34**: 23–9.
66 Poen JC, Hoppe RT, Horning SJ. High-dose therapy and autologous bone marrow transplantation for relapsed/refractory Hodgkin's disease: the impact of involved field radiotherapy on patterns of failure and survival. *Int J Radiat Oncol Biol Phys* 1996; **36**: 3–12.
67 Tsang RW, Gospodarowicz MK, Sutcliffe SB, Crump M, Keating A. Thoracic radiation therapy before autologous bone marrow transplantation in relapsed or refractory Hodgkin's disease. PMH Lymphoma Group Toronto Autologous BMT Group. *Eur J Cancer* 1999; **35**: 73–8.
68 Friedberg JW, Neuberg D, Monson J, Jallow H, Nadler LM, Freedman AS. The impact of external beam radiation therapy prior to autologous bone marrow transplantation in patients with non-Hodgkin's lymphoma. *Biol Blood Marrow Transplant* 2001; **7**: 446–53.
69 Moormeier JA, Williams SF, Kaminer LS *et al.* Autologous bone marrow transplantation followed by involved field radiotherapy in patients with relapsed or refractory Hodgkin's disease. *Leuk Lymphoma* 1991; **5**: 243–8.
70 Bierman P, Freeman M, Barrios S *et al.* An apparent advantage with the use of consolidative radiation therapy (XRT) following autologous transplantation for Hodgkin's disease (HD). *Proc Am Soc Blood Marrow Transplant* 1995; **1**: 66.
71 Brasacchio R, Constine L, Rapoport A *et al.* Dose escalation of consolidation radiation therapy (involved field) following autologous bone marrow transplant for recurrent Hodgkin's disease and lymphoma. *Intl J Radiat Oncol Biol Phys* 1996; **36** (Suppl. 1): 171.
72 Toren A, Nagler R, Nagler A. Involved field radiation post autologous stem cell transplantation in lymphoma patients is associated with major haematological toxicities. *Med Oncol* 1998; **15**: 113–8.
73 Schenkein DP, Dixon P, Desforges JF *et al.* Phase I/II study of cyclophosphamide, carboplatin, and etoposide and autologous hematopoietic stem-cell transplantation with post-transplant interferon alfa-2b for patients with lymphoma and Hodgkin's disease. *J Clin Oncol* 1994; **12**: 2423–31.
74 Robinson N, Benyunes MC, Thompson JA *et al.* Interleukin-2 after autologous stem cell transplantation for hematologic malignancy: a phase I/II study. *Bone Marrow Transplant* 1997; **19**: 435–42.
75 Benyunes MC, Higuchi C, York A *et al.* Immunotherapy with interleukin 2 with or without lymphokine-activated killer cells after autologous bone marrow transplantation for malignant lymphoma: a feasibility trial. *Bone Marrow Transplant* 1995; **16**: 283–8.
76 Miller JS, Tessmer-Tuck J, Pierson B *et al.* Low dose subcutaneous interleukin-2 after autologous transplantation generates sustained *in vivo* natural killer cell activity. *Biol Blood Marrow Transplant* 1997; **3**: 34–44.
77 Nagler A, Ackerstein A, Or R *et al.* Immunotherapy with recombinant human interleukin-2 and recombinant interferon-α in lymphoma patients postautologous marrow or stem cell transplantation. *Blood* 1997; **89**: 3951–9.
78 Nagler A, Ackerstein A, Czyz J *et al.* Lymphokine-mediated immunotherapy with recombinant interleukin-2 (rIL-2) and recombinant interferon alpha (IFN-α) versus no immunotherapy following autologous peripheral blood stem cell transplantation (ASCT) for Hodgkin's disease (HD): an interim analysis of a multicenter two-arm randomized study. *Exp Hematol* 2001; **29** (Suppl. 1): 63.
79 Czyż J, Hellmann A, Dziadziusko R *et al.* High-dose chemotherapy with autologous stem cell transplantation is an effective treatment of primary refractory Hodgkin's disease: retrospective study of the Polish Lymphoma Research Group. *Bone Marrow Transplant* 2002; **30**: 29–34.
80 Or R, Ackerstein A, Nagler A. Allogeneic cell-mediated and cytokine-activated immunotherapy for malignant lymphoma at the stage of minimal residual disease after autologous stem cell transplantation. *J Immunother* 1998; **21**: 447–53.
81 Desch CE, Lasala MR, Smith TJ, Hillner BE. The optimal timing of autologous bone marrow transplantation in Hodgkin's disease patients after a chemotherapy relapse. *J Clin Oncol* 1992; **10**: 200–9.
82 Longo DL, Duffey PL, Young RC *et al.* Conventional-dose salvage combination chemotherapy in patients relapsing with Hodgkin's disease after combination chemotherapy: the low probability for cure. *J Clin Oncol* 1992; **10**: 210–8.
83 Lazarus HM, Rowlings PA, Zhang M-J *et al.* Autotransplants for Hodgkin's disease in patients never achieving remission: a report from the Autologous Blood and Marrow Transplant Registry. *J Clin Oncol* 1999; **17**: 534–45.
84 Sweetenham JW, Carella AM, Taghipour G *et al.* High-dose therapy and autologous stem-cell transplantation for adult patients with Hodgkin's disease who do not enter remission after induction chemotherapy: results in 175 patients reported to the European Group for Blood and Marrow Transplantation. *J Clin Oncol* 1999; **17**: 3101–9.
85 Josting A, Rueffer U, Franklin J, Sieber M, Diehl V, Engert A. Prognostic factors and treatment outcome in primary progressive Hodgkin lymphoma: a report from the German Hodgkin Lymphoma Study Group. *Blood* 2000; **96**: 1280–6.
86 Ahmed T, Lake DE, Beer M *et al.* Single and double autotransplants for relapsing/refractory Hodgkin's disease: results of two consecutive trials. *Bone Marrow Transplant* 1997; **19**: 449–54.
87 Reece DE, Barnett MJ, Sheperd JD *et al.* High-dose cyclophosphamide, carmustine (BCNU), and etoposide (VP16-213) with or without cisplatin (CBV + P) and autologous transplantation for patients with Hodgkin's disease who fail to enter a complete remission after combination chemotherapy. *Blood* 1995; **86**: 451–6.
88 Prince HM, Crump M, Imrie K *et al.* Intensive therapy and autotransplant for patients with an incomplete response to front-line therapy for lymphoma. *Ann Oncol* 1996; **7**: 1043–9.
89 Moreau P, Fleury J, Brice P *et al.* Early intensive therapy with autologous stem cell transplantation in advanced Hodgkin's disease: retrospective analysis of 158 cases from the French Registry. *Bone Marrow Transplant* 1998; **21**: 787–93.
90 Josting A, Reiser M, Rueffer U, Salzberger B, Diehl V, Engert A. Treatment of primary progressive Hodgkin's and aggressive non-Hodgkin's lymphoma: is there a chance for cure? *J Clin Oncol* 2000; **18**: 332–9.
91 Lister TA, Crowther D, Sutcliffe SB *et al.* Report of a committee convened to discuss the evaluation and staging of patients with Hodgkin's disease: Cotswolds meeting. *J Clin Oncol* 1989; **7**: 1630–6.
92 Fung H, Nademanee A, Kashyap A *et al.* Evaluation of prognostic factors in patients (PTS) with Hodgkin disease (HD) in first relapse (REL) treated by autologous stem cell transplantation (ASCT): duration of first remission does not predict the transplant outcome. *Blood* 1997; **90** (Suppl. 1): 594a.
93 Kottaridis PD, Peniket AJ, Perry AR *et al.* The length of the first complete remission (1–6 months; 7–12 months; >12 months) does not predict outcome following BEAM and autotransplantation for Hodgkin's disease in first relapse. *Blood* 1997; **90** (Suppl. 1): 114a.
94 Bierman PJ, Vose JM, Armitage JO. Autologous transplantation for Hodgkin's disease: coming of age? *Blood* 1994; **83**: 1161–4.
95 Haioun C, Lepage E, Gisselbrecht C *et al.* Survival benefit of high-dose therapy in poor-risk aggressive non-Hodgkin's lymphoma: final analysis of the prospective LNH87-2 protocol-A Groupe d'Etude des Lymphomes de l'Adulte study. *J Clin Oncol* 2000; **18**: 3025–30.
96 Proctor SJ, Taylor P, Donnan P, Boys R, Lennard A, Prescott RJ. A numerical prognostic index for clinical use in identification of poor-risk patients with Hodgkin's disease at diagnosis. *Eur J Cancer* 1991; **27**: 624–9.
97 Carella AM, Carlier P, Congiu A *et al.* Autologous bone marrow transplantation as adjuvant treatment for high-risk Hodgkin's disease in first complete remission after MOPP/ABVD protocol. *Bone Marrow Transplant* 1991; **8**: 99–103.
98 Carella AM, Prencipe E, Pungolino E *et al.* Twelve years experience with high-dose therapy and autologous stem cell transplantation for high-risk Hodgkin's disease patients in first remission after MOPP/ABVD chemotherapy. *Leuk Lymphoma* 1996; **21**: 63–70.
99 Schmitz N, Hasenclever D, Brosteanu O *et al.* Early high-dose therapy to consolidate patients with high-risk Hodgkin's disease in first complete remission? Results of an EBMT/GHSG matched-pair analysis. *Blood* 1995; **86** (Suppl. 1): 439a.
100 Nademanee A, Molina A, Fung H *et al.* High-dose chemo/radiotherapy and autologous bone marrow or stem cell transplantation for poor-risk advanced-stage Hodgkin's disease during first partial or complete remission. *Biol Blood Marrow Transplant* 1999; **5**: 292–8.
101 Delain M, Cartron G, Bout M *et al.* Intensive therapy with autologous stem cell transplantation as first-line therapy in poor-risk Hodgkin's disease and analysis of predictive factors of outcome. *Leuk Lymphoma* 1999; **34**: 305–13.
102 Fleury J, Legros M, Colombat P *et al.* High-dose therapy and autologous bone marrow transplantation in first complete or partial remission for poor prognosis Hodgkin's disease. *Leuk Lymphoma* 1996; **20**: 259–66.
103 Williams CD, Goldstone AH, Pearce R *et al.* Autologous bone marrow transplantation for pediatric Hodgkin's disease: a case-matched comparison with adult patients by the European Bone Marrow

Transplant Group Registry. *J Clin Oncol* 1993; **11**: 2243–9.

104 Baker KS, Gordon BG, Gross TG *et al*. Autologous hematopoietic stem-cell transplantation for relapsed or refractory Hodgkin's disease in children and adolescents. *J Clin Oncol* 1999; **17**: 825–31.

105 Frankovich J, Donaldson SS, Lee Y *et al*. High-dose therapy and autologous hematopoietic cell transplantation in children with primary refractory and relapsed Hodgkin's disease: atopy predicts idiopathic diffuse lung injury syndromes. *Biol Blood Marrow Transplant* 2001; **7**: 49–57.

106 Kobrinsky NL, Sposto R, Shay NR *et al*. Outcomes of treatment of children and adolescents with recurrent non-Hodgkin's lymphoma and Hodgkin's disease with dexamethasone, etoposide, cisplatin, cytarabine, and L-asparaginase, maintenance chemotherapy, and transplantation: Children's Cancer Group study CCG-5912. *J Clin Oncol* 2001; **19**: 2390–6.

107 Miller CB, Piantadosi S, Vogelsang GB *et al*. Impact of age on outcome of patients with cancer undergoing autologous bone marrow transplant. *J Clin Oncol* 1996; **14**: 1327–32.

108 Kusnierz-Glaz CR, Schlegel PG, Wong RM *et al*. Influence of age on the outcome of 500 autologous bone marrow transplant procedures for hematologic malignancies. *J Clin Oncol* 1997; **15**: 18–25.

109 Spina M, Gabarre J, Rossi G *et al*. Stanford V regimen and concomitant HAART in 59 patients with Hodgkin disease and HIV infection. *Blood* 2002; **100**: 1984–8.

110 Gabarre J, Azar N, Autran B, Katlama C, Leblond V. High-dose therapy and autologous haematopoietic stem-cell transplantation for HIV-1-associated lymphoma. *Lancet* 2000; **355**: 1071–2.

111 Krishnan A, Molina A, Zaia J *et al*. Autologous stem cell transplantation for HIV-associated lymphoma. *Blood* 2001; **98**: 3857–9.

112 Kang EM, de Witte M, Malech H *et al*. Nonmyeloablative conditioning followed by transplantation of genetically modified HLA-matched peripheral blood progenitor cells for hematologic malignancies in patients with acquired immunodeficiency syndrome. *Blood* 2002; **99**: 698–701.

113 Wingard JR, Curbow B, Baker F, Piantadosi S. Health, functional status, and employment of adult survivors of bone marrow transplantation. *Ann Intern Med* 1991; **114**: 113–8.

114 Vose JM, Kennedy BC, Bierman PJ, Kessinger A, Armitage JO. Long-term sequelae of autologous bone marrow or peripheral stem cell transplantation for lymphoid malignancies. *Cancer* 1992; **69**: 784–9.

115 Chao NJ, Tierney DK, Bloom JR *et al*. Dynamic assessment of quality of life after autologous bone marrow transplantation. *Blood* 1992; **80**: 825–30.

116 Whedon M, Stearns D, Mills LE. Quality of life of long-term adult survivors of autologous bone marrow transplantation. *Oncol Nurs Forum* 1995; **20**: 1527–35.

117 Andrykowski MA, Greiner CB, Altmaier EM *et al*. Quality of life following bone marrow transplantation: findings from a multicentre study. *Br J Cancer* 1995; **71**: 1322–9.

118 Forrest DL, Nevill TJ, Connors JM *et al*. Long-term follow-up of 100 patients undergoing high-dose chemotherapy (HDCT) and autologous stem cell transplantation (ASCT) for Hodgkin's disease (HD). *Blood* 1997; **90** (Suppl. 1): 593a.

119 André M, Henry-Amar M, Blaise D *et al*. Treatment-related deaths and second cancer risk after autologous stem-cell transplantation for Hodgkin's disease. *Blood* 1998; **92**: 1933–40.

120 Milligan DW, Ruiz De Elvira C, Kolb H-J *et al*. Secondary leukaemia and myelodysplasia after autografting for lymphoma: results from the EBMT. *Br J Haematol* 1999; **106**: 1020–6.

121 Harrison CN, Gregory W, Vaughan Hudson G *et al*. High-dose BEAM chemotherapy with autologous haemopoietic stem cell transplantation for Hodgkin's disease is unlikely to be associated with a major increased risk of secondary MDS/AML. *Br J Cancer* 1999; **81**: 476–83.

122 Miller JS, Arthur DC, Litz CE, Neglia JP, Miller WJ, Weisdorf DJ. Myelodysplastic syndrome after autologous bone marrow transplantation: an additional late complication of curative cancer therapy. *Blood* 1994; **83**: 3780–6.

123 Traweek ST, Slovak ML, Nademanee AP, Brynes RK, Niland JC, Forman SJ. Clonal karyotypic hematopoietic cell abnormalities occurring after autologous bone marrow transplantation for Hodgkin's disease and non-Hodgkin's lymphoma. *Blood* 1994; **84**: 957–63.

124 Darrington DL, Vose JM, Anderson JR *et al*. Incidence and characterization of secondary myelodysplastic syndrome and acute myelogenous leukemia following high-dose chemoradiotherapy and autologous stem-cell transplantation for lymphoid malignancies. *J Clin Oncol* 1994; **12**: 2527–34.

125 Krishnan A, Bhatia S, Slovak ML *et al*. Predictors of therapy-related leukemia and myelodysplasia following autologous transplantation for lymphoma: an assessment of risk factors. *Blood* 2000; **95**: 1588–93.

126 Metayer C, Curtis RE, Sobocinski KA *et al*. Myelodysplastic syndrome (MDS) and leukemia after autotransplantation for lymphoma a multicenter case–control study. *Blood* 2002; **101**: 2015–23.

127 Chao NJ, Nademanee AP, Long GD *et al*. Importance of bone marrow cytogenetic evaluation before autologous bone marrow transplantation for Hodgkin's disease. *J Clin Oncol* 1991; **9**: 1575–9.

128 Abruzzese E, Radford JE, Miller JS *et al*. Detection of abnormal pretransplant clones in progenitor cells of patients who developed myelodysplasia after autologous transplantation. *Blood* 1999; **94**: 1814–9.

129 Pedersen-Bjergaard J, Pedersen M, Myhre J, Geisler C. High risk of therapy-related leukemia after BEAM chemotherapy and autologous stem cell transplantation for previously treated lymphomas is mainly related to primary chemotherapy and not to the BEAM-transplantation procedure. *Leukemia* 1997; **11**: 1654–60.

130 Wheeler C, Khurshid A, Ibrahim J *et al*. Incidence of post-transplant myelodysplasia/acute leukemia in non-Hodgkin's lymphoma patients compared with Hodgkin's disease patients undergoing autologous transplantation following cyclophosphamide, carmustine, and etoposide (CBV). *Leuk Lymphoma* 2001; **40**: 499–509.

131 Bhatia S, Louie AD, Bhatia R *et al*. Solid cancers after bone marrow transplantation. *J Clin Oncol* 2001; **19**: 464–71.

132 Schimmer AD, Quatermain M, Imrie K *et al*. Ovarian function after autologous bone marrow transplantation. *J Clin Oncol* 1998; **16**: 2359–63.

133 Brice P, Pautier P, Marolleau JP, Castaigne S, Gisselbrecht C. Pregnancy after autologous bone marrow transplantation for malignant lymphomas. *Nouv Rev Fr Hematol* 1994; **36**: 387–8.

134 Gulati SC, Van Poznak C. Pregnancy after bone marrow transplantation. *J Clin Oncol* 1998; **16**: 1978–85.

135 Schimmer AD, Ali V, Keith Stewart A, Imrie K, Keating A. Male sexual function after autologous blood or marrow transplantation. *Biol Blood Marrow Transplant* 2001; **7**: 279–83.

136 Vose JM, Bierman PJ, Anderson JR *et al*. Progressive disease after high-dose therapy and autologous transplantation for lymphoid malignancy: clinical course and patient follow-up. *Blood* 1992; **80**: 2142–8.

137 Varterasian M, Ratanatharathorn V, Uberti JP *et al*. Clinical course and outcome of patients with Hodgkin's disease who progress after autologous transplantation. *Leuk Lymphoma* 1995; **20**: 59–65.

138 Bolwell BJ, Kalaycio M, Goormastic M *et al*. Progressive disease after ABMT for Hodgkin's disease. *Bone Marrow Transplant* 1997; **20**: 761–5.

139 Little R, Wittes RE, Longo DL, Wilson WH. Vinblastine for recurrent Hodgkin's disease following autologous bone marrow transplant. *J Clin Oncol* 1998; **16**: 584–8.

140 Kaiser U, Weide R, Wolf M. Successful salvage treatment for relapse after autologous stem cell transplantation in a patient with Hodgkin's disease: a case report. *Ann Hematol* 1999; **78**: 33–5.

141 Shamash J, Lee SM, Radford JA *et al*. Patterns of relapse and subsequent management following high-dose chemotherapy with autologous haematopoietic support in relapsed or refractory Hodgkin's lymphoma: a two center study. *Ann Oncol* 2000; **11**: 715–9.

142 Vandenberghe E, Pearce R, Taghipour G, Fouillard L, Goldstone AH. Role of a second transplant in the management of poor-prognosis lymphomas: a report from the European Blood and Bone Marrow Registry. *J Clin Oncol* 1997; **15**: 1595–600.

143 Lin TS, Avalos BR, Penza SL, Marcucci G, Elder PJ, Copelan EA. Second autologous stem cell transplant for multiply relapsed Hodgkin's disease. *Bone Marrow Transplant* 2002; **29**: 763–7.

144 Tsai T, Goodman S, Saez R *et al*. Allogeneic bone marrow transplantation in patients who relapse after autologous transplantation. *Bone Marrow Transplant* 1997; **20**: 859–63.

145 Freytes CO, Loberiza FR, Rizzo JD *et al*. Allogeneic transplantation in patients that relapsed after autologous transplantation for lymphoma: a report from the International Bone Marrow Transplant Registry. *Proc Am Soc Clin Oncol* 2002; **21**: 414a.

146 Pettengell R, Morgenstern GR, Woll PJ *et al*. Peripheral blood progenitor cell transplantation in lymphoma and leukemia using a single apheresis. *Blood* 1993; **82**: 3770–7.

147 Ager S, Scott MA, Mahendra P *et al*. Peripheral blood stem cell transplantation after high-dose therapy in patients with malignant lymphoma: a retrospective comparison with autologous bone marrow transplantation. *Bone Marrow Transplant* 1995; **16**: 79–83.

148 Brunvand MW, Bensinger WI, Soll E *et al*. High-dose fractionated total-body irradiation, etoposide and cyclophosphamide for treatment of malignant lymphoma: comparison of autologous bone marrow and peripheral blood stem cells. *Bone Marrow Transplant* 1996; **18**: 131–41.

149 Brice P, Marolleau JP, Pautier P *et al*. Hematologic recovery and survival of lymphoma patients after autologous stem-cell transplantation: comparison of bone marrow and peripheral blood progenitor cells. *Leuk Lymphoma* 1996; **22**: 449–56.

150 Weisdorf D, Daniels K, Miller W *et al.* Bone marrow vs. peripheral blood stem cells for autologous lymphoma transplantation: a prospective randomized trial. *Blood* 1993; **82** (Suppl. 1): 444a.

151 Schmitz N, Linch DC, Dreger P *et al.* Randomised trial of filgrastim-mobilised peripheral blood progenitor cell transplantation versus autologous bone-marrow transplantation in lymphoma patients. *Lancet* 1996; **347**: 353–7.

152 Smith TJ, Hillner BE, Schmitz N *et al.* Economic analysis of a randomized clinical trial to compare filgrastim-mobilized peripheral-blood progenitor-cell transplantation and autologous bone marrow transplantation in patients with Hodgkin's and non-Hodgkin's lymphoma. *J Clin Oncol* 1997; **15**: 5–10.

153 Vellenga E, van Agthoven M, Croockewit AJ *et al.* Autologous peripheral blood stem cell transplantation in patients with relapsed lymphoma results in accelerated haematopoietic reconstitution, improved quality of life and cost reduction compared with bone marrow transplantation: the Hovon 22 study. *Br J Haematol* 2001; **114**: 319–26.

154 van Agthoven M, Vellenga E, Fibbe WE, Kingma T, Uyl-de Groot CA. Cost analysis and quality of life assessment comparing patients undergoing autologous bone marrow transplantatin for refractory or relapsed non-Hodgkin's lymphoma or Hodgkin's disease: a prospective randomized trial. *Eur J Cancer* 2001; **37**: 1781–9.

155 Bierman P, Vose J, Anderson J *et al.* Comparison of autologous bone marrow transplantation (ABMT) with peripheral stem cell transplantation (PSCT) for patients (PTS) with Hodgkin's disease (HD). *Blood* 1993; **10** (Suppl. 1): 445a.

156 Majolino I, Pearce R, Taghipour G, Goldstone AH. Peripheral-blood stem-cell transplantation versus autologous bone marrow transplantation in Hodgkin's and non-Hodgkin's lymphomas: a new matched-pair analysis of the European Group for Blood and Marrow Transplantation Registry Data. *J Clin Oncol* 1997; **15**: 509–17.

157 Perry AR, Peniket AJ, Watts MJ, Leverett D, Goldstone AH, Linch DC. Peripheral blood stem cell versus autologous bone marrow transplantation for Hodgkin's disease: equivalent survival outcome in a single-centre matched-pair analysis. *Br J Haematol* 1999; **105**: 280–7.

158 Janssen W, Smilee R, Elfenbein G. A prospective randomized trial comparing blood- and marrow-derived stem cells for hematopoietic replacement following high-dose chemotherapy. *J Hemother* 1995; **4**: 139–40.

159 Weisdorf D, Burroughs J, Miller J *et al.* G-CSF vs. GM-CSF primed bone marrow stem cells (BMSC) or peripheral blood stem cells (PBSC) for autotransplantation: a randomized comparison of engraftment and relapse. *Blood* 1996; **88** (Suppl. 1): 395a.

160 Damiani E, Fanin R, Silvestri F *et al.* Randomized trial of autologous filgrastim-primed bone marrow transplantation versus filgrastim-mobilized peripheral blood stem cell transplantation in lymphoma patients. *Blood* 1997; **90**: 36–42.

161 Appelbaum FR, Thomas ED. Bone marrow transplantation for malignant lymphoma. *Eur J Cancer Clin Oncol* 1987; **23**: 263–6.

162 Horowitz MM, Gale RP, Sondel PM *et al.* Graft-versus-leukemia reactions after bone marrow transplantation. *Blood* 1990; **75**: 555–62.

163 Chopra R, Wotherspoon AC, Blair S *et al.* Detection and significance of bone marrow infiltration at the time of autologous bone marrow transplantation in Hodgkin's disease. *Br J Haematol* 1994; **87**: 647–9.

164 Gajewski JL, Phillips GL, Sobocinski KA *et al.* Bone marrow transplants from HLA-identical siblings in advanced Hodgkin's disease. *J Clin Oncol* 1996; **14**: 572–8.

165 Milpied N, Fielding AK, Pearce RM *et al.* Allogeneic bone marrow transplant is not better than autologous transplant for patients with relapsed Hodgkin's disease. *J Clin Oncol* 1996; **14**: 1291–6.

166 Peniket AJ, Ruiz de Elvira MC, Taghipour G *et al.* Allogeneic transplantation for lymphoma produces a lower relapse rate than autologous transplantation but survival is worse because of higher treatment related mortality: a report of 764 cases from the EBMT lymphoma registry. *Blood* 1997; **90** (Suppl. 1): 255a.

167 Anderson JE, Litzow MR, Appelbaum FR *et al.* Allogeneic, syngeneic, and autologous marrow transplantation for Hodgkin's disease: the 21-year Seattle experience. *J Clin Oncol* 1993; **11**: 2342.

168 Appelbaum FR, Sullivan KM, Thomas ED *et al.* Allogeneic marrow transplantation in the treatment of MOPP-resistant Hodgkin's disease. *J Clin Oncol* 1985; **3**: 1490–4.

169 Phillips GL, Reece DE, Barnett MJ *et al.* Allogeneic marrow transplantation for refractory Hodgkin's disease. *J Clin Oncol* 1989; **7**: 1039–45.

170 Dann EJ, Daugherty CK, Larson RA *et al.* Allogeneic bone marrow transplantation for relapsed and refractory Hodgkin's disease and non-Hodgkin's lymphoma. *Bone Marrow Transplant* 1997; **20**: 369–74.

171 Lundberg JH, Hansen RM, Chitambar CR *et al.* Allogeneic bone marrow transplantation for relapsed and refractory lymphoma using genotypically HLA-identical and alternative donors. *J Clin Oncol* 1991; **9**: 1848–59.

172 Porter DL, Connors JM, Van Deerlin V *et al.* Graft-versus-tumor induction with donor leukocyte infusions as primary therapy for patients with malignancies. *J Clin Oncol* 1999; **17**: 1234–43.

173 Branson K, Chopra R, Kottaridis PD *et al.* Role of nonmyeloablative allogeneic stem-cell transplantation after failure of autologous transplantation in patients with lymphoproliferative malignancies. *J Clin Oncol* 2002; **20**: 4022–31.

174 Nagler A, Slavin S, Varadi G, Naparstek E, Samuel S, Or R. Allogeneic peripheral blood stem cell transplantation using a fludarabine-based low intensity conditioning regimen for malignant lymphoma. *Bone Marrow Transplant* 2000; **25**: 1021–8.

175 McSweeney PA, Niederwieser D, Shizuru JA *et al.* Hematopoietic cell transplantation in older patients with hematologic malignancies: replacing high-dose cytotoxic therapy with graft-versus-tumor effects. *Blood* 2001; **97**: 3390–400.

176 Carella AM, Champlin R, Slavin S, McSweeney P, Storb R. Mini-allografts: ongoing trials in humans. *Bone Marrow Transplant* 2000; **25**: 345–50.

177 Robinson SP, Goldstone AH, Mackinnon S *et al.* Chemoresistant or aggressive lymphoma predicts for a poor outcome following reduced-intensity allogeneic progenitor cell transplantation; an analysis from the Lymphoma Working Party of the European Group for Blood and Bone Marrow Transplantation. *Blood* 2002; **100**: 4310–6.

178 Anderlini P, Giralt S, Andersson B *et al.* Allogeneic stem cell transplantation with fludarabine-based, less intensive conditioning regimens as adoptive immunotherapy in advanced Hodgkin's disease. *Bone Marrow Transplant* 2000; **26**: 615–20.

179 Kottaridis PD, Milligan DW, Chopra R *et al. In vivo* CAMPATH-1H prevents graft-versus-host disease following nonmyeloablative stem cell transplantation. *Blood* 2000; **96**: 2419–25.

180 Dey BR, McAfee S, Sackstein R *et al.* Successful allogeneic stem cell transplantation with non-myeloablative conditioning in patients with relapsed hematologic malignancy following autologous stem cell transplantation. *Biol Blood Marrow Transplant* 2001; **7**: 604–12.

181 Carella AM, Cavaliere M, Lerma E *et al.* Autografting followed by nonmyeloablative immunosuppressive chemotherapy and allogeneic peripheral-blood hematopoietic stem-cell transplantation as treatment of resistant Hodgkin's disease and non-Hodgkin's lymphoma. *J Clin Oncol* 2000; **18**: 3918–24.

182 Spitzer G, Dicke KA, Litam J *et al.* High-dose combination chemotherapy with autologous bone marrow transplantation in adult solid tumors. *Cancer* 1980; **45**: 3075–85.

183 Fielding AK, Philip T, Carella A *et al.* Autologous bone marrow transplantation for lymphomas: a 15 year European Bone Marrow Transplant Registry (EBMT) experience of 3325 patients. *Blood* 1994; **84** (Suppl. 1): 536a.

184 Wheeler C, Antin JH, Churchill WH *et al.* Cyclophosphamide, carmustine, and etoposide with autologous bone marrow transplantation in refractory Hodgkin's disease and non-Hodgkin's lymphoma: a dose finding study. *J Clin Oncol* 1990; **8**: 648–56.

185 Weaver CH, Appelbaum FR, Petersen FB *et al.* High-dose cyclophosphamide, carmustine, and etoposide followed by autologous bone marrow transplantation in patients with lymphoid malignancies who have received dose-limiting radiation therapy. *J Clin Oncol* 1993; **11**: 1329.

186 Gianni AM, Bregni M, Siena S *et al.* High-dose chemotherapy and autologous bone marrow transplantation compared with MACOP-B in aggressive B-cell lymphoma. *N Engl J Med* 1997; **336**: 1290–7.

187 Bierman PJ, Vose JM, Leichner PK *et al.* Yttrium 90-labeled antiferritin followed by high-dose chemotherapy and autologous bone marrow transplantation for poor-prognosis Hodgkin's disease. *J Clin Oncol* 1993; **11**: 698–703.

188 Fitoussi O, Simon D, Brice P *et al.* Tandem transplant of peripheral blood stem cells for patients with poor-prognosis Hodgkin's disease or non-Hodgkin's lymphoma. *Bone Marrow Transplant* 1999; **7**: 747–55.

189 Brice P, Divine M, Simon D *et al.* Feasibility of tandem autologous stem-cell transplantation (ASCT) in induction failure or very unfavorable (UF) relapse from Hodgkin's disease (HD). *Ann Oncol* 1999; **10**: 1485–8.

190 Fung HC, Stiff P, Nademanee A *et al.* Tandem autologous stem cell transplantation (ASCT) for patients (pts) with primary progressive (prog) or poor risk recurrent (recur) Hodgkin's lymphoma (HL). *Proc Am Soc Clin Oncol* 2002; **20**: 414a.

Autologous Hematopoietic Cell Transplantation for Non-Hodgkin's Lymphoma

Sandra J. Horning & James O. Armitage

The non-Hodgkin's lymphomas (NHL) are a heterogeneous group of lymphoid malignancies that collectively represent the fifth most common form of cancer in the USA [1]. The projected incidence in 2001 will exceed 56,000 cases [1]. A subset of these patients will be cured with standard cytotoxic therapies but most will not. Dose escalation of selected chemotherapeutic agents alone or in combination with total body irradiation (TBI), supported by hematopoietic cell transplantation (HCT), may overcome tumor cell resistance to standard treatments in a proportion of patients. In this chapter the application of high-dose therapy and autologous HCT in NHL is reviewed according to histologic subtype and clinical features. High-dose regimen, stem cell source, immunotherapy, complications and future directions are discussed.

NHL classification

The classification of lymphoma continues to evolve with more than 30 subtypes described in the new World Health Organization Lymphoma Classification [2]. Lymphomas are categorized according to their B- or T-cell and putative natural killer (NK) cell lineage, microscopic appearance, immunologic and genetic features, and clinical presentation. The major diagnoses and their frequency using the nomenclature in the Working Formulation are detailed in Table 88.1. Two entities, diffuse large B-cell lymphoma (DLCL) and follicular lymphoma dominate, comprising nearly half of all lymphoid neoplasms. The majority of lymphomas are of B-lineage, a characteristic that influences the selection of primary and subsequent treatments targeting the pan-B-cell antigen, CD20. Because of their distinct clinical features, this review focuses on treatment results according to NHL subtype.

NHL clinical features

DLCL, the most common NHL, occurs over a broad age range. At diagnosis, there is a relatively equal distribution of limited (stage I–II) or disseminated (stage III–IV) disease, according to the Ann Arbor staging convention. Patients with limited disease are frequently cured with combination chemotherapy such as the CHOP (cyclophosphamide, doxorubicin, vincristine, prednisone) regimen, alone or with radiation therapy but the majority of patients with advanced stage disease will relapse after CHOP treatment [3]. A prognostic factor index, established by an international group of clinicians, has been found to be a particularly robust predictor of outcome in patients with DLCL treated with doxorubicin-containing combination chemotherapy [4]. The age-adjusted International Prognostic Factors Index (IPI), developed for patients under the age of 60 years, is outlined in Table 88.2 [4]. The index sums the number

Table 88.1 Major categories of lymphoma.

WHO classification	Working formulation	Frequency (%)
B-lineage		
Large B-cell lymphoma	Diffuse large cell (G)	30.6
Follicular lymphoma	Follicular small cleaved (B)	22.0
	Follicular mixed (C)	
	Follicular large cell (D)	
Small lymphocytic lymphoma/chronic lymphocytic leukemia	Small lymphocytic (A)	6.7
MALT (mucosa-associated lymphoid tissue) lymphoma	–	7.6
Mantle cell lymphoma	–	6.0
Primary mediastinal large B-cell lymphoma	Diffuse large cell (G)	2.4
Burkitt-like lymphoma	Small noncleaved, non-Burkitt (J)	2.1
Burkitt's lymphoma	Small noncleaved, Burkitt (J)	<1.0
T-lineage		
Peripheral T-cell lymphoma	–	7.0
Anaplastic large cell lymphoma	–	2.4
Lymphoblastic lymphoma	Lymphoblastic lymphoma	1.7
Mycosis fungoides	Mycosis fungoides ("miscellaneous")	<1.0

Table 88.2 Age-adjusted international prognostic factors index.

Risk category	Distribution of patients (%)	Risk factors (n)*	CR (%)	Survival at 5 years (%)	
				Disease-free	Overall
Low	22	0	92	79	83
Low intermediate	32	1	78	51	69
High intermediate	32	2	57	30	46
High	14	3	46	27	32

CR, complete remission.
*Risk factors include: elevated serum lactate dehydrogenase, Eastern Cooperative Oncology Group performance status ≥2, Ann Arbor stage III–IV disease.

of adverse factors, which includes performance status, stage and lactate dehydrogenase, and predicts the ability to achieve a complete remission (CR), the durability of remission and overall survival. The IPI has been used to select poor-risk patients for primary consolidation with autologous HCT. Recently, incorporation of the anti-CD20 chimeric monoclonal antibody, rituximab, with CHOP improved survival in older patients with DLCL [5]. The efficacy and safety of rituximab provides multiple opportunities for integration into transplantation therapy as described below.

Follicular lymphomas are disorders of the middle-aged and are nearly always widely disseminated at diagnosis. The natural history is long relative to other NHL, with median survival of about 10 years [6]. Although highly responsive to chemotherapy and irradiation at diagnosis, follicular lymphomas regularly recur and transform to a more aggressive NHL with an increasing risk over time from diagnosis [6]. In addition to traditional cytotoxic approaches based on alkylating agents, radiation therapy and purine analogs, CD20-targeted immunotherapy has emerged as an important treatment option [7–9]. However, no treatment is known to be curative. The relatively long natural history, older patient age and number of active therapies, including allogeneic HCT options, challenge the integration of high-dose treatments supported by autologous HCT in the follicular lymphomas. Optimal timing and appropriate patient selection require an assessment of anticipated benefits and risks.

There are a number of less common lymphoid neoplasms, listed in Table 88.1 according to B- or T-cell lineage. Small lymphocytic lymphomas overlap with chronic lymphocytic leukemia and, as such, are further discussed in Chapter 81. Mantle cell lymphoma presents as disseminated disease, predominantly in older males. Standard cytotoxic therapy is palliative at best and median survival of about 3 years has been reported in multiple series [10,11]. Peripheral T-cell lymphomas present a particular challenge to lymphoma classification. They are relatively rare, the histologic features are quite heterogeneous and the neoplastic population can be difficult to recognize because of the lack of a reliable immunophenotypic marker of T-cell malignancy [2]. Although potentially curable disorders, peripheral T-cell lymphomas are biologically aggressive and relapses are more common than in B-cell lymphomas [12–14]. Anaplastic lymphoma, which expresses the CD30 (Ki-1) antigen, provides an exception to these T-cell disorders [15,16]. This histologic subtype had the most favorable prognosis at 5 years of all those considered in the International Lymphoma Classification Project [17].

The majority of patients with lymphoblastic lymphoma and Burkitt's lymphoma comprise children, adolescents and young adults. Lymphoblastic lymphoma overlaps with acute lymphoblastic leukemia of T-lineage and is best approached with therapy directed toward that disorder [18]. Mediastinal disease is common at diagnosis and involvement of the bone marrow and central nervous system occurs early in the disease course. Burkitt's lymphoma is a rapidly progressive disorder that requires intensive multiagent chemotherapy. Treatment is extremely successful in both children and adults with appropriate management, even in patients with marrow and central nervous system disease [19,20]. Expert pathologists have difficulty in distinguishing high-grade Burkitt-like lymphoma from DLCL and Burkitt's lymphoma [17]. Despite this histopathologic uncertainty, a highly curable subgroup can be defined on the basis of prognostic factors.

In theory, high-dose therapy and autologous HCT could be employed at any time in the disease course in patients with lymphomas lacking a defined curative therapy. For patients with lymphomas potentially curable with current therapy, autologous HCT might be considered at relapse or as primary therapy for selected cases with high-risk features. A discussion of the results of autologous HCT as primary or subsequent therapy in multiple histologic and clinical settings follows.

Rationale for high-dose therapy in lymphoma

Experimental data demonstrated that survival of murine lymphoma cells *in vivo* was inversely proportional to dosage of alkylating agents administered [21]. This observation suggested that lymphoid tumor resistance in humans might be relative rather than absolute as well. Retrospective analyses in clinical studies have demonstrated an association between dose intensity and outcome in patients with DLCL [22]. However, the failure of modest increases in dose intensity to improve outcomes in previously untreated DLCL implies that much greater dose escalation will be necessary for a significantly favorable impact [23]. The basis for high-dose therapy and autologous HCT is that resistance to standard therapy may be overcome by escalation of doses of drugs or radiation beyond limiting marrow toxicity but within limits of acceptable morbidity and mortality caused by other organ toxicity. Other principles of chemotherapy in human lymphoma apply, such as the use of cytotoxics with different mechanisms of antineoplastic activity and limited overlapping toxicity and the requirement for multiple courses of treatment in the setting of high tumor burden.

The initial report of successful high-dose therapy and transplantation in 1978 was from the National Cancer Institute, where BACT (carmustine, cytarabine, cyclophosphamide and thioguanine) chemotherapy followed by autologous bone marrow transplantation (BMT) eradicated lymphoma in some patients previously considered incurable [24]. This experience appeared to verify the preclinical experience and spawned the current widespread clinical application of this approach.

Diffuse aggressive lymphoma

In 1987, Philip *et al.* [25] reported a cure rate of 35–40% in patients with relapsed chemotherapy-sensitive diffuse aggressive lymphoma (Fig. 88.1). These results were confirmed in 1995 in the multinational PARMA trial in which patients were randomized to receive second-line chemotherapy with cisplatin, cytarabine and dexamethasone (DHAP) with radiotherapy or DHAP consolidated with high-dose BEAC (carmustine,

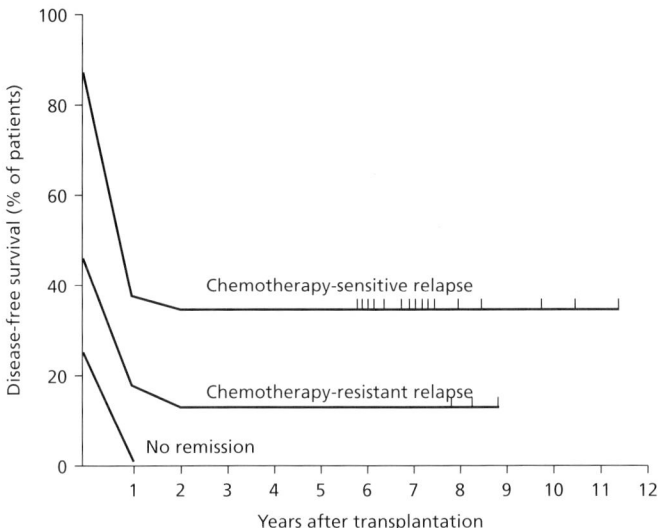

Fig. 88.1 Updated disease-free survival after high-dose therapy and autologous blood and marrow transplant (ABMT) for relapsed or refractory intermediate and high-grade non-Hodgkin's lymphoma (NHL). Patients are segregated according to chemotherapy-sensitive relapse ($n = 44$), chemotherapy-resistant relapse ($n = 22$) and failure to achieve a complete remission with primary treatment ($n = 34$). Tick marks represent censored data. (Reprinted by permission of the author and publisher from Armitage [26].)

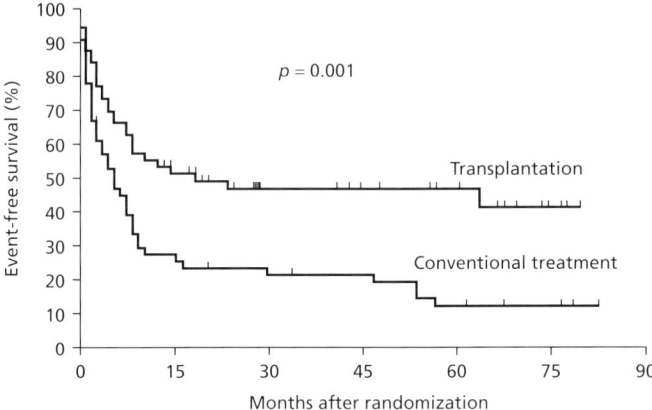

Fig. 88.2 Event-free survival of chemotherapy-sensitive patients with recurrent intermediate- and high-grade non-Hodgkin's lymphoma (NHL) treated with high-dose therapy and autologous blood and marrow transplant (ABMT) ($n = 49$) and patients treated with conventional chemotherapy ($n = 54$). The data are based on an intent-to-treat analysis. Tick marks represent censored data. (Reprinted by permission of the authors and publisher from Philip et al. [27].)

etoposide, cytarabine, cyclophosphamide) *plus* autologous BMT and radiotherapy [27]. The 5-year event-free survival was 46% for transplanted patients vs. 12% for chemotherapy-only patients ($p = 0.001$) (Fig. 88.2). The overall survival at 5 years was 53% in the transplant group vs. 32% in the conventional treatment group ($p = 0.038$). The criteria for entry into this trial included age <60 years, achievement of a CR after primary treatment, and no known marrow or central nervous system involvement with lymphoma at study entry. Only patients who responded to second-line DHAP chemotherapy, about half of the total entered on study, were subsequently randomized.

The PARMA investigators conducted subsequent retrospective analyses to identify factors prognostic of outcome. Relapse within 1 year of diagnosis and elevated lactate dehydrogenase at relapse were associated with inferior survival [28]. The IPI at relapse was significantly predictive for survival in the salvage chemotherapy group but not in the transplanted group [29]. Retrospective analyses of factors prognostic for outcome in another chemotherapy-sensitive relapsed population demonstrated that CR immediately prior to transplant predicted longer survival and remission duration [30].

In the original series of Philip et al. [26] patients refractory to initial therapy who were progressing prior to high-dose treatment did not enjoy durable responses to transplantation (Fig. 88.1). Similarly, patients with lymphoma who had responded to primary treatment but proved resistant to second-line regimens had a minimal cure rate (<15%). When all the factors in the PARMA study are considered, they apply to less than one-third of the total group of patients with DLCL who fail primary treatment [27]. In agreement with this observation, a consortium of Italian centres reported that only 20% of 474 patients with first relapse of DLCL received consolidation with HCT [31]. Therefore, initiatives to improve outcomes and offer potentially curative therapy to a greater proportion of patients are needed. Strategies include more effective salvage chemotherapy, mobilization of tumor-free stem cells, more effective preparatory regimens and application of immunotherapy in the peri-transplant period as discussed elsewhere in this chapter.

Theoretically, a larger proportion of patients will have relative rather than absolute drug resistance early in the disease course. Thus, the early application of high-dose therapy and autologous HCT may benefit a larger proportion of poor-risk patients. Gulati et al. [32] and Nademanee et al. [33] were among the first to report the potential benefit of high-dose therapy and autologous BMT as a consolidation to CR achieved with combination chemotherapy. Subsequently, this concept was tested in multiple clinical trials, as outlined in Table 88.3. These trials differ in patient selection, pathologic subtype, choice and extent of induction therapy, time of and selection for randomization, and statistical power to observe treatment effects. Prior to the consensus achieved in the IPI, clinical studies incorporated a variety of risk factors. The Groupe d'Etude des Lymphomes de Adulte (GELA) conducted a phase III study in which patients with intermediate and high-grade lymphoma with one or more unfavorable prognostic factors in first CR were randomized to receive sequential chemotherapy or high-dose CBV (cyclophosphamide, carmustine, etoposide) and autologous BMT [41]. At 5 years, there was no significant difference in event-free or overall survival in the study arms but, upon review, only 49% of participants had high-intermediate and high-risk disease as defined by the IPI (Table 88.2). Subsequent retrospective analysis of these data limited to the poor-risk subsets demonstrated an 8-year disease-free survival rate with CBV and transplantation (55%) superior to that of sequential chemotherapy (39%; $p = 0.02$) [34]. Of note, these results were achieved in poor-risk patients who achieved CR with induction chemotherapy, representing 61% of the total population.

Favorable outcomes with high-dose therapy and autologous transplantation were reported in several other randomized studies initiated prior to the adoption of the IPI. Gianni et al. [35] randomized patients to a weekly chemotherapy combination or high-dose sequential chemotherapy, in which maximal tolerated doses of individual drugs were delivered in several phases prior to a final phase of high-dose therapy and autologous HCT. By retrospective analysis, 96% of patients on the high-dose sequential arm had high intermediate or high IPI risk disease. In this rather small trial, event-free survival at 5 years was 76% for patients receiving high-dose sequential therapy, compared to 49% for those receiving standard therapy ($p = 0.004$). The Italian Cooperative Study Group initiated a study of etoposide doxorubicin, cyclophosphamide, vincristine, prednisone (VACOP) chemotherapy alone or followed by HCT [36], also prior to the IPI consensus. No statistical differences were seen in the treatment arms but, in retrospective analysis, a benefit in disease-free survival (CR patients only) was noted for high intermediate and high IPI risk patients who were transplanted.

Table 88.3 Autologous transplantation in first remission for diffuse aggressive lymphoma.

Group/analysis	Patient population	Time of randomization	n	Therapy	PFS (%)	p	Overall survival (%)	p	Time (years)	Reference
GELA/subset	First CR; aggressive NHL; retrospective HI-H IPI	CR	111 125	A/NCVB × 4 + sequential CT A/NCVB × 4, MTX + CBV and AHCT	39 55	0.02	49 64	0.04	8	[34]
Italian Coop/subset	Aggressive NHL; retrospective HI-H IPI	Study entry	36 34	VACOP-B VACOP-B + and AHCT	37 65	0.08	55 68	0.7	6	[36]
Milano/prospective	B-cell diffuse large cell lymphoma; 96% HI-H IP	Study entry	50 48	MACOP-B High-dose sequential and AHCT	49 76	0.004	81 55	0.09	7	[35]
EORTC/prospective	Aggressive NHL 29–36% HI-H IPI	CR/PR after 3 cycles	96 98	CHVmP/BV × 8 CHVmP/BV × 6 + BEAC and AHCT	56 61	n.s.	77 68	n.s.	5	[37]
German HGLSG/prospective	Aggressive NHL Abnormal LDH ~75% HI-H IPI	CR/PR/MR after 2 cycles	154 158	CHOEP × 5 CHOEP × 3 + BEAM and AHCT	49 59	0.22	63 62	0.68	3	[38]
GELA/prospective	Aggressive NHL HI-H IPI	Study entry	181 189	ACVB × 4 + Sequential CT CEOP × 1, ECVBP × 2 + BEAM and AHCT	51 39	0.01	60 46	0.007	5	[39]
Multinational/prospective	Aggressive NHL HI-HIPI	Study entry	232 235	CHOP × 6–8 CHOP × 3 + BEAM and AHCT	n.r. n.r.		54 50	n.s.	5	[40]

ACVB, doxorubicin, cyclophosphamide, vindesine, bleomycin; AHCT, autologous hematopoietic cell transplantation; BEAC, carmustine, etoposide, cytarapine and cyclophosphamide; BEAM, carmustine, etoposide, doxorubicin and melphalan; CBV, cyclophosphamide, carmustine, etoposide; CEOP, cyclophosphamide, epotoside, vincristine, prednisone; CHOP, cyclophosphamide, doxorubicin, vincristine and prednisone; CHVmP/BV, cyclophosphamide, doxorubicin, teniposide, prednisone, bleomycin and vincristine; CT, computerized tomography; ECVBP, epirubicin, cyclophosphamide, vindesine, bleomycin, prednisone; EORTC, European Organization for Research and Treatment of Cancer; GELA, Groupe d'Etude des Lymphomes de Adulte; HGLSG, high grade lymphoma study group; HI-H IPI, high-intermediate and high-risk international prognostic index; LDH, lactate dehydrogenase; MACOP-B, methotrexate, doxorubicin, cyclophosphamide, vincristine, prednisone; MR, minimal response; MTX, methotrexate; NCVB, mitoxantrone, cyclophosphamide, vindesine, bleomycin; NHL, non-Hodgkin's lymphoma; n.s., not significant; n.r., note reported; PFS, progression-free survival; PR, partial remission; VACOP-B, etoposide doxorubicin, cyclophosphamide, vincristine, prednisone.

In other randomized efforts that included DLCL patients of variable risk for treatment failure, there were no significant differences between standard and transplantation treatment arms. The European Organization for the Research and Treatment of Cancer (EORTC) conducted a trial in advanced diffuse aggressive lymphoma, randomly assigning patients to eight cycles of standard chemotherapy (CHVmP/BV [cyclophosphamide, doxorubicin, teniposide, prednisone, bleomycin, vincristine]) vs. six cycles plus high-dose chemotherapy and autologous HCT [37]. This trial was stopped early with 194 randomized patients because the results indicated that the transplant arm was not more effective than standard treatment. Only a minority of patients in this trial was in the high-intermediate or high-risk category but subset analysis failed to detect any differences in the treatment arms according to the IPI. The German High Grade Lymphoma Study Group assigned patients with an elevated lactate dehydrogenase who responded to two cycles of CHOEP (cyclophosphamide, doxorubicin, vincristine, etoposide, prednisone) chemotherapy to three further cycles or one cycle *plus* HCT [38]. Event-free survival at 4 years was 49% for conventional chemotherapy and 59% for transplantation ($p = 0.22$) and no difference in overall survival was observed. When analyzed for high-intermediate and high-risk IPI and exclusion of Burkitt's and lymphoblastic histology, there was a trend toward longer event-free survival with HCT. Together, these results demonstrated the need for prospective studies of high-intermediate and high-risk diffuse aggressive lymphoma as identified by the IPI, comparing chemotherapy alone with chemotherapy followed by HCT.

The GELA studied a shortened and intensified induction regimen with three cycles of escalated epirubicin, cyclophosphamide, vindesine, bleomycin and prednisone, designed to boost the complete remission rate, prior to autologous HCT [39]. This study was prematurely closed because of inferior results in the transplant arm (Table 88.3). In a multinational trial, no difference in overall survival was observed with three cycles of CHOP followed by BEAM (carmustine, etoposide, doxorubicin, melphalan) and autologous HCT compared with 6–8 cycles of CHOP chemotherapy in high- and high-intermediate IPI risk patients [40]. The failure to confirm the advantage for autologous HCT seen in the retrospective analyses may be related to early randomization without selection for response, inadequate duration of induction therapy, inclusion of histologic subtypes other than diffuse large cell, or other factors. The US cooperative groups are testing the hypothesis that high-intermediate and high-risk patients who respond to a full course of CHOP would benefit from immediate autologous HCT vs. an autologous HCT at relapse [42].

Whereas patients in partial remission after primary therapy are rarely cured with further conventional chemotherapy, dose escalation, theoretically, may result in a durable response in drug-sensitive subjects. A prospective phase III comparison of high-dose therapy and autologous BMT vs. DHAP chemotherapy for patients in partial response (defined as 50–80% reduction in measurable disease after two-thirds of planned therapy) was conducted in multiple institutions in Italy [43]. Although the rate of disease progression was much lower in the high-dose group (4%) than in the DHAP group (41%), the number of patients in the trial was too small to achieve statistically significant differences in overall and progression-free survival. A group of Dutch investigators studied the impact of high-dose cyclophosphamide (CY) and TBI plus autologous BMT vs. further chemotherapy in patients with a partial response (defined as 25–90% reduction in measurable disease) after three cycles of CHOP chemotherapy [44]. The majority of patients on either study arm achieved a CR. No significant differences in overall, disease-free or event-free survival were seen. Furthermore, the disease-free survival in both study arms was not different from patients in CR after three cycles of CHOP. These negative results may, in part, be related to the definition of partial remission used in patient selection. With current sophisticated imaging techniques, radiographic abnormalities, many of which do not represent viable tumor, are commonly noted after induction chemotherapy.

A number of groups tested the efficacy and safety of intensified high-dose therapy in diffuse aggressive lymphoma. Results with application of the high-dose sequential therapy regimen in recurrent or refractory patients were not encouraging in the Stanford University experience [45]. Tandem transplantation applied to high-intermediate or high IPI risk patients did not improve results over those achieved in the original GELA study [46] whereas Ballestrero *et al.* [47] reported promising results in high-risk patients receiving an intensive three-step treatment with tandem transplantation. Intensive induction therapies supported by growth factors and HCT have been assessed by other European groups in high-risk patients; unfortunately, early treatment failures were observed in more than half of patients [48,49]. An expert panel has reported an evidence-based review of the role of cytotoxic therapy with transplantation in DLCL which includes areas of needed research [50]. The application of targeted immunotherapy is an important new area of investigation directed toward improved outcomes in high-risk untreated or relapsed DLCL.

Follicular lymphoma

The database for high-dose therapy and autologous HCT in follicular lymphoma primarily represents results of prospective phase II trials or retrospective analyses. In those series with mature follow-up (Table 88.4), the median disease-free survival for patients with recurrent follicular lymphoma was approximately 4 years, with a continuous relapse pattern, and about two-thirds of patients were alive at 4 years. Freedman *et al.* [51] updated results in 153 patients who received CY/TBI and purged bone marrow in second or subsequent remission; 69% were alive a median time of 12 years from diagnosis. While this median survival is longer than that reported with conventional treatment, patients in this study had favorable characteristics including age less than 60 years, minimal tumor burden and sensitive disease. In most clinical series, patients received chemotherapy and TBI prior to transplantation. The retrospective series from Stanford University reported significantly longer disease-free survival and overall survival for patients treated with chemotherapy and TBI compared with chemotherapy alone [54]. Favorable prognostic factors in these studies included exposure to three or fewer treatment regimens prior to transplantation and molecular remission, defined as continued absence of cells with Bcl2/IgH (immunoglobulin heavy chain) rearrangement in the blood and marrow [51–54].

In lieu of randomized trial results, freedom from recurrence and survival for patients treated with CY and TBI *plus* purged autologous bone marrow were compared with chemotherapy controls matched for remission status by investigators at St. Bartholomew's hospital [52,58]. A statistically significant advantage in disease-free survival was found for autologous HCT compared with chemotherapy but this did not translate into an overall survival benefit, partly because of the occurrence of secondary myelodysplasia (MDS) and acute leukemia in transplanted patients [52,59] (see below). The GELA compared results for patients with follicular lymphoma, recurrent after treatment on prospective trials, who underwent high-dose therapy with autologous HCT or standard treatment [60]. At 5 years, freedom from second failure and survival were significantly longer for transplanted patients <65 years. In a multicentre phase III European trial, patients with recurrent follicular lymphoma were randomly assigned to chemotherapy, high-dose therapy and an unpurged autologous graft, or high-dose therapy and a purged autologous graft [61]. With 89 randomized patients and 44 months' follow-up, the progression-free survival was superior for either transplant arm compared with chemotherapy ($p = 0.01$) [62]. In this trial, no difference was seen in overall survival between the treatments but the small sample size precluded definitive statements regarding either survival or purging.

Table 88.4 High-dose therapy and autologous transplantation in follicular lymphoma.

Group [Reference]	High-dose regimen	Stem cell source	Survival (%) Progression-free	Overall	Years
Relapsed/recurrent					
DFCC [51]	CY/TBI	Purged marrow	42	66	8
St. Bartholomew's [52]	CY/TBI	Purged marrow	63	69	5
University of Nebraska [53]	CY/TBI BEAC	Unpurged marrow	44	65	4
Stanford University [54]	TBI/VP16/CY BCNU/VP16/CY	Purged PBPC	44	60	4
First remission					
DFCC [55]	CY/TBI	Purged marrow	59	84	4
Stanford University [56]	TBI/VP16/CY	Purged marrow	76	92	5
Italian GITMO [57]	High dose sequential	Unpurged PBPC	60	85	4

BEAC, carmustine, etoposide, cytarabine and cyclophosphamide; BCNU, carmustine; CY, cyclophosphamide; DFCC, Dana Farber Cancer Center; GITMO, Gruppo Italiano Trapianti Midollo Osseo; PBPC, peripheral blood progenitor cell; TBI, total body irradiation; VP16, etoposide.

Several groups reported experiences with high-dose therapy and autologous HCT in follicular lymphoma patients in first remission [55,56,63]. The Dana Farber Cancer Center (DFCC) and Stanford University studies were similar in design, incorporating chemotherapy and TBI and antibody-purged bone marrow (Table 88.4) [55,56]. Disease-free survival was extended compared to remission duration expected with chemotherapy and overall survival was excellent in both studies. As with the transplantation studies performed in patients with relapsed follicular lymphoma, late toxicity in the form of MDS or acute myeloid leukemia (AML) was seen in both studies. An Italian multicentre group reported 67% disease-free survival at 4 years in untreated follicular lymphoma patients treated with high-dose sequential chemotherapy and unpurged autologous peripheral blood progenitor cells (PBPCs) [63]. In 47% of autologous grafts, no residual tumor cells were detected by molecular analysis. In their report outlining prognostic factors, Voso *et al.* [64] found that fewer than eight sites of involvement and transplantation in first remission were favorable determinants of the success of autologous HCT in follicular lymphoma. These phase II studies support a definitive assessment of first remission transplantation such as the German Low-Grade Lymphoma Study Group's randomized multicenter trial comparing chemotherapy *plus* autologous transplantation vs. chemotherapy plus interferon.

The long and variable natural history of follicular lymphoma and the variety of therapeutic options contribute to the difficulty in interpreting the results of autologous HCT in first remission and after relapse. Investigators from Kiel, Germany, reported superior outcomes with autologous HCT in first remission but no difference in overall survival when corrected for initial time from diagnosis [65]. In all of the studies described, the most favorable outcomes were reported in patients with minimal tumor burden and continued sensitivity to standard drug therapy. Relapse of disease has been the major cause of failure after high-dose therapy and autologous HCT in all published series. This problem may be favorably impacted by the incorporation of antibody-based therapies for *in vivo* purging or as part of the induction, preparatory or post-transplant regimen as discussed below.

Transformation to a diffuse aggressive lymphoma is common in follicular lymphoma and portends a grave prognosis. Selected patients with transformation may benefit from high-dose therapy and autologous HCT. Friedberg *et al.* [66] reported a 46% disease-free survival at 36 months in transformed lymphoma patients. Results were superior for patients who had transformed within 18 months of diagnosis. A similar disease-free survival at 4 years (49%) was reported in 17 transformed lymphoma patients transplanted at Stanford University [52]. In a series of 27 transformed patients from St. Bartholomew's hospital, 19 were alive and disease-free at 2.4 years after HCT. Relapses occurred with follicular as well as transformed lymphoma [67]. Williams *et al.* [68] reporting from the European Bone Marrow Transplant Registry, found that outcomes with autologous HCT in transformed lymphoma patients were not different from those reported for *de novo* DLCL in relapse. In this report, as well as that from Chen *et al.* [69] there was a relatively high transplant-related mortality related to advanced age and previous therapy. Together, these data indicate that selected patients with transformed disease have curative potential with high-dose therapy and autologous HCT.

Mantle cell lymphoma

The absence of curative therapy and 3-year median survival have fostered interest in high-dose therapy and autologous HCT for patients with mantle cell lymphoma in first and subsequent remission. Table 88.5 describes the published data from several series employing high-dose therapy and autologous HCT in mantle cell lymphoma. In the DFCC series, the disease-free survival was 31% at 4 years for eight first remission patients and 20 relapsed patients treated with CY and TBI followed by purged autologous bone marrow [70]. An estimated event-free survival of 36% at 2 years was achieved in 40 patients transplanted at the University of Nebraska [72]. Patients receiving less than three prior therapies survived longer but, similar to those with more extensive treatment, experienced a continuous pattern of relapse. Early autologous transplantation, as a consolidation to first remission, resulted in superior outcomes in several studies. In a joint analysis from two German transplant centres, the 2-year event-free survival and overall survival for 34 mantle cell patients transplanted after standard induction, intensive chemotherapy for mobilization and radiochemotherapy were 77% and 100%, respectively, compared to 30% ($p = 0.007$) and 54% ($p = 0.0016$), respectively, for transplantation after relapse [73]. The results for first remission transplant also yielded longer event-free and overall survival when calculated from diagnosis. The combined autologous HCT experience at the City of Hope National Medical Center and Stanford University confirmed these results [71]. At 3 years, survival was 93% for 27 first remission patients compared to 64% for 42 patients transplanted beyond first remission. At 3 and 5 years, the disease-free survival was 77% and 50%, respectively,

Table 88.5 High-dose therapy and autologous transplantation in mantle cell lymphoma.

Group [Reference]	n	Status	High-dose regimen	Stem cell source	Survival (%) Progression-free	Overall	Years
DFCC [70]	8	CR1	CY/TBI	Purged marrow	53	NR	5
	20	>CR1			0	NR	
City of Hope/ Stanford [71]	27	CR1	TBI/VP16/CY	Unpurged PBPC or purged PBPC	77	93	3
	42	>CR1	BCNU/VP16/CY		39	64	
University of Nebraska [72]	40	>CR1	CY/TBI BEAC, BEAM	Unpurged marrow or PBPC	35	65	2
University of Kiel [73]	34	Remission 1	CY/TBI	Unpurged PBPC	77	100	2
	12	>Remission 1			30	54	

BCNU, carmustine; BEAC, carmustine, etoposide, cytarabine and cyclophosphamide; BEAM, carmustine, etoposide, doxorubicin and melphalan; CR, complete remission; CY, cyclophosphamide; DFCC, Dana Farber Cancer Center; NR, not reported; PBPC, peripheral blood progenitor cell; TBI, total body irradiation; VP16, etoposide.

in first remission patients, demonstrating an ongoing risk of relapse. In preliminary analysis of a prospective randomized trial conducted by the European Mantle Cell Lymphoma Intergroup, a highly significant difference was observed in the 4-year event-free survival favoring consolidative myeloablative therapy and autologous transplantation, with only 17% of patients relapsing compared with 53% who received consolidative interferon [74].

These data indicate that autologous HCT may improve prognosis in mantle cell lymphoma when performed as part of an intensive first-line treatment strategy. However, based upon the continuous pattern of relapse, first remission autologous transplants do not appear to be curative in the majority of patients. Alternative strategies for increasing the success of this approach include alternative induction therapy, enhancing the preparatory regimen and combining rituximab during mobilization or after transplant. Khouri et al. [75] have reported a high remission rate with the hyper-CVAD (fractionated cyclophosphamide, vincristine, doxorubicin, decadron, methotrexate, cytarabine) regimen for cytoreduction prior to high-dose therapy and autologous HCT. A high CR rate was reported with the induction regimen of CHOP followed by DHAP with or without rituximab, allowing a large proportion of patients to proceed to HCT in mantle cell lymphoma [76]. Gopal et al. [77] studied high-dose 131-I tositumomab, a murine anti-CD20 radioimmunoconjugate, in combination with etoposide and cyclophosphamide as a chemoradioimmunotherapy preparatory regimen for HCT for relapsed mantle cell lymphoma. At 3 years, 61% of relapsed or refractory patients were alive and progression-free. Molecular remissions have been achieved in mantle cell lymphoma with rituximab incorporated in hematopoietic cell mobilization or following transplantation for mantle cell lymphoma [78–80]. As with follicular lymphoma, achievement of molecular remission in the stem cell graft was a very strong prognostic factor for survival in mantle cell lymphoma [81].

T-cell and high-grade lymphomas

There is a paucity of data regarding the efficacy of high-dose therapy and autologous HCT in T-cell lymphomas, which represent only about 15–20% of NHL in Western countries. Reports often combine multiple T-cell subtypes, including lymphoblastic and the more favorable anaplastic large cell lymphoma. Vose et al. [82] reported similar disease-free and overall survival in 17 T-cell NHL, including three lymphoblastic and 24 B-lineage lymphomas. In a retrospective analysis of 36 T-cell lymphoma patients, 29 of whom received autologous HCT and seven of whom received allogeneic HCT, Rodriguez et al. [83] observed a 3-year survival of 36%. These results were quite favorable given the poor prognosis for peripheral T-cell lymphomas. Blystad et al. [84] reported a series of 41 chemosensitive T-cell lymphoma patients who received autologous HCT in Norway and Sweden. Seventeen patients were in first partial or complete remission. The overall survival at 4 years was 79% for the 14 anaplastic large cell patients and 44% for the other 27 patients. These data confirm other reports of successful autologous transplantation in T-cell anaplastic large cell lymphoma in relapse or initial remission [85–87]. However, the prognosis for this subtype is known to be heterogeneous, with a particularly favorable outlook for cases that express the ALK protein, such that further evaluation is necessary to determine which, if any, patients with primary disease are candidates for high-dose therapy and autologous HCT [3].

Because lymphoblastic and Burkitt's lymphoma are uncommon in adults, the reports of high-dose therapy and autologous HCT have generally included only small numbers of patients. Consolidation of first remission in lymphoblastic lymphoma with autologous HCT or further chemotherapy was studied in a randomized trial in Europe in which there was a trend toward longer relapse-free survival with autologous HCT but no difference in overall survival [88]. Registry data were reported in 128 lymphoblastic lymphoma patients treated with autologous transplantation. At 5 years, 56% had relapsed and 39% were alive [89]. As anticipated, patients with marrow involvement and those transplanted at relapse had a less favorable outlook. Because these high-grade lymphomas involve the bone marrow when advanced in stage or recurrent, resembling their lineage-associated acute lymphoblastic leukemia counterparts, many investigators favor allogeneic transplantation for poor-risk patients. The registry data showed fewer relapses after allogeneic transplantation in lymphoblastic lymphoma but overall survival was inferior to autologous HCT at 6 months and not significantly different thereafter [89]. Jost et al. [90] delivered high-dose therapy and autologous HCT following weekly chemotherapy appropriate for DLCL; their disappointing results emphasize the importance of an appropriate induction regimen prior to high-dose treatment. In contrast, Bouabdallah et al. [91] reported superior outcomes with a leukemia induction therapy prior to either autologous or allogeneic transplantation. Thus, selection of appropriate induction chemotherapy and prognostic factors, variables that influence the rate of cure with primary chemotherapy as well, influence the transplant results.

Fewer data are available for Burkitt's lymphoma and autologous transplantation. An overall survival of 72% at 3 years was observed in registry data compiled on 70 patients transplanted in first remission [92]. These data compare favorably with conventional treatment but excellent survival (73%) at 2 years was recently reported with the use of intensive pediatric induction protocols in adult Burkitt's lymphoma patients [21]. With this approach, the poorest risk patients maintained an estimated survival of 59% at 2 years. Autologous transplantation in recurrent Burkitt's lymphoma has been generally unsuccessful and is definitely not recommended for chemo-resistant patients.

High-dose regimens

Selected high-dose regimens commonly used with autologous HCT are defined in Table 88.6 (preparatory regimens are discussed in detail in Chapters 12 and 13). Based on the ability to escalate doses with acceptable extramedullary toxicity, the alkylating agents are prominently featured. Variables include the use of TBI and the individual drugs, doses and schedules. Additional chemotherapeutic agents that have been safely escalated prior to transplantation in NHL include ifosfamide, carboplatin and mitoxantrone. The CY and TBI combination has been widely utilized in NHL, particularly in the low-grade lymphomas. Several investigators have suggested that the combination of TBI, VP16 and CY may yield superior results in NHL [93–95,97–99]. In fact, because of nonoverlapping toxicities, the maximal single tolerated doses of VP16 and CY can be used in the combination. Excellent single institution results with TBI, VP16 and CY were confirmed in a cooperative group trial [95]. Several investigators have augmented the CBV regimen, which is widely employed for Hodgkin's disease as well as NHL [96,97]. In addition to higher total doses, the drugs have been given as single doses rather than prolonged infusions [99]. The importance of schedule was suggested by preclinical data in which single large doses were superior to multiple doses delivered over a longer time period [100].

The rate of relapse was similar in 221 patients receiving autologous HCT at Stanford University following radiation-containing or chemotherapy-only preparatory regimens selected on the basis of prior therapy [99]. However, a TBI-containing regimen was associated with improved outcome in a retrospective analysis of follicular lymphoma patients at that institution [101]. In contrast, better results with multiagent chemotherapy were obtained in a large registry series of DLCL patients transplanted in Spain when compared with the CY/TBI combination [102]. In the absence of randomized trials, the superiority of one regimen over another cannot be assessed. Based upon differences in the sensitivity of indolent and aggressive lymphoma to radiation therapy, it is quite possible that outcomes following transplantation might be disparate. Because of toxicity considerations, particularly pneumonitis, TBI should be avoided in patients who have received prior radiotherapy or for whom peri-transplant radiotherapy is planned [98]. There is disagreement in the literature regarding a higher risk of secondary leukemia associated with TBI as discussed below.

Gianni *et al.* [35] introduced a novel delivery of high-dose chemotherapy for NHL and other malignancies. In order to give each drug in single agent maximal tolerated dose, the agents were sequentially delivered, some with growth factor support. Whereas this approach was superior to standard chemotherapy in untreated DLCL patients, the toxicity of the approach precluded its use for relapsed patients in the Stanford University experience [45]. The high-dose sequential approach has been modified to include more cycles of standard induction chemotherapy and to incorporate high-dose cytarabine [103]. Multiple cycles of high-dose therapy and sequential chemotherapy with repeated HCT have also been studied [48,104]. The efficacy and safety of this approach relative to standard myeloablative conditioning approaches have not been definitively studied.

Press *et al.* [105] pioneered the use of high-dose radioimmunotherapy in conjunction with autologous HCT. In this approach, discussed further in Chapter 15, a radioisotope is linked to a monoclonal antibody, targeting the tissue of interest and, theoretically, sparing normal tissues. After demonstrating the safety and efficacy of iodine-131 (131-I) linked to the anti-CD20 antibody tositumomab, Press *et al.* [106] combined the radioimmunoconjugate with etoposide and cyclophosphamide followed by autologous HCT in a phase 1–2 study. Based upon these encouraging results, a randomized trial of conventional TBI vs. targeted radioimmunotherapy is in progress for B-cell NHL. In addition, as noted above, Gopal *et al.* [77] achieved encouraging results in recurrent and refractory mantle cell lymphoma with 131-I tositumomab, etoposide and cyclophosphamide and autologous HCT. Subsequently, Vose *et al.* [107] safely escalated 131-I tositumomab with full-dose BEAM prior to transplantation. The feasibility of a dose-escalated 131-I and rituximab conjugate with autologous transplantation for mantle cell lymphoma has also been demonstrated [108]. Yttrium-90 (90-Y) is an alternate isotope with pure beta-emitting properties. Investigators have successfully escalated doses of 90-Y chelated with ibritumomab, a murine anti-CD20 antibody, in combination with etoposide and cyclophosphamide or the BEAM regimen [109,110]. These new approaches may allow intensification without significant additional acute toxicity.

Stem cell source and manipulation

Tumor contamination of the autologous graft is particularly likely in follicular, mantle cell and the high-grade lymphomas. It is unclear if transplanted lymphoma cells are clonogenic or to what extent they contribute to relapse. In a series of elegant studies in which t(15;19) cells in the bone marrow were detected by polymerase chain reaction (PCR) methodology, Gribben *et al.* [111] provided convincing evidence that the ability to purge the marrow *ex vivo* with monoclonal antibodies and complement correlated with disease-free survival. In support of their observations in follicular lymphoma, the DFCC group also demonstrated that the failure of immunologic purging in mantle cell lymphoma correlated with disease recurrence [81]. Additionally, Sharp *et al.* [112] found that the

Table 88.6 High-dose therapy used with autologous transplantation in NHL.

Regimen	Drugs, dose(s) and schedule	References
CY/TBI	CY 60 mg/kg × 2 TBI 200 cGy/fraction × 6 over 3 days	[51,55]
TBI/VP16/CY	TBI 1200 cGy in 8–10 fractions VP16 60 mg/kg CY 100 mg/kg*	[93–96]
BEAC	BCNU 300 mg/m^2 VP16 200 mg/m^2 × 4 days CY 35 mg/kg × 4 days	[26]
CBV	CY 1500 mg/m^2 × 4 days BCNU 300 mg/m^2 VP16 250 mg/m^2 × 4 days	[34]
Augmented CBV	CY 100 mg/kg* BCNU 15 mg/kg* or 450–550 mg/m^2* VP16 60 mg/kg	[95–97]

BCNU, carmustine; BEAC, carmustine, etoposide, cytarabine and cyclophosphamide; CBV, cyclophosphamide, carmustine and etoposide; CY, cyclophosphamide; TBI, total body irradiation; VP16, etoposide.
*Based on ideal body weight or adjusted ideal body weight.

ability to culture tumor cells from histologically negative bone marrow in patients with NHL was associated with statistically inferior disease-free survival. Although these observations may simply be surrogates for the ability of lymphoma cells to succumb to or survive cytotoxic therapy, they support the use of a purified graft (see Chapter 19).

Patients with follicular lymphoma were found to have better overall survival if they received a purged rather than unpurged autologous graft in a case–control analysis conducted by the European Bone Marrow Transplant Registry [113]. The European CUP trial, described above, lacked the sample size necessary to demonstrate a difference related to purging [59]. In addition, purging technology often failed to eliminate molecular evidence of disease from the marrow [111]. With the transition from bone marrow to blood hematopoietic cell harvests, the significance of lymphoma contamination was again evaluated, yielding inconsistent results for molecular evidence of disease and *in vitro* culture growth of lymphoma [114,115].

Randomized trials demonstrated that transplantation of growth factor-mobilized hematopoietic cells from the peripheral blood resulted in earlier engraftment and lowered costs, while obviating the need to harvest marrow under anesthesia [116,117]. On the basis of these trials and a plethora of supporting data from single institutions, peripheral blood hematopoietic cell (PBHC) collections replaced bone marrow harvests for use after high-dose therapy in NHL. Early experience from the University of Nebraska suggested that autologous peripheral blood HCT in lymphoma patients resulted in fewer relapses than bone marrow transplants, but this finding was not confirmed in a subsequent randomized trial [114,118]. Patients receiving peripheral blood, as expected, had faster engraftment but there was no difference in event-free survival.

As a result of enrichment of CD34$^+$ cell numbers, mobilization of PBHC with chemotherapy in addition to growth factors has been adopted in many centres. In a randomized trial, Boston investigators found no differences in time to engraftment, resource utilization, tumor contamination or therapeutic outcome for patients mobilized with growth factors with or without high-dose CY [119]. These results confirm other reports indicating no improvement in engraftment kinetics above a target threshold [120,121]. A potential advantage of higher CD34 cell number enabled by mobilization with chemotherapy and growth factors relates to techniques that have been developed for purging limited volumes of enriched cells which yield PCR-negative products [120]. Commercial systems for the positive selection of CD34$^+$ cells, resulting in several logs of tumor cell depletion, have been applied alone or in combination with negative selection [122,123]. Delayed immune reconstitution and increased risk of infection are potential concerns associated with the use of highly purified autologous grafts.

Vose *et al.* [124] reported excellent engraftment but an unacceptably high rate of significant infections after transplantation with highly purified CD34$^+$ Thy1$^+$ hematopoietic stem cells in patients with recurrent indolent lymphoma. Similarly, a high frequency of life-threatening infections was observed after positive or negative selection in a report from Altes *et al.* [125]. Dreger *et al.* [126] found that CD34 selected autologous grafts were associated with rapid engraftment although recovery of CD4$^+$ and naive T cells were delayed relative to historical controls, differences that might be of greater importance with adjuvant immunotherapy. In a cohort analysis from Seattle, the risk of noncytomegalovirus viral infections and bacterial infections were significantly higher in recipients of CD34$^+$ selected autografts [127]. Other groups have observed little alteration in immune reconstitution or clinical effects with CD34 selection devices, perhaps relating to technical differences as well as the pre-transplantation therapy exposure in different patient populations. The incorporation of rituximab immunotherapy with conventional salvage chemotherapy or as part of the mobilization procedure offers an alternative to positive or negative selection procedures as discussed below.

Immunotherapy and autologous transplantation

There has been long-standing interest in the use of immunotherapy in the post-transplantation period, a strategy that would take advantage of the minimal residual disease state and potentially boost cure rates. A multicentre randomized trial of post-transplantation IL-2 is in progress. However, the delivery of nonspecific immunotherapy such as interferon and IL-2 has been complicated by toxicity. Several groups have incorporated rituximab, which has independent activity in all B-cell lymphomas and a favorable safety profile, in the peri-transplant period. At Stanford University, rituximab was administered to diffuse aggressive lymphoma patients weekly for four courses at 6 weeks and 6 months after autologous HCT [128]. The treatment was tolerated well and, at 3 years, the event-free and overall survival compared favorably to historical controls, providing a rationale for an ongoing cooperative group trial. The ability of rituximab to purge tumor cells from the graft was studied in follicular and mantle cell lymphoma by several groups, based on the rationale that rituximab has selective activity in the blood and marrow compartment. Magni *et al.* [78] successfully purged 93% of cases to PCR-negativity with CY *plus* rituximab compared to 40% of control patients treated with chemotherapy alone. In indolent lymphoma, Flinn *et al.* [129] administered single doses of rituximab as an *in vivo* purge prior to PBHC collection and upon engraftment. Ladetto *et al.* [63] demonstrated the feasibility of incorporating rituximab into a high-dose sequential chemotherapy, prior to mobilization and post-transplantation. Mangel *et al.* [80] incorporated rituximab before PBHC collection and at 2 and 6 months post-transplantation in a phase II trial in mantle cell lymphoma. The combination of rituximab and granulocyte macrophage-colony stimulating factor (GM-CSF) was tolerated well in NHL patients after autologous transplantation, several of whom were observed to have radiographic responses [130]. Overall, the toxicity profile with rituximab and autologous transplantation has been quite favorable. Transient neutropenia without significant infection was seen in a subset of patients and delayed immunoglobulin recovery was reported in the Stanford University series [128,131]. Of greater concern is a report of two cases of progressive multifocal leukoencephalopathy in remission after high-dose chemotherapy and peri-transplant rituximab [132].

Preparatory regimens with monoclonal antibodies conjugated to radioisotopes are being tested in clinical trials. Idiotype vaccination following autologous transplantation has been shown to stimulate specific anti-idiotype immune responses in B-cell lymphoma patients [133]. The use of immunotherapy with autologous transplantation is a rapidly expanding field and has been reviewed recently [134].

Complications

The early mortality associated with autologous transplantation has been reduced to 10% or less, allowing more opportunity to observe late effects such as second malignancies (see Chapter 70). Many groups have reported therapy-related MDS and AML after high-dose therapy and autologous stem cell transplantation and the topic has been extensively reviewed [56,135–146]. As with conventional therapy, the relative risk of MDS and AML after high-dose therapy is associated with cumulative exposure to cytotoxic therapy, including the treatment antecedent to the preparatory regimen [147]. In the literature, the reported estimated actuarial risk of secondary MDS and AML ranged from 4 to 36.5% at 4–10 years after autografting for NHL [145]. Cytopenia, particularly refractory anemia, is the most common presentation of therapy-related MDS or AML. The complex cytogenetic abnormalities seen in this setting are usually characteristic of alkylating agent damage with deletions or loss of chromosomes 5 and 7 [56,135–143]. Median survivals following this complication are brief, usually less than 12 months, although occasional patients have been successfully allografted [56,139,144,145].

Risk factors for MDS and AML include older age [56,135,140], the extent of prior therapy with alkylating agents [137,144,145], TBI in the conditioning regimen [135,142,143], peripheral blood as the stem cell source [140,141,144] and fewer number of cells infused [139,141]. The use of pretransplant fludarabine and mobilization of peripheral blood stem cells with high-dose etoposide have also been associated with secondary AML and MDS [56,141]. Metayer et al. [144] conducted a case–control study of 56 patients with MDS or AML and 168 matched controls within a cohort of 2739 patients receiving autotransplants for Hodgkin's disease or NHL from 12 transplant centres. Significant risks were associated with the intensity of pretransplant therapy, particularly the extent of mechlorethamine or chlorambucil compared with cyclophosphamide. Regimens containing TBI doses ≤12 Gy did not appear to elevate the AML/MDS risk. The use of PBHC was associated with a nonsignificant increased risk ($p = 0.12$) compared to bone marrow grafts. Data regarding the numbers of stem cells infused were not available.

Pederson-Bjergaard et al. [138] have argued that antecedent chemotherapy is the most important risk factor for the subsequent development of MDS/AML after high-dose therapy and autologous HCT for lymphoma. In addition to the preceding discussion, this observation is supported by a very brief latency period in some cases. Further, an association between occult cytogenetic abnormalities in stem cell harvests and secondary MDS/AML suggests that high-dose therapy might have accelerated the clinical appearance of this complication [148,149]. However, secondary MDS/AML has been reported in patients with DLCL and follicular lymphoma receiving high-dose therapy and autologous HCT in consolidation of first remission, whereas secondary AML/MDS is extremely rare after a single course of chemotherapy [62,148]. At this time, the risks of secondary AML/MDS need to be considered together with the potential benefits of high-dose therapy and autologous HCT in each NHL disease setting. Assessment of occult karyotypic abnormalities in bone marrow aspirates should be routine prior to transplantation; deletions of chromosomes 5 and 7 and balanced translocations of chromosome 11 are considered by many to be a contraindication to autologous HCT [149].

Complications of cytotoxic therapy on male and female reproductive function, as with myelotoxicity, represent cumulative drug and radiation exposure. Premature menopause and male and female sterility frequently complicate significant alkylating agent exposure. In a large experience from England and Wales, pregnancies following autologous or allogeneic HCT were likely to be successful [150]. Cataracts may complicate TBI; risk factors include single rather than fractionated irradiation, high dose rate, older age and use of steroids [151]. Most of the information regarding this side-effect comes from the allogeneic HCT literature.

Every patient must be considered on an individual basis, as per their total treatment history, in the assessment of risk for complications. This subject is fully reviewed in Chapter 69.

Future directions

Relapse of disease remains the major cause of treatment failure with high-dose therapy and autologous HCT in NHL. The incorporation of targeted immunotherapy in the peri-transplant period promises to have a major impact on this challenging problem. Preliminary data indicate that rituximab is an effective means of *in vivo* purging of circulating lymphoma cells [78]. The administration of rituximab in the post-transplant, minimal disease setting yielded promising results [128]. Extensions of this strategy include the potentiation of rituximab cytotoxicity with cytokines, adoptive immunotherapy, or both [130,152]. Improved understanding of the mechanism of rituximab cytotoxicity and genetic variability in this regard could lead to more individualized approaches to its use as a single agent or in combination with chemotherapy [153,154].

Several studies have now demonstrated that radioimmunotherapy may be incorporated in the preparatory regimen in place of TBI with excellent tolerability [106,155]. The targeted delivery of radiotherapy may provide both greater efficacy and safety. Further, early studies suggest that radioimmunotherapy can be used incrementally with full doses of standard myeloablative regimens [107,110].

As discussed in Chapters 81 and 85, nonmyeloablative regimens followed by allogeneic HCT are being actively investigated in several subtypes of NHL. It is anticipated that the graft-vs.-lymphoma effect will vary among different histologic subtypes and that the underlying proliferative rates of different lymphomas will influence the success of this approach. Combination treatment with autologous transplantation followed by nonmyeloablative allogeneic HCT has been applied successfully in myeloma and deserves investigation in NHL (see Chapter 80).

The heterogeneity of NHL complicates interpretation of the literature and clinical investigation. It is increasingly apparent that molecular profiling can identify important subtypes of a single entity, such as DLCL [156]. Further understanding of this variability, preferably through prospective analyses, will lead to identification of prognostic factors and drive efforts toward rational risk-adapted therapies. Risk groups have been identified according to early response to treatment but computed tomography is frequently not definitive. Positron emission tomography scans provide functional images that may prove useful in identifying first remission candidates for autologous HCT or assigning patients to risk-adapted therapies [157]. Definitive evaluation of these new diagnostics and therapeutics requires an ongoing commitment to clinical trials that, in turn, promise to improve the outlook for patients with NHL.

References

1 Bal DG. Cancer statistics 2001: quo vadis or whither goest thou? *CA Cancer J Clin* 2001; **51**: 11–14, 2.

2 Jaffe ES, Harris NL, Stein H, Vardiman JR eds. *Pathology and Genetics of Tumours of Haematopoietic and Lymphoid Tissues: World Health Organization Classification of Tumors.* Lyon: ARC Press, 2001.

3 Fisher RI, Gaynor ER, Dahlberg S et al. Comparison of a standard regimen (CHOP) with three intensive chemotherapy regimens for advanced non-Hodgkin's lymphoma. *N Engl J Med* 1993; **328**: 1002–6.

4 International Non-Hodgkin's Lymphoma Prognostic Factors Project. A predictive model for aggressive non-Hodgkin's lymphoma. *N Engl J Med* 1993; **329**: 987–94.

5 Coiffier B. Rituximab in combination with CHOP improves survival in elderly patients with aggressive non-Hodgkin's lymphoma. *Semin Oncol* 2002; **29**: 18–22.

6 Horning SJ. Natural history of and therapy for the indolent non-Hodgkin's lymphomas. *Semin Oncol* 1993; **20**: 75–88.

7 McLaughlin P, Grillo-López AJ, Link BK et al. Rituximab chimeric anti-CD20 monoclonal antibody therapy for relapsed indolent lymphoma: half of patients respond to a four-dose treatment program. *J Clin Oncol* 1998; **16**: 2825–33.

8 Kaminski MS, Zelenetz A, Press O, Saleh M. Multicenter, phase III study of iodine-131 tositumomab (anti-B1 antibody) for chemotherapy-refractory low grade or transformed low grade non-Hodgkin's lymphoma. *Blood* 1998; **92** (Suppl. 1): 290a.

9 Witzig TE, White CA, Gordon LI et al. Final results of a randomized controlled study of the Zevalin radioimmunotherapy regimen versus a standard course of rituximab immunotherapy for B-cell NHL. *Blood* 2000; **96**: 831a [Abstract].

10 Weisenburger DD, Armitage JO. Mantle cell lymphoma: an entity comes of age. *Blood* 1996; **87**: 4483–94.

11 Fisher RI, Dahlberg S, Nathwani BN et al. A clinical analysis of two indolent lymphoma entities:

mantle cell lymphoma and marginal zone lymphoma (including the mucosa-associated lymphoid tissue and monocytoid B-cell subcategories): a Southwest Oncology Group study. *Blood* 1995; **85**: 1075–82.

12 Ascani S, Zinzani PL, Gherlinzoni F et al. Peripheral T-cell lymphomas: clinico-pathologic study of 168 cases diagnosed according to the REAL Classification. *Ann Oncol* 1997; **8**: 583–92.

13 Coiffier B, Brousse N, Peuchmaur M et al. Peripheral T-cell lymphomas have a worse prognosis than B-cell lymphomas: a prospective study of 361 immunophenotyped patients treated with the LNH-84 regimen. The Groupe d'Etude des Lymphomes Agressives (GELA). *Ann Oncol* 1990; **1**: 45–50.

14 Ansell SM, Habermann TM, Kurtin PJ et al. Predictive capacity of the International Prognostic Factor Index in patients with peripheral T-cell lymphoma. *J Clin Oncol* 1997; **15**: 2296–301.

15 Tilly H, Gaulard P, Lepage E et al. Primary anaplastic large-cell lymphoma in adults: clinical presentation, immunophenotype, and outcome. *Blood* 1997; **90**: 3727–34.

16 Zinzani PL, Bendandi M, Martelli M et al. Anaplastic large-cell lymphoma: clinical and prognostic evaluation of 90 adult patients. *J Clin Oncol* 1996; **14**: 955–62.

17 The Non-Hodgkin's Lymphoma Classification Project. A clinical evaluation of the International Lymphoma Study Group classification of non-Hodgkin's lymphoma. *Blood* 1997; **89**: 3909–18.

18 Picozzi VJ Jr, Coleman CN. Lymphoblastic lymphoma. *Semin Oncol* 1990; **17**: 96–103.

19 Soussain C, Patte C, Ostronoff M et al. Small non-cleaved cell lymphoma and leukemia in adults: a retrospective study of 65 adults treated with the LMB pediatric protocols. *Blood* 1995; **85**: 664–74.

20 Mead GM, Sydes MR, Walewski J et al. An international evaluation of CODOX-M and CODOX-M alternating with IVAC in adult Burkitt's lymphoma: results of United Kingdom Lymphoma Group LY06 study. *Ann Oncol* 2002; **13**: 1264–74.

21 Bruce WR, Meeker BE, Valeriote FA. Comparison of sensitivity of normal hematopoietic and transplanted lymphoma colony-forming cells to chemotherapeutic agents administered *in vivo*. *J Natl Cancer Inst* 1965; **37**: 233–45.

22 Kwak LW, Halpern J, Olshen RA, Horning SJ. Prognostic significance of actual dose intensity in diffuse large-cell lymphoma: results of a tree-structured survival analysis. *J Clin Oncol* 1990; **8**: 963–77.

23 Meyer RM, Quirt IC, Skillings JR et al. Escalated as compared with standard doses of doxorubicin in BACOP therapy for patients with non-Hodgkin's lymphoma. *N Engl J Med* 1993; **329**: 1770–6.

24 Appelbaum FR, Deisseroth AB, Graw RG Jr. et al. Prolonged complete remission following high dose chemotherapy of Burkitt's lymphoma in relapse. *Cancer* 1978; **41**: 1059–63.

25 Philip T, Armitage JO, Spitzer G et al. High-dose therapy and autologous bone marrow transplantation after failure of conventional chemotherapy in adults with intermediate-grade or high-grade non-Hodgkin's lymphoma. *N Engl J Med* 1987; **316**: 1493–8.

26 Armitage JO. Bone marrow transplantation. *N Engl J Med* 1994; **330**: 827–838.

27 Philip T, Guglielmi C, Hagenbeek A et al. Autologous bone marrow transplantation as compared with salvage chemotherapy in relapses of chemotherapy-sensitive non-Hodgkin's lymphoma. *N Engl J Med* 1995; **333**: 1540–5.

28 Guglielmi C, Gomez F, Philip T et al. Time to relapse has prognostic value in patients with aggressive lymphoma enrolled onto the Parma trial. *J Clin Oncol* 1998; **16**: 3264–9.

29 Blay J, Gomez F, Sebban C et al. The International Prognostic Index correlates to survival in patients with aggressive lymphoma in relapse: analysis of the PARMA trial. Parma Group. *Blood* 1998; **92**: 3562–8.

30 Prince HM, Imrie K, Crump M et al. The role of intensive therapy and autologous blood and marrow transplantation for chemotherapy-sensitive relapsed and primary refractory non-Hodgkin's lymphoma: identification of major prognostic groups. *Br J Haematol* 1996; **92**: 880–9.

31 Guglielmi C, Martelli M, Federico M et al. Risk-assessment in diffuse large cell lymphoma at first relapse: a study by the Italian Intergroup for Lymphomas. *Haematologica* 2001; **86**: 941–50.

32 Gulati SC, Shank B, Black P et al. Autologous bone marrow transplantation for patients with poor-prognosis lymphoma. *J Clin Oncol* 1988; **6**: 1303–13.

33 Nademanee A, Schmidt GM, O'Donnell MR et al. High-dose chemoradiotherapy followed by autologous bone marrow transplantation as consolidation therapy during first complete remission in adult patients with poor-risk aggressive lymphoma: a pilot study. *Blood* 1992; **80**: 1130–4.

34 Haioun C, Lepage E, Gisselbrecht C et al. Survival benefit of high-dose therapy in poor-risk aggressive non-Hodgkin's lymphoma: final analysis of the prospective LNH87-2 protocol—a Groupe d'Etude des Lymphomes de l'Adulte study. *J Clin Oncol* 2000; **18**: 3025–30.

35 Gianni AM, Bregni M, Siena S et al. High-dose chemotherapy and autologous bone marrow transplantation compared with MACOP-B in aggressive B-cell lymphoma. *N Engl J Med* 1997; **336**: 1290–7.

36 Santini G, Salvagno L, Leoni P et al. VACOP-B versus VACOP-B plus autologous bone marrow transplantation for advanced diffuse non-Hodgkin's lymphoma: results of a prospective randomized trial by the Non-Hodgkin's Lymphoma Cooperative Study Group. *J Clin Oncol* 1998; **16**: 2796–802.

37 Kluin-Nelemans HC, Zagonel V, Anastasopoulou A et al. Standard chemotherapy with or without high-dose chemotherapy for aggressive non-Hodgkin's lymphoma: randomized phase III EORTC study. *J Natl Cancer Inst* 2001; **93**: 22–30.

38 Kaiser U, Uebelacker I, Abel U et al. Randomized study to evaluate the use of high-dose therapy as part of primary treatment for "aggressive" lymphoma. *J Clin Oncol* 2002; **20**: 4413–9.

39 Gisselbrecht C, Lepage E, Molina T et al. Shortened first-line high-dose chemotherapy for patients with poor-prognosis aggressive lymphoma. *J Clin Oncol* 2002; **20**: 2472–9.

40 Linch DC, Yung L, Smith P et al. A randomized trial of CHOP × 6–8 vs. CHOP × 3 + BEAM + ASCT in 457 patients with poor prognosis histologically aggressive non-Hodgkin's lymphoma. *Ann Oncol* 2002, **13**: 28 [Abstract].

41 Haioun C, Lepage E, Gisselbrecht C et al. Comparison of autologous bone marrow transplantation with sequential chemotherapy for intermediate-grade and high-grade non-Hodgkin's lymphoma in first complete remission: a study of 464 patients. Groupe d'Etude des Lymphomes de l'Adulte. *J Clin Oncol* 1994; **12**: 2543–51.

42 Fisher RI. Autologous stem-cell transplantation as a component of initial treatment for poor-risk patients with aggressive non-Hodgkin's lymphoma: resolved issues vs. remaining opportunity. *J Clin Oncol* 2002; **20**: 4411–12.

43 Martelli M, Vignetti M, Zinzani PL et al. High-dose chemotherapy followed by autologous bone marrow transplantation versus dexamethasone, cisplatin, and cytarabine in aggressive non-Hodgkin's lymphoma with partial response to front-line chemotherapy: a prospective randomized Italian multicenter study. *J Clin Oncol* 1996; **14**: 534–42.

44 Verdonck LF, van Putten WL, Hagenbeek A et al. Comparison of CHOP chemotherapy with autologous bone marrow transplantation for slowly responding patients with aggressive non-Hodgkin's lymphoma. *N Engl J Med* 1995; **332**: 1045–51.

45 Johnston LJ, Stockerl-Goldstein KE, Hu WW et al. Toxicity of high-dose sequential chemotherapy and purged autologous hematopoietic cell transplantation precludes its use in refractory/recurrent non-Hodgkin's lymphoma. *Biol Blood Marrow Transplant* 2000; **6**: 555–62.

46 Haioun C, Mounier N, Quesnel B et al. Tandem autotransplant as first-line consolidative treatment in poor-risk aggressive lymphoma: a pilot study of 36 patients. *Ann Oncol* 2001; **12**: 1749–55.

47 Ballestrero A, Clavio M, Ferrando F et al. High-dose chemotherapy with tandem autologous transplantation as part of the initial therapy for aggressive non-Hodgkin's lymphoma. *Int J Oncol* 2000; **17**: 1007–13.

48 Bouabdallah R, Stoppa AM, Coso D et al. Clinical outcome after front-line intensive sequential chemotherapy (ISC) in patients with aggressive non-Hodgkin's lymphoma and high-risk International Prognostic Index (IPI 3): final analysis of survival in two consecutive ISC trials. *Ann Oncol* 2001; **12**: 513–17.

49 van Imhoff GW, van der Holt B, MacKenzie MA et al. Additional intensified CHOP in up-front high dose sequential chemotherapy and auto-PSCT for high-risk aggressive NHL: results from two consecutive phase II trials by HOVON. *Ann Oncol* 2002; **13**: 76 [Abstract].

50 Hahn T, Wolff SN, Czuczman M et al. The role of cytotoxic therapy with hematopoietic stem cell transplantation in the therapy of diffuse large cell B-cell non-Hodgkin's lymphoma: an evidence-based review. *Biol Blood Marrow Transplant* 2001; **7**: 308–31.

51 Freedman AS, Neuberg D, Mauch P et al. Long-term follow-up of autologous bone marrow transplantation in patients with relapsed follicular lymphoma. *Blood* 1999; **94**: 3325–33.

52 Apostolidis J, Gupta RK, Grenzelias D et al. High-dose therapy with autologous bone marrow support as consolidation of remission in follicular lymphoma: long-term clinical and molecular follow-up. *J Clin Oncol* 2000; **18**: 527–36.

53 Bierman PJ, Vose JM, Anderson JR et al. High-dose therapy with autologous hematopoietic rescue for follicular low-grade non-Hodgkin's lymphoma. *J Clin Oncol* 1997; **15**: 445–50.

54 Cao TM, Horning S, Negrin RS et al. High-dose therapy and autologous hematopoietic-cell

transplantation for follicular lymphoma beyond first remission: the Stanford University experience. *Biol Blood Marrow Transplant* 2001; **7**: 294–301.

55 Freedman AS, Gribben JG, Neuberg D *et al*. High-dose therapy and autologous bone marrow transplantation in patients with follicular lymphoma during first remission. *Blood* 1996; **88**: 2780–6.

56 Horning SJ, Negrin RS, Hoppe RT *et al*. High-dose therapy and autologous bone marrow transplantation for follicular lymphoma in first complete or partial remission: results of a phase II clinical trial. *Blood* 2001; **97**: 404–9.

57 Ladetto M, Corradini P, Vallet S *et al*. High rate of clinical and molecular remissions in follicular lymphoma patients receiving high-dose sequential chemotherapy and autografting at diagnosis: a multicenter prospective study by the Gruppo Italiano Trapianto Midollo Osseo (GITMO). *Blood* 2002; **100**: 1559–65.

58 Rohatiner AZ, Johnson PW, Price CG *et al*. Myeloablative therapy with autologous bone marrow transplantation as consolidation therapy for recurrent follicular lymphoma. *J Clin Oncol* 1994; **12**: 1177–84.

59 Micallef IN, Lillington DM, Apostolidis J *et al*. Therapy-related myelodysplasia and secondary acute myelogenous leukemia after high-dose therapy with autologous hematopoietic progenitor-cell support for lymphoid malignancies. *J Clin Oncol* 2000; **18**: 947–55.

60 Brice P, Simon D, Bouabdallah R *et al*. High-dose therapy with autologous stem-cell transplantation (ASCT) after first progression prolonged survival of follicular lymphoma patients included in the prospective GELF 86 protocol. *Ann Oncol* 2000; **11**: 1585–90.

61 Schouten HC, Kvaloy S, Sydes M, Qian W, Fayers PM. The CUP trial: a randomized study analyzing the efficacy of high dose therapy and purging in low-grade non-Hodgkin's lymphoma (NHL). *Ann Oncol* 2000; **11**: 91–4.

62 Schouten HC, Quian W, Sydes MR *et al*. High dose therapy improves progression-free survival in relapsed follicular non-Hodgkin's lymphoma: results from the randomized European CUP trial. *Ann Oncol* 2002; **13**: 26 [Abstract].

63 Colombat P, Cornillet P, Deconinck E *et al*. Value of autologous stem cell transplantation with purged bone marrow as first-line therapy for follicular lymphoma with high tumor burden: a GOELAMS phase 2 study. *Bone Marrow Transplant* 2000; **26**: 971–7.

64 Voso MT, Martin S, Hohaus S *et al*. Prognostic factors for the clinical outcome of patients with follicular lymphoma following high-dose therapy and peripheral blood stem cell transplantation (PBSCT). *Bone Marrow Transplant* 2000; **25**: 957–64.

65 Seyfarth B, Kuse R, Sonnen R *et al*. Autologous stem cell transplantation for follicular lymphoma: no benefit for early transplant? *Ann Hematol* 2001; **80**: 398–405.

66 Friedberg JW, Neuberg D, Gribben JG *et al*. Autologous bone marrow transplantation after histologic transformation of indolent B-cell malignancies. *Biol Blood Marrow Transplant* 1999; **5**: 262–8.

67 Foran JM, Apostolidis J, Papamichael D *et al*. High-dose therapy with autologous haematopoietic support in patients with transformed follicular lymphoma: a study of 27 patients from a single centre. *Ann Oncol* 1998; **9**: 865–9.

68 Williams CD, Harrison CN, Lister TA *et al*. High-dose therapy and autologous stem-cell support for chemosensitive transformed low-grade follicular non-Hodgkin's lymphoma: a case-matched study from the European Bone Marrow Transplant Registry. *J Clin Oncol* 2001; **19**: 727–35.

69 Chen CI, Crump M, Tsang R, Stewart AK, Keating A. Autotransplants for histologically transformed follicular non-Hodgkin's lymphoma. *Br J Haematol* 2001; **113**: 202–8.

70 Freedman AS, Neuberg D, Gribben JG *et al*. High-dose chemoradiotherapy and anti-B-cell monoclonal antibody-purged autologous bone marrow transplantation in mantle-cell lymphoma: no evidence for long-term remission. *J Clin Oncol* 1998; **16**: 13–18.

71 Molina A, Kraft D, Carter N *et al*. Autologous stem cell transplantation for mantle cell lymphoma: a report of 69 patients from City of Hope and Stanford. *Proc Am Soc Hematol* 2002; **100**: 182a [Abstract].

72 Vose JM, Bierman PJ, Weisenburger DD *et al*. Autologous hematopoietic stem cell transplantation for mantle cell lymphoma. *Biol Blood Marrow Transplant* 2000; **6**: 640–5.

73 Dreger P, Martin S, Kuse R *et al*. The impact of autologous stem cell transplantation on the prognosis of mantle cell lymphoma: a joint analysis of two prospective studies with 46 patients. *Hematol J* 2000; **1**: 87–94.

74 Hiddemann W, Dreyling M, Pfreundschuh M *et al*. Myeloablative radiochemotherapy followed by autologous blood stem cell transplantation leads to a significant prolongation of the event-free survival in patients with mantel cell lymphoma (MCL): results of a prospective randomized European Intergroup Study. *Proc Am Soc Hematol* 2002; [Abstract].

75 Khouri IF, Romaguera J, Kantarjian H *et al*. Hyper-CVAD and high-dose methotrexate/cytarabine followed by stem-cell transplantation: an active regimen for aggressive mantle-cell lymphoma. *J Clin Oncol* 1998; **16**: 3803–9.

76 Lefrere F, Delmer A, Suzan F *et al*. Sequential chemotherapy by CHOP and DHAP regimens followed by high-dose therapy with stem cell transplantation induces a high rate of complete response and improves event-free survival in mantle cell lymphoma: a prospective study. *Leukemia* 2002; **16**: 587–93.

77 Gopal AK, Rajendran JG, Petersdorf SH *et al*. High-dose chemo-radioimmunotherapy with autologous stem cell support for relapsed mantle cell lymphoma. *Blood* 2002; **99**: 3158–62.

78 Magni M, Di Nicola M, Devizzi L *et al*. Successful *in vivo* purging of CD34-containing peripheral blood harvests in mantle cell and indolent lymphoma: evidence for a role of both chemotherapy and rituximab infusion. *Blood* 2000; **96**: 864–9.

79 Lazzarino M, Arcaini L, Bernasconi P *et al*. A sequence of immuno-chemotherapy with rituximab, mobilization of *in vivo* purged stem cells, high-dose chemotherapy and autotransplant is an effective and nontoxic treatment for advanced follicular and mantle cell lymphoma. *Br J Haematol* 2002; **116**: 229–35.

80 Mangel J, Buckstein R, Imrie K *et al*. Immunotherapy with rituximab following high-dose therapy and autologous stem-cell transplantation for mantle cell lymphoma. *Semin Oncol* 2002; **29**: 56–69.

81 Andersen NS, Donovan JW, Borus JS *et al*. Failure of immunologic purging in mantle cell lymphoma assessed by polymerase chain reaction detection of minimal residual disease. *Blood* 1997; **90**: 4212–21.

82 Vose JM, Peterson C, Bierman PJ *et al*. Comparison of high-dose therapy and autologous bone marrow transplantation for T-cell and B-cell non-Hodgkin's lymphomas. *Blood* 1990; **76**: 424–31.

83 Rodriguez J, Munsell M, Yazji S *et al*. Impact of high-dose chemotherapy on peripheral T-cell lymphomas. *J Clin Oncol* 2001; **19**: 3766–70.

84 Blystad AK, Enblad G, Kvaloy S *et al*. High-dose therapy with autologous stem cell transplantation in patients with peripheral T-cell lymphomas. *Bone Marrow Transplant* 2001; **27**: 711–16.

85 Fanin R, Sperotto A, Silvestri F *et al*. The therapy of primary adult systemic CD30-positive anaplastic large cell lymphoma: results of 40 cases treated in a single center. *Leuk Lymphoma* 1999; **35**: 159–69.

86 Fanin R, Ruiz de Elvira MC, Sperotto A, Baccarani M, Goldstone A. Autologous stem cell transplantation for T and null cell CD30-positive anaplastic large cell lymphoma: analysis of 64 adult and paediatric cases reported to the European Group for Blood and Marrow Transplantation (EBMT). *Bone Marrow Transplant* 1999; **23**: 437–42.

87 Deconinck E, Lamy T, Foussard C *et al*. Autologous stem cell transplantation for anaplastic large-cell lymphomas: results of a prospective trial. *Br J Haematol* 2000; **109**: 736–42.

88 Sweetenham JW, Santini G, Qian W *et al*. High-dose therapy and autologous stem-cell transplantation versus conventional-dose consolidation/maintenance therapy as post-remission therapy for adult patients with lymphoblastic lymphoma: results of a randomized trial of the European Group for Blood and Marrow Transplantation and the UK Lymphoma Group. *J Clin Oncol* 2001; **19**: 2927–36.

89 Levine JE, Harris RE, Loberiza FR Jr *et al*. A comparison of allogeneic and autologous bone marrow transplant for lymphoblastic lymphoma. *Blood* 2002; **27**: 27.

90 Jost LM, Jacky E, Dommann-Scherrer C *et al*. Short-term weekly chemotherapy followed by high-dose therapy with autologous bone marrow transplantation for lymphoblastic and Burkitt's lymphomas in adult patients. *Ann Oncol* 1995; **6**: 445–51.

91 Bouabdallah R, Xerri L, Bardou VJ *et al*. Role of induction chemotherapy and bone marrow transplantation in adult lymphoblastic lymphoma: a report on 62 patients from a single center. *Ann Oncol* 1998; **9**: 619–25.

92 Sweetenham JW, Pearce R, Taghipour G *et al*. Adult Burkitt's and Burkitt-like non-Hodgkin's lymphoma: outcome for patients treated with high-dose therapy and autologous stem-cell transplantation in first remission or at relapse—results from the European Group for Blood and Marrow Transplantation. *J Clin Oncol* 1996; **14**: 2465–72.

93 Horning SJ, Negrin RS, Chao JC *et al*. Fractionated total-body irradiation, etoposide, and cyclophosphamide plus autografting in Hodgkin's disease and non-Hodgkin's lymphoma. *J Clin Oncol* 1994; **12**: 2552–8.

94 Weaver CH, Petersen FB, Appelbaum FR *et al*. High-dose fractionated total-body irradiation, etoposide, and cyclophosphamide followed by autologous stem-cell support in patients with malignant lymphoma. *J Clin Oncol* 1994; **12**: 2559–66.

95 Stiff PJ, Dahlberg S, Forman SJ et al. Autologous bone marrow transplantation for patients with relapsed or refractory diffuse aggressive non-Hodgkin's lymphoma: value of augmented preparative regimens—a Southwest Oncology Group trial. *J Clin Oncol* 1998; **16**: 48–55.

96 Stockerl-Goldstein KE, Horning SJ, Negrin RS et al. Influence of preparatory regimen and source of hematopoietic cells on outcome of autotransplantation for non-Hodgkin's lymphoma. *Biol Blood Marrow Transplant* 1996; **2**: 76–85.

97 Weaver CH, Appelbaum FR, Petersen FB et al. High-dose cyclophosphamide, carmustine, and etoposide followed by autologous bone marrow transplantation in patients with lymphoid malignancies who have received dose-limiting radiation therapy. *J Clin Oncol* 1993; **11**: 1329–35.

98 Gulati S, Yahalom J, Acaba L et al. Treatment of patients with relapsed and resistant non-Hodgkin's lymphoma using total body irradiation, etoposide, and cyclophosphamide and autologous bone marrow transplantation. *J Clin Oncol* 1992; **10**: 936–41.

99 Blume KG, Forman SJ. High-dose etoposide (VP16)-containing preparatory regimens in allogeneic and autologous bone marrow transplantation for hematologic malignancies. *Semin Oncol* 1992; **19**: 63–6.

100 Skipper HE, Schabel FM Jr, Mellett LB et al. Implications of biochemical, cytokinetic, pharmacologic, and toxicologic relationships in the design of optimal therapeutic schedules. *Cancer Chemother Rep* 1970; **54**: 431–50.

101 Cao TM, Negrin RS, Hu WW et al. High dose chemotherapy and autologous transplantation for follicular lymphoma: a report from the Stanford experience. *Blood* 2000; **96**: 2074A.

102 Caballero MD, Perez-Simon JA, Iriondo A et al. High-dose therapy in diffuse large cell lymphoma: results and prognostic factors in 452 patients from the GEL-TAMO Spanish Cooperative Group. *Ann Oncol* 2003; **14**: 140–51.

103 Tarella C, Cuttica A, Caracciolo D et al. High-dose sequential (HDS) chemotherapy for high-risk non-Hodgkin's lymphoma: long-term analysis and future developments. *Ann Hematol* 2001; **80**: B123–6.

104 Long GD, Negrin RS, Hoyle CF et al. Multiple cycles of high dose chemotherapy supported by hematopoietic progenitor cells as treatment for patients with advanced malignancies. *Cancer* 1995; **76**: 860–8.

105 Press OW, Eary JF, Appelbaum FR et al. Phase II trial of 131-I-B1 (anti-CD20) antibody therapy with autologous stem cell transplantation for relapsed B-cell lymphomas. *Lancet* 1995; **346**: 336–40.

106 Press OW, Eary JF, Gooley T et al. A phase I–II trial of iodine-131-tositumomab (anti-CD20), etoposide, cyclophosphamide, and autologous stem cell transplantation for relapsed B-cell lymphomas. *Blood* 2000; **96**: 2934–42.

107 Vose JM, Bierman PJ, Lynch JC et al. Radioimmunotherapy with Bexxar combined with high-dose chemotherapy followed by autologous hematopoietic stem cell transplantation for refractory non-Hodgkin's lymphoma: synergistic results with no added toxicity. *Proc Am Soc Clin Oncol* 2001; **20**: 6a [Abstract].

108 Behr TM, Griesinger F, Riggert J et al. High-dose myeloablative radioimmunotherapy of mantle cell non-Hodgkin lymphoma with the iodine-131-labeled chimeric anti-CD20 antibody C2B8 and autologous stem cell support: results of a pilot study. *Cancer* 2002; **94**: 1363–72.

109 Nademanee A, Molina A, Forman SJ et al. A phase I–II trial of high-dose radioimmunotherapy with Zevalin in combination with high-dose etoposide and cyclophosphamide followed by autologous stem cell transplant in patients with poor-risk or relapsed B-cell non-Hodgkin's lymphoma. *Proc Am Soc Hematol* 2002; **11**: 182a [Abstract].

110 Winter JN, Inwards DJ, Erwin W et al. Zevalin dose-escalation followed by high-dose BEAM and autologous peripheral blood progenitor cell transplant in non-Hodgkin's lymphoma: early outcome results. *Proc Am Soc Hematol* 2002; **11**: 411a [Abstract].

111 Gribben JG, Freedman AS, Neuberg D et al. Immunologic purging of marrow assessed by PCR before autologous bone marrow transplantation for B-cell lymphoma. *N Engl J Med* 1991; **325**: 1525–33.

112 Sharp JG, Kessinger A, Mann S et al. Outcome of high-dose therapy and autologous transplantation in non-Hodgkin's lymphoma based on the presence of tumor in the marrow or infused hematopoietic harvest. *J Clin Oncol* 1996; **14**: 214–9.

113 Williams CD, Goldstone AH, Pearce RM et al. Purging of bone marrow in autologous bone marrow transplantation for non-Hodgkin's lymphoma: a case-matched comparison with unpurged cases by the European Blood and Marrow Transplant Lymphoma Registry. *J Clin Oncol* 1996; **14**: 2454–64.

114 Vose JM, Sharp G, Chan WC et al. Autologous transplantation for aggressive non-Hodgkin's lymphoma: results of a randomized trial evaluating graft source and minimal residual disease. *J Clin Oncol* 2002; **20**: 2344–52.

115 Demirkazik A, Kessinger A, Armitage JO et al. Progenitor and lymphoma cells in blood stem cell harvests: impact on survival following transplantation. *Bone Marrow Transplant* 2001; **28**: 207–12.

116 Hartmann O, Le Corroller AG, Blaise D et al. Peripheral blood stem cell and bone marrow transplantation for solid tumors and lymphomas: hematologic recovery and costs—a randomized, controlled trial. *Ann Intern Med* 1997; **126**: 600–7.

117 Schmitz N, Linch DC, Dreger P et al. Randomized trial of filgrastim-mobilised peripheral blood progenitor cell transplantation versus autologous bone-marrow transplantation in lymphoma patients. *Lancet* 1996; **347**: 353–7.

118 Vose JM, Anderson JR, Kessinger A et al. High-dose chemotherapy and autologous hematopoietic stem-cell transplantation for aggressive non-Hodgkin's lymphoma. *J Clin Oncol* 1993; **11**: 1846–51.

119 Narayanasami U, Kanteti R, Morelli J et al. Randomized trial of filgrastim versus chemotherapy and filgrastim mobilization of hematopoietic progenitor cells for rescue in autologous transplantation. *Blood* 2001; **98**: 2059–64.

120 Negrin RS, Kusnierz-Glaz CR, Still BJ et al. Transplantation of enriched and purged peripheral blood progenitor cells from a single apheresis product in patients with non-Hodgkin's lymphoma. *Blood* 1995; **85**: 3334–41.

121 Dazzi C, Cariello A, Rosti G et al. Is there any difference in PBPC mobilization between cyclophosphamide plus G-CSF and G-CSF alone in patients with non-Hodgkin's lymphoma? *Leuk Lymphoma* 2000; **39**: 301–10.

122 McQuaker IG, Haynes AP, Anderson S et al. Engraftment and molecular monitoring of $CD34^+$ peripheral-blood stem-cell transplants for follicular lymphoma: a pilot study. *J Clin Oncol* 1997; **15**: 2288–95.

123 Paulus U, Dreger P, Viehmann K, von Neuhoff N, Schmitz N. Purging peripheral blood progenitor cell grafts from lymphoma cells: quantitative comparison of immunomagnetic $CD34^+$ selection systems. *Stem Cells* 1997; **15**: 297–304.

124 Vose JM, Bierman PJ, Lynch JC et al. Transplantation of highly purified $CD34^+$ $Thy-1^+$ hematopoietic stem cells in patients with recurrent indolent non-Hodgkin's lymphoma. *Biol Blood Marrow Transplant* 2001; **7**: 680–7.

125 Altes A, Sierra J, Esteve J et al. $CD34^+$-enriched $CD19^+$-depleted autologous peripheral blood stem cell transplantation for chronic lymphoproliferative disorders: high purging efficiency but increased risk of severe infections. *Exp Hematol* 2002; **30**: 824–30.

126 Dreger P, Viehmann K, von Neuhoff N et al. Autografting of highly purified peripheral blood progenitor cells following myeloablative therapy in patients with lymphoma: a prospective study of the long-term effects on tumor eradication, reconstitution of hematopoiesis and immune recovery. *Bone Marrow Transplant* 1999; **24**: 153–61.

127 Crippa F, Holmberg L, Carter RA et al. Infectious complications after autologous CD34-selected peripheral blood stem cell transplantation. *Biol Blood Marrow Transplant* 2002; **8**: 281–9.

128 Horwitz SM, Breslin S, Negrin RS et al. Rituximab following high dose chemotherapy and autografting in B-cell non-Hodgkin's lymphoma (NHL): preliminary results of a phase I–II trial. *Proc Am Soc Clin Oncol* 2000; **19**: 51a [Abstract].

129 Flinn IW, O'Donnell PV, Goodrich A et al. Immunotherapy with rituximab during peripheral blood stem cell transplantation for non-Hodgkin's lymphoma. *Biol Blood Marrow Transplant* 2000; **6**: 628–32.

130 Rapoport AP, Meisenberg B, Sarkodee-Adoo C et al. Autotransplantation for advanced lymphoma and Hodgkin's disease followed by post-transplant rituxan/GM-CSF or radiotherapy and consolidation chemotherapy. *Bone Marrow Transplant* 2002; **29**: 303–12.

131 Horwitz SM, Breslin S, Negrin RS et al. Adjuvant rituximab after autologous peripheral blood stem cell transplant results in delayed immune reconstitution without increase in infectious complication. *Blood* 2000; **96**: 1657A.

132 Goldberg SL, Pecora AL, Alter RS et al. Unusual viral infections (progressive multifocal leukoencephalopathy and cytomegalovirus disease) after high-dose chemotherapy with autologous blood stem cell rescue and peri-transplantation rituximab. *Blood* 2002; **99**: 1486–8.

133 Davis TA, Hsu FJ, Caspar CB et al. Idiotype vaccination following ABMT can stimulate specific anti-idiotype immune responses in patients with B-cell lymphoma. *Biol Blood Marrow Transplant* 2001; **7**: 517–22.

134 Aksentijevich I, Flinn IW. Monoclonal antibody therapy with autologous peripheral blood stem cell transplantation for non-Hodgkin's lymphoma. *Cancer Control* 2002; **9**: 99–105.

135 Darrington DL, Vose JM, Anderson JR et al. Incidence and characterization of secondary myelodysplastic syndrome and acute myelogenous leukemia following high-dose chemoradiotherapy

and autologous stem-cell transplantation for lymphoid malignancies. *J Clin Oncol* 1994; **12**: 2527–34.
136 Miller JS, Arthur DC, Litz CE *et al.* Myelodysplastic syndrome after autologous bone marrow transplantation: an additional late complication of curative cancer therapy. *Blood* 1994; **83**: 3780–6.
137 Stone RM, Neuberg D, Soiffer R *et al.* Myelodysplastic syndrome as a late complication following autologous bone marrow transplantation for non-Hodgkin's lymphoma. *J Clin Oncol* 1994; **12**: 2535–42.
138 Pedersen-Bjergaard J, Pedersen M, Myhre J, Geisler C. High risk of therapy-related leukemia after BEAM chemotherapy and autologous stem cell transplantation for previously treated lymphomas is mainly related to primary chemotherapy and not to the BEAM-transplantation procedure. *Leukemia* 1997; **11**: 1654–60.
139 Friedberg JW, Neuberg D, Stone RM *et al.* Outcome in patients with myelodysplastic syndrome after autologous bone marrow transplantation for non-Hodgkin's lymphoma. *J Clin Oncol* 1999; **17**: 3128–35.
140 Bhatia S, Ramsay NK, Steinbuch M *et al.* Malignant neoplasms following bone marrow transplantation. *Blood* 1996; **87**: 3633–9.
141 Krishnan A, Bhatia S, Slovak ML *et al.* Predictors of therapy-related leukemia and myelodysplasia following autologous transplantation for lymphoma: an assessment of risk factors. *Blood* 2000; **95**: 1588–93.
142 Milligan DW, Ruiz De Elvira MC, Kolb HJ *et al.* Secondary leukaemia and myelodysplasia after autografting for lymphoma: results from the EBMT. EBMT Lymphoma and Late Effects Working Parties. European Group for Blood Marrow Transplantation. *Br J Haematol* 1999; **106**: 1020–6.
143 Hosing C, Munsell M, Yazji S *et al.* Risk of therapy-related myelodysplastic syndrome/acute leukemia following high-dose therapy and autologous bone marrow transplantation for non-Hodgkin's lymphoma. *Ann Oncol* 2002; **13**: 450–9.
144 Metayer C, Curtis RE, Vose J *et al.* Myelodysplastic syndrome and acute myeloid leukemia after autotransplantation for lymphoma: a multicenter case–control study. *Blood* 2002; **10**: 10.
145 Pedersen-Bjergaard J, Andersen MK, Christiansen DH. Therapy-related acute myeloid leukemia and myelodysplasia after high-dose chemotherapy and autologous stem cell transplantation. *Blood* 2000; **95**: 3273–9.
146 Armitage JO. Myelodysplasia and acute leukemia after autologous bone marrow transplantation. *J Clin Oncol* 2000; **18**: 945–6.
147 Levine EG, Bloomfield CD. Leukemias and myelodysplastic syndromes secondary to drug, radiation, and environmental exposure. *Semin Oncol* 1992; **19**: 47–84.
148 Traweek ST, Slovak ML, Nademanee AP *et al.* Myelodysplasia and acute myeloid leukemia occurring after autologous bone marrow transplantation for lymphoma. *Leuk Lymphoma* 1996; **20**: 365–72.
149 Chao NJ, Nademanee AP, Long GD *et al.* Importance of bone marrow cytogenetic evaluation before autologous bone marrow transplantation for Hodgkin's disease. *J Clin Oncol* 1991; **9**: 1575–9.
150 Salooja N, Szydlo RM, Socie G *et al.* Pregnancy outcomes after peripheral blood or bone marrow transplantation: a retrospective survey. *Lancet* 2001; **358**: 271–6.
151 Belkacemi Y, Labopin M, Vernant JP *et al.* Cataracts after total body irradiation and bone marrow transplantation in patients with acute leukemia in complete remission: a study of the European Group for Blood and Marrow Transplantation. *Int J Radiat Oncol Biol Phys* 1998; **41**: 659–68.
152 Friedberg JW, Neuberg D, Gribben JG *et al.* Combination immunotherapy with rituximab and interleukin 2 in patients with relapsed or refractory follicular non-Hodgkin's lymphoma. *Br J Haematol* 2002; **117**: 828–34.
153 Maloney DG, Smith B, Rose A. Rituximab: mechanism of action and resistance. *Semin Oncol* 2002; **29**: 2–9.
154 Cartron G, Dacheux L, Salles G *et al.* Therapeutic activity of humanized anti-CD20 monoclonal antibody and polymorphism in IgG Fc receptor FcgammaRIIIa gene. *Blood* 2002; **99**: 754–8.
155 Liu SY, Eary JF, Petersdorf SH *et al.* Follow-up of relapsed B-cell lymphoma patients treated with iodine-131-labeled anti-CD20 antibody and autologous stem-cell rescue. *J Clin Oncol* 1998; **16**: 3270–8.
156 Rosenwald A, Wright G, Chan WC *et al.* The use of molecular profiling to predict survival after chemotherapy for diffuse large-B-cell lymphoma. *N Engl J Med* 2002; **346**: 1937–47.
157 Kostakoglu L, Coleman M, Leonard JP *et al.* PET predicts prognosis after one cycle of chemotherapy in aggressive lymphoma and Hodgkin's disease. *J Nucl Med* 2002; **43**: 1018–27.

Anthony S. Stein & Stephen J. Forman

Autologous Hematopoietic Cell Transplantation for Acute Myeloid Leukemia

The first successful autologous hematopoietic cell transplantation (HCT) for acute leukemia (acute lymphoblastic leukemia) was reported in 1959 [1] and for acute myeloid leukemia (AML) in 1977 [2,3]. Subsequently autologous HCT utilizing previously collected and cryopreserved marrow to reconstitute normal hematopoiesis after intensive antitumor therapy has been successfully accomplished in patients with refractory malignancy. Studies in patients with refractory AML who had a syngeneic donor showed that long-term relapse-free survival could be obtained after intensive chemoradiotherapy followed by infusion of hematopoietic cells [4]. In principle, these studies raised the question of whether long-term remission of AML could be achieved with autologous marrow utilizing cells collected during first or second hematologic remission. As is true for all other indications for autologous HCT, the development of cryobiologic methods for the safe preservation and storage of marrow cells provided the technologic basis for the widespread clinical application of autologous HCT for patients with AML (see Chapter 47).

Initially, autologous HCT for AML applied the same clinical approach previously used for patients undergoing allogeneic HCT. Patients with advanced disease were treated with high-dose chemoradiotherapy and followed by infusion of their own marrow, usually collected during remission, instead of marrow from a human leukocyte antigen (HLA) matched sibling donor. Although this approach produced a high remission rate, few, if any, cures resulted [5–7]. Similar to the strategy with allogeneic HCT, autologous HCT was then used earlier in the clinical course of disease to enable high-dose consolidation therapy for patients who were in complete remission and lacked a histocompatible sibling donor.

Since the mid-1970s, interest in autologous HCT for AML has increased substantially in transplant centers around the world. This increase has been caused, in part, by the only limited success of standard-dose chemotherapy in achieving long-term disease-free survival (DFS) for the vast majority of adults with AML [8–10]. The expanded knowledge of the cellular and molecular biology of AML have allowed refinements in the interpretation of clinical results for AML in trials utilizing either chemotherapy or HCT. This chapter reviews the biology of AML, the techniques of autologous HCT, the results of trials during various stages of disease and comparisons to chemotherapy and allogeneic HCT. Potential innovations in the use of HCT in the treatment of patients with AML are also reviewed. Based on this information, the suggested role of autologous HCT for the current management of AML is outlined.

Biology of AML

Historically, the classification of AML has been based on morphologic and clinical observations [11,12]. The nuclear and cytoplasmic appearance of the cells, the presence of Auer rods and the pattern of histochemical staining provided a reasonably reproducible classification that also offered some limited prediction about clinical behavior and outcome. Despite their differences, the therapeutic approach was similar in all morphologic variants of AML.

The identification of molecular events involved in the pathogenesis of human tumors has refined the classification of many tumors, including the acute leukemias. These studies have helped define biologic subgroups of tumors with predictable clinical and biologic characteristics. In some instances, tumor-specific genetic lesions involved in transformation have been defined that can serve as targets for therapeutic agents. In AML a large number of leukemia-specific cytogenetic abnormalities have been identified and the involved genes cloned. These studies have helped elucidate the molecular pathways that may be involved in cellular transformation (leukemogenesis). In addition, the monitoring of patients after chemotherapy or transplantation has been made feasible by the development of polymerase chain reaction (PCR) based technologies designed to assess the presence of minimal residual disease (MRD), both in the stem cell product and in the patient after high-dose therapy. Table 89.1 lists the consistent cytogenetic abnormalities found in AML and the unique genes produced by these translocations. Although many patients (50%) do not have detectable structured cytogenetic changes in their leukemic cells at diagnosis, some show molecular abnormalities of the mixed-lineage leukemia (MLL) gene [13]. These assays have led to the concept that AML is a heterogenous disease with its variants best defined by

Table 89.1 Consistent cytogenetic abnormalities in acute myeloid leukemia (AML).

Cytogenetic abnormality	Frequent AML subtype	Critical genes
t(8;21)(q22;q22)	AML-M2, M1, M4	*AML1/ETO*
inv(16)(p13q22)	AML-M4Eo, M4	*CBFβ/MYH11*
t(16;16)(p13;q22)		
t(15;17)(q21;q11)	AML-M3	*PML/RARα*
t(11;17)(q23;q11)	AML-M3-variant	*PLZF/RARα*
11q23 reciprocal translocations, del11(q23)	AML-M4, M5	*MLL*
t(9;11)(p22;q23)		*MLL/AF9*
t(11;19)(q23;p13)		*MLL/ENL*
inv(3)(q21;q26)	AML-M1	*EVI1*
t(3;3)(q21;q26)		
t(6;9)(q21;q26)	AML	*DEK/CAN*

the molecular defects. Whereas in previous trials both allogeneic and autologous HCT patients were often treated as homogenous groups, recent phase 2 and 3 trials incorporated the new information on the biology of AML in the analysis of outcome in order to better understand the results of therapeutic interventions.

Prognostic factors in AML

Many investigators have attempted to identify those patients with AML in first remission who have a poor prognosis when treated with chemotherapy for whom alternative strategies, including allogeneic or autologous HCT, should be considered (Table 89.2).

These investigators have evaluated pretransplant characteristics that are predictive for DFS after initial treatment for AML. Five variables that have consistently been found to predict for poor DFS are older age [14]; high white blood cell (WBC) count at diagnosis [15]; dysmyelopoiesis [16–18]; need for more than one cycle of induction chemotherapy to achieve complete remission (CR) [14]; and, most importantly, adverse cytogenetic abnormalities [19]. In addition, other adverse risk factors have included certain types of AML according to the French–American–British (FAB) classification and marrow blast expression of CD34 [20] or multidrug-resistant gene (*MDR1*) [21,22]. All investigators now agree that patients with FAB M3 disease have a favorable prognosis when treatment includes anthracycline and all *trans* retinoic acid (ATRA), whereas outcome in patients with AML of M0, M1, M5, M6 or M7 phenotype tends to be worse [23,24]. In addition, patients with secondary AML, or those with a background of myelodysplastic morphology or a history of myelodysplasia, have poor remission-induction rates and are often offered allogeneic transplantation at diagnosis [16–18]. More recently, the presence of FLT3 receptor mutation have been demonstrated in 20–25% of patients with AML [25,26]. This feature predicts for increased relapse rate and may be particularly valuable in further classifying patients with normal cytogenetics into favorable and unfavorable risk groups [27,28]. This knowledge may further contribute to the stratification of therapy within this heterogeneous subgroup of patients.

These prognostic factors have also been applied to patients who are undergoing autologous HCT for AML in first CR. The data indicate that similar to standard chemotherapy, a high WBC count at diagnosis, the requirement of more than one cycle of chemotherapy to achieve CR [29] and certain cytogenetic abnormalities of the leukemia at diagnosis are also predictive of outcome after autologous HCT [30–32]. More recently, an analysis within the UK Medical Research Council (MRC) AML 10 and 12 trials demonstrated that the relapse risk was significantly higher and DFS and overall survival (OS) were worse in patients with FLT3 mutations undergoing autologous or allogeneic HCT [33].

Preparative regimens in HCT for AML

The high-dose chemoradiotherapy regimens that have been utilized for autologous HCT are derived from those used in allogeneic HCT. These regimens provide both cytoreduction to eliminate endogenous tumor and adequate immunosuppression to facilitate allogeneic engraftment. In the setting of autologous HCT, no immunosuppression is required and the goal of the preparative regimen is to provide maximum therapy to eradicate malignant disease, limited only by nonhematologic toxicity. The most common preparative regimens utilized in autologous HCT are listed in Table 89.3.

These regimens can be divided into those utilizing total body irradiation (TBI) and those that use chemotherapy alone. The most common non-TBI regimen utilizes busulfan (BU) and cyclophosphamide (CY) as originally developed by Santos *et al.* [37] and subsequently modified by Tutschka *et al.* [38]. These investigators lowered the CY dose to 120 mg/kg (BU/CY2), reducing the toxicity of the regimen without compromising relapse-free survival.

The most common radiation-based regimens utilize fractionated TBI (FTBI) in combination with CY or other chemotherapeutic agents. The importance of the dose of radiation in preventing a recurrence was demonstrated in a randomized trial in recipients with AML in first remission of allogeneic sibling marrow grafts comparing 12.0 Gy to 15.75 Gy. The 3-year probability of relapse was 35% for the 12 Gy group and 12%

Table 89.2 Poor prognostic factors in patients with acute myeloid leukemia (AML) treated with chemotherapy.

1 Older age
2 Poor-risk cytogenetics
3 High WBC at diagnosis
4 CD34 expression
5 MDR1 expression
6 FAB M0, M1, M5, M6, M7
7 Secondary AML (therapy related or following myelodysplastic syndrome)
8 Dysplastic morphology at diagnosis
9 Extramedullary disease at diagnosis
10 More than one cycle of induction chemotherapy to achieve complete remission
11 *FLT3* receptor mutations

FAB, French–American–British classification; WBC, white blood cell count.

Table 89.3 Preparative regimens used for autologous hematopoietic cell transplantation (HCT) for acute myeloid leukemia (AML).

Regimen [Reference]	Description
Cyclophosphomide, TBI [34]	CY, 60 mg/kg × 2, + TBI, 10 Gy
Cyclophosphomide, FTBI [35]	CY, 60 mg/kg × 2
	FTBI, 10–1320 Gy
BAVC [36]	BCNU, 800 mg/m^2 × 1
	AMSA, 150 mg/m^2 × 3
	VP16, 150 mg/m^2 × 3
	Ara-C, 300 mg/m^2
Busulfan, cyclophosphamide [37]	Busulfan, 4 mg/kg × 4
	Cyclophosphamide, 50 mg/kg × 4
Busulfan, cyclophosphamide [38]	Busulfan, 4 mg/kg × 4
	Cyclophosphamide, 60 mg/kg × 2
Busulfan, VP16 [39,40]	Busulfan, 4 mg/kg × 4
	VP16, 60 mg/kg × 1
FTBI, VP16, cyclophosphamide [29]	FTBI, 12 Gy
	VP16, 60 mg/kg × 1
	Cyclophosphamide, 75 mg/kg × 1
Busulfan, VP16, cyclophosphamide [41–43]	Busulfan 4 mg/kg × 4
	VP16, 60 mg/kg × 1 or 30 mg/kg × 1
	Cyclophosphamide, 60 mg/kg × 2
Busulfan, cyclophosphamide, FTBI [44]	Busulfan, 10.6 mg/kg
	Cyclophosphamide, 60 mg/kg
	FTBI, 12 Gy
^{131}I-labeled anti-CD45 [45] Antibody cyclophosphamide TBI	^{131}I (estimated marrow dose, 4–30 Gy) Cyclophosphamide, 120 mg/kg
	TBI, 12 Gy

BAVC, BCNU, amsacrine (AMSA), VP16 and Ara-C; FTBI, fractionated total body irradiation; TBI, total body irradiation.

for the 15.75 Gy group. Although DFS was equivalent because of increased toxicity in the group of patients who received this high dose of radiation, the decreased relapse rate with the higher radiation dose demonstrated the dose–response characteristics for AML [46].

There have been few randomized trials comparing TBI-based regimens with those that employ only chemotherapeutic agents. One randomized trial of autologous HCT performed at the University of Minnesota compared FTBI/CY to BU/CY and showed no difference in DFS in patients in first CR (2-year estimate: 69% vs. 55% log–rank; $p = 0.52$). However, patients who were transplanted beyond first remission had significantly improved DFS when irradiation was a component of the regimen (2-year estimate: 38% vs. 7% log–rank; $p = 0.04$) [47]. Blaise et al. [48] compared these two regimens for patients with AML in first remission treated with allogeneic HCT and found an increased DFS and OS, and decreased relapse and transplantation-related mortality with TBI/CY. This was confirmed in a long-term follow up of this study [48,49]. A South-West Oncology Group (SWOG) trial of allogeneic HCT for patients with advanced leukemia compared FTBI VP16 prospectively to BU and CY and showed a trend favoring the radiation-based regimen [50].

Other investigators have modified the preparative regimen, substituting drugs that appear to be more myeloid cell specific in their antitumor activity. There has been considerable interest in the role of etoposide (VP16) for treatment of leukemias and as an agent in the HCT preparative regimens [51]. In some systems, this topoisomerase II inhibitor is synergestic with other alkylating agents. Given that the immunosuppressive properties of CY are not needed in the autologous setting, studies have been conducted substituting etoposide for CY in combination with BU. Investigators from the University of California, San Francisco evaluated this regimen in 58 patients with AML in first or second remission, all of whom received purged autologous grafts. For patients in first remission, the actuarial relapse rate was 22% and the 3-year DFS was 78% [39]. In a follow-up study the same investigators used the same preparative regimen with peripheral hematopoietic cells with similar DFS but with an improved toxicity profile [52].

Given that relapse is the main obstacle for success in autologous HCT, other investigators have added etoposide to a regimen that contained TBI and CY. A phase 1 study from Seattle demonstrated that for autologous HCT, 44 mg/kg VP16 and 103 mg/kg CY followed by 12 cGy TBI can be given safely [53]. In a phase 2 trial from the City of Hope National Medical Center, investigators showed that in patients in first CR, 60 mg/kg VP16 could be added to FTBI 12 Gy and 75 mg/kg CY, followed by infusion of unpurged marrow. This regimen resulted in a DFS of 61% with a probability of relapse of 33%, with most patients developing moderate to severe mucositis and skin toxicity [29].

Others have attempted to improve BU and CY regimens by addition of VP16. In one study, although the DFS was 44% at 2 years, the regimen was associated with increased pulmonary hemorrhage, veno-occlusive disease (VOD) and a high incidence of severe reversible skin toxicity [41,42]. In a dose-dependent study comparing 30 mg/kg or 45 mg/kg VP16 in combination with 30 mg/kg BU/CY, VP16 was associated with less toxicity and a better overall survival as a result of lower transplant-related mortality [43].

Busulfan, when administered as part of a preparatory regimen, is given orally and has been shown to be associated with wide variations in the area-under-the-curve (AUC) achieved in patients given the same dose of drug. Investigators in Seattle conducted a trial in patients with chronic myeloid leukemia (CML) utilizing targeted levels of BU with dose adjustments based on drug levels achieved after the first dose. This study showed that there was a dose–response effect for BU in CML, with patients who achieved >900 ng/mL having a low relapse rate but those achieving a lower level suffering a higher rate of relapse [54]. In older patients with myelodysplasia (>55 years) the use of oral BU/CY with pharmokinetic (PK) guided dose adjustment to achieve steady-state concentration plasma levels of 600–900 ng/mL (AUC of approximately 900–1350 µmol/min) yielded longer DFS than did oral BU/CY without PK monitoring or with the use of CY/TBI [55]. At the City of Hope National Medical Center, patients with advanced leukemia were treated on a phase 1–2 study of busulfan/FTBI and VP16. Patients with an AUC of >500 µmol/min had a trend to an improved DFS [56]. Whether such a dose–response effect exists for BU in AML will require similar PK studies in patients undergoing autologous or allogeneic HCT.

A retrospective comparison in a series of allogeneic recipients of intravenous vs. oral busulfan in patients treated with a regimen of BU/CY2 for hematologic malignancies showed that the rate of hepatic VOD was significantly lower ($p = 0.002$) and the 100-day survival rate significantly higher ($p = 0.002$) in patients treated with intravenous busulfan than in patients treated with oral busulfan [57]. The parenteral administration of busulfan allows for predictable exposure without PK monitoring and is not compromised by erratic gastric absorption [58]. If one elects to use PK monitoring and targeted dosing, the intravenous or the oral route of administration has the ability to use test dose PK data to predict steady-state levels and perform individualized dose adjustments accurately.

The observation that leukemic cells demonstrate a dose–response to radiation therapy suggests that the cure rate for leukemia might improve if the radiation could be delivered selectively to marrow and other sites of leukemic involvement while sparing nonhematopoietic organs. Radio immunoconjugates that emit beta-particles such as ^{131}I-anti-CD33, ^{90}Y-anti-CD33, ^{131}I-anti-CD45 and ^{188}Re-anti-CD66c, deliver significant doses of radiation to the bone marrow and may be particularly effective when used as part of a conditioning regimen for HCT. Investigators from Seattle, utilizing I^{131}-labeled anti-CD45 antibody, were able to deliver an estimated 3.5–7.5 Gy to the liver, 4–30 Gy to the bone marrow and 7–60 Gy to the spleen followed by 120 mg/kg CY and 12 Gy TBI [45]. Initial studies in patients receiving allogeneic HCT for advanced leukemia or AML in first remission suggest that this approach is very tolerable and potentially efficacious (see Chapter 15). Clinical trials investigating ^{90}Y-HuM195 as part of preparative regimens for autologous and non-myeloablative allogeneic HCT are being conducted.

Knowing whether any of these regimens is superior to the more conventional regimens (FTBI/CY) would require a randomized study, with the patient population balanced for appropriate biologic and clinical characteristics of their leukemia.

Source of hematopoietic stem cells: marrow vs. mobilized peripheral blood cells and importance of the quality of the autograft

The major early morbidity and mortality encountered with autologous HCT are related to tissue damage caused by the preparative regimen (mucositis, enteritis, interstitial pneumonia, VOD) or infections and bleeding caused by delayed hematopoietic recovery. Autologous peripheral blood hematopoietic cell (PBHC) transplantation was initiated in patients with AML in the mid 1980s as studies failed to detect tumor cells in the peripheral blood of leukemic subjects during the early recovery phase from induction/consolidation chemotherapy [59–61]. Studies have demonstrated improved hematopoietic recovery and diminished toxicity in patients who received "primed" PBHCs. In general, these studies have shown that the duration of neutropenia and thrombocytopenia in patients treated with myeloablative therapy is shorter than with bone marrow hematopoietic cells (BMHCs) [61–63]. Although the approach with PBHCs leads to more rapid hematopoietic reconstitution, decreased post-transplant complications and shorter hospital stay, its full impact initially on DFS was unclear. Laporte et al. [64] have reported four patients transplanted with chemotherapy mobilized PBHCs and observed that three

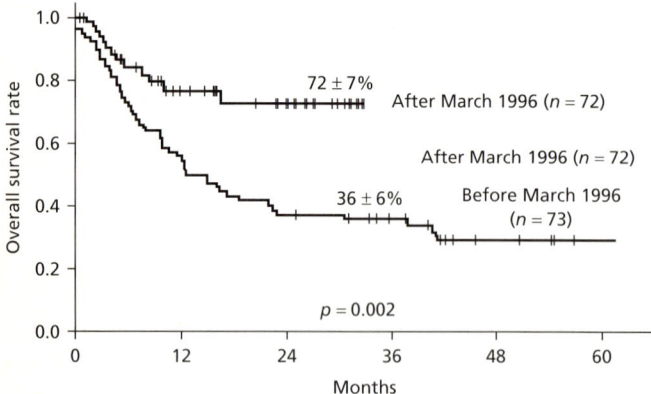

Fig. 89.1 Recent improvement of overall survival rates in patients >60 years with acute myeloid leukemia (AML) autografted in first remission (CR1). European Group for Blood and Marrow Transplantation study.

patients exhibited a very early relapse, a phenomenon that was usually not observed in patients transplanted with bone marrow. In a nonrandomized study, Körbling et al. [65] have reported that 14 of the 20 patients transplanted with PBHCs relapsed, contrasting with only 11 of the 23 patients transplanted with purged BMHCs. Mehta et al. [66] reported four consecutive patients transplanted with PBHCs, who experienced early relapse. In these early studies, patients received leukapheresis immediately following CR before any consolidation therapy was administered.

A single institution study comparing PBHCs collected postchemotherapy and BMHCs showed equivalent DFS but quicker hematologic recovery and reduced need for transfusions in favor of PBHCs [67].

In a large retrospective analysis the European Group for Blood and Marrow Transplantation (EBMT) retrospectively reviewed the data of 1393 patients undergoing PBHC transplant or purged or unpurged BMHCs. The 2-year overall survival among the three groups were similar; however, the 2-year leukemia-free survival (LFS) was $44 \pm 6\%$ for PBHCs vs. $57 \pm 3\%$ for purged BMHCs ($p = 0.01$). However, some patient characteristics differed significantly between the two groups (age, interval between diagnosis and CR1 or between CR1 and HCT), demonstrating the need for a prospectively randomized study comparing purged BMHCs vs. PBHCs [68].

Several studies indicate a better outcome in patients receiving a higher dose of hematopoietic cells following allogeneic or autologous transplants. Patients receiving higher doses of marrow submitted to purging by mafosfamide experienced a lower treatment-related mortality (TRM) ($p = 0.005$) rate and a higher LFS ($p = 0.005$) and OS ($p = 0.001$) rate [69]. Patients autografted with unmanipulated PBHCs who received higher doses of $CD34^+$ cells infused/kg correlated to better peripheral blood counts after HCT [70]. The most significant improvement in LFS utilizing PBHCs and reduced-intensity preparative regimens is seen in patients >60 years and who were transplanted after March 1996 (Fig. 89.1) [71]. The results to date suggest that the use of PBHCs for AML has improved the rate of engraftment, reduced morbidity and mortality with no influence on relapse rate.

Purging

Rationale

Autologous HCT was first attempted in patients with leukemia in relapse utilizing marrow that had been collected while the patients were in CR. In these studies, a high rate of CR was attained but all patients relapsed [5–7]. Although the advanced stage of disease at the time of HCT appeared to be the major contributor to treatment failure, the concern about the high likelihood of reinfusing leukemic cells, even from a remission marrow, led to the development of methods designed to eradicate tumor cells from autologous marrow (see Chapters 19 and 20). The goal was to achieve clinical results similar to those attained with syngeneic transplantation in which relapse occurs only as a consequence of the residual disease that is present in the patient after recovery from high-dose chemoradiotherapy. Intuitively, it would seem that all sources of autologous hematopoietic cells from patients with hematologic malignancies might contain cells that contribute to relapse. Studies of grafts have documented the presence of tumor cells including lymphoma, breast cancer, myeloma and acute leukemia (see Chapter 22).

The success of autologous HCT for AML depends in part on whether any clonogenic cells that remain in the reinfused graft can cause relapse. Although laboratory studies show the efficacy of purging to reduce tumor cell contamination, the benefit of purging of leukemic cells in human HCT has remained controversial. So far, no prospective randomized trials are available to indicate the value of purging. As shown in many studies (see Chapters 19 and 20), purging with either chemotherapy or antibodies reduces the number of clonogenic leukemia cells but usually delays engraftment, thus increasing the risk of complications and increasing cost.

There are also other observations that make the interpretation of a purging benefit difficult to assess. For instance, patients undergoing syngeneic HCT for AML in first remission experience relapse rates of 50–60% [72], similar to those seen in autologous HCT, indicating that the major obstacle to success is still the inability to eliminate the body burden of leukemic cells rather than reinfusion of viable clonogenic cells.

In a rat model for AML it appeared that most primitive normal hematopoietic cells were significantly less vulnerable to the freezing and thawing procedure as compared with clonogenic leukemic cells [73]. It was also found that the injected leukemic cells lodge at sites unfavorable for growth and that, in addition, previous supralethal high-dose chemoradiotherapy significantly hampered the regrowth of subsequent injected low number of leukemic cells, most probably because of damage to the marrow microenvironment [74]. In human studies, it was found that the recovery for AML colony-forming units (CFUs) was significantly lower than normal CFUs, indicating that cryopreservation per se may have a purging effect [75]. Some studies have documented that the infusion of autologous hematopoietic cells can contribute to relapse. Brenner et al. [76] incubated one-third of harvested marrow from two children undergoing autologous HCT with the LNL-6 retroviral vector, which contained the selectable neomycin-resistant gene, a procedure that marked approximately 5% of cultured progenitor cells. Patients underwent HCT using both marked and unmarked marrow. At the time of relapse, some of the leukemic cells contained the neomycin-resistant gene, demonstrating that these leukemic cells survived within the reinfused marrow graft and contributed to relapse (see Chapter 11).

Retrospective analyses from the Autologous Blood and Marrow Transplant Registry (ABMTR) reviewed 294 patients with AML who underwent autologous HCT in first-remission. In a multivariate analysis, patients who received a 4-hydroperoxycyclophosphamide (4-HC) purged transplant had a significantly lower rate of treatment failure. The adjusted 3-year probability of LFS was 56% (range 47–64%) and 31% (range 18–45%) after 4-HC purged and unpurged transplantation in first remission, respectively. Corresponding probabilities in second remission were 39% (range 25–33%) and 10% (range 1–29%) [77]. Retrospective analysis of multicenter EBMT registry data show that the relapse rate is significantly lower after autologous HCT in patients transplanted with purged compared to unpurged marrow when the remission duration is <6 months, the time to attain first remission exceeds 40 days and patients are autografted after TBI conditioning regimen [78]. In addition, the plateau in DFS was attained earlier in recipients of chemically purged marrow, suggesting a more effective elimination of AML cells that are capable of causing a late relapse [79].

Chao et al. [40], in a retrospective analysis, compared a cohort of 20 patients transplanted without purging to a subsequent cohort of 30 patients whose marrow was purged with 4-HC, and demonstrated a DFS of 33% vs. 56%. However, no significant difference was found between the two groups when analyzed by log–rank test because the patients were transplanted sequentially, with varying follow-up times.

Even though there is evidence that 4-HC purging may decrease relapse rates, the data have never been convincing enough to generate approval of the drug by the Food and Drug Administration and currently it is not commercially available. The major limitation to its use is its association with a marked delay in engraftment resulting in prolonged hospital stay and increased expense and mortality. Currently, ongoing trials are exploring the feasibility of purging PBHC with cyclophosphamide derivatives to determine whether this can improve the rate of engraftment compared to purged bone marrow.

Approaches to purging

The observations discussed above have led to many studies designed to reduce the leukemic cell contamination of marrow or PBHCs. Most studies that have utilized *in vitro* purging have employed pharmacologic agents. This technique allows exposure of leukemic cells to higher concentrations of drugs *in vitro* and exploits a differential sensitivity of hematopoietic stem cells and leukemic cells to these agents (see Chapter 20 for pharmacologic basis and mechanism).

Studies performed in the USA have utilized 4-HC while those in Europe have used mafosfamide. Both compounds hydrolyze in aqueous solutions to form 4-HC, the primary product of CY activation, which is then metabolized intracellularly to the active agent, phosphormoride mustard. In human studies, the maximum concentration of 4-HC for *in vitro* tumor cell depletion of the marrow is 100 μg/mL [80]. Other investigators, in order to overcome resistance of leukemic cells, have utilized combination chemotherapy with 4-HC, most commonly with VP16 (see Chapter 20) [81–83].

Monoclonal antibody (MAB) purging has targeted differentiation antigens on hematopoietic cells. The CD33 antigen is expressed by leukemic blasts from 90% of patients with AML. Although CD33 is also present on normal myeloid precursor cells, the early hematopoietic cells that provide long-term engraftment express CD34 but do not express CD33. In one trial, 12 patients, 10 of whom were in second remission, underwent HCT with marrow depleted *in vitro* with anti-CD33 MAB and complement. Four patients marrow remained disease-free 34–57 months after transplant. Delayed engraftment was observed for both neutrophils and platelets [84].

Other investigators have utilized either a combination of anti-CD15 and anti-CD14 MABs or CD15 alone. The majority of AML samples react with these MABs (91% with CD15 and 77% with CD14). These MABs are cytotoxic in the presence of rabbit complement and react with antigens that are later in differentiation but still provide significant depletion of clonogenic leukemia cells.

One hundred and thirty-eight patients have undergone HCT with CD15 MAB purging of marrow. Patients transplanted in first CR and treated with CY/TBI had a 5-year DFS of 57%, whereas those treated with BU/CY had a 5-year DFS of 45%. Of those patients in second and third remission, 23% treated with the CY/TBI regimen and 28% with BU/CY became long-term survivors. The median time to 500 neutrophils was 32 days for patients in first remission, with platelet recovery to >20,000/μL occurring by day 67 [85].

Other methods that have been used for *in vitro* purging of AML include physical separation methods based on the differential size and density of leukemic cells compared to hematopoietic precursors. There was no evidence that marrow separated by albumin density gradient centrifugation improved DFS and this technique is generally not in use [86]. Similar observations have been made for elutriation [87]. Other investigators have used long-term culture, based on the laboratory observation that leukemic cells decline and are replaced by apparently normal hematopoietic cells in culture. This technique is labor intensive and requires special equipment. It is also associated with delayed hematopoietic recovery [88]. Others have used interleukin 2 (IL-2) incubation of hematopoietic cells from marrow or blood as a mechanism for tumor cell purging. Like the long-term culture approach, this technique is associated with a significant delay in hematopoietic recovery [89].

In an attempt to render the autograft procedure safer and less expensive, many teams now favor PBHC transplants. Initially, PBHCs were collected after remission induction chemotherapy which resulted in a high relapse rate. Subsequently, investigators have utilized high-dose consolidation chemotherapy to reduce the leukemic cell burden, with collection of PBHCs early after hematologic recovery (*in vivo* purging). An EBMT study showed that patients autografted with PBHCs collected after two consolidation courses had an improved DFS and decreased relapse rate [68,90]. Tallman et al. [91] reported on a large retrospective analysis of ABMTR and the International Bone Marrow Transplant Registry (IBMTR) to determine whether pretransplant consolidation chemotherapy affects outcome of autologous HCT for AML in first CR. The risk of relapse and treatment failure were significantly less in patients receiving consolidation prior to HCT. However, there was no difference in outcome between standard- and high-dose cytarabine groups. A retrospective analysis by the EBMT group also did not find that the dosage of cytarabine influenced the relapse incidence [92]. In both these studies no analysis was performed based on cytogenetic risk groups.

Several investigators have reported results of collecting PBHCs after a single cycle of high-dose cytarabine [29], or high-dose cytarabine and VP16 [52] or an anthracycline [93,94], demonstrating comparable results with PBHCs collected after two consolidation courses.

The optimal number of cycles of consolidation and type of consolidation therapy prior to autologous HCT remains to be defined in further studies. Prolonging the time to transplant by increasing the number of consolidation treatments entails the risk of patient drop-out from toxicity as well as relapse in high-risk patients who might benefit from transplantation. The type and dosage of therapy may need to be individualized according to the biologic characteristics of the AML.

Immunotherapy after HCT

The comparison of transplantation from identical twins to allogeneic sibling transplants supports the concept that the higher relapse rates following syngeneic (or autologous) HCT are because of the lack of the allogeneic graft-vs.-leukemia (GVL) effect. Based on observations utilizing cytokines that can augment *in vitro* and *in vivo* immune activity, some investigators have used IL-2 systemically after autologous HCT. Varying regimens of IL-2 have had mixed results in the post-autologous transplant setting. Investigators at the City of Hope National Medical Center treated patients post-autologous HCT with a short course of moderate-dose IL-2 and demonstrated this treatment can be given safely with no increased mortality [94]. A phase 1–2 trial employing the same IL-2 regimen as this study, demonstrated a 25% disease-free plateau for patients transplanted from AML beyond first CR [95,96]. Using sequential IL-2 over a period of 2 months post-ABMT, Blaise et al. [97] reported 3-year relapse probabilities of 59 ± 11% for 22 AML patients in first CR; these results did not differ from those obtained without post-graft immunotherapy. A study from Schiller *et al.* [98] evaluated the role of IL-2 mobilized peripheral stem cells and found no difference in LFS when compared to matched historical controls. The Cancer and Acute Leukemia Group B (CALGB) is currently conducting a phase 3 study of prolonged low-dose IL-2 after HCT for AML. Other immunotherapy trials include the use of cyclosporine post-HCT to induce autologous graft-vs.-host disease (GVHD), but this has not resulted in a survival advantage in those patients developing GVHD [99–101]. A randomized study comparing Roquinimex (oral immunomodulator that has IL-2-like effects in stimulating natural killer [NK] cells) to placebo post-HCT showed no benefit in the Roquinimex-treated group and failed to show enhancement of NK cells in the regenerating bone marrow [102]. Studies of other post-transplant immunomodulator strategies such as vaccinations are in their early stages of development.

Results of autologous HCT for AML in first complete remission

Table 89.4 summarizes the results of trials of autologous HCT in patients with AML in first CR by HCT source, unpurged marrow [29,90,103–108], PBHCs [43,65,93,94,109] or purged marrow [42,55,57,85,110–112] and have reported DFS for patients transplanted in first CR of between 34% and 70%, 35% and 74%, and 41% and 76%, respectively. Although each trial demonstrated the potential efficacy of the approach chosen, many of the studies have been criticized for including patients who had widely varying induction therapies, types and number of consolidation cycles before autologous HCT, duration of CR before transplant, relatively short follow-up times and differences in graft manipulation and preparative regimens. In many of these studies, similar to many reports of allogeneic HCT for AML in first remission, a number of patients who otherwise would have been candidates for autologous HCT suffered a relapse prior to HCT and were not part of the subsequent analysis, thus creating a time bias toward more favorable candidates. Figure 89.2 shows a survival curve for the intent-to-transplant patients with AML who were entered on study after achieving a first CR, with *in vivo* purged primed PBHCs (single cycle high-dose cytarabine and idarubicin) and post-HCT IL-2 who received a radiation-based conditioning regimen. Figure 89.3 shows their DFS by cytogenetic risk group [94]. Other studies have reported data for all patients from initiation of induction therapy, thus overcoming potential bias inherent in many other trials [111,113].

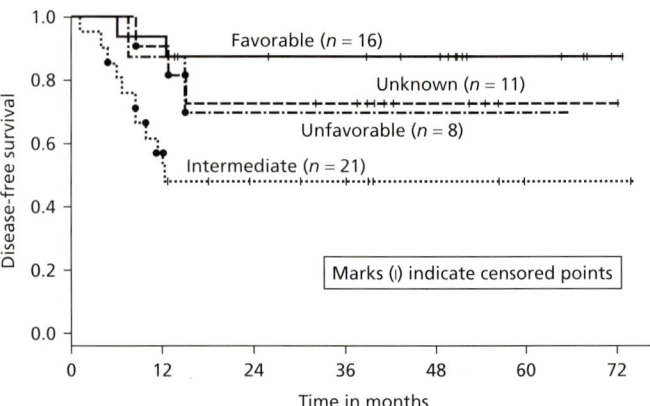

Fig. 89.3 Disease-free survival (DFS) for intent-to-treat patients with acute myeloid leukemia (AML) in first complete remission (CR) with autologous hematopoietic cell transplantation (HCT) based on cytogenetics [94]. (Reprinted with permission from the American Society of Clinical Oncology.)

Autologous HCT for patients with MDS, or AML following MDS

Myelodysplastic syndromes (MDSs) form a heterogeneous group of disorders with variable prognoses, which are curable only by allogeneic transplantation (see Chapter 79). Survival for patients with refractory anemia with excess blasts, refractory anemia with excess blasts in transformation, therapy-related MDS or secondary AML is very poor, with a median of <12 months from diagnosis [114,115]. Some of these patients achieve a remission with intensive chemotherapy but the median duration of these remissions is usually very short [114,116]. Interest in the development of autologous HCT for MDS has emerged from laboratory and clinical observations, indicating the presence of normal hematopoietic cells in the marrow of these patients who achieve a remission. Some patients with MDS and a well-characterized cytogenetic abnormality have achieved both a morphologic and cytogenetic remission after chemotherapy [114] suggesting the presence, as in *de novo* AML, of hematopoietic cells that are capable of normal hematopoietic reconstitution. Stem cell cultures in patients who achieve remission demonstrate polyclonal hematopoiesis [117,118].

Several groups of investigators have reported their results with autologous HCT for patients with MDS that had evolved into AML [105,119–121]. In this group of patients, it appears that DFS at 2 years is approximately half that achieved by autologous HCT for *de novo* AML [122]. The patients with MDS reported in this series are highly selected for the following characteristics:
1 they achieved a hematologic remission for their secondary AML;
2 the cytogenetic abnormality often disappeared at the time of achievement of remission; and
3 adequate numbers of hematopoietic cells could be collected, providing the opportunity for high-dose therapy and stem cell reinfusion.

de Witte *et al.* [123] reported their results of an intent-to-treat autologous HCT trial for patients without a donor with MDS or AML following MDS using PBHCs mobilized during the recovery phase of consolidation. Those with a donor treated with allogeneic HCT showed a 4-year DFS from CR of 27% and 31%, respectively. Figure 89.4(a) shows the overall survival of 184 evaluable patients and Fig. 89.4(b) shows the DFS rate from the time of achieving a CR [123].

Patients with MDS/AML who are not eligible for allogeneic HCT and who achieve both a morphologic and cytogenetic remission could be treated with post-remission autologous HCT, potentially improving their overall survival. In these studies, the main cause of treatment failure

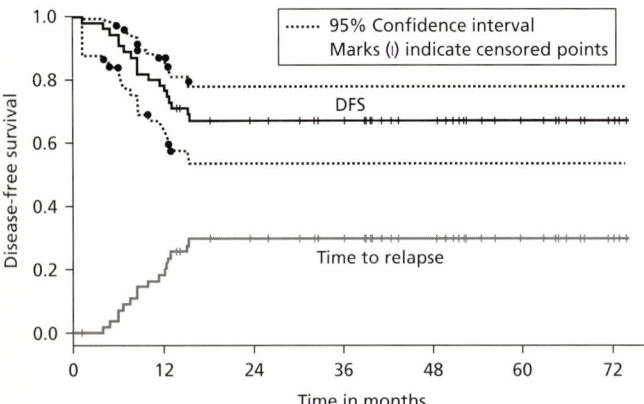

Fig. 89.2 Disease-free survival (DFS) and time to relapse for intent-to-treat patients with acute myeloid leukemia (AML) in first complete remission (CR) with autologous hematopoietic cell transplantation (HCT) [94]. (Reprinted with permission from the American Society of Clinical Oncology.)

Table 89.4 Autologous transplantation for acute myeloid leukemia (AML) in first remission.

Author [Reference]	No. patients	Median age (yr)	Age range (yr)	Median duration of CR1 at BMT (mo) (range)	Preparatory regimen	Actuarial Relapse Rate (%)	Actuarial DFS (%)	Comments
Unpurged bone marrow stem cells								
Carella et al. [103]	55	37	(12–62)	5 (1–12)	CY, 60 mg/kg × 2 days; TBI, 10 Gy single dose	36	51.1	Post-remission therapy 1–6 courses DAT
Beelen et al. [104]	20	40	(16–53)	6 (2.5–13.5)	BU/CY 120	38	55	Variable induction Rx, variable consolidation Rx + maintenance, Rx before BMT
McMillan et al. [105]	76 (26 double autografts)	40	(16–57)	5 (1–12)	BACCT	48	48	Variable no. of cycles of consolidation treatment before BMT 0–6
						30	67	
Stein et al. [29]	60 (intent to HCT) 44 (actual HCT)	39	(16–55)	4.6 (2.5–9.7)	FTBI/VP16/CY	44	49	Single course of HD Ara-C before BMT
						33	61	
Miggiano et al. [106]	51	36	(15–59)	8 (4–20)	BU/CY	23.5	70.6	Patients transplanted late in first remission
					BU/CY 200			
Mehta et al. [90]	74	31	(5–53)	118.5 days (5–346 days)	Melphalan/TBI	40.5	34.2	Patients who received two or more consolidation treatments had statistically improved DFS
Burnett et al. [107]	54	36	(15–54)	5+ (2+ to 17+)	CY/TBI	44	51	
Löwenberg et al. [108]	32	40	(16–58)	3–8	CY/TBI, 8 Gy	60	35	
Unpurged peripheral blood cells								
Sanz et al. [109]	24	40	(14–62)	4 (2–5)	BU/CY 200	60	35	Consolidated with 7 + 3
Körbling et al. [65]	20	41	(5–48)	3.5 (2–12)	TBI, 14.4 Gy/CY 200	54	35	Consolidated with Ara-C + daunorubicin
Schiller et al. [93]	59	45	(18–64)	3 (1.5–7)	TBI, 11.25 Gy/CY 120	54	42	Consolidated with HD Ara-C/mitoxantrone
Stein et al. [94]	56 (intent to HCT) 47 (actual HCT)	44	(18–61)	3.7 (2.3–10.4)	FTBI/VP16/CY	30	68	Consolidated with HD Ara-C/idarubicin and received post-ASCT IL-2
							74	
Linker et al. [52]	128	39	(18–65)	Not given	BU/VP16	24	55	Consolidated with HD Ara-C/VP16
Purged bone marrow								
Körbling et al. [55]	22	35	(17–50)	4 (2–6)	FTBI (12.1–16.7 Gy)/ CY, 200 mg/kg	36	61	
Chao et al. [40]	34	40	(2–60)	3 (1.2–7)	BU/VP16	62	32	Unpurged marrow
						28	57	Purged marrow
Linker et al. [39]	32	39	(17–59)	3 (1.5–5.5)	BU/VP16	22	76	
Linker et al. [39]	50	37	(17–59)	3 (1–10)	BU/VP16	27 ± 12	70 ± 12	No consolidation
Cassileth et al. [110]	39	36	(18–51)	2 (0.5–6)	BU/CY 200	33	54	
LaPorte et al. [111]	64	36	(16–53)	150 days (41–694 days)	FTBI/CY	25	58	
Ball et al. [85]	23	45	(2–59)	138 days (24–421 days)	BU/CY or FTBI/CY	43	57	FTBI/CY
						55	45	BU/CY
Yeager (Johns Hopkins) [112]	48	25	(4–56)	2.5+ (1.5+ to 15+)	BU/CY	49	41	High-risk patients with poor prognostic factors

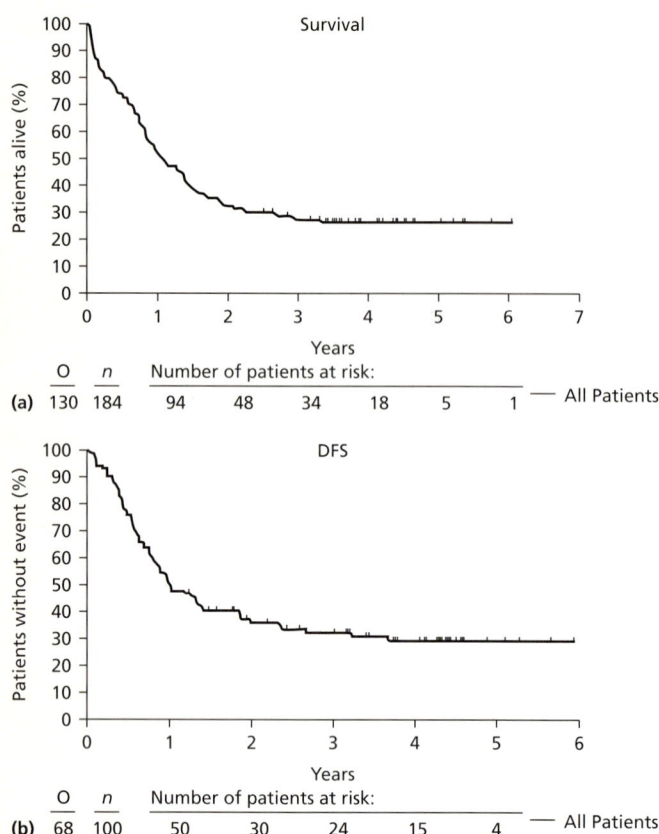

Fig. 89.4 (a) Survival of all 184 patients; and (b) disease-free survival of 100 patients who achieved complete remission (CR).

following transplant was not graft failure or post-transplant complications but the high risk of leukemic relapse.

Role of autologous HCT for acute promyelocytic leukemia

The use of combined ATRA and chemotherapy has led to improved outlook for acute promyelocytic leukemia (APL). Sanz et al. [124] developed a predictive model based on WBC and platelet counts at diagnosis. The 3-year Kaplan–Meier estimates of relapse free survival were 100%, 90% and 75% for low-, intermediate- and high-risk groups, respectively. Based on these excellent results, even for the poor-risk group there is no role for autologous HCT for APL in first molecular remission.

Most reports of APL patients transplanted in second CR were published prior to the introduction of arsenic trioxide into clinical use. In relapsed APL patients, it is now possible to obtain a CR with arsenic trioxide or with retreatment with ATRA with or without chemotherapy [125–127]. However, many patients relapse without post-remission therapy.

The outcome of autologous HCT for APL utilizing a molecularly negative graft is excellent. Meloni et al. [128] report on 15 patients who underwent HCT in second CR. All seven patients who underwent HCT with persistent PCR-detectable minimal residual disease in their marrow cells relapsed within 9 months after transplant, whereas only one patient with negative PCR relapsed, which confirms the value of PCR positivity during remission as a predictor of relapse in APL. Sanz et al. [129] reported a patient with APL in second remission and in molecular remission in the marrow just prior to conditioning, who received PBHC-bearing cells with the PML/RARβ transcript. This patient was disease free at 22 months, suggesting that autologous PBHC transplantation may

be worth pursuing in patients with APL despite the presence of positive PCR in the graft. Linker et al. [130] reported on seven patients undergoing autologous HCT after in vivo purging for APL in second remission. With a median follow up of 5.4 years, all seven patients remained in remission (Fig. 89.4). A recent survey from EBMT was reported in abstract form. One hundred and fifty-one patients underwent autologous HCT while 127 underwent allogeneic HCT for APL in second remission. OS, LFS, relapse rate and TRM for autologous and allogeneic HCT were 48% ± 12% and 58% ± 11%, 45% ± 10% and 57% ± 10%, 44% ± 10% and 15% ± 9%, 25% ± 12% and 33% ± 9%, respectively [131].

For patients in second remission whose marrow is PCR-negative, an autologous HCT procedure would be recommended, reserving an allogeneic HCT for APL in second remission for patients who show persistent PCR evidence of disease in the bone marrow.

Autologous HCT in second remission of AML

The role of autologous HCT in second remission of AML is better defined than in first remission, as the cure rate with conventional chemotherapy for such patients is extremely low. Most HCT studies in second remission have utilized either chemically or immunologically purged marrow (Table 89.5). Trials using marrow purged with 4-HC, mafosfamide or MAB [35,39,85,111,112,132,133] have demonstrated a DFS of 19–56% and relapse rates of 25–73%. A number of these trials included third remission patients as well. Two trials using unpurged marrrow have demonstrated a DFS of 42–48%. In both these trials, the median duration of first remission was 11.5–14 months and in one series 30% of patients had FAB classification M3 [134,135]. Other investigators have used consolidation therapy with high-dose cytosine arabinoside (Ara-C)/VP16 as in vivo purging followed by autologous HCT and with a median follow-up of 5.7 years; event-free survival (EFS) is projected at 52%. The most significant prognostic factor for outcome in this study was the cytogenetic information at the time of diagnosis. All seven patients with t(15;17) remained in remission, whereas EFS for 21 other patients is 38% (Fig. 89.5) [130]. The same approach has been tested by CALGB in 50 patients treated in second remission. With a median follow-up of 2.2 years, the EFS was 25% overall and 30% for patients <60 years. The CALGB study confirmed the excellent results for patients with APL, having projected EFS of 74% compared to 22% in other patients. The most important prognostic factor for patients undergoing autologous HCT for second remission is the duration of first remission. Patients with first remission >12 months appear to have improvements in DFS and OS [136].

A retrospective analysis by the EBMT comparing allogeneic HCT with autologous HCT for patients in second remission demonstrated that the TRM was higher following allogeneic HCT (32% vs. 20%; p = 0.02) and the relapse incidence lower (42% vs. 63%; p = 0.001). However, the LFS was not significantly different (allogeneic HCT 39%, autologous HCT 30%; p = 0.22) [137]. Investigators in Seattle have compared autologous HCT to HCT from unrelated donors for advanced leukemia. Patients were matched for disease and disease stage, as well as age, and were treated at the same institution during the same period of time. The relapse rates were lower with unrelated donor HCT but DFS was not statistically different between the two types of transplants [138]. This analysis indicates that autologous HCT is a reasonable alternative treatment for patients who do not have a suitable donor and for older patients who achieve a second remission and may not be candidates for allogeneic HCT.

Management of relapse after autologous HCT

The major cause of failure following autologous HCT is relapse. Patients undergoing autologous HCT using purged or unpurged marrow in first

Table 89.5 Autologous HCT with marrow treated *ex vivo* for AML in second or subsequent remission or early relapse.

Author [Reference]	No. patients	Median age (range)	Remission status at BMT	Duration of first CR median (range) (months)	Actuarial relapse rate (%)	Actuarial DFS (%)	Comments
Rosenfeld et al. [132]	24	33 (10–61)	CR2 = 7 CR3 = 8 CR4 = 1 ER = 8	13.5 (2–51) 3 (1–9)	73	19	BU/CY 200 + Ara-C or CY/TBI, marrow purged with 4-HC
Körbling et al. [35]	30	35 (17–53)	CR2 = 23 CR3 = 5 CR4 = 2		65	34	Mafosfamide purging TBI/CY
Linker et al. [39]	26	38 (15–58)	CR2 = 19 CR3 = 2 Refractory = 5	11 (1–40)	25	56	4-HC purging BU/VP16
Linker et al. [130]	31	35 (15–58)	CR2 = 23 CR3 = 2 Refractory = 6	8 months (1 patient CR1 >2 year)	35 ± 20	52 ± 20 0	4-HC purging BU/VP16
LaPorte et al. [111]	20	31.5 (17–53)	CR2		48 ± 12	34 ± 11	TBI/CY, mafosfamide
Ball et al. [85]	115	39 (5–64) 35 (17–67)	CR2 + 3 = 87 Rel = 28	Length of first CR main prognostic factor	56 65 54	23 28 37	TBI/CY BU/CY BU/CY Purged with AML –2 –23 PM81
Yeager (Johns Hopkins) [112]	98	30 (1–56)	CR2 = 82 CR3 = 16		58 55	30 27	4-HC BU/CY
Smith et al. (Johns Hopkins) [133]	69	27 (1–62)	CR2 = 60 CR3 = 9	12 months (1–78)	55 44	30 22	

CR, complete remission; ER, early relapse.

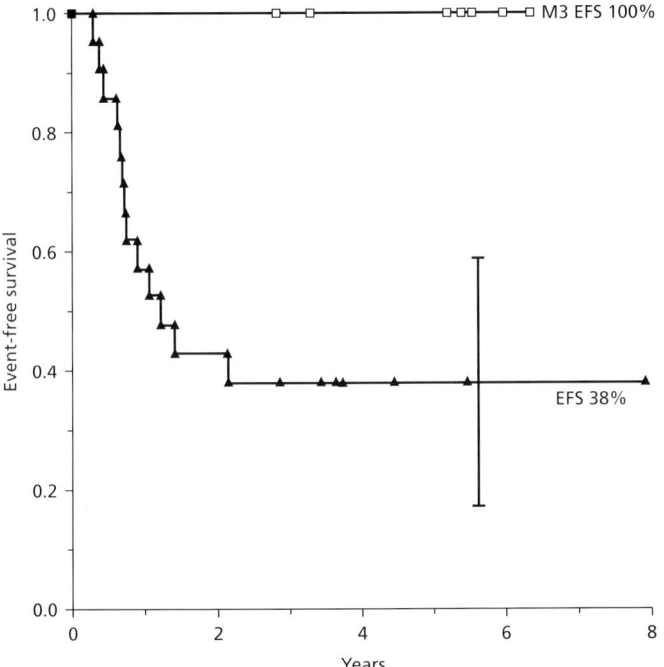

Fig. 89.5 Event-free survival (EFS) for patients with acute myeloid leukemia (AML) in second remission undergoing peripheral blood hematopoietic cell (PBHC) transplantation in second remission, t(15;17) vs. others. (Reprinted by permission of the author and publisher from [130].)

remission have relapse rates of 23–60% and 28–52%, respectively. Those patients transplanted in first relapse or second remission have relapse rates up to 73%. Once patients relapse following autologous HCT, the prognosis is poor and response to further therapy is low because of the cumulative organ toxicity of prior treatments and the chemoresistance of the leukemic cells.

Investigators have explored the option of second autologous HCT for patients who relapse after autologous HCT. Mehta et al. [139] reported four patients with AML who relapsed 12–23 months after HCT who underwent a second autologous HCT procedure in second remission. Three of four patients were alive and in remission 6–7 years after second autologous HCT. De la Rubia et al. [140] reported on the use of a second HCT procedure for patients who relapsed after their initial HCT. They treated 18 patients, 17 in untreated relapse (back-up bone marrow had been harvested in first remission). Eleven percent died of treatment-related complications and 36% of patients remained in remission at 3 years. The major prognostic factor was the interval between the first transplant and relapse. Patients who relapsed at an interval 7 months from their first transplant had DFS of 52%, compared to 20% for those relapsing <7 months from their first transplant ($p = 0.02$).

Investigators from Seattle evaluated the outcome of allogeneic HCT in 24 patients with AML who relapsed post-autologous HCT. The estimated 2-year nonrelapse mortality, relapse and DFS were 30%, 25% and 46%, respectively. Age >17 years, relapse at the time of second transplantation and the use of a chemotherapy-only preparative regimen for the second HCT procedure each appeared to be associated with an increased risk of failure [141].

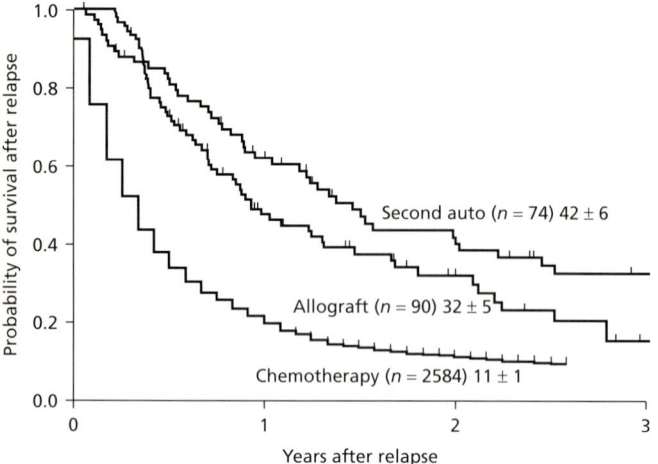

Fig. 89.6 Survival in patients with acute leukemia who relapsed after autograft and thereafter were treated with an allograft, chemotherapy or with a second autograft. (Reprinted by permission of the author and publisher from [142].)

The EBMT evaluated the role of chemotherapy, autologous HCT and allogeneic HCT as salvage therapy following relapse after an autologous HCT. Two years after relapse following first autograft, the OS for allogeneic HCT, autologous HCT and chemotherapy were $32 \pm 5\%$, $42 \pm 6\%$ and $11 \pm 1\%$, respectively (Fig. 89.6) [142]. Factors associated with a better survival were age <26 year, first remission vs. second or subsequent remission, no TBI during conditioning before first autograft, long interval from CR to first autograft and, most of all, longer interval from first autograft to relapse (>5 months). Those patients receiving a graft from an HLA-compatible related or unrelated donor had a 2-year probability of survival of $37 \pm 7\%$ vs. $13 \pm 8\%$ for those receiving HLA-mismatched marrow [143].

Investigators at City of Hope National Medical Center reported on the outcome of 28 patients (11 with AML) who relapsed following an autologous HCT who were then treated with an allogeneic or matched unrelated HCT using a reduced-intensity regimen (fludarabine/melphalan) and cyclosporine/mycophenolate mofetil (MMF) for GVHD prophylaxis. The day 100 nonrelapse mortality was 21% and the 1-year probability of DFS was 56%. This study demonstrates that allogeneic HCT following autologous HCT utilizing reduced-intensity conditioning is feasible [144].

Whether active intervention or supportive therapy is chosen for an individual patient depends on the patient's performance status, duration of remission, extent of disease present, type of previous therapy and patient preference. A second transplant could be considered, preferably in young patients who relapse >7 months after autografting. If a HLA-related or unrelated identical donor is available, an allogeneic HCT should be considered using a reduced-intensity preparative regimen. If a matched related or unrelated donor is not available then a second autologous HCT procedure should be considered.

Allogeneic vs. autologous HCT vs. standard chemotherapy for AML in first remission

Reports of many clinical trials with adequate long-term follow-up have shown that patients treated with allogeneic HCT for AML in first remission have the lowest relapse rates and a 5-year DFS of 45–65% (see Chapter 75). With improvements in post-remission chemotherapy and autologous HCT, investigators have performed randomized studies to determine how best to manage patients with AML in first remission. In all the study designs, the randomization to allogeneic HCT was determined by a "genetic randomization"; i.e. patients who had an HLA-matched related donor would proceed to allogeneic HCT and those without a donor would receive the alternative therapy. These trials have usually been restricted to patients <50 years of age.

The European Organization for Research and Treatment of Cancer (EORTC) and the Gruppo Italiano Malattie Ematologiche Maligne dell'-Adulto (GIMEMA) conducted the first large phase 3 study between 1986 and 1993. All patients received induction chemotherapy followed by one cycle of intermediate-dose Ara-C and amsacrine consolidation treatment. Patients with both HLA-matched siblings and who were <46 years of age were assigned to allogeneic HCT, whereas the other patients were randomized between autologous HCT or high-dose Ara-C/daunorubicin consolidation treatment. The preparatory regimens for autologous and allogeneic HCT were either CY/TBI or BU/CY and the majority of patients received unpurged autologous marrow. GHVD prophylaxis consisted mainly of cyclosporine (CSP) alone or in combination with methotrexate (MTX). T-cell depletion was used for 17% of the patients. Ultimately, 144 patients received allogeneic HCT, 95 autologous HCT and 104 consolidation chemotherapy. The drop-out rate was particularly severe in the group randomized to autologous BMT where only 74% of randomized patients received the treatment compared to 86% receiving allogeneic BMT and 83% receiving chemotherapy. The 4-year estimates of DFS were 55%, 48% and 30%, respectively, with a statistically significant improvement in DFS for allogeneic HCT and autologous HCT as compared to chemotherapy. However, no difference was seen in OS between the three treatment groups. This finding is attributed to better salvage therapy for patients who relapsed while on chemotherapy, with HCT being used in those patients who achieved a second remission. The outcome analysis in this study was not based on cytogenetics [145].

In the US Intergroup Study between 1990 and 1995 patients received induction therapy with standard dose Ara-C plus idarubicin. Patients in complete remission then received a consolidation cycle with idarubicin and Ara-C. Patients with a histocompatible sibling were assigned to allogeneic HCT, and the remainder were randomized between autologous HCT using 4-HC-purged marrow or one course of high-dose Ara-C (3 g/m² every 12 hours for 6 days). The 4-year DFS for chemotherapy, autologous HCT and allogeneic HCT was 35%, 37% and 42%, respectively. In this study the patients assigned to the autologous BMT group, only 54% of the patients received the autologous BMT. The relapse incidence was lowest in the allogeneic BMT arm at 29% compared to 48% for autologous BMT and 61% for chemotherapy. The TRM was highest in the allogeneic BMT arm at 21% compared to 14% for autologous BMT and 3% for chemotherapy [146].

The analysis by cytogenetics for this study showed that patients with favorable cytogenetics did significantly better after autologous HCT or allogeneic HCT than after chemotherapy alone. Patients with unfavorable cytogenetics did better with allogeneic transplantation, and patients in the intermediate category had similar results between the three treatment arms [147].

The Medical Research Council Leukemia Working Parties (MRC 10) conducted a clinical trial between 1988 and 1995 to determine whether the addition of autologous BMT to intensive consolidation chemotherapy improved RFS for patients with AML in first remission. After three courses of intensive consolidation chemotherapy, bone marrow was harvested from patients who lacked a donor. These patients were then randomized to receive, after one additional course of chemotherapy, no further treatment or an autologous BMT with unpurged bone marrow after preparation with TBI/CY. In this study only 66% of patients randomized to autologous BMT received the intended therapy. On an intent-to-treat analysis, the number of relapses was substantially lower in the group assigned to transplant (37% vs. 58%; $p = 0.0007$) which resulted in superior DFS at 7 years (54% vs. 40%; $p = 0.04$) (Fig. 89.7). The TRM in the autologous BMT group was 12%. When analyzed according to

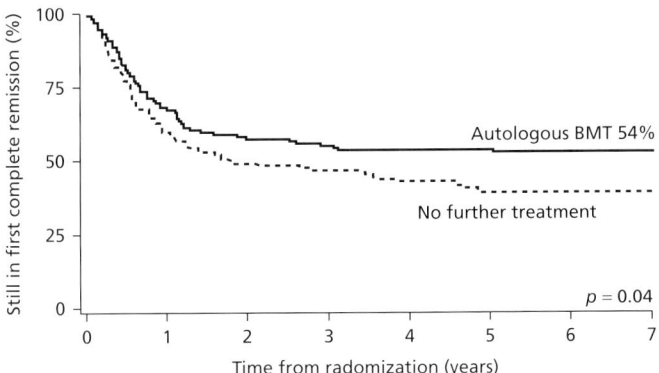

Fig. 89.7 Disease-free survival comparing autologous bone marrow transplantation vs. no further chemotherapy.

cytogenetic risk group, autologous BMT reduced the relapse rate in the favorable group from 49% to 25% ($p = -0.02$) and in the intermediate-risk group from 59% to 40% ($p = 0.04$). The relapse rate in the poor-risk group was reduced from 73% to 56%, but this was not statistically significant. However, because patients in the good-risk group allocated to chemotherapy only who relapsed could be efficiently salvaged with an autograft, the OS was not different [148]. If survival was partitioned into two time periods, there was no difference in the first 2 years ($p = 0.8$) because of excess mortality in the BMT group; however, beyond 2 years, a significant benefit for autologous BMT emerged ($p = 0.006$) as a result of decreased relapse rate [149].

Table 89.6 summarizes the results of studies that compared autologous HCT, allogeneic HCT and chemotherapy. Table 89.7 lists studies of allogeneic HCT compared to autologous HCT. These large prospective studies were designed to determine the role of autologous HCT compared to intensive chemotherapy and allogeneic HCT in the management of patients with AML. Despite these efforts, a decade later this issue still has not been resolved. The following important points have emerged from these studies.

1 In all four randomized studies, autologous transplants provide better antileukemic activity than intensive chemotherapy, as seen by the decrease in the relapse rate (Table 89.8).

2 The superior antileukemic effect of autologous transplants could have been negated by the higher procedural mortality of autologous transplants (14% in the US Intergroup and 18% in the MRC AML 10 study). Current use of peripheral blood as source of stem cells has lowered procedural mortality to <5%.

3 The significant drop-out rate of patients, particularly those assigned to the autologous HCT group where up to half the patients randomized to an autologous HCT never received one.

4 Most studies demonstrate a lower relapse rate and improved DFS in patients treated with allogeneic HCT, especially for patients with poor-risk cytogenetics.

5 When these studies were designed over a decade ago, AML was considered as a single entity and the number of patients for these studies was determined based on this consideration. With the identification of prognostic groups based on cytogenetics, it has become crucial to analyze these results based on cytogenetic risk groups. There are practical limitations in having trials where the intervention can be evaluated in every cytogenetic subgroup, as AML is a rare disease with more than 20 non-random chromosomal abnormalities.

Timing of autologous HCT for AML

With improved results for post-remission chemotherapy in some patients [50], an increasing number of physicians and patients delay transplants until the time of first relapse. For these patients it is often a difficult decision as to whether to proceed directly to transplant at the time of relapse or to undergo reinduction therapy with autologous HCT reserved for those patients who achieve a second remission.

This question was addressed in a study from Seattle with 98 patients in first remission who had marrow harvested with the intent of performing autologous HCT at the first sign of relapse. In this study, 65 of 98 patients relapsed and underwent HCT. The 4-year probability of RFS was 13% and the 4-year probability of survival for all 65 patients was 8%. Patients who survived had a longer first remission, and no patient with a peripheral blast count >5.4 × 10^9/L at the time of transplant survived [153]. This study again demonstrated the limited clinical benefit of HCT for patients in relapse.

If this approach is to be followed, patients require close observation, including frequent marrow examinations and molecular monitoring of

Table 89.6 Comparative trials comparing allogeneic and autologous hematopoietic cell transplantation (HCT) and chemotherapy.

Author [Reference]	Treatment	No. patients	Disease-free survival (%)	p	Overall survival (%)	p	Relapse (%)	p
Zittoun et al. [145]	Allo	168	55 + 4		59 + 4	0.43	24	n.r.
	Auto	128	48 + 5	0.05	56 + 5		41	
	Chemotherapy	126	30 + 4		46 + 5		57	
Harousseau et al. [150]	Allo	67	45	n.s.			38	n.s.
	Auto	67	47				44	
	Chemotherapy	61	53				43	
Reiffers et al. [151]	Allo	20	66	0.004	11 (1–40)		18	0.002
	Auto	12	41				50	
	Chemotherapy	20	16				83	
Cassileth et al. [146]	Allo	120	42	0.70	46	0.10		
	Auto	111	37		47			
	Chemotherapy	118	35		54			

Allo, allogeneic HCT; Auto, autologous HCT; n.r., not reported; n.s., not significant.

Table 89.7 Comparative trials comparing autologous hematopoietic cell transplantation (HCT) to allogeneic HCT.

Author [Reference]	Treatment	No. patients	Disease-free survival (%)	p	Overall survival (%)	p	Relapse (%)	p	Comments
Ferrant et al. [152]	Auto	33	31	0.028	28	0.0098	48	0.40	Treatment-related mortality in autologous HCT was 27%
	Allo	24	64		71		33		
Carella et al. [103]	Auto	55	49				43		Retrospective analysis
	Allo	104	52				29		
Cassileth et al. [146]	Auto	39	54 ± 16				33		No consolidation in chemotherapy given
	Allo	19	42 ± 22				23		
Löwenberg et al. [108]	Auto	32	35	n.s.	37	0.05	60	0.03	
	Allo	23	51		66		34		
Mitus et al. [113]	Auto	53			45	0.54	50	0.04	DFS by actual therapy was 62% in both groups of patients
	Allo	31			56		20		
Gorin et al. [137]	Auto	598	42 ± 3	0.006			52 ± 3	$<10^4$	Retrospective study
	Allo	516	55 ± 3				25 ± 3		

DSF, disease-free survival; n.s., not significant.

Table 89.8 Relapse following allogeneic transplant, autologous transplant and chemotherapy.

Study	Allogeneic transplant (%)	Autologous transplant (%)	Chemotherapy (%)
GIMEMA, 1995	24	40	57
GOELAM, 1997	28	45	55
MRC, 1998	19	35	53
ECOG/SWOG, 1998	29	48	61

ECOG, Eastern Cooperative Oncology Group; GIMEMA, Gruppo Italiano Malattie dell'Adulto; GOELAM, Groupe Ouest Est Leucémies Aiguës Myéloblastiques; MRC, Medical Research Council; SWOG, South-West Oncology Group.

blood during the first 2 years after marrow storage, so that relapse can be detected while patients are in good condition and with a minimal burden of leukemic cells.

Complications following autologous HCT for AML

A major morbidity and mortality encountered with autologous HCT utilizing purged or unpurged marrow grafts has been associated with delayed hematopoietic recovery, leading to prolonged transfusional support and infectious complications. The use of PBHCs has reduced the risk of these complications, as the duration of neutropenia and thrombocytopenia in patients treated with myeloablative therapy followed by infusions of mobilized PBHCs is shorter than that with unprimed marrow. Linker et al. [52] have shown that the use of PBHCs have modified the toxicity of the BU/VP16 regimen with marked reduction in mucositis, skin toxicity and hyperbilirubinemia. The use of PBHCs and related intensity conditioning regimens have enabled the EBMT and other investigators to extend the age limit up to 75 years for patients with AML and other malignancies and age should not be an exclusion for autografting [71].

The major early complication of autologous HCT for AML is infection, usually bacterial or fungal (see Chapters 51 and 52). The risk is directly related to the duration of neutropenia and the degree of organ injury associated with the preparative regimen. Although patients are immunodeficient for a variable period of time after autologous HCT, the risk of viral infections, particularly cytomegalovirus (CMV) and varicella-zoster virus (VZV), is reduced compared to that of recipients of allogeneic grafts (see Chapters 53 and 55) [154,155]. In an analysis of 159 autologous HCT recipients, in the pre-ganciclovir era, investigators in Seattle found that the probability of developing CMV reactivation by day 100 after transplantation was 61% in seropositive individuals. Despite this high rate of reactivation of endogenous viral infection, CMV pneumonia developed in only 11 patients and was fatal in nine, indicating that aggressive treatment with antiviral therapy is indicated when CMV disease is documented in such patients [155].

Late complications

Secondary malignancies

Most surveys of patients undergoing autologous HCT for treatment of AML have not, as yet, documented an increase in incidence of secondary malignancies. The follow-up for those patients is shorter than for allogeneic recipients and all long-term survivors should be followed for the development of new malignancies. The incidence of secondary acute leukemia, although difficult to assess, appears to be substantially lower in patients who are undergoing transplantation for AML than in those receiving similar preparative regimens for lymphoma and Hodgkin's disease. This finding has been attributed directly to the type of prior therapy that is utilized in patients with Hodgkin's disease and lymphoma (alkylating agents, topoisomerase I and II inhibitors) as opposed to patients with acute leukemia.

In principle, patients who receive marrow grafts incubated with cytotoxic agents may be at risk for secondary leukemia. Despite this concern, the experience to date is probably sufficient to indicate that the occurrence of secondary hematopoietic tumors is not dramatically increased in the recipients of chemotherapy-treated autologous grafts (see Chapter 20). Some investigators have studied the development of new cytogenetic abnormalities at the time of relapse in patients undergoing autologous

HCT who had received chemotherapy-purged marrow grafts. Although cytogenetic changes unrelated to the original abnormality can be detected, the new cytogenetic changes involve all chromosomes except Y, with a predominance of chromosomes 1, 3, 6 and 7. The abnormalities were not seen in the original leukemia and all were of a transitory nature [156].

Fertility

One of the major complications of higher dose chemoradiotherapy for the treatment of acute leukemia is infertility and sexual dysfunction, a frequent concern expressed by young patients who are being evaluated for HCT (see Chapters 39, 40 and 69). A potential benefit of utilization of radiolabeled antibodies as a substitute for TBI could be preservation of fertility; however, clinical data are lacking.

Future directions

The major limitation to the success of autologous HCT in all stages of disease is relapse. Given the contribution of the body burden of disease as well as contamination of the graft to relapse, improvements in the results of HCT will require improvements in both the preparative regimen and in modification of the graft to be infused.

Among the strategies that appear promising to decrease the contribution of residual disease in the patient are radioimmunotherapy designed to target the body burden of leukemia and the more rational use of chemotherapeutic agents in the preparative regimen (see Chapters 12 and 16). Although the body burden of leukemia appears to be the major contributor to relapse after autologous HCT, it is clear that the leukemic contamination of the hematopoietic cell graft can be a cause of treatment failure. The question of whether purging of PBHCs by chemotherapy will allow accelerated recovery while at the same time reducing leukemic cell contribution will require gene marking studies. Refinements in the procurement (timing), isolation and enrichment and expansion of hematopoietic cells may reduce the contribution of contaminating cells to relapse after transplant.

There has been considerable interest in attempting to mimic, in patients undergoing autologous HCT, the contributions of the GVL effect associated with allogeneic transplant. This GVL effect is a significant component of the therapeutic effect of allogeneic HCT, particularly in patients treated for advanced disease (see Chapters 28, 29 and 84). Investigators are exploring means to incorporate a GVL effect in the setting of autologous HCT by the use of post-transplant IL-2, CSP or other agents (see Chapters 29 and 30). The identification of antigen-specific cytotoxic T lymphocytes (CTLs) and the ability of these CTLs to mediate lysis of human tumors could lead to a strategy of infusion of T-cell clones that specifically react with the structural genes created by the translocated chromosomes in patients with AML (see Chapter 29). This strategy could provide a specific GVL effect that might reduce the risk of relapse from residual disease.

Conclusions

The past 10 years have witnessed the development of autologous HCT as an important treatment modality for patients with AML treated during first or subsequent remission. This increase in clinical progress has been paralleled by an increased knowledge of the molecular biology of leukemogenesis and the application of molecular techniques to classify and treat patients with both primary and secondary AML. In addition, the ease and accessibility of mobilized PBHCs have further increased the use of autologous HCT. The studies reviewed in this chapter indicate that for patients with AML who lack a histocompatible sibling donor or who are >45–50 years of age, autologous transplant in first remission remains a reasonable therapeutic option, particularly for those patients who have either standard- or poor-risk cytogenetics for which chemotherapy is unlikely to be curative. As further cytogenetic information and other risk factor analyses from large intergroup comparative HCT and chemotherapy trials become available, these data will assist in refining decisions about who should be transplanted in first remission, what type of donor transplant should be performed or whether the transplant should be delayed beyond first remission.

For those patients not transplanted in first remission who do not have a related or unrelated donor, consideration should be given to storage of their bone marrow or PBHCs in order to perform an autologous HCT procedure either in early first relapse or in second remission. This step preserves an opportunity for patients to achieve long-term survival despite having suffered a leukemic relapse.

References

1 McGovern JJ Jr, Russell PS, Atkins L, Webster EW. Treatment of terminal leukemic relapse by total-body irradiation and intravenous infusion of stored autologous bone marrow obtained during remission. *N Engl J Med* 1959; **260**: 675–83.

2 Gorin NC, Stachowiak J, Hirsch-Marie F *et al.* Greffe de moelle autologue après thèrapeutique dèfinitive entrainant une rèmission complète dans un cas de leucémie aiguë myéloblastique chimiorésistante. *Nouv Presse Med* 1977; **6**: 2741–5.

3 Gorin NC, Najman A, Duhamel G. Autologous bone marrow transplantation in acute myelocytic leukemia. *Lancet* 1977; **1**: 1050.

4 Fefer A, Cheever MA, Thomas ED *et al.* Bone marrow transplantation for refractory acute leukemia in 34 patients with identical twins. *Blood* 1981; **57**: 421–30.

5 Dicke KA, Spitzer G, Peters L *et al.* Autologous bone-marrow transplantation in relapsed adult acute myelogenous leukemia. *Lancet* 1979; **1**: 514–7.

6 Herve P, Rozenbaum A, Plouvier E *et al.* Autologous bone marrow transplantation in acute myeloid leukemia in relapse or in complete remission. *Cancer Treat Rep* 1982; **66**: 1983–5.

7 Herzig GP. Autologous marrow transplantation in cancer therapy. In: Brown EB, ed. *Progress in Hematology*. New York: Grune & Stratton, 1981: 1.

8 Embury SH, Elias L, Heller PH *et al.* Remission maintenance therapy in acute myelogenous leukemia. *West J Med* 1977; **126**: 267–72.

9 Wiernik PH, Serpick A. A randomized clinical trial of daunorubicin and a combination of prednisone, vincristine, 6-mecaptopurine, and methotrexate in adult acute nonlymphocytic leukemia. *Cancer* 1972; **32**: 2023–6.

10 Burke PJ, Karp JE, Braine HG *et al.* Timed sequential therapy of human leukemia based upon the response of leukemic cells to hormonal growth factors. *Cancer Res* 1977; **37**: 2138–46.

11 Bennett JM, Catoversusky D, Daniel MT. *et al.* Proposed revised criteria for the classification of acute myeloid leukemia: a report for the French–American–British Cooperative Group. *Ann Intern Med* 1985; **103**: 620–5.

12 Cheson BD, Cassileth PA, Head DR *et al.* Report of National Cancer Institute sponsored workshop on definitions and diagnosis and response in acute myeloid leukemia. *J Clin Oncol* 1990; **8**: 813–9.

13 Caliguri MA, Strout MP, Lawrence D *et al.* Rearrangement of ALL1 (MLL) in acute myeloid leukemia with normal cytogenetics. *Cancer Res* 1998; **58**: 55–9.

14 Mayer Rj Davis RB, Schiffer CA *et al.* Intensive post-remission chemotherapy in adults with acute myeloid leukemia. *N Engl J Med* 1994; **331**: 896–903.

15 Dutcher JP, Schiffer CA, Wiernik PH. Hyperleukocytosis in adult nonlymphocytic leukemia: impact on remission rate and duration, and survival. *J Clin Oncol* 1987; **5**: 1364–72.

16 Brito-Babapulle F, Catoversusky D, Galton DAG. Clinical and laboratory features of *de novo* acute myeloid leukemia with trilineage myelodysplasia. *Br J Haematol* 1987; **66**: 445–50.

17 Goasguen JE, Matsuo T, Cox C *et al.* Evaluation of the dysmyelopoiesis in 336 patients with *de novo* acute myeloid leukemia: major importance of dysgranulopoiesis for remission and survival. *Leukemia* 1992; **6**: 520–5.

18 Kuriyama K, Tomonaga M, Matsuo T *et al.* Poor response to intensive chemotherapy in *de novo* myeloid leukemia with trilineage myelodysplasia. *Br J Haematol* 1994; **86**: 767–73.

19 Bloomfield CD, Lawrence D, Byrd JC et al. Frequency of prolonged remission duration after high-dose cytarabine intensification in acute myeloid leukemia varies by cytogenetic subtype. *Cancer Res* 1998; **58**: 4173–9.

20 Geller RB, Zahurak M, Hurwitz CA et al. Prognostic importance of immunophenotyping in adults with acute myelocytic leukemia: the significance of the stem-cell glycoprotein CD34 (My 10). *Br J Haematol* 1990; **76**: 340–7.

21 List AF. Role of multidrug resistance and its pharmacologic modulation in acute myeloid leukemia. *Leukemia* 1996; **10**: 937–42.

22 Leith CP, Chen IM, Kopecky KJ et al. Correlation of multidrug resistance (MDR) protein expression with functional dye/drug efflux in acute myeloid leukemia by multiparameter flow cytometry: identification of discordant CD34+/MDR1/Efflux+ and MDR1+/Efflux cases. *Blood* 1995; **86**: 2329–42.

23 Bennett JM, Begg CB. Eastern Cooperative Oncology Group study of the cytochemistry of adult acute myeloid leukemia by correlation of subtypes with response and survival. *Cancer Res* 1981; **41**: 4833–7.

24 Löffler H, Gassmann W, Jürgensen CH et al. Clinical aspects of acute myelogenous leukemia of the FAB-types M3 and M4eo. *Haematol Blood Transfus* 1994; **36**: 519–24.

25 Nakao M, Yokota S, Iwai T et al. Internal tandem duplication of the *flt3* gene found in acute myeloid leukemia. *Leukemia* 1996; **10**: 1911–18.

26 Yokota S, Kiyoi H, Nakao M et al. Internal tandem duplication of the *FLT3* gene is preferentially seen in acute myeloid leukemia and myelodysplastic syndrome among various hematological malignancies: a study on a large series of patients and cell lines. *Leukemia* 1997; **11**: 1605–9.

27 Kottaridis PD, Gale RE, Frew ME et al. The presence of a *FLT3* internal tandem duplication in patients with acute myeloid leukemia (AML) adds important prognostic information to cytogenetic risk group and response to the first cycle of chemotherapy: analysis of 854 patients from the UK Medical Research Council AML 10 and 12 trials. *Blood* 2001; **98**: 1752–9.

28 Whitman SP, Archer KJ, Feng L et al. Absence of the wild type allele predicts poor prognosis in adult de novo acute myeloid leukemia with normal cytogenetics and the internal tandem duplication of *FLT3*: a cancer and leukemia group B study. *Cancer Res* 2001; **61**: 7233–9.

29 Stein AS, O'Donnell MR, Chai A et al. In vivo purging with high-dose cytarabine followed by high-dose chemoradiotherapy and reinfusion of unpurged bone marrow for adult acute myelogenous leukemia in first complete remission. *J Clin Oncol* 1996; **14**: 2206–16.

30 Ferrant A, Labopin M, Frassoni F et al. Karyotype in acute myeloblastic leukemia: prognostic significance for bone marrow transplantation in first remission: a European group for blood and marrow transplantation study. *Blood* 1997; **90**: 2931–8.

31 Schouten HC, Van Putten WLJ, Hagemeijer A et al. The prognostic significance of chromosomal findings in patients with acute myeloid leukemia in a study comparing the efficacy of autologous and allogeneic bone marrow transplantation. *Bone Marrow Transplant* 1991; **8**: 377–81.

32 Stein AS, O'Donnell MR, Slovak M et al. Do cytogenetics predict outcome of autologous bone marrow transplantation (ABMT) for acute myelogenous leukemia (AML) in first remission? *Blood* 1996; **88** (Suppl. 1): 485a [Abstract].

33 Kottaridis PD, Gale RE, Holt M et al. Consolidation of AML therapy with autograft and allograft procedures does not negate the poor prognostic impact of *FLT3* internal tandem duplications: results from the UK MRC AML 10 and 12 trials. *Blood* 2002; **100** (Suppl. 1): 75a [Abstract].

34 Carella AM, Gozza E, Santini G et al. Autologous unpurged bone marrow transplantation for acute non-lymphoblastic leukemia in first complete remission. *Bone Marrow Transplant* 1988; **3**: 537–41.

35 Körbling M, Hunstein W, Fliedner TM et al. Disease-free survival after autologous bone marrow transplantation in patients with acute myelogenous leukemia. *Blood* 1989; **74**: 1898–904.

36 Meloni G, Fabritis PD, Petti M, Mandelli F. BAVC regimen and autologous bone marrow transplantation in patients with acute myelogenous leukemia in second remission. *Blood* 1990; **75**: 2282–5.

37 Santos GW, Tutschka PJ, Brookmeyer R et al. Marrow transplantation for acute non-lymphocytic leukemia after treatment with busulfan and cyclophosphamide. *N Engl J Med* 1983; **309**: 1347–53.

38 Tutschka PJ, Copelan EA, Klein J. Bone marrow transplantation for leukemia following a new busulfan cyclophosphamide regimen. *Blood* 1987; **70**: 1382–8.

39 Linker CA, Ries CA, Damon LE, Rugo HS, Wolff JL. Autologous bone marrow transplantation for acute myeloid leukemia using busulfan plus etoposide as a preparative regimen. *Blood* 1993; **81**: 311–8.

40 Chao NJ, Stein AS, Long GD et al. Busulfan/etoposide: initial experience with a new preparative regimen for autologous bone marrow transplantation in patients with acute non-lymphoblastic leukemia. *Blood* 1993; **81**: 319–23.

41 Vaughan WP, Dennison JD, Reed EC et al. Improved results of allogeneic bone marrow transplantation for advanced hematologic malignancy using busulfan, cyclophosphamide and etoposide as cytoreductive and immunosuppressive therapy. *Bone Marrow Transplant* 1991; **8**: 489–95.

42 Crilley P, Topolsky D, Styler MJ et al. Extramedullary toxicity of a conditioning regimen containing busulfan, cyclophosphamide and etoposide in 84 patients undergoing autologous and allogeneic bone marrow transplantation. *Bone Marrow Transplant* 1995; **15**: 361–5.

43 Kröger N, Zabelina T, Sonnenberg S et al. Dose-dependent effect of etoposide in combination with busulfan plus cyclophosphamide as conditioning for stem cell transplantation in patients with acute myeloid leukemia. *Bone Marrow Transplant* 2000; **26**: 711–6.

44 Demirer T, Buckner CD, Appelbaum FR et al. Busulfan, cyclophosphamide and fractionated total body irradiation for autologous or syngeneic marrow transplantation for acute and chronic myelogenous: phase I dose escalation of busulfan based on targeted plasma levels. *Bone Marrow Transplant* 1996; **17**: 491–5.

45 Matthews DC, Appelbaum FR, Eary JF et al. Development of a marrow transplant regimen for acute leukemia using targeted hematopoietic irradiation delivered by ^{131}I-labeled anti-CD45 antibody, combined with cyclophosphamide and total body irradiation. *Blood* 1995; **85**: 1122–31.

46 Clift RA, Buckner CD, Appelbaum FR et al. Allogeneic marrow transplantation in patients with acute myeloid leukemia in first remission: a randomized trial of two irradiation regimens. *Blood* 1990; **76**: 1867–71.

47 Dusenberry KE, Steinbuch M, McGlave P et al. Autologous bone marrow transplantation in acute myeloid leukemia: the University of Minnesota experience. *Int J Radiat Oncol Biol Phys* 1996; **36**: 335–43.

48 Blaise D, Maraninchi D, Archimbaum E et al. Allogeneic bone marrow transplantation for acute myeloid leukemia in first remission: a randomized trial of busulfan/cytoxan vs. cytoxan/total body irradiation as preparative regimen: a report from the Groupe d'Eludes de la Greffe de Moelle Osseuse. *Blood* 1992; **79**: 2578–82.

49 Blaise D, Maraninchi D, Michallet M et al. Long-term follow-up of a randomized trial comparing the combination of cyclophosphamide with total body irradiation or busulfan as conditioning regimen for patients receiving HLA-identical marrow grafts for acute myeloablastic leukemia in first complete remission. *Blood* 2001; **97**: 3669–71.

50 Blume KG, Kopecky KJ, Henslee-Downey JP et al. A prospective randomized comparison of total body irradiation/etoposide vs. busulfan/cyclophosphamide as preparatory regimens for bone marrow transplantation in patients with leukemia who were not in first remission: a South-West Oncology Group study. *Blood* 1993; **81**: 2187–93.

51 Blume KG, Forman SJ. High dose busulfan/etoposide as a preparative regimen for second bone marrow transplants in hematologic malignancies. *Blut* 1987; **55**: 49–53.

52 Linker CA, Ries CA, Damon LE et al. Autologous stem cell transplantation for acute myeloid leukemia in first remission. *Biol Blood Marrow Transplant* 2000; **6**: 50–7.

53 Petersen FB, Buckner CD, Appelbaum FR et al. Etoposide, cyclophosphamide and fractionated total body irradiation as a preparative regimen for marrow transplantation in patients with advanced hematological malignancies: a phase I study. *Bone Marrow Transplant* 1992; **10**: 83–8.

54 Slattery JT, Clift RA, Buckner CD et al. Marrow transplantation for chronic myeloid leukemia: the influence of plasma busulfan levels on the outcome of transplantation. *Blood* 1997; **89**: 3055–60.

55 Deeg HJ, Storer B, Slattery JT et al. Conditioning with targeted busulfan and cyclophosphamide for hemopoietic stem cell transplantation from related and unrelated donors in patients with myelodysplastic syndrome. *Blood* 2002; **100**: 1201–7.

56 Stein A, O'Donnell MR, Parker P et al. Phase I–II study of escalating doses of busulfan (BU) in combination with fractionated total body irradiation (FTBI) and etoposide (VP16) as a preparative regimen for allogeneic bone marrow transplant (BMT) for patients with advanced leukemias. *Blood* 1998; **92** (Suppl. 1): 517a [Abstract].

57 Kashyap A, Wingard J, Cagnoni P et al. Intravenous vs. oral busulfan as part of a busulfan/cyclophosphamide preparative regimen for allogeneic hematopoietic stem cell transplantation: decreased incidence of hepatic venoocclusive disease (HVOD), HVOD-related mortality, and overall 100-day mortality. *Biol Blood Marrow Transplant* 2002; **8**: 493–500.

58 Andersson BS, Kashyap A, Gian V et al. Conditioning therapy with intravenous busulfan and cyclophosphamide (IV BuCy2) for hematologic malignancies prior to allogeneic stem cell trans-

plantation: a phase II study. *Biol Blood Marrow Transplant* 2002; **8**: 145–54.
59 To LB, Haylock DN, Kimber RJ, Juttner CA. High levels of circulating hemopoietic stem cells in very early remission from acute non-lymphoblastic leukemia and their collection and cryopreservation. *Br J Hematol* 1984; **58**: 399–410.
60 Bernard Ph, Reiffers J, Verzon G et al. Collection of circulating hematopoietic cells after chemotherapy in acute non-lymphocytic leukaemia. *Br J Hematol* 1985; **61**: 577–8.
61 Reiffers J, Bernard P, David B et al. Successful autologous transplantation with peripheral blood haematopoietic cells in a patient with acute leukaemia. *Exp Hematol* 1986; **14**: 312–5.
62 Sanz MA, de la Rubia J, Sanz GF et al. Busulfan plus cyclophosphamide followed by autologous blood stem cell transplantation for patients with acute myeloblastic leukemia in first complete remission: a status report from a single institution. *J Clin Oncol* 1993; **11**: 1661–7.
63 Reiffers J, Stoppa AM, Attal M, Michallet M. Is there a place for blood stem cell transplantation for the younger adult patient with acute myelogenous leukemia? *J Clin Oncol* 1994; **12**: 1100–1.
64 Laporte JP, Gorin NC, Feuchtenbaum J et al. Relapse after autografting with peripheral blood stem cells. *Lancet* 1987; **11**: 1393.
65 Körbling M, Fliedner TM, Holle R et al. Autologous blood stem cell (ABSCT) vs. purged bone marrow transplantation (pABMT) in standard risk AML: influence of source and cell composition of the autograft on hematopoietic reconstitution and disease-free survival. *Bone Marrow Transplant* 1991; **7**: 343–9.
66 Mehta J, Powles R, Singhal S, Treleaven J. Peripheral blood stem cells transplantation may result in increased relapsed of acute myeloid leukaemia due to reinfusion of a higher number of malignant cells. *Bone Marrow Transplant* 1995; **15**: 652–3.
67 Visani G, Lemoli RM, Tosi P et al. Use of peripheral blood stem cells for autologous transplantation in acute myeloid leukemia patients allows faster engraftment and equivalent disease-free survival compared with bone marrow cells. *Bone Marrow Transplant* 1999; **24**: 467–72.
68 Reiffers J, Labopin M, Sanz M et al. Autologous blood cell vs. marrow transplantation for acute myeloid leukemia in complete remission: an EBMT retrospective analysis. *Bone Marrow Transplant* 2000; **25**: 1115–9.
69 Gorin NC, Labopin M, Laporte JP et al. Importance of marrow dose on engraftment and outcome in acute leukemia: models derived from patients autografted with mafosfamide purged marrow at a single institution. *Exp Hematol* 1999; **27**: 1822–30.
70 Duggan PR, Guo D, Luider J et al. Predictive factors for long-term engraftment of autologous blood stem cells. *Bone Marrow Transplant* 2000; **26**: 1299–304.
71 Gorin NC, Labopin M, Prichard P et al. Feasibility and recent improvement of autologous stem cell transplantation for acute myelocytic leukemia in patients over 60 years of age: importance of the source of stem cells. *Br J Hematol* 2000; **110**: 887–93.
72 Gale RP, Horowitz MM, Ash RC et al. Identical-twin bone marrow transplants for leukemia. *Ann Intern Med* 1994; **120**: 646–52.
73 Hagenbeek A, Martens ACM. Cryopreservation of autologous marrow grafts in acute leukemia: survival of *in vivo* clonogenic leukemic cells and normal hematopoietic stem cells. *Leukemia* 1989; **3**: 535–7.
74 Hagenbeek A, Martens ACM. Reinfusion of leukemic cells with the autologous marrow graft: preclinical studies on lodging and regrowth of leukemia. *Leuk Res* 1985; **9**: 1389–95.
75 Allieri MA, Lopez M, Douay L, Mary JY, Nguyen L, Gorin NC. Clonogenic leukemic progenitor cells in acute myelocytic leukemia are highly sensitive to cryopreservation: possible purging effect for autologous bone marrow transplantation. *Bone Marrow Transplant* 1991; **7**: 101–5.
76 Brenner MK, Rill DR, Moen RC et al. Gene-marking to trace origin of relapse after autologous bone marrow transplantation. *Lancet* 1993; **341**: 85–6.
77 Miller CB, Rowlings PA, Zhang MJ et al. The effect of graft purging with 4-hydroperoxycyclophosphamide in autologous bone marrow transplantation for acute myelogenous leukemia. *Exp Hematol* 2001; **29**: 1336–46.
78 Gorin NC, Aegerter P, Auvert B et al. Autologous bone marrow transplantation for acute myelocytic leukemia in first remission: a European survey of the role of marrow purging. *Blood* 1990; **75**: 1606–14.
79 Gorin NC, Labopin M, Meloni G et al. Autologous bone marrow transplantation for acute myeloblastic leukemia in Europe: further evidence of the role of marrow purging by mafosfamide. *Leukemia* 1991; **5**: 896–904.
80 Kaiser H, Stuart RK, Brookmeyer R et al. Autologous bone marrow transplantation in acute leukemia: a phase I study of *in vitro* treatment of marrow with 4-hydroperoxycyclophosphamide to purge tumor cells. *Blood* 1985; **65**: 1504–10.
81 Kushner BH, Kwon JH, Gulati SC, Malaspina HC. Preclinical assessment of purging with VP16–213: key role for long-term marrow cultures. *Blood* 1987; **69**: 65–71.
82 Stiff PJ, Koester AR. *In vitro* chemoseparation of leukemic cells from murine bone marrow using VP16–213: importance of stem cell assays. *Exp Hematol* 1987; **15**: 263–8.
83 Gulati S, Acaba L, Yahalom J et al. Autologous bone marrow transplantation for acute myelogenous leukemia using 4-hydroperoxycyclophosphamide and VP16 purged bone marrow. *Bone Marrow Transplant* 1992; **10**: 129–34.
84 Robertson MJ, Soiffer RJ, Freedman AS et al. Human bone marrow depleted of CD33-positive cells mediates delayed but durable reconstitution of hematopoiesis: clinical trial of MY9 monoclonal antibody-purged autografts for the treatment of acute myeloid leukemia. *Blood* 1992; **79**: 2229–36.
85 Ball ED, Wilson J, Phelps V, Neudorf S. Autologous bone marrow transplantation for acute myeloid leukemia in remission or first relapse using monoclonal antibody-purged marrow. results of phase II studies with long-term follow-up. *Bone Marrow Transplant* 2000; **25**: 823–9.
86 Zander AR, Verma DS, Spitzer G et al. Autologous bone marrow transplantation in acute leukemia. *Int J Radiat Oncol Biol Phys* 1979; **5**: 1709–10.
87 Keny PC, Rubin P, Contine LS, Frantz C, Nakissa N, Gregory P. Characterization of the biophysical properties of human tumor and bone marrow cells as a preliminary step to the use of centrifugal elutriation in autologous bone marrow transplantation. *Int J Radiat Oncol Biol Phys* 1984; **10**: 1913–22.
88 Chang J, Morgenstern GR, Coutinho LH et al. The use of bone marrow cells grown in long-term culture for autologous bone marrow transplantation in acute myeloid leukemia: an update. *Bone Marrow Transplant* 1989; **4**: 5–9.
89 Klingerman HG, Eaves CJ, Barnett MJ et al. Transplantation of patients with high-risk acute myeloid leukemia in first remission with autologous marrow cultured with interleukin-2 followed by interleukin-2 administration. *Bone Marrow Transplant* 1994; **14**: 389–96.
90 Mehta J, Powles R, Singhal S et al. Autologous bone marrow transplantation for acute myeloid leukemia in first remission: identification of modifiable prognostic factors. *Bone Marrow Transplant* 1995; **16**: 499–506.
91 Tallman MS, Perez W, Keating A et al. Pretransplant consolidation chemotherapy decreases leukemia relapse after autologous stem cell transplantation (ASCT) for acute myeloid leukemia (AML) in first complete remission (CR). *Blood* 2001; **98** (Suppl. 1): 859a [Abstract].
92 Cahn JY, Labopin M, Sierra J et al. No impact of high-dose cytarabine on the outcome of patients transplanted for acute myeloblastic leukemia in first remission. Acute Leukaemia Working Party of the European Group for Blood and Marrow Transplantation (EBMT). *Br J Haematol* 2000; **110** (2): 308–14.
93 Schiller G, Lee M, Miller T et al. Transplantation of autologous peripheral blood progenitor cells procured after high-dose cytarabine-based consolidation chemotherapy for adults with acute myelogenous leukemia in first remission. *Leukemia* 1997; **11**: 1533–9.
94 Stein AS, O'Donnell MR, Slovak ML et al. Interleukin-2 following autologous stem cell transplant for adult patients with acute myeloid leukemia in first complete remission. *J Clin Oncol* 2002; **21**: 615–23.
95 Robinson N, Benganes MC, Thompson JA et al. Interleukin-2 after autologous stem cell transplantation for hematologic malignancy: a phase I/II study. *Bone Marrow Transplant* 1997; **19**: 425–42.
96 Fefer A, Robinson N, Benyunes MC et al. Interleukin-2 therapy after bone marrow or stem cell transplantation for hematologic malignancies. In: De Vita VT Jr, Hellman S, Rosenberg SA, eds. *Cancer Journal from Scientific American*, Vol. 2, Suppl 1. Seattle, Washington: 1997: S48–S53.
97 Blaise D, Attal M, Pico JL et al. The use of sequential high-dose recombinant interleukin-2 regimen after autologous bone marrow transplantation does not improve the disease transplanted in first complete remission. *Leuk Lymphoma* 1997; **25**: 469.
98 Schiller G, Wong S, Lowe T et al. Transplantation of IL-2 mobilized autologous peripheral blood progenitor cells for adults with acute myelogenous leukemia in first remission. *Leukemia* 2001; **15**: 757–63.
99 Jones RJ, Vogelsang GB, Hess AD et al. Induction of graft versus host disease after autologous bone marrow transplantation. *Lancet* 1989; **8**: 754–7.
100 Yeager AM, Vogelsang GB, Jones RJ et al. Induction of cutaneous graft versus host disease by administration of cyclosporine to patients undergoing autologous bone marrow transplantation for acute myeloid leukemia. *Blood* 1992; **79**: 3031–5.
101 Baron F, Gothot A, Salmon JP et al. Clinical course and predictive factors for cyclosporin-induced autologous graft versus host disease after autolo-

gous haematopoietic stem cell transplantation. *Br J Hematol* 2000; **111**: 745–53.
102 Simonsson B, Tötterman T, Hokland P *et al.* Roquinimex (Linomide) vs. placebo in AML after autologous bone marrow transplantation. *Bone Marrow Transplant* 2000; **25**: 1121–7.
103 Carella AM, Frassoni F, Van Lint MT *et al.* Autologous and allogeneic bone marrow transplantation in acute myeloid leukemia in first complete remission: an update of the Genoa experience with 159 patients. *Ann Hematol* 1992; **64**: 128–31.
104 Beelen DW, Quabeck K, Graeven U *et al.* Acute toxicity and first clinical results of intensive post-induction therapy using a modified busulfan and cyclophosphamide regimen with autologous bone marrow rescue in first complete remission of acute myeloid leukemia. *Blood* 1989; **74**: 1507–16.
105 McMillan AK, Goldstone AH, Linch DC *et al.* High-dose chemotherapy and autologous bone marrow transplantation in acute myeloid leukemia. *Blood* 1990; **76**: 480–8.
106 Miggiano MC, Gherlinzoni F, Rosti G *et al.* Autologous bone marrow transplantation in late first complex remission improves outcome in acute myelogenous leukemia. *Leukemia* 1996; **10**: 402–9.
107 Burnett AK, Pendry K, Rawlinson PS *et al.* Autograft to eliminate minimal residual disease in AML in first remission: update on the Glasgow experience. *Bone Marrow Transplant* 1990; **6** (Suppl. 1): 59–60.
108 Löwenberg B, Verdonch LJ, Dekker AW *et al.* Autologous bone marrow transplantation in acute myeloid leukemia in first remission: results of a Dutch prospective study. *J Clin Oncol* 1990; **8**: 287–94.
109 Sanz MA, Rubia J, Sanz GE *et al.* Busulfan plus cyclophosphamide followed by autologous blood stem cell transplantation for patients with acute myeloblastic leukemia in first complete remission: a report from a single institution. *J Clin Oncol* 1993; **11**: 1661–7.
110 Cassileth PA, Andersen J, Lazarus HM *et al.* Autologous bone marrow transplant in acute myeloid leukemia in first remission. *J Clin Oncol* 1993; **11**: 314–9.
111 LaPorte J, Lopez DM, Labopin M *et al.* One hundred twenty five adult patients with primary acute leukemia autografted with marrow purged by mafosfamide: a 10-year single institution experience. *Blood* 1994; **84**: 3810–8.
112 Yeager AM. Autologous bone marrow transplantation for acute myeloid leukemia. In: Forman SJ, Blume KG, Thomas ED, eds. *Bone Marrow Transplantation*. Oxford: Blackwell Scientific Publications, 1994: 709–30.
113 Mitus AJ, Miller KB, Schenkein DP *et al.* Improved survival for patients with acute myelogenous leukemia. *J Clin Oncol* 1995; **13**: 560–9.
114 de Witte T, Sucin T, Peetermans M *et al.* Intensive chemotherapy for poor prognosis myelodysplasia (MDS) and secondary acute myelogenous leukemia following MDS of more than 6 months duration: a pilot study by the Leukemia Cooperative Group of the European Organization for Research and Treatment in Cancer (EORTC-LCG). *Leukemia* 1995; **9**: 1805–11.
115 Kantarjian HM, Keating MJ, Walters RS *et al.* Therapy-related leukemia and myelodysplastic syndrome: clinical, cytogenetic, and prognostic features. *J Clin Oncol* 1986; **4**: 1748–57.

116 de Witte T, Muus P, De Pauw B, Haanen C. Intensive antileukemic treatment of patients younger than 65 years with myelodysplastic syndromes and secondary acute myelogenous leukemia. *Cancer* 1990; **66**: 831–7.
117 Delforge M, Demuynck H, Vandengerghe P *et al.* Polyclonal primitive hematopoietic progenitors can be detected in mobilized peripheral blood from patients with high-risk myelodysplastic syndromes. *Blood* 1995; **86**: 3660–7.
118 Carella AM, Dejana A, Lerna E *et al. In vivo* mobilization of karyotypically normal peripheral blood progenitor cells in high-risk MDS, secondary or therapy-related acute myelogenous leukemia. *Br J Haematol* 1996; **95**: 127–30.
119 Geller RB, Vogelsang GB, Wingard JR *et al.* Successful marrow transplantation for acute myelocytic leukemia following therapy for Hodgkin's disease. *J Clin Oncol* 1988; **6**: 1558–61.
120 Öberg G, Simonsson B, Smedmyr B *et al.* Is hematological reconstitution seen after ABMT in MDS patients? *Bone Marrow Transplant* 1989; **4** (Suppl. 2): 52.
121 Laporte JP, Isnard F, Lesage F *et al.* Autologous bone marrow transplantation with marrow purged by mafosfamide in seven patients with myelodysplastic syndromes in transformation (AML-MDS): a pilot study. *Leukemia* 1993; **7**: 2030–3.
122 de Witte T, Van Biezen A, Hermans J *et al.* Autologous bone marrow transplantation for patients with myelodysplastic syndrome (MDS) or acute myeloid leukemia following MDS. *Blood* 1997; **90**: 3853–7.
123 de Witte T, Suciu S, Verhoef G *et al.* Intensive chemotherapy followed by allogeneic or autologous stem cell transplantation for patients with myelodysplastic syndromes (MDSs) and acute myeloid leukemia following MDS. *Blood* 2001; **98**: 2326–31.
124 Sanz M, Coco F, Martin G *et al.* Definition of relapse risk and role of nonanthracycline drugs for consolidation in patients with acute promyelocytic leukemia: a joint study of the PETHEMA and GIMEMA cooperative groups. *Blood* 2000; **96**: 1247–53.
125 Shen ZX, Chen GQ, Li XS *et al.* Use of arsenic trioxide (As_2O_3) in the treatment of acute promyelocytic leukemia (APL). II. Clinical efficacy and pharmacokinetics in relapsed patients. *Blood* 1997; **89**: 3354–60.
126 Soignet SL, Maslak P, Wang ZG *et al.* Complete remission after treatment of acute promyelocytic leukemia with arsenic trioxide. *N Engl J Med* 1998; **339**: 1341–8.
127 Niu C, Yan H, YuT *et al.* Studies on treatment of acute promyelocytic leukemia with arsenic trioxide: remission induction, follow-up and molecular monitoring in 11 newly diagnosed and 47 relapsed APL patients. *Blood* 1999; **94**: 3315–24.
128 Meloni G, Diverio D, Vignetti M *et al.* Autologous bone marrow transplantation for acute promyelocytic leukemia in second remission: prognostic relevance of pre-transplant minimal residual disease assessment by reverse-transcription polymerase chain reaction of the *pml/rarα* fusion gene. *Blood* 1997; **90**: 1321–5.
129 Sanz MA, de la Rubia J, Bonanad S *et al.* Prolonged molecular remission after PML/RAR alpha-positive autologous peripheral blood stem cell transplantation in acute promyelocytic leukemia: is relevant pretransplant minimal residual disease in the graft? *Leukemia* 1998; **12**: 992–5.

130 Linker CA, Damon LE, Ries CA *et al.* Autologous stem cell transplantation for advanced acute myeloid leukemia. *Bone Marrow Transplant* 2002; **29**: 297–301.
131 Sanz M, Arcese W, de la Rubia J *et al.* Stem cell transplantation (SCT) for acute promyelocytic leukemia in the ATRA era: a survey of the European Blood and Marrow Transplantation Group (EBMT). *Blood* 2000; **96** (Suppl. 1): 522a [Abstract].
132 Rosenfeld C, Shadduck RK, Pzepiorka D *et al.* Autologous bone marrow transplantation with 4-hydroperoxycyclophosphamide purged marrow for acute nonlymphocytic leukemia in late remission or early relapse. *Blood* 1989; **74**: 1159–64.
133 Smith BD, Jones RJ, Lee SM *et al.* Autologous bone marrow transplantation with 4-hydroperoxycyclophosphamide purging for acute myeloid leukaemia beyond first remission: a 10-year experience. *Br J Haematol* 2002; **117**: 907–13.
134 Chopro R, Goldstone AH, McMillan AK *et al.* Successful treatment of acute myeloid leukemia beyond first remission with autologous bone marrow transplantation using busulfan/cyclophosphamide and unpurged marrow: the British autograft group experience. *J Clin Oncol* 1991; **9**: 1840–7.
135 Meloni G, Vignetti M, Avvisati G *et al.* BAVC regimen for acute myelogenous leukemia in second complete remission. *Bone Marrow Transplant* 1996; **18**: 693–8.
136 Linker C, George S, Hurd D *et al.* Autologous stem cell transplantation for acute myeloid leukemia in second remission: CALGB 9620. *Blood* 2001; **98** (Suppl. 1): 689a [Abstract].
137 Gorin NC, Labopin M, Fouillard L *et al.* Retrospective evaluation of autologous bone marrow transplantation vs. allogeneic bone marrow transplantation from an HLA identical related donor in acute myelocytic leukemia. A study of the European Cooperative Group for Blood and Marrow Transplantation (EBMT). *Bone Marrow Transplant* 1996; **18**: 111–7.
138 Buca A, Anasetti C, Anderson G *et al.* Unrelated donor or autologous marrow transplantation for treatment of acute leukemia. *Blood* 1994; **83**: 3077–84.
139 Mehta J, Powles R, Treleaven J *et al.* Outcome of acute leukemia relapsing after bone marrow transplantation: utility of second transplants and adoptive immunotherapy. *Bone Marrow Transplant* 1997; **19**: 709–19.
140 de la Rubia J, Sanz GF, Martin G *et al.* Autologous bone marrow transplantation for patients with acute myeloblastic leukemia in relapse after autologous blood stem cell transplantation. *Bone Marrow Transplant* 1996; **18**: 1167–73.
141 Radich J, Gooley T, Sanders J *et al.* Second allogeneic transplantation after failure of first autologous transplantation. *American Society for Blood and Marrow Transplantation* 2000: 272–9.
142 Ringden O, Labopin M, Gorin NC *et al.* The dismal outcome in patients with acute leukemia who relapse after an autograft is improved if a second autograft or a matched allograft is performed. *Bone Marrow Transplant* 2000; **25**: 1053–8.
143 Ringden O, Labopin M, Frassoni F *et al.* Allogeneic bone marrow transplant or second autograft in patients with acute leukemia who relapse after an autograft. *Bone Marrow Transplant* 1999; **24**: 389–96.

144 Cohen S, Fung H, Stein A *et al*. Reduced intensity allogeneic stem cell transplantation for patients who have failed a prior autologous stem cell transplant. *Blood* 2002; Suppl. 1: 177a [Abstract].

145 Zittoun RA, Mandelli F, Willemze R *et al*. Autologous and allogeneic bone marrow transplantation compared with intensive chemotherapy in acute myelogenous leukemia. *N Engl J Med* 1995; **332**: 271–323.

146 Cassileth PA, Harrington DP, Appelbaum FR *et al*. Chemotherapy compared with autologous or allogeneic bone marrow transplantation in the management of acute myeloid leukemia in first remission. *N Engl J Med* 1998; **339**: 1649–66.

147 Slovak M, Kopecky K, Cassileth P *et al*. Karyotypic analysis predicts outcome of preremission therapy in adult acute myeloid leukemia: a South-West Oncology Group/Eastern Cooperative Oncology Group study. *Blood* 2002; **96**: 4075–83.

148 Burnett AK, Goldstone AH, Stevens RM *et al*. Randomised comparison of addition of autologous bone-marrow transplantation to intensive chemotherapy for acute myeloid leukaemia in first remission: results of MRC AML 10 trial. *Lancet* 1998; **351**: 700–8.

149 Burnett AK. Evaluating the contribution of allogeneic and autologous transplantation to the management of acute myeloid leukemia in adults. *Cancer Chemother Pharmacol* 2001; **48** (Suppl. 1): S53–8.

150 Harousseau JL, Cahn JY, Pignon B *et al*. Comparison of autologous bone marrow transplantation and intensive chemotherapy as postremission therapy in adult acute myeloid leukemia. *Blood* 1997; **90**: 2978–86.

151 Reiffers J, Gaspard MH, Maraninchi D *et al*. Comparison of allogeneic or autologous bone marrow transplantation and chemotherapy in patients with acute myeloid leukemia in first remission: a prospective controlled trial. *Br J Haematol* 1989; **72**: 57–63.

152 Ferrant A, Doyen C, Delannoy A *et al*. Allogeneic or autologous bone marrow transplantation for acute non-lymphocytic leukemia in first remission. *Bone Marrow Transplant* 1991; **7**: 303–9.

153 Schiffman K, Clift R, Appelbaum FR *et al*. Consequences of cryopreserving first remission autologous marrow for use after relapse in patients with acute myeloid leukemia. *Bone Marrow Transplant* 1993; **11**: 227–32.

154 Wingard JR, Sostrin MB, Vriesendorp HM *et al*. Interstitial pneumonitis following autologous bone marrow transplantation. *Transplantation* 1988; **46**: 61–5.

155 Reusser P, Fisher LD, Buckner CD *et al*. Cytomegalovirus infection after autologous bone marrow transplantation: occurrence of cytomegalovirus disease and effect on engraftment. *Blood* 1990; **75**: 1888–94.

156 Perot C, van den Akker J, Laporte JP *et al*. Multiple chromosome abnormalities in patients with acute leukemia after autologous bone marrow transplantation using total body irradiation and marrow purged with mafosfamide. *Leukemia* 1993; **7**: 509–15.

90

Charles A. Linker

Autologous Hematopoietic Cell Transplantation for Acute Lymphoblastic Leukemia

Significant progress has been made in the treatment of acute lymphoblastic leukemia (ALL), and the disease can now be approached with curative intent in both children and adults. Although chemotherapy remains the mainstay of treatment for the majority of patients, some patients require intensified therapy supported by hematopoietic cell transplantation (HCT) in order to increase their chance of long-term disease-free survival (DFS) and cure. The results of chemotherapy treatment of ALL in children are particularly favorable, and >70% of children diagnosed with this disease are now cured. Only a small fraction of children with ALL have such high-risk features that intensified treatment with HCT is indicated early during the course of their disease. More commonly, treatment with HCT is reserved for children who relapse after primary treatment with chemotherapy. The results of treatment of ALL in adults with chemotherapy are less satisfactory, and overall cure rates have been in the range of 30–40%. In adults, a higher proportion of patients present with high-risk features that predict very poor outcomes with chemotherapy, and these patients are appropriate candidates for early intervention with intensified treatment involving HCT. Adults with ALL who relapse after primary chemotherapy treatment have a dismal outcome with standard chemotherapy, and the necessity for treatment with HCT is straightforward.

Allogeneic HCT is generally the preferred form of HCT for high-risk patients with ALL (reviewed in Chapters 77 and 78). The primary advantage of transplantation using an allogeneic donor is the lack of contamination of the stem cell graft with leukemia cells. This problem of residual disease at the time of transplantation is particularly prominent in ALL, and the presence and amount of residual disease at the time of prior transplantation have been shown to be important prognostic factors for outcome after transplantation. A second advantage of allogeneic HCT is the antileukemic affect of allogeneic T cells derived from the donor, termed the graft-vs.-leukemia (GVL) effect. Although the GVL effect is less significant in ALL than in other diseases such as acute and chronic myeloid leukemia (AML and CML), it is present none the less. However, several factors reduce the magnitude of the positive impact of allogeneic HCT in the treatment of high-risk and relapsed ALL. Most important is the problem of finding a suitably human leukocyte antigen (HLA) matched donor. A fully HLA-matched sibling donor is available in fewer than one-third of cases. The availability of alternate allogeneic donors including matched unrelated donors, partially mismatched donors and cord blood donors increases the percentage of patients who have suitable grafts for allogeneic HCT, but many still lack a possible donor. Second, the application of allogeneic HCT is restricted by age constraints, with better results in children and young adults than in older adults, and with limited applicability to adults >50–60 years. Third, treatment-related mortality (TRM) from causes other than leukemia relapse remains a daunting problem and reduces the enthusiasm for allogeneic HCT in situations where other less toxic therapies produce acceptable results. Finally, there are constraints on the intensity of the preparative regimen that can be safely used in the setting of allogeneic HCT without an unacceptable increase in TRM. Because relapsed ALL is a particularly chemotherapy- and radiation-resistant form of cancer, these constraints on treatment intensity are problematic.

Autologous HCT has been extensively studied as a treatment option for patients with high-risk and relapsed ALL. In contrast to the limited applicability of the allogeneic HCT, all patients up to the age of 60 years who have achieved a remission are potential candidates and can serve as their own donors. With current supportive care, the morbidity and mortality of the procedure are low, and the autologous HCT setting allows for substantial intensification of the preparative regimen. At present, the results of treatment with autologous HCT for ALL vary considerably and there remains controversy regarding the appropriate role of this treatment. Improvements in treatment outcome will be necessary to expand the role of this treatment.

Adult acute lymphoblastic leukemia

Standard treatment for adult ALL

With intensification of induction therapy, complete remission (CR) rates for adults aged <60 years with ALL have increased from 70% to 85–90% [1–8]. Optimal remission induction therapy includes daunorubicin, vincristine, prednisone and L-asparaginase. The addition of cyclophosphamide has a modest effect in increasing initial CR rate but does not impact long-term outcome [9]. Lower CR rates are seen in adults >60 years (60–70%) and in those with the Philadelphia chromosome (Ph) (70%) [3–5,9–11]. For adults <60 years who achieve initial remission, most large studies show 5-year DFS of 35–40% [1,3–10]. Recently, small studies using intensified chemotherapy have reported 5-year DFS of 50% [2], and it is hoped that these results will be confirmed.

Prognostic factors in adult ALL

There is a strong consensus that age, white blood cell count (WBC), immunophenotype, time to achieving CR and cytogenetics are the most important prognostic factors predicting long-term DFS in adult ALL [1–12]. Even among adults <60 years, adults <30 years fare significantly better, with long-term DFS of 50–60% as opposed to 30%. WBC is another important prognostic feature and is more important in patients with B-precursor ALL than for those with T-lineage disease. For patients with B-precursor ALL, WBC <30,000/µL is associated with significantly better outcome than those with WBC 30,000–99,000/µL, and WBC

≥100,000/µL has generally been associated with a dismal prognosis. Among patients with T-cell disease WBC is of lesser significance [12], with WBC ≥100,000/µL only modestly reducing long-term event-free survival (EFS) from 49% to 40% ($p = 0.02$) as reported in a recent large study [8,13].

The prognostic significance of immunophenotype has changed during the past two decades, and this change appears to be treatment-related. Twenty percent of adults with ALL present with a T-cell phenotype. In prior years, when less intensive therapy was used, patients with T-cell disease had an inferior outcome. At present, T-cell phenotype is a favorable prognostic feature predicting long-term EFS of 50–60%, as opposed to 30–35% for those with B-lineage disease [1,3,6,8,12]. One large recent study of T-cell ALL identified phenotypic subtypes as being of paramount prognostic importance in this group [13]. The majority of patients with T-cell ALL have a thymic phenotype with expression of CD2, and these patients have long-term EFS of 50–60%. Prethymic T-cell disease (CD2 negative) and mature T-cell disease have a less favorable prognosis with prethymic T-cell disease having EFS <20% compared to 55% for the thymic phenotype ($p = 0.005$). Patients with prethymic disease were older and less often presented with mediastinal mass, consistent with previous observations that outcome in T-cell ALL was more favorable in younger patients and in those with mediastinal masses [5].

With increasing application of cytogenetics and molecular diagnostic studies, cytogenetics has emerged as a very powerful prognostic factor in adult ALL [14–17]. The most important subgroup is that of patients with Ph-positive (Ph+) ALL, characterized by the cytogenetic marker t(9;22) and the molecular marker BCR-ABL [1–3,6,8,11,14–17]. Ph+ ALL is almost exclusively seen in the common ALL phenotype expressing both CD19 and CD10, and is generally associated with increasing age and higher WBC. Overall, Ph+ ALL accounts for 20% of all adult ALL and at least 30% of B-lineage ALL. More cases are detected with fluorescence *in situ* hybridization (FISH) and molecular probes for BCR-ABL than by conventional cytogenetics [8]. Patients with Ph+ ALL have a somewhat lower CR rate (70%) than other patients, and their long-term outcome with conventional therapy remains dismal. One recent study of 175 Ph+ ALL patients reported long-term EFS of 6% without transplantation [11]. The translocation t(4;11) involving the *MLL* gene on 11q23 is seen in approximately 5% of ALL patients and as is associated with markedly elevated WBC [8,18]. These patients also have a poor outcome with standard therapy and appear to benefit from intensification of therapy [14]. Monosomy 7 is rarely seen in ALL, but when it occurs also confers a poor prognosis [17]. One recent report suggests that trisomy 8 is another adverse prognostic factor in adult ALL [17]. The translocation t(8;14) and its variants characterizes the Burkitt's subtype of ALL, which comprises 1–2% of adult ALL. The outcome for patients with this disease has improved markedly with the development of new intensive chemotherapy regimens which are substantially different from most adult ALL regimens [19–21]. Patients with this disease are now considered and treated separately from the bulk of ALL.

Time to achieving complete remission is another very powerful prognostic factor. Although some patients not in remission at the end of a first induction course at 4 weeks may attain remission after a second induction course, their long-term outcome is very poor [1,2,6–8]. Patients who still fail to achieve complete remission after two induction courses have an even worse prognosis.

The combination of these prognostic factors can be used to construct distinct risk groups within adult ALL (Table 90.1). Approximately one-third of patients fall into a favorable-risk group with a very high CR rate (>90%) and anticipated long-term DFS ≥70%. With this favorable outcome using conventional chemotherapy, it is hard to justify the application of either allogeneic or autologous HCT in the primary treatment of these patients. Another third of patients can be identified as falling into a

Table 90.1 Risk groups in adult acute lymphoblastic leukemia (ALL).

Favorable

No adverse cytogenetics

Achieve remission with first induction course
and
B-lineage, age <30 years and WBC <30,000/µL
or
T-lineage, CD2+ and age <30 years

Intermediate

No adverse cytogenetics

Achieve remission with first induction course
and
B-lineage, age ≥30 years or WBC 30,000–99,000/µL
or
T-lineage, CD2– or age ≥30 years

Poor

Adverse cytogenetics [t(9;22), t(4;11) or other 11q23,–7]
or
Failure to achieve a complete remission with one course of induction therapy
or
B-lineage, WBC ≥100,000/µL

WBC, white blood cell count.

poor-risk group. The outcome for these patients is extremely unfavorable with few long-term survivors using chemotherapy alone. Intensification of nonablative chemotherapy does not appear to have benefited this patient group, and all of these patients are good candidates for intervention with HCT while in first remission. The remaining third of patients with adult ALL have intermediate-risk disease. The long-term DFS of such patients has generally been 30–40% when treated with chemotherapy but may be improved to as much as 50% with recent intensified programs. For this group of patients, decision-making regarding post-treatment therapy is controversial and the role of transplantation as primary therapy remains to be determined.

New prognostic factors are now being established in adult ALL. Early response to prednisone, with circulating blast count <1000/µL after 7 days of treatment, has been established as important prognostic marker in pediatric ALL [22,23]. One recent large report from the Italian group (Gruppo Italiano Malattie Ematologiche Maligne dell'Adulto [GIMEMA]) involving 778 patients showed a significant effect on DFS for this parameter in adults [9]. Long-term DFS was 36% in responders vs. 24% in prednisone nonresponders ($p = 0.0004$).

Recent studies appear to show strong prognostic significance of measurement of minimal residual disease (MRD) in adults with ALL. A subgroup of patients enrolled on the Medical Research Council (MRC) UK ALL XII trial evaluated for MRD were recently reported [24]. Patients with B-lineage ALL were studied to identify clonal markers in the VDJ region of the immunoglobulin gene, and 77% of patients were evaluable using a DNA fingerprinting technique. The presence of MRD above a threshold level between 0 and 2 months was prognostically significant, predicting a decrease in EFS from 70% to 20% ($p = 0.016$). When evaluated at 3–5 months, the presence of MRD was even more significant, predicting a decrease in EFS from 75% to 10% ($p = 0.0001$). Another recent report on the import of MRD studied 126 "standard risk" patients among those participating in the ongoing German (GMALL [German Multicenter Study Group for Adult ALL] 06/99) trial [25]. Ninety-four percent (118 of 126) of patients were evaluable with clonal rearrangements in either immunoglobulin or T-cell-receptor genes. In this initial report 50 patients had MRD analysis

Table 90.2 Clinical trials of autologous hematopoietic cell transplantation (HCT) for adults with acute lymphoblastic leukemia (ALL) in first remission (CR1).

Group/author [Reference]	Risk status	n	EFS (%)
EBMT [27]		1366	36
Gorin [27]		233	41
IBMTR [27]		172	40
LALA 87 [28,29]		95	34
Hunault et al. [30]	HR	82	36
Attal et al. [31]		77	26
Powles et al. [32]		77	52
Martin et al. [33]	Ph+	34	20
Linker et al. [34]	HR	24	48

EBMT, European Group for Blood and Marrow Transplantation; EFS, event-free survival; HR, high risk; IBMTR, International Bone Marrow Transplant Registry; LALA, French Group on Therapy for Adult ALL; Ph+, Philadelphia chromosome-positive.

correlated with clinical outcome, and at the end of induction therapy MRD level $>10^{-4}$ was associated with a marked increase in relapse rate ($p = 0.0004$). Other studies of MRD in adult ALL have been performed using flow cytometry [26]. While results of MRD studies have not been incorporated in risk stratification in adult ALL, these initial studies appear very convincing, and MRD may become a standard test for risk stratification in the future.

Clinical studies of autologous HCT for adult ALL in first remission

Several groups have reported outcomes for large series of adults with ALL undergoing autologous HCT in first remission (CR1) (Table 90.2). Gorin et al. [35] reported on 233 such patients with long-term leukemia-free survival (LFS) in 41%. In this series, the most important prognostic factor was the time interval between achieving complete remission and proceeding to transplant. Patients transplanted at an interval >9 months had LFS of 70%. LFS fell to 55% for patients transplanted between 7 and 9 months and to 35% for patients transplanted at an interval <6 months ($p = 0.01$). Similar results were reported in another study in which time from remission to transplant of >3 months was associated with improved outcomes ($p = 0.002$) [36]. Whether the effect of this time interval represented the drop-out of high-risk patients who relapsed before transplantation, or whether it represents the effect of consolidation therapy administered prior to HCT in reducing tumor burden ("in vivo purging") cannot be determined. The European Group for Blood and Marrow Transplantation (EBMT) registry reported on 1366 patients treated in first remission with an EFS of 36% [27]. The International Bone Marrow Transplant Registry (IBMTR) has reported on 172 ALL CR1 patients with EFS of 40% [27]. Overall, these large registry studies establish a baseline of expected outcome when autologous HCT is applied to adult ALL patients in CR1. However, lacking full description of the prognostic factors of these patients, and not knowing the indication for the choice of transplant as treatment, it is hard to assess the role of autologous HCT or to compare the outcome data to those expected with chemotherapy or other treatments.

One randomized trial has been completed which reports a comparison between the outcome of adults with ALL in first remission treated with chemotherapy vs. autologous HCT. In this French LALA (French Group on Therapy for Adult ALL) 87 study, adults up to age 60 were treated with induction therapy including cyclophosphamide, daunorubicin (or zororubicin) plus vincristine and prednisone [28]. Patients under age 40 with HLA-matched sibling donors were allocated to allogeneic bone marrow transplantation (BMT). The remaining patients received consolidation treatment with modest doses of daunorubicin, cytarabine and asparaginase, and patients remaining in remission after one consolidation course were randomized to receive either continued chemotherapy or autologous BMT. Bone marrow was harvested after a second course of the same modest consolidation and was purged either with mafosphamide or monoclonal antibodies. Both patient groups received a total of three courses of consolidation therapy and then received either maintenance chemotherapy or autologous BMT using a standard preparative regimen of total body irradiation (TBI) and 120 mg/kg cyclophosphamide. Of the 116 young patients with matched sibling donors, 98 received the intended allogeneic transplant, with 14 of the 18 drop-outs resulting from early relapse. Of the 262 remaining patients, 191 were randomized, 96 to chemotherapy and 95 to autologous bone marrow transplantation (ABMT). Only 63 (66%) of the patients randomized to the ABMT arm received the intended ABMT, with 19 of the 32 drop-outs resulting from early relapse. The results of this trial were initially reported in 1993 and have since been updated [27–29]. With long-term follow-up, there is no significant difference in overall survival (OS) between the two groups: 34% for ABMT vs. 29% for chemotherapy. When the patients were retrospectively analyzed according to subgroup, there was no difference in OS either among the standard-risk group (49% vs. 40%) or the high-risk group (16% vs. 11%). OS in the allogeneic BMT arm was not different in the standard-risk group (49%) but appeared superior (44%) in the high-risk group. This trial has been very influential because it represents the only randomized trial of use of autologous HCT in adult ALL to date. However, the large withdrawal rate in the group randomized to ABMT confounds the analysis.

A large trial involving collaboration between Eastern Cooperative Oncology Group (ECOG) and the MRC is ongoing and should provide valuable information on the relative merits of chemotherapy vs. autologous and allogeneic HCT [37]. The French LALA 94 trial has also randomized patients with high-risk ALL in first remission, and a preliminary report (excluding Ph+ patients) indicates an advantage to the autologous HCT arm, with EFS of 24% vs. 0% [27].

Several trials have reported comparisons between allogeneic and autologous HCT using availability of matched sibling donor as a "genetic randomization". Attal et al. [31] studied 126 patients in first remission. Forty-three patients with matched sibling donors were identified and 41 of these proceeded to allogeneic HCT. The remaining 77 patients were assigned to autologous HCT, and 64 received the intended treatment. After induction therapy, patients received post-remission chemotherapy with methotrexate and proceeded to transplant using unpurged bone marrow and a standard preparative regimen of TBI plus cyclophosphamide. EFS was 26% in the autologous arm vs. 68% in the allogeneic arm ($p = 0.001$). The Hemato Oncologie voor Volwassenen Nederland (HOVON) 18 ALL trial assigned patients <50 years with matched sibling donors to allogeneic HCT and patients lacking donors plus those aged 50–60 years to autologous HCT following a consolidation course with high-dose cytarbine plus etoposide [38]. Five-year DFS favored the allogeneic arm with DFS of 53% vs. 36% ($p = 0.05$). Of note is that the majority of patients in the autologous HCT arm received peripheral blood grafts rather than bone marrow, and TRM was 3%, lower than that in most trials.

A number of other studies have been reported on the use of autologous HCT for adults with ALL in first remission with EFS of 25–52% [30,32, 40–49]. Powles et al. [37,42] reported relatively favorable overall results in 77 patients with EFS of 52%, but noted that the presence of risk factors adversely affected outcome, and that patients with very high-risk disease fared very poorly. In contrast, the recent Groupe Ouest Est d'etude des Leucenies et Autres Maladies du Song (GOELAMS) 02 trial, which enrolled only high-risk patients, reported encouraging results with overall DFS of 46% [30]. The treatment strategy used in this study was different from many previous trials, in that more intensive post-remission therapy was given prior to autologous HCT, which was performed at a median of 5 months after achieving remission. These favorable results may be because of the contribution of pretransplant chemotherapy or to the lack of inclusion of patients who relapsed prior to transplant.

A pilot study reported from the University of California at San Francisco (UCSF) in collaboration with both Stanford University Medical Center and City of Hope National Medical Center focuses on very high-risk patients in first remission as well as patients in second remission [34]. High-risk first remission status was defined as the presence of adverse cytogenetics (Ph+, 11q23 abnormalities or –7), failure to achieve remission with first induction cycle, or B-lineage disease with WBC ≥100,000/μL. Patients received intensive consolidation therapy with high-dose 2 g/m^2 cytarabine twice a day for 4 days concurrent with 40 mg/kg etoposide. Peripheral blood grafts were collected during hematologic recovery from this consolidation therapy and were purged *in vitro* using a panel of monoclonal antibodies plus complement [50]. The preparative regimen was intensive, including TBI 1320 cGy, 100 mg/kg cyclophosphamide plus 60 mg/kg etoposide. Twenty-four patients have been treated including 18 high-risk CR1 and six patients in second remission (CR2). One patient died during consolidation and four relapsed prior to transplant. Adequate CD34$^+$ cell doses were easily collected, with a CD34$^+$ cell dose of 29×10^6/kg (median) collected in one (median) apheresis. Nineteen patients were treated with autologous HCT; one died in remission and eight relapsed. With median follow-up of 2.8 years (range 1.1–6.1 years), the projected 3-year EFS of all patients is 48 ± 21% with a relapse rate of 47%. The 3-year EFS of transplanted patients is 60% with a relapse rate of 36%. Although the patient numbers are small, the anticipated outcome of these patients with standard treatment was dismal, and the overall treatment program may have been of benefit.

Treatment of adult ALL in relapse

The treatment of adults with relapsed ALL is very problematic. In the current era, most adults with ALL are treated with intensive multiagent chemotherapy and at the time of relapse have high degrees of drug resistance. The rate of achieving CR2 is low, remissions are of short duration and long-term survival in CR2 is very poor with standard chemotherapy treatment [51]. The group from M.D. Anderson reported on a large group of 314 patients treated in first relapse [52]. Overall, 96 patients (26%) entered a second remission, but only 24 (7%) of these proceeded to transplant. The major prognostic factors predicting favorable outcome were age <40 years, CR1 duration >1 year and absence of peripheral blasts. However, even in the most favorable group, characterized by the presence of all of these factors, the CR rate was only 47% and 5-year OS was 5%. Other groups have reported a similar experience in treating adults in first relapse [53–56]. An Italian group (Associazione Italiana di Ematologia ed Oncologia Padiatrica) reported on 61 patients in first relapse [53,54]. Thirty-four patients (56%) achieved remission but only nine patients (15%) proceeded to transplant. One group reported a better experience, with 79 of 96 patients achieving complete remission and 43 (45%) proceeding to transplant [48].

Clinical studies of autologous HCT for adult ALL in second remission

There is a large amount of registry-based information on the use of autologous HCT to treat adults with ALL in CR2 (Table 90.3). The EBMT has reported on 455 adults with LFS of 21% [26]. Similarly, the IBMTR has reported on 241 patients with LFS of 20% [27]. Soiffer *et al.* [57] described 22 adults in second or subsequent remission (11 CR2 and 11 with more advanced disease) treated with autologous HCT. Bone marrow grafts were purged *in vitro* with monoclonal antibodies and an intensive

Table 90.3 Clinical trials of autologous hematopoietic cell transplantation (HCT) for adults with acute lymphoblastic leukemia (ALL) in second remission (CR2).

Group/author [Reference]	n	EFS (%)
EBMT [27]	455	21
IBMTR [27]	241	20
Soiffer *et al.* [57]	22	20
Weisdorf *et al.* [144]	–	0

EBMT, European Group for Bone and Marrow Transplantation; EFS, event-free survival; IBMTR, International Bone Marrow Transplant Registry.

preparative regimen using 1400 cGy TBI was used. The overall EFS was 20%, which was similar to results in that institution using allogeneic HCT for the same patient population. It was noted that all long-term survivors were below the age of 28 years (the median for the entire group), with 45% EFS in younger adults vs. 0% in older patients. A review of autologous HCT performed at the University of Minnesota and the Dana-Farber Cancer Institute reported no long-term survivors over the age of 18 years [50]. Several other studies indicate very poor outcomes in a similar patient group [48–58,143,144]. It is difficult to reconcile the substantial salvage rate of 20% reported in the large registry reports with more recent data that seem much less favorable.

Clinical studies of HCT for adult Ph+ ALL

Adults with Ph+ ALL fare very poorly with conventional chemotherapy, with long-term survival of <10% [11]. Treatment with allogeneic HCT produces the best results and is the treatment of choice for these patients. The IBMTR reported an EFS of 38% for 67 patients with Ph+ ALL in CR1 treated with allogeneic HCT [55]. Patients with more advanced stage disease had an EFS of approximately 30%. The groups at the City of Hope National Medical Center and at Stanford University Medical Center have updated their combined results on 47 patients with Ph+ ALL treated with allogeneic HCT using an intensive preparative regimen including fractionated TBI plus high-dose etoposide [56]. Overall 5-year DFS was 50%, 62% in 23 patients in CR1, which was superior to the 38% DFS in patients with more advanced disease ($p = 0.02$). Other groups have reported EFS in the range of 40–50% for patients in first remission including a small series from Seattle using unrelated donor transplants with LFS of 49% [56–58]. A recent report of the ongoing MRC/ECOG trial reported superior outcome in patients allocated to allogeneic transplant compared to those randomized between chemotherapy and autologous HCT, with EFS of 54% vs. 34% ($p = 0.04$) [40].

Autologous HCT has been used to treat patients with Ph+ ALL lacking allogeneic transplant options. The EBMT has reported on 92 patients in CR1 with 3-year EFS of 18% and on 18 patients in CR2 with a 3-year EFS of 13% [35]. Others have reported on small groups of patients with EFS of approximately 20% [59–61]. The German (GMALL) group have recently updated their important experience on 40 patients with Ph+ ALL (34 CR1, six CR2) treated with a comprehensive and intensive approach including autologous HCT [27,33,62]. Most patients were treated with an intensive consolidation regimen including high-dose cytarabine plus mitoxantrone followed by high-dose methotrexate. Bone marrow or peripheral blood stem cells were purged *in vitro* using a combination of monoclonal antibodies (against CD10 and CD19) and immunomagnetic beads. They used an intensive preparative regimen including 1440 cGy plus cyclophosphamide and etoposide, preceded in some cases by autologous HCT with melphalan and thiotepa. Finally, some patients received post-transplant therapy with either maintenance chemotherapy or interferon alpha and interleukin 2 (IL-2). With median follow-up of 7.3 years (range 2.4–9.5 years), long-term EFS was 20% for patients in CR1 and 0% for CR2 ($p = 0.014$). Patients in CR1 who received intensive chemotherapy prior to transplant and/or maintenance chemotherapy had a superior outcome, with EFS of 38% vs. 0% ($p = 0.02$). This report confirms the substantial salvage rate of Ph+ ALL patients with an autologous HCT approach, and suggests that pretransplant cytoreduction therapy may contribute to a successful outcome. Although the results are inferior to those achieved with allogeneic HCT, they indicate an opportunity for long-term survival for patients who are not candidates for allogeneic HCT.

Evaluation of MRD status using polymerase chain reaction (PCR) probes for BCR-ABL may be useful in identifying patients who may benefit from autologous HCT for Ph+ ALL. Recent data from the ongoing LALA 94 trial also demonstrate the predictive value of MRD prior to transplant. Patients without allogeneic donors (who were scheduled to receive autologous HCT) who were MRD-negative after consolidation therapy had 2-year OS of 56%, as opposed to 12% for those who were PCR-positive ($p = 0.01$) [27].

Imatinib mesylate is a new agent that has shown a remarkable efficacy in the treatment of Ph+ ALL as well as CML [63]. It is hoped that the combination of intensive chemotherapy plus imatinib mesylate may be able to increase the proportion of patients who are PCR-negative prior to transplant, and that this response may translate to improved outcomes of both autologous and allogeneic HCT for this disease. The Cancer and Leukaemia Group B (CALGB) and South-West Oncology Group (SWOG) have recently activated a trial to test a treatment strategy using imatinib mesylate both before and after autologous and allogeneic HCT for Ph+ ALL.

Comparison of allogeneic to autologous HCT for adult ALL

The role of allogeneic HCT as treatment for ALL is reviewed in detail in Chapters 77 and 78. The role of allogeneic HCT as initial therapy for adult ALL remains controversial. An early report in which data from the IBMTR were compared to results of chemotherapy appeared to show no difference in outcome [64,65]. An analysis of the LALA 87 trial showed no advantage for allogeneic HCT [65,66]. The IBMTR has reported on 1005 patients with ALL in first remission treated with allogeneic HCT with an overall LFS of 54% [27]. However, without knowing the risk stratification of the patients involved, it is difficult to make conclusions from this data. An updated report from the IBMTR shows a favorable effect in LFS in patients aged <30 years (53% vs. 30%; $p = 0.02$), whereas there was no difference in patients aged >30 years (30% vs. 26%) [67]. For patients with high-risk ALL who are destined to do poorly with conventional chemotherapy, allogeneic HCT clearly has a role and is the treatment of choice. Treatment with allogeneic HCT can salvage approximately 20% of patients with ALL who fail to enter remission with initial therapy [68,69] as well as 35–40% of patients with Ph+ ALL in first remission [70–74].

When matched sibling donors are available, allogeneic HCT is preferable over autologous HCT as treatment for high-risk ALL. For patients lacking suitable allogeneic donors and facing unacceptably poor outcomes with standard chemotherapy, a choice must be made between autologous HCT and allogeneic HCT using alternative donors, most commonly a matched unrelated donor. This choice remains a difficult one and no clear answer is provided by the literature. Patients with high-risk ALL, especially those in second remission, have a very short anticipated duration of remission and there may not be sufficient time to locate a matched unrelated donor. Many patients will not find such a donor or will relapse prior to transplant. In addition, the high TRM (40–60%) for adults with advanced ALL undergoing this procedure remains problematic. Weisdorf et al. [58] analyzed data on 712 patients aged <50 years who received HCT during the years 1989–98, comparing 517 patients who underwent unrelated donor (URD) allogeneic HCT facilitated by the National Marrow Donor Program (NMDP) to 195 patients who received autologous HCT and were reported to the Autologous Blood and Marrow Transplant Registry (ABMTR). There was no advantage to one form of HCT over the other for either CR1 or CR2 patients. For patients in CR1, TRM was higher for URD transplantation, 42% vs. 20% ($p = 0.004$); the relapse rate was lower, 14% vs. 49% ($p < 0.001$); and 5-year DFS was equivalent, 44% vs. 31% ($p = 0.46$). For patients in CR2, similar results were found, with URD patients having higher TRM, 40% vs. 9% ($p < 0.001$); lower relapse rate of 25% vs. 64% ($p = 0.001$); and similar 5-year DFS, 36% vs. 27% ($p = 0.11$). Similar results were seen in an analysis comparing EBMT vs. International Marrow Unrelated Search and Transplant (IMUST) data [76]. For a mixed group of adults and pediatric patients, no difference in outcome was seen comparing autologous and unrelated donor transplant with LFS of 53% at 2 years in both groups. The TRM was much higher in the unrelated transplant group at 44% vs. 15%. However, no separate analysis was provided for adult patients. The Seattle group similarly reported no significant difference in outcome of a mixed group of adult and pediatric patients with ALL treated with autologous vs. unrelated donor allogeneic HCT [77]. Although these data can serve as guidelines for decision-making, in the absence of more detailed information on the patient characteristics and the indication for transplant it is hard to make firm recommendations from these comparative data. In general, URD transplant is a more attractive option for younger patients with the highest risk disease.

Pediatric ALL

Standard therapy and prognostic factors in pediatric ALL

The treatment of childhood ALL is one of the major success stories in oncology. Complete remissions are achieved in 95–97% of patients, and approximately 75% of all patients are now cured with standard chemotherapy [22,78–82]. The major risk factors have traditionally been age, WBC, phenotype and cytogenetics [22,83]. Patients aged <1 year are usually considered in the category of infant ALL and treated as a separate group. A high proportion of these infants have the cytogenetic abnormality t(4;11) or other abnormalities involving 11q23. For infants with ALL, long-term EFS of 25% is expected, although the intensification of treatment may improve this outcome to nearly 40% [84]. Children with WBC <10,000/μL have the most favorable prognosis with EFS >80% in children aged 1–9 years and 70% in those >10 years [85]. Children with WBC between 10,000 and 50,000/μL have an intermediate prognosis with EFS of 75% if aged 1–9 years and 60% if >10 years. WBC >50,000 is associated with an inferior prognosis with EFS of 65% for those aged 1–9 years and 40% for those >10 years. Many investigators consider WBC ≥100,000/μL to constitute a separate risk group with a very poor prognosis warranting HCT in first remission. Patients with T-cell disease represent 15% of children with ALL. Most fall into a high-risk category on the basis of age and WBC, but the T-cell phenotype confers a somewhat adverse prognosis even for patients with standard risk.

Children with hyperdiploidy (chromosome number >50, often measured as a DNA index >1.16) have a very favorable prognosis [22,77]. The subgroup of patients with hyperdiploidy combined with trisomy for chromosomes 10 and 17 has a particularly favorable outcome with long-term EFS of >95% [84]. The Philadelphia chromosome, which is seen in more than 20% of adults with ALL is seen in approximately 3% of children with ALL and confers a very poor prognosis [86–88]. Within the

Ph+ group there appear to be favorable prognostic features including age <10 years, WBC <50,000/μL and rapid response to prednisone [66]. Compared to patients with Ph– ALL, the complete remission rate is much lower (82% vs. 97%) and overall EFS is inferior with 5-year EFS of 28%. Even the most favorable group of Ph+ patients has 3-year EFS of <50%. Approximately 1% of noninfant children with ALL have the t(4;11) translocation, which is a poor prognostic factor [89], as is near-haploid cytogenetics [90]. In the past, the t(1;19) translocation had been an independent risk factor but this effect has been reduced with intensification of therapy [22].

Rapid responsiveness to prednisone has emerged as a very important new prognostic factor in pediatric ALL [22,78]. Patients are initially treated for 7 days with prednisone, with prednisone response documented by a peripheral blast count <1000/μL by day 7. Approximately 10% of patients have poor prednisone response, and this is an independent risk factor predicting EFS of <50%. Similarly, response in the bone marrow at both day 7 and day 14 of induction is highly predictive of outcome [91].

Measurement of MRD has also emerged as a powerful prognostic factor in childhood ALL. Cave et al. [92] studied 226 patients for whom they constructed probes for rearrangements of the immunoglobulin or T-antigen-receptor genes, and 79% of patients were evaluable. The presence of MRD at the end of induction therapy predicted an EFS of 20% vs. 80% in those without residual disease ($p = 0.004$). The group at St. Jude's Hospital used flow cytometry to assess MRD, and this technique was applicable to 58% of the population [93]. The presence of MRD at the end of induction predicted a relapse rate of 43% vs. 10% in those who were MRD-negative ($p = 0.001$). Most recently, the Berlin–Frankfurt–Munich (BFM) group has applied flow cytometry in its MRD assessment and has developed a technique applicable to 97% of patients (105 of 108) [94]. After 12 weeks of therapy, the persistence of MRD $>10^{-4}$ was associated with 3-year EFS of 0% as opposed to 90% of patients who were MRD-negative ($p = 0.04$). For patients with a specific molecular abnormality, such as the *ALL1/AF4* fusion gene in patients with the t(4;11) translocation, detection of MRD using specific probes has been shown to strongly correlate with outcome [95].

Current practice is that treatment of pediatric ALL is based on a risk-adapted strategy [22]. Patients with favorable-risk ALL are treated with a nonintensive regimen, omitting anthracyclines from induction and omitting cranial irradiation from central nervous system (CNS) prophylaxis. Maintenance therapy includes antimetabolites alone. This favorable group has an anticipated EFS of >80%. Recently, patients with intermediate-risk disease are treated with intensified chemotherapy, which appears to have resulted in improved outcome to an EFS of 70–80%. Management of high-risk ALL remains controversial. Approximately 10% of children with noninfant ALL are identified as being very high-risk and are suitable candidates for intensive interventions with HCT during first remission [96,97]. Such patients include those with t(9;22) and t(4;11), those failing to go into remission with initial therapy and those with WBC ≥100,000/μL.

Clinical studies of autologous HCT for pediatric ALL in first remission

Few children with ALL are candidates for HCT in first remission, and allogeneic HCT would be the treatment of choice if a suitable donor were available. The role of autologous transplant for children in first remission is therefore limited. None the less, the EBMT has reported EFS of 50% in 219 children treated with autologous HCT in first remission [26]. Lacking the information on the indication for transplant in these children, it is difficult to make recommendations based on these data. Other groups of investigators have treated small numbers of high-risk children with ALL with autologous HCT in CR1 [98–100].

Treatment of relapsed pediatric ALL

Relapse is not as dire an event for children with ALL as it is for adults. Compared to adults, the chance of achieving second remission is far greater and long-term outcome is better. The recent MRC UK ALL R1 study demonstrated a remission rate of 95% in 189 children with relapsed ALL [101,102]. Long-term EFS is seen in 28–46% of patients [101–103]. There are striking differences in the outcome of children in first relapse, depending on duration of their first remission and on whether the relapse involves the bone marrow (with or without other sites) or occurs in an isolated extramedullary site such as the CNS or testes [101–103]. For patients with bone marrow relapse, the peripheral blood blast count has also been reported to be of prognostic significance [104]. Patient groups divided into absolute peripheral blasts counts of <1000/μL, 1–10,000/μL and >10,000/μL had EFS of 64%, 32% and 10%, respectively ($p = 0.001$). Relapse with T-cell phenotype also appears to have a much worse prognosis, regardless of the site of relapse [103,105].

The two major prognostic features, time to and site of relapse, can be used to construct groups with strikingly different prognosis when treated with chemotherapy [100–102]. Patients with early (defined as <2 years) relapse in the bone marrow have a very poor prognosis with most data showing <10% long-term survival (range 2–12%). Late bone marrow relapses are associated with long-term EFS of 40–50%, and patients with early isolated extramedullary relapses have EFS of approximately 35% (range 28–38%) [106]. The small number of patients who suffer a late isolated extramedullary relapse do particularly well with long-term EFS of approximately 70% (range 56–83%) [107–109]. Taken together, it has been proposed that children with ALL in the first relapse are deemed high-risk if they have either early bone marrow relapse or T-cell disease; intermediate-risk if they have either early extramedullary or late bone marrow relapses; or low-risk if found to have an isolated and late extramedullary relapse.

Clinical studies of autologous HCT for pediatric ALL in second remission

The abovementioned risk groups of relapsed childhood ALL must be considered in evaluating the results of autologous HCT in second remission (Table 90.4) [103,110–121]. The EBMT has reported an EFS of 37% in

Table 90.4 Clinical trials of autologous hematopoietic cell transplantation (HCT) for pediatric acute lymphoblastic leukemia (ALL).

Group/author [Reference]	n	EFS (%)
Early bone marrow relapse		
Messina et al. [110]	65	18
Billet et al. [111]	36	20
Borgmann et al. [103]	33	19
Maldonado et al. [112]	18	33
Late bone marrow relapse		
Billet et al. [111]	95	50
Maldonado et al. [112]	23	56
Borgmann et al. [103]	19	41
Early extramedullary relapse		
Borgmann et al. [103]	22	25
Messina et al. [113]	19	56
Maldonado et al. [112]	14	42

EFS, event-free survival.

628 children transplanted in CR2 [26]. However, lacking details of patient characteristics, it is difficult to form recommendations from this information.

A small number of studies have reported outcomes using autologous HCT to treat early bone marrow relapse in childhood ALL (Table 90.4). Billet et al. [112,118] reported on 36 such patients with long-term EFS of 20%, and others have described EFS of 18–33% [110,112]. In a matched-pair analysis, Borgmann et al. [103] reported EFS of 17% in 33 such patients, which was identical to the outcome for 33 matched historical chemotherapy-treated patients. One group of patients who fare particularly poorly with chemotherapy and who appear to benefit from autologous HCT are children with relapsed T-cell ALL. Even with small numbers of patients, Borgmann et al. [103] reported improved outcome with autologous HCT compared to chemotherapy with EFS of 45% vs. 14% ($p = 0.02$). Overall, is not clear that treatment with autologous transplant is superior to chemotherapy, although the EFS in most of these studies exceeds the <10% EFS seen with chemotherapy alone.

Results using autologous HCT for treatment of late bone marrow relapse are better than for early relapse. Billet and Ritz [111] reported EFS of 50% in 95 patients and Maldonado et al. [112] an EFS of 56% in 23 patients. These results appear somewhat better than usual results with chemotherapy treatment. However, Borgmann et al. [95] reported an EFS of 41% in 19 such patients, which was not superior to outcome with 19 matched chemotherapy control patients. The optimal treatment for this group of patients remains unclear.

For patients with early isolated extramedullary relapse, Messina et al. [113] reported on 19 patients with EFS of 56%. These results were superior in multivariable analysis to historical control patients treated with chemotherapy alone ($p = 0.01$). Maldonado et al. [112] reported EFS of 42% in 14 such patients. However, Borgmann et al. [114] reported EFS of only 25% in 22 such patients, a result which was not different from matched chemotherapy patients. Overall results in this patient subgroup are conflicting, and there is no clear treatment of choice. Patients with late isolated extramedullary relapse treated with autologous HCT do well, but given the favorable results with chemotherapy alone, it is hard to show superiority for transplant [114].

In summary, at this time there is no subgroup of relapsed childhood ALL patients (other than perhaps T-cell ALL) in which autologous HCT is clearly the treatment of choice. The question can only be answered by prospective randomized trials. Unfortunately, in the recent UK ALL-R1 trial, only 15 of 164 eligible patients (9%) accepted randomization between autologous HCT and chemotherapy [101]. It appears unlikely that future trials will have a much greater success rate in randomization, and the question of the role of autologous HCT in this setting may remain unanswered.

Improving the autologous HCT procedure

Autologous HCT is not a uniform procedure, and it is likely that many of the decisions regarding both patient selection and treatment components of the procedure have an important effect on outcome. There is a great need for improvement in the results of autologous HCT for ALL, and these improvements may come from some of the areas considered below.

Patient selection

Patient selection is a critical factor in determining the success of autologous HCT for ALL. One should probably not use this treatment for favorable-risk patients, as it would be extremely difficult to demonstrate further improvement in outcome. Application of autologous HCT should first focus on high-risk patients who are destined to fare poorly with chemotherapy and who do not have a suitably matched donor for allogeneic HCT. Once autologous HCT is more solidly validated as an effective treatment for this patient group, it would be appropriate to consider its use for intermediate-risk patients. For patients identified as being at high-risk for relapse, it is desirable to treat them as early in their course as possible, before increasing drug and radiation resistance make any form of treatment futile.

In the future, results of MRD analysis may be useful in selecting appropriate patients for autologous HCT. Data from the ongoing MRC UK ALL XII trial showed that eight of nine patients who were MRD-negative prior to transplant remained in remission as opposed to one of seven who were MRD-positive [24]. When the stem cell product was analyzed, all six patients with MRD-negative stem cell products remained in remission vs. only one of seven patients whose stem cell products contained abnormal cells. An analysis of adult patients with Ph+ ALL showed similar findings with MRD-negative status highly predictive of successful outcome [35]. In the future, results of MRD analysis may be used to help choose between autologous and unrelated donor transplant for patients lacking matched sibling donors.

Chemotherapy prior to HCT

It is well-established that many patients with ALL have measurable levels of disease prior to transplantation, and that this level correlates with outcome after autologous [123] as well as allogeneic HCT [124,125]. Data showing the striking prognostic significance of the interval from remission to transplant may also be interpreted as showing an effect of consolidation therapy in reducing tumor burden prior to transplant [35,36], although the withdrawal of high-risk patients because of early relapse almost certainly contributes to this effect. The encouraging data of one group [28] using autologous HCT as a late intensification after prior intensive consolidation may also represent the favorable impact of pretransplant chemotherapy, as can the German data on autologous HCT for Ph+ ALL [33,62] and the favorable results of autologous HCT in children at the Dana-Farber Cancer Center [103,106].

Prior consolidation therapy has been demonstrated to be an important prognostic factor for outcome after autologous HCT for AML. One group has shown that patients receiving two or more consolidation treatments prior to HCT had a much more favorable outcome than those receiving less pretransplant therapy [126]. An analysis from the ABMTR also shows a strong positive effect of prior consolidation therapy with cytarabine on outcome after autologous transplant for AML [127]. Similarly, the positive effect of ABMT as late consolidation in the MRC trial of AML in CR1 may be related to the use of prior multiagent chemotherapy [128]. Several pilot studies are in progress using intensive chemotherapy prior to autologous HCT for ALL, and more data on this point will be forthcoming.

Preparative regimens

In the absence of the GVL effect, the efficacy of autologous HCT for ALL (and other diseases) depends entirely on the high-dose therapy given as the preparative regimen. While it is possible that intensification of the preparative regimen will lead to improved disease control, there are very limited data on this point. In the setting of allogeneic transplant, it has been demonstrated for both AML and CML in randomized trials that increased doses of TBI result in decreased relapse rates [129,130]. However, in the allogeneic transplant setting, this positive effect was counterbalanced by an increase in TRM related to graft-vs.-host disease, likely related to the increased tissue damage caused by the more intensive regimens. In the autologous HCT setting, and particularly with the rapid engraftment now available with the use of peripheral blood grafts, it is possible that preparative regimens can be intensified without an increase in mortality rate.

The use of TBI-based as opposed to chemotherapy-based regimens has been reported to be superior in some settings in ALL. The EBMT reported improved LFS for patients receiving a TBI-based regimen for autologous HCT for ALL with LFS of 39% vs. 23% ($p = 0.007$) [27]. An Italian group also reported superior outcomes for children with ALL undergoing autologous HCT who received TBI compared to chemotherapy regimens, with EFS of 48% vs. 15% [110]. In allogeneic HCT for children with ALL, the IBMTR has reported better outcomes with TBI-based compared to busulfan-based regimens with a trend to decrease in relapse (35% vs. 41%; $p = 0.07$) and significant decreases in TRM (15% vs. 23%; $p = 0.02$) and improvements in LFS (50% vs. 35%; $p = 0.005$) [131].

Even among patients receiving TBI-based regimens, there is a great deal of variation in both the TBI dose as well as in the chemotherapy drugs and regimens. The pediatric group at the Memorial Sloan-Kettering Cancer Research Center used high doses of TBI of 1375–1500 cGy for allogeneic transplant for pediatric ALL [132]. It is possible that the intensity of the regimen was responsible for the unusually good outcome they reported. In the adult autologous HCT setting, the German group used a TBI dose of 1440 cGy in combination with both etoposide and cyclophosphamide, and has reported the most convincing data on the usefulness of autologous HCT in the treatment of Ph+ ALL [33,62]. It has been suggested that the addition of etoposide is particularly useful in the treatment of ALL, and several groups have combined TBI with etoposide, sometimes with cyclophosphamide in addition [71,133]. Our pilot study at UCSF used an intensive preparative regimen combing 1320 cGy TBI with 60 mg/kg etoposide plus 100 mg/kg cyclophosphamide [34]. In the setting of peripheral blood progenitor cell transplantation and rapid engraftment, this regimen is quite tolerable in patients up to the age of 60 years.

It is to be hoped that more attention will be paid to this important area and that we will learn whether increasing the intensity of the preparative regimen improves outcomes. At the present time, the use of radioimmunoconjugates to deliver ablative doses of radiation is limited to selected centres, but the concept of targeting increased doses of radiation while limiting nonhematologic toxicities is attractive [134].

In vitro purging

The role of bone marrow purging in autologous HCT for ALL remains undefined, as it is in almost all diseases. While there is clear evidence from gene marking studies that a graft containing tumor cells can contribute to relapse following autologous transplant [135], most investigators feel that the primary reason for treatment failure is the failure to eradicate systemic disease. Retrospective data have suggested a positive role for purging. Granena et al. [43], in a mixed population of children and adults, reported improved outcome from purged as opposed to unpurged bone marrow. The effect was particularly notable for patients in CR1 where relapses were reduced from 86% to 35% ($p = 0.005$) and LFS improved from 12% to 52% ($p = 0.016$). In vitro data examining the persistence of leukemia colony-forming units (CFU-L) after purging with 4-hydroperoxycyclophosphamide (4-HC) showed a correlation between persistent disease and the risk of relapse [136]. An analysis of patients with T-cell ALL whose graft was purged with either 4-HC or mafosfamide showed a trend to improved 5-year LFS of 40% vs. 26% ($p = 0.09$) [137]. However, the use of such chemotherapy-based purging has clear risks including delayed engraftment, and chemical marrow purging in the setting of ALL has been shown by the EBMT to result in an increase in TRM in adults from 7% to 16% in CR1 and from 12% to 26% in CR2 [27]. With a demonstration of an adverse affect and with controversy regarding the positive effect of 4-HC or mafosphamide purging, the enthusiasm for this procedure has waned.

In the past, the vast majority of ABMT procedures for ALL have been performed using monoclonal antibodies, usually combined with complement but sometimes based on immunomagnetic beads or other techniques [138]. More recently, one group of investigators has used the anti-CD52 antibody, Campath, for in vitro purging of bone marrow and seen no significant compromise of engraftment [139]. Campath 1-H has been commercially approved by the Federal Drug Administration (FDA), based on its effectiveness in the treatment of refractory chronic lymphocytic leukemia [140]. Future clinical trials in the USA using antibody-based purging will be hampered by the lack of FDA approval and commercial availability of other possibly effective antibodies. The anti-CD20 monoclonal antibody rituximab is of limited value in ALL because of the low expression of the target antigen CD20 in ALL. The contribution of purging to the successful outcome of autologous HCT for ALL remains uncertain.

Peripheral blood grafts

The use of hematopoietic peripheral blood cells has largely replaced the use of bone marrow as a source of hematopoietic cells in most areas of autologous HCT. The primary advantages are rapidity of engraftment, reduced transfusion requirements, reduced length of hospitalization and reduction in overall morbidity and mortality. It is possible that this more rapid engraftment may allow the intensification of preparative regiments without undue morbidity, but this remains to be tested.

The German (GMALL) group has reported that reduced tumor contamination may be another advantage of peripheral blood stem cell over bone marrow [27,62]. In the setting of Ph+ ALL, there was a 3-log reduction in the disease burden in blood as opposed to bone marrow. Although purging efficiency with monoclonal antibodies was reduced in peripheral blood compared to bone marrow, the final cell product still had 1 log less tumor cells in blood as opposed to bone marrow.

The reduction in tumor burden seen in peripheral blood cell grafts may partially reflect the in vivo purging effect of the chemotherapy used in order to mobilize such stem cells. The German ALL group used an intensive consolidation and mobilization regimen including high-dose cytarabine plus mitoxantrone [33,62]. Several other groups have also used aggressive regimens including high-dose cytarabine immediately prior to blood cell collection. One group reported that collection of $CD34^+$ cells was much more efficient in patients with ALL compared to those with AML, with median $CD34^+$ cell doses of 17×10^6/kg in ALL patients, compared to 1.4×10^6/kg in patients with AML [45]. This improved $CD34^+$ cell collection efficiency with 98% of patients ($n = 64$) meeting collection goals, allowed 75% of patients to receive the intended transplant. Our pilot study similarly demonstrated high $CD34^+$ cell yields after consolidation with high-dose cytarabine plus etoposide [34]. Other groups of investigators have reported faster engraftment with the use of peripheral blood grafts compared to marrow for autologous HCT for ALL, with reduced TRM, 0 of 42 with blood cells vs. 6 of 35 with bone marrow cells ($p = 0.005$) [32]. One pediatric transplant group mobilized blood cells during recovery from chemotherapy and performed in vitro purging using both positive and negative selection, with encouraging preliminary results [117]. The strategy of using peripheral blood cells, particularly if collected immediately following intensive consolidation therapy, seems an attractive option that may improve outcomes of autologous HCT for ALL by reducing tumor burden both in the patient and in the blood cell graft.

Post-transplant therapies

ALL is notable among malignancies for the importance of prolonged maintenance therapy in producing long-term outcomes. Even in the era of intensive post-remission therapy, attempts by the BFM group to shorten the duration of maintenance chemotherapy led to increases in relapse rate [22]. It has been suggested that maintenance chemotherapy might add to the effectiveness of autologous HCT for ALL. Some investigators have added low-dose maintenance chemotherapy with methotrexate and 6-mercaptopurine to autologous HCT programs and have shown that this concept is feasible [32]. Other groups have added post-transplant asparaginase or other forms of post-transplant chemotherapy [141]. For patients with Ph+ ALL, it is hoped that imatinib mesylate may contribute to disease control after autologous HCT. This strategy is currently being tested by CALGB and SWOG.

Post-transplant immunotherapy has been attempted using nonspecific immunostimulation with IL-2. Two studies failed to show a positive effect of IL-2 but do not provide a definitive answer to this question. One study [142] compared 28 patients treated to historical control and a second study [31] randomized a total of 60 patients of whom only 22 of 30 patients scheduled to receive IL-2 actually received the drug. Other groups have considered using tumor vaccine strategies after autologous HCT.

Conclusions

At the present time, the role of autologous HCT in the treatment of ALL remains undefined. In adult ALL, there is no patient group in whom autologous HCT has been identified as the treatment of choice. However, for patients who are destined to fare poorly with chemotherapy, such as patients with high-risk first remission disease and all patients in second remission, autologous transplant seems an appropriate strategy when patients lack suitable allogeneic donors. For children with ALL, there is no patient group in which autologous HCT has been demonstrated as the treatment of choice. Future studies should be directed towards applying autologous HCT in a risk-adapted fashion to appropriate patients with high-risk ALL. Improvements are needed in the way autologous HCT is conducted. Strategies that may be helpful include intensification of pre-transplant chemotherapy (or the use of imatinib mesylate for Ph+ ALL) to reduce minimal residual disease prior to HCT and help generate MRD-negative grafts. The use of peripheral blood grafts may also reduce the infused tumor burden and may facilitate engraftment, thereby allowing intensification of the preparative regimen.

References

1 Linker CA, Leavitt LJ, O'Donnell M et al. Treatment of adult acute lymphoblastic leukemia with intensive cyclical chemotherapy: a follow-up report. Blood 1991; 78: 2814–22.

2 Linker CA, Damon L, Ries C et al. Intensified and shortened cyclical chemotherapy for adult acute lymphoblastic leukemia. J Clin Oncol 2002; 20: 2264–71.

3 Larson RA, Dodge RK, Burns PC et al. A five-drug remission induction regimen with intensive consolidation for adults with acute lymphoblastic leukemia: Cancer Leukemia Group B Study 8811. Blood 1995; 85: 2025–37.

4 Larson RA, Dodge RK, Linker CA et al. A randomized controlled trial of filgrastim during remission induction and consolidation chemotherapy for adults with acute lymphoblastic leukemia: CALG Study 9111. Blood 1998; 92: 1556–64.

5 Larson RA, Dodge RK, Bloomfield CD et al. Treatment of biologically determined subsets of acute lymphoblastic leukemia in adults: Cancer and Leukemia Group B studies. In: Buchner Thiddemann W, Wormann B et al. eds. Acute Leukemia VI Prognostic Factors and Treatment Strategies. Berlin: Springer-Verlag, 1997: 677–86.

6 Finiewicz KJ, Larson RA. Dose-intensive therapy for adult acute lymphoblastic leukemia. Semin Oncol 1999; 26: 6–20.

7 Hoelzer D, Thiel H, Loffler H et al. Prognostic factors in a multicenter study for treatment of acute lymphoblastic leukemia in adults. Blood 1988; 71: 123–31.

8 Gokbuget N, Hoelzer D, Arnold R et al. Treatment of adult ALL according to protocols of the German multicenter study group for adult ALL (GMALL). Hematol Oncol Clin North Am 2000; 14: 1307–25.

9 Annino L, Vegna ML, Camera A et al. Treatment of adult acute lymphoblastic leukemia (ALL): long-term follow-up of the GIMEMA ALL 0288 randomized study. Blood 2002; 99: 863–71.

10 Kantarjian HM, O'Brien S, Smith TL et al. Results of treatment with hyper-CVAD, a dose-intensive regimen, in adult acute lymphoblastic leukemia. J Clin Oncol 2000; 18: 547–61.

11 Gleibner B, Gokbuget N, Bartram CR et al. Leading prognostic relevance of the BCR-ABL translocation in adult acute B-lineage lymphoblastic leukemia: a prospective study of the German Multicenter Trial Group and confirmed polymerase chain reaction analysis. Blood 2002; 99: 1536–43.

12 Boucheix C, David B, Sebban C et al. Immunophenotype of adult acute lymphoblastic leukemia, clinical parameters, and outcome: an analysis of a prospective trial including 562 tested patients (LALA 87). Blood 1994; 84: 1603–12.

13 Hoelzer D, Arnold R, Buechner T et al. Characteristics, outcome and risk factors in adult T-lineage acute lymphoblastic leukemia (ALL). Blood 1999; 94 (Suppl. 1): 659a [Abstract].

14 Bloomfield CD, Goldman AI, Alimena G et al. Chromosomal abnormalities identify high-risk and low-risk patients with acute lymphoblastic leukemia. Blood 1986; 67: 415–20.

15 Groupe Francais de Cytogenetique Hematologique. Cytogenetic abnormalities in adult acute lymphoblastic leukemia: correlations with hematologic findings and outcome. A collaborative study of the Group Francais de Cytogenetique Hematologique. Blood 1996; 87: 3135–42.

16 Secker-Walker LM, Prentice HG, Durrant J et al. Cytogenetics adds independent prognostic information in adults with acute lymphoblastic leukaemia on MRC trial UK ALL XA. Br J Haematol 1997; 96: 301–10.

17 Wetzler M, Dodge RK, Mrozek K et al. Prospective karyotype analysis in adult acute lymphoblastic leukemia: the Cancer Leukemia Group B Experience. Blood 1999; 93: 3983–93.

18 Ludwig WD, Rieder H, Bartram CR et al. Immunophenotypic and genotypic features, clinical characteristics, and treatment outcome of adult pro-B acute lymphoblastic leukemia: results of the German multicenter trials GMALL 3/87 and 4/89. Blood 1998; 92: 1898–909.

19 Soussain C, Patte C, Ostronoff M et al. Small noncleaved cell lymphoma and leukemia in adults: a retrospective study of 65 adults treated with the LMB pediatric protocols. Blood 1995; 85: 664–74.

20 Hoelzer D, Wolf-Dieter L, Thiel E et al. Improved outcome in adult B-cell acute lymphoblastic leukemia. Blood 1996; 87: 495–508.

21 Lee EJ, Petroni GR, Schiffer CA et al. Brief-duration high-intensity chemotherapy for patients with small noncleaved cell lymphoma or FAB L3 acute lymphocytic leukemia: results of the Cancer and Leukemia Group B study 9251. J Clin Oncol 2001; 19: 4014–22.

22 Pui CH. Childhood leukemias. N Engl J Med 1995; 332: 1618–29.

23 Dordelmann M, Reiter A, Borkhardt A et al. Prednisone response is the strongest predictor of treatment outcome in infant acute lymphoblastic leukemia. Blood 1999; 94: 1209–17.

24 Mortuza FY, Papaioannou M, Moreira IM et al. Minimal residual disease tests provide an independent predictor of clinical outcome in adult acute lymphoblastic leukemia. J Clin Oncol 2002; 20: 1094–104.

25 Bruggemann M, Droese J, Raff T et al. Prognostic significance of minimal residual disease in adult standard risk patients with acute lymphoblastic leukemia. Blood 1998; 92 (Suppl. 1): 314a [Abstract].

26 Ciudad J, San Miguel JF, Lopez-Berges MC et al. Prognostic value of immunophenotypic detection of minimal residual disease in acute lymphoblastic leukemia. J Clin Oncol 1998; 16: 3774–81.

27 Gorin NC. Autologous stem cell transplantation in acute lymphocytic leukemia. Stem Cells 2002; 20: 3–10.

28 Fiere D, Lepage E, Sebban C et al. Adult lymphoblastic leukemia: a multicentric randomized trial testing bone marrow transplantation as post-remission therapy. J Clin Oncol 1993; 11: 1990–2001.

29 Dhedin N, Thomas X, Huguet F et al. No superiority of autologous stem cell transplantation over chemotherapy alone in adult Ph-negtive ALL in first complete remission: a long-term follow-up report combining results of LALA 85, 87 and 94 trials. Blood 2002; 100 (Suppl. 1): 217a [Abstract].

30 Hunault M, Harousseau JL, Delain M et al. Improved outcome of high risk acute lymphoblastic leukemia (ALL) with late high dose therapy: a GOELAMS's trial. Blood 1998; 92 (Suppl. 1): 803a [Abstract].

31 Attal M, Blaise D, Marit G et al. Consolidation treatment of adult acute lymphoblastic leukemia: a

prospective, randomized trial comparing allogeneic vs. autologous bone marrow transplantation and testing the impact of recombinant interleukin-2 after autologous bone marrow transplantation. *Blood* 1995; **86**: 1619–28.

32. Powles R, Sirohi B, Trealeaven J *et al*. The role of post-transplantation maintenance chemotherapy in improving the outcome of autotransplantation in adult acute lymphoblastic leukemia. *Blood* 2002; **100**: 1641–7.

33. Martin H, Fauth F, Atta J *et al*. Singe versus double autologous BMT/PBSCT in patients with BCR-ABL-positive acute lymphoblastic leukemia. *Blood* 1994; **84** (Suppl. 1): 580a [Abstract].

34. Linker C, Damon L, Navarro W *et al*. Autologous stem cell transplantation for high-risk adult acute lymphoblastic leukemia (ALL). *Blood* 1998; (Suppl. 1): 689a [Abstract].

35. Gorin N, Aegerter P, Auvert B. Autologous bone marrow transplantation (ABMT) for acute leukemia in remission. an analysis on 1322 cases. *Bone Marrow Transplant* 1990; **4**: 3–5.

36. Sierra J, Granena A, Garcia J *et al*. Autologous bone marrow transplantation for acute leukemia: results and prognostic factors in 90 consecutive patients. *Bone Marrow Transplant* 1993; **12**: 517–23.

37. Rowe JM, Richards SM, Burnett AK *et al*. Favorable results of allogeneic bone marrow transplantation (BMT) for adults with Philadelphia chromosome-negative (Ph–) acute lymphoblastic leukemia (ALL) in first complete remission (CR): results from the international ALL trial (MRC UKALL XII/ECOG E2993). *Blood* 1998; **92** (Suppl. 1): 481a [Abstract].

38. Dekker AW, van der Veer MB, van der Holt B *et al*. Post-remission treatment with autologous stem cell transplantation (Auto-SCT) or allogeneic stem cell transplantation (Allo-SCT) in adults with acute lymphoblastic leukemia (ALL): a phase II clinical trial (HOVON 18 ALL). *Blood* 1998; **92** (Suppl. 1): 859a [Abstract].

39. Martin TG, Linker CA. Autologous stem cell transplantation for acute lymphocytic leukemia in adults. *Hematol Oncol Clin North Am* 2001; **15**: 121–43.

40. Powles R, Mehta J, Singhal S *et al*. Autologous bone marrow or peripheral blood stem cell transplantation followed by maintenance chemotherapy for adult acute lymphoblastic leukemia in first remission: 50 cases from a single center. *Bone Marrow Transplant* 1995; **16**: 241–7.

41. Muroi K, Suzuki T, Amemiya Y *et al*. Autologous peripheral blood stem cell transplantation for adults with B-lineage acute lymphoblastic leukemia: a pilot study. *Leuk Lymphoma* 2000; **38**: 103–11.

42. Buccisano F, Del Poeta G, Venditi A *et al*. Dose-intensive, ARA-C/mitoxantrone-based chemotherapy followed by hematopoietic stem cell transplantation for adult acute lymphoblastic leukemia. *Blood* 1992; **80** (Suppl. 1): 84a [Abstract].

43. Granena A, Castellsague X, Badell I *et al*. Autologous bone marrow transplantation for high risk acute lymphoblastic leukemia: clinical relevance of *ex vivo* bone marrow purging with monoclonal antibodies and complement. *Bone Marrow Transplant* 1999; **24**: 621–7.

44. Bassan R, Lerede T, Di Bona E *et al*. Induction-consolidation with an idarubicin-containing regimen, unpurged marrow autograft, and post-graft chemotherapy in adult acute lymphoblastic leukaemia. *Br J Hematol* 1999; **104**: 755–62.

45. Ewing J, Robertson J, Ryder D *et al*. Peripheral blood stem cell transplantation in first remission acute leukemia: a single center intention to treat cohort study. *Blood* 1998; **92** (Suppl. 1): 427a [Abstract].

46. Vey N, Blaise D, Stoppa AM *et al*. Bone marrow transplantation in 63 adult patients with acute lymphoblastic leukemia in first complete remission. *Bone Marrow Transplant* 1994; **14**: 383–8.

47. Gilmore MJML, Hamon MD, Prentice HG *et al*. Failure of purged autologous bone marrow transplantation in high risk acute lymphoblastic leukemia in first complete remission. *Bone Marrow Transplant* 1991; **8**: 19–26.

48. Doney K, Buckner CD, Fisher L *et al*. Autologous bone marrow transplantation for acute lymphoblastic leukemia. *Bone Marrow Transplant* 1993; **12**: 315–21.

49. Abdallah A, Egerer G, Goldschmidt H *et al*. Continuous complete remission in adult patients with acute lymphocytic leukaemia at a median observation of 12 years after autologous bone marrow transplantation. *Br J Haematol* 2001; **112**: 1012–5.

50. Negrin RS, Kusnierz-Glaz CR, Still BJ *et al*. Transplantation of enriched and purged peripheral blood progenitor cells from a single apheresis product in patients with non-Hodgkin's lymphoma. *Blood* 1995; **85**: 3334–41.

51. Bassan R, Lerede T, Barbui T. Strategies for the treatment of recurrent acute lymphoblastic leukemia in adults. *Haematologica* 1996; **81**: 20–36.

52. Thomas DA, Kantarjian H, Smith TL *et al*. Primary refractory and relapsed adult acute lymphoblastic leukemia. *Cancer* 1999; **86**: 1216–30.

53. Giona F, Annino L, Testi AM *et al*. Management of advanced acute lymphoblastic leukemia in children and adults: results of the ALL R-87 protocol. *Leuk Lymphoma* 1998; **32**: 89–95.

54. Giona F, Annino L, Rondelli R *et al*. Treatment of adults with acute lymphoblastic leukaemia in first bone marrow relapse: results of the ALL R-87 protocol. *Br J Haematol* 1997; **98**: 896–903.

55. Freund M, Diedrich H, Ganser A *et al*. Treatment of relapsed or refractory adult acute lymphocytic leukemia. *Cancer* 1992; **69**: 709–16.

56. Martino R, Bellido M, Brunet S *et al*. Intensive salvage chemotherapy for primary refractory for first relapsed adult acute lymphoblastic leukemia: results of a prospective trial. *Haematologica* 1999; **84**: 505–10.

57. Soiffer RJ, Roy DC, Gonin R *et al*. Monoclonal antibody-purged autologous bone marrow transplantation in adults with lymphoblastic leukemia at high risk of relapse. *Bone Marrow Transplant* 1993; **12**: 243–51.

58. Weisdorf DJ, Billett AL, Hannan P *et al*. Autologous versus unrelated donor allogeneic marrow transplantation for acute lymphoblastic leukemia. *Blood* 1997; **90**: 2962–8.

59. Morishima Y, Miyamura K, Kojima S *et al*. Autologous BMT in high risk patients with CALLA-positive ALL: possible efficacy of *ex vivo* marrow leukemia cell purging with monoclonal antibodies and complement. *Bone Marrow Transplant* 1993; **11**: 255–9.

60. Dunlop LC, Powles R, Singhal S *et al*. Bone marrow transplantation for Philadelphia chromosome-positive acute lymphoblastic leukemia. *Bone Marrow Transplant* 1996; **17**: 365–9.

61. Stockschlader M, Hegewisch-Becker S, Kruger W *et al*. Bone marrow transplantation for Philadelphia chromosome-positive acute lymphoblastic leukemia. *Bone Marrow Transplant* 1995; **16**: 663–7.

62. Atta J, Fauth F, Keyser M *et al*. Purging in BCR-ABL-positive acute lymphoblastic leukemia using immunomagnetic beads: comparison of residual leukemia and purging efficiency in bone marrow vs. peripheral blood stem cells by semiquantitative polymerase chain reaction. *Bone Marrow Transplant* 2000; **25**: 97–104.

63. Kantarjian HM, Cortes J, O'Brien S *et al*. Imatinib mesylate (STI571) therapy for Philadelphia chromosome-positive chronic myelogenous leukemia in blast phase. *Blood* 2002; **99**: 3547–53.

64. Horowitz MM, Messerer D, Hoelzer D *et al*. Chemotherapy compared with bone marrow transplantation for adults with acute lymphoblastic leukemia in first remission. *Ann Intern Med* 1991; **115**: 13–18.

65. Zhang MJ, Hoelzer D, Horowitz MM *et al*. Long-term follow-up of adults with acute lymphoblastic leukemia in first remission treated with chemotherapy or bone marrow transplantation. *Ann Intern Med* 1995; **123**: 428–31.

66. Sebban C, Lepage E, Vernant JP *et al*. Allogeneic bone marrow transplantation in adult acute lymphoblastic leukemia in first complete remission: a comparative study. *J Clin Oncol* 1994; **12**: 2580–7.

67. Oh H, Gale RP, Zhang MJ *et al*. Chemotherapy versus HLA-identical sibling bone marrow transplants for adults with acute lymphoblastic leukemia in first remission. *Bone Marrow Transplant* 1998; **22**: 253–7.

68. Biggs JC, Horowitz MM, Gale RP *et al*. Bone marrow transplants may cure patients with acute leukemia never achieving remission with chemotherapy. *Blood* 1992; **80**: 1090–3.

69. Forman SJ, Schmidt GM, Nademanee AP *et al*. Allogeneic bone marrow transplantation as therapy for primary induction failure for patients with acute leukemia. *J Clin Oncol* 1991; **9**: 1570–4.

70. Barrett AJ, Horowitz MM, Ash RC *et al*. Bone marrow transplantation for Philadelphia chromosome-positive acute lymphoblastic leukemia. *Blood* 1992; **79**: 3067–70.

71. Synder DS. Allogeneic stem cell transplantation for Philadelphia chromosome-positive acute lymphoblastic leukemia. *Biol Blood Marrow Transplant* 2000; **6**: 597–603.

72. Radich JP. Philadelphia chromosome-positive acute lymphocytic leukemia. *Hematol Oncol Clin North Am* 2001; **15**: 21–36.

73. Sierra J, Radich J, Hansen JA *et al*. Marrow transplants from unrelated donors for treatment of Philadelphia chromosome-positive acute lymphoblastic leukemia. *Blood* 1997; **90**: 1410–4.

74. Kroger N, Kruger W, Wacker-Backhaus G *et al*. Intensified conditioning regimen in bone marrow transplantation for Philadelphia chromosome-positive acute lymphoblastic leukemia. *Bone Marrow Transplant* 1998; **22**: 1029–33.

75. Weisdorf DJ, Bishop M, Dharan B *et al*. Autologous versus allogeneic unrelated donor transplantation for acute lymphoblastic leukemia: comparative toxicity and outcomes. *Biol Blood Marrow Transplant* 2002; **8**: 213–20.

76. Ringden O, Laboin M, Gluckman E *et al*. Donor search or autografting in patients with acute leukemia who lack an HLA-matched sibling? A matched-pair analysis. *Bone Marrow Transplant* 1997; **19**: 963–8.

77. Busca A, Anasetti C, Anderson G *et al*. Unrelated

78 Schrappe M, Reiter A, Ludwig WD et al. Improved outcome in childhood acute lymphoblastic leukemia despite reduced use of anthracyclines and cranial radiotherapy: results of trial ALL-BFM 90. *Blood* 2000; **95**: 3310–21.

79 LeClerc JM, Billet AL, Gelber RD et al. Treatment of childhood acute lymphoblastic leukemia: results of Dana-Farber ALL consortium protocol 87–01. *J Clin Oncol* 2002; **20**: 237–46.

80 Chessells JM, Bailey C, Richards SM et al. Intensification of treatment and survival in all children with lymphoblastic leukaemia: results of UK Medical Research Council trial AKALL X. *Lancet* 1995; **345**: 143–8.

81 Mahoney DH, Shuster JJ, Nitschke R et al. Intensification with intermediate-dose intravenous methotrexate is effective therapy for children with lower risk B-precursor acute lymphoblastic leukemia: a pediatric oncology group study. *J Clin Oncol* 2000; **18**: 1285–94.

82 Lange BJ, Bostrom BC, Cherlow JM et al. Double-delayed intensification improves event-free survival for children with intermediate-risk acute lymphoblastic leukemia: a report from the Children's Cancer Group. *Blood* 2002; **99**: 825–32.

83 Heerema NA, Sather HN, Sensel MG. Prognostic impact of trisomies of chromosomes 10, 17, and 5 among children with acute lymphoblastic leukemia and high hyperdiploidy (>50 chromosomes). *J Clin Oncol* 2000; **18**: 1876–87.

84 Reaman GH, Sposto R, Sensel MG et al. Treatment outcome and prognostic factors for infants with acute lymphoblastic leukemia treated on two consecutive trials of the Children's Cancer Group. *J Clin Oncol* 1999; **17**: 445–55.

85 Smith M, Arthur D, Camitta B et al. Uniform approaches to risk classification and treatment assignment for children with acute lymphoblastic leukemia. *J Clin Oncol* 1996; **14**: 18–24.

86 Beyermann B, Adams HP, Henze G et al. Philadelphia chromosomes in relapsed childhood acute lymphoblastic leukemia: a matched-pair analysis. *J Clin Oncol* 1997; **15**: 2231–7.

87 Schrappe M, Arico M, Harbott J et al. Philadelphia chromosome-positive (Ph+) childhood acute lymphoblastic leukemia: good initial steroid response allows early prediction of a favorable treatment outcome. *Blood* 1998; **92**: 2730–41.

88 Arico M, Valsecchi MG, Camitta B et al. Outcome of treatment in children with Philadelphia chromosome-positive acute lymphoblastic leukemia. *N Engl J Med* 2000; **342**: 998–1006.

89 Behm FG, Raimondi SC, Frestedt JL et al. Rearrangment of the *MLL* gene confers a poor prognosis in childhood acute lymphoblastic leukemia, regardless of presenting age. *Blood* 1996; **87**: 2870–7.

90 Heerema NA, Nachman JB, Sather HN et al. Hypodiploidy with less than 45 chromosomes confers adverse risk in childhood acute lymphoblastic leukemia: a report from the Children's Cancer Group. *Blood* 1999; **94**: 4036–46.

91 Steinherz PG, Gaynon PS, Breneman JC et al. Cytoreduction and prognosis in acute lymphoblastic leukemia: the importance of early marrow response: report from the Children's Cancer Group. *J Clin Oncol* 1996; **14**: 389–98.

92 Cave H, van der Werff ten Bosch J, Suciu S et al. Clinical significance of minimal residual disease in childhood acute lymphoblastic leukemia. *N Engl J Med* 1998; **339**: 591–8.

93 Coustan-Smith E, Sancho J, Hancock ML et al. Clinical importance of minimal residual disease in childhood acute lymphoblastic leukemia. *Blood* 2000; **96**: 2691–6.

94 Dworzak MN, Froschl G, Printz D et al. Prognostic significance and modalities of flow cytometric minimal residual disease detection in childhood acute lymphoblastic leukemia. *Blood* 2002; **99**: 1952–8.

95 Cimino G, Elia L, Cristina M et al. A prospective study of residual-disease monitoring of the ALL1/AF4 transcript in patients with t(4;11) acute lymphoblastic leukemia. *Blood* 2000; **95**: 96–101.

96 Ikuta K, Tsuchida M, Manabe A et al. Role of stem cell transplantation (SCT) for children with acute lymphoblastic leukemia with very high risk features in first remission: a Tokyo children's cancer study group (TCCSG) study L95-14. *Blood* 1998; **92** (Suppl. 1): 116a [Abstract].

97 Wheeler KA, Richards SM, Bailey CC et al. Bone marrow transplantation versus chemotherapy in the treatment of very high-risk childhood acute lymphoblastic leukemia in first remission: results from Medical Research Council UKALL X and XI. *Blood* 2000; **96**: 2412–8.

98 Marco F, Bureo E, Ortega JJ et al. High survival rate in infant acute leukemia treated with early high-dose chemotherapy and stem cell support. *J Clin Oncol* 2000; **18**: 3256–61.

99 Houtenbos I, Bracho F, Davenport V et al. Autologous bone marrow transplantation for childhood acute lymphoblastic leukemia: a novel combined approach consisting of *ex vivo* marrow purging, modulation of multi-drug resistance, induction of autograft vs. leukemia effect, and post-transplant immuno- and chemotherapy (PTIC). *Bone Marrow Transplant* 2001; **27**: 145–53.

100 Auclerc MF, Oudot C, Perel Y et al. Children with acute lymphoblastic leukemia (ALL) and leukemic induction failure can be salvaged in 30% of the cases: results of the FRALLE 93 cohort. *Blood* 1998; **92** (Suppl. 1): 116a [Abstract].

101 Lawson SE, Harrison G, Richards S et al. The UK experience in treating relapsed childhood acute lymphoblastic leukaemia: a report on the Medical Research Council UKALLR 1 study. *Br J Haematol* 2000; **108**: 531–43.

102 Wheeler K, Richards S, Bailey C et al. Comparison of bone marrow transplant and chemotherapy for relapsed childhood acute lymphoblastic leukaemia: the MRC UKALL X experience. *Br J Haematol* 1998; **101**: 94–103.

103 Borgmann A, Schmid H, Hartmann R et al. Autologous bone-marrow transplants compared with chemotherapy for children with acute lymphoblastic leukaemia in a second remission: a matched-pair analysis. *Lancet* 1995; **346**: 873–6.

104 Buhrer C, Hartmann R, Fengler R et al. Peripheral blast counts at diagnosis of late isolated bone marrow relapse of childhood acute lymphoblastic leukemia predict response to salvage chemotherapy outcome. *J Clin Oncol* 1996; **14**: 2812–7.

105 Uderzo C, Conter V, Dini G et al. Treatment of childhood acute lymphoblastic leukemia after the first relapse: curative strategies. *Haematologica* 2000; **85**: 47–53.

106 Rivera GK, Hudson MM, Liu Q et al. Effectiveness of intensified rotational combination chemotherapy for late hematologic relapse of childhood acute lymphoblastic leukemia. *Blood* 1996; **88**: 831–7.

107 Winick NJ, Smith SD, Shuster J et al. Treatment of CNS relapse in children with acute lymphoblastic leukemia: a Pediatric Oncology Group study. *J Clin Oncol* 1993; **11**: 271–8.

108 Ribeiro RC, Rivera GK, Hudson M et al. An intensive re-treatment protocol for children with an isolated CNS relapse of acute lymphoblastic leukemia. *J Clin Oncol* 1995; **13**: 333–8.

109 Ritchey AK, Pollock BH, Lauer SJ et al. Improved survival of children with isolated CNS relapse of acute lymphoblastic leukemia: a Pediatric Oncology Group study. *J Clin Oncol* 1999; **17**: 3745–52.

110 Messina C, Cesaro S, Rondelli R et al. Autologous bone marrow transplantation for childhood acute lymphoblastic leukaemia in Italy. *Bone Marrow Transplant* 1998; **21**: 1015–21.

111 Billet AL, Ritz J. Autologous hematopoietic cell transplantation for acute lymphoblastic leukemia. In: Thomas ED, Blume KG, Foreman SJ, eds. *Hematopoietic Cell Transplantation*, 2nd edn. Boston, MA: Blackwell Science, 1999: 978–89.

112 Maldonado MS, Heredia CD, Badell I et al. Autologous bone marrow transplantation with monoclonal antibody purged marrow for children with acute lymphoblastic leukemia in second remission. *Bone Marrow Transplant* 1998; **22**: 1043–7.

113 Messina C, Valsecchi MG, Arico M et al. Autologous bone marrow transplantation for treatment of isolated central nervous system relapse of childhood acute lymphoblastic leukemia. *Bone Marrow Transplant* 1998; **21**: 9–14.

114 Borgmann A, Hartmann R, Schmid H et al. Isolated extramedullary relapse in children with acute lymphoblastic leukemia: a comparison between treatment results of chemotherapy and bone marrow transplantation, *Bone Marrow Transplant* 1995; **15**: 515–21.

115 Vaidya SJ, Atra A, Bahl S et al. Autologous bone marrow transplantation for childhood acute lymphoblastic leukemia in second remission: long-term follow-up. *Bone Marrow Transplant* 2000; **25**: 599–03.

116 Uderzo C, Rondelli R, Dini G et al. High-dose vincristine, fractionated total-body irradiation and cyclophosphamide as conditioning regimen in allogeneic and autologous bone marrow transplantation for childhood acute lymphoblastic leukaemia in second remission: a 7-year Italian multicentre study. *Br J Haematol* 1995; **89**: 790–7.

117 Balduzzi A, Gaipa G, Bonanomi S et al. Purified autologous grafting in childhood acute lymphoblastic leukemia in second remission: evidence for long-term clinical and molecular remissions. *Leukemia* 2001; **15**: 50–6.

118 Billett AL, Kornmehl E, Tarbell NJ et al. Autologous bone marrow transplantation after a long first remission for children with recurrent acute lymphoblastic leukemia. *Blood* 1993; **81**: 1651–7.

119 Feig SA, Harris RE, Sather HN. Bone marrow transplantation vs. chemotherapy for maintenance of second remission of childhood acute lymphoblastic leukemia: a study of the Children's Cancer Group (CCG-1884). *Med Pediatr Oncol* 1997; **29**: 534–40.

120 Kersey JH, Weisdorf D, Nesbit ME et al. Comparison of autologous and allogeneic bone marrow transplantation for treatment of high-risk refractory acute lymphoblastic leukemia. *N Engl J Med* 1987; **317**: 461–7.

121 Parsons SK, Castellino SM, Lehmann LE *et al*. Relapsed acute lymphoblastic leukemia: similar outcomes for autologous and bone marrow transplantation in selected children. *Bone Marrow Transplant* 1996; **17**: 763–8.

122 Schmid H, Henze G, Schwerdtfeger R *et al*. Fractionated total body irradiation and high-dose VP-16 with purged autologous bone marrow rescue for children with high risk relapsed acute lymphoblastic leukemia. *Bone Marrow Transplant* 1993; **12**: 597–602.

123 Uckun FM, Kersey JH, Haake R *et al*. Pretransplantation burden of leukemic progenitor cells as a predictor of relapse after bone marrow transplantation for cute lymphoblastic leukemia. *N Engl J Med* 1993; **329**: 1296–1301.

124 Knechtli CJC, Goulden NJ, Hancock JP *et al*. Minimal residual disease status before allogeneic bone marrow transplantation is an important determinant of successful outcome for children and adolescents with acute lymphoblastic leukemia. *Blood* 1998; **92**: 4072–9.

125 Uzunel M, Mattsson J, Jaksch M *et al*. The significance of graft-versus-host disease and pretransplantation minimal residual disease status to outcome after allogeneic stem cell transplantation in patients with acute lymphoblastic leukemia. *Blood* 2001; **98**: 1982–4.

126 Sirohi B, Powles R, Singhal S *et al*. The impact of consolidation chemotherapy on the outcome of autotransplantation for acute myeloid leukemia in first remission: a single center experience of 118 adult patients. *Blood* 2001; **98** (Suppl. 1): 690a [Abstract].

127 Tallman MS, Perez W, Keating A *et al*. Pre-transplant consolidation chemotherapy decreases leukemia relapse after autologous stem cell transplantation (ASCT) for acute myeloid leukemia (AML) in first complete remission (CR). *Blood* 2001; **98** (Suppl. 1): 859a [Abstract].

128 Burnett A, Goldstone AH, Stevens RM *et al*. Randomized comparison of addition of autologous bone-marrow transplantation to intensive chemotherapy for acute myeloid leukaemia in first remission: results of MRC AML 10 trial. *Lancet* 1998; **351**: 700–8.

129 Clift RA, Buckner CD, Appelbaum FR *et al*. Allogeneic marrow transplantation in patients with acute myeloid leukemia in first remission: a randomized trial of two irradiation regimens. *Blood* 1990; **76**: 1867–71.

130 Clift RA, Buckner CD, Appelbaum FR *et al*. Allogeneic marrow transplantation in patients with chronic myeloid leukemia in the chronic phase: a randomized trial of two irradiation regimens. *Blood* 1991; **77**: 1660–5.

131 Davies S, Ramsay KC, Klein JP *et al*. Comparison of preparative regimens in transplants for children with acute lymphoblastic leukemia. *J Clin Oncol* 2000; **18**: 340–7.

132 Boulad F, Steinherz P, Reyes B *et al*. Allogeneic bone marrow transplantation vs. chemotherapy for the treatment of childhood acute lymphoblastic leukemia in second remission: a single-institution study. *J Clin Oncol* 1999; **17**: 197–207.

133 Synder DS, Chao NJ, Amylon MD *et al*. Fractionated total body irradiation and high-dose etoposide as a preparatory regimen for bone marrow transplantation for 99 patients with acute leukemia in first complete remission. *Blood* 1993; **82**: 2920–8.

134 Matthews DC, Appelbaum FR, Eary JF *et al*. Phase I study of ^{131}I-anti-CD45 antibody plus cyclophosphamide and total body irradiation for advanced acute leukemia and myelodysplastic syndrome. *Blood* 1999; **94**: 1237–47.

135 Brenner MK, Rill DR, Moen RC *et al*. Gene-marking to trace origin of relapse after autologous bone-marrow transplantation. *Lancet* 1993; **341**: 85–6.

136 Miller CB, Zehnbauer BA, Piantadosi S *et al*. Correlation of occult clonogeneic leukemia drug sensitivity with relapse after autologous bone marrow transplantation. *Blood* 1991; **78**: 1125–31.

137 Labopin M, Gorin NC. Autologous bone marrow transplantation in 2502 patients with acute leukemia in Europe: a retrospective study. *Leukemia* 1992; **6** (Suppl. 1): 95–9.

138 Uckun FM, Kersey JH, Haake R *et al*. Autologous bone marrow transplantation in high-risk remission B-lineage acute lymphoblastic leukemia using a cocktail of three monoclonal antibodies (BA-1/CD24, BA-2/CD9, and BA-3/CD10) plus complement and 4-hydroperoxycyclophosphamide for *ex vivo* bone marrow purging. *Blood* 1992; **79**: 1094–104.

139 Mehta J, Powles R, Treleaven J *et al*. Autologous transplantation with CD52 monoclonal antibody-purged marrow for acute lymphoblastic leukemia: long-term follow-up. *Leuk Lymphoma* 1997; **25**: 479–86.

140 Keating MJ, Flinn I, Jain V *et al*. Therapeutic role of alemtuzumab (Campath-1H) in patients who have failed fludarabine: results of a large international study. *Blood* 2002; **99**: 3554–61.

141 Graham ML, Asselin BL, Herndon JE *et al*. Toxicity, pharmacology and feasibility of administration of PEG-L-asparaginase as consolidation therapy in patients undergoing bone marrow transplantation for acute lymphoblastic leukemia. *Bone Marrow Transplant* 1998; **21**: 879–85.

142 Blaise D, Attal M, Pico JL *et al*. The use of a sequential high dose recombinant interleukin 2 regimen after autologous bone marrow transplantation does not improve the disease-free survival of patients with acute leukemia transplanted in first complete remission. *Leuk Lymphoma* 1997; **25**: 459–78.

143 Martino R, Bellido M, Brunet S *et al*. Allogeneic or autologous stem cell transplantation following salvage chemotherapy for adults with refractory or relapsed acute lymphoblastic leukemia. *Bone Marrow Transplant* 1998; **21**: 1023–7.

91

Ravi Bhatia & Philip B. McGlave

Autologous Hematopoietic Cell Transplantation for Chronic Myeloid Leukemia

Introduction

Chronic myeloid leukemia (CML) results from the malignant transformation of a hematopoietic stem cell [1]. Malignant cells are characterized by the Philadelphia (Ph) chromosome resulting from a translocation involving the c-*bcr* gene located on chromosome 22 and the c-*abl* gene located on chromosome 9 [2,3]. The protein product of the resulting *bcr-abl* oncogene, p210$^{bcr-abl}$ has increased tyrosine kinase activity compared with p145^{abl} and has been shown to play an important role in malignant transformation [4,5].

CML occurs most frequently in the fifth and sixth decade of life [6]. It is an invariably lethal disorder in the absence of disease modifying treatment. An initial chronic phase (CP) of disease lasts a median of 3–4 years and is invariably followed by transformation to accelerated phase (AP) and blast crisis (BC). Treatment with standard chemotherapy can reduce elevated blood counts and control symptoms during CP but does not alter the disease course. Therapy with interferon-alpha (IFN-α), either alone or in combination with cytosine arabinoside, can induce hematological remissions in more than 80% of patients. Major (including complete) cytogenetic remissions are seen in 10–25% of patients [7–12]. Major cytogenetic responses are associated with prolongation of survival. However IFN therapy is limited by the low frequency of patients who achieve major cytogenetic responses, and by poor tolerance of chronic therapy.

Imatinib mesylate (STI571, Gleevec®), a recently developed inhibitor of the p210$^{bcr-abl}$ tyrosine kinase, induces complete responses in patients with all stages of disease [13–17]. In patients with CP CML, a complete cytogenetic remission (CCR) is seen in ~70% of newly diagnosed patients and ~40% of patients resistant to or intolerant of prior IFN treatment. It is not known if responses will be durable and associated with prolongation of survival. Limited follow-up suggests that the frequency of relapse is low in CP disease, but is increased in advanced phase CML.

Allogeneic hematopoietic cell transplantation (HCT) from a related or unrelated donor is the only treatment that has been proven to result in long-term disease-free survival in CML [18,19]. Although reduced intensity conditioning regimens with reduced toxicity may allow this treatment approach to be applicable to a wider group of patients [20,21], a significant number of patients will not be eligible for allogeneic transplant because of the lack of a suitably matched donor or advanced age. Transplantation of autologous Ph-negative (Ph$^-$) hematopoietic cells following myeloablative therapy is a potential approach to restoring Ph$^-$ hematopoiesis in CML patients. In this chapter we will describe the clinical experience with and the current status of autologous HCT in CML and discuss novel strategies under development to improve results from this procedure.

Rationale for autologous HCT

Several lines of experimental evidence indicate the presence of residual normal, polyclonal progenitors in the bone marrow (BM) and blood of some CML patients. Ph$^-$ progenitors, including polyclonal primitive progenitors, can be detected following *in vitro* culture of marrow from selected patients with CML [22]. Benign progenitors have also been selected from CML marrow on the basis of cell surface phenotype [23–26]. Several lines of clinical evidence also confirm the presence of benign progenitors in CML marrow. CML patients at presentation are known to have coexistent Ph-positive (Ph$^+$) and Ph$^-$ hematopoietic cell populations in their marrow [6]. Cytogenetic remissions were obtained in some CML patients receiving high doses of busulfan, or high-dose combination chemotherapy [27–30]. A fraction of patients treated with IFN-α can achieve CCRs with restoration of Ph$^-$ hematopoiesis [11]. The persistence of residual Ph$^-$ stem cells in CML patients, including patients with advanced disease, has been recently highlighted by the high rate of cytogenetic responses seen in patients treated with imatinib mesylate [14]. These observations support the hypothesis that benign stem cells capable of reconstituting hematopoiesis after autologous transplantation can be obtained from the marrow or peripheral blood of at least some CML patients.

Other factors have also played a role in the initiation of studies evaluating the efficacy of autologous HCT in CML. Assuming that transformation from CP to BC depends on the acquisition of additional random mutagenic events, measures to reduce the numbers of Ph$^+$ stem cells could theoretically delay transformation. In addition, transplantation of Ph$^-$ and Ph$^+$ cells into human and xenogeneic animal models appears to favor the engraftment of the Ph$^-$ clone [31,32]. Engraftment of the Ph$^+$ stem cells could be diminished as a result of defects in adhesion and migration, characteristic of Ph$^+$ progenitors [33–35]. In addition, reduction of both normal and leukemic cells to low levels favors regeneration of normal stem cells, at least in the short term, because of differences in proliferation and differentiation kinetics between Ph$^-$ and Ph$^+$ progenitors [29,36,37]. These considerations have led to several clinical trials exploring the safety and efficacy of autologous HCT in patients with CML. Several approaches to target malignant CML progenitors selectively (negative selection) or to select benign progenitors (positive selection) from blood and marrow of CML patients have been evaluated in these studies (discussed below).

Clinical experience with autologous HCT in CML

Autologous HCT with unselected cells

The initial studies with autologous transplants were performed on CML patients in BC. Autologous marrow or peripheral blood cryopreserved during CP was infused following high-dose chemotherapy with or without total body irradiation after development of transformation [38–40]. Although CP CML could be reestablished in most patients, it was usually short-lived with recurrence of advanced disease and death occurring within 6 months to 1 year. However, in a few patients transient partial cytogenetic responses were achieved following transplantation.

Subsequently, the efficacy of autologous HCT for patients in CP CML was evaluated. The Hammersmith group in London performed unmanipulated autologous peripheral blood mononuclear cell transplants in 21 CP CML patients between 1984 and 1992 [41,42]. The 5-year survival of the autografted patients (56%) was significantly higher compared with 636 age-matched controls treated with conventional chemotherapy (28%). Encouragingly, some degree of Ph⁻ hematopoiesis was observed in nine patients. Forty-nine patients receiving autologous HCT for CML in CP were entered in the European Group for Blood and Marrow Transplantation (EBMT) registry between 1989 and 1991 [43]. Fifteen of 34 evaluable patients had a major cytogenetic response (MCR; >65% Ph⁻ cell) and 10 of these patients had a CCR lasting for 6–36 months after transplant. The actuarial survival at 3 years was 81.5 ± 15%, higher than was expected with conventional chemotherapy. The Bordeaux group performed transplants on 72 patients between 1980 and 1996 using peripheral blood hematopoietic cells (PBHCs) collected at diagnosis without mobilization [46]. No problems with engraftment were seen. Of 20 patients who were transplanted in CP for IFN-α resistance or high Sokal score [44,45], five patients achieved MCR and the 5-year survival was 75%. However, patients with AP ($n = 32$) and BC ($n = 20$) demonstrated a short median survival (10.4 months) after transplantation [46].

These studies suggest that transplantation of unmanipulated autologous marrow or blood grafts can lead to cytogenetic responses in a small proportion of CML patients (Table 91.1). However responses are transient. These studies also raise the possibility that autologous HCT may extend survival for CML patients with CP disease. It should be noted that for these and subsequently described studies that CCR has been usually described as the absence of the t(9;22) translocation on routine cytogenetic analysis or, in some cases, *BCR-ABL*⁺ cells within normal limits for the assay by fluorescence *in situ* hybridization (FISH). The sensitivity of these assays for detection of small numbers of residual leukemia cells is 1–5%. In contrast the sensitive reverse transcription-polymerase chain reaction (RT-PCR) assay, which can detect as few as 1 in 10^6 residual leukemic cells, almost invariably detects residual leukemia cells in patients post-autologous HCT.

Autologous HCT following *ex vivo* purging of malignant progenitors

Several groups have tried to improve results of autologous HCT with unmanipulated grafts and to increase the frequency of cytogenetic responses following autologous HCT by attempting to purge malignant progenitors from the autograft prior to transplantation (Table 91.2).

Ex vivo marrow culture

Long-term culture of CML marrow results in decline in Ph⁺ progenitors and selective maintenance of Ph⁻ hematopoietic cells [22]. The Vancouver group conducted a trial of autologous HCT using cultured marrow cells in CML patients [47]. Eighty-seven patients were screened to confirm sufficient yield of benign progenitors. Thirty-six of these patients

Table 91.1 Autologous hematopoietic cell transplantation (HCT) with unpurged blood or marrow.

Study [Ref.]	Patients transplanted	Cytogenetic response CR	PR (% Ph⁺)	Survival (median range, in months)
Advanced phase				
Haines *et al.* 1984 [38]	51*	0	3 (14–67)	26 (0.5–35)
Reiffers *et al.* 1991 [39]	47*	0	14 (<90%)	24 (4–49)
Khouri *et al.* 1996 [40]	48†	5	5 (<30%)	5.5 (4–13)
Pigneux *et al.* 1999 [46]	52†	1	2	25% at 3 years
Chronic phase				
Hoyle *et al.* 1994 [41]; Mughal *et al.* 1993 [42]	21	2	9	82 (9–105)
Reiffers *et al.* 1994 [43]	49	10	5 (<35%)	81% at 3 years
Khouri *et al.* 1996 [40]	22	3	2	34
Pigneux *et al.* 1999 [46]	20	1	4	75% at 5 years

*Blast crisis.
†Accelerated phase and blast crisis.
CR, complete response; Ph⁺, Philadelphia chromosome-positive; PR, partial response.

(41%) were eligible for the study. Twenty-two patients, 16 in CP and six with advanced disease, underwent autologous transplantation with *ex vivo*-cultured marrow. BM nucleated cells were cultured in tissue culture flasks in long-term BM culture medium (α-medium supplemented with horse serum and fetal calf serum, glutamine, inositol, 2-mercaptoethanol and hydrocortisone) at 37°C for 3 days and then at 33°C for another 7 days. At the end of the 10 days, nonadherent and adherent cells were removed, combined, washed and filtered and resuspended in medium containing autologous serum and reinfused. Thirteen of 16 evaluable patients became 100% Ph⁻ while three patients had a MCR (75–94%). However, Ph⁺ metaphases reappeared in patients experiencing compete cytogenetic remission within 4–36 months following HCT in all but one patient. Thirteen of 16 CP patients and three of six patients with advanced disease were alive 1.0–5.7 years following HCT. Four of seven patients subsequently treated with low-dose IFN-α entered CCR. Five of the 22 patients experienced delayed or partial engraftment requiring infusion of untreated "back up" cells. Similar results have been reported by the Manchester group [48].

Granulocyte macrophage colony-stimulating factor (GM-CSF)

The Johns Hopkins University group made the observation that myeloid growth factors may deplete CML progenitors *in vitro* by inducing their terminal differentiation [49]. A clinical trial was initiated in which small, dense cells were isolated by counterflow centrifugal elutriation (which allows cell separation based on cell size-density characteristics) and incubated in GM-CSF for 72 h prior to autologous HCT. After autografting all patients received GM-CSF daily for 2 months. Thirteen patients who had failed prior IFN treatment were enrolled (eight in CP and five in AP) [50]. There were three transplant-related deaths, all in AP patients. Of the remaining 10 patients, nine patients engrafted with 100 Ph⁻ hematopoiesis. All patients developed a cytogenetic relapse at a median of 6 months (range 4–22 months).

Antisense oligodeoxynucleotides (AS-ODNs) directed against *BCR-ABL*

Inhibition of p210^BCR-ABL expression with AS-ODNs against the *BCR-ABL* breakpoint junction results in inhibition of growth of Ph⁺ cells in *in*

Table 91.2 Autologous hematopoietic cell transplantation (HCT) with an *ex vivo* purged graft.

Study [Ref.]	Purging method	No. of patients transplanted	Cytogenetic response CR	PR (% Ph⁺)	Graft failure	Survival (median, range)
Barnett *et al.* 1994 [47]	Marrow culture	22	13	3 (<25%)	5	CP 81% 3 years; AP 50% 3 years
Coutinho *et al.* 1997 [48]	Marrow culture	9	4	3	2	1–87+ months
Gladstone *et al.* 1999 [50]	GM-CSF, marrow culture	13	9	0	0	6 (4–22)
de Fabritiis *et al.* 1998 [54]	Antisense to *BCR-ABL*	8	2	0	0	42–86+ months
Luger *et al.* 2002 [55]	Antisense to *myb*	24	2	3	8	2–71+ months
Roy *et al.* 2001 [56]	Photodynamic treatment	8	4	0	2	82% at 15 month
Carlo-Stella *et al.* 1994 [57]	Mafosfamide	10	6	1 (25%)	0	NA
McGlave *et al.* 1990 [58]	IFN-γ	44	10	12 (5–85%)	15	CP 71% 3 years; AP 15% 3 years

AP, accelerated phase; CP, chronic phase; CR, complete response; GM-CSF, granulocyte macrophage colony-stimulating factor; IFN-γ, interferon-gamma; NA, not applicable; Ph⁺, Philadelphia chromosome-positive; PR, partial response.

vitro and *in vivo* experiments [51–53]. De Fabritiis and colleagues performed autologous HCT on eight patients with CML at the time of transformation to AP or during second CP [54]. Patients were selected on the basis of results obtained *in vitro* at diagnosis. BM cells were exposed *in vitro* to junction-specific *BCR-ABL* AS-ODNs. The reinfused treated cells engrafted and reconstituted hematopoiesis in all patients. A CCR was seen in two patients and a minimal or no response in the other six. Four patients developed BC 7–39 months after reinfusion, one died from unrelated BMT complications 30 months after HCT, and three are in persistent second CP 14–26 months after HCT. Although this approach appears to be feasible, definite conclusions about the benefit derived from this purging procedure cannot be made from this small pilot study.

AS-ODNs directed against c-*myb*

Luger and colleagues have explored the use of AS-ODNs to the protooncogene c-*MYB* for purging of CML marrow [55]. c-*MYB* may play an important role in leukemogenesis, possibly through regulating *myc* expression. Normal cells appear to be more tolerant of *MYB* deprivation than malignant cells. This feature together with the very short half-life of c-*MYB* messenger RNA (mRNA) and protein make it an attractive target to test ODN therapy approach. In a trial of this approach, patients were screened prior to enrollment for sequence-specific sensitivity to the anti-*myb* ODNs. CD34⁺ selected marrow cells were exposed to ODN for either 24 h ($n = 19$) or 72 h ($n = 5$). Purging resulted in reduction of *MYB* RNA levels and a reduction of *BCR-ABL* expressing long-term culture initiating cells in approximately half the patients. Eight patients received back-up marrow because of poor recovery of counts post-transplant. These included five of 19 patients receiving marrow purged for 24 h and three of five patients receiving marrow purged for 72 h. Engraftment concerns in the latter group resulted in a return to the original 24-h purging protocol. Day 100 cytogenetics in 14 patients who engrafted without infusion of unmanipulated "back-up" marrow revealed that two patients had CCR, three patients had an MCR and eight remained 100% Ph⁺. These results raise the possibility that effective delivery of ODNs directed to critical proteins of short half-life may lead to development of more effective nucleic acid drugs and enhanced clinical utility of these compounds in the future.

Photodynamic purging

A dibromo-rhodamine derivative (TH9402) was developed as an agent that was highly cytotoxic to CML cells after photoactivation, resulting in the 5-log depletion of a CML cell line in preclinical studies. Roy *et al.* [56] reported results of a phase 1 trial of photodynamic therapy-mediated purging of autologous peripheral blood hematopoietic stem cell grafts. Peripheral blood hematopoietic stem cells were mobilized with an idarubicin, cytosine arabinoside and etoposide regimen from 13 CML patients (nine in CP, four in AP) who had failed IFN treatment. Grafts underwent immunomagnetic selection of CD34⁺ cells followed by either no further treatment ($n = 5$) or increasing dose-intensity of TH9402 photodynamic therapy ($n = 8$). Photodynamic therapy was effective in depleting CML progenitor cells. No residual *BCR-ABL*⁺ colonies were seen in the purged product at the highest dose. Two patients required reinfusion of untreated stored cells because of poor engraftment. Four patients achieved CCR and the overall disease-free survival at 15 months was 82%. As with some of the other purging strategies discussed above, the results of this small pilot study are encouraging, but definite conclusions about clinical efficacy are not possible.

4-hydroxyperoxycyclophosphamide (mafosfamide)

Rizzoli and colleagues, demonstrated that the cyclophosphamide derivative mafosfamide selectively kills malignant CML progenitors and enriches Ph⁻ stroma-adherent progenitors in a subset of CML patients [57]. Ten patients (five in CP, five in advanced phase), preselected on the basis of *in vitro* testing, were transplanted with autologous marrow cells treated *ex vivo* with mafosfamide. Recovering marrow metaphases were 100% Ph⁻ in six of nine evaluable patients. However, cytogenetic remissions were transient with a median duration of 6.5 months. Only one patient remains Ph⁻ while five patients developed BC after a median follow-up of 16 months.

Interferon-gamma (IFN-γ)

Using *in vitro* progenitor assays, McGlave *et al.* [58] demonstrated that exposure to IFN-γ for 36 h led to significantly greater inhibition of CML compared with normal colony forming cell growth. This led to a trial of autologous HCT with marrow cultured for 36 h *ex vivo* in the presence of 1000 μ/mL IFN-γ in 22 CP and 22 AP CML patients [58]. Regenerating marrow metaphases were 100% Ph⁻ in 10 of 39 (26%) evaluable patients and 11–95% Ph⁻ in an additional 12 patients (32%). However, in all but three evaluable patients the percentage of Ph⁻ marrow metaphases had dropped to 10% or less within 12 months of transplant. The projected 3-year survival for CP patients was 71% and for patients with CML in AP it was 15%. Fifteen patients experienced delayed or partial engraftment requiring infusion of untreated, cryopreserved "backup" peripheral blood cells obtained prior to HCT.

The above results suggest that *ex vivo* purging of Ph$^+$ progenitors from the autograft is possible and may be associated with an increased frequency of cytogenetic remission post-transplant. However, improved outcomes following purging could also be the result of selection of patients likely to have a more favorable outcome. Further, even in this selected group, cytogenetic remissions are of relatively short duration indicating the need for better purging strategies, new preparative regimens to better reduce the burden of residual leukemic cells in the patient and/or improved post-transplant antileukemic therapies to maintain remissions. Of note, a sizable fraction of patients receiving marrow treated *ex vivo* experienced delayed or partial engraftment. This observation may reflect the presence of limited numbers of benign stem cells in the graft and/or the loss or damage of viable, benign stem cells in the course of the purging process.

Autologous HCT following *in vivo* selection by priming and mobilization

Mobilization of peripheral blood stem cells (PBSCs) after chemotherapy

An alternative approach to obtain a graft enriched for benign progenitors has been to treat CML patients with high-dose combination chemotherapy. Chemotherapy regimens like those used in remission induction therapy of acute myeloid leukemia can result in transient cytogenetic remissions in up to 50% of CP CML patients. This may be related to differential kinetics of regeneration of Ph$^-$ and Ph$^+$ progenitors in CML patients [29,36]. The Swedish CML group treated 97 newly diagnosed CML patients, with sequential remission inducing therapies [59]. When a CCR was induced, marrow was harvested for autologous HCT. All patients were initially treated with hydroxyurea and IFN-α for at least 6 months. Those who did not achieve CCR were then treated with one to three courses of different intensive combination chemotherapies. Remissions were eventually achieved in the marrow of 23 of 97 patients. Fifteen patients were autografted in CCR and three in partial remission. Nine of 16 evaluable patients are Ph$^-$ 1–32 months from transplant. These results again suggest that autografting of a selected group of CML patients with good cytogenetic responses to intensive treatment is associated with a high incidence of cytogenetic responses following HCT.

The Genoa group has developed an autologous HCT strategy for CML based on the expected enrichment of Ph$^-$ progenitors in the peripheral blood of patients in the early phase of recovery following combination chemotherapy [60,61]. Therapy with the intensive regimen of idarubicin, cytosine arabinoside and etoposide (ICE), resulted in 100% Ph$^-$ apheresis collections in 12 out of 24 CP (50%) and five out of 22 advanced phase (23%) patients. Collections that were more than 50% Ph$^-$ were obtained in an additional three CP and three advanced phase patients. Sixty-four percent of patients treated within the 1st year from diagnosis had 100% Ph$^-$ apheresis collections. Thirteen of 16 patients receiving 100% Ph$^-$ autologous PBHCs following intensive chemo-radiotherapy engrafted and were alive, and five patients remained Ph$^-$ 5–29 months after transplant. Hematopoiesis was polyclonal in all four female recipients tested by evaluation of X-chromosome inactivation patterns. Updated results for autologous transplantation of Ph$^-$ grafts were recently reported for 30 patients [62]. CCR was achieved on recovery post-transplant in 16 patients and MCR in an additional 10 patients. No transplant-related mortality was seen. Twenty-eight patients were alive at 6–76 months post-transplant (median 24 months). Eight patients were in CCR at a median of 20 months post-transplant and eight in MCR at a median of 22 months post-transplant [63].

Several other groups have attempted to use chemotherapy to induce Ph$^-$ hematopoiesis prior to harvesting marrow or peripheral blood for autografting. As shown in Table 91.3, these studies suggest that complete and partial cytogenetic responses are induced in a subset of patients, but that there is considerable variability in the results obtained and the results in general have not been as predictable or as compelling as those originally described. In addition, this procedure may be associated with significant toxicity and recovery may occasionally be delayed resulting in insufficient progenitor cell yield to allow transplantation [64–68].

It is also possible that differences in the chemotherapy regimens used could play a role in the variability of collection of Ph$^-$ PBHC products [69]. However, several studies suggest that less intensive chemotherapy regimens with reduced toxicity are equally effective in mobilizing Ph$^-$ PBSC products as the more intensive regimens. For example a regimen using high doses of hydroxyurea (3.5 g/m^2 for 7 days) has been reported to be very well tolerated and has at least comparable efficacy in mobilizing Ph$^-$ PBSC products as the more intensive regimens [70]. Janssen *et al*. [71] have reported that a second course of intensive chemotherapy does not improve Ph$^-$ PBHC collection. It is possible that some of the variability observed in different studies could result from differences in patient selection. Several groups have reported a higher frequency of Ph$^-$ collections from patients treated earlier in the disease course [63,64,72,73]. Hughes *et al*. [74] reported that Ph$^-$ collections were confined to a good prognosis group (Sokal score <1). Within the low Sokal score group, other risk factors such as low premobilization white blood cell counts and low white blood cell nadir correlated with Ph$^-$ mobilization [74].

The level of Ph$^-$ cells in the autograft may predict for cytogenetic response post-transplant. Talpaz *et al*. [75] demonstrated a direct correlation between the level of Ph$^-$ cells in the inoculum and the percentage of Ph$^-$ marrow cells recovered 17–55 weeks following autologous HCT. Verfaillie *et al*. [73] reported that, whereas the cytogenetic status of the autograft predicted cytogenetic status of marrow at recovery, the cytogenetic status at 3–12 months post-transplant correlated better with number of Ph$^-$ HLA-DR CD34$^+$ cells in the autograft. It was also noted that mobilized PBHC collections yielded larger number of HLA-DR CD34$^+$ cells than steady state or primed BM. Corsetti *et al*. [76] reported that quantitative competitive RT-PCR was useful for measuring residual leukemia load in PBHCs that are Ph$^-$ by routine cytogenetic analysis, and that this approach may allow for selection of the best PBHC products for reinfusion. It remains to be determined whether cytogenetic response post-transplant is related to reduced Ph$^+$ contamination of the PBHC product or whether a good response to conventional chemotherapy identifies patients who are likely to respond well to the more intensive therapy used in transplant conditioning regimens.

In conclusion, *in vivo* purging using high-dose chemotherapy may reduce the leukemic load in the autograft in selected patients, which in turn may be associated with superior achievement of Ph$^-$ hematopoiesis post-transplant. However, results are quite variable and this approach may be associated with significant toxicity. It is also unclear whether this approach is associated with improved survival in CML patients.

Mobilization of PBSCs from patients treated with IFN-α

An alternative method of *in vivo* purging has employed collection of PBHCs following induction of cytogenetic responses by treatment with IFN-α. Archimbaud *et al*. [77] mobilized PBHCs from 30 CML patients receiving IFN-α therapy, with varying degrees of cytogenetic remission, using granulocyte colony-stimulating factor (G-CSF). IFN was continued through G-CSF administration and PBHC collection. Patients underwent one to four (median three) apheresis. Median total CD34$^+$ cells/kg were $3.4(0–140) \times 10^6$. No patient had a significant increase in the percentage

Table 91.3 Autologous hematopoietic cell transplantation (HCT) with an *in vivo* purged autograft.

Study [Ref.]	In vivo purging					Autologous transplantation				
	Chemotherapy regimen	No. of patients studied	Ph⁻ status of collections	Inadequate PBSC collection	Toxic deaths	No. of patients transplanted	Cytogenetic response	Graft failure	Toxic deaths	Survival: range (median; months)
Carella et al. 1996, 1997 [60,61]	ICE	49	CCR 24, MCR 6	NA	NA	23	CCR 13, MCR 3	2	2	1–48+
Carella et al. 1999 [63]	ICE	30	CCR 22, MCR 8	0	0	30	CCR 16, MCR 10	0	0	6–76 (24)
Verfaillie et al. 1998 [73]	CY, MAC	44	MCR 11	8	2	35	MCR 13	1	1	3–35+
Chalmers et al. 1997 [64]; Singer et al. 1998 [68]	IA	43	CCR 16, MCR 6	NA	2	32	MCR 72%	2	3	26–138 (52)
Hughes et al. 1997 [74]	CY,	23	MCR 7	2	0	Not reported				NA
Fischer et al. 1998 [72]	ICE/IA	57	CCR 8, MCR 10	0	1	31	CCR 3, MCR 4	0	0	NA
Waller et al. 1998 [66]	ICE ± IL-2	17	CCR 14, MCR 2	1	0	16	CCR 6, MCR 4	0	0	(18+)
Morton et al. 1999 [67]	ICE	21	CCR 3, MCR 6	2	0	4	CCR 1, MCR 2	0	0	NA
Sureda et al. 1999 [65]	ICE	20	CCR4, MCR 9	0	0	6	0	0	0	3–16 (7.5)
Janssen et al. 2000 [71]	IA (cycle 1) AmA (cycle 2)	19	CCR 3, MCR 5 after cycle 1 CCR 1, MCR 6 after cycle 2	1	1	7	MCR 4	0	0	25–44 (33)
Pratt et al. 1998 [70]	HU	18	6 CCR	3	0	7	MCR 2	1	NA	13–25+
Talpaz et al. 1995 [75]	DC, FMC, ICE	21	CCR 3, MCR 7	NA	NA	21	CCR 5, MCR 5	NA	NA	1–21+
Simonsson et al. 1996 [59]	HU/IFN-α, DC, MEA, AmA	160	CCR 31	NA	8	30	CCR 13	NA	1	3–64+

AmA, amsacrine, cytosine arabinoside; CCR, complete cytogenetic remission (100 Ph⁻); CY, cyclophosphamide; DC, daunorubicin, cytosine arabinoside; FMC, fludarabine, mitoxantrone, cytosine arabinoside; HU, hydroxyurea; IA, idarubicin, cytosine arabinoside; ICE, idarubicin, cytosine arabinoside, etoposide; IFN-α, interferon-alpha; IL-2, interleukin 2; MAC, mitoxantrone, cytosine arabinoside, cyclophosphamide; MCR, major cytogenetic remission (<35% Ph⁻); MEA, mitoxantrone, etoposide, cytosine arabinoside; NA, not available; PBSC, peripheral blood stem cell.

of Ph+ cells in the BM under G-CSF therapy. The percentage of Ph+ cells in apheresis products tended to decrease between the first and the last apheresis procedure. Fourteen patients who were not responsive to IFN-α underwent autologous transplantation. Nine patients had a major cytogenetic response after HCT, which correlated with the amount of Ph− cells reinfused with the graft. Other investigators have reported similar results [78,79].

The Italian Cooperative Study Group on CML conducted a prospective study of combined treatment with IFN-α followed by autologous HCT [80]. Two hundred and seventy-two patients who were previously untreated were enrolled between 1989 and 1991. Nine million IFN-α units were administered daily for at least 1 year. BM harvesting and autografting was done in patients with more than 25% Ph− cells. Of the 76 patients (28%) who were eligible, marrow was harvested in 37 (14%) and 23 (8%) autografted. There was one death from infection. Five patients progressed to BC, six were alive and in complete hematological response (CHR) and 11 in CCR. Eight years after registration, progression-free survival of autografted patients was 65%.

In conclusion, growth factor induced mobilization of PBHCs appears to be feasible and well tolerated, allowing the harvest of adequate numbers of cells without discontinuation of IFN-α during the collection process. There is no evidence that G-CSF treatment resulted in cytogenetic progression or relapse. The cytogenetics of the PBHCs product in general reflects BM cytogenetics and complete and durable cytogenetic remissions can be obtained. However, treatment is applicable to only a small, selected group of patients.

Mobilization of PBHCs from patients treated with imatinib mesylate

Treatment with imatinib mesylate results in CCR in a high proportion of CML patients [14,15]. PBHCs collected from patients while in CCR may provide a source of BCR-ABL^- stem cells for autologous HCT in case of subsequent relapse.

Maziarz et al. [81] reported on a trial of growth factor mobilization of PBHCs in 11 CML patients treated with imatinib mesylate. Patients were either refractory, or intolerant to IFN, or in AP. Six patients received G-CSF alone at 10 μg/kg/day while five required dose escalation of G-CSF or combination with GM-CSF. Two patients required remobilization efforts. Imatinib mesylate treatment was continued during G-CSF administration and PBHC collection. Peripheral blood CD34+ counts were monitored to assess onset of hematopoietic cell procurement. The minimal target dose of CD34+ progenitors (2×10^6/kg) was achieved after a median of three collections (range: 3–5). The median CD34+ collected was 2.68×10^6/kg (range: 0.78–7.95). PBHC products were Ph− in all five of the five patients evaluated. FISH analysis showed the bcr-abl gene to be absent in three, <5% in three and <10% in four of the 10 patients evaluated. Qualitative PCR for bcr-abl was negative in one, indeterminate in one and positive in seven of the nine patients evaluated. IFN-α treatment for >2 years appeared to be associated with poorer mobilization. Therefore CD34+ PBHCs can be successfully mobilized with growth factors from patients treated concurrently with imatinib mesylate.

At the City of Hope National Medical Center, PBHCs were collected from 17 patients [82]. All patients were in CCR (Ph− on karyotyping and BCR-ABL^+ cells within normal limits on FISH) on imatinib mesylate treatment. Fifteen patients were in CP and two patients were in AP. The median time from diagnosis to collection was 35 months (range 9–90 months). The median duration of imatinib mesylate treatment was 15 months (8–32 months). G-CSF (10 μg/kg/day) was administered daily and PBHC collection initiated on day +5 with a targeted minimum of 2×10^6 CD34+ cells/kg. Imatinib mesylate treatment was continued during G-CSF administration and PBHC collection. The median number of CD34+ cells (10^6/kg) collected was 2.31 (0.69–4.27) with a median of three phereses collections (range: 1–13). The target number of CD34+ cells was collected in 15 of the 17 patients. The number of CD34+ cells collected correlated inversely with time from diagnosis but not with duration of prior imatinib mesylate treatment. PBHCs were Ph− on karyotyping and BCR-ABL^- by FISH in 12 of 16 evaluable patients. Additional chromosomal abnormalities in Ph− cells (insertion+(3;4) and del(10)) were detected on karyotypic analysis of PBHC collections from two patients. The abnormal clones were not detected on earlier BM examination. BCR-ABL^+ CD34+ cells were detected in PBHC collections from eight of 11 evaluable patients. These results support the feasibility of collection of Ph− PBHC from patients in CCR on imatinib mesylate treatment, but also indicate that additional strategies may be required to further deplete BCR-ABL^+ progenitors from PBHC collections.

Post-transplant antileukemic treatment

Interferon-alpha (IFN-α)

IFN-α has been used to reverse cytogenetic relapse following allogeneic HCT. Boiron et al. [83] reported the results of autologous HCT for 45 CML patients registered with the EBMT group who failed to achieve or maintain a hematological or cytogenetic response to IFN-α. Thirty of the 45 patients received IFN-α after autografting. For 42 evaluable patients, the probabilities of being in major or CCR at 24 months were 44 ± 16% and 27 ± 13%, respectively. Nine of 30 patients receiving IFN-α post-transplant achieved CCR. These results suggest that autologous HCT may be associated with restoration of sensitivity to IFN-α in at least some CML patients who were insensitive to IFN-α before HCT. Other investigators have also reported reversal of cytogenetic relapse in autologous transplant recipients with IFN-α treatment. These results indicate that IFN-α may have a role in maintaining cytogenetic remissions achieved after HCT.

Roquinimex

Roquinimex is an immunomodulatory agent known to enhance T cell, natural killer (NK) cell and macrophage activity. A phase II trial of roquinimex was initiated in CML patients post-autologous BMT [84]. Patients received unmanipulated BM and received oral roquinimex twice weekly following neutrophil engraftment. Seventeen patients (11 CP, four AP, two second CP) were enrolled. Toxicity consisted of musculoskeletal aches, peripheral edema and skin changes including graft-vs.-host disease like rash and eccrine sweat gland necrosis. All CP patients achieved a hematological response. Seven of 11 patients had a major cytogenetic response for 1 year or longer and four patients had a CCR at 2 or more years after HCT. Cytogenetic responses post-transplant often developed over a period of time and do not appear to represent engraftment with Ph− cells. These clinical and cytogenetic data are encouraging and suggest antileukemia activity of roquinimex in Ph+ CML.

GM-CSF and hydroxyurea

Carlo-Stella et al. [85] studied the effect of prolonged (5–9 months) low-dose GM-CSF therapy (1 μg/kg/day subcutaneously) post-transplant in five CML patients resistant to IFN-α therapy who were autografted with unmanipulated marrow or PBHC. GM-CSF was discontinued and hydroxyurea was given for 2 days each week. Two patients engrafted with 81% and 100% Ph− hematopoiesis, Ph− hematopoiesis was no longer detectable at 9 months. Interestingly, two patients had late appearing Ph− hematopoiesis that either increased or cycled post-transplant. The late appearance of Ph− hematopoiesis was interpreted as supporting an antileukemic activity of the GM-CSF/hydroxyurea regimen.

Table 91.4 Approaches to improve survival after autologous hematopoietic cell transplantation for chronic myeloid leukemia (CML).

Residual malignant stem cells in the graft: improved "purging" strategies	Residual disease in the host: improved post-transplant therapies
In vivo purging	*Immunological*
Imatinib	Adoptive immunotherapy:
Imatinib in combination with	NK, CIK cells
other therapies	BCR-ABL junction peptides
Ex vivo purging	Other antigenic targets:
Targeting *BCR-ABL* expression:	WT1
Antisense oligonucleotides CML66	PR1
Ribozymes	Dendritic cell therapy:
SiRNA	Autologous
Targeting *BCR-ABL* kinase activity:	Peptide pulsed or transduced
Imatinib mesylate	*Pharmacological*
New kinase inhibitors	Imatinib mesylate
Combinations	Imatinib combinations
Phenotypic separation	
Ex vivo culture based strategies	

Potential approaches to improving the outcome for autologous HCT in CML

Although cytogenetic remissions are observed following autologous HCT for CML, they occur in only a subset of patients and are usually short lived. Relapse of CML post-transplant may reflect the presence of residual leukemic cells in the autograft, persistence of leukemic cells in the patient following pretransplant conditioning therapy, or both. Retroviral marking studies using the *NEO* resistance gene to mark a portion of CD34$^+$ marrow cells obtained from CML patients recovering from high-dose chemotherapy prior to autografting confirmed that sufficient malignant cells can remain in the autograft to contribute to systemic relapse [86]. Therefore, improved methods for purging the autograft of malignant stem cells are required. Studies of allogeneic transplant for CML clearly indicate the importance of a graft-vs.-leukemia effect to prevent and treat relapse in CML after transplant. Even if the autograft was completely purged of Ph$^-$ stem cells, relapse is likely to occur in the absence of additional antileukemic treatment delivered post-transplant. The ability of autologous HCT to achieve durable disease-free survival in the future will depend on the development of improved methods for graft purging, better preparative regimens to reduce the residual leukemic burden, as well as improved antileukemic therapy that can be delivered following HCT to treat residual disease. Several such approaches are being tested or are under consideration (Table 91.4), as discussed below.

Improved purging techniques

Purging techniques that have been employed in clinical trials so far are limited to being applicable to only a small number of CML patients in early CP, resulting in incomplete depletion of malignant stem cells and being associated with problems related to engraftment, likely reflecting damage to normal stem cells. Therefore, alternative purging approaches to purging are being explored.

Targeting *BCR-ABL* oncogene expression

AS-ODNs directed against the *BCR-ABL* breakpoint have been evaluated for purging autografts in a pilot clinical trial [54]. However, this strategy is associated with several problems including inadequate intracellular penetration, nonspecific interactions with other mRNAs and/or proteins and variable or incomplete reduction of *BCR-ABL* RNA or protein levels. Advances in AS-ODN design and improved technology for their delivery to the correct cellular compartment may allow improved targeting of *BCR-ABL* [87–90]. Another approach is to use multiunit ("hammerhead") ribozymes, which bind to *BCR-ABL* mRNA and cleave three sites that lie in close proximity to the junction points [91]. This approach may have theoretically improved specificity or efficacy compared with the use of AS-ODNs but, as with AS-ODNs, there are problems related to delivery. Another issue is that inhibition of *BCR-ABL* expression for a short period of time may not result in elimination of CP CML progenitors. Transduction of a *BCR-ABL* AS-ODNs or ribozyme-producing gene in hematopoietic stem cells allows extended exposure of CML progenitors to the antisense sequences, but is limited by the level of transduction efficiency that can be achieved [92]. Recently, short interfering RNA (siRNA) technology has been described as a potent method for specific targeting of *BCR-ABL* gene expression [93]. Advances in gene targeting may allow improved suppression of *BCR-ABL* gene expression in the future and lead to improved autologous HCT strategies.

Tyrosine kinase inhibitors

The enhanced constitutive tyrosine kinase activity of p210$^{BCR-ABL}$ fusion protein plays a critical role in *BCR-ABL* mediated transformation. As discussed earlier, imatinib mesylate, an inhibitor of Abl protein-tyrosine kinases, has shown remarkable preclinical and clinical activity in CML [13,14,94]. Recently, additional agents with more potent activity against the p210$^{BCR-ABL}$ kinase have been described and are undergoing preclinical evaluation [95]. However, the use of these agents for purging of CML autografts may be limited by incomplete suppression of Ph$^+$ progenitor growth following short-term exposure. However, the combination of imatinib mesylate with other antileukemic agents may result in enhanced killing of CML cells applicable either to *in vivo* treatment approaches, or to more effective purging of Ph$^+$ progenitors from CML autografts [96,97].

Phenotypic separation of benign progenitors

In normal hematopoiesis, primitive progenitors can be identified on the basis of CD34 antigen expression and absent or low expression of HLA-DR, lack of CD38 expression, expression of Thy1 or exclusion of the dye rhodamine-123. Verfaillie *et al.* [23,24] demonstrated that primitive progenitors in the CD34$^+$ HLA-DR-cell fraction obtained from a high proportion of patients in early CP (<1 year after diagnosis) generate progeny that are nonmalignant by cytogenetics and RT-PCR and lack the *BCR-ABL* rearrangement at the genomic level. However, the CD34$^+$ HLA-DR-population is markedly reduced and contaminated with malignant cells in late CP (>1 year from diagnosis) and advanced phase patients. This observation suggests that the proportion of benign primitive progenitors available to reconstitute hematopoiesis after autologous HCT dwindles with time, or with development of advanced disease. Selection of CD34$^+$ HLA-DR cells in some patients with early CP CML may offer a source of leukemia-free cells for autografting. This approach has been limited by technical difficulties in obtaining and expanding sufficient numbers of this rare cell population for autologous HCT.

Ex vivo culture based purging strategies

CML hematopoietic progenitors demonstrate enhanced proliferation and terminal differentiation and reduced self-renewal in response to hematopoietic growth factor stimulation [37,49,98]. Pilot studies have demonstrated the feasibility of autologous HCT using marrow cells purged by *ex vivo* long-term culture or *ex vivo* GM-CSF treatment of the autograft [47,48,50]. However *ex vivo* culture based purging results in elimination of malignant progenitors in only a limited number of CML patients and may be associated with damage and/or depletion of normal stem cells.

Modifications in this technique will be necessary to make it more widely applicable. Further optimization of growth factor combinations and duration of *ex vivo* culture may improve elimination of malignant stem cells and preservation of normal stem cells [37]. In addition, differences between CML and normal marrow progenitors in adhesion to stroma and fibronectin [33,34] and in response to growth regulatory chemokines, such as macrophage inflammatory protein-1α (MIP-1α) [99,100], could be exploited to enhance selection of Ph⁻ progenitors.

Improved antileukemic therapy to prevent recurrence after HCT

The higher frequency of relapse in CP CML patients who receive syngeneic or T-lymphocyte-depleted allogeneic grafts from healthy siblings indicates that the preparatory regimen is often not sufficient to eliminate all malignant CML stem cells from the host [101,102]. Therefore, selection of a benign progenitor population is not expected to be sufficient to establish durable cytogenetic and hematological remissions. Additional post-transplant treatments will be required to maintain remissions that may be achieved in CML patients following autologous HCT.

Adoptive immunotherapy

The requirement for an immunologically mediated "graft-vs.-leukemia effect" to suppress the expansion of persistent malignant clones suggests that malignant CML progenitors are susceptible to targeting by the immune system [101,102]. *In vitro* studies indicate that interleukin 2 (IL-2) stimulation generates cells with cytolytic activity against CML, suggesting that systemic administration of IL-2 could have useful antileukemic effects in the post-transplant phase [103,104]. NK cells may be responsible for some of the effects attributed to IL-2. $CD3^+CD56^+$ cells, termed cytokine induced killer (CIK) cells generated from CML patients are Ph⁻ and are able to suppress the growth of CML Ph⁺ marrow cells in the marrow and spleen of severe combined immunodeficiency syndrome (SCID) mice [105]. IL-2 activated natural killer (ANK) cells from CML patients have been demonstrated to suppress CML progenitors in a dose dependent manner while sparing normal progenitors [106]. Clinical studies suggest that autologous ANK cell infusions are safe [107]. These observations support the testing of ANK cells or CIK cells to prevent relapse of CML after autologous HCT.

BCR-ABL junction peptides

Studies demonstrating that a specific cytotoxic or helper T-lymphocyte response can be generated in human leukocyte antigen (HLA)-matched healthy donors against $p210^{BCR-ABL}$ breakpoint-derived peptides suggest that it may be possible to generate specific T-cell responses targeted towards malignant CML cells [108–116]. b3a2 peptides have been shown to stimulate autologous antileukemic cytotoxic T lymphocyte (CTL) responses [110,114]. CTLs generated in this manner can be shown to lyse syngeneic cell lines incubated with exogenously supplied peptide. However, it has been harder to demonstrate that these CTLs are able to lyse leukemia cells. The ability of the joining region segment to serve as a T-cell target may depend on whether major histocompatibility complex (MHC) on target cells present the peptide at a concentration high enough to stimulate CTLs [114,117,118].

Other antigenic targets

An alternative strategy is to generate CTLs directed towards other antigenic targets that may be expressed at abnormally high levels or be abnormally expressed in leukemic cells. One such target is the *WT1* gene product. Gao *et al.* [119,120] developed HLA-A0201-restricted CTLs that killed leukemic cell lines and inhibited colony formation by transformed $CD34^+$ cells but not normal $CD34^+$ cells, suggesting that *WT1* is a target for CTLs with high degree of specificity for leukemic progenitor cells. CML66 is a unique tumor-associated antigen of unknown function initially cloned from a CML complementary DNA (cDNA) expression library [121]. In normal individuals CML66 expression is restricted to the testes and heart and no expression is seen in normal hematopoietic tissues. CML66-specific antibodies are detected in patient serum, and high titers correlate with immune-induced remission after donor lymphocyte infusion. PR1 is an HLA-A2.1-restricted peptide from proteinase 3, which shows increased cytoplasmic expression in CML blasts. PR1 can be used to elicit CTLs from normal individuals that show HLA-restricted cytotoxicity and colony inhibition of myeloid leukemia cells that overexpress proteinase 3. Molldrem *et al.* [122–124] used a PR1-HLA-A2 specific tetramer to identify PR1 specific CTLs. They showed that tetramer sorted allogeneic CTLs could lyse CML blasts, indicating that these cells may be useful for leukemia-specific adoptive immunotherapy.

Dendritic cell (DC) therapy

Dendritic cells (DCs), which are the most potent antigen-presenting cells, are being actively studied for vaccine development. DCs can be generated from mononuclear cells and $CD34^+$ cells of patients with CML [125–127]. *Ex vivo* generated DCs of malignant clonal origin in CML constitutively express *BCR-ABL* and, possibly, other yet undefined leukemia-associated antigens [128]. These CML-derived DCs are capable of stimulating T lymphocytes that were cytotoxic to autologous CML targets but not to MHC-matched normal marrow targets [128,129]. Further studies have shown that DCs from CML patients may have decreased and/or considerably increased heterogeneous activity when tested with allogeneic T cells in a mixed lymphocyte reaction [130]. Measures to enhance T-cell-stimulatory activity that are being explored include transduction with vectors expressing IL-2 [131], IL-7 [132], or exposure to IFN-α [130]. Clinically applicable methods to generate autologous $BCR-ABL^+$ DCs from monocyte precursors in CML patients have been developed [127,132,133]. In a preliminary study, Fujii *et al.* [133] vaccinated a CP CML patient following autologous PBSC transplantation with autologous DCs. *In vitro* studies indicated that DCs generated from G-CSF mobilized PBHC were Ph⁺ and could elicit an antigen-specific immune response, which included vigorous cytotoxicity specific to CML cells. Infusion of leukemic DCs to this patient resulted in a decrease in the number of Ph⁺ cells in blood and marrow and induced T-cell responses, which appeared to include tumor-reactive, activated T cells.

Another approach is to use DCs from healthy individuals after pulsing with *BCR-ABL* peptides to elicit antigen-specific MHC class I and II restricted immune responses [116]. Alternatively, the use of viral vectors allows the introduction of proteins containing multiple epitopes, increasing the chance that a particular MHC will bind to the relevant antigen and elicit an immune response. Sun *et al.* [134] constructed a recombinant adeno-associated virus vector containing an 835-bp cDNA fragment encoding the b3a2 fusion region with flanking sequences and used it to express the *BCR-ABL* fusion region within primary human DCs. Peripheral blood mononuclear cells from normal healthy subjects were primed and restimulated *in vitro* with autologous DCs transduced with the *BCR-ABL* fusion region containing vector and with empty vector (negative control) or DCs pulsed with a peptide corresponding to the fusion domain (positive control). *BCR-ABL* transduced DCs primed autologous T cells in an antigen-specific MHC-restricted fashion to levels comparable with positive control. Both cytotoxic $CD4/TH1^+$ and $CD8^+$ responses were detected in this system. Cytotoxicity against *BCR-ABL* expressing tumor cell lines was also seen. This construct may serve as a candidate vaccine for gene-based antigen specific immunotherapy.

Imatinib mesylate

Imatinib mesylate has been successfully used to treat relapse following

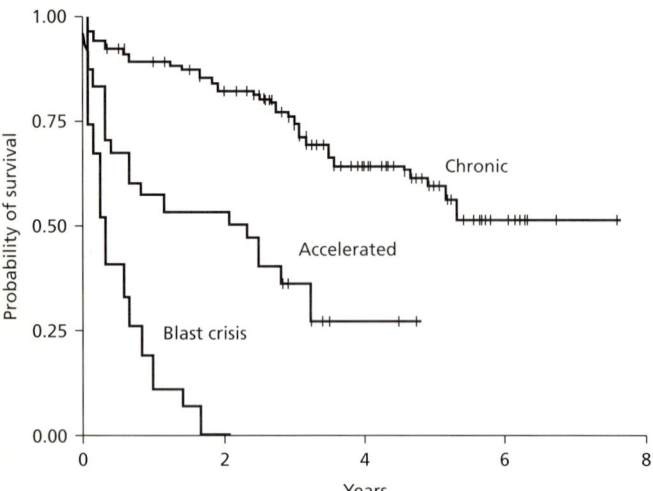

Fig. 91.1 Autologous transplantation for chronic myeloid leukemia (CML). Survival by disease stage. Survival for patients receiving autologous transplantation. Chronic phase (chronic; $n = 141$); accelerated phase (accelerated; $n = 30$); blast crisis (BC; $n = 27$). Reproduced with permission from Bhatia et al. [137].

allogeneic HCT, including patients who failed prior DLI [135]. It is reasonable to think that administration of imatinib mesylate, alone or in combination with other therapeutic modalities, post-autologous HCT could enhance and/or prolong cytogenetic responses.

Status of autologous HCT for CML

Results of autologous HCT as currently practised

The results of clinical trials of autologous HCT for CML suggest that this procedure can induce cytogenetic remissions in a subset of patients and may be associated with longer than expected patient survival. McGlave et al. [136] compiled the results of 200 consecutive autologous transplants performed with purged or unpurged marrow or blood grafts at eight different transplant centers in Europe and North America between June 1984 and January 1992. One hundred and twenty-five patients were alive at the end of the study (median follow-up of 42 months, range 1–91 months). The median survival time of 142 patients with CP CML was not reached, for patients with AP it was 35.9 months and for patients in BC it was 4.1 months. An updated survival analysis from this series is shown in Fig. 91.1 [137]. The survival probability for CP patients was 0.66 ± 0.09 at 4 years. The majority of surviving autologous transplant recipients have evidence of cytogenetic or hematological relapse, indicating that this process does not lead to elimination of malignant progenitors. It is not possible to make any definite conclusions regarding the effect of autologous HCT on survival of CML patients because of the absence of controlled clinical trials. However, such trials are unlikely in the near future because of the advent of imatinib mesylate as a very effective treatment for CML.

Autologous HCT in the context of imatinib mesylate

In the past autologous transplant was considered as a treatment option for CML patients who did not have a suitable matched allogeneic related or unrelated donor. Future trials of autologous HCT must be considered in the context of the remarkable efficacy of imatinib mesylate for the treatment of CML. In spite of the impressive efficacy of imatinib mesylate in inducing cytogenetic remissions, the long-term benefits of imatinib mesylate treatment are not yet known. In patients with CML in AP and BC, relapses are observed even after induction of CCR [13,16,17]. Relapses have been infrequent in patients with CP disease, but follow-up is limited [15,51–53]. Patients in CCR on imatinib treatment continue to demonstrate evidence of residual leukemia cells and some patients may be at risk of relapse. Therefore, for patients who have received imatinib mesylate and achieved CCR, pilot studies have been initiated for PBHC to be collected and stored to be used for autologous HCT in case of later cytogenetic or hematological progression [81]. Transplantation of a cytogenetically normal autograft may result in restoration of normal hematopoiesis post-transplant in these patients. In addition a significant percentage of patients shows evidence of sensitivity to imatinib mesylate and achieve partial CR but not CCR with imatinib mesylate treatment. For these patients, *in vivo* purging followed by autologous HCT may be effective in reducing the leukemia burden and improving the degree of cytogenetic response achieved in these patients.

The future of autologous HCT for CML

The ability of autologous HCT to achieve durable disease-free survival will depend on the future development of improved methods for graft purging, better preparative regimens to reduce the residual leukemic burden, as well as improved antileukemic therapy that can be delivered following HCT to treat residual disease. The clinical application of some of the novel methods reviewed is in this chapter expected to allow for better purging of the autograft and more effective elimination of residual leukemia than has been possible so far, and may result in long-term restoration of Ph^- hematopoiesis. The ability of imatinib mesylate to induce cytogenetic responses in the majority of CML patients in CP will allow purging procedures to be performed on cell populations greatly depleted of Ph^+ stem cells, and may allow significant chance of success. Moreover, systemic administration of imatinib mesylate, alone or in combination with other therapeutic modalities may allow for improved maintenance of cytogenetic remission status. Pilot studies to evaluate the efficacy and safety of these approaches will probably be initially limited to patients who fail to achieve optimal responses to imatinib mesylate. If successful, subsequent clinical trials should evaluate the use of such strategies earlier in the course of treatment of the disease, especially if better predictors of sustained responsiveness to imatinib mesylate treatment become available.

References

1 Fialkow PJ, Jacobson RJ, Papayannopoulou T. Chronic myelocytic leukemia. Clonal origin in a stem cell common to the granulocyte, erythrocyte, platelet and monocyte/macrophage. *Am J Med* 1977; **63**: 125–30.

2 Rowley JD. A new consistent chromosome abnormality in chronic myelogenous leukemia identified by quinacrine fluorescence and Giemsa staining. *Nature* 1973; **243**: 209–13.

3 DeKlein A, Van Kessel AG, Grosveld G et al. A cellular oncogene is translocated to the Philadelphia chromosome in chronic myelocytic leukemia. *Nature* 1982; **300**: 765–7.

4 Daley GQ, Van Etten RA, Baltimore D. Induction of chronic myelogenous leukemia in mice by the $p210^{bcr/abl}$ gene of the Philadelphia chromosome. *Science* 1990; **247**: 824–7.

5 Daley GQ, Baltimore D. Transformation of an interleukin 3-dependent hematopoietic cell line by the chronic leukemia-specific $p210^{bcr/abl}$ protein. *Proc Natl Acad Sci U S A* 1988; **85**: 9312–6.

6 Sawyers CL. Chronic myeloid leukemia. *N Engl J Med* 1999; **340**: 1330–40.

7 Allan NC, Richards SM, Shepherd PC. UK Medical Research Council randomised, multi-centre trial of interferon-α_{n1} for chronic myeloid leukaemia: improved survival irrespective of

cytogenetic response. The UK Medical Research Council's Working Parties for Therapeutic Trials in Adult Leukaemia. *Lancet* 1995; **345**: 1392–7.
8. Interferon α versus chemotherapy for chronic myeloid leukemia. A meta-analysis of seven randomized trials: Chronic Myeloid Leukemia Trialists' Collaborative Group. *J Natl Cancer Inst* 1997; **89**: 1616–20.
9. Randomized study on hydroxyurea alone versus hydroxyurea combined with low-dose interferon-α$_{2b}$ for chronic myeloid leukemia. The Benelux CML Study Group. *Blood* 1998; **91**: 2713–21.
10. Hehlmann R, Heimpel H, Hasford J et al. Randomized comparison of interferon-α with busulfan and hydroxyurea in chronic myelogenous leukemia. The German CML Study Group. *Blood* 1994; **84**: 4064–77.
11. Kantarjian HM, Giles FJ, Sm OB, Talpaz M. Clinical course and therapy of chronic myelogenous leukemia with interferon-α and chemotherapy. *Hematol Oncol Clin North Am* 1998; **12**: 31–80.
12. Guilhot F, Chastang C, Michallet M et al. Interferon α-2b combined with cytarabine versus interferon alone in chronic myelogenous leukemia. French Chronic Myeloid Leukemia Study Group. *N Engl J Med* 1997; **337**: 223–9.
13. Druker BJ, Sawyers CL, Kantarjian H et al. Activity of a specific inhibitor of the *BCR-ABL* tyrosine kinase in the blast crisis of chronic myeloid leukemia and acute lymphoblastic leukemia with the Philadelphia chromosome. *N Engl J Med* 2001; **344**: 1038–42.
14. Druker BJ, Talpaz M, Resta DJ et al. Efficacy and safety of a specific inhibitor of the *BCR-ABL* kinase in chronic myeloid leukemia. *N Engl J Med* 2001; **344**: 1031–7.
15. Kantarjian H, Sawyers C, Hochhaus A et al. Hematologic and cytogenetic responses to imatinib mesylate in chronic myelogenous leukemia. *N Engl J Med* 2002; **346**: 645–52.
16. Sawyers CL, Hochhaus A, Feldman E et al. Imatinib induces hematologic and cytogenetic responses in patients with chronic myelogenous leukemia in myeloid blast crisis: results of a phase II study. *Blood* 2002; **99**: 3530–9.
17. Talpaz M, Silver RT, Druker BJ et al. Imatinib induces durable hematologic and cytogenetic responses in patients with accelerated phase chronic myeloid leukemia: results of a phase 2 study. *Blood* 2002; **99**: 1928–37.
18. Clift RA, Appelbaum FR, Thomas ED. Treatment of chronic myeloid leukemia with marrow transplantation. *Blood* 1993; **82**: 1954–6.
19. McGlave PB, Shu XO, Wen W et al. Unrelated donor marrow transplantation for chronic myelogenous leukemia: 9 years' experience of the national marrow donor program. *Blood* 2000; **95**: 2219–25.
20. Niederwieser D, Maris M, Shizuru JA et al. Low-dose total body irradiation (TBI) and fludarabine followed by hematopoietic cell transplantation (HCT) from HLA-matched or mismatched unrelated donors and postgrafting immunosuppression with cyclosporine and mycophenolate mofetil (MMF) can induce durable complete chimerism and sustained remissions in patients with hematological diseases. *Blood* 2003; **101**(4): 1620–9.
21. Storb RF, Champlin R, Riddell SR, Murata M, Bryant S, Warren EH. Non-myeloablative transplants for malignant disease. *Hematology (Am Soc Hematol Educ Program)* 2001: 375–91.
22. Coulombel L, Kalousek DK, Eaves CJ, Gupta CM, Eaves AC. Long-term marrow culture reveals chromosomally normal hematopoietic progenitor cells in patients with Philadelphia chromosome-positive chronic myelogenous leukemia. *N Engl J Med* 1983; **308**: 1493–8.
23. Verfaillie CM, Miller WJ, Boylan K, McGlave PB. Selection of benign primitive hematopoietic progenitors in chronic myelogenous leukemia on the basis of HLA-DR expression. *Blood* 1992; **79**: 1003–10.
24. Verfaillie CM, Bhatia R, Miller W et al. *BCR/ABL*-negative primitive progenitors suitable for transplantation can be selected from the marrow of most early-chronic phase but not accelerated-phase chronic myelogenous leukemia patients. *Blood* 1996; **87**: 4770–9.
25. Leemhuis T, Leibowitz D, Cox G, Silver R, Srour EF, Tricot G et al. Identification of *BCR/ABL*-negative primitive hematopoietic progenitor cells within chronic myeloid leukemia marrow. *Blood* 1993; **81**: 801–7.
26. Delforge M, Boogaerts MA, McGlave PB, Verfaillie CM. *BCR/ABL*$^-$ CD34$^+$ HLA-DR$^-$ progenitor cells in early chronic phase, but not in more advanced phases, of chronic myelogenous leukemia are polyclonal. *Blood* 1999; **93**: 284–92.
27. Radojkovic M, Ristic S, Colovic M, Todoric B, Krtolica K. Busulfan-induced loss of Ph chromosome in chronic myeloid leukemia. *Med Oncol* 2001; **18**: 227–9.
28. Mandigers CM, Mensink EJ, Geurts van Kessel A et al. A long-lasting complete hematologic and cytogenetic remission of chronic myelogenous leukemia after treatment with busulfan alone. *Ann Hematol* 1996; **72**: 371–3.
29. Goto T, Nishikori M, Arlin Z et al. Growth characteristics of leukemic and normal hematopoietic cells in Ph$^+$ chronic myelogenous leukemia and effects of intensive treatment. *Blood* 1982; **59**: 793–808.
30. Carella AM, Dejana A, Lerma E et al. In vivo mobilization of karyotypically normal peripheral blood progenitor cells in high-risk MDS, secondary or therapy-related acute myelogenous leukaemia. *Br J Haematol* 1996; **95**: 127–30.
31. Sirard C, Lapidot T, Vormoor J, Cashman JD, Doedens M, Murdoch B et al. Normal and leukemic SCID-repopulating cells (SRC) coexist in the bone marrow and peripheral blood from CML patients in chronic phase, whereas leukemic SRC are detected in blast crisis. *Blood* 1996; **87**: 1539–48.
32. Wang JC, Lapidot T, Cashman JD et al. High level engraftment of NOD/SCID mice by primitive normal and leukemic hematopoietic cells from patients with chronic myeloid leukemia in chronic phase. *Blood* 1998; **91**: 2406–14.
33. Gordon MY, Dowding CR, Riley GP, Goldman JM, Greaves MF. Altered adhesive interactions with marrow stroma of hematopoietic progenitor cells in chronic myelogenous leukaemia. *Nature* 1984; **328**: 342–4.
34. Verfaillie CM, McCarthy JB, McGlave PB. Mechanisms underlying abnormal trafficking of malignant progenitors in chronic myelogenous leukemia: decreased adhesion to stroma and fibronectin but increased adhesion to the basement membrane components laminin and collagen type IV. *J Clin Invest* 1992; **90**: 1232–9.
35. Salgia R, Quackenbush E, Lin J et al. The *BCR/ABL* oncogene alters the chemotactic response to stromal-derived factor-1α. *Blood* 1999; **94**: 4233–46.
36. Clarkson BD, Strife A, Wisniewski D, Lambek C, Carpino N. New understanding of the pathogenesis of CML. A prototype of early neoplasia. *Leukemia* 1997; **11**: 1404–28.
37. Petzer AL, Eaves CJ, Barnett MJ, Eaves AC. Selective expansion of primitive normal hematopoietic cells in cytokine-supplemented cultures of purified cells from patients with chronic myeloid leukemia. *Blood* 1997; **90**: 64–9.
38. Haines ME, Goldman JM, Worsley AM et al. Chemotherapy and autografting for chronic granulocytic leukaemia in transformation: probable prolongation of survival for some patients. *Br J Haematol* 1984; **58**: 711–21.
39. Reiffers J, Trouette R, Marit G et al. Autologous blood stem cell transplantation for chronic granulocytic leukaemia in transformation: a report of 47 cases. *Br J Haematol* 1991; **77**: 339–45.
40. Khouri IF, Kantarjian HM, Talpaz M et al. Results with high-dose chemotherapy and unpurged autologous stem cell transplantation in 73 patients with chronic myelogenous leukemia: the M.D. Anderson experience. *Bone Marrow Transplant* 1996; **17**: 775–9.
41. Hoyle C, Gray R, Goldman J. Autografting for patients with CML in chronic phase: an update. Hammersmith BMT Team LRF Centre for Adult Leukaemia. *Br J Haematol* 1994; **86**: 76–81.
42. Mughal T, Hoyle C, Goldman JM. Autografting for patients with chronic myeloid leukaemia: the Hammersmith experience. *Stem Cells* 1993; **11** (Suppl. 3): 20–2.
43. Reiffers J, Goldman J, Meloni G, Cahn JY, Faberes C, Apperley J. Autologous transplantation in chronic myelogenous leukemia: European results. Chronic Leukemia Working Party EBMT. *Bone Marrow Transplant* 1994; **14** (Suppl. 3): S51–4.
44. Confirmation and improvement of Sokal's prognostic classification of Ph$^+$ chronic myeloid leukemia: the value of early evaluation of the course of the disease. The Italian Cooperative Study Group on Chronic Myeloid Leukaemia. *Ann Hematol* 1991; **63**: 307–14.
45. Prospective confirmation of a prognostic classification for Ph$^+$ chronic myeloid leukaemia. The Italian Cooperative Study Group on Chronic Myeloid Leukaemia. *Br J Haematol* 1988; **69**: 463–6.
46. Pigneux A, Faberes C, Boiron JM et al. Autologous stem cell transplantation in chronic myeloid leukemia: a single center experience. *Bone Marrow Transplant* 1999; **24**: 265–70.
47. Barnett MJ, Eaves CJ, Phillips GL et al. Autografting with cultured marrow in chronic myeloid leukemia: results of a pilot study. *Blood* 1994; **84**: 724–32.
48. Coutinho LH, Chang J, Brereton ML et al. Autografting in Philadelphia-positive (Ph$^+$) chronic myeloid leukaemia using cultured marrow: an update of a pilot study. *Bone Marrow Transplant* 1997; **19**: 969–76.
49. Bedi A, Griffin CA, Barber JP et al. Growth factor-mediated terminal differentiation of chronic myeloid leukemia. *Cancer Res* 1994; **54**: 5535–8.
50. Gladstone DE, Bedi A, Miller CB et al. Philadelphia chromosome-negative engraftment after autologous transplantation with granulocyte-macrophage colony-stimulating factor for chronic myeloid leukemia. *Biol Blood Marrow Transplant* 1999; **5**: 394–9.
51. Szczylik C, Skorski T, Nicolaides NC et al. Selective inhibition of leukemia cell proliferation

52 Ratajczak MZ, Kant JA, Luger SM et al. In vivo treatment of human leukemia in a SCID mouse model with c-myb antisense oligodeoxynucleotides. Proc Natl Acad Sci U S A 1992; **89**: 11,823–7.

53 de Fabritiis P, Amadori S, Calabretta B, Mandelli F. Elimination of clonogenic Philadelphia-positive cells using BCR-ABL antisense oligodeoxynucleotides. Bone Marrow Transplant 1993; **12**: 261–5.

54 de Fabritiis P, Petti MC, Montefusco E et al. BCR-ABL antisense oligodeoxynucleotide in vitro purging and autologous bone marrow transplantation for patients with chronic myelogenous leukemia in advanced phase. Blood 1998; **91**: 3156–62.

55 Luger SM, O'Brien SG, Ratajczak J et al. Oligodeoxynucleotide-mediated inhibition of c-myb gene expression in autografted bone marrow: a pilot study. Blood 2002; **99**: 1150–8.

56 Roy DC, Bioileau J, Laplante J et al. Phase I study of autologous progenitor cell transplantation (PCT) with a photodynamic approach for patients with chronic myelogenous leukemia (CML). Blood 2001; **96**(11) (Suppl. 1): 583a [Abstract].

57 Carlo-Stella C, Mangoni L, Almici C et al. Autologous transplant for chronic myelogenous leukemia using marrow treated ex vivo with mafosfamide. Bone Marrow Transplant 1994; **14**: 425–32.

58 McGlave PB, Arthur D, Miller WJ, Lasky L, Kersey J. Autologous transplantation for CML using marrow treated ex vivo with recombinant human interferon γ. Bone Marrow Transplant 1990; **6**: 115–20.

59 Simonsson B, Oberg G, Bjoreman M et al. Intensive treatment in order to minimize the Ph-positive clone in CML. Danish–Swedish CML Group. Bone Marrow Transplant 1996; **17** (Suppl. 3): S63–4.

60 Carella AM, Chimirri F, Podesta M et al. High-dose chemo-radiotherapy followed by autologous Philadelphia chromosome-negative blood progenitor cell transplantation in patients with chronic myelogenous leukemia. Bone Marrow Transplant 1996; **17**: 201–5.

61 Carella AM, Cunningham I, Lerma E et al. Mobilization and transplantation of Philadelphia-negative peripheral-blood progenitor cells early in chronic myelogenous leukemia. J Clin Oncol 1997; **15**: 1575–82.

62 Carella AM. Autografting with non-clonal mobilized hematopoietic progenitor cells in CML. Leukemia 2000; **14**: 954–5.

63 Carella AM, Lerma E, Corsetti MT et al. Autografting with Philadelphia chromosome-negative mobilized hematopoietic progenitor cells in chronic myelogenous leukemia. Blood 1999; **93**: 1534–9.

64 Chalmers EA, Franklin IM, Kelsey SM et al. Treatment of chronic myeloid leukaemia in first chronic phase with idarubicin and cytarabine: mobilization of Philadelphia-negative peripheral blood stem cells. Br J Haematol 1997; **96**: 627–34.

65 Sureda A, Petit J, Brunet S et al. Mini-ICE regimen as mobilization therapy for chronic myelogenous leukaemia patients at diagnosis. Bone Marrow Transplant 1999; **24**: 1285–90.

66 Waller CF, Heinzinger M, Rosenstiel A, Lange W. Mobilization and transplantation of Philadelphia chromosome-negative peripheral blood progenitor cells in patients with CML. Br J Haematol 1998; **103**: 227–34.

67 Morton J, Mollee P, Taylor K et al. Safe mobilization of normal progenitors in advanced chronic myeloid leukaemia with intensive chemotherapy and granulocyte-colony stimulating factor. Leuk Res 1999; **23**: 177–83.

68 Singer IO, Franklin IM, Clark RE et al. Autologous transplantation in chronic myeloid leukaemia using peripheral blood stem cells. Br J Haematol 1998; **102**: 1359–62.

69 Fischer T, Neubauer A, Mohm J et al. Outcome of peripheral blood stem cell mobilization in advanced phases of CML is dependent on the type of chemotherapy applied. Ann Hematol 1998; **77**: 21–6.

70 Pratt G, Johnson RJ, Rawstron AC, Barnard DL, Morgan GJ, Smith GM. Autologous stem cell transplantation in chronic myeloid leukaemia using Philadelphia chromosome negative blood progenitors mobilised with hydroxyurea and G-CSF. Bone Marrow Transplant 1998; **21**: 455–60.

71 Janssen JJ, van Rijn RS, van der Holt B et al. Mobilization of haemopoietic progenitors in CML. A second course of intensive chemotherapy does not improve Ph-negativity in stem cell harvests. Bone Marrow Transplant 2000; **25**: 1147–55.

72 Fischer T, Neubauer A, Mohm J et al. Chemotherapy-induced mobilization of karyotypically normal PBSC for autografting in CML. Bone Marrow Transplant 1998; **21**: 1029–36.

73 Verfaillie CM, Bhatia R, Steinbuch M et al. Comparative analysis of autografting in chronic myelogenous leukemia: effects of priming regimen and marrow or blood origin of stem cells. Blood 1998; **92**: 1820–31.

74 Hughes TP, Grigg A, Szer J et al. Mobilization of predominantly Philadelphia chromosome-negative blood progenitors using cyclophosphamide and rHUG-CSF in early chronic-phase chronic myeloid leukaemia: correlation with Sokal prognostic index and haematological control. Br J Haematol 1997; **96**: 635–40.

75 Talpaz M, Kantarjian H, Liang J et al. Percentage of Philadelphia chromosome (Ph)-negative and Ph-positive cells found after autologous transplantation for chronic myelogenous leukemia depends on percentage of diploid cells induced by conventional-dose chemotherapy before collection of autologous cells. Blood 1995; **85**: 3257–63.

76 Corsetti MT, Lerma E, Dejana A et al. Cytogenetic response to autografting in chronic myelogenous leukemia correlates with the amount of BCR-ABL positive cells in the graft. Exp Hematol 2000; **28**: 104–11.

77 Archimbaud E, Michallet M, Philip I et al. Granulocyte colony-stimulating factor given in addition to interferon-α to mobilize peripheral blood stem cells for autologous transplantation in chronic myeloid leukaemia. Br J Haematol 1997; **99**: 678–84.

78 Reiffers J, Taylor K, Gluckman E et al. Collection of Ph-negative progenitor cells with granulocyte-colony stimulating factor in patients with chronic myeloid leukaemia who respond to recombinant α-interferon. Br J Haematol 1998; **102**: 639–46.

79 Hernandez-Boluda JC, Carreras E, Cervantes F et al. Collection of Philadelphia-negative stem cells using recombinant human granulocyte colony-stimulating factor in chronic myeloid leukaemia patients treated with α-interferon. Haematologica 2002; **87**: 17–22.

80 Meloni G, Russo D, Baccarani M et al. A prospective study of α-interferon and autologous bone marrow transplantation in chronic myeloid leukemia. The Italian Co-operative Study Group on Chronic Myeloid Leukemia. Haematologica 1999; **84**: 707–15.

81 Maziarz RT, Chauncey TR, Capdeville R et al. Growth factor mobilization of CD34[+] PBSC in CML patients treated with imatinib (STI571). Blood 2001; **98**: 738a [Abstract].

82 Bhatia R, Slovak ML, McDonald T et al. PBSC collected from patients in complete cytogenetic remission on imatinib mesylate treatment are Ph[−] by standard criteria but are contaminated with BCR/ABL[+] progenitor cells. Blood 2002; **100**: 109a [Abstract].

83 Boiron JM, Cahn JY, Meloni G et al. Chronic myeloid leukemia in first chronic phase not responding to α-interferon: outcome and prognostic factors after autologous transplantation. EBMT Working Party on Chronic Leukemias. Bone Marrow Transplant 1999; **24**: 259–64.

84 Rowe JM, Rapoport AP, Ryan DH et al. Treatment of chronic myelogenous leukemia with autologous bone marrow transplantation followed by roquinimex. Bone Marrow Transplant 1999; **24**: 1057–63.

85 Carlo-Stella C, Regazzi E, Andrizzi C et al. Use of granulocyte-macrophage colony-stimulating factor (GM-CSF) in combination with hydroxyurea as post-transplant therapy in chronic myelogenous leukemia patients autografted with unmanipulated hematopoietic cells. Haematologica 1997; **82**: 291–6.

86 Deisseroth AB, Zu Z, Claxton D et al. Genetic marking shows that Ph[+] cells present in autologous transplants of chronic myelogenous leukemia (CML) contribute to relapse after autologous bone marrow in CML. Blood 1994; **83**: 3068–76.

87 Clark RE. Antisense therapeutics in chronic myeloid leukaemia: the promise, the progress and the problems. Leukemia 2000; **14**: 347–55.

88 Rowley PT, Kosciolek BA, Kool ET. Circular antisense oligonucleotides inhibit growth of chronic myeloid leukemia cells. Mol Med 1999; **5**: 693–700.

89 Clark RE, Grzybowski J, Broughton CM et al. Clinical use of streptolysin-O to facilitate antisense oligodeoxyribonucleotide delivery for purging autografts in chronic myeloid leukaemia. Bone Marrow Transplant 1999; **23**: 1303–8.

90 Spiller DG, Giles RV, Grzybowski J et al. Improving the intracellular delivery and molecular efficacy of antisense oligonucleotides in chronic myeloid leukemia cells: a comparison of streptolysin-O permeabilization, electroporation, and lipophilic conjugation. Blood 1998; **91**: 4738–46.

91 Snyder DS, Wu Y, McMahon R et al. Ribozyme-mediated inhibition of a Philadelphia chromosome-positive acute lymphoblastic leukemia cell line expressing the p190 bcr-abl oncogene. Biol Blood Marrow Transplant 1997; **3**: 179–84.

92 Zhao RC, McIvor RS, Griffin JD et al. Gene therapy for chronic myelogenous leukemia (CML): a retroviral vector that renders hematopoietic progenitors methotrexate-resistant and CML progenitors functionally normal and nontumorigenic in vivo. Blood 1997; **90**: 4687–98.

93 Scherr M, Battmer K, Winkler T, Heidenreich O, Ganser A, Eder M. Specific inhibition of bcr-abl gene expression by small interfering RNA. Blood 2003; **101**(4): 1566–9.

94 Druker B, Tamura S, Buchdunger E et al. Effects

 by BCR-ABL antisense oligodeoxynucleotides. Science 1991; **253**: 562–5.

of a selective inhibitor of the Abl tyrosine kinase on the growth of *Bcr-Abl* positive cells. *Nature Med* 1996; **2**: 561–6.

95. Wisniewski D, Lambek CL, Liu C *et al*. Characterization of potent inhibitors of the *Bcr-Abl* and the c-kit receptor tyrosine kinases. *Cancer Res* 2002; **62**: 4244–55.

96. Topaly J, Zeller WJ, Fruehauf S. Synergistic activity of the new *ABL*-specific tyrosine kinase inhibitor STI571 and chemotherapeutic drugs on *BCR-ABL*-positive chronic myelogenous leukemia cells. *Leukemia* 2001; **15**: 342–7.

97. Thiesing JT, Ohno-Jones S, Kolibaba KS *et al*. Efficacy of STI571, an *abl* tyrosine kinase inhibitor, in conjunction with other antileukemic agents against *bcr-abl*-positive cells. *Blood* 2000; **96**: 3195–9.

98. Bhatia R, Munthe HA, Williams AD *et al*. Increased sensitivity of chronic myelogenous leukemia primitive hematopoietic progenitors to growth factor induced cell division and maturation. *Exp Hematol* 2000; **12**: 1401–12.

99. Cashman J, Clark-Lewis I, Eaves A *et al*. Stromal-derived factor 1 inhibits the cycling of very primitive human hematopoietic cells *in vitro* and in NOD/SCID mice. *Blood* 2002; **99**: 792–9.

100. Cashman JD, Eaves CJ, Sarris AH *et al*. MCP-1, not MIP-1α, is the endogenous chemokine that cooperates with TGF-β to inhibit the cycling of primitive normal but not leukemic (CML) progenitors in long-term human marrow cultures. *Blood* 1998; **92**: 2338–44.

101. Horowitz MM, Gale RP, Sondel PM *et al*. Graft-versus-leukemia reactions after bone marrow transplantation. *Blood* 1990; **75**: 555–62.

102. Gale RP, Horowitz MM, Ash RC *et al*. Identical-twin bone marrow transplants for leukemia. *Ann Intern Med* 1994; **120**: 646–52.

103. Verma UN, Bagg A, Brown E *et al*. Interleukin-2 activation of human bone marrow in long-term cultures: an effective strategy for purging and generation of anti-tumor cytotoxic effectors. *Bone Marrow Transplant* 1994; **13**: 115–23.

104. Klingemann HG, Neerunjun J, Schwulera U *et al*. Culture of normal and leukemic bone marrow in interleukin-2: analysis of cell activation, cell proliferation, and cytokine production. *Leukemia* 1993; **7**: 1389–93.

105. Hoyle C, Bangs CD, Chang P *et al*. Expansion of Philadelphia chromosome-negative CD3+ CD56+ cytotoxic cells from chronic myeloid leukemia patients: *in vitro* and *in vivo* efficacy in severe combined immunodeficiency disease mice. *Blood* 1998; **92**: 3318–27.

106. Cervantes F, Pierson BA, McGlave PB *et al*. Autologous activated natural killer cells suppress primitive chronic myelogenous leukemia progenitors in long-term culture. *Blood* 1996; **87**: 2476–85.

107. Miller JS. The biology of natural killer cells in cancer, infection, and pregnancy. *Exp Hematol* 2001; **29**: 1157–68.

108. Cheever MA, Chen W, Disis ML *et al*. T-cell immunity to oncogenic proteins including mutated ras and chimeric *bcr-abl*. *Ann N Y Acad Sci* 1993; **690**: 101–12.

109. ten Bosch GJ, Toornvliet AC, Friede T *et al*. Recognition of peptides corresponding to the joining region of p210$^{BCR-ABL}$ protein by human T cells. *Leukemia* 1995; **9**: 1344–8.

110. Greco G, Fruci D, Accapezzato D *et al*. Two *bcr-abl* junction peptides bind HLA-A3 molecules and allow specific induction of human cytotoxic T lymphocytes. *Leukemia* 1996; **10**: 693–9.

111. Bocchia M, Korontsvit T, Xu Q *et al*. Specific human cellular immunity to *bcr-abl* oncogene-derived peptides. *Blood* 1996; **87**: 3587–92.

112. Pawelec G, Max H, Halder T *et al*. *BCR/ABL* leukemia oncogene fusion peptides selectively bind to certain *HLA-DR* alleles and can be recognized by T cells found at low frequency in the repertoire of normal donors. *Blood* 1996; **88**: 2118–24.

113. Mannering SI, McKenzie JL, Fearnley DB *et al*. *HLA-DR1*-restricted *bcr-abl* (b3a2)-specific CD4+ T lymphocytes respond to dendritic cells pulsed with b3a2 peptide and antigen-presenting cells exposed to b3a2 containing cell lysates. *Blood* 1997; **90**: 290–7.

114. Norbury LC, Clark RE, Christmas SE. $\beta_3\alpha_2$ *BCR-ABL* fusion peptides as targets for cytotoxic T cells in chronic myeloid leukaemia. *Br J Haematol* 2000; **109**: 616–21.

115. Pinilla-Ibarz J, Cathcart K, Korontsvit T *et al*. Vaccination of patients with chronic myelogenous leukemia with *bcr-abl* oncogene breakpoint fusion peptides generates specific immune responses. *Blood* 2000; **95**: 1781–7.

116. Osman Y, Takahashi M, Zheng Z *et al*. Generation of *bcr-abl* specific cytotoxic T-lymphocytes by using dendritic cells pulsed with *bcr-abl* ($\beta_3\alpha_2$) peptide: its applicability for donor leukocyte transfusions in marrow grafted CML patients. *Leukemia* 1999; **13**: 166–74.

117. Clark RE, Dodi IA, Hill SC *et al*. Direct evidence that leukemic cells present HLA-associated immunogenic peptides derived from the BCR-ABL$\beta_3\alpha_2$ fusion protein. *Blood* 2001; **98**: 2887–93.

118. Cheever MA, Disis ML, Bernhard H *et al*. Immunity to oncogenic proteins. *Immunol Rev* 1995; **145**: 33–59.

119. Gao L, Bellantuono I, Elsasser A *et al*. Selective elimination of leukemic CD34+ progenitor cells by cytotoxic T lymphocytes specific for *WT1*. *Blood* 2000; **95**: 2198–203.

120. Bellantuono I, Gao L, Parry S *et al*. Two distinct HLA-A0201-presented epitopes of the Wilms' tumor antigen 1 can function as targets for leukemia-reactive CTL. *Blood* 2002; **100**: 3835–7.

121. Yang XF, Wu CJ, McLaughlin S *et al*. CML66, a broadly immunogenic tumor antigen, elicits a humoral immune response associated with remission of chronic myelogenous leukemia. *Proc Natl Acad Sci U S A* 2001; **98**: 7492–7.

122. Molldrem JJ, Lee PP, Wang C *et al*. Evidence that specific T lymphocytes may participate in the elimination of chronic myelogenous leukemia. *Nat Med* 2000; **6**: 1018–23.

123. Molldrem JJ, Lee PP, Wang C *et al*. A PR1-human leukocyte antigen-A$_2$ tetramer can be used to isolate low-frequency cytotoxic T lymphocytes from healthy donors that selectively lyse chronic myelogenous leukemia. *Cancer Res* 1999; **59**: 2675–81.

124. Molldrem JJ, Clave E, Jiang YZ *et al*. Cytotoxic T lymphocytes specific for a nonpolymorphic proteinase 3 peptide preferentially inhibit chronic myeloid leukemia colony-forming units. *Blood* 1997; **90**: 2529–34.

125. Smit WM, Rijnbeek M, Van Bergen CA *et al*. Generation of dendritic cells expressing *bcr-abl* from CD34-positive chronic myeloid leukemia precursor cells. *Hum Immunol* 1997; **53**: 216–23.

126. Heinzinger M, Waller CF, von den Berg A *et al*. Generation of dendritic cells from patients with chronic myelogenous leukemia. *Ann Hematol* 1999; **78**: 181–6.

127. Zheng C, Pisa P, Stromberg O *et al*. Generation of dendritic cells from peripheral blood of patients at different stages of chronic myeloid leukemia. *Med Oncol* 2000; **17**: 270–8.

128. Choudhury A, Gajewski JL, Liang JC *et al*. Use of leukemic dendritic cells for the generation of antileukemic cellular cytotoxicity against Philadelphia chromosome-positive chronic myelogenous leukemia. *Blood* 1997; **89**: 1133–42.

129. Muller L, Provenzani C, Pawelec G. Generation of chronic myelogenous leukemia-specific T cells in cytokine-modified autologous mixed lymphocyte/tumor cell cultures. *J Immunother* 2001; **24**: 482–92.

130. Wang C, Al-Omar HM, Radvanyi L *et al*. Clonal heterogeneity of dendritic cells derived from patients with chronic myeloid leukemia and enhancement of their T-cells stimulatory activity by IFN-α. *Exp Hematol* 1999; **27**: 1176–84.

131. Dietz AB, Bulur PA, Erickson MR *et al*. Optimizing preparation of normal dendritic cells and *bcr-abl*+ mature dendritic cells derived from immunomagnetically purified CD14+ cells. *J Hemather Stem Cell Res* 2000; **9**: 95–101.

132. Westermann J, Kopp J, Korner I *et al*. Bcr/abl+ autologous dendritic cells for vaccination in chronic myeloid leukemia. *Bone Marrow Transplant* 2000; **25** (Suppl. 2): S46–9.

133. Fujii S, Shimizu K, Fujimoto K *et al*. Analysis of a chronic myelogenous leukemia patient vaccinated with leukemic dendritic cells following autologous peripheral blood stem cell transplantation. *Jpn J Cancer Res* 1999; **90**: 1117–29.

134. Sun JY, Krouse RS, Forman SJ *et al*. Immunogenicity of a p210$^{BCR-ABL}$ fusion domain candidate DNA vaccine targeted to dendritic cells by a recombinant adeno-associated virus vector *in vitro*. *Cancer Res* 2002; **62**: 3175–83.

135. Kantarjian HM, O'Brien S, Cortes JE *et al*. Imatinib mesylate therapy for relapse after allogeneic stem cell transplantation for chronic myelogenous leukemia. *Blood* 2002; **100**: 1590–5.

136. McGlave PB, de Fabritiis P, Deisseroth A *et al*. Autologous transplants for chronic myelogenous leukaemia: results from eight transplant groups. *Lancet* 1994; **343**: 1486–8.

137. Bhatia R, Verfaillie CM, Miller JS, McGlave PB. Autologous transplantation therapy for chronic myelogenous leukemia. *Blood* 1997; **89**(8): 2623–34.

92 Laurence Catley & Kenneth Anderson

Autologous Hematopoietic Cell Transplantation for Multiple Myeloma

Multiple myeloma is a malignant hematologic disorder that until now has remained almost universally fatal. The overall median survival is 3 years. It represents approximately 1% of all malignancies and 13% of hematologic malignancies in adults. In the USA about 13,200 cases of myeloma were diagnosed in the year 2000, and 11,200 people died from the disease. The incidence of myeloma increases with age. The mean age of affected men is 62 years (75% aged <70 years) and for women 61 years (79% aged <70 years). The National Cancer Institute (NCI) Surveillance, Epidemiology and End Results (SEER) [1] program reports that age-adjusted incidence between 1973 and 1999 was 5.6 cases/100,000 for all races. The incidence was lower in the white population at 5.1/100,000 than the black population at 11.5/100,000. The incidence is slightly higher in males than females, but lower in American Indians, Alaskan natives, Asians or Pacific Islanders.

Biology of multiple myeloma

The causes of multiple myeloma remain unknown, but there is evidence that the pathogenesis of multiple myeloma is a multistep process [2]. The malignant cells are derived from plasma cells that have undergone the processes of somatic hypermutation and isotype switch recombination in the germinal centers of lymph nodes, but have subsequently migrated and expanded in the bone marrow. Genetic abnormalities are common and varied. Illegitimate switch recombination (recombination events containing sequences from only one switch region) involving the immunoglobulin heavy chain (IgH) switch region appears to be the most frequent genetic abnormality in multiple myeloma [3]. Cytogenetics is informative in about 30–50% of patients using metaphase-band karyotyping methods [4,5], but chromosomal aneuploidy has been detected in almost 90% of patients with multiple myeloma using interphase fluorescence *in situ* hybridization (FISH) [6]. Karyotypic 14q32 (IgH locus) translocations have been identified at a variable frequency (10–60% in different studies) but, in the majority of cases, the partner chromosome has not been identified. Illegitimate switch recombinations into the IgH switch regions have been identified in 15 of 21 myeloma cell lines, including seven of eight lines that have been karyotyped without revealing a detectable 14q32 translocation. Abnormalities of specific oncogenes have also been identified. For example, using specific FISH probes, karyotypic abnormalities of the c-*myc* or l-*myc* locus have been identified in 19 of 20 multiple myeloma cell lines, and approximately 50% of advanced primary multiple myeloma tumors [7]. Dysregulation of cyclin D1 occurs in approximately 30% of multiple myeloma tumors in which a 14q32 translocation can be detected [8]. Intrinsic cell survival mechanisms involved in malignant transformation and resistance to drug-induced apoptosis include upregulation of antiapoptotic proteins bcl-xL, bcl-2 and mcl-1 [9], and activation of growth and survival transcription factors nuclear factor kappa B (NF-κB) and Akt via the mitogen-activated protein kinase (MAPK) pathway and phosphatidylinositol 3 (PI3)-kinase signaling. Chemotherapy itself induces drug resistance by activation of NF-κB [10] and upregulation of bcl-2 in multiple myeloma cells [11].

In addition to intrinsic genetic abnormalities in malignant plasma cells, interactions between the malignant plasma cells and the stromal cells of the bone marrow microenvironment have an important role in the proliferation of malignant cells, as well as resistance to drug-induced apoptosis. Multiple myeloma is predominantly localized to the bone marrow, where the malignant plasma cells adhere to bone marrow stromal cells (BMSCs). Molecules on the surface membrane of myeloma cells have an important role in the growth and survival of myeloma cells. β_1 integrins, specifically VLA-4 ($\alpha_4\beta_1$) and VLA-5 ($\alpha_5\beta_1$), are typically expressed on multiple myeloma cells [12]. Adhesion of multiple myeloma cells to the extracellular matrix protein fibronectin via β_1 integrins results in upregulation of the cyclin-dependent kinase inhibitor p27 and cell cycle arrest, increasing resistance to cytotoxic agents such as doxorubicin and melphalan [13]. In addition, β_1 integrin-mediated adhesion of multiple myeloma cells to fibronectin confers protection against drug-induced apoptosis and triggers NF-κB-dependent transcription and secretion of interleukin 6 (IL-6). CD40 is a 45–50-kDa glycoprotein surface membrane molecule originally identified in B lymphocytes and some B-cell malignancies, and has an important role in the proliferation and differentiation of B lymphocytes [14]. CD40 is also expressed on multiple myeloma patient cells and in multiple myeloma cell lines [15–18]. CD40 ligation on multiple myeloma cells upregulates the expression of cell surface accessory molecules, as well as secretion of transforming growth factor-β1 (TGF-β1) [19] and IL-6 [20]. CD40 ligand, present on T cells, increases endogenous IL-6 secretion by multiple myeloma and stromal cells through activation of NF-κB [21], and also increases expression of bcl-2, contributing to drug resistance.

Importantly, when multiple myeloma cells adhere to BMSCs there is a significant upregulation of cytokines such as IL-1β, IL-6 [21,22], TGF-β1 [23], insulin-like growth factor-1 (IGF-1) [24] and vascular endothelial growth factor (VEGF) [25]. IL-6, a very important multiple myeloma growth and survival factor [13,26–29] produced predominantly by BMSCs but also myeloma cells [25], contributes to the development of drug resistance in myeloma [30]. Autocrine stimulation by IL-6 occurs in some cell lines derived from patients with multiple myeloma [31]. High concentrations of IL-6 upregulate bcl-xL [32] through activation of signal transduction and activation of transcription 3 (STAT-3), contributing to resistance against drug-induced apoptosis. VEGF is produced both from BMSCs and multiple myeloma cells, and is important to both plasma cell proliferation and migration [33,34]. VEGF-mediated multiple myeloma cell migration is associated with β_1 integrin- and protein kinase C alpha (PKCα)-dependent PI3-kinase activation, as well as tumor cell proliferation via a PKCα-independent Raf-1–MEK–extracellular signal-regulated protein kinase pathway. TGF-β1 is produced in multiple myeloma by both tumor cells and BMSCs, with related tumor cell growth [23]. IGF-1 is secreted by myeloma cells, and can also act as a growth factor in human multiple myeloma.

IL-1β has osteoclast activating activity, and although not produced by normal plasma cells, is produced by malignant plasma cells in multiple myeloma [35–38]. Osteolytic lesions are a characteristic feature of multiple myeloma, and occur because of an increase in osteoclast activity resulting in increased bone resorption without compensatory new bone formation [39]. Receptor activator of NF-κB (RANK), is expressed by osteoclasts, and upregulation of RANK on osteoclasts occurs in multiple myeloma. RANK ligand (RANKL) overexpression by BMSCs also contributes to the high rate of bone resorption observed in multiple myeloma [40] by binding and activating its receptor, RANK [39]. Myeloma cells also express RANKL [41,42]. Osteoprotegrin (OPG), the inhibitor of RANK, is secreted by BMSCs, but is downregulated in multiple myeloma [40,43]. This myeloma-related stromal cell–osteoclast interaction activates osteoclast activity, resulting in increased osteolysis, while simultaneously contributing to drug resistance in the malignant plasma cells [29].

In addition to contributing to the upregulation of cytokines in multiple myeloma, the malignant plasma cells characteristically produce a single abnormal serum monoclonal protein called paraprotein, or M-protein, which is a type of immunoglobulin with a constant isotype and light-chain restriction. The paraprotein is uniform in migration pattern when subjected to electropheresis. The isotype is IgG in 53% of patients, IgA in 25% and IgD in 1%. Approximately 15% of cases are Bence Jones myeloma, in which immunoglobulin light chain only is expressed by the malignant clone. This light chain can be detected in concentrated urine as Bence Jones protein. Using more sensitive techniques such as nephelometry, the light chain can also be detected in serum [44]. In 1% of cases there is no paraprotein production.

Clinical features

The diagnosis of multiple myeloma can be made in the presence of paraprotein in the serum or urine, lytic bone lesions and >10% plasma cells in the bone marrow smear differential in the absence of causes of secondary marrow plasmacytosis such as ongoing infection or an autoimmune process. The clinical manifestations of multiple myeloma result predominantly from marrow failure, immunosuppression, lytic lesions of the axial skeleton and long bones, and renal failure. The immunosuppression is multifactorial in etiology, resulting from neutropenia, poor antigen-presenting cell function and T-cell function, together with reduced production of normal immunoglobulin and poor immunoglobulin function in the presence of paraprotein. The overgrowth of myeloma cells in the bone marrow results in marrow failure. Thus, defects of both innate and acquired immunity occur. Renal failure occurs in nearly 25% of myeloma patients, brought about by deposition in the kidney of abnormal light chain, cryoglobulin, amyloid, infection, urate nephropathy, hypercalcemia and hyperviscosity. Anemia develops in the majority of myeloma patients, secondary to plasma cell infiltration of the marrow and anemia of chronic disease. Hyperviscosity is sometimes present secondary to high paraprotein levels.

Multiple myeloma is often preceded by a premalignant monoclonal expansion of plasma cells called monoclonal gammopathy of undetermined significance (MGUS). MGUS is diagnosed when a paraprotein is detected during routine testing or during investigation of an unrelated disorder but other criteria for myeloma are not met. MGUS is reported to be present in 1% of the adult population aged >50 years, increasing to 10% of adults aged >75 years. The risk of progression from MGUS to multiple myeloma or related disorders is about 1% per year [45]. There is currently no reliable method to predict who will go on to develop myeloma, or how to prevent this progression.

Staging and prognosis

Untreated, the average survival of patients with multiple myeloma is approximately 6 months. Since the introduction of melphalan and glucocorticoid steroids in the 1960s, the average survival with treatment has been extended to 3 years. Various prognostic factors have been identified. The Durie–Salmon staging system devised in 1975 was based upon parameters of tumor burden [46]. Patients with stage IA had a low tumor burden, and a median survival of more than 5 years, compared to those with stage IIIB, who had a high tumor burden and a median survival of about 15 months. β_2-microglobulin, the light chain of the class I major histocompatibility antigen, has been of major prognostic significance, but only during the first 2 years of follow-up, and it did not provide a good predictor for long-term survival [47,48]. The combination of C-reactive protein (CRP) and β_2-microglobulin was also of prognostic importance. The median duration of survival was 6 months for patients with CRP and β_2-microglobulin >6 mg/L, but 54 months when both values were <6 mg/L.

Over the last two decades, advances in biologic techniques have allowed for subgroup analysis based upon chromosomal abnormalities detected by metaphase karyotype and interphase FISH. Cytogenetic analyses have been useful prognostic indicators. The Groupe Française de Cytogenetique Hematologique reviewed conventional metaphase banding karyotype analyses performed in 208 patients with multiple myeloma before treatment with either conventional therapy (137 patients) or autologous hematopoietic cell transplantation (AHCT) (71 patients). A total of 138 (66%) patients displayed complex chromosomal abnormalities. A multivariate analysis including stage, β_2-microglobulin, bone marrow plasmacytosis, treatment type, chromosome 13q abnormalities, hyperdiploidy and hypodiploidy showed that a hypodiploid karyotype was the first independent factor for overall survival ($p < 0.001$), followed by treatment approach [49].

The true incidence of chromosomal abnormalities in multiple myeloma is much higher than that detected by metaphase analysis. Whereas metaphase cytogenetics is informative in about 30–50% of patients, FISH explores 100% of patients [4,5]. Using interphase FISH, chromosomal aneuploidy has been detected in almost 90% of patients with multiple myeloma [6]. Cytogenetic analysis using interphase FISH does not require cellular mitosis, and is therefore not influenced by the proliferative properties of the cell population. Therefore, although it has been demonstrated that some chromosomal abnormalities correlate with a short survival, especially chromosomal 13 abnormalities and hypodiploidy, these studies may not reflect the prognostic value of the sole chromosomal changes, but also include prognostic value of proliferation because metaphase analyses are acquired while cells pass through mitosis. The routine use of FISH should therefore increase the specificity as well as the sensitivity of cytogenetic analysis with regard to providing prognostic information.

Interphase FISH analysis with selected probes has helped to define prognostic subgroups. Investigators from Austria have reported that 13q14 deletion by FISH was associated with a significantly lower rate of response to conventional dose chemotherapy of 40.8% compared with 78.6% ($p = 0.009$) and a shorter overall survival of 24.2 months compared with >60 months ($p < 0.005$) in patients without the deletion [50]. Patients with a 13q14 deletion were more likely to have stage III disease ($p = 0.022$), higher serum levels of β_2-microglobulin ($p = 0.059$) and a higher percentage of bone marrow plasma cells ($p = 0.085$) than patients with a normal 13q14 status. Although correlated with increased proliferative activity, deletions of 13q14 represented an independent adverse prognostic feature in multiple myeloma. Interphase FISH for 17p13 and 11q also provided prognostically relevant information in addition to that provided by standard prognostic factors for patients with multiple myeloma who were treated with conventional-dose chemotherapy [51]. By FISH, the deletion of 13q14 occurred in 40 patients (44.9%), deletion of 17p13 in 22 (24.7%) and 11q abnormalities in 14 (15.7%; including seven with t[11;14]). Associations with poor response to induction treatment, and with short median overall survival times, included deletions of 13q14 and 17p13. Short median overall time was also observed for patients with 11q abnormalities. According to the number of unfavorable cytogenetic features (deletion of 13q14, deletion of 17p13 and aberrations of 11q) that were present in each patient (0, 1, 2 or 3), patients with significantly different overall times could be discriminated from one another (102.4 vs. 29.6 vs. 13.9 months, respectively; $p < 0.001$).

Response to chemotherapy has also been identified as an important prognostic indicator. Patients with a rapid response to therapy and a high plasma cell labeling index had a much shorter duration of response and survival [52]. For example, patients whose M-protein value decreased by ≥ 0.6 g/dL within 2 months after beginning chemotherapy had a median survival of 13 months [53]. In combination with the development of new therapies, and in particular high-dose therapy and autologous hematopoietic cell rescue, more prognostic information has been documented and is discussed below.

Conventional chemotherapy

Since the 1960s, when the introduction of melphalan in combination with glucocorticoid steroids extended the median survival of multiple myeloma from 6 months to 3 years, melphalan has remained an important first-line treatment option for multiple myeloma. Melphalan is a bifunctional nitrogen mustard-derived alkylating agent, and the L-isomer of the phenylalanine derivative of mechlorethamine [54–57]. As an alkylating agent, melphalan interferes with DNA replication and RNA transcription, and ultimately results in the disruption of nucleic acid function. Absorption of melphalan from the gut is incomplete and extremely variable. The pharmacokinetics of orally administered melphalan have been studied extensively in adults [54–57]. Oral bioavailability is variable, and low oral bioavailability is a result of poor absorption from the gut [58,59]. The areas under the plasma concentration–time curves following oral administration are 25–89% of those following intravenous administration. Melphalan is 60–90% bound to plasma proteins, mainly albumin and to a lesser extent to α1-acid glycoprotein, but interactions between melphalan and immunoglobulins are negligible. The cellular uptake of melphalan appears to occur by an active transport system [60–62]. Melphalan undergoes rapid chemical degradation and has little if any active metabolism [59]. Inactive mono- and dihydroxy metabolites appear in plasma within minutes of drug administration. Twenty to 50 percent of the orally administered dose of melphalan is excreted in feces within 6 days but no melphalan, or melphalan derivatives, are found in the gut after intravenous administration [63]. About 20–35% of an oral dose is excreted in urine as the drug and its inactive metabolites within 24 h, and approximately 10% is excreted in urine unchanged within 24 h. At conventional low doses of melphalan, such as the commonly used schedule of 0.15–0.25 mg/kg over 4 days every 4–6 weeks, the dose-limiting toxicity is bone marrow suppression. Because of the variability of oral bioavailability, peripheral blood examination is commonly performed 3 weeks after administration to determine biologic activity and adjust the dose if necessary.

Although conventional oral therapy with melphalan and prednisone has extended the median survival of multiple myeloma, the response rates to melphalan and prednisone have been only 50–60%. Complete remissions are rare, and myeloma remains incurable with conventional chemotherapy. Cellular drug efflux mediated by P-glycoprotein [64], as well as decreased cellular uptake [65] appear to contribute to mechanisms of melphalan resistance in malignant cells. Infusional vincristine, Adriamycin and dexamethasone (VAD) was introduced in 1984 in an attempt to overcome drug resistance by using prolonged infusions of combination chemotherapy [66]. The VAD regimen consisted of daily doses of 0.4 mg vincristine and 9 mg/m^2 doxorubicin by intravenous infusion for 4 consecutive days, and 40 mg dexamethasone given orally on days 1–4 on even cycles and on days 1–4, 9–12 and 17–20 on odd cycles of VAD. Approximately 50% of patients with alkylating agent-resistant myeloma achieved a marked and rapid tumor cytoreduction of 75–90% after treatment with VAD. In patients with refractory multiple myeloma, intermittent high-dose dexamethasone achieved a response rate of 27%, similar to that achieved with the VAD regimen [67]. However, among patients who were relapsing, VAD chemotherapy induced remissions in 11 of 17 patients (65%), whereas dexamethasone alone induced remissions in only four of 19 patients (21%). The median survival of 22 months in all patients responding to either treatment was longer than that from any previous program for treatment of resistant myeloma.

Other investigators have since reported objective response rates between 40% and 70% with high-dose glucocorticoids in combination with vincristine and Adriamycin [68–71]. As with oral melphalan and prednisone, hematologic toxicity was also dose-limiting in the VAD regimen, but significant nonhematologic toxicity was also observed, in particular neurotoxicity, alopecia and infusion-site thrombophlebitis. Neither overall response rates to induction chemotherapy nor overall survival has been significantly improved with VAD or other forms of infusion chemotherapy compared to melphalan and prednisone. In 1998, an overview of 6633 patients from 27 randomized trials found no difference, either overall or within any subgroup, in mortality between combination chemotherapy vs. melphalan and prednisone [72]. The 5-year survival rate reported in the SEER database remains unchanged at 28%. Although VAD is commonly used prior to autologous harvest and hematopoietic cell transplantation, there is also evidence that dexamethasone alone is almost as effective as VAD [68], and some centers now commence therapy with dexamethasone alone to avoid the increased toxicity of vincristine and Adriamycin.

To assess high-dose therapy in multiple myeloma in a randomized setting, the first major studies included established conventional chemotherapy regimens such as oral melphalan and prednisone, or alternating cycles of combinations of chemotherapeutic agents such as VMCP and BVAP [73]. The VMCP regimen included 1 mg vincristine intravenously on day 1, 5 mg/m^2 melphalan orally days 1–4, 110 mg/m^2 cyclophosphamide orally on days 1–4 and 60 mg/m^2 prednisone orally on days 1–4. The BVAP regimen included 1 mg vincristine intravenously on day 1, 30 mg/m^2 carmustine intravenously on day 1, 30 mg/m^2 doxorubicin intravenously on day 1 and 60 mg/m^2 prednisone orally on days 1–4. These alternating cycles of VMCP and BVAP were administered at 3-week intervals for 12 months. Other combinations used have included BCNU, vincristine, melphalan, cyclophosphamide, prednisone; vincristine, BCNU, Adriamycin, dexamethasone (BVMCP/VBAD); cyclophosphamide, vincristine, doxorubicin, methylprednisolone (C-VAMP); Adriamycin, BCNU, cyclophosphamide and melphalan (ABCM); or vincristine, Adriamycin and dexamethasone (VAD) [73–77]. These regimens have been compared to high-dose therapy and AHCT. In subsequent randomized studies comparing single transplantation to tandem transplantation, VAD [78–82], or a VAD-like regimen [83], has been predominantly used as induction therapy prior to high-dose therapy.

The use of thalidomide to treat multiple myeloma has become increasingly common in recent years. Thalidomide as salvage post-AHCT for multiple myeloma has resulted in a total response rate of 32% [84,85]. As induction therapy, in 28 patients with previously untreated asymptomatic myeloma, and in 40 consecutive patients with previously untreated symptomatic myeloma treated with thalidomide in addition to dexamethasone for at least 3 months, the response rate was 36% for patients treated with thalidomide alone and 72% for patients treated with thalidomide with dexamethasone, the latter including complete remission in 16% of patients [86]. The median time to remission was 4.2 months with thalidomide alone and 0.7 months with thalidomide/dexamethasone. In addition, thalidomide in combination with dexamethasone has been used during induction therapy to overcome early drug resistance prior to high-dose therapy [87] without impairing subsequent hematopoietic cell collection [88]. A total of 32 of 50 patients (64%) responded to dexamethasone in combination with thalidomide, and 31 patients (62%) proceeded to hematopoietic cell collection after four cycles of therapy [89]. Therefore, the use of thalidomide before or after AHCT, alone or in combination with dexamethasone, appears at least as effective as the more established cytotoxic therapies, without negatively affecting subsequent hematopoietic cell mobilization and harvest. A randomized trial is currently accruing patients to directly compare the relative efficacy of thalidomide with or without dexamethasone as initial therapy prior to AHCT for multiple myeloma [89]. However, the results of this trial should be examined before the combination of thalidomide and dexamethasone can be regarded as first-line therapy.

There is evidence to support the concept that alkylating agents may adversely affect peripheral blood hematopoietic cell (PBHC) mobilization, and that duration of therapy may adversely affect subsequent progenitor cell harvest and post-AHCT engraftment [90–92]. Prolonged exposure to chemotherapy is generally avoided prior to transplantation because of potential toxicity to hematopoietic cells and subsequent difficulty with hematopoietic cell harvesting and engraftment (see section on Source of hematopoietic stem cells). The use of nonalkylating agent-containing regimens such as VAD, dexamethasone alone, or the combination of thalidomide and dexamethasone should be considered for multiple myeloma patients who are potential candidates for high-dose intensified chemotherapy. As an alternative, PBHC should be collected early from patients who may eventually be treated with oral or intravenous melphalan so that effective salvage treatment can be performed at a later stage.

In the 1990s there have been significant improvements in supportive care. The widespread use of bisphosphonates, in particular pamidronate, has been shown to significantly reduce the rate of skeletal events in patients with multiple myeloma, as well as effectively treat hypercalcemia, reduce bone pain and improve quality of life [93–97]. Newer, more potent bisphosphonates are currently being explored [98]. Erythropoietin is being used increasingly, and reduces transfusion requirements in patients with multiple myeloma and anemia [99–102]. Kyphoplasty is a recently developed surgical technique, which has significantly improved the quality of life for patients with compression fractures and multiple myeloma [103]. However, myeloma has remained mostly incurable, apart from the few patients who have been cured by allogeneic transplantation (see Chapter 80).

High-dose therapy

The conventional standard dose of oral or intravenous melphalan is usually about 0.25 mg/kg for 4 days every 4–6 weeks. At these doses, peak melphalan plasma concentrations of 0.625 μM are achieved. The availability of intravenous melphalan made dose escalation possible. Dose escalation to >100 mg/m^2 results in peak concentrations of 40–50 μM [57,104,105]. The principal toxicities in patients receiving >100 mg/m^2 of intravenous melphalan are mucositis, colitis and diarrhea. Melphalan doses up to 290 mg/m^2 have been associated with severe nausea, vomiting, mouth ulceration, decreased consciousness, seizures, muscular paralysis and cholinomimetic effects. The maximum doses used in the high-dose setting are generally around 200 mg/m^2.

High-dose therapy using melphalan without autologous marrow support for multiple myeloma was first reported in 1983 by the Royal Marsden Hospital in London [106]. This regimen was associated with some complete remissions. One previously untreated patient with plasma-cell leukemia and eight patients with myeloma (four previously untreated) were given high-dose 100–140 mg/m^2 melphalan intravenously. All patients responded to the treatment. Three of the five previously untreated patients achieved complete biochemical and bone marrow remissions. Subsequently, autologous marrow support was added to the regimen to reduce toxicity, and the treatment was intensified by the addition of 850 cGy total body irradiation (TBI) [107]. High-dose 140 mg/m^2 melphalan was later evaluated in 58 patients under the age of 63 years with multiple myeloma [108]. Among previously untreated patients 11 of 41 (27%) entered a complete remission and 21 (51%) entered a partial remission, which lasted a median of 19 months. In a subsequent study, high-dose 1 g/m^2 methyl prednisolone daily for 5 days was added to high-dose melphalan but response rates were similar. Profound myelosuppression, moderate nausea, vomiting, mucositis and diarrhea with reversible alopecia occurred in all patients.

During the 1980s, hematopoietic support using allogeneic marrow transplantation did result in some cures, but was associated with a very high early mortality of >40% [109]. By contrast, autologous transplantation was much safer, with a treatment-related mortality of <10%, and was more readily available. Therefore, in the last 15 years high-dose chemotherapy with autologous hematopoietic rescue has become a common procedure for eligible patients with this disease, and multiple myeloma has become the second most common indication for autologous transplantation after non-Hodgkin's lymphoma [110–113].

Over the last two decades, many different conditioning regimens (high-dose chemotherapy combinations) have been assessed for the treatment of multiple myeloma. High-dose 140 mg/m^2 melphalan plus 8 Gy TBI was used as the conditioning regimen in the Intergroupe Français du Myélome (IFM90) randomized multicenter trial to compare conventional chemotherapy to high-dose therapy and autologous transplantation, and was associated with an early mortality of only 2.7%. By contrast, a more intensive schedule investigated in Toronto, using 160 mg/m^2 melphalan with 12 Gy fractionated TBI and 60 mg/kg etoposide was associated with a 100-day treatment-related mortality of 12%. This early mortality predominantly reflected the development of interstitial pneumonitis in 28% of patients, of whom seven of 28 (25%) died. In a nonrandomized trial with 5 years' follow-up, there was increased morbidity and mortality without increasing overall survival beyond that reported with less toxic regimens [114].

In 1994, the Royal Marsden Group reported a 70% complete remission rate with low extrahematologic toxicity in newly diagnosed patients treated with high-dose 200 mg/m^2 melphalan [115]. This conditioning regimen has been used increasingly during the 1990s. The Spanish registry reported 259 patients treated between January 1989 and November 1995 with myeloablative high-dose therapy followed by autologous PBHC transplantation [116]. The conditioning regimens consisted of high-dose melphalan alone in 37% patients, melphalan plus TBI in 28%, busulfan plus melphalan in 22%, busulfan plus cyclophosphamide in 10% and cyclophosphamide plus TBI in 3%. There were 4% toxic deaths. The only independent factors associated with a longer survival were the number of chemotherapy courses prior to autologous PBHC transplantation and the pretransplantation response status. The conditioning regimen

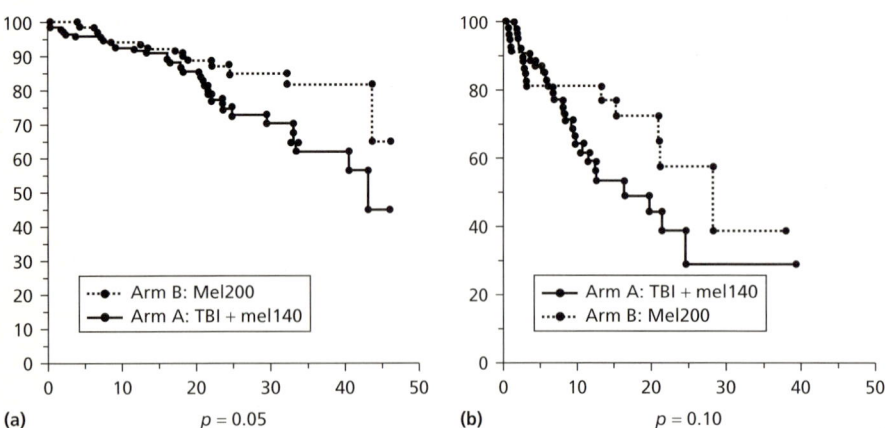

Fig. 92.1 (a) IFM95 comparison of 200 mg/m² melphalan vs. 8 Gy total body irradiation (TBI) plus 140 mg/m² melphalan as conditioning regimens: overall survival according to treatment arm. The 45-month survival was 65.8% in arm B vs. 45.5% in arm A ($p = 0.05$). (From [120] with permission.) (b) IFM95: overall survival after relapse according to treatment arm. There was a trend toward a better outcome for patients treated with 200 mg/m² melphalan compared with 8 Gy TBI plus 140 mg/m² melphalan as conditioning regimens. Post-relapse treatment was not standardized. Half the patients in arm B received a second cycle of intensive therapy with autologous hematopoietic cell transplantation (AHCT), compared with only 25% in arm A. (From [120] with permission.)

and method of stem cell mobilization had no significant impact on overall survival and progression-free survival. Of 248 patients evaluable, 51% had a complete remission and 40% had a partial response. The median duration of progression-free survival and overall survival after transplantation was 23 and 35 months, respectively. An update in 2000 showed that between 1991 and 1999 the proportion of patients receiving high-dose melphalan alone had increased to 52%, compared to melphalan plus TBI in 17%, busulfan plus melphalan in 23%, busulfan plus cyclophosphamide in 4% and cyclophosphamide plus TBI in 3% [117]. The median duration of overall survival and progression-free survival after transplantation was 47 months and 37 months, respectively. Significant factors affecting overall survival and progression-free survival were low β_2-microglobulin at diagnosis, <2 lines of chemotherapy pretransplant, <12 months from diagnosis, complete response after transplantation and interferon maintenance post-transplant.

The main high-dose chemoradiotherapy regimens used in the Spanish registry have been compared in a retrospective analysis [118,119]. A total of 472 myeloma patients treated with 200 mg/m² melphalan (MEL200), 135 patients treated with 140 mg/m² melphalan plus TBI (MEL140 + TBI), 186 patients treated with 12 mg/kg busulfan plus 140 mg/m² melphalan (BU/MEL) and 28 patients treated with 14 mg/kg busulfan followed by cyclophosphamide 120 mg/kg (BU/CY) were evaluated. There were no significant differences with respect to either transplant-related mortality or hematologic recovery between the four conditioning regimens. In patients with measurable disease at time of transplantation, BU/MEL achieved a 51% complete remission vs. 31–43% in the other groups ($p = 0.007$). The response rate for patients in partial response at the time of AHCT was 100% with BU/MEL vs. 93–86% in the other groups, which was statistically significant. The median overall survival for the BU/MEL group was 57 months, vs. 45 months for the MEL200 group and 39 months for the MEL140 + TBI and BU/CY groups. The median event-free survival was longer in the BU/MEL group at 30 months vs. 22 months in the MEL200 group, 23 months in the BU/CY group and 20 months in the MEL140 + TBI groups. The differences in overall and event-free survival did not reach statistical significance in either the univariate analysis or the multivariate analysis adjusted with other prognostic factors. The investigators concluded that the four different conditioning regimens, commonly used for AHCT in multiple myeloma, had similar antimyeloma activities, but that the trend for better results observed with BUMEL warranted a prospective trial.

In 1995 the French group, Intergroupe Français du Myélome (IFM) group, initiated a randomized study comparing high-dose 200 mg/m² melphalan vs. high-dose 140 mg/m² melphalan plus TBI in 282 patients with newly diagnosed multiple myeloma [120]. High-dose 200 mg/m² melphalan was significantly less toxic, and was associated with a shorter duration of neutropenia and thrombocytopenia, a lower incidence of grade ≥3 mucositis, and no toxic deaths vs. five deaths in the TBI group. Although the response rates and the event-free survival were identical, overall survival was superior in the high-dose 200 mg/m² melphalan group, apparently because of a better salvage after relapse (Fig. 92.1a,b). Current evidence therefore supports the use of high-dose 200 mg/m² melphalan in preference to high-dose 140 mg/m² melphalan plus TBI as the conditioning regimen for AHCT in multiple myeloma.

In nonrandomized retrospective analyses, however, the Italian Multiple Myeloma Study Group (MMSG) has compared 100 mg/m² vs. 200 mg/m² melphalan as consolidation after induction therapy [121]. Eighty-one patients enrolled from diagnosis, with a median age of 63 years, were treated with 100 mg/m² melphalan as initial consolidation therapy, and compared with 81 pair mates with a median age of 50 years treated with 200 mg/m² melphalan. The treatment-related mortality was comparable at 4% and 7%, complete remission 43% vs. 63%, event-free survival 30.4 months vs. 32.6 months and overall survival 56.8 months vs. 52.5 months, respectively. Therefore, although 100 mg/m² melphalan appears to be associated with a lower rate of complete remission, in terms of overall survival it may be as effective as 200 mg/m² melphalan. The results of the study also suggest that older patients can be safely treated with 100 mg/m² melphalan, with equivalent efficacy to 200 mg/m² melphalan. However, the data are from a nonrandomized retrospective case-match investigation, and should be confirmed with an appropriate prospective randomized trial to show that these two doses are equivalent for treatment of multiple myeloma.

The combination of melphalan and busulfan has also been reported from Italy, with a complete remission rate of 31% [122]. After a median follow-up of 55 months, the median duration of event-free survival and overall survival was 21 and 57 months, respectively, with a 24% and 48% probability of being event-free and alive after 6 years. A number of other non-TBI-containing regimens have been reported. The combination of 42 mg/m² idarubicin, 16 mg/kg busulfan and 60 mg/m² melphalan as a conditioning regimen has been used to treat to 28 patients (median age 55 years) with chemosensitive disease, followed by AHCT and subcutaneous recombinant granulocyte colony-stimulating factor (G-CSF) until neutrophil recovery [123,124]. The most severe toxicity was oral mucositis, which resolved with hematopoietic reconstitution. The overall response and complete remission rate was 52% and 40%, respectively. Thirty-six patients were alive and 19 were progression-free at a median of 20 months (range 12–36 months) from transplantation. The 3-year projected probability of progression-free survival for patients transplanted after first-line treatment was 60%. A prospective multicenter randomized study of the European Organization for Research and Treatment of Cancer–Gruppo Italiano Malattie Ematologiche Maligne dell'Adulto

Table 92.1 Trials of high-dose therapy conditioning regimens.

	Number of patients	Complete remission (%)	Median overall survival (months)
Comparative studies			
Mel 140 mg/m^2 + 8 Gy TBI *vs.* Mel 200 mg/m^2 [120]*	282	43 vs. 55	43 vs. not reached
Mel 100 mg/m^2 *vs.* Mel 200 mg/m^2 [121]†	162	43 vs. 63	56.8 vs. 52.5
Non-comparative controlled studies			
Thiotepa 750 mg/m^2 + BU 10 mg/kg + CY 120 mg/m^2 [126]	120	52, 5‡	48, 35‡
Mel 60 mg/kg + BU 16 mg/kg [122]	52	31	57
Mel 180 mg/m^2 + Mitoxantrone 60 mg/m^2 [125]	20	40	44.6
Ida 42 mg/m^2 + BU 16 mg/kg + Mel 60 mg/m^2 [123,124]	28	40	Short follow-up

BU, busulphan; CY, cyclophosphamide; Ida, idarubicin; Mel, melphalan; TBI, total body irradiation.
*Prospective randomized trial.
†Nonrandomized pair-mate analysis.
‡Outcomes for chemosensitive and primary refractory disease, respectively.

(EORTC-GIMEMA) cooperative group is currently accruing patients to evaluate the efficacy of busulfan and melphalan vs. busulfan and melphalan in combination with idarubicin.

High-dose cyclophosphamide, etoposide, mitoxantrone and melphalan have been used in 20 patients, with a response rate of 90% and complete remission rate of 40%. At 40 months follow-up the event-free survival and overall survival was 25.5 and 44.6 months, respectively [125]. Thiotepa 250 mg/m^2 for 3 days, 10 mg/kg busulfan and 120 mg/kg cyclophosphamide with mesna (TBC) has been evaluated for efficacy and safety prior to autologous hematopoietic cell transplantation in 120 patients with multiple myeloma [126]. Fifty-four patients had chemosensitive disease and 66 had refractory disease at the time of transplantation. The overall response rate was 81% and the complete remission rate was 26%. Patients with chemosensitive disease had a complete remission rate of 52% vs. 5% for patients with refractory disease. By multivariable analysis, disease status at transplantation was the factor most likely associated with long survival. The estimated median survival was 48, 35 and 9 months for patients with chemosensitive, primary refractory or refractory relapse disease, respectively. Treatment-related mortality was 5%. Therefore, comparisons between TBC and other alternative regimens in prospective studies appear warranted.

The feasibility of two consecutive AHCTs (tandem transplantation) to increase response rates and improve overall survival in multiple myeloma was demonstrated in the early 1990s [127]. The European Bone Marrow Transplant (EMBT) Myeloma Registry, established in 1987, contains data on more than 8000 AHCTs performed since 1983, and supports the use of non-TBI-containing regimens in tandem transplantation [109,128]. In an historical comparison, melphalan alone in tandem transplants has been superior to combinations with either TBI or cyclophosphamide in the second of the tandem transplants [129]. At present, investigators in Europe are accumulating follow-up data from four major prospective randomized trials to compare single vs. tandem transplantation [79,80,82,83]. These trials utilize a combination of TBI and non-TBI-containing regimens, and this should be considered when analysing the results of the trials (Table 92.1).

In summary, many different conditioning regimens have been used for AHCT in multiple myeloma. Whereas many trials have compared different combinations of standard therapy and found them to be similar in efficacy to oral melphalan and prednisone [72], only one prospective randomized trial has directly compared two different conditioning regimens prior to AHCT with the finding that high-dose 200 mg/m^2 melphalan alone was superior to high-dose 140 mg/m^2 melphalan plus TBI as the conditioning regimen for AHCT in multiple myeloma [120]. Five trials designed to compare standard chemotherapy vs. high-dose therapy [74–77,130] and four trials to compare single vs. tandem AHCT [79,80,82,83] have used a variety of different conditioning regimens as discussed below. It has not been shown that all conditioning regimens are equal, and this should be remembered when considering the results of various trials. Any differences reported by investigators between standard therapy, single transplantation and tandem transplantation should be regarded as applying only to the particular regimens used in the particular study reported.

Patient selection for high-dose therapy

Over the last three decades, AHCT has been limited to patients up to 65 years of age with normal renal function, and with a World Health Organization performance status 0–2 (0, asymptomatic; 1, restricted in physically strenuous activity but ambulatory and able to carry out work; 2, ambulatory and capable of all self-care but unable to carry out any work; 3, capable of only limited self-care, confined to bed or chair >50% of waking hours; 4, completely disabled, cannot carry out any self-care, totally confined to bed or chair). The issue of age limit is important, because the median age of multiple myeloma patients at diagnosis is currently over 60 years. The introduction of hematopoietic growth factors has profoundly modified the practice of AHCT. With PBHCs collected after priming with G-CSF or granulocyte macrophage colony-stimulating factor (GM-CSF), AHCT has become safer and can be offered to older patients. Nevertheless, in the French IFM90 randomized study comparing conventional chemotherapy to myeloablative therapy and autologous bone marrow transplantation [73], 26 patients did not undergo high-dose therapy because of premature death, poor performance status, abnormal renal function or insufficient amounts of hematopoietic cells. Overall, 12 of 67 (18%) patients aged ≤60 years, compared to 14 of 33 (42%) of patients aged >60 years, did not undergo transplantation in this study.

In a retrospective case-match analysis, the Arkansas group has compared the outcome of 49 patients ≥65 years with 49 younger pair mates selected from a cohort of 550 patients treated with high-dose therapy [131]. The complete remission rate was higher in younger patients (40% vs. 20%) and the transplant-related mortality appeared to be higher in older patients (8% vs. 2%). However, the event-free survival and overall survival were comparable. The same group recently published the results of AHCT in 70 patients over the age of 70 years [132]. Although AHCT appeared feasible in this age subgroup, the use of higher doses of melphalan of 200 mg/m² was too toxic, resulting in 16% deaths. The dose for this age group was subsequently decreased to 140 mg/m², and 44% of these patients actually received tandem AHCT. It has also been demonstrated that two or three courses of 100 mg/m² melphalan supported by PBHC support are feasible on an outpatient basis in patients up to 75 years of age [133]. Subsequently, in a nonrandomized case-match analysis 71 patients with a median age of 64 years were treated with two courses of 100 mg/m² melphalan supported by PBHC, and compared to 71 pair mates treated with conventional oral melphalan and prednisone [121]. The complete remission rate was 47% after 100 mg/m² melphalan vs. 5% after oral melphalan and prednisone. The median event free-survival was 34 months in the 100 mg/m² melphalan vs. 17.7 months in the oral melphalan and prednisone group, and the median overall survival was >56 months for 100 mg/m² melphalan vs. 48 months for oral melphalan and prednisone ($p<0.01$), revealing that intensive therapy may be superior in terms of complete remission rate, event-free survival and overall survival for older patients. The Italian MMSG investigators compared melphalan and prednisone vs. two courses of intermediate-dose 100 mg/m² melphalan, followed by AHCT in patients up to the age of 70 years [74]. Melphalan 200 mg/m² improved the response rate and event-free survival in patients with myeloma, and was well-tolerated in elderly patients, with similar toxicity to melphalan and prednisone.

Investigators from the UK reported the outcome and transplant-related morbidity of a cohort of patients >65 years of age, with a median of 67 years (range 65–74 years), compared with 17 younger pair mates with a median age of 55 years (range 31–64 years) [134]. In this study, patients received high-dose 200 mg/m² melphalan infused over 30 min if the glomerular filtration rate was >40 mL/min. In one patient with poor renal function, 16 mg/kg busulfan was used. All patients received autologous hematopoietic cell rescue. High-dose therapy was tolerated equally in both elderly patients and the matched pairs, with comparable times to neutrophil and platelet recoveries. The treatment-related mortalities appeared unusually high in both groups, however, although they were similar at 17.6% and 11.7%, respectively. The median overall survival of 3.59 years in the elderly patients was similar to 3.01 years in the younger pair mates. There was no difference in relapse rate, overall survival or myelotoxicity between the groups.

The issue of renal impairment and autologous transplantation is particularly pertinent to multiple myeloma because of the high rate of renal dysfunction in patients with this disease [135–137]. The pharmacokinetics and marrow toxicity of parenteral melphalan in dogs, before and after induction of renal failure with subtotal nephrectomy, have been analyzed [138]. The surgical procedure decreased the creatinine clearance by an average of 62% ($p = 0.001$). Following nephrectomy, there was an increase in both the terminal-phase plasma half-life and renal clearance of intravenous melphalan ($p = 0.02$) to 75% over prenephrectomy values. The lowest neutrophil counts following intravenous melphalan averaged $4.9 \times 10^3/mm^3$ prenephrectomy and $0.9 \times 10^3/mm^3$ postnephrectomy, respectively ($p = 0.002$). The mean lowest recorded platelet counts after 1 mg/kg melphalan were $115 \times 10^3/mm^3$ in the prenephrectomized dogs, and $9.7 \times 10^3/mm^3$ in those postnephrectomy. The investigators suggested the starting dose of melphalan be decreased by at least 50% when used in myeloma patients with renal failure. In 1982, a separate study in myeloma patients found that renal insufficiency significantly increased melphalan-induced myelosuppression during the initial 10 weeks of treatment in 295 patients with multiple myeloma [139]. Patients with renal insufficiency had a significantly higher frequency of severe leukopenia and thrombocytopenia following intravenous melphalan than did patients with normal renal function (50% vs. 15%, respectively; $p = 0.007$). Reduction of intravenous melphalan dose to 50% in patients with elevated blood urea nitrogen (BUN) reduced the frequency of these complications to levels that were not significantly different from those observed in patients with normal renal function.

However, pharmacokinetics have been studied in patients after the administration of 100 mg/m² melphalan, and were not adversely affected by impaired renal function [140]. The median half-life, area-under-the-concentration-curve (AUC) and clearance of melphalan was 1.1 h, 5.5 mg/h/L and 27.5 L/h, respectively, in patients with a creatinine clearance of <40 mL/min compared to 1.9 h, 7.9 mg/h/L and 23.6 L/h, for those patients whose clearance was >40 mL/min. The plasma half-life and AUC varied by a factor of 10, and melphalan clearance by a factor of 5, between patients with the lowest and highest values. However, these large variations in melphalan elimination were not caused by patient or disease characteristics, and it was concluded that the presence of renal failure did not require dose reduction of melphalan in autologous transplantation. Renal insufficiency also had no apparent negative impact on the quality of PBHC collections, and did not adversely affect post-transplantation engraftment, transfusion requirements, incidence of severe mucositis or overall survival. No transplant-related deaths were observed. However, renal failure was associated with longer duration of fever and hospitalization.

Pharmacokinetic studies have also been performed in eight patients after receiving high-dose intravenous 180 mg/m² melphalan [104]. Plasma levels of melphalan declined in a biexponential fashion with a mean terminal half-life ($t_{1/2\beta}$) of 61 min (range 40.3–132.8 min). These kinetic parameters are similar to those reported from studies using lower doses of melphalan. The estimated peak concentrations ranged from 5.45 to 16.57 µg/mL. Plasma levels were lower than the limit of quantification of the method used (20 ng/mL) by 24 h after drug administration. A weak correlation was found between melphalan clearance and creatinine clearance ($p <0.05$). No relationships were found between the pharmacokinetics of melphalan, myelosuppression or nonhematologic toxicities [105]. Investigators of another study of 81 multiple myeloma patients with renal failure at the time of AHCT [136] reported that renal failure had no impact on the quality of PBHC collection, and did not affect engraftment. AHCT was feasible even in patients on dialysis. However, hematologic toxicities were more severe and more frequent after 200 mg/m² melphalan than after 140 mg/m² melphalan. A retrospective study from the Spanish Bone Marrow Transplant Registry showed a high transplant-related mortality (29%) in patients with renal failure at the time of transplantation [135]. Reversal of renal failure has been achieved with high-dose 140 mg/m² melphalan and 200 mg/m² followed by AHCT in 59 patients still on dialysis (median duration of dialysis was 4 months) at the time of AHCT [141]. Twelve of 37 (32%) patients treated within 6 months of dialysis, compared with only one of 22 patients (5%) on dialysis for >6 months, became dialysis-independent ($p = 0.01$), suggesting that significant renal failure can be reversed by AHCT if applied early in the disease course, within 6 months of dialysis.

In summary, compromised renal function at presentation should not exclude patients from high-dose therapy programs, but renal failure may be associated with increased hematologic toxicity, and the impact of renal failure at the time of AHCT requires further study. In addition, the results of numerous studies have shown that advanced age up to 75 years by itself should not be an exclusion criterion from autologous transplantation programs, but dose adjustment of high-dose regimens may be indicated to reduce morbidity.

Source of hematopoietic stem cells

As in other malignancies, PBHCs have replaced bone marrow as the source of hematopoietic cells in AHCT for multiple myeloma because of easier accessibility and faster hematopoietic recovery, but the superiority of PBHCs with regard to relapse rate, event-free survival and long-term overall survival has never been demonstrated. Variables affecting PBHC mobilization and speed of engraftment have been analyzed [90]. There is a significant correlation between the number of $CD34^+$ cells (representing primitive hematopoietic progenitors) infused and hematopoietic reconstitution. The minimum dose of $CD34^+$ cells to ensure safe engraftment is 2×10^6/kg.

The optimal regimen for mobilizing PBHCs is unclear. Some investigators use cyclophosphamide plus G-CSF to increase the number of PBHCs, and possibly to reduce graft contamination and the tumor cell mass. The use of cyclophosphamide at a dose of 4 g/m^2 decreases hematologic and extrahematologic toxicity with an equivalent $CD34^+$ cell collection efficiency, compared to a higher dose of 7 g/m^2 [142]. Hematopoietic cells have also been successfully harvested after marrow recovery from cyclophosphamide, Adriamycin, vincristine and prednisone (CHOP) [75], dexamethasone, cyclophosphamide, etoposide and cisplatin (DCEP) [143] and dexamethasone, paclitaxel, etoposide, cyclophosphamide and G-CSF (d-TEC) [144]. The addition of stem cell factor (SCF) to G-CSF after cyclophosphamide for PBHC mobilization has resulted in a significant increase in $CD34^+$ cell yield and a concomitant reduction in the number of leukapheresis required to collect an optimal harvest of 5×10^6 $CD34^+$ cells/kg [145,146]. However, the majority of patients achieve sufficient mobilization with G-CSF following chemotherapy, so SCF is not routinely used.

To investigate the possibility that prior exposure to chemotherapy significantly impacts hematopoietic cell collection and hematopoietic recovery, the engraftment pattern of 225 patients in Arkansas with newly diagnosed or refractory multiple myeloma has been analyzed [90]. A highly significant correlation was observed between the number of $CD34^+$ cells/kg infused and recovery of both granulocytes ($p = 0.0001$) and platelets ($p = 0.0001$) [90]. After correction for the proportion of patients with $\geq 2 \times 10^6$/kg $CD34^+$ PBHCs cells infused, and with ≤ 12 months of prior therapy, no difference in engraftment kinetics was seen between patients receiving PBHCs only and those also receiving bone marrow. In the presence of growth factors that stimulate granulocytes, granulocyte recovery to $>0.5 \times 10^9$ within 21 days occurred in 97% of patients irrespective of the dose of $CD34^+$ cells infused. However, platelet recovery was much more variable. The threshold dose of $CD34^+$ cells necessary for platelet engraftment resulting in a peripheral blood platelet count $>50 \times 10^9$/L by day 21 was $\geq 2.0 \times 10^6$/kg $CD34^+$ cells for patients with ≤ 24 months of chemotherapy before transplantation. More than 5×10^6/kg $CD34^+$ cells were required to assure rapid platelet recovery in patients with ≥ 24 months exposure to prior chemotherapy. $CD34^+$ cell number therefore appeared to represent only a surrogate marker of a heterogeneous population of cells, with exposure to cytotoxic agents affecting the capacity of $CD34^+$ cells to replenish platelets more than their ability to differentiate into mature neutrophils. If $>5 \times 10^6$/kg $CD34^+$ cells were infused, platelet recovery to $>50 \times 10^9$/L before day 14 was achieved in 94% of patients, irrespective of the duration of prior therapy. However, 72% of patients who received >24 months of prior therapy failed to mobilize enough $CD34^+$ cells to ensure rapid platelet engraftment. Adequate levels of $CD34^+$ cells were obtained in 97%, 85% and 28% of patients with ≤ 12, 13–24 and >24 months of prior therapy, respectively. In addition, exposure to even ≤ 6 months of alkylating agents significantly delayed platelet recovery post-transplantation. There was a highly significant decrease ($p = 0.0001$) in the proportion of patients with early platelet recovery after more extensive exposure to alkylating agents. These data support the concept that prolonged exposure to chemotherapy prior to transplantation should be avoided because of potential toxicity to hematopoietic cells and subsequent difficulty with hematopoietic cell harvesting and engraftment.

An adequate number of PBHCs can be collected from most patients after a VAD-based regimen, even those who are refractory to therapy or in relapse. Investigators from Italy have analyzed the effects of prior chemotherapy on hematopoietic mobilization and subsequent engraftment after high-dose therapy [92]. In a retrospective analysis, 89 patients with relapsed or refractory multiple myeloma underwent $CD34^+$ PBHC collection between 1993 and 2000. Patients were divided into three groups according to their previous treatment: 37 patients had received VAD-based conventional chemotherapy, 39 had received oral melphalan and prednisone therapy and 13 had been treated with high-intermediate intravenous-dose melphalan with autologous PBHC support. The number of prior melphalan and prednisone courses was not a predictor of mobilization. Instead, the type of previous chemotherapy had the strongest influence in uni- and multivariate analyses. Fifty-nine patients achieved an adequate collection of at least 2×10^6 $CD34^+$ cells/kg. An adequate collection was obtained in 34 of 37 (92%) of patients treated with conventional nonalkylating therapy, in 22 of 39 (56%) of patients treated with oral melphalan and in three of 13 (23%) of patients who had received intravenous melphalan. These differences were statistically significant ($p < 0.05$). In a separate study, 68 patients (median age 65) from diagnosis were treated with 3 g/m^2 cyclophosphamide mobilization followed by 60 mg/m^2 melphalan and AHCT. Three courses were effectively delivered at 6-month intervals, but repeated melphalan infusions hampered subsequent $CD34^+$ harvests [147]. These data suggest that the type of prior therapy, in particular higher doses of melphalan, is important in determining subsequent hematopoietic cell yields. Investigators from Germany have reported that up to six courses of VAD chemotherapy made no significant impact on PBHC mobilization, with successful yields sufficient for at least one autograft in all 26 patients analyzed [91]. However, there was a strong negative correlation between the duration of melphalan treatment and peak $CD34^+$ values in leukapheresis products as well as total harvest yields. In contrast to the Arkansas data discussed in the previous section, harvest yields of $>2.0 \times 10^6$ $CD34^+$ cells/kg represented an independent marker of progenitor cell function with regard to short- and long-term engraftment.

The Arkansas group has analyzed the results of 117 multiple myeloma patients who were mobilized with 10–16 μg/kg G-CSF alone, without concomitant cytotoxic cytoreduction. The only factor significantly affecting optimal PBHC procurement was duration of preceding conventional chemotherapy ($p = 0.002$). Seventy-five percent of patients attained a granulocyte count of 0.5×10^9/L by day 13. However, platelet recovery to both 20×10^9/L and 50×10^9/L varied widely. On univariate analysis, factors influencing platelet recovery were the number of $CD34^+$ cells/kg infused, age, β_2-microglobulin levels, response to preceding therapy, bone marrow plasmacytosis and duration of prior therapy. On multivariate analysis, important factors included the number of $CD34^+$ cells/kg infused ($p = 0.007$), β_2-microglobulin levels ($p = 0.0001$) and older age ($p = 0.002$). The investigators concluded that patients with high tumor burden, such as patients with β_2-microglobulin levels >2.5 mg/L, may therefore benefit from chemotherapy for mobilization both in terms of cytoreduction and adequate PBHC mobilization resulting in accelerated engraftment [148]. Notably, previous therapy with alkylating agents had minimal impact on engraftment, despite duration of prior therapy being the only factor having an impact on adequate PBHC yield. In addition, the weekly administration of alkylating agent cyclophosphamide as part of the induction chemotherapy C-VAMP did not affect subsequent PBHC collection in patients with myeloma [149].

In conclusion, evidence supports the concept that prior therapy with alkylating agents adversely affects hematopoietic cell mobilization, and that duration of therapy may have an adverse effect on subsequent progenitor cell harvest and engraftment post-AHCT. In addition, patients with more advanced disease may have a higher levels of contamination with clonogenic plasma cells in the apheresis product [150–152]. Therefore, when planning to perform AHCT it would appear desirable to collect AHCs early in disease, and particularly before the use of prolonged courses of chemotherapy. However, long-term storage of hematopoietic cells may pose logistical problems, and hematopoietic cells are generally stored for patients only when AHCT is intended at a later date.

The feasibility of collecting PBHCs in previously untreated myeloma patients without any prior cytoreductive therapy has been demonstrated [153]. Overall, the collections were inferior to those performed after induction chemotherapy, but it was possible to harvest enough hematopoietic cells for one autograft at the time of diagnosis in 75% of myeloma patients. Although the plasma cell content of the collections was 0.1–64.7 $\times 10^6$ cells/kg (median 0.49), in other reports the level of plasma cell contamination in the graft did not appear to significantly contribute to the relapse rate [154,155]. Protocols have been developed to give high-dose therapy and AHCT as induction chemotherapy, to be followed by several courses of maintenance combination chemotherapy infusions to further reduce tumor burden [156,157]. However, peripheral blood progenitor harvests at presentation are currently experimental and are not routinely performed prior to cytoreductive induction chemotherapy.

As discussed in the section on conventional therapies, thalidomide has been effective in patients with newly diagnosed myeloma, especially in combination with dexamethasone [87–89]. When used during induction therapy, thalidomide appeared to subsequently dampen the $CD34^+$ cell response to mobilization but not overall hematopoietic cell yield or subsequent hematopoietic engraftment [158]. This use of thalidomide during induction harnessed the potential benefit of thalidomide without compromising hematopoietic cell harvest and subsequent AHCT, and also avoided the increased thrombogenic risk observed with combinations of chemotherapy with thalidomide [159]. A randomized trial is currently accruing patients to directly compare the relative efficacy of thalidomide with or without dexamethasone as initial therapy prior to AHCT for multiple myeloma, and the results of this trial should be examined before the combination of thalidomide and dexamethasone can be regarded as standard first-line induction therapy [89].

The problem of autologous graft contamination by tumor cells has been extensively addressed. Evidence from syngeneic transplants supports the concept that graft contamination significantly contributes to relapse post-AHCT. High-dose therapy followed by syngeneic transplants has demonstrated an improved disease-free survival but a nonsignificant improvement in overall survival compared to autologous transplantation. In a nonrandomized analysis, 25 patients with multiple myeloma received bone marrow grafts ($n = 24$) or PBHCs ($n = 1$) from twin donors [110]. The outcome was compared in a case-matched analysis to 125 patients who underwent autologous transplantation and 125 patients who underwent allogeneic transplantation. Seventeen patients (68%) receiving twin transplants entered complete remission, which was not significantly different from that of autologous (48%) or allogeneic (58%) transplants. The median overall and progression-free survival for the twins was 73 and 72 months, respectively. There was a trend towards better overall survival of 73 vs. 44 months ($p = 0.1$), and the progression-free survival was significantly better at 72 vs. 25 months ($p = 0.0094$) with syngeneic than with autologous transplantation. Three of 17 patients who entered complete remission following transplantation relapsed, but this relapse rate was significantly lower following syngeneic transplantation than following autologous transplantation, and was similar to the relapse rate with allogeneic transplantation. The lower relapse risk following syngeneic transplantation compared to autologous transplantation may be a result of reinfusion of malignant cells in some patients treated with this modality, or possibly to the presence of a graft-vs.-myeloma effect in some syngeneic transplants. Therefore, data from syngeneic transplantations are consistent with graft contamination by tumor cells contributing to relapse. Although overall survival was not statistically improved by syngeneic transplantation compared to autologous transplantation, the number of patients in this study was small and there was a trend toward improved survival in the syngeneic transplantation group.

Many attempts have been made to eradicate tumor contamination from autologous harvests. Anti-B-cell monoclonal antibodies have been used to remove malignant cells [160] and immunomagnetic-based enrichment of $CD34^+$ cells has been used, with a marked reduction in myeloma cells without affecting engraftment kinetics [151,161]. Positively selected $CD34^+$ cells can provide effective hematopoietic support for one or two subsequent courses of myeloablative therapy. However, removal of tumor cells does not seem to improve the serologic or molecular complete remission rate, event-free survival or overall survival of multiple myeloma patients [162]. Selection of $CD34^+$ PBHCs has been compared to unselected PBHCs in four multicenter trials [83,154,163,164]. These trials failed to show any benefit of $CD34^+$ selected PBHCs. Moreover, in two studies, the incidence of opportunistic infections appeared to be higher in the $CD34^+$ selected PBHC arm [83,164]. No correlation between the number of reinfused malignant plasma cells and eventual outcome was found when flow cytometry was used to detect plasma cells in peripheral blood and PBHC harvests [165]. In a randomized study reported by the EBMT, processing autografts of multiple myeloma patients by $CD34^+$ selection resulted in an overall 2-log reduction of tumor cells [154]. Polymerase chain reaction (PCR) analysis, based on the clonally rearranged IgH-chain locus and limiting dilution, was performed to quantify the myeloma cells in the grafts and follow-up bone marrow samples. At 25 months of follow-up, the number of tumor cells in the graft, as estimated by PCR, did not predict for remission duration after autografting. However, the number of tumor cells in the bone marrow after transplantation (at 3–6 months) may have a predictive value. In summary, transplantation with $CD34^+$ selected autografts is of no benefit for multiple myeloma patients.

Purging by negative selection using monoclonal magnetic microbeads against CD19, CD56 and CD138 has been evaluated [166]. Sixty newly diagnosed multiple myeloma patients were treated with a double transplantation procedure and randomized to receive either unmanipulated or *in vitro* purged PBHCs. Hematologic engraftment and immunologic reconstitution were rapid without treatment-related mortality. Using PCR, the level of minimal residual disease was compared between PBHC before and after *in vitro* purging, and *in vivo* after transplantation. A median of one tumor cell per 10^2 normal cells (range 10^1–10^5) was detected in the unmanipulated aphereses products, with a 3–4-log reduction after manipulation *in vitro*. A mean 3-log depletion of neoplastic plasma cells was achieved, so that PCR negativity was recorded in 11 of the 14 cases analyzed with a conventional dot-blot hybridization test. However, despite this tumor debulking, all patients remained PCR positive *in vivo*. At 3 years, the estimated event-free survival was 40% in the control arm and 72% in the experimental arm ($p = 0.05$), whereas the estimated overall survival was 83% in both arms. This study did not have the power to demonstrate a difference in clinical outcome between the two groups. However, within the limit of a small number of patients, an improved event-free survival was observed among patients transplanted with a purged graft, despite the fact that in this group a lower complete remission rate was achieved with VAD and cyclophosphamide.

In conclusion, the possible benefit of the use of purged PBHCs has not yet been confirmed in a specifically designed clinical trial. Overall survival has not been improved, despite extensive graft purging [83,155,162–164,166,167] or the use of syngeneic marrow [110]. No correlation between the number of reinfused malignant plasma cells and eventual outcome has been made, and current evidence suggests that relapse after autologous transplantation is mainly a result of residual disease *in vivo*, although relapse may be delayed in the setting of effective graft purging. Therefore, more effective therapy to eradicate tumor *in vivo* during induction therapy, conditioning prior to AHCT and post-transplant are needed to improve long-term results with ACHT for the treatment of multiple myeloma.

Timing of transplantation

The optimal timing of transplants remains to be determined. The large randomized trials from the IFM90 [73], MMSG [74], the French Myélome Auto Greffe (MAG) [75], the Spanish Programa para el Tratamiento de Hemopatías Malignas (PETHEMA) [76] and the British Medical Research Council (MRC) VII [77,168] all entered patients from diagnosis, and there was no significant delay between induction chemotherapy and high-dose therapy. A nonrandomized single arm study was conducted in the Mayo Clinic in Rochester, Minnesota, to examine the outcome of delayed AHCT for the management of relapsed or refractory myeloma compared to AHCT for the management of primary VAD-refractory disease [169,170]. To exclude lead-time bias, this study included only patients whose hematopoietic cells were collected within 12 months of diagnosis. The median number of months from diagnosis to bone marrow transplantation was 7.4 months for the patients refractory to VAD chemotherapy and 24 months for patients who received transplantation at first progression. The complete response rate to subsequent AHCT was 34%, comparable to complete response rates reported from centers where patients receive transplants in plateau phase. There were no differences in the complete response rates between patients with primary refractory disease who were transplanted early vs. patients who were transplanted later for relapsing disease either off therapy or still on therapy. The median survival from initial diagnosis and from day of transplantation was 51 and 20 months, respectively. The post-transplant progression-free survival was short at 11.4 months, compared to progression-free survival in excess of 2 years reported in other studies in patients who receive transplants early.

The French MAG group has conducted a randomized trial comparing early AHCT after three or four monthly courses of vincristine, doxorubicin and methylprednisolone (VAMP) vs. late AHCT performed as rescue treatment, in case of disease progression on VMCP, in case of disease resistance after six courses of VMCP, or in case of relapse in responders [171]. A median of eight courses of VMCP was given in the late high-dose therapy group (range 1–20). The study was designed to have a power of 80% to detect a 20% reduction in the mortality rate among early AHCT, compared with late AHCT patients, and all comparisons were on an intent-to-treat basis. Early AHCT significantly improved progression-free survival, but overall survival was not significantly different between the two arms. After a median follow-up of 58 months, estimated median overall survival was 64.6 months in the early AHCT group and 64 months in the late group, and the survival curves were not different. Median event-free survival was 39 months in the early AHCT group whereas median time between randomization and failure of combination chemotherapy was 13 months in the late group. The average time without symptoms, treatment and treatment toxicity was 27.8 months for early AHCT and 22.3 for late AHCT. AHCT with PBHC transplantation achieved a median overall survival exceeding 5 years in young patients with symptomatic multiple myeloma, whether performed early as first-line therapy or late as rescue treatment. Therefore, early AHCT may be preferred because it is associated with a shorter period of chemotherapy and patients transplanted before evidence of progression attained a prolonged progression-free survival of 39 vs. 13 months, which was associated with an improved quality of life. Furthermore, the Arkansas group has reported that transplantation within the first 12 months after diagnosis is a favorable prognostic factor [172,173].

In conclusion, early AHCT appears to offer some advantage to late AHCT in terms of progression-free survival and time without chemotherapy or symptoms, but overall survival does not appear to be affected by delaying transplantation until there is evidence of disease progression.

Conventional chemotherapy compared to high-dose therapy and autologous transplantation

The encouraging early results achieved with myeloablative therapy and AHCT in multiple myeloma have been directly compared with conventional chemotherapy in five prospective randomized clinical trials (Table 92.2). The French Cooperative Group IFM90 compared conventional chemotherapy to 140 mg/m^2 melphalan plus 8 Gy TBI. The MMSG [74] and MRC Myeloma VII Trial [77] compared conventional chemotherapy to high-dose 200 mg/m^2 melphalan. The French Cooperative Group MAG91 trial compared conventional chemotherapy to a combination of melphalan and busulfan without the use of TBI [75]. A study designed by the Spanish Cooperative Group PETHEMA included a second randomization of patients receiving high-dose therapy, to melphalan plus TBI or to 200 mg/m^2 melphalan alone [76].

The IFM was the first to conduct a randomized multicenter trial to compare conventional chemotherapy to high-dose therapy and autologous transplantation in patients up to the age of 65 years (Fig. 92.2) [73]. In the IFM90 trial, autologous bone marrow transplantation (ABMT) significantly improved the response rate, as 38% of patients enrolled in the ABMT arm achieved a complete remission or a very good partial response vs. 14% of patients enrolled in the conventional chemotherapy arm ($p < 0.001$). With a median follow-up of 7 years, ABMT significantly improved 7 years' event-free survival (16% vs. 8%, median 28

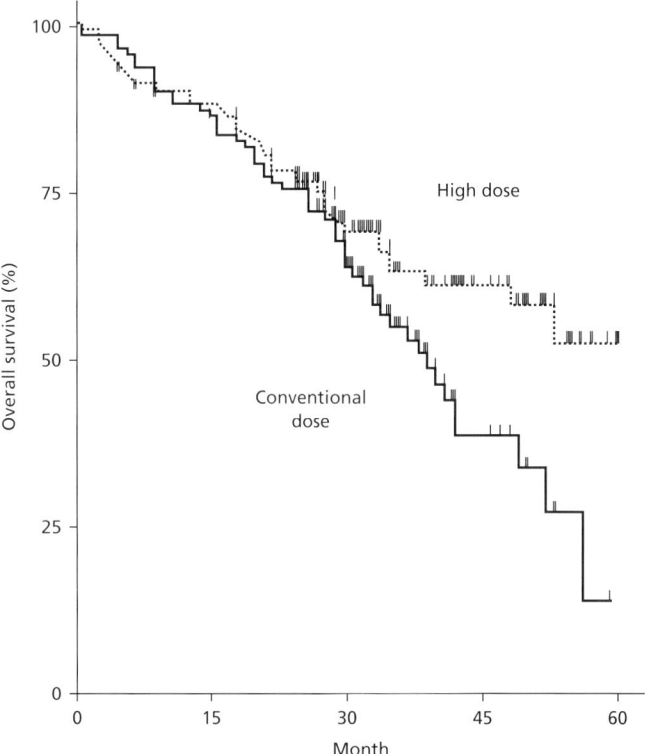

Fig. 92.2 IFM90 comparison of autologous bone marrow transplantation vs. conventional chemotherapy: overall survival according to treatment arm. With a median follow-up of 7 years [174], autologous hematopoietic cell transplantation (ABMT) significantly improved 7 years' event-free survival (16% vs. 8%, median 28 months vs. 18 months; $p = 0.01$) and 7 years' overall survival (43% vs. 25%, median 57 months vs. 44 months; $p = 0.03$). (From [73] with permission.)

Table 92.2 Randomized studies comparing conventional chemotherapy vs. high-dose therapy.

Trial	Number of patients	Median follow-up	Therapy CC	HDT	Complete remission rate (%) CC	HDT	Median overall survival (months) CC	HDT	p
IFM90 [73]	200	7 years	VMCP*/VBAP†	Mel/TBI‡	5	22	44	57	0.03§
MAG91 [75]	190	56 months	VAD¶/VMCP*	Mel‖ vs. Mel††/Bu‡‡	NE	NE	50	55	0.98**
MRCVII [77]	407	42 months	ABCM§§	Mel 200‖	9	44	42	55	0.04§
PETHEMA [76]	164	42 months	BVMCP¶¶/VBAD‖‖	Mel/TBI‡ or Mel 200‖	11	30	64	72	0.4**
MMSG [74]	195	24 months	MP***	Mel 100 × 2†††	6	26	NR	NR	NA

CC, conventional chemotherapy; HDT, high-dose therapy; IFM, Intergroupe Francaise du Myeloma; MAG, Myelome Auto Greffe; MMSG, Multiple Myeloma Study Group; MRC, Medical Research Council; NA, not applicable; NE, not evaluated; NR, not reached; PETHEMA, Programa para el Tratamiento de Hemopatias Malignas.
*Vincristine, melphalan, cyclophosphamide and prednisone.
†Vincristine, carmustine, doxorubicin and prednisone.
‡Melphalan 140 mg/m^2 plus 8 Gy total body irradiation.
§Survival benefit for HDT.
¶Vincristine, Adriamycin and dexamethasone.
‖Melphalan 200 mg/m^2.
**No survival benefit for HDT.
††Melphalan 140 mg/m^2.
‡‡Busulphan 16 mg/kg.
§§Adriamycin, BCNU, cyclophosphamide and melphalan.
¶¶BCNU, vincristine, melphalan, cyclophosphamide and prednisone.
‖‖Vincristine, BCNU, Adriamycin and dexamethasone.
***Oral melphalan and prednisone.
†††Melphalan 100 mg/m^2 × 2.

months vs. 18 months; $p = 0.01$) and 7 years' overall survival (43% vs. 25%, median 57 months vs. 44 months; $p = 0.03$). The MRCVII study was designed to compare conventional combination chemotherapy ABCM every 6 weeks to plateau vs. 200 mg/m^2 melphalan in patients aged <65 years [77,168]. This study accrued 407 patients, 203 to the standard arm and 204 to the intensive arm, between October 1993 and October 2000. Seventy-five patients randomized to the high-dose therapy actually received AHCT. In addition, 15% of patients randomized to conventional therapy eventually received AHCT. The intensive treatment group response rates were much better, with 86% of patients achieving a partial response or better (44% complete response, 42% partial response) compared to 50% in the standard group (9% complete response, 41% partial response). After 42 months' follow-up, on an intention-to-treat basis there was a statistically significant overall survival benefit of 12 months for patients treated in the intensive arm (median 54.8 months vs. 42.3 months; $p = 0.04$). The median progression-free survival was improved in the intensive group at 31.6 months compared with 19.6 months in the standard group ($p \leq 0.01$) [77]. There was a trend towards a greater survival benefit in the group of patients with poor prognosis as defined by high β_2-microglobulin. Therefore, both the IFM90 and MRCVII trials have shown a significant benefit for patients treated with high-dose therapy and AHCT in terms of progression-free survival as well as overall survival compared to patients treated with conventional therapy.

The French group MAG randomized 190 patients aged 55–65 years to receive conventional chemotherapy or high-dose therapy [75]. Although the results in the high-dose therapy group at 5 years' follow-up appeared comparable to those achieved in the IFM90 trial, there was no significant difference in overall survival between the two arms. However, in this trial there was an unexpectedly long survival in the conventional chemotherapy arm (median 55 months with high-dose therapy vs. 50 months with conventional chemotherapy). Furthermore, 17 patients in the conventional chemotherapy arm received AHCT at the time of relapse, illustrating the potential for transplantation to be used as salvage therapy. The design of the Spanish PETHEMA trial was different from the French and UK trials, because only patients responding to initial conventional chemotherapy were randomized [76]. In this trial, the complete remission rate was significantly higher in the high-dose therapy arm. Although the median event-free survival and overall survival was longer in the high-dose therapy arm (42 months vs. 33 months, and 72 months vs. 64 months, respectively), the differences were not significant at 42 months' follow-up.

The MMSG is currently accruing patients up to the age of 70 years to a prospective randomized controlled trial comparing combination melphalan and prednisone vs. two courses of intermediate-dose 100 mg/m^2 melphalan, followed by AHCT [74]. A total of 195 previously untreated patients under the age of 70 entered the study between October 1997 and December 2000. Patients were randomly assigned to receive either 100 mg/m^2 melphalan or melphalan and prednisone. The 100 mg/m^2 melphalan regimen included 3 g/m^2 cyclophosphamide followed by PBHC collection, and two courses of 100 mg/m^2 melphalan with PBHC support were then delivered. Patients relapsing after melphalan and prednisone were rescued with 100 mg/m^2 melphalan. After a median follow-up of 17 months, an interim analysis was conducted. The response rate among the patients who received 100 mg/m^2 melphalan was 83% including complete responses in 26% vs. 51% (complete responses in 6%) in the group treated with melphalan and prednisone ($p < 0.04$). The median event-free survival was 27 months for 100 mg/m^2 melphalan and 18 months for melphalan and prednisone ($p < 0.01$). The median overall survival has not been reached yet. Treatment-related mortality was 3% after 100 mg/m² melphalan and 2% after melphalan and prednisone. Therefore, 100 mg/m² melphalan improved the response rate and event-free survival in patients with myeloma, and was well-tolerated in elderly patients with similar toxicity to melphalan and prednisone.

Overall, there has been a low toxic death rate for AHCT at <3%. Compared to conventional chemotherapy, AHCT clearly improves the complete remission rate. The median event-free survival has been prolonged by 9–13 months (Table 92.2). A significant benefit has been seen in terms of overall survival in the MRCVII and IFM90 trials. In the MAG91, MMSG and PETHEMA trials, the survival benefit was less striking, partly because the follow-up is currently shorter, and partly because AHCT has been used as salvage treatment in a significant number of patients at the time of failure in the conventional chemotherapy arms. In addition, survival was unexpectedly good in the conventional chemotherapy arms of the MMSG and PETHEMA trials. AHCT has therefore proven to be of benefit, at least in fit younger patients. Analyses of large AHCT series with extended follow-up shows that long-term survival is achieved in only a small minority of patients [175,176], but some patients with no initial adverse prognostic factors enjoy prolonged event-free survival and are possibly cured by aggressive strategies including tandem AHCT [177]. There is evidence that AHCT can be delayed until disease progression occurs without reducing the potential benefit in overall survival, but this may be associated with longer periods of treatment with conventional chemotherapy, and reduced quality of life overall. Therefore, current evidence supports AHCT as recommended first-line consolidation therapy for all newly diagnosed patients with multiple myeloma. Age and renal failure should not be exclusion criteria, but consideration of a potentially increased post-AHCT morbidity in these patients should be made when planning the procedure.

Tandem transplantation

Almost 10 years ago the Arkansas group showed the feasibility of two consecutive AHCTs, because of the use of growth factors and of PBHCs instead of bone marrow [127]. In their first report of a large number of patients, 73% of patients actually received two AHCTs, and the complete remission rate increased from 24% after the first transplantation to 43% after two transplants [178]. This experience has now been extended to more than 1000 patients [172]. Treatment-related mortality was low at 2.7% with the first, and 4.8% with second AHCT. Forty-four percent of patients achieved complete remission, which lasted a median of 2.4 years. The 5-year projected event-free and overall survival was 25% and 40%, respectively.

A study from the Netherlands has shown the feasibility of administering a tandem high-dose therapy regimen using whole blood for rescue after the first regimen, and leukapheresis, harvested between the two high doses, for rescue after the second high dose [179]. The first high-dose therapy used high-dose 140 mg/m² melphalan. Patients who did not progress after 3–6 months were again mobilized, leukapheresed and treated with 16 mg/kg busulfan and 120 mg/kg cyclophosphamide (BU/CY) followed by AHCT. Sixty-six patients qualified for harvesting after high-dose melphalan. Forty-nine patients actually received BU/CY. There were four toxic deaths. The median overall survival from diagnosis for patients receiving high-dose melphalan was 49 months compared to 84 months for patients also receiving BU/CY. Selection bias existed because only patients who did not progress received the second AHCT, and this approach therefore requires further evaluation in a prospective randomized trial. As an alternative to tandem AHCT as initial consolidation therapy, investigators at the Royal Marsden Group recently evaluated the outcome of 96 patients treated with a second AHCT for relapse after the first. The median interval between the two AHCT procedures was 3.2 years. Although the overall survival was comparable to that achieved with tandem AHCT in other studies [180], the Marsden study was not a prospective randomized trial. Prospective randomized studies comparing two AHCTs up front vs. one early AHCT followed by a second at the time of progression are needed to eliminate potential bias, and to determine the role of second transplantation as salvage therapy, rather than initial consolidation therapy.

Several large prospective randomized multicenter phase 3 studies are now ongoing to compare single vs. double high-dose therapy and AHCT as initial therapy for multiple myeloma. The results are summarized in Table 92.3. The MAG95 [83], IFM94 [78,79] and Dutch–Belgium Haematology Oncology Group (HOVON) [82] studies all use TBI-containing regimens, whereas the Italian study Bologna 96 (University of Bologna) uses non-TBI containing regimens [80,81].

In 1994, the IFM initiated a randomized trial (IFM94) comparing one vs. two transplants [78,79]. From October 1994 to March 1997, 403 untreated patients under the age of 60 years were enrolled at 45 centers. At diagnosis they were randomized to receive either a single or double AHCT. The first transplantation was prepared with 140 mg/m² melphalan and the second with 140 mg/m² melphalan and 8 Gy TBI. Overall, 399 patients were evaluable. Out of 199 patients assigned to the single AHCT arm, 177 (89%) actually received the planned transplantation and there were three toxic deaths. Out of 200 patients randomized to the double transplantation arm, 156 (78%) actually received two transplants and there were five toxic deaths. There was no significant difference in the complete remission rate between single and double transplantation arms. Forty-two percent of patients who received single transplantation achieved complete response or very good partial response (>90% reduction of paraprotein by electrophoresis) vs. 50% after double AHCT ($p = 0.15$). With a median follow-up of 5 years, the 7-year probability of event-free survival was 10% for single vs. 20% for double transplantation ($p < 0.03$) [79]. The 7-year post-diagnosis overall survival was 21% for single vs. 42% for double transplantation ($p < 0.01$). Prognostic features associated with longer survival were low β_2-microglobulin at diagnosis ($p < 0.01$), young age ($p < 0.05$), low lactic dehydrogenase (LDH) at diagnosis ($p < 0.01$)) and treatment arm ($p < 0.05$). In conclusion, the final analysis of the IFM94 trial demonstrates that high dose therapy improves the overall survival in multiple myeloma and could be recommended for patients aged <60 years. Notably, the overall survival curves separated only after 4 years.

An interim analysis on an intent-to-treat basis was performed after a median of 30 months' follow-up on the first 220 patients who were enrolled in the Bologna96 trial study between January 1996 and December 1999 [81]. The complete remission rate was 21% for patients randomized to single transplantation ($n = 110$) and 24% for patients randomized to double transplantation ($n = 110$). With a median follow-up of 3 years, no statistically significant difference in overall survival was observed between the two groups (median 56 months for single transplantation vs. 60 months for double transplantation). Compared to single transplantation, double transplantation conferred a significantly longer median remission duration of 27 vs. 44 months ($p = 0.005$), resulting in extended median event-free survival of 34 months for patients randomized to double transplantation vs. 25 months for those assigned to single transplantation ($p = 0.05$). An overall response rate of 80% was achieved, effecting prolonged duration of remission compared to a single AHCT. The investigators concluded these preliminary results suggest that timely application of double ACHT was a safe and effective treatment strategy for newly diagnosed patients with multiple myeloma, but mature data derived from the final analysis of the trial must be awaited before definite conclusions can be given.

The HOVON trial was designed to detect a 15% increase (from 40% to 55%) in 2 years event-free survival after randomization in the

Table 92.3 Randomized studies comparing single vs. tandem autologous transplants.

Trial	Number of patients	Median follow-up (months)	Single transplant	Double transplant		Median overall survival (months)		
				HDT 1	HDT 2	Single	Double	p
IFM94 [78,79]	399	60	Mel 140/TBI*	Mel 140‡	Mel 140/TBI*	50	58	0.02†
HOVON [82]	255	33	Mel 70§ × 2¶	Mel 70§ × 2¶	Cyclo/TBI‖	48	44	0.2**
Bologna [80,81]	178	30	Mel 200††	Mel 200††	Mel 120/Bu‡‡	No difference		NA
MAG95 [83]	193	40	Mel 140‡/Cyclo/TBI‖ §§	Mel 140‡	Mel 140/TBI*/Etop‖‖§§	No difference		NA

HDT, high-dose therapy; HOVON, Dutch–Belgian Haematology Oncology Group; IFM, Intergroupe Francaise du Myeloma; MAG, Myelome Auto Greffe; NA, not applicable.
*Melphalan 140 mg/m² plus 8 Gy total body irradiation.
†Survival benefit for double HDT.
‡Melphalan 140 mg/m².
§Melphalan 70 mg/m² × 2.
¶No autologous rescue given.
‖Total body irradiation plus cyclophosphamide.
**No survival benefit for double HDT.
††Melphalan 200 mg/m².
‡‡Melphalan 120 mg/m² plus busulphan 12 mg/kg.
§§TBI-containing regimens supported by unselected or CD34-enriched hematopoietic stem cells.
‖‖Etoposide 30 mg/kg.

myeloablative group compared to the standard therapy group. A total of 170 patients were required in each treatment group and 178 events had to be observed. An analysis performed in November 2001 included only 129 patients in the intensified chemotherapy group and 132 patients in the myeloablative treatment group [82]. A total of 261 eligible patients with stage II/III multiple myeloma under the age of 66 years were randomized after remission induction therapy with VAD to receive intensified chemotherapy. Conditioning regimens used were 140 mg/m² melphalan divided into two doses of 70 mg/m² without hematopoietic cell rescue ($n = 129$) or the same regimen followed by a myeloablative regimen consisting of cyclophosphamide and TBI with AHCT ($n = 132$). Interferon-2α was given as maintenance. Seventy-nine percent of patients received assigned therapy. The response rate (complete remission plus partial response) was 88% in the intensified chemotherapy group vs. 95% in the myeloablative treatment group. The complete remission rate was significantly higher after myeloablative therapy (13% vs. 29%; $p = 0.002$). After a median follow-up of 33 months, the event-free survival was not different between both treatments (median 21 months vs. 22 months; $p = 0.28$). Although the time to progression was significantly longer after myeloablative treatment (25 months vs. 31 months; $p = 0.04$), the overall survival was not different between the two groups (50 vs. 47 months; $p = 0.41$).

In 1996, the MAG initiated a multicenter trial of patients aged <56 years with newly diagnosed symptomatic myeloma (MAG95) [83]. Patients were randomly assigned from presentation to receive either single transplantation or tandem transplantation. In addition, all patients were independently randomized to be transplanted with either unselected or CD34+ enriched PBHCs. The conditioning regimen for the single transplantation consisted of 140 mg/m² melphalan and 60 mg/kg cyclophosphamide with 12 Gy TBI. The double transplantation arm was prepared with 140 mg/m² melphalan for the first transplantation, and 140 mg/m² melphalan combined with 30 mg/kg etoposide with 12 Gy TBI prior to the second. A total of 230 patients were included. An interim intent-to-treat analysis was performed in 2001 including 193 patients with a median follow-up of 40 months. There was no difference in treatment-related mortality at 9% vs. 7% in single vs. double transplantation arms, respectively. Response rates were 42% vs. 37%, respectively. There was no apparent benefit for CD34+ selection. This preliminary analysis showed no difference in relapse and mortality between single vs. double transplantation, but there was an increase in infections in the CD34+ selected group.

In conclusion, the IFM94 trial is the most mature study comparing single to tandem transplantation for multiple myeloma, and shows an overall survival benefit for tandem transplantation over single transplantation of around 20% after 6 years of follow-up. Taking into account the survival curves in IFM94 trial did not separate until after 4 years, the follow-up in the HOVON trial, as well as MAG95 and Bologna96 trials, is only 27–40 months, and therefore too early to draw final conclusions regarding overall survival. The HOVON trial was designed to show a 15% increase in event-free survival at 2 years in the intensified group, but there was no difference in event-free survival even at 33 months. After a median of 30 months follow-up, the Bologna96 trial complete remission rates were not improved by tandem transplantation, but there was a significantly longer median remission duration of 44 months vs. 27 months ($p = 0.005$). Finally, the response rates in MAG95 were similar between single and tandem transplantation, there was no apparent benefit for CD34+ selection, and preliminary analysis showed no difference in relapse and mortality between single vs. double transplantation, although there was an increase in infections in the CD34+ selected group. In conclusion, tandem transplantation may be associated with a prolonged overall and disease-free survival for a minority of patients, but at present tandem transplantation is not established therapy for all patients. Certain subsets of patients may be more likely to benefit from tandem transplantation, and final analyses of all current multicenter studies is therefore awaited before definitive recommendations regarding the role of tandem transplantation in multiple myeloma can be made.

Although allografting has historically offered the only possibility of cure in patients with multiple myeloma, until now it has been accompanied by high early mortality rates of >40% [109]. Recently, the possibility of autologous transplantation followed by allogeneic transplantation with a reduced-dose conditioning regimen has proven to be not only feasible, with low early mortality, but also potentially more effective than either therapy alone [181]. A German study has reported 17 patients with multiple myeloma who were autografted with 200 mg/m^2 melphalan. A median of 119 days after the autotransplant, patients received a dose-reduced conditioning regimen consisting of 180 mg/m^2 fludarabine, 100 mg/m^2 melphalan and 3×10 mg/kg antithymocyte globulin, followed by an allograft from related, mismatched related or unrelated donors, to induce a graft-vs.-myeloma effect. All patients engrafted and complete donor chimerism was detected after a median of 30 days. The mortality rate at day 100 was 11%, and the complete remission rate was increased from 18% after autografting to 73% after allografting. With a median of 17 months' follow-up from the allograft, 13 patients (68%) remain alive.

In a separate study, investigators from Seattle, City of Hope, Stanford and University of Leipzig have also explored the possibility of combining the safety and cytoreductive effects of high-dose melphalan and AHCT with the curative potential of nonmyeloablative allogeneic hematopoietic transplantation from HLA-matched siblings mediating graft-vs.-myeloma effects [182]. Thirty-two patients with a median age of 55 years (range 39–71 years) with previously treated stage II/III myeloma, including 43% with refractory or relapsed disease, received 200 mg/m^2 melphalan followed by autologous hematopoietic rescue. Forty to 120 days later, patients received 200 cGy TBI, immunosuppression with mycophenolate mofetil and cyclosporine, and unmodified PBHC allografts from HLA-identical siblings. One patient died on day 31 from cytomegalovirus (CMV) pneumonia, and 31 of the 32 patients received nonmyeloablative allogeneic HCT with a median of 0 days of hospitalization, neutropenia and thrombocytopenia. All patients engrafted with a median of 90% donor T-cell chimerism by day 28 after allografting, and 99% by day 84, with no graft rejection. With a median of 423 days follow-up after autologous, and 328 days after nonmyeloablative allogeneic hematopoietic transplantation, the overall survival was 81%. The mortality at day 100 was 6% (one death after autologous HCT, and one from progressive disease after allogeneic HCT). Forty-five percent of patients developed acute grade II–IV graft-vs.-host disease (GVHD) (grade II in all but three cases), and 55% developed chronic GVHD requiring therapy. The overall response rate was 84%, with 53% complete remission, 31% partial response and only two progressions at the time of writing. Despite being used in a relatively older group of patients with regard to allogeneic transplantation in multiple myeloma, this novel two-step tandem autograft–allograft approach has dramatically reduced the acute toxicities of allogeneic hematopoietic transplantation while maintaining the potent potential benefit of a graft-vs.-myeloma effect. These studies provide the rationale for a comparative study between this two-step allogeneic approach and standard AHCT for the therapy of myeloma.

Prognostic features following AHCT

Various prognostic features have been identified with regard to outcome following AHCT. Immunoglobulin subtype, plasmablastic morphology, cytogenetics, β_2-microglobulin, CRP, response to induction therapy and disease status at transplantation have all been identified as prognostic factors [183,184]. Different responses according to immunoglobulin subtype have been reported [185]. The outcome of 61 newly diagnosed patients with Bence Jones myeloma presenting between May 1986 and December 1997 was compared with the outcome of 153 IgG and 39 IgA multiple myeloma patients who were similarly treated. Response to chemotherapy infusions and high-dose therapy was comparable between the three subtypes, but a significantly higher proportion of patients with Bence Jones myeloma failed to receive high-dose therapy compared to patients with IgG and IgA myeloma (53% vs. 78% vs. 74%, respectively). Complete remission post-induction was achieved in 9.4% of patients with Bence Jones myeloma, 13.7% with IgG myeloma and 15.4% with IgA myeloma. Complete remission post-AHCT was achieved in 57% of patients with Bence Jones myeloma, 45% with IgG myeloma and 58% with IgA myeloma. The overall and event-free survival was significantly longer for patients with IgG myeloma, whose overall survival was 4.5 years and event-free survival was 2.1 years, compared to patients with Bence Jones myeloma whose overall survival was 2.8 years and event-free survival was 1.2 years. However, among those patients who achieved complete remission there was no difference in overall survival and event-free survival between patients with IgG and Bence Jones myeloma. In contrast to IgG myeloma where age and β_2-microglobulin were significant prognostic factors, Cox analysis on presentation features of Bence Jones myeloma identified performance status and urine total protein as having significant impact on overall survival.

Plasmablastic morphology at the time of transplantation has been reported as an adverse prognostic factor [186]. The overall survival from the time of transplantation was significantly shorter for patients who had features of plasmablastic morphology compared with patients who did not, with a median survival time of 5 months vs. 24 months, respectively. Increased microvessel density (MVD) has been established as a feature of multiple myeloma [187,188], and may be a poor prognostic factor [189]. Previous studies have shown a decrease in MVD after chemotherapy, including AHCT, corresponding to disease response. The progression-free survival in patients who achieved a reduction in MVD after chemotherapy was significantly longer than in patients without a decrease in MVD [190]. However, a separate study found no difference in MVD at the time of complete or partial response, compared to values prior to transplantation [191].

The Rochester group have reported abnormal bone marrow metaphase cytogenetics in 43% of patients prior to AHCT [192,193]. The overall survival measured from time of transplantation was significantly better in patients with normal cytogenetics than in those with abnormal cytogenetics, with a median survival of 25 vs. 12 months. The progression-free survival was also prolonged, with median times of 12 months vs. 7 months. Overall survival measured from time of diagnosis was also longer, with median survival of 62 months vs. 39 months. The median plasma cell labeling index was 1.5% in patients with abnormal cytogenetics and 0.2% in those with normal cytogenetics. Therefore, abnormal bone marrow cytogenetics using conventional karyotype methods predicted poor survival after blood cell transplantation for myeloma. In addition, there was also a significant correlation between abnormal cytogenetics and high plasma cell labeling index, suggesting that certain cytogenetic abnormalities may be associated with increased proliferation.

Multivariate analysis of 231 patients with newly diagnosed multiple myeloma treated with tandem transplantation at Arkansas showed superior event-free survival and overall survival in the absence of 11q breakpoints and/or partial or complete deletion of chromosome 13, and with β_2-microglobulin ≤ 4 mg/L at diagnosis [173]. When combining these factors, a subgroup of patients with a very poor prognosis was identified. Patients with unfavorable cytogenetics and β_2-microglobulin >4 mg/L had a median survival of only 2.1 years, compared to 7 years for the remaining patients. Using a larger cohort of 1000 consecutive patients, including previously treated patients, the independent favorable features were mainly absence of chromosome 13 deletion using conventional cytogenetics, β_2-microglobulin level ≤ 2.5 mg/L, CRP ≤ 4 mg/L and <12 months of prior conventional chemotherapy [172]. Plateaus of the event-free survival and overall survival curves were noted in 45% and 60% of patients with all these favorable characteristics. In a recent retrospective analysis of 110 patients treated with high-dose therapy, the IFM showed that the detection of chromosome 13 abnormalities by FISH was the most powerful adverse prognostic factor [194]. The combination of FISH analysis, β_2-microglobulin and IgA isotype produce a very powerful staging system in the context of high-dose therapy. Again, patients with a high β_2-microglobulin level and chromosome 13 abnormalities had a very poor prognosis. The cytogenetic abnormalities present prior to AHCT in 1000 patients with multiple myeloma receiving melphalan-based tandem autotransplants have been reported [195]. Cytogenetic abnormalities were present in 33% of all pre-AHCT samples. Most cytogenetic abnormalities were associated with the poor prognostic factors of high β_2-microglobulin and LDH, but not with elevation of CRP and IL-6.

A comparison between the prognostic implications of metaphase karyotypic abnormalities of chromosome 13 vs. deletion of 13q14 detected by FISH (FISH 13) was made in the first 231 patients treated with tandem AHCT at Arkansas. Overall, karyotypic chromosome 13 abnormalities were detected in 14% of patients, and significantly correlated with tumor burden, proliferative activity and LDH. FISH 13 was also present in 46% of patients without metaphase karyotype chromosome 13 abnormalities. Both event-free survival and overall survival were significantly shorter in patients with chromosome 13 abnormalities, FISH 13, LDH ≥190 units/L, β_2-microglobulin ≥4 mg/L and CRP ≥4.0 mg/L. Although present in considerably fewer patients, chromosome 13 abnormalities were associated with a higher rate of relapse and death (61% and 43%, respectively) at 3 years, than FISH 13 (38% and 35%; $p = 0.02$ and 0.1, respectively) [196]. The prognostic value of chromosomal rearrangements in 168 consecutive patients with newly diagnosed multiple myeloma receiving intensive chemotherapy within clinical trials of the IFM have also been analyzed using interphase FISH, with probes specific for chromosomal changes of chromosome 13, illegitimate rearrangements of the IgH gene t(14q32), translocations t(4;14), t(11;14) and t(14;16) [197]. Patients with t(4;14) displayed a short event-free survival and short overall survival, whereas those with t(11;14) displayed long survival. Patients with neither t(4;14) nor t(11;14) had an intermediate outcome. Importantly, chromosome 13 abnormalities significantly influenced the prognosis of patient with neither t(4;14) nor t(11;14), but had less influence on patients with t(4;14) or t(11;14). Interphase FISH analysis therefore provides additional information to standard metaphase karyotype, and consistent application of FISH can be expected to provide more valuable prognostic information in the future. Application of the study of molecular cytogenetics using gene expression profiling to the study of myeloma has made some progress, but the full impact of this new technique is yet to be fully realized [174,198].

The prognostic significance of response to therapy has been evaluated in many studies. Although a study from the Mayo Clinic in Rochester has reported no difference in long-term outcome between patients who achieved complete remission following AHCT and those who did not [199], a number of studies have found, as with responses to melphalan and prednisone, response to induction chemotherapy may also be an important prognostic factor for outcome following AHCT. The Royal Marsden Hospital in London has reported prognosis according to response to induction using vincristine, doxorubicin, methylprednisolone with or without cyclophosphamide/verapamil (VAMP, C-VAMP or V-VAMP) followed by consolidation with high-dose therapy and interferon maintenance [200]. Post-induction therapy, 38 (14%) of patients achieved complete remission, 155 (55%) achieved a partial response, 63 (22%) had no response and 24 (9%) died. Of 280 patients, 209 (75%) received high-dose therapy, with an even distribution between complete remission, partial response and nonresponding patients. The median overall survival for patients who achieved complete remission, partial response and no response post-induction was 7.9 years, 4.4 years and 2.7 years, respectively ($p = 0.001$). The median event-free survival for patients who achieved complete remission, partial response and no response post-induction was 3.3 years, 2.3 years and 1.3 years, respectively ($p < 0.0001$). Patients who achieved complete remission post-induction therapy ($n = 38$) had a longer event-free survival of 3.3 years vs. 2.8 years for those who achieved complete remission after high-dose therapy ($n = 72$; $p = 0.05$), although the overall survival was comparable from the time of induction therapy. Of patients who had no response to induction chemotherapy, 40% achieved a complete remission after high-dose melphalan, indicating a significant potential benefit to patients who do not respond to induction chemotherapy [201].

Reports from the M.D. Anderson Center have shown that overall survival was similar for all patients achieving complete remission, regardless of whether complete remission was achieved with conventional chemotherapy or following high-dose therapy [202,203]. However, the achievement of complete remission post-high-dose therapy was a very important prognostic factor. Patients who achieved complete remission post-high-dose therapy had a median survival 10 months longer than patients who remained in partial response post-transplant [202]. Patients who failed to achieve complete remission after transplantation generally had a worse prognosis than those who achieved complete remission prior to high-dose therapy. To identify those patients in partial response after induction therapy who were likely to achieve complete remission post-high-dose therapy, a retrospective analysis was performed of 68 consecutive patients with multiple myeloma of high to intermediate tumor mass, who had responded to VAD or dexamethasone-based therapy [202]. These patients were compared to 50 similar patients who did not undergo transplantation. Overall, with high-dose therapy the complete remission rate was increased from 6 to 37%, with a median survival prolonged by 10 months in patients who achieved complete remission after high-dose therapy. For patients not in complete remission prior to high-dose therapy, 67% of those with a rapid reduction in tumor burden (half-life <0.5 months) and with low residual disease prior to therapy (myeloma protein <1.0 g/dL) achieved complete remission post-transplant. However, only 23% of patients with slow reduction in tumor burden and high residual disease prior to high-dose therapy entered complete remission post-transplant. Investigators from Italy have also confirmed that patients responding early to VAD were more likely to enter complete remission post-high-dose therapy [204]. It has been reported that treatment with transplantation for primary refractory disease may offer a superior outcome when compared to treatment for relapsed myeloma [205].

The achievement of complete remission has also been reported as a good prognostic factor using tandem transplantation [172]. The IFM90 study analysis reported the 5-year probability of survival after diagnosis was 72% among 51 patients who had complete or very good partial responses, 39% among 81 patients who had partial responses and 0 among 46 patients who did not have even partial responses ($p < 0.001$). Therefore, the achievement of complete remission status also appears to be an important prognostic factor in tandem transplantation. For those patients who do achieve complete remission prior to high-dose therapy, it will be necessary to determine who is most likely to benefit from subsequent high-dose therapy. More sensitive methods of minimal residual disease assessment may be of benefit, such as quantitative PCR [206]. Altogether, response to therapy appears to correlate with prognosis, with better response correlating with better prognosis.

Prognostic factors from the time of relapse following AHCT have been analyzed [207]. A total of 150 patients with newly diagnosed secretory myeloma achieved complete remission after initial chemotherapy with vincristine, doxorubicin, and methylprednisolone with or without cyclophosphamide (VAMP/C-VAMP) followed by high-dose therapy and interferon maintenance. Ninety-eight patients relapsed, with either reappearance of Bence-Jones protein or paraprotein. Median overall survival after relapse was 23 months from date of relapse. Twenty-three percent achieved a second complete remission, and the median overall survival from time of relapse of these patients was 55 months vs. 20 months in other patients ($p = 0.02$). The patients were divided into three risk groups from date of relapse: good risk if age <55 years and good performance status; intermediate risk if either age <55 years or good performance status; and poor risk if age >55 years and poor performance status. The median overall survival for each group was 3.7 years, 2.1 years and 1.3 years, respectively. The 5-year probability of overall survival in the good-risk category was 46%.

In summary, features associated with a better prognosis following AHCT include the presence of t(11;14) and a good response to initial therapy, especially achievement of complete remission. Poor prognosis is associated with plasmablastic morphology, raised β_2-microglobulin, raised LDH, raised CRP, hypodiploidy, t(4;14) and abnormalities of chromosome 13. Chromosome 13 abnormalities detected by FISH appear to be less important in the presence of either t(4;14) or t(11;14). From the time of relapse following AHCT, age <55 years, good performance status and achievement of complete remission have been associated with longer survival.

Secondary myelodysplasia and acute myeloid leukemia

The risk of secondary myelodysplasia and acute myeloid leukemia post-transplant has been analyzed by the Arkansas group [208]. A total of 188 patients were examined. Seventy-one patients had no more than one cycle of standard chemotherapy pretransplant therapy, and were enrolled in a program designed to avoid alkylating agents (group 1). The other group consisted of 117 patients with more prolonged exposure to conventional therapy (group 2). The median duration of pretransplant therapy in group 1 was 7.6 months, and was significantly shorter than the 24 months of in group 2. Seven patients developed myelodysplasia post-transplant, all of whom belonged to the second group. These results suggest that prolonged standard-dose alkylating agent therapy prior to transplantation, rather than the autotransplant-supported myeloablative treatment, is associated with the development of myelodysplasia or acute myeloid leukemia.

Maintenance therapy

In a retrospective analysis of the EBMT registry, post-AHCT maintenance with interferon alfa was associated with improved progression-free survival and overall survival in patients responding to high-dose therapy [209]. Only one randomized study of maintenance therapy post-AHCT has been completed to date [210]. This trial compared interferon alfa following recovery from high-dose therapy vs. no further therapy. With a median follow-up of 77 months, the median progression-free survival was significantly longer at 42 months vs. 27 month for the control arm. Progression-free survival and overall survival were highly significant after 52 months of follow-up, but ceased to be significantly prolonged at 77 months' follow-up. Therefore, although interferon delays relapse, most patients ultimately do relapse. However, only 85 patients were accrued to this trial, and the results should therefore be interpreted with caution. The confidence intervals were wide (99%CI: 74% odds reduction to 10% odds increase), so a greater or lesser benefit for interferon in the context of high-dose therapy, compared with other forms of chemotherapy, cannot be ruled out.

In the IFM90 trial, interferon alfa was to be administered to all patients after high-dose therapy, but there was no plateau of the event-free survival curve [73]. More randomized evidence is needed if this issue is to be addressed reliably. The results of a large ongoing intergroup trial in the USA are awaited. However, cure of patients with multiple myeloma with a single course of high-dose therapy followed by interferon alfa is unlikely. New strategies to control minimal residual disease after AHCT are necessary. They include the use of maintenance chemotherapy, thalidomide, bisphosphonates and immunotherapy (vaccination with idiotype, DNA or tumor associated antigens, immunotherapy with idiotype pulsed dendritic cells or dendritic/tumor fusion cells). These strategies are currently under evaluation. At present, significant clinical responses have been observed in only a few patients.

Novel therapies

More recently, there have been exciting new developments in novel therapies for multiple myeloma [211]. Thalidomide has been shown to have efficacy in patients who relapse after autologous transplantation, but is associated with significant toxicity including peripheral neuropathy, constipation and somnolence. Immunomodulatory analogs of thalidomide are now available which are more potent and better tolerated than thalidomide [212–214]. Another exciting new prospect is the proteasome inhibitor PS-341 [215], which showed significant efficacy in a phase 2 clinical trial for multiple myeloma [216]. At present, these novel therapies have been primarily used to treat patients who relapse after transplantation. Because of their efficacy and tolerability, these agents are now being evaluated in earlier stage patients, as initial therapy or treatment of first relapse. If these agents achieve durable responses, the role of AHCT may need reevaluation.

References

1 National Cancer Institute. *Surveillance, Epidemiology and End Results*. 2002.
2 Hallek M, Bergsagel PL, Anderson KC. Multiple myeloma: increasing evidence for a multistep transformation process. *Blood* 1998; **91**: 3–21.
3 Bergsagel PL, Chesi M, Nardini E, Brents LA, Kirby SL, Kuehl WM. Promiscuous translocations into immunoglobulin heavy chain switch regions in multiple myeloma. *Proc Natl Acad Sci U S A* 1996; **93**: 13931–6.
4 Sawyer JR, Waldron JA, Jagannath S, Barlogie B. Cytogenetic findings in 200 patients with multiple myeloma. *Cancer Genet Cytogenet* 1995; **82**: 41–9.
5 Lai JL, Zandecki M, Mary JY *et al*. Improved cytogenetics in multiple myeloma: a study of 151 patients including 117 patients at diagnosis. *Blood* 1995; **85**: 2490–7.
6 Drach J, Schuster J, Nowotny H *et al*. Multiple myeloma: high incidence of chromosomal aneuploidy as detected by interphase fluorescence *in situ* hybridization. *Cancer Res* 1995; **55**: 3854–9.
7 Shou Y, Martelli ML, Gabrea A *et al*. Diverse karyotypic abnormalities of the c-*myc* locus associated with c-*myc* dysregulation and tumor progression in multiple myeloma. *Proc Natl Acad Sci U S A* 2000; **97**: 228–33.
8 Chesi M, Bergsagel PL, Brents LA, Smith CM, Gerhard DS, Kuehl WM. Dysregulation of cyclin D1 by translocation into an IgH gamma switch region in two multiple myeloma cell lines. *Blood* 1996; **88**: 674–81.
9 Derenne S, Monia B, Dean NM *et al*. Antisense strategy shows that *Mcl*-1 rather than *Bcl*-2 or *Bcl*-x (L) is an essential survival protein of human myeloma cells. *Blood* 2002; **100**: 194–9.
10 Wang CY, Cusack JC Jr, Liu R, Baldwin AS Jr. Control of inducible chemoresistance: enhanced anti-tumor therapy through increased apoptosis by inhibition of NF-κB. *Nat Med* 1999; **5**: 412–7.
11 Tu Y, Xu FH, Liu J *et al*. Upregulated expression of *BCL*-2 in multiple myeloma cells induced by exposure to doxorubicin, etoposide, and hydrogen peroxide. *Blood* 1996; **88**: 1805–12.
12 Jensen GS, Belch AR, Mant MJ, Ruether BA, Yacyshyn BR, Pilarski LM. Expression of multiple beta 1 integrins on circulating monoclonal B cells in patients with multiple myeloma. *Am J Hematol* 1993; **43**: 29–36.
13 Damiano JS, Cress AE, Hazlehurst LA, Shtil AA, Dalton WS. Cell adhesion mediated drug resistance (CAM-DR): role of integrins and resistance to apoptosis in human myeloma cell lines. *Blood* 1999; **93**: 1658–67.
14 Westendorf JJ, Ahmann GJ, Armitage RJ *et al*. CD40 expression in malignant plasma cells: role in stimulation of autocrine IL-6 secretion by a human myeloma cell line. *J Immunol* 1994; **152**: 117–28.
15 Tai YT, Podar K, Mitsiades N *et al*. CD40 induces human multiple myeloma cell migration via phosphatidylinositol 3-kinase/AKT/NF-κB signaling. *Blood* 2003; **101**: 2762–9.
16 Tai YT, Podar K, Gupta D *et al*. CD40 activation induces p53-dependent vascular endothelial growth factor secretion in human multiple myeloma cells. *Blood* 2002; **99**: 1419–27.

17 Tong AW, Zhang BQ, Mues G, Solano M, Hanson T, Stone MJ. Anti-CD40 antibody binding modulates human multiple myeloma clonogenicity in vitro. *Blood* 1994; **84**: 3026–33.

18 Pellat-Deceunynck C, Bataille R, Robillard N et al. Expression of CD28 and CD40 in human myeloma cells: a comparative study with normal plasma cells. *Blood* 1994; **84**: 2597–603.

19 Urashima M, Chauhan D, Hatziyanni M et al. CD40 ligand triggers interleukin-6 mediated B cell differentiation. *Leuk Res* 1996; **20**: 507–15.

20 Urashima M, Chauhan D, Uchiyama H, Freeman GJ, Anderson KC. CD40 ligand triggered interleukin-6 secretion in multiple myeloma. *Blood* 1995; **85**: 1903–12.

21 Chauhan D, Uchiyama H, Akbarali Y et al. Multiple myeloma cell adhesion-induced interleukin-6 expression in bone marrow stromal cells involves activation of NF-κB. *Blood* 1996; **87**: 1104–12.

22 Chauhan D, Uchiyama H, Urashima M, Yamamoto K, Anderson KC. Regulation of interleukin 6 in multiple myeloma and bone marrow stromal cells. *Stem Cells* 1995; **13** (Suppl. 2): 35–9.

23 Urashima M, Ogata A, Chauhan D et al. Transforming growth factor-beta1: differential effects on multiple myeloma versus normal B cells. *Blood* 1996; **87**: 1928–38.

24 Georgii-Hemming P, Wiklund HJ, Ljunggren O, Nilsson K. Insulin-like growth factor I is a growth and survival factor in human multiple myeloma cell lines. *Blood* 1996; **88**: 2250–8.

25 Gupta D, Treon SP, Shima Y et al. Adherence of multiple myeloma cells to bone marrow stromal cells upregulates vascular endothelial growth factor secretion: therapeutic applications. *Leukemia* 2001; **15**: 1950–61.

26 Kawano M, Hirano T, Matsuda T et al. Autocrine generation and requirement of BSF-2/IL-6 for human multiple myelomas. *Nature* 1988; **332**: 83–5.

27 Uchiyama H, Barut BA, Chauhan D, Cannistra SA, Anderson KC. Characterization of adhesion molecules on human myeloma cell lines. *Blood* 1992; **80**: 2306–14.

28 Uchiyama H, Barut BA, Mohrbacher AF, Chauhan D, Anderson KC. Adhesion of human myeloma-derived cell lines to bone marrow stromal cells stimulates interleukin-6 secretion. *Blood* 1993; **82**: 3712–20.

29 Damiano JS, Dalton WS. Integrin-mediated drug resistance in multiple myeloma. *Leuk Lymphoma* 2000; **38**: 71–81.

30 Chauhan D, Pandey P, Hideshima T et al. SHP2 mediates the protective effect of interleukin-6 against dexamethasone-induced apoptosis in multiple myeloma cells. *J Biol Chem* 2000; **275**: 27845–50.

31 Hitzler JK, Martinez-Valdez H, Bergsagel DB, Minden MD, Messner HA. Role of interleukin-6 in the proliferation of human multiple myeloma cell lines OCI-My 1–7 established from patients with advanced stage of the disease. *Blood* 1991; **78**: 1996–2004.

32 Puthier D, Derenne S, Barille S et al. Mcl-1 and Bcl-xL are coregulated by IL-6 in human myeloma cells. *Br J Haematol* 1999; **107**: 392–5.

33 Podar K, Tai YT, Davies FE et al. Vascular endothelial growth factor triggers signaling cascades mediating multiple myeloma cell growth and migration. *Blood* 2001; **98**: 428–35.

34 Podar K, Tai YT, Lin BK et al. Vascular endothelial growth factor-induced migration of multiple myeloma cells is associated with beta 1 integrin- and phosphatidylinositol 3-kinase-dependent PKC alpha activation. *J Biol Chem* 2002; **277**: 7875–81.

35 Torcia M, Lucibello M, Vannier E et al. Modulation of osteoclast-activating factor activity of multiple myeloma bone marrow cells by different interleukin-1 inhibitors. *Exp Hematol* 1996; **24**: 868–74.

36 Carter A, Merchav S, Silvian-Draxler I, Tatarsky I. The role of interleukin-1 and tumour necrosis factor-alpha in human multiple myeloma. *Br J Haematol* 1990; **74**: 424–31.

37 Yamamoto I, Kawano M, Sone T et al. Production of interleukin 1 beta, a potent bone resorbing cytokine, by cultured human myeloma cells. *Cancer Res* 1989; **49**: 4242–6.

38 Cozzolino F, Torcia M, Aldinucci D et al. Production of interleukin-1 by bone marrow myeloma cells. *Blood* 1989; **74**: 380–7.

39 Mundy GR. Metastasis to bone: causes, consequences and therapeutic opportunities. *Nat Rev Cancer* 2002; **2**: 584–93.

40 Roux S, Meignin V, Quillard J et al. RANK (receptor activator of nuclear factor-κB) and RANKL expression in multiple myeloma. *Br J Haematol* 2002; **117**: 86–92.

41 Sezer O, Heider U, Jakob C, Eucker J, Possinger K. Human bone marrow myeloma cells express RANKL. *J Clin Oncol* 2002; **20**: 353–4.

42 Sezer O, Heider U, Jakob C et al. Immunocytochemistry reveals RANKL expression of myeloma cells. *Blood* 2002; **99**: 4646–7.

43 Giuliani N, Bataille R, Mancini C, Lazzaretti M, Barille S. Myeloma cells induce imbalance in the osteoprotegerin/osteoprotegerin ligand system in the human bone marrow environment. *Blood* 2001; **98**: 3527–33.

44 Bradwell A, Mead G, Carr-Smith H, Drayson M. Detection of Bence Jones myeloma and monitoring of myeloma chemotherapy using serum immunoassays specific for free immunoglobulin light chains. *Blood* 2001; **98**: 157a [Abstract].

45 Kyle RA, Therneau TM, Rajkumar SV et al. A long-term study of prognosis in monoclonal gammopathy of undetermined significance. *N Engl J Med* 2002; **346**: 564–9.

46 Durie BG, Salmon SE. A clinical staging system for multiple myeloma: correlation of measured myeloma cell mass with presenting clinical features, response to treatment, and survival. *Cancer* 1975; **36**: 842–54.

47 Cuzick J, Cooper EH, MacLennan IC. The prognostic value of serum beta 2 microglobulin compared with other presentation features in myelomatosis. *Br J Cancer* 1985; **52**: 1–6.

48 Cuzick J, De Stavola BL, Cooper EH, Chapman C, MacLennan IC. Long-term prognostic value of serum beta 2 microglobulin in myelomatosis. *Br J Haematol* 1990; **75**: 506–10.

49 Smadja NV, Bastard C, Brigaudeau C, Leroux D, Fruchart C. Hypodiploidy is a major prognostic factor in multiple myeloma. *Blood* 2001; **98**: 2229–38.

50 Zojer N, Konigsberg R, Ackermann J et al. Deletion of 13q14 remains an independent adverse prognostic variable in multiple myeloma despite its frequent detection by interphase fluorescence in situ hybridization. *Blood* 2000; **95**: 1925–30.

51 Konigsberg R, Zojer N, Ackermann J et al. Predictive role of interphase cytogenetics for survival of patients with multiple myeloma. *J Clin Oncol* 2000; **18**: 804–12.

52 Boccadoro M, Marmont F, Tribalto M et al. Early responder myeloma: kinetic studies identify a patient subgroup characterized by very poor prognosis. *J Clin Oncol* 1989; **7**: 119–25.

53 Hansen OP, Jessen B, Videbaek A. Prognosis of myelomatosis on treatment with prednisone and cytostatics. *Scand J Haematol* 1973; **10**: 282–90.

54 Chang SY, Alberts DS, Melnick LR, Walson PD, Salmon SE. High-pressure liquid chromatographic analysis of melphalan in plasma. *J Pharm Sci* 1978; **67**: 679–82.

55 Alberts DS, Chang SY, Chen HS et al. Kinetics of intravenous melphalan. *Clin Pharmacol Ther* 1979; **26**: 73–80.

56 Alberts DS, Chang SY, Chen HS, Larcom BJ, Jones SE. Pharmacokinetics and metabolism of chlorambucil in man: a preliminary report. *Cancer Treat Rev* 1979; **6** (Suppl.): 9–17.

57 Pallante SL, Fenselau C, Mennel RG et al. Quantitation by gas chromatography-chemical ionization-mass spectrometry of phenylalanine mustard in plasma of patients. *Cancer Res* 1980; **40**: 2268–72.

58 Alberts DS, Chang SY, Chen HS, Evans TL, Moon TE. Oral melphalan kinetics. *Clin Pharmacol Ther* 1979; **26**: 737–45.

59 Alberts DS, Chang SY, Chen HS, Larcom BJ, Evans TL. Comparative pharmacokinetics of chlorambucil and melphalan in man. *Recent Results Cancer Res* 1980; **74**: 124–31.

60 Begleiter A, Lam HP, Goldenberg GJ. Mechanism of uptake of nitrosoureas by L5178Y lymphoblasts in vitro. *Cancer Res* 1977; **37**: 1022–7.

61 Goldenberg GJ, Lee M, Lam HY, Begleiter A. Evidence for carrier-mediated transport of melphalan by L5178Y lymphoblasts in vitro. *Cancer Res* 1977; **37**: 755–60.

62 Goldenberg GJ, Lam HY, Begleiter A. Active carrier-mediated transport of melphalan by two separate amino acid transport systems in LPC-1 plasmacytoma cells in vitro. *J Biol Chem* 1979; **254**: 1057–64.

63 Tattersall MH, Jarman M, Newlands ES, Holyhead L, Milstead RA, Weinberg A. Pharmaco-kinetics of melphalan following oral or intravenous administration in patients with malignant disease. *Eur J Cancer* 1978; **14**: 507–13.

64 Larrivee B, Averill DA. Melphalan resistance and photoaffinity labelling of P-glycoprotein in multidrug-resistant Chinese hamster ovary cells: reversal of resistance by cyclosporin A and hyperthermia. *Biochem Pharmacol* 1999; **58**: 291–302.

65 Goldenberg GJ. The role of drug transport in resistance to nitrogen mustard and other alkylating agents in L518Y lymphoblsts. *Cancer Res* 1975; **35**: 1687–92.

66 Barlogie B, Smith L, Alexanian R. Effective treatment of advanced multiple myeloma refractory to alkylating agents. *N Engl J Med* 1984; **310**: 1353–6.

67 Alexanian R, Barlogie B, Dixon D. High-dose glucocorticoid treatment of resistant myeloma. *Ann Intern Med* 1986; **105**: 8–11.

68 Alexanian R, Dimopoulos MA, Delasalle K, Barlogie B. Primary dexamethasone treatment of multiple myeloma. *Blood* 1992; **80**: 887–90.

69 Abrahamson GM, Bird JM, Newland AC et al. A randomized study of VAD therapy with either concurrent or maintenance interferon in patients with newly diagnosed multiple myeloma. *Br J Haematol* 1996; **94**: 659–64.

70 Samson D, Gaminara E, Newland A et al. Infusion of vincristine and doxorubicin with oral dexa-

methasone as first-line therapy for multiple myeloma. *Lancet* 1989; **2**: 882–5.
71 Aitchison RG, Reilly IA, Morgan AG, Russell NH. Vincristine, Adriamycin and high dose steroids in myeloma complicated by renal failure. *Br J Cancer* 1990; **61**: 765–6.
72 Myeloma Trialists' Collaborative Group. Combination chemotherapy versus melphalan plus prednisone as treatment for multiple myeloma: an overview of 6633 patients from 27 randomized trials. *J Clin Oncol* 1998; **16**: 3832–42.
73 Attal M, Harousseau JL, Stoppa AM *et al*. Autologous bone marrow transplantation versus conventional chemotherapy in multiple myeloma: a prospective, randomized trial. *N Engl J Med* 1996; **335**: 91–7.
74 Palumbo A, Bringhen S, Rus C *et al*. A prospective randomized trial of intermediate dose melphalan (100 mg/m^2) versus oral melphalan/prednisone: an interim analysis. *Blood* 2001; **98**: 849a [Abstract].
75 Fermand J, Ravaud P, Katsahian S *et al*. High dose therapy and autologous stem cell transplantation versus conventional treatment in multiple myeloma: results of a randomized trial in 190 patients 55–65 years of age. *Blood* 1999; **94**: 396a [Abstract].
76 Blade J, Sureda A, Ribera J *et al*. High-dose therapy autotransplantation versus continued conventional chemotherapy in multiple myeloma in patients responding to initial chemotherapy. Results of a prospective randomized trial from the Spanish Cooperative Group PETHEMA. *Blood* 2001; **98**: 815a [Abstract].
77 Morgan G, Davies F, Hawkins K *et al*. The MRC Myeloma VII Trial of standard versus intensive treatment in patients <65 years of age with multiple myeloma. *Blood* 2002; **98**: 178a [Abstract].
78 Attal M, Harousseau J, Facon T. Single versus double transplant in myeloma: a randomized trial of the Intergroupe Francais du Myeloma (IFM). *Proceedings of the VIIIth International Myeloma Workshop, 2001*, Banff, Canada [Abstract].
79 Attal M, Harousseau JL, Facon T *et al*. Double autologous transplantation improves survival of multiple myeloma patients: final analysis of a prospective randomized study of the intergroupe francophone du myeloma (IFM94). *Blood* 2002; **100**: 5a [Abstract].
80 Cavo M, Tosi P, Zamagni E *et al*. The Bologna96 clinical trial of single versus double PBSC transplantation for previously untreated multiple myeloma: results of an interim analysis. *Proceedings of the VIIIth International Myeloma Workshop, 2001*, Banff, Canada [Abstract].
81 Cavo M, Tosi P, Zamagni E *et al*. The "Bologna 96" clinical trial of single vs. double autotransplants for previously untreated multiple myeloma patients. *Blood* 2002; **100**: 179a [Abstract].
82 Segeren CM, Sonneveld P, van der Holt B *et al*. Overall and event-free survival are not improved by the use of myelo-ablative therapy following intensified chemotherapy in previously untreated mutliple myeloma patients: a prospective randomized phase III study. *Blood* 2003; **101**: 2144–51.
83 Fermand J-P, Marolleau J-P, Alberti C *et al*. Single versus tandem high dose therapy supported with autologous stem cell transplantation using unselected or CD34 enriched ABSC: preliminary results of a two by two designed randomized trial in 230 young patients with multiple myeloma. *Blood* 2001; **98**: 815a [Abstract].
84 Singhal S, Mehta J, Desikan R *et al*. Antitumor activity of thalidomide in refractory multiple myeloma. *N Engl J Med* 1999; **341**: 1565–71.
85 Raje N, Anderson K. Thalidomide: a revival story. *N Engl J Med* 1999; **341**: 1606–9.
86 Weber D, Rankin K, Gavino M, Delasalle K, Alexanian R. Thalidomide alone or with dexamethasone for previously untreated multiple myeloma. *J Clin Oncol* 2003; **21**: 16–9.
87 Patriarca F, Fili C, Sperotto A *et al*. Thalidomide overcomes VAD chemoresistance and allows PBSC collection in three multiple myeloma patients. *Bone Marrow Transplant* 2001; **27**: S104.
88 Rajkumar S, Hayman S, Gertz M *et al*. Combination therapy with thalidomide plus dexamethasone (Thal/dex) for newly diagnosed myeloma. *Blood* 2002; **98**: 849a [Abstract].
89 Rajkumar SV, Hayman S, Gertz MA *et al*. Combination therapy with thalidomide plus dexamethasone for newly diagnosed myeloma. *J Clin Oncol* 2002; **20**: 4319–23.
90 Tricot G, Jagannath S, Vesole D *et al*. Peripheral blood stem cell transplants for multiple myeloma: identification of favorable variables for rapid engraftment in 225 patients. *Blood* 1995; **85**: 588–96.
91 Goldschmidt H, Hegenbart U, Wallmeier M, Hohaus S, Haas R. Factors influencing collection of peripheral blood progenitor cells following high-dose cyclophosphamide and granulocyte colony-stimulating factor in patients with multiple myeloma. *Br J Haematol* 1997; **98**: 736–44.
92 Boccadoro M, Palumbo A, Bringhen S *et al*. Oral melphalan at diagnosis hampers adequate collection of peripheral blood progenitor cells in multiple myeloma. *Haematologica* 2002; **87**: 846–50.
93 McCloskey EV, Dunn JA, Kanis JA, MacLennan IC, Drayson MT. Long-term follow-up of a prospective, double-blind, placebo-controlled randomized trial of clodronate in multiple myeloma. *Br J Haematol* 2001; **113**: 1035–43.
94 McCloskey EV, MacLennan IC, Drayson MT, Chapman C, Dunn J, Kanis JA. A randomized trial of the effect of clodronate on skeletal morbidity in multiple myeloma. MRC Working Party on Leukaemia in Adults. *Br J Haematol* 1998; **100**: 317–25.
95 Bloomfield DJ. Should bisphosphonates be part of the standard therapy of patients with multiple myeloma or bone metastases from other cancers? An evidence-based review. *J Clin Oncol* 1998; **16**: 1218–25.
96 Berenson JR, Lichtenstein A, Porter L *et al*. Long-term pamidronate treatment of advanced multiple myeloma patients reduces skeletal events. Myeloma Aredia Study Group. *J Clin Oncol* 1998; **16**: 593–602.
97 Berenson JR, Lichtenstein A, Porter L *et al*. Efficacy of pamidronate in reducing skeletal events in patients with advanced multiple myeloma. Myeloma Aredia Study Group. *N Engl J Med* 1996; **334**: 488–93.
98 Mundy GR, Yoneda T, Hiraga T. Preclinical studies with zoledronic acid and other bisphosphonates: impact on the bone microenvironment. *Semin Oncol* 2001; **28**: 35–44.
99 San Miguel JF, Garcia-Sanz R. Recombinant human erythropoietin in the anaemia of multiple myeloma and non-Hodgkin's lymphoma. *Med Oncol* 1998; **15** (Suppl. 1): S29–34.
100 Mittelman M, Zeidman A, Fradin Z, Magazanik A, Lewinski UH, Cohen A. Recombinant human erythropoietin in the treatment of multiple myeloma-associated anemia. *Acta Haematol* 1997; **98**: 204–10.
101 Osterborg A, Boogaerts MA, Cimino R *et al*. Recombinant human erythropoietin in transfusion-dependent anemic patients with multiple myeloma and non-Hodgkin's lymphoma: a randomized multicenter study. The European Study Group of erythropoietin (epoetin beta) treatment in multiple myeloma and non-Hodgkin's lymphoma. *Blood* 1996; **87**: 2675–82.
102 Cazzola M, Messinger D, Battistel V *et al*. Recombinant human erythropoietin in the anemia associated with multiple myeloma or non-Hodgkin's lymphoma: dose finding and identification of predictors of response. *Blood* 1995; **86**: 4446–53.
103 Dudeney S, Lieberman IH, Reinhardt MK, Hussein M. Kyphoplasty in the treatment of osteolytic vertebral compression fractures as a result of multiple myeloma. *J Clin Oncol* 2002; **20**: 2382–7.
104 Hersh MR, Ludden TM, Kuhn JG, Knight WA 3rd. Pharmacokinetics of high dose melphalan. *Invest New Drugs* 1983; **1**: 331–4.
105 Pinguet F, Martel P, Fabbro M *et al*. Pharmacokinetics of high-dose intravenous melphalan in patients undergoing peripheral blood hematopoietic progenitor-cell transplantation. *Anticancer Res* 1997; **17**: 605–11.
106 McElwain TJ, Powles RL. High-dose intravenous melphalan for plasma-cell leukaemia and myeloma. *Lancet* 1983; **2**: 822–4.
107 Barlogie B, Hall R, Zander A, Dicke K, Alexanian R. High-dose melphalan with autologous bone marrow transplantation for multiple myeloma. *Blood* 1986; **67**: 1298–301.
108 Selby PJ, McElwain TJ, Nandi AC *et al*. Multiple myeloma treated with high dose intravenous melphalan. *Br J Haematol* 1987; **66**: 55–62.
109 Bjorkstrand B. European Group for Blood and Marrow Transplantation Registry studies in multiple myeloma. *Semin Hematol* 2001; **38**: 219–25.
110 Gahrton G, Svensson H, Bjorkstrand B *et al*. Syngeneic transplantation in multiple myeloma: a case-matched comparison with autologous and allogeneic transplantation. European Group for Blood and Marrow Transplantation. *Bone Marrow Transplant* 1999; **24**: 741–5.
111 Gahrton G, Svensson H, Cavo M *et al*. Progress in allogeneic bone marrow and peripheral blood stem cell transplantation for multiple myeloma: a comparison between transplants performed between 1983–93 and 1994–98 at European Group for Blood and Marrow Transplantation centres. *Br J Haematol* 2001; **113**: 209–16.
112 Gratwohl A, Passweg J, Baldomero H, Hermans J. Blood and marrow transplantation activity in Europe. European Group for Blood and Marrow Transplantation (EBMT). *Bone Marrow Transplant*, 1999; **24**: 231–45.
113 Gratwohl A, Passweg J, Baldomero H, Hermans J. Blood and marrow transplantation activity in Europe. European Group for Blood and Marrow Transplantation (EBMT). *Bone Marrow Transplant* 1998; **22**: 227–40.
114 Abraham R, Chen C, Tsang R *et al*. Intensification of the stem cell transplant induction regimen results in increased treatment-related mortality without improved outcome in multiple myeloma. *Bone Marrow Transplant* 1999; **24**: 1291–7.
115 Cunningham D, Paz-Ares L, Milan S *et al*. High-dose melphalan and autologous bone marrow transplantation as consolidation in previously untreated myeloma. *J Clin Oncol* 1994; **12**: 759–63.

116 Alegre A, Diaz-Mediavilla J, San-Miguel J et al. Autologous peripheral blood stem cell transplantation for multiple myeloma: a report of 259 cases from the Spanish Registry. Spanish Registry for Transplant in MM (Grupo Espanol de Trasplante Hematopoyetico; GETH) and PETHEMA. Bone Marrow Transplant 1998; 21: 133–40.

117 Alegre Amor A, Lahuerta JJ, Sanz-Rodriguez C et al. Autologous peripheral blood stem cell (APB-SCT) in multiple myeloma (MM): the Spanish multicentre experience. Bone Marrow Transplant 2001; 27: S242.

118 Lahuerta JJ, Grande C, Blade J et al. Myeloablative treatments for multiple myeloma: update of a comparative study of different regimens used in patients from the Spanish registry for transplantation in multiple myeloma. Leuk Lymphoma 2002; 43: 67–74.

119 Lahuerta JJ, Martinez-Lopez J, Grande C et al. Conditioning regimens in autologous stem cell transplantation for multiple myeloma: a comparative study of efficacy and toxicity from the Spanish Registry for Transplantation in Multiple Myeloma. Br J Haematol 2000; 109: 138–47.

120 Moreau P, Facon T, Attal M et al. Comparison of 200 mg/m^2 melphalan and 8 Gy total body irradiation plus 140 mg/m^2 melphalan as conditioning regimens for peripheral blood stem cell transplantation in patients with newly diagnosed multiple myeloma: final analysis of the Intergroupe Francophone du Myelome 9502 randomized trial. Blood 2002; 99: 731–5.

121 Boccadoro M, Palumbo A, Triolo S et al. High-dose and conventional chemotherapy. Proceedings of the VIIIth International Myeloma Workshop, 2001, Banff, Canada, S37: 63–4 [Abstract].

122 Tribalto M, Amadori S, Cudillo L et al. Autologous peripheral blood stem cell transplantation as first line treatment of multiple myeloma: an Italian Multicenter Study. Haematologica 2000; 85: 52–8.

123 Capria S, Petrucci MT, Ferrazza G et al. High-dose idarubicin, busulphan and melphalan conditioning regimen for autograft in multiple myeloma. Bone Marrow Transplant 2001; 27: 456 [Abstract].

124 Meloni G, Capria S, Trasarti S et al. High-dose idarubicine, busulphan and melphalan as conditioning for autologous blood stem cell transplantation in multiple myeloma: a feasibility study. Bone Marrow Transplant 2000; 26: 1045–9.

125 Ballestrero A, Ferrando F, Miglino M et al. Three-step high-dose sequential chemotherapy in patients with newly diagnosed multiple myeloma. Eur J Haematol 2002; 68: 101–6.

126 Shimoni A, Smith TL, Aleman A et al. Thiotepa, busulfan, cyclophosphamide (TBC) and autologous hematopoietic transplantation: an intensive regimen for the treatment of multiple myeloma. Bone Marrow Transplant 2001; 27: 821–8.

127 Vesole DH, Barlogie B, Jagannath S et al. High-dose therapy for refractory multiple myeloma: improved prognosis with better supportive care and double transplants. Blood 1994; 84: 950–6.

128 Bjorkstrand B, Svensson H, Ljungman P et al. 2522 autotransplants in multiple myeloma: a registry study from the European group for blood and marrow transplantation (EBMT). Blood 1997; 90: 419a [Abstract].

129 Desikan KR, Tricot G, Dhodapkar M et al. Melphalan plus total body irradiation (MEL-TBI) or cyclophosphamide (MEL-CY) as a conditioning regimen with second autotransplant in responding patients with myeloma is inferior compared to historical controls receiving tandem transplants with melphalan alone. Bone Marrow Transplant 2000; 25: 483–7.

130 Attal M, Harousseau JL, Stoppa AM et al. A prospective, randomized trial of autologous bone marrow transplantation and chemotherapy in multiple myeloma. Intergroupe Francais Myelome. N Engl J Med 1996; 335: 91–7.

131 Siegel DS, Desikan KR, Mehta J et al. Age is not a prognostic variable with autotransplants for multiple myeloma. Blood 1999; 93: 51–4.

132 Badros A, Barlogie B, Siegel E et al. Autologous stem cell transplantation in elderly multiple myeloma patients over the age of 70 years. Br J Haematol 2001; 114: 600–7.

133 Palumbo A, Triolo S, Argentino C et al. Dose-intensive melphalan with stem cell support (MEL100) is superior to standard treatment in elderly myeloma patients. Blood 1999; 94: 1248–53.

134 Sirohi B, Powles R, Treleaven J et al. The role of autologous transplantation in patients with multiple myeloma aged 65 years and over. Bone Marrow Transplant 2000; 25: 533–9.

135 San Miguel JF, Lahuerta JJ, Garcia-Sanz R et al. Are myeloma patients with renal failure candidates for autologous stem cell transplantation? Hematol J 2000; 1: 28–36.

136 Badros A, Barlogie B, Siegel E et al. Results of autologous stem cell transplant in multiple myeloma patients with renal failure. Br J Haematol 2001; 114: 822–9.

137 Sirohi B, Powles R, Mehta J et al. The implication of compromised renal function at presentation in myeloma: similar outcome in patients who receive high-dose therapy. A single-center study of 251 previously untreated patients. Med Oncol 2001; 18: 39–50.

138 Alberts DS, Chen HG, Benz D, Mason NL. Effect of renal dysfunction in dogs on the disposition and marrow toxicity of melphalan. Br J Cancer 1981; 43: 330–4.

139 Cornwell GG 3rd, Pajak TF, McIntyre OR, Kochwa S, Dosik H. Influence of renal failure on myelosuppressive effects of melphalan. Cancer Leukemia Group B Experience. Cancer Treat Rep 1982; 66: 475–81.

140 Tricot G, Alberts DS, Johnson C et al. Safety of autotransplants with high-dose melphalan in renal failure: a pharmacokinetic and toxicity study. Clin Cancer Res 1996; 2: 947–52.

141 Lee C, Barlogie B, Zangari M et al. Dialysis-dependent renal failure in patients with myeloma can be reversed by high-dose myeloablative therapy and autotransplant. Blood 2002; 100: 431a [Abstract].

142 Fitoussi O, Perreau V, Boiron JM et al. A comparison of toxicity following two different doses of cyclophosphamide for mobilization of peripheral blood progenitor cells in 116 multiple myeloma patients. Bone Marrow Transplant 2001; 27: 837–42.

143 Lazzarino M, Corso A, Barbarano L et al. DCEP (dexamethasone, cyclophosphamide, etoposide, and cisplatin) is an effective regimen for peripheral blood stem cell collection in multiple myeloma. Bone Marrow Transplant 2001; 28: 835–9.

144 Bilgrami S, Bona RD, Edwards RL et al. Dexamethasone, paclitaxel, etoposide, cyclophosphamide (d-TEC) and G-CSF for stem cell mobilisation in multiple myeloma. Bone Marrow Transplant 2001; 28: 137–43.

145 Facon T, Harousseau JL, Maloisel F et al. Stem cell factor in combination with filgrastim after chemotherapy improves peripheral blood progenitor cell yield and reduces apheresis requirements in multiple myeloma patients: a randomized, controlled trial. Blood 1999; 94: 1218–25.

146 Harousseau JL. Optimizing peripheral blood progenitor cell autologous transplantation in multiple myeloma. Haematologica 1999; 84: 548–53.

147 Palumbo A, Triolo S, Baldini L et al. Dose-intensive melphalan with stem cell support (CM regimen) is effective and well tolerated in elderly myeloma patients. Haematologica 2000; 85: 508–13.

148 Desikan KR, Tricot G, Munshi NC et al. Preceding chemotherapy, tumour load and age influence engraftment in multiple myeloma patients mobilized with granulocyte colony-stimulating factor alone. Br J Haematol 2001; 112: 242–7.

149 Sirohi B, Powles R, Singhal S et al. Administration of weekly cyclophosphamide as part of infusional induction chemotherapy (C-VAMP) does not affect subsequent peripheral blood stem cell collection in patients with myeloma. Bone Marrow Transplant 2001; 27: P450 [Abstract].

150 Lemoli RM, Cavo M, Fortuna A. Concomitant mobilization of plasma cells and hematopoietic progenitors into peripheral blood of patients with multiple myeloma. J Hematother 1996; 5: 339–49.

151 Lemoli RM, Fortuna A, Motta MR et al. Concomitant mobilization of plasma cells and hematopoietic progenitors into peripheral blood of multiple myeloma patients: positive selection and transplantation of enriched CD34$^+$ cells to remove circulating tumor cells. Blood 1996; 87: 1625–34.

152 Demirer T, Buckner CD, Bensinger WI. Optimization of peripheral blood stem cell mobilization. Stem Cells 1996; 14: 106–16.

153 Powles R, Sirohi B, Kulkarni S et al. Feasibility of collecting peripheral blood stem cells in previously untreated myeloma patients without any prior cytoreductive therapy. Bone Marrow Transplant 2001; 27: S251 [Abstract].

154 Bakkus MHC, Everaert T, Bouko Y et al. Long-term follow-up of the randomised phase III study of the EBMT of tumour cell depletion by CD34 selection in multiple myeloma patients: does quantitative MRD analysis have a predictive value? Bone Marrow Transplant 2001; 27: S39.

155 Bensinger WI. Should we purge? Bone Marrow Transplant 1998; 21: 113–5.

156 Rokicka-Piotrowicz M, Urbanowska E, Torosian T et al. Early mobilisation, Mel 100, autologous transplantation, and VAD remission maintenance for very high-risk multiple myeloma: pilot study. Bone Marrow Transplant 2001; 27: S97 [Abstract].

157 Powles R, Sirohi B, Goyal S et al. Intensive treatment with high-dose melphalan as initial therapy in newly-diagnosed patients with multiple myeloma: key to attain rapid complete remission. Bone Marrow Transplant 2001; 27: S97 [Abstract].

158 Munshi N, Desikan R, Anaissie E et al. Peripheral blood stem cell collection after CAD + G-CSF as part of total therapy II in newly diagnosed multiple myeloma: influence of thalidomide administration. Blood 1999; 94: 578a [Abstract].

159 Zangari M, Anaissie E, Barlogie B et al. Increased risk of deep-vein thrombosis in patients with mul-

tiple myeloma receiving thalidomide and chemotherapy. *Blood* 2001; **98**: 1614–5.
160 Anderson KC, Andersen J, Soiffer R *et al.* Monoclonal antibody-purged bone marrow transplantation therapy for multiple myeloma. *Blood* 1993; **82**: 2568–76.
161 Abonour R, Scott KM, Kunkel LA *et al.* Autologous transplantation of mobilized peripheral blood CD34+ cells selected by immunomagnetic procedures in patients with multiple myeloma. *Bone Marrow Transplant* 1998; **22**: 957–63.
162 Lemoli RM, Martinelli G, Zamagni E *et al.* Engraftment, clinical, and molecular follow-up of patients with multiple myeloma who were reinfused with highly purified CD34+ cells to support single or tandem high-dose chemotherapy. *Blood* 2000; **95**: 2234–9.
163 Stewart AK, Vescio R, Schiller G *et al.* Purging of autologous peripheral-blood stem cells using CD34 selection does not improve overall or progression-free survival after high-dose chemotherapy for multiple myeloma: results of a multicenter randomized controlled trial. *J Clin Oncol* 2001; **19**: 3771–9.
164 Goldschmidt H, Bouko Y, Bourhis JH *et al.* CD34+ selected PBPCT: results in an increased infective risk without prolongation of event free survival in newly diagnosed myeloma. A randomised study from the EBMT. *Blood* 2000; **96**: 558a [Abstract].
165 Boccadoro M, Omede P, Dominietto A *et al.* Multiple myeloma: the number of reinfused plasma cells does not influence outcome of patients treated with intensified chemotherapy and PBPC support. *Bone Marrow Transplant* 2000; **25**: 25–9.
166 Barbui AM, Galli M, Dotti G *et al.* Negative selection of peripheral blood stem cells to support a tandem autologous transplantation programme in multiple myeloma. *Br J Haematol* 2002; **116**: 202–10.
167 Tricot G, Gazitt Y, Leemhuis T *et al.* Collection, tumor contamination, and engraftment kinetics of highly purified hematopoietic progenitor cells to support high dose therapy in multiple myeloma. *Blood* 1998; **91**: 4489–95.
168 Child JA, Morgan GJ, Davies FE *et al.* High-dose chemotherapy with hematopoietic stem-cell rescue for multiple myeloma. *N Engl J Med* 2003; **348**: 1875–83.
169 Gertz MA, Lacy MQ, Inwards DJ *et al.* Early harvest and late transplantation as an effective therapeutic strategy in multiple myeloma. *Bone Marrow Transplant* 1999; **23**: 221–6.
170 Gertz MA, Lacy MQ, Inwards DJ *et al.* Delayed stem cell transplantation for the management of relapsed or refractory multiple myeloma. *Bone Marrow Transplant* 2000; **26**: 45–50.
171 Fermand J-P, Ravaud P, Chevret S *et al.* High-dose therapy and autologous peripheral blood stem cell transplantation in multiple myeloma: up-front or rescue treatment? Results of a multicenter sequential randomized clinical trial. *Blood* 1998; **92**: 3131–6.
172 Desikan R, Barlogie B, Sawyer J *et al.* Results of high-dose therapy for 1000 patients with multiple myeloma: durable complete remissions and superior survival in the absence of chromosome 13 abnormalities. *Blood* 2000; **95**: 4008–10.
173 Barlogie B, Jagannath S, Desikan KR *et al.* Total therapy with tandem transplants for newly diagnosed multiple myeloma. *Blood* 1999; **93**: 55–65.
174 Anderson KC, Shaughnessy JD Jr, Barlogie B, Harousseau JL, Roodman GD. Multiple myeloma. *Hematology* (Am Soc Hematol Educ Program) 2002: 214–40.
175 Barlogie B, Jagannath S, Naucke S *et al.* Long-term follow-up after high-dose therapy for high-risk multiple myeloma. *Bone Marrow Transplant* 1998; **11**: 1101–7.
176 Moreau P, Misbahi R, Milpied N *et al.* Long-term results (12 years) of high-dose therapy in 127 patients with *de novo* multiple myeloma. *Leukemia* 2002; **16**: 1838–43.
177 Tricot G, Spencer T, Sawyer J *et al.* Predicting long-term (>5 years) event-free survival in multiple myeloma patients following planned tandem autotransplants. *Br J Haematol* 2002; **116**: 211–7.
178 Vesole DH, Tricot G, Jagannath S *et al.* Autotransplants in multiple myeloma: what have we learned? *Blood* 1996; **88**: 838–47.
179 Huijgens PC, Dekker-Van Roessel HM, Jonkhoff AR *et al.* High-dose melphalan with G-CSF-stimulated whole blood rescue followed by stem cell harvesting and busulphan/cyclophosphamide with autologous stem cell transplantation in multiple myeloma. *Bone Marrow Transplant* 2001; **27**: 925–31.
180 Sirohi B, Powles R, Singhal S, Treleaven J, Kulkarni S, Sankpal S. Second high-dose melphalan autograft for myeloma patients relapsing after one autograft: results equivalent to tandem transplantation. *Bone Marrow Transplant* 2002; **29** (Suppl. 2): S12 [Abstract].
181 Kroger N, Schwerdtfeger R, Kiehl M *et al.* Autologous stem cell transplantation followed by a dose-reduced allograft induces high complete remission rate in multiple myeloma. *Blood* 2002, 2001; **100**: 755–60.
182 Maloney DG, Sahebi F, Stockerl-Goldstein KE *et al.* Combining an allogeneic graft-vs.-myeloma effect with high-dose autologous stem cell rescue in the treatment of multiple myeloma. *Blood* 2001; **98**: 434a [Abstract].
183 Lokhorst HM, Sonneveld P, Verdonck LF. Intensive treatment for multiple myeloma: where do we stand? *Br J Haematol* 1999; **106**: 18–27.
184 Rajkumar SV, Fonseca R, Lacy MQ *et al.* β_2-microglobulin and bone marrow plasma cell involvement predict complete responders among patients undergoing blood cell transplantation for myeloma. *Bone Marrow Transplant* 1999; **23**: 1261–6.
185 Sirohi B, Powles R, Kulkarni S *et al.* Comparison of new patients with Bence Jones, IgG and IgA myeloma receiving sequential therapy: the need to regard these immunologic subtypes as separate disease entities with specific prognostic criteria. *Bone Marrow Transplant* 2001; **28**: 29–37.
186 Rajkumar SV, Fonseca R, Lacy MQ *et al.* Plasmablastic morphology is an independent predictor of poor survival after autologous stem-cell transplantation for multiple myeloma. *J Clin Oncol* 1999; **17**: 1551–7.
187 Sezer O, Niemoller K, Jakob C, Heider U. Angiogenesis in multiple myeloma. *Leuk Res* 2002; **26**: 701–2.
188 Vacca A, Ribatti D, Roncali L *et al.* Bone marrow angiogenesis and progression in multiple myeloma. *Br J Haematol* 1994; **87**: 503–8.
189 Sezer O, Niemoller K, Eucker J *et al.* Bone marrow microvessel density is a prognostic factor for survival in patients with multiple myeloma. *Ann Hematol* 2000; **79**: 574–7.
190 Sezer O, Niemoller K, Kaufmann O *et al.* Decrease of bone marrow angiogenesis in myeloma patients achieving a remission after chemotherapy. *Eur J Haematol* 2001; **66**: 238–44.
191 Rajkumar SV, Fonseca R, Witzig TE, Gertz MA, Greipp PR. Bone marrow angiogenesis in patients achieving complete response after stem cell transplantation for multiple myeloma. *Leukemia* 1999; **13**: 469–72.
192 Rajkumar S, Fonseca R, Lacy M *et al.* Abnormal cytogenetics predict poor survival after high-dose therapy and autologous blood cell transplantation in multiple myeloma. *Bone Marrow Transplant* 1999; **24**: 497–503.
193 Rajkumar SV, Fonseca R, Dewald GW *et al.* Cytogenetic abnormalities correlate with the plasma cell labeling index and extent of bone marrow involvement in myeloma. *Cancer Genet Cytogenet* 1999; **113**: 73–7.
194 Facon T, Avet-Loiseau H, Guillerm G *et al.* Chromosome 13 abnormalities identified by FISH analysis and serum beta2-microglobulin produce a powerful myeloma staging system for patients receiving high-dose therapy. *Blood* 2001; **97**: 1566–71.
195 Jacobson J, Barlogie B, Shaughnessy J *et al.* The telling role of cytogenetic abnormalities in predicting clinical outcome of 1000 patients with multiple myeloma after tandem transplants. *Blood* 2003; **120**: 734a [Abstract].
196 Shaughnessy J, Tian E, Sawyer J *et al.* Prognostic impact of cytogenetic and interphase fluorescence *in situ* hybridization-defined chromosome 13 deletion in multiple myeloma: early results of total therapy II. *Br J Haematol* 2003; **120**: 44–52.
197 Moreau P, Facon T, Leleu X *et al.* Recurrent 14q32 translocations determine the prognosis of multiple myeloma, especially in patients receiving intensive chemotherapy. *Blood* 2002; **100**: 1579–83.
198 Shaughnessy JD Jr, Barlogie B. Integrating cytogenetics and gene expression profiling in the molecular analysis of multiple myeloma. *Int J Hematol* 2002; **76** (Suppl. 2): 59–64.
199 Rajkumar SV, Fonseca R, Dispenzieri A *et al.* Effect of complete response on outcome following autologous stem cell transplantation for myeloma. *Bone Marrow Transplant* 2000; **26**: 979–83.
200 Sirohi B, Powles R, Kulkarni S *et al.* Maximal response to infusional chemotherapy prior to autotransplantation influences outcome of patients with newly diagnosed multiple myeloma. *Bone Marrow Transplant* 2001; **27**: S246 [Abstract].
201 Singhal SPR, Sirohi B, Treleaven J, Mehta J. Response to induction chemotherapy is not essential to obtain survival benefit from high-dose melphalan and autotransplantation in myeloma. *Blood* 2001; **98**: 816a [Abstract].
202 Alexanian R, Weber D, Giralt S *et al.* Impact of complete remission with intensive therapy in patients with responsive multiple myeloma. *Bone Marrow Transplant* 2001; **27**: 1037–43.
203 Alexanian R, Weber D, Delasalle K, Giralt S, Champlin R. Frequency and impact of complete remission in patients with multiple myeloma of low tumor mass who received intensive therapy supported by autologous stem cell transplantation. *Blood* 2001; **98**: 850a [Abstract].
204 Patriarca F, Sperotto A, Damiani D *et al.* Early chemosensitivity to VAD predicts a favourable outcome after autologous stem cell transplantation in multiple myeloma. *Haematologica* 2002; **87**: 779–81.

205 Rajkumar SV, Fonseca R, Lacy MQ *et al.* Autologous stem cell transplantation for relapsed and primary refractory myeloma. *Bone Marrow Transplant* 1999; **23**: 1267–72.

206 Cremer FW, Ehrbrecht E, Kiel K *et al.* Evaluation of the kinetics of the bone marrow tumor load in the course of sequential high-dose therapy assessed by quantitative PCR as a predictive parameter in patients with multiple myeloma. *Bone Marrow Transplant* 2000; **26**: 851–8.

207 Rao S, Powles R, Sirohi B *et al.* Relapse following complete remission: outcome predictors in patients with secretory myeloma. *Bone Marrow Transplant* 2001; **27**: 463 [Abstract].

208 Govindarajan R, Jagannath S, Flick JT *et al.* Preceding standard therapy is the likely cause of MDS after autotransplants for multiple myeloma. *Br J Haematol* 1996; **95**: 349–53.

209 Bjorkstrand B, Svensson H, Goldschmidt H *et al.* Alpha-interferon maintenance treatment is associated with improved survival after high-dose treatment and autologous stem cell transplantation in patients with multiple myeloma: a retrospective registry study from the European Group for Blood and Marrow Transplantation (EBMT). *Bone Marrow Transplant* 2001; **27**: 511–5.

210 Cunningham D, Powles R, Malpas J *et al.* A randomized trial of maintenance interferon following high-dose chemotherapy in multiple myeloma: long-term follow-up results. *Br J Haematol* 1998; **102**: 495–502.

211 Hideshima T, Chauhan D, Podar K, Schlossman RL, Richardson P, Anderson KC. Novel therapies targeting the myeloma cell and its bone marrow microenvironment. *Semin Oncol* 2001; **28**: 607–12.

212 Hideshima T, Chauhan D, Shima Y *et al.* Thalidomide and its analogs overcome drug resistance of human multiple myeloma cells to conventional therapy. *Blood* 2000; **96**: 2943–50.

213 Davies FE, Raje N, Hideshima T *et al.* Thalidomide and immunomodulatory derivatives augment natural killer cell cytotoxicity in multiple myeloma. *Blood* 2001; **98**: 210–6.

214 Richardson PG, Schlossman RL, Weller E *et al.* Immunomodulatory drug CC-5013 overcomes drug resistance and is well tolerated in patients with relapsed multiple myeloma. *Blood* 2002; **100**: 3063–7.

215 Hideshima T, Richardson P, Chauhan D *et al.* The proteasome inhibitor PS-341 inhibits growth, induces apoptosis, and overcomes drug resistance in human multiple myeloma cells. *Cancer Res* 2001; **61**: 3071–6.

216 Richardson PG, Barlogie B, Berenson J *et al.* A phase 2 study of bortezomib in relapsed, refractory myeloma. *N Engl J Med* 2003; **348**: 2609–17.

93

Raymond L. Comenzo & Morie A. Gertz

Autologous Hematopoietic Cell Transplantation for AL Amyloidosis

Introduction

Amyloidosis is the term for a group of diseases in which abnormal proteins self-assemble to form extracellular deposits of insoluble non-branching linear fibrils that are 7–10 nm in width, vary in length and resist proteolysis [1–3]. It appears that medical and forensic investigators at autopsy recognized such deposits over 3 centuries ago: some thought the deposited material was a fatty substance, hence the term "lardaceous disease" [4]. In 1854, the pathologist Virchow described the deposits in post-mortem liver tissue with the botanical term "amyloid," meaning starch, since the deposits had an apparent starch-like affinity for iodine. Virchow's misnomer has been perpetuated [5].

The deposits appear amorphous and ground-glass-like under the light microscope, eosinophilic with hematoxylin-eosin stain. When stained with Congo red, the deposits exhibit a characteristic apple-green birefringence in polarized light, an important observation first reported in 1927 (Plate 93.1, *facing p. 296*) [6]. A century after Virchow, the characteristic β-pleated-sheet configuration and fibrillar nature of amyloid were identified (Plate 93.1) [7,8]. In the 1970s, it was established that all of the variants of amyloidosis have fibril-precursor proteins, that is, normally soluble globular proteins that self-assemble and deposit as amyloid fibrils [9–12]. The immunoglobulin light chains of a patient with AL (light chain amyloid) are usually the fibril-precursor protein. They have an abnormal tertiary structure and self-assemble to form β-pleated sheets, causing the deposits to become relatively insoluble and to accumulate.

The term "primary amyloidosis" is of historic interest only and was used when the patient did not have a secondary cause or a positive family history. In the old nomenclature, primary actually referred to amyloid as being idiopathic. Today, primary actually refers to amyloidosis derived from immunoglobulin light chains and is always associated with a clonal plasma cell disorder that may or may not be multiple myeloma. Amyloidosis patients who do not have myeloma at presentation have a risk of only 0.5% of subsequent evolution to multiple myeloma. It is uncommon for the clinical course of a patient with AL to be significantly impacted by associated myeloma.

In AL, nearly three-quarters of the pathologic light chains are λ while, in contrast, in the normal repertoire and in multiple myeloma, λ light chains comprise only one-third of the light chains seen; this difference speaks to the intrinsic "amyloidogenicity" of λ light chains. AL is of particular interest to specialists in plasma cell diseases because clonal plasma cells secrete the monoclonal light chains that form deposits [13–15]. AL, then, is both a disorder of protein deposition and of clonal plasma cell proliferation [2].

In theory, treatment for AL amyloidosis could be directed at various aspects of its pathogenesis (Fig. 93.1). Approaches designed to reduce

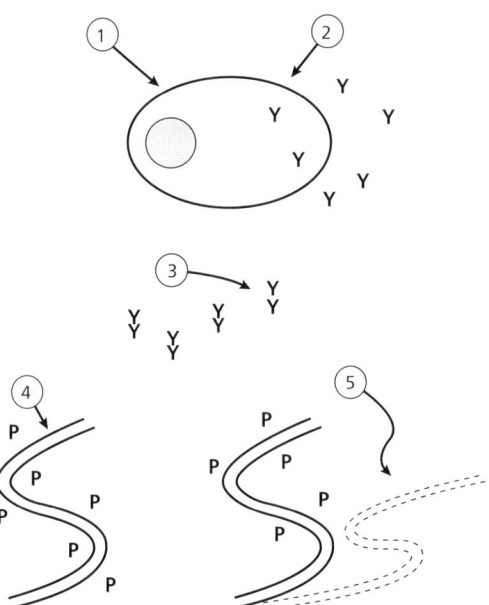

Fig. 93.1 Schematic showing theoretical remedies for amyloidosis. There are a number of points at which intervention could, in theory, control AL amyloidosis: (1) reducing the number of plasma cells with cytoreductive therapy; (2) reducing the secretion of clonal free light chains (FLCs) with drugs; (3) impairing the self-assembly and aggregation of light chains; (4) inhibiting fibril formation in tissues (p = serum amyloid P [SAP]); and (5) dissolving or enhancing the proteolysis of amyloid fibrils. Remedies that reduce the number of plasma cells include standard and high-dose chemotherapy. 4-Iodo-4-deoxydoxorubicin (I-DOX) may enhance the proteolysis of fibrils. The other possible remedies remain theoretical.

or eliminate clonal plasma cells, as in multiple myeloma, have been employed most frequently. Indeed, by the mid-1990s, limited progress had been made with standard chemotherapy in reversing the inexorable progression of this disease. At that time, after the efficacy of autologous hematopoietic cell transplantation (HCT) had been demonstrated in myeloma, the use of HCT was investigated in patients with AL.

When HCT was successful, it was observed that the production of deposits was halted and prior amyloid deposits were slowly resorbed, and that organ function, performance status and quality of life improved [16–21]. However, in the early clinical trials, transplant-related mortality was high because the viscera of AL patients were compromised by amyloid-related cardiac, gastrointestinal (GI) and neuropathic problems; these problems made AL patients distinct from other stem cell transplantation candidates [19,20]. Not surprisingly then, the evolution of HCT for AL has been characterized by refinement of patient selection and improvement of peri-transplant clinical management [22,23]. In this chapter we describe the epidemiology, pathogenesis and distinctive clinical aspects of AL and offer an approach to the evaluation of patients with AL. We also summarize the experience with HCT for AL in order to provide guidelines for current clinical research. Finally, we identify areas of promise for further work and discuss novel emerging therapies.

Epidemiology

The epidemiology of AL is difficult to define precisely, since the disease goes often undiagnosed and the data from tertiary referral centers are not necessarily representative. AL is a rare disorder with an age-adjusted incidence estimated to be 5.1–12.8 per million person-years, resulting in approximately 1275–3200 new cases annually in the USA and 255–640 cases in the UK, an incidence similar to that of chronic myelogenous leukemia or Hodgkin's disease [24]. AL appears to be more common in men based on data from tertiary centers, but the difference may be due to self-selection and referral bias. There have been no links with any race, occupation, or environmental exposures. Sixty percent of patients with AL are between 50 and 70 years of age at diagnosis [24]. The median age of patients with amyloidosis is 63 years with 2% under 40 years of age. We have seen patients as young as 26 years and as old as 89 years of age. AL is approximately one-fifth as common as multiple myeloma but it confers a worse prognosis since the median survival of patients seen at amyloid centers within 1 month of tissue diagnosis is 13.2 months [24].

Pathogenesis

The final pathway in the deposition process of amyloidosis is the formation of amyloid fibrils [25–27]. When the amyloid-subunit proteins are solubilized and deciphered by amino acid sequencing, the dominant constituent of deposits is the light-chain variable region and less frequently part of the constant region or the whole immunoglobulin [28–34]. Although the reason why some immunoglobulin light chains form amyloid remains unknown, comparisons of the primary structures of normal and AL light chains have provided a partial answer based on the stability and folding properties of pathologic light chains [35–37]. The basis for light chain amyloid formation appears to be the effects of primary structure on the conformation of immunoglobulin light chains [38–43]. Primary-structure analyses have emphasized the contribution of critical uncommon amino acid substitutions to the stability and interactive properties of misfolded or partially folded light chains [35,36]. Such partially folded intermediate forms may be prone to self-assemble aberrantly [36,37]. The identification of potentially destabilizing uncommon amino acid substitutions at unique positions in the variable regions of AL light chains has supported this hypothesis [41,42]. Purified urinary light chains from patients with AL reproduce the disease when injected into mice; purified urinary proteins from myeloma patients without AL do not cause amyloid deposits [44].

In addition, the interactions between AL light chains and passenger constituents of amyloid deposits, such as glycosaminoglycans, may also be related to these critical amino acid variations and may influence the course of AL disease by stabilizing filament and fibril formation and by enhancing the resistance of AL deposits to proteolysis [45]. Another major component of amyloid deposits is serum amyloid P (SAP) component, a member of the pentraxin protein family [46]. Of note, SAP is highly resistant to proteolysis and may act as a pathologic chaperone for amyloid fibrils [47]. SAP, however, employs a calcium-dependent binding mechanism in its interactions with amyloid fibrils. Other modifications of light chain conformation such as post-translational glycosylation may also be related to critical amino acid substitutions and may predispose light chains to self-assemble [13].

In the majority of patients with AL, free monoclonal light chains and minimal bone marrow plasmacytosis are detected, often in association with suppression of noninvolved immunoglobulin production [2]. The levels of monoclonal protein and the plasma cell infiltrates in the marrow do not increase over time as is the case in multiple myeloma. The median number of bone marrow plasma cells seen is 7%, ranging from 1% to 30%. Sixty percent of patients have marrow biopsies showing 10% or fewer clonal plasma cells [24]. Eleven percent of patients with amyloid have over 20% plasma cells with no signs of multiple myeloma. A λ light chain is present in 70%, κ in 19% and no monoclonal protein in 11%. When an immunoglobulin heavy chain was detectable in the serum, it was immunoglobulin G (IgG) in 58%, IgA in 10% and IgM in 8%. The presence of IgM amyloidosis is not well recognized; these patients usually do not have Waldenstrom's macroglobulinemia [48].

Over the past decade, a more complete understanding of the genetic endowment of AL clones has opened new research vistas [49–58]. The clones that cause AL are distinctly different from myeloma clones with respect to their repertoire of immunoglobulin light chain variable germline (Ig V_L) genes but similar in that their immunoglobulin genes are highly mutated (i.e. antigen-driven or post-germinal center clones) [51–58] and surprisingly similar to myeloma clones with respect to their cytogenetics [59,60].

The repertoire of Ig V_L genes in AL is skewed unlike that in myeloma, which is similar to the normal expressed repertoire. Nearly half of all AL clones employ one of two immunoglobulin λ light chain variable region germline genes, the *3r* (λIII) and *6a* (λVI) germline donors. There are curious differences between the degree of homology to germline in both instances; AL clones using genes derived from the *3r* germline have a significantly higher divergence from the germline sequence than those using the *6a* donor [56–58]. This difference may be related both to antigen selection and to the inherent amyloid-forming propensity of 6a light chains [55].

One of the most puzzling features of AL amyloidosis is the variety of organs that may be affected [2,24]. Although the basis of this tropism remains unknown, evaluations of the immunoglobulin light chain genetics underlying AL have suggested that some light chain variable region germline or donor genes are more likely to give one pattern of organ involvement than another [56–58]. Using the reverse-transcriptase polymerase chain reaction to clone AL light chain genes and available databases for germline gene identification, several investigators have sought to test the hypothesis that the Ig V_L genes used by AL clones influenced organ tropism [56,57]. In one series, Ig V_L germline genes were identified from 60 patients with AL and those with clones derived from the *6a* germline gene were more likely to present with dominant renal involvement while those with clones derived from the *1c*, *2a2* and *3r* genes were more likely to present with dominant cardiac and multisystem disease [56]. Despite these suggestive data, what remains unexplained in AL is how the self-assembly of misfolded light chain proteins causes progressive organ dysfunction and clinical disease at a tempo more rapid than that seen in hereditary amyloid variants. An attractive hypothesis is that partially folded light chain intermediates formed in the early stages of assemblage are directly or indirectly more toxic to cellular metabolism than the deposits themselves [59].

Interestingly, cytogenetic abnormalities commonly seen in myeloma clones are also found in AL [60,61]. Trisomies of chromosomes 7, 9, 11, 15 and 18 are seen in 33–52% of patients. Trisomy X has been seen in 13% of women and 54% of men. The aneuploidy seen in the monoclonal plasma cell population in AL supports a neoplastic nature for the disorder even when the plasma cell fraction is ≤5%. Immunoglobulin heavy chain translocations have been reported in 55% of patients with amyloidosis and abnormalities of chromosome 13 are frequent [61]. AL, then, is a plasma cell dyscrasia similar to monoclonal gammopathy of undetermined significance (MGUS) except that the M protein causes amyloidosis.

Diagnosing AL amyloidosis

The most common symptoms of amyloidosis are fatigue, dyspnea, edema, paresthesias and weight loss. The fatigue, generally caused by cardiac involvement, may be misdiagnosed as functional or stress-related since the usual features of congestive heart failure are absent. Lightheadedness is common and occurs in patients with nephrotic syndrome with hypoalbuminemia and contraction of plasma volume. Patients with cardiac amyloidosis regularly have poor diastolic filling and a reduced stroke volume leading to orthostatic hypotension but a normal echocardiographic ejection fraction. Amyloidosis patients with autonomic neuropathy will also have orthostatic hypotension, frequently associated with syncope. Amyloidosis should also be kept in mind when patients are seen with weight loss, fatigue and a monoclonal gammopathy but a bone marrow that shows a percentage of plasma cells too low to be associated with multiple myeloma.

The physical findings of amyloidosis are specific but not sensitive. Amyloid purpura are seen in only one in six patients, most commonly on the eyelids, upper face and the webbing of the neck. A palpable liver is present in one-fourth of patients and may be due to infiltration of the liver or congestion related to high right-sided cardiac pressures. Enlargement of the tongue is the most specific finding in AL but is seen in only 9% of patients. It is easily recognized because it results in dental indentations on the underside of the tongue and enlargement of the submandibular salivary glands, often misdiagnosed as enlarged submandibular lymph nodes. An occasional patient will present because of vascular claudication due to small vessel occlusion with amyloid deposits [62].

Because the symptoms and physical findings in AL are not diagnostic of amyloidosis, it is important to recognize the clinical syndromes associated with AL. The seven most common presentations of patients with AL are described in Table 93.1. When one of these clinical syndromes is seen, the next step is immunofixation of the serum and urine. A screening serum protein electrophoresis is inadequate because of the high prevalence of light chain only disease. Light chain amyloid will not produce a detectable band on the serum electrophoresis. Since many patients have significant degrees of proteinuria, a peak may be obscured in the urine as well, necessitating immunofixation [2,63]. Immunofixation will demonstrate a light chain in nearly 90% of patients. Since AL is a plasma cell dyscrasia, the finding of a monoclonal light chain in a patient with a consistent clinical syndrome would be a strong indication to pursue a biopsy for diagnosis.

Recently, the use of the free light chain (FLC) assay has demonstrated abnormal circulating FLCs even when immunofixation is negative and is a useful adjunctive test in diagnosing and monitoring patients with AL (Fig. 93.2) [64,65]. In patients who do not have a monoclonal immunoglobulin light chain in the serum or urine, the bone marrow will almost

Table 93.1 Seven presenting syndromes of systemic AL amyloidosis.

Infiltrative cardiomyopathy
Nephrotic range proteinuria
Demyelinating peripheral neuropathy
Hepatomegaly
Carpal tunnel syndrome
Tongue enlargement
Intestinal symptoms of steatorrhea or pseudo-obstruction

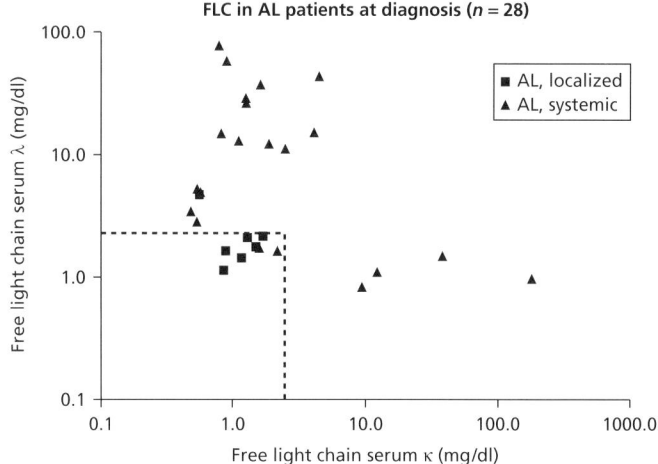

Fig. 93.2 Serum free light chain (FLC) values in newly diagnosed AL. The serum FLC assay is a sensitive measure of the fibril precursor protein in systemic AL. On this graph, the point values for 22 patients with newly diagnosed systemic and six patients with newly diagnosed localized AL are shown. Dotted lines show the normal range. Axes are logarithmic.

always demonstrate a clonal population of plasma cells either by immunohistochemistry, immunofluorescence, or flow cytometry. When combining serum and urine immunofixation, serum FLC and clonal analysis for plasma cells, all patients with AL should be recognized. If one of these features of an immunoglobulin light chain disorder cannot be detected, the diagnosis of AL is in question, and one should consider a form of amyloidosis of the non-AL type such as localized, familial, secondary, or senile [1,2].

The diagnosis of amyloidosis should be confirmed by biopsy as is standard for patients with malignancy. Patients with visceral involvement of the kidney, heart, liver, or nervous system may have the diagnosis confirmed by biopsying those viscera. The nature of amyloid, however, is that there is widespread deposition in blood vessels and soft tissues at diagnosis and less invasive biopsies will readily establish the diagnosis. Amyloid deposits are commonly seen in the subcutaneous fat and bone marrow [66–68]. The abdominal fat will contain Congophilic amyloid deposits in 70–80% of patients, although false positives can sometimes be seen due to overstaining. A bone marrow biopsy will demonstrate vascular deposits in half of the patients. The bone marrow will also allow assessment of the percentage of plasma cells in order to determine if myeloma coexists and to establish clonality. Combining the fat aspirate and bone marrow will establish the diagnosis of AL in 90% of patients. Other sites that can be safely biopsied include the minor salivary glands, the skin and the rectum.

Distinguishing AL amyloidosis

Since HCT uses myeloablative chemotherapy to eradicate the clonal population of plasma cells, it is critical that the presence of a plasma cell dyscrasia be verified. Patients with nonimmunoglobulin forms of amyloidosis will not benefit from HCT since the source of the amyloid precursor protein has nothing to do with the bone marrow or plasma cells. If a plasma cell dyscrasia cannot be verified, one must consider the possibility that the amyloidosis is localized, familial, secondary, or senile. These patients are not candidates for any form of cytotoxic therapy. The distinction between AL and non-AL forms of amyloid cannot be made on clinical grounds since localized amyloid can involve the lungs, skin and lymph nodes as can AL. Secondary forms of amyloid commonly affect the kidneys, the bowel, the liver and the heart. Familial forms of amyloid can cause peripheral neuropathy, cardiomyopathy, or nephropathy. Any patient diagnosed with amyloidosis who lacks a monoclonal protein in serum and urine and has no monoclonal population of bone marrow plasma cells should be evaluated for other types of amyloidosis [2]. HCT should not be performed.

Furthermore, concerns about whether amyloidosis is AL or another type are particularly appropriate in three situations in which patients have amyloid by tissue biopsy and a monoclonal gammopathy. First, in African-American patients over the age of 60 years, the concern of misdiagnosing AL is raised because of the increased frequency of both MGUS and hereditary amyloidosis (abnormal transthyretin, or ATTR, with isoleucine at amino acid position 122) [69]. Second, in patients with hypertension, renal amyloidosis and low-level monoclonal proteins. This concern is warranted based on a recent report of patients with the fibrinogen A α-chain variant of hereditary amyloidosis and low-level monoclonal proteins being misdiagnosed and undergoing HCT [70]. Third, in elderly patients with cardiac amyloid only and monoclonal gammopathies, the concern of misdiagnosis is based on the possible copresence of MGUS and senile cardiac amyloidosis, a disease entity that remains poorly understood and involves the deposition of normal transthyretin in the myocardium. MGUS is found in 5% of normal individuals over the age of 70 years [71]. The most practical guides to keep in mind when dealing with these concerns are: (i) that amyloidosis in the bone marrow is characteristic of AL amyloidosis (hence, the importance of Congo red staining of marrow biopsy specimens); (ii) that "vitreal floaters" on ophthalmologic examination are characteristic of hereditary ATTR variants; and (iii) that the deposits in the fibrinogen A α-chain variant often obliterate the glomeruli and stain immunohistochemically for fibrinogen.

Clinical presentations

Heart

The distribution of involved organs and frequencies of multiorgan involvement are depicted in Table 93.2. The heart is the most commonly involved organ in patients with AL, and heart involvement carries the most serious prognosis because its extent directly impacts on outcome and survival [72]. The pathophysiology is infiltration of the myocardial wall leading to restriction of ventricular filling; patients may present with disabling fatigue and unexplained weight loss as the only symptoms. The electrocardiogram will generally show low voltage with no prior history of an ischemic event. The echocardiogram will show thickening of the walls, commonly misinterpreted as concentric left ventricular hypertrophy rather than infiltration [73]. The ejection fraction is usually preserved. Thickening of the mitral and tricuspid valves due to amyloid infiltration is common and an important clinical clue [74]. In patients who have a ventricular thickness ≥15 mm, the median survival is <1 year. If the septal thickness is <15 mm, the median survival approaches 4 years. Exercise-induced syncope has been associated with a median survival of 2 months [75]. Any patient with intractable fatigue or an echocardiogram showing a thickened wall needs to have studies for the presence of a monoclonal protein in the serum or urine.

The mainstay of the treatment of cardiac amyloidosis is diuretics [76]. Many patients will have associated orthostatic hypotension and intravascular volume contraction secondary to nephrotic syndrome, making diuretic therapy difficult. The use of diuretics may precipitate syncope and can reduce renal blood flow with a resultant rise in the serum creatinine level. The high frequency of hypotension in AL makes the use of therapeutic doses of angiotensin converting enzyme (ACE) inhibitors challenging. Also, the poor flow of blood frequently leads to thrombi in the right and left ventricles. These are potential sources of embolism, which can greatly complicate the course of HCT. These thrombi occur even in patients in normal sinus rhythm. Vascular deposits in small coronary arterioles can produce angina and can be demonstrated on endomyocardial biopsy [77].

All patients with cardiac amyloidosis do not have AL. There are familial forms of amyloid cardiomyopathy, such as that noted above to be common in African-Americans [69]. There are also occasional patients who develop cardiac amyloid due to the deposition of normal transthyretin, so-called senile cardiac amyloid [63]. From a clinical standpoint, these cardiac syndromes are indistinguishable from AL except that the survival is longer.

Kidneys

The most common presentation of renal AL is proteinuria. These patients have both albuminuria as well as free monoclonal light chains in the urine. The differential diagnosis can be amyloidosis, light chain deposition disease, myeloma cast nephropathy or cryoglobulinemia [78]. Immunofixation of the urine in patients with proteinuria is important in their diagnostic evaluation. Thirty to 40% of patients with AL will have renal involvement [79]. In nondiabetic adults with nephrotic syndrome, amyloidosis can be demonstrated in 12% of renal biopsies [80]. Survival, both with standard therapy and with HCT, is impacted by the serum creatinine value at diagnosis. With standard chemotherapy, patients presenting with a creatinine value less than 1.3 mg/dL have a median survival of 25.6 months. Those with an elevated creatinine value have a median

Table 93.2 Distribution of amyloid-related organ involvement at diagnosis.

Involved organ	Frequency (%)	Symptoms
Heart	37	Heart failure Fatigue Arrhythmias Syncopes
Kidneys	30	Nephrotic-range proteinuria Lower extremity edema Hypoalbuminemia
Liver	16	Hepatomegaly Early satiety RUQ discomfort Factor X deficiency
Gastrointestinal	7	Bleeding Pseudo-obstruction Diarrhea
Nervous system	20	Paresthesias Orthostasis Weakness Urinary retention Impotence
Other	12	Soft tissue Tongue Pulmonary
One organ	57	
Two organs	30	
Three organs	6	
Four or more	1	

RUQ, right upper quadrant of the abdomen.

survival of 14.9 months. The level of 24-h urine protein excretion has no impact on survival, but patients with higher levels of proteinuria have greater morbidity associated with pretransplant conditioning including dramatic levels of fluid retention and transient acute renal failure.

Thirty percent of all patients will have proteinuria above 3 g/24 h [24]. Two-thirds of the patients have a detectable light chain in the urine and in the serum. The higher the urinary protein loss, the more likely it is to find the monoclonal light chain. Light chains are found in the urine of 86% of patients with renal AL when the daily urinary protein loss exceeds 1 g. The median survival in patients who have urinary λ light chains is 1 year compared to $2^{1}/_{2}$ years in those patients with no monoclonal protein or with free κ light chains. The type of light chain appears to have no impact on the serum creatinine value.

The major clinical consequence of renal amyloid is severe serum hypoalbuminemia. The loss of albumin results in reduced intravascular oncotic pressure and edema of the lower extremities and presacral area, and in severe cases can lead to ascites and pleural effusions. The edema generally requires diuretics for control, but diuresis may aggravate intravascular volume contraction and exacerbate hypotension. The principal long-term complication of continuous urinary protein loss in renal amyloid is tubular damage that results in endstage renal failure.

One of the goals of HCT is to eliminate the high urinary protein loss and, therefore, delay or prevent dialysis dependency. The presenting 24-h urine protein and serum creatinine predict which patients will ultimately develop end-stage renal disease in the absence of HCT. The median time from diagnosis of AL to dialysis is 15 months. Median survival from the start of dialysis is 8 months. This poor outlook justifies the use of HCT in patients with renal disease as single organ involvement. The most important extrarenal complications of AL are heart failure, cardiac arrhythmias and refractory hypotension. The extent of amyloid deposits seen on a renal biopsy do not correlate with the severity of proteinuria and hypoalbuminemia. Small amyloid deposits can be associated with advanced nephrotic syndrome. The kidneys are normal in size in amyloid in contrast to previously published literature. If amyloid does not involve the kidney at presentation, it rarely occurs during follow-up.

Renal transplantation has been performed in patients with AL, but recurrence is common. HCT for AL has been performed successfully both before and after renal allografting. If renal transplantation is undertaken in AL, strong consideration of subsequent HCT should be given. Without HCT, it is estimated that renal transplant recipients have at least a 20% chance of amyloid recurrence at 1 year.

Liver

Hepatomegaly is found by physical examination in one-fourth of amyloid patients [81,82]. Hepatomegaly may be due to amyloid-induced heart failure or direct infiltration of the hepatic parenchyma. Symptomatic liver amyloid is present in 16% of patients with AL. The most common presentations are unexplained hepatomegaly, an unexplained elevation of the serum alkaline phosphatase level and early satiety. When two organs are involved with amyloid, the most common presentation is combined hepatic and renal. Half of the patients with hepatic amyloid have >1 g of daily proteinuria. The clues that allow the recognition of hepatic amyloid are: (i) hepatomegaly out of proportion to the degree of abnormal liver function tests; (ii) a monoclonal protein in the serum or urine; (3) Howell–Jolly bodies in the peripheral blood film (splenic infiltration); and (iv) proteinuria. Most patients will have only alkaline phosphatase elevation with normal transaminases. Elevation of the bilirubin level is generally a preterminal finding. Rarely, a patient can present with splenic or hepatic rupture.

At diagnosis, in patients with hepatic involvement, the liver descends a median of 7 cm below the right costal margin; splenomegaly is seen in 11% and nephrotic syndrome in 36% of patients with hepatic involvement. Ten percent of patients, however, are diagnosed because of a significant elevation of the serum alkaline phosphatase without hepatomegaly on examination. The median elevation of the serum alkaline phosphatase value in AL patients with hepatic involvement is 2.3 times the upper limit of normal. Portal hypertension with varices and bleeding has been reported but is rarely seen [83]. Ascites is commonly found usually due to associated nephrotic syndrome, hypoalbuminemia, and congestive heart failure but is not generally associated with portal hypertension. The median survival following diagnosis is 1 year.

Radionuclide scintigraphy does not produce specific findings in hepatic amyloid and is not considered useful; the diagnosis is easily confirmed with liver biopsy with a complication rate of anywhere from 0.3% to 3.0%. The presence of hyposplenism on the peripheral blood film is specific for splenic amyloid. Technetium scanning will demonstrate a marked reduction in splenic blood flow due to amyloid infiltration.

Gastrointestinal (GI) tract

Most patients with amyloidosis will have deposits seen in GI tract biopsies [84]. Usually these are vascular deposits only and do not produce symptoms. Less than 5% of patients with AL present with symptoms referable to the GI tract. The presence of anorexia and weight loss does not correlate with the presence of GI amyloid deposits. Malabsorption with steatorrhea is seen in <5% of patients. When symptoms are present, they can include pseudo-obstruction [84,85]. Patients with advanced GI tract involvement require long-term total parenteral nutrition for management. These patients have intractable nausea and vomiting and do not respond to enteral feeding or pharmacologic interventions.

Small bowel biopsy proof of amyloidosis is obtained in only 1% of all AL patients. The most common presenting symptoms are diarrhea, anorexia, dizziness and abdominal pain. The median weight loss is 30 pounds, and 50% of patients have orthostatic hypotension. A quarter of them will have vitamin K deficiency due to malabsorption. Factor X levels are reduced in one-quarter of the patients. Intestinal involvement tends to occur in the absence of hepatic involvement. X-ray studies of the GI tract are generally not helpful. Small bowel dilatation can be seen as can thickening, nodularity, and delayed transit. CT scanning demonstrates thickening of the bowel wall. There is usually a significant delay from the onset of symptoms to the recognition of amyloid. In our experience, the median time from symptoms to histologic diagnosis is 7 months; a laparotomy may be required to establish the diagnosis. Nutritional failure is the cause of death in over half of the patients: an additional quarter die of cardiac amyloid. The diarrhea of amyloid is difficult to treat. Loperamide, diphenoxylate, octreotide and tincture of opium have all been tried with limited success. Thalidomide's constipating effect may be used to some advantage in patients who have severe diarrhea.

Amyloidosis can present as ischemic colitis. Amyloid deposits obstruct the vessels of the lamina propria and muscularis mucosa which may lead to chronic mucosal ischemia with sloughing and hemorrhage. We have seen a significant risk for GI bleeding in patients who undergo HCT. Presumably, high-dose chemotherapy leads to denuding of the intestinal mucosa, exposing amyloid-involved vessels, which rupture easily and can lead to massive bleeding. GI bleeding has been associated with an inferior outcome in HCT [86].

Nervous system

Amyloid involvement of the peripheral nerves was first described in 1938 [87]. The frequency of neuropathy in AL ranges from 15% to 20%. When patients present with dominant neuropathy, consideration needs to be given to the possibility of familial amyloidosis. The finding of a monoclonal protein in the serum or urine would suggest that the amyloidosis is AL type. The most common symptoms of amyloid neuropathy are paresthesias, muscle weakness, numbness, pain, orthostatic symptomatology, urinary retention and impotence. Syncope is seen in 12% of patients. In a quarter of patients, the peripheral neuropathy is accompanied by dysesthesias and distal burning. The lower extremities are involved before the upper extremities in 90% of patients, and two-thirds of patients have autonomic symptoms. Cranial nerve involvement occurs rarely. Carpal tunnel syndrome is seen in half of patients with amyloid peripheral neuropathy. A third of patients have significant weight loss. When patients present with amyloid peripheral neuropathy, the echocardiogram is abnormal in 44%; renal involvement is seen in only 5%.

Sural nerve biopsy demonstrates deposits in endoneurial capillaries. The median survival of patients who present with amyloid neuropathy is 25 months [87]. Standard chemotherapy treatment rarely results in clinical improvement in the neuropathic symptoms. The neuropathy is progressive over time. Marked restriction of mobility ultimately develops in three-quarters of patients and a third are ultimately bedridden. The prognostic factors for survival in patients with dominant neuropathy include the serum albumin level. A normal albumin level is associated with a median survival of 31 months while a serum albumin <3 g/dL is associated with a median survival of 18 months. HCT has been reported to have a beneficial effect on amyloid neuropathy.

There is commonly a significant diagnostic delay with amyloid neuropathy. Symptoms precede the diagnosis by a median of 29 months. Patients with a peripheral neuropathy need immunofixation of the serum or urine. Finding a monoclonal light chain limits the differential diagnosis to MGUS neuropathy, POEMS syndrome (*p*olyneuropathy, *o*rganomegaly, *e*ndocrinopathy, *M* protein, *s*kin changes), cryoglobulinemia and amyloidosis. Since amyloid preferentially causes loss of small myelinated fibers and unmyelinated fibers, an electromyogram can be normal early in the disease course. Because amyloid may deposit at the level of the nerve root leading to distal demyelination, the sural nerve biopsy can occasionally be negative.

Respiratory tract

Involvement of the respiratory tract is usually asymptomatic. Almost 40% of patients with amyloid deposits in the lungs have localized forms and do not have systemic amyloidosis [88–90]. In patients who have histologic evidence of systemic amyloidosis and lung involvement, the symptoms are overshadowed by concomitant cardiac involvement. Even when deposits are present, gas exchange in the lungs is preserved until late in the disease. Pulmonary AL presents radiographically as an interstitial or reticulonodular infiltrate with or without pleural effusion [89]. The median survival after diagnosis is 16 months [88]. Bronchoscopic lung biopsy is safe and is not associated with an increased bleeding risk.

The chest X-ray is not specific, demonstrating an interstitial process that can be misinterpreted as fibrosis. There appears to be a higher prevalence of pulmonary amyloid in patients whose amyloid is associated with an IgM monoclonal gammopathy. In patients who have dyspnea due to interstitial lung disease, low doses of prednisone produce symptomatic benefit. Pleural infiltration with amyloid can result in pleural effusions. Rarely, pulmonary hypertension can develop with right-sided cardiac failure [91].

Hemostasis

Bleeding can be a serious complication of amyloidosis. The most common manifestation of bleeding is skin purpura. Deficiency of factor X is well recognized [92]. Factor X deficiency is seen in <5% of patients and is associated with hepatic involvement. Normalization of factor X levels following transplantation for hepatic amyloidosis has been reported. Bleeding associated with factor X deficiency is generally seen only when the level falls below 25% [93]. Severe factor X deficiency is associated with increased mortality with HCT. The management of factor X deficiency prior to myeloablative chemotherapy has included splenectomy and the use of recombinant human factor VIIa [94]. A high proportion of patients have an abnormal thrombin time, not associated with clinical bleeding after myeloablative therapy.

Rarely thromboembolic disease is observed in patients with AL. At the Mayo Clinic, Minnesota, 40 AL patients with documented thromboembolic disease have been seen. Thromboembolism preceded the diagnosis of amyloid in 11 of the patients, occurred within a month of diagnosis in nine of the patients and was seen more than 1 month following the diagnosis of AL in 20 of the patients. Twenty-nine of the 40 thrombotic events were venous and 11 were arterial. Risk factors for thrombosis in amyloid patients include nephrotic syndrome, immobilization, tobacco use, heart failure and disseminated intravascular coagulation. Five of these 40 patients had activated protein C resistance. The mortality associated with thromboembolism is 20%. Forty-five percent of the patients died within a year of the thrombosis.

Prognosis

Assessing prognosis is critical because anticipating outcome is necessary to determine whether the risks of HCT are justified. The median survival of 153 patients with AL was 20 months with a 5-year survival of 20% [95]. Patients with congestive heart failure had a median survival of 8 months and a 5-year survival of 2.4%. Median survival of patients whose amyloidosis was diagnosed by liver biopsy was 9 months with a 5-year survival of 13%. The best outcome was seen in patients with amyloid neuropathy as the sole manifestation of the disease with a median survival of 40 months and a 5-year survival of 32%.

Using clinical prognostic classifications, heart failure and orthostatic hypotension are both associated with a median survival of <1 year. At some centers, the presence of orthostatic hypotension is an exclusion criterion for HCT. The most common cause of death in patients with AL is cardiac and can be either congestive cardiomyopathy or sudden death caused by arrhythmias or asystole. Clinical outcome is largely determined by the extent of cardiac involvement and echocardiography is a critical component in assessing patients with AL, particularly with regard to their suitability for HCT. In early cardiac amyloid, relaxation is abnormal. In advanced cardiac amyloid, there is restricted filling with a shortened deceleration time. Diastolic function in cardiac amyloid can be monitored serially using Doppler echocardiography. Patients can be divided into two groups on the basis of their deceleration time. At 150 ms or less, the 1-year survival is 49% compared to 92% in those with longer than 150 ms deceleration time.

The presence of heart failure, a urinary monoclonal light chain, hepatomegaly and multiple myeloma were all adverse factors affecting survival during the 1st year after diagnosis. After the first year, an increase in serum creatinine, the presence of multiple myeloma, orthostatic hypotension and a monoclonal serum protein were associated with poor survival. Recognizing these prognostic factors is important when comparing studies of therapy. Because of the morbidity associated with myeloablative chemotherapy, patients with many of these features may be excluded from HCT. An elevated creatinine has an important impact on the morbidity of HCT, and consideration of melphalan dose reduction should be given to patients with creatinine elevation.

The time between histologic diagnosis and referral for evaluation to a medical center is also an important prognostic variable. When all patients with amyloidosis seen are analyzed, the median survival is 2 years. However, when the analysis is limited to those patients seen within 30 days of diagnosis, the median survival is 13 months. This difference suggests that there is a referral bias that favors those patients who are physically able to come to a major treatment center. This information is important when interpreting the results of clinical trials originating from a single center compared to those performed in a cooperative group setting.

Therapy

Results with standard chemotherapy

The primary approach is to reduce the production of the amyloidogenic light chains with therapy directed against the plasma cell population. The same therapeutic approaches used for multiple myeloma have therefore been employed to treat AL. These include low-dose oral chemotherapy regimens, such as melphalan and prednisone (MP), single-agent dexamethasone and combination regimens, such as vincristine, BCNU, melphalan, cyclophosphamide and prednisone (VBMCP) [96–102]. These therapies, however, do not give satisfactory results, enhancing median survival from about 1 to 2 years. The conundrum of therapy is that a less toxic treatment that works gradually may be ineffective because death may occur before there is time for the amyloid deposits to regress. To add to the difficulty of selecting appropriate treatment, there have been very few randomized controlled trials in AL amyloidosis.

Oral MP was the first effective treatment for amyloidosis and has been shown in randomized controlled trials to improve survival for patients with AL as compared with placebo [96,97]. Overall median survival is prolonged from 12 to 18 months. No other standard chemotherapy has been shown to be superior. Although MP results in a response in only one-quarter of AL patients, with a median time to response of 12 months, responders do survive significantly longer than nonresponders (median 89 vs. 14 months, respectively) [96]. Patients with nephrotic syndrome fare better than do those with cardiac involvement of whom only 15–20% respond. This partly reflects the fact that MP takes approximately 1 year to produce maximum benefit. The side-effects of melphalan include myelotoxicity; in patients who survive for more than 3.5 years there is a 20% of risk of myelodysplasia, often leading to secondary leukemia [101]. Approximately 5% of patients treated with alkylating agents survive for 10 years or more [102]. These long-term survivors are predominantly patients without symptomatic cardiac involvement or peripheral neuropathy and with relatively normal renal function.

Hematopoietic cell transplantation (HCT)

Early clinical trials

Minimal progress had been made in treating AL until the mid-1990s when patients received dose-intensive intravenous melphalan and autologous HCT [16–23,103–106]. The effectiveness of HCT in reversing the AL deposits in nearly two-thirds of surviving patients has been documented by investigators at numerous centers, and amyloid scans have demonstrated resorption of AL deposits subsequent to the reduction or elimination of the clonal plasma cell disorder that causes them (Fig. 93.3) [19,103]. Such reversals result from "turning off" the clonal plasma cell factory making the fibril-precursor protein. As the deposition process is halted and the deposits resorbed, both the performance status and the quality of life of AL patients can improve [103]. Historically the most useful marker of response of the plasma cell dyscrasia to HCT has been the complete hematologic response (CR); CR occurs when immunofixation studies that were positive pre-HCT are negative post-HCT and when the presence of clonal plasma cells cannot be detected in marrow biopsies by immunohistochemical staining. Amyloid-related organ disease usually improves significantly in patients in CR post-HCT. This definition of CR, however, is undergoing revision now that the more sensitive FLC assay is available.

The experience with HCT in AL remains controversial because of treatment-related mortality (TRM) [22,23]. The average 100-day mortality of HCT in four single-center studies was 21% and in two multicenter studies it was 39%, making HCT in this population particularly morbid [19,20,103–106]. In addition, numerous deaths have been reported during stem cell mobilization, highlighting AL HCT patients as unusually prone to adverse events [103,105,106]. Transplant-related mortality was

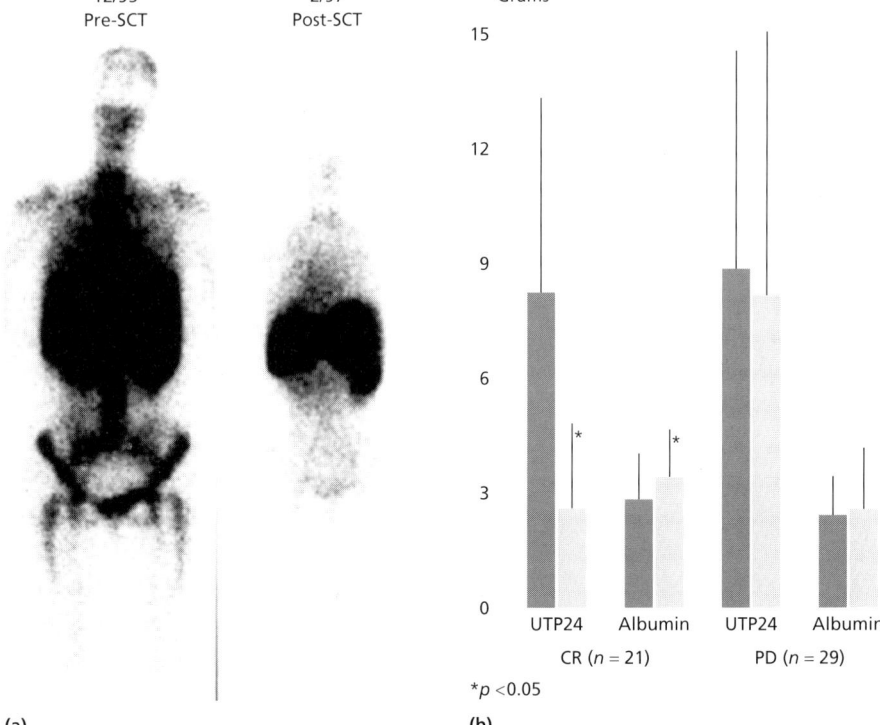

Fig. 93.3 Responses of amyloid organ involvement to hematopoietic cell transplantation (HCT). The panel of nuclear scans on the left in (a) are scintiscans employing iodine-131 labeled serum amyloid P (SAP) (courtesy of Dr Philip Hawkins). The black areas show uptake consistent with amyloid deposits that are extensive pre-HCT and markedly improved 14 months later. The graph on the right (b) depicts the responses in 50 consecutive AL patients spilling more than 1 g/day of albumin in the urine. Patients who achieved a complete response (CR, on the left) had significantly diminished daily albuminuria (UTP24) and increased serum albumin levels 1 year post-HCT ($p < 0.05$ by paired t-test). Those with persistent disease (PD) were basically unchanged. Mean values are shown and the whisker-lines represent the standard deviations.

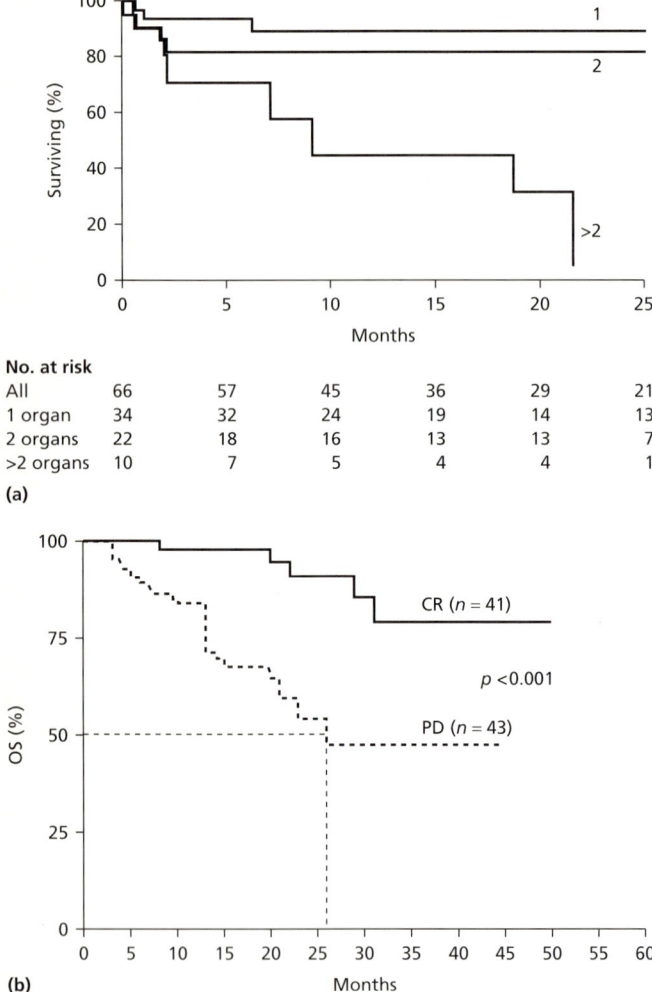

Fig. 93.4 Factors influencing survival after hematopoietic cell transplantation (HCT) for AL. These survival curves describe outcomes in two different cohorts of sequential AL patients who underwent HCT at doses of melphalan ranging from 100 to 200 mg/m². In (a) survival is shown as a function of number of organs involved with data on patients-at-risk below. In (b) survival is shown as a function of hematologic response; patients with a complete response (CR) had significantly better survival than those with persistent disease (PD).

[107]. In a multivariate analysis of survival, the two key predictors were the number of visceral organs involved and the serum creatinine level at the time of transplantation. The 30-month actuarial survival of patients transplanted was 72%. However, if more than two organs were involved at the time of transplantation, the actuarial survival was lower than 20% (Fig. 93.4a). Not only does serum creatinine predict for an adverse survival with typical high-dose chemotherapy (i.e. melphalan 140 mg/m² and total body irradiation [TBI], or melphalan at 200 mg/m²), it also predicts for the development of renal failure during the transplant procedure itself. The median creatinine level of nine patients who required dialysis during transplantation was 1.7 mg/dL [107].

The presence of cardiac amyloid also contributes significantly to peri-transplant mortality [105]. The noninvasive criteria employed to evaluate patients for cardiac involvement with AL may underestimate the incidence of cardiac deposition disease [108,109]. It is worth noting that, in the British multicenter series, three of seven cardiac patients received heart transplants prior to HCT and survived HCT without complications [19]. This therapeutic approach requires further systematic evaluation in a clinical trial [23].

In a retrospective overview of 6 years' experience with HCT for AL, Sanchorawala and colleagues at Boston Medical Center aggregated the outcomes of a series of clinical trials using a range of melphalan doses [103,106,110,111]. They succinctly describe the association between dominant cardiac amyloid, peri-transplant mortality and reduced overall survival. Seventy percent of AL patients who experienced early mortality had amyloid cardiomyopathy, and the median survival of cardiac patients was 2 years. Patients with other dominant organ involvement survived for more than 4 years with median survival not reached. The overall median survival of the entire Boston Medical Center transplant cohort was subsequently reported to be 5.5 years, and the rate of recurrence or relapse of the monoclonal gammopathy in complete responders was 5% [112].

At this time, then, it is reasonably clear that those patients with more than two major organs involved (of heart, kidneys, liver/GI tract and peripheral nervous system) and those patients with advanced cardiomyopathy are at a high risk of dying within the peri-transplant period. These patients then are poor risk candidates for HCT on high-dose regimens. However, patients with one or two organs involved and those with uncomplicated cardiac disease remain candidates for HCT on clinical trials [21–23].

Blood hematopoietic cell mobilization

Owing to the ease of collection and quicker engraftment observed with blood hematopoietic cells as compared with autologous bone marrow, most of the high-dose chemotherapy experience in AL is with mobilized blood cells. Contamination with clonotypic plasma cells has been demonstrated in the stem cell components from AL patients being collected after growth factor priming [21,110,113]. CD34+ cell selection is possible in these patients with adequate yields, but the effect on the disease course of having a positively purged apheresis product remains unknown [110]. Two-thirds of patients had amyloid identified in the bone marrow by Congo red staining, and AL deposition did not impair stem cell mobilization [103]. Currently, granulocyte colony-stimulating factor (G-CSF) mobilization is used at the majority of centers transplanting AL patients regularly and can be considered the standard approach to mobilization in this population. In addition, because of the advantages associated with prompt myeloid and thrombopoietic recovery, we recommend that the optimal dose of CD34+ cells is 5–10 × 10⁶ CD34+ cells/kg [23].

The immune recovery after autologous HCT for AL has been studied in a small number of patients [114]. At 3 months following HCT in

high in these early studies because the visceral reserve of AL patients was compromised by fibril deposition. As a rule, autologous transplant patients have hematologic malignancies but no visceral organ disease, whereas the majority of AL HCT patients possess the opposite findings. Therefore, refinement of patient selection has become a priority [22,23].

The extent of amyloid organ involvement clearly accounts for much of the transplant-related mortality. In two similar single-center trials, those with two or fewer organ-systems involved had significantly superior 100-day survival (81%, 25 of 31 patients) compared with those who had more than two systems involved (25%, four of 12 patients; p <0.01, Fisher's exact test) [103,104]. Typical post-HCT survival as a function of number of organs involved is shown in Fig. 93.4(a). The causes of TRM include GI bleeding, cardiac arrhythmias and the development of intractable hypotension and multiorgan failure. Toxic responses to transplantation occur more frequently in those patients with amyloidosis than in those who receive HCT for other indications.

Survival and amyloid-organ involvement

In 66 patients transplanted at the Mayo Clinic for AL, the TRM was 14%

patients with AL, CD4+ cells were significantly decreased and T-cell function was depressed, unlike CD8+ cells, monocytes, NK cells and B-cell number and functional activity, which had returned to baseline. These outcomes are similar to those reported for patients with other hematologic diseases after autologous HCT although the promptness of the recovery of humoral immunity is somewhat atypical [115].

Given the impaired visceral reserve, vasculopathy and coagulopathies associated with AL, it was predictable that RRT would be more prominent in AL HCT patients. It was not expected, however, that there would be significant toxicity associated with the mobilization and collection of blood stem cells [103,105]. Deaths have been reported during the mobilization of patients with symptomatic cardiac amyloid or multisystem disease at centers employing both moderate doses of cyclophosphamide (e.g. 2.5 g/m^2) and those using growth factors alone. During mobilization with G-CSF (16 µg/kg/day × 5 days) on rare occasions we, amongst others, have observed a sometimes fatal though unexplained syndrome associated with hypoxia and hypotension, which was unresponsive to supportive measures. It can occur in patients without cardiac involvement and may be due to a combination of the effects of G-CSF, activated platelets returned during leukapheresis, pulmonary shunting, cytokines, or mediators of septic hemodynamics [103,106,116]. Currently, in an attempt to minimize the risk of such toxicities, we recommend that G-CSF dosing for mobilization be given twice a day in lower doses (6 µg/kg every 12 h), with collection beginning on day 5, 2–4 h after the morning dose of G-CSF [117].

Dose-intensive regimens

Autologous hematopoietic stem cell transplantation for multiple myeloma had its origins in the work of McElwain and Powles several decades ago [118,119]. A dose–response to intravenous melphalan was documented for patients with refractory myeloma, and patients received up to 140 mg/m^2 of melphalan without growth factor or cellular support. Subsequent phase III trials and large serial cohort studies have demonstrated a survival advantage for patients receiving dose-intensive therapy vs. standard-dose alkylator-based regimens [120,121]. Melphalan has conventionally been used in doses up to 200 or 220 mg/m^2, although doses of 70, 100 and 140 mg/m^2 have also been shown to be effective with minimal TRM [122], and patients have received doses up to 280 mg/m^2 on clinical trials in combination with amifostine (G. Phillips, D. Vesole, D. Reece, unpublished observations). The efficacy of melphalan 200 mg/m^2 vs. melphalan 140 mg/m^2 plus TBI were compared in a phase III trial; both regimens were equally effective and melphalan alone was significantly less morbid [123].

The dose-intensive regimens used to treat patients with AL have been melphalan-based, and the experience parallels that in myeloma; melphalan alone is preferred to melphalan plus TBI. The CR rate, based on immunofixation criteria, is 55% at melphalan 200 mg/m^2 and 30–40% at 100 or 140 mg/m^2 [21,106]. However, the utility of the CR as previously defined has been challenged by the newly available serum FLC assay, as discussed below.

Although it is difficult to distinguish amyloid-related toxicities from RRTs, the frequency and grade of strictly defined RRTs appear to be a function of the dose of intravenous melphalan. This is indicated by the lower grade toxicities experienced by AL HCT patients treated at 100 as opposed to 200 mg/m^2 of melphalan (Table 93.3) [103,106]. Of particular note, the GI toxicity with 200 mg/m^2 of melphalan is striking, as are the higher rates of edema and bleeding. It is reasonable to conclude that amyloidosis confers on AL HCT patients an increased risk of RRTs; however, the toxicities *per se* are regimen-related and amenable to clinical management by patient selection, dose-reduction and other methods.

Table 93.3 Type and frequencies of selected treatment-related toxicities (South-West Oncology Group [SWOG] > grade 2) in AL hematopoietic cell transplantation (HCT).

Toxicity	200 mg/m^2 ($n = 23$) Frequency (% [n])*	100 mg/m^2 ($n = 27$) Frequency (% [n])†
Nausea/vomiting	83 (19)	52 (14)
Diarrhea	65 (15)	48 (13)
Mucositis	91 (21)	37 (10)
Nongastrointestinal bleeding	17 (4)	0 (0)
Gastrointestinal bleeding	22 (5)	7 (2)

*Data from Comenzo *et al.* [103].
†Data from Comenzo *et al.* [106].

RRTs and peri-transplant management

GI bleeding, cardiac complications and multiorgan failure with hypotension have been significant causes of early mortality with HCT in AL [20,22,86]. These complications have usually occurred within the first 14 days of HCT; the degree to which sepsis, autonomic dysfunction, occult chronic infections, immunologic impairments and amyloid vasculopathy contribute to these complications is unknown. The risk profile for these complications has centered on the extent of amyloid-related organ involvement, as noted above, and not on specific physiologic sequelae of organ involvement. In doing so, we should not overlook the fact that our understanding is limited despite this attribution.

In one series, 20% of patients (nine of 45) had GI bleeding, nearly half of whom (four of nine) had both upper and lower GI bleeding [86]. The most common findings on endoscopy were diffuse esophagitis and gastritis. Age, platelet nadir and CD34 count of the graft did not correlate with the risk of bleeding. Women, patients with multiorgan involvement and those on hemodialysis or with slow platelet engraftment were more likely to have GI bleeding. Patients with GI bleeding were hospitalized a median of 37 days compared with 14.5 days for those without GI bleeding ($p < 0.01$). Five of the nine patients died during the post-HCT period, one directly of GI bleeding.

GI bleeding is unusual after autologous HCT and in frequency and severity is unique to patients with AL. If amyloid extensively infiltrates the submucosa of the stomach or lower tract, the potential for severe mucositis with hemorrhage clearly must be anticipated, while neuropathic compromise of the enteric plexus often results in atony, persistent post-transplant nausea and failure to thrive. For these reasons, pre-transplant planning and peri-transplant supportive care become critical elements of the care plan. Recommendations with respect to pre and peri-transplant management have recently been described in detail [22].

Pretransplant patient evaluation should include a detailed review of GI signs and symptoms, serial stool guaiacs, endoscopic studies, to define pathology when indicated, and a complete assessment of coagulation status. Peri-transplant, proton-pump inhibitors, such as omeprazole, should be used for GI prophylaxis and, because dose-intensive intravenous melphalan can cause delayed emesis, an antiemetic regimen may be particularly useful beginning the day after the infusion of the graft. The combination of dexamethasone, lorazepam and prochlorperazine seems to be very useful. If breakthrough nausea and vomiting occur, daily granisetron is often useful.

It is important to note that major GI bleeding can present atypically as, for example, new onset atrial fibrillation or supraventricular tachycardia. In HCT patients with known GI amyloid, if stool guaiacs are positive the hemoglobin should be kept at 10 g/dL and platelets maintained over 50,000/µL. It is also important to keep in mind that visceral rupture (e.g.

splenic rupture) can also occur acutely in AL HCT patients. During the early post-transplant period, vague or atypical left-sided abdominal or shoulder pain should raise a concern about splenic hemorrhage and lead to consideration of imaging the abdomen. Splenic rupture occurring during this period has been successfully managed surgically. Other viscera, such as the esophagus or small bowel, can also perforate and present life-threatening challenges [124].

In our experience, the peri-transplant mortality in patients with cardiac amyloid and congestive heart failure, or with a history of cardiac arrhythmias, syncope or recurrent pleural effusions, approaches 100%, while patients with uncomplicated or well compensated cardiac amyloid and no other symptomatic organ involvement have a 50% peri-transplant mortality and 33% 1-year survival. At some transplant centers, it is now standard to place a pacemaker before myeloablative chemotherapy in those patients who have demonstrated bradyarrhythmias. In patients with dominant cardiac amyloid with minimal symptoms, preserved left ventricular function usually assures diuretic responsiveness. Maintenance of normal electrolyte levels in cardiac patients being diuresed is an obvious requirement.

The mortality associated with cardiac amyloid in HCT recipients is due to sudden cardiac death and to cardiopulmonary failure resulting in hypotension and hypoxia. Patients rarely, if ever, survive after ventricular arrhythmias or hypotensive bradycardic episodes begin to occur peri-HCT despite the addition of appropriate medications and use of advanced life-support measures. Hemodynamically stable tachycardias, on the other hand, occur with some frequency and are usually well tolerated; use of beta-blockade simply for control of sinus tachycardia should not be routine. Whether prophylactic pacemakers, implanted automated defibrillators, or antiarrhythmic agents, such as amiodarone, may impact peri-transplant mortality in these patients remain matters for further clinical investigation.

Clearly the management of intravascular volume and hypotension is a critical aspect of the care of AL HCT patients. Nephrotic syndrome causes salt-avidity and hypoalbuminemia and, therefore, often leads to significant edema. The risk of over-diuresis, however, may be greater than the risk of allowing some peripheral edema in the setting of clinical euvolemia. Nevertheless, intravenous fluids administered should be sodium-free whenever possible and maintaining a diuresis concurrently with melphalan administration and graft infusion is reasonable. Even mild intravascular volume-depletion may exacerbate nausea and emesis; therefore, limited hydration and a limited period of diuresis are recommended. Since a major factor causing pulmonary and peripheral edema is hypoalbuminemia, albumin infusions should be used throughout the treatment period to maintain a serum level >2.0 g/dL.

The multiorgan failure syndrome and intractable hypotension seen as a toxicity of HCT in AL patients likely reflect the limitation on visceral reserve imposed by fibril deposition. Volume-depletion, bleeding, sepsis and hypoadrenalism, followed by worsening autonomic neuropathy, are the most likely causes of hypotension post-HCT. The cellular and hormonal aspects of the syndrome remain poorly characterized. Use of morphine or fentanyl to treat mucositis can affect both blood pressure and urine output, and can complicate acyclovir prophylaxis. When renal perfusion and urine output are reduced, acyclovir toxicity may increase. Midodrine and fludrocortisone are useful treatments for orthostasis but do not work reliably in the transplant setting. It is reasonable to omit post-HCT G-CSF administration in patients with severe nephrotic syndrome because of the fluid retention associated with its use. At the time of neutrophil recovery or myeloid engraftment, it is not uncommon for patients to experience orthostasis requiring more aggressive hydration.

Monitoring response to therapy

The primary endpoint of clinical trials in this disease should remain survival from diagnosis. It will not benefit AL patients if an effective therapy is found—even one that accelerates resorption of amyloid from tissue depots—if the process of resorption itself is excessively morbid and frequently causes sudden death, for example, because of intractable arrhythmias. Therefore, one cannot overemphasize the importance of designing and conducting phase II trials with the explicit criteria of TRM and stopping rules and phase III trials that include patients representative of the population of AL patients. In such instances, the endpoint of survival should maintain primacy.

Other important endpoints in clinical trials have also usually included the response of amyloid-related organ disease and the response of the plasma cell dyscrasia [97,98,106,107]. Depending on the therapy and clinical trial design, these responses have usually been graded at specific intervals, for example, at 3 and 12 months after HCT, although continued improvement in organ function can occur over several years. The criteria for organ-disease response to therapy have been based on noninvasive testing and have usually been described as improved, stable or worsened (Table 93.4). Biopsy-based criteria do not exist and the SAP scintiscan, though likely an ideal way to monitor response to therapy, is of limited availability (Fig. 93.3a). Although scans using radiolabeled aprotinin have been shown in pilot studies to provide useful information regarding amyloid-related cardiac disease, such scans have not become widely available [125]. Therefore, we are left with noninvasive measures to evaluate response of amyloid-disease to therapy. Interestingly, a direct link between organ-system improvement and survival has been described in numerous series but a statistical algorithm for correlating improvement in specific organs with improvement in quality of life or survival has yet to be defined. In patients whose amyloid-related organ disease responds to HCT, improvements in organ function and in performance status usually occur over the 1st year post-HCT. For patients with renal involvement, this point is depicted graphically in Fig. 93.3(b), showing that patients who achieve CRs can experience significant improvement in renal disease 1-year post-HCT.

Standard criteria for hematologic responses have been modeled after myeloma response scoring. Patients whose clonal plasma disease becomes undetectable by immunofixation and whose bone marrows normalize with immunostaining for plasma cell antigens have been considered complete responders; they have no evidence of the previously identified clonal monoclonal bands on immunofixation and normal bone marrow biopsies. Patients achieving at least a 50% reduction in baseline measures of plasma cell activity have been considered partial responders. Patients not achieving either of these categories of response have been considered nonresponders from a plasma cell dyscrasia viewpoint, no matter the degree of response from an organ-involvement viewpoint. Patients who were either complete or partial responders at prior follow-up evaluation(s) but who show evidence of recurrent or progressive clonal plasma cell activity at a subsequent follow-up visit are considered in relapse.

Patients with CR after HCT are likely to have markedly reduced levels of the fibril precursor protein. That they experience reversal or stabilization of amyloid-related disease and prolonged survival as compared to those with persistent clonal plasma cell disease should come as no surprise (Fig. 93.4b). The experience at Boston Medical Center is particularly instructive with respect to the role of CRs in amyloid-related organ responses. Of 205 patients who began HCT during the second half of the 1990s, 115 (56%) survived for at least 1-year post-HCT, nearly half of whom had CR; the amyloid-related organ disease improved in approximately three quarters of all complete responders [111,112]. Furthermore, it is clear from the Boston Medical Center data and analysis, and that of others, that no other modality of therapy is as effective as HCT in achieving CRs and reversal of amyloid-related organ dysfunction, and that the relapse rate from CRs is low. How the use of the serum FLC assay will modify this view and clinical decision-making is unknown at this

Table 93.4 Criteria for amyloid-related organ responses to treatment.*

Improved	Worsened
Heart	*Heart*
• Decrease of ≥2 mm in mean left ventricular wall thickness from baseline thickness >11 mm • Two class improvement in NYHA class	• Increase ≥2 mm in wall thickness • Two class worsening in NYHA class
Kidneys	*Kidneys*
• >50% decrease in daily proteinuria without progressive renal insufficiency	• >50% increase in daily proteinuria • Progressive renal insufficiency
Liver	*Liver*
• A decrease in liver span of ≥2 cm • A concomitant decrease of alkaline phosphatase by 50%	• An increase in liver span of ≥2 cm • An increase of alkaline phosphatase by 50%
Nervous system	*Nervous system*
• Autonomic: normalization of orthostatic vital signs and symptoms, resolution of gastric atony • Peripheral neuropathy: resolution of symptoms	• Autonomic: worsening of orthostatic vital signs and symptoms, worsening of gastric atony • Peripheral neuropathy: worsening of symptoms

*If organ function neither improves nor worsens, it is graded as stable.
NYHA, New York Heart Association.

time. Suffice it to say that AL HCT patients who achieve a CR are likely to experience improvement of amyloid-related organ dysfunction and improved survival (Fig. 93.3b).

Current and future clinical research

The free light chain (FLC) assay

Scoring the response of the clonal plasma cell disease to therapy has recently become more complicated due to the availability of the FLC assay (Fig. 93.2). It is now clear that patients achieving CRs can have elevated serum FLCs for years after HCT (R.L. Comenzo, M. Fleisher; unpublished observations). The FLC assay is several logs more sensitive than immunofixation in clinical practice. Hence, the definition of a CR measured objectively by negative immunofixation electrophoresis of serum and urine has been challenged. After HCT, for example, it has frequently been observed that some patients experience worsening of amyloid-related organ disease despite apparent elimination of the monoclonal protein by immunofixation and vice-versa [27]. Indeed, the resolution of amyloid in AL patients after therapy may be a function of at least two variables: the FLC concentration and the amyloid-forming propensity of the particular FLC. We think it likely that reductions of FLC by more than 50% of baseline values will lead to improvements in amyloid disease and prolong survival irrespective of other serologic findings; this hypothesis is currently being evaluated prospectively in several centers.

Clinical trials using HCT

Continued efforts to treat AL with HCT will depend on clinical trials designed to make HCT less morbid or to answer specific questions of interest. Currently, there is a multicenter phase III trial underway under the aegis of a French myeloma intergroup. AL patients are being randomized to receive high-dose melphalan with HCT or oral therapy consisting of melphalan and dexamethasone. In addition, a risk-adapted approach to treating AL patients with intravenous melphalan (as described below) has recently been implemented in a clinical trial at Memorial Sloan-Kettering Cancer Center.

Of particular interest is the stratified randomized phase II trial recently reported in which AL patients received either HCT as initial therapy (Arm One) or two cycles of oral MP and then HCT (Arm Two) [126]. Overall survival was the primary endpoint. One hundred patients were enrolled within 1 year of diagnosis with a median age of 56 years (range 37–80 years; male : female: 1.8 : 1.0). Fifty-two patients were randomized to Arm One and 48 to Arm Two; there were no differences in age or sex between the arms. The dominant symptomatic organ was renal in 56% of patients in both arms. A substantial proportion of patients also had evidence of cardiac involvement: 34 patients in Arm One (65%) and 23 patients in Arm Two (48%). Of the 52 patients on Arm One, nine (17%) did not proceed to HCT because of disease progression/death ($n = 1$), complications or death during stem cell mobilization ($n = 4$), or patient withdrawal ($n = 4$). Of the 48 patients on Arm Two, 16 (33%) did not proceed to HCT because of progression of disease/death prior to HCT ($n = 8$), complications or death during blood cell mobilization ($n = 6$), or patient withdrawal ($n = 2$).

With 12–58 months of follow-up, median survival has not been reached for either treatment arm by Kaplan–Meier. However, survival of patients 1 year after randomization was significantly higher for those on Arm One (70% vs. 58%, $p = 0.04$). For patients with cardiac involvement, median survival was reached and was significantly longer for patients in Arm One (19.6 months vs. 5.3 months, $p = 0.02$). Overall, 35% of patients in both arms receiving HCT had CRs. Responses of the amyloid-related organ disease are still under evaluation. However, the overall incidence of disease progression, of severe complications with mobilization, or death prior to HCT was 19%—i.e. the sickest patients enrolled did not make it to HCT. This trial demonstrates that newly diagnosed patients with AL amyloidosis, eligible by minimal criteria for HCT, did not appear to benefit from initial treatment with oral MP and that, for patients with cardiac involvement, there was a survival advantage to receiving intravenous melphalan. The overall mortality due to progression of disease and toxicities of treatment was nearly 40% in the 1st year after enrollment.

Despite continued evidence for amyloid toxicities and RRTs with HCT, we are particularly encouraged by clinical HCT research employing novel biologic agents that may reduce GI toxicity. Amifostine and keratinocyte growth factor are being used with HCT to test their protective effects on mucosal surfaces and the GI tract. Myeloma and AL patients have tolerated treatment with amifostine followed by more than 200 mg/m^2 of melphalan with minimal morbidity and have survived for more than a year. Keratinocyte growth factor may also find similar applications in this patient population.

We have been guided by the experience in the early HCT trials and have concluded that the dose of intravenous melphalan should be modified based on age and organ involvement. Patients with more than two major organs involved or with advanced cardiomyopathy are at high risk of dying peri-transplant and, therefore, are poor risk candidates for HCT on high-dose regimens while patients with one or two organs involved or with uncomplicated cardiac disease remain candidates for HCT on clinical trials. We call the approach we have designed a "risk-adapted approach," based on the dose-related differences in toxicity observed in clinical trials (at 100 and 200 mg/m^2 of intravenous melphalan, Table 93.3) and on age-related differences in survival.

Patients with one or two organs involved without cardiac amyloid are considered "good risk" and would receive 200 (if <61 years old), 140 (if 61–71 years old), or 100 mg/m^2 (if >71 years old) of intravenous melphalan. Patients with one or two organs involved and cardiac amyloid that is uncomplicated are considered "intermediate risk" and would receive either 140 or 100 mg/m^2 based on age with a cut-off at 61 years of age. Patients with more than two organs involved or advanced cardiomyopathy are considered "poor risk" (i.e. not HCT candidates) and would receive investigational therapies (such as lower doses of intravenous melphalan), dexamethasone or oral MP. We have implemented this "risk-adapted approach" in a clinical trial at Memorial Sloan-Kettering Cancer Center; we are also employing the serum FLC assay and Ig V_L assessments prospectively. On this trial, after melphalan-based therapy, we provide low-dose thalidomide and dexamethasone to patients who do not achieve CRs.

HCT for AL will remain investigational until there is either a multicenter phase III trial comparing it to standard therapy in newly diagnosed patients, or a multicenter phase II trial showing reduced TRM, perhaps as the result of employing a risk-adapted approach. We believe that consensus on a risk-adapted approach will help to develop the generalized transplant expertise needed for the conduct of multicenter trials and that the results of such trials will provide further insight.

Finally, hypotheses worth examining in the context of future trials include asking whether eligibility for and outcomes with HCT vary depending on Ig V_L germline gene use, since germline gene use contributes to the organ tropism of AL, and whether hematopoietic cells in AL HCT patients contribute to post-HCT tissue-specific recovery in the liver, the heart or the gut. As the mechanism of AL and the factors responsible for amyloid resorption become better understood, we anticipate that further knowledge will be obtained as a result of the willingness of patients with AL to participate in clinical trials.

Emerging therapies

An anthracycline anticancer drug, 4′-iodo-4′-deoxydoxorubicin (I-DOX), was given serendipitously to a patient with AL amyloidosis and resulted in rapid clinical improvement [127,128]. Subsequently, this observation led to investigations into the mechanism of action of I-DOX and further tests of its clinical activity. A phase I trial was conducted and significant responses were seen in a small number of patients, unrelated to the cytotoxicity of I-DOX or its effect on the underlying plasma cell dyscrasia and M protein. The most impressive responses were seen in patients with soft-tissue or muscular amyloid deposits; no significant recovery of amyloid-related organ dysfunction was observed. Of note, I-DOX was cleared from the plasma faster in amyloid patients than in those receiving the drug in clinical trials for cancer, a phenomenon consistent with I-DOX binding to amyloid deposits. Subsequent experiments confirmed the specific targeting to all types of amyloid fibrils *in vitro* and *in vivo*. In initial phase II trials I-DOX had limited activity and a phase I/II dose-finding trial is currently underway [129,130].

Clinical trials combining I-DOX and other promising therapies with HCT or other cytoreductive treatments will need to be conducted within the next several years. Other novel non-HCT therapies for AL may emerge from efforts currently underway. For example, a transgenic mouse model has been developed carrying the human interleukin 6 gene with increased concentrations of the secondary amyloid precursor protein, serum amyloid A (SAA) protein [131]. At three months of age these mice develop renal and hepatosplenic amyloidosis and have a clinical course remarkably similar to human AA or secondary amyloidosis. The availability of such *in vivo* experimental models of AA provides a means to assess the therapeutic efficacy of new agents (such as small molecule anionic sulfates and sulfonates such as polyvinyl-sulfonate) designed to inhibit fibril formation [132].

A murine model of AL has also been developed employing human amyloid solubilized to create subcutaneous amyloidomas [133]. When these AL-bearing animals are injected with antilight chain monoclonal antibodies with specificity for an amyloid-related epitope, regression of the amyloidomas has been documented. This *in vivo* demonstration that amyloid deposits of immunoglobulin origin can be lysed by passive administration of an amyloid-specific antibody will hopefully also provide the basis for clinical trials for patients with AL [133].

In addition, the effects of SAP on amyloid fibrils have been evaluated in numerous ways; for instance, mice with the *SAP* gene knocked-out showed reduced deposition of AA amyloidosis while, in other experiments, the displacement of SAP from fibrils aided in their proteolytic degradation. Hence, SAP-related molecular dissection of deposits came to be viewed as a potentially useful therapeutic target [134]. Subsequently, a palindromic compound Ro 63–3300 was identified that literally turned the SAP dimer inside out, depleted circulating SAP and made it unavailable for binding to fibrils [136]. A phase I trial of continuous infusion of a congener of this molecule (Ro 63–8695 or CPHPC) has been performed and preliminary results indicate that CPHPC infusion was well tolerated and without toxicity [136].

Conclusions

AL amyloidosis remains a disease for which our tests, treatments and knowledge continue to evolve. Survival remains the primary endpoint for patients as well as clinical investigators. The recent availability of the FLC assay promises to improve diagnostic testing and the ability to monitor the course of therapy. Although the response rates with HCT are higher than those seen in patients treated with standard therapies, HCT for AL remains most effective in younger patients and in those with limited disease. Hopefully HCT can be risk-adapted in order to optimize benefit and limit mortality. It will remain a controversial therapy until there is a phase II trial showing low transplant-related mortality or a phase III trial establishing benefit. Solid-organ transplantation is no less controversial in this rare disorder; hopefully the combined use of hematopoietic cell and solid-organ transplantation will also be developed for systematic assessment in clinical trials.

New drugs to inhibit deposits from forming or to mobilize them from organs provide exciting prospects and are entering clinical trials at this time. As we come to understand more fully the basis of the organ-specific toxicities associated with amyloid deposition, we hope that novel cytoprotective pathways are discerned and that the promise of simple and effective drug treatment is fulfilled. The ideal treatment of AL in the future will likely involve a combination of approaches aimed at eliminating the supply of fibril-precursor light chains, inhibiting light chain self-assembly into fibrils and safely enhancing resorption of existing fibrillar deposits (Fig. 93.1). We expect that, in the future, such combinations will include minimally toxic cytoreductive HCT-based therapies that will enhance the recovery and extend the survival of most, if not all, patients with AL.

References

1. Gillmore JD, Hawkins PN, Pepys MB. Amyloidosis. A review of recent diagnostic and therapeutic developments. *Br J Haematol* 1997; **99**: 245–56.
2. Falk RH, Comenzo RL, Skinner M. The systemic amyloidoses. *N Engl J Med* 1997; **337**: 898–909.
3. Merlini G, Anesi G, Banfi G et al. AL amyloidosis: clinical and therapeutic aspects. In: Kyle RA, Gertz MA, eds. *Amyloid and Amyloidosis 1998*. Pearl River, New York: Parthenon Publishing, 1999: 142–4.
4. Kyle RA. Amyloidosis: a convoluted story. *Br J Haematol* 2001; **114**: 529–38.
5. Virchow VR. Über eine im Gehirn und Rückenmark des Menschen auf gefundene Substanz mit einer chemischen Reaction der Cellulose. *Virchow's Arch Pathol Anat* 1854; **6**: 135–8.
6. Divry P, Florkin M. Sur les propriétés optiques de l'amyloïde. *C R Seances Soc Biol Fil* 1927; **97**: 1808–10.
7. Cohen AS, Calkins E. Electron microscopic observations on a fibrous component in amyloid of diverse origins. *Nature* 1959; **183**: 1202–3.
8. Shirahama T, Cohen AS. High resolution electron microscopic analysis of the amyloid fibril. *J Cell Biol* 1967; **33**: 679–708.
9. Bonar L, Cohen AS, Skinner MM. Characterization of the amyloid fibril as a cross-β protein. *Proc Soc Exp Biol Med* 1969; **131**: 1373–5.
10. Glenner GG, Terry W, Harada M, Isersky C, Page D. Amyloid fibril proteins. Proof of homology with immunoglobulin light chains by sequence analyses. *Science* 1971; **172**: 1150–1.
11. Benditt EP, Eriksen N, Hermodson MA, Ericsson LH. The major proteins of human and monkey amyloid substance: common properties including unusual N-terminal amino acid sequences. *FEBS Lett* 1971; **19**: 169–73.
12. Costa PP, Figueira AS, Bravo FR. Amyloid fibril protein related to prealbumin in familial amyloidotic polyneuropathy. *Proc Natl Acad Sci U S A* 1978; **75**: 4499–503.
13. Buxbaum J. Mechanisms of disease: monoclonal immunoglobulin deposition. Amyloidosis, light chain deposition disease, and light and heavy chain deposition disease. *Hematol Oncol Clin North Am* 1992; **6**: 323–46.
14. Dhodapkar MV, Merlini G, Solomon A. Biology and therapy of immunoglobulin deposition diseases. *Hematol Oncol Clin North Am* 1997; **11**: 89–110.
15. Gertz MA, Lacy MQ, Dispenzieri A. Amyloidosis. *Hematol Oncol Clin North Am* 1999; **13**: 1211–33.
16. Comenzo RL, Vosburgh E, Simms RW et al. Dose-intensive melphalan with blood stem cell support for the treatment of AL amyloidosis: 1-year follow-up in five patients. *Blood* 1996; **88**: 2801–6.
17. Moreau P, Milpied N, de Faucal P et al. High-dose melphalan and autologous bone marrow transplantation for systemic AL amyloidosis with cardiac involvement. *Blood* 1996; **87**: 3063–4.
18. van Buren M, Hene RJ, Verdonck LF, Verzijlbergen FJ, Lokhorst HM. Clinical remission after syngeneic bone marrow transplantation in a patient with AL amyloidosis. *Ann Intern Med* 1995; **122**: 508–10.
19. Gillmore JD, Apperley JF, Craddock C et al. High dose melphalan and stem cell rescue for AL amyloidosis. In: Kyle RA, Gertz MA, eds. *Amyloid and Amyloidosis 1998*. Pearl River, New York: Parthenon Publishing, 1999: 60–3.
20. Moreau P, Leblond V, Baurquelot P. Prognostic factors of survival and response after high-dose therapy and autologous stem cell transplantation in systemic AL amyloidosis: a report on 21 patients. *Br J Haematol* 1998; **101**: 766–9.
21. Comenzo RL. Hematopoietic cell transplantation for primary systemic amyloidosis: what have we learned. *Leuk Lymphoma* 2000; **37**: 245–58.
22. Kyle RA. High-dose therapy in multiple myeloma and primary amyloidosis: an overview. *Semin Oncol* 1999; **26**: 74–83.
23. Comenzo RL, Gertz MA. Autologous stem cell transplantation for primary systemic amyloidosis. *Blood* 2002; **99**: 4276–82.
24. Kyle RA, Gertz MA. Primary systemic amyloidosis. Clinical and laboratory features in 474 cases. *Semin Hematol* 1995; **32**: 45–59.
25. Benson MD. Amyloidosis. In: Scriver CR, Beaudet AL, Sly WS, Valle D, eds. *The Metabolic and Molecular Bases of Inherited Disease*, 7th edn, vol. 3. New York: McGraw-Hill, 1995: 4159–91.
26. Kelly JW. Towards an understanding of amyloidosis. *Nat Struct Biol* 2002; **9**: 323–5.
27. Stevens FJ, Myatt EA, Chang CH et al. A molecular model for self-assembly of amyloid fibrils from immunoglobulin light chains. *J Biochem* 1995; **34**: 10,697–702.
28. Putnam FW, Whitley EJ, Paul C, Davidson JN. Amino acid sequence of a κ Bence Jones protein from a case of primary amyloidosis. *J Biochem* 1973; **12**: 3763–80.
29. Omtvedt LA, Haavik S, Hounsell EF, Barsett H, Slette K. The carbohydrate structure of the amyloid immunoglobulin light chain protein EPS. *Amyloid* 1995; **2**: 150–8.
30. Ramstad HM, Sletten K, Husby G. The amino acid sequence and carbohydrate composition of an immunoglobulin κ light chain amyloid fibril protein (AL) of variable subgroup I. *Amyloid* 1995; **2**: 223–8.
31. Westmark P, Sletten K, Natvig JB. Structure and antigenic behavior of κ immunoglobulin light-chain amyloid proteins. *Acta Pathol Microbiol Scand* 1981; **89**(3): 199–203.
32. Liepnieks JJ, Benson MD, Dulet FE. Comparison of the amino acid sequences of 10 κI amyloid proteins. In: Natvig JB, Forre O, Husby G et al., eds. *Amyloid and Amyloidosis*. Boston & London: Dordrecht, 1990: 153–6.
33. Pick AI, Kratzin HD, Barnikol-Watanabe S, Hilschmann N. Complete amino acid sequence of AL Bence Jones protein POL of the λI subclass. In: Natvig JB, Forre O, Husby G et al., eds. *Amyloid and Amyloidosis*. Boston & London: Dordrecht, 1990: 177–80.
34. Wally J, Kica G, Zhang Y et al. Identification of a novel substitution in the constant region of a gene coding for an amyloidogenic κ1 light chain. *Biochim Biophys Acta* 1999; **1454**: 49–57.
35. Hurle MR, Helms LR, Li L, Chan W, Wetzel R. A role for destabilizing amino acid replacements in light chain amyloidosis. *Proc Natl Acad Sci U S A* 1994; **91**: 5446–50.
36. Wetzel R. Domain stability in immunoglobulin light chain deposition disorders. *Adv Protein Chem* 1997; **50**: 183–242.
37. Stevens F, Pokkuluri PR, Schiffer M. Protein conformation and disease: pathological consequences of analogous mutations in homologous proteins. *J Biochem* 2000; **39**: 15,291–6.
38. Stevens PW, Raffen R, Hanson DK et al. Recombinant immunoglobulin variable domains generated from synthetic genes provide a system for *in vitro* characterization of light-chain amyloid proteins. *Protein Sci* 1995; **4**: 421–32.
39. Schiffer M. Molecular anatomy and pathologic expression of antibody light chains. *Am J Pathol* 1996; **148**: 1339–44.
40. Schormann N, Murell JR, Liepnieks JJ, Benson MD. Tertiary structure of an amyloid immunoglobulin light chain protein: a proposed model for amyloid fibril formation. *Proc Natl Acad Sci U S A* 1995; **92**: 9490–9.
41. Stevens FJ. Four structural risk factors identify most fibril-forming light chains. *Amyloid* 2000; **7**: 200–7.
42. Raffen R, Dieckman LJ, Szpunar M et al. Physicochemical consequences of amino acid variations that contribute to fibril formation by immunoglobulin light chains. *Protein Sci* 1999; **8**: 509–17.
43. Bellotti V, Mangione P, Merlini G. Review: immunoglobulin light chain amyloidosis is the archetype of structural and pathogenic variability. *J Struct Biol* 2000; **130**: 280–9.
44. Solomon A, Weiss DT, Kattine AA. Nephrotoxic potential of Bence Jones proteins. *N Engl J Med* 1991; **324**: 1845–51.
45. Stevens FJ, Kiselevsky R. Immunoglobulin light chains, glycosaminoglycans, and amyloid. *Cell Mol Life Sci* 2000; **57**: 441–9.
46. Skinner M, Cohen AS, Shirahama T, Cathcart ES. P-component (pentagonal unit) of amyloid: isolation, characterization and sequence analysis. *J Lab Clin Med* 1974; **84**: 604–14.
47. Tennent GA, Lovat LB, Pepys MB. Serum amyloid P component prevents proteolysis of the amyloid fibrils of Alzheimer disease and systemic amyloidosis. *Proc Natl Acad Sci U S A* 1995; **92**: 4299–303.
48. Gertz MA, Kyle RA, Noel P. Primary systemic amyloidosis. A rare complication of immunoglobulin M monoclonal gammopathies and Waldenstrom's macroglobulinemia. *J Clin Oncol* 1993; **11**: 914–20.
49. Perfetti V, Vignarelli MC, Casarini S, Ascari E, Merlini G. Biological features of the clone involved in primary amyloidosis (AL). *Leukemia* 2001; **15**: 196–202.
50. MacLennan IC, Liu YJ, Oldfield S, Zhang J, Lane PJ. The evolution of B-cell clones. *Curr Top Microbiol Immunol* 1990; **159**: 37–63.
51. Perfetti V, Ubbiali P, Vignarelli MC et al. Evidence that amyloidogenic light chains undergo antigen-driven selection. *Blood* 1998; **91**: 2948–54.
52. Sahota S, Leo R, Hamblin T, Stevenson FK. Myeloma V_L and V_H gene sequences reveal a complementary imprint of antigen selection in tumor cells. *Blood* 1997; **89**: 219–26.
53. Kosmas C, Stamatopoulos K, Stavroyianni N et al. Origin and diversification of the clonogenic cell in multiple myeloma: lessons from the immunoglobulin repertoire. *Leukemia* 2000; **14**: 1718–26.
54. Kosmas C, Viniou N-A, Stamatopoulos K et al. Analysis of the light chain variable region in multiple myeloma. *Br J Haematol* 1996; **94**: 306–17.

55 Solomon A, Frangione B, Franklin EC. Bence-Jones proteins and light chains of immunoglobulins. Preferential association of the VλVI subgroup of human light chains with amyloidosis (AL). *J Clin Invest* 1982; **70**: 453–60.

56 Comenzo RL, Zhang Y, Martinez C, Osman K, Herrera G. The tropism of organ involvement in primary systemic amyloidosis: contributions of Ig V_L germline gene use and plasma cell burden. *Blood* 2001; **98**: 714–20.

57 Abraham RS, Price-Troska DL, Gertz MA, Kyle RA, Fonseca R. Association of rearranged light chain variable region genes with organ tropism and light chain associated (AL) amyloidosis. *Blood* 2001; **98**: 151b [Abstract].

58 Perfetti V, Casarini S, Palladini G et al. Analysis of V-J expression in plasma cells from primary (AL) amyloidosis and normal bone marrow identifies 3r(III) as a new amyloid-associated germline gene segment. *Blood* 2002; **100**: 948–53.

59 Khurana R, Gillespie JR, Talapatra A et al. Partially folded intermediates as critical precursors of light chain amyloid fibrils and amorphous aggregates. *J Biochem* 2001; **40**: 3525–35.

60 Hayman SR, Bailey RJ, Jalal SM et al. Translocations involving the immunoglobulin heavy-chain locus are possible early genetic events in patients with primary systemic amyloidosis. *Blood* 2001; **98**: 2266–8.

61 Harrison CJ, Mazzullo H, Ross FM et al. Translocations of 14q32 and deletions of 13q14 are common chromosomal abnormalities in systemic amyloidosis. *Br J Haematol* 2002; **117**: 427–35.

62 Rao JK, Allen NB. Primary systemic amyloidosis masquerading as giant cell arteritis. Case report and review of the literature. *Arthritis Rheum* 1993; **36**: 422–5.

63 Gertz MA, Lacy MQ, Dispenzieri A. Amyloidosis: recognition, confirmation, prognosis, and therapy. *Mayo Clin Proc* 1999; **74**: 490–4.

64 Bradwell AR, Carr-Smith HD, Mead GP et al. Highly sensitive, automated immunoassay for immunoglobulin free light chains in serum and urine. *Clin Chem* 2001; **47**: 673–80.

65 Hawkins PN, Gallimore R, Bradwell AR, Smith L, Lachmann HJ. Highly sensitive automated immunoassay for free immunoglobulin light-chains in diagnosis and follow up of AL amyloidosis. In: Bely M, Apathy A, eds. *Amyloid and Amyloidosis: The Proceedings of the IXth International Symposium on Amyloidosis.* Budapest, Hungary: David Apathy, 2001: 227–9.

66 Libbey CA, Skinner M, Cohen AS. Use of abdominal fat tissue aspirate in the diagnosis of systemic amyloidosis. *Arch Intern Med* 1983; **143**: 1549–52.

67 Duston MA, Skinner M, Shirahama T, Cohen AS. Diagnosis of amyloidosis by abdominal fat aspiration: analysis of 4 years' experience. *Am J Med* 1987; **82**: 412–4.

68 Westermark GT, Johnson KH, Westermark P. Staining methods for identification of amyloid in tissue. *Meth Enzymol* 1999; **309**: 3–25.

69 Jacobson DR, Pastore RD, Yaghoubian R et al. Variant-sequence transthyretin (isoleucine 122) in late-onset cardiac amyloidosis in black Americans. *N Engl J Med* 1997; **336**: 466–73.

70 Lachmann HL, Booth DR, Booth SE et al. Misdiagnosis of hereditary amyloidosis as AL (primary) amyloidosis. *N Engl J Med* 2002; **346**: 1786–91.

71 Kyle RA, Therneau TM, Rajkumar SV et al. A long-term study of prognosis in monoclonal gammopathy of undetermined significance. *N Engl J Med* 2002; **346**: 564–9.

72 Klein AL, Hatle LK, Taliercio CP et al. Prognostic significance of Doppler measures of diastolic function in cardiac amyloidosis. *Circulation* 1991; **83**: 808–16.

73 Hemmingson LO, Eriksson P. Cardiac amyloidosis mimicking hypertrophic cardiomyopathy. *Acta Med Scand* 1986; **219**: 421–3.

74 Elliott PM, Mahon NG, Matsumura Y, Hawkins PN, Gillmore JD, McKenna WJ. Tissue Doppler features of cardiac amyloidosis. *Clin Cardiol* 2000; **23**: 701.

75 Chamarthi B, Dubrey SW, Cha K, Skinner M, Falk RH. Features and prognosis of exertional syncope in light-chain associated AL cardiac amyloidosis. *Am J Cardiol* 1997; **80**: 1242–5.

76 Nash KL, Brij SO, Clesham GJ. Cardiac amyloidosis and the use of diuretic and ACE inhibitor therapy in severe heart failure. *Int J Clin Pract* 1997; **51**: 384–5.

77 Al Suwaidi J, Velianou JL, Gertz MA et al. Systemic amyloidosis presenting with angina pectoris. *Ann Intern Med* 1999; **131**: 838–41.

78 Lin J, Markowitz GS, Valeri AM et al. Renal monoclonal immunoglobulin deposition disease: the disease spectrum. *J Am Soc Nephrol* 2001; **12**: 1482–92.

79 Bellotti V, Merlini G. Current concepts on the pathogenesis of systemic amyloidosis. *Nephrol Dial Transplant* 1996; **11** (Suppl. 9): 53–62.

80 Yahya TM, Pingle A, Boobes Y, Pingle S. Analysis of 490 kidney biopsies: data from the United Arab Emirates Renal Diseases Registry. *J Nephrol* 1998; **11**: 148–50.

81 Gertz MA, Kyle RA. Hepatic amyloidosis (primary [AL], immunoglobulin light chain): the natural history in 80 patients. *Am J Med* 1988; **85**: 73–80.

82 Gertz MA, Kyle RA. Hepatic amyloidosis: clinical appraisal in 77 patients. *Hepatology* 1997; **25**: 118–21.

83 Itescu S. Hepatic amyloidosis. An unusual cause of ascites and portal hypertension. *Arch Intern Med* 1984; **144**: 2257–9.

84 Friedman S, Janowitz HD. Systemic amyloidosis and the gastrointestinal tract. *Gastroenterol Clin North Am* 1998; **27**: 595–614.

85 Hayman SR, Lacy MQ, Kyle RA, Gertz MA. Primary systemic amyloidosis. A cause of malabsorption syndrome. *Am J Med* 2001; **111**: 535–40.

86 Kumar S, Dispenzieri A, Lacy MQ, Litzow MR, Gertz MA. High incidence of gastrointestinal tract bleeding after autologous stem cell transplant for primary systemic amyloidosis. *Bone Marrow Transplant* 2001; **28**: 381–5.

87 Rajkumar SV, Gertz MA, Kyle RA. Prognosis of patients with primary systemic amyloidosis who present with dominant neuropathy. *Am J Med* 1998; **104**: 232–7.

88 Utz JP, Swensen SJ, Gertz MA. Pulmonary amyloidosis. The Mayo Clinic experience from 1980 to 1993. *Ann Intern Med* 1996; **124**: 407–13.

89 Gillmore JD, Hawkins PN. Amyloidosis and the respiratory tract. *Thorax* 1999; **54**: 444–51.

90 Lim JK, Lacy MQ, Kurtin PJ, Kyle RA, Gertz MA. Pulmonary marginal zone lymphoma of MALT type as a cause of localized pulmonary amyloidosis. *J Clin Pathol* 2001; **54**: 642–6.

91 Dingli D, Utz JP, Gertz MA. Pulmonary hypertension in patients with amyloidosis. *Chest* 2001; **120**: 1735–8.

92 Greipp PR, Kyle RA, Bowie EJ. Factor-X deficiency in amyloidosis: a critical review. *Am J Hematol* 1981; **11**: 443–50.

93 Choufani EB, Sanchorawala V, Ernst T et al. Acquired factor X deficiency in patients with amyloid light-chain amyloidosis: incidence, bleeding manifestations, and response to high-dose chemotherapy. *Blood* 2001; **97**: 1885–7.

94 Boggio L, Green D. Recombinant human factor VIIa in the management of amyloid-associated factor X deficiency. *Br J Haematol* 2001; **112**: 1074–5.

95 Gertz MA, Kyle RA, Greipp PR. Response rates and survival in primary systemic amyloidosis. *Blood* 1991; **77**: 257–62.

96 Kyle R, Gertz M, Greipp P et al. A trial of three regimes for primary amyloidosis: colchicine alone, melphalan and prednisolone, and melphalan, prednisolone and colchicine. *N Engl J Med* 1997; **336**: 1202–7.

97 Skinner M, Anderson JJ, Simms R et al. Treatment of 100 patients with primary amyloidosis: a randomized trial of melphalan, prednisone, and colchicine versus colchicine alone. *Am J Med* 1996; **100**: 290–8.

98 Gertz MA, Lacy MQ, Lust JA, Greipp PR, Witzig TE, Kyle RA. Prospective randomized trial of melphalan and prednisone versus vincristine, carmustine, melphalan, cyclophosphamide, and prednisone in the treatment of primary systemic amyloidosis. *J Clin Oncol* 1999; **17**: 262–7.

99 Sezer O, Schmid P, Shweigert M et al. Rapid reversal of nephritic syndrome due to primary systemic AL amyloidosis after VAD and subsequent high-dose chemotherapy with autologous stem cell support. *Bone Marrow Transplant* 1999; **23**: 967–9.

100 Gertz MA, Lacy MQ, Lust JA, Greipp PR, Witzig TE, Kyle RA. Phase II trial of high-dose dexamethasone for untreated patients with primary systemic amyloidosis. *Med Oncol* 1999; **16**: 104–9.

101 Gertz MA, Kyle RA. Acute leukemia and cytogenetic abnormalities complicating melphalan treatment of primary systemic amyloidosis. *Arch Intern Med* 1990; **150**: 629–33.

102 Kyle RA, Gertz MA, Greipp PR et al. Long-term survival (10 years or more) in 30 patients with primary amyloidosis. *Blood* 1999; **93**: 1062–6.

103 Comenzo RL, Vosburgh E, Falk RH et al. Dose-intensive melphalan with blood stem-cell support for the treatment of AL amyloidosis: survival and responses in 25 patients. *Blood* 1998; **91**: 3662–70.

104 Gertz MA, Lacy MQ, Gastineau DA et al. Blood stem cell transplantation as therapy for primary systemic amyloidosis (AL). *Bone Marrow Transplant* 2000; **26**: 963–9.

105 Saba N, Sutton D, Ross H et al. High treatment-related mortality in cardiac amyloid patients undergoing autologous stem cell transplant. *Bone Marrow Transplant* 1999; **24**: 853–5.

106 Comenzo RL, Sanchorawala V, Fisher C et al. Intermediate-dose intravenous melphalan and blood stem cells mobilized with sequential GM + G-CFS or G-CSF alone to treat AL (amyloid light chain) amyloidosis. *Br J Haematol* 1999; **104**: 553–9.

107 Gertz MA, Lacy MQ, Dispenzieri A et al. Stem cell transplantation for the management of primary

108 Gertz MA, Grogan M, Kyle RA, Tajik AJ. Endomyocardial biopsy-proven light chain amyloidosis (AL) without echocardiographic features of infiltrative cardiomyopathy. *Am J Cardiol* 1997; **80**: 93–5.

109 Clesham GJ, Vigushin DM, Hawkins PN et al. Echocardiographic assessment of cardiac involvement in systemic AL amyloidosis in relation to whole body amyloid load measured by serum amyloid P component (SAP) clearance. *Am J Cardiol* 1997; **80**: 1104–8.

110 Comenzo RL, Michelle D, LeBlanc M et al. Mobilized CD34+ cells selected as autografts in patients with primary light-chain amyloidosis: rationale and application. *Transfusion* 1998; **38**: 60–9.

111 Sanchorawala V, Wright DG, Seldin DC et al. An overview of the use of high-dose melphalan with autologous stem cell transplantation for the treatment of AL amyloidosis. *Bone Marrow Transplant* 2001; **28**: 637–42.

112 Skinner M, Sanchorawala V, Falk RH et al. AL amyloidosis. Severity of illness, treatment decisions and outcome in 554 patients. In: Bely M, Apathy A, eds. *Amyloid and Amyloidosis: The Proceedings of the IXth International Symposium on Amyloidosis*. Budapest, Hungary: David Apathy, 2001: 221–3.

113 Perfetti V, Ubbiali P, Magni M et al. Cells with clonal light chains are present in peripheral blood at diagnosis and in apheretic stem cell harvests of primary amyloidosis. *Bone Marrow Transplant* 1999; **23**: 323–7.

114 Akpek G, Lenz G, Lee SM et al. Immunologic recovery after autologous blood stem cell transplantation in patients with AL amyloidosis. *Bone Marrow Transplant* 2001; **28**: 1105–10.

115 Guillaume T, Rubinstein DB, Symann M. Immune reconstitution and immunotherapy after autologous hematopoietic stem cell transplantation. *Blood* 1998; **92**: 1471–90.

116 Gertz MA, Lacy MQ, Bjornsson J, Litzow MR. Fatal pulmonary toxicity related to the administration of granulocyte-colony stimulating factor in systemic amyloidosis. *Am J Med* 2002; **113**: 549–55.

117 Arbona C, Prosper F, Benet I et al. Comparison between once a day vs twice a day G-CSF for mobilization of peripheral blood progenitor cells (PBPC) in normal donors for allogeneic PBPC transplantation. *Bone Marrow Transplant* 1998; **22**: 39–45.

118 McElwain TJ, Powles RL. High-dose intravenous melphalan for plasma-cell leukaemia and myeloma. *Lancet* 1983; **2**: 822–4.

119 Selby PJ, McElwain TJ, Nandi AC et al. Multiple myeloma treated with high dose intravenous melphalan. *Br J Haematol* 1987; **66**: 55–62.

120 Attal M, Harousseau JL, Stoppa AM et al. Autologous bone marrow transplantation versus conventional chemotherapy in multiple myeloma: a prospective randomized trial. *N Engl J Med* 1996; **335**: 91–7.

121 Lenhoff S, Hjorth M, Holmberg E et al. Impact on survival of high-dose therapy with autologous stem cell support in patients younger than 60 years with newly diagnosed multiple myeloma: a population-based study. Nordic Myeloma Study Group. *Blood* 2000; **95**: 7–11.

122 Lokhorst HM, Sonneveld P, Cornelissen JJ et al. Induction therapy with vincristine, adriamycin, dexamethasone (VAD) and intermediate-dose melphalan (IDM) followed by autologous or allogeneic stem cell transplantation in newly diagnosed multiple myeloma. *Bone Marrow Transplant* 1999; **23**: 317–22.

123 Moreau P, Facon T, Attal M et al. Comparison of 200 mg/m² melphalan and 8 Gy total body irradiation plus 140 mg/m² melphalan as conditioning regimens for peripheral blood stem cell transplantation in patients with newly diagnosed multiple myeloma: final analysis of the Intergroupe Francophone du Myélome 9502 randomized trial. *Blood* 2002; **99**: 731–5.

124 Schulenburg A, Kalhs P, Oberhuber G et al. Gastrointestinal perforation early after peripheral blood stem cell transplantation for AL amyloidosis. *Bone Marrow Transplant* 1998; **22**: 293–5.

125 Aprile C, Marinone G, Saponaro R et al. Cardiac and pleuropulmonary AL amyloid imaging with technetium-99m labelled aprotinin. *Eur J Nucl Med* 1995; **22**: 1393–401.

126 Sanchorawala V, Wright DG, Seldin DC et al. High-dose intravenous melphalan and autologous stem cell transplantation as initial therapy or following two cycles of oral therapy for the treatment of AL amyloidosis: results of a randomized prospective trial. *Blood* 2001; **98**: 815a [Abstract].

127 Gianni L, Bellotti V, Gianni M et al. New drug therapy for amyloidoses: resorption of AL type deposits with 4-iodo-4 deoxydoxorubicin. *Blood* 1995; **86**: 855–61.

128 Merlini G, Ascari E, Amboldi N et al. Interaction of the anthracycline 4′-iodo-4′-deoxydoxorubicin with amyloid fibrils: inhibition of fibrillogenesis. *Proc Natl Acad Sci U S A* 1995; **92**: 2959–63.

129 Merlini G, Ascari E, Amboldi N et al. Treatment of AL amyloidosis with 4′-iodo-4′-deoxydoxorubicin: an update. *Blood* 1999; **93**: 1112–3.

130 Gertz MA, Lacy MQ, Dispenzieri A et al. A multicenter phase II trial of 4′-iodo-4′deoxydoxorubicin (IDOX) in primary amyloidosis (AL). *Amyloid* 2002; **9**: 24–30.

131 Solomon A, Weiss DT, Schell M et al. Transgenic mouse model of AA amyloidosis. *Am J Pathol* 1999; **154**: 1267–72.

132 Kisilevsky R, Lemieux LJ, Fraser PE et al. Arresting amyloidosis *in vivo* using small-molecule anionic sulphonates or sulphates: implication for Alzheimer's disease. *Nat Med* 1995; **1**: 143–8.

133 Hrncic R, Wall J, Wolfenbarger DA et al. Antibody-mediated resolution of light chain-associated amyloid deposits. *Am J Pathol* 2000; **157**: 1239–46.

134 Tennent GA, Lovat LB, Pepys MB. Serum amyloid P component prevents proteolysis of the amyloid fibrils of Alzheimer disease and systemic amyloidosis. *Proc Natl Acad Sci U S A* 1995; **92**: 4299–303.

135 Pepys M, Herbert J, Hutchinson WL et al. Targeted pharmacological depletion of serum amyloid P component for treatment of human amyloidosis. *Nature* 2002; **417**: 254–9.

94 Hematopoietic Cell Transplantation for Breast Cancer

Karen H. Antman

Breast cancer mortality worldwide varies fivefold with the highest risk in northern European countries (and in countries with large numbers of decendents from northern Europe such as Canada, Australia and the USA). Breast cancer mortality is substantially lower but increasing in Asia [1]. Deaths from breast cancer have been falling in the USA, Canada and UK since about 1990 for the first time in the five decades for which such statistics are available [2]. Nevertheless, breast cancer remains the most common cancer in American women with a lifetime risk of 1 of 8, and breast cancer remains the major cause of death in 15–54-year-old American women [3,4].

Breast cancer risk, diagnosis and staging

Factors associated with a three- to fourfold increased relative risk include breast cancer in a mother or sister, early menarche or late menopause, radiation exposure especially between the ages of 10 and 40 years, nulligravida or age over 30 years at first pregnancy and prior breast cancer. Risk is especially high in known carriers of mutated BRCA 1 or 2 or Li-Fraumeni multiple familial cancer syndrome, or if both mother and a sister had breast or ovarian cancer, or either had bilateral or premenopausal breast cancer.

Current recommendations for screening asymptomatic women with no risk factors include regular bilateral mammograms with annual breast examinations for women aged 40–70 years [5]. Mammography should continue for women 70 years of age and older lacking in comorbid disease that would limit their lifetime [5].

All suspicious masses should be biopsied. About 20% of invasive cancers are not visible on mammography; thus, a normal mammogram does not preclude invasive cancer. Nevertheless, a mammogram prior to biopsy is helpful to document the size and location of any suspicious lesion and to compare with a mammogram of the biopsy specimen to insure that all microcalcifications have been removed.

The appropriate evaluation after diagnosis of breast cancer includes a complete blood count (CBC), liver function tests, a chest X-ray and a bone scan. Computerized tomography (CT) scans of the liver and magnetic resonance imaging (MRI) of the head are usually obtained for patients with symptoms or abnormal liver function tests on blood tests. The Tumor, Nodes, Metastasis (TNM) classification used for staging breast cancer is shown in Table 94.1.

Local therapy

The type of local therapy (mastectomy, lumpectomy with radiation) does not affect overall survival [6,7]. Locally advanced cancers, previously considered inoperable, have increasingly been treated with primary systemic chemotherapy followed by mastectomy, radiation or lumpectomy [8]. In two randomized studies for locally advanced disease, the overall survival and local recurrence rate was not statistically different when patients received surgery or radiotherapy following intensive induction chemotherapy [9,10].

Standard dose adjuvant chemotherapy

Most women achieve local control with mastectomy or with lumpectomy and radiation. However, relapse rates at 10 years increase proportionally to the number of positive axillary lymph nodes, from approximately 20% for patients with no involved lymph nodes and 50% for 1–3 involved lymph nodes, to >75% for ten or more axillary lymph nodes. Women with stage II disease with more than 10 positive lymph nodes, or locally advanced or inflammatory breast cancer have a very poor prognosis with conventional-dose therapy. Relapse tends to occur earlier for patients with higher numbers of lymph nodes involved, and some risk of relapse remains for at least 20 years after mastectomy [11].

Tamoxifen or an aromatose inhibitor is given for 5 years for tumors with hormone receptors [12]. The addition of chemotherapy further improves survival, although the benefit is inversely proportional to age [13]. Tamoxifen is often used alone with no chemotherapy in older postmenopausal women with small lesions and no involved lymph nodes. When both chemotherapy and tamoxifen are given, tamoxifen is best begun after completion of planned chemotherapy [14]. In one randomized trial of adjuvant anastrozole (an aromatase inhibitor) vs. tamoxifen, disease-free survival was superior for anastrozole [15].

A number of adjuvant chemotherapy regimens are accepted and range from cyclophosphamide, methotrexate and fluorouracil (CMF), generally used for older patients with 1–2 cm lesions and no involved lymph nodes, to anthracycline-containing regimens such as cyclophosphamide and doxorubicin (CA), cyclophosphamide, doxorubicin, fluorouracil (CAF) or fluorouracil, doxorubicin and cyclophosphamide (FAC) and, more recently, taxane-based regimens (Table 94.2). Four cycles of CA provides equivalent survival to six cycles of CMF [16], but CAF is superior to CMF [13]. Logically then, CAF should thus be superior to CA, although the regimens have never been directly compared.

In randomized adjuvant trials of CA followed by paclitaxel vs. no further therapy, paclitaxel improved survival in a Cancer and Leukaemia Group B (CALGB) study [22,23] but not in the National Surgical Adjuvant Breast Project (NSABP) B28 trial or in an M.D. Anderson Hospital study [24]. Docetaxel, doxorubicin and cyclophosphamide (TAC), compared with FAC, also significantly improved disease-free survival but not overall survival. Of note, survival was significantly improved in the subset of patients with 1–3 involved lymph nodes but not for those with more

Table 94.1 Tumor, Node, Metastasis (TNM) staging system for cancer of the breast.

T	**Tumor (indicates size or involvement)**
TX	Primary tumor cannot be assessed
T0	No evidence of primary tumor
Tis	Carcinoma *in situ*; intraductal carcinoma, lobular carcinoma *in situ*, or Paget's disease of the nipple with no tumor
T1	Tumor <2 cm
T1a	Tumor <0.5 cm
T1b	Tumor <0.5 cm but not >1 cm
T1c	Tumor >1 cm but not >2 cm
T2	Tumor >2 cm but not >5 cm
T3	Tumor >5 cm
T4	Tumor of any size with direct extension to chest wall* or skin†
T4a	Extension to chest wall
T4b	Edema (including *peau d'orange*), ulceration of the skin of the breast or satellite skin nodules confined to the same breast
T4c	Both of T4a and T4b
T4d	Inflammatory carcinoma
N	**Node (indicates regional lymph node involvement)**
NX	Regional lymph nodes cannot be assessed (e.g. previously removed)
N0	No regional lymph node metastases
N1	Metastases to movable ipsilateral axillary nodes
N2	Metastases to ipsilateral axillary nodes fixed to one another or to other structures
N3	Metastases to ipsilateral internal mammary lymph nodes
M	**Metastasis (indicates extent of metastasis)**
MX	Extent of metastasis cannot be determined
M0	No evidence of distant metastasis
M1	Distant metastases (including metastases to ipsilateral supraclavicular lymph nodes)

Clinical stage

I	T1, N0, M0
IIA	T0, N1, M0
	T1, N1, M0
	T2, N0, M0
IIB	T2, N1, M0
	T3, N0, M0
IIIA	T0 or T1, N2, M0
	T2, N2, M0
	T3, N1 or N2, M0
IIIB	T4, any N, M0
	Any T, N3, M0
IV	Any T, Any N, M1

*The chest wall includes the ribs, intercostal muscles and serratus anterior muscle, but not the pectoral muscle.
†Dimpling of the skin, nipple retraction or any other skin changes except those listed for T4b may occur in T1, T2, or T3 without affecting the classification.

than four involved nodes [21], the population which would be considered for high-dose studies.

Regimens containing trastuzumab (Herceptin), an accepted standard treatment in metastatic disease, are under evaluation in randomized adjuvant trials. Because the genes for her 2/erbB2 and topoisomerase 2 alpha are relatively closely linked on chromosome 17, many patients with amplification of her 2/erbB2 also have amplification of topoisomerase 2 alpha. Coamplification was associated with a favorable response to anthracycline-based treatment in one study [25].

Table 94.2 Selected conventional-dose cytotoxic drug regimens commonly used in breast cancer.

Drug	Dose	Regimen
CMF [17]		
Cyclophosphamide	100 mg/m^2 p.o.	Days 1–14
Methotrexate	40 mg/m^2 IVB	Days 1 and 8
Fluorouracil	600 mg/m^2 IVB	Days 1 and 8
FAC [18]		
Fluorouracil	500 mg/m^2 IVB	Days 1 and 8
Doxorubicin	50 mg/m^2 IVB	Day 1
Cyclophosphamide	500 mg/m^2 IVB	Day 1
CAF [19]		
Cyclophosphamide	500 mg/m^2 IVB	Day 1
Doxorubicin	50 mg/m^2 IVB	Day 1
Fluorouracil	500 mg/m^2 IVB	Day 1
CA [16,20]		
Cyclophosphamide	600 mg/m^2 IVB	Day 1
Doxorubicin	60 mg/m^2 IVB	Day 1
TAC [21]		
Taxotere	75 mg/m^2 IVB	Day 1
Doxorubicin	50 mg/m^2 IVB	Day 1
Cyclophosphamide	500 mg/m^2 IVB	Day 1

Prognostic factors for outcome with conventional treatment, in order of importance, include number of axillary lymph nodes involved by tumor, size of primary tumor, estrogen and progesterone receptor status, overexpression of c-erb B-2 (Her2/neu) oncogene, and grade of differentiation. Although patients with 1–2 cm breast cancer lesions with no tumor in lymph nodes have a survival of 90%, survival at 5 years remains 40–50% for those with 10 or more involved lymph nodes or locally advanced primary tumors, and drops to 15–20% at 10 years.

Standard-dose therapy for metastatic disease

For the 10% of patients who are initially diagnosed with metastatic breast cancer and for those who develop metastases after primary treatment, the goal of standard treatment is palliation. The median survival of 2 years has not changed appreciably in the last 50 years [26]. For patients with estrogen or progesterone receptor positive disease, considerable palliation is obtained with aromatase inhibitors for postmenopausal women or tamoxifen for premenopausal women [15,27–29].

Chemotherapy regimens are chosen to avoid drugs previously given in an adjuvant setting, particularly if the disease-free interval after adjuvant therapy was short. Thus, patients who have had adjuvant CMF generally begin an anthracycline or taxane-based regimen [30,31]. Doxorubicin-containing regimens such as CAF produce higher response rates than CMF at some cost in greater toxicity [32–36]. Those with tumors that overexpress Her2/erbB2 may receive Herceptin alone [37,38] or in combination with other chemotherapy agents [39,40]. Although standard regimens produce complete responses of up to 40% in metastatic breast cancer, the median duration of response remains 6–12 months. Conventional-dose chemotherapy-induced complete remissions that persist beyond 10 years are rare, occurring in about 1.3% of patients, as described in a large series from M.D. Anderson Hospital, Houston [41]. Successive chemotherapy regimens produce fewer responses of shorter duration.

Development of high-dose therapy regimens for breast cancer

In laboratory models of cancer, cytotoxic chemotherapy dose correlates with cure, while cumulative dose correlates with longer survival for animals who are not cured [42]. An optimal strategy may be to use high doses of chemotherapy when cure is the objective but to give many repetitive smaller doses if palliation and longer survival are the goals. A combination of repetitive cycles of high-dose cytotoxic therapy, followed by appropriate hormonal and biologic agents based on the tumor's receptors might optimally provide both the highest cure rate and the longest survival.

The initial development of bone marrow transplantation (BMT) for leukemia, and its subsequent modification to support high-dose therapies for other malignancies, began decades ago. Once the techniques of autologous and allogeneic marrow transplantation were optimized and accepted for leukemias, various groups initiated studies in lymphomas. Promising pilot studies were followed by randomized trials in relapsed Hodgkin's and non-Hodgkin's disease with significantly improved disease-free survival and survival in intermediate [43] and, very recently, low-grade lymphomas [44]. Studies in poor-risk non-Hodgkin's lymphoma in first remission showed significant benefits in disease-free survival and trends in survival [45,46]. Certainly, the question of extension of the strategy to more common invariably fatal solid tumors such as metastatic breast cancer was a reasonable research question.

Clinical trials of high-dose therapy followed by autologous hematopoietic cell transplantation (HCT) for breast cancer proceeded expeditiously and responsibly in an orderly progression of studies and publications to randomized evaluations based on the publication dates of the sequence of studies. The first phase 2 studies of combination cytotoxic chemotherapy in untreated or responding patients with metastatic disease were published between 1988 and 1992 [47–50]. Phase 2 studies in the adjuvant settings appeared in 1993 [51]. Investigators in the USA proceeded to design a randomized study based on a first-generation regimen with a high treatment-related mortality rate. Other groups, particularly the Dutch, designed their randomized study later once safer third-generation high-dose regimens became available. The first randomized study was published in 1995 [52] and the next trial 5 years later in 2000 [53]. The early emergence of this 'positive' randomized trial from South Africa [52] significantly hampered accrual onto randomized studies in the USA, where high-dose chemotherapy became available off study.

A second positive randomized high-dose study by the same South African authors reported to compare conventional CAF vs. two cycles of high-dose chemotherapy with no induction conventional-dose therapy [54] prompted an audit. Data from the two South African studies were found to have been misrepresented; discrepancies in eligibility criteria and reported data were substantial. Control group patient records were not provided for review. The title of the protocol given to the audit team suggests that the control group was treated not with CAF but rather cyclophosphamide, mitoxantrone and vincristine. Thus, the data are best considered unreliable [55].

This and the presentation of several small randomized studies with no significant benefit then further impaired accrual to the ongoing randomized studies on both sides of the Atlantic. Nevertheless, accrual on several had been substantial or complete and, after an additional 3–5 years of follow-up, additional larger studies are now being presented and a few published (Table 94.3).

Currently, 20 studies have been published in abstract or manuscript form. Most investigators, patients and insurers agree that the two discredited South African trials are uninterpretable at best, and thus they are deleted from this analysis, leaving 18 randomized studies. The studies to

Table 94.3 Eighteen randomized trials of high-dose therapy in breast cancer published to date.

Study	Number randomized
Dutch	885
Cancer & Leukaemia GroupB Intergroup	783
Anglo-Celtic	605
Easter Cooperative Oncology Group	540
Scandinavian	525
Milan HD sequential	382
French PEGASE 1	314
German Adjuvant	302
NCI Canada*	219
Philadelphia*	184
French PEGASE 3*	180
Duke CR crossover*	98
Japan COG	97
German Metastatic*	92
Dutch pilot	81
MD Anderson Hospital	78
Duke bone mets crossover*	69
French PEGASE 4*	61

*Metastatic studies.

Table 94.4 Sample sizes required for 90% power to detect various percentage differences (a = 0.05, two-sided).

Control	Test	Difference	Total n
20	24	4	4604
20	28	8	1244
20	30	10	824
20	**35**	**15**	**396**
20	40	20	238
20	50	30	116

date have a variety of different designs, schedules and regimens. Thus, the optimal regimen or schedule is unknown.

More than half of the studies randomized fewer than 300 patients and thus are underpowered, as they could not reliably exclude 15% differences. In Table 94.4, examples of various sample sizes needed to reliably detect differences of a given size with 90% power and a p-value of 0.05 are provided. In the setting of metastatic disease with perhaps 20% of patients in follow-up on standard therapy, the study would have to include almost 400 patients to reliably exclude a 15% difference (line shown in bold type). Studies randomizing about 100 patients cannot exclude differences of 30%. Because the number of events is fewer in adjuvant trials, they need to be even larger with longer follow-up to observe sufficient events to reliably detect differences of 15–30%.

Given the size of even the largest studies, subset analysis is hazardous; particularly those for metastatic disease for which even the largest study randomized only 219 patients. Thus, no firm conclusions can be drawn for either patients transplanted in partial or complete response. Finally, the studies to date have a variety of different designs, schedules and regimens. Two studies, the US and the Scandinavian adjuvant studies, compare two experimental regimens (i.e. different higher than standard dose regimens). Thus, the optimal regimen or schedule is unknown. Nevertheless, many of the studies have found statistically significant

Table 94.5 Eleven randomized high-dose breast cancer adjuvant studies. Significant and borderline significant differences are shown in bold.

	Number randomized	Toxic deaths (%)		Median years follow-up	EFS (%)			Survival (%)			Reference
		HDC	Control		HDC	Control	p	HDC	Control	p	
Dutch phase 3	885	0.9	0.2	3.5	**72**	**65**	**0.057**	NA	NA	0.31	[56]
CALGB Intergroup	783	7.4	0	5.1	61	60	0.49	70	72	0.23	[57]
Anglo-Celtic	605	1.7	0	4.0	51	54	n.s.	63	62	n.s.	[58]
ECOG	540	3.3	0	6.1	48	46	0.50	58	61	0.45	[59]
Scandinavian	525	0.7	0	2.9	**72**	**63**	**0.013**	83	77	0.12	[60]
Milan HD sequential	382	0.5	0	4.3	65	62	n.s.	76	77	n.s.	[61]
French PEGASE 01	314	0.6	0	3.0	**71**	**55**	**0.002**	85	84	0.33	[62]
German	302	2.0	0	3.7	51	41	0.095	72	67	n.s.	[63]
Japan COG	97	0	0	4.0	60	48	n.s.	67	66	n.s.	[64]
Dutch randomized phase 2	81	0	0	4.1	70	65	0.97	82	75	0.84	[65]
MD Anderson Hospital	78	2.5	0	6.5	48	62	n.s.	58	77	n.s.	[66]

CALGB, Cancer and Leukemia Group B; ECOG, Eastern Cooperative Oncology Group; HD, high dose; HDC, high-dose chemotherapy; EFS, event-free survival; NA, not available; n.s., not significant.
*Patients who relapsed on the conventional dose arm then received high-dose chemotherapy.
†Data at 6 years median follow-up.

Table 94.6 Seven randomized high-dose metastatic studies breast cancer studies. Significant and borderline significant differences are shown in bold.

	Number randomized	Toxic deaths		Median years follow-up	3-year EFS (%)			3-year survival (%)			Reference
		HDC	Control		HDC	Control	p	HDC	Control	p	
NCI Canada	223	6.2	0	1.6	**40**	**22**	**0.01**	60	59	0.96	[67]
Philadelphia Intergroup	184	1.0	0	5.6	4	3	0.31	14	13	0.62	[53,68]
French PEGASE 3	180	1.1	0	4.0	**46**	**19**	**0.0001**	38	30	0.70	[69]
Duke CR Crossover studies											
Complete responders only†	98	NA	NA	6.3	**25**	**10**	**<0.01**	33	*38	0.32	[70,71]
Bone metastases only	69	9.7	NA	4.9	**17**	**0**	**<0.01**	28	*22	NA	[72]
German	92	2.1	0	1.2	NA	NA	**0.05**	NA	NA	0.12	[73]
French PEGASE 4	61	0	0	4.4	**28**	**4**	**0.05**	61	28	0.12	[74]

EFS, event-free survival; HDC, high-dose chemotherapy; NA, not available.
*Patients who relapsed on the conventional dose arm then received high-dose chemotherapy.
†Data at 6 years median follow-up.

differences in time to relapse or disease-free survival. Follow up in the adjuvant studies is still short: 3–6 years. Significant differences in survival may or may not eventually emerge. Deaths from toxicity are variable depending on the high-dose regimens used, but are 0–2% in the majority of studies, particularly those using second- or third-generation high-dose regimens (Tables 94.5 and 94.6).

Randomized trials in the adjuvant setting

The Dutch Insurance Industry funded trial with 885 randomized patients included most women eligible at the 10 participating centers [56]. Patients received four cycles of 5-fluorouracil, epirubicin and cyclophosphamide (FEC) and then were randomized to either to cyclophosphamide, thiotepa and carboplatin (CTCb) or an additional cycle of FEC, followed by surgery, radiation and tamoxifen for 2 years. The toxic mortality was one of 443 patients on standard dose FEC and four of 442 on high-dose CTCb. At a median of 3 years follow-up, a trend ($p = 0.057$) in DFS has emerged favoring high-dose therapy. In a planned analysis of the first 284 patients with a median follow-up of 6 years, disease-free and overall survival were significantly improved with high-dose CTCb. The Netherlands Cancer Institute phase 2 pilot, which had randomized 81 women with an involved apical axillary lymph node, in a feasibility study of the same randomization design had shown no differences in disease-free and overall survival with a median follow-up of 4 years, but could not exclude differences in survival of less than 30% [65]. In fact, their 284 patient study above has a survival difference of about 10%.

In the CALGB Intergroup Study patients received four cycles of standard adjuvant CAF and then were randomized to high vs. intermediate dose cyclophosphamide, BCNU and cisplatin (CBP) [57]. Although intermediate-dose CBP is not a standard regimen, the design is a pure comparison between high- and intermediate-dose CBP. This first-generation BCNU-based high-dose regimen resulted in a high mortality (7.4%), which increased with patient age and significantly varied with the experience of the transplant center. Pulmonary and hepatic toxicity were common. With a median of 5.1 years of follow-up, fewer relapses have occurred in the high-dose arm, although neither progression-free or overall survival were significantly improved. Because the study group was selected to have a projected survival of about 25% and survival is currently around 70% in both arms, significant differences may or may not emerge as larger numbers of relapses occur.

The Anglo-Celtic I study randomized 605 women with breast cancer involving four or more involved lymph nodes (median nine) following four cycles of 75 mg/m^2 doxorubicin to CMF vs. a hematopoietic progenitor cell mobilization cycle of 4.0 g/m^2 cyclophosphamide supported by filgrastim, followed by 6.0 g/m^2 cyclophosphamide and 800 mg/m^2 thiotepa. Five women (1.7%) died of treatment-related toxicity on the high-dose arm. With a median of 4 years follow-up, event-free survival rates at 5 years for high- and conventional-dose chemotherapy are 51% and 54%, respectively. Survival is 63% and 62%, respectively [58].

In the Eastern Cooperative Oncology Group (ECOG) study, 540 patients with breast cancer involving more than 10 axillary lymph nodes were randomized to CAF for six cycles followed by either no further chemotherapy or 6 g/m^2 cyclophosphamide and 800 mg/m^2 thiotepa both by continuous intravenous infusion over 4 days. All patients received 5000 cGy to the chest wall and regional lymphatics. Those with estrogen receptor positive disease also received tamoxifen. Nine high-dose patients (3%) died of toxicity (six had received marrow- rather than blood-derived stem cells). Nine others developed acute myeloid leukemia or a myelodysplastic syndrome. At a median follow-up of 6.1 years, event-free and overall survival were similar on both arms although time to relapse was significantly better for high-dose patients [59].

The Scandinavian trial compared conventional-dose induction FEC followed either by one high-dose CTCb cycle vs. six additional cycles of escalated doses of FEC tailored to individual tolerance (up to 1800 mg/m^2 cyclophosphamide, 600 mg/m^2 5-fluorouracil and 120 mg/m^2 epirubicin per cycle). The planned and delivered cumulative doses for tailored therapy exceeds doses in the BMT arm [60]. Leukemia or myelodysplasia has developed in nine patients (3.6%) on the tailored dose arm vs. none on the marrow transplant arm. Topoisomerase-associated leukemias can occur early but alkylating agent-associated leukemias develop later than the current median follow-up of 3 years. Thus, additional cases are likely to occur. With a follow-up of just under 3 years, breast cancer relapsed in 81 patients on the tailored FEC group vs. 113 in the CTCb group ($p = 0.04$). In the tailored FEC group, 60 have died as have 82 in the CTCb group ($p = 0.12$).

The group in Milan randomized 382 women younger than 60 years with four or more positive nodes to three courses of 120 mg/m^2 epirubicin, followed by either six courses of CMF or high-dose sequential chemotherapy. High-dose therapy included the sequence of one course of 7 g/m^2 cyclophosphamide, one course of 8 g/m^2 methotrexate with leucovorin rescue, two courses of 120 mg/m^2 epirubicin and one course of 600 mg/m^2 thiotepa plus 160–180 mg/m^2 melphalan followed by HCT [61]. Stratifications included the number of involved nodes (4–9 or 9). Patients received tamoxifen for 5 years, regardless of receptor or menopausal status. One high-dose patient (0.5%) died of interstitial pneumonia. At a median follow-up of 52 months in an intent-to-treat analysis of the patients receiving conventional (197 patients) and high-dose sequential therapy (185 patients), the 5-year progression-free survival is 62% and 65%, respectively, and overall survival is 77% and 76%, respectively. A trend in favor of high-dose therapy was seen in the 112 patients younger than 36 years, and the 147 patients with 4–9 involved lymph nodes (hazard rate 0.66 and 0.69, respectively). Many patients are still receiving tamoxifen and thus follow-up analyses are required.

The French PEGASE 01 randomized 314 women aged 60 years or less with seven or more positive axillary nodes to 500 mg/m^2 5-fluorouracil, 100 mg/m^2 epirubicin, 500 mg/m^2 cyclophosphamide (FEC) followed by no further chemotherpy (155 patients) vs. 60 mg/kg/day cyclophosphamide for 2 days, 45 mg/m^2 mitoxantrone and 140 mg/m^2 melphalan (Alkeran) (CMA; 159 patients). All patients then recived radiation therapy and those with estrogen receptor positive disease received tamoxifen for 3 years. The median number of involved axillary nodes was 13. One CMA patient died of sepsis. At 3 years, disease-free survival was 55% vs. 71% ($p = 0.002$) and overall survival was 84% vs. 85% ($p = 0.33$), for conventional therapy vs. high-dose treatment, respectively [62].

The German Breast Cancer Study Group randomized 307 women with 10 or more involved axillary lymph nodes who had received four cycles of 90 mg/m^2 epirubicin and 600 mg/m^2 cyclophosphamide (EC) intravenously every 3 weeks to either a high-dose chemotherapy (152 patients) of 1500 mg/m^2 cyclophosphamide, 150 mg/m^2 thiotepa and 10 mg/m^2 mitoxantrone on 4 consecutive days, respectively, with HCT vs. three cycles of a standard-dose CMF (155 patients; 500 mg/m^2 cyclophosphamide, 40 mg/m^2 methotrexate and 600 mg/m^2 5-fluorouracil intravenously on days 1 and 8, respectively, every 4 weeks). Patients with tumors with hormone receptors received tamoxifen for 5 years. Two patients died of toxicity. With a median follow-up of 3.7 years, event-free survival is 51% vs. 41%, favoring high-dose therapy ($p = 0.095$). Survival is 72% vs. 67% [63].

The Japan Cooperative Oncology Group randomized 97 women aged 55 years or less with 10 or more positive axillary nodes to 6 g/m^2 cyclophosphamide and 600 mg/m^2 thiotepa as consolidation after six courses of 500 mg/m^2 cyclophosphamide, 40 mg/m^2 Adriamycin and 500 mg/m^2 fluorouracil every 3 weeks followed by tamoxifen. The median number of involved axillary nodes was 16 (range 10–49). The standard treatment arm included 48 patients. Of the 49 patients randomized to high-dose therapy, 15 (31%) never actually received it. No treatment-related deaths occurred. After 4 years, an analysis based on intent-to-treat relapse-free survival was 48% vs. 60% ($p = 0.42$) and overall survival was 66% vs. 67% ($p = 0.95$), for conventional therapy vs. high-dose treatment, respectively [64].

The small M.D. Anderson Cancer Center study randomized 78 patients to eight cycles of FAC with or without two cycles of high-dose cyclophosphamide, etoposide and cisplatin. Three patients randomized to conventional dose therapy underwent transplant elsewhere; six randomized to transplantation did not receive this therapy. With a median 78 months follow-up, no advantage for high-dose chemotherapy has emerged, but the study cannot exclude differences of less than 30% [66].

Summary of randomized adjuvant trials

Eight of the 11 studies randomized more than 300 patients (Table 94.5).

The US CALGB study has a significantly decreased relapse rate offset by its substantial treatment-associated mortality. The Anglo-Celtic study shows no differences to date. Disease-free survival favors the higher dose arm in the French PEGASE study and in the Scandinavian study, which compares one high-dose cycle vs. six intermediate-dose cycles.

In all studies save for the Anglo-Celtic and the M.D. Anderson hospital studies, the high-dose arm has a higher disease-free survival than the conventional-dose arm. Given that the most optimistic data project about a 2% disease-free survival after the development of metastases [41], and that the median time from relapse to death is about 2 years, event-free survival should provide an early indication of eventual survival.

Randomized trials in metastatic disease

The largest study published to date is the National Cancer Institute of Canada (NCIC) study [67]. Patients with no prior chemotherapy for metastatic breast cancer received four cycles of conventional dose anthracycline or taxane-based therapy depending on their prior adjuvant regimen. Of 386 patients entered, 223 responding patients were stratified by site of disease, estrogen and progesterone receptor status and response and were randomized to receive 2–4 additional cycles of standard chemotherapy (111 patients) or 1–2 cycles followed by high-dose 1.5 g/m^2 cyclophosphamide, 17.5 mg/m^2 mitoxantrone, 450 mg/m^2 carboplatin daily ×4 (112 patients). All estrogen receptor positive patients received hormone therapy and radiotherapy was given for solitary bone or soft tissue sites. Prior to randomization, 12% were in complete response, 45% in partial response and 43% had nonmeasurable disease. Of 112 patients randomized to high-dose therapy, 23 (21%) never received this therapy. At 19 months median follow-up, progression-free survival (40% vs. 22%) significantly favored high-dose therapy with no difference in survival.

In the Philadelphia Intergroup study, responders after 4–6 cycles of CAF or CMF chemotherapy were randomized to high-dose CTCb vs. conventional-dose chemotherapy continued until progression or for up to 24 cycles. This study randomized only 199 patients (36% of the 535 patients entered) [53]. An additional 18% of the randomized patients were deemed ineligible or did not receive their assigned treatment, leaving 164 eligible randomized patients who received their assigned treatment. Additional patients assigned to receive conventional-dose therapy underwent high-dose therapy after they relapsed. The partial/complete response rate of 7% is strikingly low. In an update with a median follow-up of 5.6 years, 27 patients were alive (16 after high-dose therapy, 11 with CMF). Survival at 5 years is 14% for high-dose therapy vs. 13% for CMF. In subset analysis, patients under the age of 43 years survived longer if treated with high-dose therapy, while those >42 years survived longer with CMF ($p = 0.02$ for interaction between treatment and age). Progression-free survival at 5 years is 4% for high-dose chemotherapy and 3% for CMF. Subgroup analysis showed a trend toward longer time to tumor progression for hormone receptor positive patients with CMF ($p = 0.05$). Given the similar survival in the two arms and the <1% mortality rate for high-dose chemotherapy, many patients might prefer a short intense treatment to up to 2 years of repetitive cycles of chemotherapy [68].

In the French PEGASE 3 trial, 308 women with metastatic breast cancer requiring first-line chemotherapy were entered and 180 responding to four cycles of 500 mg/m^2 5-fluorouracil, 500 mg/m^2 cyclophosphamide and 100 mg/m^2 epirubicin were randomized to no additional therapy [75] vs. high-dose 800 mg/m^2 thiotepa and 6000 mg/m^2 cyclophosphamide. Of 89 randomized to intensification, nine were not transplanted. One patient (1%) died of toxicity. Median age was 46 years and median follow-up was 48 months. The 1-year progression rate was 80% for conventional-dose chemotherapy vs. 54% for high-dose therapy ($p = 0.0005$). The 1-year disease-free survival was 19% vs. 46%, respectively ($p = 0.0001$), also favoring the intensive arm. The 3-year overall survival was 30% for conventional vs. 38% for high-dose therapy ($p = 0.7$) [69].

In two Duke University studies with a crossover design, 453 women with metastatic breast cancer were treated with conventional-dose doxorubicin, fluorouracil and methotrexate (AFM). Of 120 women who attained a complete remission, 98 were randomized to either immediate high-dose CBP or CBP at the time of relapse. Sixty-nine women with only metastases to bone underwent a similar randomization with crossover to high-dose therapy for women randomized to conventional treatment at the time of relapse. Significant differences in disease-free survival favor high-dose therapy in both studies. In the bone metastases study, all patients randomized to conventional therapy relapsed and then underwent high-dose therapy [72]. Although survival of the immediate BMT group in the "complete remission study" was initially reported to be shorter than for the group getting delayed BMT, with further follow-up this difference is no longer significant [70,71]. The first generation BCNU-based high-dose regimen used in this study resulted in a 9.7% mortality.

In a German study, 92 women aged <60 years with no prior treatment for metastatic breast cancer were stratified by menopausal status and hormone receptor status, and were then randomized to 6–9 courses of 60 mg/m^2 doxorubicin and 200 mg/m^2 paclitaxel every 3 weeks (44 patients) or two high-dose cycles of 4.4 g/m^2 cyclophosphamide, 45 mg/m^2 mitoxantrone and 2.5 g/m^2 etoposide, repeated after 6 weeks (48 patients). Filgrastim-mobilized hematopoietic cells were collected before and after the first course of high-dose therapy. All of the 73% who had estrogen receptor positive tumors received tamoxifen. The median age was 50 years and the median number of metastatic sites was two. Dominant disease was visceral in 86% and soft tissue in 14%. One treatment-related death (2%) occurred on the high-dose arm. Patients who relapsed after conventional-dose therapy were crossed over to high-dose therapy. At a median follow-up of 14 months, the median progression-free survival by intent-to-treat was 14.3 months vs. 10.3 months, favoring the high-dose therapy ($p = 0.05$), and survival was 28 months vs. 25 months for high- vs. conventional-dose therapy ($p = 0.39$) [73].

In the small French PEGASE 4 trial, 61 women with metastatic breast cancer responding to 4–6 courses of conventional chemotherapy were randomized to high-dose mitoxantrone, cyclophosphamide and melphalan vs. continued conventional chemotherapy [74]. The populations were well-balanced for prognostic factors except for pulmonary disease (15/32 in the intensive group vs. 4/29 in the standard group) and brain metastasis (2 vs. 0). Median event-free survival was 20 vs. 35.3 months in the standard and intensive groups ($p = 0.05$). The progression rates were 79% vs. 51% at 3 years and 91% vs. 91% at 5 years, respectively. The median overall survival was 20 and 43 months, respectively, with an overall survival rate of 18% vs. 30% at 5 years ($p = 0.12$).

Summary of randomized metastatic trials (Table 94.6)

None of these available metastatic studies randomized more than 300 patients. The Canadian study, the two French PEGASE studies and the two Duke crossover studies (i.e. six of seven studies) have significant differences in disease-free survival. Because of the crossover design of the Duke trials, survival for conventional vs. high-dose therapy cannot be compared. Based on the number of patients (~907) randomized to date, no firm conclusions can be drawn for patients with metastases, although from registry data, patients with extensive unresponsive disease do not appear to benefit [76,77]. Furthermore, analyses of even smaller subsets of patients in either partial or complete response prior to transplant would be particularly hazardous.

Autologous HCT: special situations

Are the results of high-dose therapy for metastatic breast cancer improved by a syngeneic uninvolved marrow? One potential cause for high relapse rates is marrow contamination with tumor. The Autologous Blood and Marrow Transplant Registry (ABMTR) reported data from 14 women tested at 13 centers with metastatic breast cancer for whom hematopoietic cells were collected from a healthy identical twin [78]. Their median age was 41 years (range 34–50 years). Tumors from seven women expressed estrogen receptors. Of these, three received hormonal therapy pretransplant. Twelve patients were premenopausal at diagnosis. All had received an anthracycline-based regimen; nine also had received taxane and seven radiotherapy. Two women received one chemotherapy regimen pretransplant, 10 had two or three, and two had four or five.

At transplant, four women were in complete response, five had responded partially, two had stable disease and two had progressive disease. One patient died of toxicity. Three-year survival was 63% and 3-year progression-free survival was 17%. Previous ABMTR reports have shown the 3-year survival and progression-free survival after autotransplants to be 31% and 13%, respectively. Thus, progression-free survival for women transplanted with syngeneic grafts was not strikingly better

Table 94.7 Three-year survival and 3-year progression-free survival from the Autologous Blood and Marrow Transplant Registry (ABMTR) database [78].

	Three-year survival (%)	95%CI (%)	Three-year progression-free survival (%)	95%CI (%)
Syngeneic	63	36–85	17	2–41
Autologous	31	28–34	13	10–16

CI, confidence interval.

than for women receiving autologous grafts, supporting the premise that residual cancer in the patient is the major contributor to relapse [78]. Given the number of patients studied, a medically important difference cannot be excluded (Table 94.7).

High-dose therapy for breast cancer in men

The results for the few men with breast cancer treated with high-dose therapy appear similar to those reported for women. Of 13 men treated at 10 centers reported by the ABMTR, six had stage II cancer, four had stage III and three had metastases [79]. All 12 tested tumors were estrogen receptor positive. The median age was 50 years. Of the 10 men receiving adjuvant high-dose therapy, three relapsed 3, 5 and 50 months and died at 16, 19 and 67 months post-transplant. The remaining seven were disease-free with a median follow-up of 23 months (range 6–50 months). All three men treated for metastatic breast cancer had progressive or recurrent disease at 6, 7 and 16 months post-transplant.

Allogeneic HCT for breast cancer

The role of allogeneic HCT requires that immune cells recognize breast cancer HLA-class I bound peptide antigens. In a mouse model at Washington University, St. Louis, stimulating normal peripheral blood lymphocytes against an HLA-class I matched breast cancer cell line produces tumor reactive HLA-class I restricted cytotoxic lymphocytes (CTLs) [80].

Clinical data in humans are limited. In a case report the development of circulating minor histocompatibility antigen-specific CTLs recognizing breast carcinoma targets appeared to coincide with the clinical disappearance of liver metastases, suggested a graft-vs.-tumor effect [81].

At Hadassah University Hospital, Jerusalem, patients first underwent high-dose chemotherapy and autologous HCT and then as an outpatient received HLA-matched donor peripheral blood lymphocytes (PBL) treated *in vivo* with human recombinant interleukin 2 (rIL-2). If no graft-vs.-host disease (GVHD) developed, donor PBLs were infused, again treated *in vitro* with rIL-2. Two patients developed grade I–II GVHD, one of whom was in complete response >34 months [82].

The group at M.D. Anderson conducted a trial in which 10 "poor-risk" (bone and liver metastases) women underwent HLA-identical sibling allo-peripheral blood hematopoietic cell transplants with standard GVHD prophylaxis. Two patients died of toxicity. The response rate was 60% but remission durations were short: a median of 238 days. Interestingly, in an attempt to forestall disease progression, four patients had their immunosuppression reduced and one received a donor lymphocyte infusion. Two patients had regression of liver lesions coincident with exacerbation of GVHD [83].

In a second M.D. Anderson Hospital study, five patients with metastatic breast cancer were treated with an intensity-reduced regimen followed by allogeneic HCT using 30 mg/m^2/day IV fludarabine from day –6 to –2 and 70 mg/m^2/day IV melphalan from day –3 to –2 and tacrolimus with mini-methotrexate for GVHD prophylaxis. Tacrolimus was tapered for disease progression at 100 days after HCT. On day 30, all patients had attained 100% donor-type hematolymphopoiesis. One patient who presented with metastatic disease remained in complete response. Three additional patients have had prolonged stable disease [84].

Thus, data for allogeneic HCT are preliminary. Graft-vs.-tumor strategies are most likely to be effective in the setting of minimal residual disease. The means to better control onset and extent of GVHD would improve this approach.

Research directions

Additional follow-up of these randomized trials, and the completion and presentation of unpublished randomized trials will provide more reliable information on which to base treatment decisions. Certainly, lessons from randomized high-dose trials for lymphoma should caution our early interpretation of the breast cancer randomized trials. Good-risk lymphoma patients and those with resistant disease did not appear to benefit from high-dose chemotherapy. Lymphoma studies required 4–7 years of follow-up for differences in survival to emerge; thus, any differences in a more indolent disease such as breast cancer may take longer. In one French lymphoma study, conventional-dose induction therapy significantly improved disease-free and overall survival [85]. Maintenance therapy obscures differences. We may see similar patterns in breast cancer as well.

Since the initial randomized trials were planned, the taxanes have been integrated into conventional-dose therapy for metastatic disease and are being evaluated in the adjuvant setting with impact on overall survival in one of four trials to date. Thus, although the toxicity of high-dose therapy exceeds that of conventional dose paclitaxel, the potential survival difference may also be larger. Based on data showing a correlation of dose with response for taxanes in the laboratory [86], higher doses of paclitaxel are now under study [87–89].

Some investigators postulate a threshold dose required for drug effectiveness above which survival is not improved. Because blood levels of most drugs vary about two- to fivefold, significant differences in serum levels are difficult to detect unless drug dosages are escalated substantially. This observation provides an alternative hypothesis to explain the outcomes of the four available studies of modestly increased chemotherapy doses without stem cell support. In the three studies in which no differences in outcome were detected, the dose escalations were 1.13-fold in the CALGB [22] and 1.5-fold in the two NSABP studies [90,91], probably below the level of detection. In the positive CALGB study, the dose escalation was fully twofold [75]. The dose effect was most significant in the 20% of patients whose tumors overexpressed Her2/neu, suggesting that important therapeutic differences might be missed if biologic subsets are ignored [92].

Some have criticized the further development of high-dose therapies based on a higher priority for molecularly targeted therapy. Although we all would enthusiastically welcome more effective treatments concepts for breast cancer, few currently exist. First-generation monoclonal antibodies such as Herceptin are effective for a relatively small subset of breast cancer patients and, even for these women, are unlikely to be curative as single agents. Once more effective molecularly targeted therapies are developed, their evaluation would still generally require several years. Most new treatments do not replace standard therapy but are added or integrated. Herceptin and other biologically based treatments can easily be incorporated into conventional-dose therapy prior to high-dose regimens.

The return of uncontaminated hematopoietic cells may prove necessary for improving outcome. Methods to deplete contaminating breast cancer cells are already available. Technological developments in hematopoietic cell support (including hematopoietic growth factors) have already improved methods for harvesting stem cells and provided agents to therapeutically modulate the immune response. Hematopoietic cell transplant technology is already used to deliver new biologically based therapies, and may be required for gene or immunotherapies. Sequential high-dose therapies, regimens incorporating new agents and studies of cell therapies or vaccines using dendritic cells are currently under study.

References

1. Mettlin C. Global breast cancer mortality statistics. *CA Cancer J Clin* 1999; **49**: 138–44.
2. Peto R, Boreham J, Clarke M et al. UK and USA breast cancer deaths down 25% in year 2000 at ages 20–69 years. *Lancet* 2000: **355**: 1822.
3. Jemal A, Thomas A, Murray T et al. Cancer statistics, 2002. *CA Cancer J Clin* 2002; **52**: 23–47.
4. Breast cancer statistics. *J Natl Cancer Inst* 2000; **92**: 445.
5. Screening for breast cancer: recommendations and rationale. *Ann Intern Med* 2002; **137**: 344–6.
6. Fisher B, Anderson S, Bryant J et al. Twenty-year follow-up of a randomized trial comparing total mastectomy, lumpectomy, and lumpectomy plus irradiation for the treatment of invasive breast cancer. *N Engl J Med* 2002; **347**: 1233–41.
7. Veronesi U, Cascinelli N, Mariani L et al. Twenty-year follow-up of a randomized study comparing breast-conserving surgery with radical mastectomy for early breast cancer. *N Engl J Med* 2002; **347**: 1227–32.
8. Wolff AC, Davidson NE. Preoperative therapy in breast cancer. Lessons from the treatment of locally advanced disease. *Oncologist* 2002; **7**: 239–45.
9. Perloff BM, Lesnich GJ, Chu F et al. Combination chemotherapy with mastectomy or radiotherapy for stage III breast carcinoma: a CALGB study. *J Clin Oncol* 1988; **6**: 261–9.
10. DeLena M, Varini M, Zucali R et al. Multimodality treatment for locally advanced breast cancer. *Cancer Clin Trials* 1981; **4**: 229–30.
11. Bonadonna G, Valagussa P, Moliterni A et al. Adjuvant cyclophosphamide, methotrexate, and fluorouracil in node-positive breast cancer: the results of 20 years of follow-up. *N Engl J Med* 1995; **332**: 901–6.
12. Fisher B, Dignam J, Bryant J et al. Five versus more than 5 years of tamoxifen for lymph node-negative breast cancer: updated findings from the National Surgical Adjuvant Breast and Bowel Project B-14 randomized trial. *J Natl Cancer Inst* 2001; **93**: 684–90.
13. Early Breast Cancer Trialists' Collaborative Group. Polychemotherapy for early breast cancer. An overview of the randomised trials. *Lancet* 1998; **352**: 930–42.
14. Albain KS, Green SJ, Ravdin PM et al. Adjuvant chemohormonal therapy for primary breast cancer should be sequential instead of concurrent: initial results from intergroup trial 0100 (SWOG-8814). *Proc Am Soc Clin Oncol* 2002; **21**: 37a [Abstract].
15. Anastrozole alone or in combination with tamoxifen versus tamoxifen alone for adjuvant treatment of postmenopausal women with early breast cancer: first results of the ATAC randomised trial. *Lancet* 2002; **359**: 2131–9.
16. Fisher B, Brown AM, Dimitrov NV et al. Two months of doxorubicin-cyclophosphamide with and without interval reinduction therapy compared with 6 months of cyclophosphamide, methotrexate, and fluorouracil in positive-node breast cancer patients with tamoxifen-nonresponsive tumors: results from the National Surgical Adjuvant Breast and Bowel Project B-15. *J Clin Oncol* 1990; **8**: 1483–96.
17. Tancini G, Bonadonna G, Valagussa P et al. Adjuvant CMF in breast cancer: comparative 5-year results of 12 vs. 6 cycles. *J Clin Oncol* 1983; **1**: 2–10.
18. Swenerton KD, Legha SS, Smith T et al. Prognostic factors in metastatic breast cancer treated with combination chemotherapy. *Cancer Res* 1979; **39**: 1552–62.
19. Smalley RV, Carpenter J, Bartolucci A et al. A comparison of cyclophosphamide, Adriamycin, 5-fluorouracil (CAF) and cyclophosphamide, methotrexate, 5-fluorouracil, vincristine, prednisone (CMFVP) in patients with metastatic breast cancer: a Southeastern Cancer Study Group project. *Cancer* 1977; **40**: 625–32.
20. Fisher B, Anderson S, Wickerham DL et al. Increased intensification and total dose of cyclophosphamide in a doxorubicin-cyclophosphamide regimen for the treatment of primary breast cancer: findings from National Surgical Adjuvant Breast and Bowel Project B-22. *J Clin Oncol* 1997; **15**: 1858–69.
21. Nabholtz J, Pienkowski T, Mackey J et al. Phase 3 trial comparing TAC with FAC in the adjuvant treatment of node positive breast cancer. *Proc ASCO* 2002; **21**: 141a [Abstract].
22. Henderson I, Berry D, Demetri G et al. Improved disease-free and overall survial from the addition of sequential paclitaxel but not from the escalation of doxorubicin dose level in the adjuvant chemotherapy of patients with node positive primary breast cancer. *Proc Am Soc Clin Oncol* 1998; **17**: 101a [Abstract].
23. Henderson IC, Berry DA, Demetri GD et al. Improved outcomes from adding sequential paditaxel but not from escalating doxorubicin dose in an adjuvant chemotherapy regimen for patients with node-positive primary breast cancer. *J Clin Oncol* 2003; **21**(6): 976–83.
24. Buzdar AU, Singletary SE, Valero V et al. Evaluation of paclitaxel in adjuvant chemotherapy for patients with operable breast cancer: preliminary data of a prospective randomized trial. *Clin Cancer Res* 2002; **8**: 1073–9.
25. Coon JS, Marcus E, Gupta-Burt S et al. Amplification and overexpression of topoisomerase II alpha predict response to anthracycline-based therapy in locally advanced breast cancer. *Clin Cancer Res* 2002; **8**: 1061–7.
26. Mick R, Begg CB, Antman K et al. Diverse prognosis in metastatic breast cancer: who should be offered alternative initial therapies? *Breast Cancer Res Treat* 1989; **13**: 33–8.
27. Eiermann W, Paepke S, Appfelstaedt J et al. Preoperative treatment of postmenopausal breast cancer patients with letrozole: a randomized double-blind multicenter study. *Ann Oncol* 2001; **12**: 1527–32.
28. Paridaens R, Dirix L, Beex L et al. Promising results with exemestane in the first-line treatment of metastatic breast cancer: a randomized phase 2 EORTC trial with a tamoxifen control. *Clin Breast Cancer* 2000; **1** (Suppl. 1): S19–21.
29. Ellis MJ, Coop A, Singh B et al. Letrozole is more effective neoadjuvant endocrine therapy than tamoxifen for ErbB-1- and/or ErbB-2-positive, estrogen receptor-positive primary breast cancer: evidence from a phase 3 randomized trial. *J Clin Oncol* 2001; **19**: 3808–16.
30. Nabholtz JM, Reese DM, Lindsay MA et al. Docetaxel in the treatment of breast cancer: an update on recent studies. *Semin Oncol* 2002; **29**: 28–34.
31. Biganzoli L, Cufer T, Bruning P et al. Doxorubicin and paclitaxel vs. doxorubicin and cyclophosphamide as first-line chemotherapy in metastatic breast cancer: the European Organization for Research and Treatment of Cancer 10961 Multicenter Phase 3 Trial. *J Clin Oncol* 2002; **20**: 3114–21.
32. Hayes DF, Henderson IC. CAF in metastatic breast cancer: standard therapy or another effective regimen? *J Clin Oncol* 1987; **5**: 1497–9.
33. Gianni L, Munzone E, Capri G et al. Paclitaxel by 3-hour infusion in combination with bolus doxorubicin in women with untreated metastatic breast cancer: high antitumor efficacy and cardiac effects in a dose-finding and sequence-finding study. *J Clin Oncol* 1995; **13**: 2688–99.
34. Gianni A, Siena S, Bregni M et al. Five-year results of high-dose sequential (HDS) adjuvant chemotherapy in breast cancer with ≥10 positive nodes. *Proc Am Soc Clin Oncol* 1995; **14**: 90a [Abstract].
35. Reichman B, Seidman A, Crown J et al. Paclitaxel and recombinant human granulocyte colony-stimulating factor as initial chemotherapy for metastatic breast cancer. *J Clin Oncol* 1993; **10**: 1943–51.
36. Trudeau M, Eisenhauer E, Higgins B et al. Docetaxel in patients with metastatic breast cancer: a phase 2 study of the National Cancer Institute of Canada–Clinical Trials Group. *J Clin Oncol* 1996; **14**: 422–8.
37. Cobleigh MA, Vogel CL, Tripathy D et al. Multinational study of the efficacy and safety of humanized anti-HER2 monoclonal antibody in women who have HER2-overexpressing metastatic breast cancer that has progressed after chemotherapy for metastatic disease. *J Clin Oncol* 1999; **17**: 2639–48.
38. Vogel CL, Cobleigh MA, Tripathy D et al. Efficacy and safety of trastuzumab as a single agent in first-line treatment of HER2-overexpressing metastatic breast cancer. *J Clin Oncol* 2002; **20**: 719–26.
39. Pegram MD, Lipton A, Hayes DF et al. Phase 2 study of receptor-enhanced chemosensitivity using recombinant humanized anti-p185HER2/neu monoclonal antibody plus cisplatin in patients with HER2/neu-overexpressing metastatic breast cancer refractory to chemotherapy treatment. *J Clin Oncol* 1998; **16**: 2659–71.
40. Slamon DJ, Leyland-Jones B, Shak S et al. Use of chemotherapy plus a monoclonal antibody against HER2 for metastatic breast cancer that overexpresses HER2. *N Engl J Med* 2001; **344**: 783–92.
41. Greenberg P, Hortobagyi G, Smith T et al. Long-term follow-up of patients with complete remission following combination chemotherapy for metastatic breast cancer. *J Clin Oncol* 1996; **14**: 2197–205.
42. Skipper HE. Dose intensity vs. total dose of chemotherapy: an experimental basis. In: DeVita VT, Hellman S, Rosenberg SA, eds. *Important Advances in Oncology*. Philadelphia: Lippencott, 1990: 43–64.

43. Philip T, Guglielmi C, Hagenbeek A et al. Autologous bone marrow transplantation as compared with salvage chemotherapy in relapses of chemotherapy-sensitive non-Hodgkin's lymphoma. *N Engl J Med* 1995; **333**: 1540–5 [see comments].
44. Schouten HC, Qian W, Sydes MR et al. High dose therapy improves outcome in relapsed follicular non-Hodgkin's lymphoma: results of a randomized clinical trial. *Proc Am Soc Clin Oncol* 2002; 21: 414a [Abstract].
45. Gianni AM, Bregni M, Siena S et al. High-dose chemotherapy and autologous bone marrow transplantation compared with MACOP-B in aggressive B-cell lymphoma. *N Engl J Med* 1997; **336**: 1290–7 [see comments].
46. Haioun C, Lepage E, Gisselbrecht C et al. Benefit of autologous bone marrow transplantation over sequential chemotherapy in poor-risk aggressive non-Hodgkin's lymphoma: updated results of the prospective study LNH87-2. Groupe d'Etude des Lymphomes de l'Adulte. *J Clin Oncol* 1997; **15**: 1131–7.
47. Peters W, Shpall E, Jones R et al. High-dose combination alkylating agents with bone marrow support as initial treatment for metastatic breast cancer. *J Clin Oncol* 1988; **6**: 1368–76.
48. Williams S, Mick R, Dresser R et al. High dose consolidation therapy with autologous stem cell rescue in stage IV breast cancer. *J Clin Oncol* 1989; **7**: 1824–30.
49. Dunphy FR, Spitzer G, Buzdar AU et al. Treatment of estrogen receptor-negative or hormonally refractory breast cancer with double high-dose chemotherapy intensification and bone marrow support. *J Clin Oncol* 1990; **8**: 1207–16.
50. Jones RB, Shpall EJ, Shogan J et al. The Duke AFM program: intensive induction chemotherapy for metastatic breast cancer. *Cancer* 1990; **66**: 431–6.
51. Peters W, Ross M, Vredenburgh J et al. High-dose chemotherapy and autologous bone marrow support as consolidation after standard-dose adjuvant therapy for high risk primary breast cancer. *J Clin Oncol* 1993; **11**: 1132–43.
52. Bezwoda W, Seymour L, Dansey R. High dose chemotherapy with hematopoietic rescue as primary treatment for metastatic breast cancer: a randomized trial. *J Clin Oncol* 1995; **13**: 2483–9.
53. Stadtmauer EA, O'Neill A, Goldstein LJ et al. Conventional-dose chemotherapy compared with high-dose chemotherapy plus autologous hematopoietic stem-cell transplantation for metastatic breast cancer: Philadelphia Bone Marrow Transplant Group. *N Engl J Med* 2000; **342**: 1069–76 [see comments].
54. Bezwoda WR. Randomised, controlled trial of high dose chemotherapy vs. standard dose chemotherapy for high risk, surgically treated, primary breast cancer. *Proc Am Soc Clin Oncol* 1999; **18**: 2a [Abstract].
55. Weiss RB, Rifkin RM, Stewart FM et al. High-dose chemotherapy for high-risk primary breast cancer: an on-site review of the Bezwoda study. *Lancet* 2000; **355**: 999–1003.
56. Rodenhuis S, Bontenbal M, Beex L et al. Randomized phase 3 study of high-dose chemotherapy with cyclophosphamide, thiotepa and carboplatin in operable breast cancer with four or more axillary lymph nodes. *Proc Am Soc Clin Oncol* 2000; **19**: 74a [Abstract].
57. Peters WP, Rosner G, Vredenburgh J et al. Updated results of a prospective, randomized comparison of two doses of combination alkylating agents (AA) as consolidation after CAF in high-risk primary breast cancer involving ten or more axillary lymph nodes (LN): CALGB 9082/SWOG 9114/NCIC. *Proc Am Soc Clin Oncol* 2001; **20**: 21a [Abstract].
58. Crown JP, Lind M, Gould A et al. High-dose chemotherapy with autograft support is not superior to cyclophosphamide methotrexate and 5-FU (CMF) following doxorubicin induction in patients with breast cancer and four or more involved axillary lymph nodes: the Anglo-Celtic I study. *Proc Am Soc Clin Oncol* 2002; **21**: 42a [Abstract].
59. Tallman MS, Gray R, Robert NJ et al. Conventional adjuvant chemotherapy with or without high-dose chemotherapy and autologous stem-cell transplantation in high-risk breast cancer. *N Engl J Med* 2003; **349**(1): 17–26.
60. Bergh J, Wiklund T, Erikstein B et al. Tailored fluorouracil, epirubicin, and cyclophosphamide compared with marrow-supported high-dose chemotherapy as adjuvant treatment for high-risk breast cancer: a randomised trial. Scandinavian Breast Group 9401 Study *Lancet* 2000; **356**: 1384–91.
61. Gianni A, Bonadonna G. Five-year results of the randomized clinical trial comparing standard versus high-dose myeloablative chemotherapy in the adjuvant treatment of breast cancer with >3 positive nodes (LN+). *Proc Am Soc Clin Oncol* 2001; **20**: 21a [Abstract].
62. Roche H, Pouillart P, Meyer N et al. Adjuvant high dose chemotherapy (HDC) improves early outcomes for high risk (n >7) breast cancer patients: the PEGASE 01 trial. *Proc Am Soc Clin Oncol* 2001; **20**: 26a [Abstract].
63. Zander AR, Krüger W, Kröger N et al. High-dose chemotherapy with autolgous hematopoietic stem-cell support vs. standard-dose chemotherapy in breast cancer patients with 10 or more positive lymph nodes: first results of a randomized trial. *Proc Am Soc Clin Oncol* 2002; **21**: 415a [Abstract].
64. Tokuda Y, Tajima T, Narabayashi M et al. Randomized phase 3 study of high-dose chemotherapy (HDC) with autologous stem cell support as consolidation in high-risk postoperative breast cancer: Japan Clinical Oncology Group (JCOG9208). *Proc Am Soc Clin Oncol* 2001; **20**: 38a [Abstract].
65. Rodenhuis S, Richel KJ, van der Wall E et al. Randomized trial of high-dose chemotherapy and hematopoietic progenitor cell support in operable breast cancer with extensive axillary lymph node involvement. *Lancet* 1998; **352**: 515–21.
66. Hortobagyi GN, Buzdar AU, Theriault RL et al. Randomized trial of high-dose chemotherapy and blood cell autografts for high-risk primary breast carcinoma. *J Natl Cancer Inst* 2000; **92**: 225–33.
67. Crump M, Gluck S, Stewart D et al. A randomized trial of high-dose chemotherapy (HDC) with autologous peripheral blood stem cell support (ASCT) compared to standard therapy in women with metastatic breast cancer: a National Cancer Institute of Canada (NCIC) Clinical Trials Group Study 2001; **20**: 21a [Abstract].
68. Stadtmauer EA, O'Neill A, Goldstein LJ et al. Conventional-dose chemotherapy compared with high-dose chemotherapy (HDC) plus autologous stem-cell transplantation (SCT) for metastatic breast cancer: 5-year update of the 'Philadelphia Trial'. *Proc Am Soc Clin Oncol* 2002; **21**: 43a [Abstract].
69. Biron P, Durand M, Roche H et al. High dose thiotepa, cyclophosphamide and stem cell transplantation after 4 FEC 100 compared with 4 FEC alone allowed a better disease free survival but the same overall survival in first line chemotherapy for metastatic breast cancer. Results of the PEGASE 03 French Protocol. *Proc Am Soc Clin Oncol* 2002; **21**: 42a [Abstract].
70. Peters W, Jones R, Vredenburgh J et al. A large prospective randomized trial of high-dose combination alkylating agents (CPB) with autologous cellular support as consolidation for patients with metastatic breast cancer achieving complete remission after intensive doxorubicin-based induction therapy (AFM). *Proc Am Soc Clin Oncol* 1996; **15**: 121a [Abstract].
71. Nieto Y, Nieto Y, Champlin R et al. Status of high dose chemotherapy for breast cancer: a review. *Biol Blood Marrow Transplant* 2000; **6**(5): 476–95.
72. Madan B, Broadwater G, Rubin P et al. Improved survival with consolidation high-dose cyclophosphamide, cisplatin and carmustine compared with observation in women with metastic breast cancer and only bone metastases treated with induction Adriamycin, 5-fluorouracial and methotrexate: a phase 3 prospective radomized comparative trial. *Proc ASCO* 2000; **19**: 48a [Abstract].
73. Schmid P, Samonigg H, Nitsch T et al. Randomized trial of up front tandem high-dose chemotherapy compared to standard chemotherapy with doxorubicin and paclitaxel in metastatic breast cancer. *Proc Am Soc Clin Oncol* 2002; **21**: 43a [Abstract].
74. Lotz JP, Cure H, Janvier M et al. High-dose chemotherapy with hematopoietic stem cells transplantation for metastatic breast cancer: results of the French protocol PEGASE 04. *Proc Am Soc Clin Oncol* 1999; **18**: 43a [Abstract].
75. Wood W, Budman D, Korzun A et al. Dose and dose intensity of adjuvant chemotherapy for stage II, node-positive breast carcinoma. *N Engl J Med* 1994; **330**: 1253–9.
76. Rowlings PA, Williams SF, Antman KH et al. Factors correlated with progression-free survival after high-dose therapy and hematopoietic stem cell transplantation for metastatic breast cancer. *J Am Med Assoc* 1999; **282**: 1335–43.
77. Berry DA, Broadwater G, Klein JP et al. High-dose versus standard chemotherapy in metastatic breast cancer: comparison of CALGB trials with data from the ABMTR. *J Clin Oncol* 2002; **20**(3): 743–50.
78. Williams S, Rizzo D, Wu J et al. Syngeneic stem cell transplantation for metastatic breast cancer. *Proc Am Soc Clin Oncol* 2001; **20**: 67b [Abstract].
79. McCarthy P, Hurd D, Rowlings P et al. Autotransplants in men with breast cancer. Autologous Blood Marrow Transplant Registry (ABMTR) Breast Cancer Working Committee. *Bone Marrow Transplant* 1999; **24**: 365–8.
80. Nguyen T, Naziruddin B, Dintzis S et al. Recognition of breast cancer-associated peptides by tumor-reactive, HLA-class I restricted allogeneic cytotoxic T lymphocytes. *Int J Cancer* 1999; **81**: 607–15.
81. Eibl B, Schwaighofer H, Nachbaur D et al. Evidence for a graft-versus-tumor effect in a patient treated with marrow ablative chemotherapy and allogeneic bone marrow transplantation for breast cancer. *Blood* 1996; **88**: 1501–8.
82. Or R, Ackerstein A, Nagler A et al. Allogeneic cell-mediated immunotherapy for breast cancer after autologous stem cell transplantation: a clinical pilot study. *Cytokines Cell Mol Ther* 1998; **4**: 1–6.
83. Ueno N, Randon G, Mirza N et al. Allogeneic peripheral blood progenitor cell transplantation for poor risk patients with metastatic breast cancer. *J Clin Oncol* 1998; **16**: 986–93.
84. Ueno NT, Cheng YC, Giralt SA et al. Complete donor chimerism by fludarabine/melphalan in

mini-allogeneic transplantation for metastatic renal cell carcinoma and breast cancer. *Proc Am Soc Clin Oncol* 2002; **21**: 415a [Abstract].

85 Bosly A, Sonet A, Salles G *et al*. Superiority of late over early intensification in relapsing/refractory aggressive non-Hodgkin's lymphoma: a randomized study from the GELA: LNH RP 93. *Blood* 1997; **90**: 594a.

86 Hanauske A, Degen D, Hilsenbeck S *et al*. Effects of taxotere and taxol on *in vitro* colony formation of freshly explanted human tumor cells. *Anti-Cancer Drugs* 1992; **3**: 121–4.

87 Stemmer S, Cagnoni P, Shpall E *et al*. High dose paclitaxel, cyclophosphamide and cisplatin with autologous hematopoietic progenitor cell support: a phase 1 trial. *J Clin Oncol* 1996; **14**: 1463–72.

88 Vahdat L, Papadopoulos K, Balmaceda C *et al*. Phase 1 trial of sequential high dose chemotherapy with escalating dose paclitaxel, melphalan, and cyclophosphamide, thiotepa and carboplatin with peripheral blood progenitor support in women with responding metastatic breast cancer. *Clin Cancer Res* 1998; **4**: 1689–95.

89 Hudis C, Seidman A, Baselga J *et al*. Sequential dose-dense doxorubicin, paclitaxel, and cyclophosphamide for resectable high-risk breast cancer: feasibility and efficacy. *J Clin Oncol* 1999; **17**: 93–100.

90 Wolmark N, Fisher B, Anderson S. The effect of increasing dose intensity and cumulative dose of adjuvant cyclophosphamide in node positive breast cancer. *Breast Cancer Res Treat* 1998; **46** (Suppl.): 26.

91 Fisher B, Anderson S, DeCillis A *et al*. Further evaluation of intensified and increased total dose of cyclophosphamide for the treatment of primary breast cancer: findings from National Surgical Adjuvant Breast and Bowel Project B-25. *J Clin Oncol* 1999; **17**: 3374–88.

92 Muss H, Thor A, Berry D *et al*. c-erbB-2 Expression and response to adjuvant therapy in women with node-positive early breast cancer. *N Engl J Med* 1994; **330**: 1260–6.

95
Brandon Hayes-Lattin & Craig R. Nichols

Hematopoietic Cell Transplantation in Germ Cell Tumors

Introduction

Malignant testicular tumors are the most common solid tumors among young men, with a rising annual incidence of approximately 9000 new cases in the USA. Ninety-five percent of malignant testicular tumors are germ cell tumors [1]. Germ cell tumors can also arise in extragonadal sites, such as the retroperitoneum or mediastinum, often portending a poorer prognosis.

Staging is based on pattern of spread and initial therapy is guided by the presenting stage (Tables 95.1 & 95.2) [2]. The importance of germ cell tumors in the field of oncology is highlighted by the fact that standard therapies for early stage disease routinely cure more than 95% of patients. Current research goals focus on limiting therapy while preserving high cure rates for these patients.

Before the advent of modern cisplatin-based chemotherapies, metastatic germ cell tumors were almost always fatal, but today the cure rate for metastatic disease reaches 70–80% (Table 95.3 & 95.4 [3,4]). Unfortunately, 20–30% of patients with advanced disseminated disease require additional therapy after primary cisplatin-based treatments, including salvage surgery or chemotherapy.

In an effort to better care for and study patients with metastatic disease, many prognostic models based on the pattern of disease spread and serum tumor markers at disease presentation have been employed [5–14]. In 1995, a uniform system was developed based on 5202 patients with non-seminomatous germ cell tumors and 660 patients with seminomas treated with cisplatin-containing regimens to guide decision-making and standardize patient enrollment in clinical trials (Table 95.5) [15]. Additional poor prognostic factors may include a high proliferative index or the presence and number of cytogenetic abnormalities, such as an isochromosome of the short arm of chromosome 12 [16,17].

Conventional-dose salvage approaches to patients with poor risk, recurrent, or refractory germ cell tumors lead to remission in 30–60% of patients, but only 20% gain long-term survival, leading to investigation of alternate therapies including high-dose chemotherapy with autologous hematopoietic cell transplantation (HCT) (Table 95.6). Herein, we will review the management of the small fraction of patients for whom initial treatments are incompletely effective, with emphasis on the role of high-dose chemotherapy.

Initiation of salvage therapies in germ cell tumors

The decision to pursue salvage therapy for germ cell tumor is important, and consultation with experts in the intricacies of managing this disease is recommended. Several clinical situations may mimic progressive or recurrent disease and lead to inappropriate initiation of salvage therapy.

Table 95.1 American Joint Commission on Cancer (AJCC) Staging system [2]. Tumor, node, metastasis (TNM) definitions.

Primary tumor (T)
pTX	Cannot be assessed
pT0	No evidence of tumor
pTis	Intratubular neoplasia (carcinoma *in situ*)
pT1	Limited to testis and epididymis without lymphatic/vascular invasion
pT2	Limited to testis and epididymis with lymphatic/vascular invasion, or tumor extending through the tunica albuginea with involvement of the tunica vaginalis
pT3	Invades the spermatic cord with or without lymphatic/vascular invasion
pT4	Invades the scrotum with or without lymphatic/vascular invasion

Regional lymph nodes (N)
NX	Cannot be assessed
N0	No regional lymph node metastases
N1	Metastases in a single lymph node, 2 cm or less in greatest dimension
N2	Metastases in a single lymph node, more than 2 cm but not more than 5 cm in greatest dimension; or multiple lymph nodes, none more than 5 cm in greatest dimension
N3	Metastases in a lymph node, more than 5 cm in greatest dimension

Distant metastasis (M)
MX	Cannot be assessed
M0	No distant metastasis
M1	Distant metastasis:
	M1a: nonregional nodal or pulmonary metastasis
	M1b: distant metastasis other than nonregional nodes and lungs

Serum Markers (S)
SX	Not available or not performed
S0	Marker study levels within normal limits
S1	LDH <1.5 times the upper limit of normal AND HCG (mIU/mL) <5000 AND AFP (mcg/mL) <1000
S2	LDH 1.5–10.0 times the upper limit of normal OR HCG (mIU/mL) 5000–50,000 OR AFP (mcg/mL) 1000–10,000
S3	LDH >10 times the upper limit of normal OR HCG (mIU/mL) >50,000 OR AFP (mcg/mL) >10,000

AFP, α fetoprotein; HCG, human chorionic gonadotropin; LDH, lactate dehydrogenase.

Table 95.2 American Joint Commission on Cancer (AJCC) Staging system [2]. Stage groupings.

Stage		
Stage 0		pTis, N0, M0, S0
Stage I		pT1–4, N0, M0, SX
	Stage IA	pT1, N0, M0, S0
	Stage IB	pT2–3, N0, M0, S0
	Stage IS	Any pT, N0, M0, S1–3
Stage II		Any pT, N1–3, M0, SX
	Stage IIA	Any pT, N1, M0, S0–1
	Stage IIB	Any pT, N2, M0, S0–1
	Stage IIC	Any pT, N3, M0, S0–1
Stage III		Any pT, any N, M1, SX
	Stage IIIA	Any pT, any N, M1a, S0–1
	Stage IIIB	Any pT, N1–3, M0, S2
		Any pT, any N, M1a, S2
	Stage IIIC	Any pT, N1–3, M0, S3
		Any pT, any N, M1a, S3
		Any pT, any N, M1b, any S

Table 95.3 Conventional primary therapy results.

Stage	Treatment	DFS (%)
I	Radical orchiectomy plus RPLND	95
II, III	Radical orchiectomy plus BEP × 3–4 cycles plus RPLND for partial response plus BEP × 2 cycles for residual disease	80 (good-risk) 60 (poor-risk)

BEP, bleomycin, etoposide and cisplatin therapy; DFS, disease-free survival; RPLND, retroperitoneal lymph node dissection.

Table 95.4 Conventional-dose chemotherapy regimens.

Indication	Regimen
Primary treatment of disseminated disease (Stage II–III)	BEP [3]: Bleomycin 30 U IV on days 2, 9 and 16 Etoposide 100 mg/m^2/day IV on days 1–5 Cisplatin 20 mg/m^2/day IV on days 1–5 Repeat cycle at 21-day intervals
Primary salvage treatment of relapsed disease	VeIP [4]: Vinblastine 0.11 mg/kg/day IV on days 1–2 Ifosfamide 1.2 g/m^2/day IV on days 1–5 Cisplatin 20 mg/m^2/day IV on days 1–5 Repeat cycle at 21-day intervals
	VIP [4]: Etoposide 75 mg/m^2/day IV on days 1–5 Ifosfamide 1.2 g/m^2/day IV on days 1–5 Cisplatin 20 mg/m^2/day IV on days 1–5 Repeat cycle at 21-day intervals

IV, intravenous.

Tumor markers

Management of testicular cancer has come to depend on the accurate determination and clinical interpretation of serum tumor markers. Lactate dehydrogenase (LDH) is a nonspecific marker that probably correlates with disease bulk. The most sensitive and specific markers are α fetoprotein (AFP) and β-subunit human chorionic gonadotropin (HCG). Among patients with disseminated testicular or primary retroperitoneal nonseminomatous germ cell tumors, HCG will be elevated in 75% and AFP in 40% of patients.

AFP is a glycoprotein normally produced by the fetal yolk sac or embryonal carcinoma elements of germ cell cancers, and is not detectable in normal adults. The half-life of AFP in the serum is about 5 days. False positive elevation of AFP is quite rare, with differential considerations including laboratory error, other tumor types, such as hepatoma, or liver inflammation. Any persistent elevation of AFP in a patient with seminoma is viewed as evidence of nonseminomatous elements and management should proceed as such.

β-subunit HCG is a smaller glycoprotein that is normally produced by trophoblastic tissues, such as syncytiotrophoblastic components of germ cell tumors. The HCG protein is comprised of antigenically distinct α- and β-subunits, and the serum half-life of the entire protein is 18–24 h. False elevations may occur in patients who use marijuana, and there is some crossreactivity in the radioimmunoassay with luteinizing hormone. In cases of persistently elevated HCG, patients should be asked about marijuana use and testosterone should be given to ensure that a hypogonadal state with resultant high levels of luteinizing hormone is not interfering with the measurement. If the level remains elevated, restaging procedures and investigation of sanctuary sites are in order. Pure seminoma is often associated with normal AFP and HCG levels, but some patients, particularly with advanced disease, may have low-level elevation of HCG (usually <100 mIU/mL).

The rate of disappearance of elevated tumor markers is very useful in determining response to treatment. A 10-fold decrease in serum HCG level over a 3-week period is consistent with disease eradication. Less steep declines of HCG levels usually correlate with residual disease postsurgery or the emergence of drug-resistance to chemotherapy. The reappearance of a marker elevation often precedes radiographic appearance and is an invaluable method of detecting early relapse. However, particularly among patients with HCG levels >50,000 mIU/mL, the disappearance of HCG from the serum may be unpredictable and occasionally quite prolonged. In a retrospective review of 41 patients with presenting HCG levels >50,000 mIU/mL, less than 10% had a normal HCG at the institution of the fourth course of chemotherapy [18]. However, 22 of the 41 patients (53.7%) were continuously NED (disease free) despite no further therapy. We feel Hayes-Lattin & Nichols that the optimal strategy for such patients is monthly observation with initiation of salvage therapy if and when there is serologic progression. Importantly, salvage therapy should not be initiated on the basis of a persistent HCG elevation alone, but rather reserved for the clinical setting of a well-documented rise in the markers. In cases of rising markers after standard therapy, investigation of sanctuary sites, such as the central nervous system or the contralateral testis, should be performed before initiating salvage therapy.

Radiographic abnormalities

Depending on the stage at the time of diagnosis, 20–50% of patients who undergo induction chemotherapy for disseminated germ cell tumor will have significant residual radiographic abnormalities. Post-chemotherapy surgical resection should only be considered in the setting of normalization of serum tumor markers. Resection of residual abnormalities is rarely urgent and repeat imaging of the areas of abnormality should be performed prior to surgery, as often tumors will continue to involute.

Table 95.5 International Germ Cell Consensus Classification prognostic staging system.

	Non-seminoma		Seminoma	
Good prognosis	• Testis or retroperitoneal primary *and* • No non-pulmonary visceral metastases *and* • Good markers (AFP <1000 ng/mL and HCG <5000 IU/L and LDH <1.5 × upper limit of normal)	56% of patients PFS 89% @ 5 years OS 92% @ 5 years	• Any primary site *and* • No non-pulmonary visceral metastases *and* • Normal AFP, any HCG, any LDH	90% of patients PFS 82% @ 5 years OS 86% @ 5 years
Intermediate prognosis	• Testis or retroperitoneal primary *and* • No non-pulmonary visceral metastases *and* • Intermediate markers (AFP 1000–10,000 ng/mL or HCG 5000–50,000 IU/L or LDH 1.5–10 × upper limit of normal)	28% of patients PFS 78% @ 5 years OS 80% @ 5 years	• Any primary site *and* • Non-pulmonary visceral metastases *and* • Normal AFP, any HCG, any LDH	10% of patients PFS 67% @ 5 years OS 72% @ 5 years
Poor prognosis	• Mediastinal primary *or* • Non-pulmonary visceral metastases *or* • Poor markers (AFP >10,000 ng/mL or HCG >50,000 IU/L or LDH >10 × upper limit of normal)	16% of patients PFS 41% @ 5 years OS 48% @ 5 years		

AFP, alpha-fetoprotein; HCG, human chorionic gonadotropin; LDH, lactate dehydrogenase; OS, overall survival; PFS, progression-free survival.

Table 95.6 Possible indications for high-dose chemotherapy in the management of germ cell tumors.

Salvage therapy for multiply relapsed or refractory GCT	A small proportion of (otherwise incurable) patients will be cured
Initial salvage for relapsed GCT	Single center studies suggest there may be a role. Currently being examined in European prospective randomized trial
Primary treatment for poor-risk GCT	Role is unclear. Currently being examined in North American prospective randomized trial
Treatment for failure to achieve a complete remission	Suboptimal decline/plateau in serum tumor markers (see text) Persistent clinical disease (see text)

GCT, germ cell tumor.

Patients with residual abnormalities and persistent elevations of AFP or HCG often have unresectable, viable tumor and should, therefore, be considered for salvage chemotherapy regimens rather than surgical debulking [19].

Other clinical situations may mimic progressive or recurrent disease. For example, in patients with an appropriate fall in serologic markers but with radiographic progression during induction chemotherapy, benign teratomatous portions of the tumor may be mistaken for progressive disease. This syndrome should be considered in patients whose orchiectomy specimen contained teratoma. Appropriate management of such a patient includes completion of induction chemotherapy with subsequent surgical resection of residual radiographic abnormalities and not the administration of salvage therapies.

The development of nodular lesions on chest imaging at the end or soon after completion of chemotherapy may represent bleomycin-induced pulmonary injury rather than recurrent disease. These nodules are characteristically located in a subpleural region, and the diagnosis should be considered in a patient who is otherwise responding to therapy.

Conventional salvage therapies for germ cell tumors

A unique feature in the management of germ cell tumors is the ability to achieve long-term disease-free survival (DFS) with secondary chemotherapies after initial treatment failures. The current standard for comparison for all initial salvage therapies in germ cell tumors is the combination of vinblastine, ifosfamide and cisplatin (VeIP) [4]. In one series, 135 patients with progressive disease after cisplatin and etoposide-based chemotherapy were treated with VeIP regardless of metastatic site or performance status [20]. A 50% complete response rate after chemotherapy with or without surgical resection of residual disease was seen, with a long-term overall survival (OS) rate of 32% and DFS rate of 24%. Importantly, none of the 32 patients with extragonadal nonseminomatous disease were continuously disease-free.

Salvage surgery may play a significant role in the treatment of patients with chemo-refractory germ cell tumors. Murphy *et al.* [21] retrospectively reviewed all patients felt to have progressive chemo-refractory yet resectable disease who underwent salvage surgery at Indiana University from 1977 to 1990. The majority underwent isolated retroperitoneal lymphadenectomy (69%). Thirty-eight of 48 patients (79%) were grossly disease-free after surgery and 29 (60%) obtained a serologic remission. Ten patients (21%) achieved event-free survival (EFS) for 31–89 months. Six additional patients who relapsed after surgery achieved DFS after additional surgery (four patients) or high-dose chemotherapy and autologous HCT (two patients). Notably, no patients with more than one site of metastatic disease, even when resectable, achieved long-term disease control. However, a definite potential for cure with salvage surgery was identified in selected patients with recurrent germ cell tumor.

High-dose chemotherapy for recurrent germ cell tumors

An active strategy to improve outcomes for patients with relapsed or refractory germ cell tumors is the use of high-dose chemotherapy with autologous hematopoietic cell rescue. Initial attempts at cisplatin dose-escalation (without hematopoietic stem cell support) increased toxicity without a survival advantage [22]. However, several advances have led to substantial progress towards defining the role of high-dose therapy for germ cell tumors. Drugs, such as carboplatin and etoposide, and alkylating agents, such as thiotepa or the oxazaphosphorines (ifosfamide and cyclophosphamide), demonstrated antitumor activity, dose-responsiveness and a wide dose range between dose-limiting myelotoxicity and dose-limiting extramedullary toxicities. Additional improvements in transplant procedures (hematopoietic cells from peripheral blood rather than bone marrow), supportive care (hematopoietic growth factors and selective antibiotics) and patient selection have advanced the field.

The first investigations of high-dose chemotherapy with autologous HCT for germ cell tumors involved single agent etoposide, or etoposide and cyclophosphamide [23–25]. Although some patients were refractory to these agents in standard doses, 20–40% response rates and rare long-term cures were observed.

Most modern phase I/II trials of high-dose chemotherapy have included carboplatin and etoposide, sometimes with ifosfamide, cyclophosphamide, or thiotepa (Table 95.7). Several centers intended high-dose therapy to be repeated once after recovery (tandem transplants) to maximize potential benefit. Initial investigations focused on patients with either relapse after best standard salvage chemotherapies or cisplatin-refractory germ cell tumors that were felt unlikely to be cured by any available treatment. One of the first examples was the phase I/II study of two courses of high-dose carboplatin and etoposide in patients with germ cell tumors refractory to cisplatin (defined as progression on or within 4 weeks of the last cisplatin dose), or recurrent after primary cisplatin-based therapy and a salvage regimen containing ifosfamide and cisplatin [26]. The results were updated after the first 40 patients [27]. Over half of the patients had received three or more prior regimens and 70% were considered cisplatin-refractory. Therapy consisted of carboplatin 900–2000 mg/m^2 and etoposide 1200 mg/m^2. Ifosfamide was added to the regimen in three patients. Twenty-six of 40 patients (65%) received both courses of high-dose therapy. Overall, seven of 40 patients (18%) died as a consequence of therapy, primarily due to infection. There were 12 patients (30%) who attained a complete response and 14 (35%) who achieved a partial response, for an overall response rate of 65%. Six patients (15%) were long-term disease-free survivors, and a seventh patient died at 22 months free of germ cell tumor from therapy-related acute myeloid leukemia. These results were confirmed in a phase II multi-institutional trial of similar patients receiving tandem high-dose carboplatin and etoposide where 58% completed both transplants, a 13% treatment-related mortality (TRM) was observed, nine patients (24%) achieved a complete remission (two after post-transplant surgical resections) and five patients (13%) were alive and free of disease with a minimum of 18 months follow-up [28].

Several features merit emphasis from this and similar early series. First, a portion of patients (perhaps 13–24%) with multiply recurrent germ cell tumors can achieve long-term DFS with high-dose chemotherapy and HCT. Second, nearly all relapses occur in the first 18 months post-transplant and disease status after high-dose therapy predicts long-term outcome. Third, in this series, the tandem approach was supported. In the phase I/II study, all of the long-term disease-free survivors received both transplants and eight of 12 patients in partial remission after the first transplant achieved complete remission after the second transplant [26,27]. The value of tandem cycles, however, remains to be proven in a randomized trial. Fourth, surgical salvage remained an important treatment modality after transplant, leading to complete remissions and likely contributing to cures in several patients. Lastly, patients with primary mediastinal germ cell tumors failed to respond with none of eight patients in the phase I/II study [26,27] and none of 11 patients in the phase II study [28] achieving complete remission. This is a population for whom conventional salvage therapies also have poor outcomes and such patients should be the focus of investigational approaches [29,30].

Subsequent trials of high-dose therapy began to enroll less heavily pre-treated patients and incorporate the use of peripheral blood hematopoietic cells and growth factors, which all served to shorten the duration of cytopenias. These improvements led investigators to attempt further dose escalations or add additional agents such as ifosfamide or cyclophosphamide. One trial of dose escalation involved treating 33 patients with relapsed or refractory germ cell tumors with carboplatin 1650–2100 mg/m^2 and etoposide 1200–2250 mg/m^2 for two tandem cycles [31]. The dose-limiting toxicities for this regimen were mucositis and peripheral neurotoxicity, and reversible transaminase abnormalities were common. Results were similar to earlier studies, with 20 of 33 patients (61%) completing both transplant procedures. TRM was 18%, including four patients who died prior to response evaluation. Four of the remaining 29 evaluable patients (14%) achieved complete remission and eight of 33 patients (24%) became long-term survivors.

The German Testicular Cancer Study Group added ifosfamide 0–10 g/m^2 to carboplatin 1500–2000 mg/m^2 and etoposide 1200–2400 mg/m^2 as a transplant regimen in 74 patients with relapsed or refractory germ cell tumors [32,33]. Therapy was delivered regardless of response to two proceeding cycles of reinduction standard-dose cisplatin, etoposide and ifosfamide. TRM was only 3%, but late toxicities included renal toxicity (21%), paresthesias (29%) and ototoxicity (18%). Approximately 50% of patients achieved a complete remission with this therapy, and 28 of 74 (38%) were alive from 3.2 to 5.6 years post-treatment.

In reviewing these trials, it is important to recognize the large variability in inclusion criteria, making comparisons of results difficult. A series from Margolin *et al.* [34] with a long-term DFS of 45% included 40% of patients treated during initial salvage. Ayash *et al.* [35] reported a 17% long-term DFS but included only 10% of patients treated during initial salvage and included 48% of patients with cisplatin-refractory disease including 34% who were absolutely refractory (having never achieved even stable disease on a cisplatin-containing regimen).

This heterogeneity led investigators to compile pooled data to identify prognostic variables for response and survival in male patients with relapsed or refractory germ cell tumors treated with high-dose chemotherapy [36]. Three hundred and ten patients from four centers in the USA and Europe were retrospectively evaluated and data on 283 patients were completed. Overall, the TRM was 8%. Fifty-five percent of patients achieved a favorable response (complete remission or partial remission with negative tumor markers) and 47% of those patients later relapsed. The actuarial OS rate was 51% at 1, 36% at 2 and 30% at 3 years, respectively. Multivariant analysis identified progressive disease before transplant, mediastinal nonseminomatous primary tumor, refractory or absolute refractory disease to conventional-dose cisplatin and HCG levels >1000 IU/L before transplant as independent adverse prognostic factors. Importantly, response to first-line therapy did not predict outcomes. These variables were used to identify patients with good, intermediate, or poor prognoses with predicted failure-free survival rates at 2 years after transplantation of 51%, 27% and 5%, respectively (Table 95.8).

In summary, the use of high-dose chemotherapy with autologous HCT for the treatment of relapsed or refractory germ cell tumors can produce long-term survivors in roughly 15–40% of patients. The principal toxicities include nephrotoxicity, peripheral neurotoxicity, reversible

Table 95.7 Selected Phase I/II trials: relapsed/refractory disease.

Author	Patients	Therapy	Response	Survival	Notes
Mulder et al. [25]	11 relapsed or refractory	Etoposide 2500 mg/m^2 Cyclophosphamide 7 gm/m^2 ($n = 3$) or Etoposide 2500 mg/m^2, then: Etoposide 2000 mg/m^2 Cyclophosphamide 7 gm/m^2 ($n = 8$)	RR 64% CR 18%	OS 18% @ 66–72 weeks DFS 9% @ 66 weeks TRM 0%	
Nichols et al. [26]; Broun et al. [27]	40 relapsed or refractory	Carboplatin 900–2000 mg/m^2 Etoposide 1200 mg/m^2 (Ifosfamide added for 3 pts) (tandem)	RR 65% CR 30%	OS 15% @ >24 months TRM 18%	10% initial salvage, 70% cisplatin-refractory 8 pts with mediastinal primary 26 pts received both transplants
Droz et al. [12]	17 relapsed or refractory	"salvage chemotherapy," then: Cisplatin 200 mg/m^2 Etoposide 1750 mg/m^2 Cyclophosphamide 6400 mg/m^2	CR 50%	DFS 24% @ 68–74 months TRM 6%	65% cisplatin-refractory
Nichols (ECOG) 1992 [28]	38 relapsed or refractory	Carboplatin 1500 mg/m^2 Etoposide 1200 mg/m^2 (tandem)	RR 45% CR 24%	DFS 13% @ >12 months TRM 13%	13% initial salvage, 50% cisplatin-refractory 11 pts with mediastinal primary 22 pts received both transplants
Motzer et al. [44]	13 relapsed or refractory (additional 16 initial salvage pts reported in Table 95.10)	Carboplatin 1500 mg/m^2 Etoposide 1200 mg/m^2 Cyclophosphamide 90–150 mg/kg (tandem)	CR 46%	DFS 23% @ 8–24 months TRM 3%	62% cisplatin-refractory 13 pts received both transplants
Broun et al. [31]	33 relapsed or refractory	Carboplatin 1650–2100 mg/m^2 Etoposide 1200–2250 mg/m^2 (tandem)	RR 18/29 (64%) CR 4/29 (14%)	OS 8/33 (24%) @ 10–30 months TRM 6/33 (18%)	12% initial salvage, 21% cisplatin-refractory 4 pts with mediastinal primary 20 pts received both transplants

Study	Patients	Regimen	Response	Survival	Comments
Motzer 1996 [53]	58 relapsed or refractory	Carboplatin 1500 mg/m² Etoposide 1200 mg/m² Cyclophosphamide 60–150 mg/kg (tandem)	CR 40%	OS 29% @ 10–65 months DFS 21% @ 16–65 months TRM 12%	17% initial salvage, 57% cisplatin-refractory (21% absolute) 7 pts with extragonadal primary 27 pts received both transplants
Margolin et al. [34]	20 relapsed or refractory	**1** Ifosfamide 6 gm/m² Carboplatin 1200 mg/m² Etoposide 60 mg/kg **2** Ifosfamide 9 gm/m² Carboplatin 1200 mg/m² Etoposide 60 mg/kg (tandem)	RR 60%	DFS 45% @ 23–70 months TRM 0%	40% initial salvage, 0% cisplatin-refractory 8 pts with extragonadal primary 18 pts received both transplants
Siegert et al. [32]; Beyer et al. [33]	74 relapsed or refractory	salvage cisplatin, etoposide, and ifosfamide × 2, *then*: Carboplatin 1500–2000 mg/m² Etoposide 1200–2400 mg/m² Ifosfamide 0–10 gm/m²	CR 51% (at first report)	OS 38% 3.2–5.6 years DFS 31% @ 3.2–5.6 years TRM 3%	8% initial salvage, 32% cisplatin-refractory 17 patients with extragonadal primary (5 mediastinal)
Mandanas 1998 [54]	21 relapsed or refractory	Various regimens (including cyclophosphamide and a platinum)	RR 79%	DFS 52% @ 4–10 years TRM 7%	5% initial salvage, 43% cisplatin-refractory
Ayash et al. [35]	29 relapsed or refractory	Carboplatin 1500–2100 mg/m² Etoposide 1200–2250 mg/m² (tandem)	RR 38% CR 10%	Median OS 14 months DFS 17% PFS 28% @ 31–93 months TRM 10%	10% initial salvage, 48% cisplatin-refractory (34% absolute) all testis or retroperitoneal primary 15 pts received both transplants tandems
Rick 2001 [55]	80 relapsed or refractory	salvage paclitaxel, ifosfamide, and cisplatin (TIP) × 3, *then*: (n = 23) paclitaxel, ifosfamide mobilization, *then*: Carboplatin 1500 mg/m² Etoposide 2400 mg/m² Thiotepa 450–750 mg/m² (CET)	RR 69% to TIP RR 66% to CET	OS 33% @ 22–46 months DFS 26% @ 22–46 months TRM 3%	67% initial salvage, 11% absolute cisplatin-refractory 3 pts with mediastinal primary 62 pts received both transplants

CR, complete response rate; DFS, disease-free survival; OS, overall survival; PFS, progression-free survival; RR, response rate; TRM, treatment-related mortality.

Factor	Score	Risk	2-year FFS (%)	2-year OS (%)
Progressive disease before transplant	1	Good (score 0)	51	61
Primary mediastinal tumor	1	Intermediate (score 1–2)	27	34
Cisplatin-refractory before transplant	1	Poor (score >2)	5	8
Absolute cisplatin-refractory before transplant	2			
HCG >1000 IU/L before transplant	2			

Table 95.8 Beyer Prognostic Score for survival after high-dose salvage chemotherapy.

FFS, failure-free survival; HCG, human chorionic gonadotropin; OS, overall survival.

transaminase elevations and gonadal toxicity. TRM rates ranged from 0% to 18%, with the most recent series reporting 3–5%. Patients with primary mediastinal tumors do not benefit from salvage high-dose therapy. Treatment earlier in the course of relapsed or refractory disease appears to be associated with better outcomes.

Initial salvage and primary treatment with high-dose chemotherapy for germ cell tumors

The modest results of standard-dose salvage chemotherapies (24% long-term DFS with VeIP discussed above) combined with improving rates of durable responses, decreasing morbidity and mortality associated with high-dose therapy have led to the investigation of high-dose therapy for initial salvage of relapsed germ cell tumors (Table 95.9). The largest published experience is from Indiana University, where 65 patients with relapsed or persistent testicular cancer were given initial salvage treatment with two tandem courses of carboplatin 2100 mg/m^2 and etoposide 2250 mg/m^2 followed by autologous hematopoietic cell rescue [37]. All patients had primary testicular tumors. Fifty-six of the 65 patients (86%) received at least one cycle of standard-dose salvage chemotherapy (usually VeIP) prior to transplant. Ten of 65 (15%) received *ex vivo* cytokine-stimulated, mdr-1 transduced autologous CD34-positive cells and 26 of 65 (40%) received post-transplant maintenance oral etoposide. Using the Beyer prognostic score for outcomes with high-dose therapy (Table 95.8), 61% were good risk, 31% intermediate risk and 8% poor risk. There were no treatment-related deaths. A complete remission was achieved in 28 patients (43%) with high-dose chemotherapy, in another patient with additional VeIP after only one transplant and 13 patients (20%) with post-transplant surgical resections. With follow-up ranging 16–91 months, 37 patients (57%) were continuously disease-free and 40 (60%) remain disease-free after definitive therapy.

Recently, the European Group for Blood and Marrow Transplantation (EBMT) presented preliminary data from a large, randomized trial among patients with either an incomplete response to first-line platinum-based chemotherapy or relapsing after previous complete remission [38]. Treatment consisted of either four cycles of etoposide, ifosfamide and cisplatin (VIP)/VeIP or three cycles of VIP/VeIP plus one additional cycle of high-dose cisplatin, ifosfamide and cyclophosphamide with autologous hematopoietic cell support. Overall, the response and survival rates appeared similar among 280 patients. The transplant procedure led to an overall response in 62% (including 44% complete responses), a 1-year EFS rate of 52% and a 3-year OS rate of 53% with nine toxic deaths. This outcome compared to four cycles of standard salvage therapy with an overall response rate of 58% (41% complete), a 1-year EFS rate of 48% and a 3-year OS rate of 53% with two toxic deaths. It must be noted that these data have only been presented in abstract form, without further information on the characteristics of these patients. The relatively high response rate among the VIP/VeIP control arm suggests that many of these patients may have had favorable prognostic features if treated with standard salvage chemotherapy.

A prognostic scoring system that may be of use in interpreting these results and selecting patients who may benefit from a more aggressive approach has been described (Table 95.10) [39]. One hundred and sixty four patients were treated with "conventional" platinum-based salvage chemotherapy after progression from platinum-based induction chemotherapy (with or without surgery). Multivariate analysis of prognostic factors demonstrated progression-free interval, response to induction treatment and the level of serum HCG and AFP at relapse to be significant. A poor-prognosis group was identified in which none of 30 patients survived after 3 years. In contrast, the good-prognosis group consisted of 94 patients who had a 47% 5-year survival, including 38 patients with a progression-free interval of longer than 2 years who had a 61% 5-year survival. Validation with an independent data set gave 5-year survival data for good and poor-prognosis patients of 51% and 0%, respectively.

Incorporating high-dose chemotherapy as a first-line strategy for the treatment of patients with poor-risk germ cell tumors at presentation has also been investigated. One randomized trial of high-dose chemotherapy with autologous transplant support for the treatment of patients with poor-risk germ cell tumors failed to show a benefit [40]. In this trial, patients deemed poor-risk were randomized either to receive four cycles of cisplatin 200 mg/m^2, vinblastine, etoposide and bleomycin (PVeVB), or to receive two cycles of PVeVB plus one cycle of high-dose therapy including cisplatin 200 mg/m^2 followed by autologous transplant. This study has been criticized because the four-drug regimen is not considered a standard therapy, the dose-intensity and total cisplatin dose were lower in the "high-dose" arm and a substantial number of patients randomized to the high-dose arm did not receive the assigned therapy [41,42].

One strategy for incorporating high-dose chemotherapy in the first-line therapy of patients with germ cell tumors has been to stratify poor-risk patients based on the observed decline in serum tumor markers with the first two cycles of standard chemotherapy [43]. In two published phase II trials, patients whose serum markers were either rising or not falling according to their predicted serum half-life (prolonged half-life by >7 days for AFP and >3 days for HCG) were switched to treatment with high-dose chemotherapy. The first trial of 28 patients studied standard-dose cisplatin, vinblastine, bleomycin, cyclophosphamide and dactinomycin (VAB-6) with or without two cycles of high-dose carboplatin (1500 mg/m^2) and etoposide (1200 mg/m^2) [44,45]. Twenty-two of 28 patients (79%) were treated with high-dose chemotherapy and transplantation, and the DFS of 46% at 2.5–47.0 months follow-up compared favorably to earlier conventional dose trials in similar risk patients. These results led to the second trial with a similar design [42]. This trial changed the standard therapy to VIP and increased the high-dose therapy to carboplatin (1800 mg/m^2), etoposide (1800 mg/m^2) and cyclophosphamide (150 mg/kg). Thirty patients were enrolled in this trial, and 14 (47%) went on to high-dose therapy. There were no treatment-related deaths and, again, a relatively favorable 50% long-term DFS was noted.

An alternate strategy is being tested in a phase I trial of poor-risk non-seminomatous germ cell tumors in Germany [41]. This trial is based on the front-line use of multiple high-dose cycles before drug resistance

Table 95.9 Phase I/II Trials: initial salvage/first-line therapy.

Author	Patients	Therapy	Response	Survival	Notes
Droz 1992 [56]	28 poor risk (first-line)	2 cycles mPVeBV, then: Cisplatin 200 mg/m^2 Etoposide 1750 mg/m^2 Cyclophosphamide 6400 mg/m^2	CR 61%	DFS 43% @ 7–72 months TRM 7%	9 pts with extragonadal primary 21 pts proceeded to transplant
Motzer et al. [44]; Motzer et al. [45]	28 poor risk (first-line)	VAB-6 × 2 cycles, then: VAB-6 × 2 cycles ($n = 5$) or Etoposide 1200 mg/m^2 Carboplatin 1500 mg/m^2 (tandem) ($n = 22$)	RR 96% CR 56% VAB-6 alone: CR 60% Transplant: CR 55%	OS 57% @ 2.5–47 months DFS 46% @ 2.5–47 months TRM 4%	14 of 22 received both transplants
Barnett 1993 [57]	21 poor risk or relapsed (first-line $n = 6$) (initial salvage $n = 15$)	**1** HIPE × 5–11 cycles, then: Ifosfamide 6 gm/m^2 Etoposide 3 gm/m^2 Carboplatin 1.2 gm/m^2 or **2** HIPE × 5 cycles, VIP × 1–2 cycles, then: Cyclophosphamide 7.2 gm/m^2 Etoposide 2.4 gm/m^2 Carboplatin 0.8 gm/m^2		First-line: EFS 50% Salvage: EFS 73% EFS 67% @ 6–78 months TRM 10%	Renal and Mucosal toxicity prompted regimen **2**
Broun 1994 [58]	23 relapsed (initial salvage)	VeIP or VeBP × 2 cycles, then: Etoposide 1200–2250 mg/m^2 Carboplatin 150–2100 mg/m^2	Induction: RR 87% CR 35% Transplant: RR 83% CR 56%	Transplant: OS 50% @ 10–36 months EFS 39% @ 10–33 months TRM 4% (induction)	18 pts proceeded to transplant

Table 95.9 (cont'd)

Author	Patients	Therapy	Response	Survival	Notes
Motzer et al. [42]	30 poor risk (first-line)	VIP × 2 cycles, then: VIP × 2 more cycles (n = 16) or Carboplatin 1800 mg/m² Etoposide 1800 mg/m² Cyclophosphamide 150 mg/kg (tandem) (n = 14)	initial VIP: CR 57% VIP × 4: RR 81%, CR 63% Transplant: CR 50%	OS 67% @ 15–47 months DFS 50% @ 16–47 months TRM 0%	7 pts with mediastinal primary 9 of 14 received both transplants
Bokemeyer 1998 [41]	141 poor risk (first-line)	4 cycles in 8 escalating dose levels to maximum: Cisplatin 125–150 mg/m² Etoposide 550–1250 mg/m² Ifosfamide 6–10 gm/m²		OS 78% @ 2 years PFS 73% @ 2 years Early death 8%	Transplant support used for dose levels 3–8 Analysis based on levels 1–5
Broun 1997; [59] Bhatia et al. [37]	65 relapsed (initial salvage)	Carboplatin 2100 mg/m² Etoposide 2250 mg/m² (tandem)	RR 88% CR 43% additional CR after chemo (n = 1) or surgery (n = 13)	Chemo: DFS 57% @ 16–91 months DFS 62% TRM 0%	Excluded pts with extragonadal primary 86% received initial standard chemotherapy 26 pts received both transplants gene therapy and maintenance oral etoposide used
Rosti (EBMT) et al. [38]	280 incomplete response or initial salvage	VIP/VeIP × 4 or VIP/VeIP × 3 then: Carboplatin 1000–2200 mg/m² Etoposide 1800 mg/m² Cyclophosphamide 6400 mg/m²	Chemo: RR 58% CR 41% Transplant: RR 62% CR 44%	Chemo: 1-yr EFS 48% 3-yr OS 53% TRM n = 2 Transplant: 1-yr EFS 52% 3-yr OS 53% TRM n = 9	47 pts with extragonadal primary (preliminary abstract)

CR, complete response rate; DFS, disease-free survival; HIPE, high-intensity cisplatin-etoposide; mPVeBV, modified cisplatin, vinblastine, bleomycin, etoposide; OS, overall survival; PFS, progression-free survival; RR, response rate; TRM, treatment-related morality; VAB-6, cisplatin, vinblastine, bleomycin, cyclophosphamide, dactinomycin; VeIP, vinblastine, bleomycin, cisplatin; VIP, vinblastine, ifosfamide, cisplatin; VIP, etoposide, ifosfamide, cisplatin.

Table 95.10 Fossa prognostic score for survival after standard-dose salvage chemotherapy.

Factors	Risk		
Progression-free interval <2 years	Good (<3 factors)	47% OS @ 5 yr	Progression-free >2 yr: OS 74% @ 2 yr Progression-free <2 yr: OS 45% @ 2 yr
<CR to induction therapy	Poor (3 factors)	0% OS @ 3 yr	
AFP >100 kU/L or HCG >100 IU/L			

CR, complete response rate; OS, overall survival.

develops. Patients receive four consecutive cycles of cisplatin, etoposide and ifosfamide (PEI) with granulocyte macrophage colony-stimulating factor (GM-CSF) support in the initial two dose intensity levels, or granulocyte colony-stimulating factor (G-CSF) and peripheral blood stem cell support in dose levels three to eight. Data were reported on the first 141 patients treated at dose levels one through five (cisplatin 150 mg/m^2, etoposide 1250 mg/m^2 and ifosfamide 10 g/m^2). The treatment-related death rate was 8%. After a median follow-up of 2.6 years, the 2-year survival rate was 78% and the progression-free survival rate was 73%.

In the absence of randomized trial data, a multivariate and matched-pair analysis was performed on data from three large controlled clinical trials to compare first-line high-dose chemotherapy to standard-dose chemotherapy in males with advanced, poor-risk germ cell tumors [46]. Multivariate analysis of 423 patients demonstrated superiority of first-line high-dose therapy compared to standard-dose therapy for both progression-free survival (75% vs. 62%, $p = 0.002$) and OS (81% vs. 73%, $p = 0.021$) when adjusted for available prognostic factors. A matched-pair analysis of 146 patients from each therapy estimated a 2-year OS of 82% and progression-free survival of 72% among recipients of high-dose therapy vs. 71% ($p = 0.0184$) and 59% ($p = 0.0056$), respectively, among recipients of standard-dose therapy (Figs 95.1 & 95.2 [46]).

Whether the results of these initial trials of high-dose chemotherapy in the setting of initial salvage or primary treatment of poor-risk disease represent a true therapeutic advance continues to be tested in randomized clinical trials.

Ongoing studies and future directions

Two important randomized trials are investigating the role of high-dose therapy in the treatment of patients with germ cell tumors. In Europe, initial salvage therapy has been evaluated in the trial described above and detailed results are expected soon [38]. In the USA, the issue of primary therapy for poor-risk disease is being addressed in an intergroup cooperative study by randomizing patients to receive either four cycles of bleomycin, etoposide and cisplatin (BEP) or two cycles of BEP followed by two cycles of high-dose carboplatin, etoposide and cyclophosphamide. This trial is nearing the completion of accrual and analysis is imminent.

Newer compounds with single-agent response rates are being incorporated into trials including bexarotene, paclitaxel, gemcitabine, bendamustine and oxaliplatin [47–49]. Unique dosing strategies, such as multiple cycles or alternating agents, may be incorporated in future high-dose algorithms. Adjunctive agents may reduce the toxicity of high-

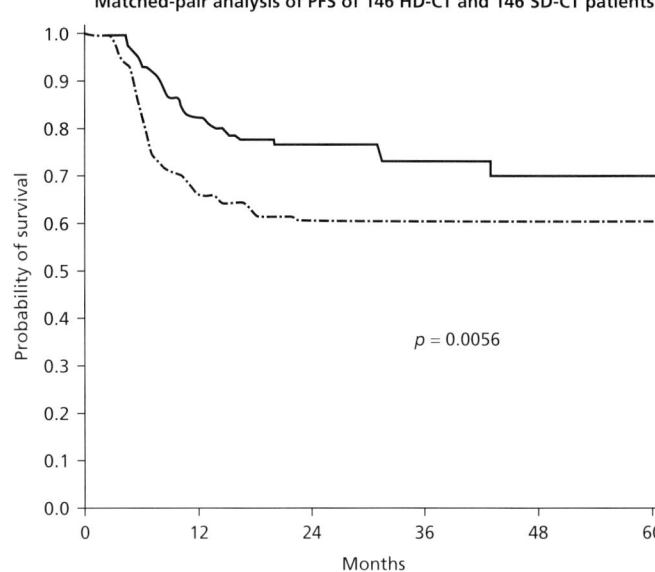

Fig. 95.1 The estimated 2-year progression-free survival (PFS) rate was greater after high-dose chemotherapy (HD-CT) vs. standard-dose chemotherapy (SD-CT) in a matched-pair analysis of 146 patients. Reproduced with permission from Bokemeyer *et al.* [46].

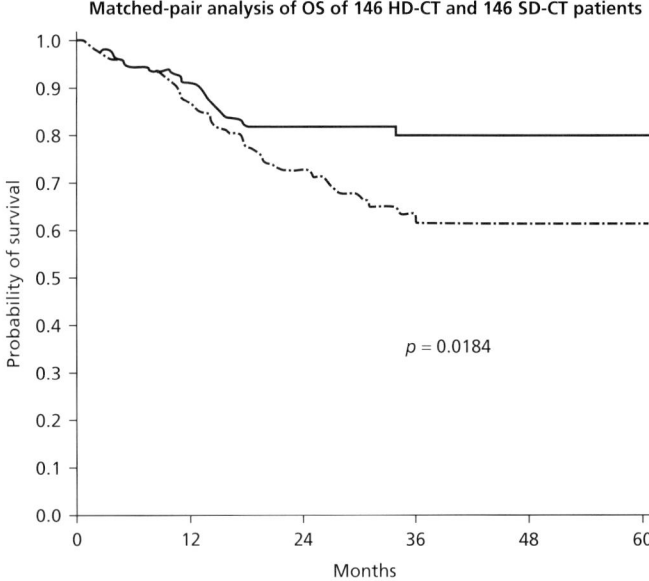

Fig. 95.2 The estimated 2-year overall survival (OS) rate was greater after high-dose chemotherapy (HD-CT) vs. standard-dose chemotherapy (SD-CT) in a matched-pair analysis of 146 patients. Reproduced with permission from Bokemeyer *et al.* [46].

dose therapy such as amifostine or keratinocyte growth factor [50]. Concern has been raised over the generation of secondary hematologic malignancies, particularly with the use of high-dose etoposide. However, in one series, the incidence of secondary leukemia among 302 recipients of autologous HCT with cumulative doses exceeding 2 g/m^2 of etoposide was only 1.3% [51]. Advances in adjuvant or maintenance therapies with oral etoposide or immunomodulators, such as interleukins, have been considered [52]. Ultimately, advances in the molecular understanding of germ cell malignancies may lead to targeted therapies.

Conclusions

High-dose carboplatin and etoposide-based chemotherapy with autologous HCT is accepted as a standard therapy for patients with germ cell tumors who have failed two prior standard-dose regimens as well as a component of salvage therapy for poor-risk patients. Study of the potential role of high-dose therapy for the treatment of initial relapse, or for primary treatment of poor-risk disease, has been slowed by the few number of patients and the relative success of standard-dose therapy. Randomized trials are underway to clarify these issues, and new treatment designs and agents are being pursued.

References

1 Bosl GJ, Motzer RJ. Testicular germ-cell cancer. *N Engl J Med* 1997; **337**: 242–53.

2 Testis. In: Greene FL, Page DL, Fleming ID *et al.* (eds.) *AJCC Cancer Staging Handbook*. New York: Springer, 2002: 347–54.

3 Williams SD, Birch R, Einhorn LH, Irwin L, Greco FA, Loehrer PJ. Treatment of disseminated germ-cell tumors with cisplatin, bleomycin, and either vinblastine or etoposide. *N Engl J Med* 1987; **316**: 1435–40.

4 Loehrer PJ Sr, Lauer R, Roth BJ, Williams SD, Kalasinski LA, Einhorn LH. Salvage therapy in recurrent germ cell cancer: ifosfamide and cisplatin plus either vinblastine or etoposide. *Ann Intern Med* 1988; **109**: 540–6.

5 Samuels ML, Holoye PY, Johnson DE. Bleomycin combination chemotherapy in the management of testicular neoplasia. *Cancer* 1975; **36**: 318–26.

6 Peckham MJ, McElwain TJ, Barrett A, Hendry WF. Combined management of malignant teratoma of the testis. *Lancet* 1979; **2**: 267–70.

7 Bosl GJ, Geller NL, Cirrincione C *et al.* Multivariate analysis of prognostic variables in patients with metastatic testicular cancer. *Cancer Res* 1983; **43**: 3403–7.

8 Prognostic factors in advanced non-seminomatous germ-cell testicular tumours. Results of a multicentre study. Report from the Medical Research Council Working Party on Testicular Tumours. *Lancet* 1985; **1**: 8–11.

9 Birch R, Williams S, Cone A *et al.* Prognostic factors for favorable outcome in disseminated germ cell tumors. *J Clin Oncol* 1986; **4**: 400–7.

10 Newlands ES, Bagshawe KD, Begent RH, Rustin GJ, Crawford SM, Holden L. Current optimum management of anaplastic germ cell tumours of the testis and other sites. *Br J Urol* 1986; **58**: 307–14.

11 Stoter G, Sylvester R, Sleijfer DT *et al.* Multivariate analysis of prognostic factors in patients with disseminated nonseminomatous testicular cancer: results from a European Organization for Research on Treatment of Cancer multiinstitutional phase III study. *Cancer Res* 1987; **47**: 2714–8.

12 Droz JP, Kramar A, Ghosn M *et al.* Prognostic factors in advanced nonseminomatous testicular cancer. A multivariate logistic regression analysis. *Cancer* 1988; **62**: 564–8.

13 Aass N, Klepp O, Cavallin-Stahl E *et al.* Prognostic factors in unselected patients with nonseminomatous metastatic testicular cancer: a multicenter experience. *J Clin Oncol* 1991; **9**: 818–26.

14 Mead GM, Stenning SP, Parkinson MC *et al.* The Second Medical Research Council study of prognostic factors in nonseminomatous germ cell tumors. Medical Research Council Testicular Tumour Working Party. *J Clin Oncol* 1992; **10**: 85–94.

15 International Germ Cell Consensus Classification. A prognostic factor-based staging system for metastatic germ cell cancers. International Germ Cell Cancer Collaborative Group. *J Clin Oncol* 1997; **15**: 594–603.

16 Sledge GW Jr, Eble JN, Roth BJ, Wuhrman BP, Fineberg N, Einhorn LH. Relation of proliferative activity to survival in patients with advanced germ cell cancer. *Cancer Res* 1988; **48**: 3864–8.

17 Dmitrovsky E, Murty VV, Moy D *et al.* Isochromosome 12p in non-seminoma cell lines: karyologic amplification of c-kit-ras^2 without point-mutational activation. *Oncogene* 1990; **5**: 543–8.

18 Zon RT, Nichols C, Einhorn LH. Management strategies and outcomes of germ cell tumor patients with very high human chorionic gonadotropin levels. *J Clin Oncol* 1998; **16**: 1294–7.

19 Sheinfeld J, Bajorin D. Management of the postchemotherapy residual mass. *Urol Clin North Am* 1993; **20**: 133–43.

20 Loehrer PJ Sr, Gonin R, Nichols CR, Weathers T, Einhorn LH. Vinblastine plus ifosfamide plus cisplatin as initial salvage therapy in recurrent germ cell tumor. *J Clin Oncol* 1998; **16**: 2500–4.

21 Murphy BR, Breeden ES, Donohue JP *et al.* Surgical salvage of chemorefractory germ cell tumors. *J Clin Oncol* 1993; **11**: 324–9.

22 Nichols CR, Williams SD, Loehrer PJ *et al.* Randomized study of cisplatin dose intensity in poor-risk germ cell tumors: a Southeastern Cancer Study Group and Southwest Oncology Group protocol. *J Clin Oncol* 1991; **9**: 1163–72.

23 Blijham G, Spitzer G, Litam J *et al.* The treatment of advanced testicular carcinoma with high dose chemotherapy and autologous marrow support. *Eur J Cancer* 1981; **17**: 433–41.

24 Wolff SN, Johnson DH, Hainsworth JD, Greco FA. High-dose VP-16-213 monotherapy for refractory germinal malignancies: a phase II study. *J Clin Oncol* 1984; **2**: 271–4.

25 Mulder PO, de Vries EG, Koops HS *et al.* Chemotherapy with maximally tolerable doses of VP16-213 and cyclophosphamide followed by autologous bone marrow transplantation for the treatment of relapsed or refractory germ cell tumors. *Eur J Cancer Clin Oncol* 1988; **24**: 675–9.

26 Nichols CR, Tricot G, Williams SD *et al.* Dose-intensive chemotherapy in refractory germ cell cancer: a phase I/II trial of high-dose carboplatin and etoposide with autologous bone marrow transplantation. *J Clin Oncol* 1989; **7**: 932–9.

27 Broun ER, Nichols CR, Kneebone P *et al.* Long-term outcome of patients with relapsed and refractory germ cell tumors treated with high-dose chemotherapy and autologous bone marrow rescue. *Ann Intern Med* 1992; **117**: 124–8.

28 Nichols CR, Andersen J, Lazarus HM *et al.* High-dose carboplatin and etoposide with autologous bone marrow transplantation in refractory germ cell cancer: an Eastern Cooperative Oncology Group protocol. *J Clin Oncol* 1992; **10**: 558–63.

29 Broun ER, Nichols CR, Einhorn LH, Tricot GJ. Salvage therapy with high-dose chemotherapy and autologous bone marrow support in the treatment of primary nonseminomatous mediastinal germ cell tumors. *Cancer* 1991; **68**: 1513–5.

30 Saxman SB, Nichols CR, Einhorn LH. Salvage chemotherapy in patients with extragonadal nonseminomatous germ cell tumors: the Indiana University experience. *J Clin Oncol* 1994; **12**: 1390–3.

31 Broun ER, Nichols CR, Mandanas R *et al.* Dose escalation study of high-dose carboplatin and etoposide with autologous bone marrow support in patients with recurrent and refractory germ cell tumors. *Bone Marrow Transplant* 1995; **16**: 353–8.

32 Siegert W, Beyer J, Strohscheer I *et al.* High-dose treatment with carboplatin, etoposide, and ifosfamide followed by autologous stem-cell transplantation in relapsed or refractory germ cell cancer: a phase I/II study. The German Testicular Cancer Cooperative Study Group. *J Clin Oncol* 1994; **12**: 1223–31.

33 Beyer J, Kingreen D, Krause M *et al.* Long-term survival of patients with recurrent or refractory germ cell tumors after high dose chemotherapy. *Cancer* 1997; **79**: 161–8.

34 Margolin BK, Doroshow JH, Ahn C *et al.* Treatment of germ cell cancer with two cycles of high-dose ifosfamide, carboplatin, and etoposide with autologous stem-cell support. *J Clin Oncol* 1996; **14**: 2631–7.

35 Ayash LJ, Clarke M, Silver SM *et al.* Double dose-intensive chemotherapy with autologous stem cell support for relapsed and refractory testicular cancer: the University of Michigan experience and literature review. *Bone Marrow Transplant* 2001; **27**: 939–47.

36 Beyer J, Kramar A, Mandanas R *et al.* High-dose chemotherapy as salvage treatment in germ cell tumors: a multivariate analysis of prognostic variables. *J Clin Oncol* 1996; **14**: 2638–45.

37 Bhatia S, Abonour R, Porcu P *et al.* High-dose chemotherapy as initial salvage chemotherapy in patients with relapsed testicular cancer. *J Clin Oncol* 2000; **18**: 3346–51.

38 Rosti G, Pico JL, Wandt H *et al.* High-dose chemotherapy (HDC) in the salvage treatment of patients failing first-line platinum chemotherapy for advanced germ cell tumors (GCT); first results of a prospective randomised trial of the European Group for Blood and Marrow Transplantation (EBMT): IT-94 study. *Proceedings of ASCO* 2002; **21**: 180a.

39 Fossa SD, Stenning SP, Gerl A *et al.* Prognostic factors in patients progressing after cisplatin-based chemotherapy for malignant non-seminomatous germ cell tumours. *Br J Cancer* 1999; **80**: 1392–9.

40 Chevreau C, Droz JP, Pico JL *et al.* Early intensified chemotherapy with autologous bone marrow transplantation in first line treatment of poor risk non-seminomatous germ cell tumours. Preliminary results of a French randomized trial. *Eur Urol* 1993; **23**: 213–7.

41 Bokemeyer C, Harstrick A, Beyer J *et al.* The use of dose-intensified chemotherapy in the treatment of metastatic nonseminomatous testicular germ cell tumors. German Testicular Cancer Study Group. *Semin Oncol* 1998; **25**: 24–32; discussion 45–8.

42 Motzer RJ, Mazumdar M, Bajorin DF, Bosl GJ, Lyn P, Vlamis V. High-dose carboplatin, etoposide, and cyclophosphamide with autologous bone marrow transplantation in first-line therapy for patients with poor-risk germ cell tumors. *J Clin Oncol* 1997; **15**: 2546–52.

43 Toner GC, Geller NL, Tan C, Nisselbaum J, Bosl GJ. Serum tumor marker half-life during chemotherapy allows early prediction of complete response and survival in nonseminomatous germ cell tumors. *Cancer Res* 1990; **50**: 5904–10.

44 Motzer RJ, Gulati SC, Crown JP et al. High-dose chemotherapy and autologous bone marrow rescue for patients with refractory germ cell tumors. Early intervention is better tolerated. *Cancer* 1992; **69**: 550–6.

45 Motzer RJ, Mazumdar M, Gulati SC et al. Phase II trial of high-dose carboplatin and etoposide with autologous bone marrow transplantation in first-line therapy for patients with poor-risk germ cell tumors. *J Natl Cancer Inst* 1993; **85**: 1828–35.

46 Bokemeyer C, Kollmannsberger C, Meisner C et al. First-line high-dose chemotherapy compared with standard-dose PEB/VIP chemotherapy in patients with advanced germ cell tumors: a multivariate and matched-pair analysis. *J Clin Oncol* 1999; **17**: 3450–6.

47 Bokemeyer C, Gerl A, Schoffski P et al. Gemcitabine in patients with relapsed or cisplatin-refractory testicular cancer. *J Clin Oncol* 1999; **17**: 512–6.

48 Bokemeyer C, Kollmannsberger C, Harstrick A et al. Treatment of patients with cisplatin-refractory testicular germ-cell cancer. German Testicular Cancer Study Group (GTCSG). *Int J Cancer* 1999; **83**: 848–51.

49 Kollmannsberger C, Gerl A, Schleucher N et al. Phase II study of bendamustine in patients with relapsed or cisplatin-refractory germ cell cancer. *Anticancer Drugs* 2000; **11**: 535–9.

50 Cronin S, Uberti JP, Ayash LJ, Raith C, Ratanatharathorn V. Use of amifostine as a chemoprotectant during high-dose chemotherapy in autologous peripheral blood stem cell transplantation. *Bone Marrow Transplant* 2000; **26**: 1247–9.

51 Kollmannsberger C, Beyer J, Droz JP et al. Secondary leukemia following high cumulative doses of etoposide in patients treated for advanced germ cell tumors. *J Clin Oncol* 1998; **16**: 3386–91.

52 Cooper MA, Einhorn LH. Maintenance chemotherapy with daily oral etoposide following salvage therapy in patients with germ cell tumors. *J Clin Oncol* 1995; **13**: 1167–9.

53 Motzer RJ, Mazumdar M, Bosl GJ, Bajorin DF, Amsterdam A, Vlamis V. High-dose carboplatin, etoposide, and cyclophosphamide for patients with refractory germ cell tumors: treatment results and prognostic factors for survival and toxicity. *J Clin Oncol* 1996; **14**: 1098–105.

54 Mandanas RA, Saez RA, Epstein RB, Confer DL, Selby GB. Long-term results of autologous marrow transplantation for relapsed or refractory male or female germ cell tumors. *Bone Marrow Transplant* 1998; **21**: 569–76.

55 Rick O, Bokemeyer C, Beyer J et al. Salvage treatment with paclitaxel, ifosfamide, and cisplatin plus high-dose carboplatin, etoposide, and thiotepa followed by autologous stem-cell rescue in patients with relapsed or refractory germ cell cancer. *J Clin Oncol* 2001; **19**: 81–8.

56 Droz JP, Pico JL, Ghosn M et al. A phase II trial of early intensive chemotherapy with autologous bone marrow transplantation in the treatment of poor prognosis no seminomatous germ cell tumors. *Bull Cancer* 1992; **79**: 497–507.

57 Barnett MJ, Coppin CM, Murray N et al. High-dose chemotherapy and autologous bone marrow transplantation for patients with poor prognosis nonseminomatous germ cell tumours. *Br J Cancer* 1993; **68**: 594–8.

58 Broun ER, Nichols CR, Turns M et al. Early salvage therapy for germ cell cancer using high dose chemotherapy with autologous bone marrow support. *Cancer* 1994; **73**: 1716–20.

59 Broun ER, Nichols CR, Gize G et al. Tandem high dose chemotherapy with autologous bone marrow tranplantation for initial relapse of testicular germ cell cancer. *Cancer* 1997; **79**: 1605–10.

96

Patrick J. Stiff

Hematopoietic Cell Transplantation in Ovarian Carcinoma

Epithelial ovarian cancer is initially one of the most chemosensitive adult solid tumors; however, like many of the hematologic malignancies, it rapidly develops drug resistance leading to death in the majority of patients with this disease. While new taxene-based systemic chemotherapy regimens appear to improve median survival, as compared to older regimens, 5–8 year survival rates have changed little since they were developed. Because of its dismal prognosis and the fact that it shares some of the features of other initially chemosensitive tumors that respond favorably to high-dose chemotherapy regimens, ovarian cancer is increasingly being targeted for trials of dose-intensive therapy. While not as extensive as it is for the hematologic malignancies, clinical trial data, including those from well-designed phase 3 trials of intraperitoneal therapy and a randomized phase 3 trial of systemic high-dose therapy are emerging to suggest that dose intensity does improve outcome in selected patients with this disease. Several comprehensive reviews of the diagnosis and management of ovarian cancer have recently been published [1–4].

Table 96.1 International Federation of Obstetrics and Gynecology (FIGO) staging/prognosis for epithelial ovarian cancer.

Stage		Percent at diagnosis	5-year survival (%)
I	Tumor limited to ovary (one or both)	25	90
II	Tumor in one or both ovaries with pelvic extension	15	75
III	Tumor in one or both ovaries with at least microscopic extension to peritoneum or regional lymph nodes	45	20
IV	Distant nonperitoneal metastases including hematogenous spread	15	5

Epidemiology and pathogenesis

In 2002, 23,300 women were diagnosed with ovarian cancer in the USA, and 13,900 died, making this tumor the deadliest gynecologic malignancy [5]. While the lifetime frequency of ovarian carcinoma is only 1/70 women as compared to 1/9 for breast cancer, the yearly death rate for women with this disease is approximately 2.5 times higher than that for breast cancer. Its incidence has not changed significantly over the past 20 years, and no shift toward earlier stage disease at presentation has been seen in the interval. Data from the Surveillance, Epidemiology and End Results (SEER) program, indicate an improvement in the 5-year survival for all patients with ovarian cancer from 1973 to 1991 of 6%, but little since then [6]. While encouraging, the major proportion of that improvement resulted from the widespread use of primary cytoreductive surgery, and the success of treating germ cell neoplasms of the ovary as compared to the earlier time point [7]. The lack of a significant improvement in the survival for women with epithelial forms of this disease has continued since 1991 because of the lack of an effective method of early detection, the absence of a premalignant form of this disease and no increase in cure rates with conventional chemotherapy.

There are three cellular origins of ovarian cancer: epithelial, comprising 85% of all tumors; sex cord/stromal cell in 13%; and germ cell in the remaining 2%. The most common form of ovarian cancer arises from the epithelial surface, and is staged as shown in Table 96.1 [8]. Approximately 75% of patients present with disease that has spread beyond the pelvis and, as a group, have an estimated 5-year survival of only 20%. The median age at onset for those with epithelial tumors is approximately 65 years, with a peak incidence above age 70 [9]. The major risk factor for the development of this disease appears to be the duration of uninterrupted ovulation [10,11]. Pregnancy, oral contraceptives and tubal ligations decrease, while nuliparity increases the risk of epithelial ovarian cancer [2–13]. The use of exogenous estrogens after menopause does not appear to increase the risk. There are no premalignant forms of ovarian cancer, and the current theory of pathogenesis is of epithelial tumors resulting from the repeated damage and repair of the ovarian epithelium during ovulation, which ultimately leads to the malignant changes. Despite the presence of a group of epithelial tumors of "low malignant potential", these do not frequently transform into malignant tumors, nor do ovarian adenomas. However, mutations of the tumor suppressor gene *p53* have been seen in benign cells of the ovarian epithelium immediately adjacent to malignant cells, suggesting that genetic changes do occur prior to the onset of malignant transformation [14]. Other oncogenes are abnormally expressed in this tumor including *p53*, c-*myc*, *HER-2/neu*, and c-*fos* and *ras*, and their presence may be associated with a poorer prognosis [15,16]. Despite a high frequency of *HER-2/neu* expression in breast cancer, only 15–30% of epithelial ovarian cancers express this oncogene [16]. Estrogen receptors are highly expressed in approximately 10% of epithelial tumors suggesting that, only in a small proportion of patients, endogenous and possibly exogenous steroids may have a role both in the pathogenesis and growth of this tumor.

Other factors involved in the pathogenesis of epithelial tumors include a "western diet" (i.e. high in saturated fats), exposure to talc powder and a strong family history, particularly with two or more affected first-degree relatives [12]. There appears to be no significant increased risk with tobacco or alcohol use. Inherited ovarian cancer associated with the *BRCA1* and *BRCA2* oncogenes is seen in approximately 5% of all cases of ovarian cancer. Of the hereditary forms of ovarian cancer, the most common is the breast–ovary syndrome. The frequency of ovarian cancer in patients with the *BRCA1* gene is approximately 63% and 85% for ovarian and breast cancer, respectively, with the frequency of ovarian cancer much lower for those with the *BRCA2* gene [17].

Epithelial tumors also arise from the peritoneal cavity and the fallopian tube. They are staged and treated similarly to epithelial tumors and, considering stage at diagnosis, have a similar prognosis. Granulosa cell tumors, the most common type of sex cord/stromal cell tumors, usually present with localized disease with patients demonstrating stigmata of hormonal excess such as that seen with precocious puberty. Patients with this form of ovarian cancer have a 5-year survival with primary therapy of 85–95% because of a lack of dissemination and chemosensitivity [18]. Germ cell tumors occur less frequently (2%), and also typically present in young women. They are also usually localized, are chemosensitive and have an overall survival rate of 80–90% [7]. Given the rarity of granulosa cell and germ cell tumors, and their high cure rate with conventional therapy, very few patients have received hematopoietic cell transplantations (HCT). Their outcome is similar to relapsed male germ cell tumors, with most performed for drug-resistant disease. Given this, the focus of this chapter is on the optimal management of epithelial ovarian cancer, including high-dose chemotherapy and HCT.

Early detection and screening

The early detection of ovarian cancer has been problematic both because of the lack of sensitive and specific screening tests that will diagnose stage I disease and the low incidence of this disease in the general population. Those with a risk of familial ovarian cancer have been recommended to have frequent screening by examination, CA 125 levels and pelvic ultrasound examinations, and to undergo a prophylactic oophorectomy after childbearing is completed [19]. However, there are no currently available methods designed to diagnose ovarian cancer at an early stage in the general population other than yearly pelvic examinations [20]. Until recently there has been little indication that it is possible to diagnose tumors at an early stage, because the low frequency of the disease in the general population requires a screening test that has both a high specificity and sensitivity. Even with a specificity of 98% and a sensitivity of 80%, it is estimated that approximately 49 unnecessary surgeries would need to be performed for every cancer diagnosis. CA 125, proposed as such a screening test, is currently not sensitive enough to be of value as it is elevated in <50% of women with stage I tumors. Einhorn *et al.* [21] screened 5550 normal females and found 175 to have an elevated CA 125. After additional testing, including surgical exploration in a number, a total of only six cancers were found, of whom only four were in either stage I or II. Transvaginal ultrasounds also do not have the sensitivity to diagnose early stage disease [20]. However, recently serum proteomic pattern changes determined by mass spectroscopy have been evaluated as a potentially more effective screening tool [22]. The cancer profile developed from samples of patients with ovarian carcinoma was tested on a "blinded" series of ovarian cancers, both early and late stage disease, and was able to classify all malignancies, including 18 stage I tumors. It also correctly identified 95% of benign lesions. If verified in larger populations, this sensitive test may facilitate the screening of large populations of both high- and low-risk patients. Whether strategies will need to include pelvic ultrasounds and/or surgery for those 5% ultimately diagnosed with a false-positive remains to be determined.

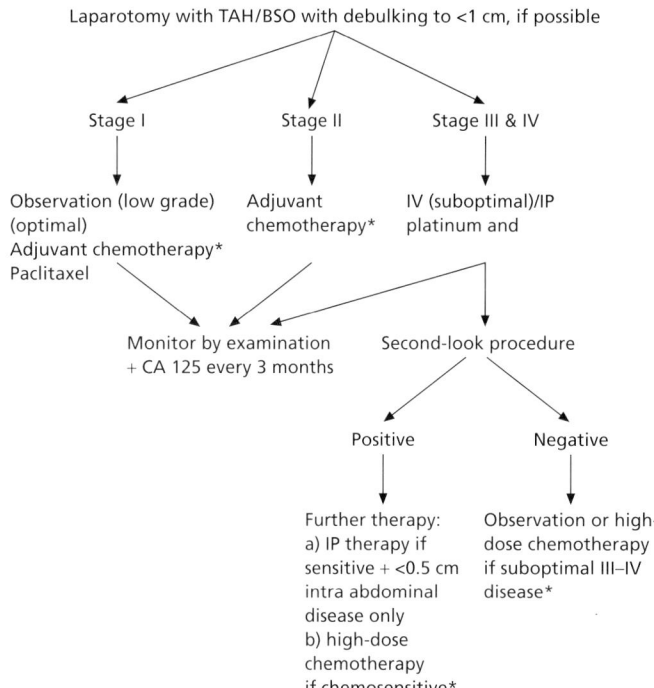

Fig. 96.1 Initial management of epithelial ovarian cancer.
IP, intraperitoneal; IV, intravenous.
*Optimal management pending results of ongoing trials.

Conventional management of ovarian cancer

Initial surgical management

The optimal initial management of ovarian cancer is well-defined for all stages of epithelial ovarian cancer (Fig. 96.1). It begins with a thorough surgical debulking, preferably by a trained gynecologic oncologist. At a minimum, a total abdominal hysterectomy, bilateral salpingo-oophorectomy and omentectomy, and removal of all enlarged pelvic and retroperitoneal lymph nodes are performed with excisional biopsies of all tumor nodules and a careful examination of the entire peritoneal cavity. As first shown by Griffiths [23], the most important prognostic factor for survival for epithelial ovarian cancer is the amount of residual tumor left after the completion of the primary surgical procedure. Based on his analysis, stage III disease is divided into two groups, based on the amount of residual disease left at the completion of the initial surgery. Patients with stage III disease and a postoperative maximum cross-sectional diameter of ≤1 cm are considered to have optimal stage III disease, while those with larger diameter residual disease are considered to have suboptimal disease. Patients with optimal stage III disease have a median survival of 40–50 months while those with suboptimal stage III have a prognosis of 25–38 months [1,2]. Most clinical trials combine suboptimal stage III with stage IV disease, and the first trial that validated the efficacy of paclitaxel as an important component in initial therapy was proven initially in patients with suboptimal stage III–IV disease [24].

Initial chemotherapy

Patients with stage IA or B, and either grade I or II are treated with surgery only, and have a 5-year progression-free survival (PFS) without chemotherapy of ≥90% [1,2]. Those with stage IC or II, or those few patients with stage IA or B with grade III tumors when treated with surgery alone, have a relapse rate of approximately 35%. Most investigators now recommend adjuvant chemotherapy with platinum and a taxene or radiotherapy including intraperitoneal phosphorus-32 (^{32}P). However, there is no consensus as to the optimal management of this patient group, and trials are ongoing to test the value of platinum-based chemotherapy.

Unlike early stage disease, patients with stage III and IV disease require postoperative chemotherapy. Unfortunately, while initially chemosensitive, 60–80% patients with advanced disease relapse after initial chemotherapy [25]. Over time, the optimal therapy for advanced stage disease has evolved from single-agent alkylating agent therapy to combination therapy with cisplatin or carboplatin and cyclophosphamide (CY) with or without doxorubicin to, most recently, platinum and paclitaxel combinations. The response rates for patients treated with platinum-based chemotherapy range from 70 to 80%, with age, histology other than clear or mucinous cell types, lack of ascites, a rapid rate of fall of serum CA 125 levels and a pathologic second-look procedure being favorable prognostic factors in addition to bulk of disease after primary surgery. The utilization of cisplatin and paclitaxel as important components of initial therapy was preceded by the demonstration of the 30% response rate for paclitaxel in chemoresistant relapsed disease [26]. In the first comparative trial, conducted by the Gynecologic Oncology Group (GOG; GOG 111), 50 mg/m^2 cisplatin plus 135 mg/m^2 paclitaxel over 24 h was compared to the standard of care at the time, 50 mg/m^2 cisplatin plus 500 mg/m^2 CY [24], there was a significant improvement in response rates (73 vs. 60%), PFS (13 vs. 18 months) and overall survival (26 vs. 38 months) for patients treated after primary surgery with the palitaxel-based arm [24]. However, because the pathologic complete remission (CR) rate was not higher for the paclitaxel/cisplatin arm, it is not surprising that longer follow-up data have not shown a survival improvement for the new combination at 7–8 years. This trial was unique in that patients treated on the cisplatin/CY arm did not have access to paclitaxel for second-line therapy as it was not commercially available at the time. Its availability would likely have led to a smaller impact on the survival advantage seen in this trial.

The follow-up trial of the GOG (GOG 132) appears to validate this conclusion. Patients with the identical clinical characteristics in this trial were randomized between the new combination of paclitaxel and cisplatin vs. paclitaxel or cisplatin alone. No difference in overall survival was seen for the combination, as compared to either cisplatin or paclitaxel alone (26.6 vs. 30.2 months vs. 26.0 months median survival) [25]. The major difference in this trial as compared to GOG 111 was that the other agent was available as second-line therapy for those failing on the single drug only arms in the later trial. The results from a subsequent multinational study testing the paclitaxel/cisplatin combination, with paclitaxel administered as a 3-h vs. 24-h infusion are supportive of the benefit of paclitaxel-containing combinations [26]. Neurotoxicity, seen typically with conventional single agent doses of cisplatin and short paclitaxel infusions, was seen more frequently in this trial as compared to GOG 111; however, there was no difference in response rate, duration of remission or overall survival for the new combination as compared to those patients treated with the cisplatin and 24-h infusional paclitaxel combination in GOG 111. However, in contrast to GOG 111, patients with optimal III and stage II disease were treated on the multinational trial. Despite their inclusion, which should have boosted the median PFS and survival for the entire group, the PFS was the same as seen in GOG 111 (16.6 months for the paclitaxel-treated group vs. 12 months for the CY/cisplatin-treated group). Taken together, there appears to be a modest benefit to paclitaxel and platinum combinations, but it appears that these regimens significantly affect the 5–7-year survival for patients with suboptimal stage III–IV disease as compared to older combinations. Ultimately, 80% of patients with suboptimal III and IV disease still die of chemoresistant disease.

When combined with paclitaxel, there is no difference in survival for patients treated with carboplatin as compared to cisplatin [27], and subsequent phase 3 studies have verified that carboplatin with paclitaxel is as effective as the original cisplatin and paclitaxel doublet, and is associated with less toxicity [28]. In addition, this regimen can be given in an outpatient setting as with less neurotoxicity seen with carboplatin compared with cisplatin, the paclitaxel can be safely given over 3 h. As a result of several recent trials, it appears that the optimal chemotherapy for patients with suboptimal stage III and IV disease is 6 monthly cycles of the combination of carboplatin at an area-under-the-curve (AUC) dosage of 5–7.5 mg/ml/min and paclitaxel given as a single 3-h infusion at a dosage of 175 mg/m^2. Pathologic CR rates, defined as an absence of disease documented by careful surgical reexploration after primary chemotherapy, occur in approximately 20–25% of patients with suboptimal and up to 40% in patients with optimal stage III disease. While associated with an improved median survival, approximately 50% of those with suboptimal stage III and IV [29] and 20% of those with optimal stage III [30], who have a pathologic CR, will relapse.

Based on synergism of cisplatin with both paclitaxel and CY, the National Cancer Institute recently performed a phase 1 trial of the three drugs in combination in patients with large bulk (>3 cm) disease [31]. Despite bulky disease, there was a 36% pathologic CR rate with a median PFS (18 months), equivalent to that seen for patients with less bulky disease. These results need confirmation but suggest that with more aggressive conventional-dose therapy, results might improve.

Patients with optimal stage III disease have also been treated with paclitaxel-based therapy. The multinational study comparing cisplatin plus CY vs. cisplatin plus paclitaxel for all stages of advanced ovarian cancer included patients with optimal stage III disease. In a subset analysis of this trial, benefit was seen for optimal stage III disease for the new combination [26]. As part of a subsequent GOG phase 3 study for optimal stage III disease that evaluated the efficacy of intraperitoneal phase 3 trial, the median survival for the control arm of systemic cisplatin and paclitaxel was 48 months, suggesting a modest benefit for the newer combination as compared retrospectively to older trials of platinum plus CY [32]. Given these results, platinum/paclitaxel combinations are the new standard of care for patients with advanced ovarian cancer yet, even for those with optimal stage III disease, only a minority are likely to be cured with conventional therapy alone.

Second-look laparotomy and interval cytoreductive surgery

Patients with normal examination, CT scans and CA 125 levels at the completion of primary chemotherapy often have residual disease that can only be documented with a second surgical procedure (laporotomy). This procedure may also improve the prognosis of those responding patients found with disease <1 cm that can be reduced to microscopic residual amounts [33,34]. However, only 25–30% of patients undergoing this procedure are in this group, and because approximately 20% of patients will have significant postoperative complications and there is no survival enhancement when additional therapy is given for persistent disease at second-look surgery, second look laporatomies have largely been abandoned except in the confines of a clinical trial. Obviously, with effective therapy for those with residual disease at second-look, the utility of this procedure would increase greatly.

Interval cytoreductive surgery, or surgery performed after several cycles of chemotherapy for patients unable to be surgically cytoreduced at their initial surgery has been associated with an improvement in survival. In the only randomized trial reported to date, the 2-year survival was 56% vs. 46% ($p = 0.01$) for those undergoing the interval surgical procedure, compared to those treated with chemotherapy alone [35]. This survival difference was apparent at follow-up times up to 5 years. A subsequent GOG-led trial that also compared interval cytoreductive surgery to chemotherapy alone for suboptimal advanced ovarian cancer has recently been completed, and appears to show no difference in outcome for those receiving the second surgical procedure. However, in contrast to the first trial, only patients who were maximally cytoreduced at their initial surgery were permitted to enter [36].

Conventional therapy for recurrent disease

A variety of both old and new agents can produce temporary responses in patients with advanced ovarian cancer [37–50]. The approach to relapsed disease has largely been based on prior responsiveness to platinum. The use of single agent carboplatin for those progressing on cisplatin results in a response rate of approximately 5%, and for those who relapse within 6 months of completing a platinum-based therapy a response rate of only 15% is seen [38,39]. In contrast, those whose remissions lasted >6 months have responses in the range of 35–40%, with those whose remission lasted >24 months having a response rate of 59%. These data have led to the definition of platinum-sensitive recurrent disease as disease that recurs after an initial platinum-induced remission of >6 months. There is currently no conventional single agent or combination chemotherapy that is superior to the reintroduction of platinum for patients with platinum-sensitive disease (Table 96.2) [37–42].

For those with platinum-resistant disease, there are a variety of agents that may produce remissions (Table 96.3) [37–51]. Paclitaxel, for those not previously treated with the agent, produces responses in approximately 25% of patients, with little difference for patients with platinum-sensitive or -resistant disease [37]. Similarly, topotecan, which produces responses in 16–20% of patients, is equally effective in platinum-resistant disease [43]. Other agents including liposomal doxorubicin [46], hexamethylmelamine [48,50], ifosfamide [49], vinorelbine [45], oral low-dose etoposide [47] and tamoxifen [51] have all been effective in a minority of patients. Median responses to any of these agents average 3–4 months, with median survivals from the onset of first relapse lasting from 5 to 12 months. Whether these agents improve median survival is doubtful, primarily because of their low response rates. These results led to the conclusion at the recent National Cancer Institute (NCI) consensus conference on ovarian cancer that current salvage chemotherapy does not improve survival and, when possible, patients should be entered on novel clinical trials [19].

High-dose therapy

There are considerable data on the application of dose intensity in ovarian cancer suggesting that high-dose therapy may be of value in improving the prognosis of this disease [52–54]. These data include favorable dose–responses both *in vitro* as well as *in vivo*, primarily for platinum compounds and other alkylating agents. This includes not only high-dose systemic therapy with HCT but also regional high-dose therapy via the intraperitoneal (IP) route using cisplatin. Ovarian cancer shares many of the features of hematologic malignancies and pediatric round cell tumors, which benefit from such high-dose therapy.

1 Chemosensitivity to conventional therapy with partial responses (PR) and CR in a high proportion of patients.
2 Occasional cures despite large bulk disease at conventional doses of therapy.
3 Disease that can be converted into a low tumor burden state with conventional modalities, even at relapse.
4 Evidence of a favorable *in vitro* dose–response for a variety of agents [55–58].
5 Active agents can be significantly dose escalated *in vivo*.
6 Synergy of active agents at high doses [59,60].
7 Clinical evidence of a favorable dose–response at high drug doses.

Dose intensity in the conventional dose range

Systemic chemotherapy

Much has been written about the lack of efficacy of dose intensity in the conventional dose range in ovarian cancer. Most trials explored only modest increases in dose intensity for patients in relapse or as part of initial therapy. Levin and Hryniuk [52] evaluated more than 30 published series in 1987, and found a correlation between platinum dose intensity and both response and survival in ovarian cancer. However, the dose intensity range where this benefit was attained varied from a dose intensity of 0.4 to 0.8, and dose intensity beyond the conventional range was not investigated [53]. Based partially on their work, trials were subsequently designed to determine if there was a continuation of the dose–response relationship beyond standard doses. However, given the toxicities of the regimens tested, most studies investigated at most a twofold increase in dose intensity of platinum therapy [54–56]. Of trials to date, only two showed an improvement in both response rates and survival. This first trial, by the Scottish Ovarian Cancer Study Group, compared CY with cisplatin at either 50 or 100 mg/m² [55]. As compared to other trials, the response rate for the low-dose arm, now considered a standard dose of cisplatin, was low at 34%, especially considering that nearly 30% of patients had early stage disease. While survival was superior, toxicity was also higher for the dose-intensive arm, with the authors not recommending the high-dose arm as standard of care. In the second trial, a small number of patients with small volume disease were treated with cisplatin at either 60 or 120 mg/m² [56]. Follow-up was short, and toxicity for the higher dose arm was again significant, caused both by

Table 96.2 Options for the management of recurrent platinum-sensitive epithelial ovarian cancer.

Therapy	PFS (months)	OS (months)
Platinum	6–9	20–24
Paclitaxel	4.5	16
Topotecan*	4.5	12
Hexamethylmelamine	5.0	16
High-dose chemotherapy with stem cell transplant	10–14	23–29

OS, overall survival; PFS, progression-free survival.
* One-third had platinum-resistant disease.

Table 96.3 Options for the management of recurrent platinum-resistant epithelial ovarian cancer.

Therapy	PFS (months)	OS (months)
Paclitaxel	4.5	12
Topotecan	3–3.5	12
Ifosfamide	–	9
Hexamethylmelamine	–	5
Liposomal doxorubicin	5.7	11
Vinorelbine	4.0	10
High-dose chemotherapy with stem cell transplant	6–7	10–12

OS, overall survival; PFS, progression-free survival.

neurotoxicity and myelosuppression. All other studies exploring up to twice conventional doses per cycle, as well as total dose given over one-half the period of conventional therapy, have been reported to show no benefit to high-dose therapy [55–58]. In one such recent report, initial therapy with single-agent carboplatin at an AUC of 12 for four cycles was compared to an AUC of 6 for six cycles; the actual dose delivered was only 22% higher for the "high-dose" arm [57]. Additional trials that combined both cisplatin and carboplatin in an attempt to increase the delivered dose of platinum but with less toxicity unfortunately delivered at most twice the conventional dose of platinum and also failed to show an improvement in response rates or durations [58]. The same results were seen when single agent cisplatin was tested at 200 mg/m^2 or carboplatin at 800 mg/m^2 in patients with relapsed disease [59,60]. Thus, while there is a dose–response below conventional doses of platinum-based chemotherapy, doubling the optimal conventional dose intensity or decreasing the frequency between courses does not improve the response rates or survival, with at times toxicity preventing a true exploration of dose intensity. These studies do not rule out the value of further dose escalations in this disease. In fact, in vitro data suggest that as the doses are increased to 5–10-fold, there is indeed additional cell killing [61–63].

Intraperitoneal chemotherapy

IP chemotherapy is another conventional approach that has been tested to explore platinum dose intensity in patients with ovarian cancer. At a standard dose of 100 mg/m^2 IP cisplatin achieves a plasma level similar to the same dose given intravenously (IV), yet achieves a local concentration 20-fold higher than plasma levels [64]. Several studies have been performed documenting the efficacy of IP cisplatin in small volume persistent or recurrent disease. While effective in relapsed disease, it is estimated that only one-third of patients are eligible based on an optimal maximum tumor bulk of <0.5 cm, lack of adhesions, platinum responsiveness and the absence of extraperitoneal spread of disease, including the retroperitoneal lymph nodes [65–67]. However, two phase 3 trials have indicated a superiority of this therapy as primary treatment for optimal stage III disease. Alberts et al. [68] reported an intergroup trial that compared IP cisplatin to the same dose (100 mg/m^2) given IV with IV CY in both groups (600 mg/m^2) for the initial management of patients with optimal stage III ovarian cancer. The trial demonstrated a 24% improvement in survival for the IP group with a median survival of 49 vs. 41 months ($p = 0.02$). In addition, there was less nephrotoxicity and neurotoxicity on the IP platinum arm. Another phase 3 IP trial has just been completed by the GOG which compared IV cisplatin and carboplatin to two doses of IV carboplatin followed by six cycles of IV paclitaxel and IP cisplatin at 135 and 100 mg/m^2, respectively [30]. Overall survival for the IP arm was 53 months, significantly longer than the 48 months for the IV platinum/paclitaxel arm. A South-West Oncology Group (SWOG) phase 2 study of both IP cisplatin and paclitaxel combined with IV paclataxel demonstrated a 2-year survival of 92% and a projected median survival >5 years, the first time survival has exceeded 5 years for optimal stage III disease [68].

In vitro studies of dose intensity

Drug resistance develops early in the treatment of ovarian cancer and, given the ease of growing ovarian cells in clonogeneic assays and the availability of multiple tumor samples from the same patient as the disease progresses, much of what is known about acquired drug resistance comes from work performed in ovarian cancer [61–63,69–71]. The cytotoxicity of platinum compounds is a result of their binding to DNA, resulting in an inhibition of DNA transcription and replication. Resistance to platinum is mediated by nucleotide excision repair enzymes, which are overexpressed in these cells. In addition, increased reduced glutathione levels are seen that lead to detoxification of alkylating agents. Of the strategies tested clinically to date, only dose-intensive chemotherapy appears to increase the cytotoxicity of platinum-resistant cells. Similar to many tumors, the rationale for dose intensity in ovarian carcinoma began with the demonstration of a favorable dose–response for agents when tested in tissue culture. In vitro studies documented a favorable dose–response to platinum, other alkylating agents and mitoxantrone, and additive or synergistic cytotoxicity for alkylating agent combinations. In particular, mitoxantrone was shown to be active at high doses for human tumors known to be platinum-resistant, explaining its incorporation into clinical trials [61].

Early hematopoietic cell transplantation trials

Single-agent trials in refractory disease

Early transplant trials demonstrated that for single alkylating agent therapy, there is a high response rate for patients with refractory relapsed ovarian cancer [72–74]. Wolff et al. treated 10 patients with high-dose thiotepa as part of a phase 1–2 trial; six responded, but details as to duration or disease characteristics were not reported [72]. While cisplatin is the most active agent for this disease, its dose-limiting toxicity, neurotoxicity, is reached at twice its conventional dose [57]. However, carboplatin can be escalated to a maximum tolerated dose (MTD) of 2000 mg/m^2, or a fivefold dose escalation as reported by Shea et al. [73]. Of the 11 patients treated on his phase 1 study with advanced ovarian cancer, seven (77%) responded, one of whom achieved a CR. Viens and Maraninchi [74] treated 14 patients with single agent high-dose melphalan for refractory disease with one lasting 18+ months. While these response rates were higher than those seen with conventional doses of each agent, validating the in vitro dose–response data, remission durations for these patients with drug-resistant disease typically lasted only several months.

Combination chemotherapy trials for refractory disease

Additional early trials consisting of platinum with one or more additional agents were reported during the same period [75–80]. All consisted of small numbers of patients, the maximum being 12, and responses and remission durations were similar to those of single agent studies. Mulder et al. [75] treated eight patients with 7 g/m^2 CY and 1–1.5 g/m^2 etoposide, with three alive at 24–56 months. These three patients, while chemoresistant, had microscopic disease at the time of transplant. Shpall et al. [76] treated a group of 12 platinum-resistant patients who had failed a median of three prior regimens, with trialkylator therapy consisting of thiotepa, CY and cisplatin. All were maximally cytoreduced surgically prior to transplant, and all received cisplatin via the IP route. Of eight evaluable patients, six (75%) had a pathologic PR, documented at a surgical procedure following the bone marrow transplantation (BMT). The median response duration was 6 months. The regimen was complicated by sepsis or severe nephrotoxicity contributing to a treatment-related mortality rate of 25%. Shea et al. [79] similarly treated eight patients with progressive disease with IP carboplatin and etoposide combined with IV thiotepa and mitoxantrone with hematopoietic cell rescue. Four of seven evaluable patients achieved a CR for a median of 6 months.

In the first multicenter trial, Broun et al. [77] treated nine patients with high-dose ifosfamide and carboplatin. There were five CRs and one that lasted for a median of 6 months. Stiff et al. [78] treated seven patients with refractory ovarian cancer with a combination of high-dose carboplatin, CY and mitoxantrone as part of a larger phase 1 trial. Mitoxantrone was chosen based on its activity for platinum-resistant disease at high doses in vitro using the tumor cloning assay [61]. This trial included a pharmacokinetic analysis that demonstrated that the mitoxantrone doses (75 mg/m^2) gave serum levels in the steepest part of the in vitro dose–response curve. All six evaluable patients (one early death) responded, with a median response duration of 7.5 months. One patient who had failed platinum-based induction therapy was progression-free at >2 years. The overall median survival was 12 months, with 29% survival at 2 years. Finally, Shea et al. [79] reported on an aggressive regimen of high-dose carboplatin, etoposide, thiotepa and mitoxantrone in eight chemoresistant patients who had failed two prior regimens. Five had a CR (63%), and overall seven of eight responded, but again the median PFS was only 6 months.

Because most centers transplanting patients with this disease in the early 1990s had treated only a few patients each on center-specific protocols, it was impossible at the time to determine whether or not there was a small group of patients with advanced disease who might benefit from such therapy. A survey of active US programs was conducted in 1992 to determine if such a subgroup could be identified [80]. Eleven programs submitted data on 153 patients. Of these, 146 (95%) received an HCT for relapsed or refractory disease, 62% of whom were platinum-resistant. The median number of prior regimens was two and, similar to the pilot studies reported above, the median number of patients treated per regimen was seven, with a maximum of 20 patients per regimen. The early death rate was 10.5%, and of the 82 with measurable disease, 71% had either a clinically defined PR (28%) or a CR (43%). While response rates for platinum-sensitive and -resistant disease were similar (87% and 85%), the CR rates were 73% and 34%, respectively. Similar to the pilot studies, the median time to progression was 6 months and 14% were progression-free at 1 year after transplant in this relapsed and refractory group. Of the seven patients transplanted in first remission, five (71%) were progression-free at 9–20+ months, with the remaining two progressing at 5 and 9 months. Compared to conventional dose salvage chemotherapy for these heavily pretreated patients, the response rates to high-dose therapy appeared to be higher, although the response durations were similar. Whether the 14% PFS rate at 1 year for relapsed disease represented a benefit could not be determined because the survey did not determine if these patients were platinum-sensitive or had a long initial remission with standard chemotherapy, both favorable prognostic factors for conventional salvage therapy.

Subsequent studies helped define the utility of high-dose chemotherapy in patients failing initial therapy, with several suggesting that disease bulk at HCT and platinum-sensitivity are important prognostic factors [81–83]. Weaver et al. [81] treated 31 patients on a phase 1–2 trial with a single cycle of high-dose melphalan (1600 mg/m^2), mitoxantrone (50 mg/m^2) and carboplatin (1000–1600 mg/m^2). The group received a median of two prior chemotherapy regimens. Fourteen (70%) achieved a CR and at a median follow-up of 20 months, 35% were progression-free and 60% were surviving. Interestingly, only one-fifth (20%) treated at carboplatin doses of 1000–1200 mg/m^2 was still disease-free at the time of the publication in contrast to 11 of 26 (42%) at the higher doses. No differences were observed for those with platinum-resistant vs. platinum-sensitive disease. Supportive of the importance of bulk, in this study, of seven in CR prior to HCT, five were in continuous CR at 9–19 months after HCT. There were three regimen-related toxic deaths (10%). The carboplatin dosage was determined on the basis of body surface area and, when converted to an AUC dose, it was noted that all deaths occurred at an AUC dosage >30 mg/ml/min. The authors concluded that AUC dosing at a target of 20–25 mg/mL/min be used in future studies rather than dosage based on body surface area.

Based on the promising results in the phase 1 trial of CY, carboplatin and mitoxantrone, a phase 2 trial of this regimen was conducted at Loyola University Medical Center in 30 patients at the MTD of 1500 mg/m^2 carboplatin, 120 mg/kg CY and 75 mg/m^2 mitoxantrone [82]. Of the 30 patients, only one-third were platinum-sensitive and 73% had bulky disease as defined by MRD >1 cm diameter at the time of HCT. The median number of conventional regimens prior to HCT was two and the median time from diagnosis to transplant was 18 months. Only three patients had both platinum-sensitive disease and <1 cm maximum tumor diameter at HCT. There was a single death (3.3%) resulting from *Aspergillus* pneumonia prior to engraftment. Of the 27 patients with measurable or evaluable disease, 89% responded with seven of eight platinum-sensitive vs. nine of 19 platinum-resistant patients obtaining a clinical CR ($p = 0.06$). The median survival for the entire group was 29 months, and median PFS was 7 months. There was a 23% survival without disease at 2 years, which included four patients who received post-HCT involved field radiotherapy. For those with platinum-sensitive disease, there was a significant improvement in PFS compared to resistant disease of 10.1 vs. 5.1 months ($p = 0.01$). A similar improvement in PFS was seen for those patients with maximum tumor diameter <1 cm at the time of HCT. The median survival for the 10 platinum-sensitive patients was not reached, with 80% surviving 1 year. Given the short overall survival for platinum-resistant patients of 10.4 months, one of the conclusions of the study was that high-dose therapy appeared not to benefit patients with platinum-resistant disease.

Multivariate analyses and comparisons to conventional chemotherapy

The first multivariate analysis of patients undergoing high-dose therapy and HCT for ovarian carcinoma was reported in 1997 on 100 patients [83]. Similar to most single center phase 2 trials, 66% were platinum-resistant and 61% had maximum tumor diameter at transplant of >1 cm. The response rates for patients with platinum-sensitive or maximal disease diameter <1 cm at HCT were higher at 94% and 97%, respectively, as compared to 81% and 78% for those with chemoresistant or more bulky disease. For the multivariate analysis, the pretransplant factors analyzed were age, remission status, platinum-sensitivity, bulk, months from diagnosis, histology, grade, number of prior regimens, response to induction therapy, transplant regimen, stage at diagnosis and response to initial conventional therapy. Post-transplant factors included time to engraftment of neutrophils and platelets, and the response to HCT (CR vs. non-CR). Pretransplant factors associated with an improvement in PFS in the univariate analysis were maximum tumor diameter at HCT, platinum sensitivity and age, while in the multivariate analysis maximum tumor diameter and platinum sensitivity alone were important. The pretransplant factors associated with an improvement in survival in the univariate analysis were age, maximum tumor diameter at transplant, platinum sensitivity, performance of a second-look laparotomy and a prior pathologic CR. In the multivariate analysis age, bulk and platinum sensitivity were the only significant factors (Table 96.4). As in the initial

Table 96.4 Multivariate analysis of factors associated with favorable outcome following autologous transplants for advanced ovarian cancer.

Factor	Loyola ($n = 100$)		ABMTR ($n = 422$)	
	PFS (p)	OS (p)	PFS (p)	OS (p)
Bulk (<1 cm)	0.0001	0.0175	n.s.*	n.s.
Platinum sensitivity	0.025	0.0330	<0.0001	<0.0001
Age <48 years	n.s.	0.001	<0.0001	<0.001
Karnofsky score >80	ND	ND	<0.0001	<0.0001
Non-clear cell	n.s.	n.s.	<0.05	<0.006

ABMTR, Autologous Blood and Marrow Transplant Registry; ND, not done; n.s., not significant; OS, overall survival; PFS, progression-free survival.
* Comparison to first complete remission group.

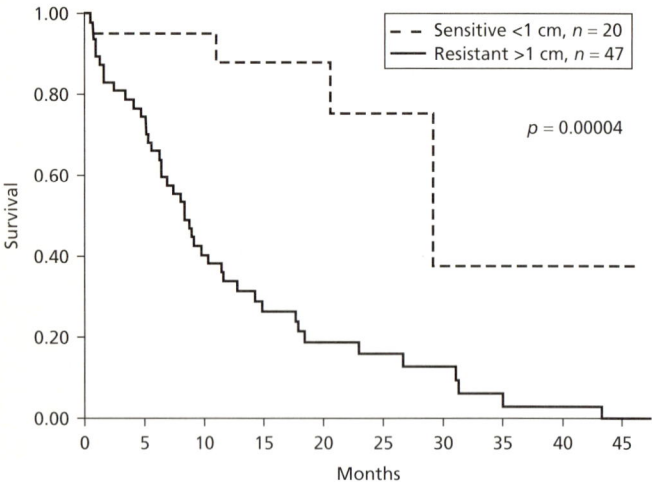

Fig. 96.2 Survival of patients undergoing high-dose chemotherapy for relapsed/refractory ovarian cancer based on platinum sensitivity and tumor bulk at transplant. (From [84].)

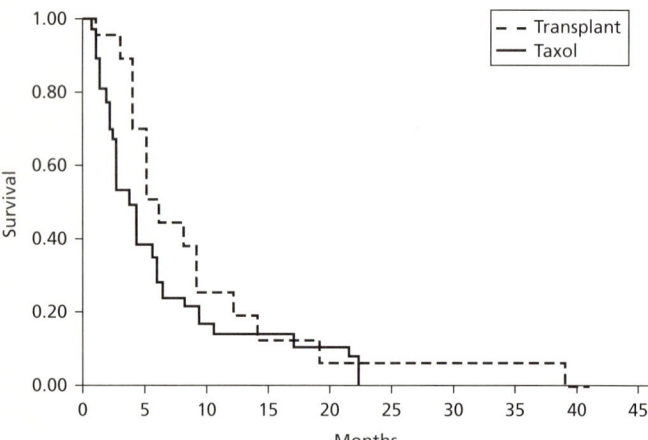

Fig. 96.3 Survival comparison of single agent paclitaxel vs. high-dose chemotherapy with autologous transplantation at first relapse: platinum-resistant disease.

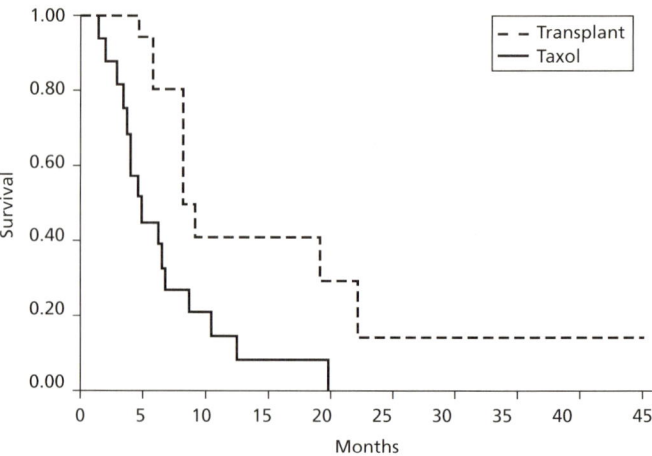

Fig. 96.4 Survival comparison of single agent paclitaxel vs. high-dose chemotherapy with autologous transplantation at first relapse: platinum-sensitive disease.

Table 96.5 Transplant or conventional salvage therapy (as in [85]) for patients with advanced ovarian carcinoma relapsing >12 months after an initial remission.

	Taxol	CAP	Transplant
Number of patients	41	38	14
Initial remission (months)	30.1	30.1	24.5
No. therapy cycles	6	6	1
Clinical CR (%)	20	32	100
Median PFS (months)	7.3	18.9	14
Median OS (months)	20.3	24.3	NR: 93% survive @ 24 months

CAP, cyclophosphamide 500 mg/m^2; Adriamycin 50 g/m^2; cisplatin 50 g/m^2; CR, complete remission; NR, not reached; OS, overall survival; PFS, progression-free survival.
Taxol: 175/m^2 3-hr infusion.
Loyola University transplant data PFS = first rise CA 125 >27 IU/mL.

phase 2 trial [82], the median survival was only 9.6 months for those with resistant disease. However, for those with both resistant disease and maximum diameter disease <1 cm, the survival was 28 months, while those with larger diameter disease had a survival of only 8.6 months. The best risk group was that with platinum-sensitivity and disease <1 cm (Fig. 96.2). This group had a PFS of nearly 19 months and a median survival of 29 months. Conventional salvage chemotherapy or surgical cytoreduction to achieve a minimal disease state prior to HCT were associated with the same post-HCT survival.

To date there have been no randomized trials comparing HCT to conventional therapy for relapsed disease. Several comparisons of conventional therapy [37,85] with this transplant database [83] have been performed to determine the relative value of transplant for patients with relapsed or refratory disease. While the disease characterstics known to be of prognostic importance for long-term remission (disease bulk, chemosensitivity) were matched, there are some differences between the groups, most notably age. These analyses have been performed only to indicate which patient groups should be studied further in phase 2 and 3 studies. Patients with platinum-resistant disease in first relapse not previously exposed to paclitaxel who are treated with this agent experience a median 4-month PFS [37], similar to the same group who received transplant (Fig. 96.3) [83]. Those with platinum-sensitive disease treated with conventional doses of paclitaxel experience a median 4.5-month PFS with paclitaxel vs. 8 months with transplant. However, while all conventionally treated platinum-sensitive patients had relapsed by 20 months, 30% of the transplanted patients were progression free, and at 3 years 18% were still progression free (Fig. 96.4). A similar analysis has been performed for those with sensitive disease whose first remission lasted >1 year before first salvage therapy was administered. Treated with either CY, doxorubicin and cisplatin or single agent paclitaxel, the median survival for these groups was 20 and 24 months, respectively [85]. Those transplanted with the same characteristics (i.e. those whose initial remission lasted >12 months) had a 93% survival at 22 months (Table 96.5) [85]. Taken together, these data—albeit from nonrandomized trials—suggest that for those with platinum-resistant, with or without bulky disease, HCT provides a similar PFS and survival to conventional therapies, and should not be pursued. However, studies should be undertaken in those with platinum-sensitive disease who, in contrast to those treated with conventional therapy, have an approximate 20% 3+ year PFS. One such phase 3 study is underway in Europe under the auspices of the European Group for Blood and Marrow Transplantation (EBMT).

Another multivariate analysis of the first 422 patients reported to the Autologous Blood and Marrow Transplant Registry (ABMTR) by 57

Table 96.6 High-dose chemotherapy following second-look surgery for advanced ovarian cancer.

Study	n	Induction	No. cycles	Preparative regimen	CR	PFS	OS (months)
Mulder [86]	11	Platinum-based	NA	Cyclophosphamide + etoposide	6/11 (55%); pathologic CR in 5	NA	23
Legros [88]	53	Cyclophosphamide, doxorubicin, cisplatin, UM 26, 8-FU	6–8	Melphalan (23) cyclophosphamide + carboplatin (30)		24 months 37	66
Viens [89]	19	Cyclophosphamide, doxorubicin, cisplatin ± hexamethylmidine	6–8	Melphalan		47% @ 2 year	–
Extra [90]	37	Platinum-based	6	Cyclophosphamide, abdominal RT, with melphalan (3) or carboplatin (14)		46% @ 3 year*	32

CR, complete remission; 8-FU, NA, not available; OS, overall survival; PFS, progression-free survival; RT, radiotherapy.
*Patients <45 years.

BMT teams was recently reported. A total of 92% of patients were beyond first remission [84]. At HCT, 38% had maximum tumor diameter disease >1 cm, and 41% were platinum-sensitive. Overall survival and PFS are similar to that previously reported from phase 2 studies for this mostly bulky or platinum-resistant group. In a multivariate analysis, lower age, higher Karnofsky score, histology (nonclear cell vs. clear cell), disease status (CR vs. non-CR) and platinum-sensitivity were important favorable prognostic factors for PFS, with all but disease status important for overall survival (Table 96.4). Patients in second CR or PR with platinum-sensitive disease had a 2-year survival of 45%, while those with chemoresistant disease had a 2-year survival of only 19%.

HCT for persistent disease at second-look laparotomy

With the suggestion that platinum sensitivity and low tumor burden are important prognostic factors for patients undergoing HCT for ovarian carcinoma, it is possible that transplanting patients at an earlier point in their disease will yield superior results. Several pilot studies have recently been reported that describe HCT at the time of second-look surgery (Table 96.6) [86–92].

Mulder et al. treated 11 patients with surgically persistent disease after a variety of induction chemotherapy regimens with high-dose 7 g/m^2 CY and 900–1000 mg/m^2 etoposide [86]. Three patients had microscopic residual disease, five had maximum tumor diameter disease ≤2 cm and three had disease >2 cm. Of the 11, five had a pathologic CR with two of six patients with stage III disease having remissions lasting 43+ and 75+ months. Dauplat et al. [87] transplanted 14 patients after a positive second-look procedure. Five had microscopic residual disease at surgery and the remainder had additional cytoreductive surgery performed. All received a single course of high-dose 140 mg/m^2 melphalan. The 3-year PFS and overall survival were 33% and 64%, respectively, and five were disease-free at the time of the report at follow-up times of 30–60 months. Legros et al. [88] subsequently reported on a total of 53 patients similarly treated, some of whom were described in the initial Dauplat report. Patients received initial chemotherapy with a platinum-based combination, and after demonstrating platinum-sensitivity, all but five (who were in a clinical CR) underwent a second-look procedure, followed by high-dose chemotherapy with either 140 mg/m^2 melphalan (23 patients) or 1600 mg/m^2 carboplatin and 6.4 g/m^2 CY (30 patients). At a median follow-up of over 6.5 years, 23% were in continuous CR and 45% were alive. Of 31 patients with no or microscopic disease at second-look, the disease-free survival (DFS) at 5 years was 26.9%. For the 19 patients in this group with a negative second-look, the 5-year DFS of 32.8% implies that the 12 patients with microscopic residual disease at second-look had a similar DFS after the HCT. For those patients with macroscopic residual disease at the initiation of their second-look surgery, the 5-year DFS was 19.2% and the 5-year survival was 33.8%. The value of HCT for those patients transplanted in a pathologic CR in this study cannot be estimated as the percentage of patients with optimal stage III is not provided. These patients have up to an 80% long-term DFS with conventional therapy alone. However, the survival of patients with a positive second-look surgery in this study does appear superior to those treated with conventional therapy only after second-look surgery. Considering that 42% of this group had suboptimal disease at diagnosis, we would expect the median survival for this group to be approximately 45 months if treated with conventional therapy rather than the 66 months reported [30,33,34].

Additional smaller trials in similar patients are supportive of this conclusion. Of the 19 patients whom Viens et al. [89] transplanted, three of 10 with maximum tumor diameter at second-look <2 cm and six of nine with a pathologic CR were alive and disease-free at a median follow-up of at least 22 months. The median overall survival from diagnosis was 47 months for the series of Extra et al. [90], despite the fact that 76% had suboptimal stage III and IV disease. Donato et al. [91] treated a total of 102 patients of whom 25 had a positive second-look and 11 were treated after three cycles of induction therapy. The majority received a novel regimen of high-dose 6.25–20 mg/m^2 topotecan, 140 mg/m^2 melphalan and 3 g/m^2 CY. Patients with nonclear cell disease in first remission as well as those in second or subsequent CR had a 6-year PFS of 22% and a survival of 55%. Although these trials were not randomized phase 3 studies, they appear to suggest a survival advantage for HCT for patients with chemosensitive disease in first remission, and did lead to phase 3 trials as indicated below. Importantly, the regimen-related fatal toxicity rate of all these studies combined is <2%.

In late 1997, the SWOG concluded a randomized phase 2 trial which compared two transplant regimens for patients in first PR (<3 cm maximum diameter disease at second-look) or at the time of first platinum-sensitive relapse, in an attempt to verify safety and efficacy of these

Table 96.7 High-dose chemotherapy followed by second look surgery in the initial management of advanced ovarian cancer.

Study	n	Suboptimal (%)	Induction	No. cycles	Preparative regimen	Pathologic CR
Benedetti-Panici [95]	35	20	Cisplatin/cyclophosphamide	2–4	Cisplatin/carboplatin/etoposide (20); carboplatin/melphalan/etoposide (15)	10/24 (42%)
Menichella [96]	13	NA	Cisplatin/cyclophosphamide	2	Cisplatin/carboplatin/etoposide	4/13 (31%)
Palmer [97]	10	40	Cisplatin/paclitaxel	5	Melphalan ± mitoxantrone	5/7 (71%)
Fennelly [101]	16	63	Cyclophosphamide/paclitaxel	2	Cyclophosphamide carboplatin × 4	5/16 (39%)

regimens [92]. Patients with clinically or pathologically persistent disease after initial chemotherapy or those relapsing >6 months after a CR were randomized to CMC (1500 mg/m^2 carboplatin, 75 mg/m^2 mitoxantrone and 120 mg/kg cyclophosphamide) or CTC (165 mg/m^2 cisplatin, 600 mg/m^2 thiotepa and 5625 mg/m^2 cyclophosphamide) followed by HCT. Of 67 randomized, the 32 and 26 eligible in the CMC and CTC arms, respectively, were matched for age, maximum tumor diameter and disease status at HCT. Low-risk disease, defined as maximum diameter disease ≤0.5 cm and platinum sensitivity was seen in approximately one-half of the patients. The median PFS was 13 and 8 months, respectively, for the CMC and CTC arms (CMC vs. CTC hazard ratio [HR] = 0.60). The median survival for the CMC and CTC arms was 29 and 22 months, respectively, and the projected 4-year survivals were 25 and 21%, respectively. Of the 67 patients there were only three toxic deaths (4.4%). In a multivariate analysis of PFS, normal CA 125 at transplant and CR to primary therapy were significant; for survival, normal CA 125 and platinum sensitivity were significant. In fact, 0% of patients with platinum-resistant disease and only 4% with an elevated CA 125 at HCT became long-term progression-free survivors. Similar to the French phase 2 studies, the median survival from transplant with low tumor burden platinum sensitivity was 32 months. The CMC regimen was recommended for phase 3 studies based both on a higher survival and lower grade IV–V toxicity.

The EBMT recently reported on their HCT transplant experience for ovarian cancer [93]. A higher proportion of patients than those reported to the ABMTR (105/254) were transplanted in first remission. For all stage III patients who underwent a transplant after initial chemotherapy, the median DFS and overall survival was 42 and 59 months, respectively. Unfortunately, the proportion transplanted with optimal vs. suboptimal stage III disease is unknown. More impressively, the median DFS and overall survival for stage IV disease transplanted in first remission were 26 and 40 months, respectively, which compares favorably to the 5–7% seem for patients treated with conventional therapy alone for stage IV disease [2].

Given improvements in the conventional therapy for advanced ovarian carcinoma and the patient selection biases inherent in these phase 2 pilot studies, the true value of HCT as consolidation therapy after a chemotherapy-induced first remission will only come from randomized trials. Under the auspices of the NCI, the GOG as well as the SWOG, Cancer and Acute Leukemia Group B (CALGB) and the Eastern Cooperative Oncology Group (ECOG) initiated a randomized phase 3 trial that compared conventional therapy to a single ablative transplant for patients in first pathologic remission. Patients with stage III disease who responded to a platinum-based regimen after 4–6 cycles and had their remission documented by a second-look procedure were randomized between six cycles of paclitaxel (175 mg/m^3 over 3 h) combined with carboplatin at an AUC of 7.5 and a single transplant using the CMC regimen. The trial closed early because of poor accrual and concern that one-half would be exposed to unproven conventional consolidation chemotherapy. However, the Group d'Investigateurs Nationaux pour l'Etude des Cancers Ovariens (GINECO) recently completed such a phase 3 trial [94]. Patients were randomized after second-look surgery if they had responsive disease to either high-dose 400 mg/m^2 carboplatin and 1500 mg/m^2/day CY for 4 days or three cycles of conventional-dose chemotherapy with the same agents monthly for 3 months at 300 mg/m^2 and 500 mg/m^2, respectively. Eligibility criteria included maximum tumor diameter <2 cm at second-look or high-risk disease with a pathologic CR. A total of 110 patients were randomized, of whom only 39% had a pathologic CR. At a median follow-up of 36 months the median DFS was 11 months for the conventional-dose arm and 22 months for the high-dose arm ($p = 0.02$). Follow-up was too short at the time of the initial report to detail survival data. In a multivariate analysis, in addition to high-dose therapy, low tumor burden at second look and prior taxene therapy were significant independent prognostic factors for PFS. Thus, as consolidation therapy for responsive disease, systemic high-dose therapy with HCT has indeed been proven to improve PFS. While some have concluded this therapy now to be a standard of care for this patient group, a confirmatory trial would be important to complete. One such trial is in the planning stages in the USA which will compare conventional therapy alone vs. conventional therapy followed by high-dose therapy and HCT. The primary endpoint will be a significant increase in the pathologic CR rate determined at the completion of assigned therapy.

High-dose chemotherapy in the initial management of ovarian cancer

Several pilot transplant studies have been reported utilizing high-dose chemotherapy immediately after or in lieu of induction chemotherapy for advanced ovarian cancer (Table 96.7). Benedetti-Panicia et al. [95] initially described the outcome of 35 previously untreated patients with stage III and IV (bulky disease in seven or 20%) with 2–4 cycles of 100–160 mg/m^2 cisplatin and 1500–1600 mg/m^2 CY, followed by hematopoietic stem cell collection by aphereis, with or without marrow harvesting. Twenty patients then received high-dose 100 mg/m^2 cisplatin, 1800 mg/m^2 carboplatin and 1800 mg/m^2 etoposide and 15 received 1200 mg/m^2 carboplatin, 900 mg/m^2 etoposide and 100 mg/m^2 melphalan and HCT. Four to 6 months after HCT, responders underwent a second-look surgery to document response. Of the 24 patients completing all therapy,

10 (42%) had a pathologic CR, including seven who had been followed for more than 3 years. As only 20% had suboptimal disease at diagnosis, these results may not be better than those achieved with the best available conventional therapy at the time the study was initiated, i.e. platinum with CY.

Similar conclusions can be drawn from smaller trials testing HCT after initial chemotherapy. Menichella et al. [96] treated 13 patients who had >0.5 cm maximum diameter residual tumor at initial surgery with two courses of cisplatin and CY, then autologous HCT with 100 mg/m^2 cisplatin, 650 mg/m^2 etoposide and 1800 mg/m^2 carboplatin. At their second-look surgery, four were in a pathologic CR (31%), with three remaining without disease at follow-up times of 108–443 days. Palmer et al. [97] treated 10 patients with five cycles of paclitaxel and cisplatin as initial chemotherapy and then high-dose 140 mg/m^2 melphalan with or without 60 mg/m^2 mitoxantrone and HCT. Six were initially optimally cytoreduced. Five of seven patients had a pathologic CR. Several studies of similar design have been undertaken in which PFS and survival are the primary endpoints. Juttner et al. [98] described 13 patients who first received a single cycle of CY to mobilize and collect hematopoietic cells, and then three cycles of conventional cisplatin and CY prior to high-dose chemotherapy. After initial chemotherapy, 11 of 13 were in remission (six in CR), and after transplant using 1200 mg/m^2 carboplatin, 900 mg/m^2 etoposide and 140 mg/m^2 melphalan, all 10 evaluable patients were in clinical CR; the other three died of toxicity. Six of the 10 remained in CR at follow-up times of 3–26 months. A similar clinical outcome was seen in patients treated with high-dose ifosfamide, carboplatin and etoposide as recently reported by Peccatori et al. [99] from Milan. In all of these studies there is not a clear description of pretreatment characteristics, therefore insight into the possible benefit of this therapy as compared to conventional options cannot be determined.

Several investigators have explored the use of multiple cycles of dose-dense subablative chemotherapy followed by HCT in lieu of conventional chemotherapy for the initial therapy of advanced ovarian carcinoma. Murakami et al. [100] treated 42 patients with two cycles of modestly dose-escalated 1600–2400 mg/m^2 CY, 80–100 mg/m^2 doxorubicin and 100–150 mg/m^2 cisplatin with HCT after primary surgery. For the 23 with microscopic residual disease after initial surgery, the 4-year survival rate was 70%, and for those with macroscopic disease the median survival was 3 years. These survival rates may not be different to those seen with conventional therapy but the dose intensity of this regimen is only twice that of conventional doses, which was not shown to be effective in improving outcome in multiple randomized trials. It is also doubtful that HCT was required for this regimen. In the largest series to date of multicycle therapy, Fennelly et al. [101] treated 16 patients (10 suboptimally debulked) with high-dose CY and paclitaxel for two cycles with cytokine support and hematopoietic cells collected by apheresis after nadir cytopenia followed by four courses of "double dose" carboplatin and CY and HCT. Of this small cohort, there were five patients with a negative second-look (38.5%). Of the 16, there was one infectious death (6.2%), and given that the cumulative period of neutropenia in this group may be as much as 3–4 times longer than that for a single transplant, the mortality rates for this type of therapy should be monitored closely as trials progress. Unpublished updates of their ongoing phase 2 trials indicated that patients with optimal stage III disease had a higher than expected frequency of a pathologic CR after this therapy; in contrast, those with suboptimal disease did not. Based on the encouraging results for optimal stage III disease, the EBMT and GOG initiated separate multicenter trials based on the program developed by Fennelly et al. The ongoing EBMT trial is a phase 3 trial in which the high-dose regimen is being compared to standard platinum-based induction therapy. PFS and survival are the primary endpoints. The GOG study, a multicenter phase 2 pilot study, had as its efficacy endpoint an increase in the expected pathologic CR rate. The trial was closed early when eight of the first nine patients (optimal stage III disease) had a positive second-look, much higher than anticipated. Another GOG pilot study has been initiated which incorporates high-dose topotecan into the multicycle dose-intensive carboplatin and paclitaxel regimen. The most mature outcome data for this three-drug regimen (topotecan, paclitaxel and carboplatin) was recently reported by Prince et al. [102]. Treating patients with high-risk advanced disease, they reported a 61% pathologic CR rate, seemingly higher than the 25% and 45% seen for suboptimal and optimal stage III–IV disease. Unlike the earlier Fennelly studies, this three-drug regimen appears to be myeloablative. It remains to be seen whether this approach will produce a superior result to that seen in the phase 3 GINECO trial [92].

Future studies

Immunotherapy may improve outcome following autologous HCT for ovarian carcinoma. Edwards et al. [103] reported on the use of interleukin 2 given IP to patients with platinum-resistant low-bulk ovarian cancer in the nontransplant setting. One-third of the 18 patients treated with disease <0.5 cm had DFS lasting for at least 7 years. This as well as other biologic approaches and gene therapy designed to eliminate small numbers of drug-resistant cells after conventional therapy will likely be tested after both conventional therapy and autologous HCT over the next several years [104].

The inclusion of paclitaxel in high-dose regimens has recently begun. It has a favorable dose–response in vitro against resistant tumor cells [63], and early phase 1 trials indicate that it can be dose escalated to 700–800 mg/m^2 have led to the development of paclitaxel-based transplant regimens at several institutions [105]. One such regimen is beginning phase 2 testing at Loyola University. Paclitaxel (700 mg/m^2 IV over 24 h on day 1) is combined with mitoxantrone (30 mg/m^2 given as a 15-min infusion on days 2, 4 and 6) and carboplatin (at an AUC 28 given as a continuous infusion over 5 days starting on day 2). The HCT is given 3 days after the completion of the final day of carboplatin. Phase 1 testing indicated that the major nonhematopoietic toxicities were similar to other regimens, with the exception of a grade I–II neuropathy that appears during the first month and then wanes over a period of several months. To date, 20 patients with suboptimal stage III–IV disease (50% with stage IV disease) were treated with the phase 2 doses of this regimen followed by HCT after the completion of initial conventional chemotherapy. Their survival after HCT seems superior to the median survival of 13 months for unselected patients with stage IV disease [106]. At a median follow-up of 26 months, there is 60% PFS and 90% survival. Whether regimens such as this are better than nonpaclitaxel-containing regimens for recurrent disease has yet to be proven.

Bone marrow contamination

Because ovarian carcinoma does not typically spread hematogenously, it is not surprising that autopsy series report only rare histologic involvement of the marrow in this disease [107]. In patients undergoing transplantation, marrow involvement histologically was not seen in large series, and marrow biopsy is now not routinely performed as a screening test. Several investigators do report that, using immunocytochemical analyses, small numbers of tumor cells are found in the marrow, but this is not a universal finding [108,109]. In the report of Cain et al. [108] the marrow was involved by tumor using immunocytochemical analyses in 23%; however, none had detectable tumor in blood stem cell concentrates, although a similar trial did not confirm this finding [109]. No clinical trial has explored purging to date.

Allogeneic transplantation

To date, only one report of allogeneic HCT in ovarian carcinoma has been published [110]. As of February 2003, only 14 cases have been registered with the IBMTR. In the only report, Bay et al. [110] treated five patients with chemoresistant disease with either marrow (four patients) or blood hematopoietic cells (one patient) from human leukocyte antigen (HLA) matched sibling donors. One received a myeloablative regimen with busulfan (BU) and cyclophosphamide (CY) and the others with BU, fludarabine and antithymocyte globulin. Graft-vs.-host disease (GVHD) prophylaxis consisted of cyclosporine alone. In the absence of GVHD, and withdrawal of cyclosporine and persistent or recurrent disease, donor lymphocyte infusion (DLI) was planned. Of the five patients, four developed acute or chronic GVHD and had a tumor regression of at least 50%. In addition, two received DLI for progressive disease of whom one responded. Three patients are alive at 4, 16 and 40 months, which is impressive considering that all had drug-resistant disease; i.e. would typically have had a 4–6 month survival with conventional therapy alone. Obviously, additional studies are appropriate, given the apparent graft-vs.-tumor effects seen in this disease.

Conclusions

Ovarian carcinoma is a tumor with a dismal outcome when treated with conventional therapy because of the rapid development of drug resistance after exposure to conventional chemotherapy. However, it is a tumor with a demonstrated *in vivo* responsiveness to high-dose chemotherapy when the agents are administered via the IP route. In fact, two phase 3 trials now indicate an improvement in survival when IP therapy is compared to conventional IV therapy. In addition, high-dose therapy and HCT at this time appears to be the only therapy capable of producing a long-term DFS in patients with relapsed chemosensitive disease. In addition, there are now data from a phase 3 trial to show that remission durations are doubled when high-dose therapy and HCT are given after the attainment of an initial chemotherapy-induced remission. Survival data from this trial and a confirmatory trial are needed before this therapy becomes standard of care in this setting. Equally impressive are early data that suggest that allogeneic HCT produces a graft-vs.-ovarian cancer effect mediated by donor lymphocytes. If true, future studies will likely test submyeloablative allogeneic HCT as a consolidation therapy for disease in first remission.

References

1 Kristensen GB, Trope C. Epithelial ovarian cancer. *Lancet* 1997; **349**: 113–7.

2 Harries M, Gore M. Chemotherapy for epithelial cancer; I and II. *Lancet Oncol* 2002; **3**: 529–45.

3 Kotz KW, Schilder RJ. High-dose chemotherapy and hematopoietic progenitor cell support for patients with epithelial ovarian cancer. *Semin Oncol* 1995; **22**: 250–62.

4 Fennelly D. The role of high-dose chemotherapy in the management of advanced ovarian cancer. *Curr Opin Oncol* 1996; **8**: 415–25.

5 Jemal A, Thomas A, Murray T, Thon M. Cancer statistics, 2002. *CA Cancer J Clin* 2002; **52**: 23–47.

6 Ries LAG, Kosary CL, Hankey BF *et al.*, eds. *SEER Cancer Statistics Review, 1973–94: Tables and Graphs* (NIH Pub 97-2789). Bethesda, MD: National Cancer Institute, 1997.

7 Williams SD, Blessing JA, Moore DH, Homesley HD, Adcock L. Cisplatin, vinblastine, and bleomycin in advanced and recurrent ovarian germ-cell tumors. *Ann Intern Med* 1989; **111**: 122.

8 International Federation of Gynecology and Obstetrics. Annual report on the results of treatment in gynecological cancer. *Int J Gynaecol Obstet* 1989; **28**: 189–90.

9 Yancik R. Ovarian cancer: age constraints in incidence, histology, disease stage at diagnosis and mortality. *Cancer* 1993; **71**: 517–23.

10 Whitemore AS. Characteristics relating to ovarian cancer risk: implications for prevention and detection. *Gynecol Oncol* 1994; **55**: S15–19.

11 Cassagrande JT, Pike MC, Russ RK, Louie EW, Roy S, Henderson BE. Incessant ovulation and ovarian cancer. *Lancet* 1979; **2**: 170–2.

12 Grene MH, Clark JW, Blaney DW. The epidemiology of ovarian cancer. *Semin Oncol* 1884; **11**: 209–26.

13 Francescho S, Parazzini F, Negri F *et al.* Pooled analysis of 3 European case–control studies of epithelial ovarian cancer. III. Oral contraceptive use. *Int J Cancer* 1991; **49**: 61–5.

14 Zheng J, Benedict WF, Xu HJ *et al.* Genetic disparity between morphologically benign cysts contiguous to ovarian carcinoma and solitary adenomas. *J Natl Cancer Inst* 1995; **87**: 1146–53.

15 Niwa K, Itoh M, Murase T *et al.* Alteration of *p53* gene in ovarian carcinoma: clinical pathological correlation and prognostic significance. *Br J Cancer* 1994; **70**: 1191–7.

16 Berchuck A, Kamel A, Whitaker R *et al.* Overexpression of *HER-2/neu* is associated with poor survival in advanced epithelial ovarian cancer. *Cancer Res* 1990; **50**: 4087–91.

17 Ford Easton DF. The genetics of breast and ovarian cancer. *Br J Cancer* 1995; **72**: 805–12.

18 Colombo N, Sessa C, Landoni F *et al.* Cisplatin, vinblastine and bleomycin combination chemotherapy in metastatic granulosa cell tumors of the ovary. *Obstet Gynecol* 1986; **67**: 265–8.

19 NIH Consensus Conference. Ovarian cancer: screening, treatment and follow-up. NIH consensus development on ovarian cancer. *J Am Med Assoc* 1995; **273**: 491–7.

20 Tenerillo MG, Park RC. Early detection of ovarian cancer. *CA Cancer J Clin* 1995; **45**: 71–87.

21 Einhorn N, Sjovvall K, Knapp RC *et al.* Prospective evaluation of serum CA 125 levels for the early detection of ovarian cancer. *Obstet Gynecol* 1992; **80**: 14–8.

22 Petricoin EF III, Andekani AM, Hitt BA *et al.* Proteomic patterns in sera identify ovarian cancer. *Lancet* 2002; **359**: 572–7.

23 Griffiths CT. Surgical resection of tumor bulk in the primary treatment of ovarian cancer. *Monogr Natl Cancer Inst* 1975; **42**: 101–4.

24 McGuire WP, Hoskins WJ, Brady MF *et al.* Cyclophosphamide and cisplatin compared with paclitaxel and cisplatin in patients with stage III and stage IV ovarian cancer. *N Engl J Med* 1996; **334**: 1–6.

25 Muggia FM, Braly PS, Brady MF *et al.* Phase III randomized study of cisplatin vs. paclitaxel vs. cisplatin and paclitaxel in patients with suboptimal stage III or IV ovarian cancer: a Gynecologic Oncology Group study. *J Clin Oncol* 2000; **18**: 105–16.

26 Piccart MJ, Bertelsen K, Stuart G *et al.* Is cisplatin-paclitaxel (P-T) the standard in first-line treatment of advanced ovarian cancer (OvCa)? The EORTC-GCCG, NOCOVA, NCI-C and Scottish intergroup experience. *Proc Am Soc Clin Oncol* 1997; **16**: 352a.

27 Alberts DS, Green S, Hannigan EV *et al.* Improved therapeutic index of carboplatin plus cyclophosphamide: final report of the South-West Oncology Group of a phase II randomized trial in stage III and IV ovarian cancer. *J Clin Oncol* 1992; **10**: 706–10.

28 Bookman MA, McGuire WP, Kilpatrick D *et al.* Carboplatin and paclitaxel in ovarian carcinoma: a phase I trial of the Gynecologic Oncology Group. *J Clin Oncol* 1996; **14**: 1895–902.

29 Gadducci A, Sartori E, Maggino T *et al.* Analysis of factors after negative second-look in patients with advanced ovarian cancer: an Italian multicentre study. *Gynecol Oncol* 1998; **68**: 150–5.

30 Creasman WT, Gall S, Bundy BN *et al.* Second-look laparotomy in the patient with minimal residual stage III ovarian cancer (a Gynecologic Oncology Group study) *Gynecol Oncol* 1989; **35**: 378–82.

31 Reed E. The chemotherapy of ovarian cancer. *Principles and Practice of Oncology* 1996; **10**: 1–12.

32 Armstrong DK, Bundy BN, Baergen R *et al.* Randomized phase III study of intravenous (IV) paclitaxel and cisplatin vs. IV paclitaxel, intraperitoneal (IP) cisplatin and IP paclitaxel in optimal stage III epithelial ovarian cancer (OC): a Gynecologic Oncology Group trial (GOG 172). *Proc Am Soc Clin Oncol* 2002; **21**: 201a.

33 Hoskins WJ, Rubin SC, Dulamey E *et al.* Influence of secondary cytoreduction at the time of second-look laparotomy on the survival of patients with epithelial ovarian cancer. *Gynecol Oncol* 1989; **34**: 365–71.

34 Willias L, Brunetto VL, Yordan E, DiSaia PJ, Creasman WT. Secondary cytoreductive surgery at second-look laparotomy in advanced ovarian cancer: a Gynecologic Oncology Group study. *Gynecol Oncol* 1997; **66**: 171–8.

35 van der Burg MEL, van Lent M, Buyse M *et al.* The effect of debulking surgery after induction

chemotherapy on the prognosis in advanced ovarian cancer. *N Engl J Med* 1995; **332**: 629–34.

36 Rose PG, Nerenstone S, Brady M *et al*. A phase III randomized study of interval secondary cytoreduction in patients with advanced stage ovarian carcinoma with suboptimal disease: a Gynecologic Oncology Group study. *Proc Am Soc Clin Oncol* 2002; **21**: 201a.

37 Thigpen JT, Blessing JA, Ball H *et al*. Phase II trial of paclitaxel in patients with progressive ovarian carcinomas after platinum based chemotherapy: a Gynecologic Oncology Group study. *J Clin Oncol* 1994; **12**: 1748–53.

38 Seltzer V, Vogl S, Kaplan B. Recurrent ovarian carcinoma: retreatment using combination chemotherapy including *cis*-diaminedichloroplatinum in patients previously responding to this agent. *Gynecol Oncol* 1985; **21**: 167–76.

39 Eisenhauer EA, Vermorken JB, van Glabbeke M. Predictors of response to subsequent chemotherapy in platinum pretreated ovarian cancer: a multivariate analysis of 704 patients. *Ann Oncol* 1997; **8**: 963–8.

40 Markman M, Rothman R, Hakes T *et al*. Second-line platinum therapy in patients with ovarian cancer previously treated with cisplatin. *J Clin Oncol* 1991; **9**: 389–93.

41 Caldas C, Morris LE, McGuire WP. Salvage therapy in epithelial ovarian cancer. *Obstet Gynecol Clin North Am* 1994; **21**: 179–94.

42 Ozols RF. Future directions in the chemotherapy of ovarian cancer. *Semin Oncol* 1997; **24** (Suppl. 15): S15–90.

43 ten Bokkel Huinik W, Gore M, Carichael J *et al*. Topotecan vs. paclitaxel for the treatment of recurrent epithelial ovarian cancer *J Clin Oncol* 1997; **15**: 2183–93.

44 Lund B, Hansen OP, Theilade K *et al*. Phase II study of gemcitabine (2′,2′-diflourodeoxycytidine) in previously treated ovarian cancer patients. *J Natl Cancer Inst* 1994; **86**: 150–33.

45 Bajetta E, DiLeo A, Biganzoli L *et al*. Phase II study of vinorelbine in patients with pretreated advanced ovarian cancer: activity in platinum-resistant disease. *J Clin Oncol* 1996; **14**: 2546–51.

46 Muggia FM, Hainsworth JD, Jeffers S *et al*. Phase II study of liposomal doxorubicin in refractory ovarian cancer: antitumor activity and toxicity modification by liposomal encapsulation. *J Clin Oncol* 1997; **15**: 987–93.

47 Rose PG, Blessing JA, Mayer AR *et al*. Prolonged oral etoposide as second-line therapy for platinum-resistant (PLATR) and platinum-sensitive (PLATS) ovarian carcinoma: a Gynecologic Oncology Group study. *Proc Am Soc Clin Oncol* 1992; **15**: 282.

48 Vergote I, Himmelmann A, Frankendal B *et al*. Hexamethylmelamine as second-line therapy in platinum-resistant ovarian cancer. *Gynecol Oncol* 1992; **47**: 282–6.

49 Markman M, Hakes T, Reichman B *et al*. Ifosfamide and mesna in previously treated advanced epithelial ovarian cancer: activity in platinum-resistant disease. *J Clin Oncol* 1992; **10**: 243–8.

50 Moore DH, Valea F, Crumpler LS, Fowler WC. Hexamethylmelamine/altretamine as second-line therapy for epithelial ovarian carcinoma. *Gynecol Oncol* 1993; **51**: 109–12.

51 van der Velden J, Gitsch G, Wain GV *et al*. Tamoxifen in patients with advanced epithelial ovarian cancer. *Int J Gynecol Cancer* 1995; **5**: 301–5.

52 Levin L, Hryniuk WM. Dose intensity analysis of chemotherapy regimens in ovarian cancer. *J Clin Oncol* 1987; **5**: 756–60.

53 Levin L, Simon R, Hryniuk W. Importance of multiagent chemotherapy regimens in ovarian carcinoma: dose intensity analysis. *J Natl Cancer Inst* 1993; **85**: 1732–42.

54 Ozols RF, Thigpen JT, Dauplat J *et al*. Advanced ovarian cancer: dose intensity. *Ann Oncol* 1993; **4** (Suppl. 4): S49–56.

55 Kaye SB, Lewis CR, Paul J *et al*. Randomized study of two doses of cisplatin with cyclophosphamide in epithelial ovarian cancer. *Lancet* 1992; **340**: 329–33.

56 Ngan HY, Choo YC, Cheung M *et al*. A randomized study of high-dose vs. low-dose cisplatinum combined with cyclophosphamide in the treatment of advanced ovarian cancer: Hong Kong ovarian carcinoma study group. *Chemotherapy* 1989; **35**: 221–7.

57 Gore ME, Mainwaring PN, MacFarlane V *et al*. Randomized study of dose intensity with single agent carboplatin in patients with advanced epithelial ovarian cancer. London Gynaecological Oncology Group. *J Clin Oncol* 1998; **16**: 2426–34.

58 Piccart MJ, Nogaret JM, Marcelis L *et al*. Cisplatin combined with carboplatin: a new way of intensification of platinum dose in the treatment of advanced ovarian cancer. *J Natl Cancer Inst* 1990; **82**: 703–7.

59 Ozols RF, Ostchego Y, Myers CE, Young RC. High-dose cisplatin in hypertonic saline in refractory ovarian cancer. *J Clin Oncol* 1985; **3**: 1246–50.

60 Ozols RF, Ostchega Y, Curt G, Young RC. High-dose carboplatin in refractory ovarian cancer patients. *J Clin Oncol* 1987; **5**: 197–201.

61 Alberts DS, Young L, Mason N, Salmon SE. *In vitro* evaluation of anticancer drugs against ovarian cancer at concentrations achievable by intraperitoneal administration. *Semin Oncol* 1985; **12** (Suppl. 4): 38–42.

62 Lidor YJ, Shpall EJ, Peters WP, Bast RC Jr. Synergistic toxicity of different alkylating agents for epithelial ovarian cancer. *Int J Cancer* 1991; **49**: 704–10.

63 Behrns BC, Hamilton TC, Masuda H *et al*. Characterization of a *cis*-diamine dichloro-platinum (II) -resistant human ovarian cancer cell line and its use in evaluation of platinum analogs. *Cancer Res* 1987; **47**: 414–18.

64 Raymond E, Hanauske A, Faivre S *et al*. Effects of prolonged vs. short-term exposure paclitaxel (Taxol) on human tumor colony-forming units. *Anticancer Drugs* 1997; **8**: 379–85.

65 Lopez JA, Krikorian JG, Reich S *et al*. Clinical pharmacology of intraperitoneal cisplatin. *Gynecol Oncol* 1985; **20**: 1–9.

66 Markman M, Reichman B, Hakes T *et al*. Responses to second-line cisplatin-based intraperitoneal therapy in ovarian cancer: influence of a prior response to intravenous cisplatin. *J Clin Oncol* 1991; **9**: 1801–5.

67 Ozols RF. Intraperitoneal salvage chemotherapy in ovarian cancer: who is left to treat? *Gynecol Oncol* 1992; **45**: 1–2.

68 Alberts DS, Liu PY, Hannigan EV *et al*. Intraperitoneal cisplatin plus intravenous cyclosphamide vs. intravenous cisplatin plus intravenous cyclophosphamide for stage III ovarian cancer. *N Engl J Med* 1996; **335**: 1950–5.

69 Rothenberg ML, Liu P, Wilczynski S *et al*. Excellent 2-yr survival in women with optimally debulked ovarian cancer treated with intraperitoneal and intravenous chemotherapapy: a SWOG/ECOG/NCIC study (S9619). *Proc Am Soc Clin Oncol* 2002; **21**: 203a.

70 Perez RP, Hamilton TC, Ozols RF, Young RC. Mechanisms and modulation of resistance to chemotherapy in ovarian cancer. *Cancer* 1993; **71**: 1571–80.

71 Teicher B, Holden SA, Jones SM, Eder JP, Herman TS. Influence of scheduling in two-day combinations of alkylating agents *in vivo*. *Cancer Chemother Pharmacol* 1989; **25**: 161–6.

72 Wolff SN, Herzig RH, Fay JW *et al*. High-dose N,N,N*-triethylenethiophosphoramide (thiotepa) with autologous bone marrow transplantation: phase I studies. *Semin Oncol* 1990; **17** (Suppl. 3): 2–6.

73 Shea TC, Flaherty M, Elias A *et al*. A phase I clinical and pharmacokinetic study of carboplatin and autologous bone marrow support. *J Clin Oncol* 1989; **7**: 651–61.

74 Viens P, Maraninchi D. High-dose chemotherapy and autologous marrow transplantation for common epithelial ovarian carcinoma. In: Armitage J, Antman K, eds. *High Dose Chemotherapy*. Baltimore: Williams & Wilkins, 1992: 729–34.

75 Mulder PO, Willemse PH, Aalders JG *et al*. High-dose chemotherapy with autologous bone marrow transplantation in patients with refractory ovarian cancer. *Eur J Can Clin Oncol* 1989; **25**: 645–9.

76 Shpall EJ, Clark-Pearson D, Soper JT *et al*. High dose alkylating agent chemotherapy with autologous bone marrow support in patients with stage III/IV epithelial ovarian cancer. *Gynecol Oncol* 1990; **38**: 386–91.

77 Broun ER, Belinson JL, Berek JS *et al*. Salvage therapy for recurrent or refractory ovarian cancer with high-dose chemotherapy and autologous bone marrow support: a Gynecologic Oncology Group pilot study. *Gynecol Oncol* 1994; **54**: 142–6.

78 Stiff PJ, McKenzie RS, Alberts DS *et al*. Phase I clinical and pharmacokinetic study of high dose mitoxantrone combined with carboplatin, cyclophosphamide and autologous bone marrow rescue: high response rate for refractory ovarian carcinoma. *J Clin Oncol* 1994; **12**: 176–83.

79 Shea T, Wiley J, Serody J *et al*. High dose chemotherapy with melphalan, VP-16, thiotepa and mitoxantrone in patients with advanced ovarian cancer. *Proc Am Soc Clin Oncol* 1995; **14**: A807.

80 Stiff P, Antman K, Broun RE. *et al*. Bone marrow transplantation for ovarian carcinoma in the United States: a survey of active programs. Proceedings of the Sixth International BMT Symposium, 1992: 1–9.

81 Weaver CH, Greco FA, Hiansworth JD *et al*. A phase I–II study of high-dose melphalan, mitoantrone and carboplatin with peripheral blood stem cell support in patients with advanced ovarian or breast carcinoma. *Bone Marrow Transplant* 1991; **20**: 847–53.

82 Stiff P, Bayer R, Camarda M *et al*. A phase II trial of high-dose mitoxantrone, carboplatin, and cyclophosphamide with autologous bone marrow rescue for recurrent epithelial ovarian carcinoma: analysis of risk factors for clinical outcome. *Gynecol Oncol* 1995; **57**: 278–85.

83 Stiff PJ, Bayer R, Kerger C *et al*. High-dose chemotherapy with autologous transplantation for

83. persistent/relapsed ovarian cancer: a multivariate analysis of survival for 100 consecutively treated patients. *J Clin Oncol* 1997; **15**: 1309–17.
84. Stiff PJ, Veum-Stone J, Lazarus HM et al. High-dose chemotherapy and autologous stem-cell transplantation for ovarian cancer: an Autologous Blood and Marrow Transplant Registry report. *Ann Int Med* 2000; **133**: 504–15.
85. Cantu MG, Buda A, Parma G et al. Randomized controlled trial of single agent paclitaxel vs. cyclophosphamide, adriamycin, and cisplatin in patient with ovarian cancer who responded to first-line platinum-based regimens. *J Clin Oncol* 2002; **20**: 1232–327.
86. Mulder PO, Willemse PHB, Alders JG et al. High-dose chemotherapy with autologous bone marrow transplantation in patients with refractory ovarian cancer. *Eur J Clin Oncol* 1989; **25**: 645–9.
87. Dauplat J, Legros M, Condat P et al. High-dose melphalan and autologous bone marrow support for treatment of ovarian carcinoma with positive second-look operation. *Gynecol Oncol* 1989; **34**: 294–8.
88. Legros M, Dauplat J, Fluery J et al. High-dose chemotherapy with hematopoietic rescue in patients with stage III to IV ovarian cancer: long-term results. *J Clin Oncol* 1997; **15**: 1302–8.
89. Viens P, Maraninchi D, Legros M et al. High-dose melphalan and autologous marrow rescue in advanced epithelial ovarian carcinomas: a retrospective analysis of 35 patients treated in France. *Bone Marrow Transplant* 1990; **5**: 227–33.
90. Extra JM, Cure H, Viens P et al. High-dose chemotherapy with autologous bone marrow transplantation in ovarian adenocarcinoma. *Bull Cancer* 1993; **80**: 156–62.
91. Donato ML, Gersherson DM, Wharton JT et al. High-dose topotecan, melphalan, and cyclophosphamide (TMC) with stem cell support: a new regimen for the treatment of advanced ovarian carcinoma. *Gynecol Oncol* 2001; **82**: 420–6.
92. Stiff PJ, Shpall EJ, Liu PY et al. Randomized phase II trial of two high-dose chemotherapy regimens with stem cell transplantation for the treatment of advanced ovarian cancer in first remission or chemosensitive relapse: a South-West Oncology Group study. *Gynecol Oncol*, 2003, in press.
93. Rosti G, Ferroite P, Ledermann J et al. High-dose chemotherapy for solid tumors: results of the EBMT. *Crit Rev Oncol Hematol* 2002; **41**: 139–40.
94. Cure H, Battista C, Guastalla JP et al. Phase III randomized trial of high-dose chemotherapy (HDC) and peripheral blood stem cells (PBSC) support as consolidation in patients with responsive low-burden advanced ovarian cancer (AOC): preliminary results of a GINECO/FNCLCC/SFGM-T study. *Proc Am Soc Clin Oncol* 2001; **19**: 20.
95. Benedetti-Panici P, Greggi S, Scambia G et al. Very high-dose chemotherapy with autologous peripheral stem cell support advanced ovarian cancer. *Eur J Cancer* 1995; **31A**: 1987–92.
96. Menichella G, Pierelli L, Foddai ML. et al. Autologous blood stem cell harvesting and transplantation in patients with advanced ovarian cancer. *Br J Haematol* 1991; **79**: 444–50.
97. Palmer PA, Schwartzberg L, Birch R, West W, Weaver CH. High dose melphalan ± mitoxantrone with peripheral blood progenitor cell support as a component of initial treatment of patients with advanced ovarian cancer. *Proc Am Soc Clin Oncol* 1995; **14**: 991.
98. Juttner CA, Davy MLJ, To LB et al. Autologous PBSC transplantation in stage 3 and 4 ovarian cancer. *Int J Cell Clone* 1992; **10** (Suppl. 1): 145.
99. Peccatori F, Colombo N, Griso C et al. Multicycle sequential high dose chemotherapy (HDCT): an effective regimen as first line treatment in poor prognosis advanced epithelial ovarian cancer (ACC). *Proc Am Soc Clin Oncol* 2001; **20**: 20.
100. Murakami M, Shinozuka T, Miyamoto T et al. The impact of autologous bone marrow transplantation on hematopoietic recovery after high-dose cyclophosphamide, doxorubicin and cisplatin chemotherapy for patients with gynecological malignancies. *Asia Oceania J Obstet Gynecol* 1993; **19**: 85–93.
101. Fennelly D, Schneider J, Bengala C et al. Escalating-dose taxol plus high-dose (HD) cyclophosphamide (C) carboplatin (CBDCA) plus C rescued with peripheral blood progenitor cells (PBP) in patients with stage IIC–IV ovarian cancer (OC). *Gynecol Oncol* 1995; **56**: 121.
102. Prince HM, Rischin D, Quinn M et al. Repetitive high-dose topotecan, carboplatin and paclitaxel with peripheral blood progenitor cell support in previously untreated ovarian cancer: results of a phase I study. *Gynecol Oncol* 2001; **81**: 216–24.
103. Edwards RP, Gooding W, Lembersky BC et al. Comparison of toxicity and survival following intraperitoneal interleukin-2 for persistent ovarian cancer after platinum: 24 h vs. 7 day infusion. *J Clin Oncol* 1997; **15**: 3399–407.
104. Bookman MA. Biologic therapy in the management of refractory ovarian cancer. *Gynecol Oncol* 1993; **51**: 113–26.
105. Stemmer SM, Cagnoni PJ, Shpall EJ et al. High-dose paclitaxel, cyclophosphamide, and cisplatin with autologous hematopoietic progenitor-cell support: a phase I trial. *J Clin Oncol* 1996; **14**: 1463–72.
106. Bonnefoi H, A'Hemrp J, Fisher C et al. Natural history of stage IV epithelial cancer. *J Clin Oncol* 1999; **17**: 767–75.
107. Dauplat J, Hacker NF, Nieberg RK et al. Distant metastases in epithelial ovarian carcinoma. *Cancer* 1987; **60**: 1561–6.
108. Cain JM, Ellis GK, Collins C et al. Bone marrow involvement in epithelial ovarian cancer by immunocytochemical assessment. *Gynecol Oncol* 1990; **38**: 442–5.
109. Genesen M, Bayer R, Feddersen R et al. Assessment of bone marrow metastases in ovarian cancer. *Proc Am Soc Clin Oncol*; 1998; **17**: 80a.
110. Bay JO, Fleury J, Choufi B et al. Allogeneic hematopoietic stem cell transplantation in ovarian cancer: results of five patients. *Bone Marrow Transplant* 2002; **30**: 95–102.

97

Katherine K. Matthay

Hematopoietic Cell Transplantation for Neuroblastoma

Neuroblastoma is a malignancy of young children derived from embryonic neural crest cells of the peripheral sympathetic nervous system. It is the most common extracranial solid tumor of childhood, with approximately 650 new cases per year in the USA, and accounts for 15% of cancer-related deaths in children [1]. Some of its unique features, such as the ability to secrete and store catecholamines, the genetic heterogeneity and the propensity to undergo differentiation either spontaneously or with various stimuli, have led to novel diagnostic and therapeutic approaches. As the therapy has become more tailored to biologic and clinical risk group, a higher proportion of children with neuroblastoma are surviving. However, nearly half of the children with neuroblastoma present after 1 year of age with metastatic disease, of whom less than 40% will survive more than 5 years, even with aggressive combination therapeutic approaches [2]. The goals of future therapy will be to increase the specificity of treatment in order to improve survival of children with advanced disease with less therapy-induced toxicity.

Clinical presentation and staging

Neuroblastoma can originate from any site in the sympathetic nervous system, presenting as a mass in the abdomen, mediastinum, neck or pelvis. The most common primary site is the adrenal gland or other abdominal sites (70%), while mediastinal tumors are more common in infants than in older children. The signs and symptoms of neuroblastoma depend on the location and extent of the primary tumor, as well as the presence of metastatic disease. Large abdominal masses may cause complaints of fullness, discomfort, vomiting or anorexia. Masses arising from the organ of Zuckerkandl in the pelvis can cause constipation and bladder dysfunction. High thoracic or cervical masses can present with unilateral ptosis, meiosis and anhidrosis (Horner's syndrome) [3]. Epidural or intradural extension of neuroblastoma occurs in 5–16% of cases of neuroblastoma. These patients may have symptoms associated with spinal cord compression including pain, bladder or bowel dysfunction, paraparesis or paraplegia. Prompt administration of chemotherapy appears to be an effective therapy for treating intraspinal neuroblastoma without the long-term sequelae associated with either radiation or surgical resection and laminectomy [4,5].

Metastatic neuroblastoma can classically present with proptosis and periorbital ecchymoses, and bone pain resulting in irritability and limp. Rapid enlargement of the liver metastases can result in respiratory compromise, particularly in neonates [6]. Skin lesions, seen almost exclusively in infants, have a bluish hue and have been given the nickname "blueberry muffin" lesions. Rarely, neuroblastoma will present with a paraneoplastic syndrome, including either watery diarrhea caused by secretion of vasoactive intestinal peptide, or opsoclonus–myoclonus–ataxia syndrome, characterized by jerky multidirectional eye movements, loss of balance and intermittent muscle jerks [7,8]. The latter syndrome is thought to be brought about by production of antineuronal antibodies that crossreact with normal brain tissue [9].

Multiple staging systems have been used for neuroblastoma, but currently most centers use the International Neuroblastoma Staging System (INSS). The INSS is a surgical staging that is quite prognostic and combines the two most common previous systems utilized by the US pediatric cooperative groups, the Pediatric Oncology Group and the Children's Cancer Group (Table 97.1) [10]. Nonmetastatic tumors are classified as INSS 1, 2A, 2B or 3, depending on the amount of gross residual tumor postsurgery, the extent of lymph node involvement and whether the tumor is invasive across the vertical midline of the body. INSS 4S is a special designation developed only for neuroblastoma, because of the unusually favorable course in infants <1 year of age with metastases limited to the liver, skin and bone marrow. Such tumors are often characterized by spontaneous differentiation and regression, and

Table 97.1 International Neuroblastoma Staging System [10].

Stage	Definition
1	Localized tumor with complete gross excision, with or without microscopic residual disease; representative ipsilateral lymph nodes negative for tumor microscopically
2A	Localized tumor with incomplete gross excision; representative ipsilateral lymph nodes negative for tumor microscopically
2B	Localized tumor with or without complete gross excision, with ipsilateral lymph nodes positive for tumor. Enlarged contralateral lymph nodes must be negative microscopically
3	Unresectable unilateral tumor infiltrating across the midline, with or without regional lymph node involvement; or localized unilateral tumor with contralateral regional lymph node involvement; or midline tumor with bilateral extension by infiltration (unresectable) or by lymph node involvement
4	Any primary tumor with dissemination to distant lymph nodes, bone, bone marrow, liver and other organs (except as defined for stage 4S)
4S	Localized primary tumor (as defined as stage 1, 2A or 2B), in patient <1 year, with dissemination limited to skin, liver and/or bone marrow (marrow involvement should be minimal with malignant cells <10% of total nucleated cells)

may be treated more than half the time with simple observation and supportive care. However, the majority of patients have stage 4 disease at diagnosis, with large primary tumors and disease that is widely metastatic, with the most frequent sites of involvement bones and bone marrow, seen in 60–80% of cases. Lung metastases are very rare in neuroblastoma, either at diagnosis or relapse, in contrast to other pediatric solid tumors [11]. Overall survival by INSS stage is excellent for patients with localized disease, with more than 95% survival at 5 years for children with stage 1, 2A and 2B with surgery as the primary treatment [12]. Children with INSS stage 3 also have a survival of 80–90%, although primary treatment includes chemotherapy as well as surgery and, in some cases, local radiation. This group is actually biologically heterogeneous, and patients with favorable biologic factors have nearly 100% survival, while those with unfavorable biology have only 50% survival [13]. Patients with INSS 4 are also biologically heterogeneous, with infants <1 year at diagnosis achieving 70% survival, compared to 40% for those >1 year at diagnosis. Furthermore, even within the infant group, patients whose tumors bear a single copy of *MYCN* oncogene have >90% event-free survival (EFS), compared to 10% for those with amplified *MYCN* tumors [14].

Risk classification and treatment approach

Risk groups with suggested treatment assignment based on recent cooperative clinical trials have been adopted by the Children's Oncology Group, with similar guidelines followed by other cooperative groups internationally. Although a myriad of clinical, laboratory and genetic characteristics have demonstrated prognostic import, current risk classification uses only a few of the most widely tested and established, readily available markers [3,15]. The risk assignment depends on age, INSS stage, *MYCN* gene copy number, histopathology and, for infants, tumor cell DNA index [10,16–20]. The risk classification and treatment guidelines are shown in Table 97.2. Low-risk tumors are managed with surgery alone, unless symptomatic cord compression or respiratory compromise necessitate a short course of chemotherapy. Patients in the low-risk

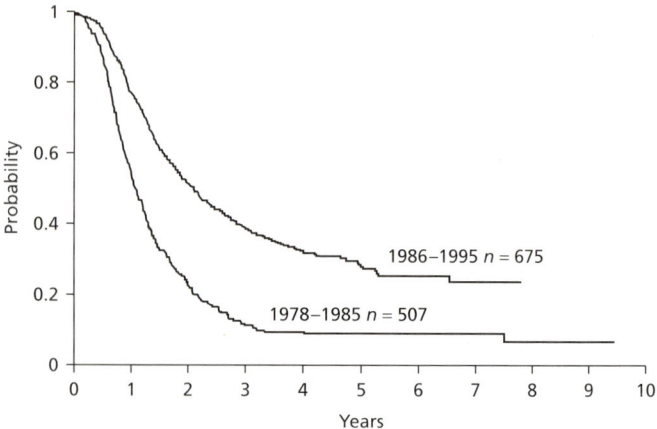

Fig. 97.1 Improving survival of children >1 year with stage 4 neuroblastoma [22].

group with stage 1 or 2 disease have an expected 4-year survival of >95% with surgery only [12], while infants with INSS 4S have >90% survival with supportive care or a short course of chemotherapy [21]. The smaller intermediate-risk group is comprised of infants with more advanced disease (but no tumor *MYCN* amplification), favorable biology stage 3 or INSS 4S with unfavorable histology or DNA index. Patients in this group are expected to have an estimated survival of >80% with standard doses of chemotherapy for 4–8 months and primary tumor resection.

The high-risk group in neuroblastoma is comprised primarily of patients with stage 4 disease who are >1 year at diagnosis, but also includes stage 3 with either tumor *MYCN* amplification or those >1 year with unfavorable histopathology, stage 2 >1 year of age with *MYCN* amplification, and stage 3, 4 and 4S infants with *MYCN* gene amplification. Despite the use of increasingly aggressive combined modality treatments, which have increased remission rates and durations, the long-term survival for INSS stage 4 disease in children who are >1 year of age at diagnosis has remained, until recently, <15% [22]. The most recent phase 3 studies indicate that the 3-year EFS of this group has now increased in the past decade to 30–40%, but is still far below the desired outcome (Fig. 97.1) [2]. The rest of this chapter focuses on the treatment of these patients, which has become increasingly dependent on dose-intensive myeloablative regimens.

Treatment of high-risk neuroblastoma

Therapy for high-risk neuroblastoma is currently divided in three phases: intensive induction treatment; marrow ablative therapy; and management of minimal residual disease. The goal of induction therapy is to achieve maximum reduction of tumor burden, including reduction of bone marrow tumor (*in vivo* purging), within a time frame that will minimize the risk of developing resistant tumor clones and clinical progression. Subsequently, very high-dose marrow ablative therapy may be used to try to overcome residual and potentially resistant tumor, followed by hematopoietic cell transplantation (HCT). The relapse rate of >40% even after such treatment [24] has led to the approach of using tumor-targeted therapies following myeloablative treatment to try to eliminate microscopic resistant clones (minimal residual disease).

Induction therapy

The introduction of platinum drugs into the combination chemotherapy may be largely responsible for improving the remission induction rate in recent years, but other important components of the induction regimen

Table 97.2 Neuroblastoma risk classification [23].

INSS	Age (days)	MYCN	Histology	Ploidy	Risk
1	Any	Any	Any	Any	Low
2A/2B	<365	Any	Any	Any	Low
	≥365	Nonamplified	Any	–	Low
	≥365	Amplified	FH	–	Low
	≥365	Amplified	UH	–	High
3	<365	Nonamplified	Any	Any	Intermediate
	<365	Amplified	Any	Any	High
	≥365	Nonamplified	FH	–	Intermediate
	≥365	Nonamplified	UH	–	High
	≥365	Amplified	Any	–	High
4	<365	Nonamplified	Any	Any	Intermediate
	<365	Amplified	Any	Any	High
	≥365	Any	Any	–	High
4S	<365	Nonamplified	FH	DI >1	Low
	<365	Nonamplified	FH	DI = 1	Intermediate
	<365	Nonamplified	UH	Any	Intermediate
	<365	Amplified	Any	Any	High

DI, DNA index; FH, favourable histology; INSS, International Neuroblastoma Staging System; UH, unfavourable histology.

include combinations with other active drugs, such as cyclophosphamide, doxorubicin, etoposide, vincristine and ifosfamide. Induction regimens used in recent large cooperative studies have shown overall response rates, including complete and partial remission (CR + PR), ranging from about 60% to 90% at the end of 5–6 months of treatment [2,25–27]. Most regimens also include surgery to residual disease, although the overall impact of complete resection on survival in stage 4 disease is still contradictory. Some studies have also investigated newer single agents in newly diagnosed neuroblastoma, using the "up-front phase 2 window". Following two courses of single agent therapy prior to induction treatment, response rates (CR + PR) of >30% were seen for ifosfamide, carboplatin, iproplatin [25] and topotecan [28]. Two agents that were less effective in this setting were epirubicin [25] and Taxol [28]. There was no evidence that the design adversely affected the outcome of patients, when compared to the patients treated with similar induction without the phase 2 window. Some pilot studies have suggested that further dose intensification of the alkylating agents and cisplatin may improve remission rates [29], but also increase the risk of second malignancy [30]. Because induction therapy contains drugs with potential late toxicity as well as the usual acute toxicities, new concerns regarding quality of life and organ function (cardiac, renal and hearing) have arisen as some children survive many years post-transplant. These toxicities are further potentiated by the common use of more platinum and alkylating agents during the myeloablative consolidation phase (see the section on Late effects below).

Local control

Recurrence in the local or regional area of primary disease is a component of relapse in a large proportion of children with high-risk neuroblastoma, in rates ranging from 20% to 80% in reports that often include local radiotherapy and myeloablative therapy [2,24,31,32]. There are both single arm studies and one randomized study that demonstrate the benefit of local control measures for children with advanced but nonmetastatic neuroblastoma [13,33–37], but the impact of resection in stage 4 disease has been mixed [38–40]. It is possible that problems with control of metastatic disease have obscured the potential value of local resection. The role of radiation therapy is also poorly established as to the best timing and optimal dose. The small patient numbers and variable rates of resection have made a randomized study difficult to perform. Only one such study has been carried out that showed better local control with the addition of 24–30 Gy of radiation in patients with stage 3 disease, but took 8 years to complete, used suboptimal chemotherapy and was begun before the refinement of biologic staging had been implemented [41]. More recent pilot studies in stage 4 disease utilizing myeloablative consolidation with radiotherapy administered to the primary tumor bed either pre- or postmyeloablative therapy suggest a lower local recurrence rate using radiotherapy in retrospective analysis, but the variability in extent of resection make these hard to interpret [32,42]. Pilot studies have also been reported using higher focal radiation via intraoperative radiotherapy in order to spare normal organs [43,44].

Evolution of myeloablative therapy

The observed linear–log relationship between drug dose and tumor cell cytotoxicity for alkylating agents suggested that if drug dose could be increased without increasing toxicity, then a multiple log increment in tumor cell killing could be achieved [45,46]. The demonstration that hematopoiesis could be restored with autologous hematopoietic cells allowed the use of much higher doses of chemotherapy with autologous bone marrow support for treatment of solid tumors [47]. The demonstration that bone marrow tumor cells could be eliminated using immunomagnetic purging [48,49] gave credence to the use of autologous marrow support in neuroblastoma, a tumor which is metastatic to bone marrow in 80% of children with high-risk stage 4 disease [11]. Early pilot studies showed that responses were seen in children with resistant neuroblastoma after high-dose chemoradiotherapy and bone marrow reinfusion [50]. Comparison of long-term survival for children >1 year of age with stage 4 neuroblastoma in the premyeloablative era, and after 1985—a time when high-dose therapy with HCT became the routine for many of these patients, showed a significant difference in outcome (Fig. 97.1) [22].

Subsequent single arm studies in the USA and Europe verified an apparent improvement in outcome for purged or nonpurged autologous bone marrow transplantation (ABMT) compared retrospectively to results for chemotherapy [24,51–55]. The single arm studies containing more than 20 patients that have been reported are summarized in Table 97.3. The 3-year EFS in these studies varied from 24% to 50%. The comparison between studies in this table is fraught with pitfalls, because EFS is sometimes estimated from time of transplant, which differs from 4 to 10 months from diagnosis, and in a few studies from time of diagnosis. The patient groups differ in whether they were comprised of only stage 4 patients >1 year at diagnosis or also included other high-risk patients. Some studies included all patients, while others only included those who achieved complete or partial remissions. In cases where the 3-year EFS was not stated in the text, it was estimated from the Kaplan–Meier curves if available; if not, another time point was reported. Finally, although we tried to avoid repetition of data, a few studies may include patients already reported in other studies, such as the overall European Group for Blood and Marrow Transplantation (EBMT) report [67].

Nonrandomized comparisons of HCT to chemotherapy

Several cooperative pediatric groups attempted statistical nonrandomized comparisons of outcome for groups of patients treated either with conventional doses of chemotherapy or myeloablative chemotherapy, total body irradiation (TBI) and purged ABMT, with differing conclusions [60,62,66,71]. Philip et al. [62] compared the LMCE1 protocol (1983–88) to the previous Lyon cooperative study, LMCE (1978–83), and showed a difference in 2-year progression-free survival of 39% vs. 12% for patients treated with myeloablative therapy and ABMT vs. standard chemotherapy.

In order to remove the bias introduced by comparing two different time periods, other reports compared concomitant groups of patients treated with either ABMT or chemotherapy by investigator or institutional choice. On the basis of two Pediatric Oncology Group (POG) studies— one a surgery plus conventional chemotherapy study (POG 8441) and the other an elective ABMT pilot protocol (POG 8340)—there was no significant prognostic benefit of switching in remission from the chemotherapy protocol to the transplant protocol ($p = 0.91$). The analysis was based on 116 patients achieving a complete or partial remission, 32 of whom received transplants on the pilot protocol [71].

The Children's Cancer Group (CCG) examined the outcome of stage IV patients >1 year of age treated with identical induction chemotherapy on a CCG pilot protocol, who then either continued on the same chemotherapy ($n = 73$) for 1 year (CCG-321P2) or proceeded to trial CCG-321P3, with myeloablative chemotherapy, TBI and purged ABMT ($n = 94$) [60]. The decision to use ABMT was nonrandom and depended on parental, investigator and institutional choice. The analysis was performed using Cox regression for censored failure-time data, treating time to ABMT as a time-varying covariate, and also by Kaplan–Meier analysis comparing EFS from time of ABMT to EFS from 8 months after diagnosis for chemotherapy patients. The advantage for ABMT vs. chemotherapy was significant for the group as a whole, with respective

Table 97.3 Event-free survival (EFS) for high-risk neuroblastoma in first remission using myeloablative therapy and HCT for studies of >20 patients. Unless otherwise stated, EFS measured from time of transplantation. (Modified from [56].)

Reference	Regimen	n	Toxic death	3-year EFS (%)
[57]	BCNU, teniposide, melphalan (total of one [n = 15] or two [n = 18] courses)	33		49 (2-year EFS)
[58]	Melphalan	24	1	40
[59]	Melphalan, TBI	54	7	32
[60,61]	1. Cisplatin, VM26, doxorubicin, melphalan, TBI	45	7	42
	2. Cisplatin, VP16, melphalan, TBI	54	5	50
	3. Carboplatin, VP16, melphalan, TBI	48	4	41
[62]	Vincristine, melphalan, TBI	62	13	30
[55]	Vincristine, melphalan, TBI	34	1	29
[63]	Cisplatin, BCNU, melphalan (or thiotepa), VP16	25	6	40
[64]	Etoposide, melphalan or cisplatin, etoposide, THP-Adriamycin, melphalan, with (n = 6) or without TBI	31	3	50
[65]	VM26 (or VP16), thiotepa, TBI	27	4	41
[66]	Melphalan ± VP16, vincristine, cisplatin, BCNU	39	7	35
[67]	European Bone Marrow Registry Data	439	60	24 (5-year EFS)
[68]	Cyclophosphamide, thiotepa	51	1	48
[2]	Carboplatin, VP16, melphalan, TBI	129	12	43
[32]	Carboplatin, VP16, melphalan, local radiation	77	4	62
[69]	Busulfan, melphalan	116	7	47
[70]	Cyclophosphamide, carboplatin	49	4	33

TBI, total body irradiation.

3-year EFS of 40% vs. 19% [60], different from the finding of Shuster et al. [71]. The advantage for ABMT was greatest for certain very high-risk subgroups, including those >2 years at diagnosis, those with bone or bone marrow metastases, those with *MYCN* gene amplification and those who had only a partial rather than complete response to the first 4–6 cycles of induction chemotherapy [60].

A smaller study by the German cooperative group evaluated 39 patients undergoing megatherapy and HCT with a variety of conditioning regimens and either allogeneic or autologous bone marrow, all with a melphalan "backbone", compared to 49 patients receiving continued chemotherapy by investigator choice. All were patients who achieved complete or partial remissions. EFS was significantly better in the transplanted patients compared to the chemotherapy group by log–rank analysis ($p = 0.005$), although the curves nearly converge by 6 years [66].

These studies, and the overall improvement in survival for high-risk neuroblastoma seen in the era after introduction of HCT, led to the few randomized comparisons discussed below.

Randomized comparison of ABMT to standard-dose chemotherapy

The European Neuroblastoma Study Group (ENSG) performed the first randomized study comparing myeloablative treatment to conventional chemotherapy [58]. This study, open from 1983 to 1985, was actually a comparison of high-dose melphalan compared to no further therapy after induction, and showed a significant advantage in progression-free survival for those patients with stage 4 disease >1 year of age at diagnosis undergoing myeloablative therapy. However, there are several problems in the application of these results. First, randomization was performed only for those patients achieving complete or good partial remission, and was not performed until approximately 10 months from diagnosis, after 10 cycles of chemotherapy. Of 84 eligible stage 4 patients, only 50 (59%) were randomized, for a variety of reasons ranging from toxic death to parental or physician preference. Thus, the applicability of these results are limited because the group as a whole excludes the highest risk patients, including the 15% who are expected to progress early in the course of induction and those who show a lesser response at the end of induction (perhaps another 20%), are not included in this study population. Second, bias may have been introduced by the high proportion of nonrandomized patients. Overall survival curves were not shown, and the large difference in EFS appears to diminish greatly after 2 years.

At the time of publication of these promising European results, the CCG launched the first large randomized study in the USA comparing high-dose chemoradiotherapy with purged ABMT to a new intensive nonmyeloablative chemotherapy intensification [2]. This study differed from that of the ENSG by performing the randomization much earlier in the course, after only two cycles of chemotherapy, at a time when 95% of the patients were still eligible. The study was also much larger, with 190 patients in each randomized group. However, it still had the problem of refusal of randomization, with a randomization rate of 70%. As ABMT was considered the experimental arm, patients who refused randomization were assigned to the chemotherapy arm, but analyzed separately. The results clearly showed a significant improvement for EFS for the patients randomly assigned to ABMT, both by an intent-to-treat analysis and also by treatment received (Fig. 97.2). As in the previous CCG non-randomized comparison, the highest risk patients, those with *MYCN* amplified tumors or those >2 years at diagnosis, had the most significant benefit. At the time of the analysis, with a median follow-up of 43 months, there was no significant difference in survival. Further follow-up will be required to see if high-dose therapy with hematopoietic support has truly made an impact on long-term survival in this disease. The other important finding from this randomized study was that there was no significant difference in toxic deaths for patients randomized to the two arms, and the hospital days were identical, helping to validate the cost-effectiveness of this treatment. At present, pilot studies have led to the approach currently used in ongoing studies, both in Europe and the USA,

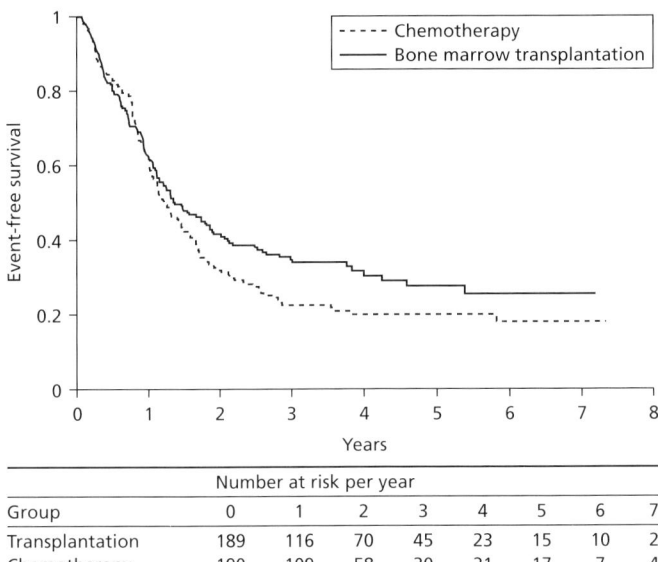

Fig. 97.2 Improved event-free survival (EFS) with myeloablative therapy compared to standard-dose chemotherapy. The difference in 3-year EFS for the 379 randomized patients was 34% vs. 22% ($p = 0.034$) [2].

of further increase in chemotherapy dose intensity by eliminating TBI, and instead using higher doses of chemotherapy and local irradiation [32].

Myeloablative regimens

The very first myeloablative regimen used in the treatment of neuroblastoma was melphalan alone, in high dose. This progressed to various combinations of other agents, including cisplatin, etoposide and doxorubicin, melphalan with busulfan, melphalan with carboplatin and etoposide. Other centers used a thiotepa base, coupled with cyclophosphamide or etoposide, or busulfan combined with cyclophosphamide. More recently, attempts have been made to incorporate topotecan into the conditioning regimen in combination with thiotepa and etoposide [72]. Few studies have tried to compare two myeloablative regimens in a randomized fashion. However, the retrospective analysis by the EBMT failed to show any difference in EFS using different high-dose regimens [54,67,73]. On the other hand, an analysis from the Institut Gustave-Roussy showed that patients treated with busulfan and cyclophosphamide appeared to have better EFS than those on other conditioning regimens at a single institution [69]. These data may depend on the chronology of the protocols as well as the fact that the busulfan regimen was compared to a combination of a variety of other regimens. The ESNG is currently testing this hypothesis in a randomized study, comparing the COG regimen of melphalan, etoposide and carboplatin to the busulfan and melphalan regimen.

Tandem transplants

Other investigators are pursuing the strategy of trying to benefit from the further increase in dose intensity obtainable with repetitive high-dose myeloablative therapies with hematopoietic cell rescue, but a randomized study is required to verify whether this approach truly improves EFS or survival [74–77]. The earlier French study of this approach included both patients in relapse and in partial response, and utilized immunomagnetic purging of autologous bone marrow and conditioning regimens of VM26, BCNU and cisplatin (or carboplatin), followed by a conditioning regimen of vincristine, melphalan and TBI, with a high toxic death rate of eight of 33 patients. Only survival figures were given, with 36% survival for the group treated in first PR [74]. The second study was for patients with less than complete or very good partial response to induction, and utilized first myeloablative therapy with BCNU, VM26 and carboplatin in 25 patients, then a final consolidation with vincristine, melphalan and TBI. There were four toxic deaths, and a rather long time to neutrophil engraftment of 31 days. Only 20 patients were able to receive both autografts. Progression-free survival at 3 years was 28% [75].

The more recent pilot studies in the USA utilized stem cells, either CD34 selected or unpurged. Grupp et al. [76] reported 39 evaluable patients who completed 70 cycles of high-dose therapy with stem cell rescue. The first myeloablative therapy employed a regimen of etoposide, carboplatin and cyclophosphamide, while the second included melphalan and TBI. An average of 7.2×10^6 CD34$^+$ cells/kg were available to support each cycle. Engraftment was rapid with median time to neutrophil engraftment of 11 days. Four patients who completed the first high-dose therapy course did not complete the second, and there were three toxic deaths. With a median follow-up of 22 months, 3-year EFS rate from diagnosis was 58%, an apparent improvement from previously reported studies. However, the follow-up is still short and the curve does not appear to have reached a plateau.

The pilot study reported by Kletzel et al. [77] has taken this strategy one step further, with a small group of patients undergoing three successive high-dose therapies followed by HCT. Preparative regimens for the first two high-dose courses with HCT consisted of carboplatin and etoposide, with a final third myeloablative course of thiotepa and cyclophosphamide. Of the initial 26 patients registered at diagnosis, 22 survived induction therapy without progression, with successful hematopoietic cell harvest and were able to proceed to high-dose therapy; of these, 19 were able to proceed to cycle 2, and only 17 to cycle 3, because of intervening toxicity. Three children had failure to engraft after the third myeloablative therapy, but the progression-free survival from diagnosis at 3 years was 57%. All patients on both of these tandem transplant studies received therapy for minimal residual disease with 13-cis-retinoic acid and, in some cases, anti-GD$_2$ monoclonal antibody.

Comparison of the multiple transplant outcomes from different studies is difficult, because of differing time to transplant, different hematopoietic cell sources and differing patient populations. The earlier studies included patients with more resistant disease, either by response status or patients with previous relapse. The two most recent US reports use an intent-to-treat analysis of EFS from diagnosis for all high-risk patients, which is harder to compare to studies that evaluate EFS from time of transplantation. However, these studies do show that repetitive transplants are feasible in the majority of patients who would be eligible for single myeloablative therapy, and suggest that EFS is not likely to be lower than in the previous studies. The possible added immunosuppressive effects, as well as the additional toxicity, hospitalization and cost will have to be evaluated and eventually justified by a prospective randomized comparison.

Targeted radionuclides as part of myeloablative therapy

Targeted radioisotope therapy using anti-GD$_2$ antibody or metaiodobenzylguanidine (MIBG) for delivery of radiation in the form of ^{131}iodine has also been tested extensively in clinical trials in relapsed neuroblastoma. Cheung et al. [78–80] have reported on the use of ^{131}I-3F8 for treatment of refractory neuroblastoma with documented responses, and now have an ongoing study for newly diagnosed patients using ^{131}I-3F8 in myeloablative doses followed by bone marrow rescue, then further treatment with cold antibody after transplant. ^{131}I-MIBG has been widely shown in European and US studies to elicit about a 30% response rate for refractory neuroblastoma [81–84]. More recently, it has also elicited responses as initial therapy for patients with regional disease [85,86]. A phase 1 dose escalation trial of ^{131}I-MIBG reported by Matthay et al. [81] determined the maximal nonmarrow-ablative dose (444 MBg/kg) and the maximal practical myeloablative dose with hematopoietic cell rescue (666 MBg/kg). In 30 patients, there was a 37% response rate and no significant toxicity other than hematologic. Based on this result, several pilot studies of ^{131}I-MIBG combined with marrow-ablative chemotherapy were undertaken, demonstrating the feasibility and engraftment using this approach [87,88]. The use of targeted radionuclides allows delivery of very large tumor doses with only minimal whole body doses of radiation [89].

Allogeneic bone marrow transplantation

Bone marrow involvement is present in >80% of patients at diagnosis, and residual tumor cells can still be detected in bone marrow samples by sensitive immunodetection methods even after several cycles of induction therapy. For this reason, allogeneic bone marrow transplantation (BMT) has been proposed as an alternative to autologous HCT. There has also been hope that the allogeneic cells will provide a further "graft-vs.-neuroblastoma" effect, although the rationale for this concept is weak, because neuroblastoma cells express little HLA class I antigens. To date, lack of evidence of any immunologic benefit, coupled with the problems with frequent lack of a HLA-compatible sibling donor and the significantly higher toxic death rates have discouraged extensive use of allogeneic transplantation. Most reports consist of fewer than 10 patients included in large groups of autologous transplants [50,59,65,90–93]. Nonrelapse death rates were generally higher than those reported for autologous transplants, in the range of 15–30%.

Two reports were found that directly compared allogeneic and autologous transplantation in neuroblastoma. The first was the CCG study from Matthay et al. [94] comparing two groups of patients in a pilot study, receiving the same induction and conditioning regimen, including 36 patients receiving an autologous purged bone marrow transplant and 20 similar patients with HLA-compatible sibling donors who received allogeneic BMT. There was no significant difference in relapse rate and an apparently higher toxicity in the allogeneic group. There were four of 20 deaths from causes other than relapse in the allogeneic group, compared to three of 36 in the autologous group (n.s.); the estimated progression-free survival was 25% for the allogeneic group vs. 49% for the autologous group ($p = 0.051$).

Ladenstein et al. [95] performed a case–control study using the EBMT Solid Tumor Registry to investigate the potential advantage of allogeneic bone marrow transplantation in high-risk neuroblastoma patients without prior disease progression. Seventeen allogeneic and 34 autologous BMT cases were matched based on a number of prognostic factors including age, sex, prior treatment duration, pregraft response status and bone and bone marrow involvement before BMT. The progression-free survival was not significantly different: 35% for autologous and 41% for allogeneic at 2 years, respectively. Nine of the allogeneic BMT patients had developed graft-vs.-host disease (GVHD): seven with grade I–II and only two with grade IV. The median donor age was very young with 74 months (range 20–240 months), which might explain the low GVHD rate.

Hematopoietic stem cell source and purging

Bone marrow involvement by neuroblastoma is extremely common in children with metastatic disease, present by light microscopy in 60–80% of children with INSS stage 4 disease at diagnosis [11]. Detection of tumor by immunocytology using a mixture of monoclonal antibodies reactive at the cell surface has recently been shown to reliably detect tumor with a sensitivity that may vary from $1/10^4$ to $1/10^6$ nucleated bone marrow cells, depending on the method used [48,96–108]. Evaluation of the efficacy of in vivo purging of tumor cells in bone marrow or blood may be a very important component of response evaluation. Assessment of tumor content may also be critical for evaluation of hematopoietic cell products, because the use of myeloablative therapy followed by HCT has been shown to be beneficial to EFS. Furthermore, because bone marrow or peripheral hematopoietic cells are necessary to reconstitute patients after myeloablative tumor therapy, an induction regimen capable of efficient tumor cell reduction in bone marrow may be important. The ability of reinfused occult tumor cells in bone marrow to cause relapse is demonstrated by the report that after infusion of unpurged autologous bone marrow marked with transduced neomycin-resistance gene, tumor cells in the recurrent neuroblastoma in all three cases showed the genetic marker [109]. The occasional reports of miliary lung relapse after autologous BMT, the site one would expect to be involved after intravenous infusion of tumor cells, supports the importance of tumor-free stem cells [110,111].

Circulating tumor cells can also be detected in the blood of up to 50% of children with INSS stage 4 neuroblastoma at diagnosis [100,106,112]. Furthermore, immunocytology has demonstrated that although marked reduction occurs in both bone marrow tumor and circulating tumor cells, contamination of bone marrow can be detected in 25% of bone marrow samples at the end of 3 months of induction chemotherapy, and in 7% of blood samples [106]. The efficacy of in vivo purging has been shown to correlate with EFS, such that patients with >0.1% tumor in bone marrow at the end of induction have a very poor outcome. Measurement of residual tumor cells in both blood and bone marrow by immunocytology and by the possibly more sensitive technique of reverse transcription-polymerase chain reaction (RT-PCR) may prove a useful surrogate marker of response and also predict impending relapse [106,112–114].

Various methods tested for ex vivo tumor cell removal from bone marrow in neuroblastoma patients include:
1 physical methods (sedimentation and filtration) [115];
2 chemical purging with 6-hydroxydopamine [116,117], Desferal [118,119] or mafosfamide [120–122]; or
3 immunologic methods with direct antibody plus complement [123–125] or immunomagnetic beads [48,126].

However, the most widely tested and validated method with 4–6 logs of tumor cell removal and no impairment of engraftment is immunomagnetic purging. The methodology was developed in the 1980s [48,126], then tested in pilot studies shortly thereafter demonstrating good engraftment [24,51,61]. This technique has been utilized in multi-institutional cooperative studies in Europe and the USA [2,127]. The large CCG study showed that bone marrow can be successfully harvested, shipped at room temperature overnight, purged using sedimentation, filtration and immunomagnetic bead separation, then cryopreserved without injury and with successful tumor cell removal and engraftment.

More recent studies have shown the feasibility of pheresis for peripheral hematopoietic cells on young children and more rapid engraftment using peripheral hematopoietic cells rather than bone marrow. There is an apparent attraction to using peripheral hematopoietic cells for HCT for solid tumors that infiltrate bone marrow, because one would expect fewer contaminating tumor cells in peripheral blood than bone marrow. None the less, up to 50% of neuroblastoma patients have circulating tumor cells at diagnosis [106], and pilot testing of peripheral blood stem cell collections have demonstrated tumor cell contamination by RT-PCR in patients who had been treated with multiple cycles of chemotherapy [97,114,128–130]. Although it is not clear what level of tumor contamination in infused grafts will cause regrowth of tumor cells, the study from the UK suggests that low levels of tumor in peripheral blood detected by RT-PCR do predict relapse [112].

Therefore, purging of peripheral blood stem cells is being studied, either by positive selection of CD34 cells, or by immunomagnetic purging using a similar method to that in bone marrow. Several studies have documented the feasibility and good engraftment after transplantation for neuroblastoma using CD34 selected hematopoietic cells [76,131–134]. There have also been several small pilot studies documenting tumor cell depletion using PCR techniques [132,135,136], despite some initial concerns that some neuroblastoma cell lines expressed CD34 antigen [137]. However, even after CD34 selection of hematopoietic cells, there have been reports of residual neuroblastoma tumor cells detected by immunocytology [138]. CD34 selection provides a relatively simple commercial method that can be utilized in most transplant centers. However, the frequency and clinical significance of tumor cell contamination must be closely monitored and studied. The other potential problem with CD34 selection is the occasional immune dysregulation, with reports of post-transplant lymphoproliferative disorders, otherwise rarely reported after autologous HCT [139,140].

The other approach under investigation for purging of hematopoietic stem cells uses a modified immunomagnetic purging method, which, after pilot testing in 20 patients with successful engraftment, is now being tested in a group-wide phase 3 Children's Oncology Group study (A3973, open September 2, 2001) for high-risk neuroblastoma. Protocol therapy consists of induction chemotherapy, hematopoietic cell harvest, radiation to the primary tumor bed, myeloablative therapy with HCT, followed by 13-*cis*-retinoic acid. Patients are randomized at the time of study registration to either purged or unpurged peripheral blood stem cells as stem cell source for myeloablative consolidation. Hematopoietic cells are harvested after the first two cycles of induction chemotherapy. For purging, the cells are sedimented with hetastarch, then excess phagocytic cells removed with carbonyl iron, followed by treatment with monoclonal antibodies attached to magnetic immunobeads and magnetic separation and cryopreservation. An aliquot of the treated product is analyzed to determine if all detectable neuroblastoma cells were removed and to quantify viable cells, colony-forming unit–granulocyte/macrophage (CFU-GM) and $CD34^+$ cells (before and after freezing). If no tumor cells are detectable and if adequate normal cells are present, the hematopoietic cells are suitable for reinfusion; if not, the product cannot be used and a second harvest or alternative therapy is necessary. Endpoints will include EFS, time to engraftment and tumor content by RT-PCR analysis before and after purging.

Treatment of minimal residual disease

Despite improvements in EFS using myeloablative therapy, the relapse rate—even for patients transplanted in complete response—remains high [2,24]. For this reason, it has become increasingly important to find new approaches to eliminate minimal residual disease with agents that will be tolerable following myeloablative therapy. Immediately after HCT, when disease is likely to be minimal, provides the ideal window of time to eradicate resistant clones that are still present using novel therapies not dependent upon standard cytotoxic mechanisms.

In vitro, both all-*trans*-retinoic acid and 13-*cis*-retinoic acid cause decreased proliferation and differentiation in neuroblastoma cell lines, including some established from refractory tumors [141–143]. A phase 2 trial in children with relapsed neuroblastoma using 13-*cis*-retinoic acid on a single daily administration schedule of 100 mg/m^2 showed responses in only two of 22 patients [144]. However, based on *in vitro* experiments with higher intermittent dosage, a phase 1 trial in children with high-risk neuroblastoma post-HCT determined that a high-dose intermittent schedule of 13-*cis*-retinoic acid following BMT had minimal toxicity, achieved levels that were effective against neuroblastoma cell lines *in vitro* and resulted in complete bone marrow responses in three of 10 patients [145]. These data indicate that 13-*cis*-retinoic acid is well-tolerated after intensive chemoradiotherapy and may have efficacy

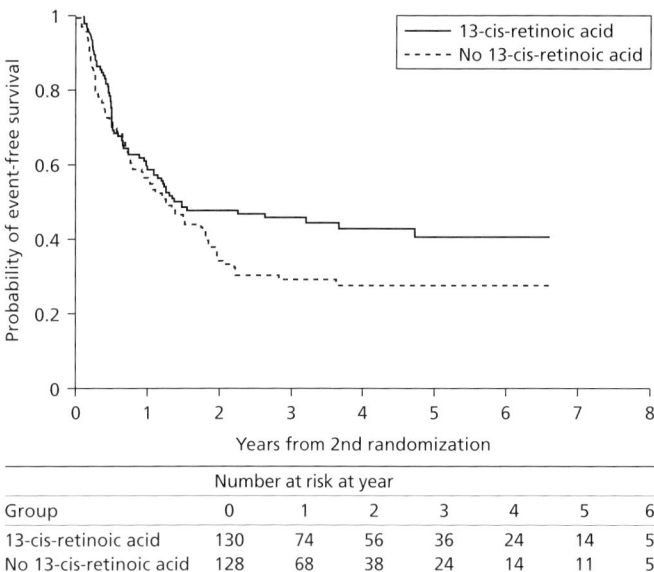

Fig. 97.3 Treatment of minimal residual disease with 13-*cis*-retinoic acid improves event-free survival (EFS) after consolidation with standard chemotherapy or myeloablative therapy ($p = 0.027$) [2].

against minimal residual disease. A subsequent phase 3 randomized trial by the CCG of children with high-risk neuroblastoma completing consolidation chemotherapy or ABMT showed that the use of oral 13-*cis*-retinoic acid following intensive therapy improves outcome. The 3-year EFS from time of randomization was significantly better for the patients randomized to 13-*cis*-retinoic acid ($46 \pm 6\%$), compared to those randomized to no further therapy ($29 \pm 5\%$; $p = 0.03$) (Fig. 97.3) [2]. Other retinoids are currently under investigation for use in minimal residual disease, such as fenretinide. In contrast to *cis*- and *trans*-retinoic acid, fenretinide does not induce maturational changes, but is cytotoxic and induces both apoptosis and necrosis [146,147]. Phase 1 studies of fenretinide in refractory neuroblastoma have been completed in the CCG and in Europe [148], and a phase 2 COG study is currently being undertaken.

Another approach to minimal residual disease post-transplant is the use of antibody-targeted therapy. Antibody therapy in relapsed neuroblastoma using murine, chimeric and humanized antibodies against the membrane ganglioside GD_2 has provided promising response and toxicity profiles which warrant the further investigation of these agents in randomized studies [149–155]. With GM-CSF or interleukin 2 (IL-2), anti-GD_2 seems to be tolerated in patients who have undergone ABMT [153,156]. A new randomized prospective trial of the use of chimeric anti-GD_2 antibody with granulocyte macrophage colony-stimulating factor (GM-CSF) and IL-2 is underway in the Children's Oncology Group. Patients who are in remission after high-dose therapy and HCT are randomized to receive either 13-*cis*-retinoic acid alone or the retinoid along with chimeric anti-GD_2 antibody (Ch14.18) and GM-CSF and IL-2. Further improvements are being tested in phase 1 trials using a fusion protein of the humanized form of the antibody, Hu14.18, and IL-2. This immunocytokine has the advantage of working simultaneously through both antibody-dependent cytotoxicity and natural killer cell mechanisms [153]. A murine neuroblastoma model showed superior activity of the immunocytokine to the physical mixture of the antibody and cytokine [157].

Other approaches to minimal residual disease in the future may utilize genetically engineered vaccines to generate immune response [158–162]. Another possible avenue would be to utilize antiangiogenic therapy post-transplantation. Angiogenesis appears to have a major role in progression of neuroblastoma, as multiple proteins associated with angiogenesis have been shown to be associated with more advanced disease or worse prognosis [163–166]. Testing in animal models suggests responsiveness to angiogenic inhibitors, particularly in minimal disease states [167].

Acute and late complications of HCT in neuroblastoma

The complications of myeloablative therapy and transplantation are similar to those of other high-dose regimens, and vary with the particular conditioning regimen. These are discussed in detail in Section IV of this book. The most common acute complications with most preparative regimens for neuroblastoma include the toxic effects of the high-dose therapy, with frequent mucositis, veno-occlusive disease (VOD), fever and infection. Potentially fatal complications include gastrointestinal hemorrhage, pneumonitis and acute respiratory distress syndrome (ARDS), severe VOD with renal failure or, rarely, intracranial hemorrhage or cardiac failure. Toxic death rates generally have ranged from 5 to 20% on autologous transplant protocols (Table 97.3). With increasing expertise, more rapid engraftment with peripheral hematopoietic cells, and the removal of TBI from most regimens, the acute toxic death rate appears to be decreasing to about 5% [32,68,69].

With more patients surviving, some of the later complications of the myeloablative therapy are becoming more troublesome. New studies examining quality of life in survivors will assume greater importance. One common complication particular to neuroblastoma is the frequent occurrence of significant hearing loss post-transplant seen in 10–20% of children. These patients receive large does of platinum compounds during induction chemotherapy and again with many of the preparative regimens. They also are exposed to other ototoxins, including aminoglycoside antibiotics, diuretics and noise exposure—all of which may exacerbate the effects of carboplatin [168,169]. Other late effects are attributable to the high-dose chemotherapy and/or TBI, and are common to many pediatric regimens. However, the developmental and growth effects are magnified, because the median age for transplant in a child with neuroblastoma would be only about 3 years. These include hormonal deficiencies resulting in growth retardation, abnormal dental development, thyroid dysfunction, sterility or delayed onset of puberty, osteochondromas and secondary malignancies. Earlier studies of transplant in neuroblastoma reported a low incidence of second malignancies, with only one patient in 129 in the CCG study [2] and two of 509 patient in the EBMT Registry report [54]. However, secondary malignancies may become a more vexing problem in children transplanted for neuroblastoma, as the high doses of alkylators and etoposide in both the induction and conditioning regimens have been shown to result in secondary leukemia [30]. Some children have now been reported to develop secondary leukemia after radiotargeted therapy for neuroblastoma [81,170]. In addition, some quite unusual second malignancies have been reported after transplantation for neuroblastoma, such as renal cell carcinoma [171,172]. Further genetic studies will improve the understanding of the etiology and eventually prevention of these cancers [173].

Conclusions

The use of myeloablative chemotherapy has been shown to increase the response rate and to improve EFS in children with advanced neuroblastoma. It is likely that this approach has also contributed to the significant overall increase in survival for children diagnosed >1 year of age with stage 4 neuroblastoma, seen over the last two decades. However, a large number of patients with long-term follow-up would be required to show definitive improvement in survival using transplantation. The tumor reduction during the transplant conditioning regimen may be further improved by eliminating TBI, using radio-immunotargeted therapy, and new noncross-resistant agents. Second, it has been shown that therapy for minimal residual disease post-transplant is also a critical component of the improvement in outcome for these patients. New targeted approaches to minimal residual disease deserve study, including genetic targeting, differentiating agents, antiangiogenic and immunologic pathways. Third, with this improved outcome, it is critical to refine the therapy of these children to reduce the serious late complications of treatment and to study health-related quality of life in the survivors.

References

1 Goodman MT, Gurney JG, Smith MA, Olshan AFP. Sympathetic nervous system tumors. In: Ries LAG, Smith MA, Gurney JG, et al. eds. *Cancer Incidence and Survival Among Children and Adolescents: USA SEER Program 1975–95*. Bethesda, MD: National Cancer Institute, SEER Program, 1999: 65–72.

2 Matthay KK, Villablanca JG, Seeger RC et al. Treatment of high-risk neuroblastoma with intensive chemotherapy, radiotherapy, autologous bone marrow transplantation, and 13-*cis*-retinoic acid: Children's Cancer Group. *N Engl J Med* 1999; **341**: 1165–73.

3 Matthay KK. Neuroblastoma: a clinical challenge and biologic puzzle. *CA Cancer J Clin* 1995; **45**: 179–92.

4 Plantaz D, Rubie H, Michon J et al. The treatment of neuroblastoma with intraspinal extension with chemotherapy followed by surgical removal of residual disease: a prospective study of 42 patients. Results of the NBL 90 Study of the French Society of Pediatric Oncology. *Cancer* 1996; **78**: 311–9.

5 Hoover M, Bowman LC, Crawford SE et al. Long-term outcome of patients with intraspinal neuroblastoma. *Med Pediatr Oncol* 1999; **32**: 353–9.

6 Hsu LL, Evans AE, D'Angio GJ. Hepatomegaly in neuroblastoma stage 4S: criteria for treatment of the vulnerable neonate. *Med Pediatr Oncol* 1996; **27**: 521–8.

7 Rudnick E, Khakoo Y, Antunes NL et al. Opsoclonus–myoclonus–ataxia syndrome in neuroblastoma: clinical outcome and antineuronal antibodies. A report from the Children's Cancer Group Study. *Med Pediatr Oncol* 2001; **36**: 612–22.

8 Russo C, Cohn SL, Petruzzi MJ, de Alarcon PA. Long-term neurologic outcome in children with opsoclonus–myoclonus associated with neuroblastoma: a report from the Pediatric Oncology Group. *Med Pediatr Oncol* 1997; **28**: 284–8.

9 Antunes NL, Khakoo Y, Matthay KK et al. Antineuronal antibodies in patients with neuroblastoma and paraneoplastic opsoclonus–myoclonus. *J Pediatr Hematol Oncol* 2000; **22**: 315–20.

10 Brodeur GM, Pritchard J, Berthold F et al. Revisions of the international criteria for neuroblastoma diagnosis, staging, and response to treatment. *J Clin Oncol* 1993; **11**: 1466–77 [see comments].

11 DuBois SG, Kalika Y, Lukens JN et al. Metastatic sites in stage IV and IVS neuroblastoma correlate with age, tumor biology, and survival. *J Pediatr Hematol Oncol* 1999; **21**: 181–9 [see comments].

12 Perez CA, Matthay KK, Atkinson JB et al. Biologic variables in the outcome of stages I and II neuroblastoma treated with surgery as primary therapy: a Children's Cancer Group study. *J Clin Oncol* 2000; **18**: 18–26.

13 Matthay KK, Perez C, Seeger RC et al. Successful treatment of stage III neuroblastoma based on prospective biologic staging: a Children's Cancer Group study. *J Clin Oncol* 1998; **16**: 1256–64.

14 Schmidt ML, Lukens JN, Seeger RC et al. Biologic factors determine prognosis in infants with stage IV neuroblastoma: a prospective Children's Cancer Group study. *J Clin Oncol* 2000; **18**: 1260–8.

15 Maris JM, Matthay KK. Molecular biology of neuroblastoma. *J Clin Oncol* 1999; **17**: 2264.

16 Seeger RC, Brodeur GM, Sather H et al. Association of multiple copies of the N-*myc* oncogene with rapid progression of neuroblastomas. *N Engl J Med* 1985; **313**: 1111–6.

17 Shimada H, Umehara S, Monobe Y et al. International neuroblastoma pathology classification for prognostic evaluation of patients with peripheral neuroblastic tumors: a report from the Children's Cancer Group. *Cancer* 2001; **92**: 2451–61.

18 Castleberry RP, Shuster JJ, Smith EI. The Pediatric Oncology Group experience with the international staging system criteria for neuroblastoma: Member Institutions of the Pediatric Oncology Group. *J Clin Oncol* 1994; **12**: 2378–81.

19 Ikeda H, Iehara T, Tsuchida Y *et al*. Experience with International Neuroblastoma Staging System and Pathology Classification. *Br J Cancer* 2002; **86**: 1110–16.

20 Bowman LC, Castleberry RP, Cantor A *et al*. Genetic staging of unresectable or metastatic neuroblastoma in infants: a Pediatric Oncology Group study. *J Natl Cancer Inst* 1997; **89**: 373–80.

21 Nickerson HJ, Matthay KK, Seeger RC *et al*. Favorable biology and outcome of stage IV-S neuroblastoma with supportive care or minimal therapy: a Children's Cancer Group study. *J Clin Oncol* 2000; **18**: 477–86.

22 Matthay KK. Neuroblastoma: biology and therapy. *Oncology* 1997; **11**: 1857–66; discussion 1869–72; 1875.

23 Matthay KK, Castleberry RP. Treatment of advanced neuroblastoma: the US experience. In: Brodeur GM, Sawada T, Tsuchida Y, Voûte PA, eds. *Neuroblastoma*. Amsterdam: Elsevier Science, 2000: 417–36.

24 Matthay KK, Atkinson JB, Stram DO, Selch M, Reynolds CP, Seeger RC. Patterns of relapse after autologous purged bone marrow transplantation for neuroblastoma: a Children's Cancer Group pilot study. *J Clin Oncol* 1993; **11**: 2226–33.

25 Castleberry RP, Cantor AB, Green AA *et al*. Phase II investigational window using carboplatin, iproplatin, ifosfamide, and epirubicin in children with untreated disseminated neuroblastoma: a Pediatric Oncology Group study. *J Clin Oncol* 1994; **12**: 1616–20 [see comments].

26 Coze C, Hartmann O, Michon J *et al*. NB87 induction protocol for stage 4 neuroblastoma in children over 1 year of age: a report from the French Society of Pediatric Oncology. *J Clin Oncol* 1997; **15**: 3433–40.

27 Kaneko M, Tsuchida Y, Uchino J *et al*. Treatment results of advanced neuroblastoma with the first Japanese study group protocol: Study Group of Japan for Treatment of Advanced Neuroblastoma. *J Pediatr Hematol Oncol* 1999; **21**: 190–7 [see comments].

28 Kretschmar CS, Kletzel K, Murray K, Smith EI, Marcus R, Castleberry R. Phase II therapy with taxol and topotecan in untreated children (>365 days) with disseminated (INSS stage 4) neuroblastoma (NB): a POG study. *Med Pediatr Oncol* 1995; **24**: 243.

29 Kushner BH, LaQuaglia MP, Bonilla MA *et al*. Highly effective induction therapy for stage 4 neuroblastoma in children over 1 year of age. *J Clin Oncol* 1994; **12**: 2607–13.

30 Kushner BH, Cheung NK, Kramer K, Heller G, Jhanwar SC. Neuroblastoma and treatment-related myelodysplasia/leukemia: the Memorial Sloan-Kettering experience and a literature review. *J Clin Oncol* 1998; **16**: 3880–9.

31 Ikeda H, August CS, Goldwein JW, Ross AJ, D'Angio GJ, Evans AE. Sites of relapse in patients with neuroblastoma following bone marrow transplantation in relation to preparatory "debulking" treatments. *J Pediatr Surg* 1992; **27**: 1438–41.

32 Villablanca JG, Matthay KK, Swift PS *et al*. Phase I trial of carboplatin, etoposide, melphalan and local irradiation (CEM-LI) with purged autologous bone marrow transplantation for children with high risk neuroblastoma. *Med Pediatr Oncol* 1999; **33**: 170.

33 Powis MR, Imeson JD, Holmes SJ. The effect of complete excision on stage III neuroblastoma: a report of the European Neuroblastoma Study Group. *J Pediatr Surg* 1996; **31**: 516–9.

34 Haase GM, Atkinson JB, Stram DO, Lukens JN, Matthay KK. Surgical management and outcome of locoregional neuroblastoma: comparison of the Children's Cancer Group and the International Staging Systems. *J Pediatr Surg* 1995; **30**: 289–95.

35 Haase GM, O'Leary MC, Ramsay NK *et al*. Aggressive surgery combined with intensive chemotherapy improves survival in poor-risk neuroblastoma. *J Pediatr Surg* 1991; **26**: 1119–23; discussion 1123–4 [see comments].

36 Halperin EC, Cox EB. Radiation therapy in the management of neuroblastoma: the Duke University Medical Center experience, 1967–84. *Int J Radiat Oncol Biol Phys* 1986; **12**: 1829–37.

37 Kaneko M, Ohakawa H, Iwakawa M. Is extensive surgery required for treatment of advanced neuroblastoma? *J Pediatr Surg* 1997; **32**: 1616–9.

38 Shorter NA, Davidoff AM, Evans AE, Ross A Jr, Zeigler MM, O'Neill JA Jr. The role of surgery in the management of stage IV neuroblastoma: a single institution study. *Med Pediatr Oncol* 1995; **24**: 287–91.

39 Matsumura M, Atkinson JB, Hays DM *et al*. An evaluation of the role of surgery in metastatic neuroblastoma. *J Pediatr Surg* 1988; **23**: 448–53.

40 La Quaglia MP, Kushner BH, Heller G, Bonilla MA, Lindsley KL, Cheung NK. Stage 4 neuroblastoma diagnosed at more than 1 year of age: gross total resection and clinical outcome. *J Pediatr Surg* 1994; **29**: 1162–5; discussion 1165–6.

41 Castleberry RP, Kun LE, Shuster JJ *et al*. Radiotherapy improves the outlook for patients older than 1 year with Pediatric Oncology Group stage C neuroblastoma. *J Clin Oncol* 1991; **9**: 789–95 [see comments].

42 Wolden SL, Gollamudi SV, Kushner BH *et al*. Local control with multimodality therapy for Stage 4 neuroblastoma. *Int J Radiat Oncol Biol Phys* 2000; **46**: 969–74.

43 Haas-Kogan DA, Fisch BM, Wara WM *et al*. Intraoperative radiation therapy for high-risk pediatric neuroblastoma. *Int J Radiat Oncol Biol Phys* 2000; **47**: 985–92.

44 Haase GM, Meagher DP Jr, McNeely LK *et al*. Electron beam intraoperative radiation therapy for pediatric neoplasms. *Cancer* 1994; **74**: 740–7.

45 Frei E 3rd, Teicher BA, Holden SA, Cathcart KN, Wang YY. Preclinical studies and clinical correlation of the effect of alkylating dose. *Cancer Res* 1988; **48**: 6417–23.

46 Keshelava N, Seeger RC, Groshen S, Reynolds CP. Drug resistance patterns in human neuroblastoma cell lines derived from patients at different phases of therapy. *Cancer Res* 1998; **58**: 5396–405.

47 Frei E 3rd, Antman K, Teicher B, Eder P, Schnipper L. Bone marrow autotransplantation for solid tumors: prospects. *J Clin Oncol* 1989; **7**: 515–26.

48 Reynolds CP, Seeger RC, Vo DD, Black AT, Wells J, Ugelstad J. Model system for removing neuroblastoma cells from bone marrow using monoclonal antibodies and magnetic immunobeads. *Cancer Res* 1986; **46**: 5882–6.

49 Kemshead JT, Heath L, Gibson FM *et al*. Magnetic microspheres and monoclonal antibodies for the depletion of neuroblastoma cells from bone marrow: experiences, improvements and observations. *Br J Cancer* 1986; **54**: 771–8.

50 August CS, Serota FT, Koch PA *et al*. Treatment of advanced neuroblastoma with supralethal chemotherapy, radiation, and allogeneic or autologous marrow reconstitution. *J Clin Oncol* 1984; **2**: 609–16.

51 Philip T, Bernard JL, Zucker JM *et al*. High-dose chemoradiotherapy with bone marrow transplantation as consolidation treatment in neuroblastoma: an unselected group of stage IV patients over 1 year of age. *J Clin Oncol* 1987; **5**: 266–71.

52 Seeger RC, Reynolds CP. Treatment of high-risk solid tumors of childhood with intensive therapy and autologous bone marrow transplantation. *Pediatr Clin North Am* 1991; **38**: 393–424.

53 Graham-Pole J, Casper J, Elfenbein G *et al*. High-dose chemoradiotherapy supported by marrow infusions for advanced neuroblastoma: a Pediatric Oncology Group study. *J Clin Oncol* 1991; **9**: 152–8.

54 Dini G, Philip T, Hartmann O *et al*. Bone marrow transplantation for neuroblastoma: a review of 509 cases: EBMT Group. *Bone Marrow Transplant* 1989; **4** (Suppl. 4): 42–6.

55 Dini G, Lanino E, Garaventa A *et al*. Myeloablative therapy and unpurged autologous bone marrow transplantation for poor-prognosis neuroblastoma: report of 34 cases. *J Clin Oncol* 1991; **9**: 962–9.

56 Matthay KK, Yamashiro D. Neuroblastoma. In: Bast RC, Kufe DW, Pollock RE, Weichselbaum RR, Holland JF, Frei E, eds. *Cancer Medicine*. London: B.C. Decker, 2000: 2185–97.

57 Hartmann O, Benhamou E, Beaujean F, Kalifa C, Lejars O, Patte C *et al*. Repeated high-dose chemotherapy followed by purged autologous bone marrow transplantation as consolidation therapy in metastatic neuroblastoma. *J Clin Oncol* 1987; **5**: 1205–11.

58 Pinkerton CR. ENSG 1-randomised study of high-dose melphalan in neuroblastoma. *Bone Marrow Transplant* 1991; **7** (Suppl. 3): 112–3.

59 Pole JG, Casper J, Elfenbein G *et al*. High-dose chemoradiotherapy supported by marrow infusions for advanced neuroblastoma: a Pediatric Oncology Group study. *J Clin Oncol* 1991; **9**: 152–8. [Published erratum appears in *J Clin Oncol* 1991; **9**: 1094.]

60 Stram DO, Matthay KK, O'Leary M *et al*. Consolidation chemoradiotherapy and autologous bone marrow transplantation versus continued chemotherapy for metastatic neuroblastoma: a report of two concurrent Children's Cancer Group studies. *J Clin Oncol* 1996; **14**: 2417–26 [see comments].

61 Seeger RC, Villablanca JG, Matthay KK *et al*. Intensive chemoradiotherapy and autologous bone marrow transplantation for poor prognosis neuroblastoma. *Prog Clin Biol Res* 1991; **366**: 527–33.

62 Philip T, Zucker JM, Bernard JL *et al*. Improved survival at 2 and 5 years in the LMCE1 unselected group of 72 children with stage IV neuroblastoma older than 1 year of age at diagnosis: is cure possible in a small subgroup? *J Clin Oncol* 1991; **9**: 1037–44.

63 Kushner BH, O'Reilly RJ, Mandell LR, Gulati SC, LaQuaglia M, Cheung NK. Myeloablative combination chemotherapy without total body irradiation for neuroblastoma. *J Clin Oncol* 1991; **9**: 274–9.

64 Ohnuma N, Takahashi H, Kaneko M *et al*. Treatment combined with bone marrow transplantation for advanced neuroblastoma: an analysis of patients who were pretreated intensively with the protocol of the Study Group of Japan. *Med Pediatr Oncol* 1995; **24**: 181–7.

65 Kamani N, August CS, Bunin N et al. A study of thiotepa, etoposide and fractionated total body irradiation as a preparative regimen prior to bone marrow transplantation for poor prognosis patients with neuroblastoma. *Bone Marrow Transplant* 1996; **17**: 911–6.

66 Hero B, Kremens B, Klingebiel T et al. Does megatherapy contribute to survival in metastatic neuroblastoma? A retrospective analysis: German Cooperative Neuroblastoma Study Group. *Klin Padiatr* 1997; **209**: 196–200.

67 Ladenstein R, Philip T, Lasset C et al. Multivariate analysis of risk factors in stage 4 neuroblastoma patients over the age of 1 year treated with megatherapy and stem-cell transplantation: a report from the European Bone Marrow Transplantation Solid Tumor Registry. *J Clin Oncol* 1998; **16**: 953–65.

68 Kletzel M, Abella EM, Sandler ES et al. Thiotepa and cyclophosphamide with stem cell rescue for consolidation therapy for children with high-risk neuroblastoma: a phase I/II study of the Pediatric Blood and Marrow Transplant Consortium. *J Pediatr Hematol Oncol* 1998; **20**: 49–54.

69 Hartmann O, Valteau-Couanet D, Vassal G et al. Prognostic factors in metastatic neuroblastoma in patients over 1 year of age treated with high-dose chemotherapy and stem cell transplantation: a multivariate analysis in 218 patients treated in a single institution. *Bone Marrow Transplant* 1999; **23**: 789–95.

70 Castel V, Canete A, Navarro S et al. Outcome of high-risk neuroblastoma using a dose intensity approach: improvement in initial but not in long-term results. *Med Pediatr Oncol* 2001; **37**: 537–42.

71 Shuster JJ, Cantor AB, McWilliams N et al. The prognostic significance of autologous bone marrow transplant in advanced neuroblastoma. *J Clin Oncol* 1991; **9**: 1045–9 [see comments].

72 Park JR, Slattery J, Gooley T et al. Phase I topotecan preparative regimen for high-risk neuroblastoma, high-grade glioma, and refractory/recurrent pediatric solid tumors. *Med Pediatr Oncol* 2000; **35**: 719–23.

73 Philip T, Ladenstein R, Lasset C et al. 1070 myeloablative megatherapy procedures followed by stem cell rescue for neuroblastoma: 17 years of European experience and conclusions. European Group for Blood and Marrow Transplant Registry Solid Tumour Working Party. *Eur J Cancer* 1997; **33**: 2130–5.

74 Philip T, Ladenstein R, Zucker JM et al. Double megatherapy and autologous bone marrow transplantation for advanced neuroblastoma: the LMCE2 study. *Br J Cancer* 1993; **67**: 119–27.

75 Frappaz D, Michon J, Coze C et al. LMCE3 treatment strategy: results in 99 consecutively diagnosed stage 4 neuroblastomas in children older than 1 year at diagnosis. *J Clin Oncol* 2000; **18**: 468–76.

76 Grupp SA, Stern JW, Bunin N et al. Tandem high-dose therapy in rapid sequence for children with high-risk neuroblastoma. *J Clin Oncol* 2000; **18**: 2567–75.

77 Kletzel M, Katzenstein HM, Haut PR et al. Treatment of high-risk neuroblastoma with triple-tandem high-dose therapy and stem-cell rescue: results of the Chicago Pilot II Study. *J Clin Oncol* 2002; **20**: 2284–92.

78 Cheung NK, Yeh SD, Gulati S et al. 131I–3F8: clinical validation of imaging studies and therapeutic applications. *Prog Clin Biol Res* 1991; **366**: 409–15.

79 Cheung NK, Munn D, Kushner BH, Usmani N, Yeh SD. Targeted radiotherapy and immunotherapy of human neuroblastoma with GD_2 specific monoclonal antibodies. *Int J Rad Appl Instrum [B]* 1989; **16**: 111–20.

80 Cheung NK, Miraldi FD. Iodine 131 labeled GD_2 monoclonal antibody in the diagnosis and therapy of human neuroblastoma. *Prog Clin Biol Res* 1988; **271**: 595–604.

81 Matthay KK, DeSantes K, Hasegawa B et al. Phase I dose escalation of ^{131}I-metaiodobenzylguanidine with autologous bone marrow support in refractory neuroblastoma. *J Clin Oncol* 1998; **16**: 229–36.

82 Klingebiel T, Berthold F, Treuner J et al. Meta-iodobenzylguanidine mIBG in treatment of 47 patients with neuroblastoma: results of the German Neuroblastoma Trial. *Med Pediatr Oncol* 1991; **19**: 84–8.

83 Lashford LS, Lewis IJ, Fielding SL et al. Phase I/II study of iodine 131 metaiodobenzylguanidine in chemoresistant neuroblastoma: a UK Children's Cancer Study Group investigation. *J Clin Oncol* 1992; **10**: 1889–96.

84 Treuner J, Gerein V, Klingebiel T et al. MIBG-treatment in neuroblastoma: experiences of the Tubingen/Frankfurt group. *Prog Clin Biol Res* 1988; **271**: 669–78.

85 Hoefnagel CA, De Kraker J, Valdes Olmos RA, Voute PA. [^{131}I]MIBG as a first line treatment in advanced neuroblastoma. *Q J Nucl Med* 1995; **39** (4 Suppl. 1): 61–4.

86 Mastrangelo R, Tornesello A, Riccardi R et al. A new approach in the treatment of stage IV neuroblastoma using a combination of [^{131}I]meta-iodobenzylguanidine (MIBG) and cisplatin. *Eur J Cancer* 1995; **31A**: 606–11.

87 Klingebiel T, Bader P, Bares R et al. Treatment of neuroblastoma stage 4 with ^{131}I-meta-iodo-benzylguanidine, high-dose chemotherapy and immunotherapy: a pilot study. *Eur J Cancer* 1998; **34**: 1398–402.

88 Yanik GA, Levine JE, Matthay KK et al. Pilot study of iodine-131-metaiodobenzylguanidine in combination with myeloablative chemotherapy and autologous stem-cell support for the treatment of neuroblastoma. *J Clin Oncol* 2002; **20**: 2142–9.

89 Matthay KK, Panina C, Huberty J et al. Correlation of tumor and whole-body dosimetry with tumor response and toxicity in refractory neuroblastoma treated with (131)I-MIBG. *J Nucl Med* 2001; **42**: 1713–21.

90 Evans AE, August CS, Kamani N et al. Bone marrow transplantation for high risk neuroblastoma at the Children's Hospital of Philadelphia: an update. *Med Pediatr Oncol* 1994; **23**: 323–7.

91 Kremens B, Klingebiel T, Herrmann F et al. High-dose consolidation with local radiation and bone marrow rescue in patients with advanced neuroblastoma. *Med Pediatr Oncol* 1994; **23**: 470–5.

92 Dopfer R, Berthold F, Einsele H et al. Bone marrow transplantation in children with neuroblastoma. *Folia Haematol Int Mag Klin Morph Blutforsch* 1989; **116**: 427–36.

93 Garaventa A, Rondelli R, Lanino E et al. Myeloablative therapy and bone marrow rescue in advanced neuroblastoma. Report from the Italian Bone Marrow Transplant Registry. Italian Association of Pediatric Hematology–Oncology, BMT Group. *Bone Marrow Transplant* 1996; **18**: 125–30.

94 Matthay KK, Seeger RC, Reynolds CP et al. Allogeneic versus autologous purged bone marrow transplantation for neuroblastoma: a report from the Children's Cancer Group. *J Clin Oncol* 1994; **12**: 2382–9.

95 Ladenstein R, Lasset C, Hartmann O et al. Comparison of auto versus allografting as consolidation of primary treatments in advanced neuroblastoma over 1 year of age at diagnosis: report from the European Group for Bone Marrow Transplantation. *Bone Marrow Transplant* 1994; **14**: 37–46.

96 Nagai J, Kigasawa H, Tomioka K, Koga N, Nishihira H, Nagao T. Immunocytochemical detection of bone marrow-invasive neuroblastoma cells. *Eur J Haematol* 1994; **53**: 74–7.

97 Moss TJ. Tumor contamination in stem cell products from patients with neuroblastoma and breast cancer. *Bone Marrow Transplant* 1996; **18** (Suppl. 1): S17.

98 Saarinen UM, Wikstrom S, Makipernaa A et al. In vivo purging of bone marrow in children with poor-risk neuroblastoma for marrow collection and autologous bone marrow transplantation. *J Clin Oncol* 1996; **14**: 2791–802.

99 Moss TJ. Sensitive detection of metastatic tumor cells in bone marrow. *Prog Clin Biol Res* 1994; **389**: 567–77.

100 Moss TJ, Cairo M, Santana VM, Weinthal J, Hurvitz C, Bostrom B. Clonogenicity of circulating neuroblastoma cells: implications regarding peripheral blood stem cell transplantation. *Blood* 1994; **83**: 3085–9.

101 Miyajima Y, Kato K, Numata S, Kudo K, Horibe K. Detection of neuroblastoma cells in bone marrow and peripheral blood at diagnosis by the reverse transcriptase-polymerase chain reaction for tyrosine hydroxylase mRNA. *Cancer* 1995; **75**: 2757–61.

102 Cheung NK, Saarinen UM, Neely JE, Landmeier B, Donovan D, Coccia PF. Monoclonal antibodies to a glycolipid antigen on human neuroblastoma cells. *Cancer Res* 1985; **45**: 2642–9.

103 Berthold F, Schneider A, Schumacher R, Bosslet K. Detection of minimal disease in bone marrow of neuroblastoma patients by immunofluorescence. *Pediatr Hematol Oncol* 1989; **6**: 73–83.

104 Moss TJ, Reynolds CP, Sather HN, Romansky SG, Hammond GD, Seeger RC. Prognostic value of immunocytologic detection of bone marrow metastases in neuroblastoma. *N Engl J Med* 1991; **324**: 219–26.

105 Moss TJ, Xu ZJ, Mansour VH et al. Quantitation of tumor cell removal from bone marrow: a preclinical model. *J Hematother* 1992; **1**: 65–73.

106 Seeger RC, Reynolds CP, Gallego R, Stram DO, Gerbing RB, Matthay KK. Quantitative tumor cell content of bone marrow and blood as a predictor of outcome in stage IV neuroblastoma: a Children's Cancer Group Study. *J Clin Oncol* 2000; **18**: 4067–76.

107 Cheung NK, Heller G, Kushner BH, Liu C, Cheung IY. Detection of metastatic neuroblastoma in bone marrow: when is routine marrow histology insensitive? *J Clin Oncol* 1997; **15**: 2807–17.

108 Reid MM, Wallis JP, McGuckin AG, Pearson AD, Malcolm AJ. Routine histological compared with immunohistological examination of bone marrow trephine biopsy specimens in disseminated neuroblastoma. *J Clin Pathol* 1991; **44**: 483–6.

109 Rill DR, Santana VM, Roberts WM et al. Direct demonstration that autologous bone marrow transplantation for solid tumors can return a multiplicity of tumorigenic cells. *Blood* 1994; **84**: 380–3.

110 Kalra R, Zoger S, Kosovich MS, Matthay KK. Radiological case of the month: miliary pulmonary neuroblastoma. *Arch Pediatr Adolesc Med* 1995; **149**: 195–6.

111 Watts RG, Mroczek-Musulman E. Pulmonary interstitial disease mimicking idiopathic pneumonia syndrome as the initial site of relapse of neuroblastoma following autologous bone-marrow transplantation: a case report. *Am J Hematol* 1996; **53**: 137–40.

112 Burchill SA, Lewis IJ, Abrams KR et al. Circulating neuroblastoma cells detected by reverse transcriptase-polymerase chain reaction for tyrosine hydroxylase mRNA are an independent poor prognostic indicator in stage 4 neuroblastoma in children over 1 year. *J Clin Oncol* 2001; **19**: 1795–801.

113 Kuroda T, Saeki M, Nakano M, Mizutani S. Clinical application of minimal residual neuroblastoma cell detection by reverse transcriptase-polymerase chain reaction. *J Pediatr Surg* 1997; **32**: 69–72.

114 Tchirkov A, Kanold J, Giollant M et al. Molecular monitoring of tumor cell contamination in leukapheresis products from stage IV neuroblastoma patients before and after positive CD34 selection. *Med Pediatr Oncol* 1998; **30**: 228–32.

115 Figdor CG, Voute PA, de Kraker J, Vernie LN, Bont WS. Physical cell separation of neuroblastoma cells from bone marrow. *Prog Clin Biol Res* 1985; **175**: 459–70.

116 Reynolds CP, Reynolds DA, Frenkel EP, Smith RG. Selective toxicity of 6-hydroxydopamine and ascorbate for human neuroblastoma *in vitro*: a model for clearing marrow prior to autologous transplant. *Cancer Res* 1982; **42**: 1331–6.

117 Kushner BH, Gulati SC, Kwon JH, O'Reilly RJ, Exelby PR, Cheung NK. High-dose melphalan with 6-hydroxydopamine-purged autologous bone marrow transplantation for poor-risk neuroblastoma. *Cancer* 1991; **68**: 242–7.

118 Hruba A, Skala JP, Matejckova S et al. [Purging of hemopoietic progenitor cells in autologous transplantation]. *Cas Lek Cesk* 1997; **136**: 151–3.

119 Skala JP, Rogers PC, Chan KW, Chao HY, Rodriguez WC. Deferoxamine as a purging agent for autologous bone marrow grafts in neuroblastoma. *Prog Clin Biol Res* 1992; **377**: 71–8.

120 Hartmann O, Valteau-Couanet D, Benhamou E et al. Stage IV neuroblastoma in patients over 1 year of age at diagnosis: consolidation of poor responders with combined busulfan, cyclophosphamide and melphalan followed by *in vitro* mafosfamide-purged autologous bone marrow transplantation. *Eur J Cancer* 1997; **33**: 2126–9.

121 Beaujean F, Hartmann O, Benhamou E, Lemerle J, Duedari N. Hemopoietic reconstitution after repeated autologous transplantation with mafosfamide-purged marrow. *Bone Marrow Transplant* 1989; **4**: 537–41.

122 Sindermann H, Peukert M, Hilgard P. Bone marrow purging with mafosfamide: a critical survey. *Blut* 1989; **59**: 432–41.

123 Saarinen UM, Coccia PF, Gerson SL, Pelley R, Cheung NK. Eradication of neuroblastoma cells *in vitro* by monoclonal antibody and human complement: method for purging autologous bone marrow. *Cancer Res* 1985; **45** (Part 2): 5969–75.

124 Juhl H, Petrella EC, Cheung NK, Bredehorst R, Vogel CW. Additive cytotoxicity of different monoclonal antibody-cobra venom factor conjugates for human neuroblastoma cells. *Immunobiology* 1997; **197**: 444–59.

125 Duerst RE, Ryan DH, Frantz CN. Variables affecting the killing of cultured human neuroblastoma cells with monoclonal antibody and complement. *Cancer Res* 1986; **46**: 3420–5.

126 Treleaven JG, Gibson FM, Ugelstad J et al. Removal of neuroblastoma cells from bone marrow with monoclonal antibodies conjugated to magnetic microspheres. *Lancet* 1984; **1**(8368): 70–3.

127 Graham-Pole J, Gee A, Emerson S et al. Myeloablative chemoradiotherapy and autologous bone marrow infusions for treatment of neuroblastoma: factors influencing engraftment. *Blood* 1991; **78**: 1607–14.

128 Mattano LAJ, Moss TJ, Emerson SG. Sensitive detection of rare circulating neuroblastoma cells by the reverse transcriptase-polymerase chain reaction. *Cancer Res* 1992; **52**: 4701–5.

129 Miyajima Y, Horibe K, Fukuda M et al. Sequential detection of tumor cells in the peripheral blood and bone marrow of patients with stage IV neuroblastoma by the reverse transcription-polymerase chain reaction for tyrosine hydroxylase mRNA. *Cancer* 1996; **77**: 1214–9.

130 Di Caro A, Bostrom B, Moss TJ et al. Autologous peripheral blood cell transplantation in the treatment of advanced neuroblastoma. *Am J Pediatr Hematol Oncol* 1994; **16**: 200–6.

131 Diaz MA, Alegre A, Benito A, Villa M, Madero L. Peripheral blood progenitor cell collection by large-volume leukapheresis in low-weight children. *J Hematother* 1998; **7**: 63–8.

132 Kletzel M, Longino R, Rademaker AW, Danner-Koptik KE, Olszewski M, Morgan ER. Peripheral blood stem cell transplantation in young children: experience with harvesting, mobilization and engraftment. *Pediatr Transplant* 1998; **2**: 191–6.

133 Civin CI, Trischmann T, Kadan NS et al. Highly purified CD34-positive cells reconstitute hematopoiesis. *J Clin Oncol* 1996; **14**: 2224–33.

134 Berenson RJ, Bensinger WI, Hill RS et al. Engraftment after infusion of CD34$^+$ marrow cells in patients with breast cancer or neuroblastoma. *Blood* 1991; **77**: 1717–22.

135 Kanold J, Yakouben K, Tchirkov A et al. Long-term results of CD34$^+$ cell transplantation in children with neuroblastoma. *Med Pediatr Oncol* 2000; **35**: 1–7.

136 Donovan J, Temel J, Zuckerman A et al. CD34 selection as a stem cell purging strategy for neuroblastoma: preclinical and clinical studies. *Med Pediatr Oncol* 2000; **35**: 677–82.

137 Voigt A, Hafer R, Gruhn B, Zintl F. Expression of CD34 and other haematopoietic antigens on neuroblastoma cells: consequences for autologous bone marrow and peripheral blood stem cell transplantation. *J Neuroimmunol* 1997; **78**: 117–26.

138 Handgretinger R, Greil J, Schurmann U et al. Positive selection and transplantation of peripheral CD34$^+$ progenitor cells: feasibility and purging efficacy in pediatric patients with neuroblastoma. *J Hematother* 1997; **6**: 235–42.

139 Ringhoffer M, Dohner K, Scheil S et al. Fatal outcome in a patient developing Epstein–Barr virus-associated lymphoproliferative disorder (EBV-LPD) without measurable disease. *Bone Marrow Transplant* 2001; **28**: 615–8.

140 Lones MA, Kirov I, Said JW, Shintaku IP, Neudorf S. Post-transplant lymphoproliferative disorder after autologous peripheral stem cell transplantation in a pediatric patient. *Bone Marrow Transplant* 2000; **26**: 1021–4.

141 Abemayor E. The effects of retinoic acid on the *in vitro* and *in vivo* growth of neuroblastoma cells. *Laryngoscope* 1992; **102**: 1133–49.

142 Melino G, Thiele CJ, Knight RA, Piacentini M. Retinoids and the control of growth/death decisions in human neuroblastoma cell lines. *J Neurooncol* 1997; **31**: 65–83.

143 Reynolds CP, Kane DJ, Einhorn PA et al. Response of neuroblastoma to retinoic acid *in vitro* and *in vivo*. *Prog Clin Biol Res* 1991; **366**: 203–11.

144 Finklestein JZ, Krailo MD, Lenarsky C et al. 13-cis-retinoic acid (NSC 122758) in the treatment of children with metastatic neuroblastoma unresponsive to conventional chemotherapy: report from the Children's Cancer Study Group. *Med Pediatr Oncol* 1992; **20**: 307–11.

145 Villablanca JG, Khan AA, Avramis VI et al. Phase I trial of 13-cis-retinoic acid in children with neuroblastoma following bone marrow transplantation. *J Clin Oncol* 1995; **13**: 894–901.

146 Delia D, Aiello A, Lombardi L et al. N-(4-hydroxyphenyl) retinamide induces apoptosis of malignant hemopoietic cell lines including those unresponsive to retinoic acid. *Cancer Res* 1993; **53**: 6036–41.

147 Maurer BJ, Metelitsa LS, Seeger RC, Cabot MC, Reynolds CP. Increase of ceramide and induction of mixed apoptosis/necrosis by N-(4-hydroxyphenyl): retinamide in neuroblastoma cell lines. *J Natl Cancer Inst* 1999; **91**: 1138–46 [see comments].

148 Basniewski PG, Reid JM, Villablanca JG, Reynolds CP, Ames MM. A phase I pharmacokinetic study of fenretinide (HPR) in chldren with high-risk solid tumors. A Children's Cancer Group (CCG) Study. *Proc Am Assoc Cancer Res* 1999; **40**: 92.

149 Cheung NK, Burch L, Kushner BH, Munn DH. Monoclonal antibody 3F8 can effect durable remissions in neuroblastoma patients refractory to chemotherapy: a phase II trial. *Prog Clin Biol Res* 1991; **366**: 395–400.

150 Cheung NK, Kushner BH, Yeh SJ, Larson SM. 3F8 monoclonal antibody treatment of patients with stage IV neuroblastoma: a phase II study. *Prog Clin Biol Res* 1994; **385**: 319–28.

151 Cheung NK, Kushner BH, Yeh SDJ, Larson SM. 3F8 monoclonal antibody treatment of patients with stage 4 neuroblastoma: a phase II study. *Int J Oncol* 1998; **12**: 1299–306.

152 Cheung NK, Kushner BH, Cheung IY et al. Anti-G (D2) antibody treatment of minimal residual stage 4 neuroblastoma diagnosed at more than 1 year of age. *J Clin Oncol* 1998; **16**: 3053–60.

153 Frost JD, Hank JA, Reaman GH et al. A phase I/IB trial of murine monoclonal anti-GD$_2$ antibody 14.G2a plus interleukin-2 in children with refractory neuroblastoma: a report of the Children's Cancer Group. *Cancer* 1997; **80**: 317–33.

154 Handgretinger R, Baader P, Dopfer R et al. A phase I study of neuroblastoma with the antiganglioside GD$_2$ antibody 14.G2a. *Cancer Immunol Immunother* 1992; **35**: 199–204.

155 Yu AL, Uttenreuther-Fischer MM, Huang CS et al. Phase I trial of a human–mouse chimeric anti-disialoganglioside monoclonal antibody ch14.18 in patients with refractory neuroblastoma and osteosarcoma. *J Clin Oncol* 1998; **16**: 2169–80.

156 Ozkaynak MF, Sondel PM, Krailo MD et al. Phase I study of chimeric human/murine anti-ganglioside G (D$_2$) monoclonal antibody (ch14.18) with granulocyte–macrophage colony-stimulating factor in children with neuroblastoma immediately after

hematopoietic stem-cell transplantation: a Children's Cancer Group Study. *J Clin Oncol* 2000; **18**: 4077–85.

157 Lode HN, Xiang R, Varki NM, Dolman CS, Gillies SD, Reisfeld RA. Targeted interleukin-2 therapy for spontaneous neuroblastoma metastases to bone marrow. *J Natl Cancer Inst* 1997; **89**: 1586–94.

158 Bowman L, Grossmann M, Rill D *et al*. IL-2 adenovector-transduced autologous tumor cells induce antitumor immune responses in patients with neuroblastoma. *Blood* 1998; **92**: 1941–9.

159 Bowman LC, Grossmann M, Rill D *et al*. Interleukin-2 gene-modified allogeneic tumor cells for treatment of relapsed neuroblastoma. *Hum Gene Ther* 1998; **9**: 1303–11.

160 Davidoff AM, Kimbrough SA, Ng CY, Shochat SJ, Vanin EF. Neuroblastoma regression and immunity induced by transgenic expression of interleukin-12. *J Pediatr Surg* 1999; **34**: 902–6; discussion 906–7.

161 Lode HN, Xiang R, Duncan SR, Theofilopoulos AN, Gillies SD, Reisfeld RA. Tumor-targeted IL-2 amplifies T cell-mediated immune response induced by gene therapy with single-chain IL-12. *Proc Natl Acad Sci U S A* 1999; **96**: 8591–6.

162 Hock RA, Reynolds BD, Tucker-McClung CL, Heuer JG. Murine neuroblastoma vaccines produced by retroviral transfer of MHC class II genes. *Cancer Gene Ther* 1996; **3**: 314–20.

163 Meitar D, Crawford SE, Rademaker AW, Cohn SL. Tumor angiogenesis correlates with metastatic disease, N-*myc* amplification, and poor outcome in human neuroblastoma. *J Clin Oncol* 1996; **14**: 405–14.

164 Canete A, Navarro S, Bermudez J, Pellin A, Castel V, Llombart-Bosch A. Angiogenesis in neuroblastoma: relationship to survival and other prognostic factors in a cohort of neuroblastoma patients. *J Clin Oncol* 2000; **18**: 27–34.

165 Erdreich-Epstein A, Shimada H, Groshen S *et al*. Integrins alpha(v)beta3 and alpha(v)beta5 are expressed by endothelium of high-risk neuroblastoma and their inhibition is associated with increased endogenous ceramide. *Cancer Res* 2000; **60**: 712–21.

166 Eggert A, Ikegaki N, Kwiatkowski J, Zhao H, Brodeur GM, Himelstein BP. High-level expression of angiogenic factors is associated with advanced tumor stage in human neuroblastomas. *Clin Cancer Res* 2000; **6**: 1900–8.

167 Stern JW, Fang J, Shusterman S *et al*. Angiogenesis inhibitor TNP-470 during bone marrow transplant: safety in a preclinical model. *Clin Cancer Res* 2001; **7**: 1026–32.

168 Sibley GS, Mundt AJ, Goldman S *et al*. Patterns of failure following total body irradiation and bone marrow transplantation with or without a radiotherapy boost for advanced neuroblastoma. *Int J Radiat Oncol Biol Phys* 1995; **32**: 1127–35.

169 Parsons SK, Neault MW, Lehmann LE *et al*. Severe ototoxicity following carboplatin-containing conditioning regimen for autologous marrow transplantation for neuroblastoma. *Bone Marrow Transplant* 1998; **22**: 669–74.

170 Garaventa A, Bellagamba O, Lo Piccolo MS *et al*. ^{131}I-metaiodobenzylguanidine (^{131}I-MIBG) therapy for residual neuroblastoma: a mono-institutional experience with 43 patients. *Br J Cancer* 1999; **81**: 1378–84.

171 Donnelly LF, Rencken IO, Shardell K *et al*. Renal cell carcinoma after therapy for neuroblastoma. *Am J Roentgenol* 1996; **167**: 915–17.

172 Kato K, Ijiri R, Tanaka Y, Kigasawa H, Toyoda Y, Senga Y. Metachronous renal cell carcinoma in a child cured of neuroblastoma. *Med Pediatr Oncol* 1999; **33**: 432–3 [Letter].

173 Megonigal MD, Cheung NK, Rappaport EF *et al*. Detection of leukemia-associated MLL-GAS7 translocation early during chemotherapy with DNA topoisomerase II inhibitors. *Proc Natl Acad Sci U S A* 2000; **97**: 2814–9.

98 Hematopoietic Cell Transplantation for Brain Tumors

Ira J. Dunkel & Jonathan L. Finlay

Introduction

Many oncologists find the management of patients with brain tumors to be a difficult and depressing task. The difficulties may in part be a consequence of the heterogeneity of these tumors. There are many distinct histopathological entities with complicated nomenclatures, and even identical tumors located in different parts of the central nervous system (CNS) may have very different clinical prognoses and treatment options. The emotional difficulties reflect the fact that the prognosis for most adults with primary malignant brain tumors has improved little in the past decade, despite advances in both neurosurgical and radiation therapy technologies. The care of these patients, however, is best addressed by multidisciplinary groups with complementary areas of expertise, and the medical oncologist can and should be a crucial part of the team.

Historically, brain tumors have been treated with neurosurgical resection and radiation therapy. Demonstration of the efficacy of chemotherapy has lagged behind that for most other types of tumors, but currently chemotherapy is being employed more frequently. Recognition of the chemo-sensitivity of many types of brain tumors, in conjunction with the still relatively guarded prognoses of many of these patients, has also logically led to exploration of the use of hematopoietic cell support as a means of increasing dose intensity. In this chapter we review the current status of high-dose chemotherapy with hematopoietic cell transplantation (HCT) for brain tumors.

High-dose chemotherapy regimens

Most multiagent high-dose chemotherapy regimens used for brain tumors include either thiotepa or melphalan. This section will describe the regimens and their toxicities, but data regarding their effectiveness will be discussed in the tumor-specific sections of the chapter that follow.

Thiotepa-based regimens

Thiotepa is an extremely lipophilic drug that achieves a 1:1 plasma to cerebrospinal fluid ratio after intravenous administration [1]. Studies in dogs demonstrated excellent penetration into normal and tumor-bearing brain tissue [2]. While a pediatric phase II trial found hematopoietic dose-limiting toxicity at 65 mg/m^2 [3], use of hematopoietic stem cells allows dose escalation to 900 mg/m^2 [4]. These properties have led several pediatric neuro-oncology groups to include thiotepa into high-dose chemotherapy regimens for malignant brain tumors.

Since 1986 the Finlay group has studied the use of high-dose chemotherapy in conjunction with HCT using three regimens (Tables 98.1–98.3). The initial regimen included thiotepa (900 mg/m^2) and etoposide (1500 mg/m^2), each divided into three daily doses. A 16% toxic mortality rate was encountered in 45 patients aged 8 months to 36 years treated on the Children's Cancer Group (CCG) protocol 9883 [4]. Subsequently the etoposide dose was decreased (750 mg/m^2) and carmustine (1,3-*bis*(2-chloroethyl)-1-nitrosourea; BCNU) (600 mg/m^2 divided over 3–4 days)

Table 98.1 Thiotepa–etoposide regimen.

Agent	Day					
	−5	−4	−3	−2	−1	0
Thiotepa (300 mg/m^2)	X	X	X			
Etoposide (250–500 mg/m^2)	X	X	X			
HCT						X

HCT, hematopoietic cell transplantation.

Table 98.2 BCNU–thiotepa–etoposide regimen.

Agent	Day								
	−8	−7	−6	−5	−4	−3	−2	−1	0
BCNU (100 mg/m^2)	XX	XX	XX						
Thiotepa (300 mg/m^2)				X	X	X			
Etoposide (250 mg/m^2)				X	X	X			
HCT									X

BCNU, 1,3-*bis*(2-chloroethyl)-1-nitrosourea (carmustine); HCT, hematopoietic cell transplantation.

Table 98.3 Carboplatin–thiotepa–etoposide regimen.

Agent	Day								
	−8	−7	−6	−5	−4	−3	−2	−1	0
Carboplatin (500 mg/m^2 or AUC = 7)	X	X	X						
Thiotepa (300 mg/m^2)					X	X	X		
Etoposide (250 mg/m^2)					X	X	X		
HCT									X

AUC, area under the curve; HCT, hematopoietic cell transplantation.

was added to the regimen, but that was found to be even more toxic in 11 patients aged 5–18 years [5]. Later, carboplatin (1500 mg/m^2 divided over 3 days, or area-under-the-curve (AUC) = 7/day via Calvert formula [6,7] for 3 days) followed by thiotepa and etoposide was used [8]. Experience and better patient selection have decreased the risk of a treatment-related death, but toxicity is still certainly an important issue, particularly for patients over 30 years of age [9]. Investigators at Columbia University, NY, modestly decreased the doses of BCNU (450 mg/m^2) and thiotepa (500–700 mg/m^2), and increased the dose of etoposide (1200–1500 mg/m^2) and noted only one treatment-related death in the 18 treated adult patients aged 19–47 years [10]. More recently, investigators at the Memorial Sloan Kettering Cancer Center (MSKCC) have used a modified regimen including thiotepa (900 mg/m^2) divided into three daily doses, topotecan (10 mg/m^2) divided into five daily doses, and carboplatin (AUC = 7/day via Calvert formula) for 3 days [11].

French investigators led by C. Kalifa have investigated a regimen that includes busulfan (BU) and thiotepa. BU has been dosed at 600 mg/m^2 divided into 16 oral doses over 4 days. Originally, thiotepa was dosed at 1050 mg/m^2 divided into three daily doses [12]. Severe neurotoxicity (drowsiness, hallucinations, coma) was seen in six patients in the original cohort of 20 patients aged 8 months to 16 years, and subsequently the dose of thiotepa was decreased to 900 mg/m^2 [13].

Thiotepa has also been used in combination with cyclophosphamide (CY). Investigators at St. Jude Children's Research Hospital, Memphis, TN treated 11 children aged 4–16 years with thiotepa (900 mg/m^2) and CY (6000 mg/m^2), both divided daily over 3 days [14]. Two patients developed interstitial pneumonitis, which was fatal in one case. No severe hepatic or neurologic toxicities were encountered. Kedar et al. [15] reported a series of nine patients aged 3–14 years treated with CY (3000–3900 mg/m^2 divided into four daily doses) and thiotepa (750–900 mg/m^2 divided into three daily doses). Two patients suffered treatment-associated toxic deaths.

Melphalan-based regimens

The Pediatric Oncology Group (POG) investigators explored a regimen that included CY (3000–6000 mg/m^2 divided into four daily doses) and melphalan (180 mg/m^2 divided into three daily doses) in 19 children aged 2–21 years with recurrent or progressive malignant brain tumors [16]. Four of the 19 died of treatment-related complications. Investigators at Duke University, NC also used those agents [17]. In their study, however, the dose of CY was fixed (6000 mg/m^2 divided into four daily doses) and the dose of melphalan escalated (75–180 mg/m^2 divided into three daily doses). Their report also included a small number of patients treated with BU (600 mg/m^2 divided into 16 oral doses over 4 days) and melphalan (140–180 mg/m^2 as a single dose), or carboplatin (2100 mg/m^2 divided into three daily doses) and etoposide (1500 mg/m^2 divided into three daily doses). In the total group of 49 patients aged 8 months to 27 years, there was one death related to toxicity, which was from pulmonary aspergillosis.

High-grade astrocytomas

Natural history with conventional therapy

High-grade astrocytomas are malignant astrocytic neoplasms that most commonly occur in the cerebral hemispheres of adults, but which may be encountered throughout the CNS of both children and adults. The prognosis for patients with a newly diagnosed anaplastic astrocytoma (AA) or glioblastoma multiforme (GBM) remains poor despite treatment with surgery, radiation therapy and conventional chemotherapy. Duncan et al. [18] treated 252 adults with supratentorial high-grade astrocytomas with radiation therapy alone from 1982 to 1987. All 17 with multifocal disease died in less than 12 months, with a median survival time of only 3 months. The 235 with unifocal disease (204 with GBM) had a median survival time of only 10 months. Patients with AA had a 36-month survival of approximately 35% and those with GBM about 15%.

Nelson et al. [19] reported the results of the Radiation Therapy Oncology Group (RTOG) trial 8302, which studied varying doses of hyperfractionated radiation therapy and adjuvant BCNU in 435 patients with high-grade astrocytomas from 1983 to 1987. The recommended dose of radiation therapy (7200 cGy) produced an overall median survival time of 12.8 months (AA patients, 49.9 months). The 18-month survival in patients with AA was approximately 75% and in patients with GBM was approximately 20%.

More recent trials have not demonstrated significant improvement. In the RTOG trial 9513, adults with GBM received radiation therapy and topotecan [20]. One-year survival was 32% and no improvement compared to patients treated on prior RTOG studies was noted. Other recent studies have used agents, such as temozolomide, irinotecan and thalidomide, but no dramatic improvement in survival has been appreciated.

Children with high-grade astrocytomas also have a poor prognosis with conventional therapies. Fifty-four children were treated with radiation therapy only (although three also received lomustine) at the Columbia-Presbytesian Medical Center, NY from 1957 to 1980 and the 5-year survival was 36% and 4%, respectively, for those with AA and GBM [21].

The CCG conducted a randomized trial (CCG-943) comparing radiation therapy alone to radiation therapy and adjuvant chemotherapy (vincristine, lomustine and prednisone) in 58 children with high-grade astrocytomas from 1976 to 1981. They demonstrated that the addition of chemotherapy improved the 5-year event-free survival (EFS) for children with GBM [22]. The subsequent randomized CCG trial (CCG-945) compared the chemotherapy-containing arm of CCG-943 to the "eight-in-one" chemotherapy regimen in 185 children with high-grade astrocytomas from 1985 to 1990 [23]. There was no difference in progression-free survival (PFS) between the two regimens. Overall, patients with AA had a 5-year PFS of 28% vs. 16% for patients with GBM. Patients with a gross total resection (>90%) fared better than did those with less radical surgery (5-year PFS for patients with AA, 42% vs. 14%, respectively, and for patients with GBM, 27% vs. 4%, respectively). Thus, perhaps apart from those who had gross total resection, the prognosis for children with newly diagnosed malignant astrocytomas remains poor.

High-dose chemotherapy with HCT

Single-agent BCNU

The earliest published studies on the treatment of high-grade astrocytomas with high-dose chemotherapy and HCT involved the use of single-agent BCNU with autologous bone marrow transplantation (BMT) in adults [24–32]. They demonstrated responses, including complete responses (CRs), in an impressive proportion of patients treated, but also substantial pulmonary, hepatic and neurological toxicity (including irreversible dementia and encephalopathy), particularly at doses above 1200 mg/m^2.

Biron et al. [33] reported the largest experience. Ninety-eight patients (89 newly diagnosed, nine with relapse) were treated with BCNU (800 mg/m^2 as a single dose) and autologous BMT and then received radiation therapy (4500 cGy) beginning on approximately day 45 after autologous BMT. The toxic mortality rate was 6.1% and the overall survival (OS) was only 10% at 36 months, with a median survival of 11 months after autologous BMT.

Overall, these experiences indicated that despite the encouraging response data, the median survival for both patients with recurrent disease and patients with newly diagnosed GBM did not improve. However, no randomized trial comparing this strategy with conventional therapy has been performed.

Other single-agent trials

Aziridinylbenzoquinone is an alkylating agent with some evidence of activity in brain tumors, but is highly marrow toxic. Abrams et al. [34] evaluated high-dose aziridinylbenzoquinone in patients with refractory CNS neoplasms but found no radiographic response in recurrent high-grade astrocytomas.

Giannone and Wolff [35] evaluated etoposide (1800–2400 mg/m^2 divided daily over 3 days) followed by autologous BMT in 16 patients with progressive astrocytomas (13 high-grade). Nonhematologic toxicity was mild. Three patients (two with high-grade astrocytomas) had objective responses, and one was a long-term survivor at 54 months. Leff et al. [36] and Long et al. [37] treated 13 patients with progressive tumors following radiation therapy (nine with high-grade astrocytomas, four with low-grade astrocytomas) with etoposide (2400 mg/m^2 divided daily over 3 days) followed by autologous BMT. They reported severe, but transient, acute neurologic toxicity including confusion, papilledema, somnolence, exacerbation of motor deficits and increased seizure activity in six patients. Two patients died of sepsis and one of pulmonary hemorrhage. Clinical improvement was seen in two of 11 patients evaluable for response, but no patient demonstrated significant radiologic improvement. The median survival time for all 13 patients was 101 days.

Ascensao et al. [38] and Ahmed et al. [39] presented the results for 16 adults with newly diagnosed high-grade astrocytomas who were treated with thiotepa (600–900 mg/m^2) followed by autologous BMT and radiation therapy (6000 cGy). Toxicity was described as minimal. Four CRs and five partial responses (PRs) were documented.

Multidrug regimens

More recent investigations have explored multidrug high-dose chemotherapy regimens. Kalifa's report of BU and thiotepa included two patients with hemispheric malignant astrocytomas [12]. Neither responded.

Heideman et al. [14] evaluated 11 children with newly diagnosed malignant astrocytomas and two children with recurrent malignant astrocytomas who were treated with thiotepa and CY. Surgery for six of the patients, including five newly diagnosed, was biopsy only. Response was evaluated on day 30, and on day 60 those patients with stable disease or better received radiation therapy. One CR and three PRs were noted. The median PFS time was 9 months, and one patient was progression free at 30 months. Two others, progression free at 23 and 24 months, died of pneumonia and shunt failure.

Kedar et al. [15] included three patients with newly diagnosed high-grade astrocytomas in a series of patients treated with CY and thiotepa. Subsequently they also received hyperfractionated radiation therapy (7560 cGy). One of the three survived disease-free, at 22 months.

The POG series using CY and melphalan included three patients with high-grade astrocytomas [16]. All died within 7 months, one from treatment-related complications and two from progressive disease. The Duke series included 10 patients with recurrent or high-risk astrocytic (nonbrain stem) tumors [17]. Of the six patients with GBM, one was an event-free survivor (duration not specified).

Finlay et al. [40] reported 10 patients with recurrent malignant astrocytomas (nine with GBM). Five received thiotepa and etoposide and five BCNU and thiotepa and etoposide, and four radiographic CRs were documented on day 28 post-autologous BMT. These promising results stimulated the CCG to investigate these regimens in a phase II trial in children with recurrent brain tumors (CCG-9883). While a 16% toxic mortality rate was encountered in the total group of 45 patients with all eligible histologies who were treated with the thiotepa and etoposide regimen, five of the 18 patients with recurrent high-grade astrocytomas were event-free survivors at 39–59 months after autologous BMT [4]. Updated data previously published in abstract form demonstrate that in 36 patients with recurrent high-grade astrocytomas treated with the three regimens, the estimated EFS 4 years after initial progression was 22% [41]. The 4-year estimated survival for patients with AA was 36% and for patients with GBM was 14%. The most powerful factor predictive of survival was the amount of residual disease present at the time of treatment, with patients having <3 cm faring significantly better than those with more bulky tumors. Investigators from France subsequently treated 22 patients aged 4–20 years with high-grade astrocytomas with the thiotepa and etoposide regimen [42]. They noted a 29% response rate, but only three patients were disease-free survivors at 54–65 months.

Because of their encouraging results in patients with recurrent disease, investigators at MSKCC performed a pilot study of the BCNU and thiotepa and etoposide regimen, followed by involved field radiation therapy, in 29 patients with newly diagnosed high-grade astrocytomas [43]. Three patients with GBM were progression-free survivors more than 5 years after autologous BMT. CCG later investigated this approach in study CCG-9922 [5]. The study needed to be closed prematurely due to an excessive rate of nonlethal grade III and IV pulmonary and neurological toxicities, but three of 11 children with GBM were progression-free survivors 2.9–5.1 years after study entry. The PFS rate at 2 years was 46% ± 14%.

HCT has also been studied in conjunction with a nonmyeloablative chemotherapy regimen. Jakacki et al. [44] used peripheral blood mononuclear cell infusions to attempt to allow more frequent cycles of procarbazine, lomustine and vincristine chemotherapy to be administered to 12 patients with newly diagnosed high-grade astrocytomas or diffuse pontine tumors. Dose intensity was successfully increased, but no improvement in survival was achieved.

Conclusions

Small trials demonstrated the feasibility of combining multiple agents at high doses with HCT. Impressive response rates have been noted, and long-term survivors of recurrent high-grade astrocytomas documented (Table 98.4).

Ependymomas

Natural history with conventional therapy

Ependymomas may arise throughout the brain and spinal cord, but usually are contiguous with the ventricular system. In children they are usually intracranial and are highly lethal while adults more commonly have spinal cord tumors that are curable with surgery alone. Histological anaplasia does not seem to be of prognostic value, but older patients and those who have had a complete surgical resection fare better than younger patients and those with an incompletely resected tumor. CCG performed a randomized trial (CCG-942) for children 2–16 years of age with posterior fossa ependymomas [45]. Forty-two patients received post-operative craniospinal radiation therapy and were randomized to receive or not to receive adjuvant chemotherapy with vincristine, lomustine and prednisone for 1 year. No difference was appreciated between the two treatment groups, and the 10-year OS rate for the entire group was 39%. A recent CCG trial (CCG-9942) treated children with completely resected ependymomas with involved-field radiation therapy only and those with incompletely resected tumors with neoadjuvant chemotherapy followed by involved-field radiation therapy.

Patients with recurrent ependymomas have a very guarded prognosis.

Table 98.4 High-dose chemotherapy with hematopoietic cell transplantation (HCT): selected results for high-grade astrocytomas.

Regimen	No. of patients	Disease status	Outcome	Ref.
Thiotepa + cyclophosphamide	13	11 Recurrent, 2 new	1 PFS (30 months)	14
Cyclophosphamide + thiotepa	3	New	1 PFS (22 months)	15
Cyclophosphamide + melphalan	3	Recurrent	0 PFS	16
Cyclophosphamide + melphalan or busulfan + melphalan or carboplatin + etoposide	6	2 Recurrent, 4 new	1 EFS (not specified)	17
Thiotepa + etoposide (± BCNU or carboplatin)	36	Recurrent	22% EFS (4 years)	
Thiotepa + etoposide	22	9 Recurrent, 13 new	3 EFS (54–65 months)	42
BCNU + hiotepa + etoposide	11	New	46% EFS (2 years)	5

BCNU, 1,3-*bis*(2-chloroethyl)-1-nitrosourea (carmustine); EFS, event-free survival; PFS, progression-free survival.

Table 98.5 High-dose chemotherapy with hematopoietic cell transplantation (HCT): results for ependymoma.

Regimen	No. of patients	Disease status	Outcome	Ref.
Busulfan + thiotepa	16	Recurrent	3 EFS (15–27 months)	47
Cyclophosphamide + melphalan	3	Recurrent	0 PFS	16
Cyclophosphamide + melphalan or busulfan + melphalan or carboplatin + etoposide	32	Recurrent, new	1 EFS (22 months), 2 EFS (22–29 months)	17
Thiotepa + etoposide (± carboplatin)	15	Recurrent	1 OS (25 months)	48

EFS, event-free survival; OS, overall survival; PFS, progression-free survival.

Goldwein *et al*. [46] reported a 29% 2-year survival following conventional salvage therapies, but noted that only seven of the 52 patients had not yet suffered a subsequent recurrence.

High-dose chemotherapy with HCT

The POG series included three children with recurrent or progressive ependymomas treated with CY and melphalan [16]. One responded but remained progression free for only 12 months. The Duke series included five patients with ependymomas, three with recurrent disease [17]. One of the three treated for recurrent disease was an event-free survivor at 22 months. The two patients treated prior to recurrence were both event-free survivors at 22 and 29 months.

Grill *et al*. [47] reported the results of a phase II trial of high dose BU (600 mg/m^2 divided into four daily doses) and thiotepa (900 mg/m^2 divided into three daily doses) followed by autologous BMT in 16 children with recurrent or refractory ependymoma. Fifteen patients were evaluable for response, and no PRs or CRs were noted. Three patients were disease-free survivors at 15–27 months after autologous BMT; all had complete resections of residual tumor and involved field radiation therapy after autologous BMT. The authors concluded that this treatment was not indicated for recurrent ependymomas.

Our group at MSKCC treated 15 children with recurrent ependymomas with the thiotepa and etoposide or the carboplatin, thiotepa and etoposide regimen with autologous BMT [48]. Five died of treatment-related toxicities, and only one patient was alive, after further disease recurrence, at 25 months after autologous BMT.

Conclusions

There is little evidence that high-dose chemotherapy with HCT using the regimens described above is beneficial for patients with recurrent ependymomas (Table 98.5).

Oligodendrogliomas

Natural history with conventional therapy

Oligodendrogliomas are usually located in the cerebral hemispheres, comprise about 5% of primary brain tumors, and are rare in children. The short-term prognosis for these patients is relatively good. Celli *et al*. [49] reported a 5-year survival of 52.4% for 105 patients but, like other authors, noted late failures and the 10-year survival was only 24%. Histology appears to be an important prognostic factor. Peterson and Cairncross [50] estimated that up to 75% of patients with nonanaplastic oligodendrogliomas survive 5 years after diagnosis, with a median survival time of 6–10 years, while those with anaplastic disease have a shorter median survival time of 3–4 years. Oligodendrogliomas have been demonstrated to be chemotherapy-sensitive tumors, with procarbazine, lomustine and vincristine being used effectively [51].

High-dose chemotherapy with HCT

One patient with a multiply recurrent anaplastic oligodendroglioma was treated with thiotepa (1125 mg/m^2 divided daily over 3 days) followed by autologous BMT [52]. No severe toxicity was encountered, and a CR was noted. A second course of the high-dose therapy was administered, but the patient died of toxicity with visceral candidiasis.

Cairncross *et al*. [53] extended this approach and presented in abstract form the results for eight adults with newly diagnosed aggressive oligodendrogliomas who were treated with procarbazine, lomustine and vincristine chemotherapy. Six, after PR or CR, or in continuing complete remission after complete surgical resection, then received thiotepa (900 mg/m^2 divided daily over 3 days) followed by HCT. No significant toxicity was encountered. Four were disease-free survivors at 7–47 months after the initiation of chemotherapy. They also treated 38 adults with recurrent aggressive oligodendrogliomas [54]. Twenty patients who

Table 98.6 High-dose chemotherapy with hematopoietic cell transplantation (HCT): results for brain stem tumors.

Regimen	No. of patients	Disease status	Outcome	Ref.
Busulfan + thiotepa	4	Recurrent	0 PFS	12
Cyclophosphamide + thiotepa	6	Newly diagnosed	1 EFS (24 months)	15
Cyclophosphamide + melphalan	1	Recurrent	0 PFS	16
Cyclophosphamide + melphalan or busulfan + melphalan or carboplatin + etoposide	2	Newly diagnosed	1 EFS (not specified)	17
Thiotepa + etoposide (± BCNU or carboplatin)	10,6	Recurrent, newly diagnosed	0 EFS, 0 EFS	60
Busulfan + thiotepa	24	Newly diagnosed	0 EFS	61

BCNU, 1,3-*bis*(2-chloroethyl)-1-nitrosourea (carmustine); EFS, event-free survival; PFS, progression-free survival.

achieved a CR or major PR to induction chemotherapy proceeded to the same high-dose thiotepa regimen. Four patients suffered treatment-related toxic deaths and four others were tumor-free survivors at a median of 42 months (range 27–77 months).

Conclusions

Oligodendrogliomas are chemotherapy-sensitive tumors. A multi-institutional trial exploring the use of high-dose thiotepa with HCT as initial therapy for patients with anaplastic oligodendroglioma has been performed but the results have not yet been published.

Brain stem tumors

Natural history with conventional therapy

Biopsy is usually not performed on diffuse pontine tumors, but autopsy series have demonstrated them to frequently be high-grade astrocytomas, and they are highly lethal malignancies. Reports regarding the use of radiation therapy, the standard therapy for this disease, indicate that only approximately 10% of patients achieve 3-year survival [55–58]. Conventional-dose chemotherapy has not been proved to be efficacious for this disease.

High-dose chemotherapy with HCT

Hara *et al.* [59] treated four children (three with unbiopsied diffuse pontine tumors) with a nitrosourea, nimustine (5–7 mg/kg) and autologous BMT. All were alive at the time of publication, but with a very short follow-up of only 3–11 months after autologous BMT. No other report of this approach has been published in the English-language medical literature.

Kalifa *et al.* [12] included four children with recurrent brain stem tumors in their phase II trial of BU and thiotepa. All died of their disease within 4–8 months.

Kedar *et al.* [15] included six patients with newly diagnosed brain stem tumors in his series of patients treated with CY and thiotepa. The patients subsequently also received hyperfractionated radiation therapy (7560 cGy). Only one of the six survived disease free, at 24 months after diagnosis.

The POG series of CY and melphalan included one child with a recurrent or progressive pontine brain stem tumor [16]. The patient died of progressive disease only 2 months later. The Duke series included two patients with brain stem tumors and noted one event-free survivor (duration not specified) [17].

The investigators at MSKCC, in conjunction with CCG, treated 16 children with diffuse pontine brain stem tumors with high-dose chemotherapy and autologous BMT [60]. Ten had recurrent or refractory disease. Six such patients received thiotepa and etoposide, two received BCNU, thiotepa and etoposide, and two received carboplatin, thiotepa and etoposide. Six newly diagnosed patients received the BCNU, thiotepa and etoposide regimen and then, 6 weeks later, were treated with hyperfractionated radiation therapy (7200–7800 cGy). Two toxic deaths occurred and there were no long-term event-free survivors. The median survival was only 4.7 months from time of autologous BMT for the patients with resistant or recurrent disease, and only 11.4 months for the newly diagnosed patients. The newly diagnosed patients did not appear to fare better than patients treated with conventional radiation therapy alone.

French investigators treated 24 children with newly diagnosed diffuse pontine tumors with external beam radiation therapy followed by high-dose BU and thiotepa [61]. Eleven others who had enrolled on study did not receive the high-dose chemotherapy, due to early progression in nine and parental refusal in two. The median survival was 10 months for the entire group, and also only 10 months for the patients who received high-dose chemotherapy. There were no long-term survivors.

Conclusions

Diffuse pontine brain stem tumors remain highly lethal despite the use of high-dose chemotherapy regimens. New approaches are desperately needed (Table 98.6).

Medulloblastoma

Natural history with conventional therapy

Medulloblastomas are neuroectodermal tumors located in the cerebellum and they most commonly occur in children. Multicenter trials performed by the CCG and the International Society of Paediatric Oncology, in conjunction with the German Society of Paediatric Oncology, noted that about 60% of children with medulloblastomas achieve 5-year EFS with neurosurgical resection, radiation therapy and chemotherapy that did not include cisplatin [62,63]. However, in single-arm studies, the addition of cisplatin chemotherapy appeared to both improve EFS and to allow the use of reduced-dose craniospinal irradiation [64]. CCG treated 65 children between 3 and 10 years of age with nonmetastatic medulloblastoma with reduced-dose craniospinal irradiation (2340 cGy) and a boost to the posterior fossa to 5580 cGy. Patients also received weekly vincristine during irradiation and, beginning 6 weeks after completion of irradiation,

Table 98.7 High-dose chemotherapy with hematopoietic cell transplantation (HCT): results for medulloblastoma.

Regimen	No. of patients	Disease status	Outcome	Ref.
Busulfan + thiotepa	20	Recurrent	50% EFS (31 months)	13
Cyclophosphamide + melphalan	8	Recurrent	2 OS (24–25 months)	16
Cyclophosphamide + melphalan or busulfan + melphalan or carboplatin + etoposide	18	Recurrent	4 EFS (27–49 months)	17
Carboplatin + thiotepa + etoposide	23	Recurrent	34% EFS (36 months)	8

EFS, event-free survival; OS, overall survival.

began a planned eight cycles of vincristine, cisplatin and lomustine chemotherapy. PFS was 79% ± 7% at 5 years. However, for patients whose medulloblastomas recur or are refractory to initial therapy, the prognosis is dismal. Reports from the Stanford University Medical Center and the Children's Hospital of Philadelphia noted no long-term survivors following recurrence [65,66].

High-dose chemotherapy with HCT

The initial report from Kalifa's group [12] of BU and thiotepa included six children with recurrent medulloblastoma. Three of the six had PRs, and three were alive at the time of publication, including two with stable disease and one who was free of disease at 24 months. The patient free of disease had not received radiation therapy prior to relapse because of young age (8 months at the time of diagnosis) and had 5000 cGy administered to the posterior fossa after autologous BMT. This group subsequently reported on 20 young children with recurrent medulloblastoma treated with high-dose BU (600 mg/m^2 divided over 4 days) and thiotepa (900 mg/m^2 divided daily over 3 days) with autologous BMT, followed by radiation therapy [13]. Thirteen had a primary-site relapse only and received radiation therapy (5000–5500 cGy) to the posterior fossa only, without craniospinal irradiation. Ten of these patients were free of disease at a median of 37 months. Of the seven with metastatic disease at recurrence, only one was free of disease at 13+ months. Overall, the 20 patients were estimated to have a 31-month EFS of 50%.

The POG series included eight children with recurrent or progressive medulloblastoma treated with CY and melphalan [16]. Three of these eight died from toxicity but they noted four responses (one CR and three PRs) and two were surviving at 24 and 25 months. The Duke series included 18 patients with recurrent medulloblastoma [17]. Fifteen received CY and melphalan, two received carboplatin and etoposide, and one received BU and melphalan. Six of the patients had primary-site recurrences only and four of them were free of disease at 27–49 months. Three of these four were over 25 years old and no failures were noted in any patient older than 24 years. In contrast, none of the 12 with metastatic disease at recurrence became an event-free survivor.

A single case report described the use of allogeneic BMT [67]. Prior to transplantation, the patient had been brought to minimal disease with conventional chemotherapy, then received BU (16 mg/kg divided over 4 days), etoposide (40 mg/kg as a single dose) and CY (120 mg/kg divided daily over 2 days) followed by transplantation of allogeneic bone marrow from an human leukocyte antigen (HLA)-matched sibling. The patient was progression free 2 years after transplantation.

The MSKCC group, in conjunction with the CCG, treated 23 patients aged 2–44 years (median, 13 years) with recurrent medulloblastoma [8]. The patients received the carboplatin, thiotepa and etoposide regimen, followed by HCT. In addition to the high-dose chemotherapy, 21 patients received other treatments: neurosurgical resection in seven, conventional chemotherapy in 17 and external-beam irradiation in 11. Three patients died of treatment-related toxicities; two of multiorgan system failure and one of *Aspergillus* infection with veno-occlusive disease. Estimates of EFS and OS were 34% ± 10% and 46% ± 11%, respectively, at 36 months after HCT. Unpublished data suggest that the addition of radiation therapy to the high-dose chemotherapy retrieval strategy was associated with a higher probability of EFS. None of the four patients with extra-neural recurrences survived, but French investigators reported two young adults with bone marrow recurrences who were treated with high-dose BU and thiotepa followed by HCT [68]. Both were event-free survivors at 20 and 27 months after relapse.

The Children's Oncology Group is currently studying the use of high-dose thiotepa-based chemotherapy with HCT in conjunction with external beam radiation therapy for patients with newly diagnosed high-risk medulloblastoma and supratentorial primitive neuroectodermal tumors (PNETs). Results are not yet available.

HCT has also been studied in conjunction with a nonmyeloablative chemotherapy regimen. Strother *et al.* [69] used peripheral blood mononuclear cell infusions to attempt to facilitate the use of intensive chemotherapy shortly after craniospinal radiation therapy. Fifty-three patients with medulloblastoma or supratentorial PNETs were treated with craniospinal radiation therapy followed by four cycles of CY (4000 mg/m^2 per cycle), cisplatin (75 mg/m^2 per cycle) and vincristine. High-risk patients also received topotecan on a phase II window. Patients were able to receive the intended dose intensity and early outcome data were very encouraging. The 2-year PFS estimates for standard and high-risk patients were 93.6% and 73.7%, respectively.

Conclusions

High-dose chemotherapy with HCT is a promising strategy for patients with recurrent medulloblastoma (Table 98.7). Patients treated after failure at the primary site only may fare better than those with metastatic disease. This approach is being studied in patients with newly diagnosed tumors.

Other primitive neuroectodermal tumors (PNETs)

Natural history with conventional therapy

PNETs that are histologically similar to medulloblastomas may arise in other locations within the CNS. A CCG trial demonstrated that children with newly diagnosed supratentorial PNET have a 45% estimated 3-year PFS with neurosurgical resection, radiation therapy and chemotherapy at standard doses [70]. Once these tumors recur, however, they are almost invariably lethal.

High-dose chemotherapy with HCT

The POG series included only one patient with a supratentorial PNET [16]. Only a minor response was noted, and the patient survived 8 months.

Table 98.8 High-dose chemotherapy with hematopoietic cell transplantation (HCT): results for primitive neuroectodermal tumors (PNETs).

Regimen	No. of patients	Disease status	Outcome	Ref.
Cyclophosphamide + melphalan	1	Recurrent	0 OS	16
Cyclophosphamide + melphalan or busulfan + melphalan or carboplatin + etoposide	5	Recurrent	2 EFS (33–34 months)	17
Thiotepa + etoposide (± carboplatin)	17	Recurrent	5 EFS (mean 8.3 years)	71

EFS, event-free survival; OS, overall survival.

The Duke series included five patients with recurrent supratentorial PNETs [17]. Neither of the two patients with pineoblastoma were event-free survivors, but two of the three patients with PNETs of other supratentorial locations were event-free survivors at 33 and 34 months.

The MSKCC group [71], in conjunction with the CCG, treated 17 patients with recurrent supratentorial PNETs with high-dose chemotherapy and HCT. Two received the thiotepa and etoposide regimen and 15 the carboplatin, thiotepa and etoposide regimen. Twelve patients died of progressive disease or complications of therapy and five patients were alive with no evidence of disease at a mean follow-up period of 8.3 years. Four of the five survivors received radiation therapy after recovery from the high-dose chemotherapy and HCT. None of the eight patients with pineoblastoma survived.

Conclusions

High-dose chemotherapy with HCT deserves further investigation in patients with recurrent PNETs (Table 98.8). Patients with nonpineal supratentorial PNETs appear to do better than those with pineoblastoma.

Germ cell tumors

Natural history with conventional therapy

Germ cell tumors, histologically identical to those that are more commonly found in the testes, ovaries, or other extraneural sites, comprise a small proportion of primary brain tumors. They usually arise in the suprasellar or pineal regions and most commonly occur in children and adolescents. Germinomas are highly curable with radiation therapy alone and may be successfully treated with chemotherapy as well, with estimated survivals of about 90% [72,73]. Nongerminomatous germ cell tumors, which express high levels of α fetoprotein from endodermal sinus tumor elements and/or the β subunit of human chorionic gonadotropin from choriocarcinomatous elements, are much more lethal. Some reports, however, suggested that the use of chemotherapy may improve the prognosis of these patients, with estimates of 2-year survival of 62% [73] and of 4-year survival of 74% being achieved [74].

High-dose chemotherapy with HCT

The Duke series included two patients with nonrecurrent CNS germ cell tumors [17]. Both tumors contained elements of endodermal sinus tumor (α fetoprotein positive). The patients were considered by the investigators to be at high risk of recurrence despite there being no evidence of disease at the time of high-dose chemotherapy by virtue of previously administered chemotherapy and radiation therapy. Both patients were event-free survivors at 22 and 30 months.

Our group at MSKCC has unpublished data regarding 13 patients with recurrent CNS germ cell tumors treated with high-dose thiotepa-based chemotherapy and HCT. Five of the six patients with germinomas are event-free survivors at a median of 48 months, while only two of seven patients with nongerminomatous germ cell tumors are event-free survivors at 22 and 35 months post-HCT.

Conclusions

There is little experience using high-dose chemotherapy with HCT for CNS germ cell tumors, but since these tumors are highly sensitive to chemotherapy, it is an appealing approach for patients with recurrent disease.

Infants

Natural history with conventional therapy

Infants are a special group of patients with a poor prognosis. The neuropsychological consequences of radiation therapy administered to young children are considered to be intolerable by most parents and pediatric neuro-oncologists and, therefore, these patients are treated with neurosurgical resection and chemotherapy in an attempt to delay or avoid radiation therapy. POG reported an estimated 2-year PFS of 37% for infants (<3 years old) with malignant brain tumors treated with this strategy [75]. For those with malignant astrocytoma, ependymoma, medulloblastoma, brain stem tumor and supratentorial PNETs, respectively, the results were 54%, 42%, 34%, 28% and 19%. Using a different chemotherapy regimen, CCG reported 55%, 26%, 22% and 0% 3-year estimated PFS for infants (<18 months old) with nonpineal supratentorial PNETs, ependymoma, medulloblastoma and pineal PNETs, respectively [76].

High-dose chemotherapy with HCT

At MSKCC we studied children <6 years old with newly diagnosed malignant brain tumors who were treated with MSKCC protocol 92-16. All patients <3 years old were eligible; those aged between 3 and 6 years were eligible if they had a high-grade astrocytoma, brain stem tumor, or a supratentorial PNET. Children 3–6 years old with medulloblastoma were eligible only if they had evidence of metastatic disease and those with ependymoma only if an incomplete resection was performed. Patients received five cycles of vincristine, cisplatin, CY and etoposide. Hematopoietic cells (either from bone marrow or, preferably, from peripheral blood) were harvested early, usually at recovery from the first cycle. If, after five cycles, disease progression had not occurred, the patients proceeded to high-dose chemotherapy with the carboplatin, thiotepa and etoposide regimen and HCT. If they had no evidence of disease prior to high-dose chemotherapy, they did not receive any radiation therapy on this protocol. If there was evidence of unresectable residual disease, then approximately 6 weeks after HCT they began involved-field radiation therapy.

For the first 62 children treated the 3-year OS and EFS estimates were 40% and 25%, respectively [77]. Patients with high-grade astrocytomas and brain stem tumors fared poorly, while those with medulloblastoma, PNETs and ependymoma achieved 2-year EFS estimates higher than 30%.

CCG investigators adopted a similar strategy in a pilot study, CCG-99703. After three cycles of induction chemotherapy and hematopoietic cell harvest, patients receive three cycles of high-dose carboplatin and thiotepa. Results are not yet available.

Our group at MSKCC has also used high-dose thiotepa-based chemotherapy for 20 young children (median age 2.9 years) whose disease had recurred after treatment with chemotherapy, but no radiation therapy, on a protocol for infants [78]. Ten became event-free survivors, with a median follow-up of 37.9 months, for a Kaplan–Meier estimate of 3-year EFS of 47% ± 14%. Seven of the event-free survivors also received radiation therapy vs. five of the 10 who had suffered an event.

Conclusions

A short duration of conventional chemotherapy followed by high-dose chemotherapy with HCT has efficacy comparable to longer duration conventional chemotherapy regimens used by POG and CCG. A randomized trial comparing these strategies may be indicated.

References

1 Heideman RL, Cole DE, Balis F et al. Phase I and pharmacokinetic evaluation of thiotepa in the cerebrospinal fluid and plasma of pediatric patients: evidence for dose-dependent plasma clearance of thiotepa. Cancer Res 1989; 49: 736–41.

2 Finlay JL, Knipple J, Turski P et al. Pharmacokinetic studies of thio-tepa in dogs following delivery by various routes. J Neurooncol 1986; 4: 110 [Abstract].

3 Heideman RL, Packer RJ, Reaman GH et al. A phase II evaluation of thiotepa in pediatric central nervous system malignancies. Cancer 1993; 72: 271–5.

4 Finlay JL, Goldman S, Wong MC et al. Pilot study of high-dose thiotepa and etoposide with autologous bone marrow rescue in children and young adults with recurrent CNS tumors. J Clin Oncol 1996; 14: 2495–503.

5 Grovas AC, Boyett JM, Lindsley K, Rosenblum M, Yates AJ, Finlay JL. Regimen-related toxicity of myeloablative chemotherapy with BCNU, thiotepa, and etoposide followed by autologous stem cell rescue for children with newly diagnosed glioblastoma multiforme: report from the Children's Cancer Group. Med Pediatr Oncol 1999; 33: 83–7.

6 Calvert AH, Newell DR, Gumbrell LA et al. Carboplatin dosage: prospective evaluation of a simple formula based on renal function. J Clin Oncol 1989; 7: 1748–56.

7 Newell DR, Pearson AD, Balmanno K et al. Carboplatin pharmacokinetics in children: the development of a pediatric dosing formula. J Clin Oncol 1993; 11: 2314–23.

8 Dunkel IJ, Boyett JM, Yates A et al. High dose carboplatin, thiotepa, and etoposide with autologous stem-cell rescue for patients with recurrent medulloblastoma. J Clin Oncol 1998; 16: 222–8.

9 Abrey LE, Rosenblum MK, Papadopoulos E, Childs BH, Finlay JL. High dose chemotherapy with autologous stem cell rescue in adults with malignant primary brain tumors. J Neurooncol 1999; 44: 147–53.

10 Papadopoulos KP, Balmaceda C, Fetell M et al. A phase I trial of high-dose BCNU, etoposide and escalating-dose thiotepa (BTE) with hematopoietic progenitor cell support in adults with recurrent and high-risk brain tumors. J Neurooncol 1999; 44: 155–62.

11 Kushner BH, Cheung NKV, Kramer K, Dunkel IJ, Calleja E, Boulad F. Topotecan combined with myeloablative doses of thiotepa and carboplatin for neuroblastoma, brain tumors, and other poor-risk solid tumors in children and young adults. Bone Marrow Transplant 2001; 28: 551–6.

12 Kalifa C, Hartmann O, Demeocq F et al. High-dose busulfan and thiotepa with autologous bone marrow transplantation in childhood malignant brain tumors: a phase II study. Bone Marrow Transplant 1992; 9: 227–33.

13 Dupuis-Girod S, Hartmann O, Benhamou E et al. Will high dose chemotherapy followed by autologous bone marrow transplantation supplant craniospinal irradiation in young children treated for medulloblastoma? J Neurooncol 1996; 27: 87–98.

14 Heideman RL, Douglass EC, Krance RA et al. High-dose chemotherapy and autologous bone marrow rescue followed by interstitial and external-beam radiotherapy in newly diagnosed pediatric malignant gliomas. J Clin Oncol 1993; 11: 1458–65.

15 Kedar A, Maria BL, Graham-Pole J et al. High-dose chemotherapy with marrow reinfusion and hyperfractionated irradiation for children with high-risk brain tumors. Med Pediatr Oncol 1994; 23: 428–36.

16 Mahoney DH Jr, Strother D, Camitta B et al. High-dose melphalan and cyclophosphamide with autologous bone marrow rescue for recurrent/progressive malignant brain tumors in children: a pilot Pediatric Oncology Group study. J Clin Oncol 1996; 14: 382–8.

17 Graham ML, Herndon JE III, Casey JR et al. High-dose chemotherapy with autologous stem-cell rescue in patients with recurrent and high-risk pediatric brain tumors. J Clin Oncol 1997; 15: 1814–23.

18 Duncan GG, Goodman GB, Ludgate CM et al. The treatment of adult supratentorial high grade astrocytomas. J Neurooncol 1992; 13: 63–72.

19 Nelson DF, Curran WJ Jr, Scott C et al. Hyperfrationated radiation therapy and bis-chlorethyl nitrosourea in the treatment of malignant glioma-possible advantage observed at 72.0 Gy in 1.2 Gy b.i.d. fractions: report of the Radiation Therapy Oncology Group protocol 8302. Int J Radiat Oncol Biol Phys 1993; 25: 193–207.

20 Fisher B, Won M, Macdonald D, Johnson DW, Roa W. Phase II study of topotecan plus cranial radiation for glioblastoma multiforme: results of the Radiation Therapy Oncology Group protocol 9513. Int J Radiat Oncol Biol Phys 2002; 53: 980–6.

21 Marchese MJ, Chang CH. Malignant astrocytic gliomas in children. Cancer 1990; 65: 2771–8.

22 Sposto R, Ertel IJ, Jenkin RDT et al. The effectiveness of chemotherapy for treatment of high grade astrocytoma in children: results of a randomized trial. J Neurooncol 1989; 7: 165–77.

23 Finlay JL, Boyett JM, Yates AJ et al. Randomized phase III trial in childhood high-grade astrocytoma comparing vincristine, lomustine, and prednisone with the eight-drugs-in-1-day regimen. J Clin Oncol 1995; 13: 112–23.

24 Hochberg FH, Parker LM, Takvorian T et al. High-dose BCNU with autologous bone marrow rescue for recurrent glioblastoma multiforme. J Neurosurg 1981; 54: 455–60.

25 Takvorian T, Parker LM, Hochberg FH et al. Autologous bone-marrow transplantation: host effects of high-dose BCNU. J Clin Oncol 1983; 1: 610–20.

26 Carella AM, Giordano D, Santini G et al. High dose BCNU followed by autologous bone marrow infusion in glioblastoma multiforme. Tumori 1981; 67: 473–5.

27 Phillips GL, Wolff SN, Fay JW et al. Intensive 1,3-bis(2-chloroethyl)-1-nitrosourea (BCNU) monochemotherapy and autologous bone marrow transplantation for malignant glioma. J Clin Oncol 1986; 4: 639–45.

28 Phillips GL, Fay JW, Herzig GP et al. Intensive 1,3-bis(2-chloroethyl)-1-nitrosourea (BCNU), nsc: 4366650 and cryopreserved autologous marrow transplantation for refractory cancer: a phase I–II study. Cancer 1983; 52: 1792–802.

29 Mortimer JE, Hewlett JS, Bay J et al. High dose BCNU with autologous bone marrow rescue in the treatment of recurrent malignant gliomas. J Neurooncol 1983; 1: 269–73.

30 Johnson DB, Thompson JM, Corwin JA et al. Prolongation of survival for high-grade malignant gliomas with adjuvant high-dose BCNU and autologous bone marrow transplantation. J Clin Oncol 1987; 5: 783–9.

31 Wolff SN, Phillips GL, Herzig GP. High-dose carmustine with autologous bone marrow transplantation for the adjuvant treatment of high-grade gliomas of the central nervous system. Cancer Treat Rep 1987; 71: 183–5.

32 Mbidde EK, Selby PJ, Perren TJ et al. High dose BCNU chemotherapy with autologous bone marrow transplantation and full dose radiotherapy for grade IV astrocytoma. Br J Cancer 1988; 58: 779–82.

33 Biron P, Vial C, Chauvin F et al. Strategy including surgery, high dose BCNU followed by ABMT and radiotherapy in supratentorial high grade astrocytomas: a report of 98 patients. In: Dicke KA, Armitage JO, Dicke-Evinger MJ, eds. Autologous Bone Marrow Transplantation: Proceedings of the Fifth International Symposium. Omaha: The University of Nebraska Medical Center, 1991: 637–45.

34 Abrams RA Jr, Casper J, Kun L et al. High-dose aziridinylbenzoquinone for patients with refractory central nervous system neoplasms: a preliminary analysis. In: Dicke KA, Spitzer G, Zander AR, Gorin NC, eds. Autologous Bone Marrow Transplantation: Proceedings of the First International Symposium. Houston: The University of Texas, MD Anderson Hospital and Tumor Institute, 1985: 227–30.

35 Giannone L, Wolff SN. Phase II treatment of central nervous system gliomas with high-dose etoposide

and autologous bone marrow transplantation. *Cancer Treat Rep* 1987; **71**: 759–61.

36 Leff RS, Thompson JM, Daly MB et al. Acute neurologic dysfunction after high-dose etoposide therapy for malignant glioma. *Cancer* 1988; **62**: 32–5.

37 Long J, Leff R, Daly M et al. Phase II trial of high-dose etoposide and autologous bone marrow transplantation for treatment of progressive glioma. Proceedings of the Annual Meeting of the American Society. *Clin Oncol* 1989; **8**: 92 [Abstract].

38 Ascensao J, Ahmed T, Feldman E et al. High-dose thiotepa with autologous bone marrow transplantation and localized radiotherapy for patients with astrocytoma grade III–IV: a promising approach. Proceedings of the Annual Meeting of the American Society. *Clin Oncol* 1989; **8**: 353a [Abstract].

39 Ahmed T, Feldman E, Helson L et al. Phase 1–2 trial of high dose thiotepa with autologous bone marrow transplantation and localized radiotherapy for patients with astrocytoma grade III–IV. Proceedings of the Annual Meeting of the American Association. *Cancer Res* 1990; **31**: 1023a [Abstract].

40 Finlay JL, August C, Packer R et al. High-dose multi-agent chemotherapy followed by bone marrow "rescue" for malignant astrocytomas of childhood and adolescence. *J Neurooncol* 1990; **9**: 239–48.

41 Dunkel IJ, Finlay JL. High-dose chemotherapy with autologous bone marrow rescue for high-grade astrocytomas. *Bone Marrow Transplant* 1994; **14**: 64s [Abstract].

42 Bouffet E, Mottolese C, Jouvet A et al. Etoposide and thiotepa followed by ABMT (autologous bone marrow transplantation) in children and young adults with high-grade gliomas. *Eur J Cancer* 1997; **33**: 91–5.

43 Papadakis V, Dunkel IJ, Cramer LD et al. High-dose carmustine, thiotepa and etoposide followed by autologous bone marrow rescue for the treatment of high risk central nervous system tumors. *Bone Marrow Transplant* 2000; **26**: 153–60.

44 Jakacki RI, Siffert J, Jamison C, Velasquez L, Allen JC. Dose-intensive, time-compressed procarbazine, CCNU, vincristine (PCV) with peripheral blood stem cell support and concurrent radiation in patients with newly diagnosed high-grade gliomas. *J Neurooncol* 1999; **44**: 77–83.

45 Evans AE, Anderson JR, Lefkowitz-Boudreaux IB et al. Adjuvant chemotherapy of childhood posterior fossa ependymoma: cranio-spinal irradiation with or without adjuvant CCNU, vincristine, and prednisone: a Children's Cancer Group study. *Med Pediatr Oncol* 1996; **27**: 8–14.

46 Goldwein JW, Glauser TA, Packer RJ et al. Recurrent intracranial ependymomas in children: survival, patterns of failure, and prognostic factors. *Cancer* 1990; **66**: 557–63.

47 Grill I, Kalifa C, Doz F et al. A high-dose busulfan-thiotepa combination followed by autologous bone marrow transplantation in childhood recurrent ependymoma: a phase II study. *Pediatr Neurosurg* 1996; **25**: 7–12.

48 Mason WP, Goldman S, Yates AJ, Boyett J, Li H, Finlay JL. Survival following intensive chemotherapy with bone marrow reconstitution for children with recurrent intracranial ependymoma. A report of the Children's Cancer Group. *J Neurooncol* 1998; **37**: 135–43.

49 Celli P, Nofrone I, Palma L et al. Cerebral oligodendroglioma: prognostic factors and life history. *Neurosurgery* 1994; **35**: 1018–34.

50 Peterson K, Cairncross JG. Oligodendroglioma. *Cancer Invest* 1996; **14**: 243–51.

51 Cairncross G, Macdonald D, Ludwin S et al. Chemotherapy for anaplastic oligodendroglioma. *J Clin Oncol* 1994; **12**: 2013–21.

52 Saarinen UM, Pihko H, Makipernaa A. High-dose thiotepa with autologous bone marrow rescue in recurrent malignant oligodendroglioma: a case report. *J Neurooncol* 1990; **9**: 57–61.

53 Cairncross G, Swinnen L, Stiff P et al. High-dose thiotepa with hematopoietic reconstitution (deferring radiation) for newly diagnosed aggressive oligodendroglioma. Proceedings of the Annual Meeting of the American Society. *Clin Oncol* 1997; **16**: 388a [Abstract].

54 Cairncross G, Swinnen L, Bayer R et al. Myeloablative chemotherapy for recurrent aggressive oligodendroglioma. *Neurooncol* 2000; **2**: 114–9.

55 Kretschmar CS, Tarbell NJ, Barnes PD et al. Pre-irradiation chemotherapy and hyperfractionated radiation therapy 66 Gy for children with brain stem tumors: a phase II study of the Pediatric Oncology Group, protocol 8833. *Cancer* 1993; **72**: 1404–13.

56 Packer RJ, Boyett JM, Zimmerman RA et al. Outcome of children with brain stem gliomas after treatment with 7800 cGy of hyperfractionated radiotherapy: a Children's Cancer Group phase I/II trial. *Cancer* 1994; **74**: 1827–34.

57 Packer RJ, Boyett JM, Zimmerman RA et al. Hyperfractionated radiation therapy (72 Gy) for children with brain stem gliomas: a Children's Cancer Group phase I/II trial. *Cancer* 1993; **72**: 1414–21.

58 Freeman CR, Krischer JP, Sanford RA et al. Final results of a study of escalating doses of hyperfractionated radiotherapy in brain stem tumors in children: a Pediatric Oncology Group study. *Int J Radiat Oncol Biol Phys* 1993; **27**: 197–206.

59 Hara T, Miyazaki S, Ishii E et al. High-dose 1-(4-amino-2-methyl-5-pyrimidinyl)-methyl-3-(2-chloroethyl)-3-nitrosourea hydrochloride (ACNU) with autologous bone marrow rescue for patients with brain stem tumors. *Childs Brain* 1984; **11**: 369–74.

60 Dunkel IJ, Garvin JH, Goldman S et al. High dose chemotherapy with autologous bone marrow rescue for children with diffuse pontine brain stem tumors. *J Neurooncol* 1998; **37**: 67–73.

61 Bouffet E, Raquin M, Doz F et al. Radiotherapy followed by high dose busulfan and thiotepa. A prospective assessment of high dose chemotherapy in children with diffuse pontine gliomas. *Cancer* 2000; **88**: 685–92.

62 Evans AE, Jenkin RDT, Sposto R et al. The treatment of medulloblastoma: results of a prospective randomized trial of radiation therapy with and without CCNU, vincristine, and prednisone. *J Neurosurg* 1990; **72**: 572–82.

63 Bailey CC, Gnekow A, Wellek S et al. Prospective randomized trial of chemotherapy given before radiotherapy in childhood medulloblastoma: International Society of Paediatric Oncology and the German Society of Paediatric Oncology: SIOP II. *Med Pediatr Oncol* 1995; **25**: 166–78.

64 Packer RJ, Goldwein J, Nicholson HS et al. Treatment of children with medulloblastomas with reduced-dose craniospinal radiation therapy and adjuvant chemotherapy: a Children's Cancer Group study. *J Clin Oncol* 1999; **17**: 2127–36.

65 Belza MG, Donaldson SS, Steinberg GK et al. Medulloblastoma: freedom from relapse longer than 8 years—a therapeutic cure? *J Neurosurg* 1991; **75**: 575–82.

66 Torres CF, Rebsamen S, Silber JH et al. Surveillance scanning of children with medulloblastoma. *N Engl J Med* 1994; **330**: 892–5.

67 Lundberg JH, Weissman DE, Beatty PA et al. Treatment of recurrent metastatic medulloblastoma with intensive chemotherapy and allogeneic bone marrow transplantation. *J Neurooncol* 1992; **13**: 151–5.

68 Millot F, Delval O, Giraud C et al. High-dose chemotherapy with hematopoietic stem cell transplantation in adults with bone marrow relapse of medulloblastoma: report of two cases. *Bone Marrow Transplant* 1999; **24**: 1347–9.

69 Strother D, Ashley D, Kellie SJ et al. Feasibility of four consecutive high-dose chemotherapy cycles with stem-cell rescue for patients with newly diagnosed medulloblastoma or supratentorial primitive neuroectodermal tumor after craniospinal radiotherapy: results of a collaborative study. *J Clin Oncol* 2001; **19**: 2696–704.

70 Cohen BH, Zeltzer PM, Boyett JM et al. Prognostic factors and treatment results for supratentorial primitive neuroectodermal tumors in children using radiation and chemotherapy: a Children's Cancer Group randomized trial. *J Clin Oncol* 1995; **13**: 1687–96.

71 Broniscer A, Nicolaides TP, Dunkel IJ et al. High-dose chemotherapy with autologous stem-cell rescue in the treatment of patients with recurrent non-cerebellar primitive neuroectodermal tumors. *Med Pediatr Oncol*, in press.

72 Matsutani M, Sano K, Takakura K et al. Primary intracranial germ cell tumors: a clinical analysis of 153 histologically verified cases. *J Neurosurg* 1997; **86**: 446–55.

73 Balmaceda C, Heller G, Rosenblum M et al. Chemotherapy without irradiation-a novel approach for newly diagnosed CNS germ cell tumors: results of an international cooperative trial. *J Clin Oncol* 1996; **14**: 2908–15.

74 Robertson PL, DaRosso RC, Allen JC. Improved prognosis of intracranial non-germinoma germ cell tumors with multimodality therapy. *J Neurooncol* 1997; **32**: 71–80.

75 Duffner PK, Horowitz ME, Krischer JP et al. Postoperative chemotherapy and delayed radiation in children less than 3 years of age with malignant brain tumors. *N Engl J Med* 1993; **328**: 1725–31.

76 Geyer JR, Zeltzer PM, Boyett JM et al. Survival of infants with primitive neuroectodermal tumors or malignant ependymomas of the CNS treated with eight drugs in 1 day: a report from the Children's Cancer Group. *J Clin Oncol* 1994; **12**: 1607–15.

77 Mason WP, Grovas A, Halpern S et al. Intensive chemotherapy and bone marrow rescue for young children with newly-diagnosed malignancies. *J Clin Oncol* 1998; **16**: 210–21.

78 Gururangan S, Dunkel IJ, Goldman S et al. Myeloablative chemotherapy with autologous bone marrow rescue in young children with recurrent malignant brain tumors. *J Clin Oncol* 1998; **16**: 2486–93.

99

Allen R. Chen & Curt I. Civin

Hematopoietic Cell Transplantation for Pediatric Patients with Solid Tumors

The most frequent pediatric solid tumors—neuroblastoma, Wilms' tumor, rhabdomyosarcoma, retinoblastoma, germ cell tumor, osteosarcoma and Ewing's sarcoma—are all chemosensitive. As a result of ongoing improvements in diagnosis, multimodal therapy and supportive care, the treatment outcome of children with cancer has steadily improved since 1960. For instance, the 5-year survival of children with Wilms' tumor has risen from <45% to >85%, for rhabdomyosarcoma from <20% to 60% and for Ewing's sarcoma from 10% to 60% [1,2].

However, subsets of patients have been defined who face a poor prognosis despite having initially responsive disease. Examples include patients >1 year of age with metastatic neuroblastoma (see Chapter 97) and patients with metastatic Ewing's sarcoma (see below). For such patients treated conventionally, the prognosis for disease-free survival (DFS) 3 years from diagnosis remains <20%.

The prognosis of recurrent or refractory pediatric solid tumors is dismal, and few patients have experienced prolonged survival. Most pediatric solid tumor patients are treated with intensive primary chemotherapy, and most recurrences occur during treatment or within 1 year of its completion. Rapid recurrence indicates the presence of tumor cells resistant to the chemotherapeutic agents used. Tumor cells often manifest substantial cross-resistance to multiple antineoplastic agents, including drugs to which the cells were never exposed.

Dose–response

Agents of most classes, including alkylators, irradiation, anthracyclines, vinca alkaloids and antimetabolites, manifest steep dose–response curves against a variety of different tumor cell types, including sarcomas. For most of these agents, there is a steep linear relationship between drug concentration and the log tumor cell kill assessed by *in vitro* colony and limiting dilution assays [3].

This steep log-linear dose–response relationship translates into important effects of chemotherapy dose on tumor response and survival in experimental tumor-bearing animals. In experiments involving osteosarcoma and mammary adenocarcinoma, sharp reductions in complete response (CR) and partial response (PR) rates accompany small (~15%) reductions in the dose of single agents of all classes, including antimetabolites (5-fluorouracil and 6-mercaptopurine), anthracycline (doxorubicin and daunorubicin), antitubule agents (vincristine) and alkylators (melphalan and cyclophosphamide [CY]). In this system, the only curative single agent is CY, at a 30% lethal dose (LD30). Various combinations of chemotherapy can produce cures at <LD10 but, even so, modest (~33%) dose reductions eliminate cures [4]. Of great relevance to pediatric oncology is a rhabdomyosarcoma xenograft model demonstrating a strong effect of the dose of melphalan on tumor response of six primary tumor cell lines, including one from a CY-resistant tumor. Importantly, melphalan at adequate doses is much more active than the standard chemotherapy combination for rhabdomyosarcoma, vincristine, actinomycin D, CY and doxorubicin [5].

Modeling of extensive experimental data indicates that the likelihood of cure correlates best with dose intensity, while the duration of PR correlates best with the total dose of chemotherapy. The maximum cumulative dose of alkylators and anthracyclines that can be administrated safely does not increase when dose intensity is reduced. It is therefore advantageous to maximize dose intensity; the maximum dose intensity is achieved by giving a single very large course of drug [6].

Dose-limiting myelotoxicity

For agents such as melphalan, carmustine (reviewed by [7]; see also Chapter 12) and carboplatin [8], whose major dose-limiting toxicity is myelosuppression, hematopoietic cell rescue may permit 3–10-fold dose escalation. Given a steep dose–response relationship, this approach may translate into several log more cell kill and improved durability of response.

Indications and outcomes

Ewing's sarcoma

Risk groups and outcomes with conventional therapy

After neuroblastoma, the most common indication for hematopoietic cell transplantation (HCT) among pediatric solid tumors is Ewing's sarcoma. The Ewing's sarcoma and primitive neuroectodermal tumor (PNET) family is defined molecularly by the expression of the cell surface glycoprotein MIC-2 and the presence of a reciprocal translocation t(11;22)(q24;q12) that results in fusion of EWS with an *ets* family transcription factor, fli-1. For these tumors, a large primary tumor >8 cm in diameter [9], fever at presentation or poor histologic response [10] are unfavorable factors. Primary pelvic location is an adverse factor, particularly in association with large tumor volume [11]. Moreover, the presence of overt metastatic disease at diagnosis portends a poor prognosis, with DFS superimposable with that of stage IV neuroblastoma patients [12,13], for whom HCT is the standard of care. Although the addition of ifosfamide and etoposide significantly improved the outcome of localized Ewing's sarcoma, neither the addition of these agents nor intensification of the ifosfamide, doxorubicin and CY improved the 4-year DFS of patients with metastatic disease, which remained 19%, and overall survival (OS) was 38% [14]. Furthermore, there is international consensus that the presence of bone and marrow metastases at diagnosis defines an

Table 99.1 Activity of high-dose melphalan regimens against measurable relapsed and refractory Ewing's tumors.

Melphalan dose (mg/m^2)	Other agents	n	CR	PR/OR	Total	Duration, months median (range)	Reference
120–215	XRT	3	2	1	3/3	12+ (3–12+)	[22]
300 mg total		1	1		1/1	4	[23]
120–225		2	1	1	2/2	6.5 (6–7)	[29]
120–210	XRT (3/8)	8	0	6	6/8	3.5 (3–7+)	[24]
140–220		9	3	2	5/9	8 (5–34)	[25]
140–200		8	1	5	6/8		[26]
180	CBP	2	1	0	1/2	12+	[30]
140–200	TBI	3	0	0	0/3		[28]
100	BU, TT	2	2	0	2/2	11.5 (6–17+)	[31]
200–300	TT	2	0	0	0/2		[32]

BU, busulfan; CBP, carboplatin; CR, complete response; OR, objective response (25–50% reduction in tumor volume); PR, partial response; TT thiotepa; XRT, local radiation therapy.

extremely poor prognosis group in whom survival with conventional chemotherapy is rare [13,15–17].

The only reported success of conventional chemotherapy for metastatic Ewing's sarcoma was the EWI-79 St. Jude regimen of CY, doxorubicin, vincristine and actinomycin D, which produced 50% 8-year survival in a cohort of 18 patients. However, the French Society of Pediatric Oncology (SFOP) could not reproduce these results, achieving only 12% 3-year DFS and 25% OS with this regimen [18], and the successor St. Jude protocol that incorporated an ifosfamide and etoposide combination achieved median survival of only 3 years [19].

The prognosis of Ewing's tumor patients who relapse after standard therapy is no better, even if their disease was initially localized. The outcome of patients who relapsed after treatment for initially localized disease on the European Intergroup Cooperative Ewing's Sarcoma Study (EICESS) and German Cooperative Ewing's Sarcoma Studies (CESS) has been analyzed. Of 272 patients registered on these studies from 1981 through 1990, 104 relapsed and, as of July 1995, 89 have died during a median observation period of 7 years from relapse. The OS 10 years from relapse was 10%. The timing of relapse carried important prognostic significance: OS was 0% for patients relapsing within 2 years of diagnosis vs. 33% for patients relapsing later [20]. Similar results for the importance of the timing of relapse were observed by the UK Children's Cancer Study Group (UKCCSG), with 4% 5-year OS for patients relapsing <2 years after diagnosis vs. 23% for patients relapsing later [13], and by the St. Jude institutional experience [21].

HCT in recurrent and refractory Ewing's tumors

The most extensive phase 2 experience with HCT in recurrent or refractory Ewing's family tumors has been based on the use of high-dose melphalan, alone or in combination with total body irradiation (TBI) or additional chemotherapy [22–28]. As a single agent, melphalan has been given at doses of 120–220 mg/m^2; some patients have received a second course of melphalan at a reduced dose, with HCT. As summarized in Table 99.1, most recurrent and refractory Ewing's tumors have responded to high-dose melphalan, but a minority of the responses were complete and the median duration of response has been short, from 3 months [26] to 8 months [25]. None the less, these studies demonstrate that high-dose melphalan is active, even against tumors refractory to intensive conventional chemotherapy.

The experience of the Institut Gustave-Roussy in Paris, France, in metastatic Ewing's sarcoma included 18 courses of high-dose chemotherapy given to 14 patients with measurable disease, nine of whom had progressive disease. Eight of the courses were based on high-dose busulfan (BU), which was combined with CY in five courses, melphalan in one course, or both in two courses. These high-dose BU-based regimens were active in these refractory and/or relapsed Ewing's sarcoma patients, with three out of eight CRs, four out of eight PRs and one minimal response [26]. High-dose thiotepa has also demonstrated activity against Ewing's sarcoma in a small number of patients [26,33].

Although the median duration of response is short, a significant subset of patients become long-term survivors. The European Blood and Marrow Transplant (EBMT) Registry has reviewed the outcome of transplants performed for Ewing's sarcoma family tumors in the presence of residual disease. From 1978 to 1996, of 411 Ewing's tumor patients whose transplants were reported to the EBMT, 210 were not in CR at the time of HCT. Of these, only 5% were patients with metastatic disease in first PR; the other patients had progressed prior to HCT. Of the patients with residual disease, 169 patients were transplanted in PR and 41 were transplanted in mixed response, no response or progressive disease (PD). The high-dose therapy produced an overall response (OR) rate of 53% and CR in 27%. For patients transplanted with residual disease, 5-year OS was 19% vs. 45% for those transplanted in CR [34].

Even more impressive long-term survival was reported in a small study conducted in Vienna, Austria and Düsseldorf, Germany at two institutions that participated in the CESS. The investigators treated 17 patients with hyperfractionated TBI, melphalan and etoposide, with or without carboplatin. The last five patients received IL-2 after HCT. Of the 17 patients treated, seven had presented with multifocal bony disease, while 10 had experienced either multiple or early relapses. In this group, the probability of long-term DFS was 45% at 6 years. In a matched historical control group, the probability of DFS was only 2% [27]. Further accrual and longer follow-up of 19 patients with early or multiple relapse confirms effective salvage in this patient population, with seven patients (37%) surviving in CR 4–12 years (median 9 years) after transplantation [35].

These results must be interpreted with caution for several reasons. First, the number of patients remains small. In addition, because the induction regimen prior to transplantation was also intensified, it is unclear what role high-dose therapy followed by HCT had in producing the improved survival. Furthermore, the study excluded patients with bulky tumor or disease progression during chemotherapy, because TBI is ineffective for high tumor burden. These selection criteria would have identified a more favorable subset of patients for HCT.

HCT as consolidation of Ewing's tumors

As yet, no randomized prospective studies of the value of HCT for high-risk Ewing's tumors have been completed. The experience reported to

EBMT has been for children with high-risk Ewing's tumors in CR. Data on 63 transplants for Ewing's sarcomas and PNETs were reported between 1982 and 1992. One-half of the patients were transplanted in first response and one-half in second response. The patients treated in first response had high-risk disease on the basis of metastases, usually to bone or marrow. Patients consolidated in first remission achieved 5-year DFS of 21%, while those treated in second CR achieved 32% 5-year DFS. Although these results are superior to the expected results with chemotherapy alone, it is unclear how the patients were selected, and the treatment regimens were heterogeneous. Several intriguing observations were made. The few patients who relapsed after primary metastatic disease fared poorly even after high-dose therapy and HCT. The outcomes of patients who received regimens without TBI ($n = 33$) were substantially better (34% DFS) than those of patients ($n = 30$) who received TBI (19% DFS). High-dose melphalan was used for 93% of patients; DFS with melphalan and BU was 51%, with etoposide 33% and with carmustine 21% [36]. As of 1996, 201 HCT procedures had been reported to EBMT for Ewing's tumor in CR at the time of transplant. The 5-year OS was 45% for those transplanted in CR [34].

The largest phase 2 studies of HCT as consolidation for high-risk Ewing's tumors have been carried out at the National Cancer Institute. Over 5 years, 91 patients were enrolled on a series of three protocols consisting of induction chemotherapy, radiation to the primary site, consolidation with 8 Gy TBI and autologous HCT. Seventy-nine percent of the patients achieved a CR with surgery, local radiation and chemotherapy were therefore eligible for HCT. Ninety percent of eligible patients proceeded to transplant, and 30% have survived long-term without progression of their disease. This proportion is higher than expected for the poor prognosis group of patients initially selected. In addition, the patients who received HCT fared much better than the concurrently treated patients who did not. However, because only patients who did not progress after chemotherapy were eligible for HCT, these improved outcomes may simply represent the effect of this patient selection bias. Lack of improvement in the outcome of the total group supports the hypothesis that selection bias, rather than enhanced efficacy, accounts for the better prognosis of the HCT patients [37].

TBI-based regimens have also been used at the University of Florida to treat patients with high-risk Ewing's tumors since 1985. For the majority of patients, a primary tumor >8 cm in diameter was the high-risk feature. The combined outcome of these regimens for patients with high-risk localized Ewing's tumors, with a primary site >8 cm in diameter, was 63% 5-year OS, better than for historical controls [38]. Although these TBI-based regimens were effective for high-risk localized Ewing's tumors, the addition of ifosfamide and etoposide at conventional doses sufficed to produce similar gains in long-term survival in patients with localized Ewing's tumors [39]. In contrast, patients with metastatic disease did not fare well on these protocols, with only 16% 5-year OS [38].

There is also considerable experience with HCT regimens based on high-dose melphalan. Used as a single agent for consolidation of first or second CR, in a limited institution series of 12 Ewing's tumor patients, it produced only 33% 2-year and 22% 4-year DFS. As in recurrent disease, relapses tended to occur early, at a median of 7 months after HCT [25]. Similar results were obtained in a contemporaneous series (1980–87) of 18 patients at the Institut Gustave-Roussy. These patients were consolidated with high-dose melphalan and carmustine, plus procarbazine in 14 patients. Thirteen of the patients received a second course of high-dose therapy (carmustine, procarbazine and melphalan in nine patients and BU with CY in four patients) 3–4 months later. Two patients died of HCT-related toxicity, and 12 patients relapsed at a median of 7 months (range 3–23 months) post-bone marrow transplantation (BMT). The 2-year DFS was 45% and the 5-year DFS was 20% [26]. The disappointing long-term survival was the impetus to improve the initial chemotherapy and to augment the high-dose alkylator regimen with synergistic chemotherapy or TBI.

Impressive results were obtained in a limited institution study in Düsseldorf and Vienna using a regimen of hyperfractionated 12 Gy TBI, 120–180 mg/m^2 melphalan and 40–60 mg/kg etoposide, with or without 1.5 g/m^2 carboplatin, given as consolidation after 5–8 months of chemotherapy per CESS protocol. Of the 17 patients treated, seven had presented with multifocal bony disease, while 10 had experienced either multiple or early relapse. In the entire group, the probability of long-term DFS was 45% at 6 years [27]. However, these results did not hold up with additional enrollment and longer follow-up. A total of 36 patients were treated with this regimen in Düsseldorf and Vienna from 1986 to 1994. For the whole group, DFS was 24% ± 7%, with median follow-up of 81 months from transplantation. However, only two of 17 (12%) patients with primary multifocal bone or marrow metastases were surviving in first remission. The only events beyond 2 years from HCT were two fatal cases of secondary myelodysplasia [35].

An analysis of the subset of patients with primary metastatic disease has been performed by the German group of the EICESS protocol in an effort to describe prognostic factors and define the role of intensification of therapy [40]. From 1990 to 1995, 177 patients with primary metastatic Ewing's sarcoma were enrolled, and because six were lost to follow-up, 171 were analyzed. Patients received a common induction regimen on the high-risk studies, but the decision to complete 12–14 courses of conventional chemotherapy vs. intensification with melphalan/etoposide/TBI HCT and/or whole lung irradiation was individualized. In this group, 61 had metastases only to lung, 64 had metastases only to bone and/or marrow, 36 had metastases to both lung and bone or marrow and 10 had metastases to other sites. The patients with disease metastatic only to lung benefited from whole lung irradiation, with 40% vs. 19% OS ($p < 0.05$) but, for this subgroup, the role of HCT was not assessed because only two patients were transplanted. Patients with bone or marrow metastases alone did unexpectedly well, with 28% DFS regardless of HCT, suggesting that the intensification of induction chemotherapy compared with historically used regimens may have been beneficial. Among patients with involvement of lung and bone or marrow, intensification strongly influenced survival, with 27% DFS among 20 patients who received either whole lung irradiation or HCT vs. 0% DFS 2 years from diagnosis ($p < 0.0001$) among 16 patients treated with conventional therapy alone [40]. There were not enough patients to assess the independent roles of HCT and whole lung irradiation. Moreover, the results need to be confirmed with an unselected patient population, because the decision to proceed with intensification was individualized in this study, and only patients in CR or PR received HCT.

However, a prospective Children's Cancer Group (CCG) study designed to evaluate this regimen of end-intensification in patients with high-risk Ewing's sarcoma with metastases to bone or marrow in first response did not demonstrate benefit over historical controls treated with a longer course of conventional chemotherapy. Patients received five cycles of induction therapy, identical to the initial treatment of the control patients. Of 32 patients, 22 achieved a CR or very good partial remission (VGPR; complete response of metastatic lesion other than possible persistent bone scan abnormalities and at least 90% resection of the primary tumor) and had peripheral blood stem cells (PBSCs) collected and thus were eligible to proceed to HCT. These patients received hyperfractionated radiation to the primary and metastatic sites, followed by the preparatory regimen of TBI, melphalan and etoposide. Of the patients who underwent HCT, three died acutely of nonrelapse causes and one died after withdrawal from protocol therapy of complications of alternative therapy. DFS for the entire cohort was 20% at 2 years from diagnosis, exactly superimposable with the results for the comparison group of patients treated with conventional chemotherapy for 27 cycles. DFS for patients undergoing HCT was 25% at 2 years from HCT but, given the selection for CR or VGPR, this result remains similar to that of the control group [41].

Moreover, the experience of the Memorial Sloan-Kettering Cancer Center in New York with the P6 protocol in 21 patients with Ewing's sarcoma metastatic to bone or marrow from 1990 to 1998 was disappointing. Although 90% of the patients achieved an initial CR or VGPR, 10 progressed rapidly on induction therapy before they could undergo HCT. Of the 11 patients who underwent HCT, eight received melphalan/TBI, and three received thiotepa and carboplatin. Only one survived long-term, with 91 months' follow-up from diagnosis [42].

There is some suggestion that regimens combining 16 mg/kg BU with 140–160 mg/m^2 melphalan may be superior. At two centers, 18 patients have been consolidated with this regimen for Ewing's tumors. High-risk features included metastatic presentation in 11, bulky primary tumors in six and second response in one patient. Twelve patients were transplanted in first CR, four in second CR, one in PR and one in PD. There was one toxic death from cytomegalovirus pneumonitis with pulmonary hemorrhage. All seven patients with localized disease and six of 11 patients with metastatic disease survived without disease progression at a median follow-up of 2 years after transplantation. The 4-year OS was 60% [43,44].

The SFOP has also studied the combination of high-dose BU and melphalan as consolidation therapy for metastatic Ewing's sarcoma. The 1988 SFOP protocol for metastatic Ewing's sarcoma used conventional-dose chemotherapy. From 1988 to 1990 this protocol accrued 25 patients and produced 12% 3-year DFS and 25% 3-year OS [18]. The 1991 SFOP protocol for metastatic Ewing's sarcoma incorporated HCT. From 1991 to 1995, this successor protocol accrued 44 patients with Ewing's sarcoma and metastases to lung ($n = 23$), bone ($n = 6$) or both sites ($n = 15$). In eight patients, the marrow was also involved. Induction chemotherapy consisted of the same regimen of CY and doxorubicin every 2 weeks as in the 1988 SFOP protocol, for five courses, followed by two courses of ifosfamide and etoposide. Patients achieving CR or VGPR of their metastatic disease were consolidated with 600 mg/m^2 BU and 140 mg/m^2 melphalan. Local therapy was administered before or after HCT. Nine of 44 patients progressed during induction chemotherapy. Thirty-four patients were transplanted: 12 in VGPR and 22 in CR. There were two transplant-related deaths and 13 patients have relapsed. Twenty patients survived without evidence of disease at a median follow-up of 30 months (range 3–50 months). For the entire cohort, 3-year DFS was 41% and OS was 62%. For those undergoing HCT, 3-year DFS was 52% and OS was 76% [45]. This is an important study. Strengths include that the entire cohort of patients with newly diagnosed metastatic disease was treated with intention-to-transplant; there are clear selection criteria for transplantation from among all patients with metastatic disease; results are presented for the entire cohort, including those excluded from transplantation; and the induction chemotherapy is the same as on the prior study, which therefore provides a valid historical control for the effect of the HCT consolidation.

Now that hundreds of transplants have been performed for Ewing's tumors over the past decade, and promising results have been obtained in phase 2 studies, it is appropriate to conduct prospective randomized controlled trials to assess the benefit of HCT for recurrent and for initially metastatic Ewing's tumors. The UKCCSG is conducting a trial randomly comparing HCT vs. chemotherapy plus whole lung irradiation in patients with Ewing's tumors and metastases only to the lung. Other patients with moderately poor prognoses, such as those who relapse during the first 2 years after diagnosis, may similarly be candidates for a prospective randomized trial of HCT vs. intensive chemotherapy. Patients with multifocal metastases and those who relapse very early may be candidates for phase 1 or 2 studies.

Rhabdomyosarcoma

Risk groups and outcomes with conventional therapy

Rhabdomyosarcoma is the most common childhood sarcoma. Although, in general, the prognosis of newly diagnosed patients is favorable, the 5-year OS of patients with metastatic presentations in the Intergroup Rhabdomyosarcoma Study (IRS) II was only 27%. Among patients with metastatic disease, only those with genitourinary primary sites had a relatively favorable prognosis, with 46% 5-year OS [46]. The outlook has not improved. In the IRS-III, which accrued patients from 1984 to 1991, patients with metastatic disease did not benefit from the addition of cisplatin or cisplatin and etoposide to their chemotherapy regimens; their 5-year DFS was 28% and OS 30% [47]. Similarly, on IRS-IV, which enrolled patients from 1992 to 1997, 3-year DFS for patients with metastatic disease from an extremity primary was only 23%. Lymph node involvement also significantly affects prognosis, with 3-year DFS below 40% in N1 disease, as compared with 70% in N0 cases ($p < 0.001$) [48].

In 1992, Koscielniak *et al.* [49] retrospectively analyzed all children with metastatic soft tissue sarcoma registered in any of the major European soft tissue sarcoma studies that accrued patients during the 1980s. Follow-up was available for 146 (95%) of the patients registered, who all had rhabdomyosarcoma, except for four patients with undifferentiated sarcoma and four patients with extraosseous Ewing's sarcoma. For the entire group, long-term OS was 18% and DFS 15%, reaching a plateau after 5 years. This analysis confirmed the advantage of patients with genitourinary primaries and showed that 16 of 20 long-term relapse-free survivors had metastases confined to one organ. This analysis was the basis for the current International Society of Pediatric Oncology strategy to test new drug combinations and the role of early consolidation with HCT in metastatic rhabdomyosarcoma. Parameningeal disease or failure to achieve CR with standard initial therapy were additional high-risk features, with <20% long-term survival [50].

Relapse after initial standard therapy defines an even higher risk population. In 1999, the IRS retrospectively analyzed the outcome of 605 patients (25.6%) whose disease relapsed or progressed after initial therapy on IRS-III (1984–91), IRS-IV pilot (1987–91) or IRS-IV (1991–97) [51]. Median survival for the entire group was only 0.82 years after first progression, and estimated 5-year OS was 17% (95%CI, 14–21%). Histology was a strong prognostic factor, with 5-year OS of 64% for botryoid tumors ($n = 19$), 26% for embryonal ($n = 313$) and 5% for alveolar or undifferentiated rhabdomyosarcoma ($n = 273$). Long-term survival in patients with alveolar or undifferentiated histology was confined to those who had group I (localized completely resected) tumors at initial diagnosis. For patients with embryonal histology, initial stage and group had similar prognostic significance, with patients with stage 1 or group I disease having 52% 5-year OS, compared to 20% for stage 2/3 group II (microscopic residual disease) and/or III (gross residual disease) patients and 12% for stage 4 patients. Among the group I or stage 1 patients with embryonal tumors, distant recurrence conferred an unfavorable prognosis, with 30% survival (95%CI, 12–49%) [51]. Unfortunately, data on salvage therapy administered after relapse were not available, so this analysis could not address the value of HCT in these patients.

HCT in recurrent and refractory rhabdomyosarcoma

In a murine xenograft model using six primary rhabdomyosarcoma cell lines, one of which was resistant to CY, there was a clear dose effect for melphalan, which demonstrated much greater activity than vincristine, actinomycin D, CY and doxorubicin, the standard chemotherapeutic agents used to treat rhabdomyosarcoma [5]. Several high-dose regimens have demonstrated activity against measurable disease refractory to standard chemotherapy, albeit in few patients (Table 99.2). Only one phase 2 study of HCT specifically for rhabdomyosarcoma has been published to

Table 99.2 Activity of high-dose regimens against measurable rhabdomyosarcoma and childhood soft-tissue sarcomas.

Agents	n	CR	PR	Total	Reference
Melphalan	1	1	0	1/1	[29]
Busulfan, cyclophosphamide	1	1	0	1/1	[52]
Melphalan				30%	[53]
Melphalan, carboplatin	2	0	1	1/2	[54]
Carboplatin, etoposide, cyclophosphamide	11 RMS 28 sarcomas	13	6	19/28	[55]
Carboplatin, etoposide, cyclophosphamide	3	0	0	0/3	[56]
Melphalan, carboplatin	6	4	0	4/6	[30]
Thiotepa	8	0	4	4/8	[33]

CR, complete response; PR, partial response; RMS, rhabdomyosarcoma.

date. Eighteen patients (six alveolar, eight embryonal, two undifferentiated and two desmoplastic small round cell tumors) were enrolled between 1986 and 1998. All had failed previous treatment with conventional multimodal therapy (six primary refractory disease, two PR of metastatic disease, 10 relapsed 1–6 times [median two times]). Thiotepa was administered as a single agent at 300 mg/m^2/day for 3 days. One patient achieved CR and five achieved PR, for an OR rate of 33%. Two patients with minimal responses were converted to CR by radiation therapy or surgery and survive 50 and 63 months without evidence of disease [57]. This response rate compares favorably to that of single agents at conventional doses in a similar patient population, but indicates the need for synergistic combinations of therapy to overcome established drug resistance in macroscopic disease.

From 1982 to 1990, 31 HCTs for relapsed and refractory soft tissue sarcoma and rhabdomyosarcoma had been reported to the EBMT. Of these, 21 were transplanted in sensitive relapse, nine in resistant relapse and one with progressive disease. All of the patients received melphalan-based preparatory regimens; some had two courses of high-dose therapy. The 5-year survival was 15%, not substantially better than the historical results [58]. The EBMT has now received reports of 98 transplants performed through 1994 in children and young adults with relapse or progression of initially localized rhabdomyosarcoma. The proportion surviving disease-free has improved marginally to 20%, and median survival remains short, only 8.3 months from HCT [59].

The German–Austrian Pediatric BMT Group in 1997 published a retrospective analysis of 36 transplants performed for childhood soft tissue sarcomas between 1986 and 1994, which included nine transplant procedures performed for relapse of initially localized tumor. Thirty-four of the 36 patients received high-dose melphalan-based regimens, usually augmented with etoposide and carboplatin. Four of nine patients transplanted in relapse survived without evidence of disease, including one patient with systemic and three patients with lymph node relapses [60]. This proportion is better than expected for patients relapsing after initial treatment for group II or III disease, but the small number of patients and unclear effects of patient selection bias preclude conclusions about the efficacy of HCT for salvage in recurrent rhabdomyosarcoma.

HCT as consolidation for high-risk rhabdomyosarcoma

In a salvage setting, high-dose regimens have demonstrated activity against rhabdomyosarcoma, but the poor durability of these responses suggests that the degree of cell kill is inadequate for elimination of resistant macroscopic disease. If so, a reasonable hypothesis is that high-dose therapy may improve long-term survival in high-risk patients when applied to consolidate a first CR. The first large-scale prospective study to evaluate this hypothesis has been conducted in Europe, using high-dose melphalan [61].

The basis for this regimen was the considerable experience accumulated by the EBMT Registry since 1984. From 1982 to 1990, 62 patients were transplanted for rhabdomyosarcoma or soft tissue sarcoma in first response, all with high-dose melphalan-based regimens. For the entire group, 5-year survival from the time of HCT was 22%, but it was 34% for 40 patients transplanted in first CR vs. 0% for 22 patients transplanted in first PR [58]. The data of EBMT were reanalyzed in 1997, including 92 transplants performed through 1994 in children and young adults with primary metastatic rhabdomyosarcoma. The proportion of patients in CR before HCT remained stable at 64%, as did DFS of 20% [59].

The 1991 prospective European intergroup study for stage 4 malignant mesenchymal tumors, MMT4-91, resulted from the amendment of MMT4-89 for patients with newly diagnosed metastatic rhabdomyosarcoma, so that institutions could chose to substitute HCT with high-dose melphalan for the fourth and final 9-week cycle of chemotherapy in patients who had achieved CR before the third cycle of therapy. Thus, there was a nearly contemporaneous control population of patients either enrolled on MMT4-89 or enrolled on MMT4-91 at centers not participating in HCT. The control group was treated with the identical aggressive initial multimodal therapy and had also achieved CR before the third cycle of therapy and continued on conventional therapy. Moreover, although patients were not randomized to HCT or conventional therapy, decisions to administer HCT consolidation were made at the center level, reducing the potential for selection bias. Unfortunately, the patient population treated with HCT ($n = 52$) in fact had poorer prognostic factors: lymph node involvement was more common (56% vs. 34%); alveolar histology was more common (44% vs. 30%); fewer patients were <10 years old (60% vs. 68%); and more patients had large tumors >5 cm diameter (73% vs. 61%) than in the control population ($n = 44$). Despite these differences and the small sample size, the median time from the end of therapy to relapse was significantly longer for the HCT group than the conventional chemotherapy group (168 vs. 104 days; $p = 0.05$). There were trends toward better 3-year event-free survival (EFS) (29.7% vs. 19.2%; $p = 0.3$) and OS (40% vs. 27.7%; $p = 0.5$) for HCT compared with conventional therapy [61].

The results of single institution protocols for high-risk rhabdomyosarcoma that incorporate HCT consolidation are similar to this aggregate experience, with DFS in stage 4 patients ranging from 14% to 28% at 3 years or more [37,62–64]. Each of these studies has shown that HCT consolidation is tolerable and that a shortened intensified course of treatment incorporating HCT for responders can at least match the long-term outcome of 1–2 years of conventional chemotherapy, but these studies do not demonstrate an unequivocal improvement in the outcome of patients with poor-prognosis rhabdomyosarcoma. Total duration of hospitalization is generally less than with conventional dose therapy. To the extent that long-term adverse effects of chemotherapy depend on cumulative doses, as opposed to peak levels, briefer more intensive therapy may not ultimately be more toxic than conventional therapy, so equal long-term survival is not necessarily a reason to abandon the strategy of HCT consolidation for high-risk rhabdomyosarcoma. Indeed, the MMT4-91 experience suggests possible improvement in long-term survival, subject to the limitations of a nonrandomized study with <100 analyzed patients. To answer this question definitively will require a larger randomized prospective trial.

Some modification of strategy may be superior to end-intensification with HCT. After HCT, a maintenance course of schedule-dependent chemotherapy not cross-resistant with the HCT may prove beneficial. Conversely, it is possible that the use of repeated peripheral blood hematopoietic cell (PBHC) rescue will allow further intensification of therapy and will result in improved survival. The use of repeated PBHC rescue to intensify nonmyeloablative therapy has been piloted in Seattle. The five most active drugs for sarcoma—vincristine, doxorubicin, cyclophosphamide, ifosfamide and etoposide—were combined in the VACIME regimen to be administered in every cycle, rather than in alternating cycles of three drugs and two drugs. Severe hematopoietic toxicity limited the delivered dose intensity [65]. Rescue with PBHCs collected during recovery from the second and fourth cycles of therapy significantly increased the delivered dose intensity compared with historical controls [66]. In this series, seven of eight patients with metastatic rhabdomyosarcoma or undifferentiated sarcoma achieved a CR of metastatic sites; there were five CRs at the primary site and three PRs. Both the CR rate and the report of three long-term survivors 39–48 months from diagnosis in this small series are encouraging. Testing in a larger population would be appropriate to assess the impact of this strategy on survival.

Wilms' tumor

Risk groups and outcomes with conventional therapy

Wilms' tumor is the exceptional childhood solid tumor that is often curable by conventional chemotherapy when metastatic at diagnosis, and even after relapse. However, high-risk groups can be defined. The National Wilms' Tumor Studies, NWTS-2 and NWTS-3, accrued 2757 untreated patients aged ≤15 years, with stage I–IV disease. The prognosis of the 367 patients (14%) who relapsed after achieving an initial CR was analyzed in 1989. Histology was an important predictor of outcome. In NWTS-3, 3-year survival after relapse was 42% with favorable histology vs. 16% with unfavorable histology. Approximately equal numbers of patients relapsed <6 months, 6–11 months and >12 months from diagnosis. Their respective 3-year survival was 18%, 30% and 41%, respectively. Among patients with favorable histology, the 3-year survival by initial stage was stage I 57%, stage II–III 36% and stage IV 17%; for patients with unfavorable histology, 3-year survival by stage was stage I 17%, stage II–III 14% and stage IV 7%. Among stage II–III patients with favorable histology, those randomized to receive three-drug initial therapy had 16% 3-year survival from relapse vs. 42% among those initially treated with two-drug regimens. Abdominal location of relapse was unfavorable when this field had been previously irradiated, precluding further radiation therapy to the site of relapse [67].

An analysis of the outcome of patients relapsing on the UKCCSG Wilms' Tumor 1 trial, which accrued 381 patients from 1980 to 1986, confirmed the negative prognostic importance of unfavorable histology, high initial stage and early relapse for long-term survival post-relapse, given salvage with ifosfamide or cisplatin and etoposide [68,69]. Taken together, these results have led to the accepted definition of a high-risk subgroup of relapsed Wilms' tumor patients whose expected 3-year survival is <20%, including those with any of the following features: unfavorable histology, relapse within 6 months of diagnosis, failure of a three-drug regimen and involvement of sites other than lung and abdomen, or involving the abdomen after irradiation.

HCT for high-risk relapse of Wilms' tumor

Limited published information is available regarding high-dose therapy for these patients. The experience collected by EBMT has been reviewed [70]. Twenty-five patients with Wilms' tumor received high-dose therapy over a 7-year period from 1984 to 1991. Twenty-one of these children had had 1–4 relapses, and four patients had stage IV disease refractory to first-line therapy. Of 11 patients transplanted in second CR, 10 had one or more high-risk features as defined above. Twenty of the 25 patients received high-dose melphalan-based regimens, although seven different regimens were used. Eight of 17 children transplanted in CR became long-term disease-free survivors. Of patients with measurable disease, five of eight achieved a CR and one of eight achieved a PR to high-dose therapy, demonstrating the activity of these regimens in refractory Wilms' tumor. However, only one of eight children with measurable disease at the time of HCT became a long-term survivor [70].

A limited institution series of 12 patients with multifocal, generally multiply recurrent Wilms' tumors were given thiotepa-based preparatory regimens. Their preparatory regimen consisted of 1200 mg/m^2 thiotepa, 1800 mg/m^2 etoposide and 50–140 mg/kg CY. One patient received 1200 mg/m^2 thiotepa and hyperfractionated 12 Gy TBI. In this preliminary report, the DFS at 18 months was 46%, suggesting benefit from high-dose thiotepa [71].

These results are sufficiently encouraging to warrant prospective evaluation, first in phase 2 trials to identify active regimens and then in a randomized comparison with chemotherapy for patients with high-risk disease. The SFOP has completed the first prospective trial of HCT for high-risk relapsed Wilms' tumor [72]. From 1988 to 1994, 31 patients underwent HCT, including 29 relapsed (second CR 16; second PR 4; third CR 3; third PR 5; fifth CR 1) and two stage IV anaplastic Wilms' tumor patients transplanted in first CR. All patients had at least one high-risk feature and were heavily pretreated with five or six chemotherapy drugs before HCT. The preparatory regimen consisted of 180 mg/m^2 melphalan, 1000 mg/m^2 etoposide and carboplatin, dosed to achieve an area-under-the-curve of 20 mg/min/mL over 5 days. Radiation therapy was delivered to sites of bulky metastatic disease after recovery from HCT. Seven patients sustained renal tubular damage, one developed veno-occlusive disease (VOD) of the liver but recovered fully, and three developed interstitial pneumonitis. Only one of nine evaluable patients failed to achieve CR after HCT. Sixteen patients relapsed at a median of 8.5 months (range 3–53 months) after HCT and 12 patients remained in continuous CR a median of 48.5 months (range 36–96 months) after HCT. DFS is $50 \pm 17\%$ and OS is $60 \pm 18\%$ at 3 years [72]. The only statistically significant prognostic factor was the number of disease progressions before HCT: in second response, DFS was $63.1 \pm 20\%$, compared with $22.2 \pm 24\%$ in third response or beyond. The results are better than historical results for high-risk patients with such advanced disease. However, over the same period, 15 patients in the participating centers with at least one adverse prognostic factor failed to undergo consolidation because of uncontrolled PD, and would need to be included in an intent-to-treat analysis to estimate survival from relapse in an unselected population.

The recently completed NWTS V pediatric salvage protocol was initially designed to incorporate HCT for patients who failed to achieve a CR after two courses of salvage induction chemotherapy. However, the study was amended to eliminate HCT. Although the results of this salvage protocol are not yet mature, the St. Jude institutional experience and the results of the CCG pilot salvage protocols suggest that new chemotherapy approaches have improved the outcome of patients with high-risk relapse even without HCT [73,74], and it would therefore be appropriate to launch an international trial to assess the value of HCT compared with conventional-dose chemotherapy in high-risk recurrent Wilms' tumor.

HCT as consolidation for Wilms' tumor

Because of the excellent curability of Wilms' tumor with conventional chemotherapy, few HCT have been reported for Wilms' tumor in first response, all for patients with stage IV disease. All five patients reported by the EBMT, including two with unfavorable histology, survive disease-free at a median of 62 months (range 14–67 months) after HCT [70], but both patients with stage IV anaplastic Wilms' tumor transplanted by the SFOP died of progressive disease [72].

Osteosarcoma

Risk groups and outcomes with conventional therapy

The most important prognostic factor in osteosarcoma is the extent of disease at diagnosis, and patients presenting with overt metastatic disease have attained only 20–30% long-term survival with excision and chemotherapy, as compared with 55–70% survival in patients with localized disease [75]. Prognosis is particularly poor in patients with distant metastases to bone or with unresectable disease with 6% vs. 35% OS in patients with metastases only to lung [76,77]. Poor histologic response, defined as <90–95% necrosis, is a negative prognostic factor, associated with 45–50% long-term survival [75,77]. P-glycoprotein expression is also associated with poorer outcomes [78] and has prognostic significance independent of histologic response [75]. Preliminary evidence suggests that high levels of vascular endothelial growth factor before therapy are associated with early metastatic relapse [79].

Survival after relapse is possible in a minority of patients, ranging from 15% to 50%, with poorer prognosis in patients who progress soon after diagnosis, with a larger number of nodules and with both bone and lung lesions at relapse [77,80].

HCT for recurrent or refractory osteosarcoma

A steep dose–response correlation has been observed for methotrexate (MTX) and doxorubicin in treating osteosarcoma and has been the basis for the design of current standard regimens, which employ high-dose MTX and dose-intensive doxorubicin; however, the cell cycle dependence of MTX and the nonhematopoietic toxicity of doxorubicin make these agents unsuitable for dose escalation in HCT cytoreductive regimens. Ironically, although Ridgeway's osteogenic sarcoma was one of the primary experimental tumor models used by Schabel et al. [4] to demonstrate the steepness of dose–response curves, particularly for CY, HCT has rarely been applied to patients with osteosarcoma. The EBMT received reports of only seven patients transplanted for osteosarcoma as of 1992. All received alkylator-based preparatory regimens. Of the five patients with measurable disease, one died of toxicity, three patients had no response and one transplanted in refractory relapse achieved a PR that was improved to CR by surgical excision of lung metastases, and remains in second CR 18 months post-HCT. The two patients transplanted in second CR relapsed 8 and 11 months after HCT [81].

The Cooperative German–Austrian–Swiss Osteosarcoma Study Group retrospectively analyzed 15 patients who received HCT for recurrent osteosarcoma. These patients had all achieved a CR when initially treated. Their sites of relapse were lung in nine patients, lung plus local in two, mediastinal in two and local only in two. All underwent resection of their recurrent disease before HCT; only two had macroscopic residual disease, and neither responded to the high-dose preparatory regimen. The preparatory regimens all incorporated a combination of etoposide with melphalan or carboplatin, or both. Six patients received two courses of HCT, first with thiotepa and CY and then with melphalan, but two of these patients died of toxicity. The 3-year OS was 29% and DFS was 20%. Both disease-free survivors received melphalan-based preparative regimens [82].

Although this poor experience is felt to reflect the poor efficacy of alkylating drugs for osteosarcoma, cisplatin and ifosfamide had good activity against osteosarcoma in phase 2 trials [83], and related agents, carboplatin and CY, can be escalated significantly as an HCT cytoreductive regimen. In a phase 1 trial of carboplatin, etoposide and CY for children with refractory or relapsed solid tumors, four patients with osteosarcoma were included, of whom three with measurable disease had major responses [55]. In addition, a patient with recurrence in bone and lung is a long-term survivor after HCT with BU and CY [84]. Therefore, larger phase 2 trials are warranted in an attempt to identify active regimens for patients with high-risk disease.

The first such trial has been conducted by SFOP. From 1992 to 1996, 11 patients with metastatic osteosarcoma were treated with 900 mg/m^2 thiotepa. All patients had undergone resection of their primary tumor but had residual metastatic disease after treatment with a median of six drugs (range 4–8 drugs) at the time of transplantation. At HCT, one patient was in first PR, two were in second PR, three each were in second and third progression, and two were in fifth progression of their disease. Toxicity was acceptable; other side-effects included vomiting and diarrhea, and one patient developed mild VOD. One patient entered CR and seven PR after HCT, for an OR rate of 73%. Residual metastases were excised in eight of 11 patients and DFS 2 years after HCT was 31%, an impressive result considering the advanced status and degree of prior therapy of this cohort [85]. Given the activity of this preparatory regimen, its use should be considered for high-risk patients.

The Italian and Scandinavian sarcoma group conducted a phase 2 study of carboplatin and etoposide with PBHC rescue in patients with high-risk recurrent osteosarcoma. They enrolled 32 patients: 21 in first relapse, eight in second relapse and three in third relapse. The patients in first relapse had multiple sites of relapse except for one, who had a very large pulmonary lesion. All patients had previously received cisplatin at conventional doses. The regimen included cyclophosphamide and etoposide for stem cell mobilization, followed by two courses of HCT with 1500 mg/m^2 carboplatin and 1800 mg/m^2 etoposide, given 4 weeks apart. Four patients received a single course of HCT because of <5 × 10^6 CD34$^+$ PBSC/kg (three patients) or VOD (one patient). The toxicity was acceptable; of 60 courses of HCT, only five were complicated by grade 3 toxicity: stomatitis in four cases and hepatic in one case. Even though all patients had previously been treated with cisplatin at conventional doses, the regimen was active: four of eight patients were converted from PR to CR by HCT. However, it was rarely curative, with 3-year OS of 20% and DFS of 12%.

Novel approaches are required for phase 2 trials in osteosarcoma, because calcified osteosarcoma lesions do not necessarily diminish in size even after effective therapy that produces complete necrosis, so conventional imaging criteria can underestimate responses. Furthermore, it is clear that chemotherapy, even at myeloablative doses, does not produce adequate local control of unresected lesions. An interesting alternative is the use of bone-seeking phosphonates to deliver radioisotopes to osteosarcoma lesions at therapeutic doses. Samarium-153 ethylene diamine tetramethylene phosphonate (^{153}Sm-EDTMP) is approved for the palliation of painful bony metastases at a conventional dose of 37 MBq/kg (1 mCi/kg). Its dose-limiting toxicity is marrow suppression. Therefore, an escalated dose of ^{153}Sm-EDTMP, 150 MBq/kg (4 mCi/kg) was given to six patients with unresectable primary or recurrent osteosarcoma with PBSC rescue. The target lesions received doses ranging from 15 to 50 Gy, with excellent pain relief, and the target lesions were controlled in half of patients [86]. Considerable further escalation of the dose of ^{153}Sm-EDTMP is feasible. A phase 1 trial demonstrated that doses up to 1.1 GBq/kg (30 mCi/kg) are tolerable, but noted prolonged platelet transfusion dependence in patients rescued with <2 × 10^6 CD34$^+$ PBSC/kg. At 1.1 GBq/kg (30 mCi/kg), because EDTMP chelates calcium, patients can develop symptomatic hypocalcemia. At this dose, the estimated red marrow dose was 30 Gy and the dose to target lesions ranged from 39 to 241 Gy; nonhematopoietic toxicities remain mild [87].

Retinoblastoma

Risk groups and outcomes with conventional therapy

Early detection of retinoblastoma is the norm, and the treatment outcome of patients with localized disease is excellent. Orbital extension is curable with multimodal therapy. In contrast, advanced central nervous system (CNS) involvement, and "trilateral retinoblastoma" [88] is incurable:

multimodal therapy including systemic and intrathecal chemotherapy and cranial irradiation has produced remissions which, however, have not been durable [89]. Hematogenous dissemination to bone, marrow, viscera and involvement of soft tissue and lymph nodes carries an extremely poor prognosis. Only ifosfamide and CY have efficacy as single agents and have produced CRs when used in two- and three-drug combinations [89]. There is a single case report of long-term survival of hematogenously disseminated retinoblastoma in a patient treated aggressively with mechlorethamine, doxorubicin, cisplatin, dacarbazine, vincristine and CY (MAD-DOC); however, 2 years later the patient developed secondary myelodysplasia requiring allogeneic BMT [90]. The patient became a long-term survivor without recurrent retinoblastoma or myelodysplasia.

HCT as consolidation for disseminated disease

There are several individual case reports [91–93] and small case series [94,95] of HCT for patients in second CR after metastatic recurrence in bone or marrow. These reports describe a total of 10 patients, of whom only two experienced further progression of their disease. The eight survivors had no evidence of disease 18–80 months after relapse.

The SFOP formally evaluated HCT for patients with high-risk retinoblastoma, using a single-arm protocol active from 1989 to 1994 [96]. The target population was patients with extraocular disease or histologic evidence of tumor at the cut end of the optic nerve or its subarachnoid space. Measurable extraocular disease had to be chemosensitive in order for patients to be eligible to proceed to HCT. During the study period, 34 high-risk patients were identified: eight with microscopic residual optic nerve involvement; 10 with extraocular disease confined to the orbit; 11 with extraocular involvement including distant bones or marrow; and five with CNS involvement. Nine patients did not proceed to HCT because of CNS progression (six patients), parental refusal (two patients) or toxicity (one patient). Therefore, 25 patients (six with optic nerve, seven with orbital disease, eight with distant bone or marrow disease and four with CNS involvement) proceeded to HCT with a preparatory regimen of 1250–1750 mg/m^2 carboplatin, 1750 mg/m^2 etoposide and 3200 mg/m^2 cyclophosphamide. Five of six patients who had measurable disease at the time of HCT achieved CR. On an intention-to-treat basis, five of eight patients with optic nerve involvement, six of 10 patients with orbital involvement, five of 11 patients with bone or marrow involvement and one of five patients with CNS involvement survived with no evidence of disease. Compared with historical results using much longer courses of conventional chemotherapy, this approach produced comparable survival for patients with optic nerve or orbital involvement, and was superior for patients with distant bone or marrow involvement [96].

Desmoplastic small cell tumor

Risk groups and outcomes with conventional therapy

Desmoplastic small cell tumor is a highly malignant abdominal small round cell tumor with epithelial, mesenchymal and neural characteristics that was initially described in 1991 [97]. It occurs in children and young adults and is probably not rare; over 101 cases have already been reported between 1989 and 1996. A balanced translocation, t(11;22)(p13;q12) results in *EWS-WT1* chimeric transcripts considered diagnostic of desmoplastic small cell tumor [98]. Tumor response was noted in 19 of 40 case reports, generally after treatment with combinations of doxorubicin, cisplatin, CY, etoposide and fluorouracil. However, the outcome has been dismal, with median survival of only 17 months (range 3–72 months); as of 1996, only seven of 101 reported patients were alive a median of 24 months (range 4–48 months) from diagnosis [99]. A series of 10 previously untreated patients has been reported from the Memorial Sloan-Kettering Cancer Center. Two of these patients underwent initial gross total resection and one died early of disease. Chemotherapy consisted of CY, doxorubicin and vincristine, alternating with ifosfamide and etoposide. All seven evaluable patients achieved a PR. After second-look surgery, there were seven CRs and two PRs [100]. Therefore, desmoplastic small cell tumors are chemosensitive, but the short duration of responses warrants attempts at consolidation.

HCT as salvage therapy

There are two reported cases of HCT as salvage therapy for recurrent or refractory desmoplastic small cell tumor. A 7-year-old boy who presented with a 10-cm mass with local extension was refractory to initial therapy per the European Study for Malignant Mesenchymal Tumors and to salvage with cisplatin and etoposide. After debulking surgery, he underwent autologous HCT in PR, but progressed despite IL-2 and abdominal irradiation [101]. A 13-year-old boy with an 8-cm abdominal mass, metastatic to liver, achieved PR to vincristine, doxorubicin, CY, ifosfamide, etoposide and second-look resection, but after continuing chemotherapy for 18 courses, he had residual liver disease. One month later, he was treated for progressive disease with HCT, using thiotepa, CY, carboplatin and etoposide. He obtained PR, but progressed 7 months after HCT [99].

HCT as consolidation

In the Memorial Sloan-Kettering Cancer Center series, the intent was to consolidate first responses of patients with initially unresectable disease with HCT. One patient with initially unresectable disease had too much toxicity from the induction chemotherapy to undergo HCT and instead received local irradiation, and was alive without recurrence more than 39 months from diagnosis. One patient died of candidiasis in CR 12 months from diagnosis. Three patients with initially unresectable disease received HCT with thiotepa and carboplatin in first response: two in CR, and one in PR. The patient transplanted in PR progressed at 15 months. The patients transplanted in CR were alive without evidence of disease 13 and 34 months from initiation of therapy [100]. In an adult population, entered on a protocol with intent to transplant in Milan, of seven patients with desmoplastic small cell tumors (DSRCT), only three achieved a PR to induction therapy with ifosfamide, vincristine and etoposide and proceeded to HCT based on melphalan and thiotepa. All progressed within 4 months [102].

Both patients with DSRCT treated with VACIME with repeated PBHC support became long-term survivors with no evidence of disease 44 and 58 months from diagnosis [63].

Case reports of HCT for pediatric solid tumors

Pleuropulmonary blastoma is a rare tumor, approximately 100 cases of which have been reported. The primary therapy is surgical excision, without adjuvant therapy. Because of the histologic resemblance to soft tissue sarcoma and Wilms' tumor, chemotherapy regimens designed for these entities have been used. Such combination chemotherapy has produced 30–40% DFS [103]. Three patients with pleuropulmonary blastoma have received melphalan-based HCT for progressive disease [104], for chemosensitive microscopic residual disease [103] and for refractory metastatic disease [105]. The patients with bulky refractory disease progressed soon after HCT, but the patient with microscopic residual disease was alive in continuous CR at 12 months after HCT.

The use of HCT for germ-cell tumors in adults is discussed in Chapter 95. A case of refractory metastatic malignant germ cell tumor which was successfully treated with high-dose carboplatin, etoposide and CY remaining in CR 3 years after transplantation suggests that this approach has curative potential in children as well as adults [106].

Esthesioneuroblastoma is a rare tumor, arising from olfactory epithelium; of over 240 cases in the literature, only 21% are pediatric. The behavior of this tumor may be more aggressive in childhood. It has been suggested that esthesioneuroblastoma may be a member of the Ewing's sarcoma family on the basis of a t(11;22) in two of three cell lines derived from metastatic esthesioneuroblastoma cases. However, unlike Ewing's tumors, esthesioneuroblastomas do not express MIC-2, and primary esthesioneuroblastomas express trisomy 8, not t(11;22) [107]. In a single institution series, long-term survival was achieved in three of five adult patients salvaged with CY-containing preparatory regimens vs. four of 17 salvaged with conventional chemotherapy [108]. One adolescent was treated for a cervical nodal recurrence with modified radical neck dissection, and consolidation with high-dose carboplatin, etoposide, melphalan and HCT, and has no evidence of disease 1 year later [109].

General considerations

Regimens

Studies that evaluate various high-dose cytoreductive regimens for solid tumors and include children or include pediatric histologies are summarized in Table 99.3. As yet there have been no prospective comparisons of regimens. Short of randomized comparisons, concurrent pilot studies in a cooperative group setting with common induction regimens and common patient selection criteria would assist in selection of a regimen to submit to a randomized comparison with conventional chemotherapy.

Role of total body irradiation

For all but the most radiosensitive tumors, the doses of radiation therapy that can be delivered as TBI are inadequate for control of bulky tumors. Indeed, doses of adjuvant radiation demonstrated to control the majority of microscopic residual disease (typically 10^6–10^8 cells) exceed the maximum tolerable doses of TBI [115]. However, the relationship between the dose of radiation and the percentage reduction in risk of recurrence appears to be linear. Extrapolating from these dose-risk data, zero reduction in risk occurs at a dose between 0 and 5 Gy, indicating that there is a low threshold, if any, for tumor cell killing by radiation [83,116]. Therefore, the modest doses of radiation feasible as TBI may be expected to control very small micrometastases (perhaps 10^2–10^4 cells).

The question of whether TBI is a necessary or desirable component of the high-dose cytoreductive regimen has been addressed retrospectively by the EBMT. For rhabdomyosarcoma patients, the addition of TBI to melphalan appears only to increase toxicity [58]. A retrospective analysis of the German–Austrian Pediatric BMT Group also found no benefit of 12 Gy hyperfractionated TBI added to melphalan, etoposide and carboplatin [60]. For Ewing's sarcomas, the EBMT Registry observed that patients receiving TBI fared worse ($n = 30$; 19% EFS) than those receiving high-dose chemotherapy alone ($n = 33$; 34% EFS); the best results were obtained with chemotherapy combinations that included BU (51% EFS) [36].

Hematopoietic cell grafts

Allogeneic vs. autologous HCT

Another question is whether there is a preferred graft for HCT. Allogeneic transplantation carries the risk of graft-vs.-host disease (GVHD) but its potential benefits include the absence of reinfused tumor cells and perhaps an immunologic antitumor effect. For rhabdomyosarcoma, the German–Austrian Pediatric BMT Group found no evidence of benefit from allogeneic HCT, as none of five allogeneic HCT recipients survived [60]. In addition, donor lymphocyte infusion (DLI) was reported to be ineffective in a case of relapsed rhabdomyosarcoma [117] but, because the patient did not have measurable disease at the time of DLI and did not develop GVHD, the possibility of an effective immune response remains untested. In contrast, for Ewing's tumors, there was a trend toward better outcome with allogeneic HCT (50% survival vs. 23% survival of entire group of 27 allografted patients at a median of 56 months) in the single

Table 99.3 Regimens evaluated against pediatric solid tumors.

Agents	Total (*n*)	Pediatric (*n*)	Diagnosis	Evaluable	CR	TR	Reference
Melphalan	3	3	ES 3	3	2	3	[22]
Melphalan	33	9	NBL 6	6	3	4	[29]
			ES 2	2	1	2	
			RMS 1	1	1	1	
Melphalan	18	18	NBL 10	10	5	7	[24]
			ES 8	8			
Melphalan	9	9	ES	9	3	5	[25]
Melphalan, TBI	13	13	ES 12, PNET 1	9	1		[28]
Melphalan, carboplatin	30	30	NBL 15				[30]
			RMS, STS 10	6	4		
			ES, PNET 4	2	1		
			Rhabdoid tumor 1				
Melphalan ± carmustine ± procarbazine	8	8	ES metastatic	8	1	3	[26]
Melphalan, TT	28	27	RMS 8	1	0	0	[32]
			GCT 6	1	1	1	
			NBL 4	3	0	0	
			Hepatoblastoma 4	4	3	4	
			ES, PNET 3	2	0	0	
			Pulmonary blastoma 1	1	1	1	
			Medulloblastoma 1	1	0	1	

Table 99.3 (cont'd)

Agents	Total (n)	Pediatric (n)	Diagnosis	Evaluable	CR	TR	Reference
BU, CY	20	20	NBL 10	10	1	3	[52]
			NHL 6	6	5	5	
			ES 3	2	0	1	
			RMS 1	1	1	1	
Dimethylbusulfan	11	5	ES 5	5	2	2	[110]
BU, CY and/or melphalan	8	8	ES metastatic	8	3	7	[26]
BU, CY	18	18	ES 7	5	0	1	[84]
			RMS 4				
			NBL 1				
			EsthesioNBL 1				
			Medulloblastoma 1			1	
			Melanoblastoma 1				
			OS 1	0			
			Hepatoblastoma 1				
			Wilms' 1			1	
Carboplatin, etoposide	30	30	NBL 16	26	1	11	[111]
			CNS 6				
			ES 1				
			OS 1				
			RMS 1				
			Lymphoma 4				
			GCT 1				
Carboplatin, etoposide, CY	27	3	GCT 15	20	9	11	[56]
			Ovarian CA 8				
			RMS 3				
			HD 1				
Carboplatin, etoposide, CY	25	25	Retinoblastoma 25	6	5	6	[96]
CY, carboplatin	43	4	ES	0	0	0	[112]
			GCT 2	1	0	1	
			OS	1	0	1	
Thiotepa	2	2	ES metastatic	2	0	1	[26]
Thiotepa	22	22	OS 7	7	0	4	[33]
			RMS 8	8	0	4	
			ES 3	3	0	2	
			NB 3	3	0	1	
			BL 1	1	0	0	
Thiotepa	11	11	OS	11	1	8	[85]
BU, etoposide, thiotepa	19	19	NBL 14	8	2	2	[113]
			ES 3	1	1	1	
			RMS 2	0	0	0	
BU, melphalan, thiotepa	28	6	ES/PNET 2	0	0	0	[114]
			NBL	1	1	1	
			Seminoma	1	0	0	
			RMS	0	0	0	
			Sarcoma	0	0	0	
BU, melphalan, thiotepa	104	6	ES 3	2	2	2	[31]
			PNET 2	2	2	2	
			NBL 1	0			

BL, Burkitt's lymphoma; CNS, brain tumor; ES, Ewing's sarcoma; GCT, germ cell tumor; GBM, glioblastoma multiforme; HD, Hodgkin's disease; NBL, neuroblastoma; NHL, non-Hodgkin's lymphoma; OS, osteosarcoma; PNET, primitive neuroectodermal tumor; RMS, rhabdomyosarcoma; STS, soft tissue sarcoma.

institution experience with (TB)I/melphalan and etoposide (with or without carboplatin) of Vienna, from 1984 to 1996 [118]. With longer follow-up, incorporating the experience from Düsseldorf, DFS after allogeneic HCT was not better than after autologous HCT for Ewing's tumors because of higher rates of nonrelapse mortality [35]. However, only few allogeneic transplants have been performed for pediatric solid tumors. This probably results largely from the role of neuroblastoma as the prototypical poor prognosis pediatric solid tumor and the clear consensus that there is no role for allogeneic transplantation in neuroblastoma [119,120]. The lack of benefit from allogeneic HCT would indicate that tumor contamination of autologous grafts is not a major source of relapse, and that alloreactive cytotoxic T lymphocytes (CTL) are not substantially effective against high-risk pediatric solid tumors. However, a potentially important biologic difference between neuroblastoma and Ewing's sarcoma is that *in vitro*, neuroblastoma cells are poor targets for CTL, whereas Ewing's sarcoma cells are excellent CTL targets and are even susceptible to lysis by melanoma tumor-infiltrating lymphocytes [121].

Source of the graft: peripheral blood hematopoietic cells vs. bone marrow

It is now recognized that mobilizing and collecting PBHCs is feasible in children despite their small size and the intensity of the pediatric chemotherapy regimens, and PBHCs produce faster engraftment [122–126] and immune reconstitution [127] than marrow. It has been suggested that mobilized PBHCs may also be free of tumor contamination [128], but we and others have found frequent contamination of mobilized PBHC grafts with tumor cells [129–132]. Therefore, purging of mobilized PBHCs is likely to be as important as purging of marrow.

Rationale for graft engineering

The question of whether the purging of autologous hematopoietic cells can improve outcome remains to be answered. A characteristic feature of Ewing's tumors is the presence of the t(11;22)(q24;q12), which results in expression of a chimeric EWS/Fli-1 transcript. This can be detected sensitively and specifically by the nested reverse transcriptase-polymerase chain reaction (RT-PCR). Using this technique, evidence of tumor contamination of blood (five of 10) and marrow (two of six) was commonly detected in (six of 12) relapsed or metastatic disease patients [131]. Both mobilized PBHC and bone marrow grafts in metastatic Ewing's tumor patients may contain tumor cells detectable by either immunocytochemistry or RT-PCR for a neural differentiation marker [132,133]. However, *in vivo* purging occurs during the course of intensive chemotherapy [66,134,135]. Moreover, while few data are available regarding the relationship between tumor contamination of the graft with survival outcomes, long-term DFS can occur in patients with Ewing's sarcoma who receive PBHC grafts containing detectable fusion transcript [102].

It is now clear on the basis of gene marking studies that neuroblastoma cells that contaminate hematopoietic cells can contribute to relapse [136]. However, retrospective analyses have not demonstrated a significant reduction in the risk of relapse by purging with monoclonal antibodies in neuroblastoma [137,138] or with mafosfamide in rhabdomyosarcoma [58]. Instead, the major determinant of long-term survival after HCT for rhabdomyosarcoma was whether CR was achieved prior to HCT [58], and 23 relapses occurred in previously known sites compared with only three in new metastatic sites [60], suggesting that tumor control in the body is the major problem. The Children's Oncology Group is now conducting a randomized trial to address definitively whether purging improves DFS in neuroblastoma.

In several patients, unusual patterns of relapse after autologous HCT, including miliary pulmonary involvement, have suggested reinfusion of clonogenic tumor cells [139–143]. Therefore, while the survival of tumor in the patient's body mandates the development of more effective cytoreductive regimens, it seems prudent to develop nontoxic methods of tumor purging. In rhabdomyosarcoma, no monoclonal antibodies are available for cytotoxic or selective purging of marrow. Therefore, some marrow grafts were purged with mafosfamide. Pharmacologic methods of purging have resulted in substantial delays in engraftment [84,144,145]. In contrast, immunomagnetic purging has had minimal effects on the rate of engraftment and has reduced the amount of detectable tumor contamination by several log [146]. A complementary approach is positive selection of hematopoietic cells based on CD34 expression. We have shown that this method is feasible [147] and our preliminary results indicate a similar degree of tumor depletion as negative immunomagnetic selection [132]. A benefit of this approach is the 2-log reduction in volume of the graft and accordingly, in the dose of dimethyl sulfoxide patients receive, which has otherwise caused children significant toxicity [148]. A further method of tumor cell depletion is achieved with *ex vivo* cytokine-supported liquid cultures, a technique that can expand a limited number of $CD34^+$ cells without expansion of endogenous solid tumor cells or exogenously mixed tumor cell lines [149].

Patterns of failure

There is consensus that after HCT for Ewing's tumors, the majority of relapses are metastatic, most commonly in lung and secondly in bone [25,26,37]. A more recent analysis indicates that bony failures often occur in involved bones outside the local radiation field, and in lesions detected by magnetic resonance imaging (MRI) or positron emission tomography (PET) scan, but not bone scan [133]. Possible solutions include to irradiate the lungs and the entire involved bone system prophylactically and to incorporate the use of MRI and/or PET scans in staging before HCT.

In contrast, failures after HCT for rhabdomyosarcoma tend to occur early, at a median of 4 months after HCT, almost always (23 of 26 cases) in previously known sites [60]. This observation argues for the use of local radiation to all previously known sites of disease.

New approaches

Tandem transplants

A substantial number of tandem transplants, in which two or more HCTs are performed with minimal recovery time between transplants, have already been performed in an attempt to improve tumor control. This approach is most likely to be effective if there is more than one active and noncross-resistant cytoreductive regimen, without cumulative toxicity. Even if a single regimen must be used twice, if a similar log cell kill may be obtained in a second course, repeated application may overcome problems of delivery of drug to the core of a bulky tumor. Whether tandem HCTs as delivered so far have been beneficial is controversial. The results of several institutional series indicate longer responses in patients receiving multiple courses of high-dose therapy [24,150,151]. However, the cumulative experience of EBMT provides no convincing evidence in favor of double transplants in Ewing's sarcoma [36]. In addition, at least with carboplatin and etoposide, no patient improved his or her response with a second course [111].

The use of PBHCs instead of BM may improve the efficacy of tandem transplants because faster hematopoietic recovery may allow greater treatment intensity. Two courses of 100 mg/m² melphalan could consistently be administered with PBHC rescue within 21–34 days (median 24 days) with no change in pharmacokinetics or pharmacodynamics [152]. A limited institution pilot study demonstrated the feasibility of tandem PBSC transplant for metastatic neuroblastoma or sarcoma, delivering 3600 mg/m² CY, 2400 mg/m² etoposide and 2000 mg/m² carboplatin followed within 28–42 days by 180 mg/m² melphalan and 12 Gy TBI in 46 of 51 eligible patients [153,154]. Of the five patients who received only one HCT, three were by patient request and two were ineligible to proceed because of liver toxicity. There were four toxic deaths (9%). Three courses of HCT have been administered to 17 of 22 patients, with one toxic death in the acute transplant period [155]. Although short-term toxicity may be acceptable, this pilot trial shows the importance of long-term follow-up, because three patients have developed pancytopenia as a late complication, two with graft failure and one with monosomy 7 associated myelodysplastic syndrome.

A novel variation is the use of double high-dose therapy with only one HCT procedure [32]. Because the dose-limiting toxicity of melphalan and thiotepa in the setting of hematopoietic cell rescue is mucosal, and the affected tissues recover relatively quickly, two cycles can be given 1 week apart and patients rescued with a single PBHC product after the second cycle. This strategy allows the safe delivery of 1000 mg/m² thiotepa and 280 mg/m² melphalan over 9 days. The indications for HCT were heterogeneous in this phase 1–2 trial, but 10 of 13 patients entering HCT in CR and six of 13 patients entering HCT with residual disease are alive with no evidence of disease 15–59 months (median 35 months) after transplantation. Of particular interest is that all three patients with hepatoblastoma who entered HCT with persistent α fetoprotein elevation achieved long-term CR [32].

Immunotherapy

Ewing's tumors are targets both for natural killer cells and for CTL. The possibility that these immunologic effector mechanisms may be clinically important in high-risk Ewing's tumors was suggested in the pilot trial of hyperfractionated TBI with melphalan and etoposide conducted in Vienna and Düsseldorf. In their initial cohort of 17 patients with very high-risk Ewing's tumors, three of four allograft recipients were disease-free survivors, along with three of five autograft recipients treated with IL-2 vs. two of eight autograft patients without IL-2 [27]. The advantage of IL-2 after autografting persisted in a larger EICESS cohort treated using the same approach: DFS was 52% for patients receiving IL-2 after HCT vs. 22% without IL-2 ($p < 0.05$) [133].

The National Cancer Institute has conducted a pilot trial of tumor-specific vaccination for Ewing's sarcoma and alveolar rhabdomyosarcoma, based on pulsing dendritic cells with the unique EWS/Fli-1 and PAX3/FKHR fusion peptides associated with the t(11;22) and t(2;13) translocations characteristic of these tumors [156]. Sixteen patients were enrolled, and 15 received at least one vaccination. Unfortunately, most patients experienced tumor progression during the first 6-week vaccination cycle, so only four patients received two or more cycles of vaccination. One of these four patients had a mixed response, and another had a fusion peptide-specific lymphocyte proliferative response. This study is important not only because of the encouraging suggestion of some immunologic activity against tumor, but also because it identifies several pitfalls of immunotherapy. These patients had severely impaired immunity and large tumor burdens, and the immature circulating dendritic cells used may actually suppress immune responses [156]. Moreover, a single peptide antigen was used, with uncertain HLA restriction and cell-surface expression, and the tumor itself may have induced tolerance or anergy in autologous lymphocytes.

The development of nonmyeloablative allogeneic HCT offers an alternative avenue to immunotherapy for pediatric solid tumors, but novel approaches may be required to demonstrate activity if this approach is beneficial only in minimal residual disease.

Conclusions

The prognosis of patients with metastatic, recurrent or refractory pediatric solid tumors is dismal. High-dose preparatory regimens with HCT have demonstrated activity against a broad spectrum of the pediatric solid tumors. HCT has produced promising results in the treatment of Ewing's tumors. Prospective randomized trials of HCT vs. conventional chemotherapy are in progress for patients with poor-prognosis Ewing's tumors and are being considered for high-risk recurrent Wilms' tumor. For less common indications, phase 1 and 2 trials are appropriate. Approaches now being investigated to improve the efficacy of HCT for pediatric solid tumors include tandem HCT, graft engineering to eliminate tumor cells, chemoprotection and immunotherapy, possibly via allogeneic HCT.

References

1 Robison LL. General principles of the epidemiology of childhood cancer. In: Pizzo PA, Poplack DG, eds. *Principles and Practice of Pediatric Oncology*, 3rd edn. Philadelphia, PA: Lippincott-Raven, 1997: 1–10.

2 Gatta G, Capocaccia R, Coleman MP, Ries LA, Berrino F. Childhood cancer survival in Europe and the United States. *Cancer* 2002; **95**: 1767–72.

3 Frei EJ, Canellos GP. Dose: a critical factor in cancer chemotherapy. *Am J Med* 1980; **69**: 585–94.

4 Schabel FM Jr, Griswold DP Jr, Corbett TH, Laster WR Jr. Increasing the therapeutic response rates to anticancer drugs by applying the basic principles of pharmacology. *Cancer* 1984; **54**: 1160–7.

5 Houghton JA, Cook RL, Lutz PJ, Houghton PJ. Melphalan: a potential new agent in the treatment of childhood rhabdomyosarcoma. *Cancer Treat Rep* 1985; **59**: 91–6.

6 Skipper HE. Dose intensity vs. total dose of chemotherapy: an experimental basis. In: Hellman S, Rosenberg SA, Devita VT, eds. *Important Advances in Oncology*. Philadelphia, PA: J.B. Lipincott, 1990: 43–64.

7 Gehan EA. Dose–response relationship in clinical oncology. *Cancer* 1984; **54**: 1204–7.

8 Shea TC, Flaherty M, Elias A *et al.* A Phase I clinical and pharmacokinetic study of carboplatin and autologous bone marrow support. *J Clin Oncol* 1989; **7**: 651–61.

9 Marcus RB Jr, Graham-Pole JR, Springfield DS *et al.* High-risk Ewing's sarcoma: end-intensification using autologous bone marrow transplantation. *Int J Radiat Oncol Biol Phys* 1988; **15**: 53–9.

10 Bacci G, Ferrari S, Bertoni F *et al.* Prognostic factors in nonmetastatic Ewing's sarcoma of bone treated with adjuvant chemotherapy: analysis of 359 patients at the Istituto Ortopedico Rizzoli. *J Clin Oncol* 2000; **18**: 4–11.

11 Hoffmann C, Ahrens S, Dunst J *et al.* Pelvic Ewing's sarcoma: a retrospective analysis of 241 cases. *Cancer* 1999; **85**: 869–77.

12 Kinsella TJ, Miser JS, Waller B *et al.* Long-term follow-up of Ewing's sarcoma of bone treated with combined modality therapy. *Int J Radiat Oncol Biol Phys* 1991; **20**: 389–95.

13 Cotterill SJ, Ahrens S, Paulussen M *et al.* Prognostic factors in Ewing's tumor of bone: analysis of 975 patients from the European Intergroup Cooperative Ewing's Sarcoma Study Group. *J Clin Oncol* 2000; **18**: 3108–14.

14 Miser JS, Krailo M, Meyers P *et al.* Metastatic Ewing's sarcoma (ES) and primitive neuroectodermal tumor (PNET) of bone: failure of new regimens to improve outcome. *Proc ASCO* 1996; **15**: 467a.

15 Cangir A, Vietti TJ, Gehan EA *et al.* Ewing's sarcoma metastatic at diagnosis: results and comparisons of two intergroup Ewing's sarcoma studies. *Cancer* 1990; **66**: 887–93.

16 Paulussen M, Braun-Munzinger G, Burdach S *et al.* Results of treatment of primary exclusively pulmonary metastatic Ewing's sarcoma: a retrospective analysis of 41 patients. *Klin Padiatr* 1993; **205**: 210–16.

17 Burdach S, Pape H, Kahn T *et al.* Myeloablative therapy, stem cell rescue and gene transfer in advanced Ewing's tumors (AET): the European intergroup consensus strategy. *Bone Marrow Transplant* 1997; **19**: S87.

18 Michon J, Oberlin O, Demeocq F *et al.* Poor results in metastatic Ewing's sarcomas (ES) treated according to the scheme of the St. Jude 1978–85 study: a study of the French Society of Pediatric Oncology. *Med Pediatr Oncol* 1993; **21**: 572a.

19 Sandoval C, Meyer WH, Parham DM *et al.* Outcome in 43 children presenting with metastatic

Ewing's sarcoma: the St. Jude Children's Research Hospital experience, 1962–92. *Med Pediatr Oncol* 1996; **26**: 180–5.
20 Paulussen M, Ahrens S, Braun-Munzinger G et al. Survival in primary disseminated or relapsed Ewing's Tumor: EICESS/CESS data. *Med Pediatr Oncol* 1996; **24**: 237a.
21 Rodriguez-Galindo C, Billups CA, Kun LE et al. Survival after recurrence of Ewing's tumors: the St. Jude Children's Research Hospital experience, 1979–99. *Cancer* 2002; **94**: 561–9.
22 Cornbleet MA, Corringham RE, Prentice HG, Boesen EM, McElwain TJ. Treatment of Ewing's sarcoma with high-dose melphalan and autologous bone marrow transplantation. *Cancer Treat Rep* 1981; **65**: 241–4.
23 McCann SR, Reynolds M, Meldrum R et al. High dose melphalan with autologous bone marrow transplantation in the treatment of metastatic Ewing's sarcoma. *Irish J Med Sci* 1983; **152**: 160–4.
24 Graham-Pole J, Lazarus HM, Herzig RH et al. High-dose melphalan therapy for the treatment of children with refractory neuroblastoma and Ewing's sarcoma. *Am J Pediatr Hematol Oncol* 1984; **6**: 17–26.
25 Pinkerton CR, Kingston J, Malpas J, McElwain TJ. High-dose melphalan with autologous marrow rescue in Ewing's sarcoma. *Bone Marrow Transplant* 1988; **3**: 85.
26 Hartmann O, Oberlin O, Beaujean F et al. Role of high-dose chemotherapy followed by bone marrow autograft in the treatment of metastatic Ewing's sarcoma in children. *Bull Cancer* 1990; **77**: 181–7.
27 Burdach S, Jurgens H, Peters C et al. Myeloablative radiochemotherapy and hematopoietic stem-cell rescue in poor-prognosis Ewing's sarcoma. *J Clin Oncol* 1993; **11**: 1482–8.
28 Stewart DA, Gyonyor E, Paterson AH et al. High-dose melphalan ± total body irradiation and autologous hematopoietic stem cell rescue for adult patients with Ewing's sarcoma or peripheral neuroectodermal tumor. *Bone Marrow Transplant* 1996; **18**: 315–8.
29 Lazarus HM, Herzig RH, Graham-Pole J et al. Intensive melphalan chemotherapy and cryopreserved autologous bone marrow transplantation for the treatment of refractory cancer. *J Clin Oncol* 1983; **1**: 359–67.
30 Shaw PJ, Pinkerton CR, Yaniv I. Melphalan combined with a carboplatin dose based on glomerular filtration rate followed by autologous stem cell rescue for children with solid tumours. *Bone Marrow Transplant* 1996; **18**: 1043–7.
31 Schiffman KS, Bensinger WI, Appelbaum FR et al. Phase II study of high-dose busulfan, melphalan and thiotepa with autologous peripheral blood stem cell support in patients with malignant disease. *Bone Marrow Transplant* 1996; **17**: 943–50.
32 Hara J, Osugi Y, Ohta H et al. Double-conditioning regimens consisting of thiotepa, melphalan and busulfan with stem cell rescue for the treatment of pediatric solid tumors. *Bone Marrow Transplant* 1998; **22**: 7–12.
33 Lucidarme N, Valteau-Couanet D, Oberlin O et al. Phase II study of high-dose thiotepa and hematopoietic stem cell transplantation in children with solid tumors. *Bone Marrow Transplant* 1998; **22**: 535–40.
34 Ladenstein R, Hartmann O, Pinkerton R et al. The impact of megatherapy (MGT) followed by stem cell reinfusion (SCR) in Ewing's tumor (ET) patients with residual disease. *Bone Marrow Transplant* 1997; **19**: S86.
35 Burdach S, van Kaick B, Laws HJ et al. Allogeneic and autologous stem-cell transplantation in advanced Ewing's tumors: an update after long-term follow-up from two centers of the European Intergroup study EICESS. Stem-Cell Transplant Programs at Düsseldorf University Medical Center, Germany and St. Anna Kinderspital, Vienna, Austria. *Ann Oncol* 2000; **11**: 1451–62.
36 Ladenstein R, Lasset C, Pinkerton R et al. Impact of megatherapy in children with high-risk Ewing's tumours in complete remission: a report from the EBMT Solid Tumour Registry. *Bone Marrow Transplant* 1995; **15**: 697–705. [Published erratum appears in *Bone Marrow Transplant* 1996; **18**: 675.]
37 Horowitz ME, Kinsella TJ, Wexler LH et al. Total-body irradiation and autologous bone marrow transplant in the treatment of high-risk Ewing's sarcoma and rhabdomyosarcoma. *J Clin Oncol* 1993; **11**: 1911–8.
38 Marcus RB, JrBerrey BH, Graham-Pole J, Mendenhall NP, Scarborough MT. The treatment of Ewing's sarcoma of bone at the University of Florida, 1969–98. *Clin Orthop* 2002; **397**: 290–7.
39 Grier H, Krailo M, Link M et al. Improved outcome in non-metastatic Ewing's sarcoma (EWS) and PNET of bone with the addition of ifosfamide and etoposide to vincristine, adriamycin, cyclophosphamide, and actinomycin: a Children's Cancer Group (CCG) and Pediatric Oncology Group (POG) report. *Proc ASCO* 1994; **13**: 421 [Abstract].
40 Paulussen M, Ahrens S, Burdach S et al. Primary metastatic (stage IV) Ewing's tumor: survival analysis of 171 patients from the EICESS studies. European Intergroup Cooperative Ewing's Sarcoma Studies. *Ann Oncol* 1998; **9**: 275–81.
41 Meyers PA, Krailo MD, Ladanyi M et al. High-dose melphalan, etoposide, total-body irradiation, and autologous stem-cell reconstitution as consolidation therapy for high-risk Ewing's sarcoma does not improve prognosis. *J Clin Oncol* 2001; **19**: 2812–20.
42 Kushner BH, Meyers PA. How effective is dose-intensive/myeloablative therapy against Ewing's sarcoma/primitive neuroectodermal tumor metastatic to bone or bone marrow? The Memorial Sloan-Kettering experience and a literature review. *J Clin Oncol* 2001; **19**: 870–80.
43 Mitchell PL, Shepherd VB, Proctor HM, Dainton M, Cabral SD, Pinkerton CR. Peripheral blood stem cells used to augment autologous bone marrow transplantation. *Arch Dis Child* 1994; **70**: 237–40.
44 Atra A, Whelan JS, Calvagna V et al. High-dose busulphan/melphalan with autologous stem cell rescue in Ewing's sarcoma. *Bone Marrow Transplant* 1997; **20**: 843–6.
45 Valteau-Couanet D, Michon J, Plouvier E et al. Treatment of metastatic Ewing's sarcomas (ES) with busulfan and melphalan consolidation high dose chemotherapy (HDCT): a study of the French Society of Pediatric Oncology (SFOP). *Med Pediatr Oncol* 1996; **24**: 238a.
46 Crist WM, Garnsey L, Beltangady MS et al. Prognosis in children with rhabdomyosarcoma: a report of the intergroup rhabdomyosarcoma studies I and II. Intergroup Rhabdomyosarcoma Committee. *J Clin Oncol* 1990; **8**: 443–52.
47 Crist W, Gehan EA, Ragab AH et al. The Third Intergroup Rhabdomyosarcoma Study. *J Clin Oncol* 1995; **13**: 610–30.
48 Neville HL, Andrassy RJ, Lobe TE et al. Preoperative staging, prognostic factors, and outcome for extremity rhabdomyosarcoma: a preliminary report from the Intergroup Rhabdomyosarcoma Study IV (1991–97). *J Pediatr Surg* 2000; **35**: 317–21.
49 Koscielniak E, Rodary C, Flamant F et al. Metastatic rhabdomyosarcoma and histologically similar tumors in childhood: a retrospective European multi-center analysis. *Med Pediatr Oncol* 1992; **20**: 209–14.
50 Atra A, Pinkerton R. Autologous stem cell transplantation in solid tumours of childhood. *Ann Med* 1996; **28**: 159–64.
51 Pappo AS, Anderson JR, Crist WM et al. Survival after relapse in children and adolescents with rhabdomyosarcoma: a report from the Intergroup Rhabdomyosarcoma Study Group. *J Clin Oncol* 1999; **17**: 3487–93.
52 Hartmann O, Benhamau E, Beaujean F et al. High-dose busulfan and cyclophosphamide with autologous bone marrow transplantation support in advanced malignancies in children: a phase II study. *J Clin Oncol* 1986; **4**: 1804–10.
53 Pinkerton R, Philip T, Bouffet E, Lashford L, Kemshead J. Autologous bone marrow transplantation in paediatric solid tumours. *Clin Haematol* 1986; **15**: 187–203.
54 Pinkerton CR, McElwain TJ. High dose carboplatin in combination regimens using autologous bone marrow rescue in neuroblastoma and soft tissue sarcoma. *Med Pediatr Oncol* 1989; **17**: 310a.
55 Wiley JM, Leventhal BG, Fresia A, Yeager AM, Strauss LC, Civin CI. High dose carboplatin (CBDCA), etoposide (VP-16) and cyclophosphamide (CY) with autologous bone marrow rescue (ABMR) in children and young asults with solid tumors results of a phase I study. *Proc ASCO* 1993; **12**: 419a.
56 Pico JL, Ibrahim A, Castagna L et al. Escalating high-dose carboplatin and autologous bone marrow transplantation in solid tumors. *Oncology* 1993; **50**: 47–52.
57 Lafay-Cousin L, Hartmann Plouvier P, Mechinaud F, Boutard P, Oberlin O. High-dose thiotepa and hematopoietic stem cell transplantation in pediatric malignant mesenchymal tumors: a phase II study. *Bone Marrow Transplant* 2000; **26**: 627–32.
58 Pinkerton CR. Megatherapy for soft tissue sarcomas: EBMT experience. *Bone Marrow Transplant* 1991; **7**: 120–2.
59 Koscielniak E, Rosti G, Hartmann O et al. High dose chemotherapy (HDC) with hematopoietic rescue (HR) in patients with rhabdomyosarcoma (RMS): an EBMT solid tumor working party survey. *Bone Marrow Transplant* 1997; **19**: S86.
60 Koscielniak E, Klingebiel TH, Peters C et al. Do patients with metastatic and recurrent rhabdomyosarcoma benefit from high-dose therapy with hematopoietic rescue? Report of the German/Austrian Pediatric Bone Marrow Transplantation Group. *Bone Marrow Transplant* 1997; **19**: 227–31.
61 Carli M, Colombatti R, Oberlin O et al. High-dose melphalan with autologous stem-cell rescue in metastatic rhabdomyosarcoma. *J Clin Oncol* 1999; **17**: 2796–803.
62 Pinkerton CR, Groot-Loonen J, Barrett A et al. Rapid VAC high dose melphalan regimen, a novel

chemotherapy approach in childhood soft tissue sarcomas. *Br J Cancer* 1991; **64**: 381–5.
63 Boulad F, Kernan NA, LaQuaglia MP et al. High-dose induction chemoradiotherapy followed by autologous bone marrow transplantation as consolidation therapy in rhabdomyosarcoma, extraosseous Ewing's sarcoma, and undifferentiated sarcoma. *J Clin Oncol* 1998; **16**: 1697–706.
64 Walterhouse DO, Hoover ML, Marymont MA, Kletzel M. High-dose chemotherapy followed by peripheral blood stem cell rescue for metastatic rhabdomyosarcoma: the experience at Chicago Children's Memorial Hospital. *Med Pediatr Oncol* 1999; **32**: 88–92.
65 Felgenhauer J, Hawkins D, Pendergrass T, Lindsley K, Conrad EU 3rd, Miser JS. Very intensive, short-term chemotherapy for children and adolescents with metastatic sarcomas. *Med Pediatr Oncol* 2000; **34**: 29–38.
66 Hawkins DS, Felgenhauer J, Park J et al. Peripheral blood stem cell support reduces the toxicity of intensive chemotherapy for children and adolescents with metastatic sarcomas. *Cancer* 2002; **95**: 1354–65.
67 Grundy P, Breslow N, Green DM, Sharples K, Evans A, Da GJ. Prognostic factors for children with recurrent Wilms' tumor: results from the Second and Third National Wilms' Tumor Study. *J Clin Oncol* 1989; **7**: 638–47.
68 Groot-Loonen JJ, Pinkerton CR, Morris-Jones PH, Pritchard J. How curable is relapsed Wilms' tumour? The United Kingdom Children's Cancer Study Group. *Arch Dis Child* 1990; **65**: 968–70.
69 Pinkerton CR, Groot-Loonen JJ, Morris-Jones PH, Pritchard J. Response rates in relapsed Wilms' tumor: a need for new effective agents. *Cancer* 1991; **67**: 567–71.
70 Garaventa A, Hartmann O, Bernard JL et al. Autologous bone marrow transplantation for pediatric Wilms' tumor: the experience of the European Bone Marrow Transplantation Solid Tumor Registry. *Med Pediatr Oncol* 1994; **22**: 11–4.
71 Warkentin PI, Brochstein JA, Strandjord SE et al. High dose therapy followed by autologous stem cell rescue for recurrent Wilms' tumor (WT). *Proc ASCO* 1993; **12**: 414a.
72 Pein F, Michon J, Valteau-Couanet D et al. High-dose melphalan, etoposide, and carboplatin followed by autologous stem-cell rescue in pediatric high-risk recurrent Wilms' tumor: a French Society of Pediatric Oncology study. *J Clin Oncol* 1998; **16**: 3295–301.
73 Dome JS, Liu T, Krasin M et al. Improved survival for patients with recurrent Wilms' tumor: the experience at St. Jude Children's Research Hospital. *J Pediatr Hematol Oncol* 2002; **24**: 192–8.
74 Abu-Ghosh AM, Krailo MD, Goldman SC et al. Ifosfamide, carboplatin and etoposide in children with poor-risk relapsed Wilms' tumor: a Children's Cancer Group report. *Ann Oncol* 2002; **13**: 460–9.
75 Saeter G, Elomaa I, Wahlqvist Y et al. Prognostic factors in bone sarcomas. *Acta Orthop Scand Suppl* 1997; **273**: 156–60.
76 Ferguson WS, Harris MB, Goorin AM et al. Presurgical window of carboplatin and surgery and multidrug chemotherapy for the treatment of newly diagnosed metastatic or unresectable osteosarcoma: Pediatric Oncology Group Trial. *J Pediatr Hematol Oncol* 2001; **23**: 340–8.
77 Bacci G, Briccoli A, Ferrari S et al. Neoadjuvant chemotherapy for osteosarcoma of the extremity: long-term results of the Rizzoli's 4th protocol. *Eur J Cancer* 2001; **37**: 2030–9.
78 Baldini N, Scotlandi K, Serra M et al. P-glycoprotein expression in osteosarcoma: a basis for risk-adapted adjuvant chemotherapy. *J Orthop Res* 1999; **17**: 629–32.
79 Kaya M, Wada T, Kawaguchi S et al. Increased pre-therapeutic serum vascular endothelial growth factor in patients with early clinical relapse of osteosarcoma. *Br J Cancer* 2002; **86**: 864–9.
80 Thompson RC Jr, Cheng EY, Clohisy DR, Perentesis J, Manivel C, Le CT. Results of treatment for metastatic osteosarcoma with neoadjuvant chemotherapy and surgery. *Clin Orthop* 2002; **397**: 240–7.
81 Colombat P, Biron P, Coze C et al. Failure of high-dose alkylating agents in osteosarcoma. Solid Tumors Working Party [Letter]. *Bone Marrow Transplant* 1994; **14**: 665–6.
82 Sauerbrey A, Bielack S, Kempf-Bielack B, Zoubek A, Paulussen M, Zintl F. High-dose chemotherapy (HDC) and autologous hematopoietic stem cell transplantation (ASCT) as salvage therapy for relapsed osteosarcoma. *Bone Marrow Transplant* 2001; **27**: 933–7.
83 Link MP, Eilber F. Osteosarcoma. In: Pizzo PA, Poplack DG eds. *Principles and Practice of Pediatric Oncology*, 3rd edn. Philadelphia: Lippincott-Raven, 1997: 889–920.
84 Graham ML, Yeager AM, Leventhal BG et al. Treatment of recurrent and refractory pediatric solid tumors with high-dose busulfan and cyclophosphamide followed by autologous bone marrow rescue. *J Clin Oncol* 1992; **10**: 1857–64.
85 Valteau-Couanet D, Kalifa C, Benhamou E et al. Phase II study of high-dose thiotepa (HDT) and hematopoietic stem cell transplantation (SCT) support in children with metastatic osteosarcoma. *Med Pediatr Oncol* 1996; **24**: 239a.
86 Franzius C, Bielack S, Flege S et al. High-activity samarium-153-EDTMP therapy followed by autologous peripheral blood stem cell support in unresectable osteosarcoma. *Nuklearmedizin* 2001; **40**: 215–20.
87 Anderson PM, Wiseman GA, Dispenzieri A et al. High-dose samarium-153 ethylene diamine tetramethylene phosphonate: low toxicity of skeletal irradiation in patients with osteosarcoma and bone metastases. *J Clin Oncol* 2002; **20**: 189–96.
88 Blach LE, McCormick B, Abramson DH, Ellsworth RM. Trilateral retinoblastoma: incidence and outcome—a decade of experience. *Int J Radiat Oncol Biol Phys* 1994; **29**: 729–33.
89 White L. Chemotherapy in retinoblastoma: current status and future directions. *Am J Pediatr Hematol Oncol* 1991; **13**: 189–201.
90 Petersen RA, Friend SH, Albert DM. Prolonged survival of a child with metastatic retinoblastoma. *J Pediatr Ophthalmol Strabismus* 1987; **24**: 247–8.
91 Saleh RA, Gross S, Cassano W, Gee A. Metastatic retinoblastoma successfully treated with immunomagnetic purged autologous bone marrow transplantation. *Cancer* 1988; **62**: 2301–3.
92 Van Riet I, Schots R, Balduc N et al. Immunomagnetic purging of bone marrow grafts for autologous transplantation in neuroblastoma. *Acta Clin Belg* 1990; **45**: 97–106.
93 Saarinen UM, Sariola H, Hovi L. Recurrent disseminated retinoblastoma treated by high-dose chemotherapy, total body irradiation, and autologous bone marrow rescue. *J Pediatr Hematol Oncol* 1991; **13**: 315–19.
94 Ekert H, Tiedemann K, Waters KD, Ellis WM. Experience with high dose multiagent chemotherapy and autologous bone marrow rescue in the treatment of twenty-two children with advanced tumors. *Aust Paediatr J* 1984; **21**: 195–201.
95 Dunkel IJ, Aledo A, Kernan NA et al. Successful treatment of metastatic retinoblastoma. *Cancer* 2000; **89**: 2117–21.
96 Namouni F, Doz F, Tanguy ML et al. High-dose chemotherapy with carboplatin, etoposide and cyclophosphamide followed by a haematopoietic stem cell rescue in patients with high-risk retinoblastoma: a SFOP and SFGM study. *Eur J Cancer* 1997; **33**: 2368–75.
97 Gerald WL, Miller HK, Battifora H, Miettinen M, Silva EG, Rosai J. Intra-abdominal desmoplastic small round-cell tumor: report of 19 cases of a distinctive type of high-grade polyphenotypic malignancy affecting young individuals. *Am J Surg Pathol* 1991; **15**: 499–513.
98 Ladanyi M, Gerald W. Fusion of the EWS and WT1 genes in the desmoplastic small round cell tumor. *Cancer Res* 1994; **54**: 2837–40.
99 Kretschmar CS, Colbach C, Bhan I, Crombleholme TM. Desmoplastic small cell tumor: a report of three cases and a review of the literature. *J Pediatr Hematol Oncol* 1996; **18**: 293–8.
100 Kushner BH, LaQuaglia MP, Wollner N et al. Desmoplastic small round-cell tumor: prolonged progression-free survival with aggressive multimodality therapy. *J Clin Oncol* 1996; **14**: 1526–31.
101 Frappaz D, Bouffet E, Dolbeau D et al. Desmoplastic small round cell tumors of the abdomen. *Cancer* 1994; **73**: 1753–6.
102 Bertuzzi A, Castagna L, Nozza A et al. High-dose chemotherapy in poor-prognosis adult small round-cell tumors: clinical and molecular results from a prospective study. *J Clin Oncol* 2002; **20**: 2181–8.
103 Bongo S, Coze C, Scheiner C, Coquet M, Devred P, Bernard JL. Pneumoblastoma in children: a clinical case and review of the literature. *Bull Cancer* 1996; **83**: 877–81.
104 Schmaltz C, Sauter S, Opitz O et al. Pleuropulmonary blastoma: a case report and review of the literature. *Med Pediatr Oncol* 1995; **25**: 479–84.
105 Bekassy AN, Garwicz S, Wiebe T, Hagerstrand I. Uncertain role of high dose chemotherapy with autologous stem cell support in pediatric pleuropulmonary blastoma (PPB) [Letter; comment]. *Med Pediatr Oncol* 1997; **28**: 75–6.
106 Devalck C, Tempels D, Ferster A et al. Long-term disease-free survival in a child with refractory metastatic malignant germ cell tumor treated by high-dose chemotherapy with autologous bone marrow rescues. *Med Pediatr Oncol* 1994; **22**: 208–10.
107 Nelson RS, Perlman EJ, Askin FB. Is esthesioneuroblastoma a peripheral neuroectodermal tumor? *Hum Pathol* 1995; **26**: 639–41.
108 Eden BV, Debo RF, Larner JM et al. Esthesioneuroblastoma: long-term outcome and patterns of failure. The University of Virginia experience. *Cancer* 1994; **73**: 2556–62.
109 Nguyen QA, Villablanca JG, Siegel SE, Crockett DM. Esthesioneuroblastoma in the pediatric age-group: the role of chemotherapy and autologous bone marrow transplantation. *Int J Pediatr Otorhinolaryngol* 1996; **37**: 45–52.

110 Kanfer EJ, Petersen FB, Buckner CD et al. Phase I study of high-dose dimethylbusulfan followed by autologous bone marrow transplantation in patients with advanced malignancy. *Cancer Treat Rep* 1987; **71**: 101–2.

111 Santana VM, Schell MJ, Williams R et al. Escalating sequential high-dose carboplatin and etoposide with autologous marrow support in children with relapsed solid tumors. *Bone Marrow Transplant* 1992; **10**: 457–62.

112 Spitzer TR, Cirenza E, McAfee S et al. Phase I–II trial of high-dose cyclophosphamide, carboplatin and autologous bone marrow or peripheral blood stem cell rescue. *Bone Marrow Transplant* 1995; **15**: 537–42.

113 Pession A, Prete A, Locatelli F et al. Phase I study of high-dose thiotepa with busulfan, etoposide, and autologous stem cell support in children with disseminated solid tumors. *Med Pediatr Oncol* 1999; **33**: 450–4.

114 Weaver CH, Bensinger WI, Appelbaum FR et al. Phase I study of high-dose busulfan, melphalan and thiotepa with autologous stem cell support in patients with refractory malignancies. *Bone Marrow Transplant* 1994; **14**: 813–9.

115 Okunieff P, Morgan D, Niemierko A, Suit HD. Radiation dose–response of human tumors. *Int J Radiat Oncol Biol Phys* 1995; **32**: 1227–37.

116 Withers HR, Peters LJ, Taylor JM. Dose–response for subclinical disease: in response to Dr Ben-Josef [letter; comment]. *Int J Radiat Oncol Biol Phys* 1995; **32**: 1267–8.

117 Moritake H, Ikuno Y, Tasaka H, Koga H, Miyazaki S, Okamura J. Donor leukocyte infusion after allogeneic bone marrow transplantation was not effective for relapsed rhabdomyosarcoma. *Bone Marrow Transplant* 1998; **21**: 725–6.

118 Ladenstein R, Peters C, Zoubek A et al. The role of megatherapy (MGT) followed by stem cell rescue (SCR) in high risk Ewing's tumors (ET): 11 years single center experience. *Med Pediatr Oncol* 1996; **24**: 237a.

119 Matthay KK, Seeger RC, Reynolds CP et al. Allogeneic versus autologous purged bone marrow transplantation for neuroblastoma: a report from the Children's Cancer Group. *J Clin Oncol* 1994; **12**: 2382–9.

120 Ladenstein R, Lasset C, Hartmann O et al. Comparison of auto vs. allografting as consolidation of primary treatments in advanced neuroblastoma over 1 year of age at diagnosis: report from the European Group for Bone Marrow Transplantation. *Bone Marrow Transplant* 1994; **14**: 37–46.

121 Shamamian P, Mancini M, Kawakami Y, Restifo NP, Rosenberg SA, Topalian SL. Recognition of neuroectodermal tumors by melanoma-specific cytotoxic T lymphocytes: evidence for antigen sharing by tumors derived from the neural crest. *Cancer Immunol Immunother* 1994; **39**: 73–83.

122 Leibundgut K, Hirt A, Luthy AR, Wagner HP, Tobler A. Single institution experience with mobilization, harvesting, and reinfusion of peripheral blood stem cells in children with a solid tumor or leukemia. *Pediatr Hematol Oncol* 1994; **11**: 215–21.

123 Suzue T, Takaue Y, Watanabe A et al. Effects of rhG-CSF (filgrastim) on the recovery of hematopoiesis after high-dose chemotherapy and autologous peripheral blood stem cell transplantation in children: a report from the Children's Cancer and Leukemia Study Group of Japan. *Exp Hematol* 1994; **22**: 1197–202.

124 Chen AR, Cohen KJ, Eby LL et al. Heterogeneous mobilization of CD34+ blood stem cells for autologous rescue in children with poor prognosis solid tumors. *Blood* 1995; **86**: 403a.

125 Diaz MA, Villa M, Alegre A et al. Collection and transplantation of peripheral blood progenitor cells mobilized by G-CSF alone in children with malignancies. *Br J Haematol* 1996; **94**: 148–54.

126 Nussbaumer W, Schonitzer D, Trieb T et al. Peripheral blood stem cell (PBSC) collection in extremely low-weight infants. *Bone Marrow Transplant* 1996; **18**: 15–7.

127 Rosillo MC, Ortuno F, Moraleda JM et al. Immune recovery after autologous or rhG-CSF primed PBSC transplantation. *Eur J Haematol* 1996; **56**: 301–7.

128 Laver J, Klann R, Kletzel M et al. Studies on the presence of tumor cells following marrow purging vs. peripheral blood collection in stem cell grafts for neuroblastoma. *Proc ASCO* 1996; **15**: 334a.

129 Moss TJ, Cairo M, Santana VM. Clonogenicity of circulating neuroblastoma cells: implications regarding peripheral blood stem cell transplantation. *Blood* 1994; **83**: 3085–9.

130 Miyajima Y, Horibe K, Fukuda M et al. Sequential detection of tumor cells in the peripheral blood and bone marrow of patients with stage IV neuroblastoma by the reverse transcription-polymerase chain reaction for tyrosine hydroxylase mRNA. *Cancer* 1996; **77**: 1214–9.

131 West DC, Grier HE, Swallow MM, Demetri GD, Granowetter L, Sklar J. Detection of circulating tumor cells in patients with Ewing's sarcoma and peripheral primitive neuroectodermal tumor. *J Clin Oncol* 1997; **15**: 583–8.

132 Leung W, Chen AR, Klann RC et al. Frequent detection of tumor cells in hematopoietic grafts in neuroblastoma and Ewing's sarcoma. *Bone Marrow Transplant* 1998; **22**: 971–9.

133 Burdach S, Nurnberger W, Laws HJ et al. Myeloablative therapy, stem cell rescue and gene transfer in advanced Ewing's tumors. *Bone Marrow Transplant* 1996; **18**: S67–8.

134 Fischmeister G, Zoubek A, Jugovic D et al. Low incidence of molecular evidence for tumour in PBPC harvests from patients with high risk Ewing's tumours. *Bone Marrow Transplant* 1999; **24**: 405–9.

135 Thomson B, Hawkins D, Felgenhauer J, Radich J. RT-PCR evaluation of peripheral blood, bone marrow and peripheral blood stem cells in children and adolescents undergoing VACIME chemotherapy for Ewing's sarcoma and alveolar rhabdomyosarcoma. *Bone Marrow Transplant* 1999; **24**: 527–33.

136 Rill DR, Santana VM, Roberts WM et al. Direct demonstration that autologous bone marrow transplantation for solid tumors can return a multiplicity of tumorigenic cells. *Blood* 1994; **84**: 380–3.

137 Evans AE, August CS, Kamani N et al. Bone marrow transplantation for high risk neuroblastoma at the Children's Hospital of Philadelphia: an update. *Med Pediatr Oncol* 1994; **23**: 323–7.

138 Ladenstein R, Lasset C, Hartmann O et al. Impact of megatherapy on survival after relapse from stage 4 neuroblastoma in patients over 1 year of age at diagnosis: a report from the European Group for Bone Marrow Transplantation. *J Clin Oncol* 1993; **11**: 2330–41.

139 Glorieux P, Bouffet E, Philip I et al. Metastatic interstitial pneumonitis after autologous bone marrow transplantation. *Cancer* 1986; **58**: 2136–9.

140 Kalra R, Xoger S, Kosovich M, Matthay K. Radiological case of the month (February): miliary pulmonary neuroblastoma. *Arch Pediatr Adolesc Med* 1995; **149**: 195–6.

141 Kushner BH, Gulati SC, Kwon J, O'Reilly RJ, Exelby PR, Cheung NV. High-dose melphalan for neuroblastoma. *Cancer* 1991; **68**: 242–7.

142 Dini G, Lanino E, Garaventa A. Myeloblative therapy and unpurged autologous bone marrow transplantation for poor-prognosis neuroblastoma: report of 34 cases. *J Clin Oncol* 1991; **9**: 962–9.

143 Matthay KK, Atkinson JB, Stram DO, Selch M, Reynolds CP, Seeger RC. Patterns of relapse after autologous purged bone marrow transplantation for neuroblastoma: a Children's Cancer Group pilot study. *J Clin Oncol* 1993; **11**: 2226–33.

144 Kushner BH, O'Reilly RJ, Mandell LR. Myeloblative combination chemotherapy without total body irradiation for neuroblastoma. *J Clin Oncol* 1991; **9**: 274–9.

145 Hartmann O, Benhamou E, Beaujean F et al. Repeated high-dose chemotherapy followed by purged autologous bone marrow transplantation as consolidation therapy in metastatic neuroblastoma. *J Clin Oncol* 1987; **5**: 1205–11.

146 Canals C, Punti C, Picon M et al. Immunomagnetic purging in autologous bone marrow transplantation: experience in 14 patients. *Prog Clin Biol Res* 1992; **377**: 289–96.

147 Civin CI, Trischmann T, Kadan NS et al. Highly purified CD34+ cells reconstitute hematopoiesis. *J Clin Oncol* 1996; **14**: 2224–33.

148 Okamoto Y, Takaue Y, Saito S et al. Toxicities associated with cryopreserved and thawed peripheral blood stem cell autografts in children with active cancer. *Transfusion* 1993; **33**: 578–81.

149 Brugger W, Scherding S, Wiesmann A, Vogel W, Kanz L. Purging in solid tumors. *Bone Marrow Transplant* 1997; **19**: S14.

150 Hartmann O, Vassal G, Valteau D, Brugieres L, Lemerle J. Autologous bone marrow transplantation in pediatric solid tumors: phase II studies. *Bone Marrow Transplant* 1991; **7** (Suppl. 3): 106–8.

151 Ghalie R, Reynolds J, Valentino LA et al. Busulfan-containing pretransplant regimens for the treatment of solid tumors. *Bone Marrow Transplant* 1994; **14**: 437–42.

152 Vassal G, Tranchand B, Valteau-Couanet D et al. Pharmacodynamics of tandem high-dose melphalan with peripheral blood stem cell transplantation in children with neuroblastoma and medulloblastoma. *Bone Marrow Transplant* 2001; **27**: 471–7.

153 Grupp SA, Stern JW, Bunin N et al. Rapid-sequence tandem transplant for children with high-risk neuroblastoma. *Med Pediatr Oncol* 2000; **35**: 696–700.

154 Grupp SA, Stern JW, Bunin N et al. Tandem high-dose therapy in rapid sequence for children with high-risk neuroblastoma. *J Clin Oncol* 2000; **18**: 2567–75.

155 Kletzel M, Katzenstein HM, Haut PR et al. Treatment of high-risk neuroblastoma with triple-tandem high-dose therapy and stem-cell rescue: results of the Chicago Pilot II Study. *J Clin Oncol* 2002; **20**: 2284–92.

156 Dagher R, Long LM, Read EJ et al. Pilot trial of tumor-specific peptide vaccination and continuous infusion interleukin-2 in patients with recurrent Ewing's sarcoma and alveolar rhabdomyosarcoma: an inter-institute NIH study. *Med Pediatr Oncol* 2002; **38**: 158–64.

100

John A. Zaia, J. Scott Cairns & John J. Rossi

AIDS and Hematopoietic Transplantation: HIV Infection, AIDS Lymphoma and Gene Therapy

The acquired immune deficiency syndrome (AIDS) is in many ways analogous to a neoplastic disorder because it is a complex disease with multiple pathogenic features, is treated with modalities that permit at least temporary clinical remission, and is subject to development of resistance to chemotherapy. Thus, similar to certain cancer therapies, it is not unusual to propose that hematopoietic cell transplantation (HCT) could have a role in the management of AIDS. Several features intrinsic to human immunodeficiency virus type 1 (HIV-1) infection contribute to the complex pathogenicity of this viral infection. These include an early infiltration and seeding of the hematopoietic tissue with HIV-infected cells; a virus replication cycle that occurs predominantly within this tissue and is coupled to cell activation and function; and virus replication that occurs in multiple cell types and tissues (e.g. thymus, brain, gut) at all stages of the disease [1,2]. There is gradual destruction of lymph nodes during the asymptomatic phase of infection and eventual loss of function of the immune system [3,4]. Confounding the pathogenic features of the disease is the genetic instability of the virus that results in HIV-1 variants in the infected individual [5], a potential constellation of drug-related adverse effects, and the difficulty of adherence to drug regimens that require significant adjustments in life style and daily activity [6]. Two factors in particular—the emergence of drug resistance [7] and the continued replication of drug-resistant HIV-1 variants in tissue [8]—undermine the clinical benefit of antiretroviral chemotherapy. In this setting, the potential for cell-based therapy to reestablish an immune system resistant to HIV-1 has been suggested [9–11]. Because HIV-1 is dependent on a variety of well-described molecular events for either infection or replication, gene-based strategies that could inhibit these events are being assessed as potentially complementary therapies for HIV-1 infection. It is the purpose of this chapter to describe the experience with HCT in AIDS and to view the current status of therapeutic approaches for HIV-1 treatment using gene-based approaches to HIV-1 infection.

HIV-1 infection

Viral genes and HIV-1 replication

As a lentivirus (a subgroup of the retrovirus family), HIV-1 shares major genetic features common to all retroviruses [12]. As shown in Fig. 100.1, these features include:

1 a promoter region known as the long-terminal repeat (LTR) located at the 3′ and 5′ end of the proviral genome;

2 two open reading frames that encode the structural proteins of the virus, namely the *gag* and *env* genes—*gag* encodes the capsid (p24, or CA), matrix (p17 or MA) and nucleocapsid (p6 or NC) proteins while *env* encodes the viral envelope proteins (gp120 and gp41); and

3 an open reading frame, *pol*, that encodes essential viral enzymes required for HIV-1 replication: protease, reverse transcriptase and integrase.

Reverse transcriptase and ribonuclease H activity are required for the conversion of the viral RNA genome to a DNA duplex, the molecular form that integrates into the host's genome. Integrase facilitates the actual integration of HIV-encoded gene sequences into host DNA. Protease is essential for processing of the Gag precursor protein (p55) to its individual Gag proteins (CA, MA, NC), which are essential for encapsidating the virion. These enzymatic functions are unique to retroviruses, making them attractive targets to suppress HIV-1 replication without impinging on normal cell function. Currently, the Food and Drug Administration (FDA) has approved 10 reverse transcriptase inhibitors and six protease inhibitors for clinical application and others are in advanced preclinical development. Integrase inhibitors have recently been described that show promise in animal studies and early phase human studies [13–15], but ribonuclease H has proven intransigent for targeted inhibition.

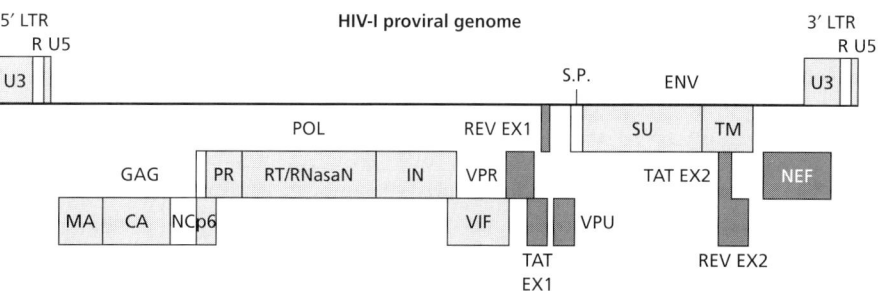

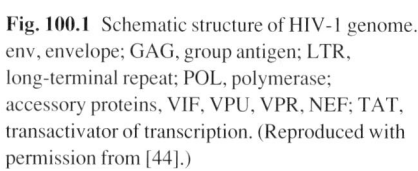

Fig. 100.1 Schematic structure of HIV-1 genome. env, envelope; GAG, group antigen; LTR, long-terminal repeat; POL, polymerase; accessory proteins, VIF, VPU, VPR, NEF; TAT, transactivator of transcription. (Reproduced with permission from [44].)

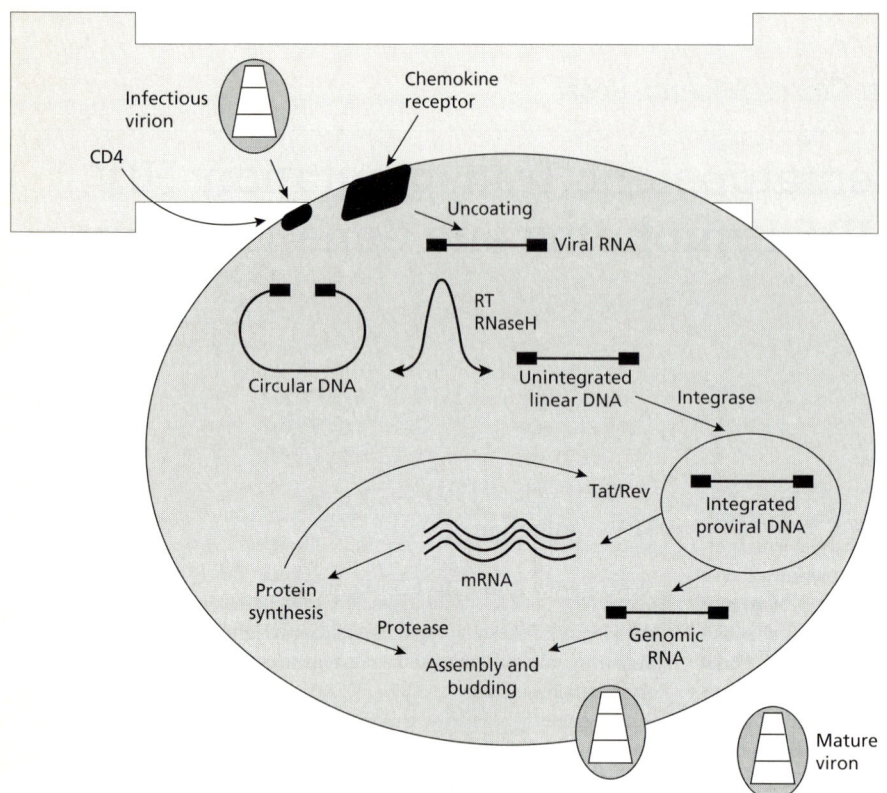

Fig. 100.2 Life cycle of HIV-1. HIV-1 binds to susceptible CD4+ T lymphocytes via the cellular CD4 receptor and enters the cell via a fusion process facilitated by a chemokine receptor. Following penetration, the viral RNA is reverse transcribed by the viral enzyme reverse transcriptase (RT) to an RNA/DNA duplex that is degraded by viral ribonuclease H (RNaseH). Second-strand complementary DNA (cDNA) is completed by the viral RT. The cDNA then migrates to the nucleus where it integrates into cellular chromosomes. Following activation by either viral regulatory proteins or cellular factors, viral transcription commences, producing Tat and Rev. Under this regulation, an internal circuit exists in which polypeptide precursors are processed by a virus-encoded protease, as shown. The mature peptides and two copies of the genomic RNA eventually migrate to the cell membrane, assemble together, and finally bud from the cell as a mature virion. All of these complex steps are potential targets for gene therapy strategies.

Virus entry into the cell

HIV-1 gains entry into susceptible cells following interaction of the viral envelope proteins and a primary cellular receptor, CD4 (Fig. 100.2) [16]. Other secondary receptors were suspected to be involved in HIV-1 interaction with and entry into target cells and, in 1996, two chemokine receptors—CXCR4 and CCR5—were demonstrated to be coreceptors required for viral entry [17,18]. Chemokines are a diverse family of peptides that bind to receptors and activate immune and/or inflammatory responses [19]. The chemokines with two consecutive cysteines are C-C chemokines, and those with an intervening amino acid are C-X-C chemokines. The chemokine receptors have seven segments traversing the cell membrane, with an extracellular segment receiving the chemokine signals and an intracellular tail interacting with heterotrimeric G-protein, leading to cellular activation [19]. Natural ligands for CCR5 such as RANTES and MIP-1α can compete with HIV-1 for binding to this receptor and inhibit HIV infection [20]. The ligand for CXCR4 is stromal-derived factor 1 (SDF-1), which can also inhibit HIV-1 infection [21]. A meta-analysis of patient cohorts has shown that only the CCR5-Ä32 and the CCR2-64I coreceptor mutations, and not the SDF-1 3′A mutation, are associated with a strong protective effect from progression of HIV-1 infection [22].

Based on these and related findings, a model has emerged that describes the sequence of events leading to HIV-1 entry. Initial virus–cell interaction occurs between the HIV-1 envelope protein (gp120) and the CD4 receptor. The gp120-CD4 complex then engages one of the chemokine receptors depending on the specific HIV-1 isolate (CCR5 for macrophage-tropic isolates or R5; CXCR4 for T-tropic or R4 strains that primarily target T lymphocytes). Many other chemokine receptors have subsequently been identified that can fulfill this coreceptor function *in vitro* [17,18,23–25], but CCR5 and CXCR4 appear to be most critical *in vivo* [23]. Formation of the HIV envelope–CD4 receptor–chemokine receptor heterotrimer complex leads to the exposure of a fusion domain contained within the HIV-1 fusion protein (gp41) [27] and, finally, the engagement of gp41 with the target cell membrane culminates in penetration of HIV-1 into the cell and movement into the nucleus [25].

Additional serum protein-based mechanisms are available for HIV entry [29–31]. Also, cell surface receptors, including mannose-binding protein on macrophages [32] and a surface protein on dendritic cells [33], interact with the HIV envelope, but do not actively promote virus fusion and entry. These molecules may improve the interaction of the virus with suboptimal concentrations of cell surface CD4 or coreceptors, or hold the virus in an extracellular or intracellular location that augments or retains viral infectivity [34,35].

Chemokine receptors have a role in leukocyte trafficking and in inflammatory responses. This raises the legitimate concern that therapeutic anti-HIV manipulations, designed to interfere with the receptors' normal cellular functions, might impinge on cellular homeostasis. However, the findings that these receptors are minimally polymorphic and that individuals with homozygous mutations exhibit no ill effects yet display relative resistance to HIV-1 infection [21,22,36–39] have fueled the search for strategies that block this very first event in HIV–cell interaction. Based on the crystal structure of HIV envelope [40,41], specific compounds that inhibit the envelope–CCR5 interaction [42], as well as the gp41-mediated fusion reaction [43], have been designed that appear promising in early stage clinical testing. It is likely that additional compounds that inhibit these early steps in the viral life cycle will be designed and developed for clinical applications.

Regulatory genes of HIV

HIV-1 is a member of the lentivirus subfamily of retroviruses. This group exhibits genomic complexity far beyond that of a prototype retrovirus, which consists of only the *gag*, *pol* and *env* genes [12]. Six additional

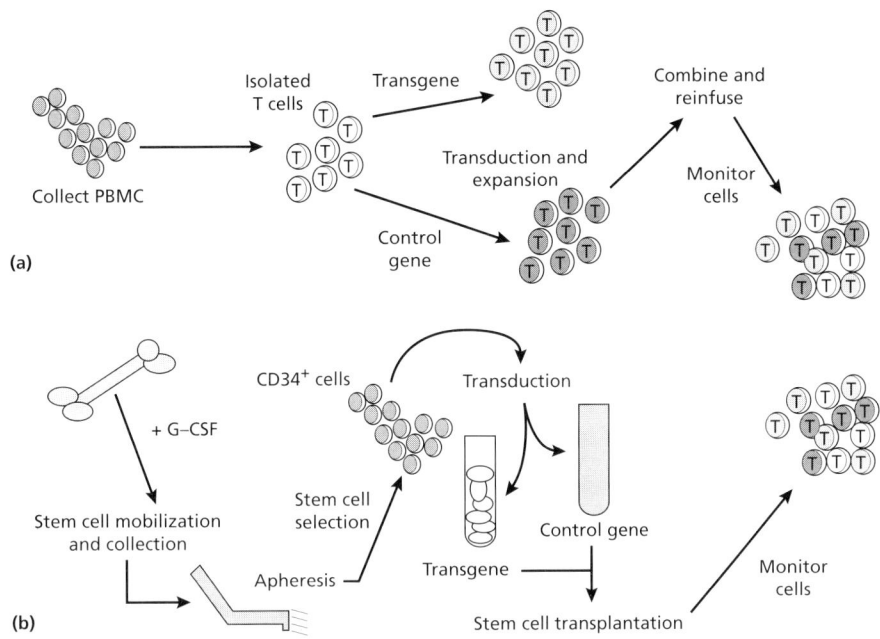

Fig. 100.3 Gene therapy strategies in clinical trials. This schema illustrates strategies for genetic manipulation of two types of cells for inhibition of HIV-1 infection: T lymphocytes and hematopoietic stem cells (HSCs). (a) The selection and expansion of T lymphocytes. T lymphocytes are selected from peripheral blood mononuclear cells (PBMCs). Transduction can be performed with vectors containing either a candidate anti-HIV-1 transgene or a control transgene. Transduced cells are then expanded *in vitro*, combined and infused. After infusion, the survival of transduced lymphocytes can be compared as a ratio of genetically marked cells. (b) The method used for gene therapy with HSC transplantation. Progenitor cells must be mobilized from marrow using a cytokine such as granulocyte colony-stimulating factor (G-CSF) and collected by leukocyte apheresis. CD34+ peripheral blood progenitor cells are then selected using immunoabsorption methods and cryopreserved. When stem cell transplantation is ready to proceed, a portion of the stored HSCs are thawed, transduced with appropriate vectors encoding candidate and control transgenes, and transplanted into an autologous recipient with the remaining untransduced HSCs. As before, progeny cells in the peripheral blood can be analyzed for relative frequency of genetically marked cells. An effective anti-HIV-1 transgene would be one that promotes enhanced survival of genetically marked cells compared to control.

regulatory genes (Fig. 100.1), with a spectrum of biologic functions have been identified in HIV-1 (seven have been identified in simian immunodeficiency virus [SIV], the simian homolog of HIV). Two of these genes, *tat* and *rev*, are required for virus replication. The Tat protein is involved early in the virus life cycle, with a primary role in transcriptional activation of the viral promoter [44]. The requirement for Tat activation appears to depend on the type and activation state of the infected cell [42]. In contrast, Rev appears to be absolutely required for HIV-1 replication. The Rev protein acts as a temporal gatekeeper later in the replication cycle, allowing transport of late messenger RNAs (mRNAs) from the nucleus to the cytoplasm where they are translated into structural proteins for assembly of progeny virus [45]. Currently, only two anti-Tat compounds have been evaluated clinically, but both have been withdrawn because of lack of clinical efficacy. No anti-Rev drugs suitable for clinical evaluation have yet been identified.

The remaining four unique genes in HIV-1 are the "accessory" genes *nef*, *vif*, *vpr* and *vpu* [46,47]. These genes are termed "accessory" based on early studies suggesting that they are dispensable for virus growth *in vitro*. However, more comprehensive studies performed *in vitro* or in experimental models that simulate *in vivo* conditions (e.g. primary T lymphocytes and macrophages infected with clinical HIV-1 isolates) identified several functions for the Nef, Vif, Vpr and Vpu proteins that are important in HIV-1 replication and pathogenesis. Moreover, each of these regulatory proteins is known to be multifunctional, having distinct roles at different stages of the virus life cycle and in pathogenic events. As such, these classes of HIV-1 regulatory proteins provide unique opportunities for conventional drug-, cell- and gene-based therapeutic strategies (reviewed in [47]).

Replication and T-lymphocyte homeostasis

Critical to the understanding of HIV-1 molecular biology and pathogenesis is the mechanism by which CD4+ lymphocyte reduction and eventual loss of immune function occurs. Proposed mechanisms of pathogenesis have evolved as the understanding of HIV-1 infection has increased. Early in the epidemic, much of the immunologic damage of AIDS was proposed to be a manifestation of autoimmune disease [48]. Later studies led to the "sink and drain" model, which uses as its basis the dynamics of HIV-1 RNA levels in the blood (viral load) and CD4+ lymphocyte turnover following the initiation of highly active antiretroviral therapy (HAART) [49,50]. Studies leading to this hypothesis demonstrated that a rise in CD4+ lymphocyte count correlated with a reduction in HIV-1 replication, and that HIV-1 infection appeared to directly destroy the CD4+ T-lymphocyte compartment. The sink and drain model postulated the direct killing ("drain") of CD4+ lymphocytes and elimination of the CD4+ lymphoid compartment ("sink") by HIV-1 infection. A hypothetical hematopoietic "faucet" dynamically replenishes this loss until the putative supply of T cells becomes exhausted, thereby resulting in overt immunodeficiency. Based on this hypothesis, antiviral agents are expected to reverse the loss of CD4+ lymphocytes and restore immune function. However, at the early stages of HIV-1 infection when CD4+ lymphocytes are in decline and the memory CD8+ lymphoid compartment is relatively increasing, both naive CD4+ and CD8+ T lymphocytes decline at the same rate [51]. Because naive CD8+ lymphocytes are not usually infected with HIV-1 and naive CD4+ lymphocytes are relatively resistant to HIV-1 infection, these declining numbers cannot be easily explained by direct killing of cells by HIV-1 [52]. Rather, HIV-1 infection appears to result in a dysregulation of T-lymphocyte homeostasis involving the peripheral pools of these cells and their altered thymic output [53].

These observations have been consolidated into a "redistribution" hypothesis, which postulates that several cytokines are released coincident with active HIV-1 infection and the ensuing cellular antiviral immunoresponse [54]. In turn, these cytokines cause trapping of T lymphocytes in peripheral lymphatic sites where they are efficiently infected by HIV-1 [55,56]. With potent anti-HIV-1 therapy, the viral load is diminished and T lymphocytes are spared from infection. As the levels of the cytokines decline, uninfected cells are released from the lymphatic tissue and enter the peripheral blood, resulting in an increase in CD4$^+$ lymphocytes, albeit a moderate one. This model also predicts that the redistribution of CD4$^+$ and CD8$^+$ lymphocytes will increase as AIDS progresses. This prediction is borne out in clinical studies, demonstrating that the initial response to potent anti-HIV-1 chemotherapy is greater in patients with advanced disease compared to that in patients at earlier stages of the disease [57].

Immune reconstitution during potent antiviral therapy

With continued chemotherapy and repression of HIV-1, naive T lymphocytes slowly increase [57]. The degree to which naive T lymphocytes can be restored and their repertoire expanded will most likely determine the success of such treatment. Reports that pretreatment perturbations in the CD4$^+$ lymphocyte immune repertoire are gradually alleviated during potent anti-HIV-1 chemotherapy [58] have not been confirmed in all studies [59]. While it appears that certain recall immune responses lost during HIV-1 disease progression may be reestablished following initiation of anti-HIV-1 chemotherapy, responses to other antigens, particularly those encoded by HIV, do not appear to be reestablished as readily. This variable recovery may be explained in part by the observation that HIV-specific CD4 cells are preferential targets for HIV infection [53]. In order to return to a situation in which T-lymphocyte homeostasis and normal immune function exist, strategies that directly influence immune reconstitution will most likely be required to effectively complement anti-HIV-1 chemotherapy.

The ability of HAART to restore antigen-specific immune functions will undoubtedly depend on a number of factors, including the time at which therapy is initiated after HIV-1 infection and the extent and duration of disease progression. Indeed, recent clinical findings indicate that the strength of immune responses to both HIV and non-HIV antigens may be proportional to the CD4$^+$ cell nadir before HAART initiation [60]. Restoration of immune functions will be strongly affected by the ability of the patient to generate new populations of naive T lymphocytes, a process believed to be largely dependent on the presence of a functional thymus. Thymic function can be affected not only by HIV-1 infection but also by age, stress and underlying medical conditions [61,62]. Understanding such person–person heterogeneity might shed light on what appear to be conflicting results concerning immune system restoration in different patient populations following potent antiviral therapy [58,59,63,64].

Cellular and anatomical reservoirs of HIV

It is now well-established that a reservoir of latently infected cells (resting memory CD4$^+$ lymphocytes) persists for prolonged periods of time, even in patients on potent antiviral therapy whose viral loads have decreased to undetectable levels [65–67]. These cells could form a pool from which HIV-1 replication can be rekindled following drug withdrawal or HIV-1 gene activation. In cases where anti-HIV-1 chemotherapy has been suspended during structured treatment interruption (STI) or following prolonged use, a rebound of replicating virus has occurred in the majority of patients studied within a few weeks [68,69]. This rapid reappearance of virus indicates that HIV-1 eradication has not occurred and implies that continuous combination therapy must be maintained at all times, possibly for the life of the patient, in order to keep HIV-1 at bay. In contrast to the demonstrated requirement for continuous drug therapy for most patients, a few reports have suggested that, in certain rare circumstances, patients can control viral rebound after withdrawal of the drugs [70,71]. The confirmation of these observations and the mechanisms responsible for long-term viral suppression in these patients following STI are subjects of intense investigation [68]. These observations notwithstanding, the hope that current antiviral drugs could lead to virus eradication seems unlikely at this point in the large majority of patients.

Clinical management

In the last several years, considerable optimism followed studies that showed dramatic reductions in HIV-1 blood levels using combination therapy of reverse transcriptase and protease inhibitors [49,50,72]. Not only are these anti-HIV-1 chemotherapy regimens effective in reducing viral load, but evidence correlates the level of virus load with disease status and progression [73,74]. Such multidrug combinations are still viewed as the first "breakthrough" in development of an effective anti-HIV-1 therapy. As a direct result of these studies, current standards of care involve the use of multiple drugs that target both HIV-1 reverse transcriptase and protease proteins [6]. Under optimal circumstances, and with careful adherence to the rigid schedule of drug administration demanded by this therapy, many patients achieve dramatic reductions in plasma viral load, often to undetectable levels. As noted, it is not clear how long these levels can remain suppressed, but many patients have maintained viral suppression for years while on continuous antiviral therapy. However, these treatments are not without associated complications, which have resulted in current guidelines for 2002 that these therapies not be initiated in patients until CD4$^+$ cells have declined to 350 cells/mL or plasma HIV RNA levels >55,000 copies/mL [6]. Further, the risk of generating drug-resistant variants increases with time on treatment. Because the presence of even low levels of HIV-1 RNA in persons receiving anti-HIV-1 treatment is associated with drug resistance [8,75], questions of long-term efficacy of these treatments remain unknown. Because drug-resistant variants can also be transmitted, an additional complication is confronted by a growing number of individuals who fail to respond to treatment altogether, as a result of primary infection with drug-resistant HIV variants. Whatever the response to treatment, chemotherapy for a lifetime is a less-than-ideal situation and, to lessen the need for continued antiviral chemotherapy, attempts have been made to transfer anti-HIV-1 genes into patients with HIV-1 (see Strategies for gene therapy of AIDS section, below). The risk of developing lymphoma is also considerably increased by HIV-1 infection, and an understanding of cancer treatment in the AIDS patient is important.

Chemotherapy and HCT in AIDS

Lymphoma and AIDS

AIDS-related lymphoma refers to both non-Hodgkin's lymphoma (NHL) and Hodgkin's disease (HD) in persons with HIV infection, and the presence of HIV-1 infection lymphoma is an AIDS-defining diagnosis [76]. The incidences of intermediate- to high-grade NHL and of HD are increased in persons with HIV-1 infection, and prior to the availability of HAART, patients with HIV infection had a 60- to 600-fold increased risk of developing NHL as compared to the general population and a 7- to 20-fold increased rate of HD [77–80]. Since the advent of potent antiviral therapy, in addition to a drop in many of the usual AIDS-related opportunistic infections, there has been a reduction in the incidence of central nervous system (CNS) lymphoma and of immunoblastic lymphoma [78]. There has been minimal, if any, change in the incidence of other forms of AIDS-related lymphoma, with 3–7 cases per 1000 HIV-1-infected patients per year [82–84]. There has been a significant increase in AIDS-related lymphoma as an AIDS-defining illness [82,84]. Nevertheless, as antiviral chemotherapy improves, the effect on the incidence of AIDS lymphoma will be affected.

Effect of HAART on incidence of AIDS lymphoma

With the availability of HAART, there has been a reduced incidence of opportunistic infections, Kaposi's sarcoma, increased CD4 counts and improved survival [85,87]. Of the many studies that have assessed the impact of HAART on the incidence of AIDS lymphoma, there are conflicting results [82,84,88–90,95–100]. Although the frequency of AIDS-defining conditions such as Kaposi's sarcoma and opportunistic infections have declined with HAART therapy, this declining trend was not observed for lymphomas [82,85]. AIDS-related lymphomas can occur in individuals with >200/mm^3 CD4 counts and without prior histories of opportunistic infections [91]. The difficulty in knowing the effect of HAART on AIDS lymphoma is because with HAART, the proportion of HIV-infected persons progressing to AIDS has declined, but the relative proportion of new AIDS cases resulting from lymphoma has increased [84]. It is likely that HAART has decreased the absolute number of new AIDS lymphoma cases by its effect on the relative number of HIV-infected patients progressing to AIDS [101]. However, AIDS-related lymphoma continues to occur as a late manifestation of the disease, and there is evidence that patients with decreased CD4 counts are now at greater risk for AIDS lymphoma [100,102].

Historical development of AIDS lymphoma treatments

Given the widespread disease presentation of AIDS lymphoma, systemic therapy is the treatment of choice [103–106]. While initial studies to treat NHL used standard-dose combination therapy regimens such as cyclophosphamide, Adriamycin, vincristine and prednisone (CHOP) and methotrexate, bleomycin, doxorubicin, cyclophosphamide, vincristine and dexamethasone (m-BACOD), the results were disappointing, with significant hematologic toxicity and opportunistic infections [107]. Trials using either attenuated doses of chemotherapy or hematopoietic growth factors were more encouraging [108], and complete remission rates of up to 65% and median survival times of 12–15 months have been reported [108,109]. None the less, treatment of AIDS-associated NHL is less successful than for similar lymphomas in the non-HIV-1 setting; e.g. up to 40% of patients do not achieve a remission and approximately 25% of patients who achieved a complete remission will ultimately relapse [110,111].

The current recommendations for antineoplastic chemotherapy during concomitant anti-HIV chemotherapy have been recently reviewed [102]. In brief, HAART therapy is usually continued during antilymphoma chemotherapy. Because of its myelosuppressive potential, however, zidovudine—a frequent component of HAART—is usually avoided in such regimens. The EPOCH regimen (etoposide, vincristine and doxorubicin for 96 h with bolus doses of cyclophosphamide and oral prednisone) used at the National Cancer Institute, suspends the use of HAART entirely in patients with AIDS lymphoma during the period of chemotherapy [112].

Using one of several conventional regimens of lymphoma chemotherapy, remission rates are increased in patients since the advent of potent anti-HIV therapy [108], but treatment of relapsed disease remains very poor, with median survival remaining <1 year [102,114,115]. Features

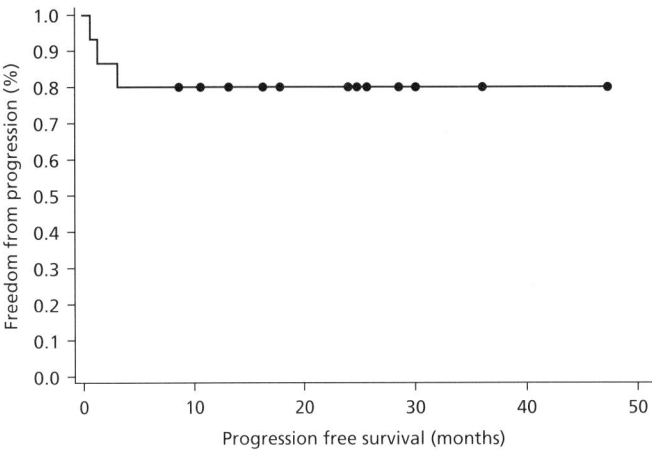

Fig. 100.4 Progression-free survival in AIDS lymphoma patients. Fifteen patients with AIDS lymphoma were treated with high-dose chemotherapy and HCT as described by Krishnan *et al.* [127]. (Reproduced with permission.)

predictive of poor survival in NHL include lower CD4 counts, prior AIDS diagnosis, stage IV disease and bone marrow involvement [116]. Studies suggest that the International Prognostic Index is the best indicator of survival [117,118]. For the high-risk patient, there is a need for alternative, more effective treatments, and thus high-dose therapy with HCT has been a method used for treatment of AIDS lymphoma.

High-dose chemotherapy and HCT for AIDS lymphoma

The superiority of high-dose chemotherapy and autologous bone marrow transplantation over salvage chemotherapy for both relapsed lymphoma and primary refractory lymphoma in the non-HIV-1 setting has been demonstrated by several trials [119–121]. This approach has now been extended to patients with "high-risk" lymphomas in first complete remission and has shown a benefit of high-dose therapy in the patients in the high intermediate and high risk groups [122,123]. As the majority of AIDS-related lymphomas fall into this category, the use of high-dose regimens in HIV-infected patients warrants further study.

Gabarre *et al.* [124] reported the first treatment of a patient with AIDS lymphoma using high-dose chemotherapy and autologous HCT. This patient was treated prior to the general availability of HAART and died of opportunistic infection. With the introduction of HAART, the ability to treat AIDS lymphoma with high-dose therapy has significantly improved. Molina *et al.* [125] and Krishnan *et al.* [126,127] have described a method of high-dose therapy and autologous HCT for high-risk AIDS lymphoma with very promising early outcomes (Fig. 100.4). Additional successful experiences have been reported by Gabarre *et al.* [128]. In the method described by Molina *et al.* [125] and by Krishnan *et al.* [126,127], patients with high-risk AIDS lymphoma, often with prior relapse, were treated with a high-dose chemotherapy regimen consisting of carmustine, etoposide and cyclophosphamide. Most recently, of 15 patients with high-risk lymphoma so treated, 12 patients had disease-free survival of 80% at a median follow-up of 24 months (range 16–54 months; Fig. 100.4) [129]. All patients engrafted at times similar to non-HIV-1 transplant recipients. Procedure-related toxicity consisted of mild hepatic toxicity and mucositis in most patients, but there were no major early opportunistic infections. One patient aged 68 years died because of cardiomyopathy and multiorgan failure. The HIV-1 load increased transiently in seven of 12 patients having serial HIV plasma levels, CD4 counts reached a nadir at a median of 4.5 months and recovered to pretransplant levels at a median of 9 months [127]. In total, for this very high-risk group, at a median follow-up of 24 months, two patients died because of relapsed lymphoma, one died of procedure-related complications and 12 remain in long-term disease-free survival. Thus, high-dose chemotherapy and HCT appears to be a promising therapy for high-risk AIDS lymphoma.

Allogeneic HCT and AIDS

It has been recognized since the 1980s that persons with AIDS can also undergo allogeneic HCT with rapid engraftment of blood cells [130–132]. In the pre-HAART era, the use of allogeneic HCT for the treatment of AIDS lymphoma was unsuccessful [130]. With the availability of HAART and reduced toxicity myeloablation, it may be feasible to treat these patients with an allogeneic HCT. Kang et al. [133] have recently described the use of a nonmyeloablative regimen for the transplantation of genetically modified cells using allogeneic HCT. In this study, two patients with AIDS and hematologic malignancies underwent reduced toxicity HCT without significant procedure-related toxicity. One patient died of relapse at 12 months post-HCT, and the other remained well and in remission, with rising CD4 counts and well-controlled HIV-1 levels. This observation clearly indicates that nonmyeloablative allogeneic HCT is feasible in patients having HAART-responsive HIV infection. The study of Kang et al. [133] also introduced genetically modified stem cells into the patient with the HCT. After 2 years, there was only low-level evidence of the transgene expression, and this finding suggests that a method of cell selection post-HCT will be necessary for successful gene therapy of AIDS using HCT. The potential for genetic approaches to control of HIV-1 rests in the understanding of HIV-1 infection and replication, and several methods have been described for control of HIV-1 using gene transfer.

Strategies for gene therapy of AIDS

General rationale

Because of the genetic instability of HIV-1 and the progressive destruction of the immune system that occurs from onset of infection, there is an urgent need for new therapeutic strategies that are multipronged, comprehensive, attack both active and quiescent forms of HIV and have long-term therapeutic outcome. Among such strategies are gene-based therapeutic approaches that can be used in concert with conventional antiretroviral drugs. Gene-based strategies aim to:
1 target viral elements in the anatomical compartments and reservoirs where the virus takes hold in the body;
2 protect $CD4^+$ T lymphocytes and other susceptible cells against HIV-1 infection or replication; and
3 restore immune function.

Highlighted here are those strategies undergoing clinical evaluation and those in advanced preclinical development.

Considerations in gene therapy

Gene therapy involves the transfer of genetic information (transgene) into human subjects to replace a missing or defective function or to produce an intracellular molecule (RNA, DNA, protein) for therapeutic purposes. This approach was made possible by the ability to copy human genes in vitro and then insert them into target cells of interest. While simple at first glance, this process is highly complex. First, the transgene must be cloned into a delivery vehicle (vector) that also provides the transcriptional regulatory elements required for gene expression. The delivery vehicle may be a viral or nonviral vector. Second, the vector must be delivered efficiently into the target cells. Most delivery methods employ a process whereby cells are removed from the patient, and the transgene is delivered to the target cells ex vivo. The modified cells are then expanded in culture and reinfused to the patient. Several approaches for direct delivery of genes to target cells in vivo, bypassing the need for expensive time-consuming ex vivo cell manipulations, are also in clinical studies, but at this point these are restricted to local tissue delivery such as skin, muscle or lung. Third, long-term stable expression of the transgene in modified cells is essential. Both integrating and nonintegrating vectors are being developed, with each having their own unique advantages and disadvantages. Vectors that can integrate the transgene into host DNA promise to produce long-lived expression, whereas nonintegrating vectors can be expected to have a shorter period of expression but will minimize the theoretical risk of insertional mutagenesis by the integrated DNA. Non-integrated vectors replicate autonomously with every cell division and partition equally to each daughter cell. Efforts to improve the technologies involved and streamline the overall process are underway, especially for:
1 the design of more efficient, safe and cost-effective gene delivery vehicles;
2 the design of delivery vehicles that do not induce immune responses which could result in the clearance of the engineered cells in vivo [134]; and
3 the design of vectors that can be targeted to specific cells or tissues and that can be used for direct in vivo delivery in infected patients.

In addition, gene therapy strategies that are nonimmunogenic (e.g. RNA-based strategies such as decoys, ribozymes, antisense approaches) and strategies based on nonpolymorphic host proteins are also being investigated and have reached the stage of clinical testing [135].

T lymphocytes as target cells for HIV-1 gene therapy

Use of genetic modification of T lymphocytes for HIV-1 treatment is based on the rationale that the transfer of a therapeutic gene into target cells, such as mature lymphocytes ($CD4^+$ T lymphocytes), and reinfusion of the altered cells will limit virus spread and delay disease progression. Most studies to date have involved the ex vivo transfer of therapeutic genes to autologous $CD4^+$ cells. Because $CD4^+$ lymphocytes are not the only cell targets for HIV-1 and because they have a finite life span, efforts are underway to isolate and engineer pluripotent hematopoietic stem cells (HSCs) while preserving their innate biologic properties. In theory, protection of even a portion of this cell population, and consequently its hematopoietic descendants, should ensure a renewable supply of HIV-1-protected cells for the life of the patient.

Cells that are susceptible to HIV-1 infection are also critical for maintaining a viable immune system: a strategy for restoring viable immune cells is therefore more likely to have a therapeutic impact if the cells can be modified to resist HIV-1 infection and to have prolonged survival. Thus, successful gene therapy approaches are intended to benefit the patient in two ways: by increasing the population of cells resistant to HIV-1 infection or replication, thereby diminishing viral load; and by expanding the population of immunocompetent T lymphocytes, which have been depleted during disease progression, thereby restoring immune function. Another application of gene therapy technologies is in the prevention of HIV-1 infection. Because HIV-1 genes can be delivered to antigen-presenting cells (e.g. dendritic cells), gene delivery is being explored for therapeutic and prophylactic vaccine strategies [136–138].

Molecular targets for HIV-1 gene therapy

A diverse array of transgenes to suppress HIV-1 functions or block the infectious cycle have been designed and tested in vitro. These can be broadly categorized in two groups: those coding for nucleic acid-based

HIV Infection, AIDS Lymphoma and Gene Therapy

Table 100.1 Transgenes for HIV-1 gene therapy.

	Reference
Protein-based	
Transdominant negative mutant	
Rev (RevM10)	[129,130]
Tat	[131]
Tat/Rev fusion (Trev)	[132]
Intrabodies (intracellular single chain antibodies)	
Anti-Tat	[133]
Anti-Env	[134,135]
Anti-Rev	[136]
Anti-Gag (MA)	[137]
Anti-RT	[138]
Intrakines	
Antichemokine receptor	[139,140]
Toxins	
Diphtheria toxin	[141,142]
HSV *tk* gene (followed by ganciclovir administration)	[143,144]
RNA-based	
Antisense	
Anti-tat	[145]
Anti-rev	[146]
Anti-gag	[147]
Ribozymes	
Hairpin	[148,149]
Hammerhead	[150]
Small inhibitory RNA	
Rev	[151]
Tat, Rev	[152]
Vif, nef, TAR, LTR	[153]
Decoys	
TAR or poly TAR	[154–156]
RRE	[157–159]
Others	
Targeted cytolytic viruses	[160,161]
CD4- and CD8-ζ chain modified T-cell receptors	[162]
HSV host shut-off protein	[163]
Interferon	[164]

suppressors; and those coding for protein-based suppressors (Table 100.1). As in drug-based therapy, the rationale for antiviral gene therapy is that inhibition of the virus at several critical functions is likely to result in more complete and effective suppression. Also, as in drug-based therapy, concerns for emergence of HIV-1 variants that resist or escape the gene-based strategy apply [5,75]. For these reasons, current gene therapy approaches use combinations of different types of transgenes with different viral and cellular targets that aim to completely neutralize HIV-1 functions at different points in the infection cycle.

RNA-based suppressors

Antisense

The binding of newly transcribed RNA-antisense molecules to mRNA sequences prevents translation of the encoded protein, thereby resulting in loss of gene function [165]. In the case of HIV, antisense molecules have been designed against a number of critical gene functions, including *tat, rev* and *integrase* (Table 100.1). These transgenes effectively block HIV-1 replication *in vitro* [140–144], and some are currently undergoing clinical evaluation [140]. An antisense vector targeted to SIV *tat* and *rev* sequences, when given to monkeys that were subsequently infected with SIV, has been reported to affect viral load in the infected primates [145]. This intriguing study is raising the possibility that a similar approach may also temper HIV-1 infection in humans.

RNA decoys

RNA decoy strategies attempt to compete with specific HIV-1 RNA elements that bind viral proteins as part of the replication cycle by overexpressing their RNA homologs. TAR (Tat-responsive) and RRE (Rev-responsive) are two such *cis*-acting RNA elements that are required for the proper function of Tat and Rev—two key HIV-1 regulatory proteins. The notion that short TAR sequences would compete with wild-type TAR for Tat binding was tested using a retrovirus delivery vector [146]. Virus replication in cells expressing a poly TAR decoy was reduced for up to 30 days after HIV-1 challenge [140,147,148]. The study of Rosenzweig *et al.* [148] is of particular relevance to HSC-based genetic therapies because transduction of $CD34^+$ blood progenitor cells with a retroviral vector encoding polymeric TAR decoy combined with an antisense-*tat* molecule permitted *in vitro* differentiation into T lymphocytes and macrophages that were relatively protected from HIV-1 infection [148]. Using a similar concept, a T-lymphocyte-derived cell line transduced with retroviral vectors expressing an RRE decoy demonstrated long-term inhibition of HIV-1 replication *in vitro*, presumably because of the interference of the RRE sequences with Rev function [36,149,150].

Because TAR and RRE RNAs also bind cellular factors, a valid concern of the decoy strategy is that overexpression of these RNA sequences may sequester not only Tat or Rev but also proteins required for normal cell function. To that end, a minimal RRE decoy of only 13-nucleotides was designed, which retained the Rev-binding domain but could no longer bind cellular factors [150]. Studies in T lymphocytes *in vitro* have indicated that the 13-nucleotide-long minimal RRE decoy is more effective in suppressing HIV-1 replication than TAR decoys [149]. Importantly, human $CD34^+$ blood progenitor cells, transduced with a retrovirus vector expressing the minimal RRE decoy, gave rise to myelomonocytic cells in long-term marrow culture that exhibited considerable resistance to infection when challenged with HIV-1 [150]. Together, these and related studies provided the conceptual basis for a clinical trial of transduced and transplanted marrow-derived HSC in HIV-1 infected children [151].

Ribozymes

Ribozymes are RNA molecules that can cleave RNA targets at specific sequences, a property that is being exploited to cleave and thus inactivate HIV-1 RNAs [152]. Ribozymes can be designed to cleave at different sites along the HIV-1 genome and to inactivate multiple genes at the same time. Such cleavage redundancy should ensure that suppression of HIV-1 can proceed, even with a loss of a ribozyme site because of mutational changes in HIV-1 sequence. Concomitant cleavage of several viral genes is also likely to be more effective in blocking virus replication than the inactivation of a single gene, analogous to combination chemotherapy directed toward inhibition of different HIV-1 functions. The first *in vitro* study suggesting the use of a "hammerhead" ribozyme to suppress HIV-1 was directed against the HIV-1 *gag* RNA sequence [153]. When human cell lines expressing this ribozyme were challenged with HIV, reduced levels of full-length *gag* RNA molecules, cleavage of the RNA at the predicted site and a decrease in p24 (Gag-derived) antigen were demonstrated. Of note, it was observed that in addition to cleaving *de novo* synthesized HIV-1 RNA, ribozymes acted directly on incoming HIV-1 RNA before the provirus could integrate into the host genome

[154]. Protecting uninfected cells with endogenous ribozyme may thus endow them with true "resistance" against HIV-1 infection. An elegant strategy attempt to colocalize endogenously synthesized HIV-1 ribozyme to the same cellular site where HIV-1 RNA accumulates during virus assembly [155], this strategy should increase the efficiency of cleaving and inactivating newly synthesized HIV-1 and may very well result in the destruction of HIV-1 RNA genome from within in a true Trojan horse approach, giving rise to noninfectious particles. Theoretically, such noninfectious particles, by maintaining the cognate conformation of all HIV-1 proteins and epitopes, may effect a secondary indirect role as therapeutic vaccines to augment immune responses in HIV-infected individuals.

A "hairpin" ribozyme that cleaves at the leader sequence at the 5' end of the HIV-1 genome conferred resistance to several HIV-1 isolates and considerable inhibitory activity was observed for up to 35 days *in vitro* [156,157]. Importantly, transduction of rhesus monkey HSCs with a hairpin ribozyme protected the emerging T lymphocytes and macrophages from SIV infection *in vitro* [158]. Subsequent refinement in the design and diversity of anti-HIV-1 hammerhead ribozymes and extensive *in vitro* studies in primary human CD4+ T-lymphocytes and in CD34+ peripheral blood progenitor cells (Fig. 100.4), has provided the scientific and technical justification to proceed with a clinical evaluation of these therapeutic concepts in HIV-infected patients.

Small inhibitory RNA

RNA interference (RNAi) targets sequence-specific downregulation of gene expression. RNA interference is a process in which double-stranded RNA (dsRNA) induces the post-transcriptional degradation of homologous transcripts, and RNAi has been observed in a variety of organisms including fungi, plants, insects, protozoans and mammals [159–165]. RNAi is initiated by exposing cells to dsRNA either via transfection or endogenous expression of viral or transposon RNAs. Double-stranded RNAs are processed by the RNAse III-like enzyme, called dicer, into 21–23 nucleotide double stranded (ds) fragments known as short interfering RNAs (siRNAs) [165,166]. These siRNAs form a complex known as the RNA-induced silencing complex (RISC), which leads to cognate target RNA destruction [167–169]. Chemically synthesized 21–23 length siRNA nucleotides duplexes with short 3' overhangs have been synthesized and are capable of mediating RNAi *in vivo* and *in vitro* [170,171]. Introduction of siRNAs allows evasion of the interferon-induced protein kinase R (PKR) and RNaseL pathways that lead to nonspecific inhibition of gene expression [170,171]. Several studies have demonstrated that the functional unit of RNAi, the siRNAs, can elicit sequence-specific target downregulation either by introduction of preformed siRNAs via transfection or by endogenous expression of 21–23 base-paired RNAs using polymerase III promoter systems [172–179]. This enabling of expression of siRNAs in mammalian cells has opened up new possibilities for therapeutic applications of siRNAs.

RNAi can be applied as a potent mechanism for inhibition of HIV-1 infection. The siRNA component of RNAi can circumvent the nonsequence-specific interferon pathways. Thus, RNAi represents an exciting, new and potentially powerful tool for anti-HIV therapy [172,178,180–182]. The recent publications demonstrating that HIV replication can be inhibited by using either synthetic or expressed siRNAs targeting either the virus, its receptor or coreceptor [172,178,180–183], have generated a great amount of interest and enthusiasm for further testing of the anti-HIV therapeutic potential of siRNAs. There are at least two different modalities by which siRNA can be used as an antiviral: transfection of the preformed siRNAs or intracellular expression of siRNAs. The latter approach may potentially be utilized in a gene therapy setting, providing intracellular immunity to hematopoietic cells susceptible to HIV-1 infection. An important question is whether or not siRNAs that are cytoplasmically localized can target destruction of incoming HIV-1 RNAs, prior to reverse transcription [178,180–182], but there is evidence that such targeting of incoming HIV can occur. Jacque *et al.* [178] demonstrated that preloading HIV-1 susceptible cells with anti-HIV-1 siRNA markedly blocked proviral DNA formation, strongly supporting the idea that siRNAs can target degradation of HIV-1 prior to completion of reverse transcription. It is also clear that RNAi can degrade post-integration genomic and subgenomic siRNAs [172,178,180–182]. Another method to inhibit proviral integration is to target either the receptor or coreceptor mRNAs [197,200]. It is also possible to target the coreceptors for HIV, namely CCR5 and CXCR4, which could prevent viral entry into protected cells. Each of these is currently under investigation as potential therapeutic targets for treatment of HIV infection.

Even though there is a great deal of enthusiasm and optimism about the potential use of RNAi as a therapeutic agent, there remain several unanswered questions about this new technology. At the time of this writing, we are aware of only a single published result demonstrating functional expression of siRNAs from an integrated retroviral vector [184]. In order to achieve good inhibition by the siRNAs, especially for antiviral inhibition, robust expression from integrated vectors is going to be required. Even though RNAi mechanisms appear to function at much lower concentrations than ribozymes or other forms of antisense, it is not yet known whether the lower amounts necessary for robust inhibition of HIV-1 can be achieved in hematopoietic cells. Recently, it has been experimentally determined that at least one form of RNAi is cytoplasmic [185]. This means that siRNAs expressed in the nucleus need to transit to the cytoplasm to become part of the RISC. The presently utilized expression systems are primarily based upon pol III promoters, with one recent exception of an engineered cytomegalovirus (CMV) promoter system for siRNA production [186]. The pol III systems, although robust, do not easily lend themselves to siRNA trafficking to the cytoplasm. The siRNAs that are functionally active via these promoters most likely passively enter the cytoplasmic compartment. To accomplish this goal, the siRNAs will have to be expressed in the context of flanking sequences that allow efficient trafficking from nucleus to cytoplasm. Successful development of siRNAs will involve designing and testing siRNAs that will be efficiently processed by dicer without activation of the PKR or RNAseL pathways. It may also be possible to achieve regulated expression of the siRNAs with inducible promoters, such as the HIV-1 LTR, if appropriate processing of the siRNA transcripts can be engineered into the system.

Protein-based suppressors

Transdominant mutant proteins

Transdominant mutant proteins act as competitors of cognate HIV-1 proteins and thus suppress normal viral functions. The most experimentally advanced transdominant protein to date is a mutant Rev protein (RevM10) [187]. RevM10 retains two Rev functions: the ability to bind RRE (see above) on the viral genome and the ability to form Rev multimers. However, it is incapable of exerting its regulatory role in transporting unspliced or singly spliced RNAs from the nucleus to the cytoplasm. Thus, susceptible cell lines that express RevM10 exhibit long-term (>30 days) resistance to HIV-1 replication [188]. *In vitro*, RevM10 expression in peripheral blood lymphocytes delayed virus replication [187–192] with no adverse effect on cell viability and normal T-lymphocyte functions [105]. Similarly, human CD34+ blood progenitor cells, transduced with RevM10, gave rise to T lymphocytes that exhibited significant resistance to challenge with HIV-1 [193]. RevM10 performed well compared with antisense or decoy strategies for *in vitro* inhibition of HIV-1 [194,195].

Based on these and other pivotal studies, clinical studies were undertaken to assess the safety of the transgene and its protective effect on transduced cells measured in cell survival relative to unprotected cells. Briefly, CD4+ lymphocytes were isolated from HIV-infected patients, and the cells were divided into two portions: one portion was transduced with a vector that expressed a functional RevM10 and the other was transduced with a negative control frame-shifted vector that produced no RevM10. The transduced cells were then mixed and returned to the respective donor. In this elegant protocol design (Fig. 100.3a), the patient provides both the positive and negative control, thereby eliminating patient–patient variations. The first human clinical study examined the potential of RevM10 to prolong the survival of transduced CD4 T-lymphocytes *in vivo* after *ex vivo* transduction, expansion and reinfusion into HIV-1 seropositive subjects. Using DNA plasmid vectors with gold particle-mediated gene delivery, a four- to fivefold survival advantage was found in cells that expressed RevM10 compared to negative control transduced cells [189]. However, the duration of engraftment was limited and transient. Although genetically modified cells were detected in one subject up to 2 months after gene transfer, the recombinant gene was not detectable in two subjects after 2 weeks [189].

In a subsequent attempt to achieve more durable engraftment, alternative gene transfer vectors and protocols for T-lymphocyte stimulation were employed [190]. These modifications included use of a retrovirus delivery vector in lieu of plasmid DNA, and CD4+ lymphocyte expansion with anti-CD3 and interleukin-2. As before, the relative survival of RevM10 transduced cells vs. cells transduced with the negative control, and relevant immune responses were analyzed. Using the above modifications, DNA and RNA polymerase chain reaction (PCR) analyses revealed that cells transduced with RevM10 retroviral vectors survived and expressed the recombinant gene for significantly longer time periods than those transduced with a negative control vector in three HIV-positive subjects tested. Rev M10-transduced cells were detected for an average of 6 months after retroviral gene transfer compared to <3 weeks for the previously reported nonviral vector delivery. In addition, immune responses were not detected either to RevM10 or to the retrovirus vector envelope (gp70) protein [190]. These findings suggest that retroviral delivery of an antiviral gene may potentially contribute to immune reconstitution in AIDS and could provide a more effective vector relative to plasmid DNA to prolong survival of CD4+ lymphocytes in HIV-infected individuals.

Another example of a transdominant protein approach is based on fusion of *tat* and *rev trans*-dominant genes that code a Tat-Rev (Trev) fusion protein. This construct has shown enhanced inhibition of HIV-1 function *in vitro* compared to either Tat transdominant protein or Rev transdominant protein alone [196,197]. A clinical protocol with Trev is about to be activated. Other transdominant protein-based strategies are in preclinical development.

Single chain antibodies

Intracellular HIV-specific single chain antibodies (intrabodies; SFv) can sequester or redirect HIV-1 proteins away from their normal subcellular compartment. *In vitro* studies with SFv, which recognizes the CD4-binding domain of gp120, trapped gp160 in the endoplasmic reticulum, prevented its transport to the cell surface and resulted in a decrease in infectious virus production [198,199]. SFv with specificity for Rev was reported to trap the protein in the cytoplasm, block the transport of unspliced and singly spliced viral RNAs from the nucleus to the cytoplasm, and inhibit virus growth *in vitro* after challenge with either laboratory or clinical HIV-1 isolates [200]. SFv that targets Tat has also been shown to be effective in inhibiting HIV-1 gene expression and replication [201]. Combinations of SFv targeted to reverse transcriptase, integrase and CCR5 have been described by Strayer *et al*. [202]. Additional transdominant protein transgenes are listed in Table 100.1.

Intracellular toxins

Intracellular toxins and conditionally toxic molecules can be used to preferentially eradicate HIV-1 infected cells [203–208]. A versatile strategy makes use of a molecule encoded by herpes simplex virus (HSV) *tk* gene that is toxic only under conditions of substrate availability. Briefly, the HSV-TK enzyme renders the host cell susceptible to ganciclovir (GCV) or aciclovir (ACV) by converting the drug to a potent inhibitor of DNA synthesis. When the *HSV-tk* gene is regulated by HIV-1 proteins, selective killing of infected cells, but not of uninfected cells, can be demonstrated *in vitro* in the presence of GCV or ACV [205,206,208]. HIV-dependent expression of attenuated diphtheria toxin similarly suggested elimination of HIV-infected cells, as measured by reduced levels of p24 and infectious virus [204,205,207]. Before diphtheria toxin and other toxin-mediated cell ablation can be applied as a gene therapy modality in humans, it will be imperative to tightly restrict expression to HIV-infected cells because even low level expression of the toxin in uninfected cells will be detrimental to the patient. A major deficiency of this approach is that these gene-modified cells do not possess a selective survival advantage and therefore cannot be enriched relative to non-modified cells. It is expected that repeated infusions of *ex vivo* modified cells will be required for therapeutic benefits. Unless an *in vivo* vector delivery system is available, the aforementioned requirement is likely to render this strategy impractical when the large HIV-infected population is considered.

An elegant approach to specifically eliminate infected cells that display HIV-1 determinants on their surface has been reported [209]. Briefly, the natural envelope gene of vesicular stomatitis virus (VSV), and in a similar study using rabies virus [210], was deleted and replaced by the CD4 and CXCR4 receptor genes required for HIV-1 entry into susceptible hosts. By so doing, the engineered VSV could specifically enter HIV-1 infected cells that displayed the viral envelope (gp120) on their surfaces. While the specificity of other toxin-mediated approaches depends on the intracellular expression of the toxin following HIV-1 infection or drug treatment, the modified VSV approach targets only HIV-1 infected cells from the outset and thus is unlikely to have an adverse effect on uninfected healthy cells. The fact that the altered VSV enters only HIV-1 infected cells also eliminates the need for selective advantage of altered cells, the lack of which is a major hurdle for other toxin-mediated strategies. Once inside the target cell, the intrinsic cytolytic activity of VSV results in the eradication of the infected cell. *In vitro*, this new form of VSV effectively controlled HIV-1 infection, reducing the virus levels to undetectable or barely detectable levels. This receptor-mediated targeting demonstrated that it is possible to deliver a vector to a specific "address", be it a cell or an anatomical site. It may thus solve a major gene therapy hurdle, namely the *in vivo* delivery of a vector to a destined cell in a therapeutic mode for any number of diseases, or in a vaccine mode for the *in vivo* delivery of a gene encoding an immunogen to antigen-presenting cells. Importantly, being able to target a vector to a specific site may pave the way to the elimination of HIV-1 reservoirs, whenever a signature cell surface marker is available that can be exploited for receptor-mediated targeting.

Altered chemokines

As indicated, HIV-1 uses the cellular CD4 receptor and a chemokine coreceptor to gain entry into susceptible lymphocytes. Several studies tested the notion that the intracellular expression of the natural ligand of the receptor would block its surface expression and thus inhibit HIV-1 entry. In one approach, the expressed chemokine (termed "intrakine") contained the "KDEL" peptide sequence. The "KDEL" sequence is an endoplasmic reticulum (ER) signal peptide that leads to the retention within the ER of a protein to which it is appended. In tissue culture experiments, these intrakines were found to trap and localize their respective receptors to the ER, thereby blocking their expression at the cell surface and rendering the modified lymphocyte resistant to HIV-1 infection [211,212]. Thus, when cells were modified to express KDEL-SDF-1, the ligand for CXCR4, the intrakine trapped the nascently synthesized CXCR4 in the ER, and the transduced cells were found to resist infection with HIV-1 isolates that use CXCR4 as a coreceptor for entry [211]. Conversely, cells that express modified RANTES or MIP-1α, the ligands for CCR5, were found to resist infection with HIV-1 isolates that use the CCR5 coreceptor isolates [212].

Strategies based on preventing the expression of chemokine coreceptors at the cell surface are particularly attractive primarily because they block the very first step in HIV-1 infection of target cells rather than blocking a viral event that occurs after the establishment of the proviral DNA in the cellular genome. Intrakine-modified cells should also have survival advantages *in vivo* in HIV-infected individuals because of their resistance to infection by certain HIV-1 isolates. Moreover, a gene-based approach that utilizes a nonpolymorphic human protein is unlikely to induce an immune response against the expressed protein. Such undesired outcome could lead to clearance by the immune system of transduced cells expressing the foreign protein.

Clearly, the advantage of one gene-based therapy over another can be ascertained only in a head-to-head comparison of the different strategies under identical conditions and variables. Data derived solely from tissue culture studies may not reflect the suppressive capacity of the transgene *in vivo*. Thus, regardless of the theoretic advantage of one given transgene relative to another, it is premature to conclude whether an advantage will be translated to clinical benefit.

Other strategies

Because HIV-1 replication can be influenced by a variety of cellular perturbations, there are many other molecular strategies for inhibiting this virus (Table 100.1). The use of the KDEL signal peptide has been used to redirect newly synthesized CD4 receptor molecules to the ER. This resulted in resistance of the transduced cells to HIV-1 infection *in vitro*, presumably because of the absence of CD4 at the cell surface for binding the viral gp160 [213]. The LTR sequence of HIV-2 has also been used to block virus replication via interference with HIV-1-specific transcriptional events [214,215]. Conditional expression of the interferon gene under transcriptional control of HIV-1 LTR activated the production of interferon upon infection of the transduced cells by HIV, and inhibited further infection as a result of the antiviral activity of interferon [216]. It is likely that other strategies will be developed that are limited only by the ingenuity of the molecular biologist.

Vectors

A number of gene delivery vehicles, both viral and nonviral, are already in use in clinical studies for diverse diseases. Several of these offering unique advantages are in preclinical development. The subject of vector transduction of hematopoietic cells is described in detail elsewhere in this volume (see Chapter 11).

Current application of gene therapy to AIDS

Current gene therapy strategies make extensive use of an *ex vivo* approach in which cells are taken from a donor, modified with the transgene of interest, expanded, and then returned to the donor. A marker gene that allows detection of the modified cells can be included. However, future gene transfer trials will most likely eliminate marker genes owing to potential toxicity of cells expressing foreign proteins [217].

T lymphocytes as targets for gene therapy

This approach uses autologous T lymphocytes as the target cells for gene modification, thereby eliminating complications caused by host-vs.-graft rejection or graft-vs.-host disease that would otherwise occur with grafts from nonidentical individuals. Using this strategy, mature $CD4^+$ lymphocytes have been genetically modified and reinfused into patients [161,189,218]. A similar strategy, in which mature $CD8^+$ lymphocytes have been modified to kill HIV-infected cells, has also been reported [134,219,220]. In either case, mature T lymphocytes have attributes that make them attractive targets for gene therapy: they are easily obtained from the donor's peripheral blood and they can be expanded to large numbers *in vitro*. Indeed, a method of cell expansion that involves cell surface stimulation, using antibodies to CD3 and CD28, promotes the expansion of cells to very high numbers [221]. Because these stimuli also transiently downregulate the expression of the chemokine receptor CCR5 [222], these cells are at a minimum temporarily resistant to infection with macrophage-tropic strains of HIV, adding another advantage for their immediate survival in an HIV-infected host.

Targeting mature T lymphocytes for gene therapy has the added advantage that the effect of the therapeutic gene can be rapidly monitored for effects on cell survival, viral load and other parameters. The transduced cells can also be selected *in vitro*, using the marker gene included in the vector, before reinfusion in the host, thereby generating a highly enriched population of genetically modified cells. For these reasons, gene therapy approaches that target mature lymphoid populations may be the method of choice for initial evaluation of new gene therapy strategies.

A negative aspect of using mature lymphocytes is that they are terminally differentiated and have limited *in vivo* growth potential and finite life span. Moreover, $CD4^+$ T lymphocytes represent only one of the cell types susceptible to HIV-1 *in vivo*. In addition, techniques used to expand $CD4^+$ lymphocytes *in vitro* can affect the expression of various surface markers and result in altered homing properties when the cells are reinfused to the host. Intense efforts are therefore underway to develop gene transfer protocols for HSCs that can give rise to all cells of the lymphoid and myeloid lineages. Conceptually then, HSCs transduced with a potent anti-HIV-1 gene should confer anti-HIV-1 protection to all hematopoietic cells lineages, including those susceptible to HIV-1 infection ($CD4^+$ T lymphocytes, monocytes, Langerhans cells, dendritic cells and others) for the life of the infected individual.

Hematopoietic stem cells as targets of gene transfer

While blood stem cells are an attractive target for gene therapy, they present a unique set of issues that are not encountered when mature T lymphocytes are used as the target cells. In addition to their low frequency, stem cells are quiescent. This relative paucity of cell replication may affect transduction strategies that rely on retroviral vectors, a class of vectors that require cell division for efficient gene transfer (see Chapter 11). As a result, current transduction methods often stimulate cell division, which may compromise the undifferentiated status, functional activity and subsequent cell lineage commitment of the transduced progenitor cells. Over recent years, newer methods of transduction have resulted in incremental improvements of vector-mediated gene transfer into $CD34^+$ cells. These include the use of recombinant fibronectin fragment CH-296 instead of stromal layers [223,224], and the combination of recombinant fl3-ligand [225,226], thrombopoietin (TPO) and stem cell factor (SCF) [227]. The critical issue is whether the vector can transduce a pluripotent stem cell, and to conclusively demonstrate that transduced $CD34^+$ cells are in fact pluripotent, it is necessary to show that cultures derived from a single transduced cell can differentiate into all hematopoietic lineages (T and B lymphocytes, monocytes, erythrocytes and others) and can result in reconstitution *in vivo* of a surrogate host. Another important factor in HSC-based gene therapy in AIDS is the functional status of the thymus—an organ required for most T-lymphocyte differentiation. While recent results suggest the presence of discernible thymic tissue in HIV-infected individuals [228], the functional integrity and capacity of this tissue to support normal T-lymphocyte differentiation is still uncertain.

The ability of stem cells to engraft in patients who have not been "preconditioned" with cytoreductive or mycloablative preparative regimens is an important issue in HSC-based gene therapy. The first successful retrovirus-based gene therapy was performed in patients with severe combined immunodeficiency (SCID) [229,230]. The initial successful outgrowth of T lymphocytes were demonstrated to contain the transgene and to be functional [229]. This clinical trial provided the first demonstration that gene transfer could cure a genetic disease, and it is a model on which anti-HIV-1 gene therapy using genetically modified HCT has been based. These results were encouraging and initiated new studies to define methods for gene transfer using HCT. The setting of autologous HCT for AIDS lymphoma is a clinical setting in which these new methods can be evaluated [127]. The comparative value of cytoreduction vs. non-myeloablative regimens, the evaluation of new vectors and stability of transgene expression, and the development of selection strategies for expansion of transduced cells *in vivo* all need to be studied. However, the initial successes in SCID patients have recently yielded retrovirus-related insertional mutagenesis with late T-cell leukemia [231]. Whether this leukemoid reaction was brought about by the interleukin γ-chain transgene, to the underlying host genetics or to the retrovirus vector is unknown, but adverse events such as these further define the problems that must be understood before stem cell-based gene therapy can be safe and efficacious.

Prospects for the future: vaccination by gene therapy using viral vectors or naked DNA in HIV-1-infected patients

Clearly, the ultimate solution to control the global spread of HIV-1 is prevention. The first gene transfer study in HIV-1 patients involved a retrovirus vector vaccine encoding HIV-1 envelope and Rev, and this clinical trial showed induction of a cellular immune response [232,233]. The direct gene transfer into muscle cells using "naked" DNA [234,235] suggested a novel approach for "therapeutic" vaccine strategy in HIV-1 infected individuals, and several such studies have been reported [230–239]. Initial studies in uninfected chimpanzees has demonstrated induction of certain immune responses and protection of uninfected animals against challenge with heterologous HIV-1 isolate [240–242]. The induced T-lymphocyte immunity is transient in duration following DNA vaccination, and it is likely that combined DNA priming and recombinant viral booster will be necessary [243].

Improved vectors and use of vaccine strategies early in infection before collapse of the immune system, e.g. in patients on potent anti-HIV-1 chemotherapy with undetectable blood levels of HIV-1 RNA, may shed light on the usefulness of therapeutic vaccines. Immunization studies may establish a novel immunization strategy, and it is likely that such a gene transfer method will have the greatest impact on control of HIV infection.

Conclusions

Assuming that both T-lymphocyte-based and HSC-based gene therapy are optimized, specific uses for each approach are likely to be identified and, in certain cases, the rationale for combined infusion of altered T cells and HSC could be established. The antiviral effects of T-lymphocyte modification can be discerned *in vivo* much faster than in T cells derived from modified HSC. Antiviral protection appears to be demonstrated in the increased survival of CD4$^+$ lymphocyte cells expressing the RevM10 transgene than in unprotected control CD4$^+$ lymphocytes [130] and by the enhanced immune function of T cells with altered T-cell receptors [220]. One application of T-lymphocyte transductions is thus for *in vivo* comparison of different and/or new antiviral genes or vectors in the same subject to establish the superiority of one approach relative to another, with T-lymphocyte survival as the criterion for success. In the era of potent anti-HIV-1 chemotherapy, candidates for such protocols are likely to represent patients who have developed resistance to currently available drugs, those who are intolerant to such therapy or have failed to have an immunologic benefit from such chemotherapy, and those who have relapsed after initial response to this treatment.

HSC-based gene therapy for AIDS requires that safe methods for transplantation be developed which are suitable for use in asymptomatic outpatients. We are far from knowing how to apply such a method. Studies are in progress to determine whether partial marrow ablation is necessary or possible in this setting. The ability to establish immune reconstitution utilizing HSC-based strategies for persons with advanced AIDS will likely require the development of adjunctive strategies, perhaps concomitant thymic tissue transplantation, cytokine replacement therapy, and other approaches related to organ failure and immune dysregulation. The integration of such modalities may yield regimens that restore and maintain immune functions sufficient to protect the host against many of the human pathogens and malignancies leading to and associated with overt AIDS. In summary, combined with improvements in T-lymphocyte expansion and related technological advancements, gene-based therapeutic protocols may eventually benefit patients who have exhausted all other options of available therapies and, importantly, add a novel modality to the arsenal of AIDS therapeutics.

References

1 Embretson J, Zupancic M, Ribas JL *et al.* Massive covert infection of helper T lymphocytes and macrophages by HIV during the incubation period of AIDS. *Nature* 1993; **362**: 359–62.

2 Pantaleo G, Graziosi C, Demarest JF *et al.* HIV infection is active and progressive in lymphoid tissue during the clinically latent stage of disease. *Nature* 1993; **362**: 355–8.

3 Fauci AS. Multifactorial nature of human immunodeficiency virus disease: implications for therapy. *Science* 1993; **262**: 1011–8.

4 Fauci AS, Pantaleo G, Stanley S, Weissman D. Immunopathogenic mechanisms of HIV infection. *Ann Intern Med* 1996; **124**: 654–63.

5 Schuitemaker H, Koot M, Kootstra NA *et al.* Biological phenotype of human immunodeficiency virus type 1 clones at different stages of infection: progression of disease is associated with a shift from monocytotropic to T-cell-tropic virus population. *J Virol* 1992; **66**: 1354–60.

6 Yeni PG, Hammer SM, Carpenter CC *et al.* Antiretroviral treatment for adult HIV infection in 2002: updated recommendations of the International AIDS Society–USA Panel. *J Am Med Assoc* 2002; **288**: 222–35.

7 Moutouh L, Corbeil J, Richman DD. Recombination leads to the rapid emergence of HIV-1 dually resistant mutants under selective drug pressure. *Proc Natl Acad Sci U S A* 1996; **93**: 6106–11.

8 Wong JK, Gunthard HF, Havlir DV *et al.* Reduction of HIV-1 in blood and lymph nodes following potent antiretroviral therapy and the virologic correlates of treatment failure. *Proc Natl Acad Sci U S A* 1997; **94**: 12574–9.

9 Bridges SH, Sarver N. Gene therapy and immune restoration for HIV disease. *Lancet* 1995; **345**: 427–32.

10 Statham S, Morgan RA. Gene therapy clinical trials for HIV. *Curr Opin Mol Ther* 1999; **1**: 430–6.

11 Buchschacher GL Jr, Wong-Staal F. Approaches to gene therapy for human immunodeficiency virus infection. *Hum Gene Ther* 2001; **12**: 1013–9.

12 Guatelli JC, Siliciano RF, Kuritzkes DR, Richman DD. Human immunodeficiency virus. In: Richman,

DD Whitley, RJ Hayden, FG eds. *Clinical Virology*. Washington D.C.: ASM Press, 2002.

13. Goldgur Y, Craigie R, Cohen GH et al. Structure of the HIV-1 integrase catalytic domain complexed with an inhibitor: a platform for antiviral drug design. *Proc Natl Acad Sci U S A* 1999; **96**: 13040–3.

14. Fujiwara T. Phase I multiple oral dose safety and pharmacokinetic study of S-1360, an HIV integrase inhibitor with healthy volunteers. XIV International AIDS Conference, Barcelona, 2002.

15. Grobler JA, Stillmock K, Hu B et al. Diketo acid inhibitor mechanism and HIV-1 integrase: implications for metal binding in the active site of phosphotransferase enzymes. *Proc Natl Acad Sci U S A* 2002; **99**: 6661–6.

16. Dalgleish AG, Beverley PC, Clapham PR, Crawford DH, Greaves MF, Weiss RA. The CD4 (T4) antigen is an essential component of the receptor for the AIDS retrovirus. *Nature* 1984; **312**: 763–7.

17. Feng Y, Broder CC, Kennedy PE, Berger EA. HIV-1 entry cofactor: functional cDNA cloning of a seven-transmembrane, G protein-coupled receptor. *Science* 1996; **272**: 872–7.

18. Dragic T, Litwin V, Allaway GP et al. HIV-1 entry into CD4+ cells is mediated by the chemokine receptor CC-CKR-5. *Nature* 1996; **381**: 667–73.

19. Premack BA, Schall TJ. Chemokine receptors: gateways to inflammation and infection. *Nat Med* 1996; **2**: 1174–8.

20. Cocchi F, DeVico AL, Garzino-Demo A, Arya SK, Gallo RC, Lusso P. Identification of RANTES, MIP-1α, and MIP-1β as the major HIV-suppressive factors produced by CD8+ T cells. *Science* 1995; **270**: 1811–5.

21. Winkler C, Modi W, Smith MW et al. Genetic restriction of AIDS pathogenesis by an SDF-1 chemokine gene variant. ALIVE Study, Hemophilia Growth and Development Study (HGDS), Multicenter AIDS Cohort Study (MACS), Multicenter Hemophilia Cohort Study (MHCS), San Francisco City Cohort (SFCC). *Science* 1998; **279**: 389–93.

22. Ioannidis JP, Rosenberg PS, Goedert JJ et al. Effects of CCR5-Delta32, CCR2-64I, and SDF-1 3′A alleles on HIV-1 disease progression: an international meta-analysis of individual-patient data. *Ann Intern Med* 2001; **135**: 782–95.

23. Raport CJ, Schweickart VL, Chantry D et al. New members of the chemokine receptor gene family. *J Leukoc Biol* 1996; **59**: 18–23.

24. Smith MW, Dean M, Carrington M et al. Contrasting genetic influence of CCR2 and CCR5 variants on HIV-1 infection and disease progression. Hemophilia Growth and Development Study (HGDS), Multicenter AIDS Cohort Study (MACS), Multicenter Hemophilia Cohort Study (MHCS), San Francisco City Cohort (SFCC), ALIVE Study. *Science* 1997; **277**: 959–65.

25. Michael NL. Host genetic influences on HIV-1 pathogenesis. *Curr Opin Immunol* 1999; **11**: 466–74.

26. Goldsmith MA, Doms RW. HIV entry: are all receptors created equal? *Nat Immunol* 2002; **3**: 709–10.

27. Chow YH, Wei OL, Phogat S et al. Conserved structures exposed in HIV-1 envelope glycoproteins stabilized by flexible linkers as potent entry inhibitors and potential immunogens. *Biochemistry* 2002; **41**: 7176–82.

28. Sherman MP, Greene WC. Slipping through the door: HIV entry into the nucleus. *Microbes Infect* 2002; **4**: 67–73.

29. Nielsen SD, Sorensen AM, Schonning K, Lund O, Nielsen JO, Hansen JE. Complement-mediated enhancement of HIV-1 infection in peripheral blood mononuclear cells. *Scand J Infect Dis* 1997; **29**: 447–52.

30. Sun J, Barbeau B, Sato S, Tremblay MJ. Neuraminidase from a bacterial source enhances both HIV-1-mediated syncytium formation and the virus binding/entry process. *Virology* 2001; **284**: 26–36.

31. Cullen BR. A new entry route for HIV. *Nat Med* 2001; **7**: 20–1.

32. Saifuddin M, Hart ML, Gewurz H, Zhang Y, Spear GT. Interaction of mannose-binding lectin with primary isolates of human immunodeficiency virus type 1. *J Gen Virol* 2000; **81**: 949–55.

33. Geijtenbeek TB, Kwon DS, Torensma R et al. DC-SIGN, a dendritic cell-specific HIV-1-binding protein that enhances trans-infection of T cells. *Cell* 2000; **100**: 587–97.

34. Stoiber H, Kacani L, Speth C, Wurzner R, Dierich MP. The supportive role of complement in HIV pathogenesis. *Immunol Rev* 2001; **180**: 168–76.

35. Kwon DS, Gregorio G, Bitton N, Hendrickson WA, Littman DR. DC-SIGN-mediated internalization of HIV is required for trans-enhancement of T cell infection. *Immunity* 2002; **16**: 135–44.

36. Liu R, Paxton WA, Choe S et al. Homozygous defect in HIV-1 coreceptor accounts for resistance of some multiply-exposed individuals to HIV-1 infection. *Cell* 1996; **86**: 367–77.

37. Samson M, Libert F, Doranz BJ et al. Resistance to HIV-1 infection in Caucasian individuals bearing mutant alleles of the CCR-5 chemokine receptor gene. *Nature* 1996; **382**: 722–5.

38. Dean M, Carrington M, Winkler C et al. Genetic restriction of HIV-1 infection and progression to AIDS by a deletion allele of the CKR5 structural gene. Hemophilia Growth and Development Study, Multicenter AIDS Cohort Study, Multicenter Hemophilia Cohort Study, San Francisco City Cohort, ALIVE Study. *Science* 1996; **273**: 1856–62.

39. Cohen OJ, Paolucci S, Bende SM et al. CXCR4 and CCR5 genetic polymorphisms in long-term nonprogressive human immunodeficiency virus infection: lack of association with mutations other than CCR5-Delta32. *J Virol* 1998; **72**: 6215–7.

40. Kwong PD, Wyatt R, Robinson J, Sweet RW, Sodroski J, Hendrickson WA. Structure of an HIV gp120 envelope glycoprotein in complex with the CD4 receptor and a neutralizing human antibody. *Nature* 1998; **393**: 648–59.

41. Kwong PD, Wyatt R, Majeed S et al. Structures of HIV-1 gp120 envelope glycoproteins from laboratory-adapted and primary isolates. *Structure Fold Des* 2000; **8**: 1329–39.

42. Takashima K, Miyake H, Furuta RA et al. Inhibitory effects of small-molecule CCR5 antagonists on human immunodeficiency virus type 1 envelope-mediated membrane fusion and viral replication. *Antimicrob Agents Chemother* 2001; **45**: 3538–43.

43. Derdeyn CA, Decker JM, Sfakianos JN et al. Sensitivity of human immunodeficiency virus type 1 to fusion inhibitors targeted to the gp41 first heptad repeat involves distinct regions of gp41 and is consistently modulated by gp120 interactions with the coreceptor. *J Virol* 2001; **75**: 8605–14.

44. Berkhout B, Silverman RH, Jeang KT. Tat transactivates the human immunodeficiency virus through a nascent RNA target. *Cell* 1989; **59**: 273–82.

45. Luznik L, Kraus G, Guatelli J, Richman D, Wong-Staal F. Tat-independent replication of human immunodeficiency viruses. *J Clin Invest* 1995; **95**: 328–32.

46. Subbramanian RA, Cohen EA. Molecular biology of the human immunodeficiency virus accessory proteins. *J Virol* 1994; **68**: 6831–5.

47. Miller RH, Sarver N. HIV accessory proteins as therapeutic targets. *Nat Med* 1997; **3**: 389–94.

48. Ziegler JL, Stites DP. Hypothesis: AIDS is an autoimmune disease directed at the immune system and triggered by a lymphotropic retrovirus. *Clin Immunol Immunopathol* 1986; **41**: 305–13.

49. Wei X, Ghosh SK, Taylor ME et al. Viral dynamics in human immunodeficiency virus type 1 infection. *Nature* 1995; **373**: 117–22.

50. Ho DD, Neumann AU, Perelson AS, Chen W, Leonard JM, Markowitz M. Rapid turnover of plasma virions and CD4 lymphocytes in HIV-1 infection. *Nature* 1995; **373**: 123–6.

51. Roederer M, Dubs JG, Anderson MT, Raju PA, Herzenberg LA. CD8 naive T cell counts decrease progressively in HIV-infected adults. *J Clin Invest* 1995; **95**: 2061–6.

52. Roederer M. Getting to the HAART of T cell dynamics. *Nat Med* 1998; **4**: 145–6.

53. Douek DC, Betts MR, Hill BJ et al. Evidence for increased T cell turnover and decreased thymic output in HIV infection. *J Immunol* 2001; **167**: 6663–8.

54. Pakker NG, Notermans DW, de Boer RJ et al. Biphasic kinetics of peripheral blood T cells after triple combination therapy in HIV-1 infection: a composite of redistribution and proliferation. *Nat Med* 1998; **4**: 208–14.

55. Mosier DE. HIV results in the frame: CD4+ cell turnover. *Nature* 1995; **375**: 193–4; discussion 198.

56. Sprent J, Tough D. HIV results in the frame: CD4+ cell turnover. *Nature* 1995; **375**: 194; discussion 198.

57. Autran B, Carcelain G, Li TS et al. Positive effects of combined antiretroviral therapy on CD4+ T cell homeostasis and function in advanced HIV disease. *Science* 1997; **277**: 112–6.

58. Gorochov G, Neumann AU, Kereveur A et al. Perturbation of CD4+ and CD8+ T-cell repertoires during progression to AIDS and regulation of the CD4+ repertoire during antiviral therapy. *Nat Med* 1998; **4**: 215–21.

59. Connors M, Kovacs JA, Krevat S et al. HIV infection induces changes in CD4+ T-cell phenotype and depletions within the CD4+ T-cell repertoire that are not immediately restored by antiviral or immune-based therapies. *Nat Med* 1997; **3**: 533–40.

60. Lange CG, Valdez H, Medvik K, Asaad R, Lederman MM. CD4+ T-lymphocyte nadir and the effect of highly active antiretroviral therapy on phenotypic and functional immune restoration in HIV-1 infection. *Clin Immunol* 2002; **102**: 154–61.

61. Bonyhadi ML, Rabin L, Salimi S et al. HIV induces thymus depletion in vivo. *Nature* 1993; **363**: 728–32.

62. Stanley SK, McCune JM, Kaneshima H et al. Human immunodeficiency virus infection of the human thymus and disruption of the thymic microenvironment in the SCID-hu mouse. *J Exp Med* 1993; **178**: 1151–63.

63. Gorochov G, Neumann AU, Parizot C, Li T, Katlama C, Debre P. Down-regulation of CD8+ T-cell expansions in patients with human immunodeficiency virus infection receiving highly active combination therapy. *Blood* 2001; **97**: 1787–95.

64. Lange CG, Lederman MM, Madero JS et al. Impact of suppression of viral replication by highly active antiretroviral therapy on immune function and phenotype in chronic HIV-1 infection. *J Acquir Immune Defic Syndr* 2002; **30**: 33–40.

65. Finzi D, Hermankova M, Pierson T et al. Identification of a reservoir for HIV-1 in patients on highly active antiretroviral therapy. *Science* 1997; **278**: 1295–300.

66. Finzi D, Blankson J, Siliciano JD et al. Latent infection of CD4+ T cells provides a mechanism for lifelong persistence of HIV-1, even in patients on effective combination therapy. *Nat Med* 1999; **5**: 512–7.

67. Chun TW, Davey RT Jr, Ostrowski M et al. Relationship between pre-existing viral reservoirs and the re-emergence of plasma viremia after discontinuation of highly active anti-retroviral therapy. *Nat Med* 2000; **6**: 757–61.

68. Frost SD. Dynamics and evolution of HIV-1 during structured treatment interruptions. *AIDS Rev* 2002; **4**: 119–27.

69. Lori F, Foli A, Lisziewicz J. Structured treatment interruptions as a potential alternative therapeutic regimen for HIV-infected patients: a review of recent clinical data and future prospects. *J Antimicrob Chemother* 2002; **50**: 155–60.

70. Vila J, Nugier F, Bargues G et al. Absence of viral rebound after treatment of HIV-infected patients with didanosine and hydroxycarbamide. *Lancet* 1997; **350**: 635–6.

71. Rosenberg ES, Altfeld M, Poon SH et al. Immune control of HIV-1 after early treatment of acute infection. *Nature* 2000; **407**: 523–6.

72. Gulick RM, Mellors JW, Havlir D et al. Treatment with indinavir, zidovudine, and lamivudine in adults with human immunodeficiency virus infection and prior antiretroviral therapy. *N Engl J Med* 1997; **337**: 734–9.

73. Mellors JW, Kingsley LA, Rinaldo CR Jr. et al. Quantitation of HIV-1 RNA in plasma predicts outcome after seroconversion. *Ann Intern Med* 1995; **122**: 573–9.

74. Mellors JW, Rinaldo CR Jr, Gupta P, White RM, Todd JA, Kingsley LA. Prognosis in HIV-1 infection predicted by the quantity of virus in plasma. *Science* 1996; **272**: 1167–70.

75. Richman DD. Clinical significance of drug resistance in human immunodeficiency virus. *Clin Infect Dis* 1995; **21** (Suppl. 2): S166–9.

76. Revision of the case definition of acquired immunodeficiency syndrome for national reporting—United States. *MMWR Morb Mortal Wkly Rep* 1985; **34**: 373–5.

77. Beral V, Peterman T, Berkelman R, Jaffe H. AIDS-associated non-Hodgkin lymphoma. *Lancet* 1991; **337**: 805–9.

78. Hessol NA, Katz MH, Liu JY, Buchbinder SP, Rubino CJ, Holmberg SD. Increased incidence of Hodgkin disease in homosexual men with HIV infection. *Ann Intern Med* 1992; **117**: 309–11.

79. Cote TR, Biggar RJ, Rosenberg PS et al. Non-Hodgkin's lymphoma among people with AIDS: incidence, presentation and public health burden. AIDS/Cancer Study Group. *Int J Cancer* 1997; **73**: 645–50.

80. Biggar RJ, Engels EA, Frisch M, Goedert JJ. Risk of T-cell lymphomas in persons with AIDS. *J Acquir Immune Defic Syndr* 2001; **26**: 371–6.

81. Appleby P, Beral V, Newton R, Reeves G. Highly active antiretroviral therapy and incidence of cancer in human immunodeficiency virus-infected adults. *J Natl Cancer Inst* 2000; **92**: 1823–30.

82. Matthews GV, Bower M, Mandalia S, Powles T, Nelson MR, Gazzard BG. Changes in acquired immunodeficiency syndrome-related lymphoma since the introduction of highly active antiretroviral therapy. *Blood* 2000; **96**: 2730–4.

83. Grulich AE. Update: cancer risk in persons with HIV/AIDS in the era of combination antiretroviral therapy. *AIDS Read* 2000; **10**: 341–6.

84. Mocroft A, Katlama C, Johnson AM et al. AIDS across Europe, 1994–98: the EuroSIDA study. *Lancet* 2000; **356**: 291–6.

85. Mocroft A, Sabin CA, Youle M et al. Changes in AIDS-defining illnesses in a London clinic, 1987–98. *J Acquir Immune Defic Syndr* 1999; **21**: 401–7.

86. Palella JF, Km D, Moorman AC et al. Declining morbidity and mortality among patients with advanced human immunodeficiency virus infection. *N Engl J Med* 1998; **338**: 853–60.

87. Goedert JJ. The epidemiology of acquired immunodeficiency syndrome malignancies. *Semin Oncol* 2000; **27**: 390–401.

88. Sparano JA, Anand K, Desai J, Mitnick RJ, Kalkut GE, Hanau LH. Effect of highly active antiretroviral therapy on the incidence of HIV-associated malignancies at an urban medical center. *J Acquir Immune Defic Syndr* 1999; **21** (Suppl. 1): S18–22.

89. Grulich AE. AIDS-associated non-Hodgkin's lymphoma in the era of highly active antiretroviral therapy. *J Acquir Immune Defic Syndr* 1999; **21** (Suppl. 1): S27–30.

90. Rabkin C, Testa M, Huang J, Von Roem J. Kaposi's sarcoma and non-Hodgkin's lymphoma incidence: trends in AIDS Clinical Trial Group Study Participants *J AIDS* 1999; **21**: S31–3.

91. Clarke CA, Glaser SL. Epidemiologic trends in HIV-associated lymphomas. *Curr Opin Oncol* 2001; **13**: 354–9.

92. Besson C, Goubar A, Gabarre J et al. Changes in AIDS-related lymphoma since the era of highly active antiretroviral therapy. *Blood* 2001; **98**: 2339–44.

93. Biggar RJ. AIDS-related cancers in the era of highly active antiretroviral therapy. *Oncology (Huntingt)* 2001; **15**: 439–48; discussion 448–9.

94. Grulich AE, Li Y, McDonald AM, Correll PK, Law MG, Kaldor JM. Decreasing rates of Kaposi's sarcoma and non-Hodgkin's lymphoma in the era of potent combination anti-retroviral therapy. *AIDS* 2001; **15**: 629–33.

95. Buchbinder SP, Holmberg SD, Scheer S, Colfax G, O'Malley P, Vittinghoff E. Combination antiretroviral therapy and incidence of AIDS-related malignancies. *J Acquir Immune Defic Syndr* 1999; **21** (Suppl. 1): S23–6.

96. Rabkin CS. AIDS and cancer in the era of highly active antiretroviral therapy (HAART). *Eur J Cancer* 2001; **37**: 1316–9.

97. Levine AM, Seneviratne L, Tulpule A. Incidence and management of AIDS-related lymphoma. *Oncology (Huntingt)* 2001; **15**: 629–39; discussion 639–40; 645–6.

98. Dal Maso L, Serraino D, Franceschi S. Epidemiology of AIDS-related tumours in developed and developing countries. *Eur J Cancer* 2001; **37**: 1188–201.

99. Little RF, Gutierrez M, Jaffe ES, Pau A, Horne M, Wilson W. HIV-associated non-Hodgkin lymphoma: incidence, presentation, and prognosis. *J Am Med Assoc* 2001; **285**: 1880–5.

100. Levine AM, Seneviratne L, Espina BM et al. Evolving characteristics of AIDS-related lymphoma. *Blood* 2000; **13**: 4084–90.

101. Mocroft A, Madge S, Johnson AM et al. A comparison of exposure groups in the EuroSIDA study: starting highly active antiretroviral therapy (HAART), response to HAART, and survival. *J Acquir Immune Defic Syndr* 1999; **22**: 369–78.

102. Levine ADTS, Zaia JA, Krishnan A. Hematologic aspects of HIV/AIDS. In: Schechter GP, Broudy VC, Williams ME, eds. *Hematology 2001: American Society of Hematology Education Program Book*. Washington D.C.: American Society of Hematology, 2001: 463–78.

103. Ioachim HL, Dorsett B, Cronin W, Maya M, Wahl S. Acquired immunodeficiency syndrome-associated lymphomas: clinical, pathologic, immunologic, and viral characteristics of 111 cases. *Hum Pathol* 1991; **22**: 659–73.

104. Levine AM, Sullivan-Halley J, Pike MC et al. Human immunodeficiency virus-related lymphoma: prognostic factors predictive of survival. *Cancer* 1991; **68**: 2466–72.

105. Sparano JA, Wiernik PH, Hu X et al. Pilot trial of infusional cyclophosphamide, doxorubicin, and etoposide plus didanosine and filgrastim in patients with human immunodeficiency virus-associated non-Hodgkin's lymphoma. *J Clin Oncol* 1996; **14**: 3026–35.

106. Seneviratne L, Espina BM, Nathwani BN, Chan JA, Brynes RK, Levine AM. Clinical, immunologic, and pathologic correlates of bone marrow involvement in 291 patients with acquired immunodeficiency syndrome-related lymphoma. *Blood* 2001; **98**: 2358–63.

107. Gill PS, Levine AM, Krailo M et al. AIDS-related malignant lymphoma: results of prospective treatment trials. *J Clin Oncol* 1987; **5**: 1322–8.

108. Levine AM, Wernz JC, Kaplan L et al. Low-dose chemotherapy with central nervous system prophylaxis and zidovudine maintenance in AIDS-related lymphoma: a prospective multi-institutional trial. *J Am Med Assoc* 1991; **266**: 84–8.

109. Kaplan LD, Kahn JO, Crowe S et al. Clinical and virologic effects of recombinant human granulocyte-macrophage colony-stimulating factor in patients receiving chemotherapy for human immunodeficiency virus-associated non-Hodgkin's lymphoma: results of a randomized trial. *J Clin Oncol* 1991; **9**: 929–40.

110. Kaplan LD, Abrams DI, Feigal E et al. AIDS-associated non-Hodgkin's lymphoma in San Francisco. *J Am Med Assoc* 1989; **261**: 719–24.

111. Kaplan LD, Straus DJ, Testa MA et al. Low-dose compared with standard-dose m-BACOD chemotherapy for non-Hodgkin's lymphoma associated with human immunodeficiency virus infection. National Institute of Allergy and Infectious Diseases AIDS Clinical Trials Group. *N Engl J Med* 1997; **336**: 1641–8.

112. Little RF, Yarchoan R, Wilson WH. Systemic chemotherapy for HIV-associated lymphoma in the era of highly active antiretroviral therapy. *Curr Opin Oncol* 2000; **12**: 438–44.

113. Navarro JT, Ribera JM, Oriol A et al. Influence of highly active anti-retroviral therapy on response to treatment and survival in patients with acquired immunodeficiency syndrome-related non-Hodgkin's lymphoma treated with cyclophosphamide, hydroxydoxorubicin, vincristine and prednisone. *Br J Haematol* 2001; **112**: 909–15.

114 Spina M, Vaccher E, Juzbasic S et al. Human immunodeficiency virus-related non-Hodgkin lymphoma: activity of infusional cyclophosphamide, doxorubicin, and etoposide as second-line chemotherapy in 40 patients. Cancer 2001; **92**: 200–6.

115 Bi J, Espina BM, Tulpule A, Boswell W, Levine AM. High-dose cytosine-arabinoside and cisplatin regimens as salvage therapy for refractory or relapsed AIDS-related non-Hodgkin's lymphoma. J Acquir Immune Defic Syndr 2001; **28**: 416–21.

116 Tirelli U, Spina M, Gaidano G, Vaccher E, Franceschi S, Carbone A. Epidemiological, biological and clinical features of HIV-related lymphomas in the era of highly active antiretroviral therapy. AIDS 2000; **14**: 1675–88.

117 Rossi G, Donisi A, Casari S, Re A, Cadeo G, Carosi G. The International Prognostic Index can be used as a guide to treatment decisions regarding patients with human immunodeficiency virus-related systemic non-Hodgkin lymphoma. Cancer 1999; **86**: 2391–7.

118 Thiessard F, Morlat C, Marimoutou S et al. Prognostic factors after non-Hodgkin's lymphoma in patients infected with the human immunodeficiency virus. Cancer 2000; **88**: 1696–1702.

119 Franken M, Estabrooks A, Cavacini L, Sherburne B, Wang F, Scadden DT. Epstein-Barr virus-driven gene therapy for EBV-related lymphomas. Nat Med 1996; **2**: 1379–82.

120 Philip T, Guglielmi C, Hagenbeek A et al. Autologous bone marrow transplantation as compared with salvage chemotherapy in relapses of chemotherapy-sensitive non-Hodgkin's lymphoma. N Engl J Med 1995; **333**: 1540–5.

121 Haioun C, Lepage E, Gisselbrecht C et al. Benefit of autologous bone marrow transplantation over sequential chemotherapy in poor-risk aggressive non-Hodgkin's lymphoma: updated results of the prospective study LNH87-2. Groupe d'Etude des Lymphomes de l'Adulte. J Clin Oncol 1997; **15**: 1131–7.

122 Nademanee A, Molina A, O'Donnell MR et al. Results of high-dose therapy and autologous bone marrow/stem cell transplantation during remission in poor-risk intermediate- and high-grade lymphoma: international index high and high-intermediate risk group. Blood 1997; **90**: 3844–52.

123 Stiff PJ, Dahlberg S, Forman SJ et al. Autologous bone marrow transplantation for patients with relapsed or refractory diffuse aggressive non-Hodgkin's lymphoma: value of augmented preparative regimens: a South-West Oncology Group trial. J Clin Oncol 1998; **16**: 48–55.

124 Gabarre J, Leblond V, Sutton L et al. Autologous bone marrow transplantation in relapsed HIV-related non-Hodgkin's lymphoma. Bone Marrow Transplant 1996; **18**: 1195–7.

125 Molina A, Krishnan AY, Nademanee A et al. High dose therapy and autologous stem cell transplantation for human immunodeficiency virus-associated non-Hodgkin lymphoma in the era of highly active antiretroviral therapy. Cancer 2000; **89**: 680–9.

126 Krishnan A, Molina A, Zaia J et al. Autologous stem cell transplantation for HIV-associated lymphoma. Blood 2001; **98**: 3857–9.

127 Krishnan A, Zaia J, Molina A. Stem cell transplantation and gene therapy for HIV-related lymphomas. J Hematother Stem Cell Res 2002; **11**: 765–75.

128 Gabarre J, Azar N, Autran B, Katlama C, Leblond V. High-dose therapy and autologous haematopoietic stem-cell transplantation for HIV-1-associated lymphoma. Lancet 2000; **355**: 1071–2.

129 Krishnan A, Molina A, Zaia J, Vasquez D, Smith D, Forman SJ. Durable remissions in HIV-related lymphoma with autologous stem cell transplantation. Blood (ASH Abstract; Philadelphia December 2002) 2002; **100**: in press.

130 Holland HK, Saral R, Rossi JJ et al. Allogeneic bone marrow transplantation, zidovudine, and human immunodeficiency virus type 1 (HIV-1) infection: studies in a patient with non-Hodgkin lymphoma. Ann Intern Med 1989; **111**: 973–81.

131 Bowden RA, Coombs RW, Nikora BH et al. Progression of human immunodeficiency virus type-1 infection after allogeneic marrow transplantation. Am J Med 1990; **88**: 49N–52N.

132 Schneider E, Lambermont M, Van Vooren JP et al. Autologous stem cell infusion for acute myeloblastic leukemia in an HIV-1 carrier. Bone Marrow Transplant 1997; **20**: 611–2.

133 Kang EM, de Witte M, Malech H et al. Non-myeloablative conditioning followed by transplantation of genetically modified HLA-matched peripheral blood progenitor cells for hematologic malignancies in patients with acquired immunodeficiency syndrome. Blood 2002; **99**: 698–701.

134 Riddell SR, Elliott M, Lewinsohn DA et al. T-cell mediated rejection of gene-modified HIV-specific cytotoxic T lymphocytes in HIV-infected patients. Nat Med 1996; **2**: 216–23.

135 Rosenberg SA, Blaese RM, Brenner MK et al. Human gene marker/therapy clinical protocols. Hum Gene Ther 1996; **7**: 1621–47.

136 Warner JF, Jolly D, Mento S, Galpin J, Haubrich R, Merritt J. Retroviral vectors for HIV immunotherapy. Ann N Y Acad Sci 1995; **772**: 105–16.

137 Bagarazzi ML, Boyer JD, Ayyavoo V, Weiner DB. Nucleic acid-based vaccines as an approach to immunization against human immunodeficiency virus type-1. Curr Top Microbiol Immunol 1998; **226**: 107–43.

138 Robinson HL. DNA vaccines for immunodeficiency viruses. AIDS 1997; **11** (Suppl. A): S109–19.

139 Alama A, Barbieri F, Cagnoli M, Schettini G. Antisense oligonucleotides as therapeutic agents. Pharmacol Res 1997; **36**: 171–8.

140 Morgan RA, Walker R. Gene therapy for AIDS using retroviral mediated gene transfer to deliver HIV-1 antisense TAR and transdominant Rev protein genes to syngeneic lymphocytes in HIV-1 infected identical twins. Hum Gene Ther 1996; **7**: 1281–306.

141 Chatterjee S, Johnson PR, Rose JA, Wong KK Jr. Dual target inhibition of HIV-1 in vitro by means of an adeno-associated virus antisense vector. Science 1992; **258**: 1485–8.

142 Manca F, Fenoglio D, Franchin E et al. Anti-HIV genetic treatment of antigen-specific human CD4 lymphocytes for adoptive immunotherapy of opportunistic infections in AIDS. Gene Ther 1997; **4**: 1216–24.

143 Peng H, Callison D, Li P, Burrell C. Long-term protection against HIV-1 infection conferred by tat or rev antisense RNA was affected by the design of the retroviral vector. Virology 1996; **220**: 377–89.

144 Biasolo MA, Radaelli A, Del Pup L, Franchin E, De Giuli-Morghen C, Palu G. A new antisense tRNA construct for the genetic treatment of human immunodeficiency virus type 1 infection. J Virol 1996; **70**: 2154–61.

145 Donahue RE, Bunnell BA, Zink MC et al. Reduction in SIV replication in rhesus macaques infused with autologous lymphocytes engineered with antiviral genes. Nature Med 1998; **4** (2): 181–6.

146 Sullenger BA, Gallardo HF, Ungers GE, Gilboa E. Overexpression of TAR sequences renders cells resistant to human immunodeficiency virus replication. Cell 1990; **63**: 601–8.

147 Lisziewicz J, Sun D, Trapnell B et al. An auto-regulated dual-function antitat gene for human immunodeficiency virus type 1 gene therapy. J Virol 1995; **69**: 206–12.

148 Rosenzweig M, Marks DF, Hempel D, Lisziewicz J, Johnson RP. Transduction of CD34+ hematopoietic progenitor cells with an antitat gene protects T-cell and macrophage progeny from AIDS virus infection. J Virol 1997; **71**: 2740–6.

149 Lee TC, Sullenger BA, Gallardo HF, Ungers GE, Gilboa E. Overexpression of RRE-derived sequences inhibits HIV-1 replication in CEM cells. New Biol 1992; **4**: 66–74.

150 Lee SW, Gallardo HF, Gilboa E, Smith C. Inhibition of human immunodeficiency virus type 1 in human T cells by a potent Rev response element decoy consisting of the 13-nucleotide minimal Rev-binding domain. J Virol 1994; **68**: 8254–64.

151 Kohn DB, Bauer G, Rice CR et al. A clinical trial of retroviral-mediated transfer of a rev-responsive element decoy gene into CD34+ cells from the bone marrow of human immunodeficiency virus-1-infected children. Blood 1999; **94**: 368–71.

152 Rossi J, Sarver N. Ribozymes and their applications. In: JR B, ed. In: Molecular Biology of Cancer. San Diego, CA: Academic Press, 1997.

153 Sarver N, Cantin EM, Chang PS et al. Ribozymes as potential anti-HIV-1 therapeutic agents. Science 1990; **247**: 1222–5.

154 Bertrand E, Castanotto D, Zhou C et al. The expression cassette determines the functional activity of ribozymes in mammalian cells by controlling their intracellular localization. RNA 1997; **3**: 75–88.

155 Westaway SK, Cagnon L, Chang Z et al. Virion encapsidation of tRNA (3Lys)-ribozyme chimeric RNAs inhibits HIV infection. Antisense Nucleic Acid Drug Dev 1998; **8**: 185–97.

156 Yu M, Ojwang J, Yamada O et al. A hairpin ribozyme inhibits expression of diverse strains of human immunodeficiency virus type 1. Proc Natl Acad Sci U S A 1993; **90**: 6340–4.

157 Gervaix A, Li X, Kraus G, Wong-Staal F. Multi-gene antiviral vectors inhibit diverse human immunodeficiency virus type 1 clades. J Virol 1997; **71**: 3048–53.

158 Rosenzweig M, Marks DF, Hempel D et al. Intracellular immunization of rhesus CD34+ hematopoietic progenitor cells with a hairpin ribozyme protects T cells and macrophages from simian immunodeficiency virus infection. Blood 1997; **90**: 4822–31.

159 Sharp PA. RNA interference. Genes Dev 2001; **15**: 485–90.

160 Bernstein E, Denli AM, Hannon GJ. The rest is silence. RNA 2001; **7**: 1509–21.

161 Hannon GJ. RNA interference. Nature 2002; **418**: 244–51.

162 Ullu E, Djikeng A, Shi H, Tschudi C. RNA interference: advances and questions. Philos Trans R Soc Lond B Biol Sci 2002; **357**: 65–70.

163 Fire A, Xu S, Montgomery MK, Kostas SA, Driver SE, Mello CC. Potent and specific genetic interference by double-stranded RNA in Caenorhabditis elegans. Nature 1998; **391**: 806–11.

164 Fire A, Albertson D, Harrison SW, Moerman DG. Production of antisense RNA leads to effective and

specific inhibition of gene expression in *C. elegans* muscle. *Development* 1991; **113**: 503–14.
165 Paddison PJ, Caudy AA, Bernstein E, Hannon GJ, Conklin DS. Short hairpin RNAs (shRNAs) induce sequence-specific silencing in mammalian cells. *Genes Dev* 2002; **16**: 948–58.
166 Bernstein E, Caudy AA, Hammond SM, Hannon GJ. Role for a bidentate ribonuclease in the initiation step of RNA interference. *Nature* 2001; **409**: 363–6.
167 Martinez J, Patkaniowska A, Urlaub H, Luhrmann R, Tuschl T. Single-stranded antisense siRNAs guide target RNA cleavage in RNAi. *Cell* 2002; **110**: 563.
168 Zamore PD. Ancient pathways programmed by small RNAs. *Science* 2002; **296**: 1265–9.
169 Nykanen A, Haley B, Zamore PD. ATP requirements and small interfering RNA structure in the RNA interference pathway. *Cell* 2001; **107**: 309–21.
170 Elbashir SM, Harborth J, Lendeckel W, Yalcin A, Weber K, Tuschl T. Duplexes of 21-nucleotide RNAs mediate RNA interference in cultured mammalian cells. *Nature* 2001; **411**: 494–8.
171 Elbashir SM, Lendeckel W, Tuschl T. RNA interference is mediated by 21- and 22-nucleotide RNAs. *Genes Dev* 2001; **15**: 188–200.
172 Lee NS, Dohjima T, Bauer G et al. Expression of small interfering RNAs targeted against HIV-1 rev transcripts in human cells. *Nat Biotechnol* 2002; **20**: 500–5.
173 Paul CP, Good PD, Winer I, Engelke DR. Effective expression of small interfering RNA in human cells. *Nat Biotechnol* 2002; **20**: 505–8.
174 Yu JY, DeRuiter SL, Turner DL. RNA interference by expression of short-interfering RNAs and hairpin RNAs in mammalian cells. *Proc Natl Acad Sci U S A* 2002; **99**: 6047–52.
175 Yang D, Buchholz F, Huang Z et al. Short RNA duplexes produced by hydrolysis with *Escherichia coli* RNase III mediate effective RNA interference in mammalian cells. *Proc Natl Acad Sci U S A* 2002; **99**: 9942–7.
176 Miyagishi M, Taira K. U6 promoter-driven siRNAs with four uridine 3′ overhangs efficiently suppress targeted gene expression in mammalian cells. *Nat Biotechnol* 2002; **20**: 497–500.
177 Brummelkamp TR, Bernards R, Agami R. A system for stable expression of short interfering RNAs in mammalian cells. *Science* 2002; **296**: 550–3.
178 Jacque JM, Triques K, Stevenson M. Modulation of HIV-1 replication by RNA interference. *Nature* 2002; **418**: 435–8.
179 Paddison PJ, Caudy AA, Hannon GJ. Stable suppression of gene expression by RNAi in mammalian cells. *Proc Natl Acad Sci U S A* 2002; **99**: 1443–8.
180 Coburn GA, Cullen BR. Potent and specific inhibition of human immunodeficiency virus type 1 replication by RNA interference. *J Virol* 2002; **76**: 9225–31.
181 Novina CD, Murray MF, Dykxhoorn DM et al. siRNA-directed inhibition of HIV-1 infection. *Nat Med* 2002; **8**: 681–6.
182 Hu W, Myers C, Kilzer J, Pfaff S, Bushman F. Inhibition of retroviral pathogenesis by RNA interference. *Curr Biol* 2002; **12**: 1301.
183 Resh M. Silence is golden for HIV-1 siRNA. *Trends Microbiol* 2002; **10**: 399.
184 Devroe E, Silver PA. Retrovirus-delivered siRNA. *BMC Biotechnol* 2002; **2**: 15.
185 Zeng Y, Cullen BR. RNA interference in human cells is restricted to the cytoplasm. *RNA* 2002; **8**: 855–60.
186 Xia H, Mao Q, Paulson HL, Davidson BL. siRNA-mediated gene silencing *in vitro* and *in vivo*. *Nat Biotechnol* 2002; **20**: 1006–10.
187 Malim MH, McCarn DF, Tiley LS, Cullen BR. Mutational definition of the human immunodeficiency virus type-1 Rev activation domain. *J Virol* 1991; **65**: 4248–54.
188 Nabel GJ, Fox BA, Post L, Thompson CB, Woffendin C. A molecular genetic intervention for AIDS: effects of a transdominant negative form of Rev. *Hum Gene Ther* 1994; **5**: 79–92.
189 Woffendin C, Ranga U, Yang Z, Xu L, Nabel GJ. Expression of a protective gene-prolongs survival of T cells in human immunodeficiency virus-infected patients. *Proc Natl Acad Sci U S A* 1996; **93**: 2889–94.
190 Ranga U, Woffendin C, Verma S et al. Enhanced T cell engraftment after retroviral delivery of an antiviral gene in HIV-infected individuals. *Proc Natl Acad Sci U S A* 1998; **95**: 1201–6.
191 Fox BA, Woffendin C, Yang ZY et al. Genetic modification of human peripheral blood lymphocytes with a transdominant negative form of Rev: safety and toxicity. *Hum Gene Ther* 1995; **6**: 997–1004.
192 Bevec D, Volc-Platzer B, Zimmermann K et al. Constitutive expression of chimeric neo-Rev response element transcripts suppresses HIV-1 replication in human CD4+ T lymphocytes. *Hum Gene Ther* 1994; **5**: 193–201.
193 Bonyhadi ML, Moss K, Voytovich A et al. RevM10-expressing T cells derived *in vivo* from transduced human hematopoietic stem-progenitor cells inhibit human immunodeficiency virus replication. *J Virol* 1997; **71**: 4707–16.
194 Bauer G, Valdez P, Kearns K et al. Inhibition of human immunodeficiency virus-1 (HIV-1) replication after transduction of granulocyte colony-stimulating factor-mobilized CD34+ cells from HIV-1-infected donors using retroviral vectors containing anti-HIV-1 genes. *Blood* 1997; **89**: 2259–67.
195 Vandendriessche T, Chuah MK, Chiang L, Chang HK, Ensoli B, Morgan RA. Inhibition of clinical human immunodeficiency virus (HIV) type 1 isolates in primary CD4+ T lymphocytes by retroviral vectors expressing anti-HIV genes. *J Virol* 1995; **69**: 4045–52.
196 Chinen J, Aguilar-Cordova E, Ng-Tang D, Lewis DE, Belmont JW. Protection of primary human T cells from HIV infection by Trev: a transdominant fusion gene. *Hum Gene Ther* 1997; **8**: 861–8.
197 Aguilar-Cordova E, Chinen J, Donehower LA et al. Inhibition of HIV-1 by a double transdominant fusion gene. *Gene Ther* 1995; **2**: 181–6.
198 Marasco WA, Haseltine WA, Chen SY. Design, intracellular expression, and activity of a human anti-human immunodeficiency virus type 1 gp120 single-chain antibody. *Proc Natl Acad Sci U S A* 1993; **90**: 7889–93.
199 Chen JD, Yang Q, Yang AG, Marasco WA, Chen SY. Intra- and extracellular immunization against HIV-1 infection with lymphocytes transduced with an AAV vector expressing a human anti-gp1 120 antibody. *Hum Gene Ther* 1996; **7**: 1515–25.
200 Duan L, Bagasra O, Laughlin MA, Oakes JW, Pomerantz RJ. Potent inhibition of human immunodeficiency virus type 1 replication by an intracellular anti-Rev single-chain antibody. *Proc Natl Acad Sci U S A* 1994; **91**: 5075–9.
201 Mhashilkar A, Bagley J, Chen S et al. Inhibition of HIV-1 Tat-mediated LTR transactivation and HIV-1 infection by anti-Tat single chain intrabodies. *EMBO J* 1995; **14**: 1542–51.
202 Strayer DS, Branco F, Landre J, BouHamdan M, Shaheen F, Pomerantz RJ. Combination genetic therapy to inhibit HIV-1. *Mol Ther* 2002; **5**: 33–41.
203 Curiel TJ, Cook DR, Wang Y, Hahn BH, Ghosh SK, Harrison GS. Long-term inhibition of clinical and laboratory human immunodeficiency virus strains in human T-cell lines containing an HIV-regulated diphtheria toxin A chain gene. *Hum Gene Ther* 1993; **4**: 741–7.
204 Brady HJ, Miles CG, Pennington DJ, Dzierzak EA. Specific ablation of human immunodeficiency virus Tat-expressing cells by conditionally toxic retroviruses. *Proc Natl Acad Sci U S A* 1994; **91**: 365–9.
205 Caruso M. Gene therapy against cancer and HIV infection using the gene encoding herpes simplex virus thymidine kinase. *Mol Med Today* 1996; **2**: 212–7.
206 Smith SM, Markham RB, Jeang KT. Conditional reduction of human immunodeficiency virus type 1 replication by a gain-of-herpes simplex virus 1 thymidine kinase function. *Proc Natl Acad Sci U S A* 1996; **93**: 7955–60.
207 Dinges MM, Cook DR, King J, Curiel TJ, Zhang XQ, Harrison GS. HIV-regulated diphtheria toxin A chain gene confers long-term protection against HIV type 1 infection in the human promonocytic cell line U937. *Hum Gene Ther* 1995; **6**: 1437–45.
208 Caruso M, Klatzmann D. Selective killing of CD4+ cells harboring a human immunodeficiency virus-inducible suicide gene prevents viral spread in an infected cell population. *Proc Natl Acad Sci U S A* 1992; **89**: 182–6.
209 Schnell MJ, Johnson JE, Buonocore L, Rose JK. Construction of a novel virus that targets HIV-1-infected cells and controls HIV-1 infection. *Cell* 1997; **90**: 849–57.
210 Mebatson T, Finke S, Weiland F, Conzelmann KK. A CXCR4/CD4 pseudotype rhabdovirus that selectively infects HIV-1 envelope protein-expressing cells. *Cell* 1997; **90**: 841–7.
211 Chen JD, Bai X, Yang AG, Cong Y, Chen SY. Inactivation of HIV-1 chemokine co-receptor CXCR-4 by a novel intrakine strategy. *Nat Med* 1997; **3**: 1110–6.
212 Yang AG, Bai X, Huang XF, Yao C, Chen S. Phenotypic knockout of HIV type 1 chemokine coreceptor CCR-5 by intrakines as potential therapeutic approach for HIV-1 infection. *Proc Natl Acad Sci U S A* 1997; **94**: 11567–72.
213 Buonocore L, Rose JK. Blockade of human immunodeficiency virus type 1 production in CD4+ T cells by an intracellular CD4 expressed under control of the viral long terminal repeat. *Proc Natl Acad Sci U S A* 1993; **90**: 2695–9.
214 Bona R, d'Aloja P, Olivetta E et al. Aberrant, non-infectious HIV-1 particles are released by chronically infected human T cells transduced with a retroviral vector expressing an interfering HIV-1 variant. *Gene Ther* 1997; **4**: 1085–92.
215 Rappaport J, Arya SK, Richardson MW, Baier-Bitterlich G, Klotman PE. Inhibition of HIV-1 expression by HIV-2. *J Mol Med* 1995; **73**: 583–9.
216 Sanhadji K, Leissner P, Firouzi R et al. Experimental gene therapy: the transfer of Tat-inducible interferon genes protects human cells against HIV-1 challenge *in vitro* and *in vivo* in severe combined immunodeficient mice. *AIDS* 1997; **11**: 977–86.
217 Su L, Lee R, Bonyhadi M et al. Hematopoietic stem cell-based gene therapy for acquired

218. Walker RE. A phase I/II pilot study of the safety of the adoptive transfer of syngeneic gene-modified cytotoxic T lymphocytes in HIV-infected identical twins. *Hum Gene Ther* 1996; **7**: 367–400.
219. Riddell SR, Greenberg PD, Overell RW et al. Phase I study of cellular adoptive immunotherapy using genetically modified CD8+ HIV-specific T cells for HIV seropositive patients undergoing allogeneic bone marrow transplant. The Fred Hutchinson Cancer Research Center and the University of Washington School of Medicine, Department of Medicine, Division of Oncology. *Hum Gene Ther* 1992; **3**: 319–38.
220. Mitsuyasu RT, Anton PA, Deeks SG et al. Prolonged survival and tissue trafficking following adoptive transfer of CD4ζ gene-modified autologous CD4+ and CD8+ T cells in human immunodeficiency virus-infected subjects. *Blood* 2000; **96**: 785–93.
221. Levine BL, Bernstein W, Craighead N et al. Ex vivo replicative potential of adult human peripheral blood CD4+ T cells. *Transplant Proc* 1997; **29**: 2028.
222. Carroll RG, Riley JL, Levine BL et al. Differential regulation of HIV-1 fusion cofactor expression by CD28 costimulation of CD4+ T cells. *Science* 1997; **276**: 273–6.
223. Moritz T, Dutt P, Xiao X et al. Fibronectin improves transduction of reconstituting hematopoietic stem cells by retroviral vectors: evidence of direct viral binding to chymotryptic carboxy-terminal fragments. *Blood* 1996; **88**: 855–62.
224. Hanenberg H, Xiao XL, Dilloo D, Hashino K, Kato I, Williams DA. Colocalization of retrovirus and target cells on specific fibronectin fragments increases genetic transduction of mammalian cells. *Nat Med* 1996; **2**: 876–82.
225. Shah AJ, Smogorzewska EM, Hannum C, Crooks GM. Flt3 ligand induces proliferation of quiescent human bone marrow CD34+CD38– cells and maintains progenitor cells in vitro. *Blood* 1996; **87**: 3563–70.
226. Kiem HP, Andrews RG, Morris J et al. Improved gene transfer into baboon marrow repopulating cells using recombinant human fibronectin fragment CH-296 in combination with interleukin-6, stem cell factor, FLT-3 ligand, and megakaryocyte growth and development factor. *Blood* 1998; **92**: 1878–86.
227. Dao MA, Hannum CH, Kohn DB, Nolta JA. FLT3 ligand preserves the ability of human CD34+ progenitors to sustain long-term hematopoiesis in immune-deficient mice after ex vivo retroviral-mediated transduction. *Blood* 1997; **89**: 446–56.
228. McCune JM, Loftus R, Schmidt DK et al. High prevalence of thymic tissue in adults with human immunodeficiency virus-1 infection. *J Clin Invest* 1998; **101**: 2301–8.
229. Cavazzana-Calvo M, Hacein-Bey S, de Saint Basile G et al. Gene therapy of human severe combined immunodeficiency (SCID) -X1 disease. *Science* 2000; **288**: 669–72.
230. Aiuti A, Vai S, Mortellaro A et al. Immune reconstitution in ADA-SCID after PBL gene therapy and discontinuation of enzyme replacement. *Nat Med* 2002; **8**: 423–5.
231. Check E. Gene therapy: shining hopes dented—but not dashed. *Nature* 2002; **420**: 735.
232. Ziegner UH, Peters G, Jolly DJ et al. Cytotoxic T-lymphocyte induction in asymptomatic HIV-1-infected patients immunized with Retrovector-transduced autologous fibroblasts expressing HIV-1IIIB Env/Rev proteins. *AIDS* 1995; **9**: 43–50.
233. Song ES, Lee V, Surh CD et al. Antigen presentation in retroviral vector-mediated gene transfer in vivo. *Proc Natl Acad Sci U S A* 1997; **94**: 1943–8.
234. Wolff JA, Malone RW, Williams P et al. Direct gene transfer into mouse muscle in vivo. *Science* 1990; **247**: 1465–8.
235. Wang B, Ugen KE, Srikantan V et al. Gene inoculation generates immune responses against human immunodeficiency virus type 1. *Proc Natl Acad Sci U S A* 1993; **90**: 4156–60.
236. Calarota S, Bratt G, Nordlund S et al. Cellular cytotoxic response induced by DNA vaccination in HIV-1-infected patients. *Lancet* 1998; **351**: 1320–5.
237. Boyer JD, Cohen AD, Vogt S et al. Vaccination of seronegative volunteers with a human immunodeficiency virus type 1 env/rev DNA vaccine induces antigen-specific proliferation and lymphocyte production of beta-chemokines. *J Infect Dis* 2000; **181**: 476–83.
238. MacGregor RR, Ginsberg R, Ugen KE et al. T-cell responses induced in normal volunteers immunized with a DNA-based vaccine containing HIV-1 env and rev. *AIDS* 2002; **16**: 2137–43.
239. Lundholm P, Leandersson AC, Christensson B, Bratt G, Sandstrom E, Wahren B. DNA mucosal HIV vaccine in humans. *Virus Res* 2002; **82**: 141–5.
240. Ugen KE, Boyer JD, Wang B et al. Nucleic acid immunization of chimpanzees as a prophylactic/immunotherapeutic vaccination model for HIV-1: prelude to a clinical trial. *Vaccine* 1997; **15**: 927–30.
241. Boyer JD, Ugen KE, Wang B et al. Protection of chimpanzees from high-dose heterologous HIV-1 challenge by DNA vaccination. *Nat Med* 1997; **3**: 526–32.
242. Boyer JD, Wang B, Ugen KE et al. In vivo protective anti-HIV immune responses in non-human primates through DNA immunization. *J Med Primatol* 1996; **25**: 242–50.
243. Shiver JW, Fu TM, Chen L et al. Replication-incompetent adenoviral vaccine vector elicits effective anti-immunodeficiency-virus immunity. *Nature* 2002; **415**: 331–5.
244. Caputo A, Rossi C, Bozzini R et al. Studies on the effect of the combined expression of anti-tat and anti-rev genes on HIV-1 replication. *Gene Ther* 1997; **4**: 288–95.
245. Levin R, Mhashilkar AM, Dorfman T et al. Inhibition of early and late events of the HIV-1 replication cycle by cytoplasmic Fab intrabodies against the matrix protein, p17. *Mol Med* 1997; **3**: 96–110.
246. Rondon IJ, Marasco WA. Intracellular antibodies (intrabodies) for gene therapy of infectious diseases. *Annu Rev Microbiol* 1997; **51**: 257–83.
247. Chang HK, Gendelman R, Lisziewicz J, Gallo RC, Ensoli B. Block of HIV-1 infection by a combination of antisense tat RNA and TAR decoys: a strategy for control of HIV-1. *Gene Ther* 1994; **1**: 208–16.
248. Kim JH, McLinden RJ, Mosca JD, Vahey MT, Greene WC, Redfield RR. Inhibition of HIV replication by sense and antisense rev response elements in HIV-based retroviral vectors. *J Acquir Immune Defic Syndr Hum Retrovirol* 1996; **12**: 343–51.
249. Lori F, Lisziewicz J, Smythe J et al. Rapid protection against human immunodeficiency virus type 1 (HIV-1) replication mediated by high efficiency non-retroviral delivery of genes interfering with HIV-1 tat and gag. *Gene Ther* 1994; **1**: 27–31.
250. Bahner I, Kearns K, Hao QL, Smogorzewska EM, Kohn DB. Transduction of human CD34+ hematopoietic progenitor cells by a retroviral vector expressing an RRE decoy inhibits human immunodeficiency virus type 1 replication in myelomonocytic cells produced in long-term culture. *J Virol* 1996; **70**: 4352–60.
251. Hamouda T, McPhee R, Hsia SC, Read GS, Holland TC, King SR. Inhibition of human immunodeficiency virus replication by the herpes simplex virus virion host shutoff protein. *J Virol* 1997; **71**: 5521–7.

101 Alan Tyndall & Alois Gratwohl

Hematopoietic Stem Cell Transplantation for Autoimmune Diseases

Autoimmune diseases (ADs) in humans represent a heterogeneous group of disorders with genetic and environmental etiologic factors. Their management involves many different subspecialties of medicine; however, there are some common themes linking ADs, one of which is the use of immunosuppression and or immune modulation strategies in their treatment. Glucocorticosteroids and immunosuppressive agents are generally employed with success. None the less, there are patients who either do not respond or require more toxic drugs to achieve or maintain clinical remission, and this subgroup poses a serious treatment dilemma.

The combination of improving hematopoietic cell transplantation (HCT) techniques, the observation in some patients receiving HCT for conventional indications that a coexisting AD also improved and animal model data suggested that HCT could be a viable option for this difficult minority of patients. This concept has led to an international collaboration and currently, worldwide, around 600 patients have received HCT as treatment of AD. This chapter summarizes the theoretical and practical background of such a treatment strategy, the results of phase 1 and 2 studies so far and how this experience has been exploited in designing the current phase 3 randomized comparative trials and ongoing science programs such as immune reconstitution.

The program of HCT in the treatment of severe AD has been evolving over the past 7 years with the first consensus statement being published in April 1995 [1] and first case report in October 1996 [2]. Since then several important events have occurred that have impacted on but not yet significantly altered the fundamental concept. These events include the increasing use of agents that modify the biologic response, e.g. antitumor necrosis factor alfa (TNF-α) in the treatment of rheumatoid arthritis (RA), the better understanding of the mechanisms of autoimmunity, especially the recognition of the role of the innate immune system, and more precise early prognostic factors in AD. In addition, with the introduction of nonmyeloablative hematopoietic stem cell transplantation (HSCT) techniques, allogeneic transplantations are being discussed as an investigational therapy for ADs. Results of the autologous HSCT programs have suggested that in favorable outcomes, adjusting an imbalance of an autoaggressive immune system may be occurring, rather than a total ablation of autoimmune inducing cells.

Autoimmune disease mechanism

Despite the heterogeneous clinical expression of AD in humans, it seems clear that most ADs share several or all of the following features. They are polyclonal, rarely with a defined inciting single antigenic epitope. By the time of clinical disease expression, there has been extensive epitope spreading and effector cell recruitment [3] and the innate immune system and tissue environment probably have a vital role in determining whether an antigen will evoke an immune reaction or anergy and/or tolerance response [4]. In addition, a genetic component is present but not sufficient and although this factor is mostly encoded within the major histocompatibility complex (MHC), multiple other genes on different chromosomes also have a role. In insulin dependent diabetes mellitus for example, at least 19 such regions are proposed [5].

Disease initiation and perpetuation probably involves activation and disturbance of specific subsets of regulatory T cells. The recent reevaluation of a subset of $CD4^+$ $CD25^+$ T cells that have suppressor activity supports this concept of dysregulation, rather than "all or nothing" events, as in malignant clonal disease [6]. Clinical expression of AD is often dependent on a mixture of inflammatory and scarring processes and when assessing the outcome of AD, a distinction between activity and damage is critical; validated activity and damage indices exist for the major ADs.

An infectious agent, including endogenous retroviruses, may trigger AD in genetically predisposed individuals at specific immunologically vulnerable periods, e.g. with changing hormonal status or during intercurrent infection. In particular, MHC complexes are both upregulated (and therefore more numerous) and have a longer half-life during infectious episodes, increasing the chance of an autoaggressive reaction trigger [7,8]. In this general model of AD, one could propose that a genetically predisposed individual experiences an event that initiates the first step toward disease. This could be damage and alteration of a self-structure, such as the effect of gliadin on the gut mucosa in celiac disease or mimicking of a self-antigen such as the heart in streptococcal-induced rheumatic fever. This initial event exposes normally hidden (cryptic) self-antigens that are then processed by antigen-presenting cells (APCs) and forwarded to the immune response system [9]. This antigen processing and presentation is controlled by proteins encoded close to the MHC complex genes, accounting in part for the genetic link with autoimmune disease. An example is the fibroblast-derived extracellular matrix protein called celiac disease autoantigen protein (Fb-CDAP) to which antireticulin and endomysial antibodies are directed in this disease. T-cell reactions to this protein are strictly regulated by the alleles *DQA1*0501* and *DQB1*0201* [10].

Presentation of self-antigens probably occurs continuously, but under normal circumstances produces either apoptosis, anergy or tolerance if presented without costimulatory molecules such as by nonprofessional APCs lacking B7-1 and B7-2 (CD80 and CD86) [11]. However, in a particular situation, such as concurrent infection, there may be upregulation of accessory molecules or increased antigen processing and MHC complex production and loading, which leads to an adequate signal to positively stimulate T cells. Alternatively, a superantigen, such as endogenous retrovirus, may be the trigger required to activate a naive autoreactive T cell, enabling it to travel from the lymph node and react in the target tissue, e.g. the islet cell of the pancreas [12]. Which T cells are needed for this autoaggressive reaction? It is known that autoreactive T cells escape thymic deletion and remain in the periphery, but with low affinity. Under the circumstances described above, these lymphocytes may be activated and induce an autoimmune process. This reaction is probably controlled by regulatory T-cell subsets, especially early in the process. Breakdown of this regulatory network over time allows clinical expression and the development of chronic AD. Reversal of this vicious circle and reinstitution of the normal regulatory network but not eradication of the last single autoreactive cell is one of the postulated mechanisms behind the concept of HCT as a therapy of AD.

The complex network nature of AD pathophysiology is reflected in the failure to obtain a cure with specific targeted therapies. Anti-CD4 monoclonal antibodies in rheumatoid arthritis were not of lasting benefit [13] and the panlymphocyte monoclonal antibody, Campath 1-H, had only a modest effect in multiple sclerosis (MS) [14]. Indeed, one-third of these Campath 1-H treated MS patients developed new autoimmune thyroid disease following the treatment, suggesting a disturbance of regulatory T cells through the treatment. Such organ-specific new AD has also been observed following autologous and allogeneic HCT in other conditions. It may in part represent passive transfer, or be caused by perturbation of regulatory networks. These organ-specific ADs tend to stabilize over time. Diffuse nonorgan-specific definite ADs such as RA or systemic lupus erythematosus (SLE) has not been described, hints for disturbed late immune function have been seen and simply more time might be required for clear assessment [15]. All these observations suggest that the beneficial and lasting effects of HCT in AD treatment could result from its impact on a broad spectrum of potential targets, including elements of the innate immune system, which targeted therapies would not affect [16].

Coincidental AD in patients receiving HCT for another indication

A number of case reports have been published over the past 20 years describing patients receiving HCT for a conventional indication (e.g. aplastic anemia or malignancy) in which a coincidental AD improved or even fully remitted, initial reports being with allogeneic HCT (Table 101.1). Many of these patients have remained free of both diseases: the hematologic and the autoimmune disease. In some patients relapse occurred, and in one such patient relapse with donor-type lymphocytes was observed [26]. More recent reports have included response following autologous HCT, emphasizing the fact that genetic predisposition alone is not sufficient for AD expression (Table 101.2) [3].

There are also case reports of transfer of AD through allogeneic HCT, including myasthenia gravis, thyroid disease, insulin dependent diabetes mellitus, celiac disease and psoriasis with arthritis [35]. In one patient, production of autoantibodies (anti Clq) but not clinical disease occurred in a recipient following HSCT from a donor with known SLE, but clinical disease did not develop [36].

In interpreting these case reports it is important to remember that there is selection bias, not all cases have been published and details of AD severity or extent are often lacking, all making it difficult to determine the clinical relevance of the outcome. It is difficult to separate the benefit derived from the HCT itself and the immunosuppression obtained from the preparative regimens and/or graft-vs.-host disease (GVHD) prophylaxis. In addition, it should be stated that the presence of an AD in a suitable donor is not an absolute contraindication, because the AD does not automatically develop in the recipient, and a risk–benefit analysis should be made of the AD vs. the target disease. There is sufficient evidence in these reports to assume some modification of the AD process following HSCT, justifying further clinical trials.

Table 101.1 Coincidental autoimmune disease (AD) and allogeneic hematopoietic cell transplantation (HCT).

Disease for which transplant performed	AD present	Outcome of AD	Patient outcome	Reference
SAA	RA	Remission	Died	[17]
SAA	RA	Remission	Died	[17]
SAA	RA	Remission	Died	[17]
SAA	RA	Remission	Well	[17]
SAA	RA	Partial remission	Well	[18]
SAA	RA	Remission	Well	[19]
SAA	RA	Remission	Well	[19]
AML	Psoriasis	Remission	Well	[20]
CML	Psoriasis	Remission	Well	[21]
AML	Ulcerative colitis	Remission	Well	[21]
ALL	Autoimmune hepatitis	Remission	Well	[22]
CML	Multiple sclerosis	Remission	Well	[23]
Various	Hyperthyroidism	No recurrence	Alive	[24]
	IDDM	No recurrence		
	SLE, RA	No recurrence		
	Crohn's disease	No recurrence		
	Vasculitis	No recurrence		
	Dermatitis herpetiformis	No recurrence		
MALT lymphoma	Sjögren's syndrome	No effect	Alive	[25]

ALL, acute lymphoblastic leukemia; AML, acute myeloid leukemia; CML, chronic myeloid leukemia; IDDM, insulin dependent diabetes mellitus; MALT, mucosa associated lymphoid tissue; RA, rheumatoid arthritis; SAA, severe aplastic anemia; SLE, systemic lupus erythematosus.

Table 101.2 Coincidental autoimmune disease (AD) and autologous hematopoietic stem cell (HSC) transplantation.

Disease for which transplant performed	AD present	Outcome of AD	Patient outcome	Reference
NHL	NHL	Remission	Well	[27]
Ovarian cancer	Ovarian cancer	Relapse	Alive	[28]
NHL	NHL	Relapse	Died	[28]
NHL	NHL	Relapse	Alive	[28]
NHL	NHL	Relapse	Alive	[28]
NHL	NHL	Remission	Alive	[29]
CML	CML	Remission	Alive	[30]
NHL	NHL	Remission	Alive	[31]
NHL	NHL	Relapse	Alive	[32]
NHL	NHL	Relapse	Alive	[32]
AML	AML	Relapse	Alive	[32]
Plasma cell leukemia	Plasma cell leukemia	Relapse	Alive	[32]
NHL	NHL	Remission	Alive	[33]
Hodgkin's	Hodgkin's	Remission	Alive	[34]

AML, acute myeloid leukemia; CML, chronic myeloid leukemia; NHL, non-Hodgkin's lymphoma.

Animal models

Support for the concept of HSCT in the treatment of AD is found in animal models. Since the original observation by Denman *et al.* [37] in 1969 that SLE could be transfered from a susceptiple to a nonsusceptible strain through allogeneic bone marrow transplantation and later Morton *et al.* [38], many proof of concept observations have been published. This has recently been extensively reviewed [39,40]. In interpreting these data it is important to distinguish models in which AD is genetically and inevitably programmed, e.g. the MLR/lpr mouse and those in which a genetic component plus a trigger are required, e.g. the buffalo rat and adjuvant arthritis. The latter is more similar to human AD, as reflected in concordance rates between identical twins, i.e. 6–14% in ulcerative colitis, 15% in SLE, 18% in RA and 25% in MS and around 50% in Crohn's disease and insulin dependent diabetes mellitus. In addition, it is important to distinguish between HCT performed to prevent AD occurring, or HCT to treat established AD.

Most models show that as with human AD, the autoimmune process has been active at a cellular level often long before the clinical features become manifest. These data have been summarized by van Bekkum [41] whose work in adjuvant arthritis and later experimental allergic encephalomyelitis demonstrated that not just allogeneic but also autologous HCT could treat, cure and prevent AD [42]. In addition a significant peripheral immunologic tolerance was induced, especially in the arthritis model. It is hoped such immunomodulation will also occur in humans, and that HCT will induce more than just profound immunosuppression. It should be noted that in none of these models has a specific autoimmune cell clone been demonstrated.

Treatment of human autoimmune disease with HCT

Currently, around 600 patients worldwide have received an HCT as treatment of an AD alone, 468 of whom are registered in the European Group for Blood and Marrow Transplantation (EBMT) and the European League Against Rheumatism (EULAR) database (Table 101.3). The majority of patients have had either MS or systemic sclerosis (SSc), also called scleroderma. This observation reflects the fact that there is no effective alternative option in these disorders. However, as experience grew, other ADs were transplanted, mostly in the context of combined phase 1 and 2 trials and following the consensus guidelines developed at international meetings early in the program [43,44].

Table 101.3 European Group for Blood and Marrow Transplant (EBMT) and European League Against Rheumatism (EULAR) autoimmune disease autologous hematopoietic cell transplantation (HCT) database. Status at August 2002.

Disease and disease category	n
Neurologic disorders	
Multiple sclerosis	135
Myasthenia gravis	2
Polyneuropathy	2
Amyotrophic lateral sclerosis	2
Rheumatologic disorders	
Systemic sclerosis	72
Rheumatoid arthritis	72
Juvenile idiopathic arthritis	51
Systemic lupus erythematosus	55
Dermatomyositis	7
Mixed connective tissue disease	4
Morbus Behçet	3
Psoriatic arthritis	2
Ankylosing spondylitis	2
Sjögren's syndrome	1
Vasculitides	
Wegener's granulomatosis	3
Cryoglobulinemia	4
Not classified	2
Hematologic immunocytopenias	
Immune thrombopenia	12
Pure red cell aplasia	4
Autoimmune hemolytic anemia	4
Thrombotic thrombocytopenic anemia	3
Evans' syndrome	2
Gastrointestinal	
Enteropathy	2
Inflammatory bowel disease	1
Other	6
Total	453

Table 101.4 Conditioning regimens used with HCT in autoimmune diseases.

Conditioning regimen	n
Cyclophosphamide	115
Cyclophosphamide ± ATG ± other drugs	110
Cyclophosphamide + radiation ± other drugs or ATG	43
Busulfan ± cyclophosphamide ± ATG ± other drugs	25
BEAM ± ATG	80
Other/missing	66
Total	439

ATG, antithymocyte globulin; BEAM, BCNU, etoposide, cytosine arabinoside and melphalan; TBI, total body irradiation (includes some patients with total lymphoid irradiation).

The quintessence of these guidelines was as follows.
1 *HCT regimens*. A limited number of protocols only should be employed (Table 101.4). This was mostly followed, and allowed some comparison of intensity vs. toxicity/benefit to be drawn (see section on Outcome below).
2 *Patient selection*. Patients should have had failed conventional therapy and have a poor prognosis concerning life or vital organ function. There should be enough reversible or maintainable vital organ function to ensure a decent quality of life if the immunologic and/or inflammatory process were arrested or reversed.
3 *The patient should have sufficient capacity to withstand the HCT procedure*. As the program proceeded, certain clinical parameters and treatment-related factors emerged as being associated with unacceptable risk, such as a mean pulmonary artery pressure >50 mmHg in SSc, high disability scores in MS and total body irradiation (TBI) without lung shielding in SSc. This experience was then exploited in the design of the phase 3 randomized studies.

In the EBMT/EULAR database, the most commonly transplanted diseases are MS, SSc, RA, juvenile idiopathic arthritis (JIA) and SLE, the data coming from over 100 transplant centers in more than 20 countries. There were long-lasting responses in all disease categories, but they were achieved at a price, the overall actuarially adjusted transplant-related mortality (TRM) being 7% [45]. This mortality rate was higher than the predicted 3% for autologous HCT overall and reflects the baseline morbidity and multiorgan involvement of many AD patients compared with breast cancer patients undergoing high-dose chemotherapy and HSCT, for example. There is a marked difference between AD groups with a TRM of 12.5% in SSc and only one patient with RA. There are also different rates and types of response. In RA, JIA and SLE more patients responded early but later relapsed than for MS and SSc.

Mobilization was in some cases associated with complications such as granulocyte colony-stimulating factor (G-CSF) induced disease flare, resulting in death in one case [46], or organ toxicity, infection and death from cyclophosphamide (CY) [47]. Many patients improved significantly after the mobilizing dose of cyclophosphamide that, combined with G-CSF, was considered the optimal regimen. In some patients, failure to mobilize enough CD34 cells was later successfully followed by either a second peripheral mobilization or a bone marrow harvest.

Multiple sclerosis

MS takes several clinical forms, the most common being relapsing and/or remitting, in which the functional state of the patient recovers between attacks. This may become a progressive disease over time, with no periods of recovery, and it is then called secondary progressive MS. Less frequently, the disease course may be slow and progressive from the onset, known as primary progressive, thought to be possibly more a degenerative disease. There is no effective therapy for either of the progressive forms.

The severity of MS is measured commonly by a composite functional scale, the Kurtzke Expanded Disability Status Scale (EDSS; Table 101.5). Such an assessment requires an experienced examiner, usually a neurologist, and grades impairment in different functional systems, with 0 being no impairment and 10 being death from MS. As a rough guide, an EDSS of ≤2.5 implies minimal impairment, ≥6.5 meaning constant bilateral walking aids and 8 being bed- and wheelchair-bound.

Table 101.5 Kurtzke Expanded Disability Status Scale (EDSS) for multiple sclerosis (simplified—a correct assessment in multiple domains requires a training in neurologic examination and experience with the EDSS).

0.0	Normal neurologic examination. All grades and functional systems (FS)
1.0	No disability, minimal signs in FS (e.g. grade 1)
1.5	No disability, minimal signs in >1 FS
2.0	Minimal disability in one FS (one FS grade 2, other 0 or 1)
1.5	Minimal disability in two FS (two FS grade 2, others 0 or 1)
3.0	Moderate disability in one FS, moderate disability in 3 or 4 FS, fully ambulant
3.5	Fully ambulant but one FS grade 3 plus others significant grades
4.0	Fully ambulant 500 m and independent, up to 12 h a day, no aids, several severe FS grades
4.5	Ambulant 300 m without aids, works a full day, some dependence in some FS
5.0	Ambulant 200 m without aids, difficulty to work full day, FS grades 5
5.5	Ambulant 100 m without aids, unable to work a full day
6.0	Intermittent or unilateral walking aid for 100 m
6.5	Constant bilateral walking aids for 20 m
7.0	Wheelchair-bound (<5 m assisted). Able to transfer and use wheelchair alone. Sometimes severe pyramidal grade 5
7.5	Few steps, unable to use nonmotorized wheelchair alone, unable to transfer
8.0	Bed- and chair-bound, self-care functions retained (arm function retained), sitting out of bed most of the day
8.5	Bedridden, some self-care arm function retained
9.0	Totally bedridden, can communicate and eat
9.5	Totally dependent, unable to communicate or eat
10	Death from multiple sclerosis

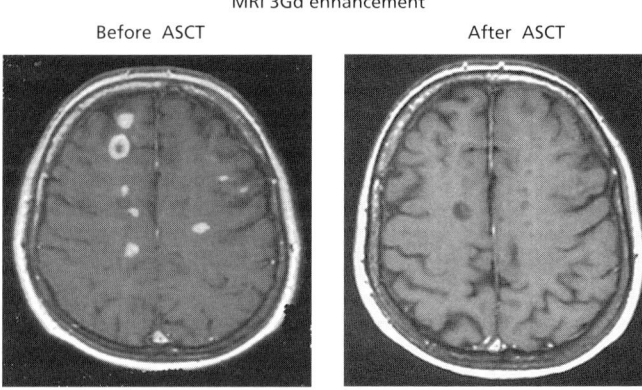

Fig. 101.1 Pre- and post-transplant magnetic resonance imaging (MRI) in multiple sclerosis. The pretransplant MRI shows marked contrast medium enhancement in several lesions, indicating active inflammatory disease. Posttransplant there is vastly reduced inflammation, but a left periventricular area of opacity, a "black hole" indicating a degree of neuronal degereneration. (With permission from [49].)

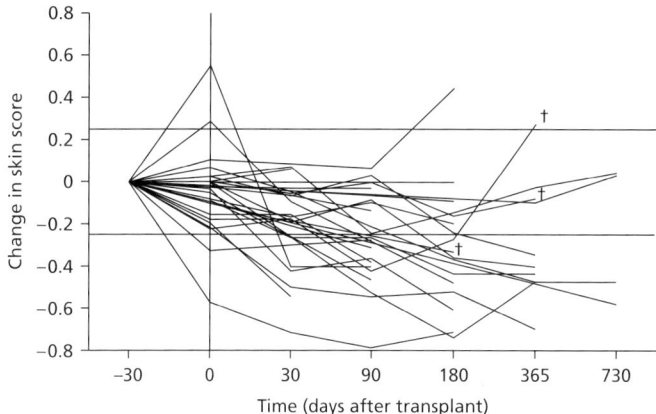

Fig. 101.2 Percentage change in skin scores in systemic sclerosis (SSc) after autologous hematopoietic stem cell transplantation (HSCT). Percentage changes in skin scores, measured by the modified Rodnan method, were compared with pretransplant levels at set time points. Note improvement occurring after mobilization in some. (Reproduced from [50] with kind permission from the BMJ Publishing Group.)

An analysis of the first 85 autografted MS patients showed a 3-year progression-free survival of 78% of the secondary progressive cases, which is better than the available agent interferon beta with 60%. There was a risk of death from any cause at 3 years of 10% (± 7%; 95%CI) [48]. The median follow-up was 16 months (range 3–59 months). Fewer positive responses were seen in primary progressive MS (66% ± 23%). Impact was more marked on the inflammatory process, as illustrated by the magnetic resonance imaging (MRI) changes (Fig. 101.1), considered a surrogate marker of MS. In a 10-patient subgroup analysis from one center, the gadolinium enhancing MRI lesions reduced from a median number of seven lesions (range 1–38 lesions) to zero after a median 15 months' (range 4–30 months) follow-up [49]. However, more long-term follow-up is required in this chronic disease, given that following arrest of inflammation, neuronal degeneration may well continue with accompanying functional deterioration.

The majority of MS cases received a peripheral stem cell transplantation, being mobilized with CY (mostly 4 g/m^2) and G-CSF. There was a suggestion that G-CSF alone could induce a flare of the MS [46], being less when combined with CY. Conditioning was mostly with carmustine, etoposide, cytosine arabinoside and melphalan (BEAM) alone (16%) or BEAM plus antithymocyte globulin (ATG; 47%). Other regimens included CY plus TBI and busulfan/CY. In a retrospective comparison, no advantage of T-cell purging was observed.

Systemic sclerosis

SSc is a multiorgan AD with immunologic, vascular and collagen overproduction components. There are two major forms: diffuse skin SSc (skin involvement proximal to the elbows and knees) associated with interstitial lung disease, systemic hypertension and positive Scl70 (antitopoisomerase I) antibodies; limited skin SSc, previously called the CREST syndrome after the major involved organs (calcinosis, Raynaud's, esophagus, sclerodactyly, telangiectasis), is associated more with pulmonary hypertension and the anticentromere antibody (ACA). There may be overlapping features, and treatment is directed toward the specific clinical problem that is most disturbing, e.g. Raynaud's phenomenon or reflux esophagitis. There is no known treatment that alters the basic disease process.

In the first 45 patients, an improvement of ≥25% in the skin score (measured by the modified Rodnan method) was seen in 70% of patients (Fig. 101.2) with a TRM of 17% [50]. Several protocols were used, mostly either CY-based conditioning (4 g/m^2 CY mobilization and 200 mg/kg body weight CY) or radiation 8 Gy and 120 mg/kg body weight CY. With further patient recruitment, TRM fell to 12.5%, considered to be related to more careful patient selection. Lung function tended to stabilize and some factors were identified as potentially hazardous for HCT, e.g. pulmonary hypertension >50 mmHg mean pulmonary arterial pressure, severe cardiac involvement, severe pulmonary fibrosis and uncontrolled systemic hypertension. When such patients were excluded from the analysis, the TRM was 7%, considered acceptable given the predicted 50% 5-year mortality of this subgroup. A long-term follow-up evaluation of this cohort showed no further transplant-related deaths and trend to durable remissions (EBMT database).

A multicenter US study of 19 SSc patients utilizing a regimen of 120 mg/kg CY, 8 Gy TBI, 90 mg/kg body weight equine ATG and a CD34 selected graft showed a sustained benefit in 12 patients at median follow-up of 14.7 months [51]. Four patients died, three from treatment-related causes and one from disease progression. In two cases, a fatal regimen-related pulmonary toxicity occurred, which was not seen in the subsequent 11 cases in whom lung shielding was employed. Twelve patients had a sustained and significant improvement of skin score and functional status to a degree not previously seen with other treatment modalities. A randomized controlled trial is being planned.

Rheumatoid arthritis

Of the 63 patients with RA transplanted, an analysis of the first 51 showed significant improvement, with 78% achieving an ACR 50 response (EBMT and IBMTR database; unpublished data). The ACR 50 is a composite score of clinical (e.g. tender joint count) and laboratory (e.g. erythrocyte sedimentation rate) parameters that should improve by at least 50%. Most of the patients had failed at least three conventional disease-modifying antirheumatic drugs (DMARDs), such as methotrexate or sulfasalazine, before the transplant. Some degree of relapse was seen in 73% of patients post-transplant, but was in most cases relatively easy to control with drugs that had proven ineffective pretransplant. The median follow-up was 18 months (range 6–40 months) and the majority of patients received a conditioning regimen of 200 mg/m^2 CY alone and received peripherally harvested stem cells after either G-CSF or CY/G-CSF (equal numbers) mobilization. A multicenter trial in Australia failed to show any advantage of T-cell depletion using CD34 selection of the graft [50].

Juvenile idiopathic arthritis

A total of 51 children with JIA, mostly the systemic form called Still's disease, have been registered. Most of these cases were treated in two Dutch centers using bone marrow and a conditioning protocol of 200 mg/kg body weight CY, 4 Gy TBI and ATG [52; N. Wulffraat, personal communication].

In the whole group there were 15 complete remissions and three partial remissions reported. In those attaining remission, the corticosteroid dose could be reduced and some patients experienced puberty and catch-up growth. Three patients died from macrophage activation syndrome, also known as the hemophagocytic syndrome, thought to be related to intercurrent infection or uncontrolled systemic activity of the disease at the time of transplantation. Protocols were modified accordingly such that systemic activity was controlled with methylprednisolone intravenously before transplantation. Since this change, no further acute deaths have occurred.

Systemic lupus erythematosus

Of the 55 registrations in the EBMT/EULAR database, most had either renal and/or central nervous system (CNS) involvement, and 21 had failed conventional CY treatment. A peripheral stem cell source after mobilization with CY and G-CSF was used for the majority of patients. Twenty-three patients received conditioning with CY and ATG, 11 received CY plus TBI and four other regimens were employed. An unselected graft was used in 29, with CD34 selection in 19. There were five procedure-related deaths and one from progressive disease, resulting in an actuarially adjusted TRM of 10% (range 2–20%). In those patients with sufficient data for analysis, 72% achieved a "remission", defined as a SLE disease activity index (SLEDAI) of ≤3 and steroid reduction to <10 mg/day. Of those achieving remission, 32% relapsed to some degree and were in most cases easily controlled by standard agents that had previously been ineffective.

Traynor et al. [53] reported on nine patients with severe SLE, who were mobilized in a transplant protocol. One died as a result of infection following mobilization and another patient died 3 months later from active lupus of the CNS, having not proceeded to transplant. The seven remaining were free of signs of active lupus at a median follow-up of 25 months post-transplant. The high-dose chemotherapy consisted of 200 mg/kg CY, 1 g methylprednisolone and 90 mg/kg equine ATG. Eligible patients had World Health Organization (WHO) class III–IV glomerulonephritis, or lupus cerebritis or transverse myelitis, or lupus vasculitis involving the heart or lung parenchyma—all unresponsive to at least six cycles of intravenous CY; or lupus-associated life-threatening severe cytopenias unresponsive to standard-dose CY; or catastrophic antiphospholipid syndrome. Of the seven patients, two were referred because of progressive lung disease and hypoxia at rest, but were not ventilator-dependent. One patient with alveolar hemorrhage was oxygen-dependent and required intermittent ventilator support. Four had WHO class III–IV glomerulonephritis and nephrotic syndrome. Five had a creatine clearance below the normal range. All had uncontrolled hypertension requiring four antihypertensive agents, two had myocardial hypokinesis and two had seizures immediately pretransplant.

Refractory autoimmune cytopenia

Refractory cytopenias represent a highly heterogeneous group. The mechanisms appear to be more clearly defined with putative antibodies directed against epitopes on one or more hematopoietic cell lines. Complete responses were published very early in a few patients with idiopathic thrombocytopenic purpura (ITP) and followed soon by failures. A total of nine patients are included in the database, two of whom attained complete remissions. The largest series of 14 patients with ITP is from the National Institutes of Health (NIH) [54]. All had severe refractory ITP not responding to at least three treatment regimens and all had undergone splenectomy. Eight showed a clear hematologic response and six a sustained complete remission beyond 2 years. None died of transplant-related complications. Conditioning was with CY and all received a CD34 selected graft.

The other patients with cytopenias were heterogeneous: pure red cell aplasia (PRCA; $n = 4$), autoimmune hemolytic anemia ($n = 2$) and Evans' syndrome ($n = 1$). Median age was 31 years (range 4–45 years) and median time to transplantation was 93 months (range 12–236 months). Most received peripheral blood graft mobilized with either growth factors ($n = 7$) or CY plus growth factors ($n = 6$). Two patients received bone marrow grafts. Conditioning regimens included CY alone ($n = 3$), CY with other drugs or ATG ($n = 9$), melphalan ($n = 2$) or were fludarabine-based ($n = 2$). Twelve grafts were T-cell depleted. Median follow-up of surviving patients was 30 months (range 5–53 months). Three patients died within 100 days after transplantation, two of hemorrhage and one from progressive hemolysis. Six patients showed a response to treatment and two obtained complete remissions (one from Evans' and one from PRCA).

The numbers of cases with vasculitis, Behçet's disease, relapsing polychondritis and other ADs are too small to draw meaningful conclusions, with further phase 1 and 2 standardized protocol pilot studies proceeding.

Prospective randomized controlled clinical trials

There is now sufficient information from phase 1–2 trials that HCT can induce lasting remissions in patients with severe autoimmune disorders. Remissions can be obtained with a variety of conditioning regimens and with grafts from bone marrow or peripheral blood using technologies that are used in HCT for other disease categories. However, there is considerable morbidity and mortality of the same type and extent as observed in HCT for advanced malignancies. There is not more than level 3 evidence about the usefulness of this approach and there are no studies so far to prove superiority above conventional approaches. It is therefore the primary international target to conduct appropriate prospective randomized studies, while still continuing to collect observational data and to continue phase 1–2 trials in those disease categories in which there are fewer patients and data.

Criteria for moving to phase 3 randomized controlled trials are the following:

1 enough information is available from phase 1–2 trials;
2 inherent mortality of the disease justifies the risk of the procedure;
3 prognostic factors of the disease are known to define patients at high risk for disease progression;
4 HCT morbidity and mortality is acceptably low;
5 risk of disease progression after HSCT is low; and
6 little or no alternative conventional therapy is available.

An international consensus meeting concluded that such criteria are currently sufficiently met for SSc, MS and RA.

Autologous Stem Cell Transplantation International Scleroderma Trial (ASTIS)

Diffuse skin SSc (scleroderma) patients are selected who have <4 years of diffuse skin involvement and evidence of progressive organ involvement or life-threatening disease. The primary endpoint on which the trial is powered is event-free survival at 2 years, events being arbitrarily but precisely defined to capture irreversible and severe end organ failure or death. Exclusion criteria are based on the phase 1 and 2 data to avoid an unacceptably high TRM risk together with a minimal chance of clinically significant improvement.

The treatment arm is mobilization with 4 g/m^2 CY and G-CSF, followed by 200 mg/kg body weight CY conditioning plus ATG and a CD34 selected graft. The control arm is monthly intravenous pulse 750 mg/m^2 CY for 12 months. Each arm is expected to accrue 100 patients.

The ASTIS trial is active, and further details are available on the website: http://www.astistrial.com. So far there has been no transplant-related death.

A similar study is being planned by a US consortium, using as treatment arm 120 mg/kg CY, 90 mg/kg equine ATG and 8 Gy TBI with lung shielding (P. McSweeney, personal communication).

Autologous Stem Cell Transplantation International Multiple Sclerosis Trial (ASTIMS)

Secondary progressive MS patients with an EDSS score between 3.5 and 6.5 will be randomized to either HCT (BEAM and ATG followed by an unmanipulated graft reconstitution) or the control arm of mitoxantrone. The primary endpoint is progression-free survival at 3 years, and it is planned that each arm recruits 80 patients. Further details are available on the EBMT website: www.ebmt.org.

Autologous Stem Cell Transplantation International Rheumatoid Arthritis Trial (ASTIRA)

Active RA patients who have failed at least four DMARDs including methotrexate and anti-TNF-α programs with a disease duration between 2 and 15 years will all receive hematopoietic cell mobilization with 4 g/m^2 CY and G-CSF. Randomization will then occur to either continued conventional therapy with either methotrexate or leflunomide or conditioning with 200 mg/m^2 CY and ATG. The graft will not be manipulated, and maintenance therapy with methotrexate or leflunomide will be given. The primary endpoint is the number of patients reaching a good or moderate EULAR response and/or ACR 20 at 6 months. Sixteen patients in each arm are required, calculated on a >50% difference in the two groups and the trial is activated. Further details are available from the EBMT website: www.ebmt.org.

In SLE, a phase 2 study is being planned to assess the role, if any, of post-transplant maintenance (e.g. mycophenolate mofetil) therapy to retain remission.

The results of phase 1–2 trials in JIA using CY alone vs. CY and TBI suggested no advantage of the TBI (N. Wulffraat, personal communication). Further phase studies will be performed to assess the optimal regimen for a phase 3 study.

Open issues

Allogeneic hematopoietic stem cell transplantation

The international guidelines stipulated that autologous HSCT should be the prefered approach. So far this recommendation has been mostly adhered to with only a few allogeneic HCTs for AD alone being in refractory cytopenias. Arguments not to use allogeneic HCT remain the same. Treatment-related toxicity is high, GVHD cannot yet be avoided and might interfere with the pre-exisiting disease without the potential benefits of added "graft-vs.-autoimmunity". Unlike the situation in malignancy, there is no as yet defined clone of autoaggressive cells to be eradicated. Furthermore, incomplete or slowed immune reconstitution after allogeneic HSCT might lead to late development of a donor-type AD, even more so in predisposed patients.

It remains an open issue whether reduced intensity conditioning regimens might alter the perspectives. Such regimens have been shown to reduce early mortality. So far, they have not reduced risk of GVHD and long-term follow-up is required. Still, there is consensus that it might be appropriate, under carefully selected conditions, to begin the planning of phase 1–2 studies to evaluate the role of allogeneic HCT. Conditioning with CY with or without ATG as used for aplastic anemia for many years might be the most appropriate choice.

Immune reconstitution

A centralized international initiative has begun to gather and share data on immune reconstitution in order to adjust later protocols and/or better understand the immunopathology of the types of ADs being transplanted. So far, anecdotal data have not produced an immune cell phenotypic pattern that predicts either remission or relapse. As already known, the CD8$^+$ CD45 RO$^+$ "memory cell" compartment expands post-transplantion, with later appearance of CD8$^+$ and CD4$^+$ CD45RA$^+$ "naive" T cells. CD19$^+$ and CD20$^+$ B cells and natural killer (NK) cells reconstitute within weeks to months, but CD4$^+$ cells may take months to years, depending on the severity of the conditioning and T-cell depletion.

Early data seem to indicate potential histologic markers of response and relapse in the RA synovium [55], but further work is required and ongoing. The finding of T-cell receptor excision circles in T cells exiting the thymus has allowed a more detailed analysis of normal and autoaggressive T-cell reactions following HCT for AD [56]. Studies are currently underway to determine if lymphocytes involved in synovial inflammation during relapse after transplantation are recent thymic emigrants or expanded unpurged mature cells (J. Isaacs, personal correspondence).

Gene marking

In allografting it is relatively easy to identify donor and recipient cells, but with autografting HCT, gene marking would be needed to identify those cells (e.g. lymphocytes) that originate from the graft product and those that arise from cells remaining in the patient after conditioning.

The problem of gene marking is well known: if a gene product expressed on the surface of the cell is used, then it may change the function of the cell, and in any case a significant loss of gene expression and indeed persistence may and does occur during multiple cell divisions. If one adds to this issue the phenomenon of massive nonspecific recruitment of immunocompetent cells during an immune reaction, the interpretation of finding gene marked cells in a lesion would be very difficult.

Aplasia-inducing therapy without HCT

Hematopoietic stem cells resist the cytotoxic effects of CY and therefore, theoretically, a HCT is not needed following aplasia induction and G-CSF supported reconstitution. Such a strategy has been successfully employed in aplastic anemia and has also been applied in SLE [57]. Early results are encouraging, but a significant number of patients have not had conventional pulse CY therapy and the time to reconstitution, especially for platelets, was prolonged compared to the rescue maneuver with HCT. Both procedures remain research-based rather than standard therapy.

New autoimmune disease indications

Theoretically, any severe active autoimmune disease could be a potential candidate for HCT, with the selection being determined by frequency of the type of AD and lack of response to conventional alternatives.

Inflammatory bowel disease (IBD) is now being explored with coincidental cases and anecdotal successful cases as primary disease indications have been presented at scientific meetings [21,24,33,34]. A combined gastroenterologic and hematologic consensus statement was published in an attempt to avoid a proliferation of protocols and to reduce toxicity in this group of often very ill patients [58]. It is to be hoped that these early phase 1 and 2 pilot studies will eventually lead to randomized phase 3 trials, given the relatively high frequency of IBD.

Many other rarer and life-threatening conditions such as relapsing polychondritis [59] and Behçet's pulmonary aneurysm have been successfully treated [60], but will never be so common as to justify a large multicenter randomized trial. Proof of concept in other more frequent ADs will remain the justification to proceed in these rarer conditions.

Conclusions

The role of HCT in the treatment of severe therapy-refractory AD remains experimental, with data on around 600 patients being sufficiently encouraging to proceed to randomized prospective trials in the major diseases: SSc, RA, MS and soon JIA and SLE. An impressive international collaboration has and is reducing duplication of effort with shared databases, protocols, patient selection criteria and endpoints. The concept of adjusting an imbalance in the complex immune network rather than total eradication of clonal autoimmunity is emerging. Further clinical trials are required to establish the place, if any, HCT has in such treatment, and concomitant studies continue to explain the pathophysiologic mechanisms of these immune modulating strategies.

References

1. Marmont ATA, Gratwohl A, Vischer T. Haematopoietic precursor cell transplants for autoimmune diseases. *Lancet* 1995; **345**: 978.
2. Tamm M, Gratwohl A, Tichelli A, Perruchoud AP, Tyndall A. Autologous haemopoietic stem cell transplantation in a patient with severe pulmonary hypertension complicating connective tissue disease. *Ann Rheum Dis* 1996; **55**: 779–80.
3. Davidson A, Diamond B. Autoimmune diseases. *N Engl J Med* 2001; **345**: 340–50.
4. Medzhitov R, Janeway CA Jr. Decoding the patterns of self and nonself by the innate immune system. *Science* 2002; **296**: 298–300.
5. Tisch R, McDevitt H. Insulin-dependent diabetes mellitus. *Cell* 1996; **85**: 291–7.
6. Shevach EM. CD4+ CD25+ suppressor T cells: more questions than answers. *Nat Rev Immunol* 2002; **2**: 389–400.
7. Cella M, Engering A, Pinet V, Pieters J, Lanzavecchia A. Inflammatory stimuli induce accumulation of MHC class II complexes on dendritic cells. *Nature* 1997; **388**: 782–7.
8. Viola A, Lanzavecchia A. T cell activation determined by T cell receptor number and tunable thresholds. *Science* 1996; **273**: 104–6.
9. Lehmann PV, Forsthuber T, Miller A, Sercarz EE. Spreading of T-cell autoimmunity to cryptic determinants of an autoantigen. *Nature* 1992; **358**: 155–7.
10. Maki M. Coeliac disease and autoimmunity due to unmasking of cryptic epitopes? *Lancet* 1996; **348**: 1046–7.
11. Kamradt T, Mitchison NA. Tolerance and autoimmunity. *N Engl J Med* 2001; **344**: 655–64.
12. Conrad B, Weissmahr RN, Boni J, Arcari R, Schupbach J, Mach B. A human endogenous retroviral superantigen as candidate autoimmune gene in type I diabetes. *Cell* 1997; **90**: 303–13.
13. Panayi GS. Targeting of cells involved in the pathogenesis of rheumatoid arthritis. *Rheumatology (Oxford)* 1999; **38** (Suppl. 2): 8–10.
14. Coles AJ, Wing M, Smith S et al. Pulsed monoclonal antibody treatment and autoimmune thyroid disease in multiple sclerosis. *Lancet* 1999; **354**: 1691–5.
15. Trendelenburg M, Gregor M, Passweg J, Tichelli A, Tyndall A, Gratwohl A. "Altered immunity syndrome": a distinct entity in long-term bone marrow transplantation survivors? *Bone Marrow Transplant* 2001; **28**: 1175–6.
16. Matzinger P. The danger model: a renewed sense of self. *Science* 2002; **296**: 301–5.
17. Baldwin JL, Storb R, Thomas ED, Mannik M. Bone marrow transplantation in patients with gold-induced marrow aplasia. *Arthritis Rheum* 1977; **20**: 1043–8.
18. Jacobs P, Vincent MD, Martell RW. Prolonged remission of severe refractory rheumatoid arthritis following allogeneic bone marrow transplantation for drug-induced aplastic anaemia. *Bone Marrow Transplant* 1986; **1**: 237–9.
19. Lowenthal RM, Cohen ML, Atkinson K, Biggs JC. Apparent cure of rheumatoid arthritis by bone marrow transplantation. *J Rheumatol* 1993; **20**: 137–40.
20. Eedy DJ, Burrows D, Bridges JM, Jones FG. Clearance of severe psoriasis after allogeneic bone marrow transplantation. *Br Med J* 1990; **300**: 908.
21. Yin JA, Jowitt SN. Resolution of immune-mediated diseases following allogeneic bone marrow transplantation for leukaemia. *Bone Marrow Transplant* 1992; **9**: 31–3.
22. Vento S, Cainelli F, Renzini C, Ghironzi G, Concia E. Resolution of autoimmune hepatitis after bone-marrow transplantation. *Lancet* 1996; **348**: 544–5.
23. McAllister LD, Beatty PG, Rose J. Allogeneic bone marrow transplant for chronic myelogenous leukemia in a patient with multiple sclerosis. *Bone Marrow Transplant* 1997; **19**: 395–7.
24. Nelson JL, Torrez R, Louie FM, Choe OS, Storb R, Sullivan KM. Pre-existing autoimmune disease in patients with long-term survival after allogeneic bone marrow transplantation. *J Rheumatol Suppl* 1997; **48**: 23–9.
25. Ferraccioli G, Damato R, De Vita S, Fanin R, Damiani D, Baccarani M. Haematopoietic stem cell transplantation (HSCT) in a patient with Sjögren's syndrome and lung MALT lymphoma cured lymphoma not the autoimmune disease. *Ann Rheum Dis* 2001; **60**: 174–6.
26. McKendry RJ, Huebsch L, Leclair B. Progression of rheumatoid arthritis following bone marrow transplantation: a case report with a 13-year follow-up. *Arthritis Rheum* 1996; **39**: 1246–53.
27. Salzman TJ, Jackson C. Clinical remission of myasthenia gravis in a patient after high dose therapy and autologous stem cell transplantation with CD34+ stem cells. *Blood* 1994; **94** (Suppl.): 206a.
28. Euler HH, Marmont AM, Bacigalupo A et al. Early recurrence or persistence of autoimmune diseases after unmanipulated autologous stem cell transplantation. *Blood* 1996; **88**: 3621–5.
29. Snowden JA, Patton WN, O'Donnell JL, Hannah EE, Hart DN. Prolonged remission of long-standing systemic lupus erythematosus after autologous bone marrow transplant for non-Hodgkin's lymphoma. *Bone Marrow Transplant* 1997; **19**: 1247–50.
30. Meloni G, Capria S, Vignetti M, Mandelli F, Modena V. Blast crisis of chronic myelogenous leukemia in long-lasting systemic lupus erythematosus: regression of both diseases after autologous bone marrow transplantation. *Blood* 1997; **89**: 4659.
31. Jondeau K, Job-Deslandre C, Bouscary D, Khanlou N, Menkes CJ, Dreyfus F. Remission of nonerosive polyarthritis associated with Sjögren's syndrome after autologous hematopoietic stem cell transplantation for lymphoma. *J Rheumatol* 1997; **24**: 2466–8.
32. Cooley HM, Snowden JA, Grigg AP, Wicks IP. Outcome of rheumatoid arthritis and psoriasis following autologous stem cell transplantation for hematologic malignancy. *Arthritis Rheum* 1997; **40**: 1712–5.
33. Kashyap A, Forman SJ. Autologous bone marrow transplantation for non-Hodgkin's lymphoma resulting in long-term remission of coincidental Crohn's disease. *Br J Haematol* 1998; **103**: 651–2.
34. Musso M, Porretto F, Crescimanno A, Bondi F, Polizzi V, Scalone R. Crohn's disease complicated by relapsed extranodal Hodgkin's lymphoma: prolonged complete remission after unmanipulated PBPC autotransplant. *Bone Marrow Transplant* 2000; **26**: 921–3.
35. Minchinton RM, Waters AH, Kendra J, Barrett AJ. Autoimmune thrombocytopenia acquired from an allogeneic bone-marrow graft. *Lancet* 1982; **2**: 627–9.
36. Sturfelt G, Lenhoff S, Sallerfors B, Nived O, Truedsson L, Sjoholm AG. Transplantation with allogenic bone marrow from a donor with systemic lupus erythematosus (SLE): successful outcome in the recipient and induction of an SLE flare in the donor. *Ann Rheum Dis* 1996; **55**: 638–41.
37. Denman AM, Russell AS, Denman EJ. Adoptive transfer of the diseases of New Zealand black mice to normal mouse strains. *Clin Exp Immunol* 1969; **5**: 567–95.
38. Morton JI, Siegel BV. Transplantation of autoimmune potential. I. Development of antinuclear antibodies in H-2 histocompatible recipients of bone marrow from New Zealand black mice. *Proc Natl Acad Sci U S A* 1974; **71**: 2162–5.
39. van Bekkum DW. Stem cell transplantation in experimental models of autoimmune disease. *J Clin Immunol* 2000; **20**: 10–16.
40. Ikehara S. Treatment of autoimmune diseases by hematopoietic stem cell transplantation. *Exp Hematol* 2001; **29**: 661–9.

41 van Bekkum DW. Conditioning regimens for the treatment of experimental arthritis with autologous bone marrow transplantation. *Bone Marrow Transplant* 2000; **25**: 357–64.

42 Knaan-Shanzer S, Houben P, Kinwel-Bohre EP, van Bekkum DW. Remission induction of adjuvant arthritis in rats by total body irradiation and autologous bone marrow transplantation. *Bone Marrow Transplant* 1991; **8**: 333–8.

43 Tyndall A, Gratwohl A. Blood and marrow stem cell transplants in auto-immune disease: a consensus report written on behalf of the European League Against Rheumatism (EULAR) and the European Group for Blood and Marrow Transplantation (EBMT). *Bone Marrow Transplant* 1997; **19**: 643–5.

44 McSweeney PA, Nash RA, Storb R, Furst DE, Gauthier J, Sullivan KM. Autologous stem cell transplantation for autoimmune diseases: issues in protocol development. *J Rheumatol Suppl* 1997; **48**: 79–84.

45 Gratwohl A, Passweg J, Gerber I, Tyndall A. Stem cell transplantation for autoimmune diseases. *Best Pract Res Clin Haematol* 2001; **14**: 755–76.

46 Openshaw H, Stuve O, Antel JP et al. Multiple sclerosis flares associated with recombinant granulocyte colony-stimulating factor. *Neurology* 2000; **54**: 2147–50.

47 Burt RK, Fassas A, Snowden J et al. Collection of hematopoietic stem cells from patients with autoimmune diseases. *Bone Marrow Transplant* 2001; **28**: 1–12.

48 Fassas AS, Passweg JR, Anagnostopoulos A et al. Hematopoietic stem cell transplantation for multiple sclerosis: a retrospective multicenter study. *J Neurol* 2002; **249**: 1088–97.

49 Mancardi GL, Saccardi R, Filippi M et al. Autologous hematopoietic stem cell transplantation suppresses Gd-enhanced MRI activity in MS. *Neurology* 2001; **57**: 62–8.

50 Binks M, Passweg JR, Furst D et al. Phase I/II trial of autologous stem cell transplantation in systemic sclerosis: procedure related mortality and impact on skin disease. *Ann Rheum Dis* 2001; **60**: 577–84.

51 McSweeney PA, Nash RA, Sullivan KM et al. High-dose immunosuppressive therapy for severe systemic sclerosis: initial outcomes. *Blood* 2002; **100**: 1602–10.

52 Barron KS, Wallace C, Woolfrey CEA et al. Autologous stem cell transplantation for pediatric rheumatic diseases. *J Rheumatol* 2001; **28**: 2337–58.

53 Traynor AE, Schroeder J, Rosa RM et al. Treatment of severe systemic lupus erythematosus with high-dose chemotherapy and haemopoietic stem-cell transplantation: a phase I study. *Lancet* 2000; **356**: 701–7.

54 Huhn RDFP, Nakamura R, Read EJ et al. High-dose cyclophosphamide with autologous lymphocyte-depleted peripheral blood stem cell (PBSC) support for treatment of refractory chronic autoimmune thrombocytopenia. *Blood* 2002; **101**: 71–7.

55 Bingham S, Veale D, Fearon U et al. High-dose cyclophosphamide with stem cell rescue for severe rheumatoid arthritis: short-term efficacy correlates with reduction of macroscopic and histologic synovitis. *Arthritis Rheum* 2002; **46**: 837–9.

56 Douek DC, Vescio RA, Betts MR et al. Assessment of thymic output in adults after haematopoietic stem-cell transplantation and prediction of T-cell reconstitution. *Lancet* 2000; **355**: 1875–81.

57 Brodsky RA, Petri M, Smith BD et al. Immunoablative high-dose cyclophosphamide without stem-cell rescue for refractory severe autoimmune disease. *Ann Intern Med* 1998; **129**: 1031–5.

58 Hawkey CJ, Snowden JA, Lobo A, Beglinger C, Tyndall A. Stem cell transplantation for inflammatory bowel disease: practical and ethical issues. *Gut* 2000; **46**: 869–72.

59 Rosen O, Thiel A, Massenkeil G et al. Autologous stem-cell transplantation in refractory autoimmune diseases after *in vivo* immunoablation and *ex vivo* depletion of mononuclear cells. *Arthritis Res* 2000; **2**: 327–36.

60 Hensel M, Breitbart A, Ho AD. Autologous hematopoietic stem-cell transplantation for Behçet's disease with pulmonary involvement. *N Engl J Med* 2001; **344**: 69.

102

Robert S. Negrin

Prevention and Therapy of Relapse following Autologous Hematopoietic Cell Transplantation

Introduction

Autologous bone marrow (BM) and peripheral blood progenitor cell (PBPC) transplantation have proven to be effective therapies for a number of hematologic malignancies. Randomized clinical trials in non-Hodgkin's lymphoma (NHL) and multiple myeloma (MM) have demonstrated that autologous hematopoietic cell transplantation (aHCT) is the treatment choice for patients with these malignancies at certain stages of disease [1,2]. In addition, treatment of patients with other disease entities such as Hodgkin's disease (HD), acute leukemia, neuroblastoma, germ cell tumors and selected solid tumors have also shown promising results with enhanced disease-free and overall survival as compared to historical control groups of patients treated with standard therapies. The development of strategies for the mobilization of hematopoietic stem cells in the form of PBPCs has resulted in a reduction in mortality risk due to more rapid hematologic recovery. Patients can now be offered aHCT earlier in the course of their disease which will likely result in improved overall results. Autologous HCT has emerged as a very effective means of achieving a state of minimal residual disease (MRD) focusing efforts on strategies to treat MRD which are likely to have a significant impact on improvement in overall results. A variety of strategies based on immunological interventions, including the use of cytokines, cellular and monoclonal antibody therapies have moved to the forefront of investigation in this field. This chapter will focus on these strategies for the treatment and, more importantly, the prevention of relapse in the setting of aHCT.

Significance of relapse following autologous transplantation

Relapse following autologous transplantation is an ominous clinical event, which predicts a very poor prognosis for that individual patient. Every effort should be made to thoroughly document relapse since some patients may continue to have abnormal blood or radiographic studies following aHCT. Therefore, a diagnosis of relapse often requires clear evidence of progression on radiographic studies or tissue diagnosis including BM evaluation or biopsy of suspicious lesions. Since patients who undergo aHCT clearly understand and fear relapse, it is critically important to not declare that a patient has relapsed until there is definitive evidence of progressive disease since patients are highly sensitized to this risk. In addition, some patients may continue to have disease responses following completion of therapy and therefore it is important to utilize serial staging studies after adequate follow-up has occurred since these studies can occasionally be misleading unless symptoms present which require investigation.

Following aHCT for most hematological malignancies relapse generally occurs soon after transplantation with approximately 75% of those patients who eventually relapse doing so within the 1st year and >95% of patients who ultimately relapse do so within 3 years. Since relapse is the most frequent cause of treatment failure following aHCT, clearly the major goal is prevention since treatment of relapse is rarely effective. In one large study 283 patients with acute leukemias, MM and NHL who relapsed following aHCT between 1989 and 1994 were analyzed [3]. Chemotherapy and radiation therapy were administered to 229 patients. Of the treated patients, 24% achieved complete remission (CR) and 19% achieved partial remission (PR) following therapy. However, overall median survival from relapse was only 5 months. For patients given salvage therapy, median survival was 7 months and for those patients who responded to salvage therapy median survival was 15 months. In this study, only six patients were alive for a period of time longer than that between the transplant and relapse clearly documenting that the outcome for these patients was extremely poor. In another study of 58 patients with NHL who relapsed following aHCT, the median time to subsequent relapse was only 4.8 months and median survival following relapse was 10 months [4]. Approximately one-third of patients who were retreated with salvage chemotherapy did have a response although these responses were relatively short-lived.

The use of second myeloablative transplants following failure of an autologous transplant has been relatively unsuccessful. These procedures are often associated with very high treatment-related mortality (TRM) which has been prohibitive, ranging between 50% and nearly 90% [5,6]. Several groups have reported results of myeloablative allogeneic transplants for patients who relapse following autologous transplantation. One of the larger series of patients reported included 59 patients in Seattle who relapsed after aHCT for acute myeloid leukemia (AML) ($n = 24$), acute lymphoblastic leukemia (ALL) ($n = 13$), NHL ($n = 18$), MM ($n = 3$) and CML ($n = 1$) [7]. Donors included human leukocyte antigen (HLA)-matched-related siblings, mismatched-related donors and matched-unrelated donors. In this retrospective evaluation, the non-relapse mortality at 2 years was 51%. Twenty-six percent of patients suffered another relapse after the second transplant procedure. The few patients who appeared to benefit were mainly children under the age of 17 at the time of the second transplant, those that achieved CR with salvage chemotherapy prior to second transplant and those who had a diagnosis of AML. A study from the European Group for Blood and Marrow Transplantation evaluated patients who had failed autografting for acute leukemia between 1981 and 1996 which revealed 2-year survival of only 11% for those individuals treated with chemotherapy [8]. Patients treated with allogeneic transplantation had a 2-year survival of 32% although with very high TRM. In a multivariate analysis, the factors that predicted for better survival included an interval from the autograft to relapse of >5 months and patient age <26 years. Some smaller studies have been more positive where one group reported a disease-free survival (DFS) of 43% in 27 relapsed patients with leukemia treated with a second myeloablative allogeneic transplant [9]. Additional experiences have been sobering with survival at 1 year of only 16% with TRM of 71% [10]. A special case can be made for children who appear to fare somewhat better. For example, in a study of 23 children with secondary AML or NHL treated with an allogeneic transplant procedure following a failed autograft for relapse or graft failure, nine patients were alive and disease-free between 1.7 and 6.7 years at the time of the report with a 4-year DFS rate of 39% [11].

With the development of strategies for nonmyeloablative allogeneic transplantation, there has been renewed interested in exploring this treatment concept in patients who have relapsed following aHCT. Cautious optimism is based upon the observations documented above that some patients can be salvaged with allogeneic transplantation suggesting that graft-vs.-tumor (GVT) effects are capable of controlling disease even in an advanced clinical setting. Therefore, the advantage of nonmyeloablative allogeneic transplantation is reduced TRM, hopefully with preserved GVT effects. This strategy has been explored in several relatively small clinical trials with limited follow-up demonstrating that patients who fail aHCT can tolerate nonmyeloablative allogeneic transplantation with a likely reduced risk of TRM. Initial studies from Israel of 12 patients who failed prior autologous transplantation for hematologic malignancies who had an HLA-matched donor and received a preparative regimen of fludarabine, busulfan and antithymocyte globulin (ATG) with cyclosporine (CSP) prophylaxis resulted in only one patient succumbing to toxicity [12]. Unfortunately, five patients have relapsed but six patients are disease-free with a maximum follow-up of 23 months. In another study of 14 patients who relapsed following aHCT, 10 received preparation with fludarabine and cyclophosphamide with four of these patients alive at a median follow-up of slightly more than 1 year [13]. An alternative strategy of cyclophosphamide, ATG and thymic irradiation with a short course of CSP was utilized to treat 13 patients with hematologic malignancies who failed autologous transplantation. If these patients did not develop graft-vs.-host disease (GVHD) prophylactic donor lymphocyte infusions (DLI) was administered 5–6 weeks following transplantation. Of the 13 patients treated, grade II–IV GVHD developed in nine patients therefore DLI was not administered to them. In this relatively small group of patients, DFS at 2 years was 37.5% and overall survival (OS) at 2 years was 45%, again demonstrating that this strategy can be employed with some success in this high-risk clinical setting [14]. In another study of 45 patients of whom 26 had failed prior autologous transplantation and all patients being at very high-risk of disease relapse, a nonmyeloablative approach using thiotepa, fludarabine and cyclophosphamide was utilized with planned reinfusions of DLI for patients without GVHD [15]. Cyclosporine and methotrexate were used for GVHD prophylaxis. TRM was 13% and patients were able to tolerate the procedure; however, median follow-up of the entire group was short at approximately 1 year precluding accurate evaluation of relapse risk. These studies document that nonmyeloablative allogeneic transplantation can be attempted in patients who fail aHCT with acceptable risk and at least some short-term efficacy. Clearly, longer-term follow-up is required to more definitively answer the important question of whether a significant percentage of patients benefit from this therapy.

The strategy of autologous transplantation followed by planned nonmyeloablative allogeneic transplant in an effort to prevent rather than treat relapse is under active investigation in a number of different diseases. Early results indicate that this treatment approach is effective in some disease settings, for example MM, resulting in acceptable mortality with a high percentage of patients achieving CR [16]. This general concept is discussed in detail elsewhere (Chapters 85 and 86).

Alternative approaches not involving chemotherapy or transplantation have been explored in relapsed patients with selective diseases in an effort to treat disease relapse. For example, patients with MM have been treated with thalidomide, which has significant biological activity in this disease [17]. An initial case report of a patient who had failed aHCT and was treated with thalidomide demonstrated biological activity [18]. Other studies include an evaluation of 11 patients who relapsed following autologous transplantation where thalidomide was dose-escalated starting at 100 mg/day as tolerated to a maximum dose of 800 mg/day. At a median dose of 600 mg/day treatment was complicated by constipation, lethargy and leukopenia. Four patients (36%) had a >50% reduction in paraprotein and another four patients responded with a >25% reduction for a total response rate of 72%, demonstrating considerable activity of thalidomide in this clinical setting. Unfortunately five of these eight patients later relapsed with a median follow-up of only 5 months [19]. In a larger study of 65 patients of which 26 individuals had relapsed after aHCT, 17 (28.3%) had a >50% reduction in paraprotein; however, 46.6% of these patients progressed relatively soon thereafter [20]. These studies demonstrate that thalidomide has biological activity with an acceptable safety profile in the clinical setting of patients with relapsed MM who have failed autologous transplantation. Additional preliminary studies in which investigators used thalidomide and dexamethasone following autologous HCT suggest efficacy in an effort to prevent rather than treat relapse [21]. The strategy of utilizing thalidomide and dexamethasone following autologous transplantation for patients with MM to reduce the risk of relapse will now be explored in a larger clinical trial, directly compared to autologous followed by nonmyeloablative allogeneic transplantation for patients who have HLA-matched sibling donors to determine which strategy is more effective in controlling disease and prolonging DFS (Bone Marrow Transplantation Clinical Trials Network).

An alternative approach for patients who have failed aHCT and do not have an HLA-matched sibling donor is to perform partially matched-related donor transplantation. Since most patients have a haploidentical donor, this type of therapy can be considered. In one study 17 patients underwent T-cell-depleted bone marrow transplantation (BMT) from partially matched sibling donors and five patients (29%) survived at a median of 68 months (range 42–84 months). Again, age <18 and fewer organ toxicities were somewhat predictive of improved survival [22]. Current strategies of haploidentical transplantation include intensive conditioning which is difficult to tolerate for patients who have failed autologous transplants [23]. Strategies for pursuing nonmyeloablative haploidentical transplantation are only beginning to be performed where some success has been achieved [24]. In one study of haploidentical nonmyeloablative transplantation, five patients were treated and responses were noted; however, most of the patients ultimately developed GVHD. Another approach has been to use cyclophosphamide following infusion of the PBPC graft in an effort to reduce T-cell alloreactivity. Early clinical trials have demonstrated the feasibility of this strategy were engraftment was achieved with acceptable toxicity and less GVHD than would be expected when crossing HLA barriers [25].

A small number of patients who relapsed following autografting have undergone transplantation with umbilical cord blood cells, which offers the opportunity of obtaining donor cells for patients who do not have HLA-matched-related donors. To date, several case reports have appeared in the literature describing patients with leukemia who have relapsed following autologous transplantation and received an umbilical cord blood graft with some evidence of response; namely, that their remission lasted longer than the time from transplant to relapse [26,27]. Further studies will be needed to determine whether this approach is an effective strategy.

Clearly, the treatment of patients who have suffered a relapse following aHCT is a challenging clinical arena with relatively few successes and a high risk for toxicity. Since the majority of patients have objective clinical responses and achieve a state of MRD following aHCT strategies aimed at preventing relapse are more likely to improve overall outcome.

Strategies to reduce relapse risk following autologous transplantation

A variety of different strategies can be envisioned to reduce the risk of relapse following aHCT. These are summarized in Table 102.1 and include improved patient selection, more effective preparative regimens, use of multiple transplants, improved purging strategies, radiation therapy to sites of previous disease, post-transplantation cytokines and immunotherapies. With the development of mobilized PBPCs and reduction in transplant-related morbidity and mortality following aHCT, patients can be considered earlier in the course of their disease for transplantation. For example, in patients with NHL the strategy of identifying patients with high-risk disease who are likely to relapse and to institute aHCT during first remission is an attractive approach [28–30]. Preliminary evidence supports this type of intervention, which is currently the subject of several randomized clinical phase III trials.

Enhanced preparative regimens

The use of more dose-intensive preparative regimens has been explored in several clinical settings. With the development of mobilized PBPCs adequate stem cells can routinely be collected to perform multiple transplant procedures. Despite significant toxicity and expense, up to four transplant procedures have been performed [31–33]. Interestingly, in patients with metastatic breast cancer with a high risk of relapse overall results were identical to that achieved with a single transplant [33]. Nevertheless, the use of tandem transplants has been utilized in patients with MM [34]. Randomized studies comparing a single to tandem transplantation are underway.

The use of radiolabeled monoclonal antibodies (MABs), as well as more intensive chemotherapy-based regimens, have been utilized in an effort to reduce relapse risk and improve outcomes. The interpretation of these studies is complicated by the early phase and exploratory nature of most of these trials and the lack of suitable control groups. Nonetheless, a particularly attractive approach includes the use of radiolabeled MABs to deliver radiation to sites of disease. This topic is discussed in detail elsewhere in this book (Chapter 15); however, a number of studies are of special note. The use of iodine-131 (^{131}I)-labeled MABs has been explored in the setting of combining this reagent with conventional autologous transplantation preparation. Both anti-CD45 and anti-CD20 MAB have been used in inpatients with leukemia, myelodysplastic syndrome (MDS) or B-cell NHL, respectively. In a phase I distribution study of I^{135} anti-CD45 combined with total body irradiation (TBI) and cyclophosphamide, 44 patients with advanced leukemia and MDS were treated of which 37 (84%) had favorable biodistribution of the radioactive nuclide defined by higher estimated dose to the BM and spleen than normal organs. In this study, 34 patients then received a therapeutic dose of between 76 and 612 mCi of I^{135} anti-CD45 MAB in an effort to deliver an estimated dose to the liver of 3.5–12.5 Gy in 12 dose levels. The maximally tolerated dose was 10.5 Gy which was limited by grade III/IV mucositis at the highest dose level. Seven of 25 AML and MDS patients and three of nine ALL patients were alive and disease-free at a median follow-up of >16 months [35]. A similar strategy was employed using ^{131}I tositumomab (anti-CD20) combined with etoposide (VP16) and cyclophosphamide in patients with relapsed B-cell NHL. In this study of 52 patients, a trace dosimetric dose was used initially followed by a calculated dose of ^{131}I to deliver a target dose of radiation of between 20 and 27 Gy to normal organs. Following "washout" of the reagents, patients were then treated with VP16 and cyclophosphamide. In this study, excellent OS and progression-free survival (PFS) at 2 years of 83% and 68% was observed, which appeared to be superior to that achieved with historical controls treated at the same institution [36]. A difficulty with the use of ^{131}I is the requirement for isolation of the patient until the decay of the reagent. Another radionuclide conjugated MAB includes rhenium-188 labeled anti-CD66 monoclonal antibody which was followed by a full-dose preparative regimen to treat 36 patients with advanced stage malignancies of whom four had received prior autologous transplants. One-hundred-day mortality was acceptable at 6%; however, late renal toxicity occurred in 17% of patients. Although this study was relatively small, relapse rates appeared low [37]. Additional studies using other radiolabeled conjugates with a variety of other radioisotopes and characteristics, which may result in the targeting of radiation therapy to sites of disease, are under active exploration.

Involved field radiotherapy following autologous transplantation

The majority of patients who relapse following aHCT do so at sites of previous disease. This observation has suggested that residual disease within the patient rather than reinfused tumor cells is the source of relapse for the majority of patients. The question of whether conventional radiation therapy delivered to involved fields following aHCT will reduce relapse risk has been pursued in a number of studies. Definitive trials have been difficult to perform due to the heterogeneity of patients, eligibility criteria and treatment plans which have hampered the interpretation of results. Nonetheless, a variety of studies have suggested that involved field radiotherapy following autologous transplantation is likely to be beneficial. In one study of 54 patients with relapsed HD who underwent autologous transplantation, 20 patients received involved field radiation therapy either prior to ($n = 7$) or after ($n = 13$) high-dose therapy [38]. Of these 54 patients, 25 patients (46.3%) eventually relapsed of which the majority (17/25 or 68%) relapsed at sites of prior disease. Patients treated with involved field radiation therapy had a lower risk of relapse at sites of prior disease (26.3% vs. 42.8%, $p = <0.05$). In addition, 21 patients had persistent disease after transplantation and 10 of these patients received involved field radiation therapy, all of whom converted to CR. Importantly, those patients with persistence of disease following transplantation had better OS if treated with involved field radiotherapy. In fact, those patients who were treated with radiation therapy for persistent disease had a similar outcome as compared to those patients who achieved CR without the use of radiation therapy. Since persistence of disease clearly defines a high-risk group, this finding is particularly compelling [38]. In another retrospective review of patients with HD who were potentially eligible to be treated with involved field radiation therapy, the toxicity of this approach was evaluated [39]. In this study of 23 patients, three (13%) died of treatment-related complications and eight patients (35%) developed grade III or grade IV complications following treatment with radiation therapy demonstrating that this form of treatment is not without significant toxicity. Nonetheless, the OS of this cohort of patients was

Table 102.1 Strategies to reduce relapse risk following autologous transplantation.

Improved patient selection
Targeted preparative regimens
Multiple transplants
Improved in vivo and ex vivo purging
Involved field radiotherapy
Immunotherapy

61%, which appears favorable. Radiation therapy can, however, also result in other severe complications including the development of transverse myeopathy [40].

Further evidence of efficacy of involved field radiotherapy comes from a review of 100 patients with relapsed or refractory HD treated at Stanford University [41]. Twenty-four patients received involved field radiotherapy immediately before or after aHCT. At a median follow-up of 40 months, patients who received radiation therapy had excellent local control of disease further suggesting that this modality may reduce relapse at sites of previous disease, which is the most common site for failure. Therefore, despite the lack of randomized trials, it is our recommendation that involved field radiotherapy be utilized in those patients whose prior or persistent disease can be encompassed in two treatment fields.

Improved purging strategies

The concern that clonogenic tumor cells may be present within the BM or PBPC innoculum and contribute to disease relapse has been persistent. Despite the lack of positive results from randomized clinical trials demonstrating improved outcomes for patients who receive a purged graft, substantial indirect evidence supports the concept that obtaining a tumor-free graft is important in improving clinical outcomes. This evidence includes retrospective analysis of improved outcomes for patients whose grafts are effectively depleted of tumor cells [42,43] as well as gene-marking studies documenting that transfer of tumor cells within the graft can contribute to disease relapse [44,45]. Strategies to deplete tumor cells from the BM or PBPCs include depletion techniques with MABs or chemotherapy as well as positive stem cell selection [46–49]. The topic of purging is extensively discussed elsewhere in this book (Chapters 19 and 20).

Rationale for immunotherapy following autologous transplantation

The rationale for utilizing immunotherapeutic treatment strategies following aHCT is based on several important observations. First, the demonstration that GVT effects play a major role in reducing relapse rates following allogeneic transplantation is beyond dispute. The cellular populations responsible for GVT effects are not known with certainty, although both T cells and natural killer (NK) cells have been implicated [50,51]. The use of post-transplant immunotherapy in the aHCT setting is based upon the hypothesis that cellular populations capable of eradicating autologous tumor cells can be activated and effective in controlling minimal tumor burden. Second, following autologous transplantation is an ideal clinical setting to test the potential efficacy of immunotherapy since the majority of patients are effectively treated to a state of MRD in which immunotherapy is more likely to be effective, yet a significant percentage of patients will likely relapse in a relatively short-time interval. Third, the precursor cells required for expansion and activation are readily available and the techniques and expertise required for cell manipulation are well-established in transplant laboratories. Fourth, the rapid expansion of knowledge in basic immunology, effector cell biology and identification of recognition structures provides insights for novel treatment strategies. Some of these strategies are listed in Table 102.2 and include the use of cytokines, MABs, cellular immunotherapy, and vaccination strategies.

Cytokines

A number of cytokines have been identified that have profound stimulatory activities on key effector cell populations resulting in the expansion and activation of such cell populations. Animal models have been

Table 102.2 Immunotherapeutic approaches to treat minimal residual disease (MRD).

Cytokines
IL-2
IL-2 and IFN
SCF and IL-2
Flt ligand and IL-2
IL-15

Antibody based therapies
Monoclonal antibodies
   Anti-CD20
   Anti-Her2/*neu*
   Radiolabeled antibodies
Bispecific antibodies

Cellular therapies
NK cells
Cytolytic cell lines
CIK cells
CTLs

Vaccination strategies
DCs
Tumor vaccines

CIK, cytokine induced killer; CTL, cytotoxic lymphocytes; DC, dendritic cell; IFN, interferon; IL, interleukin; NK, natural killer; SCF, stem cell factor.

developed that demonstrate efficacy. Such cytokines include but are not limited to the interleukins (IL) 2, 12 and 15. Translation to the clinic is complicated by availability of drug, dose, schedule and toxicity. IL-2 has been extensively evaluated in the post-aHCT setting and is currently the subject of clinical phase III trials. Since the use of IL-2 is extensively reviewed elsewhere in this book (see Chapter 28) only larger more definitive studies will be discussed here. Clearly, IL-2 has resulted in significant toxicities including hypotension, weight gain, the vascular leak syndrome and even death [52]. These toxicities are dose and schedule related. More recent studies have demonstrated that lower dose administration schedules have been developed which are reasonably well tolerated. IL-2 has been studied extensively in patients with acute leukemia and NHL following aHCT.

Several studies have demonstrated a profound impairment of IL-2 production following recovery from autologous BMT [53,54]. Nevertheless, peripheral blood (PB) lymphocytes isolated from patients following aHCT were capable of responding to exogenous IL-2 *in vitro* leading to the hypothesis that this impairment in function could be restored by the administration of IL-2 following transplantation. Indeed, phase I studies utilizing a variety of different doses and schedules of IL-2 were able to demonstrate that CD56$^+$ NK cells were expanded and activated in the PB of treated patients [55–57].

Phase II studies have been performed in the setting of aHCT for AML where Benyunes *et al.* [58] reported 14 patients who were treated with either IL-2 alone or IL-2 plus *ex vivo* activated peripheral blood mononuclear cells (PBMCs). Thirteen patients experienced mild to moderate toxicity, which was reversible; however, one patient died of multiorgan failure. At a median of 34 months only three patients had relapsed with a probability of DFS of 71% which was promising. A similar result was obtained in another small study of 18 patients with AML in first CR who underwent aHCT followed by IL-2 therapy [59]. Again significant

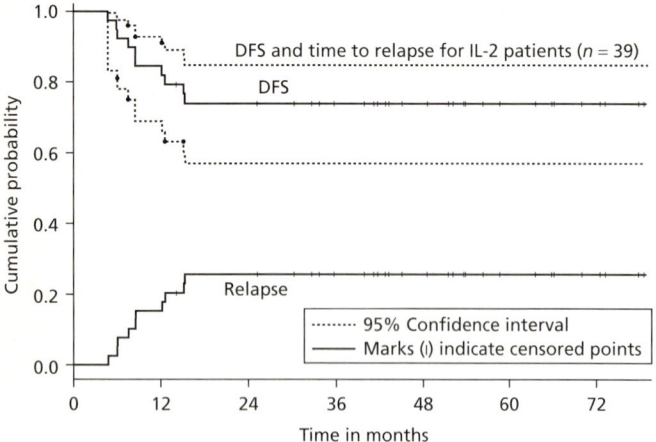

Fig. 102.1 Disease-free survival (DFS) and time to relapse for 39 patients treated with interleukin 2 (IL-2) following autologous transplantation. Reproduced with permission from Stein et al. [60].

reversible toxicity was experienced in all but one patient. At a median follow-up of 32 months following transplantation DFS was 71%.

A larger phase II trial in the setting of aHCT for patients with AML in first CR was performed at the City of Hope National Medical Center, Duarte, CA [60]. In this study 56 patients in first CR were treated with a single consolidation therapy cycle with cytosine arabinoside and idarubicin with the intent of proceeding to aHCT followed by IL-2 at a dose of 9×10^6 IU/m^2/days for 4 days followed by 10 days of 1.6×10^6 IU/m^2/day. An intention-to-treat analysis was performed where 84% of patients received aHCT and 68% subsequently received IL-2. At a median of 39 months of follow-up the 2-year probability of DFS is 68% (95%CI 55–80%) (Fig. 102.1 [60]). Of the patients who received all planned therapy DFS at 2 years was 74% (95%CI 57–85%). Even patients with unfavorable cytogenetics fared reasonably well with this treatment program [60]. These excellent results deserve extension to a phase III study to determine the relative role of IL-2 in the apparent improvement in DFS.

Less success has been achieved in the treatment of patients with ALL with IL-2 following aHCT. In a randomized study in adults with ALL, patients in first CR who had an HLA-matched sibling donor underwent allogeneic BMT whereas those individuals without donors were treated with high-dose therapy and aHCT and were then randomized to receive either IL-2 or no additional therapy [61]. The dosage of IL-2 utilized was 12×10^6 IU/m^2/day for 5 days during the first cycle, followed by four additional cycles of 2 days of treatment administered every other week. In this study, 60 patients underwent aHCT and were randomized. The 3-year post-BMT probability of continuous complete remission (CCR) was similar in the two groups of patients randomized to receive IL-2 or no additional therapy (29% vs. 27%, p = n.s.).

IL-2 has also been utilized after aHCT in patients with NHL. In an initial study of 11 patients with NHL IL-2 was administered at a median of 42 days following aHCT [62]. Although significant toxicity was observed including fever and fluid retention the treatment was tolerated reasonably well and resulted in a significant and persistent increase in NK cells in the PB for up to 6 months following therapy. There was an increase in NK functional activity of blood samples isolated from these patients against a NK-sensitive cell line.

In another study 56 patients with either NHL (n = 32) or HD (n = 24) were treated with a combination of IL-2 (3–6 IU/m^2/day) and interferon-alpha (IFN-α) for 5 days/week for 4 successive weeks [63]. The side-effects were substantial with 86% of patients developing grade II–III level toxicities which gradually resolved with cessation of treatment. In this study 80% of the treated patients were alive and free of disease with a follow-up of 34 (range 7–78) months which compared favorably to a historical cohort of patients treated in a similar fashion except for no post-transplantation cytokines (p <0.01). Randomized clinical trials are underway to confirm and extend these findings.

Due to the toxicity of IL-2 alternative doses and schedules have been explored. The utilization of prolonged treatment with low-dose IL-2 has been promising [64]. In a small study of 12 patients (6 patients with breast cancer and 6 with NHL) IL-2 dose escalation between the doses of 0.25 and 0.5×10^6 U/m^2/day administered subcutaneously (SQ) were evaluated over a treatment period of 84 days [65]. The 0.25×10^6 dose was better tolerated with 75% of the planned doses administered as compared to 48% with the higher dose. Dose limiting toxicities included a decline in performance status and thrombocytopenia. Even at the lower dose there was a 10-fold increase in CD3$^-$CD56^{bright} NK cells which were functional *in vitro*. In a comparison of intravenous vs. SQ dosing the latter administration was found to be associated with fewer infections with similar increases in CD56$^+$ cells in the PB [66]. These studies have demonstrated that IL-2 can be administered over a prolonged period of time with acceptable toxicity and with increases in functional NK cells. Further studies, preferably in randomized fashion, are required to demonstrate the efficacy of this treatment strategy. Some of these trials are currently ongoing under the auspices of the South-West Oncology Group.

Additional cytokines such as IL-12 and IL-15 have been effective in activating NK cells both *in vitro* and *in vivo* which could be utilized instead of, or in combination with, IL-2. Clinical trials have been initiated with IL-12 in the nontransplant setting [67–69]. Significant toxicities were encountered; however, doses and schedules have been developed which are tolerable. Other groups of investigators have explored the combination of early acting growth factors such as stem cell factor (SCF) or Flt ligand with IL-2 which results in the activation of early progenitor cells which mature into NK cells [70]. Clinical trials with SCF and IL-2 have been initiated; however, the toxicity of both agents, especially SCF, is considerable. The combination of Flt ligand and IL-2 may have potent synergistic effects in expanding NK cells from progenitor cell populations. Clinical trials designed to explore this finding have been initiated [71].

Antibody based therapies

Monoclonal antibodies (MABs)

MABs are attractive reagents for immunotherapy due to their high degree of specificity. It has been relatively difficult to develop MABs that are truly tumor-specific so more generic lineage restricted agents have been developed which cross-react with tumor cells such as anti-CD20 (Rituximab®) for the treatment of B-cell NHL and anti-Her2/*neu* (Herceptin®) for the treatment of some breast cancer patients. Anti-CD20 MAB have been explored in the setting of aHCT for two purposes, namely with mobilization chemotherapy in an effort to reduce contamination of the collected PBPCs and the treatment of MRD in the post-transplant setting. Results from studies exploring these two indications will be summarized below.

Anti-CD20 MAB have been combined with chemotherapy (typically cyclophosphamide) and growth factors (granulocyte colony-stimulating factor [G-CSF] or granulocyte macrophage colony-stimulating factor [GM-CSF]) given at the time of mobilization of PBPCs. In one study of 25 patients Rituximab® was administered at the dosage of 375 mg/m^2 3 days prior to administration of cyclophosphamide and G-CSF [72]. Twenty-three of the patients achieved a minimal dose of $>2 \times 10^6$ CD34$^+$ cells/kg and of the seven patients with disease detectable with molecular assays, six of these patients were found to not have detectable tumor cells in the apheresis product as assessed by polymerase chain reaction (PCR). These patients also received a second course of Rituximab® following

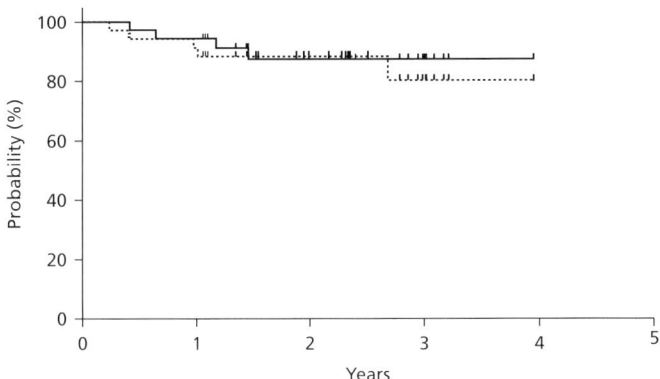

Fig. 102.2 Disease-free survival (DFS) for patients with B-cell non-Hodgkin's disease (NHL) treated with anti-CD20 monoclonal antibody following autologous transplantation. Reproduced with permission from Horwitz et al. [76].

aHCT. All patients engrafted in a timely fashion, yet interestingly six patients developed transient neutropenia at approximately day 100 [72]. In a second study 10 patients with relapsed follicular NHL and mantle cell lymphoma (MCL) were treated with Rituximab® in addition to cyclophosphamide and vincristine for mobilization. All marker positive patients were rendered PCR⁻ by the treatment in both blood and BM [73]. In this study mobilization of PBPCs was achieved with the combination of cytosine arabinoside and Rituximab® which resulted in adequate collection of $CD34^+$ cells. Autografting was then pursued followed by additional doses of antibody.

The addition of Rituximab® to a regimen of dexamethasone, carmustine, etoposide, cytarabine and melphalan (DEXABEAM) was found to be well tolerated with excellent PFS and OS of 77% and 95%, respectively, in a study of 27 patients with B-cell NHL [74]. Rituximab® has also been utilized in the setting of chronic lymphocytic leukemia (CLL) where in a preliminary study of five patients a reduction but not complete removal of $CD5^+/CD19^+$ cells was achieved [75]. Clearly, these studies are preliminary in nature and the role of antibody therapy is not definitively demonstrated, although it is clear that this agent can be added to the transplant regimens with acceptable toxicity.

Anti-CD20 MAB have also been utilized in the post-transplantation setting in an effort to treat MRD and reduce relapse risk. In a study from Stanford University, 35 patients with B-cell NHL undergoing aHCT were treated with Rituximab® (375 mg/m²/week for 4 weeks) starting around day +42 following transplantation and then again for a second 4-week treatment at 6 months. Of the 35 patients enrolled in the study 29 received all planned treatments. At 24 months estimated OS was 85% and freedom from progression was 86%. Only 4/35 patients have relapsed (Fig. 102.2 [76]). These transplant results are superior to historical experience and suggest that Rituximab® in the post-transplantation setting utilized at a time of MRD may reduce the risk of disease relapse. Interestingly, 19 patients (54%) developed grade 3–4 neutropenia, which resolved either spontaneously or with G-CSF treatment. The finding of isolated neutropenia remains unexplained. A randomized clinical trial to test the hypothesis that Rituximab® is effective in reducing the risk of relapse following aHCT for recurrent intermediate grade B-cell NHL is underway. Other anti-B-cell MABs such as 1D10, which recognizes a variant of major histocompatibility complex (MHC) class II found on a number of malignancies including B-cell NHL are also under clinical investigation.

Bispecific antibodies

The exquisite specificity of MABs and the presence of two variable binding regions have led to the concept of combining one binding site to a tumor associated antigen and the other to an effector cell in an effort to enhance target cell recognition. Resulting bispecific antibodies have been produced either by heterohybridomas or recombinant DNA technologies and utilized in preclinical animal models and early clinical trials. One such bispecific antibody combines CD3–1D10 which enhanced the *in vitro* lysis of B-cell tumors in the presence of activated T cells [77]. Other bispecific antibodies directed against myeloid leukemia cells have been shown to redirect $CD3^+$ T cells towards their own malignant cells [78]. Anti-CD3xHer2/*neu* bispecific antibodies have been used to couple activated T cells to ovarian and breast carcinomas expressing this tumor-associated antigen and to result in rapid clearance of malignant cells in a severe combined immunodeficiency syndrome (SCID) model [79]. Early clinical trials using this treatment approach are underway in a variety of disease settings [80].

Cellular therapy following autologous transplantation

The strategy of expanding and activating effector cell populations *ex vivo* followed by reinfusion following aHCT is attractive since, as stated above, the majority of patients are in a state of MRD, the progenitor cells are readily available and the expertise for cell manipulation is present in most clinical transplantation laboratories. However, the challenges of expanding biologically active cells for clinical use are substantial. Nevertheless a variety of strategies are under development supported by animal modeling which, if successful, could substantially improve the outcomes for patients undergoing aHCT.

IL-2 activated stem cell products

Activation of BM or mobilized PBPCs with IL-2 *ex vivo* followed by reinfusion of the activated cells as both the source of hematopoietic stem cells and immune effector cells is a strategy based upon animal investigations which has resulted in engraftment and GVT effects [81]. Effective purging of malignant cells was achieved without substantial toxicity to hematologic precursors [82,83]. A clinical trial has been pursued in 36 patients with hematologic malignancies where the cells were incubated with IL-2 for 24 h prior to infusion. Thereafter, patients received low-dose IL-2 by continuous intravenous infusion until hematologic recovery and then for additional maintenance cycles. In this setting the IL-2 administered after transplantation was found to retard hematologic recovery and was therefore discontinued. Of 24 patients with NHL, 9 remain in CCR and, of 12 acute leukemia patients treated, five remained in CCR at the time of publication [84].

IL-2 activated NK cells

Several groups have explored the use of IL-2 activated NK cells following aHCT. In these clinical trials PBMCs are extracted from the patient generally by apheresis and then incubated *ex vivo* for several days in the presence of IL-2. The resultant cells are then reinfused into the patient. Since the majority of animal models have indicated that exogenous IL-2 is also required for an *in vivo* effect this cytokine is administered following the infusion of cells. The requirement for IL-2 has made these studies difficult to interpret since this treatment alone may increase toxicity on the one hand and have a biological effect on the other. Benyunes and colleagues have performed several feasibility trials using this approach in patients with hematologic malignancies following transplantation [58]. As previously discussed, 16 patients with NHL and five patients with AML underwent treatment with IL-2 activated NK cells and intravenous administration of IL-2. The treatment was generally well tolerated, although in some patients there was difficulty in performing the apheresis due to low platelet counts.

An additional 12 patients (11 NHL and one with breast cancer) were treated in the immediate post-transplant period with IL-2 activated NK cells followed by IL-2 [85]. Patients tolerated the treatment reasonably well and had increases in circulating NK cells in the blood. To further assess the toxicity of these treatment approaches, a small study of 15 patients was reported where five patients received no further therapy following aHCT, five patients were treated with IL-2 at a dose of 2×10^6 IU/m^2/day for 4 days by continuous intravenous infusion and five additional patients were treated with autologous IL-2 activated NK cells and IL-2. All patients had stable grafts and there were no significant differences in severe toxicities further documenting that this form of treatment is reasonably well tolerated [86].

Due to the difficulties of obtaining adequate numbers of cells, the relatively poor expansion of NK cells, the modest *in vitro* antitumor effects and the difficulty in interpreting results with the coadministration of IL-2, studies have focused on the effects of IL-2 alone. As discussed above, promising phase II results have been obtained and phase III studies are ongoing. Other populations of effector cells have been explored which avoid some of these problems.

Natural killer (NK) cell lines

Several different cell lines have been established which have phenotypic and functional properties similar to NK cells except that these cell lines can be propagated long-term in culture. These cell lines have broad antitumor cytotoxicity against tumor cell lines *in vitro* and in animal models *in vivo*. The human cytotoxic TALL-104 cell line developed from a child with acute T-cell lymphoblastic leukemia has been extensively evaluated. This cell line has been continuously cultured, has the cell surface phenotype of $\alpha\beta TCR^+$, $CD3^+$, $CD4^-$, $CD8^+$, $CD16^-$, and $CD56^+$, lyses a broad array of tumor targets yet spares certain normal tissues [87]. TALL-104 cells have been effective in both murine and canine models of malignancy without the coadministration of IL-2 [88,89]. Biodistribution of TALL-104 cells following intravenous infusion was evaluated using ^{111}In labeling techniques. In these studies the cells were visualized in the lungs for the first 2 h followed by distribution to the liver, spleen and kidneys [90]. This approach has been extended to clinical trials in 15 patients with metastatic breast cancer where from 10^6 to 10^8 TALL-104 cells were administered for 5 consecutive days followed by monthly maintenance infusions. Toxicity was acceptable except for one episode of grade IV hepatic necrosis. Of the 15 patients treated, nine patients progressed within 1 month, five patients had stable disease, one patient had documented improvement in liver metastases and one patient had clinical improvement in bone pain [91].

Another cell line which has been adapted to continuous growth in culture termed NK-92 has phenotypic and functional features of NK cells ($CD2^+$, $CD3^-$, $CD8^-$, $CD16^-$, $CD56^+$). NK-92 cells lyse a broad array of tumor cell lines [92]. NK-92 cells have been used to simulate tumor cell purging of intentionally contaminated PBPC grafts where K562 erythroleukemia cells were successfully eliminated without any significant effects on hematopoietic progenitor cells [93]. NK-92 cells have also been shown to effectively recognize fresh acute leukemia blasts [94]. Clinical trials using this cell line have also been initiated. A significant limitation of the use of these cytolytic lines may be the short *in vivo* survival of the effector cells in allogeneic hosts.

A third cell line termed NKL was established from the PB of a patient with large granular lymphocytic leukemia. This cell line has the cell surface phenotype of $CD3^-$, $CD16^+$, $CD56^+$ typical of NK cells [95]. Due to the cell surface expression of CD16 these cells are capable of antibody dependent cellular cytotoxicity based killing mechanisms.

Cytokine induced killer (CIK) cells

An alternative population of effector cells which share properties with both T cells and NK cells can be expanded by the timed addition of interferon-gamma (IFN-γ), antibodies to CD3 and IL-2 [96,97]. These cells termed cytokine induced killer (CIK) cells, expand rapidly, demonstrate cytotoxic activity both *in vitro* and *in vivo* independent of coadministration of IL-2. CIK cells were shown to be superior to IL-2 activated NK cells in protecting SCID mice from an otherwise lethal challenge of NHL [98]. Following culture of cells under these conditions for 14–21 days there is a dramatic expansion of $CD3^+$ T cells with approximately 20–50% of the cells coexpressing the NK cell marker CD56 such that the population of $CD3^+CD56^+$ cells may expand up to 1000-fold. The addition of IFN induces IL-12 production from resident monocytes, which also provide costimulatory signals through LFA-3/CD2 resulting in the expansion of $CD3^+CD56^+$ cells [99]. The $CD3^+CD56^+$ population of cells was shown to have the greatest cytotoxic activity and these cells were derived from T cell and not NK cell precursors [98]. CIK cells produce a variety of T-helper type 1 subset (T_H1)-type cytokines, such as IFN, TNF-α and GM-CSF, as well as up-regulate several key molecules required for effector function such as perforin, granzymes and Fas ligand. CIK cells have broad cytolytic activity against a variety of cell lines of hematologic origin such as OCI-Ly-3 and SU-DHL-4 (NHL), K562 (erythroleukemia) and Daudi (T-cell NHL). In addition, CIK cells have been shown to have *in vitro* cytolytic activity against autologous myeloid but generally not lymphoid leukemic blasts [100,101]. Further studies utilizing a SCID model of chronic myeloid leukemia (CML) demonstrated that autologous CIK cells, which were Philadelphia chromosome negative (Ph^-), resulted in clearance of autologous Ph^+ CML cells and, in some instances, Epstein–Barr virus (EBV)-induced lymphoma assessed by molecular studies of tissues and human hematopoietic colonies extracted from these animals [102]. A population of murine-derived CIK cells have been generated using the same culture conditions which have similar phenotypic, cytokine production and cytotoxic function. These cells protect syngeneic animals from an otherwise lethal challenge of the B-cell lymphoma Bcl_1 [103]. Further studies have been performed utilizing syngeneic murine CIK cells in a novel bioluminescence model, which allows for the quantitative assessment of tumor burden or lymphocyte homing and survival following the introduction of the light-emitting luciferase gene. Following gene-marking, the CIK cells could be visualized following intravenous injection. Initially the cells were found in the lungs, however, by 24 h there was distribution to other sites including the liver and spleen and by 3 days infiltration of a subcutaneous tumor nodule was evident. The cells persisted at the tumor site for an additional 9 days associated with resolution of the malignancy [104]. This novel system allows for the dissection of all of the steps required for an effective cell population including intravenous injection, exit from the lungs, homing to tumor and eradication of disease.

CIK cells have been expanded from patients with a variety of malignancies by culturing mobilized PBPCs with similar phenotypic and functional properties as compared to cells expanded from normal donors [100]. Based upon these preclinical data, a phase I clinical trial was performed to assess feasibility and safety [105]. In this study nine patients were enrolled based upon the entry criteria of advanced disease without other curative therapeutic options, adequate end organ and hematologic function and informed consent. All of these patients had failed a prior aHCT procedure. Seven patients had NHL and two patients had HD. A dose escalation format was utilized starting at a cell dose of 1×10^9 cells with two other dose levels of 5×10^9 and 1×10^{10} cells. Patients were allowed to receive more than one dose if there were no grade III or IV toxicities and no progression of disease. The planned cell dose was achieved in 19 of 21 infusions. Toxicity was minimal indicating the feasibility and tolerability of this treatment strategy. Although disease response was not the endpoint, two patients attained partial responses and two patients had disease stability, one for over 18 months.

A similar strategy was utilized in a randomized study of patients with hepatomas where following surgical resection patients were randomized to receive the cellular therapy or no additional treatment [106]. Those patients who received the T-cell based therapy had a significantly enhanced relapse-free survival as compared to untreated controls.

Another small phase I study of CIK cells transfected with the *IL-2* gene also demonstrated the feasibility and tolerability of clinical treatment [107]. Further studies of CIK cells are planned in patients with HD and AML following aHCT in an effort to reduce disease relapse.

Cytotoxic T lymphocytes (CTLs)

The enhanced specificity of CTLs that recognize target cells through interaction between the T-cell receptor and peptides expressed in the context of MHC molecules have made this treatment strategy an attractive goal. Developing T cells with antitumor activity has been challenging. Several different strategies have been employed including expanding tumor infiltrating T cells or attempting to expand and activate T cells directed against particular antigens [108]. One approach has been to isolate and expand CTLs against EBV-associated proteins in an effort to treat or reduce the risk of EBV-associated lympoproliferative disorders (EBV-LPD) [109]. These studies demonstrated that cell lines directed against EBV-associated antigens could be expanded *ex vivo* and the infused CTL lines were effective in reducing the risk of EBV-LPD [110]. Since EBV antigens are expressed in approximately 50% of patients with HD further studies have been performed in an effort to treat chemo-resistant disease. EBV-specific CTLs are currently under exploration both in the setting of patients with HD who have relapsed following transplantation and following autologous transplantation in an effort to reduce disease relapse. In a preliminary report 13 patients with HD of whom nine had active disease and four were in CR following aHCT were enrolled. CTL lines directed against EBV-associated antigens, including LMP2a, which is expressed on HD cells, were successfully generated from nine of 13 patients. The CTL lines were gene-marked and infused into three patients with recurrent disease. The CTLs persisted *in vivo* for more than 13 weeks in some instances and were associated with antiviral effects in the treated patients [111]. Further studies are ongoing, especially in patients following aHCT where patients are in a state of MRD.

Another strategy has been to genetically engineer T cells to express chimeric antibody receptors which direct the cells towards lineage specific proteins. For example, CTLs have been engineered to express antibody against CD19 or CD20 for patients with B-cell ALL or NHL [112]. These elegant strategies offer the possibility of enhanced biological activity. Phase I/II studies are underway to explore the feasibility and potential efficacy of this treatment strategy.

CTLs have also been generated *ex vivo* following exposure to dendritic cells (DCs) pulsed with antigens derived from tumor tissues. DCs are the most potent and effective antigen-presenting cells (APCs) which express all of the cell surface determinants required for generating an effective immune response such as MHC, adhesion and costimulatory molecules [113]. DCs can be directly isolated from the blood, expanded from mononuclear or CD34+ cells by the timed addition of cytokines such as IL-4, GM-CSF and CD40 ligand. CD34+ cells from patients with leukemia have also been used as APCs in an effort to generate a tumor specific CTL response [114]. Following isolation DCs are pulsed with tumor-derived antigens such as peptides, proteins, RNA or tumor lysates (Fig. 102.3). The source of DCs, optimal material for cell pulsing, route of administration and dose all remain significant issues that need to be resolved. Nevertheless,

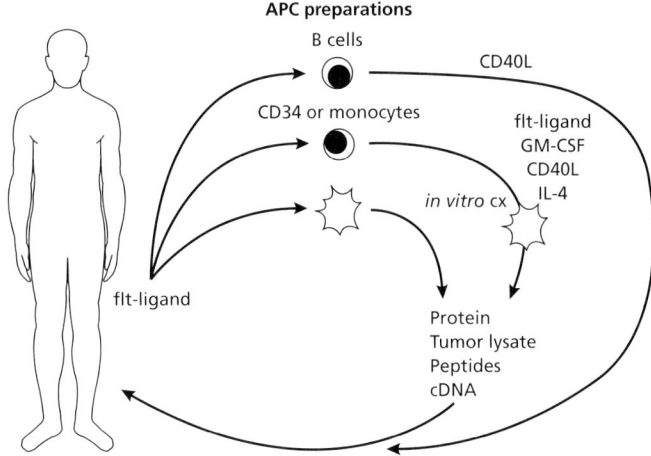

Fig. 102.3 Strategies for presentation of tumor antigens to generate antitumor immunological responses.

this strategy holds significant appeal due to the potential of generating tumor specific immune responses.

One potential target structure that has been extensively evaluated is the idiotype (Id) protein which is a tumor specific antigen in patients with B-cell malignancies such as NHL and MM. Treatment of patients with MM may be more suitable because the Id-protein can be readily isolated from PB. The monoclonal Id protein isolated by standard protein purification strategies has been used to pulse DCs, which can be used as a way of stimulating T cells *ex vivo* or infused directly into patients as a vaccine. Following Id-pulsing of DCs in two patients with MM, CTLs were generated that were shown to be capable of lysing the pulsed DCs and autologous MM targets [115]. These CTLs were generated following repetitive exposure of T cells to Id-pulsed DCs in the presence of IL-2 and IL-7. The CTLs were primarily CD8+ T cells, MHC class I restricted and functioned through a perforin mediated mechanism. Other target structures have also been utilized in an effort to generate CTLs directed against tumor targets including proteinase 3 which is over-expressed in patients with AML and CML, *bcr-abl* for patients with CML and subtypes of ALL and Her2/*neu* for patients with subtypes of breast cancer to name a few [116–118]. An alternative approach has been to use tumor cell lysates or RNA to pulse the DCs and allow the immune system to recognize tumor specific determinants [119–121]. For example, tumor cells were isolated from patients with MM and a tumor lysate prepared by repetitive freeze-thaw cycles. Following exposure to DCs the resultant APCs were used to generate CTLs after pulsing *in vitro*. Both cytolytic CD4+ and CD8+ T cells could be generated which killed autologous DCs and primary MM cells. These CTLs were class-I restricted, produced cytokines upon exposure to pulsed DCs and functioned through a perforin mediated mechanism [121]. Interestingly, CTLs from two of four patients had a weak response to Id. These studies have demonstrated the feasibility of developing CTLs that are reactive with tumor tissue, but their clinical utility has yet to be assessed.

An alternative approach has been to isolate DCs either directly from the PB or expanded from CD34+ precursor cells, pulse with antigen and then directly infuse these cells as a vaccine into patients. Significant antitumor responses have been observed following the infusion of Id-pulsed DCs in patients with recurrent NHL in the nontransplant setting [122]. A similar strategy was pursued in 12 patients with NHL following aHCT. Idiotype was rescued from the patient's lymphoma cells, coupled to keyhole limpet hemocyanin (KLH) and used to pulse autologous DC followed by reinfusion into the patients 2–12 months following transplantation. KLH responses were observed in all patients indicating that patients are capable of responding to such a vaccination strategy after aHCT [123]. Importantly, 10 of 12 patients mounted either a humoral or cellular anti-Id response and seven of the patients have enjoyed prolonged clinical remissions of 3–11 years. A significant challenge limiting the application of this strategy was the difficulty in isolating Id from patients with NHL since many patients had already received salvage chemotherapy and were in remission such that tumor tissue was inaccessible. Nonetheless, further studies are warranted.

A similar strategy has been employed in patients with MM since this disease is also characterized by the production of Id protein; however, unlike patients with NHL, the Id protein is readily accessible in PB [124]. A clinical trial has been initiated in patients with MM following transplantation as these patients benefit from high-dose therapy, but few, if any, will be cured of their disease. In one study, 26 patients with MM underwent high-dose chemotherapy and autologous transplantation followed by two infusions of Id-pulsed DCs and subcutaneous boosts of Id coupled to KLH. The infusions of the DCs and Id-KLH were generally well tolerated with only transient and minor side-effects. Twenty-four of 26 patients generated a KLH-specific response as assessed by cellular proliferation in the presence of antigen. However, only four patients developed an Id-specific immune response, of which three were in CR prior to the infusions [125,126]. A similar strategy was utilized to treat an additional three patients with this disease where CD8$^+$ T cells could be detected in the PB of vaccinated patients. Cells from one patient were found to be capable of lysing autologous myeloma cells and to be class I restricted [127]. These studies demonstrate the feasibility and tolerability of this treatment strategy; however, they also raise caution that at least in MM a CR may be required to achieve an immunological response. This requirement may be due to the high circulating quantities of Id in patients who do not achieve a CR. Possibly other antigens, cell dose or vaccination strategies may be more effective in generating tumor specific immune responses. Additional studies are required to further document response rates and to determine what clinical benefits are achieved in responding patients.

Immunomodulation therapies

Several other strategies have been explored in an effort to stimulate an immune response following aHCT. One approach, documented with well constructed animal studies has been the observation that following treatment with CSP an immunological reaction similar to GVHD is generated upon withdrawal of the immunosuppressive drug (see Chapter 30). CTLs have been isolated from rodents treated in this fashion that are reactive with class II determinants expressed on tumor cell targets [128].

This strategy has been extended to phase I/II clinical trials. In one study, 51 women with metastatic breast cancer who underwent aHCT were treated with escalating doses of CSP of 1, 2.5 and 3.75 mg/kg/day for 28 days starting on the day of BM infusion. A clinical syndrome similar to skin GVHD developed in a high proportion of patients in a dose-dependent fashion [129]. Laboratory studies on the CD8$^+$ T cells isolated from these patients demonstrated that the cells were $\alpha\beta$TCR$^+$, recognized MHC determinants which could be blocked with an antibody directed against a peptide from the invariant chain [130]. A similar strategy was employed to treat 40 patients with NHL following aHCT. DFS was reported to be 77% at 2 years of follow-up in this cohort of patients [131]. A phase I clinical trial combining CSP and IFN was reported where the CSP was utilized at a dose of 1 mg/kg/day starting on day 0 followed by IFN-γ at a dose of 0.025 mg/m^2 every other day upon early recovery of the white blood cell count for a total of 10 doses. Sixteen patients with hematologic malignancies were treated of whom seven were alive and free of disease at a median of 3 years follow-up [132]. These cumulative results appear favorable; however, randomized clinical trials will be necessary to fully evaluate the potential benefits of this treatment approach.

Conclusions

Autologous HCT has emerged as an effective treatment strategy for patients with a variety of hematologic malignancies and selected patients with solid tumors. With the development of mobilized PBPCs the safety of aHCT has clearly been enhanced. The majority of patients achieve a state of MRD yet relapse remains the most significant cause of treatment failure. A variety of strategies, detailed in this chapter, are under active preclinical and clinical investigation in an effort to reduce the risk of relapse. The virtual explosion of information concerning normal immune function, tumor recognition and escape mechanisms has resulted in strategies which are likely to have a significant impact on the risk of disease relapse. Following aHCT appears to be an ideal clinical setting in which to test these treatment approaches.

References

1 Philip T, Guglielmi C, Hagenbeek A et al. Autologous bone marrow transplantation as compared with salvage chemotherapy in relapses of chemotherapy-sensitive non-Hodgkin's lymphoma [see comments]. N Engl J Med 1995; 333: 1540–5.

2 Attal M, Harousseau JL, Stoppa AM et al. A prospective, randomized trial of autologous bone marrow transplantation and chemotherapy in multiple myeloma. Intergroupe Francais Myelome. N Engl J Med 1996; 335: 91–7.

3 Johnsen HE, Bjorkstrand B, Carlson K et al. Outcome for patients with leukemia, multiple myeloma and lymphoma who relapse after high dose therapy and autologous stem cell support. Leuk Lymphoma 1996; 24: 81–91.

4 Vaishampayan U, Du Karanes CW, Varterasian M, al-Katib A. Outcome of relapsed non-Hodgkin's lymphoma patients after allogeneic and autologous transplantation. Cancer Invest 2002; 20: 303–10.

5 Tsai T, Goodman S, Saez R et al. Allogeneic bone marrow transplantation in patients who relapse after autologous transplantation. Bone Marrow Transplant 1997; 20: 859–63.

6 di Grazia C, Raiola AM, Van Lint MT et al. Conventional hematopoietic stem cell transplants from identical or alternative donors are feasible in recipients relapsing after an autograft. Haematologica 2001; 86: 646–51.

7 Radich JP, Gooley T, Sanders JE, Anasetti C, Chauncey T, Appelbaum FR. Second allogeneic transplantation after failure of first autologous transplantation. Biol Blood Marrow Transplant 2000; 6: 272–9.

8 Ringden O, Labopin M, Gorin NC et al. The dismal outcome in patients with acute leukaemia who relapse after an autograft is improved if a second autograft or a matched allograft is performed. Acute Leukaemia Working Party of the European Group for Blood and Marrow Transplantation (EBMT). Bone Marrow Transplant 2000; 25: 1053–8.

9 Blau IW, Basara N, Bischoff M et al. Second allogeneic hematopoietic stem cell transplantation as treatment for leukemia relapsing following a first transplant. Bone Marrow Transplant 2000; 25: 41–5.

10 Martinez C, Carreras E, Rovira M et al. Allogenic stem cell transplantation as salvage therapy for patients relapsing after autologous transplantation: experience from a single institution. Leuk Res 2001; 25: 379–84.

11 Hale GA, Tong X, Benaim E et al. Allogeneic bone marrow transplantation in children failing prior autologous bone marrow transplantation. Bone Marrow Transplant 2001; 27: 155–62.

12 Nagler A, Or R, Naparstek E, Varadi G, Slavin S. Second allogeneic stem cell transplantation using nonmyeloablative conditioning for patients who relapsed or developed secondary malignancies following autologous transplantation. Exp Hematol 2000; 28: 1096–104.

13 Porter DL, Luger SM, Duffy KM et al. Allogeneic cell therapy for patients who relapse after autologous stem cell transplantation. Biol Blood Marrow Transplant 2001; 7: 230–8.

14 Dey BR, McAfee S, Sackstein R et al. Successful allogeneic stem cell transplantation with nonmyeloablative conditioning in patients with relapsed hematologic malignancy following autologous stem cell transplantation. Biol Blood Marrow Transplant 2001; 7: 604–12.

15 Corradini P, Tarella C, Olivieri A et al. Reduced-intensity conditioning followed by allografting of hematopoietic cells can produce clinical and molecular remissions in patients with poor-risk hematologic malignancies. Blood 2002; 99: 75–82.

16 Maloney DG, Molina AJ, Sahebi F et al. Nonmyeloablative allografting following cytoreductive autografts for the treatment of patients with multiple myeloma. Blood, in press.

17 Singhal S, Mehta J, Desikan R et al. Antitumor activity of thalidomide in refractory multiple myeloma. N Engl J Med 1999; 341: 1565–71.

18 Zomas A, Anagnostopoulos N, Dimopoulos MA. Successful treatment of multiple myeloma relapsing after high-dose therapy and autologous transplantation with thalidomide as a single agent. Bone Marrow Transplant 2000; 25: 1319–20.

19 Tosi P, Ronconi S, Zamagni E et al. Salvage therapy with thalidomide in multiple myeloma patients relapsing after autologous peripheral blood stem cell transplantation. Haematologica 2001; 86: 409–13.

20 Tosi P, Zamagni E, Cellini C et al. Salvage therapy with thalidomide in patients with advanced relapsed/refractory multiple myeloma. Haematologica 2002; 87: 408–14.

21 Alexanian R, Weber D, Giralt S, Delasalle K. Consolidation therapy of multiple myeloma with thalidomide-dexamethasone after intensive chemotherapy. Ann Oncol 2002; 13: 1116–9.

22 Godder KT, Metha J, Chiang KY et al. Partially mismatched related donor bone marrow transplantation as salvage for patients with AML who failed autologous stem cell transplant. Bone Marrow Transplant 2001; 28: 1031–6.

23 Aversa F, Tabilio A, Velardi A et al. Transplantation for high-risk acute leukemia with high doses of T-cell-depleted hematopoietic stem cells from full-haplotype incompatible donors. N Engl J Med 1998; 339: 1186–93.

24 Sykes M, Preffer F, McAfee S et al. Mixed lymphohaemopoietic chimerism and graft-versus-lymphoma effects after non-myeloablative therapy and HLA-mismatched bone-marrow transplantation. Lancet 1999; 353: 1755–9.

25 O'Donnell PV, Luznik L, Jones RJ et al. Nonmyeloablative bone marrow transplantation from partially HLA-mismatched related donors using posttransplantation cyclophosphamide. Biol Blood Marrow Transplant 2002; 8: 377–86.

26 Gian VG, Moreb JS, Abdel-Mageed A, Weeks FM, Scornick JC, Wingard JR. Successful salvage using mismatched umbilical cord blood transplant in an adult with recurrent acute myelogenous leukemia failing autologous peripheral blood progenitor cell transplant. A case history and review. Bone Marrow Transplant 1998; 21: 1197–200.

27 Shimokawa T, Ohashi H, Takaue Y, Kawano Y, Abe T, Kuroda Y. Successful umbilical cord blood transplantation in an infant with ALL failing initial autologous peripheral blood stem cell transplantation. Med Pediatr Oncol 2002; 38: 60–1.

28 Gianni AM, Bregni M, Siena S et al. High-dose chemotherapy and autologous bone marrow transplantation compared with MACOP-B in aggressive B-cell lymphoma [see comments]. N Engl J Med 1997; 336: 1290–7.

29 Nademanee A, Molina A, O'Donnell MR et al. Results of high-dose therapy and autologous bone marrow/stem cell transplantation during remission in poor-risk intermediate- and high-grade lymphoma: international index high and high-intermediate risk group. Blood 1997; 90: 3844–52.

30 Haioun C, Lepage E, Gisselbrecht C et al. Comparison of autologous bone marrow transplantation with sequential chemotherapy for intermediate-grade and high-grade non-Hodgkin's lymphoma in first complete remission: a study of 464 patients. Groupe d'Etude des Lymphomes de l'Adulte [see comments]. J Clin Oncol 1994; 12: 2543–51.

31 Long GD, Negrin RS, Hoyle C et al. Multiple cycles of high dose chemotherapy supported by hematopoietic progenitor cells as treatment for patients with advanced malignancies. Cancer 1995; 76: 860–8.

32 Schilder RJ, Shea TC. Multiple cycles of high-dose chemotherapy for ovarian cancer. Semin Oncol 1998; 25: 349–55.

33 Hu WW, Negrin RS, Stockerl-Goldstein K et al. Four-cycle high-dose therapy with hematopoietic support for metastatic breast cancer: no improvement in outcomes compared with single-course high-dose therapy. Biol Blood Marrow Transplant 2000; 6: 58–69.

34 Barlogie B, Jagannath S, Vesole DH et al. Superiority of tandem autologous transplantation over standard therapy for previously untreated multiple myeloma. Blood 1997; 89: 789–93.

35 Matthews DC, Appelbaum FR, Eary JF et al. Phase I study of ^{131}I-anti-CD45 antibody plus cyclophosphamide and total body irradiation for advanced acute leukemia and myelodysplastic syndrome. Blood 1999; 94: 1237–47.

36 Press OW, Eary JF, Gooley T et al. A phase I/II trial of iodine-131-tositumomab (anti-CD20), etoposide, cyclophosphamide, and autologous stem cell transplantation for relapsed B-cell lymphomas. Blood 2000; 96: 2934–42.

37 Bunjes D, Buchmann I, Duncker C et al. Rhenium 188-labeled anti-CD66 (a, b, c, e) monoclonal antibody to intensify the conditioning regimen prior to stem cell transplantation for patients with high-risk acute myeloid leukemia or myelodysplastic syndrome: results of a phase I–II study. Blood 2001; 98: 565–72.

38 Mundt AJ, Sibley G, Williams S, Hallahan D, Nautiyal J, Weichselbaum RR. Patterns of failure following high-dose chemotherapy and autologous bone marrow transplantation with involved field radiotherapy for relapsed/refractory Hodgkin's disease. Int J Radiat Oncol Biol Phys 1995; 33: 261–70.

39 Pezner RD, Nademanee A, Forman SJ. High-dose therapy and autologous bone marrow transplantation for Hodgkin's disease patients with relapses potentially treatable by radical radiation therapy. Int J Radiat Oncol Biol Phys 1995; 33: 189–94.

40 Chao MW, Wirth A, Ryan G, MacManus M, Liew KH. Radiation myelopathy following transplantation and radiotherapy for non-Hodgkin's lymphoma. Int J Radiat Oncol Biol Phys 1998; 41: 1057–61.

41 Poen JC, Hoppe RT, Horning SJ. High-dose therapy and autologous bone marrow transplantation for relapsed/refractory Hodgkin's disease: the impact of involved field radiotherapy on patterns of failure and survival. Int J Radiat Oncol Biol Phys 1996; 36: 3–12.

42 Miller CB, Zehnbauer BA, Piantadosi S, Rowley SD, Jones RJ. Correlation of occult clonogenic leukemia drug sensitivity with relapse after autologous bone marrow transplantation. Blood 1991; 78: 1125–31.

43 Gribben JG, Freedman AS, Neuberg D et al. Immunologic purging of marrow assessed by PCR before autologous bone marrow transplanation for B-cell lymphoma. N Engl J Med 1991; 325: 1525–33.

44 Brenner MK, Rill DR, Moen RC et al. Gene-marking to trace origin of relapse after autologous bone-marrow transplantation. Lancet 1993; 341: 85–6.

45 Deisseroth AB, Zu Z, Claxton D et al. Genetic marking shows that Ph+ cells present in autologous transplants of chronic myelogenous leukemia (CML) contribute to relapse after autologous bone marrow in CML. Blood 1994; 83: 3068–76.

46 Negrin RS, Kiem HP, Schmidt-Wolf IG, Blume KG, Cleary ML. Use of the polymerase chain reaction to monitor the effectiveness of ex vivo tumor cell purging. Blood 1991; 77: 654–60.

47 Negrin RS, Pesando J. Detection of tumor cells in purged bone marrow and peripheral blood mononuclear cells by polymerase chain reaction amplification of bcl-2 translocations. J Clin Oncol 1994; 12: 1021–7.

48 Vescio R, Schiller G, Stewart AK et al. Multicenter phase III trial to evaluate CD34+ selected versus unselected autologous peripheral blood progenitor cell transplantation in multiple myeloma. Blood 1999; 93: 1858–68.

49 Negrin RS, Atkinson K, Leemhuis T et al. Transplantation of highly purified CD34+Thy-1+ hematopoietic stem cells in patients with metastatic breast cancer. Biol Blood Marrow Transplant 2000; 6: 262–71.

50 Kolb HJ, Schattenberg A, Goldman JM et al. Graft-versus-leukemia effect of donor lymphocyte transfusions in marrow grafted patients. Blood 1995; 86: 2041–50.

51 Ruggeri L, Capanni M, Urbani E et al. Effectiveness of donor natural killer cell alloreactivity in mismatched hematopoietic transplants. Science 2002; 295: 2097–100.

52 Siegel JP, Puri RK. Interleukin-2 toxicity. J Clin Oncol 1991; 9: 694–704.

53 Welte KG, Ciobanu N, Moore MAS, Gulati S, O'Reilly RJ, Mertelsmann R. Defective interleukin-2 production in patients after bone marrow transplantation and in vitro restoration of defective T lymphocyte proliferation by highly purified interleukin-2. Blood 1984; 64: 380–5.

54 Cayeux S, Meuer S, Pezzutto A et al. T-cell ontogeny after autologous bone marrow transplantation: failure to synthesize interleukin-2 (IL-2) and lack of CD2- and CD3-mediated proliferation by both CD4− and CD8+ cells even in the presence of exogenous IL-2. Blood 1989; 74: 2270–7.

55 Blaise D, Olive D, Stoppa AM et al. Hematologic and immunologic effects of the systemic administration of recombinant interleukin-2 after autologous bone marrow transplantation. Blood 1990; 76: 1092–7.

56 Higuchi CM, Thompson JA, Petersen FB, Buckner CD, Fefer A. Toxicity and immunomodulatory effects of interleukin-2 after autologous bone marrow transplantation for hematologic malignancies. Blood 1991; 77: 2561–8.

57 Bosly A, Guillaume T, Brice P et al. Effects of escalating doses of recombinant human interleukin-2 in correcting functional T-cell defects following autologous bone marrow transplantation for lymphomas and solid tumors. *Exp Hematol* 1992; **20**: 962–8.

58 Benyunes MC, Massumoto C, York A et al. Interleukin-2 with or without lymphokine-activated killer cells as consolidative immunotherapy after autologous bone marrow transplantation for acute myelogenous leukemia. *Bone Marrow Transplant* 1993; **12**: 159–63.

59 Hamon MD, Prentice HG, Gottlieb DJ et al. Immunotherapy with interleukin 2 after ABMT in AML. *Bone Marrow Transplant* 1993; **11**: 399–401.

60 Stein AS, O'Donnell MR, Slovak ML et al. Interleukin-2 following autologous stem cell transplant for adult patients with acute myeloid leukemia in first complete remission. *J Clin Oncol* 2003; **21**: 615–23.

61 Attal M, Blaise D, Marit G et al. Consolidation treatment of adult acute lymphoblastic leukemia: a prospective, randomized trial comparing allogeneic versus autologous bone marrow transplantation and testing the impact of recombinant interleukin-2 after autologous bone marrow transplantation. *Blood* 1995; **86**: 1619–28.

62 Lauria F, Raspadori D, Ventura MA et al. Immunologic and clinical modifications following low-dose subcutaneous administration of rIL-2 in non-Hodgkin's lymphoma patients after autologous bone marrow transplantation. *Bone Marrow Transplant* 1996; **18**: 79–85.

63 Nagler A, Ackerstein A, Or R, Naparstek E, Slavin S. Immunotherapy with recombinant human interleukin-2 and recombinant interferon-alpha in lymphoma patients postautologous marrow or stem cell transplantation. *Blood* 1997; **89**: 3951–9.

64 Soiffer RJ, Murray C, Cochran K et al. Clinical and immunologic effects of prolonged infusion of low-dose recombinant interleukin-2 after autologous and T-cell-depleted allogeneic bone marrow transplantation. *Blood* 1992; **79**: 517–26.

65 Miller JS, Tessmer-Tuck J, Pierson BA et al. Low dose subcutaneous interleukin-2 after autologous transplantation generates sustained *in vivo* natural killer cell activity. *Biol Blood Marrow Transplant* 1997; **3**: 34–44.

66 Lopez-Jimenez J, Perez-Oteyza J, Munoz A et al. Subcutaneous versus intravenous low-dose IL-2 therapy after autologous transplantation: results of a prospective, non-randomized study. *Bone Marrow Transplant* 1997; **19**: 429–34.

67 Atkins MB, Robertson MJ, Gordon M et al. Phase I evaluation of intravenous recombinant human interleukin 12 in patients with advanced malignancies. *Clin Cancer Res* 1997; **3**: 409–17.

68 Motzer RJ, Rakhit A, Schwartz LH et al. Phase I trial of subcutaneous recombinant human interleukin-12 in patients with advanced renal cell carcinoma. *Clin Cancer Res* 1998; **4**: 1183–91.

69 Robertson MJ, Cameron C, Atkins MB et al. Immunological effects of interleukin 12 administered by bolus intravenous injection to patients with cancer. *Clin Cancer Res* 1999; **5**: 9–16.

70 Fehniger TA, Carson WE, Mrozek E, Caligiuri MA. Stem cell factor enhances interleukin-2-mediated expansion of murine natural killer cells *in vivo*. *Blood* 1997; **90**: 3647–53.

71 Yu H, Fehniger TA, Fuchshuber P et al. Flt3 ligand promotes the generation of a distinct CD34+ human natural killer cell progenitor that responds to interleukin-15. *Blood* 1998; **92**: 3647–57.

72 Flinn IW, O'Donnell PV, Goodrich A et al. Immunotherapy with rituximab during peripheral blood stem cell transplantation for non-Hodgkin's lymphoma. *Biol Blood Marrow Transplant* 2000; **6**: 628–32.

73 Lazzarino M, Arcaini L, Bernasconi P et al. A sequence of immuno-chemotherapy with Rituximab, mobilization of *in vivo* purged stem cells, high-dose chemotherapy and autotransplant is an effective and non-toxic treatment for advanced follicular and mantle cell lymphoma. *Br J Haematol* 2002; **116**: 229–35.

74 Flohr T, Hess G, Kolbe K et al. Rituximab *in vivo* purging is safe and effective in combination with CD34-positive selected autologous stem cell transplantation for salvage therapy in B-NHL. *Bone Marrow Transplant* 2002; **29**: 769–75.

75 Berkahn L, Simpson D, Raptis A, Klingemann HG. In vivo purging with rituximab prior to collection of stem cells for autologous transplantation in chronic lymphocytic leukemia. *J Hematother Stem Cell Res* 2002; **11**: 315–20.

76 Horwitz SM, Negrin RS, Blume KG et al. Rituximab as adjuvant to high dose therapy and autologous hematopoietic cell transplantation for aggressive non-Hodgkin's lymphoma. *Blood*, in press.

77 Link BK, Weiner GJ. Production and characterization of a bispecific IgG capable of inducing T-cell-mediated lysis of malignant B cells. *Blood* 1993; **81**: 3343–9.

78 Kaneko T, Fusauchi Y, Kakui Y et al. A bispecific antibody enhances cytokine-induced killer-mediated cytolysis of autologous acute myeloid leukemia cells. *Blood* 1993; **81**: 1333–41.

79 Scheffold C, Kornacker M, Scheffold YC, Contag CH, Negrin RS. Visualization of effective tumor targeting by CD8+ natural killer cells redirected with bispecific antibody F(ab′)2HER2xCD3. *Cancer Res* 2002; **62**: 5785–91.

80 James ND, Atherton PJ, Jones J, Howie AJ, Tchekmedyian S, Curnow RT. A phase II study of the bispecific antibody MDX-H210 (anti-HER2xCD64) with GM-CSF in HER2+ advanced prostate cancer. *Br J Cancer* 2001; **85**: 152–6.

81 Agah R, Malloy B, Kerner M, Mazumder A. Generation and characterization of IL-2 activated bone marrow cells as a potent graft vs. tumor effector in transplantation. *J Immuno* 1989; **143**: 3093–9.

82 Verma UN, Bagg A, Brown E, Mazumder A. Interleukin-2 activation of human bone marrow in long-term cultures: an effective strategy for purging and generation of anti-tumor cytotoxic effectors. *Bone Marrow Transplant* 1994; **13**: 115–23.

83 Klingemann HG, Deal H, Reid D, Eaves CJ. Design and validation of a clinically applicable culture procedure for the generation of interleukin-2 activated natural killer cells in human bone marrow autografts. *Exp Hematol* 1993; **21**: 1263–70.

84 Margolin KA, Van Besien K, Wright C et al. Interleukin-2-activated autologous bone marrow and peripheral blood stem cells in the treatment of acute leukemia and lymphoma. *Biol Blood Marrow Transplant* 1999; **5**: 36–45.

85 Lister J, Rybka WB, Donnenberg AD et al. Autologous peripheral blood stem cell transplantation and adoptive immunotherapy with activated natural killer cells in the immediate posttransplant period. *Clin Cancer Res* 1995; **1**: 607–14.

86 deMagalhaes-Silverman M, Donnenberg A, Lembersky B et al. Posttransplant adoptive immunotherapy with activated natural killer cells in patients with metastatic breast cancer. *J Immunother* 2000; **23**: 154–60.

87 Cesano A, Visonneau S, Cioe L, Clark SC, Rovera G, Santoli D. Reversal of acute myelogenous leukemia in humanized SCID mice using a novel adoptive transfer approach. *J Clin Invest* 1994; **94**: 1076–84.

88 Cesano A, Visonneau S, Jeglum KA et al. Phase I clinical trial with a human major histocompatibility complex nonrestricted cytotoxic T-cell line TALL-104 in dogs with advanced tumors. *Cancer Res* 1996; **56**: 3021–9.

89 Cesano A, Visonneau S, Pasquini S, Rovera G, Santoli D. Antitumor efficacy of a human major histocompatibility complex nonrestricted cytotoxic T-cell line TALL-104 in immunocompetent mice bearing syngeneic leukemia. *Cancer Res* 1996; **56**: 4444–52.

90 Cesano A, Visonneau S, Tran T, Santoli D. Biodistribution of human MHC non-restricted TALL-104 killer cells in healthy and tumor bearing mice. *Int J Oncol* 1999; **14**: 245–51.

91 Visonneau S, Cesano A, Porter DL et al. Phase I trial of TALL-104 cells in patients with refractory metastatic breast cancer. *Clin Cancer Res* 2000; **6**: 1744–54.

92 Gong JH, Maki G, Klingemann HG. Characterization of a human cell line NK-92 with phenotypical and functional characteristics of activated natural killer cells. *Leukemia* 1994; **8**: 652–8.

93 Klingemann HG, Miyagawa B. Purging of malignant cells from blood after short *ex vivo* incubation with NK-92 cells [letter; comment]. *Blood* 1996; **87**: 4913–4.

94 Yan Y, Steinherz P, Klingemann HG et al. Antileukemia activity of a natural killer cell line against human leukemias. *Clin Cancer Res* 1998; **4**: 2859–68.

95 Robertson MJ, Cochran KJ, Cameron C, Le JM, Tantravahi R, Ritz J. Characterization of a cell line, NKL, derived from an aggressive human natural killer cell leukemia. *Exp Hematol* 1996; **24**: 406–15.

96 Schmidt-Wolf IG, Lefterova P, Mehta BA et al. Phenotypic characterization and identification of effector cells involved in tumor cell recognition of cytokine-induced killer cells. *Exp Hematol* 1993; **21**: 1673–9.

97 Schmidt-Wolf IGH, Negrin RS, Kiem HP, Blume KG, Weissman IL. Use of a SCID mouse/human lymphoma model to evaluate cytokine-induced killer cells with potent antitumor cell activity. *J Exp Med* 1991; **174**: 139–49.

98 Lu PH, Negrin RS. A novel population of expanded human CD3+CD56+ cells derived from T cells with potent *in vivo* antitumor activity in mice with severe combined immunodeficiency. *J Immunol* 1994; **153**: 1687–96.

99 Lopez R, Waller E, Lu P, Negrin R. CD58/LFA-3 and IL-12 provided by activated monocytes are critical in the *in vitro* expansion and function of CD56+ T cells. *Canc Immunol Immunother* 2001; **49**: 629–40.

100 Alvarnas JC, Linn YC, Hope EG, Negrin RS. Expansion of cytotoxic CD3+CD56+ cells from peripheral blood progenitor cells of patients

undergoing autologous hematopoietic cell transplantation. *Biol Blood Marrow Transplant* 2001; **7**: 216–22.

101 Linn YC, Lau LC, Hui KM. Generation of cytokine-induced killer cells from leukaemic samples with *in vitro* cytotoxicity against autologous and allogeneic leukaemic blasts. *Br J Haematol* 2002; **116**: 78–86.

102 Hoyle C, Bangs CD, Chang P, Kamel O, Mehta B, Negrin RS. Expansion of Philadelphia chromosome-negative CD3$^+$CD56$^+$ cytotoxic cells from chronic myeloid leukemia patients: *in vitro* and *in vivo* efficacy in severe combined immuno-deficiency disease mice. *Blood* 1998; **92**: 3318–27.

103 Baker J, Verneris MR, Ito M, Shizuru JA, Negrin RS. Expansion of cytolytic CD8$^+$ natural killer T cells with limited capacity for graft-versus-host disease induction due to interferon gamma production. *Blood* 2001; **97**: 2923–31.

104 Edinger M, Cao Y, Verneris MR, Bachmann MH, Contag CH, Negrin RS. Revealing lymphoma growth and the efficacy of immune cell therapies using *in vivo* bioluminescence. *Blood* 2003; **101**: 640–8.

105 Leemhuis T, Wells S, Horn P, Scheffold C, Edinger M. Autologous cytokine-induced killer cells for the treatment of relapsed Hodgkin's disease and non-Hodgkin's lymphoma. *Blood* 2000; **96**: 839a [Abstract].

106 Takayama T, Sekine T, Makuuchi M *et al*. Adoptive immunotherapy to lower postsurgical recurrence rates of hepatocellular carcinoma: a randomised trial. *Lancet* 2000; **356**: 802–7.

107 Schmidt-Wolf IG, Finke S, Trojaneck B *et al*. Phase I clinical study applying autologous immunological effector cells transfected with the interleukin-2 gene in patients with metastatic renal cancer, colorectal cancer and lymphoma. *Br J Cancer* 1999; **81**: 1009–16.

108 Rosenberg SA, Packard BS, Aebersold PM *et al*. Use of tumor-infiltrating lymphocytes and interleukin-2 in the immunotherapy of patients with metastatic melanoma. A preliminary report. *N Engl J Med* 1988; **319**: 1676–80.

109 Rooney CM, Smith CA, Ng CYC *et al*. Use of gene-modified virus-specific T lymphocytes to control Epstein-Barr-virus related lymphoproliferation. *Lancet* 1995; **345**: 9–13.

110 Rooney CM, Smith CA, Ng CY *et al*. Infusion of cytotoxic T cells for the prevention and treatment of Epstein–Barr virus-induced lymphoma in allogeneic transplant recipients. *Blood* 1998; **92**: 1549–55.

111 Roskrow MA, Suzuki N, Gan Y *et al*. Epstein-Barr virus (EBV)-specific cytotoxic T lymphocytes for the treatment of patients with EBV-positive relapsed Hodgkin's disease. *Blood* 1998; **91**: 2925–34.

112 Jensen M, Tan G, Forman S, Wu AM, Raubitschek A. CD20 is a molecular target for scFvFc: zeta receptor redirected T cells. Implications for cellular immunotherapy of CD20$^+$ malignancy. *Biol Blood Marrow Transplant* 1998; **4**: 75–83.

113 Engleman EG. Dendritic cells in the treatment of cancer. *Biol Blood Marrow Transplantation* 1996; **2**: 115–7.

114 Choudhury A, Gajewski JL, Liang JC *et al*. Use of leukemic dendritic cells for the generation of antileukemic cellular cytotoxicity against Philadelphia chromosome-positive chronic myelogenous leukemia. *Blood* 1997; **89**: 1133–42.

115 Wen YJ, Barlogie B, Yi Q. Idiotype-specific cytotoxic T lymphocytes in multiple myeloma: evidence for their capacity to lyse autologous primary tumor cells. *Blood* 2001; **97**: 1750–5.

116 Molldrem J, Dermime S, Parker K *et al*. Targeted T-cell therapy for human leukemia: cytotoxic T lymphocytes specific for a peptide derived from proteinase 3 preferentially lyse human myeloid leukemia cells. *Blood* 1996; **88**: 2450–7.

117 Brugger W, Brossart P, Scheding S *et al*. Approaches to dendritic cell-based immunotherapy after peripheral blood stem cell transplantation. *Ann N Y Acad Sci* 1999; **872**: 363–71.

118 Westermann J, Kopp J, Korner I *et al*. Bcr/abl$^+$ autologous dendritic cells for vaccination in chronic myeloid leukemia. *Bone Marrow Transplant* 2000; **25** (Suppl. 2): S46–9.

119 Nair SK, Heiser A, Boczkowski D *et al*. Induction of cytotoxic T cell responses and tumor immunity against unrelated tumors using telomerase reverse transcriptase RNA transfected dendritic cells. *Nat Med* 2000; **6**: 1011–7.

120 Pawlowska AB, Hashino S, McKenna H, Weigel BJ, Taylor PA, Blazar BR. *In vitro* tumor-pulsed or *in vivo* Flt3 ligand-generated dendritic cells provide protection against acute myelogenous leukemia in nontransplanted or syngeneic bone marrow-transplanted mice. *Blood* 2001; **97**: 1474–82.

121 Wen YJ, Min R, Tricot G, Barlogie B, Yi Q. Tumor lysate-specific cytotoxic T lymphocytes in multiple myeloma: promising effector cells for immunotherapy. *Blood* 2002; **99**: 3280–5.

122 Hsu FJ, Benike C, Fagnoni F *et al*. Vaccination of patients with B-cell lymphoma using autologous antigen-pulsed dendritic cells. *Nature Med* 1996; **2**: 52–8.

123 Davis TA, Hsu FJ, Caspar CB *et al*. Idiotype vaccination following ABMT can stimulate specific anti-idiotype immune responses in patients with B-cell lymphoma. *Biol Blood Marrow Transplant* 2001; **7**: 517–22.

124 Reichardt VL, Okada CY, Stockerl-Goldstein KE, Bogen B, Levy R. Rationale for adjuvant idiotypic vaccination after high-dose therapy for multiple myeloma. *Biol Blood Marrow Transplant* 1997; **3**: 157–63.

125 Reichardt VL, Okada CY, Liso A *et al*. Idiotype vaccination using dendritic cells after autologous peripheral blood stem cell transplantation for multiple myeloma: a feasibility study. *Blood* 1999; **93**: 2411–9.

126 Liso A, Stockerl-Goldstein KE, Auffermann-Gretzinger S *et al*. Idiotype vaccination using dendritic cells after autologous peripheral blood progenitor cell transplantation for multiple myeloma. *Biol Blood Marrow Transplant* 2000; **6**: 621–7.

127 Li Y, Bendandi M, Deng Y *et al*. Tumor-specific recognition of human myeloma cells by idiotype-induced CD8$^+$ T cells. *Blood* 2000; **96**: 2828–33.

128 Geller RB, Esa AH, Beschorner WE, Frondoza CG, Santos GW, Hess AD. Successful *in vitro* graft-versus-tumor effect against an Ia-bearing tumor using cyclosporine-induced syngeneic graft-versus-host disease in the rat. *Blood* 1989; **74**: 1165–71.

129 Kennedy MJ, Vogelsang GB, Beveridge RA *et al*. Phase I trial of intravenous cyclosporine to induce graft-versus-host disease in women undergoing autologous bone marrow transplantation for breast cancer. *J Clin Oncol* 1993; **11**: 478–84.

130 Hess AD, Bright EC, Thoburn C, Vogelsang GB, Jones RJ, Kennedy MJ. Specificity of effector T lymphocytes in autologous graft-versus-host disease: role of the major histocompatibility complex class II invariant chain peptide. *Blood* 1997; **89**: 2203–9.

131 Gryn J, Johnson E, Goldman N *et al*. The treatment of relapsed or refractory intermediate grade non-Hodgkin's lymphoma with autologous bone marrow transplantation followed by cyclosporine and interferon. *Bone Marrow Transplantation* 1997; **19**: 221–6.

132 Vogelsang G, Bitton R, Piantadosi S *et al*. Immune modulation in autologous bone marrow transplantation: cyclosporine and gamma-interferon trial. *Bone Marrow Transplant* 1999; **24**: 637–40.

Section 7

Allogenic Transplantation for Inherited Disease

103 Guido Lucarelli & Reginald A. Clift

Marrow Transplantation in Thalassemia

Introduction

Thalassemia syndromes are widely distributed throughout the Mediterranean, Middle Eastern and Asian countries, and occur with a substantial incidence worldwide in populations that originated in these regions. Weatherall and Clegg have stated that the thalassemias probably represent the most common single gene disorder to cause a major public health problem in the world [1]. There are more than 200,000 β-homozygous thalassemia patients in the Mediterranean area alone. In certain areas, such as Greece, the Mediterranean littoral of Italy, Iran, Southern Russia, India and South-east Asia, where 10–15% of the population carry the β-thalassemia gene, the homozygous birthrate is between 1 : 150 and 1 : 200. According to the World Health Organization, approximately 180 million people are heterozygous for one of several forms of genetic disorder of hemoglobin synthesis [2]. Thalassemia major is one of the major scourges of mankind.

Defective synthesis of the β chains of adult hemoglobin A leads to an imbalance in chain production with the accumulation of free α chains in red cell precursors and red blood cells (RBCs). This accumulation causes intramedullary destruction of red cell precursors and markedly ineffective erythropoiesis that results in severe hemolytic anemia. Many patients with homozygous β-thalassemia die in childhood, from chronic anemia and its complications if insufficiently transfused, or from iron overload if transfused without adequate iron chelation therapy. Currently recommended non-transplant therapy is available in most countries and consists of hypertransfusion to maintain hemoglobin levels between 10 and 12 g/dL together with chelation therapy aimed at preventing iron accumulation as a consequence of the transfusion therapy. To be effective, chelation therapy should consist of continuous subcutaneous infusion for at least 12 h daily. The successful implementation of this treatment regimen has improved life expectancy up to and beyond the second decade of life, and has dramatically improved the quality of life for children with thalassemia. However, transfusion therapy is limited by the availability of "clean" blood and the chelation regimen is painful, tedious and very expensive, so that consistent compliance is difficult to maintain. For these reasons, the impact of this treatment on long-term survival is unclear.

Thalassemia major is most common in third world countries where the cost of instituting and maintaining hypertransfusion and chelation programs on a national scale is prohibitive. An alternative approach in dealing with this major public health problem is to invest heavily in preventive measures such as genetic counseling and prenatal diagnosis with induced termination of affected pregnancies. Religious and social constraints conspire to restrict the wider application of such measures, which may ameliorate but cannot eliminate this public health problem.

Future treatment of the thalassemic patient may be easier and improved if orally administered iron chelators become available but, after several trials of potentially useful oral chelators, none is currently acceptable. If such agents are eventually developed, hazards associated with transfusion therapy will remain. Eventually, revising the underlying genetic malformation will treat thalassemia, like all the single gene disorders, and this revision may be achieved by genetic manipulation of the hematopoietic stem cell (HSC). Although thalassemia is a disease with a well-defined genetic target, there are many daunting obstacles to success in this endeavor. Genetic engineering studies have had some limited success in animals and in the treatment of adenosine deaminase deficiency in humans, and autologous marrow transplantation will probably be the vehicle for the genetic treatment of thalassemia. Regimens derived from experience in eliminating leukemic marrow will probably be used to overcome the competitive advantage of rapidly proliferating, genetically abnormal cells [3]. Much additional research will be necessary before clinical trials are warranted in this area (this topic is addressed in Chapters 10 and 11).

It is against this background that allogeneic hematopoietic cell transplantation (HCT) has been used in attempts at curing thalassemia. The first successful marrow transplant for thalassemia was reported in 1982 by Thomas and his colleagues [4], and the first reports of series of transplants were by Lucarelli et al. [5,6].

Conventional therapy

Infants with thalassemia major who receive no treatment will die in early infancy from congestive heart failure or other complications of severe anemia. Red cell transfusion therapy designed to avert this outcome will reduce mortality derived directly from anemia but patients will develop complications resulting from severe and accelerating hemolytic anemia driven by almost completely ineffective erythropoiesis. These complications include cardiomegaly, massive hypersplenism and severe bone malformations resulting from marrow extension. In 1964, Wolman reported that patients maintained at a higher baseline hemoglobin level had less severe complications and were in better health than those maintained at lower hemoglobin levels [7]. Stimulated by this observation, Piomelli and his colleagues studied a transfusion regimen designed to prevent the baseline hemoglobin from falling below 10 g/dL. When this hypertransfusion regimen was instituted in infancy and rigorously implemented, cardiomegaly and bone malformation was greatly reduced, although normalization of growth was not achieved and the development of hypersplenism was not prevented [8]. The target hemoglobin level of 10 g/dL was designed to depress endogenous erythropoiesis and thereby avoid marrow hypertrophy with accompanying marrow space extension. This objective was partially achieved, but complete suppression of endogenous red cell production requires that hemoglobin be maintained at levels greater than 13 g/dL [9]. There are major obstacles in the way of achieving such levels. Raising the baseline hemoglobin level from 10 g/dL to 11 g/dL requires a 20% increase in the red cell transfusion requirement [10], and there are many reasons for minimizing transfusion in patients with thalassemia.

Hypertransfusion regimens have a major impact on iron traffic and distribution in patients with severe hemolytic anemia. The complications of iron overload such as endocrine deficiency, hepatic and pancreatic damage, and heart disease are the principal causes of death in patients with thalassemia receiving this form of therapy. The transfusion of 165 mL of packed red cells per kilogram per year is associated with an annual iron intake of approximately 180 mg/kg [11]. The adverse consequences of this intensive therapy include cardiopathy, diabetes and other endocrine disorders such as hypothyroidism, hypoparathyroidism and hypogonadism with consequent impairment of growth and sexual maturity. Because of these complications, attempts have been made to enhance iron mobilization and excretion by the use of chelating agents. The agent presently used is deferoxamine, which is not currently available in a form suitable for oral administration [12]. Since the maintenance of steady plasma levels of this agent is essential for the effective management of iron traffic, it must be continuously administered either intravenously or subcutaneously. The most common regimen is continuous subcutaneous administration with the aid of a portable infusion pump for 8–10 h daily [13]. This therapy, when rigorously adhered to, substantially reduces, but does not eliminate, the iron overload of patients on hypertransfusion therapy.

The diagnosis of β-thalassemia is usually made within the 1st year of life, and red cell transfusions are usually initiated soon after. Transfusions are usually required every 15–21 days in order to maintain a hemoglobin level between 10 and 12 g/dL. There are two common reasons for the failure of conventional therapy in the treatment of thalassemia. The first is an inadequate supply of safe blood even in well-developed countries, and the second is irregular and discontinuous administration of deferoxamine that is usually due to the high cost of chelation therapy and poor patient compliance.

The development of a regimen of hypertransfusion combined with regular iron chelation has transformed the prognosis for thalassemic children [14]. If good compliance is obtained, patients rarely die from anemia but children with thalassemia will be sick mainly because of complications arising from treatment with blood transfusions. Their clinical state depends primarily on the degree of iron overload but is compounded by exposure to hepatitis viruses and other blood-borne infectious agents. There is a dearth of good follow-up data, and the cohort of patients that has received this treatment since early infancy is only now in young adulthood. The first patient treated with the regimen is in his thirties. Statistics are not available which assess the outcome of treatment on the basis of intent to treat. It is abundantly clear that compliance rates for chelation therapy vary enormously and, even with strong parental support, many children find this cumbersome and unpleasant therapy completely unacceptable, particularly as they grow older.

In summary, patients with homozygous β-thalassemia, if properly transfused and chelated, have a reduced, but not abolished, organ iron overload. In children with poor compliance with the prescribed treatment regimen, iron overload is more severe creating endocrine, cardiac and hepatic lesions. Several authors have reported a high incidence of growth retardation due to impairment of the pituitary–gonadal axis, and of diabetes mellitus due to iron deposits in the pancreas as well as liver disease due to iron overload and viral hepatitis [13,15–17]. In the majority of centers treating thalassemia, adequate chelation with deferoxamine was initiated in 1976–77, and all observations reported by clinicians treating thalassemia refer to groups of patients heterogeneous for age and duration of chelation therapy.

In 1989, Gabutti et al. described the situation for patients who had not received optimal chelation therapy in a report of complications in a group of 183 20-year-old patients [13]. Of these, 20% had cardiac disease, 43% had diabetes, 26% had liver disease, 28% had hypothyroidism and 22% had hypoparathyroidism. Sixty percent of these patients had more than one complication, which is indicative of a very poor prognosis with a 50% probability of death within 10 years of the appearance of the first complication. It is certain that patients who have received regular chelation therapy will have less iron overload than those reported by Gabutti et al., together with a significantly improved survival. Unfortunately there is no way of determining from the literature what the complication rate will be in a population of patients entered into a study of modern chelation therapy. Therefore it is impossible to draw conclusions on the contemporary frequency of complications due to iron overload.

The difficulties in achieving compliance with hypertransfusion/chelation regimens are greater in patients of low economic and educational status. Moreover, thalassemia is most common in developing and third world countries where delivery of such therapy (or of marrow transplantation) to a significant proportion of the affected population is problematic.

Bone marrow transplantation

At present, allogeneic HCT is the only rational therapeutic modality for the eradication of β-thalassemia major [18]. It is a form of gene therapy that uses allogeneic stem cells as vectors for genes essential for normal hematopoiesis. Eventually the vector may well be autologous stem cells transformed by the insertion of normal genes but there is no indication that this approach will be a clinical option in the foreseeable future. All of the transplant procedures in Seattle and Pesaro discussed in this chapter were performed with bone marrow and the term bone marrow transplantation (BMT) is used for these procedures.

The first two transplant procedures for the treatment of thalassemia with marrow from matched related donors were performed in December 1981, in Seattle, WA, and in Pesaro, Italy. The Seattle approach was based on the assumption that the risks associated with BMT would be increased by the iron overload and by sensitization to human leukocyte antigens (HLAs) induced by hypertransfusion. Therefore, it was decided that early clinical studies would be conducted in very young patients who had received very few transfusions. On December 3, 1981 a 14-month-old child with β-thalassemia major who had been transfused with a total of 250 mL of packed RBCs received BMT from his HLA-identical sister in Seattle [4]. The treatment was completely successful.

The Pesaro approach was based on an assessment that restricting transplants to untransfused patients was impracticable. On December 17, 1981 the Pesaro team performed a transplant in a 16-year-old thalassemic patient who had received 150 RBC transfusions, using marrow from his HLA identical brother. This patient rejected the graft and was the first of an extensive series of transplants for thalassemia that provides most of the data supporting this chapter.

Preparatory regimens

Preparatory regimens for BMT of patients with diseases other than aplastic anemia must achieve two objectives. One is elimination of the (disordered) marrow and the other is establishment of a tolerant environment that will permit transplanted marrow to survive and thrive. Total body irradiation (TBI) can accomplish both these objectives, but there are many reasons to avoid the use of this marrow-ablative modality. These include the known growth-retarding effects of TBI in young children and the increased risk of secondary malignancies which has been reported in patients treated for leukemia [19], lymphoma and aplastic anemia [20,21]. These hazards are particularly objectionable in very young patients with potential for a long life span. The risk of these toxicities has not yet been fully explored for cytotoxic regimens that do not involve TBI. There is a considerable body of experience with the use of busulfan (BU) and its derivatives in ablating marrow in patients undergoing HCT for the treatment of non-malignant conditions such as the Wiskott–Aldrich syndrome [22,23] and inborn errors of metabolism [24]. Cyclophosphamide (CY) is an agent that is well established as providing immunosuppression adequate for allogeneic engraftment of patients with aplastic anemia [25,26]. Experience in the use of chemotherapy-only transplant regimens for the treatment of malignancy [27–32] has been pivotal in developing regimens appropriate for the treatment of thalassemia by transplantation.

BU is an alkylating agent with exquisite specificity for the most primitive precursors of the myeloid–erythroid axis. It has been used in low doses for more than 30 years for the treatment of patients with chronic myeloid leukemia, and its toxicity and effectiveness have been well-documented in that setting. Studies in rodents demonstrated that marrow-lethal doses of BU have minor toxicity to the lymphoid system and cause little immunosuppression [33]. Canine studies of transplants between dog leukocyte antigen (DLA) -identical littermates demonstrated 50% engraftment after BU alone and 95% engraftment when antithymocyte serum was added to the conditioning regimen [34]. Clinical experience with the use of BU in very high doses was delayed due to the lack of an acceptable preparation suitable for intravenous use. Santos *et al*. reported the first clinical trials of very high-dose BU in the context of BMT [29]. In these studies, patients with acute myeloid leukemia (AML) received allogeneic marrow transplants after immunosuppression with CY (200 mg/kg over 4 days), and oral BU (16 mg/kg over 4 days) was administered as additional antitumor therapy. Early results with this therapy were encouraging, and in successful attempts to reduce early transplant-related toxicity, Tutschka *et al*. reduced the CY dose to 120 mg/kg over 2 days [35].

Further, CY has been a component of most conditioning regimens for transplanting patients with hematologic malignancies. Santos *et al*. reported on its use in high doses (200 mg/kg over 4 days) as the sole antitumor agent in patients receiving allogeneic transplants for leukemia and demonstrated that it was sufficiently immunosuppressive to permit sustained allogeneic engraftment [27]. Also, CY is most commonly employed for the treatment of lymphoid malignancies and solid tumors, and it has been used as a component of combination chemotherapy for the treatment of acute leukemia. It is not considered a highly effective agent against myeloid malignancies, although single drug studies are not available in this context. The dose-limiting toxicity of CY is to the heart and not to the marrow. Mice, monkeys and humans recover hematopoiesis promptly after the highest doses of CY because CY does not eliminate HSCs. Therefore CY alone is not an appropriate conditioning modality for BMT for the treatment of thalassemia because the thalassemic marrow would recover rapidly. On the other hand, BU is an agent which has a good possibility of eradicating a diseased erythron but when used alone is not likely to be sufficiently immunosuppressive to permit sustained allogeneic engraftment. In summary, a combination of BU and CY can eradicate the thalassemia and facilitate sustained allogeneic engraftment.

Disease eradication

Many of the hematopoietic manifestations of thalassemia resemble those of hematopoietic malignancy. The disease is characterized by extreme marrow hyperplasia with aggressive extension of a rapidly proliferating erythron into intra- and extra-medullary areas not usually occupied by marrow. This results in major bone remodeling together with marked hepatomegaly and splenomegaly. By analogy with the behavior of malignant tissue, it might be supposed that this large mass of rapidly proliferating hematopoietic tissue would be more difficult to eradicate than normal hematopoietic tissue, and more likely to recur after transplantation.

Although post-transplant thalassemic recurrence is a problem, it occurs in circumstances that differ from those usually observed with leukemic relapse. The most common presentation of leukemic relapse is return of host-type leukemia in the presence of a persisting immune system of donor origin. In contrast, the recurrence of thalassemia usually occurs in the context of a return of host type immune and hematologic reconstitution. Thus, this event has aspects of both relapse and rejection and it is customary to speak of this phenomenon as rejection.

Engraftment

Most patients undergoing transplantation for the treatment of thalassemia have been transfused repeatedly. Experience with BMT for the treatment of aplastic anemia in heavily transfused patients demonstrated that a history of many pretransplant transfusions increased the probability of graft rejection [36,37]. There is a substantial incidence of graft rejection in thalassemia patients after most preparatory regimens for marrow grafting, and this seems to be related to the stage of disease at the time of transplant. As discussed above, in most cases of graft rejection the thalassemic marrow will regrow and subsequent survival will be long (albeit with thalassemia). Occasionally, patients will reject grafts without recurrence of thalassemia. Unless rescued by a second transplant such patients will die from the consequences of marrow aplasia.

The treatment of patients after graft rejection will differ depending on whether the rejection is accompanied by regeneration of host type hematopoiesis or by marrow aplasia. The Pesaro experience with this situation is discussed below.

Transplant-related morbidity and mortality

A BMT is a dangerous undertaking. Regimens capable of eradicating a diseased marrow and facilitating persistent engraftment are necessarily toxic, and the consequences of successful allogeneic marrow engraftment include acute and chronic graft-vs.-host disease (GVHD), syndromes associated with severe immune incompetence. Both prophylaxis against GVHD and methods for its treatment are immunosuppressive. Transplant associated toxicity may be aggravated by GVHD and by measures aimed at the prevention of this complication. Such toxicity can be categorized either as regimen-related toxicity (RRT) or as GVHD.

In studies of BMT for the treatment of hematologic malignancies, RRT from the preparative regimens has been well-described [38,39]. The lungs and liver are the organs most at risk for toxicity induced by TBI and BU while the heart is the main site of CY-induced damage. Increasing patient age, previous exposure to cytotoxic agents and the presence of latent viruses such as hepatitis C and cytomegalovirus adversely influence these toxicities. Patients transplanted for the treatment of thalassemia derive benefit from the fact they are usually young and without prior exposure to cytotoxic agents. However, because of previous intensive transfusion therapy they will have a high probability of carrying harmful viruses and have organ damage induced by extreme iron overload.

Clinical transplant experience

The Seattle experience

The Seattle team transplanted five patients using a regimen of a single dose of 5 mg/kg of dimethylbusulfan (DMB), a relatively soluble derivative of BU which can be administered parenterally, followed by CY 200 mg/kg over 4 days, with methotrexate (MTX) administered over 102 days as prophylaxis against acute GVHD [40–42]. Two of these patients died within the first 100 days after transplant from veno-occlusive disease (VOD) of the liver and from adenovirus interstitial pneumonia (IP),

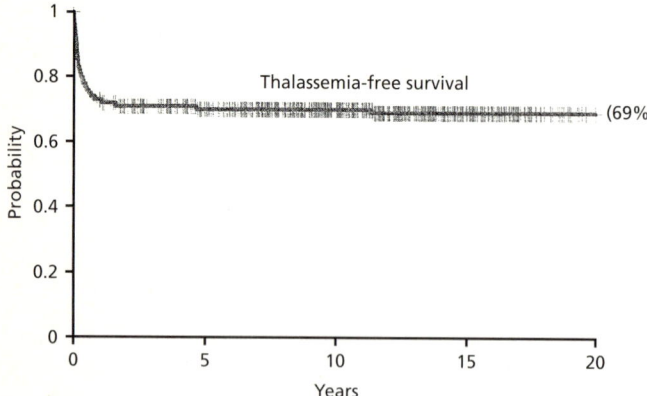

Fig. 103.1 Estimates of thalassemia-free survival of 915 patients who were transplanted for the treatment of thalassemia in Pesaro between December 1981 and June 2001.

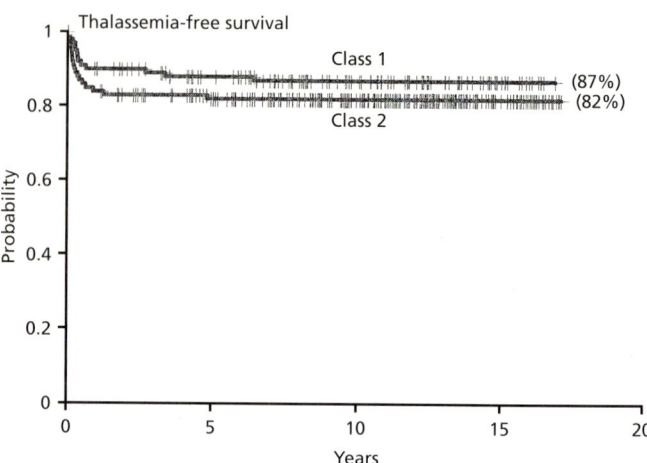

Fig. 103.2 Estimates of thalassemia-free survival for patients less than 17 years old transplanted through July 2001, categorized by risk category. One hundred and forty patients were in class 1 and 325 patients were in class 2. The categorization into risk classes is described in the text.

and three survive at more than 16, 18 and 18 years after transplant with normal hematopoiesis and Karnofsky performance scores of 100. After the Pesaro group had demonstrated the feasibility of using oral BU in very young children, the Seattle group prepared six additional patients for transplantation from matched related donors with BU 14 mg/kg, CY 200 mg/kg and GVHD prophylaxis consisting of a short course of MTX and cyclosporine (CSP). All six patients are alive at more than 2, 2, 4, 10, 13 and 13 years. One of these patients has had recurrence of thalassemia (Karnofsky performance score 90) and the others are well with Karnofsky performance scores of 100.

The Pesaro experience

By far the largest body of experience in the treatment of thalassemia with BMT has been accumulated in Pesaro. From December 1981 to June 2001, 915 patients with homozygous β-thalassemia received marrow transplants. The thalassemia-free survival of the entire group of patients (aged 1 through 35 years at the time of the transplantation) is reported in Fig. 103.1. For 880 patients, the donors were HLA identical (853 siblings, 27 parents), 29 were HLA partially matched relatives and six were HLA identical unrelated donors. Most patients were treated with one of two types of regimen: One, used for 547 patients, prescribed BU 14 mg/kg and CY 200 mg/kg and the other used BU with a lower dose of CY for patients believed to be especially susceptible to the toxic complications associated with this high dose of CY.

In early experience, the best results were obtained in younger patients [5,43,44]. Of the first six patients older than 16 years, four died of GVHD related causes within the first 100 days, one died of infection on day 235 and one had recurrence of thalassemia on day 48 and died of consequent cardiac damage more than 6 years after transplantation. In view of this experience, early studies concentrated on patients under the age of 17 years.

Children and adolescents

Results in young patients were very encouraging, and in 1990 Lucarelli and his colleagues reported their experience through August 1988 in treating 222 consecutive patients under the age of 16 years [6]. All these patients received HLA-identical marrow, in 10 cases from parents and in the other cases from siblings, after conditioning with regimens containing BU 14 mg/kg and CY 200 mg/kg. One hundred and forty-one donors were heterozygous for β-thalassemia and 81 donors were normal homozygotes. Five different regimens were used to prevent acute GVHD.

Analysis of the influence of pretransplant characteristics on the outcome of transplantation was conducted in 116 patients who were all treated with exactly the same regimen. It was demonstrated that hepatomegaly and portal fibrosis were associated with a significantly reduced probability of survival. In multivariate analysis a history of poor compliance with the chelation regimen could not be distinguished from hepatomegaly as a predictor of survival and rejection-free survival. The influence of pretransplant characteristics on the outcome of transplantation was reexamined in late 1989 [45] by which time 161 patients <17 years of age had been treated with the same regimen. The quality of chelation was characterized as regular when deferoxamine therapy was initiated no later than 18 months after the first transfusion and administered subcutaneously for 8–10 h continuously for at least 5 days each week. The chelation variable was defined as irregular for any deviation from this criterion. The degree of hepatomegaly (greater than or not greater than 2 cm), the presence or absence of portal fibrosis in the pretransplant liver biopsy and the quality of chelation (regular or irregular) given through the years before transplant were identified as variables permitting the categorization of patients into three risk classes. Class 1 patients had none of these adverse risk factors, class 3 patients had all three and class 2 patients had one or two adverse risk factors. This analysis confirmed the prognostic significance for transplant outcome of risk class and the strong influence of the quality of chelation therapy.

By the end of July 2001, 511 patients <17 years of age had received HLA-identical transplants using regimens containing BU 14 mg/kg and CY 200 mg/kg. There were 140 class 1 patients, 325 class 2 patients and 46 class 3 patients. The probabilities of thalassemia-free survival for class 1 and for class 2 patients are reported in Fig. 103.2. The probabilities of survival, thalassemia-free survival, rejection and non-rejection mortality for class 1 patients were 89%, 87%, 1% and 11%, respectively, and for class 2 patients they were 85%, 82%, 4% and 13%, respectively.

The probabilities of survival, thalassemia-free survival, rejection and non-rejection mortality for the 46 patients in class 3 were 53%, 51%, 7% and 42%, respectively, calculated at 15 years (Fig. 103.3). In an attempt to improve results in these class 3 patients, new treatment regimens were devised using BU 14 mg/kg and lower doses of CY (160 or 120 mg/kg). Experience with these regimens in 121 class 3 patients <17 years of age is depicted in Fig. 103.4.

In April 1997, a new preparative regimen (Protocol 26) was adopted for class 3 patients <17 years of age in an attempt to decrease the 28% rejection rate without a corresponding increase in reappearance of the thalassemic clone. This protocol involved an intensified preparation with 3 mg/kg of azathioprine and 30 mg/kg hydroxyurea daily from day −45

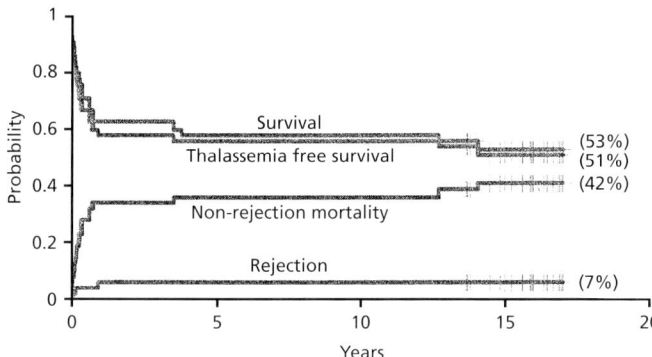

Fig. 103.3 Estimates of survival, thalassemia-free survival, rejection and non-rejection mortality for 46 patients younger than 17 years in class 3 who were treated with busulfan (BU) 14 mg/kg and cyclophosphamide (CY) 200 mg/kg.

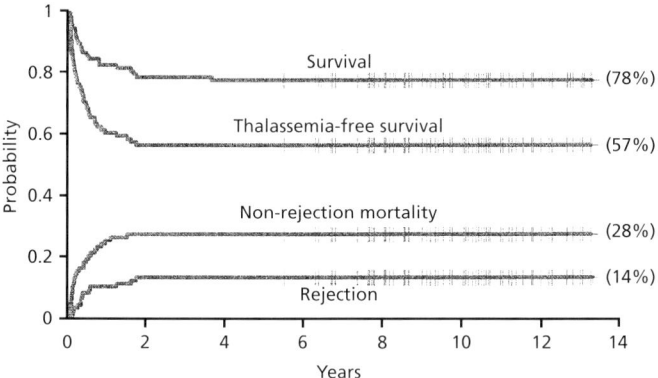

Fig. 103.4 Estimates of survival, thalassemia-free survival, non-rejection mortality and rejection for 121 patients younger than 17 years in class 3 who were treated with busulfan (BU) 14 mg/kg and cyclophosphamide (CY) 120 mg/kg or 160 mg/kg.

from the transplant, fludarabine 20 mg/m^2 from day −17 through day −11, followed by the administration of BU 14 mg/kg total dose and CY 160 mg/kg total dose. Continuous 24-h infusions of 40 mg/kg of deferoxamine via central venous catheter were initiated on day −45 and a regimen of hypertransfusion with RBCs was used to keep the level of hemoglobin between 14 and 15 g/dL. Protocol 26 was devised on the assumption that preparation with BU 14 mg/kg and CY 160 mg/kg was inadequate to eradicate thalassemic hematopoiesis in class 3 patients <17 years of age. Results obtained in 25 such patients treated with Protocol 26 are reported in Fig. 103.5.

Adult patients

From October 1988 through March 2002, 121 patients older than 16 years (adult thalassemics) received transplants from matched donors. The median age for this population was 20 years (range 17–35 years, 25th percentile = 18 years, 75th percentile = 24 years). All these patients received BU 14 mg/kg. Twenty-one patients were in class 2 and these received BU 14 mg/kg and CY 200 mg/kg. The other patients were in class 3 and 29 of these received BU 14 mg/kg and CY 120 mg/kg, 59 received BU 14 mg/kg and CY 160 mg/kg and, more recently, 12 received BU 14 mg/kg and CY 90 mg/kg.

Figure 103.6 describes the probabilities of survival, thalassemia-free survival, rejection and non-rejection mortality for the entire group of 121 adult patients. For the 21 class 2 adults, the probabilities of survival and of thalassemia-free survival were both 76%.

Transplantation provided what is probably a permanent cure for the marrow defect in nearly all these patients but prolonged follow-up is nec-

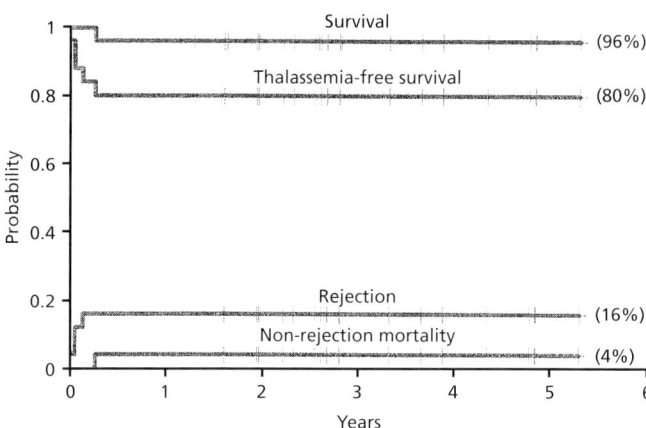

Fig. 103.5 Estimates of survival, thalassemia-free survival, non-rejection mortality and rejection for 25 patients younger than 17 years in class 3 who were treated with the regimen prescribed by protocol 26 (described in text).

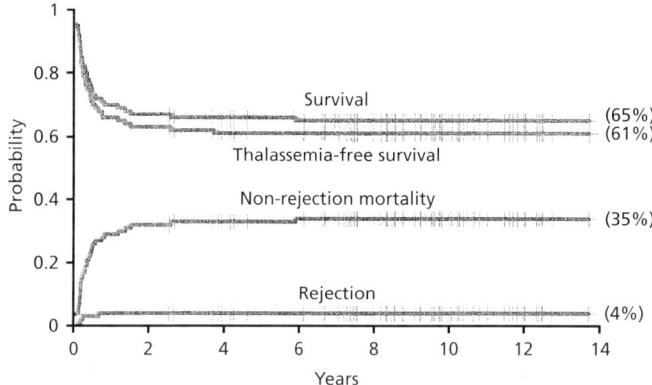

Fig. 103.6 Estimates of survival, rejection-free survival, non-rejection mortality and rejection for 121 patients older than 16 years who were treated with busulfan (BU) 14 mg/kg. Twenty-one class 2 patients received cyclophosphamide (CY) 200 mg/kg; 100 class 3 patients received 90, 120 or 160 mg/kg as described in the text.

essary to determine the long-term outcome. It is reasonable to hope that removal of the continuing cause for extramedullary organ damage will modify disease progression and permit healing of the damaged organs.

Management of patients with rejection or disease recurrence

Patients with engraftment failure and without functioning marrow have a bleak prospect because an early second transplant with a second course of conditioning is usually not a reasonable option. However, occasionally patients have late graft failure without thalassemia recurrence and in this situation second transplant attempts with intensive conditioning may provide the only treatment option to offer a chance of prolonged survival.

Patients who reject their grafts and have a return of host hematopoiesis do not have an urgent need for second transplants, and such interventions can be delayed until the toxic effects of the conditioning regimen for the first transplants have ameliorated. At least a year should be allowed to elapse between the first and second transplant. The Pesaro team has performed 15 such transplants, always from the same donor used for the first transplants, between 5 months and 2½ years after the first transplant, using regimens containing CY 200 mg/kg with or without total lymphoid irradiation. Nine patients rejected again and three of these died. Two patients died of other causes. Ten patients survive of whom six have thalassemia and four are free from thalassemia at 2.6, 4.2, 5.0 and 7.4 years after transplant.

Some patients develop persistent mixed chimerism (MC) without graft rejection.

Mixed chimerism (MC) after BMT in thalassemia

Ablation of all host HSCs is usually considered necessary to establish conditions for stable and complete marrow engraftment of donor stem cells (complete chimerism [CC]). However, we have observed that MC is not unusual in transplanted thalassemic patients. Further, MC may be transient (TMC) when it evolves into CC or graft rejection, or persistent (PMC) when the coexistence of donor and recipient cells is longer than 2 years, with hemoglobin levels sufficient for a good quality of life without RBC transfusion [46]. When PMC was detected using sensitive techniques [47], it could be demonstrated in all the nucleated hemopoietic cell subpopulations of the marrow and peripheral blood. In informative situations, all circulating mature RBCs were of the same blood group as the donor, even when 70% of burst forming units—erythroid (BFU-E) was of host origin.

In a group of 335 mostly consecutive patients, all with 2 or more years of post-transplant follow-up, the incidence of MC was 32.2% at 2 months after HCT. This proportion decreased to 10.1% at 2 years after transplantation. Within this group there were 185 class 1 or 2 patients, all treated with the same pretransplant conditioning regimen (BU 14 mg/kg and CY 200 mg/kg). For these patients, the incidence of MC at 2 months after the transplant was 21%, while it was 54.9% in the group of the remaining 150 patients (who were treated with BU 14 mg/kg and CY 120 mg/kg or 160 mg/kg). The incidence of PMC 2 years after transplant was 10.1% in each of the two groups of patients, although they were not homogeneous for the preparative regimen. Graft rejection did not occur in any of the 227 patients with CC early after HCT whereas graft rejection occurred in 35 of the 108 patients (32.4%) with MC detected during the first 2 months after HCT.

Rejection was related to the number of residual host cells (RHCs) present in patients with TMC early after HCT. Andreani and colleagues reported a classification scheme for MC [47] in which the presence of <10% RHCs was designated as level 1, RHCs between 10% and 25% was categorized as level 2 and RHCs >25% was categorized as level 3. Of the 108 patients who at 2 months after the transplant were MC, 61 patients had level 1, 27 patients had level 2 and 20 patients had level 3 chimerism. In the group of level 1 patients, 57% eventually developed CC, 13% rejected the transplant and 30% became PMCs. In the group of level 2 patients, 44% became CC, 41% rejected the transplant and 15% remained PMCs. Eighteen of the 20 patients with level 3 MC rejected the transplant, while only two developed PMC. It is interesting to observe that, of the 227 patients with CC 2 months after BMT, 4% showed the presence of PMC at 2 years after the transplant. This may be because the number of RHCs early after HCT in these patients was below the limit of sensitivity of the test.

Thirty-four ex-thalassemic patients after transplant have maintained PMC for 2–13 years and are transfusion independent with hemoglobin levels ranging from 8.3 g/dL to 14.7 g/dL. Fifteen of these patients showed level 3 persistence with large numbers of recipient precursor cells. In some patients, the proportion of donor engrafted cells decreased to levels usually predictive of complete rejection. The Pesaro team observed, however, that change in the donor/recipient distribution over time is a characteristic of patients with PMC. This finding suggests that while high numbers of RHCs in a recipient early after HCT reliably predict rejection, the same proportion of RHCs present after 2 years or later from HCT is consistent with a state of reciprocal tolerance between donor and recipient. It is not known why MC is transient in some patients, and remains persistent in others. Clones of T regulatory cells may develop in some patients with PMC and establish a state of reciprocal tolerance. Further studies are needed of the mechanisms underlying this state of tolerance to permit the design of protocols that will produce it predictably. The discovery of this phenomenon has potential importance for the future use of gene therapy and for the adoption of less toxic conditioning regimens as preparation for transplantation. The finding that patients can have major clinical benefit in the presence of a high level of thalassemic hematopoiesis should be of great interest to students of gene therapy. Also, these findings suggest that patients with a high risk of rejection can be identified soon after transplantation permitting the application of pre-emptive treatment strategies aimed at preventing rejection.

The use of alternative related donors

Between 60% and 70% of patients with hemoglobinopathies lack matched sibling donors. The curative potential of transplantation for hemoglobinopathies has encouraged the use of hematopoietic cell donations from donors other than matched related donors (alternative donors).

Recently, the Pesaro team analyzed the results of transplantation from alternative related donors for 29 patients with thalassemia major [48]. Six of the donors were relatives and HLA-phenotypically identical with the recipients, two were mismatched relatives, 13 were mismatched siblings and eight were mismatched parents. Of the mismatched donors, 15 were mismatched for one antigen, five for two antigens and three for three antigens. Most patients in this study received antilymphocyte globulin (ALG) or irradiation in addition to BU and CY in an attempt to improve the prospect for successful engraftment. Unfortunately, the patients receiving these transplants had a high incidence of graft failure (55%) with a consequent low probability of thalassemia-free survival. No relationship between survival and the degree of HLA disparity could be demonstrated in this small series of cases.

The use of unrelated donors

Results of HCT from unrelated donors for the treatment of malignant disease have improved steadily, mainly due to the introduction of high-resolution molecular techniques for histocompatibility testing and improvements in the management of post-transplant complications. These results have stimulated the use of HCT from unrelated donors for the treatment of hemoglobinopathies. The Cagliari, Pavia, and Pesaro transplant centers have recently reported results obtained in 32 thalassemic patients (aged 2–28 years) who received bone marrow from unrelated donors selected for similarity with the recipients for extended HLA haplotypes [49]. Four patients were class 1, 11 were class 2 and 17 were class 3 candidates with respect to the outcome of BMT. Twenty-eight patients received BU 14 mg/kg and thiotepa 10 mg/kg. Of these 28 patients, the class 1 and the class 2 patients received BU 14 mg/kg, thiotepa 10 mg/kg and CY 200 mg/kg, and the class 3 patients received BU 14 mg/kg, thiotepa 10 mg/kg and CY 160 mg/kg or CY 120 mg/kg if they were >16 years of age. Prophylaxis against GVHD was with CSP and a short course of MTX. The probability of thalassemia-free survival was 66% for the entire group and the mortality from causes other than rejection was 25%. Although the difference was not significant, five of the six patients who died belonged to class 3. The incidences of grade 2–4 acute and of chronic GVHD were 41% and 25%, respectively. Patients who shared at least one extended haplotype had less acute or chronic GVHD and better survival. Updating the observations of these three centers to 44 patients, the probabilities of survival, thalassemia-free survival, rejection and non-rejection mortality are 79%, 68%, 12% and 23%, respectively. These data are encouraging and show that the results of HCT from well-selected unrelated donors might be comparable to those of HLA identical sibling transplants, especially in patients with less advanced disease.

Experience at other transplant centers

Many reports describe the experience of other groups in transplanting patients for the treatment of thalassemia (Table 103.1 [50–58]). In Italy

Table 103.1 Transplants for thalassemia. Reports from centers other than Pesaro.

Center [Ref.]	Patients	Survival	Disease-free survival
Pescara [50]	102	0.91	0.87
Cagliari [51]	37	0.88	0.88
USA [52]	68	0.94/0.81*	0.81/0.57*
UK [53]	50	0.90	0.76
Tehran [54]	60	0.83	0.73
Vellore [55]	50	0.76	0.68
Malaysia [56]	28	0.86	0.75
Hong Kong [57]	25	0.86	0.83
Bangkok [58]	21	0.76	0.53

*By risk category, survival = best risk/worst risk.

the Pescara group has been particularly active, reporting 102 patients transplanted through August 1996 [50].

Management of the ex-thalassemic patient after BMT

After transplantation, ex-thalassemic patients still carry the clinical complications acquired during years of transfusion and chelation therapy. Among the issues requiring long-term management in such patients are iron overload, chronic hepatitis, liver fibrosis and endocrine dysfunction.

There is no reason to expect that BMT will eliminate the excess iron acquired during years of thalassemia, since spontaneous iron elimination occurs very slowly. In our experience, serum ferritin and transferrin saturation spontaneously return to normal levels only in class 1 patients [59]. Persisting tissue iron overload can cause significant morbidity and mortality similar to that seen in hereditary hemochromatosis [60]. Thus iron removal is indicated in all transplanted thalassemic patients who have evidence of persisting iron overload, and initiating a sequence of phlebotomies or restarting chelation with deferoxamine at 18 months post-HCT achieves this best.

Excess iron can be completely removed from the body and a body iron content within the normal range can be achieved. The necessary duration of treatment is directly correlated with the magnitude of the iron overload, and ranges from a few months to several years [61]. In most ex-thalassemics, reduction or normalization of the iron pool results in marked improvement in serum levels of liver enzymes and in the histological activity index [61]. The serum aminotransferases and the histological activity index normalized after iron depletion in about half of the patients who were seropositive for hepatitis C virus (HCV), suggesting that iron is a cofactor of HCV for liver disease [62]. Ex-thalassemics with early cardiac involvement, characterized by systolic and/or diastolic dysfunction, show complete regression of these subclinical cardiac abnormalities after iron depletion [63].

Infection with the HCV is common in thalassemic patients, particularly in those transfused before second generation enzyme-linked immunosorbent assay (ELISA) tests became available for detecting HCV in donated blood. In thalassemia, liver damage due to HCV infection is exacerbated by iron overload, and liver disease is a recognized cause of mortality and morbidity. All the donors in this series of patients were HCV seronegative. After HCT, approximately 10–15% of HCV-infected patients become HCV seronegative [64]. This may reflect complete elimination of the virus, but we cannot be sure of this. However, seropositivity has not returned in these patients. The chronic risk of conditions associated with HCV infection, such as chronic hepatitis, cirrhosis and hepatocellular carcinoma, persists in the remaining patients. The precise risk of developing one of these complications is uncertain. Transplanted thalassemics have a long, probably normal life expectancy and mild chronic liver disease has to be considered in this perspective. Chronic HCV infection and transplant-related complications are probably the only factors that may limit survival in ex-thalassemics. Thus, avoidance of progression of liver damage to cirrhosis must be a primary goal.

There are long-term complications that arise from the allogeneic transplant procedure itself, and a small proportion of patients develop chronic GVHD that occasionally may be severely disabling.

The role of transplantation in the treatment of thalassemia

The results of transplantation from HLA-identical family members are clear. Class 1 patients have a very high probability of cure with a very low early and late morbidity and mortality. There is no reason to deny these patients the advantages of a life free from daily tedious, expensive and uncomfortable therapy. We still do not know the probability that a patient receiving conventional therapy will deteriorate into a worse risk category, but the fact is that transplant centers are confronted with patients in risk classes 2 and 3 who represent failures of conventional treatment every day. Delaying transplantation until the patient is in a risk category beyond class 1 substantially reduces the probability of transplant success and jeopardizes the reversibility of liver and cardiac damage. We therefore believe that all patients with β-thalassemia who have HLA-identical related donors should be transplanted as soon as possible. Patients without such donors who have well-selected unrelated donors should also be considered for HCT, especially if they have less advanced disease.

References

1 Weatherall DJ, Clegg JB. *The Thalassaemia Syndromes*, 3rd edn. Oxford: Blackwell Scientific Publications, 1981.
2 Anonymous. Community control of hereditary anemias. *Bull World Health Organization* 1981; **61**: 63.
3 Thomas ED. Marrow transplantation and gene transfer as therapy for hematopoietic diseases. *Molecular Biology of Homo Sapiens. Cold Spring Harbor Symposia on Quantitative Biology* 1986; **51**(2): 1009–12.
4 Thomas ED, Buckner CD, Sanders JE et al. Marrow transplantation for thalassaemia. *Lancet* 1982; **ii**: 227–9.
5 Lucarelli G, Galimberti M, Polchi P et al. Marrow transplantation in patients with advanced thalassemia. *N Engl J Med* 1987; **316**: 1050–5.
6 Lucarelli G, Galimberti M, Polchi P et al. Bone marrow transplantation in patients with thalassemia. *N Engl J Med* 1990; **322**: 417–21.
7 Wolman IJ. Transfusion therapy in Cooley's anemia. Growth and health as related to long-range hemoglobin levels, a progress report. *Ann NY Acad Sci* 1964; **119**: 736–47.
8 Piomelli S, Danoff SJ, Becker MH, Lipera MJ, Travis SF. Prevention of bone malformations and cardiomegaly in Cooley's anemia by early hypertransfusion regimen. *Ann NY Acad Sci* 1969; **165**: 427–36.
9 Piomelli S, Hart D, Graziano J, Karpatkin M, McCarthy K. Current strategies in the management of Cooley's anemia. *Ann NY Acad Sci* 1985; **445**: 256–67.
10 Piomelli S, Graziano J, Karpatkin M et al. Chelation therapy, transfusion requirement, and iron balance in young thalassemic patients. *Ann NY Acad Sci* 1980; **344**: 409–17.
11 Gabutti V, Piga A. Results of long-term iron-chelating therapy. *Acta Haematol* 1996; **95**(1): 26–36.
12 Hershko C, Weatherall DJ. Iron chelating therapy. *Clin Laboratory Sci* 1988; **26**: 303–45.
13 Gabutti V, Piga A, Sacchetti L et al. Quality of life and life expectancy in thalassemic patients with complications. In: Buckner CD, Gale RP, Lucarelli G, eds. *Advances and Controversies in Thalassemia Therapy*. New York: Alan R Liss, 1989: 35–41.
14 Piomelli S. Cooley's anemia management: 25 years of progress. In: Buckner CD, Gale RP, Lucarelli G,

15 Politis C. Complications of blood transfusions in thalassemia. In: Buckner CD, Gale RP, Lucarelli G, eds. *Advances and Controversies in Thalassemia Therapy.* New York: Alan R Liss, 1989: 67–76.

16 Manenti F, Galimberti M, Lucarelli G et al. Growth and endocrine function after bone marrow transplantation for thalassemia. In: Buckner CD, Gale RP, Lucarelli G, eds. *Advances and Controversies in Thalassemia Therapy.* New York: Alan R Liss, 1989: 273–80.

17 De Sanctis V, Galimberti M, Lucarelli G, Polchi P, Ruggiero L, Vullo C. Gonadal function after allogeneic bone marrow transplantation for thalassaemia. *Arch Dis Child* 1991; **66**: 517–20.

18 Slavin S, Or R, Cividalli G et al. Bone marrow transplantation in β-thalassemia with prevention of graft-vs.-host disease. In: Fucharoen S, Rowley PT, Paul NW, eds. *Birth Defects: Original Article Series. Thalassemia: Pathophysiology and Management.* Vol. 23, Part 5B. New York: Alan R Liss, 1988: 313–6.

19 Witherspoon RP, Fisher LD, Schoch G et al. Secondary cancers after bone marrow transplantation for leukemia or aplastic anemia. *N Engl J Med* 1989; **321** (12): 784–9.

20 Socié G, Henry-Amar M, Cosset JM, Devergie A, Girinsky T, Gluckman E. Increased incidence of solid malignant tumors after bone marrow transplantation for severe aplastic anemia. *Blood* 1991; **78**: 277–9.

21 Witherspoon RP, Storb R, Pepe M, Longton G, Sullivan KM. Cumulative incidence of secondary solid malignant tumors in aplastic anemia patients given marrow grafts after conditioning with chemotherapy alone [Letter]. *Blood* 1992; **79**: 289–92.

22 Parkman R, Rappeport J, Geha R et al. Complete correction of the Wiskott–Aldrich syndrome by allogeneic bone-marrow transplantation. *N Engl J Med* 1978; **298**: 921–7.

23 Kapoor N, Kirkpatrick D, Oleske J et al. Reconstitution of normal megakaryocytopoiesis and immunologic functions in Wiskott–Aldrich syndrome by marrow transplantation following myeloablation and immunosuppression with busulfan and cyclophosphamide. *Blood* 1981; **57**: 692–6.

24 Hobbs JR, Hugh-Jones K, Shaw PJ, Downie CJC, Williamson S. Engraftment rates related to busulphan and cyclophosphamide dosages for displacement bone marrow transplants in fifty children. *Bone Marrow Transplant* 1986; **1**: 201–8.

25 Thomas ED, Buckner CD, Storb R et al. Aplastic anaemia treated by marrow transplantation. *Lancet* 1972; **i**: 284–9.

26 Storb R, Champlin RE. Bone marrow transplantation for severe aplastic anemia. *Bone Marrow Transplant* 1991; **8**: 69–72.

27 Santos GW, Sensenbrenner LL, Burke PJ et al. Marrow transplantation in man following cyclophosphamide. *Transplant Proc* 1971; **3**: 400–4.

28 Tutschka PJ, Elfenbein GJ, Sensenbrenner LL et al. Preparative regimens for marrow transplantation in acute leukemia and aplastic anemia. Baltimore experience. *Am J Ped Hematol Oncol* 1980; **2**: 363–70.

29 Santos GW, Tutschka PJ, Brookmeyer R et al. Marrow transplantation for acute nonlymphocytic leukemia after treatment with busulfan and cyclophosphamide. *N Engl J Med* 1983; **309**: 1347–53.

30 Appelbaum FR, Storb R, Ramberg RE et al. Allogeneic marrow transplantation in the treatment of preleukemia. *Ann Intern Med* 1984; **100**: 689–93.

31 Tutschka PJ, Copelan EA, Kapoor N. Replacing total body irradiation with busulfan as conditioning of patients with leukemia for allogeneic marrow transplantation. *Transplant Proc* 1989; **21**: 2952–4.

32 Tutschka PJ, Copelan EA, Kapoor N, Avalos BR, Klein JP. Allogeneic bone marrow transplantation for leukemia using chemotherapy as conditioning. Six-year results of a single institution trial. *Transplant Proc* 1991; **23**: 1709–10.

33 Floersheim GL, Elson LA. Restoration of hematopoiesis following a lethal dose of dimethyl myleran by isologic bone marrow transplantation in mice. Experiments on modification of intolerance to homologous bone marrow by 6-mercaptopurine, amino-chlorambucil and cortisone. *Acta Haematol* 1961; **26**: 233–45.

34 Storb R, Weiden PL, Graham TC, Lerner KG, Nelson N, Thomas ED. Hemopoietic grafts between DLA-identical canine littermates following dimethyl myleran. Evidence for resistance to grafts not associated with DLA and abrogated by antithymocyte serum. *Transplantation* 1977; **24**: 349–57.

35 Tutschka PJ, Copelan EA, Klein JP. Bone marrow transplantation for leukemia following a new busulfan and cyclophosphamide regimen. *Blood* 1987; **70**: 1382–8.

36 Storb R, Thomas ED, Buckner CD et al. Marrow transplantation in thirty 'untransfused' patients with severe aplastic anemia. *Ann Intern Med* 1980; **92**: 30–6.

37 Storb R, Prentice RL, Thomas ED et al. Factors associated with graft rejection after HLA-identical marrow transplantation for aplastic anaemia. *Br J Haematol* 1983; **55**: 573–85.

38 Bearman SI, Appelbaum FR, Buckner CD et al. Regimen-related toxicity in patients undergoing bone marrow transplantation. *J Clin Oncol* 1988; **6**: 1562–8.

39 Bearman SI, Appelbaum FR, Back A et al. Regimen-related toxicity and early posttransplant survival in patients undergoing marrow transplantation for lymphoma. *J Clin Oncol* 1989; **7**: 1288–94.

40 Thomas ED, Sanders JE, Buckner CD et al. Marrow transplantation for thalassemia. *Ann NY Acad Sci* 1985; **445**: 417–27.

41 Thomas ED, Lucarelli G. Marrow transplantation for thalassemia major. In: Fucharoen S, Rowley PT, Paul NW, eds. *Birth Defects: Original Article Series. Thalassemia: Pathophysiology and Management.* Vol. 23, Part 5B. New York: Alan R Liss, 1988: 303–6.

42 Storb R, Anasetti C, Appelbaum F et al. Marrow transplantation for severe aplastic anemia and thalassemia major. *Semin Hematol* 1991; **28**(3): 235–9.

43 Lucarelli G, Polchi P, Izzi T et al. Allogeneic marrow transplantation for thalassemia. *Exp Hematol* 1984; **12**: 676–81.

44 Lucarelli G, Polchi P, Galimberti M et al. Marrow transplantation for thalassemia following busulphan and cyclophosphamide. *Lancet* 1985; **i**: 1355–7.

45 Lucarelli G, Galimberti M, Polchi P et al. Bone marrow transplantation in thalassemia. *Hematol Oncol Clin North Am* 1991; **5**(3): 549–56.

46 Andreani M, Nesci S, Lucarelli G et al. Long-term survival of ex-thalassemic patients with persistent mixed chimerism after bone marrow transplantation. *Bone Marrow Transplant* 2000; **25**(4): 401–4.

47 Andreani M, Manna M, Lucarelli G et al. Persistence of mixed chimerism in patients transplanted for the treatment of thalassemia. *Blood* 1996; **87**(8): 3494–9.

48 Gaziev D, Galimberti M, Lucarelli G et al. Bone marrow transplantation from alternative donors for thalassemia: HLA-phenotypically identical relative and HLA nonidentical sibling or parent transplants. *Bone Marrow Transplant* 2000; **25**(8): 815–21.

49 La Nasa G, Giardini C, Argiolu F et al. Unrelated donor bone marrow transplantation for thalassemia: the effect of extended haplotypes. *Blood* 2002; **99**(12): 4350–6.

50 Di Bartolomeo P, Di Girolamo G, Olioso P et al. The Pescara experience of allogenic bone marrow transplantation in thalassemia. *Bone Marrow Transplant* 1997; **19** (Suppl. 2): 48–53.

51 Argiolu F, Sanna MA, Cossu F et al. Bone marrow transplant in thalassemia. The experience of Cagliari. *Bone Marrow Transplant* 1997; **19** (Suppl. 2): 65–7.

52 Clift RA, Johnson FL. Marrow transplants for thalassemia. The USA experience. *Bone Marrow Transplant* 1997; **19** (Suppl. 2): 57–9.

53 Roberts IAG, Darbyshire PJ, Will AM. BMT for children with β-thalassemia major in the UK. *Bone Marrow Transplant* 1997; **19** (Suppl. 2): 60–1.

54 Ghavamzadeh A, Bahar B, Djahani M, Kokabandeh A, Shahriari A. Bone marrow transplantation of thalassemia, the experience in Tehran (Iran). *Bone Marrow Transplant* 1997; **19** (Suppl. 2): 71–3.

55 Dennison D, Srivastava A, Chandy M. Bone marrow transplantation for thalassaemia in India. *Bone Marrow Transplant* 1997; **19** (Suppl. 2): 70.

56 Lin HP, Chan LL, Lam SK, Ariffin W, Menaka N, Looi LM. Bone marrow transplantation for thalassemia. The experience from Malaysia. *Bone Marrow Transplant* 1997; **19** (Suppl. 2): 74–7.

57 Li CK, Yuen PMP, Shing MK et al. Stem cell transplant for thalassaemia patients in Hong Kong. *Bone Marrow Transplant* 1997; **19** (Suppl. 2): 62–4.

58 Issaragrisil S, Suvatte V, Visuthisakchai S et al. Bone marrow and cord blood stem cell transplantation for thalassemia in Thailand. *Bone Marrow Transplant* 1997; **19** (Suppl. 2): 54–6.

59 Lucarelli G, Angelucci E, Giardini C et al. Fate of iron stores in thalassemia after bone marrow transplantation. *Lancet* 1993; **342**: 1388–91.

60 Niederau G, Fischer R, Purschel A, Stremmel W, Haussinger D, Strohmeyer G. Long-term survival in patients with hereditary hemochromatosis. *Gastroenterology* 1996; **110**(4): 1107–19.

61 Angelucci E, Muretto P, Lucarelli G et al. Phlebotomy to reduce iron overload in patients cured of thalassemia by bone marrow transplantation. Italian Cooperative Group for Phlebotomy Treatment of Transplanted Thalassemia Patients. *Blood* 2002; **90**(3): 994–8.

62 Angelucci E, Muretto P, Lucarelli G et al. Treatment of iron overload in the 'ex-thalassemic'. Report from the phlebotomy program. *Ann NY Acad Sci* 1998; **30**(850): 288–93.

63 Mariotti E, Angelucci E, Agostini A, Baronciani D, Sgarbi E, Lucarelli G. Evaluation of cardiac status in iron-loaded thalassemia patients following bone marrow transplantation: improvement in cardiac function during reduction in body iron burden. *Br J Haematol* 1998; **103**(4): 916–21.

64 Erer B, Angelucci E, Lucarelli G et al. Hepatitis C virus infection in thalassemia patients undergoing allogeneic bone marrow transplantation. *Bone Marrow Transplant* 1994; **14**: 369–72.

104

Mark C. Walters

Hematopoietic Cell Transplantation for Sickle Cell Disease

Sickle cell disease (SCD) is caused by a single point mutation in codon 6 of the β-globin chain. This mutation directs an amino acid substitution of valine for glutamic acid, which promotes the formation of long hemoglobin polymers under hypoxic conditions [1–3]. This propensity for polymer formation deforms the red blood cell and causes significant alterations in red cell integrity, rheologic properties and lifespan [4–7]. It is probably directly or indirectly responsible for the vasculopathy that forms in virtually all body organs. It is estimated that this heritable disorder of hemoglobin affects 1/375 African-Americans in the USA and approximately 2000 infants are identified annually by neonatal screening programs in the USA [8]. However, it has far-reaching public health effects worldwide; in Africa alone, it is estimated that 120 000 infants with SCD are born annually [9].

Since a national effort to establish and sustain comprehensive centers for sickle cell anemia 30 years ago, a generation of children and adults have benefited from advances in supportive and interventional therapies and access to services that grew from this commitment to improve care [10,11]. As a result, today the vast majority of infants diagnosed with sickle cell anemia by state newborn screening programs and enrolled in comprehensive care programs will survive to adulthood, at a rate that appears indistinguishable from African-Americans who do not inherit this disorder [12]. Thus, the key features of sickle cell anemia are shifting from events characterized by a series of life-threatening acute episodes in childhood, each having the potential for early mortality [13], to ongoing complex management issues of a chronic illness of adulthood, characterized by an inexorable accrual of significant health problems that adversely affect the quality of life [14].

Against this backdrop, attitudes about the role of hematopoietic cell transplantation (HCT) are also shifting [15]. Initially performed in those who had coexistent hematologic malignancies, these first cases served primarily to demonstrate that allogeneic transplantation had the potential for cure of sickle cell anemia [16]. The next phase of investigations targeted symptomatic patients for enrollment and focused on characterizing the consequences of transplantation and the quality of cure among those who survived free of sickle erythropoiesis [17–19]. As a consequence, in standard practice today, transplantation is reserved almost exclusively for those who have clinical features that portend a poor outcome or significant sickle-related morbidity, in part because of the toxicity of this intensive therapy. However, follow-up studies after transplantation confirm the sustained benefit of donor erythropoiesis which acts to improve significantly the quality of life among those who survive with stable engraftment of donor cells [18,20].

The current challenge is to integrate HCT into the care of individuals with SCD in an era when established therapeutic interventions are readily available, and new therapeutic options are being developed. As for malignant disorders, there are ongoing efforts to better define the role of transplantation for SCD as new targeted and supportive therapies become available. These analyses are difficult in the absence of randomized prospective trials comparing therapeutic alternatives. Still, some discussion of the pathophysiology, clinical features, supportive therapy and advances in predicting disease severity is necessary in an attempt to define when and for whom to pursue HCT for SCD.

Pathophysiology and clinical features of sickle cell disease

The clinical hallmark of SCD is vaso-occlusion. The phenomenon of vaso-occlusion originates in sickle hemoglobin, which, in the deoxygenated state, tends to form polymers that deform the red blood cell and diminish its biochemical and structural integrity [21–23]. While the causal relationship between sickle hemoglobin and vaso-occlusion is not disputed, the contributing factors and sequence of events that ultimately impair the flow of blood in microvessels are complex and still incompletely understood. The deoxygenated sickle polymer induces cellular potassium and water efflux, caused both by acidification and cellular swelling, which activate the potassium–chloride cotransport efflux pathway [24], and by cellular membrane distortion, which, with the accompanying transient calcium influx, activates the calcium-dependent Gardos channel pathway of potassium and water efflux [25,26]. The resulting cellular dehydration increases the cell density and sickle hemoglobin concentration, thereby promoting sickle hemoglobin polymerization.

Sickle hemoglobin polymerization induces perturbations in erythrocyte cellular membranes which promote adhesive interactions with vascular endothelial cells [27,28]. These interactions impact factors that control the vascular tone of blood vessels, and generally elicit vasoconstriction [29]. Other cellular blood components are affected by these events, importantly granulocytes and activated platelets that interact with adhesive sickle erythrocytes and endothelial cells [30–33]. Reticulocytes released prematurely from marrow also express membrane proteins that promote erythrocyte–endothelial interactions [34]. These cellular interactions ultimately generate the release of cytokines which promote an inflammatory response and amplify the cascade of vaso-occlusion and tissue injury. None of these factors alone can explain vaso-occlusion, although they may contribute singly or in combination. As a result, the cause and severity of vaso-occlusion may vary from event to event, and from individual to individual.

While the clinical expression of SCD is heterogeneous, it is characterized by clinical and subclinical vaso-occlusive episodes that occur in virtually all body organs. Organs that are particularly susceptible to injury early in life are the spleen, bones, lungs and brain. The most frequent complication is a painful vaso-occlusive 'crisis', the most common reason for hospitalization among patients with SCD. Pain, which may last for days or weeks, is most frequently located in the chest, back, abdomen or extremities, and multiple sites can be affected during a single episode. Until its spontaneous resolution, treatment remains largely supportive. Acute chest syndrome is a common pulmonary complication of SCD that affects 15% to >50% of patients [35–37], and is the second most frequent reason for hospitalization. The classical clinical triad of chest pain, fever and a new radiographic infiltrate suggests its diagnosis [38]. The aetiology of acute chest syndrome is varied [36]; causative agents include bacterial infection, atypical bacterial infection resulting from *Chlamydia pneumoniae* and *Mycoplasma pneumoniae*, respiratory viral infection, pulmonary thromboembolism [39], bone marrow/fat embolism [40] and rib infarction [41]. SCD is a common cause of stroke in childhood and occurs in approximately 6–12% of affected individuals [42]. Intervention with regular transfusions to reduce sickle hemoglobin (HbS) levels to ≤30% effectively reduces the risk of recurrent stroke [43], but without this therapy recurrent stroke occurs in 70–90% of patients [44]. Subtle manifestations of neurovascular disease develops in many patients. Silent cerebral infarction was observed in 17% of patients with sickle cell anemia (HbSS) who were evaluated in the Cooperative Study of Sickle Cell Disease (CSSCD) [45,46]. These subclinical events caused characteristic changes that were detectable with cerebral magnetic resonance imaging (MRI) and correlated with deficits in neuropsychologic testing.

A comprehensive discussion of all the clinical complications of sickle cell disease is beyond the scope of this chapter; however, this brief description supports the notion that SCD is a serious life-threatening hematologic disorder that significantly reduces the quality of life for many individuals. These clinical observations provide the rationale to conduct clinical trials of HCT as a curative intervention for SCD. Its clinical severity remains an important stimulus for the development of novel transplantation and other approaches that might transform the outlook for individuals who inherit this disease.

Predictors of disease severity as potential indicators of HCT eligibility

Paradoxically, knowing the genotype of SCD, which can be ascertained readily by pre- and postnatal evaluation, does not by itself confer the ability to predict the severity of an individual's clinical course with any degree of certainty [47]. This can complicate decisions about whether to employ therapeutic measures that are accompanied by risk of toxicity, as risk–benefit considerations should balance toxicity risks of the intervention against those of the underlying sickle cell anemia [48]. As a rule, SCD is a chronic illness characterized by recurrent episodes of vaso-occlusive complications that affect the quality of life and shorten lifespan. However, there are individuals who experience a milder course and, ideally, should be spared unnecessary exposure to potentially toxic interventions. Thus, the discovery and characterization of modifiers that influence the phenotype of sickle cell anemia have been the subject of intense study [49]. Knowledge of these would permit clinicians to apply interventions such as HCT according to a risk-based algorithm, as has been applied for childhood acute lymphoblastic leukemia and other malignant disorders.

To date, the most important modifier of clinical expression is the fetal hemoglobin (HbF) level. HbF interferes with sickle polymer formation and thus protects from the characteristic changes in erythrocyte deformability and lifespan that accompany deoxygenation and polymerization [50]. Significant elevations in HbF expressed in a pancellular distribution are sufficient to eliminate virtually all aspects of the sickle phenotype, as occurs naturally in the sickle hereditary persistence of fetal hemoglobin (HPFH) syndromes [5,51]. Alternatively, even incremental elevations in HbF level confer a clinical benefit and reduce the risk of having frequent painful vaso-occlusive crises [52]. Polymorphisms associated with alterations in HbF expression among those who inherit sickle cell anemia (HbSS) have been described [53–55], and these designated β-globin haplotypes purportedly modulate the sickle phenotype, although their utility in reliably predicting individual disease severity remains limited. Other loci outside the human β-globin locus that affect HbF expression have been described [56,57]. Several studies have shown that these factors are heritable, and that there are additive genetic and environmental influences that affect the level of fetal cells (F-cells), and correspondingly HbF [58]. There is also evidence that the pharmacologic response to agents that induce HbF expression is a heritable trait [59]. Not surprisingly, pharmacologic manipulation of HbF expression has been an active area of basic and clinical research.

The search for other genetic polymorphisms or molecular markers of disease severity is ongoing, but none have yet proved suitable to screen candidates for interventions like HCT. However, several studies have suggested genes that, alone or in combination, are likely to influence SCD severity [60,61]. Factors that influence sickle erythrocyte–endothelial interactions include proteins that promote adherence such as von Willebrand's factor, membrane proteins in the vascular endothelium and red blood cells (RBCs) that anchor these interactions, and interactions between RBC erythrocyte membrane proteins and the subendothelial matrix that may be exposed by vascular endothelial injury [27,28,62,63]. Examples of RBC–endothelial factors involved in these interactions include CD36 [33,64], aggregated membranous Band 3 [65] and integrin very-late activation antigen-4 (VLA4) receptors ($\alpha_4\beta_1$) [64,66] in the RBC membrane and endothelial integrins such as vascular cell adhesion molecule-1 (VCAM-1; a ligand for the RBC $\alpha_4\beta_1$ receptor) [34,66,67] and $\alpha V\beta_3$ integrin [68,69]. The expression of these membrane proteins and inflammatory cytokines such as tumour necrosis factor alfa (TNF-α) that affect the expression of VCAM-1 might also be considered for their influence on disease severity [70].

Another burgeoning area of investigation that implicates erythrocyte–endothelial interactions are the determinants of vascular tone and the effect of nitric oxide (NO) on the sickle vasculature. NO has a cytoprotective effect and downregulates expression of VCAM-1 [71], and increases arteriolar diameter, thereby lowering mean arteriolar pressure [72]. Together, these appear to have an important inhibitory effect on vaso-occlusion [73]. NO is synthesized by endothelial NO synthase, with arginine as a substrate, and is bound avidly by hemoglobin [74]. NO synthase is induced in endothelial cells by TNF-α and interleukin 1 (IL-1), depleting arginine levels and, in the end, has the opposite effect by actually lowering NO levels in the post-capillary venules [75,76]. In addition, these inflammatory mechanisms unleash an NO scavenger function by superoxide radicals that are generated by activated leukocytes [32]. These mechanisms together may deplete NO and thereby promote vasoconstriction and sickle erythrocyte–endothelial interactions. The genetic control of these epistatic events may improve our understanding of how to predict SCD severity, and these are targets of therapeutic drug development.

Similar strategies have been employed to explore epistatic factors that might increase the risk of specific sickle-related complications such as stroke. Clinically, overt stroke affects 5–10% of all SCD patients, with an additional 17% who develop subclinical vascular events that portend a risk of subsequent stroke and impair neuropsychologic performance [42,45,46,77]. Polymorphisms associated with thrombosis that include factor V Leiden, methylene-tetrahydrofolate reductase (MTHFR) deficiency and prothrombin 20210 A have not been associated with a higher stroke risk in sickle cell anemia [78–81]. However, elevated leukocyte count and lowered hemoglobin concentration have been linked to stroke, and suggest that endothelial injury and leukostasis might follow the increased or turbulent flow that accompanies anemia [42,77]. α-Thalassemia is associated with increased hemoglobin level demonstrated protection from stroke in some studies, but not in other multivariable analyses [42,82]. Surprisingly, HbF levels appear to have no effect on stroke risk. Recently, evaluations of human leukocyte antigen (HLA) associations with stroke revealed that selected class II alleles were most strongly associated with stroke risk (*DRB1*0301* and *0302* with odds ratio [OR] = 5.8; $p = 0.007$) and protection from stroke (*DRB1*1501* and *1503* with OR = 0.21; $p = 0.019$) [83,84]. To a lesser extent, class I alleles (HLA-B) were also associated with stroke risk. These observations suggest that the HLA system contributes to the pathophysiology of cerebral vasculopathy in sickle cell anemia, as has been described in moyamoya [85]. There is speculation that the inflammatory response which accompanies endothelial injury caused by vaso-occlusion is regulated in part by the HLA genes, and that specific alleles or groups of alleles are more likely to elicit a cascade of events that cause cerebral arterial occlusion.

Clinical indicators of sickle cell disease severity

Parallel with efforts to identify genetic or epistatic predictors of adverse outcomes, clinical predictors have been investigated. An analysis by the CSSCD identified predictors of adverse outcomes, defined as death, stroke and recurrent episodes of pain and acute chest syndrome (≥2 and ≥1 event(s)/year for 3 consecutive years, respectively) before 10 years of age [86,87]. These predictors included the onset of early dactylitis defined as pain and tenderness, with or without swelling, in the hands, feet, or both, before 1 year of age, leukocytosis and severe anemia (Hb level <7 g/dL during the second year of life) (Fig. 104.1). While these features may be clinical manifestations of the expression of genetic and epigenetic factors that synergistically magnify the impact of sickling, the complexity of linking these as yet undefined but potentially measurable modifiers to a clinical severity index remains elusive. However, if these predictors had reproducible and meaningful utility, they might provide a means for identifying and treating presymptomatic children with high-risk features by transplantation and thereby reduce the risk of graft rejection.

Recent research efforts have focused on methods to identify sickle cell patients at risk for specific complications such as stroke and acute chest syndrome, screen them before the event occurs and employ an intervention to prevent the adverse sickle-related complication. The most progress in developing this approach has occurred in the area of stroke prevention, and it is also a potential application for HCT. The central nervous system (CNS) injury associated with SCD, appropriately, has been a focus of intense investigation. While stroke is an overt manifestation of CNS injury which affects approximately 5–10% of patients, a more pervasive and subtle injury caused by endothelial damage and ischemia is increasingly apparent among children, and a more detailed view of the

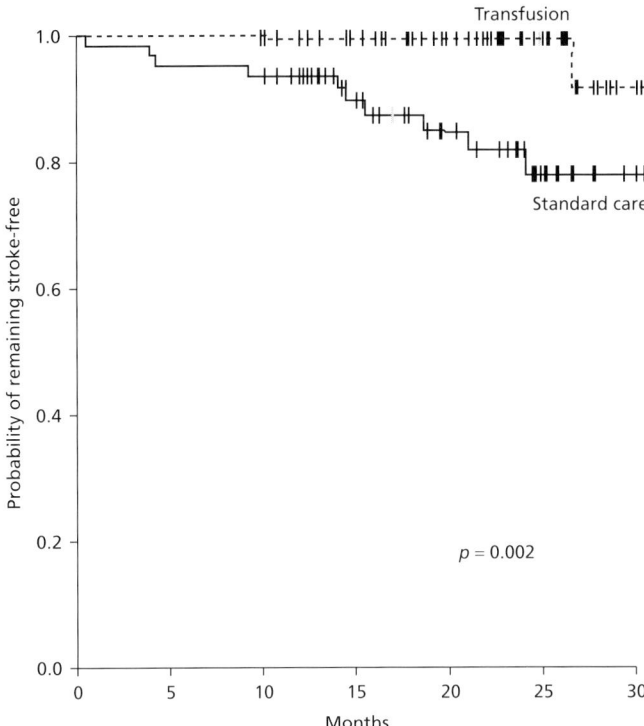

Fig. 104.2 Kaplan–Meier estimate of the probability of not having a stroke among patients receiving long-term transfusion and patients receiving standard care [90]. The *p*-value was calculated by proportional hazards regression analysis. Tick marks indicate the lengths of observation of patients who did not have a stroke. One patient in the standard care group who had an intracerebral hematoma was excluded from the analysis.

problem among adults is very likely to emerge [42,77]. Prospective investigations by MRI have documented that CNS lesions progress in number and that these injuries correlate with functional abnormalities measured by neuropsychologic testing instruments [46,88]. Silent neurovascular lesions have predictive value with regard to stroke but have perhaps optimal predictive value when combined with transcranial Doppler evaluations [89–91]. The utility of RBC transfusions in preventing stroke and silent cerebral infarction among these high-risk patients has been demonstrated, and the duration of transfusion is the subject of a current multicenter clinical investigation (Fig. 104.2) [90,91]. Stabilization of neurovascular disease as measured by cerebral MRI has been observed after successful allogeneic transplantation, raising the possibility that it too might be employed to prevent stroke and halt progression of CNS

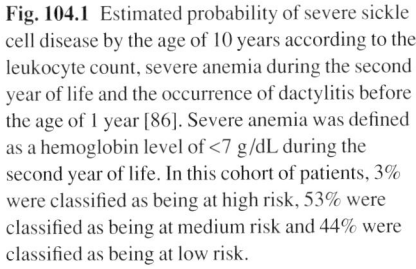

Fig. 104.1 Estimated probability of severe sickle cell disease by the age of 10 years according to the leukocyte count, severe anemia during the second year of life and the occurrence of dactylitis before the age of 1 year [86]. Severe anemia was defined as a hemoglobin level of <7 g/dL during the second year of life. In this cohort of patients, 3% were classified as being at high risk, 53% were classified as being at medium risk and 44% were classified as being at low risk.

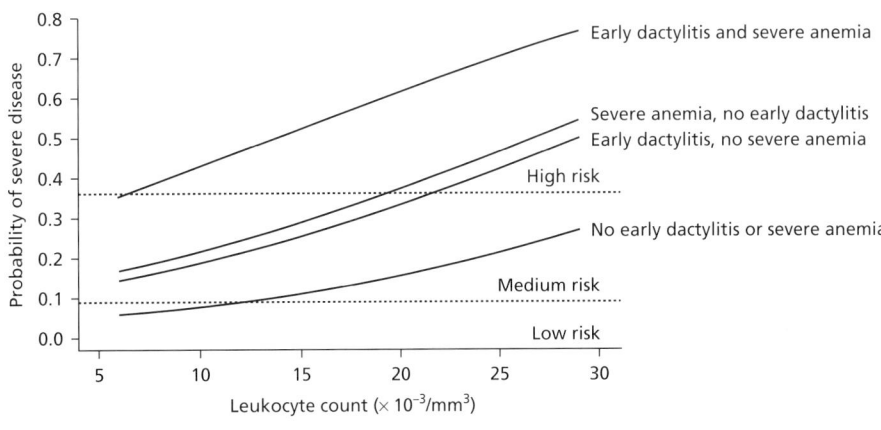

Table 104.1 Comparison of cerebral magnetic resonance angiography (MRA) in hematopoietic cell transplantation (HCT) recipients and untreated controls [93].

Patient group	n	Mean arterial diameter (mm)		Paired t-test
		First MRA (± SD)	Second MRA (± SD)	
Untreated SCD	64 vessels in 11 patients	3.4 (±1.1)	3.3 (±1.2)	n.s.
HCT recipients	22 vessels in four patients	2.9 (±1.3)	3.3 (±1.0)	0.04

HCT, hematopoietic cell transplantation; MRA, magnetic resonance angiography; n.s., not significant; SCD, sickle cell disease; SD, standard deviation.
The average follow-up between first and second MRA was 30.3 months (±9.9 months) in the untreated and 19.3 months (±10.4 months) in the HCT patients. The same six vessels were measured in all patients except in one HCT recipient who had chronic occlusion of the left internal carotid artery.

injury [18,92]. This partial recovery from pre-existing vascular injury also has been reported and improved cerebral arterial cross-sectional diameter noted in one study involving a small number of subjects after transplantation (Table 104.1) [93]. Together these observations strongly suggest that patients who have stable engraftment of donor cells after transplantation also benefit by protection from subsequent CNS vascular events.

Current indications for HCT

While the newer considerations for early identification of high-risk patients discussed above appear promising for future application, in standard practice, transplantation for SCD currently is reserved almost exclusively for those who have clinical features that portend a poor outcome or significant sickle-related morbidity, in part because of the toxicity of this intensive therapy [94]. These clinical indications, which were adapted from the multicenter investigation of bone marrow transplantation for SCD, are listed in Table 104.2. In addition, these criteria have been applied almost exclusively to children, where the risk–benefit ratio is most advantageous in terms of years-of-life gained among those who survive with sustained engraftment of donor cells. Less certain is how to apply inclusion criteria to adults with sickle cell anemia, where the experience of transplantation is much more limited but for whom the risk of significant transplantation-related toxicity remains substantial. For all patients, clinicians must carefully weigh therapeutic alternatives to HCT, with particular attention to safety, efficacy, availability and the cost of the intervention [95–98]. Unfortunately, prospective clinical trials that compare HCT to other therapeutic interventions for SCD have not been conducted, and therapeutic decision-making is hampered by this limitation, particularly with regard to understanding the impact of therapies on long-term outcomes. Although a comprehensive discussion is beyond the scope of this chapter, a brief discussion of therapeutic alternatives to HCT for SCD follows.

Treatment options

The foundation of supportive care begins with newborn screening and early diagnosis to facilitate education about life-threatening complications, which include infection prevention and treatment [99]. In addition, management of acute and chronic pain, and transfusions for selected indications remain mainstays of supportive care [100,101]. Increasingly, however, RBC transfusions are used to treat and prevent specific complications such as stroke and acute chest syndrome, and in preparation for operative procedures that utilize general anesthesia (Table 104.3) [37,43,102]. The utility of chronic RBC transfusions in preventing debilitating complications is amply documented [103], but chronic RBC transfusion exposures may cause pathogen exposures, iron overload and alloimmunization to minor blood group antigens [104–106]. Automated exchange transfusions appear to mitigate the risk of iron overload without altering the therapeutic effect of transfusions [107,108], and extended RBC phenotype donor–recipient matching may reduce the frequency of RBC alloimmunization [109,110]. The effect of chronic transfusions on long-term outcome in sickle cell anemia has not been studied.

A pharmaceutical alternative to HCT is hydroxyurea (HU), which has a favourable cost and safety profile, and thus is readily available to most adult patients [111,112]. It acts by increasing HbF levels and thereby inhibits sickle hemoglobin polymerization and vaso-occlusion. In addition, the myelosuppressive effect of HU on neutrophil, monocyte and reticulocyte levels in the blood is in part responsible for the ameliorative effect of this agent. Another property of HU is its effect to increase NO

Table 104.2 Indications of hematopoietic cell transplantation (HCT) for sickle cell disease.

Patients with sickle cell disease (SS or Sβ-thalassemia) <16 years of age
One or more of the following complications:
   Stroke or CNS event lasting >24 h
   Recurrent acute chest syndrome
   Recurrent vaso-occlusive painful episodes or recurrent priapism
   Impaired neuropsychologic function with abnormal cerebral MRI and angiography
   Stage I or II sickle lung disease
   Sickle nephropathy (GFR 30–50% of predicted normal)

CNS, central nervous system; GFR, glomerular filtration rate; MRI, magnetic resonance imaging.

Table 104.3 Indications for red blood cell (RBC) transfusions for sickle cell disease.

Acute chest syndrome
Prevention of recurrent strokes:
   Severe acute anemia or chronic symptomatic anemia of renal disease
   Stroke prevention in asymptomatic children with abnormal TCD velocity
   In preparation for surgery with general anesthesia
   Refractory leg ulcers
   Refractory recurrent severe painful episodes
   Selected obstetrical complications
   Sustained acute priapism
   Severe splenic or hepatic sequestration syndrome

TCD, transcranial Doppler.

levels, and that the vasodilatation associated with NO may contribute to its beneficial effect [113]. The clinical efficacy of HU was proved in a prospective randomized double-blind placebo-controlled trial which enrolled 299 patients, and which was prematurely halted because of a statistically significant 44% reduction in painful crises among those who were randomized to receive HU [114]. There was a 34% reduction in the number of RBC transfusions administered, and a 50% reduction in the number of episodes of acute chest syndrome. While there was no apparent reduction in the rate of stroke, more recent studies have suggested that HU might act as a suitable alternative to RBC transfusions for the prevention of stroke recurrence among those, who, for one reason or other are unable to receive chronic RBC transfusions [115,116]. However, this notion is challenged by a rate of recurrent stroke among HU recipients that exceeds the incidence reported during chronic RBC transfusions [117]. Taken together, HU is an important therapeutic agent that appears to improve the quality of life in many patients. Several pediatric trials have suggested that, as in adults, HU appears safe and beneficial in children [118–122]. Long-term assessments of its safety when treatment is initiated early in life are ongoing.

Newer agents focus on rheologic abnormalities of sickle erythrocytes as therapeutic targets for inhibiting vaso-occlusion. A nonionic surfactant that, when given intravenously, reduces blood viscosity by interfering with RBC–endothelial interactions has been observed to effect a modest reduction in the duration of painful vaso-occlusive episodes [123]. NO, whose precursor is L-arginine, causes vasodilatation and relaxation by its action on vascular smooth muscle. Its use in acute chest syndrome suggests the potential for a reduction in pulmonary arterial pressure and thus clinical improvement after administration of it or its precursor, L-arginine [74,124–126]. Another area of active investigation is to block sickling-induced cation fluxes that contribute to cellular dehydration, as a strategy to counteract the tendency of the dense sickle RBC to potentiate other factors which promote vaso-occlusion [127]. Agents such as dipyridamole and clotrimazole have shown preclinical evidence that they effectively reduce cellular dehydration by inhibiting cation influx by separate pathways [128,129]. These agents share in common with HU the potential for safety, efficacy and wide availability. However, unlike HCT, these interventions ameliorate but do not eliminate the clinical expression of sickle cell anemia. The discussion that follows focuses on the current results of HCT for SCD, its late effects and prospects for making this curative approach more widely available.

Current results of HCT for sickle cell disease

The worldwide experience of transplantation for SCD is summarized in Table 104.4 [94,131,132]. In these studies and their collective experience, the transition of transplantation from an experimental intervention reserved for the most ill patients to one in which increasingly younger children with early signs of sickle-related morbidity are targeted has been observed. Several series in Europe and North America have reported very similar results after HLA-identical sibling transplantation [19,20,139,140]. The principal aim of these multicenter clinical studies was to define more completely the risks and benefits of this therapy, and to characterize the natural history of those surviving free of SCD. The results of transplantation were best when performed in children with SCD who had HLA-identical sibling donors. Even though many children who received allografts had significant sickle-related complications, such as stroke and recurrent episodes of acute chest syndrome, the disease-free survival was very good, approximately 80–85% in several series. However, 5–10% of patients died of complications related to transplantation, with graft-vs.-host disease (GVHD) and its treatment noted as the leading cause of death. In the multicenter investigation of HCT for SCD, 59 children who ranged in age between 3.3 and 15.9 years (median 9.9 years)

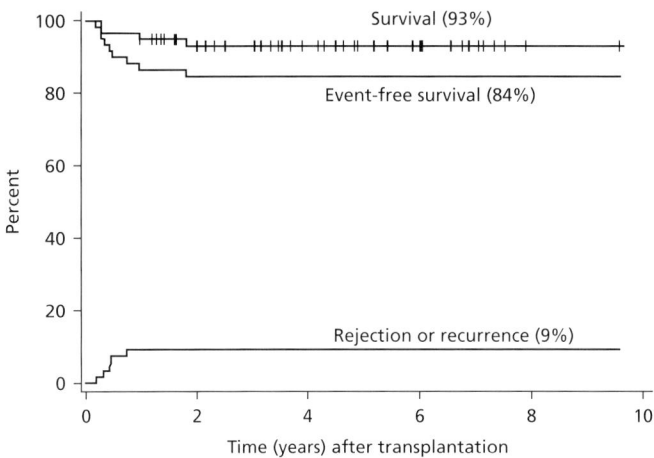

Fig. 104.3 Kaplan–Meier estimates of survival and event-free survival after bone marrow transplantation for sickle cell disease—multicenter investigation. Outcome after transplantation for 59 children with advanced symptomatic sickle cell disease [20]. Kaplan–Meier estimates for survival and event-free survival following marrow transplantation are shown. An event was defined as death, graft rejection or recurrence of sickle cell disease. A cumulative incidence curve for graft rejection and return of sickle cell disease is also depicted.

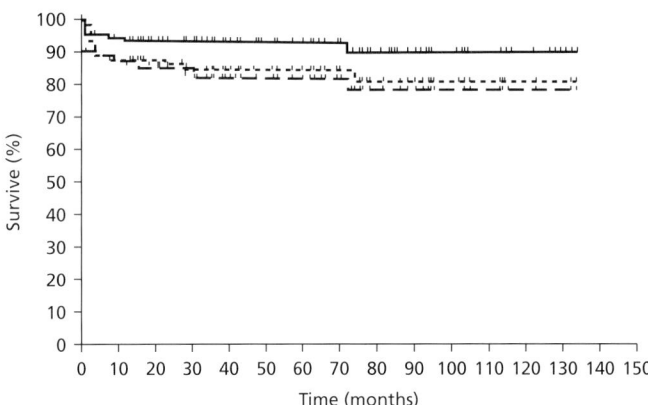

Fig. 104.4 Kaplan–Meier estimates of survival and event-free survival after bone marrow transplantation for sickle cell disease—European centers [19]. Overall survival (upper curve), disease-free survival (middle curve) and event-free survival (lower curve) are depicted among 101 patients after HCT for sickle cell disease in Europe. The results were 88%, 80% and 76%, respectively.

received HLA-identical sibling allografts between September 1991 and April 2000. Patients received a myeloablative combination of busulfan (BU), cyclophosphamide (CY) and horse antithymocyte globulin before HCT, and most received a combination of methotrexate (MTX) and cyclosporine (CSP) after HCT to prevent GVHD. Fifty-five children survive, 50 free of the underlying sickle cell anemia. The Kaplan–Meier probabilities of survival and disease-free survival are 93% and 84%, respectively (Fig. 104.3). Results among 101 patients who received myeloablative HLA-identical sibling HCT in Europe were remarkably similar, with an overall survival probability of 88% and disease-free survival of 80% (Fig. 104.4) [19]. In response to these observations, today most clinicians consider transplantation as a reasonable treatment option for patients who have significant sickle-related complications.

Among patients who had stable engraftment of donor cells after HCT, none experienced subsequent clinical vaso-occlusive events. Evaluation of the effects of transplantation on sickle cell-related organ damage is

Table 104.4 Worldwide experience of hematopoietic cell transplantation (HCT) for sickle cell disease.

Location	Regimen	n	Median age years (range)	Survival (%)	Deaths	Graft rejection/ recurrent SCD (%)	Stable mixed chimerism	Disease-free survival (%)	aGVHD	cGVHD	Seizures
Belgium [19]	BU;CY (30) BU;CY,TLI (6) BU;CY,ATG (14)	36	8.6 (1.7–23)	34 (94)	2	4	6*	30 (83)†	15‡	8	18
		14	2.0 (0.9–15)	14 (100)	0	1	–	13 (93)	5	2	
Pesaro [130]	BU;CY (17) BU;CY,ATG (2)	19	7 (4–38)	14 (74)	5	1	5	13 (68)	4	2	1
France [92,139,140]	BU;CY (12) BU;CY,ATG (48)	60	8.8 (2.2–22)	54 (90)	6§	4	–	50 (83)	6/26#	2/26#	7
Multicenter [17,18,20]	BU;CY,ATG	59	9.9 (3.3–15.9)	55 (94)	4	5	10	50 (85)	11 (grade I–III)	5	13
Other USA/Europe [16,133,138]	BU;CY,ATG (13) CY/TBI (3)	16¶	–	13 (81)	3	1	–	12 (80)†	2	1	1
Total		201§		182 (91)	19	16 (8)	11%	166 (83)	25%	12%	25%

aGVHD, acute graft-vs.-host disease; ATG, anti thymocyte globulin; BU, busulfan; cGVHD, chronic graft-vs.-host disease; CY, cyclophosphamide; SCD, sickle cell disease; TLI, total lymphoid irradiation; TBI, total body irradiation.
*Three had >30% recipient cells.
†One patient was disease-free after a second HCT.
‡Only one patient had >grade II GVHD.
§Three French patients were reported in two series, one of whom died after HCT.
¶One patient had Morquio's disease and two had acute leukemia concomitantly.
#Data on GVHD only available for 26 patients.

ongoing but suggests stabilization and, in some cases, improvement in pre-existing sickle vasculopathy [18,19]. Several groups have reported recovery of splenic function and stabilization of CNS disease and bony abnormalities after HCT [140–143]. In addition, in most patients, pulmonary disease remained stable as evaluated by pulmonary function testing, and improved linear growth was observed. Preliminary results suggest that most patients have excellent quality of life after HCT. Taken together, these observations confirm the curative potential of HCT for SCD.

To date, these promising results in children have not been extended to older patients with SCD. Anecdotal reports of transplantation for adults with sickle cell anemia suggest a poor outcome [94]. Results from a multicenter national trial included two patients who were 16 and 28 years of age (M.C. Walters, unpublished data). Unfortunately, both patients experienced substantial transplant-related adverse events and died of multiorgan failure as a result of sepsis and GVHD. These preliminary results warrant the development of novel approaches in adults with SCD to reduce the toxicity of HCT. If, in the setting of HCT for adults, the use of mobilized peripheral blood hematopoietic cells (PBHCs) in lieu of bone marrow is deemed advantageous, the administration of granulocyte colony-stimulating factor (G-CSF) and collection of PBHCs from sickle cell trait donors appears safe [144].

Complications after HCT

The problem of disease recurrence after transplantation, however, remains a key obstacle to success. The cumulative incidence of graft rejection accompanied by autologous recovery was approximately 10% in several published series [19,20,139]. In the multicenter investigation of transplantation for SCD, there was an association between graft rejection and the pretransplant administration of iron chelation therapy, suggesting that pretransplant exposures to blood products promoted an immunologic response that interfered with donor engraftment [20]. This contrasts with graft rejection rates that are very low among recipients with hematologic malignancies who undergo HLA-identical sibling transplantation [145]. Thus, the high frequency of graft rejection observed in sickle cell patients implies that immunologic barriers which might include suppression of host natural killer (NK) cells and T lymphocytes are not reliably overcome by myeloablative pretransplantation therapy. The problem of rejection might be approached by several different strategies. If sensitization to minor histocompatibility antigens mediated by host memory T cells is a key determinant of rejection, targeting younger patients with few or even no transfusion exposures might optimize outcomes. When transfusions are necessary in transplant candidates, it is important to administer gamma-irradiated leukocyte-reduced blood products to reduce the risk of sensitization to minor histocompatibility antigens [146]. Alternatively, it is possible that targeted immunosuppressive therapy that inhibits the host-vs.-graft (HVG) reaction before and after transplantation, either with or in lieu of myeloablative pretransplantation conditioning, might be employed to promote engraftment. Finally, the identification and enrichment of donor cellular populations that facilitate engraftment without causing GVHD is another strategy that could be pursued.

One complication distinctive of SCD and HCT is an increased risk of adverse neurologic events after HCT (Table 104.4). In particular, patients with a history of stroke had an increased risk of intracranial hemorrhage after HCT [147]. Four of seven initial patients in the multicenter investigation had adverse events including two episodes of intracranial hemorrhage, which led to incorporation of measures to prevent CNS complications after transplantation. These measures included anticonvulsant prophylaxis with phenytoin initiated with BU dosing and continued for 6 months following transplantation (or until CSP was discontinued), strict control of hypertension, prompt repletion of magnesium deficiency and maintenance of hemoglobin concentrations between 9 and 11 g/dL and platelet counts >50,000/mm^3. By implementing these measures, the problem of intracranial hemorrhage was eliminated in the multicenter investigation; however, patients continued to experience self-limited seizures, particularly in the setting of hypertension, relative hyperviscosity caused by transfusion or if receiving CSP. There were no long-term sequelae associated with these events [133,148]. Anticonvulsant prophylaxis in a European series similarly did not appear to reduce the seizure incidence after HCT (38% vs. 35% among those who received, or did not receive prophylaxis, respectively) [19].

The risk of malignancy after conditioning regimens using chemotherapy rather than total body irradiation is predicted to be low and was reported to be <1% in the cohort transplanted for α-thalassemia major [149,150]. However, the development of myelodysplastic syndrome and myeloid leukemia in one SCD patient after HCT was associated with the administration of intensive immunosuppression for chronic GVHD [19].

Growth and development after HCT for sickle cell disease

Several series of patients have been evaluated for linear growth after HCT. In an interim analysis of the multicenter study, 26 surviving children who were 6.9–19.2 years of age (median 14.7 years) after HCT were studied. All had normal thyroid function after HCT. The mean and median standard deviation scores (SDSs) were calculated at annual timepoints after transplantation as shown in Fig. 104.5 [18]. The median SDS score was −0.7 before transplantation, improved to −0.4 by 24 months after transplantation and was −0.2 after 48 months, although there was no significant change in the mean SDS scores for the cohort. This trend of normalized linear growth was also observed in a European cohort where growth was reported to be normal or improved except in two patients with chronic GVHD who were receiving corticosteroids.

Gonadotropin and sex hormone levels of surviving patients have also been monitored, and these confirm the toxic effect of BU on gonadal function. Among seven surviving females in the multicenter study who were >13 years of age after HCT, an interim analysis showed that five had primary amenorrhea and five had corresponding elevated luteinizing hormone (LH) and follicle-stimulating hormone (FSH) levels that were associated with decreased serum estradiol levels in four patients. One

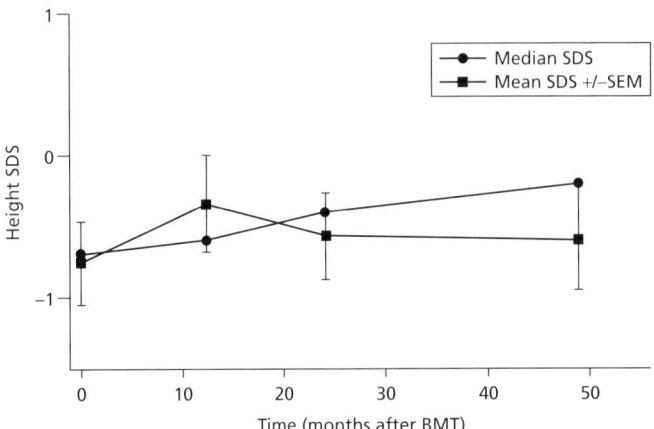

Fig. 104.5 Height standard deviation scores (SDS) after bone marrow transplantation for sickle cell disease [18]. Linear growth among individuals after transplantation for sickle cell disease is depicted. Height determinations were converted to the corresponding number of standard deviations from age- and sex-adjusted norms. By using such SDS, a child with average height would have a SDS of zero. Error bars represent standard error of the mean (SEM).

individual receiving hormonal replacement therapy had elevated LH and FSH levels and a normal serum estradiol. One post-pubertal female had normal serum FSH and estradiol levels. Of seven males who were >13 years of age, none of four tested had elevated serum LH or FSH levels. However, two males who were 14 and 16 years of age had low testosterone levels that were correlated with gonadotropin levels in the prepubertal range. Among six evaluable prepubertal girls in the Belgian cohort, five had primary amenorrhea with elevated serum LH and FSH [19]. Two post-pubertal females developed secondary amenorrhea. Testicular function was also adversely affected in four of six evaluable boys who demonstrated decreased testosterone and elevated FSH levels. It is anticipated that many if not most of the females will require hormonal replacement therapy after HCT.

Stable mixed chimerism after HCT for sickle cell disease

Stable mixed hematopoietic chimerism has been observed after conventional myeloablative transplantation for hemoglobinopathies. This condition has the potential for considerable ameliorative effect, an observation that has been particularly well-documented for β-thalassemia major and also other hereditary disorders [151–156]. Approximately 10% of children with SCD and thalassemia major developed stable mixed chimerism after conventional HLA-identical sibling HCT [20,152]. In the multicenter investigation of bone marrow transplantation (BMT) for sickle cell anemia, 13 of 50 patients with clinically successful allografts developed stable mixed chimerism. The level of donor chimerism, measured ≥6 months after transplantation in peripheral blood, varied between 90% and 99% in eight patients. Five additional patients had a lower proportion of donor cells (range 11–74%). Among these five patients, hemoglobin levels varied between 11.2 and 14.2 g/dL (median 11.3 g/dL; mean 12.0 g/dL). In patients who had donors with a normal hemoglobin genotype, the HbS fractions were 0%, 0% and 7%, which corresponded to donor chimerism levels of 67%, 74% and 11%, respectively (Fig. 104.6). Among patients who had donors with sickle trait, the HbS fractions were 36% and 37%, which corresponded to donor chimerism levels of 25% and 60%, respectively. Thus, allograft recipients with stable mixed chimerism had HbS levels similar to donor levels, and only one patient required an RBC transfusion >90 days after transplantation. None of the patients experienced painful events or other clinical complications related to SCD after transplantation. These observations are consistent with the idea that chimerism even with a minority of donor cells might have a curative effect, and that full engraftment of donor cells is not a requirement for successful HCT.

Nonmyeloablative HCT for sickle cell disease

Several groups have attempted to extend the early encouraging results after nonmyeloablative HCT for hematologic malignancies in adults to patients with SCD. In addition, murine models of sickle cell anemia have been utilized in nonmyeloablative HCT investigations, which appear to support the notion that this approach affords a significant benefit even when stable mixed chimerism develops after HCT [157,158]. However, the clinical application of nonmyeloablative HCT for SCD remains limited and incompletely defined. There have been two approaches: one utilizing a minimally toxic regimen first developed in a large animal model and translated successfully into human trials for older adult patients with hematologic malignancies and a second, reduced-intensity regimen that retains a moderate degree of the myelosuppressive effect of transplantation [159,160]. Representative examples of the two regimens are presented in Table 104.5. The former causes minimal myelosuppression and thus can be administered in the outpatient setting. This minimally toxic regimen relies on post-grafting immunosuppression to prevent graft-vs.-host (GVH) and HVG reactions and thereby promotes engraftment of donor cells. In contrast, the latter approach relies on reduced intensity preparation to suppress the HVG reaction and promote

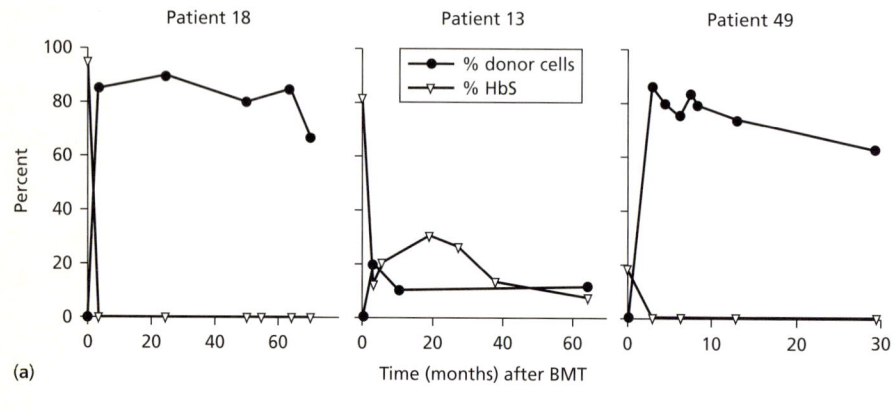

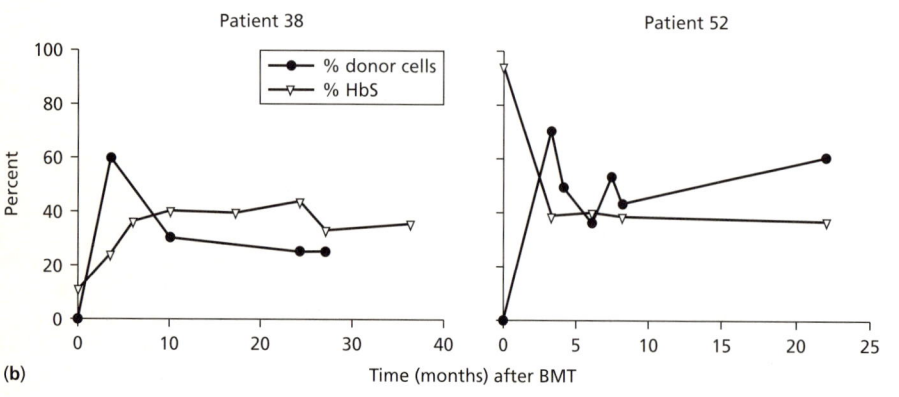

Fig. 104.6 Serial determinations of donor chimerism and sickle hemoglobin (HbS) fractions after transplantation [20]. (a) The fraction of donor cells in the blood (closed circles) and HbS fraction (open triangles) are depicted at regular intervals after transplantation with a period of follow-up extending to >5 years after transplantation. The relationship between donor chimerism and the HbS fraction is shown. Patients 13, 18 and 49 who had HbAA donors are shown. (b) HbS and chimerism studies from patients 38 and 52 who had HbAS donors are shown.

Table 104.5 Results of nonmyeloablative HLA-identical sibling HCT for sickle cell anemia [161–165].

	Minimal toxicity conditioning regimen	Reduced intensity conditioning regimen
Patients	10*	7†
Patient age years (median)	10 (range 3–28)	22 (range 7–56)
Conditioning regimen (dose)	FLU (90–150)/TBI (200) (5)	FLU (175)/BU (8)/ATG/TLI (500) (4)
	FLU (125–150)/ATG/TBI (200) (5)	FLU (120)/MEL (140)/ATG (2)
		FLU (120)/CY (120) (1)
Source of stem cells	Marrow (8); PBHC (2)	Marrow (2); PBHC (3); CBSC (1)
Induction of mixed chimerism	Yes (transient in 7)	Yes
Graft rejection/disease recurrence	7	1
GVHD	Acute 1 (grade I), chronic 0	Acute 3 (grade II–IV), chronic 3 (2 fatal)
Deaths	0	2
Event-free survival	3	4

ATG, antithymocyte globulin; CBSC, cord blood stem cell; CY, cyclophosphamide; EFS, event-free survival; FLU, fludarabine; GVHD, graft-vs.-host disease; MEL, melphalan; PBHC, peripheral blood hematopoietic cell; TBI, total body irradiation; TLI, total lymphoid irradiation.
*Includes two patients with thalassemia major.
†Includes one patient with thalassemia major.

engraftment. This reduced intensity regimen is associated with hospitalization and accompanied by a risk of regimen-related toxicity, albeit at a reduced level.

A survey of the experience to date utilizing these two alternative nonmyeloablative regimens is presented in Table 104.5 (R. Iannone et al., in press) [161–165]. All patients received HLA-identical sibling allografts, utilizing either G-CSF mobilized PBHCs or bone marrow. All 10 recipients of a minimally toxic regimen developed mixed chimerism initially, but tolerance was not sustained after post-grafting immunosuppression was discontinued in seven of 10 patients. However, most patients were treated in the outpatient setting, none developed life-threatening transplant-related complications, and GVHD occurred infrequently and was mild in this predominantly pediatric cohort. Patients reverted to a sickle cell anemia phenotype after nonfatal graft rejection. Alternatively, those who received reduced intensity conditioning regimens benefited from augmented pregrafting immunosuppression that facilitated engraftment of donor cells, and only one of the seven recipients experienced graft rejection. Acute and chronic GVHD occurred more frequently in this older cohort and, in particular, among those who received PBHC allografts and developed full donor chimerism. Thus, the problem of transplant-related mortality was not eliminated by the reduced intensity conditioning regimen, especially among older recipients.

The observations of mixed chimerism after nonmyeloablative preparation also confirmed the clinical benefit of this condition, even when it was transitory. This benefit is illustrated by two patients who had initial engraftment of donor cells that resulted in mixed hematopoietic chimerism, although the level of donor chimerism declined after post-grafting immunosuppression was withdrawn [166]. Despite the decline, the HbS fraction remained <30% during the period when there was a low level of donor chimerism. The unexpectedly high HbA levels may reflect an enrichment of normal donor RBCs because of their longer lifespan. However, it is also possible that a selective advantage for donor erythroid cells began at an earlier stage of erythroid development, even before significant hemoglobinization of the maturing erythrocyte had occurred. To investigate this, serial blast-forming unit–erythroid (BFU-E) and colony-forming unit–granulocyte/macrophage (CFU-GM) colonies were obtained from marrow samples, and donor contribution was determined. In both patients, there was overrepresentation of donor erythroid progenitors compared with myeloid counterparts (Fig. 104.7). These findings suggested that the clinical benefits of mixed chimerism after nonmyeloablative transplantation for sickle cell anemia resulted from an extended lifespan of mature donor erythrocytes and a selective advantage for donor erythroid progenitors in the marrow. Thus, it appears possible to achieve a clinical benefit even when the cellular compartment expressing normal hemoglobin represents a fraction of all marrow cells. A multicenter collaborative clinical trial to define an effective nonmyeloablative regimen for children with symptomatic SCD is ongoing.

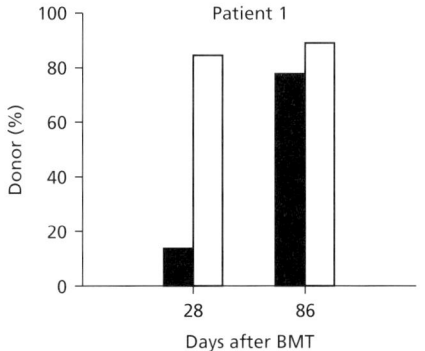
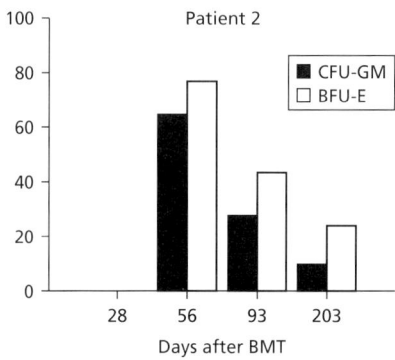

Fig. 104.7 Bone marrow chimerism after nonmyeloablative hemaotpoietic cell transplantation (HCT) for sickle cell disease [166]. The percentage of donor progenitor colonies in the bone marrow (burst-forming unit–erythroid [BFU-E; open bars] and colony-forming unit–granulocyte/macrophage [CFU-GM; closed bars]) after transplantation is depicted in two patients.

Alternative stem cell sources

The utilization of alternatative stem cell sources is an obvious but unproven method to expand HCT for SCD. Almost all transplantation cases to date have utilized bone marrow from HLA-identical siblings, and thus the experience of unrelated and HLA-mismatched related donor transplantation for sickle cell anemia is very limited. Cord blood hematopoietic cells (CBHCs) are a source of hematopoietic stem cells undergoing investigation to support transplantation for SCD. CBHCs have several unique properties that make them potentially useful in this setting. The lower incidence of severe GVHD associated with HLA-mismatched CBHC transplantation would make it very useful in this setting. However, abrogation of the allogeneic effect combined with a limiting number of hematopoietic stem cells that might act to increase the risk of engraftment failure also would be important considerations in HCT for SCD.

Early reports of successful CBHC transplantation for hemoglobinopathies, using related CBHC donors, have been extended and confirmed by recent experience from the Eurocord registry [167]. Forty-four patients (median age 5 years; range 1–20 years) with thalassemia ($n = 33$) or SCD ($n = 11$) received CBHC transplantation from a related donor. All but two donors, who were mismatched at a single HLA-A antigen, were HLA-identical sibling donors. Twenty-six patients received BU and CY, either alone ($n = 8$), or in combination with antithymocyte globulin or antilymphocyte globulin ($n = 18$). In 17 patients, a conditioning regimen that contained either BU and CY, or BU and fludarabine (FLU) was augmented by thiotepa (TT). One patient received a combination of BU, CY and FLU. None of the patients died, and 36 of 44 children survived disease-free, with a median follow-up of 24 months (range 3–76 months) after transplantation. Four patients experienced grade II acute GVHD, and two of 39 patients at risk developed limited chronic GVHD. The 2-year probabilities of event-free survival were 79% and 90% among patients with thalassemia and SCD, respectively (Fig. 104.8).

One patient with SCD and seven of 33 patients with thalassemia experienced disease recurrence after CBHC transplantation. Three of five patients had sustained donor engraftment after a second conventional BMT from the same sibling donor. The impact of the conditioning regimen and the use of MTX to prevent GVHD were considered in a univariate analysis of their associations with disease-free survival. This analysis showed that patients given MTX as part of GVHD prophylaxis had a significantly lower probability of surviving event-free compared to those who did not receive it (55% vs. 90%, respectively; $p = 0.005$). It also showed that receiving a non-MTX-containing regimen favourably affected the probability of myeloid recovery among all patients ($p = 0.04$) and in thalassemia patients ($p = 0.06$). In addition, pretransplant conditioning with BU and CY alone was associated with a lower probability of engraftment ($p = 0.0003$). Among thalassemia patients, the combinations of BU, TT and CY, or BU, TT and FLU in the conditioning regimen were associated with a significantly higher probability of surviving event-free (94% for BU, TT, CY or BU, TT, FLU vs. 62% for BU/CY; $p = 0.03$). These results suggest that outcomes after CBHC transplantation from sibling donors for hemoglobinopathies are similar to observations after BMT, with the potential for a lower rate of GVHD. The results also suggest that the problem of graft rejection is affected by the composition of pre- and post-grafting immunosuppressive regimens. To test these hypotheses, a prospective multicenter clinical trial of CBHC transplantation from HLA-identical donors has been initiated.

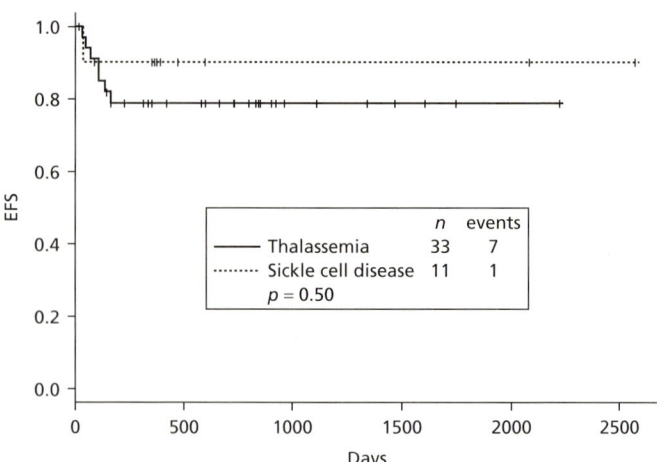

Fig. 104.8 Kaplan–Meier estimate of the probability of event-free-survival (EFS) after sibling donor cord blood hematopoietic cell (CBHC) transplantation for sickle cell anemia and thalassemia [167]. Eleven patients with sickle cell anemia and 33 with thalassemia major received sibling donor cord blood stem cell (CBSC) grafts after myeloablative conditioning therapy. The event-free survival probabilities are depicted.

Conclusions

Since the first report of successful HCT for sickle cell anemia nearly 20 years ago, this curative therapy has emerged as an important option in treating individuals who inherit this disorder. While its curative potential distinguishes it from therapeutic alternatives such as RBC transfusions and HU, the acute and late toxicities of transplantation raise concerns about its wider use. These concerns are being addressed by ongoing efforts to develop nonmyeloablative transplantation regimens for sickle cell anemia. However, an optimal regimen has not yet been identified. Ultimately, the future of transplantation for SCD will revolve around efforts to better understand the barriers to engraftment and how to overcome them. If these obstacles are eliminated, the possibility of transplantation from alternative stem cell sources such as CBHCs may become routine, thereby making transplantation available to more patients.

References

1 Pauling LIH, Singer SJ, Wells IC. Sickle cell anemia: a molecular disease. *Science* 1949; **110**: 543–8.
2 Ingram V. Gene mutations in human hemoglobin: the chemical difference between normal and sickle cell hemoglobin. *Nature* 1957; **180**: 326.
3 Noguchi CT, Schechter AN. The intracellular polymerization of sickle hemoglobin and its relevance to sickle cell disease. *Blood* 1981; **58**: 1057–68.
4 Bensinger TA, Gillette PN. Hemolysis in sickle cell disease. *Arch Intern Med* 1974; **133**: 624–31.
5 Brittenham GM, Schechter AN, Noguchi CT. Hemoglobin S polymerization: primary determinant of the hemolytic and clinical severity of the sickling syndromes. *Blood* 1985; **65**: 183–9.
6 Self F, McIntire LV, Zanger B. Rheological evaluation of hemoglobin S and hemoglobin C hemoglobinopathies. *J Lab Clin Med* 1977; **89**: 488–97.
7 Mohandas N, Evans E. Rheological and adherence properties of sickle cells: potential contribution to hematologic manifestations of the disease. *Ann N Y Acad Sci* 1989; **565**: 327–37.
8 Force ANST. Serving the family from birth to the medical home: newborn screening—a blueprint for the future. *Pediatrics* 2000; **106** (Suppl.): 383–427.
9 Fleming AF. The presentation, management and prevention of crisis in sickle cell disease in Africa. *Blood Rev* 1989; **3**: 18–28.
10 Health supervision for children with sickle cell disease. *Pediatrics* 2002; **109**: 526–35.
11 Mentzer WC, Kan YW. Prospects for research in hematologic disorders: sickle cell disease and thalassemia. *J Am Med Assoc* 2001; **285**: 640–2.

12 Centers for Disease Control and Prevention. Mortality among children with sickle cell disease identified by newborn screening during 1990–94, California, Illinois, and New York. *J Am Med Assoc* 1998; **279**: 1059–60.

13 Platt OS, Brambilla DJ, Rosse WF et al. Mortality in sickle cell disease: life expectancy and risk factors for early death. *N Engl J Med* 1994; **330**: 1639–44.

14 Wierenga KJ, Hambleton IR, Lewis NA. Survival estimates for patients with homozygous sickle-cell disease in Jamaica: a clinic-based population study. *Lancet* 2001; **357**: 680–3.

15 van Besien K, Koshy M, Anderson-Shaw L et al. Allogeneic stem cell transplantation for sickle cell disease: a study of patients' decisions. *Bone Marrow Transplant* 2001; **28**: 545–9.

16 Johnson FL, Look AT, Gockerman J, Ruggiero MR, Dalla-Pozza L, Billings FT. Bone-marrow transplantation in a patient with sickle-cell anemia. *N Engl J Med* 1984; **311**: 780–3.

17 Walters MC, Patience M, Leisenring W et al. Bone marrow transplantation for sickle cell disease. *N Engl J Med* 1996; **335**: 369–76.

18 Walters MC, Storb R, Patience M et al. Impact of bone marrow transplantation for symptomatic sickle cell disease: an interim report. *Blood* 2000; **95**: 1918–24.

19 Vermylen C, Cornu G, Ferster A et al. Haematopoietic stem cell transplantation for sickle cell anemia: the first 50 patients transplanted in Belgium. *Bone Marrow Transplant* 1998; **22**: 1–6.

20 Walters MC, Patience M, Leisenring W et al. Stable mixed hematopoietic chimerism after bone marrow transplantation for sickle cell anemia. *Biol Blood Marrow Transplant* 2001; **7**: 665–73.

21 Hebbel RP. Beyond hemoglobin polymerization: the red blood cell membrane and sickle disease pathophysiology. *Blood* 1991; **77**: 214–37.

22 Asakura T, Mattiello JA, Obata K et al. Partially oxygenated sickled cells: sickle-shaped red cells found in circulating blood of patients with sickle cell disease. *Proc Natl Acad Sci U S A* 1994; **91**: 12589–93.

23 Mozzarelli A, Hofrichter J, Eaton WA. Delay time of hemoglobin S polymerization prevents most cells from sickling *in vivo*. *Science* 1987; **237**: 500–6.

24 Brugnara C, Bunn HF, Tosteson DC. Regulation of erythrocyte cation and water content in sickle cell anemia. *Science* 1986; **232**: 388–90.

25 Sugihara T, Hebbel RP. Exaggerated cation leak from oxygenated sickle red blood cells during deformation: evidence for a unique leak pathway. *Blood* 1992; **80**: 2374–8.

26 Joiner CH, Morris CL, Cooper ES. Deoxygenation-induced cation fluxes in sickle cells. III. Cation selectivity and response to pH and membrane potential. *Am J Physiol* 1993; **264**: C734–44.

27 Hebbel RP. Perspectives series: cell adhesion in vascular biology. Adhesive interactions of sickle erythrocytes with endothelium. *J Clin Invest* 1997; **99**: 2561–4.

28 Hebbel RP, Yamada O, Moldow CF, Jacob HS, White JG, Eaton JW. Abnormal adherence of sickle erythrocytes to cultured vascular endothelium: possible mechanism for microvascular occlusion in sickle cell disease. *J Clin Invest* 1980; **65**: 154–60.

29 Setty BN, Chen D, Stuart MJ. Sickle cell vaso-occlusive crisis is associated with abnormalities in the ratio of vasoconstrictor to vasodilator prostanoids. *Pediatr Res* 1995; **38**: 95–102.

30 Brittain HA, Eckman JR, Swerlick RA, Howard RJ, Wick TM. Thrombospondin from activated platelets promotes sickle erythrocyte adherence to human microvascular endothelium under physiologic flow: a potential role for platelet activation in sickle cell vaso-occlusion. *Blood* 1993; **81**: 2137–43.

31 Hofstra TC, Kalra VK, Meiselman HJ, Coates TD. Sickle erythrocytes adhere to polymorphonuclear neutrophils and activate the neutrophil respiratory burst. *Blood* 1996; **87**: 4440–7.

32 Dias-Da-Motta P, Arruda VR, Muscara MN et al. The release of nitric oxide and superoxide anion by neutrophils and mononuclear cells from patients with sickle cell anaemia. *Br J Haematol* 1996; **93**: 333–40.

33 Sugihara K, Sugihara T, Mohandas N, Hebbel RP. Thrombospondin mediates adherence of CD36+ sickle reticulocytes to endothelial cells. *Blood* 1992; **80**: 2634–42.

34 Gee BE, Platt OS. Sickle reticulocytes adhere to VCAM-1. *Blood* 1995; **85**: 268–74.

35 Castro O, Brambilla DJ, Thorington B et al. The acute chest syndrome in sickle cell disease: incidence and risk factors. The Cooperative Study of Sickle Cell Disease. *Blood* 1994; **84**: 643–9.

36 Vichinsky EP, Neumayr LD, Earles AN et al. Causes and outcomes of the acute chest syndrome in sickle cell disease. National Acute Chest Syndrome Study Group. *N Engl J Med* 2000; **342**: 1855–65.

37 Vichinsky EP, Styles LA, Colangelo LH, Wright EC, Castro O, Nickerson B. Acute chest syndrome in sickle cell disease: clinical presentation and course. Cooperative Study of Sickle Cell Disease. *Blood* 1997; **89**: 1787–92.

38 Sprinkle RH, Cole T, Smith S, Buchanan GR. Acute chest syndrome in children with sickle cell disease: a retrospective analysis of 100 hospitalized cases. *Am J Pediatr Hematol Oncol* 1986; **8**: 105–10.

39 Durant JR, Cortes FM. Occlusive pulmonary vascular disease associated with hemoglobin SC disease: a case report. *Am Heart J* 1966; **71**: 100–6.

40 Vichinsky E, Williams R, Das M et al. Pulmonary fat embolism: a distinct cause of severe acute chest syndrome in sickle cell anemia. *Blood* 1994; **83**: 3107–12.

41 Rucknagel DL, Kalinyak KA, Gelfand MJ. Rib infarcts and acute chest syndrome in sickle cell diseases. *Lancet* 1991; **337**: 831–3.

42 Ohene-Frempong K, Weiner SJ, Sleeper LA et al. Cerebrovascular accidents in sickle cell disease: rates and risk factors. *Blood* 1998; **91**: 288–94.

43 Pegelow CH, Adams RJ, McKie V et al. Risk of recurrent stroke in patients with sickle cell disease treated with erythrocyte transfusions. *J Pediatrics* 1995; **126**: 896–9.

44 Powars D, Wilson B, Imbus C, Pegelow C, Allen J. The natural history of stroke in sickle cell disease. *Am J Med* 1978; **65**: 461–71.

45 Moser FG, Miller ST, Bello JA et al. The spectrum of brain MR abnormalities in sickle-cell disease: a report from the Cooperative Study of Sickle Cell Disease. *Am J Neuroradiol* 1996; **17**: 965–72.

46 Armstrong FD, Thompson RJ Jr, Wang W et al. Cognitive functioning and brain magnetic resonance imaging in children with sickle cell disease. Neuropsychology Committee of the Cooperative Study of Sickle Cell Disease. *Pediatrics* 1996; **97**: 864–70.

47 Nagel RL. Severity, pathobiology, epistatic effects, and genetic markers in sickle cell anemia. *Semin Hematol* 1991; **28**: 180–201.

48 Platt OS, Guinan EC. Bone marrow transplantation in sickle cell anemia: the dilemma of choice. *N Engl J Med* 1996; **335**: 426–8.

49 Nagel RL. Pleiotropic and epistatic effects in sickle cell anemia. *Curr Opin Hematol* 2001; **8**: 105–10.

50 Poillon WN, Kim BC, Rodgers GP, Noguchi CT, Schechter AN. Sparing effect of hemoglobin F and hemoglobin A2 on the polymerization of hemoglobin S at physiologic ligand saturations. *Proc Natl Acad Sci U S A* 1993; **90**: 5039–43.

51 Noguchi CT, Rodgers GP, Serjeant G, Schechter AN. Levels of fetal hemoglobin necessary for treatment of sickle cell disease. *N Engl J Med* 1988; **318**: 96–9.

52 Platt OS, Thorington BD, Brambilla DJ et al. Pain in sickle cell disease: rates and risk factors. *N Engl J Med* 1991; **325**: 11–16.

53 Steinberg MH, Hsu H, Nagel RL et al. Gender and haplotype effects upon hematological manifestations of adult sickle cell anemia. *Am J Hematol* 1995; **48**: 175–81.

54 Powars DR, Meiselman HJ, Fisher TC, Hiti A, Johnson C. β-S gene cluster haplotypes modulate hematologic and hemorheologic expression in sickle cell anemia: use in predicting clinical severity. *Am J Pediatr Hematol Oncol* 1994; **16**: 55–61.

55 Nagel RL, Fleming AF. Genetic epidemiology of the β-S gene. *Baillière's Clin Hematol* 1992; **5**: 331–65.

56 Chang YC, Smith KD, Moore RD, Serjeant GR, Dover GJ. An analysis of fetal hemoglobin variation in sickle cell disease: the relative contributions of the X-linked factor, β-globin haplotypes, α-globin gene number, gender, and age. *Blood* 1995; **85**: 1111–17.

57 Miyoshi K, Kaneto Y, Kawai H et al. X-linked dominant control of F-cells in normal adult life: characterization of the Swiss type as hereditary persistence of fetal hemoglobin regulated dominantly by gene(s) on X chromosome. *Blood* 1988; **72**: 1854–60.

58 Garner C, Tatu T, Reittie JE et al. Genetic influences on F cells and other hematologic variables: a twin heritability study. *Blood* 2000; **95**: 342–6.

59 Steinberg MH. Determinants of fetal hemoglobin response to hydroxyurea. *Semin Hematol* 1997; **34** (Suppl. 3): 8–14.

60 Nagel RL. Sickle cell anemia is a multigene disease: sickle painful crises, a case in point. *Am J Hematol* 1993; **42**: 96–101.

61 Embury SH, Clark MR, Monroy G, Mohandas N. Concurrent sickle cell anemia and α-thalassemia: effect on pathological properties of sickle erythrocytes. *J Clin Invest* 1984; **73**: 116–23.

62 Hoover R, Rubin R, Wise G, Warren R. Adhesion of normal and sickle erythrocytes to endothelial monolayer cultures. *Blood* 1979; **54**: 872–6.

63 Wick TM, Moake JL, Udden MM, Eskin SG, Sears DA, McIntire LV. Unusually large von Willebrand factor multimers increase adhesion of sickle erythrocytes to human endothelial cells under controlled flow. *J Clin Invest* 1987; **80**: 905–10.

64 Joneckis CC, Ackley RL, Orringer EP, Wayner EA, Parise LV. Integrin $\alpha_4\beta_1$ and glycoprotein IV (CD36) are expressed on circulating reticulocytes in sickle cell anemia. *Blood* 1993; **82**: 3548–55.

65 Thevenin BJ, Crandall I, Ballas SK, Sherman IW, Shohet SB. Band 3 peptides block the adherence of

65 sickle cells to endothelial cells *in vitro*. *Blood* 1997; **90**: 4172–9.
66 Swerlick RA, Eckman JR, Kumar A, Jeitler M, Wick TM. α4β1-integrin expression on sickle reticulocytes: vascular cell adhesion molecule-1-dependent binding to endothelium. *Blood* 1993; **82**: 1891–9.
67 Setty BN, Stuart MJ. Vascular cell adhesion molecule-1 is involved in mediating hypoxia-induced sickle red blood cell adherence to endothelium: potential role in sickle cell disease. *Blood* 1996; **88**: 2311–20.
68 Kaul DK, Tsai HM, Liu XD, Nakada MT, Nagel RL, Coller BS. Monoclonal antibodies to αVβ3 (7E3 and LM609) inhibit sickle red blood cell–endothelium interactions induced by platelet-activating factor. *Blood* 2000; **95**: 368–74.
69 Kumar A, Eckman JR, Wick TM. Inhibition of plasma-mediated adherence of sickle erythrocytes to microvascular endothelium by conformationally constrained RGD-containing peptides. *Am J Hematol* 1996; **53**: 92–8.
70 Lutty GA, Taomoto M, Cao J et al. Inhibition of TNF-α-induced sickle RBC retention in retina by a VLA-4 antagonist. *Invest Ophthalmol Vis Sci* 2001; **42**: 1349–55.
71 De Caterina R, Libby P, Peng HB et al. Nitric oxide decreases cytokine-induced endothelial activation: nitric oxide selectively reduces endothelial expression of adhesion molecules and proinflammatory cytokines. *J Clin Invest* 1995; **96**: 60–8.
72 Kaul DK, Liu XD, Fabry ME, Nagel RL. Impaired nitric oxide-mediated vasodilation in transgenic sickle mouse. *Am J Physiol Heart Circ Physiol* 2000; **278**: H1799–806.
73 Stuart MJ, Setty BN. Sickle cell acute chest syndrome: pathogenesis and rationale for treatment. *Blood* 1999; **94**: 1555–60.
74 Morris CR, Kuypers FA, Larkin S, Vichinsky EP, Styles LA. Patterns of arginine and nitric oxide in patients with sickle cell disease with vaso-occlusive crisis and acute chest syndrome. *J Pediatr Hematol Oncol* 2000; **22**: 515–20.
75 Lopez BL, Barnett J, Ballas SK, Christopher TA, Davis-Moon L, Ma X. Nitric oxide metabolite levels in acute vaso-occlusive sickle-cell crisis. *Acad Emerg Med* 1996; **3**: 1098–103.
76 Francis RB Jr, Haywood LJ. Elevated immunoreactive tumor necrosis factor and interleukin-1 in sickle cell disease. *J Natl Med Assoc* 1992; **84**: 611–5.
77 Kinney TR, Sleeper LA, Wang WC et al. Silent cerebral infarcts in sickle cell anemia: a risk factor analysis: the Cooperative Study of Sickle Cell Disease. *Pediatrics* 1999; **103**: 640–5.
78 Rahimy MC, Krishnamoorthy R, Ahouignan G, Laffan M, Vulliamy T. The 20210A allele of prothrombin is not found among sickle cell disease patients from West Africa. *Thromb Haemost* 1998; **79**: 444–5.
79 Kahn MJ, Scher C, Rozans M, Michaels RK, Leissinger C, Krause J. Factor V Leiden is not responsible for stroke in patients with sickling disorders and is uncommon in African Americans with sickle cell disease. *Am J Hematol* 1997; **54**: 12–5.
80 De Castro LRH, Howe JG, Smith BR. Thrombophilic genotypes do not adversely affect the course of sickle cell disease (SCD). *Blood* 1998; **92**: 161a.
81 Zimmerman SA, Ware RE. Inherited DNA mutations contributing to thrombotic complications in patients with sickle cell disease. *Am J Hematol* 1998; **59**: 267–72.
82 Adams RJ, Kutlar A, McKie V, Carl E, Nichols FT, Liu JC et al. Alpha thalassemia and stroke risk in sickle cell anemia. *Am J Hematol* 1994; **45** (4): 279–82.
83 Styles LA, Hoppe C, Klitz W, Vichinsky E, Lubin B, Trachtenberg E. Evidence for HLA-related susceptibility for stroke in children with sickle cell disease. *Blood* 2000; **95**: 3562–7.
84 Hoppe C, Cheng S, Grow M et al. A novel multilocus genotyping assay to identify genetic predictors of stroke in sickle cell anaemia. *Br J Haematol* 2001; **114**: 718–20.
85 Kitahara T, Okumura K, Semba A, Yamaura A, Makino H. Genetic and immunologic analysis on moya-moya. *J Neurol Neurosurg Psychiatry* 1982; **45**: 1048–52.
86 Miller ST, Sleeper LA, Pegelow CH et al. Prediction of adverse outcomes in children with sickle cell disease. *N Engl J Med* 2000; **342**: 83–9.
87 Miller ST, Sleeper LA, Pegelow CH et al. Prediction of adverse outcomes in the newborn cohort of the Cooperative Study of Sickle Cell Disease (CSSCD): extended follow-up to 18 years. *Blood* 2000; **96**: 12a.
88 Pegelow CH, Macklin EA, Moser FG et al. Longitudinal changes in brain magnetic resonance imaging findings in children with sickle cell disease. *Blood* 2002; **99**: 3014–8.
89 Miller ST, Macklin EA, Pegelow CH et al. Silent infarction as a risk factor for overt stroke in children with sickle cell anemia: a report from the Cooperative Study of Sickle Cell Disease. *J Pediatr* 2001; **139**: 385–90.
90 Adams RJ, McKie VC, Hsu L et al. Prevention of a first stroke by transfusions in children with sickle cell anemia and abnormal results on transcranial doppler ultrasonography. *N Engl J Med* 1998; **339**: 5–11.
91 Pegelow CH, Wang W, Granger S et al. Silent infarcts in children with sickle cell anemia and abnormal cerebral artery velocity. *Arch Neurol* 2001; **58**: 2017–21.
92 Bernaudin F. Resultats et indications actuelles de l'allogreffe de moelle dans la drepanocytose. *Pathol Biol (Paris)* 1999; **47**: 59–64.
93 Steen RG, Helton KJ, Horwitz EM et al. Improved cerebrovascular patency following therapy in patients with sickle cell disease: initial results in four patients who received HLA-identical hematopoietic stem cell allografts. *Ann Neurol* 2001; **49**: 222–9.
94 Hoppe CC, Walters MC. Bone marrow transplantation in sickle cell anemia. *Curr Opin Oncol* 2001; **13**: 85–90.
95 Woods K, Karrison T, Koshy M, Patel A, Friedmann P, Cassel C. Hospital utilization patterns and costs for adult sickle cell patients in Illinois. *Public Health Rep* 1997; **112**: 44–51.
96 Nietert PJ, Abboud MR, Silverstein MD, Jackson SM. Bone marrow transplantation vs. periodic prophylactic blood transfusion in sickle cell patients at high risk of ischemic stroke: a decision analysis. *Blood* 2000; **95**: 3057–64.
97 Wayne AS, Schoenike SE, Pegelow CH. Financial analysis of chronic transfusion for stroke prevention in sickle cell disease. *Blood* 2000; **96**: 2369–72.
98 Nietert PJ, Silverstein MD, Abboud MR. Sickle cell anaemia: epidemiology and cost of illness. *Pharmacoeconomics* 2002; **20**: 357–66.
99 *The Management of Sickle Cell Disease*, 4th edn, C. Lenfart, ed. National Institutes of Health, 2002.
100 Bunn HF. Pathogenesis and treatment of sickle cell disease. *N Engl J Med* 1997; **337**: 762–9.
101 Steinberg MH. Management of sickle cell disease. *N Engl J Med* 1999; **340**: 1021–30.
102 Vichinsky EP, Haberkern CM, Neumayr L et al. A comparison of conservative and aggressive transfusion regimens in the perioperative management of sickle cell disease: the Preoperative Transfusion in Sickle Cell Disease Study Group. *N Engl J Med* 1995; **333**: 206–13.
103 Styles LA, Vichinsky E. Effects of a long-term transfusion regimen on sickle cell-related illnesses. *J Pediatrics* 1994; **125**: 909–11.
104 Wayne AS, Kevy SV, Nathan DG. Transfusion management of sickle cell disease. *Blood* 1993; **81**: 1109–23.
105 Vichinsky EP, Earles A, Johnson RA, Hoag MS, Williams A, Lubin B. Alloimmunization in sickle cell anemia and transfusion of racially unmatched blood. *N Engl J Med* 1990; **322**: 1617–21.
106 Vichinsky E. Consensus document for transfusion-related iron overload. *Semin Hematol* 2001; **38** (1 Suppl. 1): 2–4.
107 Singer ST, Quirolo K, Nishi K, Hackney-Stephens E, Evans C, Vichinsky EP. Erythrocytapheresis for chronically transfused children with sickle cell disease: an effective method for maintaining a low hemoglobin S level and reducing iron overload. *J Clin Apheresis* 1999; **14**: 122–5.
108 Kim HC, Dugan NP, Silber JH et al. Erythrocytapheresis therapy to reduce iron overload in chronically transfused patients with sickle cell disease. *Blood* 1994; **83**: 1136–42.
109 Vichinsky EP, Luban NL, Wright E et al. Prospective RBC phenotype matching in a stroke-prevention trial in sickle cell anemia: a multicenter transfusion trial. *Transfusion* 2001; **41**: 1086–92.
110 Ambruso DR, Githens JH, Alcorn R et al. Experience with donors matched for minor blood group antigens in patients with sickle cell anemia who are receiving chronic transfusion therapy. *Transfusion* 1987; **27**: 94–8.
111 Steinberg MH, Rodgers GP. Pharmacologic modulation of fetal hemoglobin. *Medicine (Baltimore)* 2001; **80**: 328–44.
112 Atweh GF, Schechter AN. Pharmacologic induction of fetal hemoglobin: raising the therapeutic bar in sickle cell disease. *Curr Opin Hematol* 2001; **8**: 123–30.
113 Glover RE, Ivy ED, Orringer EP, Maeda H, Mason RP. Detection of nitrosyl hemoglobin in venous blood in the treatment of sickle cell anemia with hydroxyurea. *Mol Pharmacol* 1999; **55**: 1006–10.
114 Charache S, Terrin ML, Moore RD et al. Effect of hydroxyurea on the frequency of painful crises in sickle cell anemia. Investigators of the Multicenter Study of Hydroxyurea in Sickle Cell Anemia. *N Engl J Med* 1995; **332**: 1317–22.
115 Ware RE, Steinberg MH, Kinney TR. Hydroxyurea: an alternative to transfusion therapy for stroke in sickle cell anemia. *Am J Hematol* 1995; **50**: 140–3.
116 Sumoza A, De Bisotti R, Sumoza D, Fairbanks V. Hydroxyurea (HU) for prevention of recurrent stroke in sickle cell anemia (SCA). *Am J Hematol* 2002; **71**: 161–5.
117 Ware RE, Zimmerman SA, Schultz WH. Hydroxyurea as an alternative to blood transfusions for the prevention of recurrent stroke in children with sickle cell disease. *Blood* 1999; **94**: 3022–6.

118. Scott JP, Hillery CA, Brown ER, Misiewicz V, Labotka RJ. Hydroxyurea therapy in children severely affected with sickle cell disease. *J Pediatr* 1996; **128**: 820–8.
119. Wang WC, Wynn LW, Rogers ZR, Scott JP, Lane PA, Ware RE. A 2-year pilot trial of hydroxyurea in very young children with sickle-cell anemia. *J Pediatr* 2001; **139**: 790–6.
120. Kinney TR, Helms RW, O'Branski EE et al. Safety of hydroxyurea in children with sickle cell anemia: results of the HUG-KIDS study, a phase I/II trial. Pediatric Hydroxyurea Group. *Blood* 1999; **94**: 1550–4.
121. Ferster A, Tahriri P, Vermylen C et al. Five years of experience with hydroxyurea in children and young adults with sickle cell disease. *Blood* 2001; **97**: 3628–32.
122. Wang WC, Helms RW, Lynn HS et al. Effect of hydroxyurea on growth in children with sickle cell anemia: results of the HUG-KIDS Study. *J Pediatr* 2002; **140**: 225–9.
123. Orringer EP, Casella JF, Ataga KI et al. Purified poloxamer 188 for treatment of acute vaso-occlusive crisis of sickle cell disease: a randomized controlled trial. *J Am Med Assoc* 2001; **286**: 2099–106.
124. Gladwin MT, Schechter AN, Shelhamer JH, Ognibene FP. The acute chest syndrome in sickle cell disease: possible role of nitric oxide in its pathophysiology and treatment. *Am J Respir Crit Care Med* 1999; **159**: 1368–76.
125. Gladwin MT, Schechter AN. Nitric oxide therapy in sickle cell disease. *Semin Hematol* 2001; **38**: 333–42.
126. Stuart MJ, Setty BN. Acute chest syndrome of sickle cell disease: new light on an old problem. *Curr Opin Hematol* 2001; **8**: 111–22.
127. Joiner CH, Franco RS. The activation of KCL cotransport by deoxygenation and its role in sickle cell dehydration. *Blood Cells Mol Dis* 2001; **27**: 158–64.
128. Brugnara C, Gee B, Armsby CC et al. Therapy with oral clotrimazole induces inhibition of the Gardos channel and reduction of erythrocyte dehydration in patients with sickle cell disease. *J Clin Invest* 1996; **97**: 1227–34.
129. Joiner CH, Jiang M, Claussen WJ, Roszell NJ, Yasin Z, Franco RS. Dipyridamole inhibits sickling-induced cation fluxes in sickle red blood cells. *Blood* 2001; **97**: 3976–83.
130. Giardini C, Galimberti M, Lucarelli G et al. Bone marrow transplantation in sickle cell disorders in Pesaro. *Bone Marrow Transplant* 1997; **19** (Suppl. 2): 106–9.
131. Mentzer WC. Bone marrow transplantation for hemoglobinopathies. *Curr Opin Hematol* 2000; **7**: 95–100.
132. Cornu G, Vermylen C, Ferster A et al. Hematopoietic stem cell transplantation in sickle cell anemia. *Arch Pediatr* 1999; **6** (Suppl. 2): 345s–7s.
133. Abboud MR, Jackson SM, Barredo J, Holden KR, Cure J, Laver J. Neurologic complications following bone marrow transplantation for sickle cell disease. *Bone Marrow Transplant* 1996; **17**: 405–7.
134. Abboud MR, Jackson SM, Barredo J, Beatty J, Laver J. Bone marrow transplantation for sickle cell anemia. *Am J Pediatr Hematol Oncol* 1994; **16**: 86–9.
135. Johnson FL, Mentzer WC, Kalinyak KA, Sullivan KM, Abboud MR. Bone marrow transplantation for sickle cell disease: the United States experience. *Am J Pediatr Hematol Oncol* 1994; **16**: 22–6.
136. Kalinyak KA, Morris C, Ball WS, Ris MD, Harris R, Rucknagel D. Bone marrow transplantation in a young child with sickle cell anemia. *Am J Hematol* 1995; **48**: 256–61.
137. Mentzer WCPS, Wara W et al. Successful bone marrow transplant in a child with sickle cell anemia and Morquio's disease. *Blood* 1990; **76**: 69a.
138. Milpied NHJ, Garand R, David A. Bone-marrow transplantation in a patient with sickle-cell anaemia. *Lancet* 1988; **2**: 328–9.
139. Bernaudin F, Souillet G, Vannier JP et al. Report of the French experience concerning 26 children transplanted for severe sickle cell disease. *Bone Marrow Transplant* 1997; **19** (Suppl. 2): 112–5.
140. Bernaudin F, Vernant J-P, E.Vilmer et al. Results of myeloablative allogenic stem cell transplant (SCT) for severe sickle cell disease (SCD) in France. *Blood* 2002; **100**: 5a.
141. Hernigou P, Bernaudin F, Reinert P, Kuentz M, Vernant JP. Bone-marrow transplantation in sickle-cell disease: effect on osteonecrosis—a case report with a 4-year follow-up. *J Bone Joint Surg Am* 1997; **79**: 1726–30.
142. Ferster A, Bujan W, Corazza F et al. Bone marrow transplantation corrects the splenic reticuloendothelial dysfunction in sickle cell anemia. *Blood* 1993; **81**: 1102–5.
143. Walters MC, Patience M, Leisenring W et al. Updated results of bone marrow transplantation (BMT) for sickle cell disease (SCD): impact on CNS disease. *Blood* 2002; **100**: 45a.
144. Kang EM, Areman EM, David-Ocampo V et al. Mobilization, collection, and processing of peripheral blood stem cells in individuals with sickle cell trait. *Blood* 2002; **99**: 850–5.
145. Anasetti C, Amos D, Beatty PG et al. Effect of HLA compatibility on engraftment of bone marrow transplants in patients with leukemia or lymphoma. *N Engl J Med* 1989; **320**: 197–204.
146. Bean MA, Graham T, Appelbaum FR et al. Gamma-irradiation of pretransplant blood transfusions from unrelated donors prevents sensitization to minor histocompatibility antigens on dog leukocyte antigen-identical canine marrow grafts. *Transplantation* 1994; **57**: 423–6.
147. Walters MC, Sullivan KM, Bernaudin F et al. Neurologic complications after allogeneic marrow transplantation for sickle cell anemia. *Blood* 1995; **85**: 879–84.
148. Ferster A, Christophe C, Dan B, Devalck C, Sariban E. Neurologic complications after bone marrow transplantation for sickle cell anemia [Letter]. *Blood* 1995; **86**: 408–9.
149. Gaziev D, Lucarelli G, Galimberti M et al. Malignancies after bone marrow transplantation for thalassemia. *Bone Marrow Transplant* 1997; **19** (Suppl. 2): 142.
150. Baronciani D, Angelucci E, Polchi P et al. An unusual marrow transplant complication: cardiac myxoma. *Bone Marrow Transplant* 1998; **21**: 825.
151. Guffon N, Souillet G, Maire I, Straczek J, Guibaud P. Follow-up of nine patients with Hurler syndrome after bone marrow transplantation. *J Pediatrics* 1998; **133**: 119–25.
152. Andreani M, Nesci S, Lucarelli G et al. Long-term survival of ex-thalassemic patients with persistent mixed chimerism after bone marrow transplantation. *Bone Marrow Transplant* 2000; **25**: 401–4.
153. Amrolia PJ, Vulliamy T, Vassiliou G et al. Analysis of chimaerism in thalassaemic children undergoing stem cell transplantation. *Br J Haematol* 2001; **114**: 219–25.
154. Le Deist F, Blanche S, Keable H et al. Successful HLA nonidentical bone marrow transplantation in three patients with the leukocyte adhesion deficiency. *Blood* 1989; **74**: 512–6.
155. Fischer A, Landais P, Friedrich W et al. Bone marrow transplantation (BMT) in Europe for primary immunodeficiencies other than severe combined immunodeficiency: a report from the European Group for BMT and the European Group for Immunodeficiency. *Blood* 1994; **83**: 1149–54.
156. Horwitz ME, Barrett AJ, Brown MR et al. Treatment of chronic granulomatous disease with non-myeloablative conditioning and a T-cell-depleted hematopoietic allograft. *N Engl J Med* 2001; **344**: 881–8.
157. Iannone R, Luznik L, Engstrom LW et al. Effects of mixed hematopoietic chimerism in a mouse model of bone marrow transplantation for sickle cell anemia. *Blood* 2001; **97**: 3960–5.
158. Kean LS, Durham MM, Adams AB et al. A cure for murine sickle cell disease through stable mixed chimerism and tolerance induction after nonmyeloablative conditioning and major histocompatibility complex-mismatched bone marrow transplantation. *Blood* 2002; **99**: 1840–9.
159. Carella AM, Champlin R, Slavin S, McSweeney P, Storb R. Mini-allografts: ongoing trials in humans [Editorial]. *Bone Marrow Transplant* 2000; **25**: 345–50.
160. Sandmaier BM, McSweeney P, Yu C, Storb R. Nonmyeloablative transplants: preclinical and clinical results. *Semin Oncol* 2000; **27**: 78–81.
161. Schleuning M, Stoetzer O, Waterhouse C, Schlemmer M, Ledderose G, Kolb HJ. Hematopoietic stem cell transplantation after reduced-intensity conditioning as treatment of sickle cell disease. *Exp Hematol* 2002; **30**: 7–10.
162. Krishnamurti L, Blazar BR, Wagner JE. Bone marrow transplantation without myeloablation for sickle cell disease. *N Engl J Med* 2001; **344**: 68.
163. van Besien K, Bartholomew A, Stock W et al. Fludarabine-based conditioning for allogeneic transplantation in adults with sickle cell disease. *Bone Marrow Transplant* 2000; **26**: 445–9.
164. Horan JJ, Liesveld P, Rochon et al. *Hematopoietic Stem Cell Transplantation for Sickle Cell Disease and Thalassemia after Low Dose TBI, Fludarabine and Rabbit ATG*. Washington DC: National Sickle Cell Disease Program, 2002.
165. Iannone R, Casella JF, Fuchs EJ et al. Failure of a minimally toxic non-myeloablative regimen to establish stable mixed chimerism after transplantation for sickle cell anemia and β-thalassemia. *Blood* 2002; **100**: 46a.
166. Walters M, Woolfrey A, Torok-Storb B et al. Enrichment of donor erythroid cells after non-myeloablative bone marrow transplantation (BMT) for sickle cell anemia (SCA). *Blood* 2001; **98**: 490a.
167. Locatelli F, Rocha V, Reed W et al. Related cord blood transplant in patients with thalassemia and sickle cell disease. *Blood* 2003; **101**: 351–7.

105

Trudy N. Small, Wilhelm Friedrich & Richard J. O'Reilly

Hematopoietic Cell Transplantation for Immunodeficiency Diseases

Introduction

Since the last edition of this chapter in 1999, multiple advances in the diagnosis and treatment of severe combined immunodeficiency syndrome (SCID) and other congenital immunodeficiencies have been achieved, most notably the successful correction of X-linked SCID by infusion of genetically modified autologous stem cells containing the common cytokine gamma chain gene (γc) [1,2]. Transfer of a normal immune system to children affected with SCID or Wiskott–Aldrich syndrome (WAS) by transplantation of bone marrow (BM) derived from human leukocyte antigen (HLA)-matched siblings was first reported in 1968 by the groups of Gatti et al. [3] and Bach et al. [4], respectively. In 1995, Buckley reviewed the outcome of transplants for the treatment of immunodeficiency disorders reported worldwide from 1968 through 1994. Of the 515 children transplanted for SCID, long-term survival was demonstrated in 89%, 60% and 69% of recipients of HLA-matched-related ($n = 103$), T-cell-depleted mismatched-related ($n = 372$) or unrelated ($n = 16$) hematopoietic cell transplants (HCT), respectively [5]. Series including more recently transplanted patients have shown survival rates of 90–100% for patients with SCID or WAS transplanted with hematopoietic stem cells (HSCs) from an HLA-identical sibling and 50–80% for patients transplanted with alternative donors (reviewed in [6]). In this chapter, the results of HCT for congenital immunodeficiency disorders will be updated, the genetic mutations giving rise to SCID and combined immunodeficiency syndrome (CID) summarized, and the current dilemmas facing physicians caring for children with primary immunodeficiencies, particularly those lacking an HLA-matched sibling donor, discussed.

Severe combined immunodeficiency syndrome (SCID)

SCID refers to a heterogeneous group of lethal, congenital disorders that result in the inability of T and B lymphocytes to mount an antigen specific response (reviewed in [5,7]). In the general population, it occurs in approximately 1/100,000 live births. In Athabascan-speaking Native Americans, an incidence of 1/2000 live births has been reported [8]. Infants with this disorder typically present at 3–8 months of age due to the decrease in protection afforded by passively transferred maternal antibodies. Signs and symptoms often include failure to thrive, thrush, diarrhea, recurrent otitis media, and/or interstitial pneumonia secondary to *Pneumocystis carinii*, cytomegalovirus (CMV), respiratory syncytial virus (RSV), parainfluenza, adenovirus, or influenza (reviewed in [7]). In native Americans, oral and genital ulcers are a distinct clinical feature [8]. Two unusual presentations at the Memorial Sloan Kettering Cancer Center (MSKCC) include one child with a severe noninfectious cardio-myopathy which resolved following unmodified HLA-matched-related transplant and two siblings, born 10 years apart, who developed intractable seizures associated with an encephalopathy which developed shortly before ($n = 1$) or after ($n = 1$) infusion of unmodified HLA-matched sibling transplant without prior conditioning. Despite a brain biopsy in the younger sister, an infectious etiology could not be found. The possibility that an encephalopathy is part of a rare SCID/CID syndrome is suggested by the neurologic degeneration of unclear etiology reported in 16 children receiving gammaglobulin therapy for a variety of immunodeficiency disorders [9].

Prior to the identification of the multiple genetic defects which can give rise to SCID, children with this disorder were grouped primarily according to the phenotype of their circulating lymphocytes, mode of inheritance and presence or absence of adenosine deaminase (ADA), an enzyme known to be associated with SCID [10]. Within this early classification, three major forms of SCID were identified (reviewed in [7]), consisting of:

1 "classical SCID", characterized by severe T and B lymphopenia and agammaglobulinemia;

2 the more common SCID with B lymphocytes, profound T lymphopenia and varying levels of nonspecific serum immunoglobulins; and

3 ADA-deficient SCID, which may present with either of the preceding lymphoid phenotypes (reviewed in [11]).

Less common forms of SCID include:

(a) reticular dysgenesis [12], in which the severe immunodeficiency is associated with absent to low numbers of circulating neutrophils, preserved red cell and platelet production, and deafness [13];

(b) Omenn's syndrome [14], typified by scaling erythroderma, leukocytosis, eosinophilia, hepatosplenomegaly and lymphadenopathy due to infiltration with Langerhans and reticulum cells [15];

(c) SCID with short-limbed dwarfism and ectodermal dysplasia [16] (reviewed in [17]); and

(d) SCID with nonfunctional T lymphocytes associated with capping defects [18], CD8 deficiency [19,20], abnormal expression of the CD7 cell surface glycoprotein [21] or T-cell receptor-CD3 complex [22].

As shown in Table 105.1, cytokine receptor defects, including those within the α chain of the interleukin 2 (IL-2) [23], IL-7 [24,25], or β chain of the IL-2/IL-15 receptor [26] can give rise to SCID, as can mutations within the *Artemis* gene, a DNA repair enzyme [27,28], or the *CD45* gene, a tyrosine kinase involved in T-cell signaling [29].

Whereas ADA deficiency [11,30], short-limbed dwarfism [16,17], Omenn's syndrome [14], capping defects [18], CD8 deficiency [19,20] and SCID associated with mutations within the *Artemis* gene [8,27,28] or the IL-7Rα [24,25] are inherited as autosomal recessive disorders, classical SCID, SCID with B cells and reticular dysgenesis (reviewed in

Table 105.1 Mutations associated with severe combined immunodeficiency syndrome (SCID).

Defect	Function	Common phenotype	Chromosomal location	Year published
ADA	Purine salvage enzyme	$T^- B^- NK^+$	20q12–13	1972
TCR abnormalities	T-cell signaling γc Common cytokine (IL-2,4,7,15,21)	$T_{low} B^+ NK^+$	11q23	1987
	γc gene	$T^- B^+ NK^-$	Xq13	1993
ZAP 70	Tyrosine kinase	CD8 deficiency	2q12	1994
Jak-3	Tyrosine kinase, signaling through γc	$T^- B^+ NK^-$	19p13	1995
RAG-1, RAG-2, Omenn's syndrome	Recombinase activating genes: initiation of VDJ recombination	$T^- B^- NK^+$, $T^+ B^- NK^+$	11p13	1996
IL-7-Rα	Cytokine receptor	$T^- B^+ NK^+$	5p13	1998
Artemis	DNA repair enzyme	$T^- B^- NK^+$	10p	1998
CD45	Tyrosine kinase T, B cell receptor signal transduction	$T_{low} B^+ NK$	Chr 1	2000
IL-2R/IL-15β subunit	Cytokine receptor signaling	$T_{low} B^+ NK^-$	Unknown	2001

ADA, adenosine deaminase; Jak-3, Janus kinase 3; IL, interleukin; NK, natural killer; TCR, T-cell receptor; γc gene, gamma chain gene.

[7,31]) can be inherited as either an autosomal recessive or X-linked disease. Despite the heterogeneity of this disorder, the distribution of SCID phenotypes within large series performed within the USA and Europe has been surprisingly similar, with X-linked SCID comprising approximately 50% of cases, classical SCID 25%, ADA deficiency 15% and SCID with nonfunctional T cells or reticular dysgenesis accounting for about 10% and 2% of cases, respectively [32–35].

Whereas first trimester diagnosis of ADA deficiency has been possible since 1975 by measuring enzyme activity in cultured amniocytes [36] or in chorionic villi (reviewed in [11,37]), antenatal diagnosis of other forms of SCID until recently required fetal blood sampling to determine the presence or absence of T cells [38]. The elucidation of many of the genetic mutations which give rise to SCID (reviewed in [39–41]; Table 105.1), such as those within the common cytokine receptor γ chain (X-linked SCID [42–44]), ADA deficiency (reviewed in [11]), Janus kinase 3 (Jak-3, autosomal recessive SCID with B cells) [45–47], ZAP-70 (CD8 deficiency with nonfunctional T cells [48–50], reviewed in [51]), recombination activation genes, RAG-1/RAG-2 (classical SCID, Omenn's syndrome [52]) and the Artemis gene [27,28], has increased the proportion of infants who can be diagnosed in utero [53–55]. Early identification and transplantation in the neonatal period has been associated with survival rates of 90% or greater, due to transplantation prior to the development of severe opportunistic infections and more rapid immunologic reconstitution [56,57]. In a study by Myers et al. [57], long-term survival was observed in 21 of 22 of infants transplanted within the first 3 months of life, compared to 51 of 67 children transplanted at 3.5 months of age or older.

The limitation of classifying children with SCID by the presence of T, B, and/or natural killer (NK) cells, is that multiple defects can present with the same phenotype (i.e. defects within the γc gene or Jak-3, Table 105.1) and patients, even siblings, with identical mutations can present with different lymphoid phenotypes [58–60]. In 1997, Buckley and colleagues [33] evaluated 108 consecutive infants on the basis of genetic defect rather than phenotype alone. The inciting mutation could be identified in 68% of patients. Forty-six percent of patients had a mutation within the common cytokine receptor γc gene, 15% in the gene encoding ADA and 7% within the Jak-3 gene. Of the remaining 35 patients, 21 had an unknown autosomal recessive disorder, 12 males had unknown defects, one patient had reticular dysgenesis and one patient had cartilage hair hypoplasia. Analysis of transplantation outcome on the basis of genetic mutation in 89 infants who received an unmodified ($n = 12$) or soy bean agglutinin and E-rosette depletion (SBA- E-) (E$^-$) T-cell-depleted mismatched-related ($n = 77$) bone marrow transplantation (BMT) at Duke University Medical Center [61], showed similar survival rates (79–100%) regardless of SCID mutation, except in a small number of males with an unknown type of SCID, of whom only one of four survived. In contrast, a European study analysing the impact of SCID phenotype on outcome following HLA-mismatched T-cell depleted parental BMT demonstrated superior disease-free survival (DFS) in patients with B-cell positive SCID compared to B negative SCID, 60% vs. 35%, respectively [62].

Unmodified HLA-matched and mismatched-related HCT for SCID

The first successful human allogeneic HCT was performed in an infant with SCID who remains alive and well more than 3 decades following an HLA-matched sibling transplant [3]. Transplantation of unmodified (non-T-cell depleted) BM from an HLA-identical sibling remains the treatment of choice for infants with SCID [5,6,61,63–65]. In the majority of patients, even those with functional NK cells or a marginal phytohemagglutan A (PHA) response, pretransplant cytoreduction is not necessary to ensure engraftment [61,63] (reviewed in [5,6]). Prophylaxis for graft-vs.-host disease (GVHD) is generally not given due to the low incidence of significant GVHD [5,6,57,61,65], although some centers T-cell-deplete the BM graft prior to infusion [8,61]. The basis for the low incidence of acute and chronic GVHD may be the young age of the donor/recipient pair and the absence of tissue injury due to lack of cytoreduction. Of eight consecutive recipients of an unmodified HLA-matched BMT transplanted at MSKCC since 1987, none have developed GVHD despite lack of prophylaxis and infusion of unmanipulated BM containing a median (range) of 5.97 [2,5,5–10] × 10^8 total nucleated cells/kg.

Over the last 25 years, results of HLA-matched transplants for SCID have improved from the 48% long-term survival reported in 1979 [66] to 80–100% in more recent single center studies [5,6,61,63]. Thirty recipients of an HLA-matched sibling HCT for SCID at the Hôpital Necker-Enfants Malades, Paris, from 1971 to 1992 achieved an 80% long-term survival [65]. Of 12 HLA-matched sibling BMTs performed at Duke University Medical Center from 1980 to 1998, five of which were T-cell depleted prior to infusion, 100% survival was observed [61]. Ten of 11 recipients of an HLA-matched sibling transplant at MSKCC from 1980 through 2001 survive with T- and B-cell reconstitution, a median (range) of 79+ (8.1–247.5) months post-BMT. Eleven consecutive recipients of an HLA-matched sibling BMT at the Children Hospital of Los Angeles survive long-term with normal T immunity [64], and five of five Athabascan-speaking Native Americans who received an unmodified HLA-matched-related transplant survive a median (range) of 102+ (2–146) months post-HCT [7].

Multiple factors have contributed to the improved outcome of HLA-matched HCT for SCID, primarily earlier transplantation [56,57,61] and better prevention and treatment of the infectious complications associated with this disorder [67–71]. Fatal opportunistic infections in the peri-transplant period have been dramatically reduced by the availability of rapid, sensitive assays (polymerase chain reaction, shell vial, direct and indirect fluorescence) capable of detecting viruses, such as CMV, RSV, adenovirus and influenza, allowing early antiviral therapy prior to the development of lower respiratory tract disease [67–71]. Whereas interstitial pneumonia secondary to *Pneumocystis carinii* [69] and viruses [70] were the leading cause of death in patients with SCID transplanted before 1980 (reviewed in [5,35]), effective strategies to prevent and treat many of these opportunistic pathogens (CMV, RSV, *Pneumocystis carinii*, *Candida*, herpes viruses) are now available [67–71].

For most variants of SCID, unmodified, HLA-matched marrow can be administered without cytoreduction and will result in engraftment of donor T and B lymphocytes, permitting full reconstitution of immunologic function. Following infusion of BM from an HLA-matched sibling, normal numbers of circulating T cells rapidly develop, often within 2–4 weeks (Fig. 105.1) and T-cell mitogen and specific antigen responses are rapidly restored [6,35,61,64,65,72,73]. Specific B-cell function develops in most children by 1 year post-transplant, allowing cessation of monthly intravenous gammaglobulin therapy and subsequent reimmunization [6,35,61,64,65,68].

There are, however, some variants of SCID, such as those with ADA-SCID who often require multiple HLA-matched transplants to achieve engraftment [74,75]. For these patients, the administration of immunosuppressive drugs may be indicated to ensure engraftment of lymphoid progenitors. For SCID variants, such as reticular dysgenesis [76], which involve more than the lymphoid lineage, preparative regimens incorporating both myeloablative and immunosuppressive agents have been required to insure rapid and full hematopoietic and lymphoid chimerism.

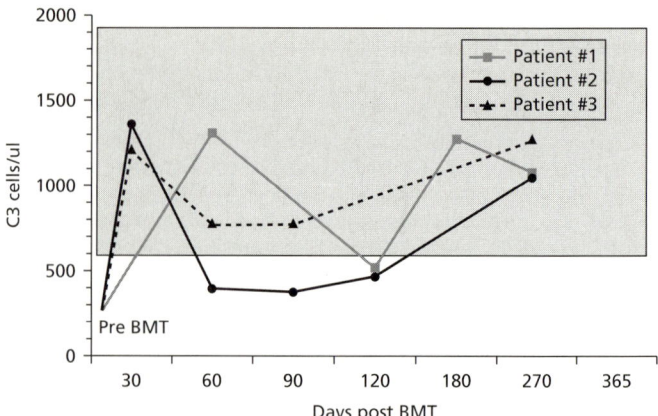

Fig. 105.1 CD3 recovery post-unmodified human leukocyte antigen (HLA)-matched sibling bone marrow transplantation (BMT) for severe combined immunodeficiency syndrome (SCID), $n = 3$. Reproduced with permission from the National Marrow Donor Program.

The use of unmodified mismatched-related BMT for SCID as well as for hematologic malignancies has been associated with poor results due to the development of severe acute and extensive chronic GVHD [77]. A review by Kenny and Hitzig published in 1979 [66] demonstrated that only two of nine recipients of an unmodified HLA-mismatched transplant survived long-term. Similarly, only seven of 21 SCID patients who received an HLA nonidentical transplant prior to 1983 were long-term survivors [78]. Current results of T-cell-depleted mismatched-parental HCT in many large transplant centers around the world obviate the need to risk the potential for severe GVHD associated with an unmodified mismatched-related or mismatched-unrelated HCT if a suitable parental donor is available.

HLA-nonidentical-related T-cell-depleted HCT for SCID

In 1973 Keightly *et al.* [79] reported the successful use of a fully mismatched fetal liver graft to reconstitute a patient with ADA deficiency. A review of this modality by O'Reilly *et al.* [80] in 1983 indicated that of 105 fetal liver transplants, 22 resulted in durable engraftment of fetal lymphoid cells and only 20% of patients survived more than 1 year after HCT. While the few SCID patients who have attained long-term immunologic reconstitution following fetal liver transplantation demonstrate that fully allogeneic hematopoietic cells lacking mature T cells can be used to achieve functional immune reconstitution without lethal GVHD, results with this approach have been inferior to those achieved with either T-cell depleted haplotype-disparate parental HCT or unmodified transplants from histocompatible unrelated donors.

The success of T-cell-depleted mismatched-related transplants for SCID depends on the degree and method of T-cell depletion (TCD) (reviewed in [81]) which impacts on the risk of graft failure, GVHD, and post-transplant complications, such as Epstein–Barr virus-associated lympoproliferative disorders (EBV-LPD). The T-cell depleted techniques which have been utilized SBA- E- [82,83], E-rosetting alone [84], antibody-mediated techniques, such as OKT3 [85] or Campath 1M [86,87] and, more recently, CD34-selection of granulocyte colony-stimulating factor (G-CSF) mobilized PBSC, with and without further T-cell depleted by E-rosetting or monoclonal antibody treatment [88].

In 1983, successful correction of SCID by T-cell-depleted mismatched-related BMT was reported in three infants transplanted with haploidentical parental SBA- E- BM [83]. These children required neither pretransplant cytoreduction nor post-transplant GVHD prophylaxis. Long-term stable donor T-cell chimerism with normal T-cell function was achieved in all three, without the development of acute or chronic

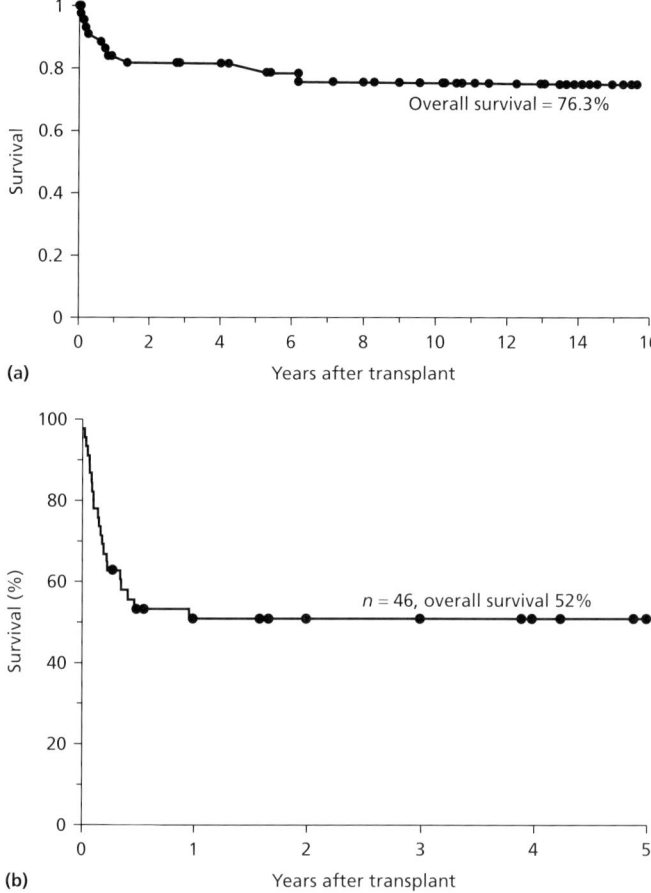

Fig. 105.2 (a) Overall survival of SBA- E- mismatched T-cell-depleted bone marrow transplantation (BMT) for severe combined immunodeficiency syndrome (SCID) performed 1987–2001 at Memorial Sloan Kettering Cancer Center (MSKCC), $n = 44$. (b) Unrelated SCID transplant procedures 1987–2001. Reproduced with permission from the National Marrow Donor Program.

GVHD. Of the 60 children who have received an SBA- E- (E⁻) mismatched-parental BMT at MSKCC from 1980 to 2001, 75% remain alive with T-cell immune reconstitution, a median (range) of 153.3+ (8.7–258.7) months post-transplant (Fig. 105.2a). The incidence of grade II acute or chronic GVHD has remained less than 10% (reviewed in [6,35,61]). Similar results with haploidentical SBA- E- BMT for the treatment of SCID have been reported from other centers including, the University of Ulm, Germany, [35,89], the University of California Medical Center at San Francisco [34] and Duke University Medical Center, NC [61]. In the recently published series from the latter institution, a 78% long-term survival was reported.

Other T-cell depleted techniques, such as Campath 1M plus complement or E-rosetting alone, have been associated with long-term survival rates of 52% to 70%. Single center studies performed at the Hôpital Necker-Enfants Malades, Paris, with marrow T-cell depleted by E-rosetting alone was associated with a 70% survival [65]. Seventeen infants with SCID transplanted at the Royal Victoria Infirmary in London from 1986 through 1996 with marrow T-cell depleted with Campath 1M plus complement achieved a 64% long-term survival [87]. In 1998, results of mismatched-related transplants for SCID performed in 18 European centers from 1982 and 1993 [90] demonstrated long-term survival in 52% of patients, with T- and B-cell reconstitution in 93% and 64% of survivors, respectively. Thirty percent of patients in the latter report, which included a variety of TCD techniques, developed acute GVHD of grade II or higher. At 6, 12 and 24 months post-BMT, 40%, 26% and 18% of these patients had evidence of chronic GVHD, respectively.

To date, few studies have been published on the specific use of T-cell depleted PBSC transplantation for the treatment of SCID. Lanfranchi *et al.* [88] explored the use of frozen T-cell depleted PBSC plus T-cell depleted BM in nine patients with primary immunodeficiency disease, including four with SCID, three with Omenn's syndrome and two with CID. This approach was undertaken primarily to determine whether high cell doses could overcome the increased incidence of graft failure observed in patients with CID who possess abnormally low but residual T-cell function. Patients were cytoreduced with 16 mg/kg busulfan (BU), 200 mg/kg cyclophosphamide (CY), and 10 mg/kg of thiotepa. In the majority of cases, the BM was T-cell depleted by Campath 1M and the PBSC by CD34 selection followed by E-rosetting. Although the follow-up is short (mean 7.5+ months), six of the seven patients transplanted for SCID survive. Although all four patients with SCID engrafted, one died of a disseminated CMV infection.

From 1995 to 2002, the author (W. Friedrich) at Ulm, Germany, performed 34 T-cell-depleted mismatched-parental PBSC for the treatment of ADA-SCID ($n = 2$), B⁻ T⁻ SCID ($n = 8$), Omenn's syndrome ($n = 3$), B⁺ SCID ($n = 19$), B⁺ T⁺ ($n = 1$) and reticular dysgenesis ($n = 1$). The T-cell depleted peripheral blood cell transplantation (PBCT) contained a median of 0.35×10^5 CD3/kg and 17×10^6 CD34 cells/kg. The majority of patients received cytoreduction (26 out of 34 patients), most with BU/CY. To date, 27 patients are alive and well, a median (range) of 42.4 (2.63–88.1) months post-CD34 selected T-cell depleted PBSC, none with GVHD. There were two graft failures, one in a patient with a mutation within the *Artemis* gene, the other in a B⁺ T⁺ SCID/CID, both of whom did not receive cytoreduction. There were seven deaths, all due to infection, one following graft failure. Of the surviving patients, one is too early to evaluate for the extent of immune reconstitution, 19 patients have full T- and B-cell reconstitution, five patients have T-cell reconstitution only and one patient has full T- and partial B-cell reconstitution. The majority of patients are mixed chimeras. *De novo* acute or chronic GVHD were not observed in any of the surviving patients. The overall survival rate in this group of SCID patients following T-cell-depleted mismatched CD34⁺ selected transplantation is 78%, similar to the experience in SCID patients after rigorous T-cell depleted BMT. As with marrow grafts, complete engraftment and reconstitution by donor cells remained highly dependent on prior use of myelosuppression, and even infusion of purified CD34⁺ cells at significant numbers did not facilitate full donor chimerism. Time to develop effective T-cell immunity post-TCD mismatched PBSCT ranged from 3 to 6 months, similar to that observed after T-cell depleted BMT (Fig. 105.3). Thus, the use of purified blood CD34 cells at high numbers does not appear to enhance the functional maturation of donor T cells.

Several studies have addressed factors that influence long-term survival following T-cell-depleted mismatched-related HCT for SCID. Younger age was associated with a better outcome [56,57,61,65,90], particularly in the neonatal period [56,57,61]. As seen in earlier studies [66], interstitial pneumonia [72,90], particularly antecedent CMV or adenoviral infections, has impacted negatively on survival (reviewed in [35]). Failure to develop T-cell function by 6 months post-transplant or the presence of chronic GVHD for more than 6 months post-HCT confers an increased mortality [90]. In the MSKCC series (reviewed in [35]), as well as that from the University of Ulm, Germany, [89], NK⁺ SCID patients who did not receive pretransplant cytoreduction had a poorer outcome primarily due to graft failure. Although not all studies have shown an association between NK function and graft resistance [61], this may relate to differences in the genetic basis giving rise to NK⁺ SCID in the transplant population evaluated.

For rarer forms of SCID, such as Omenn's syndrome, results of T-cell-depleted mismatched-related transplantation have varied depending on

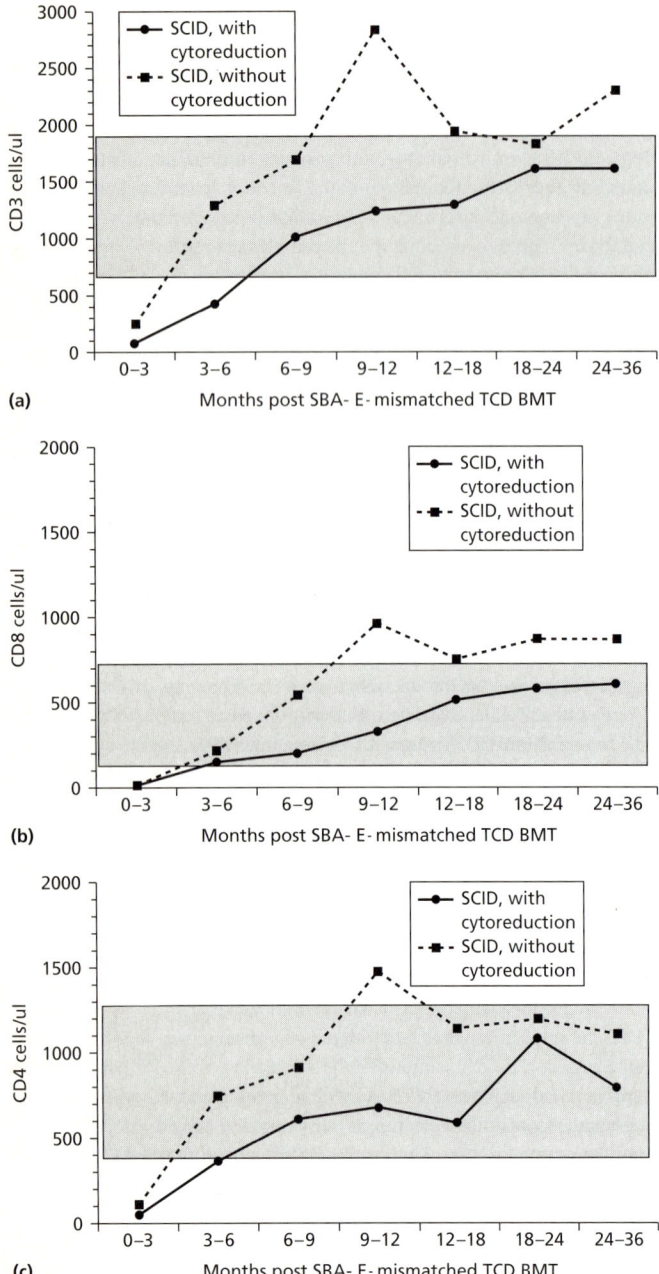

Fig. 105.3 (a) Median CD3 recovery following soy bean agglutinin (SBA)-E- mismatched-related bone marrow transplantation (BMT) for severe combined immunodeficiency syndrome (SCID), n = 60. (b) Median CD8 cells/μL recovery following SBA- E- mismatched-related BMT for SCID, n = 60. (c) Median CD4 cells/μL recovery following SBA- E- mismatched-related bone marrow transplantation (BMT) for SCID, n = 60. Reproduced with permission from the National Marrow Donor Program.

the method of TCD utilized and the cytoreduction employed. Although all three children with Omenn's syndrome who received a mismatched-related HCT T-cell depleted *in vitro* with anti-CD5 ricin died [91], three of four children with Omenn's syndrome survive following an E- T-cell-depleted mismatched-related HCT [92], as do three recipients of an SBA- E- mismatched-related BMT performed at MSCKCC. Of 10 infants with reticular dysgenesis who received a haplo-identical T-cell depleted BMT in Europe from 1979 to 1999 [93], the only three patients who survived were among the five children cytoreduced with 16 mg/kg of BU combined with CY. Transplantation without prior cytoreduction, or with less intensive regimens, resulted in absent or incomplete engraftment and subsequent death.

Following an SBA- E- mismatched-related BMT, the majority of patients will develop normal numbers of CD3, CD8, and CD4 T cells by 3–6 months post-HCT (Fig. 105.3a–c), irrespective of whether cytoreduction is employed (reviewed in [5,35,57,61,94]). The PHA response will normalize by 6 months post-transplant in approximately 50% of patients, and 80% of patients will have normal T-cell mitogen and antigen specific responses by 6–12 months [5,35,57,61,65,94]. Myers *et al.* [57] have shown that infants who receive an SBA- E- mismatched-parental BMT within 28 days of life develop higher numbers of CD45RA+ and T-cell receptor excision circle (TREC) positive T cells, and more robust T-cell proliferative responses within the first 3 years post-transplant than infants transplanted at later time points. Surprisingly, Muller *et al.* [94] did not find any differences in the pattern of naive CD4+CD45RA+ T-cell reconstitution in patients who received an unmodified HLA-matched sibling vs. a T-cell-depleted mismatched-related HCT for SCID. In patients not given pretransplant cytoreduction prior to an SBA- E- mismatched-parental HCT there is a dramatic increase in the percentage and absolute numbers of CD3+CD45RA, TREC positive T cells within the 1st year following HCT followed by a marked decline in the subsequent 5–12 years [95]. Although this observation [95] demonstrates the ability of the hypoplastic SCID thymus [96] to support robust thymopoiesis, it raises concerns about the long-term ability of these patients to generate naive thymic dependent T cells [95].

In a large European study of mismatched-T-cell depleted HCT recipients using a variety of TCD techniques, the median time to develop normal T-cell proliferative responses to tetanus toxoid was 8.7 months [90]. Of the 116 patients in this study who survived at least 6 months post-HCT only 43% of those with absent T-cell function at 6 months (n = 21) ultimately developed normal T-cell responses, compared to 71% of those patients with normal or near-normal T-cell function 6 months post-transplant [90]. The quality and kinetics of T-cell reconstitution in the European series correlated with SCID phenotype, with a higher percentage of B+ SCIDs exhibiting normal T-cell function at all time points >6 months post-HCT [90] compared to B− SCID.

Reconstitution of specific antibody formation following an SBA- E- mismatched-related HCT as with other TCD techniques is generally only observed in patients given pretransplant cytoreduction, which impacts on the degree of donor B-cell engraftment (reviewed in [5,35,61,64,65,68,90]). In the MSKCC series, normal antibody responses following immunization were observed in all patients engrafted with donor B cells, compared to less than 10% of patients with exclusively host B cells (reviewed in [5,35]). Forty-five of 72 infants transplanted at Duke University Medical Center [61], NC, required prolonged gammaglobulin therapy, the majority of whom received an SBA- E- T-cell-depleted mismatched-related marrow graft without prior cytoreduction. This contrasts to the smaller study by Dror *et al.* [34] which showed that despite absence of circulating donor B cells, six patients developed specific antibody responses 1.5–10.0 years following an SBA- E- mismatched-related BMT. In a single center study by Haddad *et al.* [73], donor B-cell engraftment was documented in four of five and three of 17 recipients of an unmodified HLA-matched or T-cell-depleted mismatched-related BMT, respectively. Ten of 18 patients with host B cells remained on intravenous immunoglobulin (IVIg) more than 2 years post-BMT. In this study, in contrast to the combined MSKCC-ULM experience, cytoreduction with 8 mg/kg BU and 200 mg/kg CY did not promote donor B-cell engraftment nor the development of specific antibody production [73].

Despite the success of T-cell-depleted mismatched-related HCT for patients lacking an HLA-matched sibling donor, several problems clearly remain (reviewed in [5,35,61,90]), namely:

1 graft failure in some series in those patients with NK cell function or minimal T-cell function [35,89];
2 GVHD following less rigorous TCD techniques [32,62,63,65,84,87,88];
3 EBV-LPD, due to dysregulated B-cell proliferation prior to T-cell development [97,98];
4 lack of donor NK cell engraftment which has been associated with epidermodysplasia verruciformis both in MSKCC and other series [99];
5 autoimmune disorders due to dysregulated B-cell function [100,101]; and
6 hypogammaglobulinemia, despite successful T-cell reconstitution in patients not given cytoreduction [5,35,61,62,64,65,73,90].

In patients with inadequate gammaglobulin replacement, exacerbated by immunoglobulin A (IgA) deficiency generally observed in these patients, severe chronic lung disease has been observed [5,35].

An ongoing debate at many centers performing T-cell depleted-mismatched HCT for SCID is whether, even in the absence of factors which increase the risk of graft rejection, all children with SCID should be cytoreduced to ensure B cell as well as NK cell reconstitution. If so, the level of cytoreduction necessary to ensure B-cell engraftment, the long-term side-effects of this cytoreduction and how early cytoreduction can safely be given to newborns, particularly those diagnosed *in utero* is unclear. Whereas some infants will develop at least partial donor B-cell chimerism and specific B-cell function with doses of BU <16 mg/kg, BU and CY <200 mg/kg, not all will [73]. It is possible that nonmyeloblative therapy such as BU combined with fludarabine or melphalan will be more readily tolerated and will allow full immunologic reconstitution. These newer cytoreductive regimens are definitely worthy of further exploration, particularly in children who present with organ toxicity at the time of diagnosis and/or HCT.

Unmodified unrelated BMT for SCID

The first unrelated HCT for the treatment of SCID, performed by O'Reilly and colleagues in 1973, utilized a one antigen HLA class I disparate female donor into an HLA-A1 homozygous male infant [102]. Following a series of transplants from this donor, durable lymphoid engraftment and full immunologic reconstitution was achieved, although severe chronic GVHD ensued. This patient unfortunately succumbed to metastatic squamous cell carcinoma of the skin 9 years following transplantation.

In 1992, eight recipients of an unmodified unrelated marrow transplant for the treatment of SCID were reported by Filipovich *et al.* [103]. Seven of the eight children were cytoreduced with BU/CY, and antithymocyte globulin (ATG), and all eight children received immunosuppressive drugs to prevent GVHD. Six of eight children survived with immunologic reconstitution 1.0–3.8+ years after BMT, with significant GVHD developing in only in one patient. An update of the international experience of unrelated BMT for SCID ($n = 24$) performed prior to 1994 was published [104]. In this series, children with X-linked or ADA+ SCID were not given cytoreduction. Of those given cytoreduction, most received BU, CY, ATG and GVHD prophylaxis with cyclosporine (CSP) A and methotrexate (MTX). Early death prior to engraftment was seen in four patients, and graft failure in two patients. The estimated 3-years survival was 61%. Grade II–IV GVHD occurred in 17% of engrafted patients [104]. Nine children with SCID received an unmodified unrelated BMT at the Hospital for Sick Children at Toronto, Canada, between December 1987 and August 1997 [105] following cytoreduction with BU/CY. CSP, methylprednisolone (MP), with or without short course MTX, was given to prevent GVHD. Donors were identified at a mean (range) of 4.7 (1–13) months. Despite antecedent pneumonia in four of the nine SCID patients, six survive a median (range) of 54.5+ (18–72) months post-unrelated transplant. Death in the other three patients was due to graft failure ($n = 1$) or grade III GVHD ($n = 2$). T-cell reconstitution occurred in all six patients. B-cell reconstitution was documented in four patients.

When comparing results of unmodified unrelated HCT to haplo-identical T-cell depleted related BMT, the years of transplant must be noted as most large haplo-identical T-cell depleted BMT series for SCID include patients transplanted prior to 1987, whereas trials of unrelated HCT were initiated after 1987 paralleling the establishment and growth of unrelated donor registries. Multiple studies have demonstrated the effect of decade of transplant on survival due to advances in antimicrobial therapy, TCD, cytoreductive regimens, and treatment and prevention of GVHD (reviewed in [6,35]). The only valid comparison of stem cell sources are therefore those performed during similar time frames utilizing similar supportive care. Although graft rejection and an increase in EBV-LPD were reported in earlier studies of T-cell depleted haplo-identical BMT for SCID, particularly in patients who failed to engraft [97,99], these complications currently occur in <5% of recipients of T-cell depleted-mismatched transplants (reviewed in [6,35], R.J. O'Reilly, manuscript in preparation). Comparison of the transplant outcome in 44 recipients of an SBA- E- mismatched-parental BM for SCID performed at MSKCC from 1987 through November 2001 with that of 46 infants who received an unmodified unrelated HCT facilitated through the National Marrow Donor Program (NMDP) [106] during the same time period for SCID reveals that 77% of children transplanted with a mismatched-parental BMT survive compared to 55% recipients of an unrelated transplant (Fig. 105.2b).

For children with SCID, if cytoreduction is going to be utilized, the advantage of unmodified unrelated HCT over rigorous T-cell-depleted mismatched-parental BMT, is unclear, as consistent engraftment and specific T- and B-cell immunity has been reproducibly observed in children with SCID given T-cell depleted haplo-identical parental BM following similar cytoreduction. In the time needed to identify a suitable unrelated donor (minimum 1 month), the infectious risk imposed on an infant with SCID is not justified unless the parental donor would impose an undue risk of infection, such as active CMV or Hepatitis B or C infection. In contrast, as will be detailed in the following sections, for children with CID [105] or those with WAS [107], the results of unmodified unrelated HCT have been superior to those with T-cell-depleted mismatched-related HCT, due to lack of graft failure, GVHD, and EBV-LPD, which commonly complicate T-cell-depleted mismatched-related BMT for these immunodeficiency disorders (reviewed in [35]).

Umbilical cord blood cell (CBC) transplants for SCID

Although over 1000 CBC transplants have been performed worldwide [108] (reviewed in [109]), there are only a limited number of studies citing specific outcome data of CBC transplants for the treatment of SCID. The largest series, reported by Knutsen and Wall in 2000 [110], described eight infants with severe T-cell immunodeficiency disease that received an unrelated CBC transplant, seven of whom engrafted. The one graft failure occurred in a patient with reticular dysgenesis cytoreduced with BU/CY. This patient successfully engrafted after infusion of cord blood from a second unrelated donor when given a total body irradiation (TBI) conditioning regimen. Despite significant HLA-mismatching between cord blood donor and recipient in this group of eight patients, five patients developed grade I acute GVHD and only one patient developed severe GVHD involving the skin and gut. T- and B-cell immunity recovered at 60–100-days post-transplant [61]. Buckley *et al.* have successfully used unrelated cord blood transplantation to rescue three children with X-linked SCID who rejected a T-cell-depleted mismatched-related BMT given in the absence of cytoreduction. In two of these cases, BU/CY was given prior to CBC transplantation. In addition to the above cases, successful correction of Omenn's syndrome ($n = 1$) and X-linked SCID ($n = 2$) by unrelated CBC transplant have been reported, as well correction of

T⁻ B⁻ NK⁺ SCID by HLA-matched sibling CBC transplant [111–113]. Although these results are promising, further studies are needed to determine whether CBC is superior to other hematopoietic cell sources in children lacking an HLA-matched sibling donor, particularly if cytoreduction is needed, engraftment is slow and immunosuppression to prevent GVHD is required.

In utero HCT for SCID

In 1995, Flake reported [114] the first successful *in utero* transplant performed in a child with X-linked SCID who was diagnosed at 12-weeks gestation. This infant received a series of three infusions of CD34⁺ selected paternal BM cells providing 114.0, 8.9 and 6.2×10^6/kg fetal weight CD34⁺ cells, containing an estimated total cell dose of $<5.2 \times 10^5$ CD3⁺ cells/kg fetal weight. The cells were injected under ultrasound guidance into the abdomen of the fetus between 15.0 and 18.5 weeks gestation. At birth, 3 and 6 months of age, circulating T cells were of donor origin while B cells, NK cells, monocytes and granulocytes were of host origin. The engrafted paternal T cells were tolerant to the patient when tested by mixed lymphocyte culture and responded normally to T-cell mitogens. Follow-up at 4 years demonstrated persistent engraftment of donor cells with specific T and B-cell function [115–117]. In 1996, Wengler et al. [118] published an article about another successful *in utero* HCT performed in an infant with X-linked SCID utilizing paternal G-CSF mobilized PBC, T-cell depleted PBSC infused at 21 weeks and again at 22 weeks gestation. Cells were T-cell depleted by CD34 selection followed by rosetting with sheep red blood cells. This infant was delivered at 38 weeks by cesarean section, healthy, without evidence of GVHD. Cord blood analyzed at birth contained 300 CD3⁺ T cells/μL, with a predominance of naive CD45RA CD4⁺ T cells, expressed the γ chain of the IL-2 receptor, were of paternal origin by HLA typing, and responded normally to PHA and OKT3. At 3.5 months of age, T-cell numbers and function were normal, although B cells analyzed at this early time point remained of host origin. In 1997, Gil and colleagues [119] performed an *in utero* transplant for T⁻, B⁺ NK⁺ autosomal recessive SCID using CD34 selected paternal BM injected intraperitoneally at 23 weeks gestation followed by a second infusion of T-cell depleted BM and *ex vivo* generated BM stromal cells. This patient rapidly developed normal T-cell function. Although intravenous gammaglobulin therapy was required until 5 months of age due to low serum levels of IgG, specific antibody production following immunization with hepatitis B to which the donor was not immune was subsequently documented [120].

Although these cases demonstrate the feasibility of inducing T-cell reconstitution before birth through an antenatal T-cell depleted graft, comparison of this treatment with other modalities is difficult due to the small numbers of such transplants and the limited data on the long-term quality and kinetics of T and, particularly, B-cell reconstitution.

Gene therapy for SCID

Despite long-term survival in up to 70–80% of patients with SCID who lack an HLA-identical donor using a variety of transplant techniques as detailed above, engraftment without cytoreduction is not universal, not all engrafted patients sustain normal T-cell function and B-cell reconstitution is generally not restored unless cytoreduction is utilized. The identification of many of the genetic defects responsible for SCID paved the way for trials of gene therapy utilizing genetically modified autologous lymphocytes or HSC in an effort to correct the defect without the need for cytoreduction or risk of GVHD (reviewed in [121]). Although ADA deficiency was the first genetic disease to be treated by gene therapy [121–125], its efficacy has been limited by the variable levels of circulating transduced cells achieved. In addition, the clinical benefit directly attributable to gene therapy in this disorder has been difficult to interpret due to the concomitant administration of polyethylene glycol conjugated ADA which may also negate any survival advantage of ADA⁺ transduced cells (reviewed in [121]). In 2000, Cavazzana-Calvo and colleagues demonstrated the successful correction of X-linked SCID with γc-transduced CD34⁺ HSC as sole therapy [1,2]. Immunologic reconstitution in five recipients of this therapy treated at a median (range) of 8 (1–11) months of age was published in 2002 [2]. Although transduced CD3⁺ T cells could not be detected in one patient, rapid clinical improvement occurred in the other four patients in whom circulating transduced T cells were demonstrated. The number of CD3⁺ cells normalized in these latter four patients between 3 and 5 months post-therapy, and specific antibody production was detected in three of the four patients. Unfortunately, one of the 11 children with X-linked SCID treated with genetically modified cells by the French group recently developed a T-cell leukemia [126], which carries the transgene inserted into an oncogene on chromosome 11. Although this development has resulted in a reexamination of the risk of retroviral gene therapy and malignant transformation due to insertional mutagenesis, the successful reconstitution of normal T- and B-cell function in nine treated patients without the use of cytoreduction, remains a remarkable achievement. Only with future studies will the risk of this therapy compared to the risk of graft rejection, complications of cytoreduction, GVHD, and/or incomplete immune reconstitution with unrelated or mismatched HCT be determined.

Aiuti and colleagues recently described the results of gene therapy in two children with ADA deficiency that had not received treatment with pegylated bovine (PEG)-ADA [127]. These children were treated with nonmyeloblative doses of BU in an effort to provide the ADA retrovirally transduced CD34⁺ autologous stem cells with an initial survival advantage. Follow-up of 14 months in one patient revealed ADA⁺ myeloid, T, B and NK cells with antigen-specific T- and B-cell function. A frequency of 70% vector-containing T cells was evident at 11+ months of follow-up. In the second patient high levels of transduced T cells were observed, although only low levels of transduced B cells were detected.

The success of gene therapy in patients with X-linked SCID and in some patients with ADA deficiency provide proof of the potential of gene therapy in the treatment of immunodeficiency disorders. The ability to correct other SCID disorders *in vitro* and/or in animal models, such as ZAP-70 [128,129], Jak-3 [130] and RAG-2 deficiency [131] will likely lead to the development of clinical trials to correct a variety of SCID disorders by infusion of genetically modified autologous CD34⁺ stem cells.

Combined immunodeficiency syndrome (CID)

Combined immunodeficiency syndrome (CID), including Nezelof syndrome [132], refers to a heterogenous group of patients with recurrent severe acute and chronic infections associated with profound but not absolute deficiencies of T- and B-cell function (reviewed in [133]). In this group of disorders, T-lymphocyte numbers may be normal or reduced. Although antigen specific responses to pathogens are not detectable, proliferative responses to nonspecific mitogens and allogeneic cells, while markedly abnormal, are not absolutely deficient as they are in patients with SCID. In several CID syndromes, B cells are prominent and immunoglobulin classes may be normal or increased. However, specific antibody production is usually absent (reviewed in [133]). Patients with CID associated with the hyper-IgM syndrome have low serum levels of IgG, IgA and IgE with normal to elevated IgM levels due to impaired T–B cell interaction (reviewed in [134]). These patients often have neutropenia of unclear etiology, autoimmune phenomena and a propensity to viral encephalitis [134]. They suffer from recurrent sinopulmonary infections, opportunistic infections, such as *Pneumocystis carinii* pneumonia (PCP), and persistent cryptosporidium infections resulting in chronic cholangitis, cirrhosis and hepatocellular carcinoma. Without HCT, patients with this disorder rarely survive past the 3rd decade of life.

The pathogenetic basis for many of the CID syndromes are known. A subset of patients with ZAP-70 deficiency [20], Omenn's syndrome [14,15], or ADA deficiency (reviewed in [11]) will present with partial rather than complete absence of T- and B-cell function. Other causes of CID syndromes due to defective cytokine production, response, receptor expression or lack of cell surface molecules involved in cell contact, antigen presentation, activation, and/or proliferation include:

- Defective IL-1 responsiveness [135].
- Defective transcription of multiple cytokine genes [136].
- Abnormal IL-2 production [137,138] or IL-2r expression [139].
- Abnormal T-cell receptor CD3 complex [22].
- Nucleoside phosphorylase deficiency [140].
- Bare lymphocyte syndrome (BLS)[141–143], a series of genetic disorders resulting in defective transcription and expression of HLA class I and/or class II determinants on the surface of lymphoid and hematopoietic cells.
- Leukocyte function-associated antigen-1 (LFA-1) deficiency [144,145].
- X–linked hyper-IgM syndrome: CD40 ligand deficiency [146,147].
- Autosomal hyper-IgM syndrome: defective CD40 expression [148] or abnormal *AID* gene, an activation-induced cytidine deaminase gene [149].

Experience in the use of HCT for CIDs has been much more limited than for SCID. Prior to 1991, experience with HLA-matched BMT for CID was extremely poor. Three patients with Nezelof syndrome transplanted with marrow derived from an HLA-matched sibling engrafted and survived after HLA-matched sibling BMT with ($n = 1$) or without prior cytoreduction ($n = 2$) [150]. Although early results of transplantation for nucleoside phosphorylase (NP) deficiency were quite dismal, successful transplantation in this disorder using a BU and fludarabine conditioning regimen has recently been achieved [151]. In 1994, Fischer *et al.* [152] reported the European experience for CID, which included eight children with BLS, three of whom survived with a functional graft, two patients with NP deficiency, both of whom rejected their transplant, and eight children with CID of unknown etiology, five of whom were alive and well at the time of the report. Of the seven children with BLS who underwent HLA-matched-related BMT at the Hôpital Necker Enfants Malades, Paris, from 1981 to 1993 [153], six of six patients cytoreduced with BU/CY engrafted. Although two engrafted patients succumbed to viral infections early in post-transplant, four recovered immune function and survive at 0.6+ 2.0+ 5.0+ and 11.0+ years post-BMT. The one patient in this series who failed to engraft was cytoreduced with ATG and CY (50/kg) and subsequently with CY (50 mg/kg), 1-(2-chloroethyl)-3-cyclohexyl-1-nitrosurea (CCNU) (300 mg/m^2), procarbazine (280 mg/kg) and ATG due to initial graft failure. Successful HLA-matched transplantation for X–linked hyper-IgM syndrome has also been reported [154].

Early studies in CID patients who lacked an HLA-identical-related donor demonstrated a high incidence of graft failure following T-cell-depleted mismatched-related HCT and long-term survival rates of less than 10% (reviewed in [35]). More encouraging results were reported when anti-LFA-1 monoclonal antibody was combined with BU/CY cytoreduction [155]. Of 11 recipients of a T-cell-depleted mismatched-related HCT reported by Fischer *et al.* [155], seven patients, including three with BLS, engrafted and achieved long-term survival with immunologic reconstitution. In a single center analysis of HLA haplotype disparate BMT for BLS, three patients were cured, one improved with partial engraftment and eight failed to engraft [153].

These results clearly indicated the need for other transplant options for patients lacking an HLA-matched-related donor. To date, results of unmodified unrelated HCT have been promising. Seven patients with combined immunodeficiency, including three with Omenn's syndrome received unmodified unrelated BMT at the Hospital for Sick Children in Toronto, Canada, between December 1987 and August 1997 [105]. Acceptable donors were identified at a mean (range) of 4.7 (1–13) months and were HLA-A, B matched by serology and HLA-DRβ1 matched in six of seven cases. All patients were cytoreduced with BU/CY and received CSP, MP, with or without short course MTX to prevent GVHD. Currently, five of the sive patients are alive, doing well, with documented specific T and B-cell function, with a median follow-up of >4 years. The three children transplanted for Omenn's syndrome, two of whom had PCP prior to transplant, are alive and well at 6+ 20+ and 101+ months. Grade II or greater GVHD was observed in four of seven patients, which was fatal in two. In order to avoid the risk of GVHD, six patients with the hyper-IgM syndrome received a T-cell-depleted unrelated BMT, following which four are alive and well with normal immune function [156]. Younger age at transplant, now possible through prenatal diagnosis [157], was associated with better outcome following HCT for this disorder [156].

Wiskott–Aldrich syndrome (WAS)

Wiskott–Aldrich syndrome (WAS) is an X-linked disorder characterized by thrombocytopenia, immunodeficiency and eczema [158–160] (reviewed in [161]). In 1994, Derry *et al.* [162] identified the mutated gene responsible for WAS, which maps to chromosome Xp11.22–11.23. The wild type gene consists of a 12 exons and encodes a 501 amino acid, 53 kDa intracellular protein (WAS protein or WASp), expressed in most hematopoietic cells. WASp is involved in cytoskeletal organization (reviewed in [163]) and plays an essential role in T and NK cell activation [163–165]. Derry and colleagues identified three separate mutations within this X-linked gene [162] in four patients, two of whom were related. Since then at least 167 independent mutations, spanning all 12 exons of the gene, have been reported to an international study group formed in an effort to correlate genetic mutations with function, clinical severity, and treatment outcomes [166]. To date, the majority of mutations accounting for WAS are single base-pair missense or nonsense mutations, which occur in exons 2, 1, 4 and 7 [166].

Although all patients with WAS are thrombocytopenic, the level of T- and B-cell immunodeficiency, and subsequent risk of autoimmune phenomena (nephropathy, vasculitis) and lymphoid malignancies can be quite variable. Shcherbina *et al.* [167] demonstrated that the clinical heterogeneity observed in WAS patients is due to variable expression of WASp in lymphoid cells, allowing subdivision of patients into Group A with mild clinical disease (low levels of WASp protein in peripheral blood mononuclear cells [PBMCs], higher levels in Epstein–Barr virus immortalized B lymphoblastoid cell lines [EBV-BLCLs], with near normal levels of WASp RNA); Group B, moderate severity (low levels of WASp in both the PBMCs and EBV-BLCLs associated with similarly low levels of WASp RNA); Group C, variable clinical severity (lack of expression of WASp in peripheral B cells and EBV-derived cell lines but WASp positive circulating T cells); and Group D, severe disease (WASp-negative PBMCs and EBV-BLCLs). Knowledge of the pattern of WASp expression in individual patients can be used to determine which patients lacking an HLA-matched-related donor should be treated with supportive care alone [168], be early candidates for unrelated HCT [114] or, potentially, gene therapy in view of successful gene transfer and WASp expression *in vitro* and in animal models [169,170].

HCT for Wiskott–Aldrich syndrome (WAS)

In 1968, Bach *et al.* [4], reported correction of the immunologic abnormalities associated with WAS following HLA-matched sibling transplantation. Despite the use of high dose CY, this patient did not demonstrate engraftment of hematopoietic elements and remained thrombocytopenic. In 1978, Parkman et al. [171] corrected the immunologic and hematologic defects in a child with WAS by administering an HLA-matched marrow graft following myelosuppressive and immunosuppressive cytoreduction consisting of TBI, procarbazine, and ATG. These authors hypothesized that myeloablation as well as immunosuppression was required to correct disorders involving nonlymphoid lineages providing "space" in which progenitor cells could proliferate and develop. Subsequently, Kapoor et al. [172] demonstrated that BU/CY provided a myeloablative and immunosuppressive regimen adequate to insure full hematopoietic chimerism, correcting both the lymphoid and platelet defects in a series of children with WAS. A worldwide review from 1968 through 1997 reported that 57 of 65 children with WAS survived long-term after HLA-matched BMT [5]. Single center studies of HLA-identical related BMT from Brochstein et al. [173], Ozsahin et al. [174] and Rimm and Rappeport [175] have recorded long-term survival rates of 80% ($n = 10$), 91% ($n = 11$) and 88% ($n = 8$), respectively. Successful HLA-matched-related cord blood transplant for WAS, following BU/CY has also been reported [176].

For patients without an HLA-matched sibling, transplants from closely matched-unrelated donors have provided excellent results. Of 30 patients with WAS who received an unrelated unmodified BMT prior to July of 1994, the overall actuarial survival was 67% [177]. Analysis of these transplantation results demonstrated that children <2 years of age at the time of transplant had a much better prognosis with 21 of 23 surviving (actuarial survival at 3 years of 91%). Acute grade II–IV GVHD occurred in 50% of patients, with the highest incidence and severity observed in patients >5 years of age. An additional four children with WAS was reported by Lenarsky et al. [178] who received an unmodified unrelated BM were alive with 3–17+ months post-BMT.

In 2001, Filipovich et al. [107] summarized and compared the results of 170 transplants reported to the International Bone Marrow Transplant Registry and/or the National Marrow Donor Registry (1968–96) including 58 patients transplanted from HLA-matched siblings, 48 from other relatives and 67 patients from unrelated donors. Transplant outcome differed according to donor type with the probability of 5 years survival of 87% (74–93%) with an HLA-identical sibling donor, 52% (37–65%) with other related donors and 71% (58–80%) with unrelated donors [107]. For recipients of unrelated HCT, the best outcomes were observed in boys transplanted when <5 years of age. Of 55 boys with WAS who received an unrelated HCT (1987–2001) facilitated through the NMDP, approximately 85% of males transplanted at <5 years of age survive, compared to 30% transplanted over 5 years of age (Fig. 105.4). Early diagnosis, including prenatal diagnosis [179], will likely add to the improved results observed with unrelated HCT currently achieved. Still problematic is the child with WAS without a matched sibling who lacks a suitable unrelated marrow or cord blood donor [6,173]. A review of 25 patients who received a T-cell-depleted mismatched-related transplant, nine (36%) are alive and well with full ($n = 7$) or partial ($n = 2$) immune reconstitution. Failures included graft rejection despite intensive cytoreduction, EBV-LPD and GVHD. Of the 25 patients, 20% experienced graft failure and 36% developed EBV-LPD [169]. In addition, 45% of engrafted patients developed grade II–IV GVHD. The increased incidence of GVHD in these patients despite even rigorous TCD is unusual. In the MSKCC series published by Brochstein et al. [173] only one of six recipients of an HLA-mismatched SBA- E- BMT now survives, 10+ years since his T-cell-depleted mismatched-related BMT [175]. Three of the six patients in this series developed grade II–III GVHD compared to <10% of SCID patients durably engrafted with SBA- E- haploidentical transplants after identical pretransplant cytoreduction [173] (reviewed in [35]). This finding suggests that the target cell populations which trigger GVHD may be different in these two patient groups.

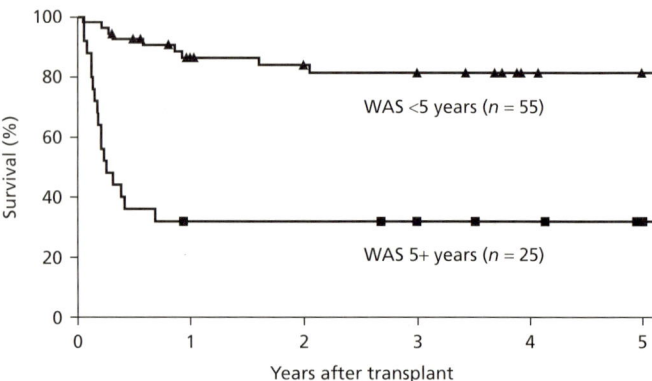

Fig. 105.4 Transplant procedures from unrelated donors for patients with Wiscott–Aldrich syndrome (1987–November 2001). Reproduced with permission from the National Marrow Donor Program.

Several advances, including adoptive immunotherapy and anti-B-cell antibodies for the treatment and/or prevention of EBV-LPD [180–184], alternative methods of transplantation, including T-cell depleted BM plus CD34 selected T-cell depleted PBSC to overcome graft rejection, and GVHD [185] are likely to improve results of T-cell depleted haploidentical BMT for this disease. The decision to transplant a child with WAS with T-cell depleted haplotype mismatched-HSC is likely to remain an area of controversy until results are markedly improved, particularly in patients determined to have mild disease on the basis of WASp expression in circulating lymphoid cells [167]. Other therapeutic options, including gene therapy, are likely to be further aggressively explored [169,170].

Conclusion

The heterogeneity of SCID and CID syndromes often requires a customized approach for individual patients in order to yield optimal transplantation results. The best transplant modality for patients lacking an HLA-matched sibling, including those which involve genetically modified autologous stem cells, will depend on which regimen confers the most durable and complete immunologic reconstitution with the least toxicity [186]. Advances in TCD, cytoreductive regimens (including nonmyeloablative regimens [187]) and gene therapy guarantee that the next 5–10 years will bring exciting trials for these rare but informative conditions.

References

1 Cavazzana-Calvo M, Hacein-Bey S, de Saint Basile G et al. Gene therapy of human severe combined immunodeficiency (SCID)-X1 disease. Science 2000; **288**: 699–72.

2 Hacein-Bey-Abina S, Le Deist F, Carlier F et al. Sustained correction of X-linked severe combined immunodeficiency by ex vivo gene therapy. N Engl J Med 2002; **346**: 1185–93.

3 Gatti RA, Meeuwissen HJ, Allen HD, Hong R, Good RA. Immunological reconstitution of sex-linked lymphopenic immunological deficiency. Lancet 1968; **2**: 1366–9.

4 Bach FH, Albertini RJ, Anderson JL et al. Bone marrow transplantation in a patient with the Wiskott–Aldrich syndrome. Lancet 1968; **2**: 1364–6.

5 Buckley RH. Bone marrow reconstitution in primary immunodeficiency. Clin Immunol Principles Prac 1995; **2**: 1813–30.

6 Small TN. Hematopoietic stem cell transplantation for severe combined immunodeficiency disease. Immunol Allergy Clin North Am 2000; **20**: 207–20.

7 Buckley RH. Primary immunodeficiency diseases

due to defects in lymphocytes. *N Eng J Med* 2000; **343**: 1313–23.

8 O'Marcaigh AS, DeSantes K, Hu D *et al.* Bone marrow transplantation for T-B-severe combined immunodeficiency disease in Athabascan-speaking native Americans. *Bone Marrow Transplant* 2001; **27**: 703–9.

9 Ziegner UH, Kobayashi RH, Cunningham-Rundles C *et al.* Progressive neurodegeneration in patients with primary immunodeficiency disease on IVIG treatment. *Clin Immunol* 2002; **102**: 19–24.

10 Giblett ER, Anderson JE, Cohen F, Pollara B, Meuwissen HJ. Adenosine deaminase deficiency in two patients with severe impaired cellular immunity. *Lancet* 1972; **2**: 1067–9.

11 Hershfield MS. Immunodeficiency caused by adenosine deaminase deficiency. *Immunol Allergy Clin North Am* 2000; **20**: 161–76.

12 DeVaal OM, Seynhaeve V. Reticular dysgenesis. *Lancet* 1959; **2**: 1123–5.

13 Small TN, Wall DA, Kurtzberg J, Cowan MJ, O'Reilly RJ, Friedrich W. Association of reticular dysgenesis (thymic alymphoplasia and congenital aleukocytosis) with bilateral sensorineural deafness. *J Pediatr* 1999; **135**: 387–9.

14 Omenn G. Familial reticuloendotheliosis. *N Engl J Med* 1965; **273**: 427–32.

15 Ruco LP, Stoppacciaro A, Pezzella F *et al.* The Omenn syndrome: histological, immunohistochemical and ultrastructural evidence for a partial T cell deficiency evolving in an abnormal proliferation of T lymphocytes and $S-100^+/T_6^+$ Langerhanslike cells. *Virchow's Arch* 1985; **407**: 69–82.

16 Gatti RA, Platt N, Pomerance HH *et al.* Hereditary lymphopenic agammaglobulinemia associated with a distinctive form of short-limbed dwarfism and ectodermal dysplasia. *J Pediatr* 1969; **75**: 675–84.

17 Masse J-F, Perusse R. Ectodermal dysplasia. *Arch Dis of Childhood* 1994; **71**: 1–2.

18 Gelfand EW, Oliver JM, Schuurman RK, Matheson DS, Dosch HM. Abnormal lymphocyte capping in a patient with severe combined immunodeficiency disease. *N Engl J Med* 1979; **301**: 1245–9.

19 Roifman CM, Hummel D, Martinez-Valdez H *et al.* Depletion of $CD8^+$ cells in human thymic medulla results in selective immune deficiency. *J Exp Med* 1989; **170**: 2177–82.

20 Monafo WJ, Polmar SH, Neudorf S, Mather A, Filipovich AH. A hereditary immunodeficiency characterized by $CD8^+$ T lymphocyte deficiency and impaired lymphocyte activation. *Clin Exp Immunol* 1992; **90**: 390–3.

21 Jung LKL, Fu SM, Hara T, Kapoor N, Good RA. Defective expression of T cell associated glycoprotein in severe combined immunodeficiency. *J Clin Invest* 1986; **77**: 940–6.

22 Alarcon B, Regueiro JR, Arnaiz-Villena A, Terhorst C. Familial defect in the surface expression of the T-cell receptor-CD3 complex. *N Engl J Med* 1988; **319**: 1203–9.

23 Roifman CM, Dadi HK. Human interleukin-2 receptor alpha deficiency. *Immunol Allergy Clin North Am* 2000; **20**: 39–50.

24 Puel A, Ziegler SF, Buckley RH, Leonard WJ. Defective IL7R expression in T^-, B^+, NK^+ severe combined immunodeficiency. *Nat Genet* 1998; **20**: 394–7.

25 Roifman CM, Zhang J, Chitayat D, Sharfe N. A partial deficiency of interleukin-7Rα is sufficient to abrogate T-cell development and cause severe combined immunodeficiency. *Blood* 2000; **96**: 2803–7.

26 Gilmour KG, Fujii H, Cranston T, Davies EG, Kinnon C, Gaspar HB. Defective expression of the interleukin-2–15 receptor β subunit leads to natural killer cell-deficient form of severe combined immunodeficiency. *Blood* 2001; **98**: 877–9.

27 Moshous D, Callebaut C, de Chasseval R *et al.* Artemis, a novel DNA double-strand Break repair/V (D) J recombination protein, is mutated in human severe combined immune deficiency. *Cell* 2001; **105**: 177–86.

28 Li L, Moshous D, Zhou Y *et al.* A founder mutation in Artemis, an SNM1-like protein, causes SCID in Athabascan-speaking Native Americans. *J Immunol* 2002; **168**: 632–9.

29 Kung C, Pingel JT, Heikinheimo M *et al.* Mutations in the tyrosine phosphatase CD45 gene in a child with severe combined immunodeficiency disease. *Nature Med* 2000; **6**: 343–5.

30 Parkman R, Gelfand EW, Rosen FS, Sanderson A, Hirschhorn R. Severe combined immunodeficiency and adenosine deaminase deficiency. *N Engl J Med* 1975; **14**: 714–9.

31 Ownby DR, Pizzo S, Blackmon L, Gall SA, Buckley RH. Severe combined immunodeficiency with leukopenia (reticular dysgenesis) in siblings. Immunologic and histopathologic findings. *J Pediatr* 1976; **89**: 382–7.

32 Fischer A, Landais P, Friedrich W *et al.* European experience of bone-marrow transplantation for severe combined immunodeficiency. *Lancet* 1990; **336**: 850–4.

33 Buckley RH, Schiff RI, Schiff SE *et al.* Human severe combined immunodeficiency: genetic, phenotypic, and functional diversity in one hundred and eight infants. *J Pediatrics* 1997; **130**: 378–87.

34 Dror Y, Gallagher RM, Wara DW *et al.* Immune reconstitution in severe combined immunodeficiency disease after lectin-treated, TCD haploidentical bone marrow transplantation. *Blood* 1993; **81**: 2021–30.

35 O'Reilly RJ, Small TN, Friedrich W. Hematopoietic cell transplant for immunodeficiency diseases. In: Thomas ED, Blume KG, Forman SJ, eds. *Hematopoietic Cell Transplantation*, 2nd edn. Malden, MA: Blackwell Science, 1999: 1154–72.

36 Hirschhorn R, Beratis N, Rosen FS, Parkman R, Stern R, Polmar S. Adenosine deaminase deficiency in a child diagnosed prenatally. *Lancet* 1975; **1**: 73–5.

37 Dooley R, Fairbanks LD, Simmonds HA *et al.* First trimester diagnosis of adenosine deaminase deficiency. *Prenat Diagn* 1987; **7**: 561–5.

38 Durandy A, Dumez Y, Guy-Grand D, Ourv C, Henrion R, Griscelli C. Prenatal diagnosis of severe combined immunodeficiency. *J Pediatr* 1982; **101**: 995–7.

39 Jones AM, Gaspar HB. Immunogenetics. changing the face of immunodeficiency. *J Clin Path* 2000; **53**: 60–5.

40 Gaspar HB, Gilmour KC, Jones AM. Severe combined immunodeficiency disease-molecular pathogenesis and diagnosis. *Arch Dis Child* 2001; **84**: 169–73.

41 Buckley RH. Primary cellular immunodeficiencies. *J Allergy Clin Immunol* 2002; **109**: 747–57.

42 Noguchi M, Yi H, Rosenblatt HM *et al.* Interleukin-2 receptor gamma chain mutation results in X-linked severe combined immunodeficiency in humans. *Cell* 1993; **73**: 147–57.

43 Puck JM, Deschenes SM, Porter JC *et al.* The interleukin-2 receptor gamma chain maps to Xq13.1 and is mutated in X-linked severe combined immunodeficiency, SCIDX1. *Human Mol Genet* 1993; **2**: 1099–104.

44 Puck JM, Pepper AE, Henthorn PS *et al.* Mutation analysis of IL2RG in human X-linked severe combined immunodeficiency. *Blood* 1997; **89**: 1968–77.

45 Russell SM, Tayebi N, Nakajima H *et al.* Mutation of *Jak3* in a patient with SCID. Essential role of *Jak3* in lymphoid development. *Science* 1995; **270**: 797–800.

46 Macchi P, Villa A, Gillani S *et al.* Mutations of *Jak-3* gene in patients with autosomal severe combined immunodeficiency disease (SCID). *Nature* 1995; **377**: 65–8.

47 Schumacher RF, Mella P, Badolato R *et al.* Complete genomic organization of the human *JAK3* gene and mutation analysis in severe combined immunodeficiency by single-strand conformation polymorphism. *Hum Genet* 2000; **106**: 73–9.

48 Arpaia E, Shahar M, Dadi H, Cohen A, Roifman CM. Defective T cell receptor signaling and $CD8^+$ thymic selection in humans lacking Zap-70 kinase. *Cell* 1994; **76**: 947–58.

49 Elder ME, Lin D, Clever J *et al.* Human severe combined immunodeficiency due to a defect in ZAP-70, a T cell tyrosine kinase. *Science* 1994; **264**: 1596–9.

50 Chan AC, Kadlecek TA, Elder ME, Filipovich AH. ZAP-70 deficiency in an autosomal recessive form of severe combined immunodeficiency. *Science* 1994; **264**: 1599–601.

51 Sharfe N, Arpaia E, Roifman CM. CD8 lymphopenia caused by Zap-70 deficiency. *Immunol Allergy Clin North Am* 2000; **20**: 2077–98.

52 Schwarz K, Gauss GH, Ludwig L *et al. RAG* mutations in human B cell-negative SCID. *Science* 1996; **274**: 97–9.

53 Puck JM, Middelton L, Pepper AE. Carrier and prenatal diagnosis of X-linked severe combined immunodeficiency: mutation detection methods and utilization. *Hum Genet* 1997; **99**: 628–33.

54 Schumacher RF, Mella P, Lalatta F *et al.* Prenatal diagnosis of *JAK3* deficient SCID. *Prenat Diagn* 1999; **19**: 653–6.

55 Villa A, Bozzi F, Sobacchi C *et al.* Prenatal diagnosis of *RAG*-deficient Omenn syndrome. *Prenat Diagn* 2000; **20**: 56–9.

56 Kane L, Gennery AR, Crooks BN, Flood TJ, Abinun M, Cant AJ. Neonatal bone marrow transplantation for severe combined immunodeficiency. *Arch Dis Child Fetal Neonatal Ed* 2000; **85**: F110–3.

57 Myers LA, Patel DD, Puck JM, Buckley RH. Hematopoietic stem cell transplantation for severe combined immunodeficiency in the neonatal period leads to superior thymic output and improved survival. *Blood* 2002; **99**: 872–8.

58 Corneo B, Moshous D, Gungor T *et al.* Identical mutations in *RAG1* or *RAG2* genes leading to defective V (D) J recombinase activity can cause either T-B-severe combined immune deficiency or Omenn syndrome. *Blood* 2001; **97**: 2772–6.

59 Villa A, Sobacchi C, Notarangelo LD *et al.* V (D) J recombination defects in lymphocytes due to *RAG* mutations: severe immunodeficiency with a spectrum of clinical presentations. *Blood* 2001; **97**: 81–8.

60 Umetsu DT, Schlossman CM, Ochs HD, Hershfield MS. Heterogeneity of phenotype in two

siblings with adenosine deaminase deficiency. *J Allergy Clin Immunol* 1994; **93**: 543–50.
61 Buckley RH, Schiff SE, Schiff RI *et al*. Hematopoietic stem-cell transplantation for the treatment of severe combined immunodeficiency. *N Engl J Med* 1999; **340**: 508–16.
62 Bertrand Y, Landais P, Friedrich W *et al*. Influence of severe combined immunodeficiency phenotype on the outcome of HLA non-identical, T-cell-depleted bone marrow transplantation: a retrospective European survey from the European group for bone marrow transplantation and the European society for immunodeficiency. *J Pediatr* 1999; **134**: 740–8.
63 Fischer A, Friedrich W, Levinsky R *et al*. Bone marrow transplantation for immunodeficiencies and osteopetrosis. European survey: 1968–85. *Lancet* 1986; **2**: 1080–3.
64 Wijnaendts L, Le Deist F, Griscelli C, Fischer A. Development of immunologic functions after bone marrow transplantation in 33 patients with severe combined immunodeficiency *Blood* 1989; **89**(74): 2212–9.
65 Stephan JL, Vlekova V, Le Deist F *et al*. Severe combined immunodeficiency: a retrospective single-center study of clinical presentation and outcome in 117 patients. *J Ped* 1993; **123**: 564–72.
66 Kenny AB, Hitzig WH. Bone marrow transplantation for severe combined immunodeficiency. *Eur J Pediatr* 1979; **131**: 155–77.
67 Dini G, Castagnola E, Comoli P, van Tol MJ, Vossen JM. Infections after stem cell transplantation in children. State of the art and recommendations. *Bone Marrow Transplant* 2001; **28** (Suppl. 1): S18–21.
68 Sullivan KM, Dykewicz CA, Longworth DL *et al*. Preventing opportunistic infections after hematopoietic stem cell transplantation: the Centers for Disease Control and Prevention, Infectious Diseases Society of America and the American Society for Blood and Marrow Transplantation Practice: guidelines and beyond. *Hematology (Am Soc Hematol Educ Program)* 2001; 392–421.
69 Leggiardi RJ, Winkelstein JA, Hughes WT. Prevalence of *Pneumocystis carinii* pneumonitis in severe combined immunodeficiency disease. *J Pediatr* 1981; **99**: 96–8.
70 Crooks BN, Taylor CE, Turner AJ *et al*. Respiratory viral infections in primary immune deficiencies: significance and relevance to clinical outcome in a single BMT unit. *Bone Marrow Transplant* 2000; **26**: 1097–102.
71 Small TN, Casson A, Sharp F *et al*. Respiratory syncytial virus infection following hematopoietic stem cell transplant. *Bone Marrow Transplant* 2002; **29**: 321–7.
72 Smogorzewska EM, Brooks J, Annett G *et al*. T cell depleted haploidentical bone marrow transplantation for the treatment of children with severe combined immunodeficiency. *Arch Immunol Ther Exp* 2000; **48**: 111–8.
73 Haddad E, Le Deist F, Aucouturier P *et al*. Long-term chimerism and B-cell function after bone marrow transplantation in patients with severe combined immunodeficiency with B cells: a single-center study of 22 patients. *Blood* 1999; **94**: 2923–30.
74 Biggar WD, Park BY, Good RA. Compatible bone marrow transplant and immunologic reconstitution of combined immunodeficiency disease. *Birth Defects* 1975; **11**: 385–90.

75 Junker AK, Chan KJ, Massing BG. Clinical and immune recovery from Omenn syndrome after bone marrow transplantation. *J Pediatr* 1989; **114**: 596–600.
76 Levinsky RJ, Tiedman K. Successful bone-marrow transplantation for reticular dysgenesis. *Lancet* 1983; **1**: 671–3.
77 Beatty PG, Clift RA, Michelson EM *et al*. Marrow transplantation from related donors other than HLA-identical siblings. *N Engl J Med* 1985; **313**: 765–71.
78 Ziegner UH, Ochs HD, Schanen C *et al*. Transplantation of hematopoietic cells for lethal congenital immunodeficiencies. *Birth defects* 1983; **19**: 129–37.
79 Keightly RG, Lawton AA, Cooper M. Successful fetal liver transplantation in a child with severe combined immunodeficiency. *Lancet* 1975; **2**: 850–3.
80 O'Reilly RJ, Pollack MS, Kapoor N *et al*. Fetal liver transplantation in man and animals. In: Gale RP, ed. *Recent Advances in Bone Marrow Transplantation*. New York: Alan R. Liss, 1983: 799–830.
81 Kernan NA. T-cell depletion for the prevention of graft versus host disease. In: Thomas ED, Blume KG, Forman SJ, eds. *Hematopoietic Cell Transplantation*, 2nd edn. Malden, MA: Blackwell Science, 1999: 186–96.
82 Reisner Y, Itsicovitch L, Meshorer A, Sharon N. Hematopoietic stem cell transplantation using mouse bone marrow and spleen cells fractionated by lectins. *PNAS* 1978; **75**: 2933–6.
83 Reisner Y, Kapoor N, Kirkpatrick D *et al*. Transplantation for severe combined immunodeficiency HLA-A, B, D, Dr incompatible parental marrow fractionated by soybean agglutinin and sheep red blood cells. *Blood* 1983; **61**: 341–8.
84 Fischer A, Durandy A, De Villartay JP *et al*. HLA-haploidentical bone marrow transplantation for severe combined immunodeficiency using E-rosette fractionation and cyclosporine. *Blood* 1986; **67**: 444–9.
85 Hayward AR, Murphy S, Githens J, Troup G, Ambruso D. Failure of a pan-reactive anti-T cell antibody, OKT3, to prevent graft versus host disease in severe combined immunodeficiency. *J Pediatr* 1982; **100**: 665–8.
86 Morgan G, Linen DC, Knott LT *et al*. Successful haploidentical mismatched bone marrow transplantation in severe combined immunodeficiency: T-cell removal using CAMPATH-1 monoclonal antibody and E-rosetting. *Br J Haematol* 1986; **62**: 421–30.
87 Dickinson AM, Reid MM, Abunum M *et al*. *In vitro* T cell depletion using Campath 1M for mismatched BMT for severe combined immunodeficiency (SCID). *Bone Marrow Transplant* 1997; **19**: 323–9.
88 Lanfranchi A, Verardi R, Tettoni K *et al*. Haploidentical peripheral blood and marrow stem cell transplantation in nine cases of primary immunodeficiency. *Haematologica* 2000; **85** (Suppl.): 41–6.
89 Friedrich W, Goldmann SF, Ebell W, Blütters-Sawatzki R. Severe combined immunodeficiency: treatment by bone marrow transplantation in 15 infants using HLA-haploidentical donors. *Eur J Pediatr* 1985; **144**: 125–30.
90 Haddad E, Landais P, Friedrich W *et al*. Long-term immune reconstitution and outcome after HLA-nonidentical T-cell-depleted bone marrow transplantation for severe combined immunodeficiency: a European retrospective study of 116 patients. *Blood* 1998; **91**: 3646–53.
91 Loechelt BJ, Shapiro RS, Jyonouchi H, Filipovich AH. Mismatched bone marrow transplantation for Omenn syndrome. A variant of severe combined immunodeficiency. *Bone Marrow Transplant* 1995; **16**: 381–5.
92 Gomez L, Le Deist F, Blanche S, Cavazzana-Calvo M, Griscelli C, Fischer A. Treatment of Omenn syndrome by bone marrow transplantation. *J Pediatr* 1995; **127**: 76–81.
93 Bertrand Y, Muller SM, Casanova JL, Morgan G, Fischer A, Friedrich W. Reticular dysgenesis. HLA non-identical bone marrow transplants in a series of 10 patients. *Bone Marrow Transplant* 2002; **29**: 759–62.
94 Muller SM, Kohn T, Schulz AS, Debatin KM, Friedrich W. Similar pattern of thymic-dependent T-cell reconstitution in infants with severe combined immunodeficiency after human leukocyte antigen (HLA)-identical and HLA-nonidentical stem cell transplantation. *Blood* 2000; **96**: 4344–9.
95 Patel DD, Gooding ME, Parrott RE, Curtis KM, Haynes BF, Buckley RH. Thymic function after haematopoietic stem-cell transplantation for the treatment of severe combined immunodeficiency. *N Eng Med J* 2000; **342**: 1325–32.
96 Burzy MS, Schulte-Wisserman H, Gilbert E, Horowitz SD, Pellet J, Hong R. Thymic morphology in immunodeficiency diseases. Results of the thymic biopsies. *Clin Immunol Immunopathol* 1979; **12**: 31–51.
97 Kapoor N, Jung LKL, Engelhard D *et al*. Lymphoma in a patient with severe combined immunodeficiency with adenosine deaminase deficiency, following unsustained engraftment of histoincompatible TCD bone marrow. *J Pediatr* 1986; **108**: 435–8.
98 Gross TG, Steinbuch M, DeFor T *et al*. B cell lymphoproliferative disorders following hematopoietic stem cell transplantation: risk factors, treatment, and outcome. *Bone Marrow Transplant* 1999; **23**: 251–8.
99 Descamps V, Blanchet-Bardon C, Petit A, Baccard M, Fisher A, Dubertret L. Epidermodysplasia verruciformis (EV) after bone marrow transplantation for the treatment of severe combined immunodeficiency: a model to understand the specific immunodeficiency of EV? *Ann Dermatol Venereol* 1991; **118**: 847–50.
100 Horn B, Viele M, Mentzer W, Mogck N, DeSantes K, Cowan M. Autoimmune hemolytic anemia in patients with SCID after T cell-depleted BM and PBSC transplantation *Bone Marrow Transplant* 1999; **24**: 1009–13.
101 Arkwright PD, Abinun M, Cant AJ. Autoimmunity in human primary immunodeficiency diseases. *Blood* 2002; **99**: 2694–702.
102 O'Reilly RJ, Dupont B, Pahwa S *et al*. Reconstitution in severe combined immunodeficiency by transplantation of marrow from an unrelated donor. *N Engl J Med* 1977; **297**: 1311–8.
103 Filipovich AH, Shapiro RS, Ramsay NKC *et al*. Unrelated donor bone marrow transplantation for correction of lethal congenital immunodeficiencies. *Blood* 1992; **80**: 270–6.
104 Filipovich AH. Stem cell transplantation from unrelated donors for correction of primary immunodeficiencies. Organ and bone marrow transplantation. 1996; **16**: 377–93.

105 Dalal I, Reid B, Doyle J et al. Matched unrelated bone marrow transplantation for combined immunodeficiency. *Bone Marrow Transplant* 2000; **25**: 613–21.

106 National Marrow Donor Program (NMDP) database.

107 Filipovich AH, Stone JV, Tomany SC et al. Impact of donor type on outcome of bone marrow transplantation for Wiskott–Aldrich syndrome: collaborative study of the International Bone Marrow Transplant Registry and the National Marrow Donor Program. *Blood* 2001; **97**: 1598–603.

108 Rubinstein P, Carrier C, Scaradavou A et al. Outcomes among 562 recipients of placental-blood transplants from unrelated donors. *N Engl J Med* 1998; **26**(339): 1565–77.

109 Gluckman E, Rocha V, Chastang C. Peripheral stem cells in bone marrow transplantation. Cord blood stem cell transplantation. *Baillieres Best Pract Res Clin Haematol* 1999; **12**: 279–92.

110 Knutsen AP, Wall DA. Umbilical cord blood transplantation in severe T-cell immunodeficiency disorders: two-year experience. *J Clin Immunol* 2000; **20**: 466–76.

111 Benito A, Diaz MA, Alonso F, Fontan G, Madero L. Successful unrelated umbilical cord blood transplantation in a child with Omenn's syndrome. *Pediatr Hematol Oncol* 1999; **16**: 361–6.

112 Ziegner UH, Ochs HD, Schanen C et al. Unrelated umbilical cord stem cell transplantation for X-linked immunodeficiencies. *J Pediatr* 2001; **138**: 570–3.

113 Toren A, Nagler A, Amariglio N et al. Successful human umbilical cord blood stem cell transplantation without conditioning in severe combined immune deficiency. *Bone Marrow Transplant* 1999; **23**: 405–8.

114 Flake AW. Successful treatment of XSCID by *in utero* transplantation of CD34 enriched paternal bone marrow cells. *Blood* 1995; **86**: 125a [Abstract].

115 Flake AW, Zanjani ED. *In utero* hematopoietic stem cell transplantation. Ontogenetic opportunities and biologic barriers. *Blood* 1999; **94**: 2179–91.

116 Flake A, Roncarolo M, Puck J et al. Treatment of X-linked severe combined immunodeficiency by *in utero* transplantation of paternal bone marrow. *New Engl J Med* 1996; **335**: 1806–145.

117 Flake A, Zanjani ED. Treatment of Severe Combined Immunodeficiency. *N Eng J Med* 1999; **341**: 291–2.

118 Wengler G, Lanfranchi A, Frusca T et al. In-utero transplantation of parental CD34 haematopoietic progenitor cells in a patient with X-linked severe combined immunodeficiency (SCIDX1). *The Lancet* 1996; **348**: 1484–7.

119 Gil J, Porta F, Bartolome J et al. Immune reconstitution after *in utero* bone marrow transplantation in a fetus with natural killer cells. *Transplant Proc* 1999; **31**: 2581.

120 Bartome J, Porta F, Lafranchi A et al. B cell function after haploidentical *in utero* bone marrow transplantation in a patient with severe combined immunodeficiency. *Bone Marrow Transplant* 2002; **29**: 625–8.

121 Cavazzana-Calvo M, Hacein-Bey S, Yates F, de Villartay JP, Le Deist F, Fischer A. Gene therapy of severe combined immunodeficiencies. *J Gene Med* 2001; **3**: 201–6.

122 Blaese RM. T lymphocyte-directed gene therapy for ADA-SCID. Initial trials results after 4 years. *Science* 1995; **270**: 475–80.

123 Bordignon C. Gene therapy in peripheral blood lymphocytes and bone marrow in ADA-immunodeficient patients. *Science* 1995; **270**: 470–5.

124 Kohn D. Engraftment of gene-modified umbilical cord blood cells in neonates with adenosine deaminase deficiency. *Nat Med* 1995; **1**: 1017–23.

125 Auiti A, Vai S, Mortello GC et al. Immune reconstitution in ADA-SCID after *PBL* gene therapy and discontinuation of enzyme replacement. *Nat Med* 2002; **8**: 423–5.

126 Buckley RH. Gene therapy for SCID: a complication after remarkable progress. *Lancet* 2002; **360**: 1185–6.

127 Aiuti A, Slavin S, Aker M et al. Correction of ADA-SCID by stem cell gene therapy combined with nonmyeloablative conditioning. *Science* 2002; **296**: 2410–3.

128 Taylor N, Bacon KB, Smith S et al. Reconstitution of T cell receptor signaling in ZAP-70-deficient cells by retroviral transduction of the *ZAP-70* gene. *J Exp Med* 1996; **184**: 2031–6.

129 Otsu M, Steinberg M, Ferrand C et al. Reconstitution of lymphoid development and function in ZAP-70-deficient mice following gene transfer into bone marrow cells. *Blood* 2002; **100**: 1248–56.

130 Bunting KD, Sangster MY, Ihle JN, Sorrentino BP. Restoration of lymphocyte function in Janus kinase 3-deficient mice by retroviral-mediated gene transfer. *Nat Med* 1998; **4**: 58–64.

131 Yates F, Malassis-Seris M, Stockholm D et al. Gene therapy of $RAG-2^{-/-}$ mice: sustained correction of the immunodeficiency. *Blood* 2002; **100**: 3942–9.

132 Lawlor GJ, Ammann AJ, Wright WC, La Franchi SH, Bilstrom D, Steihm ER. The syndrome of cellular immunodeficiency with immunoglobulins (type Nezelof 1964). *J Pediatr* 1974; **84**: 183–92.

133 Rosen F. The primary immunodeficiencies. *N Engl J Med* 1995; **333**: 431–40.

134 Levy J, Espanol-Boren T, Thomas C et al. Clinical spectrum of X–linked hyper IgM syndrome. *J Pediatr* 1997; **131**: 47–54.

135 Chu E, Rosenwasser LJ, Dinareud CA, Rosen FS, Geha RS. Immunodeficiency with defective T-cell response to interleukin-1. *PNAS* 1984; **81**: 4945–9.

136 Chatila T, Castigli E, Pahwa R et al. Primary combined immunodeficiency resulting from defective transcription of multiple T-cell lymphokine genes. *PNAS* 1990; **87**: 10,033–7.

137 Disanto JP, Keever CA, Small TN, Nichols GL, O'Reilly RJ, Flomenberg N. Absence of interleukin-2 production of a severe combined immunodeficiency disease syndrome with T-cells. *J Exp Med* 1990; **171**: 1697–704.

138 Weinberg K, Parkman R. Severe combined immunodeficiency due to a specific defect in the production of IL-2. *N Engl J Med* 1990; **322**: 1718–23.

139 Weinberg KI, Parr T, Annett GM et al. Severe combined immunodeficiency (SCID) due to defective interleukin-2 receptor alpha (IL-2R alpha). *Pediatr Res* 1989: 170a [Abstract].

140 Markert ML. Purine nucleoside phosphorylase deficiency. *Immunodeficiency Rev* 1991; **3**: 45–81.

141 Touraine JL, Betuel H, Souillet G, Jeune M. Combined immunodeficiency disease associated with absence of cell surface HLA-A and B antigens. *J Pediatr* 1978; **93**: 47–51.

142 Klein C, Lisowska-Grospierre B, Le Deist F, Fischer A, Griscelli C. Major histocompatibility complex class II deficiency. Clinical manifestations, immunologic features, and outcome. *J Pediatr* 1993; **123**: 921–8.

143 Mach B, Steimle V, Reith W. MHC class II-deficient combined immunodeficiency. A disease of gene regulation. *Imm Rev* 1994; **138**: 207–21.

144 Diamond MS, Staunton DE, de Fougerolles AR et al. ICAM-1 (CD54): a counter-receptor for Mac 1 (CD11b/CD18). *J Cell Biol* 1990; **111**: 3129–39.

145 Springer TA, Dustin ML, Kishimoto TK, Martin SD. The lymphocyte function associated with LFA-1, CD2, and LFA-3 molecules: cell adhesion receptors of the immune system. *Ann Rev Immunol* 1987; **5**: 223–52.

146 Korthauer U, Graf D, Mages HW. Defective expression of T-cell CD40L causes X-linked immunodeficiency with hyper IgM. *Nature* 1993; **361**: 539–41.

147 DiSanto JP, Bonnefoy JY, Gauchat JF et al. *CD40L* mutations in X-linked immunodeficiency with hyper IgM. *Nature* 1993; **361**: 541–3.

148 Ferrari S, Gilliani S, Insalaco A et al. Mutations of *CD40* gene cause an autosomal recessive form of immunodeficiency with hyer IgM. *PNAS* 2001; **98**: 12614–9.

149 Revy P, Muto T, Levy Y et al. Activation-induced cytidine deaminase (AID) deficiency causes the autosomal recessive form of the Hyper-IgM syndrome (HIGM2). *Cell* 2000; **102**: 565–75.

150 Businco L, Rossi P, Paganelli R et al. Immunologic reconstitution with bone marrow transplantation and thymic hormones in two patients with severe pure T cell defects. *Birth defects* 1983; **19**: 281–5.

151 Classen CF, Shulz AS, Sigl-Kraetzig M et al. Successful HLA-identical bone marrow transplantation in a patient with PNP deficiency using busulfan and fludarabine for conditioning. *Bone Marrow Transplant* 2001; **28**: 93–6.

152 Fischer A, Landais P, Friedrich W et al. Bone marrow transplantation (BMT) in Europe for primary immunodeficiencies other than severe combined immunodeficiency: a report from the European group for BMT and the European group for immunodeficiency. *Blood* 1994; **83**: 1149–54.

153 Klein C, Cavazzana-Calvo M, Le Deist F et al. Bone marrow transplantation in major histocompatibility complex class II deficiency: a single-center study of 19 patients. *Blood* 1995; **85**: 580–7.

154 Duplantier JE, Seyama K, Day NK et al. Immunologic reconstitution following bone marrow transplantation for X–linked hyper IgM syndrome. *Clin Immunol* 2001; **98**: 313–8.

155 Fischer A, Friedrich W, Fasth A et al. Reduction of graft failure by a monoclonal antibody (anti-LFA-1 CD11a) after HLA non-identical bone marrow transplantation in children with immunodeficiencies, osteropetrosis, and Fanconi's anemia: a European group for Immunodeficiency/European group for bone marrow transplantation report. *Blood* 1991; **77**: 249–56.

156 Khawaja K, Gennery AR, Flood TJ, Abinun M, Cant AJ. Bone marrow transplantation for CD40 ligand deficiency: a single center experience. *Arch Dis Child* 2001; **84**: 508–11.

157 DiSanto JP, Markiewicz S, Gauchat JF, Bonnefoy JY, Fischer A, de Saint Basile G. Brief report. Prenatal diagnosis of X-linked hyper-IgM syndrome. *N Engl J Med* 1994; **330**: 969–73.

158 Aldrich RA, Steinberg AGI, Campbell DC. Pedigree demonstrating a sex-linked recessive condition characterized by draining ears, eczemat-

158. ous dermatitis and bloody diarrhea. *Pediatrics* 1954; **113**: 133–8.
159. Cooper MD, Chase HP, Lowman JT, Krivit W, Good RA. The Wiskott–Aldrich syndrome. An immunologic deficiency disease involving the afferent limb of immunity. *Am J Med* 1968; **44**: 499–513.
160. Blaese RM, Strober W, Brown RS, Waldmann RA. The Wiskott–Aldrich syndrome: a disorder with possible defect in antigen processing or recognition. *Lancet* 1968; **1**: 1056–61.
161. Nonoyama S, Ochs HD. Wiskott–Aldrich syndrome. *Curr Allergy Asthma Rep* 2001; **1**: 430–7.
162. Derry JMJ, Ochs HD, Francke U. Isolation of a novel gene mutated in Wiskott–Aldrich syndrome. *Cell* 1994; **78**: 63–44.
163. Snapper SB, Rosen FS. The Wiskott–Aldrich syndrome protein (WASP). Roles in signaling and cytoskeletal organization. *Annu Rev Immunol* 1999; **17**: 905–29.
164. Silvin C, Belisle B, Abo A. A role for Wiskott–Aldrich syndrome protein in T-cell receptor-mediated transcriptional activation independent of actin polymerization. *J Biol Chem* 2001; **276**: 21,450–7.
165. Orange JS, Ramesh N, Remold-O'Donnell E *et al.* Wiskott–Aldrich syndrome protein is required for NK cell cytotoxicity and co-localizes with actin at NK cell-activating immunologic synapses. *Proc Natl Acad Sci U S A* 2002; **99**: 11351–6.
166. Schwarz K. WASPbase. A database of WAS- and XLT-causing mutations. *Immunol Today* 1996; **17**: 496–502.
167. Shcherbina A, Rosen FS, Remold-O'Donnell E. WASP levels in platelets and lymphocytes of Wiskott–Aldrich syndrome patients correlate with cell dysfunction. *J Immunol* 1999; **163**: 6314–20.
168. Mullen CA, Anderson KD, Blaese RM. Splenectomy and/or bone marrow transplantation in the management of the Wiskott–Aldrich syndrome: long-term follow-up of 62 cases. *Blood* 1993; **82**: 2961–6.
169. Huang M-M, Wong A, Weinberg KI, Francke U, Kohn DB. Expression of human Wiskott–Aldrich syndrome protein in patients' primary hematopoietic cells and EBV-transduced cell lines after retroviral vector-mediated gene transduction. *Blood* 1997; **90**: 263a [Abstract].
170. Strom TS, Li X, Cunningham JM, Nienhuis AW. Correction of the murine Wiskott–Aldrich syndrome phenotype by hematopoietic stem cell transplantation. *Blood* 2002; **99**: 4626–8.
171. Parkman R, Rappaport J, Geha R *et al.* Complete correction of the Wiskott–Aldrich syndrome by marrow transplantation. *N Eng J Med* 1978; **298**: 921–7.
172. Kapoor N, Kirkpatrick D, Blaese RM *et al.* Reconstitution of normal megakaryocytopoiesis and immunological functions in Wiskott–Aldrich syndrome by marrow transplantation following myeloablation and immunosuppression with busulfan and cyclophosphamide. *Blood* 1981; **57**: 692–6.
173. Brochstein JA, Gillio AP, Ruggiero M *et al.* Marrow transplantation from human leukocyte antigen-identical or haploidentical donors for correction of Wiskott–Aldrich syndrome. *J Pediatr* 1991; **119**: 907.
174. Ozsahin H, LeDeist F, Benkerrou M *et al.* Bone marrow transplantation in 26 patients with Wiskott–Aldrich syndrome from a single center. *J Pediatr* 1996; **129**: 238–44.
175. Rimm IJ, Rappeport JM. Bone marrow transplantation for the Wiskott–Aldrich syndrome: long-term follow-up. *Transplant* 1990; **50**: 617–20.
176. Wagner JE, Kernan NA, Steinbuch M, Broxmeyer HE, Gluckman E. Allogeneic sibling umbilical-cord-blood transplantation in children with malignant and non-malignant disease. *Lancet* 1995; **346**: 214–9.
177. Filpovich AH. Stem cell transplantation from unrelated donors for correction of primary immunodeficiencies. *Organ Bone Marrow Transplant* 1996; **16**: 377–93.
178. Lenarsky C, Weinberg K, Kohn DB, Parkman R. Unrelated donor BMT for Wiskott–Aldrich syndrome. *Bone Marrow Transplant* 1993; **12**: 145–7.
179. Giliani S, Fiorini M, Mella P *et al.* Prenatal molecular diagnosis of Wiskott–Aldrich syndrome by direct mutation analysis. *Prenat Diagn* 1999; **19**: 36–40.
180. Rumelhart AL, Trigg ME, Horowitz SD, Hong R. Monoclonal antibody T-cell-depleted HLA-haploidentical bone marrow transplantation for Wiskott–Aldrich syndrome. *Blood* 1990; **75**: 1031–5.
181. Straathof KC, Savoldo B, Heslop HE, Rooney CM. Immunotherapy for post-transplant lymphoproliferative disease. *Br J Haematol* 2002; **118**: 728–40.
182. O'Reilly RJ, Small TN, Papadopoulos E, Lucas K, Lacerda J, Koulova L. Adoptive immunotherapy for Epstein–Barr virus-associated lymphoproliferative disorders complicating marrow allografts. *Springer Semin Immunopathol* 1998; **20**: 455–91.
183. Benkerrou M, Jais J-P, Leblond V *et al.* Anti-b-cell monoclonal antibody treatment of severe post-transplant B-lymphoproliferative disorder: prognostic factors and long-term outcome. *Blood* 1998; **92**: 3137–47.
184. Faye A, Quartier P, Reguerre Y *et al.* Chimaeric anti-CD20 monoclonal antibody (rituximab) in post-transplant B-lymphoproliferative disorde following stem cell transplantation in children. *Br J Haematol* 2001; **115**: 112–8.
185. Martelli MF, Aversa F, Bachar-Lustig E *et al.* Transplants across human leukocyte antigen barriers. *Semin Hematol* 2002; **39**: 48–56.
186. Handgretinger R, Koscielniak E, Niethammer D, Cavazzana-Calvo M, Hacein-Bey-Abina S, Fischer A. Gene therapy for severe combined immunodeficiency disease. *N Eng J Med* 2002; **347**: 613–4.
187. Amrolia P, Gaspar HB, Hassan A *et al.* Non-myeloablative stem cell transplantation for congenital immunodeficiencies. *Blood* 2000; **96**: 1239–46.

106

Peter F. Coccia

Hematopoietic Cell Transplantation for Osteopetrosis

Osteopetrosis is a rare inherited disorder characterized by generalized skeletal sclerosis which occurs in various mammals including humans [1,2]. Osteopetrosis is a result of the dysfunction of osteoclasts, the multinucleated giant cells that resorb bone and mineralized cartilage [3–5]. The osteoclast is a specialized macrophage polykaryon derived from the hematopoietic stem cell (HSC) [4,5]. Some variants of osteopetrosis in laboratory animals and humans can be corrected by hematopoietic cell transplantation (HCT) [1,6–10]. An extensive annotated bibliography updated to April 2002 concerning various aspects of osteopetrosis can be found at http://www.osteo.org.

In this chapter, osteopetrosis in humans is characterized. The origin and function of the osteoclast is described briefly. Studies of HCT in laboratory animals with congenital osteopetrotic mutations and transgenic mutations are reviewed. The role of HCT and other therapeutic modalities in the treatment of infantile malignant osteopetrosis are detailed and future directions discussed.

Osteopetrosis in humans

Historically, two major forms of osteopetrosis have been described. The benign or "adult" form is inherited in an autosomal dominant pattern and is associated with minimal disability and a normal life expectancy. The malignant or "infantile" form is inherited in an autosomal recessive pattern and has widespread systemic manifestations. However, both forms have been found to be clinically heterogeneous and other specific variants of osteopetrosis have been reported [1].

The adult benign autosomal dominant form was first described by the German radiologist Albers-Schönberg in 1904 [11] by roentgenographic demonstration of the characteristic dense radiopaque bones (Albers-Schönberg syndrome or marble bone disease). Diagnosis is usually made in late childhood or adulthood by roentgenographic demonstration of diffuse skeletal sclerosis which increases over time. Infants with this disorder rarely have dense bones. Most patients are asymptomatic and have a normal life expectancy. Minimal disability has been reported, secondary to an increased susceptibility to fractures and, occasionally, bone pain, osteomyelitis of the mandible and cranial nerve palsies [12]. This autosomal dominant form has been extensively studied and two distinct types have been described based on clinical, radiologic, histologic and biochemical criteria [13–15]. Type I is rarer; fractures are uncommon, bones are uniformly dense and osteoclasts are reduced in number and size [13,14,16]. More families with type II have been reported; fractures are frequent, bone density is more variable and osteoclasts are increased in number, large and highly multinucleated [13–16]. Recently, type II autosomal dominant osteopetrosis has been mapped to chromosome 16p13.3 [17].

A number of variants have been described with autosomal recessive inheritance, in addition to the infantile malignant variant which is the subject of this chapter. Carbonic anhydrase II deficiency, a syndrome with mild osteopetrosis, renal tubular acidosis, cerebral calcification and a profound deficiency of carbonic anhydrase isoenzyme II has been documented in multiple kindreds [18,19]. Another variant is a rare syndrome of severe osteopetrosis with parathyroid hormone resistance and induction of bone resorption with administration of bovine parathyroid hormone [20]. Other variants of osteopetrosis [1,2] and other disorders that cause increased skeletal mass continue to be described [21,22]. These include transient infantile osteopetrosis [23–25], osteopetrosis lethal *in utero*, intermediate forms [26,27] and post-infectious osteopetrosis.

Infantile malignant osteopetrosis

The classic form of infantile malignant osteopetrosis is characterized by autosomal recessive inheritance and is almost always diagnosed in early infancy [28–32]. The inability to resorb and remodel bone because of osteoclast dysfunction, in the presence of normal bone formation by osteoblasts, results in the deposition of excessive mineralized osteoid and cartilage [33]. All bones are uniformly dense, sclerotic and radiopaque. Medullary cavities are absent on long bone radiographs [22,34,35]. Bone biopsies reveal encroachment of medullary cavities by bone and mineralized cartilage, thick trabeculae and decreased medullary spaces. The residual medullary cavities are occupied with large numbers of nonfunctional osteoclasts and there is usually increased marrow fibrosis [29,30,36–38]. Osteoclasts are reported to be normal in size in some patients [36,37] and increased in size in others, with the large osteoclasts having increased numbers of nuclei [36,38]. Electron microscopy of osteoclasts has been reported to demonstrate normal ruffled borders (described below) at the bone junction in some cases [36,38,39] and decreased or complete absence of ruffled borders in others [30,36–39].

Encroachment of marrow spaces leads to extramedullary hematopoiesis, progressive hepatosplenomegaly and hypersplenism. The result is anemia with reticulocytosis, leukoerythroblastosis and thrombocytopenia. Encroachment of cranial nerve foramina leads to retinal atrophy which progresses to blindness [40–44], auditory nerve damage and oculomotor and facial nerve palsies [45]. Defective bone resorption also leads to progressive macrocephaly, frontal bossing, hypertelorism, exophthalmos and other craniofacial abnormalities. Hydrocephalus, ventricular enlargement, increased intracranial pressure, cerebral vascular occlusive complications [46] and seizures are also reported [30,45,47]. Nasal stuffiness is a common presenting symptom, which is secondary to progressive narrowing and obstruction of nasal airways [28,48].

Obstructive sleep apnea has also been reported [49]. Excessive tearing may occur secondary to nasolacrimal duct stenosis [50].

Seizures and tetany in the neonatal period secondary to hypocalcemia have been reported in a few cases [30,51]. Rarely, diagnosis may be obscured in the neonate secondary to maternal vitamin D deficiency [52]. Other reported complications are osteomyelitis of the mandible and maxilla [53,54], retarded tooth eruption [55] and rampant caries. Sclerotic bones are brittle and pathologic fractures occur frequently [56]. Linear growth is retarded and dwarfism has been reported in survivors to the second decade. Neuropsychologic and developmental evaluation reveals a wide range of cognitive, adaptive and language skills with routinely delayed gross motor development [57].

Infections are common in children with infantile malignant osteopetrosis. Various subtle defects in neutrophil and monocyte function have been reported [8,29,58–60]. Included are defects in phagocytosis [8], decreased intracellular killing [8,58], decreased natural killer cell function [58,59], abnormal nitro blue tetrazolium reduction by both neutrophils and monocytes [59,60] and decreased response to stimuli of neutrophil activation [2,60]. Children become progressively severely debilitated and, until recently, survival beyond the first decade was not reported. Infection, bleeding and severe anemia are the usual reported causes of death. Improvements in supportive care, antibiotics and ready availability of blood components have prolonged survival in recent years [30]. It has been recently reported that these children are at high risk for anesthetic morbidity and mortality [61].

A variant of infantile malignant osteopetrosis has been described that is associated with neuronal storage of ceroid lipofuscin. Children with this disorder have features of infantile malignant osteopetrosis but, in addition, are severely retarded, demonstrate chorioretinal degeneration and progressive generalized neurodegeneration. Findings include cerebral atrophy, ventricular dilatation, hypotonia or hypertonia, central apnea and seizures. The disorder is invariably fatal before 2 years of age and is unresponsive to therapy [1,30,62–66].

Gerritsen *et al.* [30] reported on 33 patients in 26 sibships seen in Paris, France and Leiden, Holland between 1972 and 1988 and summarized the major findings of an additional 59 cases reported in the literature to 1990. About 30% of children survived at 6 years of age, with survivors to the second or third decade having poor quality of life. About 75% developed visual impairment secondary to optic atrophy in the first year of life, most in the first 3 months. About 75% also developed hematologic abnormalities in the first year of life, which was an unfavorable prognostic sign, especially when associated with early visual impairment. The eight children with both visual and hematologic impairment before the age of 3 months died before 1 year of age.

An important caveat to consider in evaluating complications in patients with infantile malignant osteopetrosis is that some reported series may include patients with the variant with neuronal storage disease, patients with carbonic anhydrase II deficiency and patients with the autosomal dominant and intermediate forms of osteopetrosis.

Osteoclast and bone resorption

There is extensive information in the literature concerning the origin, structure and function of the osteoclast and its role in bone resorption [3–5,7,67,68]. A brief overview is provided to clarify issues important to an understanding of the pathophysiology of osteopetrosis and the role of HCT in its correction.

The cell of origin of the osteoclast is the pluripotent HSC. The colony-forming unit–granulocyte/macrophage (CFU-GM) is likely the committed progenitor cell of origin of the osteoclast, as well as the circulating monocyte, the tissue macrophage and the foreign body giant cell [69]. Differentiation into the osteoclast lineage occurs prior to macrophage commitment [69]. Osteoclasts are thought to form from repeated asynchronous fusions of post-mitotic mononuclear precursors which migrate to skeletal sites via vascular pathways. Bone resorbing osteoclasts have from 1 to >20 nuclei.

Degradation of bone mineral complexes and collagenous bone matrix requires activation of the osteoclast. Activation involves elaboration of cytoplasmic infoldings of the plasma membrane next to the bone surface, which is known as the ruffled border. Once the ruffled border is formed, plasma and lysosomal membranes fuse and lysosomal contents including cathepsin K and other proteases, carbonic anhydrase isoenzyme II and acid hydrolases are released to the extracellular space. Bone resorption is confined to a small area of osteoclast–bone interface by a circumferential seal of the plasma membrane which is defined as the clear zone. Bone is first solubilized by hydrochloric acid at pH 4.5 and then the organic matrix digested by the proteases. The products of resorption are then endocytosed for additional intracellular processing [5].

Differentiation, maturation, fusion, activation, inhibition and function are controlled by lymphokines, monokines and hormones including macrophage colony-stimulating factor (M-CSF), osteoprotegerin ligand (OPGL), various interleukins, parathyroid hormone, 1,25 dihydroxyvitamin D, calcitonin, prostaglandins and glucocorticoids [4,5,68,70]. Osteoblasts, the bone-forming cells of mesenchymal origin that synthesize bone matrix, and marrow stromal cells both express M-CSF and OPGL and have important roles in the development, activation and regulation of osteoclasts [67,71].

Osteopetrotic mutations in laboratory animals

Congenital osteopetrosis is a well-known condition in a variety of mammalian species [6,7,72–74]. There are eight well-studied mutations in common laboratory animals, including the mouse, rat and rabbit (Table 106.1). In all variants, the mode of inheritance is autosomal recessive. All variants demonstrate osteoclast hypofunction, generalized skeletal sclerosis, absent or poorly developed marrow cavities, delayed tooth eruption, reduced size of osseous foramina, defective bone modelling and remodeling, and weak bone susceptible to pathologic fracture. All mutants are resistant to the hypercalcemic effects of parathyroid hormone and 1,25 dihydroxyvitamin D, and all have increased blood levels of 1,25 dihydroxyvitamin D. All of these characteristics are shared with the infantile malignant form described above.

An additional mutation in the Norway rat, microphthalmia blanc (mib/mib), has been characterized [75–77]. Affected mutants have a mild transient osteopetrosis at birth with reduced osteoclast numbers. Skeletal sclerosis gradually resolves, osteoclast numbers increase and survival is normal. Children with a syndrome of transient infantile osteopetrosis have been described [23–25].

The major differences among the variants that have been described in the current literature are compiled in Table 106.1. Included are remarkable differences in osteoclast numbers, from virtually absent in the tl/tl rat to significant hyperplasia in the ia/ia rat and humans; differences in osteoclast size, from primarily mononuclear forms in the mi/mi mouse to very large with many nuclei in the op/op rat; and differences in the appearance of the ruffled border at the osteoclast–bone interface, from absent to normal in the various mutants. Disease severity as measured by survival past infancy and known effective treatments are also detailed in Table 106.1.

The development of osteopetrosis is an *in utero* event [7]. The defect may be intrinsic to the osteoclast or in the microenvironment supporting the development and activation of the osteoclasts in the animal models and the various human variants. In all cases, the failure of the osteoclast to resorb calcified cartilage during bone development leads to persistent primary spongiosa characterized by cores of calcified cartilage within bone. This resorption failure prevents or delays development of the bone

Table 106.1 Mammalian osteoporosis. (Modified, expanded and updated from numerous reports and reviews [6,7,72–74].)

Mutation	Symbol	Osteoclasts No.	Size	Ruffled borders	Survival	Effective treatment
Mouse						
Gray–lethal	gl/gl	↓	↓	+	Lethal	HCT
Microphthalmia	mi/mi	N	↓↓	–	Normal	HCT
Osteosclerosis	oc/oc	? ↓,↑	↓	–	Lethal	None
Osteopetrosis	op/op	↓↓	↓	+	Normal	M-CSF
Rat						
Incisors–absent	ia/ia	↑↑	N	–	Normal	HCT
Osteopetrosis	op/op	↓	↑↑	+	Lethal	HCT
Toothless	tl/tl	↓↓	↓	? ±	? Reduced, normal	M-CSF
Rabbit						
Osteopetrosis	os/os	↓	N	–	Lethal	None
Human						
Infantile malignant	—	↑↑	N,↑	±	Lethal	HCT

↑↓, increases or decreases with respect to normal littermates/control subjects.
+, presence of ruffled borders.
–, absence of ruffled borders.
?, conflicting reports in the literature.
HCT, hematopoietic cell transplantation; M-CSF, macrophage colony-stimulating factor; N, same as normal littermate/control.

marrow cavity and is responsible for the distinctive radiographic appearance of homogeneously dense bones. The severity of the disease and potential therapeutic interventions depend on the etiology of the osteoclast dysfunction in the various osteopetrotic syndromes.

In addition to spontaneous mutations, various induced mutations have produced transgenic mice by targeted disruptions of protooncogenes [5,6,74]. These loss of function or "knockout" experiments have resulted in abnormalities in either the production or function of osteoclasts and the mutant mice have severe osteopetrosis. Examples of induced mutations that result in abnormal osteoclast production or maturation include the targeted disruption of c-*fos* which yields mice with abundant bone marrow macrophages but no osteoclasts [78] and PU.1, a hematopoietic transcription factor, which produces mice deficient in both macrophages and osteoclasts and which die from septicemia within 24–48 h of birth [79]. Additional mutants that fail to generate osteoclasts include those with deficient nuclear factor kappa B1 (NF-κB1) and NF-κB2 [80] and with deficient OPGL [70,81]. Mutations that result in abnormal osteoclast function include the disruption of c-*src*, a tyrosine kinase, yielding mice with normal osteoclast numbers, absent ruffled borders and defective bone resorption [82,83]. Mice produced with a deficiency in tumor necrosis factor receptor-associated factor 6 (TRAF6) have impaired osteoclast function [84]. Transgenic mice with specific resorption defects have also been created. Cathepsin K-deficient mice lack a cysteine proteinase necessary to degrade bone matrix [85,86]. Atp6i-deficient mice have an extracellular acidification defect and cannot solubilize bone mineral [87].

Hematopoietic cell transplantation in animal models

In a series of elegant experiments, Walker [88,89] demonstrated that osteopetrosis can be cured in the gl/gl and mi/mi mouse mutants by either temporary parabiosis or HCT. Infusions of marrow or spleen cells from normal littermates into lethally irradiated osteopetrotic mice resulted in complete correction of osteopetrosis and normal survival. Conversely, infusion of spleen cells from osteopetrotic mice to lethally irradiated normal littermates led to the development of osteopetrosis [89]. Similar experiments have demonstrated complete correction after HCT in the ia/ia [90] and op/op [91] rat mutations.

Correction or induction of osteopetrosis in these four strains by HCT suggests defects intrinsic to the osteoclast progenitor or the osteoclast itself. Studies in the mi/mi mouse that demonstrate bone resorbing osteoclasts are of donor origin after transplantation support this viewpoint [92,93]. Beige mice that have giant lysosomes in their hematopoietic cells were used as stem cell donors for transplants into irradiated mi/mi mice. After transplant, giant lysosomes were present in the functional osteoclasts of the recipients.

Experimental HCT in animal models has been very consistent in its approach. In most reported studies, the preparative regimen has utilized a single fraction of total body irradiation (TBI) of 600 cGy for recipient osteopetrotic mutants or 900 cGy for recipient normal littermates delivered by a cobalt-60 source. This dose is considered marrow lethal for each group. Marrow or spleen cells at $10–50 \times 10^6$ nucleated cells/animal are given intravenously or intraperitoneally 2 h later. Donors are highly inbred littermates, full engraftment is routine and graft-vs.-host disease (GVHD) has not been reported.

HCT from normal littermates has also been reported to cure osteopetrosis in transgenic mutants [5,7,72]. Complete correction has been reported in the c-*src* [82], c-*fos* [78], NF-κB1 and NF-κB2 [80] and the PU.1 [79] variants. In the newborn PU.1 negative mutant, HCT is performed soon after birth utilizing 4-week-old PU.1-positive donor animals in germ-free environments. HCT should be successful in all mutants that have osteopetrosis secondary to an induced mutation which results in a defect in the hematopoietic stem cell but not in mutants that have defects in the microenvironment.

In four other spontaneous mutants (oc/oc mouse, op/op mouse, tl/tl rat, os/os rabbit) HCT is not able to correct osteopetrosis. This observation suggests that the defects in these mutants are not intrinsic to the osteoclast progenitor or the osteoclast. Both the op/op mouse and the tl/tl rat have been found to be severely deficient in M-CSF and daily treatment with recombinant human M-CSF remarkably improves bone resorption in both mutants [7,72,94]. The op/op mouse has a nonlethal point mutation within the coding region of the M-CSF gene [95], absent M-CSF and markedly reduced monocytes, macrophages and osteoclasts. The osteopetrosis progressively corrects over time. Treatment with M-CSF results in normalization of monocytes, macrophages and osteoclasts and rapid correction of osteopetrosis [96,97]. Granulocyte macrophage colony-stimulating factor (GM-CSF) treatment restores monocytes and macrophages but fails to stimulate osteoclast development or correct osteopetrosis [98]. The tl/tl rat also has reduced monocytes, macrophages and osteoclasts but does not demonstrate skeletal improvement with age and has a reduced lifespan. Bioassay reveals reduced M-CSF activity and treatment with M-CSF improves osteopetrosis and prolongs survival [67,72,99].

The genetic defect in the oc/oc mouse spontaneous mutation has recently been identified [100]. The defective gene encodes an H^+-ATPase necessary for acidification and appears to be a defect similar to the Atp6i deficient transgenic mouse model [87]. While this lethal mutation is intrinsic to the osteoclast, successful HCT has not been reported. The lethal mutation in the os/os rabbit has not been identified. Effective therapies have not been reported for either the oc/oc mouse or the os/os rabbit [7,72,73].

Treatment of infantile malignant osteopetrosis

Historically, treatment of infantile malignant osteopetrosis has consisted of supportive care measures and attempts to control mineral intake. Anemia and thrombocytopenia were treated with transfusions and occasionally splenectomy. Dietary manipulations to reduce calcium intake, increase phosphate intake, or both, were employed in an attempt to mobilize bone calcium but without success. Attempts to induce bone resorption with infusions of parathyroid hormone, vitamin D and calcitonin were also unsuccessful. Treatment with corticosteroids results in decreased hepatosplenomegaly, decreased leukoerythroblastosis, increased hemoglobin and platelet counts, and decreased need for transfusion. However, there is no significant effect on the underlying process and patients deteriorate when corticosteroids are discontinued [101]. Treatment with corticosteroids and a low-calcium high-phosphate diet has been reported to ameliorate symptoms and improve bone density in four infants but this observation has not been confirmed by other investigators [102].

Hematopoietic cell transplantation

Reports of successful correction of osteopetrosis in mouse and rat mutants in the mid 1970s by HCT led to attempts to utilize allogeneic HCT to treat children with infantile malignant osteopetrosis. In the past 25 years, numerous reports have appeared in the literature concerning HCT for osteopetrosis. Certainly, the published material underrepresents the number of transplants performed because investigators tend not to publish their failures.

In 1977, Ballet et al. [103] reported the first HCT procedure for osteopetrosis. A 3-month-old girl was transplanted without immunosuppression with marrow from a human leukocyte antigen (HLA) identical 2-year-old sister. Although durable engraftment was not demonstrated, radiologic and other evidence for significant bone resorption was documented. O'Reilly et al. [104] speculated that extended short-term engraftment may have occurred because the patient and her donor were part of a highly inbred family. This speculation was confirmed recently with the report that the family is a carbonic anhydrase II deficiency kindred [19]. The investigators also reported three other children given transplants without immunosuppression from less well-matched donors [105]. None of the recipients showed evidence of engraftment or clinical improvement.

In 1980, Coccia et al. [8] reported a 5-month-old girl transplanted from her HLA-identical mixed leukocyte culture compatible brother after preparation with 200 mg/kg cyclophosphamide (CY) and modified 400 cGy TBI with head and lung shielding. Engraftment was documented by chromosomal analysis. Anemia, thrombocytopenia, leukoerythroblastosis and metabolic abnormalities corrected within 12 weeks of HCT. Comparison of bone biopsies before HCT and at 13 weeks after HCT revealed complete correction (Fig. 106.1). Serial X-rays demonstrated bony remodeling and new nonsclerotic bone formation (Fig. 106.2). Fluorescent Y-body analysis after HCT showed that nuclei were of donor origin (male) in osteoclasts (Fig. 106.3) but nuclei in osteoblasts remained of recipient origin (female). Subsequent follow-up showed progressive loss of her graft [33]. Dense new bone formation can be

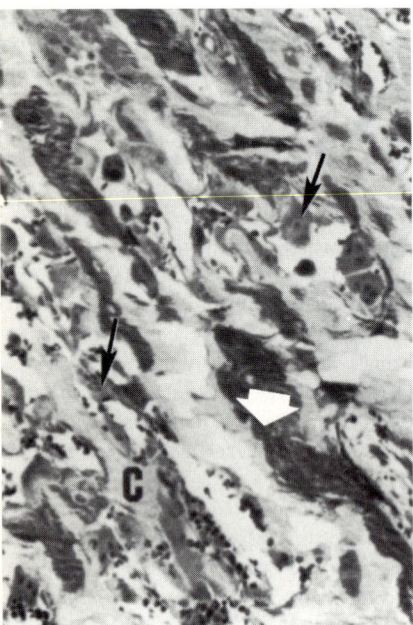
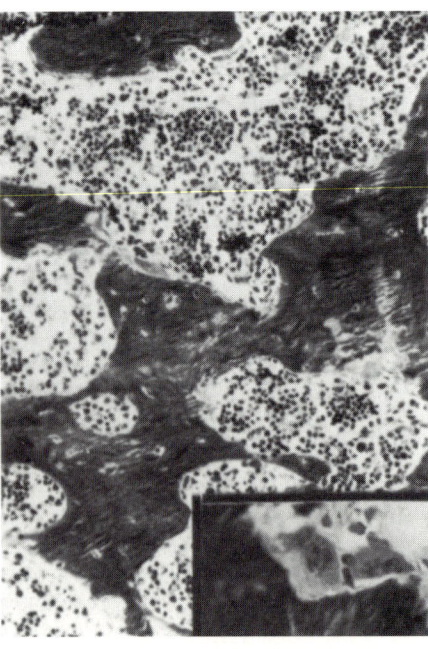

Fig. 106.1 Bone histology before bone marrow transplantation (BMT) (a) and 13 weeks after BMT (b). The biopsy specimen studied before BMT had the characteristic features of osteopetrosis. The trabecular matrix mass was markedly increased and composed of mineralized cartilage (C) as well as bone (white arrow). Numerous nonresorbing osteoclasts (black arrows) were present in the residual marrow space and contained few hematopioetic precursors (undecalcified; modified Masson, × 100). The biopsy specimen obtained 13 weeks after BMT revealed virtual normalization of the bone and marrow. The trabecular matrix mass was residual cartaginous bars. The marrow space contained abundant normal hematopioetic precursors, and the osteoclasts—the number of which was markedly reduced—were actively resorbing bone, as evidenced by their presence in resorption bays (insert) (undecalcified; modified Mason, × 100, insert × 450). (Reprinted by permission of the *New England Journal of Medicine*, from [8].)

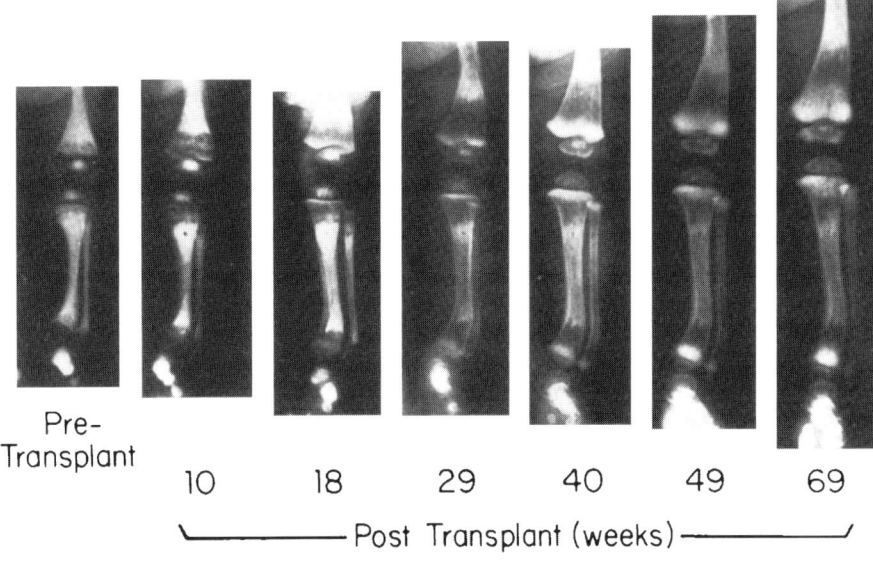

Fig. 106.2 Representative radiographs of the left leg obtained before bone marrow transplantation (BMT) and 10–69 weeks after BMT. Before BMT, the bones were very dense. The fraying of the ends of the long bones is typical of rachitic change. Ten weeks after transplantation, metaphyseal and periosteal remodeling and new bone formation of nearly normal density were seen; the rachitic changes were resolving. The provisional zone of calcification was reestablished at 18 and 29 weeks, there was a marked increase in the thickness of normal appearing new bone as a result of longitudinal and appositional growth. Metaphyses and epiphyses had a normal appearance. No evidence of rickets was seen. Dense remnants of the original bone were seen with the normally increased density, suggesting recurrence of the osteopetrotic process. Marrow cavities have not been replaced by dense bone. The small round hole seen in the proximal tibia within the dense remnant of original bone is at the site of a trephine needle biopsy performed 6 weeks after BMT.

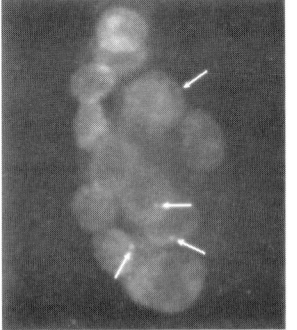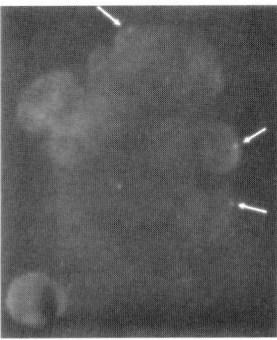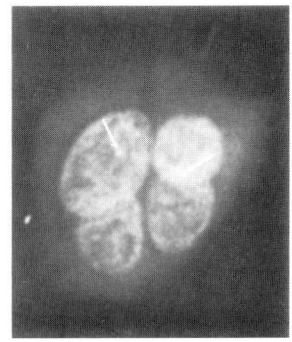

Fig. 106.3 Osteoclasts with fluorescent Y bodies after BMT. The osteoclasts were stained with quinacrine dihydrochloride. Arrows indicate the Y bodies in nuclei that are seen in this focal plane (fluorescence microscopy, × 1000; right panel enlarged for clarity). (Reprinted by permission of the *New England Journal of Medicine*, from [8].)

appreciated on the last three panels of Fig. 106.2 but with preservation of bone marrow cavities. Since 18 months after HCT, no male karyotypes have been detected in peripheral blood or marrow cells. Over 24 years have now passed since HCT and her bones are extremely sclerotic and she is short, but no other evidence of osteopetrosis remains. While her visual acuity is diminished, she has normal hearing, intelligence and pubertal development. She is a college graduate and gainfully employed. She has no hepatosplenomegaly, and blood counts and chemistries are normal. In this patient, it appears that once marrow cavities and foramina were remodeled, the correction was permanent in spite of sclerotic new bone formation.

Our HCT group has subsequently transplanted six additional infants. Three of six became long-term survivors. Donors were a one HLA-B antigen mismatched mother [106], a phenotypically identical father and an HLA-matched sibling. All three patients engrafted promptly and are fully chimeric with complete correction of all manifestations of osteopetrosis. Two had severe optic atrophy pretransplant and remain blind. The third, with mild atrophy, has preservation of vision. They are now 19, 15 and >4 years after HCT and have normal development and intelligence.

Sorell et al. [58] and O'Reilly et al. [104] reported three children: one with transient engraftment, one with complete correction and one with partial correction. Both engrafted children have durable mixed chimerism. Detailed case reports describe an additional five patients successfully engrafted from HLA matched siblings in two cases and mismatched relatives in three cases [107–110]. Three patients have shown complete correction [107,109]. The fourth patient received a T-depleted transplant, demonstrated sustained engraftment and correction of osteopetrosis, but died of an *Aspergillus* brain abscess 9 months after HCT [108]. The fifth patient was transplanted from a phenotypically HLA identical father [110]. Restriction fragment length polymorphism analysis demonstrated mixed chimerism and slow progressive loss of the graft, recurrence of osteopetrotic bone formation but correction of other manifestations of osteopetrosis similar to the previously described case [8,33].

Gerritsen et al. [9] have reported a detailed summary of the outcome of 69 patients receiving HCTs for osteopetrosis between 1976 and 1994 in Europe, Saudi Arabia and Costa Rica. The 69 children received 83 HCTs at 17 centres. Median age was 3 months (range 1–81 months). Four patients, previously reported, were transplanted without conditioning [103,105]. Of the remaining 65 patients, 19 had matched sibling donors, nine had five or six antigen HLA-matched family donors, seven had six antigen HLA-matched unrelated donors, and the remaining 30 had family donors with two or more nonidentical HLA antigens. Most patients were prepared with busulphan (BU) and CY. Many of the patients with HLA disparate donors received additional immunosuppression. All 19 children with matched sibling donors engrafted while only 30 of 42 with other donors engrafted. Engraftment was not evaluable in the remaining patients because of early death. Survival with osteoclast function is shown in Fig. 106.4. Persistent osteoclast function was documented in 37 of 41 evaluable cases. Severe hypercalcemia developed in seven of 29 evaluable recipients. Six of seven with hypercalcemia underwent HCT after 2 years of age. At the time of the report, 39 of 69 patients reported had died. Of the 30 survivors, 25 have osteoclast function and most are healthy apart from visual disability in some. The authors conclude that HCT is the treatment of choice in children with matched sibling donors; that early

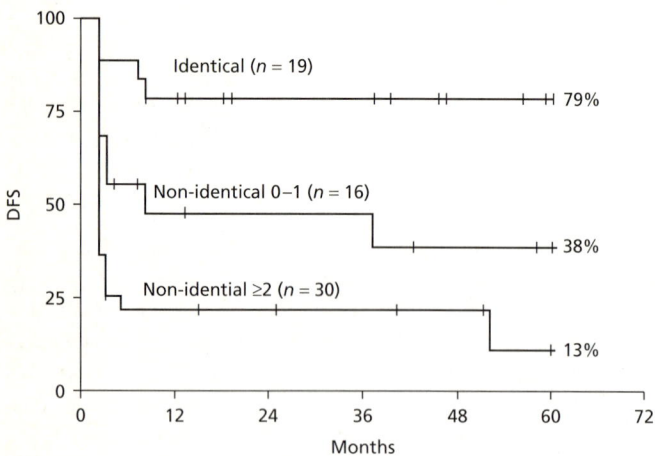

Fig. 106.4 Survival with osteoclast function in 65 patients with juvenile osteopetrosis after myeloblative conditioning and bone marrow transplantation (BMT). There were 19 patients with a genotypically HLA identical sibling donor (identical). Nine of the patients received a BMT from a related donor who was phenotypically HLA identical or with one nonidentical HLA antigen, and seven of the patients received a transplant from a related donor with two or more nonidentical BMT from an unrelated phenotypically HLA identical donor (nonidentical 0–1). Thirty patients received a HLA antigens (nonidentical ≥2). DFS, disease-free survival. (Reprinted with permission from [9].)

HCT is important if vision is to be preserved [30]; and that hypercalcemia is a worrisome complication, especially in older recipients. The authors express concern with the poor outcome (13%) in patients with family donors with two or more disparate antigens and recommend search for an unrelated phenotypically HLA identical donor. However, in children with early hematologic and visual impairment, they recommend HCT from the best available family donor as these children may not survive the search process to identify a matched unrelated donor [30].

Solh et al. [111] reported on eight patients transplanted: six with sibling donors and two with parental donors. Six engrafted, and three survived with complete correction. Jabado et al. [112] described two of nine patients who received HCT from HLA nonidentical T-cell-depleted grafts were successfully transplanted. Some patients in both series are likely part of the report of Gerritsen et al. [9].

Three additional single center experiences have been recently described. The University of Minnesota team reported HCT in 10 children with eight engrafting and five surviving: three with full or partial donor chimerism and two with autologous recovery [113]. An Israeli team reported 13 children from four related families belonging to one Bedouin tribe: nine received HCT, seven engrafted, four survived and are fully chimeric with normal bone resorption [114]. Prenatal molecular diagnosis by linkage analysis of markers on chromosome 11q12–13 identified three fetuses with osteopetrosis and two underwent HCT as infants [115,116]. A German team reported five of seven infants alive with complete resolution of osteopetrosis at a median of 4 years after HCT utilizing purified CD34+ T-cell-depleted mobilized peripheral blood from HLA haploid identical parents [117]. This encouraging result is a remarkable improvement in the outcomes reported previously by the European Group for Bone Marrow Transplantation (EBMT) [9] and the International Bone Marrow Transplant Registry (IBMTR) [10] for HLA haplotype mismatched HCT.

There were 153 patients registered up to late 2001 with the IBMTR by 55 transplant teams worldwide, who had HCT for osteopetrosis between 1978 and 2001. Many represent cases cited above. Year of transplant was before 1990 in 32 and 1990–2001 in 121. The group comprises 87 males and 66 females. Age at HCT was 1–136 months (median 6 months).

Donors were 50% matched siblings, 28% alternate related and 22% unrelated. Most (77%) were prepared with BU- and CY-containing regimens. Three-year probability of survival was 54 ± 11% for matched siblings, 47 ± 15% for alternate related and 35 ± 17% for unrelated donors (data provided by the IBMTR Statistical Center; not reviewed by the Advisory Committee).

Transplantation issues

In general, HCT for osteopetrosis is similar to HCT for other nonmalignant inherited disorders detailed in this book. However, there are certain unique issues that must be understood to select appropriate patients and donors and to improve outcomes.

Pretransplant evaluation

The typical infant with osteopetrosis presents with anemia and thrombocytopenia. Transfusion may be necessary, and red cell and platelet survival may be short secondary to hypersplenism. A course of corticosteroid therapy may stabilize the patient hematologically and temporarily reduce transfusion requirements [101]. Some patients present with or develop severe bone pain, progressive debilitation and poor oral intake, requiring narcotic analgesics and hyperalimentation prior to HCT. Evaluation for optic atrophy including funduscopic examination, visual evoked-response electroencephalograms [42] and optic foramina imaging should be completed quickly, as early optic nerve decompression may preserve vision [40,43,44]. Baseline evaluation of calcium and/or phosphorus homeostasis, alkaline and acid phosphatase levels [8] and parathyroid hormone studies [20] should be obtained. Early correction of hypocalcemia may prevent or resolve seizures [30,51]. Baseline imaging studies should include long bone radiographs, measurements of liver and spleen size, and cranial CT or MRI scans [22,34,35,47,118].

It is recommended that an open wedge bone biopsy from the anterior or posterior iliac crest be obtained to confirm the diagnosis [8,36–39]. Trephine needle biopsies are usually not adequate for evaluation. Marrow aspiration is rarely successful. Light microscopic analysis of osteoclast number, size, nucleation and morphology should be performed. Marrow cellularity and the degree of myelofibrosis should be determined. In the clinical research setting, quantitative histomorphometry [37–39] and electron microscopic analysis of osteoclasts for the presence, size and frequency of ruffled borders, clear zones and alkaline phosphatase activity at the membrane–matrix interface should be evaluated [36–39]. Recipient and donor cytogenetic or molecular studies to assess the degree of hematopoietic chimerism after HCT are essential. Careful evaluation before HCT yields important information that contributes to the better understanding of human osteopetrosis. An example is the report demonstrating an osteoblast defect in two cases of osteopetrosis [119]. HCT in two infant girls corrected the osteoblast defect and the osteoblasts remained of recipient origin, suggesting that the donor osteoclasts provided a suitable microenvironment for osteoblast function.

It has been reported and frequently cited that patients with either advanced marrow fibrosis [120] or markedly increased marrow osteoclasts, "hyperosteoclastic state" [38,39], have more severe disease and poor response to HCT because of poor engraftment. Caution must be exercised in interpreting these data. The type (open wedge vs. trephine needle), location, depth and quality of the biopsy all influence interpretation. Also, biopsies in infants tend to have more osteoclasts and less fibrosis than in older children where accumulation of bone, cartilage and fibrosis obliterate marrow spaces and displace osteoclasts [38].

The experience of our HCT group does not support this pessimistic view for HCT. The first case we transplanted had markedly increased marrow osteoclasts and minimal fibrosis (Fig. 106.1) [8,33]. She engrafted promptly and, interestingly, all longitudinal and appositional new bone formation was of normal density, but a sclerotic core of original bone persisted (Fig. 106.2). The next patient successfully transplanted had small densely fibrotic marrow cavities with minimal increase in osteoclasts [106]. She also engrafted promptly, but new bone formation was of the same density as the original bone. Her long bones gradually decreased in density over 4–6 months, and no sclerotic core was seen. Normal marrow cavities were identified radiologically only when the overall bone density was normal. The subsequent two children had moderate fibrosis and increased numbers of large abnormal appearing osteoclasts. Both engrafted promptly. New bone formation was of normal density, and the dense core of original bone progressively decreased in density to normal over several months.

Infants with early neurologic degeneration may have osteopetrosis associated with neuronal storage of ceroid lipofuscin [1,9,30,62–66]. They should not be considered as candidates for HCT as the storage disease progresses in spite of correction of the osteopetrosis [9,30,64,111,121].

HCT in other variants of osteopetrosis is controversial. Dini et al. [27] report HCT in two children at 5 and 12 years of age with a variant of mild autosomal recessive osteopetrosis. Both had severe optic atrophy and dense bones but no significant hematologic or other complications of osteopetrosis. They each engrafted, developed severe hypercalcemia, had subsequent normalization of bone density but remained blind without catch-up growth and are alive and well 5 and 6 years after HCT, respectively. Carbonic anhydrase II deficiency syndrome produces mild osteopetrosis, renal tubular acidosis, cerebral calcification, mental retardation, growth failure and dental complications [18,19]. Hematologic complications are not reported and cranial nerve compression is usually mild. While HCT should correct bone manifestations, it will not improve renal insufficiency or central nervous system (CNS) complications [19]. McMahon et al. [122] recently reported HCT in two children aged 9 months and 4 months from related Irish families with severe progressive visual and hearing loss. Both successfully engrafted, normalized bone density and stabilized vision and hearing. HCT did not correct the metabolic acidosis, the renal lesions or the development delays. HCT may have delayed onset of cerebral calcifications. In both of the above reports, it remains questionable whether correction of only the skeletal problems warrants the risks and morbidity of HCT.

Donor selection

An HLA matched nonaffected sibling is the preferred donor. If a matched sibling is unavailable, it is possible that a matched or minimally mismatched parental or extended family donor can be identified. Obligate heterozygote relatives are suitable donors. Because progression of the disease is relatively slow in many cases, unrelated donor search and unrelated marrow or cord blood HCT are reasonable options (see Chapter 43). However, if infants have early visual and hematologic impairment, rapid identification of a donor is essential [9,30]. Cord blood HCT [121,123] and haploid identical parent donors utilizing purified peripheral blood stem cells [117] may both be reasonable options if HCT is considered urgent and a closely matched family donor is unavailable.

Preparative regimens and engraftment

Most reported patients have been prepared with BU at either 2 mg/kg/day × 4 days [104,109] or 4 mg/kg/day × 4 days [9,107,110,111] followed by CY at a dose of 50 mg/kg/day × 4 days. Engraftment was prompt with the development of full hematopoietic chimerism in most children. Failure of engraftment has been reported only with mismatched donors, T-cell-depleted grafts or, most commonly, with both [9,112]. Additional immunosuppression is probably advisable in these situations. Second HCT is sometimes necessary [9]. Late graft failure has been reported in at least three well-studied patients [8,58,110]. Hepatosplenomegaly dramatically regresses after HCT but redevelops with engraftment, probably as temporary sites of extramedullary hematopoiesis. When marrow cavities develop, the spleen again regresses. In one case, liver and spleen size were maximal at 12 weeks after HCT but were normal in size by 22 weeks with concomitant appearance of medullary cavities in long bones on radiographs [8].

Evaluation after HCT

Serial reevaluations to document engraftment and bone resorption are important to assess efficacy of therapy. Studies to assess the extent of hematopoietic chimerism and, in cases of mixed chimerism, to document sustained engraftment or late graft failure are vital for long-term patient management. Second transplants may not be necessary in some cases of late graft failure as discussed above.

Marrow aspirations and biopsies at 3–6 months after HCT are valuable to assess bone resorption, marrow cavity formation and marrow cellularity. Serial long bone radiographs are the best indicators of sustained correction of osteopetrosis in most cases.

Complications after HCT

The only unusual complication after HCT referable to osteopetrosis is hypercalcemia. A 30-month-old male child (A.E. Gluckman, personal communication) received a marrow graft in 1980 from his HLA identical sister after preparation with CY and 400 cGy modified TBI. He engrafted rapidly and developed mild acute GVHD. The child demonstrated both histologic and radiologic improvement and grew 5 cm in the first 2 months after HCT. Severe hypercalcemia developed on day +60 and was refractory to saline diuresis, furosemide, corticosteroids, calcitonin and dialysis. Death with hypercalcemia occurred on day +165.

O'Reilly et al. [104] described two additional cases of severe hypercalcemia in patients 15 months and 10 years old at time of HCT who responded to prolonged intensive saline diuresis (6–10 weeks). They speculate that this is a problem in older patients who have massive bony deposition of calcium which is released with rapid resorption of bone after HCT [104]. The speculation was confirmed by Gerritsen et al. [9] who reported seven cases of severe hypercalcemia with six >2-year-olds at the time of HCT. The current availability of agents that selectively inhibit calcium resorption from bone should provide effective options to control this serious complication. Bisphosphonate derivatives selectively inhibit osteoclast mediated bone resorption [124]. These agents also can induce osteoclast apoptosis in murine osteoclasts [4,5]. Side-effects of concern are myelosuppression and nausea. Titration of these agents should allow controlled resorption of sclerotic bone without severe life-threatening hypercalcemia.

An illustrative example is a 9-month-old male (E. Chang and P.F. Coccia, personal observation) who received an HLA matched sibling donor HCT for infantile osteopetrosis, rapidly developed complete hematopoietic chimerism without GVHD and promptly demonstrated new bone formation of normal density. At 6 months after HCT, serum calcium was 12.7 mg/dL. He responded poorly to saline diuresis and furosemide and 4 weeks later serum calcium was 13.8 mg/dL. He received 0.5 mg/kg pamidronate IV with a rapid decline to 12.3 mg/dL. Four weeks later serum calcium was 14.8 mg/dL and after 0.75 mg/kg pamidronate IV was 10.8 mg/dL within 3 days. Again 4 weeks later he received 1.5 mg/kg IV of Aredia for a serum calcium of 14.0 mg/dL and all subsequent serum calcium determinations have been normal. The child remains fully chimeric with complete resolution of all manifestations of osteopetrosis 4 years after HCT.

Other therapeutic options

No other curative therapies have been reported for infantile malignant osteopetrosis. One patient treated with high-dose calcitriol (1,25 dihydroxyvitamin D) for 3 months while being maintained on a low-calcium diet demonstrated increased bone matrix and mineral turnover [125]. Osteoclasts developed ruffled borders. Markedly improved monocyte resorption of bone was demonstrated *in vitro*, but only slight clinical improvement was demonstrated. Additional patients have been treated and demonstrated stabilization of disease findings [2].

Recombinant human interferon-gamma (INF-γ) [126,127] has been utilized to treat children with infantile osteopetrosis. INF-γ increases superoxide production which is reported to be deficient in granulocytes, transformed B lymphocytes and osteoclasts of osteopetrotic patients [60,128,129]. INF-γ was administered three times a week to eight children by subcutaneous injection for 6 months in the initial report [126]. Improved bone resorption was documented biochemically, trabecular bone volume decreased on bone biopsy, osteoclasts developed ruffled borders and radionucleotide marrow scans improved. Patients demonstrated significant increases in hemoglobin concentration and platelet counts and transfusion requirements decreased. No changes in bone density on radiographs were reported. In a more recent report, 14 patients were treated for 6 months and 11 of 14 for 18 months [127]. All 11 patients treated for 18 months stabilized or improved. None of the 14 patients treated for at least 6 months died. All patients had biochemical evidence of increased bone resorption and bacterial infections were decreased in the entire group. The authors suggest that treatment with INF-γ provides a reasonable therapeutic option for patients who are not candidates for HCT and an opportunity to stabilize patients awaiting HCT. Two patients receiving INF-γ have subsequently been reported to develop fatal acute respiratory distress syndrome after receiving a platelet transfusion [130].

A recent clinical trial of INF-γ1b plus calcitriol demonstrated that patients with infantile osteopetrosis experienced fewer infections, had 50% reduction in bone mass and increases in optic nerve foramina and auditory canals [2]. While children receiving the calcitrol and INF-γ demonstrate clinical improvement, the underlying disease process remains unchanged.

Treatment of infantile malignant osteopetrosis with M-CSF has been suggested in view of the observations in the op/op mouse [94–98] and tl/tl rat [94,99]. Measurement of M-CSF in 13 patients with osteopetrosis demonstrated normal to increased levels in all patients [131]. Further, in six patients studied, the M-CSF present was biologically active. While it is unlikely that infantile malignant osteopetrosis will be corrected by M-CSF administration, pharmacologic levels of M-CSF may stimulate osteoclast function and improve bone resorption.

In patients undergoing evaluation for HCT treatment with combinations including low-dose corticosteroids [101], high-dose calcitrol [125], INF-γ [126,127] and, possibly, M-CSF may be beneficial, especially if there are delays in finding a suitable donor. These strategies may stabilize the patient, decrease transfusion requirements and produce fewer side-effects than a trial of prolonged high-dose corticosteroids [101] or parathyroid hormone [20].

Future directions

Allogeneic HCT remains the only curative therapy available for children with infantile malignant osteopetrosis. All reported survivors with sustained full hematopoietic chimerism are cured. Prenatal diagnosis of infantile malignant osteopetrosis may be possible in some cases at 20–25 weeks of gestation either radiographically [132] or by ultrasonography [133]. It is speculated that measurement of creatinine kinase brain isoenzyme (BB-CK) in serum obtained by cordocentesis may provide a means for early *in utero* testing [134,135]. Prenatal linkage analysis [116] and mutational analyses [136] may be informative in known osteopetrotic kindreds. These methods are useful only in cases where there is a prior affected sibling but, if the decision is made to carry the pregnancy to term, may allow the earlier identification of a suitable donor, earlier HCT and, possibly, preservation of vision. Potentially, *in utero* transplantation could also be a consideration (see Chapter 44).

The etiology of the bone resorption defect in infantile malignant osteopetrosis has until very recently remained obscure. The finding of increased numbers of multinucleated osteoclasts in essentially all patients studied suggests the disorder is not one of stem cell differentiation, maturation or cell fusion. Osteoclast hyperplasia suggests a disorder of function and explains the observed increases in humoral stimulators of bone resorption. Possible etiologies include defective activation by these humoral stimulators because of an abnormal receptor on the cell surface, defective recognition of effete bone or digestive incompetence secondary to abnormalities in intracellular enzyme systems [33]. Two areas of current investigation may dramatically increase our understanding of the mechanisms of osteoclast dysfunction in osteopetrosis and elucidate the specific mutations present in the human osteopetrosis variants.

The first area is the development of methods to generate osteoclasts *in vitro* by a variety of coculture techniques in both animals [137] and humans [5,129,138–140]. Osteoclasts can be obtained in large numbers from both bone marrow and peripheral blood of osteopetrosis patients. M-CSF and OPGL stimulate differentiation of macrophages to osteoclasts *in vitro*. Bone resorption by these osteoclasts has been studied *in vitro* and demonstrated to be severely reduced in patients with osteopetrosis [138–140]. In all reported cases of infantile malignant osteopetrosis studied, abundant osteoclasts can be obtained which appear to have intrinsic defects that have not yet been fully characterized.

The second area involves the recent advances in gene linkage analysis and mutational analysis in the study of inherited human disorders. Initial attempts to find correlates of induced mutations in transgenic murine models to human osteopetrosis were unsuccessful. Excluded were c-*src* [82,83,141], c-*fos* [78,142], PU.1 [79,142] and NF-κB [80,142]. Gene linkage analysis has demonstrated, in a kindred with high bone mass inherited as an autosomal dominant trait, the linkage of a gene at chromosome 11q12–13 [143,144]. A point mutation in the *LDL* receptor-related protein 5 gene has been recently described in this kindred [145,146]. The mapping of autosomal recessive osteopetrosis to 11q12–13 [115,116] in two consanguineous Bedouin kindreds correlated to the position predicted by comparative mapping of the naturally occurring oc/oc murine mutation [100]. That both studies determined linkage at 11q12–13 in an asymptomatic adult autosomal dominant condition and a severe infantile autosomal recessive remains unexplained. Mutations of a cathepsin K gene in pycnodysostosis [147], an autosomal recessive osteosclerosing skeletal disorder, in a nonconsanguineous family has been reported [148]. Transgenic cathepsin K-deficient mice have severe osteopetrosis [85,86].

Most exciting are the recent observations that mutations in *OC116*, the gene encoding the a3 subunit of the vacuolar H$^+$-ATPase were found in five of 10 children studied with infantile malignant osteopetrosis [149]. This is a defect similar to the *Atp6i* deficient transgenic mouse model [87] and the natural occurring oc/oc mouse mutant [100]. Frattini et al. [150] found similar mutations in a 116-kDa subunit of the vacuolar H$^+$-ATPase protein pump in osteoclasts of five of nine patients with infantile osteopetrosis. In a follow-up study, the *ATP6i* gene was sequenced in 44 osteopetrosis families and 21 of 44 families had *ATP6i* mutations [136]. The patients with *ATP6i* mutations are clinically indistinguishable from those without the mutations. The discovery of this genetic defect has also made it possible to perform accurate prenatal diagnosis by mutation analysis in affected families. One of 12 families studied has been found with a mutational loss of the CIC-7 chloride channel [151]. Like the *ATP6i* mutations, the osteoclasts in this patient have a defective proton pump and cannot acidify the osteoclast–bone interface, which is necessary to resorb bone mineral.

The above studies delineate the etiology of infantile malignant osteopetrosis in approximately 50% of cases studied as a defect in acidification at the osteoclast–bone interface. Carbonic anhydrase II deficiency, which results in mild osteopetrosis with renal tubular acidosis, results from an inability to generate carbonic acid which supplies the H^+-ATPase with its substrate [19]. The oc/oc mouse natural mutation, the *Atp6i* transgenic murine mutant, carbonic anhydrase II mutations in humans, and the *ATP6i* and the CIC-7 chloride channel mutations in humans all result in an inability to generate hydrochloric acid at the osteoclast–bone interface, an example of digestive incompetence secondary to abnormal osteoclast enzymes [5,16,19,100,136,151]. In the next few years, it is likely that biochemical, molecular and genetic studies will explain the genotype and phenotype of the various autosomal recessive and dominant osteopetrotic syndromes. Eventually, gene therapy may be possible (see Chapters 10 and 11).

Further studies will also improve our understanding of the complex interactions between osteoblasts which synthesize bone matrix, and osteoclasts which resorb bone matrix and bone mineral [5,68,71]. Osteogenesis imperfecta is a genetic disorder caused by production of defective type I collagen by osteoblasts. Children develop osteopenia, multiple fractures, severe bony deformities and short stature. As a result, at least in part, of the success of HCT for osteopetrosis, attempts have been made to perform HCT in this disorder with the hope that engraftment of both hematopoietic and mesenchymal stem cells would occur. Prior studies have shown that osteoblasts [8,119] and mesenchymal cells [152] remain of host origin after HCT. A clinical trial has been undertaken in an attempt to engraft mesenchymal precursor cells that would generate osteoblasts capable of modifying abnormal bone structure [153,154]. Short-term engraftment of some osteoblasts has been documented with improvement in bone structure and function but whether engraftment of long-lived osteoblast progenitors with self-renewal potential will occur remains uncertain.

Studies of HCT in laboratory animals and humans have contributed greatly to our knowledge of osteoclast ontogeny and function. Their role in understanding the mechanism and regulation of bone resorption may also benefit the many patients with disorders of excessive bone resorption. Osteoporosis [4,5,68,71,145,146,155], an endemic disease, can result from both increased osteoclast activity (post-menopausal) or decreased bone formation by osteoblasts (senile) [4,155]. The hypercalcemia of multiple myeloma and malignant tumors metastatic to bone is secondary to the production of cytokines and hormones which activate osteoclasts to resorb bone. Paget's disease of bone, periodontal disease and abnormal fracture healing are additional examples of disorders with excessive bone resorption. Many insights into the prevention and treatment of these conditions can certainly be gained from the study of osteopetrosis, a disease of deficient bone resorption.

References

1. Whyte MP. *Osteopetrosis: Connective Tissue and its Heritable Disorders*. New York: Wiley-Liss, 2002: 789–807.
2. Key LLJ, Ries WL. *Osteopetrosis: Principles of Bone Biology*. San Diego, CA: Academic Press, 2002: 1217–27.
3. Hall BK. *The Osteoclast*. Boca Raton, FL: CRC Press, 1991.
4. Roodman GD. Advances in bone biology: the osteoclast. *Endocr Rev* 1996; **17**: 308–32.
5. Teitelbaum SL. Bone resorption by osteoclasts. *Science* 2000; **289**: 1504–8.
6. Popoff SN, Schneider GB. Animal models of osteopetrosis: the impact of recent molecular developments on novel strategies for therapeutic intervention. *Mol Med Today* 1996; **2**: 349–58.
7. Felix R, Hofstetter W, Cecchini MG. Recent developments in the understanding of the pathophysiology of osteopetrosis. *Eur J Endocrinol* 1996; **134**: 134–56.
8. Coccia PF, Krivit W, Cervenka J *et al*. Successful bone-marrow transplantation for infantile malignant osteopetrosis. *N Engl J Med* 1980; **302**: 701–8.
9. Gerritsen EJ, Vossen JM, Fasth A *et al*. Bone marrow transplantation for autosomal recessive osteopetrosis: a report from the Working Party on Inborn Errors of the European Bone Marrow Transplantation Group. *J Pediatr* 1994; **125**: 896–902.
10. Fasth A, Porras O. Human malignant osteopetrosis: pathophysiology, management and the role of bone marrow transplantation. *Pediatr Transplant* 1999; **3**: 102–7.
11. Albers-Schönberg H. Roentgenbilder einer seltenen Knochener-krankung. *Münch Med Wochenschr* 1904; **51**: 365–8.
12. Johnston CC Jr, Lavy N, Lord T, Vellios F, Merritt AD, Deiss WP. Osteopetrosis: a clinical, genetic, metabolic, and morphologic study of the dominantly inherited, benign form. *Medicine* 1968; **47**: 149–67.
13. Bollerslev J, Marks SC Jr, Pockwinse S *et al*. Ultrastructural investigations of bone resorptive cells in two types of autosomal dominant osteopetrosis. *Bone* 1993; **14**: 865–9.
14. Brockstedt H, Bollerslev J, Melsen F, Mosekilde L. Cortical bone remodeling in autosomal dominant osteopetrosis: a study of two different phenotypes. *Bone* 1996; **18**: 67–72.
15. Benichou AD, Laredo JD, de Vernejoul M-C. Type II autosomal dominant osteopetrosis (Albers-Schönberg disease): clinical and radiological manifestations in 42 patients. *Bone* 2000; **26**: 87–93.
16. de Vernejoul MC, Benichou O. Human osteopetrosis and other sclerosing disorders: recent genetic developments. *Calcif Tissue Int* 2001; **69**: 1–6.
17. Benichou O, Cleiren E, Gram J, Bollerslev J, de Vernejoul M-C, Van Hul W. Mapping of autosomal dominant osteopetrosis type II (Albers-Schönberg disease) to chromosome 16p13.3. *Am J Human Genet* 2001; **69**: 647–55.
18. Sly WS, Whyte MP, Sundaram V *et al*. Carbonic anhydrase II deficiency in 12 families with the autosomal recessive syndrome of osteopetrosis with renal tubular acidosis and cerebral calcification. *N Engl J Med* 1985; **313**: 139–45.
19. Sly WS, Shah GN. The carbonic anhydrase II deficiency syndrome: osteopetrosis with renal tubular acidosis and cerebral calcification. In: Scriver CR, Beaudet AL, Sly WS, Valle D eds. *The Metabolic and Molecular Bases of Inherited Disease*. New York: McGraw-Hill, 2001: 5331–43.
20. Glorieux F, Pettifor J, Marie P, Delvin EE, Travers R, Shephard N. Induction of bone resorption by parathyroid hormone in congenital malignant osteopetrosis. *Metab Bone Dis Relat Res* 1981; **3**: 143–50.
21. Whyte MP. Skeletal disorders characterized by osteosclerosis or hyperostosis. In: Avioli LV, Krane SM eds. *Metabolic Bone Disease*. San Diego: Academic Press, 1997: 697–778.
22. Van Hul W, Vanhoenacker F, Balemans W, Janssens K, De Schepper AM. Molecular and radiological diagnosis of sclerosing bone dysplasias. *Eur J Radiol* 2001; **40**: 198–207.
23. Monaghan BA, Kaplan FS, August CS, Fallon MD, Flannery DB. Transient infantile osteopetrosis. *J Pediatr* 1991; **118**: 252–6.
24. Iacobini M, Migliaccio S, Roggini M *et al*. Apparent cure of a newborn with malignant osteopetrosis using prednisone therapy. *J Bone Miner Res* 2001; **16**: 2356–60.
25. Nadvi SZ, Kottamasu SR, Bawle E, Abella E. Physiologic osteosclerosis versus osteopetrosis of the newborn. *Clin Pediatr* 1999; **38**: 235–8.
26. Totan M, Albayrak D. Osteopetrosis: improvement of hematologic findings with age. *Indian J Pediatr* 1999; **66**: 809–12.
27. Dini G, Floris R, Garaventa A *et al*. Long-term follow-up of two children with a variant of mild autosomal recessive osteopetrosis undergoing bone marrow transplantation. *Bone Marrow Transplant* 2000; **26**: 219–24.
28. Loria-Cortes R, Quesada-Calvo E, Cordero-Chaverri C. Osteopetrosis in children: a report of 26 cases. *J Pediatr* 1977; **91**: 43–7.
29. Reeves J, Arnaud S, Gordon S *et al*. The pathogenesis of infantile malignant osteopetrosis: bone mineral metabolism and complications in five infants. *Metab Bone Dis Relat Res* 1981; **3**: 135–42.
30. Gerritsen EJ, Vossen JM, van Loo IH *et al*. Autosomal recessive osteopetrosis: variability of findings at diagnosis and during the natural course. *Pediatrics* 1994; **93**: 247–53.

31 al-Rasheed SA, al-Morhij O, al-Jurayyan N et al. Osteopetrosis in children. *Int J Clin Pract* 1998; **52**: 15–8.

32 Wilson CJ, Vellodi A. Autosomal recessive osteopetrosis: diagnosis, management and outcome. *Arch Dis Child* 2000; **83**: 449–52.

33 Coccia PF. Cells that resorb bone. *N Engl J Med* 1984; **310**: 456–8.

34 Kolawole TM, Hawass ND, Patel PJ, Mahdi AH. Osteopetrosis: some unusual radiological features with a short review. *Eur J Radiol* 1988; **8**: 89–95.

35 Cheow HK, Steward CG, Grier DJ. Imaging of malignant infantile osteopetrosis before and after bone marrow transplantation. *Pediatr Radiol* 2001; **31**: 869–75.

36 Teitelbaum SL, Coccia PF, Brown DM, Kahn AJ. Malignant osteopetrosis: a disease of abnormal osteoclast proliferation. *Metab Bone Dis Relat Res* 1981; **3**: 99–105.

37 Helfrich MH, Aronson DC, Everts V et al. Morphologic features of bone in human osteopetrosis. *Bone* 1991; **12**: 411–9.

38 Shapiro F, Key LL, Anast C. Variable osteoclast appearance in human infantile osteopetrosis. *Calcif Tissue Int* 1988; **43**: 67–76.

39 Cournot G, Trubert-Thil CL, Petrovic M et al. Mineral metabolism in infants with malignant osteopetrosis: heterogeneity in plasma 1,25-dihydroxyvitamin D levels and bone histology. *J Bone Miner Res* 1992; **7**: 1–10.

40 Haines SJ, Erickson DL, Wirtschafter JD. Optic nerve decompression for osteopetrosis in early childhood. *Neurosurgery* 1988; **23**: 470–5.

41 Kerr NC, Wang WC, Mohadjer Y, Haik BG, Kaste SC, Horwitz EM. Reversal of optic canal stenosis in osteopetrosis after bone marrow transplant. *Am J Ophthalmol* 2000; **130**: 370–2.

42 Thompson DA, Kriss A, Taylor D et al. Early VEP and ERG evidence of visual dysfunction in autosomal recessive osteopetrosis. *Neuropediatrics* 1998; **29**: 137–44.

43 Hwang JM, Kim IO, Wang KC. Complete visual recovery in osteopetrosis by early optic nerve decompression. *Pediatr Neurosurg* 2000; **33**: 328–32.

44 Siatkowski RM, Vilar NF, Sternau L, Coin CG. Blindness from bad bones. *Surv Ophthalmol* 1999; **43**: 487–90.

45 Lehman RAW, Reeves JD, Wilson WB, Wesenberz RL. Neurological complications of infantile osteopetrosis. *Ann Neurol* 1977; **2**: 378–84.

46 Tasdemir HA, Dagdemir A, Celenk C, Albayrak D. Middle cerebral arterial occlusion in a child with osteopetrosis major. *Eur Radiol* 2001; **11**: 145–7.

47 Curé JK, Key LL, Shankar L, Gross AJ. Petrous carotid canal stenosis in malignant osteopetrosis: CT documentation with MR angiographic correlation. *Radiology* 1996; **199**: 415–21.

48 Stocks RM, Wang WC, Thompson JW, Stocks MC II, Horwitz EM. Malignant infantile osteopetrosis: otolaryngological complications and management. *Arch Otolaryngol Head Neck Surg* 1998; **124**: 689–94.

49 Stocks R, Cannon CB, Wang WC, Horwitz EM, Thompson JW. Reversal of obstructive sleep apnea in osteopetrosis following bone marrow transplantation. *Clin Pediatr (Phila)* 2002; **41**: 55–7.

50 Orengo SD, Patrinely JR. Dacryocystorhinostomy in osteopetrosis. *Ophthalmic Surg* 1991; **22**: 396–8.

51 Srinivasan M, Abinun M, Cant A, Tan K, Oakhill A, Steward CG. Malignant infantile osteopetrosis presenting with neonatal hypocalcaemia. *Arch Dis Child Fetal Neonatal Ed* 2000; **83**: F21–F23.

52 Popp D, Zieger B, Schmitt-Graff A, Nutzenadel W, Schaefer F. Malignant osteopetrosis obscured by maternal vitamin D deficiency in a neonate. *Eur J Pediatr* 2000; **159**: 412–5.

53 Bakeman RJ, Abdelsayed RA, Sutley SH, Newhouse RF. Osteopetrosis: a review of the literature and report of a case complicated by osteomyelitis of the mandible. *J Oral Maxillofac Surg* 1998; **56**: 1209–13.

54 Barbaglio A, Cortelazzi R, Martignoni G, Nocini PF. Osteopetrosis complicated by osteomyelitis of the mandible: a case report including gross and microscopic findings. *J Oral Maxillofac Surg* 1998; **56**: 393–8.

55 Jälevik B, Fasth A, Dahllöf G. Dental development after successful treatment of infantile osteopetrosis with bone marrow transplantation. *Bone Marrow Transplant* 2002; **29**: 537–40.

56 Armstrong DG, Newfield JT, Gillespie R. Orthopedic management of osteopetrosis: results of a survey and review of the literature. *J Pediatr Orthop* 1999; **19**: 122–32.

57 Charles JM, Key LL. Developmental spectrum of children with congenital osteopetrosis. *J Pediatr* 1998; **132**: 371–4.

58 Sorell M, Kapoor N, Kirkpatrick D et al. Marrow transplantation for juvenile osteopetrosis. *Am J Med* 1981; **70**: 1280–7.

59 Reeves JD, Augusut CS, Humbert JR, Weston WL. Host defense in infantile osteopetrosis. *Pediatrics* 1979; **64**: 202–6.

60 Beard CJ, Key L, Newburger PE et al. Neutrophil defect associated with malignant infantile osteopetrosis. *J Lab Clin Med* 1986; **108**: 498–505.

61 Burt N, Haynes GR, Bailey MK. Patients with malignant osteopetrosis are at high risk of anesthetic morbidity and mortality. *Anesth Analg* 1999; **88**: 1292–7.

62 Takahashi K, Naito M, Yamamura F et al. Infantile osteopetrosis complicating neuronal ceroid lipofuscinosis. *Pathol Res Pract* 1990; **186**: 697–706.

63 Ruben JB, Morris RJ, Judisch GF. Chronioretinal degeneration in infantile malignant osteopetrosis. *Am J Ophthalmol* 1990; **110**: 1–5.

64 Abinun M, Newson T, Rowe PW, Flood TJ, Cant AJ. Importance of neurological assessment before bone marrow transplantation for osteopetrosis. *Arch Dis Child* 1999; **80**: 273–4.

65 Jagadha V, Halliday WC, Becker LE, Hinton D. The association of infantile osteopetrosis and neuronal storage disease in two brothers. *Acta Neuropathol (Berl)* 1988; **75**: 233–40.

66 Rees H, Ang LC, Casey R, George DH. Association of infantile neuroaxonal dystrophy and osteopetrosis: a rare autosomal recessive disorder. *Pediatr Neurosurg* 1995; **22**: 321–7.

67 Marks SCJ. The structural basis for bone cell biology. *Acta Med Dent Helv* 1997; **2**: 141–57.

68 Boyce BF, Hughes DE, Wright KR, Xing L, Dai A. Recent advances in bone biology provide insight into the pathogenesis of bone diseases. *Lab Invest* 1999; **79**: 83–94.

69 Hayase Y, Muguruma Y, Lee MY. Osteoclast development from hematopoietic stem cells: apparent divergence of the osteoclast lineage prior to macrophage commitment. *Exp Hematol* 1997; **25**: 19–25.

70 Burgess TL, Qian Y, Kaufman S et al. The ligand for osteoprotegerin (PGL) directly activates mature osteoclasts. *J Cell Biol* 1999; **145**: 527–38.

71 Ducy P, Schinke T, Karsenty G. The osteoblast: a sophisticated fibroblast under central surveillance. *Science* 2000; **289**: 1501–4.

72 Popoff S, Marks SJ. The heterogeneity of the osteopetroses reflects the diversity of cellular influences during skeletal development. *Bone* 1995; **17**: 437–45.

73 Seifert MF, Popoff SN, Jackson ME, MacKay CA, Cielinski M, Marks SCJ. Experimental studies of osteopetrosis in laboratory animals. *Clin Orthop* 1993; **294**: 23–33.

74 Athanasou NA, Sabokbar A. Human osteoclast ontogeny and pathological bone resorption. *Histol Histopathol* 1999; **14**: 635–47.

75 Cielinski MJ, Marks SC Jr. Neonatal reductions in osteoclast number and function account for the transient nature of osteopetrosis in the rat mutation microphthalmia blanc (mib). *Bone* 1994; **15**: 707–15.

76 Opdecamp K, Vanvooren P, Rivièr M et al. The rat microphthalmia-associated transcription factor gene (*Mitf*) maps at 4q34–q41 and is mutated in the *mib* rats. *Mamm Genome* 1998; **9**: 617–21.

77 Weilbaecher KN, Hershey CL, Takemoto CM et al. Age-resolving osteopetrosis: a rat model implicating microphthalmia and the related transcription factor TFE3. *J Exp Med* 1998; **187**: 775–85.

78 Grigoriadis AE, Wang ZQ, Cecchini MG et al. c-Fos: a key regulator of osteoclast-macrophage lineage determination and bone remodeling. *Science* 1994; **266**: 443–8.

79 Tondravi MM, McKercher SR, Anderson K et al. Osteopetrosis in mice lacking haematopoietic transcription factor PU.1. *Nature* 1997; **386**: 81–4.

80 Iotsova V, Caamaño J, Loy J, Yang Y, Lewin A, Bravo R. Osteopetrosis in mice lacking NF-κB1 and NF-κB2. *Nat Med* 1997; **3**: 1285–9.

81 Kong YY, Yoshida H, Sarosi I et al. OPGL is a key regulator of osteoclastogenesis, lymphocyte development and lymph-node organogenesis. *Nature* 1999; **397**: 315–23.

82 Soriano P, Montgomery C, Geske R, Bradley A. Targeted disruption of the c-*src* proto-oncogene leads to osteopetrosis in mice. *Cell* 1991; **64**: 693–702.

83 Meyerson G, Dahl N, Pahlman S. Malignant osteopetrosis: c-*src* kinase is not reduced in fibroblasts. *Calcif Tissue Int* 1993; **53**: 69–70.

84 Lomaga MA, Yeh WC, Sarosi I et al. TRAF6 deficiency results in osteopetrosis and defective interleukin-1, CD40, and LPS signaling. *Genes Dev* 1999; **13**: 1015–24.

85 Saftig P, Hunziker E, Wehmeyer O et al. Impaired osteoclastic bone resorption leads to osteopetrosis in cathepsin-K-deficiency mice. *Proc Natl Acad Sci U S A* 1998; **95**: 13453–8.

86 Gowen M, Lazner F, Dodds R, Kapadia R, Feild J, Tavaria M et al. Cathepsin K knockout mice develop osteopetrosis due to a deficit in matrix degradation but not mineralization. *J Bone Miner Res* 1999; **14**: 1654–63.

87 Li YP, Chen W, Liang Y, Li E, Stashenko P. Atp6i-deficient mice exhibit severe osteopetrosis due to loss of osteoclast-mediated extracellular acidification. *Nat Genet* 1999; **23**: 447–51.

88 Walker DG. Bone resorption restored in osteopetrotic mice by transplants of normal bone marrow and spleen cells. *Science* 1975; **190**: 784–5.

89 Walker DG. Spleen cells transmit osteopetrosis in mice. *Science* 1975; **190**: 785–7.

90 Marks SC Jr. Studies of the cellular cure for osteopetrosis by transplanted cells: specificity of the cell types in *ia* rats. *Am J Anat* 1978; **151**: 383–7.

91 Milhaud G, Labat ML, Graf B et al. Démonstration cinétique, radiographique et histologique du la guérison de l'osteopetrose congenitale du rat. *C R Acad Sci Hebd Seances Acad Sci D* 1975; **280**: 2485–8.

92 Ash P, Loutit JF, Townsend KMS. Osteoclasts derived from haematopoietic stem cells. *Nature* 1980; **283**: 669–70.

93 Marks SCJ, Walker DG. The hematogenous origin of osteoclasts: experimental evidence from osteopetrotic (microphthalmic) mice treated with spleen cells from beige mouse donors. *Am J Anat* 1981; **16**: 1–10.

94 Shalhoub V, Jackson ME, Paradise C, Stein GS, Lian JB, Marks SC Jr. Heterogeneity of colony stimulating factor-1 gene expression in the skeleton of four osteopetrotic mutations in rats and mice. *J Cell Physiol* 1996; **166**: 340–50.

95 Yoshida H, Hayashi S, Kunisada T et al. The murine mutation osteopetrosis is in the coding region of the macrophage colony stimulating factor gene. *Nature* 1990; **345**: 442–4.

96 Sundquist KT, Cecchini MG, Marks SC Jr. Colony-stimulating factor-1 injections improve but do not cure skeletal sclerosis in osteopetrotic (*op*) mice. *Bone* 1995; **16**: 39–46.

97 Umeda S, Takahashi K, Naito M, Shultz LD, Takagi K. Neonatal changes of osteoclasts in osteopetrosis (*op/op*) mice defective in production of functional macrophages colony-stimulating factor (M-CSF) protein and effects of M-CSF on osteoclast development and differentiation. *J Submicrosc Cytol Pathol* 1996; **28**: 13–26.

98 Nilsson SK, Lieschke GJ, Garcia-Wijnen CC et al. Granulocyte-macrophage colony-stimulating factor is not responsible for the correction of hematopoietic deficiencies in the maturing op/op mouse. *Blood* 1995; **86**: 66–72.

99 Seifert MF. Abnormalities in bone cell function and endochrondral ossification in the osteopetrotic toothless rat. *Bone* 1996; **19**: 329–38.

100 Scimeca J-C, Franchi A, Trojani C et al. The gene encoding the mouse homologue of the human osteoclast-specific 116-kDa V-ATPase subunit bears a deletion in osteosclerotic (oc/oc) mutants. *Bone* 2000; **26**: 207–13.

101 Reeves JD, Huffer WE, August CS, Hathaway WE, Koerper M, Walters CE. The hematopoietic effects of prednisone therapy in four infants with osteopetrosis. *J Pediatr* 1979; **94**: 210–4.

102 Dorantes LM, Mejia AM, Dorantes S. Juvenile osteopetrosis: effects on blood and bone of prednisone and a low calcium, high phosphate diet. *Arch Dis Child* 1986; **61**: 666–70.

103 Ballet JJ, Griscelli C, Coutris C, Milhaud G, Maroteaux P. Bone marrow transplantation in osteopetrosis. *Lancet* 1977; **2**: 1137.

104 O'Reilly RJ, Brochstein J, Dinsmore R, Kirkpatrick D. Marrow transplantation for congenital disorders. *Semin Hematol* 1984; **21**: 188–221.

105 Ballet JJ, Griscelli C. Lymphoid cell transplantation in human osteopetrosis. In: Horton JE, Tarpley TM, Davis WF eds. *Mechanisms of Localized Bone Loss*. Arlington, VA: Information Retrieval, 1978: 399–414.

106 Warkentin PI, Strandjord SE, Schacter B et al. Successful bone marrow transplantation (BMT) for infantile malignant osteopetrosis (OP) using a mismatched parental donor. *Blood* 1985; **66**: 255a.

107 Sieff CA, Chessells JM, Levinsky RJ et al. Allogeneic bone-marrow transplantation in infantile malignant osteopetrosis. *Lancet* 1983; **1**: 437–41.

108 Orchard PJ, Dickerman JD, Mathews CH et al. Haploidentical bone marrow transplantation for osteopetrosis. *Am J Pediatr Hematol Oncol* 1987; **9**: 335–40.

109 Kaplan FS, August CS, Fallon Dalinka M, Axel L, Haddad JG. Successful treatment of infantile malignant osteopetrosis by bone-marrow transplantation. *J Bone Joint Surg Am* 1988; **70**: 617–23.

110 Schroeder RF, Johnson FL, Silberstein MJ et al. Longitudinal follow-up of malignant osteopetrosis by skeletal radiographs and restriction fragment length polymorphism analysis after bone marrow transplantation. *Pediatrics* 1992; **90**: 986–9.

111 Solh H, Da Cunha AM, Giri N et al. Bone marrow transplantation for infantile malignant osteopetrosis. *J Pediatr Hematol Oncol* 1995; **17**: 350–5.

112 Jabado N, Le Deist F, Cant A et al. Bone marrow transplantation from genetically HLA-nonidentical donors in children with fatal inherited disorders excluding severe combined immunodeficiencies: use of two monoclonal antibodies to prevent graft rejection. *Pediatrics* 1996; **98**: 420–8.

113 Eapen M, Davies SM, Ramsay NK, Orchard PJ. Hematopoietic stem cell transplantation for infantile osteopetrosis. *Bone Marrow Transplant* 1998; **22**: 941–6.

114 Kapelushnik J, Shalev C, Yaniv I et al. Osteopetrosis: a single centre experience of stem cell transplantation and prenatal diagnosis. *Bone Marrow Transplant* 2001; **27**: 129–32.

115 Heaney C, Shalev H, Elbedour K et al. Human autosomal recessive osteopetrosis maps to 11q13, a position predicted by comparative mapping of the murine osteosclerosis (oc) mutation. *Hum Mol Genet* 1998; **7**: 1407–10.

116 Shalev H, Mishori-Dery A, Kapelushnik J et al. Prenatal diagnosis of malignant osteopetrosis in Bedouin families by linkage analysis. *Prenat Diagn* 2001; **21**: 183–6.

117 Schulz AS, Classen CF, Mihatsch WA et al. HLA-haploidentical blood progenitor cell transplantation in osteopetrosis. *Blood* 2002; **99**: 3458–60.

118 Cure JK, Key LL, Goltra DD, VanTassel P. Cranial MR imaging of osteopetrosis. *Am J Neuroradiol* 2000; **21**: 1110–15.

119 Lajeunesse D, Busque L, Menard P, Brunette MG, Bonny Y. Demonstration of an osteoblast defect in two cases of human malignant osteopetrosis: correction of the phenotype after bone marrow transplant. *J Clin Invest* 1996; **98**: 1835–42.

120 Blazar BR, Teitelbaum SL, Fallon MD et al. Malignant osteopetrosis (OP): observations on the disease spectrum. *Pediatr Res* 1984; **18**: 291A.

121 Locatelli F, Beluffi G, Giorgiani G et al. Transplantation of cord blood progenitor cells can promote bone resorption in autosomal recessive osteopetrosis. *Bone Marrow Transplant* 1997; **20**: 701–5.

122 McMahon C, Will A, Hu P, Shah GN, Sly WS, Smith OP. Bone marrow transplantation corrects osteopetrosis in the carbonic anhydrase II deficiency syndrome. *Blood* 2001; **97**: 1947–50.

123 Adler IN, Stine KC, Kurtzburg J et al. Dual-energy X-ray absorptiometry in osteopetrosis. *South Med J* 2000; **93**: 501–3.

124 Rodan GA, Martin TJ. Therapeutic approaches to bone diseases. *Science* 2000; **289**: 1508–14.

125 Key L, Carnes D, Cole S et al. Treatment of congenital osteopetrosis with high-dose calcitriol. *N Engl J Med* 1984; **310**: 409–15.

126 Key LL Jr, Ries WL, Rodriguiz RM, Hatcher HC. Recombinant human interferon gamma therapy for osteopetrosis. *J Pediatr* 1992; **121**: 119–24.

127 Key LL Jr, Rodriguiz RM, Willi SM et al. Long-term treatment of osteopetrosis with recombinant human interferon gamma. *N Engl J Med* 1995; **332**: 1594–9.

128 Yang S, Ries WL, Key LLJ. Superoxide generation in transformed B-lymphocytes from patients with severe, malignant osteopetrosis. *Mol Cell Biochem* 1999; **199**: 15–24.

129 Madyastha PR, Yang S, Ries WL, Key LLJ. IFN-γ enhances osteoclast generation in cultures of peripheral blood from osteopetrotic patients and normalizes superoxide production. *J Interferon Cytokine Res* 2000; **20**: 645–52.

130 Madyastha PR, Jeter EK, Key LL Jr. Cytophilic immunoglobulin G binding on neutrophils from a child with malignant osteopetrosis who developed fatal acute respiratory distress mimicking transfusion-related acute lung injury. *Am J Hematol* 1996; **53**: 196–200.

131 Orchard PJ, Dahl N, Aukerman SL, Blazar BR, Key LL Jr. Circulating macrophage colony-stimulating factor is not reduced in malignant osteopetrosis. *Exp Hematol* 1992; **20**: 103–5.

132 Ogur G, Ogur E, Celasun B et al. Prenatal diagnosis of autosomal recessive osteopetrosis, infantile type, by X-ray evaluation. *Prenat Diagn* 1995; **15**: 477–81.

133 Sen C, Madazli R, Aksoy F, Ocak V. Antenatal diagnosis of lethal osteopetrosis. *Ultrasound Obstet Gynecol* 1995; **5**: 278–80.

134 Whyte MP, Chines A, Silva DP Jr, Landt Y, Ladenson JH. Creatine kinase brain isoenzyme (BB-CK) presence in serum distinguishes osteopetroses among the sclerosing bone disorders. *J Bone Miner Res* 1996; **11**: 1438–43.

135 Bollerslev J, Ueland T, Landaas S, Marks SCJ. Serum creatine kinase isoenzyme BB in mammalian osteopetrosis. *Clin Orthop* 2000; **377**: 241–7.

136 Sobacchi C, Frattini A, Orchard P et al. The mutational spectrum of human malignant autosomal recessive osteopetrosis. *Hum Mol Genet* 2001; **10**: 1767–73.

137 David JP, Neff M, Chen Y, Rincon M, Horne WC, Baron R. A new method to isolate large numbers of rabbit osteoclasts and osteoclast-like cells; application to the characterization of serum response element binding proteins during osteoclast differentiation. *J Bone Miner Res* 1998; **13**: 1730–8.

138 Teti A, Migliaccio S, Taranta A et al. Mechanisms of osteoclast dysfunction in human osteopetrosis: abnormal osteoclastogenesis and lack of osteoclast-specific adhesion structures. *J Bone Miner Res* 1999; **14**: 2107–17.

139 Flanagan AM, Sarma U, Steward CG, Vellodi A, Horton MA. Study of the nonresorptive phenotype of osteoclast-like cells from patients with malignant osteopetrosis: a new approach to investigating pathogenesis. *J Bone Miner Res* 2000; **15**: 352–60.

140 Helfrich MH, Gerritsen EJA. Formation of nonresorbing osteoclasts from peripheral blood mononuclear cells of patients with malignant juvenile osteopetrosis. *Br J Haematol* 2001; **112**: 64–8.

141 Bernard F, Casanova JL, Cournot G et al. The protein tyrosine kinase p60c-Src is not implicated in the pathogenesis of the human autosomal recessive form of osteopetrosis: a study of 13 children. *J Pediatr* 1998; **133**: 537–43.

142 Yang S, Sun G, Ries W, Key LL. Pu.1, c-*fos*, and NF-κB are not defective in osteopetrotic B cells: a

143 Johnson ML, Gong G, Kimberling W, Recker SM, Kimmel DB, Recker RB. Linkage of a gene causing high bone mass to human chromosome 11 (11q12–13). *Am J Hum Genet* 1997; **60**: 1326–32.

144 Whyte MP. Searching for gene defects that cause high bone mass. *Am J Hum Genet* 1997; **60**: 1309–11.

145 Little RD, Carulli JP, Del Mastro RG *et al.* A mutation in the LDL receptor-related protein 5 gene results in the autosomal dominant high-bone-mass trait. *Am J Hum Genet* 2002; **70**: 11–19.

146 Johnson ML, Picconi JL, Recker RR. The gene for high bone mass. *Endocrinologist* 2002; **12**: 445–53.

147 Gelb BD, Brömme D, Desnick RJ. Pycnodysostosis: cathepsin K deficiency. In: Scriver CR, Beaudet AL, Sly WS, Valle D eds. *The Metabolic and Molecular Bases of Inherited Disease*. New York: McGraw-Hill, 2002: 3453–68.

148 Ho N, Punturieri A, Wilkin D *et al.* Mutations of CTSK result in pycnodysostosis via a reduction in cathepsin K protein. *J Bone Miner Res* 1999; **14**: 1649–53.

149 Kornak U, Schulz A, Friedrich W *et al.* Mutations in the a3 subunit of the vacuolar H^+-ATPase cause infantile malignant osteopetrosis. *Hum Mol Genet* 2000; **9**: 2059–63.

150 Frattini A, Orchard PJ, Sobacchi C *et al.* Defects in TCIRG1 subunit of the vacuolar proton pump are responsible for a subset of human autosomal recessive osteopetrosis. *Nat Genet* 2000; **25**: 343–6.

151 Kornak U, Kasper D, Bosl MR *et al.* Loss of the ClC-7 chloride channel leads to osteopetrosis in mice and man. *Cell* 2001; **104**: 205–15.

152 Koc ON, Peters C, Aubourg P *et al.* Bone marrow-derived mesenchymal stem cells remain host-derived despite successful hematopoietic engraftment after allogeneic transplantation in patients with lysosomal and peroxisomal storage diseases. *Exp Hematol* 1999; **27**: 1675–81.

153 Horwitz EM, Prockop DJ, Gordon PL *et al.* Clinical responses to bone marrow transplantation in children with severe osteogenesis imperfecta. *Blood* 2001; **97**: 1227–31.

154 Horwitz EM, Gordon PL, Koo WKK *et al.* Isolated allogeneic bone marrow-derived mesenchymal cells engraft and stimulate growth in children with osteogenesis imperfecta: implications for cell therapy of bone. *Proc Natl Acad Sci U S A* 2002; **99**: 8932–7.

155 Lazner F, Gowen M, Pavasovic D, Kola I. Osteopetrosis and osteoporosis: two sides of the same coin. *Hum Mol Genet* 1999; **8**: 1839–46.

107

Charles Peters

Hematopoietic Cell Transplantation for Storage Diseases

Introduction

The storage diseases represent a diverse group of lysosomal and peroxisomal disorders. Single gene defects involving a lysosomal hydrolytic enzyme or vital peroxisomal function lead to these devastating diseases and their systemic abnormalities affecting multiple organs including the brain. Progressive loss of neurodevelopmental milestones and/or neurologic function is common. Shortened life-expectancy is often due to cardiopulmonary disease. Evaluation of affected infants, children, adolescents, or adults must be multidisciplinary and comprehensive. Treatment options depend upon the stage of disease and rate of progression. They include hematopoietic cell transplantation (HCT), enzyme replacement therapy (ERT), substrate depletion and, hopefully, gene therapy.

Lysosomes are cellular organelles that contain large numbers of hydrolytic enzymes; peroxisomes are subcellular organelles that catalyze metabolic functions primarily related to lipid metabolism including fatty acid β-oxidation. In 1968, Fratantoni and Neufeld established the basis of our understanding of transferable lysosomal enzymes by demonstrating metabolic cross-correction of defects in cocultures of fibroblasts from Hurler and Hunter syndrome patients [1]. Metabolic correction of lysosomal storage disorders is based upon mannose 6-phosphate receptor-mediated endocytosis of secreted enzyme or by direct transfer of enzyme from adjacent cells (Fig. 107.1) [2–5]. It is likely that both mechanisms provide enzymatic correction following HCT. Receptor-mediated endocytosis occurs when a lysosomal hydrolase bearing a mannose 6-phosphate residue is secreted by the donor cell and binds to the host cell receptor. Enzyme is internalized into the cytoplasm and transferred to the lysosomal compartment [2–5]. Variability in receptor-mediated enzyme endocytosis in various cells and tissues may affect hydrolase uptake after HCT [6]. For example, monocytes and tissue macrophages have receptors for *N*-acetylglucosamine and mannose while glial cells have receptors for sialic acid [7]. Direct transfer of enzyme to the intracellular space occurs independently of receptor-mediated endocytosis and requires cell–cell contact [3,8,9]. A variety of adhesion molecules are involved in this process [3,9].

X-linked adrenoleukodystrophy (X-ALD) is a peroxisomal disorder of very long chain fatty acid (VLCFA) β-oxidation. Rather than metabolic cross-correction, the likely mechanism by which HCT effectively halts the cerebral demyelination of X-ALD is by replacement with metabolically normal cell populations rather than transfer of biochemical mediators from normal donor cells; decreased perivascular inflammation also contributes. The benefit from normalization of plasma VLCFA is unclear.

A crucial question in HCT for storage diseases with central nervous system (CNS) involvement is whether donor-derived cells enter the CNS and achieve metabolic correction. Microglia are mononuclear phago-

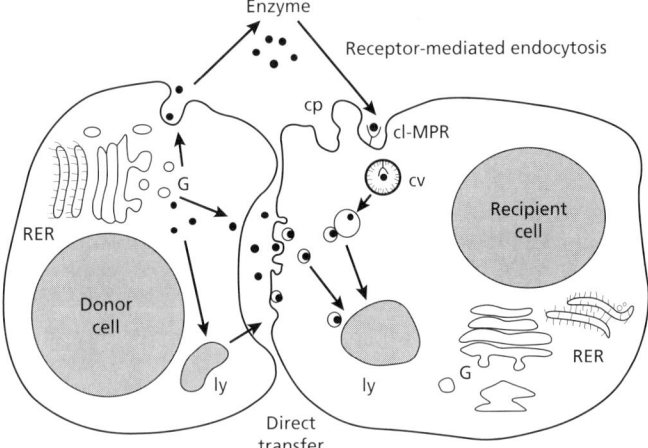

Fig. 107.1 Receptor-dependent and -independent mechanisms of intracellular transport of lysosomal hydrolases. Enzyme secreted by the donor cell bears mannose 6-phosphate (M6P) and is bound to cation-independent M6P receptors (ci-MPR) as coated pits (cp) on the cell surface. These undergo endocytosis as coated vesicles (cv), which deliver the hydrolase to the lysosomes (ly) by the endocytic pathway. The receptor-independent pathway involves direct transfer of enzyme without coated vesicles and involves intercellular adhesion molecules. G, Golgi apparatus; RER, rough endoplasmic reticulum. Reproduced with permission from Bou-Gharios *et al.* [3].

cytes in the CNS [10,11]. They account for 5–10% of non-neuronal cells in the brain. Activated microglia are involved in antigen presentation and responses to inflammation, infection, or CNS injury [12,13]. Also known as CNS macrophages, these cells are hematopoietically derived. In humans, repopulation with donor-derived microglia requires approximately 1 year. The kinetics of microglial repopulation after HCT is considerably slower than that of other tissue macrophages such as pulmonary alveolar macrophages and Kupffer cells [14,15] (Figs 107.2 & 107.3 [16]). This may explain, in part, the ineffectiveness of HCT to stabilize or prevent neurologic deterioration in rapidly progressing storage diseases.

HCT for lysosomal and peroxisomal disorders

General considerations and observations

Lysosomal storage disorders represent a group of more than 40 genetically distinct, biochemically related, inherited diseases. For most of these disorders, there are either naturally occurring animal models, or genetically manipulated (i.e. "knockout") animals. The extent to which the

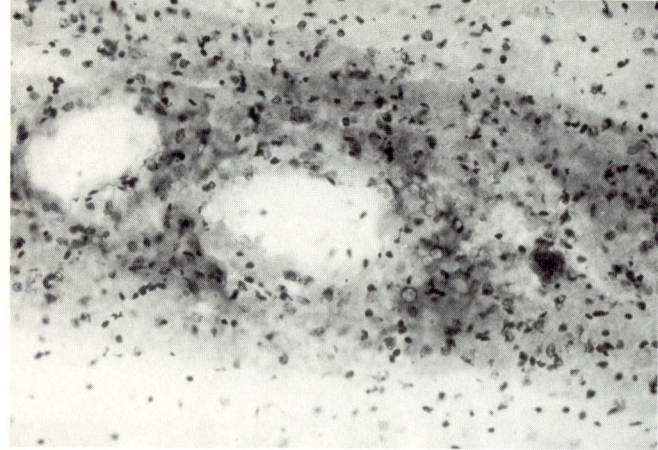

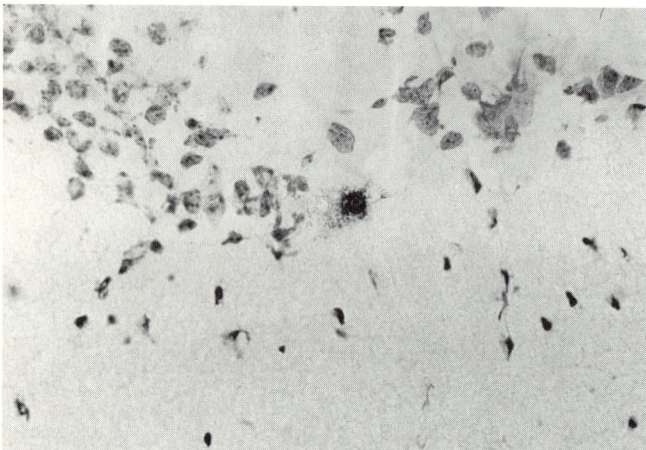

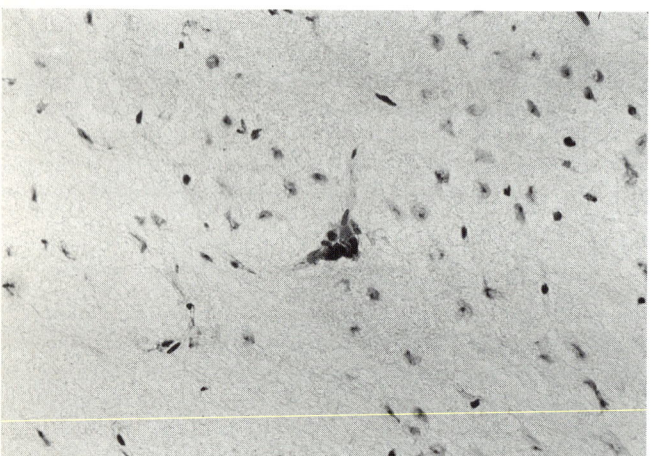

Fig. 107.2 Congenic Ly-5.1 donor mononuclear cells in the perivascular region (A, ×1300) and in the parenchymal (B, ×3130; C, ×2088) of brains of Ly-5.2 mice 60 days after bone marrow transplantation. Donor cells are stained brown by the benzidine reaction. The extended processes of the cells in the parenchyma are characteristic of ameboid (activated) microglia. Reproduced with permission from Yeager [16].

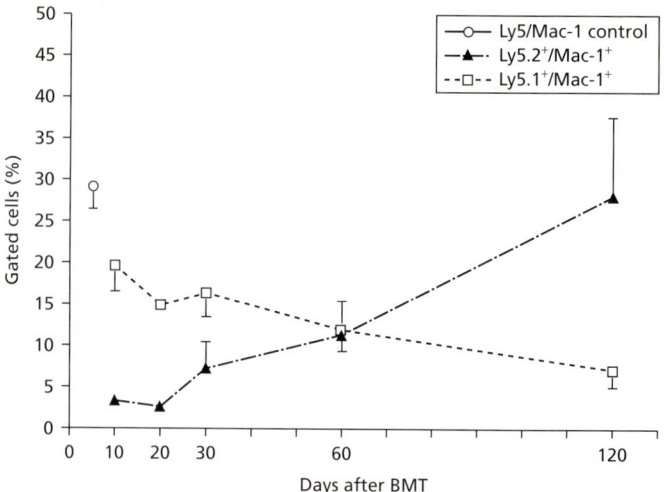

Fig. 107.3 Kinetics of the repopulation of central nervous system (CNS) macrophages after congenic bone marrow transplantation (BMT). Donor Ly-5.1$^+$/Mac-1$^+$ (solid triangles) and recipient Ly-5.2$^+$/Mac-1$^+$ (open squares) macrophages were quantified by two-color flow cytometry of suspensions of brain tissues obtained from recipient Ly-5.2 mice at selected times after congenic hematopoietic cell transplantation with Ly-5.1 cells. Mice received bone marrow transplants at age 10 days, 24 h after administration of busulfan (80 mg/kg). The level of Ly-5$^+$/Mac-1$^+$ cells in the brains of untreated 120-day-old Ly-5.1 or Ly-5.2 mice is shown for reference (open circle). (Reproduced by permission from Yeager AM. Hematopoietic cell transplantation for storage diseases. In: Thomas ED, Blume KG, Forman SJ (eds) *Hematopoietic Cell Transplantation*, 2nd edn. Boston: Blackwell Science, 1999: 1184.).

preclinical animal model approximates the human disease process varies considerably. These models have been informative for the evaluation of treatment modalities including HCT, ERT and gene transfer.

The requisites to diagnose a lysosomal or peroxisomal disorder are clearly defined. For most patients, the diagnosis is made following evaluation of specific signs and/or symptoms rather than on the basis of a family history. The potential informative nature of the family history is most evident in X-ALD. Thorough evaluation of patients with lysosomal and peroxisomal disorders is essential prior to making a decision regarding the most appropriate therapy. In some instances, DNA-based analysis of the specific mutation may be informative. If the decision to perform HCT is made, a choice regarding donor and stem cell source must be made. In addition to the evaluation of HLA matching, determination of the donor's enzyme activity level for the disease being treated can be informative. Choice of a preparative regimen should take into account the underlying disease process and the risk for regimen-related toxicities. Pharmacokinetic and pharmacogenomic features may influence how a patient will tolerate the HCT process. Close patient monitoring and long-term, multidisciplinary, coordinated follow-up should focus on HCT- and disease-related complications.

Mucopolysaccharidoses

The mucopolysaccharidoses are a group of lysosomal disorders caused by deficiency of degradative enzymes of glycosaminoglycans (GAGs) [17]. Glycosaminoglycans, such as heparan, dermatan, keratan and chondroitin sulfates, individually, or in combination, accumulate or are "stored" intracellularly and lead to cellular, tissue and organ dysfunction. These GAGs are typically excreted in urine and are often detected in the initial diagnostic screening tests. The genes and the complementary DNAs (cDNAs) encoding most of these enzymes have been cloned leading to the characterization of their primary structures, production of recombinant enzymes, and identification of disease-causing mutations. The mucopolysaccharidoses disorders and their respective enzyme deficiency are presented in Table 107.1. There are many shared clinical features among the mucopolysaccharidoses disorders including chronic, progressive courses; multiorgan system involvement; organomegaly, dysostosis multiplex and facial dysmorphia. Hearing, vision, pulmonary and cardiovascular

Table 107.1 Inborn errors of metabolism: lysosomal and peroxisomal storage diseases, mode of inheritance, enzyme deficiency, indications for hematopoietic cell transplantation (HCT) and comments.

Disease (abbreviation) Mode of inheritance Enzyme deficiency	Is HCT indicated?	Comments
Mucopolysaccharidoses		
Hurler syndrome (MPS I) Autosomal recessive α-L-iduronidase	Yes	Preservation of intelligence and improved cardiopulmonary status, skeletal deformities persist
Hunter syndrome (MPS II) X-linked iduronate sulfatase	No	Intelligence and somatic status continue to deteriorate despite HCT for severe MPS II
Sanfilippo syndrome (MPS III) Autosomal recessive MPS IIIA, sulfamidase MPS IIIB, α-*N*-acetylglucosaminidase MPS IIIC, acetyl-CoA: α-glucosaminide acetyltransferase MPS IIID, *N*-acetylglucosamine 6-sulfatase	No	Intelligence continues to deteriorate despite HCT
Morquio syndrome (MPS IV) Autosomal recessive MPS IVA, *N*-acetylgalactosamine 6-sulfatase MPS IVB, β-galactosidase	No	Skeletal deformities persist despite HCT
Maroteaux–Lamy syndrome (MPS VI) Autosomal recessive Arylsulfatase B	Yes	Significant somatic improvement especially cardiopulmonary
Sly syndrome (MPS VII) Autosomal recessive β-Glucuronidase	Yes	Effective in two cases
Leukodystrophies		
Cerebral X-adrenoleukodystrophy (cerebral X-ALD) X-linked ALD protein	Yes	Neuropsychologic and neurologic function can be preserved after HCT
Globoid-cell leukodystrophy (GLD) Autosomal recessive Galactocerebrosidase	Yes	Dramatic improvements in neurologic, neuropsychologic and neurophysiologic function have been noted after HCT, including cases of infantile onset
Metachromatic leukodystrophy (MLD) Autosomal recessive Arylsulfatase A	Yes	Stabilization of CNS in juvenile and adult onset cases; however, PNS disease typically progresses, especially in late infantile cases
Multiple sulfatase deficiency Autosomal recessive Multiple sulfatases: Arylsulfatases A, B and C Iduronate sulfatase Heparan-*N*-sulfamidase *N*-acetylgalactosamine-6-sulfate sulfatase *N*-acetylglucosamine-6-sulfate sulfatase	Possibly	HCT experience in one case
Glycoprotein disorders		
α-Mannosidosis Autosomal recessive α-Mannosidase	Yes	Significant improvement in somatic aspects, including bones, after HCT
Fucosidosis Autosomal recessive Fucosidase	Probably	Experience still limited; however, HCT appears to stabilize CNS

(Continued)

Table 107.1 (*cont'd*)

Disease (abbreviation) Mode of inheritance Enzyme deficiency	Is HCT indicated?	Comments
Aspartylglucosaminuria Autosomal recessive Aspartylglucosaminidase Other lysosomal disorders	Yes	HCT may be effective in small number of cases
Glycogen storage disease, type II (Pompe disease) Autosomal recessive Acid maltase	No	Enzyme replacement trials in progress
Mucolipidosis II (I-cell disease) Autosomal recessive Phosphotransferase	Possibly	Limited HCT primarily in patients with end-stage disease
Wolman disease Autosomal recessive Acid lipase	Possibly	Two survivors of HCT
Farber lipogranulomatosis Autosomal recessive Ceramidase	Possibly	Limited HCT experience
Niemann–Pick Autosomal recessive Types A and B, acid sphingomyelinase Type C, defective cellular trafficking of exogenous cholesterol	Possibly	HCT not effective for type A, can be effective for type B, possibly effective for type C
Gaucher 1 Autosomal recessive Glucocerebrosidase	Possibly	HCT can ameliorate the somatic disease in type, although primary therapy is enzyme replacement It is not indicated for type 2 but is probably effective in type 3
Fabry X-linked α-Galactosidase A	No	Enzyme replacement trials in progress
Neuronal ceroid lipofuscinosis (NCL) Autosomal recessive NCL 1, palmitoyl protein thioesterase NCL 2, transpeptidase	Possibly	Limited HCT experience for infantile (NCL 1) and late infantile (NCL 2) forms
G_{M1} gangliosidosis Autosomal recessive β-Galactosidase	Possibly	
Galactosialidosis Autosomal recessive β-Galactosidase and neuraminidase	Possibly	
G_{M2} gangliosidoses (Tay–Sachs, Sandhoff, G_{M2} activator deficiency) Autosomal recessive Tay–Sachs, β-hexosaminidase A Sanhoff, β-hexosaminidase A and β-hexosaminidase B G_{M2} activator deficiency, G_{M2} activator	No	Generally, too rapidly progressive, e.g. Tay–Sachs

CNS, central nervous system; PNS, peripheral nervous system.

function are often affected. Severe cognitive deficits with mental retardation are observed in Hurler syndrome (mucopolysaccharidosis [MPS] IH), the severe form of Hunter syndrome (MPS IIA), and Sanfilippo syndrome (MPS III). All of the mucopolysaccharidoses disorders, with the exception of the Hunter syndrome which is X-linked, are inherited in an autosomal recessive manner. While many mutations have been identified and found to be associated with a severe phenotype for the various mucopolysaccharidoses disorders, a precise correlation between all genotypes and phenotypes remains elusive. Enzyme assays are available for diagnosis, including prenatal evaluation, for all mucopolysaccharidoses disorders. Definitive identification of heterozygotes by enzyme determination is often not possible. Characterization of the mutation(s) within a family can be informative. In addition to naturally occurring disease models observed in dogs, cats, rats, mice and goats, there are mouse models created by targeted gene disruption. The biochemical and pathologic features of these "knockout" animal models can be similar to the human disease condition.

To date, HCT represents the only effective long-term therapy for selected mucopolysaccharidoses disorders. Mucopolysaccharidoses disorders that benefit from HCT include Hurler, Maroteaux–Lamy (MPS VI), and Sly (MPS VII) syndromes; unfortunately, unequivocal benefit particularly for the CNS or the skeletal system has not been shown for Hunter (MPS II), Sanfilippo (MPS III) and Morquio (MPS IV) syndromes.

Hurler syndrome (MPS IH)

Preclinical models

Naturally occurring preclinical models of MPS I include the dog and cat as well as the murine model generated by targeted disruption of the murine α-L-iduronidase (*IDUA*) gene [17]. In the Plott hound, HCT leads to normalization of tissue GAGs [18]. Despite low IDUA enzyme activity in the CNS, GAG is cleared from neurons and glial cells with decreased meningeal thickening [19,20]. Improvements in corneal clouding [21] and cardiac valvular thickening [22] were also noted. Compared to untransplanted littermates, skeletal abnormalities were ameliorated to some degree [23]. Detailed identification and characterization of the molecular lesion causing MPS I in cats has also been performed [24]. More recently, the development of the MPS I mouse by targeted disruption of the murine *IDUA* gene [25] has led to further insights into the pathogenesis of Hurler syndrome [26], particularly the skeletal and CNS manifestations. Analysis of the CNS revealed the novel finding of progressive neuronal loss in the cerebellum and increased levels of G_{M2} and G_{M3} gangliosides in brain tissue.

Clinical experience

Hurler syndrome represents the most severe phenotype of the three MPS I entities. A variety of approaches have been used to assess severity of the phenotype including genotyping, IDUA enzyme kinetics, immunoquantification, *in vitro* turnover studies [27], mutational analysis [28] and quantification of urinary GAGs [29]. While the *W402X* and *Q70X* mutations have been recognized as the most common mutations in MPS IH patients [30,31], numerous other mutations have been observed in patients with MPS IH, further underscoring the genetic and clinical heterogeneity of MPS I [32]. MPS IH is characterized by progressive mental retardation, hydrocephalus, frequent ear infections, rhinorrhea, auditory impairment, corneal clouding, sleep apnea [33,34], cardiopulmonary disease (including thickened valves, coronary artery narrowing, pulmonary hypertension and congestive heart failure) [35], hepatosplenomegaly and severe skeletal abnormalities, termed dysostosis multiplex [36]. These result in substantial morbidity and early death in untreated MPS IH patients yielding a median survival of 5 years with few children surviving beyond 12 years [37]. During the 2 decades since the first allogeneic HCT for MPS IH [38], over 300 MPS IH patients have been transplanted. Large HCT experiences with both unrelated [39], and related donors [40] have provided guidance for patient selection and timing of HCT and a realistic assessment of the effects of HCT on various organs and tissues in MPS IH. While it is difficult to provide a precise estimate of long-term engrafted survival for Hurler HCT patients, the likelihood is as high as 80% using bone marrow or umbilical cord blood [41,42]. When performed early in the disease course in conjunction with intensive speech therapy, HCT can preserve intellectual function and prevent the severe phenotypic manifestations associated with "classic" Hurler syndrome. The mechanism by which progressive mental retardation occurs in Hurler syndrome remains unclear; however, increasing atrophy and ventricular size on brain magnetic resonance imaging (MRI) appear to be associated with decreased ability to learn (E.G. Shapiro, personal communication). Generally, with successful HCT, children with MPS IH have not required ventriculoperitoneal shunting to treat hydrocephalus [43,44]. While age, cardiopulmonary and neurodevelopmental status are important determinants of outcome in Hurler patients following HCT, other contributing factors include quality and quantity of developmental services and therapies (e.g. speech therapy) as well as the number and severity of specific post-HCT complications such as GVHD, infections and organ toxicities [39,40,45]. HCT is able to preserve neurocognitive development in Hurler children with relatively normal intellectual function [29,46–48]. While a goal of first HCT is to achieve durable, full donor chimerism, in some cases this is not possible. Following related donor HCT, 30 out of 54 Hurler patients (56%) survived with donor-derived engraftment; engrafted survival was 75% for matched-sibling donor HCTs and 35% for other related donor HCTs [40]. Following unrelated donor HCT, 15 out of 40 Hurler patients (38%) survived with donor-derived engraftment [39]. While significant progress has been made over the past 5–10 years with respect to the safety of HCT and achieving full donor chimerism in Hurler patients, further investigation is needed. Nevertheless, if needed, a timely second HCT can be well-tolerated and beneficial in stabilizing neuropsychological function [49]. It has been shown that busulfan pharmacokinetics are not altered in children with inherited metabolic storage diseases, including Hurler syndrome, and that the rates of donor-derived engraftment are not different in these patients compared to children with other diseases [50]. There continues to be considerable discussion regarding the optimal stem cell source and IDUA enzyme activity level for HCT. While levels of IDUA can be measured in the white blood cells of marrow donors as well as in umbilical cord blood [51], the latter remains problematic since a satisfactory white blood cell sample from the umbilical cord blood unit is often not available to be analyzed in a timely manner. The nature of the preparative regimen including less intensive therapy has also being critically reviewed [52], as well as the use of haploidentical peripheral blood hematopoietic cells [53]. Centers, including the University of Minnesota caring for large numbers of high-risk Hurler patients based upon their age and/or cardiopulmonary status [54], have been examining the capability of reduced intensity regimens followed by umbilical cord blood or peripheral blood hematopoietic cell transplantation to achieve significant, stable long-term donor chimerism while minimizing regimen- and disease-related toxicities.

With successful donor-derived engraftment, Hurler patients can experience favorable long-term HCT outcomes. These outcomes include stabilization of the CNS with preservation of neurocognitive function and motor development within the range of normal and capacity for independence in activities of daily living. Careful neuropsychological and neuroradiologic assessments are required [55–57].

Hepatosplenomegaly, impaired joint mobility and upper airway obstruction with sleep apnea [58] resolve within months of the HCT; GAG disappears from hepatocytes and Kupffer cells [59]. Corneal clouding stabilizes or slowly resolves in many patients; ocular pressures may normalize; however, for many patients, electroretinogram abnormalities are evident long-term [60–62]. HCT does not reverse the progressive, profound conductive and sensorineural hearing abnormalities observed in many Hurler patients, although between 30% and 40% of children do show stabilized or improved auditory acuity after HCT [37]. Heart failure and tachyarrhythmias are corrected by 1 year after successful HCT [63,64]. Myocardial muscle function is stabilized or improved and coronary artery patency has been demonstrated up to 14 years after HCT [65]. The long-term outcome of cardiac valvular thickening and insufficiency require continued monitoring. However, some disease features show much poorer response due to poor penetration of IDUA into the relevant tissue. Principal among these are the skeletal abnormalities also known as dysostosis multiplex [66]. Successfully transplanted children often require major orthopedic surgical procedures for genu valgum, acetabular hip dysplasia, kyphoscoliosis, carpal tunnel syndrome and trigger digits by 6 years of age [67–70]. Interestingly, stabilization of the upper cervical spine has been observed in the long-term outcomes of many donor-engrafted Hurler patients [71]. However, severe spinal cord injury has been observed 6 years after successful HCT [72]. Orthopedic problems merit careful monitoring and appropriate, timely intervention, although the optimal timing of the latter remains under evaluation.

The decision of whether to proceed with HCT for patients with Hurler syndrome is a complex one. Factors include the child's neurocognitive developmental status with emphasis on the potential for growth, the presence or absence of hydrocephalus with or without a ventriculo-peritoneal shunt and a history of pulmonary and airway difficulties such as frequent pneumonias, chronic hypoxia, sleep apnea and cardiac failure. It is mandatory that a comprehensive pretransplant evaluation be performed and that detailed information be provided to families with particular attention to disease aspects that are typically refractory to HCT such as the skeletal abnormalities, some ocular and auditory features and cardiac aspects. Long-term, coordinated, comprehensive monitoring and follow-up together with close collaboration with educators and therapists (e.g. physical, occupational and speech) is paramount.

Hurler–Scheie and Scheie syndromes (MPS IH/S and MPS IS)

Hurler–Scheie syndrome demonstrates an intermediate phenotype betweez Hurler and Scheie syndromes with normal to mildly delayed neurocognitive development and survival beyond the 1st decade and often into the 3rd decade [17]. While there is no definitive animal model for MPS IH/S or MPS IS, it is felt that the IDUA-deficient dog is more consistent with MPS IH/S than MPS IH. HCT for this model has been discussed [18]. A 10-year-old child with MPS IH/S underwent HCT and demonstrated resolution of hepatosplenomegaly, amelioration of facial features, stabilization of cardiac function, improved joint range of motion, with persistent and progressive skeletal abnormalities, and unchanged corneal clouding though visual acuity improved. Neurocognitive function was preserved at the below average level [73]. While HCT can successfully treat MPS IH/S or MPS IS as well, such patients typically are treated with IDUA ERT [74].

Future directions for MPS I

Timely diagnosis of children with MPS I is uncommon. Through the development and implementation of newborn screening methods, timely diagnosis would be possible, although these efforts are in their infancy [75]. For some patients with MPS I (e.g. Hurler/Scheie and Scheie syndromes), long-term ERT may be an effective therapy [74,76,77]. A Hurler fibroblast cell line heterozygous for the *IDUA* stop mutations *Q70X* and *W402X* showed a significant increase in IDUA activity when cultured in the presence of gentamicin, resulting in the restoration of 2.8% of normal IDUA activity [78]. The clinical significance remains unclear; in the meantime, efforts continue toward gene therapy of Hurler syndrome [79–81]. It is not clear at this time what the degree of benefit of ERT will be for Hurler syndrome patients. Based upon large animal model experience there is no evidence that exogenous ERT will convey benefit directly to the CNS across the blood–brain barrier [17]. Symptomatic improvements, however, could be anticipated with ERT.

Hunter syndrome (MPS II)

There are two distinct clinical phenotypes of MPS II; the more common severe form presents before the age of 3 years with profound neurocognitive and developmental delay and shares clinical similarities with MPS IH, including facial dysmorphia, progressive conductive and sensorineural hearing loss, upper airway obstruction with sleep apnea, cardiopulmonary dysfunction, hepatosplenomegaly, joint stiffness and short stature. Dysostosis multiplex is less severe and corneal clouding is absent in Hunter syndrome. The attenuated form of MPS II is associated with less neurocognitive impairment and, in some cases, normal intelligence; survival can extend into the 5th and 6th decades in contrast with MPS IIA and its shortened life expectancy of 1–2 decades. While HCT seems to help patients with MPS IIA and B with respect to organomegaly, airway obstruction and cardiac function, boys with MPS IIA still have demonstrated profound neurocognitive disabilities despite early, successful HCT [55,82–87]. The failure of HCT to favorably alter the long-term neurocognitive outcome in MPS IIA suggests that enzyme is not being effectively delivered to essential components of the CNS. In cases of transplanted MPS IIB patients there have been somatic benefits and intellectual function has remained intact as expected based upon the natural history of the disorder. Ethical issues continue to arise in the face of limited somatic benefit and minimal to absent neurocognitive gains in patients with MPS IIB undergoing HCT [88].

Sanfilippo syndrome, types A, B, C, and D (MPS III)

Neurobehavioral manifestations are the hallmarks of all four types of MPS III. Characteristic findings include extreme hyperactivity, aggressive behaviors, attention deficits and progressive neurocognitive delay often associated with expressive language disabilities. As in MPS II, HCT is able to effectively treat the various somatic aspects of MPS III; however, the uniformly poor neurocognitive and developmental outcomes despite fully donor-engrafted marrow transplants performed early in the disease (Fig. 107.4) [55,89–92] has been attributed to the reduced efficiency in uptake of the MPS III-specific hydrolases and therefore diminished substrate clearance (Fig. 107.2) [93]. The Nubian goat model of MPS IIID is characterized by the development of neurologic complications in the neonatal period; however, HCT has not been evaluated in this animal model [94].

Morquio syndrome (MPS IV)

The two distinct biochemical forms of MPS IV have similar clinical features including severe dysostosis multiplex, dwarfism, atlantoaxial instability, short trunk and hyperextensible joints with ligamentous laxity. Corneal clouding is mild, hepatosplenomegaly moderate, cardiac abnormalities are unusual and intelligence is preserved [17]. HCT is unable to ameliorate the severe skeletal deformities. Therefore, this shortcoming of HCT and the MPS IV clinical features, make HCT a suboptimal intervention for this disease [95–97]. Recently, a mouse model of MPS IV developed through targeted mutagenesis of the *N*-acetylgalactosamine-6-sulfate sulfatase gene was reported [98]. No studies have been described as yet using this model.

Maroteaux–Lamy syndrome (MPS VI)

The principal clinical features of children with MPS VI are dysostosis multiplex with severe short stature, corneal clouding, pulmonary problems related to decreased intrathoracic volume and limited expansion due to hepatosplenomegaly, and cardiac valvular abnormalities [17]. While intelligence is felt to be preserved in this disorder, data from the University of Minnesota document neurocognitive deficits in some children with MPS VI [99]. HCT has been used successfully to treat MPS VI for 2 decades [100–102] with resolution of hepatosplenomegaly, airway obstruction and sleep apnea with the prevention of further cardiopulmonary deterioration, and improved joint mobility. Visual acuity improved in

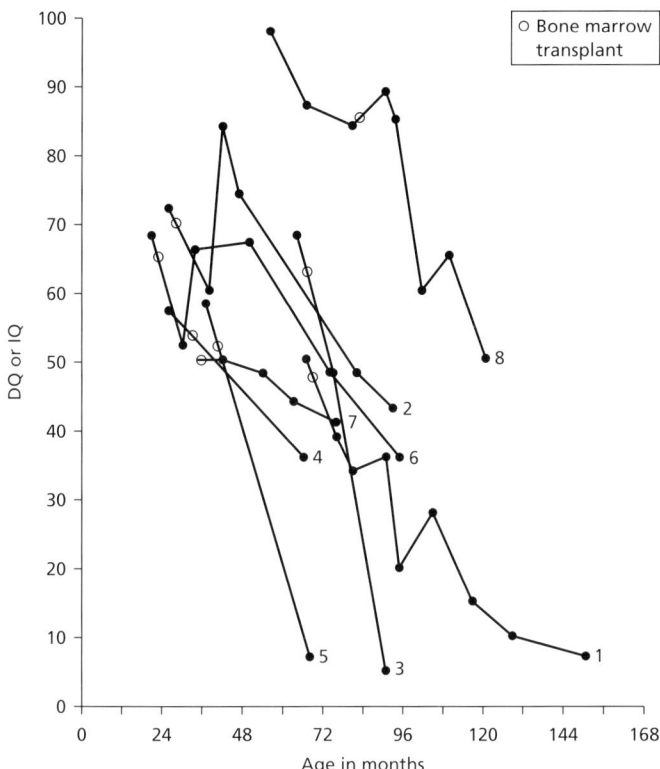

Fig. 107.4 Decline in intellectual function (developmental quotient or intelligence quotient) in eight children with mucopolysaccharidosis III (Sanfilippo syndrome). Reproduced with permission from Klein et al. [90].

some cases [85,100,101] though corneal haze did not necessarily resolve. As in other MPS disorders, HCT has not been able to treat effectively the skeletal abnormalities and consequently these successfully transplanted children still required orthopedic surgical interventions including medial femoral epiphyseal stapling for genu valgum and osteotomies of the femoral heads for acetabular hip dysplasia.

HCT leads to the resolution of corneal clouding and improved facies, gait, movement of the head and neck [103] and bone histopathology [104] in Siamese cats with MPS VI. The use of HCT in neonatal rats with MPS VI was associated with high peri-transplant mortality and does not treat the dysostosis multiplex [105]. Genetically manipulated mice with deficiency of arylsulfatase B have only a slight reduction in life span and maintain fertility; HCT has not been studied in this model.

Sly syndrome (MPS VII)

The use of HCT for MPS VII is limited by the rarity of the disorder and the predilection toward hydrops fetalis, although there are attenuated adult forms [17]. The neonatal form of MPS VII is one of the few lysosomal storage diseases with clinical manifestations *in utero* or at birth [106]. MPS VII, in certain circumstances, can be ameliorated by HCT provided that the neuropsychological and clinical status of the patient is good at the time of HCT [107]. In this case report, the 12-year-old MPS VII patient experienced major improvements in motor function and pulmonary function with diminished upper respiratory tract and middle ear infections leading to an improved quality of life.

The two preclinical models of MPS VII, the naturally occurring β-glucuronidase-deficient mouse and dog, have been studied extensively following HCT as well as ERT. HCT has led to an increased life span and correction of the metabolic defect [108] including a reduction in hearing loss [109]. Combined early ERT and HCT have been shown to convey long-term benefits [110]. Other therapeutic modalities tested included HCT and neural stem cell transplantation as well as a variety of viral-mediated gene therapies [111]. Due to the high mortality of early neonatal HCT using a myeloablative preparative regimen, nonmyeloablative regimens as well as multiple infusions of bone marrow have been tried with success in reducing bone pathology, GAG storage and improving both visceral organs and hematopoietic tissues [112]. In the canine MPS VII model, HCT led to improved echocardiographic findings as well as histopathologic and ultrastructural changes [113].

Cerebral X-linked adrenoleukodystrophy (cerebral X-ALD)

X-ALD is a peroxisomal disorder that predominantly affects males, although 40% or more of female heterozygous carrier exhibit mild to moderate signs of the disease. The minimum frequency of X-ALD in the USA is estimated to be 1/16,800 in the total population and 1/21,000 males [114]. In males, the clinical spectrum of X-ALD ranges from the rapidly progressive childhood or juvenile onset cerebral form (cerebral X-ALD), which typically leads to severe disability and death within 2–5 years from the onset of symptoms, to the milder adrenomyeloneuropathy (AMN), which usually manifests between 20 and 30 years of age, mainly affecting the spinal cord, and may allow survival into the 8th decade, to pure Addison's disease with its adrenal insufficiency [115,116]. X-ALD is characterized by impaired β-oxidation of VLCFA and reduced function of very long chain fatty acyl-CoA synthase. The principal biochemical abnormality is the accumulation of VLCFAs, particularly in brain and adrenal cortex. The *ALD* gene, identified in 1993 [116,117], is now referred to as *ABCD1* and codes for a peroxisomal membrane protein, termed ALD protein, which is a member of the adenosine triphosphate (ATP)-binding cassette transporter superfamily. Cerebral X-ALD is characterized by an inflammatory dysmyelinating process that appears to be immunologically mediated [118,119] with CD8 cytotoxic T cells operative in the early stages of dysmyelination during cytolysis of oligodendrocytes. Despite the X-linked inheritance pattern, the various phenotypes co-occur frequently within the same family or kindred. The illness does not manifest clinically before the age of 3 years. Biochemical or genetic studies can diagnose it at birth or prenatally; however, those tests do not permit phenotype prediction. Approximately 40% of boys with X-ALD will develop cerebral X-ALD during childhood or adolescence [120]. The importance of testing for X-ALD in all males in the pediatric age range with Addison's disease cannot be overstated [121]. Clinical manifestations of cerebral X-ALD depend upon the pattern and extent of dysmyelination. More than 80% of boys exhibit a parietal-occipital distribuation, approximately 15% will demonstrate predominantly frontal lobe lesions and <5% will have abnormality evident primarily in the fronto–pontine–corticospinal tracts [122]. Characteristic clinical features of these three patterns of dysmyelination are as follows:

(a) parieto–occipital–graphomotor, spatial perception and visual memory difficulties, visual agnosia ending in cortical blindness;

(b) frontal "acquired" attention deficit hyperactivity disorder-like presentation, behavioral disinhibition, verbal fluency problems, memory and new learning difficulties;

(c) fronto–pontine–corticospinal-corticospinal signs in the extremities.

A complete evaluation of a boy with cerebral X-ALD includes a thorough neurologic examination; comprehensive neuropsychological assessment with particular attention to the performance IQ, which is a sensitive indicator of deficits in visual perceptual and spatial processing, speed and efficiency of task completion and novel problem solving; and a MRI of the brain. Boys diagnosed with X-ALD due to a family history, merit careful, complete serial monitoring beginning at age 3 years and continuing into adolescence with the objective being to detect cerebral dysmyelination at an early stage and to intervene with HCT in a timely and presumably effective manner. To date, MRI scanning of the brain with gadolinium is the most effective tool to perform serial monitoring. It is strongly recommended that scans be performed at least every 6 months and more often if there is evidence of the earliest stages of dysmyelination. This is particularly relevant for boys under 10 years of age with X-ALD who have the highest risk for developing childhood onset rapidly progressive cerebral dysmyelination. However, under no circumstances should HCT be performed in the absence of cerebral disease.

Based upon the long-term outcomes of HCT for cerebral X-ALD, the worldwide HCT experience for this disease and knowledge of the natural history, the following guidelines can be promulagated:

1 The MRI severity score and gadolinium enhancement are highly predictive of the likelihood of disease progression, e.g. MRI severity score ≥3 and/or gadolinium enhancement in boys under 10 years of age is associated with approximately 90% likelihood of severe, progressive dysmyelination [123–126].

2 Boys with advanced disease manifested by low performance intelligence quotient (PIQ)—a very sensitive neuropsychological parameter for visual processing—i.e. PIQ <80, neurologic impairments and high MRI severity score (≥13) are poor candidates for HCT.

3 Boys with early stage cerebral X-ALD defined by a MRI score ≥3 and ≤7, typically without neurologic and neuropsychological abnormalities, are the best candidates for HCT.

The 5–10-year follow-up of 12 boys with cerebral X-ALD shows the long-term beneficial effect of HCT when HCT is done at an early stage of disease [125,127]. The likelihood of survival at 5 years following HCT for cerebral X-ALD from the worldwide experience of 124 transplanted patients was 58% (Fig. 107.5a); it was 67% following related-donor HCT and 51% after unrelated-donor HCT (Fig. 107.5b) [128]. Outcome measures included neuroradiologic assessment of dysmyelination, neurologic examination and neurocognitive testing, including verbal intelligence and performance (nonverbal) abilities. The typical boy with cerebral X-ALD has parietal-occipital dysmyelination and is diagnosed due to clinical symptomatology (i.e. not at an early stage of disease). He has relatively spared verbal intelligence, language and reading (if vision is intact), visual processing difficulties, neurologic impairments in one or more of the following areas—vision, hearing, speech and gait; and an MRI severity scores that is always >7 and often ≥13. The HCT- and disease-specific outcomes in these boys have been discouraging, with many dying of progressive X-ALD [122,123,129]. For survivors, there are permanent, severe neurologic and neuropsychologic sequelae; quality of life is compromised. As currently practiced, HCT has been of very limited benefit for these boys with advanced stage cerebral X-ALD.

Alternative therapies are under investigation and may shed light on the mechanism by which the cerebral dysmyelination process can be prevented, halted, or perhaps reversed. These therapies include Lorenzo's oil [130,131], immunosuppression, lovastatin [132], 4-phenylbutyrate [133] and coenzyme Q-10.

Globoid-cell leukodystrophy (GLD)

Globoid-cell leukodystrophy (GLD) is an autosomal recessive disorder. The severe, rapidly progressive infantile form of GLD (i.e. Krabbe disease) is the most common type with an incidence of 1/100,000 in the general population, although there is also a late-onset form of GLD that is 10-fold less common. Decreased ability to degrade galactolipids found almost exclusively in myelin leads to injury to the CNS and peripheral nervous system (PNS), the presence of globoid cells and decreased myelin stemming from the toxicity of psychosine and accumulation of galactosylceramide. Distinguishing early-onset from late-onset GLD is primarily a clinical assessment based upon the age of onset (i.e. <2 years or >2 years of age). A MRI of the brain is also able to distinguish early-

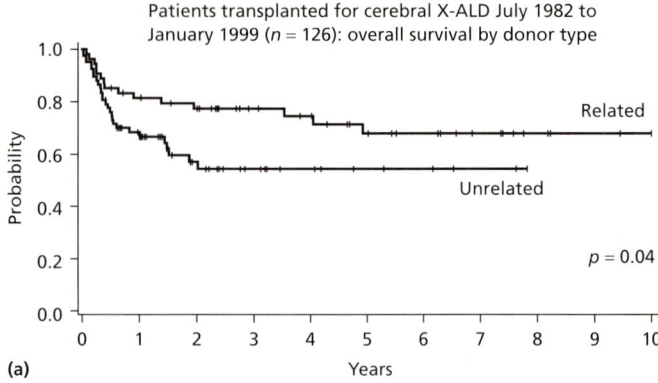

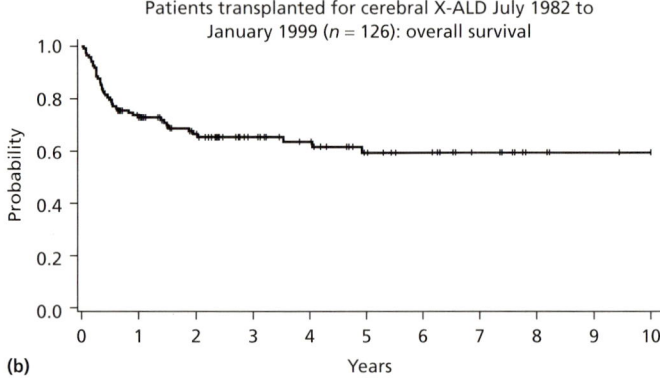

Fig. 107.5 Kaplan–Meier probability of survival following hematopoietic cell transplantation (HCT) for cerebral X-linked adrenoleukodystrophy (X-ALD). The likelihood of survival at 5 years following HCT for cerebral X-ALD from the worldwide experience of 126 transplanted patients was 58% (b); it was 67% following related donor HCT and 51% after unrelated donor HCT (a). Reproduced with permission from Peters *et al.* [128].

onset from late-onset disease, with the former characterized by cerebellar white matter involvement, deep gray matter involvement and cerebral atrophy [134]. Murine, canine and nonhuman primate models of GLD have been studied to better understand the pathophysiology of the disorder and its response to such treatment as HCT [135]. HCT has been studied extensively in the naturally occurring mouse model of GLD, namely the twitcher mouse [136] that most closely resembles human Krabbe disease [137]. HCT in the twitcher mouse leads to prolonged survival, clinical improvements, attenuation of hind limb paralysis, remyelination of peripheral nerves and the CNS, and stabilization of motor nerve conduction velocities in mice prior to onset of symptoms but not in symptomatic animals [138–142]. After HCT, enzyme is present in the CNS and non-neural tissues, and levels of psychosine are reduced in the CNS. Bone marrow transplantation has led to disappearance of globoid cells in the CNS; however, postnatal transplant was not curative for twitcher mice, primarily due to the fact that repopulation of the CNS and the PNS is not fast enough to stabilize and halt the rapidly progressive dysmyelination [143–146]. With appropriate timing and the use of HCT, GLD can be effectively treated in symptomatic late-onset cases leading to normalization of cerebrospinal fluid protein, stabilization of the neurologic examination, neuropsychologic function and the extent of dysmyelination on MRI [147]. However, to date, classic infantile-onset GLD, which is characterized by profound psychomotor retardation, failure to thrive, spasticity, seizures, optic atrophy and cortical blindness, if diagnosed antenatally, can only be ameliorated if HCT is performed in the neonatal period [147,148]. The late-onset forms are characterized by loss of vision, progressive spasticity of the lower extremities, neurocognitive decline, albeit in some cases very slowly, and localized neuropsychological deficits, gait disturbances, long-tract signs, extremity weakness, which can be asymmetric, and difficulties with coordination and balance. Persistence or progression of PNS abnormalities is expected despite successful HCT for late-onset GLD.

Metachromatic leukodystrophy (MLD)

MLD is an autosomal recessive inherited disorder of myelin metabolism characterized by accumulation of cerebroside sulfate in white matter of the CNS and PNS. MLD is one of the more common lysosomal storage disorders with an estimated incidence of 1/25,000–1/40,000 with a gene frequency of 0.5% [149,150]. Documentation of deficient leukocyte arylsulfatase A enzyme activity and elevation of urinary sulfatides are both needed to ensure an accurate diagnosis of MLD and to exclude the possibility of the pseudodeficiency state [151]. The arylsulfatase A pseudodeficiency allele is common in the general population with nearly 30% being carriers. Furthermore, in MLD kindreds, up to 15% of family members are heterozygous for the arylsulfatase A pseudodeficiency allele. MLD may have its onset at any age. The late infantile form is recognized in the 1st or 2nd year of life due to loss of motor milestones, abnormal speech and loss of neurocognitive skills culminating in dementia and death within several years, usually by the age of 10 years. HCT does not reverse or even stabilize dysmyelination in this rapidly progressive form of MLD when children are already symptomatic. Even in the few cases of presymptomatic HCT for late infantile MLD, the results have been disappointing, although cognitive but not motor function has been preserved in some patients. All children who were transplanted prior to the development of symptoms have since become wheelchair-bound and totally dependent in activities of daily living. Late-onset forms of MLD with disease manifesting during school age, adolescence or adulthood present with progressive motor signs and symptoms, including gait disturbance, clumsiness, tremor and dysarthria. Gradual decline in neurocognitive function is also observed. Neurocognitive and neurobehavioral symptoms predominate in those patients whose disease first manifests itself in the late teenage years or in early to middle adulthood. In fact, many such cases are misdiagnosed as schizophrenia or major psychosis. New onset attention deficit hyperactivity disorder in school age children is typical and they are often treated for years until mental decline is observed. Attention deficits, impulsive behavior, disinhibition, impulsivity, loss of spatial skills, memory loss and personality changes together with features of frontal lobe dysfunction often progress over years to decades. PNS disease is variably present. This indolent course in adult cases and the potential for intervening at an appropriate stage of disease for juvenile onset cases permits the effective use of HCT for these forms of MLD. HCT succeeds in stabilizing CNS disease and function while having little to no beneficial effect on the PNS [152–166].

Other leukodystrophies: Pelazeus–Merzbacher, Zellweger syndrome, vanishing white matter disease

To date, there has been neither experience with HCT nor a rationale developed for its use for the following leukodystrophies: Pelazeus–Merzbacher [167], Zellweger syndrome [168,169] and vanishing white matter disease [170,171].

Glycoprotein metabolic disorders

Fucosidosis

Fucosidosis, an autosomal recessive disorder, is characterized by, in severely affected patients, onset of psychomotor retardation in the 1st year of life, growth retardation, dysostosis multiplex and increased sweat chloride [172]. Detailed studies of a valid animal model for this disorder, namely the springer spaniel, include the use of HCT after total lymphoid irradiation to correct the enzymatic deficiency [173]. There is very limited experience with HCT in children with fucosidosis [174–176]. Due to disease variability, a definitive conclusion regarding the benefits of HCT cannot be reached at this time.

Gaucher disease, types 1, 2 and 3

Gaucher disease is an autosomal recessive lysosomal glycolipid storage disorder characterized by the accumulation of glucosylceramide [177]. Three clinical phenotypes of Gaucher disease have been identified based upon the presence and severity of neurological disease. Type 1, the most common with a prevalence of 1/40,000, is distinguished from types 2 and 3 disease by the absence of primary CNS involvement. Type 2, the acute neuronopathic form of Gaucher disease, has an early onset with severe CNS involvement and death usually occurs in the first 2 years of life. Type 3, subacute neuronopathic Gaucher disease, demonstrates neurologic manifestations of later onset and greater chronicity than those seen in type 2 Gaucher disease. Classically described as the Norrbottnian form of Gaucher disease from a northern region of Sweden, type 3 disease is associated with a life expectancy that extends into the 3rd–5th decades. Hepatosplenomegaly, bone lesions and, occasionally, involvement of lungs and other organs occur in all forms of Gaucher disease. Characteristic substrate-filled macrophages (i.e. Gaucher cells) are abundant in bone marrow. The quality of life of Gaucher patients can be improved by a variety of medical and surgical interventions including exogenous ERT, joint replacement and splenectomy. The accumulation of glucosylceramide and many of the associated clinical manifestations can be reversed by ongoing infusions of modified acid β-glucosidase (alglucerase). ERT has been used extensively and effectively in type 1 disease and to a lesser extent and with much less efficacy for type 2 and 3 patients. Issues of intravenous access and associated complications, patient comfort and lifestyle, as well as resources have led to a critical review of the risks and benefits of ERT. Infusions of alglucerase are effective in type 1 Gaucher disease and lead to regression of hepatosplenomegaly and normalization of hematologic parameters [178,179], although at a significant cost, depending upon patient weight and dosing schedule, that could prove prohibitive (e.g. from $380,000 to >$750,000/year) [180]. Furthermore, evidence is accumulating that some organs or tissues, such as the lungs, lymphoid tissue and the nervous system, derive little benefit from ERT. In fact, progressive dementia and myoclonic encephalopathy has been observed in type 3 Gaucher patients treated long-term with ERT [181]. HCT is effective in alleviating most disease manifestations of Gaucher including arresting further neuropsychological deterioration in type 3 (Norrbottnian) disease [182–186] and greatly reducing skeletal problems in severe early-onset type 1 disease [154,187–189]. HCT is not currently regarded as first line treatment due to the low morbidity of ERT [178,179]. This approach may change in type 3 disease as ERT results are scrutinized and if HCT techniques improve. The only indication for HCT is in type 3 Gaucher patients who deteriorate neurologically and/or have pulmonary compromise while receiving ERT [181].

α-Mannosidosis

α-Mannosidosis is an autosomal recessive lysosomal storage disease [190]. Defective glycoprotein degradation leads to excretion of mannose-rich oligosaccharides in urine and accumulation of oligosaccharides in various tissues, including CNS, liver and bone marrow. The infantile form of α-mannosidosis closely resembles Hurler syndrome and includes the onset of symptoms before the age of 12 months, macrocephaly, facial dysmorphia, hepatosplenomegaly, dysostosis multiplex, loss of previously acquired developmental skills and recurrent infections. There is progressive deterioration leading to early demise in the 1st or 2nd decade of life. Walkley et al. [191] demonstrated that HCT is effective in the feline model of mannosidosis. The first reported case of α-mannosidosis undergoing HCT was reported by Will and colleagues [192]. A subsequent successful case of HCT with long-term survival was reported by Wall et al. [193] with description of the resolution of sinopulmonary infections and organomegaly, improved dysostosis multiplex and stabilization of neurocognitive function. More recently, three surviving, fully engrafted patients with α-mannosidosis transplanted at the University of Minnesota were demonstrating a very good to excellent quality of life with preservation of normal neurocognitive and cardiopulmonary function [194]. α-mannosidosis patients have experienced pulmonary complications from 10 to 20 weeks after HCT. No infectious etiologies have been identified; it appears that selected storage disease patients are at increased risk for pulmonary complications including hemorrhage and/or bronchiolitis obliterans. This may be attributed to release of lysosomal storage material from damaged parenchymal cells following HCT and the resultant inflammatory response. Generally, patients transplanted early in their disease course prior to the onset of significant disease-related complications are the best candidates for HCT.

Aspartylglucosaminuria (AGU)

AGU is caused by deficiency of aspartylglucosaminuridase leading to interruption of the orderly breakdown of lysosomal glycoproteins [190]. As a consequence of abnormal glycoprotein catabolism, patients with AGU exhibit severe cell injury, especially in the CNS. The relatively uniform phenotype observed in AGU patients should make effective evaluation of treatment trials feasible. The medical center in Helsinki, Finland has experience with HCT in three patients with follow-up ranging from 1 to over 5 years including serial MRI, biochemical and clinical examinations [195]. Transplanted patients' MRIs of the brain with at least 2 years of follow-up showed nearly normal gray-white matter relationships, and improved neuropsychological function had also occurred [196]. However, more recently, longer-term follow-up has raised questions about the efficacy of HCT in these patients with respect to their ultimate neurodevelopmental outcomes [197].

Miscellaneous disorders

Neuronal ceroid lipofuscinosis (NCL)

Two forms of NCL, i.e. NCL 1 and 2, are recognized as true lysosomal enzyme storage disorders, implying that HCT might be effective therapy [198]. However, this has not been borne out by presymptomatic patients with NCL 2 who have been transplanted or by the existing animal model studies [199–202]. Additional clinical experience is needed to determine whether the natural history of NCL 2 is too rapidly progressive for HCT to be beneficial.

Niemann–Pick disease, types A, B, and C

Niemann–Pick disease types A and B are lysosomal storage disorders resulting from deficient acid sphingomyelinase enzyme activity [203]. Niemann–Pick type A is a rapidly progressive disorder of infancy characterized by failure to thrive, hepatosplenomegaly, neurodegeneration and death, often by 2–3 years of age. HCT has not been effective in preventing the inexorable neurodevelopmental decline [204]. Niemann–Pick type B is a phenotypically variable disorder that is usually diagnosed in childhood due to marked hepatosplenomegaly. HCT appears to effectively treat the somatic manifestations of Niemann–Pick type B disease [205].

Niemann–Pick disease type C is an autosomal recessive lipidosis resulting from an unique error in cellular trafficking of exogenous cholesterol and is associated with lysosomal accumulation of unesterified cholesterol [206]. A case has been reported of a 3-year-old girl with Niemann–Pick type C disease who underwent allogeneic HLA-identical sibling donor bone marrow transplantation that engrafted. She survived with improvement in somatic disease features including hepatosplenomegaly, marrow and lung infiltration; however, her neurological status continued to deteriorate [207]. It is therefore unclear at this time whether HCT has a role in the effective treatment of the CNS in Niemann–Pick disease type C.

Mucolipidosis, type II (I-cell disease)

Mucolipidosis type II or I-cell disease is an autosomal recessive disorder characterized by severe, progressive psychomotor retardation and by many of the clinical features and radiologic features observed in Hurler syndrome such as facial dysmorphia, severe skeletal abnormalities, hernias, gingival hyperplasia, corneal haze, cardiac abnormalities and frequent respiratory tract infections. Important differences exist however. I-cell disease patients do not demonstrate mucopolysacchariduria and the deficient enzyme is a phosphotransferase that is responsible for the targeting of lysosomal enzymes to lysosomes [208]. Historical experience with HCT for this disorder existed initially only in patients with end-stage cardiopulmonary disease [85,209,210]. Over the past 5 years, three patients ranging in age from 0.3 to 1.7 years have been transplanted at the University of Minnesota, all are alive and fully donor-engrafted and making developmental progress, albeit at slower than normal rates [194]. Good cardiopulmonary function has been observed in two of the three patients; the third has developed pulmonary hypertension.

Gangliosidoses: G_{M2} (Tay–Sachs, Sandhoff, G_{M2} activator deficiency) and G_{M1}

The G_{M2} gangliosidoses are a group of inherited disorders caused by excessive accumulation of ganglioside G_{M2} and related glycolipids in lysosomes, especially in neurons [211]. With infantile onset, the rapidly progressive neurodegenerative disease leads to death by 4 years (classic Tay–Sachs, Sandhoff, and G_{M2} activator deficiency), while later onset subacute or chronic forms show more slowly progressive neurologic conditions compatible with survival into late childhood, adolescence, or even adulthood. HCT does not appear to successfully correct these disorders; however, future therapy that combines a direct CNS intervention with systemic therapy such as HCT may prove beneficial for these disorders [44,211]. Deficiency of lysosomal β-galactosidase is manifested clinically as two different diseases, G_{M1} gangliosidosis and Morquio B (MPS IVB, discussed previously) [212]. G_{M1} gangliosidosis can have its onset in infancy, childhood/adolescence, or adulthood. The clinical course is generally of progressive neurologic deterioration. The role of HCT for G_{M1} gangliosidosis remains unclear since most cases are too advanced at time of diagnosis for benefit to be derived from HCT. HCT may be helpful in later onset cases at an early stage of the disease process.

Wolman syndrome

Wolman syndrome is an autosomal recessive disorder due to deficient enzyme activity of acid lipase resulting in massive accumulation of cholesteryl esters and triglycerides in most body tissues [213]. The disease occurs in infancy and is typically fatal in the 1st year of life. HCT has been performed in a small number of Wolman patients. A patient who underwent HCT in 1996 at the University of Minnesota has become a long-term survivor [214].

Farber disease

Infantile ceramidase deficiency (Farber disease) is a rare, progressive lysosomal storage disorder characterized by lipogranulomata in subcutaneous tissues, painful periarticular swelling, psychomotor retardation and varying degrees of organ involvement of the eyes, lungs and liver [215]. Depending on the presence and degree of CNS involvement, Farber disease patients are classified into three subtypes. Patients with types 2 and 3 have little, if any, CNS manifestations. In selected type 2/3 cases, particularly those treated early, HCT may be effective [216,217].

Novel, developing therapies and future directions: ERT, substrate depletion, alternative stem cell and gene therapy

Alternative and complementary therapies to HCT for these inherited metabolic storage disorders are either in place or being developed. ERT has been available for patients with Gaucher disease type 1 for over a decade [218]. More recently, enzyme replacement has been making the transition from clinical trial to proven therapy for Fabry, Pompe, Niemann–Pick type B and selected mucopolysaccharidoses including MPS I, II and VI. In the case of Fabry disease, ERT produced a reduction of severe neuropathic pain, stabilization of renal disease, and improved vascular function and structure [219]. In Pompe disease, a fatal cardiac and skeletal muscle disorder due to acid maltase deficiency, ERT has improved cardiac function and structure and increased overall muscle strength [219–221]. Important lessons from these experiences include the variability of the clinical response to ERT depending upon the disease, the organ or tissue, the dose of enzyme and the schedule of administration. Of particular importance is the observation that there is limited-to-no penetration of exogenous, intravenous enzyme into the nervous system. In the area of substrate depletion or deprivation, a number of disorders have been investigated including Gaucher, G_{M2}, Fabry and cystinosis. Drugs that slow the rate of formation of accumulating glycolipids are being developed. One such agent is N-butyldeoxynojirimycin (OGS-918) and is showing promise in Gaucher disease patients. While benefits have been observed in these various disorders, the extent of amelioration has been limited in both degree and scope.

Alternative stem cells, including both embryonic and adult stem cells, are under investigation for both transplantation and gene transfer/therapy protocols. This is important in light of the observation that bone marrow-derived mesenchymal stem cells remain host-derived despite successful hematopoietic engraftment after allogeneic transplantation in patients with lysosomal and peroxisomal storage diseases [222]. Verfaillie and colleagues have identified a class of cells which they have termed multipotent adult progenitor cells in postnatal human and rodent bone marrow that copurify with mesenchymal stem cells [223]. These cells are recovered from bone marrow mononuclear cells depleted of $CD45^+$ and glycophorin A^+ cells. Differentiation potential has included osteoblasts, chondrocytes, adipocytes, stroma cells, skeletal myoblasts and endothelial cells [224]. Further studies have demonstrated that the multipotent adult progenitor cell is a progenitor of angioblasts with subsequent differentiation into cells that express endothelial cell markers [225]. There is evidence that human postnatal bone marrow stem cells exhibit neural phenotypes, including expression of astrocyte, oligodendrocyte and neuronal markers [226]. Differentiation into functional hepatocyte-like cells has been observed as well [227]. Verfaillie and colleagues [228] also report that multipotent adult progenitor cells differentiate at the single cell level, not only into mesenchymal cells, but also into cells with visceral mesoderm, neuroectoderm and endoderm characteristics *in vitro*.

The scope of gene transfer applications in therapy for human diseases has expanded greatly over the past 15 years and includes the genetic storage diseases. Hematopoietic stem cells have been considered to be excellent targets for therapeutic gene transfer due to their ability to self-renew as well as differentiate into multiple cell lineages. The storage diseases such as Gaucher disease, Hurler syndrome, MLD and other enzyme deficiency states may be amenable to treatment by gene transfer into hematopoietic stem cells due to enzyme production, release and uptake leading to metabolic cross-correction [229].

References

1 Fratantoni JC, Hall CW, Neufeld EF. The defect in Hurler and Hunter syndromes. II. Deficiency of specific factors involved in mucopolysaccharide degradation. *Proc Natl Acad Sci U S A* 1969; **64**: 360–6.

2 Neufeld EF. Lysosomal storage diseases. *Annu Rev Biochem* 1991; **60**: 257–80.

3 Bou-Gharios G, Abraham D, Olsen I. Lysosomal storage diseases. Mechanisms of enzyme replacement therapy. *Histochem J* 1993; **25**: 593–605.

4 Chao HH-J, Waheed A, Pohlmann R, Hille A, von Figura K. Mannose-6-phosphate receptor dependent secretion of lysosomal enzymes. *EMBO J* 1990; **9**: 3507–13.

5 Pfeffer SR. Targeting of proteins to the lysosome. *Curr Top Microbiol Immunol* 1991; **170**: 43–65.

6 Rodman JS, Mercer RW, Stahl PD. Endocytosis and trancytosis. *Curr Opin Cell Biol* 1990; **2**: 664–72.

7 Jenkins HG, Martin J, Dean MF. Receptor-mediated uptake of β-glucuronidase into primary astrocytes and C6 glioma cells from rat brain. *Brain Res* 1988; **462**: 265–74.

8 Olsen I, Dean MF, Harris G, Muir H. Direct transfer of a lysosomal enzyme from lymphoid cells to deficient fibroblasts. *Nature* 1981; **291**: 244–7.

9 Olsen I, Oliver T, Muir H, Smith R, Partridge T. Role of cell adhesion in contact-dependent transfer of a lysosomal enzyme from lymphocytes to fibroblasts. *J Cell Sci* 1986; **85**: 231–44.

10 Perry VH, Gordon S. Macrophages and the nervous system. *Int Rev Cytol* 1991; **125**: 203–44.

11 Krivit W, Sung JH, Shapiro EG, Lockman LA. Microglia: the effector cell for resonstitution of the central nervous system following bone marrow transplantation for lysosomal and peroxisomal storage diseases. *Cell Transplant* 1995; **4**: 385–92.

12 Giulian D. Ameboid microglia as effectors of inflammation in the central nervous system. *J Neurosci Res* 1987; **18**: 155–71.

13 Hickey WF. Migration of hematogenous cells through the blood–brain barrier and the initiation of CNS inflammation. *Brain Pathol* 1991; **1**: 97–105.

14 Kennedy DW, Abkowitz JL. Kinetics of central nervous system microglial and macrophage engraftment: analysis using a transgenic bone marrow transplantation model. *Blood* 1997; **90**: 986–93.

15 Yeager AM, Shinn C, Hart C, Pardoll DM. Repopulation by donor-derived macrophages in the murine central nervous system (CNS) after congenic bone marrow transplantation (BMT): a quantitative study. *Blood* 1992; **80** (Suppl. 1): 269a [Abstract].

16 Yeager AM. Hematopoietic cell transplantation for storage diseases. In: Thomas ED, Blume KG, Forman SJ, eds. *Hematopoietic Cell Transplantation*, 2nd edn. Malden, MA: Blackwell Science, 1999: 1183–4.

17 Neufeld EF, Muenzer J. The mucopolysaccharidoses. In: Scriver CR, Beaudet AL, Sly WS, Valle D, eds. *The Metabolic and Molecular Bases of Inherited Disease*, 8th edn. New York: McGraw-Hill, 2001: 3421–52.

18 Brieder MA, Shull RM, Constantopoulos G. Long-term effects of bone marrow transplantation in dogs with mucopolysaccharidosis I. *Am J Pathol* 1989; **134**: 677–92.

19 Shull RM, Hastings NE, Selcer RE et al. Bone marrow transplantation in canine mucopolysaccharidosis I. Effects within the central nervous system. *J Clin Invest* 1987; **79**: 435–43.

20 Shull RM, Brieder MA, Constantopoulos G. Long-term neurological effects of bone marrow transplantation in a canine lysosomal storage disease model. *Pediatr Res* 1988; **24**: 347–52.

21 Constantopoulos G, Scott JA, Shull RM. Corneal opacity in canine MPS I. Changes after bone mar-

22 Gompf RE, Shull RM, Brieder MA, Scott JA, Constantopoulos GC. Cardiovascular changes after bone marrow transplantation in dogs with mucopolysaccharidosis I. *Am J Vet Res* 1990; **51**: 2054–60.

23 Shull RM, Walker MA. Radiographic findings in a canine model of mucopolysaccharidosis I. Changes associated with bone marrow transplantation. *Invest Radiol* 1988; **23**: 124–30.

24 He X, Li CM, Simonaro CM et al. Identification and characterization of the molecular lesion causing mucopolysaccharidosis type I in cats. *Mol Genet Metab* 1999; **67**: 106–12.

25 Clarke LA, Russell CS, Pownall S et al. Murine mucopolysaccharidosis type I targeted disruption of the murine α-L-iduronidase gene. *Hum Mol Genet* 1997; **6**: 503–11.

26 Russell C, Hendson G, Jevon G et al. Murine MPS I insights into the pathogenesis of Hurler syndrome. *Clin Genet* 1998; **53**: 349–61.

27 Bunge S, Clements PR, Byers S, Kleijer WJ, Brooks DA, Hopwood JJ. Genotype-phenotype correlations in mucopolysaccharidosis type I using enzyme kinetics, immunoquantitation and *in vitro* turnover studies. *Biochim Biophys Acta* 1998; **1407**: 249–56.

28 Beesley CE, Meaney CA, Greenland G et al. Mutational analysis of 85 mucopolysaccharidosis type I families: frequency of known mutations, identification of 17 novel mutations and *in vitro* expression of missense mutations. *Hum Genet* 2001; **109**: 503–11.

29 Guffon N, Souillet G, Maire I et al. Follow-up of nine patients with Hurler syndrome after bone marrow transplantation. *J Pediatr* 1998; **133**: 119–25.

30 Scott HS, Bunge S, Gal A, Clarke LA, Hopwood JJ. Molecular genetics of mucopolysaccharidosis type I. Diagnostic, clinical and biological implications. *Hum Mutat* 1995; **6**: 288–302.

31 Whitley CB, Krivit W, Ramsay NKC et al. Mutation analysis and clinical outcome of patients with Hurler syndrome (mucopolysaccharidosis type I-H) undergoing bone marrow transplantation. *Am J Hum Genet* 1993; **53** (Suppl.): 101a [Abstract].

32 Beck M. Variable clinical presentation in lysosomal storage disorders. *J Inherit Metab Dis* 2001; **24** (Suppl. 2): 47–51.

33 Leighton SE, Papsin B, Vellodi A, Dinwiddie R, Lane R. Disordered breathing during sleep in patients with mucopolysaccharidoses. *Int J Pediatr Otorhinolaryngol* 2001; **58**: 127–38.

34 Shih SL, Lee YJ, Sheu CY, Blickman JG. Airway changes in children with mucopolysaccharidoses. *Acta Radiol* 2002; **43**: 40–3.

35 Dangel JH. Cardiovascular changes in children with mucopolysaccharide storage diseases and related disorders, clinical and echocardiographic findings in 64 patients. *Eur J Pediatr* 1998; **157**: 534–8.

36 Peters C, Steward CG. Hematopoietic cell transplantation for inherited metabolic diseases. An overview of outcomes and practice guidelines. *Bone Marrow Transplant* 2003; **31**: 229–39.

37 Krivit W, Lockman LA, Watkins PA, Hirsch J, Shapiro EG. The future for treatment by bone marrow transplantation for adrenoleukodystrophy, metachromatic leukodystrophy, globoid cell leukodystrophy, and Hurler syndrome. *J Inherit Metab Dis* 1995; **18**: 398–412.

38 Hobbs JR, Hugh-Jones K, Barrett AJ et al. Reversal of clinical features of Hurler's disease and biochemical improvement after treatment by bone-marrow transplantation. *Lancet* 1981; **2**: 709–12.

39 Peters C, Balthazor M, Shapiro EG et al. Outcome of unrelated donor bone marrow transplantation in 40 children with Hurler syndrome. *Blood* 1996; **87**: 4894–902.

40 Peters C, Shapiro EG, Anderson J et al. Hurler syndrome. II. Outcome of HLA-genotypically identical sibling and HLA-haploidentical related donor bone marrow transplantation in fifty-four children. The Storage Disease Collaborative Study Group. *Blood* 1998; **91**: 2601–8.

41 Peters C, Orchard PJ, Defor TE et al. Hematopoietic cell transplantation for Hurler syndrome: the University of Minnesota experience from 1983 to 2001 *Blood* 2001; **98**: 667a [Abstract].

42 Staba S, Martin PL, Ciocci GH, Allison-Thacker J, Kurtzberg J. Correction of Hurler syndrome with unrelated umbilical cord blood transplantation. *Blood* 2001; **98**: 667a [Abstract].

43 Whitley CB, Belani KG, Chang PN et al. Long-term outcome of Hurler syndrome following bone marrow transplantation. *Am J Hum Genet* 1993; **46**: 209–18.

44 Krivit W, Sung JH, Lockman L et al. Bone marrow transplantation for the treatment of lysosomal and peroxisomal diseases: focus on central nervous system reconstitution. In: Rich RR, Fleisher TA, Schwartz BD, eds. *Principles of Clinical Immunology*. St Louis: Mosby, 1995: 1852–64.

45 Phipps S, Mulhern R. Developmental outcome of unrelated donor bone marrow transplantation in children with Hurler syndrome. *Blood* 1997; **89**: 732–4.

46 Peters C, Shapiro EG, Krivit W. Hurler syndrome. Past, present, and future. *J Pediatr* 1998; **133**: 7–9.

47 Fleming DR, Henslee-Downey PJ, Ciocci G et al. The use of partially HLA-mismatched donors for allogeneic transplantation in patients with mucopolysaccharidosis-I. *Pediatr Transplant* 1998; **2**: 299–304.

48 Peters C, Shapiro EG, Krivit W. Neuropsychological development in children with Hurler syndrome following hematopoietic stem cell transplantation. *Pediatr Transplant* 1998; **2**: 250–4.

49 Grewal SS, Krivit W, Defor TE et al. Outcome of second hematopoietic cell transplantation in Hurler syndrome. *Bone Marrow Transplant* 2002; **29**: 491–6.

50 Jacobson P, Park JJ, DeFor TE et al. Oral busulfan pharmacokinetics and engraftment in children with Hurler syndrome and other inherited metabolic storage diseases undergoing hematopoietic cell transplantation. *Bone Marrow Transplant* 2001; **27**: 855–61.

51 deGasperi R, Raghavan SS, Sosa MG et al. Measurements from normal umbilical cord blood of four lysosomal enzymatic activities: α-L-iduronidase (Hurler), galactocerebrosidase (globoid cell leukodystrophy), arylsulfatase A (metachromatic leukodystrophy), arylsulfatase B (Maroteaux–Lamy). *Bone Marrow Transplant* 2000; **25**: 541–4.

52 Rosales F, Peylan-Ramu N, Cividalli G et al. The role of thiotepa in allogeneic bone marrow transplantation for genetic diseases. *Bone Marrow Transplant* 1999; **23**: 861–5.

53 Kapelushnik J, Mandel H, Varadi G, Nagler A. Fludarabine-based protocol for haploidentical peripheral blood stem cell transplantation in Hurler syndrome. *J Pediatr Hematol Oncol* 2000; **22**: 433–6.

54 Drew B, Peters C, Rimell F. Upper airway complications in children after bone marrow transplantation. *Laryngoscope* 2000; **110**: 1446–51.

55 Shapiro EG, Lockman LA, Balthazor M, Krivit W. Neuropsychological outcomes of several storage diseases with and without bone marrow transplantation. *J Inherit Metab Dis* 1995; **18**: 413–29.

56 Blaser SI, Clarke JTR, Becker LE. Neuroradiology of lysosomal disorders. *Neuroimaging Clin N Am* 1994; **4**: 283–98.

57 Takahashi Y, Sukegawa K, Aoki M et al. Evaluation of accumulated mucopolysaccharides in the brain of patients with mucopolysaccharidosis by ^{1}H-magnetic resonance spectroscopy before and after bone marrow transplantation. *Pediatr Res* 2001; **49**: 349–55.

58 Malone BN, Whitley CB, Duvall AJ et al. Resolution of obstructive sleep apnea in Hurler syndrome after bone marrow transplantation. *Int J Pediatr Otorhinolaryngol* 1988; **15**: 23–31.

59 Resnick JM, Krivit W, Snover DC et al. Pathology of the liver in mucopolysaccharidosis: light and electron microscopic assessment before and after bone marrow transplantation. *Bone Marrow Transplant* 1992; **10**: 273–80.

60 Summers CG, Purple RL, Krivit W et al. Ocular changes in the mucopolysaccharidoses after bone marrow transplantation. A preliminary report. *Ophthalmology* 1989; **96**: 977–84.

61 Christiansen SP, Smith TJ, Henslee-Downey PJ. Normal intraocular pressure after a bone marrow transplant in glaucoma associated with mucopolysaccharidosis type I-H. *Am J Ophthalmol* 1990; **109**: 230–1.

62 Gullingsrud EO, Krivit W, Summers CG. Ocular abnormalities in the mucopolysaccharidoses after bone marrow transplantation. *Ophthalmology* 1998; **105**: 1099–105.

63 Braunlin EA, Hunter DW, Krivit W et al. Evaluation of coronary artery disease in the Hurler syndrome by angiography. *Am J Cardiol* 1992; **69**: 1487–9.

64 du Cret RP, Weinberg EJ, Jackson CA et al. Resting Tl-201 scintigraphy in the evaluation of coronary artery disease in children with Hurler syndrome. *Clin Nucl Med* 1994; **19**: 975–8.

65 Braunlin EA, Rose AG, Hopwood JJ et al. Coronary artery patency following long-term successful engraftment 14 years after bone marrow transplantation in the Hurler syndrome. *Am J Cardiol* 2001; **88**: 1075–7.

66 Field RE, Buchanan JA, Copplemans MG et al. Bone-marrow transplantation in Hurler's syndrome. Effect on skeletal development. *J Bone Joint Surg Br* 1994; **76**: 975–81.

67 Masterson EL, Murphy PG, O'Meara A et al. Hip dysplasia in Hurler's syndrome: orthopaedic management after bone marrow transplantation. *J Pediatr Orthop* 1996; **16**: 731–3.

68 Odunusi E, Peters C, Krivit W et al. Genu valgum deformity in Hurler syndrome after hematopoietic stem cell transplantation: correction by surgical intervention. *J Pediatr Orthop* 1999; **19**: 270–4.

69 Van Heest AE, House J, Krivit W et al. Surgical treatment of carpal tunnel syndrome and trigger digits in children with mucopolysaccharide storage disorders. *J Hand Surg Am* 1998; **23**: 236–43.

70 Krivit W, Shapiro EG, Balthazor M. Hurler syndrome. Outcomes and planning following bone marrow transplantation. In: Steward C, Hobbs JR, eds. *Correction of Genetic Diseases by Transplantation (COGENT)*, 3rd edn. London: COGENT Press, 1995: 25–40.

71. Hite S, Peters C, Krivit W. Correction of odontoid dysplasia following bone marrow transplantation and engraftment in Hurler syndrome (MPS 1H). *Pediatr Radiol* 2000; **30**: 464–70.
72. Kachur E, Del Maestro R. Mucopolysaccharidoses and apinal cord compression: case report and review of the literature with implications of bone marrow transplantation. *Neurosurgery* 2000; **47**: 223–8.
73. Navarro C, Dominguez C, Costa M, Ortega JJ. Bone marrow transplant in a case of mucopolysaccharidosis I Scheie phenotype: skin ultrastructure before and after transplantation. *Acta Neuropathol* 1991; **82**: 33–8.
74. Kakkis ED, Muenzer J, Tiller GE et al. Enzyme-replacement therapy in mucopolysaccharidosis I. *N Engl J Med* 2001; **344**: 182–8.
75. Chamoles NA, Blanco MB, Gaggioli D, Casentini C. Hurler-like phenotype. Enzymatic diagnosis in dried blood spots on filter paper. *Clin Chem* 2001; **47**: 2098–102.
76. Zhaol KW, Faull KF, Kakkis ED, Neufeld EF. Carbohydrate structures of recombinant human α-L-iduronidase secreted by Chinese hamster ovary cells. *J Biol Chem* 1997; **272**: 22,758–65.
77. Wraith JE. Enzyme replacement therapy in mucopolysaccharidosis type I. Progress and emerging difficulties. *J Inherit Metab Dis* 2001; **24**: 245–50.
78. Keeling KM, Brooks DA, Hopwood JJ, Li P, Thompson JN, Bedwell DM. Gentamicin-mediated suppression of Hurler syndrome stop mutations restores a low level of α-L-iduronidase activity and reduces lysosomal glycosaminoglycan accumulation. *Hum Mol Genet* 2001; **10**: 291–9.
79. Fairbairn LJ, Lashford LS, Spooncer E et al. Towards gene therapy of Hurler syndrome. *Cas Lek Cesk* 1997; **136**: 27–31.
80. Huang MM, Wong AYuX, Kakkis E, Kohn DB. Retrovirus-mediated transfer of the human α-L-iduronidase cDNA into human hematopoietic progenitor cells leads to correction in trans of Hurler fibroblasts. *Gene Ther* 1997; **4**: 1150–9.
81. Baxter MA, Wynn RF, Deakin JA et al. Retrovirally mediated correction of bone marrow-derived mesenchymal stem cells from patients with mucopolysaccharidosis type I. *Blood* 2002; **99**: 1857–9.
82. Warkentin PI, Dixon MS, Schafer I, Strandjord SE, Coccia PF. Bone marrow transplantation in Hunter syndrome: a preliminary report. *Birth Defects Orig Artic Ser* 1986; **22**: 31–9.
83. Bergstrom SK, Quinn JJ, Greenstein R, Ascensao J. Long-term follow-up of a patient transplanted for Hunter's disease type IIB. A case report and literature review. *Bone Marrow Transplant* 1994; **14**: 653–8.
84. Coppa GV, Gabrielli O, Zampini L et al. Bone marrow transplantation in Hunter syndrome. *J Inherit Metab Dis* 1995; **18**: 91–2.
85. Imaizumi M, Gushi K, Kurobane I et al. Long-term effects of bone marrow transplantation for inborn errors of metabolism: a study of four patients with lysosomal storage disorders. *Acta Paediatr Jpn* 1994; **36**: 30–6.
86. McKinnis EJ, Sulzbacher S, Rutledge JC, Sanders J, Scott CR. Bone marrow transplantation in Hunter syndrome. *J Pediatr* 1996; **129**: 145–8.
87. Vellodi A, Young E, Cooper A, Lidchi V, Winchester B, Wraith JE. Long-term follow-up following bone marrow transplantation for Hunter disease. *J Inherit Metab Dis* 1999; **22**: 638–48.
88. Peters C, Krivit W. Hematopoietic cell transplantation for mucopolysaccharidosis IIB (Hunter syndrome): an ethical commentary. *Bone Marrow Transplant* 2000; **25**: 1097–9.
89. Bordigoni P, Vidalilbet M, Lena M, Maire I, Gelot S. Bone marrow transplantation for Sanfilippo syndrome. In: Hobbs JR, ed. *Correction of Certain Genetic Diseases by Transplantation*. London: COGENT Press, 1989: 114–9.
90. Klein KA, Krivit W, Whitley CB et al. Poor cognitive outcome of eleven children with Sanfilippo syndrome after bone marrow transplantation and successful engraftment. *Bone Marrow Transplant* 1995; **15** (Suppl. 1): S176–81.
91. Vellodi A, Young E, New M, Pot-Mees C, Hugh-Jones K. Bone marrow transplantation for Sanfilippo disease type B. *J Inherit Metab Dis* 1992; **15**: 911–8.
92. Gungor N, Tuncbilek E. Sanfilippo disease type B. A case report and review of the literature on recent advances in bone marrow transplantation. *Turk J Pediatr* 1995; **37**: 157–63.
93. O'Brien JS, Miller AI, Loverde AW, Veath ML. Sanfilippo disease type B. Enzyme replacement and metabolic correction in cultured fibroblasts. *Science* 1973; **181**: 753–5.
94. Thompson JN, Jones MZ, Dawson G, Huffman PS. N-acetylglucosamine 6-sulfatase deficiency in a Nubian goat. A model of Sanfilippo syndrome type D (mucopolysaccharidosis IIID). *J Inherit Metab Dis* 1992; **15**: 760–8.
95. Kato S, Kubota C, Yabe H et al. Bone marrow transplantation in Morquio's disease. In: Hobbs JR, ed. *Correction of Certain Genetic Diseases by Transplantation*. London: COGENT Press, 1989: 120–6.
96. Desai S, Hobbs JR, Hugh-Jones K et al. Morquio's disease (mucopolysaccharidosis type IV) treated by bone marrow transplant. *Exp Hematol* 1983; **2** (Suppl. 13): 98–100.
97. Kato S, Yabe H, Yabe M et al. Bone marrow transplantation in children. *Tokai J Exp Clin Med* 1986; **11** (Suppl.): 43–7.
98. Tomatsu S, Orii KO, Vogler C et al. Mouse model of Morquio A syndrome produced by targeted mutagenesis. Seventh International Symposium on MPS and Related Disorders, 2002: 37.
99. Delaney K, Gray R, Charnas L, Peters C, Abel S, Shapiro EG. Neuropsychological characteristics of MPS VI with and without treatment. Thirtieth Annual Meeting of the International Neuropsychological Society, 2002.
100. Krivit W, Pierpont ME, Ayaz K et al. Bone marrow transplantation in the Maroteaux–Lamy syndrome (mucopolysaccharidosis type VI). Biochemical and clinical status 24 months after transplantation. *N Engl J Med* 1984; **311**: 1606–11.
101. Krivit W. Maroteaux–Lamy syndrome. Treatment by allogeneic bone marrow transplantation in six patients and potential for autotransplantation bone marrow gene insertion. *Int Pediatr* 1992; **7**: 47–52.
102. Herskhovitz E, Young E, Rainer J et al. Bone marrow transplantation for Maroteaux–Lamy syndrome (MPS VI): long-term follow-up. *J Inherit Metab Dis* 1999; **22**: 50–62.
103. Gasper PW, Thrall MA, Wenger DA et al. Correction of feline arylsulphatase B deficiency (mucopolysaccharidosis VI) by bone marrow transplantation. *Nature* 1984; **312**: 467–9.
104. Norrdin RW, Moffat KS, Thrall MA, Gasper PW. Characterization of osteopenia in feline mucopolysaccharidosis VI and evaluation of bone marrow transplantation therapy. *Bone* 1993; **14**: 361–7.
105. Simonaro CM, Haskins ME, Kunieda T, Evans SM, Visser JM, Schuchman EH. Bone marrow transplantation in newborn rats with mucopolysaccharidosis type VI. Biochemical, pathological, and clinical findings. *Transplantation* 1997; **63**: 1386–93.
106. Machin GA. Hydrops revisited. Literature review of 1414 cases published in the 1980s. *Am J Med Genet* 1992; **34**: 366–90.
107. Yamada Y, Kato K, Sukegawa K et al. Treatment of MPS VII (Sly disease) by allogeneic BMT in a female with homozygous A619V mutation. *Bone Marrow Transplant* 1998; **21**: 629–34.
108. Birkenmeier EH, Barker JE, Vogler CA et al. Increased life span and correction of metabolic defects in murine mucopolysaccharidosis type VII after syngeneic bone marrow transplantation. *Blood* 1991; **78**: 3081–92.
109. Sands MS, Erway LC, Vogler C, Sly WS, Birkenmeier EH. Syngeneic bone marrow transplantation reduces the hearing loss associated with murine mucopolysaccharidosis type VII. *Blood* 1995; **86**: 2033–40.
110. Sands MS, Vogler C, Torrey A et al. Murine mucopolysaccharidosis type VII. Long term therapeutic effects of enzyme replacement and enzyme replacement followed by bone marrow transplantation. *J Clin Invest* 1997; **99**: 1596–605.
111. Vogler C, Barker J, Sands MS, Levy B, Galvin N, Sly WS. Murine mucopolysaccharidosis VII. Impact of therapies on the phenotype, clinical course, and pathology in a model of a lysosomal storage disease. *Pediatr Dev Pathol* 2001; **4**: 421–33.
112. Soper BW, Lessard MD, Vogler CA et al. Nonablative neonatal marrow transplantation attenuates functional and physical defects of β-glucuronidase deficiency. *Blood* 2001; **97**: 1498–504.
113. Sammarco C, Weil M, Just C et al. Effects of bone marrow transplantation on the cardiovascular abnormalities in canine mucopolysaccharidosis VII. *Bone Marrow Transplant* 2000; **25**: 1289–97.
114. Bezman L, Moser AB, Raymond GV et al. Adrenoleukodystrophy: incidence, new mutation rate, and results of extended family screening. *Ann Neurol* 2001; **49**: 512–7.
115. Moser HW. Adrenoleukodystrophy: phenotype, genetics, pathogenesis and therapy. *Brain* 1997; **120**: 1485–508.
116. Mosser J, Douar AM, Sarde CO et al. Putative X-linked adrenoleukodystrophy gene shares unexpected homology with ABC transporters. *Nature* 1993; **361**: 726–30.
117. Mosser J, Lutz Y, Stoeckel ME et al. The gene responsible for adrenoleukodystrophy encodes a peroxisomal membrane protein. *Hum Mol Genet* 1994; **3**: 265–71.
118. Powers JM, Liu Y, Moser AB, Moser HW. The inflammatory myelinopathy of adreno-leukotrophy: cells, effector molecules and pathogenetic implications. *J Neuropathol Exp Neurol* 1992; **51**: 630–43.
119. Ito M, Blumberg BM, Mock DJ et al. Potential environmental and host participants in the early white matter lesion of adreno-leukodystrophy: morphologic evidence for CD8 cytotoxic T cells, cytolysis of oligodendrocytes, and CD1-mediated lipid antigen presentation. *J Neuropathol Exp Neurol* 2001; **60**: 1004–19.

120. Moser HW, Smith KD, Watkins PA. X-linked adrenoleukodystrophy. In: Scriver CR, Beaudet AL, Sly WS, Valle D, eds. *The Metabolic and Molecular Bases of Inherited Disease*, 8th edn. New York: McGraw-Hill, 2001: 3257–302.

121. Ronghe MD, Barton J, Jardine PE et al. The importance of testing for adrenoleukodystrophy in males with idiopathic Addison's disease. *Arch Dis Child* 2002; **86**: 185–9.

122. Loes DJ, Hite S, Moser H et al. Adrenoleukodystrophy: a scoring method for brain MR observations. *AJNR Am J Neuroradiol* 1994; **15**: 1761–6.

123. Loes DJ, Stillman AE, Hite S et al. Childhood cerebral form of adrenoleukodystrophy: short-term effect of bone marrow transplantation on brain MR observations. *AJNR Am J Neuroradiol* 1994; **15**: 1767–71.

124. Melhem ER, Loes DJ, Georgiades CS, Raymond GV, Moser HW. X-linked adrenoleukodystrophy. The role of contrast-enhanced MR imaging in predicting disease progression. *AJNR Am J Neuroradiol* 2000; **21**: 839–44.

125. Shapiro EG, Krivit W, Lockman L et al. Long-term effect of bone-marrow transplantation for childhood-onset cerebral X-linked adrenoleukodystrophy. *Lancet* 2000; **356**: 713–8.

126. Moser HW, Loes DJ, Melhem ER et al. X-linked adrenoleukodystrophy: overview and prognosis as a function of age and brain magnetic resonance imaging abnormality. A study involving 372 patients. *Neuropediatrics* 2000; **31**: 227–39.

127. Aubourg P, Blanche S, Jambaque I et al. Reveral of early neurologic and neuroradiologic manifestations of X-linked adrenoleukodystrophy by bone marrow transplantation. *N Engl J Med* 1990; **322**: 1860–6.

128. Peters C, Abel S, DeFor TE et al. The worldwide hematopoietic cell transplant experience for childhood onset cerebral X-linked adrenoleukodystrophy (COCALD). *Blood* 2000; **96**: 842a [Abstract].

129. Shapiro EG, Lockman L, Balthazor M. Neuropsychological and neurological function and quality-of-life before and after bone marrow transplantation for adrenoleukodystrophy. In: Ringden O, Hobbs JR, Steward C, eds. *Correction of Genetic Diseases by Transplantation (COGENT)*, 4th edn. London: COGENT Press, 1997: 52–62.

130. Moser HW, Raymond GV, Kohler W. et al. Evaluation of the preventive effect of glyceryl tioleate-trierucate ("Lorenzo's oil") therapy in X-linked adrenoleukodystrophy: results of two concurrent trials, in press.

131. Van Geel BM, Assies J, Haverkort EB et al. Progression of abnormalities in adrenomyeloneuropathy and neurologically asymptomatic X-linked adrenoleukodystrophy despite treatment with "Lorenzo's oil." *J Neurol Neurosurg Psychiatry* 1999; **67**: 290–9.

132. Singh I, Khan M, Key L et al. Lovastatin for X-linked adrenoleukodystrophy. *N Engl J Med* 1998; **339**: 702–3.

133. Kemp S, He-Ming W, Lu JF et al. Gene redundancy and pharmacologic gene therapy: implications for X-linked adrenoleukodystrophy. *Nat Med* 1998; **4**: 1261–8.

134. Loes DJ, Peters C, Krivit W. Globoid cell leukodystrophy: distinguishing early onset from late-onset disease using a brain MR imaging scoring method. *AJNR Am J Neuroradiol* 1999; **20**: 316–23.

135. Wenger DA. Murine, canine and non-human primate models of Krabbe disease. *Mol Med Today* 2000; **6**: 449–51.

136. Suzuki K, Suzuki K. The twitcher mouse. A model for Krabbe disease and for experimental therapies. *Brain Pathol* 1995; **5**: 249–58.

137. Krabbe K. A new familial infantile form of diffuse brain sclerosis. *Brain* 1916; **39**: 74–114.

138. Yeager AM, Brennan S, Tiffany C, Moser HW, Santos GW. Prolonged survival and remyelination after hematopoietic cell transplantation in the twitcher mouse (murine globoid cell leukodystrophy). *Science* 1984; **225**: 1052–4.

139. Yeager AM, Shinohara M, Shinn C. Hematopoietic cell transplantation after administration of high-dose busulfan in murine globoid cell leukodystrophy (the twitcher mouse). *Pediatr Res* 1991; **29**: 302–5.

140. Kondo A, Hoogerbrugge PM, Suzuki K, Poorthuis BJHM, van Bekkum DW, Suzuki K. Pathology of the peripheral nerve in the twitcher mouse following bone marrow transplantation. *Brain Res* 1988; **460**: 178–87.

141. Suzuki K, Hoogerbrugge PM, Poorthuis BJHM, van Bekkum DW, Suzuki K. The twitcher mouse. Central nervous system pathology after bone marrow transplantation. *Lab Invest* 1988; **58**: 302–9.

142. Toyoshima E, Yeager AM, Brennan S, Santos GW, Moser HW, Mayer RF. Nerve conduction studies in the twitcher mouse (murine globoid cell leukodystrophy). *J Neurol Sci* 1986; **74**: 307–18.

143. Hoogerbrugge PM, Suzuki K, Susuki K et al. Donor-derived cells in the central nervous system of twitcher mice after bone marrow transplantation. *Science* 1988; **239**: 1035–8.

144. Ichioka T, Kishimoto Y, Brennan S, Santos GW, Yeager AM. Hematopoietic cell transplantation in murine globoid cell leukodystrophy (the twitcher mouse). Effects on levels of galactosylceramidase, psychosine, and galactocerebrosides. *Proc Natl Acad Sci U S A* 1987; **84**: 4259–63.

145. Yeager AM, Shinn C, Shinohara M, Pardoll DM. Hematopoietic cell transplantation in the twitcher mouse. The effects of pretransplant conditioning with graded doses of busulfan. *Transplantation* 1993; **56**: 185–90.

146. Igisu H, Suzuki K. Progressive accumulation of toxic metabolite in a genetic leukodystrophy. *Science* 1984; **224**: 753–5.

147. Krivit W, Shapiro EG, Peters C et al. Hematopoietic stem-cell transplantation in globoid-cell leukodystrophy. *N Engl J Med* 1998; **338**: 1119–26.

148. Kurtzberg J, Richards K, Wenger D et al. Correction of Krabbe disease with neonatal hematopoietic stem cell transplantation. *Biol Blood Marrow Transplant* 2002; **8**: 97a [Abstract].

149. von Figura K, Gieselman V, Jaeken J. Metachromatic leukodystrophy. In: Scriver CR, Beaudet AL, Sly WS, Valle D, eds. *The Metabolic and Molecular Bases of Inherited Disease*, 8th edn. New York: McGraw-Hill, 2001: 3695–724.

150. Kolodny EH. Metachromatic leukodystrophy and multiple sulfatase deficiency: sulfatide lipidosis. In: Rosenberg RN, Prusiner SB, DiMauro S, Barchi RL, eds. *The Molecular and Genetic Basis of Neurological Diseases*, 2nd edn. Boston: Butterworth-Heinemann, 1997: 433–42.

151. Tylki-Szymanska AT, Czartoryska B, Lugowska A. Practical suggestions in diagnosing metachromatic leukodystrophy in probands and in testing family members. *Eur Neurol* 1998; **40**: 67–70.

152. Krivit W, Shapiro EG, Lockman LA et al. Bone marrow transplantation treatment for globoid cell leukodystrophy, metachromatic leukodystrophy, adrenoleukodystrophy, and Hurler syndrome. In: Moser HW, ed. *Handbook of Clinical Neurology: Neurodystrophies and Neurolipidoses*, Vol. 22. Amsterdam: Elsevier Science, 1996: 87–106.

153. Krivit W, Lockman LA, Watkins PA, Hirsch J, Shapiro EG. The future for treatment by bone marrow transplantation for adrenoleukodystrophy, metachromatic leukodystrophy, globoid cell leukodystrophy, and Hurler syndrome. *J Inher Metab Dis* 1995; **18**: 398–412.

154. Hoogerbrugge PM, Brouwer OF, Bordigoni P et al. Allogeneic bone marrow transplantation for lysosomal storage diseases. *Lancet* 1995; **345**: 1398–402.

155. Krivit W, Lipton ME, Lockman LA et al. Prevention of deterioration in metachromatic leukodystrophy by bone marrow transplantation. *Am J Med Sci* 1987; **294**: 80–5.

156. Krivit W, Shapiro EG, Kennedy W et al. Treatment of late infantile metachromatic leukodystrophy by bone marrow transplantation. *N Engl J Med* 1990; **322**: 28–32.

157. Dhuna A, Toro C, Torres F, Kennedy WR, Krivit W. Longitudinal neurophysiologic studies in a patient with metachromatic leukodystrophy following bone marrow transplantation. *Arch Neurol* 1994; **49**: 1088–92.

158. Stillman AE, Krivit W, Shapiro EG, Lockman L, Latchaw RE. Serial MR after bone marrow transplantation in two patients with metachromatic leukodystrophy. *AJNR Am J Neuroradiol* 1994; **15**: 1929–32.

159. Shapiro EG, Lipton ME, Krivit W. White matter dysfunction and its neuropsychological correlates: a longitudinal study of a case of metachromatic leukodystrophy treated with bone marrow transplant. *J Clin Exp Neuropsychol* 1992; **14**: 610–24.

160. Pridjian G, Humbert J, Willis J, Shapira E. Presymptomatic late-infantile metachromatic leukodystrophy treated with bone marrow transplantation. *J Pediatr* 1994; **125**: 755–8.

161. Guffon N, Souillet G, Maire I, Dorche C, Mathieu M, Guiband P. Juvenile metachromatic leukodystrophy: neurological outcome 2 years after bone marrow transplantation. *J Inher Metab Dis* 1995; **18**: 159–61.

162. Shapiro EG, Lockman LA, Knopman D, Krivit W. Characteristics of the dementia in late-onset metachromatic leukodystrophy. *Neurology* 1994; **44**: 662–5.

163. Navarro C, Fernandez JM, Dominguez C, Fachal C, Alvarez M. Late juvenile metachromatic leukodystrophy treated with bone marrow transplantation: a 4-year follow-up study. *Neurology* 1996; **46**: 254–6.

164. Kapaun P, Dittmann RW, Granitzny B et al. Slow progression of juvenile metachromatic leukodystrophy 6 years after bone marrow transplantation. *J Child Neurol* 1999; **14**: 222–8.

165. Yeager AM, Moser HW, Forte KJ et al. Allogeneic bone marrow transplantation provides biochemical improvement and stabilizes the neurocognitive status in the adult form of metachromatic leukodystrophy. *Blood* 1994; **86**: 974a [Abstract].

166. Solders G, Celsing G, Hagenfeldt L, Ljungman P, Isberg B, Ringden O. Improved peripheral nerve conduction, EEG and verbal IQ after bone marrow transplantation for adult metachromatic leukodystrophy. *Bone Marrow Transplant* 1998; **22**: 1119–22.

167. Seitelberger F, Urbarits S, Nave K-A. Pelizaeus–Merzbacher disease. In: Vinken PJ, Bruyn GW, eds. *Handbook of Clinical Neurology, Neurodystrophies*

and *Neurolipidoses*. Amsterdam: Elsevier, 1996: 559–79.
168. Wilson GN, Holmes RG, Custer J *et al*. Zellweger syndrome: diagnostic assays, syndrome delineation, and potential therapy. *Am J Med Genet* 1986; **24**: 69–82.
169. Goldfischer S, Moore CL, Johnson AB *et al*. Peroxisomal and mitochondrial defects in the cerebro–hepato–renal syndrome. *Science* 1973; **182**: 62–4.
170. Leegwater PA, Vermeulen G, Konst AA *et al*. Subunits of the translation initiation factor eIF2B are mutant in leukoencephalopathy with vanishing white matter. *Nat Genet* 2001; **29**: 383–8.
171. van der Knaap MS, Barth PG, Gabreels FJ *et al*. A new leukoencephalopathy with vanishing white matter. *Neurology* 1997; **48**: 845–55.
172. Thomas GH. Disorders of glycoprotein: α-mannosidosis, β-mannosidosis, fucosidosis, and sialidosis. In: Scriver CR, Beaudet AL, Sly WS, Valle D, eds. *The Metabolic and Molecular Bases of Inherited Disease*, 8th edn. New York: McGraw-Hill, 2001: 3507–34.
173. Taylor RM, Farrow BRH, Stewart GJ, Healy PJ. Enzyme replacement in nervous tissue after allogenic bone-marrow transplantation for fucosidosis in dogs. *Lancet* 1986; **2**: 772–4.
174. Miano M, Lanino E, Gatti R *et al*. Four-year follow-up of a case of fucosidosis treated with unrelated donor bone marrow transplantation. *Bone Marrow Transplant* 2001; **27**: 747–51.
175. Krivit W, Peters C, Shapiro EG. Bone marrow transplantation as effective treatment of central nervous system disease in globoid cell leukodystrophy, metachromatic leukodystrophy, adrenoleukodystrophy, mannosidosis, fucosidosis, aspartylglucosaminuria, Hurler, Maroteaux–Lamy, and Sly syndromes, and Gaucher disease type III. *Curr Opin Neurol* 1999; **12**: 167–76.
176. Vellodi A, Cragg H, Winchester B *et al*. Allogeneic bone marrow transplantation for fucosidosis. *Bone Marrow Transplant* 1995; **15**: 153–8.
177. Beutler E, Grabowski GA. Gaucher disease. In: Scriver CR, Beaudet AL, Sly WS, Valle D, eds. *The Metabolic and Molecular Bases of Inherited Disease*, 8th edn. New York: McGraw-Hill, 2001: 3635–68.
178. Barton NW, Brady RO, Dambrosia JM *et al*. Replacement therapy for inherited enzyme deficiency-macrophage targeted glucocerebrosidase for Gaucher's disease. *N Engl J Med* 1991; **324**: 1464–70.
179. Figueroa ML, Rosenbloom BE, Kay AC *et al*. A less costly regimen of alglucerase to treat Gaucher's disease. *N Engl J Med* 1992; **327**: 1632–6.
180. Beutler E. Gaucher disease. New molecular approaches to diagnosis and treatment. *Science* 1992; **256**: 794–9.
181. Schiffmann R, Heyes MP, Aerts JM *et al*. Prospective study of neurological responses to treatment with macrophage-targeted glucocerebrosidase in patients with type 3 Gaucher's disease. *Ann Neurol* 1997; **42**: 613–21.
182. Erikson A, Groth CG, Mansson JE *et al*. Clinical and biochemical outcome of marrow transplantation for Gaucher disease of the Norrbottnian type. *Acta Paediatr Scand* 1990; **79**: 680–5.
183. Ringden O, Groth CG, Erikson A *et al*. Long-term follow-up of the first successful bone marrow transplantation in Gaucher disease. *Transplantation* 1988; **46**: 66–70.
184. Ringden O, Groth CG, Erikson A *et al*. Ten years' experience of bone marrow transplantation for Gaucher disease. *Transplantation* 1995; **59**: 864–70.
185. Svennerholm L, Erikson A, Groth CG *et al*. Norrbottnian type of Gaucher disease—clinical, biochemical and molecular biology aspects: successful treatment with bone marrow transplantation. *Dev Neurosci* 1991; **13**: 345–51.
186. Tsai P, Lipton JM, Sahdev I *et al*. Allogenic bone marrow transplantation in severe Gaucher disease. *Pediatr Res* 1992; **31**: 503–7.
187. Rappeport JM, Ginns EI. Bone-marrow transplantation in severe Gaucher's disease. *N Engl J Med* 1984; **311**: 84–8.
188. Hobbs JR, Jones KH, Shaw PJ *et al*. Beneficial effect of pre-transplant splenectomy on displacement bone marrow transplantation for Gaucher's syndrome. *Lancet* 1987; **1**: 1111–5.
189. Starer F, Sargent JD, Hobbs JR. Regression of the radiological changes of Gaucher's disease following bone marrow transplantation. *Br J Radiol* 1987; **60**: 1189–95.
190. Aula P, Jalanko A, Peltonen L. Aspartylglucosaminuria. In: Scriver CR, Beaudet AL, Sly WS, Valle D, eds. *The Metabolic and Molecular Bases of Inherited Disease*, 8th edn. New York: McGraw-Hill, 2001: 3535–50.
191. Walkley S, Thrall M, Dobrenis K *et al*. Bone marrow transplantation corrects the enzyme defect in neurons of the central nervous system in a lysosomal storage disease. *Proc Natl Acad Sci U S A* 1994; **91**: 2970–4.
192. Will A, Cooper A, Hatton C, Sardharwalla IB. Evans DI, Stevens RF. Bone marrow transplantation in the treatment of α-mannosidosis. *Arch Dis Child* 1987; **62**: 1044–9.
193. Wall DA, Grange DK, Goulding P, Daines M, Luisiri A, Kotagal S. Bone marrow transplantation for the treatment of α-mannosidosis. *J Pediatr* 1998; **133**: 282–5.
194. Peters C, Grewal S, Orchard P. *et al*. Hematopoietic cell transplantation (HCT) is effective treatment for mucolipidosis II (MLII) and α-mannosidosis (MAN). *Am J Hum Genet* 2002; **71**: 579a [Abstract].
195. Autti T, Santavuori P, Raininko R *et al*. Bone marrow transplantation in aspartylglucosaminuria: MRI of brain suggests normalizing myelination. In: Ringden O, Hobbs JR, Steward C, eds. *Correction of Genetic Diseases by Transplantation (COGENT)*, 4th edn. London: COGENT Press, 1997: 92.
196. Autti T, Rapola J, Santavuori P *et al*. Bone marrow transplantation in aspartylglucosaminuria-histopathological and MRI study. *Neuropediatrics* 1999; **30**: 283–8.
197. Arvio M, Sauna-Aho O, Peippo M. Bone marrow transplantation for aspartylglucosaminuria. Follow-up study of transplanted and non-transplanted patients. *J Pediatr* 2001; **138**: 288–90.
198. Santavuori P, Lauronen L, Kirveskari E *et al*. Neuronal ceroid lipofuscinoses in childhood. *Neurol Sci* 2000; **21**: S35–41.
199. Lake BD, Steward CG, Oakhill A *et al*. Bone marrow transplantation in late infantile Batten disease and juvenile Batten disease. *Neuropediatrics* 1997; **28**: 80–1.
200. Lipman RD, Donohue LR, Hoppe P *et al*. Evidence that lysosomal storage proteolipids is a cell autonomous process in the motor neuron degeneration (mnd) mouse, a model of neuronal ceroid lipofuscinosis. *Neurosci Lett* 1996; **219**: 111–4.
201. Westlake VJ, Jolly RD, Jones BR *et al*. Hematopoietic cell transplantation in fetal lambs with ceroid-lipofuscinosis. *Am J Med Genet* 1995; **57**: 365–8.
202. Deeg HJ, Shulman HM, Albrechtsen D *et al*. Batten's disease: failure of allogeneic bone marrow transplantation to arrest disease progression in a canine model. *Clin Genet* 1990; **37**: 264–70.
203. Schuchman EH, Desnick RJ. Niemann–Pick disease types A and B. Acid sphingomyelinase deficiencies. In: Scriver CR, Beaudet AL, Sly WS, Valle D, eds. *The Metabolic and Molecular Bases of Inherited Disease*, 8th edn. New York: McGraw-Hill, 2001: 3589–610.
204. Bayever E, Kamani N, Ferreira P *et al*. Bone marrow transplantation for Niemann–Pick type IA disease. *J Inherit Metab Dis* 1992; **15**: 919–28.
205. Vellodi A, Hobbs JR, O'Donnell NM *et al*. Treatment of Niemann–Pick disease type B by allogeneic bone marrow transplantation. *Br Med J (Clin Res Ed)* 1987; **295**: 1375–6.
206. Patterson MC, Vanier MT, Suzuki K *et al*. Niemann–Pick disease type C. A cellular cholesterol lipidosis. In: Scriver CR, Beaudet AL, Sly WS, Valle D, eds. *The Metabolic and Molecular Bases of Inherited Disease*, 8th edn. New York: McGraw-Hill, 2001: 3611–34.
207. Hsu YS, Hwu WL, Huang SF *et al*. Niemann–Pick disease type C (a cellular cholesterol lipidosis) treated by bone marrow transplantation. *Bone Marrow Transplant* 1999; **24**: 103–7.
208. Kornfeld S, Sly WS. I-cell disease and pseudo-Hurler polydystrophy: disorders of lysosomal enzyme phosphorylation and localization. In: Scriver CR, Beaudet AL, Sly WS, Valle D, eds. *The Metabolic and Molecular Bases of Inherited Disease*, 8th edn. New York: McGraw-Hill, 2001: 3469–82.
209. Kurobane I, Inoue S, Gotoh Y *et al*. Biochemical improvement after treatment by bone marrow transplantation in I-cell disease. *Tohoku J Exp Med* 1986; **150**: 63–8.
210. Yamaguchi K, Hayasaka S, Hara S *et al*. Improvement in tear lysosomal enzyme levels after treatment with bone marrow transplantation in a patient with I-cell disease. *Ophthalmic Res* 1989; **21**: 226–9.
211. Gravel RA, Kaback MM, Proia RL, Sandhoff K, Suzuki K, Suzuki K. The G_{M2} gangliosidoses. In: Scriver CR, Beaudet AL, Sly WS, Valle D, eds. *The Metabolic and Molecular Bases of Inherited Disease*, 8th edn. New York: McGraw-Hill, 2001: 3827–76.
212. Suzuki Y, Oshima A, Nanba E. β-Galactosidase deficiency (β-galactosidosis): G_{M1} gangliosidosis and Morquio B disease. In: Scriver CR, Beaudet AL, Sly WS, Valle D, eds. *The Metabolic and Molecular Bases of Inherited Disease*, 8th edn. New York: McGraw-Hill, 2001: 3775–809.
213. Assmann G, Seedorf U. Acid lipase deficiency. Wolman disease and cholesteryl ester storage disease. In: Scriver CR, Beaudet AL, Sly WS, Valle D, eds. *The Metabolic and Molecular Bases of Inherited Disease*, 8th edn. New York: McGraw-Hill, 2001: 3551–72.
214. Krivit W, Peters C, Dusenbery K *et al*. Wolman disease successfully treated by bone marrow transplantation. *Bone Marrow Transplant* 2000; **26**: 567–70.
215. Moser HW, Linke T, Fensom AH, Levade T, Sandhoff K. Acid ceramidase deficiency: Farber lipogranulomatosis. In: Scriver CR, Beaudet AL, Sly WS, Valle D, eds. *The Metabolic and*

Molecular Bases of Inherited Disease, 8th edn. New York: McGraw-Hill, 2001: 3573–88.
216 Vormoor J, Ehlert K, Bielack S *et al.* Successful allogeneic stem cell transplantation in infantile ceramidase deficiency (Farber Disease) type 2/3. *Blood* 2002; **100**: 457–8.
217 Yeager AM, Uhas KA, Coles CD, Davis PC, Krause WL, Moser HW. Bone marrow transplantation for infantile ceramidase deficiency (Farber disease). *Bone Marrow Transplant* 2000; **26**: 357–63.
218 Barton NW, Brady RO, Dambrosia JM *et al.* Replacement therapy for inherited enzyme deficiency—macrophage-targeted glucocerebrosidase for Gaucher disease. *N Engl J Med* 1991; **324**: 1464–70.
219 Schiffmann R, Brady RO. New prospects for the treatment of lysosomal storage diseases. *Drugs* 2002; **62**: 733–42.
220 Kaye EM. Lysosomal storage diseases. *Curr Treat Options Neurol* 2001; **3**: 249–56.
221 Kaye EM. Therapeutic approaches to lysosomal storage diseases. *Curr Opin Pediatr* 1995; **7**: 650–4.
222 Koc ON, Peters C, Aubourg P *et al.* Bone marrow-derived mesenchymal stem cells remain host-derived despite successful hematopoietic engraftment after allogeneic transplantation in patients with lysosomal and peroxisomal storage diseases. *Exp Hematol* 1999; **27**: 1675–81.
223 Jiang Y, Vaessen B, Lenvik T, Blackstad M, Reyes M, Verfaillie C. Multipotent progenitor cells can be isolated from postnatal murine bone marrow, muscle, and brain. *Exp Hematol* 2002; **30**: 896–904.
224 Reyes M, Lund T, Lenvik T, Aguiar D, Koodie L, Verfaillie CM. Purification and *ex vivo* expansion of postnatal human marrow mesodermal progenitor cells. *Blood* 2001; **98**: 2615–25.
225 Reyes M, Dudek A, Jahagirdar B, Koodie L, Marker PH, Verfaillie CM. Origin of endothelial progenitors in human postnatal bone marrow. *J Clin Invest* 2002; **109**: 337–46.
226 Zhao LR, Duan WM, Reyes M, Keene CD, Verfaillie CM, Low WC. Human bone marrow stem cells exhibit neural phenotypes and ameliorate neurological deficits after grafting into the ischemic brain of rats. *Exp Neurol* 2002; **174**: 11–20.
227 Schwartz RE, Reyes M, Koodie L *et al.* Multipotent adult progenitor cells from bone marrow differentiate into functional hepatocyte-like cells. *J Clin Invest* 2002; **109**: 1291–302.
228 Jiang Y, Jahagirdar BN, Reinhardt RL *et aal*. Pluripotency of mesenchymal stem cells derived from adult marrow. *Nature* 2002; **418**: 41–9.
229 McIvor RS. Gene therapy of genetic diseases and cancer. *Pediatr Transplant* 1999; **3** (Suppl. 1): 116–21.

108 Rajni Agarwal

Hematopoietic Cell Transplantation for Macrophage and Granulocyte Disorders

Introduction

The human body is equipped with a complex immune system to defend against a wide variety of microbes ranging from viruses to bacterial and fungal organisms. First in the line of defense are two phagocytic systems, namely the monocyte–macrophage system and the granulocyte system. The primary cells of these two systems, monocytes and granulocytes, arise from a common committed progenitor in the bone marrow [1,2]. Any quantitative or qualitative defect in the elements of these systems will result in inadequate host defense against infections. This chapter will discuss the various disorders affecting these phagocyte systems and the role of HCT in their treatment.

Macrophage system overview

The monocyte–macrophage system includes a differentiation continuum from monoblasts to promonocytes to monocytes, with eventual migration of the monocytes into tissues (lungs, liver, skin, spleen and brain) to form fixed tissue macrophages, which perform specialized functions suited for the specific location. The life span of monocytes varies between 3 and 6 days. The tissue macrophage does not usually undergo cell division. However, if the cell proliferation regulatory controls are lost or altered, uncontrolled proliferation and accumulation of macrophages in multiple organs may result. One example is hemophagocytic lymphohistiocytosis (HLH), as described later in this chapter.

The functions of the monocyte–macrophage system are manifold [3]. The mononuclear phagocytes play an important role both as phagocytic and immunoregulatory cells. Macrophages secrete a variety of antimicrobial agents, including lysozyme, neutral proteases, acid hydrolases and cytokines. For example, interleukin 1 (IL-1), secreted by macrophages, stimulates vigorous production of hydrogen peroxide and toxic oxygen metabolites not only by the macrophages but also by the neutrophils. The pattern of the inflammatory response in the monocyte–macrophage system is similar to that seen in the granulocyte system. The activation of macrophages in response to insults such as infection is central to their role in host defense. Intact chemotactic mechanisms result in the accumulation of free macrophages at the site of insult. Defective mononuclear phagocytic chemotaxis may result in an inadequate host defense against infection such as seen in mucocutaneous candidiasis. Macrophages also process and present antigens to lymphocytes and secrete cytokines important for the development of lymphocytes and the regulation of their replication. The immune responses are mediated via secretory products that have pleotropic effects affecting nearly all cell types. Macrophages also participate in removing immune complexes from the circulation.

Granulocyte system overview

The inflammatory cascade of the granulocyte system has two major components: (i) vasodilatation and increased vascular permeability to phagocyte products, and (ii) "leukocytic events." The leukocytic events include several sequential steps, some of them overlapping in nature: (i) margination; (ii) adhesion to the endothelial surface; (iii) migration, which includes "rolling and diapedesis"; (iv) phagocytosis and intracellular degranulation and killing; and (v) release of leukocyte products.

Initially, pro-inflammatory cytokines, such as tumor necrosis factor-alpha (TNF-α), IL-1, IL-6 and interferon-gamma (IFN-γ), are released, resulting in vasodilatation and increased vascular permeability. Immunoglobulins and complement thereby gain access to tissues to produce phagocytic activation and microbial opsonization. A redundancy of chemoattractants is generated to ensure that the leukocytes will be attracted to the site of insult in adequate numbers. The chemoattractant molecules also up-regulate certain adhesion receptors on the leukocytes as well as promote recruitment of cytoskeletal actin.

Following margination or peripheral orientation of white cells in the moving blood stream, the white cells adhere in great numbers to the endothelial surface and eventually migrate to the infected or the injured site. The initial step in the migration of white cells, often referred to as "rolling" or "tethering," is mediated by a family of glycoprotein adhesion molecules called selectins (L, E and P selectins). Some of the rolling leukocytes become firmly attached to the vascular endothelium via β-integrin adhesion receptors on the leukocytes. The integrins are the glycosylated heterodimers of noncovalently linked β and α chains. The type of β-integrin is determined by the type of the β subunit in the complete molecule. One important β-integrin is the $β_2$-integrin. Three different $β_2$-integrin molecules result when the same $β_2$-integrin subunit (CD18) is linked with different α subunits (CD11a, CD11b and CD11c). Defective adhesion has been noted in an inherited heterogeneous defect called leukocyte adhesion deficiency type I (LAD-I). In this disorder, mutations in the common $β_2$-integrin subunit are the underlying cause of defective chemotaxis. Two patients have been described with the absence of neutrophil receptors for E-selectin resulting in defective adhesion. This disorder is called LAD type II.

The migration of the adhered or firmly attached white cells at the endothelial surface into the site of injury or infection involves the presence of a chemotactic gradient that creates directional movement of the cells. The phagocytes move by extending pseudopodia, containing a branching network of actin filaments as well as the contractile protein myosin. Defects in neutrophil motility involving actin have been noted in neutrophil actin deficiency syndromes. Once in the tissues, the

Table 108.1 Hematopoietic cell transplantation (HCT) for macrophage and granulocyte disorders.

Macrophage disorders
Hemophagocytic lymphohistiocytosis

Granulocyte disorders
Quantitative disorders:
   Kostmann syndrome
   Reticular dysgenesis
   Cyclic neutropenia
   Cartilage hair dysplasia
   Dyskeratosis congenita
   Swachman–Diamond syndrome

Qualitative disorders:
   Neutrophil actin deficiency: abnormal chemotaxis
   Leukocyte adhesion (CD11/18) deficiency: abnormal adhesion
   Chediak–Higashi syndrome: abnormal granulation
   Chronic granulomatous disease: abnormal oxidation
   Griscelli syndrome

accumulated leukocytes recognize the opsonized targets by attaching to the latter via opsonin receptors on leukocyte surfaces. The major humoral opsonins that coat microbes include immunoglobulin M (IgM), IgG_1, IgG_3, C3b and C3bi. In LAD-I, ingestion of C3bi-opsonized microbes is also impaired. Once the leukocyte–opsonin interaction has occurred, the process of engulfment is initiated.

As the final step, the engulfed material is destroyed through intracellular cytocidal and digestive activity. This process involves oxygen-independent (in the hypoxic necrotic environment of tissue injury) and oxygen-dependent pathways of microbial killing. In the oxygen-independent pathway, numerous cationic antimicrobial proteins contained within the neutrophil azurophilic granules are utilized. These antimicrobial proteins include defensins and serpocidins. In addition, the azurophilic and specific granules also contain other degradation enzymes such as lysozymes and hydrolases. Deficiencies in neutrophil granule proteins or defects in granule formation or degranulation are associated with recurrent bacterial infections as seen in Chediak–Higashi syndrome (CHS). The oxygen-dependent pathway of intracellular microbial killing, often referred to as the "respiratory burst oxidase" or NADPH pathway, utilizes the generation of superoxide radicals through mitochondrial based reactions. Mutations in the oxidase subunit result in the well-known disease entity of chronic granulomatous disease (CGD).

In addition to normally *functioning* granulocytes, adequate *numbers* of granulocytes are necessary for normal host defense. Granulocytopenia due to congenital defects, malignancy, or after the administration of chemotherapeutic agents results in increased susceptibility to bacterial infections.

The congenital disorders that affect the monocyte–macrophage and granulocyte systems often present in early childhood with recurrent, severe and often life-threatening infections. This chapter will address the various disorders of macrophages and granulocytes and the role of hematopoietic cell transplantation (HCT) as an important treatment modality (Table 108.1).

General considerations for HCT

Timing of HCT

The timing of intervention in the phagocytic disorders with HCT depends on the nature of the disease, presence of serious infections and the status of organ function. Even though the risks attendant to HCT may be a concern, a "wait and see" approach may not be in the patient's best interest. The timing of HCT should be determined by the prognosis and the anticipated risk of life-threatening infections or irreversible organ damage. The disorders with a variable clinical course need to be approached differently as opposed to disorders where delayed intervention with HCT might result in high mortality despite the provision of optimal supportive care. For example, in cyclical neutropenia, low counts can be managed with granulocyte colony-stimulating factor (G-CSF) and without intervention with HCT. On the other hand, in severe forms of reticular dysgenesis, early intervention with HCT is warranted [4]. The course of CGD can be extremely variable. However, certain phenotypes of CGD can be more severe than others [5].

Choice of donor for HCT

Since the disorders discussed in this chapter affect young children, genotypically identical sibling donors may not be available for more than 20–30% of patients, leaving 70–80% of HCT candidates without an ideally matched related donor. Since many of these disorders occur in children of consanguineous parents, an extensive family search should be conducted to identify a suitable related donor. The siblings or any other related potential donor should be tested, if technically possible, for the presence of the disease in question before they are considered to serve as donors. Many congenital disorders of the phagocyte system are transmitted as autosomal recessive conditions. The carrier-state does not result in serious clinical disease and heterozygous individuals may qualify as donors. One possible exception would be X-linked CGD, where severely imbalanced "Lyonization" may result in clinically significant disease [6]. The data for donor choice for HCT in HLH indicate that preference should be given to sibling donors. However, the sibling should be screened to rule out the presence of any occult disease. If all the available tests including natural killer (NK)-cell activity are normal, the sibling may be used as a donor. The caveat should be kept in mind that no definite tests exist to exclude the carrier-state. In the event that the sibling is suspected to be a carrier, a search for a matched unrelated donor should be performed [7]. Identification of such a donor may require several months and HCT risks may rise during the search process. In some cases, the transplantation of T-cell-depleted haploidentical grafts from parent donors have been successfully performed. However, the difficulties and risks with these HCT procedures remain a major concern.

Preparative regimens

Most of the HCT procedures for phagocytic disorders have been performed utilizing a myeloablative approach. The two major chemotherapeutic agents in use are busulfan (BU) and cyclophosphamide (CY). CY, under certain circumstances, is used in combination with total body irradiation (TBI). It remains the physician's choice to use a particular regimen, as both radiation-based and nonradiation-based regimens are relatively well tolerated by children. Since the introduction of hyperfractionated TBI, many of the previously observed long-term effects have diminished. Recent experiences suggest that lower doses of TBI may result in prolonged mixed and eventual complete donor chimerism and might be effective and less toxic in HCT procedures for some disorders [8]. More data need to be generated to prove the usefulness of this approach for children with conditions discussed in this chapter. At this time, nonmyeloablative regimens seem to be attractive and should be explored. The nonmyeloablative approach can be especially useful where mixed chimerism could restore adequate cellular function, for example, in patients with CGD.

Macrophage disorders

Hemophagocytic lymphohistiocytosis (HLH)

HLH is the most frequent disorder of the macrophage system. In HLH (familial or secondary), excessive accumulation of tissue macrophages can result in organ dysfunction/enlargement. The excessive "cell eating" behavior of the macrophages seen in HLH results in cytopenias. Abnormal proliferation and accumulation of macrophages at specific anatomic sites may result in signs and symptoms pertinent to those sites. For example, central nervous system (CNS) involvement may result in serious clinical manifestations including hypotonia or hypertonia, convulsions, hemiplegia/tetraplegia, or blindness. It includes two different conditions: (i) primary or familial HLH, an autosomal recessive disorder, and (ii) secondary HLH which includes an infection-associated hemophagocytic syndrome and a malignancy-associated hemophagocytic syndrome. HCT procedures have been performed only for primary HLH.

Primary HLH has been reported from all continents and all ethnic groups. In a retrospective study the incidence of the disease in Swedish children was estimated to be 0.12/100,000 children per year [9]. Since primary HLH is an autosomal recessive disorder, an increased incidence has been reported in families with consanguinity [10]. Most patients develop symptoms in early life, with about 70% of children presenting in the 1st year of life. However, the age of presentation may be up to 8 years. The age of onset is usually similar among multiple affected siblings. However, on occasions a difference of >3 years in age at diagnosis has been noted in this group of patients.

The diagnosis of HLH may be difficult. Diagnostic guidelines have been developed based on clinical, laboratory and histopathologic criteria. The clinical manifestations vary widely. The most common early findings are fever, hepatomegaly and splenomegaly. Although serious CNS involvement may occur in the disease, it is not included in the clinical criteria of diagnosis. The laboratory findings include cytopenias, hypertriglyceridemia and/or hypofibrinogenemia. Markedly reduced or absent NK cell and T-cell activity have been found to be associated with primary HLH [11]. Although low or absent NK-cell activity is not included in the current diagnostic guidelines, the association between this parameter and HLH is of great interest due to its potential diagnostic value. It has been found that almost all children with verified familial disease have extremely low or absent NK-cell activity, and this value only normalizes after successful HCT. By contrast, those patients with secondary HLH who have low NK-cell activity at presentation normalize their NK-cell activity as the symptoms subside. The differentiation of familial HLH from *secondary HLH* may be difficult, as about half of the patients present with infections and the family history at the time of presentation may or may not be helpful. In this situation, testing of NK-cell activity and its normalization pattern may help in distinguishing primary from secondary disease. This observation makes it mandatory to test for NK-cell activity prior to the initiation of HCT. Histologic criteria of diagnosis include infiltration of the bone marrow, lymph nodes, liver and spleen with non-malignant lymphocytes and histiocytes, in addition to evidence for hemophagocytosis in these tissues [12].

If not treated, primary HLH is rapidly fatal with a median survival of about 2 months [13]. Several treatment strategies with cytotoxic agents have been tried in the past without much success. The most effective of these moderately effective strategies was the combination of Vinblastine and steroids. Recently, the treatment of HLH has included etoposide (VP16) in combination with other agents [14]. Approximately 60% of patients have also received CNS treatment with intrathecal methotrexate and/or cranial irradiation [10].

More recently, immunosuppressive drugs such as cyclosporine (CSP) and antithymocyte globulin (ATG) have been shown to be temporarily effective in HLH [15]. The probability of survival at 5 years was only 10%, with all patients ultimately succumbing to their disease. In 1994, the Histiocyte Society developed a treatment protocol (HLH-94) designed for treatment of primary HLH [16]. The protocol includes initial treatment with CSP, VP16 and steroids.

Fischer *et al.* [17] achieved the first major breakthrough in the treatment of this fatal disease by performing a successful allogeneic HCT procedure which resulted in the patient's cure. Since then, several reports have been published describing the efficacy of HCT using related or unrelated donors. Most of the reports have come from single HCT centers or from transplant registries [10–21]. The current consensus indicates that HCT should be performed after an initial 8 weeks of treatment with chemotherapy, if a suitable donor is available. Patients without a donor continue to receive chemotherapy. It is preferred that the patient should be in a stable or quiescent disease state before an HCT procedure is contemplated. Although the definitive results from this approach are not yet available, the preliminary data appear promising.

An human leukocyte antigen (HLA)-matched sibling donor is preferred in this disorder. This donor choice is based on results from the familial HLH registry [10]. However, one caveat should be kept in mind when selecting a sibling donor: a healthy appearing sibling may develop HLH later and therefore transfer the disease to the recipient. So far, the published reports on sibling donor HCT for HLH have not described this as a frequent problem. As mentioned earlier, the presence of extremely low or absent NK-cell activity should be used as a guide to reject a sibling donor for HCT in primary HLH. In the event that a suitable sibling donor is not available, an unrelated donor should be sought. The disease-free survival (DFS) in one series of HCT was approximately 45% in recipients of grafts from both sibling and unrelated donors [20].

The preparative regimens in most of the published cases have consisted of myeloablative doses of chemotherapeutic drugs. Most centers have used high dose BU, CY and VP16 as the conditioning regimen. In a few patients, additional immunosuppression has been provided by ATG or the anti-leukocyte function-associated antigen-1 (LFA-1) monoclonal antibody. These regimens have been well tolerated by children with HLH. TBI has not been favored, as histiocytes may not be sensitive to this measure.

Following HCT, patients usually achieve full donor chimerism. However, repeated analyses should be performed at regular intervals. In some cases, a mixed chimeric state can persist with low quantities of donor cells present in the graft. Whether this phenomenon indicates persistence or recurrence of the disease is unclear [22]. In patients with declining levels of donor cells, follow-up studies are important as a progressive decrease in donor cells may indicate early relapse and the need for further intervention.

Overall, the major causes of death following HCT for HLH are transplant-related complications including graft failure, infections and graft-vs.-host disease (GVHD). In a few cases, progression of CNS disease has occurred within weeks after the HCT. Active or poorly controlled CNS disease before HCT initiation has led to deterioration after transplantation. The relapse rate for the underlying disease has been reported in the range of 0–55% [19–21]. Actuarial 5-year DFS in HLH patients who underwent HCT has been compared with those HLH patients who did not receive a transplant. The DFS was reported to be 66% in HLH patients who were transplanted vs. only 10% in those patients who did not receive HCT (Fig. 108.1) [10].

Recent data from the International Bone Marrow Transplant Registry (IBMTR) indicate that 23 patients with HLH have received unrelated donor grafts [23]. The preparative regimen for these patients consisted of BU, CY, VP16 and ATG. Follow-up data has been reported for 16 patients. Sixty-two percent of the donors were fully matched and 38% were mismatched for one antigen. Projected overall survival is 51% at 4 years. The causes of death include infection, GVHD and graft rejection.

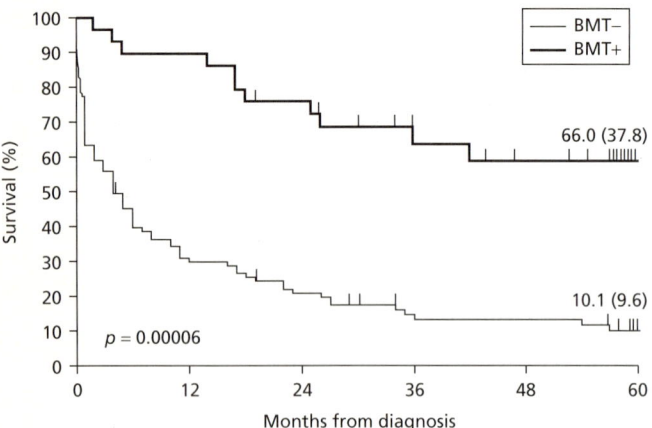

Fig. 108.1 Kaplan–Meier survival estimates of 122 children with hemophagocytic lymphohistiocytosis (HLH) treated with or without bone marrow transplantation (BMT). Reproduced with permission from Arico et al. [10].

In summary, the etiology of HLH remains unclear and diagnosis of this disease is often difficult. The use of HCT in this disease has provided the best results and remains the treatment of choice as chemotherapy alone is not curative. Therapy to achieve disease control before HCT should be attempted since the transplant outcome appears to be improved when patients are in a clinical remission.

Granulocyte disorders

The granulocyte disorders discussed here include *quantitative* disorders (where the number of granulocytes is low) and *qualitative* disorders (where the function of granulocytes is altered). Both groups of disorders are very heterogeneous and vary widely in clinical severity.

Quantitative granulocyte disorders

Clinically significant neutropenia is a condition where circulating neutrophils are <500/μL. Severe neutropenia is defined as an absolute neutrophil count of <200/μL. Severe neutropenia is often associated with life-threatening infections, especially if it is prolonged or is associated with other causes for immune deficiency. Neutropenia is common to a heterogeneous group of disorders resulting from decreased production or release of maturing myeloid cells from the bone marrow. Neutropenia may be congenital or secondary. This part of the chapter will cover the intrinsic maturation and differentiation defects of the early myeloid precursors.

Kostmann syndrome (KS)

KS, also known as congenital neutropenia, is an inherited disorder with an undefined inheritance pattern. It occurs with an estimated frequency of 1–2 cases per million, with equal gender distribution. A persistent absolute neutrophil count (ANC) of 0.2×10^9/L or less is required to make the diagnosis. Recurrent bacterial infections usually occur in the 1st year of life. Typically, these patients experience recurrent pneumonia, otitis media, gingivitis and perineal or urinary tract infections. Until recently, 50% of these patients died as a result of infection before 1 year of age and only 30% survived beyond 5 years of age [24].

The biology of KS is not completely understood. At the cellular level, a maturation arrest of myelopoiesis at the promyelocyte or myelocyte stage occurs, resulting in neutropenia [25]. Contrary to the earlier suggestions of defective G-CSF production or defective response of the cells to G-CSF, current data indicate normal or even increased endogenous G-CSF biological profile and activity in the cells of patients with KS. *In vitro* measurements of colony-forming unit–granulocyte/macrophages (CFU-GMs) also appear to be normal. No G-CSF receptor mutations from birth have been noted in KS patients. These mutations have, however, appeared in those KS patients who develop leukemia later in life. This observation suggests that these mutations are acquired and do not have a causal relationship with the underlying disease. This finding may be useful to predict the risk of leukemia in these patients. The finding that >95% of patients with KS respond to G-CSF therapy in doses in the range of 3–10 μg/kg/day also supports the hypothesis that normal G-CSF responsiveness exists in KS patients. In the 5% who are G-CSF nonresponders, the defect has not been elucidated.

Seven to nine percent of patients with KS will eventually develop myelodysplastic syndrome or secondary leukemia. This ominous finding has been linked to point mutations in the G-CSF receptor gene [26,27]. Also, cytogenetic abnormalities such as monosomy 7 have been noted in these patients. In light of these findings, KS can be considered a preleukemic condition.

G-CSF receptors are expressed in normal or even increased numbers on myeloid cells from patients with KS. Not surprisingly, therefore, treatment with cloned G-CSF has improved the prognosis in KS patients [28,29]. The myeloid progenitors in these patients retain the capacity for normal differentiation to mature myeloid cells in response to pharmacologic doses of G-CSF, which induces receptor transduction in the precursor cells [30]. Most of the patients with KS are therefore now treated continuously with recombinant G-CSF, resulting in an increase in the number of mature myeloid cells in the circulation and a concomitant decrease in the incidence of serious infections. In 1994, a Severe Chronic Neutropenia International Registry (SCNIR) was established and data on 304 patients with congenital neutropenia (KS) were collected and published [31]. Greater than 95% of patients responded to G-CSF treatment. Those patients who do not respond to G-CSF doses of 120 μg/kg/day still suffer from bacterial infections and are classified as G-CSF nonresponders or refractory to this treatment.

The G-CSF nonresponders and those patients who develop cytogenetic and G-CSF receptor mutations during the course of the disease are considered candidates for HCT. The monitoring for cytogenetic and G-CSF receptor mutations during the disease course is therefore emphasized for timely intervention with HCT. A limited number of patients with KS, including those documented in the IBMTR registry, have undergone HCT procedures using HLA-matched sibling donors. One patient received CY as a single preparative agent and attained only partial lymphoid engraftment for 6 months [30]. Another patient received an HLA-identical sibling donor transplant at 20 months of age after conditioning with procarbazine, TBI and antithymocyte serum. This patient is reported to be alive and disease-free 20 years after the HCT procedure [32]. The clinical course of this patient is depicted in Fig. 108.2 [32]. Recently, an unrelated-donor transplant procedure was performed in a G-CSF nonresponder [33]. The preparative regimen contained TBI, VP16 and CY. ATG was administered to prevent graft rejection. The patient engrafted promptly and the pre-existing pulmonary abscesses resolved [33]. At the time of writing (2002), the patient was 23 months after HCT and doing well.

Reticular dysgenesis (RD)

RD is a rare congenital disorder characterized by severe combined immunodeficiency and agranulocytosis manifesting with life-threatening fulminant infections. The term "reticular dysgenesis" was introduced in 1959 when two male twins were reported with this syndrome who subsequently died of the disease [34]. An autopsy was performed on these patients and the findings showed depletion of lymphocytes and Hassall's corpuscles in the thymus, absent lymph nodes, tonsils and Payers patches, and lack of myeloid activity in the bone marrow [34]. At the molecular

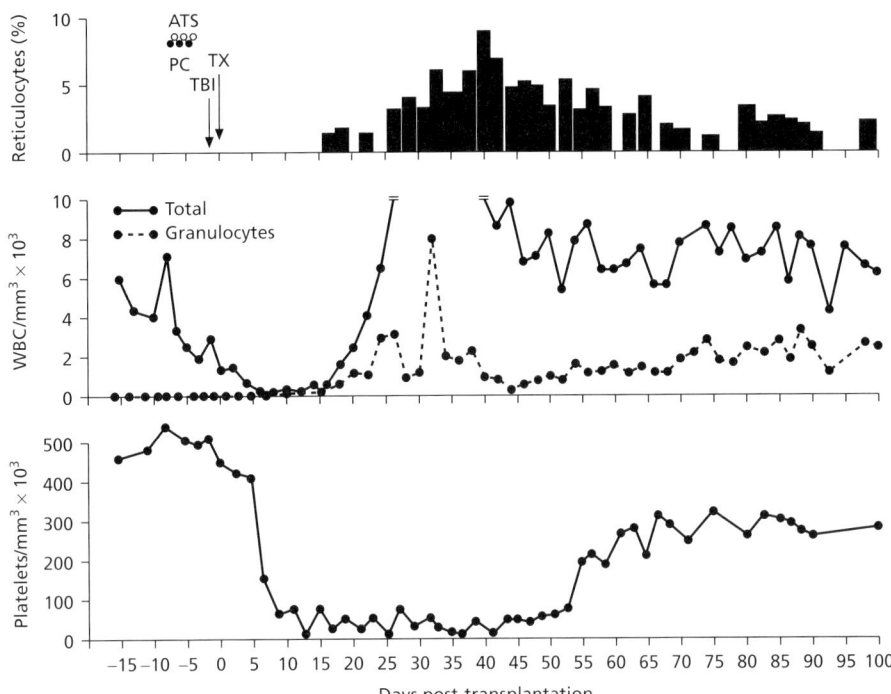

Fig. 108.2 Clinical course of a patient receiving transplant for infantile agranulocytosis (Kostmann syndrome). Note presence of granulocytes following transplantation. ATS, antithymocyte serum; PC, procarbazine; TBI, total body irradiation; TX, transplant. Reproduced with permission from Rappeport et al. [32].

level, the primary defect in RD has not yet been identified. At the cellular level, a maturation arrest in the myeloid lineage beyond the promyelocyte stage has been observed, along with a global impairment of lymphoid maturation. However, erythropoiesis and megakaryopoiesis are normal in RD, indicating the existence of a functional pluripotent hematopoietic stem cell pool in these patients. These observations are utilized to make a diagnosis of RD using established clinical and laboratory data: agranulocytosis, lymphocytopenia, bone marrow finding of early myeloid maturation arrest, failure of in vitro assays to produce mature granulocytes from precursors, lack of lymphocyte function and thymic aplasia.

Untreated patients die from infections within the first days or weeks of life. Prior to 1983, nine cases with this disorder were reported. Survival ranged from 3 days to 17 weeks [4,35–38]. In 1983, a cure was reported for RD following an HCT procedure (bone marrow graft) from an HLA-identical sibling [39]. A preparative regimen of BU and CY was used and the patient achieved full hematopoietic and lymphoid reconstitution. Since this initial report, several others have been published on successful HCT in RD patients using HLA-identical, T-cell depleted HLA-haploidentical and umbilical cord blood grafts [40–47]. Umbilical cord blood from an unrelated donor has also been used in one patient who failed to engraft initially but fully engrafted after a second unrelated cord blood transplantation procedure [46].

A challenging feature of HCT for RD is not only the choice of the donor but also the intensity of the conditioning treatment to obtain both lymphoid and myeloid reconstitution. This observation has been repeatedly substantiated from data on HLA-haploidentical transplants. A T-cell-depleted haploidentical graft has been reported successful following administration of a fully ablative regimen with BU, CY and ATG [44]. Another report using haploidentical donors described two patients who were retransplanted successfully after failing to engraft with reduced intensity conditioning only when an intensive myeloablative regimen consisting of 700 cGy of TBI was utilized prior to the second HCT procedure [45]. In a recent report, 10 patients receiving HLA-haplo-identical grafts were studied. Half of them were given intensive BU/CY myeloablative conditioning while the other half received either low dose BU with CY, or ATG and CY without BU [47]. Three of the five patients who had received intensive myeloablative conditioning survive with lymphoid and myeloid reconstitution. In the group that did not receive the intensive preparatory regimen, all patients failed to demonstrate stable engraftment of donor hematopoietic stem cells. This finding, again, indicates the paramount importance of using intensive conditioning prior to HCT in RD patients.

Cyclic neutropenia

Cyclic neutropenia is usually a familial disorder in which patients have regular cyclic fluctuations in the number of blood neutrophils. The genetic transmission is autosomal dominant with variable expression [48]. The gene responsible for cyclic neutropenia has been identified [49]. Clinical signs and symptoms include recurrent bouts of fever, malaise, periodontitis, mucosal ulcers, sore throat and lymphadenopathy. Most patients live full lives, with a gradual amelioration of the symptoms. Ten percent of patients experience frequent serious infections. The laboratory investigation reveals periods of severe neutropenia (<200 neutrophils/μL) lasting for 3–10 days alternating with periods of normal neutrophil counts. The cyclic fluctuation occurs usually every 21 days with a range of 14–36 days. For each individual patient the cycle length is constant. Bone marrow precursors also reveal concomitant cyclic oscillations. Bone marrow myeloid precursor cells are present in highest numbers at the time of the nadir of peripheral neutropenia. Therapy with G-CSF improves the neutrophil count and reduces the frequency of symptoms.

Clinical manifestations of cyclic neutropenia do not justify the use of HCT. However, HCT has contributed towards a better understanding of this disorder. In an autosomal recessive collie dog model cyclic neutropenia can be corrected by HCT [50]. To date, no human transplants have been reported for cyclic neutropenia. In one patient who was transplanted with an allogeneic donor graft with cyclic neutropenia, the disease was found to have transferred to the recipient after the HCT procedure [51].

Cartilage-hair hypoplasia

Cartilage-hair hypoplasia, an autosomal recessive disorder, is encountered primarily in the Amish and Finnish populations. The abnormal gene for cartilage-hair hypoplasia is located on the short arm of chromosome

9 [52]. Characteristic findings include short-limbed dwarfism, fine hair, moderate to severe neutropenia (ANC 100–2000/μL) and defects of cell mediated immunity [53,54]. The combination of neutropenia and cellular immunity defects lead to recurrent bacterial and viral infections, especially reactivation of varicella-zoster infection in these patients. Allogeneic HCT has been used to correct the hematologic and immunologic defects of cartilage-hair hypoplasia [55,56]. As expected, the phenotypic hair and bony abnormalities have not been corrected by HCT. So far, six patients with cartilage-hair hypoplasia have been reported to have undergone HCT. One of the six patients was conditioned with CY, cytosine arabinoside and thioguanine and achieved complete donor lymphoid engraftment, but other hematopoietic lines achieved only partial donor chimerism [56]. The remaining five patients received BU and CY and achieved full donor chimerism for lymphoid as well as all other hematologic parameters [56]. The experience with allogeneic HCT is still limited. Severely affected patients, however, seem to benefit from the procedure.

Dyskeratosis congenita (DC)

DC, a rare congenital syndrome, was originally described in 1906. The majority of patients are males, and the defective gene has been linked to chromosome Xq28 [57]. In DC, like in Fanconi anemia, associated DNA repair defects have been noted. Clinically, this disorder is characterized by reticulated hyperpigmentation of the skin, nail dystrophy, and leukoplakia of the mucus membranes. Immunohematologic manifestations include neutropenia, refractory anemia, thrombocytopenia and defective cell mediated immunity [58,59]. Allogeneic bone marrow transplantation has been used successfully to correct the hematologic abnormalities [60]. It is noted that patients with this syndrome require less intensive conditioning [59]. However, late complications associated with the HCT procedure have been observed [61]. The late complications may be multiple and involve multiple systems. Commonly seen HCT-associated late complications in DC include pulmonary fibrosis with respiratory failure and endothelial damage/activation syndromes, such as renal microangiopathy and veno-occlusive disease of the liver. In a published report of five patients with DC-associated severe aplastic anemia who had received HCT using HLA-identical related donor grafts, four patients died 2–8 years later with renal microangiopathy, veno-occlusive disease of the liver, Evans' syndrome, or invasive aspergillosis [61]. One patient alive at the time of writing (1998) had developed anemia, polyarthritis, pulmonary fibrosis and gastrointestinal malabsorption syndrome 7.5 years after the HCT procedure. In view of the occurrence of late HCT-associated complications, it is important that a complete baseline evaluation of kidneys, liver, respiratory tract and the endothelial parameters be performed prior to the initiation of HCT in these patients.

Shwachman–Diamond syndrome (SDS)

SDS is an autosomal recessive disorder characterized by exocrine pancreatic insufficiency, metaphyseal dysostosis and bone marrow hypoplasia [24]. Cyclic or persistent neutropenia is a common finding. However, in 10–25% of patients, trilineage pancytopenia may also be seen. Recurrent bacterial infections occur early in childhood and can contribute to early mortality. Progression to myelodysplasia and transformation to acute leukemia are seen in patients who have pancytopenia as the predominant finding. Overall survival without any treatment varies with different subpopulations. In patients without hypoplasia and leukemic transformation, the projected 50% survival rate is 35 years. However, this expectation is reduced to 24 years in patients with pancytopenia and further decreased to 10 years in those with leukemic transformation [24].

Conceivably, HCT would be the only curative treatment option for the bone marrow dysfunction in SDS. However, mixed results have been observed with allogeneic HCT as a therapeutic approach for SDS patients with hematologic abnormalities. So far, 15 patients with SDS have been reported to have received HCT [62–66]. The primary indications in these patients were either myelodysplastic syndrome or marrow aplasia. Six patients received HLA-matched sibling donor grafts while seven patients were transplanted with unrelated-matched grafts and two patients received mismatched-related grafts. Myeloablative conditioning with different chemotherapeutic agents with or without TBI (BU/CY in six patients and CY/TBI in nine patients) was used in these patients. Forty percent of the transplanted patients died due to the transplantation-related complications, including organ toxicity, graft rejection, GVHD and infections. Available follow-up was from 9 months to 3 years. As expected, the patients with marrow aplasia had a relatively better survival than the patients with myelodysplastic syndrome or leukemic transformation.

Qualitative neutrophil disorders

The major role of neutrophils is to defend the host against a variety of infectious agents. To accomplish this task the neutrophils must first sense infection, migrate to the site of infection (chemotaxis), adhere to the membranes of the blood vessel wall and then destroy the offender (phagocytosis) through the release of granules which take part in the activation of oxygen-dependent and oxygen-independent pathways of microbial killing. The presence of these different components of the microbial killing cascade are essential for the appropriate function of neutrophils. In the qualitative disorders discussed below, neutrophilia is usually present in response to infection. However, one or more of the functional components of the neutrophil attack may be faulty.

Neutrophil actin abnormality

This neutrophil abnormality is a rare inherited autosomal recessive disorder in which defective granulocyte motility leads to inadequate chemotaxis, resulting in serious recurrent infections. Granulocyte counts are, however, either normal or elevated. This disorder was initially described in an infant in 1974, who had failed to form abscesses during recurrent life-threatening infections with gram-positive and gram-negative organisms [67]. A Rebuck skin window had failed to reveal normal migration. Although actin levels are normal in the affected neutrophils, the polymerization of actin is defective, leading to poor or absent migration to the chemotactic stimuli. After the initial report, more children have been reported with neutrophil actin deficiency or its variants [68].

Allogeneic HCT has been attempted in a few patients with this disorder [68,69]. According to the published reports, one of three patients survived and was cured. The successfully treated patient had received a myeloablative regimen with BU, CY and ATG. The other two patients engrafted but died due to treatment-related complications, namely infections. It is possible to correct the defect in neutrophil actin abnormality by HCT using a heterozygous histocompatible sibling donor. Since the disease course is very aggressive, supportive care alone is usually not sufficient to allow prolonged survival of these patients.

Leukocyte adhesion deficiency type I (LAD-I)

First described in 1974, LAD-I is a rare heterogeneous autosomal recessive disorder in which neutrophil adhesion, chemotaxis and ingestion of the C3bi-opsonized microbes is impaired [70]. The neutrophils fail to migrate in the Rebuck skin window and also exhibit defects in adhesion and phagocytosis when tested for these functions. It is usually detected in early childhood as a result of frequent life-threatening bacterial and fungal infections, delayed umbilical cord separation and neutrophilia. The infections are mostly localized in the skin, subcutaneous tissues, middle ear and oropharynx.

At the molecular level, the basic defect is in the β_2-integrin adhesion molecule (CD11/CD18). The CD11/CD18 glycoprotein family consists of three heterodimeric proteins each composed of α and β chains.

Translocation of α and β chains to the cell surface requires assembly of the αβ heterodimer. The mutations in CD11/18 deficiency have been found in the β_2 chain, and prevent the assembly of the αβ heterodimer and thereby translocation of the heterodimer to the cell surface [71]. The cells with the mutated glycoprotein are unable to adhere or migrate in response to chemotactic stimulation. Since the β_2 chain is constant for each family and is normally present on the surface of the leukocytes, flow cytometric analysis with pertinent monoclonal antibodies can help identify those affected by the disorder. A severe clinical phenotype with <0.3% of the normal amount of β_2-integrins is more commonly seen as compared to a moderate variant in which β_2-integrin levels of 2.5–11.0% of normal are observed.

Since most of the children with LAD experience severe infections and die early in the course of their disease, early diagnosis and treatment, possibly with HCT, should be attempted. Several reports describe the course of HCT in patients with LAD-I. So far, 14 patients have been reported to have received HCT. Of these 14, five patients underwent HLA-matched sibling donor HCT and nine patients received grafts from two antigen mismatched or haplo-identical related donors [72,73]. In this study of 14 patients, the majority achieved either full or mixed chimerism. In most of the patients with mixed chimerism, although a variable number of donor cells were noted, there was no increased incidence of infections. In one patient with only 2–15% donor cells, mild gingivitis was observed after HCT. Two patients with initial immunologic graft rejection achieved full chimerism after treatment with anti-CD-2 or LFA-I monoclonal antibody. More recently, there have been reports of successful unrelated donor transplants utilizing fully matched and one antigen mismatched donors [74,75]. Although the follow-up is short for these patients, engraftment was prompt and the patients fared well.

In addition to CD11/18-integrins, there are other leukocyte adhesion molecules called selectins. Defect in these molecules may also result in significant disease. Two patients have been described with the absence of neutrophil receptors for E-selectin resulting in defective adhesion. This disorder is called LAD type II. To date, HCT has not yet been reported in patients with selectin deficiency.

Chediak–Higashi syndrome (CHS)

CHS is an autosomal recessive disorder. Clinically, it is characterized by partial ocular and cutaneous albinism, an increased susceptibility to bacterial infections and compromised platelet function. Partial albinism and photophobia are usually noted in early infancy, and increased respiratory and cutaneous infections soon become apparent. Decreased platelet function leads to a bleeding tendency. Other organ systems involved include hair, adrenal glands, pituitary gland and peripheral nerves [76]. There is an initial stable phase followed by an accelerated phase. The stable phase of the disease may or may not be associated with serious infections while the accelerated phase may be complicated by fulminant infections, massive hepatosplenomegaly, lymphadenopathy, anemia, neutropenia and thrombocytopenia [77]. The accelerated phase is uniformly fatal and no long-term survivors have been reported. In some patients the diagnosis of CHS is not apparent until the accelerated phase has developed.

Although phagocytosis *per se* occurs at a higher than normal rate in neutrophils of patients with CHS, and the postphagocytic metabolic burst is normal [78], myeloid cells in these patients produce abnormal lysosomes and granules [79]. This abnormality leads to defective microbial killing and persistent infections. The molecular defect has been reported to be an abnormal calcium uptake pump in CHS lysosomes [79] resulting in an inefficient and incomplete postphagocytic delivery of lysosomal enzymes into the phagosomes. This defect results in delayed intracellular destruction of bacteria by the Chediak-Higashi leukocytes [80]. In addition, the cellular response to chemotactic stimuli also appears to be defective.

In the laboratory, light and electron microscopy can be used to diagnose CHS by demonstrating abnormal granules and lysosomes. Neutrophils contain giant azurophilic granules along with abnormal lysosomes. Monocytes and macrophages show abnormal lysosomes. Both lymphocytes and NK cells have giant cytoplasmic granules, and NK function is decreased. In platelets, the content of dense granules is decreased leading to abnormal platelet function. The bone marrow of these patients displays ineffective myelopoiesis with increased M : E ratio and a left shift.

The first HCT procedure for CHS using a sibling donor was performed in a patient in accelerated phase [81]. CY alone was used as the preparative regimen. The patient, however, did not achieve sustained engraftment, probably due to inadequate preparation. The patient relapsed into an accelerated phase and a second transplant procedure from the same donor was attempted using a preparative regimen containing CY and TBI. This strategy resulted in stable engraftment. Another patient who was in the stable phase of the disease was similarly treated with CY and TBI, resulting in full donor engraftment and correction of the functional defect [82]. A series of 10 other patients has been published [83]. Two patients were in stable disease and eight patients were in the accelerated phase of CHS. Seven patients received HCT from fully matched sibling donors and three received one antigen mismatched or haploidentical donor grafts. The preparative regimen included BU, CY and VP16 in eight patients. One patient received additional cytosine arabinoside. Three of the seven long-term survivors achieved full donor chimerism while four patients demonstrated mixed chimerism. In one patient with low level of donor chimerism, persistent bacterial infections were seen. As expected, in none of these patients were the cutaneous, ocular and neurologic manifestations corrected.

Recently, a case report described a 10-month-old girl who underwent a matched-sibling donor transplant using a BU/CY regimen. She is now 7 years post-HCT and doing well, although chimerism studies indicate that she only has 20% donor cells. Her mixed chimerism is stable and she has been free of infections [84].

It is clear that HCT can be used successfully to treat patients with CHS in both the stable and accelerated phases. HCT should be considered in the early stages as soon as the diagnosis is established. Patients with stable-phase disease are expected to tolerate the procedure better than those treated in the advanced phase, when serious organ damage may already have taken place. If matched sibling donors are not available, unrelated donors can be considered. As evident from the discussion above, many patients developed mixed chimerism in spite of an aggressive preparatory regimen. Most of these mixed chimeric patients do not progress to the accelerated phase of CHS and continue to do well.

Chronic granulomatous disease (CGD)

CGD is a rare clinical syndrome resulting from defective neutrophil function. Both autosomal recessive and X-linked patterns of inheritance have been described. Although the carriers are usually asymptomatic, females with extreme "Lyonization" may be affected. The median age at presentation of the disease is 7 years (range: from 0.4 years to 15.0 years). Clinically, the course of CGD is extremely variable. Some patients present within their 1st year of life while others may present later. Most patients suffer from recurrent bacterial and fungal infections. Those presenting later in life may have fewer life-threatening infections than those who present early. The most common bacterial infections are from catalase-positive bacteria, such as *Staphylococcus aureus* and enteric bacilli. *Aspergillus* is the most common fungal infection. Infections are usually cutaneous or sino-pulmonary. Lymphadenitis is also seen in these patients, as well as hepatic abscesses. Serious and persistent infections may lead to formation of granulomas in vital organs.

In CGD, neutrophils are characterized by defective respiratory burst formation during phagocytosis and an inability to generate superoxide.

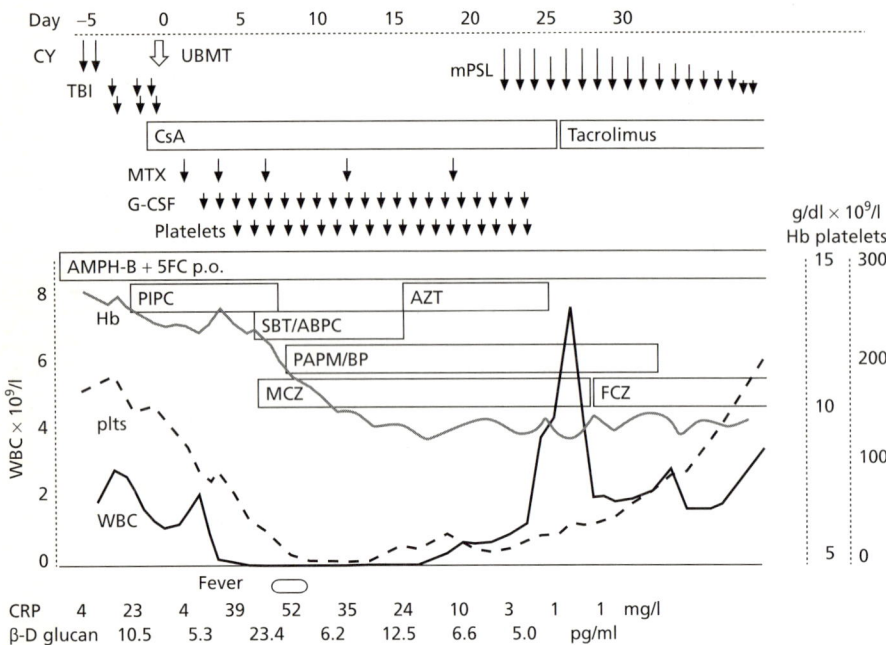

Fig. 108.3 Clinical course of a patient with chronic granulomatous disease (CGD) treated with unrelated donor bone marrow transplantation. AMPH-B, amphotericin B; AZT, aztreonam; CRP, C-reactive protein; 5 FC, flucytosine; FCZ, fluconazole; MCZ, miconazole; mPSL, methylprednisolone; PAPM/BP, panipenem/betamipron; PIPC, piperacillin; SBT/ABPC, sulbactam Na/cefoperazone Na. Reproduced with permission from Watanabe *et al.* [100].

The impaired superoxide production usually occurs transiently in each phagosome and leads to recurrent bacterial and fungal infections. Those bacteria that have their own mechanism to produce hydrogen peroxide and generate HOCl via the myeloperoxidase pathway of the phagocytic cell pose little problem. However, microbes, such as catalase-positive bacteria, can produce very low amounts of hydrogen peroxide in the phagocytic vacuoles. This defect results in insufficient production of HOCl to contribute to significant bacterial killing, culminating in recurrent infections with these bacteria [85].

The molecular basis of CGD has been well defined. The respiratory burst defects are due to mutations in one of the four subunits of the NADPH oxidase complex. Of the four subunits, two are membrane associated while the other two are located in the cytosol [86]. The gene for one of the membrane-associated subunits is located on the X chromosome, while the others are encoded by genes on chromosomes 1, 7 and 16. The disease is classified according to the underlying respiratory burst unit defect. In two large studies of 140 pediatric patients, defects in the X-linked gene for the gp91^{phox} subunit of cytochrome-b accounted for 62% of the cases. The remainder were found to be due to autosomal recessive defects in p47^{phox} (27%), p67^{phox} (5%) and p22^{phox} (6%). The nitroblue-tetrazolium (NBT) test is a very important laboratory tool to detect the disease and also to detect the carrier-state.

With the availability of excellent supportive care, the overall survival of patients with CGD has improved, with life expectancy now extending into the 30 years range. Although prophylaxis with trimethoprim-sulfamethoxazole has improved the outcome in these patients by decreasing bacterial infections [87–89], resistant fungal infections still result in early mortality.

Allogeneic HCT may be appropriate in CGD patients with frequent serious infections despite aggressive medical management. The availability of excellent supportive care with improved outcomes and the extreme variability in the disease course makes selection of appropriate patients for HCT very difficult. Pretransplant evaluation is still of critical importance. The older patients are anticipated to have a higher incidence of HCT-related complications, including graft failure and/or rejection. Tissue damage due to chronic inflammation should be carefully evaluated. Hepatic abscesses, ileocecal inflammation and gastrointestinal obstruction can influence the outcome of HCT. These patients should also be evaluated for other associated disease entities such as antibody negative collagen vascular disease, retinitis pigmentosa, Macleod red cell syndrome and Duchenne muscular dystrophy. A significantly higher mortality in patients with the X-linked recessive form of the disease has been reported and should be considered while selecting candidates [89]. Also, the possibility of extreme "Lyonization" should be kept in mind while considering related donors.

The number of reports of successful HCT in patients with CGD has increased during the last 2 decades [90–97]. Most of these HCT procedures have been performed using HLA-matched related donors. With such donors, nonmyeloablative preparative regimens containing CY or CY with antithymocyte serum were used initially. This often resulted in autologous recovery with recurrence of the disease. In one case, 1–2% cells from the donor could be identified for about 3 years after which time these cells also disappeared [98]. This observation of autologous recovery suggested the necessity for using ablative conditioning. Subsequently, CGD patients have been treated with CY and reduced doses of BU (8 mg/kg). This strategy has produced better outcomes resulting in persistent mixed chimerism (10–23%) for periods of up to 6 years [99].

Recently, reports of successful unrelated HLA-matched HCT with myeloablative conditioning have appeared in the literature [100]. Figure 108.3 illustrates the course of an 18-year-old patient with CGD who received an unrelated HCT [100]. This patient was diagnosed with CGD at 1 year of age and suffered repeated life-threatening infections despite prophylactic antibiotics and granulocyte transfusions. The patient had also been treated with IFN-γ. The patient subsequently developed an *Aspergillus* infection. Eventually, an unrelated donor HCT procedure was performed successfully in this patient.

Although fully ablative conditioning regimens have led to more success in obtaining sustained donor hematopoietic reconstitution with long-term survival, the attendant increased risk of acutely worsening infections and regimen-related toxicity cannot be ignored, especially in older patients. Other complications of HCT in CGD patients include a high risk of graft failure and an increased risk of GVHD. Repeated infections over a long period of time in the older patients may result in significant organ damage and, therefore, may predispose to a higher risk of HCT-related complications. Therefore, active infections or inflammation should be treated in a timely and appropriate fashion as described below. The increased risk of GVHD in the CGD patients may also be due to the occurrence of repeated infections and/or inflammation, resulting in the sustained elevation of TNF-α levels [101–103]. Administration of TNF-α-antagonists has been proposed to neutralize the circulating TNF-α [104].

Recently, a study of 27 CGD patients has been reported evaluating complications (including GVHD) and survival according to different risk factors (infection and/or inflammation) present at the time of HCT [105]. Twenty-five patients received grafts from compatible sibling donors and the remaining two patients received their HCT from HLA-matched unrelated donors. All patients were treated with myeloablative conditioning. In this study, an overall survival of 23 out of 27 patients has been reported with 22 of the 23 survivors cured of CGD (median follow-up of 2 years). Moreover, a slightly higher incidence of severe GVHD (grade III–IV) was found in those patients who had pre-existing overt infections and/or active inflammatory conditions prior to the HCT (four of 11 patients). Of the 16 patients who did not have any overt infection/inflammation, only three patients developed GVHD, which was mild (grade II) in all three. Also, the myeloablative conditioning used in the study did not cause significant organ toxicity in the majority of the patients who did not have pre-existing infections. It is therefore important to identify the presence and nature of the infected foci clinically, by laboratory means and by using the appropriate radiological methods (such as computed tomography [CT], positron emission tomography [PET] and combined PET/CT) to institute appropriate therapy [106]. The active infections/inflammation should be treated aggressively using antimicrobials with intracellular action in combination with G-CSF-primed granulocyte transfusions [107]. This aggressive treatment should be initiated before and continued during the HCT procedure.

In conclusion, patients with CGD can be cured with sibling donor or unrelated donor HCT. However, thorough pretransplant evaluation of patients with severe disease, treatment of active infections and inflammation prior to and during HCT, selection of appropriate timing for the procedure, and an optimal conditioning regimen are necessary to attain good results.

Since CGD results from single gene defects in proteins expressed in myeloid cells, this disorder can be considered as an excellent candidate for gene replacement therapy targeted to the hematopoietic cells. Gene replacement therapy could theoretically be useful in patients, even if as few as 10–20% NBT positive cells resulted. This concept is supported by the fact that the female carriers in the X-linked variant of CGD have as low as 10% NBT positive cells and are asymptomatic. So far, this approach has been limited to *in vitro* experiments where reconstitution of the respiratory burst activity has been displayed in Epstein–Barr-virus-transformed lymphocytes [108]. The *in vivo* attempts to mediate gene transfer into long-lived human hematopoietic cells have been limited by a lack of appropriate viral vectors to carry out gene transfer.

Griscelli syndrome (GS)

GS is an autosomal recessive disorder that affects both lymphoid and myeloid cells, characterized by lymphoid and NK-cell dysfunction with clinical manifestations of partial albinism and immunodeficiency [109,110]. The disorder is uniformly fatal and is also characterized by an abnormal regulation of the immune system resulting in an accelerated lymphohistiocytic phase along with macrophage hyperactivation as seen in HLH. Variable granulocyte dysfunction may coexist. Two different gene loci, *RAB27A* and *MYO5A*, have been identified in patients with GS [111]. The GTP-binding protein RAB27A is involved in the control of immune regulation and appears to be a key effector of cytotoxic degranulation. Also, all patients with mutations in the *RAB27A* gene have developed HLH. Patients with the *MYO5A* defect appear to have a milder clinical phenotype.

A systematic diagnostic approach is essential in suspected cases of GS. The diagnostic steps should include clinical, laboratory and histopathologic assessment as mentioned in diagnostic guidelines for HLH. The NK-cell activity should also be tested. Finally, mutation analysis of the *RAB27A* gene should also be performed to confirm the diagnosis. This systematic approach is very important to identify those patients who have worse prognosis and need timely intervention with the HCT. Patients with the *MYO5A* mutation are generally not candidates for HCT.

Allogeneic HCT is the only known curative treatment in GS. Although the data are limited due to the rarity of the disease, several reports of HCTs performed in GS patients using sibling, matched related as well as matched unrelated donors exist [110,112–114]. In one report of three patients who received matched sibling grafts [110,112], two patients died due to transplant-related complications. The third patient achieved full chimerism with normal immune and hematopoietic function. In another published case of a 6-month-old patient with GS, mobilized peripheral blood hematopoietic cells from her phenotypically HLA-identical mother were used [113]. In this patient, the conditioning included BU, CY and VP16. The patient received a CD34$^+$ cell dose of 15.4×10^6/kg along with a CD3$^+$ cell dose of 17.6×10^3/kg of recipient body weight. Three months after the transplant procedure was performed, a lymphoproliferative syndrome occurred and was successfully treated. Twenty-six months after HCT, the patient has shown mixed chimerism (52% donor cells) and is clinically well. A recent case report has shown successful HCT in a patient with GS using a matched unrelated donor graft [114]. In this patient, myeloablative doses of BU were used along with thiotepa and fludarabine as conditioning prior to the HCT. The number of nucleated cells infused was 7.8×10^8/kg of recipient body weight. Engraftment in this patient was prompt and the patient is well 30 months post-HCT with complete donor chimerism and normal blood cell counts.

In summary, in addition to a systematic diagnostic approach, an early intervention with HCT in GS patients with the *RAB27A* gene mutation is recommended. If a sibling donor is not available, an immediate search for an unrelated donor should be performed. If no histocompatible donors are available, strong consideration for a haploidentical HCT should be given, as the condition is rapidly fatal.

Conclusion

The major disease manifestation of the phagocytic disorders described in this chapter is the occurrence of recurrent, often life-threatening infections resulting in vital organ damage and increased morbidity and mortality if appropriate intervention is not instituted in a timely fashion.

The outcome of HCT in phagocytic disorders has improved during the last decade. In addition to the high-quality supportive care after HCT and improved GVHD prevention, the factors that affect a successful outcome with HCT include early diagnosis, the nature or severity of the disease, pre-existing serious infections, other pre-existing comorbidities and the status of vital organ functioning at transplantation. For example, early diagnosis and HCT is essential in some of these disorders, such as LAD and CHS, due to the aggressive and fatal nature of these disorders. An efficient pretransplant evaluation therefore is important.

Allogeneic HCT remains the procedure of choice for most of the diseases discussed in this chapter. An HLA-matched sibling is the preferred donor. However, if such a sibling is unavailable, a search for a histocompatible-matched unrelated or haploidentical related donor should not be delayed. In specific cases, such as X-linked CGD with severely imbalanced "Lyonization," or in primary HLH, the risk/benefit ratio should be assessed before choosing a sibling vs. an unrelated donor. In primary HLH, data indicate that patients receiving HCT from unrelated donors with one antigen mismatch may have survival results approaching those of HCT from closely matched unrelated donors. Current data suggest a better outcome with a myeloablative approach except in DC, where less intensive conditioning may be indicated due to the presence of DNA repair defects. The limited data on HCT in RD indicate that the use of intensive myeloablative conditioning regimens, irrespective of the type of donor graft used, is necessary to attain successful engraftment with subsequent lymphoid as well as myeloid reconstitution in the recipient.

References

1 Ackerman SK, Douglas SD. Purification of human monocytes on microexudat-coated surfaces. *J Immunol* 1978; **120**: 1372–4.

2 Ackerman SK, Douglas SD. Monocytes. In: Carr I, ed. *The Reticuloendithelial System*, vol. 1. New York: Plenum Press, 1980: 297–328.

3 Douglas SD, Yoder MC. The mononuclear phagocyte and dendritic cell systems. In: ER Stiehm, ed. *Immunologic Disorders in Children*, 4th edn. Philadelphia, PN: WB Saunders & Co, 1996: 113–32.

4 Ownby DR, Pizzo S, Blackmon L et al. Severe combined immunodeficiency with leukopenia (reticular dysgenesis) in siblings: immunologic and histopathologic findings. *J Pediatr* 1976; **89**: 382–7.

5 Babior BM, Woodman RC. Chronic granulomatous disease. *Semin Hematol* 1990; **27**: 247–59.

6 Cazzola M, Scchi F, Pagani A et al. X-linked chronic granulomatous disease in an adult woman, evidence for cell selection favoring neutrophils expressing the mutant allele. *Haematologica* 1985; **70**: 291–5.

7 Blanche S, Caniglia M, Girault D, Landman J, Griscelli C, Fischer A. Treatment of hemophagocytic lymphohistiocytosis with chemotherapy and bone marrow transplantation: a single center study of 22 cases. *Blood* 1991; **78**: 51–4.

8 McSweeny PA, Dietger N, Shizuru JA et al. Hematopoietic cell transplantation in older patients with hematologic malignancies: replacing high-dose cytotoxic therapy with graft-versus-tumor effects. *Blood* 2001; **97**: 3390–400.

9 Henter J-I, Sodder O, Ost A, Elinder G. Incidence and clinical features of familial hemophagocytic lymphohistiocytosis in Sweden. *Acta Pediatr Scand* 1991; **80**: 428–35.

10 Arico M, Janka G, Fischer A et al. Hemophagocytic lymphohistiocytsis: diagnosis treatment and prognostic factors. Report of 122 children from the International Registry. *Leukemia* 1996; **10**: 197–203.

11 Katakoa Y, Todo S, Morioka Y et al. Impaired natural killer activity and expression of interlukin-2 receptor antigen in familial erythrophagocytic lymphohistiocytosis. *Cancer* 1990; **65**(9): 1937–41.

12 Goldberg JC, Nezlof C. Familial lymphohistiocytosis: the pathologists view. *Pediatr Hematol Oncol* 1989; **6**: 199–204.

13 Janka GE. Familial erythrophagocytic lymphohistiocytosis. *Eur J Pediatr* 1983; **140**: 221–30.

14 Fischer A, Virelizier JL, Arenzana-Seisdedoss F et al. Treatment of four patients with erythrophagocytic lymphohistiocytosis by a combination of VP-16-213, steroids, intrathecal methotraxate and cranial irradiation. *Pediatrics* 1985; **76**: 263–8.

15 Loechelt BJ, Egeler M, Filipovich AH, Jyonouchi H, Shapiro RS. Immunosuppression. Preliminary results of alternative maintenance therapy for familial hemophagocytic lymphohistiocytosis. *Med Pediatr Oncol* 1994; **22**: 325–8.

16 Henter J-I, Arico M, Egeler M et al. A treatment protocol for hemophagocytic lymphohistiocytosis. *Med Pediatr Oncol* 1997; **28**: 342a [Abstract].

17 Fischer A, Cerf-Bensussan N, Blanche S et al. Allogeneic bone marrow transplantation for erythrophagocytic lymphohistiocytosis. *J Pediatr* 1986; **108**: 267–70.

18 Fischer A, Landais P, Friedrich W et al. Bone marrow transplantation (BMT) in Europe for primary immunodeficiencies other than severe combined immunodeficiency: a report from the European groups for BMT and the European groups for immunodeficiency. *Blood* 1994; **83**: 1149–54.

19 Bolme P, Henter J-I, Winiarski J et al. Allogeneic bone marrow transplantation for hemophagocytic lymphohistiocytosis in Sweden. *Bone Marrow Transplant* 1995; **15**: 331–5.

20 Baker KS, Delaat CA, Shapiro RS, Gross TG, Steinbuch M, Filipovich AH. Successful correction of hemophagocytic lymphohistiocytosis with related and unrelated bone marrow transplantation. *Blood* 1995; **86** (Suppl. 1): 387a [Abstract].

21 Baker KS, Delaat CA, Steinbuch M et al. Sucessful correction of hemophagocytic lymphohistiocytosis with related or unrelated bone marrow transplantation. *Blood* 1997; **89**: 3857–63.

22 Landman-Parker J, LeDeist F, Blaise A, Brison O, Fischer A. Partial engraftment of donor bone marrow cells associated with long term remission of hemophagocytic lymphohistiocytosis. *Br J Haematol* 1993; **85**: 37–41.

23 Baker K, Gross TG, Delaat CA et al. Unrelated donor stem cell transplantation for life-threatening hemophagocytic disorders: preliminary results from the national marrow donor program pilot study IBMTR. *Biol Blood Bone Marrow Transplant* 2002; **8**: 97a [Abstract].

24 Alter BP. The bone marrow failure syndromes. In: Nathan DJ, Oski FA, eds. *Hematology in Infancy and Childhood*, 3rd edn. Philadelphia: WB Saunders & Co., 1993: 159–241.

25 Kostmann R. Infantile genetic agranulocytosis. A review with presentation of ten new cases. *Acta Pediatr Scand* 1975; **64**: 362–8.

26 Tschan CA, Pilz C, Zeidler C et al. Time course of increasing numbers of mutations in the granulocyte colony-stimulating factor receptor gene in a patient with congenital neutropenia who developed leukemia. *Blood* 2001; **97**: 1882–4.

27 Jeha S, Chan KW, Aprikyan AG et al. Spontaneous remission of granulocyte colony-stimulating factor-associated leukemia in a child with severe congenital neutropenia. *Blood* 2000; **96**: 3647–9.

28 Dale DC, Bonilla MA, Davis MW et al. A randomized controlled phase III trial of recombinant human granulocyte colony-stimulating factor (filgastrim) for the treatment of severe chronic neutropenia. *Blood* 1993; **81**: 2496–502.

29 Glasser L, Duncan BR, Corrigan JJ. Measurement of serum granulocyte colony-stimulating factor in a patient with congenital agranulocytosis (Kostmann syndrome). *Am J Child* 1991; **145**: 925–8.

30 Pahwa RN, O'Reilly RJ, Broxmeyer HE et al. Partial correction of neutrophil deficiency in congenital neutropenia following bone marrow transplantation (BMT). *Exp Hematol* 1977; **5** (Suppl. 2): 45–6.

31 Zeidler C, Boxer L. Management of Kostmann syndrome in the G-CSF era. *Br J Haematol* 2000; **109**(3): 490–5.

32 Rappeport JM, Parkman R, Newburger P, Camitta BM, Chusid MJ. Correction of infantile agranulocytosis (Kostmann syndrome) by allogeneic bone marrow transplantation. *Am J Med* 1980; **68**: 605–9.

33 Toyoda H, Azuma E, Hori H et al. Successful unrelated BMT in a patient with Kostmann syndrome complicated by pretransplant pulmonary bacterial abscesses. *Bone Marrow Transplant* 2001; **28**: 413–5.

34 De Vaal OM, Seynhaeve V. Reticular dysgenesia. *Lancet* 1959; **ii**: 1123–5.

35 Gitlin D, Vawter G, Craig JM. Thymic alymphoplasia and congenital aleukocytosis (reticular dysgenesis). *Pediatrics* 1964; **33**: 184–92.

36 Alonso K, Dew JM, Strake WR. Thymic alymphoplasia and congenital aleukocytosis (reticular dysgenesis). *Arch Pathol* 1972; **94**: 179–83.

37 Haas RJ, Neithammer D, Goldmann SF et al. Congenital immunodeficiency and agranulocytosis (reticular dysgenesis). *Acta Paediatr Scand* 1977; **66**: 279–83.

38 Espanol T, Compte J, Alvarez C et al. Reticular dysgenesis: a report of two brothers. *Clin Exp Immunol* 1979; **38**: 615–20.

39 Levinsky R, Teidman K. Successful bone marrow transplantation for reticular dysgenesis. *Lancet* 1983; **1**: 671–3.

40 Friedrich W, Goldmann SF, Ebell W et al. Severe combined immunodeficiency: treatment by bone marrow transplantation in 15 infants using HLA haplo-identical donors. *Eur J Pediatr* 1985; **144**: 125–30.

41 Roper M, Parmely RT, Crist WM et al. Severe congenital leucopenia (reticular dysgenesis). *Am J Dis Child* 1985; **139**: 832–5.

42 Fischer A, Landais P, Friedrich W et al. European experience of bone marrow transplantation for severe combined immunodeficiency. *Lancet* 1990; **336**: 850–4.

43 Bujan W, Ferster A, Sariban E, Friedrich W. Effect of recombinant human granulocyte colony-stimulating factor in reticular dysgenesis [Letter]. *Blood* 1993; **82**: 1684.

44 Haas A, Wells J, Chin T, Steim ER. Successful treatment of reticular dysgenesis with haploidentical bone marrow transplant (BMT). *Clin Res* 1986; **34**: 127a [Abstract].

45 De Santes KB, Lai SS, Cowen MJ. Haploidentical bone marrow transplants for two patients with reticular dysgenesis. *Bone Marrow Transplant* 1996; **17**: 1171–3.

46 Knutsen AP, Wall DA. Umbilical cord blood transplantation in severe T-cell immunodeficiency disorders: 2-year experience. *J Clin Immunol* 2000; **20**: 466–76.

47 Bertrand Y, Muller SM, Casanova JL et al. Reticular dysgenesis: HLA non-identical bone marrow

transplants in a series of 10 patients. *Bone Marrow Transplant* 2002; **29**: 759–62.
48. Dale DC, Graw RG. Transplantation of allogeneic bone marrow in canine cyclic neutropenia. *Science* 1974; **183**: 83–4.
49. Horwitz M, Benson KF, Person RE *et al*. Mutations in *ELA-2*, encoding neutrophil elastase, define a 21-day biologic clock in cyclic hematopoeisis. *Nat Genet* 1999; **23**: 433–6.
50. Jones JB, Yang TJ, Dale JB, Lange RD. Canine cyclic hematopoiesis: marrow transplantation between littermates. *Br J Hematol* 1975; **30**: 215–23.
51. Krance RA, Spruce WE, Forman SJ *et al*. Human cyclic neutropenia transferred by allogeneic bone marrow grafting. *Blood* 1982; **60**: 1263–6.
52. Sulisalo T, Sistonen P, Hastbacka J *et al*. Cartilage-hair hypoplasia gene assigned to chromosome 9 by linkage analysis. *Nat Genet* 1993; **3**: 338–41.
53. Makiti O, Kaitila I. Cartilage-hair hypoplasia: clinical manifestations in 108 Finnish patients. *Eur J Pediatr* 1993; **152**: 211–7.
54. Lux SE, Johnston RB Jr, August CS *et al*. Chronic neutropenia and abnormal cellular immunity in cartilage-hair hypoplasia. *N Engl J Med* 1970; **282**: 231–6.
55. O'Reilly RJ, Brochstein J, Dinsmore R, Kirkpatric D. Marrow transplantation for congenital disorders. *Semin Hematol* 1984; **21**: 188–221.
56. Berthet F, Siegrist CA, Ozsahin H *et al*. Bone marrow transplantation in cartilage hair hypoplasia: correction of immune deficiency but not of chondroplasia. *Eur J Pediatr* 1996; **155**: 286–90.
57. Connor JM, Gatherer D, Gray F *et al*. Assignment of the gene for dyskeratosis congenital to Xq28. *Hum Genet* 1986; **72**: 348–51.
58. Ogden GR, Connor E, Chisolm DM. Dyskeratosis congenital. Report of a case and review of literature. *Oral Surg Oral Med Oral Pathol* 1988; **65**: 586–91.
59. Putterman C, Safadi R, Zlotogora J *et al*. Treatment of the hematological manifestations of dyskeratosis congenital. *Ann Hematol* 1993; **66**: 209–12.
60. Mehmoud HK, Shaefer VW, Schmidt CG *et al*. Marrow transplantation for pancytopenia in dyskeratosis congenital. *Blut* 1985; **51**: 57–60.
61. Vanderson R, Agnes D, Gerard S *et al*. Unusual complications after bone marrow transplantation for dyskeratosis congenital. *Br J Hematol* 1998; **103**: 243–8.
62. Okcu F, Roberts WM, Chan KW. Bone marrow transplantation in Shwachman–Diamond syndrome. Report of two cases and review of literature. *Bone Marrow Transplant* 1998; **21**: 849–51.
63. Faber J, Lauener R, Wick F *et al*. Shwachman–Diamond syndrome: early bone marrow transplantation in a high risk patient and new clues to pathogenesis. *Eur J Pediatr* 1999; **158**: 995–1000.
64. Arseniev L, Diedrich H, Link H. Allogeneic bone marrow transplantation in a patient with Shwachman–Diamond syndrome. *Ann Hematol* 1996; **72**: 83–4.
65. Cesaro S, Guariso G, Calore E *et al*. Successful unrelated bone marrow transplantation for Shwachman–Diamond syndrome *Bone Marrow Transplant* 2001; **27**: 97–9.
66. Hsu JW, Vogelsang G, Jones RJ *et al*. Bone marrow transplantation in Shwachman–Diamond syndrome. *Bone Marrow Transplant* 2002; **30**: 255–8.
67. Boxer LA, Hedly-White T, Stossel TP. Neutrophil actin dysfunction and abnormal neutrophil behavior. *N Engl J Med* 1974; **291**: 1093–9.
68. Coats TD, Torkildson JC, Torres M, Church JA, Howard TH. An inherited defect of neutrophil motility and microfilamentous cytoskeleton associated with abnormalities in 47-KD and 89-KD proteins. *Blood* 1991; **78**: 1338–46.
69. Camitta BM, Quesenberry PJ, Parkman R *et al*. Bone marrow transplantation for an infant with neutrophil dysfunction. *Exp Hematol* 1977; **5**: 109–11.
70. Skubitz KM. Qualitative disorders of leukocytes. In: Lee GR, Forester J, Lukens J *et al.*, eds. *Wintrob's Clinical Hematology*, 10th edn. Baltimore, MD: Lippincott, William & Wilkins, 1999: 1889–907.
71. Larson RS, Springer TA. Structure and function of leukocyte integrins. *Immunol Rev* 1990; **114**: 181–217.
72. Todd RF, Freyer DR. The CD11/CD18 leukocyte glycoprotein deficiency. *Hematol Oncol Clin North Am* 1988; **2**: 13–31.
73. Le Deist F, Blanche S, Keable H *et al*. Successful HLA non-identical bone marrow transplantation in three patients with leukocyte adhesion deficiency. *Blood* 1989; **74**: 512–6.
74. Hattori H, Tsuruta S, Horikoshi Y *et al*. Successful human leukocyte antigen mismatched related bone marrow transplantation in a 6 year old boy with leukocyte adhesion deficiency syndrome. *Pediatr Int* 2001; **43**: 306–9.
75. Mancias C, Infante AJ, Kamani NR. Matched unrelated donor bone marrow transplantation in leukocyte adhesion deficiency. *Bone Marrow Transplant* 1999; **24**: 1261–3.
76. Davis WC, Douglas SD. Defective granule formation and function in the Chediak–Higashi syndrome in man and animals. *Semin Hematol* 1972; **9**: 431–50.
77. Blume RS, Bennett JM, Yankee RA *et al*. Defective granulocyte regulation in the Chediak–Higashi syndrome. *N Engl J Med* 1968; **279**: 1009–11.
78. Root RK, Rosenthal AS, Balestra DJ. Abnormal bactericidal, metabolic and lysosomal functions of Chediak–Higashi syndrome leukocytes. *J Clin Invest* 1972; **51**: 649–65.
79. Styrt BS, Pollack CR, Klempner MS. An abnormal calcium uptake pump in Chediak–Higashi neutrophil lysosomes. *J Leukoc Biol* 1988; **44**: 130–5.
80. Stossel TP, Root RK, Vaughen M. Phagocytosis in chronic granulomatous disease and Chediak–Higashi syndrome. *N Engl J Med* 1972; **286**: 120–3.
81. Griscelli C, Virelizier JL. Bone marrow transplantation in a patient with Chediak–Higashi syndrome. In: Wedgewood RJ, Rosen FS, Paul NW, eds. *Primary Immunodeficiency Diseases*. New York: Alan R Liss, 1983: 333–4.
82. Virelizier JL, Lagrue A, Durandy A. Reversal of natural killer defect in a patient with Chediak–Higashi syndrome after bone marrow transplantation. *N Eng J Med* 1982; **306**: 1055–6.
83. Haddad E, Le Deist F, Blanche S *et al*. Treatment of Chediak–Higashi syndrome by allogeneic bone marrow transplant. Report 10 of cases. *Blood* 1995; **85**: 3328–33.
84. Trigg ME, Schugar R. Chediak–Higashi syndrome: hematopoietic chimerism corrects genetic defect. *Bone Marrow Transplant* 2001; **27**: 1211–3.
85. Curnutte JT. Chronic granulomatous disease: the solving of clinical riddle at the molecular level. *Clin Immunol Pathol* 1993; **67**: S2–15.
86. Roos D. The genetic basis of chronic granulomatous disease. *Immunol Rev* 1994; **138**: 121–57.
87. Mouy R, Fischer A, Vilmer E *et al*. Severity and prevention of infections in chronic granulomatous disease. *J Pediatr* 1989; **114**: 555–60.
88. Finn A, Hadzic N, Morgan G *et al*. Prognosis of chronic granulomatous disease. *Arch Dis Child* 1990; **65**: 942–5.
89. Winkelstein JA, Marino MC, Johnston RB *et al*. Chronic granulomatous disease report on a national registry of 368 patients. *Medicine* 2000; **79**: 155–69.
90. Di Barolomeo P, DiGirolamo G, Angrilli F *et al*. Reconstitution of normal neutrophil function in chronic granulomatous disease by bone marrow transplantation. *Bone Marrow Transplant* 1989; **4**: 695–700.
91. Zintl F, Hermann J, Fuchs D *et al*. Correction of fatal genetic diseases using bone marrow transplantation *Kinderarztl Prax* 1991; **59**: 10–5.
92. Hobbs JR, Monteil M, McClsukey DR, Jurges E, El Tumi M. Chronic granulomatous disease 100% corrected by displacement bone marrow transplantation from a volunteer unrelated donor. *Eur J Pediatr* 1992; **151**: 806–10.
93. Ozsahin H, von Planta M, Muller I *et al*. Successful treatment of invasive aspergillosis in chronic granulomatous disease by bone marrow transplantation, granulocyte colony-stimulating factor-mobilized granulocytes and liposomal amphotericin B. *Blood* 1998; **92**: 2719–24.
94. Ho CM, Vowels MR, Lockwood L *et al*. Successful bone marrow transplantation in a child with X-linked chronic granulomatous disease. *Bone Marrow Transplant* 1996; **18**: 213–5.
95. Calvino MC, Maldonado MS, Otheo E *et al*. Bone marrow transplantation in chronic granulomatous disease. *Eur J Pediar* 1996; **155**: 877–9.
96. Akioka S, Itoh H, Ueda I *et al*. Donor lymphocyte infusion at unstable mixed chimerism in an allogeneic BMT recipient for chronic granulomatous disease. *Bone Marrow Transplant* 1998; **22**: 609–11.
97. Leung TF, Chik KW, Li CK *et al*. Bone marrow transplantation for chronic granulomatous disease: long term follow up with review of literature. *Bone Marrow Transplant* 1999; **24**: 567–70.
98. Goudemand J, Anssens R, Delmas-Marsalet Y, Farriaux JP, Fontain G. Essai de traitement d'uncas de granulmatose familiale chronique par greffe de moelle osseuse allogenique. *Arch Franc Ped* 1976; **33**: 121–9.
99. Rappaport JM, Newberger PE, Goldblum RM, Goldman AS, Nathan DG, Parkman R. Allogeneic bone marrow transplantation for chronic granulomatous disease. *J Pediatr* 1982; **101**: 951–6.
100. Watanabe C, Yajima S, Taguchi T *et al*. Successful unrelated bone marrow transplantation for a patient with chronic granulomatous disease and associated resistant pneumonitis and *Aspergillus* osteomyelitis. *Bone Marrow Transplant* 2001; **28**: 83–7.
101. Morgenstern DE, Giffard MAC, Lin Li L *et al*. Absence of respiratory burst in X-linked chronic granulomatous disease and inflammatory response to *Aspergillus* fumigatus. *J Exp Med* 1997; **185**: 207–18.
102. Van Deventer SJH. Tumor necrosis factor and Crohn's disease. *Gut* 1997; **40**: 443–8.
103. Middleton PG, Taylor PR, Jackson G *et al*. Cytokine gene polymorphisms associating with severe acute graft-versus-host disease in HLA-identical sibling transplants. *Blood* 1998; **92**: 3943–8.

104 Cavazzana-Calvo M, Stephan JL, Sarnacki S et al. Attenuation of graft-versus-host disease and graft rejection by *ex vivo* immunotoxin elimination of alloreactive T cells in an H-2 haplotype disparate mouse combination. *Blood* 1994; **83**: 288–98.

105 Seger RA, Gungor T, Belohradsky BH et al. Treatment of chronic granulomatous disease with myeloablative conditioning and an unmodified hemopoietic allograft: a survey of the European experience 1985–2000. *Blood* 2002; **100**: 4344–50.

106 Gungor T, Engel-Bicik I, Eich G et al. Diagnostic and therapeutic impact of whole body positron emission tomography (PET) using fluorine-18-fluoro-2-deoxy-D-glucose (FDG) in children with chronic granulomatous disease. *Arch Dis Child* 2001; **85**: 341–5.

107 Ozsahin H, von Planta M, Muller I et al. Successful treatment of invasive aspergillosis in chronic granulomatous disease by bone marrow transplantation, granulocyte colony stimulating factor-mobilized granulocytes, and liposomal amphotericin-B. *Blood* 1998; **92**: 2719–24.

108 Volpp B, Lin Y. *In vitro* molecular reconstitution of the respiratory burst in B lymphoblasts from p47-*phox*/deficient chronic granulomatous disease. *J Clin Invest* 1993; **91**: 201–7.

109 Griscelli C, Durandy A, Guy-Grand D, Daugillard F, Herzog C, Prunieras M. A syndrome associating partial albinism and immunodeficiency. *Am J Med* 1978; **65**: 691–702.

110 Klein C, Phillipe N, Le Deist F et al. Partial albinism with immunodeficiency (Griscelli syndrome). *J Pediatr* 1994; **125**: 886–95.

111 Pastural E, Barrat FJ, Dugourcq-Lagelouse R et al. Griscelli disease maps to chromosome 15q21 and is associated with mutations in the myosine *Va* gene. *Nat Genet* 1997; **16**: 289–92.

112 Schneider LC, Berman RS, Shea CR, Perez-Atayde AR, Weinstein H, Geha RS. Bone marrow transplantation for the syndrome of pigmentary dilution and lymphohistiocytosis (Griscelli disease). *J Clin Immunol* 1990; **10**: 146–53.

113 Schuster F, Stachel DK, Schmid I et al. Griscelli syndrome: report of the first peripheral blood stem cell transplant and the role of mutations in the *RAB27A* gene as an indication for BMT. *Bone Marrow Transplant* 2001; **28**: 409–12.

114 Arico M, Zecca M, Santoro N et al. Successful treatment of Griscelli syndrome with unrelated donor allogeneic hematopoietic stem cell transplantation. *Bone Marrow Transplant* 2002; **29**: 995–8.

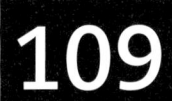

John E. Wagner, Margaret L. MacMillan & Arleen D. Auerbach

Hematopoietic Cell Transplantation for Fanconi Anemia

Introduction

Fanconi anemia (FA) is a genetically and phenotypically heterogeneous autosomal recessive disorder characterized by congenital malformations, progressive marrow failure and marked predisposition to malignancy. While the basic biochemical defects responsible for the syndrome are only now beginning to be elucidated, animal models and longitudinal studies evaluating the phenotypic consequences of specific mutations provide clues about the function of FA genes. In this chapter we will briefly review what is known about the pathogenesis and pathology of this congenital disorder as well as provide the reader with outcomes of the various treatment strategies, focusing on the results of allogeneic hematopoietic cell transplantation (HCT). To date, allogeneic HCT continues to be the only proven treatment modality with the potential of correcting the hematologic defect common to most, if not all, patients with FA.

History

In 1927, Fanconi described a family in which three male children between the ages of 5 and 7 years had pancytopenia and birth defects [1]. Based on his observations in this family and others, Fanconi's chief criteria for the diagnosis of FA were pancytopenia, hyperpigmentation, skeletal malformations, small stature, urogenital abnormalities and familial occurrence. According to Fanconi, Naegeli suggested in 1931 that the term "Fanconi's anemia" be used to describe such patients [2]. Fanconi's observations formed the basis for the chief criteria for diagnosis of FA for many years. Consideration of FA in the differential diagnosis of a patient manifesting clinical features of the syndrome depends on the clinician's concept of the FA phenotype. Most cases reported in textbooks and in the literature prior to the present decade present a clinical picture similar to the original cases described by Fanconi. Diagnosis of FA in these cases was usually made when aplastic anemia (AA) or leukemia developed in individuals with characteristic physical abnormalities. Literature reviews have thus been biased toward the most severe clinical phenotype. In a study comparing the frequencies of congenital anomalies among FA probands and their affected siblings, Glanz and Fraser [3] observed that there was a significant reduction in the incidence of congenital anomalies among the affected siblings compared to probands. Affected siblings with milder phenotypic features were identified following the diagnosis of FA in another affected family member and not because of their phenotypic presentation. Patients with "Fanconi-like" marrow failure who completely lacked congenital malformations, previously described as having the Estren–Dameshek syndrome [4], were found in the same sibships as "classical" FA. Delay in diagnosis in the majority of FA patients is still the standard for all, regardless of race, even in patients with congenital malformations [5,6]. The diagnosis is frequently missed until the onset of marrow failure, indicating the need for an increased awareness among physicians of the wide array of clinical features associated with the syndrome.

Clinical features

The FA phenotype is extremely variable; congenital malformations may range from none to many [7], and may involve any of the major organ systems (Table 109.1). Abnormalities involving central nervous system, gastrointestinal system and skeletal system in addition to radial-ray defects (i.e. radius and thumb abnormalities) have been added to the original FA phenotype [6]. FA patients may present with **V**ertebral anomalies, **A**nal atresia, **C**ardiac abnormalities, **T**racheo-**E**sophageal fistula, **R**enal anomalies, and radial **L**imb (VACTERL), and may also include hydrocephalus. These abnormalities comprise the VACTERL syndromes; thus there is considerable overlap of the phenotype in FA with these syndromes. Other syndromes with phenotypic overlap with FA include Holt–Oram syndrome, thrombocytopenia absent radius (TAR) syndrome, Baller–Gerold syndrome, Saethre–Chotzen syndrome (TWIST mutation), Dubowitz syndrome, velocardiofacial syndrome, Diamond–Blackfan anemia, dyskeratosis congenita and Nijmegen breakage syndrome.

More than 1000 cases of FA have been reported in varying detail in the world's literature; an analysis of these cases clearly demonstrates that FA patients not only have morphological abnormalities in many cases but are at progressively increasing risk of cancer as they age [8–12]. The International Fanconi Anemia Registry (IFAR) was established at The Rockefeller University in 1982 to collect clinical, genetic and hematologic information from a large number of FA patients over time to study the full spectrum of clinical features of the disease. The primary source of case material for the IFAR is physician reporting. Diagnosis of FA was confirmed in all cases by study of chromosomal breakage induced by diepoxybutane (DEB). Using the IFAR and its collection of clinical information on 754 DEB-confirmed FA patients from North America ascertained over a 20-year time period, correlations between genotype and phenotype are now possible [10].

Based on the clinical information in the IFAR, congenital malformations associated with FA are even more variable than previously recognized [6]. From a developmental standpoint, it is interesting that radial ray abnormalities in FA patients can be bilateral or unilateral. Even patients with bilateral abnormalities usually exhibit asymmetry, with limbs having different specific anomalies (Fig. 109.1). Notably, approximately one-third of FA patients do not manifest major congenital malformations. However, these patients frequently (but not always) have alterations in

Table 109.1 List of congenital malformations in Fanconi anemia (FA).

Congenital malformation	Frequency (%)
Skin pigmentation (café-au-lait spots, hyper- and hypopigmentation)	71
Thumb and radius (thenar hypoplasia, clinodactyly of fifth digit, syndactyly of fingers, hyperextensible thumbs, arachnodactyly, absence or hypoplasia of radius)	59
Skeletal (dysplastic ulna, micrognathia, frontal bossing, spina bifida, Klippel–Feil syndrome, vertebral anomalies, Sprengel's deformity)	31
Kidney and urinary tract (ectopic, horseshoe, rotated, hypoplastic or absent, dysplastic, hydronephrosis, hydroureter, reflux)	57
Genital (*males*: micropenis, undescended or atrophic or absent testes, hypospadius, phimosis, azospermia; *females*: bicornate uterus, aplasia or hypoplasia of vagina and uterus, atresia of vagina, uterus and ovary)	50 (males)
Cardiac (patent ductus arteriosis, ventricular septal defect, pulmonic or aortic stenosis, coarcation of the aorta, double aortic arch, cardiomyopathy, tetrology of Fallot)	29
Ears (deafness [usually conductive], atresia or dysplasa, canal stenosis)	Unknown
Eyes (microophthalmia, short or almond shaped palpebral fissures, ptosis, epicanthal folds, hyper- and hypotelorism)	47
Nose (flattened nasal bridge, nasal pit)	1
Gastrointestinal (esophageal atresia, duodenal atresia, anal atresia)	7
Central nervous system (CNS) (microcephaly, hydrocephalus, Bell's palsy, CNS arterial malformations, abnormal pituitary, absent corpus callosum, hyperreflexia)	1
Growth retardation (short stature)	67

growth as is observed in FA patients who manifest birth defects. Other very common findings are skin pigmentation abnormalities, hypoplastic thenar eminence and/or microophthalmia. Increased awareness of the facial anomalies as well as the complete spectrum of minor malformations seen in these patients should enable an earlier diagnosis to be made among patients without major congenital anomalies [7].

FA is usually associated with abnormal growth parameters both prenatally and postnatally. Short stature is a well-recognized feature of the syndrome and is often secondary to hormonal deficiencies. The mean stature of FA patients in the IFAR is near the 5th centile with weight and head circumference often ≤5th centile. A prospective study of 54 patients with FA, 30 males and 24 females from 47 unrelated families, showed that endocrinopathies are a common feature of FA, primarily manifesting as glucose/insulin abnormalities, growth hormone insufficiency and hypothyroidism [13]. Although short stature is a feature of FA, it is notable that 23 patients (43%) were within two standard deviations, and five (9%) were above the mean height for the general population. Expectedly, patients with endocrine dysfunction are more likely to have short stature. These data indicate that short stature is an integral feature of FA, but also that addition of endocrinopathies magnifies the growth failure in a significant proportion of patients. The finding of abnormal endogenous growth hormone secretion may demonstrate an underlying hypothalamic–pituitary dysfunction that results in poor growth. Since correction of growth hormone or thyroid hormone deficiency may improve final height outcome and quality of life, endocrine evaluations are recommended for all FA children well before use of androgens and HCT if possible.

Infertility is common. Approximately half of all female patients with FA are infertile. Menopause usually starts during the 4th decade. However, 15% of females cited in the literature or reported to the IFAR who reached at least 16 years of age and were not receiving androgen therapy had at least one pregnancy [14]. While pregnancy is possible in some females, it is often associated with complications such as rapid and marked progression of marrow failure, preeclampsia and premature labour. In contrast, males are very rarely fertile [15]. Genital malformations and hypoplastic gonads are common findings in males with FA. Results of semen analyses typically reveal very low or absent sperm counts as well as evidence of abnormal spermatogenesis.

Hematologic abnormalities occur in virtually all patients with FA at a median age of 7 years (range: birth to 41 years) (Fig. 109.2) [8,10,16]. Based on clinical data in the IFAR ($n = 754$ patients), the cumulative incidence of bone marrow failure by age 40 years was 90%. Initial hematologic findings were diverse. Thrombocytopenia was often associated with elevated levels of fetal hemoglobin and macrocytosis and usually preceded onset of anemia or neutropenia. Notably, some patients presented with myelodysplastic syndrome (MDS) or acute myeloid leukemia (AML) without prior diagnosis of AA. Of the 754 IFAR FA patients, 120 (16%) patients experienced MDS and/or AML (Plate 109.1, *facing p. 296*). The cumulative incidence of MDS or AML by age 40 years was 33% [10]. Based on a survey of FA patients performed by Rosenberg *et al.* [9], the median age of onset of leukemia was 11.3 years. Thrombocytopenia and pancytopenia were often associated with decreased marrow cellularity. Actuarial risk of clonal cytogenetic abnormalities during marrow failure was 67% by 30 years of age. Among the most frequent clonal abnormalities are duplications and triplications of the long arm of chromosome 1, gains of portions of the long arm of chromosome 3, and monosomy 7 or loss of material from the long arm of chromosome 7. Deletions of 5q, 11q, rearrangements of 6p and gains of chromosomes 8 and 21 have also been noted by different groups (Plate 109.2, *facing p. 296*) ([16,17], B. Hirsch, unpublished data). In addition, AML in FA patients rarely involves the chromosomal rearrangements commonly observed in non-FA patients with AML (e.g. t[9;11], t[8;21], t[6;9], t[11;19], inv 6). Frequently, abnormal karyotypes in FA AML are complex. Thus, many of the early descriptions of these karyotypes included designations of "marker" or "add," referring to structurally abnormal chromosomes that could not be completely identified by G- or R-banding. Recent advances in single and multicolor fluorescence *in situ* hybridization (FISH) and utilization of these and other molecular/cytogenetic techniques as adjuncts to conventional cytogenetic analysis now permits more definitive characterization of clones with the possibility of identifying new specific recurrent abnormalities (Fig. 109.3).

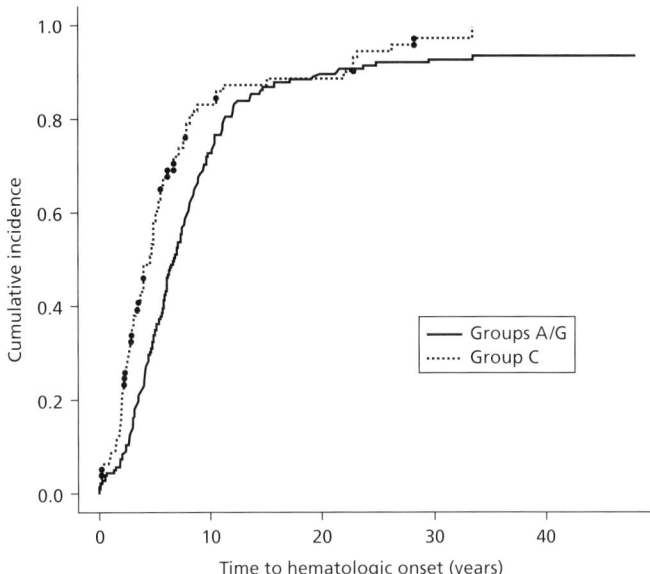

Fig. 109.2 Cumulative incidence of hematologic abnormalities over time in patients with FA-A/-G and FA-C. Of 754 FA patients within the International Fanconi Anemia Registry (IFAR) database, 601 (80%) experienced bone marrow failure with earlier onset in FA-C patients. Reproduced with permission from *Blood* 2002: DOI 10.1182/blood-2002-07-2170: p. 32. See also Plate 109.1.

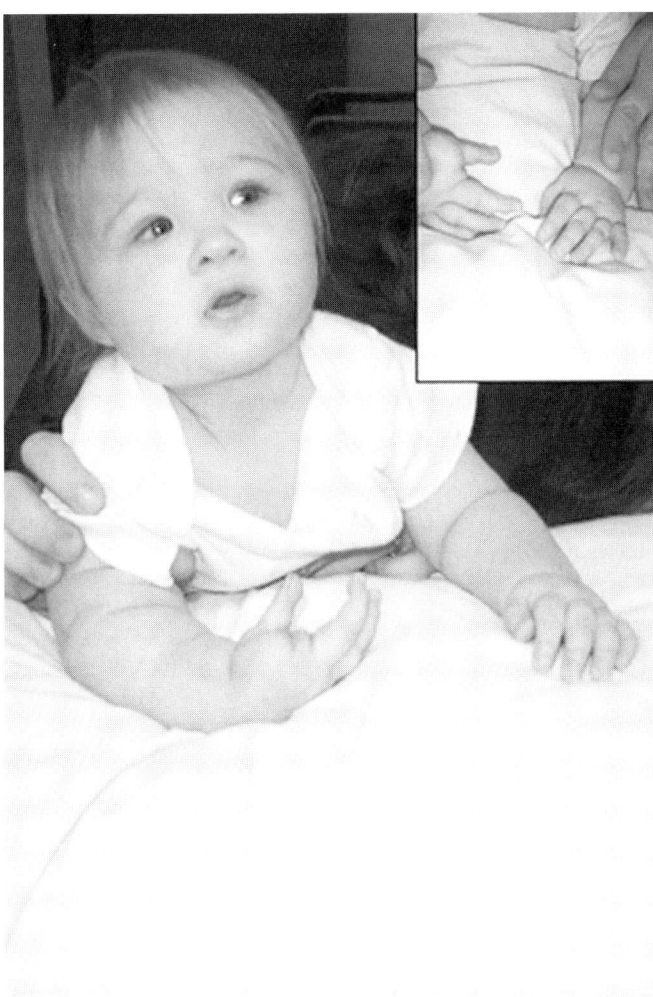

Fig. 109.1 A $1^{1}/_{12}$-year-old female who demonstrates many of the physical features associated with Fanconi anemia (FA). Before policization of the right index finger, the right hand exhibited a hypoplastic radius and absent thumb; the left hand had a hypoplastic thumb only. The patient exhibits growth retardation, microophthalmia, microcephaly and café-au-lait spots; she also has a kidney abnormality.

Clearly, early and accurate diagnosis of FA is important. Patients diagnosed early in life may have earlier endocrine intervention to optimize growth and development as well as more frequent monitoring of the hematologic profile. While investigational, harvesting of hematopoietic stem cells (HSCs) at a time when the marrow cellularity approaches normal and before the development of clonal cytogenetic abnormalities, MDS or leukemia, may be warranted. Harvested autologous HSCs could be useful for patients undergoing allogeneic HCT (as a "back-up" in the event of graft failure) or for future gene therapy and protocols incorporating an infusion of multipotent adult stem cells (MASCs). Until recently, storage of autologous HSCs has rarely been possible since most patients are diagnosed at the time of marrow failure.

Diagnostic tests

Due to considerable overlap of the FA phenotype with that of a variety of genetic and nongenetic diseases, diagnosis of FA is often difficult and unreliable on the basis of clinical manifestations alone. While FA should be strongly suspected if there are phenotype features consistent with the diagnosis plus an elevated mean corpuscular volume (MCV) for age, patients with FA may not have any clinical manifestations. Schroeder *et al.* [18] first suggested the use of spontaneous chromosomal breakage as a cellular marker for FA, but longitudinal studies of chromosome instability in FA patients showed this finding to be inconsistent. In contrast, hypersensitivity of FA cells to the clastogenic (chromosome-breaking) effect of cross-linking agents provides a reliable cellular marker for the diagnosis of this disorder (Fig 109.3). DEB and mitomycin C (MMC) are the agents most widely used for FA diagnosis. Extensive experience with MMC and DEB testing has demonstrated the sensitivity, specificity and reproducibility of the results [19–21]. Cross-linker hypersensitivity can be used to identify the preanemic patient as well as the patient with AA, MDS, or leukemia who may or may not have the physical stigmata associated with FA. It is recommended that all patients exhibiting any congenital malformation known to be associated with FA or AA at any age, or any patient with MDS with complex cytogenetic abnormalities, have a peripheral blood sample tested for cross-linker hypersensitivity [6]. Because of the lack of concordance of FA phenotype among affected siblings, *all siblings* of FA patients should also be screened. Data from DEB testing indicate that there is great variability in the degree of hypersensitivity in FA patients, although there is no overlap with the normal range [19]. In approximately 25% of FA patients, DEB testing will reveal two populations of phytohemagglutan A (PHA)-stimulated peripheral blood lymphocytes, one demonstrating an FA phenotype and the other a normal one [22]. The clinical significance of this type of mosaicism is unclear and is currently under investigation. Thus far, no correlation has been discerned between the degree of cross-linker hypersensitivity and the severity of the phenotype in FA patients or individual patient sensitivity to chemoradiotherapy ([23], J.E. Wagner & A.D. Auerbach, unpublished data). Whether the presence of mosaicism is associated with a milder disease course is currently unknown.

Importantly, the clinician should know that the chromosomal breakage test could also be applied to the study of fetal cells obtained by chorionic villous sampling (CVS), amniocentesis, or percutaneous umbilical blood

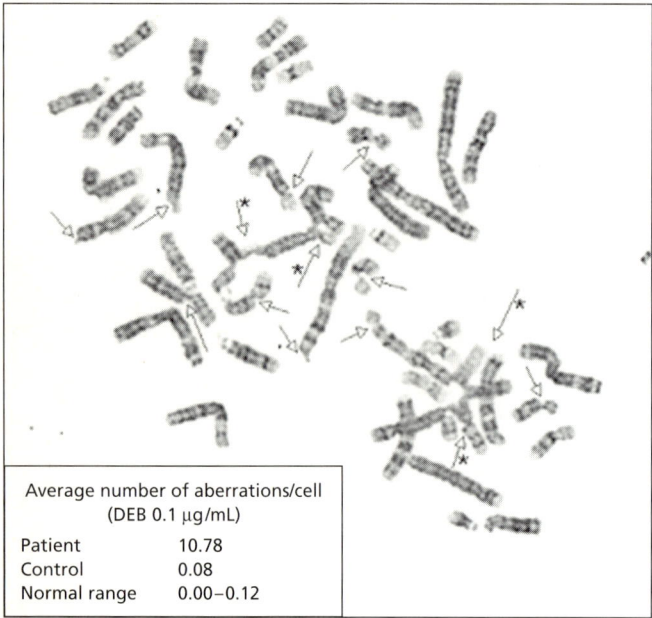

Fig. 109.3 Diepoxybutane (DEB) test. Metaphase cell from a Fanconi anemia (FA) patient after treatment with DEB *in vitro*. Arrows designate chromatid gaps and/or breaks; asterisks designate radial figures. This cell has nine gap/breaks and two multiradial figures. Figure courtesy of Betsy Hirsch, Ph.D., Director of the Cytogenetics Laboratory of the Fairview-University Medical Center, Minneapolis, MN.

sampling. If the specific mutation is known within the family, testing for the presence of the mutation on limited quantities of uncultured cells is possible and more rapid. Alternative diagnostic methods for FA, such as by cell-cycle analysis using flow cytometric methods on lymphocytes exposed to cross-linking agents, are sometimes used as a research tool [24,25]. While it is clear that duration of the G2/M phase is increased in FA cells as compared to unaffected cells, clinical diagnostic laboratories do not often use this method. Further, it has been reported that measurement of serum α fetoprotein levels may be a sensitive and reliable test for FA [26]. Due to the fact that false negative results occur at least 10% of the time (J.E. Wagner and M.L. MacMillan, unpublished data), it should only be considered supportive evidence for the diagnosis and does not obviate or replace the need for chromosomal breakage studies.

Complementation groups and gene cloning

Eight complementation groups (FA-A through FA-G, including FA-D1 and FA-D2) have been described [27–30]; complementation groups FA-A (~65%), FA-C (~15%) and FA-G (~10%) account for complementation group assignments for the majority of FA patients. The genes responsible for the defect in seven of these FA complementation groups have been identified [30–36]. These all encode unique proteins, which do not exhibit any known functional domains. The recent finding by Howlett *et al.* [37] of biallelic mutations in *BRCA2* in the reference cell line for FA-B and well as FA-D1, in addition to several other cell lines from FA patients typed as FA-D1, or untyped, suggests that *BRCA2* is the *FANCD1* gene. Support for this comes from a study showing that among cells from the eight FA complementation groups, FA-D1 cells uniquely showed impaired DNA damage-induced nuclear Rad51 foci formation, a characteristic of *BRCA2*-deficient cells [38]. Whether complementation group FA-B is a separate complementation group is still uncertain, as studies suggest that the FANCB protein functions upstream to FANCD2, while the FANCD1/BRCA2 protein functions downstream to FANCD2. Studies of additional FA-B patients are required to resolve this issue.

FANCC, the first FA gene discovered, encodes multiple transcripts, due to alternative splicing and polyadenylation signals. Each transcript shares the same 1674 nucleotide coding sequence, encoding a 558 amino acid protein (63 kDa) that shows no homologey to known proteins. A variety of *FANCC* mutations have been identified; the most common is IVS4 + 4 A > T. In North America, this mutation is found only in patients of Ashkenazi Jewish ancestry and accounts for approximately 85% of FA mutations in this population [39,40]. The carrier frequency for the IVS4 mutation in Ashkenazi Jews is one in 89. Two other relatively common *FANCC* mutations are 322delG and R548X, both found in FA patients of Northern European ancestry [23,41,42].

Like *FANCC*, *FANCA* also expresses multiple transcripts, with a major species of 5.5 kb, encoding a 4368 nucleotide coding sequence. The predicted FANCA protein is a 1455 amino acid peptide (~163 kDa) that, like FANCC, shares no significant homologey with any known protein. Sequence analysis has identified two overlapping nuclear localization signals, as well as a partial leucine zipper consensus domain, but neither of these domains has yet been demonstrated to be functional [32,33]. The *FANCA* gene contains 43 exons spanning approximately 80 kb, ranging from 34 to 188 base pairs [43]. *FANCA* mutation analysis reveals a large number of different mutations, indicating that *FANCA* is both highly polymorphic and may be hypermutable [44]. There are many private or semiprivate mutations, as well as ethnic specific mutations, making large-scale screening for *FANCA* mutations difficult [44–50].

The gene for FA-G complementation group (*FANCG*) was the third FA gene to be cloned, and was found to be identical with human *XRCC9*, which maps to 9p13 [34]. The complementary DNA (cDNA) is predicted to encode a polypeptide of 622 amino acids, with no sequence similarities to any other known protein or motifs that could point to a molecular function for *FANCG/XRCC9*. Four pathogenic mutations in *FANCG* were originally described; three were in patients of German ancestry and one was in a consanguineous Lebanese family. *FANCG* has subsequently been shown to be highly polymorphic, and to exhibit ethnic specific mutations in Korean/Japanese, Portuguese-Brazilian, French-Acadian and Northern European FA families, as well as many private mutations [51–53].

Notably, only a few FA patients have been described in the literature belonging to groups FA-B, FA-D1, FA-D2, FA-E and FA-F. Further information regarding FA mutations can be obtained from the Fanconi Anemia Mutation Database at http://www.rockefeller.edu/fanconi/mutate.

Complementation group assignment and mutation analysis

Once a patient is diagnosed as affected with FA, identification of the specific complementation group should be undertaken for reasons outlined below. Molecular diagnosis for FA complementation group C (FA-C) has been performed since 1994 by mutation screening using allele-specific assays. Assays for six *FANCC* mutations (in order of gene frequency: IVS4, 332delG, Q13X, R548X, R185X, L554P) [23] should be performed on all newly diagnosed FA patients, as these six mutations account for >85% of *FANCC* mutated alleles in Caucasian individuals. This can provide: (i) a means for rapid assignment of FA patients to group C; (ii) carrier identification for FA-C families; and (iii) prenatal diagnosis for high-risk couples that are known carriers of *FANCC* mutations. In contrast, this approach has been extremely difficult in those with *FANCA* mutations. Although 65% of FA patients are in complementation group FA-A, only two common mutations have been identified in *FANCA*: 1115–1118delTTGG and 3788–3790delTCT [44]. Upon diagnosis, FA patients should be screened for these two mutations with mutation-specific assays as this provides a rapid method of identifying the geno-

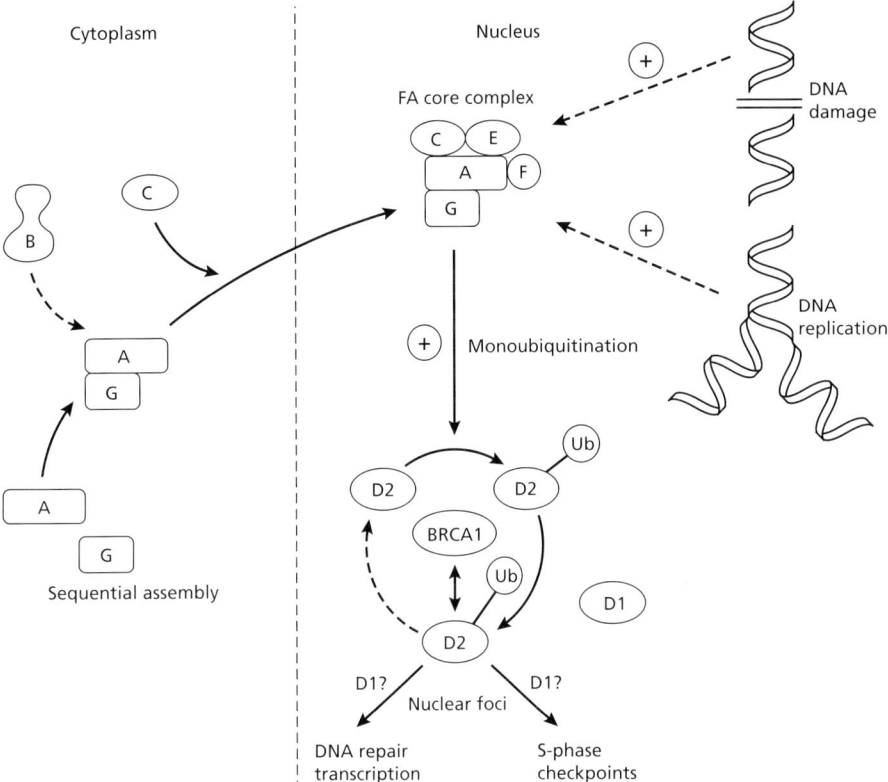

Fig. 109.4 Model of the Fanconi anemia (FA) pathway. The model shows the sequential assembly of the FA core complex in the cytoplasm and nucleus. The defect in FA-B cells indicates that FANCB might function in an early stage of this assembly process. DNA replication or DNA damage might activate the complex, either directly or indirectly, leading to the activation of FANCD2 by monoubiquination [68] and its targeting to nuclear foci. The FANCD1 protein might participate at this point. The association of BRCA1 at these sites could lead to as yet undefined downstream events, such as DNA repair or the activation of DNA synthesis (S) checkpoints. In this model, the core complex, which consists of FANCA, FANCC, FANCF, FANCG and FANCE, is the sensor for DNA damage and participates by activating FANCD2 through ubiquination. FANCD2 then facilitates repair. Reproduced with permission from *Nature Rev Genet* **2**; 2001, 446–59.

type for approximately 5% of all FA patients. Mutation screening for other mutations is limited by the large size and complexity of the *FANCA* gene and the high proportion of patients with large genomic deletions, private mutations and polymorphisms. In addition, the large size and structure of the recently identified genes, *FANCD2* and *FANCD1*, make it very difficult to identify the defective gene in newly diagnosed FA patients using mutation analysis alone.

The complementation group, however, can be determined by correction of cross-link hypersensitivity of the patient cells by transduction with retroviral vectors containing the normal *FANCA*, *FANCC*, *FANCD2*, *FANCE*, *FANCF*, or *FANCG* cDNAs. The method of cross-link hypersensitivity correction is similar to that established for testing for cross-link hypersensitivity on lymphoblastoid cell lines or peripheral blood-derived patient T cells [54,55]. After the complementation group has been determined by retroviral typing, denaturing high-performance liquid chromatography (DHPLC) can provide accurate mutation screening for FA [56]. DHPLC analysis [57] using the WAVE® DNA Fragment Analysis System (Transgenomic, San Jose, CA) provides an automated, rapid method to detect variation in DNA sequence, mainly base substitutions, microdeletions and microinsertions. This has been shown to provide accurate mutation detection for FA patients ([53,56–58], A.D. Auerbach, unpublished data).

Proposed functions of FA genes

The fundamental defect in FA cells is still undefined. Defects in DNA repair, cell-cycle checkpoints, oxygen metabolism, and induction of apoptosis have all been described in FA cells. The published data have been marked by contradictory results, which can be attributed partially to inconsistencies in experimental conditions, including variations in administration and dosage of DNA cross-linking agents administered, complementation group of the FA cells used, and the use of primary cells vs. transformed cell lines. FA genes were expected to be involved in DNA repair, but the discovery that the FANCC protein localized to the cytoplasm [59–61] initially brought skepticism to that view. However, it was soon shown that FANCC accumulates in both the cytoplasm and the nucleus [62]. Although the first FA gene was cloned 10 years ago, the biochemical function of FA proteins is only recently being elucidated. The FA genes all encode unique proteins, which do not exhibit any known functional domains. Recent studies of post-translational modifications of FANCD2 suggest that FA proteins function in regulating discrete cellular signalling pathways. Formation of a complex by several FA proteins, including FANCA, FANCC, FANCE, FANCF and FANCG [63–67], has been shown to be essential for the monoubiquitination of FANCD2 in response to DNA damage, causing this protein to translocate to nuclear foci containing BRCA1, suggesting a role for FANCD2 in DNA repair functions (Fig. 109.4) [68]. Phosphorylation of FANCD2 by ATM, a protein mutated in the chromosomal instability syndrome Ataxia Telangiectasia, is an independent post-translational modification, which is required for activation of FANCD2 [69]. Most recently, biallelic mutations in *BRCA2* in FA-D1 and FA-B patients suggest that *BRCA2* may be the gene that is responsible for FA in these patients, although further confirmation of the pathogenicity of these mutations is needed [37]. Whereas heterozygous carriers of *BRCA2* mutations have increased risk of early onset breast and ovarian cancer, inheritance of a mutated allele from each parent may lead to the birth of a child with features of FA.

Monoubiquitination of FANCD2 can be detected by immunoblotting with FANCD2 antibody [68]. Protein extracts from normal cells show both unmodified (FANCD2-S) and the monoubiquitinated (FANCD2-L) forms of the protein, while extracts from cells from FA complementation groups FA-A, -C, -E, -F and -G show only the unmodified lower FANCD2-S (short) form. It has been suggested that Western blotting to detect the presence or absence of the FANCD2-L form be used as a diagnostic screen for FA, and as an assay to detect complementation group after transduction by cDNA containing retroviral vectors [70]. While this may be a useful adjunct to standard tests of hypersensitivity to the clastogenic and cell-cycle changes induced by cross-linking agents, there are insufficient data at this time to determine its sensitivity, specificity and reproducibility for diagnosis, especially for patients that cannot be complemented by any of the cloned genes, and for mosaic patients. Analysis of chromosomal breakage after DEB treatment enables estimation of the percentage of cross-link-resistant cells, indicating the degree of mosaicism. As this may influence outcome for FA patients, it is important to apply a diagnostic test where this can be determined.

Although the FANCC protein participates in the FA nuclear complex responsible for monobiquitination of FANCD2, abundant levels of endogeneous FANCC are also found in the cytoplasm, and there is strong evidence that the cytoplasmic form interacts with other cytoplasmic proteins in control of apoptosis [59–62]. FANCC binds to a number of cytosolic proteins *in vitro*, including the mitotic cyclin-dependent kinase cdc2 [71,72], the molecular chaperone GRP94 [73], NADPH cytochrome p450 reductase [74] and the signal transducer and activator of transcription STAT1 [75,76]. FANCC is also suggested to have a role as a redox regulator of glutathione *S*-transferase P1 (GSTP1) [77]. Most recently, evidence indicates that the molecular chaperone heat shock protein 70 (Hsp 70) interacts with FANCC to protect hematopoietic cells from cytotoxicity and prevent apoptosis in hematopoietic cells exposed to interferon gamma (IFN-γ) and tumor necrosis factor-alpha (TNF-α) [78,79]. Together these protect cells against a variety of environmental factors, including oxidative stress and radiation, and act together to suppress double-stranded RNA-dependent protein kinase (PKR) activity and caspase 3 activation [80]. This interaction of FANCC and Hsp70 in suppression of PKR activity appears to be independent of the multimeric FA complex [79].

Another FANCC-interactive protein is the transcriptional repressor FAZF, a protein containing a conserved amino terminal BTB/POZ protein interaction domain and three C-terminal Krüppel-like zinc fingers [81]. FAZF is thought to affect growth and differentiation of primitive hematopoietic cells [82]. Further experiments are required to elucidate the role of FAZF in hematopoiesis, as well as to determine whether it interacts with other FA proteins that are part of the FA nuclear protein complex. A variety of studies have also suggested that other FA proteins in the complex, such as FANCA, may have direct interactions with additional proteins such as BRCA1 [83] and BRG1, a component of the SWI/SNF complex involved in chromatin remodeling [84]. Preliminary data suggest "cross-talk" between the FA protein complex and other protein complexes in addition to the FA protein FANCD2. With the possibility that there may be multiple FA pathways, the exact role of FA proteins in DNA repair, cell-cycle checkpoints, oxygen metabolism and induction of apoptosis still remains to be elucidated.

Genotype-phenotype correlations for FA-A, FA-C and FA-G

The heterogeneous nature of FA makes an understanding of the correlation between genotype and phenotype important in the clinical management of FA patients. IFAR data [10] confirm that specific complementation groups play a significant role in both the timing of bone marrow failure and survival in these patients. FA-C patients have a significantly earlier onset of bone marrow failure (Fig. 109.2) and poorer survival compared to FA-A and FA-G patients. Subdividing the FA-C group based on the region of the gene that is mutated reveals that patients with intron 4 or exon 14 mutations have an earlier onset of bone marrow failure and poorer survival compared to patients with exon 1 mutations, confirming the earlier findings of Gillio *et al.* and Yamashita *et al.* [23,85]. As reported by Gillio *et al.* [23], patients with *FANCC* genotypes can be divided into three clinical groups: (i) patients with the IVS4 mutation; (ii) patients with at least one exon 14 mutation (R548X or L554P); and (iii) patients with at least one exon 1 mutation (322delG or Q13X) and no known exon 14 mutation. IVS4 and exon 14 subgroups are associated with a severe phenotype manifested by multiple major congenital malformations, early onset of hematologic disease and poorer survival compared to exon 1 patients and to the non-FA-C IFAR population (Fig. 109.5) [10].

The ability to correlate genotype with outcome has considerable clinical significance. For the first time, the pace of hematologic abnormalities and survival can be predicted in patients with specific genotypes. This knowledge aids the family and clinician in timing the various treatment options. For example, patients with *FANCC* IVS4 or exon 14 mutations should be followed closely for early marrow failure and development of clonal cytogenetic abnormalities. The need for allogeneic HCT is likely to occur in the first 5–10 years of life. Because of the high risk of early MDS and AML in patients with these mutations, genotype itself is used as an eligibility criterion for related or unrelated HCT even prior to the development of severe hematologic manifestations. In contrast, patients with milder phenotypes usually defer aggressive therapy until cytopenias develop.

Somatic mosaicism

In addition to genotype, the presence of somatic mosaicism may be important in predicting the clinical course of the patient with FA. It is currently estimated that 25% of FA patients will exhibit two populations of T cells, one that is sensitive to the clastogenic effects of DNA cross-linking agents and one that is resistant. T-cell mosaicism has been reported for various diseases, such as severe combined immune deficiency, Duchenne

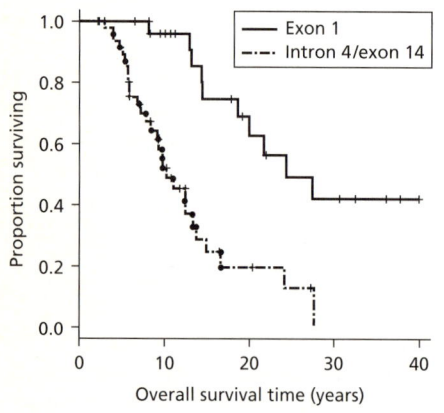
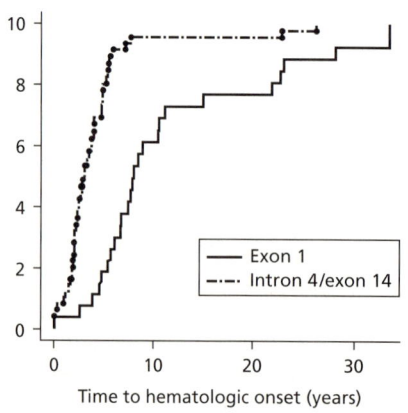

Fig. 109.5 Within complementation group C patients ($n = 78$ in the International Fanconi Anemia Registry [IFAR] database) marrow failure occurs at an earlier time point in patients with at least one intron 4 (IVS4 + 4 A > T) or at least one exon 14 (*R548X* or *L554P*) mutation ($n = 50$) compared to patients with at least one exon 1 mutation (*322delG* and *QX13*) and no mutations in exon 14 or intron 4 ($n = 27$). (a) Cumulative incidence of bone marrow failure over time in patients with exon 1 and intron 4/exon 14 mutations of *FANCC*. (b) Probability of survival over time in patients with exon 1 and intron 4/exon 14 mutations of *FANCC*. At age 15 years, the probability of survival is 74.5% and 24.7%, respectively. Reproduced with permission from [10].

muscular dystrophy, tyrosinemia, epidermolysis bullosa and Bloom syndrome [86–90]. In each of these cases, restoration of the normal allele was demonstrated only in the lymphoid lineage. The question now is whether there is any clinical significance of somatic mosaicism in patients with FA.

Gregory *et al.* [91] recently demonstrated somatic mosaicism in the HSC population. In this study, loss of the maternal *FANCA* mutation in the HSC was confirmed by the presence of revertant myeloid and erythroid precursors as well as T and B lymphocytes. Although not definitive, the data suggested that back mutation in a single HSC was the most likely mechanism for the revertant mosaicism in this patient. Other potential mechanisms that account for somatic mosaicism include mitotic gene conversion, intragenic mitotic recombination and the introduction of compensatory mutations. Regardless of the mechanism, spontaneous genetic reversion would be a rare event. If the event occurs during embryogenesis, then it would be predicted that somatic mosaicism would be found in all tissues. If the event occurs at a later time point, somatic mosaicism will be restricted to specific tissues. In the case illustrated above, 100% of skin fibroblasts exhibited the maternal FANCA mutation as would be predicted based on the subject's clinical findings of short stature and radial ray defects. While it would be predicted that hematopoiesis would be clonal, this has not been confirmed. However, in a second case, clonal hematopoiesis has been confirmed (J.E. Wagner, S.M. Davies & A.D. Auerbach, unpublished data). Like the first case, hematopoietic progenitors were insensitive to low doses of MMC, paralleling the dose–response curve of progenitors from an unaffected donor (Fig. 109.6).

It is important to recognize that somatic mosaicism originating in a pluripotential stem cell can be viewed as "spontaneous" or "natural" gene therapy. The clinical course of the patients described above may be relevant and instructive with regard to the future potential of HSC gene therapy for this disease. The main premise of gene therapy in FA patients is that corrected FA cells will have a proliferative advantage over non-corrected cells. In both cases described above, hematopoietic function was distinctly better than that in affected siblings. In both cases, these patients were detected on testing as possible bone marrow donors. However, in the first case, the possibility that HSC gene correction alone may not be sufficient is also illustrated. In this case, residual FA HSCs became dysplastic with eventual suppression of normal hematopoiesis. Therefore, the risk of malignant transformation of residual FA HSCs is an open question. The clinical course observed in the first patient suggests that it may be necessary to eradicate residual nonreverted stem cells in those with somatic mosaicism (and uncorrected stem cells after gene therapy) using low-dose chemotherapy to reduce the risk of developing MDS or AML.

The success of this approach has been suggested by Battaile *et al.* [92]. The hypothesis that normal HSCs will preferentially expand *in vivo*, particularly in the presence of chemotherapy agents, was tested in a murine model. On mixing of wild type with *FANCC* knockout HSCs, the ratio of normal to FA HSC remained stable over months. After a single injection of MMC, selection of normal cells was rapid and robust. Under these conditions, even a very small number of wild type HSCs were able to significantly repopulate the hematopoietic system. These results suggest that selective pressure must be applied not only to eradicate the risk of malignant transformation of residual FA cells in patients with somatic mosaicism or in recipient of genetically corrected HSC but to promote clonal expansion of corrected cells to rapidly restore normal hematopoiesis.

In addition, it is unclear as to the effect of somatic mosaicism on the need for and success of HCT. While it is unclear whether the clinical course differs in FA patients with T-cell mosaicism, it is clear that a proportion of patients eventually develop marrow failure and require HCT.

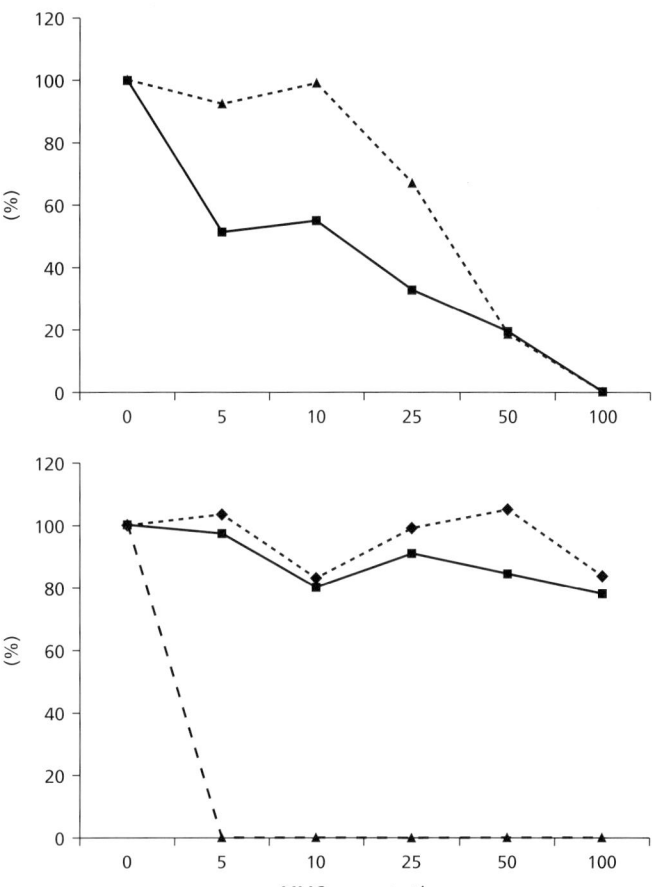

Fig. 109.6 Mitomycin C (MMC) dose–response curves. Marrow mononuclear cells were plated in methylcellulose containing differing concentrations of MMC (0, 5, 10, 25, 50 and 100 mM). After 2 weeks in culture, colonies were enumerated and compared to the number of colonies in the untreated control. Results demonstrate that colony-forming cell (CFC) MMC resistance in patients 1 and 2. Panel A (Patient 1) demonstrates partial resistance; Panel B (Patient 2) demonstrates complete MMC resistance comparable to marrow CFCs from a normal healthy volunteer. The dashed line in panel B reveals marked MMC sensitivity of marrow progenitors obtained from the patient's affected sibling.

As discussed in the Initial trials 1995–98 subsection in the Results of alternative donor HCT at the University of Minnesota section, p. 1495, the presence of a DEB-resistant population of T cells is associated with a higher risk of graft rejection. This would suggest that low-dose conditioning administered to FA patients might be insufficient for eradicating DEB-resistant cells. Further work is required to confirm these observations.

In summary, clinical data suggest that, first, T-cell mosaicism may be a risk factor for graft rejection in recipients of unrelated marrow [93] (also see Initial trials 1995–98, p. 1495). Second, HSC mosaicism may be associated with an altered "natural history" and stable hematopoietic function. Therefore, it is useful that the clinician caring for FA patients determine if T-cell and HSC somatic mosaicism exists.

Proposed mechanisms of marrow failure and leukemogenesis

While patients with FA have an extraordinary predisposition for the development of marrow failure and leukemia, the pathogenesis and pathophysiology of these disease entities are unclear. Because the prognosis of FA patients with AML is exceedingly poor, understanding the pathogenesis of this complication and development of assays to predict its occurrence could improve the timing of HCT and/or the collection of autologous HSC for genetic modification.

Murine models have been developed for four FA genes, *Fancc*, *Fanca*, *Fancg* and *Fancd2*, providing insights as to the mechanisms of marrow failure [94–106]. The phenotype of the two homozygous *Fancc* mutant animals is similar in the two murine models. Lymphocytes from these animals demonstrate the classic hypersensitivity to bifunctional crosslinking agents and G2/M cell-cycle abnormalities, although skeletal and urinary system birth defects, pancytopenia and increased cancer susceptibility have not been observed. While the peripheral blood appears normal, mice with an exon 9 deletion demonstrate age-dependent decreases in progenitor cell frequencies and hypersensitivity to IFN-γ mediated by *fas*-induced apoptosis [94]. Whitney *et al.* [94] suggest that the FANCC protein may directly or indirectly suppress an IFN-γ mediated mitotic inhibitory pathway.

Wang *et al.* [103] studied the function of constitutively expressed normal human FANCC protein in mouse hematopoietic cells. HSC from FANCC over-expressing transgenic mice were resistant to the cytolytic effect of a *fas*-triggering antibody, suggesting the *fas*-mediated apoptosis is involved in the pathogenesis of marrow failure in FA. Antisense oligonucleotides complementary to FANCC messenger RNA (mRNA) inhibited the *in vitro* clonal growth of normal erythroid and granulocyte-macrophage progenitor cells, even in the presence of exogenous growth factors. In contrast, peripheral blood $CD34^+$ cells isolated from a FA-C patient and infected with *FANCC* cDNA exhibited a 5–10-fold increase in the number of progenitor colonies *in vitro*. These results suggest that the *FANCC* gene plays a direct role in the survival of hematopoietic progenitor cells. It has been proposed that FANCC regulates an apoptotic pathway during hematopoiesis and may respond to an apoptotic pathway induced by DNA damage [104–106].

Bagby *et al.* [107] have considered the possibility that marrow failure was mediated by insufficient production of hematopoietic growth factors secondary to the FA mutation. While no abnormalities were noted in stromal production of stem cell factor (SCF) or macrophage colony-stimulating factor (M-CSF), production of interleukin 6 (IL-6), granulocyte macrophage colony-stimulating factor (GM-CSF) and granulocyte colony-stimulating factor (G-CSF) was variable. Because these responses were variable between affected siblings, the abnormalities observed are not likely to be the direct effect of the inherited mutation. Abnormal levels and responses to cytokines have also been reported in patients with FA [108,109].

Alternatively, it has been postulated that marrow failure results from absent or defective hematopoietic stem and/or progenitor cells or is a manifestation of malignant transformation. Assays of marrow obtained from patients with FA with or without marrow failure indicate abnormalities in production of hematopoietic progenitor cells [110]. The role of impaired production of hematopoietic growth factors by the marrow microenvironment appears unlikely as detailed above. Butturini and Gale [111] evaluated the proliferative capacity of hematopoietic progenitors in long-term marrow culture in eight patients with FA and marrow failure. Notably, an adherent layer formed in the cultures from seven of eight individuals and large numbers of differentiated myeloid cells were generated within 1–2 weeks. At 5 weeks, the adherent layer retained the capacity to initiate secondary long-term marrow cultures but growth of colony-forming unit–granulocyte/macrophage (CFU-GM) was impaired.

Together these data suggest that early hematopoietic precursors are present in the marrow of patients with FA despite marrow failure clinically. The question remains as to why these cells proliferate *in vitro* and not *in vivo*. Notably the size and morphology of CFU-GM was reported as abnormal. Addition of growth factors, androgens and hydrocortisone did not affect growth *in vitro*. Butturini and Gale [111] list several possible explanations for these observations: (i) culture conditions supply nutrients not present *in vivo*; (ii) absence of toxins *in vitro* (e.g. oxygen toxicity); and (iii) *in vivo* exogenous suppression directly or indirectly by a "preleukemic" clone.

Rathburn *et al.* [104] have proposed that marrow failure in patients with FA results from the accumulated losses of HSC caused by repeated episodes of low IFN-γ released in response to recurrent minor inflammatory stimuli. The capacity of IFN-γ to induce TNF-α gene expression is increased in the serum of children with FA [113]. Whitney *et al.* [94] postulate that the apoptotic phenotype in hematopoietic stem and progenitor cells creates an environment for the selection of IFN-γ resistant clones. Their findings argue that therapies designed to correct the abnormal pattern of IFN-γ sensitivity in FA cells may prevent or delay the onset of marrow failure and development of MDS and leukemia. This remains to be confirmed.

Nontransplant treatment strategies

Androgens

Primary treatment for patients with FA has long included androgens with or without prednisone. Androgen therapy (most commonly oxymetholone initiated at 2 mg/kg/day) was first evaluated in patients with FA by Shahidi and Diamond [114] with hematologic improvement in all six treated patients. Subsequent series confirmed these observations [115,116] with an overall response rate of approximately 50%. Patients responding to androgens do so within several months of drug initiation if a response is to occur [117]. While a significant proportion of patients may respond to androgens, many in turn develop toxicity (e.g. hepatic adenomata) or resistance, necessitating withdrawal with subsequent return to marrow failure. Others respond with prolonged improvement in blood counts. Notably, Macdougall *et al.* [5] reported a low rate of response to androgens (25%) in 25 black South African children. While there were no apparent differences in clinical, hematologic and cytogenetic characteristics of FA in black South African children as compared to those in other ethnic groups, mortality appeared to be higher (68%) at an earlier age (mean 9.8 ± 2.7 years). Reasons for altered response to androgens are unknown. Alter and Young [117] reported that androgen therapy prolonged survival by an average of 3 years after the onset of aplasia compared to those not on androgens, based on an analysis of data from the literature. Although unproven, it has been suggested that prednisone may promote vascular stability and decrease bleeding tendency in those with severe thrombocytopenia [117]. Whether the addition of prednisone (5–10 mg every other day) augments the response seen with oxymetholone is unknown. Further, it is unknown whether alternate androgen formulations offer advantages in terms of reduced toxicity and masculinization side-effects as compared to oxymetholone. This is of particular interest to adolescent females who frequently discontinue androgen therapy due to such side-effects.

Ideally, androgen therapy should be initiated at the onset of marrow hypoplasia and peripheral blood cytopenia. Although there has not been a formal analysis to determine the response rate between those treated at the earliest vs. advanced stages of marrow aplasia, early treatment may preempt the need for red cell or platelet transfusions, or the development of significant infectious complications. In addition, the patient should be prescribed folic acid and occasionally iron supplementation. Once a response has been documented, the oxymetholone dose should be tapered slowly but rarely discontinued. Interestingly, except in South African Afrikaaners, few patients have been successfully tapered off without recurrence of marrow aplasia and peripheral blood cytopenia [117]. During treatment, the patient must be monitored frequently for peliosis hepatis, hepatic adenomata and hepatocellular carcinoma (Plate 109.3, *facing p. 296*) by ultrasound, computerized tomography and/or magnetic resonance imaging and α fetoprotein levels. If any of these complications occurs, alternative therapies, such as hematopoietic growth factors or HCT, should be investigated. Reports on the use of antithymocyte globulin (ATG), cyclosporine, high-dose methylprednisolone and other immunosuppressants have been anecdotal [117]. Individual patients appear to have responded to such therapy with augmentation in peripheral blood counts, albeit temporary. Overall, immunosuppressive therapy has not been expected to be effective in patients with FA in contrast to patients with acquired severe AA.

Antioxidants

Shahidi and others have recommended the use of antioxidants to potentially reduce free radical oxygen toxicity that may play a role in the pathogenesis of the progressive marrow failure and epitheliod malignancy observed in patients with FA [118]. Daily intake of beta-carotene, vitamin C, vitamin E and selenium has been suggested. Whether such therapy alters the natural history of marrow failure or risk of hematologic or nonhematologic malignancy (i.e. cervical carcinoma or head and neck cancers) is unknown.

Hematopoietic growth factor therapy

To date, only two pilot studies [119,120] have been reported on the safety and efficacy of myeloid growth factor therapy in the treatment of neutropenia in patients with FA. While GM-CSF and G-CSF have both been used successfully to increase the neutrophil counts with little systemic toxicity, it is unknown whether such therapy will alter the risk of MDS, development of clonal cytogenetic abnormalities or risk of leukemia. More recently, erythropoietin has been used to increase red cell counts and decrease the need for red cell transfusions. Reports to date have been anecdotal and no formal study has been published. Due to the fact that many patients have highly elevated endogenous erythropoietin levels, it is unclear whether the addition of exogenous erythropoietin will be beneficial. At this point, carefully controlled studies are needed to determine the usefulness of exogenous erythropoietin and, potentially, IL-11 alone or in combination with G-CSF or GM-CSF on peripheral blood cytopenias. Preliminary experiences suggest that erythropoietin may be only rarely effective (R. Harris, personal observations) and IL-11 may be too toxic (pseudotumor cerebri [$n = 2$] and transient blindness [$n = 1$] in four patients; R. Harris and J. Wagner, unpublished observations). The effect of hematopoietic growth factors, perhaps in comparison to oxymetholone, on the natural history of the disease in terms of survival, time interval to transfusion dependence and risk of MDS and AML needs to be evaluated systematically.

Supportive care

Most commonly, patients will require blood product support for treatment of thrombocytopenia and anemia. Epsilon-aminocaproic acid is useful in patients with thrombocytopenia and bleeding, and hematopoietic growth factor therapy and antibiotics are often needed in patients with neutropenia and fever. For the patient not pursuing allogeneic HCT as a treatment option, such combination therapy can aid in sustaining life for years. Risk of iron overload should be minimized by early chelation therapy, keeping in mind that many patients even without a history of red cell transfusions will often have elevated iron levels (J. Wagner, unpublished observations). For the patient considering allogeneic HCT, use of red cell and platelet transfusions should be minimized to reduce the risk of alloimmunization. If transfusions are required, an effort should be made to transfuse only irradiated, cytomegalovirus-negative (or filtered) red cell or single donor platelet products from unrelated volunteer donors (i.e. not a family member). Whether specific, selected volunteer donors should be identified to limit exposure to human leukocyte antigens (HLAs) has not been proven.

Neutropenia is a frequent complication even early in the course of the disease. While most often there is a gradual decline over years to decades, transient severe marrow suppression from viral infection (e.g. varicella) has long been observed. Viral-induced neutropenia may be severe but is often transient, lasting <1–2 months even if untreated. Prolonged neutropenia, however, must be investigated and treated. The role of prophylactic antibiotics in this setting should be considered but has not yet been tested. Prolonged use of antibiotics such as Bactrim® for treatment of chronic otitis media or urinary tract infections, however, probably should be discouraged due to its marrow suppressive effect.

Hematopoietic cell transplantation (HCT)

While some of the above therapies have been used to ameliorate the progressive marrow failure found in most patients with FA, HCT is the only treatment with curative potential. Early experiences with HCT for the treatment of FA were negative. Poor outcome was primarily the result of excessive regimen-related toxicity (RRT) and severe acute graft-vs.-host disease (GVHD) [121–123]. Early transplants used conditioning regimens previously devised for patients with acquired AA, administering cyclophosphamide (CY) at a dose of 200 mg/kg with or without irradiation. Severe toxicity was noted with this regimen with a high proportion of patients dying early after transplantation with impaired cardiac function, infection, severe mucositis, gastrointestinal hemorrhage, hemorrhagic cystitis and skin toxicity [121].

Lowering the dose CY (i.e. to 150 mg/kg and then to 100 mg/kg) in a limited number of patients was unsuccessful in ameliorating RRT. This clinical experience prompted *in vitro* laboratory studies that confirmed the hypersensitivity of FA cells to CY [124,125] and also stimulated a clinical study of individual sensitivity to irradiation to determine a more appropriate conditioning regimen for FA patients [122]. In this study, Gluckman *et al.* [26] tested the *in vitro* radiation sensitivity and DNA repair capacity in eight FA patients as compared to 20 normal controls. The skin of patients and controls was exposed to 8 Gy and 10 Gy irradiation at two separate sites. The sites were then followed for signs of hyperpigmentation and/or desquamation. Cell repair capacity was considered normal if the skin reaction to a single 10 Gy dose was the same as that to 6 Gy in two doses. The results showed moderate radiosensitivity in five FA patients and increased radiosensitivity in three. Two cases showed evidence of reduced DNA repair capacity. As a result of these *in vitro* tests demonstrating hypersensitivity to radiation and alkylating agents, Gluckman *et al.* [126] proposed the use of low-dose CY (20 mg/kg) and thoraco-abdominal irradiation ([TAI], 500 cGy) in the treatment of FA patients in an attempt to reduce toxicity and improve survival. Notably, radiation was administered as a single fraction because evidence of a DNA repair defect suggested that there was little benefit to be gained from fractionation. These modifications led to markedly reduced RRT with excellent hematologic recovery.

HLA-identical sibling donor HCT

HLA-identical sibling donor HCT for the treatment of marrow failure in FA patients

Today, HCT from HLA-identical sibling donors is generally associated with an excellent outcome if performed early in life prior to the development of MDS or leukemia (Table 109.2) [123,127–133]. Gluckman [130] reported the experience at the Hôpital St. Louis in Paris, France, between 1976 and 1992, using CY 20 mg/kg and TAI 500 cGy. As postulated, Gluckman [130] observed a low incidence of RRT and an overall

Table 109.2 Clinical results in recipients of radiation-based regimens followed by human leukocyte antigen (HLA)-identical sibling donor hematopoietic cell transplantation (HCT).

Reference	Conditioning regimen	GVHD prophylaxis	No of cases	Median patient age (range)	Sustained engraftment	Acute GVHD (grades III–IV)	Outcome
Hows et al. 1989 [123]	CY 20 mg/kg + TBI 6 Gy ($n = 8$)	CSP ($n = 8$) TCD ($n = 2$)	8	8 years (6–14 years)	7/8	4/8	7/8 alive (4 months–5 years)
Di Bartolomeo et al. 1992 [127]	CY 20 mg/kg + TBI 5 Gy ($n = 5$)	CSP ($n = 1$) CSPA + MTX ($n = 4$)	5	13 years (7–14 years)	5/5	1/5	5/5 alive (18 months–5.5 years)
Kohli-Kumar et al. 1994 [128]	CY 20 mg/kg + TAI 4 Gy + ATG 120 mg/kg ($n = 17$)	CSP + ATG ($n = 17$)	17	7.7 years (1.5–10.0 years)	16/17	0.17	17/17 alive (6 months–6.3 years)
Gluckman et al. 1995 (IBMTR study) [129]	Varied	MTX + other 12% CSP + other 62% MTX + CSP 21% TCD 5%	151	10 years (1–36 years)	92%	42% (Grades II–IV)	65% alive at 5 years
Gluckman, 1993 [130]	CY 20 mg/kg + TAI 5 Gy	CSP	45*	N/A	2/45	N/A	76% alive at 5 years
Socié et al. 1998 [131]	CY 20 mg/kg + TAI 5 Gy ($n = 45$) CY 40 mg/kg + TAI 5 Gy Gy ($n = 5$)	CSP	50†	N/A	46/49	10/49	74% at 4.5 years
Ayas et al. 2001 [132]	CY 20 mg/kg, TAI 4 Gy + ATG 160 mg/kg	CSP + ATG ($n = 13$) CSP, MTX + ATG ($n = 6$)	19	8.7 years (3–15 years)	19	0	14/19 alive (1.7 months–4 years)
DuFour et al. 2001 [133]	CY 20 mg/kg + TAI 5–6 Gy ($n = 12$) CY 20–80 mg/kg, TBI 3–6 Gy ($n = 10$)‡ CY 100–200 ($n = 5$)	CSP ($n = 18$) CSP + MTX ($n = 8$) MTX alone ($n = 1$)	27‡	9 years (2.5–19.5 years)	23/25	2/25	81% at 3 years

*Includes unspecified number of patients receiving sibling donor umbilical cord blood HCT.
†Includes one patient who received a one antigen mismatched sibling bone marrow. Four patients received HLA-identical sibling donor umbilical cord blood HCT.
ATG, antithymocyte globulin; CSP, cyclosporine A; CY, cyclophosphamide; GVHD, graft-vs.-host disease; MTX, methotrexate; TAI, thoraco-abdominal irradiation; TBI, total body irradiation; TCD, T-cell depletion.
‡Includes two patients who received phenotypic identical parental donor HCT.

probability of survival of 75.6%. Reducing the immunosuppressive intensity of the conditioning regimen, however, raised the possibility that insufficient doses of preparative therapy would lead to increased risk of graft failure and mixed chimerism. In 19 FA patients, an extensive analysis of hematopoietic reconstitution was undertaken [131]. Notably, all but one successfully engrafted. Using minisatellite probes to distinguish host from donor cells, donor cell engraftment was complete in 12 patients, absent in one patient and mixed in six patients. This partial mixed hematopoietic chimerism was transient. Mixed chimerism was concordant between peripheral blood lymphocytes and neutrophils in all but one and was documented at least through day 120. Similarly, Auerbach and colleagues have observed a persistence of DEB+ cells for months after HCT with no untoward effects (A.D. Auerbach, unpublished observations).

As shown in Table 109.2, Kohli-Kumar et al. [128] reported the results of HCT in 17 patients aged 1.5–10.0 years with HLA-identical sibling donors. With a modification of the Hôpital St. Louis regimen (i.e. addition of ATG pre- and post-transplantation and lower dose TAI, 400 cGy), 16 of the 17 patients engrafted with no patient developing grades II–IV acute GVHD. With a median follow-up of 27 months (range: 6–75 months), all patients were alive at the time of the report.

Data from the largest review to date, using the database of the International Bone Marrow Transplant Registry (IBMTR), are summarized in Table 109.2 [129]. The 2-year probability of survival was 66% (58–73%) for recipients of HLA-identical sibling hematopoietic cells ($n = 151$) with 91% of survivors having a Karnofsky performance score >90% at last follow-up. Graft failure was observed in 8% (5–14%); grade II–IV acute GVHD was observed in 42% (34–50%); and chronic GVHD was observed in 44% (34–53%) among patients surviving >90 days with evidence of engraftment. Interstitial pneumonitis was observed in 12% (8–19%) of patients. Importantly, age at transplant, pretransplant platelet count, conditioning regimen and GVHD prophylaxis were identified in multivariate analysis as factors that correlated with survival after HLA-identical sibling donor HCT. Older age and lower pretransplant platelet

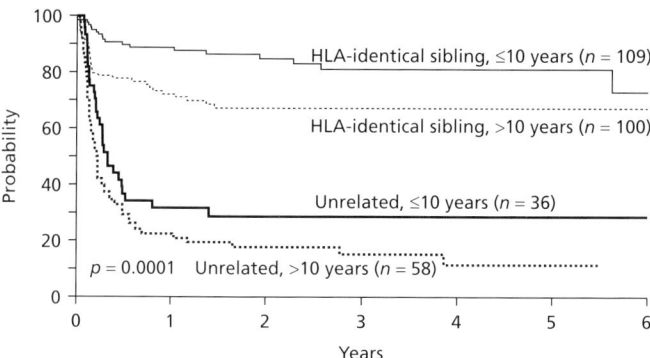

Fig. 109.7 Probability of survival after human leukocyte antigen (HLA)-identical sibling donor hematopoietic cell transplantation (HCT) in patients with Fanconi anemia (FA) as reported to the International Bone Marrow Transplant Registry (IBMTR). Reproduced with permission from IBMTR/Autologous Blood and Marrow Transplant Registry (ABMTR) [134].

count were associated with lower rates of survival, mostly as a result of increased graft failure and chronic GVHD. While lower platelet count may reflect longer standing disease or greater transfusion exposure, the reason for the importance of pretransplant platelet count is unclear. Transplant conditioning regimen also had an important impact on outcome. Use of pretransplant ATG was a favorable factor, with less acute and chronic GVHD and lower mortality. Additionally, patients receiving low-dose CY (15–25 mg/kg plus limited field or total body irradiation [TBI]) as preparative therapy had a significantly lower risk of treatment failure than did patients receiving higher dose CY (>100 mg/kg) without radiation. Recently, updated results of IBMTR data were reported on survival of FA patients transplanted with HLA-identical sibling donor HSC (Fig. 109.7 [134]). Among 209 patients transplanted between 1994 and 1999 from matched siblings, the 3-year survival was $81 \pm 9\%$ in 109 patients aged <10 years of age and $69 \pm 10\%$ in 100 older patients.

Dufour et al. [133] reported the results of 27 consecutive Italian patients who received HLA-matched sibling bone marrow transplantation for FA in 10 Italian centers of the Associazione Italiana Ematologia ed Oncologia Pediatrica (AEIOP), Gruppo Italiano Trapianti di Midollo Osseo (GITMO). As shown in Table 109.2, 22 patients received low-dose CY (median 20 mg/kg) and TAI or TBI (median dose 5 Gy), including five patients who received high-dose CY (120 mg/kg). Sustained neutrophil engraftment was achieved in 92% patients. RRT was more prevalent in patients who received high-dose CY. Overall, severe toxicity (>grade II) was observed in 18.5% patients and was fatal in three patients. The Kaplan–Meier estimate of grade II–IV acute GVHD at 36 months was 40% and was significantly associated with the presence of genital malformations and the use of high-dose CY conditioning. Three-year probability of survival was 81% and was not affected by any studied variables, including number of malformations or conditioning regimen.

Although most centers use preparative regimens based on CY and radiation, small numbers of patients with FA have been conditioned with alternative nonirradiation regimens with some success (Table 109.3) [123,135–145]. Flowers et al. [139] reported the largest series to date using a chemotherapy-based regimen in FA patients transplanted with related donor marrow. All patients received higher dose CY (140 mg/kg and 200 mg/kg) with or without ATG and no irradiation. Sustained neutrophil engraftment was observed in 36 of the 39 (92%) evaluable patients. Grade II–IV acute GVHD developed in 14 of the 39 (36%) evaluable patients. Chronic GVHD developed in 11 of the 29 (38%) evaluable patients. As previously observed by Hows et al. [123] and Gluckman [130], toxicity with higher dose CY was considerable with grade II–IV mucositis in 36 of the 40 (90%) patients and hemorrhagic cystitis in 12 of the 39 (31%) patients. Other toxicities included generalized erythroderma ($n = 4$), hepatic veno-occlusive disease ($n = 4$) and cardiomyopathy ($n = 3$). As a result, 25 of the 41 patients (61%) were alive with a median follow-up of 3.1 years (range: 0.1–21.8 years) at the time of the report. While these results are encouraging, too few patients and patient heterogeneity prevent any detailed comparison between irradiation- and nonirradiation-containing regimens. The rationale for developing effective preparative regimens without irradiation stems in part from concerns that FA patients are at increased susceptibility of tissue DNA damage and the risk of a solid tumor, particularly of the aeroesophageal tract.

Fludarabine (FLU), an antimetabolite, is a highly effective immunosuppressive agent frequently used in pretransplant conditioning therapy [146–149]. As FLU is not a DNA cross-linking agent, it was hypothesized to be a relatively safe agent in patients with FA and yet to be sufficiently immunosuppressive to allow a high probability of engraftment without the coadministration of irradiation. In two published case reports from Israel [143,150], FLU-based preparative therapy consisting of CY (10 mg/kg), FLU (150 mg/m^2) and ATG (40–50 mg/kg) was administered to two FA patients. One patient had refractory anemia with excess blasts in transformation (RAEB-T) and the other had AA. Myeloid engraftment was achieved on day +12 and day +28. At the time of the reporting, both patients remain alive and well more than 10 months after HCT.

The two largest single center experiences on the use of a FLU based regimen are at the Charite Hospital (Berlin, Germany) and the University of Minnesota (Table 109.3) [144,145]. At the University of Minnesota, between April 2000 and July 2002, seven patients (median age 12.1 years; range: 3.6–22.5) received CY (20 mg/kg), FLU (175 mg/m^2) and ATG (150 mg/kg) followed by the infusion of a T-cell depleted bone marrow ($n = 6$) or umbilical cord blood [UCB] graft ($n = 1$) for the treatment of FA associated AA ($n = 6$) or RAEB-T ($n = 1$) [144]. No grade III–IV toxicity was observed. Primary neutrophil recovery and engraftment was observed in 100%. One patient, however, experienced secondary graft failure. This patient was transplanted with HLA-matched maternal bone marrow and demonstrated graft rejection on day 28. A second transplant procedure (using the same donor) after CY 5 mg/kg/day for 4 days and total lymphoid irradiation resulted in permanent engraftment. Of note, the one patient with RAEB-T relapsed 6 months after transplantation. After failing to respond to three donor lymphocyte infusions, a second transplant procedure after CY 10 mg/kg/day for 4 days and TBI 450 cGy was performed using the same donor. Although engraftment was achieved, a second relapse occurred 7 months after second transplantation. Notably, no patient developed grade II–IV acute or chronic GVHD.

In summary, FLU-based preparative regimens are associated with comparable engraftment rates as irradiation-based regimens for related donor HCT despite incorporation of marrow T-cell depletion in the protocol. Long-term follow-up, however, is required before determining whether such an approach will reduce late effects, particularly the risks of malignancy, sterility and endocrinopathies. Preliminary results suggest that irradiation-based preparative regimens may be required for FA patients with advanced MDS or leukemia.

HLA-identical sibling donor HCT for the treatment of MDS and leukemia in FA patients

Experience in the treatment of FA patients who have developed leukemia is limited; untreated patients generally die of disease progression within months to a year of diagnosis. Clinical experience with chemotherapy in

Table 109.3 Clinical results in recipients of alternative nonradiation cytoreductive therapies followed by human leukocyte antigen (HLA)-identical sibling donor hematopoietic cell transplantation (HCT).

Reference	Conditioning regimen	No. of cases	Engrafted	Outcome (range)
Barrett et al. 1977 [135]	CY 200 mg/kg + Procarb + ATG	1	1/1	Alive >11 months
Kersey et al. 1979 [136]	CY 200 mg/kg + 6MP 1 g/m^2	1	1/1	Died, day 35 (GVHD)
Holl et al. 1981 [137]	CY 200 mg/kg + Procarb 25 mg/kg + ATG	1	1/1	Alive >4.5 years
Flowers et al. 1992 [138]	CY 100 mg/kg + BU 14 mg/kg	1	1/1	Died, day 41 (sepsis)
Ratanatharathorn et al. 1993 [140]	BU 8 mg/kg + TLI 5 Gy	2	2/2	1 alive >20 months, 1 died, day 45 (HUS, ARDS)
Flowers et al. 1996 [139]	CY 200 mg/kg ($n = 17$) CY 135–50 mg/kg ($n = 8$) CY 140 mg/kg + ATG ($n = 9$) CY 120 mg/kg ($n = 7$)	41*	92%	25/41 alive (median 3.1 years)
Maschan et al. 1997 [141]	BU 8 mg/kg + CY 40 mg/kg	1	1/1	Alive >17 months
De Mederios et al. 1999 [142]	CY 100 mg/kg ($n = 16$)	16	16	88% alive (mean 1.6 years)
Aker et al. 1999 [143]	FLU 180 mg/m^2 + CY 20 mg/kg + ATG	1**	1/1	Alive >11 months
MacMillan et al. 2002 [144]	FLU 140 mg/m^2 + CY 40 mg/kg + ATG	7	7	7 Alive >10 months
Ebell 2002 [145]	FLU 75–180 mg/m^2 + ATG + OKT3	7	5	5/7 Alive

ARDS, adult respiratory distress syndrome; ATG, antithymocyte globulin; BU, busulfan; CY, cyclophosphamide; FLU, fludarabine; GVHD, graft-vs.-host disease; HUS, hemolytic uremic syndrome; 6MP, 6 mercaptopurine; MTX, methotrexate; Procarb, procarbazine; TLI, total lymphoid irradiation.
*Includes those patients who received HLA matched ($n = 1$), one antigen mismatched ($n = 1$), or two antigens.
**Patient received an HLA-identical sibling donor umbilical cord blood transplant.

these patients is scant, although there are anecdotal reports of responses to chemotherapy and HCT (Table 109.4) [123,138,140,141,145,146,150–153]. These data indicate that long-term survival is possible in these patients and they should be considered candidates for HCT. The apparent successful eradication of the malignant clone in these patients with generally reduced doses of chemotherapy suggests that the malignant cells carry a similar hypersensitivity to alkylating agents and irradiation, characteristic of nonmalignant cells in patients with FA. However, there are currently no laboratory studies available addressing this point, which would be of great interest in planning future therapy. Despite successful engraftment after non-TBI based preparative therapy, patients with MDS and excessive blasts or AML may be at high risk of relapse after HCT. TBI or other novel approach should be considered. Further, it is unclear whether chemotherapy should be administered prior to transplantation. There are no reports in the literature to suggest that such therapy is helpful; local experience does not support the use of cytoreduction prior to HCT due to extremely high risk of severe toxicity and peri-transplant mortality (J. Wagner, unpublished observations). Limited experience, however, prevents any conclusion. Due to the inherent hypersensitivity to DNA cross-linking agents, treatment plans must be adjusted accordingly and a source of HSCs must be available in the likely event of persistent pancytopenia. FLU, cytosine arabinoside and reduced doses of anthracyclines have been tolerated in most cases.

Summary of HCT from HLA-matched sibling donors in FA patients

Together these results suggest: (i) that the optimum time for HCT is when the patient is <10 years of age, has had <20 red cell and/or platelet transfusions, and is prior to the development of MDS or leukemia; and (ii) that the optimal therapy should include lower dose therapy (perhaps without irradiation if there is no advanced MDS or AML) for patients with FA and HLA-identical sibling donors. Patients with severe organ dysfunction or older age (age >35 years) should delay or avoid HCT since such individuals would be at higher risk for transplant-related morbidity and mortality.

Alternative donor HCT for FA patients

The majority of FA patients do not have an HLA-identical unaffected sibling donor. Therefore, family members with varying degrees of HLA-mismatch have been used as alternative donors with some degree of success. Published data are summarized in Table 109.5 [93,121,123,129,138,154–157]. For the IBMTR, Gluckman et al. [121] combined the outcomes of 29 mismatched family member donor HCT recipients with 19 unrelated donor HCT recipients. The data show significantly reduced survival compared with recipients of HLA-identical sibling donor transplants, as might be expected, and a remarkably high incidence of graft failure at 24%. These data suggest that the reduced doses of conditioning therapy commonly used for FA patients is insufficient to achieve donor cell engraftment of HLA-disparate grafts.

Recently, updated results of IBMTR data were reported on survival in recipients of FA patients transplanted with alternative donor HSC [134]. Among 94 patients transplanted between 1994 and 1999, the 3-year survival was 30 ± 16% in 36 patients aged <10 years of age and 16 ± 10% in 58 older patients.

Table 109.4 Clinical results in recipients with myelodysplastic syndrome (MDS) and acute myeloid leukemia (AML) and human leukocyte antigen (HLA)-identical sibling donors.

Reference	Conditioning regimen	GVHD prophylaxis	No. of cases	Patient age (years)	Sustained engraftment	Acute GVHD (grades III–IV)	Outcome
Hows et al. 1989 [123]	CY 20 mg/kg TBI 6 Gy	CSP ($n = 2$) TCD ($n = 1$)	2	14 & 23 years	1/1 evaluable	1/1 evaluable	0/2 surviving 50 days
Flowers et al. 1992 [138]	CY 120 mg/kg TBI 12 Gy ($n = 3$)	MTX + CSP	3	12, 19 & 22 years	3/3	1/3	1/3 surviving >8 years
Ratanatharathorn et al. 1993 [140]	BU 8 mg/kg TLI 5 Gy	CSP + MP	1	17 years	1/1	0/1	1/1 surviving >20 months
Philpott et al. 1994 [151]	CY 40 mg/kg TBI 6 Gy Campath I-G	CSP Campath I-G	1	35 years	1/1	0/1	1/1 surviving >18 months
Ikushima et al. 1995 [152]	CY 100 mg/kg TBI 6 Gy ALG	CSP + MTX	1	14 years	1/1	0/1	1/1 surviving >30 months
Maschan et al. 1997 [141]	BU 8 mg/kg CY 40 mg/kg	CSP	1	11 years	1/1	0/1	1/1 surviving >17 months
Kapelushnick et al. 1997 [150]	FLU 150 mg/m^2 CY 20 mg/kg ATG	CSP	1	12 years	1/1	0/1	1/1 surviving >10 months
McCloy et al. 2001 [153]	FLU 120 mg/m^2 CY 40 mg/kg ATG	CSP	1	12 years	1/1	0/1	1/1 surviving >22 months
MacMillan et al. 2002 [144]	FLU 140 mg/m^2 CY 40 mg/kg ATG	CSP TCD	1	23 years	1/1	0/1	1/1 surviving >14 months (relapsed at 6 months)
Ebell 2002 [145]	FLU 180 mg/m^2 ATG OKT3	CSP	2	6 & 11 years	2/2	0/2	0/2 surviving

ALG, antilymphocyte globulin; ATG, antithymocyte globulin; BU, busulfan; CSP, cyclosporine; CY, cyclophosphamide; FLU, fludarabine; GVHD, graft-vs.-host disease; MP, methylprednisolone; MTX, methotrexate; TBI, total body irradiation; TCD, T-cell depletion; TLI, total lymphoid irradiation.

In 2000, the results of a retrospective multicenter study of 69 unrelated donor HCT facilitated through the European Group for Blood and Marrow Transplantation (EBMT) and the European Fanconi Anemia Registry were reported by Guardiola et al. [156]. The 3-year probability of survival was 33%. The primary causes of death were acute GVHD ($n = 18$), primary or secondary graft failure ($n = 13$), chronic GVHD ($n = 4$), infections ($n = 11$) and veno-occlusive disease of the liver ($n = 1$). Malformations (≥ 3), use of androgens prior to HCT, positive recipient cytomegalovirus serology and the use of a female donor were associated with poor survival.

More recently, an analysis of 91 transplants performed at 27 transplant centers between May 1990 and May 2001 was performed by the National Marrow Donor Program (NMDP) [157]. The median age was 12 years and most had a Karnofsky performance score >80% at the time of transplant. A TBI-based regimen was used in the vast majority of patients; however, 22 patients received FLU (18 in combination with TBI and four without TBI). GVHD prophylaxis included T-cell depletion in half and a cyclosporine-based regimen in most of the remaining patients. In 83 patients surviving at least 21 days, the overall incidence of neutrophil recovery was 78% at a median of 13 days after transplantation. In multivariate analysis, HLA mismatch and higher cell dose (for those received T-replete grafts) were associated with higher rates of engraftment. The overall incidence of grade III–IV GVHD was 25%. In univariate analysis, the incidence of grade III–IV acute GVHD was significantly less in recipients of T-cell-depleted marrow. With a median follow up of 1 year, the overall probability of survival at 2 years after transplantation was 23%. Demographic and treatment factors associated with improved survival include younger recipient age, Karnofsky performance status $\geq 80\%$, no prior history of androgen use and use of FLU in the preparative regimen.

Because of the high risk of treatment-related mortality, unrelated donor HCT conventionally has not been recommended prior to treatment with other modalities. While patients with FA should undergo HCT prior to the development of leukemia or a transfusion requirement, early use of androgens and hematopoietic growth factors at the onset of marrow failure with close follow-up has been recommended. Whether the recommendation on the use of androgens should be changed due to its potential deleterious effect on HCT is currently being debated. [156,157]

Results of alternative donor HCT at the University of Minnesota

Initial trials 1995–98

In an attempt to improve upon engraftment results, a prospective TBI

Table 109.5 Clinical results in recipients of cyclophosphamide (CY) and irradiation followed by alternative donor hematopoietic cell transplantation (HCT).

Reference	Conditioning regimen	GVHD prophylaxis	No. of cases	Median patient age (range)	Sustained engraftment	Acute GVHD (grades III–IV)	Outcome
Hows et al. 1989 [123]	CY 20 mg/kg + TBI 6 Gy	CSP ($n = 5$) TCD ($n = 4$)	5	12 years (5–13 years)	3/5	1/4 evaluable	1/5 surviving >4 years
Flowers et al. 1992 [138]	CY 120 mg/kg + TBI 12 Gy ($n = 1$); BU 14 mg/kg + CY 100 mg/kg ($n = 1$)	MTX + CSP	2	14 & 23 years	2/2	1/2	0/2 surviving beyond day 43
Gluckman et al. 1995 [129]	Varied	Varied	29	9 years	24% graft failure	51% (Grades II–IV)	29% surviving 2 years
Davies et al. 1996 [154]	CY 40 mg/kg + TBI 4.0–4.5 Gy	MTX + CSP ($n = 5$) MTX + Pred + XomaZyme ($n = 2$)	7	7.5–28.0 years	4.5 evaluable	2/4 evaluable	3 surviving >2.5* years
Dini et al. 1997 [155]	CY 40 mg/kg + TAI 5 Gy ($n = 4$) + Ara-C 18 mg/m^2 ($n = 1$); CY 40 mg/kg + TBI 5 Gy ($n = 1$)	Varied	6	n.r.	6/6	n.r.	3/6 surviving 3 months–4 years
Guardiola et al. 2000 [156]	CY 20 mg/kg + TAI ($n = 5$) or TBI ($n = 7$) ± anti-T-cell antibody CY 40 mg/kg + TAI ($n = 14$) or TBI ($n = 30$) ± anti-T-cell antibody Other + irradiation ($n = 13$)	CSP alone ($n = 9$) CSP + Pred ± anti-T-cell antibody ($n = 36$) CSP + MTX ± anti-T-cell antibody ($n = 20$) TCD alone ($n = 26$) None ($n = 4$)	69	10.8 years (4.0–37.4 years)	83%†	34%	33% at 3 years
Wagner et al. 2001 [157]	Varied	Varied	83	11.9 years (2–49 years)	79%	26%	22% at 2 years
MacMillan et al. 2000 [93]	CY 40 mg/kg + TBI 4.5–6.0 Gy	TCD + CSP	29	12.1 years (3.7–48.5 years)	63%	2/18	34% at 1 year

*Updated survival.
†Probability of secondary graft failure was 19%.
Ara-C, cytosine arabinoside; BU, busulfan; CSP, cyclosporine; CY, cyclophosphamide; GVHD, graft-vs.-host disease; MTX, methotrexate; n.r., not reported specifically for Fanconi anemia patients; Pred, prednisone; TAI, thoraco-abdominal irradiation; TBI, total body irradiation; TCD, T-cell depletion.

dose escalation study was performed at the University of Minnesota [93]. Between June 1993 and July 1998, 29 FA patients (median age 12.1 years [range: 3.7–48.5 years]) were enrolled. All patients were treated with CY 40 mg/kg, TBI 450 cGy or 600 cGy ATG followed by HCT from an alternative donor bone marrow ($n = 25$) or UCB ($n = 4$). Patients were eligible for this study if they had: (i) confirmed positive DEB test; (ii) progressive marrow failure with impending transfusion requirement (e.g. platelet count consistently <20,000/µL, hemoglobin <8 g/dL or absolute neutrophil count <500/µL) despite androgen therapy and/or growth factor; (iii) MDS with progressive clonal abnormality or leukemia; (iv) confirmed HLA-A, -B, -DRB1-matched or 1-antigen mismatched related or unrelated marrow or HLA-A, -B, -DRB1-matched or 1–3 antigen mismatched UCB donor; (v) adequate organ (kidney, liver, lung, heart) function; and (vi) absence of active bacterial, fungal and viral infection.

For the entire cohort of 29 patients, the probability of neutrophil recovery was 61% (95%CI 43–79%) and did not differ among preparative therapies, suggesting that engraftment is not improved by increasing the intensity of TBI and ATG. In univariate analysis, factors associated with increased graft failure in bone marrow recipients were the presence of T-cell somatic mosaicism ($p = 0.04$) and lower cell dose (< median of 3.4×10^7 nucleated cells/kg, $p = 0.05$). Three of the four patients who received UCB grafts were evaluable for engraftment. One patient failed to engraft and two patients engrafted 26 and 31 days after HCT. There was no correlation between number of major congenital malformations (≤1 [$n = 10$] vs. >1 [$n = 17$]) and rate of neutrophil engraftment ($p = 0.56$).

As previously noted, 25% of patients exhibited DEB-resistance [22], with approximately 10% having more than 50% of their lymphocytes DEB-resistant (i.e. having significant T-cell mosaicism, J. Wagner and A. Auerbach, personal observations). Of the 25 patients evaluable for myeloid engraftment after CY/TBI/ATG, seven of 12 patients with T-cell somatic mosaicism (i.e. >10% DEB-resistant T cells) experienced primary graft failure in contrast to three of 13 patients without T-cell somatic mosaicism failing to engraft. The probabilities of neutrophil recovery for patients with and without T-cell somatic mosaicism were 42% (95%CI 14–70%) and 83% (95%CI 61–100%), respectively ($p = 0.05$) indeed suggesting that T-cell mosaicism increased the risk of graft rejection. In an analysis of the distribution of DEB results in patients who achieved durable engraftment vs. those who failed to engraft, there was a statistically significant difference in the proportion of DEB-resistant T cells. The

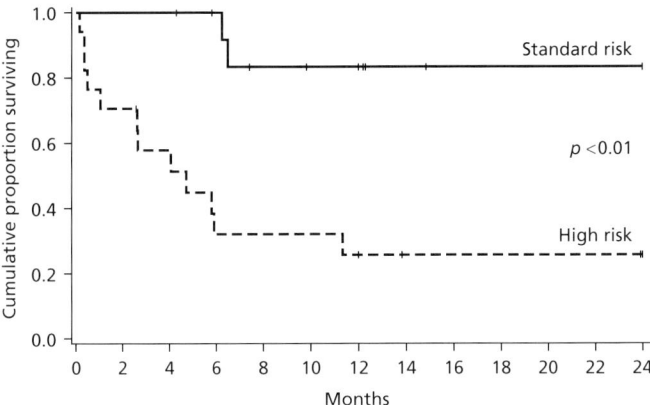

Fig. 109.8 Probability of survival after alternate donor hematopoietic cell transplantation (HCT) for the treatment of patients with Fanconi anemia (FA) at the University of Minnesota. Standard risk is defined as defined as patients <18 years of age, in early stages of marrow disease (aplastic anemia or early myelodysplastic syndrome) and absence of infection with a human leukocyte antigen (HLA)-matched bone marrow or 0–1 HLA-antigen mismatched umbilical cord blood donor. All recipients received fludarabine (FLU), cyclophosphamide (CY) and total body irradiation (TBI).

proportion of DEB-resistant T cells was a median of 72% (range: 35–100%) and 96% (range: 58–100) for patients with and without primary or secondary graft failure ($p < 0.01$). These data suggested that CY/TBI/ATG might be insufficient for the complete eradication of DEB-resistant host lymphocytes that contribute to the risk of graft failure. These results argued for the use of better immune suppressive agents to overcome graft rejection.

Current trial 1999–2002

In order to provide additional immunosuppression to overcome the high risk of graft failure, particularly in patients with somatic mosaicism, FLU was added to the CY/TBI 450 cGy/ATG preparative regimen for alternate donor recipients (Fig. 109.8). All patients received HLA-A, -B and -DRB1 matched ($n = 19$) or 1 antigen mismatched ($n = 6$) marrow or HLA 0–2 antigen mismatched UCB ($n = 6$). As of August 1, 2002, 31 subjects had been enrolled. Notably, the addition of FLU did not alter the toxicity profile of the CY/TBI 450 cGy/ATG regimen. Four patients died prior to day 21 due to infection ($n = 3$) or RRT ($n = 1$). Of 28 patients surviving 21 days, including 10 with marked T-cell somatic mosaicism, all achieved complete neutrophil recovery and engraftment. Incidences of grade II–IV and grade III–IV acute GVHD were 30% and 6%, respectively. Incidence of chronic GVHD was 12%. When stratified on the basis of risk group, patients with standard risk features (defined as <18 years of age, HLA-matched (at intermediate level typing at A and B, and high level typing at DR) bone marrow or 0–1 HLA-antigen mismatched UCB), early stage disease [AA or early MDS] and absence of infection), demonstrated 83% (95%CI, 62–100%, $n = 19$) survival at 2 years. In contrast, those with high-risk features demonstrated a significantly reduced survival of 26% (95%CI 4–48%, $n = 12$, $p = 0.01$) at 2 years. In either case, outcomes have been markedly superior to that reported by the IBMTR and NMDP, as previously described in Alternative donor HCT for FA patients, p. 1494. Again, there is no association between the number of congenital malformations and survival. Further, androgen therapy, the number of transfusions, or the presence of T-cell somatic mosaicism no longer appear as risk factors for engraftment or survival. These results suggest that patients with standard risk features should consider alternative donor HCT at an earlier time point (i.e. prior to the development of advanced MDS or AML, or serious infections).

Summary of HCT from alternative donors for FA patients

In summary, the overall outcome of HCT using alternate donors has markedly improved over time. Similar results have been observed at other institutions. In a recent summary of the experience at Children's Hospital of Cincinnati using a similar TBI/FLU/CY-based regimen (R. Harris, unpublished observations), nine of 13 children (median age 7 years: range 1–15) are alive with a median follow up of 19 months (range: 14–41). In contrast to the protocol at the University of Minnesota, eight of 13 patients received T-cell-depleted peripheral blood grafts. Sustained engraftment was observed in six of eight patients and none developed acute GVHD. Of the five deaths, infection was the cause in four. Clearly, the greatest challenge currently lies with reducing the risk of infection and the late effects of transplantation, not graft failure and GVHD, as previously had been observed.

More recently, some groups have considered the use of non-TBI containing regimens in the setting of unrelated donor HCT for FA patients. Preliminary data suggest that busulfan (1–2 mg/kg total dose) in combination with FLU/ATG/OKT3 is tolerable and sufficient for engraftment. Engraftment has been observed in 12 of 13 recipients of T-replete peripheral blood ($n = 9$) or marrow ($n = 4$) grafts with low rates of GVHD (W. Ebell, Charite Hospital, Berlin, Germany, unpublished data). This strategy is encouraging and needs to be explored further.

To date there have been a number of observations regarding risk factors for engraftment, GVHD and survival in FA patients transplanted with alternative donor HSC (summarized in Table 109.6). While it is not surprising that age, organ function and Karnofsky performance status are indeed predictive of survival, it is noteworthy that more recent analyses suggest that the number of malformations (≥ 3 sites), prior exposure to androgens and absence of FLU in the preparative therapy predicts poorer survival. The current challenges include: (i) determining the optimal time for HCT (proposed process shown in Fig. 109.9); (ii) predicting individual patient sensitivity to chemoradiotherapy; and (iii) understanding the effect of the mosaic phenotype on the natural history of the disease. With markedly improved rates of survival in the current era of HCT in FA, emphasis is now being placed on improving quality of life by reducing late effects, particularly the risks of malignancy, sterility and endocrinopathies. Improvements in therapy are likely to proceed more rapidly if patients are treated according to common protocols and data are shared between institutions.

Cancer risk after HCT for FA patients

Long-term follow-up studies indicate that although successful HCT may cure the hematological complications of FA, patients are still at high risk for malignancy after HCT [10,11,158–160]. In an analysis of 700 patients with FA ($n = 79$) or AA ($n = 621$) treated with allogeneic HCT in Seattle or Paris, the Kaplan–Meier estimate for developing any malignancy by 20 years after transplantation was 14% [158]. Among patients with FA, a single hazard peak for solid tumors occurred between 8 and 9 years after HCT. The Kaplan–Meier estimate of developing any malignancy by 20 years after HCT was 42% (95%CI, 10–74%), with all being solid tumors, while no lympho-hematopoietic malignancies were seen as in patients with severe AA. In the multivariate analysis of the 700 patients with marrow failure (FA and non-FA), the diagnosis of FA (relative risk [RR] 11.2, $p = 0.0001$) and treatment with azathioprine (RR 11.7, $p = 0.0001$) were independent predictors of secondary malignancy, while use of irradiation was not. Importantly, for those transplanted, patients were 17–29 years of age at the time of solid tumor diagnosis. The role of HCT in the development of late solid tumors in patients with FA, however, remains speculative.

Table 109.6 Summary of risk factors.

Outcome	Variable	p-value
Neutrophil	Age at transplant <10 years*	0.001
	Serum AST/ALT >2 × normal prior to HCT	<0.001
Engraftment	Male donor	<0.04
	Absence of 3-lineage cytopenia prior to HCT	<0.06
	T-cell somatic mosaicism†	0.05
	Stem cell dose	0.05
	HLA mismatch‡	0.05
	Recipient CMV serostatus	0.05
	T-replete unrelated donor BMT	0.003
	Fludarabine containing preparative therapy§	0.001
Acute GVHD	T-replete stem cells*	0.04
	Serum AST/ALT >2 × normal prior to HCT	<0.04
	Malformation of urogenital tract and/or kidneys	<0.02
	Limb malformations	<0.04
	HLA mismatch‡	0.0005
	Recipient CMV serostatus	0.02
	T-cell-depleted unrelated marrow	<0.0001
Survival	Extensive malformations (≥3 sites)*	0.005
	Serum AST/ALT >2 × normal prior to HCT	0.005
	Positive recipient CMV serostatus	0.02
	Stem cell dose†	0.03
	Age‡ (increment in decades)	0.002
	Karnofsky score prior to HCT	0.03
	Androgen therapy prior to HCT	0.04
	Fludarabine in conditioning regimen	0.003

*Guardiola *et al.* 2000 [156]
†MacMillan *et al.* 2000 [93]
‡Wagner *et al.* 2001 [157]
§Engraftment occurred in 15/15 recipients of T-cell-depleted marrow if conditioned with fludarabine.
ALT, alanine aminotransferase; AST, aspartate aminotransferase; BMT, bone marrow transplantation; CMV, cytomegalovirus; GVHD, graft-vs.-host disease; HCT, hematopoietic cell transplantation; HLA, human leukocyte antigen.

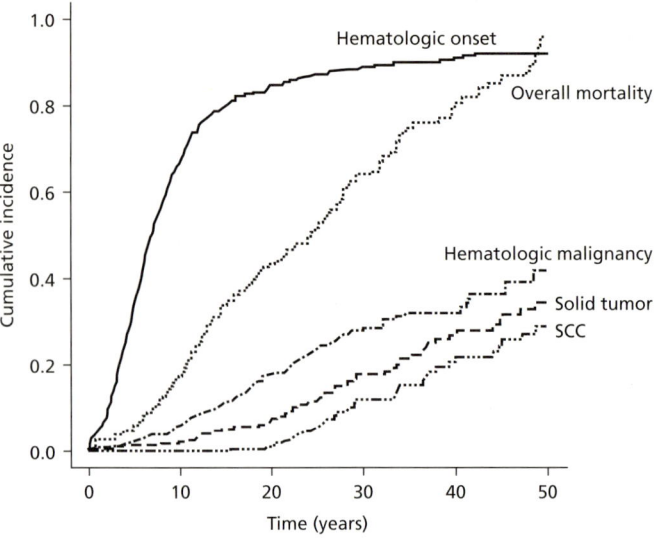

Fig. 109.10 Relative risk of solid tumors. Cumulative incidence of hematological disease, hematological malignancy, solid tumor and squamous cell carcinoma; and probability of overall mortality in patients with Fanconi anemia (FA). Reproduced with permission from [10].

Increased susceptibility to AML and solid tumors has long been recognized in children and adults with FA. However, the incidence and relative risk of these events has been difficult to quantify until recently. Two studies have recently been reported that address cancer risk in this patient population. Rosenberg *et al.* [9] assembled a survey cohort in the USA and in Canada. Questionnaires included demographics, physical malformations and age of cancer onset. Cancer diagnoses were confirmed by medical records, pathology reports and/or death certificates. In order to calculate the cancer risk relative to the general population, results in FA patients were compared to the observed numbers of cancers by age and type to those in established cancer registries. In this study 27 cancers were observed in 23 individuals of the 145 returning the questionnaire [9]. There were nine cases of leukemia and 18 cases of solid tumors. The median age of subjects at leukemia diagnosis was 11.3 years (range: 3–24

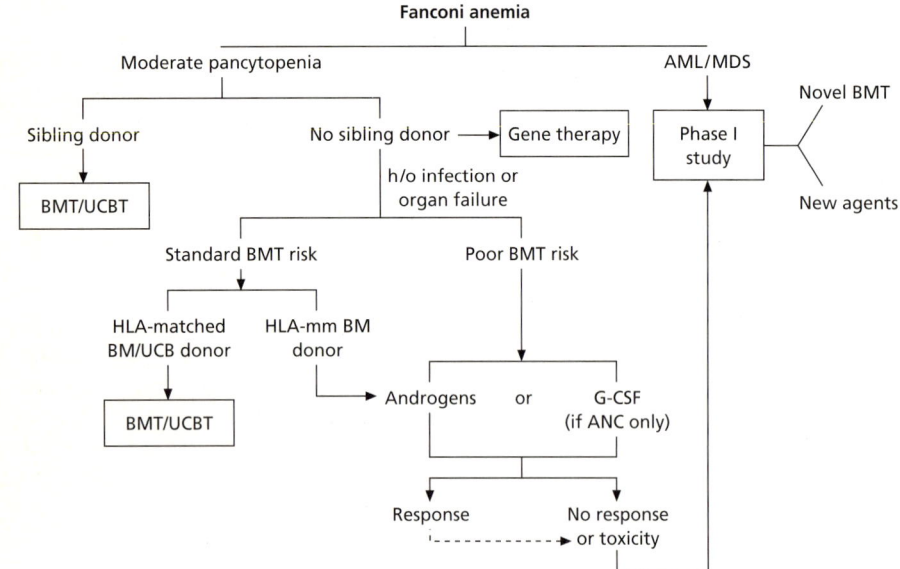

Fig. 109.9 Proposed treatment algorithm.

Table 109.7 Observed cancers (O), ratio of observed to expected cancers (O/E), and 95% confidence intervals (95%CI) among North American respondents with Fanconi anemia. Reproduced with permission from [9].

Type of cancer	O[†]	O/E[‡]	95%CI[§]
Leukemia (AML)	9	785*	360–1490
Head and neck	6	706*	260–1540
Esophagus	2	2362*	265–8530
Liver	2	386*	45–1395
Vulva	3	4317*	870–12,615
Cervix	2	179*	20–645
Osteosarcoma	1	79	1–440
Soft tissue sarcoma	1	49	0.6–270.0
Brain	1	17	0.2–95.0
Total cancers	27	50*	35–80
Total solid tumors	18	48*	30–80

*$p < 0.05$ that true O/E ratio equals 1.0 (exact two-sided tests).
†Twenty-seven cancers observed in 23 patients. Two patients had two solid tumors (cervix and vulva, and vulva and oesophagus) and one had three solid tumors (oesophagus, liver and cervix).
‡Expected cancer incidence rates calculated from the Connecticut Tumor Registry.
§Limits of the 95%CIs rounded to the nearest 5 for values ≥10.
AML, acute myeloid leukemia.

years) in contrast to 28.9 years (range: 7–45 years) at solid tumor diagnosis. Compared to the general population, these data suggest a 785-fold higher risk of leukemia and 48-fold higher risk of solid tumor in patients with FA. Importantly, the observed-to-expected ratio of solid tumors of the head and neck, oesophagus and vulva is 706, 2362 and 4317, respectively. Further, the RR of solid tumor was low until age 28 years. By age 28, 34 and 48 years the risk was 9%, 22% and 29%, respectively. As shown in Fig. 109.10, the rise in RR of solid tumors is nonlinear with no plateau.

A report of IFAR results further highlights the susceptibility of FA patients to both benign and malignant tumor development [10]. The cumulative incidence of hematologic neoplasms and solid tumors by age 40 is 33% and 28%, respectively. Evaluation of the types of neoplasms that FA patients developed revealed a wide array of different solid neoplasms (Table 109.7), with a marked predisposition toward squamous cell carcinoma, especially of the upper aerodigestive and anogenital regions. The increase in the cumulative incidence of head and neck cancer in FA patients compared to the Surveillance, Epidemiology and End Results (SEER) population is 500-fold [10].

A critical question is whether treatment consisting of chemotherapy and irradiation in combination with HCT alters the underlying cancer risk in FA patients. In the study by Rosenberg et al. [9], there appeared to be a trend toward higher risk in HCT recipients. In the IFAR study [10], the statistical analysis of the relationship between HCT and solid neoplasm development could not be performed due to the small number of HCT patients who developed solid tumors. Notably, the percentage of patients who had undergone HCT and developed solid neoplasms (2.7%) was actually less than the percentage of patients without HCT who developed solid neoplasms (13%) [10]. While not conclusive, these results suggest that the underlying chromosomal instability characteristic of FA appears to play the critical role in the development of solid tumors with an as yet underdetermined effect by HCT therapy.

Based on these observations, there are four key conclusions:

1 The risk of solid tumor does not appear to be affected by chemo-radiotherapy and HCT, although this remains unproven.
2 Solid tumors begin to appear at 5 years of age with more than a linear rise in risk without plateau.
3 As survival rates improve with HCT and death from marrow failure and leukemia are reduced, a greater proportion of FA patients will be "at risk" as they enter the 3rd and 4th decades of life.
4 Rigorous screening and cancer prevention programs are critical to the survival of FA patients particularly after the age of 20 years.

Future directions

Improved understanding the function of the FA genes has already profoundly affected our understanding of apoptosis, DNA repair and regulation of normal hematopoiesis. Additionally, there is a concerted effort by numerous investigators to find novel therapies that can potentially alter the natural history of the disease with better risk. In contrast to reports in the past, HCT now has an improved capacity to correct the hematologic manifestations of this syndrome with lower risk. Nonetheless, risk of morbidity and mortality is still present and new therapeutic strategies should be explored such as the development of safer preparative therapies and potentially safer methods of gene correction. In addition, recent developments in assisted reproduction technologies can now permit couples at high risk of having a child with FA to conceive a child free of the disease and with a desired HLA type. Although complicated by numerous ethical and legal issues, the use of preimplantation genetic diagnosis (PGD) is growing rapidly.

Gene therapy

The possibility of using gene transfer methods for correcting genetic diseases of HSCs has received much attention. Seven FA genes have been cloned and the sequences for these genes have been placed in the public domain. Currently, gene vector technology is being used in the laboratory to test whether a patient belongs to one of these seven complementation groups [54,55]. Once the complementation group is known, mutation screening for a particular family is targeted. This technology will rapidly expand our ability to predict the pace of disease progression and risk of hematological malignancy as well as identify which patients are appropriate for gene transfer studies.

The availability of FA genes has spurred considerable interest in the development of gene therapy for this disease for two reasons: (i) few FA patients have HLA genotypic-identical HSC donors; and (ii) the risks of morbidity and mortality after unrelated donor HCT in specific high-risk subpopulations are substantial. An alternative treatment would be the infusion of genetically corrected HSCs. Retroviral transduction of *FANCA, C* or *G* cDNA into primary FA cells has already been shown to correct cross-linking agent hypersensitivity and chromosomal instability in hematopoietic colony forming cells as well as improve progenitor cell survival as compared to uninfected cells.

While there have been numerous reports [161–163] demonstrating that recombinant virus transduction of FA cDNA into FA CD34+ hematopoietic progenitor cells improves clonogenic potential with phenotypic correction of CFC *in vitro*, as shown by resistance to MMC-induced cell death, loss of susceptibility to chromosomal breakage and restoration of cell cycle kinetics, clinical trials of gene transfer have been disappointing. Liu et al. [161] reported the clinical results in four FA-C patients treated with autologous hematopoietic progenitor cells transduced with the *FANCC* gene. In this study, a G1FASvNa.52 retroviral vector containing the *FANCC* and neomycin resistance coding sequences was used. After infusion, *FANCC* transgene was present transiently in the peripheral blood and BM. Function of the *FANCC* transgene was suggested by a marked increase in hematopoietic CFC, including colonies in the presence of MMC, after successive infusions of transduced cells. Despite a growth advantage *in vitro*, there has been only transient evidence of gene corrected HSCs amplification *in vivo*.

A great deal remains to be learned regarding gene therapy in the treatment of FA. Optimization of HSC mobilization, collection and gene transduction, as well as long-term expression and safety questions, has yet to be elucidated. More recent work suggests that lentiviral vectors might be a strategy for efficient gene correction of quiescent HSCs. Recently, Galimi *et al.* [164] have demonstrated correction of $FANCA^{-/-}$ and $FANCC^{-/-}$ mice. Long-term repopulating hematopoietic progenitor cells were transduced by a single exposure of unfractionated bone marrow mononuclear cells to lentivectors carrying normal *FANCA* or *FANCC* genes. Notably, no cell purification or cytokine prestimulation was necessary reducing the risk of nonspecific HSC loss, especially important in this setting where there are few HSCs available. Resistance to clastogenic agents was fully restored by lentiviral transduction, which allowed for subsequent *in vivo* selection of the corrected cells by exposure to low-dose CY.

While gene therapy may not be readily applicable to FA patients today, it is a particularly attractive candidate disease for such a therapeutic approach owing to an inherent selective advantage. Therefore, the hematologist should consider autologous HSC collection early in the course of the disease, optimally at a time preceding the development of marrow hypoplasia and MDS, as previously stated.

Multipotent adult stem cells

Embryonic stem cells are pluripotent cells derived from the inner cell mass of the blastocyst that can be propagated indefinitely in the undifferentiated state or differentiated into all cell lineages at least *in vivo*. Recently, pluripotent mesenchymal stem cells have also been isolated from adult marrow, termed MASCs [165]. After injection into an early blastocyst, single MASC have contributed to most, if not all, somatic cell types. Irrespective of their origin, embryonic stem cells and MASCs hold great promise for the treatment of many degenerative and inherited diseases. For example, MASCs from a closely HLA-matched healthy donor could be used alone or in combination with HSCs. Autologous MASCs could be genetically modified and then be used to the treatment of diseases such as FA and cancer. In the setting of FA, MASCs will likely be used as a strategy to enhance tissue repair after chemoradiotherapy. Alternatively, genetically corrected MASCs from the FA patient him/herself could be used as source of HSCs. Due to their proliferative capacity, MASCs can be genetically corrected with high efficiency. Gene correction of MASCs followed by differentiation into HSC is being explored as a particularly attractive strategy for treating the bone marrow failure common to most patients with FA.

Preimplantation genetic diagnosis (PGD)

For couples with a child with FA, counseling must include a discussion of PGD [166,167]. If appropriate for the couple, the first step is to obtain the complementation group assignment and specific mutation if possible (although not mandatory). For couples wishing to have a child that is HLA identical with the existing child with FA, the second step is to obtain HLA typing on the mother, father and affected child. Afterward, it is important to identify a team experienced in *in vitro* fertilization (IVF) that understands the specific goals of the couple. Importantly, the IVF procedure does not have to be performed at the location of the PGD team or transplant center. As with IVF for infertile couples, the procedure first requires daily injections to stimulate follicle maturation. After retrieval, each ovum is fertilized. After 2–3 days, at the 8–10 cell stage, a single cell is removed and tested for FA and HLA. Embryos that are free of disease and HLA identical (if appropriate) are identified and implanted at that time or at a future time, depending upon the desire of the family (Plate 109.4, *facing p. 296* [168]).

Due to the risk of error (albeit very low), CVS or amniocentesis must be performed to confirm that the fetus is healthy and HLA identical. Prior to delivery, arrangements are made for collection and shipment of the UCB from the HLA identical healthy sibling to the transplant center. Prior to transplantation the newborn donor is evaluated for FA and HLA a third time, due to the critical importance of these tests to the child being transplanted.

Procedural steps

- Conference with transplant physician and genetic counselor.
- Obtain complementation group assignment and mutation analysis.
- HLA type mother, father and child affected with FA (if appropriate).
- Referral to IVF center
- CVS/amniocentesis to confirm health and HLA status of fetus.
- UCB collection and harvesting.
- Confirmatory testing on umbilical cord blood/newborn baby.
- Transplantation of HLA-matched umbilical cord blood.

While the breadth of applicability remains to be identified and as the debate regarding the use of PGD to select embryos with desirable characteristics continues [169], it is clear from the number of referrals that there is a significant interest in using this technology. In addition to being aware of such technology, transplant physicians need to be intimately involved from the outset, as the patient's condition may not allow sufficient time for the delivery of the healthy HLA genotypic-identical sibling donor.

Summary

Clearly, all patients with FA should be followed routinely by a hematologist, even prior to the onset of marrow failure. To better understand the natural history of this disease and the significance of cytogenetic clonal abnormalities, patients must have marrow examinations annually and more frequently after the onset of marrow failure and/or development of clonal hematopoiesis. Moreover, the hematologist must be aware of the importance of family genetic counseling, the availability of prenatal diagnosis and PGD. However, the hematologist must also be aware that the availability of predictive testing has led to complex ethical issues, such as deliberate conception of a fetus and, more recently, embryo selection for the possibility of providing an unaffected HLA-identical sibling HSC donor. These and other ethical issues are discussed in detail elsewhere [169].

For those treated by HCT, ideally, preparative regimens would be tailored to individual patient sensitivities. An effort to individualize dosage of CY has been made by Yabe *et al.* [170]. These investigators exposed cultured FA patient lymphocytes to CY metabolites in *in vitro* culture prior to HCT. Cells were studied for chromosomal fragility and the number of chromosomal aberrations per cell scored. The dose of CY to be used in conditioning was determined according to the number of aberrations with patients with high numbers of aberrations receiving lower doses of drug. Five patients treated in this manner with related donors all achieved engraftment and survive 2–4 years after HCT. However, no recent reports of such studies have been identified. Whether HCT is prescribed or not, standardized treatment programs should be made available to all hematologists with outcome reported to a central registry. Such information will clearly aid in the development of new therapies as well as understanding the role of HCT in the treatment of FA.

References

1 Fanconi G. Familiäre infantile perniziosaartige Anämie (perniziöses Blutbild und Konstitution). *Jahrb Kinderh* 1927; **117**: 257–80.
2 Fanconi G. Familial constitutional panmyelocytopathy, Fanconi's anemia (FA). I. Clinical aspects. *Semin Hematol* 1967; **4**: 233–40.
3 Glanz A, Fraser FC. Spectrum of anomalies in Fanconi anaemia. *J Med Genet* 1982; **19**: 412–6.
4 Estren S, Dameshek W. Familial hypoplastic anemia of childhood. Report of eight cases in two families with beneficial effect of splenectomy in one case. *Am J Dis Child* 1947; **73**: 671–87.
5 Macdougall LG, Greeff MC, Rosendorff J, Bernstein R. Fanconi anemia in black African children. *Am J Med Genet* 1990; **36**: 408–13.
6 Giampietro PF, Adler-Brecher B, Verlander PC, Pavlakis SG, Davis JG, Auerbach AD. The need for more accurate and timely diagnosis in Fanconi anemia: a report from the International Fanconi Anemia Registry. *Pediatrics* 1993; **91**: 1116–20.
7 Giampietro PF, Verlander PC, Davis JG, Auerbach AD. Diagnosis of Fanconi anemia in patients without congenital malformations: An International Fanconi Anemia Registry study. *Am J Med Genet* 1997; **68**: 58–61.
8 Alter BP, Young NS. The bone marrow failure syndromes. In: Nathan DG, Orkin SH, eds. *Hematology of Infancy and Childhood*, 4th edn. Philadelphia: WB Saunders & Co., 1998: 237–335.
9 Rosenberg PS, Greene MH, Alter BP. Cancer incidence in persons with Fanconi's anemia. *Blood* 2003; **101**: 822–6.
10 Kutler DI, Singh B, Satagopan J et al. A. 20-year perspective of The International Fanconi Anemia Registry (IFAR). *Blood* 2003; **101**: 1249–56.
11 Kutler DI, Auerbach AD, Satagopan J. et al. High incidence of head and neck squamous cell carcinoma (HNSCC) in patients with Fanconi anemia (FA). *Arch Otolaryngol* 2003; **129**: 106–12.
12 Auerbach AD, Joenje H, Buchwald M. Fanconi anemia. In: Vogelstein B, Kinzler KW, eds. *The Genetic Basis of Human Cancer*, 2nd edn. New York, McGraw-Hill, 2002: 289–306.
13 Wajnrajch MP, Gertner JM, Huma Z et al. Evaluation of growth and hormonal status in patients referred to the International Fanconi Anemia Registry. *Pediatrics* 2001; **107**: 744–54.
14 Alter BP, Frissora CL, Halperin DS et al. Fanconi's anaemia and pregnancy. *Br J Haematol* 1991; **77**: 410–8.
15 Liu JM, Auerbach AD, Young NS. Fanconi anemia presenting unexpectedly in an adult kindred with no dysmorphic features. *Am J Med* 1991; **91**: 555–7.
16 Butturini A, Gale RP, Verlander PC, Adler-Brecher B, Gillio A, Auerbach AD. Hematologic abnormalities in Fanconi anemia. An International Fanconi Anemia Registry study. *Blood* 1994; **84**: 1650–5.
17 Maarch O, Jonveaux P, Le Coniat M, Derre J, Berger R. Fanconi anemia and bone marrow clonal chromosomal abnormalities. *Leukemia* 1996; **10**: 1700–4.
18 Schroeder TM, Anschultz F, Knoff A. Spontane Chromosomenaberrationen bei familiärer Panmyelopathie. *Humangenetik* 1964; **1**: 194–6.
19 Auerbach AD, Rogatko A, Shroeder-Kurth TM. International Fanconi Anemia Registry. Relation of clinical symptoms to diepoxybutane sensitivity. *Blood* 1989; **73**: 391–6.
20 Auerbach AD. Fanconi anemia diagnosis and the diepoxybutane (DEB) test. *Exp Hematol* 1993; **21**: 731–3.
21 Auerbach AD. Diagnosis of Fanconi anemia by diepoxybutane analysis. In: Dracopoli, NC, Haines, JL, Korf, BR et al. *Current Protocols in Human Genetics*. New York: Current Protocols, 1994: 8.1.7–12.
22 Lo Ten Foe JR, Kwee ML, Rooimans MA et al. Somatic mosaicism in Fanconi anaemia: molecular basis and clinical significance. *Eur J Hum Genet* 1997; **5**: 137–48.
23 Gillio AP, Verlander PC, Batish SD, Giampietro PF, Auerbach AD. Phenotypic consequences of mutations in the Fanconi-anemia *FAC* gene: an International Fanconi anemia Registry study. *Blood* 1997; **90**: 105–10.
24 Berger R, Le Coniat M, Gendron MC. Fanconi anemia. Chromosome breakage and cell cycle studies. *Cancer Genet Cytogenet* 1993; **69**: 13–6.
25 Seyschab H, Friedl R, Sun Y et al. Comparative evaluation of diepoxybutane sensitivity and cell cycle blockage in the diagnosis of Fanconi anemia. *Blood* 1995; **85**: 2233–7.
26 Cassinat B, Guardiola P, Chevret S et al. Constitutive elevation of serum α-fetoprotein in Fanconi anemia. *Blood* 2000; **96**: 859–63.
27 Strathdee CA, Duncan AM, Buchwald M. Evidence for at least four Fanconi anaemia genes including *FACC* on chromosome 9. *Nature Genet* 1992; **1**: 196–8.
28 Joenje H, Oostra AB, Wijker M et al. Evidence of at least eight Fanconi anemia genes. *Am J Hum Genet* 1997; **61**: 940–4.
29 Joenje H, Levitus M, Waisfisz Q et al. Complementation analysis in Fanconi anemia: assignment of the reference FA-H patient to group A. *Am J Hum Genet* 2000; **67**: 759–62.
30 Timmers C, Taniguchi T, Hejna J et al. Positional cloning of a novel Fanconi anemia gene, *FANCD2*. *Mol Cell* 2001; **7**: 241–8.
31 Strathdee CA, Gavish H, Shannon WR, Buchwald M. Cloning of cDNAs for Fanconi's anaemia by functional complementation. *Nature* 1992; **358**: 763–7.
32 Lo Ten Foe JR, Rooimans MA, Bosnoyan-Collins L et al. Expression cloning of a cDNA for the major Fanconi anaemia gene, *FAA*. *Nature Genet* 1996; **14**: 320–3.
33 The Fanconi Anaemia/Breast Cancer Consortium. Positional cloning of the Fanconi anaemia group A gene. The Fanconi Anaemia/Breast Cancer Consortium. *Nature Genet* 1996; **14**: 324–8.
34 De Winter JP, Waisfisz Q, Rooimans MA et al. The Fanconi anemia group G gene is identical with human *XRCC9*. *Nature Genet* 1998; **20**: 281–3.
35 De Winter JP, Rooimans MA, van Der Weel L et al. The Fanconi anaemia gene *FANCF* encodes a novel protein with homology to ROM. *Nature Genet* 2000; **24**: 15–6.
36 De Winter JP, Léveillé F, van Berkel CGM et al. Isolation of a cDNA representing the Fanconi anemia complementation group E gene. *Am J Hum Genet* 2000; **67**: 1306–8.
37 Howlett N, Toshiyasu T, Olson S et al. Biallelic inactivation of *BRCA2* in Fanconi anemia. *Science* 2002; **297**: 606–9.
38 Godthelp BC, Artwert F, Joenje H, Zdzienicka MZ. Impaired DNA damage-induced nuclear Rad51 foci formation uniquely characterizes Fanconi anemia group D1. *Oncogene* 2002; **21**: 5002–5.
39 Whitney MA, Saito H, Jakobs PM, Gibson RA, Moses RE, Grompe M. A common mutation in the *FACC* gene causes Fanconi anaemia in Ashkenazi Jews. *Nat Genet* 1993; **4**: 202–5.
40 Verlander PC, Kaporis AG, Liu Q, Zhang Q, Seligsohn U, Auerbach AD. Carrier frequency of the IVS + 4 A > T mutation of the Fanconi anemia gene *FAC* in the Ashkenazi Jewish population. *Blood* 1995; **86**: 4034–8.
41 Verlander PC, Lin JD, Udono MU et al. Mutation analysis of the Fanconi anemia gene *FACC*. *Am J Hum Genet* 1994; **54**: 595–601.
42 Gibson RA, Morgan NV, Goldstein LH et al. Novel mutations and polymorphisms in the Fanconi anaemia group C gene. *Hum Mutat* 1996; **8**: 140–8.
43 Ianzano L, D'Apolito M, Centra M et al. The genomic organization of the Fanconi anemia group A (FAA) gene. *Genomics* 1997; **41**: 309–14.
44 Levran O, Erlich T, Magdalena N et al. Sequence variation in the Fanconi anemia gene, *FAA*. *Proc Natl Acad Sci U S A* 1997; **94**: 13,051–6.
45 Savino M, Ianzano L, Strippoli P et al. Mutations of the Fanconi anemia group A gene (*FAA*) in Italian patients. *Am J Hum Genet* 1997; **61**: 1246–53.
46 Levran O, Doggett NA, Auerbach AD. Identification of Alu-mediated deletions in the Fanconi anemia gene *FAA*. *Hum Mutat* 1998; **12**: 145–52.
47 Tachibana A, Kato T, Ejima Y et al. The *FANCA* gene in Japanese Fanconi anemia: reports of eight novel mutations and analysis of sequence variability. *Hum Mutat* 1999; **13**: 237–44.
48 Morgan NV, Tipping AJ, Joenje H, Mathew CG. High frequency of large intragenic deletions in the Fanconi anemia group A gene. *Am J Hum Genet* 1999; **65**: 1330–41.
49 Tamary H, Bar-Yam R, Shalmon L et al. Fanconi anaemia group A (FANCA) mutations in Israeli non-Ashkenazi Jewish patients. *Br J Haematol* 2000; **111**: 338–43.
50 Tipping AJ, Pearson T, Morgan NV et al. Molecular and genealogical evidence for a founder effect in Fanconi anemia families of the Afrikaner population of South Africa. *Proc Natl Acad Sci U S A* 2001; **98**: 5734–9.
51 Yamada T, Tachibana A, Shimizu T, Mugishima H, Okubo M, Sasaki MS. Novel mutations of the *FANCG* gene causing alternative splicing in Japanese Fanconi anemia. *J Hum Genet* 2000; **45**: 159–66.
52 Demuth I, Wlodarski M, Tipping AJ et al. Spectrum of mutations in the Fanconi anaemia group G gene, *FANCG/XRCC9*. *Eur J Hum Genet* 2000; **8**: 861–8.
53 Auerbach AD, Greenbaum J, Pujara K et al. The spectrum of mutations in the Fanconi anemia gene *FANCG*. An International Fanconi Anemia Registry (IFAR) study. *Hum Mutat* 2003; **21**: 158–68.
54 Pulsipher M, Kupfer GM, Naf D et al. Subtyping analysis of Fanconi anemia by immunoblotting and retroviral gene transfer. *Mol Med* 1998; **4**: 468–79.
55 Hanenberg H, Batish SD, Pollok KE et al. Phenotypic correction of primary T cells from patients with Fanconi anemia with retroviral vectors as a diagnostic tool. *Exp Hematol* 2002; **30**: 410–20.

56 Xiao W, Oefner PJ. Denaturing high-performance liquid chromatography: a review. *Hum Mutat* 2001; **17**: 439–74.

57 Rischewski J, Schneppenheim R. Screening strategies for a highly polymorphic gene. DHPLC analysis of the Fanconi anemia group A gene. *J Biochem Biophys Methods* 2001; **47**: 53–64.

58 Auerbach AD, Levran O, Pujara K et al. Genetic classification of African-American Fanconi anemia patients in the International Fanconi Anemia Registry (IFAR). *Blood* 2001; **98**: 216–17a.

59 Youssoufian H. Localization of Fanconi anemia C protein to the cytoplasm of mammalian cells. *Proc Natl Acad Sci U S A* 1994; **91**: 7975–9.

60 Yamashita T, Barber DL, Zhu Y, Wu N, D'Andrea AD. The Fanconi anemia polypeptide FACC is localized to the cytoplasm. *Proc Natl Acad Sci U S A* 1994; **91**: 6712–6.

61 Youssoufian H, Auerbach AD, Verlander PC, Steimle V, Mach B. Indentification of cytosolic proteins that bind to the Fanconi anemia polypeptide FACC in vitro. Evidence of a multimeric complex. *J Biol Chem* 1995; **270**: 9876–82.

62 Hoatlin ME, Christianson TA, Keeble WW et al. The Fanconi anemia group C gene product is located in both the nucleus and cytoplasm of human cells. *Blood* 1998; **91**: 1418–25.

63 Kupfer GM, Naf D, Suliman A, Pulsiper M, D'Andrea AD. The Fanconi aneamia proteins, FAA and FAC, interact to form a nuclear complex. *Nat Genet* 1997; **17**: 487–90.

64 Garcia-Higuera I, Kuang Y, Denham J, D'Andrea AD. The Fanconi anemia proteins FANCA and FANCG stabilize each other and promote the nuclear accumulation of the Fanconi anemia complex. *Blood* 2000; **96**: 3224–30.

65 de Winter JP, van Der Weel L, de Groot J et al. The Fanconi anemia protein FANCF forms a nuclear complex with FANCA, FANCC, and FANCG. *Hum Mol Genet* 2000; **9**: 2665–74.

66 Medhurst AL, Huber PAJ, Waisfisz Q, de Winter JP, Mathew CG. Direct interactions of the five known Fanconi anemia proteins suggest a common functional pathway. *Hum Mol Genet* 2001; **10**: 423–9.

67 Siddique MA, Nakanishi K, Taniguchi T, Grompe M, D'Andrea AD. Function of the Fanconi anemia pathway in Fanconi anemia complementation group F and D1 cells. *Exp Hematol* 2001; **29**: 1448–55.

68 Garcia-Higuera I, Taniguchi T, Ganesan S et al. Interaction of the Fanconi anemia proteins and BRCA1 in a common pathway. *Mol Cell* 2001; **7**: 249–62.

69 Taniguchi T, Garcia-Higuera I, Xu B et al. Convergence of the Fanconi anemia and ataxia telangiectasia signaling. *Cell* 2002; **109**: 459–72.

70 Shimamura A, Montes de Oca R, Svenson JL et al. A novel diagnostic screen for defects in the Fanconi anemia pathway. *Blood* 2002; **100**: 4649–54.

71 Kupfer GM, Yamashita T, Naf D, Suliman A, Asano S, D'Andrea AD. The Fanconi anemia polypeptide, FAC, binds to the cyclin-dependent kinase, cdc2. *Blood* 1997; **90**: 1047–54.

72 Kruyt FAE, Dijkmans LM, Arwert F, Joenje H. Involvement of the Fanconi's anemia protein FAC in a pathway that signals to the cyclin B/cdc2 kinase. *Cancer Res* 1997; **57**: 2244–51.

73 Hoshino T, Wang J, Devetten MP et al. Molecular chaperone GRP94 binds to the Fanconi anemia group C protein and regulates its intracellular expression. *Blood* 1998; **91**: 4379–86.

74 Kruyt FA, Hoshino T, Liu JM, Joseph P, Jaiswal AK, Youssofian H. Abnormal microsomal detoxification implicated in Fanconi anemia group C by interaction of the FAC protein with NADPH cytochrome P-450 reductase. *Blood* 1998; **92**: 3050–6.

75 Pang Q, Fagerlie S, Christianson TA et al. The Fanconi anemia protein FANCC binds to and facilitates the activation of STAT1 by γ interferon and hematopoietic growth factors. *Mol Cell Biol* 2000; **20**: 4724–35.

76 Pang Q, Christianson TA, Keeble W et al. The Fanconi anemia complementation group C gene product: structural evidence of multifunctionality. *Blood* 2001; **98**: 1392–401.

77 Cumming RC, Lightfoot J, Beard K, Youssoufian H, O'Brien PJ, Buchwald M. Fanconi anemia group C protein prevents apoptosis in hematopoietic cells through redox regulation of GSTP1. *Nat Med* 2001; **7**: 814–9.

78 Pang Q, Keeble W, Christianson TA, Faulkner GR, Bagby GC. FANCC interacts with Hsp70 to protect hematopoietic cells from IFN-γ/TNF-α-mediated cytotoxicity. *EMBO J* 2001; **20**: 4478–89.

79 Pang Q, Christianson TA, Keeble K, Koretsky T, Bagby GC. The anti-apoptotic function of Hsp70 in the PKR-mediated death signaling pathway requires the Fanconi anemia protein, FANCC. *J Biol Chem*, in press.

80 Rathburn RK, Christianson TA, Faulkner GR et al. Interferon-γ-induced apoptotic responses of Fanconi anemia group C hematopoietic progenitor cells involve caspase 8-dependent activation of caspase 3 family member. *Blood* 2000; **96**: 4204–11.

81 Hoatlin ME, Zhi Y, Ball H et al. A novel BTB/POZ transcriptional repressor protein interacts with the Fanconi anemia group C protein and PLZF. *Blood* 1999; **94**: 3737–47.

82 Dai MS, Chevallier N, Stone S et al. The effects of the Fanconi anemia zinc finger (FAZF) on cell cycle, apoptosis, and proliferation are differentiation stage-specific. *J Biol Chem* 2002; **277**: 26,327–34.

83 Folias A, Matkovic M, Bruun D et al. BRCA1 interacts directly with the Fanconi anemia protein FANCA. *Hum Mol Genet* 2002; **11**: 2591–7.

84 Otsuki T, Furukawa Y, Ikeda K et al. Fanconi anemia protein, FANCA, associates with BRG1, a component of the human SWI/SNF complex. *Hum Mol Genet* 2001; **10**: 2651–60.

85 Yamashita T, Wu N, Kupfer G et al. Clinical variability of Fanconi anemia (type C) results from expression of an amino terminal truncated Fanconi anemia complementation group C polypeptide with partial activity. *Blood* 1996; **87**: 4424–32.

86 Stephan V, Wahn V, Le Deist F et al. X-linked severe combined immunodeficiency due to possible spontaneous reversion of the genetic defect in T cells. *New Engl J Med* 1996; **335**: 1563–7.

87 Hirschhorn R, Yang DR, Israni A, Huie ML, Ownby DR. Somatic mosaicism for a newly identified splice-site mutation in a patient with adenosine deaminase-deficient immunodeficiency and spontaneous clinical recovery. *Am J Hum Genet* 1994; **55**: 59–68.

88 Jonkman MF, Scheffer H, Stulp R et al. Revertant mosaicism in epidermolysis bullosa caused by mitotic gene conversion. *Cell* 1997; **88**: 543–51.

89 Ellis NA, Lennon DJ, Proytcheva M, Alhadeff B, Henderson EE, German J. Somatic intragenic recombination within the mutated locus BLM can correct the sister-chromatid exchange phenotype of Bloom syndrome cells. *Am J Hum Genet* 1995; **57**: 1019–27.

90 Kvittingen EA, Rootwelt H, Berger R, Brandtzaeg P. Self-induced correction of the genetic defect in tyrosinemia type I. *J Clin Invest* 1994; **94**: 1657–61.

91 Gregory JJ, Wagner JE, Verlander PC et al. Somatic mosaicism in Fanconi anemia: evidence of genotypic reversion in lymphohematopoietic stem cells. *Proc Natl Acad Sci U S A* 2001; **98**: 2532–7.

92 Battaile KP, Bateman R, Mortimer D et al. In vivo selection of wild-type hematopoietic stem cells in a murine model of Fanconi anemia. *Blood* 1999; **94**: 2151–8.

93 MacMillan ML, Auerbach AD, Davies SM et al. Hematopoietic cell transplantation in patients with Fanconi anaemia using alternate donors: results of a total body irradiation dose escalation trial. *Br J Haematol* 2000; **109**: 121–9.

94 Whitney MA, Royle G, Low MJ et al. Germ cell defects and hematopoietic hypersensitivity to γ-interferon in mice with a targeted disruption of the Fanconi anemia C gene. *Blood* 1996; **88**: 49–58.

95 Chen M, Tomkins DJ, Auerbach W et al. Inactivation of Fac in mice produces inducible chromosomal instability and reduced fertility reminiscent of Fanconi anaemia. *Nature Genet* 1996; **12**: 448–51.

96 Cheng NC, van de Vrugt H, van der Valk MA et al. Mice targeted disruption of the Fanconi anemia homolog *Fanca*. *Hum Mol Genet* 2000; **9**: 1805–11.

97 Haneline LS, Gobbett TA, Ramani R et al. Loss of *Fancc* function results in decreased hematopoietic stem cell repopulating ability. *Blood* 1999; **94**: 1–8.

98 Haneline LS, Broxmeyer HE, Cooper S et al. Multiple inhibitory cytokines induce deregulated progenitor growth and apoptosis in hematopoietic cells from Fac$^{-/-}$ mice. *Blood* 1998; **98**: 4092–8.

99 Carreau M, Gan OI, Doedens M, Dick JE, Buchwald M. Hematopoietic compartment of Fanconi anemia group C null mice contains fewer lineage-negative CD34$^+$ primitive hematopoietic cells and shows reduced reconstitution ability. *Exp Hematol* 1999; **27**: 1667–74.

100 Carreau M, Gan OI, Liu L et al. Bone marrow failure in the Fanconi anemia group C mouse model after DNA damage. *Blood* 1998; **91**: 2737–44.

101 Otsuki T, Wang J, Demuth I, Digweed M, Liu JM. Assessment of mitomycin C sensitivity in Fanconi anemia complementation group C gene (*Fac*) knock-out mouse cells. *Int J Hematol* 1998; **67**: 243–8.

102 Otsuki T, Nagakura S, Wang J, Bloom M, Grompe M, Liu JM. Tumor necrosis factor-α CD95 ligation suppress erythropoiesis in Fanconi anemia C gene knockout mice. *J Cell Physiol* 1999; **179**: 79–86.

103 Wang J, Youssoufian H, Lo Ten Foe JR et al. Overexpression of the Fanconi anemia group C gene (*FAC*) protects hematopoietic progenitors from fas-mediated apoptosis. *Blood* 1996; **88**: 548a.

104 Rathburn RK, Faulkner GR, Ostroski MH et al. Inactivation of the Fanconi anemia group C gene augments interferon-α-induced apoptotic responses in hematopoietic cells. *Blood* 1997; **90**: 974–85.

105 Segal GM, Magenis RE, Brown M et al. Repression of Fanconi anemia gene (*FACC*) expression inhibits growth of hematopoietic progenitor cells. *J Clin Invest* 1994; **4**: 846–52.

106 Cumming RC, Liu JM, Youssoufian H, Buchwald M. Suppression of apoptosis in hematopoietic

factor-dependent progenitor cell lines by expression of the *FAC* gene. *Blood* 1996; **8**: 4558–67.
107 Bagby GC, Segal GM, Auerbach AD, Onega T, Keeble W, Heinrich MC. Constitutive and induced expression of hematopoietic growth factor genes by fibroblasts from children with Fanconi anemia. *Exp Hematol* 1993; **21**: 1419–26.
108 Bagnara GP, Strippoli P, Bonsi L et al. Effect of stem cell factor on colony growth from acquired and constitutional (Fanconi) aplastic anemia. *Blood* 1992; **80**: 382–7.
109 Lyman SD, Seaberg M, Hanna R et al. Plasma/serum levels of flt3 ligand are low in normal individuals and highly elevated in patients with Fanconi anemia and acquired aplastic anemia. *Blood* 1995; **86**: 4091–6.
110 Daneshbod-Skibba G, Martin J, Shahidi NT. Myeloid and erythroid colony growth in non-anaemic patients with Fanconi's anaemia. *Br J Hematol* 1980; **44**: 33–8.
111 Butturini A, Gale RP. Long-term bone marrow culture in persons with Fanconi anemia and bone marrow failure. *Blood* 1994; **83**: 336–9.
112 Rathbun RK, Faulkner GR, Ostroski MH et al. Inactivation of the Fanconi anemia group C gene augments interferon γ-induced apoptotic responses in hematopoietic cells. *Blood* 1997; **90**: 974–85.
113 Schultz JC, Shahidi NT. Tumor necrosis factor-α overproduction in Fanconi's anemia. *Am J Hematol* 1993; **42**: 196–201.
114 Shahidi NT, Diamond LK. Testosterone-induced remission in aplastic anemia. *Am J Dis Child* 1959; **98**: 293–302.
115 Sanchez-Medal L. The hemopoietic action of androstanes. *Prog Hematol* 1971; **7**: 111–36.
116 Najean Y. Androgen therapy in aplastic anemia in childhood. In: *Congenital Disorders of Erythropoiesis. Ciba Foundation Symposium 37*. Amsterdam: Elsevier, 1976: 354–63.
117 Alter BP, Young NS. The bone marrow failure syndromes. In: Nathan D, Oski F, eds. *Hematology of Infancy and Childhood*, 4th edn. Philadelphia: Saunders & Co., 1993: 216–316.
118 Shahidi NT. Potential benefits of vitamins for FA patients. In: Frohnmayer D, Frohnmayer L, eds. *Fanconi Anemia, a Handbook for Families and Physicians*, 2nd edn. Eugene, OR: Fanconi Anemia Research Fund Inc., 57–60.
119 Rackoff WR, Orazi A, Robinson CA et al. Prolonged administration of granulocyte colony-stimulating factor (filgrastim) to patients with Fanconi anemia: a pilot study. *Blood* 1996; **88**: 1588–93.
120 Guinan EC, Lopez KD, Huhn RD, Felser JM, Nathan DG. Evaluation of granulocyte-macrophage colony-stimulating factor for treatment of pancytopenia in children with Fanconi anemia. *Pediatrics* 1994; **124**: 144–50.
121 Gluckman E, Devergie A, Schaison G et al. Bone marrow transplantation in Fanconi anemia. *Br J Haematol* 1980; **45**: 557–64.
122 Gluckman E, Devergie A, Dutreix J. Radiosensitivity in Fanconi anaemia: application to the conditioning regimen for bone marrow transplantation. *Br J Haematol* 1983; **54**: 431–40.
123 Hows JM, Chapple M, Marsh JCW et al. Bone marrow transplantation for Fanconi's anaemia: the Hammersmith experience 1977–89. *Bone Marrow Transplant* 1989; **4**: 629–34.
124 Berger R, Bernheim A, Gluckman E, Gisselbrecht C. In vitro effect of cyclophosphamide metabolites on chromosomes of Fanconi anaemia patients. *Br J Haematol* 1980; **45**: 565–8.
125 Auerbach AD, Adler B, O'Reilly RJ, Kirkpatrick D, Chaganh RS. Effect of procarbazine and cyclophosphamide on chromosomal breakage in Fanconi anemia cells: relevance to bone marrow transplantation. *Cancer Genet Cytogenet* 1983; **9**: 25–36.
126 Gluckman E, Berger R, Dutreix J. Bone marrow transplantation for Fanconi anemia. *Semin Hematol* 1984; **21**: 20–6.
127 Di Bartolomeo P, Di Girolamo G, Olioso P et al. Allogeneic bone marrow transplantation for Fanconi anemia. *Bone Marrow Transplant* 1992; **10**: 53–6.
128 Kohli-Kumar M, Morris C, DeLaat C et al. Bone marrow transplantation in Fanconi anemia using matched sibling donors. *Blood* 1994; **84**(6): 2050–4.
129 Gluckman E, Auerbach AD, Horowitz MM et al. Bone marrow transplantation for Fanconi anemia. *Blood* 1995; **86**: 2856–62.
130 Gluckman E. Bone marrow transplantation in Fanconi's anemia. *Stem Cells* 1993; **11**: 180–3.
131 Socié G, Gluckman E, Raynal R et al. Bone marrow transplantation for Fanconi anemia using low dose cyclophosphamide/thoraco-abdominal irradiation as conditioning regimen: chimerism study by the polymerase chain reaction. *Blood* 1993; **82**: 2249–56.
132 Ayas M, Solh H, Mustafa MM et al. Bone marrow transplantation from matched siblings in patients with Fanconi anemia utilizing low-dose cyclophosphamide, thoracoabdominal radiation and anti-thymocyte globulin. *Bone Marrow Transplant* 2001; **27**: 139–43.
133 DuFour C, Rondelli R, Locatelli F et al. Stem cell transplantation from HLA-matched related donor for Fanconi's anaemia: a retrospective review of the multicentric Italian experience on behalf of AIEOP-GITMO. *Br J Haematol* 2001; **112**: 796–805.
134 *IBMTR/ABMTR Newsletter* 1 February 2002; **9**(1).
135 Barrett AJ, Brigden WD, Hobbs JR et al. Successful bone marrow transplant for Fanconi's anaemia. *Br Med J* 1977; **1**: 420–2.
136 Kersey JH, Krivit W, Nesbit ME et al. Combined cyclophosphamide-total lymphoid irradiation compared to other forms of immunosuppression for human marrow transplantation. In: Baum SJ, Ledney GD, eds. *Experimental Hematology Today 1979*. New York: Springer-Verlag, 1979: 179–84.
137 Holl RA, Dooren LJ, Vossen JMJJ, Roos MTL, Schelleke PTA. Bone marrow transplantation in children with severe aplastic anemia. Reconstitution of cellular immunity. *Transplantation* 1981; **32**: 418–23.
138 Flowers MED, Doney KC, Storb R et al. Marrow transplantation for Fanconi anemia with or without leukemic transformation: an update of the Seattle experience. *Bone Marrow Transplant* 1992; **9**: 167–73.
139 Flowers ME, Zanis J, Pasquini R et al. Marrow transplantation for Fanconi anemia: conditioning with reduced doses of cyclophosphamide without radiation. *Br J Haematol* 1996; **92**: 699–706.
140 Ratanatharathorn V, Karanes C, Uberti J et al. Busulfan-based regimens and allogeneic bone marrow transplantation in patients with myelodysplastic syndromes. *Blood* 1993; **81**: 2194–9.
141 Maschan AA, Kryzanovskii OI, Yourlova MI et al. Intermediate-dose busulfan and cyclophosphamide as a conditioning regimen for bone marrow transplantation in a case of Fanconi anemia in myelodysplastic transformation. *Bone Marrow Transplant* 1997; **19**: 385–7.
142 De Mederios CR, Zanis-Neto J, Pasquini R. Bone marrow transplantation for patients with Fanconi anemia. Reduced doses of cyclophosphamide without irradiation as conditioning. *Bone Marrow Transplant* 1999; **24**: 849–52.
143 Aker M, Varadi G, Slavin S, Nagler A. Fludarabine-based protocol for human umbilical cord blood transplantation in children with Fanconi anemia. *J Pediatr Hematol Oncol* 1999; **21**: 237–9.
144 MacMillan ML, Weisdorf DJ, Slungaard A et al. High probability of survival in standard risk patients with Fanconi anemia (FA) after alternate donor hematopoietic cell transplantation (HCT). *Blood* 2002; **100**: 857a [Abstract].
145 Ebell W. Transplant results and observations from our transplant expert in Germany. *FA Family Newsletter* 2002; **32**: 5.
146 Terenzi A, Aristei C, Aversa F et al. Efficacy of fludarabine as an immunosuppressor for bone marrow transplantation conditioning: preliminary results. *Transplant Proc* 1996; **28**: 3101.
147 Slavin S, Nagler A, Naparstek E et al. Non-myeloablative stem cell transplantation and cell therapy as an alternative to conventional bone marrow transplantation with lethal cytoreduction for the treatment of malignant and non malignant hematologic diseases. *Blood* 1998; **91**: 756–63.
148 Nagler A, Or E, Naparstek G et al. Matched unrelated bone marrow transplantation (BMT) using a non-myeloablative conditioning regimen. *Blood* 1998; **92**: 289a [Abstract].
149 Spitzer T, McAfee S, Sackstein R et al. Induction of mixed chimerism and potent anti-tumor responses following non-myeloablative conditioning therapy and HLA-matched and mismatched donor bone marrow transplantation (BMT) for refractory hematologic malignancies (HM). *Blood* 1998; **92**: 519a [Abstract].
150 Kapelushnick J, Or R, Slavin S, Nagler A. A fludarabine-based protocol for bone marrow transplantation in Fanconi's anemia. *Bone Marrow Transplant* 1997; **20**: 1109–10.
151 Philpott NJ, Marsh JCW, Kumaran TO et al. Successful bone marrow transplant for Fanconi anaemia in transformation. *Bone Marrow Transplant* 1994; **14**: 151–3.
152 Ikushima S, Hibi S, Todo S et al. Successful allogeneic bone marrow transplantation in a case with myelodysplastic syndrome which developed following Fanconi anemia. *Bone Marrow Transplant* 1995; **16**: 621–4.
153 McCloy M, Almeida A, Daly P, Vulliamy T, Roberts IA, Dokal I. Fludarabine based stem cell transplantation protocol for Fanconi's anemia in myelodysplastic transformation. *Br J Haematol* 2001; **112**: 427–9.
154 Davies SM, Khan S, Wagner JE et al. Unrelated donor bone marrow transplantation for Fanconi anemia. *Bone Marrow Transplant* 1996; **17**: 43–7.
155 Dini G, Miano M, Mazzalari E et al. Unrelated donor marrow transplantation for genetic diseases. *Bone Marrow Transplant* 1997; **19**: 176–82.
156 Guardiola P, Pasquini R, Dokal I et al. Outcome of 69 allogeneic stem cell transplantations for Fanconi anemia using HLA-matched unrelated donors: a study on behalf of the European Group

157 Wagner JE, Auerbach AD, Gandham S et al. Unrelated donor hematopoietics cell transplantation (UD-HCT) for Fanconi Anemia (FA): impact of patient age, Pretransplant performance status, prior androgens and fludarabine based conditioning on survival. *Blood* 2001; **98**: 814a [Abstract].

158 Deeg HJ, Socié G, Schoch G et al. Malignancies after marrow transplantation for aplastic anemia and Fanconi anemia: a joint Seattle and Paris analysis of results in 700 patients. *Blood* 1996; **87**: 386–92.

159 Socie G, Devergie A, Girinski T et al. Transplantation of Fanconi's anaemia: long-term follow-up of fifty patients transplanted from a sibling donor after low dose cyclophosphamide and thoracoabdominal irradiation for conditioning. *Br J Haematol* 1998; **103**: 249–55.

160 Reed K, Ravikumar TS, Gifford RR, Grage TB. The association of Fanconi's anemia and squamous cell carcinoma. *Cancer* 1983; **52**: 926–8.

161 Liu JM, Kim S, Read EJ et al. Engraftment of hematopoietic progenitor cells transduced with the Fanconi anemia group C gene (*FANCC*). *Hum Gene Ther* 1999; **10**: 2337–46.

162 Walsh CE, Mann MM, Emmons RVB, Wang S, Liu JM. Transduction of CD34-enriched human peripheral and umbilical cord blood progenitors using a retroviral vector with the Fanconi anemia group C gene. *J Invest Med* 1995; **43**: 379–85.

163 Walsh C, Fu K, Brecher M, Kirby S, DiBartolomeo P, Jacobs P. Retroviral mediated gene transfer for group A Fanconi anemia patients. Fanconi Anemia Research Fund Scientific Symposium 2000: 46a.

164 Galimi F, Noll M, Kanazawa Y et al. Gene therapy of Fanconi anemia: preclinical efficacy using lentiviral vectors. *Blood* 2002; **100**: 2732–6.

165 Jiang Y, Jahagirdar B, Reinhardt RL et al. Pluripotency of mesenchymal stem cells derived from adult marrow. *Nature* 2002; 418: 41–9.

166 Verlinsky Y, Rechitsky S, Schoolcraft W, Strom C, Kuliev A. Preimplantation diagnosis for Fanconi anemia combined with HLA matching. *JAMA* 2001; **285**: 3130–3.

167 Belkin L. "The Made-to-Order Savior." *New York Times Magazine*, July 1 2001: pp. 36–42; 48; 62–3.

168 Verlinsky Y, Kuliev A, eds. *An Atlas of Preimplantation Genetic Diagnosis* New York: Parthenon, 2000: 92.

169 Robertson JA, Kahn JP, Wagner JE. Conception to obtain hematopoietic stem cells. *Hastings Center Report* 2002; **32**: 34–40.

170 Yabe M, Yabe H, Matsuda M et al. Bone marrow transplantation for Fanconi anemia. Adjustment of the dose of cyclophosphamide for preconditioning. *Am J Pediatr Hematol Oncol* 1993; **15**: 377–82.

Section 8

The Future

110 Ernest Beutler

Hematopoietic Cell Transplantation in the 21st Century

The past 35 years of hematopoietic cell transplantation (HCT) have been marked by gradually improving results. The advances that have been made are detailed in this volume. Rather than transplanting everything that is aspirated from the bone marrow we now try to isolate the cell types that are needed for optimal results. Better antibiotics are available now than 35 years ago, although the ability of microorganisms to adapt to what we design has somewhat blunted the advantage. Antiviral agents to suppress cytomegalovirus infections are available where there were none before. Cytokines have appeared on the scene, allowing recovery of the marrow to advance a few precious and sometimes critical days. Ever improving immunosuppressive drugs help to stay the attack of allogeneic lymphocytes on their new host, but graft-vs.-host disease (GVHD) is still very much with us. Autologous transplantation, a modality that did not seem to make sense in the treatment of leukemia, has shown itself to be useful in some circumstances, particularly when allogeneic donors were not available. "Mini-transplants" afford the benefits of stem cell transplantation to many patients who could not have tolerated a standard allogeneic transplant. Yet, that progress has not been nearly as rapid as some of us had hoped 35 years ago nor as we had predicted over the years. The mortality rate in the patient transplanted with allogeneic marrow has decreased only slightly and the cure rate for acute leukemia is not appreciably higher now than it was then. It is always hazardous to predict the future in science. In a very real sense, if we knew the future it would be the present.

There is, however, some reason to hope that progress will be more rapid in the remainder of the 21st century than it has been in the latter third of the 20th century. Often medical progress arises from chance observations or from tedious clinical trials designed empirically to find out the best way to treat patients. There is, of course, usually an underlying hypothesis, and in the fog of incomplete understanding, successful results often arise from a faulty theoretical basis. The fruits of this approach are not to be despised. Witting or unwitting empiricism has given us liver extract for the treatment of pernicious anaemia, quinine for malaria, aspirin for fever and vascular disease and, indeed, penicillin, for neither Fleming nor Chain had the faintest idea of how the substance elaborated by *Penicillium notatum* killed microorganisms. HCT, as it stands today, owes much to the systematic, empiric approach. The yield from empiricism is necessarily low but the science of marrow transplantation was hemmed in by an incomplete understanding of many basic biologic processes, particularly that of immune recognition and the regulation of cell growth and differentiation. Our ignorance of these areas persists, but will probably yield to the powerful methods of investigation of gene function and control. It is such understanding that will allow the field to leap forward in the 21st century.

The transplanted cells

The amplification of hematopoietic stem cells

The proper inoculum in transplantation is the hematopoietic stem cell in numbers sufficient to repopulate the recipient marrow rapidly. Surface markers have been the main means for attempting to identify these primitive cells, and such markers are clearly a crude way of assessing the biologic destiny of the cells that are harvested.

In the 21st century better markers or selection in culture will become available. It should be possible to isolate more specifically from the peripheral blood those cells that are needed. But that will not be enough. It should also be possible to expand these cells so that one becomes 100,000. It is generally believed that this goal can be reached by stimulating surface receptors with the proper sequence and combination of cytokines. Maybe so, and perhaps all that is required is one new factor that will solve the problem. On the other hand, stem cells have not evolved to actively self-renew, and very probably they lack the receptors needed to trigger the rapid replication that is desired. Instead, better understanding of transcriptional and translational regulation within cells will provide a way to stimulate division without triggering differentiation. In the 21st century, we will learn what gene(s) must be activated to force stem cells into division without maturation, and stem cells harvested from patients will be transduced with genes that accomplish this task. Of course the action of these genes would have to be stopped after the cells had been amplified to the desired number, otherwise the recipient would be endowed with the dubious blessing of a continuously proliferating stem cell population, a situation uncomfortably like that of acute leukemia. Thus, either an inducible "stop" mechanism must be engineered into the cells or they must be under the control of a promoter that can be turned off and on at will by the administration of an appropriate drug. In the 20th century techniques for tissue specific knockouts [1] and for drug-inducible transgenes [2,3] have already been developed. In the 21st century, such mechanisms may be employed to give stem cells wanted properties for a limited period of time (Fig. 110.1). Later in the century the direction of differentiation may be manipulated in a beneficial way. Give drug A to a patient who is thrombocytopenic after transplantation and induce those genes that direct differentiation towards platelets. Has the patient developed an infection with excessive consumption of granulocytes? No problem. Drug B diverts differentiation toward granulocytes because a drug-B inducible promoter drives the genetic program that diverts differentiation into that direction.

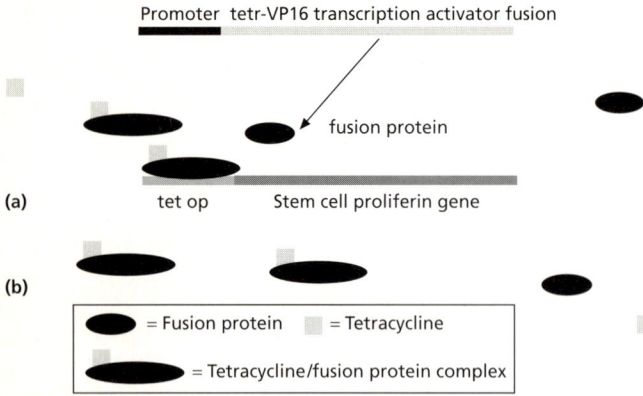

Fig. 110.1 In the 21st century the stem cell proliferin gene is cloned. Transcription of this gene causes stem cells to divide into two stem cells every 2–4 h. Normal human stem cells have been transduced with this gene fused to the bacterial *Tet* operon (b) and with a constitutively active promoter driving a fusion gene consisting of tetr+, a tet activator, the activating domain of the herpes simplex virus protein VP16(a). The conformation of the activator is changed when it binds tetracycline (tet), so that it binds to the tet operon (tet op) tetr. Binding to the operon results in transcription of the stem cell proliferin gene. The fusion protein is constantly produced, but its conformation in the absence of tetracycline is such that it cannot bind to the operator and activate transcription of the gene. When tetracycline is given the VP16 transcription activator drives the stem cell proliferin gene and causes amplification of the stem cells.

The universal donor line

At present each donor must be carefully matched to the recipient or the recipient's own cells must be used. Often a matched donor cannot be found, and autotransplantation is limited in its potential as a treatment for aplastic anaemia (where the needed cells may be absent) or for acute leukemia (where many or all of the cells may be malignant). Even when a matched donor is found, the approach envisioned for amplification of the cells may be difficult and excessively costly to perform each time a transplant is done.

How much better it would be if there could be a universal donor cell line, neatly packaged and stabilized in sealed vials and distributed by the pharmaceutical industry. Implementation of this technology depends upon understanding of how the body distinguishes self from nonself. If the line is sufficiently primitive it considers the recipient to be "self" because it will be educated in the patient's thymus in the same way that the patient's own cells are educated. Conversely, the recipient's immune system must not reject the inoculated cells. This might be accomplished by providing that patient with an immunomodulatory treatment, based on the advanced knowledge of the 21st century, or using such knowledge to make certain that the universal cell line was not antigenic (see The recipient immune system, below). Once these goals are achieved they would represent a quantum leap in the cost, convenience and safety of stem cell transplantation. No longer would there be a search for a matching donor. It would no longer be necessary to process individually cells harvested for each recipient. Instead, a commercially available source of compatible, molecularly engineered cells could serve as the inoculum used to repopulate the marrow.

The transplant recipient

Currently, preparation of the patient for allogeneic transplantation has been a major cause of morbidity and mortality. Cytoreduction or cytoablation has been necessary for three reasons: (i) to provide numerical superiority of the transplanted cells over the endogenous cells; (ii) to compromise the immune system of the recipient to allow the graft to be accepted, even though immunologically foreign except in identical twins; and (iii) to destroy tumor cells when a malignancy is being treated.

Numerical superiority of transplanted cells

Modifying the transplanted cells in such a way that they have a proliferative advantage over those of the host could be an effective strategy for replacing host cells with donor cells. This could be achieved by implementing the *in vivo* expansion technique that is envisioned as a means of allowing the inoculum of donor cells to be a small one. Critical to the success of this type of genetic manipulation is, as noted above, the ability to stop proliferation of the cells. If the transplanted cells enjoy enough of a growth advantage, cytoreduction would not be required. The transplanted cells would simply replace those of the host.

The recipient immune system

A great deal of effort has been expended to understand how the immune system distinguishes self from nonself. Fragments of the mechanism have been unraveled but there is still no clear understanding of the overall process, and it is this process that is responsible for two of the major barriers encountered in HCT, viz. immune rejection of the graft and GVHD. It seems likely that only a few of the millions of different clones of immunocytes recognize the foreign antigens in the transplanted cells. It is only these cells that need be eliminated. Various strategies have been used to produce immune tolerance. For example, immune stimulation followed by chemotherapy that kills only dividing cells should have a selective effect. But presumably because our understanding is incomplete, specific immune tolerance has not yet been achieved. If it can be achieved in this century, cytoreduction may not be necessary for transplantation to succeed and GVHD would be a thing of the past.

The elimination of malignant cells

Until now the most common indication for transplantation has been the treatment of malignant disease. One of the goals of cytoreduction in these circumstances is the elimination of tumor cells. If chemotherapy of tumors becomes so specific in the 21st century to obviate the need for ablation of the marrow, then transplantation for such disorders would no longer be necessary (see The demise of marrow transplantation, below). It is possible, however, that it will be the transplant itself that will deliver the lethal blow against the neoplasm. Perhaps the cells that are infused will be engineered in such a way as to be able to distinguish between normal host cells and tumor. In this event cytoreduction would not be needed, even in patients with malignant disease.

Transplantation in 2099; a case report

A 12-year-old girl is brought to her pediatrician because of pallor and slight bruising. The hemoglobin is 50 g/L, the platelet count 20,000/μL, and granulocytes 100/μL. A diagnosis of aplastic anaemia is quickly established. The pediatrician calls the pharmacy of the Health Maintenance Organization (HMO) and orders one vial of PolyStem™ polyvalent stem cells, which are immediately injected intravenously, providing a dose of 100,000 stem cells engineered to divide but not to differentiate as long as the inducing drug is given. The child is permitted to return home given TetraP™ and is carefully observed for fever and/or bleeding. Daily blood counts are stable. The doubling time of the cells is 6 h, so that in 4 days the inoculum of stem cells has expanded to 10^{10} cells. It is now time to stop their proliferation by discontinuing TetraP™. This silences the gene that caused proliferation of the infused stem cells. Normal differentiation is a consequence of this induced genetic change, but since the platelet count has gradually declined to 8000/μL the physician decides to give a small dose of Thromboproliferin™, which induces the gene(s) that have been engineered into the stem cells to cause differentiation into megakaryocytes. The platelet count rises rapidly, and within 3 days it is 50,000/μL. The hemoglobin and granulocyte counts rise as well. Only a small dose of Thromboproliferin™ was used, so that some differentiation into the erythroid and myeloid line occurs as well.

Adjusted for inflation, the total cost of the procedure was $30,000. Twenty-thousand dollars of this was for the engineered polyvalent stem cells (PolyStem™). (Notably, in the previous week the widely watched television program "60 Moments" had featured an exposé of the profiteering by the manufacturer of these cells. The reporter had calculated that the cost of producing one vial of these self-proliferating cells was only $20, including culture medium, vial and labor. The fact that it had required an investment of $2,000,000,000 and 10 years of repeated, frustrating failures to develop the product had conveniently been forgotten. Also forgotten was the fact that three other biotechnology firms, BMT Inc., Cells Unlimited, Inc. and HemoStem, Inc. had filed for bankruptcy in August 2078, December 2082 and June of 2084 when they failed in their attempts to develop a universal donor cell line.)

The demise of transplantation

Some day, perhaps in the 21st century, perhaps in the 22nd century, HCT will no longer be performed. This will happen for one of two reasons, which I designate "The bad scenario" and "The good scenario."

The bad scenario

It is 2037 and virtually everyone in America has prepaid health care. The American people had gradually been led to believe that state-of-the-art health care can be delivered at a relatively low price because of the managerial talents of highly paid executives in the health care industry. Physicians, on the other hand, find themselves caught between their employers, the highly profitable health care delivery industry, on the one hand, and their patients and their attorneys, on the other. Lawsuits proliferate. Physicians and their HMOs are inundated by litigation arising from failure to make diagnoses because expensive tests were not ordered or because of failure to give costly treatments to patients with far advanced neoplasms. It finally becomes apparent that, even to the lawmakers in Washington, D.C., the cost of cutting-edge care for everyone, regardless of age and regardless of diagnosis, is beyond the gross national product. Physicians, caught between their employers and the demands of their patients, go on strike. They insist that there must be guidelines that they can follow that will protect them from attack by the legal profession. By this time, the cost of stem cell transplantation has begun to increase, after a period of decreasing costs. This increase is largely due to stringent regulations by governmental agencies. Several unfortunate episodes have led to even greater regulation. Technicians who prepare stem cells are required to undergo 3 years of special training and to obtain a license. Extensive records are required in preparation of stem cells, and all stem cell harvesting facilities must undergo inspection every 3 months, at their own expense. Even if all this is overcome and patients are transplanted, it has become impossible to perform controlled trials. In the 21st century members of Congress are even less well educated in science than they were in the 20th century. They are frantic about the ethical implications of infusing stem cells into a patient. The distinction between embryonic stem cells and the stem cells that come from the marrow of an adult donor seems to have been lost on them. In any case, stringent regulations regarding the use of stem cells apply to HCT as well as to all other forms of stem cell transfer. All protocols must be approved by a committee of bioethicists that meets in Washington three times annually. But there is more. Because of concern that full disclosure must be given to each patient entering a protocol, it is mandated that no patient is entered into a protocol for 3 weeks after the initial explanation has been given to the patient. During this time an interview with a biomedical ethicist is required to make certain that the patient understands, in full, all of the risks and all of the alternatives methods of management. Unfortunately, in the context of a rapidly relapsing patient with acute leukemia such a delay is impossible, and thus some of the most pressing problems facing the transplanter cannot be studied. Finally, strict guidelines for racial balance of all participants in a study are enforced. For example, if an insufficient number of African-American patients have not been entered into a protocol, all further accession must be stopped until the mandated balance is achieved. Adherence to all of these rules is monitored by inspectors who closely follow the conduct of all approved protocols. As it turns out, the inspectors have little to do. There are so many barriers to the performance of a good clinical study that evidence-based medicine has all but disappeared and most medicine, HCT included, is practiced according to published guidelines based on the impressions of the experts who serve on the committees that create guidelines.

Health economists are enlisted by government to calculate cost/benefit ratios for the whole range of therapeutic procedures. Stem cell transplantation does not do well in this analysis. Part of the reason is that clinicians who perform transplantation have mixed high-risk experimental procedures with those that are clearly beneficial, but the high cost of transplantation is another reason. The economists find that in terms of quality-adjusted life years saved, treatment of hemochromatosis, of Hodgkin's disease, of diabetes mellitus and of clubfoot rank far above stem cell transplantation. Stem cell transplantation is no longer reimbursable! It is a research procedure. Unfortunately the National Institute of Health (NIH) has its problems, too. In the latter part of the 20th century the average successful bioscientist trained 100 postdoctoral fellows. Although a friendly congress increased funding by 3% per year, some of which was eaten by inflation, most of these trainees cannot be accommodated by the system. In a partly politically driven policy, the NIH decides that no program should have more than $200,000 per year support. This egalitarian policy provides employment for many of the trainees produced. Unfortunately, it prevents funding of any meaningful stem cell transplantation program.

In the absence of resources, stem cell transplantation dies!

The good scenario

The American people and their representatives in congress begin to realize that cutting-edge medical care has a high cost. They realize that corporate profits and high executive salaries contribute little or nothing to the health care system. A single payer system is initiated, but it is clear that national resources cannot provide everything for everyone. Priorities must be set; and they are. Stem cell transplantation is approved for well-documented indications. Congress realizes that progress requires an investment of resources and a 1% tax for clinical research is established. This greatly increases the NIH budget. In the meanwhile, training programs have been greatly curtailed, so that only the most talented and most motivated qualify. Of course, more scientists are still trained than are needed but the excess is 20% rather than 1000% as in the latter part of the 20th century. There are, of course, more demands for funds than resources but merit is the only consideration. Experimental programs in stem cell transplantation are of high quality and they are supported by research grants, not misappropriated clinical funds. The public and the congress have come to recognize that the motivations of the vast majority of clinical investigators are to help patients, and that the ethical standards of all but very few investigators are very high. Biomedical ethicists, still on the scene, begin to recognize this, and encourage the conduct of well-designed studies. They understand that impeding such studies by concerns of things that might happen, and never have, is injurious to the common good. Indeed, they begin to emphasize the fact that not carrying out human research is unethical, because it harms those who may become ill in the future.

Stem cell transplantation thrives, as do other aspects of clinical research.

Sooner or later all of the diseases that have been treated by stem cell transplantation—malignancies, genetic diseases, aplastic anaemia—are understood at a molecular level. Effective treatments are devised. Stem cell transplantation becomes an anachronism. Surprisingly soon medical students view it with amusement and a sense of superiority, similar to our disdain of bleeding and purging in the treatment of the ailments of mankind.

Stem cell transplantation is no more.

References

1 Camilli A, Beattie DT, Mekalanos JJ. Use of genetic recombination as a reporter of gene expression. *Proc Natl Acad Sci U S A* 1994; **91**: 2634–8.
2 Efrat S, Fusco-DeMane D, Lemberg H, al Emran O, Wang X. Conditional transformation of a pancreatic beta-cell line derived from transgenic mice expressing a tetracycline-regulated oncogene. *Proc Natl Acad Sci U S A* 1995; **92**: 3576–80.
3 Gossen M, Bujard H. Tight control of gene expression in mammalian cells by tetracycline-responsive promoters. *Proc Natl Acad Sci U S A* 1992; **89**: 5547–51.

Index

Notes: This index is arranged in letter-by-letter order. Entries in *italics* refer to figures, those in **bold** refer to tables. Abbreviations used in subentries are the same as those listed in the list of Abbreviations (p. xxii). Please also note that as the subject of this book is hematopoietic cell transplantation (HCT), all entries refer to this unless otherwise indicated.

To save space in this index, the following abbreviations have been used:

ALL	acute lymphoblastic leukemia
AML	acute myeloid leukemia
CLL	chronic lymphocytic leukemia
CML	chronic myeloid leukemia
CMV	cytomegalovirus
EBV-LPD	Epstein–Barr virus-associated lymphoproliferative disorder
GVHD	graft-*vs.*-host disease
GVLE	graft-*vs.*-leukemia effect
GVTE	graft-*vs.*-tumor effect
JMML	juvenile myelomonocytic leukemia
MDS	myelodysplastic syndrome
mHA	minor histocompatibility antigens
MHC	major histocompatibility complex
MTD	maximum tolerated dose
PBHCs	peripheral blood hematopoietic cells
PNH	paroxysmal nocturnal hemoglobinuria
SOS	sinusoidal obstruction syndrome
TBI	total body irradiation

A

AABB *see* American Association of Blood Banks (AABB)
AastromReplicell™ Cell Production System 101
ABCM regimen, multiple myeloma therapy 1264
abdomen
　abscesses 791
　GVHD, acute 790
　　management 792
　infection, management of 792
　pain 789–792
Abelcet **693**
ABMTR *see* Autologous Blood/Marrow Transplant Registry (ABMTR)
ABO blood group
　incompatibility **824**, 824–825
　　allogeneic transplants, recombinant erythropoietin 615
　　immune mechanisms 824
　　management 825–827
　transfusions 834
　　platelet 836
　typing, cord blood 552
abscesses, abdomen 791
accelerated hyperfractionated radiotherapy regimens 182
acetaminophen (paracetamol) 899
　dose **900**

acquired immunodeficiency syndrome (AIDS) *see* AIDS
activation-induced cell death (AICD), GVHD 356
active control phase 3 trials 421
acute lymphoblastic leukemia (ALL)
　adults *see* acute lymphoblastic leukemia (ALL), adults
　allogeneic transplants 1058
　　advantages 1238
　　HLA-partially matched related donors 1119
　　survival 1121
　　relapse management 1150, 1153–1154, *1154*, 1155, 1157
　　unrelated 1133, 1144
　autologous transplants 1238–1249
　　chemotherapy, previous 1244
　　GVLE 1238
　　patient selection 1244
　　PBHCs 1245
　　post-transplant therapies 1245–1246
　　preparative regimens 1244–1245
　　in vitro purging 1241–1242, 1245
　children *see* acute lymphoblastic leukemia (ALL), children
　CNS relapse management 1061
　diagnosis/classification 1055–1056
　　immunophenotyping 1055, **1056**
　　morphology 1055, 1056–1057
　drawbacks 1238

　epidemiology 1055
　GVLE 1062
　immunophenotypes
　　children 1079
　　classification 1055, **1056**
　　prognostic factors 1239
　mature B-cell 1056
　minimal residual disease detection post-HCT **278**, 280
　Philadelphia chromosome (*Bcr-Abl* gene fusion) 86, 1055–1056, 1056, **1056**
　　adults 1241–1242
　　allogeneic transplants 1060–1061, *1061*
　　childhood 1067
　　in children *see* acute lymphoblastic leukemia (ALL), children
　　monitoring after therapy 1063
　　prognosis 1057, 1239
　　relapse risk 279–280
　　therapy identification 1242
　prognosis 1056–1058, **1057**
　　by cytogenic subset **1058**
　　remission status *1059*
　relapse
　　rates 1150
　　risk detection 276
　transplantation in
　　HSC and/or progenitor cells 88
　　radioimmunotherapy and 202–203
　treatment outcomes **1057**

1511

acute lymphoblastic leukemia (ALL), adults 1238–1242
  allogeneic transplants 1058–1063
    autologous transplants vs. 1242
    cell source 1063
    first remission **1059**, 1059–1060, *1060*
      failure 1061, *1061*
    with Philadelphia chromosome (*Bcr–Abl* gene fusion) 1060–1061, *1061*
    post-transplant monitoring 1063
    regimen development 1062–1063
    relapse management 1061–1062
    second remission 1058, **1059**
    unrelated, for advanced 1058–1059
  autologous transplants 1238–1242
    allogeneic vs. 1242
    chemotherapy vs. 1240
    clinical studies **1240**, 1240–1241
      second remission **1241**
    with Philadelphia chromosome (*Bcr-Abl* gene fusion) 1241–1242
    in relapse 1241
    in second remission 1241
      clinical trials **1241**
  children vs. 1067–1069
  pre-B-cell markers 1068
  prognostic factors 1238–1240, **1239**
  recovery rates 1238
  standard treatment 1238
  T-cell markers 1068
acute lymphoblastic leukemia (ALL), children 1067–1083
  adults vs. 1067–1069
  allogeneic transplants 1067–1079
    conditioning regimen selection 1073–1074, *1074*
    cord blood transplantation 1076–1078, **1077**, 1078
    Down syndrome children 1078–1079
    first remission 1069, **1069**
    HLA-partially matched related donors 1075
    infants 1078
    post-transplant relapse 1079
    second remission 1069
    selection criteria 1072, **1073**
    sibling donors 1069, **1069**, **1070**, **1071**, *1076*
    survival rates *1075*, *1076*
    timing 1069–1073
    unrelated donor 1072–1073, 1075–1076, *1076*, **1077**
  autologous transplants 1243–1244
    clinical trials **1243**
    in first remission 1243
    GVLE clinical trials 410
    in second remission 1243–1244
  classification 1067
    genotypes **1068**
    NCI/Rome standard criteria 1070
    prognostic value 1067
  diagnosis 1067

  epidemiology 1068
  hyperdiploidy 1068, 1242
  Philadelphia chromosome (*Bcr-Abl* gene fusion) 1068–1069, 1242–1243
  prognosis 1070, *1072*
  pre-B-cell markers 1068
  prognostic factors 1239, 1242–1243
    therapy response 1071
  recovery rates 1238
  risk factors 1242
  T-cell markers 1068
acute myeloid leukemia (AML)
  biology 1221–1222
  chromosome rearrangement 86
  classification 1221
  cytogenetics 1025–1026, **1221**, 1221–1222
    survival *1026*
  extramedullary involvement 1030
  in Fanconi anemia 1484
  gene marking trials 122
  HCT
    allogeneic *see* acute myeloid leukemia (AML), allogeneic transplants
    autologous *see* acute myeloid leukemia (AML), autologous transplants
    radioimmunotherapy and 202–203
    relapse **278**, 280–281
      increased following T-cell depletion 226
    TBI and 185–186
  immunosuppressive agents, randomized controlled trials **642**
  mouse models 86
  multiple myeloma, autologous transplants 1277
  myeloid progenitors 86
  prognosis 1025
  refractory 1030, *1030*
  remission
    effects on treatment *1031*
    long-term 86
  therapy-related (t-AML) 963–969
    autologous transplants in non-Hodgkin's lymphoma 1215–1216
    clinical presentations 963
    clinicopathological syndromes 963–964
    diagnosis 964
    DNA repair mechanisms, defective 966
    genetics 965–967
    hematopoietic abnormalities 967
    p53 gene mutation 966–967
    pathogenesis 964–967, **965**, *965*
    prediction 968–969
    probability *963*
    prognosis 967–968
    risk factors 964
    risk reduction 969
    telomeric shortening 967
    topoisomerase II inhibitor-related AML 963–964

acute myeloid leukemia (AML), allogeneic transplants
  adults 1025–1039
    alternative treatments vs. 1028, *1028*, **1029**
    cell source 1027, 1031–1032
    consolidation therapy 1026–1027
    cord blood cells 1032, *1032*
    future directions 1034–1035
    GVHD prophylaxis 1027–1028
    HCT score 1027
    HLA-matched related donors 1032, **1033**
    nonmyeloablative **1033**
    preparatory regimen 1027
    primary induction failure 1030–1031
    prognosis 1025
    reduced intensity regimens 1032–1033
    relapse *1032*
      first 1028, 1029
      following treatment 1033–1034
      resistant 1030–1031
    remission
      first 1025–1028, *1026*, *1032*
      second 1028, 1029, *1032*
      status *1031*
    unrelated donors 1031–1032
  children 1040–1054
    adoptive immunotherapy 1048
    alternative donor 1046, *1047*
    biological randomization 1042
    bone marrow 1046–1047
    chemotherapy trials **1041**
    chemotherapy vs. 1042–1045
    classification 1040
    conditioning regimen 1044–1045
      survival **1045**
    disease status/outcome *1047*
    genetic conditions associated 1040
    GVHD 1045
    GVL 1045
    historical background 1040–1042
    HLA-matched related 1047–1048
    incidence 1040
    infants 1045
    late effects 1049
    management algorithm *1044*
    presentations 1040
    relapse 1048, *1049*
    risk 1041
    risk factors 1040
    second procedure 1048
    survival rates 1040–1041, *1041*, **1041**, *1041*, **1041**, 1044
    T-cell depletion (TCD) 1046–1047
    treatment options **1042**, 1042–1045, **1043**, 1049
      beyond relapse 1045–1047
      chemotherapy 1045
    umbilical cord blood 1047
complete remission (CR), first 1028, 1030
  autologous vs. 1229, *1230*, 1230–1231, **1231**, **1232**

survival *1026, 1027*
  treatment options 1028, *1028*, **1029**
  complete remission (CR), second 1028, 1030
  GVHD, prophylaxis 1027–1028
  HLA-partially matched related donors 1119, *1124*
    natural killer cell activity 1127
    survival 1121
  preparatory regimens 1027
  primary induction failure 1030–1031
  relapse 1030–1031, 1150, 1153, *1153*, 1155, 1157
  sibling donor HCT, in Fanconi anemia **1495**
  unrelated donor 1144
acute myeloid leukemia (AML), autologous transplants 1221–1237
  cell source 1223–1224
  complications 1232–1233
    fertility 1233
    MDS 1226–1228
    secondary malignancies 1232–1233
  future work 1223
  GVLE 1225–1226, 1233
  history 1221
  HSC and/or progenitor cells 88
  immunotherapy after treatment 1225–1226
  minimal residual disease 1221
  PBHCs 1232
    purging 1225
  preparative regimens **1222**, 1222–1223
  prognostic factors 1222, **1222**
  purging 1224–1225, 1226
    bone marrow trial 254–255
      disease free survival 255
  relapse
    detection 277
    management 1228–1230
  remission, first complete 1226
    allogeneic *vs.* 1229, *1230*, 1230–1231, **1231, 1232**
    survival rates *1226*, **1227**, *1228*
  remission, second 1228, **1229**, *1229*, **1229**, *1229*
    survival rates 1224, *1224*
    second remission *1229*
  timing 1231–1232
acute promyelocytic leukemia (APL)
  autologous transplants 1228
  relapse detection 277
acute renal failure (ARF), cryopreserved cells and 608
acyclovir
  CMV prophylaxis 712–713
  EBV infections 749
  HSV, resistance to 727
  HSV prophylaxis 730, **730**
  metabolism 741
  toxicity 743
  varicella-zoster virus infection 741–742
    efficacy 742
    prophylaxis *744*, 744–745
addiction *see* substance abuse

addressins, adoptive T-cell immunotherapy 395
adeno-associated virus (AAV) 113
adenosine deaminase (ADA) -deficient SCID
  see severe combined immune deficiency (SCID)
adenosine triphosphate (ATP), bone marrow purging 256
adenosine triphosphate (ATP)-binding cassette family, multidrug resistance gene
  see multidrug resistance 1 gene (P-glycoprotein/*MDR-1*)
adenovirus
  CNS infection 813
  gene therapy vectors 113, 120
    clinical trials 120, **120**
    transient expression 120
  immunity 757
  infections 757–758
    liver 781–782
    treatment 758, **762**
  serotypes 120
  virology 757
adhesion molecules 56, *56*
  adoptive T-cell immunotherapy 395
  antigen presentation 354–355
  homing/retention role 56–57, *57*
  PBHC mobilization 576–577, 581–582
  proliferation/survival effects 57
adipocytes
  hematopoietic microenvironment 54
  transdifferentiation 76
administrative director 466
adoptive cellular immunotherapy/transfer 5, 380–404
  AML in children 1048
  antigen overexpression 391–392
  genetic modification 393–396
    affinity improvement 394
    function enhancement 394–395
    safety improvement 395–396
    specificity changes 394
    specificity transfer *393*, 393–394
  GVLE, evidence for 370–371
  leukemias 387–390
  recurrence prevention 1257
  see also donor lymphocyte infusion (DLI); *individual diseases/disorders*
adrenal glands, complications in 948–949
Adriamycin, combination regimens
  ABCM 1264
  BCNU/cyclophosphamide/melphalan 1264
  dexamethasone/vincristine *see* VAD therapy
adult hematopoiesis 53, *56*
advanced directives 494
AEIOP *see* Associazione Italiana Ematologia ed Oncologia Pediatrica (AEIOP)
age
  ALL prognosis 1057
  children *see* children
  elderly patients, Hodgkin's disease 1198
  GVHD 637
  HLA-partially matched related HCT 1120

immune reconstitution 855
MDS prognosis 1086
outcome 11
quality of life issues 511
survival, aplastic anemia *997*
treatment outcome 456–457
agnogenic myeloid metaplasia (AMM)
  allogeneic transplants 1090–1092
  autologous transplants 1092
  definition 1090
  survival *1091*
  transplant-related mortality (TRM) *1091*
AIDS 1369–1384
  allogeneic transplants 1374
  autologous transplants 1373–1374
  CMV infections 811
  gene therapy 1374–1379
    antisense 1375
    applications 1378
    considerations 1374
    future 1379
    intracellular toxins 1377
    protein-based **1375**, 1376–1377, 1376–1378
    rationale 1374
    ribozymes 1375–1376
    RNA-based **1375**, 1375–1376
    RNA decoys 1375
    RNAi 1376
    single chain antibodies 1377
    strategies *1371*, 1374–1379
    targets 1374–1375, **1375**, 1378
      chemokines, altered 1377–1378
      HSCs 1378–1379
      ribozymes 1375–1376
      T-cells 1374, 1378
    transdominant mutant proteins 1376–1377
    transgenes **1375**
    vaccination 1379
    vectors 1378
  lymphoma 1372–1374, *1373*
  meningoencephalitis 813
  multifocal leukoencephalopathy 813
  therapy
    antiviral drug neurotoxicity 818
    chemotherapy/HCT 1372–1374
    HAART 1198, 1371, 1373
  see also HIV-1 infection
airway complications *see* pulmonary complications
AJCC (American Joint Commission on Cancer), tumor staging **1308, 1309**
albumin, cryoprotection 604
albumin, serum, allogeneic transplants, multiple myeloma 1098
alcohol dependence, treatment outcome 457–458
alemtuzumab *see* Campath 1$_M$
alkylating agent(s) 161–163
  CLL sensitivity 1105
  dose–cytotoxicity relationship 1335

alkylating agent(s) (cont.)
  following HCT 937
  high-dose chemotherapy 138–143, 161–163
    in vitro models 130
  lymphoma sensitivity 1105
  multiple myeloma therapy 1265
  myeloablation, neuroblastoma 1335
  secondary malignancies 963
  structure 131, 138–139
  therapy-related myelodysplastic syndromes 1084
  see also individual drugs
alkylysolipid, bone marrow purging 256
allele mismatches, HLA genes **1134**
allelic exclusion, antigen receptor genes 331
allergic reactions
  transfer in HCT 859
  transfusions 842
  see also anaphylactic reactions
allergic rhinitis, transfer in HCT 859
allogeneic MHC transduction, peripheral induced tolerance 303–304
allogeneic transplantation 11–12
  ABO incompatibility, recombinant erythropoietin 615
  age/treatment outcome 456–457
  agnogenic myeloid metaplasia 1090–1092
  AIDS 1374
  annual **9**
  autoimmune animal models 332, 335–340
    graft facilitating cells 337
    HLA-matched HSC 337
    induced disease 336
    mechanisms 338–340
    MHC disparate HSC 336–337
    nonmyeloablative 337–338
    spontaneous disease 335
    syngeneic vs. 336
  autoimmune disease 1391
  breast cancer 1304
  cell source, PBHCs see peripheral blood hematopoietic cells (PBHCs)
  cell sources 11–12
    cryopreservation 608–609
  complications 84–85
    acute leukemia following 969
    CMV, rate 703–704
    hematologic malignancy 953–954
    solid tumors 954
  erythropoietin, recombinant 613–615
  HLA typing see HLA typing
  nonmyeloablative see nonmyeloablative therapy
  ovarian cancer 1184, 1330
  performed yearly **9**
  quality of life issues 511
  relapse 1150–1163
    types 1150
  relapse management 1151–1163
    antilymphocyte serum 1133
    cytotoxic chemotherapy 1157
    DLI see donor lymphocyte infusion (DLI)

G-CSF 1158
G-CSF, recombinant 617
GM-CSF, recombinant 619
imatinib mesylate 1158
immunosuppression discontinuation 1157
interferon-alpha 1158
interleukin-2 1158
irradiation 1158
palliative care 1158
secondary HCT 1157
see also individual diseases/disorders
see also individual diseases/disorders
α–emitters 201, **201**
AmBisome **693**, 1123
  clinical studies **691**
American Association of Blood Banks (AABB) 536
  cord blood blanks 551
American Joint Commission on Cancer (AJCC), tumor staging **1308**, **1309**
American Red Cross (ARC), cord blood blanks 551
American Society for Blood/Bone Marrow Transplantation (ASBMT) 532–533
  Special Interest Group survey 464
amifostine, systemic cytoprotection 170
AML-1, hematopoiesis, genetic control 71
AML1–ETO fusion protein, AML 86
Amphotec **693**
amphotericin B deoxycholate see Fungizone
amyloidosis
  familial 1285–1286
  primary 1283
  secondary 1285
AL amyloidosis
  autologous transplants 1283–1297, 1289–1290
    clinical trials 1289–1290, 1293–1294
    gastrointestinal bleeding 1291–1292
    GI bleeding 1291–1292
    mortality 1292
    peri-transplant management 1291–1292
    pretransplant evaluation 1291–1292
    response 1289
    RRTs 1291–1292
    survival 1290, 1290
  cytogenetics 1284–1285
  diagnosis 1285
    differential, from non-AL types 1285–1286
    free light chain (FLC) assay 1285, 1293
  dose-intensive regimens 1291
  epidemiology 1284
  future research 1293–1294
  organ involvement **1286**
  pathogenesis 1284–1285
  PBHC mobilization 1290–1291
  presentation **1285**, 1286–1288
    GI tract 1287
    heart 1286
    hemostasis 1288
    kidneys 1286–1287

    liver 1287
    nervous system 1287–1288
    respiratory tract 1288
  prognosis 1288–1289
  treatment 1289–1291
    autologous transplants see above
    chemotherapy 1289
    emerging 1294
    response monitoring 1292–1293, **1293**
    theoretical 1283, 1283
    toxicity 1291, **1291**
analgesia see pain management
anaphylactic reactions
  DMSO 607
  transfusion-related 843
  see also allergic reactions
ancestrim see stem cell factor (SCF)
androgen(s)
  agnogenic myeloid metaplasia therapy 1090
  Fanconi anemia treatment 1490–1491
anemia
  animal models 566
  Fanconi's see Fanconi anemia
  transfusion 833
anergy
  immune response regulation 325
  T-cells 301
  in vitro induction 301
anergy subset skewing, autoimmune animal models 339–340
anesthetic(s)
  general 908
  local 908
  risks to donor 541
angiogenesis
  hematopoiesis association 74
  neuroblastomas 1339–1340
animal models
  autoimmune disease see autoimmune diseases (animal models)
  bone marrow transplantation 4–5
  cryopreservation efficacy 604
  GVHD see graft-vs.-host disease (GVHD), animal models
  GVLE, evidence for 369–370
  HLA-partially related donor HCT 1126–1127
  induced tolerance 307–308, 344
  low dose TBI 1170
  murine models
    Fanconi anemia 1490
    G-CSF 617–618
    GVHD, interleukin-11 effects 621
    HSC expansion studies 96–97
    nonmyeloablative therapy 1164–1165
    T-cell depletion 1164
    transplantation model 4
  SOS 777
  study cycle 414
  varicella-zoster virus pathogenesis 734–735, 735

xenogenic *see* xenogeneic animal models
*see also individual diseases/disorders;
individual treatments*
ankylosing spondylitis
   animal model 326t
   HLA associations 324t, 327
anorexia, treatment complications 774
Anthony Nolan Registry 1133
   history 624
anthracycline(s)
   cytosine arabinoside combination 1157
   high-dose chemotherapy 145–146
   mechanism of action 145–146
   metabolism/pharmacology 134, 146
   resistance 146
   see also doxorubicin
anti-adhesion molecule antibodies, peripheral induced tolerance 304–305
antiangiogenic agents, neuroblastoma 1339–1340
anti-B-cell antibodies
   lymphoma therapy 1105
   non-Hodgkin's lymphoma trials 203–204
   purging 1270
antibiotics
   choice 671–672
   neurotoxicity 818
   prophylaxis, oral complications 914
   prophylaxis during neutropenia 667
   resistance 666–668, 674–675
      mechanisms 666–668, **667**
   treatment strategies 671–674, 672, *673*
antibodies
   bacterial infection 678
   CMV infection 715
   immune reconstitution *857*
   intravenous (IVIg) *see* intravenous immunoglobulin (IVIg)
   subtypes
      multiple myeloma prognosis 1275
      see also individual subtypes
antibodies (therapeutic)
   animal models 1164–1166
   anti-idiotypes 204
   biodistribution 199, *199*, **199**
   Fab/F(ab')$_2$ fragments 200
   GVHD prophylaxis 643, 649–650
   GVHD treatment 215–216
   humanized 202
   immunotherapy following autologous transplants 1398–1399
   monoclonal 166, 198
      human antimouse antibody response 200
   pharmacology 200
   polyclonal 198
   radiolabeling 166, 198, 200–201
   selection, complement-mediated lysis 246–247
   specificity 200
   toxicity 205
   unconjugated, limitations 198

   see also monoclonal antibodies (MABs); radioimmunotherapy (RAIT); *specific agents*
antibody-mediated purging *see* purging
anti-carcinoembryonic antigen (CEA) antibody 198
   solid tumor radioimmunotherapy 205
anti-CD4 antibodies, murine studies 1164–1165
anti-CD6 antibodies
   multiple myeloma allogeneic transplants 1099
   partial T-cell depletion 1122
anti-CD8 antibodies, murine studies 1164–1165
anti-CD10 antibodies, ALL autologous transplants 1241–1242
anti-CD14 antibodies, purging 1225
anti-CD15 antibodies, purging 1225
anti-CD19 antibodies
   ALL autologous transplants 1241–1242
   purging 1270
anti-CD20 antibodies 203–204
   rituximab *see* rituximab (anti-CD20 antibody)
   tositumomab *see* tositumomab (anti-CD20 antibody)
anti-CD21 antibodies, EBV-LPD 385–386
anti-CD22 antibodies 204
   non-Hodgkin's lymphoma trials 204
anti-CD24 antibodies, EBV-LPD 385–386
anti-CD30 antibodies, Hodgkin's disease trials 205
anti-CD33 antibodies 166, 202
   leukemia trials 202
   purging 1225
anti-CD37 antibodies 203–204
   non-Hodgkin's lymphoma trials 203–204
anti-CD40 antibodies, induced tolerance 310
anti-CD45 antibodies 202–203, *203*
   animal studies 1166
   leukemia trials 202–203, *203*
   radioiodine labeled 166
   AML autologous transplants **1222**
anti-CD52 antibodies *see* Campath 1$_M$
anti-CD56 antibodies, purging 1270
anti-CD66 antibodies, leukemia trials 203
anti-CD138 antibodies, purging 1270
anticoagulant(s), in SOS 779
anticomplementary factor(s), complement-mediated lysis 247
anticonvulsant drugs 907
anticytokine therapy, GVHD treatment 216
anti-ferritin antibodies, Hodgkin's disease 198, 204
antifungal agents 692–695
   action sites *692*
   administration 690–692, **691**
   clinical studies **691**
   cytoprotection **168**
   resistance 690
anti-GD$_2$ antibody, neuroblastoma 1337, 1339

antigenemia assay, CMV detection *716*, 716–717
antigen presentation 324–325
   adhesion molecules 354–355
   CD28 markers 354–355
   CD40 304
   CD40 ligand 355
   cytotoxic T-lymphocyte antigen 4 354–355
   inducible costimulator 354–355
   mHA molecules 354
   MHC 31
   MHC molecules 31, 43, 354
   OX40 marker 355
   programmed death marker 354–355
antigen presenting cell(s) (APCs) 43
   depletion in immunological tolerance 304
   GVHD 353–354
   modification in peripheral induced tolerance 303–304
   T-cell interactions 20, **355**
anti-idiotype antibodies, immunological tolerance 302
antileukemic treatment
   posttransplant 1255
   recurrence prevention 1257–1258
antilymphocyte serum (ALS), allogeneic transplants 1133
antimetabolite drugs
   ALL therapy 1242
   high-dose chemotherapy 130
antimicrobials
   local cytoprotection 167–168, **168**
   mouth rinse 916
antioxidants, Fanconi anemia treatment 1491
antisense oligonucleotides *260*, 260–261
   bone marrow purging 256, 265–266
   clinical trials 264–266
      Bcl-2 targeting 264
      MYB targeting 264–266
   c-myb 1252
   first *vs.* second generation 261
   gene therapy, AIDS 1375
   LNAs 261
   nonsequence related toxicity 261
   Philadelphia chromosome (*Bcr-Abl* gene fusion) 1251–1252
   phosphorothioate 261, 264
   PNAs 261
   stability 260
antisense strategies *see* nucleic acid based therapies
anti-T-cell antibodies 221
   commercially available 222
   GVHD treatment 359
   induced tolerance 308–309
   peripheral induced tolerance 304–305
   see also T-cell depletion (TCD)
anti-T-cell receptor antibodies, animal studies 1166
antithrombin infusions, SOS as complication 779

antithymocyte globulin (ATG)
  combination regimens 985–987, *986*, 988–989
    busulfan/fludarabine
      Gaucher syndrome therapy 1174
      HLA-matched related HCT 1167–1168
      Hodgkin's disease 1201
      melanoma therapy 1184
      post-failed HCT 1172–1173
      retrospective studies 1172
    cyclophosphamide/thiotepa/TBI 1123
    cyclophosphamide/thymic irradiation 1173
      HLA-matched related HCT 1167–1168
      retrospective studies 1171
    fludarabine/thiotepa 1119
    prednisone 1165
    survival 990
  combined immunosuppression 641
  GVHD treatment 216, 360
  mechanism of action/targets **218**
  multiple myeloma therapy 1102
  partial T-cell depletion 1122
  randomized controlled trials **642, 644**
  T-cells, effects on 857
anti-TNF antibodies *see* infliximab
antiviral drugs
  CMV 704
    associated interstitial (CMV-IP) pneumonia 706–708
    resistance 710–711
  neurotoxicity 818
  varicella-zoster virus infections 741–744
  see also specific drugs
apheresis 545
  adverse events 543
  platelet preparation 834–835
APL *see* acute promyelocytic leukemia (APL)
aplastic anemia (AA)
  autologous transplants 981–982
  differential diagnosis 981
  dyskeratosis congenita 990
  etiology 981
    outcome 990
  Fanconi's anemia 990
  incidence 981
  nontransplant therapy 995–996
  pathophysiology 981
  PNH 981, 1002–1003
  related problems 981
  severe 981
    thoracoabdominal irradiation 192
aplastic anemia (AA), allogeneic transplants 981–1001
  conditioning regimens 982, 988–989
    CY/ATG 985–987
    nonmyeloablative 991
    survival 990
  graft rejection 983, 985–987
    incidence *983, 986*
    late 983
    overcoming 985

  primary 983
  reduction 985
HLA-matched related transplant 982–991, **983–984, 985**
  gonadal function 990–991
  graft rejection 982
  growth/development 991
  GVHD, acute 987–988
  GVHD, chronic 988, *988*
  interstitial pneumonia 988
  late effects 990–991
  long-term survival 990
  mixed donor-host hematopoietic chimerism 987
  secondary malignancy 991
  survival *986, 987*, 987–988, *988*, 988–990
    improved 988
    influences 988
HLA-nondentical related transplant 991–993, **992**
immunosuppression *vs.* 995–996, **996**
post-graft immunosuppression 988–989
  CSP 987
  MTX 985–987
  survival 990
survival *996*
  age effects *997*
unrelated donor 991–995, *993*, 993–995, **994**
apoptosis
  HSC senescence and 71
  inhibition in leukemia 86–87
  neuronal, cyclosporine-induced 816
Ara-C
  childhood ALL, allogeneic transplants 1073–1074
  melphalan combination/TBI 1074
ARC (American Red Cross), cord blood blanks 551
area-under-the curve (AUC)
  high-dose chemotherapy 130
  "safe" 136
ASBMT *see* American Society for Blood/Bone Marrow Transplantation (ASBMT)
asparaginase
  ALL therapy 1238
  cisplatin/cytarabine/dexamethasone/ etoposide combination 1198
  methotrexate/prednisolone/vincristine combination 1157
aspartylglucosaminuria (AGU) 1464
Aspergillus infections 85, 683, 686–687
  clinical syndromes 686–687
  CNS infection *812*
  epidemiology 683–684
  HLA-partially matched related HCT 1123
  immune response 687–689, *689*
Associazione Italiana Ematologia ed Oncologia Pediatrica (AEIOP)
  ALL autologous transplants 1241
  Fanconi anemia, sibling donor HCT 1483
astatine-211 **201**

ASTIMS (Autologous Stem Cell Transplantation International Multiple Sclerosis Trial) 1391
ASTIRA (Autologous Stem Cell Transplantation International Rheumatoid Arthritis Trial) 1391
ASTIS (Autologous Stem Cell Transplantation International Scleroderma Trial) 1390–1391
astrocytoma
  chemotherapy (high-dose) with HCT **1348**
  high-grade 1346–1347
  multidrug trials 1347
  single agent trials 1346–1347
autoimmune disease (AD) 324–343, 1385–1393
  animal models *see* autoimmune diseases (animal models)
  classification 326
  coincidental 1386, **1386, 1387**
  definition 324
  G-CSF exacerbation 817
  HCT treatment **1387**, 1387–1388
    allogeneic/autologous 1391
    conditioning regimens **1388**
    gene marking 1391
    guidelines 1388
    immune reconstitution 1391
    trials 1390–1391
  HLA associations 324t, 327
    in pathogenesis 327
  non-MHC susceptible genes 327–328
  pathogenesis 325–331, 328f
    genes/environment 326–327
  pathophysiology 1385–1386
  triggers 328–329, 1385
  see also individual diseases
autoimmune diseases (animal models) 326t, 329–331, 1387
  antigen receptor transgenics 331
  double transgenics 331
  HCT treatment 331–338
    allogeneic transplants *see* allogeneic transplantation
    autologous transplants *see* autologous transplantation
    congenic HCT 332
    graft types 333
    history 331–332
    preparation 332–333
    rationale 332
    syngeneic HCT treatment 332
    timing 334
  immunoregulatory transgenics 331
  induced 329–330
  MHC transgenics 330–331
  spontaneous 329
    inbred strains 326
  see also individual diseases
autoimmune hemolytic anemia, progression from CLL 1106

Autologous Blood/Marrow Transplant Registry
(ABMTR) 534
  AML
    PBHCs 1225
    purging efficacy 1224–1225
Autologous Stem Cell Transplantation
International Multiple Sclerosis Trial
(ASTIMS) 1391
Autologous Stem Cell Transplantation
International Rheumatoid Arthritis
Trial (ASTIRA) 1391
Autologous Stem Cell Transplantation
International Scleroderma Trial
(ASTIS) 1390–1391
autologous transplantation 11
  acquired disease 1189–1408
  acute promyelocytic leukemia 1228
  age/treatment outcome 457
  agnogenic myeloid metaplasia 1092
  AIDS 1373–1374
  aplastic anemia 981–982
  autoimmune animal models 332, 333–335
    purified HSCs 334
    TCD grafts 334
    translation to clinical practice 334–335
  autoimmune diseases 1391
  bone marrow *see* bone marrow
      transplantation (BMT)
  cell sources 11
  cellular therapy following 1399–1402
  chemotherapy *vs.* radiotherapy 190
  chronic myelomonocytic leukemia 1009
  CMV infections, prophylaxis 710
  complications
    CMV infection 704–705
    hematologic malignancy 954
    PNH 1005
    secondary malignancies
      prognosis 967–968
      risk reduction 969
    solid tumors 954
  erythropoietin, recombinant 613
  first attempts 3–4
  germ cell tumor 1311
  GVHD *see* graft-*vs.*-host disease (GVHD)
  immunotherapy following 1397–1399
  incidence/annual numbers **9**
  myeloablative therapy 1335
  problems 83–84
  quality of life issues 511
  recombinant GM-CSF 615–617, 618–619
  relapse following
    nonmyeloablative therapy 1395
    prevention/therapy 1394–1405
    risk reduction strategies **1396**, 1396–1397
    significance 1394–1396
    survival 1394–1395
    treatment options 1395
    treatment-related mortality 1394–1395
  residual disease detection 244–245
    cell culture 245
    immunocytochemistry 245
    molecular biology techniques 245
    sensitivity 244t
  transfusions, irradiated 841
  see also individual diseases/disorders
autosomal genes, mHA 388–389
autotransplant(s), use 11
avascular necrosis 951
azathioprine
  GVHD primary treatment 650
  randomized controlled trials **651**
aziridinylbenzoquinone, astrocytoma 1347
azoles 694

B

bacterial infections 665–682
  adjunctive measures 677–678
  airborne organisms 676
  antibiotic resistance 666–668
  autologous transplants, AML 1232
  catheter-related *676*, 676–677
  early recovery (phase I) 668–669, 669–671,
      670, *670*
  esophagus 787
  fever 674
  granulocyte transfusions 678
  growth factors 677–678
  immunosuppressed host **668**, 668–669
  late recovery (phase III) 669, **670**, *670*
    treatment 675
  liver 783
  lung 875–876
  mid-recovery (phase II) 669, **670**, *670*
  neutropenia 668–669, 669–671
    antibiotic prophylaxis 677
    first fever treatment *672*, *673*
    outpatient management 674
    subsequent fever management *673*,
      673–674
  opportunistic 666, **670**
  oral 920
  peri-anal 792
  prophylaxis 677
  secondary to varicella-zoster virus 738,
      739
  spectrum 669–671
  superinfection 671
  treatment 671–676, 672
    antibiotics **666**
    immunobiological agents 678
bacterial meningitis, chronic GVHD 811
bacterial pathogens
  antibiotic resistance 666–668, **667**
  bacteriocins 665
  biology 665
  evasion of host immune response 665–666
  extrachromosomal elements 666
  invasion 665
  spectrum 669–671
  virulence factors **666**
balancing selection, MHC evolution 48
basiliximab, mechanism of action/targets **218**
basophils, development *614*

BAVC regimen **161**
  AML **1222**
B-cell(s)
  development 78–80, *614*, 855
    bipotent progenitors 81
    IL-7 role 78
    Pax-5 78, 83
    prepro-B cells 79
    pro-B cells 79
  immune reconstitution *see* immune
      reconstitution
  immunological tolerance 303
  vaccination response 863
  V-DJ recombination 79
Bcl-2
  as apoptosis inhibitor 71
  chemotherapy resistance role 264
  HSC self-renewal 71, 72
  lymphoid cell development 78
  lymphomas 264
  targeted antisense therapy 264
BCNU (carmustine) 142–143, 164
  astrocytoma 1346–1347
  brain cancer **1345**, 1345–1346
  combination regimens **161**, 164
    ABCM 1264
    Adriamycin/cyclophosphamide/
        melphalan 1264
    BEAC *see* BEAC regimen
    BEAM *see* BEAM regimen
    CBV *see* CBV regimen
    cyclophosphamide/cytarabine/etoposide
        see BEAC regimen
    cyclophosphamide/etoposide combination
        see CBV regimen
    melphalan *see* BEAM regimen
    STAMP-I *see* STAMP-I regimen
  high-dose chemotherapy 142–143
  mechanism of action 142–143
  MTD **159**
  pharmacology **131**, 143
  resistance 142
  structure *131*
  toxicity 143
    neurotoxicity 817
Bcr–Abl gene fusion *see* Philadelphia
    chromosome (*Bcr–Abl* gene fusion)
BEAC regimen **161**, 163
  intermediate/high grade lymphoma
      therapy 1110
BEAM regimen **161**, 163
  cytoprotective agents 170
  Hodgkin's disease therapy 1191, *1193*
beclomethasone 210
Bence Jones protein 1263
β–emitters 200, **201**
beta-lactam antibiotics, resistance 666, **667**,
    668
β_2-microglobulin, in multiple myeloma 1263
  prognosis 1275–1276
bias, biostatistical methods 415
"biased coin" design 421–422

bile duct
  pain 790
  stones 774
  treatment complications
    biliary disease 783–784
    biliary strictures 795
biliary sludge syndrome 783
bilirubin, increased 775, **775**
biopsy
  bleeding at site 785–786
  chronic GVHD 292
  lip *293, 294*
  lung 874–875
biostatistical methods 414–433
  bias 415, 417, 426
  confounding factors 415
  data analysis 426–431
    "administrative" censoring 428, 429
    computing risks 430
    Cox proportional hazards model 430
    equivalency testing 427, **428**
    genetic data role 430–431
    intention-to-treat 426
    interim analysis 427
    interval-censored survival 429
    Kaplan–Meier graphs 429
    log–rank (Cox) test 429–430, **430**
    recurrence rates 427–428, *428*
    subgroup analysis 426–427
    surrogate endpoints 428
    time to an event 428–430
  database management 425–426
  dependent variables 415
  errors 417, *417*
  hierarchy of study designs 414, **415**
  independent variables 414–415
  observational study designs 414–416
    genetic data impact 416
    prospective cohort 415
    QoL/cost-effectiveness 416
    retrospective case–control 416
  odds ratio (OR) 416
  randomization 421–422
  relative risk (RR) 415, 429
  reporting results **431**, 431–432
  study cycle 414, *415*
  see also clinical trials; outcomes research
bipotent stem cells 74
bis-chloroethyl-nitrosourea see BCNU
bismuth-213 **201**
bisphosphonates, multiple myeloma therapy 1265
BK virus infections 763
  treatment **762**
bladder, delayed complications 951
bleeding
  active, treatment 836
  gastrointestinal 784–786
    acute GVHD 785
blood
  HSC migration into 73–74
  mature cells, cryopreservation effects 605
  mobilized peripheral
    cancer cells 83–84, *84*
    gene therapy 124
    HSC expansion studies 99, **100**
    HSC release/clearance 73–74, *74*
blood cells
  chimerism 236–237
    shared placental circulation 565
  hematopoiesis 73
    developmental 75
  number required 62–63
  support therapy, CMV infection **713**, 713–714
  see also specific cell types
blood group incompatibility 824–832
  complications 825
  delayed reactions 825
  management 825–827, **826**
  therapy 829
blood groups see ABO blood group; Rhesus (Rh) blood groups
Blood/Marrow Transplant Information Network (BMT InfoNet) 449, 485
Bloom syndrome, *in utero* transplantation and 573
"blueberry muffin" lesions, neuroblastoma 1333
BMI-1, HSC self-renewal 73
BMT Clinical Trials Network (BMT-CTN), multiple myeloma therapy 1101–1102
BMT Support Online 485
BMT-Talk 485
body surface area (BSA)
  drug dose 136–137
  estimation 136
body weight, drug dose 456
Bologna96 1274, **1274**
bone marrow
  chimerism
    testing 236–237
    transplantation tolerance 85
  hematopoiesis 73
  HSC expansion studies 99, **100**
    injury 63
  microenvironment 53
  "mobilized" 73
  stromal cells as therapeutics 58
  T-cell content 853
  transplantation see bone marrow transplantation (BMT); hematopoietic cell transplantation (HCT)
  tumor cell eradication see bone marrow purging
bone marrow donation
  adverse events 540–543, 542
    anesthesia risks 541
    serious *541*, 541–543
  complications 541
  death **542**, 542–543
  G-CSF 594
  infection risks 541–542
  mechanical tissue risks 542
  procedure 544–545
  symptoms **541**
Bone Marrow Donor Program (NMDP) 467
Bone Marrow Donors Worldwide (BMDW) 12, 1133
  registries submitting data **626**
bone marrow purging
  antisense strategies 256, 265–266
  complications 255
  drug resistance 255, *255*
  efficacy/treatment response 1338
  HCT advantages 83–84, *84*
  immunomagnetic purging 1338
  mutagenesis 255–256
  pharmacological 254–257
    agents 254–256
  pheretic purging 1338
bone marrow transplantation (BMT)
  allogeneic
    CLL see chronic lymphocytic leukemia (CLL), allogeneic transplants
    lymphomas see lymphoma(s), allogeneic transplants
  animal studies, advances 4–5
    problems recognized 5
  autologous
    first attempts 3–4
    neuroblastoma see neuroblastoma, HCT
    recombinant G-CSF 615
  beginnings 3
  cases per year 5
  CMV infections 702–703
  continuing development 6
  histocompatibility, advances 5
  history 3–8, *4*
    clinical studies 3–4
  irradiation protection effect 3
  leukemia 6
    studies in terminal patients 3–4
  problems 5
  renewed interest 5–6
  solid tumor treatment 1364
  successes 5–6
  thalassemia see thalassemia
  see also hematopoietic cell transplantation (HCT)
bone marrow transplant nephropathy 951
bone resorption, osteoclast function 1444
"boosting" radiotherapy 178, 184–185, 186
brain cells, transdifferentiation 76, **77**
brain tumors 1345–1353
  astrocytoma, high-grade 1346–1347
  chemotherapy, high-dose 1345–1346
    HCT with 1346–1347, 1348–1349, 1350–1352
  ependymomas 1347–1348
  germ cell 1351
  infants 1351–1352
  medulloblastoma 1349–1350
  oligodendrogliomas 1348–1349

primitive neuroectodermal tumors 1350–1351
stem 1349
BRCA genes
  in Fanconi anemia 1487
  ovarian cancer 1321
breast cancer 9
  allogeneic transplants 1304
  autologous transplants 1298–1307
    adjuvant therapy 1298–1299
      high-dose **1301**
        trials 1301–1302
      GVLE induction 410
      survival **1304**
    chemotherapy **1299**
      high-dose **1300**, 1300–1301
      high-dose mitoxantrone 138
      standard dose 1298–1299
    diagnosis 1298
    local therapy 1298
    men 1304
    metastatic
      allogeneic transplants 1184
      high-dose regimens **1301**
      standard-dose 1299–1300
      trials 1302–1303
    research directions 1304–1305
    risk 1298
    staging 1298, **1299**
bronchiolitis obliterans 947, **947**
bronchiolitis obliterans organizing pneumonia (BOOP) 947
bulky disease
  consolidative irradiation 191
  "debulking" chemotherapy 204
  radiotherapy "boosts" 185
Burkitt lymphoma
  allogeneic transplants 1106
  T-cell adoptive transfer 385
  therapy studies 1110
business manager 466
busulfan (BU) 141–142, 162–163
  AML, childhood 1044–1045
  autoimmune animal models 332–333
  BMT for thalassemia 1411
  CML 1008, 1010–1011
  combination regimens **160**, **1222**
    ATG/fludarabine *see* antithymocyte globulin (ATG), combination regimens
    Campath/fludarabine 1088–1089
    cyclophosphamide 162–163, 189, *190*
      allogeneic transplants childhood ALL 1074
      allogeneic transplants CLL 1106
      allogeneic transplants lymphoma 1106
      autologous transplants AML **1222**, 1223
      HLA-partially matched related donors 1119
      MDS 1088

multiple myeloma 1096, 1097, 1098, 1266
  TBI/cyclophosphamide *vs.* 1065
  TBI *vs.* **165**
cyclophosphamide/TBI
  autologous transplants AML **1222**
  cyclophosphamide *vs.* 1065
cyclophosphamide/thiotepa 1119
etoposide 163
  autologous transplants AML **1222**
etoposide/TBI **1222**
fludarabine 1171–1172
idarubicin/melphalan 1266–1267
melphalan 163, 1266
melphalan/thiotepa 163
drug interactions 142
high-dose chemotherapy 141–142
mechanism of action 141–142
metabolism 134, 142
monitoring 137–138, 142
MTD **159**
pharmacokinetics 162
pharmacology **131**, 142
solid tumor treatment **1363**
structure *131*
toxicity 142, 189
  hepatic veno-occlusive disease 135, 137
  neurotoxicity 142, 817
butorphanol, pain management 903
BVAP regimen, multiple myeloma therapy 1264

C
cachexia, treatment outcome 456
CALB *see* Cancer/Acute Leukaemia Group (CALGB)
calcineurin inhibitor, GVHD 23
CALGB *see* Cancer/Acute Leukaemia Group (CALGB)
calibrated phase 3 trials 421
Campath 1_M
  combination regimens
    busulfan/fludarabine 1088–1089
    fludarabine/melphalan
      HLA-matched related HCT 1170
      Hodgkin's disease 1201
      retrospective studies 1172
  GVHD therapy 360
    multiple myeloma therapy 1099
    sickle cell disease 1432–1434
Cancer/Acute Leukaemia Group (CALGB)
  AML autologous transplants 1226
  imatinib mesylate trials 1242
The Cancer Rehabilitation Evaluation System–Short Form (CARES) 513
Candida infection 683, 684–686
  biology/pathophysiology 684
  cardiovascular system 685
  CNS 685, 811
  dissemination with deep tissue infection 685
  epidemiology 683–684
  HLA-partially matched related HCT 1123

immune response 687–689
mucocutaneous infection 684–685
skin lesions 686
syndromes 684
candidate selection, psychosocial factors 498–499
candidemia 685
carbohydrate malabsorption 789
carboplatin 164
  combination regimens **161**, **162**
    BCNU/cisplatin/cyclophosphamide/thiotepa *see* STAMP-V regimen
    cyclophosphamide 164
    cyclophosphamide/mitoxantrone 164
    ifosfamide/etoposide *see* ICE regimen
    melphalan/mitoxantrone 164
    STAMP-V *see* STAMP-V regimen
  dosage adjustment based on GFR 137
  drug interactions 144
  germ cell tumor 1311, **1312–1313**
  high-dose chemotherapy 144
  MTD **159**
  pharmacology **131**, 144
  structure *131*
carcinoembryonic antigen (CEA) 198
cardiac evaluation, treatment outcome 455–456
cardiac muscle, transdifferentiation **77**
cardiac toxicity
  cyclophosphamide 140
  DMSO 607
  doxorubicin 146
cardiovascular disease, delayed complications 949–950
caregivers 503–504
  expectations 503
  quality of life issues 512
  measures **508**
CARES 513
carmustine *see* BCNU (carmustine)
cartilage-hair hypoplasia 1475–1476
case–control studies, retrospective 416
case management structure 464–465, 469
  nurse (NCM) 464–465
caspofungin 694
cataracts
  delayed complications 950
  GVHD and 188
  radiotherapy toxicity 188–189
  steroids and 188
β-catenin, HSC self-renewal 72, *72*
catheters, complications associated 887–888
  see also central venous catheters (CVC), complications of
cavernous sinus syndrome 813, *814*
CBCs *see* cord blood cells (CBCs)
CBER *see* Center for Biologic Evaluation/Research (CBER)
CBV regimen **161**, 163
  Hodgkin's disease 1201–1202
CCG *see* Children's Cancer Group (CCG)
CD4+ T-cell(s) *see* helper T-cell(s)

CD8+ T-cell(s) *see* cytotoxic T-cell(s)
CD14 marker, cells in PBHC 590
CD28 markers
   antigen presentation 354–355
   immunological tolerance 301
CD33 markers 202
CD34 markers 576
   cord blood cells 556
   PBHCs
      characterization 589, **589**
      positive selection 594
      purging 1338–1339
   positive selection 246, 605
   in vitro HSC expansion and 72
CD38 markers, cord blood cells 556
CD40 markers
   antigen presentation 304, 355
   multiple myeloma 1262
CD45 markers 202
CDAD (*Clostridium difficile* associated diarrhea) 675
CD markers, antibodies to *see individual antibodies*
cDNA expression cloning, mHA 389, *389*
CDRH (Center for Devices/Radiological Health) 531
CEBPα transcription factor 87
cell culture, minimum residual disease detection 245
cells, radiotherapy survival curve 178
   fractionation effect *179*
   leukemic cells 179–180
   lymphocytes 179
   multihit multitarget model 178, *179*
   quadratic (LQ) model 178, 180
cell surface markers
   hematopoietic microenvironment 55–56
   multiple myeloma 1262
   see also individual markers
cellular immunity *see* immune response/system
Center for Biologic Evaluation/Research (CBER)
   gene therapy trials 122
   HCT regulation 531
Center for Devices/Radiological Health (CDRH) 531
central nervous system (CNS)
   drug toxicity *see* neurotoxicity
   fungal infection 685
   infections following HCT 738, 740, 811–813, *812*, **819**
   stem cells 77, *77*
      transdifferentiation 76
   see also neurological complications
central venous catheters (CVC), complications of 887–888
   infections
      management **676**
      risk 669
      treatment 676–677
cephalosporins, resistance 666, **667**, 668
CEP regimen **162**

cerebral angiitis, post-herpes zoster 739
cerebral infarctions, post-herpes zoster 739
cerebral vasospasm 813
cerebral X-linked adrenoleukodystrophy 1461–1462, *1462*
cerebrovascular complications 813, *814*, **819**
CGD *see* chronic granulomatous disease (CGD)
Chediak–Higashi syndrome (CHS) 1477
chelation therapy 201
   thalassemia 1409
chemokine receptors
   adoptive T-cell immunotherapy 395
   homing mechanisms, cord blood transplantation 557–558
chemokines
   autologous GVHD 408
   gene therapy, AIDS 1377–1378
   homing mechanisms, cord blood transplantation 557
   HSC migration role 73
   inflammatory, GVHD 358
   PBHC mobilization 577
   see also individual chemokines
chemotherapy
   AIDS 1372–1374
   ALL
      autologous transplants, comparison of 1240
      autologous transplants, previous in 1244
   AML
      in children 1045
         HCT *vs*. 1042–1044
      consolidation therapy 1026–1027
      TBI *vs*. 1223
   CML 1250
      palliative 1008
   "debulking" 204
   gene therapy and 121
   high-dose *see* chemotherapy, high-dose
   JMML 1019, 1021
   multiple myeloma, autologous transplants *vs*. 1271–1273
   neuroblastoma, autologous transplants *vs*. 1335–1337, **1336**, *1337*
   pharmacogenomics contribution 133
   physiological effects 929
      gonadal function 938
      puberty 935–937
      thyroid function 930
   pretransplant conditioning 12
      GVHD 23
      immune system 16
      outcome 11
   relapse treatment following 1395
   resistance *see* drug(s), resistance
   solid tumor treatment 1355
      breast cancer 1298–1301
   SOS 777–778
   TBI *vs*. 189–190, *190*
   toxicity 189
      neurotoxicity 817–818

   see also myeloablative therapy; nonmyeloablative therapy; pretransplant conditioning; *specific drugs/indications*
chemotherapy, high-dose 130–157, 160–163
   advantages 161
   brain tumors **1345**, 1345–1352, **1348–1351**
   clinical trials, conduct 138
      guidelines **139**
   CML 1253
   consolidative irradiation 190–191
   dose 130–133
      body surface adjustment 136–137
      combination therapy 132
      concentration–response effects 130, *132*
      tumor heterogeneity/growth kinetics 130, 132
      tumor resistance **132**, 132–133
   drugs 138–147
      alkylating agents *see* alkylating agent(s)
      monitoring 137–138
      renal/hepatic function indices 137
      selection 138
      structural formulae *131*
   failure 132
   germ cell tumor 1311–1317
   individualization 135–138
   neuroblastoma, bone marrow transplant 1336–1337
   non-Hodgkin's lymphoma 1208, 1214, **1214**
   pharmacodynamics **131**, 135–138
      body surface adjustment 136–137
      renal/hepatic function indices 137
      therapeutic monitoring 137–138
   pharmacokinetics **131**, 135
   pharmacologic definition 130
   preclinical models 130, 132
   prognosis scoring **1314**
   sequential regimens 166
   TBI, and *see* total body irradiation (TBI)
   TBI *vs*. 160–161, 165
   variable responses 133–135
   see also drug metabolism; myeloablative therapy; pharmacogenomics; pretransplant conditioning; *specific drugs/indications*
chest wall "boost" 184
chest X ray, radiation pneumonopathy 186
chicken pox *see* varicella-zoster virus (VZV) infection
children
   ALL *see* acute lymphoblastic leukemia (ALL), children
   AML *see* acute myeloid leukemia (AML), allogeneic transplants, children
   decision to treat 490
   donors 546
      ethical issues 491
   fungal infections 684
   orofacial/dental growth 923–924
   pain, cognitive-behavioral strategies 898–899

solid tumors, HCT *see* solid tumor(s),
        pediatric patients
  see also pediatric transplant
"children conceived to give life" 492
Children's Cancer Group (CCG)
  ABMT *vs.* chemotherapy in neuroblastoma
        1335–1336
  ALL, allogeneic transplants 1070
Children's Oncology Group study,
        neuroblastoma treatment 1334
  immunomagnetic purging 1339
chimeric (DNA/RNA) oligonucleotides, gene
        silencing 259
chimerism
  in allogeneic transplants 332
  partial *see* chimerism, mixed
  types 234
chimerism, characterization 234–243
  clinical applications 236–239, **237**
    after myeloablative regimens 239
    in graft failure 238
    recurrent malignancy risk 238–239
    samples 236–237
  historical perspective 234–235
  molecular cytogenetics 235
  real-time PCR studies 236
    short tandem repeat polymorphisms *vs.*
        237
  short tandem repeat polymorphisms *235*,
        235–236, *236*
    real-time PCR studies *vs.* *237*
  variable number of tandem repeat
        polymorphisms *235*, 235–236,
        236
  see also genetic marker studies
chimerism, mixed 234
  aplastic anemia HLA-identical related
        transplant 987
  induced tolerance 307, 309, 311, 314, *314*
  induction, nonmyeloablative therapy *309*
  sickle cell disease 1424–1425, *1424–1425*
  thalassemia, bone marrow transplant 1414
  thalassemia, HCT 139
chlorambucil, CLL therapy 1107
chlorhexidine, cytoprotection **168**
cholangitis lenta 780
cholestasis 780
CHOP regimen
  combination regimens 1107–1108, 1109
    rituximab 1107, 1109
  intermediate/high-grade lymphoma therapy
        1109
  low-grade lymphoma therapy 1107
  non-Hodgkin's lymphoma 1207
  PBHC mobilization 1269
chorioretinitis, CMV 811
chromatin structure, transcription control
        82
chromosomal breakage test, Fanconi anemia
        1485–1486, *1486*
chromosome abnormalities, secondary
        malignancies 965–966

chromosome rearrangements
  ALL 1055–1056, **1056**
  Fanconi anemia 1484
  leukemic stem cells 86
  translocations
    ALL 1056
    ALL, childhood 1069
    AML 1026
    bcr-abl see Philadelphia chromosome
        (*Bcr-Abl* gene fusion)
    CML 1007
    healthy people 282
    nonrandom, PCR detection 245
  in utero 86
chronic granulomatous disease (CGD)
        1477–1479
  clinical course *1478*
  conditioning 1478–1479
  gene therapy trials 124
  molecular basis 1478
  nonmyeloablative therapy 1173
  survival 1478
chronic lymphocytic leukemia (CLL)
  allogeneic transplants 1105–1115
    GVHD 1105
    high-dose chemotherapy 1107
    indications 1106–1107
    nonmyeloablative regimens 1110–1111,
        1167
    published studies 1105–1106
    relapse therapy 1154
  classification 1107
  diagnosis 1106
  differential diagnosis 1106
  epidemiology 1106
  median survival 1107
  minimal residual disease detection post-HCT
        278
  prognosis 1107
  progression to autoimmune disease 1106
  relapse risk detection 281
  therapy
    allogeneic transplants *see above*
    chemotherapy 1107
chronic myeloid leukemia (CML) 86
  accelerated phase 1007–1008, **1008**
  allogeneic transplants 1007–1017
    arguments for 1014
    factors influencing outcome 1010
    GVHD *vs.* GVLE 1141, 1151–1152
    history 1007
    HLA-matched relatives
      accelerated phase 1012
      blast phase 1012
      chronic phase *1009*, 1009–1012,
        1010, *1011*
      factors influencing outcome 1010
      GVHD prophylaxis 1011
    HLA-partially matched relatives
        1119
      survival 1121
      imatinib 1014

    pretransplant conditioning 1010
      HLA-matched relatives 1010
      nonmyeloablative therapy 1167
    relapse management 1013–1014, 1150,
        1151–1153, 1155
      see also donor lymphocyte infusion
        (DLI)
    secondary transplant 1014
    unrelated donor 1012, 1143–1144
  autologous transplants 1250–1261
    adoptive immunotherapy 1257
    antileukemic therapy improvement
        1257–1258
    clinical experience 1251
    c-myb AS-ODNs 1252
    dendritic cell therapy 1257
    ex vivo marrow culture 1251
    ex vivo purging 1251–1253, **1252**,
        1256–1257
    future 1258
    GM-CSF 1251
    GM-CSF/hydroxyurea 1255–1256
    4-hydroperoxycyclophosphamide 1252
    imatinib mesylate 1257–1258, *1258*
    improving outcome 1256–1257
    interferon-α 1255
    interferon-γ 1252–1253
    PBHC mobilization
      chemotherapy 1253
      imatinib 1255
      interferonγ 1253, 1255
    phenotypic separation of benign
        progenitors 1256
    Philadelphia chromosome (*Bcr-Abl* gene
        fusion) targeting 1251–1252, 1256,
        1257
    photodynamic purging 1252
    posttransplant antileukemic treatment
        1255
    rationale 1250
    relapse prevention techniques
        1257–1258
    roquinimex 1255
    status 1258
    survival **1256**, *1258*
    tyrosine kinase inhibitors 1256
    unpurged **1251**
    in vivo selection by priming/mobilization
        1253–1255, **1254**
  blast crisis 1007–1008
  clinical description 1007–1008
  cytogenetics 1008
  epidemiology 1007
  gene marking trials 122
  GVLE 1012–1013
  hematopoiesis 65
  incidence 1007
  minimal residual disease detection post-HCT
        277–279, **278**
  molecular biology 1007
    Philadelphia chromosome (*Bcr-Abl* gene
        fusion) 86, 423, 1007

chronic myeloid leukemia (CML) (cont.)
   relapse
      increased following T-cell depletion 225–226
      Philadelphia chromosome (*Bcr-Abl* gene fusion) detection 277–279
      risk detection 277–279
      TBI and 185
   therapy
      allogeneic transplants *see above*
      antisense-mediated purging 265–266
      autologous transplants *see above*
      decision to undergo HCT 499
      Gleevac® 258
      imatinib mesylate 1014
      immunosuppressive agents, randomized controlled trials **642**
      interferon-alpha 1008–1009, 1158
      newly diagnosed patient 1014
      nontransplant therapies 1008–1009
      options 1014, 1250
      palliative chemotherapy 1008
      tyrosine kinase inhibitors 1143
chronic myelomonocytic leukemia (CMML)
   autologous transplants 1009
   unrelated donor HCT 1144
CID *see* combined immunodeficiency syndrome (CID)
cidofovir
   CMV infection 713
   varicella-zoster virus infections 744
cirrhosis 773–774, 794
cisplatin 164
   combination regimens **161, 162**
      asparaginase/cytarabine/dexamethasone/etoposide combination 1198
      cyclophosphamide/dexamethasone/etoposide 1269
      cytarabine/corticosteroids/etoposide 1107–1108
      cytarabine/decadrom combination 1109–1110
      DCEP regimen 1269
      STAMP-I *see* STAMP-I regimen
   dose-limiting toxicity 144
   drug interactions 143–144
   high-dose chemotherapy 143–144
   mechanism of action 143
   MTD **159**
   pharmacology **131**, 143–144
   resistance 143
   structure *131*
City of Hope National Medical Center
   ALL studies 1059–1060
   AML autologous transplants, first remission 1230
   HIV donors trial 457
   mouth care protocol **878**
   pulmonary complications of HCT 873–882
c-kit marker, cord blood cells 556

class II invariant chain peptide (CLIP), autologous GVHD 407, *407*
clinical nurse specialist 466
clinical trials
   authorization 465
   communication 431–432, 465
   conduct 423–425
      data coordinating center 424
      Data/Safety Monitoring Board 424
      discussions with patients 485–486
      genetic data impact 424–425
      genetics impact 424–425
      inclusion/exclusion criteria 417
      informing patients 417, 453
      Institutional Review Board (IRB) 424
      single *vs.* multicenter 423–424
   criticisms 419
   data analysis 426–431
      genetics impact 430–431
   database management 425–426
      genetics impact 426
   design 416–423
      dose-escalation 418–420, **419**, *419*
      genetic data impact 422–423
      genetics impact 422
      international guidelines 421
      key components **417**
      number of patients required 420, **420**
      phase 1 trials 417–420, *418*
      phase 2 trials **418**, 420–421
      phase 3 trials **418**, 421–422
      randomization 421–422
      sample size 422
      uncontrolled 420
   discussions with patients 485–486
   endpoints 420
   errors 417, *417*, 420
   gene therapy *see* gene therapy
   high-dose chemotherapy 138
      guidelines **139**
   HSC expansion studies 99–103
      bone marrow/peripheral blood 99, **100**
      UBC cells 99, 101–103
   informing patients 453
   legal requirements 417
   NIH definition 416
   outcome 416
   phases 416–417
   radioimmunotherapy/HCT 202–205
   radiotherapy 185–189
   randomized clinical trials
      antibody-mediated purging 251
      autoimmune disease 1390–1391
      PBHC allogeneic transplants 592–594
      quality of life improvement 512–513
   reporting results 431–432
      guidelines 431
      publication checklist **431**
   SOS 777–778
   T-cell depletion 223

   see also biostatistical methods; hematopoietic cell transplantation (HCT) program; outcomes research
CLIP (class II invariant chain peptide), autologous GVHD 407, *407*
CLL *see* chronic lymphocytic leukemia (CLL)
clofazimine 217
   mechanism of action/targets **218**
clonal deletion 300–301, 307
   autoimmunity pathogenesis 328
   central 300–301
   cyclosporine effects 406
   immune response regulation 325
   peripheral 301
   superantigens 300–301
clonogenic assays, minimal residual disease detection 245
   sensitivity 244t
Clostridium difficile associated diarrhea (CDAD) 675
CLPs *see* common lymphoid progenitors (CLPs)
CML *see* chronic myeloid leukemia (CML)
CMML *see* chronic myelomonocytic leukemia (CMML)
CMPs (common myeloid progenitors) 80
CMV *see* cytomegalovirus (CMV)
CMV-IP *see* cytomegalovirus-associated interstitial pneumonia (CMV-IP)
c-myb, antisense oligonucleotides 1252
coagulation factor components, transfusions 834
COBLT (NHLBI Cord Blood Transplantation Study) 551
coercion, donors 539
cognitive changes 486
   quality of life issues 510
   radiotherapy-induced 189
colon, GVHD 289
colony-forming cell (CFC) assays 73
coma 784
combined immunodeficiency syndrome (CID) 1436–1437
   pathogenic basis 1437
common lymphoid progenitors (CLPs) 78–79
   immune reconstitution 854, 859
common myeloid progenitors (CMPs) 80
comorbid conditions, treatment outcome 455–456
complement-mediated lysis *see* purging, antibody-mediated
complete remission (CR) *see individual diseases/disorders; individual treatments*
compliance, pediatric transplant 460
complications (of HCT)
   major groups 286
   see also individual diseases/disorders; individual treatments
computed tomography (CT)
   cerebrovascular complications 813, *814*
   cyclosporine/tacrolimus toxicity 815, *816*
   liver, SOS 776

conditioning *see* pretransplant conditioning
confidentiality
  donor registries 630
  paternity issues 490–492
confounding factors, biostatistical methods 415
congenic transplant(s), autoimmune animal models 332
congenital diseases/syndromes
  gene therapy trials 123–124
  nonmyeloablative therapy 1173–1174
  see also specific disorders
consent *see* informed consent
Consolidated Standards of Reporting Trials (CONSORT) 431
consolidative irradiation 185, 190–191
CONSORT (Consolidated Standards of Reporting Trials) 431
coping
  poor 500
  style **508**
coping strategies program 512
cord blood
  banking 551–552
    cryopreservation 551–552
    eligibility 551
  collection 550–551
  donor searching 552
  NETCORD/FACT standards 533
  registries 628–629, **629**
  survival 101
cord blood cells (CBCs) 12, 101, 599
  characteristics 555–556
  ex vivo expansion 555, 556–557, 558
  gene therapy 557
  GVHD 637
  for HCT 12, 531, 599
  HSC expansion studies 99, 101–103, **102**
    rationale 99, 101
  immune cells 558–559
  population 101
  source 12
cord blood cell transplantation 101, 550–564
  in adults 554
  allogeneic transplants 550, 551–552
    ALL, childhood 1076–1078, **1077**, 1078
    AML 1032, 1047
    unrelated donor 553–554
    in utero transplantation 567, 568
  autologous transplants 550
    relapse treatment following 1395
  cell homing 557–558
  cryopreserved cells for 608
  future work 554–555
  GVHD 101
    cytokine involvement 558
  history 550
  immune reconstitution 554
  related donor 552–553
  sickle cell disease 1426, 1435–1436
    survival *1426*
coronavirus infections 761

corticosteroids 209–210
  agnogenic myeloid metaplasia therapy 1090
  clinical use 210
  combination regimens
    antiviral therapy 743
    cisplatin/cytarabine/etoposide 1107–1108
  dose 210
  GVHD treatment 23, 643–645
  infections associated 706
  mechanism of action *210*, **218**
  pharmacology 209
  recommendations 210
  side effects 209, 950–951
    cataracts 188
    neurological 817
  structures *209*
  tapering, in pain management 906
  T-cell adoptive transfer 384–385
  toxicity 209, 817
cortisol *209*
cost–benefit analysis 436, 437, **437**
cost–effectiveness analysis 416, 436, 437, **437**, 438
costimulatory blockades
  induced tolerance 309–310, *310*
  peripheral induced tolerance 304
costimulatory signals, immunological tolerance 301
cost-minimization studies 436, **436**
cost of treatment *see* economics
cost–utility analysis 436, 437, **437**, 438
counseling/evaluation of donors *see* donor counseling
Cox (log-rank) analysis 429–430, **430**
Cox proportional hazards model 430
CpG motifs 266
CPPD regimen **161**
cranial irradiation, cataracts following 188–189
cranial neuropathy, post-herpes zoster 739
C-reactive protein (CRP), multiple myeloma 1263
Creutzfeldt–Jakob disease (CJD), transfusion transmitted 846
critical care, complications spectrum 873, **874**
critical illness polyneuropathy (CIPN) 814
critically ill patients
  ethical issues 494–495
  pain management 908
  prognosis 878–879, **879**
  survival studies 494–495
Crohn's disease 769
crossmatching, donor selection 1117–1118
CRP (C-reactive protein), multiple myeloma 1263
cryobiology 600–602
cryoprecipitate, transfusions 834
cryopreservation 599–612
  acid-citrate-dextrose 607
    reactions to 608
  allogeneic transplants 608–609
  autologous transplants, AML 1223

  cells, effect on 600–602
    mechanical damage 600
    osmotic stress 601
    post-thaw clumping 607
  cord blood banking 551–552
  cryoprotectants 602–604, **604**
    colligative 600–601, 602
    dimethyl sulfoxide 600–601, **601**, 602–603, **603**
    ethylene glycol **601**
    glycerol 600–601, 603
    hydroxyethyl starch 603, **603**
    mechanism of action 601–602
    serum proteins 603–604
    storage temperature and 606
    sugars 604
    toxicity 607–608
  dehydration injury 600
  engraftment and
    cryoprotectant effect **603**
    delayed engraftment 599, 608
    reduction of GVHD 608
  salts 604
  storage duration 606
  storage during transport 606–607
  technique **599**, 604–607
    cell concentration 605
    cooling/warming rates 602, **602**, **605**, 605–606
    efficacy evaluation 604
    post-thaw manipulation 607
    processing 605
    storage temperature 606–607
    "test vials" 604
  theory 600–602
    biology/chemistry 600–602
    phase-transition temperatures 601, 602
    physics 602, **602**
  tumor cell purging 609
  viral contamination 606
  vitrification 601
cryotherapy, local cytoprotection 167, **168**
Cryptococcus neoformans, CNS infection 811
CSP *see* cyclosporine (CSP)
CT *see* computed tomography (CT)
CTLA4 *see* cytotoxic T-lymphocyte antigen 4 (CTLA4)
CTLA-4-Ig
  GVHD treatment 360–361
  HLA-partially matched related HCT 1122
  partial T-cell depletion 1122
cultural background, information needs 483
current Good Tissue Practices (cGTP), HCT regulation 532
cutaneous T-cell lymphomas, allogeneic transplants 1110
C-VAMP regimen, multiple myeloma therapy 1264
CWG (Cytokine Working Group), solid tumor immunotherapy 1178
CY *see* cyclophosphamide (CY)

cyarabine/fludarabine/idarubicin combination
  HLA-matched related HCT 1167
  MDS 1088–1089
cyclic neutropenia 1475
cyclophosphamide (CY) 139–140, 164
  autoimmune animal models 332–333, 334
  bone marrow purging 254
  CML 1010–1011
  combination regimens **161**, **162**, 985–987, *986*, 988–989
    ABCM 1264
    Adriamycin/BCNU/melphalan 1264
    ATG/thiotepa/TBI 1123
    ATG/thymic irradiation *see* antithymocyte globulin (ATG), combination regimens
    BCNU/etoposide *see* CBV regimen
    BEAC *see* BEAC regimen
    busulfan *see* busulfan (BU), combination regimens
    busulfan/TBI **1222**
    busulfan/thiotepa 1119
    carboplatin 164
    carboplatin/mitoxantrone 164
    CBV *see* CBV regimen
    CHOP *see* CHOP regimen
    C-VAMP 1264
    doxorubicin/methylprednisolone/vincristine 1264
    doxorubicin/prednisone/vincristine *see* CHOP regimen
    etoposide/methotrexate/melphalan/TBI 1202
    etoposide/mitoxantrone/melphalan 1267
    etoposide/TBI
      CML autologous transplants **1222**, 1223
      Hodgkin's disease 1201–1202
    fludarabine
      melanoma therapy 1184
      renal cell carcinoma 1179, *1179*, 1182
    melphalan 1266
    mycophenolate mofetil/TBI 1201
    STAMP-I *see* STAMP-I regimen
    STAMP-V *see* STAMP-V regimen
    survival 990
    TBI 189–190
      ALL 1062
      AML **1222**, 1222–1223
      childhood ALL, allogeneic transplants 1073–1074
      CLL 1107
      Fanconi anemia alternative donor HCT 1495–1497, **1496**
      high-dose regimens 159, **159**, **160**, 165, 182, 185, 189
      MDS 1088
      multiple myeloma 1096, 1266
      murine studies 1164
    thiotepa/TBI 1074–1075
  delayed complications 951
  dose-limiting toxicity 140

Fanconi anemia, sibling donor HCT 1491–1492
  GVHD primary treatment 650
    multiple myeloma 1097
  high-dose chemotherapy 139–140, 191
  HLA-partially matched related donors 1119
  induced tolerance 308
  mechanism of action 139
  metabolism 135, *135*
  MTD **159**
  PBHC mobilization
    G-CSF with 1269
    GM-CSF with 580
    standard regimens 582
  PBHC purging, AML autologous transplants 1225
  pharmacology **131**, 135, 139–140
  pretransplant 12
    AML, childhood 1044–1045
  randomized controlled trials 642
  resistance 139
  single-agent immunosuppression 641
  solid tumor treatment 1363
  SOS 777–778
  structure *131*
  thalassemia, bone marrow transplant 1411
cyclosporine (CSP) 211–213
  autologous GVHD induction 405, 406, *406*, 407–408, **408**, 409
  clinical use 212–213
  clonal deletion effects 406
  combination regimens **211**
    methotrexate/TBI 1165
    mycophenolate mofetil 1179
    prednisolone/recombinant G-CSF 617
    prednisone 384
    TBI 1164
  drug interactions **213**, 816
  efficacy studies 213
  fertility 451
  GVHD 23, 359–360
    acute 987–988
    chronic 650
    multiple myeloma therapy 1098, 1102
    primary treatment 650
  immunosuppression 641
    combined 641, 643
  mechanism 211–213, *213*
  mechanism of action/targets **218**
  pharmacology 211–213
  posttransplant 985–987, *986*, 988–989
  survival 990
  randomized controlled trials **642**, **644**, **651**
  side-effects 212
  structure *212*
  T-cells, effects on 858
  toxicity 212, 829
    nephrotoxicity 813
    neurotoxicity 815–817
    treatment complication 780
CYP see cytochrome P450s *(CYP)*
cystitis, hemorrhagic 790

cytarabine 164
  combination regimens
    asparaginase/cisplatin/dexamethasone/etoposide 1198
    BEAC *see* BEAC regimen
    cisplatin/corticosteroids/etoposide 1107–1108
    cisplatin/decadrom combination 1109–1110
    G-CSF 1153
    TBI **160**
  MTD **159**
  regimens **161**
cytochrome P450s *(CYP)*
  2C subfamily 133–134
  2D subfamily 133
  3A subfamily 134
  taxane metabolism 134, 146–147
cytogenetics
  AL amyloidosis 1284–1285
  ALL 1239
  AML 1025–1026, *1026*, **1221**, 1221–1222
  MDS 1085–1086
  metaphase chromosomes, chimerism evaluation 234–235
  multiple myeloma 1262, 1275–1276
  residual disease detection **273**
  secondary malignancy 968
  sensitivity 272
  see also fluorescence *in situ* hybridization (FISH)
cytokine induced killer (CIK) cells 1400–1401
cytokines
  GVHD 355–356
    acute 638
    autologous 406, 408
    chronic 361–362, 647
    inflammatory 353
    prevention by blocking 361
    prevention by immunostimulation 313
  GVLE, exogenous application 375
  hematopoiesis 57–58, 72
  HSC expansion systems 97, 98, 101
  immune reconstitution 856
  immunotherapy following autologous transplants 1397–1398
  local cytoprotection 168, **168**
  lymphoid cell development 78
  PBHC mobilization *see* peripheral blood hematopoietic cells (PBHCs), mobilization
  production
    cord blood cells 558
    helper T-cells 325
  type 2, G-CSF stimulation 590
  upregulation, multiple myeloma 1262–1263
  see also specific cytokines
Cytokine Working Group (CWG), solid tumor immunotherapy 1178
cytomegalovirus (CMV)
  detection assay 712, *716*, 716–718
    choice 718, **718**

drug resistance 710–711
epidemiology 701–702
    changing pattern 702–703, **703**
HSC interactions 719
latency 382, 702
    reactivation post-HCT 733, 1100
monitoring, clinical specimens 711–712
risk analysis 705–706
strains, clinical significance 705
structure 701, *701*, *702*
vaccination 715–716
viral growth 702
virology 701–702
cytomegalovirus-associated interstitial
    pneumonia (CMV-IP) 295, 706–708
  ALL patients 1062
  clinical course *707*
  complications *709*
  histopathology *707*
  incidence 381
  treatment 706–708, **707**, **708**
    antiviral agents 706–708, **707**
    CMVIg 708
    corticosteroids 707–708
cytomegalovirus (CMV) infection 85, 701–726
  AML autologous transplants 1232
  associated syndromes 709
  clinical course 705, *707*, 856
  complications 709, *709*
    CNS infection 811
    enteritis 708–709
    liver 781
    lung *295*
    oral infection 920
  considerations 711–713
  diagnosis 716–718
  disease definitions 705
  GVHD 289
  historical incidence 703–704, **704**
  in HIV/AIDS 811
  HLA-partially matched related HCT 1123
  immune response 714
    cellular immunity 714
    effects 718–719
    escape from immune surveillance
      714–715
    humoral immunity 715
  incidence 702–703, **703**, *706*
  MHC expression 382
  MIC expression 384
  nonmyeloablative therapy 1171
  pathogenesis 718–719
  preantiviral era 703–704
  prevention 709–714, **710**
    acyclovir 712–713
    adoptive immunotherapy *see below*
    autologous transplants 710
    blood products **713**, 713–714
    effects *712*
    nonmyeloablative regimens 710
    risk-adapted 711
    routine dosing schedule 710
    stopping treatment/surveillance 710
    transfusions 840
  progressive/recurrent 718
  rate 703–704
    autologous/syngeneic recipients
      704–705
  transmission from donor to recipient 539
  treatment 705–706
    adoptive immunotherapy *see below*
    antiviral agents 704
      historical use 706–708
      ganciclovir 381, 706–708, 713, 1123
cytomegalovirus (CMV) infection, adoptive
    immunotherapy 380, 381–385,
    715–716, 1156
  clinical trials 383–385
    cytotoxic/helper T-cell clones 384–385
    cytotoxic T cell clones 383–384
  in donors 382–383
  evidence 381–382
  isolation/expansion *384*
  murine models 381
cytopenia, nutritional support 884
cytoprotection 166–170
  classification **167**
  local 167–169, **168**
    antimicrobials 167–168, **168**
    cryotherapy 167, **168**
    cytokines 168, **168**
    desrazoxane 169
    Mesna 168–169
    ursodeoxycholic acid 169
  systemic 169–170
  see also hemorrhagic cystitis; mucositis
cytoreductive conditioning
  bone marrow *see* bone marrow purging
  gene therapy and 121
  nutritional support 884
  radiotherapeutic 178, 179–180
cytosine arabinoside
  anthracycline combination 1157
  TBI combination 1062
cytotoxic chemotherapy, allogeneic transplants
    relapse management 1157
cytotoxic T-cell(s) 20–21
  adoptive immunotherapy
    CMV infection 382–383, 383–384,
      384–385
    EBV infection 386
  cellular therapy following autologous
    transplants 1401–1402
  GVHD 344
    animal models 346, 348, *348*, **349**
    autologous 409–410
  GVLE 369, 370, 373, 388
  solid tumors 1185
  recovery post cord blood transplantation
    554
  T-cell depletion, in DLI 1155–1156
cytotoxic T-lymphocyte antigen 4 (CTLA4)
  antigen presentation 354–355
  immunological tolerance 302

D
daclizumab **218**
DAH (diffuse alveolar hemorrhage) 876–877
D-Amb *see* Fungizone
Dana Farber Cancer Institute 452
database management 425–426
data coordinating center (DCC) 424
data mining, clinical trial design 423
Data/Safety Monitoring Board (DSMB) 424
  gene therapy trials 122
daunorubicin
  ALL therapy 1238
  cytoprotection 169
DCEP regimen, PBHC mobilization 1269
DCs *see* dendritic cells (DCs)
death, ethical issues 494–495
debrisoquin hydroxylase 133
Decadron, cisplatin/cytarabine combination
    1109–1110
DECAL regimen 1198
decision analysis 438–440
  ethical issues 488–489
  imatinib mesylate (Gleevac®) 439, *439*
decoy oligonucleotides, gene silencing 259,
    259, 260
defibrotide infusions, SOS treatment 779
delayed complications 944–961
  bronchiolitis obliterans 947, **947**
  cardiovascular disease 949–950
  chronic GVHD *see* graft-*vs.*-host disease
    (GVHD), chronic
  etiology 944, **945**
  follow-up recommendations **956**
  genitourinary dysfunction *see* genitourinary
    complications
  hematological problems 948
  immune dysregulation *see*
    immunosuppression
  infections *see* infection(s)
  malignancies *952*, 952–954
  musculofascial problems 950
  nervous system *see* neurological
    complications
  ocular problems 950
  pneumonitis 945
  psychosocial effects *see* psychosocial
    complications/factors
  pulmonary/airway disease *see* pulmonary
    complications
  rehabilitation 955
  skeletal complications 950–951
  solid tumor *see* solid tumor(s)
  spectrum 944, **945**
delirium
  opioids, side effects 901
  symptoms 501
Demerol 902–903
demyelinating disorders, following HCT
    814–815
dendritic cells (DCs)
  cord blood cells 558–559
  development *79*, 81–82

dendritic cells (DCs) (cont.)
  GVHD 355
  progenitors 81–82
  recurrence prevention 1257
  subpopulations, human vs. mouse 81
dental treatment see oral complications
dermatitis, autologous GVHD 406
dermatomes, localized herpes zoster 739, **739**
desmoplastic small cell tumor 1361
desrazoxane, local cytoprotection 169
dexamethasone, combination regimens
  asparaginase/cisplatin/cytarabine/etoposide combination 1198
  cyclophosphamide/etoposide/G-CSF/paclitaxel 1269
  fludarabine/mitoxantrone 1107–1108
  thalidomide 1265, 1270
  vincristine/Adriamycin see VAD therapy
DHAP regimen, intermediate/high-grade lymphoma therapy 1109–1110
DHFR see dihydrofolate reductase (DHFR)
diabetes mellitus type 1
  animal model 326t, 329
    allogeneic transplants 336–337, 337f, 338, 339
    autologous transplants 334, 335f
  HLA associations 324t, 327
Diagnostic/Statistical Manual of Mental Disorders 523
diarrhea 787–789
  acute GVHD 787–788
  before cytoreductive therapy 769–770
  fat/carbohydrate, malabsorption of 789
  intestinal infections 788–789
  long-term complications 795
  medications causing 789
  pretransplant conditioning 787
DIC (disseminated intravascular coagulopathy), transfusion 834
Dicer ribonuclease 263
diepoxybutane test, Fanconi anemia 1485–1486, *1486*
diet(s) 887
Dieulafoy lesion 785
"difficult" patient(s) 501
diffuse aggressive lymphoma, autologous transplants 1208–1211, **1210**
diffuse alveolar hemorrhage (DAH) 876–877
Diflucan see fluconazole
dihydrofolate reductase (DHFR)
  gene therapy trials 123
  inhibition 210
dimethyl myleran, autoimmune animal models 333
dimethylsulfoxide (DMSO)
  cryoprotection 600–601, 602–603
    engraftment kinetics **603**
    ethylene glycol vs. **601**
  toxicity 607–608
diphtheria, vaccination 859

discharge from hospital
  nursing issues 475, **479**
  psychosocial factors 501–502
  self-care regimen 501–502
  stress after 485
disease-free survival (DFS) see individual diseases/disorders; individual treatments
disheveled (Dsh), Wnt signaling 72, 72
disseminated intravascular coagulopathy (DIC), transfusion 834
DLI see donor lymphocyte infusion (DLI)
DMSO see dimethylsulfoxide (DMSO)
DNA
  defective repair, secondary malignancy 966
  HLA typing 1134–1135
  replication, telomeres 64
DNA hybrid capture assay, CMV detection 717
DNAzymes
  "10–23" DNA enzyme 262
  antisense therapy 260, 262–263
dog transplantation model 4–5
  problems identified 5
dominant epitopes, autoimmunity 328
donor(s) 538–549
  adverse events 539, 540–544
    disease transmission 538–539
  children 546
  counseling see donor counseling
  ethical/legal aspects 540
    coercion 539
    informed consent 490–492, 540
    minors 491
    motives 539
    as research subjects 540
    survivor guilt 503
  history 539
  partially HLA-matched related see HLA-partially matched related HCT
  PBHC 590–591
    adverse effects 591, **591**
  physical outcomes 503
  pregnancy 540
  psychosocial factors 502–503, 539
  quality of life 511, 512
  search coordinator 467
  searching, unrelated see donor registries
  second donations 545–546
  selection see donor selection
  transfusions 841–842
  unrelated see HLA-matched unrelated HCT
  viral infection 538–539
donor buffy coat cells (BC), randomized controlled trials **642**
Donor Centers 624–625
donor counseling 449–462
  advice 449–451
    against transplantation 452
  age 456–457
  clinical trials 453
  first visit to transplant center 449
  foreign patients 453

  informed consent 458
  interpretation of information given 452, **452**
  issues to address **450**, 451
  patients seeking multiple opinions 452–453
  psychological assessment 457–458, **458**
  second visit to transplant center 452
  terminology 449
  written information 449
  see also donor selection
donor lymphocyte infusion (DLI) 1151–1158
  ALL relapse 1153–1154, 1155
  AML in children 1048
  AML relapse 1153, *1153*, 1155
  CML relapse 1013–1014, *1151*, 1151–1153, 1155
    antitumor activity 1151
    cell dose 1152, *1152*
    GVHD/response 1151
    interferon-alpha 1152
    long-term survival 1152
    monitoring 1152–1153
    remission duration 1152
  complications 1013–1014
  EBV-PTLD 225
  GVHD incidence 1014
    reduction 226
  GVLE 372–373, 1156–1157
  HLA-matched 1155
  leukemia relapse 227, 387–388
  MDS relapse 1153, *1153*
  modifications 1155–1156, **1156**
    cytotoxic T cell depletion 1155–1156
    irradiation 1156
    plus interleukin-2 1156
    suicide gene-tranduction 1156
    T-cell depletion, selective 1156
    tumor-specific protein vaccination 1156
    in vitro cloning 1156
  multiple myeloma 1099, 1154
  renal cell carcinoma 1182
  solid tumors 1154
  toxicity 1154–1155
    GVHD 1154–1155
    pancytopenia 1155
    treatment-related mortality 1155
  unrelated donors 1155
  see also adoptive cellular immunotherapy/transfer
donor registries 624–631
  age limits 627
  confidentiality 630
  data 624
  development 1133
  Donor Centers 624–625
  ethical considerations 629–630
  history 624
  minorities 627, **627**
  recruitment 624–625, 625, 627, **627**
  retention of donors 627–628
    deferrals 628, **628**
    searching 628
      likelihood of finding match **627**

umbilical cord blood (UCB) registries 628–629, **629**
donor selection 449–462, 455–460, 538–540
  age 456–457
  eligibility criteria **456**
  ethnic background 457
  fertility 451
  GVHD 21
  HLA-partially matched unrelated HCT 39–40, 40, 1116–1118
    probability 1118
    vector of incompatibility 40, **40**
  immunology 21
  osteopetrosis 1449
  pediatric, considerations 458–460, **460**
    child development/compliance 460
    intensity-reduced regimens 459
    psychosocial issues 459–460
  pretransplant evaluation 459
    blood tests 538, 539
    cardiac evaluation 455–456
    crossmatching 1117–1118
    hepatic evaluation 456
    infections, previous 457
    laboratory tests 539–540
    nutritional status 456
    physical examination 539
    psychological assessment 457–458, **458**
    renal evaluation 456
    respiratory evaluation 456
    transfusion history 457
  procedure choice 451
  screening questionnaire 538
  second visit to transplant center 452
  survival 21
  treatment outcomes 453–457
    comorbid conditions 455–456
    compatibility effects 40–41
    data to present 451–452
    disease/remission status 453, *454*, 458–459
    donor-recipient compatibility 453–454
    genetic disparity 22–25
    performance status 455
  see also donor counseling
Donor Suitability rule, HCT regulation 532
do-not-resuscitate (DNR) 494
dormancy *272*, 282
dosimetry, radioimmunotherapy 201
Down syndrome patients
  AML treatment 1045
  childhood ALL, allogeneic transplants 1078–1079
  ethical issues 488
doxorubicin 164
  combination regimens **162**
    CHOP *see* CHOP regimen
    C-VAMP 1264
    cyclophosphamide/methylprednisolone/vincristine 1264
    cyclophosphamide/prednisone/vincristine *see* CHOP regimen

methylprednisolone/vincristine 1271
    VAMP regimen 1271
  cytoprotection 169
  cytotoxicity curves *132*
  mechanism of action 145–146
  pharmacology **131**, 146
    linear pharmacokinetics *136*, 146
  resistance 146
  structure *131*
  toxicity 146
drug(s)
  administration
    fixed rate infusion 903
    opioids 903–904
  complications 774–775
    diarrhea causing 789
    liver injury caused by 794
  dependence, treatment outcome 457–458
  dose, body weight 456
  metabolism of *see* drug metabolism
  pill esophagus 787
  resistance
    Bcl-2 role 264
    bone marrow purging 255
    dose-limiting toxicity 141
    gene therapy trials **120**, 123
    high-dose chemotherapy 132–133
    mechanisms **132**
  see also specific drugs
drug metabolism
  extensive *vs.* poor metabolizers 133
  genetics 133–135
    CYP2D6 (debrisoquin hydroxylase) 133
    cytochrome P450 2C subfamily 133–134
    cytochrome P450 3A subfamily 134
    ethnic variations 134
    genotype–phenotype relationship 133
    glutathione S-transferases (GST) 134
    multiple drug resistance gene 1 *(MDR1)* 123, *132*, 135
    see also pharmacogenomics
  hepatic/renal indices 137
  high-dose chemotherapy 135–138
  secondary malignancy 966
  see also pharmacokinetics
DSMB *see* Data/Safety Monitoring Board (DSMB)
d-TEC regimen, PBHC mobilization 1269
Duke University 463
Durie–Salmon staging system 1263
dyskeratosis congenita (DC) 1476
  aplastic anemia 990
  autologous GVHD 406
dysphagia, treatment complication 786–787
dysphoria, opioid side effects 901

E

EAE *see* experimental autoimmune encephalitis (EAE)
early-phase recovery *see* recovery
early thymic progenitors (ETPs) 79

Eastern Cooperative Oncology Group (ECOG) 1240
EBV *see* Epstein–Barr virus (EBV)
echinocandins 694–695
echovirus, liver infection 782
ECOG (Eastern Cooperative Oncology Group) 1240
economics
  gene therapy 122
  HCT 436, **436**, 436–438, **437**
  medical costs, direct *vs.* indirect 436
  T-cell depletion 224
educational information *see* information
elderly patients *see* age
electroencephalography (EEG), CNS infections *812*
ELISA (enzyme-linked immunosorbent assay) 675
  fungal infections 687
  varicella-zoster virus 741
embryo(s)
  hematopoiesis 53, 63, 74
  neuroblastoma 1333
  selection, ethical issues 492–493
  see also under fetus
embryonic stem cells (ES) 69, 74, 77, *77*
  ethical issues 493
EMBT *see* European Group for Blood/Marrow Transplantation (EMBT)
emotional distress
  pain 897–898
  pretransplant 499
emotional well-being, measures of **508**
encephalitis
  CMV 811
  herpes simplex 811–812
  varicella-zoster virus 812
encephalopathy
  drug-induced 815
  metabolic 813–814
endarteritis 813
endocrine functions
  delayed complications 948–949
  disruption 520
endothelial cells
  hematopoietic microenvironment 54–55
  transdifferentiation 77
energy requirements 885, **885**
engraftment 22
  allogeneic transplants
    PBHCs 592
    renal cell carcinoma therapy 1181, **1182**
  bacterial prophylaxis 667
  causes 22
  cells promoting 224–225
  documentation *see* chimerism, characterization
  manifestations 22
  nutritional support 884
  oral complications 911, **912**
  osteopetrosis 1449
  prevention 22

engraftment (cont.)
    risk 22
    thalassemia, bone marrow transplant 1411
    see also posttransplant
engraftment syndrome (ES) 877
enteral therapy 886–887
    complications 888
    parenteral therapy vs. 886
enteritis
    abdominal pain 789
    autologous transplants, AML 1223–1224
enteritis, CMV-associated 708–709
Enterococcal infections 674–675
enterovirus infections 764
enzyme-linked immunosorbent assay see
        ELISA (enzyme-linked
        immunosorbent assay)
EORTC QTC 441, *442*
eosinophils, development of *614*
ependymomas 1347–1348
    chemotherapy (high-dose) with HCT 1348,
        1348
    natural history with conventional therapy
        1347–1348
epigeneic transplantation see allogeneic
        transplantation
epipodophyllotoxins see etoposide (VP16)
epistasis, autoimmune diseases 328
epitope spreading, autoimmunity 328
Epstein–Barr virus (EBV)
    biology 749–750
    infection see Epstein–Barr virus (EBV)
        infections
    latent expression 749–750
    reactivation post-HCT 385, 733
    transfusion transmitted 845
    viral transcripts 749
Epstein–Barr virus-associated
        lymphoproliferative disorder
        (EBV-LPD) 385, 750–753
    abdominal 791
    clinical features 385, 751–752
    delayed complications 953
    diagnosis 752
    following T-cell depletion 225
    HLA-partially matched related HCT 1123
    incidence *750*, 750–752
    liver symptoms 784
    risks 750–752, **751**
    treatment 752–753
        response *752*
        see also Epstein–Barr virus (EBV)
            infections, T-cell therapy
    virological aspects 752
Epstein–Barr virus (EBV) infections 749–756
    acyclovir 749
    associated malignancies 385
        HCT 753
    following T-cell depletion 225
        HLA-partially matched related HCT 1123
        strategy 225
    immune response 750, *750*

in immunosuppression 749–750
lymphoproliferative disorder see
        Epstein–Barr virus-associated
        lymphoproliferative disorder
        (EBV-LPD)
    oral 920
    Reed–Sternberg cells 387
Epstein–Barr virus (EBV) infections, T-cell
        therapy 380, 385–387, 1156
    clinical trials 386–387
        as prophylaxis 387
        selected cells 386
        unselected cells 386
    donor frequency/specificity 386
        cytotoxic T-cells 386
        helper T-cells 386
    EBV-LPV 386, 387
    future work 387
    history 385
    rationale 385–386
erectile dysfunction 525–256
E-rosetting, sickle cell disease 1432–1434
erythrocytes
    antigens, chimerism evaluation 234–235
    components 833
    development 79, 80, *614*
    disorders **118**
    transfusions 833
        leukocyte depleted **833**, 833–834, **834**
        sickle cell disease 1420, **1420**
        thalassemia 1409
        washed 834
erythroderma, autologous GVHD 406
erythropoietin, in hematopoiesis *614*
erythropoietin, recombinant 613–615, **614**
    after allogeneic transplants 613–615
    after autologous transplants 613
    G-CSF combination 613
    GM-CSF combination 613
    multiple myeloma therapy 1265
ES see embryonic stem cells (ES)
ESHAP regimen, low-grade lymphoma therapy
        1107–1108
esophagus
    acute GVHD 787
    infections 786–787
    long-term complications 795
    pill 787
    pretransplant conditioning, toxicity 287
essential thrombocythemia (ET)
    definition 1090
    HCT 1090
essential tremor, drug-induced 815
esthesioneuroblastoma 1361–1362
The Estrogen Decision 525
etanercept, mechanism of action/targets
        218
ethical issues 488–497
    alternative stem cell sources 492–494
    children 490, 492–493
    confidentiality 491
    consent 489–490

donors 490–491, 540
    registries 629–630
embryo selection 492–493
end-of-life issues 494–495
noncoercion 491
nonmalignant disease 493–494
paternity 490–491
patient choice 488–489
payment 488–489
ethnicity
    donors 627, **627**
    HLA genes 1133–1135
    treatment access 443–444
    treatment outcome 457
etoposide (VP16) 164
    astrocytoma 1347
    autologous transplants AML 1223
    bone marrow purging 256
    combination regimens **161**, **162**
        asparaginase/cisplatin/cytarabine/
            dexamethasone 1198
        BCNU/cyclophosphamide see CBV regimen
        BCNU/cyclophosphamide/cytarabine see
            BEAC regimen
        BEAC see BEAC regimen
        busulfan see busulfan (BU), combination
            regimens
        busulfan/TBI combination **1222**
        carboplatin/ifosfamide see ICE regimen
        CBV see CBV regimen
        cisplatin/corticosteroids/cytarabine
            1107–1108
        cisplatin/cyclophosphamide/
            dexamethasone 1269
        cyclophosphamide/melphalan/
            mitoxantrone combination 1267
        cyclophosphamide/TBI see
            cyclophosphamide (CY),
            combination regimens
        ifosfamide/methotrexate/
            mitoxantrone 1107–1108
    TBI **160**
        ALL 1062
        allogeneic transplants, childhood ALL
            1074
        autologous transplants, ALL 1241
        autologous transplants, AML 1223
    germ cell tumor 1311, **1312–1313**
    high-dose chemotherapy 144–145, 191
    mechanism of action 144–145
    metabolism 134
    MTD **159**
    pharmacology **131**, 145
    resistance 145
    structure *131*
    toxicity 145
        neurotoxicity 818
ETPs (early thymic progenitors) 79
euphoria, opioid side effects 901
EUROCORD 438, 551
    childhood ALL, cord blood transplants
        1077–1078

European Bone Marrow Transplant Myeloma
    Registry 1267
European Group for Blood/Marrow
    Transplantation (EMBT) 438
  allogeneic transplants, PBHC 588
    chronic GVHD 593
    survival rates 593
  autoimmune disease treatment **1387**
  autologous transplants, ALL 1240
  autologous transplants, AML
    allogeneic vs. autologous in first remission
        1230
    first remission 1230
    PBHCs 1225
    second remission 1228
    survival rates 1224
  CLL therapy studies 1106, 1107
  cord blood guidelines 551
  lymphoma therapy studies 1106
  multiple myeloma therapy 1096, **1097**
  Registry 438
  voluntary accreditation/regulation 533
European League Against Rheumatism
    (EULAR) **1387**
European Organization for Research/Treatment
    of Cancer
  Gruppo Italiano Malattie Ematologische
      Maligne dell'Adulto, multiple
      myeloma studies 1266–1267
  Quality of Life Questionnaire-C30 (EORTC
      QLQ-C30) 513
    subscales **514**
eutectic point 601
event-free survival (EFS) see *individual*
    diseases/disorders; individual
    treatments
evidence-based medicine
  grades of recommendation **441**
  levels of evidence **441**
  outcomes research 440–441
  study cycle 414
  see also outcomes research
Ewing's sarcoma 1354–1357
  conventional therapy 1354–1355
  HCT as consolidation 1355–1357
  metastatic 1356–1357
  relapsed/refractory 1355, **1355**
  risk groups 1354–1355
  survival 1355
experimental autoimmune encephalitis (EAE)
    326t, 329–330
  allogeneic transplants 335
  autologous HCT 333–334
  syngeneic HCT 334
extracellular matrix (ECM), components 55
extrahepatic biliary obstruction 784
extraocular muscles, weakness following HCT
    818–819
extrathymic pathways, immune reconstitution
    1121
extrinsic regulators, HSC expansion studies
    98–99

ex vivo expansion
  autologous transplants in CML 1251, **1252**
  cord blood cells (CBCs) 555, 556–557,
      558
eye(s)
  cataracts see cataracts
  chronic GVHD 647
  delayed complications 950
  radiotherapy shielding 184
  radiotherapy toxicity 188–189

F
Fab/F(ab')$_2$ fragments, radioimmunotherapy
    200
facilitator cells (FCs) 84–85
FACT see Foundation for the Accreditation of
    Cellular Therapy (FACT)
FACT-BMT (Functional Assessment of Cancer
    Therapy-Bone Marrow Transplant)
    513
famciclovir, varicella-zoster virus infections
    743–744
family issues
  pediatric transplant 459–460
  vaccinations 865, **868**
FANC genes 1486
Fanconi anemia 1483–1504
  aplastic anemia 990
  clinical features 1483–1485, *1485*
    congenital abnormalities **1484**
    growth features 1484
    hematologic abnormalities 1484
    infertility 1484
  complementation groups *1485*, 1486–1489,
      1488
    assignment 1486–1487
    genotype–phenotype correlations 1488
    mutation analysis 1486–1487
    somatic mosaicism 1488–1489
  diagnostic tests 1485–1486
  differential diagnosis 1483
  gene cloning 1486–1489
    proposed functions 1487–1488
  genes, proposed functions 1487–1488
  hematopoietic growth factor production
      1490
  history 1483
  leukemogenesis 1489–1490
  marrow failure mechanisms 1489–1490
  murine models 1490
  nonmyeloablative therapy 1173
  pathogenesis *1487*
  preimplantation genetic diagnosis 1500
  treatment 1490–1491
    androgens 1490–1491
    antioxidants 1491
    future work 1499–1500
    gene therapy 125, 1499–1500
    HCT see Fanconi anemia, HCT
    hemopoietic growth factors 1491
    multipotent adult stem cells (MASC)
        1500

  supportive care 1491
  thoracoabdominal irradiation 192
  in utero transplantation 573
Fanconi anemia, HCT 1491–1500
  alternative donor 1494–1497
    clinical trials 1495–1497
    survival rates *1497*
  conditioning therapies 1491–1493
  HLA-identical sibling donor 1491–1494
    AML treatment **1495**
    bone marrow failure 1491–1493
    leukemia 1493–1494
    MDS 1493–1494, **1495**
    nonradiation cytoablation **1494**
    radiation cytoablation **1493**
    relapse rates 1494
  secondary malignancies 1497–1499
    relative risk *1498*
    risk factors **1498**
  survival rates *1493*
  treatment algorithm *1498*
Farber disease 1465
Fas ligand
  adoptive T-cell immunotherapy 396
  expression
    interferon-gamma 356–357
    tumor necrosis factor-α 356–357
  GVHD 356
fatigue
  biological mechanisms 510
  quality of life issues 509–510
fat malabsorption 789
Federal Food, Drug/Cosmetic Act (FDCA) 531
female(s)
  gonadal function following HCT 938–939
  hypothalamic-pituitary-gonad axis 522
  physiological/biological changes 522–523
  sexual dysfunction 522–523
    puberty following HCT **936**
    treatment 525
fentanyl, pain management 903
fertility see infertility
fetus
  hematopoiesis 53, *63*, 74–76, *75*, 80–81,
      566, *566*
    blood 75
    lineage commitment 80–81
    liver *63*, 74–75
    thymus 75, 79–80, 565
  immunological tolerance 565–566
  thymic organ cultures 76
  in utero transplantation see *in utero*
      transplantation (IU-HCT)
fever
  causes after engraftment **671**
  treatment strategies 671–674, *673*
FFP (fresh frozen plasma), transfusions 834
fibroblast growth factor 7 (FGF-7) see
    keratinocyte growth factor
fibroblasts 54
fibronectin 577
  hematopoietic microenvironment 55

filgrastim
  adverse events 543
    serious 544
  clinical trials 615, 616
  PBHC donation 545
  see also granulocyte colony-stimulating factor (G-CSF), recombinant; lenograstim
financial coordinator 466–467
FISH see fluorescence in situ hybridization (FISH)
FK506 see tacrolimus (FK506)
FLIC see The Functional Living Index–Cancer (FLIC)
flossing 916
flow cytometry
  ALL 275
  CMV-specific T-cells 381–382
  disadvantages 275
  residual disease detection **273**
  tumor cell detection, sensitivity 244t
Flt ligand, PBHC mobilization 577, **582**, 582, 589
fluconazole **693**, 694
  clinical studies **691**
  fungal infections 690, 1144
fludarabine
  autoimmune animal models 333
  CLL therapy 1107
  combination regimens
    ATG/busulfan see antithymocyte globulin (ATG), combination regimens
    ATG/thiotepa 1119
    busulfan 1171–1172
    busulfan/Campath 1088–1089
    Campath 1$_M$/melphalan see Campath 1$_M$, combination regimens
    CHOP 1107
    cyarabine/idarubicin see cyarabine/fludarabine/idarubicin combination
    cyclophosphamide see cyclophosphamide, combination regimens
    dexamethasone/mitoxantrone 1107–1108
    FND 1107–1108
    melphalan 1100
    TBI
      acute GVHD *1171*
      hematologic malignancy studies 1170
      melanoma therapy 1184
      multiple myeloma 1098–1099, 1102, 1170
      neutrophil/platelet changes *1170*
      non-Hodgkin's lymphoma 1170
      retrospective studies 1172
    TBI, low dose 1174
    thiotepa 1182
  Fanconi anemia HCT 1493
  neurotoxicity 818
fluorescence in situ hybridization (FISH)
  ALL cytogenetics 1239
  chimerism evaluation 235, *235*
    recurrent malignancies **238**
  clinical applications 272, 274
  CLL chromosomal aberrations 1106
  flow 65
  hypermetaphase 274
  limitations 274
  minimal residual disease detection 1150
  multiple myeloma diagnosis 1262
  probes 273
  quantitative 65
  residual disease detection 272–275, **273**, *274*
  secondary malignancy prognosis 968
  sensitivity 274
  telomere measurement 65
  tumor cell detection, sensitivity 244t
fluorescent-antibody staining of membrane antigen (FAMA) 741
FND regimen, low-grade lymphoma therapy 1107–1108
foamy virus-based vectors 112–113
focus groups 441
follicular lymphoma
  autologous transplants 1211–1212, **1212**
  DLI in relapse 1153
follow-up recommendations **956**
Food/Drug Administration (FDA), HCT regulation 531–532
foreign patient counseling 453
foscarnet
  CMV infection 713, 1123
  varicella-zoster virus infections 744
Foundation for the Accreditation of Cellular Therapy (FACT) 532–536, 551
  Accreditation Manual 533
  Accreditation Program 534–536, *535*
    annual report 535
    application 535
    common deficiencies 536
    Inspectors **535**
    on-site inspection 535–536
    potential outcomes **536**
    registration 534–535
    renewal 535
    review 535
  historical background 532–533
  standards 533–534
  Transplant Essential Data (TED) 534
Foundation for the Accreditation of hematopoietic Cell Therapy (FAHCT) see Foundation for the Accreditation of Cellular Therapy (FACT)
4-1BB marker, antigen presentation 355
fractionated radiotherapy see radiotherapy regimens
Fred Hutchinson Cancer Research Center
  body weight/treatment outcome 456
  infant ALL, allogeneic transplants 1078
  survival rates 944
free light chain (FLC) assay 1285, *1285*, 1293
freezing see cryopreservation

French-American-British (FAB) Cooperative Group
  ALL classification 1055
  AML classification 1040
  AML prognosis 1222
  MDS definition 1084, **1085**
French Bone Marrow Transplant Group Registry 1109
French Cooperative Group IFM90 1271–1272, **1272**
French Group on Therapy for Adult ALL 1060, **1060**
fresh frozen plasma (FFP), transfusions 834
frizzled (Fzd), Wnt signaling 72, *72*
fucosidosis 1463
full chimerism 234
fulminant viral hepatitis 773
Functional Assessment of Cancer Therapy–Bone Marrow Transplant (FACT-BMT) 513
Functional Assessment of Chronic Illness Therapies (FACT) 441, *442*, 443
The Functional Living Index–Cancer (FLIC) 513
  subscales **514**
fungal infections
  AML autologous transplants 1232
  emerging pathogens 684
  esophagus 786
  liver 783
    chronic 794–795
  oral 919
  pretransplant conditioning 689
  therapy, fluconazole 1144
  see also invasive fungal infections (IFIs)
Fungizone 692–694, **693**
  clinical studies **691**
  disadvantages 690

G
gallbladder, treatment complications 783–784
gallstones 774
  long-term complications 795
gamma camera, radioimmunotherapy dosimetry 201, *203*
gamma irradiation see radiation
ganciclovir
  CMV infection 381, 706–708, 713, 1123
  introduction 1144
  problems of universal therapy 711
  varicella-zoster virus infections 744
gangliosidoses 1464
gastric antral vascular ectasia (GAVE) 785
gastric motility disorders 775
gastrointestinal/hepatic complications 769–810, 775–786
  cytoreductive therapy, problems before 769–774
    fungal infections 770–771
    hepatic fibrosis/cirrhosis 773–774
    hepatitis 771–773
    infections 769–770

inflammatory bowel disease 769
   stones 774
   ulcers/tumors 769
  delayed/long term 952
   malignancy 794
  GVHD *290*, 290–292
   colon *289*
   diagnosis difficulties 290
   differential diagnosis 291–292
   histopathology 288–289, *288–290*
   infections 289
   sequence of damage 289
   treatment 210
  hepatomegaly 775–786
  infarction 791
  infections 769–770, 775
   bacterial 783
   diarrhea 788–789
   EBV-LPD 791
   fungal 770–771, 783
    chronic 794–795
   mucosal 785, 791
   viral 781
  long-term 792–793
  malignancy 784
  opioids, side effects 901
  perforation 791
  posttransplant lymphoproliferative disease *291*
  pseudo-obstruction 789–790
  recovery period, first 6 months 774–792
   abdominal pain 789–792
   abnormal liver tests 775–784
   acute GVHD 774
   bleeding 784–786
   diarrhea 787–789
   dysphagia 786–787
   infections 775
   long-term survivors 792–795
   medication/parenteral nutrition 774–775
   motility disorders 775
   nausea 774
   peri-anal pain 792
 gastrointestinal (GI) tract
  acyclovir toxicity 743
  damage *see* graft-*vs*.-host disease (GVHD)
  presentation of amyloidosis 1287
  thiotepa toxicity 141
  transdifferentiation **77**
 gastrostomy feeding 886
 gastrulation 74
 Gaucher's disease 1463
  gene therapy 125
  nonmyeloablative therapy 1174
 GAVE (gastric antral vascular ectasia) 785
 GCRC (General Clinical Research Center) 122
 G-CSF *see* granulocyte colony-stimulating factor (G-CSF)
 GeMCRIS (Genetic Modification Clinical Research Information System) 425

gemtuzumab
  AML treatment in children 1046
  SOS 287–288, 778
gender
  mismatching, GVHD 637
  quality of life issues 512
gene(s)
  cloning, Fanconi anemia 1486–1489
  duplication, HLA evolution 43
  expression
   analysis 82–83
    microarrays *see* microarray(s)
   control 82
   molecular inhibition *see* nucleic acid based therapies
  polymorphisms
   acute GVHD 638
   chronic GVHD 647
   HLAs 1133–1135
gene expression profiling, secondary malignancy 967
general anesthetic 908
General Clinical Research Center (GCRC) 122
gene therapy 118–129
  antisense oligonucleotides *see* antisense oligonucleotides
  clinical trials using HCT **120**, 121–126
   adenosine deaminase-deficient SCID 557
   adverse events 125–126
   congenital immune deficiencies 123–124
   design 423
   drug resistance transfer **120**, 123
   Fanconi anemia 125
   gene expression control 120–121
   HIV-1 infection 125
   lysosomal storage diseases 125
   pathway **121**
   practical issues 121–122
   promise 126
   see also gene therapy
  cord blood cells 557
  costs 122
  cytoreductive conditioning and 121
  early stopping rules 423
  Fanconi anemia treatment 1499–1500
  future directions 126–127
  gene augmentation 122
  gene correction 127
  gene replacement 122
  gene silencing, therapeutic potential 258
  gene transfer methods *see* gene transfer
  HIV infection *see* AIDS, gene therapy
  immunogenicity 121
  production of clinical grade vectors 122
  severe adverse event reporting 425
  sickle cell disease 1436
  targets **118**, 118–119
   hemoglobinopathies 126–127
   ongoing trials *425*
  transgene expression 120–121
  see also nucleic acid based therapies; *specific disorders*

genetically different transplant *see* allogeneic transplantation
genetically identical transplant *see* autologous transplantation
genetic data
  clinical trial conduct 424–425
  clinical trial designs 422
  ethical considerations 424
  information systems 426
  observational study designs 416
genetic disease(s) **118**
  gene therapy *see* gene therapy
  gene transfer *see* gene transfer
  HSC transplantation 118
  see also individual diseases
genetic marker studies
  applications 239
  biologic insights 239
  see also chimerism, characterization
Genetic Modification Clinical Research Information System (GeMCRIS) 425
genetic susceptibility, secondary malignancy 966–967
genetic tags 122
  clinical trials using HSCs **120**, 122
  retroviral vectors 119
genetic testing, clinical trial design 422–423
gene transfer 107–117, 119–120
  animal xenograft models 111
  committed clonogenic cells 113–114
  ex vivo HSC transduction 119, **119**
  genes introduced 107
  hematopoietic target cells
   sources 113
   viral contact 109–110
  historical background 107
  implications/outlook 114
  infection protocols 109
  pseudotype vectors 110
  receptor binding 110
  retroviral vectors 107–109, *109*, 119–120
   alternatives 111–113
   colocalization with target cell *110*, 110–111
   Fanconi anemia trials 125
   genome integration 119, 126
   HIV based 112, 126
   lentiviruses 111–112, **120**, 126
   primary immune deficiencies 124
  selection strategies 111
  sources of hematopoietic target cells 113
  target cell/viral contact 109–110
  threshold levels 119, **119**
  toxicology 111
  viral vectors 119–120
   adeno-associated virus 113
   foamy virus 112–113
   genome integration 119
    problems associated 126
   herpes virus 113
   production of clinical grade 122
   properties **112**

gene transfer
  viral vectors (cont.)
    pseudotypes 110
    receptor binding 110
    retroviruses see above
    see also individual viruses
genitourinary complications 951–952
  opioids, side effects 901
genome mapping 422
genotype–phenotype relationships, drug metabolism 133
germ cell tumor(s) 1308–1319
  autologous transplants 1311
  chemotherapy
    conventional dose **1309**, **1317**
    high-dose **1310**, 1311–1314, 1314–1317, *1317*
  multivariate analysis 1314
  prognosis **1310**, 1314, **1314**, **1317**
  radiographic abnormalities 1309–1310
  recurrent 1311–1314, **1312–1313**
  salvage therapy
    conventional 1310
    initial 1314–1317, **1315–1316**
    initiation of 1308–1310
  sites 1308
  staging **1308**, **1309**
  treatment
    chemotherapy see above
    conventional **1309**
    future directions 1317
    salvage therapy see above
  tumor markers 1309
GIMEMA see Gruppo Italiano Malattie Ematologische Maligne dell'Adulto (GIMEMA)
GITMO (Gruppo Italiano Trapianti de Midollo Osseo) 1483
glass-transition temperature (Tg) 601
GLD (globoid-cell leukodystrophy) 1462–1463
Gleevac™ see imatinib mesylate (Gleevac®)
α-globin gene therapy 126–127
β-globin gene therapy 126–127
  transgene expression 120, 126
globoid-cell leukodystrophy (GLD) 1462–1463
glomerular filtration rate (GFR), carboplatin monitoring 137
glucocorticoid(s) see corticosteroids
glucose, cryoprotection 604
glutamine 890
glutathione S-transferases (GST) 134
glycerol, cryoprotection 600–601
glycoprotein disorders **1457–1458**, 1463–1465
glycosaminoglycan(s), hematopoietic microenvironment 55
GMALL, ALL autologous transplants 1241–1242
  PBHC purging 1245
GM-CSF see granulocyte macrophage colony-stimulating factor (GM-CSF)
GOELAL 02 trial, ALL autologous transplants 1240–1241

gonads
  damage 520
  delayed complications 949, 952
  following HCT 935, 937–939, **938**
    HLA-identical related transplant 990–991
  sickle cell disease 1423–1424
Good Manufacturing Practice (GMP), gene therapy trials 122
GRACE (Group for the Collection/Expansion of Hematopoietic Cells) 551
graft failure
  chimerism characterization 238
  HLA class I genes 1136, **1137–1138**, 1138
  HLA class II genes 1136, **1137–1138**, 1138
  HLA-partially matched related HCT
    posttransplant immunosuppression 1119
    sensitization 1119
    T-cell depleted HCT 1122
    T-replete marrow grafts **1118**, 1118–1119
  HLA typing 1136–1138, 1138
graft rejection
  aplastic anemia 982, 985–991
    incidence *982, 986*
  causes 22
  conditioning regimens 985–987
  histocompatibility see histocompatibility
  HLA see histocompatibility; HLA
  late 982
  mHA 40
  natural killer cell mediated 22
  overcoming 985
  presentation 22
  prevention 22
  primary 982
  reduction 985
  risk 22
  T-cell mediated 22
  tolerance development 24–25
graft-vs.-host disease (GVHD) 635–664
  allogeneic transplants
    ALL 1062
    AML, childhood 1045
    CML, GVLE vs. 1141, 1151–1152
    cord blood cell transplantation 101, 553
      cytokine involvement 558
    GVLE association 371–372, *372*
    HLA-partially matched related 1119–1120, *1120*
    multiple myeloma 1098, 1101
    PBHC **592**
    renal cell carcinoma 1180–1181, 1182
    in utero transplantation 567–568, 571–572
  animal models 344–352
    interleukin-11 effects 621
    mHA 347–349
      CD4+ cell role 348–349
      CD8+ cell role 348, *348*, **349**
      features 348
      GVLE, separation from 349–350
      immunopathology 350
      targets 347–348

    MHC antigens class I 346
      CD4+ cells 347
      donor marrow plus CD8+ cells 346
    MHC antigens class II 345–346
      in nonirradiated hosts 347
    pathogenesis 344
    susceptibility 345
    target antigens 344
  autologous transplants 405–413, 636
    clinical studies 407–409
    cyclosporine induction 405, 406, *406*, 407–408, **408**, *409*
    effector mechanisms 408–409
    GVLE relationship 409–410
    mechanisms 405–409
    multiple myeloma 1101
    preclinical studies/animal models 405–407
    relationship with 409–410
    T-cell repertoire 408–409
  background 635
  chimerism characterization 239
  clinical features 23
    cataracts and 188
    gastrointestinal tract see gastrointestinal/hepatic complications
    liver 290, 290–292
      differential diagnosis 291–292
      histological consequences 290
    PNH 1003
  cytokine storm 23
  DLI toxicity 1154–1155
  donor effects 21
  GVLE 1177
  history 635
  HLA 1139–1141
    class I genes 1140
    class II genes 1139–1140
    typing **1135**, 1139–1141
  hyperacute 638
  immune reconstitution 25–26, 857–858, *858*
    T-cells *858*
  incidence, identical sibling transplant *13*
  initial description 4
  misdiagnosis 740
  neurological complications **819**
    CNS infection 811
    relationship 818
  oral 294, 921–922, **922**
    assessment 923
  pathogenesis/pathophysiology 353–368, *354*, 635, *635*
    alloreactivity 635
    antigen presenting cells 353–354
    cell-mediated cytotoxin mechanisms 23
    cellular effectors 356–357
    cytotoxic T cells 344
    dendritic cells 355
    donor T-cells
      activation 353–355
      cytokine secretion 355–356

effector phase 23
Fas/FasL pathway 356
helper T-cells 345, 355
inflammatory cytokines 353, 358
inflammatory effectors 357
initiation 22
interferon-gamma 355
interleukin-1 353, 357
interleukin-2 355
interleukin-6 361
interleukin-8 361
lipopolysaccharide 357–358
macrophages 357
microbial environment 636
natural killer cells 345
nitrous oxide 357
nutritional effects 889
perforin/granzyme pathway 356
preconditioning effects 353
pretransplant conditioning effects 23
TBI 353
T-cells 221
tumor necrosis factor-α 353, 357
pathology 288–294
　histopathology
　　gastrointestinal 289–290
　　liver *290*, 290–292
　　pulmonary 296–297
　　skin 288, *289*
　immunohistology 292–294
prevention 16, 311–312, 312–314, 358–361, 987
　in AML 1027–1028
　in CML 1011
　conditioning regimen reduction 359
　delayed T-cell administration 313–314
　donor T cell modulation 359–361
　　activation reduction 359–360
　　number reduction 359
　　proliferation reduction 360
　　tolerance induction 360–361
　　see also tolerance, induced
　helper T-cells
　　subset balance 312–313
　　transplantation 356
　immunostimulatory cytokine blocking 313, 361
　immunosuppression 358
　induced tolerance *see* tolerance, induced
　intravenous immunoglobulin 643
　microbiological load reduction 358
　T-cell depletion (TCD) *see* T-cell depletion (TCD)
　T-cell modification 227
　transfusion-associated 636–637, 840, 841
pulmonary 296–297
risk 23
sickle cell disease 1432, 1433
skin *see* skin
syngeneic 362
tolerance 636

transfusion-associated 636
treatment 4, 23
　anti-T-cell antibodies 359
　ATG 216, 360
　Campath 1$_M$ *see* Campath 1$_M$
　CTLA-4-Ig 360–361
　cyclophosphamide *see* cyclophosphamide (CY)
　cyclosporine *see* cyclosporine (CSP)
　immunosuppression *see* immunosuppression, GVHD
　infliximab 361
　interleukin-1 receptor antagonist 361
　intravenous immunoglobulin 215–216, 858
　methotrexate *see* methotrexate (MTX)
　mycophenolate mofetil 360
　opioids 906
　prednisolone 360, 650
　regimens **211**
　sirolimus (rapamycin) 360
　skin 906
　tacrolimus (FK506) 23, 359–360
　T-cell anergy induction 217, 227
T regulatory cells (Tregs) 356
vaccinations 858
vaginal 523
varicella-zoster reactivation post HCT 733, **734**
graft-*vs.*-host disease (GVHD), acute 22–24, 637–646, 987–988
　abdominal 790
　age 637
　cell dose 638
　cell source 637–638
　clinical features 638–639, 1119
　　diarrhea 787–788
　　esophagus 787
　　gastrointestinal tract 638–639, 774, 780, 785
　　liver 780
　cytokines 638
　defined 635
　diagnosis 639–640
　differential diagnosis 639–640
　donor-host factors 637, 640–641
　gene polymorphisms 638
　grading 443, **639**, 639–640, **640**
　HLA-partial matched donor HCT *1120*
　incidence *637*, 637–638
　PBHC allogeneic transplants 592–593
　predictive factors 637–638
　prevention 640–643
　　antibody prophylaxis 643
　　cryopreserved cells 608
　　marrow T-cell depletion 643
　prognosis 645–646
　risk factors 1119–1120
　　sex mismatching 637
　severity 639–640, *640*, **640**, *641*, 645, *646*
　survival in aplastic anemia 987, *987*

treatment 210, 643–645
　immunomodulation 638
　immunosuppression
　　combined 641, 643
　　randomized controlled trials **642**
　　single-agent 641
　primary 643–645, **644**
　salvage regimens 645
　secondary 645
　supportive care 645
graft-*vs.*-host disease (GVHD), chronic 24, 361–362, 646–654, 945
　cell source 646–647
　classification **649**
　clinical features 647, *648*
　　gastrointestinal tract 647, 648, 793
　　liver *291*, 793
　　meningitis 811
　cytokines 361–362, 647
　defined 635
　diagnosis 649
　donor-host factors 646, *646*
　gene polymorphisms 647
　grading 443, 649, *650*
　HLA-partially matched related HCT 1120
　immune abnormalities 858
　immunodeficiency 653
　incidence 646–647
　　HLA-identical siblings 988
　late infections 653, *653*
　mortality/morbidity 654, **946**, 988, *989*
　pathogenesis 646
　pathology
　　histopathology 292–294, *293*
　　immunohistology 292–294
　PBHC allogeneic transplants 593, **593**
　predictive factors 646–647
　prevention 649–650
　　antibody prophylaxis 649–650
　　antimicrobial prophylaxis 653
　　T-cell depletion 649
　prognosis 654, **654**
　　death 988
　quality of life 654
　solid tumor development 988
　staging 649, **649**
　thymic factors 649
　treatment 210, 650–653
　　immunomodulation 647
　　immunosuppression 650
　　　prolonged 650
　　　trials **651**
　　primary 650–651, *651*
　　secondary 652, *652*
　　supportive care 652–653
　vaccinations 653
graft-*vs.*-leukemia effect (GVLE) 24, 226, 369–379
　allogeneic transplants
　　ALL 1062
　　AML, childhood 1045
　　animal models 370, 1157

graft-vs.-leukemia effect (GVLE)
  allogeneic transplants (cont.)
    CML 1012–1013
      GVHD vs. 1141, 1151–1152
      DLI remission 372–373
      GVHD association 371–372, 372
      HLA-partially matched related 1120–1121
      Hodgkin's disease 1200–1201
      immunosuppression cessation/remission association 371
      PBHC 593
      relapse rate 371, 371, 372, 372
    application in relapse see donor lymphocyte infusion (DLI)
    autologous transplants
      ALL 1238
      ALL, childhood 410
      AML 1225–1226, 1233
    DLI 1156–1157
    effector cells 373–374, 1157
      cytotoxic T-cells 388
      natural killer cells 1185
    evidence 1012
      adoptive cellular immunotherapy 370–371
      animal models 369–370
    future work 375
    GVHD 1177
      absence of 226
      animal models 349–350
      association 371–372, 372
    HLA typing 1141
    induction of 374–375
    mechanisms 1157
    solid tumors see solid tumors, allogeneic transplants
    targets 373–374
    see also graft-vs.-tumor effect (GVTE)
graft-vs.-tumor effect (GVTE) 369–379
  allogeneic transplants 371–373
    DLI remission 372–373
    GVHD association 371–372, 372
    Hodgkin's disease 1200–1201
    immunosuppression cessation/remission association 371
    relapse rate 371, 371, 372, 372
  evidence
    adoptive cellular immunotherapy 370–371
    animal models 369–370
  history 1164
  neuroblastoma 1338
  susceptible diseases 1167
  see also graft-vs.-leukemia effect (GVLE)
granulocyte(s)
  development 79, 80
  disorders 1471–1472, 1474–1480
  system 1471–1472
  transfusions 839
    bacterial infection 678
    reactions 843

granulocyte colony-stimulating factor (G-CSF)
  ALL, PBHC 1063
  allogeneic transplants relapse management 1158
  autoimmunity and 817
  bone marrow donation 594
  cord blood transplantation 555–556
  cytarabine combination, AML relapse 1153
  cytoprotection 168, 168
  in Fanconi anemia 1490, 1491
  in hematopoiesis 614
  immunosuppressive effects 1124
  in murine models 617–618
  neutrophils, stimulation of 590, 592
  pancytopenia therapy 1155
  PBHC mobilization 577, 1098
    chemotherapy combination vs. 580
    CHOP regimen 1269
    clinical trials 582
    cyclophosphamide combination 1269
    DCEP regimen combination 1269
    doses 579, 588–589
    GM-CSF vs. 578, 578–579, 579
    GM-CSF with 589
    interleukin-2 combination 579–580
    interleukin-3 combination 579
    introduction 588
    multiple myeloma autologous transplants 1267, 1269
    standard regimens 582
    stem cell factor combination 579
  recombinant 614, 615–618
    after allogeneic transplants 617
    after autologous transplants 615–617
    clinical trials 615–617, 616
    cyclosporine/prednisolone combination 617
    erythropoietin combination 613
    GM-CSF vs. 618
    recombinant interleukin-3 combination 619–620
    side effects 615
    timing of treatment 617
    see also filgrastim; lenograstim
  side effects 590–591, 594
  toxicity 590
  type 2 cytokine production 590
granulocyte macrophage colony-stimulating factor (GM-CSF)
  adoptive T-cell immunotherapy 395
  allogeneic transplants 619
  autologous transplants 618–619
  CML 1251
  cytoprotection 168, 168
  in Fanconi anemia 1490, 1491
  functions 618
    in hematopoiesis 614
  hypersensitivity in JMML 1019
  PBHC mobilization 577
    chemotherapy combination vs. 580
    cyclosporine combination vs. 580

    doses 579
    G-CSF vs. 578, 578–579, 579
    G-CSF with 589
    interleukin-3 combination 579
    multiple myeloma autologous transplants 1267
    standard regimens 582
  posttransplant antileukemic treatment 1255–1256
  recombinant 614, 618–619
    clinical trials 618, 619
    erythropoietin combination 613
    G-CSF vs. 618
    interleukin-3 combination 620
    see also sargramostim
  treatment of JMML 1019
granulocytopenia, transfusions 839
Graves' disease, HLA associations 324t, 327
Griscelli syndrome (GS) 1479
GROβ, PBHC mobilization 577, 582
"ground glass" chest X ray, radiation pneumonopathy 186
Groupe Française de Cytogenetique Hematologique, multiple myeloma staging 1263
Group for the Collection/Expansion of Hematopoietic Cells (GRACE) 551
growth/development after HCT 929–943
  chemotherapy 930, 932, 935–937
    men 938
    women 938, 938
  gonadal function 937–939
    ovaries 935, 937–939
    testes 935
  height 934
  HLA-identical related transplant 991
  irradiation effects see radiotherapy, growth/development following
  Leydig cell damage 937
  orofacial growth 934, 934
  pregnancy 939
  puberty 935–937, 936, 937
  sickle cell disease 1423–1424
  thyroid function 929–934, 930
growth factors
  adverse events 543, 544
  bacterial infection 677–678
  clinically available 614
  Fanconi anemia treatment 1490, 1491
  functions 614
  fungal infections 695–696
  HSC expansion studies 96–99
  pain management 906
  recombinant 613–623
  use 545
  see also specific types
growth hormone (GH)
  deficiency following irradiation 932, 932–934, 934
  therapy 932–933, 933

Gruppo Italiano Malattie Ematologische
   Maligne dell'Adulto (GIMEMA)
   ALL prognostic factors 1239
   AML autologous transplants 1230
Gruppo Italiano Trapianti de Midolio Osseo
   (GITMO) 1483
GST (glutathione S-transferases) 134
guanine arabinoside (ARA-G), bone marrow
   purging 256
Guillain–Barré syndrome, following HCT 815,
   819
GVHD see graft-vs.-host disease (GVHD)
GVLE see graft-vs.-leukemia effect (GVLE)
GVTE see graft-vs.-tumor effect (GVTE)

H
HAART (highly-active antiretroviral therapy)
   1198, 1371, 1373
HA–1 peptide gene 388
hairpin ribozymes, antisense therapy 262
hammerhead ribozyme, antisense therapy 260,
   262
"Hayflick limit" 71
HCT see hematopoietic cell transplantation (HCT)
headaches, drug-induced 815
health care professionals
   sexual dysfunction management 524
   vaccinations 865, **868**
Health Insurance Portability/Accountability Act
   (HIPAA) 424
health-related quality of life (HRQOL) 441, 507
   see also quality of life (QOL)
Health Resources/Services Administration
   (HRSA) 536
health services research 434
   access studies 443–444
   improving HCT practice 443–444
   quality of care 444
   see also outcomes research
heart
   presentation of amyloidosis 1286
   see also under cardiac
helper T-cell(s)
   adoptive immunotherapy
      CMV infection 383, 384–385
      EBV infections 386
   antigen presentation 324–325
   GVHD
      animal models 345–346, 347, 348–349
      autologous 406
      pathophysiology 345
      prevention, subset balance in 312–313
   GVLE 373
      solid tumors 1185
   immunological tolerance 302
   recovery after PBHC allogeneic transplants
      592
   helper T-cells type 1 (T_H1) 325
      GVHD 355
         subset balance, in prevention 312–313
         transplantation, prophylaxis 356
      immune regulation 325

helper T-cells type 2 (T_H2) 325
   GVHD 355
      subset balance, in prevention 312–313
      transplantation, prophylaxis 356
   immune regulation 325
   immunological tolerance 306–307
hemangioblasts 74
hematologic diseases
   in Fanconi anemia 1484
   genetic see genetic disease
   infectious 118
      gene therapy potential **118**
   malignancies
      gene therapy potential 118, **118**
      leukemia see leukemia
      lymphoma see lymphoma
   targeted therapies 258
      gene therapy see gene therapy
      nucleic acids see nucleic acid based
         therapies
   see also specific disorders
hematologic immunocytopenia, treatment **1387**
hematologic malignancies 953–954
   GVHD 646
   immunosuppressive agents, randomized
      controlled trials **642**
   nonmyeloablative therapy see
      nonmyeloablative therapy
hematoma(s)
   abdominal pain 790
   subdural 813
hematopoiesis 63, 63–64, 74–76, 614
   angiogenesis association 74
   embryonic 63, 74
   fetal see fetus
   gene expression inhibition see nucleic acid
      based therapies
   genetic control 71–72
      AML-1 71
      transcription factors 82
   microenvironment 53–61, 54
      adhesion receptors 56, 56–57, 57
      adult 53, 54
      cellular components 53–55
      cytokines 57–58
      development 53
      ECM components 555–56
   neonatal 75, 76
   tissues 73
      see also blood cells; bone marrow; spleen
hematopoietic cells (HCs)
   amplification, future work 1507–1508
   collection, FACT standards 533–534
   cord blood 12, 599
      homing, cord blood transplantation 557–558
   osmotic tolerance 601
   peripheral blood see peripheral blood
      hematopoietic cells (PBHCs)
   processing, FACT standards 534
   redistribution, radiotherapeutic principles
      178
   repopulation, radiotherapeutic principles 178

   sources 11–12, 529–632, 531
      allogeneic transplants in AML 1031–1032
      GVHD 637–638, 646–647
      MDS prognosis 1087
   stem cells see hematopoietic stem cells
      (HSCs)
   storage
      cell loss with 599
      cryopreservation see cryopreservation
      nonfrozen 600
   transplantation see hematopoietic cell
      transplantation (HCT)
   transport 600, 606–607
hematopoietic cell transplantation (HCT) 83
   allogeneic see allogeneic transplantation
   animal studies 4–5
   applications 5–6, 9–13
      indications 9–10, **10**
      leukemia 3–4, 6, 83, 88
         see also leukemia
      long-term survivors 13
      malignant disease 9–10, **10**
      nonmalignant disease 10, **10**
      older patients 10
      patient selection 10–11
   autologous see autologous transplantation
   cases per year **5**
   cell sources see hematopoietic cells
   coincidental AD treatment 1386, **1386, 1387**
   conditions affecting outcome 453–460
   economics 436
      clinical benefit and 436–438, **437**
      cost-minimization studies **436**
   experience–outcome relationship 444
   future work 6, 1507–1510
      cell amplification 1507–1508
      malignant cell elimination 1508
      recipient immune system 1508
      transplanted cell proliferation 1508
      universal donor line 1508
   histocompatibility, advances 5
   history 3–8, 4
      clinical studies 3–4
   irradiation protection effect 3
   outcomes research see outcomes research
   practice variation 444
   problems 5
      animal studies 5
      cancer cell contamination 83–84
      opportunistic infection 85
   programs see hematopoietic cell
      transplantation program
   racial differences in access 443–444
   regimens 12–13
      choice 451
   regulation/accreditation 531–537
      American Association of Blood Banks
         (AABB) 536
      FACT see Foundation for the
         Accreditation of Cellular Therapy
         (FACT)
      governmental 531–532

hematopoietic cell transplantation (HCT)
  regulation/accreditation (*cont.*)
    National Marrow Donor Program (NMDP) 5, 438, 485, 536–537
    voluntary 532–537
  renewed interest 5–6
  stem cells *see* hematopoietic stem cell transplantation (HSCT)
  storage
    cryopreservation *see* cryopreservation
    nonfrozen 600
  successes 5–6
  support groups 485
  tandem transplant 1364–1365
  tolerance induction 85
  in utero see in utero transplantation (IU-HCT)
  volume–outcome relationship 444
  see also bone marrow transplantation (BMT)
hematopoietic cell transplantation (HCT) program
  administration 463–468, 466–467
    director/business manager 466
  authorization process 465
  charges 463, **464**
  clinical nurse specialist (CNS) 466
  clinical roles 463–466
  clinical support 463–468
  communication 465
  composition 463
  director/business manager 466
  factors affecting 463
  financial coordinator 466–467
  information provision 465
  nurse case manager (NCM) 464–465
    patient number 464, **465**
    survey 464
  nurse program manager (NPM) 463–464
  patient teaching 465
  psychosocial assessment 465
  quality indicators **464**
  search coordinator 467
  see also clinical trials
hematopoietic growth factors *see* growth factors
hematopoietic progenitor cells (HPCs) 69–75
  bipotent 79–80, 81
  definitions 77–78
  gene expression analysis 82–83
    profiles 82
  gene therapy 119
  lineage committed 77–82, 79
    alternative pathways 81
    dendritic progenitors 79, 81–82
    fetal 80–81
    isolation 77–78
    lymphoid progenitors 78–80, 79
    myeloid progenitors 79, 80
    see also specific cell lineages/progenitors
  malignant transformation 86–88, 87
    see also leukemia; leukemic stem cells
  monopotent 77–78

  mouse
    cell markers *70*
    isolation 70
    properties 70–72, *71*
  multipotent (MPP) 70, *70*, 79, *79*
  oligopotent 77, 78
  ontogeny 74–76, *75*
  transplantation
    acute leukemia 88
    HSC cotransplantation 85
hematopoietic stem cells (HSCs) 69–75
  aging/senescence 74–76, 96
    "Hayflick limit" 71
    replicative potential 63
  cell cycle/cell division 70–71
    daughter cells 62, 64
    function 64
    quantity 62–63
    telomere checkpoint 65
    transplantation and 71
  cell population 62
  definitions 69
  differentiation 69, 70, *70*, 79
    alternative pathways 81
    fetal liver *vs.* adult 80
    lineage restriction 83
    molecular control of cell fate 64, 82–83
    priming model 83
    progenitors *see* hematopoietic progenitor cells (HPCs)
    transcriptional regulation 82
    see also specific cell lineages
  embryonic *see* embryonic stem cells (ES)
  expansion 96–106
    animal models
      large animals 97
      mouse studies 71, *71*, 96–97, 97–98
      xenogeneic (human–mouse) 97–98
      xenogeneic (human–sheep) 98
    clinical trials 99–103
      bone marrow/mobilized peripheral blood 99, **100**
      cytokine-based systems 97, 98, 101
      UBC cells 99, 100–103, **102**
    extrinsic/intrinsic factors 98–99
    growth factor 96–99
    maintenance *vs.* 99
    novel approaches 98–99
    preclinical studies 96–99
    stroma induced 96–99
    in vitro 72–73
    in vivo 72
  ex vivo cultures 72, 96
    conditions 119, **119**
    proliferation 96
  gene expression analysis 82–83
  gene therapy *see* gene therapy
  genetic manipulation *see* gene transfer
  hierarchy 62
    multipotent 69
    pluripotent 69, 74, 76, 77

  totipotent 69, 76
  unipotent 69
  isolation
    history 69–70
    sources 96
    spleen colony-forming cells 69–70
    subpopulations 70, *70*
    techniques 84
  leukemic 85–87
    see also leukemia
  migration into blood 73–74
    clearance 73, *74*
    release mechanisms 73
  molecular control of fate 64
    factors involved 64
  mouse
    cell markers *70*
    HSC transplantation 83–85
    properties 70–72, *71*
  ontogeny 74–76, *75*
    embryonic 53, 63, 74
    fetal 53, 63, *63*, 74–76
    postnatal 76
    tissue organization *63*, 63–64
  progenitor cells *vs.* 69
  regeneration 63
  response to injury 63
  self-renewal 62–68, 69, 87, 96
    cytokines 72
    genetic pathways *72*, 72–73
    LT- *vs.* ST-HSCs 70
    malignant 85–86, 87
    Wnt signaling *72*, 72–73
  sources 96
    ethical issues 492–494
  subpopulations 62
    long-term HSCs 70, *70*, 79
    self-renewal of 70, 79
    short-term HSCs 70, *70*, 79
  telomeres 65, 71
    checkpoint 65
    maintenance 71
  tissue development/organisation *63*, 63–64
  transdifferentiation 76–77, **77**
  transplantation *see* hematopoietic stem cell transplantation (HSCT)
hematopoietic stem cell transplantation (HSCT) 83–85
  acute leukemia 88
  advantages, cancer cell purging 83–84, *84*
  cell cycle effects 71
  engraftment kinetics 84, *84*, 85
  expansion following *see* hematopoietic stem cells (HSCs), expansion
  facilitator cells and 84–85
  genetic diseases, limitations 118
  HCT *vs.* 83
  HPC cotransplantation 85
  neuroblastoma 1337
  number of HSCs required 84
  opportunistic infection 85
  self-renewal of different subpopulations 70

syngeneic mouse transplants 84, *85*
T-cell depletion/radiation damage 188
tolerance induction 85
hemoglobinopathies
  ethical issues in treatment 493
  gene therapy 126–127
    transgene expression control 120
  see also individual disorders
hemoglobinuria, cryopreserved cells and 608
hemolysis
  blood group incompatibility 824–832
    ABO **824**, 824–825
    delayed reactions 825
    management 825–827, **826**
    risk decreasing 825–826
    therapy 829
  DMSO-induced 608
hemophagocytic lymphohistiocytosis (HLH)
    1473–1474
  diagnosis 1473
  familial 1473
  primary 1473
  survival *1474*
  treatment options 1473
hemorrhage(s)
  oral 921
  varicella 738
hemorrhagic cystitis 790
  protection from 165
  see also cytoprotection
hemostasis, amyloidosis presentation 1288
hepatic venous pressure gradient, SOS 776
hepatitis
  donors 457, 771–772
    management algorithm *770, 771*
    viral markers 771–773
  fulminant viral 773
  human papillomavirus 729
  SOS 773
  transfusion transmitted 844
  transplant patient, management algorithm
      772
  varicella-zoster 740
hepatitis A, transfusion transmitted 844–845
hepatitis B virus (HBV)
  chronic 793
  liver infection 782
  transfusion transmitted 539, 845
  vaccination in HCT recipients 862
hepatitis C virus (HCV)
  chronic 793
  donor, management 772, 773
  liver infection 782–783
  transfusion transmitted 538–539, 845
hepatitis G virus (HGV)
  liver infection 783
  transfusion transmitted 845
Herceptin 1398
herpes simplex virus (HSV)
  gene therapy vector 113
  HSV-1 728
  HSV-2 728

reactivation post-HCT 733
virology 727
herpes simplex virus (HSV) infection
    727–731
  clinical manifestations 729
  CNS 811–812
    EEG *812*
  diagnosis 729
  epidemiology 728
    in the HCT patient 728
  genital 729
  hepatitis 729
  immunology 727–728
    in the HCT recipient 728, 856
  liver 781
  oropharyngeal 729, 920
  pathogenesis 727–728
  peri-anal 792
  pneumonia 729
  prophylaxis 730, **730**
  treatment 730, **730**
    acyclovir resistance 727
herpesvirus
  associated complications 749
  infections
    oral 920
    treatment **762**
  vectors for gene therapy 113
  see also human herpesvirus
herpesvirus type 6, CNS infection 813
herpes zoster *see* varicella-zoster virus (VZV)
    infection
heterozygosity loss analysis, secondary
    malignancy prognosis 968–969
heterozygote advantage (overdominant
    selection), MHC evolution 48
high-dose chemotherapy *see* chemotherapy,
    high-dose
high-dose radiotherapy *see* radiotherapy
highly-active antiretroviral therapy
    (HAART) 1198, 1371, 1373
HIPAA (Health Insurance Portability/
    Accountability Act) 424
histocompatibility 31–42
  advances in bone marrow transplant 5
  allogeneic cord blood transplantation
      typing 551–552
  donor compatibility, impact on outcome
      40–41
  graft rejection 40
  HLAs *see* HLAs (human leukocyte antigens)
  mHA *see* minor histocompatibility antigens
      (mHA)
  MHC *see* major histocompatibility complex
      (MHC)
HIV
  cellular/anatomical reservoirs 1372
  donors 457
  entry into cell 1370
  as gene therapy vector 111–112, *112*, 126
    clinical trials **120**, 125
    strategies *1371*

infection *see* HIV-1 infection
life cycle *1370*
regulatory genes 1370–1371, *1371*
T-cell homeostasis 1371–1372
viral genes/replication 1369, *1369*
HIV-1 infection 1369–1372
  autologous transplants, Hodgkin's disease
      1198
  clinical management 1372
    antiviral drugs 1372
      immune reconstitution 1372
      neurotoxicity 818
  CMV infections 811
  donors 457
  transmission from donor to recipient 538,
      845
  see also AIDS
HLA class I molecules **32**, 43
  functions 1116
  genes (HLA-A, -B, -C, -E, -F, -G) 31–33, **32**,
      43, 1116
    allele mismatches **1134**
    downregulation, CMV infection 714
    in graft failure 1136, **1137–1138**, 1138
    in GVHD 11, 1140
    identification 1132
    linkage disequilibrium effects 1135
    locations *32, 44*
    polymorphism *see* polymorphism (below)
    structure 34
    variation 35
  killer immunoglobulin-like receptors 1125,
      1125, 1126, 1142
  polymorphism 35, 43, *45*, 1117
    allelic diversity 43, 44
    class II molecules *vs.* 44
    class I molecules *vs.* 44
    conservation 45, *46*
    evolution 43–52
    gene duplication 43
    second exon 45–47
    structure 33, 34, *34*, 48
HLA class II molecules 43
  functions 1116
  genes (HLA-DR, -DQ, -DP) *33*, 33–34, 43,
      1116
    allele mismatches **1134**
    DRB-locus 44, **45**, 45–47, *46*, 1133–1135
    in graft failure 1136, **1137–1138**, 1138
    in GVHD 1139–1140
    hypervariable regions 44, 47
    linkage disequilibrium effects 1135
    locations *32, 44*
    polymorphism *see* polymorphism (below)
    recombination 47, 48–49, *49*
  polymorphism 43, *45*, 1117
    allelic diversity 43, 44
    class I molecules *vs.* 44
    conservation 45, *46*
    evolution 43–52
    second exon 45–47
    structure 34, *34*

HLA class III molecules 34, 43
  evolution 43
  genes 34
    locations *32*
HLA-identical related bone marrow transplant 1132
  acute GVHD 987–988
  aplastic anemia 982–991, **983–984**
  chronic GVHD 988
    incidence 988
    risk factors 988
  survival *989*, 989–990
HLA-matched HCT
  DLI 1155
  nonmyeloablative therapy, preclinical studies 1165
HLA-matched related HCT
  allogeneic transplants
    ALL, childhood 1069, **1069**, **1070**, **1071**, *1076*
    AML, adults **1032**, *1033*
    AML, children 1047–1048
  chronic phase CML *1009*, 1009–1012, *1010*, *1011*
  nonmyeloablative therapy, hematologic malignancies 1167–1171
  quality of life issues 511
  relapse treatment following autologous transplants 1395
HLA-matched unrelated HCT 1132–1149
  ALL 1133, 1144
    childhood 1072–1073, 1075–1076, *1076*, **1077**
  AML 1031–1032, 1144
  aplastic anemia *993*, 993–995, **994**
  chronic myelomonocytic leukemia (CMML) 1144
  CML 1143–1144
  DLI 1155
  donor registries *see* donor registries
  HLA barrier 1132
  in MDS 1087, 1144–1145
  nonmyeloablative therapy, hematologic malignancies 1171–1172
  quality of life issues 511
  refractory anemia 1144
  refractory anemia with excess blasts 1144
HLA-matching *see* HLA typing
HLA-partially matched related HCT 1116–1131
  acute GVHD *1120*
  bone marrow transplant, aplastic anemia 991–993, **992**
  childhood ALL 1075
  chronic GVHD 1120
  killer immunoglobulin-like receptors (KIR) 1125
  matching *see* donor selection; HLA typing
  natural killer cell action *see* natural killer cells (NKCs)
  nonmyeloablative therapy
    hematologic malignancies 1171–1172
    preclinical studies 1165, 1166

T-cell depletion 1122–1126
  characteristics 1123
  conditioning 1123, *1123*
  ex vivo depletion 1122
  graft failure risk 1122
  immunodeficiency 1124
  infections 1123–1124
  Japanese studies 1124–1125
  natural killer cells *see* natural killer cells (NKCs)
  outcomes 1123–1125
  partial depletion 1122
  PBHC 1123
  Perugia studies 1123–1124
  protocols 1123
  survival 1124
  Tübingen studies 1124
T-replete marrow grafts 1118–1122, 1128
  graft failure **1118**, 1118–1119
  GVHD 1119–1120, *1120*
  GVLE 1120–1121
  immune reconstitution 1121
  survival *1121*, 1121–1122
HLAs (human leukocyte antigens)
  advances 5
  antigen-binding cleft *34*
  characteristics 34–35
  chromosome location 31, *32*
  class I molecules *see* HLA class I molecules
  class II molecules *see* HLA class II molecules
  class III molecules *see* HLA class III molecules
  crossreactive groups **36**
  disease associations 48
    autoimmune diseases 327
  diversity 31
  evolution 43–52
    balancing selection 48
    conservation 31, 45, 48
      polymorphism sites 44, 45
    frequency-dependent selection 48
    functional 49–50
    gene duplication/divergence 43
    heterozygote advantage 48
    patterns of diversification 44, 45–47
    recombination (segmental exchange) 47–48, 48–49, *49*
    sequence convergence 47
  function 116
  genes 16, *32*
    allele mismatches **1134**
    ancestral 43
    chromosomal location 31, *32*, 44
    frequencies 1133
    hypervariable regions 44, 45, 47
    linkage disequilibrium 35
    pseudogenes 48
    racial differences 1133–1135
    structure/function 31–34
    see also specific classes
  genetic polymorphism 31, 43, 116, 1133–1135

allelic diversity 43
evolutionary conservation 44, 45
maintenance 48–49
sequence diversity 45
sites *34*
two-layer 43, *45*
in graft failure 1136, 1138
GVHD 637, *637*, 646, 1139–1141
haplotypes 34–35, *35*, **36**, 1116–1117
  DRB organization **45**
  segregation in families 1116–1117, *1117*
  see also HLA typing
inhibition, CMV infection 714–715
linkage disequilibrium 35
matching *see* HLA typing
nomenclature 34
phylogenetic analysis 44, 45, *46*, *47*, *49*
structure 17–18, 33, 34
  antigen-binding cleft *34*
  polymorphic sites *34*
  see also specific molecules
typing *see* HLA typing
upregulation, renal cell carcinoma, allogeneic transplants *1180*
varicella-zoster reactivation post HCT 733, **734**
HLA typing 11–12, 16–17, 35–41
  amplification strategies 37
  cell sources 11–12
  cellular typing 37
  clinical relevance 39, 1136–1142, **1137–1138**
    graft failure 1136–1138
    GVHD **1135**, 1139–1141
    outcome effects 1135–1136
    qualitative 1136
    quantitative 1136, 1138, 1140, **1140**
    relapse, effects on 1141
    survival, effects on **1141**, 1141–1142
  cord blood 552
  DNA typing 37, 1134–1135
  donors 12
    identification 16, 39–40
  functional assays 1142–1143
  GVLE 1141
  history 35–39, 1132–1133
  identical sibling, results of transplant *13*
  linkage disequilibrium effects 1135
  mHA 40
  mismatch **1117**
    definition 40, **40**
    effects *see* HLA-partially matched related HCT
  oligonucleotide arrays 39
  partial 12
  partially 12
  PCR 37
  reference strand mediated conformation analysis 38–39
  registries *see* donor registries
  selection of method 39

sequence-specific oligonucleotide probe hybridization 37, 38, *38*
sequence-specific primer typing 37, *37*
sequencing 38, *39*
serology 35–36
see also HLA-matched unrelated HCT
HLH *see* hemophagocytic lymphohistiocytosis (HLH)
Hodgkin's disease (HD)
  AIDS 1372
  allogeneic transplants 1106, 1200–1202
    GVLE 1200–1201
    high-dose regimens 1201–1202
    nonmyeloablative regimens 1201
    survival rates *1200*, 1201, **1201**
  autologous transplants 1191–1200
    chemotherapy *vs.* 1193
    elderly patients 1198
    HIV-associated disease 1198
    immunotherapy 204–205
    late events 1198–1199
    PBHCs 1200
    pediatric patients 1198
    posttransplant therapy 1195
      radiation 1194–1195
    pretransplant therapy
      "debulking" 1194
      radiation 1194–1195
    prognostic factors 1192–1193, **1193**
    relapse
      first *1196*, 1196–1197, **1197**
      management 1199–1200
      second *1195*, 1197
    remission
      failure *1195*, 1195–1196, **1196**
      first **1197**, *1197*, 1197–1198
      results **1192**
    secondary malignancies 1199
    timing **1195**, 1195–1198
  delayed complications 953
  high-dose chemotherapy, consolidative irradiation 190, 191
  T-cell adoptive transfer 385
holmium-166 165–166
homeobox genes
  HOX genes *see HoxB4* genes
  overexpression, HSC expansion studies 98
  stem cell fate 64
  stem cell renewal 72, 73
homing receptors, adoptive T-cell immunotherapy 395
homozygous typing cells (HTCs) 1133
Hoogsteen bonds 258
hormone replacement therapy (HRT) 486
  sexual dysfunction 525
hospitalization
  discharge *see* discharge from hospital
  psychosocial factors 500–501
HOVON
  ALL autologous transplants 1240
  multiple myeloma tandem transplantation trials 1273–1274, **1274**

*Hox*B4 genes
  HSC development 75
  HSC self-renewal 72, 73
HPCs *see* hematopoietic progenitor cells (HPCs)
HRSA (Health Resources/Services Administration) 536
HSCs *see* hematopoietic stem cells (HSCs)
human antimouse antibody (HAMA) response 200
human herpesvirus 6 (HHV-6) infection 762–763
  liver 781
human herpesvirus 7 (HHV-7) infection 763
human herpesvirus 8 (HHV-8) infection 763
  liver 781
human immunodeficiency virus (HIV) *see* HIV
human leukocyte antigens *see* HLAs (human leukocyte antigens)
human metapneumovirus infection 761
human papillomavirus (HPV) infection 729, 763
human T-lymphotrophic virus (HTLV), transfusion transmitted 845
human trials *see* clinical trials
humoral immunity, CMV infection 715
Hunter syndrome (MPS II) 1460
  gene therapy 125
Hurler–Scheie syndrome (MPS IH/S) 1460
Hurler syndrome (MPS IH) 1459–1460
  clinical experience 1459–1460
  gene therapy 125
  nonmyeloablative therapy 1174
  preclinical models 1459
  survival, untreated/HCT 1459
hydrogen peroxide, cytoprotection 168
hydromorphine (Dilaudid) 903
4-hydroperoxycyclophosphamide (4-HC) 1252
  autologous transplants
    ALL purging 1244
    AML 1224–1225, *1225*
      second remission 1226
  bone marrow purging 255
  disease free survival *255*
hydroxychloroquine 217
  mechanism of action/targets **218**
hydroxyethyl starch (HES) 603
  engraftment kinetics **603**
hydroxyurea (HU)
  agnogenic myeloid metaplasia therapy 1090
  polycythemia vera therapy 1090
  posttransplant antileukemic treatment 1255–1256
  sickle cell disease 1420–1421
hygiene care **915**, 915–916
hygromas, subdural 813
hyperdiploidy, childhood ALL 1068, 1242
hyperfractionated radiotherapy regimens *see* radiotherapy regimens
hypersensitivity, transfer in HCT 859
hypertension, varicella 738
hypertransfusion regimens, thalassemia 1410

hypoactive sexual desire disorder 524–525
hypothalamic-pituitary axis, delayed complications 949
hypothalamic-pituitary-gonad axis 520
  female 522, *522*
  male *522*
hypoxic encephalopathy 813

I
ibritumomab 166
  non-Hodgkin's lymphoma trials 204
ICBTR (International Cord Blood Transplant Registry) 550
ICE regimen **162**, 164
  Hodgkin's disease therapy 1194
  PBHC mobilization 580
    clinical trials **582**
ICH (International Conference on Harmonization), clinical trial design guidelines 421
ICOS *see* inducible costimulator (ICOS)
idarubicin
  busulfan/melphalan combination 1266–1267
  cytarabine/fludarabine combination *see* cyarabine/fludarabine/idarubicin combination
idiopathic hyperammonemia 784
IFAR *see* International Fanconi Anemia Registry (IFAR)
IFM *see* Intergroup Français du Myélome (IFM)
ifosfamide 164, *254*
  bone marrow purging 254
  combination regimens
    carboplatin/etoposide *see* ICE regimen
    etoposide/methotrexate/mitoxantrone 1107–1108
  metabolism 134
  neurotoxicity 818
  pharmacology **131**
  regimens **162**
  structure *131*
IGF-1 (insulin-like growth factor-1), multiple myeloma 1262
ignorance, immunological 325
ikaros, HSC expression 82
IL-1 *see* interleukin-1 (IL-1)
IL-2 *see* interleukin-2 (IL-2)
IL-3 *see* interleukin-3 (IL-3)
IL-4 *see* interleukin-4 (IL-4)
IL-6 *see* interleukin-6 (IL-6)
IL-7 *see* interleukin-7 (IL-7)
IL-8 *see* interleukin-8 (IL-8)
IL-10 *see* interleukin-10 (IL-10)
IL-11 *see* interleukin-11 (IL-11)
IL-12 *see* interleukin-12 (IL-12)
IL-15 (interleukin-15), *in vitro* T-cell culture 380
IL-17 (interleukin-17), PBHC mobilization 582, **582**
illegitimate switch recombination, multiple myeloma diagnosis 1262

imatinib mesylate (Gleevac®) 258, 1009
　accelerated FDA approval 427, 429
　allogeneic transplants, relapse management 1158
　arguments for 1014
　autologous transplants 1258
　　ALL 1242
　　CML 1014, 1250
　　　newly diagnosed patient 1014
　decision analysis 439, *439*
　PBHC mobilization after 1255
　recurrence prevention 1257–1258
　resistance 1009
IMBTR *see* International Bone Marrow Transplant Registry (IBMTR)
immune deficiency *see* immunodeficiency diseases
immune reconstitution 25–26, 853–861
　age effects 855
　antiretroviral therapy for AIDS 1372
　autoimmune disease 1391
　B-cells 853–854
　　antibody activity *857*
　　cord blood transplantation 554
　　functional analysis 856–857
　　PBHC allogeneic transplants 592
　　phenotypic analysis 855
　beneficial therapy 858–859
　common lymphoid progenitor cells 854, 859
　cord blood transplantation 554
　cytokines
　　analysis 856
　　interleukin-1 856
　　interleukin-2 856
　　interleukin-7 859
　　keratinocyte growth factor 859
　disease transfer 859
　enhancement 26
　extrathymic pathways 1121
　GVHD effects 25–26, 857–858, *858*
　HLA-partially matched related HCT 1121
　impaired 26
　normal ontogeny 854–855
　oral complications 911, **912**
　PBHC allogeneic transplants 592
　phenotypic analysis 855
　severe combined immunodeficiency 856
　T-cells 25, 853
　　CD3+ 855, 857
　　CD4+ 855, 858
　　CD8+ 855
　　functional analysis 856
　　GVHD effects *858*
　　positive selection 1121
　thymus 855
　vaccination 857, 859, **859**
　　in GVHD 858
immune response/system 16–30, 324–325
　adaptive response 18
　antigen presentation *see* antigen presentation
　antigens 16
　blood group incompatibility 824
　cellular
　　CMV infection 714, 718–719
　　following autologous transplants 1399–1402
　　granulocyte system 1471–1472
　　macrophage system 1471
　　see also natural killer cells (NKCs); T-cell(s)
　compromised 668–669
　donor/recipient genetic disparity, outcomes 22–25
　　engraftment 22
　　GVHD *see* graft-*vs.*-host disease (GVHD)
　　GVLE *see* graft-*vs.*-leukemia effect (GVLE)
　　tolerance development 24–25
　donor selection 21
　dysregulation, delayed 948
　fungal infection 687–689
　generation 16
　humoral immunity
　　CMV infection 715
　　see also antibodies; B-cell(s)
　induction perpetuation 324–325
　MHC 31
　normal ontogeny *854*, 854–855
　peripheral nervous system complications 814–815, **819**
　recipient, future work 1508
　regulation 324–325
　transgene products 121
　vaccination 863
　varicella-zoster virus infections 736–737
　see also individual components
immune thrombopurpuric anemia 1106
immunization *see* vaccination
immunobiological agents, bacterial infection 678
immunocytochemistry, minimal residual disease detection 245
　sensitivity 244t
immunodeficiency diseases 306–307, 1430–1442
　HLA-partially matched related HCT 1124
　nonmyeloablative therapy 1173
　primary (congenital) **118**
　　gene therapy 123–124
　in utero transplantation (IU-HCT) 572, **572**
　see also specific diseases/disorders
immunofluorescence, varicella-zoster virus infections 740–741
immunoglobulin(s) *see* antibodies
immunoglobulin A, mucosal, posttransplant 855, *856*
immunoglobulin E (IgE), posttransplant 857–858
immunoglobulin G (IgG)
　posttransplant *856*
　varicella-zoster virus specific 736
immunoglobulin M (IgM)
　posttransplant *856*
　varicella-zoster virus specific 736
immunological adjuvants, oligonucleotides 266
immunological ignorance 325
immunological purging *see* purging, antibody-mediated
immunological tolerance *see* tolerance, immunological
immunomagnetic bead depletion *see* purging, antibody-mediated
immunomodulation
　following autologous transplants 1402
　nutritional support 890
immunophenotypes *see* acute lymphoblastic leukemia (ALL)
immunostimulatory cytokines, GVHD prevention 313
immunosuppression 308–312
　discontinuation
　　allogeneic transplants relapse management 1157
　　GVLE, evidence for 371
　　remission association 371
　drugs *see* immunosuppressive drugs
　GVHD
　　prevention 358
　　prolonged in chronic 650
　　treatment 209–220
　immune response regulation 325
　induced tolerance *see* tolerance, induced
　nonmyeloablative therapy *vs.* 1167
　posttransplant 12
　　graft failure 1119
　　GVHD 1120
　　GVHD risk 23
　　MTX/CSP 985–987, *986*
　pretransplant 12
　　HLA-partially matched related HCT 1119
　radioimmunotherapy 201–202
　radiotherapy 179, 185
　survival, aplastic anemia *996*
　vs. HCT 995–996, **996**
immunosuppressive drugs 209–220
　fungal infection 688–689
　induced tolerance 308
　mechanism of action/targets **218**
　neurotoxicity 817
　new 643
　nonspecific 209–211
　randomized controlled trials **642**, **651**
　specific 211–216
　see also specific drugs
immunotherapy
　autologous transplants **1397**, 1397–1399
　　ALL 1246
　　AML 1225–1226
　　non-Hodgkin's lymphoma 1215
　CMV infection 715–716
　fungal infections 695–696
　ovarian cancer 1329
　solid tumor treatment 1365
immunotoxins *see* purging, antibody-mediated
inbreeding, osteopetrosis 1446
indications for transplant 9–10, **10**
indium-111 (^{111}In) 200

inducible costimulator (ICOS)
   antigen presentation 354–355
   immunological tolerance 301
induction chemotherapy, MDS , HCT of 1087–1088
INF-α *see* interferon-alpha (INF-α)
infants, allogeneic transplants, ALL 1078
infection(s)
   bacterial *see* bacterial infections
   catheter-related 887–888
   CNS following HCT 811–813, *812*, **819**
   delayed 945
   fungal *see* fungal infections
   GVHD 653, *653*
   HLA-partially matched related HCT 1123–1124
   intestinal 775
     mucosal 785, 791
   lung 875–876
   oral 919–921
   pathology 294–295
   previous, treatment outcome 457
   risks to donor 541–542
   in utero transplantation risk 570–571
   viral *see* viral infections
   see also specific infections/infectious agents
infectious mononucleosis *see* Epstein–Barr virus (EBV) infections
"infectious tolerance" 302, 304–305
infertility 486, 949
   autologous transplants, AML 1233
   counseling 451
   Fanconi anemia 1484
   HLA-identical related transplant 990–991
   permanent following transplant 451
INF-γ *see* interferon-gamma (INF-γ)
inflammatory bowel disease (IBD) 769
inflammatory cytokines, GVHD 353
infliximab
   GVHD treatment 361
   mechanism of action/targets **218**
influenza virus
   infections 761, **762**
   vaccination in HCT recipients 862–863
     response 864
information
   assessment of needs 483
   educational videotapes 449
   Internet 449, 465
   oral hygiene 916
   pain 898, **898**
   provision 465
   recording 484
   repeating 484
   survival 451–452
   written, for patients 449
informed consent
   donors 490–492, 540
   emotional distress 499
   ethical issues 489–490
   pediatric transplant 458
   psychosocial factors 499

innate response 18–19
inner cell mass, pluripotent stem cells 74
in situ hybridization (ISH), varicella-zoster virus detection 735, 741
INSS (International Neuroblastoma Staging System) 1333, **1333**
Institutional Review Boards (IRBs)
   clinical trial conduct 424
   gene therapy trials 122
insulin-like growth factor-1 (IGF-1), multiple myeloma 1262
integrin(s)
   cell migration
     developmental 75
     HSCs into blood 73
   hematopoietic microenvironment 56
   immunological tolerance 304–305
   multiple myeloma 1262
   PBHC mobilization 576–577, **582**
   proliferation/survival effects 57
integrin $\alpha_4\beta_1$, HSC migration 73, 75
intention-to-treat principle 426
Interactive Voice Response 515
interferon-alpha (INF-α)
   allogeneic transplants, relapse management 1158
   autologous transplants
     ALL 1242
     Hodgkin's disease 1195
   CML 1008–1009, 1158
     DLI combination 1152
     posttransplant relapse 1013
   GVHD risk factor 1155
   JMML 1021
   multiple myeloma maintenance therapy 1277
   PBSC mobilization after 1253–1254
   polycythemia vera therapy 1090
   posttransplant antileukemic treatment 1255
interferon-gamma (INF-γ)
   CML 1250, 1252–1253
   Fas expression 356–357
   GVHD 355, 409
     chronic 361–362
   host response to varicella-zoster virus 736, *737*
Intergroup Français du Myélome (IFM)
   high *vs.* lose dose melphalan 1266
   tandem transplantation trials 1273, **1274**
interleukin(s)
   autologous transplants, following 1397–1398, *1398*, 1399–1400
   in hematopoiesis *614*
interleukin-1 (IL-1)
   GVHD 353, 357
   immune reconstitution 856
   multiple myeloma 1262, 1263
interleukin-1 receptor antagonist, GVHD treatment 361
interleukin-2 (IL-2)
   activated killer cells, induced tolerance 312
   adoptive T-cell immunotherapy 395

   allogeneic transplants, relapse management 1158
   autologous transplants
     ALL 1242, 1246
     AML 1225
     Hodgkin's disease 1195
   DLI combination 1156
   GVHD 355
     autologous 406, 409
   GVLE 369, 370, 374, *374*
   GVTE 371
   immune reconstitution 856
   PBHC mobilization, G-CSF with 579–580
   T cell proliferation 325
interleukin-3 (IL-3)
   HSC self-renewal 72
   PBHC mobilization 577, 589
     G-CSF/GM-CSF with 579
   recombinant **614**, 619–620
     recombinant G-CSF combination 619–620
     recombinant GM-CSF combination 620
   synthetic receptor 620
interleukin-4 (IL-4)
   autologous GVHD 406
   chronic GVHD 361–362
   G-CSF stimulation 590
interleukin-6 (IL-6)
   in Fanconi anemia 1490
   GVHD 361
   multiple myeloma 1262
interleukin-7 (IL-7)
   immune reconstitution 859
   lymphoid cell development 78
   T-cell differentiation 854–855
interleukin-8 (IL-8)
   GVHD 361
   PBHC mobilization 577, 582, **582**
interleukin-10 (IL-10)
   autologous GVHD 408
   G-CSF stimulation 590
interleukin-11 (IL-11)
   effects 620
   PBHC mobilization 577
     clinical trials **582**
   recombinant **614**, 620–621
   systemic cytoprotection 169
interleukin-12 (IL-12)
   autologous GVHD 406
   in vitro T-cell culture 380
interleukin-15 (IL-15), *in vitro* T-cell culture 380
interleukin-17 (IL-17), PBHC mobilization 582, **582**
International Bone Marrow Transplant Registry (IBMTR) 424, 485, 534
   ALL
     allogeneic transplants 1069
     autologous transplants 1240
     remission failure 1061, **1062**
     survival rates 1058
   AML, autologous transplants PBHCs 1225

International Bone Marrow Transplant Registry
(IBMTR) (cont.)
CLL, therapy studies 1107
CML, classifications 1007, **1008**
Fanconi anemia
alternative donor HCT 1494–1497
sibling donor HCT 1492–1493
GVHD Severity Index 640, **640**, *641*, **649**
low-grade lymphoma therapy studies
1108–1109, *1109*
MDS outcomes 1085, *1086*
PBHC allogeneic transplants 588
related donor cord blood transplantation
552–553
International Conference on Harmonization
(ICH), clinical trial design guidelines
421
International Cord Blood Transplant Registry
(ICBTR) 550
International Fanconi Anemia Registry
(IFAR) 1483–1484
secondary tumor development 1499
International Neuroblastoma Staging System
(INSS) 1333, **1333**
International Prognostic Factors Index, non-
Hodgkin's lymphoma 1207–1208,
1208
International Prognostic Scoring System (IPSS),
MDS 1084, **1085**
International Society for Cellular Therapy
(ISCT) 551
International Society for Hematotherapy/Graft
Engineering (ISHAGE) 532
European collaboration 533
*International Standards for Cord Blood
Processing, Testing, Banking,
Selection/Release* (2000) 533
Internet, information 449, 485
interstitial pneumonia (IP) 295–296
autologous transplants, AML 1223–1224
CMV *see* cytomegalovirus-associated
interstitial pneumonia (CMV-IP)
HLA-identical related transplant 989
incidence, identical sibling transplant *13*
radiotherapy and 180, 186–188
interstitial pneumonia syndrome (IPS)
295–296
interstitial pneumonitis (IPN), incidence *13*
intestines *see* gastrointestinal (GI) tract
intracranial hemorrhage 813, *814*
drug-induced 815
intrahepatic coagulation, SOS 778
intramural hematomas, treatment complication
786
intraparenchymal hemorrhage, drug-induced
815
intravascular catheters *see* central venous
catheters (CVC), complications of
intravenous immunoglobulin (IVIg)
GVHD prophylaxis 643
GVHD treatment 215–216, 858
HCT recipients 854

mechanism of action/targets **218**
posttransplant 859
in utero transplantation (IU-HCT) 565–575, 572
advantages/potential **571**, 573
animal studies 566–569
human–sheep 568
mouse 566, *568*
engraftment efficiency *568*
sheep 566–567, *567*
strain combination effects 568, *569*
barriers to engraftment 568–569
host cell competition 568
immunologic 568–569, *569*
lack of space 568
cell sources 567, 568
clinical applications 569, 570–573, **572**
clinical experience/results 573
dose division/engraftment 567, *567*
fetal immunological tolerance 565–566
fetal receptive environment 566
"macrochimerism" 569
maternal/fetal risk 570–572
GVHD 567–568, 571–572
infection 570–571
procedural 570
"microchimerism" 568, 569
natural chimerism 565
osteopetrosis 1450
saturation kinetics 567, *567*
SCID 1436
strategies 569–570
competitive balance alteration 570, *571*
stromal cotransplantation 569–570, *570*
TBI enhancement 570, *572*
"window of opportunity" 567, *567*
xenogenic 568
invasive fungal infections (IFIs) 683–700
biology 684–687
children 684
classes 683
diagnostic testing 687
environmental considerations 688–690
epidemiology 683–684
immune response 687–688
immunotherapy 695–696
pathophysiology 684–687
patients, approaches 696–697
prophylaxis 688, 690, 692
vaccine 696
risks 683, *684*
immunosuppressive agents 688
treatment 688
antifungal agents 692, **693**, 694–695
administration 690, 692
clinical studies **691**
surgical approaches 696
see also fungal infections; *individual fungal
infections*
in vitro fertilization (IVF), ethical issues
492–493
involved-field (IF) boost irradiation 186
relapse reduction strategies 1396–1397

iodinated-3F8 (^{131}I-3F8), neuroblastoma 1337
iodine-131 (^{131}I), radioimmunotherapy 200, **201**
IPS (idiopathic pneumonia syndrome) 876
IPSS (International Prognostic Scoring System),
MDS 1084, **1085**
IRBs *see* Institutional Review Boards (IRBs)
iron, overload 774, 793–794
irradiation *see* radiotherapy
irradiation protection effect 3
ischemic stroke 813
ISCT (International Society for Cellular
Therapy) 551
ISHAGE *see* International Society for
Hematotherapy/Graft Engineering
(ISHAGE)
Italian Bone Marrow Transplant group,
childhood ALL, allogeneic
transplants 1072
Italian Multiple Myeloma Study Group
(MMSG) 1266
multiple myeloma autologous transplants,
high-dose *vs.* conventional **1272**,
1272–1273
itraconazole **693**, 694
clinical studies **691**
IU-HCT *see in utero* transplantation (IU-HCT)
IVIg *see* intravenous immunoglobulin (IVIg)

J
jaundice, treatment complications 775–786
JC virus infections 763
treatment **762**
JIA (juvenile idiopathic arthritis) 1390
JMML *see* juvenile myelomonocytic leukemia
(JMML)
juvenile chronic myelogenous leukemia
(JCML) *see* juvenile myelomonocytic
leukemia (JMML)
juvenile idiopathic arthritis (JIA) 1390
juvenile myelomonocytic leukemia (JMML)
1018–1024
age of onset 1018
biology 1019
chemotherapy 1019, 1021
clinical manifestations 1018–1019
cytogenetics 1019
diagnosis 1018
criteria **1018**
differential diagnosis 1019
GM-CSF 1019, 1021
HCT **1020**, 1021–1022
survival *1021*, *1022*
laboratory findings 1018–1019
neurofibromatosis type I 1018–1019
Philadelphia chromosome (*Bcr-Abl* gene
fusion) 1019
treatment 1019, 1021

K
Kaplan–Meier survival graphs 416, 429
diseases/disorders *see individual
diseases/disorders*

interval-censored survival 429
overestimation of event 430
weighted 429
Karnofsky score 455, **455**
outcome 11
karyotype analysis, multiple myeloma prognosis 1276
keratinocyte growth factor (KGF)
immune reconstitution 859
recombinant 620–621
systemic cytoprotection 169–170
KIAA0023 gene 388, 390
kidney(s)
acyclovir toxicity 743
delayed complications 951–952
evaluation, treatment outcome and 456
failure
cryopreserved cells and 608
multiple myeloma 1263, 1268
high-dose chemotherapy dose 137
presentation of amyloidosis 1286–1287
radiotherapy shielding 184
SOS 778
transdifferentiation **77**
killer immunoglobulin-like receptors (KIR)
GVLE 373
HLA class I molecules **1125**, 1142
HLA-partially matched related HCT 1125
HLA typing effects 1142
KIR *see* killer immunoglobulin-like receptors (KIR)
kit ligand *see* stem cell factor (SCF)
c-kit receptor, HSC migration role 73
Kostmann syndrome (KS) 1474, *1475*
Kurtzke extended disability status scale (EDSS) **1388**

L

LAD *see* leukocyte adhesion deficiency (LAD)
LAK *see* lymphokine-activated killing (LAK)
Lansky Play–Performance Scale 459, **459**
late-phase recovery *see* recovery
Laura Graves Foundation 624
learning difficulties 486
LEF/TCF signaling 72, *72*
legal issues, donors 540
lenograstim
adverse events 543
clinical trials 615, 616
see also filgrastim; granulocyte colony-stimulating factor (G-CSF), recombinant
lentiviruses
as gene transfer vectors *see* gene transfer
HIV *see* HIV
leridistim, PBHC mobilization **582**
leukemia(s) 85–88
apoptosis inhibition in 86–87
bone marrow transplantation 5
history 3–4
cell count 272
in Fanconi anemia 1493–1494

HCT 6, 83
graft failure after T-cell depletion 224–225
history 3–4
purified stem cells/progenitors 88
radioimmunotherapy and 202–203
unrelated donor cord blood transplantation 553–554, *554*
varicella-zoster virus reinfection following 734
mortality, IBMTR Severity Index *641*
"preleukemic disease" 87–88
radiotherapy, cell survival curve 179–180
relapse *see* relapse
secondary, autologous transplants, AML 1232–1233
stem cells *see* leukemic stem cells
targeted therapies 258
gene therapy *see* gene therapy
nucleic acids *see* nucleic acid based therapies
T-cell adoptive transfer *see* adoptive cellular immunotherapy/transfer; minor histocompatibility antigens (mHA)
see also individual diseases/disorders
leukemic stem cells 85–87
lineage 78
malignant self-renewal 85–86, *87*
malignant transformation 86–87
chromosomal rearrangements 86
final 86–87
myeloid progenitors 86–87
differentiation impairment 88–89
preleukemic 86
transplant contamination 83–84
leukemogenesis, Fanconi anemia 1489–1490
leukocyte(s)
adverse effects transfusions **833**
B-cells *see* B-cell(s)
cell survival curve, radiotherapy 179
depletion in RBC transfusions 833–834
adverse effects **833**
GVHD prevention 841
recommendations **834**
development 78–80
cytokines 78
progenitors *see* lymphoid progenitor cells
promiscuity 82–83
malignancies, delayed complications 953
NK cells *see* natural killer cells (NKCs)
T-cells *see* T-cell(s)
leukocyte adhesion deficiency (LAD) 1476–1477
gene therapy 124
leukodystrophies **1457**, 1461–1463
nonmyeloablative therapy 1174
see also individual diseases/disorders
leukopheresis, toleration of 591
lexitropsins, gene silencing 259
Leydig cell damage, following HCT 937
libido 486
life support withdrawal 494

life years (LYs), decision tree analysis 439
light microscopy, tumor cell detection **244**
limiting dilution assays (LDAs), HLA antigens 1142
linkage disequilibrium
HLA class I genes 1135
HLA class II genes 1135
HLA typing 1135
lipopolysaccharide (LPS), GVHD 357–358
lips
biopsy *293*, *294*
care 916
Listeria monocytogenes, CNS infection 811
liver
complications *see* gastrointestinal/hepatic complications
drug-induced injury 780–781
enzymes, elevation in nutritional support 888, **888**
evaluation, treatment outcome 456
fetal hematopoiesis *63*, 74–75
lineage commitment 80–81
fibrosis 773–774
hepatic capsule distention 906
injury, medication causing 794
presentation of amyloidosis 1287
SOS 776
transdifferentiation 77, **77**
veno-occlusive disease *288*
liver function tests
drug dosage adjustment 137
varicella 738
local anesthetic(s) 908
locked nucleic acids (LNAs), antisense therapy 261
log–rank (Cox) test 429–430, **430**
lomustine, regimens **161**
long-term culture initiating cells (LTC-IC) 590
long-term marrow cultures (LTMC) 96–97
lumbar puncture, pain management 907
lung(s)
BCNU toxicity 143
biopsy 874–875
disease 295–296
evaluation 456
failure 814
HCT complications *see* pulmonary complications
radiation sensitivity 180, 186–188
relapse relationship 186
shielding 184
transdifferentiation **77**
see also respiratory symptoms
lymphocytes *see* leukocyte(s)
lymphoid progenitor cells 78–80
bipotent 79–80, 81
common lymphoid progenitors (CLPs) 78–79
gene transfer and 119
early thymic progenitors (ETPs) 79
gene expression analysis 82–83

lymphokine-activated killing (LAK)
  autologous transplants, Hodgkin's disease 1195
  GVLE 369, 373
  solid tumor treatment 1178
lymphokines see cytokines
lymphoma(s)
  AIDS 1372–1374
  allogeneic transplants 1105–1115
    GVHD 1105
    GVTE 1105
    HLA-partially matched relatives 1121
    intermediate/high grade 1109–1110
    low grade 1107–1109
      survival rates 1108
    nonmyeloablative regimens 1110–1111
      survival 1111, 1111
    published studies 1105–1106
  autologous transplants
    high-grade 1213–1214
    low-grade 1108
      survival rates 1108
    T-cell 1213–1214
  Bcl-2 expression 264
  delayed complications 953
  radiotherapy
    consolidative irradiation 190–191
    TBI 186
  reclassification 1109
  recombinant G-CSF 615, 616
  relapse 191
  secondary malignancy following HCT 969–971
    late-onset 971
  targeted therapies 258, 264
    radioimmunotherapy/HCT 203–205
    rituximab treatment 258
  WHO classification 1105
  see also individual diseases/disorders
lymphoproliferation
  disorders, recombinant G-CSF therapy 616
  following XSCID gene therapy trials 125–126
Lyon cooperative study (LMCE) 1335
lysofylline, systemic cytoprotection 169
lysosomal acid hydrolase deficiency, nonmyeloablative therapy 1174
lysosomal storage disease(s) 118, 1455–1461
  considerations 1455–1456
  diagnosis 1456
  gene therapy trials 125

M
macrophage(s) 1471
  development 80
    bipotent progenitors 81
  disorders 1471–1473, **1472**, 1473–1474, 1479–1480
    considerations 1472–1473
  GVHD 357
macrophage antigen-1 (Mac-1) 577

mafosfamide 1252
  ALL autologous transplants, purging 1244
  autologous transplants, AML 1225
    second remission 1226
MAG95, multiple myeloma tandem transplantation trials 1274, **1274**
MAGE, T-cell adoptive immunotherapy 391
magnetic resonance imaging (MRI)
  cerebrovascular complications 813, *814*
  CNS infections *812*
  cyclosporine/tacrolimus toxicity 815, *816*
  liver, SOS 776
major histocompatibility complex (MHC)
  antigen presentation 31, 43, 354
    MHC–peptide interactions 49–50
  class I molecules 43, 344
    downregulation 394
    GVHD, animal models see graft-vs.-host disease (GVHD), animal models
    role in varicella-zoster virus immune evasion 736
    structure 48, *49*
    see also HLA class I molecules
  class II molecules 43, 344
    GVHD, animal models see graft-vs.-host disease (GVHD), animal models
    GVLE 373
    see also HLA class II molecules
  class III molecules 43
    see also HLA class III molecules
  evolution 43–52
    balancing selection 48
    conservation 31, 44, 45, 50
    frequency-dependent selection 48
    functional 49–50
    heterozygote advantage 48
    patterns of diversification 44, 45–47
    recombination (segmental exchange) 47–48
      intraexonic 48–49
    sequence convergence 47
  expression, CMV infection 382
  genes 16, 43
  genetic polymorphism 43
    allelic diversity 43
    conservation of sites 44
    maintenance 48–49
    sequence diversity 45
  history 31
  phylogenetic analysis 44, 45, *46, 47, 49*
  role 31
  self-tolerance 405
  see also HLAs (human leukocyte antigens); minor histocompatibility antigens (mHA)
major IE protein (IE-1) 383
male(s)
  hypothalamic-pituitary-gonad axis *522*
  physiological/biological changes 520, *522*
  puberty following HCT 936, **937**
  sexual dysfunction 521–522
    gonadal function 938, *939*
    treatment 525–526

malignant disease(s) **10**
  delayed complications 952–954
  future work 1508
  gastrointestinal/hepatic treatment complications 784
  immunosuppressive agents, randomized controlled trials **642**
  liver, long-term complications 794
  minimal residual disease detection post-HCT 281
  oral, secondary 924
  posttransplant *952*
  secondary malignancy see secondary malignancies
  see also individual diseases/disorders
malnutrition 888–889
α-mannosidosis 1463–1464
mantle cell lymphoma
  allogeneic transplants 1110
  autologous transplants 1212–1213, **1213**
  relapse management 1154
Maroteaux–Lamy syndrome (MPS VI) 1460–1461
marrow see bone marrow
MART1, T-cell adoptive immunotherapy 391
mast cell growth factor see stem cell factor (SCF)
maximum tolerated dose (MTD)
  dose-escalating phase 1 trials 418–420
  see also individual drugs
MBP (myelin-basic protein), EAE induction 329
MDM-2, T-cell adoptive immunotherapy 392
MDS see myelodysplastic syndromes (MDS)
measles–mumps–rubella (MMR) vaccine
  response HCT recipients 865
  vaccination 859
measles virus
  infections 761
  vaccination in HCT recipients 862
mechanical ventilation, prognosis **879**
mediastinal masses, ALL prognosis 1057
medical decision making, ethical issues 488–489
Medical Outcomes Study Short Form 36 (SF-36) 441
medical referral, psychosocial factors 497–498
Medical Research Council (MRC)
  AML 10 trials 1222
    allogeneic vs. autologous in first remission 1230–1231
  AML 12 trials 1222
  multiple myeloma autologous transplants 1271
    high-dose vs. conventional **1272**
  UKALL/ECOG Trial 1060, 1062
  UK ALL XII trial 1244
medications see drug(s)
medulloblastoma 1349–1350
  chemotherapy (high-dose) with HCT 1350, **1350**
  natural history with conventional therapy 1349–1350

megakaryocyte/erythrocyte progenitors (MEPs) 80
megakaryocyte growth/development factor (MGDF), recombinant 620
melanoma, allogeneic transplants 1177, 1182–1184
   GVTE 371
melphalan 140–141, 163
   brain cancer 1346
   combination regimens **161**
      ABCM 1264
      Adriamycin/BCNU/cyclophosphamide 1264
      BCNU see BEAM regimen
      BEAM see BEAM regimen
      busulfan 163, 1266
      busulfan/idarubicin 1266–1267
      busulfan/thiotepa 163
      Campath 1_M/fludarabine see Campath 1_M, combination regimens
      carboplatin/mitoxantrone 164
      cyclophosphamide 1266
      cyclophosphamide/etoposide/methotrexate/TBI 1202
      cyclophosphamide/etoposide/mitoxantrone 1267
      fludarabine 1100
      prednisone 1264
      TBI **160**
         melphalan **160**
         multiple myeloma 1096, 1265–1266, 1266
         sequential trials 165
      TBI/Ara-C (TAM) 1074
   dose-limiting toxicity 140
   high-dose chemotherapy 140–141
   mechanism of action 140
   MTD **159**
   multiple myeloma therapy 1100–1101, 1102, 1264–1268
   myeloablation in neuroblastoma 1337
   pharmacokinetics 1268
   pharmacology **131**, 140–141
   resistance 140
   solid tumor treatment 1355, 1356, 1357, 1358, 1359, **1362–1363**
   structure *131*
Memorial Sloan–Kettering Cancer Center (MSKCC)
   allogeneic transplants, ALL 1069
   allogeneic transplants, childhood ALL 1072
   autologous transplants, Hodgkin's disease 1192–1193
Memorial Symptom Assessment Scale 515
meningitis, bacterial, chronic GVHD 811
meningoencephalitis 813
meningoencephalitis, varicella 738
menopause 486, 522–523
meperidine 902–903
6-mercaptopurine, ALL autologous transplants 1246
merocyanine, bone marrow purging 256

mesenchymal associated progenitor cells (MAPCs), transdifferentiation 76
mesenchymal stem cells (MSC) 58
   transdifferentiation and 77
Mesna, local cytoprotection 168–169
messenger RNA (mRNA), translational silencing *260*, 260–266
   half-life effects 267
   processing perturbation 264
   see also nucleic acid based therapies; *specific methods*
meta-analysis, outcomes research 440, *440*
metabolic abnormalities, nutritional support 888
metabolic complications, encephalopathy 813–814, **819**
metabolic storage diseases, nonmyeloablative therapy 1174
metabolic support *see* nutritional support
metachromatic leukodystrophy (MLD) 1463
   nonmyeloablative therapy 1174
metaiodobenzylguanidine (MIBG), neuroblastoma 1337–1338
metaphase chromosomes, chimerism evaluation 234–235
metastatic breast cancer *see* breast cancer
methotrexate (MTX) 210–211
   autologous transplants, ALL 1246
   clinical use 211
   combination regimens **211**
      asparaginase/prednisolone/vincristine combination 1157
      cyclophosphamide/etoposide/melphalan/TBI combination 1202
      cyclosporine/TBI 1165
      etoposide/ifosfamide/mitoxantrone 1107–1108
   dose 211, **211**
   engraftment effects, PBHC allogeneic transplants 592
   GVHD treatment 4, 23, 360
      acute 987–988
      chronic 650
      multiple myeloma therapy 1097, 1098, 1102
   immunosuppression 641
      combined 641, 643
   low-dose, GVLE 374
   mechanism 210
   mechanism of action/targets **218**
   "mini-dose" 211
   pharmacology 210–211
   posttransplant 12, 985–987, *986*, 988–989
      survival 990
   randomized controlled trials **642**
   T-cells, effects on 853
   toxicity 211
      neurotoxicity 817
O^6-methylguanine DNA methyltransferase (MGMT), gene therapy trials 123

methylprednisolone (MP) *209*
   combination regimens
      C-VAMP 1264
      cyclophosphamide/doxorubicin/vincristine 1264
      doxorubicin/vincristine 1264, 1271
      VAMP regimen 1271
   GVHD primary treatment 643–645
   mechanism 209, 643
   randomized controlled trials **642**, **644**
   response 644
   side effects 209
   targets/mechanisms of action **218**
MG *see* myasthenia gravis (MG)
MGUS (monoclonal antibody of undetermined significance) 1263
mHA *see* minor histocompatibility antigens (mHA)
MHC *see* major histocompatibility complex (MHC)
MIC expression, CMV infection 384
microangiopathy, isolated 829
microarray(s)
   HLA typing 39
   HSC gene expression 82–83
microbiological load reduction, GVHD, prevention 358
microsatellite polymorphisms *see* short tandem repeat (STR) polymorphisms
microvessel density, multiple myeloma prognosis 1275
middle-phase recover *see* recovery
MINE regimen, low-grade lymphoma therapy 1107–1108
mini-ICE regimen, PBHC mobilization 580
minimal residual disease (MRD)
   ALL **278**, 1239–1240, 1242
      in children 1071–1072, 1242
   AML **278**, 1221
      in children 1048
   CLL **278**, 281
   CML **278**, 278–279, 1013
   detection 244–245, 272–285
      clonogenic assays 245
      conventional therapy 276–277, *277*
      genetic testing 422–423
      immunocytochemistry 245
      methods 272–276, **273**, *274*, *275*, *276*
      post-HCT 277–281
   dormancy 282
   multiple myeloma 245, 281
   non-Hodgkin's lymphoma **278**, 281
   relapse risks 1150
   research limitations 281–282
   treatment 282
   see also individual diseases/disorders
minisatellite polymorphisms, chimerism characterization 235, 235–236, *236*
minor histocompatibility antigens (mHA) 18, 40
   antigen presentation 354
   gene identification 388–390

minor histocompatibility antigens (mHA)
    gene identification (*cont.*)
        autosomal genes 388–389
        cDNA expression cloning 389, *389*
        as therapy targets 390
        Y-chromosome genes 389–390
    graft rejection 40
    GVHD, animal models *see* graft-*vs.*-host disease (GVHD), animal models
    GVLE 373
    T-cell adoptive transfer, leukemia treatment 387–390
        clinical trials 390
        isolation/proliferation *388*
mismatched HCT *see* HLA-partially matched related HCT
mitoxantrone 164
    combination regimens **161**
        carboplatin/melphalan 164
        cyclophosphamide/carboplatin 164
        cyclophosphamide/etoposide/melphalan combination 1267
        dexamethasone/fludarabine 1107–1108
        etoposide/ifosfamide/methotrexate 1107–1108
    high-dose in breast cancer 138
    MTD **159**
mixed lineage leukemia (MLL) gene 1221–1222
    childhood ALL prognosis 1078
mixed lymphocyte culture (MLC), HLA antigens 1132, 1142
MLC (mixed lymphocyte culture), HLA antigens 1132, 1142
MMF *see* mycophenolate mofetil (MMF)
MMSG *see* Italian Multiple Myeloma Study Group (MMSG)
modified Fibonacci scheme 418–429, **429**
MODS *see* multiple organ dysfunction syndrome (MODS)
MOG (myelin oligodendrocyte glycoprotein), EAE induction 329
molecular cytogenetics, chimerism characterization 235
molecular mimicry, autoimmunity 328
molgramostin *see* granulocyte macrophage colony-stimulating factor (GM-CSF)
Moloney murine leukemia virus (MuMLV) 107
monoclonal antibodies (MABs)
    antibody-mediated purging *see* purging, antibody-mediated
    bacterial infection 678
    GVHD prophylaxis 643
    immunotherapy following autologous transplants 1398–1399
    induced tolerance 308–309
    relapse reduction strategies 1396
    see also antibodies (therapeutic)
monoclonal antibody of undetermined significance (MGUS) 1263

monocytes
    development 79, 80, *614*
    recovery after PBHC allogeneic transplants 592
MOPP, doxorubicin/bleomycin/vinblastine/dacarbazine, Hodgkin's disease therapy 1197
morphine
    dose *904*
    pain management 902
morphology
    ALL classification 1055
    MDS prognosis 1085–1086
    residual disease detection **273**
Morquio syndrome (MPS IV) 1460
mortality
    identical sibling transplant *13*
    malignancy-related 654
    transplant-related 654
    see also survival
motor weakness
    following HCT 818
    post-herpes zoster 739
mouth, COH-TEAM care protocol **878**
mouthwash specimens, chimerism evaluation 236
MP *see* methylprednisolone (MP)
M-protein, multiple myeloma 1263
MRC *see* Medical Research Council (MRC)
MRD *see* minimal residual disease (MRD)
MRI *see* magnetic resonance imaging (MRI)
mRNA *see* messenger RNA (mRNA), translational silencing
MS *see* multiple sclerosis (MS)
MSKCC *see* Memorial Sloan–Kettering Cancer Center (MSKCC)
MTX *see* methotrexate (MTX)
mucolipidosis 1464
mucopolysaccharidoses 1456–1461, **1457**
    future directions 1460
mucositis
    AML autologous transplants 1223–1224
    protection from 167
        see also cytoprotection
    treatment complication 786
mucositosis, drug-induced 1340
    melphalan toxicity 140
multiattribute utility theory 437–438
multi-CSF *see* interleukin-3 (IL-3)
multidrug resistance 1 gene (P-glycoprotein/*MDR–1*) 135
    AML 1222
    gene therapy trials 123
    MCF-7^{ADR} cell expression *132*
multifocal leukoencephalopathy 813
multiple myeloma 1262–1282
    clinical features 1263
    cytogenetics 1262
    cytokine upregulation 1262–1263
    diagnosis 1264
    epidemiology 1096, 1262
    genetic abnormalities 1262, 1263–1264

minimal residual disease detection 245
relapse risk detection 281
staging/prognosis 1263–1264
surface markers 1262
survival 1264
therapy
    allogeneic transplants *see* multiple myeloma, allogeneic transplants
    autologous transplants *see* multiple myeloma, autologous transplants
    conventional chemotherapy 1264–1265
    DLI 1154
    melphalan 140–141
multiple myeloma, allogeneic transplants 1096–1104
    advantages 1096
    with autologous transplants *1101*, 1101–1102
        GVHD incidence 1101
        survival rates *1101*
        trials 1101–1102
    cell source 1098–1099
        T-cell depletion 1099
    DLI 1099
    future work 1102
    GVHD 1098
    myeloablative conditioning 1096–1098, **1097**
        after failed autologous transplantation 1099–1100
        complete remission 1096–1097
        TBI 1096
    nonmyeloablative conditioning 1098–1099, **1100**, 1100–1101
        fludarabine/TBI combination 1170
    PBHCs 1098
    prognostic factors 1098, *1099*
    relapse
        management 1154, *1154*
        risks 1099–1100
    transplant-related mortality 1096, 1098
multiple myeloma, autologous transplants 1264–1277
    with allogeneic transplants *see* multiple myeloma, allogeneic transplants
    AML, secondary 1277
    cell source 1264–1271
    chemotherapy *vs.* 1271–1273
    conditioning regimens 1265–1268
    maintenance therapy 1277
    MDS, secondary 1277
    myeloablative conditioning 1265–1268
        age studies 1267–1268
        clinical trials **1267**
        patient selection 1267–1268
    overall survival 1276
    PBHCs
        ages 1267–1268
        mobilization 1269–1270
        nonmobilization 1270
    prognostic features 1275–1277
    renal impairment 1268

tandem transplantation 1273–1275
    clinical trials 1267, **1274**
    prognosis 1276
    timing 1271, *1271*
    tumor contamination reduction 1270–1271
multiple organ dysfunction syndrome (MODS) 814
    prognosis **879**
multiple sclerosis (MS)
    animal model *see* experimental autoimmune encephalitis (EAE)
    HLA associations 324t
    MRI, pre/posttransplant *1389*
    severity scale 1388, **1388**
    treatment 1388–1389
multipotent adult stem cells (MASC) 69
    Fanconi anemia treatment 1500
mumps, vaccination in HCT recipients 862
muscle(s)
    transdifferentiation **77**
    weakness, following HCT 814–815, 818
mutagenesis, bone marrow purging 255–256
MY01G gene 388–389
myasthenia gravis (MG)
    animal model 326t
    following HCT 814, 815
MYCN oncogene, neuroblastoma 1344
Mycobacterium tuberculosis, CNS infection 811
mycophenolate mofetil (MMF) 215
    combination regimens
        cyclophosphamide/TBI 1201
        cyclosporine 1179
    GVHD treatment 360
    pharmacology 215
    toxicity 215
c-*myc* proto-oncogene 264
    mRNA half-life 277
    targeted antisense therapy 264–266
myelin-basic protein (MBP), EAE induction 329
myelin oligodendrocyte glycoprotein (MOG), EAE induction 329
myeloablative therapy 159–166, 307–308
    allogeneic transplants
        ALL, childhood 1073–1074
        multiple myeloma *see* multiple myeloma, allogeneic transplants
    autologous GVHD 406–407
    chimerism characterization 239
    CLL therapy 1110
    complications
        SOS prevention 778
        SOS treatment 779–780
    induced tolerance 307–308
    lymphoma therapy 1110
    MDS, nonmyeloablative therapy *vs.* 1088–1089
    neuroblastoma/HCT
        evolution of 1335
        regimens 1337
        targeted radionucleotides 1337–1338

nonmyeloablative therapy *vs.* 1170–1171
    relapse management 1157
    toxicity, abdominal pain 789
    see also chemotherapy, high-dose; pretransplant conditioning; tolerance, induced; *individual diseases/disorders; individual treatments*
myelodysplastic syndromes (MDS) 87–88, 1084–1089
    causes of death 1084–1085
    definition 1084–1085
    delayed complications 953–954
    Fanconi anemia 1484
        sibling donor HCT 1493–1494, **1495**
    incidence 1084
    secondary 954
        autologous transplants, multiple myeloma 1277
    therapy-related *see* myodysplasia, therapy-related (t-MDS)
myelodysplastic syndromes (MDS), HCT of allogeneic
    HLA-partially matched relative 1121
    nonmyeloablative therapy 1167
    relapse management 1153, *1153*
    sibling donor 1493–1494, **1495**
    unrelated donor 1144–1145
    autologous 1087
        AML 1226–1228
    disease-free survival (DFS) 1085, *1086*, 1087, *1089*
    immunoradiotherapy/HCT 203
    induction chemotherapy 1087–1088
    nonrelapse mortality 1085, *1086*
    preparative regimens 1088–1089
    prognostic factors 1085–1087
        age 1086
        cell source 1087
        cytogenetics 1085–1086
        morphology 1085–1086
    timings 1089
myeloid cell development 79, 80
    promiscuity 82–83
    see also individual cell types
myeloid progenitors 80
    bipotent 81
    colony-forming units 80
    common myeloid progenitors 80
        gene transfer and 119
    gene expression
        analysis 82–83
        transcription factors 87
    granulocyte/macrophage progenitors 80
    leukemic transformation 86–87
    megakaryocyte/erythrocyte progenitors 80
myeloma, multiple *see* multiple myeloma
myelomatosis *see* multiple myeloma
Myélome Auto Greffe (MAG), autologous transplants, multiple myeloma 1271
    high-dose *vs.* conventional 1272, **1272**

myeloproliferative disorders 87–88
    HCT 1089–1092
myelosuppression, polycythemia vera therapy 1090
Mylotarg *see* gemtuzumab
myodysplasia, therapy-related (t-MDS) 963–969, 1084
    clinical presentations **963**
    clinicopathological syndromes 963–964
    diagnosis 964
    DNA repair mechanisms, defective 966
    genetics 965–967
    HCT therapy of 1086–1087
        autologous in non-Hodgkin's lymphoma 1215–1216
    hematopoietic abnormalities 967
    pathogenesis 964–967, **965**, *965*
        p53 gene mutation 966–967
        telomeric shortening 967
    prediction *963*, 968–969
    prognosis 967–968
    risk factors 964
        reduction 969
    topoisomerase II inhibitor-related AML 963–964
myofibroblasts, hematopoietic microenvironment 54
myopathy
    delayed complications 950
    following HCT 814–815

N

nalbuphine, pain management 903
nasogastric feeding 886
nasojejunal feeding 886
National BMT Link 485
National Cancer Institute (NCI)
    clinical trials information 486
    solid tumor immunotherapy 1177–1178
National Gene Vector Laboratory (NGVL) 122
National Heart, Lung/Blood Institute (NHLBI), cord blood bank 550
National Institutes of Health (NIH), clinical trial definition 416
National Marrow Donor Program (NMDP) 5, 438, 485, 1133
    donor deferral 628, **628**
    history 624
    minorities **627**
    searching 628
        likelihood of matching **627**
    standards 537
    voluntary accreditation 536–537
natural killer cells (NKCs)
    cellular therapy following autologous transplants 1399–1400
    development 78–80, *79, 614*
    engraftment promotion 224–225
    graft rejection mediated by 22
    GVHD 23, 345
        autologous 409
    GVLE 369–370, 370, 373

natural killer cells (NKCs) (cont.)
　GVTE 371
　　solid tumors 1185
　　HLA-partially related donor HCT
　　　1125–1128, 1126
　　　animal models 1126–1127
　　　clone isolation 1127
　　　donor-recipient alloreactivity 1126–1128,
　　　　1127
　　immune regulation 325
　　　tolerance 306
　　interleukin-2 activation 312
　　in PBHC 590
　　recovery post cord blood transplantation
　　　554
　　response regulation 18, 18–19
　　varicella-zoster virus infection post-HCT
　　　737
natural killer cell triggering receptors
　1125–1126
Natural Menopause 525
natural suppressor (NS) cells, T-cell tolerance
　303
nausea
　long-term complications 795
　opioids, side effects 901
　TBI side-effect 185
　treatment complications 774
NCI see National Cancer Institute (NCI)
NCI/Rome standard criteria, ALL, childhood
　1070
NCL (neuronal ceroid lipofuscinosis) 1464
nephrotoxicity, acyclovir 743
nervous system
　central see central nervous system (CNS)
　delayed complications 955
　"gate control theory" 894
　peripheral see peripheral nervous system
　　(PNS)
　presentation of amyloidosis 1287–1288
NETCORD organization 533
neuroblastoma, HCT 1333–1344, 1337
　allogeneic
　　autologous vs. 1338
　　complications/quality of life 1338
　autologous
　　allogeneic vs. 1338
　　bone marrow vs. chemotherapy
　　　1335–1336, 1336, **1336**, 1336–1337,
　　　1337
　cell source 1338–1339
　clinical presentation 1333–1334
　complications/quality of life 1335, 1340
　　bone marrow involvement 1338
　induction therapy 1334–1335
　　"up-front phase 2 window" 1335
　local control 1335
　metastatic 1333
　minimal residual disease treatment 1339,
　　1339, 1339–1340
　MYCN oncogene 1344
　myeloablative therapy

　　acute/late complications 1340
　　autologous bone marrow 1335,
　　　1336–1337
　　development 1335
　　regimens 1337
　　stem cell rescue 1337
　　targeted radionucleotides 1337–1338
　purging 1338–1339
　　antibody-mediated 250
　relapse rates 1335, 1339
　risk classification 1344, **1344**
　staging 1333, **1333**
　survival 1334, 1344
　tandem transplants 1337
　treatment of high-risk disease 1334–1340
neuroendocrine system, chemotherapy/
　irradiation effects 929
neurofibromatosis type I (NF-1), JMML
　1018–1019
neurological complications 811–823, **819**, 955
　cerebrovascular 813, 814, **819**
　CNS infection 738, 739, 740, 811–813, 812,
　　819
　　see also specific infections
　differential diagnosis 818–819
　DMSO-induced 608
　GVHD relationship 818
　HCT for sickle cell disease 1423
　immune-mediated 814–815, **819**
　metabolic 813–814, **819**
　neuroendocrine dysfunction 948–949
　radiotherapy 189
　rates 811
　toxic/drug-related see neurotoxicity
　treatment **1387**
neuromuscular symptoms, chronic GVHD 648
neuronal ceroid lipofuscinosis (NCL) 1464
neuropathy 895, 907
　opioids 907
　pain management 899
　　substance abuse history 906
　treatment 907
neurotoxicity 815–818, **819**, 922–923
　acyclovir 743
　conditioning/chemotherapy agents 141,
　　817–818
　cyclosporine 815–817
　immunosuppressive drugs 817
　irradiation 189
　supportive care 818
　tacrolimus 815–817
　see also individual drugs
neutropenia
　in Fanconi anemia 1491
　fever, antifungal agents 692
　infections 668–669, 669–671
　　antibiotic prophylaxis during 667
　　fungal 683
　　treatment strategies 671–674, 672
　oral complications 911
　outpatient management 674
　scoring index **674**

neutrophil actin abnormality 1476
neutrophil-activating peptide (NAP-1) see
　interleukin-8 (IL-8)
neutrophils
　depletion see neutropenia
　development 614
　engraftment, cord blood
　　transplantation 555–556
　G-CSF stimulation 590, 592
　qualitative disorders 1476–1479
Nezelof syndrome 1436–1437
NGVL (National Gene Vector Laboratory) 122
NHL see non-Hodgkin's lymphoma (NHL)
NHLBI (National Heart, Lung/Blood Institute),
　cord blood bank 550
NHLBI Cord Blood Transplantation Study
　(COBLT) 551
nicotine dependence, treatment outcome
　457–458
Niemann–Pick disease 1464
NIH (National Institutes of Health), clinical trial
　definition 416
nitrosoureas 163
　regimens **161**
nitrous oxide (NO), GVHD 357
NKCs see natural killer cells (NKCs)
NMDP see National Marrow Donor Program
　(NMDP)
NMDP (US National Marrow Donor Program)
　12
nociceptive systems 894–895, **895**
nodular regenerative hyperplasia (NRH) 784
non-Hodgkin's lymphoma (NHL)
　AIDS 1372
　allogeneic transplants 1106
　antibody-mediated purging 250
　autologous transplants 1207–1220, **1210**,
　　1212, **1213**
　　cell source/manipulation 1214–1215
　　complications 1215–1216
　　future directions 1216
　　immunotherapy 1215
　　infections 1215
　　outcomes 1209
　　rationale 1208
　　survival 1209, 1209
　classification 1207, **1207**
　clinical features 1207–1208
　nonmyeloablative conditioning
　　fludarabine/TBI combination 1170
　　GVLE clinical trials 410
　　high-dose therapy 1214, **1214**
　　　consolidative irradiation 190–191
　　　rationale 1208
　　　survival 1209, **1212**, **1213**
　　incidence 1207
　　minimal residual disease detection post-
　　　HCT **278**
　　prognostic factors 1207–1208, **1208**
　　radioimmunotherapy/HCT 203–204
　　recombinant G-CSF 616–617
　　relapse risk detection 281

non-leukemic disease, PBHC allogeneic
    transplants 594
nonmalignant disease **10**
    ethical issues 493–494
    immunosuppressive agents, randomized
        controlled trials **642**
nonmedical costs 436
nonmyeloablative therapy 164–165, 165,
    1164–1176
    allogeneic transplants 1164
        agnogenic myeloid metaplasia 1092
        AML **1033**, 1167
        CLL 1167
        CML 1167
        Hodgkin's disease 1201
        MDS 1167
        multiple myeloma 1098–1099, **1100**,
            1100–1101
        PNH 1004–1005
        solid tumors *see* solid tumors, allogeneic
            transplants
    canine models 1165–1166
    chimerism effects, Philadelphia chromosome
        (Bcr–Abl gene fusion) 1172, *1172*
    clinical results 1166–1167
    CMV reactivation 1100
    GVHD association 1204
    hematologic malignancies 1167–1173,
        1168–1169
        HLA-matched related HCT 1167–1171
        HLA-partially matched related HCT
            1171–1172
        post failed transplants 1172–1173
        unrelated HCT 1171–1172
    high-dose chemotherapy 164–165, 165
    immunosuppression *vs.* *1167*
    mixed chimerism induction *309*
    murine models 1164–1165
    myeloablative therapy *vs.* 1170–1171
        in MDS 1088–1089
    nonmalignant disorders 1173–1174
    oral complications 923
    preclinical studies 1164–1166
        marrow space *vs.* immunosuppression
            1166
        MHC matched grafts 1165
        MHC partially matched grafts 1165,
            1166
        mixed chimerism 1165–1166
        radioimmunotherapy 1166
        TBI doses/toxicity 1165, **1165**
    regimens 991
        AML in children 1045
        CMV 710
    in relapse 1151
    sickle cell disease 1424–1425, **1425**
    solid tumors *see* solid tumors, allogeneic
        transplants
    see also chemotherapy; pretransplant
        conditioning; *individual drugs*
nonrandom chromosomal translocations, PCR
    detection 245

nonrelapse mortality (NRM) *see individual
    diseases/disorders; individual
    treatments*
non-steroidal anti-inflammatory drugs
    (NSAIDs) 899
    dose **900**
Nordic Bone Marrow Transplant group
    1069
Norwalk virus infections 764
Notch pathway
    HSC expansion studies 98–99
    HSC self-renewal 72, 73
NRH (nodular regenerative hyperplasia) 784
NSAIDs *see* non-steroidal anti-inflammatory
    drugs (NSAIDs)
nucleic acid based therapies 258–271
    antisense oligonucleotides *see* antisense
        oligonucleotides
    delivery 266
    efficacy 266–267
    gene (transcriptional) targeting 258–259
        "anti-HIV-1 genes" 125
        chimeric (DNA/RNA) oligonucleotides
            259
        decoy oligos 259, *259*
        lexitropsins 259
        polyamides 259, *260*
        triple-helix forming oligonucleotides
            (TFOs) 258–259, *259*
    hematological disease trials 258, 264–266,
        265, 267
        Bcl-2/apoptosis targeting 264
        immunological adjuvants 266
        MYB transcription factor targeting
            264–266
        PKC-α targeting 258
        Ras targeting 258
        ribozymes 263
    history 258
    mRNA (translational) targeting *260*,
        260–264
        antisense DNA (oligonucleotides) *260*,
            260–261
        DNAzymes *260*, 262–263
        mRNA processing perturbation 264
        ribozymes *260*, 261–262
        RNAi 263–264
        target abundance/half-life 267
    problems 266–277
    signal transduction targeting 266
    see also antisense oligonucleotides; gene
        therapy; *specific therapies*
nucleic acid sequence-based amplification
    (NASBA), CMV detection 717–718
nude mice 330
nurse case manager (NCM) *see* hematopoietic
    cell transplantation (HCT) program
nurse program manager (NPM) 463–464
nursing issues 469–482
    assessment 470, **470–472, 474–479**
    bone marrow harvest 471–472, **475**
    conditioning 471, **472**

    coordination of care 470, **470–472,
        474–479**
    discharge 475, **479**
    donor care 470–471, 471, **471**
    intensive care management 475
    long-term recovery 475, 479
    post-engraftment, early 474–475, **478**
    preconditioning 470, **471**
    pre-engraftment 472, 474, **477**
    prework-up 470, **470**
    relapse posttransplant 475
    staff maintenance 469–470
    symptoms **473–474**
    teaching 470, **474–479**
    transplant phase 472, **476**
    work-up 470, **470**
nutritional support 883–893
    adjustment 888–890
        experimental modifications 889–890
        glutamine 890
        GVHD 889
        immunomodulatory formulas 890
        malnourished patients 888–889
        systemic inflammatory response 889
    benefits 883
    complications 887–888
    cytopenia 884
    cytoreduction 884
    dietary prescriptions 887
    energy requirements 885, **885**
    engraftment 884
    long-term considerations 890–891
    monitoring 887, **887**
    posttransplant 886
    requirement changes 884
    during transplant 885–887
    types
        enteral therapy 886–887
        gastrostomy feeding 886
        nasogastric/nasojejunal feeding 886
        oral intake 886
        parenteral therapy *see* parenteral feeding
        total parenteral *883*
NY-ESO-1, T-cell adoptive immunotherapy
    391

O
OBA (Office of Biotechnology Activities) 122
obesity
    drug dosing 456
    pediatric transplant 459
    treatment outcome 456
observational study designs *see* biostatistical
    methods
obstructive airway disease (OAD) 877
    delayed 947
ocular sicca 950
odds ratio (OR) 416
Office of Biotechnology Activities (OBA) 122
OKT3
    partial T-cell depletion 1122
    sickle cell disease 1432–1434

oligodendroglioma(s) 1348–1349
  chemotherapy (high-dose) with HCT 1348–1349
  natural history with conventional therapy 1348
oligonucleotides
  antisense *see* antisense oligonucleotides
  arrays *see* microarray(s)
  chimeric (DNA/RNA) 259
  decoy 259, *259*
  HLA typing 39
  as immunological adjuvants 266
  triple-helix forming (TFOs) 258–259, *259*
  "walking" 266
Omenn's syndrome
  cord blood cell transplantation 1435
  HCT 1437
  pathogenic basis 1437
  T-cell depleted HCT 1433–1434
oncogenes, ovarian cancer 1321
oncogenic fusion genes/proteins 86
ophthalmoplegia, following HCT 819
opioids 899–905
  administration 903–904
  clinical practice 903–904
  commonly used 902–903
  GVHD 906
  neuropathy 907
  pain management 899–905
  pharmacodynamics 900–901
  pharmacokinetics 900, *901*
  pharmacology 900
  side effects 901–902
    physical dependence 902
    tolerance development 902
  tapering 904–905
opportunistic infection(s) 26, 666, **670**
  see also individual infections
oprelvekin *see* interleukin-11 (IL-11)
oral complications 911–928
  COH-TEAM mouth care protocol **878**
  conditioning 911, **912**
  dental treatment 912–913, 912–914
    decay management 913
    delayed complications 951
    dentures 913–914, **914**
    endodontic disease 913
    extraction 913
    orthodontic appliances 913, **914**
    periodontal disease 913
  engraftment 911, **912**
  examination 923
  gingival hyperplasia 924
  granulomatous lesions 924
  growth/development 923
  GVHD 294, 921–922, **922**, 923
    assessment 923
    chronic 647
  hemorrhage 921
  immune reconstitution 911, **912**
  infections 919–921
    bacterial 920
    early 919–920
    fungal 919
    late 920–921
    viral 919–920
  long-term follow-up 923
  malignancy, secondary 924
  management
    dental treatment *see* dental treatment *above*
    hygiene care **915**, 915–916
    mucosal care 916
    oropharyngeal mucositis 917–919, **918**
  medical information required 912
  neurotoxicity/pain 922–923
  neutropenia 911, **912**
  nonmyeloablative transplantation 923
  oropharyngeal mucositis 916–919, *917*
  posttransplant 911, **912**, 914–924
  pretransplant 911, 912, **912**
  prophylaxis 914
  relapse 924
  salivary gland hypofunction 921
  taste dysfunction 922
  temporomandibular dysfunction 914
  toxicities 914
  xerostomia 921, **921**
orofacial growth, following treatment 934–935
  strategies 935
oropharyngeal mucositis 916–919, *917*
  management 917–919, **918**
  pain management 905
osmotic stress, cryopreservation 601
osteoblast(s) 54
osteoclast(s)
  function in bone resorption 1444
  osteopetrosis *1447*
  survival *1448*
osteopenia 950–951
osteopetrosis 1443–1454
  adult 1443
  animal models 1444–1446, **1445**
    HCT 1445–1446
    knockout experiments 1445
    mutations 1444–1445
  forms 1443
  humans 1443
  infantile malignant *see below*
  osteoclast/bone resorption 1444
osteopetrosis, infantile malignant 1443–1444
  diagnosis 1443–1444
  future directions 1450–1451
  HCT 1446–1448
    complications 1449
    conditioning regimen 1449
    donor selection 1449
    engraftment 1449
    posttransplant evaluation 1449
    pretransplant evaluation 1448–1449
    survival *1448*
    transplant issues 1448
  histology *1446, 1447*
  survival 1444
  symptoms 1443–1444
  treatment 1446, 1450
  in utero transplant 1450
  variant 1444
osteoporosis 950–951
osteosarcoma 1360
ototoxicity
  cisplatin 144
  neuroblastoma treatment 1340
outcome (of HCT)
  factors leading to improved 10–11
  Karnofsky score 11
  patient age 10
  pretransplant conditioning 11
  psychosocial predictors 509
outcomes research 414, 434–446
  combining data 438–441
    decision analysis 438–440
    evidence-based medicine 440–441, **441**
    meta-analysis 440, *440*
    publication bias 440
    Q-TWiST 416, 440, *440*
    registry studies 438
  constructs 441
  definition 434
  economic analysis 436–438
    cost–benefit analysis 436, 437, **437**
    cost–effectiveness analysis 416, 436, **437**, 437, 438
    cost reduction 436, **436**
    cost–utility analysis 436, 437, **437**, 438
    multiattribute utility theory 437–438
    power 438
    standard gambles 437
    time trade-off 437
  historical aspects 434–436
  instrument (survey) development 442–443
  patient experience 441–442
    see also quality of life (QOL)
  scale development 443
  see also biostatistical methods; evidence-based medicine; health services research
outpatients, neutropenia 674
ovarian cancer 1320–1332
  bone marrow contamination 1329
  detection 1321
  epidemiology 1320–1321
  future studies 1329
  incidence **1320**
  oncogenes 1321
  pathogenesis 1320–1321
  prognosis 1320
  risk factors 1320–1321
  screening 1321
ovarian cancer management
  chemotherapy 1321–1322
    combination 1324–1325
    high-dose 1323, **1327**, **1328**, 1328–1329
    intraperitoneal 1324
    systemic 1323–1324

comparisons **1326**
conventional 1321–1323, 1323–1324
HCT
  allogeneic 1184, 1330
    clinical trials 1324–1329
    persistent disease 1327–1329
  initial *1321*, 1328–1329
  interval cytoreductive therapy 1322–1323
  multivariate analyzes **1325**, 1325–1327
  recurrent disease 1323, **1323**
  refractory disease 1324–1325, **1326**
  salvage therapy **1326**
  surgical 1321
    laparotomy 1322–1323, 1327–1329
  in vitro studies of dose density 1324
ovaries, function following HCT **935**, 937–939, **938**
overdominant selection (heterozygote advantage), MHC evolution 48
OX40 marker, antigen presentation 355
oxazophosphorines, bone marrow purging 254
oxymetholone, Fanconi anemia therapy 1490

P
p53 mutation, secondary malignancy 966–967
p65, CMV infection 383–384
paclitaxel 165
  dexamethasone/cyclophosphamide/etoposide/G-CSF combination 1269
  high-dose chemotherapy 137
  mechanism of action 146
  metabolism 146–147
  monitoring 137
  PBHC mobilization, standard regimens **582**
  pharmacology **131**, 147
    nonlinear pharmacokinetics *136*
  regimens **161**
  structure *131*
  toxicity 147
    neurotoxicity 818
PACT (Psychosocial Assessment of Candidates for Transplant Scale) 498–499
pain
  abdomen 789–792
  anatomy 894
  assessment/measurement 896–897
    categoric scale 897
    history taking 896
    numerical scales *896*, 896–897
    scales 896–897
    visual analog scales 897, *897*
  defined 895
  diagnostics 897
  emotions 897–898
  experience *895*
    factors 896
  functioning ability 897
  management *see* pain management
  neuropathic 907
  nociceptive systems 894–895, *895*
  orofacial 922–923
  patient perspectives 484
  phenomenon 895–897
  physiology 894
  procedures causing 907–908
  procedures causing pain 907–908
  sources **894**
  suffering in HCT patients 895–896
pain management 484, 894–910, 897
  clinical 905–907
  critically ill patients 908
  invasive techniques 908
  neuropathic 907
  nonopioid 899
  nonpharmacological techniques 897–899
    cognitive-behavioural strategies 898
    education 898, **898**
    information 898
    mechanisms 897–898
    pediatric considerations 898–899
  peritransplant 905
  pharmacological 899–908
    see also individual drugs
  post-engraftment 906–907
  pretransplant 905
  pseudoaddiction 905
  selection 897
  substance abuse, patients with prior history 905–906
  surgical 907
palliative care, allogeneic transplants relapse management 1158
pamidronate, multiple myeloma therapy 1265
pancreas, pain 790
pancytopenia
  DLI toxicity 1155
  neurological complications **819**
  radiotherapy side-effect 205
papovavirus infections 763–764
paracetamol *see* acetaminophen (paracetamol)
parainfluenza virus infection 760–761, **762**
paraprotein, multiple myeloma 1263
parasitic disease(s), transfusion transmitted 845–846
parental decision making 493–494
parenteral feeding 885–886
  adjustment 885–886
  complications 774–775
  disadvantages 886
  enteral feeding *vs.* 886
parotiditis, TBI side-effect 185
parovirus
  liver infection 782
  transfusion transmitted 845
paroxysmal nocturnal hemoglobinuria (PNH) 63
  allogeneic transplants 1002–1006
    conditioning 1003
    death 1003
    GVHD 1003
    nonmyeloablative transplant 1004–1005
    published reports **1003**, 1003–1004, **1004**
  aplastic anemia 981, 1002–1003
  autologous transplants 1005
  clinical diagnosis 1002–1003
  hematopoiesis 65
  nontransplant treatment 1005
  pathogenesis 1002
partial chimerism 234
parvovirus B19 infections 763–764
passenger lymphocyte syndrome 825
passive immunization **870**
paternity issues 490–492
pathology of HCT 286–299
  complication groups 286
  GVHD *see* graft-*vs.*-host disease (GVHD)
  hepatic sinusoidal obstructive syndrome *see* sinusoidal obstruction syndrome (SOS)
  infection *see* infection(s)
  interstitial pneumonia (IP) *see* interstitial pneumonia (IP)
  interstitial pneumonia syndrome (IPS) 295–296
  posttransplant evaluation 286–287
  pretransplant evaluation 286
  pulmonary disease *see* pulmonary complications
  toxicity from cytoreductive therapy 287, **287**
patient(s) 447–528
  assessment of needs 483
  autonomy 489–490
  clinical trials discussion 485–486
  communication language 483–484
  counseling *see* donor counseling
  cultural background 483
  "difficult" 501
  expectations 507
  foreign patients 453
  information *see* information
  interpretation of data 452, **452**
  nursing issues *see* nursing issues
  opinions, multiple 452–453
  pain management 484
  perspective 483–487
  procedure choice 451
  psychosocial issues *see* psychosocial complications/factors
  quality of life post-treatment 486–487
  risk perspectives 483
  selection 10–11
    ethical issues 488–489
  stress 484–485
  terminology 449
  understanding 484
patient controlled analgesia (PCA) 904
Pax-5, B-cell development 78, 83
PBHCs *see* peripheral blood hematopoietic cells (PBHCs)
PCA (patient controlled analgesia) 904
PCR (polymerase chain reaction)
  advantages/disadvantages 275
  in CML 275
    multidrug resistance monitoring 1013
  in CMV *716*, 717
  fungal infections 687

PCR (polymerase chain reaction) (cont.)
  HLA typing 37, 1132
  minimal residual disease detection **273**, 275, 1150
  quantitative 279
  real-time studies, chimerism characterization 236
  reverse transcriptase (RT-PCR) *276*
  secondary malignancy, prognosis 968–969
  tumor cell detection 245
    sensitivity 244t
  varicella-zoster virus detection 735, 741
Pediatric Cancer QOL Inventory 514
Pediatric Oncology Group (POG) studies 1335
The Pediatric Quality of Life Inventory 514
pediatric transplant
  child development/compliance 460
  considerations 458–460
  disease status/decision not to proceed 458–459
  informed consent 458
  intensity-reduced regimens 459
  issues **460**
  obesity 459
  orofacial/dental growth 923–924
  pretransplant evaluation 459
  psychosocial/family issues 459–460
  quality of life issues 512
  see also children
Pelazeus–Merzbacher 1463
penicillin resistance 666, **667**, 668
peptide nucleic acids (PNAs), antisense therapy 261
peptides, GVHD treatment 217
perforin/granzyme pathway, GVHD 356
perfosfamide *see* 4-hydroperoxycyclophosphamide (4-HC)
peripheral blood, HSC expansion studies 99, **100**
peripheral blood hematopoietic cells (PBHCs) 599
  allogeneic transplants 588–598
    characteristics/dose 589–590
    EBV risk 751
    engraftment 592
    future developments 594
    GVHD **592**, 637–638
    GVHD, acute 592–593
    GVHD, chronic 593, **593**
    HLA-partially matched related 1123
    immune cells 590
    immune recovery 592
    multiple myeloma 1098
    non-leukemic disease 594
    randomized trials 592–594
    relapse rates 593
    survival 593–594
    T-cell depleted HCT 1123
    transplant related mortality 593
    unrelated 594
  autologous transplants
    ALL 1245
    AML 1225, 1232, 1233

    Hodgkin's disease 1200
    non-Hodgkin's lymphoma 1215
    recombinant G-CSF 615, 616
  cryopreservation 599, 605
  donation
    adverse events 543–544
    death 544
    pain *543*
    procedure 545
    symptoms **543**
  MDS therapy 1087
  mobilization *see* peripheral blood hematopoietic cells (PBHCs), mobilization
  purging 1225, 1245, 1338–1339
  residual tumor cells 245–246
  solid tumor treatment 1364
  T-cell content 853
peripheral blood hematopoietic cells (PBHCs), mobilization 576–587, 588–589
  adhesion molecules 576–577, 581–582
  after chemotherapy 1253
  autologous transplants
    AML 1225
    multiple myeloma 1269–1270
  chemokines 577
    chemotherapy combinations 580
  clinical applications 577
  clinical studies **582**
  collection techniques 577–578
  cytokines 577, 578–580, 1098
    combinations **578**, *579*, 579–580
    doses *579*
    see also individual cytokines
  future work 581–583
  identification/enumeration 576
    optimal yield 578, *578*
  imatinib 1255
  side effects 590–591
  standard regimens **582**
  T-cell depletion 594
  tumor contamination 581
  yield-affecting factors 580–581, **581**
peripheral induced tolerance *see* tolerance, induced
peripheral nervous system (PNS)
  neuropathy
    drug-induced 818
    immune-mediated complications of HCT 814–815, **819**
    post-herpes zoster 739
  stem cells 77, *77*
peroxisomal disorders 1455–1461
  considerations 1455–1456
"personalized" medicine 431
  high-dose chemotherapy 135–138
PET (positron emission tomography) 201
PETHEMA *see* Programa para el Tratamiento de Hemopatías Malignas (PETHEMA), multiple myeloma autologous transplants

P-glycoprotein/*MDR-1* see multidrug resistance 1 gene (P-glycoprotein/*MDR-1*)
pharmacodynamics *see individual drugs*
pharmacogenomics
  clinical trials, impact on 423
  contribution to chemotherapy 133
  drug metabolism/transport 133–135
pharmacokinetics
  high-dose chemotherapy **131**, 135
  linear *136*
  nonlinear 135, *136*
  see also drug metabolism; *individual drugs*
pharmacologic purging, antibody-mediated purging combination 247–248
pharmacology *see specific drugs/indications*
pheretic purging 1338
Philadelphia chromosome (*Bcr–Abl* gene fusion) 75, 86, 423
  antisense
    ALL *see* acute lymphoblastic leukemia (ALL)
    autologous transplants in CML 1251–1252
  healthy people 282
  JMML 1019
  kinetics of emergence *279*
  purging techniques 1256
  quantitative studies 279
  recurrence prevention 1257
  relapse risk 277–280, 282
  RT-PCR *276*
  T-cell adoptive immunotherapy 391
PHN *see* postherpetic neuralgia (PHN)
phosphorothioate oligonucleotides, antisense therapy 261, 264
phylogenetic analysis, MHC 44, 45, *46*, *47*, *49*
phytohemagglutan A, T-cell stimulation 855
pill esophagus 787
plasmablastic morphology, multiple myeloma prognosis 1275
plasma transfusions, in GVHD 841
platelets
  development *614*
  engraftment, cord blood transplantation 555–556
  fludarabine/TBI combination *1170*
  storage 835
  transfusions 834–839
    apheresis 834–835
    blood groups 836
    concentrate-related factors 837
    concentrates from whole blood 834
    crossmatching 837
    HLA-matching 837
    outcome 836
    patient-related factors 837
    reactions 843
    refractoriness 836–839
      concentrate-related factors 837
      management 837–838
      management strategies 837–838
      patient-related factors 837

practical approach 838
  prevention 838–839
  storage 835
  thrombopoietin 839
platinating agents
  high-dose chemotherapy 143–144
  in vitro models 130
  metabolism 134
  neuroblastoma induction therapy 1334–1335
  see also carboplatin; cisplatin
pleiotropic agents 144–147
  see also individual drugs
pleural disease 877
pleuropulmonary blastoma 1361
pluripotent stem cells 69, 74, 77
PML/RARα fusion protein, AML 86
PNETs *see* primitive neuroectodermal tumors
pneumonia 811
  CMV *see* cytomegalovirus-associated interstitial pneumonia (CMV-IP)
  human papillomavirus 729
  idiopathic syndrome 876
  interstitial *see* cytomegalovirus-associated interstitial pneumonia (CMV-IP); interstitial pneumonia (IP)
  vaccination in HCT recipients 862
    response 863–864
  varicella-zoster 738, 740
pneumonitis, delayed 945
PNH *see* paroxysmal nocturnal hemoglobinuria (PNH)
polio vaccine 859
polyamides, gene silencing 259, *260*
polycomb family, HSC self-renewal 73
polycythemia vera (PV)
  definition 1089–1090
  HCT 1090
polyenes 692–694, **693**
polymers, GVHD treatment 217
polymyositis, following HCT 814
polysaccharide antigens
  response posttransplant 857
  vaccination 859
positron emission tomography (PET) 201
postherpetic neuralgia (PHN) 739, 812
  management 743
posttransplant
  autologous transplants therapy, Hodgkin's disease 1195
  energy requirements 886
  evaluation 286–287
    osteopetrosis 1449
  fungal infections 684, *684*
  immunosuppression *see* immunosuppression
  malignant disease *952*, 952–954
  oral complications 911, **912**, 914–924
  pain management 906–907
  psychosocial factors 500–501
  transfusion strategies 840
  see also engraftment
posttransplant lymphoproliferative disorder (PTLD) 969–971

B-cell 969–970
  pathogenesis 969
  prediction 970
  risk factors 969, **970**
  treatment 970
liver *291*
T-cell 971
Power of Attorney for Health Care 494
PRCA *see* pure red cell aplasia (PRCA)
pre-B-cell markers 1068
prednisolone (PSE) *209*
  combination regimens **211**
    asparaginase/methotrexate/vincristine combination 1157
    cyclosporine 384
    cyclosporine/recombinant G-CSF 617
    combined immunosuppression 641
    Fanconi anemia therapy 1490
    GVHD treatment 360, 650
    randomized controlled trials **642**, 651, **651**
prednisone *209*
  ALL therapy 1238
  combination regimens **211**
    ATG 1165
    CHOP regimen *see* CHOP regimen
    cyclophosphamide/doxorubicin/vincristine *see* CHOP regimen
    melphalan 1264
  neurological complications 817
pregnancy
  donation 540
  following HCT 939
preimplantation genetic diagnosis (PGD)
  ethical issues 492–493
  Fanconi anemia 1500
prenatal diagnosis 565
  osteopetrosis 1450, 1451
preparative regimens *see* pretransplant conditioning
pretransplant
  emotional distress 499
  evaluation 286
    neurological 819
    oral evaluation 912
    osteopetrosis 1448–1449
    pediatric transplant 459
    psychosocial factors 500
    pulmonary function 873–874, **874**
  oral complications 911, **912**
  pain management 905
  quality of life issues 509
  transfusion strategies 839–840
pretransplant conditioning 12, 158–177
  agents
    chemotherapeutic *see* chemotherapy
    radiotherapeutic *see* radiotherapy
  ALL
    autologous transplants 1244–1245
    in children 1073–1074, *1074*
  allogeneic transplants
    bone marrow transplant in thalassemia 1410–1411

in children 1073–1074, *1074*
  HLA-partially matched related graft failure 1119
    T-cell depleted HCT 1123, *1123*
AML
  in adults 1027
  autologous transplants **1222**, 1222–1223
  in children 1044–1045
aplastic anemia 982
autologous transplants
  ALL 1244–1245
  AML **1222**, 1222–1223
  multiple myeloma 1265–1268
chimerism, effects on 237
CML 1010
complications 774
  SOS prevention 778–779
cytoprotection *see* cytoprotection
evaluation 158, **158**
Fanconi anemia, HCT 1491–1493
growth/development following
  chemotherapy 932
  irradiation 932–934
GVHD 23, 353
immune system 16
infections during 668–669
  fungal infections 689
JMML 1021–1022
MDS 1088–1089
mucosal necrosis 785
multiple myeloma, autologous transplants 1265–1268
oral complications 911, **912**
osteopetrosis 1449
outcome 11
pain management 908
  substance abuse history 906
PNH 1003
psychosocial factors 500
quality of life issues 511
relapse reduction strategies 1396
toxicity 287
  diarrhea 787
  see also chemotherapy; chemotherapy, high-dose; myeloablative therapy; nonmyeloablative therapy; *individual regimens*
primary induction failure, AML 1030–1031
primary myelofibrosis *see* agnogenic myeloid metaplasia (AMM)
primate models 5
primitive germline cells (PGCs) 77
primitive neuroectodermal tumors (PNETs) 1350–1351, **1351**
procarbazine
  GVHD primary treatment 650
  single-agent immunosuppression 641
progenitor cell(s)
  cryopreservation efficacy 604
  hematopoietic *see* hematopoietic progenitor cells (HPCs)
  purging techniques 1256

progenitor cell(s) (*cont.*)
  stem cells *vs.* 69
  transdifferentiation 76
Programa para el Tratamiento de Hemopatías Malignas (PETHEMA), multiple myeloma autologous transplants 1271
  high-dose *vs.* conventional 1272, **1272**
programmed cell death *see* apoptosis
programmed death (PD-1) marker, antigen presentation 354–355
prophylaxis *see individual diseases/disorders; individual treatments*
prospective cohort studies 415
proteasome inhibitor(s) 1277
proteinase 3 (PR3) 391–392
protein kinase C-α (PKC-α), antisense therapies 266
proteoglycans 55
proteolipid protein (PLP) 329
PS-341, multiple myeloma maintenance therapy 1277
PSA, T-cell adoptive immunotherapy 391
PSE *see* prednisolone (PSE)
Pseudomonas infections 85
  HLA-partially matched related HCT 1123
psychological dependence (addiction), opioids 902
psychosocial assessment
  goals **458**
  nurse care manager (NCM) 465
  treatment outcome 457–458
Psychosocial Assessment of Candidates for Transplant Scale (PACT) 498–499
psychosocial complications/factors 484–485, 497–506, 955
  caregivers 503–504
  donors 502–503, 539
    motives 539
  measures **508**
  medical staff 504–505
  objective/subjective measures, correlations **515**
  pediatric transplant 459–460
  post-treatment 484–485
  quality of life issues, measures **508**
  recipients 497–502
  sexual dysfunction 523
Psychosocial Levels System (PLS) 498–499
PTLD *see* posttransplant lymphoproliferative disorder (PTLD)
PU.1 transcription factor
  loss of function in leukemia 87
  T-cell development 83
puberty
  complications 949
  following HCT 935–937
    boys **936**, 937
    girls **936**
Public Health Services (PHS) Act 531
pulmonary complications 295–297, 873–882, **874**

critically ill patients, prognosis 878–879
delayed 945, 947
diagnosis
  function testing 873
  infiltrates 874–875
  lung biopsy 874–875
  radiographic imaging 873–875
GVHD 296–297
  chronic 647–648
infections 295, 295–296, **296**, 875–876
  see also individual infections
mechanical ventilation 878, **879**
pretransplant assessment 873–874, **874**
pulmonary/airway disease 945
  obstructive 947
  pathology 295–296
  restrictive 945, 947
respiratory failure 878–879
specific disease 875–878
time frame 875, **875**
transfusion-related injury 842–843
upper airway complications 877–878
see also respiratory symptoms
pulmonary vascular disease 877
pure red cell aplasia (PRCA) 824–825, 826
  incidence 824, 827
  mechanism 826
  treatment 826–827
purging
  autologous transplants
    ALL 1241–1242, 1245
    AML 1224–1225, 1226
    CML 1251–1253
  bone marrow *see* bone marrow purging
  improved techniques 1256–1257
  photodynamic 1252
  relapse reduction strategies 1397
purging, antibody-mediated 244–253
  aims 244
  autologous transplants
    ALL 1244
    AML 1225
  clinical studies 249–251
  complement-mediated lysis 246f, 247–248
    antibody selection 246–247
    clinical studies/efficacy 249–250
    other methods *vs.* 247t
  efficacy assessment 248–250
    methods 249t
  immunomagnetic bead depletion 248, 1338, 1339
    efficacy/clinical studies 250
    multiple antibodies 248
    other methods *vs.* 247t
  immunotoxins 248
    clinical trials/efficacy 249, 250
    other methods *vs.* 247t
  methods 246–248, 246f, 246t
    comparisons 247t
    immunoglobulin M 246–247
    see also individual methods

monoclonal antibodies 246
  humanized 251
  outcomes 250–251, 250f
    engraftment, impact on 249t
  pharmacologic purging combination 247–248
  target antigens 246t
purine synthesis pathways *215*

Q
Q-TWiST analysis 416, 440, *440*
quality adjusted life years (QALYs), decision tree analysis 439
quality of life (QOL) 519–520
  acute treatment 509
  age effects 511
  assessment in recipients 507–518
    clinically meaningful differences 515
    internal consistency 515
    pediatric 512
    psychometrics 515
    reliability 515
    test-retest reliability 515
    validity 515
  biostatistical methods 416
  caregivers 512
  cognitive function 510, **515**
  components 507
  conditioning regimen 511
  definition of health-related 507
  dimensions 441, *442*, 507, 509, 519, *520*
  diversity 511
  donors 512
    type effect 511
  fatigue 509–510
  first year 509
  gender 512
  GVHD, chronic 654
  improvement 512–513
  instruments 441, *442*
  late effects 510–511
  long-term function 509
  measures 507, **508**, 513
    alternative 514
    formats 514–515
    generic 513
    multidimensional **508**
    parent/proxy 514
    response shift 513
    specific dimensions 513, *514*
  outcomes research 441–442
  patient expectations 507
  during phases of HCT 509
  post-treatment 486–487
    neuroblastoma 1340
  pretransplant 509
  pyramid 507
  randomized controlled trials (RCTs) 512
  relapse 511
  sexuality **508**, 520
  social function **508**

studies **521**
symptoms **508**
quantitative granulocyte disorders 1474–1476

R
RAC (Recombinant DNA Advisory Committee) 122
race *see* ethnicity
radiation
  blood components for transfusion 840–841
  CLL sensitivity 1105
  lymphoma sensitivity 1105
  secondary malignancy 963
  side effects 950
  see also total body irradiation (TBI)
radiation pneumonopathy 180, 186–188
radiographic imaging
  abnormalities in germ cell tumor 1309–1310
  pulmonary function 873–874
  see also computed tomography (CT); magnetic resonance imaging (MRI)
radioimmunoassay (RIA), varicella-zoster virus 741
radioimmunotherapy (RAIT) 199–202
  biodistribution 199, *199*, **199**
    favorable 202
  bone-seeking 165–166
  dose 201, 205
    escalation 203, 204
    monitoring 201, *203*
  external beam radiation *vs.* 201
  Fab/F(ab')$_2$ fragments 200
  HCT and 198–208
    ALL therapy 1062–1063
    AML **1222**, 1223, 1233
      second remission 1226
    future 205–206
    Hodgkin's disease trials 204–205
    leukemia trials 202–203
    neuroblastoma 1337–1338
    non-Hodgkin's lymphoma trials 203–204
    solid tumor trials 205
  historical background 198–199
  immunosuppression 201–202
  labeling 198, 200–201
  limitations 198, 205
    human antimouse antibody response 200
    toxicities 205
  neuroblastoma 1337–1338
  nonmyeloablative therapy, preclinical studies 1166
  pharmacology 200
  pretargeting 206
  radiation effects 201–202
  radioisotopes 200–201, **201**
  specificity 200
  target antigen 199–200
  trace-labeled dose 201, *203*
  see also antibodies (therapeutic)
radioisotopes 165–166, 200–201, **201**
  targeted *see* antibodies (therapeutic); radioimmunotherapy (RAIT)

radiotherapy 178–197
  basic principles 178–179, *179*
  clinical results 185–189
    chemotherapy *vs.* 189–190, *190*
    high-dose chemotherapy and 190–191
    TBI 185–189
    total lymphoid irradiation (TLI) 191–192
  CLL therapy 1107
  consolidative irradiation 185, 190–191
  cytoreduction of leukemic cells 179–180
  DLI modifications 1156
  gonadal function following 938–939, 939
  growth/development following 929, 930–931, 932, **934**, 937
    height **934**
    men 939
    rates 932
    thoracoabdominal 938–939
    women 938–939, 939
  high-dose radiation
    chemotherapy *vs.* 130
    pretransplant 12
  immunosuppression 179, 185
  irradiation protection effect 3
  irradiation syndrome, secondary phase 221
  locoregional 191
  normal tissue toxicity *180*, 180–182
    bone epiphyses 189
    brain 189
    delivery regimen effects 180, **181**, 182, **182**, *182*, 187
    immune system **181**
    lens 188–189
    lung 180, **181**, 186–188
    TLI 192
  physical considerations 182–185
    "boosting" 178, 184–185, 186
    dose rate/distance from source 182, 183
    energy 183
    homogeneity 184
    patient position *183*, 183–184
    shielding 184
    TBI stands *184*
  puberty following 937
  regimens *see* radiotherapy regimens
  relapse 185–186
  side-effects
    acute 185
    pancytopenia 205
  thoracoabdominal irradiation *see* thoracoabdominal irradiation (TAI)
  thyroid function following 930–931
  total body *see* total body irradiation (TBI)
  see also total body irradiation (TBI)
radiotherapy regimens 178, 192
  fractionated 179, 180, 182, 187
    modeling impact 182
    normal tissue toxicity and 180, **181**, 182, **182**, *182*, 187, **187**
    relapse rates 186
    single-dose *vs.* 179, *179*, **187**

hyperfractionated 180, 187, 188
    accelerated 182
    cataract reduction 188
  single-dose 179, 182, 185, 187–188
    fractionated *vs.* 179, *179*, **187**
    low-dose rate 182
  toxicity and 180, **181**, 182, **182**, *182*, 187
RAG knockout mice 330
RAIT *see* radioimmunotherapy (RAIT)
Ramsay–Hunt syndrome, post-herpes zoster 739
randomization procedures 421–422
randomized clinical trials (RCTs) *see* clinical trials
rapamycin *see* sirolimus (rapamycin)
Ras GTPase
  antisense therapies 266
  mRNA half-life 267
ras mutation, T-cell adoptive immunotherapy 391
ratio of costs to charges (RCC) 436
receptor activator of NFκB (RANK), multiple myeloma 1263
Recombinant DNA Advisory Committee (RAC) 122
recombination
  chromosome rearrangement in leukemia 86
  MHC evolution 47–48
    intraexonic 48–49
  V-DJ 79
recovery
  follow-up recommendations **956**
  immune system compromise **668**
  infections 668–669, 669–671, **670**, 671
    opportunistic *670*
    treatment 675
  relapse risk 278
Recruitment Groups 627, **627**
rectal administration, opioids 903
recurrence (of malignancies) *see* relapse
red blood cells *see* erythrocytes
Reed–Sternberg cells, EBV infections 387
reference strand mediated conformational analysis (RSCA) 38–39
refractory anemia (RA) 1144
refractory anemia with excess blasts (RAEB) 1144
refractory autoimmune cytopenia 1390
regimen related toxicity (RRT) system 158, **158**
Registration Rule, HCT regulation 532
regulatory T-cell(s) *see* T regulatory cells (Tregs)
relapse
  allogeneic transplants, GVLE, evidence for 371, *371*, 372, *372*
  AML 1028, 1030–1031
    in children 1045–1046, 1048
    following treatment 1033–1034
  autologous transplants, following *see* autologous transplantation, relapse following
  chimerism evaluation **238**
  CML 1013–1014

relapse (cont.)
  definition 272
  donor cell origins 239
  HLA typing effects 1141
  infused tumor cell contribution 249–251
  leukemias
    increased following T-cell depletion 225–227
    TBI and 185–186
  oral presentations 924
  PBHC allogeneic transplants 593
  Philadelphia chromosome (Bcr-Abl gene fusion), kinetics of emergence 279
  quality of life issues 511
  risks
    chimerism characterization 238–239
    detection 276–277
      time from transplant 278
    donor status 278–279
  treatment
    DLI 387–388
    vaccination 227–228
  see also minimal residual disease (MRD)
relative risk (RR) 415
remission
  definition 272
  status/treatment 1031
    treatment outcome 453, 454
  see also individual diseases/disorders; individual treatments
renal cell carcinoma, allogeneic transplants 1177, 1179–1182, 1180, 1181
  donor chimerism assessment 1181
  emerging role 1182
  engraftment patterns 1181, **1182**
  GVHD association 1180–1181, 1182
  HLA upregulation 1180
  mechanisms 1181–1182
  protocol 1179
  toxicities/limitations 1182
  see also solid tumors, allogeneic transplants
reoxygenation, radiotherapeutic principles 178
respiratory symptoms
  opioids, side effects 901–902
  viral infections 758–762
    isolation practices 762
  see also lung(s); pulmonary complications
respiratory syncytial virus (RSV) infection 758–760
  clinical significance 758
  incidence 758, **759**, 759
  prevention 759–760
  prognosis **760**
  risk factors 758–759
  treatment 759–760, **762**
restrictive pulmonary disease 945, 947
retching, mucosal trauma 784
reticular dysgenesis (RD) 1474–1475
retinoblastoma 1360–1361
13-cis-retinoic acid, neuroblastoma minimal residual disease treatment 1339, 1339

retrospective case–control studies 416
retroviruses
  as gene transfer vectors see gene transfer
  genome 107–108, 108
  infection 108
  lifecycle 108
  long-terminal repeats 108
  see also specific viruses
reverse transcriptase PCR (RT-PCR), HSC gene expression 82, 83
reverse transcriptase telomerase protein (hTERT) 64, 71
revised European–American classification, lymphomas 1109–1110
rhabdomyosarcoma 1357–1359
  conventional therapy 1357
  HCT as consolidation 1358–1359
  high-dose regimen **1358**
  relapse/refractory 1357–1358
  risk groups 1357
  survival 1357
Rhesus (Rh) blood groups
  cord blood typing 552
  hemolytic complications of incompatibility 825–826
  platelet transfusions 836
rheumatoid arthritis 1390
  animal model 326t
  autologous HCT 333
  HLA associations 324t
rheumatological disorders, treatment **1387**
rhinovirus infections 761
  treatment 762
rhodium-186/-188 (^{186}Rh, ^{188}Rh), radioimmunotherapy 200–201, **201**
ribozymes 261
  antisense therapy 260, 261–262
    phase I/II trials 263
  gene therapy, AIDS 1375–1376
  hairpin 262
  hammerhead 260, 262
RISC complex 263
rituximab (anti-CD20 antibody) 362
  autologous transplants
    ALL 1244
    immunotherapy following 1398–1399
  CHOP combination
    high-grade lymphoma therapy 1109
    low-grade lymphoma therapy 1107
  EBV infection 752, 753
  EBV-LPD 385–386
  non-Hodgkin's lymphoma 203–204, 1208, 1215
RNA decoy, gene therapy, AIDS 1375
RNAi see RNA interference (RNAi)
RNA interference (RNAi) 263–264
  gene therapy, AIDS 1376
  mechanism 263, 263
  vector expressed RNA 263–264
roquinimex, posttransplant antileukemic treatment 1255
rotavirus, infections 764

RSV infection see respiratory syncytial virus (RSV) infection
"runt disease" 4, 635

S
salivary gland hypofunction 921
Sandhoff 1464
Sanfilippo syndrome (MPS III) 1460
  intellectual decline 1461
sargramostim
  adverse events 543
  recombinant G-CSF vs. 618–619
  see also granulocyte macrophage colony-stimulating factor (GM-CSF)
SCF see stem cell factor (SCF)
scFvs, AIDS gene therapy 1377
Scheie syndrome (MPS IS) 1460
Schwachman–Diamond syndrome (SDS), nonmyeloablative therapy 1174
SCID see severe combined immune deficiency (SCID)
SCID-repopulating cells (SRC), HSC expansion studies 97
scopolamine, cholinergic effects 818
search coordinator 467
Seattle criteria for grading graft-vs.-host disease 639, **639**, **640**, **649**
"secondary disease" 635
secondary malignancies 962–977
  acute leukemia 969
  alkylating agent-related 963
  allogeneic transplants, HLA-identical related transplant 991
  autologous transplants, AML 1232–1233
  classification 962
  lymphoma 969–971
    late-onset 971
  neuroblastoma treatment 1340
  posttransplant lymphoproliferative disorder 969–971
  radiation-related 963
  risk factors 962, **962**
  solid tumor 971–973
  therapy-related AML 963–969
  therapy-related myodysplasia 963–969
secondary phase of irradiation syndrome 221
sedation
  critically ill patients 908
  opioids, side effects 901
  procedures, pain management 908
SEERS see Surveillance, Epidemiology/End Results (SEERS)
seizures, drug-induced 815, 817
selectin(s)
  hematopoietic microenvironment 56
  PBHCs 576–577
self-care behaviour 501
self-renewal 62–68, 69
sensitization, graft failure 1119
sequence-specific oligonucleotide probe (SSOP) hybridization 37, 38, 38
sequence-specific primer (SSP) typing 37, 37

sequencing, HLA typing 38, *39*
serum proteins, cryoprotection 603–604
severe aplastic anaemia
   immunosuppressive agents, randomized controlled trials **642**
   marrow transplant 5
severe combined immune deficiency (SCID) 1430–1436
   adenosine deaminase (ADA)-deficient 123, 124
     gene therapy trials 123, 124, 557
     in utero transplantation and 573
   allogeneic transplants 5, 1133
     animal model 336–337, 337f, 339
     nonidentical-related T-cell depleted 1432–1434
     unmodified matched/mismatched-related 1431–1432
     unmodified unrelated 1435
   animal model 330
   classification 1430–1431
   gene therapy 1436
     trials 123, 124
       candidate disorder 121
       lymphoproliferation following 125–126
   HCT
     cord blood cell transplant 1435–1436
     GVHD 1432
     immune reconstitution 856
     immunological reconstitution 1432, *1432*
     problems associated 1434–1435
     recovery *1434*
     survival 1433, *1433*
     in utero 572, 1436
   immunological tolerance 306
   incidence 1430
   murine models
     HSC expansion studies 97
     varicella-zoster virus pathogenesis 734–735, *735*
   mutations 1430–1431, **1431**
   nonmyeloablative therapy 1173
   SCID-repopulating cells 97
   signs/symptoms 1430
   X-linked *see* X-linked severe combined immune deficiency syndrome (XSCID)
sexual dysfunction 486, 519–528, 937–939
   autologous transplants, AML 1233
   females
     physiological/biological changes 522–523
     treatment 525
   health care professionals, role 524
   hypoactive sexual desire disorder 524–525
   impacting variables; physical, psychological, social 520, 521–523
   improvement, assessment, interventions 523–524
   incidence 520
   males
     physiological/biological changes 520, 522
     treatment 525–526

menopause 522–523
psychosocial variables 523
quality of life 519–520, *520*
   measures **508**
significance 520
social variables 523
study 520
see also infertility
sexual response cycle 519
   dimensions *520*
   phases 519
sheep, *in utero* transplantation 566–567, *567*
Short Form 36 Health Survey (SF36) 513
   subscales **514**
short tandem repeat (STR) polymorphisms *235*, 235–236, *236*
Shwachman–Diamond syndrome (SDS) 1476
sialomucins
   hematopoietic microenvironment 56
   proliferation/survival effects 57
sickle cell disease 1417–1430
   clinical features 1417–1418
   crisis 1418
   HCT
     alternative cell sources 1426
     complications 1423
     eligibility 1418–1419
     growth/development *1423*, 1423–1424
     indicators 1420, **1420**
     nonmyeloablative 1424–1425, **1425**
     results 1421–1423, **1422**
     stable mixed chimerism 1424, *1424*, *1425*
     survival estimates 1422, *1422*, *1426*
   leukocyte count *1419*
   pathophysiology 1417–1418
   severity predictors 1418–1419, 1419–1420, **1420**
   stroke 1418–1419, *1419*
   treatment 1420–1421
     gene therapy 126
     HCT *see above*
     hydroxyurea 1420–1421
     nonmyeloablative therapy 1174
     RBC transfusion 1420, **1420**
The Sickness Impact Profile (SIP) 513
signal transduction
   antisense therapies 266
   HSC expansion studies 98
sildenafil 256
single chain antibodies, AIDS gene therapy 1377
single-dose radiotherapy regimens *see* radiotherapy regimens
single-photon emission computed tomography (SPECT) 201
sinus 813
sinusoidal fibrosis, SOS 778
sinusoidal obstruction syndrome (SOS) 169, 775–780, 814
   animal models 777
   autologous transplants, AML 1223–1224
   clinical presentation 775–776, **776**

   abdominal pain 789
   hepatitis 773
   kidney 778
   liver *288*
   clinical studies 777–778
   course 777
   definition 775
   diagnosis 775–776
     histological findings 287–288
   differential diagnosis 287–288, 776
   drug-induced 778, 1340
     busulfan and 135
     chemotherapy 777–778
     gemtuzumab ozogamicin 287–288
     melphalan toxicity 140
   incidence 775
   nomenclature 775
   pathogenesis 777–778
   pathology 287–288
   prevention 778–779
   prognosis 777
   treatment 779–780
     radiotherapy 184
     TBI 778
sirolimus (rapamycin) 214
   GVHD treatment 360
   mechanism of action/targets **218**
   pharmacology 214
   structure *212*
   toxicity 214
skeletal complications 950–951
skeletal muscle, transdifferentiation **77**
skin
   fungal infection 686
   GVHD *289*, *293*, 293–294
     acute 638
     chronic 647
     histopathology 288
SLE *see* systemic lupus erythematosus (SLE)
Sly syndrome (MPS VII) 1461
smallpox vaccination 865
social factors *see* psychosocial complications/factors
solid tumor(s)
   adoptive immune cell transfer 1178
   chronic GVHD 988
   pathogenesis 954–955
   pediatric patients 1354–1368
     allogeneic *vs.* autologous 1362, 1364
     approaches 1364–1365
     dose-limiting myelotoxicity 1354
     dose-response 1354
     HCT case reports 1361–1364, **1362–1363**
     failure patterns 1364
     immunotherapy 1365
     prognosis 1354
     regimens **1362–1363**
   prophylaxis 955
   secondary malignancy 888–889, 971–973
     delayed complications 954
     genetic susceptibility 971–972
     pathogenesis 971–972, *972*

solid tumor(s)
  secondary malignancy (*cont.*)
    risk factors **972**
    screening 973
    treatment 972}–973
  therapy 955
solid tumors, allogeneic transplants 1177–1187
  GVLE 1177
    animal models 1178
    clinical evidence 1178
    mechanisms *1185*, 1185–1186
  immune system 1177–1178
  melanoma *see* melanoma, allogeneic transplants
  metastatic breast carcinoma 1184
  nonmyeloablative conditioning 1178–1185, **1183**
    limitations **1184**
    patient characteristics **1184**
  ovarian cancer 1184, 1330
  relapse management 1154
  see also renal cell carcinoma, allogeneic transplants
somatic correction, *in utero* transplantation and 573
somatic mosaicism, Fanconi anemia 1488–1489
somnolence syndrome, radiotherapy-induced 189
SOS *see* sinusoidal obstruction syndrome (SOS)
Southern blot, tumor cell detection 244t
South-West Oncology Group (SWOG) 1242
soy bean agglutinin (SBA-E) 1432–1434, *1433*, *1434*
SPECT (single-photon emission computed tomography) 201
sphenoid sinusitis *814*
spirituality
  measures **508**
  quality of life issues 507, 509
spleen
  "boost" radiotherapy 184–185
    relapse and 186
  colony-forming cells 69–70
  hematopoiesis 73
spleen focus-forming virus (SFFV), gene therapy trials 123
splenectomy
  agnogenic myeloid metaplasia 1090
  CLL 1107
  CML 1011
splicing
  thalassemia 264
  translational (mRNA) silencing 264
split chimerism 234
Sporonox *see* itraconazole
SSOP *see* sequence-specific oligonucleotide probe (SSOP) hybridization
SSP *see* sequence-specific primer (SSP) typing
ST1571 *see* imatinib mesylate (Gleevac®)
staging *see* individual diseases/disorders
STAMP-I regimen **161**, 163

STAMP-V regimen **161**
  sequential TBI 165
standard gambles 437
Standards for a Transfusion Service (1958) 536
Standards for Hematopoietic Progenitor Cell Collection, Processing/ Transplantation (1996) 533, 534
Stanford University Medical Center
  body weight/treatment outcome 456
  HCT program 463
Staphylococcus aureus, varicella-zoster virus, secondary to 738
Steel factor (SLF) *see* stem cell factor (SCF)
stellate cells, SOS 778
stem cell(s) *see* hematopoietic stem cells (HSCs)
stem cell factor (SCF)
  HSC self-renewal 72
  PBHC mobilization 577, 589
    clinical trials **582**
    G-CSF with 579
  recombinant **614**, 620
sterility *see* infertility
steroids *see* corticosteroids
Stomatococcus mucillaginosus infections 811
storage disorders 1455–1470
  CNS involvement 1455, *1456*
  metabolic correction 1455, *1455*
  treatment options 1455
stratified randomization 422
Streptococcus pneumoniae infection *see* pneumonia
Streptococcus pyogenes, varicella-zoster virus, secondary to 738
stress
  decision to undergo HCT 497
  post-treatment 484–485
  sources 497
  see also psychosocial complications/factors
stroke (ischemic) 813
stromal cells
  HSC expansion studies 96–99
  as therapeutics 58
stromal derived factor-1 (SDF-1), PBHC mobilization 577
subdural hematoma(s) 813
subdural hygroma(s) 813, *814*
substance abuse
  ethical issues 488
  pain management 905–907
  treatment outcome 457–458
sugars, cryoprotection 604
"suicide genes"
  adoptive T-cell immunotherapy 395–396
  DLI 1156
superantigen(s)
  autoimmune disease 339
  clonal deletion 300–301
superinfection 671
supportive care 12–13
  diverse requirements 883
  nutritional *see* nutritional support

suppressor T-cells *see* T suppressor cells
surgery
  fungal infections 696
  pain management 907
  SOS treatment 780
Surveillance, Epidemiology/End Results (SEERS) 1049
  Fanconi anemia HCT 1499
survey questions, patient's views of HCT 441
survival
  AML autologous transplants 1224, *1224*
    second remission *1229*
  analysis
    Kaplan–Meier model 416
    QoL incorporation 416
  critically ill patients 494
  HLA typing effects *989*, 989–990, **1141**, 1141–1142
    long-term 990
  information presentation 451–452
  long-term 13
    complications 13
    gastrointestinal/hepatic problems 792–795
  PBHC allogeneic transplants 593–594
  rates at FHCRC 944
  see also Kaplan–Meier survival graphs; mortality; *individual diseases/disorders; individual treatments*
survivin, T-cell adoptive immunotherapy 392
SWOG (South-West Oncology Group) 1242
syncope, TBI side-effect 185
syngeneic transplant *see* autologous transplantation
Synthokine-SC55494 620
syphilis, transfusion transmitted 844
systemic inflammatory response 889
systemic lupus erythematosus (SLE) 1390
  animal model 326t, 329
    allogeneic transplants 335
    autologous HCT 333–334
  HLA associations 324t
systemic sclerosis 1389
  skin score following HCT *1389*

T
TAAs *see* tumor-associated antigens (TAAs)
tacrolimus (FK506) 213–214
  autologous GVHD induction 406
  clinical use 214
  dose 214
  GVHD treatment 23, 359–360
  immunosuppression 641
    combined 643
  mechanism of action 211, *213*, **218**
  pharmacology 213
  prednisone combination 384
  randomized controlled trials **642**, **651**
  structure *212*
  toxicity 214
    neurotoxicity 815–817
  treatment complication 780

tamoxifen, breast cancer treatment 1298
tandem transplant, solid tumor treatment 1364–1365
Taqman 276, *276*
taste dysfunction 886, 922
taurolidine, bone marrow purging 256
taxanes
  high-dose chemotherapy 146–147
  mechanism of action 146
  metabolism 134, 146–147
  pharmacology 147
  see also paclitaxel
Tay–Sachs disease 1464
TBI *see* total body irradiation (TBI)
TCAs *see* tricyclic antidepressants (TCAs)
TCD *see* T-cell depletion (TCD)
T-cell(s)
  activation 20–21
    alloantigens 20–21
    in GVHD *see below*
    outcomes 20
    pathway investigations 211
    signal transduction 20
  antigens, interactions with 19
    antigen-presenting cell interactions 20, **355**
    major/minor antigen response 19–20
  autoimmune disease pathogenesis 327, 328f
  bone marrow, content of 853
  development/differentiation 78–80, *614*, *854*, 854–855, *855*
    bipotent progenitors 81
    fetal liver 75–76, **76**
    interleukin-7 78, 854–855
    negative selection 19, *19*
    positive selection 19, *19*
    pro-T cells 79, 83
    PU.1 83
    thymus, selection in 19
  drugs, effects of
    ATG 857
    cyclosporine 858
    methotrexate 853
  effector functions 20–21
  genetic modification *see* adoptive cellular immunotherapy/transfer
  in graft rejection 22
  in GVHD 221
    activation 353–355
      prevention of 359–360
    autologous repertoire 408–409
    modification to control 227
    prevention, reduction in proliferation 360
    treatment of 217, 227
  helper *see* helper T-cell(s)
  immune reconstitution *see* immune reconstitution
  immunological tolerance *see* tolerance, immunological
  lymphoproliferative disorders 953

autologous transplants 1213–1214
  XSCID gene therapy, following 125–126
markers in ALL 1068
maternal, in cord blood 558
PBHC, content of 853
persistence after HCT, chimerism testing 238–239
phytohemagglutinin A stimulation 855
primary response 20–21, *21*
priming 19
receptor *see* T-cell receptor
regulatory *see* T regulatory cells (Tregs)
secondary response 21, *21*
suppressor *see* T suppressor cells
transfer *see* adoptive cellular immunotherapy/transfer; donor lymphocyte infusion (DLI)
vaccination response 863
varicella-zoster virus infection (post-HCT) *736*, 736–737, *737*
in vitro culture 380
T-cell depletion (TCD)
  advantages **222**
  allogeneic transplants, autoimmune animal models 338–339
  ALL treatment in children 1075
  alternative donor HCT 223
    Fanconi anemia 1495
  AML treatment in children 1046–1047
  animal models 221
    autoimmune 334
    murine studies 1164
  complications 221
  costs 224
  delayed immune reconstitution 225
  disadvantages **222**, 224–227
  dose impact 222
  functional 227
  future 227–228
  graft failure following 185, 224–225
    strategies 224–225
  GVHD
    predictor of 1155
    prevention of 221–234, 359
      in children with AML 1046–1047
  HLA-matched relative HCT 223
  HLA-partially matched related HCT *see* HLA-partially matched related HCT, T-cell depletion
  human trials 223
  leukemic relapse 225–227
  MDS therapy 1088
  mortality 224
  organ dysfunction 223–224
  PBHC mobilization 594
  quality of life 224
  selective, DLI modifications 1156
  sickle cell disease 1432–1435
  specificity 222
  TBI immunosuppression 185, 186
    cataract reduction 188
    lung damage 188

techniques 221, **221**
  negative selection **221**
  positive selection **221**
  recombinant GM-CSF 619
T-cell receptor (TCR) 324–325
  αβ gene family 75, 76
  autologous GVHD 406–407, *407*
  development 75–76
  δ gene family 75
  γδ 855
  γ gene family 75, 76
  structure 300
  transgenic mice 566
  Vβ family 348–350
  Vγ2 75, 76
  Vγ3 75, 76
  Vγ4 75, 76
  Vγ5 75, 76
TCR *see* T-cell receptor (TCR)
TED (Transplant Essential Data) 534
teeth, following treatment *934*, 934–935
TEL-AML1 fusion proteins
  ALL 86
  ALL, childhood 1067, 1068
telomerase 64
  reverse transcriptase component (TERT) 64, 71
  see also telomeres
telomerase RNA template component (hTERC) 64
telomeres
  checkpoint 66
  hematopoietic stem cells 65, 71
  loss/shortening 64, 65
    age-related *66*
    compensation 64
    secondary malignancy 967
  structure/function 64–65
  see also telomerase
temporomandibular dysfunction (TMD) 914
"10–23" DNA enzyme 262
TERS (Transplant Evaluation Rating Scale) 498–499
testicular "boost" 184
testicular cancer *see* germ cell tumor(s)
testicular function, following HCT **935**, **938**
tetanus
  vaccination 859
  vaccination in HCT recipients, response 865
TGF-1, multiple myeloma 1262
TGF-β *see* transforming growth factor-β (TGF-β)
thalassemia(s) 1409–1416
  bone marrow transplant 1410–1415
    adults 1413, *1413*
    alternative related donor 1414
    children *1412*, 1412–1413, *1412–1413*
    clinical experience 1411–1415, *1412–1413*, **1415**
    conditioning regimens 1410–1411
    disease recurrence, management 1413–1414

thalassemia(s)
  bone marrow transplant (cont.)
    engraftment 1411
    eradication 1411
    management following 1415
    mixed chimerism 1414
    mortality/morbidity 1411
    rejection 1413–1414
    role 1415
    unrelated donor 1414
  β-thalassemia, mouse model 127
  mRNA processing 264
  therapy
    chelation 1409
    conventional 1409–1410
    gene therapy 126–127
    HCT see above
    hypertransfusion regimens 1410
    nonmyeloablative therapy 1174
    transfusions 1409–1410
thalidomide 216–217
  clinical use 217
  dexamethasone combination 1265, 1270
  mechanism of action/targets **218**
  multiple myeloma therapy 1265, 1277
  pharmacology 216
  randomized controlled trials **651**
  relapse treatment following autologous transplants 1395
  toxicity 216–217
    neurotoxicity 817
The Estrogen Decision 525
T-helper cell(s) see helper T-cell(s)
therapeutic drug level monitoring (TDM), high-dose chemotherapy 137–138
therapeutic equivalency testing 427, **428**
therapeutic ratio, radiotherapy 178–179
therapy-related myelodysplasia see myodysplasia, therapy-related (t-MDS)
thiotepa 141, 163
  astrocytoma 1347
  brain tumor **1345**, 1345–1346
  combination regimens
    ATG/cyclophosphamide/TBI 1123
    ATG/fludarabine 1119
    BCNU/carmustine/cisplatin/cyclophosphamide see STAMP-V regimen
    busulfan/cyclophosphamide 1119
    busulfan/melphalan 163
    cyclophosphamide/TBI 1074–1075
    fludarabine 1182
    STAMP-V see STAMP-V regimen
  high-dose chemotherapy 141
  mechanism of action 141
  metabolism 134, 141
  MTD **159**
  pharmacology **131**, 141
  regimens **161**
  resistance 141
  solid tumor treatment 1358, **1363**

structure *131*
toxicity, dose-limiting 141
third-party payment, ethical issues 488–489
thoracoabdominal irradiation (TAI) 192
  gonadal function following 938–939
thrombocytopenia
  cerebrovascular complications 813
  in Fanconi anemia 1491
  platelet transfusion 835–836
thrombocytopenic purpura (TTP)
  clinical presentation 827–829
  differential diagnosis 829
  HUS form 828–829
  incidence 827
  mortality 829
  therapy 829
thrombolytic therapy, SOS treatment 779
thrombopoietin (TPO)
  cord blood transplantation 555–556
  HSC self-renewal 72
  platelet transfusion, role 839
  recombinant **614**, 620
thrombotic microangiopathy (TM) 827, *828*
thrombotic thrombocytopenic purpura (TTP) 813
Thy1 marker 576
  cord blood cells 556
thymic irradiation
  ATG/cyclophosphamide combination see antithymocyte globulin (ATG), combination regimens
  see radiation; radiotherapy
thymidine kinase genes (herpes simplex), donor T cell transduction 313
thymopoiesis 79
thymus
  autologous GVHD 406–407
  development 75, 79–80
  fetal immunological tolerance 565–566
  hematopoiesis 75, 79
  immune reconstitution 855
  intrathymic injection, immunological tolerance 305
thyroid gland
  chemotherapy/irradiation effects 929–934, **930**
    growth 931
    risk factors 929
    treatment 931
    tumor 929–930
  delayed complications 948
time trade-off questions 437
TIPS (transjugular intrahepatic portosystemic shunt), SOS treatment 779–780
tissue injury
  autoimmunity 328–329
  radiation *180*, 180–182
tissue repair, radiotherapeutic principles 178
tissue-typing see HLA typing
TLI see total lymphoid irradiation (TLI)
t-MDS see myodysplasia, therapy-related (t-MDS)
TNF-α see tumor necrosis factor-α (TNF-α)

TNM (Tumor, Node, Metastasis), breast cancer staging **1299**
tolerance, immunological 16, 300–323, 302
  B-cells 303
  fetal 565–566
  MHC 405
  T-cells 300–303
    anergy 301
    clonal deletion see clonal deletion
    peripheral vs. central 305
    self-tolerance/alloantigen recognition 19–20
    suppression 301–303
  see also tolerance, induced
tolerance, induced 303–305, 305–315
  animal models 307–308, 344
  in donor inoculum 312, *314*
    interleukin-2 activated killer cells 312
    suppressive T-cells 312
  donor-specific transfusion 303–304
  GVHD prevention 360–361
  immunosuppression 305, 308–312
    anti-T cell antibodies 308–309
    B-cell 311
    costimulatory blockades 309–310, *310*
    cyclophosphamide 308
    GVHD prevention 311–312
    mixed chimerism 311
    sublethal TBI 308
  marrow-originating T cells 314–315
  myeloablative conditioning 307–308
  peripheral 303–305
    allogeneic MHC transduction 303–304
    anti-adhesion molecule antibodies 304–305
    antigen-presenting cell modification 303–304
    anti-T cell antibodies 304–305
    costimulatory blockades 304
    total lymphoid irradiation 305, 307
  see also immunodeficiency diseases; myeloablative therapy
tolerance development 24–25
  opioids 902
toothbrushing 915–916
topoisomerase II inhibitors
  high-dose chemotherapy 144–147
  secondary malignancy 963–964
  see also individual drugs
tositumomab (anti-CD20 antibody)
  non-Hodgkin's lymphoma trials 204
  radioiodine labeled 166
total body irradiation (TBI) 159–160
  allogeneic transplants
    ALL, childhood 1073–1074
    CLL 1106
    Fanconi anemia 1491–1492, **1492**
    lymphoma 1106
    multiple myeloma 1096
  autologous transplants
    ALL 1244–1245
    AML 1222–1223

chemotherapy-only regimens vs. 160–161, 165, 189–190, *190*
   AML autologous transplants 1223
clinical results 185–189
   acute side-effects 185
   immunosuppression 185
   lens toxicity 188–189
   lung toxicity 186–188
   relapse 185–186
CML 1010
combination regimens
   Ara-C/melphalan combination (TAM) 1074
   ATG/cyclophosphamide/thiotepa 1123
   busulfan/cyclophosphamide *see* busulfan (BU), combination regimens
   busulfan/etoposide combination **1222**
   cyclophosphamide *see* cyclophosphamide (CY), combination regimens
   cyclophosphamide/etoposide *see* cyclophosphamide (CY), combination regimens
   cyclophosphamide/etoposide/melphalan/methotrexate combination 1202
   cyclophosphamide/mycophenolate mofetil 1201
   cyclophosphamide/thiotepa 1074–1075
   cyclosporine 1164
   cyclosporine/methotrexate 1165
   cytarabine **160**
   cytosine arabinoside 1062
   etoposide *see* etoposide (VP16), combination regimens
   fludarabine *see* fludarabine, combination regimens
   high-dose regimens 165
   melphalan *see* melphalan, combination regimens
consolidative irradiation 190–191
fractionation 159–160
GVHD pathogenesis 353
hematopoietic failure 69
high-dose regimens, and **160**, 165
immunoradiotherapy vs. 201–202
induced tolerance 307
low dose
   animal studies 1170
   induced tolerance 305, 308
   nonmyeloablative therapy 1165, **1165**
MTD **159**
patient position *183*, 183–184
pretransplant 12
   AML, childhood 1045
scheduling, mathematical model 182
solid tumor treatment 1356, 1362
SOS 778
stands *184*
thalassemia, bone marrow transplant 1410–1411
total lymphoid irradiation and 179

toxicity, nonmyeloablative therapy 1165, **1165**
   see also radiation; radiotherapy
total lymphoid irradiation (TLI) 191–192
   peripheral induced tolerance 305, 307
   TBI and 179
total parenteral nutrition (TPN) *883*
Toxoplasma gondii, CNS infection 811, *812*
TPO *see* thrombopoietin (TPO)
tramadol, pain management 903
transcriptional gene regulation, HSCs 82
transcriptional targeting *see* nucleic acid based therapies
transcription factors
   hematopoietic 82, 87, 264
   targeted therapies 259, 264–266
transdifferentiation 76–77, **77**
transdominant mutant proteins, AIDS gene therapy 1376–1377
transforming growth factor-β (TGF-β)
   autologous GVHD 406
   cytoprotection 168
transfusions
   allergic reactions 842
   anaphylactic reactions 843
   bacterial contamination 843
   blood group compatibility 834
   CMV infection, prevention 840
   coagulation factor components 834
   complications 842–846
      nonimmunological 843
   disease transmission 843–846
      donor screening, impact *844*
      reduction strategies **844**
      risks **844**
   donor therapy 841–842
   febrile nonhemolytic reactions 842
   fresh frozen plasma 834
   granulocyte 839
      reactions 843
   GVHD 636–637
      autologous bone marrow transplant 841
      noncellular blood components 841
      prevention 636–637, 840–841
   hemolytic reactions 842
   irradiation of blood components 840–841
   leukocyte-depleted red cells *see* leukocyte(s), depletion in RBC transfusions
   platelet components *see* platelets
   posttransplant 840
   pretransplant 839–840
   pulmonary reactions 842–843
   red blood cell (RBC) *see* erythrocytes, transfusions
   status, survival 982, *982*
   strategies in HCT 839–840
   support principles before/after 833–852
   thalassemia 1409–1410
   treatment outcome/history 457
transfusion-transmitted virus (TTV) 845
   liver infection 783
transgene expression 120–121

transjugular intrahepatic portosystemic shunt (TIPS), SOS treatment 779–780
translational targeting *see* nucleic acid based therapies
translocations *see* chromosome rearrangements
Transplant Essential Data (TED) 534
Transplant Evaluation Rating Scale (TERS) 498–499
transplant registries 438
transplant-related mortality (TRM)
   agnogenic myeloid metaplasia *1091*
   allogeneic transplants
      multiple myeloma 1096, 1098
      PBHCs 593
   DLI toxicity 1155
   see also individual diseases/disorders; individual treatments
Tregs *see* T regulatory cells (Tregs)
T regulatory cells (Tregs)
   GVHD 356
   GVLE 370
   immunological tolerance 302
tricyclic antidepressants (TCAs) 899
   neuropathy 907
   pain management 899
TRM *see* transplant-related mortality (TRM)
T suppressor cells
   immunological tolerance 306
   induced tolerance 312
TTP *see* thrombocytopenic purpura (TTP)
TTP (thrombotic thrombocytopenic purpura) 813
tumor(s)
   chemotherapy resistance **132**, 132–133
   growth kinetics 130, 132
   heterogeneity 130, 132
   markers 1309
   size effects 133
   solid *see* solid tumor(s)
   staging **1308**, **1309**
   treatment complications 769
   see also specific cancers
Tumor, Node, Metastasis (TNM), breast cancer staging **1299**
tumor-associated antigens (TAAs) 198
   GVLE 369
   immunocytology 1338
   radioimmunotherapy and 199–200
   solid tumor immunotherapy 1178
   transient gene expression 120
   vaccines 375, 1178
      DLI modifications 1156
   see also specific antigens
tumor cell eradication
   bone marrow *see* bone marrow purging
   cryopreservation and 609
   radiotherapy 178, 179
   in vivo, efficacy/treatment response 1338
tumor-infiltrating lymphocytes (TILs) 1178
tumor necrosis factor-α (TNF-α)
   downregulation 590
   GVHD 353, 357, 406
   varicella-zoster virus, host response to 736, *737*

twin studies
  chimerism evaluation 239
  transplant results *13*
typhlitis 770
tyramine cellobiose 201
tyrosine kinase inhibitors
  CML therapy 1143
  purging techniques 1256

U

UCSF (University of California at San Francisco), ALL autologous transplants 1241
UDCA *see* ursodeoxycholic acid (UDCA)
UK Medical Research Council *see* Medical Research Council (MRC)
ulcer(s)
  esophageal, gastric, duodenal 785
  intestinal tract 769
ulcerative colitis, treatment complications 769
umbilical cord blood (UCB) *see* cord blood
unipotent stem cells 69
universal donor line 1508
University of California at San Francisco (UCSF), ALL autologous transplants 1241
upper airway complications 877–878
uremic encephalopathy 813
ursodeoxycholic acid (UDCA) 643
  local cytoprotection 169
US Intergroup Study, AML autologous transplants 1230
US National Marrow Donor Program (NMDP) 12
UTY gene 389–390

V

vaccination 862–874
  antifungal 696
  carers 865, **868**
  diseases 862–863
    CMV infection
      active 715–716
      passive 715
    diphtheria 859
    HIV-1 1379
    varicella-zoster virus 859
      prophylaxis 745
  immune reconstitution 857, 859, **859**
  measles–mumps–rubella vaccine 859
  passive **870**
  polio vaccine 859
  polysaccharide antigens 859
  rating system **864**, **871**
  recommendations 865, **866**, **869**
  relapse reduction strategies 227–228
    neuroblastoma 1339
  response 863–865
    in healthy persons 863
    successful 863
  tetanus 859
  tumors 1178

VAD therapy 1264
  multiple myeloma autologous transplants 1269
vagina, GVHD 523
valaciclovir
  CMV prophylaxis 713
  varicella-zoster virus infections 743–744
validity
  content 443
  convergent 443
  instrument (survey) development 442, 443
VAMP regimen, HCT *vs.*, multiple myeloma therapy 1271
vancomycin resistant enterococci (VRE) 674–675
vanishing white matter disease 1463
variable number of tandem repeat (VNTR) polymorphisms, chimerism characterization *235*, 235–236, *236*
varicella *see* varicella-zoster virus (VZV) infection
varicella vaccine
  inactivated 745, *745*
  live attenuated (Oka–Merck) 745
  prophylactic 744, 745, *745*
  vaccination 859
varicella-zoster immunoglobulin (VZIG) 744
varicella-zoster virus (VZV) 732
  detection 740–741
  infection *see* varicella-zoster virus (VZV) infection
  latency 732, 735
  vaccination in HCT recipients 863
    response 864–865
varicella-zoster virus (VZV) infection 732–748
  AML autologous transplants 1232
  antiviral therapy 741–744
    acyclovir 741–742
    cidofovir 744
    famciclovir/valaciclovir 743–744
    foscarnet 744
    ganciclovir 744
    primary (varicella, "chicken pox") 742
    reactivation/recurrent (herpes zoster) 742–743, *743*
    steroids as adjuncts to 743
    toxicity 743
    varicella-zoster immunoglobulin 742
    vidarabine 744
  clinical manifestations 732, 737–740
    atypical herpes zoster 732, 740
    disseminated herpes zoster 740, 742
    localized herpes zoster 739, **739**
    pain 906–907
    primary (varicella, "chicken pox") 737–738, *738*
    prodrome 737, 739
    reactivation/recurrent (herpes zoster) 739–740

subclinical reactivation 735, 740
complications 738
  CNS 738, 739, 743, 812–813
  pneumonia 738, 740
epidemiology 732–734, **733**, 856
  primary (varicella, "chicken pox") 732
  reactivation/recurrent (herpes zoster) 732–734
  reinfection 734
  risk factors for reactivation 733–734, **734**
  temporal pattern 733, *733*
GVHD *vs.* 740
laboratory diagnosis 740–741
latency 732, 735
liver infection 781
mortality 740
oral infection 920
pathogenesis 734–737
  animal models (SCID-hu mice) 734–735, *735*
  cell-associated viremia 734
  host response *736*, 736–737, *737*
  primary (varicella, "chicken pox") 734–735
  reactivation/recurrent (herpes zoster) 735–736
  T-cell response *736*, 736–737, *737*, 745
  viral immune evasion 736
prophylaxis 744–745
  acyclovir *744*, 744–745
  varicella vaccine 744, 745
  varicella-zoster immunoglobulin 744
vascular abnormalities, cyclosporine/tacrolimus toxicity 815
vascular cell adhesion molecule-1 (VCAM-1) 577
  hematopoietic microenvironment 55–56
vascular endothelial damage 813
vascular endothelial growth factor (VEGF), multiple myeloma 1262–1263
vasculitides, treatment **1387**
vasectomy, reverse, ethical issues 492
vasoactive mediators, SOS 778
VCAM-1 *see* vascular cell adhesion molecule-1 (VCAM11)
V-DJ recombination 79
VEGF, multiple myeloma 1262–1263
VEGF (vascular endothelial growth factor), multiple myeloma 1262–1263
veno-occlusive disease (VOD) *see* sinusoidal obstruction syndrome (SOS)
vesicular exanthem, primary varicella infection 737–738
vesicular stomatitis virus (VSV), HIV-1 elimination 1377
vesicular stomatitis virus G (VSV-G) protein, lentiviral vectors 126
veto cells, T-cell tolerance 302–303
Vfend see voriconazole
vidarabine, varicella-zoster virus infections 744

vinca alkaloids, metabolism 134
vincristine
  ALL therapy 1238
  combination regimens
    Adriamycin/dexamethasone see VAD therapy
    asparaginase/methotrexate/prednisolone 1157
    CHOP regimen see CHOP regimen
    C-VAMP 1264
    cyclophosphamide/doxorubicin/methylprednisolone 1264
    cyclophosphamide/doxorubicin/prednisone see CHOP regimen
    doxorubicin/methylprednisolone 1271
    VAMP regimen 1271
viral DNA, laboratory diagnosis 741
viral gene transfer vectors see gene transfer
viral infections 757–768
  esophagus 786–787
  immune evasion 736
  liver 781
  lung 876
  oral 919–920
  respiratory 758–762
    isolation practices 762
  transmission from donor to recipient 538–539
  see also individual viruses
viremia, nonmyeloablative therapy 1171
vitamin deficiencies 888
vitrification 601

VMCP regimen, multiple myeloma therapy 1264
vomiting
  mucosal trauma 784
  opioids, side effects 901
  TBI side-effect 185
  treatment complications 774
voriconazole **693**
  adverse effects 695
  trials 694–695
VZV see varicella-zoster virus (VZV)

W

Wegener's granulomatosis, T-cell adoptive immunotherapy 392
weight loss, long-term complications 795
West Nile virus, transfusion transmitted 846
whole body irradiation see total body irradiation (TBI)
Wilm's tumor 1359
  conventional therapy 1359
  HCT
    as consolidation 1359
    for high-risk relapse 1359
  risk groups 1359
  T-cell adoptive immunotherapy 391
Wiskott–Aldrich syndrome (WAS) 1437
  HCT 1437–1438, *1438*
  in utero transplantation 572
Wnt signaling
  β-catenin role 72
  frizzled–disheveled interaction 72, *72*

  HSC self-renewal *72*, 72–73
  LEF/TCF *72*, 72–73
Wolman syndrome 1464–1465
World Health Organization (WHO)
  AML classification 1040
  MDS definition 1084
World Marrow Donor Association (WMDA) 625
WT1 gene, T-cell adoptive immunotherapy 391

X

xenogeneic animal models
  gene transfer 111
  HSC expansion studies 97–98
  in utero 568
xerostomia 921, **921**
X-linked hyper-IgM syndrome, gene therapy 124
X-linked severe combined immune deficiency syndrome (XSCID)
  gene therapy trials 123, 124
    lymphoproliferation following 125–126
  in utero transplantation 572, 573

Y

Y-chromosome genes, mHA 389–390
yolk sac, hematopoiesis 63, 74
yttrium-90 (^{90}Y) 165–166
  radioimmunotherapy 200, **201**

Z

Zellweger syndrome 1463
"zoster sine herpete" 739